# HEMOSTASIS AND THROMBOSIS

## Basic Principles and Clinical Practice

### FIFTH EDITION

*Editors*

**Robert W. Colman, MD**
Sol Sherry Professor of Medicine
Director, Sol Sherry Thrombosis Research Center
Temple University School of Medicine
Chief of Hematology
Department of Medicine
Temple University Hospital
Philadelphia, Pennsylvania

**Victor J. Marder, MD**
Professor of Clinical Medicine
Department of Medicine, Pediatrics, and Neurology
Director, Vascular Medicine Program
Hematology/Medical Oncology Division
David Geffen School of Medicine at UCLA
Los Angeles, California

**Alexander W. Clowes, MD**
Professor
Department of Surgery
University of Washington School of Medicine
Chief of Vascular Surgery
Department of Surgery
University of Washington Medical Center
Seattle, Washington

**James N. George, MD**
Professor of Medicine
Department of Medicine
University of Oklahoma Health Sciences Center
Oklahoma City, Oklahoma

**Samuel Z. Goldhaber, MD**
Associate Professor of Medicine
Harvard Medical School
Director, Venous Thromboembolism Research Group
Director, Anticoagulation Service
Staff Cardiologist, Cardiovascular Division
Department of Medicine
Brigham and Women's Hospital
Boston, Massachusetts

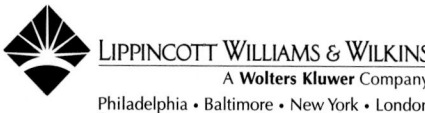

**LIPPINCOTT WILLIAMS & WILKINS**
A **Wolters Kluwer** Company
Philadelphia • Baltimore • New York • London
Buenos Aires • Hong Kong • Sydney • Tokyo

*Acquisitions Editor*: Jonathan W. Pine, Jr.
*Developmental Editor*: Keith Donnellan, Dovetail Content Solutions
*Managing Editor*: Anne E. Jacobs
*Project Manager*: Alicia Jackson
*Senior Manufacturing Manager*: Benjamin Rivera
*Associate Marketing Director*: Adam Glazer
*Creative Director*: Doug Smock
*Cover Designer*: Louis Fuiano
*Production Service*: Laserwords Private Limited
*Printer*: Quebecor World-Taunton

Printed in the United States

Library of Congress Cataloging-in-Publication Data
Hemostasis and thrombosis: basic principles and clinical practice / Robert
    W. Colman ... [et al.]. -- 5th ed.
        p. ; cm.
    Includes bibliographical references and index.
    ISBN 0-7817-4996-4
    1. Blood coagulation disorders.  2. Thrombosis.  3. Blood--Coagulation.
  4. Hemostasis.     I. Colman, Robert W.
    [DNLM:  1. Hemorrhagic Disorders.  2. Blood Coagulation Disorders.
  3. Hemostasis.  4. Thrombosis.     WH 312 H489 2006]
    RC647.C55H45 2006
    616.1'57--dc22                                        2005027296

Care has been taken to confirm the accuracy of the information presented and to describe
generally accepted practices. However, the authors, editors, and publisher are not
responsible for errors or omissions or for any consequences from application of the
information in this book and make no warranty, expressed or implied, with respect to the
currency, completeness, or accuracy of the contents of the publication. Application of the
information in a particular situation remains the professional responsibility of the
practitioner.

The authors, editors, and publisher have exerted every effort to ensure that drug
selection and dosage set forth in this text are in accordance with current recommendations
and practice at the time of publication. However, in view of ongoing research, changes in
government regulations, and the constant flow of information relating to drug therapy and
drug reactions, the reader is urged to check the package insert for each drug for any change
in indications and dosage and for added warnings and precautions. This is particularly
important when the recommended agent is a new or infrequently employed drug.

Some drugs and medical devices presented in the publication have Food and Drug
Administration (FDA) clearance for limited use in restricted research settings. It is the
responsibility of the health care provider to ascertain the FDA status of each drug or device
planned for use in their clinical practice.

To purchase additional copies of this book, call our customer service department at
(800) 638-3030 or fax orders to (301) 223-2320. International customers should call (301)
223-2300.

Visit Lippincott Williams & Wilkins on the Internet: at LWW.com. Lippincott Williams
& Wilkins customer service representatives are available from 8:30 am to 6 pm, EST.

10 9 8 7 6 5 4 3 2 1

To our emeritus editors, Drs. Jack Hirsh and Edwin W. Salzman, who played an important role in the evolution of this textbook.

To our mentors:

Dr. Colman dedicates the book to Sol Sherry, MD, DSc (Hon) whose basic studies of fibrinolysis led to thrombolytic therapy. Dr. Sherry founded the Temple University Thrombosis Center, the International Society on Thrombosis and Haemostasis, the Council on Thrombosis of the American Heart Association, and the International Society of Cardiology.

Dr. Marder cites the invaluable mentorship of Dr. C. Lockard Conley, Professor Emeritus of Medicine and former Chief of Hematology at The Johns Hopkins University School of Medicine, an incomparable clinician–scientist who has made seminal contributions to the field, and whose advice, support, and leadership by example were profoundly influential in Dr. Marder's career direction.

Dr. Clowes expresses his gratitude to Morris Karnovsky, DSc, MB, BCh, who introduced him to the field of vascular biology.

Dr. George dedicates the book to David A. Sears, MD, who guided his initial scientific career, and to Gary E. Raskob, PhD, who catalyzed his transition to patient-oriented research.

Dr. Goldhaber wishes to give special thanks to several of his mentors: Eugene Braunwald, MD, Arthur Sasahara, MD, and Peter Libby, MD.

Charles S. Abrams, MD
Associate Professor of Medicine
Division of Hematology/Oncology
Department of Medicine
University of Pennsylvania School of Medicine
Staff Physician
Division of Hematology/Oncology
Department of Medicine
University of Pennsylvania Medical Center
Philadelphia, Pennsylvania

Peter Acs, MD
Fellow
Division of Hematology/Oncology
Department of Medicine
Georgetown University Medical Center
Division of Hematology/Oncology
Department of Medicine
Lombardi Comprehensive Cancer Center
Washington, District of Columbia

Giancarlo Agnelli, MD
Professor of Internal Medicine
Department of Internal Medicine
University of Perugia
Perugia, Italy

Martine Aiach, PhD
Professor
Inserm U428, Department of Hematology
Faculty of Pharmacy, Université Paris 5
Director
Department of Biological Hematology
Hôpital Européen Georges Pompidou
Paris, France

Stylianos E. Antonarakis, MD
Professor of Medical Genetics
Geneva University Medical School
Director, Department of Genetic Medicine and Development
University Hospital of Geneva
Geneva, Switzerland

Barrie Ashby, PhD
Professor
Department of Pharmacology
Temple University School of Medicine
Philadelphia, Pennsylvania

Fedor Bachmann, MD
Emeritus Professor
Department of Medicine
University of Lausanne
Le Mont, Switzerland

S. Paul Bajaj, PhD
Professor
Department of Orthopaedic Surgery
David Geffen School of Medicine at UCLA
Los Angeles, California

Shannon M. Bates, MDCM, MSc, FRCP(C)
Assistant Professor
Department of Medicine
McMaster University
Staff, Thromboembolism Service
Department of Medicine
McMaster University Medical Centre
Hamilton, Ontario
Canada

Kenneth A. Bauer, MD
Professor
Department of Medicine
Harvard Medical School
Director, Thrombosis Clinical Research
Division of Hemostasis and Thrombosis
Beth Israel Deaconess Medical Center
Boston, Massachusetts

Kenneth L. Baughman, MD
Professor of Medicine
Harvard Medical School
Director, Advanced Heart Disease Section
Brigham and Women's Hospital
Boston, Massachusetts

Judith A. Berliner, PhD
Professor
Departments of Pathology and Medicine
University of California at Los Angeles
Los Angeles, California

Michael Claude Berndt, PhD
Professor
Department of Biochemistry and
    Molecular Biology
Monash University
Clayton, Australia

Rebecca J. Beyth, MD, MS
Baylor College of Medicine
Section of Health Services Research
Houston Center for Quality of Care and Utilization Studies
Veterans Affairs Medical Center
Houston, Texas

Morey Blinder, MD
Associate Professor
Departments of Internal Medicine and Pathology
    and Immunology
Washington University School of Medicine
St. Louis, Missouri

Susan C. Bock, PhD
Professor of Medicine and Bioengineering
Department of Medicine and Bioengineering
University of Utah
Salt Lake City, Utah

Nuala A. Booth, PhD
Professor
School of Medical Sciences
University of Aberdeen
Aberdeen, United Kingdom

Henri Bounameaux, MD
Professor of Medicine and Chairman
Department of Medicine
Faculty of Medicine, University of Geneva
Director
Division of Angiology and Hemostasis and
    Department of Medicine
University Hospitals of Geneva
Geneva, Switzerland

Lawrence F. Brass, MD, PhD
Professor and Vice Chair
Department of Medicine
University of Pennsylvania
Philadelphia, Pennsylvania

George J. Broze, Jr., MD
Professor of Medicine
Division of Hematology
Washington University
St. Louis, Missouri

George R. Buchanan, MD
Professor
Department of Pediatrics
The University of Texas Southwestern Medical Center at Dallas
Dallas, Texas

Allen P. Burke, MD
Associate Chairman
Department of Cardiovascular Pathology
Armed Forces Institute of Pathology
Washington, District of Columbia

Raphaële Buser, PhD
Post-doctoral
Department of Cell Physiology and Metabolism
University Medical Center
Geneva, Switzerland

Eric Camerer, PhD
Assistant Researcher
Cardiovascular Research Institute
University of California
San Francisco, California

Rodney M. Camire, PhD
Assistant Professor
Department of Pediatrics
University of Pennsylvania
Assistant Professor
Department of Pediatrics
Division of Hematology
The Children's Hospital of Philadelphia
Philadelphia, Pennsylvania

Christopher P. Cannon, MD
Associate Professor of Medicine
Harvard Medical School
Senior Investigator
TIMI Study Group
Associate Physician
Brigham and Women's Hospital
Boston, Massachusetts

Jonathan M. Chen, MD
Assistant Professor of Surgery
Department of Surgery
Columbia University College of Physicians
    and Surgeons
Chief, Pediatric Cardiac Surgery
Department of Cardiothoracic Surgery
New York Presbyterian Hospital–Cornell Campus
New York, New York

Beng H. Chong, MBBS, PhD, FRCP, FRACP,
    FRCP(A)
Professsor and Head
Department of Medicine, St. George Clinical
    School
The University of New South Wales
Sydney, Australia
Professor of Medicine
Division of Medicine
St. George Hospital
Kogarah, Australia

Marc Chretien, MSc
Graduate Student
Department of Laboratory Medicine
    and Pathobiology
University of Toronto
Graduate Student
Division of Cellular and Molecular Biology
Toronto General Hospital
Toronto, Ontario
Canada

Alexander W. Clowes, MD
Professor
Department of Surgery
University of Washington School of Medicine
Chief of Vascular Surgery
Department of Surgery
University of Washington Medical Center
Seattle, Washington

Désiré Collen, MD, PhD
Professor
Center for Molecular and Vascular Biology
Katholieke Universiteit Leuven
Leuven, Belgium

Robert W. Colman, MD
Sol Sherry Professor of Medicine
Director, Sol Sherry Thrombosis Research
    Center
Temple University School of Medicine
Chief of Hematology
Department of Medicine
Temple University Hospital
Philadelphia, Pennsylvania

Anthony J. Comerota, MD, FACS
Clinical Professor of Surgery
Department of Surgery
University of Michigan
Ann Arbor, Michigan
Director
Jobst Vascular Center
The Toledo Hospital
Toledo, Ohio

**Shaun R. Coughlin, MD, PhD**
Director
Cardiovascular Research Institute
Professor
Departments of Medicine and Cellular and Molecular
    Pharmacology
University of California
San Francisco, California

**Elisabeth M. Cramer, MD, PhD**
Professor of Hematology
Department of Hematology
Institut Cochin
Paris, France
Head
Department of Haematology and Immunology
Hôpital Ambroise Paré
Boulogne, France

**Bruce J. Darrow, MD, PhD**
Assistant Professor
Departments of Cardiology and Medicine
Assistant Professor
The Zena and Michael A. Wiener Cardiovascular Institute
    and the Marie-Josée and Henry R. Kravis Center for
    Cardiovascular Health
Mount Sinai School of Medicine
New York, New York

**Earl W. Davie, PhD**
Professor
Departments of Biochemistry
University of Washington
Seattle, Washington

**Thomas G. DeLoughery, MD**
Associate Professor of Medicine and Pathology
Division of Hematology/Medical Oncology
Department of Medicine
Division of Laboratory Medicine
Department of Pathology
Oregon Health & Science University
Portland, Oregon

**Gregory J. del Zoppo, MD, MS**
Associate Professor
Department of Molecular and Experimental Medicine
The Scripps Research Institute
Member
Department of Hematology/Medical Oncology
Scripps Clinic
La Jolla, California

**Xiu-Rong Dong, MD**
Carolina Cardiovascular Biology Center
University of North Carolina
Chapel Hill, North Carolina

**David M. Dudzinski, BS, JD**
Student
Department of Health Sciences and Technology
Harvard Medical School
Cardiovascular Research Center
Brigham and Women's Hospital
Boston, Massachusetts

**Harold F. Dvorak, MD**
Mallinckrodt Professor of Pathology
Department of Pathology
Harvard Medical School
Chair
Department of Pathology
Beth Israel Deaconess Medical Center
Boston, Massachusetts

**Charles S. Eby, MD**
Associate Professor
Department of Pathology and Immunology
    and Department of Medicine
Washington University School of Medicine
Medical Director
Hematology Laboratory
Barnes-Jewish Hospital
St. Louis, Missouri

**L. Henry Edmunds, Jr., MD**
Julian Johnson Professor of Cardiothoracic Surgery
Université of Pennsylvania Health System
Department of Surgery
Hospital of the University of Pennsylvania
Philadelphia, Pennsylvania

**Michelle A. Elliott, MD**
Department of Hematology
Mayo Clinic
Rochester, Minnesota

**Joseph Emmerich, MD, PhD**
Professor of Vascular Medicine
Université Paris 5
Professor of Vascular Medicine
Departments of Vascular Medicine and Hypertension
Hôpital Européen Georges Pompidou
Paris, France

**Miguel A. Escobar, MD**
Assistant Professor
Department of Internal Medicine and Pediatrics
The University of Texas Health Science Center
Associate Medical Director
Gulf States Hemophilia and Thrombophilia Center
Houston, Texas

**Suzanne G. Eskin, PhD**
Principal Research Scientist
Department of Biomedical Engineering
Georgia Institute of Technology and Emory University
    School of Medicine
Atlanta, Georgia

**Charles T. Esmon, PhD**
Lloyd Noble Chair in Cardiovascular Research
Member and Head, Cardiovascular Biology Research Program
Oklahoma Medical Research Foundation
Oklahoma City, Oklahoma
Investigator
Howard Hughes Medical Institute
Chevy Chase, Maryland

**Philip J. Fay, PhD**
Professor
Department of Biochemistry and Biophysics
University of Rochester School of Medicine
Rochester, New York

Donald I. Feinstein, MD, M(ASCP)
Professor of Medicine
Departments of Medicine and Hematology
Keck School of Medicine of the University of Southern
    California School of Medicine
Los Angeles, California

Michaëla Fontenay, MD, PhD
Maitre de Conferences des Universites
Department of Hematology
Inserm 567, Universite Paris 5
Assistant, Practicien Hospitalier
Department of Hematology
Hospital Cochin
Paris, France

Charles W. Francis, MD
Professor of Medicine and Professor of Pathology
    and Laboratory Medicine
Department of Medicine
University of Rochester School of Medicine and Dentistry
Director
Hemostasis and Thrombosis Program
University of Rochester Medical Center
Rochester, New York

Colin D. Funk, PhD
Professor
Department of Physiology and Biochemistry
Queen's University
Kingston, Ontario
Canada

David Gailani, MD
Associate Professor
Departments of Pathology and Medicine
Vanderbilt University
Medical Director, Coagulation Laboratory
Department of Pathology
Vanderbilt University Medical Center
Nashville, Tennessee

Eli V. Gelfand, MD
Clinical Fellow in Medicine
Harvard Medical School
Fellow in Cardiovascular Diseases
Beth Israel Deaconess Medical Center
Boston, Massachusetts

James N. George, MD
Professor of Medicine
Department of Medicine
University of Oklahoma Health Sciences Center
Oklahoma City, Oklahoma

Jeffrey S. Ginsberg, MD
Professor
Department of Medicine
McMaster University
Chief
Thrombosis Service
McMaster University Medical Centre
Hamilton, Ontario
Canada

David Ginsburg, MD
Professor
Departments of Medicine and Human Genetics
Investigator
Howard Hughes Medical Institute
University of Michigan
Ann Arbor, Michigan

Gregory R. Giugliano, MD, SM, FACC, FSCAI
Associate Director
Cardiac Catheterization Laboratory and
    Cardiology Research
Baystate Medical Education and Research Foundation
Springfield, Massachusetts
Assistant Professor
Tufts University School of Medicine
Boston, Massachusetts

Samuel Z. Goldhaber, MD
Associate Professor of Medicine
Harvard Medical School
Director, Venous Thromboembolism
    Research Group
Director, Anticoagulation Service
Staff Cardiologist, Cardiovascular Division
Department of Medicine
Brigham and Women's Hospital
Boston, Massachusetts

Maud B. Gorbet
Post-doctoral Fellow
Department of Chemical Engineering
McMaster University
Hamilton, Ontario
Canada

Charles S. Greenberg, MD
Professor
Departments of Medicine and Pathology
Duke University Medical Center
Attending Physician
Department of Hematology
Duke University Health System
Durham, North Carolina

Daniel L. Greenberg, MD
Research Scientist
Department of Biochemistry
University of Washington School of Medicine
Attending Physician
Department of Medicine
University of Washington Medical Center
Seattle, Washington

Lazar J. Greenfield, MD
Professor of Surgery and Chair Emeritus
Department of Surgery
University of Michigan
Ann Arbor, Michigan

Sandra L. Haberichter, PhD
Assistant Professor
Department of Pediatrics
Medical College of Wisconsin
Milwaukee, Wisconsin
Researcher
Children's Research Institute
Children's Hospital of Wisconsin
Wauwatosa, Wisconsin

Katherine A. Hajjar, MD
Professor and Chairman
Department of Cell and Developmental Biology
Weill Medical College of Cornell University
Attending Pediatrician
Department of Pediatrics
New York Presbyterian Hospital
New York, New York

Jonathan L. Halperin, MD
Robert and Harriet Heilbrunn Professor of Medicine
Department of Cardiology
Mount Sinai School of Medicine
Director, Clinical Cardiology Services
The Zena and Michael A. Wiener
    Cardiovascular Institute
The Marie-Josée and Henry R. Kravis Center for
    Cardiovascular Health
Mount Sinai Medical Center
New York, New York

Justin R. Hamilton, PhD
Research Fellow
Cardiovascular Research Institute
University of California
San Francisco, California

Roy R. Hantgan, PhD
Associate Professor
Department of Biochemistry and Molecular Medicine
Wake Forest University School of Medicine
Winston-Salem, North Carolina

Jillian A. Harrison, PhD
Post-doctoral Scientist
Department of Morphology
University of Geneva Medical Center
Geneva, Switzerland

Justin P. Hart, PhD
Student
Department of Pathology
Duke University Medical Center
Durham, North Carolina

John A. Heit, MD
Professor of Medicine
Department of Internal Medicine
Mayo Clinic College of Medicine
Director, Coagulation Laboratories and Clinic
Department of Laboratory Medicine and Pathology
Mayo Clinic
Rochester, Minnesota

Dirk F. Hendriks, PharmD, PhD
Professor
Department of Pharmaceutical Sciences
University of Antwerp
Antwerp, Belgium

Moira Jackson, PhD
Assistant Professor
Department of Anatomy and Cell Biology
University of Florida College of Medicine
Gainesville, Florida

James J. Jang, MD
Fellow
Department of Medicine
Division of Cardiology
Mount Sinai School of Medicine
New York, New York

Nancy Swords Jenny, PhD
Research Assistant Professor
Department of Pathology
University of Vermont College of Medicine
Colchester, Vermont

Hylton V. Joffe, MD
Clinical and Research Fellow in Medicine
Harvard Medical School
Clinical and Research Fellow
Department of Medicine
Brigham and Women's Hospital
Boston, Massachusetts

J. Heinrich Joist, PhD
Deceased

Janna M. Journeycake, MD
Assistant Professor
Department of Pediatrics
The University of Texas Southwestern Medical
    Center at Dallas
Dallas, Texas

Ajay K. Kakkar, BSc, PhD, FRCS
Professor and Head
Centre for Surgical Sciences
Barts and The London School of Medicine
    and Dentistry
Consultant Surgeon
Barts and The London NHS Trust
St. Bartholomew's Hospital
London, United Kingdom

William H. Kane, MD, PhD
Associate Professor of Medicine and Pathology
Divison of Hematology
Duke University Medical Center
Durham, North Carolina

Ana Kasirer-Friede, PhD
Project Scientist
Department of Medicine
Division of Hematology/Oncology
University of California
La Jolla, California

Randal J. Kaufman, PhD
Professor
Department of Biological Chemistry
University of Michigan Medical Center
Investigator
Howard Hughes Medical Institute
Ann Arbor, Michigan

Kenneth Kaushansky, MD
Helen M. Ranney Professor and Chair
Department of Medicine
University of California
Attending Physician
Department of Medicine
UCSD Medical Center
San Diego, California

Clive Kearon, MB, MRCP(I), FRCP(C), PhD
Professor
Department of Medicine
McMaster University
Head, Clinical Thromboembolism Service
Department of Medicine
Henderson General Hospital
Hamilton, Ontario
Canada

**Craig M. Kessler, MD**
Professor of Medicine and Pathology
Georgetown University Medical Center
Washington, District of Columbia

**Thomas S. Kickler MD**
Professor
Departments of Pathology, Medicine, and Oncology
Johns Hopkins University School of Medicine
Director, Hematology and Coagulation Laboratories
Department of Pathology
Johns Hopkins Hospital
Baltimore, Maryland

**Chelsea S. Kidwell, MD**
Associate Professor
Department of Neurology
Georgetown University
Medical Director, WHC Stroke Center
Washington Hospital Center
Washington, District of Columbia

**Craig S. Kitchens, MD**
Professor of Medicine
Department of Hematology/Oncology
University of Florida
Associate Chief of Staff
Veterans Healthcare Administration
North Florida/South Georgia System
Gainesville, Florida

**Walter Klepetko, MD**
Professor
Department of Cardiothoracic Surgery
Medical University of Vienna
Vienna, Austria

**Kiarash Kojouri, MD, MPH**
Resident
Hematology/Oncology Section
Department of Medicine
University of Oklahoma Health Sciences Center
Oklahoma City, Oklahoma

**Frank D. Kolodgie, PhD**
Research Scientist
Department of Cardiovascular Pathology
Armed Forces Institute of Pathology
Washington, District of Columbia

**Barbara A. Konkle, MD**
Associate Professor of Medicine
Departments of Medicine, Pathology, and Laboratory
   Medicine
Director, Penn Comprehensive Hemophilia and Thrombosis
   Program
University of Pennsylvania School of Medicine
Philadelphia, Pennsylvania

**Stavros Konstantinides, MD**
Professor of Medicine and Vice Chairman
Department of Cardiology and Pulmonology
Georg August University School of Medicine
Goettingen, Germany

**Nils Kucher, MD**
Assistant Director
Venous Thromboembolism Research Group
Harvard Medical School
Fellow in Cardiovascular Medicine
Cardiovascular Division
Brigham and Women's Hospital
Boston, Massachusetts

**Satya P. Kunapuli, PhD**
Professor
Departments of Physiology, Pharmacology
Sol Sherry Thrombosis Research Center
Temple University School of Medicine
Philadelphia, Pennsylvania

**Thomas J. Kunicki, PhD**
Associate Professor
Department of Molecular and Experimental Medicine
The Scripps Research Institute
La Jolla, California

**Juliana C. Kwok, PhD**
Research Officer
St. George Clinical School
The University of New South Wales
Research Officer
Department of Medicine
St. George Hospital
Sydney, Australia

**Thung-Shen Lai, PhD**
Assistant Professor
Department of Medicine
Duke University Medical Center
Durham, North Carolina

**Bernhard Lämmle, MD**
Professor of Hematology
Director
Division of Hematology and Central Hematology Laboratory
University Hospital, Inselspital
Bern, Switzerland

**Irene M. Lang, MD**
Professor of Vascular Biology
Department of Cardiology
Medical University of Vienna
Department of Cardiology
Allgemeines Krankenhaus
Vienna, Austria

**B. Lowell Langille, PhD**
Professor
Department of Laboratory Medicine and Pathobiology
University of Toronto
Senior Scientist
Division of Cellular and Molecular Biology
Toronto General Hospital
Toronto, Ontario
Canada

**Daniel A. Lawrence, PhD**
Professor
Department of Internal Medicine
University of Michigan
Ann Arbor, Michigan

Agnes Y. Y. Lee, MD, MSc, FRCP(C)
Associate Professor
Department of Medicine
McMaster University
Active Medical Staff
Department of Medicine
Hamilton Health Sciences Henderson General Hospital
Toronto, Ontario
Canada

Alain Leizorovicz, MD
Director
Clinical Trial Unit (EA 3736)
School of Medicine RTH Laennec
University of Lyon
Lyon, France

Judith Leurs, PhD
Post-doctoral Fellow
Department of Pharmaceutical Sciences
University of Antwerp
Wilrijk, Belgium

Marcel Levi, MD
Professor of Medicine
Department of Medicine
University of Amsterdam
Chairman
Department of Medicine
Academic Medical Center
Amsterdam, The Netherlands

Mark Levine, MD, MSc, FRCP(C)
Professor
Department of Clinical Epidemiology and Biostatistics
   and Department of Medicine
Buffett Taylor Chair, Breast Cancer Research
McMaster University
Director
Clinical Trials Methodology Group
Henderson Research Centre
Hamilton, Ontario
Canada

Klaus Ley, MD
Director, Cardiovascular Research Center,
Professor
Departments of Biomedical Engineering, Molecular
   Physiology, and Biological Physics
University of Virginia
Charlottesville, Virginia

Xiaoning Li, MS
Hematology-Oncology Section, Department of Medicine,
College of Medicine
Department of Biostatistics and Epidemiology
College of Public Health
The University of Oklahoma Health Sciences Center
Oklahoma City, Oklahoma

Peter Libby, MD
Mallinckrodt Professor of Medicine
Department of Medicine
Harvard Medical School
Chief, Cardiovascular Medicine
Department of Medicine
Brigham and Women's Hospital
Boston, Massachusetts

H. Roger Lijnen, PhD
Professor
Center for Molecular and Vascular Biology
Katholieke Universitiet Leuven
Leuven, Belgium

José Aron López, MD
Professor of Medicine
Department of Medicine/Thrombosis Research
Baylor College of Medicine
Staff Physician
Department of Hematology
Houston VA Medical Center
Houston, Texas

Susan T. Lord, PhD
Professor
Department of Pathology and
   Laboratory Medicine
University of North Carolina at Chapel Hill
Chapel Hill, North Carolina

David J. Loskutoff, PhD
Professor
Department of Cell Biology, Division
   of Vascular Biology
The Scripps Research Institute
La Jolla, California

Amir Lotfi, MD
Division of Cardiology
Baystate Medical Center
Springfield, Massachusetts

Roger L. Lundblad, PhD
Adjunct Professor of Pathology
University of North Carolina
Chapel Hill, North Carolina

Alice D. Ma, MD
Assistant Professor
Department of Medicine, Division of Hematology/Oncology
University of North Carolina
Attending Physician
Departments of Medicine and Hematology/Oncology
University of North Carolina Hospitals
Chapel Hill, North Carolina

Mark W. Majesky, PhD
Professor of Medicine and Genetics
Associate Director, Carolina Cardiovascular Biology Center
University of North Carolina
Chapel Hill, North Carolina

Kenneth G. Mann, PhD
Professor and Chairman
Department of Biochemistry
University of Vermont
Burlington, Vermont

Victor J. Marder, MD
Professor of Clinical Medicine
Department of Medicine, Pediatrics, and Neurology
Director, Vascular Medicine Program
Hematology/Medical Oncology Division
David Geffen School of Medicine at UCLA
Los Angeles, California

Guglielmo Mariani, MD
The Department of Internal Medicine
University of L'Aquila
L'Aquila, Italy

Peter W. Marks, MD, PhD
Senior Clinical Research Physician
Novartis Oncology
East Hanover, New Jersey

Neil A. Martin, MD
Professor
Division of Neurosurgery
David Geffen School of Medicine at UCLA
Chief
Division of Neurosurgery
UCLA Medical Center
Los Angeles, California

Larry V. McIntire, PhD
Wallace H. Coulter Chair
Department of Biomedical Engineering
Georgia Institute of Technology and Emory University School
    of Medicine
Atlanta, Georgia

Bernhard Meier, MD, FACC, FESC
Professor of Cardiology and Chairman
Department of Cardiology
University Hospital
Bern, Switzerland

Mark H. Meissner, MD
Associate Professor
Department of Surgery
University of Washington
Seattle, Washington

Thomas Michel, MD, PhD
Professor of Medicine
Department of Medicine
Harvard Medical School, Brigham and Women's Hospital
Boston, Massachusetts
Chief of Cardiology
Cardiology Section, Medical Service
VA Boston Healthcare System
West Roxbury, Massachusetts

Alan D. Michelson, MD
Professor of Pediatrics, Medicine, and Pathology
Department of Pediatrics
Director
Center for Platelet Function Studies
University of Massachusetts Medical School
Worcester, Massachusetts

Patrick Mismetti, MD
Unité de Pharmacologie Clinique
Université Jean Monnet
Saint Etienne, France

Jennifer L. Moen, PhD
Protocol Review Committee Coordinator
Lineberger Comprehensive Cancer Center
University of North Carolina
Chapel Hill, North Carolina

Robert R. Montgomery, MD
Professor of Pediatric Hematology
Department of Pediatrics
Medical College of Wisconsin
Senior Investigator
Blood Research Institute
BloodCenter of Wisconsin
Milwaukee, Wisconsin

James H. Morrissey, PhD
Professor
Department of Biochemistry
University of Illinois College of Medicine
Urbana, Illinois

Adam Dallas Munday, PhD
Research Fellow
Department of Biochemistry and Molecular Biology
Monash University
Clayton, Australia

Nicola J. Mutch, PhD
Post-doctoral Research Associate
Department of Biochemistry
University of Illinois
Urbana, Illinois

Ralph L. Nachman, MD
E. Hugh Luckey Distinguished Professor of Medicine,
    Chairman of Medicine and Physician-In-Chief
Weill Medical College of Cornell University
New York, New York

Thuraia Nageh, MD
Invasive Fellow
Swiss Cardiovascular Center
University Hospital
Bern, Switzerland

Michael E. Nesheim, BSc, PhD
Professor
Department of Biochemistry and Medicine
Queen's University
Kingston, Ontario
Canada

Sabrena F. Noria, MD, PhD
Resident
Department of Surgery
Toronto General Hospital
Toronto, Ontario
Canada

Alan T. Nurden, PhD
Research Director, CNRS
Institut Fédératif de la Recherche
Hôpital Cardiologique
Pessac, France

Paquita Nurden, MD
Laboratoire d'Hématologie
Hôpital Cardiologique
Pessac, France

Jeffrey W. Olin, DO
Professor of Medicine
Director, Vascular Medicine
Zena and Michael A. Wiener Cardiovascular Institute
Mount Sinai Medical Center and School of Medicine
New York, New York

Tracee S. Panetti, PhD
Assistant Professor
Sol Sherry Thrombosis Research Center
Department of Microbiology and Immunology
Temple University School of Medicine
Philadelphia, Pennsylvania

Michael S. Pepper, MBChB, PhD, MD
Professor
Department of Immunology
Faculty of Health Sciences
University of Pretoria
Director
NetCare Molecular Medicine Institute
Unitas Hospital
Pretoria, South Africa

Arnaud Perrier, MD
Professor
Department of Internal Medicine
Geneva Faculty of Medicine
Chief of Service
Division of General Internal Medicine
Department of Internal Medicine
Geneva University Hospital
Geneva, Switzerland

Salvatore V. Pizzo, MD, PhD
Professor, Chairman of Pathology
Department of Pathology
Duke University School of Medicine
Durham, North Carolina

Edward F. Plow, PhD
Chairman
Department of Molecular Cardiology
The Cleveland Clinic Foundation
Cleveland, Ohio

Eleanor S. Pollak, MD, FCAP
Assistant Professor
Department of Pathology and Laboratory Medicine
University of Pennsylvania School of Medicine
Assistant Director
Department of Pathology and Laboratory Medicine
Hospital of the University of Pennsylvania
Philadelphia, Pennsylvania

Jun Qin, PhD
Professor
Department of Molecular Medicine
Lerner College of Medicine, Case Western
    Reserve University
Staff
Department of Molecular Cardiology
Cleveland Clinic Foundation
Cleveland, Ohio

Rene Quiroz, MD, MPH
Research Fellow
Department of Medicine
Harvard Medical School
Research Fellow
Department of Medicine
Brigham and Women's Hospital
Boston, Massachusetts

Jacob H. Rand, MD
Professor
Departments of Pathology and Medicine
Albert Einstein College of Medicine
Director, Hematology, Coagulation and Protein
    Separation Laboratories
Department of Pathology
Montefiore Medical Center
Bronx, New York

A. Koneti Rao, MD
Professor of Medicine and Thrombosis
Associate Dean for MD/PhD Program
Temple University School of Medicine
Philadelphia, Pennsylvania

Frederick R. Rickles, MD
Professor
Departments of Medicine, Pediatrics, and Pharmacology
    and Physiology
The George Washington University School of Medicine
    and Health Sciences
Attending Physician
Department of Medicine
The George Washington University Hospital
Washington, District of Columbia

Paul M. Ridker, MD, MPH
Eugene Braunwald Professor of Medicine
Harvard Medical School
Director, Center for Cardiovascular Disease
    Prevention
Department of Medicine
Brigham and Women's Hospital
Boston, Massachusetts

Harold R. Roberts, MD
Sarah Graham Kenan Distinguished
    Professor
Department of Medicine and Pathology
University of North Carolina
Attending Physician
Department of Hematology/Oncology
University Hospitals
Chapel Hill, North Carolina

Eric A. Rose, MD
Director of Surgical Service
Department of Surgery
Columbia University
Chairman
Department of Surgery
Columbia University Medical Center
New York, New York

Gerald J. Roth, MD
Professor
Department of Medicine
University of Washington
Chief, Hematology Section
Department of Primary and Specialty Care
VA Puget Sound Health Care System
Seattle Division
Seattle, Washington

Zaverio M. Ruggeri, MD
Professor and Division Head
Director, Roon Research Center for Arteriosclerosis and
    Thrombosis
The Scripps Research Institute
Division of Experimental Hemostasis and Thrombosis
Department of Molecular and Experimental Medicine
La Jolla, California

J. Evan Sadler, MD, PhD
Investigator
Howard Hughes Medical Institute
Professor
Departments of Medicine, Biochemistry, and Molecular
    Biophysics
Washington University School of Medicine
St. Louis, Missouri

David C. Sane, MD
Associate Professor of Internal Medicine
Department of Internal Medicine, Section of Cardiology
Wake Forest University School of Medicine
Attending Physician
Department of Internal Medicine, Section of Cardiology
North Carolina Baptist Hospital
Winston-Salem, North Carolina

Samuel A. Santoro, MD, PhD
Dorothy B. and Theodore R. Austin Professor and Chair of
    Pathology, Professor of Biochemistry
Department of Pathology
Vanderbilt University School of Medicine
Nashville, Tennessee

Brian Savage, PhD
Staff Scientist
Department of Molecular and Experimental Medicine
The Scripps Research Institute
La Jolla, California

Jeffrey L. Saver, MD
Professor
Department of Neurology
David Geffen School of Medicine at UCLA
Director
Stroke Center
UCLA Medical Center
Los Angeles, California

Paul K. Schick, MD, FACP
Research Professor of Medicine
Department of Medicine
Division of Hematology/Oncology
Drexel University College of Medicine
Emeritus Professor of Medicine
Cardeza Foundation for Hematologic Research
Jefferson Medical College of Thomas Jefferson University
Philadelphia, Pennsylvania

Ann Marie Schmidt, MD
Gerald and Janet Carrus Professor of Surgical Science
Division of Surgical Science, Department of Surgery
Columbia University
New York, New York

Michael V. Sefton, ScD
University Professor and Director
Institute of Biomaterials and Biomedical
    Engineering
University of Toronto
Toronto, Ontario
Canada

Lisa Senzel, MD, PhD
Senior Resident
Department of Pathology
Montefiore Medical Center
Bronx, New York

Sanford J. Shattil, MD
Professor of Medicine and Chief of Hematology/
    Oncology
Department of Medicine
University of California
La Jolla, California

Daniel I. Simon, MD, FACC
Associate Professor
Department of Medicine
Harvard Medical School
Associate Director, Interventional Cardiology
Cardiovascular Division
Brigham and Women's Hospital
Boston, Massachusetts

Emer M. Smyth, PhD
Research Assistant Professor
Department of Pharmacology
University of Pennsylvania
Philadelphia, Pennsylvania

Daphne Stewart, MD
Post-doctoral
Hematology/Medical Oncology Division
David Geffen School of Medicine at UCLA
Los Angeles, California

Ayalew Tefferi, MD
Professor of Medicine
Consultant in Hematology
Department of Hematology
Mayo Clinic
Rochester, Minnesota

Arthur R. Thompson, MD, PhD
Professor of Medicine
Division of Hematology
University of Washington School of Medicine
Director of Hemophilia Care and
    Hemostasis Laboratories
Puget Sound Blood Center
Seattle, Washington

Douglas M. Tollefsen, MD, PhD
Professor
Department of Medicine
Washington University Medical School
St. Louis, Missouri

Huyen A. M. Tran, MBBS (Hons), FRACP, FRCP(A)
Clinical Fellow
Department of Medicine
McMaster University
Clinical Fellow
Department of Medicine
McMaster University Medical Centre
Hamilton, Ontario
Canada

William Vainchenker, MD, PhD
Research Director
Inserm U 362
Institut Gustave Roussy
Villejuif, France
Consultant
Hematology Polyclinique
Hospital Saint Louis
Paris, France

Sara K. Vesely, PhD
Assistant Professor
Department of Biostatistics and Epidemiology and
    Department of Medicine
University of Oklahoma Health Sciences Center
Oklahoma City, Oklahoma

Renu Virmani, MD
Chairman, Department of Cardiovascular Pathology
Armed Forces Institute of Pathology
Washington, District of Columbia

Peter N. Walsh, MD, PhD
Professor
Departments of Medicine and Biochemistry
Sol Sherry Thrombosis Research Center
Temple University School of Medicine
Physician/Scientist
Medicine, Hematology Division
Temple University Hospital
Philadelphia, Pennsylvania

Theodore E. Warkentin, MD, FRCP(C), FACP
Professor
Departments of Pathology and Molecular Medicine,
    and Department of Medicine
McMaster University
Hematologist and Associate Head, Transfusion Medicine
Hamilton Regional Laboratory Medicine Program
Hamilton Health Sciences, Hamilton General Hospital
Hamilton, Ontario
Canada

Jeffrey I. Weitz, MD, FRCP(C), FACP, FCCP
Professor
Departments of Medicine and Biochemistry
McMaster University
Director
Henderson Research Centre
Hamilton, Ontario
Canada

Gilbert C. White II, MD
Professor
Division of Hematology Oncology
Carolina Cardiovascular Biology Center
University of North Carolina School of Medicine
Chapel Hill, North Carolina

Stephan Windecker, MD
Assistant Professor of Cardiology
Director, Invasive Cardiology
Department of Cardiology
University Hospital
Bern, Switzerland

Ann K. Wittkowsky, PharmD, CACP, FASHP
Clinical Professor
Department of Pharmacy
University of Washington School of Pharmacy
Director
Anticoagulation Services
University of Washington Medical Center
Seattle, Washington

San-Pin Wu, MS
Cardiovascular Sciences
Baylor College of Medicine
Houston, Texas

Manuel Yepes, MD
Assistant Professor
Department of Neurology
Center for Neurodegenerative Diseases
Emory University School of Medicine
Atlanta, Georgia

Bin Zhang, PhD
Research Investigator
Life Sciences Institute
University of Michigan
Ann Arbor, Michigan

Lijuan Zhang, PhD
Assistant Professor
Department of Pathology and Immunology
Washington University
St. Louis, Missouri

Marc Zumberg, MD
Assistant Professor
Department of Medicine
University of Florida
Gainesville, Florida

Mary M. Zutter, MD
Professor of Pathology and Cancer Biology
Ingram Professor of Cancer Research
Department of Pathology and Cancer Biology
Vanderbilt University School of Medicine
Director of Hematopathology
Department of Pathology
Vanderbilt University Medical Center
Nashville, Tennessee

The progress in the field of hemostasis and thrombosis has accelerated. The fourth edition of this textbook was published 7 years after the third, while this—the fifth edition—debuts only 5 years after the fourth. The number of chapters has increased from 91 to 123 because of the diversity and complexity of new knowledge. For example, in the basic principles section on coagulation, the chapter on protein Z and protein Z–dependent proteases discusses the role of a new cofactor. In the fibrinolysis section, the chapter on thrombin-activatable fibrinolysis inhibitor describes a new regulatory enzyme that inhibits thrombin-activated fibrinolysis. In the platelet section, a specific chapter on thrombopoietin emphasizes its greater recognition as a hematopoietic growth factor. Individual chapters on platelet receptors for thrombin, adenosine diphosphate, collagen, and prostanoids emphasize the greater knowledge of their importance and the understanding of their molecular interactions. A new chapter on the molecular characterization of epitopes for drug-dependent antibodies demonstrates the new molecular understanding of these important mechanisms of disease. New chapters on immune and drug-induced thrombocytopenia describe new concepts of etiology and new approaches to treatment. A new enzyme, ADAMTS13, has shed new light on both von Willebrand disease and thrombotic thrombocytopenia. The section on vascular biology, added in the fourth edition to reflect the strong interaction between hemostasis, thrombosis, and the cells of the vessel wall, now includes new information on vascular embryogenesis and development. This section also highlights the inflammatory interaction of leukocytes and platelets and helps us understand advances in the fields of atherosclerosis and cancer. Changes in the clinical application section reflect the increasing emphasis on translational medicine and atherothrombosis as it relates to cardiovascular medicine. The section on venous thromboembolism has been reorganized, with new chapters on epidemiology, women's health, upper extremity thrombosis, diagnosis, risk stratification, anticoagulant therapy, thrombolysis, caval filters, thromboembolic pulmonary hypertension, paradoxical embolism, and venous thromboembolism prophylaxis.

To update cardiovascular medicine, new chapters have been written about acute coronary syndromes, percutaneous coronary intervention, peripheral vascular disease, stroke, atrial fibrillation, cardiomyopathy, and valvular heart disease. New chapters have also been written on topics of practical clinical interest to hematologists, such as management of anticoagulation clinics.

The book has undergone a number of organizational changes. A founding editor of all four previous editions, Dr. Jack Hirsh has retired. Jack placed his stamp of evidence-based medicine not only on all the many chapters that he wrote but also on the entire clinical section of the book. He has been replaced by Samuel Z. Goldhaber, MD, a cardiologist with a special interest in thrombosis, as it occurs in the setting of cardiovascular and pulmonary vascular disease. This change in the textbook's leadership has led to many new chapters and new authors.

We hope that this new edition will serve the interests of medical and graduate students, scientists, and physicians. We expect that in addition to hematologists, cardiologists, vascular medicine specialists, pulmonologists, obstetricians, pediatricians, and surgeons will find useful information in this book. Finally, we thank all the authors for their outstanding contributions.

*Robert W. Colman, MD*
*Victor J. Marder, MD*
*Alexander W. Clowes, MD*
*James N. George, MD*
*Samuel Z. Goldhaber, MD*

The hemostatic system has evolved over millions of years from a much simpler system. In the limulus, a 400 million-year-old living fossil, the entire hemostatic system is contained in one cell (the amebocyte) that, in response to endotoxin elaborated by a vibrio, engulfs the organism and forms a coagulant from intracellular constituents. This single cell can be viewed as a progenitor of the platelet and the leukocyte, serving both hemostatic and inflammatory functions. The hemostatic system that evolved in humans features extracellular coagulation proteins, many of which are still present in platelets and endothelial cells, and has, therefore, conserved a function and structural interrelationship of plasma proteins and cellular elements.

*Hemostasis and Thrombosis* reviews the biochemistry and physiology of hemostasis, as well as the pathophysiology of thrombosis, and considers the diagnosis and treatment of both. The difficulty of separating one part of the system from another is illustrated by considering one of the best known hemostatic proteins, Factor VIII, which is currently regarded as a complex of two molecules—von Willebrand protein and procoagulant Factor VIII. Von Willebrand protein is synthesized in endothelial cells and megakaryocytes and is secreted into the plasma, while the coagulant Factor VIII molecule is synthesized in other cells, possibly under the control of the von Willebrand protein. The latter influences platelet adhesion to exposed subendothelium and probably to other cells, while Factor VIII increases the rate of Factor X activation and thrombin formation, which, in turn, stimulates platelets to undergo the release reaction and to aggregate and converts fibrinogen to fibrin. An obvious requirement for hemostasis, being deficient in the coagulant portion in classic hemophilia and in both the coagulant and platelet cofactor portions in von Willebrand disease, the Factor VIII complex is probably also intimately associated with pathologic thrombus formation. Thus, an understanding of the role of Factor VIII requires a detailed knowledge of its interactions with platelets, vascular wall cells, and other plasma proteins, as well as the influence of rheologic factors on these reactions, as manifest in the opposing mechanisms of hemostasis and thrombosis.

This textbook is directed at all who wish to explore this fascinating area of biology in greater depth. We hope that it will prove to be a useful reference for the student, the physician, and the scientist who is interested in laboratory or clinical aspects of these disorders and who may wish to obtain a comprehensive discussion and complete reference source. Many authors have contributed to *Hemostasis and Thrombosis*, and some overlap of information was inevitable, but this was not actively avoided. Therefore, we hope that each chapter is complete in its own right, concentrating on either basic aspects or clinical applications of a disorder or relevant cellular or protein components.

# CONTENTS

SECTION D ■ VASCULAR BIOLOGY,
EMBRYOGENESIS, DEVELOPMENT, AND
DISORDERS

PART II ■ CLINICAL APPLICATIONS

SECTION A ■ INHERITED HEMORRHAGIC
DISORDERS

## SECTION F ■ COMPLEX THROMBOHEMORRHAGIC DISORDERS

## SECTION G ■ THERAPY, NEW DIRECTIONS, AND COMPLICATIONS IN THROMBOTIC DISORDERS

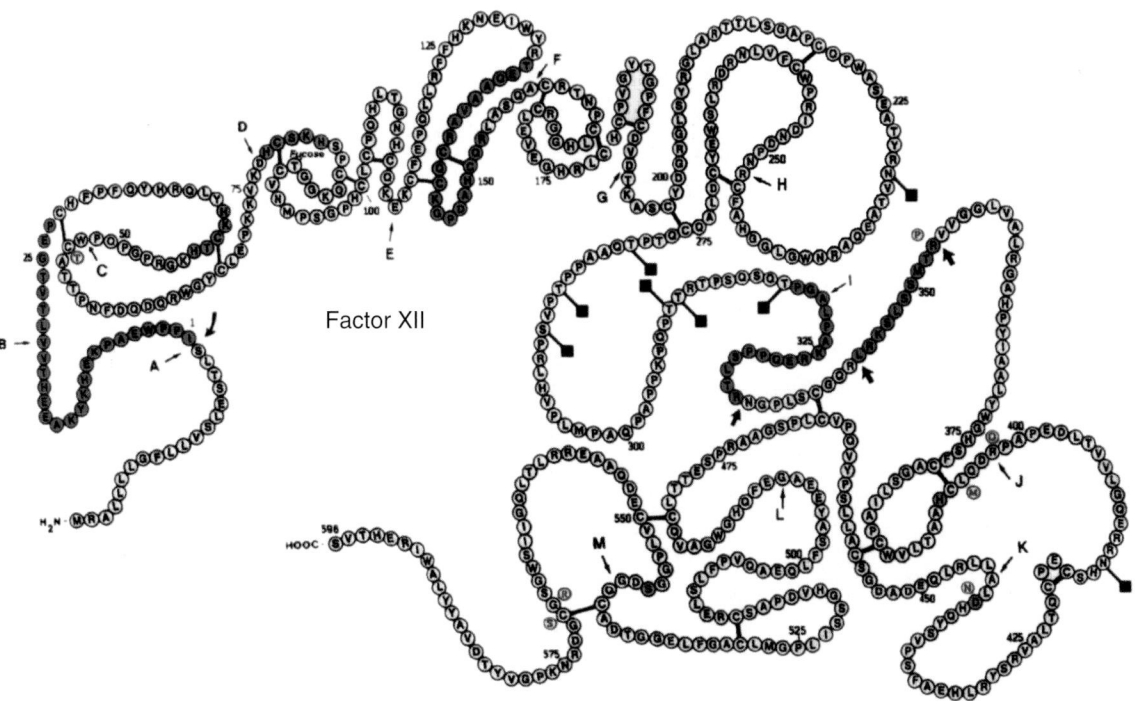

**COLOR FIGURE 6-1.** Schematic diagram of human factor XII. (FXII) The standard one-letter code is given in the *open circles*. The *solid black bars* indicate possible disulfide bonding between cysteine residues based on homologies and other proteins. The *arrows A to M* indicate positions of introns in the coding sequence. The *curved arrow* indicates the cleavage site to remove the propeptide and reveal the *N*-terminal isoleucine. The *straight arrows* are the sites of kallikrein cleavage. The *black squares* are the sites of glycosylation. The *red residues* are the catalytic triad, H393, D458, and S556. The *red letters* in *red open circles* are sites of known missense mutations leading to loss of coagulant activity. The *purple residues* are the three putative surface binding regions. The *two green regions* are $Zn^{2+}$ binding sequences.

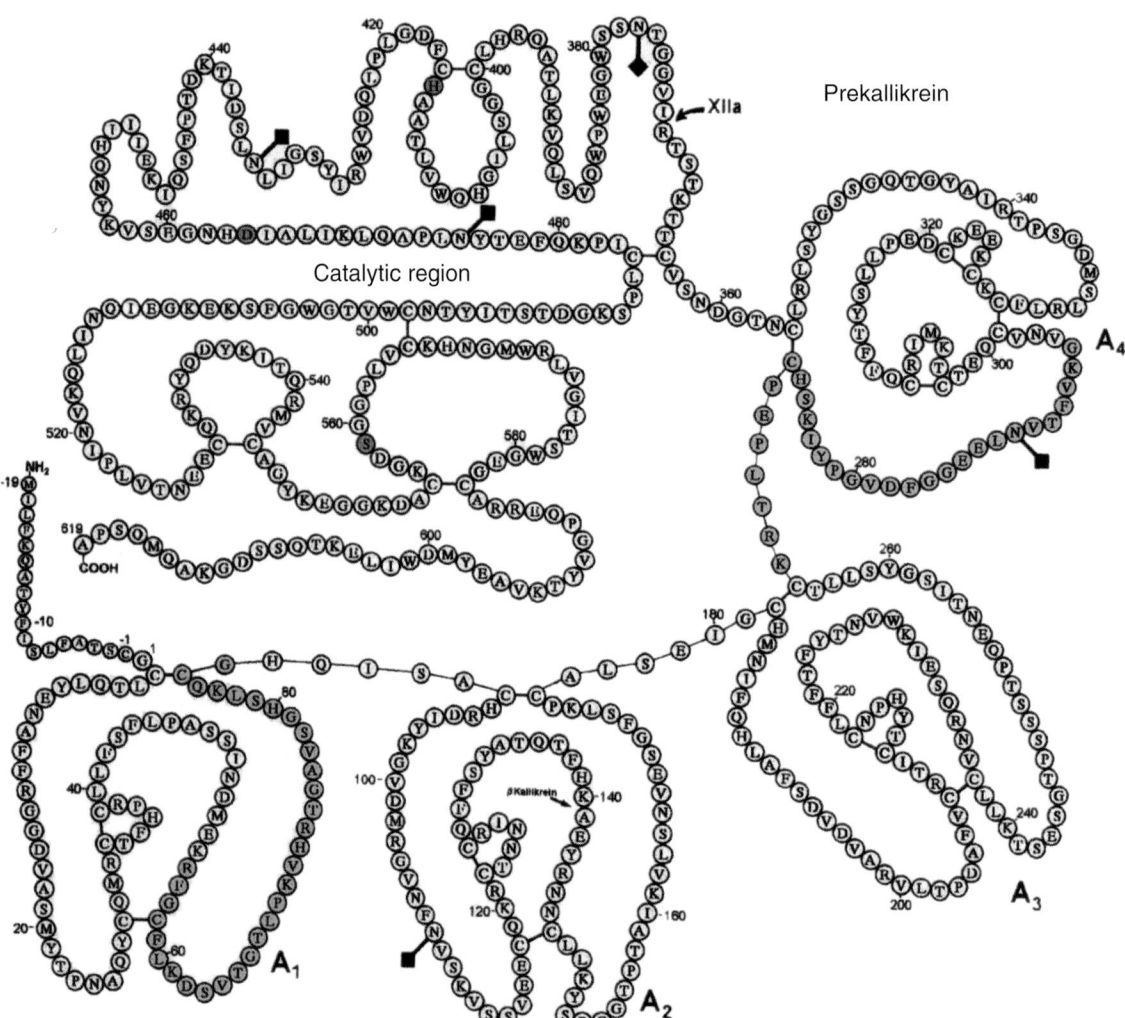

COLOR FIGURE 6-2. Schematic diagram of human prekallikrein. The four apple domains in the N-terminal portion of the molecule are labeled $A_1$ to $A_4$. The regions that bind high-molecular-weight kininogen are *yellow*. The bond cleaved by FXIIa is R371-I372. The catalytic triad, H415, D464, S559, is indicated in *red*. The sites of N- and O-glycosylation are indicated as *black squares*. The N-terminal of the propeptide is indicated $NH_2$, and the site of its cleavage to yield the mature protein is between amino acids −1 and 1. The site of kallikrein cleavage of itself to yield β-kallikrein is indicated with an *arrow*. The site of FXIIa cleavage to activate prekallikrein is indicated with a *curved arrow*. No intron location is indicated as the structure of the human kallikrein gene has not been determined.

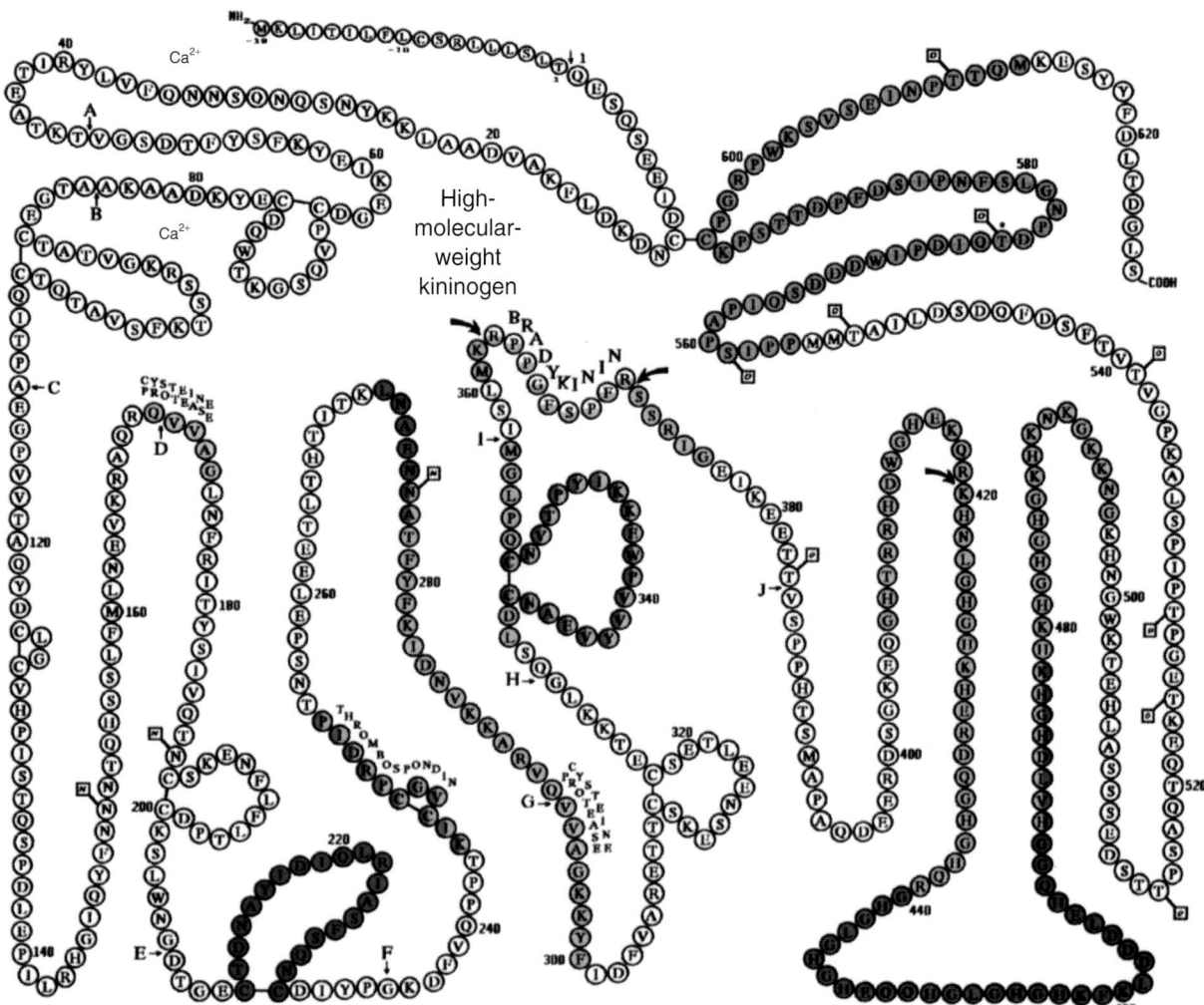

COLOR FIGURE 6-3. Primary sequence and genetic structure of human high-molecular-weight kininogen. Numbers 1 to 626 are amino acid (aa) locations with leader sequence −18 to −1. Letters A through J are the locations of the intron/exon junctions D1 (aa 1 to 113) is coded by exons 1, 2, and 3. D2 (aa 114 to 234) is coded by exons 4, 5, and 6. D3 (aa 235 to 357) is coded by exons 7, 8, and 9. D4 (aa 358 to 383) is coded by exon 10$_{BK}$. D5 (aa 384 to 502) is coded by the 5′ portion of exon 10$_{HK}$. D6 (aa 503 to 626) is coded by the 3′ portion of exon 10$_{HK}$. The *curved arrows* indicate plasma kallikrein cleavage sites. *Boxed O* is the location of an O-linked carbohydrate chain. *Boxed N* is the location of an N-linked carbohydrate chain. The *yellow* sequences (aa 170 to 174, aa 292 to 296) are binding sites for cysteine proteases. The *maroon* sequence (aa 211 to 230) is a site that inhibits calpain 2 activity. The *purple-half red* sequence (aa 244 to 254) is a binding site for both endothelial cells and thrombospondin (TSP). The *green* sequences (aa 271 to 277, aa 333 to 352, and aa 440 to 478) represent binding sites for neutrophils on D3 and D5. The *purple* sequences (aa 331 to 357, aa 361 to 376, aa 406 to 439, and aa 471 to 496) represent binding sites for endothelial cells on D3, D4, and D5. The *pink* sequence (aa 556 to 613) is the binding site for FXI, and the *chartreuse* sequence (aa 565 to 595) is the binding site for PK, both on D6. This representation was created by Dr. Robin Pixley.

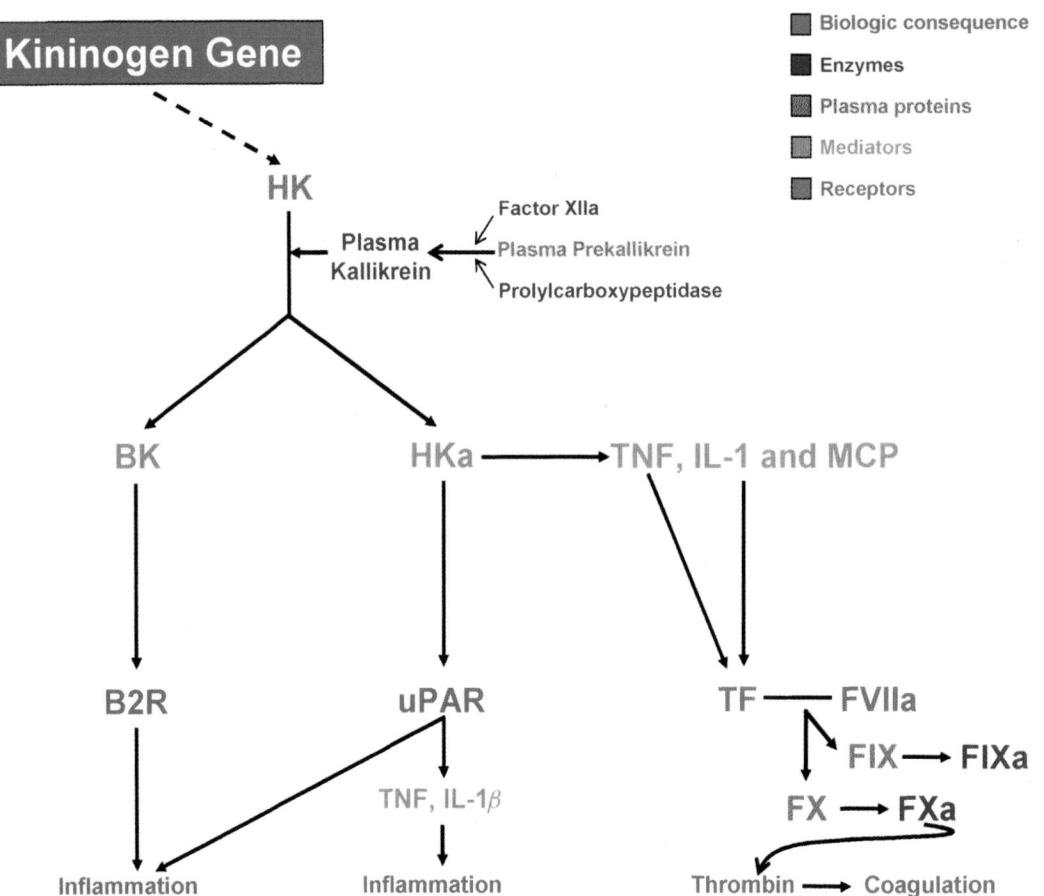

COLOR FIGURE 6-4. Role of kallikrein–kinin system in inflammation—a hypothesis. The kininogen gene codes for high-molecular-weight kininogen (HK). Factor XIIa from plasma or prolylcarboxypeptidase (an outer cell membrane enzyme) cleaves plasma prekallikrein to plasma kallikrein, which in turn hydrolyzes HK to two mediators. Bradykinin (BK), through its constitutive receptor, B2R, stimulates inflammation. HKa, through one of its receptors, uPAR, stimulates inflammation in leukocytes. TF, a receptor induced by inflammatory cytokines (IL-1, TNF), is responsible for binding and fascilitating the activation of FVII to FVIIa. TF-FVIIa activates FIX and FX, resulting in FXa, which generates thrombin.

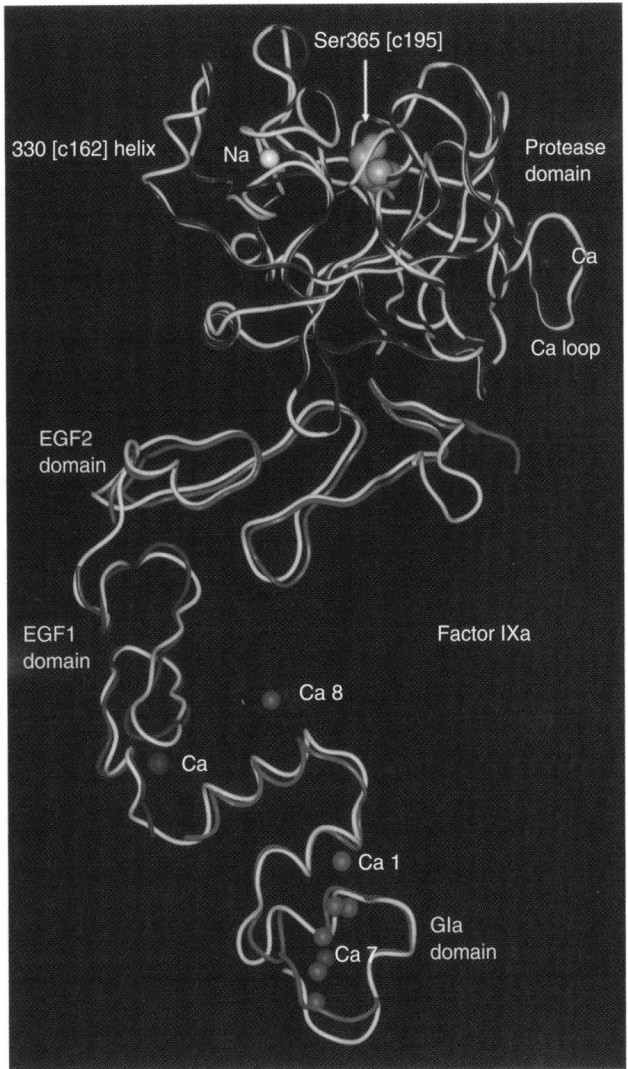

COLOR FIGURE 7-2. Schematic representation of the structure of factor IXa. Coordinates of porcine factor IXa [yellow, Protein Data Bank (PDB) code 1pfx] (66), human factor IXa EGF2 and protease domains (purple and light blue, PDB code 1rfn), human EGF1 domain (dark blue, PDB code 1edm), and the human Gla domain (magenta, PDB code 1j35) were used. The location of each domain is indicated. The location of the active site Ser365 [c195] in grey spheres (*arrow*) and the 330-helix [c162-helix] are shown, where residues are numbered from the sequence of the secreted human protein and [c] refers to the corresponding position of the prototype serine protease, chymotrypsin. The protease domain's bound $Ca^{2+}$ ion (*purple sphere*) and $Na^+$ ion (*grey sphere*), the EGF1-bound $Ca^{2+}$ ion (*dark blue sphere*), and Gla domain's bound $Ca^{2+}$ ions (*magenta spheres*) are shown. Ca1, Ca7, and Ca8 can be replaced by $Mg^{2+}$ (PDB code 1j34).

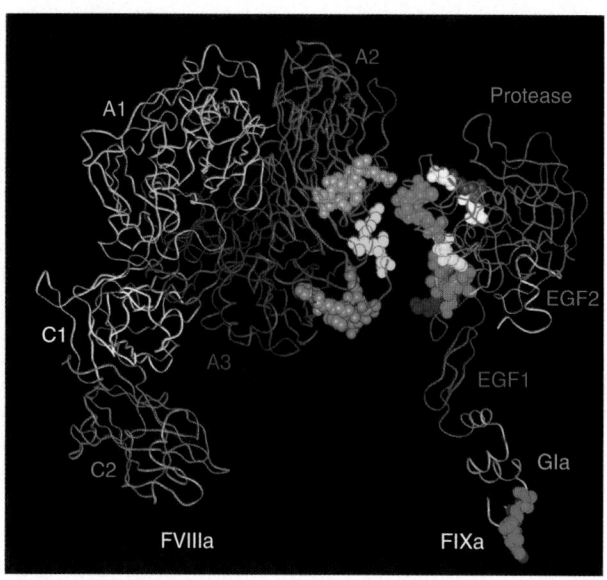

COLOR FIGURE 7-3. A model of the interaction of factor IXa with factor VIIIa. The coordinates for the factor IXa structure are from the Protein Data Bank (code 1rfn and 1pfx) and the coordinates for the A1, A2, A3, C1, and C2 subunits of factor VIIIa are from Stoilova-McPhie (HAMSTeR database) (242). Ribbon structure for each protein is depicted. The A1, A2, and A3 domains of factor VIIIa are homologous to the ceruloplasmin domains, whereas the C1 and C2 domains are homologous to the galactose oxidase lipid binding domain. The hypothesized interface residues are shown as CPK space-filling models. On the right, the factor IXa protease domain is in *green*, the EGF2 domain is in *lavender*, the EGF1 domain is in *red*, and the Gla domain is in *orange*. The A1 subunit of factor VIIIa is in *yellow*, the A2 subunit is in *magenta*, the A3 subunit is in *blue*, the C1 subunit is in *white*, and the C2 subunit is in *orange*. The factor IXa protease domain, with residues numbered as in Figure 7-2, Asn346 [c178] is in *pink*, residues of the 330-helix [c162-helix] are in *cyan*, residues 301–303 [c132–c134] are in *yellow*, Arg403 [c233] is *purple*, and Lys293 [c126] is *white*. In EGF2, residues 89–93 are *red-orange*, and residues 84–87 are *dark blue*. Residues Lys5, Leu6, Phe9, and Val10 of the factor IXa Gla domain that are involved in binding to the phospholipids surface are shown and colored by atom type in which carbons are *green*, nitrogens are *blue*, and oxygens are *red*. The protease domain residues most likely interact with the A2 subunit of factor VIIIa, whereas the EGF2 domain residues may be involved in binding to the A2 and/or the A3 subunit of factor VIIIa. In factor VIIIa, depicted on the left, the A2 subunit residues 558–565 are in orange and 707–712 are in *yellow*. The A3 subunit residues 1811–1818 are shown in *light green*. The A2 subunit residues could possibly be involved in binding to the heavy chain (protease domain), whereas the A3 subunit residues could be involved in binding to the light chain (including the EGF2 domain) of factor IXa. It should be noted that the crystal structure of a partial bovine factor Va suggests a different orientation of C1 and C2 domains such that C1 may also bind to the lipid surface (244).

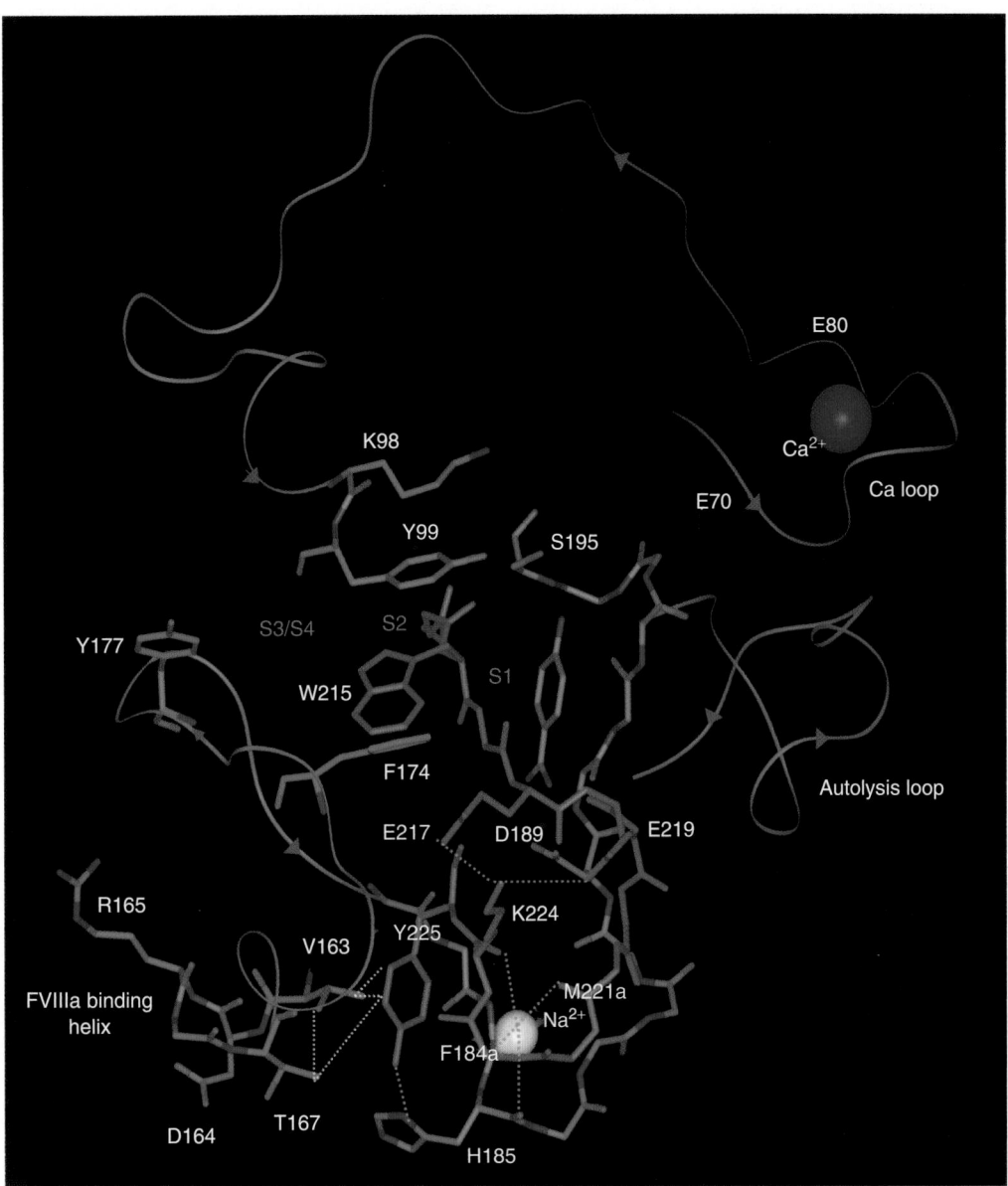

COLOR FIGURE 7-4. Relation of the Na$^+$-binding site to the S1 site and factor VIIIa binding helix in factor IXa. The two loops that bind the Na$^+$ ion, 353–359 [c183–c189] colored by atom type and 391–395 [c221–c225] colored *magenta*, and the 330-helix [c162-helix] that binds factor VIIIa are shown and colored by atom type in which carbons are *green*, nitrogens are *blue*, and oxygens are *red*. The bound Ca$^{2+}$ ion is shown as a *purple sphere*. Na$^+$ ion is shown as a *grey* sphere and is coordinated to the carbonyl O atoms of Phe353 [c184A], His354 [c185], Met391 [c221A], and Lys394 [c224]. The benzene ring of Tyr395 [c225] makes Van der Waals contacts with Val331 [c163] and Thr335 [c167]. The hydroxyl group of Tyr395 [c225] makes an H-bond with His354 [c185] and Lys394 [c224] makes H-bonds with Glu387 [c217] and Glu388 [c219]. Note that the 380 loop [c220 loop] is one residue shorter in factor IXa than in chymotrypsin. The S1 site is occupied by *p*AB and its benzamidine moiety makes H-bonds with Asp359 [c189], and the amino group of Val181 [c16] makes an H-bond with carboxylate of Asp364 [c194]. The H-bonds are shown with *cyan dashed lines* and Van der Waals contacts are shown with *white dashed lines*. Asp332 [c164] and Arg333 [c165] are two residues that are important in binding to factor VIIIa. Residues Lys265 [c98], Tyr266 [c99], Phe342 [c174], Tyr345 [c177], and Trp385 [c215] that play important roles in occupancy of the substrate at the S2/S3/S4 sites are also depicted. All residues are colored by atom type except Trp385 [c215], which is colored *magenta*. *Red* represents oxygen, *blue* represents nitrogen, and *green* represents carbon. The locations of the S2 and S3/S4 sites are also shown. The Ca$^{2+}$ loop and autolysis loop are also shown. The figure is drawn based upon the atomic coordinates (PDB code 1rfn). The numbering system used in this figure is that of chymotrypsin.

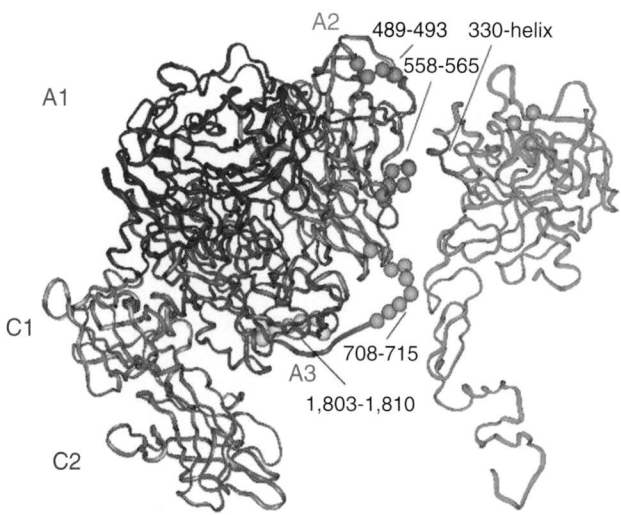

COLOR FIGURE 8-4. Molecular modeling of the factor Xase. Factor VIIIa (*left*) and factor IXa (*right*) are drawn in *ribbon* format on the basis of the five-domainal model of factor VIII (161) and the crystal structure of factor IXa (160), respectively. Factor IXa is shown in *green* with the 330 helix shown in *red*. *Spheres* indicate the α carbon positions of the active site residues. Factor VIII domains are coded as A1 (*blue*), A2 (*cyan*), A3 (*red*), and C-domains (*copper*). *Spheres* indicate α carbon positions for the indicated factor IXa–interactive sites. (Reprinted from Fay PJ, Jenkins PV. Mutating factor VIII: lessons from structure to function. *Blood Rev* 2005;19:15-27, with permission from Elsevier.)

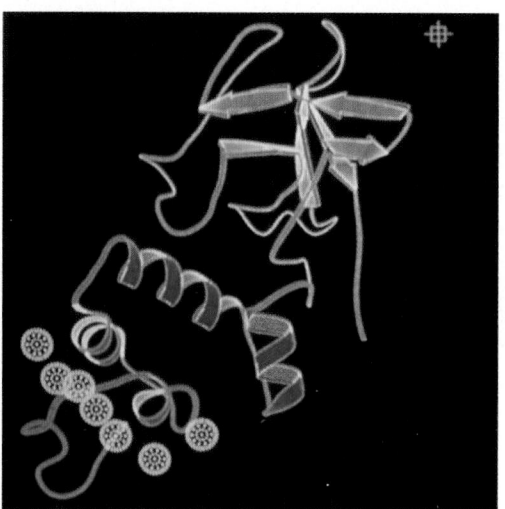

COLOR FIGURE 10-2. Orientation of the backbone peptide chain of prothrombin fragment 1. The NH$_2$-terminal segment of the molecule is oriented toward the lower left-hand quadrant (7 o'clock) of the figure. The kringle 1 segment of the molecule is in the upper right (2 o'clock). Pleated sheet segments are indicated by *arrows*. Calcium ions are identified by *orange balls*. The connecting region between the Gla domain and kringle 1 is represented by an α-helix. (Courtesy of Drs. Timothy Rydel and Alexander Tulinsky.)

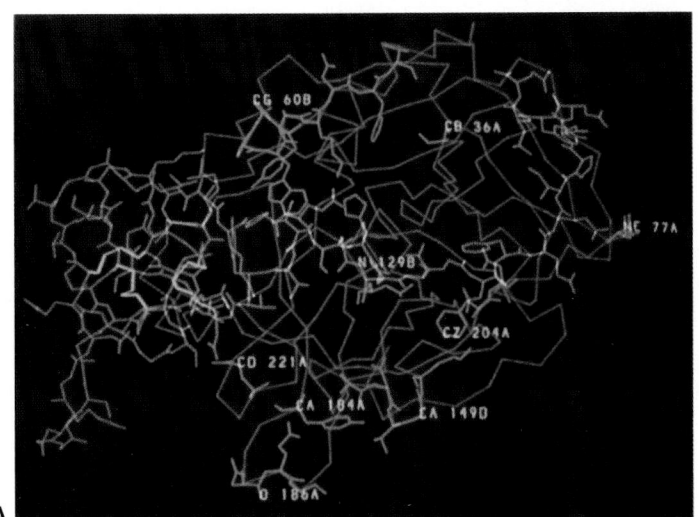
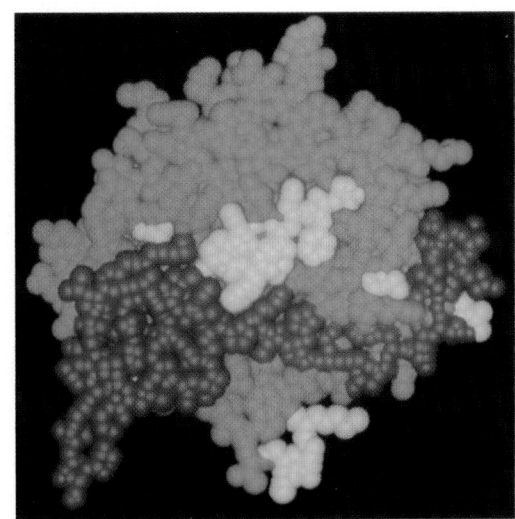

COLOR FIGURE 10-3. The α-thrombin–hirudin complex. **A:** The α-carbon backbone structure of thrombin (*light blue*) and the α-carbon backbone structure of hirudin (*red*). Disulfide bonds in the NH$_2$-terminal domain of the hirudin molecule are in *yellow*, and "insertion loops" in the thrombin molecule relative to chymotrypsinogen are represented with their appropriate side chains in *light blue*. Insertion loop residues are identified to orient the reader with respect to the identity of various insertional loops. The nomenclature used is that of Bode et al. (56) and in some instances represents an earlier stage of refinement of insertional nomenclature. There are, therefore, a few differences between nomenclature in this figure and that defined in Table 10-2. However, all nomenclature reflected in the figure is within one or two residues of the notation presented in Table 10-2. **B:** A space-filling model of the same complex; α-thrombin (*blue*), hirudin (*red*), and insertion loops (*yellow*). (From Bode W, Mayr I, Baumann U, et al. The refined 1.9 Å crystal structure of human α-thrombin: interaction with D-Phe-Pro-Arg chloromethylketone and significance of the Tyr-Pro-Pro-Trp insertion segment. *EMBO J* 1989;8:3467, with permission.)

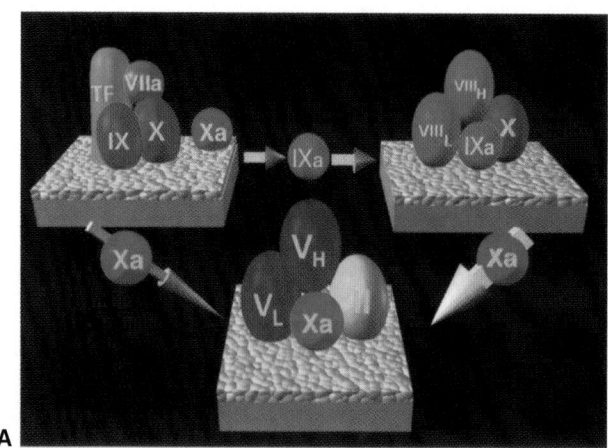

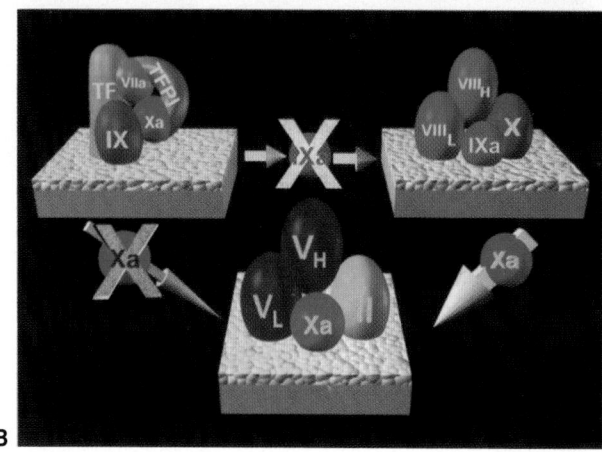

COLOR FIGURE 10-5. The procoagulant vitamin K–dependent complexes. **A:** The tissue factor–factor VIIa (extrinsic) complex triggers coagulation by activating factors IX and X. Factor Xa also cleaves factor IX and accelerates factor IXa generation. The factor VIIIa–factor IXa (intrinsic) complex activates factor X at a much higher rate than the extrinsic complex, thereby allowing formation of the factor Va–factor Xa (prothrombinase) complex and initiating explosive thrombin generation. **B:** Tissue factor pathway inhibitor (TFPI) interacts with the tissue factor–factor VIIa–factor Xa ternary complex to inhibit extrinsic complex-dependent activation of factors IX and X. Subsequent factor Xa generation occurs only via the intrinsic tenase complex.

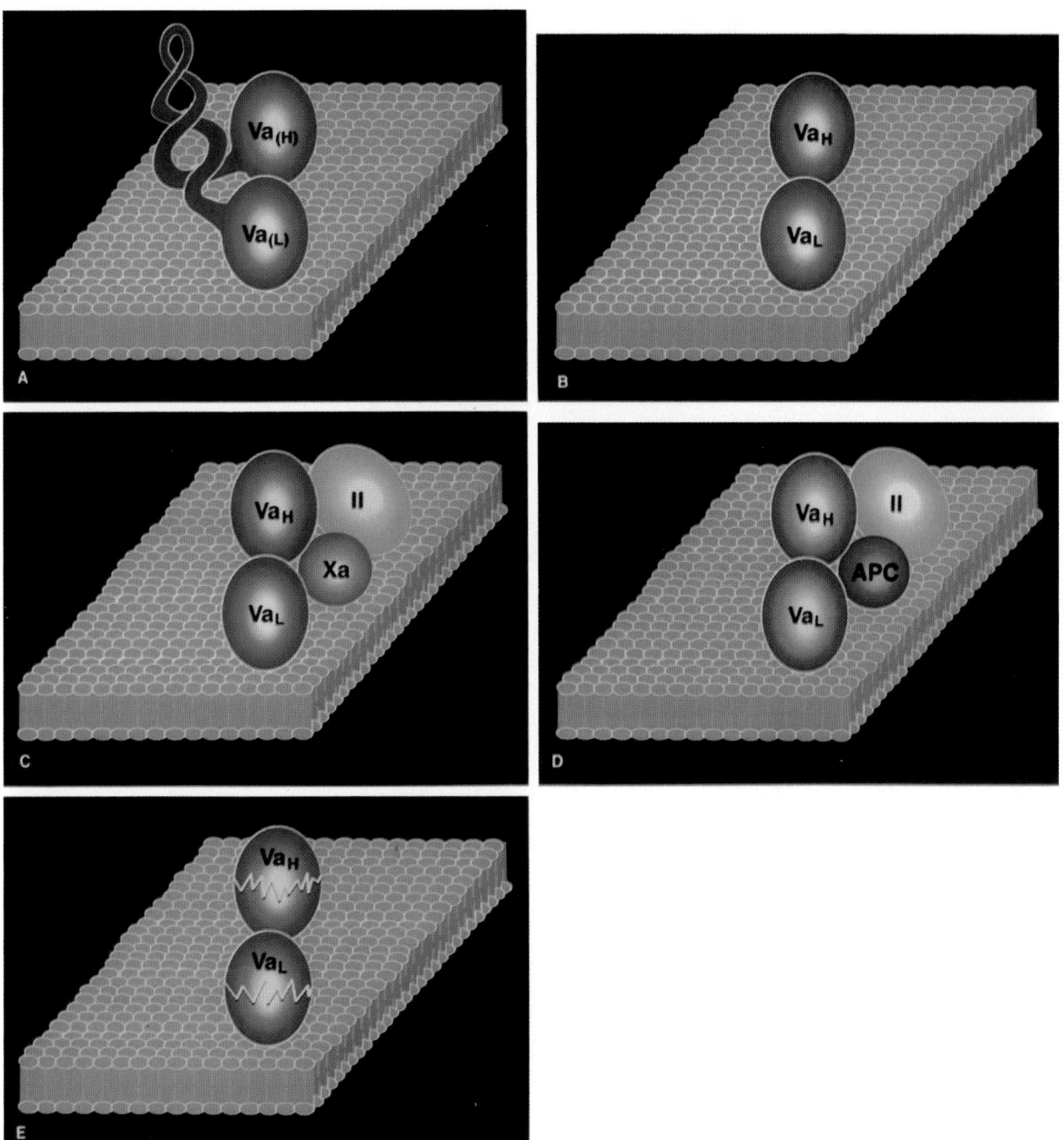

COLOR FIGURE 10-6. Assembly and expression of the prothrombinase complex. **A:** Factor V is shown as a multidomain molecule embedded in the membrane lipid bilayer predominantly through the COOH-terminal region of the molecule. **B:** Following thrombin activation, the factor Va molecule, comprising the COOH-terminal–derived peptide, Va(L), and the NH$_2$-terminal–derived peptide, Va(H), remains bound to the membrane surface through Va(L). **C:** The light chain of factor Va forms at least part of the receptor for factor Xa, which binds to membrane-bound factor Va in a 1:1 molar stoichiometry. Prothrombin, composed of fragment 1 (F1), fragment 2 (F2), and prothrombin 2 (P2) domains, interacts with Va(H) of the factor Va molecule through its F2 region. **D:** Activated protein C (APC) also appears to form a complex with Va(L) of the membrane-bound factor Va molecule. The APC–factor Va interaction is competitive with factor Xa, but unaffected by prothrombin binding. **E:** APC cleaves both chains of factor Va, eliminating the complex.

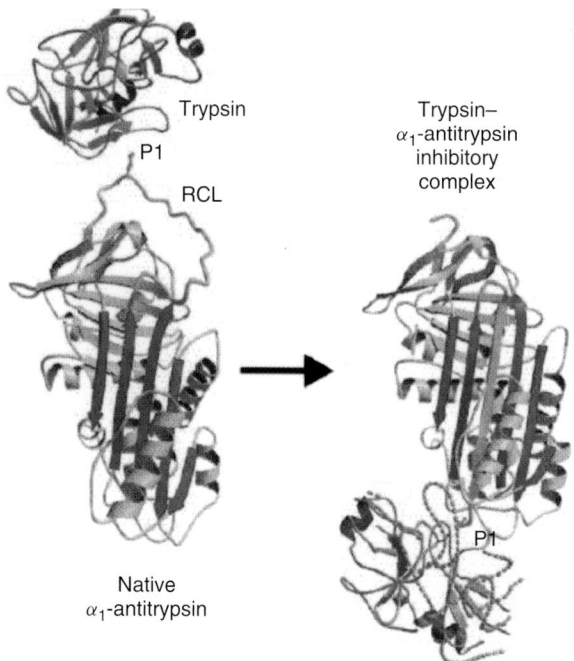

COLOR FIGURE 13-2. Serpin inhibition mechanism. **Left:** The native $\alpha_1$-antitrypsin molecule contains a 5-stranded central $\beta$-sheet (*red*) and an intact and fully exposed reactive center loop (RCL) (*yellow*) that is recognized as a substrate by target enzymes, including trypsin. **Right:** Formation of an inhibitory complex between $\alpha_1$-antitrypsin and trypsin involves: (a) trypsin recognition and cleavage of the P1–P1' peptide bond in the RCL polypeptide, (b) formation of a covalent acyl linkage between the serpin P1 residue and the enzyme active site serine, (c) expansion of the serpin central $\beta$-sheet by incorporation of the cleaved RCL polypeptide as a sixth strand, (d) translocation of the P1 residue and covalently bound enzyme from the north pole to the south pole of the serpin molecule, and (e) deformation of the translocated trypsin molecule. Target enzyme deformation in the inhibitory complex alters active-site geometry, which prevents deacylation and facilitates proteolytic destruction of disordered regions (interrupted coils). (From Huntington J, Read R, Carrell R. Structure of a serpin-protease complex shows inhibition by deformation. *Nature* 2000;407:923–926, with permission.)

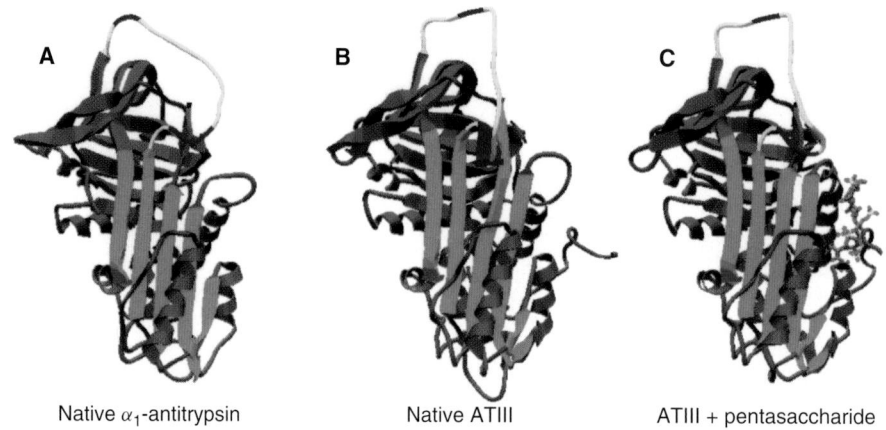

COLOR FIGURE 13-3. Structural basis for limited reactivity of native ATIII, and ATIII allosteric activation by heparin pentasaccharide. Serpin–reactive center loop (RCL) polypeptides are drawn in *yellow*, with the P1–P1' scissile bonds marked in *purple* and the P14 residues marked in *blue*. Central A $\beta$-sheets are *orange*. **A:** RCL loops of most serpins, such as $\alpha_1$-antitrypsin, are fully exposed and unconstrained by A-sheet insertion, and they inhibit their target enzymes rates of approximately $10^6$ $M^{-1}$ $sec^{-1}$. **B:** The RCL loop of native ATIII is constrained by insertion of its P14 residue into $\beta$-sheet-A, which reduces rates of native ATIII target enzyme inhibition to approximately $10^3$ $M^{-1}$ $sec^{-1}$. **C:** Heparin pentasaccharide binding to ATIII allosterically expels the RCL loop and restores FXa inhibition rates into the approximately $10^6$ $M^{-1}$ $sec^{-1}$ range. Figures are drawn using 1QLP.pbd for $\alpha_1$-antitrypsin, 1E05.pbd for native ATIII, and 1E03.pbd for ATIII pentasaccharide.

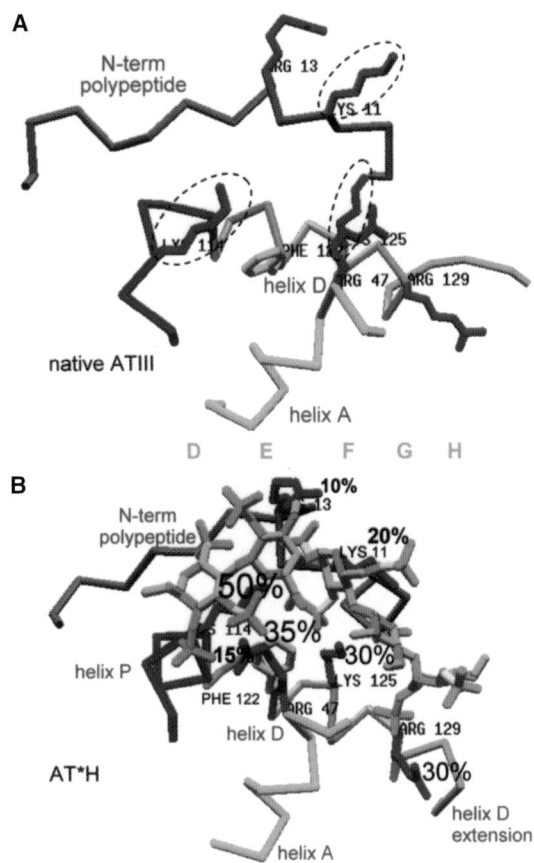

COLOR FIGURE 13-5. Pentasaccharide occupancy of the heparin binding site on ATIII induces a protein conformational change that leads to high-affinity binding of the cofactor, reactive center loop expulsion, and acceleration of FXa inhibition. (**A**) and (**B**) show pentasaccharide binding surfaces of native
ATIII (1E05.pdb) and of AT*H (1E03.pdb), respectively. Side chains of the basic residues of heparin
binding site are *blue*, and that of phenylalanine122 is *green*. **A:** Circled lysine125, 114, and 11 residues of
native ATIII (**A**) participate in cofactor recognition and in the formation of the initial weak AT–H intermediate. **B:** Pentasaccharide atoms are drawn in *aqua* (carbon), *red* (oxygen), and *yellow* (sulfur), and the
D–H sugar labels are in *aqua*. Numbers indicate the percentage of pentasaccharide-free energy of binding
that is lost upon mutation of indicated residues. Conformational changes induced by pentasaccharide
binding can be visualized by comparing the main-chain polypeptide backbones of key structural elements
in native (**A**) and AT*H (**B**) molecules. *Orange* shows elongation of helical region at arginine47 end of
helix A; *purple* shows formation of helix P at the amino-terminal end of helix D (*light blue*), and *pink*
shows elongation of helix D at its carboxy terminus.

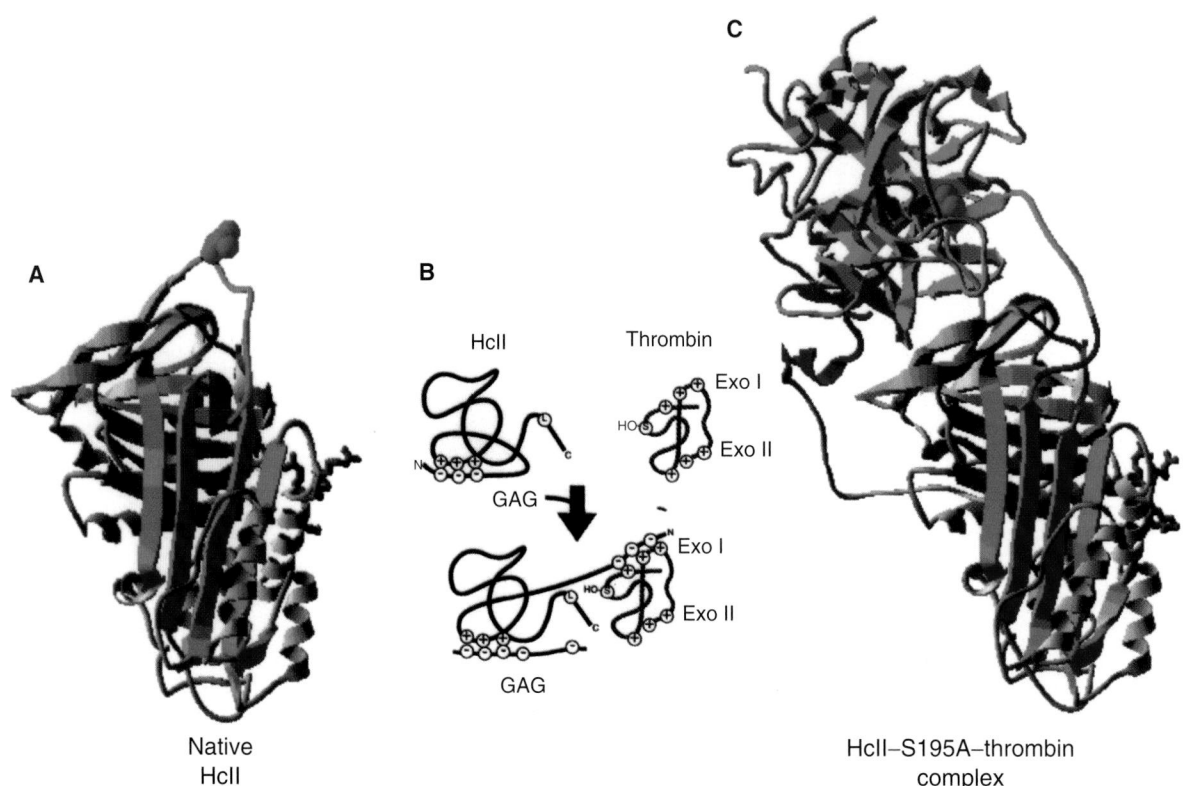

**COLOR FIGURE 13-7.** Heparin cofactor II (HcII) inhibition of thrombin. **A:** Native HcII. The reactive center loop (*orange and purple*) of native HcII is constrained because of incorporation of its C-terminal end (*purple*) into β-sheet-A (*pink*). The leucine P1 residue of the reactive center loop is shown as a *red* van der Waals surface, and side chains of positively charged residues in the GAG-binding site are drawn in *aqua*. The N-terminal hirudin-like polypeptide of HcII was not visible in this structure because perturbations caused by intermolecular contacts in the dimeric native HcII crystal structure largely prevented assignment of its location. **B:** Cartoon model of native HcII shows intramolecular binding of its N-terminal, negatively charged hirudin-like and positively charged GAG-binding domains, as inferred from mutagenesis studies. Activation occurs when cofactor heparin or dermatan sulfate molecules bind HcII and competitively displace its N-terminal domain from its GAG-binding site. This uncoupling leads to: (a) allosteric HcII conformational changes and (b) HcII N-terminal domain binding to the thrombin anion-binding exosite I, which together increase the specificity, rate, and strength of the inhibitory complex formation. **C:** S195A-thrombin–HcII Michaelis complex. In this structure, the N-terminal anionic binding site (*dark blue ribbon*) interacts with exosite I on thrombin (*green*), and the allosteric change leading to expulsion of the reactive center loop (*purple* and *orange*) from the A β-sheet has occurred. (**A** and **C:** From Protein Data Bank structures 1JMJ and 1JMO, respectively. **B:** From Tollefsen D. Heparin cofactor II. *Adv Exp Med Biol* 1997;425:35–44, with permission.)

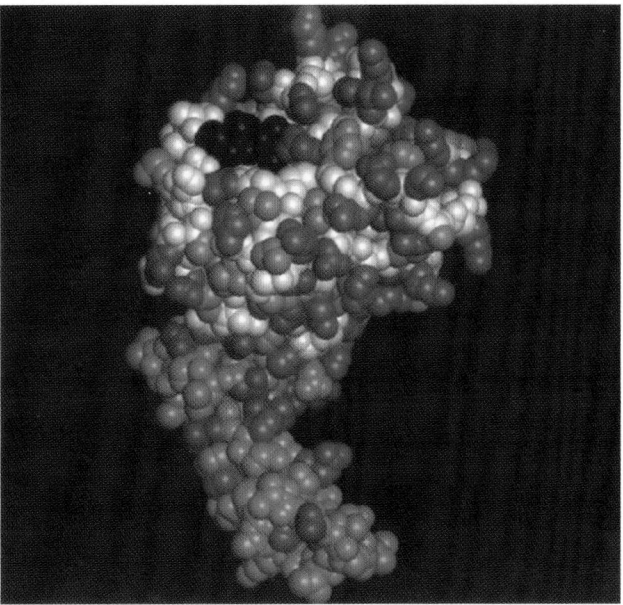

COLOR FIGURE 14-4. Space-filling model of the activated protein C crystal. The model is based on the previously determined structure of activated protein C lacking the Gla domain (128). The active site inhibitor is shown in *black*. Basic residues are in *blue*, acidic residues are *red*, and hydrophobic residues are *gold*. Other residues in the protease domain are *white*. The acidic, basic, and hydrophobic residues of the EGF domains follow the same convention, but the other residues are in *green* to set off the EGF domains from the protease domain. The three basic residues critical for activation by the thrombin–TM complex are at the top of the figure. The exosite runs just underneath these residues. The $Ca^{2+}$ binding site is to the far right of the protease domain near the acidic (*red*) residue that is almost completely hidden by the basic (*blue*) residues.

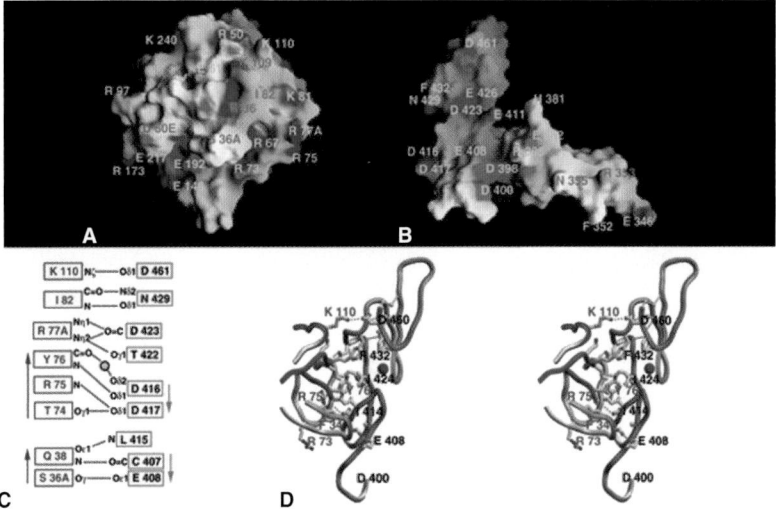

COLOR FIGURE 14-7. The thrombin-thrombomodulin interaction interface is dominated by hydrophobic contacts. Graphical representation and analysis of surface properties (GRASP) (425) electrostatic surface potentials of $\alpha$-thrombin (**A**) and TME456 (**B**). Both moieties have been slightly rotated around the *y* axis to present their interaction interfaces to the viewer. Note the overall complementarity of electrostatic potentials. **C**: Major hydrogen–bonding interactions (*dotted lines*) between thrombin and TM. **D**: Detail of the interaction interface, highlighting its primary hydrophobic character. Selected hydrogen bonds are indicated as *green spheres*. Note that single, solvent-exposed salt bridge forms between thrombin and TM (Lys110 N$\zeta$-Asp461 0$\delta$2). For clarity, only residues Asp400-Cys462 of TM and thrombin loops of the contact interface are shown. (Reprinted with permission from Fuentes-Prior P, et al. *Nature* 2000;404:518–525, copyright 2000.)

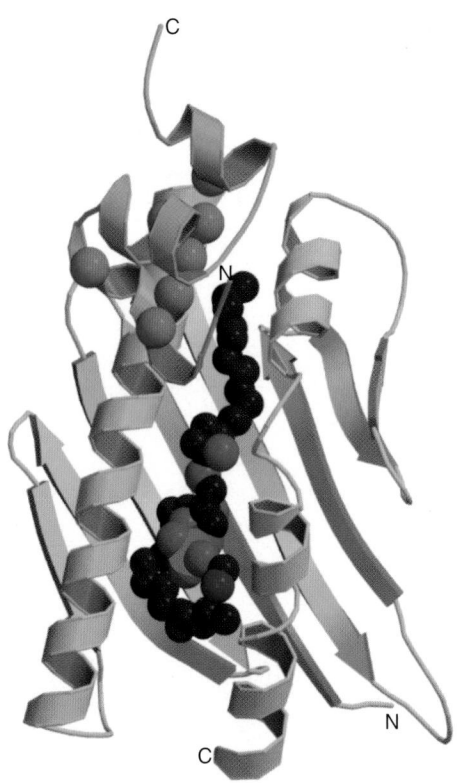

COLOR FIGURE 14-9. The rs-endothelial cell protein C receptor (EPCR) molecule with a portion of the protein C Gla domain and a lipid molecule. In EPCR (*yellow ribbon*), two α-helices and an eight-stranded β-sheet create a groove that is filled with phospholipid (the space-filling balls in the center). Binding of Ca$^{2+}$ ions (*spheres in magenta*) to the protein C Gla domain (*green ribbon*) exposes the *N*-terminal "omega" loop, which in the absence of EPCR interacts with the phospholipid surfaces on the membrane. There do not appear to be direct interactions between the protein C Gla domain and the lipid molecule located in the groove of rsEPCR. The model of the complex consists of residues 7 to 177 of rsEPCR and the first 33 residues of the protein C Gla domain (422–424). [Reprinted with permission from Oganesyan et al., *The J Biol Chem* 2002;277(28):24851–24854, copyright 2002.]

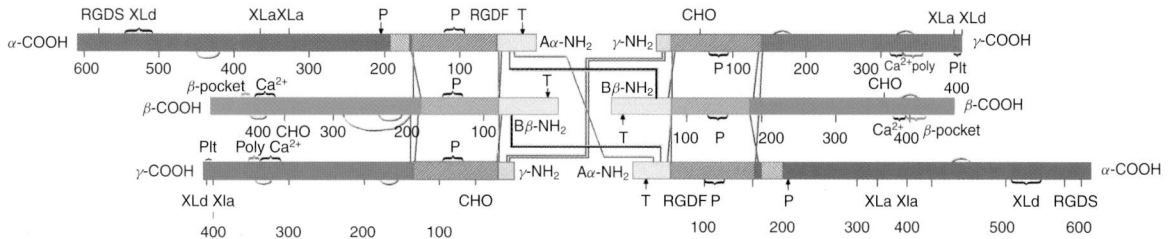

COLOR FIGURE 16-1. Schematic diagram of the six polypeptide chains of fibrinogen: The Aα, Bβ, and γ chains of human fibrinogen are represented by bars (*blue*, *green*, and *red*, respectively) that are proportional to the number of residues of each chain; the numbers beneath the rectangles define the sequence number. Note the three disulfide bonds (*yellow lines*) that connect the two halves of the molecule in an antiparallel arrangement; a twofold symmetry axis passes through the center of this region, perpendicular to the plane of the page. The seven pairs of interchain disulfide bonds are represented by *straight yellow lines* and the six pairs of intrachain disulfide bonds by *curved, yellow lines*. Thrombin cleavage sites on the Aα and Bβ chains are indicated by a *T* and an *arrow*. *Brackets* define the plasmin-sensitive regions within the coiled-coil regions; the *single arrow* with a P indicates the plasmin cleavage that releases the polar portion of the carboxyl-terminal of the α chain. The positions of lysine and glutamine residues, which have been identified as crosslink electron donor and acceptor sites, are indicated by XLd and XLa, respectively; regions of the α chain that contain lysine donor sites are identified by brackets. Regions of the β and γ chains involved in calcium binding are marked with brackets and Ca²⁺. Sequences on the γ chain that interact with GPRP, thereby defining a polymerization site involved in fibrin assembly, are indicated by poly (*red brackets*), and those involved in platelet binding by Plt. Regions on the β chain that interact with GHRP are denoted by β-pocket (*green brackets*). Sites of carbohydrate attachment are indicated by CHO. The different shadings and colors within each rectangle indicate the portions of the polypeptide chain that define the central domain (*dotted*), the coiled-coil region (*right diagonals*), the outer domains (β-domain, *solid green*; γ-domain, *solid red*), and in the case of the Aα chain, the polar region (*solid blue*). The *small, blue, left-diagonal region* on the α chain denotes its "hairpin helix".

Complete details of the sequences of each polypeptide can be found in electronic databases with the following identifiers:

FIBRINOGEN ALPHA/ALPHA-E CHAIN PRECURSOR. (GENE: FGA) FIBA_HUMAN
Primary accession number: P02671
FIBRINOGEN BETA CHAIN PRECURSOR. (GENE: FGB) FIBB_HUMAN
Primary accession number: P02675
FIBRINOGEN GAMMA-A CHAIN PRECURSOR. (GENE: FGG) FIBG_HUMAN
Primary accession number: P02679.

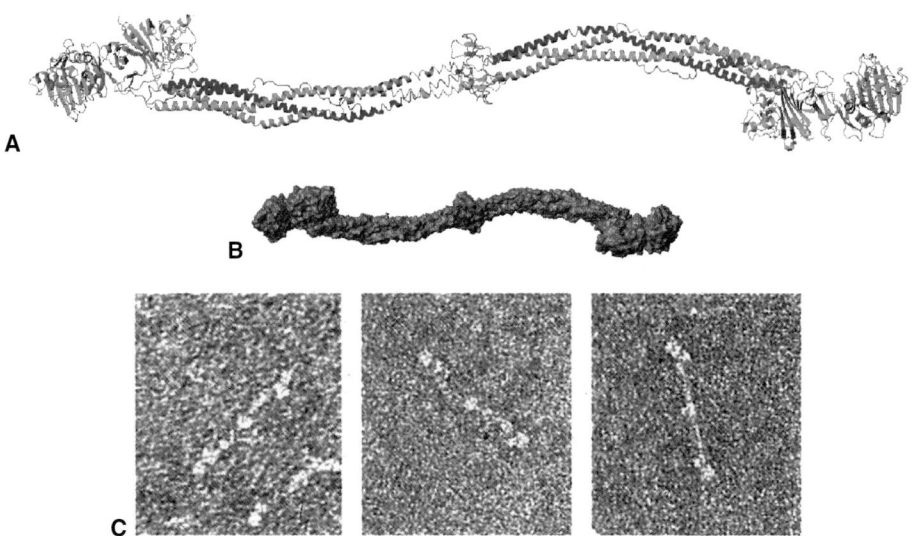

COLOR FIGURE 16-2. Fibrinogen structure determined by x-ray diffraction crystallography and electron microscopy. The **top** image depicts a color-coded chain-tracing of fibrinogen structure based on the crystal structure chicken fibrinogen reported by Yang et al. 2001 (4). The color scheme used in Figure 16-1 to represent the intact fibrinogen molecule, namely $\alpha$ chain (*blue*), $\beta$ chain (*green*), and $\gamma$ chain (*red*), is used here to represent the path of each main chain in fibrinogen. $\alpha$-helices are shown as *ribbons* and $\beta$-strands as *wide arrows*. Starting with the small globular central domain, coiled-coil regions formed by the entwined $\alpha$, $\beta$, and $\gamma$ chains extend to both the right and left, then they connect to the carboxyl-terminal $\beta$ and $\gamma$ segments that fold into independent globular domains. The $\alpha$ chain folds back on itself to form a "hairpin helix"; however, the chicken fibrinogen molecule lacks the long carboxyl-terminal segment found on human fibrinogen. This figure was prepared using the molecular graphics software MOL-MOL (69) and is patterned after Figure 1 of Yang Z, Kollman JM, Pandi L, et al. Crystal structure of native chicken fibrinogen at 2.7 A resolution. *Biochemistry* 2001;40:12515–12523. (Coordinates are available from the Protein Data Bank as entry 1JFE.PDB.) The middle panel depicts a surface representation of the fibrinogen molecule at approximately twofold smaller scale than the color-coded structural diagram. The **bottom** panel depicts images of fibrinogen obtained by electron microscopy reported by Fowler and Erickson, 1983 (70). These images are at approximately fivefold smaller scale than the color-coded fibrinogen structural diagram.

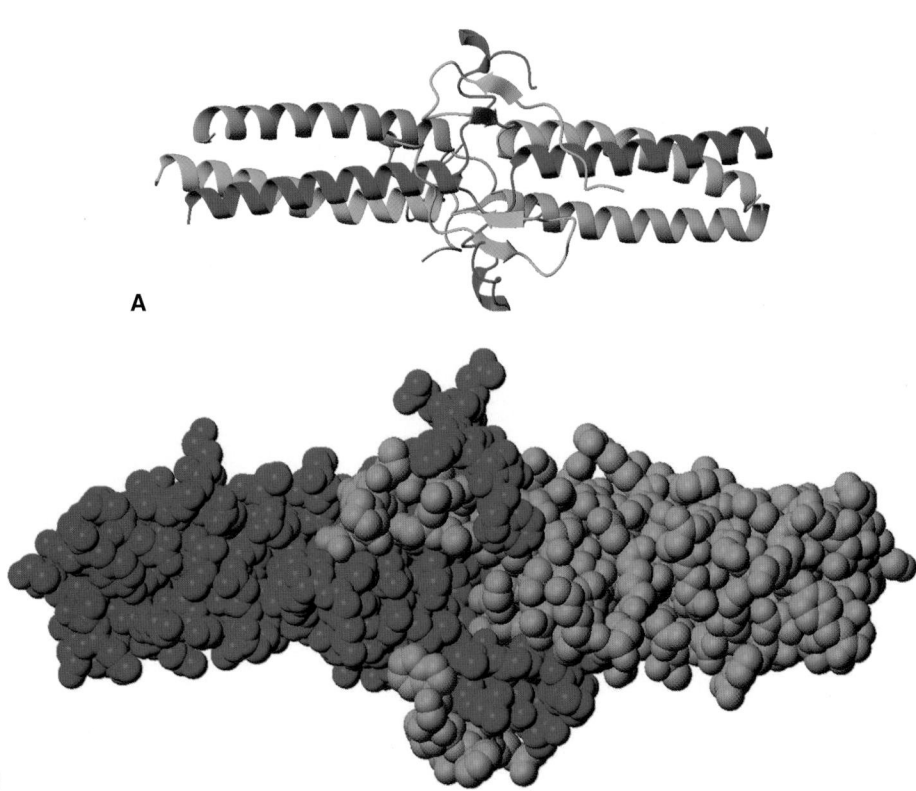

A

B

COLOR FIGURE 16-3. **A:** Structural diagram of the constituent polypeptide chains of fragment E (bovine). The color scheme used in Figure 16-1 to represent the intact fibrinogen molecule, namely $\alpha$ chain (*blue*), $\beta$ chain (*green*), and $\gamma$ chain (*red*), is used here to represent the path of each main chain in the dimeric fragment $E_5$. $\alpha$-helices are shown as *ribbons* and $\beta$-strands as *wide arrows*. This 35-kDa fragment contains the N-terminal disulfide knot and portions of the coiled-coils from the $\alpha$, $\beta$, and $\gamma$ chains but not the fibrinopeptides. Crystal structure of the central region of bovine fibrinogen (E5 fragment) at 1.4 Å resolution (coordinates are available from the Protein Data Bank as entry 1JY2.PDB). **B:** Space-filling diagram of the structure of fragment $E_5$. Note how the two halves (*red* and *blue*) of this dimeric central domain fragment form a "handshake" interface. This figure was prepared using the molecular graphics software MOLMOL (69) and is patterned after Figure 2 of Madrazo J, Brown JH, Litvinovich S, et al. Crystal structure of the central region of bovine fibrinogen (E5 fragment) at 1.4 Å resolution. *Proc Nat'l Acad Sci* 2001;98:11867–11972. (Coordinates are available from the Protein Data Bank as entry 1JY2.PDB.)

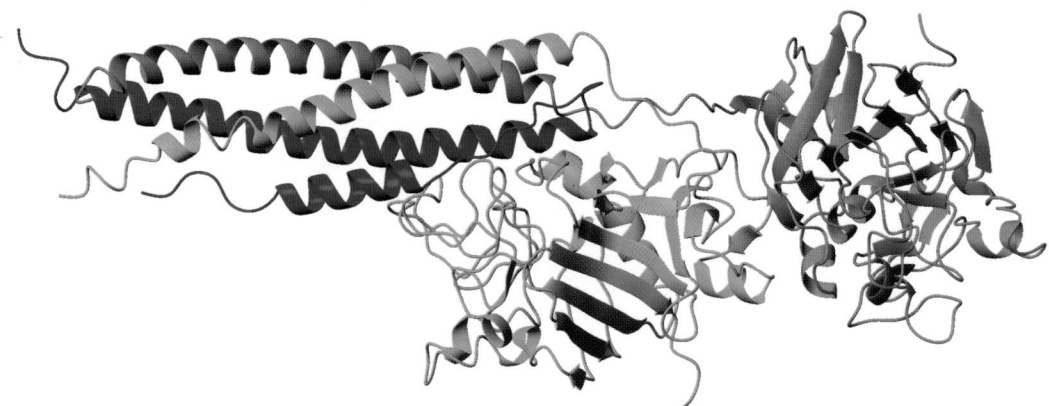

COLOR FIGURE 16-4. Structural diagram of the constituent polypeptide chains of fragment D. The color scheme used in Figure 16-1 to represent the intact fibrinogen molecule, namely α chain (*blue*), β chain (*green*), and γ chain (*red*), is used here to represent the path of each main chain in fragment D. α-helices are shown as *ribbons* and β-strands as *wide arrows*. Note the coiled-coil regions formed by the entwined α, β, and γ chains, and how the carboxyl-terminal β and γ segments fold into independent globular domains. In contrast, the α chain folds back on itself to form the "hairpin helix". This figure has been prepared using MOLMOL, molecular graphics software (69) and is patterned after Figure 2a of Spraggon G, Everse SJ, Doolittle RF: Crystal structures of fragment D from human fibrinogen and its crosslinked counterpart from fibrin. *Nature* 1997;389:455–462. (Coordinates are available from the Protein Data Bank as entry 1FZA.PDB.)

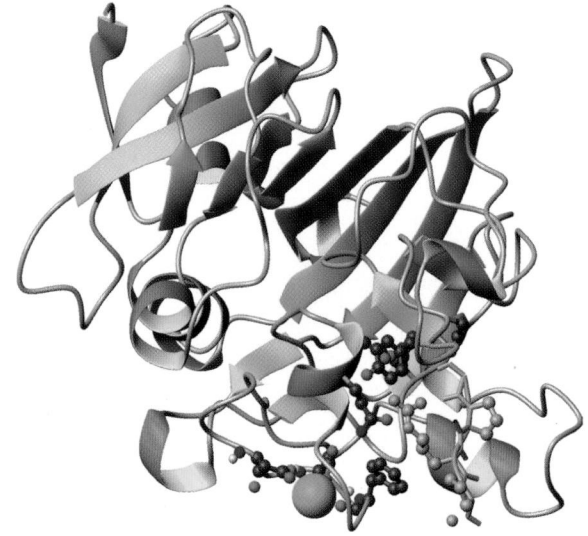

COLOR FIGURE 16-5. Structural diagram of the γ-chain carboxyl-terminal domain. The path of the main chain is represented by a tube, color-coded according to secondary structure such that *red* denotes α–helical regions, *blue* indicates regions of β-structure, and *yellow* indicates nonrepetitive structural elements. Residues that bind a calcium ion (*green*) are shown in *ball and stick* representation with *red* indicating oxygen, *blue* indicating nitrogen, and *gray* indicating carbon atoms. The same format is used to highlight residues that bind the polymerization inhibitor GPRP (*orange*). This figure has been prepared using MOLMOL molecular graphics software (69), and is patterned after Figure 4 of Pratt KP, Cote HCF, Chung DW, et al. The primary fibrin polymerization pocket: Three-dimensional structure of a 30-kDa C-terminal γ chain fragment complexed with the peptide Gly-Pro-Arg-Pro, *Proc Natl Acad Sci U S A* 1997;94:7176–7181. (Coordinates are available from the Protein Data Bank as entry 2FIB.PDB.)

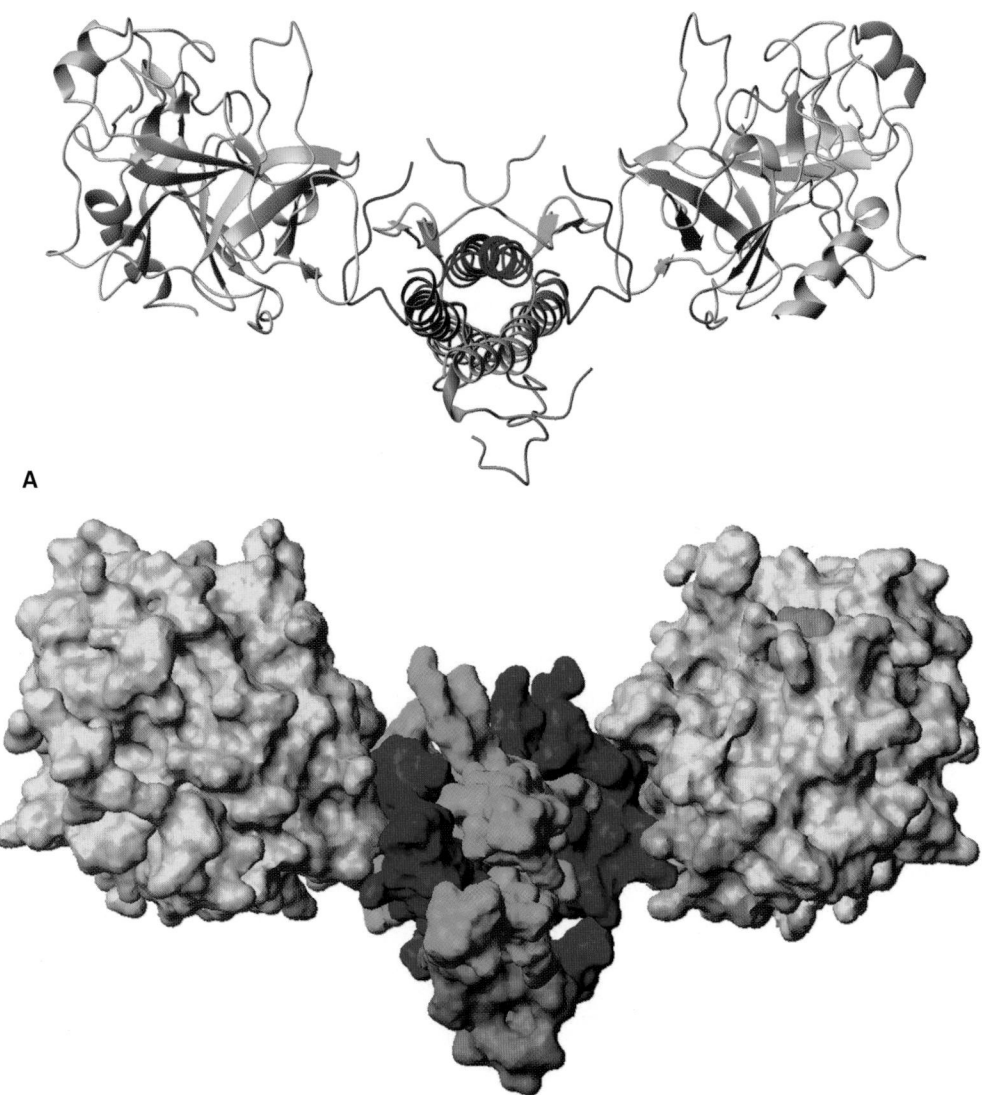

COLOR FIGURE 16-8. **A:** Structural diagram of the constituent polypeptide chains of the complex formed between fragment E and two thrombin molecules. The color scheme used in Figure 16-3 to represent the fragment E, namely α chain (*blue*), β chain (*green*), and γ chain (*red*), is also used here. The polypeptide chains of each thrombin molecule are represented by *gold lines*, with α-helices shown as *ribbons* and β-strands as *wide arrows*. This figure has been prepared using the molecular graphics software MOLMOL (69), and is patterned after Figure 1.C. of Pechik I, Madrazo J, Mosesson MW, et al. Crystal structure of the complex formed between thrombin and the central "E" region of fibrin. *Proc Nat'l Acad Sci* 2004;101:2718–2723. (Coordinates are available from the Protein Data Bank as entry 1QVH.PDB.) **B:** Space-filling diagram of the structure of the thrombin: fragment-E complex. The color-coding follows that in panel (**A**), except that the hydrophobic core of fragment E is shown in *gray*, the sites on thrombin where the inhibitor PPACK binds are shown in *magenta*, and thrombin's exosites is shown in *orange*. Note that only a portion of the exosites makes direct contact with fragment E.

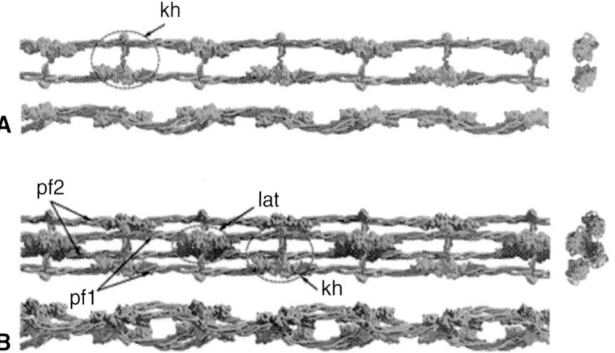

COLOR FIGURE 16-9. **A:** schematic of fibrin protofibril structure. Individual fibrin monomer molecules with the two-stranded protofibrils are shown in space-filling mode with α chains in *magenta*, β chains in *blue*, and γ chains in *green*. The *red oval* outlines the knob-hole (kh) noncovalent contacts that stabilize each protofibril. The views are presented: top, side, and end-on. **B:** Schematic of two protofibrils (pf1, pf2) laterally associated as the first step in formation of a thick fibrin fiber. Note that the lateral contacts between these aligned protofibrils (lat) are distinct from the knob-hole interaction that stabilizes the individual protofibrils. (From Yang Z, Mochalkin I, Doolittle RF. A model of fibrin formation based on crystal structures of fibrinogen and fibrin fragments complexed with synthetic peptides. *Proc Natl Acad Sci U S A* 2000;97:14156, with permission.)

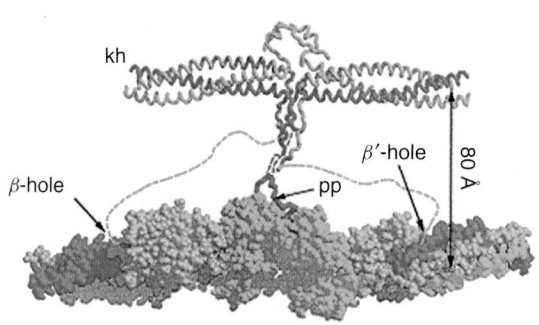

COLOR FIGURE 16-10. Schematic of the knob–hole interactions that stabilize a fibrin protofibril. The color-coding follows that in Figure 16-8. The upper molecule, the central domain of a fibrin monomer, is shown in polypeptide backbone mode with *dashed lines* corresponding to the flexible segments of the α and β chains that have not been visualized in crystal structures. The lower molecule, separated by 80 Å, is a fragment DD shown in space-filling mode. "*pp*" denotes the binding sites for the A-knob mimetic peptide Gly-Pro-Arg-Pro-amide. (From Yang Z, Mochalkin I, Doolittle RF. A model of fibrin formation based on crystal structures of fibrinogen and fibrin fragments complexed with synthetic peptides. *Proc Natl Acad Sci U S A* 2000;97:14156, with permission.)

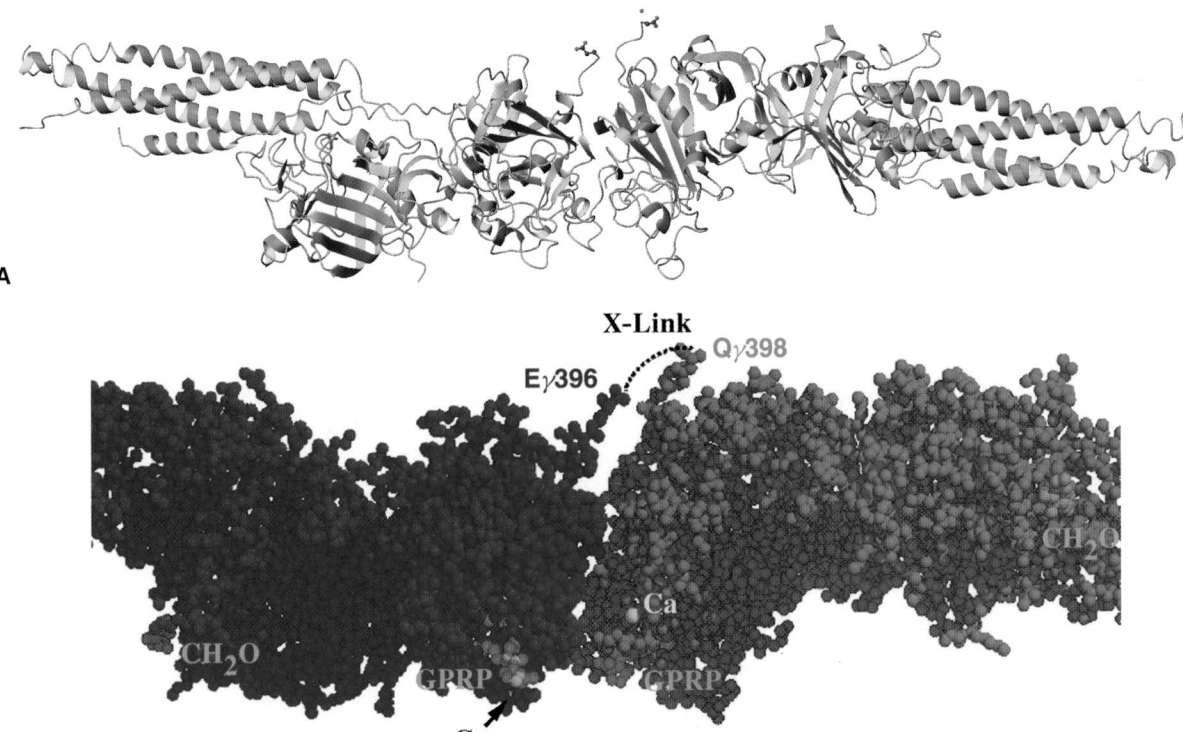

**A**

**B**

**X-Link**

E γ396   Q γ398

CH₂O

Ca

GPRP   GPRP

CH₂O

Ca

COLOR FIGURE 16-11. **A:** Structural diagram of cross-linked fragment D-Dimer. The path of each of the six constituent polypeptide chains is represented by a tube, color-coded according to secondary structure such that *red* denotes α-helical regions, *blue* indicates regions of β-structure, and *yellow* indicates nonrepetitive structural elements. Note how the γ-domains are aligned end to end in crosslinked fragment D. This figure was prepared using MOLMOL molecular graphics software (69) and is patterned after Figure 6 of Spraggon G, Everse SJ, Doolittle RF: Crystal structures of fragment D from human fibrinogen and its crosslinked counterpart from fibrin. *Nature* 1997;389:455–462. (Coordinates are available from the Protein Data Bank as entry 1FZB.PDB.) **B:** Space-filling representation of a portion of the crosslinked fragment D-Dimer shown in panel (**A**). The last carboxyl-terminal residue in each γ-chain that could be visualized in the crystal structure, γGLU396 and γGLN398 are annotated, and a *dotted line* denotes the putative path of the cross-linking site. (From Figure 6 of Spraggon G, Everse SJ, Doolittle RF: Crystal structures of fragment D from human fibrinogen and its crosslinked counterpart from fibrin. *Nature* 1997;389:455–462.)

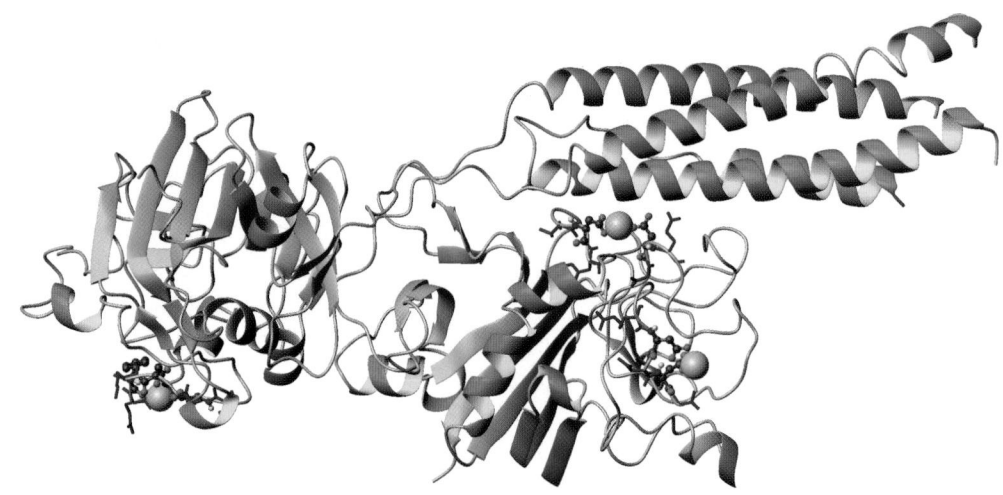

COLOR FIGURE 16-12. Structural diagram of (recombinant) fragment D. The path of the main chain is represented by a tube, color-coded according to secondary structure such that *red* denotes α–helical regions, *blue* indicates regions of β-structure and *yellow* indicates nonrepetitive structural elements. Residues that bind a calcium ion (*green*) are shown in *ball and stick* representation in which *red* indicates oxygen, *blue* indicates nitrogen, and *gray* indicates carbon atoms. This figure has been prepared using MOLMOL molecular graphics software (69) and is patterned after Figure 3 of Kostelansky MS, Betts L, Gorkun OV, et al. 2.8 A crystal structures of recombinant fragment D with and without two peptide ligands: GHRP binding to the "b" site disrupts its nearby calcium-binding site. *Biochemistry* 2002;41:12124–12132. (Coordinates are available from the Protein Data Bank as entry 1LTJ.PDB.)

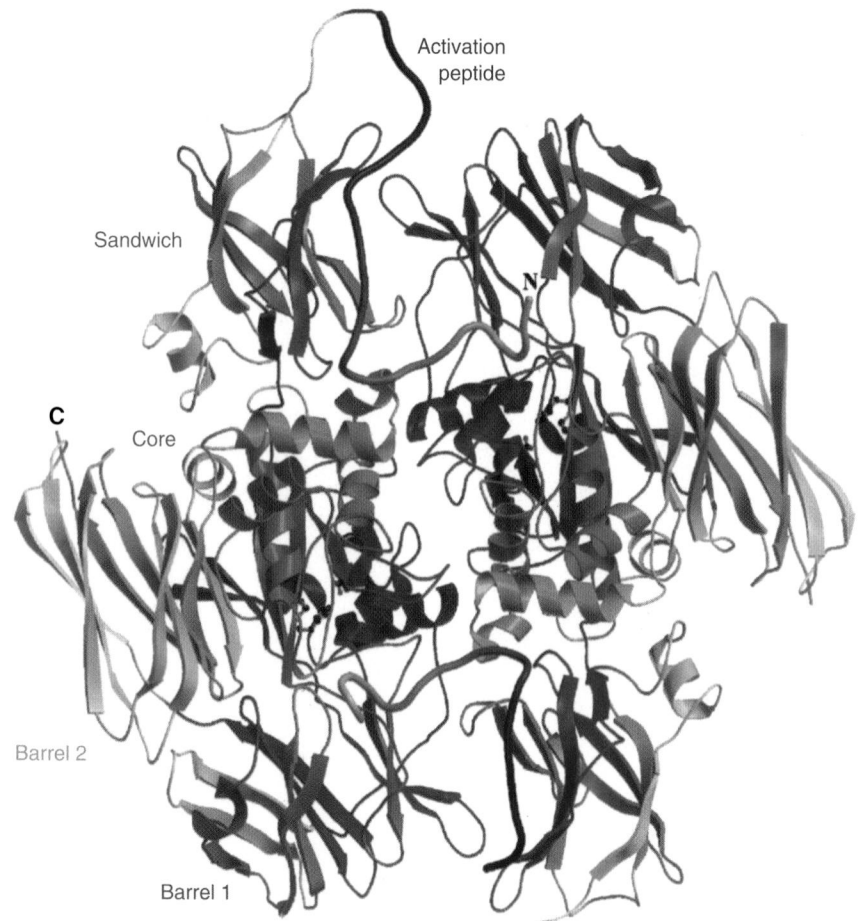

COLOR FIGURE 17-2. X-ray crystal structure of the factor XIII $A_2$-zymogen, shown in ribbon representation. The labeled structural domains are colored separately, with the colors ramped from less intense at the *N*-terminus to more intense at the *C*-terminus. Side-chain groups of the catalytic triad residues in the core domain are shown as space-filling structures. (Figure scaled to approximately 11 cm × 11 cm.)

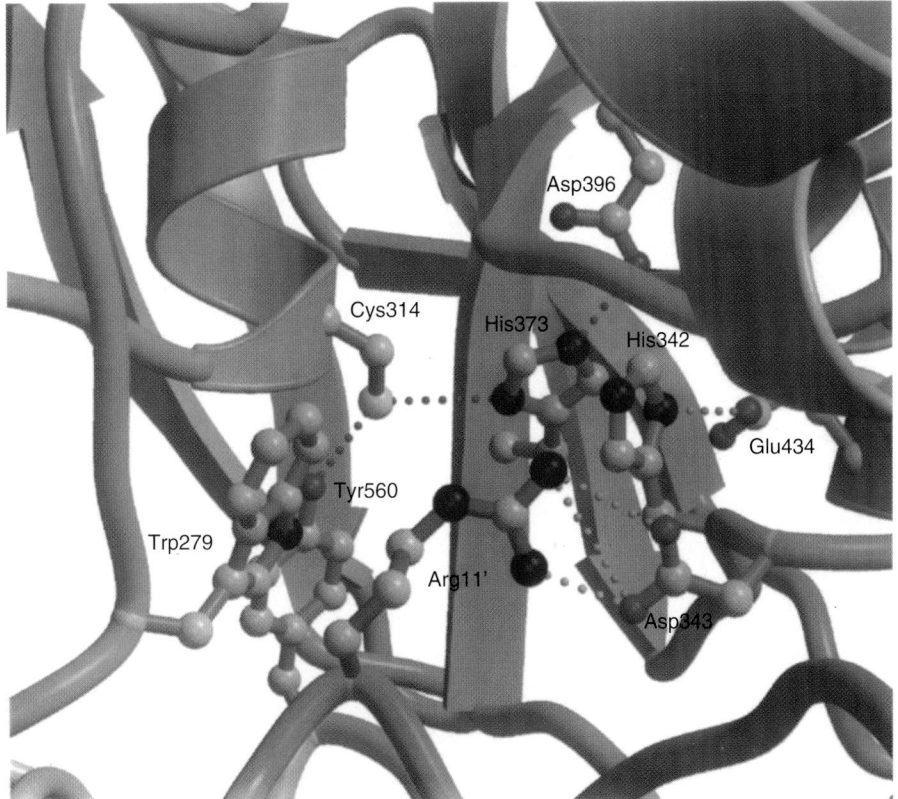

COLOR FIGURE 17-3. Close-up view of the factor XIII active site in the crystal structure of the zymogen. Side-chain groups of the Cys314-His373-Asp396 catalytic triad and of other conserved residues in the region are shown. Hydrogen-bonding interactions are represented by *dotted lines*. (Figure scaled to approximately 11 cm wide × 9.8 cm long.)

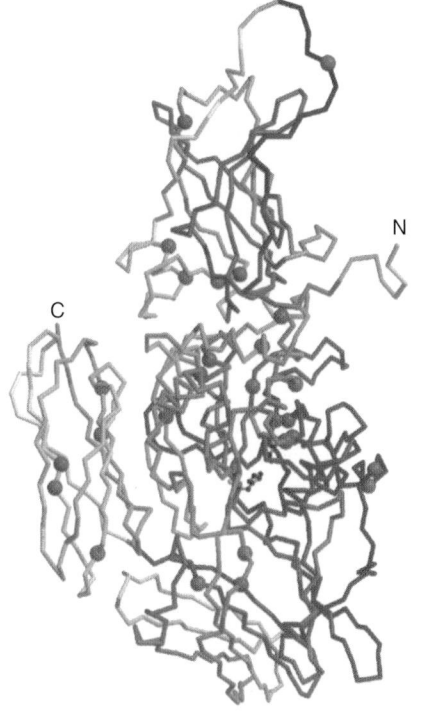

COLOR FIGURE 17-4. Distribution of the 21 amino acid residues altered by factor XIII–deficiency missense mutations. The factor XIII–A-subunit structure is shown as a backbone carbon trace colored by domain, similar to that shown in Color Figure 17-2 with labeled *N*- and *C*-termini. The 21 residues affected by deficiency mutations are represented by *red* carbon spheres; four polymorphism sites appear as *blue* carbon spheres. The side-chain groups of the Cys314, His373, Asp396 catalytic triad residues are drawn as *ball-and-stick* structures (see Fig. 17-3).

# PAI-1 structure

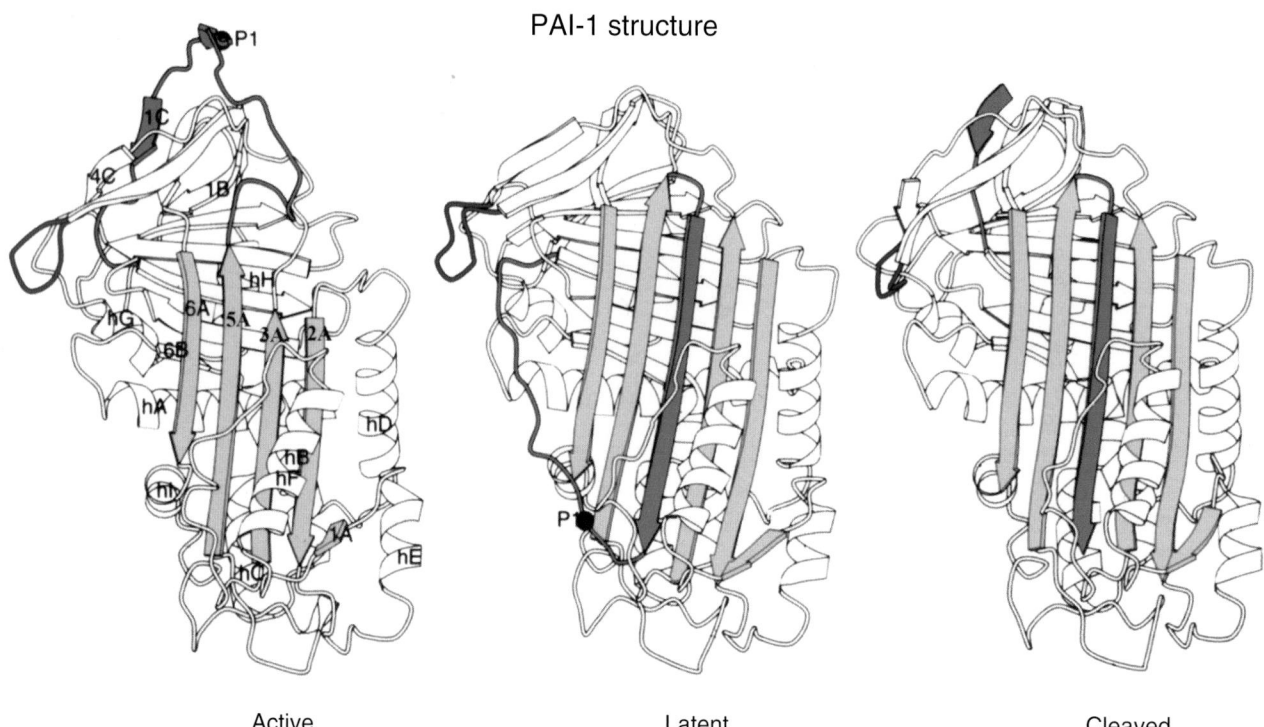

Active                    Latent                    Cleaved

COLOR FIGURE 19-1. Schematic illustration of the three conformations of plasminogen activator inhibitor-1 (PAI-1). The major β-sheet (β-sheet A) is highlighted in *light gray*, and the reactive center loop (RCL) is in *dark gray*. **A:** The active conformation of a stable mutant of PAI-1 (61). **B:** The latent conformation of PAI-1 (60). **C:** The cleaved conformation of PAI-1 (287). In both the latent and cleaved forms of PAI-1, the RCL is inserted into β-sheet A to form a new β-strand, (strand 4A). (From Sharp AM, Stein PE, Pannu NS, et al. The active conformation of plasminogen activator inhibitor 1, a target for drugs to control fibrinolysis and cell adhesion. *Structure Fold Des* 1999;7:111–118, with permission.)

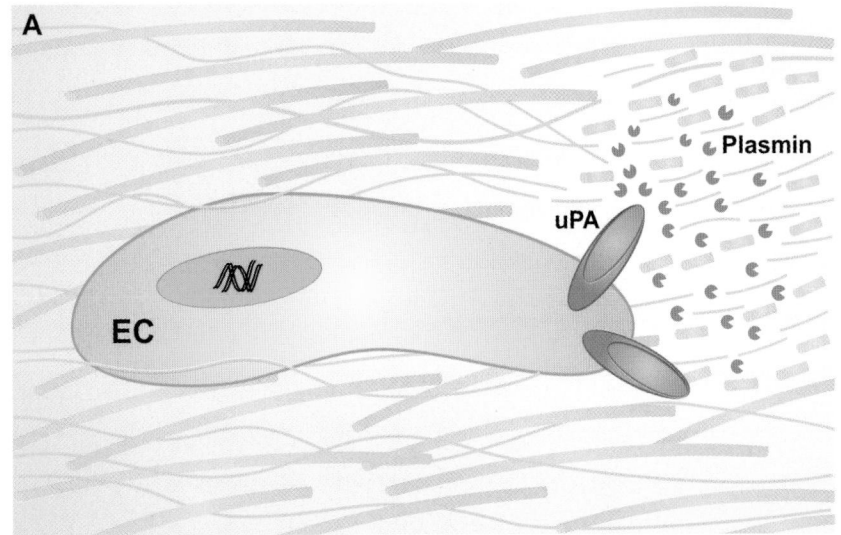

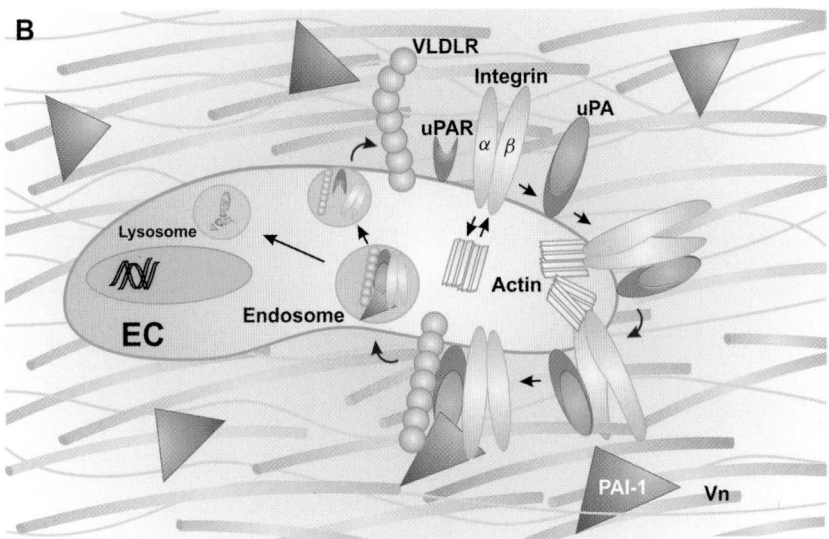

COLOR FIGURE 19-4. The evolution of our understanding of the role of plasminogen activator inhibitor-1 (PAI-1) in cell migration. **A:** Before the multiple actions of urokinase PA (uPA), urokinase-type plasminogen activator receptor (uPAR), and PAIs were fully understood, the simplest model for the function of uPA in cell migration was based solely on its ability to activate plasmin. Plasmin in turn degraded extracellular matrix (ECM) proteins, which allowed the cell to escape its matrix barrier and migrate. **B:** A model of the potential role of PAI-1 in cell migration that assumes that the cell surface receptors uPAR, integrins, and low-density lipoprotein receptor (LDL-R) family, such as the very low-density lipoprotein receptor (VLDLR), are expressed by the cell. The integrin may or may not be attached to the matrix and connected to the cytoskeleton, and uPA may be expressed by the same cell or by a nearby cell. Binding of the secreted uPA to uPAR may enhance the association of uPAR with an integrin, which may also promote adhesion. If there is also PAI in the surrounding milieu, it can then bind to the uPA present in the ternary complex. This PAI would most likely be PAI-1 because its expression is stimulated by conditions associated with cell migration and because it will specifically localize to the matrix through binding to vitronectin. The binding of PAI-1 to uPA induces the conformational change in PAI-1 that simultaneously reduces its affinity for the matrix while enhancing its affinity for the clearance receptor (Fig. 19-2). This association also promotes integrin disengagement from the matrix, and very likely from the cytoskeleton as well, and binding to the clearance receptor (VLDLR). Whether the integrin first disengages from the matrix and then binds to the clearance receptor or whether it is the association of the quaternary complex with the clearance receptor that induces the integrin to disengage is not yet clear. Regardless of the exact sequence of events, the quaternary complex is then endocytosed, and, in the endosome, the PAI–uPA complex separates from the three receptors and is targeted to the lysosome for degradation. The LDL-R, uPAR, and the integrin are then recycled back to the cell surface where the process can be repeated. This cycled attachment–detachment–reattachment of integrins is necessary for cell migration. This figure does not indicate the many potential intracellular signaling events that each one of these interactions could generate, but each one of these receptor interactions could signal the cell. The downstream consequences of these events undoubtedly also modulate cell adhesion and migration through other pathways. (From Stefansson S, Lawrence DA. Old dogs and new tricks, proteases, inhibitors, and cell migration. *Sci STKE* 2003;e24, with permission.)

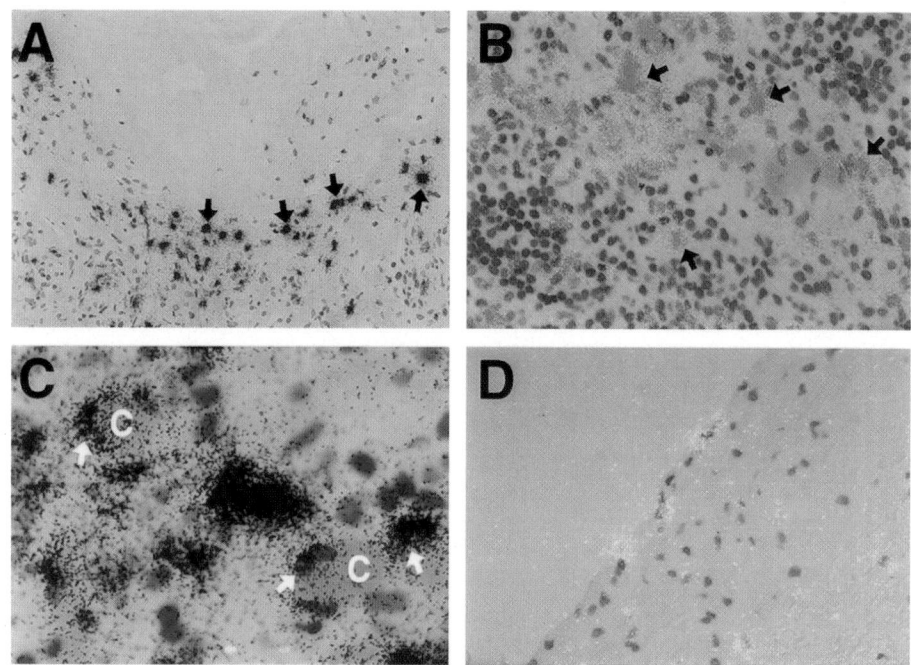

COLOR FIGURE 19-6. Plasminogen activator inhibitor-1 (PAI-1) gene expression in the abdominal aortic aneurysm wall. Tissue samples were analyzed for the expression of PAI-1 mRNA (messenger ribonucleic acid) by *in situ* hybridization. **A:** Atherosclerotic aneurysm wall. The PAI-1 transcript is expressed in cells (*arrows*) aligned at the base of the necrotic atheroma core, ×200, bright field. **B:** Atherosclerotic aneurysm wall. Macrophagelike cells expressing PAI-l mRNA (*arrows*) within the inflammatory infiltrate, ×400, epiluminescence. **C:** Atherosclerotic aneurysm wall. PAI-l mRNA expression in circumferentially arranged cells (*arrows*), which depict a cross-section of ringlike structures that are assumed to be small caliber capillaries (C) within an inflammatory infiltrate, ×1,000, bright field. **D:** Normal aorta. PAI-1 mRNA signal is detected in luminal endothelium and in a few subintimal cells, ×400, epiluminescence. (From Schneiderman J, Bordin GM, Engelberg I, et al. Expression of fibrinolytic genes in atherosclerotic abdominal aortic aneurysm wall. A possible mechanism for aneurysm expansion. *J Clin Invest* 1995;96:639–645, with permission.)

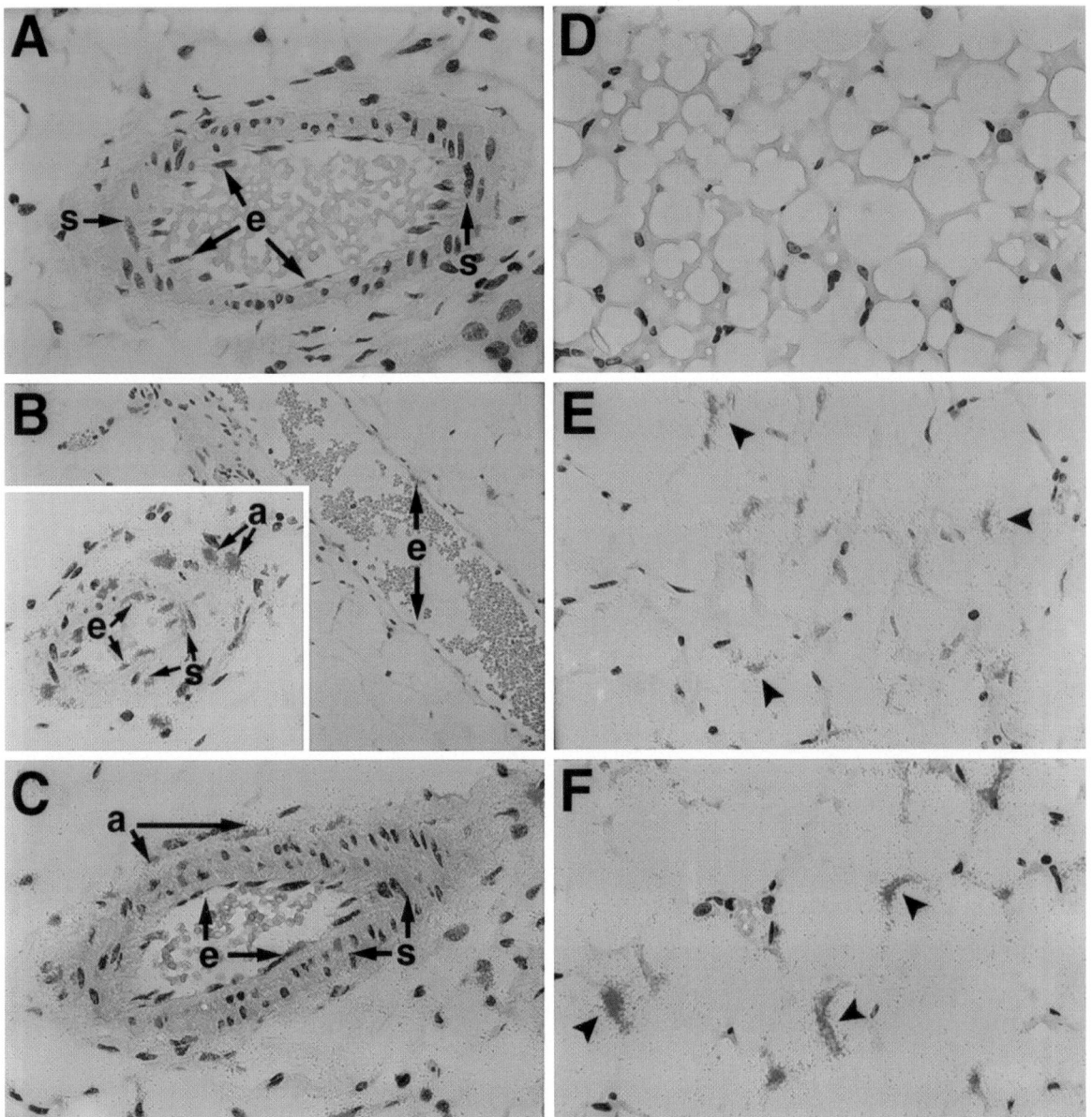

COLOR FIGURE 19-7. Localization of plasminogen activator inhibitor-1 (PAI-1) messenger ribonucleic acid (mRNA) in the adipose tissue of CB6 mice after lipopolysaccharide (LPS) or tumor necrosis factor (TNF)-α treatment. *In situ* hybridization of paraffin sections showing vasculature from epididymal fat pads of untreated mice (**A**) or from mice treated with LPS (**B**) or with TNF-α (**C**) for 3 hours. *e*, endothelial cells; *a*, adventitial cells; *s*, cells within smooth muscle layers. *In situ* hybridization on sections of epididymal fat pad–containing adipocytes and microvascular endothelial cells from untreated mice (**D**) or from mice treated with LPS (**E**) or TNF-α (**F**) for 3 hours. Some positive cells are indicated by *arrowheads*. Slides were exposed for 8 weeks at 4°C and were stained with hematoxylin and eosin. Original magnification, ×400. (From Samad F, Yamamoto K, Loskutoff DJ. Distribution and regulation of plasminogen activator inhibitor-1 in murine adipose tissue *in vivo*. Induction by tumor necrosis factor-alpha and lipopolysaccharide. *J Clin Invest* 1996;97:37–46, with permission.)

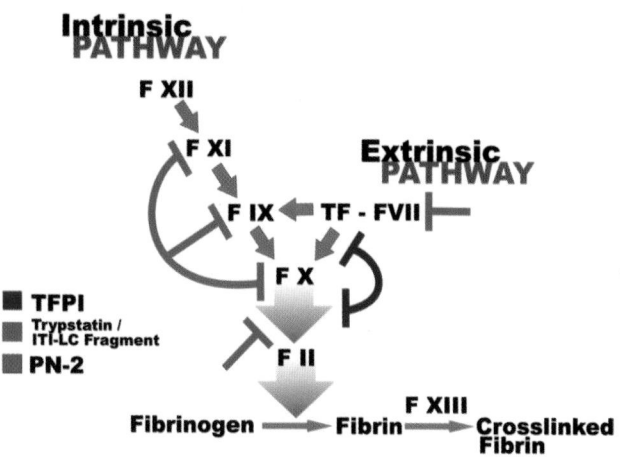

COLOR FIGURE 21-4. Kunin inhibitors and the coagulation cascade. Increasing evidence suggests that the kunins protease nexin-2 (PN-2), trypstatin/inter-α-trypsin inhibitor light chain (ITI-LC) fragment, and tissue factor pathway inhibitor (TFPI) are capable of regulating a number of factors within both the intrinsic and extrinsic coagulation pathway. Activated coagulation factors and factors V and VIII have been omitted in order to simplify this schematic.

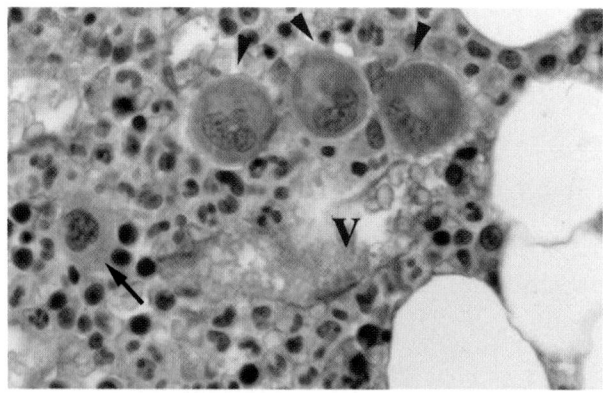

A

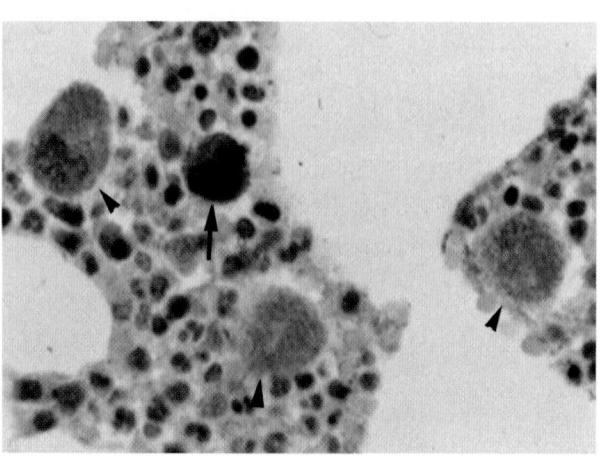

B

COLOR FIGURE 25-1. Human normal bone marrow biopsy immunostained for fibrinogen (A) and von Willebrand factor (VWF) (B) by the alkaline phosphatase–anti-alkaline phosphatase (APAAP) technique. A: Megakaryocytes (MK) are frequently located along a vascular sinusoid (V). Fibrinogen displays a centrifugal staining pattern typical of an α-granule protein endocytosed from the extracellular medium. The staining intensity is weak in the small immature MK (*arrow*) even as it is maximal in large, mature MK (*arrowheads*). B: VWF displays a centripetal staining pattern (*arrowheads*) with a stronger expression in the paranuclear region in large, mature MK. The staining intensity is maximal in the small MK (*arrow*).

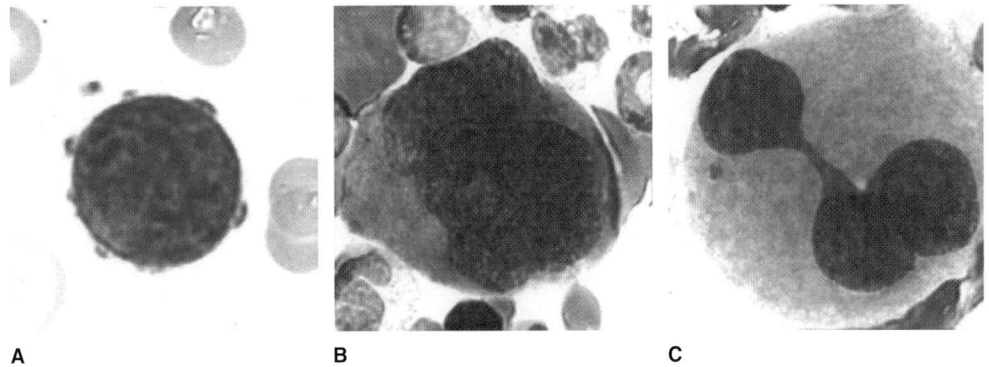

A                          B                         C

COLOR FIGURE 25-3. Light microscopic appearance of the three different maturation stages of megakaryocytes (MK) from a bone marrow smear stained by the Romanovski technique. **A:** Immature MK or megakaryoblast (type I): The relatively large size of this otherwise poorly differentiated hemoblast [high nucleus/cytoplasm (N/C) ratio, thin chromatin, and basophilic cytoplasm] allows it to be assigned to the MK lineage. **B:** MK of intermediate maturation (type II): This stage is characterized by large size, convoluted polyploid large nucleus, which is surrounded by a uniformly basophilic cytoplasm; some azurophilic granules appear toward the cell center. **C:** Mature MK (type III): In this stage, the MK appears as a large cell with a polylobulated nucleus and a uniformly granular and azurophilic cytoplasm.

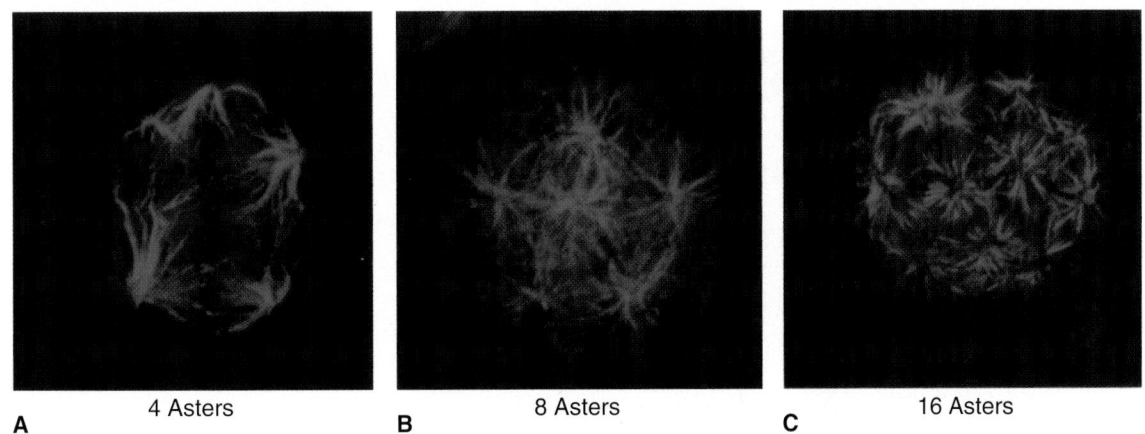

            4 Asters                   8 Asters                16 Asters

A                          B                         C

COLOR FIGURE 25-6. Immunofluorescent labeling of $\alpha$ and $\beta$ tubulin in megakaryocytes (MK) undergoing endomitosis. These images of promet aphasis of endomitosis from 4N to 8N, 8N to 16N, and 16N to 32N show the structure and assymmetry of the multipolar mitotic spindles.

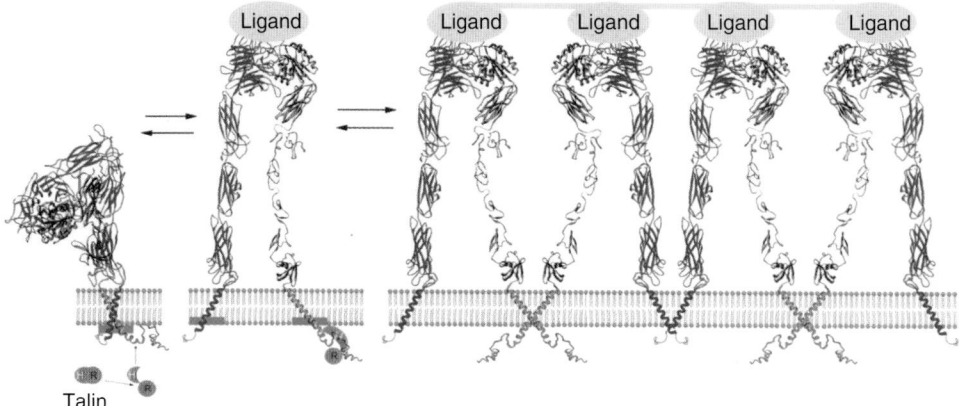

Talin

COLOR FIGURE 30-2. Model of a pathway for activation of $\alpha_{IIb}\beta_3$. Talin binding to the cytoplasmic tail of the $\beta_3$ subunit can lead to unclasping of integrin subunit tails and a membrane-associated structural change of the cytoplasmic face. This change may entail a transition from a bent conformation in its resting state to an extended conformation in which it becomes competent to bind soluble ligands. The receptors can also cluster, further enhancing their avidity for ligand. The $\alpha$-subunit is in *blue* and the $\beta$-subunit is in *red*. (Reproduced with permission from Qin J, Vinogradova O, Plow EF. Integrin bidirectional signaling: a molecular view. *PLoS Biol.* 2004;2:e169.)

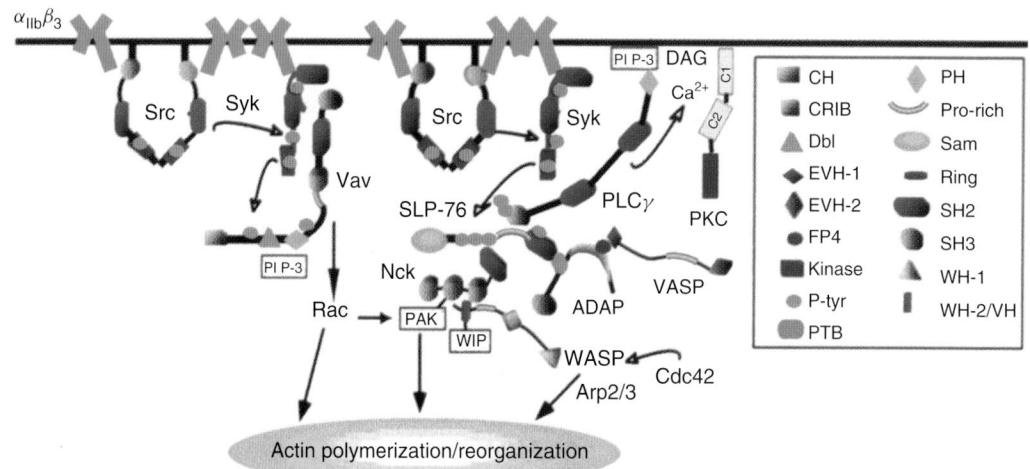

COLOR FIGURE 30-4. Cartoon depicting selected aspects of outside-in signaling in platelets. (1) Agonists induce affinity modulation, and ligand binding induces integrin clustering. (2) Ligated and clustered $\alpha_{IIb}\beta_3$ triggers early events, such as activation of Src and Syk, and (3) a cascade of signaling events lead to activation and recruitment of cytoskeletal proteins WIP, Wiskott-Aldrich syndrome protein (WASP), and Arp2/3, which can eventually nucleate actin filament growth and provoke cytoskeletal reorganization. The insert provides a key to some of the modules or domains within the proteins that mediate or regulate protein functions and/or interactions. Domain abbreviations: CH, calponin homology; P-tyr, phosphotyrosine; PTB, phosphotyrosine binding; PH, pleckstrin homology; WH, WASP homology; and VH, verprolin homology. WIP indicates WASP interacting protein; PLCγ, phospholipase Cγ. No attempt is made to show all proteins involved or all interactions of a given protein. (Reproduced with permission from Shattil SJ, Newman PJ. Integrins: dynamic scaffolds for adhesion and signaling in platelets. *Blood.* 2004;104: 1606–1615.)

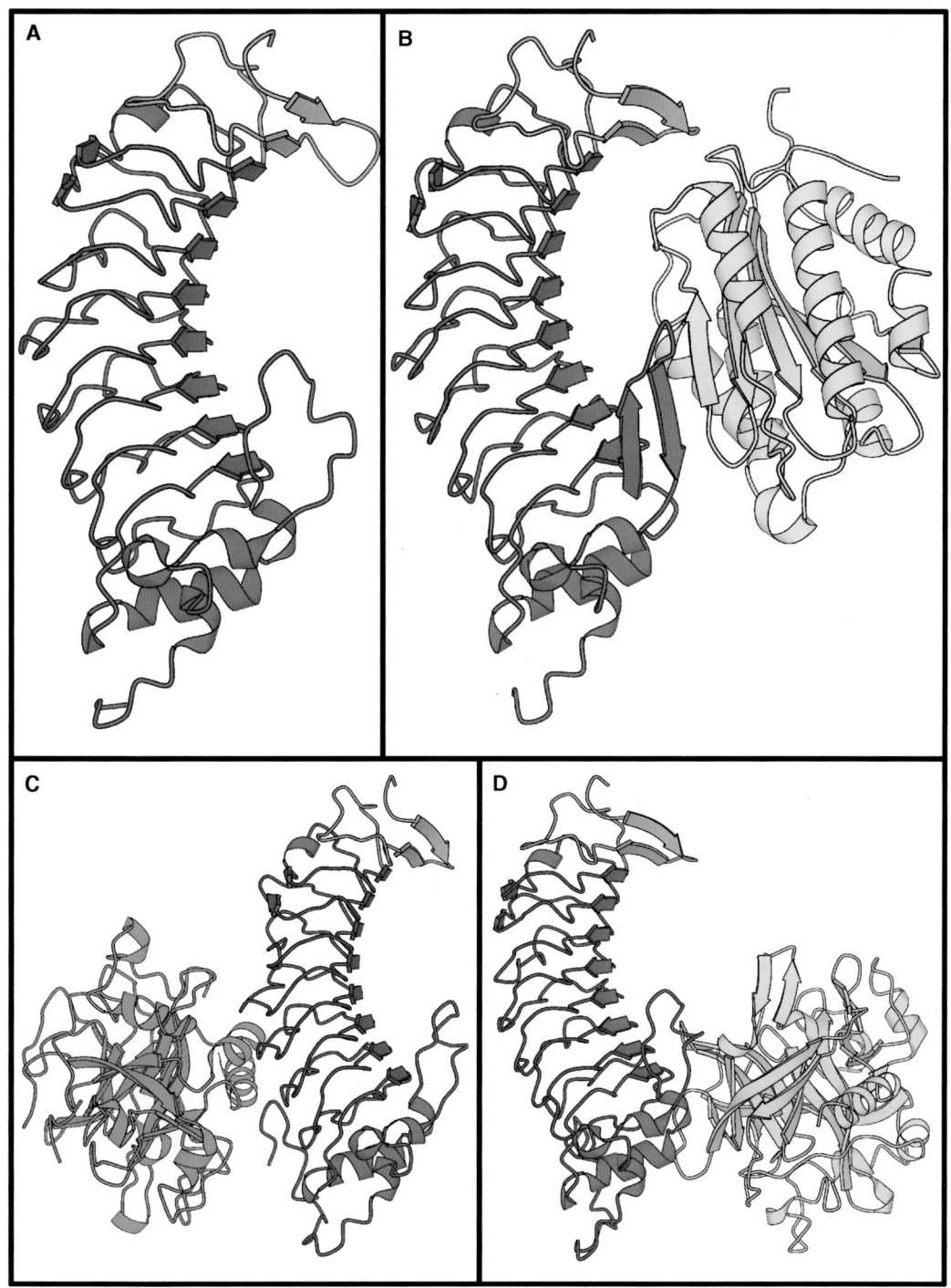

COLOR FIGURE 31-2. Summary of structural studies of GP Ibα and its binding partners. **A:** The 1.7-Å structure of the apo form of GP Ibα (pdb identifier 1P9A). The *N*-terminal "finger" is shown in *pink* and the *C*-terminal flank region in *magenta*. The eight tandem leucine-rich repeats are in *red*. **B:** The complex between GP Ibα [coloring as for part (A)] and von Willebrand factor A1 domain (*light green*) (pdb identifier 1SQ0). **C, D:** The crystal structure of GP Ibα [coloring as in (A)] in complex with thrombin reveals two possible binding sites. In panel (**C**), thrombin (*green*) is shown interacting with the sulfated tyrosine residues in the C-terminal tail of GP Ibα. In panel (**D**), thrombin (*yellow*) is interacting with the C-terminal flank (*magenta*). (Celikel R, McClintock RA, Roberts JR, et al. Modulation of α-thrombin function by distinct interactions with platelet glycoprotein Ibα. *Science* 2003;301:218–221.)

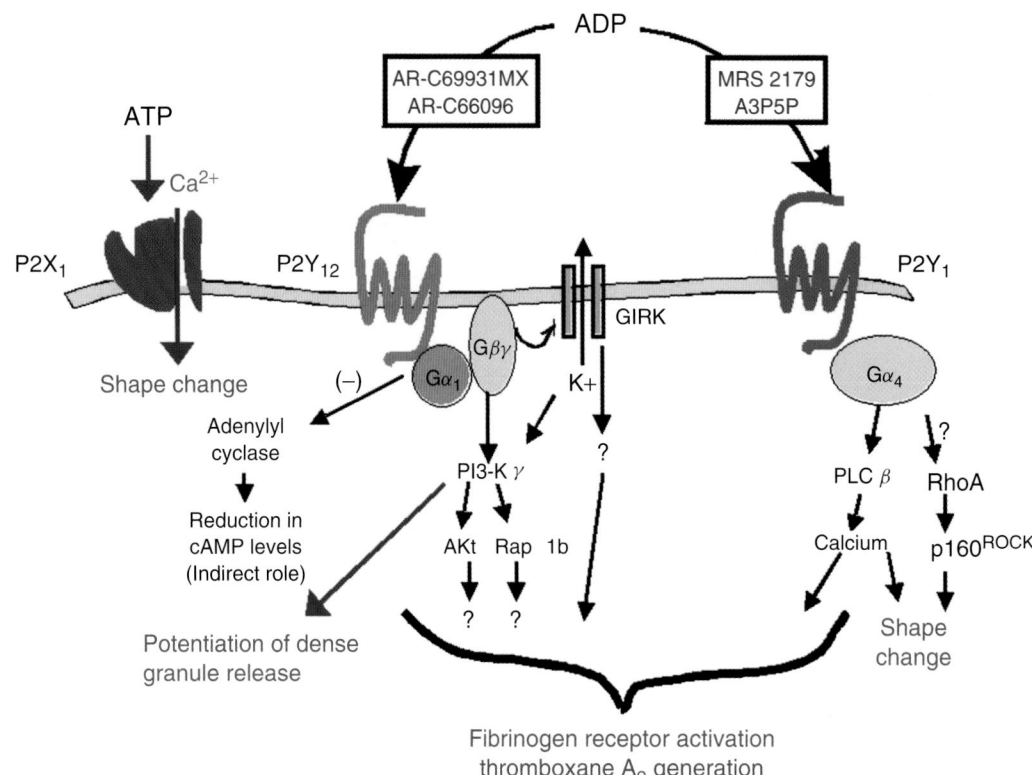

**COLOR FIGURE 32-1.** Functional roles of the platelet adenosine 5′-diphosphate (ADP) receptors. PLC, phospholipase C; GIRK, G protein–gated inwardly rectifying potassiums; ATP, adenosine 5′-triphosphate; cAMP, adenosine 3′,5′-cyclic monophosphate.

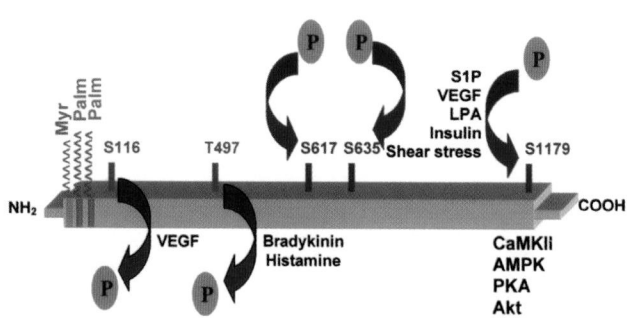

**COLOR FIGURE 42-1.** Endothelial nitric oxide synthase (eNOS) activity is regulated by agonist-mediated phosphorylation and dephosphorylation at a number of eNOS serine and threonine sites (amino acid sequence numbers refer to bovine eNOS). Phosphorylation at Ser1179 and Ser635 are believed to stimulate eNOS activity, whereas phosphorylation at Ser617 may promote calmodulin binding and therefore increase eNOS activity. Many eNOS agonists, including shear stress, vascular endothelial growth factor (VEGF), S1P, estrogen, and leptin, lead to phosphorylation at Ser1179. Phosphorylation at Ser116 or Thr497 attenuates eNOS catalytic activity. VEGF-induced dephosphorylation at Ser116 may increase eNOS activity; similarly, protein phosphatase 2A may dephosphorylate Thr497 and Ser1179. LPA, lysophosphatidic acid; AMPK, AMP-activated protein kinase.

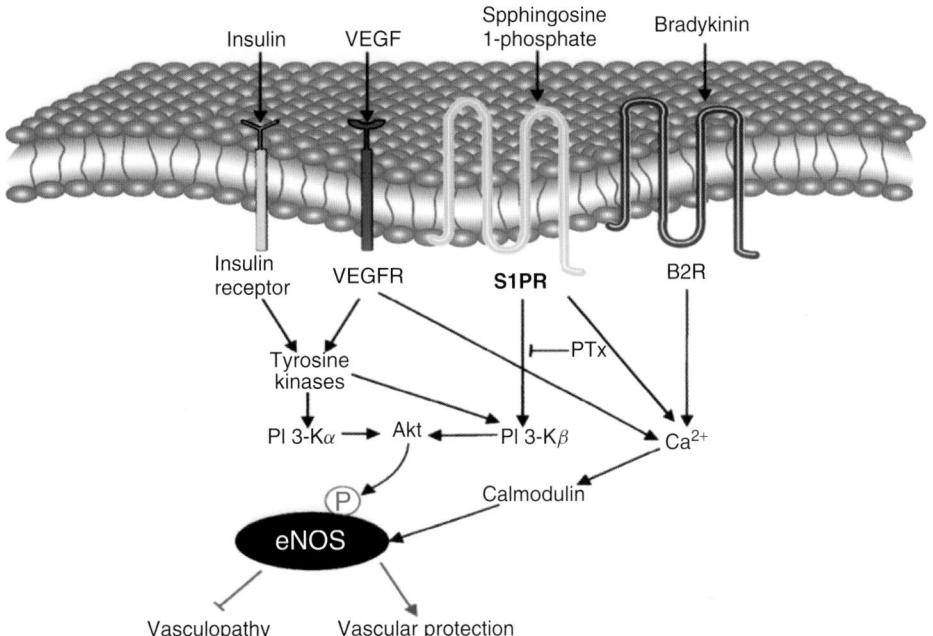

COLOR FIGURE 42-2. Diverse agonists affect various endothelial cell receptors and signaling pathways that activate endothelial nitric oxide synthase (eNOS) via calcium and/or phosphorylation. Agonists that activate eNOS by increasing intracellular calcium level include bradykinin, sphingosine 1-phosphate (S1P), and vascular endothelial growth factor (VEGF). VEGF, S1P, and insulin activate phosphoinositide-3-kinase (PI 3-K) isoforms, which then activate kinase Akt. Cross talk between the various agonist-mediated signaling pathways represents another key point of regulation. For example, VEGF induces both calcium- and phosphorylation-dependent pathways; VEGF also induces synthesis of S1P receptors. (From Igarashi J, Michel T. More sweetness than light: A search for the causes of diabetic vasculopathy. *J Clin Invest* 2001;108:1425–1427, with permission.)

Integrin activation

**A**. Inside-out
(affinity change)

**B**. Clustering
(avidity change)

**C**. Ligand-induced
conformational
change

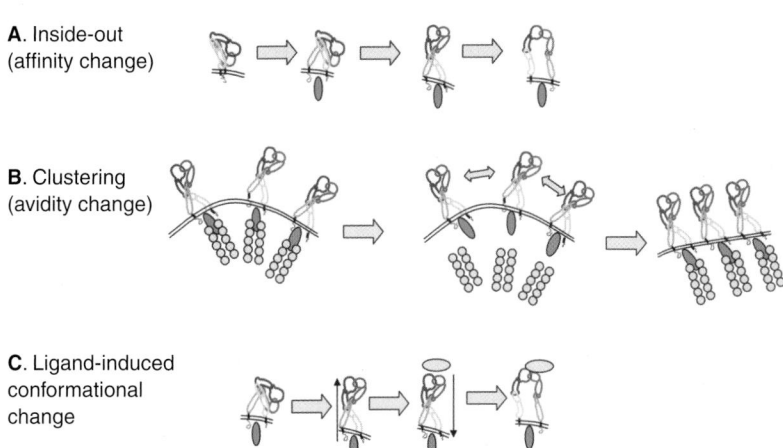

COLOR FIGURE 45-1. Regulation of integrin ligand binding activity. **A:** Integrin affinity regulation by conformational changes in the $\alpha$ and $\beta$ chains (*red* and *blue*), resulting in increased affinity for monovalent ligands. Note that cytoplasmic tails move apart during affinity regulation, probably through interaction with talin (*green ellipse*). **B:** Integrin avidity regulation by lateral mobility/clustering. Transient release of integrins from cytoskeletal anchorage (actin filaments, represented as *strings of circles*) allows integrin rearrangement and clustering in the plane of the cell membrane, resulting in increased avidity for multivalent ligands. It is not known whether the release occurs at the level of talin–actin binding. Integrins bind actin through talin and various other linker proteins (not shown). **C:** Ligand-induced activation and outside-in signaling. After activation as in **A**, inside-out signaling, *arrow up*, ligand (*blue ellipse*) binding induces outside-in signaling (*arrow down*) and bond maturation.

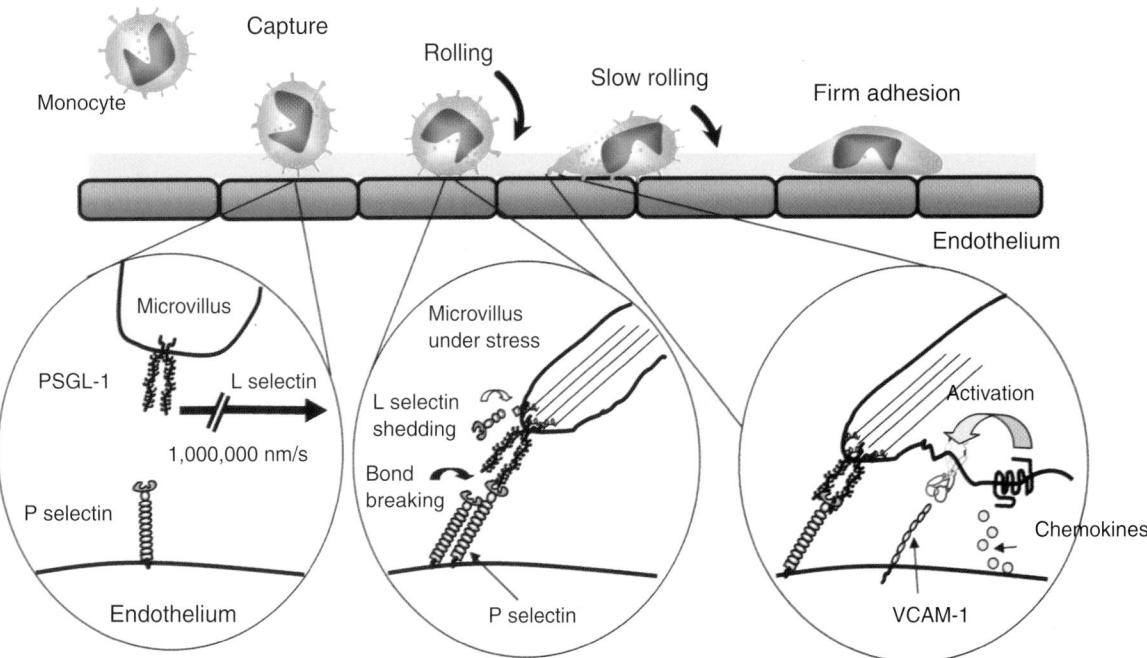

COLOR FIGURE 45-2. Sequence of monocyte capture, rolling, slow rolling, and adhesion on endothelial cells. Flow from left to right, endothelial surface layer shown in *light grey*. Primary capture or tethering is initiated by monocyte P selectin glycoprotein ligand (PSGL)-1 binding to endothelial P selectin (**left insert**). Note high velocity of monocyte (1 mm per second). The **middle insert** shows a P selectin/PSGL-1 bond at the trailing edge of a rolling monocyte. Applied stress induces faster bond breakage and may also activate cleavage of L selectin. The **right insert** shows VLA-4/vascular cell adhesion molecule (VCAM)-1–dependent bond required for slow rolling. Monocyte activation by surface-immobilized chemokine binding to chemokine receptor results in integrin affinity upregulation and firm binding to endothelial ligands such as VCAM-1 (shown here). (Modified from Mammalian Carbohydrate Recognition Systems: Functions of Selectins, Kinsley, Figure 1, Page 180, © Springer Verlag Berlin, Heidelberg 2001.)

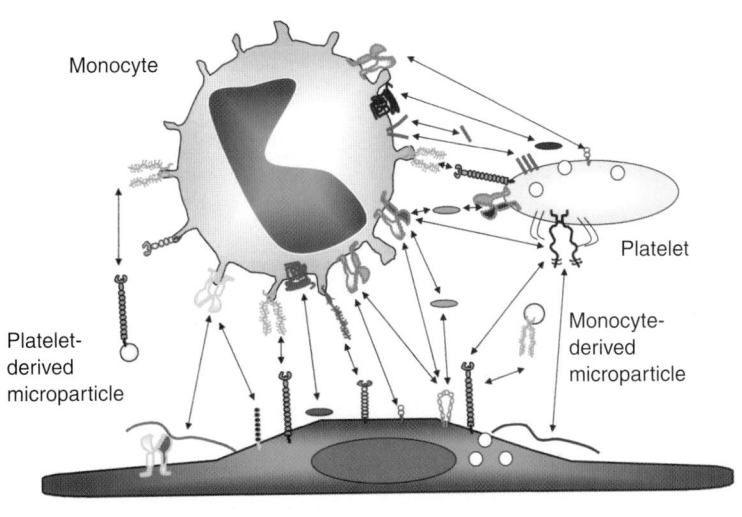

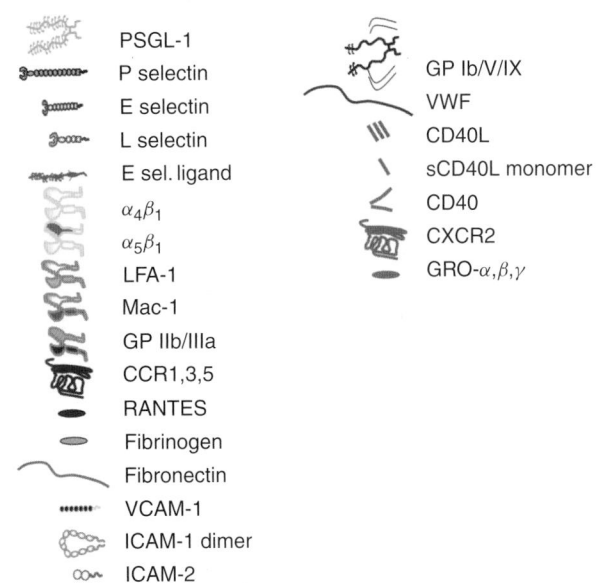

**COLOR FIGURE 45-4.** Monocyte–platelet–endothelial interactions. Each *arrow* shows a molecular interaction, legend for molecules indicated in figure. Monocyte- and platelet-derived microparticles are also shown. See text for details. PSGL, P selectin glycoprotein ligand; LFA, lymphocyte function–associated antigen; GP, glycoprotein; CCR, corresponding chemokine receptors; RANTES, regulated on activation, normal T cell expressed and secreted; VCAM, vascular cell adhesion molecule; ICAM, intercellular adhesion module; VWF, von Willebrand factor.

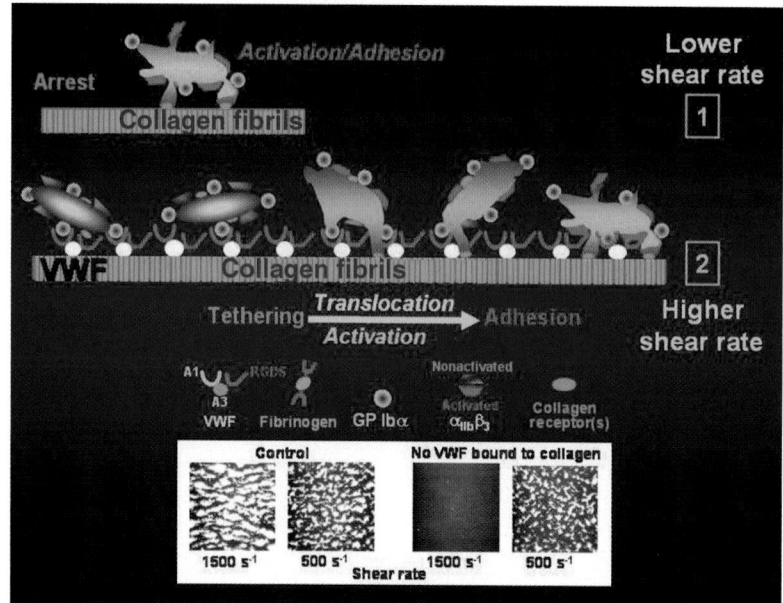

A

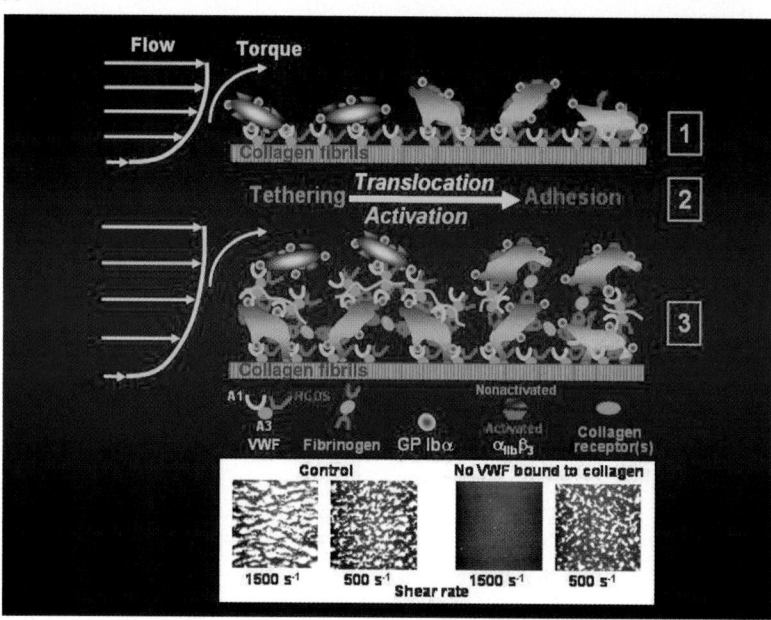

B

COLOR FIGURE 47-5. Schematic representation of the distinct biomechanical properties of bonds supporting platelet adhesion to collagen type I fibrils. *1*, lower shear rate. Initial attachment and subsequent irreversible adhesion are rapidly mediated by collagen receptors. The binding of von Willebrand factor (VWF) to collagen is not required to support thrombus formation, as shown in the **bottom panel** (VWF binding to collagen blocked by an antibody directed against VWF domain A3). *2*, higher shear rate. The first contact between platelets and the substrate is mediated by VWF bound to collagen. The VWFA1–GP Ibα bond forms rapidly and has high resistance to tensile stress (78) but a limited half-life; in the absence of other bonds, platelets detach at the tailing edge where tension is greatest and move forward with a rotational movement (rolling) because of the torque imposed by the flowing fluid. New VWFA1–GP Ibα bonds form as different regions of the membrane of rolling platelets come close to the surface; therefore platelets remain in contact with the substrate for extended periods of time while translocating at low velocity. In normal conditions, however, the initial tethering to VWF is rapidly followed by binding to collagen through specific receptors (namely, GP VI and $\alpha_2\beta_1$), and by firm adhesion, activation, and additional stable bonds being mediated by $\alpha_{IIb}\beta_3$. Note that thrombus formation on collagen exposed to a high shear rate is blocked if the interaction with VWF cannot take place (see **bottom panel**), demonstrating the role of the initial rapid tethering in permitting subsequent bonds.

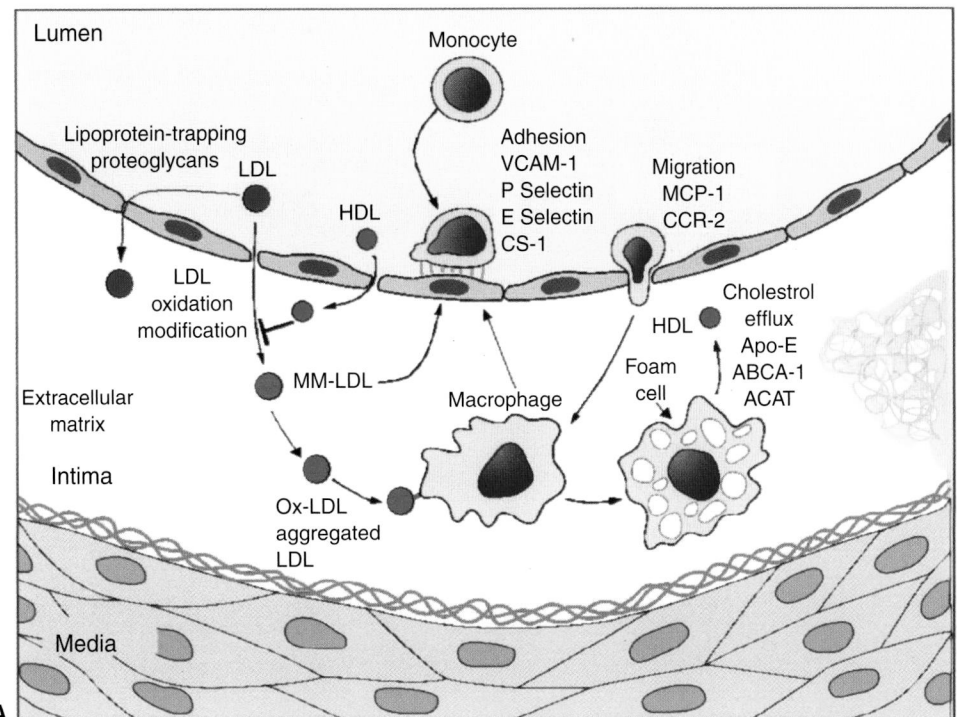

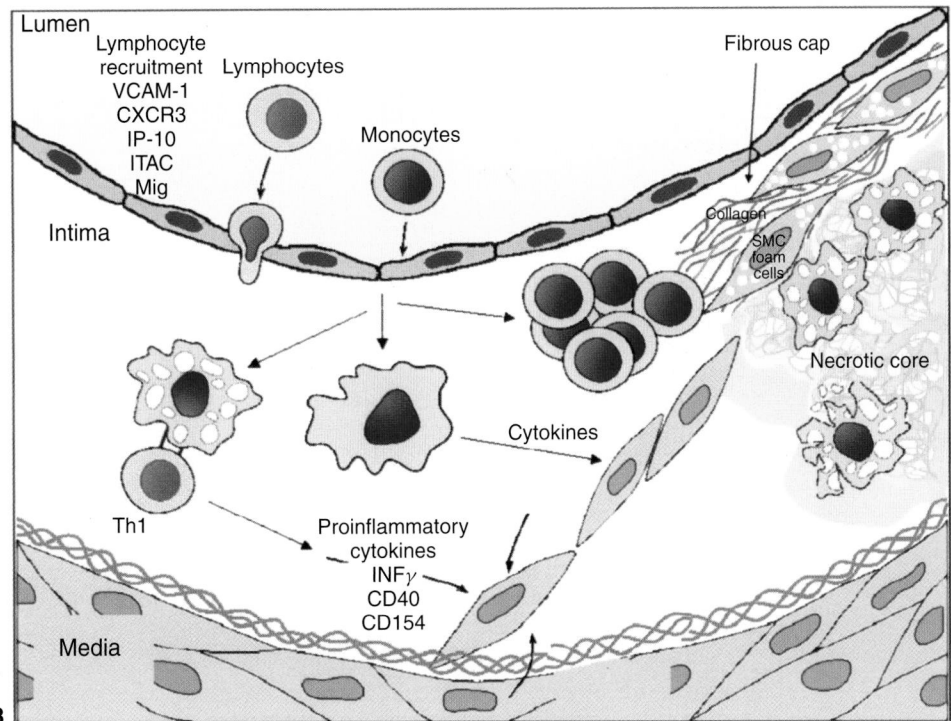

COLOR FIGURE 51-1. Stages in the development of the atherosclerotic lesion. **A:** Formation of the fatty streak. Lipoproteins enter the vessel wall and become oxidized. This oxidation can be inhibited by high density lipoproteins (HDL). Oxidized lipids increase monocyte endothelial interactions. Monocytes form foam cells by taking up highly oxidized low density lipoproteins (LDL). **B:** Development of the fibrous plaque. Monocytes and lymphocytes enter the vessel wall at the shoulder region. Smooth muscle cells (SMC) migrate from the media to the intima and proliferate in response to cytokines. They form the fibrous cap that covers dying foam cells. **C:** Plaque rupture. Monocytes that enter the lesion produce metalloproteinases that weaken the vessel wall. A break in the endothelium occurs, leading to thrombus formation by exposure to the high levels of tissue factor released from dying foam cells. These thrombi are stable because of the low levels of tissue-type plasminogen activator (tPA) and the high levels of plasminogen activator inhibitor (PAI) in the lesions. VCAM-1, vascular cell adhesion molecule-1; IP-10, Human interferon-inducible protein 10; INFγ, Interferon γ; MCP-1, monocyte chemoattractant protein-1; ACAT, acyl coenzyme A-cholesterol acyltransferase; MMPs, matrix metalloproteinases.

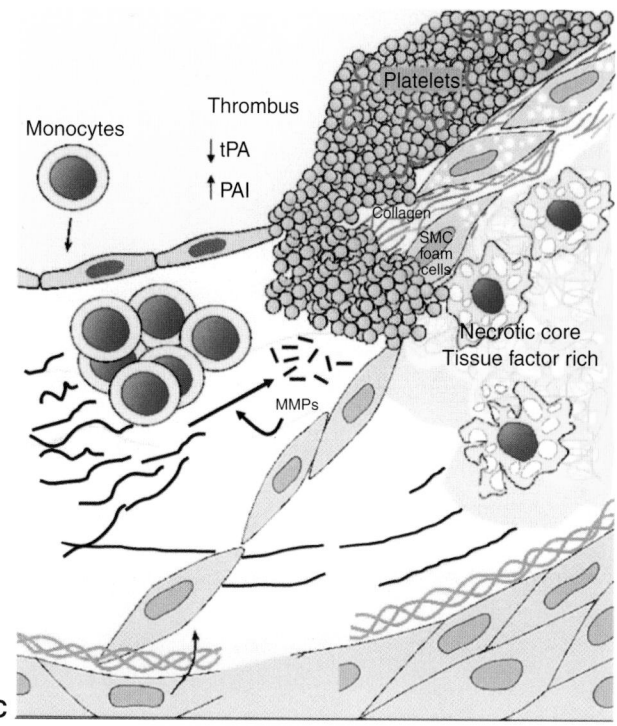

**C**

COLOR FIGURE 51-1.  Continued.

## Development of human coronary atherosclerosis

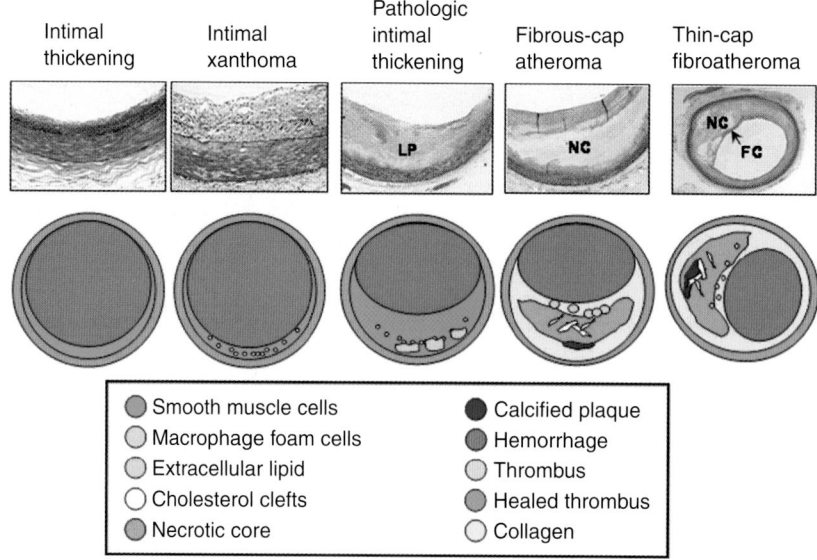

| Intimal thickening | Intimal xanthoma | Pathologic intimal thickening | Fibrous-cap atheroma | Thin-cap fibroatheroma |

Smooth muscle cells
Macrophage foam cells
Extracellular lipid
Cholesterol clefts
Necrotic core

Calcified plaque
Hemorrhage
Thrombus
Healed thrombus
Collagen

COLOR FIGURE 54-1.  Intimal thickening and intimal xanthoma: preatherosclerotic coronary lesions. Lesions are uniformly present in all populations, although intimal xanthomas (fatty streaks) are more prevalent with exposure to a standard American diet. Both lesions occur soon after birth; the intimal xanthoma (fatty streak) is known to regress. Intimal thickening consists mainly of smooth muscle cells (SMCs) in a proteoglycan matrix, whereas intimal xanthomas primarily contain macrophage-derived foam cell, T lymphocytes, and varying degrees of SMCs. Pathologic intimal thickening versus atheroma: Pathological intimal thickening (PIT) is a poorly defined entity, referred to in the literature as "intermediate" lesion. True necrosis is not apparent, and there is no evidence of cellular debris; lipid pools (LP) are seen deep in the lesion. The tissue over the lipid pools is rich in SMCs and proteoglycans—some scattered macrophages and lymphocytes may also be present. The more definitive lesions, the fibrous-cap (FC) atheroma, classically shows a necrotic core (NC) containing cholesterol esters, free cholesterol, phospholipids, and triglycerides. The FC consists of SMCs in a proteoglycan–collagen matrix, with a variable number of macrophages and lymphocytes. The TCFA (vulnerable plaque): TCFAs are lesions with large NCs containing numerous cholesterol clefts. The overlying FC is thin ($<65$ $\mu$m) and heavily infiltrated by macrophages; SMCs are rare and microvessels are generally present in the adventitia and intima. (From Virmani R, Kolodgie FD, Burke AP, et al. Lessons from sudden coronary death: a comprehensive morphological classification scheme for atherosclerotic lesions. *Arterioscler Thromb Vasc Biol* 2000;20:1262–1275, with permission.)

A nonhemodynamically limiting
thin-cap fibroatheroma

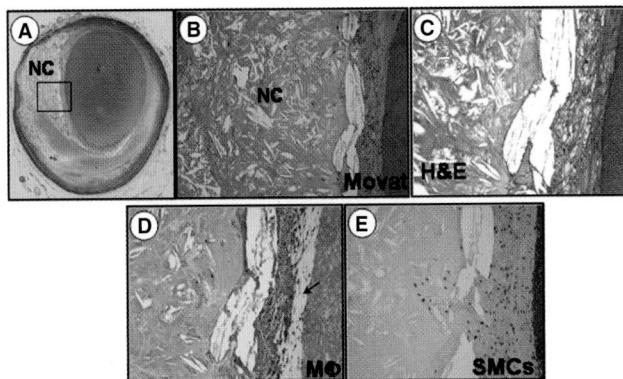

COLOR FIGURE 54-2. A nonhemodynamically limiting thin-cap fibroatheroma (TCFA). **A:** A TCFA having a necrotic core (*NC*) and an overlying thin fibrous cap (<65 $\mu$m). **B:** The high power view of the **boxed area** in A; note that an advanced NC with a large number of cholesterol clefts with surrounding loss of matrix and no cellular infiltration is seen. The fibrous cap is infiltrated by macrophages, better seen in (**C**) when stained by hematoxylin and eosin (*H&E*). (**D**) and (**E**) show macrophage (*M$\phi$*) infiltration (CD68-positive) and rare staining of smooth muscle cells (*SMCs*) ($\alpha$-actin positive) in the fibrous cap.

Fibrous-cap atheroma (late necrosis)

Thin fibrous-cap atheroma

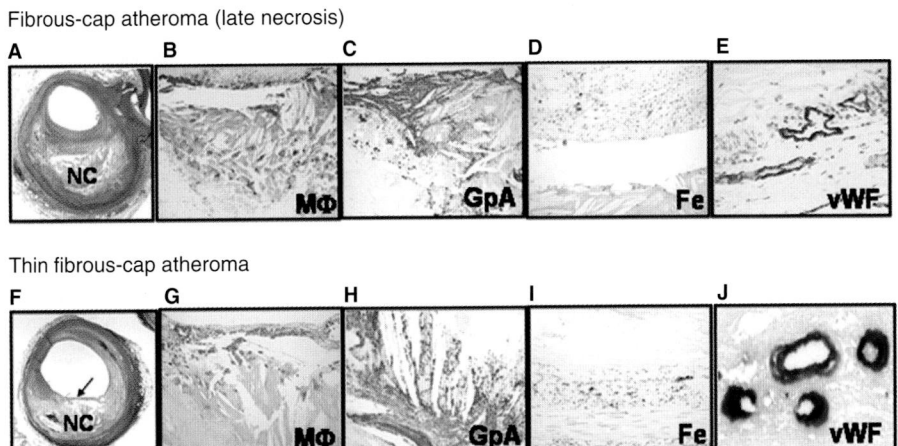

COLOR FIGURE 54-3. Late core (A–E) and thin fibrous-cap atheroma (TCFA) (F–J) showing intraplaque hemorrhage. A: Shows a low-power view of a fibrous-cap (FC) atheroma with a late necrotic core (*NC*) (Movat Pentachrome ×20). B: Intense staining of CD68-positive macrophages is seen within the NC. C: Shows extensive glycophorin A (*Gp A*)–positive erythrocyte membranes colocalized with numerous cholesterol clefts within the necrotic core (×200). D: Iron deposits (*blue*) are seen within macrophage foam cells (×200). E: Microvessels bordering the NC show perivascular von Willebrand factor (*VWF*) deposition (×400). F: Shows a low-power view of a fibroatheroma with a thin FC (*arrow*) overlying a relatively large NC (Movat Pentachrome, ×20). G: The FC is devoid of smooth muscle cells (not shown) and is heavily infiltrated by CD68-positive macrophages (*M$\phi$*, ×200). H: Intense Gp A staining of erythrocyte membranes within the NC colocalized with cholesterol clefts (×100). I: Adjacent coronary segment with accumulated iron (*blue pigment*) in a macrophage-rich region deep within the plaque (×200). J: Perivascular diffuse deposits of VWF in microvessels, indicates leaky vessels bordering the NC (×400). (From Kolodgie FD, Gold HK, Burke AP, et al. Intraplaque hemorrhage and progression of coronary atheroma. *N Engl J Med* 2003;349:2316–2325, with permission.)

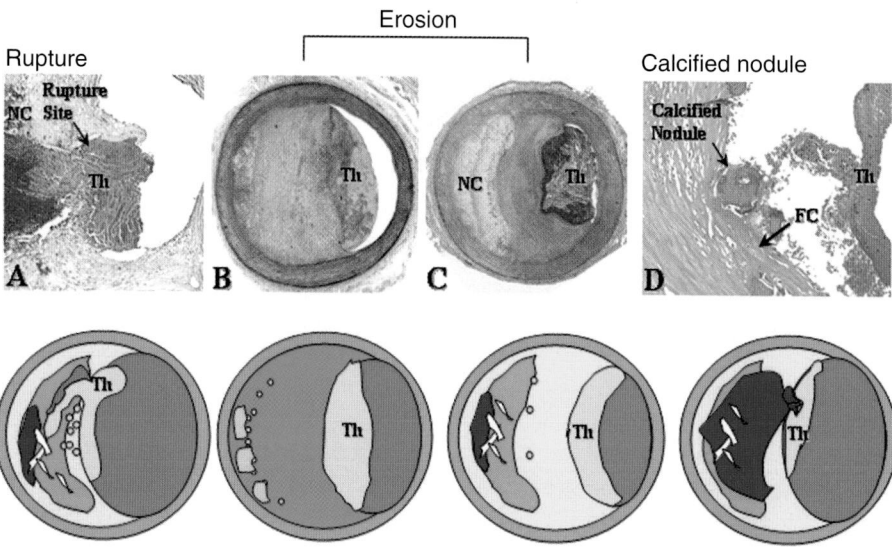

COLOR FIGURE 54-4. Atherosclerotic lesions with luminal thrombi. **A:** Ruptured plaques are thin fibrous-cap atheromas with luminal thrombi (*Th*). These lesions usually have an extensive necrotic core (*NC*) containing large numbers of cholesterol crystals and a thin fibrous-cap (FC) ($<65 \ \mu$m) infiltrated by foamy macrophages and T lymphocytes. The FC is thinnest at the site of rupture and consists of a few collagen bundles and rare smooth muscle cells. The luminal thrombus is in communication with the lipid-rich necrotic core. **B and C:** Erosions occur over lesions rich in smooth muscle cells and proteoglycans. Luminal Th overlie areas lacking surface endothelium. The deep intima of the eroded plaque often shows extracellular lipid pools, but NCs are uncommon; when present, the NC does not communicate with the luminal thrombus. Inflammatory infiltrate is usually absent, but, if present, it is sparse and consists of macrophages and lymphocytes. **D:** Calcified nodules are plaques with luminal Th showing calcified nodule protruding into the lumen through a disrupted thin FC. An endothelium is absent at the site of the thrombus, and inflammatory cells (macrophages, T lymphocytes) are absent.

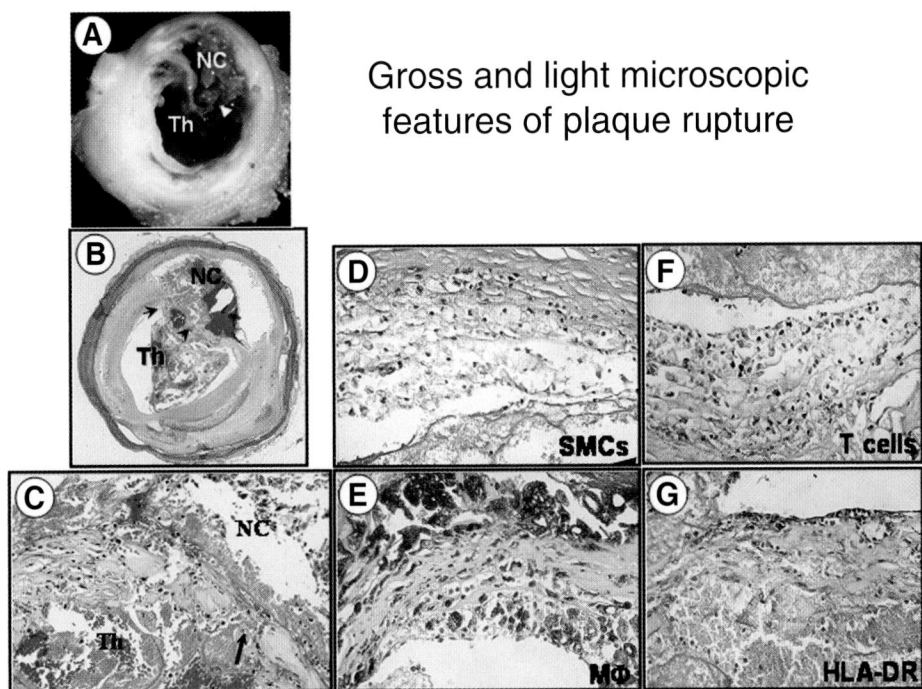

Gross and light microscopic features of plaque rupture

COLOR FIGURE 54-5. Gross photograph and histologic composition of plaque rupture. **A:** Gross photograph of a coronary artery cut in cross section showing the site of plaque rupture (*arrow*) with an underlying necrotic core (*NC*) and luminal thrombus (*Th*). **B:** Histologic section of the artery in (**A**) showing rupture site, necrotic core, and luminal thrombus. (Movat ×20) **C:** High-power view of the area of the fibrous cap disruption (*arrow*), and there is communication of the thrombus (*Th*) with the underlying NC (×200). **D:** High-power view of the thin fibrous cap (FC) showing a paucity of smooth muscle cells (α-actin, ×200). **E** and **F:** The FC is heavily infiltrated by macrophages and T lymphocytes (CD68 and CD45Ro, respectively, ×200). **G:** Shows the strong expression of HLA-DR antigens, particularly in macrophages and T cells of the FC. (From Farb A, Burke AP, Tang AL, et al. Coronary plaque erosion without rupture into a lipid core. A frequent cause of coronary thrombosis in sudden coronary death. *Circulation* 1996;93:1354–1363, with permission.)

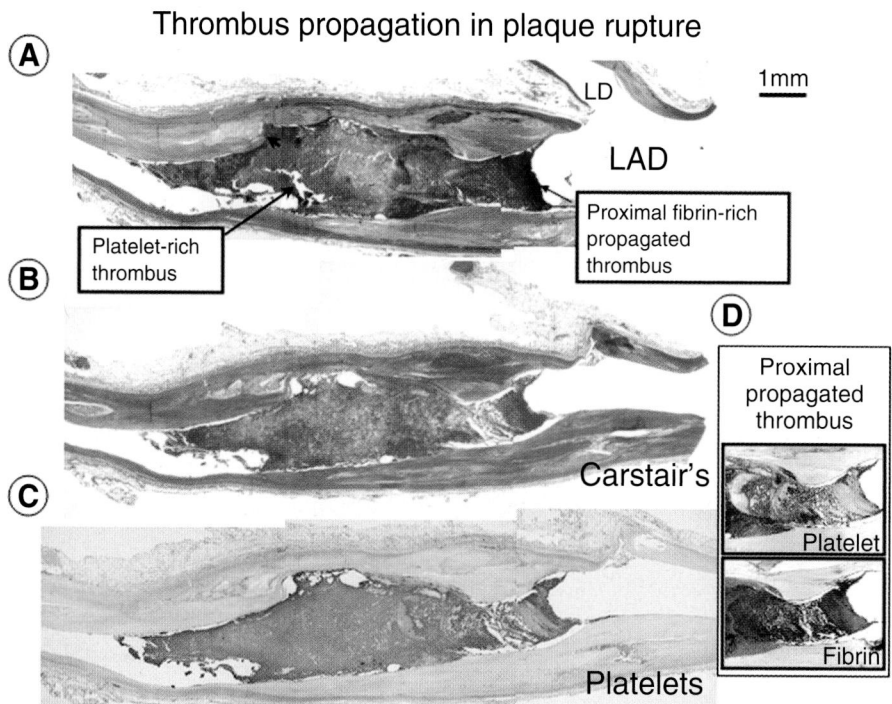

**Thrombus propagation in plaque rupture**

COLOR FIGURE 54-6. Thrombus propagation in plaque rupture. **A:** Composite of a longitudinal section of a left anterior descending (*LAD*) coronary artery with plaque rupture; the rupture site is marked by the arrowhead (Movat pentachrome, original magnification ×20). **B:** Shows the same longitudinal section as in **A** stained with Carstair method for the detection of fibrin (*dark red*) and platelets (*blue-grey*). The proximal thrombus consists predominantly of fibrin whereas the more distal portion at the rupture site is platelet-rich. **C:** The presence of platelets was further confirmed using an antibody directed against glycoprotein IIIa. **D:** Proximal propagated portion of the thrombus showing mostly fibrin; mild layered reactivity is seen for platelets.

## Angiographic and histologic representation
## of plaque rupture and erosion

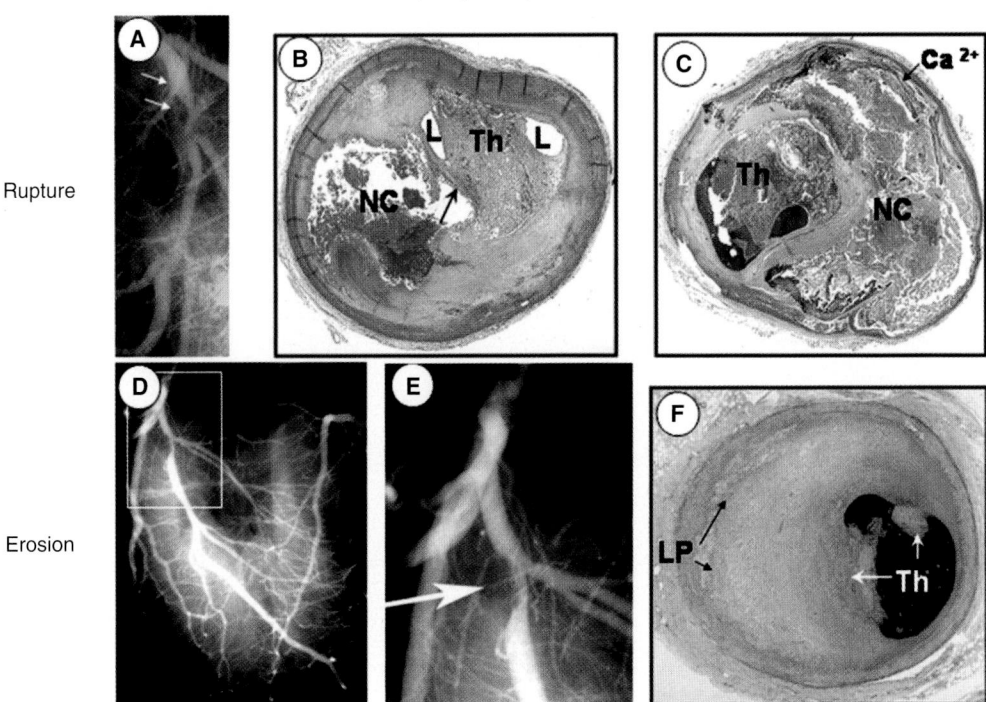

COLOR FIGURE 54-7. Angiographic and histologic representation of plaque rupture and erosion. A 43-year-old white man with no known history of risk factors was found unresponsive in the bathroom. **A:** Postmortem angiogram shows the left anterior descending (LAD) coronary artery at the origin of the left diagonal with near total occlusion. Sections taken from these sites show a plaque rupture [*arrow*, and (**B**)] with an underlying necrotic core (*NC*). The occluded artery shows an organizing thrombus with small lumens (*L*). In (**C**), the fibrous cap is intact with a large underlying NC with peripheral calcification (Ca$^{2+}$), and the lumen shows organizing thrombus (*Th*) with small lumens (*L*). At autopsy, there was a healing transmural myocardial infarction present in the distribution of the LAD. Postmortem angiogram (**D** and **E**) and corresponding photomicrograph (**F**) of a 38-year-old man, who died of sudden coronary thrombosis. A focal stenosis is present in the left anterior coronary artery (**boxed area**), which is highlighted in (**A**) and an arrow points to the area of narrowing at the take off of the left diagonal. In (**F**), acute nonocclusive luminal thrombus (*Th*) is present on the surface of an erosive plaque rich in proteoglycans, and the underlying plaque shows pathologic intimal thickening with lipid pools (*LP*). (From Farb A, Tang AL, Burke AP, et al. Sudden coronary death. Frequency of active coronary lesions, inactive coronary lesions, and myocardial infarction. *Circulation* 1995;92:1701–1709, with permission.)

### Healed plaque rupture

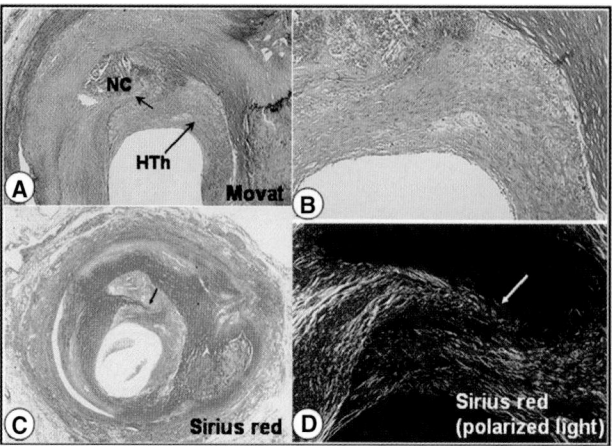

COLOR FIGURE 54-8. Healed plaque rupture. **A:** Areas of intraintimal lipid-rich core with hemorrhage and cholesterol clefts; an old area of necrosis (*NC*) is seen underlying a healed thrombus (*HTh*). **B:** Higher magnification showing extensive smooth muscle cells (SMCs) within a collagenous proteoglycan-rich neointima (healed thrombus) with clear demarcation from the fibrous region of old plaque to right. **C** and **D:** Layers of collagen by Sirius red staining. **C:** Note area of dense, dark collagen surrounding lipid hemorrhagic cores seen in corresponding view in **A. D:** Image taken with polarized light. Dense collagen (type I) that forms the fibrous cap is disrupted (*arrow*), with newer greenish type III collagen on the right and above the rupture site; (**A**) and (**B**), Movat pentachrome. (From Burke AP, Kolodgie FD, Farb A, et al. Healed plaque ruptures and sudden coronary death: evidence that subclinical rupture has a role in plaque progression. *Circulation* 2001;103:934–940, with permission.)

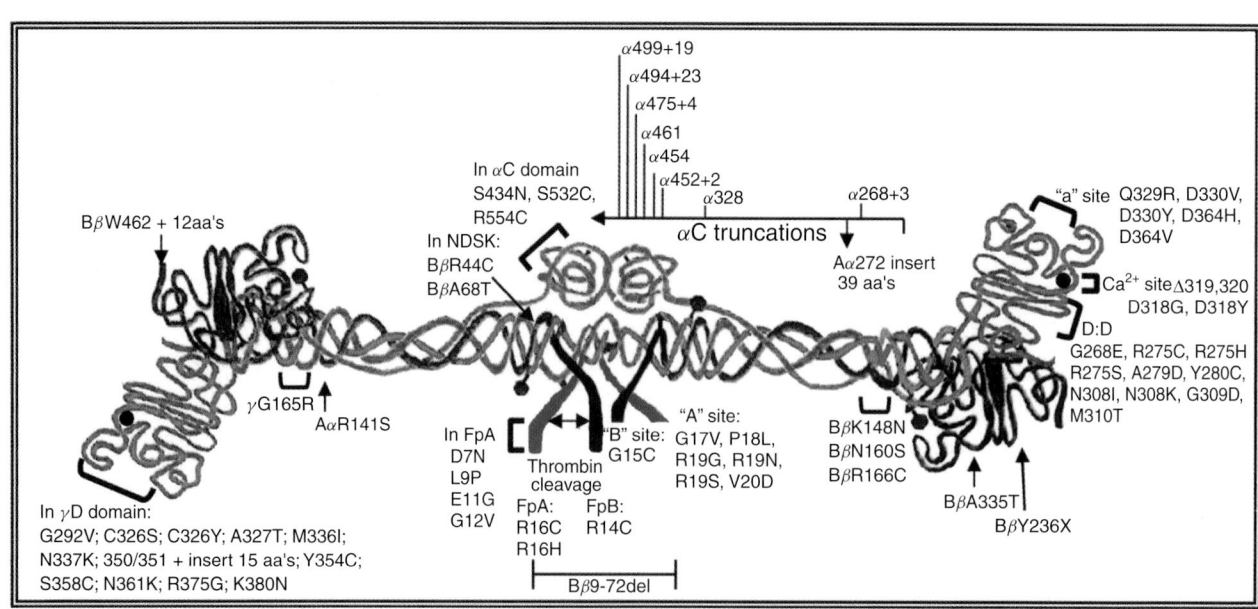

COLOR FIGURE 62-2. Schematic representation of the fibrinogen molecule with dysfibrinogens denoted. The γ, Aα, and Bβ chains are featured in *red, blue,* and *green,* respectively. Locations of dysfibrinogens are approximate based on known crystal structures of the D fragment. The N-termini of the Aα and Bβ chains are depicted with (left pair) and without (right pair) fibrinopeptides, to show the mutations within the Fp's and the exposed "A" and "B" knobs, respectively. Truncations of the αC domains are listed as the residue where the mutation occurs, followed by the number of residues added because of frameshift, before termination. *Purple* hexagons represent carbohydrate additions and *black* circles represent calcium. (From Cote HC, Lord ST, Pratt KP. γ chain dysfibrinogenemias: molecular structure–function relationships of naturally occurring mutations in the γ chain of human, fibrinogen. *Blood* 1998;92(7):2195–2212, with permission.)

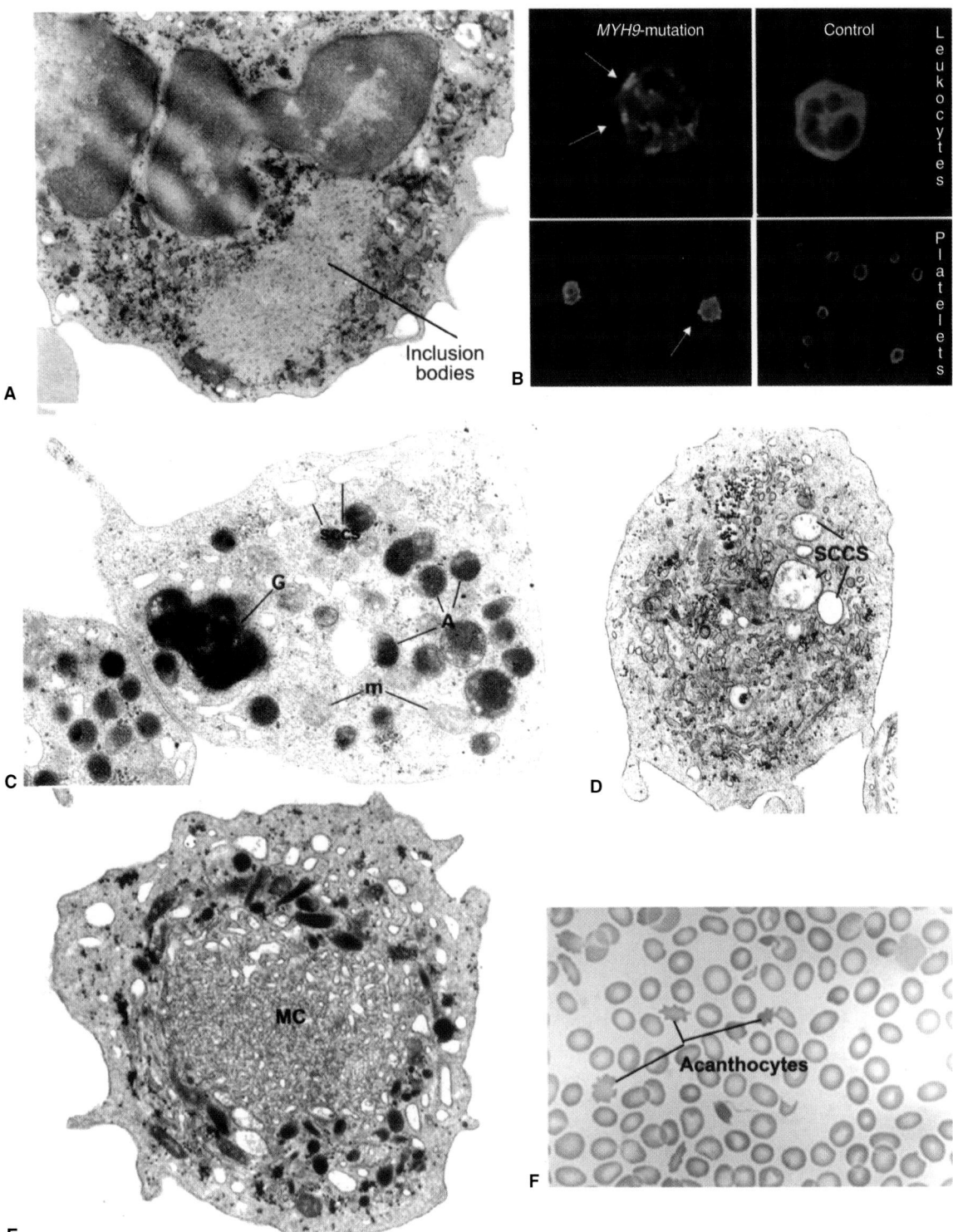

COLOR FIGURE 65-1. Composite illustration showing some of the striking ultrastructural characteristics of blood cells in selected inherited thrombocytopenias. (A) shows an electron micrograph of a Döhle-like body inclusion in a neutrophil from one of the first patients with May-Hegglin anomaly to be characterized (from Dr. A. Greinacher and courtesy of Dr. J.G. White, published from Greinacher A, Bux J, Kiefel V, et al. May-Hegglin anomaly: a rare cause of thrombocytopenia. *Eur J Pediatr* 1992;151:668, with permission). (B) shows the typical changes in NMMHC-IIA localization as detected using immunofluorescence in leukocytes and giant platelets from a patient with Sebastian syndrome (from Dr. A. Greinacher). (C) shows a typical giant α-granule in the enlarged platelets of a patient with Paris-Trusseau syndrome [from Dr. Elizabeth Cramer, published from Favier R, Jondeau K, Boutard P, et al. Paris-Trusseau syndrome: clinical, hematological, molecular data of 10 new cases. *Thromb Haemost* 2003;90:893, with permission (39)]. (D) presents a round and enlarged platelet from a Bordeaux patient with gray platelet syndrome. The absence of α-granules is to be noted. (E) shows an electron micrograph of a large round platelet with a cytoplasmic cluster of smooth endoplasmic reticulum membranes and membrane complexes, and (F) is a light microscopy slide of May-Grünweld-Giemsa stained blood cells showing dysmorphic red blood cells, both from a patient with X-linked macrothrombocytopenia due to a *GATA-1* mutation. G, giant granule; m, mitochondria; A, α-granule; SCCS, surface connected canalicular system; MC, membrane complexes. [from Kathleen Freson and Chris Van Geet, published with permission from Freson K, Devriendt K, Matthijs G, et al. Platelet characteristics in patients with X-linked macrothrombocytopenia because of a novel *GATA1* mutation. *Blood* 2001;98:85 (40)].

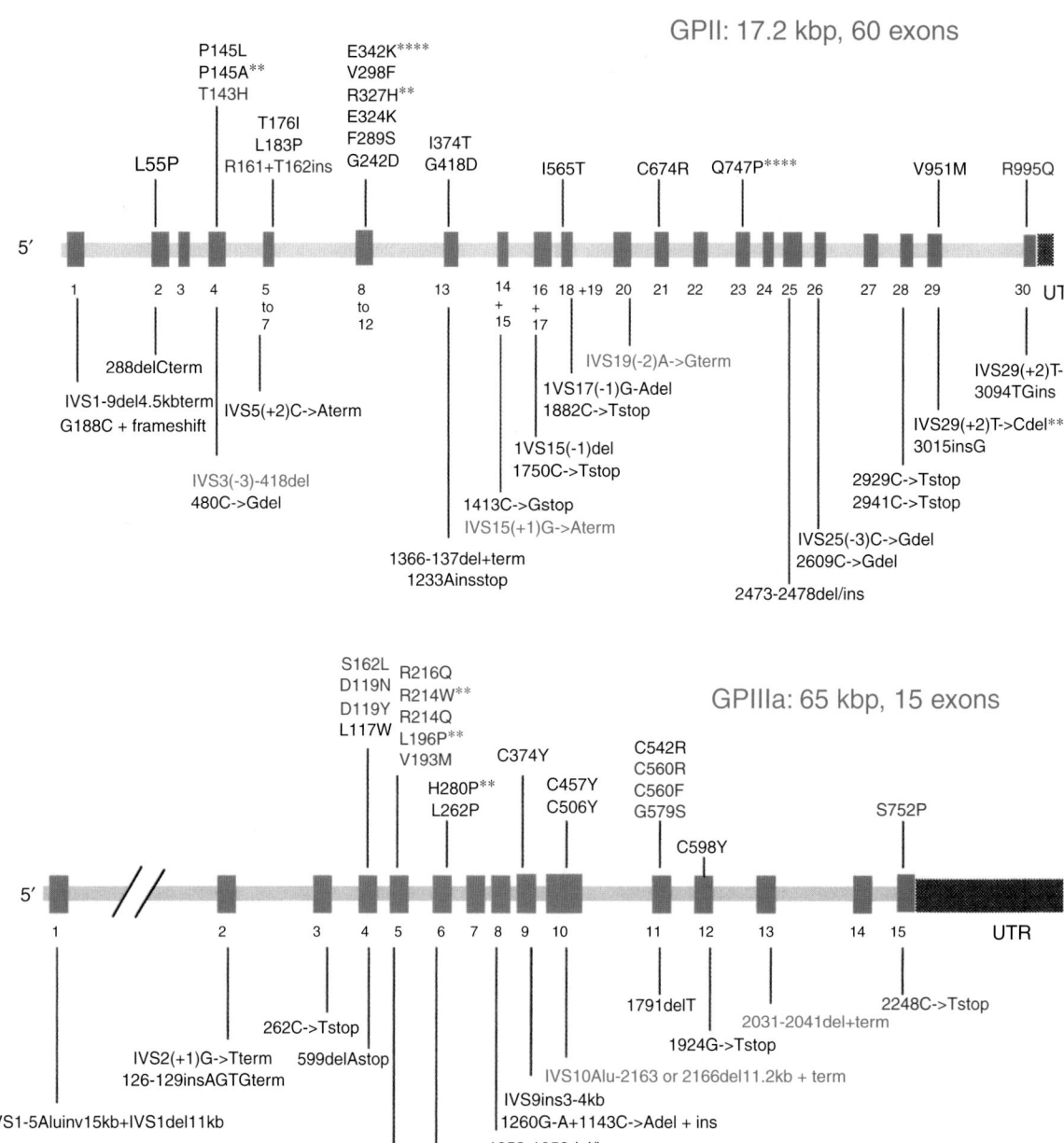

COLOR FIGURE 66-2. Schematic representation of the structure of the GP IIb and GP IIIa genes together with a representative spectrum of the types of genetic abnormalities that give rise to GT. The defects responsible for variant forms of the disease are represented by *brown* symbols; those that prevent GP IIb/IIIa complex expression are in *green*. Asterisks indicate the number of times that the same genetic defect has been described in apparently unrelated families. Mutations in *blue* refer to variant forms; those in *green* are characteristic of different ethnic groups. Note that abnormalities are distributed about equally in both genes and that no part of the gene appears to be exempt. In contrast, variant forms are more likely to have GP IIIa gene defects (see also Table 66-2). Only some of the illustrated mutations are discussed in the text. UTR, untranslated region; ins, insertion; inv, inversion; del, deletion; term, termination; stop, stop codon.

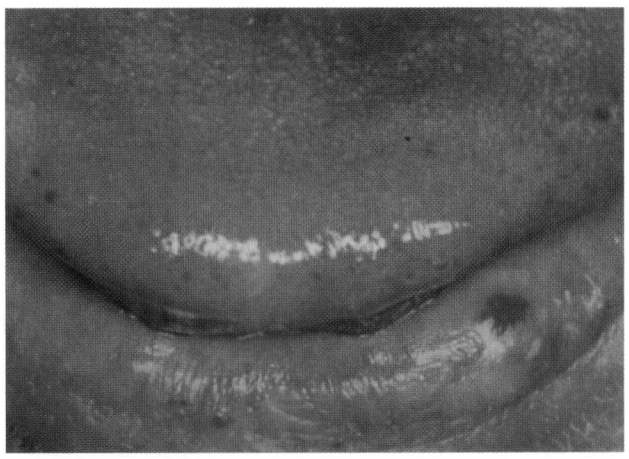

COLOR FIGURE 67-1. Telangiectases of the tongue and lower lip in a patient with hereditary hemorrhagic telangiectasia.

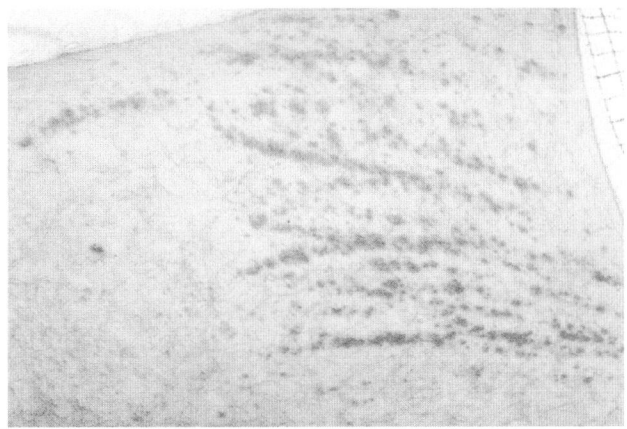

COLOR FIGURE 67-2. Scratch purpura demonstrating capillary fragility. This patient awoke and noted these linear petechiae on his thigh as the presenting sign of autoimmune thrombocytopenic purpura.

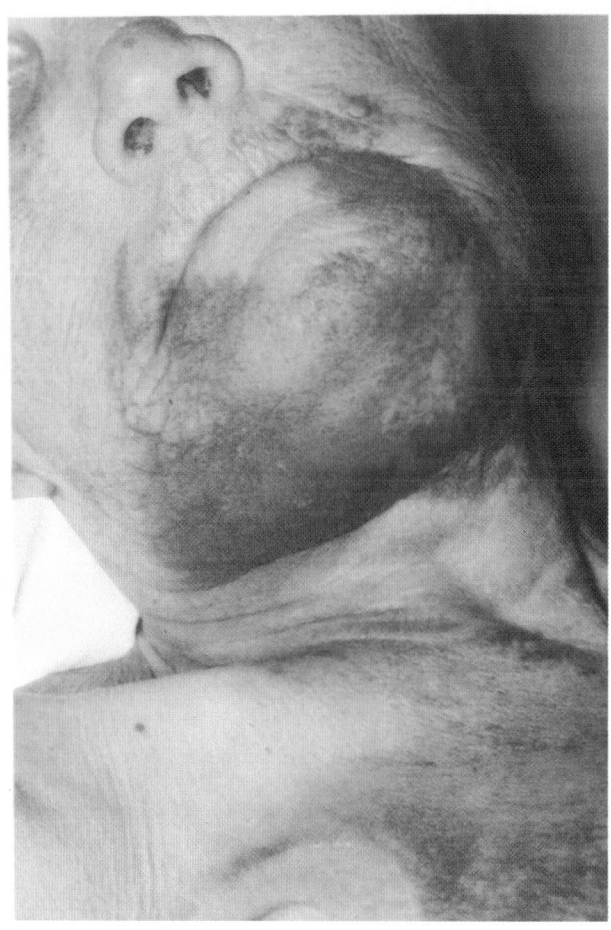

**COLOR FIGURE 67-3.** Ecchymosis in a patient with a spontaneous inhibitor to factor VIII. A small oral lesion bled into the floor of the mouth and with gravity dissected along the subcutaneous planes of the neck and chest.

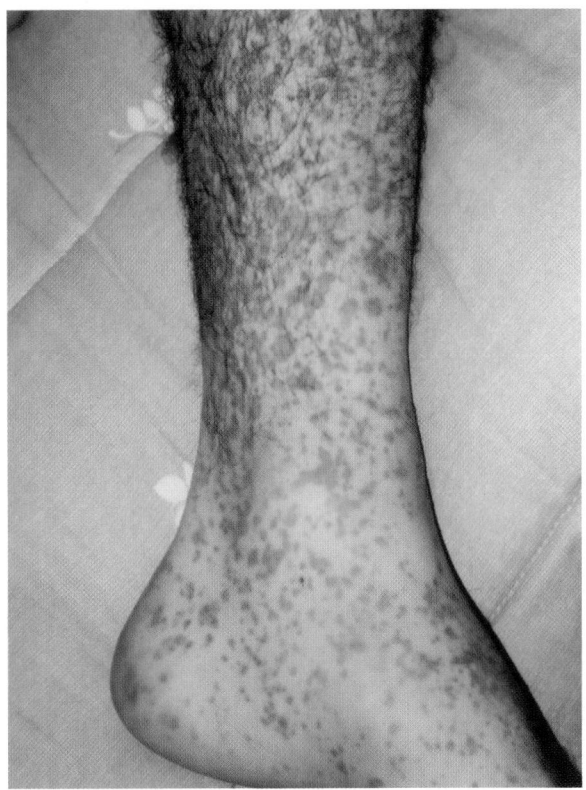

COLOR FIGURE 67-4. Cutaneous vasculitis in Henoch-Schönlein purpura (HSP). This 18-year-old boy had an upper respiratory tract infection 1 week prior. He awoke with this purpuric rash, knee pain, and vague abdominal pain. Protein and red cells were in his urine. All manifestations were cleared within 10 days without therapy.

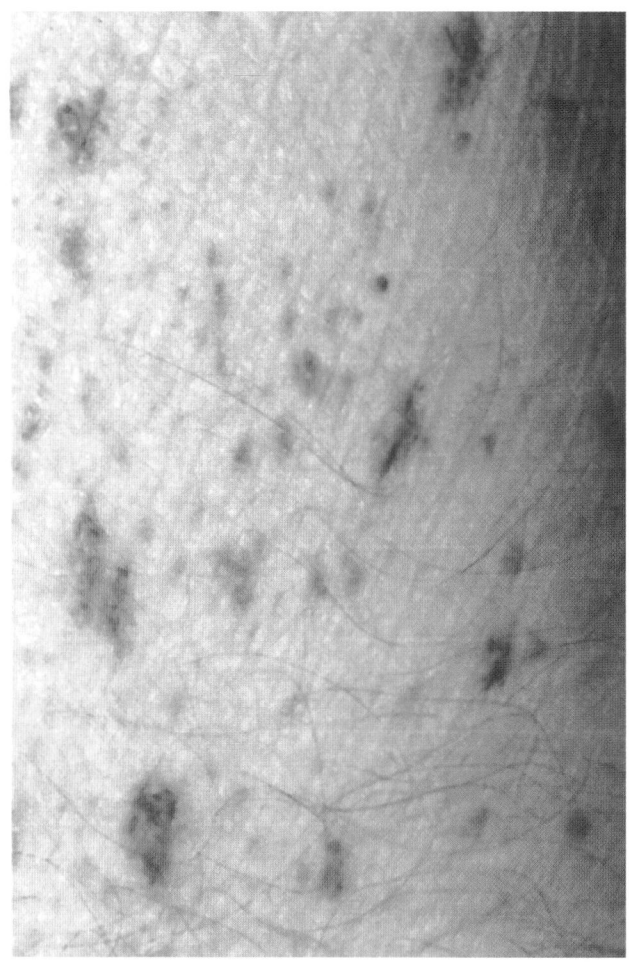

COLOR FIGURE 67-5. Perifollicular hemorrhages on the thigh in a patient with scurvy. He had subsisted on beer alone for 4 months.

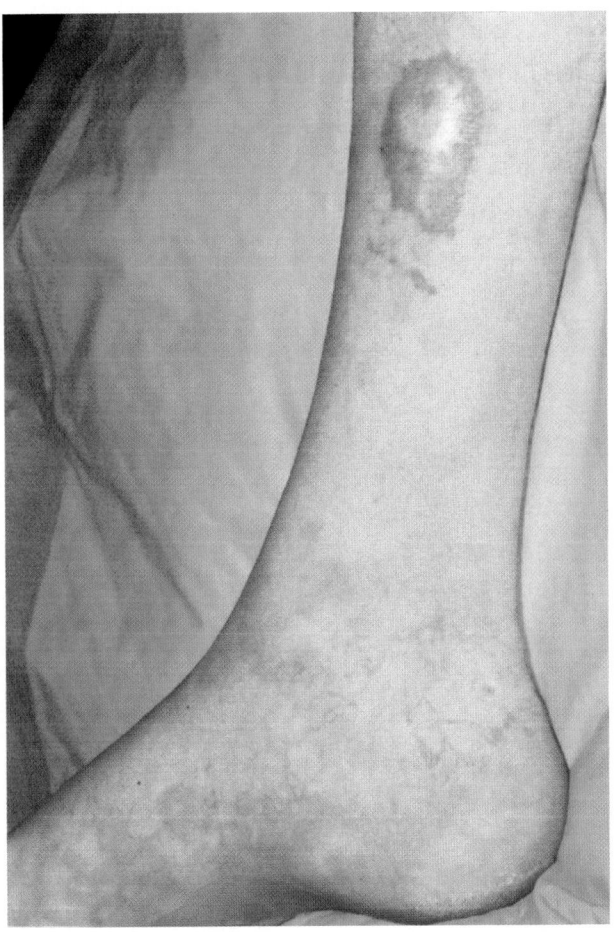

COLOR FIGURE 67-6. Expanding necrosing ("gunmetal gray") purpuric lesions of disseminated intravascular coagulation in a postsplenectomy patient with sepsis due to *Capnocytophaga*. Note the linear purpura lesion 2 cm distal to the necrotizing area; this was one of multiple scratches caused by a new pet dog and one of the presumed portals of entry for this bacterium.

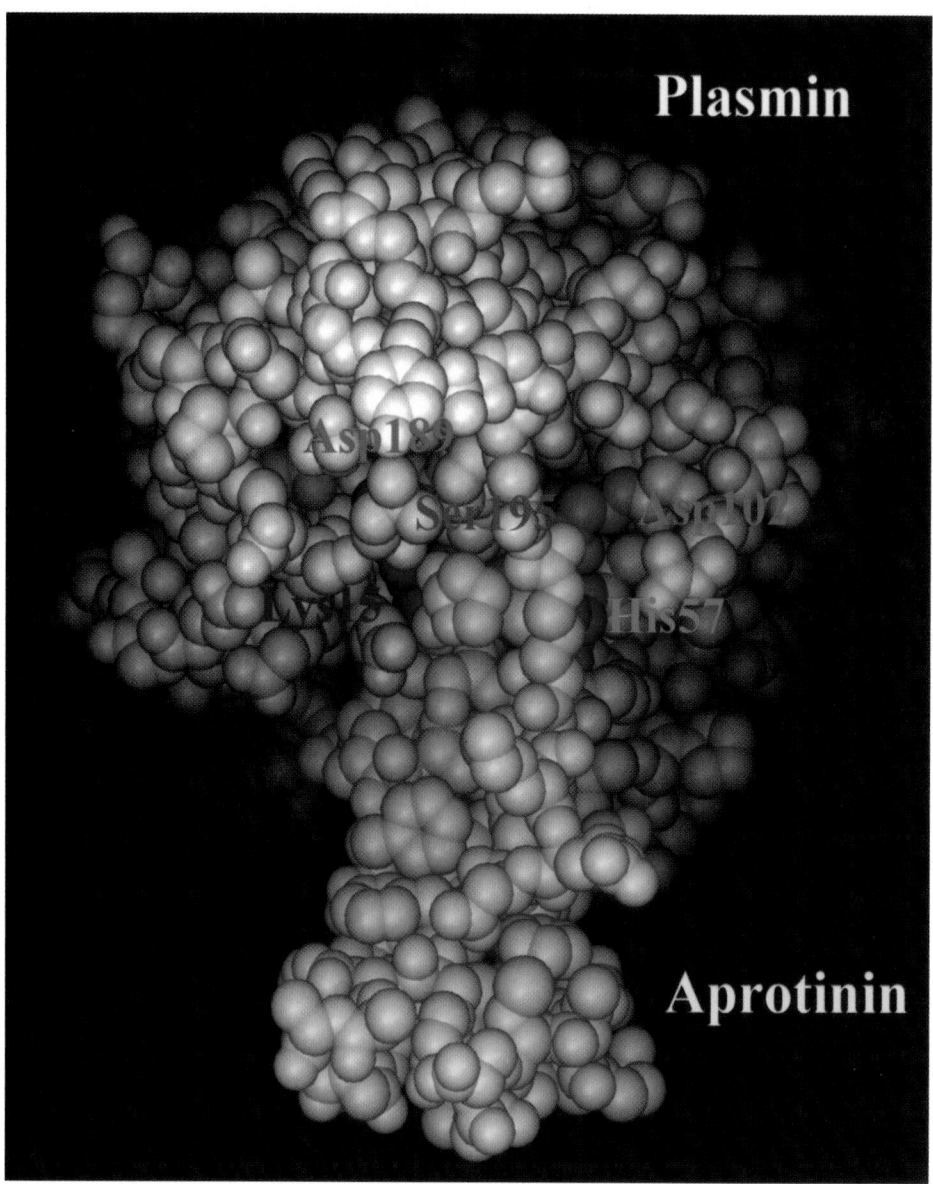

COLOR FIGURE 79-1. Modeled complex of the interaction between Aprotinin and plasmin's protease domain. The plasmin active site triads residues—His57(603), Asp102(646), and Ser195(741) are shown. Lys15 (shown in *blue*) of aprotinin inserts into the active site of the enzyme, forming a salt bridge with Asp189(736) (shown in *red*) at the base of the active site. The plasmin structure of plasmin is from Wang et al. (62) and that of aprotinin from (63). The model was built using the methodology by Bajaj et al. (64).

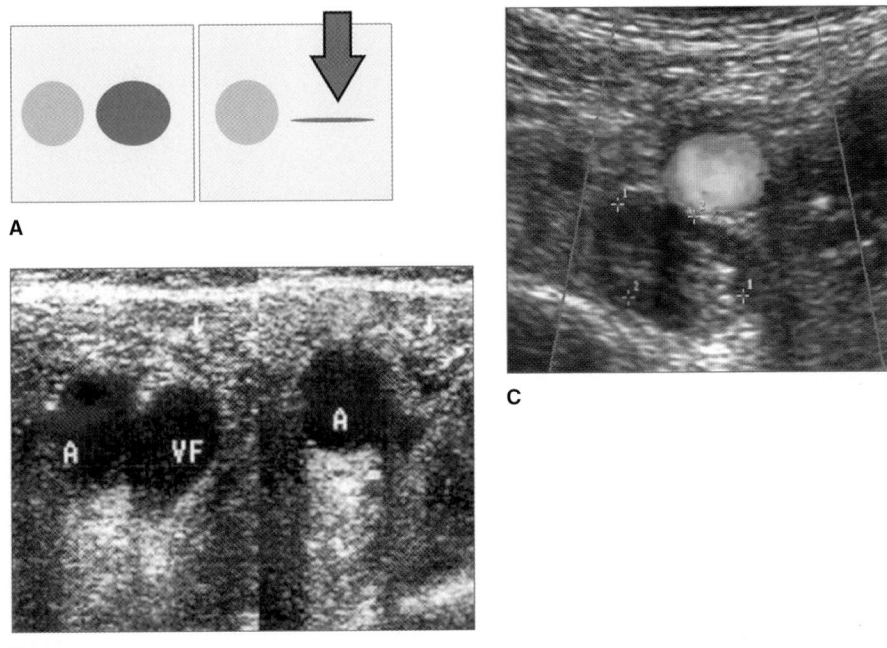

**COLOR FIGURE 87-6.** Ultrasonogram showing from the left to right, the adjacent femoral artery (*A*) and vein (*VF*), the full compressibility of the vein by the transducer, characteristic of the absence of thrombosis, and the incompressibility of the vein by the transducer, characteristic of the presence of an occluding thrombus. This procedure is called compression ultrasonography (CUS).

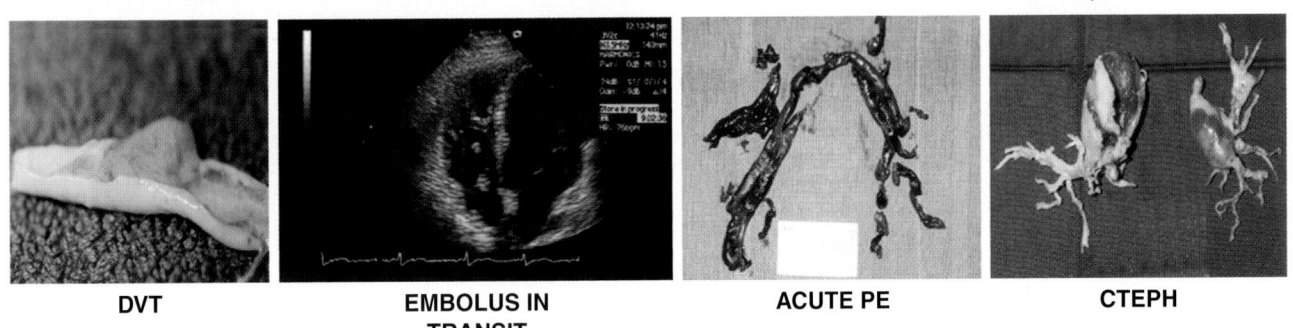

**DVT**   **EMBOLUS IN TRANSIT**   **ACUTE PE**   **CTEPH**

**COLOR FIGURE 92-1.** Spectrum of venous thromboembolism. The *arrow* illustrates the directionality of venous thromboemboli following venous blood flow from the peripheral venous bed, with the pulmonary arteries as the ultimate landing zone.

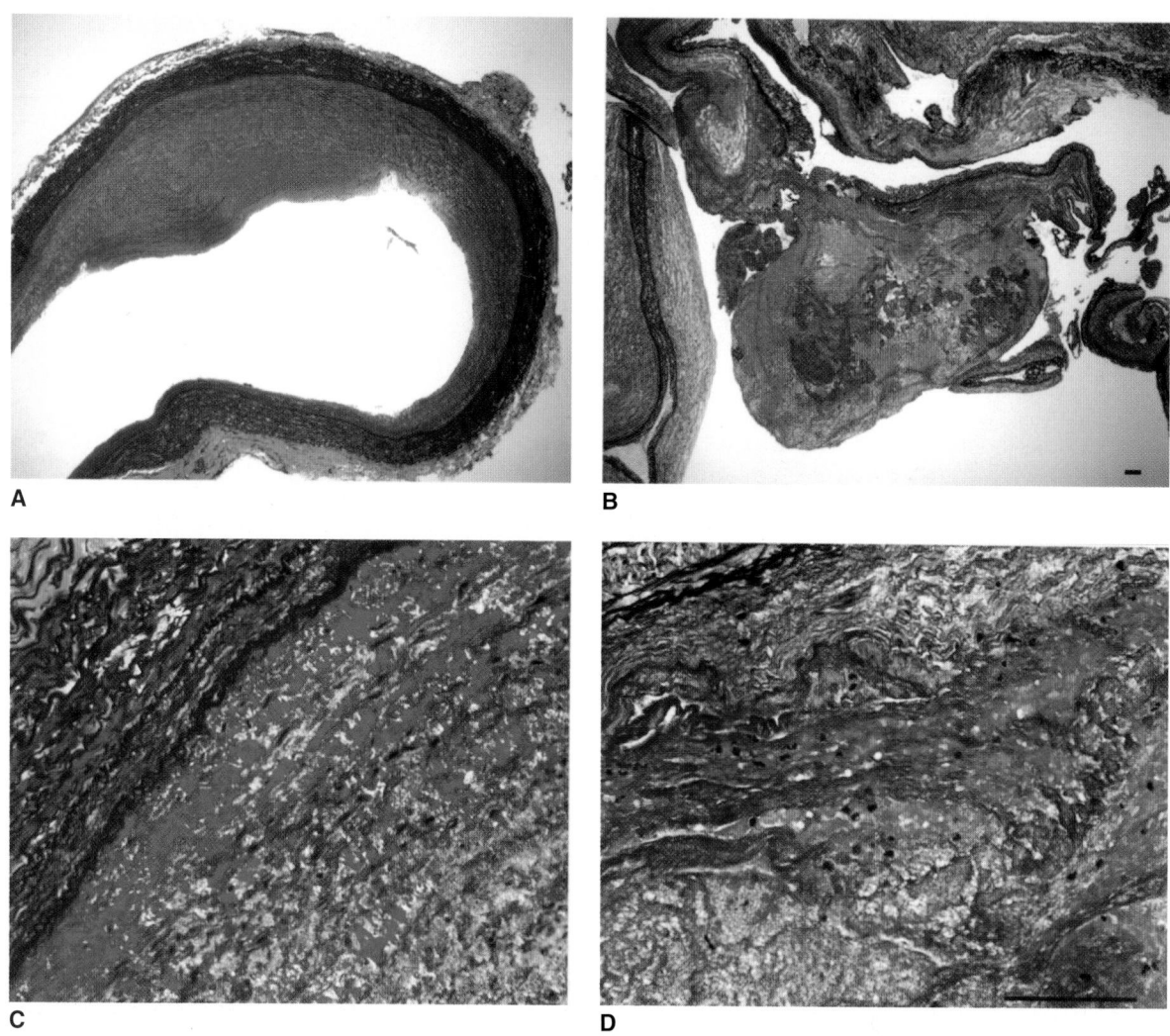

COLOR FIGURE 92-2. Trichrome stain of a representative deep venous thrombus (**A** and **C**) and a pulmonary arterial thrombus (**B** and **D**) harvested at pulmonary thromboendarterectomy (PEA). The modified trichrome stain identifies elastic fibers as *black*, collagen as *green*, fibrin as *red*, erythrocytes as *orange-yellow*, and nuclei as *blue-black*. Panels (**A**) and (**C**) show a representative example of a partly organized deep vein thrombus, with panel (**C**) (200-fold) representing a higher magnification of panel (**A**) (40-fold). Panels (**B**) and (**D**) show a representative chronic thromboembolic pulmonary hypertension (CTEPH) thrombus, with panel (**D**) representing a higher magnification of panel (**B**) (200-fold vs. 40-fold). Scale bars represent 100 $\mu$m.

# CTEPH TYPE II

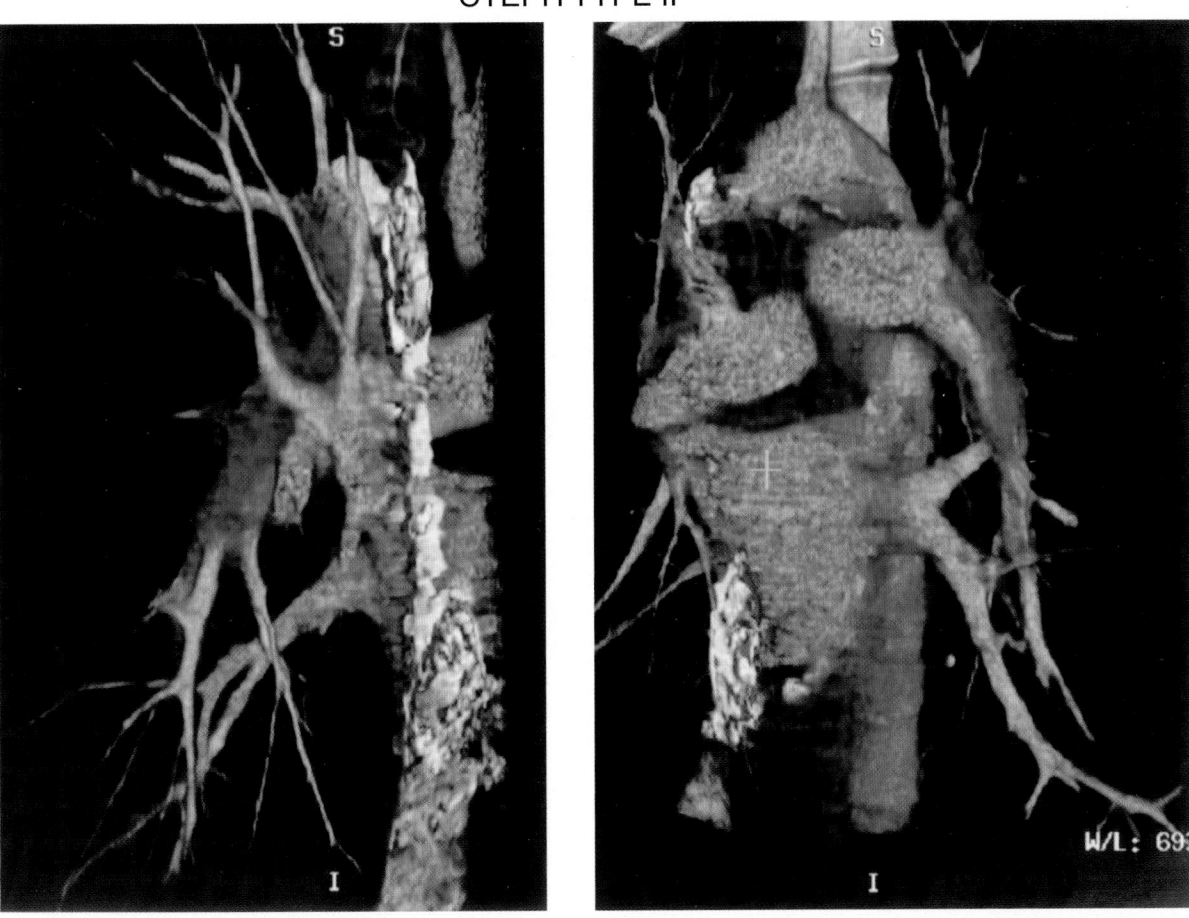

COLOR FIGURE 92-4. Representative computerized tomography images of a patient with type II chronic thromboembolic pulmonary hypertension (CTEPH). The 3-D rendering demonstrates thrombus in *red*. Pulmonary arteries and veins are imaged at the same time.

# CTEPH TYPE IV

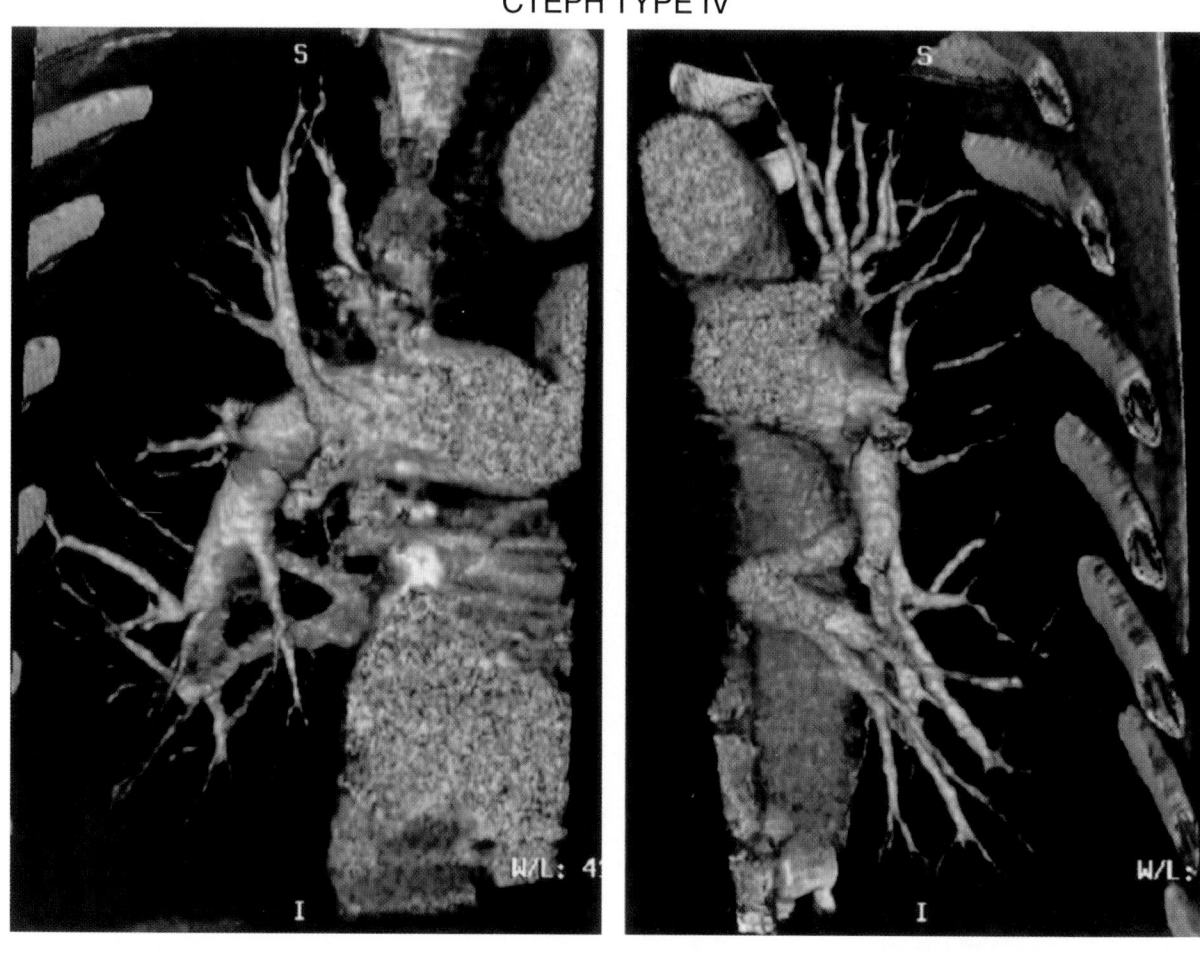

COLOR FIGURE 92-5. Representative computerized tomographic images of a patient with type IV chronic thromboembolic pulmonary hypertension (CTEPH).

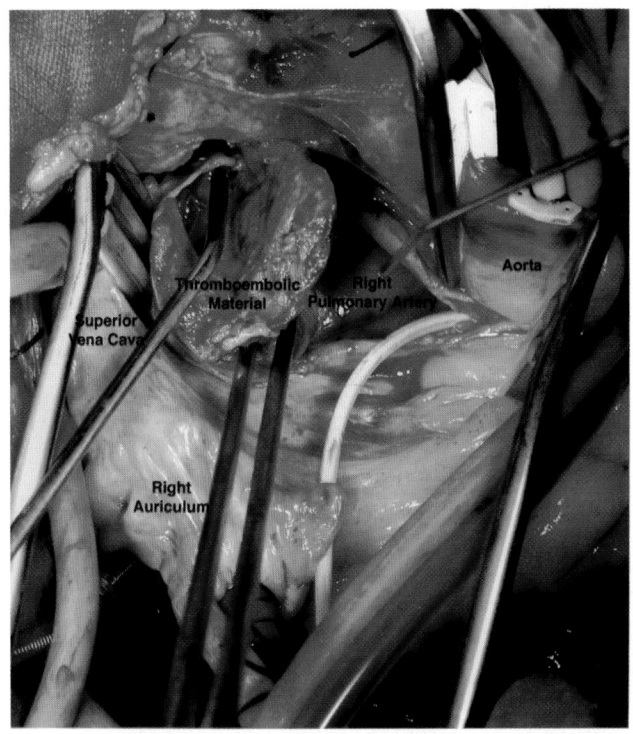

COLOR FIGURE 92-7. The typical operative field of surgical pulmonary thromboendarterectomy shows a lengthwise incised pulmonary artery with a sizeable thrombus being removed.

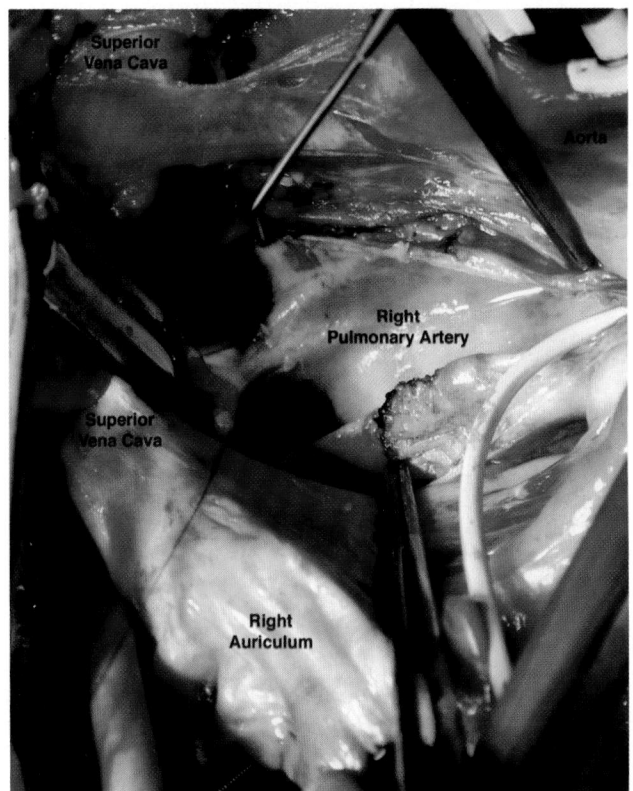

COLOR FIGURE 92-8. At the end of surgical pulmonary thromboendarterectomy, a new inner surface of the pulmonary artery is created that is devoid of fibrotic thrombus tissue. The most relevant anatomical structures are labeled in the photomicrograph.

## CTEPH classification

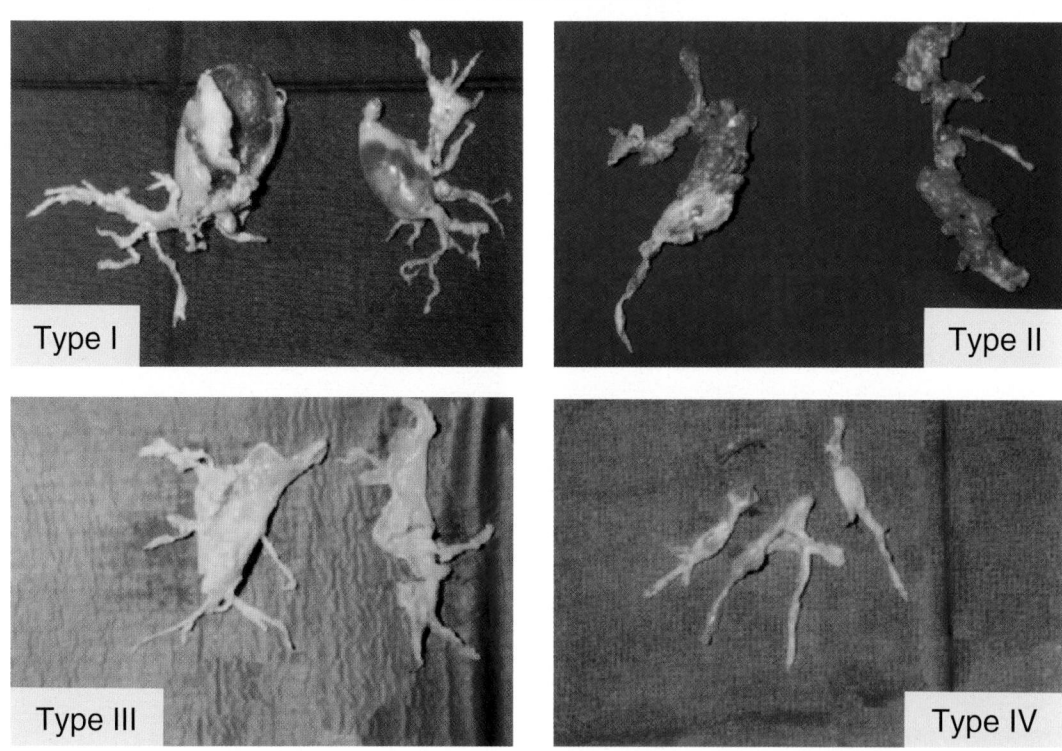

COLOR FIGURE 92-9. Surgical classification of chronic thromboembolic pulmonary hypertension. Most patients (roughly two thirds) present with type II disease. Type IV disease does not yield any thrombus at surgery in most cases. In the example that is shown, small amounts of thrombus were recovered.

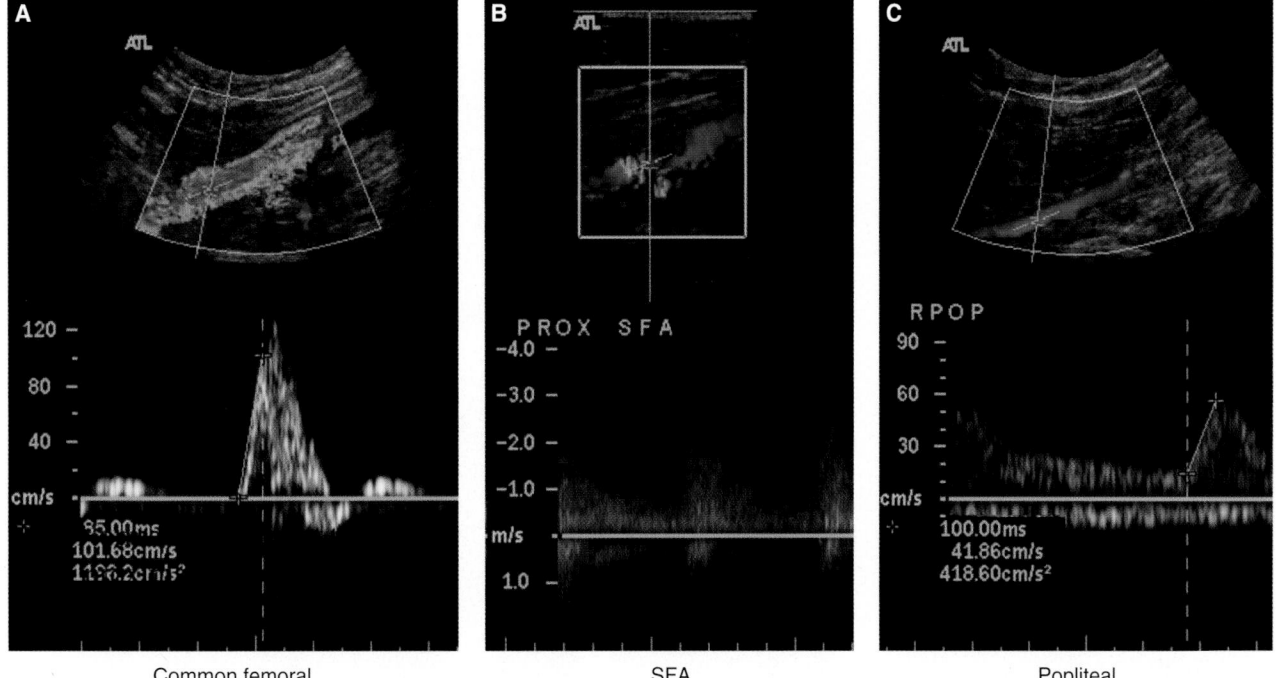

**COLOR FIGURE 101-4.** Arterial duplex in a patient with superficial femoral artery (SFA) stenosis. **A:** Normal duplex of the common femoral artery with associated triphasic velocity signal. **B:** Turbulence and substantially elevated velocity at the site of stenosis in the superficial femoral artery (SFA). **C:** Attenuated Doppler signal in the popliteal artery distal to a high-grade SFA stenosis.

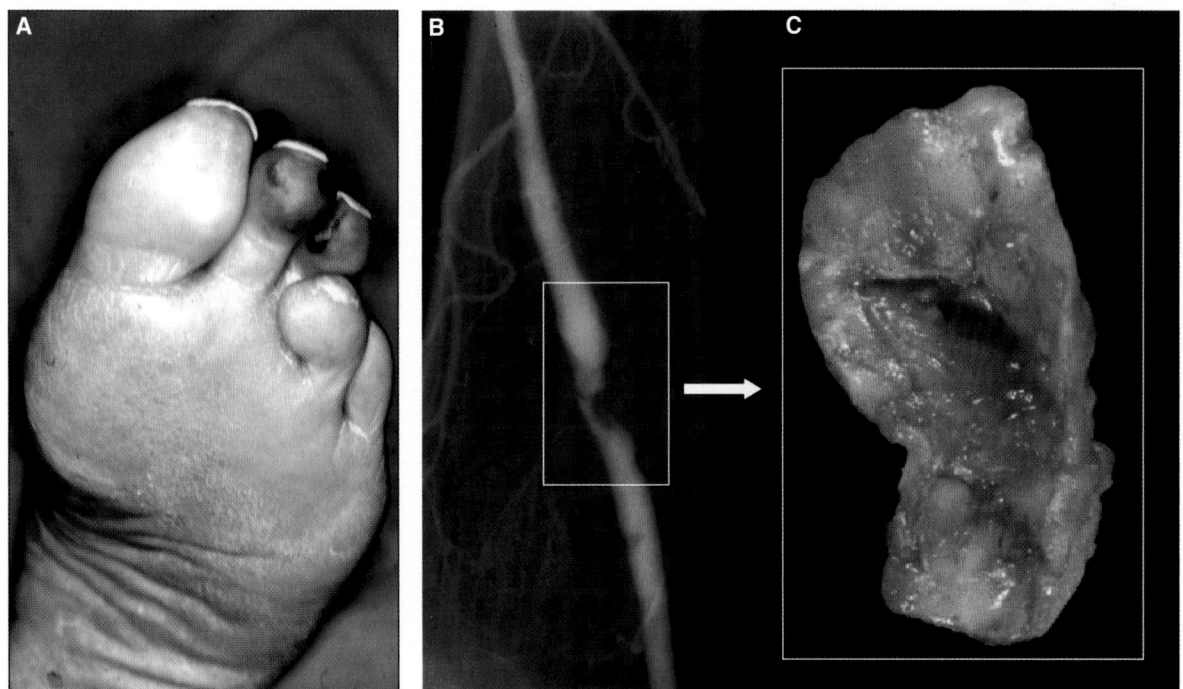

**COLOR FIGURE 101-5.** Blue toe syndrome associated with a focal superficial femoral artery (SFA) lesion. **A:** Patient presenting with painful ischemic toes but an otherwise well-perfused foot. The ABI was 0.7. **B:** Arteriogram demonstrates the culprit lesion in the SFA. **C:** Endarterectomy specimen showing ulceration and laminated platelet-fibrin thrombus on the plaque.

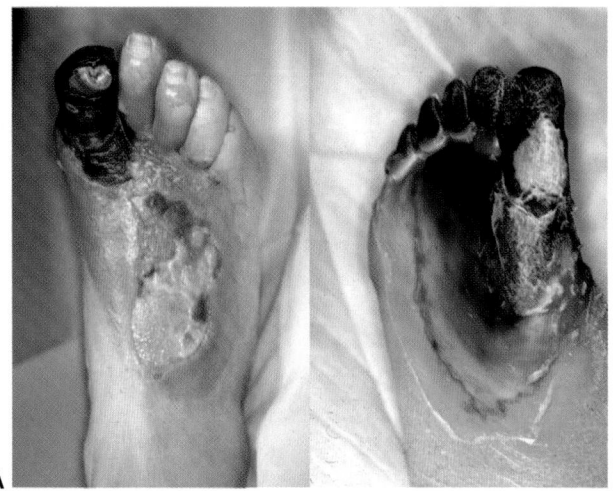

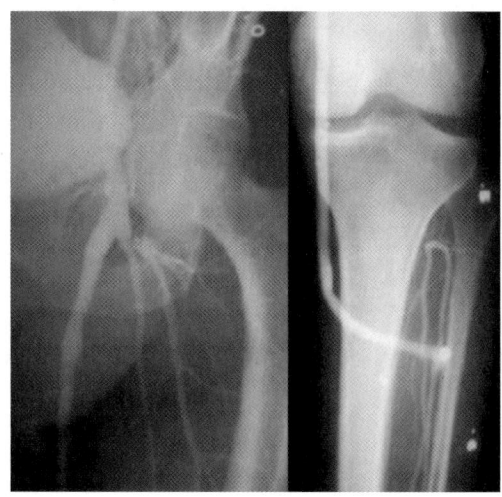

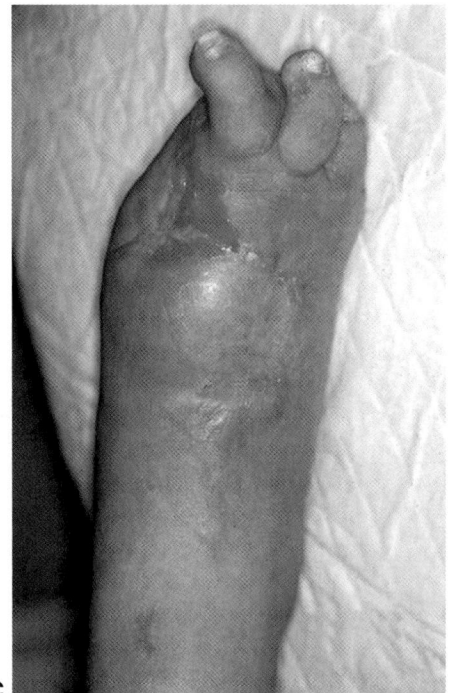

COLOR FIGURE 101-6. Femoral–tibial bypass for critical limb ischemia. Advanced gangrenous changes of a patient's foot due to multilevel infrainguinal arterial occlusive disease with poor profunda collateral flow (photo taken 5 days following revascularization; note pink foot with demarcation developing between healthy tissue and necrotic tissue) (A). B: Completion arteriogram shows a patent femoral–anterior tibial bypass using autogenous vein with the *in situ* technique. C: Clinical outcome following revascularization and eventual amputation of necrotic toes; patient ambulates normally with shoe prosthesis.

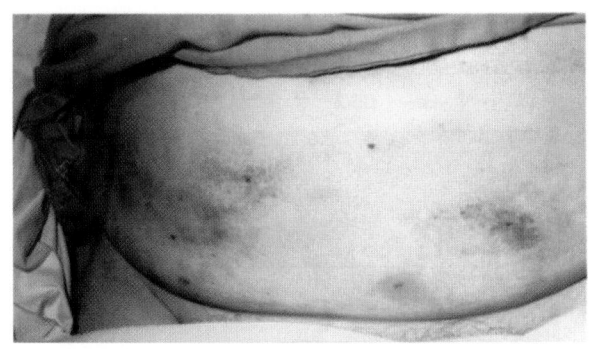

**A**

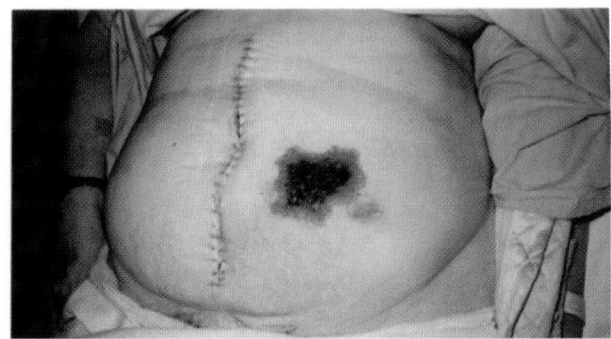

**B**

**C**

Platelet count (×10$^{-9}$/L)

Laparotomy    Skin necrosis

Subcutaneous heparin prophylaxis

Days in hospital

COLOR FIGURE 114-5. Heparin-induced skin lesions. **A:** Erythematous plaques and (**B**) skin necrosis. The serial platelet counts of the patient with skin necrosis shown in (**B**) is shown in (**C**). Note that only mild thrombocytopenia was observed despite the severe skin necrosis at the heparin injection site. [(**A**) From Warkentin TE. Heparin-induced skin lesions. *Br J Haematol* 1996;92:494–497.]

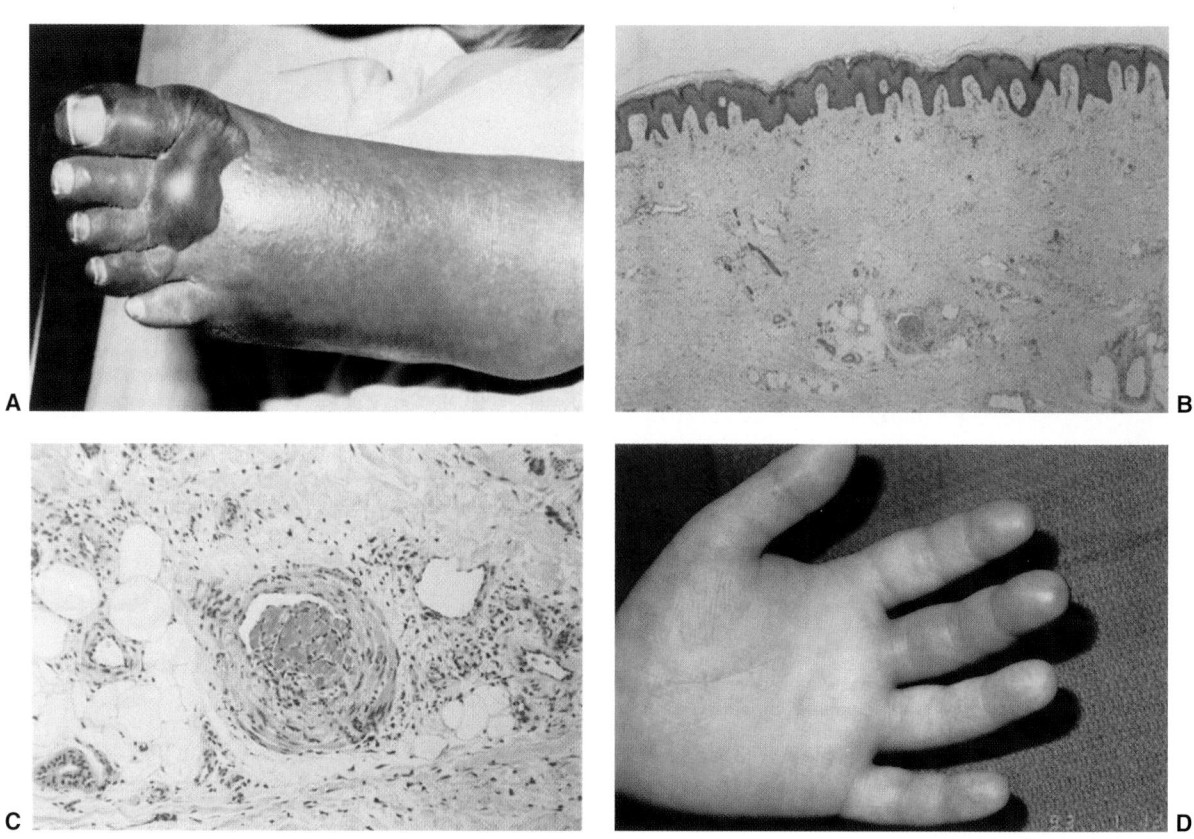

COLOR FIGURE 115-3. **A:** Warfarin-induced venous limb gangrene complicating heparin-induced thrombocytopenia (HIT). **B:** An occluding thrombus can be seen in a subcutaneous venule (original magnification, × 40). **C:** High-power view (original magnification, ×100) of the subcutaneous venule from part (**B**). **D:** Warfarin-associated phlegmasia cerulea dolens complicating HIT. [Photograph from patient 4, reported previously (5)]. (Figs. 115A-C from Warkentin TE, Elavathil LJ, Hayward CPM, et al. The pathogenesis of venous limb gangrene associated with heparin-induced thrombocytopenia. *Ann Intern Med* 1997;127:804–812, with permission.)

# PART I ■ BASIC PRINCIPLES OF HEMOSTASIS AND THROMBOSIS

# CHAPTER 1 ■ OVERVIEW OF HEMOSTASIS

ROBERT W. COLMAN, ALEXANDER W. CLOWES, JAMES N. GEORGE,
SAMUEL Z. GOLDHABER, AND VICTOR J. MARDER

Humans have evolved an intricate hemostatic system that is designed to maintain blood in a fluid state under physiologic conditions, but that is primed to react to vascular injury in an explosive manner to stem blood loss by sealing the defect in the vessel wall. Thrombosis may occur if the hemostatic stimulus is unregulated, either because the capacity of inhibitory pathways is impaired or, more commonly, because the capacity of the natural anticoagulant mechanism is overwhelmed by the intensity of the stimulus. Thrombosis may be regarded as an accident of nature that has not had time to adapt through the lengthy process of evolution to the advances of modern medicine, which allow patients to survive the hemostatic challenge of major surgery and trauma but leave them vulnerable to venous thrombosis.

The normal vascular endothelium maintains blood fluidity by inhibiting blood coagulation and platelet aggregation and promoting fibrinolysis (see Fig. 1-1). It also provides a protective barrier that separates blood cells and plasma factors from highly reactive elements in the deeper layers of the vessel wall. These components include adhesive proteins such as collagen, fibronectin, laminin, vitronectin, and von Willebrand factor (VWF), which promote platelet adhesion, and tissue factor, a membrane protein located in smooth muscle, fibroblasts, and macrophages, that triggers blood coagulation. After the vessel is severed, it constricts, thereby diverting blood from the site of injury, and the shed blood is exposed to these subendothelial structures that stimulate hemostatic plug formation by promoting platelet adhesion and aggregation and by activating blood coagulation. After platelets are stimulated by subendothelial collagen, they expose and assemble membrane glycoprotein (GP) IIb and GP IIIa, which can then bind fibrinogen and VWF, cofactors for platelet recruitment and aggregation. Secretion of proteins from $\alpha$-granules is mediated by thromboxane $A_2$ synthesis, phosphorylation of specific proteins, and intracellular calcium translocation. Protein cofactors such as factor V, secreted by platelets or derived from plasma, serve as a nidus for assembling enzyme–cofactor complexes on the platelet surface, thereby accelerating factor X and prothrombin activation. The result is thrombin formation, which augments its own production manyfold by converting factors V and VIII into activated cofactors and stimulating platelet secretion.

This explosive cellular and molecular reaction is modulated by endothelial cell elaboration of antithrombotic lipids (prostacyclin, or $PGI_2$), proteins (thrombomodulin), inorganic compounds [nitric oxide (NO)], and polysaccharides (heparan); by surface-binding enzymes such as adenosine diphosphatase (ADPase) (CD39); and by several plasma protease inhibitors, most importantly antithrombin (AT) III for factors IXa, Xa, and thrombin; C1 inhibitor, for the contact system enzymes factor XIIa, factor XIIf, and kallikrein; $\alpha_1$-antitrypsin for factor XIa; and $\alpha_2$-macroglobulin as a general backup. A major substrate of thrombin is fibrinogen, which, after initial hydrolysis, forms fibrin monomers that then undergo spontaneous polymerization to form the fibrin clot. Covalent cross-linking

by the thrombin-activated enzyme factor XIIIa increases the resistance of the clot to fibrinolysis.

Plasminogen, a plasma zymogen, is converted to plasmin by two plasminogen activators elaborated by endothelial cells. The process is modulated by at least three plasminogen activator inhibitors. Plasmin normally does not act on fibrinogen in solution because of the presence of $\alpha_2$-antiplasmin. However, plasmin on the surface of the fibrin clot is protected from the inhibitor, and fibrinolysis occurs with the formation of fibrin degradation products. Second, plasminogen activator inhibitor (PAI-1) released by endothelial cells and by platelets neutralizes tissue-type plasminogen activator (tPA) and prevents early lysis of clot. Third, thrombin activates a carboxypeptidase B proenzyme, called *thrombin-activated fibrinolytic inhibitor* (TAFI), that impairs fibrinolytic degradation of fibrin strands. Therefore, with more active coagulation and with more complete conversion of prothrombin to thrombin, not only is more fibrin formed from fibrinogen, but such fibrin is further protected from fibrinolysis by TAFI. Dissolution of the clot paves the way for the deposition of collagen, formation of fibrous tissue, and wound healing.

## ENDOTHELIUM

Normal endothelium (see Fig. 1-2) maintains blood fluidity by producing inhibitors of blood coagulation and platelet aggregation, modulating vascular tone and permeability, and providing a protective envelope, thereby separating hemostatic blood components from reactive subendothelial structures. Endothelial cells synthesize and secrete basement membrane and extracellular matrix, which contain adhesive proteins, collagen, fibronectin, laminin, vitronectin, and VWF. The endothelium inhibits blood coagulation by synthesizing and secreting thrombomodulin and heparan sulfate onto its surface; modulates fibrinolysis by synthesizing and secreting tPA, urokinase plasminogen activator (uPA), and plasminogen activator inhibitors; inhibits platelet aggregation by releasing $PGI_2$ and NO; and regulates vessel wall tone by synthesizing endothelins, which induce vasoconstriction, and $PGI_2$ and NO, which produce vasodilation.

Defective vascular function can lead to abnormal bleeding if the endothelium becomes more permeable to blood cells, if the vasoconstrictive response is impaired because of structural abnormalities of the vessel wall or extravascular supporting tissues, or if physiologic fibrinolysis is not controlled by the normal production of plasminogen activator inhibitor. Bleeding associated with endothelial injury may be mediated by immune complexes and viruses (1,2). Proteolytic enzymes released from leukocytes in inflammatory states perturb endothelial cells and alter connective tissue proteins and also could contribute to petechial hemorrhage in vasculitic disorders (3,4). Attenuation and fenestration of the vascular endothelium may contribute to the hemorrhagic manifestations

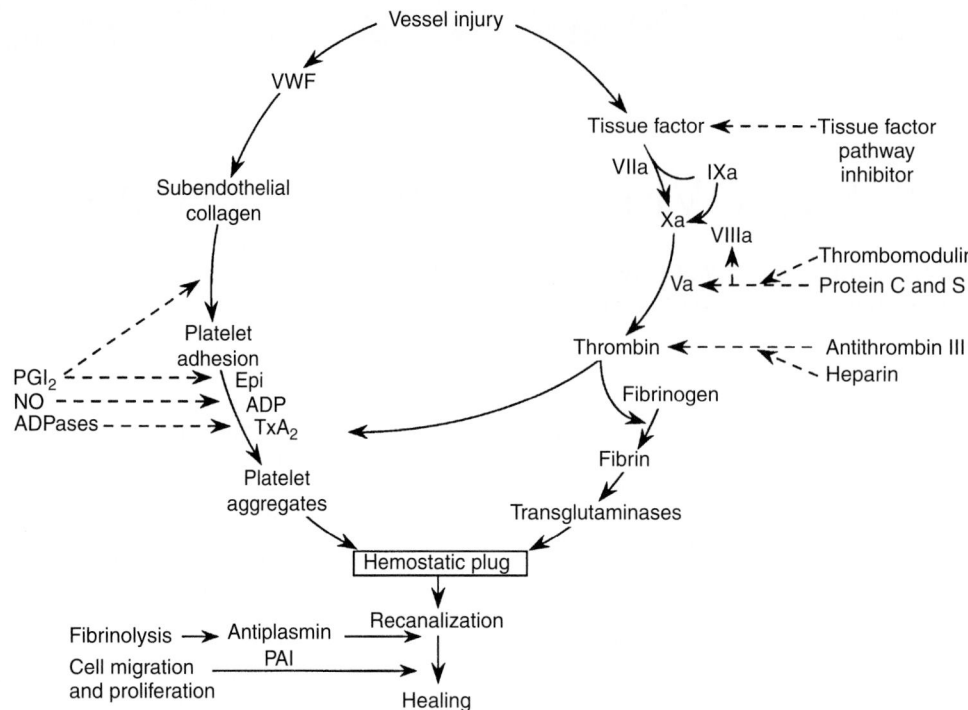

**FIGURE 1-1.** Overview of hemostasis. ADP, adenosine diphosphate; ADPase, adenosine diphosphatase; Epi, epinephrine; TxA$_2$, thromboxane A$_2$; PAI, plasminogen activator inhibitor; PGI$_2$, prostacyclin; NO, nitric oxide; VWF, von Willebrand factor.

of idiopathic thrombocytopenia purpura, which may respond to prednisone therapy promptly, even before a detectable rise in platelet count (5).

Endothelial cells lose their nonthrombogenic protective properties after they are stimulated by enzymes such as thrombin, hypoxia, fluid shear stress, oxidants; cytokines such as interleukin-1, tumor necrosis factor, and γ-interferon; synthetic hormones such as desmopressin acetate and endotoxin. Synthesis of tissue factor and PAI-1 is induced and the concentration of surface-bound thrombomodulin is reduced by cytokines and endotoxin, whereas desmopressin acetate results in the release of high-molecular-weight VWF multimers from Weibel-Palade bodies that may augment platelet adhesion to the injured vessel wall. Endothelial cells contain receptors, termed *integrins*, of the very late antigen (VLA) type, that allow binding of fibronectin ($\alpha_1\beta_1$), collagen ($\alpha_V\beta_1$), and laminin ($\alpha_3\beta_1$, $\alpha_6\beta_1$) and of the cytoadhesive type, notably the vitronectin receptor ($\alpha_2\beta_3$) (6). The stimulated endothelial cell synthesizes chemokines, such as monocyte chemoattractant protein, interleukin-8, regulated on activation normal T-cell expressed and secreted (RANTES), and GRO. Endothelial cells also contain intercellular adhesion molecules (see Chapter 45) such as ICAM-1 and ICAM-2, and VCAM-1, which act

as counterreceptors for leukocyte integrins (7,8). Before tight adhesion to the endothelium, platelets and leukocytes roll, an interaction mediated by E selectin and P selectin (which is stored in Weibel-Palade bodies).

Endothelium is heterogeneous, both metabolically and structurally (9). For instance, angiotensin-converting enzyme apparently is synthesized by most endothelial cells but is principally synthesized by aortic endothelium, not by cardiac microvessel endothelium; on the other hand, thromboxane A$_2$ is not synthesized by most endothelial cells but is synthesized by pulmonary arterial endothelium. Endothelial cell turnover is low under resting conditions but varies with location. At sites of hemodynamic stress and injury, proliferation is especially increased. Endothelial cells contain a full array of contractile proteins, but of special importance are the stress fibers involved in cell attachment and maintenance of endothelial junctional apposition by vascular endothelial (VE) cadherin and platelet–endothelial cell adhesion molecule (PECAM). Endothelial cells contain caveolae that concentrate glycosylphosphatidyl-linked proteins such as the urokinase receptor.

Endothelial cell permeability is influenced by the functional adaptations that join the cells to their neighbors. Macromolecules pass across the endothelium into the vessel wall through

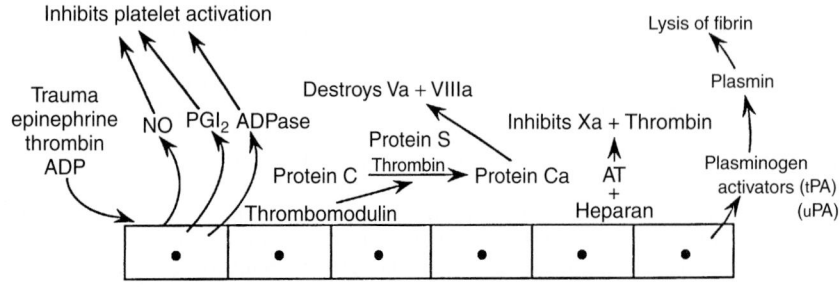

**FIGURE 1-2.** Thromboresistant properties of endothelium. The endothelial cells express adenosine diphosphatase (ADPase), and synthesize prostacyclin (PGI$_2$), thrombomodulin, heparan, and plasminogen activators, all of which inhibit hemostasis (and thrombus formation) and contribute to the maintenance of vascular patency. ADP, adenosine diphosphate; AT, antithrombin; NO, nitric oxide; tPA, tissue-type plasminogen activator; uPA, urokinase plasminogen activator.

patent intercellular junctions, by endocytosis, and through the transendothelial pores. Vessel permeability is increased by vasodilation, by induction of severe thrombocytopenia, and by high doses of heparin. Spontaneous bleeding observed with a low platelet count or after heparin infusion may be induced by increased vascular permeability.

Increased fenestration and attenuation of endothelium may account for the loss of barrier function associated with experimental thrombocytopenia. The thrombocytopenia-induced extravasation of erythrocytes, manifest clinically as petechiae, occurs principally through postcapillary venular interendothelial channels. The loss of endothelial barrier function, associated with extreme platelet depletion, may be related to a loss of serotonin and norepinephrine delivered by platelets to the microvascular milieu, as exogenous sources of either amine prevent petechial formation in severely thrombocytopenic animals or failure of platelets to plug gaps at intracellular junctions between retracted endothelial cells.

Endothelial cells are highly negatively charged, a feature that may repel the negatively charged platelets. This anionic surface, as well as other antithrombotic properties of endothelium, could be important in limiting the intravascular extension of the hemostatic reaction induced by vessel injury (10). Therefore, $PGI_2$, synthesized and released from endothelial cells close to the site of hemostatic plug formation, could inhibit intravascular platelet aggregation (11–14). Thrombomodulin and heparan sulfate, the two endothelial surface–bound thrombin inhibitors, could limit the intravascular spread of fibrin beyond the confines of the hemostatic plug (15–19). Heparan sulfate, a glycosaminoglycan, activates AT and, therefore, catalyzes the inhibition of thrombin and factor Xa. Endothelial cell–associated ADPase (CD39) cleaves adenosine diphosphate (ADP) to adenosine monophosphate (AMP), thereby modulating this stimulatory agonist (20).

Thrombomodulin binds thrombin and inhibits the ability of the enzyme to cleave fibrinogen and activate platelets and factors Va and VIIIa. Thrombomodulin also markedly enhances thrombin's ability to activate protein C. Protein C binds to endothelial cell protein C receptor, which enhances its activation (21). Protein C, in turn, inactivates factors Va and VIIIa and enhances fibrinolysis, probably by binding an inhibitor of plasminogen activators (22). Thrombin bound to thrombomodulin also is inactivated by circulating AT, a step accelerated by heparan sulfate. Protein C activity is controlled by protein C inhibitor (PAI-3) and $\alpha_1$-proteinase inhibitor and is stimulated by protein S, a cofactor (23,24). Protein S, in turn, is controlled by C4b, which forms a complex with it, thereby preventing its action (25). The enhancement of fibrinolysis by protein C also may depend on protein S (26). Therefore, the binding of thrombin with thrombomodulin results in the loss of the coagulant effect and in the enhancement of thrombin's ability to activate protein C and therefore to inhibit thrombogenesis.

The synthesis of $PGI_2$ by endothelial cells is stimulated by thrombin and other stimuli, including epinephrine and trauma (27). Other agonists, including histamine, adenosine triphosphate (ATP), bradykinin, and acetylcholine, stimulate endothelial cell guanylate cyclase, raising the levels of intracellular cyclic 3′,5′-guanosine monophosphate (cGMP), which results in the synthesis of NO. Therefore, endothelial cells exposed to appropriate stimuli synthesize and release two distinct mediators of vasodilation and inhibition of platelet function (28). Stimulated endothelial cells also synthesize a group of peptides known as *endothelins* that have counterregulatory properties, including vasoconstriction (29). Endothelial cells also elaborate plasminogen activators, which, in the presence of fibrin, promote fibrinolysis and can aggravate a bleeding tendency in susceptible patients. The bleeding tendency can be controlled by synthetic and natural fibrinolytic inhibitors (see Chapter 79). PAI-1 also is elaborated with a different time course

and in response to different stimuli (30). Deficiency of PAI-1 causes a bleeding tendency, an indication that unopposed physiologic fibrinolysis disrupts the hemostatic balance.

Endothelial cells are stimulated by cytokines and other mediators to mount a procoagulant response characterized by an increased synthesis and release of PAI-1, release of VWF, synthesis and availability of tissue factor, and reduction of cell membrane–associated thrombomodulin. The postoperative and posttraumatic fibrinolytic shutdown is associated with increased synthesis of PAI-1 and could be mediated by cytokines elaborated as a response to tissue damage (30). Thrombin bound to thrombomodulin also more efficiently activates the TAFI (31). This response protects the newly formed hemostatic plug from premature dissolution but also may contribute to the increased risk of postoperative venous thrombosis.

Chapter 41 summarizes the changing focus of the function of endothelial cells from mediating mostly antithrombotic reaction to changes based on studies of embryonic and adult development of endothelial cells into new vessels. These changes may be in response to alteration of blood flow roles as well as changes required on vascular remodeling in physiologic and pathologic changes. An explosion of studies of both vasculogenesis (origination of blood vessels) and angiogenesis (neovascularization) have delineated a large number of angiogenic stimulators and inhibitors as well as explored some of the signaling mechanisms.

The complex interplay between mediators and countermediators derived from the vessel wall, the endothelial lining, and even the vasomotor regulation of arteries and veins, affects hemostasis and wound healing. All these vascular processes act in concert with similarly complex processes in the platelet, in plasma coagulation, and in fibrinolytic and inhibitory pathways to maintain normal hemostasis. Occasionally, however, the hemostatic response is excessive and leads to intravascular thrombosis. Proteins of the hemostatic system participate in the regulation of angiogenesis, including plasminogen, AT, kininogen, platelet factor 4, and collagen. Fragmented or altered forms of these proteins show antiangiogenic activity.

# PLATELETS

Platelets are produced from bone marrow megakaryocytes, a giant cell with 8 to 32 nuclei as a result of division of nuclei without cell division (32). Recent data shows that the fragmentation is similar to apoptosis because it is a result of caspase activation within the megakaryocytes (33). The dominant growth factor is thrombopoietin, which is responsible for both DNA replication and cytoplasmic differentiation (34). Multiple transcription factors specific for the hematopoietic lineage are responsible (35).

The participation of platelets in hemostasis is a fundamental component of this physiologic process. The reactions involved include adhesion to the cut end of a blood vessel, spreading of adherent platelets on the exposed subendothelial surface, secretion of stored platelet constituents (including molecules involved in hemostasis and wound healing), and formation of large platelet aggregates (36). In addition, platelet membrane sites become available for adsorption and concentration of clotting factors, and plasma coagulation is accelerated, resulting in the formation of a fibrin network that reinforces the otherwise friable platelet plug. The firm platelet–fibrin clot subsequently retracts into a smaller volume, a process that is also platelet-dependent.

Platelets do not adhere to normal vascular endothelial cells, but an area of endothelial disruption (e.g., the cut end of a divided blood vessel) provides binding sites for the adhesive protein, VWF, through the platelet GP Ib/IX/V complex, and fibrinogen as well as fibronectin through integrin receptors (37). These adhesive proteins are thought to participate in the formation of a bridge from platelets to subendothelial connective tissue, although this may be an oversimplification.

The importance of these events is illustrated by the occurrence of hemorrhage in Bernard-Soulier disease, in which patients lack GP Ib/IX, or in von Willebrand disease, in which VWF is decreased or defective. At high-shear rates (i.e., >800 per second), comparable to those found in arteries in the microvasculature, plasma VWF is required for normal adhesion of platelets to subendothelium, perhaps as a bridge between platelets and the fibrillar surface (38). At low-shear rates, adhesion of platelets to subendothelium is normal in patients with these disorders, suggesting that other proteins can substitute for the action of VWF, at least to some extent. Signaling through GP Ib/IX/V activates GP IIb/IIIa without involvement of other receptors (39).

Other adhesive events that are involved include interactions of collagen with the platelet GP Ia/IIa (40) followed by activation of intracellular signaling pathways by platelet GP VI (41). Abnormalities in either of these platelet receptors for collagen cause bleeding defects.

Once adherent to subendothelium, platelets spread out on the surface, and additional platelets, delivered by the flowing blood, adhere first to the basal layer of adherent platelets and eventually to one another, forming a mass of aggregated platelets. A crucial event in platelet aggregation is induction of a change in the disposition of surface membrane GP IIb/IIIa (42), which acquires the capacity to bind fibrinogen, as well as VWF, fibronectin, and vitronectin (43). Fibrinogen appears to be the most important in aggregation by virtue of its divalent structure, possibly allowing it to form a bridge from platelet to platelet and thereby mediating aggregation.

The current paradigm for bidirectional signaling has been well summarized (44). Inside-out signaling from the cytoplasmic tail of this integrin to the ligand recognition site results in conformational changes leading to increased ligand affinity. An increase in the number of surface receptors is derived from fusion of the platelet $\alpha$-granule membranes with the plasma membranes. Shuttling of GP IIb/IIIa between these two membranes is responsible for acquisition of fibrinogen from plasma.

Several other integrins in the platelet membrane act as receptors for adhesive plasma proteins. These heterodimers, such as the vitronectin receptor, are present on the surface of both blood cells and endothelial cells (45). Whereas VWF and collagen can interact with resting platelets, fibrinogen forms a high-affinity bond only with an integrin GP IIb/IIIa on activated platelets (46). In the congenital disorder Glanzmann thrombasthenia, the GP IIb/IIIa complex is deficient, and the associated defect in fibrinogen binding results in a bleeding tendency (47). Likewise, the bleeding in congenital afibrinogenemia is caused in part by an abnormality of platelet aggregation.

Interaction with GP receptors in the platelet membrane also is a feature of participation in platelet aggregation by fibronectin and thrombospondin. The interaction of the latter with GP IV may act to stabilize platelet aggregates.

Of the many platelet agonists whose ability to induce aggregation and secretion has been studied *in vitro*, those having the greatest physiologic relevance are the proteolytic enzyme thrombin, ADP, collagen, arachidonic acid, and epinephrine. Epinephrine is the only one of these that does not result in a detectable change in platelet shape.

Specific receptors exist on the platelet surface for these agonists (see Fig. 1-3) (48). Many of the receptor–agonist complexes interact in the platelet membrane with coupling proteins that hydrolyze guanosine triphosphate, the G proteins. Evidently, some interact with target proteins coupled to ion-permeable channels in the platelet membrane, modulating ion flux, especially the inward movement of ionized calcium. Others are linked to protein tyrosine kinases (TK) that phosphorylate other sites on the receptor protein itself. Accompanying these biochemical events are visible effects, such as the disappearance of the equatorial band of microtubules that normally maintain the platelet's discoid shape, centralization of storage granules, and formation of pseudopodia. Stimulatory agonists lead to activation of phospholipase C, which cleaves phosphatidylinositol bisphosphate ($PIP_2$) to form inositol triphosphate ($IP_3$) and diacylglycerol. $IP_3$ reacts with receptors on calcium storage organelles known as the *dense tubular system*, analogous to the sarcoplasmic reticulum of muscle, leading to mobilization of ionized calcium and increasing its cytoplasmic concentration (49). Familial abnormalities in a G protein (50) and a phospholipase C (51) have been shown to lead to mild hemorrhagic disorders.

Many processes involved in platelet activation are calcium dependent, including phosphorylation of the light chain of myosin by a specific kinase enzyme and liberation of arachidonic acid from membrane phospholipids by the enzyme phospholipase $A_2$ (52,53). Phospholipase $A_2$ liberates arachidonic acid from phosphatidylcholine and probably other phospholipids. Arachidonic acid is converted by the enzyme cyclooxygenase to prostaglandin endoperoxides and ultimately to the potent platelet agonist thromboxane $A_2$, as well as to stable prostaglandins such as prostaglandin $D_2$. The latter inhibits platelet activation and, in a negative feedback system, may serve to modulate platelet activities. A reactive serine in cyclooxygenase is alkylated by aspirin, inactivating the enzyme permanently; this accounts for the substantial pharmacologic action on platelets of this widely used drug. High concentrations of intracellular calcium (occurring, for example, after thrombin stimulation) lead to activation of a calcium-dependent neutral cysteine protease (calpain), which may participate in remodeling of cytoskeletal proteins, cleavage of receptor proteins (54), and thrombin-induced activation of platelets.

Diacylglycerol—such as $IP_3$, a product of the action of phospholipase C—activates a ubiquitous enzyme, protein kinase C, in platelets (55). Protein kinase C phosphorylates (among other substrates) pleckstrin, a 47-kDa protein that is a marker for activation of the kinase. Phosphatases provide a negative feedback, reducing the elevation of ionized calcium by $IP_3$ (56). Diacylglycerol may be responsible for the alleged "calcium-independent" reactions occurring during platelet activation, or may act together with ionized calcium to activate protein kinase C and stimulate secretion (57).

Platelets contain several classes of granules in which intracellular constituents are sequestered, including "dense bodies" (containing serotonin, ATP, ADP, pyrophosphate, and calcium), $\alpha$-granules [containing fibrinogen, VWF, factor V, high-molecular-weight kininogen (HK), fibronectin, $\alpha_1$-antitrypsin, (A5)b-thromboglobulin, platelet factor 4, and platelet-derived growth factor], and lysosomes (containing a variety of acid hydrolases) (58). Centralization of these granules after stimulation of platelets results from activation of the platelet cytoskeletal contractile apparatus; polymerization of filamentous actin and phosphorylation of myosin are prominent reactions in platelets responding to receptor-mediated stimulation. In the presence of elevated cytoplasmic calcium, this leads to fusion of the granular envelope with the lining membranes of intracellular canaliculi and to external secretion of the granule contents.

ADP is thought to react with three receptors. The first, $P2X_1$, is an ADP-operated calcium channel with little functional effect. $P2Y_1$ mediates shape change by activating phospholipase C, whereas $P2Y_{12}$ decreases stimulated adenylate cyclase activity and reduces platelet cyclic $3',5'$-adenosine monophosphate (cAMP) (59). Both $P2Y_1$ and $P2Y_{12}$ are required for aggregation (see Chapter 32) (60). A molecular defect in $P2Y_{12}$ results in hemorrhagic defect (61). The $\alpha_2$-adrenergic receptor responsible for epinephrine interaction with platelets has been cloned and sequenced, and a thromboxane $A_2$ and $PGH_2$ receptor has been demonstrated in binding studies (62,63). All

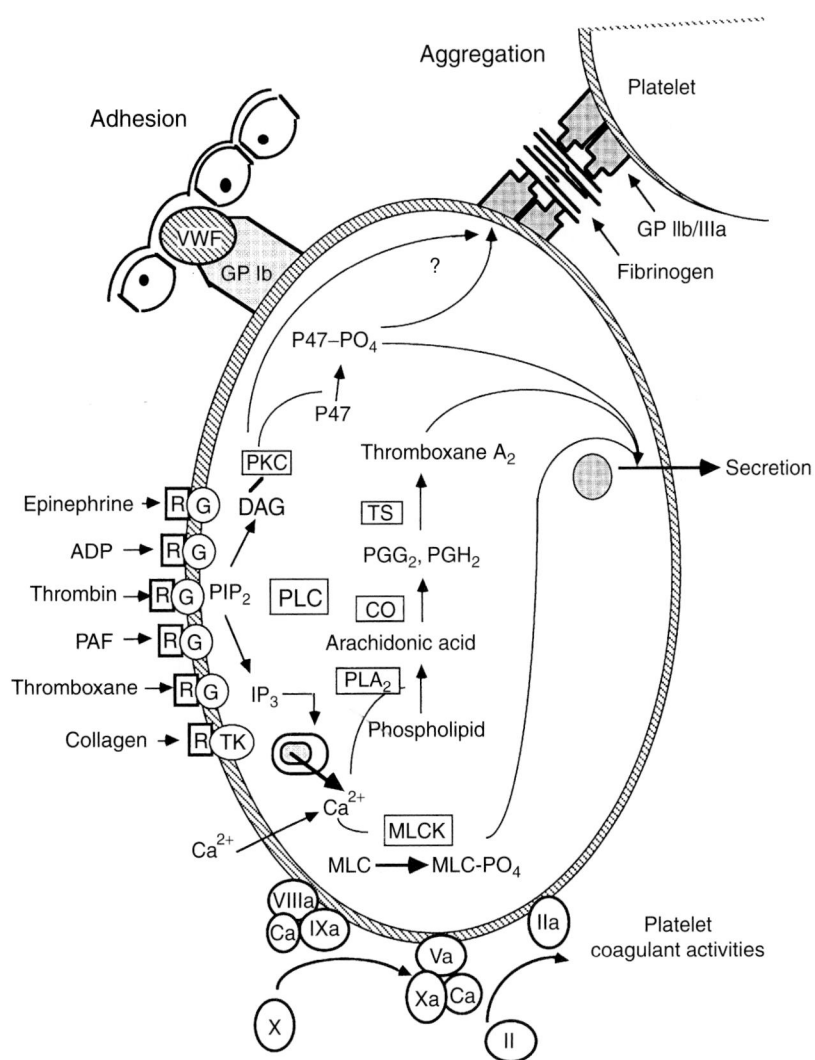

**FIGURE 1-3.** Platelet function. Adhesion to endothelial cells is mediated by glycoprotein (GP) Ib, which binds von Willebrand factor (VWF) on the endothelial cells. Aggregation is mediated by GP IIb/IIIa bridged to GP IIb/IIIa on another platelet by fibrinogen. Various agonists such as adenosine diphosphate (ADP) and platelet activating factor (PAF) are pictured as interacting with specific receptors and activating phospholipase C, probably through G proteins. This enzyme catalyzes the cleavage of phosphatidyl inositol bisphosphate ($PIP_2$) to $IP_3$, which mobilizes $Ca^{2+}$ from the dense tubular system to activate myosin light chain kinase (MLCK), which phosphorylates myosin light chain (MLC). $Ca^{2+}$ also activates phospholipase $A_2$ ($PLA_2$) to release arachidonic acid from phospholipids, which is in turn converted by cyclooxygenase (CO) to $PGG_2$ and $PGH_2$, and then by thromboxane synthetase (TS) to thromboxane $A_2$. The other product of the cleavage of $PIP_2$ is diacylglycerol (DAG), which stimulates protein kinase C (PKC) to phosphorylate the intracellular protein P47 to $P47-PO_4$. The latter, thromboxane $A_2$ and $MLC-PO_4$, together stimulate secretion of products of the dense $\alpha$- and lysosomal granules. Platelet coagulant activity is generated by coagulation factors, shown in roman numerals form "tenase" (VIII, IXa, $Ca^{2+}$) and "prothrombinase" (Va, Xa, $Ca^{2+}$), on the platelet external membrane phospholipid to convert prothrombin (II) to thrombin (IIa). (Courtesy of Dr. A. Koneti Rao.)

these receptor–agonist interactions result in unmasking of functional fibrinogen-binding sites by outside-in signaling through G proteins.

During activation, platelets expose receptors for specific plasma clotting factors, particularly activated factor V (Va), which may be either secreted and expressed by the platelet or bound from plasma. This "acquired" receptor, in conjunction with anionic phospholipids exposed on activated platelets, also functions as a binding site for factor Xa and thereby provides an efficient catalytic environment for the conversion of prothrombin to thrombin by factor Xa (64). An analogous system appears to exist for the binding of factor IXa and conversion of factor X to Xa on platelets.

Platelet activation and its effects are modulated by several regulatory substances, of which the most important is cAMP (65). Like virtually all other animal cells except human red cells, platelets contain adenylate cyclase, the enzyme that converts ATP to cAMP. Its action is powerfully stimulated by the arachidonic acid products prostaglandin $D_2$ in platelets and $PGI_2$ (prostacyclin) in endothelial cells. Platelets also contain cyclic nucleotide phosphodiesterases that cleave cAMP to AMP, modulating intracellular cAMP concentration (66). The major cAMP phosphodiesterase in platelets, PDE3A, is inhibited by cGMP. Therefore, compounds that increase cGMP also inhibit platelet activation. cAMP stimulates a protein kinase that mediates phosphorylation of an ATP-dependent calcium-pumping system that removes calcium from the cytosol. In sufficient concentration, cAMP inhibits not only platelet aggregation, secretion, and shape change but adhesion to surfaces as well.

Other checks on unbridled platelet activation exist on the surface of endothelial cells, including an ADP-destroying ectoenzyme (ADPase), and thrombomodulin, a powerful thrombin inhibitor. Endothelial cells, when stimulated by agonists such as ATP, produce NO, a potent vasodilator that inhibits platelet function by raising platelet cGMP (67). There is evidence to indicate that platelets themselves have the capacity to form NO from L-arginine and that this results in a rise in the concentration of cGMP, which is a powerful intracellular regulator of platelet activity (68).

## COAGULATION

Although it has been traditional (and useful for *in vitro* laboratory testing) to divide the coagulation system into intrinsic and extrinsic pathways, such a division does not occur *in vivo* because tissue factor–factor VIIa complex is a potent activator of both factor IX and factor X.

### Extrinsic System

The principal initiating pathway of *in vivo* blood coagulation is the extrinsic system, which involves components from both the blood and vascular elements (see Chapter 5). The crucial component is tissue factor, an intrinsic membrane protein composed of a single polypeptide chain that functions as a cofactor to factor VIII in the intrinsic system, and to factor V in the "final common pathway" (see Fig. 1-4). Tissue factor pathway inhibitor (TFPI) is a protein that in association with factor Xa inhibits the tissue factor–factor VII complex (69,70). Tissue factor synthesis in macrophages and endothelial cells is induced by endotoxin and by such cytokines as interleukin-1 and tumor necrosis factor (71,72).

The major plasma component of the extrinsic pathway is factor VII, one of a group of vitamin K–dependent proteins (including factors IX and X, prothrombin, and protein C) synthesized as prozymogens and converted (activated) to serine proteases by a limited number of proteolytic cleavages (see Fig. 1-5). Protein S, also a vitamin K–dependent protein, is a cofactor rather than a zymogen. Common to these proteins are unique γ-glutamyl carboxyl acid (Gla) residues at the N-terminal end of the molecule that require vitamin K for proper synthesis by hepatocytes. This postribosomal modification of the protein is required for calcium binding, one calcium with the two carboxyl groups of a Gla residue, thereby serving as a bridge for protein binding to the phospholipid surface.

Both factor IX and factor X are activated by the TF–FVIIa complex and by factor Xa itself. The active form is designated

factor VIIa and represents approximately 1% of total factor VII. Interaction between the intrinsic and extrinsic pathways occurs at several levels of the clotting cascade. The zymogen factor VII itself has minimal but definite protease activity and is capable of autoactivation. It converts factor VII to VIIa and then activates it, thereby displaying both positive and negative feedback effects.

The factor VIIa–tissue factor enzyme complex, which assembles on the activated monocyte or perturbed endothelial cell, has two principal substrates, factor IX (see Chapter 7) and factor X (see Chapter 10), both vitamin K–dependent proteins. Cleavage of either protein results in a serine protease, factor IXa or Xa, that remains membrane-bound. Its Gla residues facilitate further reactions if appropriate cofactors are present. The required cofactor for factor IXa to catalyze the conversion of factor X to factor Xa is factor VIII (see Chapter 8), whereas that for Xa conversion of prothrombin to thrombin is factor V (see Chapter 9).

Factor VIII exists in plasma mostly as a noncovalent complex with VWF, and its coagulant function is to accelerate factor IXa conversion of factor X to Xa. The absence of factor VIII or IX underlies the hemophilia syndromes, classic hemophilia A and hemophilia B, which produce identical hemorrhagic states. Perhaps the similarity of the hemorrhagic condition with either factor VIII or IX deficiency results from a lack in each case of a

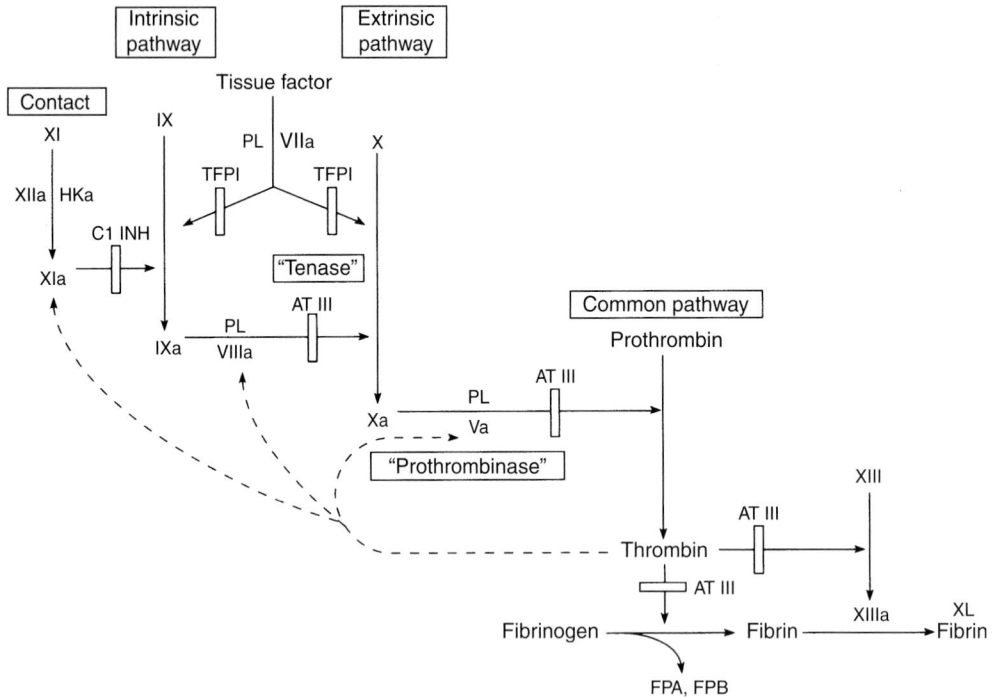

**FIGURE 1-4.** The clotting cascade. The central precipitating event is considered to involve tissue factor (TF), which, under physiologic conditions, is not exposed to the blood. With vascular or endothelial cell injury, TF acts in concert with activated factor VIIa and phospholipid (PL) to convert factor IX to IXa and factor X to Xa. The "intrinsic pathway" includes "contact" activation of factor XI by the XIIa–activated high-molecular-weight kininogen (HKa) complex. It should be noted that the contact system contributes to fibrinolysis and bradykinin formation *in vivo*. Factor XIa also converts factor IX to IXa, and factor IXa, in turn, converts factor X to Xa, in concert with factor VIIIa and PL (the "tenase" complex). However factor Xa is formed, it is the active catalytic ingredient of the "prothrombinase" complex, which includes factor Va and PL and converts prothrombin to thrombin. Thrombin cleaves fibrinopeptides (FPA, FPB) from fibrinogen, allowing the resultant fibrin monomers to polymerize, and converts factor XIII to XIIIa, which cross-links (XL) the fibrin clot. Thrombin accelerates the process (*interrupted lines*) by its potential to activate factors V and VIII, but continued proteolytic action also dampens the process by activating protein C, which degrades factor Va and VIIIa. Thrombin activation of factor XI to XIa is a proposed pathway. Natural plasma inhibitors retard clotting: C1-inhibitor (C1 INH) neutralizes factor XIIa, tissue factor pathway inhibitor (TFPI) blocks factor VIIa/TF, and antithrombin III (ATIII) blocks factors IXa and Xa and thrombin. *Arrows*, active enzymes; *filled rectangles*, sites of inhibitor action; *dashed lines*, feedback reactions.

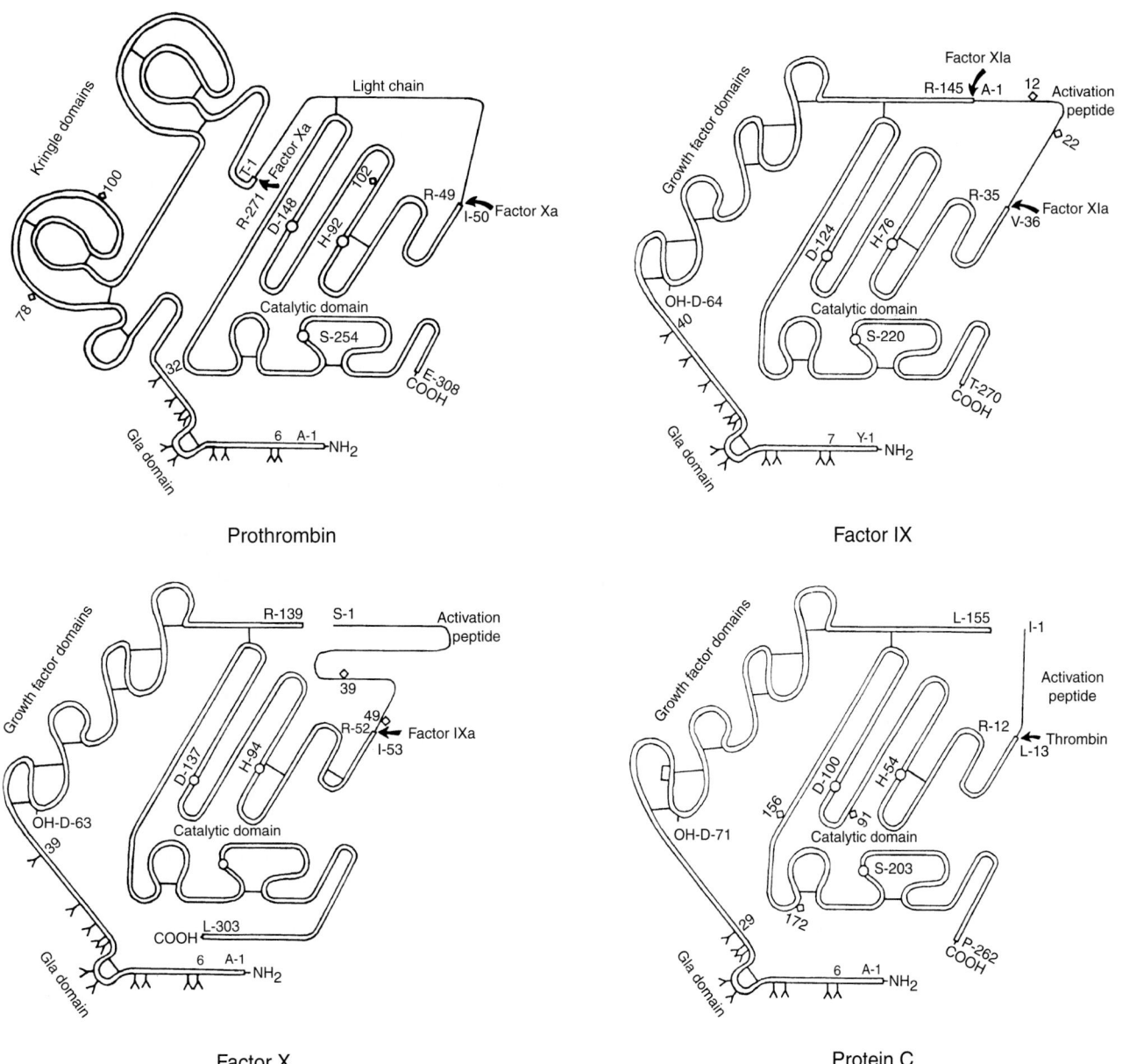

**FIGURE 1-5.** Tentative structures of human prothrombin, factor IX, factor X, and protein C. The Ys refer to the γ-carboxyglutamic acid residues present in the Gla domains. The *open diamonds* refer to potential *N*-linked carbohydrate chains. Cleavage sites and the enzymes involved during the activation of each protein are identified by *solid arrows*. Amino acids involved in catalysis (H, D, S) also are identified. Proposed disulfide bonds have been placed by analogy to those in bovine prothrombin and epidermal growth factor.

proper "tenase" complex that is crucial for factor X activation (Fig. 1-4). The severity of the clinical disorder reflects the concentration of factor VIII or IX. The most severe clinical disease, manifest by spontaneous joint hemorrhage (hemarthroses), occurs with factor VIII or factor IX levels of 0% to 1% (see Chapter 50). At factor levels of 5% to 30%, symptoms may be mild or even nonexistent, except in serious trauma such as surgery, and activity above 30% usually suffices for normal hemostasis. The presence of more than twice as much factor VIII or IX in healthy persons as is present in carriers (mean 50%) indicates that clotting proteins usually are present in excess and that deficiencies must be relatively severe to produce clinically significant effects.

The direct conversion of factor X to factor Xa by factor VIIa–tissue factor complex bypasses the need for factor VIII

or IX. Nonetheless, a congenital deficiency of factor VII or X produces a similar hemorrhagic condition, and distinguishing one from the other requires the determination of specific coagulation factor activities (see Chapter 58). A clinically definable decrease in tissue factor has not been described.

## Intrinsic System

Parallel with the extrinsic system is the intrinsic system, which could be defined as coagulation initiated by components entirely contained within the vascular system. This pathway results in the activation of factor IX by a novel dimeric serine protease, factor XIa (Fig. 1-4), providing a pathway independent of factor VII for blood coagulation. However, an important difference exists between these two pathways in the clotting cascade. Whereas the activation of factor IX by XIa requires only the presence of ionized calcium, the activation of factor IX by VIIa requires calcium and the protein cofactor, tissue factor, embedded in a cell membrane (lipid bilayer).

The role of the contact system proteins (see Chapter 6) in initiation of the intrinsic pathway of coagulation in hemostasis is questionable, because only a deficiency of factor XI is associated with a hemorrhagic tendency. These proteins participate instead in the initiation of the inflammatory response, complement activation, fibrinolysis, angiogenesis (73), and kinin formation (74), and studies show that kininogen is an anticoagulant protein *in vivo* (75). The mechanism may be the inhibition of binding of low concentrations of thrombin to platelet GP Ib/IX (76). The contact system is involved when blood interacts with a foreign surface, as in cardiopulmonary bypass. The zymogen factor XII (Hageman factor) is the first protein in the series of tightly regulated reactions (Fig. 1-4) and binds to negatively charged surfaces such as kaolin, dextran sulfate, and sulfatides. The heavy chain of factor XII binds to the surface, allowing a large increase in local concentration of the enzyme, autoactivation, and action on its substrates, prekallikrein and factor XI, to form kallikrein and factor XIa (77). In most coagulation enzymes, the light chain contains the active site residues serine, histidine, and aspartic acid, homologous to the archetypal serine protease chymotrypsin, whereas the heavy chain contains binding regions to surfaces, phospholipids, cell membrane, and connective tissue, which define the unique role of each coagulation proteolytic enzyme.

The assembly of cofactor, enzyme, and substrate is a recurrent theme in blood coagulation, resulting in maximal efficiency and speed of the molecular reactions, especially as a phospholipid or cell membrane provides the surface for efficient positioning of interacting enzyme complexes with proenzyme substrates.

Kallikrein cleaves HK to liberate the nonapeptide bradykinin, and the remaining kinin-free kininogen (activated HK) binds at least 10-fold better to surface than to the intact procofactor, thereby allowing more prekallikrein to associate with the urokinase receptor on the endothelial cell (78), enhance fibrinolysis (79), and inhibit angiogenesis (75).

Negative feedback regulation is characteristic of the coagulation system. One such reaction is factor XIa cleavage of the light chain of HK, which contains the coagulant activity, thereby destroying its cofactor activity and allowing factor XIa to dissociate from the activating surface (80). Similarly, thrombin activates factors V and VIII, but conversion of protein C to activated protein C leads to the destruction of factors Va and VIIIa. Although deficiency of any of the three proteins involved in the contact system pathway results in slow generation of thrombin and a prolonged *in vitro* partial thromboplastin time, their effect *in vivo* appears to be unrelated or the opposite. HK is an antithrombotic protein after endothelial injury (75), and a deficiency may predispose to thrombosis. Factor XII deficiency has been implicated as a risk factor in venous and perhaps arterial thrombosis (81), so it may be a natural anticoagulant. Only a deficiency of factor XI may result in a hemorrhagic disorder. Even factor XI deficiency results only in a mild disorder of hemostasis in half of the affected individuals, and it is likely that blood coagulation *in vivo* is initiated by factor IX or X through TF–VIIa mechanisms.

## Coagulation Common Pathway

Once factor Xa is formed by either the extrinsic or the intrinsic pathway, it converts prothrombin to thrombin (see Chapter 10). As with the other vitamin K–dependent factors (Fig. 1-5), prothrombin has distinct functional domains devoted to calcium binding to phospholipids (10 Gla residues at the N-terminal portion). This region resembles epidermal growth factor containing $\beta$-hydroxyaspartic acid or asparagine, which can bind $Ca^{2+}$, a region for cofactor (factor V) interaction, an activation peptide region, and a portion containing the catalytic center. Elevated prothrombin levels due to a mutation in the 3′ untranslated region, G20120A, result in a common genetic cause of the hypercoagulable state (82). After appropriate cleavage of prothrombin by factor Xa, the N-terminal Gla portion is removed, and the resultant two-chain thrombin molecule detaches from the phospholipid surface. The interaction of the four components of the prothrombinase complex (factor Xa, factor V, phospholipid, and calcium) provides a markedly increased rate of prothrombin activation—more than 300,000-fold more than that achievable with only the enzyme (factor Xa) and substrate (prothrombin). Factor V that participates in this "prothrombinase complex" on the platelet membrane probably is supplied as the result of its secretion from platelet $\alpha$-granules or fusion with the plasma membrane, and it serves as a receptor for factor Xa binding to the activated platelet (83). Because of this involvement of platelets, the bleeding manifestations of factor V deficiency may resemble those of qualitative platelet disorders. Alternative pathways for prothrombin activation by factor Xa independent of factor V have been described in malignant cells, hypoxic endothelial cells, and macrophages (84–86).

Blood coagulation proteins can be grouped according to shared properties, activities, or localization. For instance, phospholipid-oriented enzymes require vitamin K–dependent carboxylation of glutamic acid residues at their N-terminal domains, and procofactors with no enzymatic activity share an ability to facilitate attachment and interaction of clotting factors on biological surfaces. Another grouping of factors includes those that serve as a substrate for thrombin: for instance, cofactors V and VIII (activated, then inactivated), protein C (activated), prothrombin (cleaved to prethrombin), protein S (inactivated), factor XIII (to form active fibrin-stabilizing factor), and fibrinogen (liberating the fibrinopeptides). Further, deficiency of factor VIII or IX produces the same clinical disorder by virtue of their cooperation in the "tenase" complex. In addition, factor V, fibrinogen, and the adhesive proteins fibronectin, VWF, and thrombospondin are all stored in platelet $\alpha$-granules.

The mapping of the entire human genome has uncovered new relationships of old pairings of coagulation proteins. Mutations in the *LMANI* gene (87) leads to defects in the processing of both factor V and VIII in the ER–Gogli subcellular system, explaining the combined deficiency of these coagulation cofactors. Deficiency of vitamin K epoxide reductase (88) leads to warfarin resistance of factor II, VII, IX, and X. Another important new hemostatic gene recently discovered (89) is *ADAMTS*, which controls the proteolytic breakdown of VWF mutimers and *ADAMTS* deficiency, as associated with thrombotic thrombocytopenic purpura (TTP).

Plasma proteolytic inhibitors (see Chapters 11, 13, 19, and 21) serve to limit and control the extent and speed of both blood coagulation and fibrinolytic reactions (see Table 1-1).

## Inhibition of Coagulation

The major inhibitor of the contact system is C1 inhibitor, which accounts for 95% of the plasma inhibitory capacity for factor XIIa and more than 50% toward kallikrein; however, hereditary deficiency of C1 inhibitor results in angioedema rather than bleeding (90). $\alpha_1$-Antitrypsin is the major inhibitor of factor XIa, but a more critical role is its inhibition of neutrophil elastase; inhibitor deficiency results in emphysema due to the unopposed effects of elastase in the lung alveoli (91).

**TABLE 1-1**

PLASMA PROTEASE INHIBITORS OF CONTACT SYSTEM COAGULATION
AND FIBRINOLYSIS

| Inhibitor | Plasma concentration | | Molecular weight (daltons) | Major target enzymes |
|---|---|---|---|---|
| | $\mu$g/mL | nM | | |
| $\alpha_1$-Protease inhibitor | 2,500 | 45,000 | 55,000 | Factor XI, elastase |
| Antithrombin III | 290 | 4,700 | 62,000 | Factor Xa, thrombin |
| $\alpha_2$-Macroglobulin | 2,500 | 3,400 | 725,000 | Kallikrein, plasmin, thrombin |
| C1 inhibitor | 240 | 2,300 | 105,000 | Activated factor XII, kallikrein |
| $\alpha_2$-Antiplasmin | 70 | 1,050 | 67,000 | Plasmin |
| Heparin cofactor II | 40 | 600 | 65,000 | Thrombin |
| Plasminogen activator inhibitor-1 (PAI-1) | 10 | 200 | 50,000 | Tissue plasminogen activator, urokinase |
| Protein C inhibitor (PAI-3) | 5 | 10 | 53,000 | Protein C, kallikrein |
| Tissue factor pathway inhibitor | 0.1 | 0.25 | 40,000 | Factor VIIa (tissue factor), factor Xa (tissue factor) |

ATIII is the major inhibitor of factors IXa, Xa, and thrombin. Although enough ATIII is present to neutralize three times the total amount of thrombin that could form in the blood, a decrease to 40% to 50% predisposes to thrombotic disorders. That congenital ATIII deficiency is associated with a strikingly increased risk of venous thromboembolism indicates that inhibitors play a major regulatory role and that a delicate balance exists between the procoagulant and anticoagulant forces. The catalytic-site serine of thrombin reacts with an arginine in the active center of ATIII to form a covalent inactive complex. The inhibition produced by ATIII is potentiated by heparin, a sulfated polysaccharide with the highest negative charge of any naturally occurring polymer and a close relative to the heparan sulfate that exists on the endothelial surface (Fig. 1-2). Heparin binds to a basic group in ATIII to increase its rate of inactivation of thrombin. Once thrombin is bound to fibrin, it is resistant to ATIII and even more so to ATIII–heparin complex (92,93). Heparin cofactor II is a serpin (serine protease inhibitor) that selectively inactivates thrombin (not factor Xa) in the presence of heparin or dermatan sulfate (94).

Factor Xa also has a specific inhibitor, Z protease inhibitor, the action of which is markedly enhanced by protein Z, a vitamin K–dependent protein, in a phospholipid and $Ca^{2+}$-dependent manner (95).

$\alpha_2$-Macroglobulin is a secondary or backup inhibitor for many plasma coagulant and fibrinolytic enzymes, including kallikrein, thrombin, and plasmin. Because enzymes trapped in the cage structure of this inhibitor exhibit some activity, $\alpha_2$-macroglobulin–enzyme complexes may serve as a repository of enzymatic activity that is protected against other inhibitors. No clinical disorder of severe $\alpha_2$-macroglobulin deficiency has been described. $\alpha_2$-Antiplasmin is the primary inhibitor of plasmin acting to prevent a systemic fibrinogenolytic response to noxious stimuli, limiting the fibrinolytic response to thrombi in the affected region and allowing hemostatic plugs to remain intact until healing is complete (96). In the absence of $\alpha_2$-antiplasmin, hemostatic plugs dissolve before healing has occurred and a hemorrhagic state results (97). A deficiency in PAI-1 also results in a hemorrhagic tendency (98). Protein C inhibitor also is a serpin that can inactivate protein C and thereby function as a potential procoagulant molecule (99).

# FIBRIN FORMATION AND FIBRINOLYSIS

Thrombin acts on multiple substrates, including fibrinogen; factors XIII, V, and VIII; platelet membrane GP V; protein S; and protein C (see Fig. 1-6). In so doing, thrombin occupies a central role in the process of hemostatic plug formation, influencing its form, rate of formation, and limitation. Its potentiating effect on factors VIII and V produces an increase in the tenase and prothrombinase complexes (Fig. 1-4), resulting in a burst of thrombin activity and fibrin strand formation. When thrombin hydrolyzes factor V too slowly because of a point mutation at a cleavage site, the result is the most common genetic cause of thrombosis factor $V_{Leiden}$ (100). Thrombin also helps to recruit platelets into the hemostatic plug, depending on the relative influences of intrinsic or extrinsic clotting systems that are operative. When coagulation starts principally on the altered platelet surface (intrinsic system), thrombin formation is slower than when the extrinsic coagulation system is initiated by exposure to tissue factor, a membrane protein found in macrophages, activated endothelial cells, and tumor cells. In the latter situation, thrombin might have a greater influence on platelet aggregation.

The formation of fibrin strands represents the second phase in hemostasis (the first being the primary platelet aggregate). The precursor of fibrin is fibrinogen, a large glycoprotein of $M_r$ 340,000 present in high concentration in both plasma and platelet granules that interacts with other proteins, including factor XIII, fibronectin, $\alpha_2$-plasmin inhibitor, plasminogen, and plasminogen activator (101). The location and surface concentration of these modifying proteins influence the orderly process of fibrin formation, cross-linking, and fibrin lysis. Thrombin binds to the fibrinogen central domain and liberates fibrinopeptides A and B, resulting in fibrin monomer and polymer formation (102). Progressive lengthening of the polymer chain occurs by a half-overlap, side-to-side approximation of fibrin monomer molecules (see Fig. 1-7), and the two-stranded protofibrils interact laterally to form long, thin fibrin strands or short, broad sheets of fibrin (103,104). Although the degree of lateral strand association probably contributes to the tensile strength of the

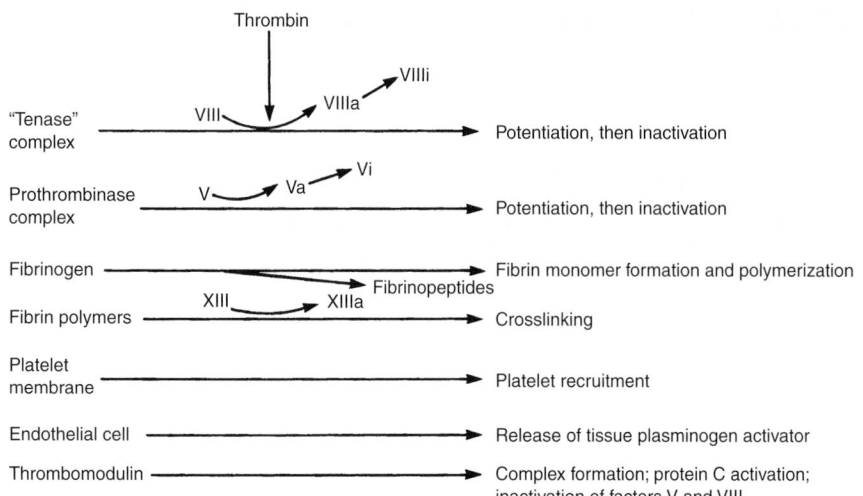

**FIGURE 1-6.** The multitude of actions of thrombin, resulting in procoagulant tendencies, potentiation of ongoing reactions, feedback inhibition, and limitation of clotting.

clot, its resistance to plasmin degradation is influenced mainly by cross-linking mediated by factor XIIIa (105). In addition, factor XIIIa, by linking $\alpha_2$-plasmin inhibitor to fibrin, may protect the clot against fibrinolysis. Factor XIII exists in plasma as a four-chain precursor molecule of $M_r$ 320,000, and after thrombin activation, the enzyme (with calcium) induces cross-linking of the fibrin polymer (106). Covalent isopeptide bonds form between lysine donors and glutamine receptors, with two $\gamma$ chains cross-linked rapidly to form $\gamma$-$\gamma$ dimers; $\alpha$ chains are cross-linked more slowly, each with two other such chains, to form a polymer network (107,108). In mature forms, the fibrin fiber contains approximately 100 protofibrils, with a somewhat random pattern of branching that links the fibers together.

The fibrin mesh binds the platelets together and contributes to their attachment to the vessel wall, mediated by binding to platelet receptor glycoproteins and by interactions with other adhesive proteins such as thrombospondin, fibronectin, and platelet fibrinogen (released from platelet granules but probably otherwise equivalent to plasma fibrinogen) (109). After attachment to platelet-binding sites, these proteins may serve as molecular bridges between plasma proteins and the platelet interior, between platelets and the vessel wall, and between plasma

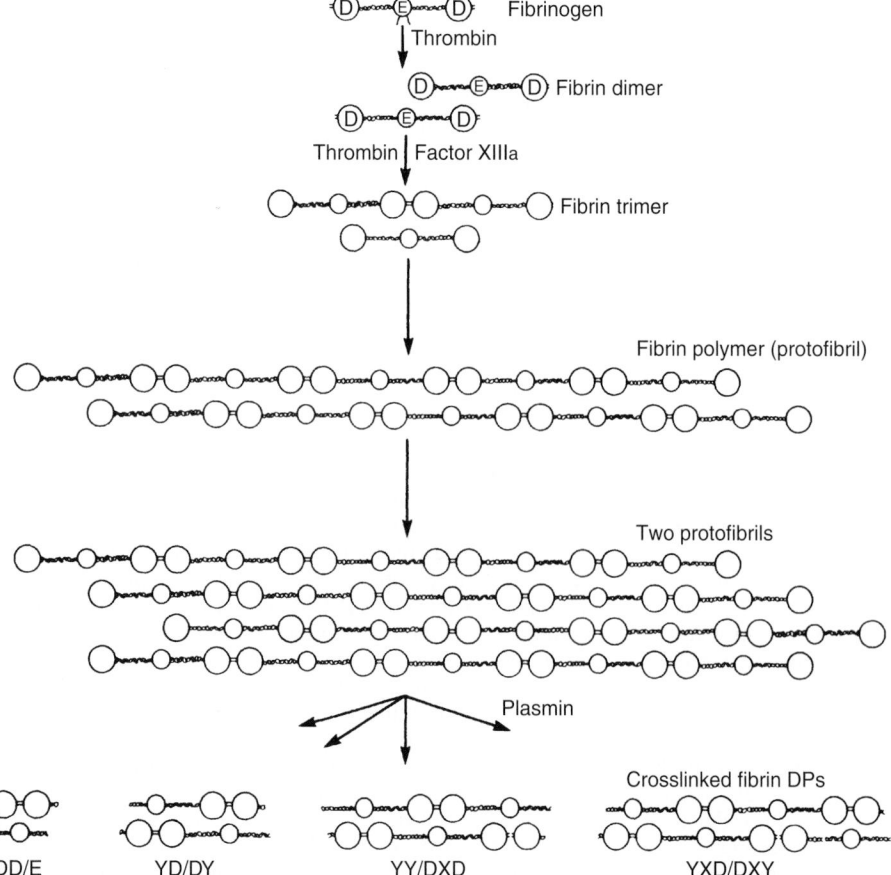

**FIGURE 1-7.** Fibrinogen and thrombin-induced fibrin monomer and polymer formation, factor XIIIa–induced fibrin cross-linking, and plasmin-induced cross-linked fibrin degradation. The *curly lines* represent coiled coils between central and terminal domains, and the *double horizontal lines* represent cross-link sites induced by factor XIIIa between $\gamma$ chains of two contiguous fragment D-domains. The central and two terminal domains of fibrinogen are included in the fragment E- and D-domains, respectively. The fibrinopeptides are indicated as *small vertical lines* connected to the central (E) domain of fibrinogen and are absent from the fibrin monomer molecules after thrombin action. Plasmin action is depicted here as limited to cleavage of the coiled coils between center (E) and terminal (D) domains, to yield the complexes noted at the bottom. These complexes consist of two noncovalently bound fragments (e.g., fragments DD and E in the DD–E complex).

fibrin fibers and the subendothelial matrix. For instance, fibronectin is cross-linked by factor XIIIa to fibrin, and its separate binding site for collagen could serve to bridge fibrin to the vessel wall (110,111). VWF also could serve as a bridge between platelet membrane GP Ib (or IIb/IIIa) and a subendothelial matrix component (112). Additionally, the platelet membrane GP IIb/IIIa could join plasma fibrinogen (or $\alpha$-granule fibrinogen) to intracellular actin, thereby mediating clot retraction and vessel wall constriction (113).

The potential for hemorrhagic or thrombotic disease that results from derangements in fibrinogen structure, concentration, or interaction with thrombin or factor XIII, is great and varied. It could, for instance, manifest as a poorly polymerizing protein, by slow or absent liberation of a fibrinopeptide, or as an inadequately cross-linked fibrin (114). The latter situation similarly could be produced by an absent or faulty factor XIII molecule, which could contribute to both a hemorrhagic condition and inadequate wound healing. The most common acquired disorders of fibrinogen are those of consumption, the disseminated intravascular coagulation (DIC) syndromes, which may reflect excessive or inappropriate coagulation or proteolytic degradation of plasma fibrinogen and can result in a variety of hemorrhagic and thrombotic manifestations, depending to a great extent on the underlying pathologic process (115).

Several distinct mechanisms for controlling and localizing hemostasis exist, including the effects of vascular flow and hemodilution, proteolytic feedback by thrombin, inhibition by plasma proteins and endothelial cell–localized activation of an inhibitory enzyme (protein C), and fibrinolysis. First, the hemostatic plug is exposed to the disruptive pull of blood flow, and small clumps of platelets that are inadequately attached to the main body of platelets or to the vessel wall can be washed free into the blood. Second, thrombin that is present in the hemostatic plug and that has already contributed to its formation by potentiating the activation of factors V and VIII ultimately inactivates these same cofactors (Fig. 1-6) in the presence of thrombomodulin, a membrane protein of endothelial cells. This complex effect of thrombin is an exquisite yet simple example of self-dampening that effectively limits the growth of the fibrin-platelet plug. Third, soluble activated coagulant proteins such as factor Xa or thrombin may diffuse away from the clot, to be bound to inhibitory plasma proteins that destroy or at least markedly decrease their coagulant potential. Principal among these inhibitors is ATIII, which forms a tight complex not only with thrombin but also with other serine protease coagulant proteins and with the fibrinolytic enzyme plasmin. However, although thrombin can be readily inactivated by ATIII in solution, thrombin's catalytic site is inaccessible to the inhibitor while the enzyme is bound to fibrin, and it may retain the ability to cleave fibrinopeptides even in the presence of heparin. Fourth, thrombin that diffuses into the endothelial cell surface may bind to a specific receptor, thrombomodulin, thereby setting into motion another restraint on local coagulation. As previously stated, the thrombin–thrombomodulin complex serves as a receptor for the vitamin K–dependent protein C (Figs. 1-2 and 1-5), which is activated and released from the endothelial cell surface. Activated protein C reacts with factors V and VIII to destroy their coagulant properties, thereby limiting the effect of thrombin. Patients with deficiencies of protein C, protein S (a cofactor of protein C), and ATIII have been described in whom the hemostatic process is not effectively limited and in whom there is a lifelong tendency for pathologic thromboembolic disease.

The last mechanism for limiting clot formation is fibrinolysis, which also constitutes a repair mechanism, along with endothelial cell regrowth and vessel recanalization. Fibrinolysis resembles the cascade mechanism of clotting factor activation in that it involves zymogen-to-enzyme conversions, feedback potentiation and inhibition, and a finely tuned balance with

inhibitors. The inactive precursor protein is plasminogen, present in plasma at twice the molar concentration of $\alpha_2$-plasmin inhibitor. During the initial period of hemostatic plug formation, platelets and endothelial cells release plasminogen activator inhibitors that facilitate fibrin formation (116). However, in response to a poorly understood but precisely timed and orchestrated sequence of stimuli, endothelial cells liberate tissue plasminogen activator (117). Both tissue plasminogen activators and prourokinase have the capacity to convert plasminogen (especially a plasminogen molecule bound to fibrin) to the serine protease-active form, plasmin (118).

As with thrombin feedback that leads to accelerated factor Xa formation, plasmin also exerts positive feedback by cleavage of an activation peptide from plasminogen (connecting Glu-plasminogen to Lys-plasminogen), rendering it more susceptible to surface binding and subsequent activation by plasminogen activators. Perhaps more critical is the markedly heightened reactivity of plasminogen after it is bound to fibrin by lysine-binding sites located on its kringle structures. Lipoprotein A with multiple kringles and histidine-rich glycoprotein also modulates fibrin–plasminogen interactions by inhibiting plasminogen binding to fibrin (119,120).

Although only a small proportion of plasma plasminogen is bound to fibrin during particulate clot formation, this is sufficient to influence subsequent physiologic fibrinolysis (121). The process is a balanced one, however, because $\alpha_2$-plasmin inhibitor also is bound to the fibrin, covalently attached by factor XIIIa action (122). The relative proportions and positions of profibrinolytic plasminogen and plasminogen activator molecules and antifibrinolytic $\alpha_2$-plasmin inhibitor molecules on the fibrin strand influence the timing and degree of clot dissolution. Clinical derangements related to the molecular disorders include a hemorrhagic disorder due to deficient or defective $\alpha_2$-plasmin inhibitor and PAI-1 (123).

Studies have elucidated an important connection between the coagulation and fibrinolytic pathways by virtue of thrombin–thrombomodulin mediation of both protein C and TAFI activation. Whereas activation of protein C leads to inactivation of factors Va and VIIIa and curtailment of further clot formation, TAFI activation promotes stabilization of fibrin and therefore persistence of formed fibrin clots. The mode of action of TAFI is to cleave C-terminal lysine residues from fibrin, thereby preventing plasminogen, plasmin, or tissue-type plasminogen activators (tPA) from binding to fibrin, and secondarily, inhibition of fibrinolysis. Clinical conditions of decreased coagulation, such as classic hemophilia, not only are deficient in thrombin and fibrin formation but, by virtue of low TAFI formation, allow fibrinolysis to proceed relatively unimpeded. The combination of less fibrin and more lysis contributes to the bleeding seen in patients with factor VIII deficiency. Similarly, patients with deficiency of contact-induced coagulation also appear to have decreased TAFI activation, perhaps by inadequate completion of clotting after initial fibrin formation. On the other hand, patients with deficiency of protein C manifest a thrombotic tendency by virtue of a failure of "feedback inhibition" of factors Va and VIIIa by thrombin. The predilection to thrombosis also may have a contribution by excessive TAFI formation due to continuously high production of thrombin. In this case, not only are thrombin and fibrin formed but such fibrin is rendered resistant to plasmin lysis by TAFI.

The enhanced fibrinolysis seen with activation of the plasma kallikrein–kinin system has now been explained. When HK is cleaved by kallikrein, bradykinin is released, which stimulates release of tPA. The cleaved HK (HKa) binds to endothelial urokinase plasminogen [urokinase plasminogen activator receptor (uPAR)] (78). The event places HKa [in complex with prekallikrein (77)] in position to bind to domains 2 and 3 of uPAR in close proximity to prourokinase bound to domain 1 of uPAR, thereby enhancing the possibility of activation of prourokinase to urokinase. PK is converted to kallikrein by the endothelial cell membrane protease prolylcarboxypeptidase (124). This localization allows kallikrein to efficiently activate prourokinase to urokinase (125) without inhibition by plasma serpins such as C1 inhibitor. Direct evidence for this is provided by a study showing that HK–PK interaction is required (79) for plasmin formation by prourokinase on the endothelial cell membrane.

Once plasmin is produced locally on the hemostatic plug, the potential for fibrin degradation exists. By an intricate balance of the simultaneous forces of coagulation and platelet aggregation, inhibition of coagulation, profibrinolytic and antifibrinolytic reactions, and cellular mechanisms for both coagulation and lysis (in leukocytes as well as in platelets and endothelial cells), the clot is gradually reduced. The neutral serine protease (elastase) released from the primary granules of neutrophils also contributes to the local fibrinolytic potential (126). The surface of the clot may be removed first, revealing fresh surfaces that are progressively attacked until the process is completed (127).

During hemostatic plug or thrombus dissolution, solubilized fibrin degradation products are liberated into the circulation, some of which represent unique cross-linked derivatives such as D-dimer that can be distinguished from fibrinogen degradation products (128). The circulating degradation products serve as diagnostic markers of thrombin or factor XIIIa, or both, plus plasmin action that reflects prior clot formation and ongoing fibrinolysis. The surface of a clot and circulating fibrin derivatives may possess a small but significant amount of active thrombin that could serve to propagate the coagulant process elsewhere in the circulation (129). Active plasmin molecules also may be released into the circulation during fibrinolysis, but just as free thrombin is neutralized by ATIII, plasmin is extremely susceptible in solution to inhibitor neutralization by $\alpha_2$-plasmin inhibitor (130). This latter reaction serves to limit fibrinogenolysis to the region of the clot, just as ATIII serves to prevent disseminated coagulation by the spread of a regional hemostatic process.

When hemostatic plug formation is defective (e.g., in hemophilia), naturally occurring fibrinolysis may aggravate bleeding; conversely, the use of epsilon aminocaproic acid aids in hemostasis. This mechanism also may apply in bleeding after dextran infusion, $\alpha_2$-antiplasmin deficiency, and factor XIII deficiency. In the latter case, the lack of cross-links leads to increased susceptibility to plasmin and to failure to cross-link antiplasmin to the fibrin clot, which also may lead to increased fibrinolysis and hemorrhage.

The entire process involving endothelial cells and platelets, clotting factors and adhesive proteins, and inhibitory mechanisms of clotting, fibrinolysis, and platelet aggregation serves to promote the right balance and location of hemostasis and recovery. This highly developed system of checks and balances allows a rapid and efficient hemostatic response to bleeding but avoids a thrombogenic response away from the site of injury or persisting beyond the time of its physiologic need. Derangement of any portion of the intricate process can produce an imbalance, sometimes only slight, with a resultant hemorrhagic or thrombotic clinical disorder. A further complicating feature of this delicate balance is therapeutic intervention, which must be carefully regulated to correct a hemostatic defect without upsetting the balance too far and thereby leading to thrombosis.

# References

1. Cines DB, Tomaski A, Tannenbaum S. Immune endothelial-cell injury in heparin-associated thrombocytopenia. *N Engl J Med* 1987;316(10): 581–589.
2. MacGregor RR, Friedman HM, Macarak EJ, et al. Virus infection of endothelial cells increases granulocyte adherence. *J Clin Invest* 1980;65(6): 1469–1477.
3. Janoff A, Sloan B, Weinbaum G, et al. Experimental emphysema induced with purified human neutrophil elastase: tissue localization of the instilled protease. *Am Rev Respir Dis* 1977;115(3):461–478.
4. LeRoy EC, Ager A, Gordon JL. Effects of neutrophil elastase and other proteases on porcine aortic endothelial prostaglandin I2 production, adenine nucleotide release, and responses to vasoactive agents. *J Clin Invest* 1984;74:1003–1010.
5. Kitchens CS. The anatomical basis of purpura. *Prog Hemost Thromb* 1982; 5:211–210.
6. Hynes RO. Integrins: a family of cell surface receptors. *Cell* 1987;48(4): 549–554.
7. Dustin ML, Garcia Aguilar J, Hibbs ML, et al. Structure and regulation of the leukocyte adhesion receptor LFA-1 and its counterreceptors, ICAM-1 and ICAM-2. *Cold Spring Harb Symp Quant Biol* 1989;54(Pt 2):753–765.
8. Hession C, Osborn L, Goff D, et al. Endothelial leukocyte adhesion molecule 1: direct expression cloning and functional interactions. *Proc Natl Acad Sci U S A* 1990;87(5):1673–1677.
9. Rosenberg RD, Aird WC. Vascular-bed—specific hemostasis and hypercoagulable states. *N Engl J Med* 1999;340(20):1555–1564.
10. Ofosu FA, Buchanan MR, Anvari N, et al. Heparin, heparan sulfate and dermatan sulfate. *Ann N Y Acad Sci* 1989;556:123.
11. Marcus AJ, Weksler BB, Jaffe EA. Enzymatic conversion of prostaglandin endoperoxide H2 and arachidonic acid to prostacyclin by cultured human endothelial cells. *J Biol Chem* 1978;253(20):7138–7141.
12. Moncada S, Vane JR. The role of prostacyclin in vascular tissue. *Fed Proc* 1979;38(1):66–71.
13. Weiss HJ, Turitto VT. Prostacyclin (prostaglandin I2, PGI2) inhibits platelet adhesion and thrombus formation on subendothelium. *Blood* 1979;53(2):244–250.
14. Weksler BB, Marcus AJ, Jaffe EA. Synthesis of prostaglandin I2 (prostacyclin) by cultured human and bovine endothelial cells. *Proc Natl Acad Sci U S A* 1977;74(9):3922–3926.
15. Busch C, Owen WG. Identification *in vitro* of an endothelial cell surface cofactor for antithrombin III. Parallel studies with isolated perfused rat hearts and microcarrier cultures of bovine endothelium. *J Clin Invest* 1982;69(3):726–729.
16. Esmon CT, Owen WG. Identification of an endothelial cell cofactor for thrombin-catalyzed activation of protein C. *Proc Natl Acad Sci U S A* 1981; 78(4):2249–2252.
17. Hatton MW, Berry LR, Regoeczi E. Inhibition of thrombin by antithrombin III in the presence of certain glycosaminoglycans found in the mammalian aorta. *Thromb Res* 1978;13(4):655–670.
18. Lollar P, Owen WG. Clearance of thrombin from circulation in rabbits by high-affinity binding sites on endothelium. Possible role in the inactivation of thrombin by antithrombin III. *J Clin Invest* 1980;66(6):1222–1230.
19. Teien AN, Abildgaard U, Hook M. The anticoagulant effect of heparan sulfate and dermatan sulfate. *Thromb Res* 1976;8(6):859–867.
20. Marcus AJ, Safier LB, Hajjar KA, et al. Inhibition of platelet function by an aspirin-insensitive endothelial cell ADPase. Thromboregulation by endothelial cells. *J Clin Invest* 1991;88(5):1690–1696.
21. Fukudome K, Esmon CT. Identification, cloning, and regulation of a novel endothelial cell protein C/activated protein C receptor. *J Biol Chem* 1994; 269:26486–26491.
22. Esmon NL, Owen WG, Esmon CT. Isolation of a membrane-bound cofactor for thrombin-catalyzed activation of protein C. *J Biol Chem* 1982; 257(2):859–864.
23. Heeb MJ, Espana F, Geiger M, et al. Immunological identity of heparin-dependent plasma and urinary protein C inhibitor and plasminogen activator inhibitor-3. *J Biol Chem* 1987;262(33):15813–15816.
24. Walker FJ. Regulation of activated protein C by protein S. The role of phospholipid in factor Va inactivation. *J Biol Chem* 1981;256(21): 11128–11131.
25. Dahlback B. Inhibition of protein Ca cofactor function of human and bovine protein S by C4b-binding protein. *J Biol Chem* 1986;261(26): 12022–12027.
26. de Fouw NJ, Haverkate F, Bertina RM, et al. The cofactor role of protein S in the acceleration of whole blood clot lysis by activated protein C *in vitro*. *Blood* 1986;67(4):1189–1192.
27. MacIntyre DE, Pearson JD, Gordon JL. Localisation and stimulation of prostacyclin production in vascular cells. *Nature* 1978;271(5645):549–551.
28. Warner TD, Mitchell JA, de Nucci G, et al. Endothelin-1 and endothelin-3 release EDRF from isolated perfused arterial vessels of the rat and rabbit. *J Cardiovasc Pharmacol* 1989;13(Suppl. 5):S85–S88; discussion S102.
29. MacCumber MW, Ross CA, Glaser BM, et al. Endothelin: visualization of mRNAs by in situ hybridization provides evidence for local action. *Proc Natl Acad Sci U S A* 1989;86(18):7285–7289.
30. Wiman B, Chmielewska J, Ranby M. Inactivation of tissue plasminogen activator in plasma. Demonstration of a complex with a new rapid inhibitor. *J Biol Chem* 1984;259(6):3644–3647.
31. Nesheim ME, Wang W, Boffa M, et al. Thrombin, thrombomodulin and TAFI in the molecular link between coagulation and fibrinolysis. *Thromb Haemost* 1997;78:386.
32. George JN. Platelets. *Lancet* 2000;355:1531–1539.
33. De Botton S, Sabri S, Daugas E, et al. Platelet formation is the consequence of caspase activation within megakaryocytes. *Blood* 2002;100(4): 1310–1317.

34. Kaushansky K. Thrombopoietin. *N Engl J Med* 1998;339(11):746–754.
35. Mikkola HK, Klintman J, Yang H, et al. Haematopoietic stem cells retain long-term repopulating activity and multipotency in the absence of stem-cell leukaemia SCL/tal-1 gene. *Nature* 2003;421(6922):547–551.
36. Ruggeri ZM, Dent JA, Saldivar E. Contribution of distinct adhesive interactions to platelet aggregation in flowing blood. *Blood* 1999; 94(1):172–178.
37. Pytela R, Pierschbacher MD, Ginsberg MH, et al. Platelet membrane glycoprotein IIb/IIIa: member of a family of Arg-Gly-Asp—specific adhesion receptors. *Science* 1986;231(4745):1559–1562.
38. Weiss HJ, Turitto VT, Baumgartner HR. Effect of shear rate on platelet interaction with subendothelium in citrated and native blood. I. Shear rate—dependent decrease of adhesion in von Willebrand's disease and the Bernard-Soulier syndrome. *J Lab Clin Med* 1978;92(5):750–764.
39. Kasirer-Friede A, Cozzi MR, Mazzucato M, et al. Signaling through GP Ib-IX-V activates alpha IIb beta 3 independently of other receptors. *Blood* 2004;103(9):3403–3411.
40. Staatz WD, Rajpara SM, Wayner EA, et al. The membrane glycoprotein Ia-IIa (VLA-2) complex mediates the Mg++-dependent adhesion of platelets to collagen. *J Cell Biol* 1989;108(5):1917–1924.
41. Howard JB. Methylamine reaction and denaturation-dependent fragmentation of complement component 3: comparison with alpha-2-macroglobulin. *J Biol Chem* 1980;255:7082–7084.
42. Shattil SJ, Kashiwagi H, Pampori N. Integrin signaling: the platelet paradigm. *Blood* 1998;91(8):2645–2657.
43. Shattil SJ, Hoxie JA, Cunningham M, et al. Changes in the platelet membrane glycoprotein IIb.IIIa complex during platelet activation. *J Biol Chem* 1985;260(20):11107–11114.
44. Hynes RO. Integrins: bidirectional, allosteric signaling machines. *Cell* 2002; 110(6):673–687.
45. Lam SC, Plow EF, D'Souza SE, et al. Isolation and characterization of a platelet membrane protein related to the vitronectin receptor. *J Biol Chem* 1989;264(7):3742–3749.
46. Bennett JS, Vilaire G. Exposure of platelet fibrinogen receptors by ADP and epinephrine. *J Clin Invest* 1979;64(5):1393–1401.
47. Nurden AT, Caen JP. The different glycoprotein abnormalities in thrombasthenic and Bernard- Soulier platelets. *Semin Hematol* 1979;16(3):234–250.
48. Colman RW. Platelet receptors. *Hematol Oncol Clin North Am* 1990;4:27–42.
49. Feinstein MB. The role of calcium in blood platelet function. In: Weiss GB, ed. *Calcium in drug action.* New York: Plenum Publishing, 1978:197–239.
50. Gabbeta J, Yang X, Kowalska MA, et al. Platelet signal transduction defect with Galpha subunit dysfunction and diminished Galphaq in a patient with abnormal platelet responses. *Proc Natl Acad Sci U S A* 1997;94(16):8750–8755.
51. Lee SB, Rao AK, Lee KH, et al. Decreased expression of phospholipase C-beta 2 isozyme in human platelets with impaired function. *Blood* 1996;88(5):1684–1691.
52. Adelstein RS, Conti MA. Phosphorylation of platelet myosin increases actin-activated myosin ATPase activity. *Nature* 1975;256(5518):597–598.
53. Pickett WC, Jesse RL, Cohen P. Initiation of phospholipase A2 activity in human platelets by the calcium ion ionophore A23187. *Biochim Biophys Acta* 1976;486(1):209–213.
54. Colman RW, Hoffman I. Calpains and hemostasis. In: Mellgren R, Murachi T, eds. *Intracellular calcium-dependent proteolysis.* CRC Press, 1990: 211–224.
55. Nishizuka Y. The role of protein kinase C in cell surface signal transduction and tumour promotion. *Nature* 1984;308(5961):693–698.
56. Berridge NJ. Inositol trisphosphate and diacylglycerol as second messengers. *Biochem J* 1984;220:345–340.
57. Rink TJ, Sanchez A, Hallam TJ. Diacylglycerol and phorbol ester stimulate secretion without raising cytoplasmic free calcium in human platelets. *Nature* 1983;305(5932):317–319.
58. Holmsen H. Platelet secretion and energy metabolism. In: Hirsh J, Marder V, Salzman E, eds. *Hemostasis and thrombosis: basic principles and clinical practice.* Philadelphia, PA: JB Lippincott Co, 1993.
59. Mills DC, Figures WR, Scearce LM, et al. Two mechanisms for inhibition of ADP-induced platelet shape change by 5'-p-fluorosulfonylbenzoyladenosine. Conversion to adenosine, and covalent modification at an ADP binding site distinct from that which inhibits adenylate cyclase. *J Biol Chem* 1985; 260(13):8078–8083.
60. Jin J, Kunapuli SP. Coactivation of two different G protein-coupled receptors is essential for ADP-induced platelet aggregation. *Proc Natl Acad Sci U S A* 1998;95(14):8070–8074.
61. Cattaneo M, Zighetti ML, Lombardi R, et al. Molecular bases of defective signal transduction in the platelet P2Y12 receptor of a patient with congenital bleeding. *Proc Natl Acad Sci U S A* 2003;100(4):1978–1983.
62. Kobilka BK, Matsui H, Kobilka TS, et al. Cloning, sequencing, and expression of the gene coding for the human platelet alpha 2-adrenergic receptor. *Science* 1987;238(4827):650–656.
63. Saussy DL Jr, Mais DE, Burch RM, et al. Identification of a putative thromboxane A2/prostaglandin H2 receptor in human platelet membranes. *J Biol Chem* 1986;261(7):3025–3029.
64. Hoyer LW, Wyshock EG, Colman RW. Coagulation cofactors: factors V and VIII. In: Colman RW, Hirsh J, Marder VJ, eds. *Hemostasis and thrombosis: basic principles and clinical practice,* 3rd ed. Philadelphia, PA: JB Lippincott Co, 1994:109–133.
65. Haslam RJ, Davidson MM, Fox JE, et al. Cyclic nucleotides in platelet function. *Thromb Haemost* 1978;40(2):232–240.
66. Colman RW. Platelet cyclic nucleotide phosphodiesterases. In: Rao GHR, ed. *Handbook of platelet physiology and pharmacology.* Boston, MA: Kluwer Academic Publishers, 1999:251–267.
67. Rapoport RM, Murad F. Endothelium-dependent and nitrovasodilator-induced relaxation of vascular smooth muscle: role of cyclic GMP. *J Cyclic Nucleotide Protein Phosphor Res* 1983;9(4-5):281–296.
68. Radomski MW, Palmer RM, Moncada S. An L-arginine/nitric oxide pathway present in human platelets regulates aggregation. *Proc Natl Acad Sci U S A* 1990;87(13):5193–5197.
69. Broze GJ Jr, Warren LA, Novotny WF, et al. The lipoprotein-associated coagulation inhibitor that inhibits the factor VII-tissue factor complex also inhibits factor Xa: insight into its possible mechanism of action. *Blood* 1988; 71(2):335–343.
70. Rao LV, Rapaport SI. Studies of a mechanism inhibiting the initiation of the extrinsic pathway of coagulation. *Blood* 1987;69:645–651.
71. Colucci M, Balconi G, Lorenzet R, et al. Cultured human endothelial cells generate tissue factor in response to endotoxin. *J Clin Invest* 1983;71(6): 1893–1896.
72. Edwards RL, Rickles FR. Macrophage procoagulants. *Prog Hemost Thromb* 1984;7:183–209.
73. Colman RW, Jameson BA, Lin Y, et al. Domain 5 of high molecular weight kininogen (kininostatin) down-regulates endothelial cell proliferation and migration and inhibits angiogenesis. *Blood* 2000;95(2):543–550.
74. Colman RW. Biologic activities of the contact factors *in vivo*: potentiation of hypotension, inflammation, and fibrinolysis, and inhibition of cell adhesion, angiogenesis, and thrombosis. *Thromb Haemost* 1999;82:1568–1577.
75. Colman RW, White JV, Scovell S, et al. Kininogens are antithrombotic proteins *in vivo*. *Arterioscler Thromb Vasc Biol* 1999;19:2245–2250.
76. Bradford HN, DeLa Cadena RA, Kunapuli SP, et al. Human kininogens regulate thrombin binding to platelets through the GP Ib-IX-V complex. *Blood* 1997;90:1508–1515.
77. Mandle R Jr, Colman RW, Kaplan AP, Identification of prekallikrein and high molecular weight kininogen as a complex in human plasma. *Proc Natl Acad Sci U S A* 1976;73:4179–4183.
78. Colman RW, Pixley RA, Najamunnisa S, et al. Binding of high molecular weight kininogen to human endothelial cells is mediated via a site within domains 2+3 of the urokinase receptor. *J Clin Invest* 1997;100:1481–1487.
79. Lin Y, Harris RB, Yan W, et al. High molecular weight kininogen peptides inhibit the formation of kallikrein on endothelial cell surfaces and subsequent urokinase-dependent plasmin formation. *Blood* 1997;90:690–697.
80. Scott CF, Silver LD, Purdon AD, et al. Cleavage of human high molecular weight kininogen by factor XIa *in vitro*. Effect on structure and function. *J Biol Chem* 1985;260:10856–10863.
81. Halbmayer WM, Mannhalter C, Feichtinger C, et al. The prevalence of factor XII deficiency in 103 orally anticoagulated outpatients suffering from recurrent venous and/or arterial thromboembolism. *Thromb Haemost* 1992;68:285–290.
82. Poort SR, Rosendaal FR, Reitsma PH, et al. A common genetic variation in the 3'-untranslated region of the prothrombin gene is associated with elevated plasma prothrombin levels and an increase in venous thrombosis. *Blood* 1996;88:3698–3703.
83. Miletich JP, Jackson CM, Majerus PW. Properties of the factor Xa binding site on human platelets. *J Biol Chem* 1978;253(19):6908–6916.
84. Gordon SG, Cross BA. A factor X-activating cysteine protease from malignant tissue. *J Clin Invest* 1981;67(6):1665–1671.
85. Maier RV, Hahnel GB. Microthrombosis during endotoxemia: potential role of hepatic versus alveolar macrophages. *J Surg Res* 1984;36(4):362–370.
86. Ogawa S, Gerlach H, Esposito C, et al. Hypoxia modulates the barrier and coagulant function of cultured bovine endothelium. Increased monolayer permeability and induction of procoagulant properties. *J Clin Invest* 1990;85(4):1090–1098.
87. Nichols WC, Seligsohn U, Zivelin A, et al. Mutations in the ER-Golgi intermediate compartment protein ERGIC-53 cause combined deficiency of coagulation factors V and VIII. *Cell* 1998;93(1):61–70.
88. Li T, Chang CY, Jin DY, et al. Identification of the gene for vitamin K epoxide reductase. *Nature* 2004;427(6974):541–544.
89. Levy GG, Nichols WC, Lian EC, et al. Mutations in a member of the ADAMTS gene family cause thrombotic thrombocytopenic purpura. *Nature* 2001;413(6855):488–494.
90. Schapira M, Scott CF, Colman RW. Protection of human plasma kallikrein from inactivation by C1 inhibitor and other protease inhibitors. The role of high molecular weight kininogen. *Biochemistry* 1981;20:2738–2743.
91. Scott CF, Schapira M, James HL, et al. Inactivation of factor XIa by plasma protease inhibitors: predominant role of alpha 1-protease inhibitor and protective effect of high molecular weight kininogen. *J Clin Invest* 1982; 69:844–852.
92. Hogg PJ, Jackson CM. Fibrin monomer protects thrombin from inactivation by heparin-antithrombin III: implications for heparin efficacy. *Proc Natl Acad Sci U S A* 1989;86:3619–3623.
93. Weitz JI, Hudoba M, Massel D, et al. Clot-bound thrombin is protected from inhibition by heparin-antithrombin III but is susceptible to inactivation by antithrombin III-independent inhibitors. *J Clin Invest* 1990;86:385–391.
94. Tollefsen DM, Majerus DW, Blank MK. Heparin cofactor II. Purification and properties of a heparin-dependent inhibitor of thrombin in human plasma. *J Biol Chem* 1982;257(5):2162–2169.
95. Broze GJ. Jr Protein Z-dependent regulation of coagulation. *Thromb Haemost* 2001;86(1):8–13.

96. Moroi M, Aoki N. Isolation and characterization of alpha2-plasmin inhibitor from human plasma. A novel proteinase inhibitor which inhibits activator-induced clot lysis. *J Biol Chem* 1976;251(19):5956–5965.

97. Koie K, Kamiya T, Ogata K, et al. Alpha2-plasmin-inhibitor deficiency (Miyasato disease). *Lancet* 1978;2(8104-5):1334–1336.

98. Schleef RR, Higgins DL, Pillemer E, et al. Bleeding diathesis due to decreased functional activity of type 1 plasminogen activator inhibitor. *J Clin Invest* 1989;83(5):1747–1752.

99. Suzuki K, Deyashiki Y, Nishioka J, et al. Characterization of a cDNA for human protein C inhibitor. A new member of the plasma serine protease inhibitor superfamily. *J Biol Chem* 1987;262(2):611–616.

100. Bertina RM, Koeleman BP, Koster T, et al. Mutation in blood coagulation factor V associated with resistance to activated protein C. *Nature* 1994;369:64–67.

101. Doolittle RF, Goldbaum DM, Doolittle LR. Designation of sequences involved in the "coiled-coil" interdomainal connections in fibrinogen: constructions of an atomic scale model. *J Mol Biol* 1978;120:311–325.

102. Blomback B, Blomback M. The molecular structure of fibrinogen. *Ann N Y Acad Sci* 1972;202:77–97.

103. Ferry JD. The mechanism of polymerization of fibrin. *Proc Natl Acad Sci U S A* 1952;38:566.

104. Hermans J, McDonagh J. Fibrin: structure and interactions. *Semin Thromb Hemost* 1982;8(1):11–24.

105. Robbins KC. A study on the conversion of fibrinogen to fibrin. *Am J Physiol* 1944;142:581–580.

106. Schwartz ML, Pizzo SV, Hill RL, et al. Human factor XIII from plasma and platelets. Molecular weights, subunit structures, proteolytic activation, and cross-linking of fibrinogen and fibrin. *J Biol Chem* 1973;248:1395–1407.

107. Folk JE, Finlayson JS. The epsilon-(gamma-glutamyl)lysine crosslink and the catalytic role of transglutaminases. *Adv Protein Chem* 1977;31:1–133.

108. McKee PA, Mattock P, Hill RL. Subunit structure of human fibrinogen, soluble fibrin, and cross-linked insoluble fibrin. *Proc Natl Acad Sci U S A* 1970;66(3):738–744.

109. Kaplan KL, Broekman MJ, Chernoff A, et al. Platelet alpha-granule proteins: studies on release and subcellular localization. *Blood* 1979;53(4):604–618.

110. Mosher DF. Action of fibrin-stabilizing factor on cold-insoluble globulin and alpha2-macroglobulin in clotting plasma. *J Biol Chem* 1976;251(6):1639–1645.

111. Ruoslahti E, Pekkala A, Engvall E. Effect of dextran sulfate on fibronectin-collagen interaction. *FEBS Lett* 1979;107(1):51–54.

112. Wagner DD, Urban-Pickering M, Marder VJ. Von Willebrand protein binds to extracellular matrices independently of collagen. *Proc Natl Acad Sci U S A* 1984;81(2):471–475.

113. Nachmias V, Sullender J, Asch A. Shape and cytoplasmic filaments in control and lidocaine-treated human platelets. *Blood* 1977;50(1):39–53.

114. McDonagh J, Carrell N. Dysfibrinogens and other disorders of fibrinogen structure and function. In: Hirsh J, Marder V, Salzman E, eds. *Hemostasis and thrombosis: basic principles and clinical practice*, 3rd ed. Philadelphia, PA: JB Lippincott Co, 1993.

115. Marder V, Colman RW, Francis CW. Consumptive thrombohemorrhagic disorders. In: Hirsh J, Marder V, Salzman E, eds. *Hemostasis and thrombosis: basic principles and clinical practice*, 3rd ed. Philadelphia, PA: JB Lippincott Co, 1993.

116. Plow EF, Collen D. The presence and release of alpha 2-antiplasmin from human platelets. *Blood* 1981;58(6):1069–1074.

117. Levin EG, Marzec U, Anderson J, et al. Thrombin stimulates tissue plasminogen activator release from cultured human endothelial cells. *J Clin Invest* 1984;74:1988–1995.

118. Lijnen HR, Collen D. Interaction of plasminogen activators and inhibitors with plasminogen and fibrin. *Semin Thromb Hemost* 1982;8(1):2–10.

119. Lijnen HR, Hoylaerts M, Collen D. Isolation and characterization of a human plasma protein with affinity for the lysine binding sites in plasminogen. Role in the regulation of fibrinolysis and identification as histidine-rich glycoprotein. *J Biol Chem* 1980;255(21):10214–10222.

120. Mao SJ, Tucci MA. Lipoprotein(a) enhances plasma clot lysis *in vitro*. *FEBS Lett* 1990;267:131–134.

121. Alkjaersig N, Fletcher NP, Sherry S. The mechanism of clot dissolution by plasmin. *J Clin Invest* 1959;38:1086–1080.

122. Sakata Y, Aoki N. Cross-linking of alpha 2-plasmin inhibitor to fibrin by fibrin-stabilizing factor. *J Clin Invest* 1980;65(2):290–297.

123. Aoki N, Moroi M, Sakata Y, et al. Abnormal plasminogen. A hereditary molecular abnormality found in a patient with recurrent thrombosis. *J Clin Invest* 1978;61(5):1186–1195.

124. Shariat-Madar Z, Mahdi F, Schmaier AH. Identification and characterization of prolylcarboxypeptidase as an endothelial cell prekallikrein activator. *J Biol Chem* 2002;277(20):17962–17969.

125. Ichinose A, Fujikawa K, Suyama T. The activation of prourokinase by plasma kallikrein and its inactivation by thrombin. *J Biol Chem* 1986;261:3486–3489.

126. Plow EF. Leukocyte elastase release during blood coagulation. A potential mechanism for activation of the alternative fibrinolytic pathway. *J Clin Invest* 1982;69(3):564–572.

127. Francis CW, Marder VJ, Martin SE. Plasmic degradation of crosslinked fibrin. I. Structural analysis of the particulate clot and identification of new macromolecular-soluble complexes. *Blood* 1980;56(3):456–464.

128. Kopec M, Teisseyre E, Dudek-Wojciechowska G. Studies on "Double D" fragment from stabilized bovine fibrin. *Thromb Res* 1973;2:283–280.

129. Francis CW, Markham RE, Barlow GH, et al. Thrombin activity of fibrin thrombi and soluble plasmic derivatives. *J Lab Clin Med* 1983;102(2):220–230.

130. Collen D. On the regulation and control of fibrinolysis. Edward Kowalski Memorial Lecture. *Thromb Haemost* 1980;43(2):77–89.

# CHAPTER 2 ■ OVERVIEW OF COAGULATION, FIBRINOLYSIS, AND THEIR REGULATION

ROBERT W. COLMAN, VICTOR J. MARDER, AND ALEXANDER W. CLOWES

Blood coagulation is a series of steps in which plasma zymogens of serine proteases are transformed into active enzymes. These enzymes act to convert their procofactor substrates to cofactors, which assemble these proteases on cell surfaces. This assembly increases the local concentration of the reactants. The sequential nature of the reactions, in which the product serves as the next enzyme, amplifies the overall velocity of the reaction. The final event is the formation of thrombin, which converts a soluble protein, fibrinogen, into an insoluble polymer, fibrin, that forms the clot. Fibrinolysis is an analogous series of transformations of zymogens to proteolytic enzymes, which, in the presence of cofactors on cell surfaces, convert plasminogen to plasmin, which can hydrolyze the fibrin clot, thereby solubilizing it. At each step, a series of protease inhibitors limits the reaction. The occurrence of these reactions at cell surfaces allows regulation at the level of binding to receptors and the participation of the phospholipids of the cell membrane.

It should be noted that the completion of the human genome project in 2003 has stimulated the addition of a new Chapter 4. An example of the importance of genomewide scans is the discovery of three new hemostasis-related genes. Combined factor VIII and V deficiency is due to mutations in an ER–Gogli protein coded for by the *LMANI* gene, also known as *ERGIC-53* (1). Major breakthroughs are identification of the gene responsible for thrombotic thrombocytopenia purpura, *ADAMTS 13* (2), and a gene related to warfarin resistance and action, vitamin K epoxide reductase (*VKORC*) (3).

Normally, no coagulation takes place in the bloodstream because of the properties of the endothelium and the inactive form of the proteins, which are either zymogens or procofactors. The initiation of the system depends on the exposure of the blood to components that are not present physiologically. These coagulation activators are revealed as a result of either mechanical injury, as is the case after a vessel is severed or after the endothelium is denuded during coronary angioplasty, or biochemical alteration, such as the release of cytokines, which in turn stimulate biosynthesis of induced receptors. Each of these events occurs in the initiation of blood coagulation and involves a single critical component, tissue factor (TF) (see Fig. 2-1). TF is a type I integral membrane receptor for coagulation factor VII (4). The extracellular portion is required for procoagulant activity, but the cytoplasmic domain is involved in signaling, important in angiogenesis and cell migration. TF is expressed constitutively on most cells (other than hepatocytes) that do not normally contact the blood, such as fibroblasts. After vascular injury, the blood contacts constitutive TF. Alternatively, endotoxin can stimulate monocytes and endothelial cells to biosynthesize the cytokines, tumor necrosis factor, and interleukin-1, which, in turn, induce the biosynthesis of TF (5,6). Factor VII binds to constitutive or

induced TF on fibroblasts and monocytes, respectively. In all healthy individuals, trace levels of factor VIIa are present in the circulation, accounting for approximately 1% of the total factor VII concentration (7). Therefore, exposure of TF to plasma results in binding of both factor VII and factor VIIa; only the TF–VIIa complexes are enzymatically active. Factor VII bound to TF is then activated by TF–VIIa, termed *autoactivation* (8). This reaction may be insufficient to ignite the full capacity of the coagulation cascade. Other coagulation factor proteases, such as factor XIIa (9) and factor Xa (10), are much more effective.

The TF–VIIa complex has two substrates, factor IX (intrinsic pathway) and factor X (extrinsic pathway). Cleavage of either protein results in a cell-bound serine protease, factor IXa or factor Xa. However, the reaction is tightly regulated by tissue factor pathway inhibitor (TFPI) (11), a protein produced by the endothelial cell and consisting of three Kunitz domains (12). The first domain binds to and inhibits TF–VIIa, and the second, factor Xa. The direct activation of factor Xa is thereby rapidly downregulated. Ligation of factor Xa is required for TFPI to inhibit TF–VIIa (11).

In the presence of TFPI, the major pathway for the propagation of coagulation then becomes the intrinsic pathway, which is activated by factor IXa. The required cofactor for factor IXa to activate factor X is factor VIIIa. Factor VIII circulates in plasma bound to von Willebrand factor, which protects this vulnerable protein from unwanted proteolytic attack. For the procofactor, factor VIII, to be converted to the active cofactor, factor VIIIa, by thrombin or factor Xa, it must dissociate from von Willebrand factor. The factor IXa–VIIIa complex is the most important activator of factor X, which helps explain the clinical severity of the deficiency of either factor IX or factor VIII and their identical clinical presentation in hemophilias B and A, respectively.

Once formed, factor Xa can catalyze the conversion of prothrombin to thrombin, but the reaction is slow. The presence of the active cofactor, factor Va, bound to a cell surface (monocyte or platelet), results in a 300,000-fold acceleration (13). The procofactor, factor V, is converted to factor Va either by factor Xa or by thrombin (14). Factor Va functions as a cofactor by binding to a cell surface and in conjunction with phospholipid binding of factor Xa to form prothrombinase. Prothrombin binds with relatively low affinity to the cell surface, primarily by the γ-carboxyglutamic acid residues. This posttranslational modification is characteristic of all proteins that require vitamin K and is catalyzed by microsomal vitamin K–dependent carboxylase. These γ-carboxyglutamic acid residues are bridged by calcium to anionic phospholipid exposed on the surface of activated cells. Prothrombinase then cleaves prothrombin into fragment 1.2 (widely used as a marker of thrombin generation) and thrombin.

Coagulation

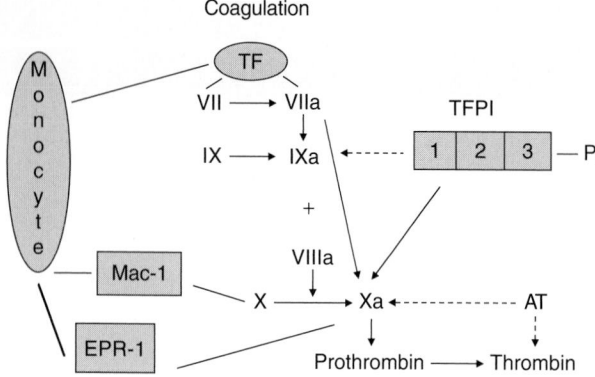

**FIGURE 2-1.** Coagulation. *Lines* indicate binding; *filled arrows*, activation of zymogens to active enzymes; *dashed arrows*, inhibition of active enzymes. a, arterial enzyme; AT, antithrombin; EPR-1, monocyte effector protease receptor-1; Mac-1, monocyte integrin $\alpha_M\beta_2$; PL, phospholipid; TF, tissue factor; TFPI, tissue factor pathway inhibitor.

The older concept of the intrinsic system was that of coagulation initiated by components contained entirely in the vascular system so that the initiation would be independent of TF. One protein, factor XIa, is capable of activating factor IX and, therefore, provides a potential mechanism for initiating the intrinsic pathway. Factor XI deficiency, even when biochemically severe (<1% of normal), is clinically mild. The major manifestation is posttraumatic bleeding (15), and only one half of the patients have some excessive bleeding. Factor XII can be activated by three plasma proteases—factor XIIa, factor XIa, and thrombin. Factor XIIa can activate factor XI in the presence of the contact system cofactor, high-molecular-weight kininogen (HK), and in the presence of a foreign surface (16), such as in cardiopulmonary bypass or hemodialysis. However, deficiency of factor XII, HK, or prekallikrein (which plays a role in activation of factor XII) does not lead to a hemorrhagic state. On the contrary, this system inhibits coagulation by blocking thrombin binding to platelets and is also profibrinolytic (17), which is discussed when fibrinolysis is considered (see Chapter 6). Factor XI also can autoactivate in the presence of a negatively charged surface such as dextran sulfate, but this is not a physiologic surface. In a purified system, factor XI is activated by thrombin (18), but HK and fibrinogen (19) both markedly decrease the rate of conversion in a plasma environment. However, both HK and prothrombin can serve as cofactors for the binding of factor XI to the surface of the activated platelet with a 5,000-fold increase in the rate of factor XI activation by thrombin (20). Therefore, positive feedback by thrombin is characteristic of the coagulation system because thrombin acts to convert both procofactors V and VIII to the active cofactors Va and VIIIa, which assemble the prothrombinase and tenase complexes, respectively.

The cellular localization of coagulation complexes is important. Activated monocytes localize the extrinsic system because they not only express TF after they are activated but also have receptors for factor X and the integrin Mac-1 ($\alpha_M\beta_2$). After factor X is converted to factor Xa, it binds to a receptor on monocytes or to factor Va, which itself binds to cells (21). Platelets bind factor XI and XIa to separate binding sites (15). Platelets secrete factor Va, which serves as a locus for binding factor Xa. Once prothrombin is cleaved, thrombin binds to protease-activated receptors (PAR) 1 (22) and 4 on platelets.

The principal substrate of thrombin is fibrinogen, which is a dimer composed of two identical heterotrimers. The A$\alpha$, B$\beta$, and $\gamma$ polypeptides, each under control of a separate gene, are arranged in a trinodular array linked by coiled-coil segments (23). The central domain consisting of N-terminals of each

chain bound in a disulfide knot is the binding site for thrombin, which cleaves off 2 mol of each of the acidic fibrinopeptides A and B, resulting in fibrin monomer formation (24). These monomers then spontaneously polymerize by side-to-side approximation to form the protofibrin and, finally, the fibrin array. The final step is cross-linking of fibrin to form $\gamma$-dimers and $\alpha$-polymers catalyzed by the transamidase, factor XIIIa (25). Factor XIIIa is derived from the precursor factor XIII by limited proteolysis by thrombin in the presence of $Ca^{2+}$ (26). The covalent cross-linking isopeptide mechanically stabilizes the molecule.

Regulation of blood coagulation is achieved by several mechanisms, including dilution and the rate of blood flow, and by the action of proteolytic inhibitors such as TFPI and antithrombin. Antithrombin is a serpin (SERine Protease INhibitor) that primarily inhibits thrombin, factor Xa, and, to a lesser extent, factor IXa. However, thrombin binding to the fibrin clot is relatively protected from antithrombin (27). The rate of the inactivation of factor Xa increases by more than 300-fold associated with a pentasaccharide derived from heparin (28). Serine proteases, such as kallikrein, factor XIIa, and factor IXa, also are inhibited, but not as potently as factor Xa or thrombin (29). Factor X is also inhibited by a 72-kDa serpin, Z protease inhibitor (ZPI), the activity of which is enhanced 1,000-fold by a vitamin K–dependent protein, protein Z, in the presence of phospholipid and $Ca^{2+}$ (30). Another major mechanism is a negative feedback initiated by thrombin binding to thrombomodulin (31) on the endothelial surface. Thrombin changes its substrate specificity and loses its ability to cleave fibrinogen and activate factor V and VIII to the active cofactors, factors Va and VIIa. Instead, it cleaves and activates protein C, which, in the presence of protein S, can inactivate factors Va and VIIIa (31). Additionally, an endothelial cell protein C receptor has been identified and characterized (32) and shown to be expressed on the endothelial cell surface. In the presence of an endothelial cell protein C receptor, the activation of protein C is enhanced 10- to 20-fold, whereas the activity of activated protein C to hydrolyze factor V is inhibited by occupying the exosite (33).

Fibrinolysis is the ultimate mechanism that counteracts the consequences of the coagulation process. The dissolution or solubilization of the fibrin clot at the correct time is crucial for the orderly process of wound healing. Fibrinolysis is required for angiogenesis as well as vessel recanalization after clot formation. Similar to coagulation, there are two activators with different localization and different cofactors (see Fig. 2-2). Endothelial cells liberate tissue-type plasminogen activator (tPA) after stimulation by thrombin (34), which binds tightly to fibrin (35); fibrin serves as a cofactor enabling efficient activation of plasminogen to plasmin by tPA. Plasminogen also binds to fibrin (35). Therefore, the substrate, fibrin, localizes both the activator and the zymogen. Plasmin cleaves fibrinogen or fibrin, or both, to produce degradation products, which inhibit thrombin action and fibrin polymerization, serving as natural anticoagulants, especially in disseminated intravascular coagulation. Plasmin exerts a positive feedback by cleavage of an N-terminal peptide from the native glu-plasminogen, converting it to lys-plasminogen, which undergoes a large conformational change (36), rendering it much more susceptible to activation.

A second plasminogen activator, urokinase plasminogen activator (uPA), is synthesized by endothelial cells, but on endothelial perturbation, prourokinase is expressed on the surface by binding to urokinase plasminogen activator receptor (uPAR), a glycerol-phosphate inositol-anchored receptor. Prourokinase can autoactivate, a process enhanced by binding to uPAR (37). Plasmin also can catalyze a positive feedback by converting prourokinase to urokinase. A potent initiating mechanism involving the contact system has been described that may account for the enhanced fibrinolysis that occurs with

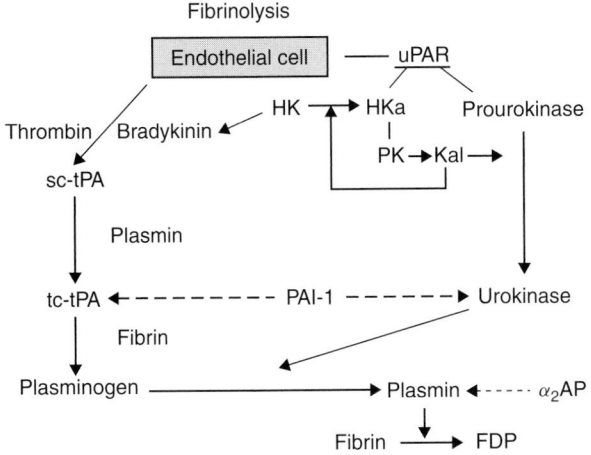

**FIGURE 2-2.** Fibrinolysis. *Lines* indicate binding; *thin arrows,* transformation or stimulation; *filled arrows,* transformation of zymogens to active enzymes; *dashed arrows,* inhibition of active enzymes. $\alpha_2$AP, $\alpha_2$ antiplasmin; FDP, fibrinogen deposition products; HK, high-molecular-weight kininogen; HKa, kinin-free kininogen; Kal, kallikrein; PAI-1, plasminogen activator inhibitor 1; PK, prekallikrein; sc-tPA, single-chain tissue-type plasminogen activator; tc-tPA, two-chain tissue-type plasminogen activator; uPAR, urokinase plasminogen activator receptor.

activation of this system (see Fig. 2-3). HK, after being cleaved, liberates bradykinin, which enhances release of tPA. The kinin-free kininogen (HKa) binds to endothelial uPAR (38) at domains 2 and/or 3 in close proximity to prourokinase. HK circulates in complex with prekallikrein (16), which is converted to kallikrein by an endothelial cell membrane–associated serine protease, prolylcarboxypeptidase (39). Kallikrein is known to activate prourokinase to urokinase (40). That this mechanism contributes to the initiation of the uPA pathway is supported by a study demonstrating that peptides that inhibit the HK–prekallikrein (or kallikrein) interaction prevent the formation of plasmin on the endothelial cell surface (41).

This system also is subject to multiple regulatory mechanisms. Lipoprotein A contains multiple kringles (42) that can compete with plasminogen. $\alpha_2$-Antiplasmin, a serpin, inhibits plasmin directly and with a rapid rate of association (43). Plasminogen activator inhibitor-1 is another serpin that inhibits both uPA and tPA. Thrombin-activated fibrinolytic inhibitor (TAFI) is a procarboxypeptidase that is activated by thrombin–thrombomodulin

complex (44). The active carboxypeptidase impairs fibrinolysis by removing lysine residues on fibrin critical to plasminogen binding (45). TAFI also inactivates two vasoactive peptides, C5a and bradykinin, and thereby downregulates vascular inflammation (46). Factor XIIIa–induced cross-linking of the fibrin matrix renders it much more resistant to plasmin action.

Coagulation and fibrinolysis are responses to vessel or cell injury. The reactions are mostly confined to the cell membranes, which increases their effective concentration by proximity on approximated receptors and by limiting their diffusion (47). The protease inhibitors exist in the plasma to prevent their propagation into the systemic circulation, and it is this process that may malfunction in thrombosis and disseminated intravascular coagulation.

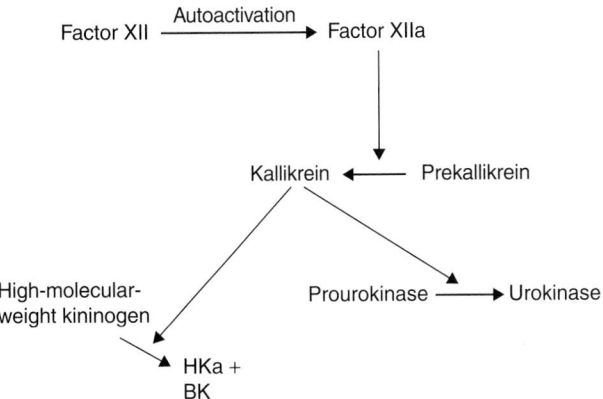

**FIGURE 2-3.** Contact system and fibrinolysis. *Horizontal arrows* indicate transformation from zymogen to active enzyme. *Vertical or diagonal arrows* indicate action of enzyme on substrate. HKa, kinin-free kininogen; BK, bradykinin.

## References

1. Nichols WC, Seligsohn U, Zivelin A, et al. Mutations in the ER-Golgi intermediate compartment protein ERGIC-53 cause combined deficiency of coagulation factors V and VIII. *Cell* 1998;93(1):61–70.
2. Levy GG, Nichols WC, Lian EC, et al. Mutations in a member of the *ADAMTS* gene family cause thrombotic thrombocytopenic purpura. *Nature* 2001;413(6855):488–494.
3. Li T, Chang CY, Jin DY, et al. Identification of the gene for vitamin K epoxide reductase. *Nature* 2004;427(6974):541–544.
4. Rao LV, Williams T, Rapaport SI. Studies of the activation of factor VII bound to tissue factor. *Blood* 1996;87:3738–3748.
5. Camerer E, Kolsto AB, Prydz H. Cell biology of tissue factor, the principal initiator of blood coagulation. *Thromb Res* 1996;81(1):1–41.
6. Geczy CL. Cellular mechanisms for the activation of blood coagulation. *Int Rev Cytol* 1994;152:49–108.
7. Morrissey JH, Macik BG, Neuenschwander PF, et al. Quantitation of activated factor VII levels in plasma using a tissue factor mutant selectively deficient in promoting factor VII activation. *Blood* 1993;81:734–744.
8. Neuenschwander PF, Fiore MM, Morrissey JH. Factor VII autoactivation proceeds via interaction of distinct protease-cofactor and zymogen-cofactor complexes. Implications of a two-dimensional enzyme kinetic mechanism. *J Biol Chem* 1993;268(29):21489–21492.
9. Radcliffe R, Bagdasarian A, Colman R, et al. Activation of bovine factor VII by Hageman factor fragments. *Blood* 1977;50:611–617.
10. Butenas S, Mann KG. Kinetics of human factor VII activation. *Biochemistry* 1996;35:1904–1910.
11. Rao LV, Rapaport SI. Studies of a mechanism inhibiting the initiation of the extrinsic pathway of coagulation. *Blood* 1987;69:645–651.
12. Broze GJ Jr, Warren LA, Novotny WF, et al. The lipoprotein-associated coagulation inhibitor that inhibits the factor VII-tissue factor complex also inhibits factor Xa: insight into its possible mechanism of action. *Blood* 1988; 71(2):335–343.
13. Nesheim ME, Taswell JB, Mann KG. The contribution of bovine Factor V and Factor Va to the activity of prothrombinase. *J Biol Chem* 1979;254: 10952–10962.
14. Colman RW. The effect of proteolytic enzymes on bovine factor V. I. Kinetics of activation and inactivation by bovine thrombin. *Biochemistry* 1969;8: 1438–1445.
15. Walsh PN. Factor XI: a renaissance. [Review] [131 refs]. *Semin Hematol* 1992;29:189–201.
16. Mandle R Jr, Colman RW, Kaplan AP. Identification of prekallikrein and high molecular weight kininogen as a complex in human plasma. *Proc Natl Acad Sci U S A* 1976;73:4179–4183.
17. Colman RW, Schmaier AH. Contact system: a vascular biology modulator with anticoagulant, profibrinolytic, antiadhesive, and proinflammatory attributes. *Blood* 1997;90:3819–3843.
18. Naito K, Fujikawa K. Activation of human blood coagulation factor XI independent of factor XII: factor XI is activated by thrombin and factor XIa in the presence of negatively charged surfaces. *J Biol Chem* 1991;266: 7353–7358.
19. Scott CF, Colman RW. Fibrinogen blocks the autoactivation and thrombin-mediated activation of factor XI on dextran sulfate. *Proc Natl Acad Sci U S A* 1992;89:11189–11193.
20. Baglia FA, Walsh PN. Prothrombin is a cofactor for the binding of factor XI to the platelet surface and for platelet-mediated factor XI activation by thrombin. *Biochemistry* 1998;37(8):2271–2281.
21. Miletich JP, Jackson CM, Majerus PW. Properties of the factor Xa binding site on human platelets. *J Biol Chem* 1978;253:6908–6916.
22. Coughlin SR, Vu TK, Hung DT, et al. Characterization of a functional thrombin receptor. Issues and opportunities. [Review]. *J Clin Invest* 1992; 89:351–355.
23. Doolittle RF, Goldbaum DM, Doolittle LR. Designation of sequences involved in the "coiled-coil" interdomainal connections in fibrinogen: constructions of an atomic scale model. *J Mol Biol* 1978;120:311–325.

24. Blomback B, Blomback M. The molecular structure of fibrinogen. *Ann N Y Acad Sci* 1972;202:77–97.
25. Schwartz ML, Pizzo SV, Hill RL, et al. Human factor XIII from plasma and platelets. Molecular weights, subunit structures, proteolytic activation, and cross-linking of fibrinogen and fibrin. *J Biol Chem* 1973;248:1395–1407.
26. Folk JE, Finlayson JS. The epsilon-(gamma-glutamyl)lysine crosslink and the catalytic role of transglutaminases. *Adv Protein Chem* 1977;31:1–133.
27. Weitz JI, Hudoba M, Massel D, et al. Clot-bound thrombin is protected from inhibition by heparin-antithrombin III but is susceptible to inactivation by antithrombin III-independent inhibitors. *J Clin Invest* 1990;86:385–391.
28. Choay J, Petitou M, Lormeau JC, et al. Structure-activity relationship in heparin: a synthetic pentasaccharide with high affinity for antithrombin III and eliciting high anti-factor Xa activity. *Biochem Biophys Res Commun* 1983;116(2):492–499.
29. Bauer KA, Rosenberg RD. Role of antithrombin III as a regulator of *in vivo* coagulation. [Review] [51 refs]. *Semin Hematol* 1991;28:10–18.
30. Broze GJ Jr. Protein Z-dependent regulation of coagulation. *Thromb Haemost* 2001;86(1):8–13.
31. Esmon CT. The roles of protein C and thrombomodulin in the regulation of blood coagulation. *J Biol Chem* 1994;264:4723.
32. Fukudome K, Esmon CT. Identification, cloning, and regulation of a novel endothelial cell protein C/activated protein C receptor. *J Biol Chem* 1994;269:26486–26491.
33. Fukudome K, Kurosawa S, Stearns-Kurosawa DJ, et al. The endothelial cell protein C receptor. Cell surface expression and direct ligand binding by the soluble receptor. *J Biol Chem* 1996;271:17491–17498.
34. Levin EG, Marzec U, Anderson J, et al. Thrombin stimulates tissue plasminogen activator release from cultured human endothelial cells. *J Clin Invest* 1984;74:1988–1995.
35. Lijnen HR, Collen D. Interaction of plasminogen activators and inhibitors with plasminogen and fibrin. *Semin Thromb Hemost* 1980;255:10214–10210.
36. Mangel WF, Lin B, Ramakrishnan V. Characterization of an extremely large ligand-induced conformational change in plasminogen. *Science* 1990;248:69.
37. Higazi A, Cohen RL, Henkin J, et al. Enhancement of the enzymatic activity of single-chain urokinase plasminogen activator by soluble urokinase receptor. *J Biol Chem* 1995;21:17375–17380.
38. Colman RW, Pixley RA, Najamunnisa S, et al. Binding of high molecular weight kininogen to human endothelial cells is mediated via a site within domains 2+3 of the urokinase receptor. *J Clin Invest* 1997;100:1481–1487.
39. Shariat-Madar Z, Mahdi F, Schmaier AH. Identification and characterization of prolylcarboxypeptidase as an endothelial cell prekallikrein activator. *J Biol Chem* 2002;277(20):17962–17969.
40. Ichinose A, Fujikawa K, Suyama T. The activation of prourokinase by plasma kallikrein and its inactivation by thrombin. *J Biol Chem* 1986;261:3486–3489.
41. Lin Y, Harris RB, Yan W, et al. High molecular weight kininogen peptides inhibit the formation of kallikrein on endothelial cell surfaces and subsequent urokinase-dependent plasmin formation. *Blood* 1997;90:690–697.
42. Mao SJ, Tucci MA. Lipoprotein(a) enhances plasma clot lysis *in vitro*. *FEBS Lett* 1990;267:131–134.
43. Moroi M, Aoki N. Isolation and characterization of alpha2-plasmin inhibitor from human plasma. A novel proteinase inhibitor which inhibits activator-induced clot lysis. *J Biol Chem* 1976;251:5956–5965.
44. Bajzar L, Morser J, Nesheim M. TAFI, or plasma procarboxypeptidase B, couples the coagulation and fibrinolytic cascades through the thrombin-thrombomodulin complex. *J Biol Chem* 1996;271(28):16603–16608.
45. Nesheim ME, Wang W, Boffa M, et al. Thrombin, thrombomodulin and TAFI in the molecular link between coagulation and fibrinolysis. *Thromb Haemost* 1997;78:386.
46. Myles T, Nishimura T, Yun TH, et al. Thrombin activatable fibrinolysis inhibitor, a potential regulator of vascular inflammation. *J Biol Chem* 2003;278(51):51059–51067.
47. Mann KG, Nesheim ME, Church WR, et al. Surface-dependent reactions of the vitamin K-dependent enzyme complexes. [Review] [172 refs]. *Blood* 1990;76:1–16.

# CHAPTER 3 ■ THE BLOOD COAGULATION FACTORS: THEIR COMPLEMENTARY DNAS, GENES, AND EXPRESSION

DANIEL L. GREENBERG AND EARL W. DAVIE

The complementary DNAs (cDNAs) and genes corresponding to all the proteins known to participate in the blood coagulation cascade have been cloned (1). Most of these coagulation proteins are synthesized in the liver and secreted into the plasma. Accordingly, the cloning of these proteins has been made possible by the isolation of liver messenger ribonucleic acid (mRNA), the preparation of cDNAs corresponding to the liver mRNA, and the insertion of these cDNAs into plasmids or phage for their amplification, identification, and sequence analysis. These experiments have provided a fruitful approach to the study of the structure, function, and biosynthesis of the coagulation proteins and the organization of their genes from both healthy individuals and patients with clotting disorders. More recently, substantial progress has been made in the understanding of the liver-specific expression of these genes. The pharmaceutical production of factors VIII, IX, and VIIa have greatly enhanced treatment options for patients with hemophilia and other clotting disorders. Additionally, animal models for gene therapy have been encouraging for both hemophilia A and B. The cDNAs and genes for these various proteins are described in this chapter, with primary emphasis on those of human origin.

## FIBRINOGEN

Fibrinogen ($M_r$ 340,000) participates in the final stages of the blood coagulation process (1). It is a complex glycoprotein consisting of two sets of three different polypeptide chains, including two $\alpha$ chains ($M_r$ 67,600), two $\beta$ chains ($M_r$ 52,300), and two $\gamma$ chains ($M_r$ 48,900) (2). Fibrinogen also contains four carbohydrate chains, including one on each of the $\beta$ and $\gamma$ chains (3,4). The $\alpha$ chain is free of carbohydrates (5). The complete amino acid sequence for human fibrinogen has been determined by amino acid sequence analysis and cDNA and genomic cloning (6–18).

A single copy of the gene for each of the three polypeptide chains of fibrinogen is present on the long arm of human chromosome 4 at q23-q32 (15). The three genes are grouped together in approximately 50 kb of DNA and range in size from 5.4 to 8.4 kb (see Fig. 3-1) (16). The three genes occur in the order of $\gamma$, $\alpha$, and $\beta$, with approximately 14 kb of DNA separating the genes for the $\gamma$ and $\alpha$ chains and approximately 13 kb of DNA separating the genes for the $\alpha$ and $\beta$ chains. The gene for the $\beta$ chain is oriented in the opposite transcriptional direction from the genes for the $\gamma$ and $\alpha$ chains (15).

The genes for the three chains of human fibrinogen have been sequenced in their entirety (16,18). The gene coding for the $\gamma$ chain is 8.5 kb long and contains nine introns (A through I) and 10 exons (see Fig. 3-2) (16–18). The introns vary considerably in size, ranging from 96 to 1,638 nucleotides (see Table 3-1). The poly(A) addition site as determined by the cDNA sequence for the $\gamma$ chain is 203 nucleotides downstream from the stop codon of TAA and follows the typical processing or polyadenylation sequence of AATAAA by 19 nucleotides (19).

The gene coding for the $\alpha$ chain of human fibrinogen is 5.4 kb long and contains four introns (A through D) and five exons (Fig. 3-2) (16). The introns range in size from 459 to 1,132 nucleotides (Table 3-1). The fifth exon is unusually large: It codes for more than 75% of the $\alpha$ chain (amino acids 153 through 625). This exon also codes for eight tandem repeats of 13 amino acids (residues 270 through 374) that are unique to the $\alpha$ chain (see Table 3-2). These repeats also typically contain the sequence of Gly-Ser-Ser, which is coded by the nucleotide sequence of GGG-AGC-TCT.

The DNA sequence coding the gene for the $\beta$ chain of fibrinogen is 8 kb long and contains seven introns and eight exons (Fig. 3-2) (16). The size and location of the introns in the gene are shown in Table 3-1. Three polyadenylation sites are present in the 3'-flanking regions, which can lead to slightly different lengths in the mRNAs. The gene for the $\beta$ chain also contains two Alu repetition sequences, including one in intron E and one in the 3'-flanking region of the gene. The location of the introns in the three chains of fibrinogen relative to the coiled-coil regions present in the intact molecule are illustrated in Figure 3-2.

Fibrinogen is synthesized primarily in the hepatic parenchymal cells, where the individual polypeptides are processed and assembled (20,21). Its synthesis is markedly increased during an acute-phase state induced by tissue damage, inflammation, or stress. Synthesis of the three chains also appears to be under coordinate control in that defibrination by injection of Malayan pit viper venom results in a coordinate increase in liver mRNA for each of the three chains (22). Studies in rats suggest that the expression of the three chains of fibrinogen is under coordinate regulation at the transcriptional level (23).

Recent epidemiologic data has indicated that high levels of circulating fibrinogen are associated with an increased risk of myocardial infarction and stroke (24,25). These studies have prompted an interest in the regulation the expression fibrinogen by hepatocytes. Fibrinogen biosynthesis is unusual in that it is an acute-phase reactant (APR) although it is constitutively expressed at a high level. Fibrinogen belongs to the class II group of APRs because it is induced by the inflammatory cytokine IL-6. Inflammatory cells contain receptors for fibrinogen and fibrinogen degradation products, and will produce IL-6 in response to these products (25,26). Glucocorticoids stimulate the synthesis of class II APRs through increasing the production of IL-6 by inflammatory cells. The IL-6 promoter contains glucocorticoid response elements that result in increased transcription of the hormone in the presence of glucocorticoids. The

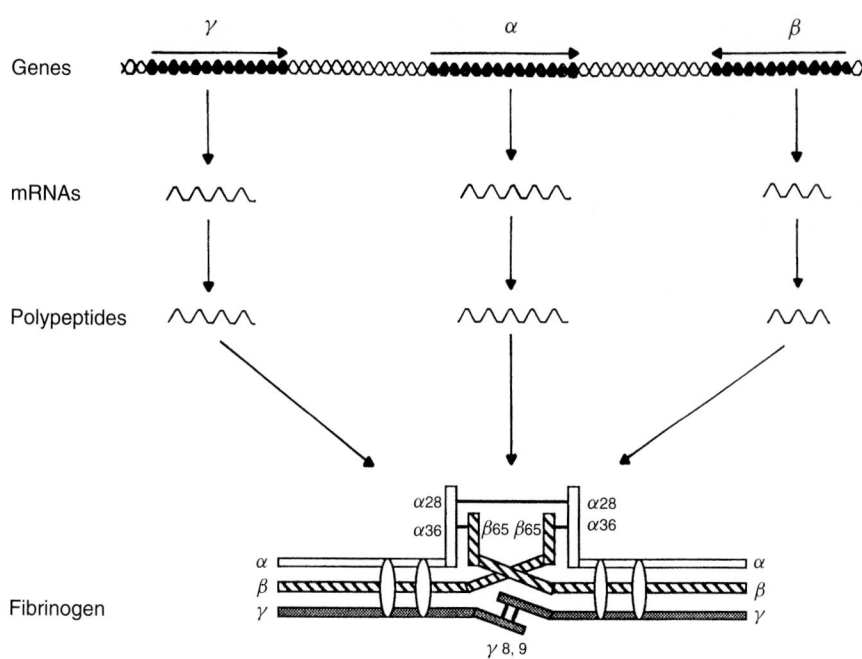

**FIGURE 3-1.** Abbreviated scheme illustrating the biosynthesis of human fibrinogen in liver. The arrangement of the $\gamma$, $\alpha$, and $\beta$ genes on human chromosome 4 is indicated by the *solid wavy lines*. The *arrows* above each gene indicate the direction of transcription. The individual messenger RNAs (mRNAs) are processed and transported from the nucleus to the cytoplasm, where they form the membrane-bound polysomes for the biosynthesis of each polypeptide chain. Additional processing of each polypeptide chain and assembly of the three chains into a mature molecule generate a fibrinogen that is secreted into the plasma. The intrachain and interchain disulfide bonds shown in the mature molecule are discussed in the text.

increased production of IL-6 by inflammatory cells then stimulates the hepatocytes to increase the synthesis of class II APRs. IL-6 enhances the gene expression of many of the type II APRs through the IL-6 activated transcription factor STAT 3 (signal transducer and activator of transcription 3) (27). In rats, activated STAT 3 binds to IL-6 response elements and is required for the upregulation of fibrinogen genes during an acute-phase response (28). However, in humans it is unclear which nuclear transcription factor(s) regulate the IL-6 response elements in the $\alpha$ and $\beta$ chains. In the human $\gamma$ chain, IL-6 activated STAT 3 bound weakly to the promoter element, and this binding decreased the functional activity of the promoter as measured by reporter gene (29). Accordingly, the mechanism of IL-6–dependent regulation of the fibrinogen gene requires further investigation.

An interesting relation is developing between fibrinogen gene expression and lipid metabolism. Oxysterols, which inhibit cholesterol synthesis by a feedback mechanism, diminish fibrinogen expression in both primary and transformed hepatic cells (30). Additionally, activation of the hepatic nuclear hormone receptor peroxisome proliferation-activated receptor-$\alpha$ (PPAR-$\alpha$) with fenofibrate, a lipid-lowering agent, reduces the IL-6–mediated induction of most, if not all, of the type II APRs (31). This suppression of IL-6–regulated APR genes produced by the liver is due to PPAR-$\alpha$–mediated downregulation of important IL-6 signal transduction proteins and the ubiquitous transcription factors CCAAT-enhancer/binding proteins (see subsequent text) (32).

The 5'-flanking regions of all three of the chains making up fibrinogen have been investigated. In keeping with the observation that fibrinogen is upregulated by IL-6, all three of the transcriptional regulatory regions of these genes contain a functional IL-6 response element (see Fig. 3-3) (33). There is a unique difference between the IL-6 responsive element in the gene for the $\gamma$ chain and those in the genes for the $\alpha$ and $\beta$ chains. In the latter two genes, the IL-6 responsive element is associated with an adjacent functional CCAAT-enhancer binding protein (C/EBP) site, which is essential for transactivation by IL-6 (35–38). However, in the gene for the $\gamma$ chain, the IL-6 response element is not associated with an active C/EBP site (34).

The genes for the $\alpha$ and $\beta$ chains are apparently expressed in a liver-specific manner by a hepatocyte nuclear factor-1

(HNF-1)–dependent mechanism. In contrast, liver-specific expression of the gene for the $\gamma$ chain is apparently mediated by an upstream stimulatory factor (USF). USF and HNF-1 are expressed in many different tissues, as well as by the liver, indicating that tissue-specific cofactors or accessory proteins are also involved. DNA binding and functional reporter gene assays have demonstrated that both HNF-1 and USF must also associate with other tissue-specific transacting proteins to achieve liver-specific expression (see subsequent text). All three fibrinogen genes contain TATA-like sequences that presumably facilitate the choice of transcription initiation sites by RNA polymerase II.

The 5'-flanking region of the gene coding for the human $\alpha$ chain has been isolated, sequenced, and characterized (36). The principal site of transcription initiation is located 55 bp upstream from the initiator methionine codon, or 13,399 bp downstream from the polyadenylation site of the gene coding for the $\gamma$ chain. The promoter and IL-6 response element lie within the region from −217 bp to the transcription start site, located at +1 bp. Although six sequences with homology to the consensus IL-6 response element are present, a single sequence of CTGGGA localized from −127 to −122 bp was shown to be a functional element in IL-6 induction (36,37). A C/EBP site is located at −142 to −134 bp. Mutation of this C/EBP site decreases IL-6 response by threefold, indicating that C/EBP is among the regulatory proteins associated with the IL-6 response. Recent studies suggest that the IL-6 response element of the $\alpha$ chain also binds to the novel transcription factor A $\alpha$-core protein, which is homologous to the mitochondrial single-stranded DNA binding protein P16 (39,40). An HNF-1 binding site, present from −59 to −47 bp, in combination with other upstream elements, is essential for liver-specific expression (36). An additional positive element (−1393 to −133 bp) and a negative element (−749 to −133 bp) have also been characterized by reporter gene assays. A series of patients with hypofibrinogenemia were recently found to be heterozygous for the single base pair substitution C to T at −1138 bp in the 5'-flanking region of the $\alpha$ chain (41). Functional *in vitro* experiments analyzing this mutation showed a corresponding reduction in hepatocyte reporter gene expression.

The 5'-flanking region containing the regulatory sequences for the liver-specific expression of the $\beta$ chain has also been partially characterized (34,35). HNF-1 binds at −91 to −79 bp

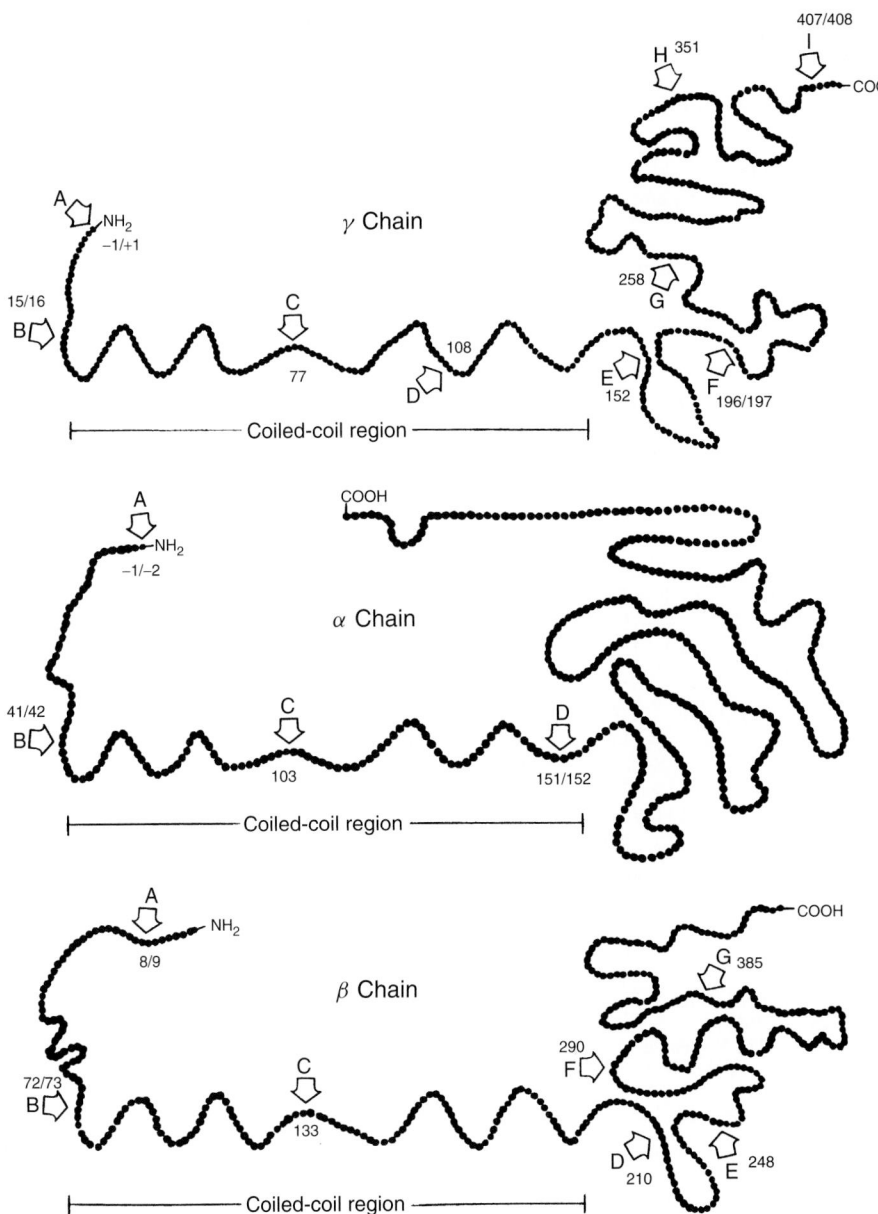

**FIGURE 3-2.** Location of the introns in the genes for the γ, α, and β polypeptide chains of human fibrinogen. The *open arrows* indicate the nine (A through I), the four (A through D), and the seven (A through G) introns present in the three genes relative to the coiled-coil region of the polypeptide chains.

relative to the transcription start site. A C/EBP site located at −132 to −124 bp, and the functional IL-6 response element is located at −142 to −137 bp. The liver-specific expression of the β chain gene appears to be mediated in part by the presence of an accessory protein designated as dimerization cofactor of HNF-1 (DCoH) (42). The IL-6 response element is located at −143 to −137 bp, adjacent to the C/EBP site, and contains the core sequence CTGGAAA. Full IL-6 response activity is dependent on C/EBP binding and other accessory or cofactors, including DCoH. Two common single-base substitution polymorphisms, one at −455 bp and the other at −854 bp, independently increase transcription of the β chain, and this is correlated with the observed increase in plasma fibrinogen in middle-aged men who have the polymorphism (43).

The 5′-flanking region of the γ chain of human fibrinogen has also been characterized for its promoter activity (33,44). Reporter gene studies and DNA-protein binding assays showed that a TATA-like sequence (−23 to −20 bp), a CCAAT-like sequence (−57 to −54 bp), and a USF binding site (−77 to −66 bp) are required for full expression in liver. Three putative IL-6 response elements with the sequence CTGG(G)AA are located at −306 to −301 bp, −146 to −140 bp, and −44 to −38 bp (33,44). The

primary functional IL-6 response element is located at −306 to −301 bp. Serum amyloid activating factor 1 binds to a site located at −273 to −259 bp and functions as an IL-6 responsive element (45). In contrast to the IL-6 response elements in the human α- and β-fibrinogen genes, the IL-6 response element of the γ chain is not C/EBP dependent (33). Supershift DNA binding studies performed with monoclonal antibodies directed against a variety of known transcription factors demonstrate that the transcription factor STAT 3 is a component of the IL-6 regulatory complex. STAT 3 has also been found to be involved in the regulation of other class II APRs, including α₂-macroglobulin (46,47). A negative regulatory region from −407 to −333 bp contains two putative negative elements with the sequence AGGA. The AGGA sequence has also been shown to be present in the silencer regions of the genes for human ε-globin, catalase, gastrin, factor IX, mouse c-myc, rat growth hormone, and chicken vimentin (48).

The transcriptional control of fibrinogen and other type II ARPs is complex, involving extracellular signals including IL-6 and other interleukins (49). The association between hyperlipidemia and hyperfibrinogenemia is intriguing and may

**TABLE 3-1**

LOCATION AND SIZE OF EXONS AND INTRONS IN THE GENES CODING FOR
THE $\gamma$, $\alpha$, AND $\beta$ CHAINS OF HUMAN FIBRINOGEN

| Exons | Nucleotide positions | Nucleotide length (bp) | Amino acids | Intron | Nucleotide positions | Nucleotide length (bp) |
|-------|---------------------|------------------------|-------------|--------|---------------------|------------------------|
| $\gamma^a$ Chain | | | | | | |
| I | 1–129 | 129 | −26 to −1 | A | 130–225 | 96 |
| II | 226–270 | 45 | 1–15 | B | 271–459 | 189 |
| III | 460–643 | 184 | 16–76 | C | 644–762 | 119 |
| IV | 763–856 | 94 | 77–108 | D | 857–2,463 | 1,607 |
| V | 2,464–2,594 | 131 | 109–151 | E | 2,595–2,897 | 303 |
| VI | 2,898–3,031 | 134 | 152–196 | F | 3,032–4,010 | 979 |
| VII | 4,011–4,195 | 185 | 197–258 | G | 4,196–5,678 | 1,483 |
| VIII | 5,679–5,956 | 278 | 259–350 | H | 5,957–7,594 | 1,638 |
| IX | 7,595–7,764 | 170 | 351–407 | I | 7,765–8,306 | 542 |
| X | 8,307–8,525 | 219 | 408–411 | | | |
| $\alpha^b$ Chain | | | | | | |
| I | 1–54 | 54 | −19 to −2 | A | 55–1,123 | 1,069 |
| II | 1,124–1,249 | 126 | −1 to 41 | B | 1,250–1,708 | 459 |
| III | 1,709–1,892 | 184 | 42–102 | C | 1,893–3,024 | 1,132 |
| IV | 3,025–3,170 | 146 | 103–151 | D | 3,171–3,755 | 585 |
| V | 3,756–5,177 | 1422 | 152–625 | | | |
| $\beta^c$ Chain | | | | | | |
| I | 1–90 | 90 | −22 to 8 | A | 91–2,764 | 2,674 |
| II | 2,765–2,956 | 192 | 9–72 | B | 2,957–3,445 | 489 |
| III | 3,446–3,629 | 184 | 73–133 | C | 3,630–4,549 | 920 |
| IV | 4,550–4,777 | 228 | 134–209 | D | 4,778–5,337 | 560 |
| V | 5,338–5,451 | 114 | 210–247 | E | 5,452–6,139 | 688 |
| VI | 6,140–6,265 | 126 | 248–289 | F | 6,266–6,473 | 208 |
| VII | 6,474–6,759 | 286 | 290–385 | G | 6,760–7,377 | 618 |
| VIII | 7,378–7,606 | 229 | 386–461 | — | — | — |

bp, base pair.
[a]Data from Rixon MW, Chung DW, Davie EW. Nucleotide sequence of the gene for the gamma chain of human fibrinogen. *Biochemistry* 1985;24:2077.
[b]Data from Chung DW, Harris JE, Davie EW. Nucleotide sequences of the three genes coding for human fibrinogen. In: Liu CY, Chien S, eds. *Advances in the experimental medicine and biology.* New York: Plenum, 1991. Data were modified slightly by deleting 2 bp in exon IV and adding them to exon V.
[c]Data from Fornace AJ Jr, Cummings DE, Comeau CM, et al. Structure of the human gamma-fibrinogen gene. *J Biol Chem* 1984;259:12826.

be mediated, in part, by nuclear hormone receptors such as PPAR-$\alpha$. Furthermore, liver-specific and ubiquitous transcription factors responsible for promoting gene transcription are themselves regulated by extracellular signals. Finally, each of the three fibrinogen chains is coordinately expressed to form heterotrimeric protein.

Transcription of the three genes coding for fibrinogen gives rise to three large RNAs that undergo considerable processing and reduction in size in the nucleus (Fig. 3-1). The processing involves a capping reaction at the 5′ end of the RNA, the addition of poly(A) at the 3′ end, and splicing out of the various introns at specific intron–exon splice junction sequences. The splice junction sequences follow the GT-AG rule and are shown in Table 3-3 for the gene for the $\gamma$ chain of fibrinogen (17,18,50). Splicing occurs between coding triplets with some introns (splice junction type O) or within coding triplets for other introns (type I or II). A similar situation exists for the genes coding for the $\alpha$ and $\beta$ chains.

After processing, the three mature mRNAs are transported into the cytoplasm for translation and polypeptide synthesis. Each of the three polypeptide chains is then synthesized on membrane-bound ribosomes with a leader or signal sequence

containing an initiating methionine residue (see Fig. 3-4) (16). The initiating methionines are located at position −19 (or −16) in the $\alpha$ chain, −30 (or −27 or −16) in the $\beta$ chain, and −26 in the $\gamma$ chain. These signal sequences that contain a hydrophobic core rich in Leu, Val, Tyr, and Phe are removed during biosynthesis by signal peptidase (51). This reaction apparently occurs on the lumen side of the rough endoplasmic recticulum as the nascent polypeptide chains are being synthesized and disulfide bonds are being formed.

The mRNA for the $\alpha$ chain of the human molecule is approximately 2,200 nucleotides long [not counting the poly(A) tail] and includes 1,875 nucleotides that code for a polypeptide chain of 625 amino acids (11,14). This polypeptide, free of its leader sequence, then undergoes additional processing by the cleavage of a carboxyl-terminal fragment of 15 amino acids. This results in a mature $\alpha$ chain of 610 residues. It is unknown whether this latter processing occurs within the hepatocyte or after secretion of the intact fibrinogen molecule into the blood. The eight internal tandem repeats of 39 nucleotides code for eight homologous repeats that are 13 amino acids long (Table 3-2) (11,14). These repeats are located in the carboxyl half of the molecule and follow the coiled-coil region of the molecule.

## TABLE 3-2

### AMINO ACID AND NUCLEOTIDE SEQUENCES FOR TANDEM REPEATS IN THE α CHAIN OF HUMAN FIBRINOGEN

| Tandem repeat number | | | | | | | | | | | | | | | Homology (%) |
|---|---|---|---|---|---|---|---|---|---|---|---|---|---|---|---|
| 1 | 270 | | | | | | | | | | | | | | |
| | Pro | Ser | Ser | Ala | Gly | Ser | Trp | Asn | Ser | Gly | Ser | Ser | Gly | | 77 |
| | CCT | AGC | AGT | GCT | GGA | AGC | TGG | AAC | TCT | GGG | AGC | TCT | GGA | | 92 |
| 2 | 283 | | | | | | | | | | | | | | |
| | Pro | Gly | Ser | Thr | Gly | Asn | Arg | Asn | Pro | Gly | Ser | Ser | Gly | | 92 |
| | CCT | GGA | AGT | ACT | GGA | AAC | CGA | AAC | CCT | GGG | AGC | TCT | GGG | | 95 |
| 3 | 296 | | | | | | | | | | | | | | |
| | Thr | Gly | Gly | Thr | Ala | Thr | Trp | Lys | Pro | Gly | Ser | Ser | Gly | | 62 |
| | ACT | GGA | GGG | ACT | GCA | ACC | TGG | AAA | CCT | GGG | AGC | TCT | GGA | | 85 |
| 4 | 309 | | | | | | | | | | | | | | |
| | Pro | Gly | Ser | Ala | Gly | Ser | Trp | Asn | Ser | Gly | Ser | Ser | Gly | | 85 |
| | CCT | GGA | AGT | GCT | GGA | AGC | TGG | AAC | TCT | GGG | AGC | TCT | GGA | | 95 |
| 5 | 322 | | | | | | | | | | | | | | |
| | Thr | Gly | Ser | Thr | Gly | Asn | Gln | Asn | Pro | Gly | Ser | Pro | Arg | | 69 |
| | ACT | GGA | AGT | ACT | GGA | AAC | CAA | AAC | CCT | GGA | AGT | CCT | AGA | | 79 |
| 6 | 335 | | | | | | | | | | | | | | |
| | Pro | Gly | Ser | Thr | Gly | Thr | Trp | Asn | Pro | Gly | Ser | Ser | Glu | | 85 |
| | CCT | GGT | AGT | ACC | GGA | ACC | TGG | AAT | CCT | GGC | AGC | TCT | GAA | | 85 |
| 7 | 348 | | | | | | | | | | | | | | |
| | Arg | Gly | Ser | Ala | Gly | His | Trp | Thr | Ser | Glu | Ser | Ser | Val | | 54 |
| | CGC | GGA | AGT | GCT | GGG | CAC | TGG | ACC | TCT | GAG | AGC | TCT | GTA | | 79 |
| 8 | 361 | | | | | | | | | | | | | | |
| | Ser | Gly | Ser | Thr | Gly | Gln | Trp | His | Ser | Glu | | Ser | Gly | | 62 |
| | TCT | GGT | AGT | ACT | GGA | CAA | TGG | CAC | TCT | GAA | | TCT | GGA | | 72 |
| Consensus sequence | | Pro | Gly | Ser | Thr | Gly | Asn | Trp | Asn | Pro Ser | Gly | Ser | Ser | Gly | |
| | | CCT | GGA | AGT | ACT | GGA | AAC | TGG | AAC | TCCT | GGG | AGC | TCT | GGA | |

A gap is inserted in tandem repeat 8 for better alignment.
Reprinted from Rixon MW, Chan WY, Davie EW, Chung DW. Characterization of a cDNA coding for the alpha-chain of human fibrinogen. *Biochemistry* 1983;22:3237–3244, with permission. Copyright 1983 American Chemical Society.

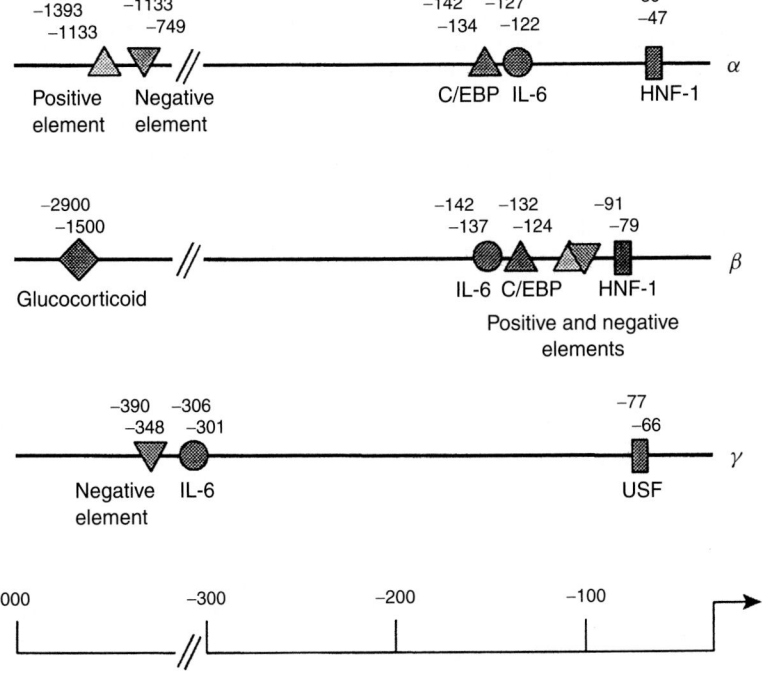

**FIGURE 3-3.** Schematic representation of the locations of the regulatory elements in the genes for the γ, α, and β chains of human fibrinogen. The liver-specific hepatocyte nuclear factor-1 (HNF-1) and upstream stimulatory factor (USF) elements are located close to the transcription sites. The CCAAT-enhancer binding protein (C/EBP)-associated interleukin-6 (IL-6) elements are similarly located in the α and β genes, whereas the IL-6 element of the γ chain is located further upstream and is not associated with a C/EBP binding site. Weak dexamethasone response has been functionally localized to an upstream region in the β gene. (From Mizuguchi J, Hu CH, Coa Z, et al. Characterization of the 5'-flanking region of the gene for the gamma chain of human fibrinogen. *J Biol Chem* 1995;270:28350, with permission.)

**TABLE 3-3**

INTRON–EXON SPLICE JUNCTION SEQUENCES AND SPLICE JUNCTION TYPES
IN THE GENE FOR THE γ CHAIN OF HUMAN FIBRINOGEN

| | Splice junction sequences | | | |
| --- | --- | --- | --- | --- |
| Intron | Exon \| 5' | Intron | 3' \| Exon | Splice junction type[a] |
| A | GCA \| GTAAGT | —TTTTAG | T | 0 |
| B | TTC \| GTAAGT | —TTTCAG | G | 0 |
| C | CAA \| GTGAGA | —TTACAG | A | I |
| D | TCG \| GTAAGG | —TTGTAG | A | II |
| E | AAG \| GTAACT | —CTCTAG | A | I |
| F | AAG \| GTAATT | —AATTAG | A | 0 |
| G | CAG \| GTACTG | —TCTCAG | T | II |
| H | AAG \| GTATGT | —TTTTAG | G | I |
| I | CAG \| GTCAGA | —TCACAG | G | 0 |
| Consensus sequence | CAAG \| GTAGAGT | —TCTCNTCAG | G | — |

[a]Data from Mount SM. A catalogue of splice junction sequences. *Nucleic Acids Res* 1982;10:459.
Reprinted from Rixon MW, Chung DW, Davie EW. Nucleotide sequence of the gene for the gamma chain
of human fibrinogen. *Biochemistry* 1985;24:2077–2086, with permission. Copyright 1985 American
Chemical Society.

The mRNA for the β chain of human fibrinogen is approximately 1,900 nucleotides long and includes 1,383 nucleotides that code for a mature polypeptide chain of 461 amino acids (12,14). The mRNA for the γ chain is approximately 1,600 nucleotides long and includes 1,233 nucleotides that code for a mature polypeptide chain of 411 amino acids. A less abundant mRNA coding for the γ' chain of 427 amino acids is also synthesized in liver (52–55). It contains an additional 90 nucleotides at the 3' end. In humans, this minor mRNA results from alternative mRNA polyadenylation within the region normally constituting the ninth intron (intron I, Fig. 3-2) (56). Translation of this mRNA generates a less prevalent γ' polypeptide chain (approximately 10% of the normal γ chain) that contains 20 different amino acids at the carboxyl-terminal end. The carboxyl-terminal sequence of the γ' chain also contains tyrosine sulfate (57). Analysis of the fibrinogen γ' chain by electrospray ionization mass spectrometry suggests that both tyrosine residues are sulfated and furthermore, this tandem sulfation may confer additional binding affinity of γ'-containing fibrinogen to thrombin (58). Both the γ and γ' polypeptides are present in the fibrinogen molecule that circulates in plasma. The γ' chain, however, is not found in fibrinogen isolated from platelets (38,59).

The addition of carbohydrate chains to fibrinogen presumably occurs in several steps, including the addition of a core carbohydrate unit in the rough endoplasmic reticulum and the remaining carbohydrate addition and processing occurring in the smooth endoplasmic reticulum and Golgi apparatus. These carbohydrate chains are all N-linked, being attached to Asn364 in the β chain and Asn52 in the γ chain.

The mechanism and sequence of assembly of the three polypeptide chains leading to the formation of the trinodular structure has been partially elucidated. In human fibrinogen, the synthesis of the β chain appears to be rate limiting, at least in Hep-G2 cells (60). The synthesis and assembly of human fibrinogen has been accomplished in a variety of mammalian cell types, including baby hamster kidney (BHK) and COS-1 cells, yeast cultures, and more recently in mammary glandular tissues for large-scale production in milk (61–65). Hence, the assembly of fibrinogen does not require hepatic-specific factors. Indeed, transient association of partially assembled fibrinogen intermediates with the ubiquitous chaperon protein BiP has been observed in HepG2, BHK, and COS-1 cells. Several pathways for fibrinogen assembly have been proposed (61,62,66). Studies from our laboratory employing stable transfected BHK cells show that the initial assembly of fibrinogen involves the formation of αγ and βγ heterodimers, followed by the addition of a third chain to form half molecules (αβγ) (67,68). The carboxyl-terminal region of the γ chain, specifically residue Ile387, appears to be critical in order to assemble the αγ and

```
                                                      -19         -16
α  chain                                              Met Phe Ser Met Arg
              -30              -27
β  chain      Met Lys Arg Met Val Ser Trp Ser Phe His Lys Leu Lys Thr Met Lys

γ  chain                  Met Ser Trp Ser Leu His Pro Arg Asn Leu Ile Leu


              -10                     -5            -1 +1
α  chain      Ile Val Cys Leu Val Leu Ser Val Val Gly Thr Ala Trp Thr Ala Asp

β  chain      His Leu Leu Leu Leu Leu Leu Cys Val Phe Leu Val Lys Ser Gln Gly

γ  chain      Tyr Phe Tyr Ala Leu Leu Phe Leu Ser Ser Thr Cys Val Ala Tyr Val
```

FIGURE 3-4. Amino acid sequence of the signal peptides of the γ, α, and β chains of human fibrinogen. Amino acids present in the amino-terminal end of the mature polypeptide chains are marked as +1.

## TABLE 3-4

### COMPARISON OF NORMAL AND SEVERAL ABNORMAL CHAINS OF HUMAN FIBRINOGEN AND THE PROPOSED NUCLEOTIDE CHANGES

| Chain | Normal fibrinogen | | Abnormal fibrinogen | | |
|---|---|---|---|---|---|
| | Amino acid | Codon | Amino acid | Codon | Identification |
| $\alpha$ | Arg19 | AG$\boxed{\text{G}}$ | Ser19 | AG$\boxed{\begin{smallmatrix}T\\C\end{smallmatrix}}$ | Detroit[a] |
| | Arg19 | A$\boxed{\text{GG}}$ | Asn19 | A$\boxed{\text{A}}\begin{smallmatrix}T\\C\end{smallmatrix}$ | Munich I[b] |
| | Arg16 | c$\boxed{\text{G}}$T | His16 | c$\boxed{\text{A}}$T | Sydney I and II[b] |
| | Arg16 | $\boxed{\text{C}}$GT | Cys16 | $\boxed{\text{T}}$GT | Zurich I[a] |
| | Gly12 | g$\boxed{\text{G}}$A | Val12 | g$\boxed{\text{T}}$A | Rouen[b] |
| | Asp7 | $\boxed{\text{G}}$AC | Asn7 | $\boxed{\text{A}}$AC | Lille[b] |
| $\beta$ | Ala335 | $\boxed{\text{G}}$CC | Thr335 | $\boxed{\text{A}}$CC | Pontoise[b] |
| $\gamma$ | Arg275 | c$\boxed{\text{G}}$c | His275 | c$\boxed{\text{A}}$c | Bergamo II[a,c] |
| | Asp330 | g$\boxed{\text{A}}$T | Val330 | g$\boxed{\text{T}}$T | Milano I[b] |

Nucleotides shown in boxes are those that have been changed by mutation.
[a]Data from Blomback M, Blomback B, Mammen EF, Prasad AS. Fibrinogen Detroit: a molecular defect in the N-terminal disulphide knot of human fibrinogen? *Nature* 1968;218:134.
[b]Data from Henschen A. Genetically abnormal human fibrinogens: a summary of 32 structurally elucidated variants. In: Peeters H, ed. Protides of the biological fluids, Vol. 33. Oxford: Pergamon, 1985.
[c]Fibrinogens Essen and Haifa also contain His at position 275 (34).
Fibrinogens Petoskey, Becetre, Louisville, Manchester, New Albany, Amiens, Bern II, Chapel Hill II, Clermont-Ferrand I, Leitchfield, Sydney I and II, and White Marsh also contain His in position 16 (34).
Fibrinogens Metz, Amsterdam I, Bergamo I, Frankfurt II and III, Paris, Stonybrook, and Schwarzach also contain Cys in position 16 (34).

$\beta\gamma$ half molecules (69). The amino acid sequences that direct the order of chain additions to form the half molecule are located in the second and first halves of the coiled-coil domain of the fibrinogen chains. In the coiled-coil region, the distribution of hydrophobic amino acids favors the formation of two stranded coiled-coils and then three stranded coiled-coils, respectively (70). The $\alpha\beta\gamma$ half molecules then dimerize to form the mature six-chain fibrinogen, $(\alpha\beta\gamma)_2$, that is secreted and circulates in the blood.

The two half molecules are covalently linked in the native protein by disulfide bonds, which are located in the amino-terminus of each monomeric chain. Analysis of the fibrinogen synthesized in transfected (BHK) cells employing various combinations of mutations revealed that $\alpha$-Cys36 and $\beta$-Cys65 form disulfide bonds between two $\alpha\beta\gamma$ half molecules rather than within the same half molecule (71). This disulfide bond has been confirmed by x-ray analysis (72). These two disulfide bonds are sufficient to hold the two half molecules together as intact fibrinogen. Disulfide bonds formed by $\gamma$-Cys8 and 9 were also sufficient to hold the two fibrinogen $\alpha\beta\gamma$ half molecules together, whereas the disulfide between the two $\alpha$-Cys28 residues failed to form in the absence of the disulfide bonds linking the $\alpha$ and $\beta$ chains and the two $\gamma$ chains.

The cloning of the cDNAs and genes for human fibrinogen has also made it possible to characterize several abnormal fibrinogens at their DNA level. Most of the amino acid changes that were initially reported were identified within the first 19 amino acids of the $\alpha$ chain (see Table 3-4) (73,74). These amino acid changes can be predicted primarily on the basis of a single nucleotide transversion or transition. Fibrinogen New York I, however, is due to the presence of an abnormal chain resulting from a deletion of amino acid residues 9 to 72 (75). This deletion, which leads to a nonclottable fibrinogen, corresponds to the second exon in the gene for the $\beta$ chain. Consequently, the abnormality in New York I may be due to a mutation at a splice junction between introns A and B or a deletion of the second exon from the gene. Several hundred mutations in the three genes coding for human fibrinogen have been identified (76–78).

# PROTHROMBIN

Prothrombin ($M_r$ 71,600) is synthesized in the liver and secreted into the blood, where it circulates as a zymogen to a serine protease (1). During the final stages of the blood coagulation process, prothrombin is converted to thrombin by the cleavage of an internal Arg271–Thr peptide bond that follows the two-kringle domains and an Arg259–Ile bond located at the beginning of the serine protease domain (see Fig. 3-5). These reactions are catalyzed by factor Xa in the presence of factor Va, calcium ions, and phospholipid. The complete amino acid sequences of human and bovine prothrombin have been established by amino acid sequence analysis and cDNA and genomic cloning (79–85). Human prothrombin is a glycoprotein (8.2% carbohydrate) containing 579 amino acids and three N-linked carbohydrate chains (83). These chains are located at Asn78 and 100 in the first kringle structure and at Asn373 in the serine protease, or catalytic, domain. Prothrombin also contains 10 residues of $\gamma$-carboxyglutamic acid in the amino-terminal region of the protein, which make up the Gla domain and two regions of internal homology called *kringle structures* (Fig. 3-5) (79,86,87). The kringle structure of 80 amino acids each are followed by 49 amino acids, of which 36 become the light chain of thrombin (Thr285–Arg259) and 260 amino acids (Ile320–Glu579) that form the catalytic or serine protease part of thrombin.

The gene for human prothrombin is present in approximately 21 kb of DNA (83,85,88,89). It contains 13 introns (A through M) (Fig. 3-5), ranging in size from 84 to 9,447 base pairs, and 14 exons ranging in size from 25 to 315 base pairs, in the coding and 3' noncoding portions of the gene (see Table 3-5). The first intron (A) is located in the prepro leader sequence at residue −17. The second intron (B) follows the Gla domain and is located between residues 37 and 38 in the mature protein, whereas the third (C) is nine residues later at residue 46. These three introns are located in positions analogous to the first three introns in the coding regions of the genes for factor VII, factor IX, factor X, and protein C (see Table 3-6) (72,90–93). The fourth intron (D) in the gene for prothrombin is located

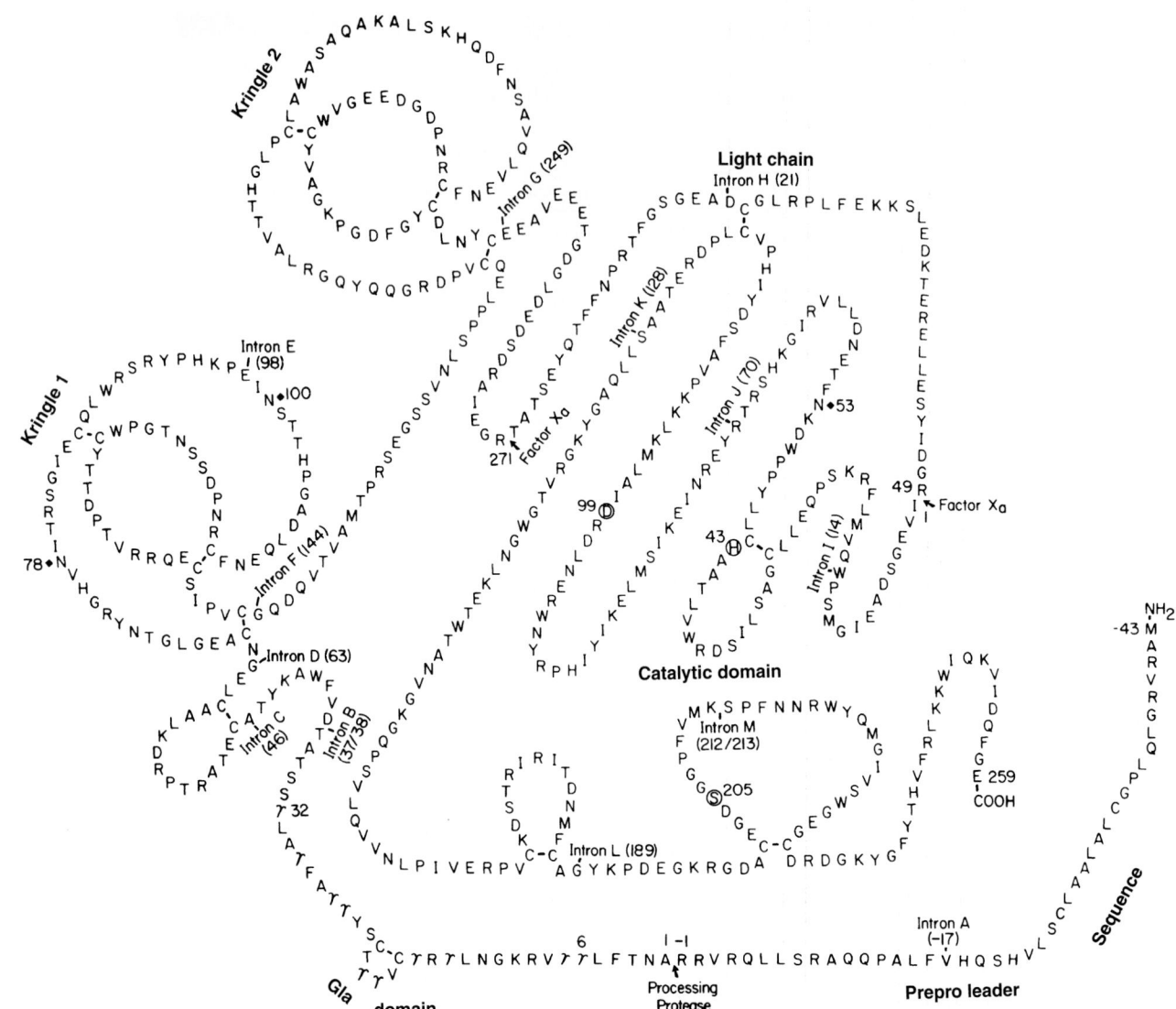

**FIGURE 3-5.** Amino acid sequence for human prepro prothrombin shows the location of the 13 introns (A through M) (62). The prepro leader sequence (numbered −43 to −1) is removed during biosynthesis by signal peptidase and a processing protease that hydrolyzes the R–A bond between −1 and 1. The Gla domain and the kringle domains are located within residues 1 through 271, which constitute fragment 1. This fragment is released from prothrombin during its conversion to thrombin by factor Xa. The light chain in thrombin is generated by the cleavage of the R319–I bond by factor Xa, and this chain is attached to the catalytic domain by a single disulfide bond. The serine protease or catalytic domain of thrombin contains 259 residues, including the three principal amino acids participating in catalysis. These three amino acids (H363, D419, and S525) are *circled*. Three potential carbohydrate-binding sites are shown by *solid diamonds*. The proposed disulfide bonds in human prothrombin have been placed by analogy to those in the bovine molecule. The single-letter code for amino acids is as follows: A, Ala; R, Arg; N, Asn; D, Asp; C, Cys; Q, Gln; E, Glu; G, Gly; H, His; I, Ile; L, Leu; K, Lys; M, Met; F, Phe; P, Pro; S, Ser; T, Thr; W, Trp; Y, Tyr; V, Val; g, g-carboxyglutamic acid.

just before the first kringle, whereas the next intron (E) is present within the first kringle. The fifth intron (F) is located immediately after kringle 1 (residue 144) and the sixth (G) immediately after kringle 2 (residue 249). The second kringle does not contain an intron, in contrast to the first kringle and the kringles in all other proteins so far studied. The seventh intron (H) occurs in the region of prothrombin that becomes the light chain of the enzyme (residue 21). The remaining five introns (I through M) are distributed throughout the heavy chain or *catalytic* domain of thrombin. They are located at positions 14, 70, 128, 189, and between 212 and 213 in the serine protease, or catalytic domain of the molecule. The sequences at the splice

junctions agree with the GT-AG rule of Breathnach and Chambon (50) and the consensus sequence of Mount (94), except for one splice site at the 5′ end of intervening sequence L (see Table 3-7).

The gene for prothrombin also contains 30 copies of Alu repetitive sequences, which make up 39% of the gene (85). This family of DNA sequences is composed of approximately 300 nucleotides, and the human haploid genome contains roughly 350,000 copies (95). This is equivalent to about one Alu sequence in every 6 kb of DNA. The precise function of these highly repetitive sequences is unknown. In the prothrombin gene, many Alu sequences are tightly clustered and include five sets of tandem repeats. Intervening sequence L (9.5 kb)

**TABLE 3-5**

LOCATION AND SIZE OF EXONS AND INTERVENING SEQUENCES IN THE GENE FOR HUMAN PROTHROMBIN

| Exon | Nucleotide positions | Length (bp) | Amino acids | Intervening sequence | Type[a] | Nucleotide positions | Length (bp) | No. of Alu repeats |
|---|---|---|---|---|---|---|---|---|
| I | +1–79 | 79+[b] | −43 to −17 | A | 1 | 80–465 | 386 | — |
| II | 466–626 | 161 | −17 to 37 | B | 0 | 627–1,285 | 659 | — |
| III | 1,286–1,310 | 25 | 38–46 | C | 1 | 1,311–1,552 | 242 | — |
| IV | 1,553–1,603 | 51 | 46–63 | D | 1 | 1,604–3,929 | 2,326 | 4 |
| V | 3,930–4,035 | 106 | 63–98 | E | 2 | 4,036–4,131 | 96 | — |
| VI | 4,132–4,268 | 137 | 98–144 | F | 1 | 4,269–6,606 | 2,338 | 3 |
| VII | 6,607–6,921 | 315 | 144–249 | G | 1 | 6,922–7,245 | 324 | — |
| VIII | 7,246–7,374 | 129 | 249–292 | H | 1 | 7,375–7,458 | 84 | — |
| IX | 7,459–7,585 | 127 | 292–334 | I | 2 | 7,586–8,742 | 1,157 | 2 |
| X | 8,743–8,910 | 168 | 334–390 | J | 2 | 8,911–9,407 | 497 | — |
| XI | 9,408–9,581 | 174 | 390–448 | K | 2 | 9,582–10,123 | 542 | 1 |
| XII | 10,124–10,305 | 182 | 448–509 | L | 1 | 10,306–19,752 | 9,447 | 20[c] |
| XIII | 19,753–19,823 | 71 | 509–532 | M | 0 | 19,824–19,969 | 146 | — |
| XIV | 19,970–20,210 | 241 | 533–poly(A) site | — | — | — | — | — |

bp, base pair.

[a]Intervening sequence placement as discussed by Mount (78), in which a type 0 indicates placement between two codons, a type 1 interrupts a codon between the first and second bases, and a type 2 occurs between the second and third bases of the codon.

[b]The length of the 5′ noncoding region of the messenger RNA for human prothrombin is unknown; therefore, the length of exon 1 is measured from the initiator methionine.

[c]This intervening sequence also has two copies of partial Kpn repeats.

Taken from Terasawa F, Okumura N, Kitano K, et al. Hypofibrinogenemia associated with a heterozygous missense mutation gamma 153 cys to arg (Matsumoto IV): *in vitro* expression demonstrates defective secretion of the variant fibrinogen. *Blood* 1999;94:4122.

contains 20 Alu repeats, five of which occur in head-to-tail orientation with no additional DNA between them. The prothrombin gene also contains two copies of partial KpnI repeats located in intervening sequence L. These partial repeats are 170 bp and 326 bp long.

The mRNA for human prothrombin is approximately 2,000 nucleotides long and includes 1,866 nucleotides that code for a prepro leader sequence of 43 amino acids and a mature polypeptide chain of 579 amino acids (Fig. 3-5) (83,85). The prepro leader sequence includes a hydrophobic stretch of amino acids (residues −37 to −26) and ends with an arginine residue just before the amino-terminal alanine that is present in the mature protein that circulates in plasma. The Arg–Ala peptide bond, however, is not cleaved by signal peptidase (51). This enzyme cleaves the prepro polypeptide chain near the middle of the prepro leader sequence at one of the small amino acid residues such as alanine, cysteine, or serine. This leaves a propiece of approximately 18 to 24 amino acids still attached to the polypeptide chain. The propiece is then cleaved by a second processing protease with a substrate preference for a basic residue at −4, −2, and −1 (96). This enzyme cleaves the arginine at position −1 (96).

A prepro leader sequence is typical of the vitamin K–dependent coagulation factors present in plasma (see Fig. 3-6), suggesting a similar processing mechanism during the biosynthesis of each of the vitamin K–dependent plasma proteins. Also, it is these homologous leader sequences that play a role in the carboxylation reaction for the vitamin K–dependent proteins that occurs on the lumen side of the rough endoplasmic reticulum (97,98). Carboxylation also occurs before the cleavage of the propiece from the mature polypeptide chains (98). The conserved Phe and Ala residues at positions −16 and −10 appear to play an important role in the recognition sequence for this carboxylase (99,100).

Like the other vitamin K–dependent coagulation factors, the liver-specific expression of prothrombin is transcriptionally regulated. The immediate 5′-flanking sequence does not contain TATA or CCAAT boxes, and the two major transcription start sites are located at −36 and −23 bp upstream of the initiator codon (101). Full tissue-specific promoter activity has been found to be located within 1,000 bp of the transcription start sites (101–103). A weak positive element lies in the region 400 bp upstream of the mRNA coding sequence, accounting for approximately 5% of the total promoter activity in HepG2 cells. A liver-specific enhancer element is located in the region between −940 and −860 bp. DNA-protein binding studies and functional reporter gene analysis with mutant promoter constructs have demonstrated that this 80-bp enhancer contains an HNF-1 binding site flanked by a G-C rich motif which binds a ubiquitous Sp1-like transacting factor (see Fig. 3-15) (101,102).

A common G to A substitution at nucleotide position 20,210 in the 3′-untranslated end of the prothrombin gene has recently been described (104). Individuals who are heterozygous for this mutation have a slightly elevated level of circulating prothrombin and have 2.8-fold increased risk for venous thrombosis relative to persons homozygous for the G allele (104). The estimated frequency of the G to A substitution is reported to be approximately 2% in the general population, with an increased frequency in southern Europeans and a decreased frequency among those of Asian or African decent (105). How this mutation causes the observed increase in expression of prothrombin and the associated increase risk of thrombosis is not clear at this time.

# FACTOR V

Factor V ($M_r$ 330,000) participates in the latter phase of the blood coagulation cascade (1). It is synthesized as a single-chain molecule in liver and megakaryocytes and circulates in blood as an inactive cofactor (106). Approximately 25% of

TABLE 3-6

COMPARISON OF INTRON LOCATION AND SPLICE
JUNCTION TYPE AND SIZE FOR HUMAN FACTORS
VII, IX, X, PROTEIN C, AND PROTHROMBIN

| Intron | Protein | Location (amino acid) | Splice type | Size (bp) |
|--------|---------|-----------------------|-------------|-----------|
| A | Prothrombin | −17 | 1 | 386 |
|   | Factor VII | −17 | 1 | 2,574 |
|   | Factor IX | −17 | 1 | 6,206 |
|   | Factor X | −17 | 1 | 6,542 |
|   | Protein C | −19 | 1 | 1,263 |
| B | Prothrombin | 37/38 | 0 | 659 |
|   | Factor VII | 38/39 | 0 | 1,919 |
|   | Factor IX | 38/39 | 0 | 188 |
|   | Factor X | 37/38 | 0 | 8,836 |
|   | Protein C | 37/38 | 0 | 1,462 |
| C | Prothrombin | 46 | 1 | 242 |
|   | Factor VII | 46 | 1 | 68 |
|   | Factor IX | 47 | 1 | 3,689 |
|   | Factor X | 46 | 1 | 874 |
|   | Protein C | 46 | 1 | 92 |
| D | Factor VII | 84 | 1 | 1,908 |
|   | Factor IX | 85 | 1 | 7,163 |
|   | Factor X | 84 | 1 | 1,447 |
|   | Protein C | 92 | 1 | 102 |
| E | Factor VII | 131 | 1 | 971 |
|   | Factor IX | 128 | 1 | 2,565 |
|   | Factor X | 128 | 1 | 2,798 |
|   | Protein C | 137 | 1 | 2,668 |
| F | Factor VII | 15/16 | 0 | 595 |
|   | Factor IX | 15/16 | 0 | 9,473 |
|   | Factor X | 15/16 | 0 | 3,224 |
|   | Protein C | 15/16 | 0 | 873 |
| G | Factor VII | 57 | 1 | 816 |
|   | Factor IX | 54 | 1 | 668 |
|   | Factor X | 55 | 1 | 1,418 |
|   | Protein C | 55 | 1 | 1,129 |

bp, base pair.
Note: The numbering system for introns F and G begins with number
1 of the heavy chain of the active molecule.
Data from Degen , Davie EW. Nucleotide sequence of the gene for
human prothrombin. *Biochemistry* 1987;25:6165–6177; O'Hara PJ,
Grant FJ, Haldeman BA, et al. Nucleotide sequence of the gene coding
for human factor VII, a vitamin K–dependent protein participating in
blood coagulation. *Proc Natl Acad Sci U S A* 1987;84:5158; Anson
DS, Choo KH, Rees DJG, et al. The gene structure of human antihaemophilic factor IX. *EMBO J* 1984;3:1053; Yoshitake S, Schach
BG, Foster DC, et al. Nucleotide sequence of the gene for human factor IX (antihemophilic factor B). *Biochemistry* 1985;24:3736; Leytus
SP, Foster DC, Kurachi K, Davie EW. Gene for human factor X, a
blood coagulation factor whose gene organization is essentially identical to that of factor IX and protein C. *Biochemistry* 1986;25:5098;
Foster DC, Yoshitake S, Davie EW. The nucleotide sequence of the
gene for human protein C. *Proc Natl Acad Sci U S A* 1985;82:4673.

the factor V in blood is present in the α-granules of platelets,
whereas the rest is present in the plasma (107). Factor V functions as a cofactor in the conversion of prothrombin to thrombin. This reaction is catalyzed by factor Xa and occurs in the
presence of calcium and phospholipid. Before its participation
in the coagulation cascade, the single-chain protein of 2,196
amino acids undergoes minor proteolysis (108). These proteolytic cleavages are catalyzed by thrombin and occur at Arg709,
Arg1018, and Arg1545.

Factor V contains several types of internal repeats that are
highly homologous to factor VIII and ceruloplasmin (see Fig. 3-7)
(108–111). Each of these proteins contains three A-domains
that are approximately 350 amino acids long. The A-domains in
factor V and factor VIII are approximately 30% identical to the
three A-domains present in ceruloplasmin (108). The second
and third A-domains of factor V and factor VIII are separated
by large connecting regions. The connecting region in factor V
is 836 amino acids long and is located between amino acids 710
and 1,545. This region is characterized by numerous N-linked
oligosaccharide chains and a high content of Thr and Ser. It also
contains two tandem repeats of 17 amino adds and 31 tandem
repeats of nine amino acids (see Fig. 3-8). The latter repeats
have a consensus sequence of [TNP]LSPDLSQT. The connecting region in factor V shows no similarity in amino acid sequence
to that in human factor VIII. Interestingly, chimeric cDNA expression constructs in which the connecting regions of factor V
and factor VIII were exchanged show that sequences within the
factor V connecting region increase the expression of the factor
VIII chimera and its corresponding mRNA by twofold in COS-
1 cells (112). In another study, the connecting region or B-
domain of factor V did not require the chaperone proteins
calnexin or calreticulin for efficient secretion, whereas the connecting region or B-domain of factor VIII was required for both
chaperone protein binding and proper secretion of factor VIII
from a Chinese hamster ovary (CHO) cell line (113). The third
A-domain in factor V, as well as factor VIII is followed by two
C-domains. Each of these C-domains is approximately 150
amino acids long. Their amino acid sequence identity with each
other is 35% to 50%.

The cDNA for factor V is approximately 7 kb in size (108).
It codes for a leader peptide of 28 amino acids and a mature
protein of 2,196 amino acids. The 3′ noncoding sequence also
contains the typical sequence of AATAAA that functions as a
polyadenylation signal (19). Little is known at the present
time regarding the transcriptional regulation of this gene.

The gene coding for human factor V is located on chromosome lq21-35 within 300 kb of the genes for the selectin family
of leukocyte adhesive molecules (114,115). The factor V gene
spans more than 80 kb of DNA and consists of 25 exons (116).
The exons range in size from 72 to 2,820 bp, whereas the 24 introns range in size from 400 bp to more than 11 kb of DNA.

The organization of the gene for human factor V shows remarkable similarity to that of human factor VIII. The latter
gene, however, contains one additional exon (i.e., 26 rather
than 25). The gene for factor VIII is also much larger than the
gene for factor V, being approximately 180 kb in size. A comparison of the genomic DNA sequences for factor V and factor VIII indicated that 21 of the intron–exon boundaries occur
at exactly the same location in the amino acid sequences of the
two genes (see Fig. 3-9) (116). Of particular interest, the connecting region of the genes coding for both factors V and VIII
are both coded by one very large exon. In factor V, this exon is
located between the twelfth and thirteenth introns, whereas in
factor VIII it is between the thirteenth and fourteenth introns.
In view of the great similarity between the amino acid sequence
and gene organization of factor V and factor VIII, it is clear
that these two proteins, as well as ceruloplasmin, evolved from
a common ancestor.

Recently, a homozygous factor $V_{Leiden}$ mutation (A for G at
nt 1691) has been shown to cause activated protein C resistance and is the major known cause of hereditary thrombophilia (117,118). This mutation results in the replacement of Gln
for Arg at amino acid residue 506 and disrupts the cleavage
site for the inactivation of factor Va by activated protein C
(119). Accordingly, the factor $V_{Leiden}$ mutation produces a cofactor, which cannot be completely inactivated by the activated
protein C complex. This leads to a continued procoagulant activity of this cofactor that confers a lifelong risk of thrombosis.

**TABLE 3-7**

**INTRON–EXON SPLICE JUNCTION SEQUENCES IN THE GENE FOR HUMAN PROTHROMBIN**

| Intron | Exon \| 5′ Intron 3′ \| (Splice junction sequences) | Exon |
|---|---|---|
| A | ATG \| GTAAGG—CCACCGCCTTTACAG | T |
| B | ACG \| GTGAGC—GCCCTTGITTTTCAG | G |
| C | CAG \| GTGAGC—CTGGGTCTTTTCCAG | C |
| D | AAG \| GTGAGC—GTGGGGTCTCCGCAG | G |
| E | TGA \| GTGAGT—AATTTCCTCTTCCAG | A |
| F | GTG \| GTAGGC—CCCCTCACCCACCAG | G |
| G | GTG \| GTGAGC—CCTGGGTCCCAACAG | A |
| H | CAG \| GTGAGG—TGGCTTGCTCTGCAG | A |
| I | TTG \| GTGTGT—TGCTGCCCCTCCCAG | G |
| J | AAG \| GTACAG—TTGGGGTCTCTGCAG | G |
| K | CAG \| GTGGGC—CTTCCTTCCCCAAAG | C |
| L | CTG \| GCAAGT—CTGTTCTCTTTCAAG | G |
| M | AAG \| GTAAGC—ATCTTTCTTCTTCAG | A |
| Consensus sequence[a] | CAAG \| GTAGAGT—TCTCTCTCTCTCTCTCTCTCTCNTCAG | G |

[a]From Degen SJF, Davie EW. Nucleotide sequence of the gene for human prothrombin. *Biochemistry* 1987;25:6165–6177, with permission.

The heterozygous state is common among whites, in whom the prevalence is up to 15%, whereas it has not been found among other human races (120).

## FACTOR VII

Factor VII is a single-chain glycoprotein ($M_r$ 50,000) that is synthesized in the liver and secreted into the blood as a zymogen composed of 416 amino acids (see Fig. 3-10) (121-124). It contains 10 $\gamma$-carboxyglutamic acid residues that are localized in the Gla domain of the protein (amino acids 1 to 35). These residues require vitamin K for their biosynthesis (125). Factor VII also contains a residue of $\beta$-hydroxyaspartic acid (amino acid 63), located in the first of the two EGF-like growth factor domains (126). The first EGF-like domain appears to be important in stabilizing the factor VIIa–tissue factor complex, as well as participating in calcium binding (127-129). The $\beta$-hydroxylation of the Asn63 is not essential for the coagulant activity of factor VIIa, because recombinant factor VII is not $\beta$-hydroxylated, but functions as well as the plasma-derived counterpart (130). Factor VIIa has another potential carbohydrate attachment site located at Asn322. The first EGF-like domain also contains novel O-linked carbohydrates at residues Ser52 and Ser60 (131-133). The Ser52 is O-glycosylated being linked to either a disaccharide (Xyl-Glc) or a trisaccharide ($Xyl_2$-Glc), in approximately equal amounts. The Ser60 contains one residue that is conjugated to fucose by O-glycosylation. Recombinant factor VII/VIIa missing either one or both O-linked Ser residues exhibits decreased tissue factor binding but similar calcium-binding relative to the wild type (129).

Factor VII is converted to a serine protease called factor VIIa by minor proteolysis. This protein, however, has little if any physiologic activity until it combines with tissue factor. The factor VIIa–tissue factor complex then converts factor X to factor Xa in the presence of phospholipids and calcium ions (1).

```
                                                      -16                     -4     -1  +1
Prothrombin  M A H V R G L Q L P G C L A L A A L C S L V H S Q H - - - V F L A P Q Q A R S L L Q R V R R   A
Factor VII   M V S Q A L R L L C L L L G L Q G C L A A - - - - - - - - V F V T Q E E A H G V L H R R R R   A
Factor IX    M Q R V N M I M A E S P G L I T I C L L G Y L L S A E C T V F L D H E N A N K I L N R P K R   Y
Factor X     M G R P L H L V L L S A S L A G L L L L G E S - - - - - - L F I R R E Q A N N I L A R V T R   A
Protein C    M W Q L T S L L L F V A T W G I S G T P A P L D S - - - - V F S S S E R A H Q V L R I R K R   A
Protein S    M R V L G G R C G A P L A C L L L V L P V S E A - - - - - N L L S K Q Q A S Q V L V R K R R   A
Protein Z    M A G C V P L L Q G L V L V L A L H R V E P S - - - - - - V F L P A S K A N D V L V R W K R   A
```

FIGURE 3-6. Prepro leader sequence of the vitamin K–dependent human plasma proteins. The putative hydrophobic core of each signal sequence is *boxed*. Highly conserved and homologous amino acid residues within the propeptide region are also *boxed*. Numbering is relative to the mature amino-termini of the proteins.

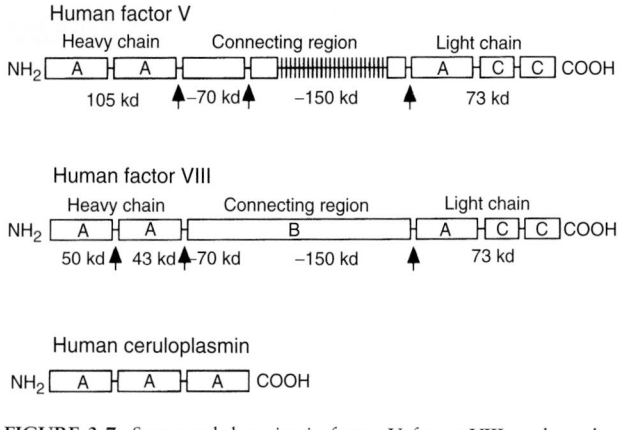

**FIGURE 3-7.** Structural domains in factor V, factor VIII, and ceruloplasmin. Thrombin cleavage is indicated by *solid arrows*. Molecular weight is based on SDS-PAGE and may not be completely accurate, due in part to the presence of carbohydrate. The identity of the domains is indicated by letters A, B, and C inside *boxes*. The 31 tandem repeats in the connecting region of factor V have a consensus sequence of [T,N,P] LSPDLSQT and are indicated by *vertical bars*. The A-domains in factor V correspond approximately to amino acids 1 through 331, 337 through 711, and 1,649 through 2,196. The C-domains in factor VIII correspond approximately to amino acids 2,020 through 2,172 and 2,173 through 2,332. The A-domains in ceruloplasmin correspond approximately to amino acids 1 through 338, 348 through 699, and 711 through 1,047. The amino acids corresponding to the heavy chain region and light chain region of factors V and VII also are indicated.

Factor VIIa also converts factor IX to factor IXa in the presence of tissue factor and calcium ions (129). Whereas it is controversial which of these two activation reactions is more important under physiologic conditions, recent *in vitro* experiments evaluating the initiation phase of blood coagulation with ultrasensitive fluorescent markers have demonstrated that factor Xa is generated almost exclusively by the factor VIIa–tissue factor complex during the initiation phase (135).

The cDNA and gene for factor VII have been isolated, and their sequence determined (90,136). The gene spans approximately 12.8 kb and consists of eight exons interrupted by seven introns. The positions of the introns with respect to the amino acid sequence are almost exactly the same as the genes coding for the other vitamin K–dependent proteins (Fig. 3-10 and Table 3-6). The types of the intron–exon boundaries are also the same as the other vitamin K–dependent proteins. The gene coding for factor VII also contains five regions of tandem repetitive sequences, and more than a quarter of the intron sequences consist of minisatellite DNA sequences, which vary in the number of copies among individuals (137).

Genetic defects leading to an abnormal factor VII have recently been identified (138). These include a replacement of Arg304 or Arg353 with Gln, resulting in reduced clotting activity (139,140). Loss of these positively charged residues presumably leads to a conformational change near the catalytic site of factor VIIa. A substitution of Phe38 to Ser (F328S) known as factor VII Central results in reduced tissue factor binding and impairs the activation of factors IX and X (141). The factor VII variant Gln-100 to Arg (Q110R) is likewise characterized by reduced tissue factor binding and procoagulant function (142). Mutations and polymorphisms that affect circulating factor VII blood levels have also been reported to occur in the 5'-flanking sequences of the factor VII gene. A polymorphism originating from a decanucleotide (CCTATATC-CT), inserted at position −323 relative to the first Met initiating codon, results in a modest reduction in factor VII levels without clinical bleeding (143). Substitution of G for T at nucleotide −61 disrupts an HNF-4 binding site in the factor VII

| | | | | | | | | | | |
|---|---|---|---|---|---|---|---|---|---|---|
| | 1139 | P | T | D | I | S | Q | M | S | P |
| | 1148 | S | S | E | H | E | V | W | Q | T |
| 1 | 1157 | V | I | S | P | D | L | S | Q | V |
| 2 | 1166 | T | L | S | P | E | L | S | Q | T |
| 3 | 1175 | N | L | S | P | D | L | S | H | T |
| 4 | 1184 | T | L | S | P | E | L | I | Q | R |
| 5 | 1193 | N | L | S | P | A | L | G | Q | M |
| 6 | 1202 | P | I | S | P | D | L | S | H | T |
| 7 | 1211 | T | L | S | P | D | L | S | H | T |
| 8 | 1220 | T | L | S | L | D | L | S | Q | T |
| 9 | 1229 | N | L | S | P | E | L | S | Q | T |
| 10 | 1238 | N | L | S | P | A | L | G | Q | M |
| 11 | 1247 | P | L | S | P | D | L | S | H | T |
| 12 | 1256 | T | I | S | L | D | F | S | Q | T |
| 13 | 1265 | N | L | S | P | E | L | S | H | M |
| 14 | 1274 | T | L | S | P | E | L | S | Q | T |
| 15 | 1283 | N | L | S | P | A | L | G | Q | M |
| 16 | 1292 | P | I | S | P | D | L | S | H | T |
| 17 | 1301 | T | L | S | L | D | F | S | Q | T |
| 18 | 1310 | N | L | S | P | E | L | S | Q | T |
| 19 | 1319 | N | L | S | P | A | L | G | Q | M |
| 20 | 1328 | P | L | S | P | D | P | S | H | T |
| 21 | 1337 | T | L | S | L | D | L | S | Q | T |
| 22 | 1346 | N | L | S | P | E | L | S | Q | T |
| 23 | 1355 | N | L | S | P | D | L | S | E | M |
| 24 | 1364 | P | L | F | A | D | L | S | Q | I |
| 25 | 1373 | P | L | T | P | D | L | D | Q | M |
| 26 | 1382 | T | L | S | P | D | L | G | E | T |
| 27 | 1391 | D | L | S | P | N | F | G | Q | M |
| 28 | 1400 | S | L | S | P | D | L | S | Q | V |
| 29 | 1409 | T | L | S | P | D | I | S | D | T |
| 30 | 1418 | T | L | L | P | D | L | S | Q | I |
| 31 | 1427 | S | P | P | P | D | L | D | Q | I |
| | 1436 | F | Y | P | S | E | S | S | Q | S |
| | 1445 | L | L | L | Q | E | F | N | E | S |
| | 1454 | F | P | Y | P | D | L | G | Q | M |
| | 1463 | P | S | P | S | S | P | T | L | N |

|  |  |  |  |  |  |  |  |  |  |
|---|---|---|---|---|---|---|---|---|---|
| | | | | | | | | T | |
| **CONSENSUS** | N | L | S | P | D | L | S | Q | T |
| | | | | | | | | P | |

**FIGURE 3-8.** Thirty-one tandem repeats of a nine amino acid sequence in the connecting region of factor V. The consensus sequence for the nine amino acid repeats is shown (**bottom**). Residues present in the consensus sequence are enclosed in *shaded boxes*. (From Mount SM. A catalogue of splice junction sequences. *Nucleic Acids Res* 1982; 10:459, with permission.)

promoter and results in factor VII deficiency (see subsequent text) (144).

The structure of the mRNA for human factor VII has been characterized as a cDNA (136). It contains approximately 2,450 nucleotides that code for a prepro leader sequence of

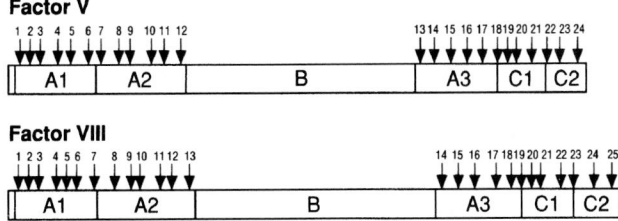

**Factor V**

1 2 3  4 5 6 7  8 9  10 11 12

| A1 | A2 | B | | A3 | C1 | C2 |

13 14 15 16 17 18 19 20 21 22 23 24

**Factor VIII**

1 2 3  4 5 6 7  8  9 10 11 12 13

| A1 | A2 | B | | A3 | C1 | C2 |

14 15 16 17 18 19 20 21 22 23 24 25

**FIGURE 3-9.** Location of the introns in the genes coding for factors V and VIII. The 24 introns in factor V and the 25 introns in factor VIII are shown with *vertical arrows*. The positions of A-, B-, and C-domains in the two proteins also are shown. (From Foster DC, Rudinski MS, Schach BG, et al. Propeptide of human protein C is necessary for gamma-carboxylation. *Biochemistry* 1987;26:7003; and Radcliffe R, Nemerson Y. Mechanism of activation of bovine factor VII: products of cleavage by factor Xa. *J Biol Chem* 1976;251:4797, with permission.)

38 amino acids and the 406 amino acids present in the mature protein circulating in blood (Fig. 3-10). A noncoding region of 1,026 nucleotides plus a poly(A) tail follows the stop codon of TAG. The noncoding region also contains the polyadenylation recognition sequence of AATAAA, which is located 40 nucleotides upstream from the poly(A) tail (19).

A second clone has also been identified for human factor VII, containing a prepro leader sequence of 60 amino acids (136). This leader sequence contains an additional 22 amino acids inserted between Val at −17 and Ala at −18 in the 38–amino acid prepro leader sequence. It has been confirmed that these 22 amino acids are encoded by an additional exon in intron A, suggesting that the two mRNA species have resulted from an alternative splicing (90). The removal of the prepro leader sequence requires signal peptidase in addition to a second processing protease that cleaves the peptide bond following the arginine at position −1 (96).

The essential transcriptional regulatory elements in the 5′-flanking region of the factor VII gene have been characterized (Fig. 3-15). The absence of a CCAAT box in the factor VII promoter contrasts with the promoter structures of factor IX, which has a functional CCAAT box and factor X, which contains a putative CCAAT box that binds the ubiquitous transcription factor NF-Y (145-147). The major transcription start site for factor VII is located approximately 50 bp upstream from the first initiation Met and is close to the binding sites for an Sp1-like transcription factor and HNF-4 (148,149). The G-C rich Sp1-like site is located at −100 to −94 whereas the HNF-4 site is located at −63 to −58. The factor VII HNF-4 recognition sequence, ACTTTG is also present in the promoters for factor X and factor IX. A naturally occurring mutation in the factor IX HNF-4 site causes the hemophilia B Leyden phenotype (see subsequent text), whereas a similar mutation in the factor VII promoter causes lifelong bleeding and virtually no detectable factor VII (144,146).

The conversion of human factor VII to factor VIIa occurs in the presence of thrombin, factor IXa, factor Xa, and factor XIIa (122,123,150-153). The activation is due to the cleavage of a single peptide bond (Arg152-I1e) (Fig. 3-10). Evidence also indicates that factor VIIa can be generated by an autocatalytic mechanism, and this mechanism may play an important role in the initiation of the extrinsic pathway of coagulation (154-156). This results in the formation of factor VIIa composed of a light chain (152 amino acids) and a heavy chain (254 amino acids), held together by a single disulfide bond between Cys135 and Cys462. The light chain contains the Gla domain followed by the two epidermal growth factor (EGF) domains, whereas the heavy chain contains the catalytic domain with the active-site residues of His193, Asp242, and Ser344.

Pharmaceutical preparations of recombinant factor VIIa are available in Europe and are being investigated for FDA approval in the United States. These preparations, NovoSeven and Novostase, are manufactured by Novo Nordisk, Denmark. In clinical studies, recombinant factor VIIa has the ability to bypass factor VIII and IX inhibitors, as well as partially correcting hemostasis in patients with other coagulopathies (157,158).

Factor VII is highly homologous in its amino acid sequence and gene organization with the other vitamin K–dependent proteins, including factor IX, factor X, and protein C. Accordingly, the vitamin K–dependent proteins represent another family of proteins that have evolved from a common ancestor by gene duplication and exon shuffling.

# FACTOR VIII (ANTIHEMOPHILIC FACTOR)

Factor VIII ($M_r$ 330,000) is a glycoprotein that participates in the middle phase of the intrinsic pathway of blood coagulation (1). It is apparently synthesized primarily in the liver and secreted into plasma, where it circulates, in part, as a complex with von Willebrand factor (VWF) (159). Factor VIII functions as a cofactor in blood coagulation in that it accelerates the conversion of factor X to factor Xa in the presence of factor IXa, calcium, and phospholipid. Factor VIII must undergo minor proteolysis by thrombin or some other serine protease before it shows cofactor activity (160–162).

Although factor VIII is synthesized as a single polypeptide chain, it circulates in plasma primarily as a two-chain molecule. This is due to the cleavage of the peptide bond at Arg1648 by a protease(s) during biosynthesis and secretion or during circulation of the molecule in plasma (see Fig. 3-11) (163,164). The coagulant activity of factor VIII as a cofactor requires additional minor proteolysis by thrombin or some other protease. This proteolitic cleavage occurs primarily at Arg740, giving rise to a heavy chain (amino acids 1 to 740) and a light chain (1,649 to 2,332); these two chains are apparently held together by calcium. The connecting polypeptide fragment (amino acids 741 to 1,648), also called the B-domain, is rich in carbohydrate and is split out by this proteolytic cleavage. Additional cleavages occur at Arg372 in the heavy chain and Arg1689 in the light chain (see Fig. 3-12). Precisely which cleavage(s) is responsible for the activation and inactivation of factor VIII by thrombin is unclear at present.

Factor VIII contains 25 potential carbohydrate attachment sites linked to asparagine. These potential N-linked carbohydrate chains are present primarily in the connecting region between the heavy and light chains generated by thrombin (Figs. 3-11 and 3-12). The presence of O-linked carbohydrate chains has not been established.

Six tyrosine sulfation sites are predicted in the factor VIII molecule, including Tyr346 in the 50-kDa fragment of the light chain; Tyr718, 719, and 723 in the 43-kDa fragment of the light chain; and Tyr1664 and 1680 in the heavy chain. Tyrosine residues in the light chain are partially sulfated in recombinant factor VIII expressed in CHO cells and the sulfation of these residues does not influence the coagulant activity of factor VIII (165). Recombinant factor VIII expressed in COS-1 cells have all six tyrosine residues sulfated (166). Both the tyrosine residues in the heavy chain are completely sulfated in all preparations of recombinant factor VIII and sulfation of Tyr1680 has been shown to be essential for the binding of factor VIII to VWF (166,167).

The mRNA for human factor VIII is approximately 9,000 nucleotides long and codes for a leader sequence of 19 amino acids and a mature protein of 2,302 amino acids (163,164,168,169). The mature polypeptide chain ending in tyrosine is followed by a stop codon of TGA and 1,802 nucleotides of noncoding sequence. A polyadenylation or processing site of AATAAA is present 19 nucleotides upstream from the polyadenylation signal (19).

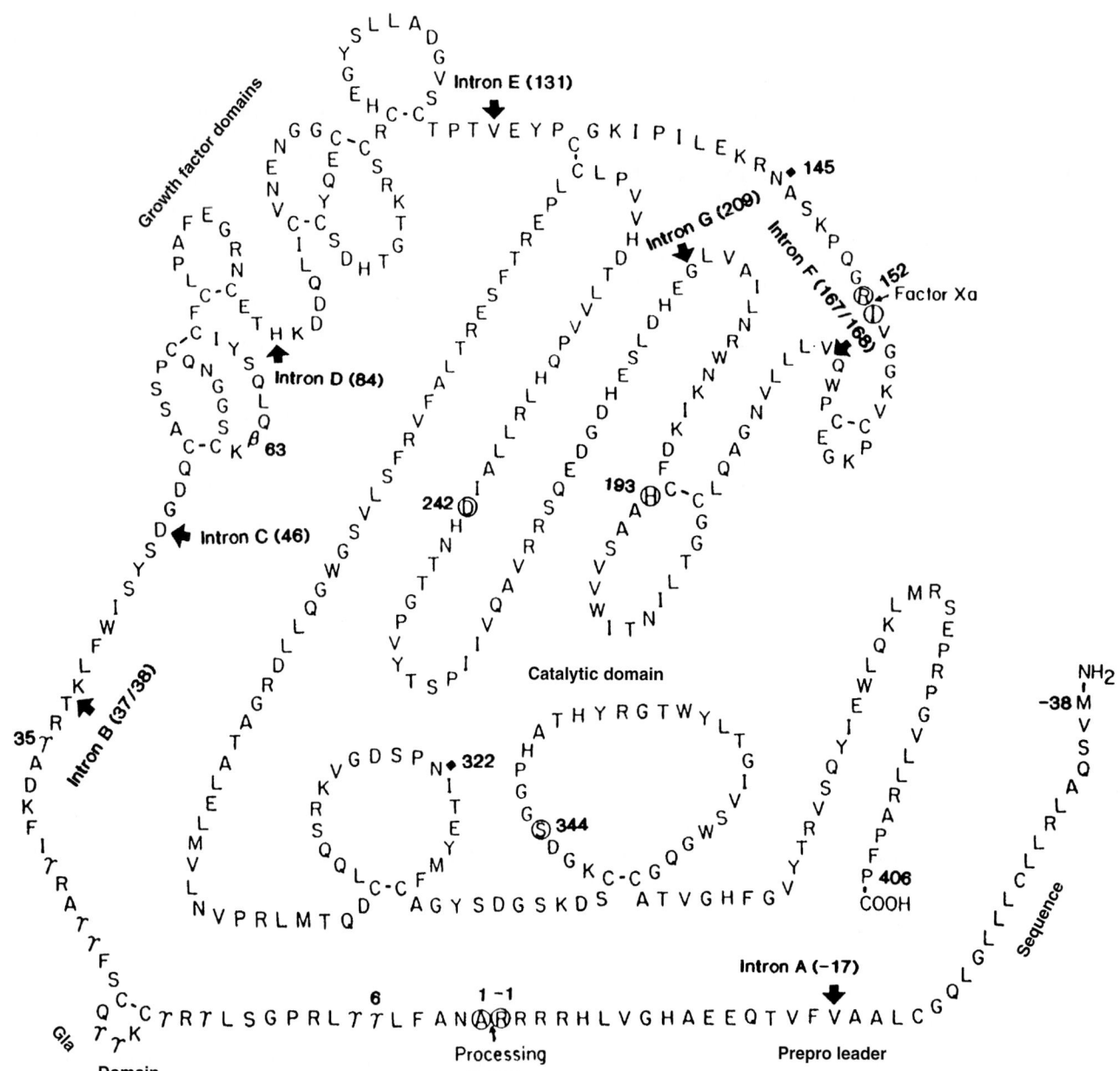

**FIGURE 3-10.** Amino acid sequence and tentative structure for human prepro factor VII. The prepro leader sequence (numbered −38 to −1) is removed during biosynthesis by signal peptidase and a processing protease that hydrolyzed the R–A bond between −1 and 1. The single cleavage site after factor VII is converted to factor VIIa by factor Xa is shown by a *solid arrow*. The Gla domain and potential growth factor domains are located within residues 1 through 152, which constitute the light chain of factor VIIa. The heavy chain or catalytic domain contains 254 residues, including the three principal amino acids participating in catalysis. These amino acids (H193, D242, and S344) are *circled*. Two potential carbohydrate-binding sites are shown by *solid diamonds*. The proposed disulfide bonds have been placed by analogy to those established in bovine prothrombin and epidermal growth factor. The single-letter code for amino acids is given in Figure 3-5; b, b-hydroxyaspartic acid.

The amino acid sequence of factor VIII as predicted by the cDNA sequence contains two types of internal homology (162,163,167,168). The first internal homology consists of a triplicated sequence located at residues 1 to 329, 380 to 711, and 1,649 to 2,019 (Figs. 3-7 and 3-11). These repeated sequences are approximately 30% homologous with each other. The second and third repeats in this triplication are separated by 983 amino acids that are very high in potential N-linked glycosylation sites. The second duplication of 150 amino acids is located in the carboxyl-terminal end of the molecule (residues 2,020 to 2,174 and 2,175 to 2,332). These two tandem repeats are approximately 40% homologous. As previously noted, a remarkable feature of the triplicated repeats is their high homology with factor V and plasma ceruloplasmin, a plasma protein that contains six copper atoms. Furthermore, the amino acids proposed for the binding of the ligand in ceruloplasmin are also present in similar positions in the first and third domain of factor VIII. Accordingly, two reports have confirmed that copper is bound to the processed and secreted factor VIII (170,171). However, it is unclear if this ligand binding stabilizes or is necessary for intersubunit interactions between the heavy and light chains.

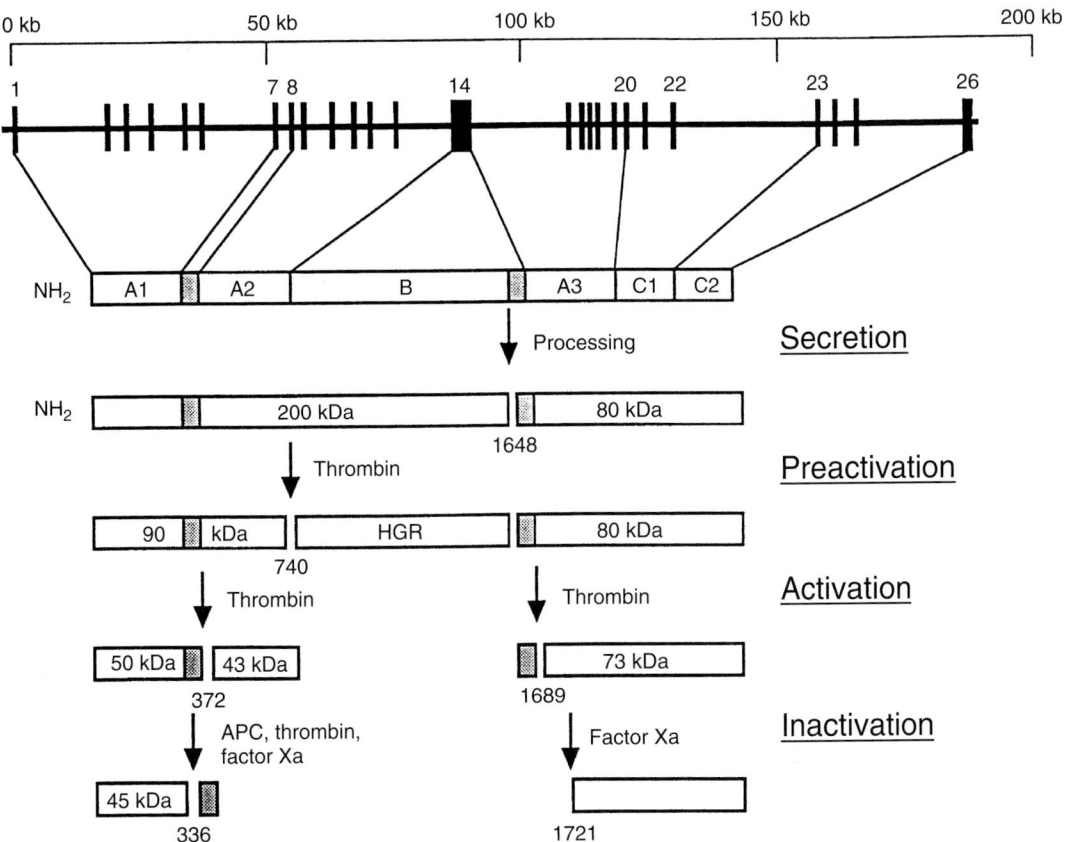

**FIGURE 3-11.** Gene organization and processing of factor VIII. Top line represents the factor VIII gene, showing the 26 exons (*vertical bars*). Factor VIII is synthesized as a single-chain precursor with domains A1, A2, B, A3, C1, and C2. On secretion from the cell, factor VIII is cleaved into a 200-kDa heavy chain and an 80-kDa light chain, apparently held together by calcium ions. The B-domain is heavily glycosylated. *Shaded regions* are rich in acidic residues. *Arrows* indicate the cleavage sites (numbered) by proteolysis during the activation and inactivation of the factor VIII molecules. kb, kilobase; kDa, kilodalton; HGR, heavily glycosylated region; APC, activated protein C.

The gene for factor VIII is located on the tip of the long arm of the X chromosome in region Xq28 (168). It contains approximately 186 kb of DNA and consists of 26 exons and 25 introns (163,164,168,169). The exons range in size from 69 to 3,106 nucleotides, whereas the introns vary in size from 200 nucleotides up to 32.4 kb. Six of the introns are very large and contain more than 14 kb of DNA and, as previously noted, the connecting region in the center of the protein is coded by one very large exon (exon 14, Fig. 3-11). Accordingly, approximately 5% of the gene is present in the exons and the remaining 95% is noncoding DNA. A start site for initiation of mRNA synthesis has been suggested from ribonuclease (RNase) mapping experiments (168). These data indicated that mRNA synthesis started most frequently at a G located 170 nucleotides upstream from the initiating methionine.

Interestingly, intron 22 of the factor VIII gene contains an independent gene oriented in the opposite direction (172). A transcript of 1.8 kb is present in many cells, and its cDNA isolated from a human liver library contains a long reading frame. A comparison of the genome and cDNA sequence has revealed that this independent gene within intron 22 itself contains no introns.

Like fibrinogen, factor VIII plasma levels increase dramatically during acute inflammatory events. Accordingly, there is considerable interest in characterizing the regulatory mechanisms involved in transcription of the corresponding mRNA. The regulation of the transcription of factor VIII has been studied in hepatocytes (173,174). Although factor VIII mRNA has been found in various nonhepatic tissues, the observation

that liver transplant results in the correction of the coagulopathy characterized by hemophilia A suggests that the liver is the major site of factor VIII synthesis (175). Full promoter activity was found to be located within the 300 bp from the initiation codon. The factor VIII regulatory region is complex in that DNA-protein binding studies show the presence of 19 binding sites distributed along the region from $-1175$ to $-9$ bp, many of which are currently being investigated (173). The functional *cis*-acting elements within the fully active factor VIII promoter that have been identified include HNF-1 ($-64$ to $-35$ bp), NF$\kappa$B ($-123$ to $-79$ bp), C/EBP$\alpha$ ($-203$ to $-149$ bp), C/EBP$\beta$ ($-275$ to $-252$ bp), and HNF-4 ($-312$ to $-279$ bp) (173,174,176). A link between inflammation and factor VIII transcription has been suggested by observations showing that the stimulation of cultured human hepatocytes with the cytokine IL-6 results in a sixfold increase of factor VIII mRNA (177). Mutation of the putative TATA sequence GATAAA ($-201$ to $-196$ bp) to GACCGA resulted in only a twofold decrease in promoter activity. Like many other genes expressed in the liver, the HNF-1 binding site is essential for factor VIII transcription in HepG2 cells (173).

A vast number of genomic DNAs from patients with hemophilia A have been analyzed using a variety of methods (178,179). These include Southern blotting, oligonucleotide hybridization, direct nucleotide sequencing, chemical or enzymatic cleavage of fragments, denaturing gradient gel electrophoresis, and single-strand gel electrophoresis. Most of these methods involve *in vitro* amplification of the genomic DNA by the polymerase chain reaction. It is particularly difficult to analyze the gene

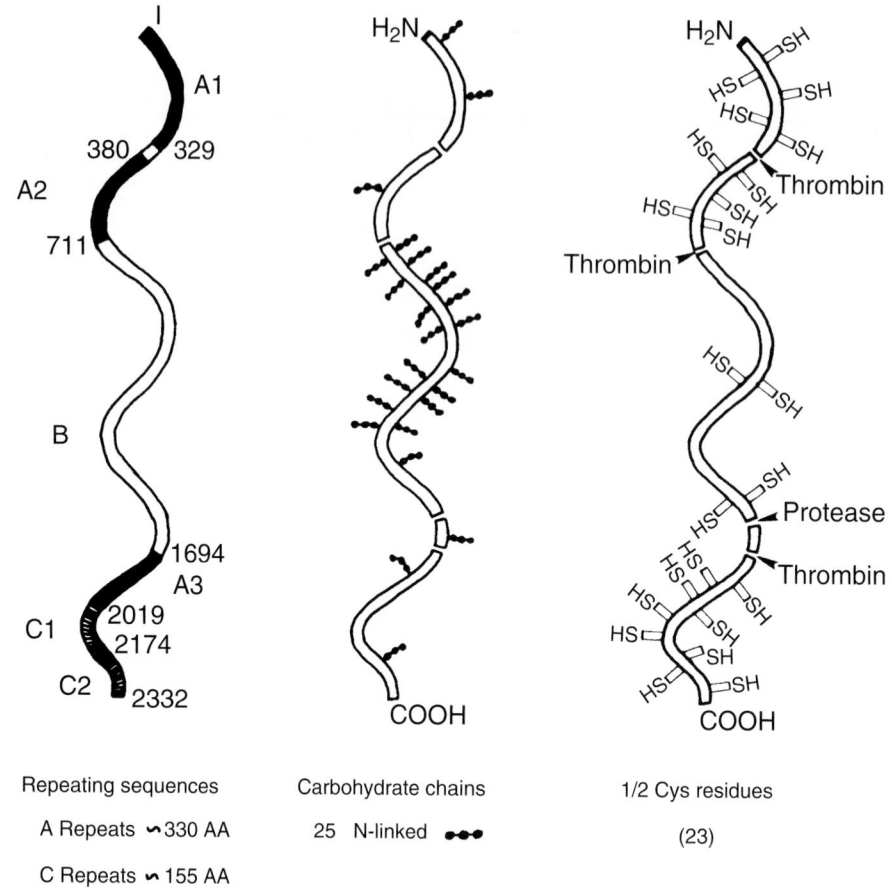

**FIGURE 3-12.** Repeating sequences, carbohydrate chains, and principal thrombin cleavage sites in human factor VIII (139,145). The three triplications (1 to 329, 380 to 711, and 1,649 to 2,019) are shown with *solid bars*, and the two duplications (2,020 to 2,174 and 2,175 to 2,332) are shown with *shaded bars* in the figure on the left. The potential N-carbohydrate attachment sites are shown by *connected dots* in the middle figure, and the thrombin or protease cleavage sites are shown by *arrowheads* in the figure on the right, along with the 23 half-Cys residues.

for human factor VIII because of its large size, complex genomic structure, heterogeneous mutations among individual cases, and high frequency of *de novo* mutations (approximately one third of patients are sporadic) (178,179).

Gross rearrangements of the gene for factor VIII, including deletions and insertions, have been found in 1% to 5% of the hemophiliacs studied (180–182). Accordingly, most of the defects in the gene for factor VIII are caused by point mutations. Most deletions and nonsense mutations (which create termination codons) lead to truncated molecules of factor VIII and cause severe hemophilia. In one case, a patient exhibited moderately severe hemophilia caused by an in-frame deletion of exon 22 encoding 52 amino acids (181,182). Most deletions appear to be the result of nonhomologous recombination between dissimilar sequences in which short sequence homologies facilitate end-joining reactions (183). Deletion breakpoints, however, are not clustered in particular regions of the factor VIII gene (180). Deletions of the factor VIII gene are also associated with a higher risk (approximately fivefold) of developing inhibitors, compared with other severe hemophiliacs without gene deletion (180).

Insertions of the transposable line 1 repetitive sequence into exon 14 have been found in two sporadic cases (184). In each case, the inserted sequence contained most of the second open reading frame for a reverse transcriptase and poly(A) sequence; moreover, a target-site duplication at the 5′ and 3′ ends flanked the insertion (185). A smaller insertion of a 5′-truncated line 1

element has also been found in a patient with hemophilia; however, it does not seems to be the cause of hemophilia A (185). A putative progenitor of this active transposable element has been isolated (186). Most cases of moderately and mildly severe hemophilia are caused by single-point mutations, which lead to impaired biosynthesis, secretion, and stability of the molecule (187). Only a few mutations have proved to be causative for functional abnormalities of factor VIII protein. These include substitutions of Arg372 and Arg1689 by Cys or His and of Tyr1680 by Phe (188–190). The mutation at residue 372 results in a molecule that is resistant to the thrombin cleavage required for activation (191,192). Tyr1680, as well as Arg1689, is included in a putative binding site of the light chain for VWF (193). As previously noted, sulfation of this residue is essential for the binding of factor VIII to VWF, which in turn prevents the degradation of factor VIII by proteolytic enzymes (165,166).

Numerous other mutations result in hemophilia A, but the precise mechanisms for the deficiency or dysfunction of the factor VIII molecule have not been identified. A substantial number of point mutations also occur at the CpG dinucleotides (194,195). These tend to be hot spots for mutations, because CpG dinucleotides provide a preferred site for cytosine methylation and 5-methylcytosine is prone to mutate to thymidine by deamination (195). Because of the extreme heterogeneity of defects in the factor VIII molecule, intragenic DNA polymorphisms, such as the BclI site in intron 18, the

XbaI site in intron 22, and a hypervariable dinucleotide repeat in intron 13, will continue to be useful in a pedigree analysis for genetic prediction (188,196).

Factor VIII, like factor IX, has been expressed in cultured mammalian cells (164,169). One of the expression vectors for factor VIII was constructed in a plasmid that included a tandem SV40 early promoter/adenovirus-2 major late promoter, followed by the cDNA for factor VIII and the hepatitis B virus surface antigen polyadenylation site (169). The plasmid also contained a murine dihydrofolate reductase cDNA transcribed by an SV40 early promoter to provide a selectable marker. The plasmid was transfected into hamster kidney cells by the calcium phosphate precipitation method to give cells that readily synthesized a 9-kb RNA and secreted factor VIII into the medium. The biologic properties of the secreted protein were characterized by its ability to reduce the clotting time of hemophilic plasma, its binding to VWF, its activation by thrombin, and its inactivation by activated protein C and antibodies directed toward factor VIII. Similar results were obtained after transfection of COS-1 cells with a slightly different mammalian expression vector (169). Accordingly, the preparation of factor VIII by methods of recombinant DNA technology for the routine treatment of patients with classic hemophilia has been accomplished. Kogenate (Bayer) and Recombinate (Baxter/Hyland) are two pharmaceutical preparations of recombinant factor VIII currently available in the United States to treat hemophilia A. Kogenate is produced in BHK cells and Recombinate is produced in CHO cells (197). Recombinant factor VIII lacking the B-domain has also been produced and is currently being used in phase II/III clinical trials (198).

Major progress is being made in the development of gene therapy for the treatment of hemophilia A. The entire factor VIII cDNA is too large to be effectively packaged into most viral vectors for gene transfer. Consequently, factor VIII cDNA with the B-domain deleted has been used (199). The ongoing research into this form of treatment continues to offer hope that someday gene therapy will make the use of exogenous factor VIII a thing of the past. This approach, however, is still plagued by the development of antibodies to factor VIII in patients with hemophilia A, as well as B.

# FACTOR IX

Factor IX and factor VIII are the two sex-linked proteins that participate in the coagulation cascade. The gene for factor IX, like factor VIII, is located on the distal region of the long arm of the X chromosome; no link, however, exists between the genes for these two proteins (200–203). The factor IX gene is in region Xq27 and is closely linked to the fragile X site (204).

Factor IX ($M_r$ 57,000) is a single-chain glycoprotein (17% carbohydrate) composed of 415 amino acids (see Fig. 3-13) (205–207). It is also a vitamin K–dependent protein and contains 12 residues of γ-carboxyglutamic acid (Gla domain) located in the amino-terminal region of the protein. The amino-terminal region of the protein also contains two potential EGF domains; as previously noted, these domains show considerable homology with the corresponding regions of factor VII, factor X, protein C, and protein S, as well as with EGF (208–211). The EGF domains are followed by an activation peptide and a catalytic domain. During the coagulation cascade, factor IX is cleaved at two internal arginine peptide bonds (Arg145–Ala and Arg180–Val), resulting in the formation of a light chain and a heavy chain; these two chains are held together by a disulfide bond (1,212). During the conversion to factor IXa, an activation glycopeptide of 35 amino acid residues is released.

The gene for human factor IX has been isolated and completely sequenced (72,91). It contains approximately 34 kb of DNA, including eight exons (I to VIII) and seven introns (A to G) located within the coding and 3′ noncoding region of the gene (Fig. 3-13). The eight exons range in size from 25 bp (exon III) to 1,935 bp (exon VIII). Exons I and II code for a prepro leader sequence and a Gla domain, whereas exons IV and V each code for EGF domains. The last three exons code for the activation peptide and the catalytic domain. The seven introns range in size from 188 nucleotides (intron B) to 9,473 nucleotides (intron F) (see Table 3-8). The introns are located in positions essentially identical to those in factor VII, factor X, and protein C (Table 3-6). The nucleotide sequences at the 5′ and 3′ splice junctions and the splice junction types are

## TABLE 3-8

LOCATION AND SIZE OF THE EXONS AND INTRONS IN THE GENE FOR HUMAN FACTOR IX

| Exon | Nucleotide positions[a] | Nucleotide length[a] (bp) | Amino acids[b] | Intron | Nucleotide positions | Nucleotide length (bp) |
|---|---|---|---|---|---|---|
| I | 1–117 | 117 | −46 to −17 | A | 118–6,325 | 6,206[c] |
| II | 6,326–6,489 | 164 | −46 to 37 | B | 6,490–6,677 | 188 |
| III | 6,678–6,702 | 25 | 38–47 | C | 6,703–10,391 | 3,689 |
| IV | 10,392–10,505 | 114 | 47–85 | D | 10,506–17,668 | 7,163 |
| V | 17,669–17,797 | 129 | 85–128 | E | 17,798–20,362 | 2,565 |
| VI | 20,363–20,565 | 203 | 128–195 | F | 20,566–30,038 | 9,473 |
| VII | 30,039–30,153 | 115 | 196–234 | G | 30,154–30,821 | 668 |
| VIII | 30,822–32,757 | 1,935 | 234–415 | — | — | — |

bp, base pair.
[a]Includes 30 nucleotides at the 5′ end and 1,390 nucleotides at the 3′ end that are not translated.
[b]Amino acids coded for each exon; negative numbers refer to amino acids in the prepro leader sequence.
[c]Includes the 50 extra nucleotides in the polymorphic DNA.
Reprinted from Yoshitake S, Schach BG, Foster DC, et al. Nucleotide sequence of the gene for human factor IX (antihemophilic factor B). *Biochemistry* 1985;24:3736–3750, with permission. Copyright 1985 American Chemical Society.

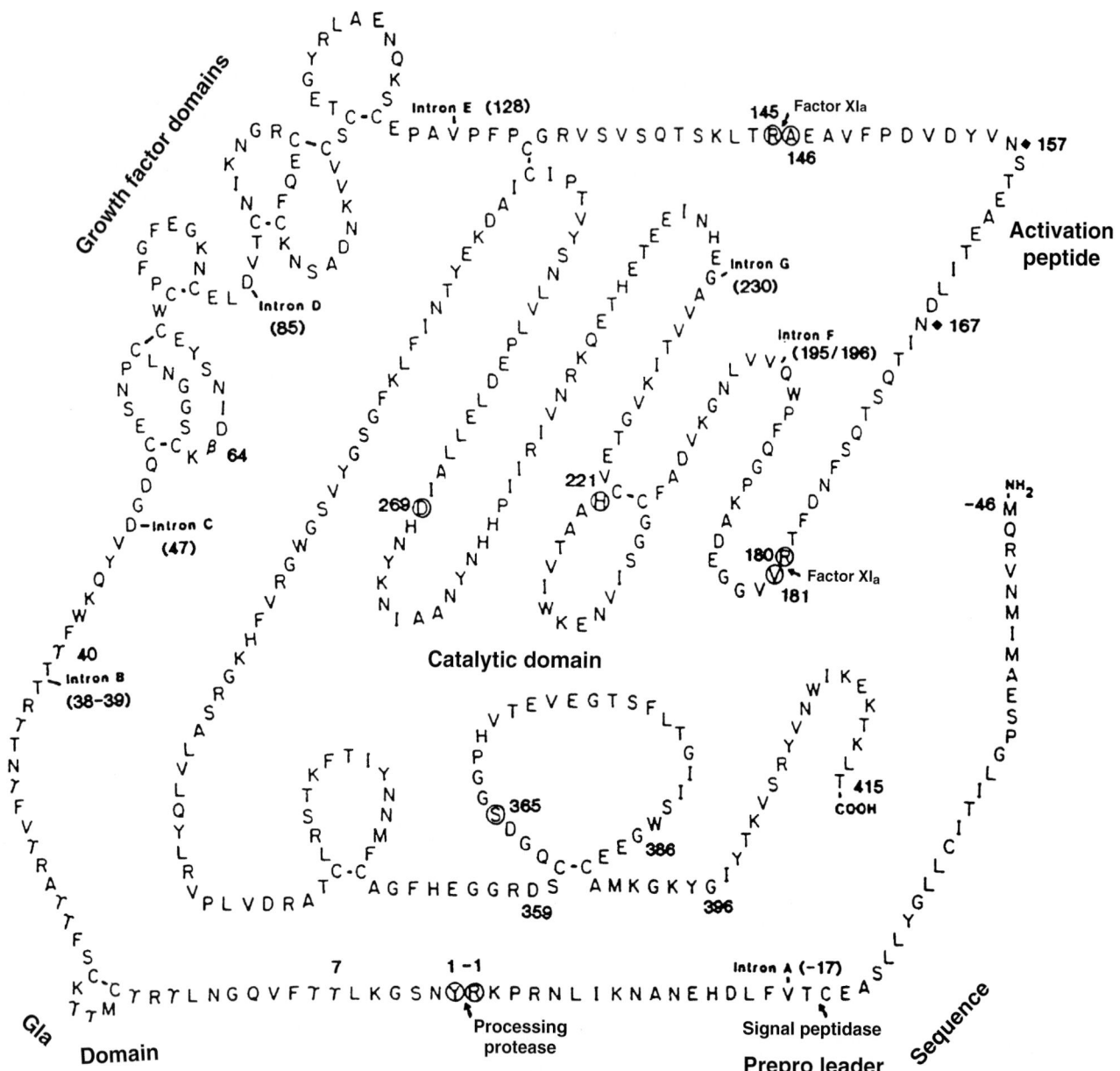

**FIGURE 3-13.** Amino acid sequence and tentative structure for human prepro factor IX show the location of the seven introns (A to G). The prepro leader sequence (numbered −46 to −1) is removed during biosynthesis by signal peptidase and a processing protease that hydrolyzes the R–Y bond between −1 and 1. The Gla domain and potential growth factor domains are located within residues 1 through 145, which constitute the light chain of factor IXa. The activation peptide of 35 residues is released from factor IX during its conversion to factor IXa by factor XIa. The amino acids at which this cleavage occurs (R–A and R–V) are *circled*. The serine protease or catalytic domain of factor IX contains 235 residues, including the three principal amino acids participating in catalysis. These three amino acids (H221, D269, and S365) also are *circled*. Two potential carbohydrate-binding sites in the activation peptide are shown by *solid diamonds*. The proposed disulfide bonds in factor IX have been placed by analogy to those in bovine prothrombin and epidermal growth factor. The single-letter code for amino acids is given in Figure 3-5; b, b-hydroxyaspartic acid.

shown in Table 3-9. They follow the typical consensus sequences of GT and AG located on the 5′ and 3′ ends of the boundary of each intron (50).

Initiation sites for the transcription of the gene for human factor IX have been examined by S1 nuclease mapping and primer extension studies. Originally, it was suggested that the initiation site for mRNA synthesis starts at an A 29 nucleotides upstream from the initiation methionine. Other studies, however, have indicated three major transcription sites, including +1, +4, and +30, as well as a minor site at +8 (213). Therefore, there may be considerable heterogeneity of transcription initiation, reflecting the absence of a well-defined or typical TATA-like promoter element in the 5′ end of the gene. The 5′ end of the gene also contains three Met codons (at −46, −41, and −39) for polypeptide initiation, but the Met at −39 is the only one conserved in the human, monkey, dog, and murine factor IX genes (214,215). This suggests that the Met at −39 is the most probable initiation site for human factor IX biosynthesis under physiologic conditions.

**TABLE 3-9**

INTRON–EXON SPLICE JUNCTION IN THE GENE FOR HUMAN FACTOR IX

| | Splice junction sequences | | | Splice junction |
| Intron | Exon \| 5' | Intron | 3' \| Exon | type[a] |
|---|---|---|---|---|
| A | CAG \| GTTTGT | —TTTCAG | \| T | 1 |
| B | ACA \| GTGAGT | —TTATAG | \| A | 0 |
| C | TTG \| GTAAGC | —TCAAAG | \| A | 1 |
| D | TAG \| GTAAGT | —TTTTAG | \| A | 1 |
| E | CAG \| GTCATA | —TTCTAG | \| T | 1 |
| F | CAG \| GTACTT | —TCACAG | \| G | 0 |
| G | CAG \| GTAAAT | —TAATAG | \| G | 1 |
| Consensus sequence | CAAG \| GTAGAGT | —TCTCNTCAG | \| G | |

[a]Data from Mount SM. A catalogue of splice junction sequences. *Nucleic Acids Res* 1982;10:459.
Reprinted from Yoshitake S, Schach BG, Foster DC, et al. Nucleotide sequence of the gene for human factor IX (antihemophilic factor B). *Biochemistry* 1985;24:3736–3750, with permission. Copyright 1985 American Chemical Society.

The transcriptional regulation of the factor IX gene has been the most extensively studied of all the vitamin K–dependent coagulation factors (Fig. 3-13). This is because a rare variant of hemophilia B, the Leyden phenotype, has been described. Hemophilia B Leyden is characterized by spontaneous correction of severe childhood hemophilia B with the onset of puberty (216). The genetic defects that confer the factor IX$_{Leiden}$ phenotype have been found to be single nucleotide substitutions within a 54-bp region of the factor IX transcriptional promoter (217–222). The developmental timing of the expression of the factor IX gene characterized by these mutations suggests that the transcription of the factor IX gene is, in part, hormonally mediated. A consensus androgen response element (ARE) has been identified between nucleotides −36 and −17 of the factor IX promoter (223,224). This sequence overlaps a functional HNF-4 binding site. Interestingly, a substitution of C for G at −26 bp causes lifelong hemophilia B, presumably by disruption of the ARE, whereas substitutions at −21 and −20 bp (A,G or C for T in the sequence ACTTTG) result in disruption of the HNF-4 binding site and the Leyden phenotype (221–223). These data suggest that androgen binding can partially overcome the negative effect of impaired HNF-4 binding to the promoter. Other Leyden mutations include nucleotide substitutions at positions −6, −5, +8, and +13 relative to the transcription start site (225). These mutations correspond to a disruption in the proximal C/EBP binding site (+1 to +18 bp) and a disruption in the binding site of an uncharacterized transactivating regulatory factor (−15 to −1 bp) (218,226). Experiments investigating the molecular mechanisms explaining Leyden-specific mutations outside the putative ARE have identified interactions between C/EBP and the hormonally regulated transcription factors D-site binding protein (DBP) and hepatic leukemia factor (227–230). Accordingly, the hormonal sensitivity of the factor IX promoter may be mediated by both direct androgen receptor binding to the promoter and the indirect regulatory effects of androgen receptor on the expression of developmentally regulated transcription factors. The factor IX promoter is complex and includes a negative regulatory or silencer activity in the region spanning −1,700 to −1,400 bp (231). This region contains the short sequence ATCCTCTCC, which has been associated with the silencer activity in several genes expressed primarily in the liver (48).

Recently Kurachi et al. have discovered a molecular mechanism for the observed phenomenon of age-related increase in blood coagulation (232,233). Through careful analysis of the expression of human factor IX mRNA in transgenic mice, they have found that the factor IX gene contains two age-related stability elements (ASE) (232,233). A short sequence from −797 to −776 bp contains an enhancer-like ASE-5' element. The other ASE element, which confers increased mRNA stability, was found in the middle of the 3'-untranslated region in an extensive stretch of dinucleotide repeating structures.

The gene for factor IX contains four Alu sequences (91). The first is located in intron A, with the next three in intron F. A fifth Alu sequence is present in the 3'-flanking region of the gene, located approximately 230 nucleotides downstream from the poly(A) adenylation site. Each of the five Alu sequences contains short, direct flanking repeats ranging from 7 to 14 nucleotides long. The gene for factor IX contains other repetitive sequences, including a KpnI repetitive element. The first KpnI repeat is present in the 5' end of the gene and contains approximately 2,600 nucleotides. Another Kpn repeat of approximately 2,000 nucleotides is present within intron D, but the boundaries of this repeat are difficult to define.

Several polymorphic sites have been found in the gene for factor IX. A major polymorphic site involving a deletion of 50 nucleotides is present within intron A; this deletion occurs with a frequency of 0.25 in the healthy white population (234). A second reported polymorphic site is a TaqI site after the fourth exon in the gene (202,235). The presence or absence of this polymorphism gives rise to Taql fragments of 1,380 and 463 nucleotides or 1,843 nucleotides. The frequency for the TaqI polymorphic site was 0.29 when 49 unrelated French men and women were studied (202). A third polymorphic site has been observed in exon VI that codes for the activation peptide (236). This polymorphic site is caused by a change of a G to an A and results in the conversion of alanine 3 (GCT) to threonine (ACT). The threonine appears to be more prevalent in the general population, with a frequency perhaps as high as 0.8. A fourth polymorphic site is present in intron C in which a G has been changed to a C results in a loss of a recognition site for endonuclease XmnI (234). This gives rise to DNA fragments of 5,119 and 6,467 or 11,586 following digestion of normal genomic

DNA with endonuclease XmnI and Southern blotting. The frequency of the XmnI polymorphism was 0.29 in a group of 72 healthy unrelated whites. These various polymorphic sites have made it possible to establish methods for carrier detection for factor IX deficiencies.

At present, many factor IX abnormalities have been defined at the protein and gene level. Factor IX Chapel Hill is due to a substitution of a His for an Arg as position 145 (Fig. 3-13) (237). Accordingly, the cleavage of a critical Arg–Ala bond by factor XIa during the coagulation process is blocked. This reduces the specific activity of factor IX Chapel Hill to approximately 8% of normal. The mutation is most likely due to a change of a G (in CGT) to an A (in CAT) in exon VI. Another factor IX abnormality has been shown to be due to a point mutation that changes an essential G in a splice junction site to a T (238). This occurs on the 5′ end of intron F (Table 3-9). Accordingly, the exon–intron junction has been changed from GAG/GTACT to GAG/TTACT. A similar mutation in the GT of a donor splice sequence in the β-globin gene has been shown to result in β-thalassemia (239). No other considerable change was observed in the gene of this patient when the apparent promoter, exons, and the 5′ noncoding region were sequenced. This mutation in the splice junction site was not observed, however, in nine other patients with factor IX deficiency. Gene deletions have also been reported in four out of five patients with antibodies to factor IX (240). Two patients had deletions of more than 18 kb of DNA coding for factor IX, whereas a third patient had a deletion of more than 9 kb. The DNA of this patient, however, still contained a portion of the factor IX gene.

The mRNA for human factor IX is approximately 2,800 nucleotides long and includes 138 nucleotides that code for a prepro leader sequence of 46 amino acids and 1,245 nucleotides that code for 415 amino adds present in the mature protein circulating in plasma (Fig. 3-13) (72,91,204). The prepro leader sequence of 46 amino acids includes two additional methionines that could also generate a prepro leader sequence of 41 or 39 amino acids. It is unknown which of these start sites is used under physiologic conditions. The stop codon of TAA in the mRNA is followed by a rather long 3′ noncoding sequence of 1,387 nucleotides and a poly(A) tail. The processing or polyadenylation sequence of AATAAA is located 16 nucleotides upstream from the poly(A) tail.

The isolation of a cDNA coding for human factor IX has made it possible to express this protein in rat hepatoma cells, chick embryo fibroblasts, and BHK cells (241–243). In these experiments, approximately 50% of the secreted factor IX was biologically active when associated with factor IX–deficient plasma. The biosynthesis of factor IX required supplementation of the culture medium with vitamin K (1 to 10 μg per mL). Recombinant factor IX is now produced as Benefix (Genetics Institute, US) for use in the treatment of hemophilia B. The full-length cDNA for human factor IX is coexpressed with the processing enzyme furin in CHO cells (244). Recombinant factor IX has procoagulant function that is indistinguishable from plasma-derived factor IX and has been extensively characterized with respect to posttranslational modifications (245).

Over the past 5 years, significant advances have been made in the development of gene therapy for the treatment of hemophilia B. Although most of the gene delivery systems target the liver, other targets have included myoblasts, primary fibroblasts, keratinocytes, capillary endothelial cells, and hematopoietic stem cells (246–250). Several gene delivery systems have been used to deliver factor IX genes to a variety of cell types *in vitro* and *in vivo*. These include viral vectors derived from retroviruses, adenoviruses, and herpes simplex viruses, as well as nonviral vectors such as naked DNA, DNA protein complexes, and liposome-encapsulated DNA (251).

One successful preclinical study of gene transfer for hemophilia B was accomplished by infusion of an amphotrophic retroviral vector encoding canine factor IX cDNA into the Chapel Hill inbred strain of hemophilia B dogs after partial hepatectomy (252). In this model, plasma factor IX concentration increased from undetectable amounts to between 1 and 10 ng per mL (approximately 0.1% of normal) (253). Accordingly, the whole blood clotting time in these animals was decreased from a pretreatment time of 45 to 55 minutes to 15 to 25 minutes after viral infusion and remained at these reduced levels for 11 months. Further investigation into the field of gene therapy for the treatment of hemophilia B is ongoing.

# FACTOR X (STUART FACTOR)

Factor X ($M_r$ 58,800) is a vitamin K–dependent glycoprotein (15% carbohydrate) that participates in the middle phase of blood coagulation (1). Like many other blood coagulation proteins, it is synthesized in the liver and secreted into the plasma as a precursor to a serine protease. The human protein is composed of a light chain ($M_r$ 16,200) and a heavy chain ($M_r$ 42,000), held together by a single disulfide bond (see Fig. 3-14) (126,254). The amino acid sequences for the heavy and light chains of factor X have been established by amino acid sequence analysis and cDNA and genomic cloning (92,255–257). The light chain of human factor X contains 11 residues of γ-carboxyglutamic acid and one residue of β-hydroxyaspartic acid (residue 63) (255). It also contains two growth factor domains that have replaced the two kringle structures present in prothrombin (79,208,209,256,257). The heavy chain of factor X contains the catalytic domain of the protein (258). The heavy chain also contains carbohydrate, and in bovine factor X, it includes an N-linked (Asn36) as well as an O-linked (Thr300) carbohydrate chain (258).

In the blood coagulation cascade, the conversion of human factor X to factor Xa involves the cleavage of an alanine-isoleucine peptide bond in the heavy chain. This liberates a small activation peptide of 52 amino acids (Fig. 3-14) (254). In the intrinsic pathway of blood coagulation, this reaction is catalyzed by factor IXa in the presence of factor VIIIa, calcium ions, and phospholipid. This same peptide bond is also cleaved by factor VIIa in the presence of tissue factor in the extrinsic pathway of blood coagulation.

The gene for human factor X is located on chromosome 13 at q32-qter in approximately 27 kb of DNA (92,259). It is 2.8 kb downstream from the gene coding for factor VII (260). The gene for human factor X contains eight exons and seven introns. The introns are located between amino acid residues −17 (intron A), 37 and 38 (B), at residue 46 (C), and at residue 84 (D) between the two potential growth factor domains (Fig. 3-14 and Table 3-6). Intron E is located at residue 128 just after the second growth factor domain and just before the disulfide bond connecting the light and heavy chains. The last two introns (F and G) are located in the heavy chain or catalytic domain of the molecule and are present between residues 15 and 16 and at residue 55. The rest of the catalytic chain, in contrast with prothrombin, is free of introns.

The gene for factor X also contains several interspersed repetitive sequences within the introns, including members from the Alu, O, and KpnI families of repetitive sequence (92,148). Genetic defects of factor X have been determined for both its deficiencies and molecular abnormalities. The first patient identified with factor X deficiency was Rufus Stuart, who had a hereditary bleeding disorder originally identified by Lewis and Ferguson and later characterized by Hougie, Barrow, and Graham (261–263). Since that time, other genetic defects resulting in factor X deficiency have been found. These include partial

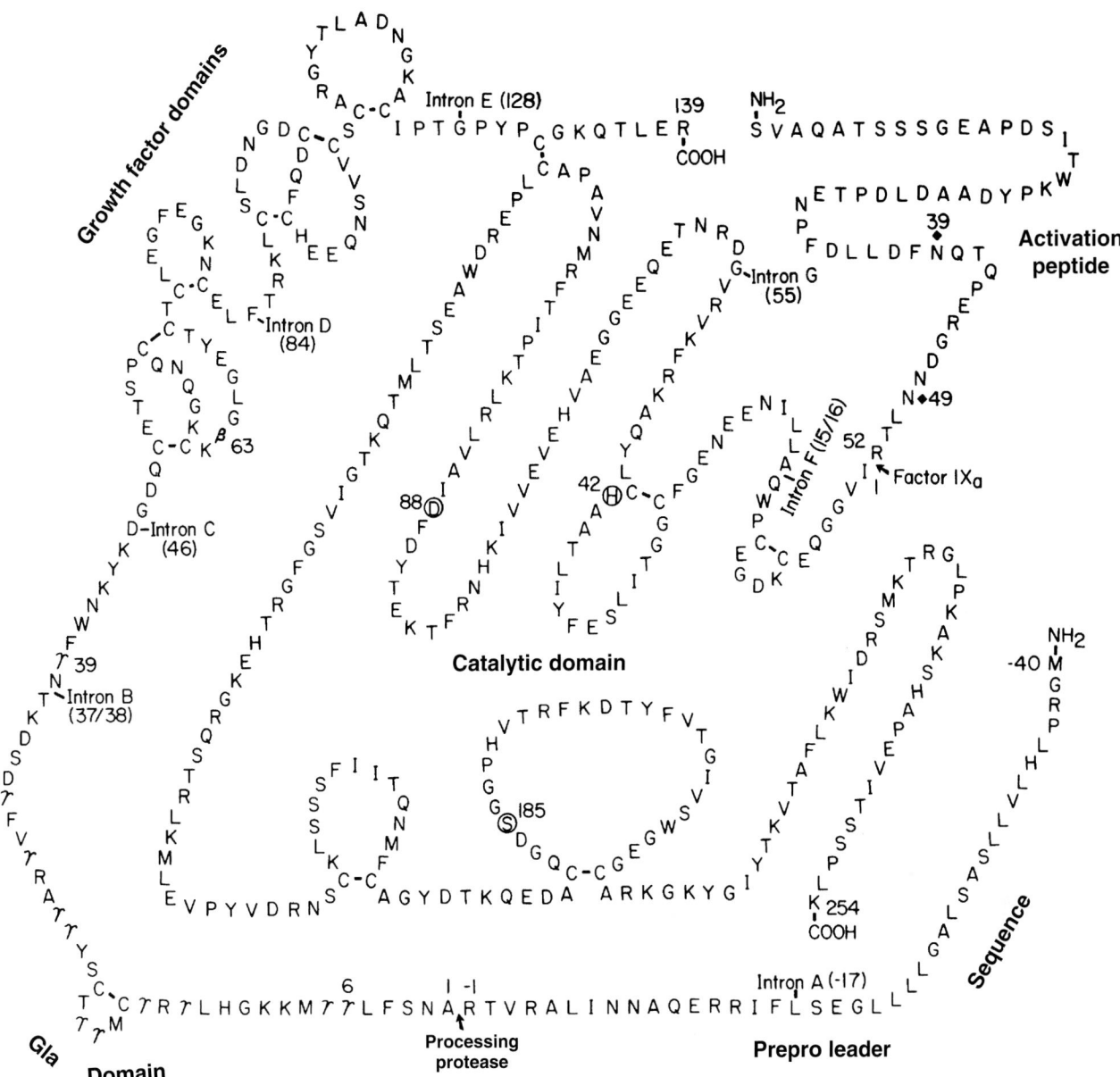

**FIGURE 3-14.** Amino acid sequence and tentative structure for human prepro factor X shows the location of the seven introns (A to G). The 5′ end of the gene and additional introns have not been identified thus far by sequence analysis. The tripeptide of Arg-Lys-Arg that connects the light chain to the heavy chain is not shown. The prepro leader sequence (numbered −40 to −1) is removed during biosynthesis by signal peptidase and a processing protease that cleaves the R–A bond between −1 and 1. The Gla domain and potential growth factor domains are located in the light chain within residues 1 through 139. The activation peptide of 52 residues is released from factor X during its conversion to factor Xa. The serine protease or catalytic domain of factor X contains 254 residues, including the catalytic triad of H42, D88, and S185, which are *circled*. Two N-linked carbohydrate attachment sites in the activation peptide are shown by *solid diamonds*. The proposed disulfide bonds in factor IX have been placed by analogy to those established in bovine prothrombin and epidermal growth factor. The single-letter code for amino acids is given in Figure 3-5; b, b-hydroxyaspartic acid.

deletions of exons VII and VIII, a deletion of a single nucleotide followed by an in-frame stop codon in exon VII, and point mutations resulting in amino acid substitutions of Arg for Gly(−20), Lys for Gla14, Ser for Pro343, Cys for Arg366 (264–269). Of interest, the substitution of Arg for Gly in the hydrophobic core of the signal peptide prevents cleavage by the signal peptidase and secretion of the mutant factor X (267).

The mRNA for human factor X is approximately 1,500 nucleotides long and includes 1,475 nucleotides that code for a prepro leader sequence of 40 amino acids, a light chain of 139 amino acids, a connecting tripeptide, and 303 amino acids that constitute the heavy chain (256,257). A very short noncoding region of 10 nucleotides is present on the 3′ end of the mRNA following the stop codon of TGA. The processing or polyadenylation sequence of ATTAAA is unusual in that it is located in the coding sequence and precedes the stop codon by one nucleotide (19).

Two transcription start sites, a major one at −26 bp and a minor one at −10 bp upstream from the initiation Met codon, are present in the human factor X 5′-flanking region (270).

Functional reporter gene experiments with the 5'-flanking sequence indicate that full liver-specific promoter activity is contained with 457-bp upstream from the translation start site (see Fig. 3-15) (260). An apparent CCAAT sequence, present at −120 to −116 bp, is required for full promoter activity. DNA-protein binding studies indicate that this sequence binds the ubiquitous transcription factor NF-Y (148). An HNF-4 functional element has been localized between −63 and −42 bp, and HNF-4 binding is required for liver-specific expression. As mentioned earlier, the core HNF-4 element ACTTTG is also located close to the transcription start site in the factor VII and X promoters. Two additional positive regulatory regions, one at −215 to −149 bp and another at −457 to −351 bp, were also identified (260). A negative or silencing region located at −457 to −351 bp unidirectionally blocks the activity of the positive promoter elements in reporter gene constructs (260). This negative regulatory region may prevent

activation of the factor VII gene, which is 2,800 bp upstream from the initiation codon of the factor X gene and is transcribed in much lower amounts.

Like the other vitamin K–dependent proteins, factor X is synthesized in the liver with a prepro leader sequence that requires two processing steps for its removal (Fig. 3-6). These reactions are catalyzed by a signal peptidase, as well as by a second processing enzyme that cleaves the arginine residue on the carboxyl end of the propiece. Additional processing in the single-chain precursor occurs between Arg139 and Ser143, leading to the removal of an internal basic tripeptide of Arg-Lys-Arg and the formation of a two-chain molecule held together by a single disulfide bond (Fig. 3-14). The activation peptide for factor X is rich in glutamic acid and aspartic acid, and this accounts in part for the marked difference in the electrophoretic mobility of factor X versus factor Xa (126). The activation peptide from human factor X also contains two

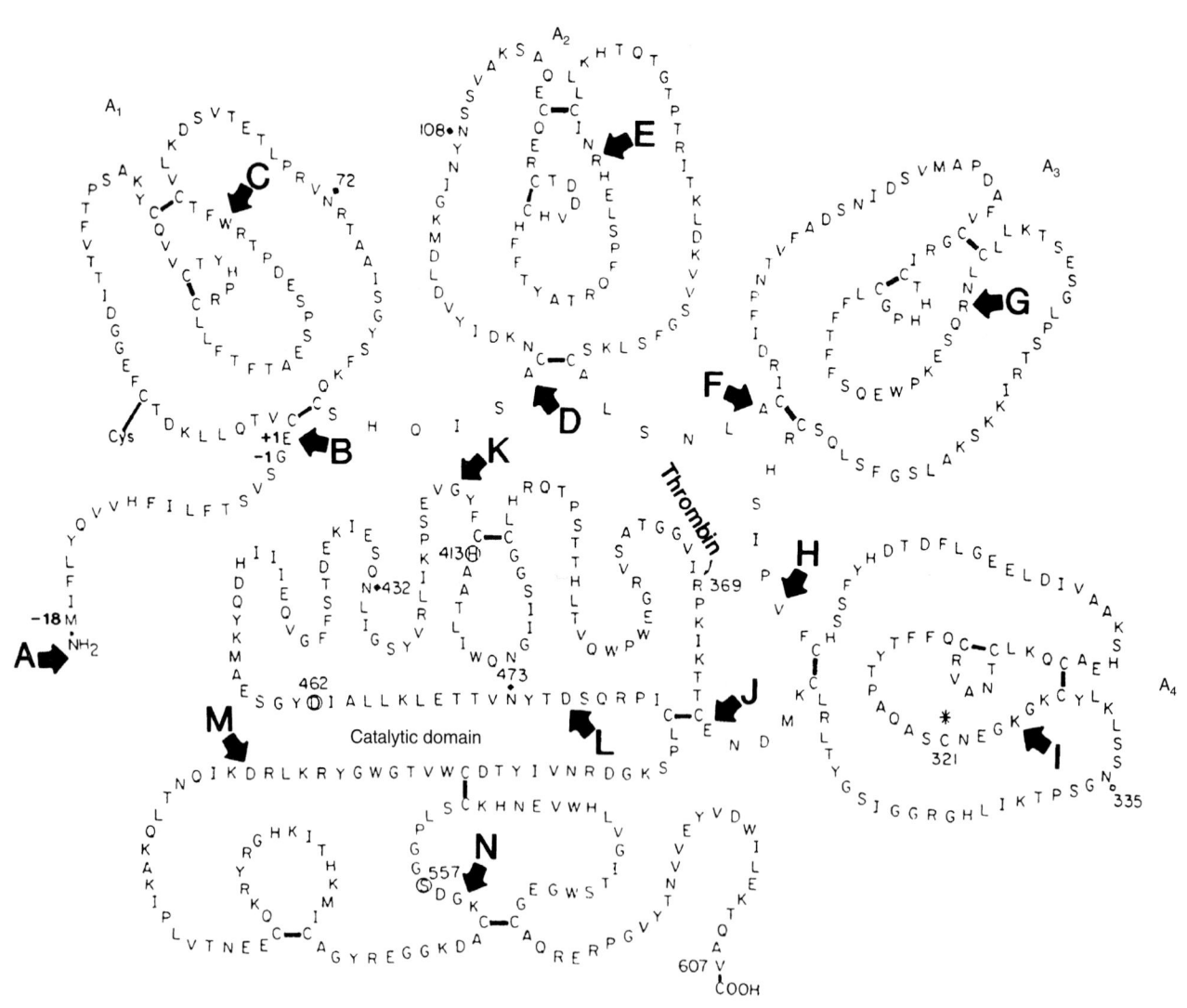

**FIGURE 3-15.** Amino acid sequence and tentative structure for human factor XI. The signal sequence (numbered −18 to −1) is removed during biosynthesis by signal peptidase by cleavage of the Gly–Glu bond between −1 and 1. Factor XI circulates in plasma as a dimer connected by a single disulfide bond linking Cys321 in both of the four Apple domains. The 14 introns (A to N) are shown by *solid arrows*. The four Apple domains (of 90 or 91 amino acids) are labeled A1, A2, A3, and A4. The site of cleavage catalyzed by thrombin during the conversion of factor XI to factor XIa is shown with a *small arrow*. The three members of the catalytic triad (H413, D462, and S557) are *circled*. The four N-linked carbohydrate chains (Asn72, Asn108, Asn432, and Asn473) are shown by *solid diamonds*. The single-letter code for amino acids is given in Figure 3-5.

potential N-linked carbohydrate-binding sites, including an Asn-Gln-Thr sequence and an Asn-Leu-Ser sequence starting with Asn39 and Asn49, respectively. It is also likely that the human molecule, analogous to the bovine molecule, contains O-linked carbohydrate in the heavy chain, but this has not yet been established.

# FACTOR XI

Factor XI ($M_r$ 143,000) is a plasma glycoprotein (5% carbohydrate) that participates in the intrinsic pathway of blood coagulation. It is synthesized in the liver and secreted into the plasma as a zymogen that circulates as a complex with high-molecular-weight kininogen (HMWK) (271). Factor XI is an unusual zymogen to a serine protease in that it contains two identical polypeptide chains linked by a single disulfide bond (Fig. 3-15) (272,273). The presence of two active catalytic sites per mole of the activated form of the protein (i.e., factor XIa) has been demonstrated by titration with antithrombin III (272).

The conversion of factor XI to factor XIa by thrombin occurs in the presence of a negatively charged material such as dextran sulfate, sulfatide, or heparin (274,275). Factor XI can also be activated *in vitro* by factor XIIa in the presence of HMWK and a negatively charged surface (276). Both of these activation reactions are due to the cleavage of the same internal Arg369-Ile peptide bond in each of the two polypeptide chains of factor XI (277). This results in the formation of a serine protease composed of two heavy chains (each 369 amino acids) and two light chains (each 23 amino acids), and these four chains are held together by three disulfide bonds. There is also evidence that factor XI is directly activated by thrombin in the presence of activated platelets (278,279). This thrombin-specific activation occurs when the dimerized form of factor XI binds to the GP Ib-$\alpha$ subunit of the GP Ib/V/IX receptor complex on the activated platelet surface (280,281).

Each heavy chain of factor XIa contains four tandem repeats of 90 (or 91) amino acids that range in identity from 23% to 34% (Fig. 3-15) (277). These tandem repeats, called *apple domains*, form separate domains in the heavy chain (277,282). Disulfide bonds link the first and sixth, second and fifth, and third and fourth half-Cys in each of the four apple domains (282). An extra half-Cys (Cys11), present in apple 1, forms a disulfide bond with another half-Cys residue, whereas Cys321 in each fourth apple domain links the two identical subunits of the protein together by a disulfide bond. The four apple domains in factor XI are also highly homologous to the four tandem repeats present in plasma prekallikrein; however, they have not yet been identified in any other protein (283,284). Present evidence indicates that factor XI is bound to HMWK through apple 1, whereas apple 2 is involved in the interaction of factor XI with factor IX (285–288).

Each of the light chains of factor XIa contains a catalytic domain with amino acid sequences that are typical of the pancreatic trypsin family of serine proteases (Fig. 3-15). This includes the catalytic triad of His413, Asp462, and Ser557. The light chain, starting with isoleucine 370, also contains the typical amino-terminal sequence of Ile-Val-Gly-Gly that is characteristic of most serine proteases.

Factor XIa is a glycoprotein with five potential N-glycosylation sites in each chain of the molecule. The presence of four carbohydrate chains, inducting two on the heavy chain (Asn72 and Asn108) and two on the catalytic or light chain (Ash432 and Asn473), have been established by amino acid sequencing techniques, whereas no carbohydrate is present on Asn335 of the heavy chain.

The cDNA for human factor XI has been isolated from a λgtll expression library prepared from human liver; the mRNA was approximately 2,100 nucleotides long (277). These data also indicated that factor XI was synthesized as a single polypeptide chain with a typical leader sequence of 18 amino acids (Fig. 3-15). Each of the two chains present in the mature molecule contained 607 amino acids. Also, the cDNA for factor XI contained a potential polyadenylation or processing sequence of AACAAA rather than the typical AATAAA (19). This sequence was located 21 nucleotides upstream from the poly(A) tail and was present in the 166 nucleotides that constitute the 3′ noncoding sequence of the mRNA.

The gene for human factor XI is approximately 23 kb and is located on the distal end of the long arm of chromosome 4 (4q35) (289,290). It contains 15 exons interrupted by 14 introns (Fig. 3-15). The first exon codes for the 5′ untranslated region, whereas exon 2 codes for the signal peptide. The four apple domains are coded by the next eight exons. Each apple domain is coded by two exons interrupted by a single intron, and these introns are located in essentially the same position within each of the four apple domains. The carboxyl-terminal region of factor XIa containing the catalytic chain is coded by five exons, four of which are located in the same positions as those in the genes for human tissue plasminogen activator and human urokinase.

Factor XI deficiency is an unusually mild bleeding tendency that occurs in either sex (291). Generally, spontaneous bleeding and hemorrhaging occur only after trauma or minor surgery. Factor XI deficiency is inherited as an autosomal recessive trait and is usually characterized by the virtual absence of factor XI coagulant activity or factor XI antigen circulating in plasma. Factor XI deficiency is found primarily in the Ashkenazi Jewish population, where the heterozygote frequency is approximately one in eight (292). These mutations occur almost entirely in two regions of the gene (288,293). The first mutation (Type II) involves a stop codon at residue 117 in the protein, where GAA, coding for Gln, is replaced by a stop codon of TAA. This mutation leads to the synthesis of a truncated polypeptide and loss of biological activity. The second principal mutation (Type III) results in an amino add substitution of Phe283 in the fourth apple domain, by Leu. This substitution results in reduced dimerization of the molecule during protein biosynthesis, with a resultant lowered secretion (294). The third, far less common mutation (Type I), disrupts normal mRNA splicing and changes a nucleotide sequence of GTAAC to ATAAC. This occurs at the last intron–exon boundary in the gene.

In more recent studies of 43 Ashkenazi Jewish patients in Israel with severe factor XI deficiency, it was found that 49% were due to the Type II mutation and 47% to Type III (293). These data indicated that these two mutations, which result in factor XI deficiency, represent an excellent example of a founder effect in the factor XI gene (295).

# FACTOR XIII

Factor XIII (fibrin-stabilizing factor) is the proenzyme for plasma transglutaminase. In the presence of fibrin, thrombin converts factor XIII to an enzyme called factor XIIIa (296,297). Because thrombin and fibrin are generated in the final stage of the coagulation process, the factor XIII activation is one of the last events in the blood coagulation cascade. Factor XIIIa catalyzes the formation of intermolecular epsilon-($\gamma$-glutamyl) lysine bonds between various protein substrates such as fibrin monomers, $\alpha_2$-plasmin inhibitor, fibronectin, and collagen (298–300). These intermolecular cross-linking reactions between various plasma and extracellular matrix proteins contribute to hemostasis, wound healing, and maintenance of pregnancy. A deficiency of factor XIII can therefore result in a lifelong bleeding tendency, delayed wound healing, and recurrent spontaneous abortion.

Factor XIII ($M_r$ 320,000) circulates in blood in association with fibrinogen (301). It is a heterotetramer composed of two $a$ subunits and two $b$ subunits ($a_2b_2$). The $a$ and $b$ dimers are held together by noncovalent bonds. The $a$ subunit contains the catalytic site with transglutaminase activity; the $b$ subunit seems to protect or stabilize the a subunit (302,303). The exact function of the $b$ subunit, however, remains unknown.

## The $a$ Subunit of Factor XIII

Although the $a$ subunit of factor XIII $M_r$ (75,000) circulates in blood as a heterotetramer ($a_2b_2$), it exists as a dimer ($a_2$) in various tissues and cells such as the placenta, prostate, uterus, platelets, and macrophages. The exact site of the biosynthesis and mechanism of secretion of the $a$ subunit into the blood has not been established. The plasma concentration of the $a$ subunit is reported to be 15 $\mu$g per mL, and essentially all of the $a$ subunit exists in a complex with the $b$ subunit (304). The plasma level of the $a$ subunit changes in various disease states (299,305). In the presence of thrombin, an activation peptide ($M_r$ 4,000) of 37 amino acids is released from the amino-terminus of each $a$ subunit of factor XIII (306,307). In the presence of calcium ions, the modified tetramer dissociates into an active $a'$ dimer and two $b$ subunits. In the latter reaction, calcium ions bind to the $a'$ dimer and unmask the active sites. The presence of fibrin accelerates the activation of factor XIII by thrombin significantly (308).

The size of the mRNA for the $a$ subunit of human factor XIII isolated from placenta is approximately 3.8 kb. Its cDNA is characterized by the absence of a typical hydrophobic leader sequence for secretion and a long 3' noncoding region of approximately 1.5 kb (307,309,310). The mature protein for the $a$ subunit starts with the acetyl-Ser-Glu-Thr sequence and consists of 731 amino acids (see Fig. 3-16). The activation of factor XIII by thrombin involves the cleavage of a peptide bond between Arg37 and Gly38. There are two putative calcium-binding sites based on the homology to the EF hand (311). The active-site Cys residue is located at position 315 within the sequence of Tyr-Gly-Gln-Cys-Trp that is identical to the active site of human and guinea pig tissue transglutaminase (312). Eight more Cys residues are present in the $a$ subunit, but none forms disulfide bridges. Although there are six potential Asn-linked glycosylation sites in the $a$ subunit, little or no carbohydrate has been detected in the molecule. An acetylated amino-terminal amino acid and the absence of glycosylation and disulfide bonds are consistent with the fact that the $a$ subunit is a cytoplasmic protein in most tissues and is secreted into circulation by apoptosis or by unknown mechanisms. These structural features of the $a$ subunit lead to its favorable expression in yeast for therapeutic purposes (313).

The gene for the $a$ subunit of human factor XIII is located on chromosome 6 at p24-25 (314,315). The gene spans more than 160 kb and includes 15 exons interrupted by 14 introns (310). The activation peptide is encoded by the second exon, the first putative calcium-binding site by the sixth, the active-site Cys by the seventh, the second putative calcium-binding site by the eleventh, and a thrombin inactivation site by the twelfth exons. Accordingly, the introns may separate the $a$ subunit into functional and structural domains (Fig. 3-16). Apparent polymorphism in amino acid residues of the $a$ subunit are found when its gene, cDNA, and protein sequences are compared (310). Several changes have also been found in the genomic DNA from patients with an $a$ subunit deficiency, although their relevance to a clotting disorder is difficult to confirm. Restriction fragment length polymorphisms have also been detected among individuals, using several restriction enzymes such as EcoRI and BamHI.

Recently the primary structures of tissue and keratinocyte transglutaminases and human erythrocyte membrane band 4.2 protein have been determined by cDNA cloning (312,316–318). The homology of the $a$ subunit of factor XIII to tissue, keratinocyte transglutaminase, and band 4.2 protein is 41%, 45%, and 27%, respectively. However, the active-site Cys residue in the band 4.2 protein is replaced by an Ala residue so that it lacks transglutaminase activity. A transglutaminase has also been purified from hemocytes of horseshoe crab, and its cDNA has been cloned (319). The horseshoe crab transglutaminase is also homologous to the members of this family, suggesting that transglutaminases are important enzymes that have been maintained during evolution. The gene for band 4.2 protein has been confirmed to have exactly the same structure as that of the $a$ subunit of factor XIII in terms of the location of its introns in the protein and the type of intron–exon junctions (320). This observation supports the idea that the members of this gene family have evolved from a common ancestry. The gene for keratinocyte transglutaminase has been localized on chromosome 14, which is different from that for the $a$ subunit of factor XIII (321).

## The $b$ Subunit of Factor XIII

The $b$ subunit of factor XIII ($M_r$ 80,000) is a plasma glycoprotein (8.5% carbohydrate) synthesized in the liver. It circulates in blood both as a complex with the $a$ dimer ($a_2b_2$) and as a free $b_2$ dimer. The concentration in plasma is reported to be 21 $\mu$g per mL (322). Expression of the $b$ subunit seems to be partially regulated by the $a$ subunit, because administering the $a$ subunit to patients with an $a$ subunit deficiency causes an increase in the plasma level of the $b$ subunit, as well as that of the $a$ subunit (323,324). Three families with the $b$ subunit deficiency have been reported (325–327). Homozygotes of the $b$ subunit deficiency present bleeding tendencies like those with the $a$ subunit deficiency. Plasma from these homozygotes has little or no $b$ subunit and significantly reduced amounts of the $a$ subunit. Furthermore, the half-life of the transfused $a$ subunit in the patient with the $b$ subunit deficiency seems to be shorter than that in the $a$ subunit deficiency (327). These findings support the idea that one role of the $b$ subunit is to protect or stabilize the $a$ subunit. Following fibrin formation, the $b$ subunit remains in serum *in vitro*, whereas the $a$ subunit of factor XIII remains firmly bound to the fibrin clot.

The mRNA for the $b$ subunit is approximately 2.3 kb long and codes for a typical hydrophobic leader sequence of 20 amino acids that is involved in secretion (328,329). The mature protein starts with the unblocked amino-terminal sequence of Glu-Glu-Lys-Pro and consists of 641 amino acids (see Fig. 3-17). Almost the entire molecule (98%) of the $b$ subunit is composed of 10 tandem repeats, called *sushi structures* (330). Each sushi structure consists of 60 to 65 amino acids and contains highly conserved Cys, Pro, Gly, Tyr, Phe, and Trp residues. Sushi structures are found in at least 26 different proteins and two cDNAs from mammalian sources (300,330). They are also present in proteins of the horseshoe crab and vaccinia virus. The $b$ subunit contains 40 Cys residues (four each in the 10 sushi structures). The first and third, and the second and fourth Cys residues in each sushi structure of the $b$ subunit are most likely linked by a disulfide bond, analogous to those determined in $\beta_2$-glycoprotein I and C4b binding protein (331,332). Three potential Asn-linked glycosylation sites are present in the $b$ subunit. An -Arg-Gly-Asp- sequence exists in the last sushi structure of the $b$ subunit, but its function is unclear.

The gene for the $b$ subunit of factor XIII is localized on chromosome 1 at bands q31-q32.1 (333). Of particular interest, many other genes coding for proteins containing multiple sushi structures are also clustered on chromosome 1 at q32 (334). The gene for the *b* subunit spans approximately 28 kb and includes 12 exons interrupted by 11 introns (329). All the intron–exon boundaries follow the GT-AG rule (19). The leader sequence is encoded by the first exon, whereas the carboxyl-terminal region of the protein and the 3′ noncoding region are encoded by the twelfth exon. Each of the 10 sushi structures is encoded by a single exon, and its 5′ and 3′ intron–exon bound-

aries are type I (329). All sushi structures in the genes for other proteins are also encoded by separate exons, with very few exceptions (333). Therefore, it seems likely that the ancestral gene coding for the sushi structure did not contain an internal intron but was duplicated during evolution. The gene for the subunit contains four Alu repeats within the introns and one in the 3′-flanking region. Other types of repetitive sequences, such as the KpnI repeats and O-family repeats, are also found in the gene for the *b* subunit.

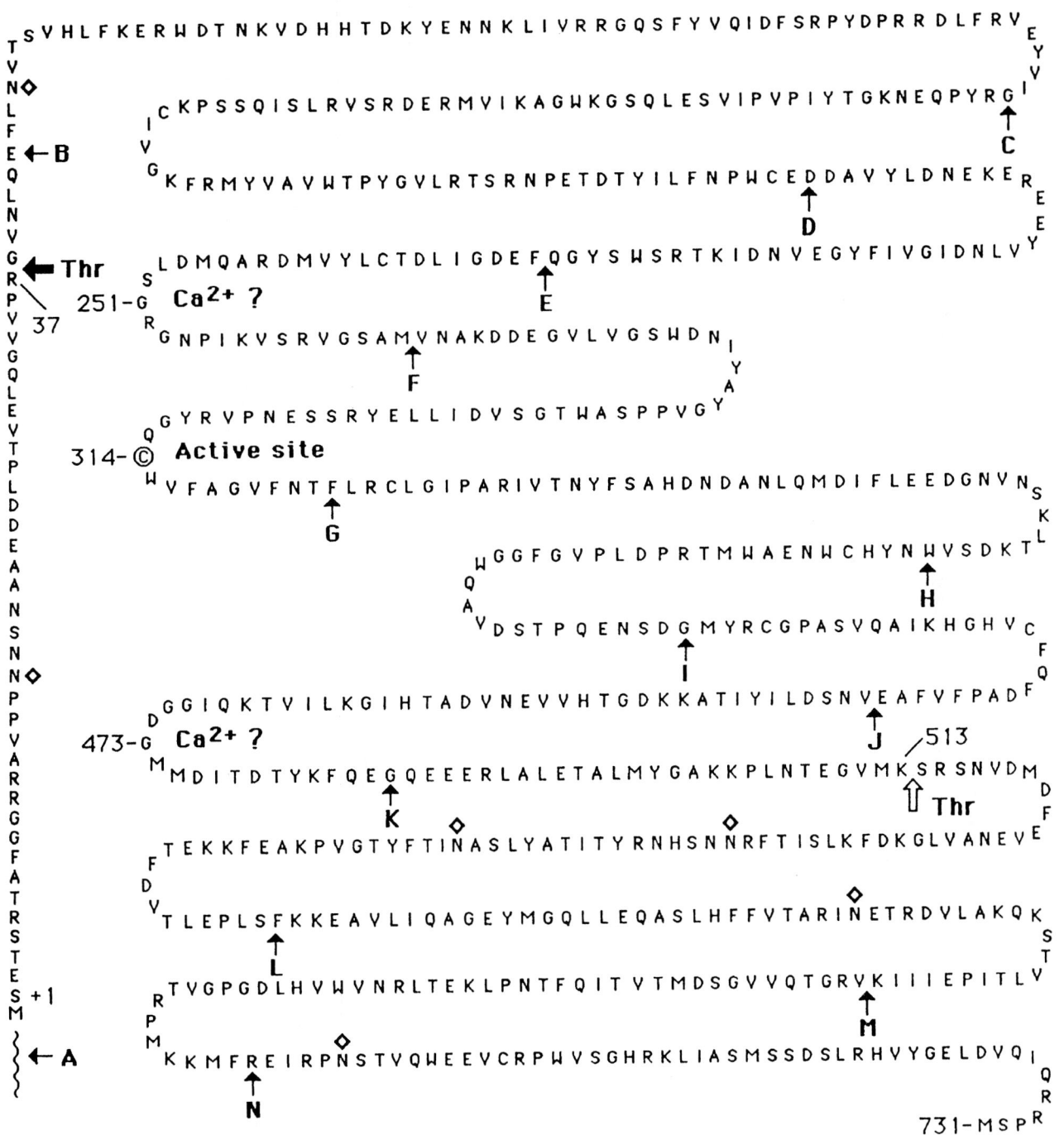

FIGURE 3-16. Amino acid sequence for the *a* subunit of human factor XIII shows the location of the 14 introns (A to N). The thrombin cleavage site at Arg37-Gly, leading to the activation of the molecule, is shown with a *solid arrow*. The various introns (A to N) are shown with *small arrows*. Potential calcium-binding sites also are shown with the active-site Cys314. A thrombin inactivation site at K513-S is shown with an *open arrow*. Potential N-glycosylation sites are identified by *open diamonds*. The single-letter code for amino acids is given in Figure 3-5.

Although the presence of polymorphisms in amino acid sequences has been suggested by isoelectric focusing technique, no mutations have been reported thus far. On the contrary, restriction fragment length polymorphisms are detected in the genomic DNAs by restriction enzymes such as BglII, EcoRI, and XbaI (334). The genetic defects of the complete *b* subunit deficiency have been determined (335). This study indicated that a nucleotide deletion destroyed an intron–exon splice junction in one allele and replacement of a Cys residue with Phe diminished a disulfide bridge in another allele.

## TISSUE FACTOR

Human tissue factor apoptotein ($M_r$ 44,000) is located in the tissue adventitia and comes into contact with blood after vascular injury (336–339). It is an integral membrane glycoprotein, tightly associated with phospholipid, containing 263 amino acids (see Fig. 3-18) (340–343). It is also a single-chain protein, synthesized with a signal peptide of 32 amino acids. The extrinsic pathway of the blood coagulation cascade is initiated when tissue factor binds to factor VII to form a one-to-one complex in the presence

of calcium ions (1,344–347). This facilitates the conversion of factor VII to factor VIIa by minor proteolysis (137,347–349). The newly formed complex of factor VII and tissue factor then converts factor X to factor Xa by the cleavage of a single peptide bond in the amino-terminal end of the heavy chain (254).

The extracellular or cellular surface domain of tissue factor is 219 residues and contains three repeating sequences of Trp-Lys-Ser. It also contains two disulfide bonds linking Cys49 with Cys57 and Cys186 with Cys209 (350). The membrane-spanning legion of tissue factor is 23 amino acids, whereas the cytoplasmic portion of the protein at the carboxyl end of the molecule is 21 residues long. The cytoplasmic portion also contains a half-Cys residue (Cys245) that is acylated by palmitic and stearic acid (350). Three potential glycosylation sites with a sequence of Asn-X-Thr/Ser (Asnll, Asn124, Asn137) are also present in the molecule (341–343).

The mRNA for human tissue factor is 2.3 kb (341–343). This includes a 5' noncoding region of 75 bp, 885 bp of coding sequence, a stop codon, and a 3' noncoding region of 1,141 bp followed by a poly(A) tail. The polyadenylation or processing signal of AATAAA is located 18 bases upstream from the poly(A) tail (9).

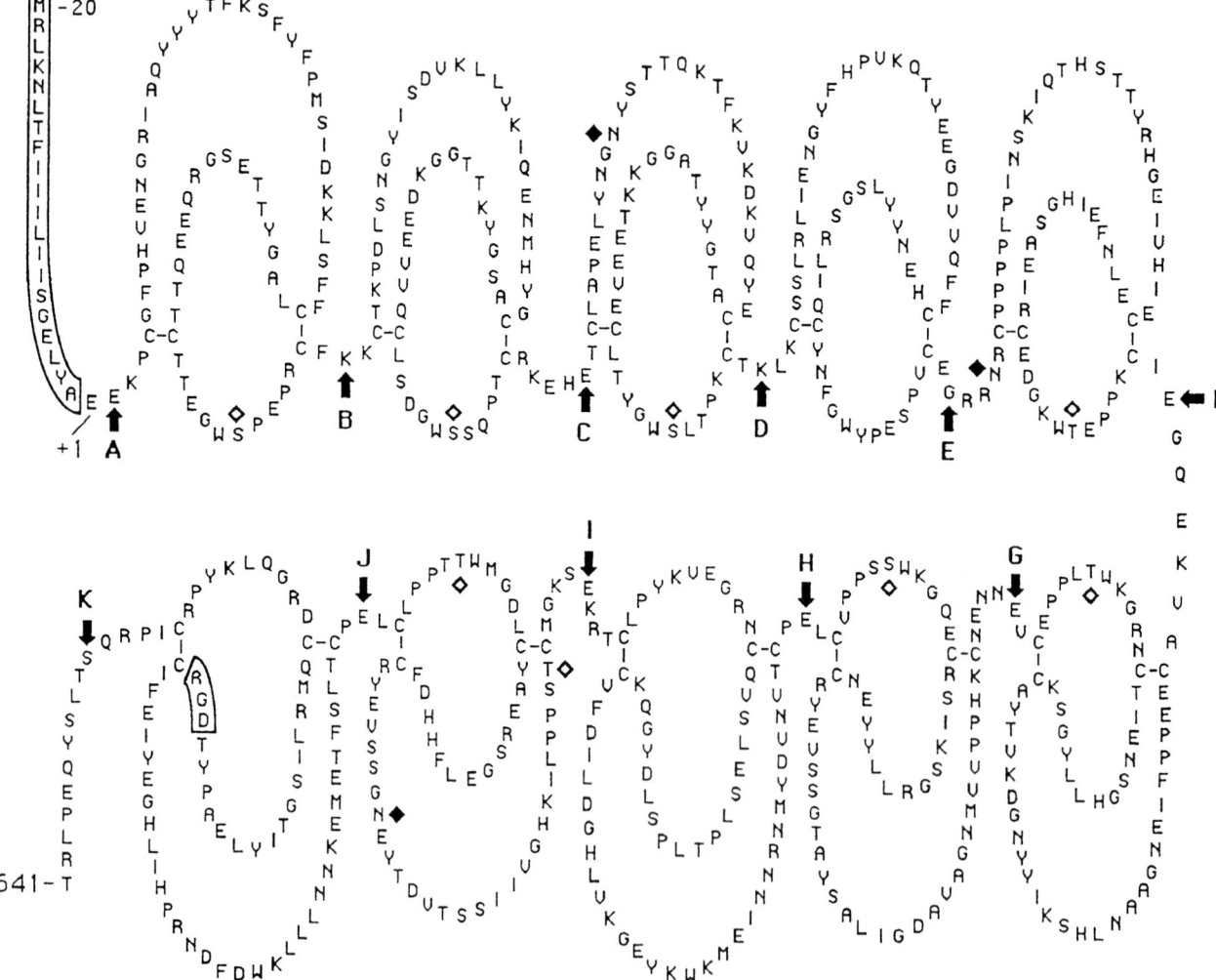

**FIGURE 3-17.** Amino acid sequence of the *b* subunit of human factor XIII and location of the 11 introns (A to K), indicated by solid arrows. Residues from −1 to −20, enclosed in a box, constitute the signal sequence. The 10 sushi domains are linked by disulfide bonds by analogy with those in b-2 glycoprotein and C4b binding protein (297,298). (From Naski MC, Lorand L, Shafer JA. Characterization of the kinetic pathway for fibrin promotion of alpha-thrombin-catalyzed activation of plasma factor XIII. *Biochemistry* 1991;30:934 and Folk JE, Finlayson JS. The epsilon-(gamma-glutamyl) lysine crosslink and the catalytic role of transglutaminases. *Adv Protein Chem* 1977;31:1, with permission.)

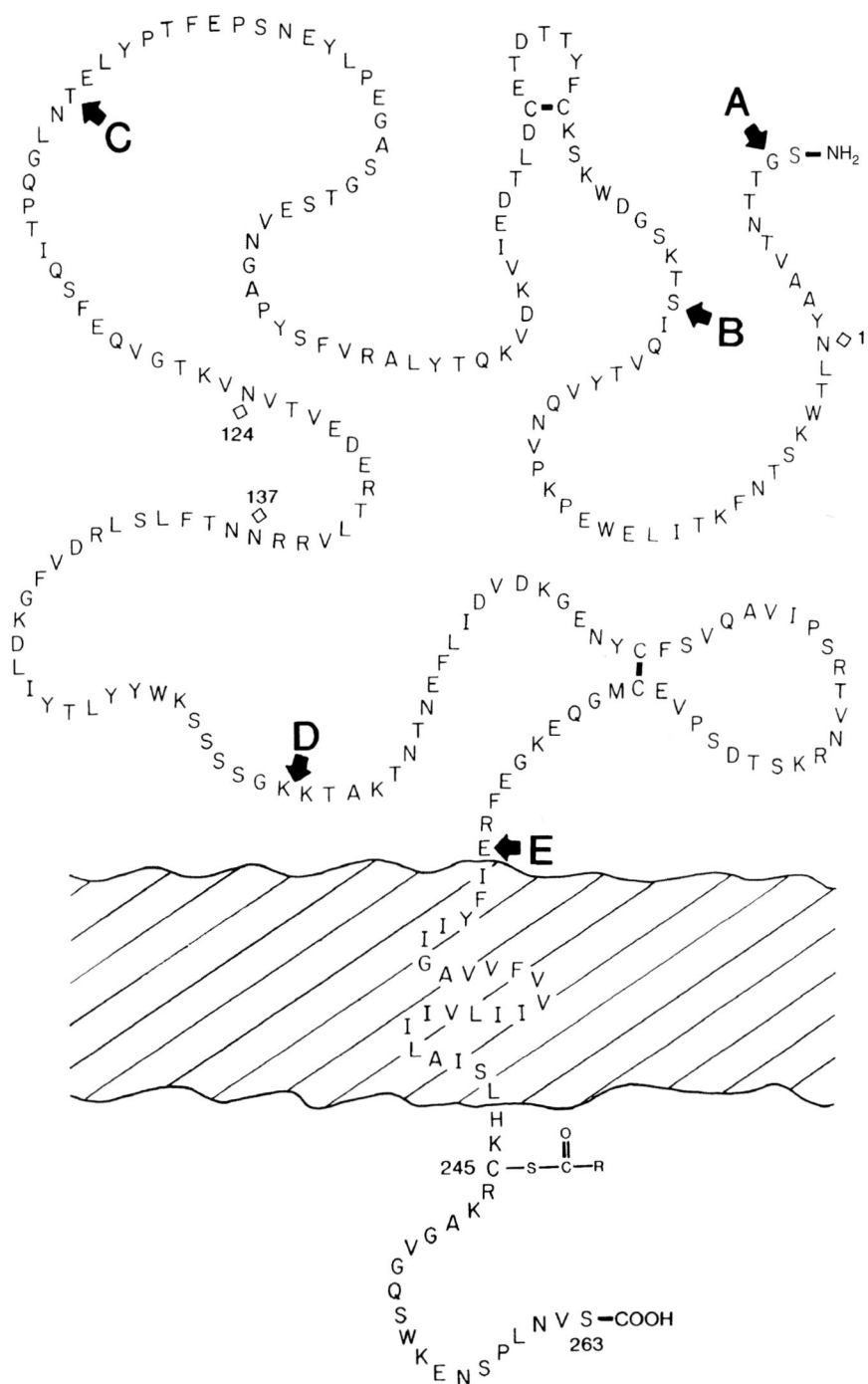

**FIGURE 3-18.** Amino acid sequence for human tissue factor, along with the locations of the introns. The *solid arrows* indicate the position of the five introns (A to E). The three potential carbohydrate-binding sites are indicated by *open diamonds*. The extracellular domain extends from residues 1 to E219, whereas the transmembrane region of 23 amino acids extends from Ile220 to Leu242. The cytoplasmic portion of the molecule is 21 residues in length and is located on the carboxyl end of the molecule. Cys245 is acylated by palmitic or stearic acid.

The gene for human tissue factor spans approximately 12.4 kb and is located on chromosome 1 (342–351). It contains six exons separated by five introns (A to E, Fig. 3-18). Each of the three Trp-Lys-Ser sequences in the apoprotein is coded by a separate exon (exons 2, 3, and 4) that may have arisen by tandem duplication. In addition to the transmembrane and cytoplasmic portions of the protein, the last exon (exon 6) also codes for a large 3′ noncoding region. The gene for human tissue factor contains three full Alu sequences, one partial Alu sequence, and

a typical TATA promoter element present 26 bp upstream from the cap site; however, the gene tacks a typical CCAAT box. Two direct repeats of ll bp and 9 bp are also present and show some sequence similarity to analogous regions flanking the genes for IL-1, tumor necrosis factor (TNF) α, and plasminogen activator inhibitor 1. Although the vascular endothelium has little or no tissue factor, it can be induced by stimulation with several agents, such as phytohemagglutinin and endotoxin, interleukin 1, TNF, phorbol esters, and thrombin (352–355). Transcription of the tissue factor gene is also increased in blood monocytes by many of the same agonists (356–358). These observations suggest that cell type–specific mechanisms are involved in tissue factor regulation. Functional studies indicate that basal tissue factor transcription is controlled by the transcription factor Sp1. A distal enhancer (−227 to −172 bp) containing two AP-1 sites and an NF-κB site mediates the induction of the tissue factor transcription in monocytic and endothelial cells (359). In human epithelial cells and vascular smooth muscle cells, the proximal enhancer region (−109 to −59 bp) is regulated, in part, by the transcription factor Egr-1 (359).

## PROTEIN C

Protein C ($M_r$ 62,000) is another plasma glycoprotein that circulates in blood as a precursor to a serine protease (360–363). This vitamin K–dependent protein plays an important regulatory role in blood coagulation. It is converted to activated protein C by thrombin in the presence of thrombomodulin, a protein present on the surface of endothelial cells (360,364–367). Activated protein C then inactivates factor Va and factor VIIIa by minor proteolysis (361,368–371). Protein S functions in the latter reaction as a cofactor (371–373).

Human protein C is composed of a heavy chain ($M_r$ 41,000) and a light chain ($M_r$ 21,000), held together by a disulfide bond (see Fig. 3-19) (374,375). The amino acid sequence for the human protein has been established by amino acid sequence analysis and cDNA and genomic cloning (93,376–379). The nine γ-carboxyglutamic acid residues and one β-hydroxyaspartic acid, which has been reported to be involved in $Ca^{2+}$ binding and anticoagulant activity, are present in the light chain (127,380). The light chain also contains two potential EGF domains. The heavy chain of protein C contains the catalytic or serine protease portion of the molecule. Human protein C contains four potential attachment sites for carbohydrate bound to asparagine. These are located at residue 97 in the light chain and residues 79, 144, and 160 in the heavy chain.

The gene for human protein C is present on chromosome 2 at q14-21 and in approximately 11 kb of DNA (93,379,381). The gene contains nine exons and eight introns. The first intron is located in the 5′ noncoding region of the gene; the other seven are present in the coding region of the gene (Fig. 3-19) (379). The introns range in size from 92 to 2,668 nucleotides, and the exons range in size from 25 to 885 nucleotides. All the intron–exon boundaries follow the GT-AG rule (50). The 5′ untranslated region of the protein C gene contains an additional short noncoding sequence corresponding to an untranslated exon. This exon is separated from the translation start codon by a 1,463-bp intronic sequence (382). This noncoding exon and the intron separating it is unique to protein C among the vitamin K–dependent coagulation factors. The rest of the introns separate the protein into several domains. Intron A is located in the prepro leader sequence. Intron B follows the Gla domain. Intron C is located just before the first potential growth factor domain. Intron D separates the two potential growth factor domains. Intron E follows the second potential growth factor domain. Introns F and G are located in the heavy chain that contains the catalytic domain. As previously noted, the seven introns in the coding regions of the gene are located in positions essentially identical to those in human factor VII, factor IX, and factor X (Table 3-6). The gene for protein C contains two Alu sequences, both in intron E.

The transcription regulation of protein C has been studied. Sufficient information for high-level expression of the gene for protein C in HepG2 cells is contained within a 1,500-bp 5′-flanking region, which includes 66 bp of the noncoding exon (see previous text) (382). The major transcription start site is located 65 bp upstream from the first intron–exon boundary or 1,515 bp upstream from the initiation Met codon

(382). Two minor transcription start sites are located at −7 and +13 bp relative to the major transcription start site. DNA binding studies and functional reporter gene analysis have demonstrated several cis elements within the protein C promoter. These elements include HNF-1 (−10 to +9 bp), HNF-3 (−25 to −11 bp), a unique liver-specific binding site (12 to +30 bp), and an Sp1 site in the noncoding exon (+58 to +65 bp). A strong silencer region is located between −162 and −82 bp and two possible liver-specific enhancer regions, which interact coordinately with promoter elements, are located between −1,462 and −162 bp (Fig. 3-15).

Several genetic defects of protein C have been found in patients with hereditary thrombophilia, including a nonsense mutation of Arg306, a replacement of Arg169 with Trp at the activation cleavage site, and the conversion of Trp402 to Cys, which may lead to instability of the molecule (383–385). Mutations have also been found within the protein C promoter that result in thrombophilia in some cases. The +3 C to T and −2 T to C mutations disrupt the HNF-1 site, and the −15 T to A and the −20 A to G mutations disrupt the HNF-3 binding site (386,387). A recent report suggests that the −2 mutations may in fact disrupt HNF-6 binding as well, suggesting that HNF-6 and HNF-1 share a common binding site (388).

The mRNA for human protein C is approximately 1,700 nucleotides long, and it includes 126 nucleotides that code for a prepro leader sequence of 42 amino acids. The mRNA also codes for a single-chain polypeptide of 419 amino acids, along with a stop codon of TAG. The 3′ noncoding sequence consists of 68 nucleotides and includes a processing or polyadenylation sequence of ATTAAA, which is located 16 nucleotides upstream from the poly(A) tail (19). The leader peptide contains an arginine located next to the alanine, which is the amino-terminal residue of the mature protein circulating in plasma. Because an Arg-Ala bond is not cleaved by signal peptidase, it is evident that protein C, like the other vitamin K–dependent proteins present in plasma, is synthesized with a prepro leader sequence (Fig. 3-19). It is likely that the signal peptidase cleaves the prepro leader sequence following the serine residue located at −18. The light and heavy chains of protein C are initially connected by a dipeptide of Lys-Arg. This dipeptide is also removed during the biosynthesis and processing or secretion of the protein by an unknown protease(s).

## PROTEIN S

Human protein S ($M_r$ 69,000) is a single-chain plasma glycoprotein (7.8% carbohydrate) that contains 10 γ-carboxylglutamic acid (Gla) residues (126,389). Accordingly, protein S requires vitamin K and a carboxylase for its biosynthesis in liver (390). In the presence of phospholipid and calcium, protein S functions as a cofactor of activated protein C in the inactivation of factors Va and VIIIa (371–373,391). The role of protein S is that of an anticoagulant, and its deficiency therefore leads to a predisposition for venous thrombosis (392–395). The concentration of protein S in human plasma is approximately 25 μg per mL (396,397). Forty percent of the human protein exists in a free form, and the remaining 60% in a stoichiometric complex with C4b-binding protein (396). Complex formation, however, does not lead to the inactivation of C4b, although it no longer functions as a cofactor (398,399). In the bovine system, another plasma protein that binds to protein S has been identified and found to "enhance" the cofactor activity of protein S in the inactivation of factor Va by activated protein C (400). This S-binding protein apparently differs from C4b-binding protein because it is a two-chain molecule composed of 94-kDa and 46-kDa subunits. The human counterpart of this new protein has not yet been reported.

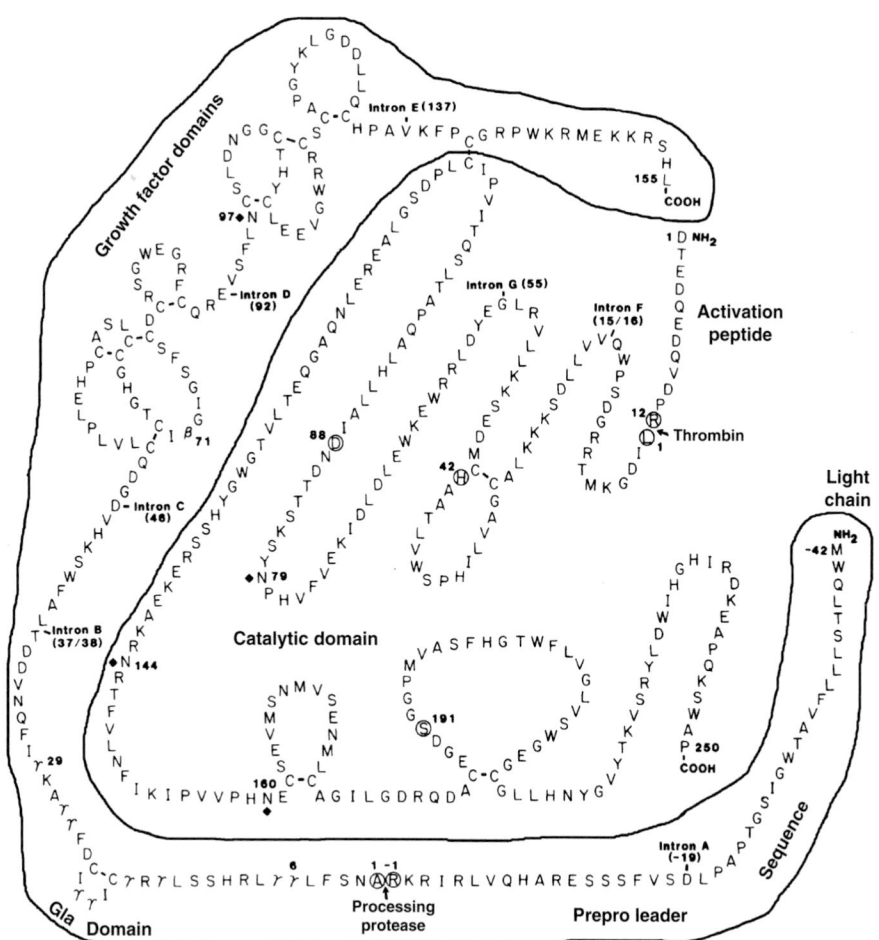

**FIGURE 3-19.** Amino acid sequence and tentative structure for human prepro protein C, showing the location of the seven introns (A to G) in the coding region of the gene (71,375). The eighth intron in the 58 noncoding sequence is not shown. The prepro leader sequence (numbered −42 to −1) is removed during biosynthesis by signal peptidase and a processing protease that cleaves the R–A bond between −1 and 1. The Gla domain and potential growth factor domains are located in the light chain within residues 1 through 155. The connecting peptide of Lys-Arg present between the light and heavy chains is not shown. The activation peptide of 12 residues is released from protein C by thrombin during its conversion to activated protein C. The amino acids (R–L) in which this cleavage occurs are *circled*. The serine protease or catalytic domain of protein C contains 250 residues, including the three principal amino acids of H42, D88, and S191 that participate in catalysis; these are also *circled*. Two potential carbohydrate-binding sites in the activation peptide are shown by *solid diamonds*. The proposed disulfide bonds in protein C have been placed by analogy to those established in bovine prothrombin and epidermal growth factor. The single-letter code for amino acids is given in Figure 3-5; b, b-hydroxyaspartic acid.

The primary structure of human protein S has been determined by cDNA cloning (401,402). The size of its mRNA is approximately 3.5 to 4.0 kb, including two polyadenylation signals at the 3′ end. As with other vitamin K–dependent proteins (Table 3-6), protein S is synthesized with a hydrophobic signal sequence and prepropeptide of 41 amino acids (see Fig. 3-20). The mature protein consists of 635 amino adds and starts with a sequence of Ala-Asn-Ser. Starting from the amino-terminus, there is a Gla domain, a thrombin-sensitive region, a short stretch of aromatic residues, four EGF domains, and a sequence homologous to steroid hormone binding globulin (SHBG, Fig. 3-20) (403). Chemical modification of the Gla residues of protein S leads to a loss of both binding capability to phospholipid and anticoagulant cofactor activity (404). The Gla domain also contains calcium-binding sites. The cleavage by thrombin of two Arg-Ser/Ala bonds in the second disulfide loop results in the release of a peptide containing residues 53 to 70 and the loss of protein S cofactor activity (403,405–407).

The first EGF domain of bovine protein S contains a β-hydroxyaspartic acid (residue 95); each of the remaining three EGF domains contains one β-hydroxyasparagine (residues 136, 178, and 217) (408). One Asp and three Asn residues at the same positions in human protein S are also very likely hydroxylated, but these residues are not required for anticoagulant cofactor activity or for binding to C4b binding protein (409). The carboxyl-terminal portion of the SHBG region is important for the binding of protein S to C4b-binding protein and for the enhancement of the anticoagulant activity of activated protein C (410). Potential Asn-linked glycosylation sites are clustered in the middle of the SHBG region. Cloning of human cDNA for protein S has made it possible to express a functional recombinant protein S in mammalian cells (411,412).

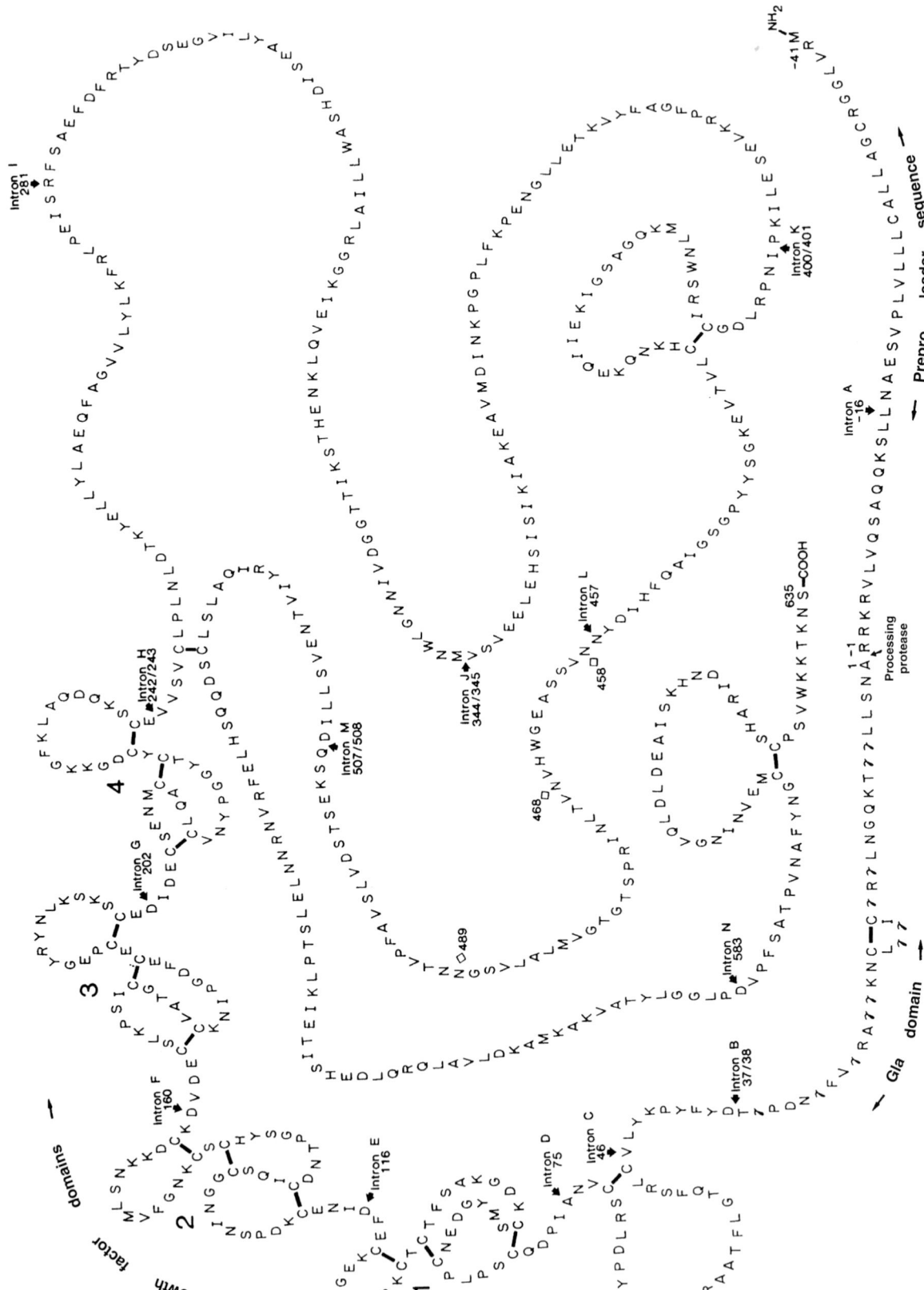

**FIGURE 3-20.** Amino acid sequence for human prepro protein S and location of the 14 introns (A to N), indicated by *solid arrows*. The prepro leader sequence includes residues −41 to −1. *Open diamonds* indicate potential carbohydrate attachment sites of the Asn-X-Ser/Thr type. Large numbers denote orders of four epidermal growth factor domains, which are followed by a region of steroid hormone–binding globulins.

The gene for human protein S has been localized to chromosome 3 (413,414). No other genes coding for the proteins involved in blood coagulation or fibrinolysis are located on chromosome 3. The structure and organization of the gene for protein S has been determined recently by several groups (415–417). It spans more than 80 kb and contains 15 exons interrupted by 14 introns. All nucleotide sequences around the intron–exon boundaries follow the AG/GT rule and the consensus sequence. There are six Alu repeats located throughout the gene. The signal sequence is encoded by the first exon, the propeptide and Gla domain by the second exon, the short stretch of aromatic residues by the third exon, and the thrombin-sensitive region by the fourth exon. Each of the four EGF domains is encoded by a single exon, while the SHBG region is encoded by seven exons as in the human SHBG gene (418). Three potential glycosylation sites are encoded within a single exon.

Two copies of the gene for human protein S have been identified, and the second gene is very likely a pseudogene (419,420). The latter spans over 55 kb and shows the absence of exon l, as well as many nucleotide substitutions, including stop codon, insertions, and deletions resulting in frameshifts and the consequent in-frame stop codons. Overall homology between the exons of the gene for protein S and those of the pseudogene is 97%, indicating that these two genes diverged recently. The pseudogene also exists in the genomes of the gorilla and chimpanzee (416).

This information allowed the characterization of various genetic defects of human protein S among individuals. A deletion of the middle portion of the gene coding for protein S has been identified in the DNA of patients with protein S deficiency (420). A dimorphism at position 460 (Ser to Pro) in one of three potential Asn-linked glycosylation sites has been detected, although the variant molecule seems to retain normal functions (421).

## References

1. Davie EW, Fujikawa K, Kisiel W. The coagulation cascade: initiation, maintenance, and regulation. *Biochemistry* 1991;30:10363–10370.
2. McKee PA, Rogers LA, Marler E, et al. The subunit polypeptides of human fibrinogen. *Arch Biochem Biophys* 1966;116:271.
3. Iwanaga S, Blomback B, Grondahl NH, et al. Amino acid sequence of the N-terminal part of gamma-chain in human fibrinogen. *Biochim Biophys Acta* 1968;160:280.
4. Topfer-Petersen E, Lottspeich F, Henschen A. Carbohydrate linkage site in the beta-chain of human fibrin. *Hoppe Seylers Z Physiol Chem* 1976;357:1509.
5. Pizzo SV, Schwartz ML, Hill RL, et al. The effect of plasmin on the subunit structure of human fibrinogen. *J Biol Chem* 1972;247:636.
6. Henschen A, Lottspiech F. Preliminary note on the completion of the beta-chain sequence. *Hoppe Seylers Z Physiol Chem* 1977;358:1643.
7. Lottspeich F, Henschen A. Amino acid sequence of human fibrin. Preliminary note on the completion of the gamma-chain sequence. *Hoppe Seylers Z Physiol Chem* 1977;358:935.
8. Doolittle RF, Watt KWK, Cottrell BA, et al. The amino acid sequence of the alpha-chain of human fibrinogen. *Nature* 1979;280:464.
9. Henschen A, Lottspeich F, Hessel B. Amino acid sequence of human fibrin; preliminary note on the completion of the intermediate part of the alpha-chain sequence. *Hoppe Seylers Z Physiol Chem* 1979;360:1951.
10. Watt KWK, Takagi T, Doolittle RF. Amino acid sequence of the beta-chain of human fibrinogen. *Biochemistry* 1979;18:68.
11. Rixon MW, Chan W-Y, Davie EW, et al. Characterization of a complementary deoxyribonucleic acid coding for the alpha-chain of human fibrinogen. *Biochemistry* 1983;22:3237.
12. Chung DW, Que BG, Rixon MW, et al. Characterization of a complementary deoxyribonucleic acid coding for the beta-chain of human fibrinogen. *Biochemistry* 1983;22:3237.
13. Chung DW, Chain W-Y, Davie EW. Characterization of a complementary deoxyribonucleic acid coding for the gamma chain of human fibrinogen. *Biochemistry* 1983;22:3250.
14. Kant JA, Lord ST, Crabtree GR. Partial mRNA sequences for human alpha, beta, and gamma fibrinogen chains: evolutionary and functional implications. *Proc Natl Acad Sci U S A* 1983;80:3953.
15. Kant JA, Fornace AJ Jr, Saxe D, et al. Evolution and organization of the fibrinogen locus on chromosome 4: gene duplication accompanied by transposition and inversion. *Proc Natl Acad Sci U S A* 1985;82:2344.
16. Chung DW, Harris JE, Davie EW. Nucleotide sequences of the three genes coding for human fibrinogen. In: Liu CY, Chien S, eds. *Advances in experimental medicine and biology.* New York: Plenum Publishing, 1991.
17. Rixon MW, Chung DW, Davie EW. Nucleotide sequence of the gene for the gamma chain of human fibrinogen. *Biochemistry* 1985;24:2077.
18. Fornace AJ Jr, Cummings DE, Comeau CM, et al. Structure of the human gamma-fibrinogen gene. *J Biol Chem* 1984;259:12826.
19. Proudfoot NJ, Brownlee GG. 3′ noncoding region sequences in eukaryotic messenger RNA. *Nature* 1976;263:211.
20. Nickerson JM, Fuller GM. *In vitro* synthesis of rat fibrinogen: identification of pre-alpha, pre-beta, and pre-gamma polypeptides. *Proc Natl Acad Sci U S A* 1981;78:303.
21. Koj A. Acute-phase reactants: their synthesis, turnover and biological significance. In: Allison AC, ed. *Structure and function of plasma proteins,* Vol. 1. London: Plenum Publishing, 1974.
22. Crabtree GR, Kant JA. Coordinate accumulation of the mRNAs for the alpha, beta and gamma chains of rat fibrinogen following defibrination. *J Biol Chem* 1982;257:7277.
23. Fowlkes DM, Mullis NT, Comeau CM. Potential basis for regulation of the coordinately expressed fibrinogen genes: homology in the 5′ flanking regions. *Proc Natl Acad Sci U S A* 1984;81:2313.
24. Meade TW. Fibrinogen and ischaemic heart disease. *Eur Heart J* 1995;16(Suppl. A):31.
25. Luc G, Bard JM, Juhan-Vague I, et al. C-reactive protein, interleukin-6, and fibrinogen as predictors of coronary heart disease: the PRIME study. *Arterioscler Thromb Vasc Biol* 2003;23(7):1255.
26. Mandl J, Csala M, Lerant I, et al. Enhancement of IL-6 production by fibrinogen degradation product D in human peripheral monocytes and perfused murine liver. *Scand J Immunol* 1995;42:175.
27. Zhing Z, Wen Z, Darnell JE. STAT 3: A STAT family member activated by tyrosine phosphorylation in response to epithelial growth factor and interleukin-6. *Science* 1994;264:95.
28. Fuller GM, Zhang Z. Transcriptional control mechanism of fibrinogen gene expression. *Ann N Y Acad Sci* 2000;936:469.
29. Duan HO, Simpson-Haidaris PJ. Functional analysis of interleukin-6 response elements on the human gamma-fibrinogen promoter: binding of hepatic STAT3 correlates negatively with transactivation potential of type II IL-6 response elements. *J Biol Chem* 2003;278(42):41270.
30. Xia H, Redman CM. Oxysterols suppress constituative fibrinogen expression. *Thromb Haemost* 2003;90(1):43.
31. Gervois P, Kleeman R, Pilon A, et al. Global suppression of IL-6 induced acute phase response gene expression after chronic *in vivo* treatment with peroxisome-proliferator-activated receptor-alpha activator fenofibrate. *J Biol Chem* 2004;279(16):16154.
32. Gervois P, Vu-Dac N, Kleeman R, et al. Negative regulation of human fibrinogen gene expression by peroxisome-proliferator-activated receptor-alpha agonists via inhibition of CCAAT box enhancer binding protein B. *J Biol Chem* 2001;276:33471.
33. Mizuguchi J, Hu CH, Coa Z, et al. Characterization of the 5′-flanking region of the gene for the gamma chain of human fibrinogen. *J Biol Chem* 1995;270:28350.
34. Kunicki TJ, Newman PJ, Amrani DL, et al. Human platelet fibrinogen: purification and hemostatic properties. *Blood* 1985;66:808.
35. Anderson GM, Shou AR, Shafer JA. Functional characterization of promoter elements involved in regulation of human B-beta fibrinogen expression. *J Biol Chem* 1993;268:22650.
36. Dalmon J, Laurent M, Courtois G. The human beta-fibrinogen promoter contains a hepatocyte nuclear factor 1-dependent interleukin-6-response element. *Mol Cell Biol* 1993;13:1183.
37. Hu CH, Harris JE, Davie EW, et al. Characterization of the 5′-flanking region of the gene for the alpha-chain of human fibrinogen. *J Biol Chem* 1995;270:28342.
38. Liu Z, Fuller GM. Detection of a novel transcription factor for the A-alpha fibrinogen in response to interlekin-6. *J Biol Chem* 1995;270:7580.
39. Liu Z, Fuller GM. Detection of a novel transcription factor for the A-alpha fibrinogen gene. *J Biol Chem* 1995;270:7580.
40. Liu Z, Fuentes NL, Jones SA, et al. A unique transcription factor for the A-alpha fibrinogen gene is related to the mitochndrial single stranded DNA binding protien P16. *Biochemistry* 1997;36:14799.
41. Okomura N, Terasawa F, Yonecawa O, et al. C to T nucleotide substitution at position −1138bp of the 5′-flanking region of the fibrinogen A alpha- chain gene. *Ann N Y Acad Sci* 2001;936:526.
42. Hansen LP, Crabtree GPT. Regulation of HNF-1 homeodomain proteins by DCoH. *Curr Opin Genet Dev* 1993;3:246.
43. Van't Hooft FM, Von Bahr SJ, Silviera A, et al. Two functional polymorphisms in the promoter region of the β-fibrinogen genes contribute to regulation of plasma fibrinogen concentration. *Arterioscler Thromb Vasc Biol* 1999;19:3063.
44. Zhung Z, Fuentes NL, Fuller GM. Characterization of the IL-6 responsive elements in the gamma fibrinogen gene promoter. *J Biol Chem* 1995;270:24287.
45. Ray A. An SAF binding site in the promoter region of the human gamma-fibrinogen gene functions as an IL-6 response element. *J Immunol* 2000;165:3411.
46. Akira S, Nishio Y, Inoue M, et al. Molecular cloning of APRF, a novel IFN-stimulated gene factor 3 p91-related transcription factor involved in gp130-mediated signaling pathway. *Cell* 1994;77:63.

47. Heroch S, Revel M, Chebath J. Il-6 signaling via four transcription factors binding palindromic enhancers of different genes. *J Biol Chem* 1994;269: 26191.

48. Sato K, Ito K, Kohara H, et al. Negative regulation of catalase gene expression in hepatoma cells. *Mol Cell Biol* 1992;12:2525.

49. Zhang Z, Fuller GM. IL-1β inhibits IL-6 mediated rat γ-fibrinogen gene expression. *Blood* 2000;96:3466.

50. Breathnach R, Chambon P. Organization and expression of eukaryotic split genes coding for proteins. *Annu Rev Biochem* 1981;50:349.

51. Blobel G, Walter P, Chang CN, et al. Translocation of proteins across membranes: the signal hypothesis and beyond. In: Hopkin CR, Duncan CJ, eds. *Secretory mechanisms*, Vol. 33. London: Cambridge University Press, 1979.

52. Haidaris PJ, Francis CW, Sporn LA, et al. Megakaryocyte and hepatocyte origins of human fibrinogen biosynthesis exhibit hepatocyte-specific expression of gamma chain-variant polypeptides. *Blood* 1989;74:743.

53. Francis CW, Marder VJ, Martin SE. Demonstration of a large molecular weight variant of the gamma chain of normal human plasma fibrinogen. *J Biol Chem* 1980;255:5599.

54. Wolfenstein-Todel C, Mosesson MW. Human plasma fibrinogen heterogeneity: evidence for an extended carboxyl-terminal sequence in a normal gamma chain variant (gamma'). *Proc Natl Acad Sci U S A* 1980;77:5069.

55. Wolfenstein-Todel C, Mosesson MW. Carboxy-terminal amino acid sequence of a human fibrinogen gamma-chain variant (gamma'). *Biochemistry* 1981;20:6146.

56. Chung DW, Davie EW. gamma and gamma' chains of human fibrinogen are produced by alternative mRNA processing. *Biochemistry* 1984;23:4232.

57. Farrell DH, Mulvihill ER, Huang S, et al. Recombinant human fibrinogen and sulfation of the gamma' chain. *Biochemistry* 1991;30:9414–9420.

58. Meh DA, Sienbenlist KG, Brennan SO, et al. The amino acid sequence in fibrin responsible for high affinity thrombin binding. *Thromb Haemost* 2001;85(3):470.

59. Forman WB, Barnhart MI. Cellular site for fibrinogen synthesis. *JAMA* 1964;187:128.

60. Roy SN, Mukhopadhyay G, Redman CM. Regulation of fibrinogen assembly: transfection of Hep-G2 cells with B beta cDNA specifically enhances synthesis of the three component chains of fibrinogen. *J Biol Chem* 1990;265:6389.

61. Roy SN, Procyk R, Kudryk BJ, et al. Assembly and secretion of recombinant human fibrinogen. *J Biol Chem* 1991;266:4758.

62. Hartwig R, Danishefsky KJ. Studies on the assembly and secretion of fibrinogen. *J Biol Chem* 1991;266:6578.

63. Farrell DH, Mulvihill ER, Huang S, et al. Recombinant human fibrinogen sulfation of the gamma' chain. *Biochemistry* 1991;30:9414.

64. Roy SN, Kudryk B, Redman CM. Secretion of biologically active recombinant fibrinogen by yeast. *J Biol Chem* 1995;270:23761.

65. Butler SP, van-Cott K, Subramanian A, et al. Current progress in the production of recombinant human fibrinogen in the milk of transgenic animals. *Thromb Haemost* 1997;78:537.

66. Zhang JZ, Redman C. Fibrinogen assembly and secretion; role of intrachain disulfide loops. *J Biol Chem* 1996;271:30083.

67. Huang S, Mulvihill ER, Farrell DH, et al. Biosynthesis of human fibrinogen: subunit interactions and potential intermediates in the assembly. *J Biol Chem* 1993;268:8919.

68. Terasawa F, Okumura N, Kitano K, et al. Hypofibrinogenemia associated with a heterozygous missense mutation gamma 153cys to arg (Matsumoto IV): in vitro expression demonstrates defective secretion of the variant fibrinogen. *Blood* 1999;94:4122.

69. Okumura N, Terasawa F, Tanaka H, et al. Analysis of fibrinogen gamma-chain truncations shows the c-terminus, particularly gamma ile 387, is essential for assembly and secretion. *Blood* 2002;99:3564.

70. Xu W, Chung DW, Davie EW. The assembly of human fibrinogen. *J Biol Chem* 1996;271:27948.

71. Huang S, Cao Z, Davie EW. The role of amino-terminal disulfide bonds in the structure and seembly of fibrin. *Biochem Biophys Res Commun* 1993; 190:488.

72. Anson DS, Choo KH, Rees DJG, et al. The gene structure of human antihaemophilic factor IX. *EMBO J* 1984;3:1053.

73. Blomback M, Blomback B, Mammen EF, et al. Fibrinogen Detroit: a molecular defect in the N-terminal disulphide knot of human fibrinogen? *Nature* 1968;218:134.

74. Henschen A. Genetically abnormal human fibrinogens: a summary of 32 structurally elucidated variants. In: Peeters H, ed. *Protides of the biological fluids*, Vol. 33. Oxford: Pergamon, 1985.

75. Liu CY, Koehn JA, Morgan FJ. Characterization of fibrinogen New York 1. *J Biol Chem* 1985;260:4390.

76. Ebert RF, ed. *Index of variant human fibrinogens*. Boca Raton, FL: CRC Press, 1991.

77. Haverkate F, Samama M. Familial dysfibrinogenemia and thrombophilia: report on a study of the SSC subcommittee on fibrinogen. *Thromb Haemost* 1995;73:151.

78. Martinez J. Congenital dysfibrinogenemia. *Curr Opin Hematol* 1997;4:357.

79. Magnusson S, Petersen TE, Sottrup-Jensen L. Complete primary structure of prothrombin: isolation, structure and reactivity of 10 carboxylated glutamic residues and regulation of prothrombin activation by thrombin. In:

Reich E, Rifkin DB, Shaw E, eds. *Proteases and biological control.* Cold Spring Harbor, NY: Cold Spring Harbor Laboratories, 1975.

80. Butkowski EJ, Elion J, Downing MR, et al. Primary structure of human prothrombin 2 and alpha-thrombin. *J Biol Chem* 1977;252:4942.

81. Thompson AR, Enfield DL, Ericsson LH, et al. Human thrombin: partial primary structure. *Arch Biochem Biophys* 1977;178:356.

82. Walz DA, Hewett-Emmett D, Seegers WH. Amino acid sequence of human prothrombin fragments 1 and 2. *Proc Natl Acad Sci U S A* 1977; 74:1969.

83. Degen DJF, MacGillivray RTA, Davie EW. Characterization of the complementary deoxyribonucleic acid and gene coding for human prothrombin. *Biochemistry* 1983;22:2087.

84. MacGillivray RTA, Davie EW. Characterization of bovine prothrombin mRNA and its translation product. *Biochemistry* 1984;23:1626.

85. Degen SJF, Davie EW. Nucleotide sequence of the gene for human prothrombin. *Biochemistry* 1987;25:6165–6177.

86. Stenflo J, Fernlund P, Egan W, et al. Vitamin K-dependent modifications of glutamic acid residues in prothrombin. *Proc Natl Acad Sci U S A* 1974; 71:2730.

87. Nelsestuen GL, Zytkovicz TH, Howard JB. The mode of action of vitamin K: identification of gamma-carboxyglutamic acid as a component of prothrombin. *J Biol Chem* 1974;249:6347.

88. Davie EW, Degen SJF, Yoshitake S, et al. Cloning of vitamin K-dependent clotting factors. In: de Bernard B, Sottocasa GL, Sandri G et al., eds. *Calcium binding proteins*, Vol. 25. Amsterdam: Elsevier Science, 1983.

89. Degen SJF, Rajput B, Reich E. Coagulation and fibrinolysis: characterization of the human prothrombin and human tissue-plasminogen activator genes. In: Peeters H, ed. *Protides of the biological fluids*, Vol. 33. Oxford: Pergamon, 1985.

90. O'Hara PJ, Grant FJ, Haldeman BA, et al. Nucleotide sequence of the gene coding for human factor VII, a vitamin K-dependent protein participating in blood coagulation. *Proc Natl Acad Sci U S A* 1987;84:5158.

91. Yoshitake S, Schach BG, Foster DC, et al. Nucleotide sequence of the gene for human factor IX (antihemophilic factor B). *Biochemistry* 1985; 24:3736.

92. Leytus SP, Foster DC, Kurachi K, et al. Gene for human factor X, a blood coagulation factor whose gene organization is essentially identical to that of factor IX and protein C. *Biochemistry* 1986;25:5098.

93. Foster DC, Yoshitake S, Davie EW. The nucleotide sequence of the gene for human protein C. *Proc Natl Acad Sci U S A* 1985;82:4673.

94. Mount SM. A catalogue of splice junction sequences. *Nucleic Acids Res* 1982;10:459.

95. Deininger PL, Jolly DJ, Rubin CM, et al. Base sequence studies of 300 nucleotide renatured repeated human DNA clones. *J Mol Biol* 1981;151:17.

96. Kawabata S-I, Davie EW. A microsomal endopeptidase from liver with substrate specificity for processing proproteins such as the vitamin K-dependent proteins of plasma. *J Biol Chem* 1992;267:10331.

97. Carlisle TL, Suttie JW. Vitamin K-dependent carboxylase: subcellular location of the carboxylase and enzymes involved in vitamin K metabolism in rat liver. *Biochemistry* 1980;19:1161.

98. Bristol JA, Ratcliffe JV, Roth DA, et al. Biosynthesis of prothrombin: intracellular localozation of the vitamin K-dependent carboxylase and the sites of gamma-carboxylation. *Blood* 1996;88:2585.

99. Furie B, Furie BC. Molecular basis of vitamin K-dependent gamma-carboxylation. *Blood* 1990;75:1753.

100. Foster DC, Rudinski MS, Schach BG, et al. Propeptide of human protein C is necessary for gamma-carboxylation. *Biochemistry* 1987;26:7003.

101. Chow BKC, Ting V, Tufero F, et al. Characterization of a novel liver-specific enhancer in the human prothrombin gene. *J Biol Chem* 1991;266: 18927.

102. Bancroft JD, McDowell SA, Degan SJ. The human prothrombin gene: transcriptional regulation in hepG2 cells. *Biochemistry* 1992;31:12469.

103. Bancroft JD, Schaefer LA, Deegan SJ. Characterization of the Alu-rich 5'-flanking region of the human prothrombin-encoding gene: identification of a positive cis-acting element that regulates liver-specifec expression. *Gene* 1990;95:253.

104. Poort SR, Rosentdall FR, Reitsma PH, et al. A common genetic variaton in the 3'-untranslated region of the prothrombin gene is associated with elevated plasma prothrombin levels and an increase in venous thrombosis. *Blood* 1966;88:3698.

105. Rosendaal FR, Doggen CJ, Zivelin A, et al. Geographic distribution of the 20210 G to A prothrombin variant. *Thromb Haemost* 1998;79:706.

106. Gewirtz AM, Keefer M, Doshi K, et al. Biology of human megakaryocyte factor V. *Blood* 1986;67:1639.

107. Tracy PB, Eide LL, Bowie EJ, et al. Radioimmunoassay of factor V in human plasma and platelets. *Blood* 1982;60:59.

108. Kane WH, Davie EW. Blood coagulation factors V and VIII: structural and functional similarities in their relationship to hemorrhagic and thrombotic disorders. *Blood* 1988;71:539.

109. Kane WH, Davie EW. Cloning of a cDNA coding for human factor V, a blood coagulation factor homologous to factor VIII and ceruloplasmin. *Proc Natl Acad Sci U S A* 1986;83:6800.

110. Kane WH, Ichinose A, Hagen FS, et al. Cloning of cDNAs coding for the heavy chain region and connecting region of human factor V, a blood coagulation factor with four types of internal repeats. *Biochemistry* 1987; 26:6508.

111. Jenny RJ, Pittman DD, Toole JJ, et al. Complete cDNA and derived amino acid sequence of human factor V. *Proc Natl Acad Sci U S A* 1987; 84:4846.
112. Pittman DD, Marquette KA, Kaufman RJ. Role of the B domain in factor VIII and factor V expression. *Blood* 1994;84:4214.
113. Pipe SW, Morris JA, Shah J, et al. Differential interaction of coagulation factor VIII and factor V with protein chaperones calnexin and calreticulin. *J Biol Chem* 1998;273:8537.
114. Wang H, Riddell DC, Guinto ER, et al. Localization of the gene encoding human factor V to chromosome 1q21:25. *Genomics* 1988;2:324.
115. Watson ML, Kingsmore SF, Johnston GI, et al. Genomic organization of the selectin family of leukocyte adhesion molecules on human and mouse chromosome 1. *J Exp Med* 1990;172:263.
116. Cripe LD, Moore KD, Kane WH. Structure of the gene for human coagulation factor V. *Biochemistry* 1992;31:3777.
117. Dahlback B, Carlsson M, Svenson PJ. Familial thrombophilia due to a previously unrecognized mechanism characterized by poor anticoagulant response to activated protein C. *Proc Natl Acad Sci U S A* 1993;90:1004.
118. Dahlback B, Hildebrand B. Inherited resistance to activated protein C is corrected by anticoagulant cofactor activity found to be a property of factor V. *Proc Natl Acad Sci U S A* 1994;91:1396.
119. Bertina RM, Koeleman BPC, Koster T, et al. Mutation in blood coagulation factor V associated with resistance to activated protein C. *Nature* 1994; 369:64.
120. Dahlback B. Resistance to activated protein C caused by the factor V R$^{506}$Q mutation is a common risk factor for venous thrombosis. *Thromb Haemost* 1997;78:483.
121. Kisiel W, Davie EW. Isolation and characterization of bovine factor VII. *Biochemistry* 1975;14:4928.
122. Radcliffe R, Nemerson Y. Activation and control of factor VII by activated factor X and thrombin: isolation and characterization of a single chain form of factor VII. *J Biol Chem* 1975;250:388.
123. Broze GJ Jr, Majerus PW. Purification and properties of human coagulation factor VII. *J Biol Chem* 1980;255:1242.
124. Bajaj SP, Rapaport SI, Brown SF. Isolation and characterization of human factor VII: activation of factor VII by factor Xa. *J Biol Chem* 1981;256:253.
125. DiScipio RG, Hermodson MA, Yates SG, et al. A comparison of human prothrombin, factor IX (Christmas factor), factor X (Stuart factor), and protein S. *Biochemistry* 1977;16:698.
126. McMullen BA, Fujikawa K, Kisiel W. The occurrence of beta-hydroxyaspartic acid in the vitamin K-dependent blood coagulation zymogens. *Biochem Biophys Res Commun* 1983;115:8.
127. Selander-Sunnerhagen M, Ullner M, Persson E, et al. How epidermal growth factor (EGF)-like domain binds calcium. *J Biol Chem* 1992;267:19642.
128. Banner DW, D'Arcy A, Chene C, et al. The crystal structure of the complex of blood coagulation factor VIIa with soluble tissue factor. *Nature* 1996;380:41.
129. Iino M, Foster DC, Kisiel W. Functional consequences of mutations of Ser-52 and Ser-60 in human blood coagulation factor VII. *Arch Biochem Biophys* 1998;352:182.
130. Thim L, Bjoern S, Christensen M, et al. Amino acid sequence and post-translational modifications of human factor VIIa from plasma and transfected baby hamster kidney cells. *Biochemistry* 1988;27:7785.
131. Iwanaga S, Nishimura H, Kawabata S, et al. A new trisaccharide sugar chain linked to a serine residue in the first EGF-like domain of clotting factors VII and IX and protein Z. *Adv Exp Med Biol* 1990;281:121.
132. Nishimura H, Kawabata S, Kisiel W, et al. Identification of a disaccharide (Xyl-Glc) and a trisaccharide (Xyl2-Glc) O-glycosidically linked to a serine residue in the first epidermal growth factor-like domain of human factors VII and IX and protein Z and bovine protein Z. *J Biol Chem* 1989; 264:20320.
133. Bjoern S, Foster DC, Thim L, et al. Human plasma and recombinant factor VII. Characterization of O-glycosylations at serine residues 52 and 60 and effects of site-directed mutagenesis of serine 52 to alanine. *J Biol Chem* 1991;266:11051.
134. Osterud B, Rapaport SI. Activation of factor IX by the reaction product of tissue factor and factor VII: additional pathway for initiating blood coagulation. *Proc Natl Acad Sci U S A* 1977;74:5260.
135. Butenas S, van t Veer C, Mann KG. Evaluation of the initiation phase of blood coagulation using ultrasensitive assays for serive proteases. *J Biol Chem* 1997;272:21527.
136. Hagen FS, Gray CL, O'Hara P, et al. Characterization of a cDNA coding for human factor VII. *Proc Natl Acad Sci U S A* 1986;83:2412.
137. O'Hara PJ, Grant FJ. The human factor VII gene is polymorphic due to variation in repeat copy number in a minisatellite. *Gene* 1988;66:147–158.
138. Tuddenham EGD, Pemberton S, Cooper DN. Inherited factor VII deficiency: genetics and molecular pathology. *Thromb Haemost* 1995;74:313.
139. O'Brien DP, Gale KM, Anderson JS, et al. Purification and characterization of factor VII 304-Gln: a variant molecule with reduced activity isolated from a clinically unaffected male. *Blood* 1991;78:132–140.
140. Green F, Kelleher C, Wilkes H, et al. A common genetic polymorphism associated with lower coagulation factor VII levels in healthy individuals. *Arterioscler Thromb* 1991;11:540–546.
141. Bharadwaj D, Iino M, Kantayianni M, et al. Factor VII central. *J Biol Chem* 1996;271:30685.
142. Kemball-Cook J, Johnson DJD, Takamiya O, et al. Coagulation factor VII Gln$^{100}$ to Arg. *J Biol Chem* 1998;273:8516.
143. Marchetti G, Patracchini P, Papachini M, et al. A polymorphism in the 5'-region of coagulation factor VII gene caused by an inserted decanucleotide. *Hum Genet* 1993;90:575.
144. Arbini A, Pollak ES, Bayleran JK, et al. Severe factor VII deficiency due to a mutation disrupting hepatocyte nuclear factor 4 binding site in the factor VII promoter. *Blood* 1997;89:176.
145. Miao CH, Leytus SP, Chung DW, et al. Liver-specific expression of the gene coding for human factor X, a blood coagulation factor. *J Biol Chem* 1992;267:7395.
146. Reijnen MJ, Sladik FM, Bertina RM, et al. Disruption of a binding site for hepatic nuclear factor 4 results in hemophilia B Leyden. *Proc Natl Acad Sci U S A* 1992;89:6300.
147. Hung HS, High KA. Liver-enriched transcription factor HNF-4 and Ubiquitious factor NF-Y are critical for expression of blood coagulation factor X. *J Biol Chem* 1996;271:2323.
148. Greenderg D, Miao CH, Ho WT, et al. Liver-specific expression of the human factor VII gene. *Proc Natl Acad Sci U S A* 1995;92:12347.
149. Pollak ES, Hung HL, Godin G, et al. Functional characterization of the human factor VII 5'-flanking region. *J Biol Chem* 1996;271:1738.
150. Seligsohn U, Osterud B, Brown SF, et al. Activation of human factor VII in plasma and in purified systems: roles of activated factor IX, kallikrein, and activated factor XII. *J Clin Invest* 1979;64:1056.
151. Radcliffe R, Nemerson Y. Mechanism of activation of bovine factor VII: products of cleavage by factor Xa. *J Biol Chem* 1976;251:4797.
152. Kisiel W, Fujikawa K, Davie EW. Activation of bovine factor VII (proconvertin) by factor XIIa (activated Hageman factor). *Biochemistry* 1977; 16:4189.
153. Radcliffe R, Bagdasarian S, Colman R, et al. Activation of bovine factor VII by Hageman factor fragments. *Blood* 1977;50:611.
154. Yamamoto M, Nakagaki T, Kisiel W. Tissue factor dependent autoactivation of human blood coagulation VII. *J Biol Chem* 1992;267:19089.
155. Pedersen AH, Lund-Hansen T, Bisgaard-Frantzen H, et al. Autoactivation of human recombinant coagulation factor VII. *Biochemistry* 1989;28: 9331.
156. Nakagaki T, Foster DC, Berkner KL, et al. Initiation of the extrinsic pathway of blood coagulation: evidence for the tissue factor-dependent autoactivation of human coagulation factor VII. *Biochemistry* 1991; 30:10819.
157. Hedner U. Dosing and monitoring NovoSeven treatment. *Haemostasis* 1996;26(Suppl. 1):150.
158. Hedner U, Feldstedt M, Glazer S. Recombinant factor VIIa. In: Lusher JM, Kessler CM, eds. *Hemophilia treatment (in) hemophilia and von Willebrand's disease in the 1990's*. Amsterdam: Elsevier Science, 1991.
159. Tuddenham EGD, Lane RS, Rotblat F, et al. Response to infusions of polyelectrolyte fractionated human factor VIII concentrate in adults with haemophilia A and von Willebrand disease. *Br J Haematol* 1982;52:259.
160. Rapaport SI, Schiffman S, Patch MJ, et al. The importance of activation of antihemophilic globulin and poraccelerin by traces of thrombin in the generation of intrinsic prothrombinase activity. *Blood* 1963; 21:221.
161. Osterud B, Rapaport SI, Schiffman S, et al. Formation of intrinsic factor X-antifactor activity, with special reference to the role of thrombin. *Br J Haematol* 1971;21:643.
162. Vehar GA, Davie EW. Preparation and properties of bovine factor VIII (antihemophilic factor). *Biochemistry* 1980;19:401.
163. Vehar GA, Keyt B, Eaton D, et al. Structure of human factor VIII. *Nature* 1984;312:337.
164. Toole JJ, Knopf LJ, Wozney JM, et al. Molecular cloning of a cDNA encoding human antihaemophilic factor. *Nature* 1984;312:342.
165. Mikkelsen J, Thomsen J, Ezban M. Heterogeneity in the tyrosine sulfation of Chinese hamster ovary cell produced recombinant FVIII. *Biochemistry* 1991;30:1533.
166. Michnick DA, Pittman DD, Wise RJ, et al. Identification of individual tyrosine sulfation sites within factor VIII required for optimal activity and efficient thrombin cleavage. *J Biol Chem* 1994;269:20095.
167. Leyte A, van Schijndel HB, Niehrs C, et al. Sulfation of Tyr1680 of human blood coagulation factor VIII is essential for the interaction of factor VIII with von Willebrand factor. *J Biol Chem* 1991;266:740.
168. Gitschier J, Wood WI, Goralka TM, et al. Characterization of the human factor VIII gene. *Nature* 1984;312:326.
169. Wood WI, Capon DJ, Simonsen CC, et al. Expression of active human factor VIII from recombinant DNA clones. *Nature* 1984;312:330.
170. Tagliavacca L, Moon N, Dunham WR, et al. Identification and functional requirement of Cu (I) and its ligands within coagulation factor VIII. *J Biol Chem* 1997;272:27428.
171. Sudhaker K, Fay PJ. Effects of copper on the strutcure and function of factor VIII subunits; evidence for an auxiliary role for copper ions in cofactor activity. *J Biol Chem* 1998;37:6874.
172. Levinson B, Kenwrick S, Lakich D, et al. A transcribed gene in an intron of the human factor VIII gene. *Genomics* 1990;7:1.
173. McGlynn LK, Mueller CR, Begbie M, et al. Role of the liver-enriched transcription factor HNF-1 in transcriptional regulation of the factor VIII gene. *Mol Cell Biol* 1996;16:1936.
174. Figueiredo MS, Brownlee GG. Cis-acting elements and transcription factors involved in the promoter activity of the human factor VIII gene. *J Biol Chem* 1995;270:11828.
175. Bontempo FA, Lewis JH, Garenc TJ, et al. Liver transplantation in hemophilia A. *Blood* 1987;69:1721.
176. Stirling D, Hannant WA, Ludlam CA. Transcriptional activation of the factor VII gene in liver cell lines by IL-6. *Thromb Haemost* 1998;79(1):74.

177. Begbie M, Notley C, Tinlin S, et al. The factor VIII gene acute phase response requires the participation of NF kappa B and C/EBP. *Thromb Haemost* 2000;84(2):216.

178. Kemball-Cook G, Tuddenham EGD, Wacey AI. The factor VIII structure and mutation resource site. HAMSTERS version 4. *Nucleic Acids Res* 1998;26:216.

179. Tuddenham EGD, Cooper DN, Gitschier J, et al. Haemophilia A: database of nucleotide substitutions, deletions, insertions and rearrangements of the factor VIII gene. *Nucleic Acids Res* 1991;19:4821.

180. Millar DS, Steinbrecher RA, Wieland K, et al. The molecular genetic analysis of haemophilia A: characterization of six partial deletions in the factor VIII gene. *Hum Genet* 1990;86:219.

181. Youssoufian H, Antonarakis SE, Aronis S, et al. Characterization of five partial deletions of the factor VIII gene. *Proc Natl Acad Sci U S A* 1987; 84:3772.

182. Youssoufian H, Kasper CK, Phillips DG, et al. Restriction endonuclease mapping of six novel deletions of the factor VIII gene in hemophilia A. *Hum Genet* 1988;80:143.

183. Woods-Samuels P, Kazazian HH Jr, Antonarakis SE. Nonhomologous recombination in the human genome: deletions in the human factor VIII gene. *Genomics* 1991;10:94.

184. Kazazian HH Jr, Wong C, Youssoufian H, et al. Haemophilia A resulting from de novo insertion of L1 sequences represents a novel mechanism for mutation in man. *Nature* 1988;332:164.

185. Woods-Samuels P, Wong C, Mathias SL, et al. Characterization of a non-deleterious L1 insertion in an intron of the human factor VIII gene as further evidence of open reading frames in functional L1 elements. *Genomics* 1989;4:290.

186. Dombroski BA, Mathias SL, Nanthakumar E, et al. Isolation of an active human transposable element. *Science* 1991;254:1805.

187. Higuchi M, Antonarakis SE, Kasch L, et al. Molecular characterization of mild-to-moderate hemophilia A: detection of the mutation in 25 of 29 patients by denaturing gradient gel electrophoresis. *Proc Natl Acad Sci U S A* 1991;88:8307.

188. Gitschier J, Kogan S, Levinson B, et al. Mutations of factor VIII cleavage sites in hemophilia A. *Blood* 1988;72:1022.

189. Pattinson JK, Millar DS, McVey JH, et al. The molecular genetic analysis of hemophilia A: a directed search strategy for the detection of point mutations in the human factor VIII gene. *Blood* 1990;76:2242.

190. Higuchi M, Wong C, Kochhan L, et al. Characterization of mutations in the factor VIII gene by direct sequencing of amplified genomic DNA. *Genomics* 1990;6:65.

191. Arai M, Inaba H, Higuchi M, et al. Direct characterization of factor VIII in plasma: detection of a mutation altering a thrombin cleavage site (Arg372:histidine). *Proc Natl Acad Sci U S A* 1989;86:4277.

192. Arai M, Higuchi M, Antonarakis SE, et al. Characterization of a thrombin cleavage site mutation (Arg1689 to Cys) in the factor VIII gene of two unrelated patients with cross-reacting material-positive hemophilia A. *Blood* 1990;75:384.

193. Foster PA, Fulcher CA, Houghten RA, et al. An immunogenic region within residues Val1670-Glu1684 of the factor VIII light chain induces antibodies which inhibit binding of factor VIII to von Willebrand factor. *J Biol Chem* 1988;263:5230.

194. Youssoufian H, Kazazian HH Jr, Phillips DG, et al. Recurrent mutations in hemophilia A give evidence for CpG mutation hot spots. *Nature* 1986; 324:380.

195. Duncan BK, Miller JH. Mutagenic deamination of cytosine residues in DNA. *Nature* 1980;287:560.

196. Lalloz MRA, McVey JH, Pattinson JK, et al. Haemophilia A diagnosis by analysis of a hypervariable dinucleotide repeat within the factor VIII gene. *Lancet* 1991;338:207.

197. Roddie PH, Ludlam CA. Recombinant coagulations factors. *Blood Rev* 1997;11:169.

198. Mikaelson M, Ericksson B, Lind P, et al. Manufacturing and characterization of a new B-domain deleted recombinant factor VIII, rVIIISQ. *Thromb Haemost* 1993;69:1205.

199. Connelly S, Kaleko M. Gene therapy for hemophilia A. *Thromb Haemost* 1997;78:31.

200. Chance PF, Dyer KA, Kurachi K, et al. Regional localization of the human factor IX gene by molecular hybridization. *Hum Genet* 1983;65:207.

201. Boyd Y, Buckle VJ, Munro EA, et al. Assignment of the haemophilia B (factor IX) locus to the q26-qter region of the X chromosome. *Ann Hum Genet* 1984;48:145.

202. Camerino G, Grzeschik KH, Jaye M, et al. Regional localization on the human X chromosome and polymorphism of the coagulation factor IX gene (hemophilia B locus). *Proc Natl Acad Sci U S A* 1984;81:498.

203. McKusick VA. On the X chromosome of man. *Q Rev Biol* 1962;37:69.

204. Camerino G, Mattei MG, Mettei JF, et al. Close linkage of fragile X-mental retardation syndrome to haemophilia B and transmission through a normal male. *Nature* 1983;306:701.

205. Kurachi K, Davie EW. Isolation and characterization of a cDNA coding for human factor IX. *Proc Natl Acad Sci U S A* 1982;79:6461.

206. Jaye M, De La Salle H, Schamber F, et al. Isolation of a human antihaemophilic factor IX cDNA clone using a unique 52-base synthetic oligonucleotide probe deduced from the amino acid sequence of bovine factor IX. *Nucleic Acids Res* 1983;11:2325.

207. Jagadeeswaran P, Lavelle DE, Kaul R, et al. Isolation and characterization of human factor IX cDNA: identification of Taq1 polymorphism and regional assignment. *Somat Cell Mol Genet* 1984;10:465.

208. Leytus SP, Chung DW, Kisiel W, et al. Characterization of a cDNA coding for human factor X. *Proc Natl Acad Sci U S A* 1984;81:3699.

209. Fung MR, Hay CW, MacGillivray RTA. Characterization of an almost full-length cDNA coding for human blood coagulation factor X. *Proc Natl Acad Sci U S A* 1985;82:3591.

210. Dayhoff MO. *Atlas of protein sequence and structure*, Vol. 5, Suppl. 3. Washington, DC: National Biomedical Research Foundation, 1978.

211. Doolittle RF, Feng DF, Johnson MS. Computer-based characterization of epidermal growth factor precursor. *Nature* 1984;307:558.

212. DiScipio RG, Kurachi K, Davie EW. Activation of human factor IX (Christmas factor). *J Clin Invest* 1978;61:1528.

213. Reijnen MJ, Bertina RM, Reitsma PH. Localization of transcription initiation sites in the human coagulation factor IX gene. *FEBS Lett* 1990; 270:207.

214. Pang C-P, Crossley M, Kent G, et al. Comparative sequence analysis of mammalian factor IX promoters. *Nucleic Acids Res* 1990;18:6731.

215. Kozak M. An analysis of 5'-noncoding sequences from 699 vertebrate messenger RNAs. *Nucleic Acids Res* 1987;15:8125.

216. Briet E, Bertina RM, Van Tilburg NA, et al. Hemophilia B Leyden: a sex linked hereditary disorder that improves after puberty. *N Engl J Med* 1982;306:782.

217. Bolton-Maggs PHB, Jones P, Rizza CR, et al. Hemophilia B Liverpool: a new British family with mild hemophilia B associated with a G to A mutation at −6 in the factor IX promoter. *Thromb Haemost* 1995;69:848.

218. Crossley M, Brownlee GG. Disruption of a C/EBP binding site in the factor IX promoter is associated with hemophilia B. *Nature* 1990;345:444.

219. Picketts DJ, D'Souza C, Bridge PJ, et al. An A to T transversion at position −5 of the factor IX promoter results in hemophilia B. *Genomics* 1992;12:161.

220. Reijnen MJ, Massdam D, Bertina RM, et al. Hemophilia B Leyden: the effect of mutations at +13 on the liver-specific transcription of the factor IX gene. *Blood Coagul Fibrinolysis* 1994;5:341.

221. Reijnen MJ, Peerlinck K, Massdam D, et al. Hemophilia B Leyden: substitution of thymine for guamine at position −21 results in a disruption of a hepatocye nuclear factor 4 binding site in the factor IX promoter. *Blood* 1993;82:151.

222. Reijnen MJ, Sladek FM, Bertina RM, et al. Disruption of a binding site for HNF-4 results in hemophilia B Leyden. *Proc Natl Acad Sci U S A* 1992; 89:6300.

223. Crossley M, Ludwig M, Stowell KM, et al. Recovery from hemophilia B Leyden: an androgen responsive element in the factor IX promoter. *Science* 1992;257:377.

224. Brody JN, Notley C, Cameron C, et al. Androgen effects on factor IX expression: *in vitro* and *in vivo* studies in mice. *Br J Haematol* 1988; 101:273.

225. Giannelli F, Green PM, Sommer SS, et al. Hemophilia B: database of point mutations and short additions and deletions; 5th ed. *Nucleic Acids Res* 1994;22:3546.

226. Picketts D, Mueller CR, Lillicrap D. Transcriptional control of the factor IX gene: analysis of five cis-acting elements and the deleterious effects of naturally occurring hemophilia B Leyden mutations. *Blood* 1994;84:2992.

227. Picketts DJ, Lillicrap DP, Mueller CR. Synergy between transcription factors DBP and C/EBP compensates for a hemophilia B Leyden factor IX mutation. *Nat Genet* 1993;3:175.

228. Birkenmeier EH, Gwynn B, Howard S, et al. Tissue-specific expression, developmemntal regulation and genetic mapping of the gene encoding CCAAT/enhancer binding protein. *Genes Dev* 1989;3:1146.

229. Mueller CR, Maire P, Schibler U. DBP, a liver-enriched transcriptional activator is expressed late in ontogeny and its tissue specificity is determined post-transcriptionally. *Cell* 1990;61:279.

230. Boccia LM, Lillicrap D, Newcombe K, et al. Binding of the Ets factor GA-binding protein to an upstream site in the factor IX promoter is a critical event in transactivation. *Mol Cell Biol* 1996;16:1929.

231. Salier JP, Hirosawa S, Kurachi K. Functional characterization of the 5'-regulatory region of the human factor IX gene. *J Biol Chem* 1990; 265:7062.

232. Kurachi S, Deyashiki Y, Takeshita J, et al. Genetic mechanisms of age regulation of human blood coagulation factor IX. *Science* 1999;285(5428):739.

233. Kurachi S, Hitomi E, Kurachi K. Age and sex dependent regulation of the factor IX gene in mice. *Thromb Haemost* 1996;76(6):965.

234. Winship PR, Anson DS, Rizza CR, et al. Carrier detection in haemophilia B using two further intragenic restriction fragment length polymorphisms. *Nucleic Acids Res* 1984;12:8861.

235. Giannelli F, Choo KH, Winship PR, et al. Characterization and use of an intragenic polymorphic marker for detection of carriers of haemophilia B (factor IX deficiency). *Lancet* 1984;1:239.

236. McGraw RA, Davis LM, Noyes CM, et al. Evidence for a prevalent dimorphism in the activation peptide of human coagulation factor IX. *Proc Natl Acad Sci U S A* 1985;82:2847.

237. Noyes CM, Griffith MJ, Roberts HR, et al. Identification of the molecular defect in factor IX Chapel Hill: substitution of histidine for arginine at position 145. *Proc Natl Acad Sci U S A* 1983;80:4200.

238. Rees DJG, Rizza CR, Brownlee GG. Haemophilia B caused by a point mutation in a donor splice junction of the human factor IX gene. *Nature (London)* 1985;314:643.

239. Weatherall DJ, Higgs DH, Wood WG, et al. Genetic disorders of human hemoglobin as models for analyzing gene regulation. *Philos Trans R Soc Lond B Biol Sci* 1984;307:247.

240. Giannelli F, Choo KH, Rees DJG, et al. Gene deletions in patients with haemophilia B and anti-factor IX antibodies. *Nature (London)* 1983; 303:181.

241. Anson DS, Austen DEG, Brownlee GG. Expression of active human clotting factor IX from recombinant DNA clones in mammalian cells. *Nature (London)* 1985;315:683.

242. De La Salle H, Altenburger W, Elkaim R, et al. Active gamma-carboxylated human factor IX expressed using recombinant DNA techniques. *Nature (London)* 1985;316:268.

243. Busby S, Kumar A, Joseph M, et al. Expression of active human factor IX in transfected cells. *Nature (London)* 1985;316:271.

244. Wasley LC, Rehemtulla A, Bristol JA, et al. PACE/Furin can process the vitamin K-dependant pro-factor IX precursor within the secretory pathway. *J Biol Chem* 1993;286:8458.

245. White GC, Beebe A, Nielsen B. Recombinant factor IX. *Thromb Haemost* 1997;78:261.

246. Dai Y, Roman M, Naviaux RX, et al. Gene therapy via primary myoblasts: long term expression of factor IX protein following transplantation *in vivo*. *Proc Natl Acad Sci U S A* 1992;89:10892.

247. Plamer TD, Thompson AR, Miller AD. Production of human factor IX in animals by genetically modified skin fibroblasts: potential therapy for hemophilia B. *Blood* 1989;73:438.

248. Gerrard AJ, Hudson DL, Brownlee GG, et al. Towards gene therapy for hemophilia B using primary human keratinocytes. *Nat Genet* 1993;3:180.

249. Yao SN, Wilson JM, Nabel EG, et al. Expression of human factor IX in rat capillary endothelial cells: toward somatic gene therapy for hemophilia B. *Proc Natl Acad Sci U S A* 1991;88:8101.

250. Hao QL, Malik P, Salazar R, et al. Expression of biologically active human factor IX in human hematopoietic cells after retroviral vector-mediated gene transduction. *Hum Gene Ther* 1995;6:873.

251. Eisensmith RC, Woo SLC. Viral vector mediated gene therapy for hemophilia B. *Thromb Haemost* 1997;78:24.

252. Kay MA, Rothenberg S, Landen C, et al. *In vivo* gene therapy for hemophilia B: sustained partial correction in factor IX deficient dogs. *Science* 1993;262:117.

253. Kay MA, Landen CN, Rothenberg SR, et al. *In vivo* hepatic gene therapy: complete allbeit transient correction of factor IX deficiency in hemophilia B dogs. *Proc Natl Acad Sci U S A* 1994;91:2353.

254. DiScipio RG, Hermodson MA, Davie EW. Activation of human factor X (Stuart factor) by a protease from Russell's viper venom. *Biochemistry* 1977;16:5253.

255. McMullen BA, Fujikawa K, Kisiel W, et al. Complete amino acid sequence of the light chain of human blood coagulation factor X: evidence for identification of residue 63 as beta-hydroxyaspartic acid. *Biochemistry* 1983; 22:2875.

256. Banyai I, Varadi A, Patthy L. Common evolutionary origin of the fibrin-binding structures of fibronectin and tissue-type plasminogen activator. *FEBS Lett* 1983;163:37.

257. Doolittle RF, Feng DF, Johnson MS. Computer-based characterization of epidermal grown factor precursor. *Nature* 1984;307:558.

258. Titani K, Fujikawa K, Enfield DL, et al. Bovine factor X1 (Stuart factor): amino acid sequence of heavy chain. *Proc Natl Acad Sci U S A* 1975; 72:3082.

259. Royle NJ, Fung MR, MacGillivray RTA, et al. The gene for clotting factor X is mapped to 13q32:qter. *Cytogenet Cell Genet* 1986;41:1185.

260. Miao CH, Leytus SP, Chung DW, et al. Liver-specific expression of the gene coding for factor X, a blood coagulation factor. *J Biol Chem* 1992; 267:7395.

261. Lewis JH, Ferguson JH. Congenital hypoprocertinemia. *Proc Soc Exp Biol Med* 1953;84:651.

262. Hougie C, Barrow EM, Graham JB. Stuart clotting defect I. *J Clin Invest* 1957;36:485.

263. Graham JB, Barrow EM, Hougie C. Stuart clotting defect II. *J Clin Invest* 1957;36:497.

264. Bernardi F, Marchetti G, Patracchini P, et al. Partial gene deletion in a family with factor X deficiency. *Blood* 1989;73:2123.

265. Wieland K, Millar DS, Grundy CB, et al. Molecular genetic analysis of factor deficiency: gene deletion and germline mosaicism. *Hum Genet* 1991;86:273.

266. Reddy SV, Zhou Z-Q, Rao KJ, et al. Molecular characterization of human factor X San Antonio. *Blood* 1989;74:1486.

267. Watzke HH, Wallmark A, Hamaguchi N, et al. Factor XIII Santo Domingo, evidence that the severe clinical phenotype arises from a mutation blocking secretion. *J Clin Invest* 1991;88:1685.

268. Watzke HH, Lechner K, Roberts HR, et al. Molecular defect (Gla + 14 (r) Lys) and its functional consequences in a hereditary factor X deficiency (Factor X "Vorarlberg"). *J Biol Chem* 1990;265:11982.

269. James HL, Girolami A, Fair DS. Molecular defect in coagulation factor X Friuli results from a substitution of serine for proline at position 343. *Blood* 1991;77:317.

270. Huang MN, Hung HL, Stanfield-Oakley SA, et al. Characterization of the human blood coagulation factor X promoter. *J Biol Chem* 1992;267:15440.

271. Thompson RE, Mandle R Jr, Kaplan AP. Association of factor XI and high-molecular-weight kininogen in human plasma. *J Clin Invest* 1977;60:1376.

272. Kurachi K, Davie EW. Activation of human factor XI (plasma thromboplastin antecedent) by XIIa (activated Hageman factor). *Biochemistry* 1977;16:5831.

273. Bouma BN, Griffin JH. Human blood coagulation factor XI: purification, properties, and mechanism of activation by activated factor XII. *J Biol Chem* 1977;252:6432.

274. Naito K, Fujikawa K. Activation of human blood coagulation factor XI independent of factor XII. *J Biol Chem* 1991;266:7353.

275. Gailani D, Broze GJ Jr. Factor XI activation in a revised model of blood coagulation. *Science* 1991;253:909.

276. Kurachi K, Fujikawa K, Davie EW. Mechanism of activation of bovine factor XI by factor XII and factor XIIa. *Biochemistry* 1980;19:1330.

277. Fujikawa K, Chung DW, Hendrickson L, et al. Amino acid sequence of human factor XI: a blood coagulation factor with four tandem repeats that are highly homologous with plasma prekallikrein. *Biochemistry* 1986; 25:2417.

278. Baglia FA, Walsh PN. Thrombin-mediated feedback activation of factor XI on the activated platelet surface is preferred over contact activation by factor XIIa or factor XIa. *J Biol Chem* 2000;275(27):20514.

279. Walsh PN. Roles of platelets and factor XI in the initiation of blood coagulation by thrombin. *Thromb Haemost* 2001;86(1):75.

280. Baglia FA, Badellino KO, Li CQ, et al. Factor XI binding to the platelet glycoprotein Ib-IX-V complex promotes factor XI activation by thrombin. *J Biol Chem* 2002;277(3):1662.

281. Baglia FA, Shrimpton CN, Lopez JA, et al. The glycoprotein Ib-V-IX complex mediates localization of factor XI to lipid rafts on the platelet membrane. *J Biol Chem* 2003;278(24):21744.

282. McMullen BA, Fujikawa K, Davie EW. Location of the disulfide bonds in human coagulation factor XI: the presence of tandem apple domains. *Biochemistry* 1991;30:2056.

283. Chung DW, Fujikawa K, McMullen BA, et al. Human plasma prekallikrein: a zymogen to a serine protease that contains four tandem repeats. *Biochemistry* 1986;25:2410.

284. McMullen BA, Fujikawa K, Davie EW. Location of the disulfide bonds in human plasma prekallikrein: the presence of four novel apple domains in the amino-terminal portion of the molecule. *Biochemistry* 1991;30:2050.

285. De la Cadena RA, Baglia FA, Johnson CA, et al. Naturally occurring human antibodies against two distinct functional domains in the heavy chain of FXI/FXIa. *Blood* 1988;72:1748.

286. Baglia FA, Jameson BA, Walsh PN. Localization of the high-molecular-weight kininogen binding site in the heavy chain of human factor XI to amino acids phenylalanine 56 through serine 86. *J Biol Chem* 1990; 265:4149.

287. Baglia FA, Jameson BA, Walsh PN. Fine mapping of the high-molecular-weight kininogen binding site on blood coagulation factor XI through the use of rationally designed synthetic analogs. *J Biol Chem* 1992;26:4247.

288. Baglia FA, Jameson BA, Walsh PN. Identification and chemical synthesis of a substrate-binding site for factor IX on coagulation factor XIa. *J Biol Chem* 1991;266:24190.

289. Asakai R, Davie EW, Chung DW. Organization of the gene for human factor XI. *Biochemistry* 1987;26:7221.

290. Kato A, Asakai R, Davie EW, et al. Factor XIII gene (FII) is located on the distal end of the long arm of chromosome 4. *Cytogenet Cell Genet* 1989; 52:77.

291. Rapaport SI, Proctor RR, Patch MJ, et al. The mode of inheritance of PTA deficiency: evidence for the existence of major PTA deficiency and minor PTA deficiency. *Blood* 1961;18:159.

292. Seligsohn U. High gene frequency of factor XI (PTA) deficiency in Ashkenazi Jews. *Blood* 1978;51:1223.

293. Asakai R, Chung DW, Davie EW, et al. Factor XI deficiency in Ashkenazi Jews in Israel. *N Engl J Med* 1991;325:153.

294. Meijers JCM, Mulvihill ER, Davie EW, et al. Apple four in human blood coagulation factor XI mediates dimer formation. *Biochemistry* 1992;31:4680.

295. Asakai R, Chung DW, Ratnoff OD, et al. Factor XI (plasma thromboplastin antecedent) deficiency in Ashkenazi Jews is a bleeding disorder that can result from three types of point mutations. *Proc Natl Acad Sci U S A* 1989;86:7667.

296. Lorand L, Konishi K. Activation of the fibrin stabilizing factor of plasma by thrombin. *Arch Biochem Biophys* 1964;105:58.

297. Naski MC, Lorand L, Shafer JA. Characterization of the kinetic pathway for fibrin promotion of alpha-thrombin-catalyzed activation of plasma factor XIII. *Biochemistry* 1991;30:934.

298. Folk JE, Finlayson JS. The epsilon-(gamma-glutamyl) lysine crosslink and the catalytic role of transglutaminases. *Adv Protein Chem* 1977;31:1.

299. Lorand L, Losowsky MS, Miloszewski KJM. Human factor XIII: fibrin-stabilizing factor. *Prog Hemost Thromb* 1980;5:245.

300. Ichinose A, Davie EW. Primary structure of human coagulation factor XIII. *Adv Exp Med Biol* 1988;231:15.

301. Greenberg CS, Shuman MA. The zymogen forms of blood coagulation factor XIII bind specifically to fibrinogen. *J Biol Chem* 1982;257:6096.

302. Schwartz ML, Pizzo SV, Hill RL, et al. Human factor XIII from plasma and platelets; molecular weights, subunit structures, proteolytic activation, and crosslinking of fibrinogen and fibrin. *J Biol Chem* 1973;248:1395.

303. Lorand L. Activation of blood coagulation factor XIIIa. *Ann N Y Acad Sci* 1986;485:144.

304. Skrzynia C, Reisner HM, McDonagh J. Characterization of the catalytic subunit of factor XIII by radioimmunoassay. *Blood* 1982;60:1089.

305. Chung D, Ichinose A. Hereditary disorders related to fibrinogen and factor XIII. In: Scriver CR, Beaudet AL, Sly WS et al., eds. *The metabolic basis of inherited disease*. New York: McGraw-Hill, 1993.

306. Takagi T, Doolittle RF, Amino acid sequence studies on factor XIII and the peptide released during its activation by thrombin. *Biochemistry* 1974; 13:750.

307. Ichinose A, Hendrickson LE, Fujikawa K, et al. Amino acid sequence of the a subunit of human factor XIII. *Biochemistry* 1986;25:6900.

308. Lewis SD, Janus TJ, Lorand L, et al. Regulation of formation of factor XIIIa by its fibrin substrates. *Biochemistry* 1985;24:6772.

309. Grundmann U, Amann E, Zettlmeissl G, et al. Characterization of cDNA coding for human factor XIIIa. *Proc Natl Acad Sci U S A* 1986;83:8024.

310. Ichinose A, Davie EW. Characterization of the gene for the a subunit of human factor XIII (plasma transglutaminase), a blood coagulation factor. *Proc Natl Acad Sci U S A* 1988;85:5829.

311. Tufty RM, Kretsinger RH. Troponin and parvalbumin calcium binding regions predicted in myosin light chain and Tr lysozyme. *Science* 1975; 187:167.

312. Ikura K, Nasu T, Yokota H, et al. Amino acid sequence of guinea pig liver transglutaminase from its cDNA. *Biochemistry* 1988;27:2898.

313. Bishop PD, Teller DC, Smith RA, et al. Expression, purification, and characterization of human factor XIII in saccharomyces cerevisiae. *Biochemistry* 1989;29:1861.

314. Weisberg LJ, Shiu DT, Greenberg CS, et al. Localization of the gene for coagulation factor XIII a-chain to chromosome 6 and identification of sites of synthesis. *J Clin Invest* 1987;79:649.

315. Board PG, Webb GC, McKee J, et al. Localization of the coagulation factor XIIIa subunit gene (F13A) to chromosome bands 6p24-p25. *Cytogenet Cell Genet* 1988;48:25.

316. Korsgren C, Lawler J, Lambert S, et al. Complete amino acid sequence and homologies of human erythrocyte membrane protein band 4.2. *Proc Natl Acad Sci U S A* 1990;87:613.

317. Phillips MA, Stewart BE, Qin Q, et al. Primary structure of keratinocyte transglutaminase. *Proc Natl Acad Sci U S A* 1990;87:9333.

318. Gentile V, Saydak M, Chiocca EA, et al. Isolation and characterization of cDNA clones to mouse macrophage and human endothelial cell tissue transglutaminases. *J Biol Chem* 1991;266:478.

319. Tokunaga F, Yamada M, Muta T, et al. Limulus type II transglutaminase: its purification, characterization, and cDNA cloning. *Thromb Haemost* 1991;65:936.

320. Korsgren C, Cohen CM. Organization of the gene for human erythrocyte membrane protein 4.2: structural similarities with the gene for the a subunit of factor XIII. *Proc Natl Acad Sci U S A* 1991;88:4840.

321. Plakowska RR, Eddy RL, Shows TB, et al. Epidermal type I transglutaminase (TGM1) is assigned to human chromosome 14. *Cytogenet Cell Genet* 1991;56:105.

322. Yorifuji H, Anderson K, Lynch GW, et al. B protein of factor XIII: differentiation between free b and complexed b. *Blood* 1988;72:11645.

323. Rodeghiero F, Morbin M, Barbui T. Subunit a of factor XIII regulated subunit b plasma concentration. *Thromb Haemost* 1981;46:621.

324. Ikematsu S. An approach to the metabolism of factor XIII. *Acta Haematol Jpn* 1981;44:1499.

325. Girolami A, Burul A, Fabris F, et al. Studies on factor XIII antigen in congenital factor XIII deficiency: a tentative classification of the disease in two groups. *Folia Haematol* 1978;105:131.

326. Capellato MG, Lazzaro AR, Marafioti F, et al. A new family with congenital factor XIII deficiency showing a deficit of both subunit a and b type I factor XIII deficiency. *Haematol* 1987;20:179.

327. Saito M, Asakura H, Yoshida T, et al. A familial factor XIII subunit b deficiency. *Br J Haematol* 1990;74:290.

328. Ichinose A, McMullen B, Fujikawa K, et al. Amino acid sequence of the b subunit of human factor XIII, a protein composed of 10 repetitive segments. *Biochemistry* 1986;25:4633.

329. Bottenus RE, Ichinose A, Davie EW. Nucleotide sequence of the gene for the b subunit of human factor XIII. *Biochemistry* 1990;29:11195.

330. Ichinose A, Bottenus RE, Davie EW. Structure of transglutaminases. *J Biol Chem* 1990;265:13411.

331. Lozier J, Takahashi N, Putnam FW. Complete amino acid sequence of human plasma beta2-glycoprotein I. *Proc Natl Acad Sci U S A* 1984; 81:3640.

332. Janatova J, Reid KBM, Willis AC. Disulfide bonds are localized within the short consensus repeat units of complement regulatory proteins: C4b-binding protein. *Biochemistry* 1989;28:4754.

333. Cordoba SR, Rey-Campos J, Dykes DD, et al. Coagulation factor XIII b subunit is encoded by a gene linked to the regulator of complement activation (RCA) gene cluster in man. *Immunogenet* 1988;28:452.

334. Webb GC, Coggan M, Ichinose A, et al. Localization of the coagulation factor XIII b subunit gene (F13B) to chromosome bands 1q31-32.1 and restriction fragment length polymorphism at the locus. *Hum Genet* 1989; 81:157.

335. Ichinose A, Izumi T, Hashiguchi T. The normal and abnormal genes of the a and b subunits in coagulation factor XIII. *Semin Thromb Hemost* 1996; 22:385.

336. Maynard JR, Heckman CA, Pitlick FA, et al. Association of tissue factor activity with the surface of cultured cells. *J Clin Invest* 1975;55:814.

337. Maynard JR, Dreyer BE, Stemerman MB, et al. Tissue-factor coagulant activity of cultured human endothelial and smooth muscle cells and fibroblasts. *Blood* 1977;50:387.

338. Weiss HJ, Turitto VT, Baumgartner HR, et al. Evidence for the presence of tissue factor activity on subendothelium. *Blood* 1989;73:968.

339. Wilcox JN, Smith KM, Schwartz SM, et al. Localization of tissue factor in the normal vessel wall and in the atheroschlerotic plaque. *Proc Natl Acad Sci U S A* 1989;86:2839.

340. Pitlick FA, Nemerson Y. Binding of the protein component of tissue factor to phospholipids. *Biochemistry* 1970;9:5105.

341. Morrissey JH, Fakhrai H, Edginton TS. Molecular cloning of the cDNA for tissue factor, the cellular receptor for the initiation of the coagulation protease cascade. *Cell* 1987;50:129.

342. Scarpati EM, Wen D, Broze GJ, et al. Human tissue factor: cDNA sequence and chromosome localization of the gene. *Biochemistry* 1987;26:5234.

343. Spicer EK, Horton R, Bloem L, et al. Isolation of cDNA clones coding for human tissue factor: primary structure of the protein and cDNA. *Biochemistry* 1987;84:5148.

344. Broze GJ Jr. Binding of human factor VII and VIIa to monocytes. *J Clin Invest* 1982;70:526.

345. Bach R, Gentry R, Nemerson Y. Factor VII binding to tissue factor in reconstituted phospholipid vesicles: induction of cooperativity by phosphatidylserine. *Biochemistry* 1986;25:4007.

346. Fair DS, MacDonald MJ. Cooperative interaction between factor VII and cell surface-expressed tissue factor. *J Biol Chem* 1987;262:11692.

347. Sakai T, Lund-Hansen T, Paborsky L, et al. Binding of human factors VII and VIIa to a human bladder carcinoma cell line (J82): implications for the initiation of the extrinsic pathway of blood coagulation. *J Biol Chem* 1989;264:9980.

348. Nemerson Y, Repke D. Tissue factor accelerates the activation of coagulation factor VII: the role of a bifunctional coagulation cofactor. *Thromb Res* 1985;40:351.

349. Rao IVM, Rapaport SI. Activation of factor VII bound to tissue factor: a key early step in the tissue factor pathway of blood coagulation. *Proc Natl Acad Sci U S A* 1988;85:6687.

350. Bach R, Konigsberg W, Nemerson Y. Human tissue factor contains thioester-linked palmitate and stearate on the cytoplasmic half-cysteine. *Biochemistry* 1988;27:4227.

351. Mackman N, Morrissey JH, Fowler B, et al. Complete sequence of the human tissue factor gene, a highly regulated cellular receptor that initiates the coagulation protease cascade. *Biochemistry* 1989;28:1755.

352. Lyberg T, Galdal KS, Evensen SA, et al. Cellular cooperation in endothelial cell thromboplastin synthesis. *Br J Haematol* 1983;53:85.

353. Nawroth PP, Handley DA, Esmon CT, et al. Interleukin 1 induces endothelial cell procoagulant while surpressing cell-surface anticoagulant activity. *Proc Natl Acad Sci U S A* 1986;83:3460.

354. Stern DM, Drillings M, Kisiel W, et al. Activation of factor IX bound to cultured bovine aortic endothelial cells. *Proc Natl Acad Sci U S A* 1984;81:913.

355. Brox JH, Osterud B, Bjorklid E, et al. II Production and availability of thromboplastin in endothelial cells: the effects of thrombin, endotoxin and platelets. *Br J Haematol* 1984;57:239.

356. Rivers RPA, Hathaway WE, Weston WL. The endotoxin-induced coagulant activity of human monocytes. *Br J Haematol* 1975;30:311.

357. Osterud B, Bjorklid E. The production and availability of tissue thromboplastin in cellular populations of whole blood exposed to various concentrations of endotoxin: as assay for detection of endotoxin. *Scand J Haematol* 1982;29:175.

358. Lybert T, Nilsson K, Prydz H. Synthesis of thromboplastin by U937 cells. *Br J Haematol* 1982;51:631.

359. Mackman N. Regulation of the tissue factor gene. *Thromb Haemost* 1997; 78:747.

360. Kisiel W. Human plasma protein C: isolation, characterization and activation by human thrombin. *J Clin Invest* 1979;64:761.

361. Marlar RA, Kleiss AJ, Griffin J. Mechanism of action of human activated protein C, a thrombin-dependent anticoagulant enzyme. *Blood* 1982; 59:1067.

362. Stenflo J. A new vitamin K-dependent protein, purification from bovine plasma and preliminary characterization. *J Biol Chem* 1976; 251:355.

363. Esmon CT, Stenflo J, Suttie JW, et al. A new vitamin K-dependent protein, a phospholipid-binding zymogen of a serine esterase. *J Biol Chem* 1976; 251:3052.

364. Kisiel W, Ericsson LH, Davie EW. Proteolytic activation of protein C from bovine plasma. *Biochemistry* 1976;15:4893.

365. Esmon CT, Owen WG. Identification of an endothelial cell cofactor for thrombin-catalyzed activation of protein C. *Proc Natl Acad Sci U S A* 1981;78:2249.

366. Owen WG, Esmon CT. Functional properties of an endothelial cell cofactor for thrombin-catalyzed activation of protein C. *J Biol Chem* 1981; 256:5532.

367. Esmon NL, Owen WG, Esmon CT. Isolation of a membrane-bound cofactor for thrombin-catalyzed activation of protein C. *J Biol Chem* 1982; 257:859.

368. Kisiel W, Canfield WM, Ericsson LH, et al. Anticoagulant properties of bovine plasma protein C following activation by thrombin. *Biochemistry* 1977;16:5824.

369. Dahlback B, Stenflo J. Inhibitory effect of activated protein C on activation of prothrombin by platelet-bound factor Xa. *Eur J Biochem* 1980; 107:331.

370. Vehar GA, Davie EW. Preparation and properties of bovine factor VIII by activated protein C and protein S. *Arch Biochem Biophys* 1987;252:322.

371. Walker FJ, Chavin SI, Fay PJ. Inactivation of factor VIII by activated protein C and protein S. *Arch Biochem Biophys* 1987;252:322.

372. Walker FJ. Regulation of activated protein C by a new protein. *J Biol Chem* 1980;255:5521.

373. Walker FJ. Regulation of activated protein C by protein S. *J Biol Chem* 1981;256:11128.

374. Fernlund P, Stenflo J. Amino acid sequence of the light chain of bovine protein C. *J Biol Chem* 1982;257:12170.

375. Stenflo J, Fernlund P. Amino acid sequence of the heavy chain of bovine protein C. *J Biol Chem* 1982;257:12180.

376. Foster D, Davie EW. Characterization of a cDNA coding for human protein C. *Proc Natl Acad Sci U S A* 1984;81:4766.

377. Long GL, Belagaje RM, MacGillivray RTA. Coding and sequencing of liver cDNA coding for bovine protein C. *Proc Natl Acad Sci U S A* 1984; 81:4766.

378. Beckmann RJ, Schmidt RJ, Santerre RF, et al. The structure and evolution of a 461 amino acid human protein C precursor and its messenger RNA, based upon the DNA sequence of cloned human liver cDNAs. *Nucleic Acids Res* 1985;13:5233.

379. Plutzky J, Hoskins JA, Long GL, et al. Evolution and organization of the human protein C gene. *Proc Natl Acad Sci U S A* 1986;83:546.

380. Drakenberg T, Fernlund P, Roepstorff P, et al. beta-Hydroxyaspartic acid in vitamin K-dependent protein C. *Proc Natl Acad Sci U S A* 1983;80:1802.

381. Kato A, Miura O, Sumi Y, et al. Assignment of the human protein C gene (PROC) to chromosome region 2q14:q21 by *in situ* hybridization. *Cytogenet Cell Genet* 1988;47:46.

382. Miao Ch, Ho WT, Greenberg DL, et al. Transcriptional regulation of the gene coding for human protein C. *J Biol Chem* 1996;271:9587.

383. Romeo G, Hassan HJ, Staempfli S, et al. Hereditary thrombophilia: identification of nonsense and missense mutations in the protein C gene. *Proc Natl Acad Sci U S A* 1987;84:2829.

384. Matsuda M, Sugo T, Sakata Y, et al. A thrombotic state due to an abnormal protein C. *N Engl J Med* 1988;319:1265.

385. Grundy C, Chitolie A, Talbot S, et al. Protein C London 1: recurrent mutation at Arg 169 (CGG:TGG) in the protein C gene causing thrombosis. *Nucleic Acids Res* 1989;17:10513.

386. Berg LP, Scopes DA, Alhaq A, et al. Disruption of a binding site for HNF-1 in the protein C gene promoter is associated with hereditary thrombophilia. *Hum Molec Genet* 1994;3:2147.

387. Spek CA, Greengard JS, Griffin JH, et al. Two mutations in the promoter region of the human protein C gene. Both cause type I protein C deficiency by disruption of two HNF-3 binding sites. *J Biol Chem* 1995; 270: 24216.

388. Spek CA, Lannoy VJ, Lemaigre FP, et al. Type I protein C deficiency caused by disruption of a hepatocyte nuclear factor (HNF)-6/HNF-1 binding site in the human protein C gene promoter. *J Biol Chem* 1998; 273:10168.

389. DiScipio RG, Davie EW. Characterization of protein S, a gamma-carboxyglutamic acid containing protein from bovine and human plasma. *Biochemistry* 1979;18:899.

390. Fair DS, Marlar RA. Biosynthesis and secretion of factor VII, protein C, protein S, and the protein C inhibitor from a human hepatoma cell line. *Blood* 1986;67:64.

391. Koedam JA, Meijers JCM, Sixma JJ, et al. Inactivation of human factor VIII by activated protein C, cofactor activity of protein S and protective effect of von Willebrand factor. *J Clin Invest* 1988;82:1236.

392. Schwarz HP, Fischer M, Hopmeier P, et al. Plasma protein S deficiency in familial thrombotic disease. *Blood* 1984;64:1297.

393. Comp PC, Nixon RR, Cooper MR, et al. Familial protein S deficiency is associated with recurrent thrombosis. *J Clin Invest* 1984;74:2082.

394. Comp PC, Esmon CT. Recurrent venous thromboembolism in patients with a partial deficiency of protein S. *N Engl J Med* 1984;311:1525.

395. Broekmans AW, Bertina RM, Reinalda-Poot J, et al. Hereditary protein S deficiency and venous thromboembolism, a study in three Dutch families. *Thromb Haemost* 1985;53:273.

396. Dahlback B. Purification of human C4b-binding protein and formation of its complex with vitamin K-dependent protein S. *Biochem J* 1983; 209:847.

397. Fair DS, Revak DJ. Quantitation of human protein S in the plasma of normal and warfarin-treated individuals by radioimmunoassay. *Thromb Res* 1984;36:527.

398. Dahlback B, Hildebrand B. Degradation of human complement C4b in the presence of the C4b-binding protein/protein S complex. *Biochem J* 1983;209:857.

399. Dahlback B. Inhibition of protein $C_a$ cofactor function of human and bovine protein S by C4b-binding protein. *J Biol Chem* 1986;261:12011.

400. Walker FJ. Identification of a new protein involved in the regulation of the anticoagulant activity of activated protein C, protein S-binding protein. *J Biol Chem* 1986;261:10941.

401. Lundwall A, Dackowski W, Chohen E, et al. Isolation and sequencing of the cDNA for human protein S, a regulator of blood coagulation. *Proc Natl Acad Sci U S A* 1986;83:6716.

402. Hoskins J, Norman DK, Beckmann RJ, et al. Cloning and characterization of human liver cDNA encoding a protein S precursor. *Proc Natl Acad Sci U S A* 1987;84:349.

403. Dahlback B, Lundwall A, Stenflo J. Localization of thrombin cleavage sites in the amino-terminal region of bovine protein S. *J Biol Chem* 1986; 261:5111.

404. Walker FJ. Properties of chemically modified protein S: effect on the conversion of gamma-methyleneglutamic acid on functional properties. *Biochemistry* 1986;25:6305.

405. Dahlback B. Purification of human vitamin K-dependent protein S and its limited proteolysis by thrombin. *Biochem J* 1983;209:837.

406. Suzuki K, Nishioka J, Hasimoto S. Regulation of activated protein C by thrombin-modified protein S. *J Biochem* 1983;94:699.

407. Walker FJ. Regulation of vitamin K-dependent protein S, inactivation by thrombin. *J Biol Chem* 1984;259:10335.

408. Stenflo J, Lundwall A, Dahlback B. beta-Hydroxyasparagine in domains homologous to the epidermal growth factor precursor in vitamin K-dependent protein S. *Proc Natl Acad Sci U S A* 1987;84:368.

409. Nelson RM, VanDusen WJ, Friedman PA, et al. beta-Hydroxyaspartic acid and beta-hydroxyasparagine residues in recombinant human protein S are not required for anticoagulant cofactor activity or for binding to C4b-binding protein. *J Biol Chem* 1991;266:20586.

410. Walker FJ. Characterization of a synthetic peptide that inhibits the interaction between protein S and C4b-binding protein. *J Biol Chem* 1989; 264:17645.

411. Grinnell BW, Walls JD, Marks C, et al. Gamma-carboxylated isoforms of recombinant human protein S with different biologic properties. *Blood* 1990;76:2546.

412. Malm J, Cohen E, Dackowski W, et al. Expression of completely gamma-carboxylated and beta-hydroxylated recombinant human vitamin K-dependent protein S with full biological activity. *Eur J Biochem* 1990; 187:737.

413. Ploos van Amstel HK, van der Zanden AL, Bakker E, et al. Two genes homologous with human protein S cDNA are located on chromosome 3. *Thromb Haemost* 1987;58:982.

414. Watkins PC, Eddy R, Fukushima Y, et al. The gene for protein S maps near the centromere of human chromosome 3. *Blood* 1988;71:238.

415. Schmidel DK, Tatro AV, Phelps LG, et al. Organization of the human protein S genes. *Biochemistry* 1990;29:7845.

416. Ploos van Amstel HK, Reitsma PH, van der Logt PE, et al. Intron-exon organization of the active human protein S gene PS alpha and its pseudogene PS beta: duplication and silencing during primate evolution. *Biochemistry* 1990;29:7853.

417. Edenbrandt CM, Lundwall A, Wydro R, et al. Molecular analysis of the gene for vitamin K-dependent protein S and its pseudogene. *Biochemistry* 1990;29:7861.

418. Gershagen S, Lundwall A, Fernlund P. Characterization of the human sex hormone binding globulin (SHBG) gene and demonstration of two transcripts in both liver and testis. *Nucleic Acids Res* 1989;17:9245.

419. Ploos van Amstel HK, Reitsma PH, Bertina RM. The human protein S locus: identification of the PS alpha gene as a site of liver protein S messenger RNA synthesis. *Biochem Biophys Res Commun* 1988;157:1033.

420. Ploos van Amstel HK, Huisman MV, Reitsma PH, et al. Partial protein S gene deletion in a family with hereditary thrombophilia. *Blood* 1989; 73:479.

421. Bertina RM, Ploos van Amstel HK, van Wijngaarden A, et al. Heerlen polymorphism of protein S, an immunologic polymorphism due to dimorphism of residue 460. *Blood* 1990;76:538.

# CHAPTER 4 ■ GENETICS OF COAGULATION

RODNEY M. CAMIRE AND ELEANOR S. POLLAK

The determination of the gene, complementary deoxyribonucleic acid (cDNA), and amino acid sequences of all of the proteins known to be involved in the hemostatic process has been completed. This task, begun in the early 1980s, has allowed for (a) deduction of amino acid sequences from the cloned cDNAs of several species, (b) characterization of gene structure and organization, (c) characterization of mutations responsible for inherited abnormalities, (d) characterization of polymorphisms useful for gene-tracking studies, (e) production of large quantities of recombinant protein for research and for therapeutic purposes, and (f) the development of animal models of hemostatic disease through transgenic and gene knockout technologies. It has also made possible the contemplation of a novel approach to the treatment of bleeding diatheses—that of gene transfer. This chapter focuses primarily on various genetic aspects of procoagulant, anticoagulant, and fibrinolytic factors involved in human blood coagulation, with emphasis on gene structure and mutations that predispose to bleeding or thrombosis. We have also focused on mutational mechanisms and how new genomic information derived from the Human Genome Project (HGP) will impact genetic analysis.

## GENOMIC ERA

The completion of the HGP in April 2003 was an enormous and basic scientific achievement (1,2). The HGP has provided and will continue to provide substantial advances in the understanding of gene structure and organization, genetic variation, comparative genomics, and genomic medicine. Genomic research, the study of the functions and interactions of all the genes in the genome, including interactions with environmental factors, offers a new and unique opportunity for understanding how diseases occur. Although the plethora of new data generated from the HGP has enormous potential, navigating and analyzing the data in a meaningful way can be a daunting task. To assist scientists, numerous Web sites, courses, and textbooks have become available, in addition to published guides (3). There are currently three major Web portals that serve as central hubs for genome-related resources (3). The first is the National Center for Biotechnology Information (NCBI) run by the National Institutes of Health (NIH) (http://www.ncbi.nlm.nih.gov/); the second is Ensembl (http://www.ensembl.org), which is a collaborative effort between the Wellcome Trust Sanger Institute and (European Molecular Biology Laboratory) EMBL's European Bioinformatics Institute; and the third is the UCSC Genome Browser (http://www.genome.ucsc.edu) developed by an academic research group at the University of California, Santa Cruz. Listed in Table 4-1 are relevant Web sites that will enable investigators to obtain genomic information, search for useful sequence features such as single nucleotide polymorphisms (SNPs) and mutations, and also perform sequence-based searching. The list is far from comprehensive and is intended to introduce the reader to the major genomic Web portals.

## Application of Genomic Information

An immediate application of genomic sequence information is to accelerate the identification of genes that are associated with human disease (4). There are several strategies to accomplish this, the most common being genetic linkage analysis (genome-wide linkage scan or homozygosity mapping) (5). In this type of analysis, the chromosomal location of a disease-causing gene can be identified. Genome-wide linkage analysis usually requires families in which several individuals are affected with the disease of interest. Evenly spaced DNA markers are used to trace the inheritance of each copy of each chromosome. Chromosomal segments that do not influence disease segregate randomly, whereas those that do will not be inherited at random. Instead, the particular copy that, in each family, carries the disease-causing mutation will be shared among affected family members more often than would be predicted by chance (6). The DNA markers that are typically used are termed microsatellites, which are di-, tri-, or tetranucleotide tandem repeats in DNA sequences and can be readily followed by simple polymerase chain reaction (PCR) techniques. Typically, the segment of the genome between identified microsatellite markers that influences the disease state is quite large: millions to tens of millions of base pairs in length, spanning dozens to hundreds of genes. However, the advent of the HGP has allowed researchers to move rapidly from large chromosomal regions to individual candidate genes because all genes identified within any linkage region are immediately available. It should be pointed out that this process formerly took months to years but can now be accomplished in a few weeks.

The development of more powerful software analysis tools as well as better DNA markers should help facilitate the identification of genes that are caused by the combined effects of multiple genes with environmental factors (i.e., thrombosis). Among such tools under development is a haplotype map of the human genome. A haplotype is a group of nearby alleles or genetic markers that are inherited together. These blocks of DNA are roughly consistent among all humans, but different individuals have different versions of the blocks, allowing identification of relation between these haplotype blocks and diseases in groups of individuals (7). The International Haplotype Map Project (HapMap; http://www.hapmap.org) aims to define the haplotype structure of human populations and the markers to identify them unambiguously. The HapMap should greatly facilitate genetic linkage studies by decreasing the number of genetic markers that need to be examined.

**TABLE 4-1**

COMPILATION OF USEFUL INTERNET RESOURCES

Major genome browsers:
   http://www.ncbi.nlm.nih.gov/mapview
   http://www.ensembl.org
   http://genome.ucsc.edu
Genome annotation:
   http://www.ncbi.nlm.nih.gov/genome/guide/build.html
   http://www.ensembl.org/Docs/wiki/html/EnsemblDocs/EnsemblDAS.html
   http://www.ensembl.org/Docs/wiki/html/EnsemblDocs/ScienceDocumentation.html
Genomic databases and resources:
   http://www.hgmd.org
   http://www.ncbi.nlm.nih.gov/Omim
   http://www.ncbi.nlm.nih.gov/SNP/
   http://snp.cshl.org
   http://www.hapmap.org
Sequence-based searching:
   http://www.ncbi.nlm.nih.gov/BLAST/
   http://www.ensembl.org/Homo_sapiens/blastview

There are now several examples in which genome-wide scans have localized or identified disease-causing genes. A notable example is the identification of the lamin A gene as being responsible for Hutchinson-Gilford progeria syndrome (8). With respect to hemostasis-related genes, there are three excellent recent examples: the gene responsible for combined factor V/factor VIII (FV/FVIII) deficiency (*ERGIC-53*, now called *LMAN1*) (9,10), the gene responsible for thrombotic thrombocytopenic purpura (*ADAMTS13*) (11), and the gene for vitamin K 2, 3-epoxide reductase (*VKORC1*) (12,13).

# MUTATIONS: MECHANISMS AND DATABASES

Alterations in a gene sequence can be neutral, detrimental, or favorable. The evolution of these alterations plays an important role in disease, including those of blood coagulation and fibrinolysis. Alterations in the gene sequence are semantically referred to as a mutation when the variation leads to a phenotypic change, a polymorphism when the genetic change is present in greater than 5% of alleles in a population, and a rare sequence variant when the change occurs in less than 5% of alleles. Therefore, distinct populations show variations not only in disease prevalence but also in the frequency of polymorphic changes. These variations prove critical in tracking the migration of a particular population. Mechanisms commonly responsible for genetic changes will be discussed in the following sections.

## Types of Genetic Mutations

### Point Mutations

A point mutation is defined as a change of a single base pair of a DNA sequence in a gene caused by the substitution of one nucleotide for another. A single codon in frame (missense mutation) may predict replacement of a single amino acid in an otherwise normal protein. When the change results in a stop codon (nonsense mutation), a truncated protein product results. Sometimes, the mutated proteins are not properly produced, secreted into the blood, or located in the physiologic site. When they do circulate in substantial amounts, the variant

protein often circulates with impaired function. When a single base change is phenotypically silent, this is commonly referred to as an SNP. Outside the actual coding region, it is even more likely that nucleotide substitutions are silent. This is because much of the sequence surrounding the coding regions is of limited importance for gene function. Notable exceptions are mutations in binding sites for transcription factors that regulate gene activity, mutations that affect splicing of the immature RNA, and mutations that may alter the stability of the RNA.

Up to approximately 50% of the single nucleotide substitutions occur as transitions within cytosine–phosphoguanine (CpG) dinucleotides, the most common hot–spot for mutation (14,15). This finding is all the more remarkable when one considers that CpG dinucleotides are underrepresented in most genes, presumably because of the evolutionary loss of these dinucleotides. The reason CpG dinucleotides are hot spots for mutation lies in the fact that these dinucleotides are sites of methylation of the cytosine residue (i.e., a CpG becomes a TpG or a CpA) (14). Methylcytosine readily deaminates to thymine spontaneously (see Fig. 4-1). After the C to T transition occurs in the reverse or "antisense" DNA strand, the sequence in its complementary coding strand is changed from G to A. Because the common (but not exclusive) codon for Arg is CGx, many CpG dinucleotide mutations are found within Arg codons, producing Arg to stop, Gln, His, Cys, or Trp mutations. When the same CpG transition occurs among different families, it often is possible to distinguish independent mutational events from founder effects through haplotype or pedigree analyses.

### Insertion/Deletion

Insertion/deletion is a type of variation that is defined as a change in the DNA sequence created by the addition or subtraction of nucleotides. When the insertion or deletion is within the triplet open reading frame and the change is a number of nucleotides that is not a multiple of three, this disruption results in a frameshift mutation. A frameshift almost inevitably results in a termination signal that changes the length and sequence of the mature RNA transcript; the message translates from the mutation onward and usually results in a premature stop codon producing a grossly abnormal protein with impaired function and viability.

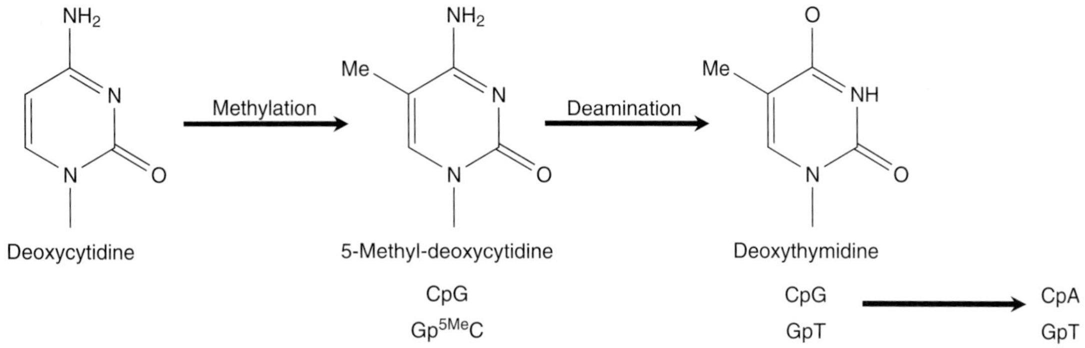

**FIGURE 4-1.** Deamination of 5-methyl-deoxycytidine. Methylation of deoxyribonucleic acid (DNA) occurs on most of the cytosine residues that are in cytosine–phosphoguanine (CpG or CG) dinucleotides. Loss of the amino group of 5-methyl-deoxycytidine changes it to deoxythymidine and represents a common mechanism of point mutations. After the C to T transition occurs in the antisense strand, the coding sequence is changed from 5'-CG-3' to 5'-CA-3' (i.e., G to A in the sense strand).

## Categorization of Mutations

Mutations themselves are commonly categorized either as recessive or dominant. Strictly speaking, a recessive mutation implies that heterozygotes (one copy of mutation) have a normal phenotype and that only homozygotes (two copies of the mutation) are phenotypically affected. Recessive-negative mutations display a predominantly recessive inheritance with a nearly infinite number of different mutations. Most known mutations in the genes encoding the coagulation and fibrinolytic genes are recessive negative. Mutations of this category come to clinical attention when present in homozygous (doubly or compound heterozygous) or hemizygous (for X-linked disorders) form. Mutations that underlie recessive-negative mutations are highly variable and may occur randomly anywhere in the gene because an almost infinite number of possibilities could impair gene function. A dominant mutation refers to a genetic change that lacks phenotypic differences between affected heterozygous and homozygous individuals.

Dominant-negative mutations show a dominant inheritance with a narrow spectrum of mutations. From the perspective of family studies, this distinction is informative in that dominant mutations should be suspected after successive generations are affected; recessive mutations normally occur only within one generation. Dominant-negative mutations are exemplified by the genes for multimeric proteins such as von Willebrand factor (VWF) and fibrinogen (16,17).

Dominant (incomplete) inheritance is usually seen when there is a mutation that causes a gain-of-function. This inheritance is much less common because there is usually only a small spectrum of mutations that will increase the function of a gene. The best known example of a gain-of-function mutation is factor $V_{Leiden}$, discussed herein. Gain-of-function mutations are clearly less heterogeneous than loss-of-function mutations. This can be explained by the fact that there are an infinite number of ways to destroy gene function, whereas few mutations lead to improvement of gene or protein function. As a result, it is easier to set up simple and effective genetic screening for gain-of-function mutations.

In reality, mutations are not always strictly dominant or recessive; the penetrance of a mutant phenotype can vary dramatically, largely because of the influence of concomitant genetic changes. Therefore, recessive-negative mutations are not always entirely recessive. For example, although homozygous protein C deficiency produces severe thrombotic disease and purpura fulminans at birth (18), heterozygotes may either experience thromboembolic disease later in life or never develop venous thrombosis (19,20).

## Normal Variants and Polymorphisms

Normal variants and polymorphisms are particularly useful in gene-tracking studies of families with a severe bleeding or thrombotic disorder. In such studies, a polymorphism is used as a marker of a defective gene when the actual gene mutation is not known. The defective gene can then be followed throughout a family. Several key family members usually are needed to follow the inheritance of both normal and defective genes. This approach has been particularly useful in genetic counseling for hemophilia A or B. Several limitations restrict the use of polymorphisms in genetic counseling (21). First, polymorphisms are not informative when key individuals are homozygous for the marker. One can try to circumvent this problem by using multiple markers for a gene. This approach is not always helpful because polymorphisms are often in linkage disequilibrium, which means that of all the possible haplotypes of a polymorphic gene, only a few occur in the population. Therefore, when an individual is homozygous for one marker in a gene, he or she is also likely to be homozygous for all other markers. Furthermore, sometimes DNA samples on key family members are unavailable, which precludes linkage studies.

When informative intragenic polymorphisms are not available for family studies, extragenic loci are sometimes used. However, the frequency of recombination (crossover) between a linked extragenic site and the mutation within the gene is between 2% and 10% per meiosis, precluding definitive carrier testing. Extragenic sites are not sufficiently linked to be reliable for prenatal diagnosis.

Polymorphisms also are increasingly popular as markers of risk factors for disease (22). In the case of coagulation proteins, most of these studies are directed at venous thrombosis and cardiovascular disease. Often, as in the case of protein C, fibrinogen, factor VII, plasminogen activator inhibitor-1 (PAI-1), and the prothrombin 20210GA variant, a particular relation exists between polymorphisms and plasma levels of the protein. Studies of these polymorphisms in (nested) case–control or family studies may help define the role of specific clotting factors in disease.

## Multifactorial Disease

Contrasting with rare monogenetic diseases are the milder and much more common multifactorial or complex diseases, such as type 2 diabetes mellitus, hypertension, coronary artery disease, and venous thrombosis. In these diseases, a multitude of genetic and environmental risk factors interact in the pathogenesis. In venous thrombotic disease, thrombotic episodes typically occur relatively late in life. In up to 50% of patients, genetic risk factors such as heterozygosity for mutations in coagulation inhibitors are found. In addition, heterozygosity for additional mutations (e.g., antithrombin, protein C, protein S, and factor $V_{Leiden}$) acts as a susceptibility factor contributing to the age of disease onset (23). Moreover, it is increasingly clear that the presence of more than one of these heterozygous susceptibility factors is not rare. Therefore, heterozygosity for recessive mutations may contribute to a disease but may lessen the risk of other diseases.

The high prevalence of the factor $V_{Leiden}$ allele predisposing patients to a risk of venous thrombosis can be explained from an evolutionary standpoint by a survival advantage in women because of a reduced rate of intrapartum hemorrhage in carriers of factor $V_{Leiden}$ (24). This prevalence becomes most apparent in extensive family or population studies. In addition, environmental/acquired challenges may reveal a genetic change that would otherwise not be detected. A salient example of this phenomenon is the discovery of a warfarin-sensitivity mutation in patients receiving warfarin therapy who are otherwise phenotypically normal (25). These risk factors often occur in combination with "environmental" risk factors such

as severe illness, surgery, or the use of oral contraceptives. It is important to note that when carriers of one genetic risk factor are compared with carriers of multiple risk factors, thrombotic symptoms tend to occur at an earlier age in the second group (26). Current therapeutic recommendations for prophylactic treatment are largely dependent on factors beyond the exact patient genotype.

## Databases of Mutations

Over the last decade, several groups have undertaken the compilation of mutations in the genes for coagulation factors that result in a measurable change in phenotype. These databases are useful for clinicians and for investigators interested in both regulation of expression and structure–function analyses of these proteins. Although many of these databases have been published in a variety of forms, most large databases are currently available on the Internet (see Table 4-2). These online databases are continually updated and typically provide useful information about the gene of interest, as well as pertinent references. Some of the hemostatic proteins currently do not have their own mutation databases; mutations in these proteins can be found at the Human Gene Mutation Database at the Institute of Medical Genetics in Cardiff, at http://www.hgmd.org/.

### TABLE 4-2

COMPILATION OF NATURALLY OCCURRING MUTATIONS IN THE GENES OF HUMAN COAGULATION FACTORS

| Genes | Database Web site |
|---|---|
| Prothrombin | www.hgmd.org; In Search enter "119894" for keyword |
| Factor X | www.hgmd.org; In Search enter "119890" for keyword |
| Factor VII | http://193.60.222.13/ |
| Factor IX | http://www.kcl.ac.uk/ip/petergreen/haemBdatabase.html |
| Factor XI | www.hgmd.org; In Search enter "119891" for keyword |
| Tissue factor | www.hgmd.org; In Search enter "119895" for keyword |
| Factor VIII | http://europium.csc.mrc.ac.uk/WebPages/Main/main.htm |
| Factor V | www.hgmd.org; In Search enter "119896" for keyword |
| Protein C | http://www.xs4all.nl/%7Ereitsma/Prot_C_home.htm |
| Thrombomodulin | www.hgmd.org; In Search enter "119613" for keyword |
| Protein S | http://www.med.unc.edu/isth/proteins.htm |
| *EPCR* | www.hgmd.org; In Search enter "PROCR" for keyword |
| *ATIII* | http://www.med.ic.ac.uk/divisions/7/antithrombin/default.htm |
| *TFPI* | www.hgmd.org; In Search enter "127364" for keyword |
| Heparin cofactor II | www.hgmd.org; In Search enter "SERPIND1" for keyword |
| Factor XII | www.hgmd.org; In Search enter "119892" for keyword |
| Prekallikrein | www.hgmd.org; In Search enter "KLKB1" for keyword |
| HMW kininogen | www.hgmd.org; In Search enter "KNG" for keyword |
| *tPA* | www.hgmd.org; In Search enter "PLAT" for keyword |
| Plasminogen | www.hgmd.org; In Search enter "PLG" for keyword |
| Plasmin inhibitor | www.hgmd.org; In Search enter "SERPINF2" for keyword |
| *PAI-1* | www.hgmd.org; In Search enter "SERPINE1" for keyword |
| *TAFI* | www.hgmd.org; In Search enter "CPB2" for keyword |
| Fibrinogen | http://www.geht.org/databaseang/fibrinogen/ |
| Factor XIII A chain | www.hgmd.org; In Search enter "F13A1" for keyword |
| Factor XIII B chain | www.hgmd.org; In Search enter "F13B" for keyword |
| *VWF* | http://www.sheffield.ac.uk/vwf/ |
| γ-Glutamylcarboxylase | www.hgmd.org; In Search enter "GGCX" for keyword |
| Epoxide reductase I | Not available |

EPCR, endothelial cell protein C receptor; TFPI, tissue factor pathway inhibitor; HMW, high-molecular-weight; tPA, tissue-type plasminogen activator; PAI-1, plasminogen activator inhibitor-1; TAFI, thrombin-activatable fibrinolysis inhibitor; VWF, von Willebrand factor.

# MOLECULAR GENETICS OF HEMOSTATIC PROTEINS

Hemostatic proteins can be divided into procoagulant serine proteases, procoagulant cofactors, anticoagulants, contact activators, and fibrinolytic factors. Other relevant proteins involved in hemostasis that are considered in this chapter are fibrinogen, factor XIII, VWF, γ-glutamyl carboxylase, and vitamin K 2,3-epoxide reductase I (VKOR). Essentially for all of the hemostatic proteins, deficiency states have been reported and lead to either bleeding or thrombosis. In certain circumstances, the deficiency states can be incompatible with life, life threatening, or in some cases the phenotypes are quite mild. The hemostatic proteins considered in this chapter and their gene symbols, identification numbers for various databases, chromosomal location, size of gene, mRNA, and cDNA sequences are shown in Table 4-3. At present, most of the hemostatic proteins have been experimentally knocked-out in mouse models. Where appropriate, these studies are discussed and a summary of each of these models is provided in Table 4-4.

## Procoagulant Serine Proteases

### Prothrombin

The vitamin K–dependent serine protease zymogen prothrombin plays a central role in the coagulation pathway. Following its activation by the prothrombinase complex (i.e., factor Xa, factor Va, calcium ions, and anionic membranes), the resulting product thrombin participates in numerous biologic processes, including the cleavage of fibrinogen to fibrin, which leads to clot formation (see Chapter 10). The gene encoding prothrombin is approximately 20 kb in length with 14 exons, and is assigned to chromosome 11p11–q12 (27). The mRNA for human prothrombin was cloned in 1983 and is approximately 2 kb in length and includes a 1,866-bp cDNA (28). The major site of synthesis of prothrombin is in the liver (29), whereas much smaller sites have been reported in the central nervous system, skeletal and smooth muscle cells, and the kidney (30–33). Prothrombin is expressed as a single polypeptide chain of 622 amino acids. Following removal of a 43–amino acid leader sequence, it is secreted into plasma as a 72-kDa protein containing 579 amino acids at a concentration of 1.4 $\mu$M (28,34).

Homozygosity or compound heterozygosity for loss-of-function mutations in the prothrombin gene leads to a bleeding diathesis. There are no known cases of a total deficiency of prothrombin, consistent with the studies in mice that indicate that a complete lack of the protein is lethal to the embryo (35,36). Prothrombin deficiency is reported to have a prevalence of approximately 1:1,000,000 to 1:2,000,000 (37). Approximately 32 different mutations are known, most of which lead to a variant protein [for a listing of mutations and references see (37,38)]. In a number of instances, these prothrombin variants have been isolated from plasma and subjected to detailed biochemical analysis. One example is thrombin Quick I, in which the genetic defect is the replacement of arginine by cysteine at position 382 (39). This arginine is found in the anion-binding exosite of thrombin (exosite I) (40). Thrombin Quick I has near normal activity with thrombin-specific low-molecular-weight (LMW) substrates; however, its activity with fibrinogen is about 100 times lower than that observed with thrombin (41).

An important development is the role of a 20210G to A polymorphism as a thrombotic risk factor (42). This polymorphism was originally found in probands with a strong personal and familial history of venous thrombosis and is associated with slightly elevated levels of prothrombin (42). Further epidemiologic data confirmed that the DNA variant is a risk factor for venous thrombosis (43–46).

Initially, the molecular mechanism for the increased prothrombin plasma levels was unclear. A recent report has indicated that the mutation, located 20 nucleotides downstream of the poly A signal, increases the posttranslational 3′ end processing efficiency, thereby leading to a higher transcription rate (47). However, this study has been called into question because prothrombin 20210G and 20210A mRNA levels were found equal in fresh liver tissue from a 20210G/A heterozygote (48). This study was able to demonstrate that the 20210A mutation affects the position of the 3′-cleavage/polyadenylation reaction, an event that may lead to its abnormal mRNA function (48). Additional studies have shown that the mutant allele influences mRNA stability; however the mechanism remains unclear (49).

An important question that remains to be answered is how moderate increases in prothrombin increase the prothrombotic tendency. It is usually assumed that prothrombin levels are sufficient and that the kinetics of prothrombin activation are not influenced by moderate fluctuations like those present in heterozygotes for the mutation. The prevalence of the 20210A allele is between 1% and 2% and is dependent somewhat on the geographic origin of the subjects (50). Homozygotes also are, therefore, relatively rare, and only a few have been described (46). No solid evidence exists to suggest that homozygosity increases the risk more than heterozygosity.

### Factor X

Factor X is a vitamin K–dependent plasma protein that plays a central role in the process of blood coagulation because it participates in both the intrinsic and extrinsic pathways. In the presence of its cofactor protein factor Va, activated factor X cleaves two peptide bonds in prothrombin to form thrombin. Factor X is synthesized primarily in the liver, but other tissues also may contribute, such as lung, heart, ovary, and small intestine (51). The gene for factor X has been cloned and is approximately 27 kb in length, contains 8 exons, and is located on chromosome 13q34-qter, 2.8 kb from the factor VII gene (52,53). The cDNA has been isolated by a number of laboratories and has an open reading frame of 1,467 nucleotides and encodes a protein of 488 amino acids (pre-profactor X) (54–56). Following proteolytic processing, mature factor X (59 kDa) is a two-chain serine protease zymogen of 445 amino acids covalently associated through a single disulfide bond and circulates in plasma at a concentration of 170 nM (57,58).

Factor X deficiency is a rare (1:1,000,000) autosomal recessive bleeding disorder. Heterozygotes are usually free of symptoms but may exhibit abnormal bleeding during surgery. There are approximately 50 factor X–deficient families reported in the literature and approximately 60 different mutations have been identified (37,59,60). Large deletions have been identified but most defects are missense mutations. The missense mutations predict replacement of a single amino acid and are often associated with detectable factor X antigen levels and mild-to-asymptomatic disease (59). Mice rendered experimentally deficient in factor X show frequent embryonic lethality, and those that survive die shortly after birth from massive intraabdominal bleeding (61).

A collection of factor X mutations has been described that appear to have differential responses to the intrinsic and extrinsic pathways. For example, factor X Vorarlberg is associated with a marked reduction of activity in the extrinsic system and a much more modest reduction of activity in the intrinsic system (62,63). A patient was found to be homozygous for a

**TABLE 4-3**

CHARACTERISTICS OF HUMAN COAGULATION FACTOR GENES

| Genes | Gene symbol | Gene ID | Ensembl gene ID | Accession no. gene | Accession no. mRNA | Chromosomal location | Exons | Size of gene | Size of mRNA | Size of cDNA |
|---|---|---|---|---|---|---|---|---|---|---|
| Prothrombin | F2 | 2147 | ENSG00000180210 | M17262 | NM_000506 | 11p11-q12 | 14 | 20.3 kb | 1,997 bp | 1,866 bp |
| Factor X | F10 | 2159 | ENSG00000126218 | AH002727 | NM_000504 | 13q34-qter | 8 | 26.7 kb | 1,502 bp | 1,467 bp |
| Factor VII | F7 | 2155 | ENSG00000057593 | J02933 | NM_000131 | 13q34-qter | 8 | 13.1 kb | 2,478 bp | 1,335 bp |
| Factor IX | F9 | 2158 | ENSG00000101981 | K02402 | NM_000133 | Xq27.1-q27.2 | 8 | 31.3 kb | 2,804 bp | 1,386 bp |
| Factor XI | F11 | 2160 | ENSG00000088926 | AH002647 | NM_000128 | 4q34-q35 | 15 | 22.6 kb | 2,217 bp | 1,878 bp |
| Tissue factor | F3 | 2152 | ENSG00000117525 | J02846 | NM_001993 | 1p22-p21 | 6 | 11.6 kb | 2,153 bp | 888 bp |
| Factor VIII | F8 | 2157 | No ensembl prediction | AH002692 | NM_000132 | Xq28 | 26 | ~186 kb | 9,030 bp | 7,056 bp |
| Factor V | F5 | 2153 | ENSG00000056213 | AH005274 | MN_000130 | 1q23 | 25 | ~80 kb | 6,914 bp | 6,675 bp |
| Protein C | PROC | 5624 | ENSG00000115718 | M11228 | NM_000312 | 2q13-q14 | 9 | 10.8 kb | 1,843 bp | 1,386 bp |
| Thrombomodulin | THBD | 7056 | ENSG00000178726 | J02973 | NM_000361 | 20p11-cen | 1 | 4.2 kb | 4,048 bp | 1,728 bp |
| Protein S | PROS1 | 5627 | ENSG00000184500 | AH002976 | NM_000313 | 3p11-q11.2 | 15 | 80 kb | 3,309 bp | 2,031 bp |
| EPCR | PROCR | 10544 | ENSG00000101000 | AF106202 | NM_006404 | 20q11.2 | 4 | 6 kb | 1,483 bp | 717 bp |
| ATIII | SERPINC1 | 462 | ENSG00000117601 | X68793 | NM_000488 | 1q23-q24 | 7 | 13.5 kb | 1,395 bp | 1,395 bp |
| TFPI | TFPI | 7035 | ENSG00000003436 | AH002869 | NM_006287 | 2q31-q32.1 | 9 | ~85 kb | 1,431 bp | 915 bp |
| Heparin cofactor II | SERPIND1 | 3053 | ENSG00000099937 | M58600 | NM_000185 | 22q11.21 | 5 | 13.6 kb | 2,217 bp | 1,500 bp |
| Factor XII | F12 | 2161 | ENSG00000131187 | AH005292 | NM_000505 | 5q33-qter | 14 | 12 kb | 2,048 bp | 1,848 bp |
| Prekallikrein | KLKB1 | 3818 | ENSG00000164344 | AH009508 | NM_000892 | 4q34-q35 | 15 | 31 kb | 2,245 bp | 1,917 bp |
| HMW kininogen | KNG | 3827 | ENSG00000113889 | AH005302 | NM_000893 | 3q26-qter | 11 | 27 kb | ~3,200 bp | 1,935 bp |
| tPA | PLAT | 5327 | ENSG00000104368 | K03021 | NM_000930 | 8p12-p11 | 14 | 32.7 kb | ~2,600 bp | 1,689 bp |
| Plasminogen | PLG | 5340 | ENSG00000122194 | J05286 | NM_000301 | 6q26-q27 | 19 | 53.5 kb | ~2,900 bp | 2,433 bp |
| Plasmin inhibitor | SERPINF2 | 5345 | ENSG00000167711 | J03830 | NM_000934 | 17p11 | 10 | ~16 kb | ~2,300 bp | 1,476 bp |
| PAI-1 | SERPINE1 | 5054 | ENSG00000106366 | M17121 | NM_000602 | 7q21.3-q22 | 9 | 12.3 kb | ~2,800 bp | 1,209 bp |
| TAFI | CPB2 | 1361 | ENSG00000080618 | AF080222 | NM_001872 | 13q14.11 | 11 | ~48 kb | ~1,700 bp | 1,272 bp |
| Fibrinogen Aα chain | FGA | 2243 | ENSG00000171560 | M64982 | NM_021871 | 4q28 | 5 | 5.4 kb | 2,182 bp | 1,935 bp |
| Fibrinogen Bβ chain | FGB | 2244 | ENSG00000171564 | M64983 | NM_005141 | 4q28 | 8 | 8.2 kb | 1,918 bp | 1,476 bp |
| Fibrinogen γ chain | FGG | 2266 | ENSG00000171557 | M10014 | NM_000509 | 4q28 | 10 | 8.4 kb | 1,559 bp | 1,314 bp |
| Factor XIII A chain | F13A1 | 2162 | ENSG00000124491 | AL133326 | NM_000129 | 6p25.3-p24.3 | 15 | >160 kb | ~4,000 bp | 2,199 bp |
| Factor XIII B chain | F13B | 2165 | ENSG00000143278 | M64554 | NM_001994 | 1q31-q31.2 | 12 | ~28 kb | ~2,200 bp | 1,986 bp |
| VWF | VWF | 7450 | ENSG00000110799 | M25716 | NM_000552 | 12p13.3 | 52 | ~178 kb | 8,923 bp | 8,442 bp |
| γ-Glutamylcarboxylase | GGCX | 2677 | ENSG00000115486 | U65896 | NM_000821 | 2p12 | 15 | 13 kb | 3,245 bp | 2,277 bp |
| Epoxide reductase I | VKORC1 | 79001 | No ensembl prediction | Not listed | NM_024006 | 16p11.2 | 3 | ~5 kb | 1,003 bp | 492 bp |

EPCR, endothelial cell protein C receptor; TFPI, tissue-factor pathway inhibitor; HMW, high-molecular-weight; tPA, tissue-type plasminogen activator; PAI-1, plasminogen activator inhibitor-1; TAFI, thrombin-activatable fibrinolysis inhibitor; VWF, von Willebrand factor.

The size of the cDNAs is defined as the number of nucleotides from the start to the stop codons. The Ensembl gene ID numbers can be accessed at: http://www.ensembl.org. The Accession numbers for the genes and mRNAs can be assessed at: http://ncbi.nlm.nih.gov/. See Table 4-1 for additional useful Web sites.

## TABLE 4-4

GENETIC MODELS OF THROMBOSIS AND HEMOSTASIS

| Gene knockout | Strain | Viable | Days of gestation | Phenotype | References |
|---|---|---|---|---|---|
| Prothrombin | C57BL/6 | No | ~9–11 | Fatal hemorrhage/yolk sac defect | 35,36 |
| Factor X | Swiss | No | ~11–13 | Partial embryonic lethal/intraabdominal bleeding | 61 |
| Factor VII | C57BL6J | No | | Fatal perinatal bleeding | 84 |
| Factor IX | C57BL/6 | Yes | | Severe bleeding following trauma | 106–108 |
| Factor XI | C57BL/6 | Yes | | Normal/prolonged aPTT | 132 |
| Tissue factor | Several | No | ~9–12 | Fatal embryonic bleeding | 142–144 |
| Factor VIII | 129sv | Yes | | Severe bleeding following trauma | 154 |
| Factor V | C57BL/6J | No | ~10 | Fatal hemorrhage/yolk sac defect | 180 |
| Protein C | Swiss | No | ~18–19 | Consumptive coagulopathy | 211 |
| Thrombomodulin | 129sv | No | ~9–10 | Embryonic lethal/yolk sac defect | 221–223 |
| EPCR | Swiss | No | ~10 | Embryonic lethal/placental thrombosis | 262 |
| ATIII | C57BL/6J | No | ~15–16 | Consumptive coagulopathy/severe hemorrhage | 285 |
| TFPI | C57BL/6 | No | ~10–13 | Intrauterine lethality | 291 |
| Heparin cofactor II | C57BL/6 | Yes | | Normal; differences observed in thrombosis model | 313 |
| tPA | C57BL/6 | Yes | | Develop normally; no macroscopic abnormalities | 357 |

*(continued)*

**TABLE 4-4**

CONTINUED

| Gene knockout | Strain | Viable | Days of gestation | | | | | | | | | | | | | | | | | | | | Phenotype | References |
|---|---|---|---|---|---|---|---|---|---|---|---|---|---|---|---|---|---|---|---|---|---|---|---|---|
| | | | 1 | 2 | 3 | 4 | 5 | 6 | 7 | 8 | 9 | 10 | 11 | 12 | 13 | 14 | 15 | 16 | 17 | 18 | 19 | | |
| Plasminogen | C57BL/6 | Yes | | | | | | | | | | | | | | | | | | | | Predispose to thrombosis; ligneous conjunctivitis | 382–384 |
| Plasmin inhibitor | C57BL6/J | Yes | | | | | | | | | | | | | | | | | | | | Develop normally; enhanced fibrinolytic potential | 394 |
| PAI-1 | C57BL/6 | Yes | | | | | | | | | | | | | | | | | | | | Develop normally; mild hyperfibrinolytic state | 419,420 |
| TAFI | C57BL/6 | Yes | | | | | | | | | | | | | | | | | | | | Normal | 432 |
| Fibrinogen A chain | C57BL/6 | Yes | | | | | | | | | | | | | | | | | | | | Wound healing defect/failure of pregnancy | 448 |
| Factor XIII A chain | C57BL/6 | Yes | | | | | | | | | | | | | | | | | | | | Develop normally; severe uterine bleeding; miscarriages | 461,462 |
| VWF | C57BL/6J | Yes | | | | | | | | | | | | | | | | | | | | Defects in hemostasis and thrombosis; model type 3VWD | 475 |
| γ-Carboxylase | C57BL/6J | No | | | | | | | | | | | | ■ | ■ | ■ | ■ | ■ | | | | Massive intraabdominal hemorrhage | 484 |

EPCR, endothelial cell protein C receptor; ATIII, antithrombin III; TFPI, tissue factor pathway inhibitor; tPA, tissue-type plasminogen activator; PAI-1, plasminogen activator inhibitor-1; TAFI, Thrombin-activatable fibrinolysis inhibitor; VWF, von Willebrand factor.

mutation in the Gla domain (Gla14 to Lys; *N*-terminal domain of factor X) and heterozygous for Glu102 to Lys in the second epidermal growth factor (EGF)–like domain. In studies of the patient plasma, activity in the extrinsic system was only 5% of normal, whereas activity in the intrinsic system was substantially higher at 25% of normal. This suggested that the mutant protein has differing rates of activation by the intrinsic and extrinsic Xases enzyme complexes. These types of data imply that factor VIIa/tissue factor and factor IXa/factor VIIIa likely have different sites of interaction with factor X, despite the fact that they cleave the same bond within the zymogen. A review of the literature demonstrates at least eight naturally occurring factor X variants that display marked differences in activity in the intrinsic and extrinsic systems (see Table 4-5) (62–70).

Factor X was originally called Stuart-Prower factor after the first individuals in whom factor X deficiency was discovered (71,72). The mutations in these two families are now known. One of the index cases of the Stuart family is homozygous for a replacement of Val by Met at position 298 (59). A descendent of the Prower case also has been sequenced. This individual was shown to be a compound heterozygote for an Asp282 to Asn and an Arg287 to Trp mutation (59). An informative historic sketch on the discovery of factor X has recently been published (73).

## Factor VII

Factor VII is a vitamin K–dependent serine protease zymogen that circulates in plasma as a single-chain polypeptide (50 kDa) of 406 amino acids at a concentration of 10 nM (74–76). Like most clotting factors, it is synthesized primarily in the liver as a 444–amino acid precursor protein. Activated factor VII, in concert with its cofactor, tissue factor, initiates the process of blood coagulation following vascular injury by activating factors IX and X (77). The cDNA and full genomic sequence of factor VII are known (78–80). The gene is relatively small (approximately 13 kb), contains 8 exons, and is located on chromosome 13q34-qter, only 2.8 kb upstream of

the factor X gene (81,82). The full-length mRNA is almost 2.5 kb, whereas the cDNA sequence is 1,335 nucleotides long.

Factor VII deficiency is a rare autosomal disorder with a prevalence of approximately 1:500,000 (37). Most studies state that there is no clear relation between reduced factor VII levels and clinical symptoms. Individuals with factor VII antigen and activity levels less than 1% display a moderate-to-severe bleeding phenotype. Mutations associated with this phenotype include frameshift, splice site, promoter, and missense mutations, with the total number of mutations now reaching more than 110 (37). The situation is less clear for mutations associated with measurable levels of factor VII activity. Many of the individuals carrying these mutations are asymptomatic. On the Internet there is a factor VII mutation database (http://www.europium.csc.mrc.ac.uk) that includes data from more than 230 individuals (83). Almost 50% of the mutations occur at CpG dinucleotides. In this respect, the spectrum of mutations in the factor VII gene is similar to the spectrum in hemophilia B.

At present, it is not entirely clear whether a complete absence of factor VII is incompatible with life. For example, investigation of the factor VII knockout mouse revealed that these organisms develop normally to term but die shortly after birth from major abdominal and intracranial hemorrhage (84). In addition, McVey et al. (85) identified a splice site mutation in the factor VII gene that was associated with a complete absence of factor VII and that resulted in fatal intracerebral hemorrhage at the age of 14 days. In contrast however, Peyvandi et al. (86) have recently reported a homozygous 2-bp deletion in the factor VII gene that was associated with a complete absence of factor VII and was nonlethal. Although it is likely that some compensatory mechanism is affecting the phenotype in this individual, this mechanism has not yet been identified.

Several mutations have been identified in the promoter region of the factor VII gene; one of the mutations appears to disrupt the Sp1 binding site, whereas the other two interfere with binding of the transcription factor HNF-4 or the binding of an unidentified protein near the transcription state site (87–89).

## TABLE 4-5

### FACTOR X VARIANTS WITH DIFFERENTIAL RESPONSES TO THE INTRINSIC AND EXTRINSIC PATHWAYS

| Variant | Mutation[e] | Intrinsic activity (%) | Extrinsic activity (%) | RVV activity (%) | Antigen (%) | Bleeding episodes | Reference |
|---|---|---|---|---|---|---|---|
| FX$_{Melbourne}$[a] | Unknown | 8 | 100 | 100 | 100 | Asymptomatic | 64 |
| FX$_{Roma}$[b] | Thr$^{318(135c)}$ to Met | 3 | 30–50 | 100 | 80 | Mild; severe following trauma | 65 |
| FX$_{Padua}$[c] | Arg251(71c) to Trp | 100 | 25–30 | 100 | 100 | Asymptomatic | 66,67 |
| FX$_{Vorarlberg}$[c] | Glu14/102 to Lys | 25 | 5 | 15 | 20 | None; mild bruising | 62 |
| FX$_{D102K/D14K}$[d] | Glu102 to Lys Glu14 to Lys | 30 | <1 | 20 | 20 | Mild bruising | 63 |
| FX$_{Tokyo}$[b] | Glu32 to Gln | 70–80 | 3 | 70–80 | 61 | Moderate bleeding | 68 |
| FX$_{St Louis II}$ | Gla7 to Gly | 3 | <1 | — | 100 | Unknown | 69 |
| FX$_{D19A}$[b] | Gla19 to Ala | 16 | <1 | 16 | 16 | Unknown | 70 |

[a]The patient is thought to be homozygous for the defect.
[b]The patient is homozygous for the defect.
[c]The patient is homozygous for Gla14 to Lys and heterozygous for Glu102 to Lys.
[d]The patient is homozygous for both mutations.
[e]The "c" following some numbers refers to the chymotrypsin numbering system.

Interest in the relation between elevated factor VII levels and an increased risk of cardiovascular disease was stimulated by the findings of the Northwick Park Heart Study (90,91). In part, these results could be confirmed in the prospective PROCAM (Prospective Cardiovascular Münster) study but only in patients with fatal events; however, the results did not reach statistical significance (92). Indeed, strong associations have been found among factor VII levels and a variety of common polymorphisms in the factor VII gene. Two examples are the decanucleotide insertion/deletion polymorphism at position −323 in the promoter region and the Arg/Gln polymorphism at codon 353 in exon 8 (93–98). The presence of the decanucleotide insert, previously reported to correlate with a 20% decrease in FVII:C per allele and with a possible cardioprotective effect, has been shown to require a haplotype including the SNP at −122 (99). The effect of a SNP (G to A) at −402, previously thought to cause an increase in FVII:C levels by itself, has been reported to be in complete allelic association with an SNP at −670 such that the critical influential polymorphism has not been definitively proved (100). The variation of the frequency of specific polymorphisms within these haplotypes in different ethnicities can aid in establishing the influential polymorphic sequences.

## Factor IX

Factor IX is a vitamin K–dependent serine protease zymogen that plays a critical role in the middle phase of blood coagulation. Activated factor IX is the serine protease component of the intrinsic Xase enzymatic complex, which is also composed of factor VIIIa, anionic membranes, and calcium ions (see Chapter 7). Factor IX is synthesized primarily in the liver and is composed of 461 amino acids. Following proteolytic processing and removal of the pre-proregion, it circulates in plasma as a single-chain 415–amino acid protein (55 kDa) at a concentration of 90 nM. The factor IX gene was cloned between 1982 and 1984 and lies on the long arm of the X chromosome, band q27 (101–105). The full gene sequence is known and is approximately 31 kb in length and has 8 exons (105). The mRNA is approximately 2.8 kb in length, whereas the cDNA is 1,386 bp long (102,105).

Loss-of-function mutations in the factor IX gene result in hemophilia B. The prevalence of this X-linked disorder is 1 in 25,000 men, whereas women are rarely affected. The fivefold difference in prevalence between hemophilia A and B is roughly equivalent to the difference in size of the coding portions of the factor VIII and IX genes. This is consistent with the fact that the chance of a given gene to be inactivated by mutation depends largely on its size. The clinical manifestation of hemophilia B is almost identical to that for hemophilia A. Several mouse models of hemophilia B have been described and have proved useful for gene therapy studies (106–108).

The first mutation in the factor IX gene was described in 1983 (109). This mutation was a deletion that showed up in a screening using Southern blotting of genomic DNA. The first point mutation in factor IX, factor IX Chapel Hill, was discovered by protein sequencing, not by DNA analysis (110). The pace of mutation detection changed dramatically after the introduction of PCR in 1987, and, at present, hundreds of different mutations are known in the factor IX gene (111).

The various mutations associated with hemophilia B are registered in an international database, and are available on the Internet (http://www.kcl.ac.uk/ip/petergreen/haemBdatabase.html). This hemophilia B mutation database focuses primarily on relatively small defects because, at most, gross gene alterations account for 5% of all hemophilia B cases. In this respect, hemophilia A and B differ significantly because, in the former disease, inversion events are the most common cause of severe disease.

In 2003, the hemophilia B database was in its twelfth edition. Some mutations appear to occur independently in patients from diverse geographic regions. These are mostly mutations at CpG dinucleotides, the most common hot spot for point mutations. Overall, approximately 50% of the independent missense mutations found in different families with hemophilia B have been transitions within a CpG dinucleotide (see database Web site for references).

Of considerable interest are the 14 different mutations in the promoter region of the factor IX gene (111). Two of these mutations are associated with conventional hemophilia B. The other promoter mutations are all associated with a certain form of hemophilia B (hemophilia B Leyden), arguably the most fascinating of all promoter mutations (112–114). The unique feature of these variants is that individuals exhibit "recovery" from severe hemophilia with the onset of puberty. Therefore, the disease is characterized by the absence of factor IX expression in childhood (factor IX levels <2%) and a gradual rise in factor IX levels after the onset of puberty (see Fig. 4-2). The increase in factor IX levels after puberty is probably related to increasing levels of testosterone (115). Mutation detection in individuals with hemophilia B Leyden has revealed a heterogeneous group of mutations, all clustered at the 5′ end of the gene.

The explanation for the absence of factor IX expression during childhood in these individuals is theoretically straightforward, inasmuch as all the mutations disrupt protein-binding sites in the 5′ flanking sequence, but the pathophysiologic basis for the gradual recovery after the onset of puberty has been more difficult to establish. Three sites appear to be involved, all of which are clustered on a 50-bp segment of DNA that includes the transcriptional start site. In the normal IX promoter, hepatocyte nuclear factor 4 (HNF-4) appears to bind to the two upstream elements, whereas the downstream element binds C/EBP (CCAAT-enhancer binding protein) or DBP (D-site binding protein) or both (116–119). The best explanation for the postpubertal recovery in hemophilia B Leyden lies in an androgen-responsive enhancer that partly overlaps

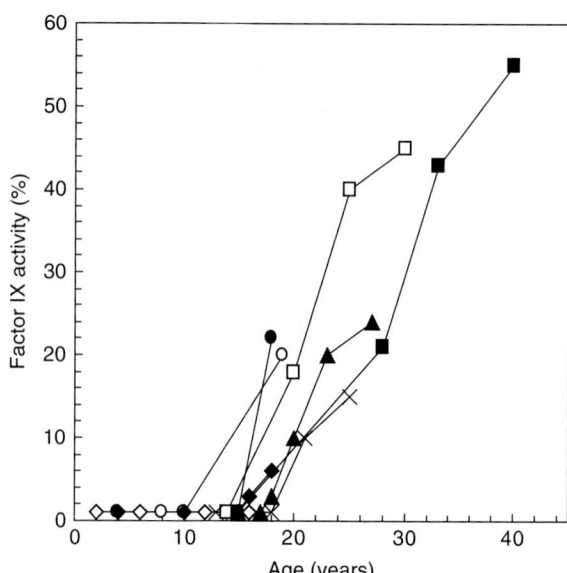

**FIGURE 4-2.** Factor IX levels measured over time in eight individuals with Leyden variant hemophilia B. These mutations in the promoter result in severe factor IX deficiency until puberty when factor IX levels rise gradually to approximately 30%. (From Briet E, Bertina RM, van Tilburg NH, et al. Hemophilia B Leyden: a sex-linked hereditary disorder that improves after puberty. *N Engl J Med* 1982;306:788–790, with permission.)

one of the HNF-4 binding sites (120,121). Strong support for this hypothesis stems from the fact that mutations in this element lead to severe hemophilia B throughout life.

The relatively recent discovery of three factor IX mutations (i.e., Ala10 to Val, Ala10 to Thr; and Asn9 to Lys) has revealed a unique type of genetic predisposition to bleeding during oral anticoagulation therapy that is attributable to increased warfarin sensitivity (25,122,123). The Ala10 and Asn9 residues are within the factor IX propeptide region and are critical for interaction with γ-glutamyl carboxylase and, therefore, γ-carboxylation; mutations at these sites impair this reaction. When receiving coumarins, patients with these variants showed a disproportionate decrease of factor IX activity approaching that of severe hemophilia B. As a consequence, these patients may have bleeding at the very beginning of oral anticoagulation. After discontinuation of treatment, the factor IX levels return to normal.

## Factor XI

Factor XI is a serine protease zymogen that contributes to hemostasis by activating factor IX (see Chapter 12). Factor XI is converted to factor XIa through proteolytic cleavage, either by factor XIIa or by thrombin. Factor XIa appears to be important for sustaining thrombin production after initial fibrin formation, which consolidates and protects fibrin clots from degradation by fibrinolysis (124). A near full-length cDNA encoding factor XI was cloned in 1986, and the structure of the factor XI gene was determined in 1987 (125,126). The gene consists of 15 exons spread over 23 kb of DNA. The factor XI gene is on chromosome 4q34-q35, adjacent to the prekallikrein gene (126). Factor XI is synthesized in the liver and circulates in plasma at a concentration of 30 nM (127,128). It is a disulfide-bond–linked dimer of two 80-kDa polypeptides of 608 amino acids each (127).

Factor XI deficiency is an autosomal disorder characterized by trauma- or surgery-induced hemorrhage and is only rarely characterized by spontaneous bleeds (129). It is usually rare in most ethnic groups but is highly prevalent among Ashkenazi Jews (130). It has been estimated that, in this population, the frequency of mutated factor XI genes may be as high as 13% (130,131). Homozygosity for factor XI deficiency is associated with a very mild bleeding tendency, even when factor XI levels are low or undetectable. This is usually consistent with factor XI–deficient mice that do not show any increased tendency to bleed (132). The inheritance pattern of factor XI deficiency is not strictly recessive because some heterozygotes also display a mild but definite bleeding tendency.

In the Ashkenazi Jewish population, three mutations dominate, all of which are associated with severely reduced levels of factor XI protein in homozygotes or compound heterozygotes (<1% to 10% of normal) (131,133). The first mutation (type I) is a G to A transition in the donor splice junction of intron 5. The type II mutation introduces a premature stop codon in exon 5 at amino acid position 117. The type III mutation is replacement of Phe283 by Leu. Proof that type III mutation is responsible for factor XI deficiency has come from *in vitro* expression studies where approximately 10 times less mutant protein than wild-type protein was secreted. The type I mutation is rare compared with the type II and III defects. The latter defects each account for more than 40% of factor XI deficiency cases among Ashkenazi Jews.

The recurrence of mutations in Jews is thought to be the result of founder effects (131). This interpretation is supported by the fact that in other ethnic groups the mutations are more diverse. More than 30 different mutations are known in factor XI, many of which are associated with decreased antigen levels. The mutations vary from splice site defects and amino acid replacements to frameshift mutations.

## Procoagulant Cofactors

### Tissue Factor

Tissue factor is a cell-associated cofactor protein for factor VIIa, and the enzyme complex is considered to be the physiologic trigger of the blood clotting system in normal hemostasis and perhaps in thrombotic disease (see Chapter 5) (77). The gene for tissue factor resides on the short arm of chromosome 1 (p21-p22) and is approximately 12 kb long and contains six exons (134,135). The size of the predominant tissue factor mRNA in cells is approximately 2.2 kb, with the cDNA being 888-bp long (134,136–138). Tissue factor is an integral membrane protein of 263 amino acids and is initially synthesized with a 32–amino acid signal peptide. Tissue factor is expressed constitutively by epithelial cells and adventitial fibroblasts surrounding blood vessels as well as by cardiomyocytes and astrocytes in the brain and is exposed to the blood following injury (139,140).

Several studies have identified binding sites for transcription factors that regulate basal and inducible tissue factor gene expression in different cell types. Basal expression appears to be regulated by the Sp1 transcription factor, whereas inducible expression is regulated by c-Fos/c-Jun, c-Rel/p65, and Egr-1 [reviewed in (141)]. Regulation of tissue factor expression by inflammatory mediators and angiogenic factors suggests that it may contribute to both inflammation and angiogenesis.

At present, there are no published missense mutations in the tissue factor gene and no known tissue factor–deficient patients, suggesting that tissue factor deficiency may be lethal. Support for this concept comes from tissue factor knockout mice that die *in utero* between days 8.5 and 10.5 (142–144). Promoter polymorphisms in the tissue factor gene, however, have been identified. A recent study investigated whether individual differences in tissue factor gene expression would predispose to thrombosis (145). Six novel promoter polymorphisms were found that were distributed over two haplotypes with equal frequencies. One of the haplotypes (TF-603A) has been linked to venous thromboembolic disease, suggesting that it might protect against thrombosis by reducing the level of circulating tissue factor; however, no link with myocardial infarction has been found (145). Further studies have shown that these polymorphisms significantly influence constitutive tissue factor gene expression in human monocytes but have no major effect on tissue factor gene expression or on whole blood clotting time (146).

### Factor VIII

Factor VIII is a metal ion–dependent pro-cofactor that circulates in plasma as a heterodimer of a heavy chain and light chain (see Chapter 8). Thrombin-activated factor VIII is the cofactor protein for factor IXa and plays a key role in the activation of factor X (147). The essential role of factor VIII in blood coagulation is evidenced by the severe bleeding diathesis associated with its deficiency (hemophilia A). The factor VIII gene was originally cloned in 1984 and is approximately 186 kb in length and has 26 exons and lies on the X chromosome (q28) (148–150). The gene encodes a mature mRNA of approximately 9 kb, and the cDNA is 7,056 nucleotides long (151,152). Preprofactor VIII has 2,351 amino acids, whereas mature factor VIII has 2,332 amino acids and circulates in plasma at a concentration of approximately 0.7 nM (151–153). A mouse model of hemophilia A was described in 1995 (154). Accounts describing the discovery of the factor VIII protein and gene have recently been published (155,156).

The first description of mutations in the factor VIII gene dates to 1985. In this paper by Gitschier et al., two nonsense mutations in the coding sequence and two partial deletions of the factor VIII gene were described (157). The finding of four distinctly different mutations in the factor VIII gene of otherwise similar patients was the first hint that a large variety of mutations exist in the factor VIII gene in patients with hemophilia. This prediction was borne out after PCR was introduced for large-scale point-mutation detection.

There is also an unusually common inversion in the factor VIII gene that is highly prevalent among patients with severe hemophilia A (158,159). This common rearrangement in the factor VIII gene was discovered in 1993 and is present in approximately 40% to 50% of all severe hemophilia A cases (158). Because it is so prevalent and relatively easy to detect, the discovery of this rearrangement has revolutionized genetic counseling for hemophilia A. It results from an unequal crossover event between a sequence in intron 22 of the factor VIII gene and one of two extragenic copies of this sequence that lie distal on the X chromosome. As can be seen in Figure 4-3, inversion of the factor VIII gene by homologous recombination leads to complete disruption of the factor VIII coding sequence and consequently to a severe form of hemophilia A. Recently, another factor VIII inversion has been identified and characterized. The inversion occurs in intron 1 and breaks the factor VIII gene, resulting in production of two chimeric mRNAs and in severe hemophilia A (160,161). The prevalence of this inversion in patients with severe hemophilia A appears to be approximately 4% to 5% (161).

The molecular pathology of the factor VIII gene is constantly being updated and reviewed in an electronic version of the hemophilia A database: http://www.europium.csc.mrc.ac.uk/WebPages/Main/main.htm (162). In 2003, there were more than 940 unique mutations in factor VIII of all types reported. More than 600 different point mutations are known for the factor VIII gene, and this number is increasing steadily as more patients are analyzed. The effect of these mutations on gene function is diverse. Severe dysfunction is produced by point mutations that introduce premature stop codons and by mutations that destroy splice junctions between introns and exons. On the other hand, these types of mutations also contain most, if not all, of the mild and moderately severe forms of hemophilia A. These are mostly missense mutations that predict replacement of the normal amino acid by another amino acid.

Gene deletions of less than 100 bp up to several hundred kilobases have been found in many severely affected patients. In fact, deletions may be present in up to 5% of patients with severe hemophilia A (163). This estimate is somewhat biased in that gross gene arrangements are readily detected by a simple Southern blot, whereas point-mutation detection requires elaborate screening of all the coding regions of the factor VIII gene (164).

Insertions are relatively uncommon in the factor VIII gene (162). As with deletions, it is important in principle to distinguish in-frame from frameshift insertions. It should be noted, however, that the insertions known to date have always been found in patients with severe symptoms with undetectable levels of factor VIII activity. In the group of large insertions are the so-called LINE (long inserted element) retrotransposons (165,166). These DNA elements comprise approximately 5% of the human genome. Intact LINEs encode a protein with reverse transcriptaselike activity and have the capacity to spread through the genome through an RNA intermediate. The LINE first identified in patients with hemophilia A was derived from an element on chromosome 22. Subsequent to the original description in hemophilia A, insertion of LINEs has been found to disrupt various other genes.

## Factor V

Activated factor V is the cofactor protein for the serine protease factor Xa in the prothrombinase complex. The precursor of factor Va is factor V, a large heavily glycosylated, single-chain protein that is homologous to factor VIII (see Chapter 9) (167). The factor V gene is located on the long arm of chromosome 1q23, not far from the antithrombin gene and is approximately 80 kb in length and contains 25 exons (168). The first factor V cDNA sequences were published in 1986–1987

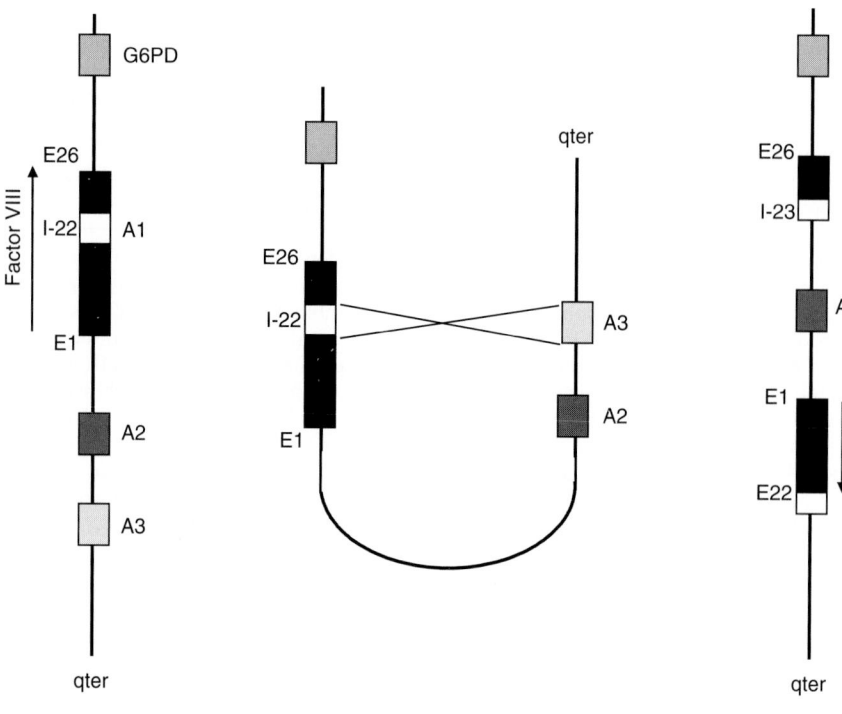

FIGURE 4-3. Factor VIII intron 22 inversion. The **left** panel depicts the normal alignment of the factor VIII gene on the X chromosome. Intron 22 (*white box*) of the factor VIII gene harbors a copy of the so-called A1 gene, whereas highly homologous A2 and A3 genes are located toward the tip of the X chromosome (indicated as qter). The **middle** panel shows alignment of the A1 gene with the A3 gene as it may occur during male spermatogenesis. When this alignment of A1 with A2 (or alternatively A3) results in a nonhomologous recombination, a rearrangement results as depicted at the **right** panel. In this rearranged X chromosome, the integrity of the factor VIII gene is completely disrupted because it is cut in two parts that are now aligned in opposite directions.

(169–171). The mRNA is approximately 7 kb, whereas the cDNA sequence is 6,675 nucleotides long. Factor V is synthesized in the liver as a 2,240–amino acid protein and is secreted after preprocessing as a 2,196 single-chain protein and circulates in plasma at a concentration of 20 nM (172–174). In addition to plasma factor V, approximately 20% of the total factor V in whole blood is contained in the α-granules of platelets (174). Although it was originally thought that megakaryocytes synthesize factor V (175,176), a more recent study has shown that most platelet-derived factor V originates from plasma through an endocytotic mechanism (177). This observation has been confirmed recently by one other laboratory (178).

Factor V deficiency is a rare recessively inherited disorder associated with a mild-to-severe bleeding tendency caused by loss-of-function mutations in the factor V gene (37). Its incidence is about 1:1,000,000 and there have been more than 200 cases described thus far. The study of the molecular basis of factor V deficiency started in 1995 with the description of factor V New Brunswick, an Ala221 to Val mutation that resulted in mild parahemophilia (179). Because factor V deficiency is so rare and the gene is large, relatively few patients have been characterized genetically. More than 15 mutations have been reported that are responsible for factor V deficiency, and they include missense mutations as well as insertions, deletions, and splice-site mutations. A compendium database of factor V mutations has been constructed by Dr. Hans L. Vos (Hemostasis and Thrombosis Research Center, Leiden University Medical Center, Leiden, The Netherlands; email: h.l.vos@lumc.nl) and is available on request via email.

There has been some discussion regarding whether complete factor V deficiency is compatible with life. Factor V knockout mice display a severe phenotype wherein approximately 50% of the embryos do not survive past midgestation and the remaining come to term normally but die within hours after birth from excessive hemorrhage (180). In contrast, there have been several recent reports describing individuals who have undetectable amounts of factor V, yet the patients are still alive (181–184). In one of these patients, the individual is homozygous for a 4-bp deletion in exon 13 and has undetectable levels of factor V antigen and activity, yet has only a very mild bleeding tendency (181). This observation suggests that there may be some, as yet undescribed, compensatory mechanism present in human blood, which either bypasses or reduces the need for factor V in generating enough thrombin for survival (167).

In some cases, factor V deficiency coinherits with factor VIII deficiency, the molecular basis for which is now clear (10). Combined factor V and VIII deficiency is a distinct autosomal recessive disorder, and the affected patients demonstrate a moderate bleeding tendency with plasma factor V and factor VIII levels in the range of 5% to 30% of normal. Approximately 50% of the families described to date are of Mediterranean origin, and the disorder is particularly prevalent among Jews of Middle Eastern and Sephardic origin (185). A major breakthrough in our understanding of this disorder came in 1997 when two groups independently linked combined factor V and VIII deficiency to a locus on chromosome 18q using homozygosity mapping (9,186). Subsequent positional cloning identified a candidate gene called *ERGIC-53* (now called *LMAN1*) in this region (10). *LMAN1* is a mannose-binding type 1 transmembrane protein localized to the endoplasmic reticulum (ER)–Golgi intermediate compartment that likely functions as a molecular chaperone of a specific subset of secreted proteins, including coagulation factors V and VIII. DNA sequence analysis identified two different mutations that accounted for all affected individuals in nine families studied (10). Subsequently, an additional 54 families have been analyzed for mutations, and a total of 17 different mutations have been identified, with all but one mutation being nonsense or frameshift alleles (187,188). However, no mutations in *LMAN1* could be found in approximately 30% of the families analyzed, suggesting that mutations in another gene may also be associated with factors V and VIII deficiency. This second gene and corresponding mutations causing factor V/VIII deficiency has been recently found, and the deficiency is termed *MCFD2* (multiple coagulation factor deficiency 2) (189). *MCFD2* is localized to the ER–Golgi intermediate compartment through a direct interaction with *LMAN1*. The phenotypes associated with mutations in *MCFD2* and *LMAN1* are indistinguishable and associated only with deficiency of factors V and VIII, although a selective delay in secretion of other proteins has been noted.

The most common genetic defect described in factor V is a gain-of-function mutation. In 1993 Dahlbäck et al. observed that plasma from individuals who experienced venous thrombotic episodes had a reduced response to activated protein C (APC), a condition that was termed *APC resistance* (190). The genetic basis of this abnormality is a G1691 to A mutation in the factor V gene, which results in a change of Arg506 to Gln at a critical APC inactivation cleavage site in factor Va (see Fig. 4-4) (191–193). The mutation was termed *factor V_{Leiden}* and is associated not with a bleeding diathesis but with an increased thrombotic risk. Subsequent biochemical studies have shown that factor Va_{Leiden} is less readily inactivated by APC, thereby enhancing the procoagulant capacities of factor V (194–196). This genetic abnormality is prevalent in approximately 3% of whites, and numerous studies have shown factor V_{Leiden} to be the most common genetic risk factor in venous thrombosis [for review see (197)]. An insightful

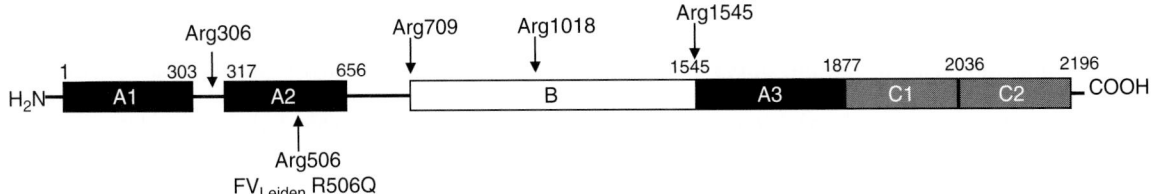

**FIGURE 4-4.** Illustration of the molecular defect called factor V_{Leiden}. Central in the figure is a schematic illustration of the domain structure of mature factor V as it circulates in plasma (A1-A2-B-A3-C1-C2). Factor V is activated by thrombin or factor Xa. The major cleavage sites for these activators are Arg709, Arg1018, and Arg1545. Activated factor V can be inactivated by activated protein C (APC). Inactivation occurs by cleavage of a site (Arg306) between domains A1 and A2, at Arg506 within the A2 domain, and at Arg679 (not shown). In factor V_{Leiden}, the codon for Arg506 at the A2 cleavage site is changed to Gln. This amino acid replacement results in loss of the A2 inactivation site and therefore in a factor Va molecule relatively resistant to APC. Mutations have also been identified at the Arg306 cleavage site: factor V_{Cambridge} and factor V_{Hong Kong}.

historic sketch on the discovery of APC resistance has recently been published by Dahlbäck (198).

Most individuals are heterozygous for factor $V_{Leiden}$, but homozygosity is also seen. Homozygotes have a higher risk for venous thrombosis than heterozygotes. Apart from true homozygosity, there also exists the so-called pseudohomozygosity for factor $V_{Leiden}$ (199,200). In this situation, one factor V allele carries the 506 mutation, whereas the other allele harbors a loss-of-function mutation. In such individuals, only factor $V_{Leiden}$ circulates in plasma, and at levels approximately 50% of normal. It is conceivable that such individuals have a thrombotic risk not unlike true homozygotes, but this has not been proved. Mutations at Arg306 also have been described and may also be associated with APC resistance and thrombotic disease (201,202). The prevalence of this variant seems to be much lower than that of factor $V_{Leiden}$. The reasons for this are unknown.

## Inhibitors of Coagulation

### Protein C

Protein C is a vitamin K–dependent plasma serine protease zymogen that plays a central role in regulating blood coagulation as an anticoagulant (see Chapter 14). Thrombin in complex with thrombomodulin on endothelial cells is the major activator of protein C. APC exerts its anticoagulant function by inactivating, via limited proteolysis, factors Va and VIIIa (197). Human protein C is encoded by a gene on chromosome 2q13-q14 and spans approximately 11 kb and contains nine exons (203–205). The protein C gene encodes mRNA transcripts of 1.8 and 1.6 kb; the difference appears to result from alternative polyadenylation signals present in the transcript (206). A notable feature of the DNA sequence of the protein C gene is that it has a high CpG content (see also later in this section). The cDNA is 1,386 nucleotide long and encodes a mature protein of 461 amino acids. Prior to secretion, a 42–amino acid pre-prosequence is removed as well as internal proteolytic cleavage, resulting in the secretion of a 419–amino acid two-chain protein (62 kDa) that circulates in plasma at a concentration of 60 nM (206,207).

Loss-of-function mutations in the protein C gene lead to protein C deficiency. The first protein C–deficient family was discovered in 1981 (208). This family was studied because some members experienced episodes of venous thrombosis, a disease that was expected to be related to low levels of protein C. After this original report, many others confirmed that heterozygosity for protein C deficiency can be found in a significant number of families with venous thrombosis.

In addition, in the early 1980s, the first reports describing homozygous deficiency appeared (209,210). This deficiency is a much more serious condition than heterozygous protein C deficiency. In homozygotes, life-threatening thrombotic symptoms often start immediately after birth and take the form of purpura fulminans. Inactivation of the protein C gene in mice leads to lethal perinatal consumptive coagulopathy and is therefore inconsistent with short-term survival (211).

More than 300 different mutations have been described for the protein C gene. Each of these mutations is assumed (or has been proved) to lead to absent or defective protein C. The mutations in the protein C gene are compiled on a regular basis and can be found on the Web site: http://www.xs4all.nl/%7Ereitsma/Prot_C_home.htm (212). The mutations cover the whole spectrum of what can be expected of loss-of-function mutations, varying from missense mutations (some leading to variant proteins that have proven useful for structure–function

analysis of plasma purified protein), promoter mutations, and RNA processing mutations to frameshift mutations.

The protein C database of mutations contains many multiple entries for certain mutations. For instance, the Arg230 to Cys mutation has been documented in 28 apparently unrelated families. Two factors are important when considering these multiple occurrences of mutations. The first is that they may result from a founder effect. In one example, the common origin of several families was traced back to the 18th century (213). The second explanation for the recurrence of mutations is that they have arisen independently. On the basis of geographic considerations or haplotyping, this has been confirmed for several mutations (213,214).

These recurrent mutations typically occur at CpG dinucleotides. When one plots the relation between specific mutations and the geographic dispersal, the observed curve closely matches the curve that is expected on the basis of the likelihood of a given mutation to occur (215). This analysis indicates that most multiple reports of mutations reflect recurrent mutation rather than founder effect.

Approximately 30% of the different protein C mutations occur in CpG dinucleotides. However, the distribution of CpG dinucleotides in the protein C gene is highly nonrandom. In exons 4, 5, and 6 especially, CpG dinucleotides are present in abundance. This relatively high CpG frequency is indicative of a so-called CpG island, in which mutation of CpGs is not favored (216). Indeed, of the more than 30 mutations in exons 4, 5, and 6, only 2 occur in a CpG dinucleotide (212).

### Thrombomodulin

Thrombomodulin is an endothelial cell surface glycoprotein receptor for thrombin. The thrombin–thrombomodulin complex initiates the protein C anticoagulant pathway by activating the zymogen protein C (see Chapter 14). Several groups have cloned and sequenced the thrombomodulin cDNA and gene (217–219). The gene is 4.2 kb in length and is located on chromosome 20p12-cen and is unusual in that it does not contain any introns and has a high GC content. The mRNA is approximately 4 kb in length, whereas the cDNA is 1,728 bp long and encodes a protein of 575 amino acids. The mature protein is 559 amino acids in length following removal of the signal sequence. An informative historic sketch on the discovery of thrombomodulin has been recently published (220).

Given its function in the protein C pathway, a hereditary deficiency of thrombomodulin is a strong candidate for pathophysiologic involvement in venous thrombosis. Although mouse embryos homozygous for the thrombomodulin deletion die in utero by E9.5 precluding detailed studies, mice genetically modified to inactivate or alter (missense mutation) the thrombomodulin gene have shown increased fibrin deposition and a prothrombotic state (221–223). Some evidence from clinical studies supports a role for thrombomodulin in thrombotic disease. For example, in the Atherosclerosis Risk in Communities (ARIC) study, soluble thrombomodulin showed a strong, graded, inverse association with and was a good predictor of incident coronary artery disease (224). A role for genetic variation in disease has been suggested by findings that mutations in the thrombomodulin gene occur in patients with thrombosis. The first mutation, a G to T mutation that predicts replacement of Asp468 by Tyr, was found in an American patient of Hispanic descent in 1995 with pulmonary embolism at age 45 years (225). Other missense mutations have been identified that correlate with thromboembolic disease, several of which have been recently biochemically characterized (226).

The Ala455 to Val polymorphism that occurs with frequencies of 0.82/0.18 in whites does not appear to be a risk factor for venous thrombosis (227). This polymorphism may, however, be associated with cardiovascular risk in certain populations and may also be associated with varicose veins through linkage with promoter mutations (228,229). Another thrombomodulin polymorphism that has been investigated with respect to arterial disease is the Ala25 to Thr substitution. The Thr allele was found to be more prevalent among patients with myocardial infarction compared to control subjects in the SMILE (Study of Myocardial Infarctions Leiden) (230). However, two subsequent investigations did not find a correlation between this polymorphism and coronary artery disease and stroke (222,231).

## Protein S

Protein S is a vitamin K–dependent glycoprotein that has an anticoagulant effect in the coagulation pathway (see Chapter 14). Protein S circulates in plasma in two forms: free (approximately 40%) and bound to C4b binding protein, a component of the complement system. Only free protein S has anticoagulant properties. Protein S acts as a cofactor for APC in the inactivation of the procoagulant factors Va and VIIIa, possibly by potentiating the binding of protein C to procoagulant phospholipid surfaces; however, the precise mechanism is not known, and, in general, the effects of protein S in modulating APC function *in vitro* tend to be minor.

The human genome contains two protein S genes, one of which is active (*PROS1*), and the other a pseudogene (*PROS2*) (232–234). The *PROS1* gene is approximately 80 kb in length and contains 15 exons and is located on chromosome 3 (3p11.1-q11.2) (235,236). The major mRNA species from *PROS1* is approximately 4 kb long, whereas the cDNA is 2,031 nucleotides in length (237,238). The protein S precursor protein is 676 amino acids long, whereas mature protein S is a single-chain glycoprotein of 635 amino acids. The *PROS2* gene is a highly homologous pseudogene of *PROS1* that contains a variety of mutations, such as stop codons and deletions that prohibit proper translation. Moreover, no transcription product of the *PROS2* gene could be identified (239).

Mutations in the protein S gene lead to protein S deficiency, an autosomal dominant trait affecting up to 5% of families with congenital thrombophilia (240). The first cases of heterozygous protein S deficiency were described in 1984; since then numerous reports have appeared (241–243). The prevalence in the general population is not known with great certainty. The clinical symptoms in heterozygous protein S deficiency are comparable to protein C deficiency and are relatively mild. Only a few cases of homozygous deficiency have been described, and these were associated with severe thrombotic disease and purpura fulminans immediately after birth (244–247). At present, a protein S–deficient mouse model has not been described.

The mutations that have been found in protein S deficiency are collated in a database of mutations (http://www.med.unc.edu/isth/proteins.htm), which was updated in 2000 (248). The current database describes the genetic findings in more than 200 patients with protein S deficiency. The spectrum of mutations is similar to what already has been discussed for hemophilia B and protein C deficiency (see section, "Factor IX and Protein C").

In total, 71 different point mutations have been noted in the protein S gene. Only five of these occur in CpG dinucleotides and are compatible with methylation-mediated deamination (14). This differs from what was found, for instance, in hemophilia B or protein C deficiency, in which approximately 30% of the point mutations occur in CpG dinucleotides. The reason for this difference is unknown.

A number of sequence variations in the protein S gene probably represent polymorphisms. Some of these variations are rare and are typical for a specific pedigree. The Heerlen polymorphism is an example of a more common sequence variant (249). This polymorphism was originally found on the "normal" allele in individuals with type I deficiency. It was detectable because the variant protein was no longer recognized by the monoclonal antibody in an enzyme-linked immunosorbent assay (ELISA). This is understandable because the polymorphism affects overall protein S structure. Ser460 is replaced by Pro, which leads to loss of a glycosylation site and circulating protein S with a lower molecular weight. Two observations indicate that the Heerlen polymorphism is neutral and of little importance. The first is that plasma-based tests failed to show differences in activity between normal protein S and Heerlen protein S. The second is that the prevalence of the Heerlen polymorphism is not increased in unexplained thrombosis. However, the neutrality of the Heerlen polymorphism has been challenged (250–252). Using a variety of protein S assays, these studies showed that the Heerlen polymorphism is associated with type III protein S deficiency. Moreover, it appears that protein S Heerlen displays a higher affinity for C4b-binding protein than normal protein S. Expression and functional characterization of the protein S Heerlen mutant protein indicates that the protein displays a reduced anticoagulant activity as a cofactor to APC in plasma-based assays, particularly when using factor $V_{Leiden}$ (253). The data suggest a possible mechanism of synergy between protein S Heerlen and factor $V_{Leiden}$ that might be involved in the pathogenesis of thrombosis in individuals carrying both mutations.

## Endothelial Cell Protein C Receptor

The endothelial cell protein C receptor (EPCR) is a cell-specific type 1 transmembrane protein that binds both protein C and APC on the cell surface and was identified in 1994 by Fukudome and Esmon (254,255). The protein was named EPCR and appears to function by augmenting protein C activation by the thrombin–thrombomodulin complex, primarily by reducing the apparent $K_m$ for protein C [for review see (256)]. A soluble form of EPCR (43 kDa) has been identified in human plasma and it circulates at a concentration of approximately 2.5 nM (257). The gene for EPCR spans about 6 kb of genomic DNA, contains 4 exons, and is localized to chromosome 20 (20q11.2) (258,259). The mRNA is approximately 1.4 kb, whereas the cDNA is 717 nucleotides in length and encodes a protein of 238 amino acids (254). In adults, EPCR is localized primarily on endothelial cells of large blood vessels, but during development it is expressed at high levels on trophoblast giant cells (260,261).

In view of the role EPCR plays in the protein C pathway, deficiencies of the protein might be expected to be thrombogenic. Although homozygous EPCR deficiency has not been described in humans, the EPCR knockout mouse has been recently reported (262). Disruption of the gene causes placental thrombosis and results in an early embryonic (E10.5) lethal phenotype, suggesting that EPCR plays a critical role in the regulation of blood coagulation.

In 2001, the first mutation in the *EPCR* gene was reported. In this study, a 23-bp insertion in the *EPCR* gene was found in survivors of myocardial infarction and deep vein thrombosis (263). When this mutation is identified in thrombophilic patients, its role in thrombosis is difficult to assess because the allelic frequency is low (264–267). Point mutations have also been described in the promoter region of the gene in four thrombophilic patients and also in coding region of the protein (Arg96 to Cys), but the involvement of these mutations in gene regulation or functional activity could not be clearly demonstrated (268,269). However, elevated levels of soluble EPCR associated with the A3 haplotype, characterized by 13 polymorphisms, appear to be associated with an increased risk of venous thrombosis (270). Further studies are clearly needed in order to evaluate the actual importance of the *EPCR* gene variations in thrombotic diseases.

## Antithrombin III

Antithrombin is the major serpin family regulator of blood-clotting proteases in plasma (see Chapter 13). This anticoagulant protein downregulates blood clotting by inhibiting thrombin, factor Xa, and factor IXa, thereby forming a stable equimolar complex with the enzymes by an unusual mechanism that is shared by other serpin family protease inhibitors (271). The stability of the complex is dependent on cleavage at Arg393 of antithrombin by the active site of the serine protease. Inhibition of protease activity is greatly accelerated by the participation of the glycosaminoglycans heparin and heparin sulfate that induce conformational changes that enhance the serpin's reactivity with the enzymes.

The relative abundance (approximately 2.5 $\mu$M; 150 $\mu$g per mL) of antithrombin and its ease of purification from plasma facilitated the deduction of most of its primary structure by Edman degradation in 1979 (272). The first cDNA sequence was cloned between 1982 and 1983 (273–275), and 10 years later the full gene sequence was published (276). The 13.5-kb gene is localized on chromosome 1q23–24 and consists of seven exons (277–279). The mRNA is approximately 1.4 kb long, whereas the cDNA is 1,395 bp long. The deduced primary structure of the protein indicates a 32–amino acid signal sequence and a mature protein of 432 amino acids.

Because of its essential role as an anticoagulant, individuals with deficiencies of antithrombin are at increased risk for thrombosis. The prevalence of this condition in the general population is approximately 1:500 (280). The prevalence in patients with a history of thromboembolic disease is approximately 5% (281). The first report of antithrombin deficiency was published in 1965 (282). Since then, numerous families with antithrombin deficiency have been described. From these studies, it is clear that antithrombin deficiency is heterogeneous with respect to genetic background and clinical manifestations.

On the basis of coagulation tests, several classification schemes have been proposed for antithrombin deficiency. The most recent classification was proposed by Lane et al. (283). In this scheme, two major types of deficiencies are recognized: type I has reduced plasma levels of a functionally normal antithrombin variant, whereas type II covers all types with dysfunctional antithrombin variants. Within type II, the defect may involve the reactive site (i.e., type II RS) or the heparin-binding site (i.e., type II HBS) or both (i.e., type II PE). It is usually believed that type II HBS mutations result in less risk of thrombosis than the other subtypes. Homozygous type I deficiency is probably not compatible with life. There is only one report of a child born to consanguine parents who had very low plasma antithrombin activity and antigen who died at 3 weeks of age of disseminated arterial and venous thrombosis. Mutational analysis was not performed (284). This is consistent with the observation that a complete antithrombin deficiency in mice is embryonically lethal (E15.5 to 16.5) (285).

The first mutation in the antithrombin gene (deletion) was characterized in 1983 (286). Since then numerous mutations have been characterized. These mutations are collated on a regular basis in a database of antithrombin mutations: http://www.med.ic.ac.uk/divisions/7/antithrombin/default.htm. The current database contains more than 250 entries (283). In 12 cases, large deletions (defined as >100 bp) have been found in the antithrombin gene that account for type I deficiency. Other types of mutations in type I deficiency are mostly frameshift mutations, premature stop codons, and splice-site mutations, but also some missense mutations. These missense mutations are believed to lead to an improper folded antithrombin that does not reach the circulation. Interestingly, in one case of an in-frame 9-bp deletion, as well as in a case of a 105-bp deletion, measurable levels of inactive, high-molecular-weight (HMW) antithrombin were found in plasma (287,288).

## Tissue Factor Pathway Inhibitor

Tissue factor pathway inhibitor (TFPI) is a trivalent 34-kDa proteinase inhibitor. The inhibitor, a Kunitz-type protein, plays an essential role in regulating coagulation through the inhibition of a quaternary complex of TFPI, factor VIIa, TF, and factor Xa. The first Kunitz domain (K1) of the TFPI protein is an *N*-terminal acidic region that inhibits factor VIIa complexed to tissue factor (TF). The second Kunitz domain (K2) inhibits factor Xa, and the third Kunitz domain (K3) contains the *C*-terminal basic region. An account of the discovery and isolation of TFPI has been published recently by Broze (289).

The gene for TFPI is approximately 85 kb, located on chromosome 2q31-q32.1, and contains 9 exons. Unlike deficiencies of other coagulation inhibitors (i.e., antithrombin, protein C, and protein S), severe deficiencies of TFPI have not been described. However, there may be a decreased threshold for thrombosis as suggested by TFPI resistance, which is defined as poor anticoagulant response to TFPI. This resistance was observed in 4.7% of controls and in 11.0% of patients with venous thrombosis (290). TFPI knockout mice were first reported in 1997 (291). Heterozygous TFPI knockout mice were phenotypically normal, despite lower levels of TFPI in a factor VIIa/TF inhibition assay. In homozygous TFPI knockout mice, embryonic lethality with signs of yolk sac hemorrhage was seen in 60% of the litter between E9.5 and E11.5 (291). Past E11.5, central nervous system (CNS) and tail hemorrhages were present, and none of the knockout mice survived to the neonatal period.

To date, five polymorphisms have been described in the TFPI gene, two in the promoter, two in the coding region, and one in intron 7 (292–295). Several of these have been assessed for their effect on the risk of venous thrombosis with conflicting results. The Pro15 to Leu polymorphism was first reported to be associated with venous thrombosis (292,296), but this was not confirmed by subsequent studies (297,298). There was no association found between the risk of venous thrombosis or coronary heart disease with either the Val264 to Met or the C-399T and T-287C promoter polymorphisms (293,299). The T-33C polymorphism in intron 7 appears to be an independent risk factor for venous thrombosis but larger independent studies are needed for verification (300).

## Heparin Cofactor II

Heparin cofactor II, a plasma serine protein inhibitor (serpin), specifically binds and inactivates thrombin in the presence of heparin, heparan sulfate, and dermatan sulfate (see Chapter 13). In so doing, it inhibits the rate of thrombin activity by 1,000-fold (301). The anticoagulant protein heparin cofactor II is highly homologous with antithrombin III, with the notable exception that the equivalent of Arg393 in antithrombin III is a Leu. Its stimulation by dermatan sulfate is unique among the serpins. A full-length cDNA for heparin cofactor II was isolated and sequenced in 1988 (302). The complete sequence of the gene, which has five exons and is nearly 13.6 kb in length, also has been determined and has been localized to chromosome 22q11.21 (303).

Heparin cofactor II, synthesized in the liver, circulates in humans at a concentration of approximately 1 $\mu$M (304). A physiologic role during pregnancy and normal placental function is suggested such that during the third trimester, heparin cofactor II levels increase to 150% (305) and thrombin heparin cofactor II levels increase fourfold (306), whereas a 50% decrease in the heparin cofactor II levels has been documented in women with preeclampsia (307).

Inherited deficiency of heparin cofactor II has been documented in at least 15 families [for review see (308)]. Heterozygous deficiency appears to predispose patients to both arterial and venous thromboembolic disorders, but solid data to support these claims still are lacking (309). In an asymptomatic person, an Arg189 to His mutation has been described (310). The variant protein retains its antithrombin activity in the presence of heparin but loses the ability to interact specifically with dermatan sulfate. Two frameshift mutations have been found in heparin cofactor II deficiency. One, an insertion of a T in exon 2, was discovered in a Japanese patient with heparin cofactor II deficiency who had coronary artery disease (311). The other mutation, a deletion of two nucleotides in exon 5, was found in two apparently unrelated Italian patients with heterozygous deficiency and thrombophilia (312). The recurrence of this mutation is probably due to a founder effect.

A knockout mouse model reveals that mice deficient in heparin cofactor II are viable and fertile without any gross abnormalities and are born at the expected mendelian frequency (313). However, in a photochemical model of induced endothelial cell injury, results suggest that HCII may inhibit thrombosis in the arterial circulation.

## Contact Activation Factors

### Factor XII

Factor XII (Hageman factor) is an activator both of the coagulation system and the kinin system. It is synthesized in the liver and circulates as an inactive zymogen. During contact activation, factor XII is proteolytically cleaved at several sites by plasma kallikrein to yield enzymatically active factor XIIa. Factor XIIa is capable of activating prekallikrein and factor XI and is therefore the first component of the contact activation system (314). Moreover, factor XII seems capable of autoactivation.

The amino acid sequence of factor XII was determined by Edman degradation between 1983 and 1985 (315,316). Factor XII cDNA was also cloned in 1985 (317). The mRNA is 2,048 nucleotides long and encodes a protein of 615 amino acids. Clones containing the factor XII gene have been isolated and characterized. The data show that the gene is 12 kb long with 14 exons and is located on chromosome 5q33-qter (318, 319). The promoter of factor XII is TATA-less and contains a functional estrogen response element modulated by HNF-4 in an estrogen-dependent manner (320).

Factor XII deficiency results in an isolated markedly prolonged activated partial thromboplastin time (apt) (>150 seconds) that corrects to normal with a 1:1 mix with normal plasma. There is no recognized bleeding tendency or clinical consequences (321–324). In fact, the original patient in whom this disorder was defined died of pulmonary embolism. This has led to the controversial proposition that factor XII levels are related to venous thrombosis (325–327).

In the first patient in whom a specific point mutation was identified, Miyata et al. found that the codon for Cys571 was changed to one for Ser (321). This Cys residue participates in the disulfide bond that stabilizes the active center Ser

in serine proteases. The mutation is therefore likely to be responsible for the moderately severe decrease of factor XII activity (3% level) in this homozygous individual. Bernardi et al. found a new TaqI site 3' to the acceptor splice junction of exon 2 (within intron 2) in five of 10 genes from five patients with severe factor XII deficiency (328). Three of the five patients were heterozygous and one was homozygous for the mutation; the fifth patient did not manifest this site on either of the factor XII genes. The defect was absent in DNA from 120 healthy individuals, suggesting that it is at least closely linked to the deficiency state. For it to be responsible for the mutation, however, the intron sequence would have to be defined to determine whether a new splice junction had been introduced.

In one large study, 31 unrelated patients from Austria, Germany, and Switzerland were screened for mutations in the factor XII gene (323). Several novel mutations were found in this cohort, including missense mutations that directly or indirectly affected the catalytic triad of factor XII. Two of the mutations reported in this study caused shifts in the reading frame of the gene. A final mutation is in the putative promoter regulatory region ($-8$ GC) of the gene and is also associated with the aberrant TaqI site just mentioned.

In the factor XII 5' untranslated region, a common C to T transition, associated with lower levels of factor XII, has been proposed to play a protective role against coronary disease as well as a role in responsiveness to therapy (329,330). In some, but not all, studies reported, low levels of factor XII coagulant activity have been associated with recurrent abortion in up to 14% of women (331).

### Prekallikrein

Normal human plasma contains two forms of prekallikrein of slightly different molecular weights of 85 kDa and 88 kDa. Plasma prekallikrein (KLKB1, previously known as KLK3) is the zymogen of a serine protease and is activated by factor XIIa. The active enzyme, kallikrein, shows proteolytic activity on a number of substrates, of which, factor XII, HMW kininogen, and urokinase are probably of physiologic importance [for review see (314)]. It circulates in plasma as a complex with HMW kininogen at a concentration of about 40 $\mu$g per mL. Recently, prolylcarboxypeptidase has been identified as a physiologic endothelial cell activator of plasma prekallikrein (332).

Both amino acid sequence analysis and cDNA cloning have been used to determine the primary structure of prekallikrein (333). The mRNA is approximately 2.2 kb long and encodes a protein of 638 amino acids (333). The human prekallikrein gene has been recently characterized, is approximately 31 kb long, contains 15 exons, and is located on chromosome 4q34–35, not far from the factor XI gene (334).

Several kindred with plasma prekallikrein deficiency (Fletcher factor deficiency) have been reported (335–338). The plasma of homozygous cases has no detectable prekallikrein activity. Despite this, affected individuals have no clear signs of a bleeding tendency or some other clinical problem. In 2003, the first reports on the genetic basis for prekallikrein deficiency were reported in two separate families (339,340).

### High-Molecular-Weight Kininogen

The plasma kininogens are the substrate for kallikrein. HMW kininogen and LMW kininogen are two related plasma proteins that derive from the same gene on chromosome 3q26-qter through alternative splicing (341–344). Normal, mature, secreted, full-length HMW kininogen is a 626–amino acid protein.

Deficiency of HMW kininogen is a rare disorder lacking a bleeding or thrombotic clinical phenotype despite an isolated prolonged aPTT of greater than 150 seconds. Activities of HMW and LMW kininogen in regulatory pathways have been revealed through structure–function analyses. Kininogens interact with numerous proteins by binding to cell surface membranes and receptors and by interacting with receptor proteases.

One of the originally described patients who was deficient in kininogen with the associated Williams trait was homozygous for a C to T transition at nucleotide 586, resulting in an Arg to stop mutation in the fifth exon (345). Fitzgerald trait has a nonsense mutation at amino acid 502, no functional HK activity, 40% of normal levels of LMW kininogen antigen activity, and 40% of normal levels of LK antigen activity (346).

Krijanovski et al. described a 6-year-old boy who, subsequent to a traumatic injury, was found to have extensive left vertebral basilar artery thrombosis and a left vertebral artery dissection. As a result of a frameshift mutation of a single base pair deletion at amino acid 480 of the mature protein, the patient had no plasma HK because of degeneration into a stop codon downstream (347).

## Fibrinolytic Factors

### Tissue-Type Plasminogen Activator

Once a clot has been formed, the fibrinolytic system comes into play to dissolve the clot in a regulated fashion. Like the coagulation system, the fibrinolytic system is a network of reactions in which zymogens are proteolytically cleaved to form active enzymes. The final step in the cascade of reactions is the activation of plasminogen to plasmin, which is the principal degrading enzyme of insoluble fibrin.

Tissue-type plasminogen activator (tPA) is a plasma serine protease that mediates plasmin generation and clot lysis by specifically cleaving clot-bound plasminogen (348). The tPA is the main endothelial cell–derived blood activator of the fibrinolytic system. The tPA gene is relatively large (i.e., 32.7 kb), contains 14 exons, and is located on chromosome 8 (p12-p11) (349–352). The *tPA* mRNA was isolated in 1983 using a human Bowes melanoma cell line (353). The mRNA is approximately 2.6 kb in length, whereas the cDNA is 1,689 bp long (353,354). The precursor form of tPA is composed of 562 amino acids, whereas the mature protein has 527 amino acids and has a molecular mass of 68 kDa. The tPA is secreted primarily by endothelial cells as a single-chain glycoprotein, but can be easily converted to the two-chain form by plasmin-mediated cleavage at Arg275 (348). In normal plasma, the antigen concentration of tPA is approximately 0.005 $\mu$g per mL (i.e., 70 pM), and most of it is present in complex with PAI-1 (355,356). A tPA knockout mouse has been described, and, surprisingly, it developed normally and did not exhibit any macroscopic abnormality (357). Microscopic examination revealed mild glomerulonephritis. An informative historic sketch on discovery of tPA has recently been published (358).

Of the numerous nucleotide sequence differences that have been identified within the *tPA* gene, the most studied is a 311-bp Alu insertion/deletion in intron 8 (359) In one study, the presence of one insertion was associated with an increased risk of myocardial infarction, whereas homozygous carriers had a twofold adjusted risk (360). These findings, however, could not be confirmed in other investigations, calling into question the role of this variation in arterial disease (361).

It has been suggested that local endothelial release rate of tPA, rather than the steady state plasma concentration, determines thrombotic potential, and genetic factors may have an influence (362). In a search for genetic variations that may effect tPA protein production, eight polymorphisms

were identified (363). One of these polymorphisms located at position −7351 within the enhancer region of the *tPA* gene was identified and was shown to be strongly correlated with endothelial tPA release rates (363). This polymorphism is within an Sp1 binding site, and the T allele was shown to inhibit Sp1 binding and was associated with less than 50% of the tPA release observed compared to the wild-type C allele. This polymorphism has recently been shown to be clinically relevant, having a strong association with first myocardial infarction and ischemic stroke (364,365).

### Plasminogen

The terminal event in the activation of the fibrinolytic system is the generation of the serine protease plasmin, which has a variety of functional properties, the most notable being dissolution of fibrin clots (348). The precursor of plasmin is plasminogen, a single chain glycoprotein of 92 kDa that circulates in plasma at a concentration of 200 $\mu$g per mL (i.e., 2 $\mu$M). The primary amino acid sequence of plasminogen was reported in 1978 (366). The plasminogen gene encodes a mRNA transcript of approximately 2.9 kb, whereas the cDNA is 2,433 bp in length and encodes a 791–amino acid mature protein with a 19–amino acid signal sequence (367, 368). The gene for plasminogen is localized on chromosome 6q26-q27 in proximity to two genes for apolipoprotein A (369,370). The gene spans 53.5 kb and contains 19 exons, making it the largest gene among the constituents of the fibrinolytic system (371).

One might expect plasminogen deficiency to reduce the capacity to remove excessive clot and, therefore, to contribute to thromboembolic disease. Plasminogen deficiency is classified into two types: type I or hypoplasminogenemia (i.e., antigen and activity reduced) and type II or dysplasminogenemia (i.e., normal antigen, dysfunctional protein). The first case of hereditary heterozygous deficiency of plasminogen (type II) linked to thrombophilia was reported by Aoki et al. in 1978 (372). Since this initial report, many other cases have been described, and it is estimated that plasminogen deficiency occurs with a prevalence of approximately 0.5% in the general population and with that of 1% to 3% in thrombosis patients (373–375). Despite this frequency, the relation between heterozygous deficiency of plasminogen and venous thromboembolism has been called into question on the basis of two pieces of evidence.

The first piece of evidence comes from family studies of patients who present with a history of thrombosis and from the evidence of plasminogen deficiency. Several studies have failed to demonstrate a relation between heterozygous plasminogen deficiency and thrombosis, suggesting that it is not a risk factor (375–378). The second piece of evidence comes from studies on the incidence of plasminogen deficiency in the general population.

Severe deficiency of plasminogen leads to occlusive hydrocephalus and congenital ligneous conjunctivitis, a rare hereditary disorder characterized by the formation of proliferative pseudomembranes on the conjunctiva and other mucosal membranes (379–381). The abnormalities in these patients reflect the important role of plasminogen in wound healing and are due to homozygous loss-of-function mutations in the plasminogen gene, such as Arg216 to His or Trp597 to Stop. None of the homozygous or heterozygous individuals developed spontaneous thrombosis, but one of the children had repeated thrombotic occlusions of an implanted catheter. Mice deficient in plasminogen, in addition to developing thrombotic complications, also develop fibrin-rich conjunctival lesions that appear indistinguishable from human ligneous conjunctivitis (382–384).

## Plasmin Inhibitor

Once plasmin is formed, it has the potential to have a profound anticoagulant effect by digesting not only fibrin but also fibrinogen as well as other coagulation factors. Within the circulation, however, rapid inhibition of free plasmin occurs with plasmin inhibitor (PI), which is a serine protease inhibitor (serpin) and which was formally called α₂-*plasmin inhibitor* or α₂-*antiplasmin* (385). PI is the primary inhibitor of plasmin and is a single-chain glycoprotein with an $M_r$ of 70,000 and circulates in plasma at a concentration of 70 μg per mL (1 μM) (386). Partial and full-length cDNA clone of PI were isolated between 1986 and 1987. The full-length mRNA is approximately 2.3 kb long, whereas the cDNA is 1,476 nucleotides long. Full-length PI is 491 amino acids long, whereas the mature inhibitor is 464 amino acids long (Met-form) (387–389). There is a second form of the inhibitor in plasma that is 12 amino acids shorter (Asn-form) (390). The PI gene contains 10 exons and is distributed over approximately 16 kb of DNA and is localized on chromosome 17p13 (391,392).

PI deficiency is a rare autosomal recessive disorder and is characterized by bleeding tendencies, with homozygous patients being generally more affected. Type I deficiency is defined as the absence or decreased concentrations of the protein, where type II is characterized by a dysfunctional protein. The first deficiency states were reported in 1978, and since then more than 13 cases have been reported [reviewed in (393)]. Most patients present with severe bleeding that appears during childhood. Heterozygotes who have approximately 50% of the normal level of PI in blood may either have a mild bleeding tendency or be asymptomatic. In contrast to patients with a severe deficiency of PI who have mild-to-severe hemorrhagic tendencies, mice that are deficient in PI have a transient enhanced endogenous fibrinolytic activity and do not have overt bleeding tendencies (394).

At present, there are seven published reports detailing the molecular basis of PI deficiency: (a) a trinucleotide insertion responsible for an additional Ala within the 353 to 357 fragment (395), (b) a frameshift mutation in exon 10 that is responsible for elongation of the protein (396), (c) a trinucleotide deletion responsible for a Glu137 deletion (397), (d) a G to A transition responsible for a Val384 to Met substitution (398), (e) a splicing donor site suppression in intron 2 (399), (f) a single T deletion at nucleotide position 332 in exon 5 that causes a frame shift and shortening of the protein (400), and (g) a splicing donor site mutation in intron 6 that leads to exon 6 skipping (401). In some of these cases, expression systems that were established to ensure the mutations were responsible for the deficiency state.

## Plasminogen Activator Inhibitor 1

PAI-1, the principal inhibitor of fibrinolysis, is a 50-kDa serpin (serine protease inhibitor) that interacts with and inhibits both tPA and urokinase plasminogen activator (uPA). PAI-1, is predominantly located in two areas, in the plasma, as secreted by endothelial cells in an active form, and in platelets, present mainly in an inactive form (402). Cofactors for PAI-1 activity include heparin, the presence of which increases PAI-1 activity toward thrombin, and vitronectin, a stabilizing factor. PAI-1 levels show diurnal variations, with a peak level in the early morning, a finding that appears to be associated with the 4G5G polymorphism (see subsequent text) (403).

The *PAI-1* gene is located on chromosome 7q21.3-q22, covers approximately 12.3 kb and consists of 9 exons and 8 introns (404–409). The *PAI-1* gene encodes two distinct species of mRNA approximately 2.3 and 3.4 kb in size. The cDNA of PAI-1 has been cloned by seven different groups and is 1,209 bp in length (410–414). The promoter of PAI-1 contains a TATA box, lacks a CAAT box, and contains numerous regulatory sequences including two enhancerlike glucocorticoid response elements and nucleotides (415). Studies have shown a correlation with a functional 4G or 5G genotype in the PAI-1 promoter. Both the 4G and 5G alleles GACACGTG(G₄ or ₅)AGT(4G/5G) bind a transcriptional activator at −675 in the PAI-1 5′ untranslated region. However, the 5G allele also binds a repressor protein in an overlapping binding site, resulting in lower levels in the 5G than in the 4G allele. Numerous correlations have shown a significantly higher prevalence of particular cardiovascular disease states with the 4G allele (416–418).

PAI-1$^{-/-}$ knockout mice are viable and show no apparent histologic or hemostatic abnormalities. Challenge with endotoxins in the knockout mice appear to induce a greater resistance to venous thrombosis and a mild hyperfibrinolytic state (419,420). Other physical challenges in this knockout mouse show tumor growth, angiogenesis, and increased responses to injury.

## Thrombin-Activatable Fibrinolysis Inhibitor

Thrombin-activatable fibrinolysis inhibitor (TAFI), also known as procarboxypeptidase B and procarboxypeptidase U, is a zymogen found in plasma that is thought to play an important role in hemostasis by linking both coagulation and fibrinolysis (421). Activated TAFI, when exposed to a fibrin clot, catalyzes the removal of C-terminal lysines, thereby diminishing the cofactor activity for plasminogen activation. This in turn reduces plasmin production on fibrin, slowing clot lysis or prolonging fibrinolysis [for review see (421)]. This inhibitor has been isolated from plasma, has been characterized by three independent laboratories, and was cloned in 1991 (422–424). The TAFI mRNA is approximately 1.7 kb in length, whereas the cDNA is 1,272 nucleotides long. The human *TAFI* gene was characterized in 1999, is located on chromosome 13q14.11, and consists of 11 exons spanning approximately 48 kb of DNA (425). TAFI is synthesized in the liver as a pre-propeptide of 423 amino acids, which includes a 22–amino acid signal sequence. It has a molecular mass of 60 kDa and circulates in plasma at a concentration of approximately 70 nM (426).

Because of its role as a negative regulator of fibrinolytic efficiency, TAFI may be considered a potential candidate in thrombotic disease. Making use of a large population-based case–control study on venous thrombosis, the Leiden Thrombophilia Study (LETS), van Tilburg et al. found that elevated TAFI antigen levels were only a mild risk factor for venous thrombosis (427). In addition, elevated TAFI levels were also found to be a mild risk factor for coronary artery disease and ischemic stroke (428,429). In contrast, however, two studies have reported that very high TAFI antigen levels are associated with a lower risk of coronary events (430,431). Although no reports have yet described individuals with TAFI deficiency, the phenotype is likely to be mild because TAFI knockout mice do not exhibit any abnormal phenotypes, even in arterial and venous injury models (432).

The first polymorphisms in the *TAFI* gene were described in 1998 and were identified following cloning of the cDNA using multiple liver libraries. One is a G to A substitution at nucleotide 505 on the cDNA sequence, leading to an Ala to Thr substitution at amino acid 147, and the other is a C to T substitution at nucleotide 678, resulting in a silent polymorphism (433). *In vitro* studies revealed that the Ala147 to Thr substitution did not adversely affect TAFI function. Other polymorphisms have now been identified: at least five in the promoter region and two in the 3′-UTR. It was found that all of these polymorphisms were in strong linkage disequilibrium with each other and with the Ala147 to Thr polymorphism (434). Together, these polymorphisms generated four main haplotypes, and it was determined that the Ala147 to Thr and the 1542C/G polymorphisms in combination showed the strongest influence on TAFI levels; however, the mechanism is not clear.

More recently, another SNP has been identified in the *TAFI* gene that appears to be associated with reduced TAFI levels. The polymorphism is a C to T change at nucleotide position 1,040 and results in a Thr325 to Ile substitution (435,436). Interestingly, however, biochemical characterization revealed that this particular mutation increases the thermal stability of the protein, resulting in enhanced activity of activated TAFI and consequently in an increased antifibrinolytic potential (436). At present, it is unclear whether this polymorphism influences thrombotic disease. However, one recent report indicates that this polymorphism may be involved in the susceptibility of patients for meningococcal disease and, in particular, may be related to mortality once meningococcal disease has been contracted (437).

## Other Important Hemostatic Proteins

### Fibrinogen

The final reaction in the coagulation cascade is the formation of an insoluble fibrin network from fibrinogen. Fibrinogen is a complex molecule, a 340-kDa glycoprotein that consists of two disulfide-linked monomers. Each of the monomers consists of three polypeptide chains encoded by three distinct genes: $A\alpha$, $B\beta$, and $\gamma$ (438). The fibrinogen to fibrin transformation is initiated after thrombin proteolytically removes two acidic peptides—fibrinopeptide A (FPA) and fibrinopeptide B (FPB)—from the $N$-terminus of the $A\alpha$ and $B\beta$ chains, respectively. Removal of these peptides exposes sites (often denoted A and B knobs) on the fibrinogen molecule that favor intermolecular reactions between fibrinogen dimers and therefore allow polymerization and formation of a fibrin network (438). Factor XIIIa stabilizes the fibrin clot by cross-linking fibrin monomers.

The cDNAs encoding the $A\alpha$, $B\beta$, and $\gamma$ chains were cloned in 1993 (439–442). The mRNA for the $A\alpha$ chain is approximately 2.2 kb nucleotides long and encodes a 625–amino acid long mature protein (439,442). The signal peptide is either 16 or 19 amino acids long, depending on whether the methionine at position −16 or −19 is used as the initiation codon. The $A\alpha$ gene also has been cloned and is approximately 5.4 kb and contains five exons (442). There is also a variant form of the $A\alpha$ chain found in plasma (<2%) that is extended by 236 amino acids and that is encoded by a sixth exon. The $B\beta$ mRNA counts 1,918 nucleotides and encodes a protein of 461 amino acids. Uncertainty also exists about the initiation codon in the $B\beta$ mRNA because methionines are found at codon −16 and −27. Genomic clones covering the entire $B\beta$ gene also have been isolated and the gene is approximately 8 kb and contains eight exons (440). The fibrinogen $\gamma$ gene is approximately 8.4 kb long and contains 10 exons. The gene encodes two slightly different forms of the $\gamma$ chain: $\gamma A$ and $\gamma B$ (443). The most abundant form is $\gamma A$, which is produced from mRNA and spliced at nucleotide 7,774 in exon 9. The $\gamma B$ mRNA is not spliced after exon 9, leading to read-through at the donor splice site and to the addition of 20 codons before a stop codon is reached. Exon 10 is not used, and polyadenylation occurs at a different site.

The genes encoding the fibrinogen chains cover approximately 50 kb and are located on chromosome 4q28 (444–446). The genes in the fibrinogen locus are linked in the order $\gamma \rightarrow A\alpha \leftarrow B\beta$ (444). The direction of transcription of the $B\beta$ gene is therefore reversed compared to the direction of

transcription of the other two genes. Transcription of the three genes occurs in a coordinated fashion, in which transcription from the $B\beta$ gene is the rate-limiting step (447).

A knockout model of fibrinogen shows that homozygous mice deficient in fibrinogen ($A\alpha$ chain–deficient) are born at the expected Mendelian frequency (448). In the neonatal period, approximately 30% of the mice manifest overt bleeding in the peritoneal cavity, skin, and soft tissues around joints. However, survival of the neonatal period is followed by a better control of the blood loss. Long-term survival in the mice deficient in fibrinogen varies and is highly dependent on genetic background; however, in pregnant mice, fatal uterine bleeding occurs around the tenth day of gestation.

Afibrinogenemia, first described in 1920, is a rare autosomal recessive disorder associated with spontaneous, postsurgical, and postpartum bleeding of variable severity (37). It is characterized by a severe deficiency of fibrinogen both in the plasma and the platelet. More than 30 afibrinogenemia-causing mutations have been reported, mostly in the $A\alpha$ and just a few in the $B\beta$ gene. It is interesting to note that the bleeding tendency in individuals with complete afibrinogenemia is not always severe and that an increased bleeding tendency may not occur after small amounts of fibrinogen circulate.

Dysfibrinogenemia is characterized by a variant form of fibrinogen, mostly because of a missense mutation that replaces an amino acid (449,450). The clinical symptoms are highly variable: some patients have a bleeding tendency, whereas others have venous thrombosis. There are also examples of individuals with increased bleeding who also experience venous thrombosis. Most patients of dysfibrinogenemia present themselves in heterozygous form. This dominant inheritance is expected from the dimeric structure of fibrinogen and the multimeric structure of fibrin. Consequently, abnormal subunits are covalently linked to normal ones, leading to an overall abnormal fibrinogen and fibrin. A large number of different mutations have been documented (>350) in dysfibrinogenemia, and they are collected and presented on an electronic database: http://www.geht.org/databaseang/fibrinogen/ (451).

Heterozygosity for dysfibrinogenemia is associated with little or no clinical symptoms. Homozygotes for dysfibrinogenemia have also been reported, and in these individuals, bleeding may be more serious, but this is not always the case. In patients with a history of venous thrombosis, the prevalence of dysfibrinogenemia is approximately 0.8% (452). Most bleeding episodes are mild to moderate and may occur postoperatively, postpartum, antepartum, and as a result of delayed wound healing. Thrombotic problems include deep venous thrombosis, thrombophlebitis, pulmonary embolism, arterial thrombosis, and joint arterial and venous thrombosis. In addition, patients who experience a thrombotic event may also have a history of bleeding (27%).

Elevated fibrinogen levels are an important risk factor for cardiovascular disease (453). This finding has raised considerable interest in defining genetic determinants of fibrinogen levels. Such determinants have indeed been found as polymorphisms that occur with a high prevalence in the population (453). The best studied are two promoter polymorphisms in the fibrinogen $B\beta$ gene, a G/A site at nucleotide −455 and a C/T variant site at −148. The two variant sites are in complete linkage equilibrium (454). Individuals homozygous for the −455A allele have, on average, 0.28 g per L higher fibrinogen levels than GG homozygotes. By extrapolation, one can calculate that the GG individuals should have a 40% higher risk for ischemic heart disease (22). It is uncertain whether this is indeed the case. It may be that the association between high fibrinogen levels and coronary disease is not one of cause and effect. Given the fact that fibrinogen is an acute-phase reactant, elevated fibrinogen levels may well reflect the inflamed state of atherosclerotic vessels.

## Factor XIII

Activated factor XIII is the final component of the blood clotting cascade and is responsible for cross-linking fibrin. Plasma factor XIII is a tetrameric molecule composed of two A subunits (83 kDa) and two B subunits (80 kDa) [for review see (455)]. Platelet factor XIII consists only of two A subunits. The factor XIII-A subunits belong to the transglutaminase family of proteins. Thrombin cleaves a peptide bond within the A chain, forming factor XIIIa, which stabilizes the fibrin clot. This is accomplished by a transglutaminase reaction forming covalent bonds between Lys and Gln side chains near the carboxyl-termini of the γγ chains (within strands) and between γα chains (within the mesh). The factor XIII-A subunit gene has been localized to chromosome 6p24-25 (F13A) and is approximately 160 kb and contains 15 exons (456,457). The mature A subunit has 731 amino acids. The factor XIII B–subunit gene (F13B) is approximately 28 kb in length, has 12 exons, and is located on chromosome 1q31-32.1 (458,459). The mature protein has 641 amino acids and contains 10 short consensus repeats known as *sushi domains* (460).

Factor XIII deficiency is a rare autosomal disorder that is associated with a severe bleeding diathesis when factor XIII levels are less than 1%. Women with inherited factor XIII deficiency have recurrent abortions and difficulty carrying a pregnancy to term. The inheritance of this disorder is not completely recessive because increased bleeding has been reported for some heterozygous individuals. In most cases, however, heterozygotes are asymptomatic.

The role of factor XIII during pregnancy and placental/uterine hemostasis was demonstrated with factor XIII-A knockout mice (461,462). Despite being able to become pregnant, knockout mice with factor XIII-A frequently died of excessive vaginal bleeding with massive placental hemorrhage and subsequent necrosis at gestational day 10. This phenotype correlates with spontaneous miscarriage in pregnant humans with factor XIII deficiency.

More than 30 mutations have been characterized in factor XIII deficiency, most of which affect the A gene. As expected, mutations that have been found are variable in nature and include missense mutations, premature stop codons, small deletions and insertions, or deletion of most of the gene.

Two mutations have been characterized in the B gene (463). One is a missense mutation (Cys430 to Phe) and the other a deletion of one nucleotide in the acceptor splice junction of exon 2. These mutations were found in a compound heterozygote with complete absence of the B subunit. Subunit A in platelets was normally present but did not prevent the bleeding tendency. Several polymorphisms of both the A and B subunit genes have been described and should prove useful in distinguishing A chain from B chain defects in family studies (455).

A common mutation in the factor XIII-A subunit has been implicated in some, but not all, studies (ARIC study) as a risk factor for vascular disease. This Val34 to Leu dimorphism, which is three amino acids from the activation site of factor XIII, is protective against myocardial infarction and predisposes to intracerebral hemorrhage (464,465). Studies show that the effect of an environmental influence, such as smoking or aspirin consumption varies between individuals with and without the Leu allele, highlighting the importance of analyzing numerous parameters when assessing genetic impacts in the multifactorial disease process of thrombosis (466).

## von Willebrand Factor

VWF is a large multimeric adhesive glycoprotein. It performs two major roles in hemostasis. At sites of vascular damage, VWF mediates adhesion of platelets to the subendothelium. VWF also plays a critical role in stabilizing the procoagulant cofactor, factor VIII. In response to numerous stimuli, VWF is released from storage granules of platelets (α-granules) and from endothelial cells (Weibel-Palade bodies) and is constitutively secreted by endothelial cells and is possibly produced in placental syncytiotrophoblasts (467). In the plasma, VWF circulates at concentrations of approximately 10 mg per mL. The VWF protein itself exists as a series of multimers that are linked by disulfide bonds located near the C-terminal end of each subunit (see Fig. 4-5).

The *VWF* gene, located on the short arm of chromosome 12 (12p13.3), is approximately 178 kb in length and contains 52 exons (468,469). A partial, highly homologous pseudogene is present on chromosome 22q11-13 and is approximately 21 to 29 kb in length (469). This pseudogene has no known function, but its presence complicates genetic analysis of von Willebrand disease (VWD). Several groups originally cloned the cDNA for VWF in 1985 to 1986 (470–473). It is almost 9,000 bp long and encodes a protein of 2,813 amino acids.

VWD is a congenital bleeding disorder caused by defects at the VWF locus. This autosomally inherited mucocutaneous bleeding disorder was first reported by Erik von Willebrand in 1926 in a large family from the Aland Islands off the coast of Finland. On the basis of phenotypic and genetic characteristics,

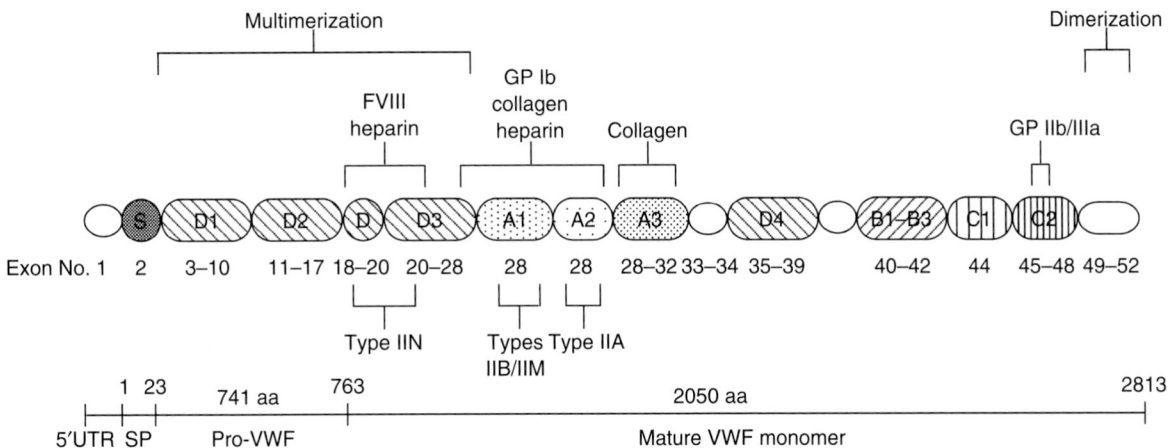

**FIGURE 4-5.** Gene organization of von Willebrand factor (VWF). The 52 exons of the *VWF* gene are shown along with the indicated protein domain regions. Potential functional binding sites with other proteins are also shown. Type II mutation hot spots between exons 18 and 28 are indicated. GP, glycoprotein.

a revised classification of VWD has been adopted (474). Type I deficiency includes patients with a partial quantitative deficiency of VWF levels in plasma. Type II deficiency refers to a qualitative deficiency. Type III VWD comprises patients with extremely low or undetectable levels of VWF. Symptomatology of VWF deficiency includes easy bruising, nosebleeds, and hematomas. Excessive menstrual bleeding and heavy bleeding following oral cavity, tooth extraction, tonsillectomy, and adenoidectomy are also common. A mouse model of VWF has been described, and it was found that these mice very closely mimic severe (type III) human VWD (475).

The inheritance of VWD varies with the type of deficiency. Type I deficiency accounts for approximately 75% of all VWD (476). Heritable variances are modest and not solely linked to the VWF locus. Notably, variation in VWF is highly linked to an individual's ABO blood type. In addition, in non–type III disease, VWF levels increase during pregnancy and during stress, such as at the time of drawing blood. Individuals with blood type O have VWF levels 25% to 35% lower than individuals of blood types A, B, or AB. Variations are influenced by polymorphisms including a $-1793G > C$ SNP. VWD is viewed as the most frequent bleeding disorder, with an estimated prevalence of 1% in the general population. The frequency of VWD is highly dependent on the criteria used in establishing the diagnosis. Experts differ on the definition of VWF type I deficiency from less than 15% levels to levels below 50% (476).

Type I and types IIA, IIB, and IIM variants are most commonly dominant. Type IIA is the most common subclass and refers to qualitative variants with decreased platelet-dependent function associated with absence of HMW forms of VWF multimers; type IIB mutations increase the affinity of cWF for platelet glycoprotein (GP) Ib; type IIM refers to variants that share decreased platelet-dependent function that is not the result of the absence of HMW forms; and finally, type IIN refers to those VWF variants with a decreased affinity for factor VIII (Fig. 4-5). Type IIN deficiency seems silent in heterozygous carriers.

Type III deficiency inherits as a recessive trait. The mode of inheritance can be understood from the underlying mutations. Mutations identified in patients with VWD are continuously collected and published electronically and are listed according to the classification mentioned previously in this section (see: http://www.sheffield.ac.uk/vwf/) (477,478). Type III describes the most severe form of VWD. This form is caused by homozygosity for complete loss-of-function mutations in the *VWF* gene. As is the case in hemophilia A and B, an almost infinite number of possible mutations leads to this phenotype. This fact, combined with the large size of the *von Willebrand* gene, underlines the difficulty in routinely identifying mutations in type III deficiency.

## γ-Glutamyl Carboxylase

γ-Glutamyl carboxylase is an integral membrane enzyme responsible for a unique posttranslational modification: the carboxylation of the γ carbon of between 9 and 13 glutamic acid residues in the *N*-terminal region of coagulation proteins factors II, VII, IX, X, and proteins C, S, and Z (479). In addition, several other proteins not known to be involved in coagulation (e.g., bone gla protein, matrix gla protein, gas 6, and proline-rich gla proteins 1 and 2) contain a signature propeptide region targeting these proteins for carboxylation through a common homology domain. It is of interest to note that the carboxylase itself is similarly carboxylated.

The γ-glutamyl carboxylase is found in the rough endoplasmic reticulum and is a 758–amino acid protein. It requires vitamin K as a cofactor to modify the affected proteins because they are secreted through the endoplasmic reticulum into the Golgi apparatus (480). Each $CO_2$ addition cycle is balanced by oxidation of vitamin K hydroquinone to vitamin K 2,3-epoxide, with a concomitant reduction of oxygen to water. The carboxylase protein is produced in the liver, where it is critical for normal hemostasis.

The gene for human γ-glutamyl carboxylase is 13 kb long, located on chromosome 2p12, contains 15 exons, and has a 217-bp sequence between the transcription and translation start sites (481,482). Similar to the genes of the vitamin K–dependent clotting proteins, the promoter lacks a TATA box and contains critical proximal functional binding sites for Sp1 required for promoter activity. A DNA sequence at −76 to −65 contains functional properties essential for the developmental expression of the carboxylase as shown with *in vivo* footprinting experimentation (483). A knockout mouse model of the carboxylase gene has been reported and reveals phenotypically normal heterozygous mice, whereas the homozygous knockout mice die of massive hemorrhage at birth and possess prenatal developmental abnormalities resembling the human syndrome of warfarin teratogenicity (484).

Hereditary combined deficiency of vitamin K–dependent proteins is a rare bleeding disorder that has only been reported in a few patients. Theoretically, this disorder may stem from functional deficiency of either the γ-glutamyl carboxylase or the vitamin K 2,3-epoxide reductase. A few mutations in the epoxide reductase gene have recently been identified (see next section), and two mutations in the γ-glutamyl carboxylase gene have been found that account for this deficiency. The first mutation was identified in 1998 and is a missense mutation in exon 9, leading to the conversion of Leu394 to Arg (485). Expression studies revealed that the mutant enzyme had approximately threefold reduced activity compared to the wild type. The second mutation is in exon 11, resulting in the conversion of Trp501 to Ser (486). Oral vitamin $K_1$ administration resulted in resolution of the clinical symptoms. To date, no insertions or deletions have been identified.

## Epoxide Reductase I

VKOR is a warfarin-sensitive enzyme that is responsible for reducing vitamin K 2,3-epoxide back to the active cofactor, vitamin K hydroquinone. Although the enzyme was first described in 1974, the gene encoding the epoxidase reductase has eluded investigators until recently (487). In 2004, the gene was identified by two separate groups using two elegant complementary techniques: (a) positional cloning in humans, rats, and mice (12) and (b) siRNA pools against individual candidate genes (13). Previous results restricting the locus of the VKOR enzyme to 16q12-21 (488), aided by the accessibility of genomic data from humans, rats, and mice, were critical in finding this long sought after gene.

The *VKOR* gene contains three exons and creates a protein 163 amino acids in length that has a relative molecular mass of 18 kDa, with at least one transmembrane domain (12,13). In humans, Rost et al. identified a homozygous point mutation (292 C to T), at a CpG mutation hotspot, in the third exon, leading to an Arg98 to Trp in two unrelated patients of Lebanese and German descent (12). In addition, they found heterozygous mutations in patients with warfarin resistance at Val29 to Leu, Val45 to Ala, Arg58 to Gly, and Leu128 to Arg. These mutations were not seen in 384 control chromosomes.

By using positional cloning and by integrating data from human, mouse, and rat species, Li et al. concluded that both vitamin K–dependent clotting factor type 2 (VKFCD-2) and warfarin resistance are due to mutations in the same protein, VKOR (13). Li et al. relied upon the NCBI database to restrict the 52 genes in the region with unknown function to 13 genes, predicting a transmembrane section. These investigators then worked to identify a cell line expressing a high level of VKOR activity so that they could systematically knock down all 13 candidate genes using siRNA. In so doing, they were able to identify the *VKOR* gene and subsequently confirm its activity in Sf9 (*Spodoptera frugiperda*) cells.

# SUMMARY

The completion of the HGP in 2003 has made gene and cDNA sequences immediately available to anyone. This genomic information should provide a powerful means of discovering hereditary factors in multifactorial/multigenic diseases such as thrombosis. However, it should be reiterated that it is not genes alone but the interplay of genetic and environmental factors also that determines phenotype. A challenge for the future will be to determine which combinations of genetic changes (i.e., SNPs) directly or indirectly influence complex disease states. Genetic tools such as the HapMap should facilitate this process. In addition, genome sequences from other animals may also prove useful in defining informative genetic changes. Many of these genomes are available or are in the process of being sequenced (see http://www.tigr.org/). These databases should also prove useful in furthering our understanding of the evolution of blood coagulation. The availability of genetic information for the hemostatic proteins has also made possible the safe and efficient production of pharmacologically relevant proteins for therapeutic purposes (i.e., recombinant factor VIIa, VIII, and IX). Furthermore, it also provides new methods for the treatment of diseases using gene therapy approaches.

## *References*

1. The International Human Genome Sequencing Consortium. Initial sequencing and analysis of the human genome. *Nature* 2001;409:860–921.
2. Collins FS, Green ED, Guttmacher AE, et al. A vision for the future of genomics research. *Nature* 2003;422:835–847.
3. Wolfsberg TG, Wetterstrand KA, Guyer MS, et al. A user's guide to the human genome. *Nature Genet* 2003;4(Suppl 1):4–79.
4. Austin CP. The impact of the completed human genome sequence on the development of novel therapeutics for human disease. *Annu Rev Med* 2004;55:1–13.
5. Lander ES, Botstein D. Homozygosity mapping: a way to map human recessive traits with the DNA of inbred children. *Science* 1987;236:1567–1570.
6. Broeckel U, Schork NJ. Identifying genes and genetic variation underlying human diseases and complex phenotypes via recombination mapping. *J Physiol* 2003;554:40–45.
7. Gabriel SB, Schaffner SF, Nguyen H, et al. The structure of haplotype blocks in the human genome. *Science* 2002;296:2225–2229.
8. Eriksson M, Brown WT, Gordon LB, et al. Recurrent de novo point mutations in lamin A cause Hutchinson-Gilford progeria syndrome. *Nature* 2003;423:293–298.
9. Nichols WC, Seligsohn U, Zivelin A, et al. Linkage of combined factors V and VIII deficiency to chromosome 18q by homozygosity mapping. *J Clin Invest* 1997;99(4):596–601.
10. Nichols WC, Seligsohn U, Zivelin A, et al. Mutations in the ER-Golgi intermediate compartment protein ERGIC-53 cause combined deficiency of coagulation factors V and VIII. *Cell* 1998;93:61–70.
11. Levy GG, Nichols WC, Lian EC, et al. Mutations in a member of the ADAMTS gene family causes thrombotic thrombocytopenic purpura. *Nature* 2001;413:488–494.
12. Rost S, Fregin A, Ivaskevicius V, et al. Mutations in VKORC1 cause warfarin resistance and multiple coagulation factor deficiency type 2. *Nature* 2004;427:537–541.
13. Li T, Chang CY, Jin DY, et al. Identification of the gene for vitamin K epoxide reductase. *Nature* 2004;427:541–544.
14. Cooper DN, Youssoufian H. The CpG dinucleotide and human genetic disease. *Hum Genet* 1988;78:151–155.
15. Ketterling RP, Vielhaber E, Sommer SS. The rates of G:C → T:A and G:C → C:G transversions at CpG dinucleotides in the human factor IX gene. *Am J Hum Genet* 1994;54:831–835.
16. Sadler JE, Gralnick HR. Commentary: a new classification for von Willebrand disease. *Blood* 1994;84:676–679.
17. Ebert RF. *Index of variant human fibrinogens*. Boca Raton, FL: KLC Press, 1994.
18. Marlar RA, Montgomery RR, Broekmans AW. Diagnosis and treatment of homozygous protein C deficiency. Report of the working party on homozygous protein C deficiency of the subcommittee on protein C and protein S, International Committee on Thrombosis and Haemostasis. *J Pediatr* 1989;114:528–534.
19. Bovill EG, Bauer KA, Dickermann JD, et al. The clinical spectrum of heterozygous protein C deficiency in a large New England kindred. *Blood* 1989;73:712–717.
20. Koster T, Rosendaal FR, Briet E, et al. Protein C deficiency in a controlled series of unselected outpatients: an infrequent but clear risk factor for venous thrombosis (Leiden Thrombophilia Study). *Blood* 1995;85:2754–2761.
21. Peake I. Molecular genetics and counseling in haemophilia. *Thromb Haemost* 1995;74:40–44.
22. Humphries SE, Panahloo A, Montgomery HE, et al. Gene-environment interaction in the determination of levels of haemostatic variables involved in thrombosis and fibrinolysis. *Thromb Haemost* 1997;78:457–461.
23. Koeleman BP, Reitsma PH, Bertina RM. Familial thrombophilia: a complex genetic disorder. *Semin Hematol* 1997;34:256–264.
24. Lindqvist PG, Svensson PJ, Dahlbäck B, et al. Factor V Q506 mutation (activated protein C resistance) associated with reduced intrapartum blood loss—a possible evolutionary selection mechanism. *Thromb Haemost* 1998;79:69–73.
25. Chu K, Wu S-M, Stanley TB, et al. A mutation in the propeptide of factor IX leads to warfarin sensitivity by a novel mechanism. *J Clin Invest* 1996;98:1619–1625.
26. Emmerich J, Rosendaal FR, Cattaneo M, et al. Combined effect of factor V$_{Leiden}$ and prothrombin 20210A on the risk of venous thromboembolism—pooled analysis of 8 case-control studies including 2310 cases and 3204 controls. Study group for pooled-analysis in venous thromboembolism. *Thromb Haemost* 2001;86:809–816.
27. Degen SJF, Davie EW. Nucleotide sequence of the gene for human prothrombin. *Biochemistry* 1987;26:6165–6177.
28. Degen SJF, MacGillivray RTA, Davie EW. Characterization of the complementary deoxyribonucleic acid and gene coding for human prothrombin. *Biochemistry* 1983;22:2087.
29. Barnhart MI. Cellular site for prothrombin synthesis. *Am J Physiol* 1960;199:360–366.
30. Aoubine MN, Ma JY, Smirnova IV, et al. A molecular mechanism for synapse elimination: novel inhibition of locally generated thrombin delays synapse loss in neonatal mouse muscles. *Dev Biol* 1996;179:447–457.
31. Glazner GW, Yadav K, Fitzgerald S, et al. Cholinergic stimulation increases thrombin activity and gene expression in cultured mouse muscles. *Dev Brain Res* 1997;99:148–154.
32. Flynn PD, Byrne CD, Baglin TP, et al. Thrombin generation by apoptotic vascular smooth muscle cells. *Blood* 1997;89:4378–4384.
33. Suzuki K, Tanaka T, Miyazawa K, et al. Gene expression of prothrombin in human and rat kidneys: basic and clinical approach. *J Am Soc Nephrol* 1999;10:S408–S411.
34. Mann KG, Elion J, Butkowski RJ, et al. Prothrombin. *Methods Enzymol* 1981;80:286–302.
35. Xue J, Wu Q, Westfield LA, et al. Incomplete embryonic lethality and fatal neonatal hemorrhage caused by prothrombin deficiency in mice. *Proc Natl Acad Sci U S A* 1998;95:7603–7607.
36. Sun WY, Witte DP, Degen JL, et al. Prothrombin deficiency results in embryonic and neonatal lethality in mice. *Proc Natl Acad Sci U S A* 1998;95:7597–7602.
37. Peyvandi F, Duga S, Akhavan S, et al. Rare coagulation deficiencies. *Haemophilia* 2002;8:308–321.
38. Akhavan S, Mannucci PM, Lak M, et al. Identification and three-dimensional structural analysis of nine novel mutations in patients with prothrombin deficiency. *Thromb Haemost* 2000;84:989–997.
39. Henriksen RA, Mann KG. Identification of the primary structural defect in the dysthrombin thrombin Quick-I: substitution of cysteine for arginine 382. *Biochemistry* 1988;27:9160.
40. Bode W, Mayr I, Bauman Y, et al. The refined 1.9 Å crystal structure of human α-thrombin: interaction with D-Phe-Pro-Arg chloromethylketone and significance of the Tyr-Pro-Trp insertion segment. *EMBO J* 1989;8:3467–3475.
41. Henriksen RA, Owen WG. Characterization of the catalytic defect in the dysthrombin, thrombin Quick. *J Biol Chem* 1987;262:4664–4669.
42. Poort SR, Rosendaal FR, Reitsma PH, et al. A common genetic variation in the 3′-untranslated region of the prothrombin gene is associated with elevated plasma prothrombin levels and an increase in venous thrombosis. *Blood* 1996;88:3698–3703.
43. Cumming AM, Keeney S, Salden A, et al. The prothrombin gene G20210A variant: prevalence in a U.K. anticoagulant clinic population. *Br J Haematol* 1997;98:353–355.
44. Ferraresi P, Marchetti G, Legnani C, et al. The heterozygous 20210 G/A prothrombin genotype is associated with early venous thrombosis in inherited thrombophilia and is not increased in frequency in artery disease. *Arterioscler Thromb Vasc Biol* 1997;17(11):2418–2422.
45. Hillarp A, Zoller B, Svensson PJ, et al. The 2010 allele of the prothrombin gene is a common risk factor among Swedish outpatients with verified deep venous thrombosis. *Thromb Haemost* 1997;78:990–992.
46. Howard TE, Marusa M, Channell C, et al. A patient homozygous for a mutation in the prothrombin gene 3′-untranslated region associated with massive thrombosis. *Blood Coagul Fibrin* 1997;8:316–319.

47. Gehring NH, Frede U, New-Yilik G, et al. Increased efficiency of mRNA 3′ end formation: a new genetic mechanism contributing to hereditary thrombophilia. *Nature Genet* 2001;28:389–392.

48. Pollak ES, Lam HS, Russell JE. The G20210A mutation does not affect the stability of prothrombin mRNA *in vivo*. *Blood* 2002;100:359–362.

49. Carter AM, Sachchithananthan M, Stasinopoulos S, et al. Prothrombin G20210A is a bifunctional gene polymorphism. *Thromb Haemost* 2002; 87:846–853.

50. Rosendaal FR, Doggen CJ, Zivelin A, et al. Geographic distribution of the 20210 G to A prothrombin variant. *Thromb Haemost* 1998;79:706–708.

51. Hung HL, High KA. Liver-enriched transcription factor HNF-4 and ubiquitous factor NF-Y are critical for expression of blood coagulation factor X. *J Biol Chem* 1996;271:2323–2331.

52. Leytus SP, Foster DC, Kurachi K, et al. Gene for human factor X a blood coagulation factor whose gene organization is essentially identical to that of factor IX and protein C. *Biochemistry* 1986;25:5098–5101.

53. Royle NJ, Fung MR, MacGillivray RTA, et al. The gene for clotting factor X is mapped to 13q32:qter. *Cytogenet Cell Genet* 1986;41:185.

54. Leytus SP, Chung DW, Kisiel W, et al. Characterization of a cDNA coding for human factor X. *Proc Natl Acad Sci U S A* 1984;81:3699–3702.

55. Fung MR, Hay CW, MacGillivray RTA. Characterization of an almost full-length cDNA coding for human blood coagulation factor X. *Proc Natl Acad Sci U S A* 1985;82:3591.

56. Kaul RK, Hildebrand B, Roberts S, et al. Isolation and characterization of human blood coagulation factor X cDNA. *Gene* 1986;41:311–314.

57. Fujikawa K, Legaz ME, Davie EW. Bovine Factors X1 and X2 (Stuart Factor). Isolation and characterization. *Biochemistry* 1972;11:4882–4891.

58. Di Scipio RG, Hermodson MA, Yates SG, et al. A comparison of human prothrombin, factor IX (Christmas Factor), factor X (Stuart Factor), and protein S. *Biochemistry* 1977;16:698–706.

59. Cooper DN, Millar DS, Wacey A, et al. Inherited factor X deficiency: molecular genetics and pathophysiology. *Thromb Haemost* 1997;78(1):161–172.

60. Peyvandi F, Menegatti M, Santagostino E, et al. Gene mutations and three-dimensional structural analysis in 13 families with severe factor X deficiency. *Br J Haematol* 2002;117:685–692.

61. Dewerchin M, Liang Z, Moons L, et al. Blood coagulation factor X deficiency causes partial embryonic lethality and fatal neonatal bleeding in mice. *Thromb Haemost* 2000;83:185–190.

62. Watzke HH, Lechner K, Roberts HR, et al. Molecular defect (Gla14 to Lys) and its functional consequences in a hereditary factor X deficiency (factor VII "Voralrlberg"). *J Biol Chem* 1990;265:11982–11989.

63. Forberg E, Huhmann I, Jimenez-Boj E, et al. The impact of Glu102Lys on the factor X function in a patient with a doubly homozygous factor X deficiency (Gla14Lys and Glu102Lys). *Thromb Haemost* 2000;83:234–238.

64. Parkin JD, Madaras F, Sweet B, et al. A further inherited variant of coagulation factor X. *Aust N Z J Med* 1974;4:561–564.

65. De Stefano V, Leone G, Ferrelli R, et al. Roma: a congenital factor variant defective at different degrees in the intrinsic and the extrinsic activation. *Br J Haematol* 1988;69:387–391.

66. Girolami A, Vicarioto M, Ruzza G, et al. Factor X Pauda: a "new" congenital factor X abnormality with a defect only in the extrinsic system. *Acta Haematol* 1985;73:31–36.

67. Girolami A, Vianello F, Cabrio L, et al. A new mutation (Arg251Trp) in the Ca2+ binding site of factor X protease domain appears to be responsible for the defect in the extrinsic pathway activation of factor X Padua. *Clin Appl Thromb Hemost* 2004;10:5–8.

68. Zama T, Murata M, Watanabe K, et al. A family with hereditary factor X deficiency with a point mutation Gla32 to Gln in the Gla domain (factor X Tokyo). *Br J Haematol* 1999;106:809–811.

69. Rudolph AE, Mullane MP, Porche-Sorbet R, et al. Factor X (St. Louis II): identification of a glycine substitution at residue 7 and characterization of the recombinant protein. *J Biol Chem* 1996;271:28601–28606.

70. Pinotti M, Marchetti G, Baroni M, et al. Reduced activation of the Gla19Ala FX variant via the extrinsic coagulation pathway results in symptomatic CRMred FX deficiency. *Thromb Haemost* 2002;88:236–241.

71. Hougie C, Barrow HM, Graham JB. Stuart clotting defect. Segregation of a hereditary hemorrhagic state from the heterozygous hereto fore called "stable factor" (SPCA, proconvertin factor VII deficiency). *J Clin Invest* 1957;36:485–493.

72. Telfer TP, Denson KW, Wright DR. A "new" coagulation defect. *Haematologica* 1956;2:308–316.

73. Graham JB. Stuart Factor: discovery and designation as factor X. *J Thromb Haemost* 2003;1:871–877.

74. Kisiel W, Davie EW. Isolation and characterization of bovine factor VII. *Biochemistry* 1975;14:4928–4934.

75. Bajaj SP, Rapaport SI, Brown SF. Isolation and characterization of human factor VII. *J Biol Chem* 1981;256:253–259.

76. Broze GJ Jr, Majerus PW. Purification and properties of human coagulation factor VII. *J Biol Chem* 1980;255:1242–1247.

77. Morrissey JH. Tissue factor: an enzyme cofactor and true receptor. *Thromb Haemost* 2001;86:66–74.

78. Hagen FS, Gray CL, O'Hara P, et al. Characterization of a cDNA coding for human factor VII. *Proc Natl Acad Sci U S A* 1986;84:2412–2416.

79. Berkner K, Busby S, Davie EW, et al. Isolation and expression of cDNAs encoding human factor VII. *Cold Spring Harb Sym* 1986;51:531–541.

80. O'Hara PJ, Grant FJ, Haldeman BA. Nucleotide sequence of the gene coding for human factor VII, a vitamin K-dependent protein participating in blood coagulation. *Proc Natl Acad Sci U S A* 1987;84:5158–5162.

81. Ott R, Pfeiffer RA. Evidence that activities of coagulation factors VII and X are linked to chromosome 13 (q34). *Hum Hered* 1984;34:123–126.

82. Miao CH, Leytus SP, Chung DW, et al. Liver-specific expression of the gene coding for human factor, a blood coagulation factor. *J Biol Chem* 1992; 267:7395–7401.

83. McVey JH, Boswell E, Mumford AD, et al. Factor VII deficiency and the FVII mutation database. *Hum Mutat* 2001;17:3–17.

84. Rosen ED, Chan JCY, Idusogie E, et al. Mice lacking factor VII develop normally but suffer fatal perinatal bleeding. *Nature* 1997;390:290–293.

85. McVey JH, Boswell EJ, Takamiya O, et al. Exclusion of the first EGF domain of factor VII by a splice site mutation causes lethal factor VII deficiency. *Blood* 1998;92:920–926.

86. Peyvandi F, Mannucci PM, Jenkins PV, et al. Homozygous 2 bp deletion in the human factor VII gene: a non-lethal mutation that is associated with a complete absence of circulating factor VII. *Thromb Haemost* 2000;84:635–637.

87. Arbini AA, Pollak ES, Bayleran JK, et al. Severe factor VII deficiency due to a mutation disrupting a hepatocyte nuclear factor 4 binding site in the factor VII promoter. *Blood* 1997;89:176–182.

88. Carew JA, Pollak ES, High KA, et al. Severe factor VII deficiency due to a mutation disrupting an Sp1 binding site in the factor VII promoter. *Blood* 1998;92:1639–1645.

89. Carew JA, Pollak ES, Lopaciuk S, et al. A new mutation in the HNF4 binding region of the factor VII promoter in a patient with severe factor VII deficiency. *Blood* 2000;96:4370–4372.

90. Meade TW, Mellows S, Brozovic M, et al. Haemostatic function and ischemic heart disease: principal results of the Northwick Park Heart Study. *Lancet* 1986;2:533–537.

91. Meade TW, Ruddock V, Stirling Y, et al. Fibrinolytic activity, clotting factor, and long-term incidence of ischemic heart disease in the Northwick Park heart study. *Lancet* 1993;342:1076–1079.

92. Heinrich J, Balleisen L, Schulte H, et al. Fibrinogen and factor VII in the prediction of coronary risk. Results from the PROCAM study in healthy men. *Arterioscler Thromb Vasc Biol* 1994;14:54–59.

93. Marchetti G, Patracchini P, Papacchini M, et al. A polymorphism in the 5′ region of coagulation factor VII gene (F7) caused by an inserted decanucleotide. *Hum Genet* 1993;90:575–576.

94. Pollak ES, Hung HL, Godin W, et al. Functional characterization of the human factor VII 5′-flanking region. *J Biol Chem* 1996;271:1738–1747.

95. Green F, Kelleher C, Wilkes H, et al. A common genetic polymorphism associated with lower coagulation factor VII levels in healthy individuals. *Arterioscler Thromb Vasc Biol* 1991;11:540–546.

96. Lane A, Cruickshank JK, Mitchell J, et al. Genetic and environmental determinants of factor VII coagulant activity in ethnic groups at differing risk of coronary heart disease. *Atherosclerosis* 1992;94:43–50.

97. Hunault M, Arbini AA, Lopaciuk S, et al. The Arg353 Gln polymorphism reduces the level of coagulation factor VII. *Arterioscler Thromb Vasc Biol* 1997;17:2825–2529.

98. Bernardi F, Marchetti G, Pinotti M, et al. Factor VII gene polymorphisms contribute about one third of the factor VII level variation in plasma. *Arterioscler Thromb Vasc Biol* 1996;16:72–76.

99. Kudaravalli R, Tidd T, Pinotti M, et al. Polymorphic changes in the 5′ flanking region of factor VII have a combined effect on promoter strength. *Thromb Haemost* 2002;88:763–767.

100. Carew JA, Basso F, Miller GJ, et al. A functional haplotype in the 5′ flanking region of the factor VII gene is associated with an increased risk of coronary heart disease. *J Thromb Haemost* 2003;1:2179–2185.

101. Kurachi K, Davie EW. Isolation and characterization of a cDNA coding for human factor IX. *Proc Natl Acad Sci U S A* 1982;79:6461–6464.

102. Choo KH, Gould KG, Rees DJG, et al. Molecular cloning of the gene for human anti-hemophilic factor IX. *Nature* 1982;299:178–180.

103. Anson DS, Choo KH, Rees DJG. The gene structure of human anti-haemophilic factor IX. *EMBO J* 1984;3:1053–1060.

104. Camerino G, Grzeschik KH, Jaye M. Regional localization on the human X chromosome and polymorphism of the coagulation factor IX gene (hemophilia B locus). *Proc Natl Acad Sci U S A* 1984;81:498–502.

105. Yoshitake S, Schach BG, Foster DC. Nucleotide sequence of the gene for human factor IX (Antihemophilic factor B). *Biochemistry* 1985;24:3736–3750.

106. Wang L, Zoppe M, Hackeng TM, et al. A factor IX-deficient mouse model for hemophilia B gene therapy. *Proc Natl Acad Sci U S A* 1997;94:11563–11566.

107. Lin HF, Maeda N, Smithies O, et al. A coagulation factor IX-deficient mouse model for hemophilia B. *Blood* 1997;90:3962–3966.

108. Kundu RK, Sangiorgi F, Wu LY, et al. Targeted inactivation of the coagulation factor IX gene causes hemophilia B. *Blood* 1998;92:168–174.

109. Giannelli F, Choo KH, Rees DJ, et al. Gene deletions in patients with haemophilia B and anti-factor IX antibodies. *Nature* 1983;303:181–182.

110. Noyes CM, Griffith MJ, Robert HR, et al. Identification of the molecular defect in factor IX Chapel Hill: substitution of histidine for arginine at position 145. *Proc Natl Acad Sci U S A* 1983;80:4200–4202.

111. Giannelli F, Green PM, Sommer SS, et al. Haemophilia B: database of point mutations and short additions and deletions—eighth edition. *Nucleic Acids Res* 1998;26:265–268.

112. Veltkamp JJ, Meilof J, Remmelts HG, et al. Another genetic variant of haemophilia B: haemophilia B Leyden. *Scand J Haematol* 1970;7: 82–90.

113. Briet E, Bertina RM, van Tilburg NH, et al. Hemophilia B Leyden: a sex-linked hereditary disorder that improves after puberty. *N Engl J Med* 1982;306:788–790.

114. Mandalaki T, Louizou C, Dimitriadou C, et al. Haemophilia B Leyden in Greece. *Thromb Haemost* 1986;56:340–342.

115. Briet E, Wijnands MC, Veltkamp JJ. The prophylactic treatment of hemophilia B Leyden with anabolic steroids. *Ann Intern Med* 1985;103(225): 226.

116. Crossley M, Brownlee GG. Disruption of a C/EBP binding site in the factor IX promoter is associated with haemophilia B. *Nature* 1990;345:444–446.

117. Reijnen MJ, Sladek FM, Bertina RM, et al. Disruption of a binding site for hepatocyte nuclear factor 4 results in hemophilia B Leyden. *Proc Natl Acad Sci U S A* 1992;89:6300–6303.

118. Picketts DJ, Mueller CR, Lillicrap D. Transcriptional control of the factor IX gene: analysis of five cis-acting elements and the deleterious effects of naturally occurring hemophilia B Leyden mutations. *Blood* 1994;84: 2992–3000.

119. Reijnen MJ, Maasdam D, Bertina RM, et al. Haemophilia B Leyden: the effect of mutations at position +13 on the liver-specific transcription of the factor IX gene. *Blood Coagul Fibrin* 1994;5:341–348.

120. Crossley M, Ludwig M, Stowell KM, et al. Recovery from hemophilia B Leyden: an androgen-responsive element in the factor IX promoter. *Science* 1992;257:377–379.

121. Morgan GE, Rowley G, Green PM, et al. Further evidence for the importance of an androgen response element in the factor IX promoter. *Br J Haematol* 1997;98:79–85.

122. Oldenburg J, Quenzel EM, Harbrecht U, et al. Missense mutations at ALA-10 in the factor IX propeptide: an insignificant variant in normal life but a decisive cause of bleeding during oral anticoagulant therapy. *Br J Haematol* 1997;98:240–244.

123. Stanley TB, Humphries J, High KA, et al. Amino acids responsible for the reduced affinities of vitamin K-dependent propeptides for the carboxylase. *Biochemistry* 1999;38:15681–15687.

124. Gailani D. Activation of factor IX by factor XIa. *Trends Cardiovasc Med* 2000;10:198–204.

125. Asakai R, Davie EW, Chung DW. Organization of the gene for human factor XI. *Biochemistry* 1987;26:7221–7228.

126. Kato A, Asakai R, Davie EW, et al. Factor XI gene (F11) is located on the distal end of the long arm of chromosome 4. *Cytogenet Cell Genet* 1989; 52:77–78.

127. Bouma BN, Griffin JH. Human blood coagulation Factor XI: purification, properties, and mechanism of activation by activated Factor XII. *J Biol Chem* 1977;252:64327–66437.

128. Gailani D, Sun M, Sun Y. A comparison of murine and human factor XI. *Blood* 1997;90:1055–1064.

129. Seligsohn U. Factor XI deficiency. *Thromb Haemost* 1993;70:68–70.

130. Seligsohn U. High gene frequency of Factor XI (PTA) deficiency in Ashkenazi Jews. *Blood* 1978;51:1223–1228.

131. Peretz H, Mulai A, Usher S, et al. The two common mutations causing factor XI deficiency in Jews stem from distinct founders: one of ancient Middle Eastern origin and another of more recent European Origin. *Blood* 1997;90:2654–2659.

132. Gailani D, Lasky NM, Broze GJ Jr. A murine model of factor XI deficiency. *Blood Coagul Fibrin* 1997;8:134–144.

133. Asakai R, Chung DW, Davie EW, et al. Factor XI deficiency in Ashkenazi Jews in Israel. *N Engl J Med* 1991;325:153–158.

134. Scarpati EM, Wen D, Broze GJ Jr. Human tissue factor: cDNA sequence and chromosome localization of the gene. *Biochemistry* 1987;26:5234–5238.

135. Mackman N, Morrissey JH, Fowler B, et al. Complete sequence of the human tissue factor gene, a highly regulated cellular receptor that initiates the coagulation protease cascade. *Biochemistry* 1989;28:1755–1762.

136. Fisher KL, Gorman CM, Vehar DP, et al. Cloning and expression of human tissue factor cDNA. *Thromb Res* 1987;48:89–99.

137. Morrissey JH, Fakhrai H, Edgington TS. Molecular cloning of the cDNA for tissue factor, the cellular receptor for the initiation of the coagulation protease cascade. *Cell* 1987;50:129–135.

138. Spicer EK, Horton R, Bloem L, et al. Isolation of cDNA clones coding for human tissue factor: primary structure of the protein and cDNA. *Proc Natl Acad Sci U S A* 1987;84:5148–5152.

139. Drake TA, Ruf W, Morrissey JH, et al. Functional tissue factor is entirely cell surface expressed on lipopolysaccharide-stimulated human blood monocytes and a constitutively tissue factor producing neoplastic cell line. *J Cell Biol* 1989;109:389–395.

140. Fleck RA, Rao LVM, Rapaport SI, et al. Localization of human tissue factor antigen by immunostaining with monospecific, polyclonal ant-human tissue factor antibody. *Thromb Res* 1990;57:765–781.

141. Mackman N. Regulation of the tissue factor gene. *Thromb Haemost* 1997; 78:747–754.

142. Bugge TH, Xiao Q, Koimbrinck KW, et al. Fatal embryonic bleeding events in mice lacking tissue factor, the cell-associated initiator of blood coagulation. *Proc Natl Acad Sci U S A* 1996;93:6258–6263.

143. Carmeliet P, Mackman N, Moons L, et al. Role of tissue factor in embryonic blood vessel development. *Nature* 1996;383:73–75.

144. Toomey JR, Kratzer KE, Lasky NM, et al. Targeted disruption of the murine tissue factor gene results in embryonic lethality. *Blood* 2004;88: 1583–1587.

145. Arnaud E, Barbalat V, Nicaud V, et al. Polymorphisms in the 5′ regulatory region of the tissue factor gene and the risk of myocardial infarction and venous thromboembolism. The ECTIM and PATHROS studies. *Arterioscler Thromb Vasc Biol* 2000;20:892–898.

146. Reny JL, Laurendeau I, Fontana P, et al. The TF-603A/G gene promoter polymorphism and circulating monocyte tissue factor gene expression in healthy volunteers. *Thromb Haemost* 2004;91:248–254.

147. Fay PJ. Activation of factor VIII and mechanisms of cofactor action. *Blood Rev* 2004;18:1–15.

148. Gitschier J, Wood WI, Goralka TM, et al. Characterization of the human factor VIII gene. *Nature* 1984;312:326–330.

149. Purrello M, Alhadeff B, Esposito D, et al. The human genes for hemophilia A and hemophilia B flank the X chromosome fragile site at Xq27.3. *EMBO J* 1985;4:725–729.

150. Tantravahi U, Murty VV, Jhanwar SC, et al. Physical mapping of the factor VIII gene proximal to two polymorphic DNA probes in human chromosome band Xq28: implications for factor VIII gene segregation analysis. *Cytogenet Cell Genet* 1986;42:75–79.

151. Vehar G, Keyt B, Eaton D, et al. Structure of human factor VIII. *Nature* 1984;312:337–342.

152. Toole JJ, Knopf JL, Wozney JM, et al. Molecular cloning of a cDNA encoding human antihaemophilic factor. *Nature* 1984;312:342–347.

153. Vehar G, Davie EW. Preparation and properties of bovine FVIII (antihemophilic factor). *Biochemistry* 1980;19:401–410.

154. Bi L, Lawler AM, Antonarakis SE, et al. Targeted disruption of the mouse factor VIII gene produces a model of haemophilia A. *Nature Genet* 1995; 10:119–121.

155. Tuddenham EGD. In search of the eight factor: a personal reminiscence. *J Thromb Haemost* 2003;1:403–409.

156. Gitschier J. Remembrances of factor VIII. Part 1: the race to the gene. *J Thromb Haemost* 2004;2:383–387.

157. Gitschier J, Wood WI, Tuddenham EG, et al. Detection and sequence of mutations in the factor VIII gene of haemophiliacs. *Nature* 1985;315: 427–430.

158. Lakich D, Kazazian HH, Antonarakis SE, et al. Inversions disrupting the factor VIII gene are a common cause of severe haemophilia A. *Nature Genet* 1993;5:236–241.

159. Naylor JA, Green PM, Rizza CR, et al. Analysis of factor VIII mRNA reveals defects in everyone of 28 haemophilia A patients. *Hum Mol Genet* 1993;2:11–17.

160. Brinke A, Tagliavacca L, Naylor J, et al. Two chimeric transcription units result from an inversion breaking intron 1 of the factor VIII gene and a region reportedly affected by reciprocal translocations in T-cell leukemia. *Hum Mol Genet* 1996;5:1945–1951.

161. Bagnall RD, Waseem N, Green PM, et al. Recurrent inversion breaking intron 1 of the factor VIII gene is a frequent cause of severe hemophilia A. *Blood* 2002;99:168–174.

162. Kemball-Cook G, Tuddenham EG, Wacey AI. The factor VIII structure and mutation resource site: HAMSTeRS version 4. *Nucleic Acids Res* 1998;26:216–219.

163. Antonarakis SE, Youssoufian H, Kazazian HH. Molecular genetics of hemophilia A in man (factor VIII deficiency). *Mol Biol Med* 1987;4:81–94.

164. Millar DS, Steinbrecher RA, Wieland K, et al. The molecular genetic analysis of haemophilia A; characterization of six partial deletions in the factor VIII gene. *Hum Genet* 1990;86:219–227.

165. Kazazian HH, Wong C, Youssoufian H, et al. Haemophilia A resulting from de novo insertion of L1 sequences represents a novel mechanism for mutation in man. *Nature* 1988;332:164–166.

166. Woods-Samuels P, Wong C, Mathias SL, et al. Characterization of a non-deleterious L1 insertion in an intron of the human factor VIII gene and further evidence of open reading frames in functional L1 elements. *Genomics* 1989;4:290–296.

167. Mann KG, Kalafatis M. Factor V: a combination of Dr. Jekyll and Mr. Hyde. *Blood* 2002;101:20–30.

168. Cripe LD, Moore D, Kane WH. Structure of the gene for human coagulation factor V. *Biochemistry* 1992;31:3777–3785.

169. Kane WH, Davie EW. Cloning of a cDNA coding for human factor V, a blood coagulation factor homologous to factor VIII and ceruloplasmin. *Proc Natl Acad Sci U S A* 1986;83:6800–6804.

170. Jenny RJ, Pittman DD, Toole JJ, et al. Complete cDNA and derived amino acid sequence of human factor V. *Proc Natl Acad Sci U S A* 1987;84: 4846–4850.

171. Kane WH, Ichinose A, Hagen FS, et al. Cloning of cDNAs coding for the heavy chain region and connecting region of human Factor V, a blood coagulation factor with four types of internal repeats. *Biochemistry* 1987; 26:6508.

172. Wilson DB, Salem HH, Mruk JS, et al. Biosynthesis of coagulation factor V by a human hepatocellular carcinoma cell line. *J Clin Invest* 1984;73:654–658.

173. Mazzorana M, Baffet G, Kneip B, et al. Expression of coagulation factor V gene by normal adult human hepatocytes in primary culture. *Br J Haematol* 1991;78:229–235.

174. Tracy PB, Eide LL, Bowie EJW, et al. Radioimmunoassay of factor V in human plasma and platelets. *Blood* 1982;60:59–63.

175. Chiu HC, Schick P, Colman RW. Biosynthesis of Factor V in isolated guinea pig megakaryocytes. *J Clin Invest* 1985;75:339–346.

176. Gewirtz AM, Keefer M, Doshi K, et al. Biology of human megakaryocyte Factor V. *Blood* 1986;67:1639–1642.

177. Camire RM, Pollak ES, Kaushansky K, et al. Secretable human platelet-derived factor V originates from the plasma pool. *Blood* 1998;92:3035–3041.

178. Christella M, Thomassen LG, Castoldi E, et al. Endogenous factor V synthesis in megakaryocytes contributes negligibly to the platelet factor V pool. *Haematologica* 2003;88:1150–1156.

179. Murray JM, Rand MD, Egan JO, et al. Factor V NewBrunswick: Ala$_{221}$-to-Val substitution results in reduced cofactor activity. *Blood* 1995; 86(5):1820–1827.

180. Cui J, O'Shea KS, Purkayastha A, et al. Fatal haemorrhage and incomplete block to embryogenesis in mice lacking coagulation factor V. *Nature* 1996;384:66–68.

181. Guasch JF, Cannegieter S, Reitsma PH, et al. Severe coagulation factor V deficiency caused by a 4 bp deletion in the factor V gene. *Br J Haematol* 1998;101:32–39.

182. Montefusco MC, Duga S, Asselta R, et al. A novel two base pair deletion in the factor V gene associated with severe factor V deficiency. *Br J Haematol* 2000;111:1240–1246.

183. Asselta R, Montefusco MC, Duga S, et al. Severe factor V deficiency: exon skipping in the factor V gene causing a partial deletion of the C1 domain. *Thromb Haemost* 2003;1:1237–1244.

184. Montefusco MC, Duga S, Asselta R, et al. Clinical and molecular characterization of 6 patients affected by severe deficiency of coagulation factor V: broadening of the mutational spectrum of factor V gene and *in vitro* analysis of the newly identified missense mutations. *Blood* 2003;102:3210–3216.

185. Seligsohn U. Combined factor V and factor VIII deficiency. In: Seghatchian J, Savidge GT, eds. *Factor VIII-von Willebrand factor*, Boca Raton: CRC Press, 1989:89–100.

186. Neerman-Arbez M, Antonarakis SE, Blouin JL, et al. The locus for combined factor V-factor VIII deficiency (F5F8D) maps to 18q21, between D18S849 and D18S1103. *Am J Hum Genet* 1997;61:143–150.

187. Neerman-Arbez M, Johnson KM, Morris MA, et al. TuMolecular analysis of the ERGIC-53 gene in 35 families with combined factor V-factor VIII deficiency. *Blood* 1999;93:2253–2260.

188. Nichols WC, Terry VH, Wheatly MA, et al. ERGIC-53 gene structure and mutation analysis in 19 combined factors V and VIII deficiency families. *Blood* 1999;93:2261–2266.

189. Zhang B, Cunningham MA, Nichols WC, et al. Bleeding due to disruption of a cargo-specific ER-to-Golgi transport complex. *Nature Genet* 2003;34:220–225.

190. Dahlbäck B, Carlsson M, Svensson PJ. Familial thrombophilia due to a previously unrecognized mechanism by poor anticoagulant response to activated protein C: prediction of a cofactor to activated protein C. *Proc Natl Acad Sci U S A* 1993;90:1004–1008.

191. Bertina RM, Koeleman BPC, Koster T, et al. Mutation in blood coagulation factor V associated with resistance to activated protein C. *Nature* 1994;369:64–67.

192. Voorberg J, Roelse J, Koopman R, et al. Association of idiopathic venous thromboembolism with single point-mutation at Arg$^{506}$ of factor V. *Lancet* 1994;343:1535–1538.

193. Greengard JS, Sun X, Xu X, et al. Activated protein C resistance caused by Arg$^{506}$Gln mutation in factor Va. *Lancet* 1994;343:1362–1363.

194. Nicolaes GAF, Tans G, Thomassen MCLGD, et al. Peptide bond cleavages and loss of functional activity during inactivation of factor Va and factor VaR560Q by activated protein C. *J Biol Chem* 1995;270:21158–21166.

195. Kalafatis M, Bertina RM, Rand MD, et al. Characterization of the molecular defect in factor V$^{R506Q}$. *J Biol Chem* 1995;270:4053–4057.

196. Heeb MJ, Kojima Y, Greengard JS, et al. Activated protein C resistance: molecular mechanisms based on studies using purified Gln506-factor V. *Blood* 1995;85(12):3405–3411.

197. Dahlbäck B. Resistance to activated protein C as risk factor for thrombosis: molecular mechanisms, laboratory investigation, and clinical management. *Sem Hematol* 1997;34(3):217–234.

198. Dahlbäck B. The discovery of activated protein C resistance. *J Thromb Haemost* 2003;1:3–9.

199. Simioni P, Scudeller A, Radossi P, et al. "Pseudo homozygous" activated protein C resistance due to double heterozygous factor V defects (factor V Leiden mutation and type I quantitative factor V defect) associated with thrombosis: report of two cases belonging to two unrelated kindreds. *Thromb Haemost* 1996;75:422–426.

200. Zehnder JL, Jain M. Recurrent thrombosis due to compound heterozygosity for factor V$_{Leiden}$ and factor V deficiency. *Blood Coagul Fibrin* 1996;7:361–362.

201. Williamson D, Brown K, Luddington R, et al. Factor V Cambridge: a new mutation (Arg$^{306}$ to Thr) associated with resistance to activated protein C. *Blood* 1998;91(4):1140–1144.

202. Chan WP, Lee CK, Kwong YL, et al. A novel mutation of Arg$^{306}$ of factor V gene in Hong Kong Chinese. *Blood* 1998;91(4):1135–1139.

203. Patracchini P, Aiello V, Palazzi P, et al. Sublocalization of the human protein C gene on chromosome 2q13-q14. *Hum Genet* 1989;81:191–192.

204. Foster DC, Yoshitake S, Davie EW. The nucleotide sequence of the gene for human protein C. *Proc Natl Acad Sci U S A* 1985;82:4673–4677.

205. Plutzky J, Hoskins JA, Long GL, et al. Evolution and organization of the human protein C gene. *Proc Natl Acad Sci U S A* 1986;83:546–550.

206. Foster DC, Davie EW. Characterization of a cDNA coding for human protein C. *Proc Natl Acad Sci U S A* 1984;81:4766–4770.

207. Griffin JH, Mosher DF, Zimmerman TS, et al. Protein C, an antithrombotic protein, is reduced in hospitalized patients with intravascular coagulation. *Blood* 1982;60:261–264.

208. Griffin JH, Evatt B, Zimmerman TS, et al. Deficiency of protein C in congenital thrombotic disease. *J Clin Invest* 1981;68:1370–1373.

209. Branson HE, Katz J, Marble R, et al. Inherited protein C deficiency and coumarin-responsive chronic relapsing purpura fulminans in a newborn infant. *Lancet* 1983;2:1165–1168.

210. Seligsohn U, Berger A, Abend M, et al. Homozygous protein C deficiency manifested by massive venous thrombosis in the newborn. *N Engl J Med* 2004;310:559–562.

211. Jalbert LR, Rosen ED, Moons L, et al. Inactivation of the gene for anticoagulant protein C causes lethal perinatal consumptive coagulopathy in mice. *J Clin Invest* 1998;102:1481–1488.

212. Reitsma PH. Protein C deficiency: summary of the 1995 database update. *Nucleic Acids Res* 1996;24:157–159.

213. Reitsma PH, Poort SR, Allaart CF, et al. The spectrum of genetic defects in a panel of 40 Dutch families with symptomatic protein C deficiency type I: heterogeneity and founder effects. *Blood* 1991;78:890–894.

214. Grundy CB, Schulman S, Krawczak M, et al. Protein C deficiency and thromboembolism: recurrent mutation at Arg 306 in the protein C gene. *Hum Genet* 1992;88:586–588.

215. Krawczak M, Reitsma PH, Cooper DN. The mutational demography of protein C deficiency. *Hum Genet* 1995;96:142–146.

216. Bird AP. CpG-rich islands and the function of DNA methylation. *Nature* 1986;321:209–213.

217. Jackman RW, Beeler DL, Fritze L, et al. Human thrombomodulin gene is intron depleted: nucleic acid sequence of the cDNA and gene predict protein structure and suggest sites of regulatory control. *Proc Natl Acad Sci U S A* 1987;84:26425–26429.

218. Suzuki K, Kusumoto H, Deyashiki Y. Structure and expression of human thrombomodulin, a thrombin receptor on endothelium acting as a cofactor for protein C activation. *EMBO J* 1987;6:1891–1897.

219. Wen DZ, Dittman WA, Ye RD, et al. Human thrombomodulin: complete cDNA sequence and chromosome localization of the gene. *Biochemistry* 1987;26:4350–4357.

220. Esmon CT, Owen WG. The discovery of thrombomodulin. *Thromb Haemost* 2003;2:209–213.

221. Healy AM, Rayburn HB, Rosenberg RD, et al. Absence of the blood-clotting regulator thrombomodulin causes embryonic lethality in mice before development of a functional cardiovascular system. *Proc Natl Acad Sci U S A* 1995;92:850–854.

222. Warner D, Catto A, Kunz G, et al. The thrombomodulin gene mutation G (127) to A (Ala25Thr) and cerebrovascular disease. *Cerebrovasc Dis* 2000; 10:359–363.

223. Healy AM, Hancock WW, Christie PD, et al. Intravascular coagulation activation in a murine model of thrombomodulin deficiency: effects of lesion size, age, and hypoxia on fibrin deposition. *Blood* 1998;92:4188–4197.

224. Salomaa V, Matei C, Aleksic N, et al. Soluble thrombomodulin as a predictor of incident coronary heart disease and symptomless carotid artery atherosclerosis in the Atherosclerosis Risk in Communities (ARIC) study: a case-cohort study. *Lancet* 1999;353:1729–1734.

225. Ohlin AK, Marlar RA. The first mutation identified in the thrombomodulin gene in a 45-year-old man presenting with thromboembolic disease. *Blood* 1995;85:330–336.

226. Kunz G, Ohlin AK, Adami A, et al. Naturally occurring mutations in the thrombomodulin gene leading to impaired expression and function. *Blood* 2002;99:3646–3653.

227. van der Velden PA, Krommenhoek-Van Es T, Allaart CF, et al. A frequent thrombomodulin amino acid dimorphism is not associated with thrombophilia. *Thromb Haemost* 1991;65:511–513.

228. Wu KK, Aleksic N, Ahn C, et al. Thrombomodulin Ala455Val polymorphism and risk of coronary heart disease. *Circulation* 2001;103:1386–1389.

229. Le Flem L, Mennen L, Aubry ML, et al. Thrombomodulin promoter mutations, venous thrombosis, and varicose veins. *Arterioscler Thromb Vasc Biol* 2001;21:445–451.

230. Doggen CJM, Kunz G, Rosendaal FR, et al. A mutation in the thrombomodulin gene, 127G to A coding for Ala25Thr, and the risk of myocardial infarction in men. *Thromb Haemost* 1998;80:743–748.

231. Norlund L, Holm J, Zoller B, et al. The Ala25-Thr mutation in the thrombomodulin gene is not frequent in Swedish patients suffering from ischemic heart disease. *Thromb Haemost* 1999;82:1367–1368.

232. Schmidel DK, Tatro AV, Phelps LG, et al. Organization of the human protein S genes. *Biochemistry* 1990;29:7845–7852.

233. Ploos van Amstel HK, Reitsma PH, van der Logt PE, et al. Intron-exon organization of the active human protein S gene PSα and its pseudogene PSβ: duplication and silencing during primate evolution. *Biochemistry* 1990;29:7853–7861.

234. Edenbrandt CM, Lundwall A, Wydro R, et al. Molecular analysis of the gene for vitamin K-dependent protein S and its pseudogene. Cloning and partial gene organization. *Biochemistry* 1990;29:7861–7868.

235. Ploos van Amstel HK, van der Zanden AL, Bakker E. Two genes homologous with human protein S cDNA are located on chromosome 3. *Thromb Haemost* 1987;58:982–987.

236. Watkins PC, Eddy R, Fukushima Y. The gene for protein S maps near the centromere of human chromosome 3. *Blood* 1988;71:238–241.

237. Lundwall A, Dackowski WR, Cohen EH, et al. Isolation and sequencing of the cDNA for human protein S, a regulator of blood coagulation. *Proc Natl Acad Sci U S A* 1986;83:6716–6720.

238. Hoskins J, Norman DK, Beckmann RJ, et al. Cloning and characterization of human liver cDNA encoding a protein S precursor. *Proc Natl Acad Sci U S A* 1987;84:349–353.

239. Ploos van Amstel HK, Reitsma PH, Bertina RM. The human S locus: identification of the PS alpha gene as a site of liver protein S messenger RNA synthesis. *Biochem Biophys Res Commun* 1988;157:1033–1038.

240. Borgel D, Gandrille S, Aiach M. Protein S deficiency. *Thromb Haemost* 1997;78:351–356.

241. Comp PC, Esmon CT. Recurrent thromboembolism in patients with a partial deficiency of protein S. *N Engl J Med* 1984;311:1525–1528.

242. Comp PC, Nixon RR, Cooper MR, et al. Familial protein S deficiency is associated with recurrent thrombosis. *J Clin Invest* 1984;74:2082–2088.

243. Schwarz HP, Fischer M, Hopmeier P, et al. Plasma protein S deficiency in familial thrombotic disease. *Blood* 1984;64:1297–1300.

244. Mahasandana C, Suvatte V, Marlar RA, et al. Neonatal purpura fulminans associated with homozygous protein S deficiency. *Lancet* 1990;335:61–62.

245. Pegelow CH, Ledford M, Young JN, et al. Severe protein S deficiency in a newborn. *Pediatrics* 1992;89:674–676.

246. Gomez E, Ledford MR, Pegelow CH, et al. Homozygous protein S deficiency due to a one base pair deletion that leads to a stop codon in exon III of the protein S gene. *Thromb Haemost* 1994;71:723–726.

247. Mahasandana C, Veerakul G, Tanphaichitr VS, et al. Homozygous protein S deficiency: 7-year follow-up. *Thromb Haemost* 1996;76:1122.

248. Gandrille S, Borgel D, Sala N, et al. Protein S deficiency: a database of mutations—summary of the first update. *Thromb Haemost* 2000;84:918.

249. Bertina RM, Ploos van Amstel HK, van Wijngaarden A, et al. Heerlen polymorphism of protein S, an immunologic polymorphism due to dimorphism of residue 460. *Blood* 1990;76:538–548.

250. Duchemin J, Gandrille S, Borgel D, et al. The Ser460 to Pro substitution of the protein S alpha (PROS1) gene is a frequent mutation associated with free protein S (type IIa) deficiency. *Blood* 1995;86:3436–3443.

251. Borgel D, Duchemin J, Alhenc-Gelas M, et al. Molecular basis for protein S hereditary deficiency: genetic defects observed in 118 patients with type I and type IIa deficiencies. The French network on molecular abnormalities responsible for protein C and protein S deficiencies. *J Lab Clin Med* 1996;128:218–227.

252. Espinosa-Parrilla Y, Navarro G, Morell M, et al. Homozygosity for the protein S Heerlen allele is associated with type I PS deficiency in a thrombophilic pedigree with multiple risk factors. *Thromb Haemost* 2000;83:102–106.

253. Giri TK, Yamazaki T, Sala N, et al. Deficient APC-cofactor activity of protein S Heerlen in degradation of factor Va$_{Leiden}$: a possible mechanism of synergism between thrombophilic risk factors. *Blood* 2000;96:523–531.

254. Fukudome K, Esmon CT. Identification, cloning, and regulation of a novel endothelial cell protein C/activated protein C receptor. *J Biol Chem* 1994;269(42):26486–26491.

255. Fukudome K, Esmon CT. Molecular cloning and expression of murine and bovine endothelial cell protein C/activated protein C receptor (EPCR). *J Biol Chem* 1995;270:5571–5577.

256. Esmon CT. The endothelial cell protein C receptor. *Thromb Haemost* 2000;83:639–643.

257. Kurosawa S, Stearns-Kurosawa DJ, Hidari N, et al. Identification of functional endothelial cell protein C receptor in human plasma. *J Clin Invest* 1997;100:411–418.

258. Simmonds RE, Lane DA. Structural and functional implications of the intron/exon organization of the human endothelial cell protein C/activated protein C receptor (EPCR) gene: comparison with the structure of SD1/major histocompatibility complex alpha1 and alpha2 domains. *Blood* 1999;94:632–641.

259. Hayashi T, Nakamura H, Okada A, et al. Organizational and chromosomal localization of the human endothelial protein C receptor gene. *Gene* 19699;238:367–373.

260. Laszik Z, Mitro A, Taylor FB, et al. Human protein C receptor is present primarily on endothelium of large blood vessels: implications for the control of the protein C pathway. *Circulation* 1997;96:3633–3640.

261. Crawley JT, Gu JM, Ferrell G, et al. Distribution of endothelial cell protein C/activated protein C receptor (EPCR) during mouse embryo development. *Thromb Haemost* 2002;88:259–266.

262. Gu JM, Crawley JCW, Ferrell G, et al. Disruption of the endothelial cell protein C receptor gene in mice causes placental thrombosis and early embryonic lethality. *J Biol Chem* 2002;277:43335–43343.

263. Biguzzi E, Merati G, Liaw PC, et al. A 23 bp insertion in the endothelial protein C receptor (EPCR) gene impairs EPCR function. *Thromb Haemost* 2001;86:945–948.

264. von Depka M, Czwallinna A, Eisert R, et al. Prevalence of a 23bp insertion in exon 3 of the endothelial cell protein C receptor gene in venous thrombophilia. *Thromb Haemost* 2001;86:1360–1362.

265. Galligan L, Livingstone W, Mynett-Johnston L, et al. Prevalence of the 23bp endothelial protein C receptor (EPCR) gene insertion in the Irish population. *Thromb Haemost* 2002;87:773–774.

266. Poort SR, Vos HL, Rosendaal FR, et al. The endothelial protein C receptor (EPCR) 23 bp insert mutation and the risk of venous thrombosis. *Thromb Haemost* 2002;88(160):162.

267. Akar N, Gokdemir R, Ozel D, et al. Endothelial cell protein C receptor (EPCR) gene exon III, 23 bp insertion mutation in the Turkish pediatric thrombotic patients. *Thromb Haemost* 2002;88:1068–1069.

268. Biguzzi E, Gu JM, Merati G, et al. Point mutations in the endothelial protein C receptor (EPCR) promoter. *Thromb Haemost* 2002;87:1085–1086.

269. Hermida J, Hurtada V, Villegas-Mendez A, et al. Identification and characterization of a natural R96C EPCR variant. *J Thromb Haemost* 2003;1:1850–1852.

270. Saponsik B, Reny JL, Gaussem P, et al. A haplotype of the EPCR gene is associated with increased plasma levels of sEPCR and is a candidate risk factor for thrombosis. *Blood* 2004;103:1311–1318.

271. Gettins PGW. Serpin structure, mechanism, and function. *Chem Rev* 2002;102:4751–4803.

272. Petersen TE, Dudek-Wojciechowska G, Sottrup-Hensen L. Primary structure of antithrombin III (heparin cofactor). Partial homology between alpha-1-antitrypsin and antithrombin III. In: Collen D, Wiman B, Verstraete M, eds. *The physiological inhibitors of coagulation and fibrinolysis*, Amsterdam: Elsevier-North Holland, 1979:43–54.

273. Bock SC, Wion KL, Vehar GA, et al. Cloning and expression of the cDNA for human antithrombin III. *Nucleic Acids Res* 1982;10(24):8113–8125.

274. Chandra T, Stackhouse R, Kidd VJ, et al. Isolation and sequence characterization of a cDNA clone of human antithrombin III. *Proc Natl Acad Sci U S A* 1983;80(7):1845–1848.

275. Prochownik EV, Markham AF, Orkin SH. Isolation of a cDNA clone for human antithrombin III. *J Biol Chem* 1983;258:8389–8394.

276. Olds RJ, Lane DA, Chowdhury V, et al. Complete nucleotide sequence of the antithrombin gene: evidence for homologous recombination causing thrombophilia. *Biochemistry* 1993;32:4216–4224.

277. Winter JH, Bennett B, Watt JL, et al. Confirmation of linkage between antithrombin III and Duffy blood group and assignment of AT3 to 1q22 to q25. *Ann Hum Genet* 1982;46:29–34.

278. Bock SC, Harris JF, Balazs I, et al. Assignment of the human antithrombin III structural gene to chromosome 1q23-25. *Cytogenet Cell Genet* 1985;39:67–69.

279. Kao FT, Morse HG, Law ML, et al. Genetic mapping of the structural gene for antithrombin III to human chromosome 1. *Hum Genet* 1984;67:34–36.

280. Tait RC, Walker ID, Perry DJ, et al. Prevalence of antithrombin deficiency in the healthy population. *Br J Haematol* 1994;87:106–112.

281. Harper PL, Luddington RJ, Daly M, et al. The incidence of dysfunctional antithrombin variants: four cases in 210 patients with thromboembolic disease. *Br J Haematol* 1991;77(3):360–364.

282. Egeberg O. Inherited antithrombin III deficiency causing thrombophilia. *Thromb Diath Haemorrh* 1965;13:516–530.

283. Lane DA, Bayston T, Olds RJ, et al. Antithrombin mutation database: 2nd (1997) update. For the plasma coagulation inhibitors subcommittee of the scientific and standardizations committee of the international society on thrombosis and haemostasis. *Thromb Haemost* 1997;77:197–211.

284. Hakten M, Deniz U, Ozbay G. Two cases of homozygous antithrombin III deficiency in a family with congenital deficiency of ATIII. In: Sinzinger H, Vinazzer H, eds. *Thrombosis and haemorrhagic disorders. Proceedings of the 5th international meeting of the Danubian league against thrombosis and haemorrhagic disorders*, Wurzburg, Germany: Schmitt and Meyer, 1989:177–181.

285. Ishiguro K, Kojima T, Kadomatsu K, et al. Complete antithrombin deficiency in mice results in embryonic lethality. *J Clin Invest* 2000;106:873–878.

286. Prochownik EV, Antonarakis S, Bauer KA, et al. Molecular heterogeneity of inherited antithrombin II deficiency. *N Engl J Med* 1983;308:1549–1552.

287. Emmerich J, Chadeuf G, Alhenc-Gelas M, et al. Molecular basis of antithrombin type I deficiency: the first large in-frame deletion and two novel mutations in exon 6. *Thromb Haemost* 1994;72:534–539.

288. Emmerich J, Vidaud D, Alhenc-Gelas M, et al. Three novel mutations of antithrombin inducing high-molecular-mass compounds. *Arterioscler Thromb* 1994;14:1958–1965.

289. Broze GJ Jr. The rediscovery and isolation of TFPI. *J Thromb Haemost* 2003;1:1671–1675.

290. Tardy-Poncet B, Tardy B, Laporte S, et al. Poor anticoagulant response to tissue factor pathway inhibitor in patients with venous thrombosis. *J Thromb Haemost* 2003;1:507–510.

291. Huang ZF, Higuchi D, Lasky N, et al. Tissue factor pathway inhibitor gene disruption produces intrauterine lethality in mice. *Blood* 1997;90:944–951.

292. Kleesiek K, Schmidt M, Gotting C, et al. A first mutation in the human tissue factor pathway inhibitor gene encoding [P151L]TFPI. *Blood* 1998;92:3976–3980.

293. Miyata T, Sakata T, Kumeda K, et al. C-399T polymorphism in the promoter region of human tissue factor pathway inhibitor (TFPI) gene does not change the plasma TFPI antigen level and does not cause venous thrombosis. *Thromb Haemost* 1998;80:345–346.

294. Moatti D, Seknadji P, Galand C, et al. Polymorphisms of the tissue factor pathway inhibitor (TFPI) gene in patients with acute coronary syndromes and in healthy subjects: impact of the V264M substitution on plasma levels of TFPI. *Arterioscler Thromb Vasc Biol* 1999;19:862–869.

295. Moatti D, Haidar B, Fumeron F, et al. A new T-287C polymorphism in the 5′ regulatory region of the tissue factor pathway inhibitor gene. Association study of the T-287C and C-399T polymorphisms with coronary artery disease and plasma TFPI levels. *Thromb Haemost* 2000;84:244–249.

296. Kleesiek K, Schmidt M, Gotting C, et al. The 536C → T transition in the human tissue factor pathway inhibitor (TFPI) gene is statistically associated with a higher risk for venous thrombosis. *Thromb Haemost* 1999;82: 1–5.

297. Gonzalez-Conejero R, Lozano ML, Corral J, et al. The TFPI 536C → T mutation is not associated with increased risk for venous or arterial thrombosis. *Thromb Haemost* 2000;83:787–788.

298. Junker R, Glahn J, Tidow N, et al. The tissue factor pathway inhibitor C536T mutation is not associated with the risk of stroke in young adults. *Thromb Haemost* 2002;87:920–921.

299. Arnaud E, Moatti D, Emmerich J, et al. No link between the TFPI V264M mutation and venous thromboembolic disease. *Thromb Haemost* 1999;82: 159–160.

300. Ameziane N, Seguin C, Borgel D, et al. The −33T → C polymorphism in intron 7 of the TFPI gene influences the risk of venous thromboembolism, independently of the factor V$_{Leiden}$ and prothrombin mutations. *Thromb Haemost* 2002;88:195–199.

301. Tollefsen DM. Insight into the mechanism of action of heparin cofactor II. *Thromb Haemost* 1995;74:1209–1214.

302. Blinder MA, Marasa JC, Reynolds CH, et al. Heparin cofactor II: cDNA sequence, chromosome localization, restriction fragment length polymorphism, and expression in *Escherichia coli*. *Biochemistry* 1988;27:752–759.

303. Herzog R, Lutz S, Blin N, et al. Complete nucleotide sequence of the gene for human heparin cofactor II and mapping to chromosomal band 22q11. *Biochemistry* 1991;30:1350–1357.

304. Tollefsen DM. Antithrombin deficiency. In: Scriver CR, Beaudet AL, Sly WS, et al, eds. *The metabolic and molecular basis of inherited disease*, New York, NY: McGraw-Hill, 2001:4455–4471.

305. Massouh M, Jatoi A, Gordon EM, et al. Heparin cofactor II activity in plasma during pregnancy and oral contraceptive use. *J Lab Clin Med* 1989; 114:697–699.

306. Liu L, Dewar L, Song Y, et al. Inhibition of thrombin by antithrombin III and heparin cofactor II *in vivo*. *Thromb Haemost* 1995;73:405–412.

307. Bellart J, Gilabert R, Cabero L, et al. Heparin cofactor II: a new marker for pre-eclampsia. *Blood Coagul Fibrin* 1998;9:205–208.

308. Tollefsen DM. Heparin cofactor II deficiency. *Arch Pathol Lab Med* 2002;126:1394–1400.

309. Bertina RM, van der Linden IK, Engesser L, et al. Hereditary heparin cofactor II deficiency and the risk of development of thrombosis. *Thromb Haemost* 1987;57:196–200.

310. Blinder MA, Andersson TR, Abildgaard U, et al. Heparin cofactor IIOslo. Mutation of Arg-189 to His decreases the affinity for dermatan sulfate. *J Biol Chem* 1989;264:5128–5133.

311. Kondo S, Tokunaga F, Kario K, et al. Molecular and cellular basis for type I heparin cofactor II deficiency (heparin cofactor II Awaji). *Blood* 1996;87:1006–1012.

312. Bernardi F, Legnani C, Micheletti F, et al. A heparin cofactor II mutation (HCII Rimini) combined with factor V$_{Leiden}$ or type I protein C deficiency in two unrelated thrombophilic subjects. *Thromb Haemost* 1996;76: 505–509.

313. He L, Vicente CP, Westrick RJ, et al. Heparin cofactor II inhibits arterial thrombosis after endothelial injury. *J Clin Invest* 2002;109:213–219.

314. Colman RW, Schmaier AH. Contact system: a vascular biology modulator with anticoagulant, profibrinolytic, antiadhesive, and proinflammatory attributes. *Blood* 1997;90:3819–3843.

315. Fujikawa K, McMullen BA. Amino acid sequence of human β-factor XIIa. *J Biol Chem* 1983;258:10924–10933.

316. McMullen BA, Fujikawa K. Amino acid sequence of the heavy chain of human α-factor XIIa (activated Hageman factor). *J Biol Chem* 1985;260: 5328–5341.

317. Cool DE, Edgell C-JS, Louie GV, et al. Characterization of human blood coagulation factor XII cDNA. Prediction of the primary structure of factor XII and the tertiary structure of β-factor XIIa. *J Biol Chem* 1985;260: 13666–13676.

318. Cool DE, MacGillivray RTA. Characterization of the human blood coagulation factor XII gene. Intron/exon gene organization and analysis of the 5′-flanking region. *J Biol Chem* 1987;262:13662–13673.

319. Royle NJ, Nigli M, Cool DE, et al. Structural gene encoding human factor XII is located at 5q-33-qter. *Somat Cell Mol Genet* 1988;14:217–221.

320. Citarella F, Misiti S, Felici A, et al. Estrogen induction and contact phase activation of human factor XII. *Steroids* 1996;61:270–276.

321. Miyata T, Kawabata S, Iwanaga S, et al. Coagulation factor XII (Hageman factor) Washington DC: inactive factor XIIa results from Cys-571— Ser substitution. *Proc Natl Acad Sci U S A* 1989;86:8319–8322.

322. Schloesser M, Hofferbert S, Bartz U, et al. The novel acceptor splice site mutation 11396(G → A) in the factor XII gene causes a truncated transcript in cross-reacting material negative patients. *Hum Mol Genet* 1995; 4(7):1235–1237.

323. Schloesser M, Zeerleder S, Lutze G, et al. Mutations in the human factor XII gene. *Blood* 1997;90:3967–3977.

324. Hovinga JK, Schaller J, Stricker H, et al. Coagulation factor XII Locarno: the functional defect is caused by the amino acid substitution Arg 353 → Pro leading to loss of a kallikrein cleavage site. *Blood* 1994;84: 1173–1181.

325. Lammle B, Wuillemin WA, Huber I, et al. Thromboembolism and bleeding tendency in congenital factor XII deficiency—a study on 74 subjects from 14 Swiss families. *Thromb Haemost* 1991;65:117–121.

326. Halbmayer WM, Mannhalter C, Feichtinger C, et al. The prevalence of factor XII deficiency in 103 orally anticoagulated outpatients suffering from recurrent venous and/or arterial thromboembolism. *Thromb Haemost* 1992;68:285–290.

327. Koster T, Rosendaal FR, Briet E, et al. John Hageman's factor and deep-vein thrombosis: Leiden thrombophilia study. *Br J Haematol* 1994;87: 422–424.

328. Bernardi F, Marchetti G, Volinia S, et al. A frequent factor XII gene mutation in Hageman trait. *Hum Genet* 1988;80:149–151.

329. Kanaji T, Okamura T, Osaki K, et al. A common genetic polymorphism (46 C to T substitution) in the 5′-untranslated region of the coagulation factor XII gene is associated with low translation efficiency and decrease in plasma factor XII level. *Blood* 1998;91:2010–2014.

330. Endler G, Mannhalter C, Sunder-Plassmann H, et al. Homozygosity for the C → T polymorphism at nucleotide 46 in the 5′ untranslated region of the factor XII gene protects from development of acute coronary syndrome. *Br J Haematol* 2001;115:1007–1009.

331. Pauer HU, Burfeind P, Kostering H, et al. Factor XII deficiency is strongly associated with primary recurrent abortions. *Fertil Steril* 2003;80: 590–594.

332. Shariat-Madar Z, Mahdi F, Schmaier AH. Identification and characterization of prolylcarboxypeptidase as an endothelial cell prekallikrein activator. *J Biol Chem* 2002;277:17962–17969.

333. Chung DW, Fujikawa K, McMullen BA, et al. Human plasma prekallikrein, a zymogen to a serine protease that contains four tandem repeats. *Biochemistry* 1986;25:2410–2417.

334. Yu H, Anderson PJ, Freedman BI, et al. Genomic structure of the human plasma prekallikrein gene, identification of allelic variants, and analysis in end-stage renal disease. *Genomics* 2000;69:225–234.

335. Wuillemin WA, Furlan M, Stricker H, et al. Functional characterization of a variant factor XII (F XII Locarno) in a cross reacting material positive F XII deficient plasma. *Thromb Haemost* 1992;67:219–225.

336. Bouma BN, Kerbiriou DM, Baker J, et al. Characterization of a variant prekallikrein, prekallikrein Long Beach, from a family with mixed cross-reacting material-positive and cross-reacting material-negative prekallikrein deficiency. *J Clin Invest* 1986;78:170–176.

337. Sollo DG, Saleem A. Prekallikrein (Fletcher factor) deficiency. *Ann Clin Lab Sci* 1985;15:279–285.

338. Colman RW. Patho-physiology of kallikrein system. *Ann Clin Lab Sci* 1980;10:220–226.

339. Shigekiyo T, Fujino O, Kanagawa Y, et al. Prekallikrein (PK) Tokushima: PK deficiency caused by a Gly401 → Glu mutation. *J Thromb Haemost* 2003;1:1314–1316.

340. Lombardi AM, Sartori MT, Cabrio L, et al. Severe prekallikrein (Fletcher factor) deficiency due to a compound heterozygosis (383Trp stop codon and Cys529Tyr). *Thromb Haemost* 2003;90:1040–1045.

341. Cheung PP, Cannizzaro LA, Colman RW. Chromosomal mapping of human kininogen gene (KNG) to 3q26–qter. *Cytogenet Cell Genet* 1992;59:24–26.

342. Takagaki Y, Kitamura N, Nakanishi S. Cloning and sequence analysis of cDNAs for human high molecular weight and low molecular weight prekininogens. Primary structures of two human prekininogens. *J Biol Chem* 1985;260:8601–8609.

343. Kitamura N, Kitagawa H, Fukushima D, et al. Structural organization of the human kininogen gene and a model for its evolution. *J Biol Chem* 1985;260:8610–8617.

344. Fong D, Smith DI, Hsieh WT. The human kininogen gene (KNG) mapped to chromosome 3q26–qter by analysis of somatic cell hybrids using the polymerase chain reaction. *Hum Genet* 1991;87:189–192.

345. Cheung PP, Kunapuli SP, Scott CF, et al. Genetic basis of total kininogen deficiency in Williams' trait. *J Biol Chem* 1993;268:23361–23365.

346. Waldmann R, Abraham JP, Rebuck JW, et al. Fitzgerald factor: a hitherto unrecognized coagulation factor. *Lancet* 1974;1:949–952.

347. Krijanovski Y, Proulle V, Mahdi F, et al. Characterization of molecular defects of Fitzgerald trait and another novel high-molecular-weight kininogen-deficient patient: insights into structural requirements for kininogen expression. *Blood* 2003;101:4430–4436.

348. Collen D. The plasminogen (fibrinolytic) system. *Thromb Haemost* 1999; 82:259–270.

349. Benham FJ, Spurr N, Povey S, et al. Assignment of tissue-type plasminogen activator to chromosome 8 in man and identification of a common restriction length polymorphism within the gene. *Mol Biol Med* 1984;2:251–259.

350. Browne MJ, Tyrrell AW, Chapman CG, et al. Isolation of a human tissue-type plasminogen-activator genomic DNA clone and its expression in mouse L cells. *Gene* 1985;33:279–284.

351. Fisher R, Waller EK, Grossi G, et al. Isolation and characterization of the human tissue-type plasminogen activator structural gene including its 5′ flanking region. *J Biol Chem* 1985;260:11223–11230.

352. Degen SJ, Rajput B, Reich E. The human tissue plasminogen activator gene. *J Biol Chem* 1986;261:6972–6985.

353. Pennica D, Holmes WE, Kohr WJ, et al. Cloning and expression of human tissue-type plasminogen activator cDNA in E. coli. *Nature* 1983;301:214–221.

354. Edlund T, Ny T, Ranby M, et al. Isolation of cDNA sequences coding for a part of human tissue plasminogen activator. *Proc Natl Acad Sci U S A* 1983;80:349–352.

355. Rijken DC, Juhan-Vague I, de Cock F, et al. Measurement of human tissue-type plasminogen activator by a two-site immunoradiometric assay. *J Lab Clin Med* 1983;101:274–284.

356. Takada Y, Takada A. Plasma levels of t-PA free PAI-1 and a complex of tPA with PAI-1 in human males and females at various ages. *Thromb Res* 1989;55:601–609.

357. Carmeliet P, Schoonjans L, Kieckens L, et al. Physiological consequences of loss of plasminogen activator gene function in mice. *Nature* 1994;368:419–424.

358. Collen D, Lijnen HR. Tissue-type plasminogen activator: a historical perspective and personal account. *J Thromb Haemost* 2004;2:541–546.

359. Ludwig M, Wohn KD, Schleuning WD, et al. Allelic dimorphism in the human tissue-type plasminogen activator (TPA) gene as a result of an Alu insertion/deletion event. *Hum Genet* 1992;88:388–392.

360. van der Bom JG, de Knijff P, Haverkate F, et al. Tissue plasminogen activator and risk of myocardial infarction. The Rotterdam study. *Circulation* 1997;95:2623–2627.

361. Iacoviello L, Di Castelnuovo A, de Knijff P, et al. Alu-repeat polymorphism in the tissue-type plasminogen activator (tPA) gene, tPA levels and risk of familial myocardial infarction (MI). *Fibrinolysis* 1996;10:13–16.

362. Jern C, Ladenvall P, Wall U, et al. Gene polymorphism of t-PA is associated with forearm vascular release rate of tPA. *Arterioscler Thromb Vasc Biol* 1999;19:454–459.

363. Ladenvall P, Wall U, Jern S, et al. Identification of eight novel single-nucleotide polymorphisms at human tissue-type plasminogen activator (t-PA) locus: association with vascular tPA release *in vivo. Thromb Haemost* 2000;84:150–155.

364. Ladenvall P, Johansson L, Jansson JH, et al. Tissue-type plasminogen activator −7,351C/T enhancer polymorphism is associated with a first myocardial infarction. *Thromb Haemost* 2002;87:105–109.

365. Jannes J, Hamilton-Bruce MA, Pilotto L, et al. Tissue plasminogen activator −7351C/T enhancer polymorphism is a risk factor for lacunar stroke. *Stroke* 2004;35;1090–1094.

366. Sottrup-Hensen L, Claeys H, Zajdel M. et al. The primary structure of human plasminogen: isolation of two lysine-binding fragments and one "mini" plasminogen (MW 38,000) by elastase-catalyzed-specific limited proteolysis. In: Davidson JF, Rowan RM, Samama MM, eds. *Progress in chemical fibrinolysis and thrombolysis*, New York: Raven Press, 1978:191–209.

367. Malinowski DP, Sadler JE, Davie EW. Characterization of a complementary deoxyribonucleic acid coding for human and bovine plasminogen. *Biochemistry* 1984;23:4243–4250.

368. Forsgren M, Raden B, Israelsson M, et al. Molecular cloning and characterization of a full-length cDNA clone for human plasminogen. *FEBS Lett* 1987;213(254):260.

369. Murray JC, Buetow KH, Donovan M, et al. Linkage disequilibrium of plasminogen polymorphisms and assignment of the gene to human chromosome 6q26-6q27. *Am J Hum Genet* 1987;40:338–350.

370. Frank SL, Klisak I, Sparkes RS, et al. The apolipoprotein(a) gene resides on human chromosome 6q26-27, in close proximity to the homologous gene for plasminogen. *Hum Genet* 1988;79:352–356.

371. Petersen TE, Martzen MR, Ichinose A, et al. Characterization of the gene for human plasminogen, a key proenzyme in the fibrinolytic system. *J Biol Chem* 1990;265:6104–6111.

372. Aoki N, Moroi M, Sakata Y, et al. Abnormal plasminogen. A hereditary molecular abnormality found in a patient with recurrent thrombosis. *J Clin Invest* 1978;61:1186–1195.

373. Tait RC, Walker ID, Islam SIAM, et al. Plasminogen levels and putative prevalence of deficiency in 400 blood donors. *Br J Haematol* 2004;77(S1):10.(abst).

374. Heijboer H, Brandjes DPM, Buller HR, et al. Deficiencies of coagulation-inhibiting and fibrinolytic proteins in outpatients with deep vein thrombosis. *N Engl J Med* 1990;323:1512–1516.

375. Demarmels-Biasiutti F, Sulzer I, Stucki B, et al. Is plasminogen deficiency a thrombotic risk factor? A study on 23 thrombophilic patients and their family members. *Thromb Haemost* 1998;80:167–170.

376. Shigekiyo T, Uno Y, Tomonari A, et al. Type I congenital plasminogen deficiency is not a risk factor for thrombosis. *Thromb Haemost* 1992;67:189–192.

377. Tait RC, Walker ID, Conkie JA, et al. Isolated familial plasminogen deficiency may not be a risk factor for thrombosis. *Thromb Haemost* 1996;76:1004–1008.

378. Shigekiyo T, Kanazuka M, Aihara K, et al. No increased risk of thrombosis in heterozygous congenital dysplasminogenemia. *Int J Hematol* 2000;72:247–252.

379. Mingers AM, Heimburger N, Zeitler P, et al. Homozygous type I plasminogen deficiency. *Semin Thromb Hemost* 1997;23:259–269.

380. Schuster V, Mingers AM, Seidenspinner S, et al. Homozygous mutations in the plasminogen gene of two unrelated girls with ligneous conjunctivitis. *Blood* 1997;90:958–966.

381. Schullek V, Zeitler P, Seregard S, et al. Homozygous and compound heterozygous type I plasminogen deficiency is a common cause of ligneous conjunctivitis. *Thromb Haemost* 2001;85:1004–1010.

382. Bugge TH, Flick MJ, Daugherty CC, et al. Plasminogen deficiency causes severe thrombosis but is compatible with development and reproduction. *Genes Dev* 1985;9(794):807.

383. Ploplis VA, Carmeliet P, Vazirzadeh S, et al. Effects of disruption of the plasminogen gene on thrombosis, growth, and health in mice. *Circulation* 1995;92:2585–2593.

384. Drew AF, Kaufman AH, Danton MJS, et al. Ligneous conjunctivitis in plasminogen deficient mice. *Blood* 1998;91:1616–1624.

385. Blomback B, Abildgaard U, van den Besselaar AM, et al. Nomenclature of quantities and units in thrombosis and haemostasis (recommendation 1993). A collaborative project of the Scientific and Standardization Committee of the International Society on Thrombosis and Haemostasis (ISTH/SSC) and the Commission. /Committee on Quantities and Units (in Clinical Chemistry) of the International Union of Pure and Applied Chemistry-International Federation of Clinical Chemistry (IUPAC-IFCC/CQU(CC)). *Thromb Haemost* 1994;71:375–394.

386. Sakata Y, Aoki N. Cross-linking of $\alpha2$-plasmin inhibitor to fibrin by fibrin-stabilizing factor. *J Clin Invest* 1980;65:290–297.

387. Sumi Y, Nakamura Y, Aoki N, et al. Structure of the carboxyl-terminal half of human alpha 2-plasmin inhibitor deduced from that of cDNA. *J Biochem* 1986;100:1399–1402.

388. Tone M, Kikuno R, Kume-Iwaki A, et al. Structure of human alpha 2-plasmin inhibitor deduced from the cDNA sequence. *J Biochem* 1987;102:1033–1041.

389. Holmes WE, Nelles L, Lijnen HR, et al. Primary structure of human alpha 2-antiplasmin, a serine protease inhibitor (serpin). *J Biol Chem* 1987;262:1659–1664.

390. Bangert K, Johnsen AH, Christensen U, et al. Different N-terminal forms of alpha 2-plasmin inhibitor in human plasma. *Biochem J* 1993;291:623–625.

391. Hirosawa S, Nakamura Y, Miura O, et al. Organization of the human alpha 2-plasmin inhibitor gene. *Proc Natl Acad Sci U S A* 1989;85:6836–6840.

392. Kato A, Hirosawa S, Toyota S, et al. Localization of the human alpha 2-plasmin inhibitor gene (PLI) to 17p13. *Cytogenet Cell Genet* 1993;62:190–191.

393. Favier R, Aoki N, De Moerloose P. Congenital alpha2-plasmin inhibitor deficiencies: a review. *Br J Haematol* 2001;114:4–10.

394. Lijnen HR, Okada K, Matsuo O, et al. Alpha2-antiplasmin gene deficiency in mice is associated with enhanced fibrinolytic potential without overt bleeding. *Blood* 1999;93:2274–2281.

395. Holmes WE, Lijnen HR, Nelles L, et al. Alpha 2-antiplasmin Enschede: alanine insertion and abolition of plasmin inhibitory activity. *Science* 1987;238:209–211.

396. Miura O, Hirosawa S, Kato A, et al. Molecular basis for congenital deficiency of alpha 2-plasmin inhibitor. A frameshift mutation leading to elongation of the deduced amino acid sequence. *J Clin Invest* 1989;83:1598–1604.

397. Miura O, Sugawara Y, Aoki N. Hereditary alpha 2-plasmin inhibitor deficiency caused by a transport-deficient mutation (alpha 2-PI-Okinawa). Deletion of Glu137 by a trinucleotide deletion blocks intracellular transport. *J Biol Chem* 1989;264:18213–18219.

398. Lind B, Thorsen S. A novel missense mutation in the human plasmin inhibitor (alpha2-antiplasmin) gene associated with a bleeding tendency. *Br J Haematol* 1999;107:317–322.

399. Yoshinaga H, Hirosawa S, Chung DH, et al. A novel point mutation of the splicing donor site in the intron 2 of the plasmin inhibitor gene. *Thromb Haemost* 2000;84:307–311.

400. Yoshinaga H, Nakahara M, Koyama T, et al. A single thymine nucleotide deletion responsible for congenital deficiency of plasmin inhibitor. *Thromb Haemost* 2002;88:144–148.

401. Hanss MML, Farcis M, Ffrench PO, et al. A splicing donor site point mutation in intron 6 of the plasmin inhibitor (alpha2 antiplasmin) gene with heterozygous deficiency and a bleeding tendency. *Blood Coagul Fibrin* 2003;14:107–111.

402. Loskutoff DJ, Sawdey M, Mimuro J. Type 1 plasminogen activator inhibitor. *Prog Hemost Thromb* 1989;9:87–115.

403. van der Bom JG, Bots ML, Haverkate F, et al. The 4G5G polymorphism in the gene for PAI-1 and the circadian oscillation of plasma PAI-1. *Blood* 2003;101:1841–1844.

404. Loskutoff DJ, Linders M, Keijer J, et al. Structure of the human plasminogen activator inhibitor 1 gene: nonrandom distribution of introns. *Biochemistry* 1987;26:3763–3768.

405. Bosma PJ, van den Berg EA, Kooistra T, et al. Human plasminogen activator-inhibitor-1 gene. Promoter and structural gene nucleotide sequences. *J Biol Chem* 1988;263:9129–9141.

406. Strandberg L, Lawrence D, Ny T. The organization of the human-plasminogen-activator-inhibitor-1 gene. Implications on the evolution of the serine-protease inhibitor family. *Eur J Biochem* 1988;176:609–616.

407. Follo M, Ginsburg D. Structure and expression of the human gene encoding plasminogen activator inhibitor, PAI-1. *Gene* 1989;84:447–453.

408. Schwartz CE, Stanislovitis P, Phelan MC, et al. Deletion mapping of plasminogen activator inhibitor, type I (PLANH1) and beta-glucuronidase (GUSB) in 7q21—q22. *Cytogenet Cell Genet* 1991;56:152–153.

409. Klinger KW, Winqvist R, Riccio A, et al. Plasminogen activator inhibitor type 1 gene is located at region q21.3-q22 of chromosome 7 and genetically linked with cystic fibrosis. *Proc Natl Acad Sci U S A* 1987;84:8548–8552.

410. Ginsburg D, Zeheb R, Yang AY, et al. cDNA cloning of human plasminogen activator-inhibitor from endothelial cells. *J Clin Invest* 1986;78:1673–1680.

411. Ny T, Sawdey M, Lawrence D, et al. Cloning and sequence of a cDNA coding for the human beta-migrating endothelial-cell-type plasminogen activator inhibitor. *Proc Natl Acad Sci U S A* 1986;83:6776–6780.

412. Pannekoek H, Veerman H, Lambers H, et al. Endothelial plasminogen activator inhibitor (PAI): a new member of the Serpin gene family. *EMBO J* 1986;5:2539–2544.

413. Andreasen PA, Riccio A, Welinder KG, et al. Plasminogen activator inhibitor type-1: reactive center and amino-terminal heterogeneity determined by protein and cDNA sequencing. *FEBS Lett* 1986;209:213–218.

414. Wun TC, Kretzmer KK. cDNA cloning and expression in E. coli of a plasminogen activator inhibitor (PAI) related to a PAI produced by Hep G2 hepatoma cell. *FEBS Lett* 1987;210:11–16.

415. Loskutoff DJ. Regulation of PAI-1 gene expression. *Fibrinolysis* 1991;5:197–206.

416. Eriksson P, Kallin B, van't Hooft FM, et al. Allele-specific increase in basal transcription of the plasminogen-activator inhibitor 1 gene is associated with myocardial infarction. *Proc Natl Acad Sci U S A* 1995;92:1851–1855.

417. Boekholdt SM, Bijsterveld NR, Moons AH, et al. Genetic variation in coagulation and fibrinolysis proteins and their relation with acute myocardial infarction: a systematic review. *Circulation* 2001;104:3063–3068.

418. Ossei-Gerning N, Mansfield MW, Stickland MH, et al. Plasminogen activator inhibitor-1 promoter 4G/5G genotype and plasma levels in relation to a history of myocardial infarction in patients characterized by coronary angiography. *Arterioscler Thromb Vasc Biol* 1997;17:33–37.

419. Carmeliet P, Kieckens L, Schoonjans L, et al. Plasminogen activator inhibitor-1 gene-deficient mice. I. Generation by homologous recombination and characterization. *J Clin Invest* 1993;92:2746–2755.

420. Carmeliet P, Stassen JM, Schoonjans L, et al. Plasminogen activator inhibitor-1 gene-deficient mice. II. Effects on hemostasis, thrombosis, and thrombolysis. *J Clin Invest* 1993;92:2756–2760.

421. Nesheim ME, Wang W, Boffa M, et al. Thrombin, thrombomodulin and TAFI in the molecular link between coagulation and fibrinolysis. *Thromb Haemost* 1997;78:386–391.

422. Eaton DL, Malloy BE, Tsai SP, et al. Isolation, molecular cloning, and partial characterization of a novel carboxypeptidase B from human plasma. *J Biol Chem* 1991;266:21833–21838.

423. Wang W, Hendriks DF, Scharpe SS. Carboxypeptidase U, a plasma carboxypeptidase with high affinity for plasminogen. *J Biol Chem* 1994;269:15937–15944.

424. Bajzar L, Manuel R, Nesheim ME. Purification and characterization of TAFI, a thrombin-activable fibrinolysis inhibitor. *J Biol Chem* 1995;270(24):14477–14484.

425. Boffa MB, Reid S, Joo E, et al. Characterization of the gene encoding human TAFI (thrombin-activable fibrinolysis inhibitor; plasma procarboxypeptidase B). *Biochemistry* 1999;38:6547–6558.

426. Bajzar L, Nesheim ME, Tracy PB. The profibrinolytic effect of activated protein C in clots formed from plasma is TAFI-dependent. *Blood* 1996;88:2093–2100.

427. van Tilburg NH, Rosendaal FR, Bertina RM. Thrombin activatable fibrinolysis inhibitor and the risk for deep vein thrombosis. *Blood* 2000;95:2855–2859.

428. Silveira A, Schatteman K, Goossens F, et al. Plasma procarboxypeptidase U in men with symptomatic coronary artery disease. *Thromb Haemost* 2000;84:364–368.

429. Santamaria A, Oliver A, Borrell M, et al. Risk of ischemic stroke associated with functional thrombin-activatable fibrinolysis inhibitor plasma levels. *Stroke* 2003;34:2387–2391.

430. Juhan-Vague I, Morange PE, Aubert H, et al. Plasma thrombin-activatable fibrinolysis inhibitor antigen concentration and genotype in relation to myocardial infarction in the north and south of Europe. *Arterioscler Thromb Vasc Biol* 2002;22:867–873.

431. Juhan-Vague I, Morange PE. Very high TAFI antigen levels are associated with a lower risk of hard coronary events: the PRIME Study. *Thromb Haemost* 2003;1:2243–2244.

432. Nagashima M, Yin ZF, Zhao L, et al. Thrombin-activatable fibrinolysis inhibitor (TAFI) deficiency is compatible with murine life. *J Clin Invest* 2002;109:101–110.

433. Zhao L, Bajzar L, Nesheim ME, et al. Identification and characterization of two thrombin-activatable fibrinolysis inhibitor isoforms. *Thromb Haemost* 1998;80:949–955.

434. Henry M, Aubert H, Morange PE, et al. Identification of polymorphisms in the promoter and the 3′ region of the TAFI gene: evidence that plasma TAFI antigen levels are strongly genetically controlled. *Blood* 2001;97:2053–2058.

435. Brouwers GJ, Vos HL, Leebeek FWG, et al. A novel, possibly functional, single nucleotide polymorphism in the coding region of the thrombin-activatable fibrinolysis inhibitor (TAFI) gene is also associated with TAFI levels. *Blood* 2001;98:1992–1993.

436. Schneider M, Boffa M, Stewart R, et al. Two naturally occurring variants of TAFI (Thr-325 and Ile-325) differ substantially with respect to thermal stability and antifibrinolytic activity of the enzyme. *J Biol Chem* 2002;277:1021–1030.

437. Kremer Hovinga JA, Franco RF, Zago MA, et al. A functional single nucleotide polymorphism in the thrombin-activatable fibrinolysis inhibitor (TAFI) gene associates with outcome of meningococcal disease. *Thromb Haemost* 2004;2:54–57.

438. Doolittle RF. X-ray crystallographic studies on fibrinogen and fibrin. *J Thromb Haemost* 2003;1:1559–1565.

439. Rixon MW, Chan WY, Davie EW, et al. Characterization of a complementary deoxyribonucleic acid coding for the alpha chain of human fibrinogen. *Biochemistry* 1993;22:3237–3244.

440. Chung DW, Que BG, Rixon MW, et al. Characterization of complementary deoxyribonucleic acid and genomic deoxyribonucleic acid for the beta chain of human fibrinogen. *Biochemistry* 1983;22:3244–3250.

441. Chung DW, Chan WY, Davie EW. Characterization of a complementary deoxyribonucleic acid coding for the gamma chain of human fibrinogen. *Biochemistry* 1983;22:3250–3256.

442. Kant JA, Lord ST, Crabtree GR. Partial mRNA sequences for human A alpha, B beta, and gamma fibrinogen chains: evolutionary and functional implications. *Proc Natl Acad Sci U S A* 1983;80:3953–3957.

443. Rixon MW, Chung DW, Davie EW. Nucleotide sequence of the gene for the gamma chain of human fibrinogen. *Biochemistry* 1985;24:2077–2086.

444. Kant JA, Fornace AJJ, Saxe D. Evolution and organization of the fibrinogen locus on chromosome 4: gene duplication accompanied by transposition and inversion. *Proc Natl Acad Sci U S A* 1985;82:2344–2348.

445. Henry I, Uzan G, Weil D, et al. The genes coding for A alpha-, B beta-, and gamma-chains of fibrinogen map to 4q2. *Am J Hum Genet* 1984;36:760–768.

446. Marion MW, Fuller GM, Elder FF. Chromosomal localization of human and rat A alpha, B beta, and gamma fibrinogen genes by in situ hybridization. *Cytogenet Cell Genet* 1986;42:36–41.

447. Roy SN, Mukhopadhyay G, Redman CM. Regulation of fibrinogen assembly. Transfection of Hep G2 cells with B beta cDNA specifically enhances synthesis of the three component chains of fibrinogen. *J Biol Chem* 1990;265:6389–6393.

448. Suh TT, Holmback K, Jensen NJ, et al. Resolution of spontaneous bleeding events but failure of pregnancy in fibrinogen-deficient mice. *Genes Dev* 1995;9:2020–2033.

449. Martinez J. Congenital dysfibrinogenemia. *Curr Opin Hematol* 1997;4:357–365.

450. Hayes T. Dysfibrinogenemia and thrombosis. *Arch Pathol Lab Med* 2002;126:1387–1390.

451. Hanss M, Biot F. A database for human fibrinogen variants. *Ann NY Acad Sci* 2001;936:89–90.

452. Mosesson MW. Dysfibrinogenemia and thrombosis. *Semin Thromb Hemost* 1999;25:311–319.

453. Voetsch B, Loscalzo J. Genetic determinants of arterial thrombosis. *Arterioscler Thromb Vasc Biol* 2004;24:216–229.

454. Thomas A, Lamlum H, Humphries S, et al. Linkage disequilibrium across the fibrinogen locus as shown by five genetic polymorphisms, G/A-455 (HaeIII), C/T-148 (HindIII/AluI), T/G + 1689 (AvaII), and BclI (beta-fibrinogen) and TaqI (alpha-fibrinogen), and their detection by PCR. *Hum Mutat* 1994;3:79–81.

455. Ariens RAS, Lai TS, Weisel JW, et al. Role of factor XIII in fibrin clot formation and effects of genetic polymorphisms. *Blood* 2002;100:743–754.

456. Board PG, Webb GC, McKee J, et al. Localization of the coagulation factor XIIa subunit gene (F13A) to chromosome bands 6p24-p25. *Cytogenet Cell Genet* 1988;48:25–27.

457. Ichinose A, Davie EW. Characterization of the gene for the a subunit of human factor XIII (plasma transglutaminase) a blood coagulation factor. *Proc Natl Acad Sci U S A* 1988;85:5829–5833.

458. Bottenus RE, Ichinose A, Davie EW. Nucleotide sequence of the gene for the b subunit of human factor XIII. *Biochemistry* 1990;29:11195–11209.

459. Webb GC, Coggan M, Ichinose A, et al. Localization of the coagulation Factor XIII b subunit gene (F13B) to chromosome bands 1q31-32.1 and restriction fragment length polymorphism at the locus. *Hum Genet* 1989;81:157–160.

460. Ichinose A, McMullen B, Fujikawa K, et al. Amino acid sequence of the b subunit of human factor XIII, a protein composed of ten repetitive segments. *Biochemistry* 1986;25:4633–4638.

461. Lauer P, Metzner HJ, Zettimeibl G, et al. Targeted inactivation of the mouse locus encoding coagulation factor XIII-A: hemostatic abnormalities in mutant mice and characterization of the coagulation deficit. *Thromb Haemost* 2002;88:967–974.

462. Koseki-Kuno S, Yamakawa M, Dickneite G, et al. Factor XIII A subunit-deficient mice developed severe uterine bleeding events and subsequent spontaneous miscarriages. *Blood* 2003;102:4410–4412.

463. Hashiguchi T, Saito M, Morishita E, et al. Two genetic defects in a patient with complete deficiency of the b-subunit for coagulation factor XIII. *Blood* 1993;82:145–150.

464. Catto AJ, Kohler HP, Bannan S, et al. Factor XIII Val 34 Leu: a novel association with primary intracerebral hemorrhage. *Stroke* 1998;29:813–816.

465. Kohler HP, Stickland MH, Ossei-Gerning N, et al. Association of a common polymorphism in the factor XIII gene with myocardial infarction. *Thromb Haemost* 1998;79:8–13.

466. Undas A, Sydor WJ, Brummel K, et al. Aspirin alters the cardioprotective effects of the factor XIII Val34Leu polymorphism. *Circulation* 2003;107:17–20.

467. Wagner DD, Olmsted JB, Marder VJ. Immunolocalization of von Willebrand protein in Weibel-Palade bodies of human endothelial cells. *J Cell Biol* 1982;95:355–360.

468. Mancuso DJ, Tuley EA, Westfield LA, et al. Structure of the gene for human von Willebrand factor. *J Biol Chem* 1989;264:19514–19527.

469. Mancuso DJ, Tuley EA, Westfield LA, et al. Human von Willebrand factor gene and pseudogene: structural analysis and differentiation by polymerase chain reaction. *Biochemistry* 1991;30:253–269.

470. Ginsburg D, Handin RI, Bonthron DT, et al. Human von Willebrand factor (VWF): isolation of complementary DNA (cDNA) clones and chromosomal localization. *Science* 1985;228:1401–1406.

471. Verweij CL, de Vries CJ, Distel B, et al. Construction of cDNA coding for human von Willebrand factor using antibody probes for colony-screening and mapping of the chromosomal gene. *Nucleic Acids Res* 1985;13:4699–4717.

472. Sadler JE, Shelton-Inloes BB, Sorace JM, et al. Cloning and characterization of two cDNAs coding for human von Willebrand factor. *Proc Natl Acad Sci U S A* 1985;82:6394–6398.

473. van Oost BA, Edgell CJ, Hay CW, et al. Isolation of a human von Willebrand factor cDNA from the hybrid endothelial cell line EA.hy926. *Biochem Cell Biol* 1986;64:699–705.

474. Sadler JE. A revised classification of von Willebrand disease. For the Subcommittee on von Willebrand Factor of the Scientific and Standardization Committee of the International Society on Thrombosis and Haemostasis. *Thromb Haemost* 1994;71:520–525.

475. Denis C, Methia N, Frenette PS, et al. A mouse model of severe von Willebrand disease: Defects in hemostasis and thrombosis. *Proc Natl Acad Sci U S A* 1998;95:9524–9529.

476. Sadler JE. Von Willebrand disease type 1: a diagnosis in search of a disease. *Blood* 2003;101:2089–2093.

477. Sadler JE, Ginsburg D. A database of polymorphisms in the von Willebrand factor gene and pseudogene. For the consortium on von Willebrand factor mutations and polymorphisms and the subcommittee on von Willebrand factor of the scientific and standardization committee of the International Society on Thrombosis and Haemostasis. *Thromb Haemost* 1993;69:185–191.

478. Federici AB, Rand JH, Bucciarelli P, et al. Acquired von Willebrand syndrome: data from an international registry. *Thromb Haemost* 2000;84:345–349.

479. Presnell SR, Stafford DW. The Vitamin K-dependent carboxylase. *Thromb Haemost* 2002;87:937–946.

480. Wu SM, Cheung W-F, Frazier D, et al. Cloning and expression of the cDNA for human gamma-glutamyl carboxylase. *Science* 1991;254:1634–1636.

481. Kuo WL, Stafford DW, Cruces J, et al. Chromosomal localization of the gamma-glutamyl carboxylase gene at 2p12. *Genomics* 1995;25:746–748.

482. Wu SM, Stafford DW, Frazier LD, et al. Genomic sequence and transcription start site for the human gamma-glutamyl carboxylase. *Blood* 1997;89:4058–4062.

483. Romero EE, Marvi U, Niman ZE, et al. The vitamin K-dependent gamma-glutamyl carboxylase gene contains a TATA-less promoter with a novel upstream regulatory element. *Blood* 2003;102:1333–1339.

484. Zhu A, Raymond R, Zheng X, et al. Abnormalities of development and hemostasis in gamma-carboxylase deficient mice. *Blood* 1998;92:152a(abstract 611).

485. Brenner B, Sanchez-Vega B, Wu SM, et al. A missense mutation in gamma-glutamyl carboxylase gene causes combined deficiency of all vitamin K-dependent blood coagulation factors. *Blood* 1998;92:4554–4559.

486. Spronk HMH, Farah RA, Buchanan GR, et al. Novel mutation in the gamma-glutamyl carboxylase gene resulting in congenital combined deficiency of all vitamin K-dependent blood coagulation factors. *Blood* 2000;96:3650–3652.

487. Suttie JW. Vitamin K dependent carboxylase. *Ann Rev Biochem* 1985;54:459–477.

488. Fregin A, Rost S, Wolz W, et al. Homozygosity mapping of a second gene locus for hereditary combined deficiency of vitamin K-dependent clotting factors to the centromeric region of chromosome 16. *Blood* 2002;100:3229–3232.

# CHAPTER 5 ■ TISSUE FACTOR STRUCTURE AND FUNCTION

JAMES H. MORRISSEY AND NICOLA J. MUTCH

Blood circulates as a liquid, but once it escapes from an injured blood vessel it must rapidly gel, or clot, to form a hemostatic plug in order to limit further blood loss. On the other hand, pathologic activation of the blood clotting system within the lumina of blood vessels is a major cause of human death and disability. This chapter focuses on the mechanism of initiation of the blood clotting system, both in normal hemostasis and in many thrombotic diseases. Two main pathways for triggering the blood clotting cascade are initially described: the intrinsic, or contact, pathway and the extrinsic, or tissue factor (TF), pathway. The intrinsic pathway is so called because it appears to be an intrinsic property of plasma; that is, when blood or plasma is placed in a glass tube, it will clot spontaneously. This pathway has also been called the *contact pathway*, which is perhaps a more accurate name because the pathway is readily activated through the contact of blood or plasma with an artificial surface, such as glass or clay. Although intensively studied, the contact pathway *per se* is no longer thought to be of primary importance in normal hemostasis because individuals in whom the contact pathway is inactive (owing to a severe congenital deficiency in one of the contact factors, such as factor XII) exhibit no bleeding tendency. On the other hand, the distinction between the contact and extrinsic pathways has become blurred with the realization that there is cross talk between the pathways: Factor IX can be activated through the TF pathway (1); it can also be activated by thrombin (2). The contact pathway is considered in detail elsewhere in this book (see Chapter 6).

The TF pathway of blood clotting is triggered when plasma comes into contact with cells that express the integral membrane protein, TF (tissue factor), on their surfaces. TF is abundant on a variety of cell types found outside the vasculature but is present only in tiny amounts within the vasculature. After vascular injury, blood is exposed to cells bearing TF, whereupon TF binds factor VII—one of the soluble clotting factors—with high affinity. It is the complex of TF and factor VII (or more accurately, the activated form of factor VII known as *factor VIIa*) that initiates the blood clotting cascade in normal hemostasis. In addition, TF is responsible for triggering the clotting cascade in a variety of thrombotic disorders. The remainder of this chapter will deal exclusively with the initiation of the blood clotting system by TF.

## OVERVIEW OF THE INITIATION OF BLOOD COAGULATION BY TISSUE FACTOR AND FACTOR VII

The clotting cascade is made up of a series of reactions involving the activation of zymogens (inert precursors of enzymes) by limited proteolysis. With the exception of thrombin, the newly generated proteases have low activity until they bind to specific protein cofactors on suitable phospholipid surfaces. Such binding events potentiate the enzymatic activity of clotting proteases by as much as several hundred-thousandfold.

The first enzyme in the clotting cascade consists of two subunits: a serine protease, factor VIIa (the catalytic subunit); and a protein cofactor, TF (the positively acting regulatory subunit). Because TF is an integral membrane protein, the complex of TF and factor VIIa (TF:VIIa) is tethered to the cell surface. Free factor VIIa is a weak enzyme, but the TF:VIIa complex is the most potent known activator of the blood clotting cascade.

All of the serine proteases of the blood clotting cascade (including factor VII) circulate in the plasma as inert zymogens. Furthermore, most protein cofactors of the clotting cascade circulate as inert procofactors. (TF is a notable exception; it does not require proteolysis to become active.) A nagging question for many years has been: How can the clotting cascade be initiated through the assembly of a collection of inert precursors? The answer appears to come from the fact that trace amounts of active factor VIIa are present in the circulation at all times.

The active forms of most serine proteases of the clotting system have extremely short plasma half-lives (measured in seconds) because plasma contains high concentrations of protease inhibitors. Free factor VIIa, however, is not reactive with plasma protease inhibitors (3). When injected into animals or humans, factor VIIa has a long circulating half-life of approximately 2 hours, similar to the 5-hour half-life of zymogen factor VII (4). Therefore, if factor VIIa is generated *in vivo*, it can circulate for considerable periods.

TF binds factor VII or VIIa with high affinity, resulting in a 1:1 complex of the two proteins on the cell surface. As depicted in Figure 5-1, once bound to TF, factor VII is rapidly converted to factor VIIa by limited proteolysis (5). So, there are two ways to form the TF:VIIa complex: through direct capture of circulating factor VIIa by TF or through capture of factor VII by TF followed by conversion of the bound factor VII to VIIa.

Once formed, the TF:VIIa complex triggers the blood clotting cascade in two ways. TF:VIIa can activate factor IX via limited proteolysis (reaction 1 in Fig. 5-2). The newly generated factor IXa then binds with a protein cofactor on a phospholipid (PL) surface to form the IXa:VIIIa complex, which catalyzes the conversion of factor X to Xa. Alternatively, TF:VIIa can directly activate factor X (see reaction 2 in Fig. 5-2). This latter mechanism predominates in most *in vitro* conditions, in which factor X is the preferred substrate for TF:VIIa.

The discussions about the mechanism of the blood clotting cascade brings us to the question: Where does the first burst of serine protease activity come from if all the enzymes and their essential cofactors circulate as inactive precursors? It turns out that trace levels of factor VIIa are present in the circulation of all normal individuals, making up approximately 1% of the

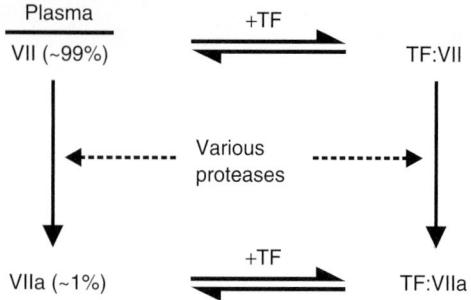

**FIGURE 5-1.** Two pathways for the formation of the tissue factor (TF) and factor VIIa complex (TF:VIIa). Plasma contains a mixture of approximately 1% active factor VIIa and 99% zymogen factor VII. Both factors, VII and VIIa, bind reversibly to TF with similarly high affinities to generate TF:VII and TF:VIIa complexes, respectively. Factor VII can be converted to factor VIIa by a variety of plasma proteases (see text), and factor VII bound to TF is an especially good substrate for conversion to factor VIIa. (From Nemerson Y, Repke D. Tissue factor accelerates the activation of coagulation factor VII: the role of a bifunctional coagulation cofactor. *Thromb Res* 1985;40:351–358, with permission.)

total factor VII concentration (but with considerable individual variation) (6). Exposure of TF to plasma therefore results in assembly of both TF:VII and TF:VIIa complexes, and only the latter are enzymatically active. However, these low initial

levels of TF:VIIa are thought to trigger enough of the clotting cascade to result in the back-activation of the rest of the bound factor VII by downstream proteases. A variety of coagulation proteases activate factor VII to VIIa *in vitro*, including factors IXa, Xa, and XIIa; thrombin; plasmin; and factor VII–activating protease (FSAP), a novel plasma protease that can activate both factor VII and plasminogen activators (5,7–13). In addition, the TF:VIIa complex can catalyze the autoactivation of factor VII bound to TF (14,15). It is currently unclear which of these proteases plays the major role in activating TF-bound factor VII during clotting, although many investigators consider factor Xa the most likely candidate.

It is also presently unclear where or how circulating factor VIIa is generated. One important clue comes from the discovery that patients with hemophilia B (who lack factor IX) have plasma factor VIIa levels that are only approximately 10% of what is considered normal (16). This finding indicates that factor IX (presumably, as factor IXa) participates in the formation of much of the circulating factor VIIa found in plasma. Another clue is the fact that factor VIIa levels rise postprandially, especially after high fat meals (17,18). This rise occurs in individuals who are deficient in factor XI or XII but not in those who are deficient in factor IX (19), suggesting that activation of factor VII may occur on lipoprotein particles, apparently involving factor IXa. Consistent with this notion, plasma factor VIIa levels are very low in patients with familial abetalipoproteinemia (20). And finally, factor VIIa levels are higher in lymph than in plasma (21), suggesting that at least some of the factor VIIa may be generated extravascularly and returned to the circulation by the lymph.

# TISSUE FACTOR PROTEIN STRUCTURE

TF is also known as *thromboplastin*, *CD142*, and *coagulation factor III*. It is a glycosylated membrane protein consisting of a single polypeptide chain of 261 or 263 amino acids (the two forms are nearly equal in abundance), with variability in length owing to microheterogeneity at the amino-terminus (22–24). The calculated molecular weight of the polypeptide chain of TF is 29,447 Da or 29,593 Da, whereas the mobility of the fully glycosylated protein on sodium dodecyl sulfate (SDS) gels suggests a molecular weight of approximately 45,000 Da (25). TF belongs to the class 2 cytokine receptor superfamily (26). Topographically, TF is a type I integral membrane protein, which means that the amino-terminus of the protein is located outside the cell, whereas the carboxy terminus is located inside the cell. The overall domain structure of TF is given diagrammatically in Figure 5-3. The extracellular portion is composed of two fibronectin type III domains, which are a variation on the immunoglobulin fold. This portion of TF has three *N*-linked carbohydrate chains (27), but they are dispensable for clotting activity because the recombinant protein produced in bacteria is fully functional (28). The extracellular domain also has two disulfide bonds (29), at least one of which is essential for activity (30).

TF has a typical hydrophobic membrane-spanning domain that anchors the protein to the cell surface. Membrane anchoring of TF is essential for full procoagulant activity, although the exact nature of the membrane anchor does not appear to be important. This observation was demonstrated by replacing the transmembrane domain of TF with that of a heterologous protein and also by expressing recombinant TF with a glycosylphosphatidylinositol membrane anchor (31). In both cases, the recombinant protein had full TF activity.

The short (23–amino acid long) cytoplasmic domain of TF contains a cysteine residue to which a fatty acyl chain (palmitate or stearate) is attached by a thioester linkage (29). In addition, the cytoplasmic domain can be phosphorylated on

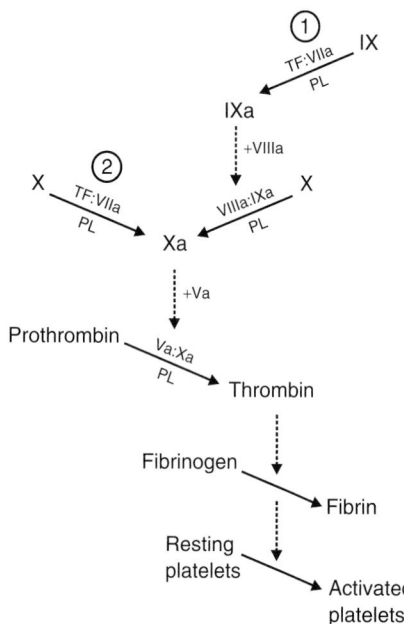

**FIGURE 5-2.** Simplified map of the blood clotting cascade initiated by the complex of tissue factor (TF) and factor VIIa (TF:VIIa). The TF:VIIa complex can initiate clotting by activating either factor IX (reaction 1) or factor X (reaction 2). Regardless of the mechanism for triggering the clotting system, all clotting pathways converge at the formation of factor Xa, which assembles on a phospholipid (PL) surface with its protein cofactor (factor Va) to catalyze the conversion of prothrombin to thrombin. Thrombin is responsible for converting fibrinogen to fibrin (again, by limited proteolysis), which spontaneously polymerizes to form a gel, or fibrin clot. In addition, thrombin is a potent activator of platelets (see Chapter 33). In this simplified clotting cascade, a number of back-activation reactions have been omitted. For example, factors Va and VIIIa circulate as inert precursors (factors V and VIII, respectively) and are activated following limited proteolysis by thrombin or factor Xa. The reactions involving hemostatically relevant factors XI and XIII, as well as all of the inhibitors of the clotting system, have also been omitted.

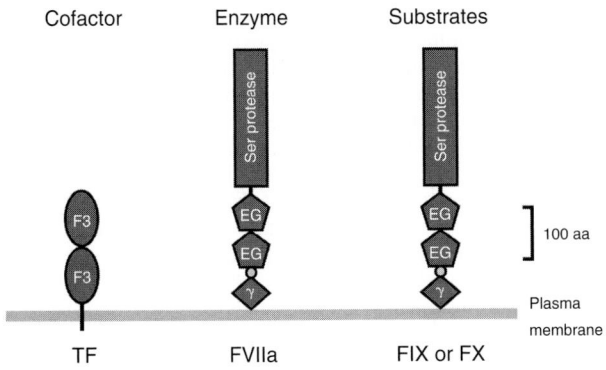

**FIGURE 5-3.** Schematic representation of the domain structure of tissue factor (TF), factor VII/VIIa (FVIIa), and factors IX and X (FIX and FX). The two fibronectin type III domains of TF are indicated as *F3*. The Gla domains of factors VII, IX, and X are indicated by γ, whereas the epidermal growth factor (EGF)–like domains are indicated by *EG* and the serine protease domains by *Ser Protease*. The aromatic stack is indicated by a small circle between the Gla and EGF domains. aa, amino acids.

serine (32). Deletion of the cytoplasmic domain has no discernible effect on TF procoagulant activity (31), making its role in blood clotting unclear, but there is increasing evidence that the cytoplasmic domain of TF may be important in some of the nonhemostatic roles of TF (see the section, "Nonhemostatic Functions for Tissue Factor and Factor VII").

TF has been purified from human brain and placenta using factor VII affinity chromatography (25,33) or, more conveniently, using monoclonal antibody-based immunoaffinity chromatography (34,35). Much larger quantities of TF can be obtained by expressing the recombinant protein in eukaryotic or prokaryotic expression systems (28). Purified TF can readily be reconstituted into phospholipid vesicles by using a variety of techniques (36–38). A water-soluble form of TF consisting of the isolated extracellular domain also has been produced (39). Soluble TF has proved useful in a large number of studies of structure and function because it is easy to produce and handle.

Several groups have determined the x-ray crystal structures of human and rabbit soluble TF (40–44). Soluble TF is an elongated and apparently rather rigid molecule in which the two fibronectin type III domains are joined at an angle of approximately 120 degrees. In addition, the x-ray crystal structures of the complex of soluble TF and factor VIIa have also been determined (discussed in the section, "Structure of the TF:VIIa Complex"). Further reference to crystal structures of TF and factor VII may be found at http://www.tf7.org/xray.htm.

## SITES OF TISSUE FACTOR EXPRESSION: NORMAL AND PATHOLOGIC

TF, being an integral membrane protein, is mainly found on the surface of cells in which it is synthesized. TF is abundant in a variety of cell types distributed throughout the body, including adventitial cells surrounding all blood vessels larger than capillaries; differentiating keratinocytes in the skin; and a number of epithelial cell types, including those present in mucous membranes and many organ capsules (45–47). The distribution of TF can be rationalized by the requirement that it be present throughout the body, ready to trigger the clotting cascade at any time and place following vascular injury. This pattern of expression has been described as a protective

"hemostatic envelope" surrounding the vasculature, organ structures, and the entire organism (45). In addition, TF is relatively abundant at anatomic sites in which the risk—or the deleterious consequences—of bleeding are high, such as the renal glomerulus and throughout the brain (45,47).

Spontaneous bleeding in patients with hemophilia occurs most commonly in anatomic locations such as the skeletal muscle and the joints, which contain especially low levels of TF (45). It is possible that patients with hemophilia bleed at these locations because direct activation of factor X by low levels of TF:VIIa is insufficient for hemostasis, and they lack the amplification step provided when TF:VIIa activates factor IX. Conversely, patients with hemophilia do not tend to bleed excessively from superficial cuts, which may be explained by the abundance of TF in the skin—exposure of large amounts of TF should allow direct activation of factor X in quantities sufficient for hemostasis.

Under normal circumstances, TF is readily detectable only in adventitial cells within the blood vessel wall; TF antigen or messenger ribonucleic acid (mRNA) is usually undetectable in vascular smooth muscle and endothelial cells (45–47). Atherosclerotic plaques, however, contain significant levels of TF mRNA and antigen, which is associated with monocytes and smooth muscle cells within the plaque (46,48–51). (As described in the section, "Tissue Factor Gene: Structure and Regulation," synthesis of TF can be induced in monocytes and smooth muscle cells by a variety of cytokines and other inflammatory mediators.) TF antigen is also present in the acellular core of atheromas, most likely derived from cells that have undergone necrosis. TF in plaques can bind factor VIIa and is fully functional (50,51). In healthy arteries, TF is separated from the lumen of the blood vessel by both the intima (i.e., the endothelium and underlying basement membrane) and the media (i.e., multiple layers of vascular smooth muscle cells). In atherosclerosis, however, blood is protected from exposure to TF by only a thin monolayer of endothelial cells—a much more dangerous situation. It is generally accepted that myocardial infarction is triggered by rupture or fissure of atherosclerotic plaques in coronary arteries (52). These events expose TF to blood within the lumen of the artery, triggering the formation of a thrombus that may occlude the vessel. Similar mechanisms are likely to precipitate other forms of arterial thrombosis, such as ischemic stroke.

TF is expressed in a variety of malignancies, where it can lead to thrombotic disease (e.g., in Trousseau syndrome). This can be caused by the expression of TF by the tumor cells themselves, by infiltrating monocytes, or by stromal cells. The association of TF with malignancy and its role in tumor pathology is reviewed in detail by Fernandez et al. (53) and in Chapter 57.

Experiments using specific inhibitors of TF:VIIa have demonstrated that the coagulopathies associated with sepsis and septic shock are mediated by TF, and furthermore that TF:VIIa contributes directly to mortality in sepsis (54,55). Mice engineered to express very low levels of TF were protected against coagulopathy and mortality following challenge with bacterial endotoxin, and this was true even when low TF expression was limited to hematopoietic cells (56). These studies underscore the importance of monocyte TF in driving the life-threatening coagulopathy of sepsis.

## TISSUE FACTOR GENE: STRUCTURE AND REGULATION

Located on chromosome 1 at p21-22 (24,57), the TF gene (locus abbreviation, *F3*) spans 12.4 kb and contains six exons interrupted by five introns (58). The first exon contains the 5′ noncoding sequence of the mRNA and also encodes the signal peptide, which directs the protein to the membrane and which is removed during biosynthesis. The first exon is located within a CpG island, a GC-rich deoxyribonucleic acid (DNA) region approximately 1 kb long that contains an unusually high density of CpG codons. The next four exons encode the extracellular domain, whereas the sixth exon encodes the transmembrane and cytoplasmic domains. The sixth exon also contains the relatively long 3' noncoding sequence, which is unusual because it includes an Alu-family repeat sequence that persists in the mature mRNA. The mRNA for TF is approximately 2.3 kb long, although in some cell types such as monocytes, minor amounts of a larger TF mRNA species (approximately 3.1 kb) are also observed (24). The longer mRNA retains the first intron and it is thought not to encode an active protein (59,60).

Another alternatively spliced form of TF mRNA, initially discovered in certain leukemia cells, lacks the fifth exon (61). If translated, it would encode a TF protein lacking a portion of the extracellular domain (normally encoded by exon 5) that is replaced by a novel amino acid sequence derived from reading exon 6 out of frame. Bogdanov et al. (62) have identified this alternatively spliced TF mRNA in a variety of normal cell types and have also discovered that the protein product of this alternatively spliced TF mRNA can be detected at low levels in plasma as an apparently soluble protein (discussed in the section, "Blood-Borne Tissue Factor").

The TF gene is inducible in a variety of cultured cells. Quiescent fibroblasts in the dermis have no detectable TF antigen (45), and serum-starved fibroblasts in culture also do not express TF. When cultured quiescent fibroblasts are stimulated with serum or with various mitogenic cytokines, transcription of the TF gene is rapidly induced (63,64).

Expression of TF on the surface of activated monocytes and macrophages is an important effector function of these cells in inflammation. Monocytes isolated from peripheral blood usually have undetectable levels of TF but will express this protein strongly after stimulation with bacterial endotoxin or certain other inflammatory mediators (65,66). This directly parallels the observation that TF is expressed in circulating monocytes following intravenous administration of endotoxin or bacteria (67). Furthermore, leukocytes (in particular, monocytes) have been shown to mediate the Schwartzman reaction in endotoxin-stimulated animals (68). As with fibroblasts, the primary level of regulation of TF gene expression in monocytes is transcriptional (69). In addition, endotoxin treatment of monocytes prolongs the half-life of TF mRNA (59).

A number of studies have focused on the regulation of TF gene expression in established cell lines of the monocytic lineage, and, in general, the findings of these studies resemble those of freshly isolated monocytes (65,66). A notable difference, however, is that established cell lines from the myeloblastic lineage frequently express TF constitutively, whereas peripheral blood monocytes express undetectable (or extremely low) quantities of TF antigen or mRNA. Again, this resembles the situation *in vivo*, in which certain leukemic cells express TF (70–72). The presence of circulating, TF-expressing leukemic cells is associated with the development of disseminated intravascular coagulation.

In cell culture, vascular endothelial cells can be induced to express TF robustly in response to a variety of inducers, including interleukin-1, tumor necrosis factor-α, and bacterial endotoxin (65,66). *In vivo*, however, TF is expressed during severe sepsis by endothelial cells in only a few, highly restricted areas, such as in the splenic microvasculature (73). This suggests that additional factors, which are not necessarily replicated *in vivo* during sepsis, may govern TF expression in cultured endothelial cells. Endothelial expression of TF has been observed *in vivo* in other conditions, including placental villitis (74) and graft rejection (75,76).

In addition to studies with fibroblasts, monocytes, and endothelial cells, induction of TF gene expression has been studied in other cell types, including vascular smooth muscle cells and keratinocytes (65,66). A variety of agents that are capable of inducing TF expression have been identified (77). Transcriptional control of TF gene expression has been studied in several cell types, including monocytic cells, fibroblasts, and vascular endothelial and smooth muscle cells. These studies have identified transcription factor binding sites flanking the promoter of the TF gene: Sp1 sites are important in basal transcription of the TF gene, whereas Egr-1 sites, AP-1 sites (binding c-Fos/c-Jun heterodimers), and a nuclear factor kappa B (NFκB) site (binding c-Rel/p65 heterodimers) are important in inducible expression of TF in response to bacterial endotoxin, serum, or phorbol ester, depending upon the cell type (78). TF gene expression is also induced by hypoxia in several cell types (79).

# FACTOR VII PROTEIN STRUCTURE

Factor VII, a glycosylated plasma protein, consists of a single polypeptide chain of 406 amino acids and has an overall molecular weight of approximately 50,000 Da (9,80,81). Synthesized by the liver, it circulates in plasma at a concentration of approximately 500 ng per mL (10 nM) (82). The domain structure of factor VII is depicted in Figure 5-3. Starting with the amino-terminus of the protein, it consists of the γ-carboxyglutamic acid–rich domain (Gla domain), the hydrophobic or aromatic stack, two epidermal growth factor (EGF)–like domains, and the serine protease domain. Complementary DNA and genomic cloning has revealed that factor VII has the same domain structure as factors IX, X, and protein C; shares considerable sequence homology with these coagulation serine proteases; and has a similar gene organization of introns and exons (83,84) (see Chapter 3).

Typical of vitamin K–dependent coagulation proteins, factor VII is synthesized with a signal peptide on its amino-terminus that directs the protein to the endoplasmic reticulum for secretion, followed by a propeptide that directs the cell to modify glutamic acid residues in the Gla domain. The signal and propeptides are removed before secretion. Two types of complementary DNA clones for human factor VII have been identified, one of which has an additional 22 amino acids in the propeptide (83). Products of alternative splicing, these two forms of factor VII mRNA encode identical mature protein and appear to be functionally equivalent.

Factor VII contains 10 γ-carboxyglutamic acid residues in its Gla domain, resulting from vitamin K–dependent modification of glutamic acid residues during biosynthesis. As with other vitamin K–dependent coagulation proteins, these γ-carboxyglutamic acid residues are essential for activity. Specifically, the Gla domain confers on factor VII the ability to bind, in a reversible and $Ca^{2+}$-dependent manner, to membranes containing negatively charged phospholipids. In the crystal structure of the TF:VIIa complex, the Gla domain contains seven bound $Ca^{2+}$ (85).

The aromatic stack of factor VII is a short amino acid sequence containing a small cluster of aromatic residues. It is adjacent to the Gla domain and, although encoded by a separate exon, is classified by some investigators as a part of the Gla domain. The two EGF domains have a typical growth factor fold and a disulfide-bonding pattern. The first EGF domain binds a single $Ca^{2+}$ with relatively high affinity (85,86), whereas the second EGF domain does not bind $Ca^{2+}$. The first EGF domain of bovine factor VII contains the modified amino acid, β-hydroxyaspartic acid, whereas this modification is absent in human factor VII (87).

The serine protease domain of factor VII is homologous to the digestive enzymes trypsin and chymotrypsin and exhibits trypsinlike substrate specificity (i.e., a preference for cleaving peptide bonds after arginine or lysine). It has a typical serine protease catalytic triad composed of His193, Asp242, and Ser344. As with many other coagulation serine proteases, the protease domain of factor VII binds a single $Ca^{2+}$ (85,88). The protease domain also binds zinc ions, which inhibit factor VIIa enzymatic activity (89,90).

Zymogen factor VII is converted to factor VIIa, the enzymatically competent form, by proteolysis of a single peptide bond between Arg152 and Ile153. The result, factor VIIa, is composed of two polypeptide chains held together by a disulfide bond. The light chain of factor VIIa, consisting of the Gla domain, aromatic stack, and both EGF domains, has 152 amino acids and a molecular weight of approximately 20,000. The heavy chain, consisting of the serine protease domain, has 254 amino acids and a molecular weight of approximately 30,000. Unlike many other coagulation zymogens, factor VII does not release an activation peptide when converted to factor VIIa.

Factor VII contains two N-linked carbohydrate chains attached to residues Asn145 and Asn322 (87). It also contains two short, O-linked carbohydrate chains attached to the first EGF domain: glucose, glucose–xylose, or glucose–(xylose)$_2$ attached to Ser52; and a single fucose attached to Ser60 (91).

Factor VII can be purified from plasma using conventional chromatography (9,80,81) or immunoaffinity chromatography (92). Recombinant human factor VII has been produced in cultured mammalian cells (87). Truncated forms of factor VII have been produced in which the Gla domain has been removed (Gla-domainless factor VII) by limited proteolysis (93,94) or by expression of the truncated recombinant protein (95). Gla-domainless factor VII may or may not contain the aromatic stack, depending on the site of cleavage. Furthermore, a form of factor VII lacking both the Gla domain and the first EGF domain has also been produced recombinantly (96–98). This truncated form of factor VII fails to bind to TF (96). A factor VII mutant has been produced in which the activation cleavage site has been mutated so that it cannot be activated by its usual activators (99). This mutant has been used to demonstrate that zymogen factor VII had no detectable enzymatic activity. In addition, the active site, serine, of factor VII (Ser344) has been mutated to alanine, generating a form of factor VIIa without enzyme activity. This has been useful in investigating the conversion of factor VII to VIIa (14).

# STRUCTURE OF THE TISSUE FACTOR AND FACTOR VIIa COMPLEX

The x-ray crystal structure of the complex of soluble TF and active site–inhibited factor VIIa has been solved to a resolution of 2.0 Å (85), and the structure of a similar complex inhibited with a modified version of bovine pancreatic trypsin inhibitor has been solved to a resolution of 2.1 Å (100). The structure of TF in these complexes is almost identical to the structure determined from crystals of soluble TF alone, confirming the relative rigidity of this molecule. Within the complex, factor VIIa is a highly elongated protein that forms extended contacts with TF (see Fig. 5-4). The main sites of contact on factor VIIa are located in the first EGF domain and the protease domain, with additional points of contact within the second EGF domain and the aromatic stack region of the Gla domain. The sites of contact on TF are located on both fibronectin type III domains and the interfacial region between them.

Several studies have used domain swapping and site-directed mutagenesis to identify the binding sites on TF and factor

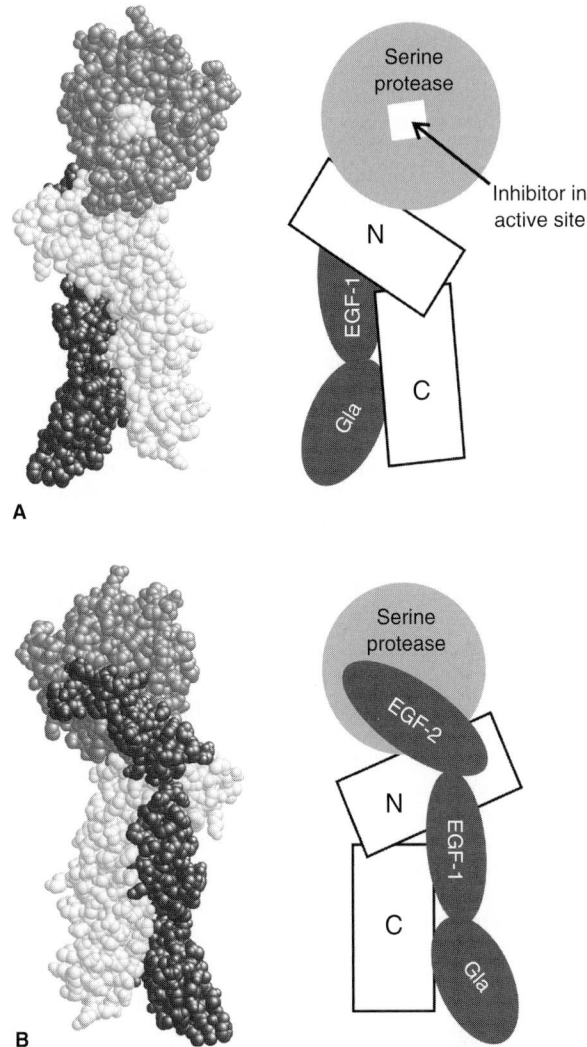

**FIGURE 5-4.** Two views of the x-ray crystal structure of the complex of soluble tissue factor (TF) and active site–inhibited factor VIIa (*left*), and diagrammatic representations of the domain organizations of TF and factor VIIa (*right*). **A:** "Front" view of the TF:VIIa complex, with the active site facing the viewer. **B:** "Back" view of the complex, with the active site facing away from the viewer. The membrane surface would be located at the bottom of each complex. TF is *white*, whereas factor VIIa is shown in *black* (light chain) and *gray* (heavy chain). In addition, the tripeptidylchlormethylketone inhibitor in the active site of factor VIIa is colored *white*. For the TF representation, N and C refer to the N-terminal and C-terminal fibronectin type III domains, respectively. For the factor VIIa representation, the Gla domain is labeled *Gla* and the epidermal growth factor–like domains are labeled *EGF-1* or *EGF-2*. The serine protease domain and the inhibitor are also labeled. The two views of the TF:VIIa complex were generated with the program RASMOL (101), using the atomic coordinates file 1DAN (85) from the Protein Data Bank. (From Sayle RA, Milner-White EJ. RASMOL: biomolecular graphics for all. *Trends Biochem Sci* 1995;20:374; Banner DW, D'Arcy A, Chène C, et al. The crystal structure of the complex of blood coagulation factor VIIa with soluble tissue factor. *Nature* 1996;380:41–46, with permission.)

VIIa that permit them to interact with each other (102–105). When analyzed in light of the crystal structure of the TF:VIIa complex, these studies have allowed the assessment of the contributions of individual amino acid side chains to the binding interactions within the TF:VIIa complex. This approach has revealed that some contacts are important for stabilizing the binding of TF to factor VIIa (chiefly with the first

EGF domain of factor VIIa), whereas others appear to be important in enhancing the enzymatic activity of factor VIIa (chiefly with the protease domain of factor VIIa). These findings are reviewed in detail elsewhere (104,105).

The portion of the Gla domain located at the bottom of the factor VIIa molecule (as shown in Fig. 5-4) contains three solvent-exposed hydrophobic residues that are proposed to be inserted into the hydrophobic core of the phospholipid bilayer. The carboxy terminus of soluble TF is also located near the bottom of the structure, as presented in Figure 5-4; in intact TF, this part of the molecule is linked to the membrane anchor by a short peptide sequence. Therefore, in the views given in Figure 5-4, the membrane surface should be located at the bottom of the complex, with TF linked to the membrane by its membrane-anchoring domain and with VIIa interacting with phospholipid head groups through the Gla domain. Fluorescence resonance energy transfer experiments indicate that the TF:VIIa complex is oriented almost perpendicular to the membrane, with the active site of factor VIIa located approximately 78 Å above the membrane surface (106,107).

# MODULATION OF FACTOR VIIa ACTIVITY BY TISSUE FACTOR

When factor VIIa binds to TF, its ability to catalyze the hydrolysis of small, peptidyl-amide or peptidyl-ester substrates is enhanced approximately 20-fold to 100-fold, depending upon the substrate (39,108–110). This is usually accomplished by an increase in the catalytic rate constant ($k_{cat}$) and, in some cases, by a decrease in the Michaelis-Menton constant ($K_m$). Binding of factor VIIa to TF causes changes within the active center for the enzyme because these substrates are far too small to make contacts with TF itself. TF therefore functions as an allosteric activator of factor VIIa.

Substrate hydrolysis by serine proteases is a multistep process (111), and the mechanism by which TF enhances the enzymatic activity of factor VIIa is not completely understood. Studies with a slowly hydrolyzed model substrate have shown that TF enhances the rate of substrate hydrolysis by factor VIIa chiefly by enhancing substrate affinity of factor VIIa rather than by altering the rates of any of the subsequent catalytic steps (112).

A wealth of structure–function studies combining site-directed mutagenesis and x-ray crystallography have enhanced the understanding of the allosteric activation of factor VIIa by TF (97,113), although many questions remain unanswered. Insights into the mechanism of allosteric activation of factor VIIa have also been obtained by designing mutants of factor VIIa that have enhanced enzymatic activity in the absence of TF (114–116). One of the most surprising results comes from the crystal structure of zymogen factor VII, which exhibits extensive β-strand reregistration relative to the crystal structures of factor VIIa (98).

Serine protease zymogens are converted to active enzymes by limited proteolysis. A key step is when the newly generated amino-terminus folds back into the protein to stabilize the oxyanion pocket (117). It has been hypothesized that free factor VIIa exists in two states in equilibrium with each other: one in which the protein is catalytically active and a second, zymogenlike state, in which the amino-terminus of the heavy chain is not properly folded back into the catalytic domain (118). There is some experimental evidence to support the view that the binding of factor VIIa to TF stabilizes factor VIIa in the catalytically active state (119). Surprisingly, however, in the crystal structure of factor VIIa obtained in the absence of TF or any inhibitor in the active site, the amino-terminus of the factor VII heavy chain was still folded back into the catalytic domain and the oxyanion pocket was intact (97).

Free factor VIIa proteolytically activates its major protein substrates, factors IX and X, extremely slowly. When factor VIIa binds to TF that has been incorporated into suitable phospholipid vesicles, its activity is enhanced many thousand-fold (120–122). (Factors IX and X will bind to phospholipid vesicles only if they contain negatively charged phospholipids, most particularly phosphatidylserine. Therefore, TF is most often reconstituted into vesicles containing a mixture of phosphatidylserine and the neutral phospholipid, phosphatidylcholine.) There are three main reasons for this rate enhancement. First, the reversible binding of factors IX and X to phospholipid surfaces raises the concentration of these substrates in the vicinity of the enzyme TF:VIIa, which reduces the apparent $K_m$. Second, TF is an allosteric activator of factor VIIa enzymatic activity. Third, TF appears to provide an extended binding site (exosite) for macromolecular substrates, which was identified by site-directed mutagenesis studies (95,123,124).

The fact that most coagulation reactions are restricted to two-dimensional surfaces substantially complicates the interpretation of their enzyme kinetics (125–127). In addition, coagulation reactions can occur *in vivo* under conditions of stasis or under conditions of considerable blood flow. Andress and Nemerson have published extensively on the effects of flow on the kinetics of factor X activation by the TF:VIIa complex (128).

It has long been known that resting, intact cells have much lower procoagulant activity than do cells that have been damaged, lysed, or treated with calcium ionophore (129). Although present on the surface of intact cells, TF becomes fully active only when the membrane properties of the cell are altered (130,131). There are several potential explanations for this phenomenon. The first is that most cells restrict the distribution of aminophospholipids (such as phosphatidylserine) to the inner leaflet of the plasma membrane (132). Exposure of negatively charged phospholipids on the outer leaflet is necessary for efficient binding of substrate (i.e., factor IX or X), so the membrane asymmetry of intact cells will tend to limit the activity of TF. When cells are lysed, damaged, or treated with calcium ionophore, phospholipid asymmetry is lost, resulting in the exposure of phosphatidylserine and phosphatidylethanolamine on the outer leaflet of the plasma membrane, thereby enhancing the activity of TF:VIIa. Another potential explanation in some cell types is that TF may associate with caveolae, areas of the cell surface with altered lipid composition (133,134). Finally, it has been proposed that dimerization or oligomerization of TF in the membrane may reduce its activity and that damage or lysis of cells may foster the formation of TF monomers with enhanced activity (135).

TF:VIIa has an extremely restricted substrate specificity; its main natural substrates appear to be factors VII, IX, and X. Factor X is the favored substrate under most *in vitro* conditions, although activation reactions taking place on intact cells can show a preference for either factor IX or factor X (122,136–138). The reasons for this are not clear. When factor IX is activated, two peptide bonds must be cleaved. TF:VIIa complex catalyzes the cleavage of one of these bonds (i.e., at Arg180) more efficiently than the other (i.e., at Arg145), and, furthermore, factor Xa and TF:VIIa complex can synergize to activate factor IX to IXa more efficiently (139).

Factor VII is a substrate for factor VIIa (140) in an autoactivation reaction enhanced by TF (14). This reaction requires that the TF:VIIa and TF:VII complexes encounter each other by lateral diffusion in the plane of the membrane (15). Factor VIIa can also catalyze the activation of factor VII on sphingosine-containing phospholipids in the absence of TF (141). Autoactivation of factor VII might be important in initiating the clotting cascade, although its precise role is yet to be elucidated.

TF:VIIa complex can catalyze the proteolysis of factors V and VIII at multiple peptide bonds (142,143). The physiologic significance of this is unclear, but it may represent a pathway for inactivation of factors V and VIII that does not require them to go through an active cofactor intermediate.

# INHIBITION OF TISSUE FACTOR AND FACTOR VIIa COMPLEX

Although free factor VIIa is essentially unreactive with any plasma protease inhibitor, two plasma inhibitors are capable of reacting with factor VIIa in the TF:VIIa complex: tissue factor pathway inhibitor (TFPI) and antithrombin (formerly known as *antithrombin III*). TFPI is composed of three Kunitz-type protease inhibitor domains, the first of which reacts with the active site of factor VIIa (but only when factor VIIa is bound to TF) (144,145). The affinity of TFPI alone for TF:VIIa complex is rather low but is enhanced by heparin (146,147). The second Kunitz domain of TFPI reacts with the active site of factor Xa, inhibiting it and enhancing the ability of TFPI to inhibit the TF:VIIa complex [reviewed by Broze (148)]. The result is a fully inhibited tetramolecular complex (TF:VIIa: TFPI:Xa). In addition to blocking the enzymatic activity of TF:VIIa, TFPI also promotes the internalization and degradation of TF:VIIa complex on the cell surface (96,149). Antithrombin can react with factor VIIa only when it is bound to TF, and the reaction rate is slow in the absence of heparin (3). TFPI-2 (which is related to TFPI) also inhibits the TF:VIIa complex (150). The roles of TFPI and antithrombin are reviewed in greater detail in Chapter 13.

Several artificial inhibitors of TF:VIIa complex have been developed. These include a potent inhibitor consisting of the light chain of factor Xa linked to the first Kunitz domain of TFPI (151), and other Kunitz-type inhibitors that have been engineered for increased reactivity with TF:VIIa (152,153). An inhibitor with enhanced potency for factor VIIa was created by linking a modified Kunitz-type inhibitor with a mutated form of soluble TF (154). In addition, an inhibitor that targets TF:VIIa complex, termed *NAPc2*, has been cloned from hookworms (155) and is being evaluated in clinical studies as a novel antithrombotic agent (156). Blocking antibodies to TF or factor VIIa have been utilized in animal models of sepsis and thrombosis, in which they reduce the severity of coagulopathy or thrombosis (54,157–159). Active site–blocked factor VIIa (factor VIIai) has also been successfully used as a selective inhibitor of TF function in animal models of thrombotic disease (55,160–163). Novel peptide inhibitors that bind to exosites on factor VII/VIIa and allosterically inhibit factor VIIa have been reported (164). Several studies have reported that blocking TF:VIIa complex is effective in decreasing thrombosis without causing bleeding side effects associated with other antithrombotic agents (162,165–167). This suggests that inhibitors directed at TF or factor VII may have advantages over conventional antithrombotic drugs, an area that will doubtless continue to be the subject of considerable research interest in the future. Indeed, several lead compounds for the development of small molecule inhibitors of TF:VIIa have recently been reported (167–169).

# DIAGNOSTIC AND THERAPEUTIC USES OF TISSUE FACTOR AND FACTOR VIIa

The commonly employed prothrombin time (PT) clotting assay uses a source of TF as the procoagulant agent. Typically, PT reagents are made from homogenates of brain, lung, or placenta (of human, rabbit, or bovine origin) and are often referred to as *thromboplastins*. Because these reagents have varying amounts of TF, phospholipids, and contaminants, they have varying potencies. A major application of the PT assay is to monitor dosage for oral anticoagulant therapy, but the results obtained with this assay may vary according to the sensitivity of the thromboplastin reagents. To control for differing thromboplastin sensitivities, a standardization system for these reagents has been developed—the international sensitivity index (ISI), which is used in conjunction with a normalization method, and the international normalized ratio (INR) for reporting prolongations of the PT in patients receiving oral anticoagulant therapy (170). Recombinant thromboplastin reagents are now commercially available that are made from purified, recombinant TF that has been reconstituted into phospholipid vesicles. Because the recombinant reagents have a defined composition, their ISI values can be adjusted readily by the manufacturer to more closely resemble international reference standards for thromboplastins (171).

A clotting test has been developed that uses soluble TF in place of full-length TF (6) to measure trace levels of circulating factor VIIa. This assay takes advantage of the fact that soluble TF does not promote the conversion of factor VII to VIIa (172), so clotting times are dependent upon the preexisting levels of plasma factor VIIa.

Soluble TF has also been used as an experimental antineoplastic agent. In this approach, soluble TF is linked to targeting molecules in order to deliver it to tumor vasculature, where it can kill tumors by infarction (173).

Recombinant human factor VIIa has been developed for use as a pharmaceutical agent, termed *eptacog alfa*, and has been marketed under the brand names NovoSeven or NiaStase. It is approved for use in treating bleeding episodes in patients with hemophilia who have intractable inhibitors (blocking antibodies) to factor VIII and who therefore fail to respond to factor VIII replacement therapy (174). It is also being investigated as a more general hemostatic agent (175). High levels of plasma factor VIIa permit the bypass of the factor VIIIa/IXa part of the clotting cascade in a manner that is not fully understood. High levels of factor VIIa may do this by enhancing the activity of TF that is exposed at sites of vascular injury or by directly activating factor X (especially in the presence of negatively charged phospholipids at the site of injury) in a TF-independent manner (176).

# ROLES OF FACTOR VII/VIIa AND TISSUE FACTOR IN PROTHROMBOTIC STATES

The blood clotting system is composed of a large number of hemostatic factors that can be subdivided into procoagulant, anticoagulant, and fibrinolytic arms. Ideally, all of these factors act in a balanced fashion so that blood clots are formed only for the purpose of stopping blood loss following injury. It is widely appreciated that certain hereditary conditions and disease states can predispose individuals to episodes of thrombosis. The altered balance of hemostatic factors in such individuals is often called *prothrombotic* or *hypercoagulable* state. Thrombosis is typically a multifactorial disease. Accordingly, alterations in the quantity or activity of a number of different hemostatic factors—including factor VII and TF—have been reported to be associated with altered risk of thrombotic disease.

Several methodologies exist for measuring plasma factor VII levels, including measurements of total factor VII mass (factor VII + VIIa), factor VII coagulant activity (FVII:C), or factor VIIa. Total factor VII mass is typically quantified by measuring factor VII antigen levels (FVII:Ag) (177) or by the coupled amidolytic assay (FVII:Am), an activity assay in which factor VII is quantitatively converted to factor VIIa (178). FVII:C assays measure the procoagulant activity of factor VII in a plasma sample in a clot-based assay. Because some of the factor VII is converted to VIIa during the test, FVII:C assays measure an aggregate of both factor VII and factor VIIa (179,180). The relative sensitivities of FVII:C assays to factor VII versus VIIa varies according to the way the assay is performed (181). Factor VIIa levels can be measured in several ways: a soluble TF-based clotting assay that measures the levels of enzymatically active factor VIIa in plasma (6), an enzyme-linked immunosorbent assay (ELISA) based on an antipeptide antibody that binds to the newly formed carboxy terminus of the factor VIIa light chain (182), or a commercial ELISA that measures the levels of active factor VIIa capable of reacting with a biotinylated enzyme inhibitor. These assays give somewhat different results, for reasons that are not entirely clear at the present time.

Elevated level of plasma factor VII (measured in a variety of ways) was initially identified as a risk factor for thrombotic disease in several epidemiologic studies. The studies include two large, prospective studies [Northwick Park Heart Study and the Prospective Cardiovascular Münster (PROCAM) study] reporting that elevated factor VII:C was a risk factor for ischemic heart disease (183,184), particularly when fatal events were analyzed in long-term follow-up (185). Other epidemiologic studies have reported correlations between elevated plasma factor VII:C or VIIa levels and angina pectoris, transient ischemic attacks, diabetes, uremia, and peripheral vascular disease (186–195). These studies are complicated by the fact that the activation state of plasma factor VII is influenced by plasma lipid levels (17,18,196,197).

On the other hand, several studies have failed to find a relation between factor VII levels and thrombotic disease (198, 199). This may be due, at least in part, to the fact that different methods for measuring factor VII:C have been employed, which exhibit different sensitivities to factor VII versus VIIa (200–202). Elevated plasma factor VIIa levels have been proposed to cause the formation of larger thrombi following plaque rupture (179,185). In this view, factor VIIa levels might not be related to the development of atherosclerosis or to the frequency of coronary events, but such levels might be important in determining whether a thrombus will be large enough to occlude the blood vessel. Indeed, population studies have reported that factor VII levels are unrelated to the degree of carotid artery thickness or other manifestations of vascular disease (203–207).

Several studies have directly investigated the relation between plasma factor VIIa levels and risk of thrombotic disease. Some studies have found significant positive correlations (208), whereas a few have found significant negative correlations (209,210) between plasma factor VIIa levels and risk of thrombotic disease in different study populations. In some studies, factor VIIa levels were found to be significantly related to the risk of thrombotic disease only in women (208,209). The relation between variation in plasma factor VIIa levels and risk of thrombotic disease is therefore currently unclear.

Naturally occurring polymorphisms have been identified in the factor VII gene. This includes a substitution of Gln for Arg353 in the protease domain of factor VII (211) as well as mutations in the promoter region of the gene (212–215). These polymorphisms are associated with variation in factor VII levels, and, furthermore, some of these markers are in strong linkage disequilibrium with each other (199,214,216). Some studies (217) have found factor VII genotype to be associated with thrombotic risk, but others (218,219) have not

obtained similar results, and this area remains controversial (199,216).

# BLOOD-BORNE TISSUE FACTOR

TF antigen has been detected at low levels in plasma and urine, and these levels increase significantly in certain pathologic states, such as disseminated intravascular coagulation, thrombotic thrombocytopenic purpura, diabetic microangiopathy, glomerulonephritis, and certain leukemias (220–223). Studies have been undertaken to identify individuals whose monocytes respond especially strongly to endotoxin challenge by expressing TF as a potential marker for hypercoagulability or tumor progression (224,225). Functional assays have demonstrated the presence of active TF in whole blood (although at low levels). Whole blood TF activity levels increase following endotoxin challenge and in other settings in which intravascular activation of the blood clotting system can occur, such as sickle cell disease (226–228).

Giesen et al. (229) reported that TF-containing microparticles, along with monocytes and granulocytes that were positive for TF antigen, accumulated in thrombi formed *ex vivo* by flowing blood over collagen-coated surfaces. Because the perfusions lasted only 5 minutes, there was clearly insufficient time for *de novo* synthesis of TF by leukocytes, and therefore this protein must have come from a preexisting source. Furthermore, these studies suggested that blood-borne TF may play an important role in thrombus formation. Subsequent studies from the same laboratory (230) and other studies have continued to demonstrate that blood-borne TF can be detected at low levels in blood and that it appears to accumulate in thrombi, where it can play an active role in thrombus propagation [reviewed by Morrissey (231), Morel et al. (232), and Giesen and Nemerson (233)].

The source of blood-borne TF is currently a matter of intense research. The TF-bearing microparticles shed from leukocytes seem to be a likely source. Monocytes are capable of synthesizing TF following exposure to inflammatory mediators, but low levels of leukocyte TF expression in nonpathologic settings could contribute to blood-borne TF microparticles. TF has been reported to exist in multiple forms intravascularly—as a soluble protein; as a membrane protein in microparticles; and on the surface of, or within, monocytes, granulocytes, and platelets (229,234–239). Not all of these reports agree with each other and, in particular, the results about the presence of TF in platelets and granulocytes is controversial (240–242). TF-bearing membrane particles could bind to the surface of granulocytes and platelets by adhesive receptors. TF in granulocytes could also result from phagocytosis of membrane fragments derived from other cell types. Transfer of TF-bearing microparticles between various blood cell types (especially between monocytes, platelets, and granulocytes) has been well documented in several studies, and there appear to be multiple mechanisms by which this can take place (236,243,244).

Recently, it has been reported that an alternatively spliced, soluble form of TF is present at low levels in plasma, and, furthermore, that it can become incorporated into growing thrombi *in vivo* and *ex vivo* (62). It is unclear how much procoagulant activity alternatively spliced TF has, but this intriguing finding suggests an alternative source of blood-borne TF that could play a role in hemostasis and thrombosis.

There are many questions surrounding blood-borne TF that remain to be answered. Where does it come from? How is it activated and incorporated into growing thrombi? How can incorporation of blood-borne TF into growing thrombi be controlled so that it does not cause the unregulated expansion of blood clots?

# HEREDITARY DEFICIENCIES IN TISSUE FACTOR

Human deficiencies in TF have not been reported, leading to the presumption that TF is essential for life. When the TF gene was inactivated in mice, heterozygotes were normal and healthy but the homozygous TF-null mice died between days E8.5 and E11.5 of embryonic development (245–247). The TF-null embryos exhibited abnormalities in the yolk sac vasculature by approximately day E9.5, and their death was attributed to bleeding from both embryonic and extraembryonic vessels (245,246) and subsequent wasting owing to insufficiency in vitelloembryonic circulation (247). Some investigators have suggested that these developmental abnormalities may be caused by a nonhemostatic role of TF that is essential for normal blood vessel development (248). Evidence supporting an involvement of TF:VIIa complex in cell signaling and angiogenesis is discussed in the section, "Nonhemostatic Functions for Tissue Factor and Factor VII." Interestingly, genetic background influences the morbidity of TF-null mice: In a 129/Sv background, all TF-null embryos died by midgestation, whereas in a C57BL/6 background, two populations of null embryos were observed, one that died at midgestation and another that died at birth (249). The latter population appears normal before birth, and one TF-null pup that was delivered by cesarean section lived for 4 weeks before dying from intracranial hemorrhage. The authors of the report of this latter study concluded that TF was essential for allowing the mice to survive the hemostatic challenges at midgestation and the trauma of birth (249).

Although TF-null mice die during embryogenesis, mice in which only the cytoplasmic domain of TF has been deleted develop normally and show no bleeding tendency (250,251). In addition, fibroblasts from these mice show normal signal transduction when factor VIIa binds to the mutant TF. On the other hand, these mice have reduced immunoinflammatory responses, macrophage function, and susceptibility to arthritis (252); and they have blunted leukocyte responses to bacterial endotoxin challenge and decreased susceptibility to death from endotoxemia (253).

TF-null mice can be rescued by using a human TF "minigene" that is expressed at only 1% the level of the endogenous murine TF gene (254). These low-TF mice develop normally but have shorter life spans than do wild-type mice. Female low-TF mice may have fatal bleeding episodes during pregnancy. Examination of the cause of premature death in low-TF mice revealed frequent cases of spontaneous hemorrhage, deposition of hemosiderin, and fibrosis in cardiac tissue (255). These mice show impaired heart contractility, which, although insufficient to induce heart failure, may contribute to the shortened life span and hemorrhage-associated death observed in these animals. Interestingly, mice engineered to express extremely low levels of factor VII also show significant hemosiderin and fibrosis in their hearts (255). Mice lacking the cytoplasmic tail of TF did not exhibit the same phenotype as low-TF mice, again excluding a role for the cytoplasmic tail in the fibrosis and early death associated with low-TF mice. TF levels are much higher in cardiac muscle than in skeletal muscle (45), suggesting that TF plays a role in protecting the myocardium from ongoing vascular damage and subsequent hemorrhage. Interestingly, TF has been implicated in cardiomyopathy as a result of increased expression of mRNA and antigen in cardiomyocytes during myocardial ischemia (256). TF-dependent thrombin generation could contribute to the inflammatory response by increasing chemokine expression and by recruiting neutrophils.

# HEREDITARY DEFICIENCIES IN FACTOR VII

Hereditary deficiency in factor VII is a rare, recessive autosomal disorder in humans (257). Individuals with severe factor VII deficiency may exhibit life-threatening bleeding episodes, although the correlation between factor VII:C levels and bleeding tendency is not particularly strong. In rare instances, persons with factor VII deficiency have even exhibited thrombotic tendencies. The molecular basis for inherited factor VII deficiency has been determined for a number of individuals, resulting in the identification of a variety of nonsense, missense, and splice-site mutations throughout the factor VII coding region, as well as a few small deletions and at least one mutation in the promoter region that causes reduced factor VII levels. An extensive list of known factor VII mutations in humans is maintained by Dr. John McVey at http://193.60.222.13/.

Factor VII–deficient mice have been produced by targeted disruption of the factor VII gene (258). These mice develop normally *in utero* but die neonatally from massive hemorrhaging. This finding parallels that of a splice-site mutation in the human factor VII gene, which results in an in-frame deletion of the region encoding the first EGF domain of factor VII in the mature mRNA (259). A human infant who is homozygous for this mutation had no detectable plasma factor VII activity and no developmental abnormalities, but died from severe postnatal bleeding. Taken together, these results indicate that a total lack of factor VII is not compatible with life.

The difference in phenotype between the TF-null and factor VII–null mice (i.e., embryonic lethality with developmental abnormalities versus postnatal lethality without developmental problems) is, on the face of it, puzzling. More recent studies have shown that factor VII–null embryos are apparently kept alive *in utero* because of leakage of small amounts of maternal factor VII across the placenta. Factor VII binds to TF with a $K_d$ of less than 30 pM (260,261), which is far lower than the plasma concentration of factor VII (approximately 10 nM), so even minuscule levels of maternally transferred factor VII could keep an embryo alive until birth. In mouse studies using mothers engineered to express extremely low levels of factor VII, the factor VII–null embryos died *in utero* and phenotypically resembled TF-null embryos (Elliot Rosen, personal communication).

# NONHEMOSTATIC FUNCTIONS FOR TISSUE FACTOR AND FACTOR VII

## Tissue Factor as a Signal Transducer

A role for TF as a signaling molecule is now well documented and appears unconnected to its role in coagulation. Initial reports established that binding of factor VIIa to TF evoked intracellular calcium responses in a variety of cell types (262,263). These observations were followed by reports of phosphorylation of several mitogen-activating protein (MAP) kinases, such as p38 and JNK, in response to binding of factor VIIa to TF (264,265). Activation of the Src family members, c-Src, Lyn, and Yes, by TF:VIIa complex in fibroblasts triggers activation of the downstream GTPases Rac and Cdc42 by phosphatidylinositol 3-kinase (266), ultimately resulting in p38 MAP kinase activation and cytoskeletal reorganization. Interestingly, these responses depend on the catalytic activity of factor VII because factor VIIai (which binds tightly to TF but which has no enzymatic activity) or blocking anti-TF antibodies abolish these effects (263–265,267).

A number of genes are upregulated in response to factor VIIa binding to TF, including genes involved in transcription and mRNA processing, such as poly(A) polymerase (268) and Egr-1 (265). Microarray analysis of the transcriptional profile of keratinocytes and fibroblasts upon association of factor VIIa and TF (267,269) demonstrated increases in mRNA levels for growth factors like connective tissue growth factor and fibroblast growth factor-5 and for inflammatory cytokines such as interleukin-1$\beta$ and interleukin-8. Several of these genes encode proteins involved in cellular reorganization and migration [e.g., Cyr61 (267) and collagenases 1 and 3 (269)]. Upregulation of the urinary-type plasminogen activator receptor (uPAR) by TF:VIIa complex has been documented in a pancreatic cancer cell line and in keratinocytes (269,270). The urokinase/uPAR system contributes to tumor invasion by facilitating matrix degradation and cell migration. The pattern of genes upregulated in response to factor VIIa binding to TF highlights a role for this system in wound healing, tissue repair, and cancer metastasis.

The mechanism by which occupation of TF by VIIa leads to intracellular signaling is the subject of intense research. TF has a short cytoplasmic domain, so it has been proposed that signaling by TF:VIIa likely involves an additional receptor. The absolute requirement for enzymatically active factor VIIa strongly suggests that signal transduction occurs by proteolysis of members of the protease-activated receptor (PAR) family. Indeed, there is a growing body of evidence that TF:VIIa can transduce signals by activation of PAR-1 and PAR-2 (271,272). However, TF:VIIa readily activates downstream coagulation proteases, such as factors IXa and Xa, and, indirectly, thrombin. Because some of these proteases are potent PAR activators, it has been a matter of some speculation whether TF:VIIa directly or indirectly activates PARs. Some groups have reported that factor X is required to generate an intracellular response through TF:VIIa (273,274). Riewald and Ruf (274) have proposed that newly activated factor X remains bound to TF:VIIa long enough for it to be presented within a ternary TF:VIIa:Xa complex to PARs. Factor Xa in this transient ternary complex is therefore proposed to activate PAR-1 and PAR-2 more efficiently than either TF:VIIa or factor Xa alone. One report has shown that the combination of factor VIIa and factor Xa, but not factor VIIa alone, strongly induced migration of breast cancer cells by MAP kinase phosphorylation (275). On the other hand, certain studies have employed specific factor Xa inhibitors, such as tick anticoagulant protein (TAP), or thrombin inhibitors, such as hirudin, in their experiments to show that neither factor Xa nor thrombin is necessary for TF signaling (264,276,277). These differences in apparent mechanism could potentially arise from the use of different cell types or different concentrations of factor VIIa. (In fact, a criticism of some studies on TF:VIIa signaling is the use of factor VIIa concentrations that are far in excess of the physiologic factor VII concentration in plasma. But other studies have employed factor VIIa at concentrations that are closer to those that can occur *in vivo*.)

Both TF and PAR-2 are specifically upregulated in response to inflammatory stimuli (278,279). Ahamed and Ruf (280) showed that phosphorylation of the TF cytoplasmic domain was induced by PAR-2 but not PAR-1 upon ternary TF:VIIa:Xa complex formation. In accordance with other reports (281), protein kinase C $\alpha$ was a prerequisite for Ser258 phosphorylation. Other coagulation proteases failed to induce phosphorylation of the TF cytoplasmic domain in endothelial cells, suggesting that PAR-2 activation distinguishes between upstream and downstream coagulation protease signaling. PAR-2 activation stimulates the Rac pathway and formation of a complex of $\beta$-arrestin and extracellular signal–regulated kinase (ERK) (282,283), which promotes cell motility. The reported effects of PAR-2 and TF suggest that these systems could act in concert to control cell migration. Indeed, it was recently demonstrated that binding of TF to factor VIIa resulted in increased cell migration in a breast cancer cell line because of specific upregulation of interleukin-8 through PAR-2 (284). Activation of PAR-2 required only TF:VIIa and not the formation of the ternary TF:VIIa:Xa complex, although the effect was potentiated by factor Xa at low factor VIIa concentrations. Interestingly, activation of PAR-2 by TF:VIIa failed to induce intracellular $Ca^{2+}$ mobilization, whereas $Ca^{2+}$ mobilization *was* observed when PAR-2 was activated with the PAR-2 agonist peptide or trypsin. Despite mechanistic differences, these reports show reciprocal activation of TF and PAR-2 and indicate a role for both TF and PAR-2 in the regulation of cell migration.

The function of the cytoplasmic domain of TF in signaling is not completely defined. It is not essential for induction of gene expression by TF:VIIa (269), but both intra- and extracellular domains of TF are required for the prometastatic function of TF, at least in some model systems (285,286). Serine residues in the cytoplasmic tail of TF are phosphorylated by protein kinase C–mediated events (32). Chimeric molecules, generated from extracellular and transmembrane parts of the interleukin-2 receptor and the cytoplasmic domain of TF, interacted with actin-binding protein-280 (ABP-280) by the cytoplasmic domain of TF (287). Ser253 and Ser258 in the cytoplasmic tail of TF were crucial for this interaction. ABP-280 is fundamental for normal cell migration and implicates TF in cytoskeletal organization. Actin filament assembly induced by TF could lead to downstream phosphorylation of focal adhesion kinase (a nonreceptor tyrosine kinase), thereby providing a template for assembly of signaling complexes involved in cell adhesion (287).

Binding of factor VIIa to TF on human fibroblasts can enhance chemotaxis by 100-fold (277). This stimulation takes place via platelet-derived growth factor-B isoform (PDGF-BB) through activation of phospholipase C. Adhesion and migration of mononuclear phagocytes on endothelial cells have been shown to be TF-dependent (288). TF-based peptides and antibodies to TF inhibited this migration. This evidence, along with the role of the TF cytoplasmic tail in binding of ABP-280 and the association of TF with PAR-2, demonstrate a possible function for TF in adhesion and migration. These findings may provide an explanation for the value of inhibiting TF:VIIa activity in reducing neointima formation in animal models with restenosis (161).

---

## Tissue Factor in Angiogenesis and Tumor Development

A role for TF in both embryonic and tumor angiogenesis has been described extensively. As discussed in the section, "Hereditary Deficiencies in Tissue Factor," genetic deficiency of TF causes embryonic lethality as a result of hemorrhage and abnormal development of the yolk sac vasculature (245–247). In contrast, mice lacking only the intracellular domain of TF display normal embryonic development and survival, so the cytoplasmic domain is not essential for embryogenesis (251). The signaling events discussed in the preceding paragraphs indicate that the cytoplasmic domain of TF may be required for certain cellular functions of TF:VIIa. It is therefore likely that TF contributes to angiogenesis by both clotting-dependent and clotting-independent pathways (289). Clotting-dependent pathways are likely to involve the production of the downstream protease thrombin, activation of PAR-1 (and possibly other PARs), and subsequent signal transduction. Clotting-independent pathways may involve phosphorylation of the cytoplasmic tail of TF (290).

A significant relation exists between TF expression and tumor vascularization (291,292). In a mouse xenograft model, transfection of tumor cells with antisense TF or injecting specific antibodies to TF reduced tumor growth and vascularization (293,294). Factor VIIai has been shown to have antimetastatic properties, demonstrating the importance of factor VIIa proteolytic activity in the metastatic process (286). Overexpression of TF in tumor cells contributes to an angiogenic phenotype by both upregulating the expression of the proangiogenic molecule vascular endothelial growth factor (VEGF) and downregulating the antiangiogenic protein thrombospondin (290,293). Significant correlations exist between expression of TF and VEGF in human tumors (291,295,296). Embryos lacking VEGF or TF have similar histopathologies (297,298). Together, these findings suggest that VEGF and TF might regulate similar functions *in vivo*. One study, using TF mutants lacking the serine residues in the cytoplasmic domain, showed that this domain of TF was essential in VEGF regulation (299). This report was not substantiated by others (300), and some investigators have suggested that upregulation of VEGF requires generation of factor Xa (301,302). Despite conflicting reports on the mechanism involved, it is clear that TF can indeed upregulate VEGF. The converse is also true, that is, VEGF upregulates TF expression by Egr-1 on endothelial cells (303). The wealth of information derived from mouse genetics and clinical studies has led to the idea that TF plays direct and indirect roles in tumor development and neovascularization.

New evidence suggests that PAR-2 could also be involved in TF-dependent angiogenesis. Belting et al. (304) report that mice lacking the cytoplasmic tail of TF exhibit enhanced PAR-2–dependent angiogenesis, suggesting a role for this domain in the negative regulation of PAR-2 signaling. This system appears to work in synergy with PDGF-BB and could potentially play a role in vascular disorders such as diabetic retinopathy. The fact that the cytoplasmic tail of TF is shown to be nonessential for embryonic vasculogenesis (251) must be considered in relation to these findings and indicates that although this system may play an important role in disease progression, it is not vital for day-to-day survival.

## References

1. Østerud B, Rapaport SI. Activation of factor IX by the reaction product of tissue factor and factor VII: additional pathway for initiating blood coagulation. *Proc Natl Acad Sci U S A* 1977;74:5260–5264.
2. Gailani D, Broze GJ Jr. Factor XI activation in a revised model of blood coagulation. *Science* 1991;253:909–912.
3. Kondo S, Kisiel W. Regulation of factor VIIa activity in plasma: evidence that antithrombin III is the sole plasma protease inhibitor of human factor VIIa. *Thromb Res* 1987;46:325–335.
4. Seligsohn U, Kasper CK, Østerud B, et al. Activated factor VII: presence in factor IX concentrates and persistence in the circulation after infusion. *Blood* 1979;53:828–837.
5. Nemerson Y, Repke D. Tissue factor accelerates the activation of coagulation factor VII: the role of a bifunctional coagulation cofactor. *Thromb Res* 1985;40:351–358.
6. Morrissey JH, Macik BG, Neuenschwander PF, et al. Quantitation of activated factor VII levels in plasma using a tissue factor mutant selectively deficient in promoting factor VII activation. *Blood* 1993;81:734–744.
7. Römisch J. Factor VII activating protease (FSAP): a novel protease in hemostasis. *Biol Chem* 2002;383:1119–1124.
8. Rao LV, Rapaport SI. Activation of factor VII bound to tissue factor: a key early step in the tissue factor pathway of blood coagulation. *Proc Natl Acad Sci U S A* 1988;85:6687–6691.
9. Radcliffe R, Nemerson Y. Activation and control of factor VII by activated factor X and thrombin: isolation and characterization of a single chain form of factor VII. *J Biol Chem* 1975;250:388–395.
10. Kisiel W, Fujikawa K, Davie EW. Activation of bovine factor VII (proconvertin) by factor XIIa (activated Hageman factor). *Biochemistry* 1977;16:4189–4194.
11. Seligsohn U, Østerud B, Brown SF, et al. Activation of human factor VII in plasma and in purified systems: roles of activated factor IX, kallikrein, and activated factor XII. *J Clin Invest* 1979;64:1056–1065.
12. Masys DR, Bajaj SP, Rapaport SI. Activation of human factor VII by activated factors IX and X. *Blood* 1982;60:1143–1150.
13. Tsujioka H, Suehiro A, Kakishita E. Activation of coagulation factor VII by tissue-type plasminogen activator. *Am J Hematol* 1999;61:34–39.
14. Nakagaki T, Foster DC, Berkner KL. Initiation of the extrinsic pathway of blood coagulation: evidence for the tissue factor dependent autoactivation of human coagulation factor VII. *Biochemistry* 1991;30:10819–10824.
15. Neuenschwander PF, Fiore MM, Morrissey JH. Factor VII autoactivation proceeds via interaction of distinct protease-cofactor and zymogen-cofactor complexes. Implications of a two-dimensional enzyme kinetic mechanism. *J Biol Chem* 1993;268:21489–21492.
16. Wildgoose P, Nemerson Y, Hansen LL, et al. Measurement of basal levels of factor VIIa in hemophilia A and B patients. *Blood* 1992;80:25–28.
17. Lefevre M, Kris-Etherton PM, Zhao G, et al. Dietary fatty acids, hemostasis, and cardiovascular disease risk. *J Am Diet Assoc* 2004;104:410–419.
18. Miller GJ. Postprandial lipaemia and haemostatic factors. *Atherosclerosis* 1998;141:S47–S51.
19. Miller GJ, Martin JC, Mitropoulos KA, et al. Activation of factor VII during alimentary lipemia occurs in healthy adults and patients with congenital factor XII or factor XI deficiency, but not in patients with factor IX deficiency. *Blood* 1996;87:4187–4196.
20. Miller GJ, Mitropoulos KA, Nanjee MN, et al. Very low activated factor VII and reduced factor VII antigen in familial abetalipoproteinaemia. *Thromb Haemost* 1998;80:233–238.
21. Miller GJ, Howarth DJ, Attfield JC, et al. Haemostatic factors in human peripheral afferent lymph. *Thromb Haemost* 2000;83:427–432.
22. Morrissey JH, Fakhrai H, Edgington TS. Molecular cloning of the cDNA for tissue factor, the cellular receptor for the initiation of the coagulation protease cascade. *Cell* 1987;50:129–135.
23. Spicer EK, Horton R, Bloem L, et al. Isolation of cDNA clones coding for human tissue factor: primary structure of the protein and cDNA. *Proc Natl Acad Sci U S A* 1987;84:5148–5152.
24. Scarpati EM, Wen D, Broze GJ Jr, et al. Human tissue factor: cDNA sequence and chromosome localization of the gene. *Biochemistry* 1987;26:5234–5238.
25. Broze GJ Jr, Leykam JE, Schwartz BD, et al. Purification of human brain tissue factor. *J Biol Chem* 1985;260:10917–10920.
26. Bazan JF. Structural design and molecular evolution of a cytokine receptor superfamily. *Proc Natl Acad Sci U S A* 1990;87:6934–6938.
27. Paborsky LR, Harris RJ. Post-translational modifications of recombinant human tissue factor. *Thromb Res* 1990;60:367–376.
28. Paborsky LR, Tate KM, Harris RJ, et al. Purification of recombinant human tissue factor. *Biochemistry* 1989;28:8072–8077.
29. Bach R, Konigsberg WH, Nemerson Y. Human tissue factor contains thioester-linked palmitate and stearate on the cytoplasmic half-cystine. *Biochemistry* 1988;27:4227–4231.
30. Rehemtulla A, Ruf W, Edgington TS. The integrity of the cysteine 186-cysteine 209 bond of the second disulfide loop of tissue factor is required for binding of factor VII. *J Biol Chem* 1991;266:10294–10299.
31. Paborsky LR, Caras IW, Fisher KL, et al. Lipid association, but not the transmembrane domain, is required for tissue factor activity. Substitution of the transmembrane domain with a phosphatidylinositol anchor. *J Biol Chem* 1991;266:21911–21916.
32. Zioncheck TF, Roy S, Vehar GA. The cytoplasmic domain of tissue factor is phosphorylated by a protein kinase C-dependent mechanism. *J Biol Chem* 1992;267:3561–3564.
33. Guha A, Bach R, Konigsberg W, et al. Affinity purification of human tissue factor: interaction of factor VII and tissue factor in detergent micelles. *Proc Natl Acad Sci U S A* 1986;83:299–302.
34. Carson SD, Ross SE, Bach R, et al. An inhibitory monoclonal antibody against human tissue factor. *Blood* 1987;70:490–493.
35. Morrissey JH, Revak D, Tejada P, et al. Resolution of monomeric and heterodimeric forms of tissue factor, the high-affinity cellular receptor for factor VII. *Thromb Res* 1988;50:481–493.
36. Carson SD, Konigsberg WH. Lipid activation of coagulation factor III apoprotein (tissue factor)—reconstitution of the protein-membrane complex. *Thromb Haemost* 1980;44:12–15.
37. Bach R, Gentry R, Nemerson Y. Factor VII binding to tissue factor in reconstituted phospholipid vesicles: induction of cooperativity by phosphatidylserine. *Biochemistry* 1986;25:4007–4020.
38. Smith SA, Morrissey JH. Rapid and efficient incorporation of tissue factor into liposomes. *J Thromb Haemost* 2004;2:1155–1162.
39. Ruf W, Rehemtulla A, Morrissey JH, et al. Phospholipid-independent and -dependent interactions required for tissue factor receptor and cofactor function. *J Biol Chem* 1991;266:2158–2166.
40. Harlos K, Martin DMA, O'Brien DP, et al. Crystal structure of the extracellular region of human tissue factor. *Nature* 1994;370:662–666.
41. Muller YA, Ultsch MH, Kelley RF, et al. Structure of the extracellular domain of human tissue factor: location of the factor VIIa binding site. *Biochemistry* 1994;33:10864–10870.
42. Huang M, Syed R, Stura EA, et al. The mechanism of an inhibitory antibody on TF-initiated blood coagulation revealed by the crystal structures

of human tissue factor, Fab 5G9 and TF•5G9 complex. *J Mol Biol* 1998; 275:873–894.

43. Muller YA, Kelley RF, de Vos AM. Hinge bending within the cytokine receptor superfamily revealed by the 2.4 Å crystal structure of the extracellular domain of rabbit tissue factor. *Protein Sci* 1998;7:1106–1115.

44. Muller YA, Ultsch MH, de Vos AM. The crystal structure of the extracellular domain of human tissue factor refined to 1.7 Å resolution. *J Mol Biol* 1996;256:144–159.

45. Drake TA, Morrissey JH, Edgington TS. Selective cellular expression of tissue factor in human tissues: implications for disorders of hemostasis and thrombosis. *Am J Pathol* 1989;134:1087–1097.

46. Wilcox JN, Smith KM, Schwartz SM, et al. Localization of tissue factor in the normal vessel wall and in the atherosclerotic plaque. *Proc Natl Acad Sci U S A* 1989;86:2839–2843.

47. Fleck RA, Rao LVM, Rapaport SI, et al. Localization of human tissue factor antigen by immunostaining with monospecific, polyclonal anti-human tissue factor antibody. *Thromb Res* 1990;59:421–437.

48. Tipping PG, Malliaros J, Holdsworth SR. Procoagulant activity expression by macrophages from atheromatous vascular plaques. *Atherosclerosis* 1989;79:237–243.

49. Ichikawa K, Nakagawa K, Hirano K, et al. The localization of tissue factor and apolipoprotein(a) in atherosclerotic lesions of the human aorta and their relation to fibrinogen-fibrin transition. *Pathol Res Pract* 1996;192:224–232.

50. Marmur JD, Thiruvikraman SV, Fyfe BS, et al. Identification of active tissue factor in human coronary atheroma. *Circulation* 1996;94:1226–1232.

51. Thiruvikraman SV, Guha A, Roboz J, et al. In situ localization of tissue factor in human atherosclerotic plaques by binding of digoxigenin-labeled factors VIIa and X. *Lab Invest* 1996;75:451–461.

52. Forrester JS, Litvack F, Grundfest W, et al. A perspective of coronary disease seen through the arteries of living man. *Circulation* 1987;75:505–513.

53. Fernandez PM, Patierno SR, Rickles FR. Tissue factor and fibrin in tumor angiogenesis. *Semin Thromb Hemost* 2004;30:31–44.

54. Taylor FB Jr, Chang A, Ruf W, et al. Lethal *E. coli* septic shock is prevented by blocking tissue factor with monoclonal antibody. *Circ Shock* 1991; 33:127–134.

55. Taylor FB Jr. Role of tissue factor and factor VIIa in the coagulant and inflammatory response to LD$_{100}$ *Escherichia coli* in the baboon. *Haemostasis* 1996;26:83–91.

56. Pawlinski R, Mackman N. Tissue factor, coagulation proteases, and protease-activated receptors in endotoxemia and sepsis. *Crit Care Med* 2004;32:S293–S297.

57. Kao FT, Hartz J, Horton R, et al. Regional assignment of human tissue factor gene (F3) to chromosome 1p21-p22. *Somat Cell Mol Genet* 1988; 14:407–410.

58. Mackman N, Morrissey JH, Fowler B, et al. Complete sequence of the human tissue factor gene, a highly regulated cellular receptor that initiates the coagulation protease cascade. *Biochemistry* 1989;28:1755–1762.

59. Brand K, Fowler BJ, Edgington TS, et al. Tissue factor mRNA in THP-1 monocytic cells is regulated at both transcriptional and posttranscriptional levels in response to lipopolysaccharide. *Mol Cell Biol* 1991;11:4732–4738.

60. van der Logt CPE, Reitsma PH, Bertina RM. Alternative splicing is responsible for the presence of two tissue factor mRNA species in LPS stimulated human monocytes. *Thromb Haemost* 1992;67:272–276.

61. Guo W, Zhu J, Wang H. Effects of all-trans retinoic acid, arsenic trioxide and daunorubicin on tissue factor expression in NB4 cells. *Zhonghua Xue Ye Xue Za Zhi* 1999;20:453–455.

62. Bogdanov VY, Balasubramanian V, Hathcock J, et al. Alternatively spliced human tissue factor: a circulating, soluble, thrombogenic protein. *Nat Med* 2003;9:458–462.

63. Mackman N, Fowler BJ, Edgington TS, et al. Functional analysis of the human tissue factor promoter and induction by serum. *Proc Natl Acad Sci U S A* 1990;87:2254–2258.

64. Ranganathan G, Blatti SP, Subramaniam M, et al. Cloning of murine tissue factor and regulation of gene expression by transforming growth factor type β1. *J Biol Chem* 1991;266:496–501.

65. Geczy CL. Cellular mechanisms for the activation of blood coagulation. *Int Rev Cytol* 1994;152:49–108.

66. Camerer E, Kolsto AB, Prydz H. Cell biology of tissue factor, the principal initiator of blood coagulation. *Thromb Res* 1996;81:1–41.

67. Li A, Chang AC, Peer GT, et al. Comparison of the capacity of rhTNF-alpha and *Escherichia coli* to induce procoagulant activity by baboon mononuclear cells *in vivo* and *in vitro*. *Shock* 1996;5:274–279.

68. Niemetz J, Fani K. Thrombogenic activity of leukocytes. *Blood* 1973;42:47–59.

69. Gregory SA, Morrissey JH, Edgington TS. Regulation of tissue factor gene expression in the monocyte procoagulant response to endotoxin. *Mol Cell Biol* 1989;9:2752–2755.

70. Andoh K, Kubota T, Takada M, et al. Tissue factor activity in leukemia cells. Special reference to disseminated intravascular coagulation. *Cancer* 1987;59:748–754.

71. Tanaka M, Yamanishi H. The expression of tissue factor antigen and activity on the surface of leukemic cells. *Leuk Res* 1993;17:103–111.

72. Tallman MS, Hakimian D, Kwaan HC, et al. New insights into the pathogenesis of coagulation dysfunction in acute promyelocytic leukemia. *Leuk Lymphoma* 1993;11:27–36.

73. Drake TA, Cheng J, Chang A, et al. Expression of tissue factor, thrombomodulin, and E-selectin in baboons with lethal *Escherichia coli* sepsis. *Am J Pathol* 1993;142:1458–1470.

74. Faulk WP, Labarrere CA, Carson SD. Tissue factor: identification and characterization of cell types in human placentae. *Blood* 1990;76:86–96.

75. Blakely ML, van der Werf WJ, Berndt MC, et al. Activation of intragraft endothelial and mononuclear cells during discordant xenograft rejection. *Transplantation* 1994;58:1059–1066.

76. Salom RN, Maguire JA, Hancock WW. Endothelial activation and cytokine expression in human acute cardiac allograft rejection. *Pathology* 1998;30:24–29.

77. Vercellotti GM. Effects of viral activation of the vessel wall on inflammation and thrombosis. *Blood Coagul Fibrinolysis* 1998;9(Suppl. 2):S3–S6.

78. Mackman N. Regulation of the tissue factor gene. *Thromb Haemost* 1997;78:747–754.

79. Yan SF, Mackman N, Kisiel W, et al. Hypoxia/hypoxemia-induced activation of the procoagulant pathways and the pathogenesis of ischemia-associated thrombosis. *Arterioscler Thromb Vasc Biol* 1999;19:2029–2035.

80. Kisiel W, Davie EW. Isolation and characterization of bovine factor VII. *Biochemistry* 1975;14:4928–4934.

81. Broze GJ Jr, Majerus PW. Purification and properties of human coagulation factor VII. *J Biol Chem* 1980;255:1242–1247.

82. Fair DS. Quantitation of factor VII in the plasma of normal and warfarin-treated individuals by radioimmuno assay. *Blood* 1983;62:784–791.

83. Hagen FS, Gray CL, O'Hara P, et al. Characterization of a cDNA coding for human factor VII. *Proc Natl Acad Sci U S A* 1986;83:2412–2416.

84. O'Hara PJ, Grant FJ, Haldeman BA, et al. Nucleotide sequence of the gene coding for human factor VII, a vitamin K–dependent protein participating in blood coagulation. *Proc Natl Acad Sci U S A* 1987;84:5158–5162.

85. Banner DW, D'Arcy A, Chène C, et al. The crystal structure of the complex of blood coagulation factor VIIa with soluble tissue factor. *Nature* 1996;380:41–46.

86. Schiodt J, Harrit N, Christensen U, et al. Two different Ca$^{2+}$ ion binding sites in factor VIIa and in des(1-38) factor VIIa. *FEBS Lett* 1992;306: 265–268.

87. Thim L, Bjoern S, Christensen M, et al. Amino acid sequence and post-translational modifications of human factor VIIa from plasma and transfected baby hamster kidney cells. *Biochemistry* 1988;27:7785–7793.

88. Sabharwal AK, Birktoft JJ, Gorka J, et al. High affinity Ca$^{2+}$-binding site in the serine protease domain of human factor VIIa and its role in tissue factor binding and development of catalytic activity. *J Biol Chem* 1995; 270:15523–15530.

89. Pedersen AH, Lund-Hansen T, Komiyama Y, et al. Inhibition of recombinant human blood coagulation factor VIIa amidolytic and proteolytic activity by zinc ions. *Thromb Haemost* 1991;65:528–534.

90. Petersen LC, Olsen OH, Nielsen LS, et al. Binding of Zn$^{2+}$ to a Ca$^{2+}$ loop allosterically attenuates the activity of factor VIIa and reduces its affinity for tissue factor. *Protein Sci* 2000;9:859–866.

91. Bjoern S, Foster DC, Thim L, et al. Human plasma and recombinant factor VII. Characterization of O-glycosylations at serine residues 52 and 60 and effects of site-directed mutagenesis of serine 52 to alanine. *J Biol Chem* 1991;266:11051–11057.

92. Jenny R, Church W, Odegaard B, et al. Purification of six human vitamin K–dependent proteins in a single chromatographic step using immunoaffinity columns. *Prep Biochem* 1986;16:227–245.

93. Higashi S, Kawabata S, Nishimura H, et al. Monoclonal antibody (VII-M31) to bovine factor VII: a specific epitope in the gamma-carboxyglutamic acid domain. *J Biochem (Tokyo)* 1990;108:654–662.

94. Nicolaisen EM, Petersen LC, Thim L, et al. Generation of Gla-domainless FVIIa by cathepsin G-mediated cleavage. *FEBS Lett* 1992;306: 157–160.

95. Huang Q, Neuenschwander PF, Rezaie AR, et al. Substrate recognition by tissue factor–factor VIIa. Evidence for interaction of residues Lys$^{165}$ and Lys$^{166}$ of tissue factor with the 4-carboxyglutamate-rich domain of factor X. *J Biol Chem* 1996;271:21752–21757.

96. Hamik A, Setiadi H, Bu GJ, et al. Down-regulation of monocyte tissue factor mediated by tissue factor pathway inhibitor and the low density lipoprotein receptor-related protein. *J Biol Chem* 1999;274:4962–4969.

97. Sichler K, Banner DW, D'Arcy A, et al. Crystal structures of uninhibited factor VIIa link its cofactor and substrate-assisted activation to specific interactions. *J Mol Biol* 2002;322:591–603.

98. Eigenbrot C, Kirchhofer D, Dennis MS, et al. The factor VII zymogen structure reveals reregistration of beta strands during activation. *Structure (Cambridge)* 2001;9:627–636.

99. Wildgoose P, Berkner KL, Kisiel W. Synthesis, purification, and characterization of an Arg$_{152}$ → Glu site-directed mutant of recombinant human blood clotting factor VII. *Biochemistry* 1990;29:3413–3420.

100. Zhang E, St Charles R, Tulinsky A. Structure of extracellular tissue factor complexed with factor VIIa inhibited with a BPTI mutant. *J Mol Biol* 1999;285:2089–2104.

101. Sayle RA, Milner-White EJ. RASMOL: biomolecular graphics for all. *Trends Biochem Sci* 1995;20:374.

102. Chang JY, Stafford DW, Straight DL. The roles of factor VII's structural domains in tissue factor binding. *Biochemistry* 1995;34:12227–12232.

103. Martin DMA, Boys CWG, Ruf W. Tissue factor: Molecular recognition and cofactor function. *FASEB J* 1995;9:852–859.

104. Edgington TS, Dickinson CD, Ruf W. The structural basis of function of the TF.VIIa complex in the cellular initiation of coagulation. *Thromb Haemost* 1997;78:401–405.

105. Jin J, Chang J, Chang J-Y, et al. Factor VIIa's first epidermal growth factor-like domain's role in catalytic activity. *Biochemistry* 1999;38:1185–1192.

106. McCallum CD, Hapak RC, Neuenschwander PF, et al. The location of the active site of blood coagulation factor VIIa above the membrane surface and its reorientation upon association with tissue factor: a fluorescence energy transfer study. *J Biol Chem* 1996;271:28168–28175.

107. McCallum CD, Su B, Neuenschwander PF, et al. Tissue factor positions and maintains the factor VIIa active site far above the membrane surface even in the absence of the factor VIIa Gla domain—a fluorescence resonance energy transfer study. *J Biol Chem* 1997;272:30160–30166.

108. Pedersen AH, Nordfang O, Norris F, et al. Recombinant human extrinsic pathway inhibitor. Production, isolation, and characterization of its inhibitory activity on tissue factor-initiated coagulation reactions. *J Biol Chem* 1990;265:16786–16793.

109. Lawson JH, Butenas S, Mann KG. The evaluation of complex-dependent alterations in human factor VIIa. *J Biol Chem* 1992;267:4834–4843.

110. Neuenschwander PF, Branam DE, Morrissey JH. Importance of substrate composition, pH and other variables on tissue factor enhancement of factor VIIa activity. *Thromb Haemost* 1993;70:970–977.

111. Kraut J. Serine proteases: structure and mechanism of catalysis. *Annu Rev Biochem* 1977;46:331–358.

112. Payne MA, Neuenschwander PF, Johnson AE, et al. Effect of soluble tissue factor on the kinetic mechanism of factor VIIa: enhancement of *p*-guanidinobenzoate substrate hydrolysis. *Biochemistry* 1996;35:7100–7106.

113. Eigenbrot C, Kirchhofer D. New insight into how tissue factor allosterically regulates factor VIIa. *Trends Cardiovasc Med* 2002;12:19–26.

114. Persson E, Kjalke M, Olsen OH. Rational design of coagulation factor VIIa variants with substantially increased intrinsic activity. *Proc Natl Acad Sci U S A* 2001;98:13583–13588.

115. Petrovan RJ, Ruf W. Role of zymogenicity-determining residues of coagulation factor VII/VIIa in cofactor interaction and macromolecular substrate recognition. *Biochemistry* 2002;41:9302–9309.

116. Soejima K, Yuguchi M, Mizuguchi J, et al. The 99 and 170 loop-modified factor VIIa mutants show enhanced catalytic activity without tissue factor. *J Biol Chem* 2002;277:49027–49035.

117. Freer ST, Kraut J, Robertus JD. Chymotrypsinogen: 2.5-Å crystal structure, comparison with α-chymotrypsin, and implications for zymogen activation. *Biochemistry* 1970;9:1997–2009.

118. Higashi S, Iwanaga S. Molecular interaction between factor VII and tissue factor. *Int J Hematol* 1998;67:229–241.

119. Higashi S, Matsumoto N, Iwanaga S. Molecular mechanism of tissue factor-mediated acceleration of factor VIIa activity. *J Biol Chem* 1996;271:26569–26574.

120. Nemerson Y, Gentry R. An ordered addition, essential activation model of the tissue factor pathway of coagulation: evidence for a conformational cage. *Biochemistry* 1986;25:4020–4033.

121. Bom VJ, Bertina RM. The contributions of Ca²⁺, phospholipids and tissue-factor apoprotein to the activation of human blood-coagulation factor X by activated factor VII. *Biochem J* 1990;265:327–336.

122. Komiyama Y, Pedersen AH, Kisiel W. Proteolytic activation of human factors IX and X by recombinant human factor VIIa: effects of calcium, phospholipids, and tissue factor. *Biochemistry* 1990;29:9418–9425.

123. Ruf W, Miles DJ, Rehemtulla A, et al. Tissue factor residues 157-167 are required for efficient proteolytic activation of factor X and factor VII. *J Biol Chem* 1992;267:22206–22210.

124. Kirchhofer D, Lipari MT, Moran P, et al. The tissue factor region that interacts with substrates factor IX and factor X. *Biochemistry* 2000;39:7380–7387.

125. Fiore MM, Neuenschwander PF, Morrissey JH. The biochemical basis for the apparent defect of soluble mutant tissue factor in enhancing the proteolytic activities of factor VIIa. *J Biol Chem* 1994;269:143–149.

126. Gentry R, Ye L, Nemerson Y. Surface-mediated enzymatic reactions: simulations of tissue factor activation of factor X on a lipid surface. *Biophys J* 1995;69:362–371.

127. Nelsestuen GL, Martinez MB. Steady state enzyme velocities that are independent of [enzyme]: an important behavior in many membrane and particle-bound states. *Biochemistry* 1997;36:9081–9086.

128. Andree HA, Nemerson Y. Tissue factor: regulation of activity by flow and phospholipid surfaces. *Blood Coagul Fibrinolysis* 1995;6:189–197.

129. Maynard JR, Dreyer BE, Stemerman MB, et al. Tissue-factor coagulant activity of cultured human endothelial and smooth muscle cells and fibroblasts. *Blood* 1977;50:387–396.

130. Drake TA, Ruf W, Morrissey JH, et al. Functional tissue factor is entirely cell surface expressed on LPS stimulated human blood monocytes and a constitutively tissue factor producing neoplastic cell line. *J Cell Biol* 1989;109:389–395.

131. Bach R, Rifkin DB. Expression of tissue factor procoagulant activity: regulation by cytosolic calcium. *Proc Natl Acad Sci U S A* 1990;87:6995–6999.

132. Bevers EM, Comfurius P, Dekkers DW, et al. Transmembrane phospholipid distribution in blood cells: control mechanisms and pathophysiological significance. *Biol Chem* 1998;379:973–986.

133. Sevinsky JR, Rao LVM, Ruf W. Ligand-induced protease receptor translocation into caveolae: a mechanism for regulating cell surface proteolysis of the tissue factor-dependent coagulation pathway. *J Cell Biol* 1996;133:293–304.

134. Mulder AB, Smit JW, Bom VJ, et al. Association of smooth muscle cell tissue factor with caveolae. *Blood* 1996;88:1306–1313.

135. Bach RR, Moldow CF. Mechanism of tissue factor activation on HL-60 cells. *Blood* 1997;89:3270–3276.

136. Almus FE, Rao LVM, Rapaport SI. Functional properties of factor VIIa/tissue factor formed with purified tissue factor and with tissue factor expressed on cultured endothelial cells. *Thromb Haemost* 1989;62:1067–1073.

137. Bom VJ, van Hinsbergh VW, Reinalda-Poot HH, et al. Extrinsic activation of human coagulation factors IX and X on the endothelial surface. *Thromb Haemost* 1991;66:283–291.

138. Rao LVM, Robinson T, Hoang AD. Factor VIIa/tissue factor-catalyzed activation of factors IX and X on a cell surface and in suspension: a kinetic study. *Thromb Haemost* 1992;67:654–659.

139. Lawson JH, Mann KG. Cooperative activation of human factor IX by the human extrinsic pathway of blood coagulation. *J Biol Chem* 1991;266:11317–11327.

140. Pedersen AH, Lund-Hansen T, Bisgaard-Frantzen H, et al. Autoactivation of human recombinant coagulation factor VII. *Biochemistry* 1989;28:9331–9336.

141. Iino M, Kisiel W. Sphingosine-containing phospholipid vesicles support human factor VII autoactivation in the absence of tissue factor. *Thromb Res* 1996;82:119–127.

142. Safa O, Morrissey JH, Esmon CT, et al. Factor VIIa/tissue factor generates a form of factor V with unchanged specific activity, resistance to activation by thrombin, and increased sensitivity to activated protein C. *Biochemistry* 1999;38:1829–1837.

143. Warren DL, Morrissey JH, Neuenschwander PF. Proteolysis of blood coagulation factor VIII by the factor VIIa-tissue factor complex: generation of an inactive factor VIII cofactor. *Biochemistry* 1999;38:6529–6536.

144. Broze GJ Jr. Tissue factor pathway inhibitor. *Thromb Haemost* 1995;74:90–93.

145. Broze GJ Jr. Tissue factor pathway inhibitor and the revised theory of coagulation. *Annu Rev Med* 1995;46:103–112.

146. Callander NS, Rao LVM, Nordfang O, et al. Mechanisms of binding of recombinant extrinsic pathway inhibitor (rEPI) to cultured cell surfaces. Evidence that rEPI can bind to and inhibit factor VIIa-tissue factor complexes in the absence of factor Xa. *J Biol Chem* 1992;267:876–882.

147. Lindahl AK, Sandset PM, Abildgaard U. The present status of tissue factor pathway inhibitor. *Blood Coagul Fibrinolysis* 1992;3:439–449.

148. Broze GJ Jr. Tissue factor pathway inhibitor and the current concept of blood coagulation. *Blood Coagul Fibrinolysis* 1995;6(Suppl 1):S7–13.

149. Rao LV, Pendurthi UR. Regulation of tissue factor-factor VIIa expression on cell surfaces: a role for tissue factor-factor VIIa endocytosis. *Mol Cell Biochem* 2003;253:131–140.

150. Petersen LC, Sprecher CA, Foster DC, et al. Inhibitory properties of a novel human Kunitz-type protease inhibitor homologous to tissue factor pathway inhibitor. *Biochemistry* 1996;35:266–272.

151. Girard TJ, MacPhail LA, Likert KM, et al. Inhibition of factor VIIa-tissue factor coagulation activity by a hybrid protein. *Science* 1990;248:1421–1424.

152. Dennis MS, Lazarus RA. Kunitz domain inhibitors of tissue factor-factor VIIa. II. Potent and specific inhibitors by competitive phage selection. *J Biol Chem* 1994;269:22137–22144.

153. Stassen JM, Lambeir A-M, Matthyssens G, et al. Characterisation of a novel series of aprotinin-derived anticoagulants. I. *In vitro* and pharmacological properties. *Thromb Haemost* 1995;74:646–654.

154. Lee GF, Lazarus RA, Kelley RF. Potent bifunctional anticoagulants: Kunitz domain-tissue factor fusion proteins. *Biochemistry* 1997;36:5607–5611.

155. Stassens P, Bergum PW, Gansemans Y, et al. Anticoagulant repertoire of the hookworm *Ancylostoma caninum*. *Proc Natl Acad Sci U S A* 1996;93:2149–2154.

156. Lee AY, Vlasuk GP. Recombinant nematode anticoagulant protein c2 and other inhibitors targeting blood coagulation factor VIIa/tissue factor. *J Intern Med* 2003;254:313–321.

157. Jang I-K, Gold HK, Leinbach RC, et al. Antithrombotic effect of a monoclonal antibody against tissue factor in a rabbit model of platelet-mediated arterial thrombosis. *Arterioscler Thromb* 1992;12:948–954.

158. Thomas WS, Mori E, Copeland BR, et al. Tissue factor contributes to microvascular defects after focal cerebral ischemia. *Stroke* 1993;24:847–853.

159. Pawashe AB, Golino P, Ambrosio G, et al. A monoclonal antibody against rabbit tissue factor inhibits thrombus formation in stenotic injured rabbit carotid arteries. *Circ Res* 1994;74:56–63.

160. Valentin S, Reutlingsperger CPM, Nordfang O, et al. Inhibition of factor X activation at extracellular matrix of fibroblasts during flow conditions: a comparison between tissue factor pathway inhibitor and inactive factor VIIa. *Thromb Haemost* 1995;74:1478–1485.

161. Jang Y, Guzman LA, Lincoff AM, et al. Influence of blockade at specific levels of the coagulation cascade on restenosis in a rabbit atherosclerotic femoral artery injury model. *Circulation* 1995;92:3041–3050.

162. Harker LA, Hanson SR, Wilcox JN, et al. Antithrombotic and antilesion benefits without hemorrhagic risks by inhibiting tissue factor pathway. *Haemostasis* 1996;26:76–82.

163. Taylor FB Jr, Chang AC, Peer G, et al. Active site inhibited factor VIIa (DEGR VIIa) attenuates the coagulant and interleukin-6 and -8, but not tumor necrosis factor, responses of the baboon to LD$_{100}$ *Escherichia coli*. *Blood* 1998;91:1609–1615.

164. Maun HR, Eigenbrot C, Lazarus RA. Engineering exosite peptides for complete inhibition of factor VIIa using a protease switch with substrate phage. *J Biol Chem* 2003;278:21823–21830.

165. Himber J, Kirchhofer D, Riederer M, et al. Dissociation of antithrombotic effect and bleeding time prolongation in rabbits by inhibiting tissue factor function. *Thromb Haemost* 1997;78:1142–1149.

166. Harker LA. Therapeutic inhibition of thrombin activities, receptors, and production. *Hematol Oncol Clin North Am* 1998;12:1211–1230.

167. Suleymanov OD, Szalony JA, Salyers AK, et al. Pharmacological interruption of acute thrombus formation with minimal hemorrhagic complications by a small molecule tissue factor/factor VIIa inhibitor: comparison to factor Xa and thrombin inhibition in a nonhuman primate thrombosis model. *J Pharmacol Exp Ther* 2003;306:1115–1121.

168. Young WB, Kolesnikov A, Rai R, et al. Optimization of a screening lead for factor VIIa/TF. *Bioorg Med Chem Lett* 2001;11:2253–2256.

169. Parlow JJ, Case BL, Dice TA, et al. Design, parallel synthesis, and crystal structures of pyrazinone antithrombotics as selective inhibitors of the tissue factor VIIa complex. *J Med Chem* 2003;46:4050–4062.

170. Poller L. International Normalized Ratios (INR): the first 20 years. *J Thromb Haemost* 2004;2:849–860.

171. Tripodi A, Arbini A, Chantarangkul V, et al. Recombinant tissue factor as substitute for conventional thromboplastin in the prothrombin time test. *Thromb Haemost* 1992;67:42–45.

172. Neuenschwander PF, Morrissey JH. Deletion of the membrane anchoring region of tissue factor abolishes autoactivation of factor VII but not cofactor function. Analysis of a mutant with a selective deficiency in activity. *J Biol Chem* 1992;267:14477–14482.

173. Huang X, Molema G, King S, et al. Tumor infarction in mice by antibody-directed targeting of tissue factor to tumor vasculature. *Science* 1997;275:547–550.

174. Lusher J, Ingerslev J, Roberts H, et al. Clinical experience with recombinant factor VIIa. *Blood Coagul Fibrinolysis* 1998;9:119–128.

175. Hedner U. Recombinant activated factor VII as a universal haemostatic agent. *Blood Coagul Fibrinolysis* 1998;9:S147–S152.

176. Hoffman M. A cell-based model of coagulation and the role of factor VIIa. *Blood Rev* 2003;17(Suppl 1):S1–S5.

177. Kitchen S, Malia RG, Preston FE. A comparison of methods for the measurement of activated factor VII. *Thromb Haemost* 1992;68:301–305.

178. Seligsohn U, Østerud B, Rapaport SI. Coupled amidolytic assay for factor VII: its use with a clotting assay to determine the activity state of factor VII. *Blood* 1978;52:978–988.

179. Hemker HC, Muller AD, Gonggrijp R. The estimation of activated human blood coagulation factor VII. *J Mol Med* 1976;1:127–134.

180. Kario K, Narita N, Matsuo T, et al. Genetic determinants of plasma factor VII activity in the Japanese. *Thromb Haemost* 1995;73:617–622.

181. Mann KG. Factor VII assays, plasma triglyceride levels, and cardiovascular disease risk. *Arteriosclerosis* 1989;9:783–784.

182. Philippou H, Adami A, Amersey RA, et al. A novel specific immunoassay for plasma two-chain factor VIIa: investigation of FVIIa levels in normal individuals and in patients with acute coronary syndromes. *Blood* 1997;89:767–775.

183. Meade TW, Mellows S, Brozovic M, et al. Haemostatic function and ischaemic heart disease: principal results of the Northwick Park Heart Study. *Lancet* 1986;2:533–537.

184. Balleisen L, Schulte H, Assmann G, et al. Coagulation factors and the progress of coronary heart disease. *Lancet* 1987;2:461.

185. Ruddock V, Meade TW. Factor-VII activity and ischaemic heart disease: fatal and non-fatal events. *Q J Med* 1994;87:403–406.

186. Broadhurst P, Kelleher C, Hughes L, et al. Fibrinogen, factor VII clotting activity and coronary artery disease severity. *Atherosclerosis* 1990;85:169–173.

187. Carvalho de Sousa J, Azevedo J, Soria C, et al. Factor VII hyperactivity in acute myocardial thrombosis: a relation to the coagulation activation. *Thromb Res* 1988;51:165–173.

188. Cortellaro M, Boschetti C, Cofrancesco E, et al. The PLAT study: hemostatic function in relation to atherothrombotic ischemic events in vascular disease patients. Principal results. *Arterioscler Thromb* 1992;12:1063–1070.

189. Hoffman C, Shah A, Sodums M, et al. Factor VII activity state in coronary artery disease. *J Lab Clin Med* 1988;111:475–481.

190. Hoffman CJ, Miller RH, Lawson WE, et al. Elevation of factor VII activity and mass in young adults at risk of ischemic heart disease. *J Am Coll Cardiol* 1989;14:941–946.

191. Kario K, Sakata T, Matsuo T, et al. Factor VII in non-insulin-dependent diabetic patients with microalbuminuria. *Lancet* 1993;342:1552.

192. Kario K, Matsuo T, Sakata T, et al. Factor VII hyperactivity and ischaemic heart disease. *Lancet* 1994;343:233.

193. Kario K, Matsuo T, Matsuo M, et al. Marked increase of activated factor VII in uremic patients. *Thromb Haemost* 1995;73:763–767.

194. Orlando M, Leri O, Macioce G, et al. Factor VII in subjects at risk for thromboembolism: activation or increased synthesis? *Haemostasis* 1987;17:340–343.

195. Suzuki T, Yamauchi K, Matsushita T, et al. Elevation of factor VII activity and mass in coronary artery disease of varying severity. *Clin Cardiol* 1991;14:731–736.

196. Hoffman CJ, Lawson WE, Miller RH, et al. Correlation of vitamin K-dependent clotting factors with cholesterol and triglycerides in healthy young adults. *Arterioscler Thromb* 1994;14:1737–1740.

197. Daae LN, Kierulf P, Landaas S, et al. Cardiovascular risk factors: interactive effects of lipids, coagulation and fibrinolysis. *Scand J Clin Lab Invest Suppl* 1993;215:19–27.

198. Hultin MB. Fibrinogen and factor VII as risk factors in vascular disease. *Prog Hemost Thromb* 1991;10:215–241.

199. Grant PJ. The genetics of atherothrombotic disorders: a clinician's view. *J Thromb Haemost* 2003;1:1381–1390.

200. Morrissey JH. Tissue factor modulation of factor VIIa activity: use in measuring trace levels of factor VIIa in plasma. *Thromb Haemost* 1995;74:185–188.

201. Miller GJ, Stirling Y, Esnouf MP, et al. Factor VII-deficient substrate plasmas depleted of protein C raise the sensitivity of the factor VII bio-assay to activated factor VII: an international study. *Thromb Haemost* 1994;71:38–48.

202. Morrissey JH. Plasma factor VIIa: measurement and potential clinical significance. *Haemostasis* 1996;26:66–71.

203. Folsom AR, Wu KK, Shahar E, et al. Association of hemostatic variables with prevalent cardiovascular disease and asymptomatic carotid artery atherosclerosis. *Arterioscler Thromb* 1993;13:1829–1836.

204. Koster T, Rosendaal FR, Reitsma PH, et al. Factor VII and fibrinogen levels as risk factors for venous thrombosis. A case-control study of plasma levels and DNA polymorphisms—the Leiden Thrombophilia Study (LETS). *Thromb Haemost* 1994;71:719–722.

205. Moor E, Silveira A, van't Hooft F, et al. Coagulation factor VII mass and activity in young men with myocardial infarction at a young age: role of plasma lipoproteins and factor VII genotype. *Arterioscler Thromb* 1995;15:655–664.

206. Sosef MN, Bosch JG, van Oostayen J, et al. Relation of plasma coagulation factor VII and fibrinogen to carotid artery intima-media thickness. *Thromb Haemost* 1994;72:250–254.

207. Vaziri ND, Kennedy SC, Kennedy D, et al. Coagulation, fibrinolytic, and inhibitory proteins in acute myocardial infarction and angina pectoris. *Am J Med* 1992;93:651–657.

208. Kalaria VG, Zareba W, Moss AJ, et al. Gender-related differences in thrombogenic factors predicting recurrent cardiac events in patients after acute myocardial infarction. *Am J Cardiol* 2000;85:1401–1408.

209. Danielsen R, Önundarson PT, Thors H, et al. Activated and total coagulation factor VII, and fibrinogen in coronary artery disease. *Scand Cardiovasc J* 1998;32:87–95.

210. Cooper JA, Miller GJ, Bauer KA, et al. Comparison of novel hemostatic factors and conventional risk factors for prediction of coronary heart disease. *Circulation* 2000;102:2816–2822.

211. Green F, Kelleher C, Wilkes H, et al. A common genetic polymorphism associated with lower coagulation factor VII levels in healthy individuals. *Arterioscler Thromb* 1991;11:540–546.

212. Marchetti G, Patracchini P, Papacchini M, et al. A polymorphism in the 5' region of coagulation factor VII gene (F7) caused by an inserted decanucleotide. *Hum Genet* 1993;90:575–576.

213. Sacchi E, Tagliabue L, Scoglio R, et al. Plasma factor VII levels are influenced by a polymorphism in the promoter region of the FVII gene. *Blood Coagul Fibrinolysis* 1996;7:114–117.

214. Humphries S, Temple A, Lane A, et al. Low plasma levels of Factor VIIc and antigen are more strongly associated with the 10 base pair promoter (−323) insertion than the glutamine 353 variant. *Thromb Haemost* 1996;75:567–572.

215. van't Hooft FM, Silveira A, Tornvall P, et al. Two common functional polymorphisms in the promoter region of the coagulation factor VII gene determining plasma factor VII activity and mass concentration. *Blood* 1999;93:3432–3441.

216. Grant PJ, Humphries SE. Genetic determinants of arterial thrombosis. *Baillieres Best Pract Res Clin Haematol* 1999;12:505–532.

217. Iacoviello L, Di Castelnuovo A, de Knijff P, et al. Polymorphisms in the coagulation factor VII gene and the risk of myocardial infarction. *N Engl J Med* 1998;338:79–85.

218. Doggen CJM, Manger Cats V, Bertina RM, et al. A genetic propensity to high factor VII is not associated with the risk of myocardial infarction in men. *Thromb Haemost* 1998;80:281–285.

219. Corral J, González-Conejero R, Lozano ML, et al. Genetic polymorphisms of factor VII are not associated with arterial thrombosis. *Blood Coagul Fibrinolysis* 1998;9:267–272.

220. Koyama T, Nishida K, Ohdama S, et al. Determination of plasma tissue factor antigen and its clinical significance. *Br J Haematol* 1994;87:343–347.

221. Wada H, Nakase T, Nakaya R, et al. Elevated plasma tissue factor antigen level in patients with disseminated intravascular coagulation. *Am J Hematol* 1994;45:232–236.

222. Asakura H, Kamikubo Y, Goto A, et al. Role of tissue factor in disseminated intravascular coagulation. *Thromb Res* 1995;80:217–224.

223. Lwaleed BA, Bass PS, Chisholm M, et al. Urinary tissue factor in glomerulonephritis: a potential marker of glomerular injury? *J Clin Pathol* 1997;50:336–340.

224. Østerud B. Cellular interactions in tissue factor expression by blood monocytes. *Blood Coagul Fibrinolysis* 1995;6(Suppl 1):S20–S25.

225. Lwaleed BA, Chisholm M, Francis JL. The significance of measuring monocyte tissue factor activity in patients with breast and colorectal cancer. *Br J Cancer* 1999;80:279–285.

226. Key NS, Slungaard A, Dandelet L, et al. Whole blood tissue factor procoagulant activity is elevated in patients with sickle cell disease. *Blood* 1998;91:4216–4223.

227. Aras O, Shet A, Bach RR, et al. Induction of microparticle- and cell-associated intravascular tissue factor in human endotoxemia. *Blood* 2004;103:4545–4553.

228. Marsik C, Quehenberger P, Mackman N, et al. Validation of a novel tissue factor assay in experimental human endotoxemia. *Thromb Res* 2003;111:311–315.

229. Giesen PLA, Rauch U, Bohrmann B, et al. Blood-borne tissue factor: another view of thrombosis. *Proc Natl Acad Sci U S A* 1999;96:2311–2315.

230. Himber J, Wohlgensinger C, Roux S, et al. Inhibition of tissue factor limits the growth of venous thrombus in the rabbit. *J Thromb Haemost* 2003;1:889–895.

231. Morrissey JH. Tissue factor: in at the start … and the finish? *J Thromb Haemost* 2003;1:878–880.

232. Morel O, Toti F, Hugel B, et al. Cellular microparticles: a disseminated storage pool of bioactive vascular effectors. *Curr Opin Hematol* 2004;11:156–164.

233. Giesen PL, Nemerson Y. Tissue factor on the loose. *Semin Thromb Hemost* 2000;26:379–384.

234. Himber J, Kling D, Fallon JT, et al. In situ localization of tissue factor in human thrombi. *Blood* 2002;99:4249–4250.

235. Ozcan M, Morton CT, Solovey A, et al. Whole blood tissue factor procoagulant activity remains detectable during severe aplasia following bone marrow and peripheral blood stem cell transplantation. *Thromb Haemost* 2001;85:250–255.

236. Rauch U, Nemerson Y. Tissue factor, the blood, and the arterial wall. *Trends Cardiovasc Med* 2000;10:139–143.

237. Siddiqui FA, Desai H, Amirkhosravi A, et al. The presence and release of tissue factor from human platelets. *Platelets* 2002;13:247–253.

238. Zillmann A, Luther T, Müller I, et al. Platelet-associated tissue factor contributes to the collagen-triggered activation of blood coagulation. *Biochem Biophys Res Commun* 2001;281:603–609.

239. Müller I, Klocke A, Alex M, et al. Intravascular tissue factor initiates coagulation via circulating microvesicles and platelets. *FASEB J* 2003;17:476–478.

240. Østerud B, Rao LVM, Olsen JO. Induction of tissue factor expression in whole blood: lack of evidence for the presence of tissue factor expression in granulocytes. *Thromb Haemost* 2000;83:861–867.

241. Imamura T, Kaneda H, Nakamura S. New functions of neutrophils in the Arthus reaction: expression of tissue factor, the clotting initiator, and fibrinolysis by elastase. *Lab Invest* 2002;82:1287–1295.

242. Østerud B. Tissue factor in neutrophils: no. *J Thromb Haemost* 2004;2:218–220.

243. Rauch U, Bonderman D, Bohrmann B, et al. Transfer of tissue factor from leukocytes to platelets is mediated by CD15 and tissue factor. *Blood* 2000;96:170–175.

244. Østerud B. The role of platelets in decrypting monocyte tissue factor. *Dis Mon* 2003;49:7–13.

245. Toomey JR, Kratzer KE, Lasky NM, et al. Targeted disruption of the murine tissue factor gene results in embryonic lethality. *Blood* 1996;88:1583–1587.

246. Bugge TH, Xiao Q, Kombrinck KW, et al. Fatal embryonic bleeding events in mice lacking tissue factor, the cell-associated initiator of blood coagulation. *Proc Natl Acad Sci U S A* 1996;93:6258–6263.

247. Carmeliet P, Mackman N, Moons L, et al. Role of tissue factor in embryonic blood vessel development. *Nature* 1996;383:73–75.

248. Carmeliet P, Moons L, Dewerchin M, et al. Insights in vessel development and vascular disorders using targeted inactivation and transfer of vascular endothelial growth factor, the tissue factor receptor, and the plasminogen system. *Ann N Y Acad Sci* 1997;811:191–206.

249. Toomey JR, Kratzer KE, Lasky NM, et al. Effect of tissue factor deficiency on mouse and tumor development. *Proc Natl Acad Sci U S A* 1997;94:6922–6926.

250. Parry GCN, Mackman N. Mouse embryogenesis requires the tissue factor extracellular domain but not the cytoplasmic domain. *J Clin Invest* 2000;105:1410–1554.

251. Melis E, Moons L, de Mol M, et al. Targeted deletion of the cytosolic domain of tissue factor in mice does not affect development. *Biochem Biophys Res Commun* 2001;286:580–586.

252. Yang YH, Hall P, Milenkovski G, et al. Reduction in arthritis severity and modulation of immune function in tissue factor cytoplasmic domain mutant mice. *Am J Pathol* 2004;164:109–117.

253. Sharma L, Melis E, Hickey MJ, et al. The cytoplasmic domain of tissue factor contributes to leukocyte recruitment and death in endotoxemia. *Am J Pathol* 2004;165:331–340.

254. Parry GC, Erlich JH, Carmeliet P, et al. Low levels of tissue factor are compatible with development and hemostasis in mice. *J Clin Invest* 1998;101:560–569.

255. Pawlinski R, Fernandes A, Kehrle B, et al. Tissue factor deficiency causes cardiac fibrosis and left ventricular dysfunction. *Proc Natl Acad Sci U S A* 2002;99:15333–15338.

256. Erlich JH, Boyle EM, Labriola J, et al. Inhibition of the tissue factor-thrombin pathway limits infarct size after myocardial ischemia-reperfusion injury by reducing inflammation. *Am J Pathol* 2000;157:1849–1862.

257. Cooper DN, Millar DS, Wacey A, et al. Inherited factor VII deficiency: molecular genetics and pathophysiology. *Thromb Haemost* 1997;78:151–160.

258. Rosen ED, Chan JC, Idusogie E, et al. Mice lacking factor VII develop normally but suffer fatal perinatal bleeding. *Nature* 1997;390:290–294.

259. McVey JH, Boswell EJ, Takamiya O, et al. Exclusion of the first EGF domain of factor VII by a splice site mutation causes lethal factor VII deficiency. *Blood* 1998;92:920–926.

260. Waxman E, Ross JBA, Laue TM, et al. Tissue factor and its extracellular soluble domain: the relationship between intermolecular association with factor VIIa and enzymatic activity of the complex. *Biochemistry* 1992;31:3998–4003.

261. Neuenschwander PF, Morrissey JH. Roles of the membrane-interactive regions of factor VIIa and tissue factor. The factor VIIa Gla domain is dispensable for binding to tissue factor but important for activation of factor X. *J Biol Chem* 1994;269:8007–8013.

262. Røttingen J-A, Enden T, Camerer E, et al. Binding of human factor VIIa to tissue factor induces cytosolic $Ca^{2+}$ signals in J82 cells, transfected COS-1 cells, Madin-Darby canine kidney cells and in human endothelial cells induced to synthesize tissue factor. *J Biol Chem* 1995;270:4650–4660.

263. Camerer E, Røttingen J-A, Iversen JG, et al. Coagulation factors VII and X induce $Ca^{2+}$ oscillations in Madin-Darby canine kidney cells only when proteolytically active. *J Biol Chem* 1996;271:29034–29042.

264. Poulsen LK, Jacobsen N, Sorensen BB, et al. Signal transduction via the mitogen-activated protein kinase pathway induced by binding of coagulation factor VIIa to tissue factor. *J Biol Chem* 1998;273:6228–6232.

265. Camerer E, Røttingen J-A, Gjernes E, et al. Coagulation factors VIIa and Xa induce cell signaling leading to up-regulation of the Egr-1 gene. *J Biol Chem* 1999;274:32225–32233.

266. Versteeg HH, Hoedemaeker I, Diks SH, et al. Factor VIIa/tissue factor-induced signaling via activation of Src-like kinases, phosphatidylinositol 3-kinase, and Rac. *J Biol Chem* 2000;275:28750–28756.

267. Pendurthi UR, Allen KE, Ezban M, et al. Factor VIIa and thrombin induce the expression of Cyr61 and connective tissue growth factor, extracellular matrix signaling proteins that could act as possible downstream mediators in factor VIIa · tissue factor-induced signal transduction. *J Biol Chem* 2000;275:14632–14641.

268. Pendurthi UR, Alok D, Rao LV. Binding of factor VIIa to tissue factor induces alterations in gene expression in human fibroblast cells: up-regulation of poly(A) polymerase. *Proc Natl Acad Sci U S A* 1997;94:12598–12603.

269. Camerer E, Gjernes E, Wiiger M, et al. Binding of factor VIIa to tissue factor on keratinocytes induces gene expression. *J Biol Chem* 2000;275:6580–6585.

270. Taniguchi T, Kakkar AK, Tuddenham EGD, et al. Enhanced expression of urokinase receptor induced through the tissue factor-factor VIIa pathway in human pancreatic cancer. *Cancer Res* 1998;58:4461–4467.

271. Siegbahn A. Cellular consequences upon factor VIIa binding to tissue factor. *Haemostasis* 2000;30(Suppl 2):41–47.

272. Riewald M, Ruf W. Orchestration of coagulation protease signaling by tissue factor. *Trends Cardiovasc Med* 2002;12:149–154.

273. Camerer E, Huang W, Coughlin SR. Tissue factor- and factor X-dependent activation of protease-activated receptor 2 by factor VIIa. *Proc Natl Acad Sci U S A* 2000;97:5255–5260.

274. Riewald M, Ruf W. Mechanistic coupling of protease signaling and initiation of coagulation by tissue factor. *Proc Natl Acad Sci U S A* 2001;98:7742–7747.

275. Jiang X, Bailly MA, Panetti TS, et al. Formation of tissue factor-factor VIIa-factor Xa complex promotes cellular signaling and migration of human breast cancer cells. *J Thromb Haemost* 2004;2:93–101.

276. Petersen LC, Thastrup O, Hagel G, et al. Exclusion of known protease-activated receptors in factor VIIa-induced signal transduction. *Thromb Haemost* 2000;83:571–576.

277. Siegbahn A, Johnell M, Rorsman C, et al. Binding of factor VIIa to tissue factor on human fibroblasts leads to activation of phospholipase C and enhanced PDGF-BB-stimulated chemotaxis. *Blood* 2000;96:3452–3458.

278. Nystedt S, Ramakrishnan V, Sundelin J. The proteinase-activated receptor 2 is induced by inflammatory mediators in human endothelial cells. Comparison with the thrombin receptor. *J Biol Chem* 1996;271:14910–14915.

279. Mechtcheriakova D, Schabbauer G, Lucerna M, et al. Specificity, diversity, and convergence in VEGF and TNF-α signaling events leading to tissue factor up-regulation via EGR-1 in endothelial cells. *FASEB J* 2001;15:230–242.

280. Ahamed J, Ruf W. Protease-activated receptor 2-dependent phosphorylation of the tissue factor cytoplasmic domain. *J Biol Chem* 2004;279:23038–23044.

281. Dorfleutner A, Ruf W. Regulation of tissue factor cytoplasmic domain phosphorylation by palmitoylation. *Blood* 2003;102:3998–4005.

282. DeFea K, Schmidlin F, Dery O, et al. Mechanisms of initiation and termination of signalling by neuropeptide receptors: a comparison with the proteinase-activated receptors. *Biochem Soc Trans* 2000;28:419–426.

283. Ge L, Ly Y, Hollenberg M, et al. A β-arrestin-dependent scaffold is associated with prolonged MAPK activation in pseudopodia during protease-activated receptor-2-induced chemotaxis. *J Biol Chem* 2003;278:34418–34426.

284. Hjortoe GM, Petersen LC, Albrektsen T, et al. Tissue factor-factor VIIa-specific up-regulation of IL-8 expression in MDA-MB-231 cells is mediated by PAR-2 and results in increased cell migration. *Blood* 2004;103:3029–3037.

285. Bromberg ME, Konigsberg WH, Madison JF, et al. Tissue factor promotes melanoma metastasis by a pathway independent of blood coagulation. *Proc Natl Acad Sci U S A* 1995;92:8205–8209.

286. Mueller BM, Ruf W. Requirement for binding of catalytically active factor VIIa in tissue factor-dependent experimental metastasis. *J Clin Invest* 1998;101:1372–1378.

287. Ott I, Fischer EG, Miyagi Y, et al. A role for tissue factor in cell adhesion and migration mediated by interaction with actin-binding protein 280. *J Cell Biol* 1998;140:1241–1253.

288. Randolph GJ, Luther T, Albrecht S, et al. Role of tissue factor in adhesion of mononuclear phagocytes to and trafficking through endothelium *in vitro*. *Blood* 1998;92:4167–4177.

289. Rickles FR, Shoji M, Abe K. The role of the hemostatic system in tumor growth, metastasis, and angiogenesis: tissue factor is a bifunctional molecule capable of inducing both fibrin deposition and angiogenesis in cancer. *Int J Hematol* 2001;73:145–150.

290. Shoji M, Abe K, Nawroth PP, et al. Molecular mechanisms linking thrombosis and angiogenesis in cancer. *Trends Cardiovasc Med* 1997;7:52–59.

291. Koomägi R, Volm M. Tissue-factor expression in human non-small-cell lung carcinoma measured by immunohistochemistry: correlation between tissue factor and angiogenesis. *Int J Cancer* 1998;79:19–22.

292. Abdulkadir SA, Carvalhal GF, Kaleem Z, et al. Tissue factor expression and angiogenesis in human prostate carcinoma. *Hum Pathol* 2000;31:443–447.

293. Zhang Y, Deng Y, Luther T, et al. Tissue factor controls the balance of angiogenic and antiangiogenic properties of tumor cells in mice. *J Clin Invest* 1994;94:1320–1327.

294. Mueller BM, Reisfeld RA, Edgington TS, et al. Expression of tissue factor by melanoma cells promotes efficient hematogenous metastasis. *Proc Natl Acad Sci U S A* 1992;89:11832–11836.

295. Shoji M, Hancock WW, Abe K, et al. Activation of coagulation and angiogenesis in cancer: immunohistochemical localization *in situ* of clotting proteins and vascular endothelial growth factor in human cancer. *Am J Pathol* 1998;152:399–411.

296. Takano S, Tsuboi K, Tomono Y, et al. Tissue factor, osteopontin, $\alpha_v\beta_3$ integrin expression in microvasculature of gliomas associated with vascular endothelial growth factor expression. *Br J Cancer* 2000;82:1967–1973.

297. Ferrara N, Carver-Moore K, Chen H, et al. Heterozygous embryonic lethality induced by targeted inactivation of the VEGF gene. *Nature* 1996;380:439–442.

298. Carmeliet P, Ferreira V, Breier G, et al. Abnormal blood vessel development and lethality in embryos lacking a single VEGF allele. *Nature* 1996;380:435–439.

299. Abe K, Shoji M, Chen J, et al. Regulation of vascular endothelial growth factor production and angiogenesis by the cytoplasmic tail of tissue factor. *Proc Natl Acad Sci U S A* 1999;96:8663–8668.

300. Bromberg ME, Sundaram R, Homer RJ, et al. Role of tissue factor in metastasis: functions of the cytoplasmic and extracellular domains of the molecule. *Thromb Haemost* 1999;82:88–92.

301. Ollivier V, Bentolila S, Chabbat J, et al. Tissue factor-dependent vascular endothelial growth factor production by human fibroblasts in response to activated factor VII. *Blood* 1998;91:2698–2703.

302. Ollivier V, Chabbat J, Herbert JM, et al. Vascular endothelial growth factor production by fibroblasts in response to factor VIIa binding to tissue factor involves thrombin and factor Xa. *Arterioscler Thromb Vasc Biol* 2000;20:1374–1381.

303. Mechtcheriakova D, Wlachos A, Holzmüller H, et al. Vascular endothelial cell growth factor-induced tissue factor expression in endothelial cells is mediated by EGR-1. *Blood* 1999;93:3811–3823.

304. Belting M, Dorrell MI, Sandgren S, et al. Regulation of angiogenesis by tissue factor cytoplasmic domain signaling. *Nat Med* 2004;10:502–509.

# CHAPTER 6 ■ CONTACT ACTIVATION (KALLIKREIN-KININ) PATHWAY: MULTIPLE PHYSIOLOGIC AND PATHOPHYSIOLOGIC ACTIVITIES

ROBERT W. COLMAN

Four proteins, namely, factor XII (FXII) (Hageman factor), prekallikrein (PK) (Fletcher factor), high-molecular-weight kininogen (Williams-Fitzgerald-Flaujeac factor), and C1-inhibitor (C1-INH), have been shown to be the major factors required for the activation and inhibition of the surface-mediated pathway, or "contact system." Recent studies have shown that the surface *in vivo* is the cell membrane of blood and endothelial cells. In this system, the zymogens, FXII and PK, are converted by limited proteolysis into the active serine proteases. High-molecular-weight kininogen (HK) is a nonenzymatic procofactor for these interconversions. Hereditary deficiencies, manifested by abnormal results of blood coagulation tests, have been described for the first three of these four proteins. Deficiency of C1-INH does not alter blood coagulation but presents as hereditary angioedema (HAE). Importantly, although the genetically determined deficiencies of FXII, PK, and HK display abnormal *in vitro* plasma coagulation, none of these deficiencies is associated with a bleeding state. Thus, none of these proteins is an essential hemostatic protein but, paradoxically, several may have an antithrombotic function. Moreover, study of FXII, PK, and HK from molecular, biochemical, physiologic, and pathophysiologic perspectives indicates a wide variety of important interactions with other plasma proteins. FXIIa activates factor XI (1), factor VII (2), and C1 component of complement (3). Plasma kallikrein activates prourokinase (4), prorenin (5), and FXII (6), and cleaves HK, thereby releasing bradykinin (BK) (7). Each protein binds to blood and vascular cells. FXII downregulates the Fc receptor on monocytes (8), releases interleukin 1 (IL-1) and IL-6 from monocytes and macrophages (9), and stimulates neutrophils (10). Plasma kallikrein activates neutrophils (11) and potentiates fibrinolysis on endothelial cells (12). HK inhibits adhesion of neutrophils to blood-compatible surfaces under flow conditions (13), enhances cellular fibrinolysis (12), and inhibits thrombin-induced platelet activation. The contact system (Kallikrein-Kinin) has counteradhesive, profibrinolytic, inflammatory, and antithrombotic properties and regulates angiogenesis. Thus, the molecular events of the contact system activation and inhibition affect a number of important plasma biochemical and cellular systems and play an important role in various pathophysiologic conditions.

This chapter first deals with the molecular biology, structure, and biochemical properties of FXII, PK, and HK. FXI, the primary function of which is related to the coagulation system, will be dealt with in detail in Chapter 11 and will be mentioned briefly only as it pertains to interactions with the proteins of the contact system. The interaction of each protein with the others is then considered in initiation, amplification, and regulation of the pathway, and the role of these proteins in other proteolytic systems is explored. The relation of these proteins to cellular elements in contact with plasma (i.e., platelets, neutrophils, monocytes, and endothelial cells) is then summarized. Finally, the clinical implications of deficiencies and activation of these proteins and their involvement in pathologic processes are presented.

## FACTOR XII (HAGEMAN FACTOR)

FXII is coded for by a single gene of 12 kilobases (kb) that maps to chromosome 5 (14,15), comprising 13 introns and 14 exons (16). A putative signal peptide sequence on the amino ($NH_2$) terminus of the zymogen is located on the first exon, followed by a region of unknown homology encoded by the second exon. A "type II" region homologous with collagen-binding properties in fibronectin is represented by exons II and IV. Exon V codes for the epidermal growth factor (EGF)–like domain, followed by the "type I" homology or the fibrin finger in fibronectin that is coded by exon VI. Exon VII encodes the second EGF-like domain, preceding a kringle structure and a proline-rich region on exons VIII–IX. The light chain of FXIIa is encoded by five exons (X–XIV), of which exon XIV is the largest, encoding 55 amino acid residues of the serine protease and 150 base pairs (bp) of the 3'-untranslated end of the messenger RNA (mRNA) (16,17).

The FXII intron/exon gene is similar in structure to the serine protease subfamily of tissue-type plasminogen activator (tPA) and urokinase plasminogen activator (uPA) genes (see Fig. 6-1). The mRNA codes for a 596–amino acid, single polypeptide chain with a molecular mass of 80 kDa. Its electrophoretic migration as a $\beta$-globulin is consistent with an isoelectric point of $6.3 \pm 0.1$ (18). FXII concentration in plasma is $31 \pm 8$ $\mu$g per mL ($0.375$ $\mu$M) (19). Human liver has been shown to express FXII mRNA, and rat hepatocytes in culture synthesize FXII (20). Postmenopausal women treated with estrogens and pregnant women have elevated plasma levels of FXII expression. In isolated livers of estrogen- and prolactin-treated rats, FXII is elevated (21). Rat FXII deoxyribonucleic acid (DNA) has been shown to have a functional estrogen promoter element that binds $17\beta$-estradiol (22). FXII, possibly by virtue of its EGF domain, displays mitogenic activity that enhances HepG2 cell proliferation (23) and stimulates a signal transduction pathway by a mitogen-induced protein kinase (24). This activity does not depend on FXIIa proteolytic activity.

Plasma proteinases, including plasma kallikrein and plasmin or autoactivation, activate FXII to FXIIa ($\alpha$FXIIa), cleaving the bond connecting Arg353–Val354 and generating a two-chain molecule composed of a heavy chain (353 residues) and a light chain (243 residues), held together by a single

107

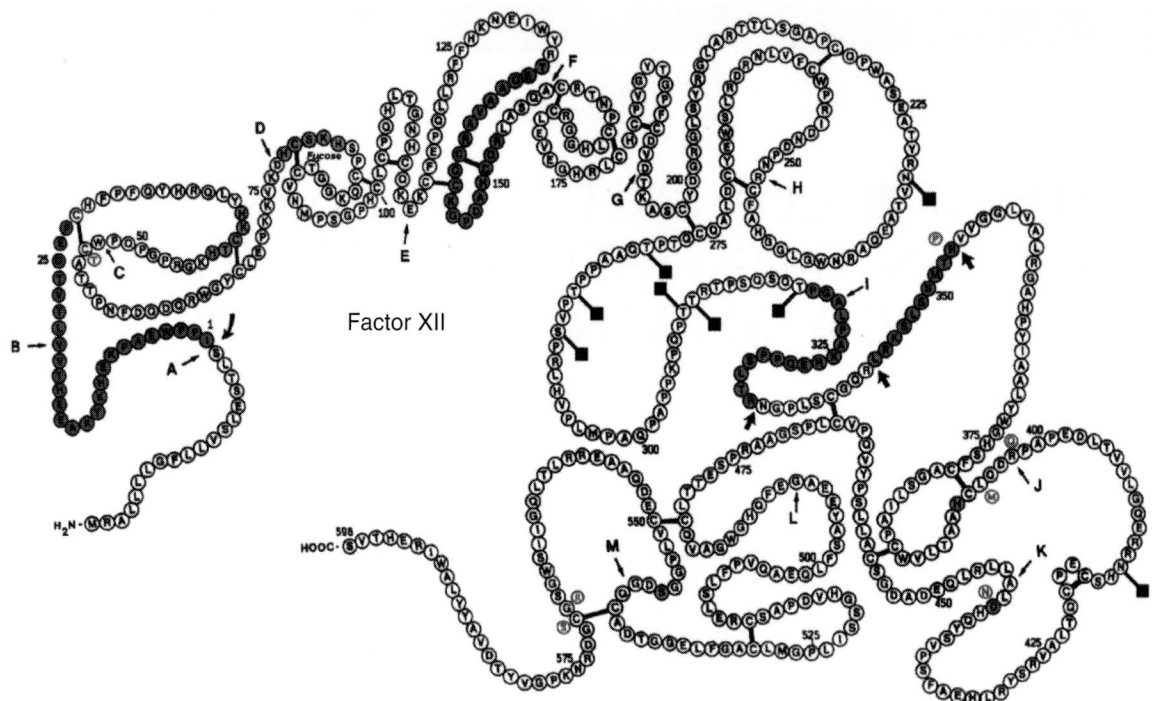

Factor XII

**FIGURE 6-1.** Schematic diagram of human factor XII. (FXII) The standard one-letter code is given in the *open circles*. The *solid black bars* indicate possible disulfide bonding between cysteine residues based on homologies and other proteins. The *arrows A to M* indicate positions of introns in the coding sequence. The *curved arrow* indicates the cleavage site to remove the propeptide and reveal the *N*-terminal isoleucine. The *straight arrows* are the sites of kallikrein cleavage. The *black squares* are the sites of glycosylation. The *red residues* are the catalytic triad, H393, D458, and S556. The *red letters* in *red open circles* are sites of known missense mutations leading to loss of coagulant activity. The *purple residues* are the three putative surface binding regions. The *two green regions* are $Zn^{2+}$ binding sequences (see Color Fig. 6-1).

disulfide bond (17). The heavy chain contains two binding sites to anionic surfaces and cells, one in the fibronectin type I region (T134-R153) and a second near the distal *N*-terminal end because one monoclonal antibody to this entire region blocks all surface-mediated activities (25,26). Studies using recombinant deletion mutants of FXII confirmed these conclusions and also indicated that a third discontinuous region on the heavy chain, located in the proline-rich region (P313–R334, L344–R353), also participated in artificial surface binding (27). Upon contact with negatively charged surfaces and on cell membranes, FXII is autoactivated (28). The binding to the surface and the cleavage during autoactivation result in different sequential conformational changes (29). The light chain of FXIIa is a typical serine proteinase containing the canonical Asp, His, Ser, and is the site for inhibition by its major plasma inhibitor, C1-INH (30).

Proteolytic activation of zymogen FXII by such enzymes as trypsin, plasmin, and kallikrein produces a group of proteases that progressively decrease in size, increase in net negative charge, decrease in clotting activity, and have altered surface binding properties while retaining the same active site (31–35). At least two proteolytic products of activated FXII have been well characterized. FXIIa and FXII fragment (β-FXIIa, $M_r$ 30,000) because of cleavage of the bonds in the light chain by plasma kallikrein between Arg334–Asn335, Arg343–Leu344, and Arg353–Val354, resulting in two polypeptide chains (9 and 243 residues in size) held together by a disulfide bond. The 80-kDa form of activated FXII has the ability to bind to negatively charged surfaces and activate FXI. Because the 28- to 30-kDa enzymatic form of FXII has no heavy chain, it has no surface-binding properties or ability to activate FXI but retains its ability to activate PK and C1 (31,32).

The autoactivation of FXII arises from binding with negatively charged surfaces (28,36,37). $Zn^{2+}$ binding to FXII induces a conformation change that makes the protein more susceptible to autoactivation when associated with negatively charged surfaces (38,39). There are four $Zn^{2+}$-binding sites, and amino acids within two have been identified (H40–H44, H78–H82) (40). Autoactivation is independent of $Zn^{2+}$ when induced by sulfatides or by low concentrations of dextran sulfate but is dependent on $Zn^{2+}$ when higher concentrations of dextran sulfate or phosphatidyl inositol phosphate are used as surfaces (41). Biologic components, which include fatty acids (42), also promote surface-dependent activation of FXII. A variety of components of basement membranes, including types I, II, and III collagen; proteoglycans; and mixtures of these substances, failed to initiate intrinsic coagulation in normal plasma. However, cerebroside sulfates (43), a biologic component of all cell membranes and certain glycosaminoglycans (44), are very potent activators of FXII. Recently, it has been shown that heat shock protein 90 contained in cytosol and membrane fractions of endothelial cells can activate PK in the presence of kininogen and $Zn^{2+}$ (45); but whether this activation occurs on the surface of endothelial cells is not known. FXII is known to bind to gC1qR (46). Moreover, FXII-dependent contact activation occurs in the presence of HK and $Zn^{2+}$ when gC1qR and cytokeratin 1 (CK1) are present on endothelial cells, and the reaction is inhibited by antibodies to these proteins (47). Further investigations have shown that FXII binds to a multiprotein assembly of urokinase receptor (uPAR), gC1qR, and cytokeratin on endothelial cells (48). The binding site on FXII is the peptide Tyr39–Arg47 from the *N*-terminal of FXII in fibronectin type II domain, previously identified (49) as a binding site to anionic surfaces. Alternative mechanisms have been sought for activation of PK *in vivo* independent of FXII. Assembly of PK bound to HK on human umbilical vein endothelial cells allows PK activation independent of FXII by a cell-associated protease (50). In further studies, a modest dependence on FXII was found but this dependence was a feedback reaction to activate additional PK to kallikrein because there was no autoactivation of FXIIa on the endothelial surface (51). The cell-associated protease was identified, purified, and found by amino acid sequencing to be prolylcarboxypeptidase (52). The purified enzyme, a serine protease, activated PK to kallikrein. The endothelial matrix also was able to bind HK and contained a PK activator (53), which was also identified as prolylcarboxypeptidase (54). These observations support an alternate initiation pathway in which the cellular activation of PK could precede FXII autoactivation. For these enzymes, FXIIa and prolylcarboxypeptidase, the question of which predominates under pathophysiologic conditions requires further study.

The major plasma protease inhibitor of FXIIa and XIIf is C1-INH. More than 90% of the inhibition of these proteases in plasma is attributed to this serpin (55–57). C1-INH binds both proteins in 1:1 stoichiometry and irreversibly inactivates them with concomitant loss of C1-INH activity. FXIIa adsorbed on a kaolin surface is protected from C1-INH inactivation (58), and recently, binding of FXIIa to endothelial cells was also found to provide protection from inactivation (59). Endothelial cells have been reported to produce a protein that inhibits the activation of FXII but not the proteolytic activity of FXIIa (60), but this moiety has not yet been identified.

# PREKALLIKREIN (FLETCHER FACTOR)

The gene structure for human PK has been determined (61) and is similar to that of rat plasma PK (62) and to the gene for human FXI (63) (with which PK is highly homologous). The human plasma PK gene is composed of 15 exons and 14 introns. The sequence identity between the human and the rat proteins is 75%. These data and the results of chromosomal localization for human plasma PK, FXI, and rat PK (all chromosome 4) genes strongly corroborate a gene duplication event from a common ancestor for both PK and FXI (64), approximately 270 million years ago. PK mRNA codes for a mature human protein of 609 amino acids with 58% identity to human FXI. Plasma PK is a fast $\gamma$-globulin with an isoelectric point of 8.7 (65) and with an estimated plasma concentration of 42 $\mu$g per mL (0.49 $\mu$M) (66). Approximately 75% of plasma PK circulates bound to HK (67,68), and only 25% circulates as free PK. By reduced or nonreduced polyacrylamide gel electrophoresis (PAGE) in sodium dodecyl sulfate (SDS), plasma PK has been found to consist of two components of $M_r$ 85,000 and 88,000 (69,70), which probably differ in the degree of glycosylation. The conversion of PK to kallikrein, its active form, is catalyzed by FXIIa on a surface to which HK is bound or by FXII fragment in the fluid phase (71). A single bond (Arg371–Ile372) is split, generating a heavy chain of 371 amino acids (53 kDa) and a light chain of 248 amino acids (36 and 33 kDa) held together by a single disulfide bond (69,72). PK has four tandem repeats in the *N*-terminal portion of the molecule due to the linking of the first and sixth, second and fifth, and third and fourth half-cysteine (1/2-Cys) residues present in each repeat (see Fig. 6-2) (73). This arrangement results in four groups of 90 or 91 amino acids that are arranged in "apple" domains (74), which, in addition to PK, are seen only in FXI. However, on the basis of homology search and structure prediction methods, the *N*-terminal domains of the plasminogen and hepatocyte growth factor family, as well as certain nematode proteins,

have been found to belong to the same molecule superfamily as the apple domains (75). The fourth repeat contains two additional 1/2-Cys residues, forming an additional disulfide bridge. In contrast, in FXI, there is only one extra 1/2-Cys, allowing interchain dimerization. Repeats 1 and 3 and repeats 2 and 4 share the highest degree of homology (76). Repeats 2 and 4 each have a carbohydrate chain linked to homologous asparagine residues 108 and 289. A short connecting region of nine amino acids follows repeat 4, culminating at the cleavage site between the light and heavy chains.

Kallikrein catalyzes an autolytic cleavage at Lys140–Ala141, resulting in $\beta$-kallikrein (77). This enzyme exhibits decreased coagulation activity, a diminished rate of cleavage of HK, and decreased ability to stimulate neutrophils. The heavy chain is required for complexing with HK (78). The HK binding domain of PK resides within the C-terminal 231 amino acids of the heavy chain (amino acids 141 to 371) (79). In addition, studies using a monoclonal antibody to PK heavy chain indicate that there is also a heavy chain site recognized by FXIIa within the same 28-kDa fragment (residues 141 to 371) but that the two subdomains are separate (80). The HK binding region in the C-terminal region is on apple 4 (Lys266–Gly295), and there is a second site for HK binding on the apple 1 domain (Phe56–Gly86) (81–83). The separation of apple domains 1 and 4 in $\beta$-kallikrein accounts for its low affinity for HK, which decreases its coagulant activity and its ability to stimulate neutrophils and release elastase (77). The third major site for HK binding to PK is on the A2 domain, more specifically amino acid residues 92 to 153 (84). Similarly, binding of factor XI to HK requires multiple apple domains on factor XI, with A2 being the most important (85).

The light chain contains the catalytic triad His415, Asp464, and Ser559. The isolated light chain retains the ability to activate FXII in solution and is also able to cleave HK, although at a slower rate. The molecule also contains 15% carbohydrate and five putative sites for *N*-asparaginyl-linked glycosylation. Heterogeneity of the carbohydrate attachments provides the basis for two light chains of 36 and 33 kDa. The light chain of kallikrein is the site for reactions with protease inhibitors (86). In plasma, kallikrein is rapidly inactivated by two protease inhibitors, $\alpha_2$-macroglobulin and C1-INH, each of which form a 1:1 stoichiometric complex with kallikrein (87), resulting in loss of both the proteolytic activity of the enzyme and the inhibitory function of C1-INH (88). Although HK and C1-INH bind to different regions of the kallikrein molecule, it has been observed that HK and its light chain protect kallikrein from inhibition by C1-INH and other plasma protease inhibitors in a purified system (89). This observation is compatible with substrate protection of an enzyme from an active site–directed inhibitor because HK is a substrate for kallikrein (90). $\alpha_2$-Macroglobulin inhibits the release of BK from kininogens, but it only partially inhibits its amidolytic activity when forming a covalent complex with kallikrein. Antithrombin III (AT-III), in the presence or absence of heparin, is an inefficient inhibitor of kallikrein. However, recent studies suggest that in the presence of HK, heparin (91) accelerates the inhibition of kallikrein by AT-III considerably. Protein C inhibitor is also a potent inhibitor of kallikrein in purified systems (92). Plasma PK mRNA is expressed in all tissues tested, with high levels in pancreas, kidney, testis, spleen, and prostate, but the highest levels in the liver (93).

# HIGH-MOLECULAR-WEIGHT KININOGEN (WILLIAMS-FITZGERALD-FLAUJEAC FACTOR)

The two plasma kininogens, HK and low-molecular-weight kininogen (LK), are the products of a gene (94,95) that maps

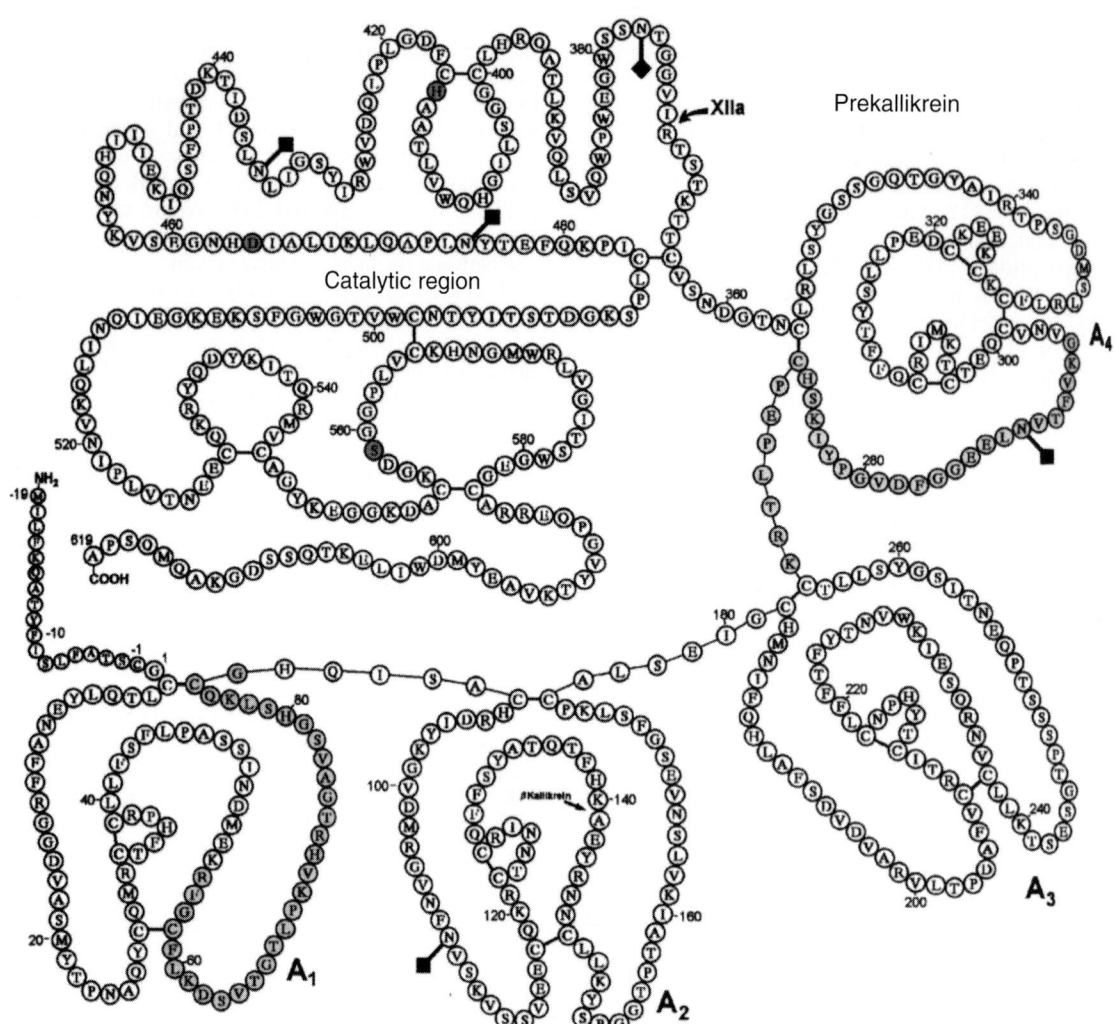

**FIGURE 6-2.** Schematic diagram of human prekallikrein. The four apple domains in the N-terminal portion of the molecule are labeled $A_1$ to $A_4$. The regions that bind high-molecular-weight kininogen are *yellow*. The bond cleaved by FXIIa is R371-I372. The catalytic triad, H415, D464, S559, is indicated in *red*. The sites of N- and O-glycosylation are indicated as *black squares*. The N-terminal of the propeptide is indicated $NH_2$, and the site of its cleavage to yield the mature protein is between amino acids −1 and 1. The site of kallikrein cleavage of itself to yield β-kallikrein is indicated with an *arrow*. The site of FXIIa cleavage to activate prekallikrein is indicated with a *curved arrow*. No intron location is indicated as the structure of the human kallikrein gene has not been determined (see Color Fig. 6-2).

to 3q26-qter. *The kininogen gene* (27 kb) consists of 11 exons and produces unique mRNAs for HK and LK, respectively, by alternative splicing (see Fig. 6-3) (95). HK and LK both contain the coding region for exons 1 to 9, a part of exon 10 containing the BK sequence and the first 12 amino acids after the C-terminal amino acid of BK. Exon 11 codes for the 4-kDa light chain of LK. Exon 10 contains the coding sequence for the 56-kDa light chain of HK. The mRNA for HK and LK are 3.5 and 1.7 kb, respectively.

The heavy chain of HK and LK consists of three tandemly repeated units designated domains 1, 2, and 3 (96,97), which are coded for by exons 1 to 3, 4 to 6, and 7 to 9, respectively. Ylinenjarvi et al. (98) have expressed kininogens' domain 2 in *Escherichia coli*, with preservation of its ability to inhibit cathepsin L and papain but with reduced affinity for calpain when compared to LK. Domain 3 has been expressed in *E. coli*, with full preservation of its ability to inhibit papain and cathepsin L (99), as well as cathepsins B and H (100), and to inhibit thrombin binding to platelets (101). Domain 4 contains BK and flanking amino acids. The light chain

which comprises domains $5_H$ and 6 of HK has been expressed in bacteria in our laboratory, with preservation of domain $5_H$ binding to artificial surfaces, heparin and platelet, neutrophil, and endothelial surfaces, and of the ability of domain 6 to bind PK and FXI (102). The function of domain $5_L$ of LK is unknown.

The molecular basis of one example of homozygous deficiency of both HK and LK, Williams trait, is a C to T substitution at nucleotide 587 that changes a CGA (Arg) codon to TGA(stop) mutation in exon 5. This point mutation prevents the synthesis of both kininogens because it occurs in the common heavy chain (103). The phenotype of this defect, total plasma kininogen deficiency, is similar to that seen in Brown Norway Katholiek rats, but, in the rat, the defect is a single-point mutation in the heavy chain, Ala163 to Thr, which results in defective hepatic secretion (104). In the rat, ovariectomy results in a reduction of hepatic kininogen mRNA levels, whereas estrogens increase the level of kininogen transcripts (105). This result is consistent with the physiologic increase in HK in human pregnancy. Murine fibroblasts are stimulated

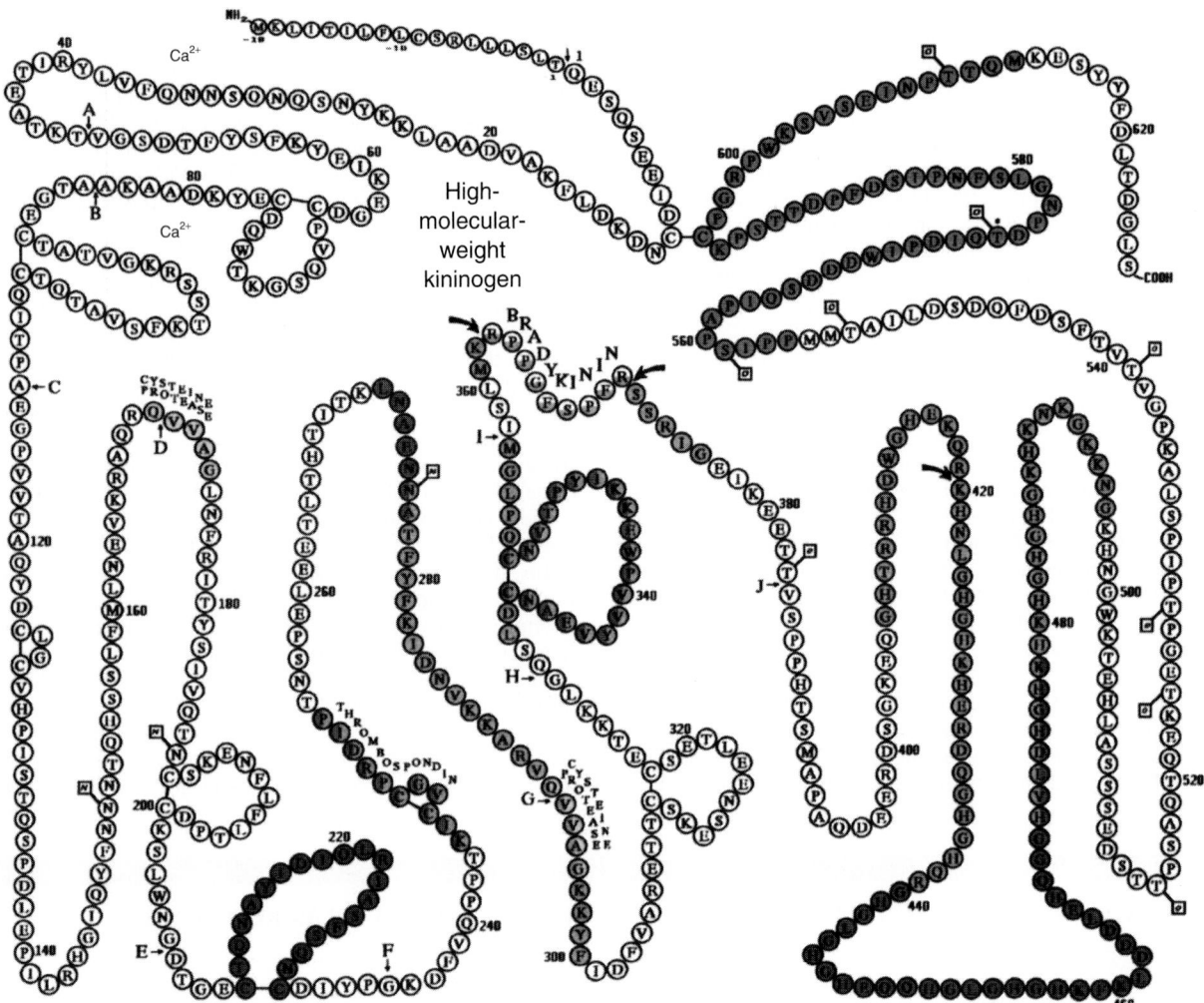

**FIGURE 6-3.** Primary sequence and genetic structure of human high-molecular-weight kininogen. Numbers 1 to 626 are amino acid (aa) locations with leader sequence −18 to −1. Letters A through J are the locations of the intron/exon junctions D1 (aa 1 to 113) is coded by exons 1, 2, and 3. D2 (aa 114 to 234) is coded by exons 4, 5, and 6. D3 (aa 235 to 357) is coded by exons 7, 8, and 9. D4 (aa 358 to 383) is coded by exon $10_{BK}$. D5 (aa 384 to 502) is coded by the 5′ portion of exon $10_{HK}$. D6 (aa 503 to 626) is coded by the 3′ portion of exon $10_{HK}$. The *curved arrows* indicate plasma kallikrein cleavage sites. *Boxed O* is the location of an O-linked carbohydrate chain. *Boxed N* is the location of an N-linked carbohydrate chain. The *yellow* sequences (aa 170 to 174, aa 292 to 296) are binding sites for cysteine proteases. The *maroon* sequence (aa 211 to 230) is a site that inhibits calpain 2 activity. The *purple-half red* sequence (aa 244 to 254) is a binding site for both endothelial cells and thrombospondin (TSP). The *green* sequences (aa 271 to 277, aa 333 to 352, and aa 440 to 478) represent binding sites for neutrophils on D3 and D5. The *purple* sequences (aa 331 to 357, aa 361 to 376, aa 406 to 439, and aa 471 to 496) represent binding sites for endothelial cells on D3, D4, and D5. The *pink* sequence (aa 556 to 613) is the binding site for FXI, and the *chartreuse* sequence (aa 565 to 595) is the binding site for PK, both on D6. This representation was created by Dr. Robin Pixley (see Color Fig. 6-3).

by cyclic adenosine monophosphate (cAMP), forskolin, prostaglandin $E_2$, and tumor necrosis factor α (TNF-α) to synthesize and secrete HK (106). In addition, mRNA for LK is expressed and upregulated by the same agonists (107). Similarly, TNF-α has been recognized to increase kininogen expression in HEP-G2 cells (108).

The two kininogen mRNAs code for LK, a 66-kDa β-globulin with a plasma concentration of 90 μg per mL (1.3 μM) (108) and an isoelectric point of 4.7 (7), and for HK, a 120-kDa α-globulin with a plasma concentration of 80 μg per mL (0.67 μM) and an isoelectric point of 4.3 (109,110). Human liver contains mRNAs for HK and LK (94,95), and human umbilical vein endothelial cells contain HK mRNA and synthesize HK (111). Human HK antigen has been quantified

in platelets, granulocytes, endothelial cells, and renal tubular cells (109,111–114). HK is composed of three globular units, domains 1 to 3, domain 5, and domain 6, in a curvilinear arrangement on electron microscopy (115), consistent with the molecular size on gel filtration of 220 kDa, indicating a high axial ratio. The location of each globular element was deduced by association with specific monoclonal antibodies and PK. Cleavage of HK by plasma kallikrein leads to a striking change in conformation in the resultant HKa, previously predicted by functional and immunologic studies. The central globular region (D5) is separated after BK liberation and forms a tetrahedral array, with associations not only with the cysteine protease inhibitory region (D1 to D3) but also with the PK binding region (D6) (115). The domains in HK are separated by disordered regions that are sensitive to cleavage by serine proteases (96,116,117). Approximation of these domains is important for certain biologic functions of kininogens such as HK binding to cells (118,119), which require both D3 and D5 amino acid sequences. LK, which binds to endothelial cells using the D3 and D4 domains, requires a particular conformation (120). Similarly, calpain inhibition requires noncontiguous primary sequences in domain 2. In contrast, proteolytic cleavage of HK-separating domains unmasks a new function—its cell antiadhesive activity (121,122) and ability to inhibit angiogenesis.

HK and LK are multidomainal proteins, each with unique activities (see Table 6-1). Domain 1 displays low-affinity calcium binding, the role of which is unknown; (123) it also contains a 20–amino acid peptide, which antagonizes the natriuretic and diuretic effect of atrial natriuretic peptide *in vivo* in rats (124). Domains 2 and 3 contain the canonical amino acid sequence, QVVAG, found in the cysteine protease inhibitors related structurally to cystatin (96). Both LK and HK are tight-binding, reversible inhibitors of cysteine proteases, with a $K_i$ of 2 and 0.5 nM, respectively, for platelet calpain (110,125). Calpain inhibitory region of kininogens is exclusively found on domain 2 (99,116,118,125), whereas papain and cathepsin L are inhibited by regions on both domains 2 and 3 (96). A molecular model of domain 2 was constructed by homology modeling using x-ray coordinates of crystalline cystatin, which is 50% identical to domain 2 (118). Peptides from domain 2 of HK were selected, stabilized by inclusion or addition of cysteine residues, and air oxidized to form disulfide-bonded loops. A peptide containing Q170-VVA-G174 blocked HK inhibition of calpain and therefore functioned as a binding

site for calpain, whereas another peptide (C211–C229) C-terminal to this peptide was a direct inhibitor of calpain ($IC_{50} = 35\ \mu M$). The molecular model predicts that these two regions probably form a continuous binding site for calpain in the three-dimensional structure of HK and LK. In contrast, the optimal inhibition of cathepsin B and H requires three loops of domain 3 (100). HK is also a substrate of calpain when there is molar excess of enzyme to inhibitor (kininogen) (110,126,127), which may occur at the cell surface. Because kininogens are extracellular or within granules in platelets, the mechanism of interaction with platelet calpain is usually cytosolic or is localized on the internal face of the cell membrane. However, when platelets are activated, calpain translocates to the external membrane, where it could be inhibited by plasma HK or externalized platelet $\alpha$-granule HK (127–129).

The heavy chain of kininogens also contains sequences in domain 3 responsible for binding to platelets (130,131), endothelial cells (132), and neutrophils (133). By using synthetic peptides corresponding to surface-exposed regions, three peptides, K244–P254, N276–I301, and L331–M357, inhibited biotin–HK binding to endothelial cells (134). Because papain inhibited HK binding to endothelial cells, the inhibitory site for cysteine proteases overlaps with the cell-binding site on domain 3, and, therefore, the portion of domain 3 that is contiguous to domain 4, the BK region, is an endothelial cell-binding site (134). Thrombospondin (TSP), a platelet $\alpha$-granule protein secreted upon platelet stimulation, also binds to HK, both to a site on the heavy chain requiring calcium ions and to the light chain independent of calcium ions (135). The interaction of

---

### TABLE 6-1

#### THE FUNCTIONS OF HIGH-MOLECULAR-WEIGHT KININOGEN AND ITS CELLULAR RECEPTORS

| Kininogen domain | Actions | Biologic function | Cell receptors involved | Cells involved |
|---|---|---|---|---|
| 1 | Inhibits atrial natriuretic factor | Antidiuretic | — | — |
| 2 | Prevents calpain-related platelet aggregation | Antithrombotic | — | Platelets |
| 3 | Prevents thrombin binding to platelets | Antithrombotic | GP Ib/IX/V | Platelets |
| 4 (Bradykinin) | Stimulates prostacyclin and NO | Antithrombotic | B2 receptor | *Endothelial cells* |
| 4 (Bradykinin) | Stimulates tPA release | Profibrinolytic | B2 receptor | *Endothelial cells* |
| 4 (RPPGF) | Prevents thrombosis by cleaving PAR-1 | Antithrombotic | Thrombin receptor (PAR-1) | Platelets |
| 5H | Prevents neutrophils from sticking to artificial surfaces | Antiadhesive | Mac-1 | Neutrophils |
| 5H | Displaces fibrinogen from neutrophils and surfaces | Antiadhesive | Mac-1 | Neutrophils |
| 5H | Prevents endothelial cells from sticking to vitronectin | Antiadhesive | Urokinase receptor | *Endothelial cells* (neutrophils) |
| 5H | Inhibits proliferation and/or stimulates apoptosis | Antiangiogenic | Urokinase receptor | *Endothelial cells* |
| 6 | Allows binding of PK and its activation | Profibrinolytic | — | — |
| 6 | Allows binding of kallikrein and activation of neutrophils | Inflammatory | — | — |

NO, nitric oxide; GP, glycoprotein; PAR-1, protease-activated receptor 1; Mac-1, integrin $\alpha M \beta_2$, CD11b/18; PK, prekallikrein; tPA, tissue-type plasminogen activator.

TSP with the heavy chain of kininogens is K244–P254 in domain 3 (136).

A critical function ascribed to domain 3 is the ability of kininogen to inhibit the activation of platelets. Puri et al. (137) showed that HK inhibited thrombin-induced platelet aggregation in a plasmatic environment and that HK inhibited thrombin binding to platelets. Jiang et al. (131) localized this activity to domain 3 and showed that the thrombin inhibitory region was not the same as the platelet-binding region because one monoclonal antibody, which did not block to cell binding, neutralized HK's ability to inhibit $\alpha$-thrombin's activation of platelets. The $\alpha$-thrombin inhibitory regions on kininogens are not the cell-binding regions. Two distinct sequences from domain 3 and domain 4 are each capable of inhibiting thrombin-induced platelet activation, although the affinities and mechanisms are different. Kunapuli et al. (102) expressed domain 3 in $E.\ coli$, G235–M357, and the recombinant GST fusion polypeptide inhibited thrombin-induced aggregation of platelets (IC$_{50}$ = 4 $\mu$M). Most of the inhibitory activity of D5 was coded for by exon 7, G235–Q292 (IC$_{50}$ = 0.2 $\mu$M). Moreover, a recombinant peptide of 23 amino acids, K270–Q292, exhibited an IC$_{50}$ of 30 $\mu$M. A synthetic heptapeptide, L271–A277 (LNAENNA), contained the minimal sequence (IC$_{50}$ = 65 $\mu$M) to inhibit $\alpha$-thrombin–induced platelet aggregation. This sequence competes for thrombin binding to platelets by mimicking a glycoprotein (GP) Ib sequence on platelets for binding thrombin, which represented the first clue that GP Ib is an HK receptor on platelets. Hasan et al. (138) indicate that domain 4 contains another site of thrombin inhibitory activity that inhibits thrombin-induced activation of platelets. Further studies indicate that BK, analogs of BK, and its breakdown products block $\alpha$-thrombin–induced platelet activation by preventing $\alpha$-thrombin from cleaving its cloned receptor (138), although the concentration required is in the low mM range. Domain 4 is the region that contains BK. Although HK is a better substrate of plasma kallikrein and LK is a better substrate of tissue kallikrein for cleavage of BK, both are substrates to both plasma and tissue kallikreins. FXIIa cleaves HK similarly to plasma kallikrein, releasing BK (139). FXIa initially cleaves HK into 76- and 46-kDa bond components. Subsequent cleavages release BK and proteolyze the 46-kDa light chain of HK to smaller, inactive fragments (140). Cleavage of LK by elastase renders the protein a better substrate of plasma kallikrein to liberate BK and Met-Lys-BK (141), although it destroys HK's procoagulant activity. One last function of domain 4 may be to serve as a cell-binding region (142). The C-terminal portion of BK and the N-terminal portion of kininogen's common light chain participate as a very low affinity ($K_d$ = 1 mM) binding site to endothelial cells. However, domain 4 probably forms a continuous binding site with domain 3 sequences, which hold HK and LK in the proper conformation for optimal cell binding. For example, intact HK binds to endothelial cells maintained at 37°C with a $K_d$ of 7 nM and $1 \times 10^7$ molecules per cell versus kinin-free kininogen that binds to endothelial cells maintained at 37°C with a $K_d$ of 30 nM and 1.0 to $2.6 \times 10^6$ molecules per cell. However, it is now known if these two forms of kininogen may bind to different receptors (see the following text).

The light chain of HK is 45 kDa and consists of two domains, domains 5 (D5$_H$) and 6. Domain 5 of HK has another cell-binding site. D5$_H$ serves as an additional cell-binding site on platelets, granulocytes, and endothelial cells. Two areas of D5$_H$ are found to participate in cell binding (143). One is on the N-terminal end of the domain and consists of sequences G402–K420 and H421–H441. These peptides inhibit HK binding with IC$_{50}$ of 792 $\mu$M and 215 $\mu$M, respectively. The other region is on the C-terminal region of D5$_H$ and is contained within the sequence, H479-H498, which inhibits HK binding (IC$_{50}$ = 0.2 to 0.8 $\mu$M). The region responsible for

binding to neutrophils on D5 is localized to H493–K520 (144). D5$_H$ was first recognized as the domain that binds to HK anionic surfaces (102,116,145). This histidine- and glycine-rich region has the ability to bind both zinc and heparin (146,147). A monoclonal antibody that blocks HK clotting and the binding of cleaved HK to anionic surfaces (116) was used in an immunoaffinity column. A 57-amino acid peptide (H441–K497) was isolated from a proteolytic digest of HK, and it inhibited coagulant activity and had the ability to bind to anionic surfaces with an IC$_{50}$ = 30 $\mu$M. D5$_H$ contains two histidine- and glycine-rich regions, one rich in lysine (H457–K502) and the other closer to the N-terminal side (K420–H458). The anionic surface binding region was found to be associated with both histidine- and glycine-rich regions of D5$_H$ using recombinant polypeptides (102). Each region displayed coagulant activity when associated with D6. The synthetic peptides, H479–H498 and H471–K494, were shown to have a high-affinity cell binding of D5$_H$. Both peptides inhibited the $in\ vitro$ procoagulant activity of HK (143). A polyclonal antibody raised to H479–H498 is also able to prolong the procoagulant activity of HK in plasma (143). Therefore, the cell-binding and the artificial surface binding regions on HK are contained within the same highly conserved region of D5$_H$. The sites for heparin binding have also been mapped to D5$_H$ and are Zn$^{2+}$ dependent (148). Fine mapping of the binding sites indicate that the N-terminal region of D5 is Zn$^{2+}$ dependent, whereas the C-terminal region is rich in lysine and independent of Zn$^{2+}$ (149). However, heparan sulfate, the glycosaminoglycan present on endothelial cells, does not seem to affect binding of HK (150). Although heparan is present, removing heparin with bacterial heparinases or blocking with an antibody to heparin sulfate does not affect the rate of kallikrein formation by assembly of FXII, HK, and PK, nor does the binding of FITC-labeled HK to endothelial cells. Finally, cleaved HK has the ability to prevent the adhesive interaction of vitronectin with tumor cells (121), endothelial cells, platelets, and monocytes, and this ability is much weaker in intact, nonproteolyzed HK. This result is consistent with the early finding that cleaved HK binds much more tightly to anionic surfaces than the uncleaved HK (151).

Domain 6 of HK has overlapping binding sites for PK (S565–K595) and FXI (P556–M613) (152–154). The affinity of PK for binding to intact HK or S565–K595 is the same (17 nM) (155,156). The PK binding site consists of a 31-residue sequence that contains predominantly $\beta$-turn elements (157). Although the 31–amino acid region (S565–K595) was shown to be sufficient for binding (158,159), more recent studies show that an N-terminally and C-terminally truncated 27-mer (W569–K595) has the essential structural elements for PK binding, and a 25-mer is sufficient (12). The procoagulant activity of HK depends both on the ability to bind to anionic surfaces via D5$_H$ and the ability of PK and FXI to bind to domain 6. Inhibition of either interaction with monoclonal antibodies directed to these regions will inhibit HK's procoagulant activity (116,160,161). HK's domain 6 serves as the acceptor protein for either FXI or PK binding to platelets, neutrophils, and endothelial cells (12,50,162, 163). PK binding to bound HK initiates a sequence of events that leads to PK activation and fibrinolysis on the endothelial cell surface independent of FXII activation (12).

# INTERACTIONS BETWEEN THE CONTACT SYSTEM PROTEINS AND CELLS

Many investigators had regarded the contact system as being biologically irrelevant because most studies had focused on its activation on artificial surfaces. However, detailed investigation of the interactions of the proteins of the contact system has led to the hypothesis that the cell membranes are the physiologic negatively charged surfaces for contact system activation. The binding sites on kininogens are similar for all cells in the intravascular compartment, but each cell has one or more characteristic receptors for kininogens (Table 6-1).

The critical protein that assembles the contact system on cell membranes is HK. Platelets, granulocytes, and endothelial cells not only contain HK and LK but also express unoccupied binding sites for HK on each of these cells (109,111,112, 127,164–166). In platelets, less than 8% of total platelet HK is tightly bound to the platelet membrane (109,127). Upon platelet activation, 40% of total platelet HK is secreted, and another 40% of the total becomes bound to TSP expressed on the activated platelet membrane (127). Although the total platelet contribution to plasma HK is only 0.23% (109,167), the local concentration of HK on or near the activated platelet membrane may exceed the plasma concentration of this protein because platelets secrete their granule contents by exocytosis. Most of the granulocyte-associated HK appears to be exogenous HK, tightly bound and nonexchangeable with the granulocyte surface (168). Granulocytes assemble all of the proteins of the contact system on bound HK (169). Neutrophil elastase secreted from granulocytes proteolyzes cell-bound HK (112). It is now believed that there is no mechanism for HK internalization by endothelial cells (119).

There is an absolute requirement for $Zn^{2+}$ for kininogen to bind to all cells. The $Zn^{2+}$-binding region of HK is in $D5_H$ (146,147). A correct fold of D5 is required for cell binding and activation of the contact system. These changes are conformational changes as determined by fluorescent spectroscopy and negative-staining electron microscopy (170). The observation that LK binding to platelets and endothelial cells also requires $Zn^{2+}$ indicates that $Zn^{2+}$ may directly interact with cellular receptors (130). Although $Ca^{2+}$ is not required for cell binding, calcium enhances the upregulation of LK binding to endothelial cells after stimulation with phorbol esters (171). When HK or LK binds to platelets, granulocytes, or endothelial cells, the affinity of binding is similar, between 7 and 52 nM. Because the plasma concentration of HK (670 nM) is more than 10-fold the $K_d$ value, all kininogen binding sites in the intravascular compartment are probably saturated *in vivo*. Unstimulated platelets have approximately 1,000 binding sites per cell, but the value is 5,000 when activated with thrombin. Granulocytes display 50,000 sites per cell. Endothelial cells average approximately 1,000,000 sites per cell at 4°C and approximately 10,000,000 sites per cell when maintained at 37°C. Therefore, the density of receptors is similar because the sites per cell are roughly proportional to the surface area. However, this does not imply that there is a single receptor on each cell; in fact, these cells probably have a minimum of two different receptors (see subsequent text).

HK binds to platelets, endothelial cells, and granulocytes, utilizing specific sequences on both their heavy and light chains (132,133,164,172). Hasan et al. have suggested that HK utilizes parts of three domains to approximate to the putative kininogen receptor(s) on endothelial cells (142). The interaction sites between HK and its putative receptor may be multiple locations, 3 in domain 3, 1 in domain 4, and 2 in domain 5 (134,142,143). The sequences of peptide L331–M357 from domain 3 and H479–498 from domain 5 are the highest-affinity binding regions on HK for endothelial cells (134,143). Recently, these same sequences were shown to be responsible for binding to uPAR (173). The binding of even a very low affinity sequence from domain 4 will block whole HK from binding to endothelial cells (142), suggesting that HK and, to a lesser extent, LK have a tight fit into its binding site(s), that is, putative receptor(s). The fact that bound HK has altered

susceptibility to kallikrein cleavage (172) indicates that a conformational alteration may allow better fit into the binding site of at least one receptor. This postulate would explain the higher affinity for HK than HKa in binding to endothelial cells. These biologic changes are predictable from the major conformational changes that take place between HK and kinin-free kininogen, as shown by increase of the latter's binding to anionic surfaces (151) and by the differences demonstrated by electron microscopy (115) and documented by circular dichroism (174). When LK is cleaved between domains 1 and 2, there is a change in the conformation of the LK, which results in decreased LK binding to endothelial cells compared with intact LK (120).

The putative receptor(s) for kininogen on endothelial cells appears to be regulated. First, the ability of cells to bind kininogen requires metabolic energy and is dependent on temperature (119) but not new protein synthesis. Second, exposure of endothelial cells to BK results in increased HK and LK binding, and this pathway is mediated by protein kinase C and the endothelial cell B1 BK receptor (171). Third, angiotensin-converting enzyme (ACE) inhibitors potentiate the effect of BK on upregulating the HK binding site on endothelial cells (171). Finally, when HK binds to endothelial cells, it initiates a series of events that allow endothelial cell-associated or matrix-associated prolylcarboxypeptidase to activate PK bound to HK (50). All of these observations indicate the likely existence of protein receptors on blood and endothelial cells.

Each cell has unique as well as common kininogen receptors. The first well-documented receptor was discovered on neutrophils. Antibody inhibition studies suggest that Mac-1 (integrin $\alpha M\beta_2$) (CD11b/18) is an HK binding site on granulocytes (133). This finding is consistent with the fact that fibrinogen is a noncompetitive inhibitor of HK binding to granulocytes (175). HK has been shown to bind directly to purified CD11b/18 and to cells transfected with the mRNA for this receptor (176). The finding that integrins such as Mac-1 are tightly associated with the urokinase receptor (177) and can enhance the binding of ligands such as vitronectin to domain 2/3 of uPAR could be relevant to the interaction of kininogens with neutrophils, which display two kininogen-binding proteins, CD11b/18 and uPAR. The finding provides a potential pathway by which kininogen binding could effect cell signaling through neutrophil integrins. Because uPAR is anchored in the membrane but has no cytoplasmic domain, CD11b/18 would provide the biochemical apparatus for signal transduction. Soluble urokinase receptor (suPAR) markedly inhibits the binding of HK, and domains 2 + 3 of this soluble receptor form a complex in a cell-free system. Mahdi et al. (173) have localized two regions on uPAR, one on the C-terminal of D2 (L166-T195) and the other on the $N$-terminal of uPAR D3 (Q215-N255). Herwald et al. have isolated a 33-kDa protein that was identified as gC1qR (179) on an HK affinity column from a human umbilical vein endothelial cell line (178). gC1qR is a known C1 receptor protein (180) that binds only HKa and peptides from domain 5 but not LK or binding peptides from domain 3. FXII blocks HK binding to gC1qR, consistent with the finding that FXII partially blocks HK binding to endothelial cells (181). HK also binds to the uPAR on endothelial cells (122) but HKa displays much higher affinity than HK because domain 5 is the major site for binding. An antibody to domain 2/3 of uPAR completely inhibits HK binding to endothelial cells, as it does vitronectin, a ligand for uPAR. In a separate mechanism, vitronectin and HKa form a bimolecular complex that inhibits the binding of each ligand to cellular receptors (182). CK1 is an additional kininogen (HK and LK) binding site, particularly on endothelial cells (183). Kininogen binding to CK1 requires $Zn^{2+}$, and all cell binding domains of kininogens interact with it. The three receptors of HK (CK, gC1qR, and uPAR) appear to be a multiprotein receptor complex because they colocalize on the endothelial cell surface, as shown by laser scanning confocal microscopy. This finding is consistent with the finding that an antibody to any of these proteins inhibits the binding of HK and FXII to endothelial cells (184). This picture has been further defined (185) by the observation that CK1 interacts with either uPAR or gC1qR, but uPAR and gC1qR do not directly bind to each other. In fact, uPAR and gC1qR compete with each other for binding to CK1. This scheme may be understood by the fact that domain 5 is highly exposed in HKa and can bind to either uPAR or gC1qR. In contrast, HK domains 3 and 5 both bind to CK1. When HK or HKa binds to endothelial cells, they may carry with them either PK or factor XI, which binds to overlapping sites on domain 6 of HK. Two papers have addressed the relative priority of the assembly of these two zymogens on cultured human endothelial cells. Baird and Walsh (186), using human umbilical cord endothelial cells (HUVEC)-coated microcarrier beads, showed that physiologic concentrations of factor XI inhibit lower levels of HK from binding, whereas PK has no effect on HK binding to endothelial cells. Mahdi et al. (187) used confluent monolayers of HUVEC as well as suspensions of HUVEC and HUVEC matrix. Their study showed that PK specifically binds to HUVEC in the presence of HK and low levels of $Zn^{2+}$. Plasma concentrations of PK completely blocked factor XI or XIa. Therefore, PK activation can contribute to the constitutive anticoagulant nature of the intravascular compartment. Experimental conditions may explain the differences in the two results just reported.

Kallikrein, but not PK, activates neutrophils. Exposure of neutrophils to concentrations of kallikrein capable of eliciting chemotaxis (188) increases aerobic glycolysis and the activity of the hexose-monophosphate shunt (11). In the presence of calcium, neutrophils aggregate in response to kallikrein, associated with stimulation of the respiratory burst in neutrophils, as indicated by an increase in oxygen uptake (11). Kallikrein also induces neutrophils to secrete human neutrophil elastase from their primary azurophilic granules (10) and potentiates superoxide formation. In plasma, human neutrophils release elastase during blood coagulation (10), but neutrophils resuspended in either PK- or FXII-deficient plasma release less than one third of the amount of elastase released in normal human plasma (10), indicating a major role for the contact system in neutrophil activation. *In vivo* chemotaxis of leukocytes in response to tissue or microvascular injury shows a significant impairment in chemotaxis in patients deficient in FXII and PK (189). The *in vitro* release of elastase from neutrophils by kallikrein requires the presence of both the active site of kallikrein (on its light chain) and an intact heavy chain (77). The need for an uncleaved heavy chain can be explained by the requirement for both apple 1 and apple 4 sequences for binding of kallikrein to HK on neutrophils. In human sepsis and experimental arthritis and enterocolitis, kallikrein would also recruit neutrophils to participate in the body defenses. FXIIa stimulates neutrophil aggregation (10) and degranulation (release of elastase). Because FXIIf will not stimulate neutrophils, a domain on the heavy chain is required. However, the catalytic mechanism present on the light chain of FXIIa is required because active site inhibitors abolish the reaction. FXIIa can downregulate FcγR1 (immunoglobulin) receptors on monocytes. This interaction requires the heavy chain but, in contrast to the effect of FXIIa on neutrophils, does not require the catalytic apparatus of the light chain (8). The site on FXII responsible for the downregulation of FcγR1 may be within the N-terminal 18 amino acids (190), and this decrease could impair the clearance of immune complexes. Toossi et al. (9) have found that, in addition to FXII-induced monocyte synthesis and secretion of IL-1 and IL-6, lipopolysaccharide (LPS)-stimulated secretion of these interleukins is also potentiated.

# BIOLOGIC FUNCTIONS OF CONTACT SYSTEM PROTEINS

Understanding of the physiologic functions of the contact system has been delayed by the observations that a deficiency of HK, PK, and FXII prolongs artificial surface-activated clotting without being associated with bleeding. Contact system activation influences vascular biology independent of its lack of effect on hemostasis. Kininogens have a number of potential biologic activities, either within the domains of intact protein or developing when the intact protein is proteolyzed by kallikreins or activated FXII (Table 6-1). This system is a potent local regulator of blood pressure through BK delivery. In contrast, the lack of hemorrhagic symptoms in HK deficiency is consistent with selective antithrombin and profibrinolytic activity. The cleavage of HK by kallikrein uncovers antiadhesive properties of the protein. HKa and kallikrein decrease urokinase-induced monocyte adhesion to plastic surfaces (191).

## Bradykinin Formation

The best known function of the plasma kininogens is the release of BK, a potent bioactive peptide (7). Both kininogens and BK contribute to vessel patency; increased blood flow; and antiadhesive, profibrinolytic, and antithrombotic activities. BK is a potent stimulator of endothelial cell prostacyclin synthesis. Prostacyclin, by stimulating adenylate cyclase to increase intracellular cAMP, is both an inhibitor of platelet function (192) as well as a vasodilator. BK stimulates endothelial nitric oxide synthetase to form NO, which upregulates guanylate cyclase, elevating cyclic guanosine monophosphate (cGMP), and therefore acting as an inhibitor of platelet function and a vasodilator (193), as well as inhibiting subendothelial smooth muscle proliferation (194). Therefore, kinins prevent vascular smooth muscle growth and proliferation in the intact endothelial cell (195,196). Conversely, vessel injury results in BK stimulating protein kinase C and mitogen-activating protein (MAP) kinases, signaling systems that enhance vascular smooth muscle growth (197,198). Therefore, BK functions to keep intact vessels patent; but with vessel injury, BK stimulates vascular repair and may contribute to atherosclerotic processes by enhancing smooth muscle proliferation and intimal hypertrophy.

BK binds to two cloned receptors, designated B1 and B2 (199,200). Both of these receptors are 7-transmembrane and G-protein–coupled. BK binding stimulates cellular signal transduction. Chronic blockade of the B2 receptor with an antagonist in developing rats results in higher blood pressures, heart rates, and increased body weights (201). ACE inhibitors are cardioprotective by elevating BK, thereby increasing NO, as well as decreasing angiotensin II formation. The cardiac protection of isolated ischemic hearts from ACE-treated animals is abolished by a B2 receptor antagonist (201). ACE-inhibitor treatment in spontaneously hypertensive rats prevents the development of hypertension and left ventricular hypertrophy, presumably by decreasing angiotensin II and increasing BK. Evidence for the latter effect is that a B2 receptor blocks or prevents these changes (202). ACE inhibitors in humans are protective against myocardial infarction by increasing myocardial blood flow and decreasing ischemic changes. The use of BK receptor blockers, although useful, may lead to erroneous conclusions to the degree to which some of these drugs may have partial agonist effects. In addition, recent evidence suggests that some antagonists may be reverse agonists; that is, they inhibit only stimulated responses but may not affect the effects of basal concentration of BK. A powerful approach, the targeted disruption of the mouse B2 BK receptor in embryonic stem cells, creating a B2 receptor knockout (B2R-KO), was achieved by Borkowski and Hess (203). The biologic responses in these B2R-KO mice has provided additional insights into the role of BK. In these animals, not only was the blood pressure decrease in response to BK completely abolished but a high Na$^+$ diet also produced an enhanced hypertensive effect as well as increased heart and kidney weight (204). These changes are accompanied by a decreased renal blood flow and increased renal vascular resistance in the B2R-KO compared to normal rat of the same genetic background (205). A possible explanation of these results is that the elimination of response to BK leads to the unopposed hypertensive action of the renin–angiotensin system (206). This hypothesis is supported by the finding that chronic inhibition of ACE by captopril in B2R-KO mice leads to an exaggerated blood pressure reduction because of interference with the unbalanced vasoconstrictor action of the renin–angiotensin system. Further evidence for this concept was obtained in a model of renovascular hypertension in which partial obstruction of one renal artery with a clip leads to an activated renin–angiotensin system in the ischemic kidney and upregulation of B2 receptors in the contralateral kidney. In the B2R-KO mice, the blood pressure rise was increased, as was the heart weight (207). Therefore, BK exerts a protective effect against excessive blood pressure elevation in renovascular hypertension. Preconditioning has been shown to protect the heart against ischemic–reperfusion injury in mice (208). The cardioprotective effect is absent in the B2R-KO mice. Therefore, an intact kallikrein–kinin system is necessary, and activation of PK to release kinins from kininogen may contribute to the effects of preconditioning.

## Regulation of Blood Pressure by Kallikreins

Little is known about what regulates the liberation of BK from kininogens by plasma and tissue kallikrein on the vascular endothelium. Regulation of these enzymes is important because they directly modulate BK liberation, which, in turn, has a direct effect on blood pressure *in vivo*. Infusion of dextran sulfate into rats results in arterial hypotension that can be prevented by an antagonist of the B2 receptor (209). Overexpression of tissue kallikrein in transgenic mice renders them chronically hypotensive. Intramuscular delivery of the gene for rat kallikrein–binding protein gene reverses hypotension in these transgenic mice (210). Rat kallikrein–binding protein (human kallistatin) is the major inhibitor of tissue kallikrein (211,212). Delivery of the tissue kallikrein gene reduced the arterial blood pressure of spontaneous hypertensive rats, and this inhibition was prevented by an infusion of kallikrein-binding protein (213). These studies show directly that BK liberated by tissue kallikrein can modulate local or systemic blood pressure. An additional level of regulation is evident from the observation that hypertension induced by chronic inhibition of nitric oxide synthetase leads to enhanced synthesis of kininogen and tissue kallikrein (214). Recently, elevation of plasma PK has been shown to be a risk marker for hypertension and nephropathy in type 1 diabetes (215).

## Thrombin Inhibition

The kininogens (precursors of BK) have been shown to selectively inhibit thrombin-induced platelet activation by at least three mechanisms. HK and LK can inhibit platelet calpain (110). Cytosolic or internal membrane–associated platelet calpain translocates to the activated platelet surface following activation by thrombin (128,129). Externalized platelet calpain is able to proteolyze GP Ib to produce glycocalicin (216) as well as other platelet surface membrane glycoproteins. Platelet calpain can aggregate platelets by cleaving a putative platelet adenosine diphosphate (ADP) receptor that exposes the platelet fibrinogen receptor (217). Therefore, inhibition of externalized platelet calpain by HK, LK, or other inhibitors of calpains results in inhibition of thrombin-mediated platelet aggregation by preventing fibrinogen binding (218). Molecular models of domain 2 have helped to identify critical sequences that can prevent α- and γ-thrombin–induced platelet aggregation without interfering with the induction of platelet activation by other platelet agonists (219,220). These peptides could serve as lead compounds to develop peptidomimetics that can specifically inhibit platelet aggregation by thrombin.

A second mechanism stemmed from detailed studies to try to ascertain the mechanism of HK inhibition of thrombin-induced platelet activation. Both kininogens were found to modulate thrombin-induced platelet secretion and aggregation (131,137). Because thrombin-induced platelet secretion is independent of and occurs before platelet aggregation, there must be mechanism(s) other than inhibition of calpain-related platelet aggregation. The discovery that HK blocked thrombin binding to platelets established a second mechanism (137). The ability to inhibit α-thrombin binding to platelets initially was localized to domain 3 of kininogen (131). However, the differential effect of a monoclonal antibody on cell-binding and α-thrombin inhibitory activity suggested that two different regions of domain 3 are involved (131). The fact that Kunapuli et al. (101) found that recombinant domain 3 (containing no residues for domain 4) inhibited thrombin aggregation of platelets with only twofold less affinity than purified HK indicates that a major site for inhibition is localized to domain 3. The effect of Leu271–Ala277 was specific because a concentration that blocked thrombin-induced aggregation did not inhibit platelet aggregation by ADP or collagen. No effect of Leu271–Ala277 was demonstrated on the amidolytic or clotting activity of thrombin. Leu271–Ala277 also failed to inhibit platelet shape change, the first event associated with an increase in intracellular calcium, an activity associated with activation of the thrombin receptor. Further, Leu271–Ala277 did not inhibit SFLLRN from aggregating platelets. Bradford et al. (221) showed that Leu271–Ala277 and Lys270–Gln292 inhibit thrombin-induced platelet activation at low thrombin concentrations by inhibiting the binding of thrombin to GP Ib/IX/V complex. First, Leu271–Ala277 shifted the dose-response curve of thrombin 10-fold, similar to the requirement of 10-fold more thrombin needed to stimulate the platelets of patients lacking GP Ib/IX (Bernard-Soulier disease). Moreover, HK failed to inhibit thrombin stimulation of platelets of patients with Bernard-Soulier disease. Further, HK binding to platelets was inhibited by antibodies to GP Ib/IX as well as ligands of GP Ib. HK inhibited binding of antibodies to GP Ib/IX complex to platelets. High-affinity (125) I-thrombin binding to platelets was inhibited by peptides from domain 3 of kininogens. Finally, the binding of thrombin to fibroblasts transfected with GP Ib/IX/V, but not expressing the 7-transmembrane receptor for thrombin, was inhibited by HK. Therefore, domain 3 peptides inhibit thrombin binding to a high-affinity site on GP Ibα. A possible reason is that the amino acid sequence NAEN appears in HK domain 3 peptides, and the ligand-binding domain of GP Ibα. It is likely that GP Ibα may serve to present thrombin to the G-protein–linked receptor, thereby decreasing the concentration of thrombin necessary to cleave the latter receptor. HK and LK, by modulating this interaction, would then inhibit thrombin-induced activation.

In a third mechanism described by Hasan et al. (138), kininogens and peptides derived from it inhibit thrombin-induced platelet activation by blocking the ability of the protease to cleave the G-protein–linked thrombin receptor PAR-1. Peptides from domain 4, BK, and related sequences were found to inhibit thrombin-induced platelet activation. Although HK, LK, and domain 3 inhibited thrombin binding to platelets, isolated domain 4, including BK (R363–R371) and M361–G376, did not inhibit binding (130,131,138), indicating that another mechanism is operative. Like HK and LK, domain 4 peptides did not inhibit the ability of thrombin to cleave a tripeptide substrate or clot fibrinogen, suggesting that these peptides did not form a complex with thrombin (119,130,131,138). Domain 4 peptides were not substrates of α-thrombin, and did not block ADP-, collagen-, or U46619-induced platelet aggregation (138). The domain 4 peptides did inhibit thrombin-induced calcium mobilization and γ-thrombin–induced platelet aggregation. The minimal sequence from domain 4 that inhibited α-thrombin–induced platelet activation was the peptide RPPGF. RPPGF is a major breakdown product of BK resulting from proteolytic cleavage by ACE with a half-life in plasma of 4.2 hours (222,223). RPPGF does not block the thrombin receptor peptide, SFLLRN, from inducing platelet activation (138). Instead, domain 4 peptides prevent α-thrombin from cleaving the hepta-spanning G-protein–coupled thrombin receptor after arginine-41, which is a requirement for thrombin activation of cells through this receptor (138). RPPGF and HK prevented thrombin from hydrolyzing the bond between the arginine and the serine on a peptide, NATLDPRSFLLR, spanning the cleavage site of the receptor. Domain 4 peptides are selective inhibitors of thrombin that prevent it from cleaving certain of its substrates. RPPGF specifically interferes with the ability of thrombin to cleave the hepta-spanning thrombin receptor that is required to activate platelets without interfering with its procoagulant activity. Bradford et al. (224) showed that FXIIa also binds to GP Ib/IX/V complex and inhibits thrombin-induced platelet aggregation, but the site is not identical to that of kininogen.

## Fibrinolysis

HK participates in cellular fibrinolysis. Even before HK deficiency was recognized, this protein has been ascribed to have a role in the fibrinolytic process (225). Contact activation has long been known to increase plasma fibrinolysis (226). Kallikrein and FXIIa cleave plasminogen directly, although much more slowly than tPA or urokinase plasminogen activator (70,227). However, plasma kallikrein has been characterized as a kinetically favorable activator of single-chain urokinase in a purified system (4). Prourokinase activation by kallikrein is most efficient on cell surfaces (12,50,122,228,229).

These studies prompted reexamination of PK assembly on endothelial cells and how it may participate in prourokinase activation. Binding of PK to HK on endothelial cells results in activation of the zymogen to kallikrein, as indicated by elaboration of amidolytic activity, changes in the structure of PK to kallikrein on reduced gel electrophoresis, and cleavage of HK. PK is activated on the endothelial cell surface by a membrane-associated serine protease, prolylcarboxypeptidase (52). The degree of PK activation is regulated by HK. Increasing HK concentrations upregulate the enzyme that activates cell-bound PK. We have shown that peptides derived from D6 of HK can downregulate plasmin formation by interfering with PK binding to HK on the endothelial cell surface (12). Increased BK increases kininogen binding, which prevents fluid-phase kallikrein from cleaving HK to liberate more BK (171). This feedback allows close linkage of PK activation and BK liberation.

Two pathways of fibrinolysis are initiated by PK activation on endothelial cells. First, kallikrein cleaves HK, liberating BK, a potent and specific agonist of endothelial cell tissue plasminogen activator secretion. Second, kallikrein converts prourokinase into two-chain urokinase, despite being in an environment where there is a molar excess of plasminogen activator inhibitor-1. Formation of urokinase results in a 4.3-fold increase in plasmin formation (12). This system for plasminogen activation on the endothelial surface is independent of FXIIa. Prourokinase activation is a pathway for cellular fibrinolysis that is either independent of or conjoined with prourokinase activation associated with its binding to its receptor (230). The binding of HK (and, thus, kallikrein) to domains 2 and 3 of the urokinase receptor (122) on the same molecule as prourokinase, which binds to domain 1 of the receptor, allows for a very efficient cleavage of the latter by kallikrein. In addition, HK can compete with vitronectin, which also binds to domains 2 and 3 of the urokinase receptor, and can displace vitronectin and its associated molecule, plasminogen activator inhibitor 1, thereby enhancing fibrinolysis.

## Antiadhesive Interactions

The antiadhesive action of HK has been observed under three different situations. First, cleaved, kinin-free kininogen (HKa) can bind and displace adhesive proteins on negatively charged surfaces occurring on biomaterials. Second, HKa can inhibit adhesive protein binding to cells. Third, HK on anionic surfaces or bound to cells can inhibit cell adhesion to protein-covered surfaces.

Vroman and Adams (231) found that within seconds after normal human plasma contacts an anionic surface, fibrinogen can be detected immunochemically within minutes, but is no longer available to the antibodies. This phenomenon is caused by the displacement of fibrinogen by HK following surface-dependent autoactivation of FXII to FXIIa (232,233). FXIIa, both directly and by forming plasma kallikrein, cleaves HK to HKa. Both cleavage of HK and the presence of HK light chain are needed to displace fibrinogen from the surface (233). This time- and surface-dependent generation of HKa, by contact activation of plasma, accounts for the "Vroman effect," or physical displacement of adherent fibrinogen from the surface (233). Extensive proteolysis, especially by FXIa (140), presents displacement of fibrinogen (233).

HK and/or HKa can displace (125) I-fibrinogen from both neutrophils and platelets (175). Asakura et al. (121) extended these results by showing that the protein present in serum, which inhibited the adhesion and spreading of human osteosarcoma cells to vitronectin-coated polystyrene plates, was HKa but not HKi, HK, or LK. Furthermore, HKa also inhibited the attachment of monocytes and platelets to extracellular matrix proteins. The spreading of bovine aortic endothelial cells on both fibrinogen and vitronectin was also inhibited by HKa (121). Monocyte attachment to vitronectin is inhibited by HKa because these two proteins compete for occupancy of domains 2 and 3 on the urokinase receptor, which is present on these cells. Neutrophils in a radial flow system at a shear rate of 20 per second adhere to a fibrinogen-coated surface linearly. We have shown that the rate of adherence to the same surface coated with HK is at least five times slower (13). The possibility of passivating anionic surfaces with HKa or selected peptides could provide new approaches to biocompatibility (234). We have recently applied these findings to inhibiting the adhesion of leukocytes to vitronectin, a component of the provisional extracellular matrix important in inflammation. We found that in addition to HKa and D5 (235), a histidine–glycine–lysine-rich peptide derived from D5, G486-K502 (236), inhibited cell adhesion to vitronectin. However, platelets do not express uPAR; therefore, this receptor cannot be a major kininogen receptor on all cells. Platelets appear to have two receptors for HK and FXII, that is, gC1qR and GP Ib/IX/V complex. Binding to the latter by HK or FXII (224) blocks thrombin binding and activation of platelets. Much attention has centered on the role of platelet–leukocyte interactions in inflammatory conditions. A new mechanism for the formation of cell aggregates is the bridging of Mac-1 on neutrophils or monocytes to GP Ib on platelets by HK (237). The activation of intravascular cells can be mediated by peptides released from contact system proteins or by the proteases formed: FXIIa and kallikrein. Kininogen binding to cells is a key event in forming of these active components. Platelet and endothelial cell–bound HK is protected from activation by exogenous plasma kallikrein (172,238). Because PK binds to HK at domain 6 separate from the binding sites (domains 3, 4, and 5), it serves as an acquired binding site for PK on cells (50,163). PK bound to HK on platelets or endothelial cells can result in its activation to kallikrein by FXIIa-dependent (228) or -independent (50) mechanisms. Both situations result in the generation of BK.

## Antiangiogenic Actions

Because of the antiadhesive and profibrinolytic action of HKa and its binding to uPAR, we postulated that HKa would inhibit angiogenesis. We found that recombinant domain 5 (kininostatin) inhibited endothelial cell proliferation stimulated by fibroblast growth factor 2 (FGF2), as well as endothelial cell migration toward vitronectin (239). Domain 5 inhibited FGF2-stimulated angiogenesis in a chicken chorioallantoic membrane (CAM). Endothelial cell migration was inhibited by a peptide 485–503, whereas proliferation was modulated by a different peptide 440–455, both from domain 5 (239). Kawasaki et al. (240) confirmed the former results and found that an octapeptide 484–491 inhibited the adhesion and invasion (migration) of tumor cells *in vitro* and metastasis *in vivo*. HGK, a sequence contained in 484–491, was also active *in vitro*. The synergism between the effects on migration and proliferation explains the potent inhibition of angiogenesis by domain 5 ($IC_{50}$ = 100 nM) and HKa (30 nM). We then investigated the mechanism by which D5 inhibited endothelial cell proliferation by FGF2 (241). Endothelial cells stimulated by FGF2 showed typical morphologic features of apoptosis after exposure to D5, confirmed by nuclear staining and DNA fragmentation. The conclusion that HKa induces endothelial cell apoptosis is consistent with the observations of other investigators (240). D5 was found to significantly reduce cyclin D1, a critical component of the cell cycle required for transition from G1 to S phase. Further evidence that HKa affected the cell cycle was that during the apoptosis produced upregulation of Cdc2 and cyclin A (242) responsible for S to G2 transition. This change has been interpreted as a compensatory change secondary to either apoptosis or cyclic D1 downregulation.

An important insight into the mechanism of action of D5 was that the apoptotic effect of HKa is regulated by extracellular matrix proteins (243). We found that the inhibitory action of HKa and D5 was dependent on the component of the provisional extracellular matrix to which the endothelial cell adheres. HKa inhibits endothelial adhesion to vitronectin but not to fibronectin. In parallel, HKa induces apoptosis when cells are grown attached to vitronectin but not fibronectin. These findings suggest that apoptosis is at least in part mediated by cell detachment, in particular, anoxis. We showed that HKa and D5 inhibited cell spreading and F-actin formation in endothelial cells attached to vitronectin, accompanied by inhibition of the downstream signaling molecules, focal adhesion

kinase, as well as paxillin. Evidence from our laboratory (244) indicates that these inhibitory effects are mediated by binding of HKa to the urokinase receptor and dissociation of integrins $\alpha_V\beta_3$ and $\alpha_5\beta_1$ to interrupt the downstream intracellular signaling including the phosphorylation of focal adhesion kinase by the Syk kinase yes and the subsequent phosphorylation of paxillin.

Endothelial cells are similar to cancer cells in that both need to invade tissues to form vessels and metastasize respectively. HKa and D5 both inhibit haptotaxis (vitronectin-mediated migration) and haptoinvasion of osteosarcoma cells (245). Moreover, the peptide responsible (H479-K493) is similar to the peptide that inhibited migration of endothelial cells (239). Recently, we have demonstrated (246) that D5 can also inhibit colon carcinoma proliferation by blocking the cell cycle at the G1-S transition.

Because HKa (247) and D5 were antiangiogenic, we postulated that intact HK would be proangiogenic, as observed for collagen and plasminogen and their proteolytic cleavage products, endostatin and angiostatin, respectively. Both HK and LK stimulated angiogenesis in the CAM (248), demonstrating that D5 is not involved in the proangiogenic effect. Inhibition of kallikrein blocked the proangiogenic activity of HK, suggesting that BK was responsible for the stimulation of neovascularization. This result is consistent with the demonstration by Parenti et al. (249) that BK promotes angiogenesis by upregulation of endogenous FGF2 in endothelial cells by the nitric oxide synthetase pathway. Furthermore, a monoclonal antibody to HK (mAb C11C1) that blocks HK binding to endothelial cells also recognizes ornithokininogen in the CAM. This finding explains the observation that mAb C11C1 inhibits HK stimulation of angiogenesis as well as FGF2- or VEGF-induced neovascularization in the CAM (248). Moreover, mAb C11C1 inhibits the growth of human fibrosarcoma on the CAM. This result suggests that mAb C11C1 may have the potential to inhibit tumor-induced angiogenesis in animal models of angiogenesis. Recently, we have demonstrated that this antibody inhibited the growth of human colon carcinoma, a xenograft in an immunoincompetent (nude) mouse (250).

# CONTACT SYSTEM IN DISEASE STATES

## Systemic Inflammatory Response Syndrome

Systemic inflammatory response syndrome (SIRS) (251) is caused by either sepsis or trauma; is manifested by hypotension, disseminated intravascular coagulation (DIC), adult respiratory distress syndrome (ARDS), and multiple organ failure; and is the result of overresponses by the host defense systems that are triggered to combat injury. The complex humoral response (252) results in the release of mediators such as monokines, particularly TNF (253) and IL-1; prostaglandins (254); neutrophil release of proteolytic enzymes such as elastase (255); and the activation of the serine protease cascades of the coagulation (256), fibrinolytic (257), complement (258), and kallikrein–kinin systems (259). SIRS may begin with a localized infection that may disseminate organisms to the blood. Bacterial cell wall components, which include endotoxins or proteoglycan polysaccharides, trigger the release of host mediators and initiate plasma protease cascades.

In sepsis, FXII and PK are cleaved and activated to enzymes that rapidly react with C1-IHN to form FXIIa–C1-INH and kallikrein–C1-INH complexes (see Table 6-2). The result is depletion of functional PK and FXII with persistence of normal levels of the corresponding antigens. Functional C1-INH also declines, but its antigen remains constant or may

## TABLE 6-2

### CLINICAL AND EXPERIMENTAL CONDITIONS ASSOCIATED WITH CONTACT SYSTEM ACTIVATION

| Disease/Experimental model | PK | HK | C1-INH | Factor XI | Factor XII | $\alpha_2$M-Kal complexes | C1-INH–Kal complexes |
|---|---|---|---|---|---|---|---|
| Sepsis (205,255,258,262,263,270) | ↓ | ↓ | ↓ | — | ↓ | ↑ | — |
| Typhoid fever (256,259,268) | ↓[a] | — | ↓[b] | — | — | — | ↑ |
| ARDS (261) | ↓ | ↓ | ↓[b] | ↔ | ↓ | — | — |
| Rocky Mountain spotted fever (269) | ↓ | — | ↑ | ↑ | ↔ | — | ↑ |
| Cardiopulmonary bypass (266,267,278,279) | — | — | — | — | — | — | ↑ |
| Hereditary angioedema (260,264,282) | ↓ | ↓ | ↓ | — | — | ↑ | — |
| Low-dose endotoxin administration (274,275) | ↓[a] | ↓ | — | ↓ | — | ↑ | — |
| Baboon *Escherichia coli* sepsis (276,277) | ↓ | ↓ | — | ↑ | — | ↑ | — |
| Rat arthritis (274,285–288) | ↓ | ↓ | — | ↓ | — | — | — |
| Rat enterocolitis (290–296) | ↓ | ↓ | — | ↓ | — | — | — |

PK, prekallikrein; HK, high-molecular-weight kininogen; C1-INH, C1-inhibitor; $\alpha_2$M-Kal, $\alpha_2$-macroglobulin-kallikrein; C1-INH–Kal, C1-INH–kallikrein; ARDS, adult respiratory distress syndrome; ↓, decreased; ↑, increased; ↔, unaffected; —, not assayed.
[a]Antigen unaffected.
[b]Antigen increased.

even increase, suggesting that it behaves as a weak acute-phase reactant. As functional C1-INH decreases, $\alpha_2$M becomes a more important inhibitor of kallikrein, and $\alpha_2$M-kallikrein complexes are formed (260). The HK coagulant activity and antigen decrease in parallel (261).

Functional FXII, PK, and C1-INH are decreased in patients with hypotensive septicemia (262) and DIC caused by septicemia or viremia. Individuals with DIC secondary to neoplasia had no significant changes in the kallikrein–kinin system. In patients with postoperative septicemia, decreased PK activity and elevated BK were associated with positive blood cultures and hypotension (263). In an experimental infection of humans with typhoid fever, all patients with the onset of fever and thrombocytopenia also showed a decrease in functional PK and C1-INH, but not immunologic levels of the same protein, and circulating kallikrein–C1-INH complexes were detected (268). In ARDS, affected patients had reduced plasma levels of FXII, PK, HK, and C1-INH activity, but there were increased levels of C1-INH antigen, which behaves as an acute-phase protein (261). In a vaccine trial, patients who develop Rocky Mountain spotted fever show decreased PK levels and increased kallikrein–C1-INH complexes (269).

Because kallikrein–C1-INH complexes are cleared rapidly in most cases of septic shock (270), we developed a "sandwich" enzyme-linked immunosorbent assay (ELISA) for $\alpha_2$M-Kal complexes. We found that in septicemic hypotension, but not in septicemia alone or liver disease, $\alpha_2$M-Kal complexes were elevated (264). In a surgical intensive care unit, PK was reduced and kininogen was cleaved in both sepsis and nonsepsis patients (265).

To address the question of whether activation of the contact system was an early event, normal human volunteers were given a low dose of *E. coli* endotoxin (0.4 ng per kg body weight). These individuals developed a hyperdynamic cardiovascular state and a "flulike" syndrome lasting 24 hours (275). Functional PK levels were significantly lower in the endotoxin group as compared with controls at 2 hours after infusion and remained low up to 24 hours. The concentration of $\alpha_2$M-Kal complexes was significantly elevated four- to fivefold in the endotoxin-treated group up to 5 hours, with a return to normal in the circulating levels of complexes by 24 hours. Therefore, a low dose of endotoxin can induce a prolonged state of contact activation.

To evaluate the role of either shock or DIC, relevant to contact activation, an established experimental baboon model of bacteremia was utilized. Two concentrations of *E. coli* were used to produce lethal and nonlethal hypotension. In the lethal group, the decline in functional levels of HK and an increase in $\alpha_2$M-Kal complexes correlated significantly with the delayed irreversible hypotension (276). In contrast, in the nonlethal group, there was a less striking decline in HK, and only slight elevation in $\alpha_2$M-Kal, and the hypotension was reversible. Therefore, hypotension correlates with activation of the contact system. To address whether the contact activation in shock and hypotension was cause or effect, a monoclonal antibody to human FXII was selected, which is able *in vitro* to inhibit FXII coagulant activity in baboon plasma by 60% and slow kininogen cleavage in dextran sulfate-activated baboon plasma. This antibody was infused into the lethal baboon group 30 minutes before the challenge with *E. coli* (277). DIC was unaffected; the decline of factor V, fibrinogen, and platelets was similar in both groups. However, contact activation was inhibited; whereas there was a marked decline in HK in the untreated group reaching 40% of the baseline levels by 300 minutes, in the treated group, HK remained stable and was significantly higher at 360 minutes. Furthermore, in the untreated group there was a progressive rise of $\alpha_2$M-Kal complexes, which was highly significant, but in the group treated with the antibody, the increase in $\alpha_2$M-Kal complexes was completely inhibited. A significant decline of mean systemic arterial pressure was observed in both groups of animals between 60 and 120 minutes, possibly resulting from the TNF-$\alpha$, which peaks at this time. Irreversible hypotension supervened in the untreated group, whereas the blood pressure showed recovery in the treated group. The treated animals survived significantly longer than untreated animals, as assessed by a Kaplan-Meier plot. Inhibition of contact system activation with a monoclonal antibody to FXII modulates the hypotension, but not the DIC, indicating the role of the contact system in sepsis.

## Cardiopulmonary Bypass

Clinical cardiopulmonary bypass (CPB) is performed in more than 800,000 individuals in the United States and in more than 2 million patients in the world each year. During CPB, there is extensive contact between blood and the synthetic surfaces of the extracorporeal circuit. Blood in the bypass circuit must be anticoagulated with heparin at 10 times the concentration necessary for treatment of venous thrombosis. The bleeding time is progressively prolonged during bypass, postoperative blood loss is increased, and a chemical and cellular "whole body inflammatory response" is triggered by blood cell interactions and plasma protein alterations. Qualitative and quantitative alterations of platelets, neutrophils, and complement and contact systems have been documented in CPB (278). Heparin, which markedly accelerates the inhibitory action of AT-III *in vitro* on thrombin and FXa, shows the inactivation of FXIIa and kallikrein in CPB. In simulated extracorporeal bypass, there is a significant increase in kallikrein–C1-INH complex formation (266) and C1–C1-INH complexes. These findings indicate that FXII activation is occurring, which cleaves both PK and C1, thereby activating both the contact and classical complement pathways (266). Aprotinin, an inhibitor of both plasmin and plasma kallikrein, can reduce blood loss after cardiac operations and decrease the elevated postoperative bleeding time. In a simulated extracorporeal bypass model, in which no plasmin is found, aprotinin decreased both kallikrein–C1-INH and C1–C1-INH complexes, resulting in a marked inhibition of the release of neutrophil elastase (267). More specific kallikrein inhibitors, Bz-Pro-Phe-boroArg-OH, Arg15-aprotinin, and Ala357-Arg358-$\alpha_1$-protease inhibitor (279), also decrease neutrophil activation, indicating a critical role for plasma kallikrein in the inflammatory responses associated with CPB.

## Hereditary Angioedema

HAE is a congenital condition associated with a quantitative deficiency or qualitative functional defect in C1 inhibitor (280,281). Acute attacks of HAE are associated with contact system activation (282) manifested by reduced plasma PK activity with normal plasma PK antigen and reduced HK activity and antigen (282). Contact activation is promoted by the low C1-INH levels, the major inhibitor of kallikrein and FXIIa. BK liberation is the major mediator of the edema seen in HAE (273). An *in vitro* model is the cold activation of FVII. This phenomenon is a result of cold inactivation of C1-INH and FXII activation in a tube with resultant factor VII activation (283). Lowering temperatures to below 37°C decreases the reactivity of C1-INH for all of its enzyme targets (284).

## Arthritis in Genetically Susceptible Rats—A Model for Human Inflammatory Arthritis

A model of acute and chronic relapsing arthritis induced by intraperitoneal injection of proteoglycan polysaccharide from group A streptococci (PG-APS) into rats (274) provided a means to investigate the role of the kallikrein–kinin system in experimental inflammatory arthritis. The mean joint diameter peaked at a maximum value of 8 on a scale of 1–10 at day 3, reflecting the acute-phase. The volume of the joint declined during days 9 through 12, but then the joint diameter spontaneously increased beginning at day 15, indicating the start of the chronic phase. The arthritis progressed with waxing and waning of individual joints, indicating reactivation leading to chronic synovitis and joint erosion. The arthropathy was consistently associated with an increase in the acute-phase protein, T-kininogen, splenic enlargement, and the development of the anemia of chronic disease. HK in rat plasma decreased on days 1, 5, and 15, and correlated inversely with joint enlargement on day 5, with $\gamma = -0.85$. PK levels decreased as early as 30 minutes after injection of PG-APS, and the levels

remained low throughout the experimental protocol, and were significantly lower than the untreated animals. When the rats were injected with PG-APS and received a specific, potent, oral plasma kallikrein inhibitor, P8720 or Bz-Pro-Phe-boroArg-OH ($K_i = 0.15$ nM), there was a significant decrease (61%) in joint swelling at 49 hours with an absence of most of the dense infiltration of neutrophils and mononuclear cells (285). P8720 prevented the decrease in plasma HK seen in the animals injected with PG-APS but not treated. The anemia, the increase in TK, and the splenic weight increase were inhibited by P8720. BK receptor type 2 antagonist also attenuated acute (286) and chronic (287) arthritis in Lewis rats. Moreover, monoclonal antibody C11C1 inhibited chronic reactive arthritis (induced by PG-APS) in a Lewis rat, presumably by blocking the proangiogenic effects of BK and/or the proinflammatory effects of HKa (288). These data indicate that contact system activation in part mediates the arthritis and that its inhibition modulates all of the manifestations of this disorder.

## Experimental Acute and Chronic Enterocolitis—A Model for Crohn Disease

The role of the contact system in inflammatory bowel disease was investigated by using a model of acute and chronic enterocolitis induced by subserosal injection of PG-APS into the wall of the distal ileum and cecum at multiple sites (289). Acute intestinal inflammation in the genetically susceptible Lewis rat and the resistant Buffalo rat is characterized by edema, hemorrhage, thickening of the bowel wall and mesentery, and adhesions. However, Lewis rats, but not Buffalo rats, spontaneously develop chronic enterocolitis with dense adhesions, thickening of intestinal wall, serosal nodules, enlarged mesenteric lymph nodes, histologic changes consisting of mononuclear cell infiltration and crypt abscesses, and a markedly elevated intestinal myeloperoxidase that persists for more than 16 weeks. Arthritis and hepatic granulomas occurred in 73% of Lewis rats examined for 14 days or more after PG-APS injection; however, only 4% of Buffalo rats developed hepatic granulomas, and arthritis was not evident in Buffalo rats. T-kininogen, the major acute-phase protein in rats, increased in the Lewis rats but not in the Buffalo rats. PK levels were significantly lower in PG-APS–treated Lewis rats compared with controls or Buffalo rats during both acute (290) and chronic (291) phases of inflammation. HK levels were significantly decreased in PG-APS–treated Lewis rats compared to the respective control group. Buffalo rats injected with PG-APS had stable plasma HK concentrations at all timepoints. We demonstrated the first direct connection of the genetic susceptibility of Lewis rats to kallikrein–kininogen–kinin cascade when we found that proteolysis of plasma HK to yield BK was faster in Lewis rats than in Buffalo rats (287). A single point mutation at nucleotide 1586 was found translating respectively to Ser511 in Buffalo and Fischer rat HK, and Asn511 in Lewis rat HK (292). This leads to unique *N* glycosylation in the light chain of HK, which correlates with the more rapid cleavage. Additional evidence for the critical role of kininogen in the mediation of chronic enterocolitis is found in the modulation of systemic and local inflammation in rats with kininogen deficiency on a Lewis genetic background (293). In another model, dextran sulfate sodium–induced colitis in kininogen-deficient rats showed less shortening of the colon, higher hematocrit, and longer survival (294). These changes are not model-specific because kallikrein–kininogen system activation was also found in indomethacin-induced enterocolitis (295). Treatment with the specific oral plasma kallikrein inhibitor, P8720, in the acute and chronic phase of enterocolitis in the Lewis rats reduced the increase of joint diameter, the gross gut score, intestinal myeloperoxidase, and

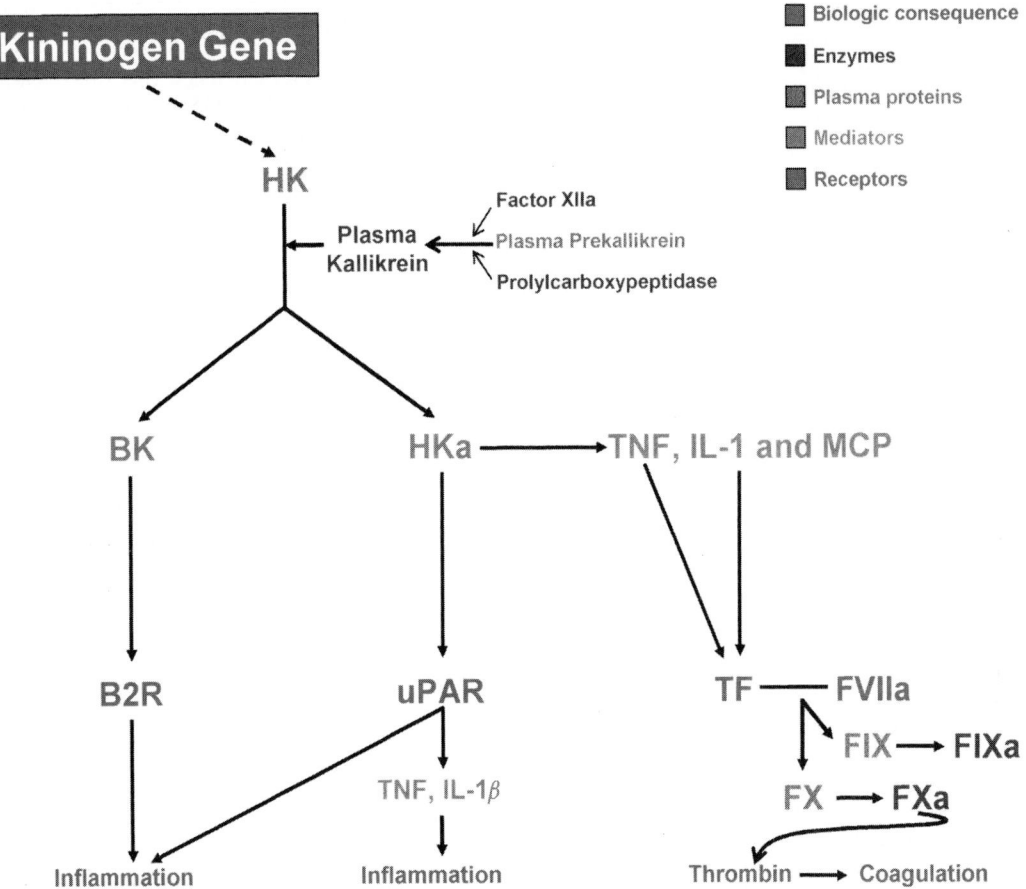

**FIGURE 6-4.** Role of kallikrein–kinin system in inflammation—a hypothesis. The kininogen gene codes for high-molecular-weight kininogen (HK). Factor XIIa from plasma or prolylcarboxypeptidase (an outer cell membrane enzyme) cleaves plasma prekallikrein to plasma kallikrein, which in turn hydrolyzes HK to two mediators. Bradykinin (BK), through its constitutive receptor, B2R, stimulates inflammation. HKa, through one of its receptors, uPAR, stimulates inflammation in leukocytes. TF, a receptor induced by inflammatory cytokines (IL-1, TNF), is responsible for binding and fascilitating the activation of FVII to FVIIa. TF-FVIIa activates FIX and FX, resulting in FXa, which generates thrombin (see Color Fig. 6-4).

IL-1 activity, and prevented the decrease of FXI and HK. The kallikrein inhibitor could block the release of BK and, thus, pain, swelling, and vasodilation as well as neutrophil activation. *In vitro*, FXIIa can stimulate IL-1 expression and IL-1 induces IL-6 expression. Because a monoclonal antibody to FXIIa blocks IL-6 release, one can surmise that contact activation is involved in the cytokine release observed in the acute and chronic phases of the enterocolitis (9,296). Demonstration of a pathogenic role of the kallikrein–kinin system in experimental enterocolitis, arthritis, and related systemic inflammation suggests a similar role in idiopathic human intestinal and joint inflammation. Selective kallikrein inhibitors may be useful in disorders like Crohn disease and rheumatoid arthritis (see Fig. 6-4).

# GENETIC ABNORMALITIES OF CONTACT FACTORS: THROMBOTIC RISK FACTORS

## Factor XII (Hageman Trait)

Human plasma FXII deficiency was first identified by Ratnoff and Colopy in 1955 in a white American male who had a markedly prolonged activated partial thromboplastin time (APTT) (297). FXII deficiency is an autosomal-recessive trait with no apparent associated clinical bleeding disorder. In fact, the index case, John Hageman, died of a pulmonary embolism after a hip fracture (298), demonstrating the lack of protection from arterial thrombotic disease in patients deficient in FXII.

There is an increased incidence of venous thrombosis in patients with congenital FXII deficiency (299–303) and in acquired thrombotic disorders such as myocardial infarction (304) and rethrombosis of coronary arteries after thrombolytic therapy (305). FXII deficiency has reportedly been associated with coronary stent thrombosis (306). Careful prospective investigations with age- and sex-matched controls will be required to determine whether FXII deficiency should be added to the ever-increasing list of inherited risk factors for thrombosis.

Recently, FXII deficiency in women has been found to be linked to recurrent miscarriage. Six of seven women with reduced FXII activity had early or midtrimester fetal losses. In 241 women with a history of recurrent miscarriage, the prevalence of FXII deficiency was 2.9% (307). Low levels of FXII but not of protein C, protein S, antithrombin, or factor XIII was a precursor of recurrent miscarriage (308). These results have been confirmed and extend to primary recurrent abortion with which FXII deficiency was strongly associated (309).

Low levels of FXII are associated with recurrent fetal loss (odds ratio, 5.4) (310) but the common genetic polymorphism (46 C/T) is not so associated (311).

Reduced levels of FXII occur in antiphospholipid antibody-syndrome patients (312) and most of these cases are associated with antibody directed to FXII (313). It is not clear whether this is a statistical association or an actual result of the antibody itself.

Individual patients of Swiss (314), Asian (315,316), and Italian origin (317) are noted to have decreased levels of FXII. In investigating the low FXII in Asians, a polymorphism 46 C to T substitution was found in the promoter region 4 bases upstream from the ATG translation initiation codon (318). The allele frequency of C to T was 0.27 to 0.73 in Asian subjects and 0.80 to 0.20 in white subjects which correlated with the mean FXII levels CC = 170%, CT = 141%, and TT = 82%. In vitro translation of FXII was less in cDNA containing 46 T than 46 C. These low levels of FXII correlated well with cardiovascular risk factors such as smoking, hypertension, and diabetes (319). The C46T polymorphism is also a determinant of factor XIIa, fibrinopeptide A and possibly factor VIIIc (320). Activated FXII correlated with the C46T but only accounted for 18% of the variance where the more common risk factors each contributed (320). Two quantitative-trait loci were found, one near the FXII gene or chromosome 5 and the other on chromosome 10. Each interacted with the 46 C/T to increase the FXII activity and the tendency for thrombosis (321). The FXII:46T decreased the odds ratio for the acute coronary syndrome to 0.4 (322). An HMGCoA reductase inhibitor, pravastin, had no benefit for the 46TT genotype but had significant benefit for 46 CC or 46 CT (323). A recent study using linkage analysis for the 46 C to T polymorphism provides new information that unravels some of the apparently conflicting data. Tirado et al. (324) demonstrated that the genotype T/T was associated with an increased risk of venous thromboembolism (adjusted odds ratio, 4.82). The plasma FXII levels between the patients and controls were virtually identical. However, when the FXII concentrations in the patients were analyzed as a function of the 46 C to T polymorphism, the homozygous TT had 62% or normal, heterozygous 94%, and the CC genotype 127% differences that were highly significant ($P < 0.00001$). Therefore, there are two effects of the polymorphism but only one is associated with disease.

Most Hageman trait plasma lacks both functional and antigenic (CRM−) FXII. Immunoreactive FXII cross-reacting material (CRM+) is present in three patients who lack functional FXII activity (325–328). The molecular basis of several types of CRM-FXII has been elucidated. In one family, a T to C transition 224 bp upstream of exon 3 leads to a G to C transversion upstream of the transcription initiator site (329). In a second family, a splice site mutation 11396 (GA) in the FXII gene results in a truncated transcript and a lack of circulatory FXII protein (330). Defects in the light chain of FXII result in disorders of the enzymatic activity of the protein. Coagulation FXII Washington DC has a Cys571-to-Ser substitution that results in complete loss of procoagulant activity (331). Coagulation FXII$_{Bern}$ is a protein that, when kallikrein-cleaved, is unable to activate FXI or PK (332). Coagulation FXII Mie-1 is a homozygous mutation in the catalytic domain Trp486 to Cys that reduces activity of FXII to antigen to less than 5% of normal. Transient expression in mammalian cells shows a markedly reduced secretion with a normal intracellular content attributed to incorrect folding (333). Two novel mutations of FXII are reported that alter the behavior of the enzyme to proteosomal degradation. Q421K mutation results in resistance to degradation but cannot exit the endoplasmic reticulum component efficiently. In contrast, R123P is susceptible to proteosome degradation and is therefore not secreted intact (334).

## Prekallikrein (Fletcher Trait)

Human plasma PK deficiency was first identified by Hathaway and colleagues in 1965 in a young girl of African American and white ancestry who had a markedly prolonged APTT. This abnormality was corrected after incubation with a surface (i.e., the rate of contact activation seemed to be impaired) (335). Subsequent patients with this deficiency, including a brother of the index case (336), have been reported in African American (337,338), white American (337,339), Nigerian (340), Mediterranean (341), Italian (342), and Austrian (343) populations, suggesting that there may be no racial predilection. PK deficiency, as in the case of FXII deficiency, is an autosomal-recessive trait with no apparent associated clinical bleeding disorder (337). Patients with this deficiency have experienced myocardial infarction, thromboembolism, or multiple cerebral thrombosis (299,344,345), again demonstrating the lack of protection from arterial thrombotic disease. Additionally, surface-mediated fibrinolysis and increased vascular permeability are also defective in plasma of these patients (346). The presence of immunoreactive PK CRM+ has been detected in 5 of 18 patients of Mediterranean origin, who lack functional PK activity (347). Both functional and antigenic (CRM−) PK lacking in Fletcher trait plasma have been most often reported in African Americans (348). Furthermore, reduced levels of PK antigen have been detected in a white family from Long Beach, California, whose members lack PK functional activity (349). A family has been recently described where the prepositus has severe deficiency of PK owing to compound heterozygosity (383 Wstop, C529Y) (350).

## High- and Low-Molecular-Weight Kininogen (Williams Trait)

Human plasma HK and LK deficiency (Williams trait) was identified by our group in 1975 in an African American with a markedly prolonged aPTT, deficiency in both HK and LK, and no kinin formation (225). In the same year, two other laboratories reported similar patients, one of African American origin (Fitzgerald trait) (311–313) and one of white French origin (Flaujeac trait) (351), both deficient only in HK. Additionally, a deficiency in HK has been reported in an American (352), an aborigine from Australia (353), a white family of Portuguese origin in which the propositus was completely deficient and four other family members were partially deficient (354), and several Japanese families (355–358). In the last group, Southern blot analysis revealed no gross defect, suggesting that a single point mutation may account for the defect (358). HK deficiency is also an autosomal-recessive trait with no apparent associated clinical bleeding disorder (351,359). In fact, we have observed deep vein thromboses and pulmonary embolus in the index case (Williams trait), demonstrating the lack of protection from thrombotic disease in a patient deficient in both HK and LK. Independent of the multiple mechanisms by which kininogens, which are selective antithrombins, modulate $\alpha$-thrombin's activation of platelets and endothelial cells in vitro and the proposed physiologic mechanism for cellular fibrinolysis caused by assembly of HK and PK on endothelium, clinical observation suggests that deficiencies of these proteins may be additional risk factors for thrombosis. We have characterized a mutation (103) in Ms. Williams, a patient who was completely deficient in both LK and HK. A C-T transition has been located at nucleotide 587 downstream from the start codon ATG, resulting in a CGA (Arg)-TGA (stop) mutation in exon 5 of the kininogen gene. Because the stop mutation is localized before the differential splice site (in exon 10), the synthesis of both LK and HK proteins is affected. The trait segregates the family as autosomal recessive. Recently, two patients from Japan were reported to have the same molecular defect associated with total kininogen deficiency (360) as in Williams trait (103), indicating that this mutation is in a CpG genetic "hot spot." Recently, a CRM−HK (<1% antigen and activity) was found to result from a stop codon at nucleotide 1597 corresponding to amino acid 532, which resulted from a single base-pair deletion in cDNA position 1492 (361). In the same study, monoclonal antibodies to heavy chain and D5 detected a short 92-kDa HK in the original Fitzgerald plasma corresponding to amino acid 1–502 (domains 1 to 5) but lacking part of domain. This was found to be caused by a 17-bp mutation in intron 9, which probably affected processing or secretion.

## High- and Low-Molecular-Weight Kininogen Deficiency in Rats—A "Knockout" Model

To date, no murine knockouts of plasma components of the contact system have been described. In the case of kininogen, this is because there are two genes for kininogen in the murine genome and both are expressed in mouse tissues (362). However, in 1979, a "natural knockout" strain of rat (Brown Norway Katholiek) congenitally deficient in plasma HK and LK was discovered (363). The defect is one of secretion, since both HK and LK protein and mRNA are present in the liver of the affected rats. The defect was shown to be a point mutation of G to A at nucleotide 487 resulting in a substitution of Ala163 to Thr in the heavy chain of HK and LK, and the secretion defect was reproduced in transfected COS-1 cells (104).

Similar to studies using B2R murine knockouts, the kininogen-deficient rats have been studied in regard to hypertension and the role of the kidney in sodium regulation. The systemic blood pressure in the deficient rats is normal and, thus, BK does not seem to regulate basal blood pressure. However, vascular sensitivity to either salt loading or angiotensin II infusion is markedly enhanced in the kininogen-deficient rats compared with normal Brown Norway rats (364). Therefore, nonpressor doses of angiotensin II cause hypertension in Brown Norway Katholiek rats (365). The effects of salt loading on the blood pressure of the kininogen-deficient rats was reversed by an infusion of bovine LK (366). Therefore, the kallikrein–kinin system plays an important role in the regulation of blood pressure in the sodium-loaded state and is a countervailing influence to the renin–angiotensin system. Because overactivity of the latter system has a detrimental effect on cardiac function, it was of interest to study the effect of preconditioning in the kininogen-deficient rat. In general, the effects were similar to those of the rat treated in B2R antagonists (208). Preconditioning reduced the ratio of infarct size to risk area following ischemia and the incidence of reperfusion arrhythmias in the normal Brown Norway rat, but not the kininogen-deficient rat. This observation provides further evidence for the critical role of kininogen (and kinins) in cardioprotection conferred by preconditioning.

The role of kinins in inflammatory reactions differs depending on the nature of the inflammation. In general, inflammation that is partially or completely dependent on the presence and activation of FXII may be mediated by kinins. It should be noted that, since activated FXII initiates the classic complement pathway by converting C1r to activated C1r, the role of complement must also be considered. One inflammatory model originally introduced to study nonsteroidal drugs in rheumatoid arthritis is that of carrageenin-induced edema. Carrageenins, sulfated polysaccharides derived from seaweed, are potent activators of FXII *in vitro*. Intraperitoneal injection of carrageenin in normal rats gave rise to increased efflux of radiolabeled albumin into the peritoneal cavity with the formation of large amounts of peritoneal fluid containing high concentrations of kinins. The same injection in kininogen-deficient rats yielded only a small volume of fluid, with markedly decreased albumin concentration and no kinins (367). Zymosan, a known activator of the alternative pathway of complement, also produced the peritoneal fluid changes but no diminution was observed in kininogen-deficient rats. These results indicate that kininogen is involved in carrageenin-induced inflammation involving FXIIa but not zymosan-induced inflammation involving the alternative complement pathway. The cause of the intense inflammation in gout is thought to be urate crystals. Uric acid induced kinin formation in normal rat plasma and intense edema when injected into the rat paw. The inflammation is markedly reduced in the kininogen-deficient rats, indicating the involvement of the kinin system in gouty arthritis (368).

The systemic inflammatory response syndrome (discussed in the preceding text) is thought to be mediated in part by kinins, resulting from activation of FXII. Ellagic acid, a known FXII activator, injected into normal rats caused congestion of spleen, liver, and lymph nodes; prolonged aPTT with a decrease in PK and HK; and prolonged hypotension as well as consumption of fibrinogen and platelets (369). When ellagic acid was injected into Brown Norway Katholiek rats, there was much less congestion of the lymphoid tissues, no consumption of PK, and the hypotension was short lived. Interestingly, these changes were strikingly similar to those seen in primate sepsis after treatment with an FXII monoclonal antibody (277). The results indicated that the vascular changes but not the DIC depends on the integrity of the kallikrein–kinin system. These conclusions were reinforced by a study of endotoxin-induced hypotension in rats. The hypotensive response in normal rats to endotoxin is biphasic, with an acute decrease with a nadir at 15 minutes followed by a delayed response occurring at 70 to 80 minutes after endotoxin administration (370). In the kininogen-deficient rat, the delayed phase attributed to platelet activity function occurs, but the acute phase is blocked. Similarly, the permeability increase in rat skin induced by endotoxin is partially inhibited in the kininogen-deficient rats, with the rest of the response inhibited by a platelet activation factor antagonist (371).

Recently this "natural knockout" in rats has been exploited to probe the nonkinin functions of kininogen. HK binds PK tightly and circulates as a bimolecular complex in plasma (67). An interesting question is whether the clearance of exogenous plasma kallikrein, its tissue uptake, or its extravasation in tissues under inflammatory conditions is influenced by its complex with HK. Using (125) I-prekallikrein, the clearance for the circulation and its extravasation was similar in normal and kininogen-deficient rats. Thus, the formation of an HK–prekallikrein complex does not influence its half-life (372). However, the splenic uptake was decreased, indicating that the binding of PK to spleen cells may require HK. Because both kininogens have been demonstrated to inhibit thrombin activation of platelets and HK is profibrinolytic, it might be predicted that a lack of kininogen might render animals (and humans) prothrombotic. To test this hypothesis, we studied a model of mild arterial injury in rats caused by mechanical de-endothelialization for 4 hours using a laser–Doppler probe to measure flow. The healthy rats occluded the vessel 90% with a mean of 180 minutes, whereas the mean of kininogen-deficient rats was approximately 35 minutes (373). Therefore, kininogen may be an antithrombotic protein.

The importance of kininogen for chronic inflammation has been demonstrated in kininogen-deficient rats in two models of enterocolitis (293,294). The proangiogenic effect of intact HK accounts for the observation that *in vivo* angiogenesis was supressed in kininogen-deficient rats (374). Evidence included decreased spontaneous angiogenesis as well as decreased FGF-2-stimulated and tumor-induced angiogenesis. Vasodilation, a component of angiogenesis, was also decreased in kininogen-deficient rats (271). Kininogen-deficient rats have also been employed to demonstrate a critical role for this protein in the hyperalgesia of nerve injury (272) and the pathogenesis of inflammatory pain (375).

# References

1. Kurachi K, Fujikawa K, Davie EW. Mechanism of activation of bovine factor XI by factor XII and factor XIIa. *Biochemistry* 1980;19:1330–1338.
2. Radcliffe R, Bagdasarian A, Colman R, et al. Activation of bovine factor VII by Hageman factor fragments. *Blood* 1977;50:611–617.
3. Ghebrehiwet B, Randazzo BP, Dunn JT, et al. Mechanisms of activation of the classical pathway of complement by Hageman factor fragment. *J Clin Invest* 1983;71:1450–1456.
4. Ichinose A, Fujikawa K, Suyama T. The activation of prourokinase by plasma kallikrein and its inactivation by thrombin. *J Biol Chem* 1986;261:3486–3489.
5. Sealey JE, Atlas SA, Laragh JH. Linking the kallikrein and renin systems via activation of inactive renin: new data and a hypothesis. *Am J Med* 1978;65:994–1000.
6. Fujikawa K, Heimark RL, Kurachi K, et al. Activation of bovine factor XII (Hageman factor) by plasma kallikrein. *Biochemistry* 1980;19:1322–1330.
7. Jacobsen S, Kriz M. Some data on two purified kininogens from human plasma. *Br J Pharmacol* 1967;29:25–36.
8. Chien P, Pixley RA, Stumpo LG, et al. Modulation of the human monocyte binding site for monomeric immunoglobulin G by activated Hageman factor. *J Clin Invest* 1988;82:1554–1559.
9. Toossi Z, Sedor JR, Mettler MA, et al. Induction of expression of monocyte interleukin 1 by Hageman factor (factor XII). *Proc Natl Acad Sci U S A* 1992;89:11969–11972.
10. Wachtfogel YT, Pixley RA, Kucich U, et al. Purified plasma factor XIIa aggregates human neutrophils and causes degranulation. *Blood* 1986;67:1731–1737.
11. Schapira M, Despland E, Scott CF, et al. Purified human plasma kallikrein aggregates human blood neutrophils. *J Clin Invest* 1982;69:1199–1202.
12. Lin Y, Harris RB, Yan W, et al. High molecular weight kininogen peptides inhibit the formation of kallikrein on endothelial cell surfaces and subsequent urokinase-dependent plasmin formation. *Blood* 1997;90:690–697.
13. Yung LL, Lim F, Khan MMH, et al. Neutrophil adhesion on surfaces preadsorbed with high molecular weight kininogen under well-defined flow conditions. *Immunopharmacology* 1996;32:19–23.
14. Citarella F, Tripodi M, Fantoni A, et al. Assignment of human coagulation factor XII (fXII) to chromosome 5 by cDNA hybridization to DNA from somatic cell hybrids. *Hum Genet* 1988;80:397.
15. Royle NJ, Nigli M, Cool D, et al. Structural gene encoding human factor XII is located at 5q33-qter. *Somat Cell Mol Genet* 1988;14:217–221.
16. Cool DE, MacGillivray RT. Characterization of the human blood coagulation factor XII gene. Intron/exon gene organization and analysis of the 5′-flanking region. *J Biol Chem* 1987;262:13662–13673.
17. Cool DE, Edgell CJ, Louie GV, et al. Characterization of human blood coagulation factor XII cDNA: prediction of the primary structure of factor XII and the tertiary structure of beta-factor XIIa. *J Biol Chem* 1985;260:13666–13676.
18. Griffin JH, Cochrane CG. Human factor XII (Hageman factor). *Methods Enzymol* 1976;45:56–65.
19. Saito H, Ratnoff OD, Pensky J. Radioimmunoassay of human Hageman factor (factor XII). *J Lab Clin Med* 1976;88:506–514.
20. Gordon EM, Gallagher CA, Johnson TR, et al. Hepatocytes express blood coagulation factor XII (Hageman factor). *J Lab Clin Med* 1990;115:463–469.
21. Gordon EM, Johnson TR, Ramos LP, et al. Enhanced expression of factor XII (Hageman factor) in isolated livers of estrogen- and prolactin-treated rats. *J Lab Clin Med* 1991;117:353–358.
22. Farsetti A, Misiti S, Citarella F, et al. Molecular basis of estrogen regulation of Hageman factor XII gene expression. *Endocrinology* 1995;136:5076–5083.
23. Schmeidler Sapiro KT, Ratnoff OD, Gordon EM. Mitogenic effects of coagulation factor XII and factor XIIa on HepG2 cells. *Proc Natl Acad Sci U S A* 1991;88:4382–4385.
24. Gordon EM, Venkatesan N, Salazar R, et al. Factor XII-induced mitogenesis is mediated via a distinct signal transduction pathway that activates a mitogen-activated protein kinase. *Proc Natl Acad Sci U S A* 1996;93:2174–2179.
25. Pixley RA, Stumpo LG, Birkmeyer K, et al. A monoclonal antibody recognizing an icosapeptide sequence in the heavy chain of human factor XII inhibits surface catalyzed activation. *J Biol Chem* 1987;262:10140–10145.
26. Clarke BJ, Cote HC, Cool DE, et al. Mapping of a putative surface-binding site of human coagulation factor XII. *J Biol Chem* 1989;264:11497–11502.
27. Citarella F, Ravon DM, Pascucci B, et al. Structure/function analysis of human factor XII using recombinant deletion mutants. Evidence for an additional region involved in the binding to negatively charged surfaces. *Eur J Biochem* 1996;238:240–249.
28. Miller G, Silverberg M, Kaplan AP. Autoactivatability of human Hageman factor (factor XII). *Biochem Biophys Res Commun* 1980;92:803–810.
29. Samuel M, Pixley RA, Villanueva MA, et al. Human factor XII (Hageman factor) autoactivation by dextran sulfate: circular dichroism, fluorescence, and ultraviolet difference spectroscopic studies. *J Biol Chem* 1992;267:19691–19697.
30. Forbes CO, Pensky J, Ratnoff OD. Inhibition of activated Hageman factor and activated plasma thromboplastin antecedent by purified C1-inhibitor. *J Lab Clin Med* 1970;76:805–809.
31. Revak SD, Cochrane CG, Bouma BN, et al. Surface and fluid phase activities of two forms of activated Hageman factor produced during contact activation of plasma. *J Exp Med* 1978;147:719–729.
32. Revak SD, Cochrane CG. The relationship of structure and function in human Hageman factor: the association of enzymatic and binding activities with separate regions of the molecule. *J Clin Invest* 1976;57:852–860.
33. Revak SD, Cochrane CG, Griffin JH. The binding and cleavage characteristics of human Hageman factor during contact activation. A comparison of normal plasma with plasmas deficient in factor XI, prekallikrein, or high molecular weight kininogen. *J Clin Invest* 1977;59:1167–1175.
34. Cochrane CG, Revak SD, Wuepper KD. Activation of Hageman factor in solid and fluid phases. A critical role of kallikrein. *J Exp Med* 1973;138:1564–1583.
35. Bagdasarian A, Talamo RC, Colman RW. Isolation of high molecular weight activators of human plasma prekallikrein. *J Biol Chem* 1973;248:3456–3463.
36. Espana F, Ratnoff OD. Activation of Hageman factor (factor XII) by sulfatides and other agents in the absence of plasma proteases. *J Lab Clin Med* 1983;102:31–45.
37. Wiggins RC, Cochrane CG. The autoactivation of rabbit Hageman factor. *J Exp Med* 1979;150:1122.
38. Schousboe I. Contact activation in human plasma is triggered by zinc ion modulation of factor XII (Hageman factor). *Blood Coagul Fibrinolysis* 1993;4:671–678.
39. Bernardo MM, Day DE, Olson ST, et al. Surface-independent acceleration of factor XII activation by zinc ions. I. Kinetic characterization of the metal ion rate enhancement. *J Biol Chem* 1993;268:12468–12476.
40. Bernardo MM, Day DE, Halvorson HR, et al. Surface-independent acceleration of factor XII activation by zinc ions. II. Direct binding and fluorescence studies. *J Biol Chem* 1993;268:12477–12483.
41. Rojkjaer R, Schousboe I. The surface-dependent autoactivation mechanism of factor XII. *Eur J Biochem* 1997;243:160–166.
42. Didisheim P, Mibasham RS. Activation of Hageman factor (factor XII) by long chain saturated fatty acids. *Thromb Diath Haemorrh* 1963;9:346.
43. Tans G, Rosing J, Griffin JH. Sulfatide-dependent autoactivation of human blood coagulation Factor XII (Hageman Factor). *J Biol Chem* 1983;258:8215–8222.
44. Hojima Y, Cochrane CG, Wiggins RC, et al. *In vitro* activation of the contact (Hageman factor) system of plasma by heparin and chondroitin sulfate E. *Blood* 1984;63:1453–1459.
45. Joseph K, Tholanikunnel BG, Kaplan AP. Heat shock protein 90 catalyzes activation of the prekallikrein-kininogen complex in the absence of factor XII. *Proc Natl Acad Sci U S A* 2002;99:896–900.
46. Joseph K, Ghebrehiwet B, Peerschke EI. Identification of the zinc-dependent endothelial cell binding protein for high molecular weight kininogen and factor XII: identity with the receptor that binds to the globular "heads" of C1q (gC1q-R). *Proc Natl Acad Sci U S A* 1996;93:8552–8557.
47. Joseph K, Shibayama Y, Ghebrehiwet B, et al. Factor XII-dependent contact activation on endothelial cells and binding proteins gC1qR and cytokeratin 1. *Thromb Haemost* 2001;85:119–124.
48. Mahdi F, Madar ZS, Figueroa CD, et al. Factor XII interacts with the multiprotein assembly of urokinase plasminogen activator receptor, gC1qR, and cytokeratin 1 on endothelial cell membranes. *Blood* 2002;99:3585–3596.
49. Citarella F, te Velthuis H, Helmer-Citterich M, et al. Identification of a putative binding site for negatively charged surfaces in the fibronectin type II domain of human factor XII—an immunochemical and homology modeling approach. *Thromb Haemost* 2000;84:1057–1065.
50. Motta G, Rojkjaer R, Hasan AAK, et al. High molecular weight kininogen regulates prekallikrein assembly and activation on endothelial cells—a novel mechanism for contact activation. *Blood* 1998;91:516–528.
51. Rojkjaer R, Hasan AA, Motta G, et al. Factor XII does not initiate prekallikrein activation on endothelial cells. *Thromb Haemost* 1998;80:74–81.
52. Shariat-Madar Z, Mahdi F, Schmaier AH. Identification and characterization of prolylcarboxypeptidase as an endothelial cell prekallikrein activator. *J Biol Chem* 2002;277:17962–17969.
53. Motta G, Shariat-Madar Z, Mahdi F, et al. Assembly of high molecular weight kininogen and activation of prekallikrein on cell matrix. *Thromb Haemost* 2001;86:840–847.

54. Moreira CR, Schmaier AH, Mahdi F, et al. Identification of prolylcarboxypeptidase as the cell matrix-associated prekallikrein activator. *FEBS Lett* 2002;523:167–170.

55. Schreiber AD, Kaplan AD, Austen FK. Inhibition by C1-INH of Hageman factor fragment activation of coagulation, fibrinolysis and kinin-generation. *J Clin Invest* 1973;52:1402.

56. DeAgostini A, Lijnen HR, Pixley RA, et al. Inactivation of factor XII active fragment in normal plasma: predominant role of C1-inhibitor. *J Clin Invest* 1984;73:1542–1549.

57. Pixley RA, Schapira M, Colman RW. The regulation of human factor XIIa by plasma proteinase inhibitors. *J Biol Chem* 1985;260:1723–1729.

58. Pixley RA, Schmaier A, Colman RW. Effect of negatively charged activating compounds on inactivation of factor XIIa by C1 inhibitor. *Arch Biochem Biophys* 1987;256:490–498.

59. Schousboe I. Binding of activated Factor XII to endothelial cells affects its inactivation by the C1-esterase inhibitor. *Eur J Biochem* 2003;270:111–118.

60. Kleniewski J, Donaldson VH. Endothelial cells produce a substance that inhibits contact activation of coagulation by blocking the activation of Hageman factor. *Proc Natl Acad Sci U S A* 1993;90:198–202.

61. Yu H, Anderson PJ, Freedman BI, et al. Genomic structure of the human plasma prekallikrein gene, identification of allelic variants, and analysis in end-stage renal disease. *Genomics* 2000;69:225–234.

62. Beaubien G, Rosinski-Chupin I, Mattei MG, et al. Gene structure and chromosomal localization of plasma kallikrein. *Biochemistry* 1991;30:1628–1635.

63. Asakai R, Davie EW, Cheung DW. Organization of the gene for human Factor XI. *Biochemistry* 1987;26:7221.

64. Veloso D, Shilling J, Shine J, et al. Recent evolutionary divergence of plasma prekallikrein and factor XI. *Thromb Res* 1986;43:153–160.

65. McConnell DJ, Mason B. The isolation of human plasma prekallikrein. *Br J Pharmacol* 1970;38:490–502.

66. Fisher CA, Schmaier AH, Addonizio VP, et al. Assay of prekallikrein in human plasma: comparison of amidolytic, esterolytic, coagulation, and immunochemical assays. *Blood* 1982;59:963–970.

67. Mandle R Jr, Colman RW, Kaplan AP. Identification of prekallikrein and high molecular weight kininogen as a complex in human plasma. *Proc Natl Acad Sci U S A* 1976;73:4179–4183.

68. Scott CF, Colman RW. Function and immunochemistry of prekallikrein-high molecular weight kininogen complex in plasma. *J Clin Invest* 1980;65:413–421.

69. Scott CF, Liu CY, Colman RW. Human plasma prekallikrein: a rapid high-yield method for purification. *Eur J Biochem* 1979;100:77–83.

70. Mandle RJ Jr, Kaplan AP. Human plasma prekallikrein: mechanism of activation by Hageman factor and participation in Hageman-factor-dependent fibrinolysis. *J Biol Chem* 1977;252:6097–6104.

71. Wuepper KD, Cochrane CG. Plasma prekallikrein: isolation, characterization, and mechanism of activation. *J Exp Med* 1972;135:1–20.

72. Mandle R Jr, Kaplan AP. Hageman factor substrates. Human plasma prekallikrein: mechanism of activation by Hageman factor and participation in Hageman factor-dependent fibrinolysis. *J Biol Chem* 1977;252:6097–6104.

73. McMullen BA, Fujikawa K, Davie EW. Location of the disulfide bonds in human coagulation factor XI: the presence of a Tandem apple domain. *Biochemistry* 1991;30:2056.

74. McMullen BA, Fujikawa K, Davie EW. Location of the disulfide bonds in human plasma prekallikrein: the presence of four novel apple domains in the amino-terminal portion of the molecule. *Biochemistry* 1991;30:2050–2056.

75. Tordai H, Banyai L, Patthy L. The PAN module: the N-terminal domains of plasminogen and hepatocyte growth factor are homologous with the apple domains of the prekallikrein family and with a novel domain found in numerous nematode proteins. *FEBS Lett* 1999;461:63–67.

76. Chung DW, Fujikawa K, McMullen BA, et al. Human plasma prekallikrein, a zymogen to a serine protease that contains four tandem repeats. *Biochemistry* 1986;25:2410–2417.

77. Colman RW, Wachtfogel YT, Kucich U, et al. Effect of cleavage of the heavy chain of human plasma kallikrein on its functional properties. *Blood* 1985;65:311–318.

78. Van der Graaf FG, Tans G, Bouma BN, et al. Isolation and functional properties of the heavy and light chains of human plasma kallikrein. *J Biol Chem* 1982;257:14300–14305.

79. Page JD, Colman RW. Localization of distinct functional domains on prekallikrein for interaction with both high molecular weight kininogen and activated factor XII in a 28-kDa fragment (amino acids 141-371). *J Biol Chem* 1991;266:8143–8148.

80. Page JD, You JL, Harris RB, et al. Localization of the binding site on plasma kallikrein for high molecular weight kininogen to both apple 1 and apple 4 domains of the heavy chain. *Arch Biochem Biophys* 1994;314:159–164.

81. Hock J, Vogel R, Linke RP, et al. High molecular weight kininogen-binding site of prekallikrein probed by monoclonal antibodies. *J Biol Chem* 1990;265:12005–12011.

82. Lin Y, Shenoy S, Harris RB, et al. Direct evidence for multi-facial contacts between high molecular weight kininogen and plasma prekallikrein. *Biochemistry* 1996;35:12945–12949.

83. Herwald H, Renne T, Meijers JCM, et al. Mapping of the discontinuous kininogen binding site of prekallikrein: a distal binding segment is located in the heavy chain domain A4. *J Biol Chem* 1996;271:13061–13067.

84. Renne T, Sugiyama A, Gailani D, et al. Fine mapping of the H-kininogen binding site in plasma prekallikrein apple domain 2. *Int Immunopharmacol* 2002;2:1867–1873.

85. Renne T, Gailani D, Meijers JC, et al. Characterization of the H-kininogen-binding site on factor XI: a comparison of factor XI and plasma prekallikrein. *J Biol Chem* 2002;277:4892–4899.

86. Schapira M, Silver LD, Scott CF, et al. New and rapid functional assay for C1 inhibitor in human plasma. *Blood* 1982;59:719–724.

87. Gigli I, Mason JW, Colman RW, et al. Interaction of plasma kallikrein with the C1 inhibitor. *J Immunol* 1970;104:574–581.

88. Schapira M, Scott CF, Colman RW. Protection of human plasma kallikrein from inactivation by C1 inhibitor and other protease inhibitors. The role of high molecular weight kininogen. *Biochemistry* 1981;20:2738–2743.

89. Schapira M, Scott CF, James A, et al. High molecular weight kininogen or its light chain protects human plasma kallikrein from inactivation by plasma protease inhibitors. *Biochemistry* 1982;21:567–572.

90. Lahiri B, Bagdasarian A, Mitchell B, et al. Antithrombin-heparin cofactor: an inhibitor of plasma kallikrein. *Arch Biochem Biophys* 1976;175:737–747.

91. Olson ST, Sheffer R, Francis AM. High molecular weight kininogen potentiates the heparin-accelerated inhibition of plasma kallikrein by antithrombin: role for antithrombin in the regulation of kallikrein. *Biochemistry* 1993;32:12136–12147.

92. Meijers JC, Kanters DH, Vlooswijk RA, et al. Inactivation of human plasma kallikrein and factor XIa by protein C inhibitor. *Biochemistry* 1988;27:4231.

93. Neth P, Arnhold M, Nitschko H, et al. The mRNAs of prekallikrein, factors XI and XII, and kininogen, components of the contact phase cascade are differentially expressed in multiple non-hepatic human tissues. *Thromb Haemost* 2001;85:1043–1047.

94. Takagaki Y, Kitamura N, Nakanishi S. Cloning and sequence analysis of cDNAs for human high molecular weight and low molecular weight prekininogens. Primary structures of two human prekininogens. *J Biol Chem* 1985;260:8601–8609.

95. Kitamura N, Kitagawa H, Fukushima D, et al. Structural organization of the human kininogen gene and a model for its evolution. *J Biol Chem* 1985;260:8610–8617.

96. Salvesen G, Parkes C, Abrahamson M, et al. Human low-Mr kininogen contains three copies of a cystatin sequence that are divergent in structure and in inhibitory activity for cysteine proteinases. *Biochem J* 1986;234:429–434.

97. Kellermann J, Lottspeich F, Henschen A, et al. Completion of the primary structure of human high-molecular-mass kininogen. The amino acid sequence of the entire heavy chain and evidence for its evolution by gene triplication. *Eur J Biochem* 1986;154:471–478.

98. Ylinenjarvi K, Prasthofer TW, Martin NC, et al. Interaction of cysteine proteinases with recombinant kininogen domain 2, expressed in Escherichia coli. *FEBS Lett* 1995;357:309–311.

99. Auerswald EA, Rossler D, Mentele R, et al. Cloning, expression and characterization of human kininogen domain 3. *FEBS Lett* 1993;321:93–97.

100. Bano B, Kunapuli SP, Bradford HN, et al. Structural requirements for cathepsin B and cathepsin H inhibition by kininogens. *J Protein Chem* 1996;15:519–525.

101. Kunapuli SP, Bradford HN, Jameson BA, et al. Thrombin-induced platelet aggregation is inhibited by the heptapeptide Leu271-Ala277 domain 3 in the heavy chain of high molecular weight kininogen. *J Biol Chem* 1996;271:11228–11234.

102. Kunapuli SP, DeLa Cadena RA, Colman RW. Deletion mutagenesis of high molecular weight kininogen light chain: identification of two anionic surface binding subdomains. *J Biol Chem* 1993;268:2486–2492.

103. Cheung PP, Kunapuli SP, Scott CF, et al. Genetic basis of total kininogen deficiency in Williams' trait. *J Biol Chem* 1993;268:23361–23365.

104. Hayashi I, Hoshiko S, Makabe O, et al. A point mutation of alanine 163 to threonine is responsible for the defective secretion of high molecular weight kininogen by the liver of brown Norway Katholiek rats. *J Biol Chem* 1993;268:17219–17224.

105. Chen LM, Chung P, Chao S, et al. Differential regulation of kininogen gene expression by estrogen and progesterone in vivo. *Biochim Biophys Acta* 1992;1131:145–151.

106. Takano M, Yokoyama K, Yayama K, et al. Murine fibroblasts synthesize and secrete kininogen in response to cyclic-AMP, prostaglandin E2 and tumor necrosis factor. *Biochim Biophys Acta* 1995;1265:189–195.

107. Takano M, Kondo J, Yayama K, et al. Expression of low-molecular-weight kininogen mRNA in human fibroblast WI38 cells. *Jpn J Pharmacol* 1996;71:341–343.

108. Scott CF, Shull B, Muller-Esterl W, et al. Rapid direct determination of low and high molecular weight kininogen in human plasma by Particle Concentration Fluorescence Immunoassay (PCFIA). *Thromb Haemost* 1997;77:109–118.

109. Schmaier AH, Zuckerberg A, Silverman C, et al. High-molecular weight kininogen. A secreted platelet protein. *J Clin Invest* 1983;71:1477–1489.

110. Schmaier AH, Bradford H, Silver LD, et al. High molecular weight kininogen is an inhibitor of platelet calpain. *J Clin Invest* 1986;77:1565–1573.

111. Schmaier AH, Kuo A, Lundberg D, et al. The expression of high molecular weight kininogen on human umbilical vein endothelial cells. *J Biol Chem* 1988;263:16327–16333.

112. Gustafson EJ, Schmaier AH, Wachtfogel YT, et al. Human neutrophils contain and bind high molecular weight kininogen. *J Clin Invest* 1989;84:28–35.

113. Proud D, Perkins M, Pierce JV, et al. Characterization and localization of human renal kininogen. *J Biol Chem* 1981;256:10634–10639.

114. Hallbach J, Adams G, Wirthensohn G, et al. Quantification of kininogen in human renal medulla. *Biol Chem Hoppe Seyler* 1987;368:1151–1155.

115. Weisel JW, Nagaswami C, Woodhead JL, et al. The shape of high molecular weight kininogen: organization into structural domains, changes with activation, and interactions with prekallikrein, as determined by electron microscopy. *J Biol Chem* 1994;269:10100–10106.

116. Schmaier AH, Schutsky D, Farber A, et al. Determination of the bifunctional properties of high molecular weight kininogen by studies with monoclonal antibodies directed to each of its chains. *J Biol Chem* 1987;262:1405–1411.

117. Vogel R, Assfalg-Machleidt I, Esterl A, et al. Proteinase-sensitive regions in the heavy chain of low molecular weight kininogen map to the inter-domain junctions. *J Biol Chem* 1988;263:12661–12668.

118. Bradford HN, Jameson BA, Adam AA, et al. Contiguous binding and inhibitory sites on kininogens required for the inhibition of platelet calpain. *J Biol Chem* 1993;268:26546–26551.

119. Hasan AA, Cines DB, Ngaiza JR, et al. High-molecular-weight kininogen is exclusively membrane bound on endothelial cells to influence activation of vascular endothelium. *Blood* 1995;85:3134–3143.

120. Hasan AA, Zhang J, Samuel M, et al. Conformational changes in low molecular weight kininogen alters its ability to bind to endothelial cells. *Thromb Haemost* 1995;74:1088–1095.

121. Asakura S, Hurley RW, Skorstengaard K, et al. Inhibition of cell adhesion by high molecular weight kininogen. *J Cell Biol* 1992;116:465–476.

122. Colman RW, Pixley RA, Najamunnisa S, et al. Binding of high molecular weight kininogen to human endothelial cells is mediated via a site within domains 2 + 3 of the urokinase receptor. *J Clin Invest* 1997;100:1481–1487.

123. Ishiguro H, Higashiyama S, Ohkubo I, et al. Heavy chain of human high molecular weight and low molecular weight kininogen binds calcium ion. *Biochemistry* 1987;26:7021–7029.

124. Croxatto HR, Silva R, Figueroa X, et al. A peptide released by pepsin from kininogen domain 1 is a potent blocker of ANP-mediated diuresis-natriuresis in the rat. *Hypertension* 1997;30:897–904.

125. Bradford HN, Schmaier AH, Colman RW. Kinetics of inhibition of platelet calpain II by human kininogens. *Biochem J* 1990;270:83–90.

126. Scott CF, Whitaker EJ, Hammond BF, et al. Purification and characterization of a potent 70-kDa thiol lysyl-proteinase (Lys-gingivain) from Porphyromonas gingivalis that cleaves kininogens and fibrinogen. *J Biol Chem* 1993;268:7935–7942.

127. Schmaier AH, Smith PM, Purdon AD, et al. High molecular weight kininogens: localization in the unstimulated and activated platelet and activation by a platelet calpain(s). *Blood* 1986;67:119–130.

128. Schmaier AH, Bradford HN, Lundberg D, et al. Membrane expression of platelet calpain. *Blood* 1990;75:1273–1281.

129. Saido T, Suzuki H, Yamazaki H, et al. In situ capture of m-calpain activation of platelets. *J Biol Chem* 1993;268:7422–7426.

130. Meloni FJ, Schmaier AH. Low molecular weight kininogen binds to platelets to modulate thrombin-induced platelet activation. *J Biol Chem* 1991;266:6786–6794.

131. Jiang YP, Muller Esterl W, Schmaier AH. Domain 3 of kininogens contains a cell-binding site and a site that modifies thrombin activation of platelets. *J Biol Chem* 1992;267:3712–3717.

132. Reddigari SR, Kuna P, Miragliotta G, et al. Human high molecular weight kininogen binds to human umbilical vein endothelial cells via its heavy and light chains. *Blood* 1993;81:1306–1311.

133. Wachtfogel YT, DeLa Cadena RA, Kunapuli SP, et al. High molecular weight kininogen binds to Mac-1 on neutrophils by its heavy chain (domain 3) and its light chain (domain 5). *J Biol Chem* 1994;269:19307–19312.

134. Herwald H, Hasan AAK, Godovac-Zimmermann J, et al. Identification of an endothelial cell binding site on kininogen domain D3. *J Biol Chem* 1995;270:14634–14642.

135. DeLa Cadena RA, Wyshock EG, Kunapuli SP, et al. Platelet thrombospondin interactions with human high and low molecular weight kininogens. *Thromb Haemost* 1994;72:125–131.

136. DeLa Cadena RA, Kunapuli SP, Walz DA, et al. Expression of thrombospondin 1 on the surface of activated platelets mediates their interaction with the heavy chains of human kininogens through Lys244-Pro254. *Thromb Haemost* 1998;79:186–194.

137. Puri RN, Zhou F, Hu CJ, et al. High molecular weight kininogen inhibits thrombin-induced platelet aggregation and cleavage of aggregin by inhibiting binding of thrombin to platelets. *Blood* 1991;77:500–507.

138. Hasan AAK, Amenta S, Schmaier AH. Bradykinin and its metabolite, Arg-Pro-Pro-Gly-Phe, are selective inhibitors of a-thrombin-induced platelet activation. *Circulation* 1996;94:517–528.

139. Wiggins RC. Kinin release from high molecular weight kininogen by the action of Hageman factor in the absence of kallikrein. *J Biol Chem* 1983;258:8963–8970.

140. Scott CF, Silver LD, Purdon AD, et al. Cleavage of human high molecular weight kininogen by factor XIa *in vitro*. Effect on structure and function. *J Biol Chem* 1985;260:10856–10863.

141. Sato F, Nagasawa S. Mechanism of kinin release from human low-molecular-mass-kininogen by the synergistic action of human plasma kallikrein and leukocyte elastase. *Biol Chem Hoppe Seyler* 1988;369:1009–1017.

142. Hasan AAK, Cines DB, Zhang J, et al. The carboxyl terminus of bradykinin and amino terminus of the light chain of kininogens comprise an endothelial cell binding domain. *J Biol Chem* 1994;269:31822–31830.

143. Hasan AAK, Cines DB, Herwald H, et al. Mapping the cell binding site on high molecular weight kininogen domain 5. *J Biol Chem* 1995;270:19256–19261.

144. Khan M, Punia N, Majluf-Cruz A, et al. The binding sites on high molecular weight kininogen (HK) to activated human neutrophils are localized to K263-Q292, Q329-M357, and H493-K520. *Blood* 1995;86:33a.

145. DeLa Cadena RA, Colman RW. The sequence HGLGHGHE-QQHGLGHGH in the light chain of high molecular weight kininogen serves as a primary structural feature for zinc-dependent binding to an anionic surface. *Prot Sci* 1992;1:151–160.

146. Retzios AD, Rosenfeld R, Schiffman S. Effects of chemical modifications of the surface- and protein-binding properties of the light chain of human high molecular weight kininogen. *J Biol Chem* 1987;262:3074–3081.

147. Bjork I, Olson ST, Sheffer RG, et al. Binding of heparin to human high molecular weight kininogen. *Biochemistry* 1989;28:1213–1221.

148. Lin Y, Pixley RA, Colman RW. Kinetic analysis of the role of zinc in the interaction of domain 5 of high-molecular weight kininogen (HK) with heparin. *Biochemistry* 2000;39:5104–5110.

149. Pixley RA, Lin Y, Isordia-Salas I, et al. Fine mapping of the sequences in domain 5 of high molecular weight kininogen (HK) interacting with heparin and zinc. *J Thromb Haemost* 2003;1:1791–1798.

150. Fernando LP, Fernando AN, Joseph K, et al. Assessment of the role of heparan sulfate in high molecular weight kininogen binding to human umbilical vein endothelial cells. *J Thromb Haemost* 2003;1:2444–2449.

151. Scott CF, Silver LD, Schapira M, et al. Cleavage of human high molecular weight kininogen markedly enhances its coagulant activity. Evidence that this molecule exists as a procofactor. *J Clin Invest* 1984;73:954–962.

152. Tait JF, Fujikawa K. Identification of the binding site for plasma prekallikrein in human high molecular weight kininogen. A region from residues 185 to 224 of the kininogen light chain retains full binding activity. *J Biol Chem* 1986;261:15396–15401.

153. Tait JF, Fujikawa K. Primary structure requirements for the binding of human high molecular weight kininogen to plasma prekallikrein and factor XI. *J Biol Chem* 1987;262:11651–11656.

154. Vogel R, Kaufmann J, Chung DW, et al. Mapping of the prekallikrein binding site of human H-kininogen by ligand screening of lambda gt11 expression libraries: mimicking of the predicted binding site by anti-idiotypic antibodies. *J Biol Chem* 1990;265:12494–12502.

155. Bock PE, Shore JD. Protein–protein interactions in contact activation of blood coagulation. Characterization of fluorescein-labeled human high molecular weight kininogen-light chain as a probe. *J Biol Chem* 1983;258:15079.

156. Bock PE, Shore JD, Tans G, et al. Protein-protein interactions in contact activation of blood coagulation. Binding of high molecular weight kininogen and the 5-(iodoacetamido) fluorescein-labeled kininogen light chain to prekallikrein, kallikrein, and the separated kallikrein heavy and light chains. *J Biol Chem* 1985;260:12434–12443.

157. Scarsdale JN, Harris RB. Solution phase conformation studies of the prekallikrein binding domain of high molecular weight kininogen. *J Protein Chem* 1990;9:647–659.

158. You JL, Scarsdale JN, Harris RB. Calorimetric and spectroscopic examination of the solution phase structures of prekallikrein binding domain peptides of high molecular weight kininogen. *J Protein Chem* 1991;10:301–311.

159. You JL, Page JD, Scarsdale JN, et al. Conformational analysis of synthetic peptides encompassing the factor XI and prekallikrein overlapping binding domains of high molecular weight kininogen. *Peptides* 1993;14:867–876.

160. Reddigari S, Kaplan AP. Monoclonal antibody to human high molecular weight kininogen recognizes its prekallikrein binding site and inhibits coagulant activity. *Blood* 1989;74:695–702.

161. Kaufmann J, Haasemann M, Modrow S, et al. Structural dissection of the multidomain kininogens. Fine mapping of the target epitopes of antibodies interfering with their functional properties. *J Biol Chem* 1993;268:9079–9091.

162. Greengard JS, Heeb MJ, Ersdal E, et al. Binding of coagulation factor XI to washed human platelets. *Biochemistry* 1986;25:3884–3890.

163. Lenich C, Pannell R, Gurewich V. Assembly and activation of the intrinsic fibrinolytic pathway on the surface of human endothelial cells in culture. *Thromb Haemostasis* 1995;74:698–703.

164. Gustafson EJ, Schutsky D, Knight L, et al. High molecular weight kininogen binds to unstimulated platelets. *J Clin Invest* 1986;78:310–318.

165. Greengard JS, Griffin JH. Receptors for high molecular weight kininogen on stimulated washed human platelets. *Biochemistry* 1984;23:6863–6869.

166. van Iwaarden F, de Groot PG, Sixma JJ, et al. High-molecular weight kininogen is present in cultured human endothelial cells: localization, isolation, and characterization. *Blood* 1988;71:1268–1276.

167. Kerbiriou-Nabias DM, Garcia FO, Larrieu MJ. Radioimmunoassays of human high and low molecular weight kininogens in plasmas and platelets. *Br J Haematol* 1984;56:273–286.

168. Figueroa CD, Henderson LM, Kaufmann J, et al. Immunovisualization of high (HK) and low (LK) molecular weight kininogens on isolated human neutrophils. *Blood* 1992;79:759.

169. Henderson LM, Figueroa CD, Muller-Esterl W, et al. Assembly of contact-phase factors on the surface of the human neutrophil membrane. *Blood* 1994;84:474–482.

170. Herwald H, Morgelin M, Svensson HG, et al. Zinc-dependent conformational changes in domain D5 of high molecular mass kininogen modulate contact activation. *Eur J Biochem* 2001;268:396–404.

171. Zini JM, Schmaier AH, Cines DB. Bradykinin regulates the expression of kininogen binding sites on endothelial cells. *Blood* 1993;81:2936–2946.

172. Meloni FJ, Gustafson EJ, Schmaier AH. High molecular weight kininogen binds to platelets by its heavy and light chains and when bound has altered susceptibility to kallikrein cleavage. *Blood* 1992;79:1233–1244.

173. Mahdi F, Shariat-Madar Z, Kuo A, et al. Mapping the interaction between high molecular weight kininogen and the urokinase plasminogen activator receptor. *J Biol Chem* 2004;279:16621–16628.

174. Villanueva GB, Leung L, Bradford H, et al. Conformation of high molecular weight kininogen: effects of kallikrein and factor XIa cleavage. *Biochem Biophys Res Commun* 1989;158:72–79.

175. Gustafson EJ, Lukasiewicz H, Wachtfogel YT, et al. High molecular weight kininogen inhibits fibrinogen binding to cytoadhesins of neutrophils and platelets. *J Cell Biol* 1989;109:377–387.

176. Sheng N, Fairbanks MB, Heinrikson RL, et al. Cleaved high molecular weight kininogen binds directly to the integrin CD11b/CD18 (Mac-1) and blocks adhesion to fibrinogen and ICAM-1. *Blood* 2000;95:3788–3795.

177. Wei Y, Lukashev M, Simon DI, et al. Regulation of integrin function by the urokinase receptor. *Science* 1996;273:1551–1555.

178. Edgell CJS, McDonald CC, Graham JB. Permanent cell lines expressing human factor VIII-related antigen established by hybridization. *Proc Natl Acad Sci U S A* 1983;80:3734.

179. Herwald H, Dedio J, Kellner R, et al. Isolation and characterization of the kininogen-binding protein p33 from endothelial cells: identity with the gC1q receptor. *J Biol Chem* 1996;271:13040–13047.

180. Ghebrehiwet B, Lim BL, Peerschke EI, et al. Isolation, cDNA cloning, and overexpression of a 33-kD cell surface glycoprotein that binds to the globular "heads" of C1q. *J Exp Med* 1994;179:1809–1821.

181. Reddigari SR, Shibayama Y, Brunnee T, et al. Human Hageman factor (factor XII) and high molecular weight kininogen compete for the same binding site on human umbilical vein endothelial cells. *J Biol Chem* 1993;268:11982–11987.

182. Chavakis T, Boeckel N, Santoso S, et al. Inhibition of platelet adhesion and aggregation by a defined region (Gly-486-Lys-502) of high molecular weight kininogen. *J Biol Chem* 2002;277:23157–23164.

183. Hasan AAK, Zisman T, Schmaier AH. Cytokeratin 1 is the major endothelial cell receptor for kininogens. *Thromb Haemost* 1997;76:141.

184. Mahdi F, Shariat-Madar Z, Todd RF 3rd, et al. Expression and colocalization of cytokeratin 1 and urokinase plasminogen activator receptor on endothelial cells. *Blood* 2001;97:2342–2350.

185. Joseph K, Tholanikunnel BG, Ghebrehiwet B, et al. Interaction of high molecular weight kininogen binding proteins on endothelial cells. *Thromb Haemost* 2004;91:61–70.

186. Baird TR, Walsh PN. Factor XI, but not prekallikrein, blocks high molecular weight kininogen binding to human umbilical vein endothelial cells. *J Biol Chem* 2003;278:20618–20623.

187. Mahdi F, Shariat-Madar Z, Schmaier AH. The relative priority of prekallikrein and factors XI/XIa assembly on cultured endothelial cells. *J Biol Chem* 2003;278:43983–43990.

188. Goetzl EJ, Austen KF. Stimulation of human neutrophil leukocyte aerobic glucose metabolism by purified chemotactic factors. *J Clin Invest* 1974;53:591–599.

189. Rebuck JW. The skin window as a monitor of leukocytic functions in contact activation factor deficiencies in man. *Am J Clin Pathol* 1983;79:405–413.

190. Chien P, Pixley RA, Ruiz P, et al. Modulation of the human monocyte FcgR1 by activated Hageman factor: mapping the functional XIIa site. *Blood* 1990;76:178a.

191. Li C, Gurewich V, Liu JN. Urokinase-type plasminogen activator-induced monocyte adhesion is modulated by kininogen, kallikrein, factor XII, and plasminogen. *Exp Cell Res* 1996;226:239–242.

192. Hong SL. Effect of bradykinin and thrombin on prostacyclin synthesis in endothelial cells from calf and pig aorta and human umbilical cord vein. *Thromb Res* 1980;18:787–795.

193. Palmer RMJ, Ferrige AG, Moncada S. Nitric oxide release accounts for the biologic activity of endothelium-derived relaxing factor. *Nature* 1987;327:524–526.

194. Boulanger C, Schini VB, Moncada S, et al. Stimulation of cyclic GMP production in cultured endothelial cells of the pig by bradykinin, adenosine diphosphate, calcium ionophore A23187 and nitric oxide. *Br J Pharmacol* 1990;101:152–156.

195. Busse R, Mulsch A. Induction of nitric oxide synthase by cytokines in vascular smooth muscle cells. *FEBS Lett* 1990;275:87–90.

196. Imai T, Hirata Y, Kanno K, et al. Induction of nitric oxide synthase by cyclic AMP in rat vascular smooth muscle cells. *J Clin Invest* 1994;93:543–549.

197. Dixon BS, Breckon R, Fortune J, et al. Effects of kinins on cultured arterial smooth muscle. *Am J Physiol* 1990;258:C299–C308.

198. Dixon BS, Sharma RV, Dickerson T, et al. Bradykinin and angiotensin II: activation of protein kinase C in arterial smooth muscle. *Am J Physiol* 1994;266:C1406–C1420.

199. McEachern AE, Shelton ER, Bhakta S, et al. Expression cloning of a rat B2 bradykinin receptor. *Proc Natl Acad Sci U S A* 1991;88:7724–7728.

200. Menke JG, Borkowski JA, Bierilo K, et al. Expression cloning of a human B1 bradykinin receptor. *J Biol Chem* 1994;269:21583.

201. Linz W, Scholkens BA. Role of bradykinin in the cardiac effects of angiotensin-converting enzyme inhibitors. *J Cardiovasc Pharmacol* 1992;20(Suppl. 9):S83.

202. Gohlke P, Linz W, Scholkens BA, et al. Angiotensin-converting enzyme inhibition improves cardiac function. Role of bradykinin. *Hypertension* 1994;23:411.

203. Borkowski JA, Hess JF. Targeted disruption of the mouse B2 bradykinin receptor in embryonic stem cells. *Can J Physiol Pharm* 1995;73:773–779.

204. Alfie ME, Yang XP, Hess F, et al. Salt-sensitive hypertension in bradykinin B2 receptor knockout mice. *Biochem Bioph Res Co* 1996;224:625–630.

205. Alfie ME, Sigmon DH, Pomposiello SI, et al. Effect of high salt intake in mutant mice lacking bradykinin-B2 receptors. *Hypertension* 1997;29:483–487.

206. Emanueli C, Angioni GR, Anania V, et al. Blood pressure responses to acute or chronic captopril in mice with disruption of bradykinin B2-receptor gene. *J Hypertens* 1997;15:1701–1706.

207. Madeddu P, Milia AF, Salis MB, et al. Renovascular hypertension in bradykinin B2-receptor knockout mice. *Hypertension* 1998;32:503–509.

208. Yang XP, Liu YH, Scicli GM, et al. Role of kinins in the cardioprotective effect of preconditioning: study of myocardial ischemia/reperfusion injury in B2 kinin receptor knockout mice and kininogen-deficient rats. *Hypertension* 1997;30:735–740.

209. Siebeck J, Cheronis JC, Fink E, et al. Dextran sulfate activates contact system and mediates arterial hypotension via B2 kinin receptors. *J Appl Physiol* 1994;77:2675.

210. Ma JX, Yang Z, Chao J, et al. Intramuscular delivery of rat kallikrein-binding protein gene reverses hypotension in transgenic mice expressing human tissue kallikrein. *J Biol Chem* 1995;270:451–455.

211. Chao J, Chai KX, Chen LM, et al. Tissue kallikrein-binding protein is a serpin. I. Purification, characterization, and distribution in normotensive and spontaneously hypertensive rats. *J Biol Chem* 1990;265:16394–16401.

212. Zhou GX, Chao L, Chao J. Kallistatin: a novel human tissue kallikrein inhibitor. Purification, characterization, and reactive center sequence. *J Biol Chem* 1992;267:25873–25880.

213. Wang C, Chao L, Chao J. Direct gene delivery of human tissue kallikrein reduces blood pressure in spontaneously hypertensive rats. *J Clin Invest* 1995;95:1710–1716.

214. Chao C, Madeddu P, Wang C, et al. Differential regulation of kallikrein, kininogen, and kallikrein-binding protein in arterial hypertensive rats. *Am J Physiol* 1996;271:F78–F86.

215. Jaffa AA, Durazo-Arvizu R, Zheng D, et al. Plasma prekallikrein: a risk marker for hypertension and nephropathy in type 1 diabetes. *Diabetes* 2003;52:1215–1221.

216. Coller BS. Effects of tertiary amine local anesthetics on von Willebrand factor-dependent platelet function: alteration of membrane reactivity and degradation of GPIb by a calcium-dependent protease(s). *Blood* 1982;60:731–743.

217. Puri RN, Zhou FX, Bradford H, et al. Thrombin-induced platelet aggregation involves an indirect proteolytic cleavage of aggregin by calpain. *Arch Biochem Biophys* 1989;271:346–358.

218. Puri RN, Zhou FX, Colman RF, et al. Cleavage of a 100 kDa membrane protein (aggregin) during thrombin-induced platelet aggregation is mediated by the high affinity thrombin receptors. *Biochem Biophys Res Commun* 1989;162:1017–1024.

219. Puri RN, Matsueda R, Umeyama H, et al. Modulation of thrombin-induced platelet aggregation by inhibition of calpain by a synthetic peptide derived from the thiol-protease inhibitory sequence of kininogens and S-(3-nitro-2-pyridinesulfenyl)-cysteine. *Biochem Biophys Res Commun* 1989;162:1017–1024.

220. Matsueda R, Umeyama H, Puri RN, et al. Design and synthesis of a kininogen-based selective inhibitor of thrombin-induced platelet aggregation. *Pept Res* 1994;7:32–35.

221. Bradford HN, DeLa Cadena RA, Kunapuli SP, et al. Human kininogens regulate thrombin binding to platelets through the GPIb-IX-V complex. *Blood* 1997;90:1508–1515.

222. Majima M, Sunahara N, Harada Y, et al. Detection of the degradation products of bradykinin by enzyme immunoassays as markers for the release of kinin *in vivo*. *Biochem Pharmacol* 1993;45:559–567.

223. Shima C, Majima M, Katori M. A stable metabolite, Arg-Pro-Pro-Gly-Phe, of bradykinin in the degradation pathway in human plasma. *Jpn J Pharmacol* 1992;60:111–119.

224. Bradford HN, Pixley RA, Colman RW. Human factor XII binding to the glycoprotein Ib-IX-V complex inhibits thrombin-induced platelet aggregation. *J Biol Chem* 2000;275:22756–22763.

225. Colman RW, Bagdasarian A, Talamo RC, et al. Human kininogen deficiency with diminished levels of plasminogen proactivator and prekallikrein associated with abnormalities of the Hageman factor-dependent pathways. *J Clin Invest* 1975;56:1650–1662.

226. Niewiarowski S, Prou-Wartelle O. Role of the contact factor (Hageman factor) in fibrinolysis. *Thromb Diath Haemorrh* 1959;3:593–598.

227. Colman RW. Activation of plasminogen by human plasma kallikrein. *Biochem Biophys Res Commun* 1969;35:273–279.

228. Loza JP, Gurewich V, Johnstone M, et al. Platelet-bound prekallikrein promotes pro-urokinase-induced clot lysis: a mechanism for targeting the factor XII dependent intrinsic pathway of fibrinolysis. *Thromb Haemost* 1994;71:347–352.

229. Gurewich V, Johnstone M, Loza JP, et al. Pro-urokinase and prekallikrein are both associated with platelets. Implications for the intrinsic pathway of fibrinolysis and for therapeutic thrombolysis. *FEBS Lett* 1993;318: 317–321.

230. Higazi A, Cohen RL, Henkin J, et al. Enhancement of the enzymatic activity of single-chain urokinase plasminogen activator by soluble urokinase receptor. *J Biol Chem* 1995;21:17375–17380.

231. Vroman L, Adams A. Possible involvement of fibrinogen and proteolysis in surface activation: a study with the recording ellipsometer. *Thromb Diath Haemorrh* 1967;18:510–524.

232. Schmaier AH, Silver L, Adams AL, et al. The effect of high molecular weight kininogen on surface-adsorbed fibrinogen. *Thromb Res* 1984;33: 51–67.

233. Brash JL, Scott CF, ten Hove P, et al. Mechanism of transient adsorption of fibrinogen from plasma to solid surfaces: role of the contact and fibrinolytic systems. *Blood* 1988;71:932–939.

234. Yung LL, Colman RW, Cooper SL. Neutrophil adhesion on polyurethanes preadsorbed with high molecular weight kininogen. *Blood* 1999;94: 2716–2724.

235. Chavakis T, Kanse SM, Lupu F, et al. Different mechanisms define the antiadhesive function of high molecular weight kininogen in integrin- and urokinase receptor-dependent interactions. *Blood* 2000;96:514–522.

236. Chavakis T, Kanse SM, Pixley RA, et al. Regulation of leukocyte recruitment by polypeptides derived from high molecular weight kininogen. *FASEB J* 2001;15:2365–2376.

237. Chavakis T, Santoso S, Clemetson KJ, et al. High molecular weight kininogen regulates platelet-leukocyte interactions by bridging Mac-1 and glycoprotein Ib. *J Biol Chem* 2003;278:45375–45381.

238. Nishikawa K, Shibayama Y, Kuna P, et al. Generation of vasoactive peptide bradykinin from human umbilical vein endothelium-bound high molecular weight kininogen by plasma kallikrein. *Blood* 1992;80:1980–1988.

239. Colman RW, Jameson BA, Lin Y, et al. Domain 5 of high molecular weight kininogen (kininostatin) down-regulates endothelial cell proliferation and migration and inhibits angiogenesis. *Blood* 2000;95:543–550.

240. Kawasaki M, Maeda T, Hanasawa K, et al. Effect of His-Gly-Lys motif derived from domain 5 of high molecular weight kininogen on suppression of cancer metastasis both *in vitro* and *in vivo*. *J Biol Chem* 2003;278: 49301–49307.

241. Guo YL, Wang S, Colman RW. Kininostatin, an angiogenic inhibitor, inhibits proliferation and induces apoptosis of human endothelial cells. *Arterioscler Thromb Vasc Biol* 2001;21:1427–1433.

242. Wang S, Hasham MG, Isordia-Salas I, et al. Upregulation of Cdc2 and cyclin A during apoptosis of endothelial cells induced by cleaved high molecular weight kininogen. *Am J Physiol* 2003;284:1917–1923.

243. Guo YL, Wang S, Cao DJ, et al. Apoptotic effect of cleaved high molecular weight kininogen is regulated by extracellular matrix proteins. *J Cell Biochem* 2003;89:622–632.

244. Cao DJ, Guo YL, Colman RW. Urokinase-type plasminogen activator receptor (uPAR) is involved in mediating the apoptotic effect of cleaved high molecular weight kininogen in human endothelial cells. *Circ Res* 2004; 94:1227–1234.

245. Kamiyama F, Maeda T, Yamane T, et al. Inhibition of vitronectin-mediated haptotaxis and haptoinvasion of MG-63 cells by domain 5 (D5(H)) of human high-molecular-weight kininogen and identification of a minimal amino acid sequence. *Biochem Biophys Res Commun* 2001;288:975–980.

246. Bior AD, Colman RW. Domain 5 of high molecular weight kininogen inhibits proliferation of HCT-116 cancer cell lines by interfering with G1/S phase of the cell cycle, a mechanism different from the effects on endothelial cells. *FASEB J* 2003;17:A677.

247. Zhang JC, Claffey K, Sakthivel R, et al. Two-chain high molecular weight kininogen induces endothelial cell apoptosis and inhibits angiogenesis: partial activity within domain 5. *Faseb J* 2000;14:2589–2600.

248. Colman RW, Pixley RA, Sainz I, et al. Inhibition of angiogenesis by antibody blocking the action of proangiogenic high-molecular-weight kininogen. *J Thromb and Haemost* 2003;1:164–170.

249. Parenti A, Morbidelli L, Ledda F, et al. The bradykinin/B1 receptor promotes angiogenesis by up-regulation of endogenous FGF-2 in endothelium via the nitric oxide synthase pathway. *FASEB J* 2001;15:1487–1489.

250. Song JS, Sainz IM, Cosenza SC, et al. Inhibition of tumor angiogenesis *in vivo* by monoclonal antibody targeted to domain 5 of high molecular weight kininogen. *Blood* 2004;104:2065–2072.

251. Bone R. Sepsis and multiple organ failure: consensus and controversy. In: Lamy M, Thijs LG, eds. *Mediators of sepsis*, New York: Springer-Verlag, 1992:3–12.

252. Waage A, Brandtzaeg P, Halstensen A. The complex patterns of cytokines in serum from patients with meningococcal septic shock: association between interleukin 6, interleukin 1, and fatal outcome. *J Exp Med* 1989; 169:333–330.

253. Beutler B, Cerami A. Cachectin: more than a tumor necrosis factor. *N Engl J Med* 1987;316:379–385.

254. Carmona RH, Tsao TC, Trunkey DD. The role of prostacyclin and thromboxane in sepsis and septic shock. *Arch Surg* 1984;119:189–192.

255. Philippe J, Dooijewaard G, Offner F, et al. Granulocyte elastase, tumor necrosis factor-a and urokinase levels as prognostic markers in severe infection. *Thromb Haemost* 1992;68:19–23.

256. Smith-Erichsen N, Aasen AO, Gallimore MJ, et al. Studies of components of the coagulation systems in normal individuals and septic shock patients. *Circ Shock* 1982;9:491–497.

257. Voss R, Borkowski G, Reitz D, et al. Endogenous fibrinolysis in septic patients. Second Vienna Shock Forum. *Prog Clin Biol Res* 1989;308: 383–387.

258. Kalter ES, Daha MR, Verhoef J, et al. Activation and inhibition of Hageman factor-dependent pathways and the complement system in uncomplicated bacteremia or bacterial shock. *J Infect Dis* 1985;151: 1019–1027.

259. Colman RW. The role of plasma proteases in septic shock. *N Engl J Med* 1989;320:1207–1209.

260. Chhibber G, Cohen A, Lane S, et al. Immunoblotting of plasma in a pregnant patient with hereditary angioedema. *J Lab Clin Med* 1990;115: 112–121.

261. Carvalho AC, DeMarinis S, Scott CF, et al. Activation of the contact system of plasma proteolysis in the adult respiratory distress syndrome. *J Lab Clin Med* 1988;112:270–277.

262. Mason JW, Colman RW. The role of Hageman factor in disseminated intravascular coagulation induced by septicemia, neoplasia, or liver disease. *Thromb Diath Haemorrh* 1971;26:325–331.

263. O'Donnell TF, Clowes GH, Talamo RC, et al. Kinin activation in the blood of patients with sepsis. *Surg Gynecol Obstet* 1976;143:539–545.

264. Kaufman N, Page JD, Pixley RA, et al. Alpha 2-macroglobulin-kallikrein complexes detect contact system activation in hereditary angioedema and human sepsis. *Blood* 1991;77:2660–2667.

265. Karsrad TS, Buo L, Aasen AD, et al. Cleavage of plasma high molecular weight kininogen in surgical ICU patients. *Intensive Care Med* 1996;22: 760.

266. Wachtfogel YT, Harpel PC, Edmunds LH Jr , et al. Formation of C1s-C1-inhibitor, kallikrein-C1-inhibitor, and plasmin-alpha 2-plasmin-inhibitor complexes during cardiopulmonary bypass. *Blood* 1989;73:468–471.

267. Wachtfogel YT, Kucich U, Hack CE, et al. Jr Aprotinin inhibits the contact, neutrophil and platelet activation systems during simulated extracorporeal perfusion. *J Thorac Cardiovasc Surg* 1993;106:1–10.

268. Colman RW, Edelman R, Scott CF, et al. Plasma kallikrein activation and inhibition during typhoid fever. *J Clin Invest* 1978;61:287–296.

269. Rao AK, Schapira M, Clements ML, et al. A prospective study of platelets and plasma proteolytic systems during the early stages of Rocky Mountain spotted fever. *N Engl J Med* 1988;318:1021–1028.

270. Nuijens JH, Huijbregts CC, Eerenberg Belmer AJ, et al. Quantification of plasma factor XIIa-Cl(-)-inhibitor and kallikrein-Cl(-)-inhibitor complexes in sepsis. *Blood* 1988;72:1841–1848.

271. Katada J, Majima M. AT(2) receptor-dependent vasodilation is mediated by activation of vascular kinin generation under flow conditions. *Br J Pharmacol* 2002;136:484–491.

272. Yamaguchi-Sase S, Hayashi I, Okamoto H, et al. Amelioration of hyperalgesia by kinin receptor antagonists or kininogen deficiency in chronic constriction nerve injury in rats. *Inflamm Res* 2003;52:164–169

273. Fields AP, Ghebrehiwet B, Kaplan AP. Kinin formation in hereditary angioedema plasma: evidence against kinin derivation from C2 and in support of "spontaneous" formation of bradykinin. *J All Clin Immun* 1983; 72:54.

274. DeLa Cadena RA, Laskin KJ, Pixley RA, et al. Role of kallikrein-kinin system in pathogenesis of bacterial cell wall-induced inflammation. *Am J Physiol* 1991;260:G213–G219.

275. DeLa Cadena RA, Suffredini AF, Page JD, et al. Activation of the kallikrein-kinin system after endotoxin administration to normal human volunteers. *Blood* 1993;81:3313–3317.

276. Pixley RA, DeLa Cadena RA, Page JD, et al. Activation of the contact system in lethal hypotensive bacteremia in a baboon model. *Am J Pathol* 1992;140:897–906.

277. Pixley RA, DeLa Cadena RA, Page JD, et al. The contact system contributes to hypotension but not disseminated intravascular coagulation in lethal bacteremia: *In vivo* use of a monoclonal anti-factor XII antibody to block contact activation in baboons. *J Clin Invest* 1993;91:61–68.

278. Colman RW, Scott CF, Pixley RA, et al. Effect of heparin on the inhibition of the contact system enzymes. *Ann NY Acad Sci* 1989;556:95–103.

279. Wachtfogel YT, Hack CE, Nuijens JH, et al. Selective kallikrein inhibitors alter human neutrophil elastase release during extracorporeal circulation. *Am J Physiol* 1995;268:H1352–H1357.

280. Donaldson VH, Evans RR. Biochemical abnormality in hereditary angioneurotic edema. *Am J Med* 1963;35:37.

281. Landerman NS. Hereditary angioneurotic edema. I. Case reports and review of the literature. *J All Clin Immun* 1962;33:316.

282. Schapira M, Silver LD, Scott CF, et al. Prekallikrein activation and high molecular weight kininogen consumption in hereditary angioedema. *N Engl J Med* 1983;308:1050–1053.

283. Seligsohn U, Osterud B, Brown SF, et al. Activation of human factor VII in plasma and in purified systems. *J Clin Invest* 1979;64:239.

284. Weiss R, Kaplan AP. The effect of C1 inhibitor upon Hageman factor autoactivation. *Blood* 1986;68:239.

285. DeLa Cadena RA, Stadnicki A, Uknis AB, et al. Inhibition of plasma kallikrein prevents peptidoglycan-induced arthritis in the Lewis rat. *FASEB J* 1995;9:446–452.

286. Uknis AB, DeLa Cadena RA, Janardham R, et al. Bradykinin receptor antagonists type 2 attenuate the inflammatory changes in peptidoglycan-induced acute arthritis in the Lewis rat. *Inflamm Res* 2001;50:149–155.

287. Sainz I, Uknis AB, Isordia-Salas I, et al. Interactions between bradykinin (BK) and cell adhesion molecule (CAM) expression in peptidoglycan-polysaccharide (PG)-PS-induced arthritis. *FASEB J* 2004;18:887–889.

288. Espinola RG, Uknis A, Sainz IM, et al. A monoclonal antibody to high molecular weight kininogen is therapeutic in a rodent model of reactive arthritis. *Am J Pathol* 2004;165:969–976.

289. Sartor RB, DeLa Cadena RA, Green KD, et al. Selective kallikrein-kinin system activation in inbred rats differentially susceptible to granulomatous enterocolitis. *Gastroenterology* 1996;110:1467–1481.

290. Stadnicki A, DeLa Cadena RA, Sartor RB, et al. Selective plasma kallikrein inhibitor attenuates acute intestinal inflammation in Lewis rat. *Dig Dis Sci* 1996;41:912–920.

291. Stadnicki A, Sartor RB, Janardham R, et al. Specific inhibition of plasma kallikrein modulates chronic granulomatous intestinal and systemic inflammation in genetically susceptible rats. *FASEB J* 1998;12:325–333.

292. Isordia-Salas I, Pixley RA, Parekh H, et al. The mutation Ser511Asn leads to N-glycosylation and increases the cleavage of high molecular weight kininogen in rats genetically susceptible to inflammation. *Blood* 2003; 102:2835–2842.

293. Isordia-Salas I, Pixley RA, Li F, et al. Kininogen deficiency modulates chronic intestinal inflammation in genetically susceptible rats. *Am J Physiol Gastrointest Liver Physiol* 2002;283:G180–G186.

294. Kamat K, Hayashi I, Mizuguchi Y, et al. Suppression of dextran sulfate sodium-induced colitis in kininogen-deficient rats and non-peptide B2 receptor antagonist-treated rats. *Jpn J Pharmacol* 2002;90:59–66.

295. Stadnicki A, Sartor RB, Janardham R, et al. Kallikrein-kininogen system activation and bradykinin (B2) receptors in indomethacin-induced enterocolitis in genetically susceptible Lewis rats. *Gut* 1998;43:365–374.

296. Jansen PM, Pixley RA, Brouwer M, et al. Inhibition of factor XII in septic baboons attenuates the activation of complement and fibrinolytic systems and reduces the release of interleukin-6 and neutrophil elastase. *Blood* 1996;87:2337–2344.

297. Ratnoff OD and Colopy JE. A familial hemorrhagic trait associated with a deficiency of a clot-promoting fraction of plasma. *J Clin Invest* 1955; 34(4):602–613.

298. Ratnoff OD, Busse RJ Jr, Sheon RP. The demise of John Hageman. *N Engl J Med* 1968;279:760.

299. Goodnough LT, Saito H, Ratnoff OD. Thrombosis or myocardial infarction in congenital clotting factor abnormalities and chronic thrombocytopenias: a report of 21 patients and a review of 50 previously reported cases. *Medicine (Baltimore)* 1983;62:248–255.

300. Mannhalter C, Fisher M, Hopmeier P, et al. Factor XII activity and antigen concentrations in patients suffering from recurrent thrombosis. *Fibrinolysis* 1987;1:259–263.

301. Lammle B, Wuillemin WA, Huber I, et al. Thromboembolism and bleeding tendency in congenital factor XII deficiency: a study on 74 subjects from 14 Swiss families. *Thromb Haemost* 1991;65:117–121.

302. Halbmayer WM, Mannhalter C, Feichtinger C, et al. The prevalence of factor XII deficiency in 103 orally anticoagulated outpatients suffering from recurrent venous and/or arterial thromboembolism. *Thromb Haemost* 1992;68:285–290.

303. von Kanel R, Wuillemin WA, Furlan M, et al. Factor XII clotting activity and antigen levels in patients with thromboembolic disease. *Blood Coagul Fibrin* 1992;3:555–561.

304. Jespersen J, Munkvad S, Pedersen OD, et al. Evidence for a role of factor XII-dependent fibrinolysis in cardiovascular diseases. *Ann N Y Acad Sci* 1992;667:454–456.

305. Munkvad S, Jespersen J, Gram J, et al. Long-lasting depression of the factor XII-dependent fibrinolytic system in patients with myocardial infarction undergoing thrombolytic therapy with recombinant tissue-type plasminogen activator: a randomized placebo-controlled study. *J Am Coll Cardiol* 1991;17:957–962.

306. Helft G, Le Feuvre C, Metzger JP, et al. Factor XII deficiency associated with coronary stent thrombosis. *Am J Hematol* 2000;64:322–323.

307. Yamada H, Kato EH, Ebina Y, et al. Factor XII deficiency in women with recurrent miscarriage. *Gynecol Obstet Invest* 2000;49:80–83.

308. Ogasawara MS, Aoki K, Katano K, et al. Factor XII but not protein C, protein S, antithrombin III, or factor XIII is a predictor of recurrent miscarriage. *Fertil Steril* 2001;75:916–919.

309. Pauer HU, Burfeind P, Kostering H, et al. Factor XII deficiency is strongly associated with primary recurrent abortions. *Fertil Steril* 2003;80:590–594.

310. Jones DW, MacKie IJ, Gallimore MJ, et al. Antibodies to factor XII and recurrent fetal loss in patients with the anti-phospholipid syndrome. *Br J Haematol* 2001;113:550–552.

311. Iinuma Y, Sugiura-Ogasawara M, Makino A, et al. Coagulation factor XII activity, but not an associated common genetic polymorphism (46C/T), is linked to recurrent miscarriage. *Fertil Steril* 2002;77:353–356.

312. Takeishi M, Mimori A, Nakajima K, et al. Reduction of factor XII in antiphospholipid antibody-positive patients with thrombotic events in the rheumatology clinic. *Clin Rheumatol* 2003;22:40–44.

313. Jones DW, Gallimore MJ, MacKie IJ, et al. Reduced factor XII levels in patients with the antiphospholipid syndrome are associated with antibodies to factor XII. *Br J Haematol* 2000;110:721–726.

314. Baumann R, Straub PW. Congenital deficiency of Hageman factor (clotting factor XII): report on the first two families found in Switzerland. *Helv Med Acta* 1968;34:313.

315. Miwa S, Asai I, Tsukada T, et al. Hageman factor deficiency: second case found in Japanese. *Acta Haematol Jpn* 1967;30:859.

316. Gordon EM, Donaldson VH, Saito H, et al. Reduced titers of Hageman factor (factor XII) in Asians. *Ann Intern Med* 1981;95:697.

317. Barbui T, Dini E. A new family with congenital factor XII deficiency. *Acta Haematol* 1975;54:345.

318. Kanaji T, Okamura T, Osaki K, et al. A common genetic polymorphism (46 C to T substitution) in the 5′-untranslated region of the coagulation factor XII gene is associated with low translation efficiency and decrease in plasma factor XII level. *Blood* 1998;91:2010–2014.

319. Ishii K, Oguchi S, Murata M, et al. Activated factor XII levels are dependent on factor XII 46C/T genotypes and factor XII zymogen levels, and are associated with vascular risk factors in patients and healthy subjects. *Blood Coagul Fibrin* 2000;11:277–284.

320. Colhoun HM, Zito F, Norman Chan N, et al. Activated factor XII levels and factor XII 46C → T genotype in relation to coronary artery calcification in patients with type 1 diabetes and healthy subjects. *Atherosclerosis* 2002;163:363–369.

321. Soria JM, Almasy L, Souto JC, et al. A quantitative-trait locus in the human factor XII gene influences both plasma factor XII levels and susceptibility to thrombotic disease. *Am J Hum Genet* 2002;70: 567–574.

322. Endler G, Mannhalter C, Sunder-Plassmann H, et al. Homozygosity for the C → T polymorphism at nucleotide 46 in the 5′ untranslated region of the factor XII gene protects from development of acute coronary syndrome. *Br J Haematol* 2001;115:1007–1009.

323. Zito F, Lowe GD, Rumley A, et al. Association of the factor XII 46C → T polymorphism with risk of coronary heart disease (CHD) in the WOSCOPS study. *Atherosclerosis* 2002;165:153–158.

324. Tirado I, Soria JM, Mateo J, et al. Association after linkage analysis indicates that homozygosity for the 46C → T polymorphism in the F12 gene is a genetic risk factor for venous thrombosis. *Thromb Haemost* 2004; 91:899–904.

325. Saito H, Scott JG, Movat HZ, et al. Molecular heterogeneity of Hageman trait (factor XII deficiency): evidence that two of 49 subjects are cross-reacting material positive (CRM+). *J Lab Clin Med* 1979;94:256.

326. Saito H, Scialla SJ. Isolation and properties of an abnormal Hageman factor (factor XII) molecule in a cross-reacting material-positive Hageman trait plasma. *J Clin Invest* 1981;68:1028.

327. Lammle B, Berrettini M, Schwarz HP, et al. Quantitative immunoblotting assay of blood coagulation factor XII. *Thromb Res* 1986;41:747.

328. Takahashi I, Saito H. A rapid purification with high recovery of factor XII (Hageman factor) on immunoaffinity column: application to an abnormal clotting factor XII (Factor XII Toronto). *J Biochem* 1988;103:641.

329. Hofferbert S, Muller J, Kostering H, et al. A novel 5′-upstream mutation in the factor XII gene is associated with a TaqI restriction site in an Alu repeat in factor XII-deficient patients. *Hum Genet* 1996;97:838–841.

330. Schloesser M, Hofferbert S, Bartz U, et al. The novel acceptor splice site mutation 11396 (G→A) in the factor XII gene causes a truncated transcript in cross-reacting material negative patients. *Hum Mol Genet* 1995; 4:1235–1237.

331. Miyata T, Kawabata SI, Iwanaga S, et al. Coagulation factor XII (Hageman factor) Washington DC: inactive factor XIIa results from Cys571 to Ser substitution. *Proc Natl Acad Sci U S A* 1989;86:8319.

332. Wuillemin WA, Huber I, Furlan M, et al. Functional characterization of an abnormal factor XII molecule (FXII Bern). *Blood* 1991;78:997.

333. Wada H, Nishioka J, Kasai Y, et al. Molecular characterization of coagulation factor XII deficiency in a Japanese family. *Thromb Haemost* 2003; 90:59–63.

334. Kanaji T, Kanaji S, Osaki K, et al. Identification and characterization of two novel mutations (Q421 K and R123P) in congenital factor XII deficiency. *Thromb Haemost* 2001;86:1409–1415.

335. Hathaway WE, Belhasen LP, Hathaway HS. Evidence for a new plasma thromboplastin factor. I. Case report, coagulation studies and physicochemical properties. *Blood* 1965;26:521.

336. Hathaway WE, Wuepper KD, Weston WL. Clinical and physiologic studies of two siblings with prekallikrein (Fletcher factor) deficiency. *Am J Med* 1976;60:654.

337. Hattersley WE, Hayse D. Fletcher factor deficiency: a report of three unrelated cases. *Br J Haematol* 1970;18:411–415.

338. Abildgaard CF, Harrison J. Fletcher factor deficiency: family study and detection. *Blood* 1974;43:641.

339. Raffoux C, Alexandre P, Perrier P, et al. HLA typing in a new family with Fletcher factor deficiency. *Hum Genet* 1982;60:71.

340. Essien EM, Ebhota MI. Fletcher factor deficiency: detection of a severe case in a population survey. *Acta Haematol* 1977;58:353.
341. Aznar JA, Espana F, Aznar J, et al. Fletcher factor deficiency: report of a new family. *Scand J Haematol* 1978;21:94.
342. Colla G, Carrea M, Sbaffi A. Fletcher factor deficiency: report of a new case. *La Ricerca Clin Lab* 1983;13:443.
343. Kyrle PA, Niessner H, Deutsch E, et al. CRM+ severe Fletcher factor deficiency associated with Graves' disease. *Haemostasis* 1984;14:302.
344. Currimbhoy Z, Vinciguerra V, Palakavongs P, et al. Fletcher factor deficiency and myocardial infarction. *Am J Clin Pathol* 1976;65:970.
345. Harris MG, Exner T, Rickard KA, et al. Multiple cerebral thrombosis in Fletcher factor (prekallikrein) deficiency: a case report. *Am J Hematol* 1985;19:387.
346. Saito H, Ratnoff OD, Donaldson VH. Defective activation of clotting, fibrinolysis and performance-enhancing systems in human Fletcher trait plasma. *Circ Res* 1974;34:641.
347. Saito H, Goodnough LT, Soria J, et al. Heterogeneity of human plasma prekallikrein deficiency (Fletcher trait): evidence that five of 18 cases are positive for crossreacting material. *N Engl J Med* 1981;305:910.
348. Sollo DG, Saleem A. Prekallikrein (Fletcher factor) deficiency. *Ann Clin Lab Sci* 1985;15:279.
349. Bouma BN, Kerbiriou DM, Baker J, et al. Characterization of a variant prekallikrein, prekallikrein Long Beach, from a family with mixed cross-reacting material-positive and cross-reacting material-negative prekallikrein deficiency. *J Clin Invest* 1986;78:170.
350. Lombardi AM, Sartori MT, Cabrio L, et al. Severe prekallikrein (Fletcher factor) deficiency due to a compound heterozygosis (383Trp stop codon and Cys529Tyr). *Thromb Haemost* 2003;90:1040–1045.
351. Wuepper KD, Miller DR, Lacombe MJ. Flaujeac trait. Deficiency of human plasma kininogen. *J Clin Invest* 1975;56:1663–1672.
352. Lutcher CL, Reid trait. A new expression of high molecular weight kininogen (HMW-kininogen) deficiency. *Clin Res* 1976;24:47A.
353. Exner T, Barber S, Naujalis J. Fitzgerald factor deficiency in an Australian aborigine. *Med J Aust* 1987;146:545–547.
354. Lefrere JJ, Horellou MH, Gozin D, et al. A new case of high-molecular-weight kininogen inherited deficiency. *Am J Hematol* 1986;22:415–419.
355. Hayashi H, Koya H, Kitajima K, et al. Coagulation factor deficiency apparently related to the Fitzgerald trait: the first cases in Japan. *Acta Med Okayama* 1978;32:81.
356. Nakamura K, Iijima H, Fukuda C. Tachibana trait: human high molecular weight kininogen deficiency with diminished levels of prekallikrein and low molecular weight kininogen. *Acta Haematol Jpn* 1985;48:1473.
357. Hayashi H, Ishimaru F, Fujita T. The fifth case of high molecular weight kininogen deficiency in Japan. *Jpn J Clin Hematol* 1988;29:2358.
358. Hayashi H, Ishimaru F, Fujita T, et al. Molecular genetic survey of five Japanese families with high molecular weight kininogen deficiency. *Blood* 1990;75:1296–1304.
359. Donaldson VH, Glueck HI, Miller MA, et al. Kininogen deficiency in Fitzgerald trait: role of high molecular weight kininogen in clotting and fibrinolysis. *J Lab Clin Med* 1976;87:327–337.
360. Ishimaru F, Dansako H, Nakase K, et al. Molecular characterization of total kininogen deficiency in Japanese patients. *Int J Hematol* 1999;69:126–128.
361. Krijanovski Y, Proulle V, Mahdi F, et al. Characterization of molecular defects of Fitzgerald trait and another novel high-molecular-weight kininogen-deficient patient: insights into structural requirements for kininogen expression. *Blood* 2003;101:4430–4436.
362. Merkoulov SM, Komar A, McCrae KR. Kininogen gene duplication in mice. *Blood* 2003;102:92b.
363. Damas J, Adam A. The kallikrein-kininogen-kinin system in the Brown Norway rat. *Biomedicine* 1979;31:249.
364. Majima M, Adachi K, Kuribayashi Y, et al. Increase in vascular sensitivity to angiotensin II and norepinephrine after four-day infusion of 0.3 M sodium chloride in conscious kininogen-deficient brown Norway Katholiek rats. *Jpn J Pharmacol* 1995;69:149–158.
365. Majima M, Mizogami S, Kuribayashi Y, et al. Hypertension induced by a nonpressor dose of angiotensin II in kininogen-deficient rats. *Hypertension* 1994;24:111–119.
366. Majima M, Yoshida O, Mihara H, et al. High sensitivity to salt in kininogen-deficient brown Norway Katholiek rats. *Hypertension* 1993;22:705–714.
367. Damas J, Bourdon V, Remacle-Volon G, et al. Kinins and peritoneal exudates induced by carrageenin and zymosan in rats. *Br J Pharmacol* 1990;101:418–422.
368. Damas J, Remacle-Volon G, Adam A. Inflammation in the rat paw due to urate crystals. Involvement of the kinin system. *Naunyn Schmiedebergs Arch Pharmacol* 1984;325:76–79.
369. Damas J, Adam A, Remacle-Volon G, et al. Studies on the vascular and hematological changes induced by ellagic acid in rats. *Agents Actions* 1987;22:270–279.
370. Ueno A, Ishida H, Oh-ishi S. Comparative study of endotoxin-induced hypotension in kininogen-deficient rats with that in normal rats. *Brit J Pharmacol* 1995;114:1250–1256.
371. Ueno A, Tokumasu T, Naraba H, et al. Involvement of bradykinin in endotoxin-induced vascular permeability increase in the skin of rats. *Eur J Pharmacol* 1995;284:211–214.
372. Kouyoumdjian M, Damas J. The fate of plasma kallikrein in normal and kininogen-deficient rats. *Arch Physiol Biochem* 1998;106:25–32.
373. Colman RW, Scovell S, Stadnicki A, et al. Kininogens are antithrombotic proteins *in vivo*. *Blood* 1997;90:29a.
374. Hayashi I, Amano H, Yoshida S, et al. Suppressed angiogenesis in kininogen-deficiencies. *Lab Invest* 2002;82:871–880.
375. Ikeda Y, Ueno A, Naraba H, et al. Evidence for bradykinin mediation of carrageenin-induced inflammatory pain: a study using kininogen-deficient Brown Norway Katholiek rats. *Biochem Pharmacol* 2001;61:911–914.

# CHAPTER 7 ■ MOLECULAR AND STRUCTURAL BIOLOGY OF FACTOR IX

S. PAUL BAJAJ AND ARTHUR R. THOMPSON

## FACTOR IX AND HEMOPHILIA B

Hemophilia B was distinguished from the more prevalent hemophilia A because mixing of plasmas from two different patients who are affected would occasionally correct the prolonged clotting times (1,2). As with hemophilia A, hemophilia B is also an X-linked disorder and was first shown in a family with the surname of Christmas (3). A serum fraction that only had the hemophilia B protein activity was prepared (4). Although *in vitro* clotting of normal plasma consumed the factor that was deficient in patients with hemophilia A (factor VIII), most of the protein that corrected deficient plasma from the patients with hemophilia B (factor IX) was not consumed, allowing its partial purification from serum. Because factor IX could be adsorbed to and be eluted from insoluble barium salts, the two types of hemophilia were distinguished in clinical laboratories by a "thromboplastin generation test" where fractions of serum (factor IX) or barium adsorbed plasma (factor VIII) was added to a patient's plasma to see which would correct the prolonged clotting time. A major advance in hemophilia screening was the use of an efficient contact phase activation system, initially with kaolin (5), which led to partial thromboplastin time-based factor assays using plasmas from patients with known, severe deficiency of hemophilia A or B. Clotting times are determined after recalcification of deficient plasma with various dilutions of patient plasma compared to the dilutions of a normal plasma pool.

Factor IX was initially isolated from bovine plasma (6) and its primary structure was determined (7). Human factor IX was isolated using similar affinity chromatography steps including insolubilized heparin (8). Antibodies raised to the isolated human protein demonstrated considerable molecular heterogeneity in hemophilia B and dysfunctional factor IX protein in patients on warfarin (9). Characterization of specific mutations responsible for hemophilia B followed cloning and sequencing of human factor IX cDNA.

## GENE STRUCTURE AND EXPRESSION

### cDNA and Gene Localization

From the bovine amino acid sequence, a series of oligonucleotides were synthesized assuming bovine–human homology, leading to cloning and sequencing the human factor IX cDNA (10,11). The factor IX gene is in the long arm of the X chromosome (12–14). Some extragenic polymorphic sites are linked (15). Physical localization is within an 8-mb yeast artificial chromosome fragment containing Xq-26 (16). The GeneBank factor IX (*F9*) genomic sequence [AL033403 (gi:3859054), from a contig NT_011786], is 34 kb and localized to Xq27.1. Its exons are oriented from the centromer to the telomere. It is 12 kb centromeric to MCF.2, a cell line derived transforming sequence. Factor IX is flanked by hypoxanthine phosphoribosyl transferase (HPRT-1), 4.2 Mb 5' in Xq26.3, and the fragile X-mental retardation syndrome loci (FMR), 9–10 Mb 3' in Xq27.3.

### Gene Structure

The factor IX gene contains eight exons (see Fig. 7-1A) (17) and the entire gene has been sequenced (18). The 5' sequence includes a Line-1 element and the major transcription start site appears to be at or near an adenine at −176 (Fig. 7-1B) (19). Upstream TATA-like and CCAAC-like boxes have been assigned as indicated. Translation begins with Met-46 (adenine +30); alternatively, Met-41 or Met-39 may serve as transcription start sites; of these three, only Met-39 is in the dog and rat sequences. The human gene includes a 1.4-kb 3' untranslated sequence that begins with TAA416 (stop codon). There is a typical polyadenylation sequence, AATAAA, followed by a predicted transcription termination sequence, CATTG (18).

Knowledge of the gene sequence led to the identification and localization of potential promoter elements and intragenic polymorphic sites and to the identification of mutations in families with hemophilia B. Hemophilia results from gross gene alterations, small deletions and insertions (usually causing frameshifts) or splice junction, and nonsense or missense single base substitutions. Mutation rates and types appear similar among different populations (21). Severe hemophilia B has been created in mice with targeted disruption of the murine factor IX gene and homologous recombination in embryonic stem cells (22–24). Phenotypic males have a severe bleeding tendency owing to the resultant partial gene deletions and alterations. They can bleed to death from tail vein section or cage injuries. These mice have provided a small animal model of hemophilia B, used extensively in preclinical studies of gene therapy for hemophilia B. Certain hemophilic missense or nonsense point mutations have been created in mice (25,26). These create models of more prevalent human genotypes seen in patients with moderately severe or severe hemophilia, to extend the types of small animal models available; gross partial gene deletions or rearrangements only account for fewer than 5% of genotypes in families with severe hemophilia B (27).

### Polymorphisms

Several polymorphic sites are within or very close to the factor IX gene (Fig. 7-1A) (15). Ethnic frequencies vary considerably and those most informative for different groups are indicated

131

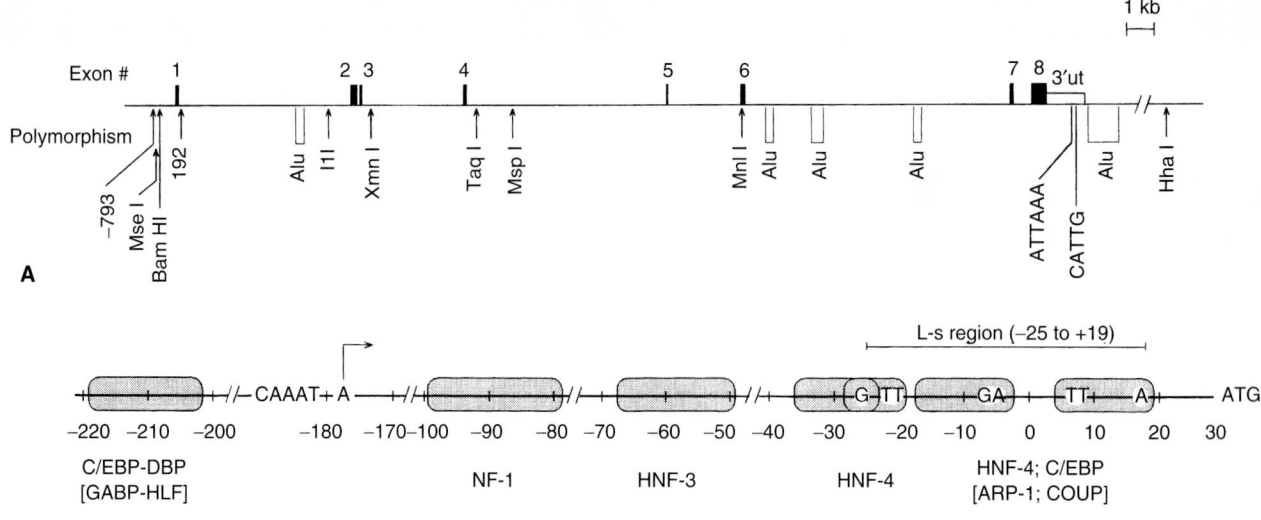

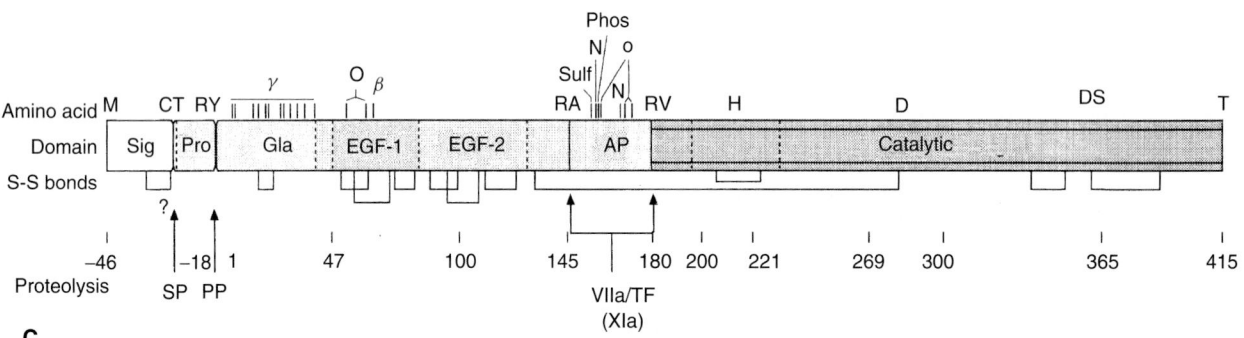

**FIGURE 7-1.** Factor IX gene and protein **A:** The factor IX gene is 34 kb and composed of eight exons; the cDNA is 2.8 kb including half as a 3′ untranslated region (18). Polymorphic sites (Table 7-1) are indicated by *arrows*, including single base variants, a 50 bp insert (I1I) and a 3′ CA repeat sequence. One Alu repeat sequence is found in intron 1, three in intron 6 and a 5th about 100 bp 3′ to the end of the gene. **B:** In the 5′ untranslated sequence, 6 or 7 sites for binding of promoter elements have been identified (19,20). The sequence is shown for three proximal binding sites flanking what was originally thought to be the transcription start site (18) through the first of three Met residues for the initiation of translation (ATG, Met-46). The proximal binding sites comprise a "Leiden-specific" region where mutations from −23 to +13 (but not −26) result in hemophilia B that improves dramatically after puberty (8 bases are shown as sites of these mutations). Transcription may begin 176 bp before the originally assigned site (*arrow*) following a TATA-like box (TCAAAT) and CCAAC-like upstream sequence (AGCCACT) (19) as shown; additional transcription start sites appear to be present, consistent with the lack of well-defined initiator and TATA elements. **C:** The factor IX protein, as transcribed intracellularly, is shown with six domains or regions. Sites of intracellular peptide bond cleavage are Cys-19–Thr-18 for a signal peptidase and Arg-1–Tyr+1 for a processing protease. It circulates as a single polypeptide zymogen, being converted to an active protease by either factors VIIa/tissue factor or factor XIa with cleavage of Arg145–Ala146 and Arg180–Val181 peptide bonds. Sites of γ carboxylation (above "*Gla*" in 7–1C), O- and N-linked glycosylation, β-hydroxylation (β), sulfation (*Sulf*) and phosphorylation (*Phos*) are also indicated. The *vertical dotted lines* indicate coding changes from one exon to the next. Disulfide bonds include Cys18–Cys23 in the Gla domain; Cys51–Cys62, Cys56–Cys71 and Cys73–Cys82 in epidermal growth factor (EGF)-1; Cys88–Cys99, Cys95–Cys109 and Cys111–Cys124 in EGF-2; Cys132–Cys289 between the connecting peptide and catalytic domain; Cys206–Cys222 (His loop), Cys336–Cys350 and Cys361–Cys389 (active center Ser loop) in the catalytic domain. A potential disulfide exists in the signal peptide, Cys-19–Cys-34. Specific residues are given above the bar in the single letter amino acid representation.

in Table 7-1. Polymorphic analyses provide linkage data to identify carriers, especially where the mutation is unknown; they can also establish the point of origin of *de novo* mutations in those families (about half) where hemophilia B is an isolated occurrence.

## Leiden-Specific and Promoter Regions

An uncommon type of hemophilia B, factor IX$_{Leiden}$ (34), is associated with a less severe phenotype after puberty. Several

## TABLE 7-1

### ETHNIC FREQUENCIES OF POLYMORPHIC ALLELES IN THE FACTOR IX GENE

| Polymorphism | | Ethnic group–allele frequencies | | |
| --- | --- | --- | --- | --- |
| Nucleotide alleles[a] | Restriction enzyme | Asian/Native American | Black American | Caucasian American/European |
| **5' UNTRANSLATED (BEYOND)** | | | | |
| G-793A | SalI[b], ASO[c] (28) | 0.5 A | – | 0.6 G |
| C-698T | MseI (29) | [0.7−] | [0.6+] | [0.7−] |
| T-561G | BamHI | 1.0 – | [0.6 −] | 0.95 – |
| **INTRON 1** | | | | |
| A192G | BstUI[b], NruI[b] | [0.8 A] | 1.0 A | 1.0 A |
| 5505-56 | (52 bp insert)[c] | 1.0 – | [0.65−] | [0.7−] |
| **INTRON 3** | | | | |
| C7076G | XmnI | 1.0 – | 0.95 – | 0.7 – |
| **INTRON 4** | | | | |
| A11113G | TaqI | 1.0 – | 0.9 – | 0.7− |
| G15625A | MspI | 1.0 + | [0.6+] | 0.8 + |
| **EXON 6** | | | | |
| A20422G | MnlI | 1.0 + | 0.9 + | [0.7+] |
| **3' UNTRANSLATED (BEYOND)** | | | | |
| G32197-T32206(8) | (GT)$_{5>6>4}$ (30) | 1.0 (GT)$_5$ | – | 0.7 (GT)$_5$ |
| A42939G 6 kb | HhaI (31) | [0.8+] | [0.6−] | [0.6−] |

In Caucasians, XmnI is informative if TaqI or MnlI are homozygous positive. When MnlI is negative (A), codon 148 is Thr; positive (G) is Ala; this polymorphism is also detected by monoclonal antibodies that require Thr148 to bind.

Frequencies are rounded to the nearest 0.05 and include some unpublished data (Thompson); boxed are those most informative for each ethnic group.

[a]Nucleotides numbering from Yoshitake, Schach BG, Foster DC, et al. Nucleotide sequence of the gene for human factor IX (antihemophilic factor B). *Biochemistry* 1985;24:3736–3750.

Polymorphic base assigned from UW-FHCRC's Variation Discovery Resource (www.pga.gs.washington.edu/) and unpublished ethnic data of Tom E. Howard, Emory University School of Medicine, Atlanta. The Web site lists 18 other dimorphic alleles with a variant frequency of over 10% including at the following bp sites (numbered according to the UW database starting ~1.5bp 5' from the Yoshitake sequence bp 1): 323 (5'ut); 3285, 4135, 5333, 5415, 6347 (intron 1); 10948, 11452 (intron 3); 15584, 16780 (intron 4); 21554 (intron 5); 26211, 29287, 31089, 31206 (intron 6); and 33641, 31524 and 35243 (3'ut); HhaI site is also numbered according to the genomic sequence used by the database.

[b]Amplification mismatch used to introduce a restriction enzyme recognition sequence (32,33).

Unless otherwise referenced, data are from Peake I. Registry of DNA polymorphisms within or close to the human factor VIII and factor IX genes. For the Factor VIII/IX Subcommittee of the Scientific and Standardization Committee of the International Society on Thrombosis and Haemostasis. *Thromb Haemost* 1992;67:277–280.

[c]Determined by restriction digest except for allele-specific oligonucleotide (ASO) hybridization (28), or electrophoresis for insert or repeat polymorphism (15,30). The intron 1 insert was reported as 50bp (Yoshitake) but includes an additional "AT" on more recent genomic sequencing.

mutations in different families occur in the 5' untranslated sequence within a "Leiden-specific" (Fig. 7-1B) region. The region extends to 5' but does not include a guanine −26 where mutations lead to severe hemophilia B that does not improve after puberty (35). The mechanism responsible for mediating a postpubertal increase in factor IX remains to be clarified but there is considerable evidence that an androgen effect on transcription is important in both humans and mice (36,37).

In analyzing 5' sequences for promoter elements, several regions are identified on footprint analysis indicating protection by peptide binding. C/enhancer binding protein (EBP)α, DBP, GABPα/b, hepatic leukemia factor (HLF), NF-1, hepatocyte nuclear factor (HNF)-3 and -4, COUP/Ear3 and ARP-1 binding sites have been demonstrated (19,20,38), and the last two appear to repress transcription by competition with proximal HNF-4 binding. C/EBPα gene knockout diminishes factor IX transcription (39). It would be of interest to determine factor IX transcription and protein levels in an adult mice model with 10% expression of their C/EBPα genes (40). Factor IX cDNA transcription is enhanced when a partial intron 1 sequence is included in the construct (41,42). This is likely due to enhanced mRNA processing.

## Expression

Expression in transfected mammalian cells (43) led to the development of a Chinese hamster ovary cell line (44) now used to produce a synthetic concentrate for patients with hemophilia B (45). Transgenic sheep (46) and pigs (47) have been prepared to express human factor IX as "bioreactors." Pigs' milk contained 2 to 3 g of factor IX per L per hour but a large fraction was inactive owing to incomplete γ carboxylation. Affinity chromatographic purification was required to first separate factor IX from the bulk of porcine milk proteins and caseins and, second ion exchange chromatography fractionated the more active factor IX species on the basis of their higher net negative charge.

Gene transfer of factor IX is an attractive target for ameliorating, if not curing hemophilia B. Murine and canine animal models have been extensively evaluated with a variety of viral and nonviral vectors (48,49). The preclinical studies were particularly encouraging with an adenoassociated viral vector (50). This led to two clinical trials in patients with hemophilia B (51). Intramuscular injections of a factor IX "minigene" using a viral promoter showed persistent expression for up to 10 months in muscle biopsies and there were no serious adverse events (52). The trial enrolled eight subjects and despite dose-escalation, circulating levels of factor IX were not convincingly demonstrated and, at best, were transient. Expression was improved in the mouse model using a muscle-specific promoter (53) or by regional perfusion as opposed to intramuscular injection (54).

The second clinical trial used a liver-specific promoter and delivery into the hepatic circulation in seven subjects with severe hemophilia B (51). One of two subjects treated at the highest dose achieved 12% factor IX clotting activity but the response disappeared after a few weeks; disappearance was associated with laboratory evidence of transient hepatic toxicity, likely from a delayed T-cell response to the viral capsid protein (55). The study is now closed and research is focusing on measures to limit vector (and transgene) immune responses.

# POSTTRANSLATIONAL PROTEIN PROCESSING

Before secretion from the hepatocyte, factor IX protein undergoes several modifications. These include γ-carboxylation, partial β-hydroxylation of a specific Asp residue, cleavage of signal and propeptides, addition of O-linked and N-linked carbohydrate, sulfation and phosphorylation.

## γ-Carboxylation

The γ-carboxylase (56) binds to specific residues of the propeptide of vitamin K–dependent proteins. There are conflicting studies showing that the N-terminal segment (57) or the C-terminal segment of γ-carboxylase binds to the propeptide of factor IX (58). The γ-carboxylase catalyzes a second carboxylation on the γ-carbon of all glutamyl residues (Glu to γ-carboxyglutamyl glutamic or Gla) within the first 40 amino acids of the mature proteins, a step essential for activity. This reaction has been shown to be processive (59); that is, γ-carboxylase binds to the propeptide and catalyzes multiple carboxylations in the Gla domain of factor IX. Notably, the Gla domain of factor IX has been shown to have an allosteric effect on propeptide binding to γ-carboxylase (60). This allosteric effect is believed to play a large role in the processive nature of γ-carboxylation of the Glu residues in factor IX. Gla residues were originally identified following alkaline hydrolysis of an amino-terminal fragment of bovine prothrombin (61). The Gla domain of human factor IX contains 12 Glas (62) and the first 10 are at homologous positions of other vitamin K–dependent proteins. Once the propeptide is cleaved from the Gla domain, these residues form eight $Ca^{2+}$ binding sites (see Fig. 7-2) as demonstrated in the crystal structure of the Gla domain of human factor IX (63,64). $Mg^{2+}$ can replace Ca-1, Ca-7, and Ca-8 but not the other $Ca^{2+}$ ions (63). In vitamin K antagonism, an inactive factor IX species circulates at mildly reduced levels (9,65).

The propeptide contains the carboxylase recognition site; site-specific mutagenesis of Phe-16 to Ala or Ala-10 to Glu inhibit γ-carboxylation (67,68). Naturally occurring Ala-10 to Thr or Val and Asn-9 to Lys mutations lead to warfarin hypersensitivity where severe depression of factor IX occurs despite

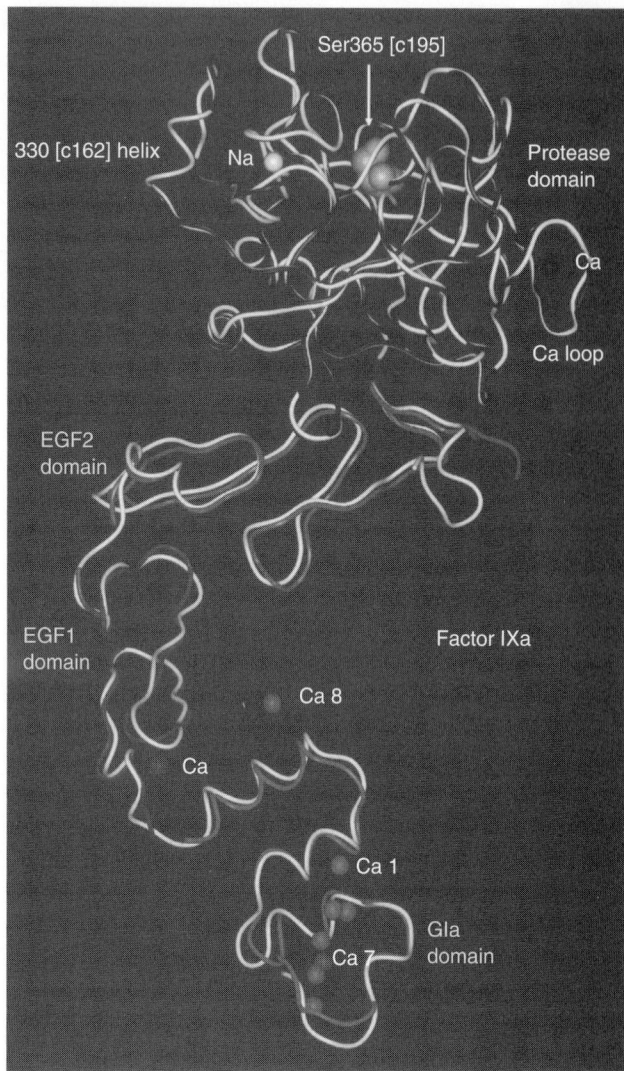

**FIGURE 7-2.** Schematic representation of the structure of factor IXa. Coordinates of porcine factor IXa [yellow, Protein Data Bank (PDB) code 1pfx] (66), human factor IXa EGF2 and protease domains (purple and light blue, PDB code 1rfn), human EGF1 domain (dark blue, PDB code 1edm), and the human Gla domain (magenta, PDB code 1j35) were used. The location of each domain is indicated. The location of the active site Ser365 [c195] in grey spheres (*arrow*) and the 330-helix [c162-helix] are shown, where residues are numbered from the sequence of the secreted human protein and [c] refers to the corresponding position of the prototype serine protease, chymotrypsin. The protease domain's bound $Ca^{2+}$ ion (*purple sphere*) and $Na^+$ ion (*grey sphere*), the EGF1-bound $Ca^{2+}$ ion (*dark blue sphere*), and Gla domain's bound $Ca^{2+}$ ions (*magenta spheres*) are shown. Ca1, Ca7, and Ca8 can be replaced by $Mg^{2+}$ (PDB code 1j34) (see Color Fig. 7-2).

mild reductions in other vitamin K–dependent proteins such that the prothrombin times are relatively normal (69–71). Synthetic propeptides with Thr-10 or Gly-10 have reduced carboxylase affinity compared to Ala-10 (69). Leu-6 is one of the most highly conserved residues throughout all the vitamin K–dependent proteins with the exception of bone Gla protein and matrix Gla protein (71). Change of this residue in factor IX to aspartate resulted in impaired γ-carboxylation in tissue culture (72). Mutation of Gly-10 to Ala and Val-6 to Leu in bone Gla protein converted its binding to γ-carboxylase from negligible to equivalent to the profactor IX (71). From the nuclear magnetic resonance (NMR) structure of a synthetic factor IX propeptide, the recognition site is likely within an α-helical sequence that includes a hydrophobic surface (73) as in prothrombin. Residues in position −15, −10, and −6 have been shown to be major players in determining the propeptide affinity for γ-carboxylase (71). The $K_m$ for binding of profactor IX is dependent upon the covalently linked propeptide, whereas high-affinity carboxylase binding to the bone-Gla protein is not (74); this is attributable to differences in highly conserved residues within the propeptide of bone Gla protein. Notably, the Gla domain also plays a role in γ-carboxylase binding to factor IX. Linkage of the propeptide to the Gla domain increased its affinity approximately 20-fold for γ-carboxylase (60). The Gla domain was also found to play a very important role in the rate of release of factor IX from γ-carboxylase as the $k_{off}$ of fully carboxylated factor IX Gla domain linked to the propeptide was found to be approximately threefold faster than the $k_{off}$ of the noncarboxylated protein segment (60). As shown with immunofluorescent subcellular localization of prothrombin species in transfected Chinese hamster ovary cells, complete carboxylation occurs in the endoplasmic reticulum before propeptide cleavage and transport to the Golgi apparatus (75).

## β-Hydroxylation

A second amino acid modification is hydroxylation by a dioxygenase of the β-carbon of Asp64 in the first epidermal growth factor–like domain (76). The dioxygenase recognizes the native conformation of the epidermal growth factor EGF1 domain of factor IX requiring the consensus sequence C-X-X-X-X-X-X-X-X-C in the main β-sheet and C-X-D/N-X-X-X-X-Y/F-X in the antiparallel β-sheet (77). In human factor IX, only about a third of the Asp64 residues are hydroxylated (78) and inhibition of hydroxylation in recombinant factor IX does not decrease activity (79). Although Asp64 contributes to a high-affinity $Ca^{2+}$ binding site (80), the hydroxyl group is not necessary for binding (81).

## Signal Peptide and Its Cleavage

Signal peptides are typically hydrophobic. One important hydrophobic residue appears to be Ile-30 because the hemophilic mutation to Asn results in severe hemophilia B with no detectable factor IX antigen (27). Signal peptide cleavage occurs at Cys-19 Thr-18. Cys-19 mutations to Gly, Arg, Tyr or Trp have been associated with hemophilia B (27). When the signal and propeptides of factor IX are substituted for those of protein C, full γ-carboxylation occurs (82). Therefore the signal and propeptide sequences are not specific among homologous vitamin K–dependent proteins.

## Propeptide Cleavage

Propeptides are cleaved by a processing protease that recognizes at least two Arg residues within the first four amino acids amino-terminal to the cleavage site. In factor IX, this sequence includes three basic residues, −Arg-4−Pro−Lys−Arg-1−Tyr+1−; hemophilic mutations at the −4, −2, and −1 positions (P4, P2, and P1) cause severe bleeding tendencies with circulating, dysfunctional factor IX antigen (27,65,83). Purified hemophilic factor IX proteins from patients with Arg-4 to Trp, Gln, or Leu react normally to antibodies that bind in the presence of $Mg^{2+}$, indicating that γ-carboxylation has occurred, but they require more than 5 mM $Ca^{2+}$ for binding to phospholipid membranes (84). Similarly, site specific mutagenesis of Arg-1 to Thr reduced cleavage by more than 99%; nonconservative mutations at Pro-3 and Leu-6 also reduced cleavage (85). Recombinant profactor

IX was isolated from an expression system with limited processing activity (86). Despite full γ-carboxylation, profactor IX could not bind to phospholipid membranes nor be activated by factor XIa unless the propeptide was cleaved by a processing protease, PACE/furin. A free amino-terminus is essential for proper conformational folding of the Gla domain and acylation of Tyr+1 is sufficient to inactivate factor IX (84).

## Glycosylation, Sulfation, and Phosphorylation

Bovine factor IX contains 26% carbohydrate (6) and humans contain 17% (87). Oligosaccharides are primarily N-linked to consensus-Asn-Xxx-Thr/Ser- sequences (4 in bovine and 2 in human). The two sites in both species are Asn157 and Asn167 in the activation peptide (18). Among factor IXs sequenced from other species, all other than human are predicted to have Asn260 (human numbers), all have Asn157, all but porcine have Asn167, and sequence of bovine, porcine, and ovine predict an Asn172 site (88). Although it appeared that cleavage of sialic acid residues inactivates factor IX (89), in vitro activity was preserved after sialic acid removal with a more specific, highly purified neuraminidase (90).

Within the first EGF-like domain, Ser53 has O-linked di- and trisaccharides [$Xyl_1$- or $Xyl_2$-Glc-O-Ser (91)] and Ser61 contains a tetrasaccharide [NeuAc-Gal-GlcNAc-Fuc-O-Ser (92)]. Ser53 is part of a consensus sequence (C-X-S-X-P-C) recognized by UDP-glucose: protein O-glucosyltransferase (93). This enzyme is believed to recognize not only the amino acid sequence but also the 3D structure in the EGF domain. Each of these oligosaccharide species is also found in a recombinant human factor IX preparation (94). Factor IX proteins from other species such as porcine do not have homologous Ser residues. Therefore, O-linked carbohydrate moieties in the first EGF-like domain are unlikely to be of functional importance.

In the activation peptide, the hydroxyl groups of Thr159 and Thr169 are glycosylated (95). Plasma-derived factor IX has an O-linked oligosaccharide at Thr172 and the activation peptide is further modified by sulfation of Tyr155 and phosphorylation of Ser158 (94). Of activation peptide modifications, only the equivalent of Ser158 phosphorylation and N-linked Asn157 glycosylation are conserved in all factor IX genes of other species sequenced. In the catalytic domains of plasma-derived or recombinant human factor IXs, there are no detectable posttranslational modifications (94,96).

# CIRCULATING LEVELS

Circulation of the zymogen in plasma depends on transcription, translation, secretion, and catabolism, processes that can be altered by certain hemophilic mutations. It remains to be established what controls a person's circulating level or why there is a threefold variation in levels among normal individuals (compared to a narrower range for other vitamin K–dependent proteins).

Relatively small differences in expression or secretion can be difficult to interpret, as seen with increased levels of an Ala+1 compared to the native Tyr+1 factor IX (97); there may also be subtle changes in specific activities. Several hemophilic missense mutations are associated with reduced levels of factor IX antigen or comparably diminished activity and antigen (27). Disordered transcription with a less stable mRNA, altered splicing, or altered protein stability in vivo as opposed to altered secretion of a transcribed protein are difficult to distinguish because hemophilic hepatocytes are required. Leaky transcription from lymphocytes cannot reliably be substituted because these are incomplete, even in normal individuals (98). For a known point mutation, transfection and expression in a mammalian cell line likely approximates the intracellular transcription, posttranslational protein processing, and secretion that normally occurs in hepatocytes.

## Alterations of Transcription

In the mammary glands of transgenic mice and sheep, alternative splicing from the Val307 codon to 131 bases 3′ to the normal stop codon occurs and accounts for low yields of expressed protein (99). The extent to which aberrant splicing occurs in factor IX hepatocyte expression has not been assessed. Among hemophilic mutations, premature termination codons, splice junctions, and frameshift mutations usually result in severe deficiencies with no detectable circulating protein. It is assumed that altered transcripts or proteins are unstable. When proteins circulate despite such a mutation, this can usually be accounted for by exon skipping. A clear example in factor IX is a partial gene deletion that removes the entire 4th exon (100). The 5th exon is in frame and although affected members have severe hemophilia with factor IX clotting activity less than 1%, their baseline antigen level is 30% due to a small protein (101). In another partial gene deletion of the 5th and 6th exons, the donor splice junction of exon 4 is not in frame with the acceptor splice junction of exon 7; trace amounts of a truncated factor IX protein were identified in the urine of these patients (102). Epitopes from the Gla and first EGF-like domains, but not those beyond the deleted fragment, were recognized by monoclonal antibodies.

Cryptic splice sites have been invoked as mechanisms for some families with hemophilia B, especially where a point mutation does not alter the predicted amino acid. For example, moderately severe hemophilia B with CAA to CAG (Gln191) is found in a patient with low activity and antigen (27). Another example may be a new donor splice site due to an A to G transition approximately 100 bp 5′ to the poly A site in the 3′ untranslated region in severe hemophilia B without detectable factor IX antigen (27). This mutation, however, could also affect a potential promoter/enhancer element; RNA studies are needed to distinguish these mechanisms.

## Secretion

The carboxyl-terminal region of factor IX was examined for mutations that may affect secretion following transfection into Hep G2 cells and transient expression (103). The hemophilic mutations Tyr404 to His, Trp407 to Arg, and Thr412 to Lys, as well as Tyr404 to Pro, Ile408 to Asn, and Thr412 to Asn had variably reduced levels of intracellular factor IX antigen that increased with proteosome inhibition. Secretion, however, was markedly impaired and remained so after inhibitors were added. Therefore the carboxyl-terminal sequence of factor IX, the most variable among the catalytic domains of different vitamin K–dependent zymogens (e.g., protein C and factors VII and X are longer), has an important structure recognized by hepatic secretion processes. The residues tested are within a carboxyl-terminal α-helical portion; mutations that increase charge or disrupt helical structure as with Pro404 will likely decrease hepatocyte secretion. Candidate subcellular interactions remain to be identified. Of note, factor X has a considerably longer carboxyl-terminal sequence; of sequenced factor IX's (see Table 7-2), the length is the same except for 2 more residues in the pufferfish and 10 more in the zebrafish.

## Developmental Changes and Sex Differences

During the second half of fetal life to the newborn period, the average factor IX level is lower than that of other vitamin K–dependent proteins and averages 40% (one SD ± 13) at term birth (110). During the first 9 months of life, a group of individual nonhemophilic children increased their factor IX levels from 39% to 65% (±18), but variability remained high. In mice, factor IX clotting activities averaged approximately twice as much in 28-month-old children versus 2-month-old animals, correlating with a similar increase in liver-specific mRNA (111). Two additional strains of mice had similar increases of factor IX mRNA with age, but unlike the previous study, increase in both clotting activity and mRNA were predominantly in male mice. Although estrogen effects from either late pregnancy or oral contraceptives often double factor VIII and von Willebrand factor levels, factor IX levels are only mildly increased, averaging 1.3-fold higher in women on oral contraceptives (112).

In transgenic mice, human factor IX levels nearly double with advanced age, owing to two specific age-related stability elements within the gene (113). The 5′ element, GAGGAAG, also contributes to liver-specific expression (114). In humans, factor IX levels were somewhat higher, averaging 107% in a series of 25 Italian centenarians (100 to 102 years old), although this was not statistically different from 104% in 51- to 69-year-old, or 96% in 20- to 51-year-old control subjects (115). The centenarians did have significantly higher levels of circulating factor IX activation peptide consistent with increased basal activation of coagulation that may reflect aging or subclinical atherosclerotic changes in the vasculature.

Some women who are carriers of hemophilia B have sufficiently low factor IX levels to be at least mildly hemophilic themselves. Although this may be due to an extreme in random X chromosome inactivation of their normal as opposed to their hemophilic factor IX gene, there are several examples in which symptomatic carriers have preferential inactivation of a normal gene X-chromosome (116–119).

## Intravascular Recovery and Survival

Factor IX is somewhat smaller than albumin and distributes in the intravascular and extravascular spaces. Therefore, human factor IX is recovered in the circulation of rodents after subcutaneous injection (120), as well as in hemophilic dogs and one patient with hemophilia, who were tested (121). Kinetic studies in patients with hemophilia B indicate variability in recoveries and survivals (122) that could be due in part to low levels of nonneutralizing antibodies to factor IX. When one group of patients received infusions of a monoclonal-purified, plasma-derived factor IX preparation versus a recombinant factor IX concentrate, survivals were identical but the recovery of the recombinant product was lower [38% vs. 53% averages (123)]. Variability occurred, as typically observed in clotting activities and even antigen levels post infusion, particularly in early time points. When [125]I-labeled factor IX was given to animals or patients with hemophilia B, however, disappearance curves tightly fit a 2-phase open kinetic model; recovery averaged 35% (124). It is possible that the radiolabeling altered the protein although recoveries of [125]I-labeled factor IX in dogs and baboons paralleled levels of factor IX activity and antigen; iodinated factor IX does allow frequent early sampling that allows more accurate calculation of recovery than less frequent and later sampling used for clotting activities. Survival data post infusion are subject to the model and methods of calculation, but are comparable to disappearance following the administration of coumarin anticoagulants (125).

Being smaller than albumin, the possibility of administration by nonvascular parenteral routes exists; as a protein, it is unlikely that it would survive digestion from an oral route. When a recombinant human factor IX concentrate was administered subcutaneously to dogs or monkeys (126), activity could

## TABLE 7-2

AMINO ACID IDENTITY WITHIN DIFFERENT FACTOR IX SPECIES
AND HOMOLOGOUS HEMOSTATIC PROTEINS

| Protein | Domain: number of amino acids (% identity with human factor IX) | | | | | | | | |
|---|---|---|---|---|---|---|---|---|---|
| Species | Signal | Propeptide | Gla | EGF-1 | EGF-2 | Connect pep | Act'n pep | Catalytic | Mature protein |
| **FACTOR IXS** | | | | | | | | | |
| FIX, man | 28 (100) | 18 (100) | 46 (100) | 38 (100) | 43 (100) | 18 (100) | 35 (100) | 235 (100) | 415 (100) |
| FIX, chimpanzee | 28 (100) | 18 (100) | 46 (100) | 38 (100) | 43 (100) | 18 (100) | 35 (100) | 235 (99.6) | 415 (99.8) |
| FIX, macaque | 28 (100) | 18 (100) | 46 (100) | 38 (100) | 43 (95) | 28 (94) | 35 (97) | 235 (99.6) | 415 (96.4) |
| FIX, dog | 21 (64) | 18 (78) | 46 (93) | 38 (89) | 43 (88) | 19 (72) | 32 (71) | 235 (91) | 413 (86) |
| FIX, cow | | | 46 (93) | 38 (89) | 43 (81) | 19 (100) | 35 (63) | 235 (85) | 416 (84) |
| FIX, pig | | | 46 (91) | 38 (87) | 43 (76) | 19 (78) | 35 (57) | 235 (92) | 416 (86) |
| FIX, sheep | | | | | | 19 | 35 (63) | 235 (88) | |
| FIX, rabbit | | 18 (89) | 46 (91) | 38 (92) | 43 (79) | 19 (83) | 35 (60) | 235 (84) | 416 (83) |
| FIX, mouse | 28 (57) | 18 (78) | 46 (91) | 38 (87) | 43 (83) | 19 (67) | 44 (63) | 235 (83) | 425 (82) |
| FIX, rat | 21[a] | | | | | 19[a] | 42 (74) | 235 (85) | |
| FIX, guinea pig | | | | | | 19[a] | 45 (49) | 235 (86) | |
| FIX, chicken | 21 (43) | 18 (39) | 46 (76) | 38 (81) | 43 (58) | 19 (50) | 50 (11) | 235 (60) | 484 (58) |
| FIX, pufferfish | 27 (24) | 18 (33) | 46 (63) | 38 (61) | 44 (44) | 21 (39) | 95 (17) | 248 (47) | 483 (47) |
| FIX, zebrafish | 19 (38) | 18 (50) | 46 (63) | 38 (47) | 45 (27) | 18 (33) | 69 (23) | 250 (42) | 492 (41) |
| Other proteins | | | | | | | | | |
| FX, man | ~ 21 (24) | ~ 18 (44) | 45 (63) | 38 (63) | 44 (50) | 12[b] (39) | 52 (9) | 254 (34) | 445 (42) |
| FVII, man | ~ 19 (24) | ~ 18 (39) | 45 (59) | 38 (66) | 47 (41) | 14 (33) | 8 (3) | 254 (29) | 419 (37) |
| Protein C, man | ~ 24 (8) | ~ 18 (39) | 45 (52) | 46 (45) | 45 (33) | 19[b] (39) | 12 (3) | 250 (29) | 417 (34) |
| eProthrombin, man | ~ 23 (19) | ~ 18 (39) | 45 (46) | Kringle -1 | Kringle -2 | 23 (6) | 49 (6) | 259 (31) | 579 |

Connect pep, peptide connecting EGF2; act'n pep, activation peptide.

Sequences are compared to human sequence (18) and from the protein database (www.ncbi.nih.gov/Entrez/protein.html), including sequence predictions from factor IX (FIX) cDNAs for canine (104), murine (105), rabbit (106), chicken (107), zebrafish (108), and (partial) sheep, rat, and guinea pig (88) species and sequence determined from isolated bovine factor IX protein (7). Note that all species have 12 Gla residues in a 46aa Gla domain, and identical half-cysteine residues indicating the same disulfide bonds (except the zebrafish is missing the 5th of 6 homologous half-cysteine residues in its second growth factor–like domain) and homologous sequence in the amino-terminus and catalytic triad of the catalytic domain. Neither teleost has an Arg at the comparable β-cleavage site between the connecting and activation peptides of other factor IXs (although the pufferfish does have an Arg–Arg sequence three residues toward its carboxyl terminus) and both fish catalytic domains have additional residues that flank the disulfide His loop (first and second variable regions) and at their carboxyl termini. Where a different number of residues exist, only those with homologous residues in human factor IX are included to calculate the "% identity."

[a]From partial signal peptide (109) or connecting peptide sequences (88).

[b]Based on expressed factor X or protein C protein before processing protease cleavage.

be recovered intravascularly. Furthermore, levels were sufficient to provide prophylaxis against spontaneous bleeding in hemophilic dogs (127). Therapeutic levels could also be achieved with intratrachial administration (128). When factor IX was conjugated to albumin, in an attempt to prolong its survival, the conjugate was cleared like factor IX and not albumin (129).

The reason for a lower initial recovery of recombinant as opposed to plasma-derived factor IX is not well understood. Minor structural differences between plasma-derived and recombinant concentrates are primarily confined to the activation peptide. Lack of phosphorylation of Ser158 and only partial sulfation of Tyr155 occur and the Chinese hamster ovary cells also N-glycosylate with a somewhat different composition at Asn157 and Asn167 than factor IX derived from human hepatocytes. These differences, however, do not readily explain why only recovery and not survival is different. Of note, deleting 23 of the 35 residues in the activation peptide, including those posttranslationally modified in preceding text, did shorten survival (130). When compared to full-length recombinant factor IX, with or without deglycosylation of Asn-linked carbohydrate, hemophilia B mice had only 17% as much of the truncated protein remaining in plasma 6 hours after injection (130).

The basis for differences in survival among different vitamin K–dependent hemostatic proteins remains to be determined. With some other protein systems, catabolism is enzymatically mediated and proteases such as chymotrypsin and neutrophil elastase inactivate factor IX in vitro by cleavages that are near to but distinct from activation cleavage sites (131). Bonds cleaved by granulocyte elastase have been identified (132). Nevertheless, there is no in vivo evidence to support intravascular enzymatic degradation of factor IX as a significant pathway for clearance in normal catabolism or pathologic states. Binding to the low density lipoprotein receptor-related protein (LRP) should accelerate clearance, although such binding appears to require the activated species, not the zymogen (133), and would be unlikely to substantially affect factor IX's catabolism.

One difference between factor IX and other vitamin K–dependent clotting factors is Lys5, near the amino-terminus in the Gla domain. Ala5 shows reduced binding to endothelial cells and enhanced initial recovery in hemophilic mice (134). This was confirmed in another study where the initial recovery was higher with an Ala5 mutant, although survival was shortened compared to the recombinant, Lys5 species (130).

# PROTEIN STRUCTURE

The 3 Å crystallographic structure of porcine factor IXa, Protein Data Bank (PDB) code 1pfx (66), and the 2.8 Å structure of the EGF2 and protease domain of human factor IXa, PDB code 1rfn (135), have been solved. A ribbon diagram of factor IXa is shown in Figure 7-2. Recently several crystal and NMR structures of various factor IXa domains have been deposited in the PDB. A brief description of each of these structures with its PDB code is given in Table 7-3. The activation peptide is present in the zymogen but is not visualized in the crystal structure of the activated species; this sequence has the greatest variability among factor IX sequences from different species, suggesting that its structure contributes little to enzymatic activity. The activation peptide is believed to dissociate from the factor IXa molecule after cleavage by factor XIa or factor VIIa/tissue factor. The signal and propeptides are cleaved before zymogen secretion; data on their structures are discussed in the preceding text, under posttranslational processing.

## Gla Domain

The Gla domain of factor IXa undergoes a transition to an ordered structure on addition of calcium or calcium and magnesium, as seen in x-ray diffracted crystals (63,64); NMR studies indicate a very similar structure for factor IX in solution (136,137). Binding of $Ca^{2+}$ or $Ca^{2+}/Mg^{2+}$ to the Gla domain is necessary to properly fold and orient the $\omega$ loop, which consists of the $N$-terminus of the Gla domain (63,64). The coordination of the $Ca^{2+}$ within the Gla domain of factor IX differs slightly from the coordinations seen in factor VII, factor X, and prothrombin (63,64). This difference in $Ca^{2+}$ coordination is not believed to be attributable to the presence of either the Fab fragment of mAb 10C12 or factor IX/factor X-binding protein because each of these bound the Gla domain at different positions (63,64). The Gla domain of factor IX binds 8 $Ca^{2+}$; five of the binding sites are internal and three are on the surface and contribute to surface charge (63,64). The three sites on the surface have been shown to bind to $Mg^{2+}$ as well (63). Of the Gla residues, 8 of the first 10 that are homologous to the other vitamin K–dependent hemostatic proteins are essential for activity. Of the 10, hemophilia B is associated with mutations in all but Gla15 (27), which coordinates to Ca-7 (63,64). Gla21 mutations result in an inactive protein (140). This is interesting because Gla21 coordinates to Ca-6 (63) and Ca-6 have been

shown to coordinate to lysophosphatidylserine, which displaces a water molecule from the coordination sphere in prothrombin fragment I (141). In contrast, the nonhomologous Gla36 and Gla40 do not contribute to activity (142); however, they provide all four ligands in coordinating to Ca-8 (63), indicating that Ca-8 is not necessary for factor IXa activity. Antibodies that bind to factor IX's Gla domain in the presence of divalent metal ions indicate there are both calcium and calcium or calcium-dependent epitopes and the latter are localized to the carboxyl-terminal end of the domain (143). Magnesium binding to the Gla domain appears important for activity (144). Comparison of immunoreactivity of factor IX's substituted with portions of the factor VII Gla domain indicates that Gla33, Thr39, and Gla40 are involved in a high affinity where a magnesium ion can bind (145). The $\omega$ loop in factor IXa is important in binding to negatively charged phospholipid surfaces. This interaction is believed to involve Lys-5 (Fig. 7-2) binding to the glycerol phosphate backbone and the carboxyl group of phosphatidylserine coordinating to Ca-5 and Ca-6 as has been shown for prothrombin fragment I (64,141).

Gla20 and Gla21 are in a conserved 4–amino acid disulfide loop that is buried with hydrophobic interactions to an aromatic stack composed of Phe41, Trp42, and Tyr45 near the carboxyl-terminal end of this domain. Hemophilic or recombinant mutations of the Cys residues also inactivate the protein (146). Recombinant factor IX without the aromatic stack could be activated by factor XIa but had a low specific activity; mutagenesis of Phe41 to Val or Asp similarly affected activity, whereas Tyr41 retained 64% of native factor IX activity (147). The Gla domain of factor IXa has been shown to be important for its activation by both factor VIIa/tissue factor (148,149) as well as by factor Xia (150). The Gla domain of factor IXa has been implicated in binding to tissue factor in the factor VIIa/tissue factor/factor IXa ternary complex; however, it has been shown to bind directly to factor XIa (150). The Gla domain of factor IXa also appears to bind to the light chain (A3-C1-C2) of factor VIIIa (151).

## Epidermal Growth Factor–like Domains

The three disulfide bonds in each EGF-like domain link 6 Cys residues in a 1-3, 2-4, and 5-6 pattern characteristic of EGF. The first of these domains extends from the aromatic stack to the second EGF-like domain; the second is angulated and lies under the catalytic domain [Fig. 7-2; (66,135)]. The two EGF domains in factor IX interact with each other through a salt

---

### TABLE 7-3

**FACTOR IXa CRYSTAL STRUCTURES AND NUCLEAR MAGNETIC RESONANCE STRUCTURES AVAILABLE THROUGH THE PROTEIN DATA BANK**

| PDB code | Factor IXa domains | Resolution | Details | Reference |
|---|---|---|---|---|
| 1pfx | Gla-EGF1-EGF2-Protease | 3.0 Å | Porcine factor IXa | 66 |
| 1rfn | EGF2-Protease | 2.8 Å | Human factor IXa | 135 |
| 1cfh | Gla | | NMR study | 136 |
| 1cfi | Gla | | NMR study | 137 |
| 1mgx | Gla | | NMR study | 136 |
| 1j35 | Gla with $Ca^{2+}$ | 1.8 Å | With binding protein | 63 |
| 1j34 | Gla with $Ca^{2+}$ and $Mg^{2+}$ | 1.55 Å | With binding protein | 63 |
| 1nl0 | Gla with $Ca^{2+}$ | 2.1 Å | With Fab 10c12 | 64 |
| 1ixa | EGF1 | | NMR study | 138 |
| 1edm | EGF1 | 1.5 Å | With $Ca^{2+}$ | 139 |

EGF, epidermal growth factor; NMR, nuclear magnetic resonance.

bridge between Glu78 and Arg94, as well as by a hydrophobic patch (152,153). This hydrophobic patch is composed of a convex hydrophobic loop near the carboxyl terminus of EGF1 that fits into a concave hydrophobic pocket near the amino-terminus of EGF2. Of note, there is more restriction of rotation between the two hydrophobic patches in factor IXa than in factor Xa (154). The interface between the EGF2 domain and the serine protease domain has extensive contacts between aromatic residues (154). The structure of the EGF fragment by 2-D–NMR (138) indicates antiparallel β-pleated sheets observed in crystals exist in solution. The first EGF domain of factor IX was crystallized with $Ca^{2+}$ bound to the $Ca^{2+}$ site, as shown in Figure 7-2 (139).

Factor IX without its Gla domain has two high-affinity calcium-binding sites (155), and one is in the first EGF-like domain (139,156,157). $Ca^{2+}$ in the EGF1 domain of factor IX coordinates to the side chains of residues Asp47, Gln50, and Asp64 and to the backbone carbonyls of residues Gly48 and Asp65 (139); Val46Glu or Gln50Glu mutations do not affect binding of $Ca^{2+}$ to the EGF1 domain (158). Tyr69 Cys produces severe hemophilia B (27); site-specific mutagenesis indicates this residue is important for activity but is not involved in calcium binding nor in β-hydroxylation (159). Gly60 Ser is a recurrent hemophilic mutation associated with a mild bleeding tendency and reduced factor IX antigen (27). Modeling predicts misfolding due to steric clash with the Cys73–Cys82 (third) disulfide bond in EGF1; the recombinant mutant contained native-like shifts in NMR patterns in the presence of calcium ions (160). Therefore, a portion of the mutant protein appears to have folded sufficiently similarly to that of the native domain to preserve activity. Pro55 to Ser or Leu also cause mild hemophilia. The Pro55 Ser factor IXa mutant is impaired in activation of factor X in the presence and absence of phospholipid or factor VIIIa and the Pro55 Leu mutant undergoes minor proteolysis between Arg318 and Ser319 in the autolysis loop of the protease domain during activation by factor VIIa/tissue factor or factor XIa (161).

Domain exchange among homologous vitamin K–dependent factors has provided further evidence for key structural elements of the EGF-like domains. Lin et al. (162) found that replacing the first EGF-like domain of factor X into factor IX had little effect on activity, whereas substitution of both EGF-like domains with those of factor X retained only 4% activity compared to wild-type factor IX. Conversely, replacing both the Gla and first EGF-like domain of factor IX into factor X led to a requirement of higher concentrations of factor Va for factor X activity (163); therefore, cofactor binding was somewhat suboptimal but did not require specific factor X sequences within the replaced segment. When the EGF-like domains of factor IX were substituted with those of protein C, the resulting activated protein C had 10% of the activity of the wild-type protein in an activated partial thromboplastin time (aPTT) assay (164). The first EGF-like domain of factor VII (where 25 of the 38 residues are identical, Table 7-2) has also been substituted for that of factor IX in a recombinant protein (165); this species is of particular interest because factor VIIa–tissue factor activates factor IX and this portion of factor VII participates in tissue factor binding. Curiously, the chimeric protein had twice the specific activity of wild-type factor IX, and enhanced binding to factor VIIIa; enhanced activity persisted after infusion into a dog with hemophilia B, and the chimeric protein had comparable survival to that of a wild-type, recombinant human protein. Use of a monoclonal antibody that recognizes the C-terminal part of the EGF1 domain, particularly Trp72 and Lys80, blocked factor IX activation by factor XIa, marginally decreased its activation by the factor VIIa/tissue factor complex, and slightly decreased the $k_{cat}$ for factor X activation in both the presence and absence of factor VIIIa (166). Further, the Fab fragment of this EGF1 monoclonal antibody, AW, has approximately 10-fold higher affinity

for factor IXa as compared to factor IX (167), indicating that the conformational changes that occur in the protease domain during activation and removal of the activation peptide are linked to the EGF1 domain. This monoclonal antibody also supports the hypothesis that the EGF1 domain of factor IXa is most likely not involved in binding to factor VIIIa. Among species, there is less homology between the second growth factor–like domain than the first (Table 7-2).

EGF1 domain of factor IX is also required for its activation by the factor VIIa/ tissue factor complex but not by factor XIa (168,169). Further studies by Zhong et al. revealed that the EGF1 domain of factor IX interacts with tissue factor in the factor VIIa/tissue factor (170). Recently, Ndonwi et al. reported that EGF1 domain of factor IXa is important for the feedback activation of factor VII/tissue factor to factor VIIa/tissue factor (171). These studies are supported by the molecular models of the ternary complexes (149,172,173).

Within the second EGF-like domain, dysfunctional hemophilic mutations (27) cluster in the loop before the second disulfide bond and the main β-pleated sheet; mutations in the third disulfide loop are predominantly associated with near-normal specific activities. The EGF2 domain has been implicated in binding to factor VIIIa, as well as in binding to the platelet surface. Each of three loops (loop 1: residues 88–99, loop 2: residues 95–109, and loop 3: residues 111–124) in the EGF2 domain of factor IXa was replaced by a comparable loop from factor VIIa and the entire EGF2 domain was replaced with the EGF2 domain from factor VIIa. These proteins showed no difference in binding to factor VIIIa; however, the $K_d$ for assembly of the factor X activating complex on the platelet surface was increased for the loop 1, loop 2, and the EGF2 replacement mutants (174). Therefore, residues 88–109 in the EGF2 domain of factor IXa is important in assembly of the factor X activating complex on the platelet surface. Further studies with these EGF2 replacement mutants showed that residues 88–109 of the EGF2 domain are important in assembly of the factor X activating complex on the platelet surface (175). In studies of factor IXa EGF2 mutants in which the Asn89-Lys91 loop and Leu84-Thr87 linker region were replaced with analogous regions from factor X or factor VII, the Asn89-Lys91 loop was found to have only a minor effect on factor X activation in the presence of factor VIIIa, whereas the Leu84-Thr87 linker region has a substantial effect on factor X activation in the presence of factor VIIIa. However, binding of the A2 subunit was marginally affected (176). Further, a decrease in factor X activation was found with the purified protein from a patient with hemophilia with an Asn92His mutation (177). Chang et al. used scanning Ala mutagenesis of the EGF2 domain and proposed that residues 89–93 are involved in binding to factor VIIIa and residues 102–108 are involved in binding to factor X (178). Therefore, the EGF2 domain most likely plays a role in factor VIIIa binding, tenase complex assembly, and mediating binding to the platelet surface. These two roles are discussed in detail in the subsequent section, "Binding Properties of Factors IX and IXa."

## Connecting and Activation Peptides

Physiologically, factor IX can be activated by either the factor VIIa/tissue factor/$Ca^{2+}$ complex or factor XIa/$Ca^{2+}$ (179,180). Factor XIa activation of factor IX is part of the sustained phase of clotting because factor VIIa/tissue factor complex is rapidly inhibited by tissue factor pathway inhibitor (TFPI-1) after generating small amounts of factor Xa and thrombin. Factor IX is activated by cleavage of the Arg145–Ala146 and Arg180–Val181 peptide bonds and release of a 35-residue activation peptide (179). Both factor VIIa/tissue factor and factor XIa cleave the Arg145-Ala146 peptide bond first followed by the Arg180-Val181 bond (96,179,181). Factor IX can also be activated *in vitro* by the factor X coagulant protein from Russells viper venom (RVV-X) (135,182,183). RVV-X cleaves the peptide bonds in the reverse order, preferring to cleave the Arg180-Val181 bond first and generating an intermediate factor IXaα, although relative rates differ between bovine and human factor IXs. Following activation, factor IXa consists of two chains, a light chain and a heavy chain, which are held together by a single disulfide bond between Cys132 to Cys289. The light chain is composed of the Gla, EGF1, and EGF2 domains, whereas the heavy chain consists of the protease domain. The homologous Cys residues are present in all factors VII, IX, and X species, although there is variability between proteins in the connecting peptide sequence that contains Cys132 (Table 7-2). Among different factor IX species, the factor IX activation peptide has considerable variability including length (Table 7-2). Furthermore, no dysfunctional missense mutations have been identified within the activation peptide sequence except at the cleavage sites. Of these, hemophilic mutations of Arg145 are relatively mild, whereas those at the β-cleavage site, Arg180, are associated with severe bleeding tendencies despite normal circulating levels of a dysfunctional antigen (27).

## Catalytic Domain

The heavy chain of factor IXa is composed of the serine protease domain, which contains the catalytic triad, His221 [c57], where [c] indicates chymotrypsin numbering, Asp269 [c102], and Ser365 [c195]. Following activation peptide cleavage, a new amino-terminus is generated, Val181 [c16]. In serine proteases, the amino group of Val181 [c16] must insert into the active site and form a salt bridge with the side chain carboxylate of Asp364 [c194] for conversion of zymogen to enzyme. This converts the hydroxyl side chain of Ser365 to a reactive species, capable of hydrolyzing the activation cleavage site of factor X. Lack of appropriate factor IX cleavage as in Arg180 or Val181 mutations leads to severe hemophilia B with normal antigen levels; Val182 is likely important for docking with the factor VIIa/tissue factor complex. Other mutations such as Gly184 to Arg, or of Gly309 allow the appropriate factor IX activation cleavages but sterically block ion pair formation (27). Among species, the regions around the amino-terminus and catalytic triad residues are highly conserved; however, fish have additional residues flanking the His221 [c57] disulfide loop and at the carboxyl terminus (Table 7-2). A longer carboxyl terminus in the mammalian proteins might diminish secretion.

As with other serine proteases, catalysis of factor X proceeds by an acyl intermediate from the peptide bond being cleaved to the active hydroxyl group of Ser365 [c195] in factor IXa with charge contributions from the other catalytic triad residues, His221 [c57] and Asp269 [c102] (Fig. 7-2). Substrate specificity is greatly restricted in factor IXa (185). This has been attributed to a variety of amino acid and loop differences that exist in factor IXa when compared with other homologous serine proteases. One of the most important variances is in the [c99] loop (185). When this loop was replaced with the c99 loop from factor X, the factor IXa protein exhibited an approximately 22-fold increase in catalytic activity toward synthetic substrates (185) and this loop was also shown to restrict catalytic activity toward factor X in the absence but not in the presence of factor VIIIa (186). In the factor IXa crystal structures 1rfn and 1pfx, Tyr266 [c99] has two different conformations. In the structure with pAB in the S1 site (PDB code 1rfn), access to the S2 site is hindered by Tyr266 [c99]; whereas, in the structure with the active site inhibitor, PPAck (D-Phe-Pro-Arg-chloromethylketone, 1pfx), Tyr266 [c99] side chain is rotated such that it is positioned to interact with Phe, which occupies the S4 site, of PPAck

(66,135). Sichler et al. have shown that Lys265 [c98] and Tyr266 [c99] are linked to the amidolytic activity of factor IXa and mutation of Tyr259 [c94], Lys265 [c98], and Tyr345 [c177] produced a factor IXa molecule with an approximately 7,000-fold increased activity and altered specificity (183). Interestingly, mutation of Tyr266 to a smaller residue leads to decreased activity, whereas mutation of Lys265 to a smaller and uncharged residue leads to increased activity; these differences are most likely due to complex changes affecting the S1–S4 sites (183).

It has also been proposed that surface loop 199–204 [c30–c40] of factor IXa is involved in macromolecular substrate interaction in the absence but not in the presence of factor VIIIa (186). However, further data that provide direct protein–protein contact interfaces between the enzyme, substrate, and cofactor are needed to verify this concept. Organophosphorous compounds such as di-isopropyl fluorophosphonate (DFP) acylate the active site Ser365 [c195] although the active site of factor IX is less accessible than that of other coagulation proteases at physiologic pH (179). A second form of active site inhibition uses peptide-cholormethylketones to alkylate the catalytic triad His221 [c57]; D-Phe-Pro-Arg-cholormethylketone was used to inhibit the porcine factor IXa preparation used in crystallization (66). Hemophilic mutations of the catalytic triad residues produce severe bleeding tendencies with normal circulating levels of dysfunctional protein (27,187). Gly207Glu is within the His221 disulfide loop and is predicted to remove a hydrogen bond that stabilizes the active site (188).

Trypsin-like serine proteases bind their substrates' Arg side chain to an S1 binding pocket with a negative charge provided by the carboxyl side chain of an Asp residue [c189] at the bottom. In factor IXa this is Asp359. Mutation of Asp359 to Gly in factor IXa causes hemophilia B (27), most likely due to defective binding and activation of its substrate, factor X. Mutations of Val307 are predicted to also disrupt this binding pocket (187). Ser360 [c190] is important in substrate binding to the S1 site because it allows an additional H-bond to be formed with the P1 Arg or Lys residue, thereby stabilizing the substrate residues (189). Mutation of Gly363 [c193] has also been reported to cause hemophilia B (27). Gly363 [c193] is involved in the formation of the oxyanion hole in factor IXa and other serine proteases. Mutation to any other residue most likely repositions the backbone amide of residue 363 [c193] such that it is pointing away from the oxyanion hole and unable to stabilize the developing oxyanion of the tetrahedral intermediate (190). Factor X binding includes secondary binding sites such as one that is partially disrupted with an Ile397Thr hemophilic mutation (191). This is a common recurrent mutation and represents a founder effect (27). A recombinant Arg338Ala was created (192) to examine a potential thrombin inactivation cleavage within the autolysis loop (193). The recombinant Ala338 protein had threefold enhanced activity but this was due to enhanced $k_{cat}$ for factor X cleavage, indicating involvement of this mutation in substrate interaction as opposed to stabilization from cleavage. Arg338 is in a Cys336-Cys350 disulfide loop and these data suggest this region can affect catalysis, possibly through interaction with factor VIIIa (194). Of note, thrombin cleavage of factor IX is inhibited by physiologic calcium binding (131). The catalytic domain's high-affinity calcium-binding site is in a loop involving Glu235 [c70] and Glu245 [c80] carboxyl groups, adjacent to the autolysis loop that contains the proteolysis site, the Arg318–Ser319 peptide bond (195). Cleavage of factor IXa in the autolysis loop generates a molecule, factor IXaγ, impaired in catalytic activity toward small synthetic substrates, as well as in factor X activation (195). Therefore, $Ca^{2+}$ most likely protects the autolysis loop from cleavage by thrombin or factor XIa. When Glu235 [c70] was replaced by Lys, 75% of activity remained as predicted from the structure of thrombin where a Lys-Glu salt bridge occurs instead of a calcium-binding site;

less than 10% factor IX reactivity remained in a recombinant species in which both Glu's were mutated to Lys (196).

As discussed in the preceding text, specificity of factor IXa's active site is more restricted than that of other hemostatic serine proteases. Nevertheless, antithrombin III with heparin rapidly inactivates factor IXa (197). The rate of antithrombin inhibition of factor IXa is increased approximately 1 million-fold by the addition of heparin (198). Heparin binding increases the reactivity of factor IXa toward both peptidyl substrates and bovine pancreatic trypsin inhibitor (BPTI) inhibition through induced conformational changes from the exosite to the active site (199). Residues Lys293 [c126], Arg333 [c165], Arg338 [c170], Lys390 [c230], and Arg393 [c233] in factor IXa are part of an exosite that binds to heparin (200). Further, the affinity of full-length factor IXa for heparin is increased approximately 10-fold by $Ca^{2+}$ indicating that $Ca^{2+}$ promotes factor IXa inhibition by the template mechanism (201).

Factor IXa activates factor X slowly in the presence of only $Ca^{2+}$; however, addition of phospholipids and factor VIIIa enhance the activation several orders of magnitude (202,203). Factor IXa has poor catalytic activity toward synthetic substrates, as well as macromolecular substrates such as factor X. Factor VIIIa binding increases the catalytic activity of factor X activation approximately $10^6$-fold with no effect on synthetic substrate hydrolysis (204,205). Several helixes and residues within the protease domain of factor IXa have been shown to be important in factor VIIIa binding. At present, strong evidence exists for the involvement of the 293-helix [c126-helix], 330-helix [c162-helix], and Asn346 [c178] in binding to factor VIIIa (206–208). Therefore, it appears that heparin may bind to or at least overlap with at least one exosite on factor IXa where factor VIIIa binds. Further, residues Phe342-Asn346 [c174-c178] of factor IXa appear to contribute to interaction with the endocytic receptor, low density LRP (133). Increasing concentrations of ethylene glycol increases the catalytic activity of factor IXa toward synthetic substrates in a bell-shaped pattern with maximal activity at approximately 35% to 45% ethylene glycol concentration (183,208) and it has been shown to bind between the Glu224 [c60] and Pro255 [c90] in factor IXa, which is believed to mimic the effects of factor X binding on the Asn264-Tyr266 [c99] loop (209). Under some conditions, factor IXa can activate factor VII (210), or factor VIII (211) but any physiologic or pathologic relevance of these reactions *in vivo* remains to be demonstrated. Nevertheless, postprandial activation of factor VII that is detected at low levels in lipemic plasmas requires factors IX but not factors XI or XII (212).

## Immunologic Epitopes

Polyclonal antibodies to factor IX contain species that only bind in the presence of calcium and predominantly recognize the Gla domain, which is in the light chain (65). Monoclonal antibodies that bind to the Gla domain (213), first EGF-like domain (167,214) activation peptide (213), and catalytic domain (215) have been characterized. Inhibitory antibodies are generated in 1% to 4 % of patients with severe hemophilia B, who are treated (216). Although alloantibodies to factor IX are far less frequently encountered in patients with hemophilia B than those to factor VIII in hemophilia A, their onset may be complicated by anaphylaxis and nephrotic syndrome (217). In 2 of 3 such patients studied, there were strong IgG1 antibodies that blotted to the heavy chain (catalytic domain) of factor IXa (218) but more sensitive studies on similar patients are required to identify any common features of epitopes involved in their immunologic responses. A recent study by Christophe et al. (219) examined eight patients with severe hemophilia who developed inhibitors to factor IXa and found

that the antibodies were primarily directed against the Gla and protease domains. The antibodies against the protease domain blocked the factor VIIIa enhancement of factor X activation, and the antibodies against the Gla domain inhibited both phospholipid binding, as well as binding to the light chain (A3-C1-C2) of factor VIIIa (219).

# BINDING PROPERTIES OF FACTORS IX AND IXa

## Phospholipid Binding

The distance from a rhodamine-labeled lipid surface to a fluorescein-labeled factor IXa active site was at least 70 Å (220). This value is consistent with the molecular dimensions of the crystallographic structure if lipid binding involves the Gla domain and the balance of the protein extends vertically above the surface (66). Electron crystallographic studies of 2D crystals of human factor IX zymogen bound to a lipid layer also support this orientation (221). Freedman et al. (136,137,222) used NMR spectroscopy to compare phospholipid binding of factor IX's Gla domain in the presence of calcium or magnesium; membrane binding was localized to the first 11 amino-terminal residues termed the $\omega$ loop. Furthermore, synthetic species with a Phe containing a photoactivatable p-benzoyl group in place of Leu6 or Phe9 (but not Phe46) showed radiation-induced crosslinking to the lipid surface that was calcium dependent. Therefore, there is direct hydrophobic interaction between amino-terminal residues and the hydrophobic lipid surface. In the presence of $Ca^{2+}$, the Gla domain folds to bind to phospholipid; however, in the absence of $Ca^{2+}$, it cannot fold properly and therefore cannot bind to the phospholipid surface. Notably, in the absence of $Ca^{2+}$, $Mg^{2+}$ can substitute and enables residues 12–47 of the Gla domain to properly fold, whereas the $\omega$ loop (residues 1–11) cannot fold properly without $Ca^{2+}$ (136,137, 222). Leu6, Phe9, and Val10 are hydrophobic residues in the factor IX $\omega$ loop that are believed to insert into the lipid membrane to anchor factor IX to the phospholipid surface (223). Further, on the basis of the crystal structure of prothrombin fragment 1 with lysophosphatidylserine (141), Lys5 in factor IX is hypothesized to bind to the glycerol phosphate backbone and Ca-5 and Ca-6 may coordinate with the carboxyl group of the serine head group (64,223). It has also been suggested that the residues 88–109 in the EGF2 domain may play a role (perhaps indirect) in binding to the phospholipid surface and assembling the tenase complex (175).

## Cell Surface Binding

Cultured endothelial cells have specific receptors that bind factors IX and IXa (224,225), allowing intrinsic factor X activation without platelets. Binding also occurs *in vivo* (226). As with phospholipids, binding involves residues 3 through 11 (227) although collagen may account for at least some of the observed binding (228). Using protein fragments to inhibit $^{125}$I labeled factor IX binding to cultured endothelial cells, determinants in the first EGF-like domain of factor IX were demonstrated, whereas binding to phospholipids was only completed with Gla domain peptides (229). From domain exchange experiments with factor IX and protein C, optimal endothelial cell binding appears to involve the entire factor IX Gla domain including its aromatic stack (230). In kinetic studies, factor VIIa activated factor IX, but not directly factor X, on an endothelial surface and factor IX activation was about one sixth as rapid as on stimulated platelets (231). *In vivo,* there is a basal low level of activity of factor VIIa on activating factors IX (232), presumably at endothelial cell surfaces. Therefore, there is good supporting evidence that factor VIIa activation of factor IX and intrinsic factor X activation on the endothelium are an important component of the hemostatic response *in vivo*. Mutation of Lys5 to Ala or Val10 to Lys considerably reduced the affinity of factor IX for endothelial cells, whereas Lys5 to Ala increased factor IX affinity for bovine vascular endothelial cells approximately threefold (227). The endothelial cell-binding site for factor IX has been shown to be two sites on collagen IV that are 50 and 98 nm from the C-terminus of collagen IV (228,233). Further, factor IX has been shown to bind *in vivo* to endothelial cell collagen IV surfaces (134) and this binding may play an important role in regulating the concentration of factor IX in the blood.

Upon activation by thrombin or the SFLLRN peptide, platelets expose 1,000-1,200 sites for factor VIIIa and factor X each (234,235) and approximately 10% of the activated platelet population expose approximately 6,000 sites per platelet for factor IXa (236). The colocalization of factor IXa, factor VIIIa, and factor X on the platelet surface increases the rate of factor X activation by approximately 24 million-fold (237). However, whether this is simply by these proteins binding to the phospholipid surface of the platelet or to protein receptors on the platelet surface is unknown. Binding of factor IXa again involves the amino-terminal ω loop sequence Gly4 through Gln11 (238), although the factor X–activating complex requires an intact second EGF-like domain of factor IX (239). Residues Cys88 to Cys109 comprise two loops in the EGF2 domain that appear to mediate binding of factor IXa to the platelet surface, as well as assembly of the tenase complex (174). There is also evidence from chemical crosslinking that the first EGF-like domain contributes a weak interaction in binding of factor X to factor IXa (240). The platelet surface is believed to be the primary site of factor XIa activation of factor IX due to platelet surface protection of factor XIa from inactivation by protease nexin 2. Factor XIa has also been shown to bind to HUVEC although this is believed to be physiologically unlikely because high-molecular-weight kininogen will most likely prevent factor XIa binding (241).

## Factor VIIIa Binding

Currently, several laboratories are actively pursuing the domains and residues in factor IXa that interact with specific regions of factor VIIIa. There are several factor IXa:factor VIIIa models that have been published (242,243). Most of the recent models only have minor differences. In the models, the protease domain of factor IXa interacts with the A2 subunit of factor VIIIa, part(s) of the EGF2/EGF1 domains interact with the A3 subunit of factor VIIIa, and the Gla domain interacts with the C2 subunit of factor VIIIa. In this model, factor IXa is "standing" somewhat straight. A model of the factor IXa:factor VIIIa complex is shown in Figure 7-3.

Binding of factor VIIIa to factor IXa's protease domain was suggested because a monoclonal antibody to factor IX was shown to inhibit activity by decreasing factor IXa binding to factor VIIIa (245). This antibody binds to a conformational epitope in the amino-terminal half of the catalytic domain (216). Mutation of charged surface residues to the homologous residue in factor X, however, failed to identify a species that had reduced factor VIIIa binding (246). Therefore, either the mutations were not sufficient to disrupt binding to other sites on factor IX, or the antibody binding inhibits interaction at other sites. Strong evidence supports the involvement of residues from the 293-helix [c126-helix], the 330-helix [c162-helix], and Asn346 [c178] in factor IXa in binding to factor VIIIa (205–207). The 330-helix [c162-helix] has been shown to bind to the 558–565 region of the A2 subunit of factor

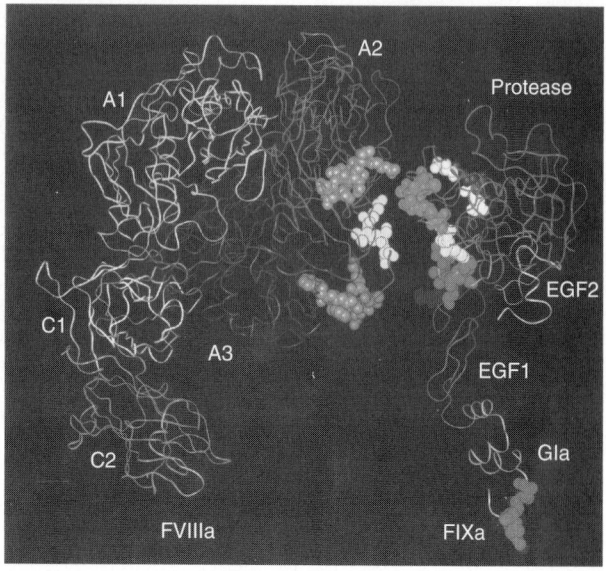

**FIGURE 7-3.** A model of the interaction of factor IXa with factor VIIIa. The coordinates for the factor IXa structure are from the Protein Data Bank (code 1rfn and 1pfx) and the coordinates for the A1, A2, A3, C1, and C2 subunits of factor VIIIa are from Stoilova-McPhie (HAMSTeR database) (242). Ribbon structure for each protein is depicted. The A1, A2, and A3 domains of factor VIIIa are homologous to the ceruloplasmin domains, whereas the C1 and C2 domains are homologous to the galactose oxidase lipid binding domain. The hypothesized interface residues are shown as CPK space-filling models. On the right, the factor IXa protease domain is in *green*, the EGF2 domain is in *lavender*, the EGF1 domain is in *red*, and the Gla domain is in *orange*. The A1 subunit of factor VIIIa is in *yellow*, the A2 subunit is in *magenta*, the A3 subunit is in *blue*, the C1 subunit is in *white*, and the C2 subunit is in *orange*. The factor IXa protease domain, with residues numbered as in Figure 7-2, Asn346 [c178] is in *pink*, residues of the 330-helix [c162-helix] are in *cyan*, residues 301–303 [c132–c134] are in *yellow*, Arg403 [c233] is *purple*, and Lys293 [c126] is *white*. In EGF2, residues 89–93 are *red-orange*, and residues 84–87 are *dark blue*. Residues Lys5, Leu6, Phe9, and Val10 of the factor IXa Gla domain that are involved in binding to the phospholipids surface are shown and colored by atom type in which carbons are *green*, nitrogens are *blue*, and oxygens are *red*. The protease domain residues most likely interact with the A2 subunit of factor VIIIa, whereas the EGF2 domain residues may be involved in binding to the A2 and/or the A3 subunit of factor VIIIa. In factor VIIIa, depicted on the left, the A2 subunit residues 558–565 are in orange and 707–712 are in *yellow*. The A3 subunit residues 1811–1818 are shown in *light green*. The A2 subunit residues could possibly be involved in binding to the heavy chain (protease domain), whereas the A3 subunit residues could be involved in binding to the light chain (including the EGF2 domain) of factor IXa. It should be noted that the crystal structure of a partial bovine factor Va suggests a different orientation of C1 and C2 domains such that C1 may also bind to the lipid surface (244) (see Color Fig. 7-3).

VIIIa (247). Isolated A2 domain enhances factor IXa activation of factor X approximately 200-fold (248), although this is less than the effect of the intact cofactor, factor VIIIa. Plasma-derived, recombinant wild-type, and two protease domain Ca²⁺-site mutants Glu235 [c70] to Lys and Glu245 [c80] to Val were compared in terms of the effect of phospholipid and apparent factor VIIIa binding (194). In native factor IX, phospholipid enhances factor IXa–VIIIa binding approximately 2000-fold. The Val245 [c80] mutant did not bind calcium, and was susceptible to cleavage at Arg318 [c150] in the autolysis loop during activation by factor XIa, but not by factor VIIa–tissue factor. The factor IXa mutant Glu245 Val also had reduced factor VIIIa binding (194); however, the Lys235 [c70] mutant was only partially affected, presumably because it allows a salt bridge to occur between Lys235 [c70] and Glu245

[c80]. However, mutation of other residues within the $Ca^{2+}$ binding loop have little or no effect on factor VIIIa binding (246). Therefore, one may infer that the $Ca^{2+}$ binding loop is not directly involved in binding to factor VIIIa, but instead imparts a structural change in conformation that favors binding to factor VIIIa (243). Proteolysis in the autolysis loop, residues 310–323 [c141–c155] of factor IXa decreases binding to factor VIIIa (194,195). Further, mutation of Lys316 [c148] to Ala or Glu (249), mutation of Arg312 [c143] to Ala (250), and proteolysis at the Lys316–Gly317 [c148–c149] peptide bond (195) substantially reduces the rate of factor X activation in both the presence and absence of factor VIIIa. Therefore, the autolysis loop of factor IXa is most likely involved in factor X binding. Proteolysis of the autolysis loop is hypothesized to affect factor VIIIa binding because the two helices important in binding to factor VIIIa, 293-helix [c126-helix] and the 330-helix [c162-helix], are each linked to the autolysis loop via a single β-strand (243). Therefore, cleavage of the autolysis loop could allow both of these helices to slightly move and be misaligned for binding to factor VIIIa (243).

There is evidence indicating that the protease domain of factor IXa contains a $Na^+$ site (251). In this proposed site, $Na^+$ is predicted to coordinate to the carbonyl groups of residues 353 [c184A], 354 [c185], 391 [c221A], and 394 [c224]. Tyr395 [c225] plays an important role in orienting the carbonyl oxygen atom of residue 394 toward the $Na^+$-coordination shell (252). As shown in Figure 7-4, the $Na^+$-site in factor IXa resembles that of factor Xa (253,254), activated protein C (255), and factor VIIa (251) but not thrombin (253). This may be due to the presence of three additional residues in the 183 loop of thrombin. As a result of this insertion, the carbonyl oxygens of this loop in thrombin are spatially distant and unable to coordinate with $Na^+$. Instead, the cavity in thrombin is filled with water molecules, two of which are optimally situated to coordinate with $Na^+$. $Na^+$ in factor IXa appears to play a role in catalysis and factor VIIIa binding (251). The two $Na^+$ binding loops are held together by an H-bond between Tyr395 [c225] and His354 [c185], and Tyr395 [c225] makes Van der Walls contacts with the 330-helix [c162-helix] that binds factor VIIIa (251). A hemophilia B mutation in which Tyr395 [c225] is changed to His has been reported (27), which could be due to impaired $Na^+$ and/or factor VIIIa binding.

There is also evidence for a specific interaction between factor IXa's EGF2 domain and factor VIIIa. The EGF2 domain (residues 88–109) has been shown to be important in assembly of the tenase complex on both a phospholipid surface, as well as on activated platelets (174,175). Further studies by Celie et al. (176) investigated the role of the EGF1/EGF2 linker region Leu84–Thr87, as well as the role of the Asn89–Lys91 loop region by substituting these regions with analogous regions from factor VIIa. Replacement of the Asn89–Lys91 loop region only decreased the activation of factor X in the presence of factor VIIIa by a small amount; however replacement of the EGF1/EGF2 linker region Leu84–Thr87 greatly decreased the activation of factor X in the presence of factor VIIIa (less effect with the A2 subunit) (176). Chang et al. (178) mutated every residue in the EGF2 domain to Ala and examined the effects of each mutation on factor VIIIa binding and factor X activation. They concluded that residues 89–94 are important in binding to factor VIIIa and residues 102–108 are involved in binding to factor X (178). Therefore, there is some discrepancy between these studies and their results that remains to be resolved. Studies pertaining to factor IXa binding to factor VIIIa have been reviewed (243). It is possible that the EGF2 domain binds to either the A2 subunit, the A3 subunit, or to both the A2 and A3 subunits of factor VIIIa. Earlier studies have shown that the 1811–1818 region of the A3 subunit of factor VIIIa may bind to factor IXa (257); however,

it is unclear as to which region of factor IXa it binds to. For factor IXa, cleavage of the Arg145–Ala146 bond appears to enhance binding of the factor VIIIa light chain (258).

The EGF1 domain may also influence factor VIIIa binding although this may not be due to a direct interaction. Several studies have emphasized the importance of $Ca^{2+}$ binding to the EGF1 domain of factor IXa in factor VIIIa binding on a phospholipid surface (80,152). However, Gln50 (residue which coordinates to $Ca^{2+}$) to Pro mutation only reduced affinity for factor VIIIa in the presence of phospholipid and not in its absence (207). Further replacement of the EGF1 domain with that of protein C resulted in approximately 80-fold decreased affinity for factor VIIIa in the presence of phospholipid and a minor difference in a system without phospholipid (207). Moreover, recent studies with a monoclonal antibody to the EGF1 domain showed that the antibody did not affect factor VIIIa binding to factor IXa (166). This monoclonal antibody also indicated that conformational changes in the protease domain of factor IXa that occur during activation may be allosterically transmitted to the EGF2 and EGF1 domains (166). However, this study and others question whether the hydrogen bond between Glu78 in the EGF1 domain and Arg94 in the EGF2 domain is crucial for the interaction of factor IXa with the light chain of factor VIIIa as hypothesized by Christophe et al. (259). Therefore, it appears that the EGF1 domain does not directly bind to factor VIIIa but rather correctly positions the EGF2 and protease domains for proper interactions.

The Gla domain may also be involved in factor VIIIa binding. Using synthesized Gla domains with Phe9, Phe25, or Val46 replaced with benzoylphenylalanine, Gla25BPA, and Gla47BPA, constructs were cross-linked to factor VIIIa, and immunoprecipitation with a C2 antibody studies indicated that the Gla domain of factor IXa interacts with the C2 domain of factor VIIIa (151). This interaction most likely involves Phe25 and Val46. Mutation of Gly12 to Arg has also been reported to disrupt factor VIIIa binding (259); however, this is most likely due to a structural impairment rather than from a direct binding effect. Therefore, more studies are needed to elucidate the exosites on factor IXa important in binding to factor VIIIa, particularly in respect to the EGF2, EGF1, and Gla domains.

# ROLE OF FACTORS IX AND IXa IN HEMOSTASIS AND THROMBOSIS

## Initiation of Clot Formation *In Vivo*

Intrinsic and extrinsic system clotting are distinct mechanisms *in vitro*, accounting for the partial thromboplastin and prothrombin times, respectively. A salient observation was that factor IX could be activated by factor VIIa–tissue factor (180) in addition to the intrinsic activator, factor XIa, and extrinsic activation of factor IX was at least the major path *in vivo* (260). The current formulation (203,261,262) is that initially, a small amount of factor VIIa is generated and with limiting amounts of tissue factor, factor IX activation is preferred to direct extrinsic factor X activation. The initiation phase of extrinsic factor IX activation is followed by a burst of intrinsically activated factor X that overwhelms the TFPI. This later stage, propagation, leads to a sufficiently high concentration of localized thrombin to clot fibrinogen. This theory accounts for the bleeding tendencies associated with factors VIII or IX deficiency and why most contact activation protein deficiencies do not have bleeding tendencies. Unexplained is the mild bleeding tendency in approximately half of the patients with even severe factor XI deficiency.

The presence of detectable factor IX activation peptide in circulating blood (260) suggests that either there is a systemic basal

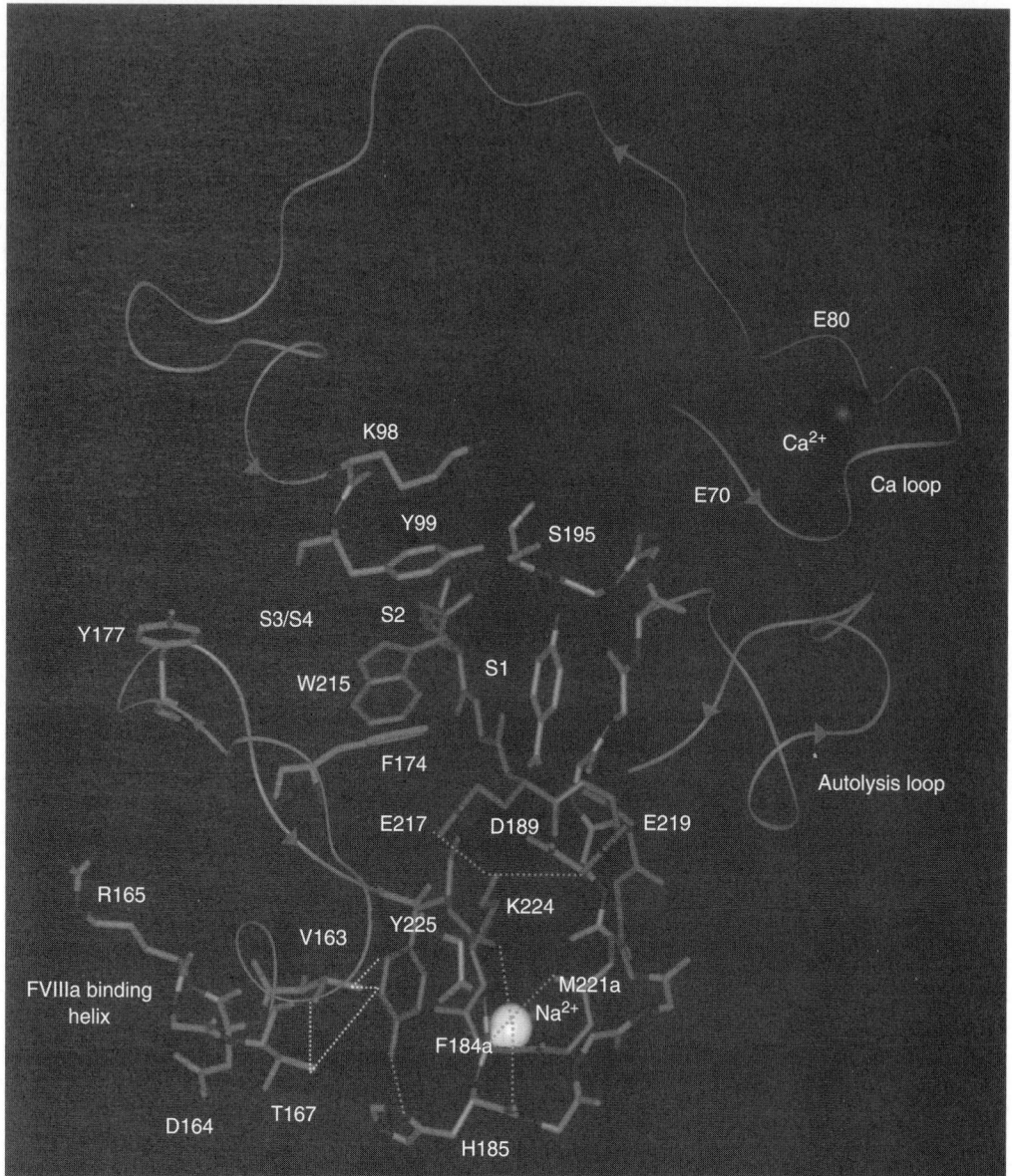

**FIGURE 7-4.** Relation of the Na$^+$-binding site to the S1 site and factor VIIIa binding helix in factor IXa. The two loops that bind the Na$^+$ ion, 353–359 [c183–c189] colored by atom type and 391–395 [c221–c225] colored *magenta*, and the 330-helix [c162-helix] that binds factor VIIIa are shown and colored by atom type in which carbons are *green*, nitrogens are *blue*, and oxygens are *red*. The bound Ca$^{2+}$ ion is shown as a *purple* sphere. Na$^+$ ion is shown as a *grey* sphere and is coordinated to the carbonyl O atoms of Phe353 [c184A], His354 [c185], Met391 [c221A], and Lys394 [c224]. The benzene ring of Tyr395 [c225] makes Van der Waals contacts with Val331 [c163] and Thr335 [c167]. The hydroxyl group of Tyr395 [c225] makes an H-bond with His354 [c185] and Lys394 [c224] makes H-bonds with Glu387 [c217] and Glu388 [c219]. Note that the 380 loop [c220 loop] is one residue shorter in factor IXa than in chymotrypsin. The S1 site is occupied by pAB and its benzamidine moiety makes H-bonds with Asp359 [c189], and the amino group of Val181 [c16] makes an H-bond with carboxylate of Asp364 [c194]. The H-bonds are shown with *cyan dashed lines* and Van der Waals contacts are shown with *white dashed lines*. Asp332 [c164] and Arg333 [c165] are two residues that are important in binding to factor VIIIa. Residues Lys265 [c98], Tyr266 [c99], Phe342 [c174], Tyr345 [c177], and Trp385 [c215] that play important roles in occupancy of the substrate at the S2/S3/S4 sites are also depicted. All residues are colored by atom type except Trp385 [c215], which is colored *magenta*. *Red* represents oxygen, *blue* represents nitrogen, and *green* represents carbon. The locations of the S2 and S3/S4 sites are also shown. The Ca$^{2+}$ loop and autolysis loop are also shown. The figure is drawn based upon the atomic coordinates (PDB code 1rfn). The numbering system used in this figure is that of chymotrypsin (see Color Fig. 7-4).

rate of coagulation ongoing or that it represents an accumulation of localized intravascular coagulation events that are controlled by inhibitory pathways. The amount of factor IXa that is inhibited is much lower than that predicted by the level of the activation peptide, favoring the latter (263). Furthermore, in model systems, it appears that picomolar amounts of factor IXa, but not factor Xa, can trigger thrombin generation without tissue factor. These data suggest that inhibition of factor

IXa would provide selective antithrombotic effects, at least in some clinical settings with increased thrombotic risk.

## Elevated Factor IX Levels and Thrombotic Risk

Factor IX antigen levels were determined in 426 patients with a first episode of deep vein thrombosis versus and compared to those in 473 matched control subjects (264). Ten percent of controls versus 20% of patients with venous thrombosis had factor IX antigen levels above 129 U per dL; the corrected relative risk was 2.0 (95% CI, 1.3 to 3.2). Although significant, this risk is less than half that of an elevated factor VIII. Its clinical significance, especially using clotting activity assays that are optimized to detect deficiencies, has not been established. Transgenic mice that overexpress human factor IX developed myocardial fibrosis due to enhanced coronary artery fibrin deposition leading to early death (265). Half of those expressing more than sevenfold elevations of factor IX died in 5 months.

## Inhibition of Factor IXa As an Antithrombotic Strategy

In dogs, inhibition of endogenous factor IXa was accomplished by the administration of an active site-inhibited factor IXa (266). Factor IXai was as antithrombotic as heparin in preventing coronary occlusion. Moreover, an abnormal hemorrhagic or bleeding response from a surgical wound was only present with heparin, not factor IXai. These data suggest a relative dissociation of anticoagulant (hemorrhagic) from antithrombotic effects that have been extended to animal models of vascular repair (267) and cardiopulmonary bypass (268). In rabbits, factor Xai is more potent than factor IXai in inhibiting venous clot formation on a cotton thread in the vena cava, whereas the two comparably inhibited thrombosis in an arterio-venous shunt model (269). Therefore inactivation of factor IXa or of intrinsic factor X activation provides a potential antithrombotic strategy that could result in a lower risk of hemorrhagic complications. In a cell-based *in vitro* model of tissue factor-initiated coagulation, factors VIIai and Xai inhibited platelet and fibrin clot formation, whereas factor IXai only inhibited the latter (270), providing a possible basis for the reduced risk of bleeding with factor IXai *in vivo*. Optimal and species-specific reagents remain to be defined, as do the clinical types of thrombotic disorders that are most responsive to this approach.

Similar antithrombotic effects have been observed with a murine monoclonal antibody that inhibits factors IX and IXa in both venous and arterial animal models; the immunoglobulin preparation has been "humanized" (271–273). Synthetic oligonucleotides (RNA aptamers) that bind to and inhibit human factor IXa in plasma were developed and an inhibitor-antidote pair, conjugated to polyethylene glycol, was examined in six patients with heparin-associated thrombocytopenia where heparin had to be discontinued despite the thrombotic setting (274). The aPTTs were reversibly prolonged by the aptamer; the clinical antithrombotic effect of this novel approach remains to be assessed.

## ACKNOWLEDGMENTS

Supported in part by the National Institutes of Health, RO1 HL36365 & RO1 HL70369, SPB, & R01HL071093, ART. Dr. Tom Howard, Emory University, is thanked for sharing unpublished ethnic data on factor IX variants.

## References

1. Aggeler PM, White SG, Glendening MB, et al. Plasma thromboplastin component (PTC) deficiency: a new disease resembling hemophilia. *Proc Soc Exp Biol Med* 1952;79:692–694.
2. Schulman I, Smith CH. Hemorrhagic disease in an infant due to deficiency of a previously undescribed clotting factor. *Blood* 1952;7:794–807.
3. Biggs R, Douglas AS, Macfarlane RG, et al. Christmas disease: a condition previously mistaken for haemophilia. *Br Med J* 1952;2:1378–1382.
4. White SG, Aggeler PM, Glendening MB. Plasma thromboplastin component (PTC), a hitherto unrecognized blood coagulation factor – case report of PTC deficiency. *Blood* 1953;8:101–124.
5. Proctor RR, Rapaport SI. The partial thromboplastin time with kaolin. A simple screening test for first stage plasma clotting factor deficiencies. *Am J Clin Pathol* 1961;36:212–219.
6. Fujikawa K, Thompson AR, Legaz ME, et al. Isolation and characterization of bovine factor IX (Christmas factor). *Biochemistry* 1973;12:4938–4945.
7. Katayama K, Ericsson LH, Enfield DL, et al. Comparison of amino acid sequence of bovine coagulation Factor IX (Christmas Factor) with that of other vitamin K-dependent plasma proteins. *Proc Natl Acad Sci U S A* 1979; 76:4990–4994.
8. Andersson LO, Borg H, Miller-Andersson M. Purification and characterization of human factor IX. *Thromb Res* 1975;7:451–459.
9. Thompson AR. Factor IX antigen by radioimmunoassay. Abnormal factor IX protein in patients on warfarin therapy and with hemophilia B. *J Clin Invest* 1977;59:900–910.
10. Choo KH, Gould KG, Rees DJ, et al. Molecular cloning of the gene for human anti-haemophilic factor IX. *Nature* 1982;299:178–180.
11. Kurachi K, Davie EW. Isolation and characterization of a cDNA coding for human factor IX. *Proc Natl Acad Sci U S A* 1982;79:6461–6464.
12. Chance PF, Dyer KA, Kurachi K, et al. Regional localization of the human factor IX gene by molecular hybridization. *Hum Genet* 1983;65:207–208.
13. Camerino G, Grzeschik KH, Jaye M, et al. Regional localization on the human X chromosome and polymorphism of the coagulation factor IX gene (hemophilia B locus). *Proc Natl Acad Sci U S A* 1984;81:498–502.
14. Boyd Y, Buckle VJ, Munro EA, et al. Assignment of the haemophilia B (factor IX) locus to the q26-qter region of the X chromosome. *Ann Hum Genet* 1984;48:145–152.
15. Peake I. Registry of DNA polymorphisms within or close to the human factor VIII and factor IX genes. For the Factor VIII/IX Subcommittee of the Scientific and Standardization Committee of the International Society on Thrombosis and Haemostasis. *Thromb Haemost* 1992;67:277–280.
16. Little RD, Pilia G, Johnson S, et al. Yeast artificial chromosomes spanning 8 megabases and 10-15 centimorgans of human cytogenetic band Xq26. *Proc Natl Acad Sci U S A* 1992;89:177–181.
17. Anson DS, Choo KH, Rees DJ, et al. The gene structure of human anti-haemophilic factor IX. *EMBO J* 1984;3:1053–1060.
18. Yoshitake S, Schach BG, Foster DC, et al. Nucleotide sequence of the gene for human factor IX (antihemophilic factor B). *Biochemistry* 1985;24: 3736–3750.
19. Kurachi K, Kurachi S. Regulatory mechanism of the factor IX gene. *Thromb Haemost* 1995;73:333–339.
20. Boccia LM, Thompson D, Newcombe K, et al. Binding of the Ets factor GA-binding protein to an upstream site in the factor IX promoter is a critical event in transactivation. *Mol Cell Biol* 1996;16:1929–1935.
21. Sommer SS, Ketterling RP. The factor IX gene as a model for analysis of human germline mutations: an update. *Hum Mol Genet* 1996;5:1505–1514.
22. Lin HF, Maeda N, Smithies O, et al. A coagulation factor IX-deficient mouse model for human hemophilia B. *Blood* 1997;90:3962–3966.
23. Wang L, Zoppe M, Hackeng TM, et al. A factor IX-deficient mouse model for hemophilia B gene therapy. *Proc Natl Acad Sci U S A* 1997;94: 11563–11566.
24. Kundu RK, Sangiorgi F, Wu LY, et al. Targeted inactivation of the coagulation factor IX gene causes hemophilia B in mice. *Blood* 1998;92:168–174.
25. Jin DY, Zhang TP, Gui T, et al. Creation of a mouse expressing defective human factor IX. *Blood* 2004;104:1733–1739.
26. Sabatino DE, Armstrong E, Edmonson S, et al. Novel hemophilia B mouse models exhibiting a range of mutations in the factor IX gene. *Blood* 2004; 104:2767–2774.
27. Giannelli F, Green PM, Sommer SS, et al. Haemophilia B: database of point mutations and short additions and deletions—eighth edition. *Nucleic Acids Res* 1998;26:265–268. Also available and updated as: http:// www.kcl.ac.uk/ip/petergreen/haemBdatabase.html; 13th edition, 2004.
28. Rai HK, Winship PR. A-793 G to A transition in the factor IX gene promoter is polymorphic in the Caucasian population. *Br J Haematol* 1996;92: 501–503.
29. Winship PR, Nichols CE, Chuansumrit A, et al. An MseI RFLP in the 5′ flanking region of the factor IX gene: its use for haemophilia B carrier detection in Caucasian and Thai populations. *Br J Haematol* 1993;84: 101–105.
30. Sommer SS, Tillotson VL, Vielhaber EL, et al. "Cryptic" dinucleotide polymorphism in the 3′ region of the factor IX gene shows substantial variation among different populations. *Hum Genet* 1994;93:357–358.
31. Reiner AP, Thompson AR. An HhaI polymorphism is present in factor IX genes of Asian subjects. *Hum Genet* 1990;86:87–88.

32. Toyozumi H, Kojima T, Matsushita T, et al. Diagnosis of hemophilia B carriers using two novel dinucleotide polymorphisms and Hha I RFLP of the factor IX gene in Japanese subjects. *Thromb Haemost* 1995;74:1009–1014.

33. Weinmann AF, Reiner AP, Thompson AR. A polymorphic MseI site 5′ to the factor IX gene varies among ethnic groups. *Hum Mol Genet* 1993;2:486.

34. Briet E, Bertina RM, van Tilburg NH, et al. Hemophilia B Leyden: a sex-linked hereditary disorder that improves after puberty. *N Engl J Med* 1982;306:788–790.

35. Morgan GE, Rowley G, Green PM, et al. Further evidence for the importance of an androgen response element in the factor IX promoter. *Br J Haematol* 1997;98:79–85.

36. Brady JN, Notley C, Cameron C, et al. Androgen effects on factor IX expression: *in-vitro* and *in-vivo* studies in mice. *Br J Haematol* 1998;101:273–279.

37. Kurachi S, Hitomi E, Kurachi K. Age and sex dependent regulation of the factor IX gene in mice. *Thromb Haemost* 1996;76:965–969.

38. Naka H, Brownlee GG. Transcriptional regulation of the human factor IX promoter by the orphan receptor superfamily factor, HNF4, ARP1 and COUP/Ear3. *Br J Haematol* 1996;92:231–240.

39. Davies N, Austen DE, Wilde MD, et al. Clotting factor IX levels in C/EBP alpha knockout mice. *Br J Haematol* 1997;99:578–579.

40. Lee YH, Sauer B, Johnson PF, et al. Disruption of the C/EBP alpha gene in adult mouse liver. *Mol Cell Biol* 1997;17:6014–6022.

41. Jallat S, Perraud F, Dalemans W, et al. Characterization of recombinant human factor IX expressed in transgenic mice and in derived trans-immortalized hepatic cell lines. *EMBO J* 1990;9:3295–3301.

42. Kurachi S, Hitomi Y, Furukawa M, et al. Role of intron I in expression of the human factor IX gene. *J Biol Chem* 1995;270:5276–5281.

43. Berkner KL. Expression of recombinant vitamin K-dependent proteins in mammalian cells: factors IX and VII. *Methods Enzymol* 1993;222:450–477.

44. Kaufman RJ, Wasley LC, Furie BC, et al. Expression, purification, and characterization of recombinant gamma-carboxylated factor IX synthesized in Chinese hamster ovary cells. *J Biol Chem* 1986;261:9622–9628.

45. Roth DA, Kessler CM, Pasi KJ, et al. Human recombinant factor IX: safety and efficacy studies in hemophilia B patients previously treated with plasma-derived factor IX concentrates. *Blood* 2001;98:3600–3606.

46. Schnieke AE, Kind AJ, Ritchie WA, et al. Human factor IX transgenic sheep produced by transfer of nuclei from transfected fetal fibroblasts. *Science* 1997;278:2130–2133.

47. Lindsay M, Gil GC, Cadiz A, et al. Purification of recombinant DNA-derived factor IX produced in transgenic pig milk and fractionation of active and inactive subpopulations. *J Chromatogr A* 2004;1026:149–157.

48. VandenDriessche T, Collen D, Chuah MK. Gene therapy for the hemophilias. *J Thromb Haemost* 2003;1:1550–1558.

49. Walsh CE. Gene therapy progress and prospects: gene therapy for the hemophilias. *Gene Ther* 2003;10:999–1003.

50. Couto LB. Preclinical gene therapy studies for hemophilia using adeno-associated virus (AAV) vectors. *Semin Thromb Hemost* 2004;30:161–171.

51. High KA. Clinical gene transfer studies for hemophilia B. *Semin Thromb Hemost* 2004;30:257–267.

52. Manno CS, Chew AJ, Hutchison S, et al. AAV-mediated factor IX gene transfer to skeletal muscle in patients with severe hemophilia B. *Blood* 2003;101:2963–2972.

53. Liu YL, Mingozzi F, Rodriguez-Colon SM, et al. Therapeutic levels of factor IX expression using a muscle-specific promoter and adeno-associated virus serotype 1 vector. *Hum Gene Ther* 2004;15:783–792.

54. Arruda VR, Stedman HH, Nichols TC, et al. Regional intravascular delivery of AAV-2-F.IX to skeletal muscle achieves long-term correction of hemophilia B in a large animal model. *Blood* 2005;105:3458–3464.

55. High KA, Manno C, Sabatino D. Immune responses to AAV and to factor IX in a phase I study of AAV-mediated, liver-directed gene transfer for hemophilia B. *Mol Ther* 2004;9:1002, abstract.

56. Wu SM, Stanley TB, Mutucumarana VP, et al. Characterization of the γ-glutamyl carboxylase. *Thromb Haemost* 1997;78:599–604.

57. Yamada M, Kuliopulos A, Nelson NP, et al. Localization of the factor IX propeptide binding site on recombinant vitamin K dependent carboxylase using benzoylphenylalanine photoaffinity peptide inactivators. *Biochemistry* 1995;34:481–489.

58. Wu SM, Mutucumarana VP, Geromanos S, et al. The propeptide binding site of the bovine γ-glutamyl carboxylase. *J Biol Chem* 1997;272:11718–11722.

59. Morris DP, Stevens RD, Wright DJ, et al. Processive post-translational modification. Vitamin K-dependent carboxylation of a peptide substrate. *J Biol Chem* 1995;270:30491–30498.

60. Lin PJ, Straight DL, Stafford DW. Binding of the factor IX gamma-carboxyglutamic acid domain to the vitamin K-dependent γ-glutamyl carboxylase active site induces an allosteric effect that may ensure processive carboxylation and regulate the release of carboxylated product. *J Biol Chem* 2004;279:6560–6566.

61. Stenflo J, Fernlund P, Egan W, et al. Vitamin K dependent modifications of glutamic acid residues in prothrombin. *Proc Natl Acad Sci U S A* 1974;71:2730–2733.

62. Fryklund L, Borg H, Andersson LO. Amino-terminal sequence of human factor IX: presence of γ-carboxyl glutamic acid residues. *FEBS Lett* 1976;65:187–189.

63. Shikamoto Y, Morita T, Fujimoto Z, et al. Crystal structure of Mg2+- and Ca2+-bound Gla domain of factor IX complexed with binding protein. *J Biol Chem* 2003;278:24090–24094.

64. Huang M, Furie BC, Furie B. Crystal structure of the calcium-stabilized human factor IX Gla domain bound to a conformation-specific anti-factor IX antibody. *J Biol Chem* 2004;279:14338–14346.

65. Thompson AR, Chen SH. Characterization of factor IX defects in hemophilia B. *Methods Enzymol* 1993;222:143–169.

66. Brandstetter H, Bauer M, Huber R, et al. X-ray structure of clotting factor IXa: active site and module structure related to Xase activity and hemophilia B. *Proc Natl Acad Sci U S A* 1995;92:9796–9800.

67. Jorgensen MJ, Cantor AB, Furie BC, et al. Recognition site directing vitamin K-dependent γ-carboxylation resides on the propeptide of factor IX. *Cell* 1987;48:185–191.

68. Rabiet M-J, Jorgensen MJ, Furie B, et al. Effect of propeptide mutations on post-translational processing of factor IX. Evidence that β-hydroxylation and γ-carboxylation are independent events. *J Biol Chem* 1987;262:14895–14898.

69. Chu K, Wu SM, Stanley T, et al. A mutation in the propeptide of factor IX leads to warfarin sensitivity by a novel mechanism. *J Clin Invest* 1996;98:1619–1625.

70. Oldenburg J, Quenzel EM, Harbrecht U, et al. Missense mutations at Ala-10 in the factor IX propeptide: an insignificant variant in normal life but a decisive cause of bleeding during oral anticoagulant therapy. *Br J Haematol* 1997;98:240–244.

71. Stanley TB, Humphries J, High KA, et al. Amino acids responsible for reduced affinities of vitamin K-dependent propeptides for the carboxylase. *Biochemistry* 1999;38:15681–15687.

72. Handford PA, Winship PR, Brownlee GG. Protein engineering of the propeptide of human factor IX. *Protein Eng* 1991;4:319–323.

73. Cheng JW, Chen C, Huang TH, et al. Conformation of the propeptide domain of factor IX. *Biochim Biophys Acta* 1995;1245:227–231.

74. Stanley TB, Wu SM, Houben RJ, et al. Role of the propeptide and gamma-glutamic acid domain of factor IX for in vitro carboxylation by the vitamin K-dependent carboxylase. *Biochemistry* 1998;37:13262–13268.

75. Bristol JA, Ratcliffe JV, Roth DA, et al. Biosynthesis of prothrombin: intracellular localization of the vitamin K-dependent carboxylase and the sites of gamma-carboxylation. *Blood* 1996;88:2585–2593.

76. Fernlund P, Stenflo J. β-hydroxyaspartic acid in vitamin K-dependent proteins. *J Biol Chem* 1983;258:12509–12512.

77. Stenflo J, Stenberg Y, Muranyi A. Calcium-binding EGF-like modules in coagulation proteinases: function of the calcium ion in module interactions. *Biochim Biophys Acta* 2000;1477:51–63.

78. McMullen BA, Fujikawa K, Kisiel W. The occurrence of β-hydroxyaspartic acid in the vitamin K-dependent blood coagulation zymogens. *Biochem Biophys Res Commun* 1983;115:8–14.

79. Derian CK, VanDusen W, Przysiecki CT, et al. Inhibitors of 2-ketoglutarate-dependent dioxygenases block aspartyl β-hydroxylation of recombinant human factor IX in several mammalian expression systems. *J Biol Chem* 1989;264:6615–6618.

80. Rees DJG, Jones IM, Handford PA, et al. The role of β-hydroxyaspartate and adjacent carboxylate residues in the first EGF domain of human factor IX. *EMBO J* 1988;7:2053–2061.

81. Sunnerhagen MS, Persson E, Dahlqvist I, et al. The effect of aspartate hydroxylation on calcium binding to epidermal growth factor-like modules in coagulation factors IX and X. *J Biol Chem* 1993;268:23339–23344.

82. Geng JP, Castellino FJ. The propeptides of human protein C, factor VII, and factor IX are exchangeable with regard to directing γ-carboxylation of these proteins. *Thromb Haemost* 1996;76:205–207.

83. Thompson AR, Schoof JM, Weinmann AF, et al. Factor IX mutations: rapid, direct screening methods for 20 new families with hemophilia B. *Thromb Res* 1992;65:289–295.

84. Wojcik EGC, Van Den Berg M, Poort SR, et al. Modification of the N-terminus of human factor IX by defective propeptide cleavage or acetylation results in a destabilized calcium-induced conformation: effects on phospholipid binding and activation by factor XIa. *Biochem J* 1997;323 (Pt 3):629–636.

85. Bristol JA, Furie BC, Furie B. Propeptide processing during factor IX biosynthesis. Effect of point mutations adjacent to the propeptide cleavage site. *J Biol Chem* 1993;268:7577–7584.

86. Bristol JA, Freedman SJ, Furie BC, et al. Profactor IX: the propeptide inhibits binding to membrane surfaces and activation by factor XIa. *Biochemistry* 1994;33:14136–14143.

87. Di Scipio RG, Hermodson MA, Yates SG, et al. A comparison of human prothrombin, factor IX (Christmas factor), factor X (Stuart factor), and protein S. *Biochemistry* 1977;16:698–706.

88. Sarkar G, Koeberl DD, Sommer SS. Direct sequencing of the activation peptide and the catalytic domain of the factor IX gene in six species. *Genomics* 1990;6:133–143.

89. Chavin SI, Weidner SM. Blood clotting factor IX. Loss of activity after cleavage of sialic acid residues. *J Biol Chem* 1984;259:3387–3390.

90. Bharadwaj D, Harris RJ, Kisiel W, et al. Enzymatic removal of sialic acid from human factor IX and factor X has no effect on their coagulant activity. *J Biol Chem* 1995;270:6537–6542.

91. Nishimura H, Kawabata S, Kisiel W, et al. Identification of a disaccharide (Xyl-Glc) and a trisaccharide (Xyl2-Glc) O-glycosidically linked to a serine

residue in the first epidermal growth factor-like domain of human factors VII and IX and protein Z and bovine protein Z. *J Biol Chem* 1989;264: 20320–20325.

92. Harris RJ, van Halbeek H, Glushka J, et al. Identification and structural analysis of the tetrasaccharide NeuAc alpha(2-*6)Gal beta(1-*4)GlcNAc beta(1-*3)FUC-alpha 1--*0-*linked* to serine 61 of human factor IX. *Biochemistry* 1993;32:6539–6547.

93. Shao L, Luo Y, Moloney DJ, et al. O-glycosylation of EGF repeats: identification and initial characterization of a UDP-glucose: protein O-glucosyltransferase. *Glycobiology* 2002;12:763–770.

94. Bond M, Jankowski M, Patel H, et al. Biochemical characterization of recombinant factor IX. *Semin Hematol* 1998;35:11–17.

95. Agarwala KL, Kawabata S, Takao T, et al. Activation peptide of human factor IX has oligosaccharides O-glycosidically linked to threonine residues at 159 and 169. *Biochemistry* 1994;33:5167–5171.

96. Bajaj SP, Rapaport SI, Russell WA. Redetermination of the rate-limiting step in the activation of factor IX by factor XIa and by factor VIIa/tissue factor. Explanation for different electrophoretic radioactivity profiles obtained on activation of 3H- and ¹²⁵I-labeled factor IX. *Biochemistry* 1983; 22:4047–4053.

97. Meulien P, Balland A, Lepage P, et al. Increased biological activity of a recombinant factor IX variant carrying alanine at position +1. *Protein Eng* 1990;3:629–633.

98. Green PM, Rowley G, Giannelli F. Unusual expression of the F9 gene in peripheral lymphocytes hinders investigation of F9 mRNA in hemophilia B patients. *J Thromb Haemost* 2003;1:2675–2676.

99. Yull F, Harold G, Wallace R, et al. Fixing human factor IX (fIX): correction of a cryptic RNA splice enables the production of biologically active fIX in the mammary gland of transgenic mice. *Proc Natl Acad Sci U S A* 1995;92: 10899–10903.

100. Vidaud M, Chabret C, Gazengel C, et al. A de novo intragenic deletion of the potential EGF domain of the factor IX gene in a family with severe hemophilia B. *Blood* 1986;68:961–963.

101. Thompson AR. Molecular biology of the hemophilias. *Prog Hemost Thromb* 1991;10:175–214.

102. Bray GL, Thompson AR. Partial factor IX protein in a pedigree with hemophilia B due to a partial gene deletion. *J Clin Invest* 1986;77:1194–1200.

103. Kurachi S, Pantazatos DP, Kurachi K. The carboxyl-terminal region of factor IX is essential for its secretion. *Biochemistry* 1997;36:4337–4344.

104. Evans JP, Watzke HH, Ware JL, et al. Molecular cloning of a cDNA encoding canine factor IX. *Blood* 1989;74:207–212.

105. Wu SM, Stafford DW, Ware J. Deduced amino acid sequence of mouse blood-coagulation factor IX. *Gene* 1990;86:275–278.

106. Pendurthi UR, Tukey RH, Rao LV. Characterization of a rabbit factor IX cDNA. *Thromb Res* 1992;65:177–186.

107. Davidson CJ, Tuddenham EG, McVey JH. 450 million years of hemostasis. *J Thromb Haemost* 2003;1:1487–1494.

108. Hanumanthaiah R, Day K, Jagadeeswaran P. Comprehensive analysis of blood coagulation pathways in teleostei: evolution of coagulation factor genes and identification of zebrafish factor VIIi. *Blood Cells Mol Dis* 2002; 29:57–68.

109. Pang C-P, Crossley M, Kent G, et al. Comparative sequence analysis of mammalian factor IX promoters. *Nucleic Acids Res* 1990;18:6731–6732.

110. Thompson AR. Radioimmunoassay of factor IX. *Methods Haematol* 1982; 5:122–136.

111. Boland EJ, Liu YC, Walter CA, et al. Age-specific regulation of clotting factor IX gene expression in normal and transgenic mice. *Blood* 1995;86: 2198–2205.

112. Briet E, van Tilburg NH, Veltkamp JJ. Oral contraception and the detection of carriers in haemophilia B. *Thromb Res* 1978;13:379–388.

113. Kurachi S, Deyashiki Y, Takeshita J, et al. Genetic mechanisms of age regulation of human blood coagulation factor IX. *Science* 1999;285:739–743.

114. Zhang K, Kurachi S, Kurachi K. New function for age-related stability element in conferring strict tissue-specific expression of human factor IX and protein C genes. *Thromb Haemost* 2002;88:537–538.

115. Mari D, Mannucci PM, Coppola R, et al. Hypercoagulability in centenarians: the paradox of successful aging. *Blood* 1995;85:3144–3149.

116. Chen SH, Schoof JM, Weinmann AF, et al. Heteroduplex screening for molecular defects in factor IX genes from haemophilia B families. *Br J Haematol* 1995;89:409–412.

117. Schroder W, Wulff K, Wollina K, et al. Haemophilia B in female twins caused by a point mutation in one factor IX gene and nonrandom inactivation patterns of the X-chromosomes. *Thromb Haemost* 1997;78:1347–1351.

118. Taylor SA, Deugau KV, Lillicrap DP. Somatic mosaicism and female-to-female transmission in a kindred with hemophilia B (factor IX deficiency). *Proc Natl Acad Sci U S A* 1991;88:39–42.

119. Wadelius C, Lindstedt M, Pigg M, et al. Hemophilia B in a 46, XX female probably caused by non-random X inactivation. *Clin Genet* 1993;43:1–4.

120. Gerrard AJ, Austen DE, Brownlee GG. Subcutaneous injection of factor IX for the treatment of haemophilia B. *Br J Haematol* 1992;81: 610–613.

121. Liles D, Landen CN, Monroe DM, et al. Extravascular administration of factor IX. Potential for replacement therapy of canine and human hemophilia B. *Thromb Haemost* 1997;77:944–948.

122. White GC III, Shapiro AD, Kurczynski EM et al. The Mononine Study Group. Variability of *in vivo* recovery of factor IX after infusion of monoclonal antibody purified factor IX concentrates in patients with hemophilia B. *Thromb Haemost* 1995;73:779–784.

123. White G, Shapiro A, Ragni M, et al. Clinical evaluation of recombinant factor IX. *Semin Hematol* 1998;35:33–38.

124. Smith KJ, Thompson AR. Labeled factor IX kinetics in patients with hemophilia-B. *Blood* 1981;58:625–629.

125. Van Oosterom AT, Kerkhoven P, Veltkamp JJ. Metabolism of the coagulation factors of the prothrombin complex in hypothyroidism in man. *Thromb Haemost* 1979;41:273–285.

126. McCarthy K, Stewart P, Sigman J, et al. Pharmacokinetics of recombinant factor IX after intravenous and subcutaneous administration in dogs and cynomolgus monkeys. *Thromb Haemost* 2002;87:824–830.

127. Russell KE, Olsen EH, Raymer RA, et al. Reduced bleeding events with subcutaneous administration of recombinant human factor IX in immune-tolerant hemophilia B dogs. *Blood* 2003;102:4393–4398.

128. Russell KE, Read MS, Bellinger DA, et al. Intratracheal administration of recombinant human factor IX (BeneFix) achieves therapeutic levels in hemophilia B dogs. *Thromb Haemost* 2001;85:445–449.

129. Sheffield WP, Mamdani A, Hortelano G, et al. Effects of genetic fusion of factor IX to albumin on *in vivo* clearance in mice and rabbits. *Br J Haematol* 2004;126:565–573.

130. Begbie ME, Gataiance S, Eltringham-Smith L, et al. Accelerated clearance of a recombinant human factor IX protein lacking activation peptide residues 155-177. *Blood* 2003;102:307a.

131. Enfield DL, Thompson AR. Cleavage and activation of human factor IX by serine proteases. *Blood* 1984;64:821–831.

132. Samis JA, Kam E, Nesheim ME, et al. Neutrophil elastase cleavage of human factor IX generates an activated factor IX-like product devoid of coagulant function. *Blood* 1998;92:1287–1296.

133. Rohlena J, Kolkman JA, Boertjes RC, et al. Residues Phe342-Asn346 of activated coagulation factor IX contribute to the interaction with low density lipoprotein receptor-related protein. *J Biol Chem* 2003;278:9394–9401.

134. Gui T, Lin HF, Jin DY, et al. Circulating and binding characteristics of wild-type factor IX and certain Gla domain mutants *in vivo*. *Blood* 2002;100:153–158.

135. Hopfner KP, Lang A, Karcher A, et al. Coagulation factor IXa: the relaxed conformation of Tyr99 blocks substrate binding. *Structure Fold Des* 1999; 7:989–996.

136. Freedman SJ, Furie BC, Furie B, et al. Structure of the metal-free gamma-carboxyglutamic acid-rich membrane binding region of factor IX by two-dimensional NMR spectroscopy. *J Biol Chem* 1995;270:7980–7987.

137. Freedman SJ, Furie BC, Furie B, et al. Structure of the calcium ion-bound gamma-carboxyglutamic acid-rich domain of factor IX. *Biochemistry* 1995; 34:12126–12137.

138. Baron M, Norman DG, Harvey TS, et al. The three-dimensional structure of the first EGF-like module of human factor IX: comparison with EGF and TGF-alpha. *Protein Sci* 1992;1:81–90.

139. Rao Z, Handford P, Mayhew M, et al. The structure of a Ca(2+)-binding epidermal growth factor-like domain: its role in protein-protein interactions. *Cell* 1995;82:131–141.

140. Wolberg AS, Li L, Cheung WF, et al. Characterization of γ-carboxyglutamic acid residue 21 of human factor IX. *Biochemistry* 1996;35:10321–10327.

141. Huang M, Rigby AC, Morelli X, et al. Structural basis of membrane binding by Gla domains of vitamin K-dependent proteins. *Nat Struct Biol* 2003;10: 751–756.

142. Gillis S, Furie BC, Furie B, et al. Gamma-carboxyglutamic acids 36 and 40 do not contribute to human factor IX function. *Protein Sci* 1997;6:185–196.

143. Cheung WF, Wolberg AS, Stafford DW, et al. Localization of a metal-dependent epitope to the amino terminal residues 33-40 of human factor IX. *Thromb Res* 1995;80:419–427.

144. Sekiya F, Yoshida M, Yamashita T, et al. Localization of the specific binding site for magnesium(II) ions in blood coagulation factor IX. *FEBS Lett* 1996;392:205–208.

145. Wojcik EG, Cheung WF, van den Berg M, et al. Identification of residues in the Gla-domain of human factor IX involved in the binding to conformation specific antibodies. *Biochim Biophys Acta* 1998;1382:91–101.

146. Wojcik EG, Simioni P, d Berg M, et al. Mutations which introduce free cysteine residues in the Gla-domain of vitamin K dependent proteins result in the formation of complexes with alpha 1-microglobulin. *Thromb Haemost* 1996;75:70–75.

147. Hughes PE, Handford PA, Austen DE, et al. Protein engineering of the hydrophobic domain of human factor IX. *Protein Eng* 1994;7:1121–1127.

148. Kirchhofer D, Lipari MT, Moran P, et al. The tissue factor region that interacts with substrates factor IX and factor X. *Biochemistry* 2000;39: 7380–7387.

149. Chen SW, Pellequer JL, Schved JF, et al. Model of a ternary complex between activated factor VII, tissue factor and factor IX. *Thromb Haemost* 2002;88: 74–82.

150. Aktimur A, Gabriel MA, Gailani D, et al. The factor IX γ-carboxyglutamic acid (Gla) domain is involved in interactions between factor IX and factor XIa. *J Biol Chem* 2003;278:7981–7987.

151. Blostein MD, Furie BC, Rajotte I, et al. The Gla domain of factor IXa binds to factor VIIIa in the tenase complex. *J Biol Chem* 2003;278:31297–31302.

152. Christophe OD, Lenting PJ, Kolkman JA, et al. Blood coagulation factor IX residues Glu78 and Arg94 provide a link between both epidermal growth factor-like domains that is crucial in the interaction with factor VIII light chain. *J Biol Chem* 1998;273:222–227.

153. Celie PH, Lenting PJ, Mertens K. Hydrophobic contact between the two epidermal growth factor-like domains of blood coagulation factor IX contributes to enzymatic activity. *J Biol Chem* 2000;275:229–234.

154. Bode W, Brandstetter H, Mather T, et al. Comparative analysis of haemostatic proteinases: structural aspects of thrombin, factor Xa, factor IXa and protein C. *Thromb Haemost* 1997;78:501–511.

155. Morita T, Kisiel W. Calcium binding to a human factor IXa derivative lacking γ-carboxyglutamic acid: evidence for two high-affinity sites that do not involve β-hydroxyaspartic acid. *Biochem Biophys Res Commun* 1985;130: 841–847.

156. Astermark J, Bjork I, Ohlin AK, et al. Structural requirements for Ca2+ binding to the γ-carboxyglutamic acid and epidermal growth factor-like regions of factor IX. Studies using intact domains isolated from controlled proteolytic digests of bovine factor IX. *J Biol Chem* 1991;266:2430–2437.

157. Handford PA, Baron M, Mayhew M, et al. The first EGF-like domain from human factor IX contains a high-affinity calcium binding site. *EMBO J* 1990;9:475–480.

158. Persson KE, Astermark J, Bjork I, et al. Calcium binding to the first EGF-like module of human factor IX in a recombinant fragment containing residues 1-85. Mutations V46E and Q50E each manifest a negligible increase in calcium affinity. *FEBS Lett* 1998;421:100–104.

159. Hughes PE, Morgan G, Rooney EK, et al. Tyrosine 69 of the first epidermal growth factor-like domain of human factor IX is essential for clotting activity. *J Biol Chem* 1993;268:17727–17733.

160. Whiteman P, Downing AK, Smallridge R, et al. A Gly → Ser change causes defective folding *in vitro* of calcium-binding epidermal growth factor-like domains from factor IX and fibrillin-1. *J Biol Chem* 1998;273:7807–7813.

161. Knobe KE, Persson KE, Sjorin E, et al. Functional analysis of the EGF-like domain mutations Pro55Ser and Pro55Leu, which cause mild hemophilia B. *J Thromb Haemost* 2003;1:782–790.

162. Lin S-W, Smith KJ, Welsch D, et al. Expression and characterization of human factor IX and factor IX-factor X chimeras in mouse C127 cells. *J Biol Chem* 1990;265:144–150.

163. Hertzberg MS, Ben-Tal O, Furie B, et al. Construction, expression, and characterization of a chimera of factor IX and factor X. The role of the second epidermal growth factor domain and serine protease domain in factor Va binding. *J Biol Chem* 1992;267:14759–14766.

164. Yu S, Zhang L, Jhingan A, et al. Construction, expression, and properties of a recombinant chimeric human protein C with replacement of its growth factor-like domains by those of human coagulation factor IX. *Biochemistry* 1994;33:823–831.

165. Chang JY, Monroe DM, Stafford DW, et al. Replacing the first epidermal growth factor-like domain of factor IX with that of factor VII enhances activity *in vitro* and in canine hemophilia B. *J Clin Invest* 1997;100:886–892.

166. Persson KE, Villoutreix BO, Thamlitz AM, et al. The N-terminal epidermal growth factor-like domain of coagulation factor IX. Probing its functions in the activation of factor IX and factor X with a monoclonal antibody. *J Biol Chem* 2002;277:35616–35624.

167. Persson KE, Knobe KE, Stenflo J. An anti-EGF monoclonal antibody that detects intramolecular communication in factor IX. *Biochem Biophys Res Commun* 2001;286:1039–1044.

168. Zhong D, Smith KJ, Birktoft JJ, et al. First epidermal growth factor-like domain of human blood coagulation factor IX is required for its activation by factor VIIa/tissue factor but not by factor XIa. *Proc Natl Acad Sci U S A* 1994;91:3574–3578.

169. Wu PC, Hamaguchi N, Yu YS, et al. Hemophilia B with mutations at glycine-48 of factor IX exhibited delayed activation by the factor VIIa-tissue factor complex. *Thromb Haemost* 2000;84:626–634.

170. Zhong D, Bajaj MS, Schmidt AE, et al. The N-terminal epidermal growth factor-like domain in factor IX and factor X represents an important recognition motif for binding to tissue factor. *J Biol Chem* 2002;277:3622–3631.

171. Ndonwi M, Broze G Jr, Bajaj SP. The first epidermal growth factor-like domains of factor Xa and factor IXa are required for the activation of the factor VII—tissue factor complex. *J Thromb Haemost* 2005;3:112–118.

172. Norledge BV, Petrovan RJ, Ruf W, et al. The tissue factor/factor VIIa/factor Xa complex: a model built by docking and site-directed mutagenesis. *Proteins* 2003;53:640–648.

173. Venkateswarlu D, Duke RE, Perera L, et al. An all-atom solution-equilibrated model for human extrinsic blood coagulation complex (sTF-VIIa-Xa): a protein-protein docking and molecular dynamics refinement study. *J Thromb Haemost* 2003;1:2577–2588.

174. Wilkinson FH, Ahmad SS, Walsh PN. The factor IXa second epidermal growth factor (EGF2) domain mediates platelet binding and assembly of the factor X activating complex. *J Biol Chem* 2002;277:5734–5741.

175. Wilkinson FH, London FS, Walsh PN. Residues 88-109 of factor IXa are important for assembly of the factor X activating complex. *J Biol Chem* 2002;277:5725–5733.

176. Celie PH, Van Stempvoort G, Fribourg C, et al. The connecting segment between both epidermal growth factor-like domains in blood coagulation factor IX contributes to stimulation by factor VIIIa and its isolated A2 domain. *J Biol Chem* 2002;277:20214–20220.

177. Nishimura H, Takeya H, Miyata T, et al. Factor IX Fukuoka. Substitution of Asn92 by His in the second epidermal growth factor-like domain results in defective interaction with factors VIIa/X. *J Biol Chem* 1993;268:24041–24046.

178. Chang YJ, Wu HL, Hamaguchi N, et al. Identification of functionally important residues of the epidermal growth factor-2 domain of factor IX by

179. DiScipio RG, Kurachi K, Davie EW. Activation of human factor IX (Christmas factor). *J Clin Invest* 1978;61:1528–1538.

180. Osterud B, Rapaport SI. Activation of factor IX by the reaction product of tissue factor and factor VII: additional pathway for initiating blood coagulation. *Proc Natl Acad Sci U S A* 1977;74:5260–5264.

181. Lawson JH, Mann KG. Cooperative activation of human factor IX by the human extrinsic pathway of blood coagulation. *J Biol Chem* 1991;266: 11317–11327.

182. Lindquist PA, Fujikawa K, Davie EW. Activation of bovine factor IX (Christmas factor) by factor XIa (activated plasma thromboplastin antecedent) and a protease from Russell's viper venom. *J Biol Chem* 1978;253:1902–1909.

183. Sichler K, Kopetzki E, Huber R, et al. Physiological FIXa activation involves a cooperative conformational rearrangement of the 99-loop. *J Biol Chem* 2003;278:4121–4126.

184. Butenas S, van 't Veer C, Mann KG. Evaluation of the initiation phase of blood coagulation using ultrasensitive assays for serine proteases. *J Biol Chem* 1997;272:21527–21533.

185. Hopfner KP, Brandstetter H, Karcher A, et al. Converting blood coagulation factor IXa into factor Xa: dramatic increase in amidolytic activity identifies important active site determinants. *EMBO J* 1997;16:6626–6635.

186. Kolkman JA, Christophe OD, Lenting PJ, et al. Surface loop 199-204 in blood coagulation factor IX is a cofactor-dependent site involved in macromolecular substrate interaction. *J Biol Chem* 1999;274:29087–29093.

187. Weinmann AF, Murphy ME, Thompson AR. Consequences of factor IX mutations in 26 families with haemophilia B. *Br J Haematol* 1998;100:58–61.

188. Lin S-W, Lin CN, Hamaguchi N, et al. Characterization of a factor IX variant with a glycine207 to glutamic acid mutation. *Blood* 1994;84: 1866–1873.

189. Sichler K, Hopfner KP, Kopetzki E, et al. The influence of residue 190 in the S1 site of trypsin-like serine proteases on substrate selectivity is universally conserved. *FEBS Lett* 2002;530:220–224.

190. Bajaj SP, Spitzer SG, Welsh WJ, et al. Experimental and theoretical evidence supporting the role of Gly363 in blood coagulation factor IXa (Gly193 in chymotrypsin) for proper activation of the proenzyme. *J Biol Chem* 1990;265:2956–2961.

191. Geddes VA, Le Bonniec BF, Louie GV, et al. A moderate form of hemophilia B is caused by a novel mutation in the protease domain of factor IX-Vancouver. *J Biol Chem* 1989;264:4689–4697.

192. Chang J, Jin J, Lollar P, et al. Changing residue 338 in human factor IX from arginine to alanine causes an increase in catalytic activity. *J Biol Chem* 1998;273:12089–12094.

193. Kisiel W, Smith KJ, McMullen BA. Proteolytic inactivation of blood coagulation factor IX by thrombin. *Blood* 1985;66:1302–1308.

194. Mathur A, Zhong D, Sabharwal AK, et al. Interaction of factor IXa with factor VIIIa. Effects of protease domain Ca2+ binding site, proteolysis in the autolysis loop, phospholipid, and factor X. *J Biol Chem* 1997;272: 23418–23426.

195. Schmidt AE, Bajaj SP. Specific cleavage at Lys148/Gly149 in the serine protease domain of human factor IXaβ by plasmin: effect on catalytic efficiency and factor VIIIa binding. In: Houghten RA, ed. *Leb1 M peptides: the wave of the future*. San Diego, CA: American Peptide Society, 2001: 965–966.

196. Hamaguchi N, Stafford D. *In vitro* mutagenesis study of two critical glutamic acids in the calcium binding loop of the factor IX heavy chain. *Thromb Haemost* 1994;72:856–861.

197. Rosenberg JS, McKenna PW, Rosenberg RD. Inhibition of human factor IXa by human antithrombin. *J Biol Chem* 1975;250:8883–8888.

198. Bedsted T, Swanson R, Chuang YJ, et al. Heparin and calcium ions dramatically enhance antithrombin reactivity with factor IXa by generating new interaction exosites. *Biochemistry* 2003;42:8143–8152.

199. Neuenschwander PF. Exosite occupation by heparin enhances the reactivity of blood coagulation factor IXa. *Biochemistry* 2004;43:2978–2986.

200. Yang L, Manithody C, Rezaie AR. Localization of the heparin binding exosite of factor IXa. *J Biol Chem* 2002;277:50756–50760.

201. Wiebe EM, Stafford AR, Fredenburgh JC, et al. Mechanism of catalysis of inhibition of factor IXa by antithrombin in the presence of heparin or pentasaccharide. *J Biol Chem* 2003;278:35767–35774.

202. van Dieijen G, Tans G, Rosing J, et al. The role of phospholipid and factor VIIIa in the activation of bovine factor X. *J Biol Chem* 1981;256: 3433–3442.

203. Kalafatis M, Egan JO, van 't Veer C, et al. The regulation of clotting factors. *Crit Rev Eukaryot Gene Expr* 1997;7:241–280.

204. McRae BJ, Kurachi K, Heimark RL, et al. Mapping the active sites of bovine thrombin, factor IXa, factor Xa, factor XIa, factor XIIa, plasma kallikrein, and trypsin with amino acid and peptide thioesters: development of new sensitive substrates. *Biochemistry* 1981;20:7196–7206.

205. Kolkman JA, Lenting PJ, Mertens K. Regions 301-303 and 333-339 in the catalytic domain of blood coagulation factor IX are factor VIII-interactive sites involved in stimulation of enzyme activity. *Biochem J* 1999;339: 217–221.

206. Lefkowitz JB, Nuss R, Haver T, et al. Factor IX Denver, ASN 346 → ASP mutation resulting in a dysfunctional protein with defective factor VIIIa interaction. *Thromb Haemost* 2001;86:862–870.

207. Mathur A, Bajaj SP. Protease and EGF1 domains of factor IXa play distinct roles in binding to factor VIIIa. Importance of helix 330 (helix 162 in

chymotrypsin) of protease domain of factor IXa in its interaction with factor VIIIa. *J Biol Chem* 1999;274:18477–18486.

208. Sturzebecher J, Kopetzki E, Bode W, et al. Dramatic enhancement of the catalytic activity of coagulation factor IXa by alcohols. *FEBS Lett* 1997;412:295–300.

209. Sichler K, Banner DW, D'Arcy A, et al. Crystal structures of uninhibited factor VIIa link its cofactor and substrate-assisted activation to specific interactions. *J Mol Biol* 2002;322:591–603.

210. Masys DR, Bajaj SP, Rapaport SI. Activation of human factor VII by activated factors IX and X. *Blood* 1982;60:1143–1150.

211. Rick ME. Activation of factor VIII by factor IXa. *Blood* 1982;60:744–751.

212. Miller GJ, Martin JC, Mitropoulos KA, et al. Activation of factor VII during alimentary lipemia occurs in healthy adults and patients with congenital factor XII or factor XI deficiency, but not in patients with factor IX deficiency. *Blood* 1996;87:4187–4196.

213. Bray GL, Weinmann AR. Calcium-specific immunoassays for factor IX: reduced levels of antigen in patients with vitamin K disorders. *J Lab Clin Med* 1986;107:269–278.

214. Smith KJ, Ono K. Monoclonal antibodies to factor IX: characterization and use in immunoassays for factor IX. *Thromb Res* 1984;33:211–224.

215. Frazier D, Smith KJ, Cheung WF, et al. Mapping of monoclonal antibodies to human factor IX. *Blood* 1989;74:971–977.

216. Ljung RC. Gene mutations and inhibitor formation in patients with hemophilia B. *Acta Haematol* 1995;94(Suppl. 1):49–52.

217. Warrier I, Ewenstein BM, Koerper MA, et al. Factor IX inhibitors and anaphylaxis in hemophilia B. *J Pediatr Hematol Oncol* 1997;19:23–27.

218. Yamamoto M, Kamisue S, Sawamoto Y, et al. Factor IX inhibition and epitope localization of factor IX inhibitor antibodies in haemophilia B patients with anaphylactoid reactions. *Haemophilia* 1997;3:189–193.

219. Christophe OD, Lenting PJ, Cherel G, et al. Functional mapping of anti-factor IX inhibitors developed in patients with severe hemophilia B. *Blood* 2001;98:1416–1423.

220. Mutucumarana VP, Duffy EJ, Lollar P, et al. The active site of factor IXa is located far above the membrane surface and its conformation is altered upon association with factor VIIIa. A fluoresence study. *J Biol Chem* 1992;267:17012–17021.

221. Stoilova S, Gray E, Barrowcliffe TE, et al. Structural determination of lipid-bound human blood coagulation factor IX. *Biochim Biophys Acta* 1998;1383:175–178.

222. Freedman SJ, Blostein MD, Baleja JD, et al. Identification of the phospholipid binding site in the vitamin K-dependent blood coagulation protein factor IX. *J Biol Chem* 1996;271:16227–16236.

223. Grant MA, Baikeev RF, Gilbert GE, et al. Lysine 5 and phenylalanine 9 of the factor IX omega-loop interact with phosphatidylserine in a membrane-mimetic environment. *Biochemistry* 2004;43:15367–15378.

224. Heimark RL, Schwartz SM. Binding of coagulation factors IX and X to the endothelial cell surface. *Biochem Biophys Res Commun* 1983;111:723–731.

225. Stern DM, Drillings M, Nossel HL, et al. Binding of factors IX and IXa to cultured vascular endothelial cells. *Proc Natl Acad Sci U S A* 1983;80:4119–4123.

226. Stern DM, Knitter G, Kisiel W, et al. In vivo evidence of intravascular binding sites for coagulation factor IX. *Br J Haematol* 1987;66:227–232.

227. Cheung WF, Hamaguchi N, Smith KJ, et al. The binding of human factor IX to endothelial cells is mediated by residues 3-11. *J Biol Chem* 1992;267:20529–20531.

228. Wolberg AS, Stafford DW, Erie DA. Human factor IX binds to specific sites on the collagenous domain of collagen IV. *J Biol Chem* 1997;272:16717–16720.

229. Ryan J, Wolitzky B, Heimer E, et al. Structural determinants of the factor IX molecule mediating interaction with the endothelial cell binding site are distinct from those involved in phospholipid binding. *J Biol Chem* 1989;264:20283–20297.

230. Prorok M, Geng JP, Warder SE, et al. The entire γ-carboxyglutamic acid- and helical stack-domains of human coagulation factor IX are required for optimal binding to its endothelial cell receptor. *Int J Pept Protein Res* 1996;48:281–285.

231. Brinkman HJ, Mertens K, Holthuis J, et al. The activation of human blood coagulation factor X on the surface of endothelial cells: a comparison with various vascular cells, platelets and monocytes. *Br J Haematol* 1994;87:332–342.

232. Bauer KA, Mannucci PM, Gringeri A, et al. Factor IXa-factor VIIIa-cell surface complex does not contribute to the basal activation of the coagulation mechanism in vivo. *Blood* 1992;79:2039–2047.

233. Cheung WF, van den Born J, Kuhn K, et al. Identification of the endothelial cell binding site for factor IX. *Proc Natl Acad Sci U S A* 1996;93:11068–11073.

234. Ahmad SS, Scandura JM, Walsh PN. Structural and functional characterization of platelet receptor-mediated factor VIII binding. *J Biol Chem* 2000;275:13071–13081.

235. Scandura JM, Ahmad SS, Walsh PN. A binding site expressed on the surface of activated human platelets is shared by factor X and prothrombin. *Biochemistry* 1996;35:8890–8902.

236. London FS, Marcinkiewicz M, Walsh PN. A subpopulation of platelets responds to thrombin- or SFLLRN-stimulation with binding sites for factor IXa. *J Biol Chem* 2004;279:19854–19859.

237. Ahmad SS, London FS, Walsh PN. The assembly of the factor X-activating complex on activated human platelets. *J Thromb Haemost* 2003;1:48–59.

238. Ahmad SS, Wong MY, Rawala R, et al. Coagulation factor IX residues G4-Q11 mediate its interaction with a shared factor IX/IXa binding site on activated platelets but not the assembly of the functional factor X activating complex. *Biochemistry* 1998;37:1671–1679.

239. Ahmad SS, Rawala R, Cheung WF, et al. The role of the second growth-factor domain of human factor IXa in binding to platelets and in factor-X activation. *Biochem J* 1995;310(Pt 2):427–431.

240. Astermark J, Hogg PJ, Stenflo J. The gamma-carboxyglutamic acid and epidermal growth factor-like modules of factor IXa beta. Effects on the serine protease module and factor X activation. *J Biol Chem* 1994;269:3682–3689.

241. Baird TR, Walsh PN. The interaction of factor XIa with activated platelets but not endothelial cells promotes the activation of factor IX in the consolidation phase of blood coagulation. *J Biol Chem* 2002;277:38462–38467.

242. Stoilova-McPhie S, Villoutreix BO, Mertens K, et al. 3-Dimensional structure of membrane-bound coagulation factor VIII: modeling of the factor VIII heterodimer within a 3-dimensional density map derived by electron crystallography. *Blood* 2002;99:1215–1223.

243. Schmidt AE, Bajaj SP. Structure-function relationships in factor IX and factor IXa. *Trends Cardiovasc Med* 2003;13:39–45.

244. Adams TE, Hockin MF, Mann KG, et al. The crystal structure of activated protein C-inactivated bovine factor Va: implications for cofactor function. *Proc Natl Acad Sci U S A* 2004;101:8918–8923.

245. Bajaj SP, Rapaport SI, Maki SL. A monoclonal antibody to factor IX that inhibits the factor VIII:Ca potentiation of factor X activation. *J Biol Chem* 1985;260:11574–11580.

246. Hamaguchi N, Bajaj SP, Smith KJ, et al. The role of amino-terminal residues of the heavy chain of factor IXa in the binding of its cofactor, factor VIIIa. *Blood* 1994;84:1837–1842.

247. Bajaj SP, Schmidt AE, Mathur A, et al. Factor IXa:factor VIIIa interaction. helix 330-338 of factor IXa interacts with residues 558-565 and spatially adjacent regions of the A2 subunit of factor VIIIa. *J Biol Chem* 2001;276:16302–16309.

248. Fay PJ, Koshibu K. The A2 subunit of factor VIIIa modulates the active site of factor IXa. *J Biol Chem* 1998;273:19049–19054.

249. Kolkman JA, Mertens K. Surface-loop residue Lys316 in blood coagulation Factor IX is a major determinant for Factor X but not antithrombin recognition. *Biochem J* 2000;350:701–707.

250. Yang L, Manithody C, Olson ST. Contribution of basic residues of the autolysis loop to the substrate and inhibitor specificity of factor IXa. *J Biol Chem* 2003;278:25032–25038.

251. Schmidt AE, Stewart JE, Mathur A, et al. Na$^+$-site in blood coagulation factor IXa: effect on catalysis and factor VIIIa binding. *J Mol Biol* 2005;350:78–91.

252. Dang QD, Di Cera E. Residue 225 determines the Na(+)-induced allosteric regulation of catalytic activity in serine proteases. *Proc Natl Acad Sci U S A* 1996;93:10653–10656.

253. Zhang E, Tulinsky A. The molecular environment of the Na+ binding site of thrombin. *Biophys Chem* 1997;63:185–200.

254. Underwood MC, Zhong D, Mathur A, et al. Thermodynamic linkage between the S1 site, the Na+ site, and the Ca2+ site in the protease domain of human coagulation factor xa. Studies on catalytic efficiency and inhibitor binding. *J Biol Chem* 2000;275:36876–36884.

255. Schmidt AE, Padmanabhan K, Underwood MC, et al. Thermodynamic linkage between the S1 site, the Na+ site, and the Ca2+ site in the protease domain of human activated protein C (APC). Sodium ion in the APC crystal structure is coordinated to four carbonyl groups from two separate loops. *J Biol Chem* 2002;277:28987–28995.

256. Lenting PJ, van de Loo JW, Donath MJ, et al. The sequence Glu1811-Lys1818 of human blood coagulation factor VIII comprises a binding site for activated factor IX. *J Biol Chem* 1996;271:1935–1940.

257. Lenting PJ, Christophe OD, Maat H, et al. Ca2+ binding to the first epidermal growth factor-like domain of human blood coagulation factor IX promotes enzyme activity and factor VIII light chain binding. *J Biol Chem* 1996;271:25332–25337.

258. Lenting PJ, ter Maat H, Clijsters PP, et al. Cleavage at arginine 145 in human blood coagulation factor IX converts the zymogen into a factor VIII binding enzyme. *J Biol Chem* 1995;270:14884–14890.

259. Larson PJ, Stanfield-Oakley SA, VanDusen WJ, et al. Structural integrity of the gamma-carboxyglutamic acid domain of human blood coagulation factor IXa is required for its binding to cofactor VIIIa. *J Biol Chem* 1996;271:3869–3876.

260. Bauer KA, Kass BL, ten Cate H, et al. Factor IX is activated in vivo by the tissue factor mechanism. *Blood* 1990;76:731–736.

261. Davie EW, Fujikawa K, Kisiel W. The coagulation cascade: initiation, maintenance, and regulation. *Biochemistry* 1991;30:10363–10370.

262. Hoffman M, Monroe DM, Oliver JA, et al. Factors IXa and Xa play distinct roles in tissue factor-dependent initiation of coagulation. *Blood* 1995;86:1794–1801.

263. Butenas S, Orfeo T, Gissel MT, et al. The significance of circulating factor IXa in blood. *J Biol Chem* 2004;279:22875–22882.

264. van Hylckama Vlieg A, van der Linden IK, Bertina RM, et al. High levels of factor IX increase the risk of venous thrombosis. *Blood* 2000;95:3678–3682.

265. Ameri A, Kurachi S, Sueishi K, et al. Myocardial fibrosis in mice with overexpression of human blood coagulation factor IX. *Blood* 2003;101:1871–1873.

266. Benedict CR, Ryan J, Wolitzky B, et al. Active site-blocked factor IXa prevents intravascular thrombus formation in the coronary vasculature

without inhibiting extravascular coagulation in a canine thrombosis model. *J Clin Invest* 1991;88:1760–1765.

267. Spanier TB, Oz MC, Minanov OP, et al. Heparinless cardiopulmonary bypass with active-site blocked factor IXa: a preliminary study on the dog. *J Thorac Cardiovasc Surg* 1998;115:1179–1188.

268. Spanier TB, Oz MC, Madigan JD, et al. Selective anticoagulation with active site blocked factor IXa in synthetic patch vascular repair results in decreased blood loss and operative time. *ASAIO J* 1997;43:M526–M530.

269. Wong AG, Gunn AC, Ku P, et al. Relative efficacy of active site-blocked factors IXa, Xa in models of rabbit venous and arterio-venous thrombosis. *Thromb Haemost* 1997;77:1143–1147.

270. Kjalke M, Monroe DM, Hoffman M, et al. Active site-inactivated factors VIIa, Xa, and IXa inhibit individual steps in a cell-based model of tissue factor-initiated coagulation. *Thromb Haemost* 1998;80:578–584.

271. Feuerstein GZ, Patel A, Toomey JR, et al. Antithrombotic efficacy of a novel murine antihuman factor IX antibody in rats. *Arterioscler Thromb Vasc Biol* 1999;19:2554–2562.

272. Toomey JR, Blackburn MN, Storer BL, et al. Comparing the antithrombotic efficacy of a humanized anti-factor IX(a) monoclonal antibody (SB 249417) to the low molecular weight heparin enoxaparin in a rat model of arterial thrombosis. *Thromb Res* 2000;100:73–79.

273. Feuerstein GZ, Toomey JR, Valocik R, et al. An inhibitory anti-factor IX antibody effectively reduces thrombus formation in a rat model of venous thrombosis. *Thromb Haemost* 1999;82:1443–1445.

274. Rusconi CP, Scardino E, Layzer J, et al. RNA aptamers as reversible antagonists of coagulation factor IXa. *Nature* 2002;419:90–94.

# CHAPTER 8 ■ FACTOR VIII AND HEMOPHILIA A

RANDAL J. KAUFMAN, STYLIANOS E. ANTONARAKIS, AND PHILIP J. FAY

The physiologic response to blood vessel injury is the sequential activation of plasma proteases within the blood coagulation cascade, leading to a localized burst of thrombin generation with subsequent conversion of soluble fibrinogen to insoluble fibrin. Thrombin generation requires the interaction of proteases, protein cofactors, and substrate zymogens that assemble in the presence of calcium on a phospholipid surface provided by damaged or activated cells. The well-coordinated balance between procoagulant and anticoagulant activities is required for normal hemostasis and to prevent pathologic thrombosis. Factor VIII is an essential component of the blood coagulation cascade. Factor VIII circulates in plasma in an inactive form that is proteolytically cleaved by factor Xa and/or thrombin to yield activated factor VIIIa. Factor VIIIa serves as a cofactor for factor IXa–mediated proteolytic activation of factor X. Subsequently, factor Xa acts in the presence of its activated cofactor, factor Va, to convert prothrombin to its active enzymatic form thrombin.

Hemophilia A was documented more than 1,700 years ago in the Talmud as a sex-linked severe bleeding disorder (1). The genetics of hemophilia A was described during the early 1800s (2), and transfusion of whole blood was shown to successfully treat a hemophilia-associated bleeding episode by 1840 (3). In 1911, Addis demonstrated that normal plasma can shorten the clotting time of hemophilic blood (4). It was 25 years later when Patek and Taylor described the role of factor VIII in hemostasis and designated the factor as "antihemophilic globulin" (5). In the 1950s, plasma concentrates, and then in 1965, cryoprecipitates, were developed for treatment of bleeding episodes associated with hemophilia A. In the early 1980s, factor VIII was purified from human plasma (6), and subsequently, the factor VIII gene was cloned (7,8). These developments dramatically increased our understanding of the structure and function of factor VIII in blood coagulation and provided monoclonal antibody purified plasma-derived factor VIII and recombinant-derived factor VIII for the treatment of hemophilia A (9,10).

The distinction between hemophilia A and von Willebrand disease was confused for many years because the autosomally inherited von Willebrand disease is associated with factor VIII deficiency, although the hereditary factor VIII deficiency of hemophilia A is an X-chromosome-linked disease. In addition, early preparations of antihemophilic factor could correct the clotting time of hemophilic plasma as well as restore platelet adhesion and aggregation defects in the plasma from patients with von Willebrand disease. It is now known that the early preparations of antihemophilic factor contained both factor VIII and von Willebrand factor (VWF). Factor VIII and VWF are two separate proteins that exist as a complex in plasma and are under separate genetic control. Factor VIII is an X-linked gene product that accelerates the activation of factor X by factor IXa in the presence of calcium and negatively charged phospholipids. VWF is a chromosome 12p gene product that is essential for platelet adhesion to subendothelium and for ristocetin-induced platelet agglutination. Because VWF and factor VIII are found in the plasma as a complex and VWF serves to stabilize factor VIII and regulate its activity, the activities of these two proteins are intimately intertwined. Early reports on the structure and function of factor VIII must be interpreted with caution because what was then identified as factor VIII protein had physical properties of VWF. Many immunoassays used were termed "factor VIII-" or "factor VIII–related antigen," although they really measured VWF. For consensus, the International Committee on Thrombosis and Haemostasis formulated nomenclature guidelines in 1985 (11): Factor VIII protein is designated VIII; factor VIII antigen is designated VIII:Ag; factor VIII procoagulant activity is designated VIII:C; von Willebrand factor is designated VWF; and von Willebrand factor antigen is designated VWF:Ag.

## FACTOR VIII PROTEIN

### Factor VIII Structure and Function

#### Factor VIII Cofactor Activity

Factor VIII acts to increase the rate of conversion of factor X to factor Xa by the protease factor IXa. The $K_m$ for factor X activation in the presence of factor IXa and calcium is decreased several orders of magnitude by phospholipid (see Table 8-1) because of concentration of enzyme and substrate on the plane of the phospholipid surface. Factor VIIIa dramatically increases the $V_{max}$ of factor X activation by factor IXa by 100,000-fold (12). Factor VIIIa accelerates the proteolysis of factor X by interaction with both factor X and factor IXa on a phospholipid surface to facilitate a conformational change in the active site of factor IXa that favors catalysis (13). In a similar manner, the homologous coagulation cofactor, activated factor V, increases the $V_{max}$ for prothrombin activation by factor Xa (Table 8-1).

The definition of factor VIII–specific activity is complicated because both thrombin and factor Xa convert the cofactor into a much more active form, factor VIIIa. However, for standardization, 1 U of factor VIII is defined as that amount of activity in 1 mL of normal pooled human plasma measured in a clotting assay using factor VIII–deficient plasma (14). Purification of factor VIII has yielded specific activities that vary between 2,300 U per mg (6) and 8,000 U per mg (15). For greater convenience and precision, factor VIII activity is measured in a factor X activation assay in the presence of factor IXa, phospholipid, and calcium ions. Factor Xa generation is measured directly by monitoring cleavage of a synthetic chromogenic substrate (16). Factor VIII antigen can be measured using factor VIII–specific antibodies in specific immunoassays (17,18).

## TABLE 8-1

### THE EFFECT OF COFACTORS ON THE RATE OF ACTIVATION OF FACTOR X AND PROTHROMBIN

| Component | $K_m$ | $V_{max}$ | Catalytic efficiency[a] |
|---|---|---|---|
| **FACTOR X ACTIVATION** | | | |
| IXa | 300 | 0.002[b] | 1 |
| IXa, Ca²⁺ | 181 | 0.011 | 8 |
| IXa, Ca²⁺, PL | 0.06 | 0.002 | $5.8 \times 10^3$ |
| IXa, Ca²⁺, PL, VIIIa | 0.06 | 500 | $1 \times 10^9$ |
| **PROTHROMBIN ACTIVATION** | | | |
| Xa | 130 | 0.61[c] | 1 |
| Xa, Ca²⁺ | 84 | 0.68 | 1.7 |
| Xa, Ca²⁺, PL | 0.06 | 2.30 | $8.3 \times 10^3$ |
| Xa, Ca²⁺, PL, Va | 0.21 | 1,900 | $2.0 \times 10^6$ |

[a]The catalytic efficiency ($V_{max}/K_m$) for a mixture is compared to that of the enzyme alone.
[b]$V_{max}$, mol factor Xa/min/mol factor IXa
[c]$V_{max}$, mol thrombin/min/mol factor Xa
Data from bovine proteins and adapted from Gilles JG, Jacquemin MG, Saint-Remy JM. Factor VIII inhibitors. *Thromb Haemost* 1997;78:641–646.

Factor VIII protein characterization was hampered by its low concentration in plasma, its heterogeneity in size, and its exquisite sensitivity to proteolysis. Two major breakthroughs were the application of immunoaffinity chromatography for the successful purification of factor VIII from porcine (6,19) and human (6,20) plasma and the cloning of the human factor VIII gene to deduce the primary structure of the factor VIII protein (7,8).

### Factor VIII Primary Structure

The deduced primary amino acid sequence of human factor VIII demonstrated that factor VIII is encoded by a large precursor protein of 2,351 amino acid residues from which a 19–amino acid signal peptide is cleaved upon translocation into the lumen of the endoplasmic reticulum (ER). Upon secretion from the cell, factor VIII is further processed to a heterodimer consisting of a carboxy terminal–derived light chain of 80,000 MW in a metal ion–dependent association with an amino-terminal–derived heavy-chain fragment ranging from 90,000 to 200,000 MW (7,8). In the plasma, this complex is stabilized by association through hydrophilic and hydrophobic interactions with a 50-fold molar subunit excess of VWF. The factor VIII amino acid sequence revealed an organization of three structural domains that occur in the order A1:A2:B:A3:C1:C2 (see Fig. 8-1) (7,8). In addition to these domains, there are three acidic amino acid–rich regions that reside at the junction of the A1/A2 (residues 331–372), A2/B (residues 700–740), and B/A3 (residues 1649–1689) domains (Fig. 8-1). The A1 (amino acid residues 1–329) and A2 (380–711) domains of factor VIII occur in the heavy chain, and the A3 (1649–2019) domain occurs in the light chain. The A-domains have 30% identity to each other and to the triplicated A-domains of ceruloplasmin and factor V and to the single A-domain of ferroxidase (7, 8,21,22). The C1 (residues 2020–2172) and C2 (residues 2173–2332) domains occur in the carboxy terminus of the factor VIII light chain and exhibit homology to milk fat globule protein and to the A, C, and D chains of discoidin 1, all proteins capable of binding glycoconjugates and negatively charged phospholipids (23,24). The B-domain is encoded by a single large exon of 3,100 nucleotides, has no known homology to other proteins, and contains 18 of the 25 potential asparagine (N)-linked glycosylation sites within factor VIII. Although the amino acid sequences between the B-domains human and murine factor VIII have diverged, they have both conserved the large number of potential N-linked glycosylation sites, although in different positions. This conservation suggests that glycosylation in the B-domain is important for factor VIII expression and/or function (25). Similarly, factor VIII and factor V have conserved a high degree of amino acid conservation between the A- and C-domains, with no detectable homology between the B-domains

Cysteine residues and disulfide bonds.

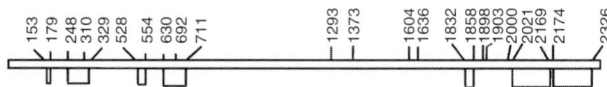

Potential Asn linked carbohydrates (total of 25) and sites of tyrosine sulfation.

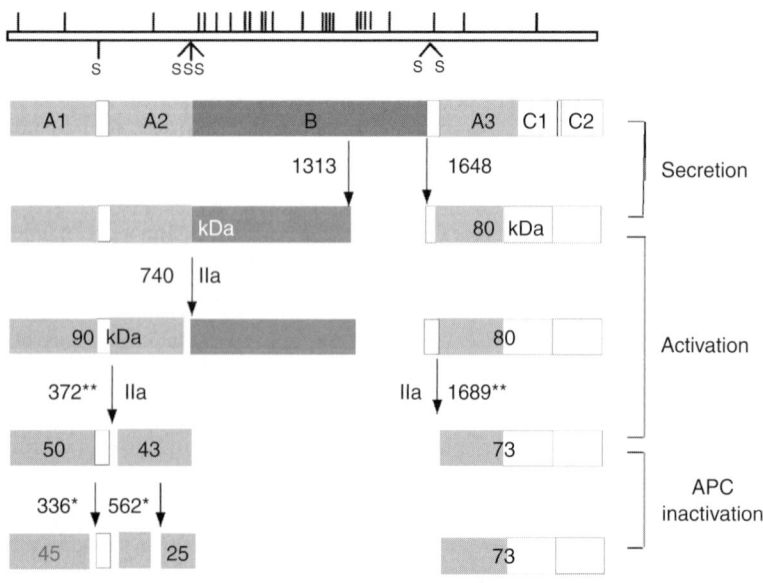

**FIGURE 8-1.** Domain structure and processing of factor VIII. The structural domains of factor VIII are depicted in the top line: (i) a triplicated A-domain of 330 amino acids; (ii) a unique B-domain of 980 amino acids; and (iii) a duplicated C-domain of 150 amino acids. The *hatched* areas represent regions enriched in acidic amino acids. The location of free cysteine residues and disulfide bonds (*brackets below line*), potential asparagine-linked glycosylation sites, and sites of tyrosine sulfation are shown (*S*). Within the Golgi compartment in the cell, factor VIII is cleaved at two sites within the B-domain to generate a 200- or a 160-kDa heavy-chain polypeptide and the 80-kDa light-chain polypeptide. The thrombin (IIa), activated protein C (APC), and factor Xa (Xa) cleavage sites are shown. Factor Xa also cleaves at all of the thrombin cleavage sites. The two cleavages required for thrombin activation (**) and the sites of proteolytic inactivation by APC (*) are shown. (Reproduced from Kaufman RJ and Antonarakis SE. Structure, biology, and genetics of factor VIII. In: Hoffman R, Benz EJ Jr, Shattil SJ et al., eds. *Hematology: basic principles and practice*, 4th ed. Philadelphia: Elsevier, 2005, with permission.)

(7,8,21,22). In addition, like the factor VIII B-domain, the B-domain of factor V is encoded by a large single exon and contains a large number of N-linked glycosylation sites. The domain organization and homologies between factors V and VIII suggests that these genes evolved from a primordial ferroxidase gene by triplication of the A-domain, insertion of the B-domain, and addition of the two C-domains to form the primordial cofactor gene. Subsequently, the factor V and factor VIII genes possibly evolved by duplication and divergence of amino acid residues within the B-domain, although the high number of N-linked glycosylation sites were preserved, whereas amino acid sequences within the A- and C-domains were conserved.

## Metal Ions in Factor VIII

Metal ion–dependent interactions appear vital for both factor VIII structure and function. Two distinct interactions have been probed by reconstitution of isolated subunits, as well as by limited studies using mutagenesis. These interactions include the binding of copper ion and calcium/manganese ions. A single copper ion was identified in factor VIII by atomic adsorption spectrometry, and this ligand is lost upon dissociation of the factor VIII chains (26). Electron paramagnetic resonance studies demonstrated that a single molecule of reduced copper ion ($Cu^+$) was present in factor VIII (27). Studies examining the reconstitution of factor VIII from isolated heavy and light chains revealed a primary role for copper in enhancing the interchain affinity (28). That study also showed that copper, which alone is insufficient to regenerate the active conformation of factor VIII, in the presence of calcium (see subsequent text) does marginally increase the specific activity of factor VIII. The site(s) involved in coordinating the Cu ion remains controversial. On the basis of homologies of the factor VIII A-domains with ceruloplasmin (8,29), three potential copper sites have been identified in the cofactor. Type 1 copper sites exist in both the A1 and A3 domains, whereas a type 2 copper site is believed to span the A1 and A3 domains.

Site-directed mutagenesis of the cysteine residues in the type 1 sites demonstrated that the type 1 site in the A1 domain (composed of ligands His265–Cys310–His315–Met320) was essential for cofactor function, whereas the type 1 site in the A3 domain was dispensable (27). That study also showed that mutation of Cys310Ser in the type 1 site in the A1 domain destroyed factor VIII activity and yielded secreted heavy and light chains that were not associated, supporting a requirement for this copper ion-binding site in heavy- and light-chain association. A Cys310Phe mutation in a patient with severe hemophilia A has been reported in the mutation database (http://europium.csc.mrc.rpms.ac.uk). On the other hand, recent studies employing fluorescence energy transfer techniques indicated the interchain affinity in the absence of copper ($K_d$ approximately 50 nM) is increased as much as 100-fold in the presence of copper ($K_d$ approximately 0.5 nM) (28). The latter analysis employed subunits that were modified with fluorophores at Cys310 (a residue within the type 1 copper site in A1 domain) and Cys2000 (a residue within the type 1 copper site in A3 domain). This observation provides indirect evidence in support of a functional role for the type 2 copper site. Therefore, the latter data support a model in which copper ion occupancy of the type 2 site bridging the A1 and A3 domains makes a direct contribution to the interchain binding affinity, whereas copper occupancy of both type 1 sites appears necessary for maximal specific activity of the cofactor.

Reconstitution studies using isolated factor VIII chains have demonstrated that copper alone is insufficient to generate cofactor activity (30,31). However, recombining purified factor VIII chains in buffers containing $Ca^{2+}$ or $Mn^{2+}$ yields active factor VIII (30,32). These ions do not contribute to the interchain affinity but rather promote cofactor activity by modulating the conformation of the heterodimer (28). $Ca^{2+}$ (33) and $Mn^{2+}$ (34) bind to both heavy and light chains of factor VIII, yet this binding appears to occur at nonidentical sites. A putative site for $Ca^{2+}$ binding is proposed in the A1 domain (residues 108–124) (33) based upon homology of this region to a site proposed for factor V (35). Site-directed mutagenesis of the homologous region in factor VIII (residues 110–126) was performed to evaluate the role of this region in metal ion coordination (36). Stimulation of cofactor activity in response to added $Ca^{2+}$ or $Mn^{2+}$ was used to determine affinity values. $Ca^{2+}$ binding affinity was greatly reduced (or lost) following substitution at Glu110, Asp116, Glu122, Asp125, or Asp126 with alanine. However, Ala-substitution at Glu113, Glu115, or Glu124 showed wild type–like activity with little or no reduction in $Ca^{2+}$ affinity. Examination of $Mn^{2+}$ affinity showed minimal effects except for the mutations at Asp116 and Asp125. Assuming that the loss of a ligand for divalent metal ion coordination results in reductions in metal ion–binding affinity, it was proposed that Glu110, Asp116, Glu122, Asp125, and Asp126 likely coordinate $Ca^{2+}$, whereas Asp116 and Asp125 may contribute to $Mn^{2+}$ coordination.

---

# Biosynthesis and Metabolism of Factor VIII

## Factor VIII Expression

Although the natural cell type that produces factor VIII has not been definitively identified, liver transplant studies in factor VIII–deficient dogs (37) and in several patients with hemophilia (38) strongly implicates that the liver and/or the reticuloendothelial system are primary sites of factor VIII synthesis. Initial immunochemical localization by light microscopic (39) or electron microscopic (40) examination detected the factor VIII antigen in hepatocytes. However, RNA hybridization analysis detected factor VIII mRNA in hepatocytes and in many other cells and tissues (41). More recent analysis of factor VIII mRNA by quantitative reverse transcription polymerase chain reaction (RT-PCR) identified highest levels in liver, followed by kidney (42). Factor VIII mRNA and protein were concentrated in hepatic sinusoidal endothelial or Kupffer cells, with considerably less in hepatocytes (42). In addition, isolated sinusoidal endothelial cells were shown to produce factor VIII (43). Because there are no known established cell lines that express factor VIII, it has not been possible to study the biosynthesis of factor VIII in its natural host cell. However, the expression of factor VIII in cultured mammalian cells transfected with the factor VIII gene allowed analysis of the biosynthesis and processing of this glycoprotein (44).

## Factor VIII Trafficking and Modification within the Cell

The factor VIII biosynthetic pathway was proposed on the basis of analysis of factor VIII expression in transfected cell lines, such as Chinese hamster ovary cells (see Fig. 8-2). On synthesis, factor VIII is translocated into the lumen of the ER, where the signal peptide is cleaved. In the ER, high mannose-containing core oligosaccharides are attached to multiple asparagine residues within the factor VIII molecule. A substantial portion of the newly synthesized factor VIII is retained in the ER through interactions with two protein chaperone systems designed to prevent the exit of unfolded proteins from the ER. First, factor VIII is bound to the most abundant ER protein, the glucose-regulated protein of 78,000 MW (GRP78), also known as immunoglobulin-binding protein (BiP) (45), (Fig. 8-2). BiP expression is induced by glucose deprivation, inhibition of N-linked glycosylation, or the presence of misfolded protein within the ER. In addition, high-level factor VIII expression can also induce transcription of the BiP gene (46). The level of BiP in the cell inversely correlates with the efficiency of factor VIII

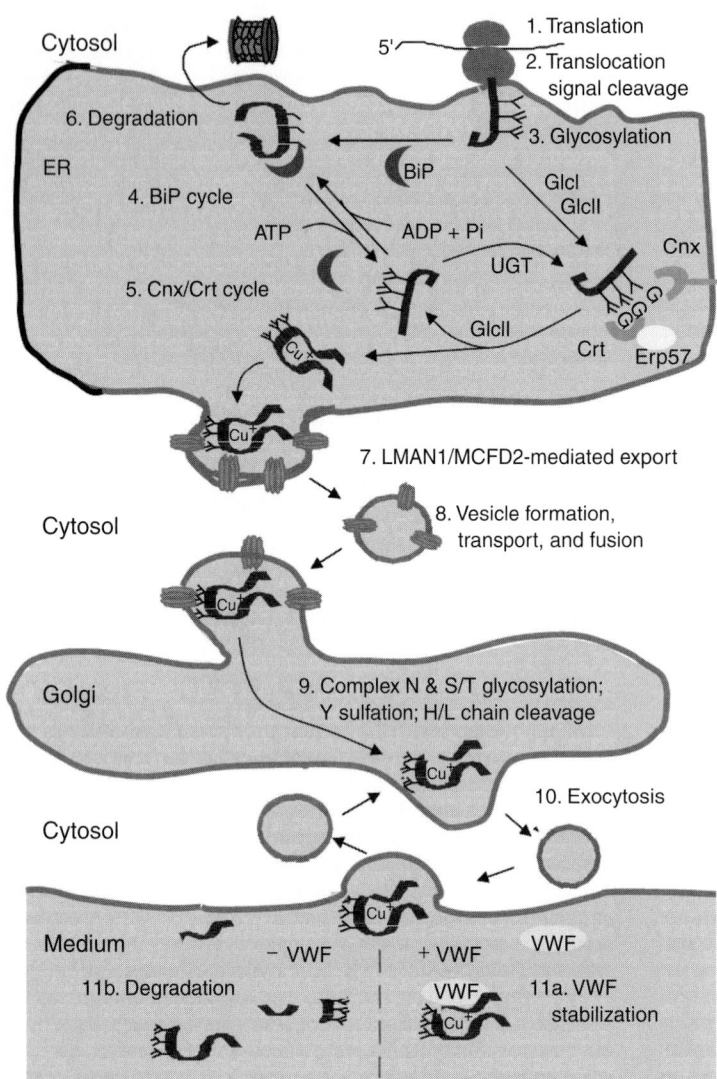

**FIGURE 8-2.** Synthesis, processing, and secretion of factor VIII in mammalian cells. The factor VIII primary translation product is translocated into the lumen of the endothelial reticulum, where the signal peptide sequence and asparagines (N)-linked glycosylation occurs. After trimming of two glucose residues from core oligosaccharides by glucosidase I and II, factor VIII may interact with calnexin (Cnx) and calreticulin (Crt) that promotes exposure to the oxidoreductase Erp57 to promote proper disulfide bond formation. Glucosidase II promotes release from Cnx and Crt. The UDP-glucose:glycoprotein glycosyltransferase (UGT) reglucosylates the high-mannose core oligosaccharides on unfolded or misfolded factor VIII molecules to regenerate the monoglucosylated glycan as a ligand for Cnx and Crt. A fraction of factor VIII binds tightly to the BiP and requires ATP binding for release. A portion of factor VIII is retrotranslocated into the cytoplasm and is degraded by the cytosolic 26S proteasome. Properly folded and processed factor VIII interacts with the LMAN1/ MCFD2 complex for transit to the Golgi apparatus. In the Golgi apparatus, additional processing occurs that includes complex modification of carbohydrate on N-linked sites, addition of carbohydrate to serine and threonine residues, sulfation of tyrosine residues, and cleavage of the protein to the mature heavy and light chains. The presence of VWF in the medium promotes heavy and light chain association and stable accumulation of factor VIII in the medium. In the absence of VWF, the individual chains do not associate and are degraded.

secretion (47,48). BiP exhibits a peptide-dependent adenosine triphosphatase activity. Factor VIII dissociation from BiP and secretion requires an unusually high level of intracellular adenosine triphosphate (ATP) (49). Because factor VIII interacts with BiP, and factor V does not, it was possible to identify a primary BiP-binding site by analysis of the secretion of factor VIII and factor V chimeric proteins. This study identified a hydrophobic β-sheet within the factor VIII A1 domain that resides adjacent to a proposed ligand, Cys310, for binding type-1 copper ion (50,51). Hydrophobic residues are preferred sites of BiP binding. Mutation of a single phenylalanine at residue 309 to serine within the hydrophobic sheet, the residue adjacent to cysteine 310, increased the secretion efficiency of factor VIII severalfold, and this correlated with a reduced requirement for ATP for secretion (50). These studies suggest that BiP may provide a role in copper ion binding to factor VIII. Finally, a portion of factor VIII forms high-molecular-weight aggregates immediately after synthesis (52). These aggregates require ATP for disassembly and secretion (52).

The second chaperone system that retains factor VIII in the ER recognizes the structure on N-linked oligosaccharides on factor VIII. It is now known that a primary determinant in the trafficking of unfolded glycoproteins in the ER is the structure of N-linked oligosaccharides. Proteins translocated into the ER become N-glycosylated upon transfer of a preassembled

core glycan (N-acetylglucosamine$_2$-mannose$_9$-glucose$_3$) from a lipid-dolichol donor in the ER membrane to nascent chains emerging in the ER lumen. Rapid trimming of the two outermost glucose residues prepares protein-bound N-glycans for association with the two homologous ER lectins calnexin (CNX) and calreticulin (CRT) and exposure to the glycoprotein-specific oxidoreductase ERp57 to catalyze proper disulfide bond rearrangement (53,54). Release from CNX/CRT depends on glucosidase II cleavage of the innermost glucose residue. Although the modalities of misfolded protein domain recognition and ER retention are not known (55,56), the enzyme UDP-glucose:glycoprotein glucosyltransferase (UGT) and the CNX/CRT chaperone system are thought to play central roles (57,58). Current models (57–62) propose that UGT reglucosylates nonnative polypeptides, thereby preventing their release from the CNX/CRT chaperone system and their exit from the ER. Factor VIII interacts with both CNX and CRT, although their roles in factor trafficking within the ER are not known (63).

Improperly folded proteins are selectively extracted from the ER and directed for degradation by the cytosolic proteasome in a process called ER-associated degradation (ERAD). A significant portion of factor VIII within the ER never transits to the Golgi compartment but rather is degraded through ERAD (Fig. 8-2). Proteolysis of intracellular factor VIII is inhibited by lactacystin, a microbiotic that specifically modifies the active site of the proteasome, although secretion of factor VIII is not improved (63). These results indicate that factor VIII within the ER is directed to the cytosolic 26S proteasomal machinery for degradation. Recently, an ER degradation enhancing mannosidase-like protein, (EDEM), was shown to recognize oligosaccharide structures trimmed by ER mannosidase I and mediate their transfer to the cytosol for ERAD (64–66). Finally, studies on combined deficiency of factors V and VIII indicate that oligosaccharides are also important for trafficking of factor VIII from the ER to the Golgi compartment through interaction with the transport complex LMAN1/MCFD2 (see subsequent text). The sum of these findings supports that oligosaccharide processing plays a central role to direct factor VIII trafficking within the secretory pathway.

The portion of factor VIII that is secretion competent transits to the Golgi apparatus, where most of the factor VIII is processed at two sites within the B-domain after residues 1313 and 1648 to generate the heavy chains (90,000–200,000 MW) and the light chain (80,000 MW). Also within the Golgi apparatus, factor VIII is further processed by (a) modification of the asparagine-linked high mannose–containing oligosaccharides to complex types, (b) addition of carbohydrate to multiple serine and threonine residues within the B-domain, and (c) addition of sulfate to six tyrosine residues within the heavy and the light chains (67).

## Interaction with von Willebrand Factor

### von Willebrand Factor Regulates Factor VIII

The levels of factor VIII and VWF in plasma are maintained at a fairly constant ratio of 1 molecule of factor VIII to 50–100 VWF subunits. For example, patients with type 1 von Willebrand disease who have a 50% reduction in VWF have a corresponding 50% reduction in factor VIII. Infusion of VWF into patients who are VWF deficient elicits an immediate rise in circulating levels of factor VIII. In addition, increase in the plasma concentration of VWF following infusion with 1-desamino-8-D-arginine vasopressin (DDAVP) elicits an increase in the plasma level of factor VIII (68). Upon infusion of VWF into a VWF-deficient pig, there was no change in the factor VIII mRNA level in the liver, although the plasma concentration of factor VIII increased by fivefold (69). These results support that VWF controls the plasma level of factor VIII by a posttranscriptional mechanism.

It is established that VWF stabilizes factor VIII in plasma. Factor VIII and VWF are cleared with a half-life of 12 hours upon infusion of the factor VIII–VWF complex into patients with hemophilia (70–72). Infusion of pure factor VIII into patients who are factor VIII deficient also exhibits clearance kinetics similar to that of factor VIII–VWF complex, presumably due to rapid binding of the factor VIII to plasma VWF (73). By contrast, infusion of pure factor VIII into patients with severe von Willebrand disease results in rapid clearance with a half-life of approximately 2 hours (70,74). Therefore, monoclonal-purified plasma- and recombinant-derived factor VIII (which both contain minimal amounts of VWF) are ineffective in the treatment of patients with severe von Willebrand disease (75). Finally, autosomally inherited factor VIII deficiency occurs in von Willebrand disease type Normandy or type 2N and results from missense mutations in the factor VIII–binding site within the first 91 amino acids of mature VWF (76,77). Therefore, the factor VIII deficiency appears to result from a defect in VWF to bind and stabilize factor VIII in plasma. These studies establish the stabilizing influence of VWF on factor VIII in the circulation; however, it is not known whether VWF also regulates factor VIII protein synthesis and/or secretion *in vivo*.

*In vitro* studies demonstrate that VWF can alter intracellular transport and secretion of factor VIII from the cell. VWF promotes the association of the light and heavy chains of factor VIII and results in stable accumulation of factor VIII activity in the conditioned medium of factor VIII–producing cultured mammalian cells (32,44). In the absence of VWF in the conditioned medium, the factor VIII heavy and light chains are secreted into the medium as dissociated chains that are subsequently degraded. *In vitro* reconstitution experiments demonstrated that VWF can directly promote reassembly of isolated heavy and light chains of factor VIII (30,32), suggesting a possible role of VWF in facilitating factor VIII assembly. The effect of VWF in promoting factor VIII heavy- and light-chain assembly and stable secretion in cell culture systems may reflect the role of VWF in regulating levels of factor VIII activity *in vivo* (70,71,73,74). The immediate rise in VWF and factor VIII observed after administration of DDAVP suggests the existence of a pool of factor VIII–VWF complex that is DDAVP releasable (78). DNA transfer experiments in cell culture and in mice have demonstrated that VWF coexpressed with factor VIII in endothelial cells or platelets can direct factor VIII into intracellular VWF storage granules (Weibel-Palade bodies or α-granules, respectively) that are released upon stimulation (79–82). Although these studies demonstrate the potential for an intracellular factor VIII–VWF complex to form and be released from the cell upon stimulation, at present there are no natural cell types that are known to express both factor VIII and VWF (83).

In addition to increasing factor VIII survival, VWF plays a critical role in directly regulating factor VIII activity (84). VWF prevents factor VIII binding to phospholipids (85) and activated platelets (86), and inhibits factor VIII from activation by factor Xa (87) and inactivation by activated protein C (APC) (88–90). On the other hand, VWF does not interfere with activation by thrombin (91,92) and actually serves as a cofactor in facilitating the thrombin-catalyzed cleavage of factor VIII light chain, thereby enhancing rates of factor VIIIa dissociation from VWF (93). It is likely that VWF mediates its inhibitory effects on factor VIII activity by preventing factor VIII interaction with phospholipids, a reaction required for both factor Xa and APC-mediated cleavage of factor VIII. However, recent evidence suggests that binding sites for VWF and APC in the factor VIII C2 domain may overlap (90), supporting a mechanism of inhibition by direct competition. It is proposed that VWF binding to platelet receptor GP Ib brings factor VIII to the vicinity of platelets adhering to damaged endothelium (86) (see Fig. 8-3). After proteolytic activation of factor VIII, factor VIIIa is released from VWF, permitting its interaction with the platelet surface.

### Factor VIII and von Willebrand Factor Interactive Sites

The affinity and stoichiometry of the factor VIII–VWF interaction have been extensively studied (84). Binding assays that immobilize VWF onto plastic have yielded stoichiometries of 1 molecule of factor VIII:50 to 100 monomers of VWF (94,95). In contrast, gel filtration, ultracentrifugation, and immobilization of VWF on colloidal gold or agarose microspheres yield stoichiometries close to 1:1 (95–98). It appears that immobilization of VWF onto plastic alters the conformation to prevent most of the sites from being occupied. To date, these *in vitro* studies have not identified the mechanism by which the stoichiometry in plasma is maintained at 1:50 (73). In contrast, the dissociation constant for the VWF–factor VIII interaction is similar for all the methods described ($K_d$ approximately 0.2 to 0.4 nM) and binding is very rapid, with the majority occurring within seconds (84,85,99).

The interaction of factor VIII with VWF is mediated by a major factor VIII–binding site within the first 272 amino acids

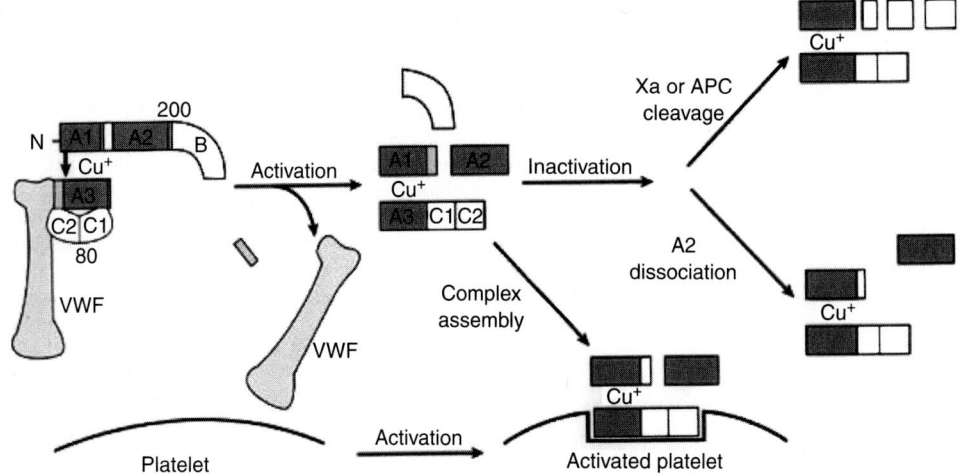

**FIGURE 8-3.** Model for thrombin activation and inactivation of factor VIII. Factor VIII is depicted as two chains in a copper ion $(Cu^+)$–dependent association. VWF is illustrated to bind the light chain of factor VIII through the acidic region and the C2 domain. Thrombin cleavage at residues 372 and 1689 releases the activated species from VWF. Inactivation may occur through dissociation of the A2 subunit or by a specific proteolytic event(s). Assembly onto an activated surface that has exposed negatively charged phospholipids promotes assembly of the factor Xase enzyme complex. VWF is shown to interact with its two platelet receptors GP Ib and $\alpha_{IIb}\beta_3$. (Reprinted from Kaufman RJ, Antonarakis SE. Structure, biology, and genetics of factor VIII. In: Hoffman R, Benz EJ Jr, Shattil SJ et al., eds. *Hematology: basic principles and practice*, 4th ed. Philadelphia: Elsevier, 2005, with permission.)

of the mature VWF molecule (100–102) with residues 78 to 96, residues approximately 53, and the amino-terminus providing crucial roles (95–97,100,103). As noted earlier, type N von Willebrand disease is caused by missense mutations within this region of VWF that result in a factor VIII deficiency due to reduced interaction of factor VIII with VWF (77). The VWF propeptide serves an essential role in multimerization of VWF (104), a process that leads to expression of the high-affinity factor VIII–binding site (97). Expression of propeptide-deleted VWF does not produce multimeric VWF, but rather produces dimeric VWF through carboxy-terminal disulfide bonds. This dimeric form of VWF binds factor VIII with a sixfold reduced affinity (97). Although the propeptide promotes generation of a high-affinity factor VIII–binding site, cleavage of the propeptide is required to expose the factor VIII–binding site (97).

High-affinity binding to VWF requires both the amino-terminal and carboxy-terminal ends of the factor VIII light chain (105–107). A VWF binding site on factor VIII was localized by monoclonal antibody inhibition to residues 1673 to 1684 (94, 108). This region is composed of a high density of acidic amino acids located at the amino-terminus of the factor VIII light chain and is removed by thrombin cleavage at residue 1689 (Fig. 8-1). Deletion of the acidic region at the amino-terminus of the light chain by site-directed mutagenesis yielded a molecule that bound VWF with a 10-fold reduced affinity, although the mutant protein had a specific activity similar to wild-type factor VIII (86, 109). These results demonstrate that the acidic region between residues 1649 and 1689 of the light chain is critical for appropriate interaction with VWF but is not required for cofactor function of factor VIII. Interestingly, an antifactor light-chain antibody that interacts with a C2 domain epitope between residues 2248 and 2285 was able to restore high-affinity VWF binding to a factor VIII molecule that had deleted the acidic region at the amino-terminus of the factor VIII light chain (109,110). Presumably, this antibody was able to induce a conformational change within the factor VIII light chain that is capable of high-affinity VWF binding. This suggests that the acidic region may not directly contact VWF, but may be required to induce a change in conformation at the carboxy-terminus of the light chain that exhibits high affinity for VWF.

Antibodies that react with residues 2248 to 2312 within the factor VIII C2 domain can inhibit factor VIII binding to VWF and to phosphatidylserine (110). This observation is consistent with the presence of a phospholipid-binding region within the C2 domain (110) and that phospholipid and VWF compete for binding to factor VIII (85,98,111). Recent evidence indicates that the two hydrophobic spikes represented by Met2199/Phe2200 and Leu2251/Leu2252 that participate in binding to phospholipid membranes (see subsequent text) also contribute to the binding of VWF. When mutated in pairs, the resulting factor VIII showed reductions of approximately 15- to 20-fold in affinity for VWF, and when all four residues were mutated, a 200-fold reduction in affinity was observed (112). The C1 domain also shows involvement in this interaction. Mutations at C1 residues Tyr2105, Arg2116, and Ser2119 show direct and/or indirect effects on binding VWF (113), the latter attributed to effects on positioning of the C1 domain relative to the A3 domain. Furthermore, an isolated C1–C2 fragment demonstrated higher affinity for VWF than isolated C2 (113). Taken together, these data suggest a complex intermolecular interaction that occurs over an extended interface involving the amino-terminal region of VWF and both ends of the factor VIII light chain.

## The Factor Xase Complex

### Interaction with Factor IXa

The proteolytically activated form of factor VIII, factor VIIIa (see subsequent section, "Regulation of Cofactor Activity"), serves as a cofactor for the serine protease factor IXa in the conversion of factor X to factor Xa. This complex of enzyme and cofactor, assembled on an anionic phospholipid surface, is referred to as the intrinsic factor Xase. The role of factor VIIIa is to increase the catalytic rate constant $(k_{cat})$ by several orders of magnitude (Table 8-1). The phospholipid surface is primarily involved in reducing molecular interactions to a two-dimensional space, thereby markedly decreasing the $K_m$ for factor X. The role of surface also appears to contribute to the $k_{cat}$ effect (114). The association of factor VIIIa and factor IXa is complex and not fully understood. At least two subunits of the factor VIIIa heterotrimer have been implicated as possessing factor IXa interactive sites. The factor VIII light chain–derived A3-C1-C2 subunit possesses a high-affinity site for factor IXa. The free light chain of factor VIII shows similar affinity for factor IXa ($K_d$ approximately 14 nM to approximately 50 nM (115,116) as is observed for factor VIIIa ($K_d$ approximately 2 to 20 nM, 117,118). This suggests minimal contribution by the factor VIII heavy chain–derived subunits, A1 and A2, to the binding energy for factor IXa interaction. This interactive site was localized to the A3 domain following studies using inhibition by a monoclonal antibody whose epitope is represented by residues 1178 to 1840 (115), and was further localized to within residues 1811 to 1818 on the basis of studies employing synthetic peptides (119). More recent studies employing a chimera where sequences of factor VIII were substituted for the homologous sequences in factor V have proposed factor VIII residues 1803 to 1810 as factor IXa-interactive (120). A number of mutations associated with hemophilia A have been identified within the Gln1778–Asp1840 region, including Arg1781His, Ser1784 Tyr, Leu1789Phe, Met1823Ile, Pro1825Ser, Thr1826Pro, and Ala1834Val/Thr (121), supporting the essential role of this high-affinity interaction in contributing to cofactor function.

On the basis of the identification of an APC cleavage site at Arg562 in the A2 subunit (122) (see subsequent section, "Inactivation of Cofactor Function") and the capacity for factor IXa to selectively protect from cleavage at this site (123,124), a factor IXa-interactive site in the A2 subunit was postulated. Synthetic peptides spanning residues 558 to 565 noncompetitively inhibited factor Xase activity (124), suggesting that these reagents block a critical interaction between cofactor and enzyme. Several natural mutations in patients with mild to moderate hemophilia A have been reported in these amino acids and include Ser558Phe, Val559Ala, Gln565Lys, and Gln565Arg (121). Kinetic evaluation of several point mutations within this region, expressed as recombinant factor VIII from BHK cells, indicated that these residues individually contributed to the overall catalytic rate for factor IXa–catalyzed activation of factor X (125). That study also showed a modest contribution of Asp560 to the interprotein binding energy. The 558–565 segment of factor VIII appears to be interactive with the 330 helix of factor IXa (126). Mutations in the helix results in a hemophilia B phenotype characterized as not showing stimulation of factor Xa generation by factor VIIIa (127). On the basis of the hypothesis that the 558 loop of A2 interacts with the 330 helix of factor IXa, Bajaj et al. (126) suggested that this interface represented an extended structure consisting of a number of potential interactions contributed by residues within and adjacent to these structures. Another A2 segment likely contributing to this interface, residues 708 to 715, is accounted for in the Bajaj model. A peptide to this sequence blocked factor VIIIa stimulation of factor IXa activity (116). That study also showed that Asp712, which is predicted in the model to form a salt bridge with Lys294 of factor IXa, likely contributes to this ionic tethering because its substitution with Ala reduced the interprotein affinity severalfold (equivalent to a stability contribution of approximately 1 kcal per mol). However, mutagenesis of several other residues predicted to directly interact with factor IXa failed to demonstrate a considerable effect on catalytic activity and/or affinity (116), suggesting that some refinement of this interface model is required.

In addition, other residues in A2, not accounted for by the Bajaj model, may also play a role in modulating factor IXa activity by mechanisms that remain to be elucidated. Mutation at Arg527, which yields a mild phenotype and shows defective stimulation of factor IXa activity (128), is located very close to the 558 loop in the model of the factor VIII A-domains. Therefore, this residue may indirectly contribute to function by stabilizing a factor IXa–interactive site. Another region in A2, residues 484 to 509, represents a major epitope for inhibitor antibodies (106), confirming an important role in factor VIII function. Ala-scanning mutagenesis of charged residues (individually or in clusters) was performed and resultant factor VIII mutants assessed for rates of factor Xa generation (129). One cluster mutant, where residues Arg489, Arg490, and Lys493 were substituted with Ala, demonstrated reduced rates of catalysis but exhibited little, if any, effects on affinity for factor IXa binding or the $K_m$ for factor X. Interestingly, these reductions in reaction rate were not observed with the single-site mutations, consistent with this region modulating $k_{cat}$ by its basic electrostatic potential. The exact mechanism by which these charged residues contribute to catalysis remains to be determined.

The isolated A2 subunit was shown to stimulate the factor IXa–catalyzed activation of factor X (130). In the presence of A2 subunit, the $k_{cat}$ (approximately 1 per minute) was approximately 100-fold greater than the value observed for factor IXa alone. However, this stimulation is fractional compared with the $k_{cat}$ in the presence of intact factor VIIIa (approximately 200 per minute). The affinity of the isolated A2 subunit for factor IXa was estimated from the factor Xa generation assay to be approximately 300 nM (130), which is a significantly weaker affinity than that observed for intact factor VIII(a) or the isolated light chain (A3-C1-C2 subunit).

## Interaction with Factor X

Little information is available on the interaction of factor VIIIa with factor X, the substrate for factor Xase. Analyses employing solid phase binding assays (131) and fluorescence anisotropy (132) localized a factor X interactive site to the acidic C-terminal region (residues 337–372) of the A1 subunit. The affinity of this association was determined to be 1 to 3 $\mu$M; however, these experiments were performed in the absence of phospholipid vesicles, which may contribute to the affinity of the interaction. Zero-length cross-linking studies revealed that the site of interaction on factor X was in the serine protease-forming domain of the heavy chain but was not in that portion of the sequence representing the activation peptide (133). Factor VIIIa reduces the Km of factor Xase for factor X by severalfold (134,135), suggesting a direct or indirect contribution to substrate affinity. Interestingly, deletion of the C-terminal region of A1 following proteolysis at Arg336 by factor Xa or APC (see subsequent text) resulted in an approximately fivefold increase in the $K_m$ for factor X (136). This increase in $K_m$ from approximately 40 nM to approximately 200 nM could potentially depress factor Xase activity in plasma because the latter $K_m$ value is approximately twice the plasma concentration of factor X. Furthermore, evidence indicates that factor X increases the affinity of factor IXa for factor VIIIa by approximately10-fold (137). Evaluation of a functional Kd for the factor VIIIa–factor IXa interaction as measured by rates of factor Xa generation yields a value of approximately 70 pM. One interpretation of these data is that the enhanced affinity for the binary interactions reflects interdependent associations involving the three proteins: cofactor, enzyme, and substrate.

From the studies mentioned in the preceding text, it appears that all three A-domains of factor VIII participate in interprotein interactions essential for the efficient conversion of substrate to product. Although progress has been made in the identification and initial characterization of intermolecular binding sites, the mechanism by which factor VIIIa modulates the active site of factor IXa to greatly stimulate factor Xa generation is not known. Fluorescence studies using active site-modified factor

IXa have yielded insights into the factor VIIIa–factor IXa inter-action. Fluorescence energy transfer studies show that binding of factor VIIIa does not markedly alter the distance separating the active site of factor IXa and the phospholipid surface (13). However, binding factor VIIIa did alter the emission intensity and anisotropy of the fluorescent probes used to modify the fac-tor IXa, indicating a change in probe environment. Duffy et al. (117) showed that the fluorescence anisotropy of active site–labeled factor IXa was increased in the presence of factor VIII and that a further incremental increase was observed upon thrombin activation of factor VIII. Although both the A1/A3-C1-C2 dimer and A2 subunit somewhat increased anisotropy of a similarly labeled factor IXa molecule, factor VIIIa–like increas-es in anisotropy values required reconstitution of the cofactor from the isolated subunits (138). Interestingly, in the absence of factor VIIIa, substrate factor X shows little effect on the anisotropy of the labeled factor IXa (139). However, inclusion of factor X produced a maximal increase in the factor VIIIa–dependent anisotropy. These results indicate that a primary role of factor VIIIa is to alter the conformation around the active site of factor IXa and its orientation relative to substrate factor X.

## Interaction with Phospholipids

Phospholipids interact with substrates, enzymes, and cofactors to play a critical role in the assembly and functional activity of the coagulation protease complexes. Negatively charged phos-pholipids are required for factor VIIIa–mediated enhancement of the activation of factor X (12,140,141). *In vivo*, the nega-tively charged phospholipids are likely provided by activated platelets and damaged endothelial cells. Factor VIII and factor V bind phosphatidylserine by both hydrophobic and electro-static interactions (142–147). However, factor V does not effi-ciently compete with the binding of factor VIII to phospholipid vesicles composed of 15% phosphatidyl-L-serine (140). Under equilibrium conditions, factor VIII can bind phospholipid vesi-cles containing 15% to 25% phosphatidylserine with an appar-ent $K_d$ of 2 to 4 nM (98,117,140). Saturation occurs between 170 and 385 moles of phospholipid per mole of factor VIII (140), although the process involves both rapid and slow inter-actions (148). Factor VIII binding to phospholipid involves stereo-selective recognition of the *o*-phospho-L-serine moiety of phosphatidylserine (98). Because the composition of phos-phatidylserine exposed on the platelet membrane surface can increase from 2% to 13% after stimulation (149), the increase in phosphatidylserine content could account for the ability for factor VIII to specifically bind the surface of thrombin-activated platelets.

Addition of negatively charged phospholipids to the factor VIII–VWF complex dissociates factor VIII from VWF (85,111). Interestingly, thrombin-treated factor VIII does not bind VWF with high affinity (91,150,151) but binds phospholipid with a 10-fold increased affinity compared with that of the procofac-tor, factor VIII (152). On basis of the capacity of the anti-C2 monoclonal antibody, ESH8, to lock the conformation of C2 into the low affinity form, this effect is thought to result from a conformational change within the C2 domain following ac-tivation. The phospholipid-binding domain within factor VIII is localized to the light chain (153,154), and antibody inhibi-tion studies suggest that the phospholipid binding site likely occurs in the C2 domain (155).

## Molecular Modeling of Factor VIII

Although the crystal structure for factor VIII is not available, a molecular model of the A-domains of factor VIII, based on the crystal structure of the homologous plasma protein ceruloplas-min, was proposed (29). In the model, the three A-domains are arranged in a triangular configuration. Each A-domain is com-posed of two "d" subdomains consisting of a β-barrel structure.

Therefore, the d1 subdomain is at the N-terminus of the A1 domain, whereas the d6 subdomain is located at the C-terminus of the A3 domain. This model comprises only the A-domains and lacks the intervening acidic regions and the B- and C-domains. This model can be used to visualize the two sites in the factor VIII A-domains that are interactive with factor IXa (see Fig. 8-4). The model suggests that the two interaction sites are in close prox-imity and located on the same face of the factor VIII molecule. Complementary sites in factor IXa are not fully known. How-ever, studies have implicated residues in the Gla domain (156), the first and second epidermal growth factor domains (EGF1 and EGF2) (157,158), and the serine protease domain (159) as con-taining factor VIII interactive regions. The crystal structure of factor IXa shows it to be an elongated molecule analogous to a tulip with the γ-carboxyglutamic acid (Gla)– rich, EGF, and ser-ine protease domains representing the bulb, stem, and flower, re-spectively (160). The Gla domain binds the protease to the phospholipid surface, whereas the active site is located high above the membrane surface ( >70 Å, 13,131). The A3-C1-C2 sub-unit of factor VIIIa associates with the phospholipid surface via residues in the C2 domain. Therefore, it is reasonable to spec-ulate that high-affinity binding sites in factors VIIIa and IXa in-volve a surface-proximal interaction between the A3 domain of factor VIIIa and the Gla-EGF domains of factor IXa. On the other hand, the A2 subunit of factor VIIIa is likely high above the surface on the basis of the five-domainal model (161). Further-more, as described earlier, the A2 subunit directly modulates the active site of factor IXa. Therefore, a surface-distal, weaker affin-ity interaction likely occurs between the A2 subunit and the ser-ine protease domain. The recent x-ray structure of the bovine factor Va A1/A3-C1-C2 dimer obtained following inactivation by APC (162) may provide added insights into the interactions of factor VIII(a) subunits, because models derived from this struc-ture would likely be superior to existing ones on the basis of structural and functional homologies of factor V and VIII.

In contrast, a high-resolution x-ray structure of the factor VIII C2 domain was determined (163). It predicts a β-sandwich

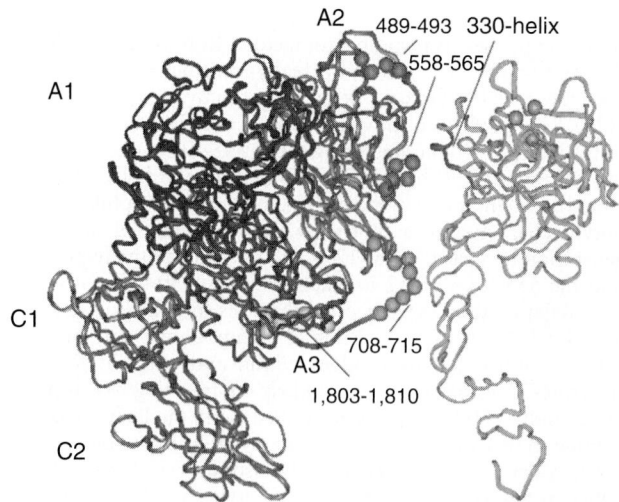

**FIGURE 8-4.** Molecular modeling of the factor Xase. Factor VIIIa (*left*) and factor IXa (*right*) are drawn in *ribbon* format on the basis of the five-domainal model of factor VIII (161) and the crystal structure of factor IXa (160), respectively. Factor IXa is shown in *green* with the 330 helix shown in *red*. *Spheres* indicate the α carbon positions of the active site residues. Factor VIII domains are coded as A1 (*blue*), A2 (*cyan*), A3 (*red*), and C-domains (*copper*). *Spheres* indicate α car-bon positions for the indicated factor IXa–interactive sites (see Color Fig. 8-4). (Reprinted from Fay PJ, Jenkins PV. Mutating factor VIII: lessons from structure to function. *Blood Rev* 2005;19:15-27, with permission from Elsevier.)

core (40 Å × 30 Å) with two pairs of hydrophobic residues extending from adjacent loops that contribute to phospholipid binding. The two hydrophobic spikes comprising Met2199/Phe2200 and Leu2251/Leu2252 are proposed to penetrate the lipid bilayer and associate with the aliphatic hydrocarbon chains. On the other hand, a ring of basic residues (Arg2215, Arg2220, Lys2227, and Lys2249) localized above the hydrophobic residues contributes electrostatic interactions. A number of point mutations resulting in hemophilia A that map to the C2 domain tend to cluster at the protein core region rather than at putative membrane-binding sites. One explanation proposed for this observation (164) is that the binding energy reflects the additive nature of several side chains at the membrane interface. For this reason, single-point mutations within this flexible region may be tolerated. Conversely, mutations within the protein core of the C2 domain could disrupt folding and interfere with secretion, thereby producing loss of function. Studies on two-dimensional crystals of factor VIII bound to phospholipid have yielded gross information (at approximately 15 Å resolution) to generate a model for the orientation of five domains: three A- and two C-domains (165). This surface-bound model of factor VIII has utility in assembling and modeling complex structures such as the factor Xase complex. Unfortunately, these models do not consider what changes occur upon activation of factor VIII to factor VIIIa. However, these three-dimensional models do provide a basis for predictions of intramolecular and intermolecular interactions.

## Regulation of Cofactor Activity

### Activation of Cofactor Function

Upon treatment of intact factor VIII with thrombin or factor Xa, there is a rapid, greater than 30-fold increase and subsequent first-order decay of procoagulant activity. However, the maximal activation by thrombin is greater than that observed with factor Xa (166). The activation coincides with proteolysis of both the heavy and light chains of factor VIII, as depicted in Figure 8-1. Cleavage within the heavy chain at Arg740 generates a 90,000 MW polypeptide that is subsequently cleaved at Arg372 to generate polypeptides of 50,000 MW and 43,000 MW (167). These polypeptides are designated as the A1 (residues 1–372) and A2 (residues 373–740) subunits, respectively, owing to their domainal derivations. Concomitantly, the 80,000 MW light chain is cleaved at Arg1689 to generate a 73,000 MW polypeptide (168) designated as the A3-C1-C2 subunit (residues 1690–2332). Regions rich in acidic amino acids that contain the posttranslational modified amino acid tyrosine-sulfate border each of these cleavage sites (169). The tyrosine-sulfate residues enhance thrombin cleavage at adjacent sites but do not affect factor Xa cleavage (170). These observations suggest that thrombin selectively utilizes tyrosine sulfate residues to facilitate interaction and/or cleavage. In support of this contention is data showing that a mutation at a tyrosine sulfation site (Tyr346 to Cys) yielded a factor VIII that was defective in activation by thrombin (171). In addition, recent results support a primary role of the factor VIII C2 domain in containing an interactive site for thrombin (172) and factor Xa (173) docking, leading to subsequent catalysis.

Significant data support that thrombin anion-binding exosites I and II are involved in recognition of factor VIII. For example, thrombin activation of factor VIII is inhibited by either heparin, a molecule that interacts with anion-binding exosite II, or hirugen, a peptide that contains tyrosine sulfate and binds the anion-binding exosite I of thrombin (174,175). Mutagenesis studies confirmed the roles for these exosites in cleaving the procofactor. Substitution of Arg residues 93, 97, and 101 with Ala yields a thrombin molecule possessing a triple mutation, designated thrombin RA, that did not bind heparin (176) and was slow to activate factor VIII (175). A single-point mutation in thrombin, Arg98Ala, possessed approximately 40% the activity of wild-type thrombin (177). Interestingly, this mutation showed disparate activities relative to the scissile bonds. Although similar rates of cleavage of light chain (Arg1689–Ser1690) were observed for the mutant and wild-type enzymes, the mutant protein showed only approximately 30% of the wild-type activity directed toward cleaving factor VIII at the Arg372 to Ser373 site (177). This result suggested that the relative contribution of distinct interactive sites varies depending upon the location of the cleavage site. Similarly, evaluation of an extensive collection of point mutations in exosite 1 identified several critical residues involved in this interaction (177). Specifically, Ala-scanning mutagenesis at six sites (Lys21, His66, Lys65, Arg68, Arg70, and Tyr71) showed less than 50% in activation compared to the wild-type procofactor. Two of these mutations, Arg68Ala and Tyr71Ala, showed reduced activity in cleaving the thrombin-sensitive bonds in the light chain and at the junction of the A1 and A2 domains.

Numerous studies have correlated the appearance of the 50,000, 43,000, and 73,000 MW polypeptides with peak factor VIII activity (167,178,179). Mutagenesis studies showed that cleavages after residues 740 and 1648 were not required for cofactor activity (180,181). In contrast, mutation at either Arg372 or Arg1689 yielded molecules that were not cleaved by thrombin at the mutated site and were not susceptible to thrombin activation (180). The importance of cleavage at residues 372 and 1689 for factor VIII activation was demonstrated *in vivo* by the identification of patients with hemophilia A having missense mutations that prevent cleavage at either Arg372 or Arg1689 (182–185). These findings indicate that activation requires cleavage at both residues 372 and 1689, but does not appear to require a specific sequential order for cleavage at these sites. Cleavage at Arg1689 releases factor VIII from the inhibitory influence of VWF (186) and appears to additionally increase the activity of factor VIIIa (187,188). Cleavage at Arg372 is essential to expose a functional factor IXa–interactive site(s) in the A2 domain that is cryptic in the inactivated molecule (189).

Factor VIIIa is a heterotrimer of A1, A2, and A3-C1-C2 subunits (188,190,191). The A1 and A3-C1-C2 subunits retain the metal ion linkage and can be isolated as a stable A1/A3-C1-C2 dimer. Conversely, the A2 subunit is associated with the A1/A3-C1-C2 dimer in a primarily electrostatic interaction and readily dissociates from the dimer at physiologic pH and ionic strength (see subsequent text). However, under appropriate reaction conditions, factor VIIIa can be reconstituted from isolated A1/A3-C1-C2 dimer and A2 subunit (190,191). The affinity of A2 subunit for the A1/A3-C1-C2 was measured following functional assay (192,193), as well as physical assay employing surface plasmon resonance (194) or fluorescence energy transfer (136). In human factor VIIIa, the affinity of A2 subunit for the A1/A3-C1-C2 dimer ($K_d$ approximately 260 nM at physiologic pH) is increased 10-fold under slightly acidic conditions ($K_d$ approximately 30 nM at pH = 6.0) (192). The subunit structure of porcine factor VIIIa generated following factor Xa cleavage was identified (195). This cofactor form is somewhat more complex than thrombin-activated factor VIIIa and consists of five subunits resulting from additional cleavages at Arg219 within the A1 domain and Arg490 within the A2 domain. Factor Xase composed of factor Xa–activated factor VIIIa shows reduced catalytic efficiency compared with thrombin-derived factor VIIIa, possessing a reduced $k_{cat}$ and increased $K_m$ (195), likely a reflection of this altered subunit structure.

Little information is available about residues in the A2 subunit and A1/A3-C1-C2 dimer that are involved in the intersubunit interactions. Earlier studies suggested that the C-terminal region of the A1 subunit participated in the retention of A2 subunit following cleavage at the A1–A2 junction. A2 subunit did not appear to bind the A1/A3-C1-C2 dimer in which the A1 subunit has been truncated at residue 336 (122,194). Furthermore, a synthetic peptide corresponding to factor VIII residues 337 to 372 inhibited the association of A2 subunit with the A1/A3-C1-C2 dimer (196) as measured in a functional assay. However, recent results showed similar affinity of A2 subunit for an A1 subunit truncated at Arg336 (197), suggesting that this C-terminal region of A1 may function in orienting A2 within the factor Xase complex (136) rather than contributing substantially to the intersubunit binding energy. Complementary interactive sites in A2 subunit are poorly defined. Analyses using peptide inhibition of functional assays and binding as measured by fluorescence energy transfer suggested three segments in A2 (residues 373–395, 418–428, and 518–533) that interact with the A1/A3-C1-C2 dimer (198).

Furthermore, a number of missense mutations have been reported that give rise to a one-stage/two-stage discrepancy (199–203) wherein the one-stage assay yields a greater activity value than the two-stage assay, an indicator that the cofactor possesses increased lability, likely a result of an increased dissociation rate of A2 subunit. These mutations occur in A1, A2, and A3 domains of factor VIII and many lie at the interdomainal interfaces with the A2 domain. In many cases, these mutations increase A2 domain rate of dissociation by three- to fourfold (199–203). This observation suggests these residues may directly participate in interactions involving A2 subunit retention following cleavage at the A1–A2 boundary during cofactor activation. Alternatively, mutations at these residues may lead to detrimental interactions at the interface that facilitate A2 dissociation.

Aside from identification of cleavage sites, the structural alterations that transform "procofactor" factor VIII into active cofactor, factor VIIIa, are not well characterized. Circular dichroism spectral analyses indicate that purified factor VIIIa shows considerable reduction in random coil and increase in β-sheet structures compared with factor VIII (118); however, it is unclear what contribution the B-domain makes to these gross conformational differences. Zero-length cross-linking studies suggest formation of a new salt bridge between the N-terminal half of A2 subunit and the C-terminal region of A1 subunit following thrombin cleavage (204). Taken together, these results suggest that activation of factor VIII resulting of limited proteolytic cleavage is accompanied by changes in the protein conformation.

## Inactivation of Cofactor Function

Factor Xase has been regarded as "self-damping" (205), and the labile nature of this complex reflects the decay of factor VIIIa. The affinity of A2 subunit for the A1/A3-C1-C2 dimer ($K_d$ approximately 260 nM; 192,193) greatly exceeds the concentration of factor VIII in plasma (approximately 1 nM). Therefore, one would predict that activation of factor VIII would be followed by immediate and near complete dissociation of A2 subunit. The dissociation rate constant for loss of A2 subunit in human factor VIIIa (approximately 0.35 per minute) is markedly faster than that observed with porcine factor VIIIa (approximately 0.12 per minute), indicative of a higher affinity interaction in the latter (193). Indeed, that study showed that reconstitution of factor VIIIa using porcine A2 subunit plus human A1/A3-C1-C2 yielded a hybrid factor VIIIa molecule possessing threefold higher specific activity than factor VIIIa reconstituted from the human subunits.

However, an effect opposing dissociation of subunits is the capacity for factor IXa to stabilize the labile factor VIIIa heterotrimer. Lollar et al. (206) determined that at low factor VIIIa (<1 U per mL) and factor IXa (5 nM) and in the presence of

phospholipid, porcine factor VIIIa was stabilized from spontaneous decay. More recently, it was determined that factor IXa transiently enhanced the reconstitution of factor VIIIa from isolated subunits by a mechanism consistent with reducing the intersubunit dissociation rate constant (207). One mechanism by which factor IXa stabilizes factor VIIIa may involve interaction of the enzyme with sites on the A2 subunit and A3 domain to in effect tether the labile subunits. However, it was observed in that study that prolonged reaction of factor VIIIa with factor IXa resulted in proteolysis in the A1 subunit and subsequent inactivation of the cofactor. Sequence analysis revealed that factor IXa cleaved the A1 subunit at Arg336 (208,209), thereby altering interaction of A1 with the A2 subunit to yield a low activity conformation. A secondary, slow reacting site at Arg1719 was also identified; however, cleavage at this site is not inactivating (210). This factor VIII–directed proteolytic activity coupled with the inter-factor VIIIa subunit stabilizing activity provides factor IXa mechanisms for regulating its own activity by modulating the activity of its cofactor. Therefore, a situation of "reciprocal regulation" appears to exist and may influence the activity of intrinsic factor Xase.

Contributions of cofactor dissociation and cleavage to the decay of factor Xase have been modeled using a recombinant factor VIII possessing an Arg336 to Ile substitution that is resistant to cleavage by factor IXa (210). This analysis showed that the decay of factor Xase primarily resulted from A2 subunit dissociation when reactant concentrations were below the Kd for the factor VIIIa–factor IXa interaction, whereas factor IXa–catalyzed proteolysis of the A1 subunit primarily accounted for the decay of activity at higher reactant levels. This factor IXa–catalyzed cleavage of the cofactor was inhibited by factor X, possibly by a steric mechanism given the close proximity of the cleavage site to the factor X interactive site [residues 336-372; (131)]. Therefore, decay of factor Xase by proteolysis may be blocked until conditions of substrate depletion exist. Modeling of the coagulation cascade reactions predicts the formation of low concentrations of factor IXa (211). Furthermore, mathematical simulations of clotting require inclusion of constraints associated with factor Xase lability (211). On the basis of these models, the weak affinity inter-factor VIIIa subunit interaction may be a primary regulator of factor Xase activity. For this reason, there is high interest in developing novel factor VIII forms with enhanced intersubunit stability. Using recombinant DNA technology, novel factor VIII molecules have been constructed possessing covalent attachment of the A2 domain to the light chain of factor VIII and have yielded factor VIIIa molecules that were stable following thrombin activation (109,212).

APC is a potent anticoagulant, and its importance as a regulator of blood coagulation is apparent from predisposition to thrombosis in individuals with protein C deficiency [see ref. (213) for review]. The anticoagulant effect is phospholipid- and $Ca^{2+}$-dependent and results from the selective inactivation of factor Va and factor VIIIa. Cleavage of factor VIIIa occurs at Arg562 (122), bisecting the A2 subunit and Arg336 (122,167) preceding the C-terminal acidic region of the A1 subunit. The former cleavage occurs within a factor IXa interactive site and has been shown to effect the factor VIIIa–dependent modulation of the factor IXa active site, as judged by fluorescence anisotropy (132). The latter cleavage likely influences the affinity of the A1/A3-C1-C2 dimer for A2 subunit, as well as affecting the interaction of factor VIIIa with substrate factor X. APC-catalyzed cleavage appears to be ordered. Using the bovine enzyme, the A2 subunit is cleaved initially (122), whereas the human enzyme cleaves the A1 subunit initially (214). Factor IXa selectively protects cleavage of factor VIIIa at Arg562; however, this effect is abrogated by inclusion of protein S (123), a cofactor for APC. APC-catalyzed inactivation of factor VIIIa maybe secondary to its inactivation by subunit dissociation. Comparison of rates of cofactor inactivation attributable to APC action suggest factor Va is the primary substrate, because most factor VIIIa activity loss was not the result of proteolysis (214). Furthermore, studies using a reconstituted coagulation model show greater degradation of factor Va compared with factor VIIIa by the APC pathway (215).

APC resistance is one of the major causes of hereditary thrombophilia as a consequence of an Arg-to-Gln mutation in the APC cleavage site in factor V at residue 506 (216–218). The APC-resistant phenotype was first reported as a poor anticoagulant response to APC in an activated partial thromboplastin time assay (called the APC resistance ratio) (216). It is possible that APC-resistant mutations in factor VIII may also lead to hereditary thrombophilia. Analysis of mutant factor VIII protein demonstrated that cleavage at either Arg336 or Arg562 only partially inactivated factor VIII and that resistance to cleavage at both Arg336 and Arg562 was necessary to detect a poor anticoagulant response in an activated partial thromboplastin time assay (219). These results show that a single mutation in either factor APC cleavage site to yield cleavage resistance would not be detected as a poor anticoagulant response *in vitro*. In addition, a search did not identify any mutations at Arg336 or 562 in factor VIII in 125 patients with venous thrombosis (220). The sum of these studies indicates that it is unlikely mutations in factor VIII APC cleavage sites will result in thrombophilia.

Factor Xa also catalyzes inactivating cleavages in factor VIIIa, and because this protease is a product of factor Xase, suggests a potential to participate in its downregulation. Factor Xa cleaves factor VIIIa at Arg336 (167) and Lys36 (221) in the A1 subunit. Loss of activity because of cleavage at the latter site is less well understood than cleavage at Arg336 but appears to result in an altered conformation of this subunit affecting interaction with A2 subunit (221). The interaction of protease with the factor VIII substrate appears to require residues in the C2 domain (173) and the C-terminal region of A1 subunit (221). Binding to the latter site may make use of a heparin-binding exosite (221) recently identified in factor Xa (222). Overall, the relative contributions of spontaneous A2 subunit dissociation and proteolysis mediated by APC, factor Xa, or factor IXa in limiting factor VIIIa *in vivo* remain unclear.

## Modulation by Biological Membranes

Procoagulant activity is profoundly affected by the presence of cellular surfaces. Upon platelet activation by thrombin, the platelet surface exhibits procoagulant activity. This activity results from the exposure of negatively charged phospholipids and possibly specific receptors for the coagulation factors. Negatively charged phospholipids are usually confined to the inner leaflet of cellular membranes (223,224) and are exposed upon cellular lysis at sites of injury. Inactivated platelets exhibit binding sites for factor Va and Xa (225–227). Platelet activation is associated with exposure of factor VIII and factor IXa binding sites (135,228–230). There are approximately 400 factor VIII sites per activated platelet ($K_d$ approximately 4 nM), and factor V cannot compete with factor VIII binding (228). Factor VIIIa binds to an additional 300 to 400 sites with approximately twofold enhanced affinity ($K_d$ approximately 2 nM) (231). Coordinate binding effects on the platelet surface involving factors VIIIa, IXa, and X have been observed [see (232) for review]. For example, in the presence of saturating, active site-modified factor IXa, factor X binds platelets with approximately 25-fold greater affinity ($K_d$ approximately 5 nM) in the presence of factor VIIIa, forming a stoichiometric complex (233). These results suggest that factor VIIIa binds platelets with high affinity and presents substrate factor X to factor IXa. The specificity in binding of factor VIII suggests that a specific protein receptor for factor VIII is involved. In addition, the kinetics of thrombin generation mediated by the prothrombinase complex on pure phospholipid surfaces compared to activated platelets suggests that a specific saturable receptor exists for prothrombinase and probably also for the factor Xa–generating enzyme complex (234). However, a classical membrane receptor has not yet been identified.

Platelet binding is mediated by the factor VIII light chain and is inhibited by the presence of VWF. A factor VIII mutant protein that cannot bind VWF with high affinity retains its ability to bind platelets (86). Therefore, the VWF-binding site and the platelet-binding site appear to be distinct within the factor VIII molecule. Isolated factor VIII domains and monoclonal antibodies have been used to probe platelet-binding interactions. Results from these studies [reviewed in (232)] provided evidence for a platelet receptor-binding site within C2 domain residues 2303 to 2332 and an additional binding site contained within C2 residues 2248 to 2285 that increases the affinity and stoichiometry of factor VIIIa binding in the presence of factors IXa and X. Studies using isolated, recombinant C2 domain showed an approximately sevenfold weaker affinity for the platelet membrane than that observed for intact factor VIIIa, suggesting that other light chain domains (A3 and/or C1) may contribute to the affinity of this interaction.

The anticoagulant properties of the endothelial cell surface is maintained by several independent mechanisms: (a) heparin sulfate on the surface of endothelial cells accelerates the inactivation of thrombin by antithrombin III; (b) thrombomodulin expressed on endothelial cells alters the proteolytic specificity of thrombin so that it activates protein C; (c) endothelial cells secrete prostacyclin, an inhibitor of platelet aggregation, and tissue plasminogen activator, an initiator of fibrinolysis. The endothelium also exhibits dramatic procoagulant activities. Activated endothelial cells induce expression of tissue factor and can mediate the activation of factor X. Endothelial cells contain high-affinity receptors for factor IX or IXa and for factor X (235,236). At present, it is not known if specific binding sites for factor VIII exist on endothelial cells. Therefore, the endothelial cell surface may positively or negatively influence factor VIII activity through the generation of APC or by the binding of factor IXa and X to initiate assembly of the factor X activating complex.

## Factor VIII Clearance from the Circulation

In the circulation, factor VIII(a) catabolism is mediated by low density lipoprotein receptor-related protein (LRP) (237–239), a hepatic clearance receptor. LRP is a large cell surface receptor that is ubiquitously expressed in a variety of tissues and is present on a wide range of cell types, including hepatocytes, smooth muscle cells, and monocytes. It is a member of the low density lipoprotein (LDL) receptor family of endocytotic receptors and recognizes a wide range of distinct ligands.

Factor VIII interacts with LRP through at least three distinct sites, one localized within the C2 domain (237), one localized to within residues 1804 to 1834 of the A3 domain (120), and the other within residues 484 to 509 in the A2 domain (238). Therefore, the presence of multiple binding sites allows for uptake of factor VIII, as well as factor VIIIa subunits A1/A3-C1-C2 and A2 that have undergone dissociation. A recent report described construction of a chimeric factor V/factor VIII molecule wherein factor VIII residues 1811 to 1818 were replaced with the homologous residues in factor V (120). Although LRP binding was reduced markedly, cofactor activity was largely eliminated. The presence of an LRP interaction site in C2 suggests that this interaction would be blocked when factor VIII is associated with VWF. Indeed, the association of factor VIII with VWF reduced its binding to LRP by more than 90% (237).

It has been established that LRP contributes to the cellular uptake and subsequent lysosomal delivery of factor VIII *in vitro*

(237,238). *In vivo*, the factor VIII half-life was prolonged in mice by a bolus administration of purified receptor-associated protein (RAP), a protein that inhibits ligand binding to LRP, or by deletion of LRP (238,240). In VWF knockout mice, LRP blockade increased factor VIII levels similar to that obtained by providing VWF (241). The affinity of the factor VIII–LRP interaction [$K_d$ values of approximately 60 to 120 nM, (237,238) relative to the circulating concentration of factor VIII (approximately 1 nM)] has led investigators to suggest mechanisms that would contribute to the concentration of factor VIII(a) on the cell surface. Cell-surface heparan sulfate proteoglycans (HSPG) demonstrate high affinity for factor VIII and an HSPG-binding site was localized to residues 558 to 565 within the A2 domain (242).

# MOLECULAR BASIS FOR HEMOPHILIA A

## Hemophilia A

The gene for factor VIII is located on the human X chromosome, and therefore hemophilia A is a classic example of X-linked recessive inheritance. It occurs almost exclusively in men because they have only one X chromosome; women with one abnormal copy of the factor VIII gene are carriers, because the other X chromosome contains a normal copy of the gene. The frequency of the disorder is 1 in 5,000 to 10,000 male births, and there is no particular ethnic group that has unusually lower or higher incidence of the disease. Severe hemophilia A was in the past a genetically lethal disease in which affected men produced few offspring. Therefore, nearly one third of the mutant alleles would be lost in each generation. Haldane, in 1935, predicted that in order to maintain a constant frequency in the population, about one third of cases would be the result of novel mutations. The prediction was proven to be correct because a large number of different mutations exist in the factor VIII gene and many patients carry a *de novo* mutation not present in the X chromosome of their mothers. One notable exception to the Haldane prediction is the case of the common inversion of factor VIII (see subsequent text).

The severity and frequency of bleeding in the patients correlates with the level of factor VIII activity in plasma (243). Approximately 50% to 60% of patients have severe hemophilia A with factor VIII activity less than 2% of normal; these patients have frequent spontaneous bleeding into joints, muscles, and internal organs. Moderately severe hemophilia A occurs in approximately 25% to 30% of patients; the factor VIII activity is 2% to 10% of normal, and there is bleeding after minor trauma. Mild hemophilia occurs in 15% to 20% of patients and is associated with factor VIII activity of 20% to 30% where bleeding occurs only after a major trauma or surgery. Individuals with factor VIII activity greater than 30% do not have symptoms of hemophilia A. Of particular interest for understanding the mechanism factor VIII action is a category of patients with a considerable amount of factor VIII protein in their plasma (at least 30% of normal) but in whom the protein is nonfunctional. Approximately 5% of patients belong to this category, termed CRM (cross-reacting material) positive (244). CRM-reduced is another category in which the factor VIII antigen and activity are equally reduced.

## Factor VIII Gene Structure

The factor VIII gene is 186 kb long (approximately 0.1% of the DNA of the X chromosome) and contains 26 exons and 25 introns. The nucleotide sequence of the exons, intron–exon boundaries, 5′ and 3′ untranslated regions, has been determined (8,205). The exon length varies from 69 to 262 nucleotides except for exon 14, which is 3,106 nucleotides, and the last exon 26, which has 1,958 nucleotides (see Fig. 8-5). There are some large intervening sequences, including IVS22, which is 32 kb long.

The factor VIII mRNA is approximately 9 kb, of which the coding sequence is 7,053 nucleotides. There is a CpG island within IVS22 that is associated with two additional transcripts. One transcript of 1.8 kb is produced abundantly in a wide variety of cells. The orientation of this transcript is opposite to that of factor VIII and contains no intervening sequence (245). This 1,739 nt long cDNA, termed factor VIII–associated gene A (F8A), is conserved in the mouse (246). The second transcript [factor VIII–associated gene B (F8B)] of 2.5 kb is transcribed in the same direction as factor VIII and, after a short exon that may encode for 8 amino acids, it utilizes exons 23 to 26 of the factor VIII gene (247). The two transcripts F8A and F8B originate within 122 bases from each other. The sequences of F8A and F8B, along with a few kilobases of surrounding DNA, are also present in two other areas of the X chromosome approximately 400 kb telomeric to factor VIII gene (245,248). The function of these transcripts and their potential protein products is unknown. Transgenic mice with a deletion of the F8B gene showed eye abnormalities that included anterior segment dysgenesis, absent or abnormal lens, persistence of the primary vitreous, Harderian gland tumors, and ectopic pigmented cells, suggesting that migration of neural crest cells might have been perturbed during eye development (249).

The promoter (5′ flanking) region of factor VIII has been studied in liver-derived cell lines. More than 12 protein binding sites distributed up to 1 kb upstream of the transcription start site have been identified. A region up to approximately 300 nucleotides contains all the necessary elements for maximal promoter activity (250). The putative TATA box is not essential for factor VIII promoter activity. Liver-enriched transcription factors such as hepatocyte nuclear factor (HNF)1, NFκB, C/enhancer binding protein (EBP)$\alpha$, and C/EBP$\beta$ interact with the factor VIII promoter region (250).

The factor VIII gene maps on the long arm of the X chromosome in the most distal band Xq28. Haldane and Smith (251) reported linkage of hemophilia A with color blindness, and Boyer and Graham (252) demonstrated close linkage of hemophilia A with polymorphisms at the G6PD locus. The order of these loci and the direction of transcription, as revealed by the genome analysis of Xq28, is Xcen-G6PD-3′F8-5′F8-Xqter (248). The distance from factor VIII gene to the Xq telomere was estimated to be approximately 1 Mb. In the most recent sequence assembly of the human genome sequence (http://www.ensembl.org), the F8 gene maps approximately 153.6 Mb of the X chromosome (nucleotides 153,627,773 to 153,814,702 bp); the Xqter is at 154.8 Mb. The next centromeric gene is MPP1 that ends 30 kb upstream, whereas the next telomeric gene (on the opposite strand) is FUNDC2, which ends just 4 kb downstream.

## Factor VIII Gene Defects

The factor VIII gene of more than 4,500 patients with hemophilia A has been examined for molecular defects using a variety of methods. A database of mutations in the factor VIII gene has been created and is constantly updated (http://europium.csc.mrc.ac.uk/usr/WWW/WebPages/main.dir/main.htm and 253). The human gene mutation database (HGMD; http://www.hgmd.org) also provides a comprehensive list of the F8 mutations. In this latter database, each pathogenic mutation was entered once regardless of the recurrences in different families. Figure 8-6 depicts the different kinds of mutations found in

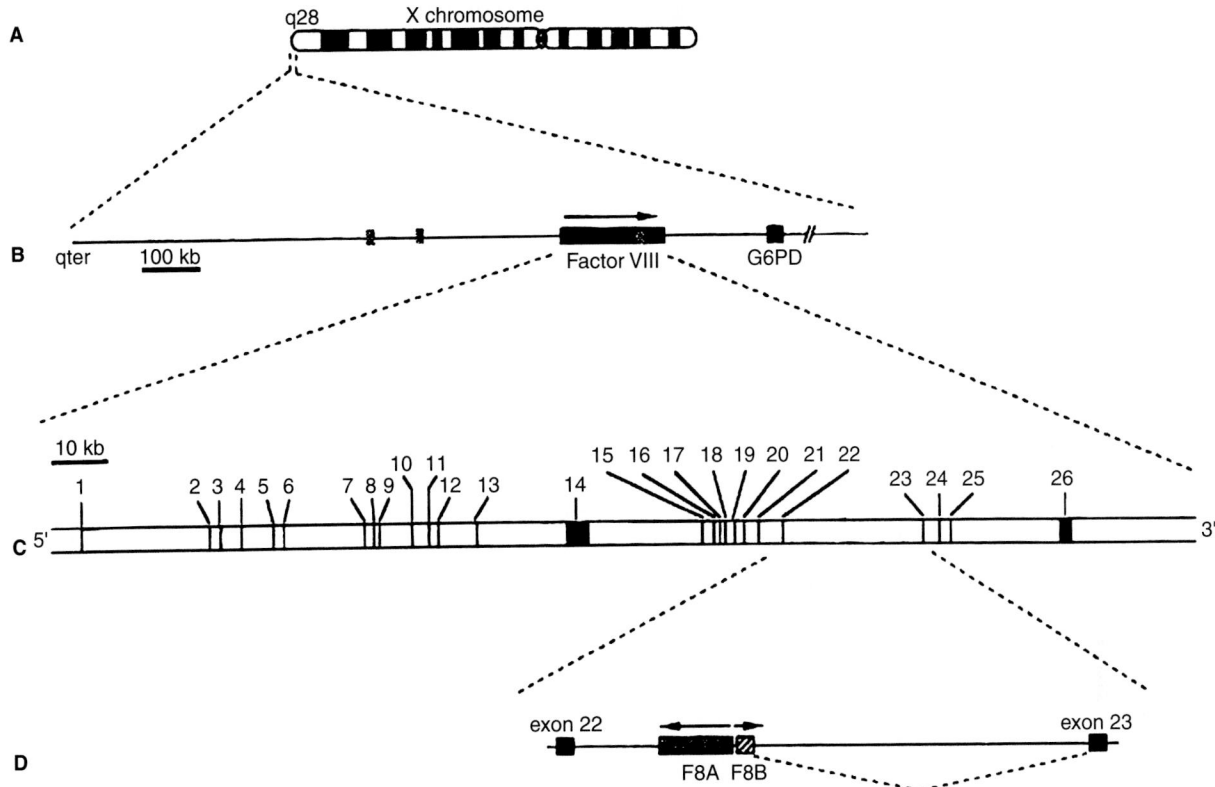

**FIGURE 8-5.** Chromosomal localization and structure of the factor VIII gene. The factor VIII gene is located on the X-chromosome (**A**), approximately 1,000 kb from the Xqter (**B**). It is 186 kb long and contains 26 exons (**C**). In the large intron 22, there are two nested genes, the intronless F8A and F8B, which utilizes the exon 23 of the factor VIII gene as its second exon (**D**). There are three copies of the F8A–F8B sequences on Xq28, as shown by the *gray boxes* (**B**). See text for further discussion of the gene structure. (Reprinted from Kaufman RJ and Antonarakis SE. Structure, biology, and genetics of factor VIII. In: Hoffman R, Benz EJ Jr, Shattil SJ et al., eds. *Hematology: basic principles and practice,* 4th ed. Philadelphia: Elsevier, 2005, with permission.)

patients with hemophilia A from the studies of references (254,255) as updated after the identification of the common inversion by Lakich et al. (256). These studies were selected because they are the first in which almost all mutations have been

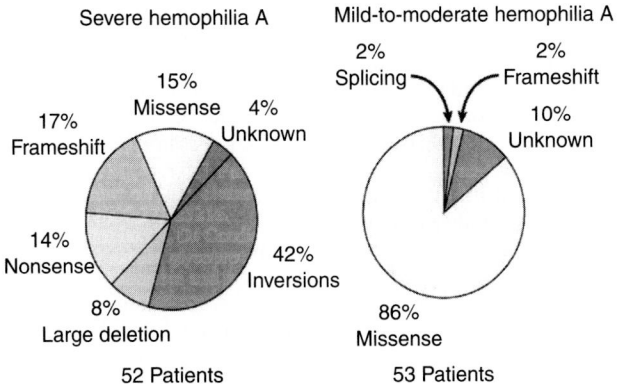

**FIGURE 8-6.** Factor VIII gene defects in severe and mild to moderate hemophilia A. The frequency of gene defects in severe and mild to moderate hemophilia A are shown as identified from studies in which all mutations were identified in a given sample (254,255,273). (Reprinted from Kaufman RJ and Antonarakis SE. Structure, biology, and genetics of factor VIII. In: Hoffman R, Benz EJ Jr, Shattil SJ et al., eds. *Hematology: basic principles and practice,* 4th ed. Philadelphia: Elsevier, 2005, with permission.)

identified in a given sample. The HGMD on the December 13, 2004, release contained 844 different pathogenic F8 mutations that cause hemophilia A of variable severity (see Table 8-2). The hemophilia A mutation database on the November 12, 2004, release contained 1,012 unique pathogenic mutations (Table 8-2). The total number of point mutations in the database (including all multiple occurrences) is 1,392. The clinical severity of these mutations was mild in 34% patients, moderate in 18%, severe in 33% patients, and unreported in 14% cases. Both databases contained complete lists of references and personal communications about the pathogenic F8 mutations.

Even after extensive search for mutations in patients with well-documented X-linked hemophilia A, there are approximately 5% to 10% of patients in whom the pathogenic molecular defect remains uncharacterized. The mutations in these cases could reside in unknown functional genomic elements within or close to F8 gene. Such functional elements have been recently recognized by comparative analysis of the human genome with that of the mouse (257).

### Gross DNA Rearrangements

**The Common Partial Inversion in the Factor VIII Gene.** Lakich et al. in 1993 and Naylor et al. in 1993 (256,258) found that approximately 40% of patients with severe hemophilia A have a partial inversion of the factor VIII gene (the gene up to and including exon 22 is inverted). The inversion is due to homologous recombination between the region that includes the F8A gene in intron 22 and one of the two other homologous

**TABLE 8-2**

PATHOGENIC F8 MUTATIONS CAUSING HEMOPHILIA
IN SELECTED DATABASES

- Human Gene Mutation Database 13th December 2004
  (unique mutations regardless of recurrence)
  http://www.hgmd.org

  | | |
  |---|---:|
  | Nucleotide substitution: missense codon | 426 |
  | Nucleotide substitution: nonsense codon | 92 |
  | Nucleotide substitution: splicing error | 51 |
  | Nucleotide substitution: regulatory | 0 |
  | Small deletions (up to 20 bp) | 119 |
  | Small insertions (up to 20 bp) | 38 |
  | Small indels (insertion/deletions) | 5 |
  | Gross deletions | 87 |
  | Gross insertions and duplications | 7 |
  | Complex rearrangements (including inversions) | 9 |

- The hemophilia A mutation database 12th November 2004
  (unique mutations)
  http://europium.csc.mrc.ac.uk/usr/WWW/WebPages/main.
  dir/main.htm

  | | |
  |---|---:|
  | Nucleotide substitution: missense codon | 501 |
  | Nucleotide substitution: nonsense codon | 108 |
  | Nucleotide substitution: splicing error | 62 |
  | Nucleotide substitution: regulatory | 0 |
  | Small deletions (up to 50 bp) | 163 |
  | Small insertions (up to 50 bp) | 58 |
  | Gross deletions | 120 |

regions located more than 400 kb 5′ (telomeric) to the factor VIII gene (256) (see Fig. 8-7). The regions of homology are each 9.5 kb long, and there is more than 98% nucleotide sequence identity among them (259). Depending upon which extragenic copy of gene A is involved in the crossing-over event, two main types of inversions are recognized. Type 1 inversion affects the distal, whereas type 2 inversion the proximal copy (256). In addition, a rare type 3 results from an inversion occurring in individuals carrying more than two extragenic copies of gene A. The inversions originate almost exclusively in male meiosis (260). Because the mutation occurs very rarely in female germ cells, nearly all mothers of patients with inversions are carriers of factor VIII deficiency. A consortium analysis of 2,093 patients with severe hemophilia A revealed an inversion of factor VIII in 890 or 43% (261). Inversion type 1 accounts for 83% and type 2 for 16% of the inversion cases; the type 3 patterns were observed in only 1% of the cases. Other, more rare rearrangements that involve intron 22 have been described. The discovery of this mutation is of considerable clinical significance because it accounts for approximately 25% of all patients with hemophilia A and greater than 40% of those with severe disease. It is of interest that a similar intron 22 inversion has been detected in the Chapel Hill colony of factor VIII–deficient dogs; these animals are frequently used for gene therapy trials (262).

A second inversion of similar mechanism has been identified in intron 1 of the F8 gene (257,263). This inversion is mediated by a 1,041-bp duplicon that maps within intron 1 and approximately 140 kb telomerically near the VBP1 gene. The two copies of the duplicon differ by only one nucleotide and are in opposite orientation. The inversion is caused by intrachromosome or intrachromatid homologous recombination that results in splitting of exon 1 from the remainder of F8 and severe hemophilia A. The frequency of that inversion in intron 1 accounts for 2% to 4.8% of patients with severe hemophilia A (263).

**Large Deletions.** In approximately 5% of the patients with hemophilia A, there are large (more than 100 nucleotides) deletions in the factor VIII gene (264). The mutation database contains 120 different deletions (see http://europium.csc.mrc. ac.uk/WebPages/Main/main.htm). Patients with the same breakpoints are rare, suggesting that factor VIII gene does not contain sequences that are prone to become deletion breakpoints. Deletions almost always produce severe hemophilia A; however, a deletion of exon 22 and another deletion of exons 23 to 24 were associated with moderate disease probably because of in-frame joining (after mRNA splicing) of exons 21 and 23 in one case and exons 22 and 25 in the other, to produce proteins lacking 52 and 98 amino acids, respectively. Few deletion breakpoints have been characterized by nucleotide sequencing and do not occur in repetitive elements such as Alu sequences. There is usually 2 to 4 nucleotide homology at the junction point, and the deletion mechanism is probably by nonhomologous recombination (265). A total of 43 of the 96 patients (45%) with deletions for which data were available have developed inhibitors (antibodies against factor VIII) after treatment.

**Insertion of Retrotransposons.** *De novo* insertion of long interspersed nuclear element (LINE) repetitive elements in the human genome was first reported in the factor VIII gene in two cases of severe *de novo* hemophilia A (266). In one case, a 3.8 kb portion of a LINE element was inserted in exon 14 of factor VIII. The full-length "active" LINE element responsible for this insertion maps on chromosome 22q11 and probably encodes for a reverse transcriptase. The *de novo* insertion in the second case was a 2.1 kb portion of a LINE element and occurred in a different site of exon 14. LINE elements comprise approximately 20% of the human genome, and there are approximately 850,000 copies (267). The full length of the element is 6.5 kb, and most of the copies in the human genome are partial and defective. The consensus sequence of LINE element contains two open reading frames, the second of which predicts a protein with amino acid homology to viral reverse transcriptase. Approximately 3,000 LINE copies are full length and are potential transposable elements. Some of these are probably transcribed and then reinserted as double-stranded DNA into a new genomic site. The master gene produces an mRNA that is probably reverse-transcribed (possibly by a reverse transcriptase encoded by itself), and the double-stranded nucleic acid is then reinserted into an A-rich region of the genome. LINEs likely integrate into genomic DNA by a process called target-primed reverse transcription (268). The proposed mechanism of LINE retrotransposition is as follows: an active LINE is transcribed in the nucleus and is subsequently transported to and translated in the cytoplasm. The two LINE proteins, ORF1 and ORF2, complex with their LINE transcript in ribonucleoprotein particles. The complex is then transported to recipient DNA sequences where target-primed reverse transcription occurs. The new, integrated LINE copy is usually truncated at its 5′ end. L1s have shaped mammalian genomes through a number of mechanisms. First, they have greatly expanded the genome both by their own retrotransposition and by providing the machinery necessary for the retrotransposition of other mobile elements, such as Alu sequences. Second, they have shuffled non-L1 sequence throughout the genome by a process termed transduction. Accidents of retrotransposition could cause diseases.

**Duplications.** Two duplications have been described in the factor VIII gene. In one, there was a duplication of 23 kb of IVS22 inserted between exons 23 to 25 (269). This rearrangement found in two female siblings was apparently unstable and led to deletion of exons 23 to 25 in the male offspring of one of the women. In the second case, there was an in-frame duplication of exon 13 in a patient with mild hemophilia A (270).

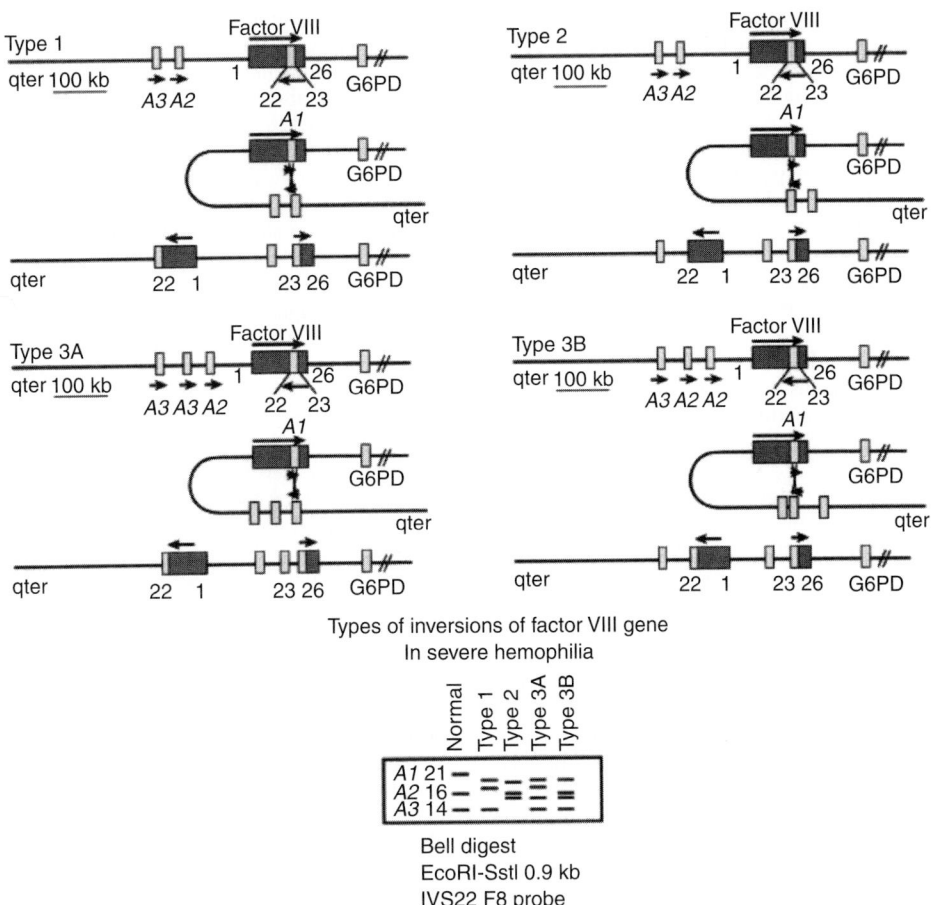

**FIGURE 8-7.** Factor VIII gene inversions in hemophilia A. Owing to intrachromosomal crossing-over between the homologous regions A1, A2, and A3, there is an inversion of factor VIII sequences encompassing exons 1 to 22. The various types of inversion (types 1, 2, 3A, and 3B) are shown. These inversions are easily recognizable after Southern blot analysis using part of the homologous regions as probe (*bottom of the figure*). (Reproduced from Kaufman RJ and Antonarakis SE. Structure, biology, and genetics of factor VIII. In: Hoffman R, Benz EJ Jr, Shattil SJ et al., eds. *Hematology: basic principles and practice*, 4th ed. Philadelphia: Elsevier, 2005, with permission.)

**Chromosomal Rearrangement Breakpoints Involving the Factor VIII Gene.** A complex *de novo* translocation of chromosomes X and 17 [46,X,t(X;17)] was reported in a woman with severe hemophilia A (271). The normal X, always late replicating, contained a normal factor VIII gene. The der(17) contained a deleted factor VIII gene that lacked exons 1 to 15; exons 16 to 26 were present in another autosome. One of the breakpoints of the complex rearrangement was therefore between exons 15 and 16 of the factor VIII gene.

## Point Mutations and Small (<100 bp) Deletion/Insertions

**Small Deletions or Insertions.** Small deletions or insertions in the coding region of factor VIII gene that result in frameshifts and cause severe hemophilia A have been reported in more than 200 unrelated patients (253; see http://europium.csc.mrc.ac.uk/usr/WWW/WebPages/main.dir/main.htm and www.hgmd.org for tables and references). The database contains 163 small deletions (1 to 23 nucleotides) among 892 independent point mutations recorded (18%). There are 58 small insertions (1 to 31 nucleotides) (6.5% of the total point mutations). More than one third of the small deletions and half of the insertions were found as expected in the large exon 14. Most small deletions/insertions occur in DNA regions of short direct repeats. Consistent with

this observation are the multiple occurrences of identical mutations in short nucleotide repeats. There are, for example, more than 50r recurrent deletions or insertions of 1 bp (adenine) in a string of 9, as in codons 1191 to 1194 of exon 14. The most plausible mechanism for small deletions or insertions mediated by the presence of direct nucleotide repeats is the slipped mispairing model. Almost all of the mutations that result in translation frameshifts cause severe hemophilia A. An exception was observed in a family with moderately severe hemophilia A that had a deletion of a single nucleotide T within an $A_8TA_2$ sequence of exon 14. A small amount of functional factor VIII protein was detected in the patient's plasma. There was evidence for a partial correction of the defect because of (i) DNA replication/RNA transcription errors resulting in restoration of the reading frame and/or (ii) "ribosomal frameshifting" resulting in the production of normal factor VIII polypeptide and, therefore, in a milder than expected hemophilia A. All of these mechanisms probably were promoted by the longer run of adenines, $A_{10}$ instead of $A_8TA_2$, after the delT (272).

**Nonsense Mutations.** There are 235 independent nonsense mutations in 105 different codons that are included in the point mutation database, comprising 17% of the total number of 1,373 nucleotide substitutions (253; see http://europium.csc.mrc.ac.uk/usr/WWW/WebPages/main.dir/main.htm for table and references). Remarkably, 119 of the 235

(51%) independent nonsense mutations are CGA to TGA (Arg to Stop) substitutions due to the hypermutability of CpG dinucleotide. In two samples of 52 patients with severe hemophilia A (255,273) in which all point mutations have been characterized, the number of nonsense codons were seven, that is, 13.5% (7 of 52) of the total severe mutations or 29% (7 of 24) of the severe point mutations.

**CpG Dinucleotide Hypermutability.** The study of point mutations in factor VIII led to the discovery of a mutation hotspot at CpG dinucleotides in which there is a common substitution CG to TG if the mutation occurs in the sense strand or CG to CA if the mutation occurs in the antisense strand (274). The mutations probably occur because, in mammalian DNA, most CpG dinucleotides are methylated (at the 5 carbon of cytosine) by methyltransferase; the subsequent spontaneous deamination of the 5-methylcytosine produces a TpG dinucleotide. The mutation usually occurs in tissues in which the gene is not expressed (275). There are 540 independent mutations in 46 sites that conform to the CG to TG rule (40%). There are 35 sites in which recurrent mutation at CpG dinucleotides has occurred. An unbiased estimate of the frequency of CG to TG mutation may be obtained from studies in which all point mutations have been characterized in a given sample of patients (254,255,273,276). In these studies, a total of 84 point mutations have been characterized, and 32 are of the CG to TG rule (38%). It has been estimated that in the factor VIII gene, CG to TG or CA mutations are 10 to 20 times more frequent than mutations of CG to any other dinucleotide (277). The mutation hotspot has subsequently been observed in a wide variety of other human genes related to disease phenotypes. For example, 45% of pathogenic mutations in 11 X-linked disorders (1,712 out of 3,840) obey the CG to TG hypermutability (278).

**Exon Skipping Due to Nonsense Mutations.** An important observation concerning nonsense mutations has been made in the factor VIII gene and independently in the fibrillin and ornithine aminotransferase genes (273,279). In some cases, a nonsense codon mutation can lead to abnormal RNA processing in which the exon containing the mutation is skipped. In one case of E1987X in exon 19, all detectable mRNA lacked exon 19. In the second case of R2116X in exon 22, there was approximately 50% of mRNA without exon 22, whereas the remaining 50% of mRNA was of normal size. The junctions of exons 18 to 20 and 21 to 23 do not result in translational frameshift. This phenomenon is termed nonsense-mediated altered splicing (NAS), and its underlying mechanism is unclear. It was recently recognized that any nucleotide substitution in exons (nonsense, missense, or translationally silent point mutation) that disrupts a splicing enhancer or silencer may affect either the pattern or efficiency of mRNA splicing (280,281).

**Missense Mutations.** Missense mutations that result in amino acid substitutions, are important for understanding the function of the protein and the pathophysiology of the disease. A total of 501 missense mutations in 1,138 unrelated patients are included in the database; some of them are schematically presented in Figure 8-8 (see http://europium.csc.mrc.ac.uk/usr/WWW/WebPages/main.dir/main.htm for table and references). These mutations are spread throughout the gene except for exon 14 that encodes for domain B, which is devoid of amino acid substitutions that cause hemophilia A. Despite the wealth of amino acid substitutions found, the mode of action of most these mutations in producing reduced factor VIII activity in plasma is unknown. Several mutations have been identified that alter specific factor VIII molecular interactions and result in CRM positive hemophilia A. First, there are mutations in patients with CRM-positive hemophilia A that affect the thrombin cleavage sites. Mutations R372H, R372C, and S373L have been shown *in vitro* to abolish this cleavage in the heavy chain (182, 185,282). Mutations R1689C and R1689H abolish thrombin

cleavage at the light chain (184,254) and result in CRM-positive hemophilia A. Second, the Y1680F substitution at the site of tyrosine sulfation that is required for high-affinity VWF interaction has been observed in patients with moderate, CRM reduced hemophilia A (283). The Y1680F mutant factor VIII has lost high-affinity binding to VWF, presumably because the Phe residue cannot be sulfated (170,284). Finally, two other CRM-positive mutations produce severe hemophilia A by creating new N-glycosylation sites in the protein (285). The first I566T creates a new such site at N564 (NQI to NQT) in the A2 domain. The second new site is in the A3 domain; the mutation is M1772T, changing the N1770 (NIM to NIT). In both cases, factor VIII is present at normal levels in plasma, but it is completely inactive. When the plasma of either patient is deglycosylated, factor VIII activity is restored to a significant degree. Inhibition assays using synthetic peptides corresponding to residues 558 to 565, previously shown to be a factor IXa–interaction site, provided support that the defect in the I566T mutant factor VIII is caused by steric hindrance for the interaction with factor IXa (286). Missense mutations S558P, V559A, D560A, and Q565R modulate FIXa enzymatic activity. The stability of activated FVIII is affected by mutations such as R531H, A284E, S289L, N694I, R698W, and R698L.

**Splicing Errors.** Only 62 potential splicing errors have been found (http://europium.csc.mrc.ac.uk/usr/WWW/WebPages/main.dir/main.htm). There are 12 mutations in the invariant AG of the acceptor splice site and 12 in the invariant GT of the donor splice site in various introns; the majority are associated, as expected, with severe disease. All the other mutations are within the donor or acceptor splice-site consensus, and two are in cryptic sites. No formal proof that the mutations cause abnormal splicing has been obtained. In addition, it is likely that mutations within exons that affect splice enhancers may cause abnormal splicing and hemophilia A (280).

**Promoter Mutations.** No examples of mutations in the 5′ untranslated region of factor VIII gene have been reported to date. If such mutations do occur, they are probably infrequent because two laboratories failed to find any nucleotide substitutions in 530 nucleotides of the 5′ flanking region of factor VIII in 227 patients with hemophilia A (283). Alternatively, mutations in regulatory regions may cause mild reductions in factor VIII gene expression that do not result in hemophilia A. Finally, certain *cis*-acting regulatory regions may not be yet known, and therefore, the mutation searches do not target these elements.

## Combined Factors V and VIII Deficiency

Combined factors V and VIII deficiency is an autosomal recessive disease that was described in 1954 by Oeri et al. (287). To date, a total of 89 patients in 58 families have been reported, where 24 of the families are from the Mediterranean region. Patients with this disorder exhibit factor V and factor VIII antigen levels in the range of 5% to 30% that correlates with the activity measurements. Bleeding is similar to that observed in other coagulation factor deficiencies. The levels of all other plasma proteins that have been measured appear normal in these patients, including those of the homologous copper ion–binding protein ceruloplasmin. Although there have been several reports of individuals who simultaneously inherited mutations in both the factor VIII and factor V gene (288), this is rare (approximately 1 per $10^{10}$).

Although it was originally proposed that combined deficiency of factors V and VIII resulted from a loss of protein C inhibitor (289), more recently, homozygosity mapping and positional cloning approaches were used to identify the defective gene as *LMAN1* (Mannose-binding lectin), encoding the protein ERGIC-53 (endoplasmic reticulum and Golgi intermediate compartment 53-kDa protein). Haplotype analysis among

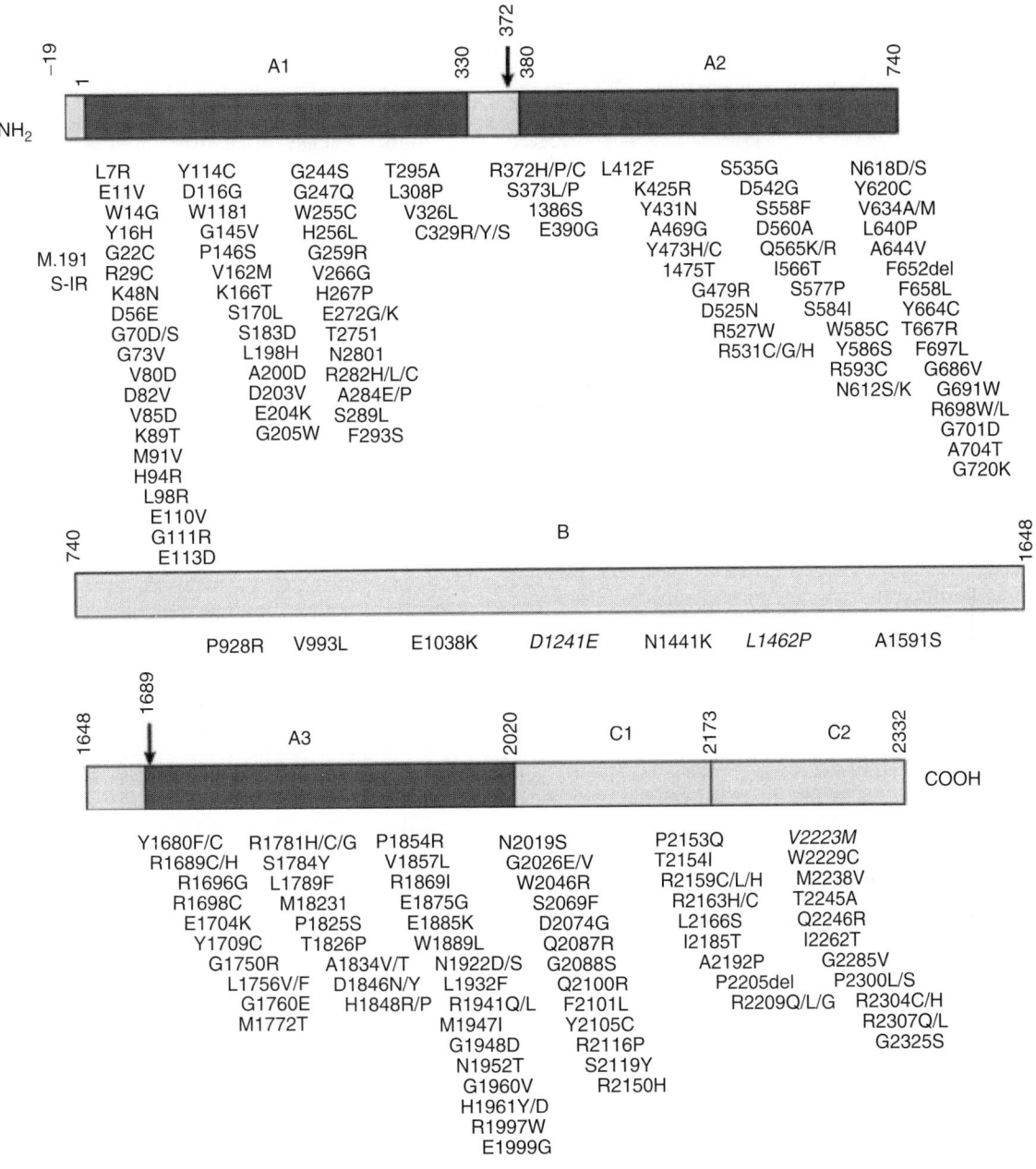

**FIGURE 8-8.** Missense mutations in the factor VIII gene. The structural domains of the protein are shown and the amino acid substitutions are depicted using the one-letter code for amino acids. For example, E11V indicates a Glu to Val substitution at amino acid residue 11; similarly, R282H/L/C indicates that Arg282 is substituted by His, Leu, or Cys in different patients. (Reproduced from Kaufman RJ and Antonarakis SE. Structure, biology, and genetics of factor VIII. In: Hoffman R, Benz EJ Jr, Shattil SJ et al., eds. *Hematology: basic principles and practice,* 4th ed. Philadelphia: Elsevier, 2005, with permission.)

these families suggested that two independent founders gave rise to two mutations in all of the original nine unrelated families studied. DNA sequence analysis of additional patients has identified the following mutations: a Met1Thr substitution; three nonsense mutations in codons 202, 302, and 456; four splicing errors in the donor splice sites of introns 5, 7, and 9; six small deletions, and three small insertions (290,291).

*LMAN1* encodes a 53,000-MW transmembrane protein of the ER-Golgi intermediate compartment (hence, ERGIC-53) that has mannose-binding capability and that cycles between the ER and the Golgi compartment (292,293). Analysis of lymphocytes from patients with factors V and VIII deficiency demonstrated a complete lack of LMAN1 protein (294). Factor VIII directly interacts with LMAN1, and cells that are defective in LMAN1 are selectively defective in the secretion of factor V and factor VIII (295,296).

However, approximately 30% of individuals with combined deficiency of factor V and factor VIII had normal levels of LMAN1. Recently, inactivating mutations in *MCFD2* (multiple coagulation factor deficiency 2) were demonstrated to cause a phenotype identical to that caused by mutations in *LMAN1* (297). *MCFD2* encodes a protein that interacts with LMAN1 to form a specific receptor for transport of factors V and VIII. The elucidation of defects in LMAN1 or MCFD2 as the cause for combined factor V and VIII deficiency supports the hypothesis that the selective loss of factors V and VIII in the plasma is due to defective intracellular transport and secretion unique to these two coagulation factors. Both factor VIII and factor V contain an unusually heavily glycosylated B-domain, suggesting that LMAN1 may interact with the B-domain to facilitate their intracellular transport and secretion.

# THE FUTURE FOR HEMOPHILIA A THERAPY

## Factor VIII Inhibitors

One of the major limitations with present factor VIII replacement therapy is the development of inhibitory antibodies to factor VIII (known as inhibitors) in approximately 10% to 20% of patients with severe hemophilia A (298,299). The etiology of inhibitor development is unknown (300). Studies attempting to relate inhibitor development with HLA haplotypes have had little success. Epitope mapping has shown specificities against the heavy or light chain or both in different patients (266,268). Studies established that the most common factor VIII epitopes that induce inhibitory antibodies are localized to the A2 domain (residues 373–740), the C2 domain (residues 2173–2332), and possibly the A3 domain (106,301–304). Lollar et al. prepared chimeric molecules that had amino acid residues between 484 and 508 in human factor VIII replaced by the respective porcine residues. The resultant factor VIII displayed less reactivity to antifactor VIII inhibitory antibodies (106).

The analysis of many factor VIII mutations and their association with inhibitor development may uncover some rules, if such exist, concerning the contribution of the nature of the mutations to inhibitor formation. In the consortium analysis of more than 900 patients with factor VIII inversions, 130 patients out of 642 studied had developed inhibitors (20%); in the control population of patients with severe hemophilia A without inversions, 131 out of 821 patients had developed inhibitors (16%) (261). These results are not statistically different, suggesting that factor VIII inversions are not a predisposing factor for inhibitor development.

Most of the reported inhibitor cases have nonsense mutations, deletions, or inversions in their factor VIII gene. Among 164 patients with missense mutations and inhibitor status information, 54 had developed inhibitors (33%). Among 758 patients with missense mutations and inhibitor status information, 55 had developed inhibitors (7%). There are, however, 41 missense mutations reported in the database that are associated with low levels of inhibitors. Among the nonsense mutations, R1941X is associated with inhibitors in 10/14 cases; R2147X in 5/17, R2209X in 6/19, K1827X in 2/2, and R1696X in 2/2 cases. Other nonsense mutations, however, (for example, eight cases with R336X or nine cases with R2116X), were rarely associated with inhibitors. In these cases, exon skipping may provide a protein merely lacking 20 to 50 amino acids (exon skipping has been detected for R2116X mutation 273 in which inhibitors have never been observed). Among the 41 missense mutations, inhibitors have been recurrently observed in Arg593, Arg1997, Glu1999, Tyr2105, Arg2150, Arg2209, Trp2229, and Pro2300. A relatively high incidence of inhibitors occurs in missense mutations in the region between residue 1940 and the C-terminus. Gross deletions of the factor VIII gene result in two fold to threefold increased incidence of inhibitors compared to patients without detectable deletions (305). However, no clear picture has emerged as to the correlation between the size or the breakpoints of the deletions and the development of inhibitors.

## Genetic Diagnosis

The molecular elucidation of the defects in the factor VIII gene in many patients with hemophilia A has dramatically changed the practice of diagnosis of carriers and affected fetuses. The discovery of the common partial inversion of the factor VIII gene (256) provided a means of diagnosis using Southern blot analysis. This defect accounts for approximately 45% of severe hemophilia A. The diagnosis of the exact molecular defect in the remaining families is still not practical even in most laboratories. Because of the enormous variety of the remaining mutations, DNA diagnosis is limited to indirect detection using linked DNA polymorphisms; however, a small number of diagnostic laboratories provide sequence analysis of all exons and intron–exon junctions of the FVIII gene. For the linkage studies, the affected factor VIII gene is marked within the family using polymorphic markers both within (256,306–309) and outside (310,311) the gene. Nearly all families are informative, but 20% to 30% for extragenic polymorphisms only. In those families, the chance of error is 2% to 5%, depending on the polymorphism used. When an intragenic polymorphism is used, the chance of error is negligible (<1%).

The indirect detection of mutant genes is not feasible when only one male offspring is available and the carrier status of the mother is unknown. In these cases, direct detection of molecular defect should be employed, but few diagnostic service laboratories are dealing with the direct detection of nucleotide substitutions. The situation has dramatically changed with the simple test to recognize the common partial inversion of factor VIII, which accounts for approximately 45% of cases of severe hemophilia A. Most laboratories use Southern blot analysis for the detection of the inversion. A method of long-distance polymerase chain reaction (LD-PCR) has been developed for the rapid detection of the inversion (312,313), but it is not widely used because of false-negative results. Other than the detection of the inversion, few laboratories deal with the remaining molecular defects. Further technical improvements are needed to make the analysis faster and less costly. The availability of high-density oligonucleotide arrays (314) for the factor VIII gene will permit the rapid detection of most of the missense mutations in patients with moderately severe and mild hemophilia A.

## Animal Models for Hemophilia A

There are both small and large animal models available to evaluate improved therapeutic regimens for hemophilia A and to study the role of factor VIII *in vivo*. Several dogs have been diagnosed with spontaneous mutations in the factor VIII gene, and two colonies have been established that are frequently used for research. The founder of the Chapel Hill hemophilia A dog colony was an Irish Setter with severe hemophilia A that has an inversion in the factor VIII gene inside intron 22, analogous to the common deletion in humans (262). The founder of the Queen's University hemophilia A dog colony was a miniature Schnauzer and likely has a similar genetic defect (315). The affected dogs have spontaneous bleeding into soft tissues and joints and have prolonged *in vitro* whole blood and plasma clotting times. The cuticle bleeding time test is a unique *in vivo* clotting assay in which the nail is cut to the quick and time to stop bleeding is measured. This test is frequently used to test efficacy of therapeutic regimens in the dog model (316).

A mouse with severe factor VIII deficiency was created by targeted insertion of a neomycin resistance gene into either exon 16 or exon 17 of the murine factor VIII gene (317). The two strains of resulting affected mice have less than 1% factor VIII activity and bleeding after minor trauma, a phenotype similar to that observed in severe hemophilia A (317). However, affected mice do not bleed spontaneously. Heterozygous female mice show, as expected, factor VIII levels that are approximately 50% of normal. Affected female mice were also produced; when bred with affected male mice, they survived pregnancy and delivery. RT-PCR of liver mRNA indicated that the factor VIII deficiency in the exon 16 knockout mice is due to truncated protein, whereas in exon 17 knockout mice, it is due to either truncated or partially deleted protein (318). Assay of cryoprecipitate from the plasma of affected mice using two anti-mouse factor VIII monoclonal antibodies failed to detect any factor VIII. The mice with hemophilia A provide an excellent animal model for gene therapy experiments and the study of factor VIII inhibitors.

## Gene Therapy

Although prophylactic treatment of hemophilia A can reduce the frequency and severity of bleeding, this therapy is limited by availability and high cost of factor VIII, the short half-life of factor VIII *in vivo*, and difficulties associated with frequent administration. In addition, development of inhibitory antibodies is a serious problem in approximately 20% of patients. Hemophilia A has been discussed as a logical candidate disease gene for gene therapy for several reasons (319). First, the factor VIII gene and protein are well characterized. Second, the levels of factor VIII that would have considerable therapeutic benefit can be as low as 10 ng per mL, or approximately 10% of normal plasma values. Third, expression of factor VIII does not need to be regulated and only requires that the protein be delivered to the plasma in a biologically active form. Finally, the immunologic response to factor VIII administered by intravenous infusion into patients with hemophilia A is well characterized and provides a foundation for understanding immunologic responses that may develop with gene therapy. However, several features of factor VIII have limited development of gene therapy protocols for hemophilia A, compared to factor IX for hemophilia B. First, the factor VIII gene is large, greater than 180 kb, and the cDNA is greater than 7 kb, too large to effectively package into most available viral vectors for gene transfer. As a consequence, most studies to date have used a B-domain deleted factor VIII that is only 4.5 kb (320,321). Second, accumulation of factor VIII mRNA (322–324) and secretion of the protein are inefficient (44,45). Deletion of the B-domain does not affect function, activity, or immunogenicity, but the levels of mRNA expression and protein expression are dramatically improved (92,325). Finally, factor VIII is susceptible to proteolysis and requires VWF to prevent its degradation (44).

Although initial progress in hemophilia A gene therapy was made through use of adenoviral vectors to deliver the factor VIII gene, hepatotoxicity due to an immunologic response to the virus limits utility. More recent progress has been made using adeno-associated virus and lentivirus as delivery vectors. A number of reports have now described either partial and/or persistent correction of hemophilia A in both murine and canine models (326–335).

Over the last several years, three phase 1 clinical trials have been conducted for hemophilia A (336,337). The first trial involved introducing a factor VIII expression plasmid into autologous fibroblasts *ex vivo* and subsequent injection of the expanded fibroblasts into the greater omentum. Four of the six patients showed an improvement in factor VIII concentration (0.5% to 3.5% increase) or had decreased spontaneous bleeding episodes. However, the factor VIII levels decreased to the pretreatment levels in all patients after 10 months (338). In the second trial, the B-domain–less factor VIII cDNA in an amphotropic murine leukemia retrovirus was given by peripheral vein infusion in 13 patients. There was no considerable change in the bleeding tendency, and none of the patients have

sustained concentrations of factor VIII above 0.01 IU per mL (339). The third trial involved a modified adenovirus containing the factor VIII cDNA. One patient was recruited, and sustained concentrations of factor VIII of approximately 0.01 IU per mL were observed over several months (336,337). Clearly, considerably more work is needed to achieve a safe and effective gene therapy protocol. The use of lentiviral and adenoassociated viruses (AAV) and the development of more efficient nonviral DNA-mediated delivery methods are now being explored for the development of alternative and improved clinical trials (326). However, the potential benefit of gene therapy needs to be compared with the current safe and effective replacement therapy by intravenous infusion of purified and recombinant factor VIII protein. The benefit from gene therapy versus the potential risks should be carefully considered before any clinical trial is considered (340–342).

## References

1. Rosner F. Hemophilia in the Talmud and rabbinic writings. *Ann Intern Med* 1969;70:833–837.
2. Otto JC. An account of an hemorrhagic disposition existing in certain families. *Clin Orthop Relat Res* 1996;328:4–6.
3. Lane S. Haemorrhagid diathesis. Successful transfusion of blood. *Lancet* 1840;1:185–188.
4. Addis T. The pathogenesis of hereditary hemophilia. *J Pathol Bacteriol* 1911;15:426–452.
5. Patek AJ, Taylor FHL. Hemophilia II: Some properties of a substance obtained from normal human plasma effective in accelerating the coagulation of hemophilic blood. *J Clin Invest* 1937;16:113–124.
6. Fulcher CA, Zimmerman TS. Characterization of the human factor VIII procoagulant protein with a heterologous precipitating antibody. *Proc Natl Acad Sci U S A* 1982;79:1648–1652.
7. Toole JJ, Knopf JL, Wozney JM, et al. Molecular cloning of a cDNA encoding human antihaemophilic factor. *Nature* 1984;312:342–347.
8. Vehar GA, Keyt B, Eaton D, et al. Structure of human factor VIII. *Nature* 1984;312:337–342.
9. Lusher JM, Arkin S, Abildgaard CF et al. Kogenate Previously Untreated Patient Study Group. Recombinant factor VIII for the treatment of previously untreated patients with hemophilia A. Safety, efficacy, and development of inhibitors. *N Engl J Med* 1993;328:453–459.
10. Bray GL, Gomperts ED, Courter S et al. The Recombinate Study Group. A multicenter study of recombinant factor VIII (recombinate): safety, efficacy, and inhibitor risk in previously untreated patients with hemophilia A. *Blood* 1994;83:2428–2435.
11. Marder VJ, Mannucci PM, Firkin BG, et al. Standard nomenclature for factor VIII and von Willebrand factor: a recommendation by the International Committee on Thrombosis and Haemostasis. *Thromb Haemost* 1985;54:871–872.
12. van Dieijen G, Tans G, Rosing J, et al. The role of phospholipid and factor VIIIa in the activation of bovine factor X. *J Biol Chem* 1981;256:3433–3442.
13. Mutucumarana VP, Duffy EJ, Lollar P, et al. The active site of factor IXa is located far above the membrane surface and its conformation is altered upon association with factor VIIIa. A fluorescence study. *J Biol Chem* 1992;267:17012–17021.
14. Rizza CR, Rhymes IL. Coagulation assay of VIIIc and IXa. In: Bloom AL, ed., *The hemophilias*, Vol. 5. Edinburgh, New York: Churchill Livingstone, 1982.
15. Hamer RJ, Koedam JA, Beeser-Visser NH, et al. Human factor VIII: purification from commercial factor VIII concentrate, characterization, identification and radiolabeling. *Biochim Biophys Acta* 1986;873:356–366.
16. Suomela H, Blomback M, Blomback B. The activation of factor X evaluated by using synthetic substrates. *Thromb Res* 1977;10:267–281.
17. Nordfang O, Ezban M, Nilsson P, et al. Radioimmunoassay for quantitative measurement of factor VIII-heavy chain. *Br J Haematol* 1988;68:307–312.
18. Girma JP, Fressinaud E, Houllier A, et al. Assay of factor VIII antigen (VIII:CAg) in 294 haemophilia A patients by a new commercial ELISA using monoclonal antibodies. *Haemophilia* 1998;4:98–103.
19. Fass DN, Knutson GJ, Katzmann JA. Monoclonal antibodies to porcine factor VIII coagulant and their use in the isolation of active coagulant protein. *Blood* 1982;59:594–600.
20. Rotblat F, O'Brien DP, O'Brien FJ, et al. Purification of human factor VIII:C and its characterization by Western blotting using monoclonal antibodies. *Biochemistry* 1985;24:4294–4300.
21. Jenny RJ, Pittman DD, Toole JJ, et al. Complete cDNA and derived amino acid sequence of human factor V. *Proc Natl Acad Sci U S A* 1987;84:4846–4850.
22. Koschinsky ML, Funk WD, van Oost BA, et al. Complete cDNA sequence of human preceruloplasmin. *Proc Natl Acad Sci U S A* 1986;83:5086–5090.

23. Poole S, Firtel RA, Lamar E, et al. Sequence and expression of the discoidin I gene family in Dictyostelium discoideum. *J Mol Biol* 1981;153:273–289.

24. Stubbs JD, Lekutis C, Singer KL, et al. cDNA cloning of a mouse mammary epithelial cell surface protein reveals the existence of epidermal growth factor-like domains linked to factor VIII-like sequences. *Proc Natl Acad Sci U S A* 1990;87:8417–8421.

25. Elder B, Lakich D, Gitschier J. Sequence of the murine factor VIII cDNA. *Genomics* 1993;16:374–379.

26. Bihoreau N, Pin S, de Kersabiec AM, et al. Copper-atom identification in the active and inactive forms of plasma-derived FVIII and recombinant FVIII-delta II. *Eur J Biochem* 1994;222:41–48.

27. Tagliavacca L, Namdvo Moon N, Dunham WR, et al. Identification and functional requirement of Cu(I) and its ligands within coagulation factor VIII. *J. Boil Chem* 1997;272(43):27428–27434.

28. Wakabayashi H, Koszelak ME, Mastri M, et al. Metal ion-independent association of factor VIII subunits and the roles of calcium and copper ions for cofactor activity and inter-subunit affinity. *Biochemistry* 2001;40:10293–10300.

29. Pemberton S, Lindley P, Zaitsev V, et al. A molecular model for the triplicated A domains of human factor VIII based on the crystal structure of human ceruloplasmin. *Blood* 1997;89:2413–2421.

30. Fay PJ. Reconstitution of human factor VIII from isolated subunits. *Arch Biochem Biophys* 1988;262:525–531.

31. Sudhakar K, Fay PJ. Effects of copper on the structure and function of factor VIII subunits: evidence for an auxiliary role for copper ions in cofactor activity. *Biochemistry* 1998;37:6874–6882.

32. Wise RJ, Dorner AJ, Krane M, et al. The role of von Willebrand factor multimers and propeptide cleavage in binding and stabilization of factor VIII. *J Biol Chem* 1991;266:21948–21955.

33. Wakabayashi H, Schmidt KM, Fay PJ. Ca(2+) binding to both the heavy and light chains of factor VIII is required for cofactor activity. *Biochemistry* 2002;41:8485–8492.

34. Wakabayashi H, Zhen Z, Schmidt KM, et al. Mn2+ binding to factor VIII subunits and its effect on cofactor activity. *Biochemistry* 2003;42:145–153.

35. Zeibdawi AR, Pryzdial EL. Mechanism of factor Va inactivation by plasmin. Loss of A2 and A3 domains from a Ca2+-dependent complex of fragments bound to phospholipid. *J Biol Chem* 2001;276:19929–19936.

36. Wakabayashi H, Freas J, Zhou Q, et al. Residues 110-126 in the A1 domain of factor VIII contain a Ca2+ binding site required for cofactor activity. *J Biol Chem* 2004;279:12677–12684.

37. Marchioro TL, Hougie C, Ragde H, et al. Hemophilia: role of organ homografts. *Science* 1969;163:188–190.

38. Lewis JH, Bontempo FA, Spero JA, et al. Liver transplantation in a hemophiliac. *N Engl J Med* 1985;312:1189–1190.

39. Kelly DA, Summerfield JA, Tuddenham EG. Localization of factor VIIIC antigen in guinea-pig tissues and isolated liver cell fractions. *Br J Haematol* 1984;56:535–543.

40. Zelechowska MG, van Mourik JA, Brodniewicz-Proba T. Ultrastructural localization of factor VIII procoagulant antigen in human liver hepatocytes. *Nature* 1985;317:729–730.

41. Wion KL, Kelly D, Summerfield JA, et al. Distribution of factor VIII mRNA and antigen in human liver and other tissues. *Nature* 1985;317: 726–729.

42. Hollestelle MJ, Thinnes T, Crain K, et al. Tissue distribution of factor VIII gene expression *in vivo*—a closer look. *Thromb Haemost* 2001;86:855–861.

43. Do H, Healey JF, Waller EK, et al. Expression of factor VIII by murine liver sinusoidal endothelial cells. *J Biol Chem* 1999;274:19587–19592.

44. Kaufman RJ, Wasley LC, Dorner AJ. Synthesis, processing, and secretion of recombinant human factor VIII expressed in mammalian cells. *J Biol Chem* 1988;263:6352–6362.

45. Dorner AJ, Bole DG, Kaufman RJ. The relationship of N-linked glycosylation and heavy chain-binding protein association with the secretion of glycoproteins. *J Cell Biol* 1987;105:2665–2674.

46. Dorner AJ, Wasley LC, Kaufman RJ. Increased synthesis of secreted proteins induces expression of glucose-regulated proteins in butyrate-treated Chinese hamster ovary cells. *J Biol Chem* 1989;264:20602–20607.

47. Dorner AJ, Wasley LC, Kaufman RJ. Overexpression of GRP78 mitigates stress induction of glucose regulated proteins and blocks secretion of selective proteins in Chinese hamster ovary cells. *EMBO J* 1992;11:1563–1571.

48. Dorner AJ, Krane MG, Kaufman RJ. Reduction of endogenous GRP78 levels improves secretion of a heterologous protein in CHO cells. *Mol Cell Biol* 1988;8:4063–4070.

49. Dorner AJ, Wasley LC, Kaufman RJ. Protein dissociation from GRP78 and secretion are blocked by depletion of cellular ATP levels. *Proc Natl Acad Sci U S A* 1990;87:7429–7432.

50. Swaroop M, Moussalli M, Pipe SW, et al. Mutagenesis of a potential immunoglobulin-binding protein-binding site enhances secretion of coagulation factor VIII. *J Biol Chem* 1997;272:24121–24124.

51. Tagliavacca L, Moon N, Dunham WR, et al. Identification and functional requirement of Cu(I) and its ligands within coagulation factor VIII. *J Biol Chem* 1997;272:27428–27434.

52. Tagliavacca L, Wang Q, Kaufman RJ. ATP-dependent dissociation of non-disulfide-linked aggregates of coagulation factor VIII is a rate-limiting step for secretion. *Biochemistry* 2000;39:1973–1981.

53. Zapun A, Darby NJ, Tessier DC, et al. Enhanced catalysis of ribonuclease B folding by the interaction of calnexin or calreticulin with ERp57. *J Biol Chem* 1998;273:6009–6012.

54. Dejgaard S, Nicolay J, Taheri M, et al. The ER glycoprotein quality control system. *Curr Issues Mol Biol* 2004;6:29–42.

55. Ritter C, Helenius A. Recognition of local glycoprotein misfolding by the ER folding sensor UDP-glucose:glycoprotein glucosyltransferase. *Nat Struct Biol* 2000;7:278–280.

56. Taylor SC, Ferguson AD, Bergeron JJ, et al. The ER protein folding sensor UDP-glucose glycoprotein-glucosyltransferase modifies substrates distant to local changes in glycoprotein conformation. *Nat Struct Mol Biol* 2004;11:128–134.

57. Ellgaard L, Molinari M, Helenius A. Setting the standards: quality control in the secretory pathway. *Science* 1999;286:1882–1888.

58. Parodi AJ. Protein glucosylation and its role in protein folding. *Annu Rev Biochem* 2000;69:69–93.

59. Schrag JD, Procopio DO, Cygler M, et al. Lectin control of protein folding and sorting in the secretory pathway. *Trends Biochem Sci* 2003;28:49–57.

60. Cabral CM, Liu Y, Sifers RN. Dissecting glycoprotein quality control in the secretory pathway. *Trends Biochem Sci* 2001;26:619–624.

61. Kleizen B, Braakman I. Protein folding and quality control in the endoplasmic reticulum. *Curr Opin Cell Biol* 2004;16:343–349.

62. Helenius A, Aebi M. Roles of N-linked glycans in the endoplasmic reticulum. *Annu Rev Biochem* 2004;73:1019–1049.

63. Pipe SW, Morris JA, Shah J, et al. Differential interaction of coagulation factor VIII and factor V with protein chaperones calnexin and calreticulin. *J Biol Chem* 1998;273:8537–8544.

64. Eriksson KK, Vago R, Calanca V, et al. EDEM contributes to maintenance of protein folding efficiency and secretory capacity. *J Biol Chem* 2004;279:44600–44605.

65. Molinari M, Calanca V, Galli C, et al. Role of EDEM in the release of misfolded glycoproteins from the calnexin cycle. *Science* 2003;299:1397–1400.

66. Oda Y, Hosokawa N, Wada I, et al. EDEM as an acceptor of terminally misfolded glycoproteins released from calnexin. *Science* 2003;299:1394–1397.

67. Kaufman RJ. Post-translational modifications required for coagulation factor secretion and function. *Thromb Haemost* 1998;79:1068–1079.

68. Mannucci PM. Desmopressin (DDAVP) in the treatment of bleeding disorders: the first 20 years. *Blood* 1997;90:2515–2521.

69. Kaufman RJ, Dorner AJ, Fass DN. von Willebrand factor elevates plasma factor VIII without induction of factor VIII messenger RNA in the liver. *Blood* 1999;93:193–197.

70. Tuddenham EG, Lane RS, Rotblat F, et al. Response to infusions of polyelectrolyte fractionated human factor VIII concentrate in human haemophilia A and von Willebrand's disease. *Br J Haematol* 1982;52:259–267.

71. Douglas AS. Antihemophilic globulin assay following plasma infusions in hemophilia. *J Lab Clin Med* 1958;51:850–859.

72. Over J, Sixma JJ, Bruine MH, et al. Survival of 125 iodine-labeled factor VIII in normals and patients with classic hemophilia. Observations on the heterogeneity of human factor VIII. *J Clin Invest* 1978;62:223–234.

73. Weiss HJ, Sussman, II, Hoyer LW. Stabilization of factor VIII in plasma by the von Willebrand factor. Studies on posttransfusion and dissociated factor VIII and in patients with von Willebrand's disease. *J Clin Invest* 1977;60:390–404.

74. Brinkhous KM, Sandberg H, Garris JB, et al. Purified human factor VIII procoagulant protein: comparative hemostatic response after infusions into hemophilic and von Willebrand disease dogs. *Proc Natl Acad Sci U S A* 1985;82:8752–8756.

75. Morfini M, Mannucci PM, Tenconi PM, et al. Pharmacokinetics of monoclonally-purified and recombinant factor VIII in patients with severe von Willebrand disease. *Thromb Haemost* 1993;70:270–272.

76. Nishino M, Girma JP, Rothschild C, et al. New variant of von Willebrand disease with defective binding to factor VIII. *Blood* 1989;74:1591–1599.

77. Mazurier C. von Willebrand disease masquerading as haemophilia A. *Thromb Haemost* 1992;67:391–396.

78. Casonato A, Pontara E, Zerbinati P, et al. DDAVP infusion: a possible useful tool in the diagnosis of the haemophilia A carrier state. *Blood Coagul Fibrinolysis* 1991;2:679–680.

79. Rosenberg JB, Foster PA, Kaufman RJ, et al. Intracellular trafficking of factor VIII to von Willebrand factor storage granules. *J Clin Invest* 1998;101:613–624.

80. Yarovoi HV, Kufrin D, Eslin DE, et al. Factor VIII ectopically expressed in platelets: efficacy in hemophilia A treatment. *Blood* 2003;102: 4006–4013.

81. Rosenberg JB, Greengard JS, Montgomery RR. Genetic induction of a releasable pool of factor VIII in human endothelial cells. *Arterioscler Thromb Vasc Biol* 2000;20:2689–2695.

82. Wilcox DA, Shi Q, Nurden P, et al. Induction of megakaryocytes to synthesize and store a releasable pool of human factor VIII. *J Thromb Haemost* 2003;1:2477–2489.

83. Kaufman RJ. Good things come in small packages for hemophilia. *J Thromb Haemost* 2003;1:2472–2473.

84. Vlot AJ, Koppelman SJ, Bouma BN, et al. Factor VIII and von Willebrand factor. *Thromb Haemost* 1998;79:456–465.

85. Andersson LO, Brown JE. Interaction of factor VIII-von Willebrand Factor with phospholipid vesicles. *Biochem J* 1981;200:161–167.

86. Nesheim M, Pittman DD, Giles AR, et al. The effect of plasma von Willebrand factor on the binding of human factor VIII to thrombin-activated human platelets. *J Biol Chem* 1991;266:17815–17820.

87. Koedam JA, Hamer RJ, Beeser-Visser NH, et al. The effect of von Willebrand factor on activation of factor VIII by factor Xa. *Eur J Biochem* 1990;189:229–234.

88. Koedam JA, Meijers JC, Sixma JJ, et al. Inactivation of human factor VIII by activated protein C. Cofactor activity of protein S and protective effect of von Willebrand factor. *J Clin Invest* 1988;82:1236–1243.

89. Fay PJ, Coumans JV, Walker FJ. von Willebrand factor mediates protection of factor VIII from activated protein C-catalyzed inactivation. *J Biol Chem* 1991;266:2172–2177.

90. Nogami K, Shima M, Nishiya K, et al. A novel mechanism of factor VIII protection by von Willebrand factor from activated protein C-catalyzed inactivation. *Blood* 2002;99:3993–3998.

91. Hamer RJ, Koedam JA, Beeser-Visser NH, et al. The effect of thrombin on the complex between factor VIII and von Willebrand factor. *Eur J Biochem* 1987;167:253–259.

92. Pittman DD, Alderman EM, Tomkinson KN, et al. Biochemical, immunological, and *in vivo* functional characterization of B-domain-deleted factor VIII. *Blood* 1993;81:2925–2935.

93. Hill-Eubanks DC, Lollar P. von Willebrand factor is a cofactor for thrombin-catalyzed cleavage of the factor VIII light chain. *J Biol Chem* 1990; 265:17854–17858.

94. Leyte A, Verbeet MP, Brodniewicz-Proba T, et al. The interaction between human blood-coagulation factor VIII and von Willebrand factor. Characterization of a high-affinity binding site on factor VIII. *Biochem J* 1989; 257:679–683.

95. Vlot AJ, Koppelman SJ, van den Berg MH, et al. The affinity and stoichiometry of binding of human factor VIII to von Willebrand factor. *Blood* 1995;85:3150–3157.

96. Lollar P, Parker CG. Stoichiometry of the porcine factor VIII-von Willebrand factor association. *J Biol Chem* 1987;262:17572–17576.

97. Bendetowicz AV, Morris JA, Wise RJ, et al. Binding of factor VIII to von Willebrand factor is enabled by cleavage of the von Willebrand factor propeptide and enhanced by formation of disulfide-linked multimers. *Blood* 1998;92:529–538.

98. Gilbert GE, Drinkwater D, Barter S, et al. Specificity of phosphatidylserine-containing membrane binding sites for factor VIII. Studies with model membranes supported by glass microspheres (lipospheres). *J Biol Chem* 1992;267:15861–15868.

99. Vlot AJ, Koppelman SJ, Meijers JC, et al. Kinetics of factor VIII-von Willebrand factor association. *Blood* 1996;87:1809–1816.

100. Bahou WF, Ginsburg D, Sikkink R, et al. A monoclonal antibody to von Willebrand factor (vWF) inhibits factor VIII binding. Localization of its antigenic determinant to a nonadecapeptide at the amino terminus of the mature vWF polypeptide. *J Clin Invest* 1989;84:56–61.

101. Foster PA, Fulcher CA, Marti T, et al. A major factor VIII binding domain resides within the amino-terminal 272 amino acid residues of von Willebrand factor. *J Biol Chem* 1987;262:8443–8446.

102. Takahashi Y, Kalafatis M, Girma JP, et al. Localization of a factor VIII binding domain on a 34 kilodalton fragment of the N-terminal portion of von Willebrand factor. *Blood* 1987;70:1679–1682.

103. Jorieux S, Gaucher C, Pietu G, et al. Fine epitope mapping of monoclonal antibodies to the NH2-terminal part of von Willebrand factor (vWF) by using recombinant and synthetic peptides: interest for the localization of the factor VIII binding domain. *Br J Haematol* 1994;87:113–118.

104. Wise RJ, Pittman DD, Handin RI, et al. The propeptide of von Willebrand factor independently mediates the assembly of von Willebrand multimers. *Cell* 1988;52:229–236.

105. Saenko EL, Shima M, Rajalakshmi KJ, et al. A role for the C2 domain of factor VIII in binding to von Willebrand factor. *J Biol Chem* 1994;269: 11601–11605.

106. Healey JF, Lubin IM, Nakai H, et al. Residues 484-508 contain a major determinant of the inhibitory epitope in the A2 domain of human factor VIII. *J Biol Chem* 1995;270:14505–14509.

107. Saenko EL, Scandella D. The acidic region of the factor VIII light chain and the C2 domain together form the high affinity binding site for von Willebrand factor. *J Biol Chem* 1997;272:18007–18014.

108. Foster PA, Fulcher CA, Houghten RA, et al. An immunogenic region within residues Val1670-Glu1684 of the factor VIII light chain induces antibodies which inhibit binding of factor VIII to von Willebrand factor. *J Biol Chem* 1988;263:5230–5234.

109. Pipe SW, Kaufman RJ. Characterization of a genetically engineered inactivation-resistant coagulation factor VIIIa. *Proc Natl Acad Sci U S A* 1997; 94:11851–11856.

110. Shima M, Scandella D, Yoshioka A, et al. A factor VIII neutralizing monoclonal antibody and a human inhibitor alloantibody recognizing epitopes in the C2 domain inhibit factor VIII binding to von Willebrand factor and to phosphatidylserine. *Thromb Haemost* 1993;69:240–246.

111. Lajmanovich A, Hudry-Clergeon G, Freyssinet JM, et al. Human factor VIII procoagulant activity and phospholipid interaction. *Biochim Biophys Acta* 1981;678:132–136.

112. Gilbert GE, Kaufman RJ, Arena AA, et al. Four hydrophobic amino acids of the factor VIII C2 domain are constituents of both the membrane-binding and von Willebrand factor-binding motifs. *J Biol Chem* 2002;277: 6374–6381.

113. Liu ML, Shen BW, Nakaya S, et al. Hemophilic factor VIII C1- and C2-domain missense mutations and their modeling to the 1.5-angstrom human C2-domain crystal structure. *Blood* 2000;96:979–987.

114. Gilbert GE, Arena AA. Activation of the factor VIIIa-factor IXa enzyme complex of blood coagulation by membranes containing phosphatidyl-L-serine. *J Biol Chem* 1996;271:11120–11125.

115. Lenting PJ, Donath MJ, van Mourik JA, et al. Identification of a binding site for blood coagulation factor IXa on the light chain of human factor VIII. *J Biol Chem* 1994;269:7150–7155.

116. Jenkins PV, Dill JL, Zhou Q, et al. Contribution of factor VIIIa A2 and A3-C1-C2 subunits to the affinity for factor IXa in factor Xase. *Biochemistry* 2004;43:5094–5101.

117. Duffy EJ, Parker ET, Mutucumarana VP, et al. Binding of factor VIIIa and factor VIII to factor IXa on phospholipid vesicles. *J Biol Chem* 1992;267: 17006–17011.

118. Curtis JE, Helgerson SL, Parker ET, et al. Isolation and characterization of thrombin-activated human factor VIII. *J Biol Chem* 1994;269:6246–6251.

119. Lenting PJ, van de Loo JW, Donath MJ, et al. The sequence Glu1811-Lys1818 of human blood coagulation factor VIII comprises a binding site for activated factor IX. *J Biol Chem* 1996;271:1935–1940.

120. Bovenschen N, Boertjes RC, van Stempvoort G, et al. Low density lipoprotein receptor-related protein and factor IXa share structural requirements for binding to the A3 domain of coagulation factor VIII. *J Biol Chem* 2003;278:9370–9377.

121. Kemball-Cook G, Tuddenham EG, Wacey AI. The factor VIII Structure and Mutation Resource Site: HAMSTeRS version 4. *Nucleic Acids Res* 1998;26:216–219.

122. Fay PJ, Smudzin TM, Walker FJ. Activated protein C-catalyzed inactivation of human factor VIII and factor VIIIa. Identification of cleavage sites and correlation of proteolysis with cofactor activity. *J Biol Chem* 1991; 266:20139–20145.

123. Regan LM, Lamphear BJ, Huggins CF, et al. Factor IXa protects factor VIIIa from activated protein C. Factor IXa inhibits activated protein C-catalyzed cleavage of factor VIIIa at Arg562. *J Biol Chem* 1994;269:9445–9452.

124. Fay PJ, Beattie T, Huggins CF, et al. Factor VIIIa A2 subunit residues 558-565 represent a factor IXa interactive site. *J Biol Chem* 1994;269: 20522–20527.

125. Jenkins PV, Freas J, Schmidt KM, et al. Mutations associated with hemophilia A in the 558-565 loop of the factor VIIIa A2 subunit alter the catalytic activity of the factor Xase complex. *Blood* 2002;100:501–508.

126. Bajaj SP, Schmidt AE, Mathur A, et al. Factor IXa:factor VIIIa interaction. Helix 330-338 of factor IXa interacts with residues 558-565 and spatially adjacent regions of the a2 subunit of factor VIIIa. *J Biol Chem* 2001;276: 16302–16309.

127. Mathur A, Bajaj SP. Protease and EGF1 domains of factor IXa play distinct roles in binding to factor VIIIa. Importance of helix 330 (helix 162 in chymotrypsin) of protease domain of factor IXa in its interaction with factor VIIIa. *J Biol Chem* 1999;274:18477–18486.

128. Mertens K, van Wijngaarden A, Bertina RM, et al. The functional defect of factor VIII Leiden, a genetic variant of coagulation factor VIII. *Thromb Haemost* 1985;54:650–653.

129. Jenkins PV, Dill JL, Zhou Q, et al. Clustered basic residues within segment 484-510 of the factor VIIIa A2 subunit contribute to the catalytic efficiency for factor Xa generation. *J Thromb Haemost* 2004;2:452–458.

130. Fay PJ, Koshibu K. The A2 subunit of factor VIIIa modulates the active site of factor IXa. *J Biol Chem* 1998;273:19049–19054.

131. Lapan KA, Fay PJ. Localization of a factor X interactive site in the A1 subunit of factor VIIIa. *J Biol Chem* 1997;272:2082–2088.

132. Regan LM, O'Brien LM, Beattie TL, et al. Activated protein C-catalyzed proteolysis of factor VIIIa alters its interactions within factor Xase. *J Biol Chem* 1996;271:3982–3987.

133. Lapan KA, Fay PJ. Interaction of the A1 subunit of factor VIIIa and the serine protease domain of factor X identified by zero-length cross-linking. *Thromb Haemost* 1998;80:418–422.

134. Gilbert GE, Arena AA. Partial activation of the factor VIIIa-factor IXa enzyme complex by dihexanoic phosphatidylserine at submicellar concentrations. *Biochemistry* 1997;36:10768–10776.

135. Rawala-Sheikh R, Ahmad SS, Ashby B, et al. Kinetics of coagulation factor X activation by platelet-bound factor IXa. *Biochemistry* 1990;29: 2606–2611.

136. Nogami K, Wakabayashi H, Schmidt K, et al. Altered interactions between the A1 and A2 subunits of factor VIIIa following cleavage of A1 subunit by factor Xa. *J Biol Chem* 2003;278:1634–1641.

137. Mathur A, Zhong D, Sabharwal AK, et al. Interaction of factor IXa with factor VIIIa. Effects of protease domain Ca2+ binding site, proteolysis in the autolysis loop, phospholipid, and factor X. *J Biol Chem* 1997;272: 23418–23426.

138. O'Brien LM, Medved LV, Fay PJ. Localization of factor IXa and factor VIIIa interactive sites. *J Biol Chem* 1995;270:27087–27092.

139. Lollar P, Parker ET, Curtis JE, et al. Inhibition of human factor VIIIa by anti-A2 subunit antibodies. *J Clin Invest* 1994;93:2497–2504.

140. Gilbert GE, Furie BC, Furie B. Binding of human factor VIII to phospholipid vesicles. *J Biol Chem* 1990;265:815–822.

141. Kemball-Cook G, Barrowcliffe TW. Interaction of factor VIII with phospholipids: role of composition and negative charge. *Thromb Res* 1992; 67:57–71.

142. Bloom JW, Nesheim ME, Mann KG. Phospholipid-binding properties of bovine factor V and factor Va. *Biochemistry* 1979;18:4419–4425.

143. Andersson LO, Thuy LP, Brown JE. Affinity chromatography of coagulation factors II, VIII, IX and X on matrix-bound phospholipid vesicles. *Thromb Res* 1981;23:481–489.

144. Pusey ML, Nelsestuen GL. Membrane binding properties of blood coagulation Factor V and derived peptides. *Biochemistry* 1984;23:6202–6210.

145. Krieg UC, Isaacs BS, Yemul SS, et al. Interaction of blood coagulation factor Va with phospholipid vesicles examined by using lipophilic photoreagents. *Biochemistry* 1987;26:103–109.

146. Lecompte MF, Krishnaswamy S, Mann KG, et al. Membrane penetration of bovine factor V and Va detected by labeling with 5-iodonaphthalene-1-azide. *J Biol Chem* 1987;262:1935–1937.

147. Atkins JS, Ganz PR. The association of human coagulation factors VIII, IXa and X with phospholipid vesicles involves both electrostatic and hydrophobic interactions. *Mol Cell Biochem* 1992;112:61–71.

148. Bardelle C, Furie B, Furie BC, et al. Membrane binding kinetics of factor VIII indicate a complex binding process. *J Biol Chem* 1993;268:8815–8824.

149. Bevers EM, Comfurius P, Zwaal RF. Changes in membrane phospholipid distribution during platelet activation. *Biochim Biophys Acta* 1983; 736:57–66.

150. Hamer RJ, Koedam JA, Beeser-Visser NH, et al. Factor VIII binds to von Willebrand factor via its Mr-80,000 light chain. *Eur J Biochem* 1987; 166:37–43.

151. Lollar P, Hill-Eubanks DC, Parker CG. Association of the factor VIII light chain with von Willebrand factor. *J Biol Chem* 1988;263:10451–10455.

152. Saenko EL, Scandella D, Yakhyaev AV, et al. Activation of factor VIII by thrombin increases its affinity for binding to synthetic phospholipid membranes and activated platelets. *J Biol Chem* 1998;273:27918–27926.

153. Kemball-Cook G, Edwards SJ, Sewerin K, et al. Factor VIII procoagulant protein interacts with phospholipid vesicles via its 80 kDa light chain. *Thromb Haemost* 1988;60:442–446.

154. Bloom JW. The interaction of rDNA factor VIII, factor VIIIdes-797-1562 and factor VIIIdes-797-1562-derived peptides with phospholipid. *Thromb Res* 1987;48:439–448.

155. Arai M, Scandella D, Hoyer LW. Molecular basis of factor VIII inhibition by human antibodies. Antibodies that bind to the factor VIII light chain prevent the interaction of factor VIII with phospholipid. *J Clin Invest* 1989;83:1978–1984.

156. Blostein MD, Furie BC, Rajotte I, et al. The Gla domain of factor IXa binds to factor VIIIa in the tenase complex. *J Biol Chem* 2003;278:31297–31302.

157. Christophe OD, Lenting PJ, Kolkman JA, et al. Blood coagulation factor IX residues Glu78 and Arg94 provide a link between both epidermal growth factor-like domains that is crucial in the interaction with factor VIII light chain. *J Biol Chem* 1998;273:222–227.

158. Chang YJ, Wu HL, Hamaguchi N, et al. Identification of functionally important residues of the epidermal growth factor-2 domain of factor IX by alanine-scanning mutagenesis. Residues Asn(89)–Gly(93) are critical for binding factor VIIIa. *J Biol Chem* 2002;277:25393–25399.

159. Bajaj SP, Rapaport SI, Maki SL. A monoclonal antibody to factor IX that inhibits the factor VIII:Ca potentiation of factor X activation. *J Biol Chem* 1985;260:11574–11580.

160. Brandstetter H, Bauer M, Huber R, et al. X-ray structure of clotting factor IXa: active site and module structure related to Xase activity and hemophilia B. *Proc Natl Acad Sci U S A* 1995;92:9796–9800.

161. Stoilova-McPhie S, Villoutreix BO, Mertens K, et al. 3-Dimensional structure of membrane-bound coagulation factor VIII: modeling of the factor VIII heterodimer within a 3-dimensional density map derived by electron crystallography. *Blood* 2002;99:1215–1223.

162. Adams TE, Hockin MF, Mann KG, et al. The crystal structure of activated protein C-inactivated bovine factor Va: Implications for cofactor function. *Proc Natl Acad Sci U S A* 2004;101:8918–8923.

163. Pratt KP, Shen BW, Takeshima K, et al. Structure of the C2 domain of human factor VIII at 1.5 A resolution. *Nature* 1999;402:439–442.

164. Fuentes-Prior P, Fujikawa K, Pratt KP. New insights into binding interfaces of coagulation factors V and VIII and their homologues lessons from high resolution crystal structures. *Curr Protein Pept Sci* 2002;3:313–339.

165. Stoylova SS, Lenting PJ, Kemball-Cook G, et al. Electron crystallography of human blood coagulation factor VIII bound to phospholipid monolayers. *J Biol Chem* 1999;274:36573–36578.

166. Lollar P, Knutson GJ, Fass DN. Activation of porcine factor VIII:C by thrombin and factor Xa. *Biochemistry* 1985;24:8056–8064.

167. Eaton D, Rodriguez H, Vehar GA. Proteolytic processing of human factor VIII. Correlation of specific cleavages by thrombin, factor Xa, and activated protein C with activation and inactivation of factor VIII coagulant activity. *Biochemistry* 1986;25:505–512.

168. Pittman DD, Tomkinson KN, Michnick D, et al. Posttranslational sulfation of factor V is required for efficient thrombin cleavage and activation and for full procoagulant activity. *Biochemistry* 1994;33:6952–6959.

169. Pittman DD, Wang JH, Kaufman RJ. Identification and functional importance of tyrosine sulfate residues within recombinant factor VIII. *Biochemistry* 1992;31:3315–3325.

170. Michnick DA, Pittman DD, Wise RJ, et al. Identification of individual tyrosine sulfation sites within factor VIII required for optimal activity and efficient thrombin cleavage. *J Biol Chem* 1994;269:20095–20102.

171. Mumford AD, Laffan M, O'Donnell J, et al. A Tyr346 → Cys substitution in the interdomain acidic region a1 of factor VIII in an individual with factor VIII:C assay discrepancy. *Br J Haematol* 2002;118:589–594.

172. Nogami K, Shima M, Hosokawa K, et al. Factor VIII C2 domain contains the thrombin-binding site responsible for thrombin-catalyzed cleavage at Arg1689. *J Biol Chem* 2000;275:25774–25780.

173. Nogami K, Shima M, Hosokawa K, et al. Role of factor VIII C2 domain in factor VIII binding to factor Xa. *J Biol Chem* 1999;274:31000–31007.

174. Barrow RT, Healey JF, Lollar P. Inhibition by heparin of thrombin-catalyzed activation of the factor VIII-von Willebrand factor complex. *J Biol Chem* 1994;269:593–598.

175. Esmon CT, Lollar P. Involvement of thrombin anion-binding exosites 1 and 2 in the activation of factor V and factor VIII. *J Biol Chem* 1996;271: 13882–13887.

176. Ye J, Rezaie AR, Esmon CT. Glycosaminoglycan contributions to both protein C activation and thrombin inhibition involve a common arginine-rich site in thrombin that includes residues arginine 93, 97, and 101. *J Biol Chem* 1994;269:17965–17970.

177. Myles T, Yun TH, Hall SW, et al. An extensive interaction interface between thrombin and factor V is required for factor V activation. *J Biol Chem* 2001;276:25143–25149.

178. Fulcher CA, Roberts JR, Zimmerman TS. Thrombin proteolysis of purified factor viii procoagulant protein: correlation of activation with generation of a specific polypeptide. *Blood* 1983;61:807–811.

179. Fay PJ, Anderson MT, Chavin SI, et al. The size of human factor VIII heterodimers and the effects produced by thrombin. *Biochim Biophys Acta* 1986;871:268–278.

180. Pittman DD, Kaufman RJ. Structure-function relationships of factor VIII elucidated through recombinant DNA technology. *Thromb Haemost* 1989;61:161–165.

181. Pittman DD, Kaufman RJ. Proteolytic requirements for thrombin activation of anti-hemophilic factor (factor VIII). *Proc Natl Acad Sci U S A* 1988;85:2429–2433.

182. Gitschier J, Kogan S, Levinson B, et al. Mutations of factor VIII cleavage sites in hemophilia A. *Blood* 1988;72:1022–1028.

183. O'Brien DP, Tuddenham EG. Purification and characterization of factor VIII 1,689-Cys: a nonfunctional cofactor occurring in a patient with severe hemophilia A. *Blood* 1989;73:2117–2122.

184. Arai M, Higuchi M, Antonarakis SE, et al. Characterization of a thrombin cleavage site mutation (Arg 1689 to Cys) in the factor VIII gene of two unrelated patients with cross-reacting material-positive hemophilia A. *Blood* 1990;75:384–389.

185. Arai M, Inaba H, Higuchi M, et al. Direct characterization of factor VIII in plasma: detection of a mutation altering a thrombin cleavage site (arginine-372—histidine). *Proc Natl Acad Sci U S A* 1989;86:4277–4281.

186. Hill-Eubanks DC, Parker CG, Lollar P. Differential proteolytic activation of factor VIII-von Willebrand factor complex by thrombin. *Proc Natl Acad Sci U S A* 1989;86:6508–6512.

187. Regan LM, Fay PJ. Cleavage of factor VIII light chain is required for maximal generation of factor VIIIa activity. *J Biol Chem* 1995;270: 8546–8552.

188. Lollar P, Parker CG. Subunit structure of thrombin-activated porcine factor VIII. *Biochemistry* 1989;28:666–674.

189. Fay PJ, Mastri M, Koszelak ME, et al. Cleavage of factor VIII heavy chain is required for the functional interaction of a2 subunit with factor IXA. *J Biol Chem* 2001;276:12434–12439.

190. Fay PJ, Haidaris PJ, Smudzin TM. Human factor VIIIa subunit structure. Reconstruction of factor VIIIa from the isolated A1/A3-C1-C2 dimer and A2 subunit. *J Biol Chem* 1991;266:8957–8962.

191. Pittman DD, Millenson M, Marquette K, et al. A2 domain of human recombinant-derived factor VIII is required for procoagulant activity but not for thrombin cleavage. *Blood* 1992;79:389–397.

192. Fay PJ, Smudzin TM. Characterization of the interaction between the A2 subunit and A1/A3-C1-C2 dimer in human factor VIIIa. *J Biol Chem* 1992;267:13246–13250.

193. Lollar P, Parker ET, Fay PJ. Coagulant properties of hybrid human/porcine factor VIII molecules. *J Biol Chem* 1992;267:23652–23657.

194. Persson E, Ezban M, Shymko RM. Kinetics of the interaction between the human factor VIIIa subunits: effects of pH, ionic strength, Ca2+ concentration, heparin, and activated protein C-catalyzed proteolysis. *Biochemistry* 1995;34:12775–12781.

195. Parker ET, Pohl J, Blackburn MN, et al. Subunit structure and function of porcine factor Xa-activated factor VIII. *Biochemistry* 1997;36:9365–9373.

196. Fay PJ, Haidaris PJ, Huggins CF. Role of the COOH-terminal acidic region of A1 subunit in A2 subunit retention in human factor VIIIa. *J Biol Chem* 1993;268:17861–17866.

197. Koszelak Rosenblum ME, Schmidt K, Freas J, et al. Cofactor activities of factor VIIIa and A2 subunit following cleavage of A1 subunit at Arg336. *J Biol Chem* 2002;277:11664–11669.

198. Koszelak ME, Huggins CF, Fay PJ. Sites in the A2 subunit involved in the interfactor VIIIa interaction. *J Biol Chem* 2000;275:27137–27144.

199. Duncan EM, Duncan BM, Tunbridge LJ, et al. Familial discrepancy between the one-stage and two-stage factor VIII methods in a subgroup of patients with haemophilia A. *Br J Haematol* 1994;87:846–848.

200. Rudzki Z, Duncan EM, Casey GJ, et al. Mutations in a subgroup of patients with mild haemophilia A and a familial discrepancy between the one-stage and two-stage factor VIII:C methods. *Br J Haematol* 1996;94: 400–406.

201. Pipe SW, Eickhorst AN, McKinley SH, et al. Mild hemophilia A caused by increased rate of factor VIII A2 subunit dissociation: evidence for nonproteolytic inactivation of factor VIIIa *in vivo*. *Blood* 1999;93:176–183.

202. Pipe SW, Saenko EL, Eickhorst AN, et al. Hemophilia A mutations associated with 1-stage/2-stage activity discrepancy disrupt protein-protein

interactions within the triplicated A domains of thrombin-activated factor VIIIa. *Blood* 2001;97:685–691.

203. Hakeos WH, Miao H, Sirachainan N, et al. Hemophilia A mutations within the factor VIII A2-A3 subunit interface destabilize factor VIIIa and cause one-stage/two-stage activity discrepancy. *Thromb Haemost* 2002; 88:781–787.

204. O'Brien LM, Huggins CF, Fay PJ. Interacting regions in the A1 and A2 subunits of factor VIIIa identified by zero-length cross-linking. *Blood* 1997;90:3943–3950.

205. Jesty J. Analysis of the generation and inhibition of factor Xa. Area under generation curves is independent of enzyme generation rate. *J Biol Chem* 1990;265:17539–17544.

206. Lollar P, Knutson GJ, Fass DN. Stabilization of thrombin-activated porcine factor VIII:C by factor IXa phospholipid. *Blood* 1984;63:1303–1308.

207. Lamphear BJ, Fay PJ. Factor IXa enhances reconstitution of factor VIIIa from isolated A2 subunit and A1/A3-C1-C2 dimer. *J Biol Chem* 1992; 267:3725–3730.

208. Lamphear BJ, Fay PJ. Proteolytic interactions of factor IXa with human factor VIII and factor VIIIa. *Blood* 1992;80:3120–3126.

209. O'Brien DP, Johnson D, Byfield P, et al. Inactivation of factor VIII by factor IXa. *Biochemistry* 1992;31:2805–2812.

210. Fay PJ, Beattie TL, Regan LM, et al. Model for the factor VIIIa-dependent decay of the intrinsic factor Xase. Role of subunit dissociation and factor IXa-catalyzed proteolysis. *J Biol Chem* 1996;271:6027–6032.

211. Hockin MF, Jones KC, Everse SJ, et al. A model for the stoichiometric regulation of blood coagulation. *J Biol Chem* 2002;277:18322–18333.

212. Gale AJ, Pellequer JL. An engineered interdomain disulfide bond stabilizes human blood coagulation factor VIIIa. *J Thromb Haemost* 2003;1: 1966–1971.

213. Dahlback B. The discovery of activated protein C resistance. *J Thromb Haemost* 2003;1:3–9.

214. Lu D, Kalafatis M, Mann KG, et al. Comparison of activated protein C/protein S-mediated inactivation of human factor VIII and factor V. *Blood* 1996;87:4708–4717.

215. van 't Veer C, Mann KG. Regulation of tissue factor initiated thrombin generation by the stoichiometric inhibitors tissue factor pathway inhibitor, antithrombin-III, and heparin cofactor-II. *J Biol Chem* 1997;272: 4367–4377.

216. Dahlback B, Hildebrand B. Inherited resistance to activated protein C is corrected by anticoagulant cofactor activity found to be a property of factor V. *Proc Natl Acad Sci U S A* 1994;91:1396–1400.

217. Dahlback B. Resistance to activated protein C as risk factor for thrombosis: molecular mechanisms, laboratory investigation, and clinical management. *Semin Hematol* 1997;34:217–234.

218. Bertina RM, Koeleman BP, Koster T, et al. Mutation in blood coagulation factor V associated with resistance to activated protein C. *Nature* 1994; 369:64–67.

219. Amano K, Michnick DA, Moussalli M, et al. Mutation at either Arg336 or Arg562 in factor VIII is insufficient for complete resistance to activated protein C (APC)-mediated inactivation: implications for the APC resistance test. *Thromb Haemost* 1998;79:557–563.

220. Roelse JC, Koopman MM, Buller HR, et al. Absence of mutations at the activated protein C cleavage sites of factor VIII in 125 patients with venous thrombosis. *Br J Haematol* 1996;92:740–743.

221. Nogami K, Wakabayashi H, Fay PJ. Mechanisms of factor Xa-catalyzed cleavage of the factor VIIIa A1 subunit resulting in cofactor inactivation. *J Biol Chem* 2003;278:16502–16509.

222. Rezaie AR. Heparin-binding exosite of factor Xa. *Trends Cardiovasc Med* 2000;10:333–338.

223. Bevers EM, Comfurius P, van Rijn JL, et al. Generation of prothrombin-converting activity and the exposure of phosphatidylserine at the outer surface of platelets. *Eur J Biochem* 1982;122:429–436.

224. Zwaal RF. Membrane and lipid involvement in blood coagulation. *Biochim Biophys Acta* 1978;515:163–205.

225. Miletich JP, Jackson CM, Majerus PW. Properties of the factor Xa binding site on human platelets. *J Biol Chem* 1978;253:6908–6916.

226. Kane WH, Lindhout MJ, Jackson CM, et al. Factor Va-dependent binding of factor Xa to human platelets. *J Biol Chem* 1980;255:1170–1174.

227. Tracy PB, Nesheim ME, Mann KG. Coordinate binding of factor Va and factor Xa to the unstimulated platelet. *J Biol Chem* 1981;256: 743–751.

228. Nesheim ME, Pittman DD, Wang JH, et al. The binding of 35S-labeled recombinant factor VIII to activated and unactivated human platelets. *J Biol Chem* 1988;263:16467–16470.

229. Muntean W, Leschnik B, Haas J. Factor VIII coagulant moiety binds to platelets by binding to phospholipids of the platelet membrane. *Thromb Res* 1987;45:345–354.

230. Gilbert GE, Sims PJ, Wiedmer T, et al. Platelet-derived microparticles express high affinity receptors for factor VIII. *J Biol Chem* 1991;266:17261–17268.

231. Ahmad SS, Scandura JM, Walsh PN. Structural and functional characterization of platelet receptor-mediated factor VIII binding. *J Biol Chem* 2000;275:13071–13081.

232. Ahmad SS, London FS, Walsh PN. The assembly of the factor X-activating complex on activated human platelets. *J Thromb Haemost* 2003;1:48–59.

233. Ahmad SS, Walsh PN. Coordinate binding studies of the substrate (factor X) with the cofactor (factor VIII) in the assembly of the factor X activating

complex on the activated platelet surface. *Biochemistry* 2002;41: 11269–11276.

234. Nesheim ME, Furmaniak-Kazmierczak E, Henin C, et al. On the existence of platelet receptors for factor V(a) and factor VIII(a). *Thromb Haemost* 1993;70:80–86.

235. Stern DM, Drillings M, Kisiel W, et al. Activation of factor IX bound to cultured bovine aortic endothelial cells. *Proc Natl Acad Sci U S A* 1984; 81:913–917.

236. Stern DM, Drillings M, Nossel HL, et al. Binding of factors IX and IXa to cultured vascular endothelial cells. *Proc Natl Acad Sci U S A* 1983;80: 4119–4123.

237. Lenting PJ, Neels JG, van den Berg BM, et al. The light chain of factor VIII comprises a binding site for low density lipoprotein receptor-related protein. *J Biol Chem* 1999;274:23734–23739.

238. Saenko EL, Yakhyaev AV, Mikhailenko I, et al. Role of the low density lipoprotein-related protein receptor in mediation of factor VIII catabolism. *J Biol Chem* 1999;274:37685–37692.

239. Turecek PL, Schwarz HP, Binder BR. *In vivo* inhibition of low density lipoprotein receptor-related protein improves survival of factor VIII in the absence of von Willebrand factor. *Blood* 2000;95:3637–3638.

240. Bovenschen N, Herz J, Grimbergen JM, et al. Elevated plasma factor VIII in a mouse model of low-density lipoprotein receptor-related protein deficiency. *Blood* 2003;101:3933–3939.

241. Schwarz HP, Lenting PJ, Binder B, et al. Involvement of low-density lipoprotein receptor-related protein (LRP) in the clearance of factor VIII in von Willebrand factor-deficient mice. *Blood* 2000;95:1703–1708.

242. Sarafanov AG, Ananyeva NM, Shima M, et al. Cell surface heparan sulfate proteoglycans participate in factor VIII catabolism mediated by low density lipoprotein receptor-related protein. *J Biol Chem* 2001;276: 11970–11979.

243. Hoyer LW. Molecular pathology and immunology of factor VIII (hemophilia A and factor VIII inhibitors). *Hum Pathol* 1987;18:153–161.

244. Lazarchick J, Hoyer LW. Immunoradiometric measurement of the factor VIII procoagulant antigen. *J Clin Invest* 1978;62:1048–1052.

245. Levinson B, Kenwrick S, Lakich D, et al. A transcribed gene in an intron of the human factor VIII gene. *Genomics* 1990;7:1–11.

246. Levinson B, Bermingham JR Jr., Metzenberg A, et al. Sequence of the human factor VIII-associated gene is conserved in mouse. *Genomics* 1992; 13:862–865.

247. Levinson B, Kenwrick S, Gamel P, et al. Evidence for a third transcript from the human factor VIII gene. *Genomics* 1992;14:585–589.

248. Freije D, Schlessinger D. A 1.6-Mb contig of yeast artificial chromosomes around the human factor VIII gene reveals three regions homologous to probes for the DXS115 locus and two for the DXYS64 locus. *Am J Hum Genet* 1992;51:66–80.

249. Valleix S, Jeanny JC, Elsevier S, et al. Expression of human F8B, a gene nested within the coagulation factor VIII gene, produces multiple eye defects and developmental alterations in chimeric and transgenic mice. *Hum Mol Genet* 1999;8:1291–1301.

250. McGlynn LK, Mueller CR, Begbie M, et al. Role of the liver-enriched transcription factor hepatocyte nuclear factor 1 in transcriptional regulation of the factor V111 gene. *Mol Cell Biol* 1996;16:1936–1945.

251. Haldane JBS, Smith CAB. A new estimate of the linkage between the genes for colourblindness and haemophilia A. *Ann Eugen* 1947;14:10–31.

252. Boyer SH, Graham JB. Linkage between the X chromosome loci for G6PD eletrophoretic variation and hemophilia A. *Am J Hum Genet* 1965;17: 320–324.

253. Wacey AI, Kemball-Cook G, Kazazian HH, et al. The haemophilia A mutation search test and resource site, home page of the factor VIII mutation database: HAMSTeRS. *Nucleic Acids Res* 1996;24:100–102.

254. Higuchi M, Antonarakis SE, Kasch L, et al. Molecular characterization of mild-to-moderate hemophilia A: detection of the mutation in 25 of 29 patients by denaturing gradient gel electrophoresis. *Proc Natl Acad Sci U S A* 1991;88:8307–8311.

255. Higuchi M, Kazazian HH Jr, Kasch L, et al. Molecular characterization of severe hemophilia A suggests that about half the mutations are not within the coding regions and splice junctions of the factor VIII gene. *Proc Natl Acad Sci U S A* 1991;88:7405–7409.

256. Lakich D, Kazazian HH Jr, Antonarakis SE, et al. Inversions disrupting the factor VIII gene are a common cause of severe haemophilia A. *Nat Genet* 1993;5:236–241.

257. Dermitzakis ET, Reymond A, Lyle R, et al. Numerous potentially functional but non-genic conserved sequences on human chromosome 21. *Nature* 2002;420:578–582.

258. Naylor J, Brinke A, Hassock S, et al. Characteristic mRNA abnormality found in half the patients with severe haemophilia A is due to large DNA inversions. *Hum Mol Genet* 1993;2:1773–1778.

259. Naylor JA, Buck D, Green P, et al. Investigation of the factor VIII intron 22 repeated region (int22h) and the associated inversion junctions. *Hum Mol Genet* 1995;4:1217–1224.

260. Rossiter JP, Young M, Kimberland ML, et al. Factor VIII gene inversions causing severe hemophilia A originate almost exclusively in male germ cells. *Hum Mol Genet* 1994;3:1035–1039.

261. Antonarakis SE, Rossiter JP, Young M, et al. Factor VIII gene inversions in severe hemophilia A: results of an international consortium study. *Blood* 1995;86:2206–2212.

262. Lozier JN, Dutra A, Pak E, et al. The Chapel Hill hemophilia A dog colony exhibits a factor VIII gene inversion. *Proc Natl Acad Sci U S A* 2002;99:12991–12996.

263. Bagnall RD, Waseem N, Green PM, et al. Recurrent inversion breaking intron 1 of the factor VIII gene is a frequent cause of severe hemophilia A. *Blood* 2002;99:168–174.

264. Antonarakis SE, Kazazian HH Jr. The molecular basis of hemophilia A in man. *Trends Genet* 1988;4:233–237.

265. Woods-Samuels P, Kazazian HH Jr, Antonarakis SE. Nonhomologous recombination in the human genome: deletions in the human factor VIII gene. *Genomics* 1991;10:94–101.

266. Kazazian HH Jr, Wong C, Youssoufian H, et al. Haemophilia A resulting from de novo insertion of L1 sequences represents a novel mechanism for mutation in man. *Nature* 1988;332:164–166.

267. Lander ES, Linton LM, Birren B, et al. Initial sequencing and analysis of the human genome. *Nature* 2001;409:860–921.

268. Ostertag EM, Kazazian HH Jr. Biology of mammalian L1 retrotransposons. *Annu Rev Genet* 2001;35:501–538.

269. Gitschier J. Maternal duplication associated with gene deletion in sporadic hemophilia. *Am J Hum Genet* 1988;43:274–279.

270. Murru S, Casula L, Pecorara M, et al. Illegitimate recombination produced a duplication within the FVIII gene in a patient with mild hemophilia A. *Genomics* 1990;7:115–118.

271. Migeon BR, McGinniss MJ, Antonarakis SE, et al. Severe hemophilia A in a female by cryptic translocation: order and orientation of factor VIII within Xq28. *Genomics* 1993;16:20–25.

272. Young M, Inaba H, Hoyer LW, et al. Partial correction of a severe molecular defect in hemophilia A, because of errors during expression of the factor VIII gene. *Am J Hum Genet* 1997;60:565–573.

273. Naylor JA, Green PM, Rizza CR, et al. Analysis of factor VIII mRNA reveals defects in everyone of 28 haemophilia A patients. *Hum Mol Genet* 1993;2:11–17.

274. Youssoufian H, Kazazian HH Jr, Phillips DG, et al. Recurrent mutations in haemophilia A give evidence for CpG mutation hotspots. *Nature* 1986;324:380–382.

275. Cooper DN, Youssoufian H. The CpG dinucleotide and human genetic disease. *Hum Genet* 1988;78:151–155.

276. Diamond C, Kogan S, Levinson B, et al. Amino acid substitutions in conserved domains of factor VIII and related proteins: study of patients with mild and moderately severe hemophilia A. *Hum Mutat* 1992;1:248–257.

277. Youssoufian H, Antonarakis SE, Bell W, et al. Nonsense and missense mutations in hemophilia A: estimate of the relative mutation rate at CG dinucleotides. *Am J Hum Genet* 1988;42:718–725.

278. Antonarakis SE. CpG dinucleotides and human disorders. In: Antonarakis SE, ed. *Encyclopedia of the human genome.* London: Nature Publishing Group, 2003:950–956. 1 vol.

279. Dietz HC, Valle D, Francomano CA, et al. The skipping of constitutive exons *in vivo* induced by nonsense mutations. *Science* 1993;259:680–683.

280. Liu HX, Cartegni L, Zhang MQ, et al. A mechanism for exon skipping caused by nonsense or missense mutations in BRCA1 and other genes. *Nat Genet* 2001;27:55–58.

281. Cartegni L, Chew SL, Krainer AR. Listening to silence and understanding nonsense: exonic mutations that affect splicing. *Nat Rev Genet* 2002;3:285–298.

282. O'Brien DP, Pattinson JK, Tuddenham EG. Purification and characterization of factor VIII 372-Cys: a hypofunctional cofactor from a patient with moderately severe hemophilia A. *Blood* 1990;75:1664–1672.

283. Higuchi M, Wong C, Kochhan L, et al. Characterization of mutations in the factor VIII gene by direct sequencing of amplified genomic DNA. *Genomics* 1990;6:65–71.

284. Leyte A, van Schijndel HB, Niehrs C, et al. Sulfation of Tyr1680 of human blood coagulation factor VIII is essential for the interaction of factor VIII with von Willebrand factor. *J Biol Chem* 1991;266:740–746.

285. Aly AM, Higuchi M, Kasper CK, et al. Hemophilia A due to mutations that create new N-glycosylation sites. *Proc Natl Acad Sci U S A* 1992;89:4933–4937.

286. Amano K, Sarkar R, Pemberton S, et al. The molecular basis for crossreacting material-positive hemophilia A due to missense mutations within the A2-domain of factor VIII. *Blood* 1998;91:538–548.

287. Oeri J, Matter M, Isenschmid H, et al. Angeborener mangel an factor V (parahaemophilie) verbunden mit echter haemophilie A bein zwei brudern. *Med Probl Paediatr* 1954;1:575.

288. Ozsoylu S. Combined congenital deficiency of factor V and factor VIII [letter]. *Acta Haematol* 1983;70:207–208.

289. Marlar RA, Griffin JH. Deficiency of protein C inhibitor in combined factor V/VIII deficiency disease. *J Clin Invest* 1980;66:1186–1189.

290. Nichols WC, Terry VH, Wheatley MA, et al. ERGIC-53 gene structure and mutation analysis in 19 combined factors V and VIII deficiency families. *Blood* 1999;93:2261–2266.

291. Neerman-Arbez M, Johnson KM, Morris MA, et al. Molecular analysis of the ERGIC-53 gene in 35 families with combined factor V-factor VIII deficiency. *Blood* 1999;93:2253–2260.

292. Schweizer A, Fransen JA, Bachi T, et al. Identification, by a monoclonal antibody, of a 53-kD protein associated with a tubulo-vesicular compartment at the cis-side of the Golgi apparatus. *J Cell Biol* 1988;107:1643–1653.

293. Arar C, Carpentier V, Le Caer JP, et al. ERGIC-53, a membrane protein of the endoplasmic reticulum-Golgi intermediate compartment, is identical to MR60, an intracellular mannose-specific lectin of myelomonocytic cells. *J Biol Chem* 1995;270:3551–3553.

294. Nichols WC, Seligsohn U, Zivelin A, et al. Mutations in an endoplasmic reticulum-Golgi intermediate compartment protein cause combined deficiency of coagulation factors V and VIII. *Cell* 1998;93:61–70.

295. Cunningham MA, Pipe SW, Zhang B. et al. LMAN1 is a molecular chaperone for the secretion of coagulation factor VIII. *J Thromb Haemost* 2003;1:2360–2367.

296. Moussalli M, Pipe SW, Nichols WC, et al. Mistargeting of the lectin Ergic-53 to the endoplasmic reticulum impairs the secretion of the coagulation factors V and VIII. *Blood* 1998;92:474a.

297. Zhang B, Cunningham MA, Nichols WC, et al. Bleeding due to disruption of a cargo-specific ER-to-Golgi transport complex. *Nat Genet* 2003;34:220–225.

298. Hoyer LW. Hemophilia A. *N Engl J Med* 1994;330:38–47.

299. Sultan Y, French Hemophilia Study Group. Prevalence of inhibitors in a population of 3435 hemophilia patients in France. *Thromb Haemost* 1992;67:600–602.

300. Gilles JG, Jacquemin MG, Saint-Remy JM. Factor VIII inhibitors. *Thromb Haemost* 1997;78:641–646.

301. Gilles JG, Arnout J, Vermylen J, et al. Anti-factor VIII antibodies of hemophiliac patients are frequently directed towards nonfunctional determinants and do not exhibit isotypic restriction. *Blood* 1993;82:2452–2461.

302. Scandella D, DeGraaf Mahoney S, Mattingly M, et al. Epitope mapping of human factor VIII inhibitor antibodies by deletion analysis of factor VIII fragments expressed in Escherichia coli. *Proc Natl Acad Sci U S A* 1988;85:6152–6156.

303. Zhong D, Saenko EL, Shima M, et al. Some human inhibitor antibodies interfere with factor VIII binding to factor IX. *Blood* 1998;92:136–142.

304. Fulcher CA, de Graaf Mahoney S, Roberts JR, et al. Localization of human factor FVIII inhibitor epitopes to two polypeptide fragments. *Proc Natl Acad Sci U S A* 1985;82:7728–7732.

305. Millar DS, Steinbrecher RA, Wieland K, et al. The molecular genetic analysis of haemophilia A; characterization of six partial deletions in the factor VIII gene. *Hum Genet* 1990;86:219–227.

306. Wion KL, Tuddenham EG, Lawn RM. A new polymorphism in the factor VIII gene for prenatal diagnosis of hemophilia A. *Nucleic Acids Res* 1986;14:4535–4542.

307. Antonarakis SE, Waber PG, Kittur SD, et al. Hemophilia A. Detection of molecular defects and of carriers by DNA analysis. *N Engl J Med* 1985;313:842–848.

308. Gitschier J, Drayna D, Tuddenham EG, et al. Genetic mapping and diagnosis of haemophilia A achieved through a BclI polymorphism in the factor VIII gene. *Nature* 1985;314:738–740.

309. Antonarakis SE, Copeland KL, Carpenter RJ Jr, et al. Prenatal diagnosis of haemophilia A by factor VIII gene analysis. *Lancet* 1985;1: 1407– 1409.

310. Harper K, Winter RM, Pembrey ME, et al. A clinically useful DNA probe closely linked to haemophilia A. *Lancet* 1984;2:6–8.

311. Oberle I, Camerino G, Heilig R, et al. Genetic screening for hemophilia A (classic hemophilia) with a polymorphic DNA probe. *N Engl J Med* 1985;312:682–686.

312. Liu J, Liu Q, Liang Y, et al. PCR assay for the inversion causing severe Hemophilia A and its application. *Chin Med J (Engl)* 1999;112:419–423.

313. Bowen DJ, Keeney S. Unleashing the long-distance PCR for detection of the intron 22 inversion of the factor VIII gene in severe haemophilia A. *Thromb Haemost* 2003;89:201–202.

314. Chee M, Yang R, Hubbell E, et al. Accessing genetic information with high-density DNA arrays. *Science* 1996;274:610–614.

315. Hough C, Kamisue S, Cameron C, et al. Aberrant splicing and premature termination of transcription of the FVIII gene as a cause of severe canine hemophilia A: similarities with the intron 22 inversion mutation in human hemophilia. *Thromb Haemost* 2002;87:659–665.

316. Giles AR, Tinlin S, Greenwood R. A canine model of hemophilic (factor VIII:C deficiency) bleeding. *Blood* 1982;60:727–730.

317. Bi L, Lawler AM, Antonarakis SE, et al. Targeted disruption of the mouse factor VIII gene produces a model of haemophilia A. *Nat Genet* 1995;10:119–121.

318. Bi L, Sarkar R, Naas T, et al. Further characterization of factor VIII-deficient mice created by gene targeting: RNA and protein studies. *Blood* 1996;88:3446–3450.

319. Connelly S, Kaleko M. Gene therapy for hemophilia A. *Thromb Haemost* 1997;78:31–36.

320. Toole JJ, Pittman DD, Orr EC, et al. A large region (approximately equal to 95 kDa) of human factor VIII is dispensable for *in vitro* procoagulant activity. *Proc Natl Acad Sci U S A* 1986;83:5939–5942.

321. Eaton DL, Wood WI, Eaton D, et al. Construction and characterization of an active factor VIII variant lacking the central one-third of the molecule. *Biochemistry* 1986;25:8343–8347.

322. Lynch CM, Israel DI, Kaufman RJ, et al. Sequences in the coding region of clotting factor VIII act as dominant inhibitors of RNA accumulation and protein production. *Hum Gene Ther* 1993;4:259–272.

323. Hoeben RC, Fallaux FJ, Cramer SJ, et al. Expression of the blood-clotting factor-VIII cDNA is repressed by a transcriptional silencer located in its coding region. *Blood* 1995;85:2447–2454.

324. Koeberl DD, Halbert CL, Krumm A, et al. Sequences within the coding regions of clotting factor VIII and CFTR block transcriptional elongation. *Hum Gene Ther* 1995;6:469–479.

325. Berntorp E. Second generation, B-domain deleted recombinant factor VIII. *Thromb Haemost* 1997;78:256–260.

326. Park F, Ohashi K, Kay MA. Therapeutic levels of human factor VIII and IX using HIV-1-based lentiviral vectors in mouse liver. *Blood* 2000;96: 1173–1176.

327. Moayeri M, Ramezani A, Morgan RA, et al. Sustained phenotypic correction of hemophilia A mice following oncoretroviral-mediated expression of a bioengineered human factor VIII gene in long-term hematopoietic repopulating cells. *Mol Ther* 2004;10:892–902.

328. Gallo-Penn AM, Shirley PS, Andrews JL, et al. Systemic delivery of an adenoviral vector encoding canine factor VIII results in short-term phenotypic correction, inhibitor development, and biphasic liver toxicity in hemophilia A dogs. *Blood* 2001;97:107–113.

329. Roy S, Shirley PS, Connelly S, et al. *In vivo* evaluation of a novel epitopetagged human factor VIII-encoding adenoviral vector. *Haemophilia* 1999; 5:340–348.

330. Connelly S, Mount J, Mauser A, et al. Complete short-term correction of canine hemophilia A by *in vivo* gene therapy. *Blood* 1996;88:3846–3853.

331. Connelly S, Gardner JM, Lyons RM, et al. Sustained expression of therapeutic levels of human factor VIII in mice. *Blood* 1996;87:4671–4677.

332. Connelly S, Gardner JM, McClelland A, et al. High-level tissue-specific expression of functional human factor VIII in mice. *Hum Gene Ther* 1996;7:183–195.

333. Connelly S, Smith TA, Dhir G, et al. *In vivo* gene delivery and expression of physiological levels of functional human factor VIII in mice. *Hum Gene Ther* 1995;6:185–193.

334. Chuah MK, Schiedner G, Thorrez L, et al. Therapeutic factor VIII levels and negligible toxicity in mouse and dog models of hemophilia A following gene therapy with high-capacity adenoviral vectors. *Blood* 2003;101: 1734–1743.

335. VandenDriessche T, Vanslembrouck V, Goovaerts I, et al. Long-term expression of human coagulation factor VIII and correction of hemophilia A after *in vivo* retroviral gene transfer in factor VIII-deficient mice. *Proc Natl Acad Sci U S A* 1999;96:10379–10384.

336. Nathwani AC, Davidoff AM, Tuddenham EG. Prospects for gene therapy of haemophilia. *Haemophilia* 2004;10:309–318.

337. Lozier J. Gene therapy of the hemophilias. *Semin Hematol* 2004;41: 287–296.

338. Roth DA, Tawa NE Jr, O'Brien JM, et al. Nonviral transfer of the gene encoding coagulation factor VIII in patients with severe hemophilia A. *N Engl J Med* 2001;344:1735–1742.

339. Powell JS, Ragni MV, White GC II, et al. Phase 1 trial of FVIII gene transfer for severe hemophilia A using a retroviral construct administered by peripheral intravenous infusion. *Blood* 2003;102:2038–2045.

340. Negrier C. Gene therapy for hemophilia? Yes. *J Thromb Haemost* 2004; 2:1234–1235.

341. Giangrande PL. Gene therapy for hemophilia? No. *J Thromb Haemost* 2004;2:1236–1237.

342. Dimichele D, Miller FG, Fins JJ. Gene therapy ethics and haemophilia: an inevitable therapeutic future? *Haemophilia* 2003;9:145–152.

# CHAPTER 9 ■ FACTOR V

WILLIAM H. KANE

Quick (1) first reported that a labile factor in plasma was necessary for the rapid conversion of prothrombin to thrombin. At approximately the same time, Owren (2) identified a patient with a severe bleeding disorder who lacked this factor. This protein, which was the fifth coagulation factor to be discovered, was designated factor V by Owren (2). Subsequent work has established that activated factor V functions as a nonenzymatic cofactor in the prothrombinase complex, which consists of factor Xa, factor Va, calcium, and a phospholipid membrane surface (3). The observation that a factor V mutation is the most common risk factor for venous thrombosis (4) has further focused attention on this protein and has led to many recent advances in the field. This chapter focuses primarily on studies reported during the last 10 years. More comprehensive reviews of earlier work are available (3,5–8).

## GENE STRUCTURE

The gene for human factor V has been localized to human chromosome 1q21-25 (9). Genomic clones encoding human factor V have been isolated from lung fibroblast and monocyte λ-phage genomic libraries (10). The Sanger Centre chromosome 1 mapping group sequenced a P1-derived artificial chromosome clone, PAC 86F14, which contains the entire human factor V gene (GenBank accession Z99572). The human factor V gene spans approximately 80 kilobases (kb) of DNA and consists of 25 exons (see Fig. 9-1). The exons range in size from 72 to 286 base pairs (bp) with the exception of exon 13, which spans 2820 bp. The 24 introns in the factor V gene range in size from 448 bp to 11.4 kb. Characterization of the exon structure of murine factor V genomic clones containing exons 7 to 13 was identical to the human gene (11,12). At the present time, there is no evidence for alternative splicing of factor V transcripts, and the mechanisms responsible for the control of factor V gene transcription and translation remain unknown.

## PROTEIN STRUCTURE

### cDNA and Predicted Amino Acid Sequence

Human factor V cDNAs have been isolated from adult liver, fetal liver, and HepG2 cDNA libraries (13–15). The cDNA for human factor V is approximately 7 kb in size and encodes a mature protein of 2,196 amino acids. Analysis of the predicted amino acid sequence revealed that the protein contains several types of internal repeats organized with the following domain structure: A1-A2-B-A3-C1-C2. The A-type domains contain approximately 350 amino acids each, the B-type domain contains approximately 836 amino acids, and the C-type domains contain approximately 150 amino acids each. Complete or partial cDNA clones have also been characterized for bovine (16), porcine (17), murine (12), chicken (18), and puffer fish (18)

factor V. The predicted amino acid sequences are approximately 60% to 90% identical except in the B-domain, where only 16% to 50% of the amino acid residues are conserved (18) (see subsequent text).

Human factor V contains 19 cysteine residues, which are conserved except for a single free cysteine in the B-domain that is not present in bovine factor V (Fig. 9-1). The disulfide bonding of the cysteines in the heavy and light chains of bovine factor Va has been determined by Xue et al. (19,20). One of the two free cysteine residues in the heavy chain of bovine factor Va is reactive with dithiobis-(nitrobenzoic acid) (DTNB) (21). A second sulfhydryl group, corresponding to Cys2113 in human factor V light chain, is also reactive with sulfhydryl modifying agents (21–23).

Factor V is a glycoprotein (24,25) that contains both N-linked and O-linked carbohydrate moieties. The primary sequence of human factor V encodes 26 strong (N-X-S/T) and 11 weak (N-X-S/T-P) potential N-linked oligosaccharide attachment sites (Fig. 9-1). Many, but not all, of these sites are clustered in the B-domain. The use of individual asparagine acceptor sites has not been determined except for Asn2181 in the light chain that is partially glycosylated (26,27).

Factor V has also been shown to contain tyrosine sulfate (28). Consensus tyrosine sulfation sites are clustered near thrombin cleavage sites that release the heavy and light chains during activation of factor V (Fig. 9-1). Tyrosine sulfate has been implicated in the interaction of thrombin with a number of proteins, including the thrombin inhibitor hirudin (29). The sulfation of recombinant factor V can be inhibited by sodium chlorate, resulting in a molecule with reduced specific activity and impaired thrombin activation (30). The exact locations of tyrosine sulfate in human factor V have not yet been determined. Factor V can be phosphorylated by a casein kinase II–like kinase expressed in activated platelets (31,32). This modification accelerates the inactivation of the molecule by activated protein C (APC) (32). The phosphorylation site has been localized to Ser692 in human factor Va (32).

### Homologies with Other Proteins

The primary sequence of human factor V is 40% identical to human coagulation factor VIII, except in the B-domain, where there is no similarity (33,34). The exon–intron organization of the genes encoding these coagulation factors is almost identical (10,34). The genes for factors V and VIII are composed of 25 and 26 exons, respectively. The gene for factor V spans approximately 80 kb, whereas the gene for factor VIII is considerably larger—approximately 180 kb—because six of the introns in the factor V gene are much smaller than the corresponding introns in the factor VIII gene. Human factor V also shares 56% amino acid identity with the snake venom protein pseutarin C, except in the B-domain, which is largely truncated in the snake venom protein (35).

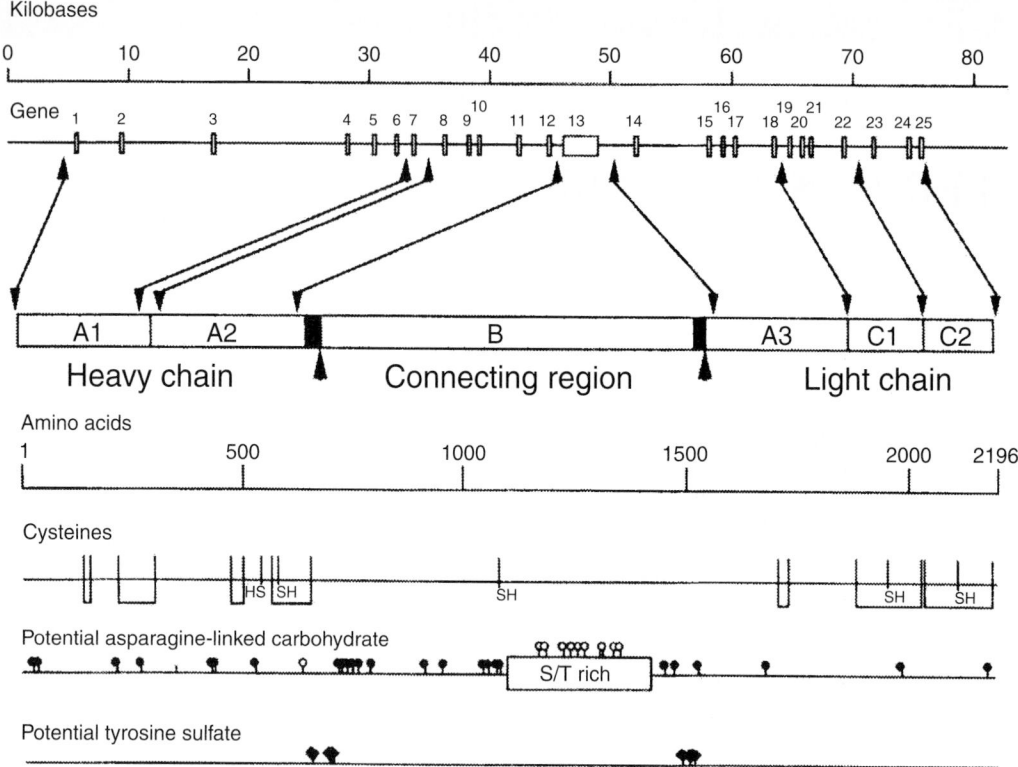

**FIGURE 9-1.** Features of the factor V gene and predicted amino acid sequence. The top line shows the scale for factor V genomic sequences in kilobases. The second line shows the intron–exon organization of the factor V gene with the exons being represented by the *open boxes*. The number of each exon is indicated and the intron sequences are represented by the *thin lines*. The domain structure encoded by the factor V cDNA is shown by the boxes labeled A1, A2, B, A3, C1, and C2. The correlation between the exon–intron structure of the factor V gene and the protein domains are shown by the *lines with arrows* at each end. The thrombin cleavage sites at Arg709 and Arg1545 are indicated by the *solid arrows*. The acidic regions adjacent to these cleavage sites are indicated by the *black boxes*. The scale in amino acids is shown in the fourth line. The fifth line shows the positions of the cysteine residues in the predicted amino acid sequence for human factor V indicated by the *vertical lines*. The predicted sulfhydryl groups in human factor V are indicated by -SH, and the connecting *horizontal lines* indicate the disulfide bonds. The sixth line indicates the presence of potential asparagine-linked carbohydrate. Strong acceptor sites are indicated by the *solid circles* and *vertical lines*; weak acceptor sites are indicated by the *open circles* and *vertical lines*. A region within the B-domain spanning greater than 200 amino acids that contains greater than 30% serine and threonine is indicated by the *box* labeled *S/T rich*. The seventh line shows the location of potential tyrosine sulfation sites, which are indicated by the *solid diamonds* and *vertical lines*.

Factor V and factor VIII contain three A-type domains, approximately 350 amino acids in length, which are approximately 30% identical to each other and to the triplicated A-type domains in the copper binding proteins ceruloplasmin (36) and hephaestin (37). Both factor V (38) and factor VIII (39) have been shown to contain a single copper ion.

The C-type domains in factor V and factor VIII are approximately 150 amino acids in length and are homologous with discoidin I, a lectin that mediates cell adhesion and migration in the single cell organism *Dictyostelium discoideum* (13–15,40). One or two copies of discoidin domains have been found in a growing family of proteins that have been implicated in cell adhesion and/or developmental processes (41).

The connecting region or B-domain of human factor V contains two tandem repeats of a 17–amino acid sequence and 31 tandem repeats of a nine–amino acid sequence (see Fig. 9-2) (13–15). The consensus sequences for these two types of repeats are SQDTGSPSXMRPWEDXP and [T,N,P]LSPDLSQT. Comparison of the sequences of the human, porcine, bovine, and murine factor V B-domains reveals that only 28% of the amino acid residues are conserved in all four species (12). Furthermore, there are several gaps present in the aligned sequences, many of

which correspond to regions containing a different number of tandem repeats. The entire B-domain of factor V is encoded within a single exon, exon 13, in both humans (10) and mice (12). Similarly, the B-domain of factor VIII is also encoded in a single exon (34). There has been relatively little selective pressure to conserve amino acid sequences in the B-domains, which are released during cofactor activation. The significance of the tandem repeat structures that are present in the B-domain of factor V but not factor VIII remains to be determined.

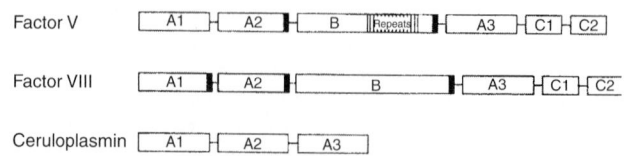

**FIGURE 9-2.** Protein modules in factor V and related proteins. Structural domains in factor V, factor VIII, and ceruloplasmin are indicated by the labeled boxes (see text). The acidic regions adjacent to thrombin cleavage sites in factor V and factor VIII are indicated by the *black boxes.*

## Structure and Physical Properties

Factor V circulates in the plasma as a single-chain glycoprotein with an approximate molecular weight of 330,000 kDa (24, 42–44). Adams et al. (45) have recently solved the structure of APC inactivated bovine factor Vai (A1/A3-C1-C2) (see Fig. 9-3). This structure, together with the structure of the triplicated A-domains in ceruloplasmin (46) has been used to generate a molecular model for factor Va (45). In this model, the triplicated A-domains of factor Va are arranged in a pseudo-threefold axis similar to ceruloplasmin. In factor Va, the three A-domains sit on a platform formed by the two C-domains, which are aligned in an edge-to-edge fashion.

The locations of the high-affinity binding sites for both calcium and copper have been identified in the factor Vai structure (45). The high-affinity $Ca^{2+}$ binding site is located in the A1 domain of factor Va with ligands Asp111 and Asp112 along with the main chain carbonyl oxygens of Lys93 and Glu108 (45,47). The $Cu^{2+}$ binding site is located in the A3 domain of bovine factor Va with ligands His1802, His1804, and Asp1844 arranged in a trigonal planar coordination geometry (45). Neither binding site is involved directly in bridging the heavy and light chains. Occupancy of the high-affinity $Ca^{2+}$ binding site is necessary for stable association of the factor Va heavy and light chains (47,48). The functional importance of $Cu^{2+}$ in factor V is not known; however, the binding of $Cu^{2+}$ to factor VIIIa stabilizes the noncovalent association of factor VIIIa subunits (49).

The structure of the factor V B-domain has not yet been determined. The ultrastructure of factor V and factor Va has been studied using electron microscopy (50,51). Factor V contains a globular core 10 to 12 nm in diameter, which corresponds to the factor Va heavy and light chain. Extending from the globular core is a rodlike tail of up to 50 nm in length that corresponds to the B-domain. Thrombin activation of factor V removes the tail structure from the globular domain leading to activation of the molecule.

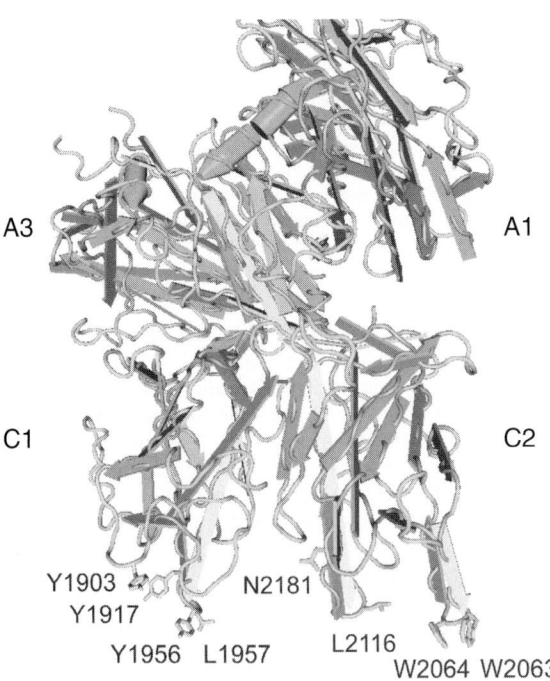

A3    A1

C1    C2

Y1903    N2181
Y1917
Y1956  L1957    L2116
W2064 W2063

**FIGURE 9-3.** Structure of bovine factor Vai solved by Adams et al. (45). Domains and selected hydrophobic amino acid residues implicated in membrane binding are labeled. Alternative glycosylation at Asn2181 results in the glycoforms factor Va₁ and factor Va₂.

# STRUCTURE–FUNCTION RELATIONSHIPS

## Activation of Factor V

As a single-chain protein, factor V expresses very little, if any, procoagulant activity (52). Procoagulant activity is expressed following limited proteolysis at discrete sites in the molecule. Thrombin activates human factor V by cleavage at Arg709, Arg1018, and Arg1545 (see Fig. 9-4) (15). Thrombin-activated factor V is a calcium-dependent heterodimer consisting of a 105-kDa heavy chain (A1-A2) and a 73-kDa light chain (A3-C1-C2) (43,48,53–55). The B-domain is not necessary for procoagulant activity and is released during activation by thrombin (53,54,56). The use of snake venom proteases and factor V mutants has provided important insights into the functions of the individual thrombin cleavage sites (57–61). Thrombin cleavage at Arg709 is kinetically favored over cleavage at Arg1018 and Arg1545. Thrombin cleavage at Arg709 results in little or no increase in cofactor activity (57,58,60). Cleavage at both Arg709 and Arg1018 releases the amino-terminal portion of the B-domain resulting in further partial activation of the cofactor (57,60). Cleavage at Arg1545 and release of the carboxyl-terminal fragment of the B-domain from the light chain fragment is required for maximal activation (57,58,60,61). Cleavage at Arg709 and Arg1018 is necessary for maximal rates of factor V activation by thrombin (57,58). Factor V mutants, in which cleavage at Arg709 and/or Arg1018 are blocked, are resistant to thrombin cleavage at Arg1545. In contrast, these mutants can be fully activated by the snake venom protease RVV-V, which cleaves factor V at Arg1018 and Arg1545 (57,61). These observations indicate that release of the B-domain from the heavy chain is not absolutely required for maximal expression of procoagulant activity.

Thrombin cleavage of factor V at Arg709 and Arg1545 requires interactions with anion-binding exosite-1 on thrombin (62–64). An acidic region in factor V, Asp695-Tyr698, is required for efficient thrombin cleavage at Arg709 (65). The sequence of this peptide (DYDYQ) contains the consensus sequence for tyrosine sulfation and is the likely site of sulfation in the factor Va heavy chain (28). Tyrosine sulfation of factor V has been previously shown to be required for efficient thrombin cleavage at both Arg709 and Arg1545 (30). The factor V B-domain contains a similar acidic region Glu1508-Tyr1515, which is the likely site of sulfation in the factor V B-domain (28,30). This peptide (EDDYAEIDY) may also play a role in binding to exosite-1 and facilitating thrombin cleavage at Arg1545. Consistent with this hypothesis, deletion of the entire factor V B-domain (amino acids 710–1545) results in a molecule that is resistant to thrombin cleavage and activation (66). In contrast, factor V molecules with deletions of amino acid residues 811 to 1491 (57,67,68) or 709 to 1476 (69) were efficiently cleaved by thrombin and fully activated.

Characterization of the B-domain deletion mutant lacking amino acid residues 811 to 1492 indicates that deletion of the B-domain results in a partially (67) or fully (68) active single-chain cofactor. Mutation of the thrombin cleavage sites at Arg709 and Arg1545 confirmed that the enhanced activity was not due to cleavage at these sites (57,68). Mutation of the individual thrombin cleavage sites demonstrated that the activity of the single-chain cofactor was not affected by thrombin cleavage at Arg709 and that cleavage at Arg1545 resulted in a fully active cofactor (57). These results suggest the presence of the B-domain in factor V is necessary to inhibit constitutive cofactor activity. Removal of portions of the B-domain leads to partial activation of the cofactor; however, cleavage at Arg1545 is essential for complete activation of factor V (57). Consistent with this

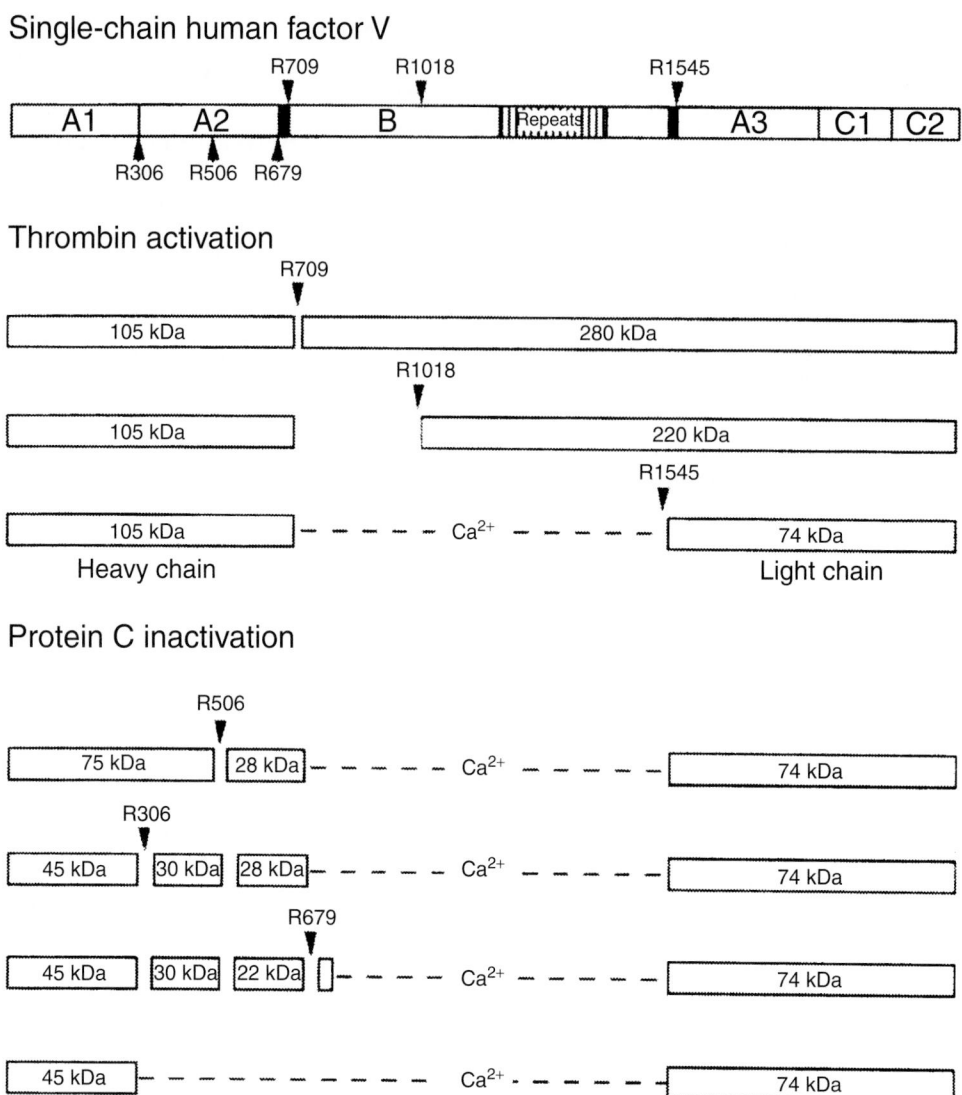

**FIGURE 9-4.** Proteolytic activation and inactivation of human factor V. The domains present in single-chain human factor V are indicated by the labeled *boxes*. The locations of the cleavage sites for thrombin and APC are indicated by the *arrows* at the top and bottom of the figure, respectively. The apparent molecular mass of the intermediates and final products following activation by thrombin and inactivation by APC are indicated. The orders of bond cleavage shown are favored kinetically but do not exclude other pathways. The heavy chain and light chain of thrombin-activated factor Va form a calcium-dependent heterodimer. The activation fragments released from the connecting region during thrombin activation and from the A2 domain, following inactivation by APC, are not shown.

observation, thrombin cleavage at Arg1545 appears to be required for optimal factor Xa binding affinity (60,61).

Factor V can also be activated by factor Xa (58,70). Factor Xa cleaves factor V at Arg709, Arg1018, and Arg1545 to produce activation products similar to thrombin-activated factor Va (58). There are a number of significant differences between the activation of factor V by thrombin and by factor Xa. First, activation of factor V by factor Xa requires an anionic phospholipid membrane surface (70,71). Second, the activation of factor V by factor Xa appears to be less efficient because enzyme substrate ratios of 1:10 are needed for efficient activation (58,70). Third, the acidic spacer region and the other cleavage sites in the B-domain of factor V do not appear to be required for optimal factor Xa cleavage at Arg1545 (69). Fourth, tyrosine sulfation does not appear to be required for efficient cleavage at Arg709 or Arg1545 (30). Finally, at high factor Xa concentrations, factor Xa also cleaves the factor Va light chain at Arg1761 and Arg1765 (58,60).

The relative importance of thrombin- and factor Xa–catalyzed activation of factor V has been evaluated in purified systems (72–74). In the presence of high concentrations of tissue factor–factor VIIa (5 nM), both factor Xa and thrombin were responsible for factor V activation (72). In contrast, when clotting was initiated in the presence of low concentrations of tissue factor–factor VIIa (1.25 pM), no factor V activation was observed in the absence of thrombin. Thorelli et al. (59) found that mutation of the thrombin cleavage sites at Arg709 and/or Arg1545 resulted in impaired thrombin generation in purified systems when clotting was initiated with low concentrations of tissue factor. These mutations had little effect on thrombin generation when clotting was initiated in the presence of high concentrations of tissue factor, suggesting that other proteolytic cleavages may contribute to the generation of cofactor activity under these conditions. Using biophysical and biochemical approaches to establish second-order rate constants and numerical simulations incorporating the various pathways of factor V activation, Orfeo et al. (74) concluded that direct activation of factor V by factor Xa at physiologically relevant concentrations does not appear to be a significant contributor to factor Va formation.

Several other enzymes have also been shown to activate factor V. In contrast to the activators discussed previously, these enzymes can only partially activate factor V. The proteolytic cleavage patterns are complex, and the locations of individual cleavage sites have in many cases not been completely defined. Platelet calpain is capable of partially activating factor V, producing proteolytic cleavage products distinct from those obtained with thrombin (75). Furthermore, the factor V released from activated platelets is partially activated and is more sensitive to activation by factor Xa than is plasma factor V (76,77). Monocyte-derived cathepsin G cleaves factor V at Tyr696, Phe1031, and Leu1518, resulting in a 103-kDa heavy chain and an 80-kDa light chain (78). Human neutrophil elastase cleaves factor V at Thr678, Ile708, Ile819, and Ile1484, resulting in a 102-kDa heavy chain and a 90-kDa light chain (78). Plasmin has been reported to both activate and inactivate human factor V (79,80). Finally, a protease (NN) purified from the venom of the snake *Naja nigricollis nigricollis* cleaves factor V at Asp697, Asp1509, and Asp1514, resulting in a 100-kDa heavy chain and a 80-kDa light chain (61).

## Function of Factor Va in the Prothrombinase Complex

The procoagulant activity of factor Va is manifested by its ability to markedly enhance the activation of prothrombin to thrombin by the serine proteinase factor Xa in the presence of calcium ions and a procoagulant phospholipid surface (3). Factor V contributes to the amplification of prothrombin activation by (a) stabilizing the enzyme (factor Xa)–cofactor–(factor Va)–substrate (prothrombin) complex and by (b) altering the kinetic mechanism of prothrombin activation (3,81). Steady-state kinetic measurements of thrombin formation comparing the activity of factor Xa alone with that observed using binary and ternary combinations of the protease factor Va and phospholipid membrane surface have been used to investigate the mechanism for the enhanced activity of the prothrombinase complex (52,82–84). The acceleration of prothrombin activation by phospholipids results from a 100-fold decrease in the $K_m$ for prothrombin (82,84). In the presence of membranes with a low content of phosphatidylserine and a low affinity for prothrombin, factor Va also lowers the $K_m$ for prothrombin (84). However, the major contribution of factor Va is a 3,000-fold increase in the $V_{max}$ for prothrombin activation (52,82, 84). The observed increase in $V_{max}$ is due in part to the fact that factor Va acts as a receptor for factor Xa resulting in an increased concentration of factor Xa at the membrane surface. However, the main effect of factor Va is to enhance the catalytic efficiency $k_{cat}$ of prothrombin activation. The molecular basis for this enhanced catalytic efficiency remains poorly understood. The activation of prothrombin can proceed by two pathways, depending on the order of bond cleavage at Arg271 and Arg320. In the absence of factor Va, factor Xa slowly converts prothrombin to thrombin through the reaction intermediates fragment 1.2 and prethrombin 2 (85). However, in the presence of factor Va, prothrombin activation proceeds exclusively through the intermediate meizothrombin (86–89). This shift in the reaction pathway could result from effects of factor Va on the orientation of factor Xa and prothrombin (90). Additionally, factor Va may lead to conformation changes in factor Xa exosites involved in substrate recognition (91–93). Recent data also demonstrates channeling of $\alpha$-thrombin activation intermediates during activation of prothrombin by the prothrombinase complex that minimizes the appearance of intermediates in solution (94–96).

## Interaction of Factor Va with Phospholipid Membranes

Formation of the prothrombinase complex requires the presence of a membrane surface to which the individual components will bind and subsequently assemble into a functional complex. Activated platelets, platelet microparticles, and damaged vascular cells provide this surface *in vivo* (97). The interaction of factor V with cellular surfaces appears to be mediated, at least in part, by binding to acidic phospholipids (e.g., phosphatidylserine). These phospholipids are normally sequestered in the inner leaflet of the cellular membrane, facing the cytoplasm, but become exposed following platelet activation and microparticle formation (97). Synthetic phospholipid vesicles have been used as a model system to study these interactions. Factor Va binds to phospholipid vesicles containing 25% phosphatidylserine and 75% phosphatidylcholine with a $K_d$ of approximately $10^{-9}$ M (21,98). Binding to phospholipid membranes does not require cofactor activation or the presence of calcium ions (21,99).

High-affinity binding of factor Va to a phospholipid membrane surface requires the presence of phosphatidylserine because poor binding is observed using vesicles containing only phosphatidylcholine (21). Each molecule of factor Va binds to approximately 10 phosphatidylserine molecules (21). The affinity of factor Va for phospholipid membranes decreases as the phosphatidylserine content of the membrane drops below 15% (100). The interaction of factor Va with phosphatidylserine shows high specificity and is not simply caused by the electrostatic potential of the phospholipid membrane. Therefore, the procoagulant activity of phosphatidylserine is not diminished significantly when the surface charge of the membrane is made positive by incorporation of stearylamine (101). Furthermore, optimal binding of factor Va to the membrane depends on the stereochemical configuration of the polar headgroup of phosphatidylserine (102). Factor Va binds to membranes containing L-$\alpha$-glycerophosphoryl-L-serine with approximately 25-fold higher affinity than to the L-$\alpha$-glycerophosphoryl-D-serine isomer. Membranes containing phosphatidylcholine alone bind factor Va with low affinity and a $K_d$ of $3 \times 10^{-6}$ M (103). This suggests the interaction of factor Va with neutral phospholipids in the membrane may also contribute considerably to the total free energy of binding (100,103). The interaction of factor Va with phospholipids membranes appears to involve both hydrophobic (104,105) and electrostatic interactions (106–108).

The primary membrane-binding sites for factor V are contained within the light chain fragment (A3-C1-C2) (109,110). Membrane-binding sites for PS membranes have been identified in the C1 (111,112) and C2 (112–118) domains of factor V. The structures factor Va-C2 (22) and APC-inactivated factor Vai (A1/A3-C1-C2) (45) have been solved and provide important insights into the membrane-binding mechanism. The factor V C1 and C2 domains are each composed of a common distorted jelly-roll $\beta$-barrel structure with three variable loops, or "spikes," located at the membrane-binding surface (22,45). The C1 and C2 domains in factor Va are aligned in an edge-to-edge orientation, making it possible for the variable loops in both domains to interact with a membrane surface (45). In contrast, the factor V A3 domain, which has also been proposed to interact with phospholipids membranes (21,118), rests on top of the platform formed by the C1 and C2 domains (45).

The factor V C2 domain provides most of the free energy associated with the binding of factor Va to phospholipids membranes (119). Spike-1 in the factor V C2 domain consists of a $\beta$-hairpin structure with the solvent-exposed indole side chains of Trp2063/Trp2064 located at the apex (22). These indole side chains insert into the membrane bilayer (120) and are required for high-affinity binding of factor Va to phospholipids membranes (116,119). Spike-3 within the factor V C2 domain also contains a β-hairpin structure with the solvent-exposed side chain of Leu2116 at the apex. The role of Leu2116 in membrane binding remains to be clarified; however, the groove formed by spike-1 and spike-3 has been proposed to contain a stereospecific PS-binding pocket (22). The isolated factor V C2 domain binds one molecule of soluble PS (C6PS) (23). The binding of C6PS to the isolated factor V C2 domain can be blocked by 5,5-dithiobis(2-nitrobenzoate) (DTNB) modification of Cys2113, which is located near the proposed PS-binding site (23,26). Partial glycosylation of the factor V C2 domain modulates the affinity of factor Va for membranes containing phosphatidylserine (26,98,121,122). Factor Va exists as two isoforms, factor $Va_1$ and $Va_2$, because of partial glycosylation at Asp2181 (26,27), which is located near the membrane-binding site (22,45). Glycosylation of the C2 = × 8 domain reduces the affinity of factor $Va_1$ for negatively charged phospholipid membranes up to 50-fold compared to factor $Va_2$ (26,98,121,122). As a result of this difference in membrane-binding affinity, factor $Va_1$ expresses decreased cofactor activity compared to factor $Va_2$ when prothrombin is activated on membranes containing low concentrations of phosphatidylserine (98,121).

The factor V C1 domain also contributes to membrane binding. Spike-3 in the factor V C1 domain contains a β-hairpin structure with the solvent-exposed side chains of Tyr1956/Leu1957 located at the apex (45,111). Alanine substitutions for Tyr1956/Leu1957 reduce the affinity of factor Va for 25% PS membranes by 12-fold (111). The ability of both factor Va mutants (W2063,W2064)A and (Y1956,L1957)A to form a productive prothrombinase complex is markedly reduced on 5% PS membranes, but only minimally affected on 25% PS membranes (111,116,119). However, combined mutation of C1 and C2 domain hydrophobic residues, (Y1956,L1957,W2063,W2064)A, effectively blocks prothrombinase complex assembly on 25% PS membranes (112).

## Interaction of Factor Va with Factor Xa

Factor Va interacts with factor Xa in the presence of calcium ions on a phospholipid membrane surface to accelerate the conversion of prothrombin to thrombin. Factor Xa binds to phospholipids membranes; however, the affinity of this interaction is low ($K_d$ 0.1 μM) (123), and physiologic concentrations of factor Xa probably do not exceed 0.15 nM (124). In the absence of membranes, factor Xa binds to factor Va, but the affinity of this interaction is also low ($K_d$ 1 μM) (125). However, when factor Va is bound to a membrane surface containing acidic phospholipids, the affinity of factor Xa binding increases by more than three orders of magnitude (21,52,123,126–128). The high affinity of factor Xa for factor Va on the membrane surface ($K_d$ 1 nM) appears to be due to additive factor Xa–factor Va (129) and factor Xa membrane interactions (130). Binding of factor Xa to factor Va allosterically alters the active site of factor Xa and, in addition, repositions the active site of the enzyme to the proper distance above the membrane for prothrombin activation (90). The binding of factor Xa to factor Va also results in modulation of the binding of prothrombin to substrate binding exosites distinct from the active site of factor Xa (131,132). Recent studies also suggest that PS may allosterically regulate interactions between factor Va and factor Xa (133).

The interaction between factor Va and factor Xa involves discontinuous epitopes on both the heavy chain (134–140) and the light chain (134,135,141) of the activated cofactor. Synthetic peptides have been used to identify binding sites involving residues 311 to 325 (136), 323 to 331 (138,139), and 493 to 506 (137) in the heavy chain. Site-directed glycosylation has also been used to demonstrate that regions surrounding residues 467, 511, and 652 in the heavy chain and residue 1683 in the light chain are important for factor Xa binding to factor Va (142). The ability of factor Va to bind to factor Xa is lost when factor Va is proteolytically cleaved by APC (140). APC cleavage of factor Va at Arg506 decreases the affinity of the cofactor for factor Xa (143), whereas APC cleavage at Arg306 leads to a total loss of factor Xa binding (144). Membrane-dependent cleavage of factor Va at Lys309, Lys310, and Arg313 by plasmin also prevents factor Xa binding (80). Removal of the carboxyl-terminal region of the factor Va heavy chain 684-709 results in reduced affinity for factor Xa (145).

## Interaction of Factor Va with Prothrombin

The interaction between factor Va and prothrombin is mediated by the heavy chain of the cofactor, and this interaction is independent of calcium ions (146). Prothrombin does not bind to factor V, indicating that the cofactor must be activated before it will bind prothrombin (140). Sedimentation equilibrium analysis revealed that the factor Va heavy chain and prothrombin form a 1:1 complex with a dissociation constant of 10 μM (146). Proteolysis of the factor Va heavy chain by APC results in the loss of its ability to bind prothrombin (140). A prothrombin-binding site has been localized to an acid peptide containing residues 697 to 709 at the carboxyl terminus of the factor Va heavy chain (61,65). The binding of prothrombin to factor Va appears to involve proexosite-1 in the catalytic domain of prothrombin (147) as well as the kringle 1 and kringle 2 domains (148).

## Inactivation of Factor Va

### Protein C Cleavage Sites

Activation of the protein C pathway leads to inactivation of factor Va and downregulation of the prothrombinase complex. APC is a vitamin K–dependent serine protease that inactivates factor Va by limited proteolysis of the factor Va heavy chain (140,149). Efficient inactivation of factor Va requires a protein cofactor, protein S (150,151), and a phospholipid (144,152,153) or platelet membrane surface (154,155). APC cleaves human factor Va heavy chain at Arg306, Arg506, and Arg679 (Fig. 9-4) (156). The APC cleavage sites at Arg306 and Arg506 are conserved in bovine (16), porcine (17), and murine (12) factor V. The APC cleavage site corresponding to Arg679 is not conserved in bovine factor Va; however, the bovine protein can be cleaved at Arg662 (144). In porcine and murine factor Va, the cleavage sites corresponding to Arg679 and Arg662 are both conserved. There is an additional APC cleavage site present at Lys994 in the B-domain of human factor V (156). This cleavage site is conserved in porcine and murine factor V, but not in the bovine protein. Binding sites for APC have been localized to the factor Va light chain (157,158).

### Kinetics of Activated Protein C Catalyzed Cleavage

Characterization of factor $V_{Leiden}$ ($FV_{Leiden}$) has helped to define the roles of the APC cleavage sites at Arg306 and Arg506. $FV_{Leiden}$ lacks the APC cleavage site at Arg506 due to substitution of glutamine at this position (R506Q). Several groups have isolated factor V from patients homozygous for this mutation and have studied inactivation of the molecule by APC (143,159–162). APC-catalyzed inactivation of factor Va isolated from normal individuals is characterized by an initial rapid loss of activity followed by a second, slower phase that results in complete inactivation of the cofactor (143). In contrast, APC-catalyzed inactivation of $FVa_{Leiden}$ occurs slowly, at a rate similar to the second phase of inactivation of normal factor Va. Therefore, the initial rapid phase of factor Va inactivation correlates with APC cleavage at Arg506. Both heavy-chain fragments generated following APC cleavage at Arg506 remain associated with the factor Va light chain (143). APC cleavage at Arg506 results in a partial loss of cofactor activity because of a 50-fold decrease in the affinity of the cofactor for factor Xa (143). The amount of residual cofactor activity measured following APC cleavage at Arg506 is variable depending on the concentration of factor Xa present in the assay. The second, slow phase of inactivation seen during inactivation of factor Va and $FVa_{Leiden}$ correlates with APC cleavage at Arg306. APC cleavage at Arg306 releases the heavy-chain fragment corresponding to the A2 domain (amino acids 307–709), generating an A1/A3C1C2 heterodimer that expresses no cofactor activity (163). Initially, it was thought that APC cleavage at Arg506 was required for exposure of the APC cleavage site at Arg306 (156). However, subsequent studies characterizing the inactivation of $FVa_{Leiden}$ have demonstrated that APC cleavage at Arg506 is kinetically favored but not required for cleavage at Arg306 (143,159). Kinetic analysis of APC cleavage at Arg506 revealed a $k_{cat}$ of 0.9 per second with a $K_m$ of 20 nM, whereas analysis of APC cleavage at Arg306 revealed a $k_{cat}$ of 0.37 per second with a much higher $K_m$ of 190 nM (143). The role of APC cleavage at Arg679 has not been completely defined. APC cleavage at Arg679 occurs more slowly than APC cleavage at Arg506 or Arg306 and appears to play a minor role in the inactivation of normal factor Va (143,159). The importance of APC cleavage at Arg506 has been confirmed in studies characterizing tissue factor–initiated prothrombin activation in plasma (164) and in a reconstituted system using purified components (165). In these studies, the amount of thrombin formed in the presence of $FV_{Leiden}$ was found to be significantly increased compared to the native protein.

Rapid inactivation of factor Va by APC requires a phospholipid membrane surface containing phosphatidylserine (144). At low concentrations of phosphatidylserine, phosphatidylethanolamine selectively promotes the inactivation of factor Va by APC (152,166). Rapid cleavage of factor Va by APC at Arg306 is completely membrane dependent (144). APC cleavage of factor Va at Arg506 can occur in the absence of phospholipid membranes (156); however, the membranes do enhance the rate of this cleavage (143). In contrast, the slow cleavage of factor Va at Arg679 does not appear to be enhanced on the membrane surface (143,156). Factor Va exists as two isoforms, factor $Va_1$ and factor $Va_2$, that differ in their affinity for phospholipid membranes (98) (see preceding text). Factor $Va_1$ has a lower affinity for phospholipid membranes and is inactivated by APC at a slower rate than factor $Va_2$ (121). The phospholipid requirements for APC-catalyzed factor Va inactivation and of expression of factor Va procoagulant activity were found to differ significantly (121). Therefore, the thrombin-forming capacity of factor $V_1$ was found to be sevenfold higher than factor $V_2$ when examined in the presence of factor Xa, prothrombin, APC, protein S, and a membrane surface similar to that of activated platelets (121).

Protein S is a vitamin K–dependent plasma protein that acts as a cofactor promoting inactivation of factor Va by APC. Protein S was shown to selectively promote APC cleavage of factor Va at Arg306 while having no effect on the rate of APC cleavage at Arg506 (161). Biophysical studies have demonstrated that protein S repositions the active site of APC from 94 Å to 84 Å above the membrane surface, providing a structural explanation for the enhanced rate of APC cleavage at Arg306 (167,168). Protein S may also directly inhibit prothrombinase in the absence of APC through direct interactions with factor Xa and factor Va (169–171).

Formation of the prothrombinase complex by addition of factor Xa protects factor Va from inactivation by APC (172). Rosing et al. (161) demonstrated that factor Xa selectively

inhibits APC cleavage at Arg506 while having no effect on the rate of APC cleavage at Arg306. These findings suggest that the binding sites for factor Xa and APC overlap. The inhibitory effects of factor Xa can be partially overcome in the presence of protein S because of the enhanced rate of APC cleavage at Arg306 (161). In the presence of both factor Xa and protein S, therefore, inactivation of factor Va and $FVa_{Leiden}$ proceed at similar rates because the contribution of APC cleavage at Arg506 to inactivation of the cofactor is minimal under these conditions (161). These observations may explain the relatively mild prothrombotic risk associated with the $FV_{Leiden}$ mutation.

In the initial studies characterizing patients who were resistant to APC, Dahlbäck hypothesized that the molecular defect in these patients was the deficiency of a cofactor for APC that was designated APC cofactor II (173). This cofactor was subsequently identified to be factor V (174). However, the discovery by Bertina et al. (4) that most APC-resistant patients express a factor V molecule lacking the APC cleavage site at Arg506 suggested the resistance of $FV_{Leiden}$ to APC inactivation was due directly to delayed inactivation of the protein by APC. Detailed studies carried out by several groups characterizing inactivation of $FV_{Leiden}$ by APC have confirmed this proposed mechanism (see preceding text). The potential role of factor V as a cofactor for the inactivation of factor Va has been difficult to study because factor V can be cleaved by thrombin, factor Xa, and APC. However, factor VIIIa is inactivated by APC in the presence of protein S and phospholipid membranes (175), and recent studies have confirmed that factor V enhances the rate of inactivation of factor VIIIa (176–178). The structural requirements for the APC cofactor activity expressed by factor V have been further defined using assays measuring the rate of APC-catalyzed inactivation of factor VIIIa. The APC cofactor activity of factor V is lost following activation of factor V by thrombin (176). Thrombin cleavage at Arg709 and Arg1018 has no effect on APC cofactor activity (179); however, cleavage at Arg1545 by either thrombin (179) or Russell viper venom (178,179) results in a total loss of APC cofactor activity. The carboxyl-terminal region of the B-domain appears to be required for expression of APC cofactor activity (179). Therefore, a factor V deletion mutant lacking amino acids 709 to 1476 of the B-domain expresses normal APC cofactor activity, whereas deletion of the entire B-domain (amino acids 710–1545) results in a complete loss of APC cofactor activity (179). Proteolysis of single-chain factor V by APC appears to be required for optimal expression of APC cofactor II activity (178,180). Lu et al. (177) found that all of the single-chain factor V had been cleaved by APC at the beginning of the factor VIIIa inactivation assay. Varadi et al. (178) observed that factor $V_{Leiden}$ expressed 10-fold less APC cofactor II activity compared to the native protein. Thorelli et al. (180) confirmed that mutation of the APC cleavage site at Arg506 resulted in poor APC cofactor II activity and demonstrated that mutation of the other APC cleavage sites at Arg306 and Arg679 had no effect. These observations suggest that the proteolytic regulation of the procoagulant and anticoagulant functions of factor V are complex due to the activities of partially cleaved intermediates (180). Therefore, APC cleavage of factor V at Arg506 leads to expression of APC cofactor activity. Subsequent cleavage by thrombin at Arg709 and Arg1018 results in a molecule that expresses both APC cofactor activity and procoagulant activity. Complete activation by thrombin results in a molecule that still retains significant procoagulant activity. The importance of factor V APC cofactor activity in regulating thrombin generation has been confirmed in studies characterizing tissue factor–initiated prothrombin activation in plasma (181). Further studies are required to confirm the physiologic importance of factor V cleavage products in regulating the activity of factor VIII activity *in vivo* and to determine whether the APC cofactor activity of factor V also plays a role in regulation of the prothrombinase complex.

# BIOSYNTHESIS AND PROCESSING

Factor V circulates in plasma at a concentration of approximately 10 $\mu$g per mL (30 nM). In addition to circulating in the plasma compartment, approximately 20% of the factor V in blood is contained in platelet $\alpha$-granules (182). The storage of factor V within platelets appears to be important because, when platelets aggregate to form the primary hemostatic plug, they also provide both a surface for assembly of the prothrombinase complex as well as high local concentrations of released platelet factor V (183). The main site of factor V biosynthesis appears to be the liver because plasma factor V levels are decreased in advanced liver disease. Factor V mRNA has been detected in human liver (15), and the protein is expressed in HepG2 cells (12) and in primary cultures of normal adult human hepatocytes (184). Human megakaryocytes also have been shown to contain factor V mRNA (185,186), and factor V is expressed in both guinea pig (187) and human megakaryocytes (186,188). However, recent evidence suggests that in humans, most or all of platelet factor V originates from the plasma pool (189,190). Platelet fibrinogen, albumin, and IgG have been shown to originate from the plasma through endocytosis (191). However, uptake of factor V by megakaryocytes has not yet been demonstrated, and the origin of platelet factor V in humans remains controversial (192). In contrast to humans, the murine platelet factor V compartment is derived exclusively from primary biosynthesis within cells of marrow origin, presumably megakaryocytes (193). Furthermore, in the mouse, either the platelet or plasma factor V pool is sufficient for basal hemostasis (194). The synthesis of factor V by several other cell types, including bovine aortic endothelial cells (195), bovine vascular smooth muscle cells (196), and human mesangial cells (197), has also been reported. The physiologic importance of synthesis at these sites remains to be determined.

Little is known about regulation of factor V gene expression (10). As reviewed in preceding text, factor V undergoes a number of important posttranslational modifications, including glycosylation (24,198,199), sulfation (28,30), and phosphorylation (31,32). Asparagine-linked glycosylation is required for efficient secretion of factor V (25), and deletion of the heavily glycosylated B-domain results in increased levels of protein expression (67). During biosynthesis, factor V interacts with calreticulin, a protein chaperone that preferentially interacts with glycoproteins containing monoglucosylated N-linked oligosaccharides during transit through the secretory pathway (200). The combined deficiency of factor V and factor VIII has been found to be caused by defects in two proteins localized to the endoplasmic reticulum-Golgi intermediate compartment (201–205). These findings suggest that the transport and secretion of both factor V and factor VIII may require specific interactions with molecular chaperones (205). The plasma clearances of factor V– and factor V–derived peptides have been studied in the baboon (206). The half-life of single-chain factor V was found to be approximately 13 hours. The isolated factor Va heavy chain and light chain were each cleared very rapidly with half-lives of less than 20 minutes. In contrast, the 150-kDa B-domain activation peptide that is released following thrombin was cleared very slowly, with a half-life of greater than 60 hours.

# INTERACTIONS OF FACTOR V WITH VASCULAR CELLS

Activated human platelets promote the conversion of prothrombin to thrombin by the prothrombinase complex (207). Following platelet activation, factor V is secreted from platelet $\alpha$-granules (208) and phosphatidylserine is expressed on the surface of activated platelets, allowing assembly of the prothrombinase complex (97). Platelet factor V is heterogeneous because of proteolysis within the B-domain (76,77,209). The protease and cleavage sites have not been identified; however, these cleavages result in both partial activation of the cofactor and increased susceptibility of the cofactor to activation by factor Xa (76,77,209). Recent N-terminal sequencing and MALDI-TOF analysis of platelet-derived factor V/Va peptides have identified the presence of a full-length heavy chain subunit, as well as a light chain formed by cleavage at Tyr1543 rather than at Arg1545, accounting for the intrinsic levels of cofactor activity (77). Platelet factor V/Va was also found to be uniquely modified on Thr402 with an N-acetylglucosamine or N-acetylgalactosamine (77). Furthermore, Ser691 in platelet factor V/Va was found to be unmodified and resistant to phosphorylation by either casein kinase II or activated platelets (77). Platelet factor V is stored in a complex with another $\alpha$-granule protein, multimerin 1 (210). Approximately 25% of platelet factor V is covalently linked to multimerin 1 through a disulfide linkage involving Cys1085 in the factor V B-domain (211). A multimerin 1 binding site has been localized to the factor V C2 domain, which overlaps with the binding site for phosphatidylserine (212). The dissociation of platelet factor V-multimerin 1 complexes following factor V activation suggests a role for multimerin 1 localizing factor V on the platelet surface before prothrombinase assembly (212). Platelet factor V may also be cleaved and partially activated by calpain during platelet activation (75). The majority of factor V circulates in the plasma as a single-chain procofactor (182). However, the release of partially active platelet factor V is thought to be an important stimulus for thrombin formation during the early phases of hemostasis (76,77). Following the activation of human platelets with thrombin, factor V can be cross-linked to actin in the platelet cytoskeleton by factor XIIIa (213). Factor XIIIa catalyzes the incorporation of synthetic amines into the factor V B-domain and forms cross-links leading to the production of homo- (214,215) and hetero-polymers (213) containing factor V. The physiologic importance of these reactions requires further study; however, it is possible that they provide an additional mechanism for localizing factor V to the surface of activated platelets. The nature of the membrane-binding sites for factor Va and the prothrombinase complex have not been completely defined (54,216). Exposure of phosphatidylserine on the surface of intact platelets and platelet microparticles appears to be required for expression of these binding sites (97); however, additional platelet membrane proteins may also be required. The surface of activated platelets also promotes the inactivation of factor Va by APC (154,155). Compared to plasma-derived factor Va, platelet factor V is resistant to complete inactivation by APC (77,217). The molecular basis for the impaired inactivation of platelet factor V by APC is not yet known. These differences may be due to differential phosphorylation of the factor Va heavy chain by a platelet kinase (77,218). Assembly of the prothrombinase complex has also been demonstrated on the surface of activated endothelial cells (219,220) and on monocytes (221). Inactivation of factor Va by APC occurs more rapidly on endothelial cell surfaces than on the surface of activated platelets (222,223).

# MOLECULAR GENETICS

## Factor V Deficiency

Congenital factor V deficiency, also called parahemophilia, is a rare disorder that has an estimated incidence of 1 in $10^6$. More than 200 cases have been reported in the literature (224).

Parahemophilia is characterized by low levels of functional factor V activity in plasma and platelets and is inherited in an autosomal recessive manner. Clinical manifestations include ecchymoses, epistaxis, oral bleeding, menorrhagia, and bleeding following surgery or trauma. Rare patients have also been reported who have had thromboembolic events, including deep and superficial venous thromboses, pulmonary embolism, stroke, and myocardial infarction (225). Most patients with congenital factor V deficiency have low antigenic levels of factor V; however, approximately 17% of patients were found to have a discrepancy between their functional and antigenic levels (226). Plasma factor V levels have not correlated well with the hemorrhagic tendency, and several authors have suggested that the severity of bleeding symptoms may be more closely correlated with platelet than with plasma factor V levels (183,227). The molecular basis for factor V deficiency has been established in more than 35 patients (see Table 9-1). Factor V$_{New Brunswick}$ (A221V) is a missense mutation in the factor V heavy chain that results in the expression of a factor V molecule with reduced specific activity caused by an increased rate of dissociation of the heavy and light chains of factor Va (228,229). Several missense or splicing mutations have been shown to result in impaired secretion of factor V (230–232). Five patients have been described with severe factor V deficiency caused by homozygous nonsense or frameshift mutations in the B-domain (233–236). These mutations predict the synthesis of truncated factor V molecules lacking a portion of the B-domain and all of the light chain. In contrast, factor V–deficient mice generated by homologous recombination have a phenotype characterized by fatal hemorrhage and an incomplete block in embryogenesis (11). Transgenic rescue of these factor V–deficient mice indicates that factor V levels of

## TABLE 9-1

FACTOR V GENE MUTATIONS

| Exon | Domain | Mutation | Type | Genotype | % FV activity | % FV antigen | Phenotype | Reference |
|------|--------|----------|------|----------|---------------|--------------|-----------|-----------|
| 4 | A1 | nt 675 del A | Frameshift | CompHet | 1 | 2 | FV deficiency | 282 |
| 4 | A1 | G119stop | Nonsense | Het | | | FV deficiency Pseudohomozygous FV I359T | 280 |
| 6 | A1 | A221V | Missense | Comp Het | 10 | 39 | FV deficiency Mild bleeding | 228,229 |
| 6 | A1 | K310stop | Nonsense | Het | | | FV deficiency heterozygote | 233 |
| 7 | A1-A2 | R306G | Missense | Het | 100 | | APC sensitive APC cleavage site | 264 |
| 7 | A1-A2 | R306T | Missense | Het | 100 | | APC cleavage site APC resistance Impaired APC cofactor | 265 |
| 7 | A2 | nt 1131 del 8 | Frameshift | Comp Het | 1 | 3 | FV deficiency | 233 |
| 8 | A2 | I359T | Missense | Het | | | New N-glycosylation site APC resistance Impaired APC cofactor | 280,281 |
| 8 | A2 | G392C | Missense | Comp Het | <1 | 1 | FV deficiency | 283 |
| | | IVS8 2A > G | Splicing | Hom | 1.6 | 7 | FV deficiency | 284 |
| 10 | A2 | C472G | Missense | Comp Het | <1 | 2 | FV deficiency | 230 |
| 10 | A2 | R506stop | Nonsense | Het | | | FV deficiency heterozygote | |
| 10 | A2 | R506Q | Missense | Het/Hom | 100 | 100 | APC resistance APC cleavage site | 4 |
| 10 | A2 | Nt 1701 G > T | Splicing | Hom | <1 | 8 | FV deficiency | 286 |
| 11 | A2 | Y530S | Missense | | | | FV deficiency | 287 |
| 12 | A2 | C585R | Missense | Het | | | FV deficiency heterozygote | 233 |
| 13 | B | nt2238 del AG | Frameshift | Comp Het | <1 | 1.5 | FV deficiency | 284 |
| 13 | B | R712stop | Nonsense | Het | | | FV deficiency Pseudohomozygous FV R506Q | 230,288 |
| 13 | B | Q773stop | Nonsense | Hom | 1 | | FV deficiency | 233 |
| 13 | B | nt 2952 del T | Frameshift | Comp Het | <1 | 1 | FV deficiency | 289 |
| 13 | B | 1299 | Missense | Het | | | FV deficiency Pseudohomozygous FV R506Q | 212 |

*(continued)*

**TABLE 9-1**

CONTINUED

| Exon | Domain | Mutation | Type | Genotype | % FV activity | % FV antigen | Phenotype | Reference |
|------|--------|----------|------|----------|---------------|--------------|-----------|-----------|
| 13 | B | 3706 2 bp insertion | Frameshift | Het | | | FV deficiency Pseudohomozygous FV R506Q | 290 |
| 13 | B | nt 2833 del AC | Frameshift | Hom | <1 | 1 | FV deficiency | 234 |
| 13 | B | nt 2856 ins 4 bp | Frameshift | Het | | | FV deficiency Pseudohomozygous FV R506Q | 291 |
| 13 | B | R1002 stop | Nonsense | Comp Het | <1 | <1 | FV deficiency | 230 |
| 13 | B | R1133 stop | Nonsense | Hom | <1 | <1 | FV deficiency | 235 |
| 13 | B | Nt 3706 ins TC | Frameshift | Het | | | FV deficiency Pseudohomozygous FV R506Q | 290,292 |
| 13 | B | nt4013 del4 bp | Frameshift | Hom | <1.6 | <0.3 | FV deficiency | 236 |
| 13 | B | nt 4294 del C | Frameshift | Hom | <1 | 3 | FV deficiency | 233 |
| 14 | A3 | nt 4888 del G | Frameshift | Comp Het | <1 | 1 | FV deficiency | 283 |
| 14 | A3 | R1606 stop | Nonsense | Comp Het | <1 | <1 | FV deficiency | 230 |
| 15 | A3 | Nt 5128 ins A | Frameshift | Comp Het | <1 | 2 | FV deficiency | 230 |
| 15 | A3 | Y1702C | Missense | Hom/Het | 1 | 3 | FV deficiency | 230,230, 233, 293, 294 |
| 16 | A3 | G5493 ins G | Frameshift | Comp Het | <1 | 1 | FV deficiency | 289 |
| 16 | A3 | nt 5509 G > A | Splicing | | | | FV deficiency Pseudohomozygous FV R506Q | 258 |
| 17 | A3 | nt 5682 del T | Frameshift | Het | | | FV deficiency Pseudohomozygous FV R506Q | 295 |
| 17 | A3 | V1813M | Missense | Comp Het | <1 | 5 | FV deficiency | 230 |
| 18 | A3 | W1854 stop | Nonsense | Hom | 2 | 1 | FV deficiency | 230 |
| 21 | C1 | nt6122 | Frameshift | Comp Het | <1 | <1 | FV deficiency | 230 |
| | | IVS19 + 3 A > T | Splicing | Hom | <1 | <1 | FV deficiency | 232 |
| 23 | C2 | P2070L | Missense | Hom | | | FV deficiency | 296 |
| 23 | C2 | G2079V | Missense | Comp Het | <1 | 1.5 | FV deficiency | 284 |
| 23 | C2 | R2074C | Missense | Hom | 4 | 2 | FV deficiency | 231,297 |
| 23 | C2 | R2074H | Missense | Hom | 2 | 2 | FV deficiency | 298 |
| 24 | C2 | Nt 6581 del 21 bp, nt 6613 del G | Frameshift | Het | | | FV deficiency Pseudohomozygous FV R506Q | 295 |

less than 0.1% are sufficient for survival (237). Survival of patients with homozygous nonsense mutations may be explained by ribosomal slippage and trace expression of factor V (237,238).

## Combined Factor V–Factor VIII Deficiency

Combined deficiencies of factor V and factor VIII have been observed more commonly than could be explained by the chance association of hemophilia A and factor V deficiency (239). More than 81 families have been reported, and the frequency of this disorder in non-Ashkenazi Jews has been estimated to be as high as 1 in $10^5$ (239). Characteristics of this disorder include autosomal recessive inheritance, frequent familial consanguinity, quantitative factor deficiencies (5% to 30%), and a bleeding diathesis similar to parahemophilia or mild hemophilia A (239,240). The molecular basis for this disorder has recently been established by

positional cloning (205). Mutations in two different genes, LMAN1 (201) and MCFD2 (204), can lead to combined deficiency of factor V and factor VIII. The products of these two genes form a stable complex localized to the secretory pathway in cells and most likely function to transport newly synthesized factor V and factor VIII from the endoplasmic reticulum to the Golgi (204).

## Deficiency of Platelet Factor V

Several bleeding disorders have been identified in which there is a deficiency of platelet factor V with normal levels of factor V circulating in plasma. Patients with storage pool disease or gray platelet syndrome are deficient in platelet α-granules and release decreased amounts of platelet factor V (241,242). Patients with the Quebec platelet disorder have a deficiency of platelet factor V (227) that is associated with megakaryocytic expression and storage of urokinase-type plasminogen activator, intraplatelet generation of plasmin, and degradation of $\alpha$-granule proteins (243–246). In addition, these patients also have mild thrombocytopenia and an impaired aggregation response to epinephrine, collagen, and adenosine 5'-diphosphate (ADP) (243).

## Factor V Inhibitors

Antibodies directed against factor V can result in acquired factor V deficiency (247). These antibodies may arise spontaneously, but they more commonly arise following exposure to trace amounts of bovine factor V present in thrombin preparations that are used for local hemostasis (248). Bleeding complications in these patients are variable, and platelet transfusions may be useful for treatment because they provide a source of factor V that is sequestered from the antibody (249,250). Anti–factor V antibodies have been detected in the platelets of a patient with a factor V inhibitor, suggesting that inhibitor antibodies can be incorporated into platelet $\alpha$-granules *in vivo* (251). One inhibitor has been shown to bind to the heavy chain of factor Va and interfere with factor Xa binding to the cofactor (134). In a second study, factor V inhibitors from 12 patients were characterized, and all were found to bind to the factor Va light chain (252). Factor V antibodies from the eight patients who experienced bleeding complications were all found to bind to the phosphatidylserine-binding site in the factor V C2 domain and interfere with membrane binding (252–254).

## Activated Protein C Resistance

Resistance to APC is the most common inherited risk factor for venous thrombosis (255,256). A single nucleotide substitution in exon 10 of the factor V gene (G1691A) is found in nearly all cases of inherited APC resistance (4,257) (Table 9-1). The mutant protein (FV R506Q, $FV_{Leiden}$) lacks the APC cleavage site at Arg506$^n$. Consequently, $FV_{Leiden}$ is both resistant to inactivation by APC and deficient in APC cofactor activity (see preceding text). Patients who are heterozygous for this mutation have an approximately five- to 10-fold increased risk of venous thrombosis (256). The risk of venous thrombosis is increased 50- to 100-fold in patients homozygous for $FV_{Leiden}$ (256). This risk is further amplified by other genetic and environmental risk factors. Patients have been identified who are pseudohomozygous for $FV_{Leiden}$ (258). These patients are compound heterozygotes for $FV_{Leiden}$ and factor V deficiency (258) (Table 9-1). As a result, only $FV_{Leiden}$ is expressed, and these patients have a laboratory and clinical phenotype similar to patients homozygous for this mutation (258). On the basis of haplotype analysis of factor V gene polymorphisms, it has been concluded that the $FV_{Leiden}$ mutation arose on a single Caucasoid ancestor approximately 21,000 to 34,000 years ago (259). In Europe, the frequency of the $FV_{Leiden}$ allele varies significantly, ranging from 2% in Italy and Spain to as high as 15% in parts of Sweden. The mutation is not found in native Africans and Southeast Asians (259). The widespread presence of this mutation in Caucasian populations may reflect a selective advantage related to an increased risk of life-threatening bleeding in premodern times (206). Supporting this notion are the observations that heterozygosity for the $FV_{Leiden}$ mutation reduces intrapartum blood loss (260) and ameliorates the bleeding tendency in patients with hemophilia A (261). $FV_{Leiden}$ has also been found to be associated with a survival advantage in patients with severe sepsis and in mouse endotoxemia (262). Conversely, the risk of venous thrombosis in patients heterozygous for $FV_{Leiden}$ is relatively low in the absence of other risk factors, particularly before the age of reproduction (263).

Two factor V mutations have been identified in which the APC cleavage site at Arg306 has been mutated to either glycine (264) or threonine (265). In light of the critical role that APC cleavage at Arg306 plays in the inactivation of factor Va (156), it is surprising that mutations at Arg306 result in only a mild degree of resistance to APC (266,267). This observation may be explained by the presence of alternative cleavage sites near Arg306, which are cleaved by APC much more slowly than Arg306 or Arg506 (268). Mutations at Arg306 are much less common than $FV_{Leiden}$, and it is not clear whether these mutations are associated with an increased risk of venous thrombosis (269–271).

A common factor V gene haplotype marked by the H1299R (R2) polymorphism is also associated with mild APC resistance (272,273). This haplotype encodes several amino acid substitutions in the A2, B, A3, and C2 domains of factor V. The R2 allele is associated with a 20% decrease in plasma factor V levels (272). Expression studies have demonstrated that the R2194G polymorphism is largely responsible for the impaired secretion of factor V (274,275). There is no difference between the rates of APC inactivation of $FVa_{R2}$ and native FVa. However, the APC cofactor activity of $FV_{R2}$ is reduced by approximately 25% (181,276). The molecular basis for the reduced APC cofactor activity of $FV_{R2}$ remains to be elucidated. Epidemiologic studies on the importance of the R2 allele have so far been inconclusive (277). Several factor V polymorphisms, including D79H, M2120T, and D2194G, are associated with mildly decreased plasma factor V levels and may lead to increased resistance to APC in $FV_{Leiden}$ carriers through a pseudohomozygous mechanism (278,279).

Finally, a novel missense mutation in factor V, I359T, has recently been reported to be associated with thrombosis and resistance to APC (280). This mutation creates an additional *N*-linked glycosylation site in factor V at Asn357. The presence of this additional carbohydrate chain significantly reduces the rate of APC cleavage at Arg306 but not at Arg506 (281). In addition, the I359T mutant expressed reduced APC cofactor activity, similar to $FV_{Leiden}$. The prothrombotic tendency was observed only in individuals who were pseudohomozygous for the I359T mutation. The failure to observe this mutation in the DNA of a pool of healthy blood donors suggests that FV I359T is not a polymorphic allele (280).

## References

1. Quick AJ. On the constitution of prothrombin. *Am J Physiol* 1943; 140:212.
2. Owren PA. The coagulation of blood: investigations on a new clotting factor. *Acta Med Scand* 1947;194(Suppl. 194):1–327.
3. Mann KG, Jenny RJ, Krishnaswamy S. Cofactor proteins in the assembly and expression of blood clotting enzyme complexes. *Annu Rev Biochem* 1988;57:915–956.
4. Bertina RM, Koeleman BPC, Koster T, et al. Mutation in blood coagulation factor V associated with resistance to activated protein C. *Nature* 1994;369:64–67.
5. Colman RW. Factor V. *Prog Hemost Thromb* 1976;3:109–143.
6. Kane WH, Davie EW. Blood coagulation factors V and VIII: structural and functional similarities and their relationship to hemorrhagic and thrombotic disorders. *Blood* 1988;71:539–555.
7. Mann KG, Kalafatis M. Factor V: a combination of Dr. Jekyll and Mr. Hyde. *Blood* 2003;101(1):20–30.
8. Nicolaes GA, Dahlbäck B. Factor V and thrombotic disease: description of a janus-faced protein. *Arterioscler Thromb Vasc Biol* 2002;22(4):530–538.
9. Wang H, Riddell DC, Guinto ER, et al. Localization of the gene encoding human factor V to chromosome 1q21-25. *Genomics* 1988;2:234.
10. Cripe LD, Moore KD, Kane WH. Structure of the gene for human coagulation factor V. *Biochemistry* 1992;31:3777–3785.
11. Cui JS, O'Shea KS, Purkayastha A, et al. Fatal haemorrhage and incomplete block to embryogenesis in mice locking coagulation factor V. *Nature* 1996;384:66–68.
12. Yang TL, Cui J, Rehumtulla A, et al. The structure and function of murine factor V and its inactivation by protein C. *Blood* 1998;91:4593–4599.
13. Kane WH, Davie EW. Cloning of a cDNA coding for human factor V, a blood coagulation factor homologous to factor VIII and ceruloplasmin. *Proc Natl Acad Sci U S A* 1986;83:6800–6804.

14. Kane WH, Ichinose A, Hagen FS, et al. Cloning of cDNAs coding for the heavy chain region and connecting region of human factor V, a blood coagulation factor with four types of internal repeats. *Biochemistry* 1987; 26:6508–6514.

15. Jenny RJ, Pittman DD, Toole JJ, et al. Complete cDNA and derived amino acid sequence of human factor V. *Proc Natl Acad Sci U S A* 1987;84: 4846–4850.

16. Guinto ER, Esmon CT, Mann KG, et al. The complete cDNA sequence of bovine coagulation factor V. *J Biol Chem* 1992;267:2971–2978.

17. Healey JF, Lubin IM, Lollar P. The cDNA and derived amino acid sequence of porcine factor VIII. *Blood* 1996;88:4209–4214.

18. Davidson CJ, Hirt RP, Lal K, et al. Molecular evolution of the vertebrate blood coagulation network. *Thromb Haemost* 2003;89(3):420–428.

19. Xue J, Kalafatis M, Mann KG. Determination of the disulfide bridges in factor Va light chain. *Biochemistry* 1993;32:5917–5923.

20. Xue J, Kalafatis M, Silveira JR, et al. Determination of the disulfide bridges in factor Va heavy chain. *Biochemistry* 1994;33:13109–13116.

21. Krishnaswamy S, Mann KG. The binding of factor Va to phospholipid vesicles. *J Biol Chem* 1988;263:5714–5723.

22. Macedo-Ribeiro S, Bode W, Huber R, et al. Crystal structures of the membrane-binding C2 domain of human coagulation factor V. *Nature* 1999; 402(6760):434–439.

23. Srivastava A, Quinn-Allen MA, Kim SW, et al. Soluble phosphatidylserine binds to a single identified site in the C2 domain of human factor Va. *Biochemistry* 2001;40(28):8246–8255.

24. Kane WH, Majerus PW. Purification and characterization of human coagulation factor V. *J Biol Chem* 1981;256:1002–1007.

25. Pittman DD, Tomkinson KN, Kaufman RJ. Post-translational requirements for functional factor V and factor VIII secretion in mammalian cells. *J Biol Chem* 1994;269:17329–17337.

26. Kim SW, Ortel TL, Quinn-Allen MA, et al. Partial glycosylation at asparagine-2181 of the second C-type domain of human factor V modulates assembly of the prothrombinase complex. *Biochemistry* 1999;38(35): 11448–11454.

27. Nicolaes GA, Villoutreix BO, Dahlbäck B. Partial glycosylation of asn(2181) in human factor V as a cause of molecular and functional heterogeneity. Modulation of glycosylation efficiency by mutagenesis of the consensus sequence for N-linked glycosylation [In Process Citation]. *Biochemistry* 1999; 38(41):13584–13591.

28. Hortin GL. Sulfation of tyrosine residues in coagulation factor V. *Blood* 1990;76:946–952.

29. Braun PJ, Dennis S, Hofsteenge J, et al. Use of site-directed mutagenesis to investigate the basis for specificity of hirudin. *Biochemistry* 1988;27: 6517–6522.

30. Pittman DD, Tomkinson KN, Michnick D, et al. Posttranslational sulfation of factor V is required for efficient thrombin cleavage and activation and for full procoagulant activity. *Biochemistry* 1994;33:6952–6959.

31. Kalafatis M, Rand MD, Jenny RJ, et al. Phosphorylation of factor Va and factor VIIIa by activated platelets. *Blood* 1992;81:704–719.

32. Kalafatis M. Identification and partial characterization of factor Va heavy chain kinase from human platelets. *J Biol Chem* 1998;273:8459–8466.

33. Vehar GA, Keyt B, Eaton DL, et al. Structure of human factor VIII. *Nature* 1984;312:337–342.

34. Gitschier J, Wood WI, Goralka TM, et al. Characterization of the human factor VIII gene. *Nature* 1984;312:326–330.

35. Rao VS, Swarup S, Kini RM. The nonenzymatic subunit of pseutarin C, a prothrombin activator from eastern brown snake (*Pseudonaja textilis*) venom, shows structural similarity to mammalian coagulation factor V. *Blood* 2003; 102(4):1347–1354.

36. Ortel TL, Takahashi N, Putnam FW. Structural model of human ceruloplasmin based on internal triplication, hydrophilic/hydrophobic character, and secondary structure of domains. *Proc Natl Acad Sci U S A* 1984;81: 4761–4765.

37. Vulpe CD, Kuo YM, Murphy TL, et al. Hephaestin, a ceruloplasmin homologue implicated in intestinal iron transport, is defective in the sla mouse. *Nat Genet* 1999;21(2):195–199.

38. Mann KG, Lawler CM, Vehar GA, et al. Coagulation Factor V contains copper ion. *J Biol Chem* 1984;259:12949–12951.

39. Tagliavacca L, Moon N, Dunham WR, et al. Identification and functional requirement of Cu(I) And its ligands within coagulation factor VIII. *J Biol Chem* 1997;272:27428–27434.

40. Poole S, Firtel RA, Lamar E, et al. Sequence and expression of the discoidin I gene family in *Dictyostelium discoideum*. *J Mol Biol* 1981;153: 273–289.

41. Baumgartner S, Hofmann K, Chiquet-Ehrismann R, et al. The discoidin domain family revisited: new members from prokaryotes and a homology-based fold prediction. *Protein Sci* 1998;7:1626–1631.

42. Nesheim ME, Myrmel KH, Hibbard L, et al. Isolation and characterization of single chain bovine factor V. *J Biol Chem* 1979;254:508–517.

43. Dahlbäck B. Human coagulation factor V purification and thrombin-catalyzed activation. *J Clin Invest* 1980;66:583–591.

44. Katzmann JA, Nesheim ME, Hibbard LS, et al. Isolation of functional human coagulation factor V by using a hybridoma antibody. *Proc Natl Acad Sci U S A* 1981;78:162–166.

45. Adams TE, Hockin MF, Mann KG, et al. The crystal structure of activated protein C-inactivated bovine factor Va: Implications for cofactor function. *Proc Natl Acad Sci U S A* 2004;101(24):8918–8923.

46. Zaitseva I, Zaisev V, Card G, et al. The X-ray structure of human serum ceruloplasmin at 3.1 Å: Nature of the copper centres. *J Biol Inorg Chem* 1996;1:15–23.

47. Sorensen KW, Nicolaes GA, Villoutreix BO, et al. Functional properties of recombinant factor V mutated in a potential calcium-binding site. *Biochemistry* 2004;43(19):5803–5810.

48. Guinto ER, Esmon CT. Formation of a calcium-binding site on bovine activated factor V following recombination of the isolated subunits. *J Biol Chem* 1982;257:10038–10043.

49. Wakabayashi H, Koszelak ME, Mastri M, et al. Metal ion-independent association of factor VIII subunits and the roles of calcium and copper ions for cofactor activity and inter-subunit affinity. *Biochemistry* 2001; 40(34):10293–10300.

50. Mosesson MW, Church WR, DiOrio JP, et al. Structural model of factors V and Va based on scanning transmission electron microscope images and mass analysis. *J Biol Chem* 1990;265:8863–8868.

51. Fowler WE, Fay PJ, Arvan DS, et al. Electron microscopy of human factor V and factor VIII: Correlation of morphology with domain structure and localization of factor V activation fragments. *Proc Natl Acad Sci U S A* 1990;87:7648–7652.

52. Nesheim ME, Taswell JB, Mann KG. The contribution of bovine Factor V and Factor Va to the activity of prothrombinase. *J Biol Chem* 1979;254: 10952–10962.

53. Esmon CT. The subunit structure of thrombin-activated factor V. Isolation of activated factor V, separation of subunits, and reconstitution of biological activity. *J Biol Chem* 1979;254:964–973.

54. Kane WH, Majerus PW. The interaction of human coagulation factor Va with platelets. *J Biol Chem* 1982;257:3963–3969.

55. Laue TM, Johnson AE, Esmon CT, et al. Structure of bovine blood coagulation factor Va. Determination of the subunit associations, molecular weights, and asymmetries by analytical ultracentrifugation. *Biochemistry* 1984;23:1339–1348.

56. Suzuki K, Dahlbäck B, Stenflo J. Thrombin-catalyzed activation of human coagulation factor V. *J Biol Chem* 1982;257:6556–6564.

57. Keller FG, Ortel TL, Quinn-Allen MA, et al. Thrombin-catalyzed activation of recombinant human factor V. *Biochemistry* 1995;34:4118–4124.

58. Thorelli E, Kaufman RJ, Dahlbäck B. Cleavage requirements for activation of factor V by factor Xa. *Eur J Biochem* 1997;247:12–20.

59. Thorelli E, Kaufman RJ, Dahlbäck B. Cleavage requirements of factor V in tissue-factor induced thrombin generation. *Thromb Haemost* 1998;80: 92–98.

60. Steen M, Dahlbäck B. Thrombin-mediated proteolysis of factor V resulting in gradual B-domain release and exposure of the factor Xa-binding site. *J Biol Chem* 2002;277(41):38424–38430.

61. Kalafatis M, Beck DO, Mann KG. Structural requirements for expression of factor Va activity. *J Biol Chem* 2003;278(35):33550–33561.

62. Esmon CT, Lollar P. Involvement of thrombin anion-binding exosites 1 and 2 in the activation of factor V and factor VIII. *J Biol Chem* 1996;271: 13882–13887.

63. Dharmawardana KR, Olson ST, Bock PE. Role of regulatory exosite I in binding of thrombin to human factor V, factor Va, factor Va subunits, and activation fragments. *J Biol Chem* 1999;274:18635–18643.

64. Myles T, Yun TH, Hall SW, et al. An extensive interaction interface between thrombin and factor V is required for factor V activation. *J Biol Chem* 2001;276(27):25143–25149.

65. Beck DO, Bukys MA, Singh LS, et al. The contribution of amino acid region ASP695-TYR698 of factor V to procofactor activation and factor Va function. *J Biol Chem* 2004;279(4):3084–3095.

66. Pittman DD, Marquette KA, Kaufman RJ. Role of the B domain for factor VIII and factor V expression and function. *Blood* 1994;84:4214–4225.

67. Kane WH, Devore-Carter D, Ortel TL. Expression and characterization of recombinant human factor V and a mutant lacking a major portion of the connecting region. *Biochemistry* 1990;29:6762–6768.

68. Toso R, Camire RM. Removal of B-domain sequences from factor V rather than specific proteolysis underlies the mechanism by which cofactor function is realized. *J Biol Chem* 2004;279(20):21643–21650.

69. Marquette KA, Pittman DD, Kaufman RJ. The factor V B-domain provides two functions to facilitate thrombin cleavage and release of the light chain. *Blood* 1995;86:3026–3034.

70. Monkovic DD, Tracy PB. Activation of human factor V by factor Xa and thrombin. *Biochemistry* 1990;29:1118–1128.

71. Foster WB, Nesheim ME, Mann KG. The factor Xa-catalyzed activation of factor V. *J Biol Chem* 1983;258:13970–13977.

72. Lawson JH, Kalafatis M, Stram S, et al. A model for the tissue factor pathway to thrombin. I. An empirical study. *J Biol Chem* 1994;269: 23357–23366.

73. Butenas S, Vantveer C, Mann KG. Evaluation of the initiation phase of blood coagulation using ultrasensitive assays for serine proteases. *J Biol Chem* 1997;272:21527–21533.

74. Orfeo T, Brufatto N, Nesheim ME, et al. The factor V activation paradox. *J Biol Chem* 2004;279(19):19580–19591.

75. Bradford HN, Annamalai A, Doshi K, et al. Factor V is activated and cleaved by platelet calpain: comparison with thrombin proteolysis. *Blood* 1988;71:388–394.

76. Monkovic DD, Tracy PB. Functional characterization of human platelet-released factor V and its activation by factor Xa and thrombin. *J Biol Chem* 1990;265:17132–17140.

77. Gould WR, Silveira JR, Tracy PB. Unique *in vivo* modifications of coagulation factor V produce a physically and functionally distinct platelet-derived cofactor: characterization of purified platelet-derived factor V/Va. *J Biol Chem* 2004;279(4):2383–2393.

78. Camire RM, Kalafatis M, Tracy PB. Proteolysis of factor V by cathepsin G and elastase indicates that cleavage at Arg1545 optimizes cofactor function by facilitating factor Xa binding. *Biochemistry* 1998;37:11896–11906.

79. Lee CD, Mann KG. Activation/Inactivation of human factor V by plasmin. *Blood* 1989;73:185–190.

80. Kalafatis M, Mann KG. The role of the membrane in the inactivation of factor Va by plasmin. Amino acid region 307-348 of factor V plays a critical role in factor Va cofactor function. *J Biol Chem* 2001;276(21):18614–18623.

81. Mann KG, Nesheim ME, Church WR, et al. Surface-dependent reactions of the vitamin K–dependent enzyme complexes. *Blood* 1990;76:1–16.

82. Rosing J, Tans G, Govers Riemslag JW, et al. The role of phospholipids and factor Va in the prothrombinase complex. *J Biol Chem* 1980;255:274–283.

83. Nesheim ME, Tracy RP, Mann KG. "Clotspeed," a mathematical simulation of the functional properties of prothrombinase. *J Biol Chem* 1984;259:1447–1453.

84. van Rijn JL, Govers Riemslag JW, Zwaal RF, et al. Kinetic studies of prothrombin activation: effect of factor Va and phospholipids on the formation of the enzyme-substrate complex. *Biochemistry* 1984;23:4557–4564.

85. Krishnaswamy S, Church WR, Nesheim ME, et al. Activation of human prothrombin by human prothrombinase. Influence of factor Va on the reaction mechanism. *J Biol Chem* 1987;262:3291–3299.

86. Tans G, Janssen-Claessen T, Hemker HC, et al. Meizothrombin formation during factor Xa-catalyzed prothrombin activation. Formation in a purified system and in plasma. *J Biol Chem* 1991;266:21864–21873.

87. Krishnaswamy S, Mann KG, Nesheim ME. The prothrombinase-catalyzed activation of prothrombin proceeds through the intermediate meizothrombin in an ordered, sequential reaction. *J Biol Chem* 1986;261:8977–8984.

88. Rosing J, Zwaal RFA, Tans G. Formation of meizothrombin as intermediate in factor Xa-catalyzed prothrombin activation. *J Biol Chem* 1986;261:4224–4228.

89. Orcutt SJ, Krishnaswamy S. Binding of substrate in two conformations to human prothrombinase drives consecutive cleavage at two sites in prothrombin. *J Biol Chem* 2004;279(52):54927–54936.

90. Husten EJ, Esmon CT, Johnson AE. The active site of blood coagulation factor Xa. Its distance from the phospholipid surface and its conformational sensitivity to components of the prothrombinase complex. *J Biol Chem* 1987;262:12953–12961.

91. Krishnaswamy S, Vlasuk GP, Bergum PW. Assembly of the prothrombinase complex enhances the inhibition of bovine factor Xa by tick anticoagulant peptide. *Biochemistry* 1994;33:7897–7907.

92. Betz A, Krishnaswamy S. Regions remote from the site of cleavage determine macromolecular substrate recognition by the prothrombinase complex. *J Biol Chem* 1998;273:10709–10718.

93. Boskovic DS, Troxler T, Krishnaswamy S. Active site-independent recognition of substrates and product by bovine prothrombinase: a fluorescence resonance energy transfer study. *J Biol Chem* 2004;279(20):20786–20793.

94. Boskovic DS, Bajzar LS, Nesheim ME. Channeling during prothrombin activation. *J Biol Chem* 2001;276(31):28686–28693.

95. Wu JR, Zhou C, Majumder R, et al. Role of procoagulant lipids in human prothrombin activation. 1. Prothrombin activation by factor X(a) in the absence of factor V(a) and in the absence and presence of membranes. *Biochemistry* 2002;41(3):935–949.

96. Weinreb GE, Mukhopadhyay K, Majumder R, et al. Cooperative roles of factor V(a) and phosphatidylserine-containing membranes as cofactors in prothrombin activation. *J Biol Chem* 2003;278(8):5679–5684.

97. Zwaal RF, Comfurius P, Bevers EM. Lipid-protein interactions in blood coagulation. [Review] [151 refs]. *Biochim Biophys Acta* 1998;1376:433–453.

98. Rosing J, Bakker HM, Thomassen MCLGD, et al. Characterization of two forms of human factor Va with different cofactor activities. *J Biol Chem* 1993;268:21130–21136.

99. Bloom JW, Nesheim ME, Mann KG. Phospholipid-binding properties of bovine factor V and factor Va. *Biochemistry* 1979;18:4419–4425.

100. Cutsforth GA, Koppaka V, Krishnaswamy S, et al. Insights into the complex association of bovine factor $V_a$ with acidic-lipid-containing synthetic membranes. *Biophys J* 1996;70:2938–2949.

101. Rosing J, Speijer H, Zwaal RF. Prothrombin activation on phospholipid membranes with positive electrostatic potential. *Biochemistry* 1988;27:8–11.

102. Comfurius P, Smeets EF, Willems GM, et al. Assembly of the prothrombinase complex on lipid vesicles depends on the stereochemical configuration of the polar headgroup of phosphatidylserine. *Biochemistry* 1994;33:10319–10324.

103. Koppaka V, Lentz BR. Binding of bovine factor $V_a$ to phosphatidylcholine membranes. *Biophys J* 1996;70:2930–2937.

104. Lecompte MF, Krishnaswamy S, Mann KG, et al. Membrane penetration of bovine factor V and Va detected by labeling with 5-iodonaphthalene-1-azide. *J Biol Chem* 1987;262:1935–1937.

105. Krieg UC, Isaacs BS, Yemul SS, et al. Interaction of blood coagulation factor Va with phospholipid vesicles examined by using lipophilic photoreagents. *Biochemistry* 1987;26:103–109.

106. Pusey ML, Nelsestuen GL. Membrane binding properties of blood coagulation Factor V and derived peptides. *Biochemistry* 1984;23:6202–6210.

107. van de Waart P, Bruls H, Hemker HC, et al. Interaction of bovine blood clotting factor Va and its subunits with phospholipid vesicles. *Biochemistry* 1983;22:2427–2432.

108. Pusey ML, Mayer LD, Wei GJ, et al. Kinetic and hydrodynamic analysis of blood clotting factor V-membrane binding. *Biochemistry* 1982;21:5262–5269.

109. Tracy PB, Mann KG. Prothrombinase complex assembly on the platelet surface is mediated through the 74,000-dalton component of factor Va. *Proc Natl Acad Sci U S A* 1983;80:2380–2384.

110. Saenko EL, Scandella D, Yakhyaev AV, et al. Activation of factor VIII by thrombin increases its affinity for binding to synthetic phospholipid membranes and activated platelets. *J Biol Chem* 1998;273(42):27918–27926.

111. Saleh M, Peng W, Quinn-Allen MA, et al. The factor V C1 domain is involved in membrane binding: identification of functionally important amino acid residues within the C1 domain of factor V using alanine scanning mutagenesis. *Thromb Haemost* 2004;91(1):16–27.

112. Peng W, Quinn-Allen MA, Kane WH. Mutation of hydrophobic residues in the factor Va C1 and C2 domains blocks membrane-dependent prothrombin activation. *J Thromb Haemost* 2005;3(2):351–354.

113. Ortel TL, Devore-Carter D, Quinn-Allen MA, et al. Deletion analysis of recombinant human factor V. Evidence for a phosphatidylserine binding site in the second C-type domain. *J Biol Chem* 1992;267:4189–4198.

114. Ortel TL, Quinn-Allen MA, Charles LA, et al. Characterization of an acquired inhibitor to coagulation Factor V. Antibody binding to the second C-type domain of Factor V inhibits the binding of Factor V to phosphatidylserine and neutralizes procoagulant activity. *J Clin Invest* 1992;90:2340–2347.

115. Ortel TL, Quinn-Allen MA, Keller FG, et al. Localization of functionally important epitopes within the second C-type domain of coagulation factor V using recombinant chimeras. *J Biol Chem* 1994;269:15898–15905.

116. Kim SW, Quinn-Allen MA, Camp T, et al. Identification of functionally important amino acid residues within the C2 domain of human factor V using alanine scanning mutagenesis. *Biochemistry* 2000;39:1951–1958.

117. Nicolaes GA, Villoutreix BO, Dahlbäck B. Mutations in a potential phospholipid binding loop in the C2 domain of factor V affecting the assembly of the prothrombinase complex. *Blood Coagul Fibrinolysis* 2000;11(1):89–100.

118. Kalafatis M, Rand MD, Mann KG. Factor Va-membrane interaction is mediated by two regions located on the light chain of the cofactor. *Biochemistry* 1994;33:486–493.

119. Peng W, Quinn-Allen MA, Kim SW, et al. Trp$^{2063}$ and Trp$^{2064}$ in the factor Va C2 domain are required for high-affinity binding to phospholipid membranes but not for assembly of the prothrombinase complex. *Biochemistry* 2004;43(14):4385–4393.

120. Majumder R, Quinn-Allen MA, Kane WH, et al. The phosphatidylserine binding site of factor Va C2 domain accounts for membrane binding but does not contribute to assembly or activity of the human factors Xa-Va complex. *Biochemistry* 2005;44(2):711–718.

121. Hoekema L, Nicolaes GAF, Hemker HC, et al. Human factor Va$_1$ and factor Va$_2$: Properties in the procoagulant and anticoagulant pathways. *Biochemistry* 1997;36:3331–3335.

122. Koppaka V, Talbot WF, Zhai X, et al. Roles of factor v-a heavy and light chains in protein and lipid rearrangements associated with the formation of a bovine factor v-a-membrane complex. *Biophys J* 1997;73:2638–2652.

123. Krishnaswamy S, Jones KC, Mann KG. Prothrombinase complex assembly. Kinetic mechanism of enzyme assembly on phospholipid vesicles. *J Biol Chem* 1988;263:3823–3834.

124. Rand MD, Lock JB, Van't Veer C, et al. Blood clotting in minimally altered whole blood. *Blood* 1996;88:3432–3445.

125. Pryzdial ELG, Mann KG. The association of coagulation factor Xa and factor Va. *J Biol Chem* 1991;266:8969–8977.

126. Nesheim ME, Eid S, Mann KG. Assembly of the prothrombinase complex in the absence of prothrombin. *J Biol Chem* 1981;256:9874–9882.

127. Lindhout T, Govers Riemslag JW, van de Waart P, et al. Factor Va–factor Xa interaction. Effects of phospholipid vesicles of varying composition. *Biochemistry* 1982;21:5494–5502.

128. Krishnaswamy S. Prothrombinase complex assembly. Contributions of protein–protein and protein–membrane interactions toward complex formation. *J Biol Chem* 1990;265:3708–3718.

129. Boskovic DS, Giles AR, Nesheim ME. Studies of the role of factor Va in the factor Xa-catalyzed activation of prothrombin, fragment 1·2-prothrombin-2, and dansyl-L-glutamyl-glycyl-L-arginine-meizothrombin in the absence of phospholipid. *J Biol Chem* 1990;265:10497–10505.

130. Nelsestuen GL, Broderius M. Interaction of prothrombin and blood-clotting factor X with membranes of varying composition. *Biochemistry* 1977;16:4172–4177.

131. Walker RK, Krishnaswamy S. The influence of factor Va on the active site of factor Xa. *J Biol Chem* 1993;268:13920–13929.

132. Krishnaswamy S, Betz A. Exosites determine macromolecular substrate recognition by prothrombinase. *Biochemistry* 1997;36:12080–12086.

133. Majumder R, Weinreb G, Zhai X, et al. Soluble phosphatidylserine triggers assembly in solution of a prothrombin-activating complex in the absence of a membrane surface. *J Biol Chem* 2002;277(33):29765–29773.

134. Annamalai AE, Rao AK, Chiu HC, et al. Epitope mapping of functional domains of human factor Va with human and murine monoclonal antibodies. Evidence for the interaction of heavy chain with factor Xa and calcium. *Blood* 1987;70:139–146.

135. Kalafatis M, Xue J, Lawler CM, et al. Contribution of the heavy and light chains of factor Va to the interaction with factor Xa. *Biochemistry* 1994;33:6538–6545.

136. Kojima Y, Heeb MJ, Gale AJ, et al. Binding site for blood coagulation factor Xa involving residues 311-325 in factor Va. *J Biol Chem* 1998;273:14900–14905.

137. Heeb MJ, Kojima Y, Hackeng TM, et al. Binding sites for blood coagulation factor Xa and protein S involving residues 493-506 in factor Va. *Protein Sci* 1996;5:1883–1889.

138. Kalafatis M, Beck DO. Identification of a binding site for blood coagulation factor Xa on the heavy chain of factor Va. Amino acid residues 323-331 of factor V represent an interactive site for activated factor X. *Biochemistry* 2002;41(42):12715–12728.

139. Singh LS, Bukys MA, Beck DO, et al. Amino acids Glu323, Tyr324, Glu330, and Val331 of factor Va heavy chain are essential for expression of cofactor activity. *J Biol Chem* 2003;278(30):28335–28345.

140. Guinto ER, Esmon CT. Loss of prothrombin and of factor Xa–factor Va interactions upon inactivation of factor Va by activated protein C. *J Biol Chem* 1984;259:13986–13992.

141. Tucker MM, Foster WB, Katzmann JA, et al. A monoclonal antibody which inhibits the factor Va:factor Xa interaction. *J Biol Chem* 1983;258:1210–1214.

142. Steen M, Villoutreix BO, Norstrom EA, et al. Defining the factor Xa-binding site on factor Va by site-directed glycosylation. *J Biol Chem* 2002;277(51):50022–50029.

143. Nicolaes GAF, Tans G, Thomassen MCLGD, et al. Peptide bond cleavages and loss of functional activity during inactivation of factor Va and factor Va$^{R506Q}$ by activated protein C. *J Biol Chem* 1995;270:21158–21166.

144. Kalafatis M, Mann KG. Role of the membrane in the inactivation of factor Va by activated protein C. *J Biol Chem* 1993;268:27246–27257.

145. Bakker HM, Tans G, Thomassen MCLGD, et al. Functional properties of human factor Va lacking the Asp$^{683}$-Arg$^{709}$ domain of the heavy chain. *J Biol Chem* 1994;269:20662–20667.

146. Luckow EA, Lyons DA, Ridgeway TM, et al. Interaction of clotting factor V heavy chain with prothrombin and prethrombin 1 and role of activated protein C in regulating this interaction: Analysis by analytical ultracentrifugation. *Biochemistry* 1989;28:2348–2354.

147. Anderson PJ, Nesset A, Dharmawardana KR, et al. Role of proexosite I in factor Va-dependent substrate interactions of prothrombin activation. *J Biol Chem* 2000;275(22):16435–16442.

148. Deguchi H, Takeya H, Gabazza EC, et al. Prothrombin kringle 1 domain interacts with factor Va during the assembly of prothrombinase complex. *Biochem J* 1997;321:729–735.

149. Kisiel W, Canfield WM, Ericsson LH, et al. Anticoagulant properties of bovine plasma protein C following activation by thrombin. *Biochemistry* 1977;16:5824–5831.

150. Walker FJ. Regulation of activated protein C by a new protein. A possible function for bovine protein S. *J Biol Chem* 1980;255:5521–5524.

151. Walker FJ. Regulation of activated protein C by protein S. The role of phospholipid in factor Va inactivation. *J Biol Chem* 1981;256:11128–11131.

152. Smirnov MD, Ford DA, Esmon CT, et al. The effect of membrane composition on the hemostatic balance. *Biochemistry* 1999;38:3591–3598.

153. Bakker HM, Tans G, Janssen-Claessen T, et al. The effect of phospholipids, calcium ions and protein S on rate constants of human factor Va inactivation by activated human protein C. *Eur J Biochem* 1992;208:171–178.

154. Solymoss S, Tucker MM, Tracy PB. Kinetics of inactivation of membrane-bound factor Va by activated protein C. Protein S modulates factor Xa protection. *J Biol Chem* 1988;263:14884–14890.

155. Tans G, Rosing J, Thomassen MC, et al. Comparison of anticoagulant and procoagulant activities of stimulated platelets and platelet-derived microparticles. *Blood* 1991;77:2641–2648.

156. Kalafatis M, Rand MD, Mann KG. The mechanism of inactivation of human factor V and human factor Va by activated protein C. *J Biol Chem* 1994;269:31869–31880.

157. Krishnaswamy S, Williams EB, Mann KG. The binding of activated protein C to factors V and Va [published erratum appears in J Biol Chem 1987 Feb 5;262(4):1926]. *J Biol Chem* 1986;261:9684–9693.

158. Walker FJ, Scandella D, Fay PJ. Identification of the binding site for activated protein C on the light chain of factors V and VIII. *J Biol Chem* 1990;265:1484–1489.

159. Kalafatis M, Bertina RM, Rand MD, et al. Characterization of the molecular defect in factor V$^{R506Q}$. *J Biol Chem* 1995;270:4053–4057.

160. Heeb MJ, Kojima Y, Greengard JS, et al. Activated protein C resistance: molecular mechanisms based on studies using purified Gln$^{506}$-factor V. *Blood* 1995;85:3405–3411.

161. Rosing J, Hoekema L, Nicolaes GAF, et al. Effects of protein S and factor Xa on peptide bond cleavages during inactivation of factor Va and factor Va$^{R506Q}$ by activated protein C. *J Biol Chem* 1995;270:27852–27858.

162. Aparicio C, Dahlbäck B. Molecular mechanisms of activated protein C resistance – Properties of factor V isolated from an individual with homozygosity for the Arg$^{506}$ to Gin mutation in the factor V gene. *Biochem J* 1996;313:467–472.

163. Mann KG, Hockin MF, Bean KJ, et al. Activated protein c cleavage of factor va leads to dissociation of the a2 domain. *J Biol Chem* 1997;272:20678–20683.

164. Nicolaes GF, Thomassen MD, Tans G, et al. Effect of activated protein C on thrombin generation and on the thrombin potential in plasma of normal and APC-resistant individuals. *Blood Coagul Fibrinolysis* 1997;8:28–38.

165. Van't Veer C, Kalafatis M, Bertina RM, et al. Increased tissue factor-initiated prothrombin activation as a result of the Arg$^{506}$ → Gln mutation in factor V$^{LEIDEN}$. *J Biol Chem* 1997;272:20721–20729.

166. Smirnov MD, Esmon CT. Phosphatidylethanolamine incorporation into vesicles selectively enhances factor Va inactivation by activated protein C. *J Biol Chem* 1994;269:816–819.

167. Yegneswaran S, Wood GM, Esmon CT, et al. Protein S alters the active site location of activated protein C above the membrane surface. *J Biol Chem* 1997;272:25013–25021.

168. Yegneswaran S, Smirnov MD, Safa O, et al. Relocating the active site of activated protein C eliminates the need for its protein S cofactor – A fluorescence resonance energy transfer study. *J Biol Chem* 1999;274:5462–5468.

169. Hackeng TM, Van't Veer C, Meijers JCM, et al. Human protein S inhibits prothrombinase complex activity on endothelial cells and platelets via direct interactions with factors Va and Xa. *J Biol Chem* 1994;269:21051–21058.

170. Heeb MJ, Rosing J, Bakker HM, et al. Protein S binds to and inhibits factor Xa. *Proc Natl Acad Sci U S A* 1994;91:2728–2732.

171. Sere KM, Rosing J, Hackeng TM. Inhibition of thrombin generation by protein S at low procoagulant stimuli: implications for maintenance of the hemostatic balance. *Blood* 2004;104(12):3624–3630.

172. Nesheim ME, Canfield WM, Kisiel W, et al. Studies of the capacity of factor Xa to protect factor Va from inactivation by activated protein C. *J Biol Chem* 1982;257:1443–1447.

173. Dahlbäck B, Carlsson M, Svensson PJ. Familial thrombophilia due to a previously unrecognized mechanism characterized by poor anticoagulant response to activated protein C: prediction of a cofactor to activated protein C. *Proc Natl Acad Sci U S A* 1993;90:1004–1008.

174. Dahlbäck B, Hildebrand B. Inherited resistance to activated protein C is corrected by anticoagulant cofactor activity found to be a property of factor V. *Proc Natl Acad Sci U S A* 1994;91:1396–1400.

175. Fay PJ, Smudzin TM, Walker FJ. Activated protein C-catalyzed inactivation of human factor VIII and factor VIII$_a$. Identification of cleavage sites and correlation of proteolysis with cofactor activity. *J Biol Chem* 1991;266:20139–20145.

176. Shen L, Dahlbäck B. Factor V and protein S as synergistic cofactors to activated protein C in degradation of factor VIIIa. *J Biol Chem* 1994;269:18735–18738.

177. Lu DS, Kalafatis M, Mann KG, et al. Comparison of activated protein C protein S-mediated inactivation of human factor VIII and factor V. *Blood* 1996;87:4708–4717.

178. Varadi K, Rosing J, Tans G, et al. Factor V enhances the cofactor function of protein S in the APC-mediated inactivation of factor VIII: influence of the factor VR506Q mutation. *Thromb Haemost* 1996;76:208–214.

179. Thorelli E, Kaufman RJ, Dahlbäck B. The C-terminal region of the factor V B-domain is crucial for the anticoagulant activity of factor V. *J Biol Chem* 1998;273:16140–16145.

180. Thorelli E, Kaufman RJ, Dahlbäck B. Cleavage of factor V at Arg 506 by activated protein C and the expression of anticoagulant activity of factor V. *Blood* 1999;93:2552–2558.

181. Castoldi E, Brugge JM, Nicolaes GA, et al. Impaired APC cofactor activity of factor V plays a major role in the APC resistance associated with the factor V Leiden (R506Q) and R2 (H1299R) mutations. *Blood* 2004;103(11):4173–4179.

182. Tracy PB, Eide LL, Bowie EJ, et al. Radioimmunoassay of factor V in human plasma and platelets. *Blood* 1982;60:59–63.

183. Miletich JP, Majerus DW, Majerus PW. Patients with congenital factor V deficiency have decreased factor Xa binding sites on their platelets. *J Clin Invest* 1978;62:824–831.

184. Mazzorana M, Baffet G, Kneip B, et al. Expression of coagulation factor V gene by normal adult human hepatocytes in primary culture. *Br J Haematol* 1991;78:229–235.

185. Gewirtz AM, Shen YM. Effect of phorbol myristate acetate on c-myc, beta-actin, and FV gene expression in morphologically recognizable human megakaryocytes: a kinetic analysis employing in situ hybridization. *Exp Hematol* 1990;18:945–952.

186. Gewirtz AM, Shapiro C, Shen YM, et al. Cellular and molecular regulation of factor V expression in human megakaryocytes. *J Cell Physiol* 1992;153:277–287.

187. Chiu HC, Schick PK, Colman RW. Biosynthesis of factor V in isolated guinea pig megakaryocytes. *J Clin Invest* 1985;75:339–346.

188. Gewirtz AM, Keefer M, Doshi K, et al. Biology of human megakaryocyte factor V. *Blood* 1986;67:1639–1648.

189. Camire RM, Pollak ES, Kaushansky K, et al. Secretable human platelet-derived factor V originates from the plasma pool. *Blood* 1998;92:3035–3041.

190. Christella M, Thomassen LG, Castoldi E, et al. Endogenous factor V synthesis in megakaryocytes contributes negligibly to the platelet factor V pool. *Haematologica* 2003;88(10):1150–1156.

191. Handagama P, Rappolee DA, Werb Z, et al. Platelet alpha-granule fibrinogen, albumin, and immunoglobulin G are not synthesized by rat and mouse megakaryocytes. *J Clin Invest* 1990;86:1364–1368.

192. Colman RW. Where does platelet factor V originate? *Blood* 1999;93:3152.

193. Yang TL, Pipe SW, Yang A, et al. Biosynthetic origin and functional significance of murine platelet factor V. *Blood* 2003;102(8):2851–2855.

194. Sun H, Yang TL, Yang A, et al. The murine platelet and plasma factor V pools are biosynthetically distinct and sufficient for minimal hemostasis. *Blood* 2003;102(8):2856–2861.

195. Cerveny TJ, Fass DN, Mann KG. Synthesis of coagulation factor V by cultured aortic endothelium. *Blood* 1984;63:1467–1474.

196. Rodgers GM. Vascular smooth muscle cells synthesize, secrete and express coagulation factor V. *Biochim Biophys Acta* 1988;968:17–23.

197. Ono T, Liu N, Kasuno K, et al. Coagulation process proceeds on cultured human mesangial cells via expression of factor V. *Kidney Int* 2001;60(3):1009–1017.

198. Bruin T, Sturk A, ten Cate JW, et al. The function of the human factor V carbohydrate moiety in blood coagulation. *Eur J Biochem* 1987;170:305–310.

199. Silveira JR, Kalafatis M, Tracy PB. Carbohydrate moieties on the procofactor factor V, but not the derived cofactor factor Va, regulate its inactivation by activated protein C. *Biochemistry* 2002;41(5):1672–1680.

200. Pipe SW, Morris JA, Shah J, et al. Differential interaction of coagulation factor VIII and factor V with protein chaperones calnexin and calreticulin. *J Biol Chem* 1998;273:8537–8544.

201. Nichols WC, Seligsohn U, Zivelin A, et al. Mutations in the ER-Golgi intermediate compartment protein ERGIC-53 cause combined deficiency of coagulation factors V and VIII. *Cell* 1998;93:61–70.

202. Neerman-Arbez M, Johnson KM, Morris MA, et al. Molecular analysis of the ERGIC-53 gene in 35 families with combined factor V factor VIII deficiency. *Blood* 1999;93:2253–2260.

203. Nichols WC, Terry VH, Wheatley MA, et al. ERGIC-53 gene structure and mutation analysis in 19 combined factors V and VIII deficiency families. *Blood* 1999;93:2261–2266.

204. Zhang B, Cunningham MA, Nichols WC, et al. Bleeding due to disruption of a cargo-specific ER-to-Golgi transport complex. *Nat Genet* 2003;34(2):220–225.

205. Zhang B, Ginsburg D. Familial multiple coagulation factor deficiencies: new biologic insight from rare genetic bleeding disorders. *J Thromb Haemost* 2004;2(9):1564–1572.

206. Rand MD, Hanson SR, Mann KG. Factor V turnover in a primate model. *Blood* 1995;86:2616–2623.

207. Tracy PB. Regulation of thrombin generation at cell surfaces. *Semin Thromb Hemost* 1988;14:227–233.

208. Chesney CM, Pifer D, Colman RW. Subcellular localization and secretion of factor V from human platelets. *Proc Natl Acad Sci U S A* 1981;78:5180–5184.

209. Viskup RW, Tracy PB, Mann KG. The isolation of human platelet factor V [published erratum appears in Blood 1987 Jul;70(1):339]. *Blood* 1987;69:1188–1195.

210. Hayward CP, Furmaniak-Kazmierczak E, Cieutat AM, et al. Factor V is complexed with multimerin in resting platelet lysates and colocalizes with multimerin in platelet alpha-granules. *J Biol Chem* 1995;270:19217–19224.

211. Hayward CP, Fuller N, Zheng S, et al. Human platelets contain forms of factor V in disulfide-linkage with multimerin. *Thromb Haemost* 2004;92(6):1349–1357.

212. Jeimy SB, Woram RA, Fuller N, et al. Identification of the MMRN1 binding region within the C2 domain of human factor V. *J Biol Chem* 2004;279(49):51466–51471.

213. Wang DL, Annamalai AE, Ghosh S, et al. Human platelet factor V is crosslinked to actin by FXIIIa during platelet activation by thrombin. *Thromb Res* 1990;57:39–57.

214. Francis RT, McDonagh J, Mann KG. Factor V is a substrate for the transamidase factor XIIIa. *J Biol Chem* 1986;261:9787–9792.

215. Huh MM, Schick BP, Schick PK, et al. Covalent crosslinking of human coagulation factor V by activated factor XIII from guinea pig megakaryocytes and human plasma. *Blood* 1988;71:1693–1702.

216. Tracy PB, Nesheim ME, Mann KG. Coordinate binding of factor Va and factor Xa to the unstimulated platelet. *J Biol Chem* 1981;256:743–751.

217. Camire RM, Kalafatis M, Simioni P, et al. Platelet-derived factor Va/Va Leiden cofactor activities are sustained on the surface of activated platelets despite the presence of activated protein C. *Blood* 1998;91:2818–2829.

218. Rand MD, Kalafatis M, Mann KG. Platelet coagulation factor Va: the major secretory platelet phosphoprotein. *Blood* 1994;83:2180–2190.

219. Rodgers GM, Shuman MA. Prothrombin is activated on vascular endothelial cells by factor Xa and calcium. *Proc Natl Acad Sci U S A* 1983;80:7001–7005.

220. Hamilton KK, Hattori R, Esmon CT, et al. Complement proteins C5b-9 induce vesiculation of the endothelial plasma membrane and expose catalytic surface for assembly of the prothrombinase enzyme complex. *J Biol Chem* 1990;265:3809–3814.

221. Allen DH, Tracy PB. Human coagulation factor V is activated to the functional cofactor by elastase and cathepsin G expressed at the monocyte surface. *J Biol Chem* 1995;270:1408–1415.

222. Hockin MF, Kalafatis M, Shatos M, et al. Protein c activation and factor va inactivation on human umbilical vein endothelial cells. *Arterioscler Thromb Vasc Biol* 1997;17:2765–2775.

223. Oliver JA, Monroe DM, Church FC, et al. Activated protein C cleaves factor Va more efficiently on endothelium than on platelet surfaces. *Blood* 2002;100(2):539–546.

224. Girolami A, Simioni P, Scarano L, et al. Hemorrhagic and thrombotic disorders due to factor V deficiencies and abnormalities: an updated classification. [Review] [41 refs]. *Blood Rev* 1998;12:45–51.

225. Manotti C, Quintavalla R, Pini M, et al. Thromboembolic manifestations and congenital factor V deficiency: a family study. *Haemostasis* 1989;19:331–334.

226. Chiu HC, Whitaker E, Colman RW. Heterogeneity of human factor V deficiency. Evidence for the existence of antigen-positive variants. *J Clin Invest* 1983;72:493–503.

227. Tracy PB, Giles AR, Mann KG, et al. Factor V (Quebec): a bleeding diathesis associated with a qualitative platelet Factor V deficiency. *J Clin Invest* 1984;74:1221–1228.

228. Murray JM, Rand MD, Egan JO, et al. Factor V$_{New\ Brunswick}$: Ala$_{221}$-to-Val substitution results in reduced cofactor activity. *Blood* 1995;86:1820–1827.

229. Steen M, Miteva M, Villoutreix BO, et al. Factor V New Brunswick: Ala221Val associated with FV deficiency reproduced *in vitro* and functionally characterized. *Blood* 2003;102(4):1316–1322.

230. Montefusco MC, Duga S, Asselta R, et al. Clinical and molecular characterization of 6 patients affected by severe deficiency of coagulation factor V: broadening of the mutational spectrum of factor V gene and *in vitro* analysis of the newly identified missense mutations. *Blood* 2003;102(9):3210–3216.

231. Duga S, Montefusco MC, Asselta R, et al. Arg2074Cys missense mutation in the C2 domain of factor V causing moderately severe factor V deficiency: molecular characterization by expression of the recombinant protein. *Blood* 2003;101(1):173–177.

232. Asselta R, Montefusco MC, Duga S, et al. Severe factor V deficiency: exon skipping in the factor V gene causing a partial deletion of the C1 domain. *J Thromb Haemost* 2003;1(6):1237–1244.

233. van Wijk R, Nieuwenhuis K, van den BM, et al. Five novel mutations in the gene for human blood coagulation factor V associated with type I factor V deficiency. *Blood* 2001;98(2):358–367.

234. Montefusco MC, Duga S, Asselta R, et al. A novel two base pair deletion in the factor V gene associated with severe factor V deficiency. *Br J Haematol* 2000;111(4):1240–1246.

235. van Wijk R, Montefusco MC, Duga S, et al. Coexistence of a novel homozygous nonsense mutation in exon 13 of the factor V gene with the homozygous Leiden mutation in two unrelated patients with severe factor V deficiency. *Br J Haematol* 2001;114(4):871–874.

236. Guasch JF, Cannegieter S, Reitsma PH, et al. Severe coagulation factor V deficiency caused by a 4 bp deletion in the factor V gene. *Br J Haematol* 1998;101:32–39.

237. Yang TL, Cui J, Taylor JM, et al. Rescue of fatal neonatal hemorrhage in factor V deficient mice by low level transgene expression. *Thromb Haemost* 2000;83(1):70–77.

238. Young M, Inaba H, Hoyer LW, et al. Partial correction of a severe molecular defect in hemophilia A, because of errors during expression of the factor VIII gene. *Am J Hum Genet* 1997;60:565–573.

239. Seligsohn U, Zivelin A, Zwang E. Combined factor V and factor VIII deficiency among non-Ashkenazi Jews. *N Engl J Med* 1982;307:1191–1195.

240. Seligsohn U, Zivelin A, Zwang E. Decreased factor VIII clotting antigen levels in the combined factor V and VIII deficiency. *Thromb Res* 1984;33:95–98.

241. Baruch D, Lindhout T, Dupuy E, et al. Thrombin-induced platelet factor Va formation in patients with a gray platelet syndrome. *Thromb Haemost* 1987;58:768–771.

242. Weiss HJ, Lages B. Platelet prothrombinase activity and intracellular calcium responses in patients with storage pool deficiency, glycoprotein IIb-IIIa deficiency, or impaired platelet coagulant activity–a comparison with Scott syndrome. *Blood* 1997;89:1599–1611.

243. Hayward CP, Rivard GE, Kane WH. An autosomal dominant, qualitative platelet disorder associated with multimerin deficiency, abnormalities in platelet factor V, thrombospondin, von Willebrand factor, and fibrinogen and an epinephrine aggregation defect. *Blood* 1996;87:4967–4978.

244. Hayward CPM, Cramer EM, Kane WH, et al. Studies of a second family with the quebec platelet disorder–evidence that the degradation of the alpha-granule membrane and its soluble contents are not secondary to a defect in targeting proteins to alpha-granules. *Blood* 1997;89:1243–1253.

245. Kahr WH, Zheng S, Sheth PM, et al. Platelets from patients with the Quebec platelet disorder contain and secrete abnormal amounts of urokinase-type plasminogen activator. *Blood* 2001;98(2):257–265.

246. Sheth PM, Kahr WH, Haq MA, et al. Intracellular activation of the fibrinolytic cascade in the Quebec Platelet Disorder. *Thromb Haemost* 2003;90(2):293–298.

247. Ortel TL. Clinical and laboratory manifestations of anti-factor V antibodies. *J Lab Clin Med* 1999;133(4):326–334.

248. Zehnder JL, Leung LLK. Development of antibodies to thrombin and factor V with recurrent bleeding in a patient exposed to topical bovine thrombin. *Blood* 1990;76:2011–2016.

249. Chediak J, Ashenhurst JB, Garlick I, et al. Successful management of bleeding in a patient with factor V inhibitor by platelet transfusions. *Blood* 1980;56:835–841.

250. Nesheim ME, Nichols WL, Cole TL, et al. Isolation and study of an acquired inhibitor of human coagulation factor V. *J Clin Invest* 1986;77:405–415.

251. Ajzner E, Balogh I, Haramura G, et al. Anti-factor V auto-antibody in the plasma and platelets of a patient with repeated gastrointestinal bleeding. *J Thromb Haemost* 2003;1(5):943–949.

252. Ortel TL, Moore KD, Quinn-Allen MA, et al. Inhibitory anti-factor V antibodies bind to the factor V C2 domain and are associated with hemorrhagic manifestations. *Blood* 1998;91:4188–4196.

253. Ortel TL, Quinn-Allen MA, Charles LA, et al. Characterization of an acquired inhibitor to coagulation factor V. Antibody binding to the second C-type domain of factor V inhibits the binding of factor V to phosphatidylserine and neutralizes procoagulant activity. *J Clin Invest* 1992; 90:2340–2347.

254. Izumi T, Kim SW, Greist A, et al. Fine mapping of inhibitory anti-factor V antibodies using factor V C2 domain mutants. Identification of two antigenic epitopes involved in phospholipid binding. *Thromb Haemost* 2001; 85(6):1048–1054.

255. Svensson PJ, Dahlbäck B. Resistance to activated protein C as a basis for venous thrombosis. *N Engl J Med* 1994;330:517–522.

256. Martinelli I. Risk factors in venous thromboembolism. *Thromb Haemost* 2001;86(1):395–403.

257. Zoller B, Svensson PJ, He X, et al. Identification of the same factor V gene mutation in 47 out of 50 thrombosis-prone families with inherited resistance to activated protein C. *J Clin Invest* 1994;94:2521–2524.

258. Guasch JF, Lensen RP, Bertina RM. Molecular characterization of a type I quantitative factor V deficiency in a thrombosis patient that is "pseudo homozygous" for activated protein C resistance. *Thromb Haemost* 1997; 77:252–257.

259. Zivelin A, Griffin JH, Xu X, et al. A single genetic origin for a common Caucasian risk factor for venous thrombosis. *Blood* 1997;89:397–402.

260. Lindqvist PG, Svensson PJ, Dahlbäck B, et al. Factor V Q506 mutation (activated protein C resistance) associated with reduced intrapartum blood loss—a possible evolutionary selection mechanism. *Thromb Haemost* 1998; 79:69–73.

261. Nichols WC, Amano K, Cacheris PM, et al. Moderation of hemophilia A phenotype by the factor V R506Q mutation. *Blood* 1996;88:1183–1187.

262. Kerlin BA, Yan SB, Isermann BH, et al. Survival advantage associated with heterozygous factor V Leiden mutation in patients with severe sepsis and in mouse endotoxemia. *Blood* 2003;102(9):3085–3092.

263. Koeleman BP, Reitsma PH, Bertina RM, Familial thrombophilia: a complex genetic disorder. [Review] [100 refs]. *Semin Hematol* 1997;34:256–264.

264. Chan WP, Lee CK, Kwong YL, et al. A novel mutation of Arg306 of factor V gene in Hong Kong Chinese. *Blood* 1998;91:1135–1139.

265. Williamson D, Brown K, Luddington R, et al. Factor V Cambridge: a new mutation (Arg[306] Thr) associated with resistance to activated protein C. *Blood* 1998;91:1140–1144.

266. Norstrom E, Thorelli E, Dahlbäck B. Functional characterization of recombinant FV Hong Kong and FV Cambridge. *Blood* 2002;100(2):524–530.

267. van der Neut KM, Dirven RJ, Tans G, et al. The activated protein C (APC)-resistant phenotype of APC cleavage site mutants of recombinant factor V in a reconstituted plasma model. *Blood Coagul Fibrinolysis* 2002;13(3):207–215.

268. van der Neut KM, Dirven RJ, Vos HL, et al. Factor Va is inactivated by activated protein C in the absence of cleavage sites at Arg-306, Arg-506, and Arg-679. *J Biol Chem* 2004;279(8):6567–6575.

269. Chan WP, Lee CK, Kwong YL, et al. A novel mutation of Arg306 of factor V gene in Hong Kong Chinese. *Blood* 1998;91(4):1135–1139.

270. Franco RF, Elion J, Tavella MH, et al. The prevalence of factor V Arg(306)- > Thr (factor V Cambridge) and factor V Arg(306)- > Gly mutations in different human populations. *Thromb Haemost* 1999;81:312–313.

271. Franco RF, Maffei FH, Lourenco D, et al. Factor V Arg306 → Thr (factor V Cambridge) and factor V Arg306 → Gly mutations in venous thrombotic disease. *Br J Haematol* 1998;103(3):888–890.

272. Lunghi B, Iacoviello L, Gemmati D, et al. Detection of new polymorphic markers in the factor V gene: association with factor V levels in plasma. *Thromb Haemost* 1996;75:45–48.

273. Bernardi F, Faioni EM, Castoldi E, et al. A factor V genetic component differing from factor V R506Q contributes to the activated protein C resistance phenotype. *Blood* 1997;90:1552–1557.

274. Yamazaki T, Nicolaes GA, Sorensen KW, et al. Molecular basis of quantitative factor V deficiency associated with factor V R2 haplotype. *Blood* 2002;100(7):2515–2521.

275. van der Neut KM, Dirven RJ, Vos HL, et al. The R2-haplotype associated Asp2194Gly mutation in the light chain of human factor V results in lower expression levels of FV, but has no influence on the glycosylation of Asn2181. *Thromb Haemost* 2003;89(3):429–437.

276. Hoekema L, Castoldi E, Tans G, et al. Functional properties of factor V and factor Va encoded by the R2-gene. *Thromb Haemost* 2001;85(1):75–81.

277. Castaman G, Faioni EM, Tosetto A, et al. The factor V HR2 haplotype and the risk of venous thrombosis: a meta-analysis. *Haematologica* 2003; 88(10):1182–1189.

278. Bossone A, Cappucci F, D'Andrea G, et al. The factor V (FV) gene ASP79HIS polymorphism modulates FV plasma levels and affects the activated protein C resistance phenotype in presence of the FV Leiden mutation. *Haematologica* 2003;88(3):286–289.

279. van der Neut KM, Dirven RJ, Poort SR, et al. Characterization of an immunologic polymorphism (D79H) in the heavy chain of factor V. *J Thromb Haemost* 2004;2(6):910–917.

280. Mumford AD, McVey JH, Morse CV, et al. Factor V I359T: a novel mutation associated with thrombosis and resistance to activated protein C. *Br J Haematol* 2003;123(3):496–501.

281. Steen M, Norstrom EA, Tholander AL, et al. Functional characterization of factor V-Ile359Thr: a novel mutation associated with thrombosis. *Blood* 2004;103(9):3381–3387.

282. Hou LH, Xie F, Liu XE, et al. A novel mutation causes congenital factor V deficiency. *Zhonghua Xue Ye Xue Za Zhi* 2003;24(9):455–459.

283. Fu Q, Wu W, Ding Q, et al. Type I coagulation factor V deficiency caused by compound heterozygous mutation of F5 gene. *Haemophilia* 2003;9(5): 646–649.

284. Fu QH, Zhou RF, Liu LG, et al. Identification of three F5 gene mutations associated with inherited coagulation factor V deficiency in two Chinese pedigrees. *Haemophilia* 2004;10(3):264–270.

285. Mirochnik O, Halim-Kertanegara N, Henniker AJ, et al. A novel factor V null mutation at Arg 506 causes a false positive Factor V Leiden result [letter]. *Thromb Haemost* 1999;82(3):1198–1199.

286. Schrijver I, Koerper MA, Jones CD, et al. Homozygous factor V splice site mutation associated with severe factor V deficiency. *Blood* 2002;99(8): 3063–3065.

287. Xie F, Cheng F, Zhu X. Studies on hereditary deficiency of coagulation factor V. *Zhonghua Xue Ye Xue Za Zhi* 2001;22(9):453–456.

288. Lunghi B, Castoldi E, Mingozzi F, et al. A novel factor V null mutation detected in a thrombophilic patient with pseudo-homozygous APC resistance and in an asymptomatic unrelated subject [letter]. *Blood* 1998;92: 1463–1464.

289. Ajzner EE, Balogh I, Szabo T, et al. Severe coagulation factor V deficiency caused by 2 novel frameshift mutations: 2952delT in exon 13 and 5493insG in exon 16 of factor 5 gene. *Blood* 2002;99(2):702–705.

290. Castoldi E, Kalafatis M, Lunghi B, et al. Molecular bases of pseudo-homozygous APC resistance: the compound heterozygosity for FV R506Q and a FV null mutation results in the exclusive presence of FV Leiden molecules in plasma. *Thromb Haemost* 1998;80:403–406.

291. Zehnder JL, Hiraki DD, Jones CD, et al. Familial coagulation factor V deficiency caused by a novel 4 base pair insertion in the factor V gene: factor v stanford. *Thromb Haemost* 1999;82:1097–1099.

292. Simioni P, Scudeller A, Radossi P, et al. "Pseudo homozygous" activated protein C resistance due to double heterozygous factor V defects (factor V Leiden mutation and type I quantitative factor V defect) associated with thrombosis: report of two cases belonging to two unrelated kindreds. *Thromb Haemost* 1996;75:422–426.

293. Castoldi E, Simioni P, Kalafatis M, et al. Combinations of 4 mutations (FV R506Q, FV H1299R, FV Y1702C, PT 20210G/A) affecting the prothrombinase complex in a thrombophilic family. *Blood* 2000;96(4): 1443–1448.

294. Castoldi E, Lunghi B, Mingozzi F, et al. A missense mutation (Y1702C) in the coagulation factor V gene is a frequent cause of factor V deficiency in the Italian population. *Haematologica* 2001;86(6):629–633.

295. Dargaud Y, Trzeciak MC, Meunier S, et al. Two novel factor V null mutations associated with activated protein C resistance phenotype/genotype discrepancy. *Br J Haematol* 2003;123(2):342–345.

296. Asselta R, Tenchini ML, Holme R, et al. The discovery of Mary's mutation. *J Thromb Haemost* 2003;1(2):397–398.

297. Bossone A, D'Angelo F, Santacroce R, et al. Factor V Arg2074Cys: a novel missense mutation in the C2 domain of factor V. *Thromb Haemost* 2002; 87(5):923–924.

298. Schrijver I, Houissa-Kastally R, Jones CD, et al. Novel factor V C2-domain mutation (R2074H) in two families with factor V deficiency and bleeding. *Thromb Haemost* 2002;87(2):294–299.

# CHAPTER 10 ■ THROMBIN

NANCY SWORDS JENNY, ROGER L. LUNDBLAD, AND KENNETH G. MANN

The enzyme thrombin has long been recognized for its multiple functions in blood coagulation as well as for its more recently defined roles in tissue repair, development, and pathogenic processes (1–6). Thrombin originates from prothrombin, a circulating zymogen precursor protein. Prothrombin and thrombin are members of the family of vitamin K–dependent blood clotting proteins characterized by an NH$_2$-terminal "Gla domain," which contains several γ-carboxyglutamic acid residues. Prothrombin, $M_r$ = 72,000, is the most abundant of these proteins, circulating at a plasma concentration of 1 to 2 μM (7,8). The human prothrombin molecule (see Fig. 10-1) is synthesized primarily in the liver. Low levels of prothrombin expression have been reported in brain, diaphragm, stomach, kidney, spleen, intestine, and in uterine, placental, and adrenal tissues (9,10). The 21-kb-long prothrombin gene, located on chromosome 11p11-q12, has been extensively characterized (11–14). Of the 26,929 base pairs (bp) of continuous sequence that has been determined, 6,544 bp are upstream from the methionine initiator, 20,241 bp span the site of initiation of transcription to the site of polyadenylation, and 145 bp constitute the 3′ flanking region (14). The gene is organized into 14 exons and 13 introns (14) and is transcribed as a pre-propeptide containing 622 amino acids (11,12). The 43–amino acid pre-propeptide region mediates posttranslational processing to generate the mature protein molecule of 579 amino acids containing 10 γ-carboxyglutamic (Gla) residues in the 40–amino acid NH$_2$-terminal Gla domain region and 3 asparagine-linked glycosylation sites (Fig. 10-1).

Thrombin and prothrombin are also members of the large family of serine proteases and their zymogen precursors that includes chymotrypsin and chymotrypsinogen and trypsin and trypsinogen. The parent molecule of the serine protease family is historically considered to be bovine α-chymotrypsin (16,17). The nomenclature used in this chapter refers to the structure of the mature, secreted human prothrombin molecule. However, other nomenclature systems are also used to denote bovine prothrombin (the numbering system has the superscript "b") and chymotrypsinogen (the numbering system has the superscript "c").

Studies of partial primary structures of bovine (8) and human (18,19) prothrombins and the complete primary structure and glycosylation sites of human prethrombin 2 (residues 272 to 579), the immediate precursor of thrombin (20), led to initial observations about the structure–function relation of the molecule. MacGillivray and Davie (21) later isolated the cDNA for bovine prothrombin and deduced the primary structure for the bovine molecule. Subsequently, Degen et al. (11) determined the cDNA sequence and gene structure for the human prothrombin molecule. The mature human prothrombin molecule consists of four distinct domains (Fig. 10-1): the Gla domain (residues 1 to 40), the kringle 1 domain (residues 65 to 143), the kringle 2 domain (residues 170 to 248), and the serine protease precursor domain (residues 321 to 579), which is homologous to other members of the serine protease family.

## PROTHROMBIN FRAGMENT 1 (GLA DOMAIN AND KRINGLE 1)

Thrombin cleaves its zymogen prothrombin at residue 155, separating the Gla domain and kringle 1 region from the COOH-terminal domains of the molecule. This fragment is termed *prothrombin fragment 1*. Subsequent cleavage of prothrombin fragment 1 by chymotrypsin at residue 40 separates the Gla and kringle 1 domains (22). The Gla domains of the vitamin K–dependent blood clotting proteins mediate the metal ion– and membrane-binding capabilities of these proteins and are essential for protein function. The Gla domain of prothrombin contains 10 γ-carboxyglutamic acids (Fig. 10-1) as a consequence of a vitamin K–dependent modification of preprothrombin in the liver. The vitamin K–dependent carboxylase assists in modifying the γ-hydrogen position of a glutamic acid residue, thereby forming a γ-carboxyglutamic acid. Coincident with generation of the modified amino acid, the reduced hydroquinone form of vitamin K is oxidized to the epoxide form of the vitamin. Reductase activity present in the liver regenerates the reduced form of vitamin K (23,24). The 10 γ-carboxyglutamic acid residues in prothrombin are responsible for binding calcium ions that, in turn, induce a significant conformational transition in the molecule (25,26). In the absence of calcium ions, the Gla domain is completely disordered (27,28). When calcium ions are present, however, the amino acid residues of the Gla domain are arranged in an ordered structure (29). The initial structural observations obtained by metal ion–dependent fluorescence and circular dichroism were confirmed in the studies of the crystal structure of bovine prothrombin fragment 1 (thrombin cleavage at residue 156[b]). The positions of the first 35 amino acids in the calcium ion–free structure of bovine prothrombin fragment 1 are not represented because of the random orientation of the residues (27,28). When calcium ions are infused into the crystal, the crystal distorts and fractures because of the large conformational change in the Gla domain (29). The calcium ion–induced conformational change that occurs in prothrombin fragment 1 has been illustrated for other vitamin K–dependent proteins—factor VII, factor X, and protein C—as well (30).

Calcium binding and the attendant conformational changes are requirements for prothrombin fragment 1 and prothrombin, and, presumably, for other members of the family of vitamin K–dependent proteins, to bind to membranes containing acidic phospholipids (31). Once bound to the membrane surface, prothrombin is effectively presented as a substrate for activation by the prothrombinase complex. The phospholipid bilayer is believed to serve not only as a surface for condensing the proteins involved in thrombin generation but also as a functional element of the prothrombinase complex (32).

The importance of the Gla domain has been demonstrated using partially carboxylated prothrombins isolated from the blood of warfarin-treated cows. The absence of carboxylation of as few as two of the appropriate glutamic acid residues results in

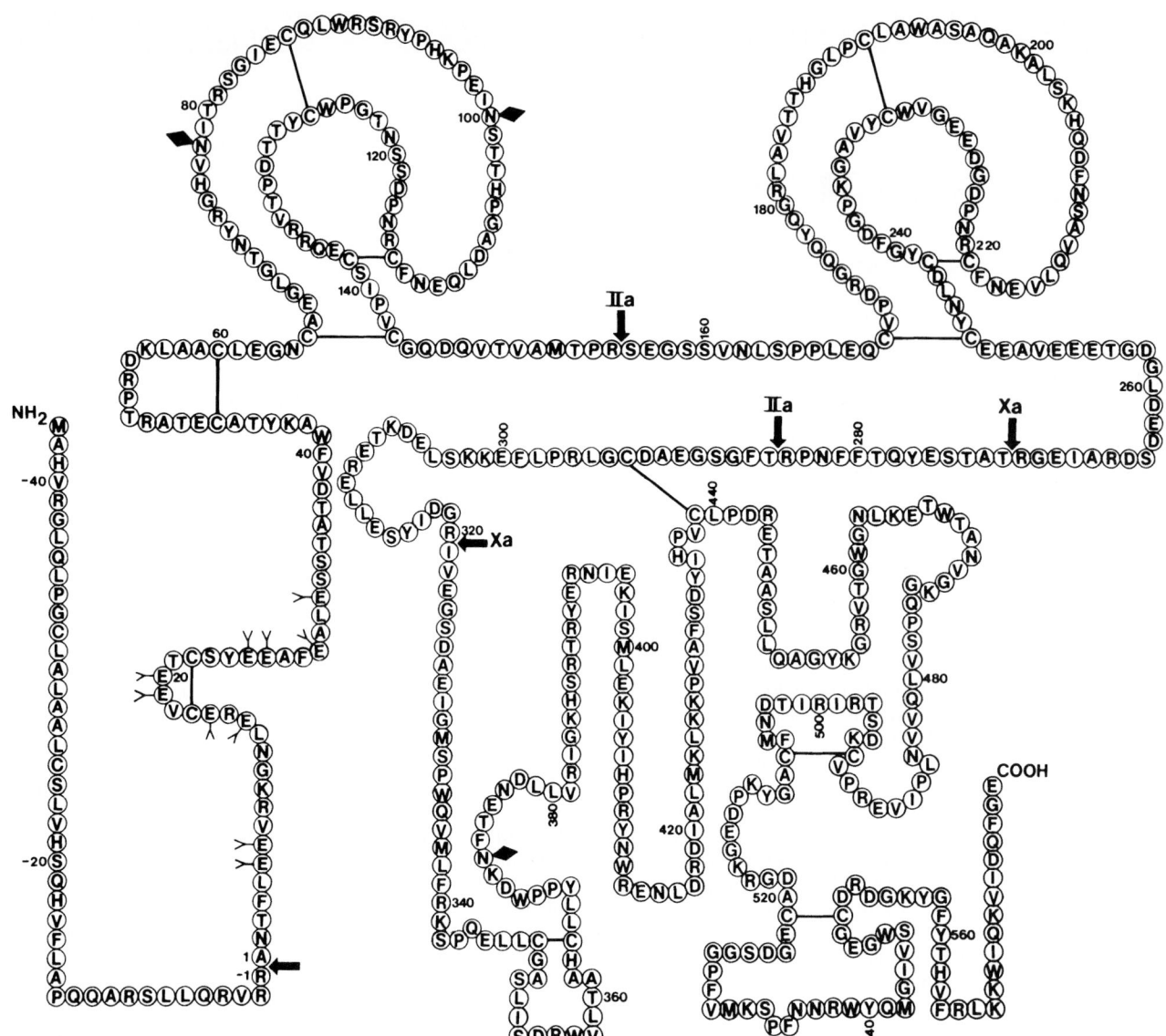

**FIGURE 10-1.** Primary sequence of human pre-prothrombin as deduced by Degan et al. (12). Ys correspond to γ-carboxyglutamate. *Closed triangles* correspond to an asparagine-linked carbohydrate side chain. The organization of the two kringles of prothrombin uses the format described by Magnusson and colleagues (8). The organization of the thrombin peptide chain segments is according to the model developed by Elion and associates (15). Sites of cleavage of pre-prothrombin by the signal peptidase and of prothrombin by thrombin and by factor Xa are indicated by *arrows*. (From Degen SJ, Davie EW. Nucleotide sequence of the gene for human prothrombin. *Biochemistry* 1987;26:6165; Magnusson S, Petersen TE, Scottrup-Jensen L. Complete primary structure of prothrombin: isolation, structure and reactivity of 10 carboxylated glutamic acid residues and regulation of prothrombin activation by thrombin. In: Reich E, Rifkin DB, Shaw E, eds. *Proteases and biological control*. Cold Spring Harbor, NY: Cold Spring Harbor Laboratory, 1975:123–149; Elion J, Downing MJ, Butkowski RJ. Structure of human thrombin: comparison with other serine proteases. In: Lundblad RL, Fenton JW, Mann KG, eds. *Chemistry and biology of thrombin*. Ann Arbor, MI: Ann Arbor Science Publishers, 1977, with permission.)

a prothrombin molecule that is an ineffective substrate for the prothrombinase complex (33). γ-Carboxyglutamic acid–deficient prothrombins fail to undergo the calcium ion–dependent conformational transitions required for binding to acidic phospholipids and for effective presentation to the prothrombinase complex. The likely mode of action of warfarin at the chemical level is to block the reduction reactions required to regenerate the vitamin K hydroquinone form from the epoxide form, thereby blocking vitamin K–dependent reactions. The reduction in the level of γ-carboxylation blocks the membrane-binding properties of the vitamin K–dependent proteins, thereby reducing their ability to function properly.

The prothrombin fragment 1 portion of the prothrombin molecule also contains the kringle 1 domain of prothrombin.

Kringles have been identified as common motifs in many plasma proteins including prothrombin, plasminogen, tissue plasminogen activator, urokinase, factor XII, and apolipoprotein A (34–36). A unique activity has not yet been definitively associated with the kringle 1 region of prothrombin, although some reports suggest a possible role in the interaction of prothrombin with factor Va in the prothrombinase complex (37,38).

The kringle 1 domain of bovine prothrombin (residues 66[b] to 144[b]) is noteworthy for being the first blood coagulation protein fragment structure to be determined by x-ray crystallography (27). The folding of the kringle is largely determined by close van der Waals contacts between the interloop cysteine disulfide bonds (Cys87[b] to Cys127[b] and Cys115[b] to Cys139[b]).

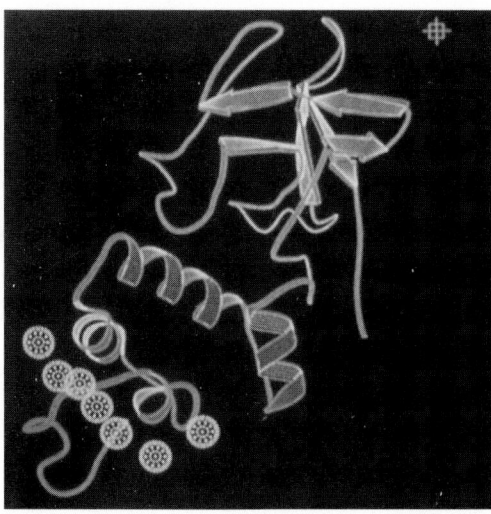

**FIGURE 10-2.** Orientation of the backbone peptide chain of prothrombin fragment 1. The NH$_2$-terminal segment of the molecule is oriented toward the lower left-hand quadrant (7 o'clock) of the figure. The kringle 1 segment of the molecule is in the upper right (2 o'clock). Pleated sheet segments are indicated by *arrows*. Calcium ions are identified by *orange balls*. The connecting region between the Gla domain and kringle 1 is represented by an $\alpha$-helix (see Color Fig. 10-2). (Courtesy of Drs. Timothy Rydel and Alexander Tulinsky.)

These cysteine residues are buried in the interior of the molecule and are inaccessible to solvent. Figure 10-2 illustrates the backbone arrangement for both the Gla and kringle 1 domains in the calcium ion–dependent conformation of prothrombin fragment 1 (27–29). As predicted by hydrodynamic studies, the overall structure of prothrombin fragment 1 is highly asymmetric. The calcium ions (orange balls) are tightly bound to the $\gamma$-carboxyglutamic acid residues in the Gla domain in an almost linear array (Fig. 10-2). It is likely that several of these metal ions interact with acidic phospholipids on a membrane surface. The tightly interwoven disulfide-linked structure of the kringle 1 domain is visible in the upper right of Figure 10-2. The interconnecting region between kringle 1 and the Gla domain is an $\alpha$-helix and is quite prominent in the structure.

# PROTHROMBIN FRAGMENT 2 (KRINGLE 2)

The kringle 2 domain of prothrombin is found in prothrombin fragment 2 (residues 156 to 274). Kringle 2 is similar to kringle 1 in terms of amino acid sequence and presumably in terms of structure as well. Unlike kringle 1, however, kringle 2 has several interesting functional assignments. The kringle 2 domain binds calcium ions and appears to be the primary region in prothrombin that mediates the interaction of the prothrombin molecule with the cofactor, factor Va, in the prothrombinase complex (39–41). The precise effect of this interaction on the overall function of the prothrombinase complex still remains unclear (42). The interaction between the kringle 2 domain of prothrombin and factor Va may be responsible for altering the conformation of prothrombin, making the cleavage sites on prothrombin more accessible to factor Xa, the enzyme component of the prothrombinase complex (42).

The fragment 2 region of prothrombin also noncovalently associates with thrombin with a dissociation constant of approximately 10 nM (43,44). On account of the tight association, it is unlikely that free thrombin is found in plasma. The

active thrombin species in the biologic milieu may actually consist of a prothrombin fragment 1.2–$\alpha$-thrombin complex or a prothrombin fragment 2–$\alpha$-thrombin complex. Chemical modification and x-ray crystallographic studies have shown that prothrombin fragment 2 interacts with exosite II, or the heparin-binding region, of thrombin (45–49). The interaction involves the formation of salt bridges between the inner loop of kringle 2 and exosite II of thrombin (50). This interaction has been reported to have multiple effects on thrombin function. Prothrombin fragment 2 has been reported to inhibit thrombin inactivation by antithrombin III (ATIII) by blocking the interaction between thrombin and ATIII (51), alter the active site and exosite I regions of thrombin (52), enhance thrombin activity toward small peptide substrates (43), inhibit the ability of thrombin to cleave fibrinogen (53), and influence protein C activation (54).

# PRETHROMBIN 2 AND THROMBIN

Prethrombin 2 (residues 272 to 579) contains the sequence of the enzyme $\alpha$-thrombin. The human and bovine prethrombin 2 peptides share considerable homology. Cleavage of prethrombin 2 by factor Xa at residue 320 (323[b]) yields the two-chain active enzyme composed of an A chain of 49 residues and a B chain of 259 residues. Once the active site is generated, human thrombin cleaves its own A chain at Arg284, generating the stable form of human $\alpha$-thrombin with an A chain of 36 residues (55).

Comparison of bovine $\alpha$-chymotrypsin, the parent molecule of the serine protease family, and human $\alpha$-thrombin shows that nearly one third of the amino acid residues are totally conserved in both proteins, as are the positions of the disulfide bonds connecting the two chains of human $\alpha$-thrombin and the three chains of bovine $\alpha$-chymotrypsin. (The three-chain structure of $\alpha$-chymotrypsin is attributable to excision of residues 148[c] to 159[c] during the activation process.) However, key differences are observed in human $\alpha$-thrombin relative to $\alpha$-chymotrypsin (see Table 10-1) (15). There is a deletion of the residue corresponding to $\alpha$-chymotrypsin position 218[c]. Additionally, human thrombin has segments of residues that can be represented as major insertions or "loops" and minor insertions of one or two amino acids (15) (Table 10-1). The NH$_2$-terminal portion of the $\alpha$-thrombin A chain (residues 285 to 292) has no counterpart in $\alpha$-chymotrypsin. The general positions of the insertions were confirmed upon determination of the crystal structure of human FPR-ck-$\alpha$-thrombin.[1] The positions of the insertions have likewise been identified with respect to the three-dimensional structure of the human $\alpha$-thrombin molecule (56,57). The COOH-terminus of the $\alpha$-thrombin A chain contains a 13-residue insertion (residues 307 to 319) called the *A loop* (15). The three-dimensional structural model of $\alpha$-thrombin shows that the A loop is on the backside of the molecule relative to the active site. Removal of the A loop from bovine thrombin does not appear to effect the fibrinogen-clotting activity (58), and this insertion is not likely to contribute to fibrinogen interactions. The A loop is also on the opposite side of the $\alpha$-thrombin molecule relative to the hirudin-binding site. Positions 343 and 393, however, are two single amino acid substitutions that appear to play a prominent role in hirudin binding. The insertion composed of residues 367 to 375, or the "B loop," caps the active site

---

[1]FPR-ck-$\alpha$-thrombin is $\alpha$-thrombin modified at its active site histidine with the d-Phe-Pro-Arg chloromethyl ketone. The modified protein is irreversibly inactivated.

## TABLE 10-1

INSERTIONS IN THROMBIN RELATIVE TO CHYMOTRYPSIN

| Human prothrombin numbering | Chymotrypsinogen numbering | Notes |
|---|---|---|
| 271–284 | 1 U–1 I | Deleted in stable form of human α-thrombin |
| 285–292 | 1 H–1 A | Not well ordered in crystal of FRP-ck-α-thrombin; found in different location in hirudin-thrombin |
| 307–319 | 14 A–14 M | Exposed loop, the "A loop," with extensive salt-bridge–stabilized structure at the NH₂-end; the COOH-terminal end of this loop appears to be flexible |
| 343 | 37 A | Contributes to hirudin binding |
| 367–375 | 60 A–60 I | Contains carbohydrate implicated in chemotactic activity; peptide has growth factor activity; this loop, the "B loop," caps the active site of thrombin |
| 393 | 77 A | Contributes to hirudin binding |
| 414 | 97 A | Protrudes from molecule |
| 447–449 | 129 A–129 C | |
| 470–474 | 149 A–149 E | Site of extensive proteolysis, flexible; the "γ loop," or "C loop" |
| 510 | 184 A | Highly exposed loop; water molecules plentiful in this region of structure |
| 513–516 | 186 A–186 D | The "E loop" |
| 535–536 | 204 A–204 B | Large 1–6 turn |
| 549–550 | 218 | Loop similar to trypsin |
| 553 | 221 A | |
| 578–579 | 245 A–245 B | |

of α-thrombin (15). This insertion also contains the single carbohydrate adduct found in α-thrombin and is the region of α-thrombin that mediates the chemotactic and growth factor properties of the molecule (5,6). The "E loop" represents an insertion composed of residues 513 to 516 and is located near the bottom of the active site pocket (15). Many of the water molecules identified in the crystal structure are near this loop structure (15). The position of the "C loop" or "γ loop," residues 470 to 474, varies considerably between the FPR-ck-α-thrombin and the hirudin–α-thrombin structures, indicating that this segment of α-thrombin is mobile in solution (15). The C or γ loop is also susceptible to proteolysis.

Different numbering systems have been developed for prothrombin on the basis of bovine or human amino acid sequence or on the sequences of prethrombin 2, bovine α-thrombin, human α-thrombin, or chymotrypsinogen. The various systems have caused some confusion. In this text, we are using the nomenclature system based on the human prothrombin sequence, with residue 1 considered to be the first residue of the secreted prothrombin product. Bovine prothrombin contains a one–amino acid insertion near its NH₂-terminus at position three relative to human prothrombin, and the bovine prothrombin numbering system differs from the human by one residue. Other studies make use of the chymotrypsinogen numbering system (56). This approach is valuable in making direct comparisons between the members of the serine protease family. Table 10-1, which lists the insertions in human α-thrombin relative to chymotrypsinogen, indicates the numbering systems on the basis of both chymotrypsinogen and human prothrombin.

Although substantial differences exist between α-thrombin and α-chymotrypsin, the serine protease family is characterized by specific structural features present in both these molecules. The four disulfide bridges in α-thrombin are entirely homologous with the equivalent disulfide bridges in chymotrypsin (see Table 10-2). The serine protease family is also characterized by specific structural features associated with the "charge-relay system." The essential residues for this system in chymotrypsin, His57ᶜ, Asp102ᶜ, and Ser195ᶜ are

## TABLE 10-2

EQUIVALENT DISULFIDE BRIDGES IN THROMBIN AND CHYMOTRYPSIN

| Designation | Chymotrypsin | Thrombin |
|---|---|---|
| Histidine loop | Cys42–Cys58 | Cys348–Cys364 |
| Methionine loop | Cys168–Cys182 | Cys493–Cys507 |
| Serine loop | Cys191–Cys220 | Cys521–Cys551 |
| A–B chain bridge | Cys1–Cys122 | Cys293–Cys439 |
| B–C chain bridge | Cys136–Cys201 | — |

entirely equivalent to His363, Asp419, and Ser525 in human α-thrombin. The α-thrombin active site serine, Ser525, and the sequence surrounding it are highly conserved in the active site regions of chymotrypsin and the other serine proteases. Additionally, the B chain of human α-thrombin contains a sodium ion binding site, which is most likely involved in allosteric regulation of the active site of the enzyme (59). The sequence of the sodium ion binding site is highly homologous to the sequences of the sodium ion binding sites in the other serine proteases involved in blood coagulation—factor VII, factor IX, factor X, and protein C (59).

Other structural similarities between α-thrombin and chymotrypsin are also observed. When chymotrypsinogen is cleaved, a conformational change occurs that allows the new NH₂-terminal residue, Ile16ᶜ, to form a salt bridge with Asp194ᶜ, in turn leading to a conformational change in the region of the active site serine, Ser195ᶜ, generating a functional enzyme (60,61). A similar bond is formed in thrombin following factor Xa cleavage of prethrombin 2 at Arg320. The new NH₂-terminal residue of the human protein, Ile321, forms a salt bridge with Asp524. The accompanying conformational transition results in a 30-Å distance between Ile321 and Arg320 in the active enzyme α-thrombin. When Ile321 is modified with nitrous acid, preventing salt bridge formation, the resulting thrombin product has no activity (62).

# SUBSTRATE/INHIBITOR BINDING SITES

Thrombin possesses at least four distinct binding sites for substrates, inhibitors, cofactors, and sodium ions. The sodium ion binding site appears to help determine whether thrombin acts as a procoagulant and recognizes fibrinogen as a substrate (presence of sodium ions) or acts as an anticoagulant and recognizes protein C as a substrate (absence of sodium ions). The other three sites, exosite I, exosite II, and the active site, recognize a variety of molecules and account for the diverse functions of thrombin (63).

The sodium ion binding site is contained within a cylindrical cavity formed by three antiparallel β-sheets of the human α-thrombin B chain. The site is more than 15 Å from the catalytic site. The cavity containing the sodium ion binding site bisects the α-thrombin molecule from the active site to the opposite surface and contains Asp419 of the charge-relay system. The sequence of the sodium ion binding site is highly conserved in thrombins from different species and is homologous to the equivalent sites in other serine proteases. The transition triggered when human α-thrombin binds sodium ions is thought to be responsible for altering the specificity of the enzyme. In the presence of sodium ions, α-thrombin recognizes and cleaves fibrinogen acting as a procoagulant. When no sodium is bound, α-thrombin has increased specificity for substrates like protein C, which have an acidic residue in the P3 position, and acts as an anticoagulant. The change in enzyme specificity allows α-thrombin to act in a dual role, as both a procoagulant and anticoagulant enzyme (59,63).

Exosite I, the fibrinogen binding site, is an anion-binding electropositive site, distinct from, but acting in concert with, the active site (63). Exosite I also binds the COOH-terminal domain of hirudin, the hirudinlike region of the thrombin

receptor protease-activated receptor (PAR)-1, and the fifth and sixth epidermal growth factor–like domains of thrombomodulin (63). Detailed information about this region is available because of x-ray crystallographic studies of the α-thrombin–hirudin complex. Hirudin demonstrates a high affinity interaction with α-thrombin to form a stable, noncovalent complex with a dissociation constant in the range of $2 \times 10^{-14}$ M (64,65). Hirudin is believed to bind to both exosite I and the active site of thrombin (65–67). Figure 10-3 illustrates the space-filling and carbon backbone models of the α-thrombin–hirudin complex. In the α-carbon backbone model (Fig. 10-3A), the structure of α-thrombin is blue and the structure of hirudin is red. The structure also shows the tightly knitted disulfide bonds of hirudin (yellow) and inserted residues in the α-thrombin backbone structure relative to chymotrypsin (light blue). In the space-filling model, (Fig. 10-3B), the α-thrombin structure is blue, the hirudin structure is red, and prominent insertions are yellow.

In solution, the COOH-terminal domain of hirudin is disordered (68,69). However, in the α-thrombin–hirudin complex, (Fig. 10-3), the COOH-terminal of hirudin interacts with the large groove in the α-thrombin molecule and extends across the face of the molecule to interact with exosite I (Fig. 10-3B), which is distant from the active site (Fig. 10-3A) of α-thrombin. The interaction of α-thrombin and hirudin is stabilized by electrostatic, polar, and hydrophobic interactions that account for the very high affinity interaction between the two proteins.

The NH$_2$-terminus of hirudin also penetrates into the active site of thrombin. Ile1 of hirudin is hydrogen bonded to the active site serine, Ser525, of α-thrombin. However, hirudin does not interact with the α-thrombin S$_1$ subsite that accommodates arginyl substrates. In contrast to the COOH-terminal domain, the structure of the NH$_2$-terminal domain of hirudin does not appear to be altered considerably upon interaction

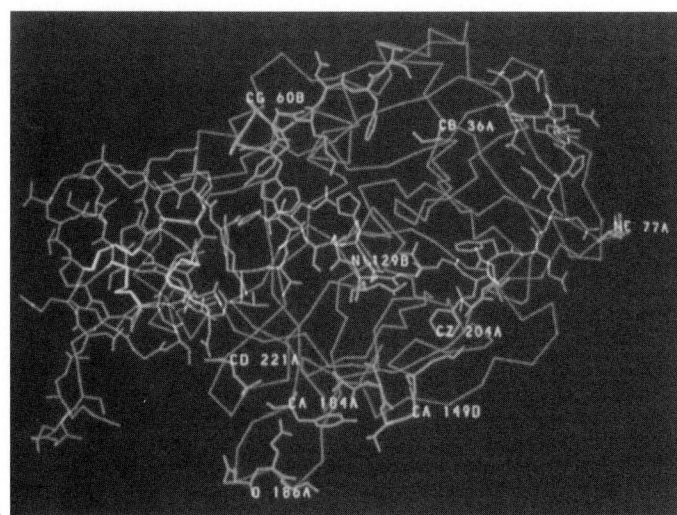
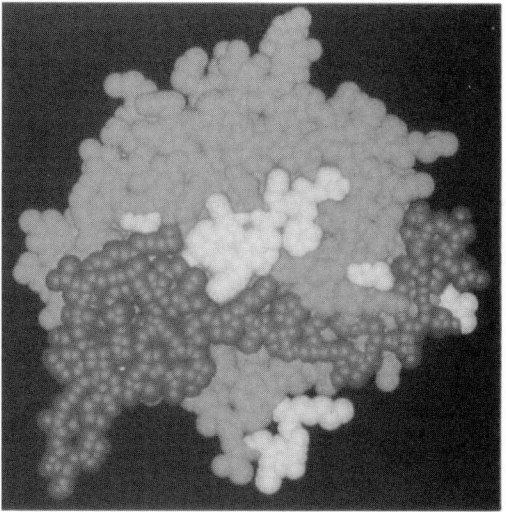

**FIGURE 10-3.** The α-thrombin–hirudin complex. **A:** The α-carbon backbone structure of thrombin (*light blue*) and the α-carbon backbone structure of hirudin (*red*). Disulfide bonds in the NH$_2$-terminal domain of the hirudin molecule are in *yellow*, and "insertion loops" in the thrombin molecule relative to chymotrypsinogen are represented with their appropriate side chains in *light blue*. Insertion loop residues are identified to orient the reader with respect to the identity of various insertional loops. The nomenclature used is that of Bode et al. (56) and in some instances represents an earlier stage of refinement of insertional nomenclature. There are, therefore, a few differences between nomenclature in this figure and that defined in Table 10-2. However, all nomenclature reflected in the figure is within one or two residues of the notation presented in Table 10-2. **B:** A space-filling model of the same complex; α-thrombin (*blue*), hirudin (*red*), and insertion loops (*yellow*) (see Color Fig. 10-3). (From Bode W, Mayr I, Baumann U, et al. The refined 1.9 Å crystal structure of human α-thrombin: interaction with D-Phe-Pro-Arg chloromethylketone and significance of the Tyr-Pro-Pro-Trp insertion segment. *EMBO J* 1989;8:3467, with permission.)

with α-thrombin. Very little of the NH₂-terminal domain of hirudin (Fig. 10-3, red) is actually in contact with α-thrombin.

One of the dominant features of the α-thrombin molecule resolved from studies of the x-ray crystal structures of FPR-ck-α-thrombin and the α-thrombin–hirudin complex is the groove that extends across the face of the molecule beginning at the active site (56,57). The COOH-terminal tail of hirudin interacts with this groove, and it is likely that most macromolecular substrates, such as fibrinogen, have secondary binding sites associated with this groove or other similar exosites on the surface of α-thrombin (57,70).

Exosite II, a second electropositive, anion-binding site, is found on the side opposite of the α-thrombin molecule compared to exosite I, which binds hirudin and fibrinogen. Exosite II is responsible for binding highly sulfated polysaccharides like heparin, the COOH-terminal domain of the B chain of thrombin, and the chondroitin sulfate moiety of thrombomodulin (63). The fourth defined binding site on the α-thrombin molecule, the active site region, interacts with substrate molecules that include protein C and AT-III (63).

The insertions and deletions in the α-thrombin sequence, compared to factor VIIa, factor IXa, factor Xa, trypsin, and chymotrypsin, are unquestionably responsible for the selectivity of α-thrombin toward its macromolecular substrates and its functions as a hydrolytic serine protease (71). The primary binding site for substrates on the α-thrombin molecule, the active site, is similar to the active sites of trypsin and chymotrypsin. However, unlike the two pancreatic enzymes trypsin and chymotrypsin, α-thrombin also has secondary binding sites, exosites I and II, that confer the unique specificity associated with the enzyme. The S1 binding site of trypsin is defined by Asp189$^c$, which interacts with arginyl or lysyl P₁ residues of substrates in the bottom of the trypsin-binding pocket (72). Human α-thrombin also has an aspartic acid residue, Asp521, in the corresponding position in its binding pocket, as does bovine factor Xa. Chymotrypsin has a hydrophobic binding pocket similar to trypsin but lacks the aspartic acid residue in the S₁ position. Chymotrypsin instead has a methionine residue in the equivalent position.

Although the primary binding sites of α-thrombin and trypsin are similar, the nature of the specificity of α-thrombin is more complex because of the active site region and the exosites. In chymotrypsin, the NH₂-terminal segment of the substrate peptide bond P₁ to P₃ forms an antiparallel sheet with the S₁ to S₃ sequence of the enzyme. After the S₃ position, the chymotrypsin structure bends sharply away from the substrate and does not interact with the substrate beyond the substrate P₃ position. In α-thrombin, however, the binding site is far more extensive. The α-thrombin cleavage sites on various macromolecular substrates, presented in Table 10-3, often occur after the sequence X-Pro-Arg. In three cleavage sites on human and bovine prothrombins, the residues Gly-Ser are found at subsites P₃′ and P₄′ (Table 10-3). In addition, phenylalanine at the P₉ position in the fibrinogen Aα chain is highly conserved among various species and is required for specificity in the fibrinogen–α-thrombin interaction (73,74). The fibrinogen-binding site extends from the P₉ to at least the P₃′ site, and perhaps as far as the P₈′ to P₃₅′ site (75). There may also be multiple secondary binding sites for fibrinogen (76). α-Thrombin binding interactions with substrates are far larger in scope than equivalent interactions between trypsin and its substrates.

The specificity of α-thrombin toward the arginyl–glycyl bonds of the Aα and Bβ chains of fibrinogen is most likely a result of the primary, rather than the tertiary, structure of fibrinogen (101). α-Thrombin can cleave fibrinopeptides isolated from the Aα and Bβ chains, and the sequence of fibrinopeptide A is highly conserved among different species. Synthetic peptide analogs of fibrinopeptides A and B also act as inhibitors of α-thrombin. The first 51 amino acids of the Aα chain of fibrinogen appear to be responsible for the interactions with the

binding sites on α-thrombin (102). The primary binding site appears to be located in the NH₂-terminal sequence of the Aα between residues 1 and 23, with secondary binding interactions mediated by residues 34 to 44 and 45 to 51.

In addition to the exosites and active site region implicated in specific substrate binding, there also appears to be an apolar binding site near the catalytic center of human α-thrombin (70). This site binds ρ-chlorobenzylamino-ε-aminocaproyl agarose and proflavine and lies near the entrance to the specificity pocket. In α-thrombin, the site is lined by Ile499, Trp547, His363, Tyr367, and Trp370. The corresponding residues in chymotrypsin are Ile174$^c$, Trp215$^c$, His57$^c$, Tyr60$^c$A, and Trp60$^c$D.

# DEGRADED FORMS OF THROMBIN

Preparations of α-thrombin are often subject to relatively specific cleavages resulting in forms of stable, degraded thrombins with altered reactivity (103–105). These forms have been labeled β- and γ-thrombins (see Fig. 10-4). The degradation of α-thrombin may be autocatalytic but is more likely the result of the presence of contaminating proteases in some preparations of α-thrombin because stable preparations of α-thrombin have been observed. In addition, the cleavage reactions that give rise to β- and γ-thrombins sometimes occur after lysine residues, and lysine is not a preferred cleavage site for α-thrombin (Table 10-3).

The cleavage sites that give rise to bovine β-thrombin have been identified (106). The A chain of bovine α-thrombin (residues 275$^b$ to 323$^b$) is proteolyzed at two sites, Lys287$^b$ and Lys304$^b$, leaving only a remnant of the A chain. At least two cleavages, Lys388$^b$ and Arg396$^b$, also occur in the B chain (residues 324$^b$ to 582$^b$) upon degradation to β-thrombin. As a consequence of proteolysis of the B chain, the peptide segment containing the active site histidine, His366$^b$, and the segment containing the other residues of the charge–relay system, Arg422$^b$ and Ser528$^b$, are no longer covalently attached (106). The loss of association of the charge–relay complex, which includes the active site serine, does not appear to affect the ability of bovine β-thrombin to bind fibrinogen. Both bovine α-thrombin and β-thrombin bind fibrinogen with essentially equal affinity (107). However, the ability of bovine β-thrombin to cleave fibrinogen is greatly reduced compared to α-thrombin (103,107,108).

Degradation of human α-thrombin has likewise been specifically described (109,110). The B chain of the stable form of human α-thrombin (residues 321 to 579) is proteolyzed at Arg382 and Asn394, giving rise to human β-thrombin (Fig. 10-4). Cleavage of the B chain at Arg443 and Lys474 deletes another segment of the B chain, giving rise to human γ-thrombin (Fig. 10-4). The peptide deleted in γ-thrombin is the "γ" or "C loop" and is an extremely mobile part of the thrombin structure. The degraded forms of human α-thrombin retain at least some ability to cleave small peptide substrates (111,112), factor XIII (113), ATIII (114), and prothrombin (115). However, the activities of human β- and γ-thrombins toward fibrinogen, thrombospondin, and protein C are very limited (108,114,116).

# MEIZOTHROMBIN

Figure 10-4 depicts the prothrombin molecule and the proteolytic processing required to obtain the various forms of thrombin. In addition to the α-, β-, and γ-thrombins, there are two larger active species: meizothrombin and meizothrombin des-fragment 1 (117). Meizothrombin was first identified as a product of *Echis carinatus* venom protease cleavage of human

## TABLE 10-3

### SITES OF CLEAVAGE BY THROMBIN ON VARIOUS PROTEINS

| Protein | Subsite $P_9$ $P_8$ $P_7$ $P_6$ $P_5$ $P_4$ $P_3$ $P_2$ $P_1$ | $\alpha$lla $P_1'$ $P_2'$ $P_3'$ $P_4'$ $P_5'$ $P_6'$ $P_7'$ $P_8'$ $P_9'$ | Reference |
|---|---|---|---|
| Fibrinogen (A$\alpha$), human | Phe-Leu-Ala-Glu-Gly-Gly-Gly-Val-Arg (16) | Gly-Pro-Arg-Val-Val-Glu-Arg-His | 77 |
| | Glu-Gly-Gly-Gly-Val-Arg-Gly-Pro-Arg (19) | Val-Val-Glu-Arg-His-Gln-Ser-Ala | 78 |
| Fibrinogen (B$\beta$), human | Asn-Glu-Glu-Gly-Phe-Phe-Ser-Ala-Arg (14) | Gly-His-Arg-Pro-Leu-Asp-Lys | 77 |
| Factor XIII, human | Thr-Val-Glu-Leu-Glu-Glu-Val-Pro-Arg (36) | Gly-Val-Asx-Leu-Glx-Glx | 79 |
| Factor XIII, bovine | Val-Glu-Leu-Gln-Gly-Leu-Val-Pro-Arg (37) | Gly-Phe-Asx, Pro-Glx-Glx | 79 |
| Factor VIII, human | Asn-Ser-Pro-Ser-Phe-Ile-Gln-Ile-Arg (372) | Ser-Val-Ala-Lys-Lys-His-Pro-Lys-Thr | 80 |
| Factor VIII | Leu-Ser-Asn-Asn-Ala-Ile-Gly-Pro-Arg (740) | Ser-Phe-Ser-Gln-Asn-Ser-Arg-His-Pro | 80 |
| Factor VIII | Gln-Asn-Phe-Val-The-Gln-Ser-Lys-Arg (1,313) | Ala-Leu-Lys-Gln-Phe-Arg-Leu-Pro-Leu | 80 |
| Factor VIII | Asp-Glu-Asp-Glu-Asn-Gln-Ser-Pro-Arg (1,689) | Ser-Phe-Gln-Lys-Lys-The-Arg-His-Tyr | 80 |
| Factor V, human | Arg-Leu-Ala-Ala-Ala-Leu-Gly-Ile-Arg (709) | Ser-Phe-Arg-Asn-Ser-Ser-Leu-Asn-Gln | 81 |
| Factor V | Thr-His-His-Ala-Pro-Leu-Ser-Pro-Arg (1,018) | Thr-Phe-His-Pro-Leu-Arg-Ser-Glu-Ala | 81 |
| Factor V | Asp-Asn-Ile-Ala-Ala-Trp-Tyr-Leu-Arg (1,545) | Ser-Asn-Asn-Gly-Asn-Arg-Arg-Asn-Tyr | 81 |
| Factor VII, human | Arg-Asn-Ala-Ser-Lys-Pro-Gln-Gly-Arg (152) | Ile-Val-Gly-Gly-Lys-Val-Cys-Pro-Lys | 82 |
| Factor VII, bovine | Arg | Gly-Val-Thr-Ala | 83 |
| Prothrombin, human | Gln-Val-Thr-Val-Met-Val-Thr-Pro-Arg (155) | Ser-Glu-Gly-Ser-Ser-Val-Asn-Leu | 18,84 |
| | Arg-Pro-Leu-Thr-Phe-Phe-Asn-Pro-Arg (286) | Thr-Phe-Gly-Ser-Gly-Glu-Ala-Asn | 55 |
| Prothrombin, bovine | Arg-Val-Thr-Val-Glu-Val-Thr-Pro-Arg (156) | Ser-Gly-Gly-Ser-Thr-Thr-Ser-Gln | 8,85 |
| Protein C, human | Asp-Gln-Gly-Asp-Gln-Val-Asp-Pro-Arg (169) | Leu-Ile-Asp-Gly-Lys-Met-Thr-Arg-Arg | 86 |
| Protein C, bovine | Asp-Gln-Lys-Asp-Gln-Leu-Asp-Pro-Arg (171) | Ile-Val-Asp-Gly-Gln-Glu-Ala-Gly-Trp | 87 |
| Protein S, human | Pro-Asp-Leu-Arg-Ser-Cys-Val-Asn-Arg (74) | Ile-Pro-Asn-Gln-Cys-Ser-Pro-Leu-Pro | 88 |
| Secretin, porcine | Phe-Thr-Ser-Glu-Leu-Ser-Arg-Leu-Arg (14) | Asp-Ser-Ala-Arg-Leu-Gln-Arg-Leu | 89 |
| Chorionic $\beta$-subunit, human | NH$_2$-Ser-Lys-Glu-Pro-Leu-Arg-Pro-Arg (8) | Cys-Arg-Pro-Ile-Asn-Ala-Thr-Leu | 90 |
| | Leu-Pro-Gln-Val-Val-Cys-Asn-Tyr-Arg (60) | Asp-Val-Arg-Phe-Glu-Ser-Ile-Arg | 90 |
| | Ser-Ile-Arg-Leu-Pro-Gly-Cys-Pro-Arg (74) | Gly-Val-Asn-Pro-Val-Val-Ser-Tyr | 90 |
| | Leu-Ser-Cys-Gln-Cys-Ala-Leu-Cys-Arg (94) | Arg-Ser-Thr-Thr-Asp-Cys-Gly-Gly | 90 |
| Chymotrypsinogen, bovine | Gln-Pro-Val-Leu-Ser-Gly-Leu-Ser-Arg (15) | Ile-Val-Asn-Gly-Glu-Glu-Ala-Val | 91 |
| Lysozyme, egg white | Gly-Thr-Asp-Val-Gln-Ala-Trp-Ile-Arg (125) | Gly-Cys-Arg-Leu-COOH | 92 |
| Cholecystokinin, pancreozymin, porcine | NH$_2$-Lys-Ala-Pro-Ser-Gly-Arg (6) | Val-Ser-Met-Ile-Lys-Asn-Leu-Gln | 93 |
| Growth hormone, human | Gly-Arg-Leu-Glu-Asp-Gly-Ser-Pro-Arg (133) | Thr-Gly-Gln-Ile-Phe-Lys-Gln-Thr | 94 |
| Growth hormone, bovine | Arg-Glu-Leu-Glu-Asp-Gly-Thr-Pro-Arg (131) | Ala-Gly-Gln-Ile-Leu-Lys-Gln-Thr | 94 |
| Growth hormone, ovine | Arg-Glu-Leu-Glu-Asp-Val-Thr-Pro-Arg (52) | Ala-Gly-Gln-Ile-Leu-Lys-Gln-Thr | 94 |
| Actin, rabbit skeletal muscle | Gly-Phe-Ala-Gly-Asp-Asp-Ala-Pro-Arg (28) | Ala-Val-Phe-Pro-Ser-Ile-Val-Gly | 95 |
| | Phe-Pro-Ser-Ile-Val-Gly-Arg-Pro-Arg (39) | His-Gln-Gly-Val-Met-Val-Gly-Met | 95 |
| | Leu-Thr-Glu-Ala-Pro-Leu-Asn-Pro-Lys (113) | Ala-Asn-Arg-Glu-Lys-Met-Thr-Gln | 95 |
| Apolipoprotein-C-III-1 | Ser-Gln-Gln-Val-Ala-Ala-Gln-Gln-Arg (40) | Gly-Trp-Val-Thr-Asp-Gly-Phe-Ser | 96 |
| Troponin C | Ala-Gly-Glu-Leu-Ala-Glu-Ile-Phe-Arg (120) | Ala-Ser-Gly-Gln-His-Val-Thr-Asp | 97 |
| Thrombin receptor, PAR-1 | Ala-Thr-Asn-Ala-Thr-Leu-Asp-Pro-Arg (41) | Ser-Phe-Leu-Leu-Arg-Asn-Pro-Asn-Asp | 98 |
| Thrombin receptor, PAR-4 | Trp-Val-Leu-Ala-Thr-Gln-Ala-Pro-Arg (47) | Leu-Pro-Ser-Thr-Met-Leu-Leu-Met-Asn | 99 |
| TAFI | Ile-Ser-Asn-Asp-Thr-Val-Ser-Pro-Arg (92) | Ala-Ser-Ala-Ser-Tyr-Tyr-Glu-Gln-Tyr | 100 |

PAR, protease-activated receptor; TAFI, thrombin-activatable fibrinolysis inhibitor.

prothrombin at Arg320 (118). Meizothrombin is autolytically cleaved at Arg156, releasing prothrombin fragment 1 (the Gla domain and kringle 1 region) from the molecule, generating meizothrombin des-fragment 1 (117). Subsequent autolytic cleavage at Arg283 gives rise to the stable form of human $\alpha$-thrombin (Fig. 10-4). Meizothrombin is now recognized as an obligate intermediate in normal prothrombin activation and the first product produced by the prothrombinase complex during the activation of prothrombin (119,120).

Although meizothrombin is an intermediate product with a brief life span, it is thought to play a variety of important roles in the coagulation response. Meizothrombin is also present after fibrin clot formation and likely participates in the regulation of vascular tone as well (121). Meizothrombin is a potent vasoactive agent and acts on the adrenergic receptor. The ability of meizothrombin to induce vascular constriction is approximately five to seven times that of $\alpha$-thrombin (106,122).

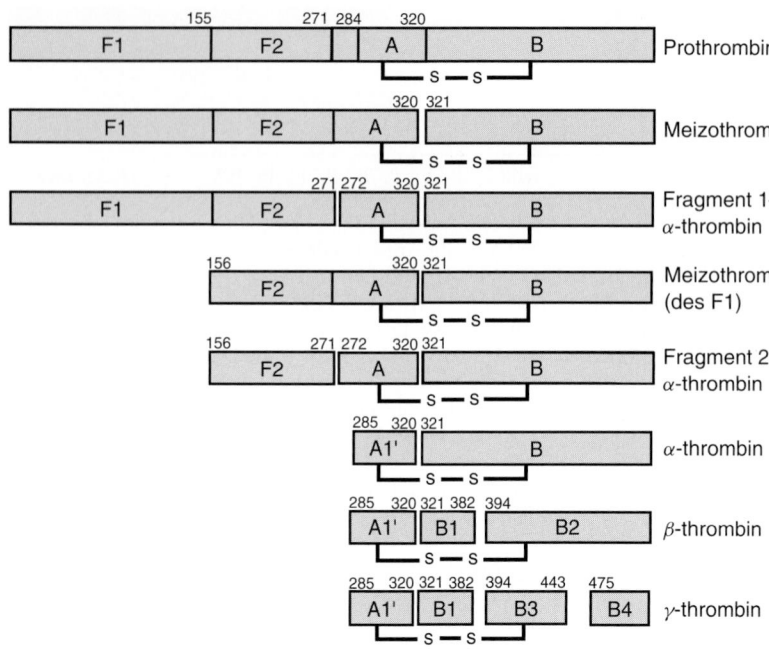

FIGURE 10-4. Prothrombin and the various active species derived from prothrombin. Prothrombin fragments 1 and 2 and the A and B chains of α-thrombin are identified. Cleavages at positions 155 and 284 are catalyzed by thrombin, whereas the cleavages at positions 271 and 320 are catalyzed by factor Xa. The cleavage sites associated with human α-, β-, and γ-thrombin are also identified.

Meizothrombin activity toward fibrinogen and platelets, however, is greatly reduced compared to that of α-thrombin (117,123). Meizothrombin does have the ability to cleave other α-thrombin substrates. Meizothrombin and α-thrombin have comparable activity toward protein C, factor V, factor XI, and small peptide substrates (117,123–127). Recombinant meizothrombin has been reported to produce factor Va at a slightly faster rate than α-thrombin, indicating that meizothrombin likely contributes to factor V activation *in vivo* (126). Meizothrombin-catalyzed activation of factor XI may likewise function in the propagation of coagulation through potentiation of the factor XI–dependent feedback loop in the intrinsic pathway (127). Meizothrombin also has significant anticoagulant properties and is a better activator of protein C than α-thrombin is (124,128). Meizothrombin, therefore, downregulates production of both meizothrombin and α-thrombin (128). The ability of meizothrombin to activate protein C is a key factor early in the procoagulant response when the concentration of α-thrombin is low and the concentration of meizothrombin is relatively high (125,128).

Meizothrombin and β- and γ-thrombins have been identified in the multiple products produced as a consequence of clot formation in whole human blood (121). Although the degraded forms of thrombin may not play major roles in normal hemostasis, meizothrombin, the active intermediate leading to α-thrombin formation, likely contributes to hemostasis at several levels. Meizothrombin functions in a procoagulant capacity to generate factor Va and factor XIa. Meizothrombin also mediates the anticoagulant response through the generation of activated protein C and functions as a potent vasoconstrictor in the regulation of vascular tone.

# NATURAL MUTATIONS THAT LEAD TO DEFECTIVE DYSTHROMBINS

Congenital disorders of prothrombin are very rare (estimated at 1 in 2,000,000 individuals) and are characterized by either reduced synthesis of prothrombin (i.e., hypoprothrombinemia or type I prothrombin deficiency) or by synthesis of a dysfunctional prothrombin molecule (i.e., dysprothrombinemia or type II prothrombin deficiency). Patients homozygous for hypoprothrombinemia have markedly decreased prothrombin levels—1% to 25% of normal—and generally manifest clinical bleeding diatheses (129). Heterozygous patients, with prothrombin levels of approximately 50% of normal, demonstrate only mild, if any, bleeding tendencies (129). Patients with dysprothrombinemia have a wide range of bleeding problems, with the severity of the problem correlating with the amount of activity of the dysfunctional thrombin molecule produced on activation of the abnormal prothrombin.

A number of thrombin mutants have been identified that are associated with bleeding diatheses in humans. In the dysprothrombins Barcelona, Madrid, and Dharan, Arg271 is replaced by a cysteine, resulting in the loss of a factor Xa cleavage site required for normal prothrombin activation and generating a modified meizothrombin (130–132). Dysprothrombin Padua I results from an arginine to histidine mutation, also at position 271, with loss of the activation cleavage site (133). The Arg320 to His mutation in prothrombin San Antonio removes a factor Xa cleavage site at Arg320-Ile321 (134).

Dysprothrombins Himi I and Himi II are characterized by Met337 to Thr and Arg388 to His mutations, respectively. Both replacements are associated with altered thrombin reactivity, most likely because of impaired interactions with fibrinogen (135). The Arg418 to Trp mutation in thrombin Tokushima also impairs fibrinogen-clotting activity of the molecule (136). Likewise, thrombins Salakta and Frankfurt, characterized by a Glu466 to Ala mutation, demonstrate reduced fibrinogen-clotting activity (137,138). Prothrombin Greenville contains an Arg517 to Gln mutation that results in reduced fibrinogen clotting-activity as well (139). The mutation at this residue likely distorts the structure of the sodium ion binding site and interferes with the transition between the procoagulant and anticoagulant forms of thrombin (139). Prothrombin Scranton, a Lys556 to Thr mutation, results in alteration of another key residue involved in sodium binding. Carriers of this mutation have reduced clotting activity but there are no reported bleeding diatheses (140).

The Quick dysprothrombins are the result of two mutations in the same individual, leading to two defective gene products and two defective thrombin molecules. In prothrombin Quick I, Arg382 is replaced by a cysteine (141). Dysthrombin Quick I shows poor reactivity with fibrinogen—less than 2% of the activity of normal thrombin—but is able to efficiently hydrolyze small peptide substrates (141). The x-ray model of thrombin (Fig. 10-3) indicates that Arg382 is associated with the prominent groove extending from the active site. Modification of this residue probably interferes with binding of fibrinogen to its secondary binding sites. The same Arg382 to Cys mutation is also observed in prothrombin Corpus Christi (132). In addition, an Arg382 to His mutation has been observed (142). A substitution of Gly558 to Val is found in prothrombin Quick II (143). This residue is conserved in trypsinlike serine proteases and forms part of the substrate-binding site for the $P_1$ residue (arginine) of the substrate. Dysthrombin Quick II has no reactivity toward substrates that contain an arginine residue in the $P_1$ position (143), and examination of the crystal structure of thrombin confirms that the Gly558 to Val substitution interferes with $P_1$ subsite binding.

A patient with a severe bleeding diathesis and two mutations in the prothrombin protein has also been identified (129). The first mutation, Cys138 to Tyr, disrupts the disulfide bond between Cys138 and Cys114 in the kringle 1 domain and introduces a free sulfhydryl group. This mutation most likely results in an unstable protein that is rapidly degraded. The second mutation, Trp357 to Cys, is located on the thrombin B chain. Trp357 is highly conserved in the serine protease family. The presence of the free sulfhydryl due to this mutation may likewise lead to protein instability and rapid degradation (129). Dysprothrombin Carora, Tyr44 to Cys, is also associated with abnormal folding of the protein and lack of circulating antigen because of a block in secretion or rapid degradation (144). Additional mutations that destabilize the kringle 1, Asp118 to Tyr, and kringle 2 regions, Arg220 to Cys, have been identified (142).

Mutations in the propeptide, Arg1 to Gln and Arg2 to Trp, are believed to affect cleavage of the propeptide from the Gla domain (142). Three other recently identified mutations, Gly330 to Ser, Ser354 to Arg, and Arg538 to Cys, likely affect the association of the α-thrombin A and B chains, thereby altering catalytic function (142). An Arg457 to Gln mutation designated as prothrombin Puerto Rico I removes a salt bridge that links the A and B chains of α-thrombin. This mutation not only appears to affect α-thrombin generation but also destabilizes the circulating prothrombin molecule (145). A homozygous deletion mutation of one of the contiguous Lys9–Lys10 residues in the A chain of α-thrombin likewise results in severe prothrombin deficiency and bleeding diatheses (142).

---

# NATURAL SUBSTRATES FOR THROMBIN

Proteolysis of fibrinogen to generate a fibrin clot and arrest blood flow due to injury is one of α-thrombin's major functions. However, in addition to the clotting reaction itself, α-thrombin is involved in several other proteolytic processes that maintain hemostasis. α-Thrombin also cleaves protein C, factor VII, factor V, factor VIII, factor XI, factor XIII, the human thrombin receptors PAR-1, PAR-3, and PAR-4, and thrombin-activatable fibrinolysis inhibitor (TAFI).

The fibrin clot is derived from α-thrombin cleavage of plasma fibrinogen. Fibrinogen circulates as a symmetrical dimer composed of Aα, Bβ, and γ polypeptide chains that are associated noncovalently as well as by disulfide bonds (146–149). Several α-thrombin–dependent cleavages are required for fibrin

clot formation (149). α-Thrombin cleavage of the Aα chain at Arg16 releases fibrinopeptide A (FPA) and generates fibrin I. The release of two FPA fragments initiates formation of overlapping fibrils (150). α-Thrombin cleavage of the Bβ chain at Arg14 releases fibrinopeptide B (FPB) fragments, thereby forming fibrin II. FPB release initiates lateral strand association (151,152).

Further strengthening of the clot and resistance to plasmin degradation is provided by factor XIIIa, the product of α-thrombin activation of zymogen factor XIII. Factor XIIIa provides essential crosslinks to stabilize the fibrin clot by catalyzing the formation of intermolecular γ-glutamyl ε-lysyl amide bonds between fibrin molecules (153). Additionally, factor XIIIa cross-links factor V molecules by the B region (154,155), cross-links factor V to actin (156), cross-links fibrin to fibronectin (157) and von Willebrand factor (VWF) (158), cross-links fibronectin to collagen (158), and cross-links α2-antiplasmin to fibrin (159). The activation of factor XIII is a multistep process requiring α-thrombin cleavage of the a subunit of the $a_2b_2$ tetramer comprising plasma factor XIII. (Factor XIII is also found in platelets, but the platelet form lacks the b subunit.) After proteolytic cleavage, a 37-residue NH$_2$-terminal peptide is removed from factor XIII, calcium ions bind to the molecule, the a subunit dissociates, and an active site sulfhydryl group is exposed in the cleaved a′ subunit (153,160). Factor XIIIa then acts in concert with α-thrombin to create a stable fibrin clot.

The activation of factor XI by α-thrombin is likewise of major importance in procoagulant events and provides a positive feedback mechanism to support enhanced α-thrombin generation (161). Although factor XIIa is also able to activate factor XI (162), the predominant activator of factor XI is most likely α-thrombin (163). The active enzyme, factor XIa, cleaves factor IX to form factor IXa, the enzyme component of the intrinsic tenase complex. The intrinsic tenase complex provides high levels of factor Xa for prothrombinase complex assembly and α-thrombin production. This feedback loop ensures that adequate levels of vital enzymes, factors IXa and Xa, are available to support the α-thrombin generation required for stable clot formation (161).

α-Thrombin activation of the cofactors and factors V and VIII is also well documented (81, 164–166). Factors V and VIII are highly homologous proteins, as are their cofactor products (81). Both thrombin exosites I and II are involved in α-thrombin recognition of the procofactor substrates, although exosite II plays less of a role in factor V recognition (167–169). Isolated factor V, $M_r = 330,000$, is essentially a procofactor and has less than 1/400th the activity of α-thrombin-activated factor V (170). The generation of cofactor activity in factor V occurs concomitantly with three specific cleavages (Table 10-3) in the single chain factor V molecule to generate factor Va composed of a heavy chain derived from the NH$_2$-terminus of factor V and a light chain derived from the COOH-terminus of factor V. Factor Va serves as a cofactor for factor Xa, the serine protease responsible for activating prothrombin to α-thrombin.

Factor VIII, also a procofactor, is initially synthesized as a single chain molecule, $M_r = 380,000$ (171,172). However, factor VIII is proteolyzed during processing and/or circulation at several sites in the molecule producing a collection of heavy chains of various sizes associated with a light chain. In circulation, factor VIII is complexed with the large multimeric protein VWF (173). The activation of factor VIII by α-thrombin results in cleavage of the VWF binding site and in the release of the factor VIII/VIIIa molecule from the complex (174). Additional α-thrombin cleavages (Table 10-3) in the released factor VIII/VIIIa protein produce the factor VIIIa cofactor that consists of three chains. Factor VIIIa serves as a cofactor for factor IXa, the serine protease that activates factor X to factor Xa.

α-Thrombin may play a role in activation of factor VII as well (175). Factor VII is cleaved at Arg152 to generate the active enzyme factor VIIa (82). However, under conditions chosen to mimic those *in vivo*, most factor VIIa is thought to be generated by membrane-bound factor Xa (176).

Protein C, a vitamin K–dependent serine protease zymogen, is activated by α-thrombin to generate the enzyme activated protein C (APC) (177,178). When α-thrombin binds to the cell-membrane–presented anticoagulant cofactor thrombomodulin, the reactivity of α-thrombin is changed so that it no longer recognizes fibrinogen as a substrate or serves in a procoagulant role (179,180). The altered reactivity is thought to be attributable to the influence of sodium ions on the α-thrombin structure (59,63). The α-thrombin–thrombomodulin complex cleaves protein C (Table 10-3), giving rise to the potent anticoagulant APC. APC has the capacity to inactivate both factor Va and factor VIIIa (179,181). Protein S, a vitamin K–dependent glycoprotein, functions as a cofactor for APC in the inactivation of factors Va and VIIIa (182,183). α-Thrombin cleavage of protein S at Arg74 results in removal of the Gla domain and loss of cofactor activity (184).

TAFI, also known as plasma carboxypeptidase B or carboxypeptidase U, $M_r = 46,000$, is a single-chain 401–amino acid protein (100,185). TAFI is cleaved by α-thrombin, the α-thrombin–thrombomodulin complex, or plasmin at Arg92 (Table 10-3) generating a $M_r = 35,000$ product (i.e., activated TAFI or TAFIa). TAFI is activated by α-thrombin alone, only in the presence of very high levels of α-thrombin such as levels immediately following clot formation (186). The α-thrombin–thrombomodulin complex is believed to be the primary physiologic activator of TAFI in a calcium ion–dependent reaction (186–188). The mechanism of TAFI activation by the α-thrombin–thrombomodulin complex is similar to protein C activation; however, more of the thrombomodulin structure is required (189,190) and different regions of α-thrombin are involved (191,192).

TAFIa has carboxypeptidase B–like activity and serves to link the coagulation and fibrinolytic cascades (187,188). TAFIa prolongs clot lysis through several mechanisms. TAFIa cleaves COOH-terminal lysine and arginine residues on fibrin, reducing the ability of fibrin to enhance tissue plasminogen activator–dependent plasminogen activation (193). At elevated concentrations, TAFIa also directly inhibits the enzyme plasmin and blocks plasmin-dependent clot lysis (193). The profibrinolytic effect of APC is also attributed to TAFI. APC cleavage of factor Va inhibits prothrombin conversion to α-thrombin, thereby reducing the α-thrombin–dependent generation of TAFIa (194). The prolongation of clot lysis by TAFIa likely contributes to the prothrombotic tendencies associated with APC resistance in factor $V_{Leiden}$ (195).

In addition, TAFI is a substrate for transglutaminases such as factor XIII. TAFI is cross-linked to fibrin and incorporated into the fibrin clot (196). TAFIa likely serves to protect the clot from premature lysis (196–198). Premature clot lysis in factor VIII–, IX–, X–, or XI–deficient plasmas is alleviated by increased levels of TAFIa (197,198).

Examination of the fibrinogen- and fibrin-derived products produced during the blood clotting event indicates that key α-thrombin–dependent processes involved in stable clot formation—fibrinogen cleavage, factor XIII activation, and TAFI activation—likely occur simultaneously (199). Significant levels of FPA fragments are released because of α-thrombin cleavage of the Aα chains of fibrinogen before visible clot formation. FPA release is coincident with activation of factor XIIIa, allowing cross-linking of the γ chains of fibrinogen and fibrin I. γ–γ Cross-linking is almost complete before the α-thrombin cleavage, releasing FPB fragments from the Bβ chains of the fibrinogen/fibrin I molecules. Subsequent to FPB release, a carboxypeptidase B–like enzyme (presumably TAFIa) cleaves the FPB fragments, generating des-Arg FPB. These events unfold in such a way that the initial clot is heterogeneous and consists of both fibrinogen and fibrin I cross-linked by intermolecular bonds. Fibrin II and TAFIa are generated subsequent to initial clot formation, serving to create a more stable, mature clot (199).

α-Thrombin also interacts with a variety of cellular receptors (200). α-Thrombin has been recognized for years as the most potent activator of platelets (201) and induces a number of responses in other cell types as well (202–206). Many of these responses are elicited through α-thrombin binding to a receptor and initiating a signal transduction mechanism. The interactions between α-thrombin and the human platelet thrombin receptors, PAR-1 and PAR-4, however, are dependent on a more unusual activation mechanism where the receptors are also substrates for α-thrombin by intramolecular ligand activation (98,206,207). PAR-1, a member of the family of G protein–coupled receptors, is a 425–amino acid transmembrane protein with a large $NH_2$-terminal extracellular domain (98,207). α-Thrombin cleaves the $NH_2$-terminal extension of PAR-1 at Arg 41 (Table 10-3) producing a "tethered ligand." The new $NH_2$-terminus created by this cleavage binds back to the receptor effecting its activation (98,207). PAR-1 interacts with two sites on α-thrombin, the active site, which binds the cleavage recognition domain of PAR-1, and exosite I, which binds the hirudinlike domain of PAR-1 (206,207). PAR-4, also a G protein–coupled receptor, is a 385–amino acid protein that shares 33% amino acid sequence homology with PAR-1 (99). PAR-4 activation requires 10 to 100 times higher α-thrombin levels than PAR-1 activation (99,208,209). Unlike PAR-1, PAR-4 lacks a hirudinlike sequence that can interact with the α-thrombin anion-binding exosite and facilitate receptor cleavage (99,208,209). PAR-4 is cleaved by α-thrombin at Arg47 (Table 10-3), producing a tethered ligand similar to that produced during the activation of PAR-1 (99).

α-Thrombin is believed to activate human platelets by cleaving and activating both PAR-1 and PAR-4 (99,208,210,211). Initiation of platelet activation by this pathway likely occurs through PAR-1 activation at low α-thrombin levels. PAR-1 activation triggers a rapid and transient increase in intracellular calcium. PAR-4 activation requires higher α-thrombin levels; however, the increase in levels of intracellular calcium in response to PAR-4 activation is more sustained than that initiated by PAR-1 (208,209,211–213). PAR-1 and PAR-4 likely act in combination as a dual mechanism for governing the variety of α-thrombin–induced effects in human platelets (208).

The contribution of other platelet α-thrombin receptors, particularly the glycoprotein (GP) Ib/IX/V complex, is still not fully understood. GP Ib is a heterodimer composed of disulfide-linked α and β subunits. GP Ibα contains a high-affinity binding site for α-thrombin (214). Removing or blocking this domain decreases platelet responses to α-thrombin (215–218). Although PAR-1 and PAR-4 provide the predominant response to α-thrombin on human platelets, other α-thrombin interactions such as those with GP Ibα may contribute to activation of PAR-1 or influence other platelet receptor interactions with α-thrombin (211).

PAR-1 is also present on T lymphocytes, monocytes, and endothelial cells and mediates the hormonelike actions of α-thrombin on these cells (206,219–221). Other members of the PAR family—PAR-2 and PAR-3—do not have clearly established roles. PAR-2 is not activated by α-thrombin (211). PAR-3 is required for normal thrombin-dependent platelet activation in mice (208,222); however, its role in the human system appears to be primarily in cellular development because of high expression levels in human megakaryocytes (223).

# FACTOR Xa AND PROTHROMBIN ACTIVATION

Prothrombin is activated to α-thrombin in a membrane-dependent process that includes the actions of the serine protease factor Xa, its cofactor factor Va, and divalent calcium ions assembled into a complex on a membrane. The fully assembled complex is termed *prothrombinase* (224). *In vivo*, the membrane surface is thought to be provided primarily by platelets, although other circulating blood cells such as monocytes and lymphocytes and vascular endothelial cells may contribute as well (225). Most basic laboratory studies have made use of synthetic vesicles composed of phosphatidyl choline and phosphatidyl serine (PCPS) that function in a manner similar to that of cellular membranes. Examination of the properties of the membrane-dependent procoagulant and anticoagulant complexes have focused largely on the prothrombinase complex, which has served as a model for complex formation and function of the vitamin K–dependent complex enzymes.

The membrane dependency of the procoagulant and anticoagulant complexes is the result of multiple factors. Modeling of prothrombinase complex assembly and function suggests that the membrane serves as a protective environment to shield proteases from inactivation by circulating inhibitors (226). Vitamin K–dependent proteins such as factor X/Xa, factor IX/IXa, and prothrombin bind to the phospholipid surface by a calcium ion–dependent process that involves the $NH_2$-terminal Gla residues of the proteins and anionic lipids on the surface (44,227,228). Anionic phospholipid, but not calcium ions, is also required for plasma-derived cofactors such as factor Va to associate with the membrane surface (229). In addition, the membrane likely serves to limit the degrees of freedom of the interacting molecules and to restrict them to reactions in two dimensions rather than three dimensions in the solution phase (226,229,230). The general mechanism for procoagulant complex assembly and function begins with zymogen conversion to active serine proteases. Plasma-derived cofactors are proteolyzed to generate functional cofactors (i.e., factors Va and VIIIa), or integral membrane cofactors (i.e., tissue factor) are expressed to initiate complex assembly. Membrane surface is presented concomitantly as a consequence of vascular damage and/or cellular activation events (231), providing the necessary surface for complex assembly.

The generation of factor Xa, the enzyme component of the prothrombinase complex, is vital to α-thrombin formation. Factor Xa is derived from a two-chain circulating zymogen, factor X, or Stuart factor. Factor X is activated by excision of a small peptide from its heavy chain (232) by either the intrinsic (i.e., factor VIIIa–factor IXa complex) or extrinsic (i.e., tissue factor–factor VIIa) tenase (see Fig. 10-5A). Factor Xa is a trypsin-like enzyme with specificity for the sequence Ile-Glu-Gly-Arg. Although factor X is activated by two separate multiprotein complexes, the combined action of both complexes is required for adequate clot formation (Fig. 10-5A). Under certain circumstances, such as high tissue factor concentration, the extrinsic tenase can provide sufficient levels of factor Xa to bypass the need for factor Xa activation by the intrinsic tenase complex. High levels of factor VIIa have been used clinically to arrest bleeding episodes in hemophilias A and B (factor VIII and factor IX deficiencies, respectively) (233,234). However, normal physiologic levels of factor VIIa do not compensate for deficiencies in the intrinsic tenase pathway.

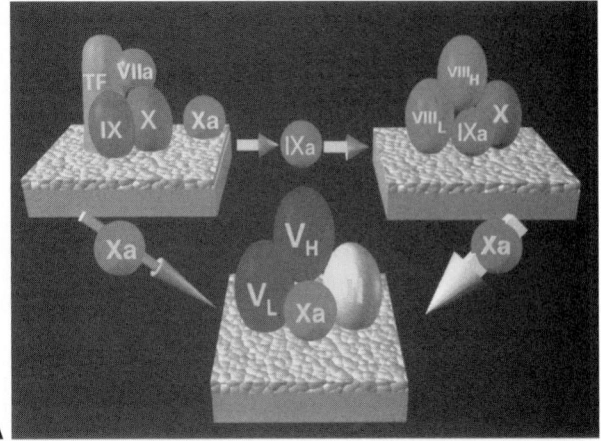

A

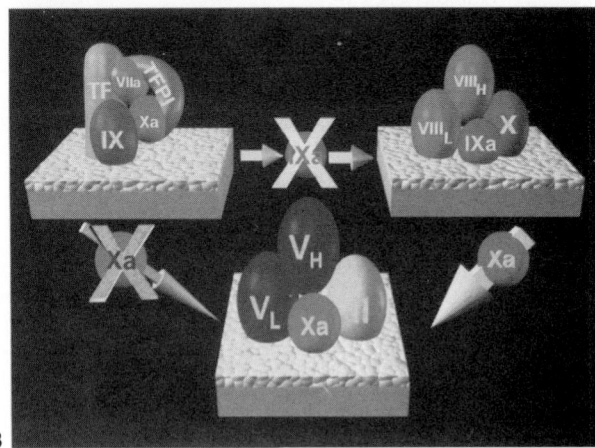

B

**FIGURE 10-5.** The procoagulant vitamin K–dependent complexes. **A:** The tissue factor–factor VIIa (extrinsic) complex triggers coagulation by activating factors IX and X. Factor Xa also cleaves factor IX and accelerates factor IXa generation. The factor VIIIa–factor IXa (intrinsic) complex activates factor X at a much higher rate than the extrinsic complex, thereby allowing formation of the factor Va–factor Xa (prothrombinase) complex and initiating explosive thrombin generation. **B:** Tissue factor pathway inhibitor (TFPI) interacts with the tissue factor–factor VIIa–factor Xa ternary complex to inhibit extrinsic complex-dependent activation of factors IX and X. Subsequent factor Xa generation occurs only via the intrinsic tenase complex (see Color Fig. 10-5).

The intrinsic tenase complex is highly homologous to the prothrombinase complex. Complex formation between the cofactor, factor VIIIa, and the serine protease component, factor IXa, in the presence of divalent calcium ions and a phospholipid membrane serves to stabilize factor VIIIa (235, 236) and considerably enhances the rate of factor Xa generation. The fully assembled complex activates factor X at a rate of approximately $10^9$-fold greater than factor IXa alone (see Table 10-4) (229,237).

The extrinsic tenase comprises an integral membrane-protein cofactor, tissue factor, and a serine protease, factor VIIa. Although the assembly and activity of the intrinsic tenase complex are not membrane- and divalent cation–dependent (238,239), the membrane surface is required for effective presentation of the substrates factor X and factor IX (Table 10-4) (240–243). The generation of the enzyme factor VIIa is also somewhat unusual. Factor VII is activated by factors IXa, Xa, XIIa, and α-thrombin as well as by autoactivation upon association with tissue factor (244–247). Circulating factor VIIa may likewise play a role in activation of the zymogen factor VII.

RELATIVE EFFICIENCIES OF THE PROCOAGULANT ENZYMES AND THEIR
RESPECTIVE COFACTOR-ENZYME COMPLEXES

| Enzyme | Substrate | $K_m$ ($\mu$M) | $k_{cat}$/min | $k_{cat}$/$K_m$ M/min | Efficiency ratio |
|---|---|---|---|---|---|
| VIIa | IX | NA | NA | — | — |
| VIIa/TF/PCPS/Ca$^{2+}$ | IX | 0.243 | 15.6 | $6.42 \times 10^7$ | — |
| VIIa | X | 4.87 | 0.024 | $4.93 \times 10^3$ | — |
| VIIa/TF/PCPS/Ca$^{2+}$ | X | 0.45 | 69.0 | $1.53 \times 10^8$ | $3.10 \times 10^4$ |
| IXa | X | 299.0 | 0.002 | 6.69 | — |
| IXa/VIIIa/PCPS/Ca$^{2+}$ | X | 0.063 | 500.0 | $7.94 \times 10^9$ | $1.19 \times 10^9$ |
| Xa | II | 131.0 | 0.6 | $4.58 \times 10^3$ | — |
| Xa/Va/PCPS/Ca$^{2+}$ | II | 1.0 | 1800.0 | $1.80 \times 10^9$ | $3.93 \times 10^5$ |

$k_{cat}$, turnover number; $K_m$, the Michaelis constant; $k_{cat}$/$K_m$, efficiency of the free enzyme or cofactor–enzyme complex; TF, tissue factor; PCPS, phosphatidyl choline/phosphatidyl serine; II, prothrombin; NA, not applicable.

From Jenny NS, Mann KG. Coagulation cascade: an overview. In: Loscalzo J, Schafer AI, eds. *Thrombosis and hemorrhage*, 2nd ed. Baltimore, MD: Williams & Wilkins, 1994:3–27, with permission.

The roles of the intrinsic and extrinsic tenase complexes in factor Xa generation have been well characterized. Studies of the extrinsic tenase demonstrate that in the presence of both factor X and factor IX, factor IX appears to be the preferred substrate and the rate of factor Xa generation is decreased (229,248). The extrinsic tenase is therefore proposed to act as a "trigger" of blood coagulation and initiate procoagulant events by providing low levels of factor Xa and essential levels of factor IXa. Factor IXa forms the intrinsic tenase with factor VIIIa on a membrane surface and produces factor Xa at a rate that is 50-fold greater than the extrinsic tenase. The extrinsic tenase complex is also subject to inhibition by tissue factor pathway inhibitor (TFPI) that binds the tissue factor–factor VIIa–factor Xa ternary complex and blocks production of both factor Xa and factor IXa (see Fig. 10-5B) (249). The increased rate of factor Xa generation by the factor VIIIa–factor IXa complex should overcome circulating inhibitors of factor Xa (i.e., AT-III and TFPI) and the dynamic APC inhibition system, permitting the formation of the prothrombinase complex.

Factor Xa requires an additional protein species, factor Va, for efficient activation of prothrombin (Table 10-4). Factor Va is the cofactor form of the circulating procofactor factor V. Single-chain factor V can be proteolyzed by a variety of enzymes including $\alpha$-thrombin, factor Xa, and plasmin (170,250–254). The active factor Va produced by $\alpha$-thrombin is the best characterized species and is composed of two polypeptide chains. The $M_r$ = 94,000 heavy chain is obtained from the NH$_2$-terminus of factor V, and the $M_r$ = 74,000 light chain is derived from the COOH-terminus of the factor V molecule. The heavy and light chains of factor Va are noncovalently associated through divalent calcium ion bridging between the chains. A large portion of factor V, corresponding to nearly 50% of the total mass of factor V, is excised from the middle of the molecule upon activation. No function has yet been established for the activation peptide, or B-domain, of factor V.

The functions of the heavy and light chains of factor Va have been determined from studies of the isolated chains and by binding and immunochemical techniques. The heavy chain appears to mediate the binding of both prothrombin and factor Xa (255,256). The light chain also contributes to factor Xa binding and recognizes acidic phospholipids mediating membrane-protein association (81,255–259). In the overall interaction associated with construction of the prothrombinase complex, factor Va serves as an anchor that secures factor Xa on the membrane surface through interactions between the factor Xa light chain and both the heavy and light chains of factor Va. The dissociation constant for the factor Xa-PCPS interaction is 110 nM (260), whereas the dissociation constant for the factor Va-factor Xa-PCPS interaction is approximately 1 nM (227). The membrane–protein and protein–membrane interactions inherent in complex formation stabilize the complex and allow for functional complex assembly at biologically relevant concentrations of factor Va and factor Xa (Table 10-4).

The sequence of events in the procoagulant response leading to $\alpha$-thrombin production include the conversion of factor X to factor Xa. Factor V may be proteolyzed by factor Xa to generate a species of factor Va; however, this reaction occurs at a relatively slow rate, and its relevance in producing factor Va and factor Xa to form the prothrombinase complex is uncertain. The assembled complex cleaves prothrombin at two sites (Fig. 10-1) to produce $\alpha$-thrombin, which is the most important activator of factor V and other procoagulant procofactors and zymogens.

The series of events that lead to prothrombinase complex assembly, function, and inactivation is shown in Figure 10-6. The factor V molecule is represented as a three-lobed structure in which the NH$_2$- and COOH-terminal domains are joined by the central B-domain (Fig. 10-6A). The COOH-terminal domain, or light chain (L), is responsible for mediating the factor V–membrane association. Activation of factor V by $\alpha$-thrombin gives rise to the preassembled factor Va molecule through excision of the B-domain. The light chain of factor Va (L) is embedded in the membrane and the heavy chain (H) is noncovalently associated with the light chain (Fig. 10-6B). Factor Xa interacts with both the light and heavy chains of factor Va, whereas prothrombin interaction is mediated by the membrane, the heavy chain of factor Va, and the active site of factor Xa (Fig. 10-6C). The fragment 1 region of prothrombin, containing the NH$_2$-terminal Gla domain, associates with anionic phospholipids in the membrane, and the fragment 2 region of prothrombin, which contains kringle 2, interacts with the heavy chain of factor Va. The fully assembled prothrombinase complex cleaves the prothrombin molecule at two sites (Fig. 10-1), generating the active $\alpha$-thrombin product.

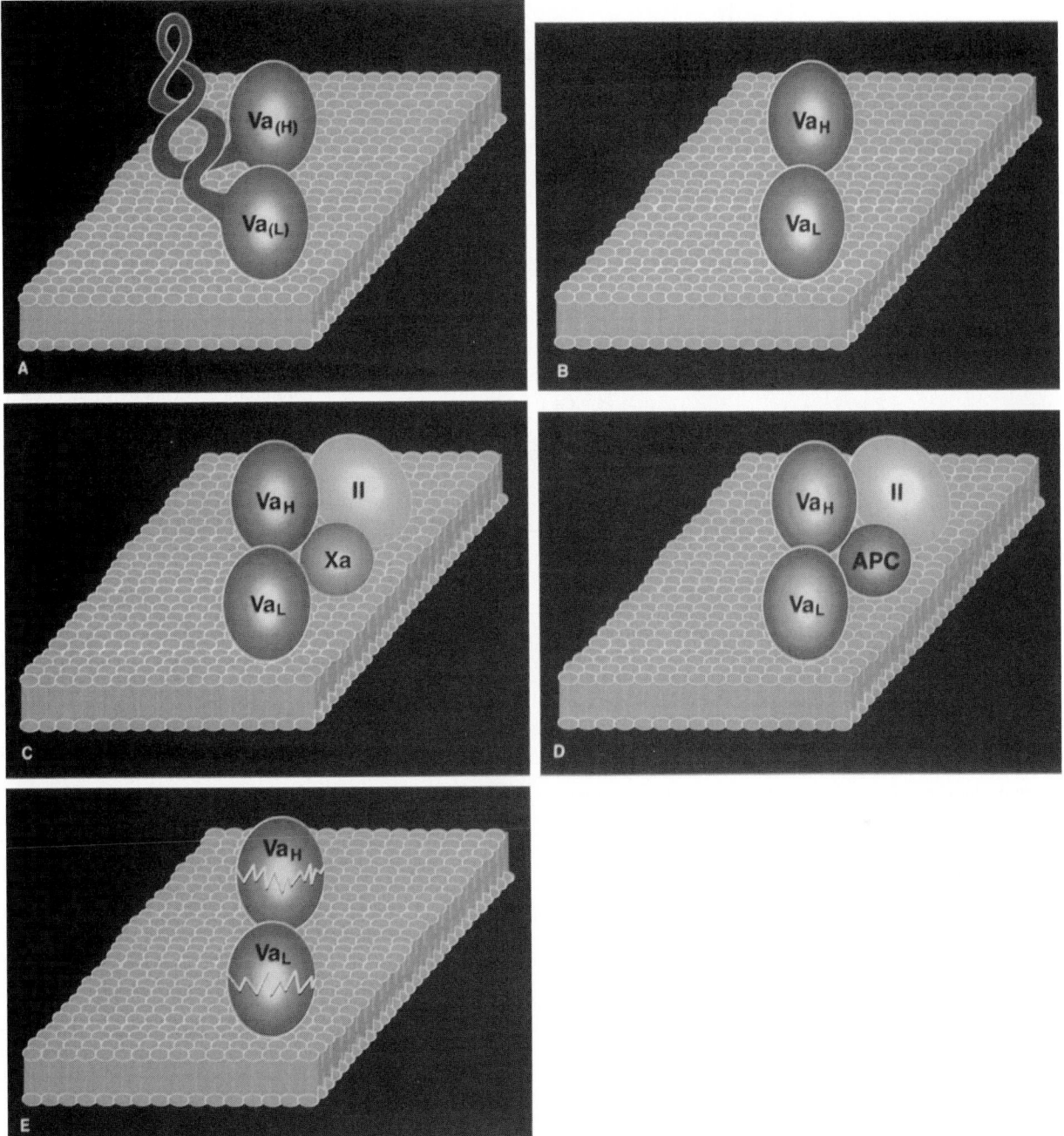

**FIGURE 10-6.** Assembly and expression of the prothrombinase complex. **A:** Factor V is shown as a multidomain molecule embedded in the membrane lipid bilayer predominantly through the COOH-terminal region of the molecule. **B:** Following thrombin activation, the factor Va molecule, comprising the COOH-terminal–derived peptide, Va(L), and the NH$_2$-terminal–derived peptide, Va(H), remains bound to the membrane surface through Va(L). **C:** The light chain of factor Va forms at least part of the receptor for factor Xa, which binds to membrane-bound factor Va in a 1:1 molar stoichiometry. Prothrombin, composed of fragment 1 (F1), fragment 2 (F2), and prothrombin 2 (P2) domains, interacts with Va(H) of the factor Va molecule through its F2 region. **D:** Activated protein C (APC) also appears to form a complex with Va(L) of the membrane-bound factor Va molecule. The APC–factor Va interaction is competitive with factor Xa, but unaffected by prothrombin binding. **E:** APC cleaves both chains of factor Va, eliminating the complex (see Color Fig. 10-6).

α-Thrombin also participates in inactivation of the prothrombinase complex. The α-thrombin–thrombomodulin complex activates protein C to APC, which competes with factor Xa for binding to membrane-associated factor Va (Fig. 10-6D). Bound factor Xa blocks the binding of APC to factor Va. However, if factor Xa dissociates from the prothrombinase complex, APC can bind. Once bound to factor Va on the membrane surface, APC cleaves and inactivates factor Va (Fig. 10-6E). APC cleaves both the heavy and light chains of factor Va, although the cleavages associated with the heavy chain play the dominant role in inactivation of the molecule (261,262).

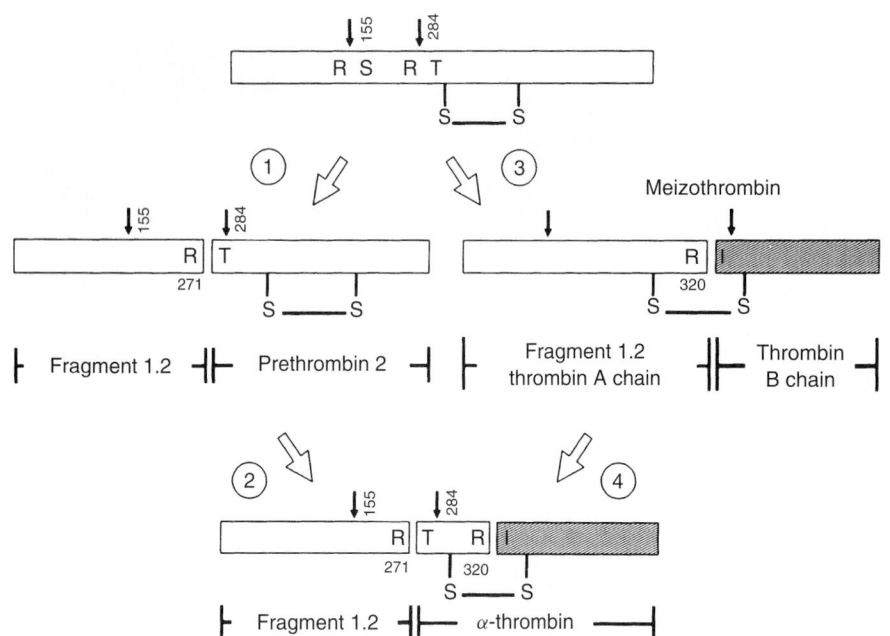

FIGURE 10-7. The pathways for activation of human prothrombin. The thrombin cleavage sites at 155 and 284 are identified, as well as the factor Xa cleavages at positions 271 and 320. Prothrombinase-catalyzed activation of human prothrombin occurs by virtue of cleavage 3, followed by 4 to produce fragment 1.2 and α-thrombin as the final products of the reaction. When factor Xa is used as the catalyst for prothrombin activation, cleavage 1 is followed by cleavage 2 to produce the same ultimate products, but at a much slower rate.

Two pathways for prothrombin activation are illustrated in Figure 10-7. Prothrombin can be activated by factor Xa alone at a very slow rate. In the presence of factor Xa and calcium ions, the initial cleavage (step 1) occurs at Arg271, giving rise to prothrombin fragment 1.2 and prethrombin 2. Cleavage of prethrombin 2 at Arg320 (step 2) gives rise to prothrombin fragment 1.2 and α-thrombin, which associate noncovalently. Additional cleavages by α-thrombin may occur at residues 155 and 284 during the activation process. The cleavage at Arg284 in the human α-thrombin A chain results in removal of residues 1 to 13 of the NH$_2$-terminus of α-thrombin. The stable form of human α-thrombin is therefore a des1-13 truncated molecule.

The activation of prothrombin by prothrombinase proceeds with the reverse order of bond cleavage as compared to factor Xa acting alone. The initial cleavage of prothrombin by prothrombinase (step 3) occurs at Arg320, giving rise to meizothrombin. Meizothrombin is an enzyme with some of the same activities demonstrated for the final product, α-thrombin. Meizothrombin is subsequently cleaved at Arg271 (step 4), generating prothrombin fragment 1.2 and α-thrombin. In addition to the difference in the mechanism of activation, the activation rates are also quite disparate. The rate of α-thrombin generation by prothrombinase is 300,000-fold faster than the rate for factor Xa alone at potential physiologic concentrations of the proteins (Table 10-4) (263).

Prothrombin is also commonly activated by a venom protease isolated from *Echis carinatus* (264–266). The venom protease cleaves the prothrombin molecule at the Arg320–Ile321 bond, generating a meizothrombin product identical to that formed by the initial prothrombinase cleavage of prothrombin. Subsequent autoproteolytic steps result in removal of residues 1 to 284 from the meizothrombin molecule and generation of the stable human α-thrombin molecule (267,268).

*In vivo*, the activity of the prothrombinase complex must be tightly regulated to ensure that adequate, but limited, levels of α-thrombin are produced. Two reaction systems, one covalent and one proteolytic, appear to be largely responsible for attenuating the activity of the prothrombinase complex. ATIII-heparin (or heparan sulfate) is a potent inhibitor of blood coagulation and inhibits both factor Xa and α-thrombin via covalent interactions (269,270). α-Thrombin also binds to thrombomodulin on the vascular cell surface and activates protein C to APC. APC cleaves factor Va and the proteolyzed cofactor can no longer bind factor Xa or prothrombin. However, the inactivated factor Va and unproteolyzed active factor Va have equivalent membrane-binding capacities. As a consequence of this equivalence, the inactivated cofactor remains on the membrane-binding site and blocks further prothrombinase formation.

The membrane surface plays a key role in the inactivation of factor Va. When bound to a membrane surface, factor Va is rapidly and completely inactivated by APC through a sequential series of cleavages in the heavy chain domain (261,271). The cleavage of human factor Va at Arg306 is lipid dependent and is required for complete inactivation of factor Va (261). In the absence of the membrane surface, APC-mediated cleavages at Arg506 and Arg679 in the human factor Va heavy chain still occur, but without the additional cleavage at Arg306, factor Va retains considerable cofactor activity (approximately 60% of its original activity) (261). The membrane dependence of APC inactivation is linked to the association of APC with the membrane via its Gla domain. This effect is clearly demonstrated for protein C Vermont in which Glu20 is mutated to Ala and Val34 to Met (272). The loss of the γ-carboxylation site at Glu20 is primarily responsible for the increased risk of arterial and venous thrombosis associated with protein C Vermont (273). The active enzyme, APC Vermont, still cleaves factor Va at Arg506 and Arg679, but no lipid-dependent cleavage at Arg306 is observed (274). Factor Va still retains considerable cofactor activity in the absence of cleavage at Arg306, thereby prolonging prothrombinase activity and α-thrombin generation.

α-Thrombin is the essential enzyme product of the reactions that provide for hemostasis. The other procoagulant proteins (i.e., factors VII, IX, X, V and VIII, and tissue factor), and anticoagulant proteins (i.e., AT-III, protein C, protein S, TFPI, and thrombomodulin), in combination with cellular membrane–binding sites, function to govern the production and inactivation of α-thrombin (275). Studies of human physiology generally describe the "normal" state as a range of 50% to 150% of the average plasma levels for the host of procoagulant and anticoagulant proteins (276,277). However, many epidemiologic studies demonstrate considerable thrombotic risk associated with variations in the concentrations of some of these proteins within the "normal" range (278). In synthetic and whole blood *ex vivo* model systems, prothrombin and ATIII levels appear to have the most significant effect on α-thrombin generation. Increased levels of ATIII dramatically reduce α-thrombin generation by inhibiting α-thrombin activity and by preventing the positive feedback loops (factor V and factor VIII activation and factor XIa generation) required to promote efficient prothrombin activation. Conversely, decreased levels of ATIII allow for higher levels of prothrombin activation and a prolongation of α-thrombin activity, thereby promoting the risk of thrombosis. Increased levels of prothrombin also directly lead to increased α-thrombin generation (275). *In vivo* evidence for this effect is provided by the prothrombin gene mutation G20210A. The G → A transition at nucleotide position 20210 in the 3′-untranslated region of the prothrombin gene leads to elevated plasma levels of prothrombin (279) and is strongly associated with an increased risk for venous thrombosis (280–283).

Factors V, VIII, IX, and X; protein C; protein S; and TFPI have little effect on α-thrombin generation when individually present at a minimum of 25% of the average plasma level. Increased individual levels (>100%) of these proteins likewise have no substantial effect on α-thrombin production (275).

When mechanisms that localize or constrain the normal hemostatic response to injury malfunction, clinical intervention may be necessary to avoid potentially fatal consequences. In contrast to indirect α-thrombin inhibitors such as heparins and vitamin K antagonists, direct α-thrombin inhibitors bind to α-thrombin and prevent interaction with its substrates. Several direct α-thrombin inhibitors are used in prevention and treatment of venous and arterial thrombosis (284,285). The first clinically utilized direct inhibitor was hirudin, a 65–amino acid polypeptide originally isolated from the medicinal leech, *Hirudo medicinalis*. Hirudin forms a 1:1 stoichiometric complex with α-thrombin, binding both the active site and exosite I with high affinity. The recombinant form of hirudin lacks a sulfate group on Tyr63 and is termed *desulfatohirudin* (Desirudin). Bivalirudin (Hirulog; Angiomax) is a 20–amino acid hirudin analog that consists of an NH$_2$-terminal domain that interacts with the α-thrombin active site, a linker region, and a COOH-terminal region that interacts with exosite I (286). Argatroban (Novastan) is synthetic hirudin analog designed to interact only with the α-thrombin active site (287). A fibrinopeptide A mimetic, Melagatran, likewise interacts with the α-thrombin active site (284). Melagatran is also administered as a proform, ximelagatran (Exanta), which is metabolized to the active inhibitor *in vivo*. Selective PAR-1 antagonists that mimic the tethered ligand generated upon α-thrombin cleavage of the receptor are also currently being studied for clinical efficacy in prevention and treatment of thrombosis (288,289).

# SUMMARY

The process of blood coagulation was first described as a sequential series of proteolytic actions (290,291). However, the nature of hemostasis is perhaps better described as threshold-limited, complex, intertwined processes that include physical, cellular, and biochemical events. α-Thrombin plays a central role in the overall maintenance of blood fluidity and contributes to reactions at all levels (see Fig. 10-8).

α-Thrombin has direct effects on coagulation through activation of platelets, formation of fibrin clots, and activation of various zymogens and cofactors in the coagulation cascade. α-Thrombin activity extends from the coagulation process to anticoagulation and stimulation of fibrinolytic reactions. α-Thrombin's roles continue into the tissue repair

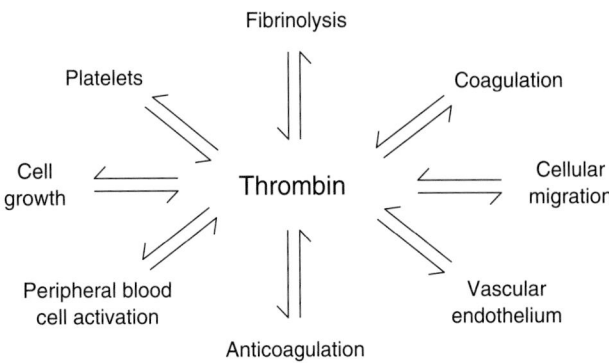

**FIGURE 10-8.** The multiple roles of thrombin.

and remodeling phase necessary to regenerate damaged vascular tissue. α-Thrombin is a potent mitogen (292–297) and stimulates cell division in smooth muscle cells (205,293,298), macrophages (6), and endothelial cells (6,299). The proliferative effects of α-thrombin result from direct activation of mitogenic pathways (297) and/or α-thrombin-mediated secretion of a variety of growth factors. The combination of α-thrombin and growth factors often demonstrates a synergistic effect on cellular proliferation (300–304). α-Thrombin also induces the release of cytokines (305–309), vasoactive compounds (310–313), and chemoattractants (313) from cells in the vicinity of tissue damage. The processes involved in development of atherosclerosis are likewise highly α-thrombin–dependent (314). α-Thrombin increases the permeability of the vascular endothelium (315), promotes neutrophil adhesion to endothelial cells (316), induces contraction of smooth muscle cells (317), induces release of serotonin from platelet stores (98,318), and stimulates macrophage chemotaxis (6).

α-Thrombin also appears to be involved in the growth and metastasis of tumors. α-Thrombin promotes angiogenesis (319,320) and angiogenesis is in turn required for tumor progression (321). α-Thrombin may promote angiogenesis in part by potentiating vascular endothelial growth factor (VEGF)–mediated angiogenesis (322). VEGF is a key angiogenic factor specific for endothelial cells and induces cellular migration, proliferation, and tube formation (322,323).

The wide range of functions for α-thrombin continue to expand. α-Thrombin has been reported to initiate bone resorption (324), contribute to strokes and Alzheimer disease by inducing apoptosis of astrocytes and neurons (325–327), regulate neurite outgrowth (328), and play a key role in muscle development (329–335). In light of our limited knowledge of some of the less well-studied coagulation proteins, it is likely that multiple roles will be established for these proteins as well.

# ACKNOWLEDGMENTS

We would like to acknowledge the intellectual contributions of Dr. Ruth Ann Henriksen to elements of this chapter dealing with thrombin. We would also like to thank Drs. Wolfram Bode and Alexander Tulinsky for making x-ray coordinates available for direct inspection and Drs. Tim Rydel and Alexander Tulinsky for providing Figures 10-2 and 10-3. We would like to thank Drs. Matthew Rand and Jeffrey Lawson for their assistance in clarifying nomenclatures for thrombin amino acid residues. Finally, Dr. Mann would like to acknowledge the research support of the National Heart, Lung, and Blood Institute for the last 36 years.

# *References*

1. Schmidt A. *Zur Blutlehre.* Leipzig: FCW Vogel, 1892.
2. Morawitz P. Die chemie der blutgerrinnung. *Ergebn Physiol* 1905;4:307.
3. Fuld E, Spiro K. Der Einfluß einiger gerrinnungshemmender Agentien auf das Vogel plasma. *Beitr Chem Phys Pathol (Hofmeister's)* 1904;5:171.
4. Xue J, Westfield LA, Tuley EA, et al. Incomplete embryonic lethality and fatal neonatal hemorrhage caused by prothrombin deficiency in mice. *Proc Natl Acad Sci U S A* 1998;95:7603.
5. Bar-Shavit R, Kahn A, Mudd MS, et al. Localization of a chemotactic domain in human thrombin. *Biochemistry* 1984;23:397.
6. Bar-Shavit R, Kahn AJ, Mann KG, et al. Identification of a thrombin sequence with growth factor activity on macrophages. *Proc Natl Acad Sci U S A* 1986;83:976.
7. McDuffie FC, Giffin C, Niedringhaus R, et al. Prothrombin, thrombin and prothrombin fragments in plasma of normal individuals and of patients with laboratory evidence of disseminated intravascular coagulation. *Thromb Res* 1979;16:759.
8. Magnusson S, Petersen TE, Scottrup-Jensen L. Complete primary structure of prothrombin: Isolation, structure and reactivity of ten carboxylated glutamic acid residues and regulation of prothrombin activation by thrombin. In: Reich E, Rifkin DB, Shaw E, eds. *Proteases and biological control.* Cold Spring Harbor, NY: Cold Spring Harbor Laboratory, 1975:123–149.
9. Chow BK, Ting V, Tufaro F, et al. Characterization of a novel liver-specific enhancer in the human prothrombin gene. *J Biol Chem* 1991;266:18927.
10. Bancroft JD, McDowell SA, Degen SJ. The human prothrombin gene: transcriptional regulation in HepG2 cells. *Biochemistry* 1992;31:12469.
11. Degen SJ, MacGillivray RT, Davie EW. Characterization of the complementary deoxyribonucleic acid and gene coding for human prothrombin. *Biochemistry* 1983;22:2087.
12. Degen SJ, Davie EW. Nucleotide sequence of the gene for human prothrombin. *Biochemistry* 1987;26:6165.
13. Bancroft J, Schaefer LA, Degen SJF. Characterization of the Alu-rich 5′-flanking region of the human prothrombin-encoding gene: identification of a positive cis-acting element that regulates liver-specific expression. *Gene* 1990;95:253.
14. Degen SJF. The prothrombin gene and its liver-specific expression. *Semin Thromb Hemost* 1992;18:230.
15. Elion J, Downing MJ, Butkowski RJ. Structure of human thrombin: comparison with other serine proteases. In: Lundblad RL, Fenton JW, Mann KG, eds. *Chemistry and biology of thrombin.* Ann Arbor, MI: Ann Arbor Science Publishers, 1977.
16. Hartley BS. Proteolytic enzymes. *Ann Rev Biochem* 1960;29:45.
17. Birktoft JJ, Blow DM. Structure of crystalline chymotrypsin. V. The atomic structure of tosyl-α-chymotrypsin at 2 Å resolution. *J Mol Biol* 1972;68:187.
18. Walz DA, Hewett-Emmett D, Seegers WH. Amino acid sequence of human prothrombin fragments 1 and 2. *Proc Natl Acad Sci U S A* 1977;74:1969.
19. Thompson AR, Enfield DL, Ericsson LH, et al. Human thrombin: partial primary structure. *Arch Biophys Acta* 1977;178:356.
20. Butkowski RJ, Elion J, Downing MR, et al. Primary structure of human prethrombin 2 and α-thrombin. *J Biol Chem* 1977;252:4942.
21. MacGillivray RTA, Davie EW. Characterization of bovine prothrombin mRNA and its translation product. *Biochemistry* 1984;23:1626.
22. Morita T, Jackson CM. Preparation and properties of derivatives of bovine factor X and factor Xa from which the γ-carboxyglutamic acid containing domain has been removed. *J Biol Chem* 1986;261:4015.
23. Stenflo J, Fernlund P, Egan W, et al. Vitamin K dependent modifications of glutamic acid residues in prothrombin. *Proc Natl Acad Sci U S A* 1974;71:2730.
24. Suttie JW. Vitamin K-dependent carboxylase. *Ann Rev Biochem* 1985;54:459.
25. Nelsestuen GL, Broderius M, Martin G. Role of γ-carboxyglutamic acid: an unusual protein transition required for the calcium-dependent binding of prothrombin to phospholipid. *J Biol Chem* 1976;251:5648.
26. Prendergast FG, Mann KG. Differentiation of metal ion-induced transitions of prothrombin fragment 1. *J Biol Chem* 1977;252:840.
27. Park CH, Tulinsky A. Three-dimensional structure of the kringle sequence: structure of prothrombin fragment 1. *Biochemistry* 1986;25:3977.
28. Tulinsky A, Park CH, Skrzypczak-Jankun E. Structure of prothrombin fragment 1 refined at 2.8 Å resolution. *J Mol Biol* 1988;202:885.
29. Soriano-Garcia M, Park CH, Tulinsky A, et al. Structure of Ca$^{+2}$ prothrombin fragment 1 including the conformation of the Gla domain. *Biochemistry* 1989;28:6805.
30. Church WR, Boulanger LL, Messier TL, et al. Evidence for a common metal ion-dependent transition in the 4-carboxyglutamic acid domains of several vitamin K-dependent proteins. *J Biol Chem* 1989;264:17882.
31. Dombrose FA, Gitel SN, Zawalich K, et al. The association of bovine prothrombin fragment 1 with phospholipid: quantitative characterization of the Ca$^{2+}$ ion-mediated binding of prothrombin fragment 1 to phospholipid vesicles and a molecular model for its association with phospholipid. *J Biol Chem* 1979;254:5027.
32. Kung C, Hayes E, Mann KG. A membrane-mediated catalytic event in prothrombin activation. *J Biol Chem* 1994;264:25838.
33. Malhotra OP, Nesheim ME, Mann KG. The kinetics of activation of normal and γ-carboxyglutamic acid-deficient prothrombins. *J Biol Chem* 1985;260:279.
34. Patthy L. Evolution of the proteases of blood coagulation and fibrinolysis by assembly from modules. *Cell* 1985;41:657.
35. McLean JW, Tomlinson JE, Kuang WJ, et al. cDNA sequence of human apolipoprotein(a) is homologous to plasminogen. *Nature* 1987;330:132.
36. Castellino FJ, Beals JM. The genetic relationships between the kringle domains of human plasminogen, prothrombin, tissue plasminogen activator, urokinase, and coagulation factor XII. *J Mol Evol* 1987;26:358.
37. Deguchi H, Takeya H, Gabazza EC, et al. Prothrombin kringle 1 domain interacts with factor Va during the assembly of prothrombinase complex. *Biochem J* 1997;321:729.
38. Sugo T, Nakamikawa C, Tanabe S, et al. Activation of prothrombin by factor Xa bound to the membrane surface of human umbilical vein endothelial cells: its catalytic efficiency is similar to that of prothrombinase complex on platelets. *J Biochem (Tokyo)* 1995;117:244.
39. Bajaj SP, Butkowski RJ, Mann KG. Prothrombin fragments. Ca$^{2+}$ binding and activation kinetics. *J Biol Chem* 1975;250:2150.
40. Esmon CT, Jackson CM. The conversion of prothrombin to thrombin. IV. The function of the fragment 2 region during activation in the presence of factor V. *J Biol Chem* 1974;249:7791.
41. Kotkow KJ, Dietcher SR, Furie B, et al. The second kringle domain of prothrombin promotes factor Va-mediated prothrombin activation by prothrombinase. *J Biol Chem* 1995;270:4551.
42. Krishnaswamy S, Walker RK. Contribution of the prothrombin fragment 2 domain to the function of factor Va in the prothrombinase complex. *Biochemistry* 1997;36:3319.
43. Myrmel KH, Lundblad RL, Mann KG. Characteristics of the association between prothrombin fragment 2 and α-thrombin. *Biochemistry* 1976;15:1767.
44. Nesheim ME, Abbott T, Jenny R, et al. Evidence that the thrombin-catalyzed feedback cleavage of fragment 1.2 at Arg$_{154}$-Ser$_{155}$ promotes the release of thrombin from the catalytic surface during the activation of prothrombin. *J Biol Chem* 1988;263(2):1037.
45. Arni RK, Padmanabhan K, Padmanabhan KP, et al. Structures of the noncovalent complexes of human and bovine prothrombin fragment 2 with human PPACK-thrombin. *Biochemistry* 1993;32:4727.
46. Arni RK, Padmanabhan K, Padmanabhan KP, et al. Structure of the noncovalent complex of prothrombin kringle 2 with PPACK-thrombin. *Chem Phys Lipids* 1994;67/68:59.
47. Church FC, Pratt CW, Noyes CM, et al. Structural and functional properties of human α-thrombin, phosphopryidoxylated α-thrombin, and γ$_T$-thrombin. Identification of lysyl residues in α-thrombin that are critical for heparin and fibrin(ogen) interactions. *J Biol Chem* 1989;264:18419.
48. Bode W, Turk D, Karshikov A. The refined 1.9-Å X-ray crystal structure of D-Phe-Pro-Arg chloromethylketone-inhibited human α-thrombin: structure analysis, overall structure, electrostatic properties, detailed active-site geometry, and structure-function relationships. *Protein Sci* 1992;1:426.
49. Sheehan JP, Sadler JE. Molecular mapping of the heparin-binding exosite of thrombin. *Proc Natl Acad Sci U S A* 1994;91:5518.
50. Liaw PCY, Fredenburgh JC, Stafford AR, et al. Localization of the thrombin-binding domain on prothrombin fragment 2. *J Biol Chem* 1998;273:8932.
51. Walker FJ, Esmon CT. The effect of prothrombin fragment 2 on the inhibition of thrombin by antithrombin III. *J Biol Chem* 1979;254:5618.
52. Bock PE. Active-site-selective labeling of blood coagulation proteinases with fluorescence probes by the use of thioester peptide chloromethyl ketones. II. Properties of thrombin derivatives as reporters of prothrombin fragment 2 binding and specificity of the labeling approach for other proteinases. *J Biol Chem* 1992;267:14974.
53. Jakubowski HV, Kline MD, Owen WG. The effect of bovine thrombomodulin on the specificity of bovine thrombin. *J Biol Chem* 1986;261:3876.
54. Liu L-W, Rezaie AR, Carson CW, et al. Occupancy of anion binding exosite 2 on thrombin determines Ca$^{2+}$ dependence of protein C activation. *J Biol Chem* 1994;269:11807.
55. Downing MR, Butkowski RJ, Clark MM, et al. Human prothrombin activation. *J Biol Chem* 1975;250:8897.
56. Bode W, Mayr I, Baumann U, et al. The refined 1.9Å crystal structure of human α-thrombin: interaction with D-Phe-Pro-Arg chloromethylketone and significance of the Tyr-Pro-Pro-Trp insertion segment. *EMBO J* 1989;8:3467.
57. Rydel TJ, Ravichandran KG, Tulinsky A, et al. The structure of a complex of recombinant hirudin and human α-thrombin. *Science* 1990;249:277.
58. Hageman TC, Endres GF, Scheraga HA. Mechanism of action of thrombin on fibrinogen: on the role of the A chain of bovine thrombin in specificity and in differentiating between thrombin and trypsin. *Arch Biochem Biophys* 1975;171:327.
59. DiCera E, Guinto ER, Vindigni A, et al. The Na$^+$ binding site of thrombin. *J Biol Chem* 1995;270:22089.
60. Freer ST, Kraut J, Robertus JD, et al Chymotrypsinogen: 2.5-Å crystal structure, comparison with α-chymotrypsin, and implications for zymogen activation. *Biochemistry* 1970;9:1997.

61. Weber LD, Tulinsky A, Johnson JD, et al. Expression of functionality of α-chymotrypsin. The structure of a fluorescent probe-α-chymotrypsin complex and the nature of its pH dependence. *Biochemistry* 1979;18:1297.

62. Magnusson S, Hofmann T. Inactivation of bovine thrombin by nitrous acid. *Can J Biochem* 1970;48:432.

63. Tulinsky A. Molecular interactions of thrombin. *Semin Thromb Hemost* 1996;22:117–124.

64. Stone SR, Hofsteenge J. Kinetics of the inhibition of thrombin by hirudin. *Biochemistry* 1986;25:4622.

65. Stone SR, Braun PJ, Hofsteenge J. Identification of regions of α-thrombin involved in its interaction with hirudin. *Biochemistry* 1987;26:4617.

66. Braun PJ, Dennis S, Hofsteenge J, et al. Use of site-directed mutagenesis to investigate the basis for the specificity of hirudin. *Biochemistry* 1988;27:6517.

67. Chang JY, Ngai PK, Rink H, et al. The structural elements of hirudin which bind to the fibrinogen recognition site of thrombin are exclusively located within its acidic C-terminal tail. *FEBS Lett* 1990;261:287.

68. Folkers PJ, Clore GM, Driscoll PC, et al. Solution structure of recombinant hirudin and the Lys47 → Glu mutant: a nuclear magnetic resonance and hybrid geometry-dynamical simulated annealing study. *Biochemistry* 1989;28:2601.

69. Haruyama H, Wuthrich K. Conformation of recombinant desulfatohirudin in aqueous solution determined by nuclear-magnetic resonance. *Biochemistry* 1989;28:4301.

70. Berliner LJ, Shen YY. Physical evidence for an apolar binding site near the catalytic center of human α-thrombin. *Biochemistry* 1977;16:4622.

71. Furie B, Bing DH, Feldman RJ, et al. Computer-generated models of blood coagulation factor Xa, factor IXa, and thrombin based upon structural homology with other serine proteases. *J Biol Chem* 1982;257:3875.

72. Schecheter I, Berger A. On the size of the active site in proteases. I. Papain. *Biochem Biophys Res Commun* 1967;27:157.

73. Liem RK, Scheraga HA. Mechanism of action of thrombin on fibrinogen. III. Partial mapping of the active sites of thrombin and trypsin. *Arch Biochem Biophys* 1973;158:387.

74. Liem RK, Scheraga HA. Mechanism of action of thrombin on fibrinogen IV. Further mapping of the active sites of thrombin and trypsin. *Arch Biochem Biophys* 1974;160:333.

75. Scheraga HA. Active-site mapping of thrombin. In: Lundblad RL, Fenton JW, Mann KG, eds. *The chemistry and biology of thrombin*. Ann Arbor, MI: Ann Arbor Press, 1977:145–158.

76. Gorman JJ. Inhibition of human thrombin assessed with different substrates and inhibitors. Characterization of fibrinopeptide binding interaction. *Biochim Biophys Acta* 1975;412:273.

77. Blomback B. The N-terminal disulphide knot of human fibrinogen. *Br J Haematol* 1969;17:145.

78. Iwanaga S, Wallen P, Grandahl NY. On the primary structure of human fibrinogen, isolation and characterization of N-terminal fragments from plasmic digests. *Eur J Biochem* 1964;8:189.

79. Takagi T, Doolittle RF. Amino acid sequence studies on factor XIII and the peptide released during its activation by thrombin. *Biochemistry* 1974;13:750.

80. Eaton D, Rodriguez H, Vehar GA. Proteolytic processing of human factor VIII. Correlation of specific cleavages by thrombin, factor Xa, and activated protein C with activation and inactivation of factor VIII coagulant activity. *Biochem* 1986;25:505.

81. Mann KG, Jenny RJ, Krishnaswamy S. Cofactor proteins in the assembly and expression of blood clotting enzyme complexes. *Ann Rev Biochem* 1988;57:915.

82. Hagen FS, Gray CL, O'Hara P, et al. Characterization of a cDNA coding for human factor VII. *Proc Natl Acad Sci U S A* 1986;83:2412.

83. Radcliffe R, Nemersen Y. Bovine factor VII. *Methods Enzymol* 1976;45:49.

84. Elion J, Butkowski RJ, Downing MR, et al. Primary structure of human fragment 2. *Circulation* 1976;54:118.

85. Heldebrant CM, Noyes C, Kingdon HS, et al. The activation of prothrombin III: the partial amino acid sequences at the amino terminal of prothrombin and the intermediates of activation. *Biochem Biophys Res Commun* 1973;54:155.

86. Foster D, Davie EW. Characterization of a cDNA coding for human protein C. *Proc Natl Acad Sci U S A* 1984;81:4766.

87. Long GL, Belagaje RM, MacGillivray RTA. Cloning and sequencing of liver cDNA coding for bovine protein C. *Proc Natl Acad Sci U S A* 1984;81:5653.

88. Mutt V, Magnusson S, Jorpes JE, et al. Structure of porcine secretin. Degradation with trypsin and thrombin. Sequence of the tryptic peptides. The C-terminal residue. *Biochemistry* 1965;4:2358.

89. Morgan FJ, Birken S, Canfield RE. The amino acid sequence of human chorionic gonadotropin. The α subunit and β subunit. *J Biol Chem* 1975;250:5247.

90. Engel A, Alexander B. Activation of chymotrypsinogen-A by thrombin preparations. *Biochemistry* 1966;5:3590.

91. Mutt V, Jorpes JE. Structure of porcine cholecystokinin-pancreozymin. 1. Cleavage with thrombin and with trypsin. *Eur J Biochem* 1968;6:156.

92. Lundblad RL, Kingdon HS, Mann KG. Thrombin. *Methods Enzymol* 1976;45:156.

93. Graf L, Barat E, Borvendeg J, et al. Action of thrombin on ovine, bovine and human pituitary growth hormones. *Eur J Biochem* 1976;64:333.

94. Muszbek L, Gladner JA, Laki K. The fragmentation of actin by thrombin: isolation and characterization of split products. *Arch Biochem Biophys* 1975;167:99.

95. Sparrow JT, Pownall HJ, Hsu F, et al. Lipid binding by fragment of apolipoprotein C-III-1 obtained by thrombin cleavage. *Biochemistry* 1977;16:5427.

96. Leavis PC, Rosenfeld S, Lu RC. Cleavage of a specific bond in troponin C by thrombin. *Biochim Biophys Acta* 1978;535:281.

97. Jenny NS, Mann KG. Coagulation cascade: an overview. In: Loscalzo J, Schafer AI, eds. *Thrombosis and hemorrhage*, 2nd ed. Baltimore, MD: Williams & Wilkins, 1994:3–27.

98. Vu T-KH, Hung DT, Wheaton VI, et al. Molecular cloning of a functional thrombin receptor reveals a novel proteolytic mechanism of receptor activation. *Cell* 1991;64:1057.

99. Xu W-F, Andersen H, Whitmore TE, et al. Cloning and characterization of human protease-activated receptor 4. *Proc Natl Acad Sci U S A* 1998;95:6642.

100. Eaton DL, Malloy BE, Tsai SP, et al. Isolation, molecular cloning, and partial characterization of a novel carboxypeptidase B from human plasma. *J Biol Chem* 1991;266:2183.

101. Blombäck B, Blombäck M, Hessel B, et al. Structure of N-terminal fragments of fibrinogen and specificity of thrombin. *Nature* 1967;215:1445.

102. Hogg H, Blombäck B. The mechanism of the fibrinogen-thrombin relation. *Thromb Res* 1978;12:953.

103. Seegers WH, McCoy L, Kipfer RK, et al. Preparation and properties of thrombin. *Arch Biochem Biophys* 1968;128:194.

104. Mann KG, Batt CW. The molecular weights of bovine thrombin and its primary autolysis products. *J Biol Chem* 1969;244:6555.

105. Rosenberg RD, Waugh DF. Multiple bovine thrombin components. *J Biol Chem* 1970;245:5049.

106. Lundblad RL, Noyes C, Mann KG, et al. The covalent differences between bovine α- and β-thrombin: a structural explanation for the changes in catalytic activity. *J Biol Chem* 1979;254:8524.

107. Lundblad RL, Uhteg LC, Vogel CN, et al. Preparation and partial characterization of two forms of bovine thrombin. *Biochem Biophys Res Commun* 1975;66:482.

108. Lundblad RL, Nesheim ME, Straight DL, et al. Bovine α- and β-thrombin. Reduced fibrinogen-clotting activity of β-thrombin is not a consequence of reduced affinity for fibrinogen. *J Biol Chem* 1984;259:6991.

109. Fenton JW, Landis BH, Walz DA. Human thrombins. In: Lundblad RL, Fenton JW, Mann KG, eds. *The chemistry and biology of thrombin*. Ann Arbor, MI: Ann Arbor Press, 1977:43–70.

110. Boissel J-P, Le Bonniec B, Rabiet M-J, et al. Covalent structures of β and γ autolytic derivatives of human α-thrombin. *J Biol Chem* 1984;259:5691.

111. Lottenberg R, Hall JA, Fenton JW II, et al. The action of thrombin on peptide ρ-nitroanilide substrates: hydrolysis of Tos-Gly-Pro-Arg-ρNA and D-Phe-Pip-Arg-ρNA by human α and γ and bovine α and β-thrombins. *Thromb Res* 1982;28:313.

112. Witting JI, Miller TM, Fenton JW II. Human α- and γ-thrombin specificity with tripeptide ρ-nitroanalide substrates under physiologically relevant conditions. *Thromb Res* 1987;46:567.

113. Lorand L, Credo RB. Thrombin and fibrin stabilization. In: Lundblad RL, Fenton JW, Mann KG, eds. *Chemistry and biology of thrombin*. Ann Arbor, MI: Ann Arbor Press, 1977:311–323.

114. Bezeaud A, Denninger MH, Guillin MC. Interaction of human α-thrombin and γ-thrombinwith antithrombin III, protein C and thrombomodulin. *Eur J Chem* 1985;153:491.

115. Seegers WH, McCoy LE, Walz DA, et al. Isolation of thrombin-E and the evolution of enzyme activity from prothrombin. *Experientia* 1974;30:1130.

116. Takahashi K, Aiken M, Fenton JW II, et al. Thrombospondin fragmentation by α-thrombin and resistance to γ-thrombin. *Biochem* 1984;224:673.

117. Doyle M, Mann KG. Multiple active forms of thrombin. IV. Relative activities of meizothrombin. *J Biol Chem* 1990;265:10693.

118. Morita T, Iwanaga S, Suzuki T. The mechanism of activation of bovine prothrombin by an activator isolated from *Echis carinatus* venom and characterization of the new active intermediates. *J Biochem (Tokyo)* 1976;79:1089.

119. Krishnaswamy S, Mann KG, Nesheim ME. The prothrombinase-catalyzed activation of prothrombin proceeds through the intermediate meizothrombin in an ordered, sequential reaction. *J Biol Chem* 1986;261:8977.

120. Krishnaswamy S, Church WR, Nesheim ME, et al. Activation of human prothrombin by human prothrombinase. Influence of factor Va on the reaction mechanism. *J Biol Chem* 1987;262:3291.

121. Bovill EG, Tracy RP, Hayes TE, et al. Evidence that meizothrombin is an intermediate product in the clotting of whole blood. *Arterioscler Thromb Vasc Biol* 1995;15:754.

122. Thompson LP, Doyle MF, Mann KG, et al. Sensitivity of rabbit arteries to meizothrombin is greater than that to α-thrombin. *J Vasc Med Biol* 1989;1:347.

123. Stevens WK, Côté HCF, MacGillivray RTA, et al. Calcium ion modulation of meizothrombin autolysis at Arg55-Asp56 and catalytic activity. *J Biol Chem* 1996;271:8092.

124. Côté HCF, Bajzar L, Stevens WK, et al. Functional characterization of recombinant human meizothrombin and meizothrombin (desF1). *J Biol Chem* 1997;272:6194.

125. Rosing J, Zwaal RFA, Tans G. Formation of meizothrombin as intermediate in factor Xa-catalyzed prothrombin activation. *J Biol Chem* 1986;261: 4224.

126. Tans G, Nicolaes GAF, Thomassen MCLGD, et al. Activation of human factor V by meizothrombin. *J Biol Chem* 1994;269:15969.

127. von dem Borne PA, Mosnier LO, Tans G, et al. Factor XI activation by meizothrombin: stimulation by phospholipid vesicles containing both phosphatidylserine and phosphatidylethanolamine. *Thromb Haemost* 1997;78:834.

128. Hackeng TM, Tans G, Koppelman SJ, et al. Protein C activation on endothelial cells by prothrombin activation products generated *in situ*: meizothrombin is a better protein C activator than α-thrombin. *Biochem J* 1996;319:399.

129. Poort SJ, Michiels JJ, Reitsma PH, et al. Homozygosity for a novel missense mutation in the prothrombin gene causing a severe bleeding disorder. *Thromb Haemost* 1994;72:819.

130. Rabiet MJ, Furie BC, Furie B. Molecular defect of prothrombin Barcelona: substitution of cysteine for arginine at residue 273. *J Biol Chem* 1986;261:15045.

131. Diuguid DL, Rabiet MJ, Furie BC, et al. Molecular defects of factor IX Chicago-2 (Arg 145 → His) and prothrombin Madrid (Arg 271 → Cys): arginine mutations that preclude zymogen activation. *Blood* 1989;74:193.

132. O'Marcaigh AS, Nichols WL, Hassinger NL, et al. Genetic analysis and functional characterization of prothrombin Corpus Christi (Arg328-Cys), Dharhan (Arg271-His), and hypoprothrombinemia. *Blood* 1996;88: 2611.

133. James HL, Kim DJ, Zheng D-A, et al. Prothrombin Padua I: incomplete activation due to an amino acid substitution at a factor Xa cleavage site. *Blood Coagul Fibrinolysis* 1994;5:841.

134. Sun WY, Burkart MC, Holahan JR, et al. Prothrombin San Antonio: a single amino acid substitution at factor Xa activation site (Arg320 to His) results in dysprothrombinemia. *Blood* 2000;95:711.

135. Morishita E, Saito M, Kumabashiri I, et al. Prothrombin Himi: a compound heterozygote for two dysfunctional prothrombin molecules (Met-337 → Thr and Arg-388 → His). *Blood* 1992;80:2275.

136. Miyata T, Morita T, Inomoto T, et al. Prothrombin Tokushima, a replacement of arginine-418 by tryptophan that impairs the fibrinogen clotting activity of derived thrombin Tokushima. *Biochemistry* 1987;26:1117.

137. Miyata T, Aruga R, Umeyama H, et al. Prothrombin Salakta: substitution of glutamic acid-466 by alanine reduces the fibrinogen clotting activity and the esterase activity. *Biochemistry* 1992;31:7457.

138. Friezner Degen SJ, McDowell SA, Sparks LM, et al. Prothrombin Frankfurt: a dysfunctional prothrombin characterized by substitution of Glu-466 by Ala. *Thromb Haemost* 1995;73:203.

139. Henrikson RA, Dunham CK, Miller LD, et al. Prothrombin Greenville, Arg[517] → Gln, identified in an individual heterozygous for dysprothrombinemia. *Blood* 1998;91:2026.

140. Sun WY, Smirnow D, Jenkins ML, et al. Prothrombin Scranton: substitution of an amino acid residue involved in the binding of Na⁺ (Lys-556 to Thr) leads to dysprothrombinemia. *Thromb Haemost* 2001;85:651.

141. Henriksen RA, Mann KG. Identification of the primary structure defect in the dysthrombin thrombin quick I. *Biochemistry* 1988;92:9160.

142. Akhavan S, Mannucci PM, Lak M, et al. Identification and three-dimensional structural analysis of nine novel mutations in patients with prothrombin deficiency. *Thromb Haemost* 2000;84:989.

143. Henriksen RA, Mann KG. Substitution of Val for Gly-558 in the congenital dysthrombin, thrombin quick II, alters primary substrate specificity. *Biochemistry* 1989;28:2078.

144. Sun WY, Ruiz-Saez A, Burkart MC, et al. Prothrombin Carora: hypoprothrombinemia caused by a substitution of Tyr-44 by Cys. *Br J Haematol* 1999;105:670.

145. Lefkowitz JB, Weller A, Nuss R, et al. A common mutation, Arg457 → Gln, links prothrombin deficiencies in the Puerto Rican population. *J Thromb Haemost* 2003;1:2381.

146. Shafer JA, Higgins DL. Human fibrinogen. *Crit Rev Clin Lab Sci* 1988; 26:1.

147. Doolittle RF. Fibrinogen and fibrin. *Annu Rev Biochem* 1984;53:195.

148. Blombäck B, Blombäck M, Edman P, et al. Human fibrinopeptides. Isolation, characterization and structure. *Biochim Biophys Acta* 1966;28:115.

149. Mossesson MW. The roles of fibrinogen and fibrin in hemostasis and thrombosis. *Semin Hematol* 1992;29:177.

150. Spraggon G, Everse SJ, Doolittle RF. Crystal structures of fragment D from human fibrinogen and its crosslinked counterpart from fibrin. *Nature* 1997;389:455.

151. Hantgan R, McDonagh J, Hermans J. Fibrin assembly. *Ann N Y Acad Sci* 1983;408:344.

152. Lorand L, Jeong JM, Radek JT, et al. Human plasma factor XIII: subunit interactions and activation of zymogen. *Methods Enzymol* 1993; 222:22.

153. Lorand L, Konishi K. Activation of the fibrin-stabilizing factor of plasma by thrombin. *Arch Biochem Biophys* 1964;105:58.

154. Francis RT, McDonagh J, Mann KG. Factor V is a substrate for the transamidase factor XIIIa. *J Biol Chem* 1986;261:9787.

155. Huh MM, Schick BP, Schick PK, et al. Covalent crosslinking of human coagulation factor V by activated factor XIII from guinea pig megakaryocytes and human plasma. *Blood* 1988;71:1693.

156. Wang DL, Anjanayaki E, Annamalai E, et al. Human platelet factor V is crosslinked to actin by FXIIIa during platelet activation by thrombin. *Thromb Res* 1990;57:39.

157. Iwanaga S, Suzuki K, Hashimoto S. Bovine plasma cold-insoluble globulin: gross structure and function. *Ann N Y Acad Sci* 1978;312:56.

158. Mosher DF, Schad PE. Cross-linking of fibronectin to collagen by blood coagulation factor XIIIa. *J Clin Invest* 1979;64:781.

159. Sakata Y, Aoki N. Cross-linking of alpha 2-plasmin inhibitor to fibrin by fibrin-stabilizing factor. *J Clin Invest* 1980;65:290.

160. Yee VC, Pedersen LC, Trong IL, et al. Three-dimensional structure of a transglutaminase: human blood coagulation factor XIII. *Proc Natl Acad Sci U S A* 1994;91:7296.

161. Gailani D, Broze GJ Jr. Factor XI activation in a revised model of blood coagulation. *Science* 1991;253:909.

162. Fujikawa K, Chung DW, Hendrickson LE, et al. Amino acid sequence of human factor XI, a blood coagulation factor with four tandem repeats that are highly homologous with plasma prekallikrein. *Biochemistry* 1986;25:2417.

163. Butenas S, van't Veer C, Mann KG. Evaluation of the initiation phase of blood coagulation using ultra sensitive assays for serine proteases. *J Biol Chem* 1997;272:21527.

164. Fay PJ. Subunit structure of thrombin-activated human factor VIIIa. *Biochim Biophys Acta* 1988;952:181.

165. Lollar P, Parker CG. Subunit structure of thrombin-activated porcine factor VIII. *Biochemistry* 1989;28:666.

166. Jenny RJ, Pittman DD, Toole JJ, et al. Complete cDNA and derived amino acid sequence of human factor V. *Proc Natl Acad Sci U S A* 1987;84:4846.

167. Esmon CT, Lollar P. Involvement of thrombin anion-binding exosites 1 and 2 in the activation of factor V and factor VIII. *J Biol Chem* 1996;271: 13882.

168. Dharmawardana KR, Bock PE. Demonstration of exosite I-dependent interactions of thrombin with human factor V and Va involving the factor Va heavy chain: analysis by affinity chromatography employing a novel method for active-site-selective immobilization of serine proteases. *Biochemistry* 1998;37:13143.

169. Dharmawardana KR, Olson ST, Bock PE. Role of regulatory exosite I in binding of thrombin to human factor V, factor Va, factor Va subunits, and activation fragments. *J Biol Chem* 1999;274:18635.

170. Nesheim ME, Mann KG. Thrombin-catalyzed activation of single chain bovine factor V. *J Biol Chem* 1979;254:1326.

171. Toole JJ, Knopf JL, Wozney JM, et al. Molecular cloning of a cDNA encoding human antihaemophilic factor. *Nature* 1984;312:342.

172. Vehar GA, Keyt B, Eaton D, et al. Structure of human factor VIII. *Nature* 1984;312:337.

173. Hoyer LW. The factor VIII complex: structure and function. *Blood* 1981;58:1.

174. Lollar P, Hill Eubanks DC, Parker CG. Association of the factor VIII light chain with von Willebrand factor. *J Biol Chem* 1988;263:10451.

175. Radcliffe R, Nemerson Y. Activation and control of factor VII by activated factor X and thrombin. Isolation and characterization of a single chain form of factor VII. *J Biol Chem* 1975;250:388.

176. Butenas S, Mann KG. Kinetics of human factor VII activation. *Biochemistry* 1996;35:1904.

177. Kisiel W, Canfield WM, Ericsson LH, et al. Anticoagulant properties of bovine plasma protein C following activation by thrombin. *Biochemistry* 1977;16:5824.

178. Walker FJ. Regulation of bovine activated protein C by protein S: the role of the cofactor protein in species specificity. *Thromb Res* 1981;22:321.

179. Esmon CT. The roles of protein C and thrombomodulin in the regulation of blood coagulation. *J Biol Chem* 1989;264:4743.

180. Walker FJ, Fay PJ. Regulation of blood coagulation by the protein C system. *FASEB J* 1992;6:2561.

181. Esmon C, Owen W. Identification of an endothelial cell cofactor for thrombin catalyzed activation of protein C. *Proc Natl Acad Sci U S A* 1981;78:2249.

182. Walker FJ, Chavin SI, Fay PJ. Inactivation of factor VIII by activated protein C and protein S. *Arch Biochem Biophys* 1987;252:322.

183. Walker FJ. Regulation of activated protein C by a new protein. A possible function for bovine protein S. *J Biol Chem* 1980;255:5521.

184. Walker FJ. Regulation of vitamin K-dependent protein S. Inactivation by thrombin. *J Biol Chem* 1984;259:10335.

185. Boffa MB, Wang W, Bajzar L, et al. Plasma and recombinant thrombin-activatable fibrinolysis inhibitor (TAFI) and activated TAFI compared with respect to glycosylation, thrombin/thrombomodulin-dependent activation, thermal stability, and enzymatic properties. *J Biol Chem* 1998;273:2127.

186. Nesheim M. Thrombin and fibrinolysis. *Chest* 2003;124(Suppl 3):33S.

187. Bajzar L, Manuel R, Nesheim ME. Purification and characterization of TAFI, a thrombin-activatable fibrinolysis inhibitor. *J Biol Chem* 1995; 270:14477.

188. Bajzar L, Morser J, Nesheim M. TAFI, or plasma procarboxypeptidase B, couples the coagulation and fibrinolytic cascades through the thrombin-thrombomodulin complex. *J Biol Chem* 1996;271:16603.

189. Wang W, Nagashima M, Schneider M, et al. Elements of the primary structure of thrombomodulin required for efficient thrombin-activatable fibrinolysis inhibitor activation. *J Biol Chem* 2000;275:22942.

190. Kokame K, Zheng X, Sadler JE. Activation of thrombin-activatable fibrinolysis inhibitor requires epidermal growth factor-like domain 3 of thrombomodulin and is inhibited competitively by protein C. *J Biol Chem* 1998;273:12135.

191. Hall SW, Nagashimi M, Zhao L, et al. Thrombin interacts with thrombomodulin, protein C, and thrombin-activatable fibrinolysis inhibitor via specific and distinct domains. *J Biol Chem* 1999;274:25510.

192. Bell R, Stevens WK, Jia Z, et al. Fluorescence properties and functional roles of tryptophan residues 60d, 96, 148, 207, and 215 of thrombin. *J Biol Chem* 2000;275:29513.

193. Wang W, Boffa MB, Bajzar L, et al. A study of the mechanism of inhibition of fibrinolysis by activated thrombin-activable fibrinolysis inhibitor. *J Biol Chem* 1998;273:27176.

194. Bajzar L, Nesheim ME, Tracy PB. The profibrinolytic effect of activated protein C in clots formed from plasma is TAFI-dependent. *Blood* 1996;88:2093.

195. Bajzar L, Kalafatis M, Simioni P, et al. An antifibrinolytic mechanism describing the prothrombotic effect associated with factor VLeiden. *J Biol Chem* 1996;271:22949.

196. Valnickova Z, Enghild JJ. Human procarboxypeptidase U, or thrombin-activable fibrinolysis inhibitor, is a substrate for transglutaminases. *J Biol Chem* 1998;273:27220.

197. Broze GJ Jr, Higuchi DA. Coagulation-dependent inhibition of fibrinolysis: role of carboxypeptidase-U and the premature lysis of clots from hemophilic plasma. *Blood* 1996;88:3815.

198. von dem Borne PA, Bajzar L, Meijers JCM, et al. Thrombin-mediated activation of factor XI results in thrombin-activatable fibrinolysis inhibitor-dependent inhibition of fibrinolysis. *J Clin Invest* 1997;99:2323.

199. Brummel KE, Butenas S, Mann KG. An integrated study of fibrinogen during blood coagulation. *J Biol Chem* 1999;274:22862.

200. Coughlin SR. Sol Sherry lecture in thrombosis. How thrombin 'talks' to cells. Molecular mechanisms and roles *in vivo*. *Arterioscler Thromb Vasc Biol* 1998;18:514.

201. Davey M, Luscher E. Actions of thrombin and other coagulant and proteolytic enzymes on blood platelets. *Nature* 1967;216:857.

202. Hattori R, Hamilton KK, Fugate RD, et al. Stimulated secretion of endothelial VWF is accompanied by rapid redistribution to the cell surface of the intracellular granular membrane protein GMP-140. *J Biol Chem* 1989;264:7768.

203. Daniel TO, Gibbs VC, Milfay DF, et al. Thrombin stimulates *c-sis* gene expression in microvascular endothelial cells. *J Biol Chem* 1986;261:9579.

204. Colotta F, Sciacca FL, Sironi M, et al. Expression of monocyte chemotactic protein-1 by monocytes and endothelial cells exposed to thrombin. *Am J Pathol* 1994;144:975.

205. McNamara CA, Sarembok IJ, Gimple LW, et al. Thrombin stimulation of smooth muscle cell proliferation is mediated by a proteolytic receptor-mediated mechanism. *J Clin Invest* 1992;91:94.

206. Hou L, Howells GL, Kapas S, et al. The protease-activated receptors and their cellular expression and function in blood-related cells. *Br J Haematol* 1998;101:1.

207. Vu T-KH, Wheaton VI, Hung DT, et al. Domains specifying thrombin-receptor interaction. *Nature* 1991;353:674.

208. Kahn ML, Zheng Y-W, Huang W, et al. A dual thrombin receptor system for platelet activation. *Nature* 1998;394:690.

209. Nakanishi-Matsui M, Zheng Y-W, Sulcinen DJ, et al. PAR3 is a cofactor for PAR4 activation by thrombin. *Nature* 2000;404:609.

210. Kahn ML, Nakanishi-Matsui M, Shapiro MJ, et al. Protease-activated receptors 1 and 4 mediate activation of human platelets by thrombin. *J Clin Invest* 1999;103:879.

211. Brass LF. Thrombin and platelet activation. *Chest* 2003;124(Suppl. 3):18S.

212. Covic L, Gresser AL, Kuliopulos A. Biphasic kinetics of activation and signaling for PAR1 and PAR4 thrombin receptors in platelets. *Biochemistry* 2000;39:5458.

213. Shapiro MJ, Weiss EJ, Faruqi TR, et al. Protease-activated receptors 1 and 4 are shut off with distinct kinetics after activation by thrombin. *J Biol Chem* 2000;275:25216.

214. De Cristofaro R, De Candia E, Rutella S, et al. The Asp(272)-Glu(282) region of platelet glycoprotein Ib alpha interacts with the heparin-binding site of α-thrombin and protects the enzyme from the heparin-catalyzed inhibition by antithrombin III. *J Biol Chem* 2000;275:3887.

215. De Marco L, Mazzucato M, Masotti A, et al. Function of glycoprotein Ibα in platelet activation induced by alpha-thrombin. *J Biol Chem* 1991;266:23776.

216. Harmon JT, Jamieson GA. Platelet activation by thrombin in the absence of the high-affinity thrombin receptor. *Biochemistry* 1988;27:2151.

217. Mazzucato M, De Marco LD, Masotti A, et al. Characterization of the initial α-thrombin interaction with glycoprotein Ib alpha in relation to platelet activation. *J Biol Chem* 1998;273:1880.

218. De Candia E, Hall SW, Rutella S, et al. Binding of thrombin to glycoprotein Ib accelerates the hydrolysis of PAR-1 on intact platelets. *J Biol Chem* 2001;276:4692.

219. Howells GL, Macey MG, Curtis MA, et al. Peripheral blood lymphocytes express the platelet-type thrombin receptor. *Br J Haematol* 1993;84:156.

220. Joseph S, MacDermott J. The N-terminal thrombin receptor fragment SFLLN, but not catalytically inactive thrombin-derived agonists, activate U937 monocytic cells: evidence for receptor hydrolysis in thrombin-dependent signaling. *Biochem J* 1993;290:571.

221. Garcia JGN, Patterson C, Bahler C, et al. Thrombin receptor activating peptides induce Ca²⁺ mobilization, barrier dysfunction, prostaglandin synthesis, and platelet-derived growth factor mRNA expression in cultured endothelium. *J Cell Physiol* 1993;150:4876.

222. Ishihara H, Connolly AJ, Zheng D, et al. Protease-activated receptor 3 is a second thrombin receptor in humans. *Nature* 1997;386:502.

223. Schmidt VA, Nierman WC, Maglott DR, et al. The human proteinase-activated receptor-3 (PAR-3) gene. Identification within a PAR gene cluster and characterization in vascular endothelial cells and platelets. *J Biol Chem* 1998;273:15061.

224. Mann KG. The assembly of blood clotting complexes on membranes. *Trends Biochem Sci* 1987;12:229.

225. Tracy PB, Eide LL, Mann KG. Human prothrombinase complex assembly and function on isolated peripheral blood cell populations. *J Biol Chem* 1985;260:2119.

226. Mann KG, Krishnaswamy S, Lawson JH. Surface-dependent hemostasis. *Semin Hematol* 1992;29:213.

227. Mann KG. Prothrombin. *Methods Enzymol* 1976;45:123.

228. Nelsestuen GL, Kisiel W, DiScipio RG. Interaction of vitamin K-dependent proteins with membranes. *Biochemistry* 1978;17:2134.

229. Mann KG, Nesheim ME, Church WR, et al. Surface-dependent reactions of the vitamin K-dependent enzyme complexes. *Blood* 1990;76:1.

230. Krishnaswamy S. Prothrombinase complex assembly: contributions of protein-protein and protein-membrane interactions towards complex formation. *J Biol Chem* 1990;265:3708.

231. Mann KG. Biochemistry and physiology of blood coagulation. *Thromb Haemost* 1999;82:165.

232. Fujikawa K, Lagaz ME, Davie EW. Bovine factor X-1 and X-2 (Stuart factor) isolation and characterization. *Biochemistry* 1972;11:4882.

233. Hedner U, Glazer S, Pingel K, et al. Successful use of recombinant factor VIIa in patient with severe haemophilia A during synovectomy. *Lancet* 1988;2:1193.

234. Hedner U. Recombinant activated factor VII as a universal hemostatic agent. *Blood Coagul Fibrinolysis* 1998;(Suppl 1):S147.

235. Lamphear BJ, Fay PJ. Factor IXa enhances reconstitution of factor VIIIa from isolated A2 subunit and A1/A3-C1-C2 dimer. *J Biol Chem* 1992;267:3725.

236. Curtis JE, Helgerson SL, Parker ET, et al. Isolation and characterization of thrombin-activated human factor VIII. *J Biol Chem* 1994;269:6246.

237. Ahmad SS, Rawala-Sheikh R, Walsh PN. Components and assembly of the factor X activating complex. *Semin Thromb Hemost* 1992;18:311.

238. Nemerson Y. Tissue factor and hemostasis. *Blood* 1988;71:1.

239. Lawson JH, Butenas S, Mann KG. The evaluation of complex-dependent alterations in human factor VIIa. *J Biol Chem* 1992;267:4834.

240. Krishnaswamy S, Field KA, Edgington TS, et al. Role of the membrane surface in the activation of human coagulation factor X. *J Biol Chem* 1992;267:26110.

241. Ruf W, Rehetulla A, Morrissey JH, et al. Phospholipid-independent and dependent interactions required for tissue factor receptor and cofactor function. *J Biol Chem* 1991;266:16256.

242. Fiore MM, Neuenschwander PF, Morrissey JH. The biochemical basis for the apparent defect of soluble mutant tissue factor in enhancing the proteolytic activities of factor VIIa. *J Biol Chem* 1994;269:143.

243. Rezaie AR, Neuenschwander PF, Morrissey JH, et al. Analysis of the functions of the first epidermal growth factor-like domain of factor X. *J Biol Chem* 1993;268:8176.

244. Nemerson Y, Repke D. Tissue factor accelerates the activation of coagulation factor VII: the role of a bifunctional coagulation cofactor. *Thromb Res* 1985;40:351.

245. Nemerson Y, Esnouf MP. Activation of a proteolytic system by a membrane lipoprotein: mechanism of action of tissue factor. *Proc Natl Acad Sci U S A* 1973;70:310.

246. Seligsohn U, Osterud B, Brown SF, et al. Activation of human factor VII in plasma and in purified systems: roles of activated factor IX, kallikrein, and activated factor XII. *J Clin Invest* 1979;64:1056.

247. Neuenschwander PF, Fiore MM, Morrissey JH. Factor VII autoactivation proceeds via interaction of distinct protease-cofactor and zymogen-cofactor complexes. Implications of a two-dimensional enzyme kinetic mechanism. *J Biol Chem* 1993;268:21489.

248. Lawson JH, Mann KG. Cooperative activation of human factor IX by the human extrinsic pathway of blood coagulation. *J Biol Chem* 1991;266:11317.

249. Broze GJ Jr, Gerard TJ, Novotny WF. Regulation of coagulation by a multivalent Kunitz-type inhibitor. *Biochemistry* 1990;29:7539.

250. Nesheim ME, Foster WB, Hewick R, et al. Characterization of factor V activation intermediates. *J Biol Chem* 1984;259:3187.

251. Suzuki K, Dahlback B, Stenflo J. Thrombin-catalyzed activation of human coagulation factor V. *J Biol Chem* 1982;257:6556.

252. Foster BW, Nesheim ME, Mann KG. The factor Xa-catalyzed activation of factor V. *J Biol Chem* 1983;258:13970.

253. Monkovic DD, Tracy PB. Activation of human factor V by factor Xa and thrombin. *Biochemistry* 1990;29:1118.

254. Lee CD, Mann KG. Activation/inactivation of human factor V by plasmin. *Blood* 1989;73:185.

255. Kalafatis M, Xue J, Lawler CM, et al. Contribution of the heavy and light chains of factor Va to the interaction with factor Xa. *Biochemistry* 1994; 33:6538.

256. Chattopadhyay A, James HL, Fair DS. Molecular recognition sites on factor Xa which participate in the prothrombinase complex. *J Biol Chem* 1992;267:12323.

257. Kalafatis M, Rand MD, Mann KG. Factor Va-membrane interaction is mediated by two regions located on the light chain of the cofactor. *Biochemistry* 1994;33:486.

258. Ortel TL, Devore-Carter D, Quinn-Allen M, et al. Deletion analysis of recombinant human factor V. Evidence for a phosphatidylserine binding site in the second C-type domain. *J Biol Chem* 1992;267:4189.

259. Kalafatis M, Jenny RJ, Mann KG. Identification and characterization of a phospholipid-binding site of bovine factor Va. *J Biol Chem* 1990;265: 21580.

260. Krishnaswamy S, Jones KC, Mann KG. Prothrombinase complex assembly: kinetic mechanism of enzyme assembly on phospholipid vesicles. *J Biol Chem* 1988;263:3823.

261. Kalafatis M, Rand MD, Mann KG. The mechanism of inactivation of human factor V and human factor Va by activated protein C. *J Biol Chem* 1994;269:31869.

262. Guinto ER, Esmon CT. Loss of prothrombin and of factor Xa-factor Va interactions upon activation of factor Va by activated protein C. *J Biol Chem* 1984;259:13986.

263. Nesheim ME, Taswell JB, Mann KG. The contribution of bovine factor V and factor Va to the activity of prothrombinase. *J Biol Chem* 1979;254: 10952.

264. Morita T, Iwanaga S. Purification and properties of prothrombin activator from the venom of *Echis carinatus. J Biochem* 1978;83:559.

265. Rhee M-J, Morris S, Kosov DP. Role of meizothrombin and meizothrombin-(des F1) in the conversion of prothrombin to thrombin by the *Echis carinatus* venom coagulant. *Biochemistry* 1982;21:3437.

266. Fortova H, Dyr JE, Vodrazka Z, et al. Isolation of the prothrombin-converting enzyme from fibrinogenolytic enzymes of *Echis carinatus* venom by chromatographic and electrophoretic methods. *J Chromatogr* 1983;259:473.

267. Morita T, Iwanaga S. Prothrombin activator from *Echis carinatus* venom. *Methods Enzymol* 1980;80:303.

268. Doyle MF, Haley PE. Meizothrombin: active intermediate formed during prothrombinase-catalyzed activation of prothrombin. *Methods Enzymol* 1993;222:299.

269. Bjork I, Lindahl U. Mechanism of the anticoagulant action of heparin. *Mol Cell Biochem* 1982;48:161.

270. Rosenberg RD. Chemistry of the hemostatic mechanism and its relationship to the action of heparin. *Fed Proc* 1977;36:10.

271. Kalafatis M, Mann KG. Role of the membrane in the inactivation of factor Va by activated protein C. *J Biol Chem* 1993;268:27246.

272. Bovill EG, Tomczak JA, Grant B, et al. Protein C$_{VERMONT}$: symptomatic type II protein C deficiency associated with two Gla domain mutations. *Blood* 1992;79:1456.

273. Lu D, Bovill EG, Long GL. Molecular mechanism for familial protein C deficiency and thrombosis in protein C$_{Vermont}$ (Glu20 → Ala and Val34 → Met). *J Biol Chem* 1994;269:29032.

274. Lu D, Kalafatis M, Mann KG, et al. Loss of membrane-dependent factor Va cleavage: a mechanistic interpretation of the pathology of protein C$_{VERMONT}$. *Blood* 1994;84:687.

275. Butenas S, van't Veer C, Mann KG. "Normal" thrombin generation. *Blood* 1999;94:2169.

276. Andrew M, Paes B, Milner R, et al. Development of the human coagulation system in the full-term infant. *Blood* 1987;70:165.

277. Andrew M, Vegh P, Johnston M, et al. Maturation of the hemostatic system during childhood. *Blood* 1992;80:1998.

278. Woodward M, Lowe GD, Rumley A, et al. Epidemiology of coagulation factors, inhibitors and activation markers: the third Glasgow MONICA survey. II. Relationships to cardiovascular risk factors and prevalent cardiovascular disease. *Br J Haematol* 1997;97:785.

279. Poort SR, Rosendaal FR, Reitsma PH, et al. A common genetic variation in the 3′-untranslated region of the prothrombin gene is associated with elevated plasma prothrombin levels and an increase in venous thrombosis. *Blood* 1996;88:3698.

280. Reuner KH, Ruf A, Grau A, et al. Prothrombin gene G$_{20210}$ → A transition is a risk factor for cerebral venous thrombosis. *Arterioscler Thromb Vasc Biol* 1998;18:1765.

281. Hillarp A, Zöller B, Svensson PJ, et al. The 20210 A allele of the prothrombin gene is a common risk factor among Swedish outpatients with verified deep venous thrombosis. *Thromb Haemost* 1997;78:990.

282. Ferraresi P, Marchetti G, Legnani C, et al. The heterozygous 20210 G/A prothrombin genotype is associated with early venous thrombosis in inherited thrombophilias and is not increased in frequency in artery disease. *Arterioscler Thromb Vasc Biol* 1997;17:2418.

283. Margaglione M, Brancaccio V, Guiliani N, et al. Increased risk for venous thrombosis in carriers of the prothrombin G → A$^{20210}$ gene variant. *Ann Intern Med* 1998;129:89.

284. Heit JA. The potential role of direct thrombin inhibitors in the prevention and treatment of venous thromboembolism. *Chest* 2003;124(Suppl. 3):40S.

285. Weitz JI. A novel approach to thrombin inhibition. *Thromb Res* 2003; 109:S17.

286. Silverstein MD, Heit JA, Mohr DN, et al. Trends in the incidence of deep vein thrombosis and pulmonary embolism: a 25-year population-based study. *Arch Intern Med* 1998;158:585.

287. Hursting MJ, Alford KL, Becker JC, et al. Novastan (brand of argatroban): a small-molecule, direct thrombin inhibitor. *Semin Thromb Haemost* 1997;23:503.

288. Chackalamannil S. G-protein coupled receptor antagonists-1: protease activated receptor-1 (PAR-1) antagonists as novel cardiovascular therapeutic agents. *Curr Top Med Chem* 2003;3:1115.

289. Ahn HS, Chackalamannil S, Boykow G, et al. Development of proteinase-activated receptor 1 antagonists as therapeutic agents for thrombosis, restenosis and inflammatory diseases. *Curr Pharm Des* 2003;9:2349.

290. Davie EW, Ratnoff OD. Waterfall sequence for intrinsic blood clotting. *Science* 1964;145:1310.

291. MacFarlane RG. An enzyme cascade in the blood clotting mechanism and its function as a biochemical amplifier. *Nature* 1964;202:498.

292. Fenton JW II. Regulation of thrombin generation and functions. *Semin Thromb Hemost* 1988;14:234.

293. Bar-Shavit R, Benezra M, Elder M, et al. Thrombin immobilized to extracellular matrix is a potent mitogen for vascular smooth muscle cells: Nonenzymatic mode of action. *Cell Regul* 1990;1:453.

294. Berk BC, Taubman MB, Cragoe EJ Jr, et al. Thrombin signal transduction mechanisms in rat vascular smooth muscle cells. Calcium and protein kinase C-dependent and -independent pathways. *J Biol Chem* 1990;265: 17334.

295. Michel MC, Brass LF, Williams A, et al. Alpha 2-adrenergic receptor stimulation mobilizes intracellular Ca2+ in human erythroleukemia cells. *J Biol Chem* 1989;264:4986.

296. He CJ, Rondeau E, Metcalf RL, et al. Thrombin increases proliferation and decreases fibrinolytic activity of kidney glomerular epithelial cells. *J Cell Physiol* 1991;146:131.

297. Glenn KC, Carney DH, Fenton JW II, et al. Thrombin active site regions required for fibroblast binding and initiation of cell division. *J Biol Chem* 1980;255:6609.

298. Herbert JM, Lamarche I, Dol F. Induction of vascular smooth muscle cell growth by selective activation of the thrombin receptor: effect of heparin. *FEBS Lett* 1992;301:155.

299. Sago H, Iinuma K. Cell shape change and cytosolic Ca2+ in human umbilical-vein endothelial cells stimulated with thrombin. *Thromb Haemost* 1992;67:331.

300. Cherington PV, Pardee AB. Synergistic effects of epidermal growth factor and thrombin on the growth stimulation of diploid Chinese hamster fibroblasts. *J Cell Physiol* 1980;105:25–32.

301. Gospodarowicz D, Brown KD, Birdwell CR, et al. Control of proliferation of human vascular endothelial cells. Characterization of the response of human umbilical vein endothelial cells to fibroblast growth factor, epidermal growth factor, and thrombin. *J Cell Biol* 1978;77:774.

302. Zetter Br, Antoniades HN. Stimulation of human vascular endothelial cell growth by a platelet-derived growth factor and thrombin. *J Supramol Struct* 1979;11:361.

303. Weiss RH, Nuccitelli R. Inhibition of tyrosine phosphorylation prevents thrombin-induced mitogenesis, but not intracellular free calcium release, in vascular smooth muscle cells. *J Biol Chem* 1992;267:5608.

304. Weiss RH, Maduri M. The mitogenic effect of thrombin in vascular smooth muscle cells in largely due to basic fibroblast growth factor. *J Biol Chem* 1993;268:5724.

305. Harlan JM, Thompson PJ, Ross RR, et al. Alpha-thrombin induces release of platelet-derived growth factor-like molecule(s) by cultured human endothelial cells. *J Cell Biol* 1986;103:1129.

306. Vlodavsky I, Folkman J, Sullivan R, et al. Endothelial cell-derived basic fibroblast growth factor: synthesis and deposition into subendothelial extracellular matrix. *Proc Natl Acad Sci U S A* 1987;84:2292.

307. Ross R, Glomset J, Karlya B, et al. A platelet-dependent serum factor that stimulates the proliferation of arterial smooth muscle cells *in vitro. Proc Natl Acad Sci U S A* 1974;71:107.

308. Majesky MW, Kindmer V, Twardzik DR, et al. Production of transforming growth factor $\beta_1$ during repair of arterial injury. *J Clin Invest* 1991; 88:904.

309. Clinton SK, Dinarello CA, Cannon JG, et al. Induction *in vitro* of interleukin-1 (IL-1) gene expression in rabbit aortic tissue. *Circulation* 1988;78(Suppl. II):II–65.

310. Douglas SA, Louden C, Vickery-Clark LM, et al. A role for endogenous endothelin-1 in neointimal formation after rat carotid artery balloon angioplasty. Protective effects of the novel nonpeptide endothelin receptor antagonist SB 209670. *Circ Res* 1994;75:190.

311. Sigal SL, Gillman J, Sarembock IJ, et al. Effects of serotonin-receptor blockade on angioplasty-induced vasospasm in an atherosclerotic rabbit model. *Arterioscler Thromb* 1991;11:770.

312. Mugge A, Heistad DD, Densen P, et al. Activation of leukocytes with complement C5a is associated with prostanoid-dependent constriction of large arteries in atherosclerotic monkeys *in vivo. Atherosclerosis* 1992; 95:211.

313. Seino Y, Ikeda U, Ikeda M, et al. Interleukin 6 gene transcripts are expressed in human atherosclerotic lesions. *Cytokine* 1994;6:87.

314. McNamara CA, Sarembock IJ, Bachhuber BG, et al. Thrombin and vascular smooth muscle cell proliferation: implications for atherosclerosis and restenosis. *Semin Thromb Hemost* 1996;22:139.

315. Malik AB, Fenton JW II. Thrombin-mediated increase in vascular endothelial permeability. *Semin Thromb Hemost* 1992;18:193.

316. Sugama Y, Malik AB. Thrombin receptor 14-amino acid peptide mediates endothelial hyperactivity and neutrophil adhesion by P-selectin-dependent mechanism. *Circ Res* 1992;71:1015.

317. Hollenberg MD, Yang SG, Laniyonu AA, et al. Action of thrombin receptor polypeptide in gastric smooth muscle: identification of a core pentapeptide retaining full thrombin-mimetic intrinsic activity. *Mol Pharmacol* 1992;42:186.

318. Vouret-Craviari V, Van Obberghen-Schilling E, Rasmussen UB, et al. Synthetic alpha-thrombin receptor peptides activate G protein-coupled signaling pathways but are unable to induce mitogenesis. *Mol Cell Biol* 1992;3:95.

319. Tsopanoglou NE, Pipili-Synetos E, Maragoudakis ME. Thrombin promotes angiogenesis by a mechanism independent of fibrin formation. *Am J Physiol* 1993;264:C1302.

320. Haralabopoulos GC, Grant DS, Kleinman HK, et al. Thrombin promotes endothelial cell alignment in Matrigel *in vitro* and angiogenesis *in vivo*. *Am J Physiol* 1997;273:C239.

321. Folkman J. Tumor angiogenesis. *Adv Cancer Res* 1985;43:175.

322. Tsopanoglou NE, Maragoudakis ME. On the mechanism of thrombin-induced angiogenesis. Potentiation of vascular endothelial growth factor activity on endothelial cells by up-regulation of its receptors. *J Biol Chem* 1999;274:23969.

323. Ferrara N, Davis-Smyth T. The biology of vascular endothelial growth factor. *Endocr Rev* 1997;18:4.

324. Gustafson GT, Lerner U. Thrombin, a stimulator of bone resorption. *Biosci Rep* 1983;3:255.

325. Donovan FM, Pike CJ, Cotman CW, et al. Thrombin induces apoptosis in cultured neurons and astrocytes via a pathway requiring tyrosine kinase and RhoA activities. *J Neurosci* 1997;17:5316.

326. Turgeon VL, Lloyd ED, Wang S, et al. Thrombin perturbs neurite outgrowth and induces apoptotic cell death in enriched chick spinal motoneuron cultures through caspase activation. *J Neurosci* 1998;18:6882.

327. Smirnova IV, Shang SX, Citron BA, et al. Thrombin is an extracellular signal that activates intracellular death protease pathways inducing apoptosis in model motor neurons. *J Neurobiol* 1998;36:L64.

328. Gurwitz D, Cunningham DD. Thrombin modulates and reverses neuroblastoma neurite outgrowth. *Proc Natl Acad Sci U S A* 1988;85:3440.

329. Chinni C, de Niese MR, Tew DJ, et al. Thrombin, a survival factor for cultured myoblasts. *J Biol Chem* 1999;274:9169.

330. Liu Y, Fields RD, Festoff BW, et al. Proteolytic action of thrombin is required for electrical activity-dependent synapse reduction. *Proc Natl Acad Sci U S A* 1994;91:10300.

331. Zoubine MN, Ma JY, Smirnova IV, et al. A molecular mechanism for synapse elimination: novel inhibition of locally generated thrombin delays synapse loss in neonatal mouse muscle. *Dev Biol* 1996;179:447.

332. Citron BA, Smirnova IV, Zoubine MN, et al. Quantitative PCR analysis reveals novel expression of prothrombin mRNA and regulation of its levels in developing mouse muscle. *Thromb Res* 1997;87:303.

333. Glazner GW, Yadav K, Fitzgerald S, et al. Cholinergic stimulation increases thrombin activity and gene expression in cultured mouse muscle. *Brain Res Dev Brain Res* 1997;99:148.

334. Suidan HS, Niclou SP, Dreessen J, et al. The thrombin receptor is present in myoblasts and its expression is repressed upon fusion. *J Biol Chem* 1996;271:29162.

335. Abraham LA, Jenkins AL, Stone SR, et al. Expression of the thrombin receptor in developing bone and associated tissues. *J Bone Miner Res* 1998;13:818.

# CHAPTER 11 ■ PROTEIN Z AND PROTEIN Z–DEPENDENT PROTEASE INHIBITOR

GEORGE J. BROZE, JR.

In 1977, Prowse and Esnouf identified an additional vitamin K–dependent protein circulating in bovine plasma and named it protein Z (PZ) because it was the last of the vitamin K–dependent proteins to elute during anion exchange chromatography (1). PZ serves as a cofactor for the inhibition of factor Xa by another plasma protein called protein Z–dependent protease inhibitor (ZPI) (2). ZPI is a member of the serpin superfamily of proteinase inhibitors and not only inhibits factor Xa in a PZ–dependent fashion, but also inhibits factor XIa in the absence of PZ (3,4). The physiologic importance of the regulation of coagulation by PZ and ZPI is not yet clear and is the focus of ongoing research.

## PROTEIN Z

### Structure

The human counterpart to bovine PZ was isolated in 1984 (5). Mature human PZ is a 62,000–molecular weight, 360–amino acid, single-chain glycoprotein whose structure is very similar to the other vitamin K–dependent proteins, factors VII, IX, X, and protein C (see Fig. 11-1) (5–7). A prepro-leader sequence directs the vitamin K–dependent γ-carboxylation of 13 glutamic acid residues within an N-terminal γ-carboxyglutamic acid (Gla) domain that is followed by two epidermal growth factor (EGF)–like domains and a C-terminal pseudocatalytic domain. PZ contains five potential N-linked glycosylation sites (Fig. 11-1). In the first EGF-like domain, a disaccharide or trisaccharide is attached to Ser53, and Asp64 is probably a β-hydroxyaspartic acid residue (8,9). Two "extra" cysteine residues are present in PZ, but it is not determined whether they form a disulfide bond. In contrast to other coagulation factors that are serine proteinase zymogens, in PZ, the region around the typical "activation site" is absent and the histidine and serine residues of the canonical catalytic triad have been replaced with lysine and aspartic acid residues, respectively (7,9). The active site aspartic acid residue is conserved. Therefore, like protein S, PZ does not serve a proteolytic function.

The PZ gene is at chromosome 13q34, the location where the genes for factor VII and factor X reside side by side (10). It spans 14 kb and consists of nine exons, including an alternatively spliced exon that inserts a unique peptide of 22 amino acids in the prepro-leader sequence of PZ. The exon–intron organization of the PZ gene is identical to that of factors VII, IX, X, and protein C, indicating that these genes were derived from a common ancestor during evolution (Fig. 11-1) (10). Several polymorphisms have been identified in the PZ gene, including one in the promoter (a-13g) and one in exon 8 that leads to Arg255His replacement in the encoded protein (11).

A polymorphism in intron A (g103a) and a polymorphism in intron F (g79a), which is in a high degree of linkage disequilibrium with the a-13g and Arg255His polymorphisms, are associated with reduced plasma levels of PZ (12,13).

## Properties

The range of PZ plasma levels in normal individuals is very broad (95% interval of 32% to 168% of the mean) and appears to be influenced predominantly by heritable factors (13–15). Reported mean concentrations of PZ in adult plasmas have varied from 1.2 to 2.9 $\mu$g per mL, but the reason for this discrepancy is not obvious. PZ circulates in plasma complexed with ZPI (see subsequent text).

Similar to other coagulation factors, the liver appears to be the major source of PZ. The level of PZ is reduced in individuals with severe liver disease and is low in newborn infants (16,17). Oral contraceptive use substantially increases PZ levels (18). Plasma PZ is reportedly increased with chronic hemodialysis and reduced in the nephrotic syndrome (19,20). Whether PZ behaves as a negative acute-phase reactant is controversial (19,21). Immunoreactive PZ has been detected in atherosclerotic plaques (22).

In contrast to other plasma vitamin K–dependent proteins, the coumarin class of oral anticoagulants dramatically affects levels of PZ. For example, in patients on stable warfarin therapy, levels of antigenic and γ-carboxylated PZ are 8% ± 4% and 1% ± 2%, respectively, in comparison to levels of antigenic and γ-carboxylated protein C of 53 ± 8 and 28 ± 6 (14). The interaction of PZ with phospholipid vesicles also differs distinctively from that of the other vitamin K–dependent coagulation factors. Although the ultimate binding affinity of PZ is comparable to that of the other proteins, its association (3.4 $10^{-5}$ per second M) and dissociation (0.06 per second) rate constants are markedly slower (23).

Despite its isolation, the physiologic function of PZ remained an enigma for many years. Bovine PZ was shown to interact with diisopropylphosphoryl (DIP)-inactivated thrombin ($K_d$ = 0.15 $\mu$M) and mediate the binding of DIP-thrombin to phospholipids (24). Human PZ, however, binds thrombin poorly ($K_d$ = 8.9 $\mu$M) and has a minimal impact on thrombin's association with phospholipids (25). Additional studies showed that the enhanced binding of thrombin to bovine PZ requires the 36–amino acid C-terminal extension present in bovine but absent in human PZ (25). Thrombin cleavage of bovine PZ at Arg365 releases this C-terminal peptide (25,26).

Subsequently, it was noted that the procoagulant activity of factor Xa in a one-stage plasma coagulation assay was reduced if factor Xa was first incubated with PZ (2). This inhibitory effect of PZ required the presence of phospholipids

215

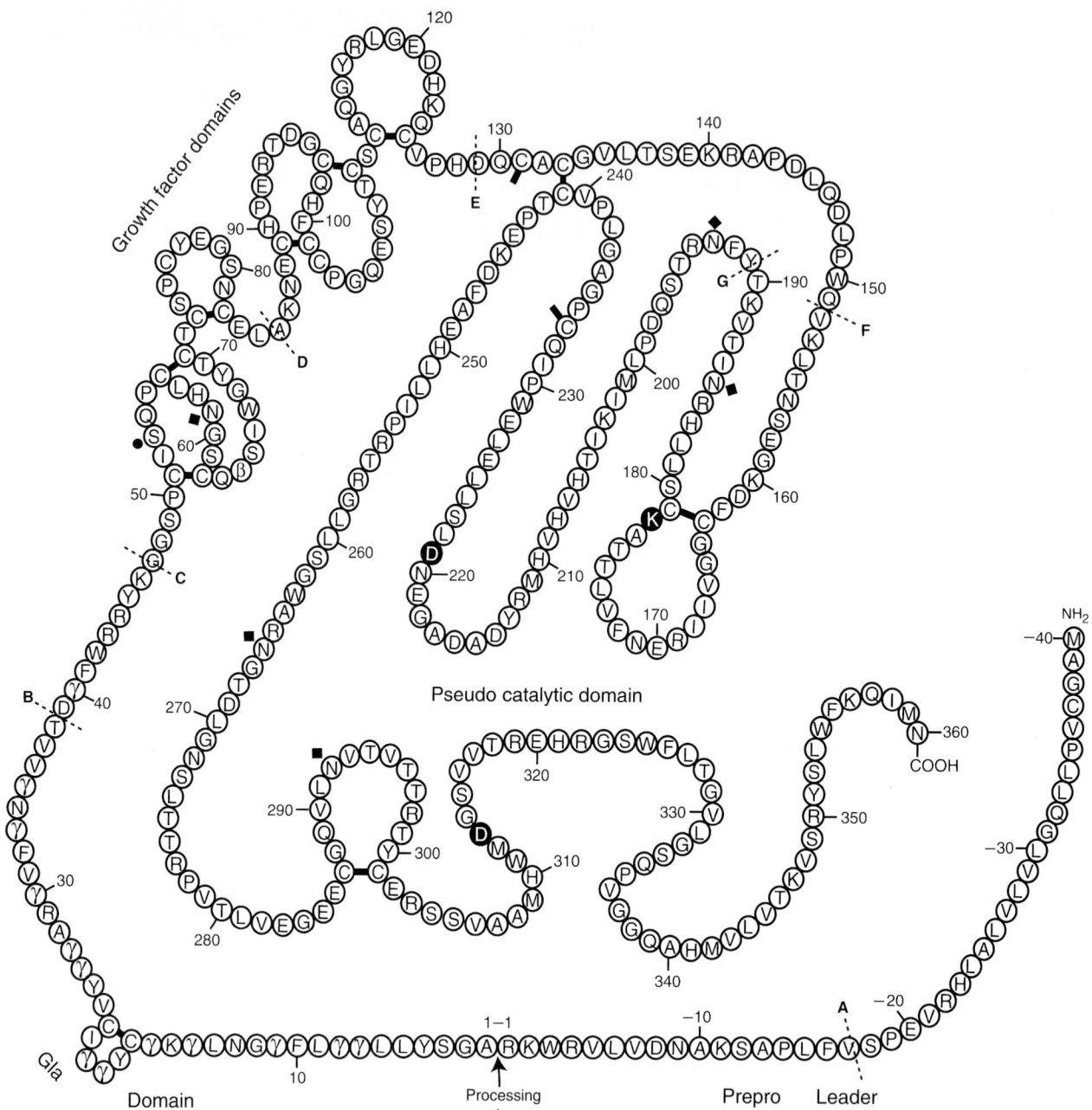

**FIGURE 11-1.** Amino acid sequence of protein Z. Disulfide bonds have been placed by analogy to other vitamin K–dependent proteins. Cysteine residues at positions 131 and 233 are not present in the homologous vitamin K–dependent proteins. *Solid diamonds* indicate potential N-linked glycosylation sites. The *solid circle* denotes site of a disaccharide or trisaccharide linked to Ser53. *Shaded* residues are sites of amino acids involved in the catalytic triad of serine proteases. *Dashed lines* indicate intron–exon boundaries (27). γ, γ-carboxyglutamic acid; β, potential β-hydroxyaspartic acid at residue 64. (Modified from Ichinose A, Davie E. The blood coagulation factors: their cDNAs, genes, and expression. In: Colman R, Hirsh J, Marder V, et al., eds. *Hemostasis and thrombosis: basic principles and clinical practice.* Philadelphia, PA: JB Lippincott Co, 1994:19–54, with permission.)

and Ca$^{2+}$ ions and was time dependent, apparently reflecting the slow association of PZ with phospholipids (23). PZ that was proteolytically cleaved at Arg43, thereby separating its Gla domain from the remainder of the molecule, lacked inhibitory activity (2). These results suggested that an interaction between factor Xa and PZ occurs at the phospholipid surface, and additional studies showed that the inhibitory effect of PZ on factor Xa activity in the one-stage coagulation assay was due, at least in part, to a plasma ZPI that recognizes the factor Xa–PZ complex (2).

# PROTEIN Z–DEPENDENT PROTEASE INHIBITOR

## Structure

ZPI was isolated from human plasma in 1998 and shown to be a previously unidentified, 72,000–molecular weight, single-chain glycoprotein (2). ZPI cDNA is 2.44 kb in length and has

◇

| | | | | | | | | | | | | | | | | | | | | | | | | | | | | | | | | | | | | | | | | | | | | | |
|---|---|---|---|---|---|---|---|---|---|---|---|---|---|---|---|---|---|---|---|---|---|---|---|---|---|---|---|---|---|---|---|---|---|---|---|---|---|---|---|---|---|---|---|---|---|---|
ZPI | E R G T E A V A G I L S E I T A Y S M P P - - - V I K V D R P F H F M I Y E E T S G M L L F L G R V V N P T L L
RASP-1 | E R G T E V V S G T V S E I T A Y C M P P - - - V I K V D R P F H F I I Y E E M S R M L L F L G R V V N P T V L
α1AT | E K G T E A A G A M F L E A I P M S I P P - - - E V K F N K P F V F L M I E Q N T K S P L F M G K V V N P T Q K
AT | E E G S E A A A S T A V V I A G R S L N P N R V T F K A N R P F L V F I R E V P L N T I I F M G R V A N P C V K
HC-II | E E G T Q A T T V T T V G F M P L S T Q V - - - R F T V D R P F L F L I Y E H R T S C L L F M G R V A N P S R S
PN-1 | E D G T K A S A A T T A I L I A R S S P P - - - W F I V D R P F L F F I R H N P T G A V L F M G Q I N K P

**FIGURE 11-2.** Carboxy-terminal sequences of protein Z–dependent protease inhibitor (ZPI) and other serpins. *Diamond* denotes $P_1$–$P_1'$ cleavage site. Residues identical to ZPI are indicated in *bold* type. Rasp-1, rat regeneration-associated serpin protein; $\alpha_1$AT, $\alpha_1$-antitrypsin; AT, antithrombin; HC-II, heparin cofactor-II; and PN-1, protease nexin-1.

a relatively long 5′ region (466 nt) that contains six potential ATG translation start codons (3). ATGs 1 to 4 are followed by short, open reading frames, whereas ATG5 and ATG6 are in an uninterrupted open reading frame that includes the encoded ZPI protein. *In vitro* experiments show that ATG6 is sufficient for the expression of rZPI in cultured Chinese hamster ovary (CHO) cells. Northern analysis suggests that the liver is the major site of ZPI synthesis (3). The predicted 423 residue amino acid sequence of mature ZPI is 25% to 35% homologous with members of the serpin superfamily of protease inhibitors and is 78% identical to the amino acid sequence predicted by a previously described cDNA isolated from rat liver, regeneration-associated serpin protein-1 (rasp-1) (28). Therefore, ZPI is likely the human homolog of rat rasp-1, which was identified as a gene whose transcription is increased following subtotal hepatectomy in rats (28). Alignment of the amino acid sequence of ZPI with those of other serpins predicts that Tyr387 is the $P_1$ residue at the reactive center of the ZPI molecule (see Fig. 11-2). Consistent with this notion, rZPI(Tyr387Ala), an altered form of ZPI in which tyrosine 387 has been changed to alanine, lacks PZ-dependent factor Xa inhibitory activity (3).

## Properties

Although less marked than PZ, plasma levels of ZPI also span a broad range (95% interval 46% to 154% of the mean) with a mean concentration of ZPI of approximately 4.0 μg per mL (9). PZ and ZPI form a complex and in pooled normal plasma, which contains excess ZPI, all the PZ appears to be bound to ZPI (29). Therefore, an early report that found a $t_{1/2}$ of 2 to 3 days for PZ in plasma was likely studying the clearance of the PZ–ZPI complex (14). The plasma level of ZPI is related to the level of PZ: Oral contraceptive use raises both PZ (approximately 35%) and ZPI (approximately 17%) levels, whereas warfarin treatment reduces PZ (approximately 92%) and ZPI (approximately 53%) levels (18). This interrelation of plasma concentrations of PZ and ZPI might be explained if the rate of clearance of the PZ–ZPI complex differs from that of PZ or ZPI alone. Alternatively, the synthesis, secretion, or extraplasma localization of one of these proteins may be affected by the presence of the other.

## PROTEIN Z AND PROTEIN Z–DEPENDENT PROTEASE INHIBITOR FUNCTION

### Factor Xa Inhibition

In the presence of phospholipids and $Ca^{2+}$, the rate of factor Xa inhibition by ZPI is enhanced greater than 1,000-fold ($t_{1/2}$ <10 seconds vs. 210 minutes) by preincubation of factor Xa with PZ (3,4). Indirect evidence strongly suggests that the inhibitory process involves the formation of a stoichiometric complex of factor Xa-ZPI-PZ at the phospholipid surface (3,4). Heparin does not affect ZPI-mediated inhibition of factor Xa in the presence of PZ. The combination of PZ and ZPI dramatically delays the initiation and reduces the ultimate rate of thrombin generation in mixtures containing prothrombin, factor V, phospholipids, and $Ca^{2+}$ (4). In similar mixtures containing factor Va, however, PZ and ZPI do not inhibit thrombin generation. Therefore, the anti–factor Xa action of PZ and ZPI presumably must precede the activation of factor V and the formation of the prothrombinase complex. With coagulation induced in plasma by factor IXa, the presence of PZ delays the onset and the extent of thrombin production (30).

PZ is not the only protein that has been shown to function as a cofactor to enhance the inhibitory activity of a serpin toward an enzyme. Thrombomodulin increases the rate of thrombin inhibition by protein C inhibitor approximately 140-fold (31). This effect of thrombomodulin reportedly depends primarily on the interaction between thrombin and thrombomodulin. Vitronectin increases the rate of thrombin inhibition by plasminogen activator inhibitor-1 (PAI-1) approximately 200-fold (32). Vitronectin appears to produce this enhancement by both binding PAI-1, thereby inducing a conformational change at its reactive center, and through a protein–protein interaction with thrombin. Similarly, the cofactor action of PZ presumably involves its ability both to bind and to bring ZPI to the phospholipid surface, as well as its ability to interact with factor Xa at this surface (2,29).

Two potential pathways for PZ–dependent factor Xa inhibition by ZPI are shown in Figure 11-3. On the left, PZ and

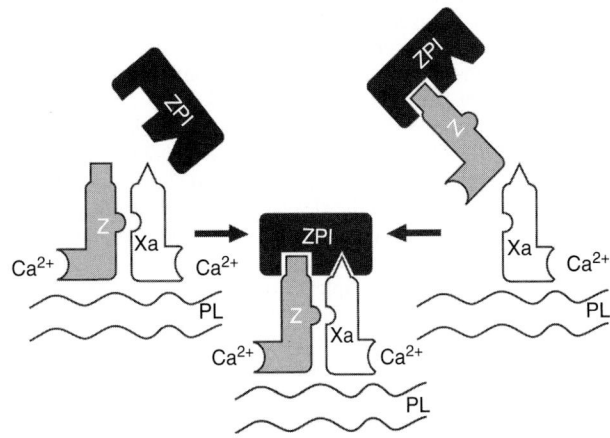

**FIGURE 11-3.** Two pathways for the inhibition of factor Xa by protein Z–dependent protease inhibitor (ZPI) with protein Z (PZ). On the left, ZPI binds to a preformed PZ–factor Xa complex at the phospholipid surface. On the right, the circulating PZ–ZPI complex binds to factor Xa at the phospholipid surface. Both pathways result in a final inhibitory complex containing PZ-factor Xa-ZPI. PL, phospholipid surface; $Ca^{2+}$ denotes $Ca^{2+}$-dependent binding of factor Xa and PZ to the phospholipid surface (33). (Reproduced from Broze G, Jr. Protein Z and thrombosis. *Lancet* 2001;357:900–901, with permission.)

factor Xa first form a complex at the phospholipid surface, and this complex is subsequently recognized by ZPI. On the right, a preformed PZ–ZPI complex is directed to the phospholipid surface by its PZ moiety and binds factor Xa. The final result of either pathway is the formation of a $Ca^{2+}$-dependent complex at the phospholipid surface that contains PZ, factor Xa, and ZPI. Because PZ circulates bound to ZPI, the pathway on the right presumably reflects the inhibitory mechanism that occurs in the plasma milieu.

## Factor XIa Inhibition

ZPI also inactivates factor XIa in a reaction that does not require the presence of PZ, phospholipids, or $Ca^{2+}$, and that is not affected by the presence of high-molecular-weight kininogen (4). Heparin increases the rate and extent of factor XIa inhibition produced by ZPI (4), whereas factor XIa inhibition by ZPI is reduced when ZPI is bound to PZ (29). An apparent interaction between factor XIa and ZPI can be detected in the plasma milieu (see subsequent text), suggesting that ZPI competes effectively with other factor XIa inhibitors (e.g., $\alpha_1$-antitrypsin, $C_1$ esterase inhibitor, antithrombin) and the substrate factor IX in plasma for the active site of factor XIa.

## Instability of Protein Z–Dependent Protease Inhibitor–Proteinase Complexes

As is typical for members of the serpin superfamily of proteinase inhibitors, ZPI is proteolytically cleaved during its inhibition of factor Xa and factor XIa with a reduction in its size from 72 kDa to 68 kDa. The N-terminal amino acid sequences of the peptides (4.2-kDa) released from ZPI following its interaction with factor Xa and factor XIa are identical, SMPPVIKVDRPF, and correspond to the amino acid sequence in the ZPI molecule following Tyr387 (4). Therefore, the reactive center of ZPI that is involved in its inactivation of both factors Xa and XIa is Tyr387-Ser388 ($P_1$-$P_1'$).

The factor Xa–ZPI and factor XIa–ZPI inhibitory complexes, however, are dramatically less stable than other protease-serpin complexes. In contrast to the thrombin–antithrombin interaction, for example, the factor Xa–ZPI and factor XIa–ZPI complexes do not survive sodium dodecyl (lauryl) surfate-polyacrylamide gel electrophoresis (SDS-PAGE) but can be detected in the less denaturing conditions of native-PAGE (without SDS) (4). Dissociation of the thrombin–antithrombin complex is very slow (approximately $2.5 \times 10^{-6}$ per second) and appears to proceed exclusively through the cleavage of antithrombin (34). Dissociation of the factor Xa–ZPI complex is much more rapid (approximately $1.7 \times 10^{-4}$ per second) and likely also occurs through the cleavage of ZPI (4). In this regard, therefore, ZPI behaves as a very poor substrate for the factor Xa-PZ- phospholipid-$Ca^{2+}$ complex and for factor XIa. In view of the instability of the complexes of factor Xa and factor XIa with ZPI, it seems likely that these proteinases would ultimately be transferred from ZPI to alternative proteinase inhibitors.

## Consumption of Protein Z–Dependent Protease Inhibitor During Coagulation

Serum produced from plasma *in vitro* by the induction of coagulation with kaolin, phospholipids, and $Ca^{2+}$, or tissue factor and $Ca^{2+}$, contains little ZPI functional activity. Western blot analysis shows that during coagulation of plasma *in vitro*, ZPI is proteolytically cleaved at its C-terminus with reduction in its apparent molecular weight from 72 kDa to 68 kDa (4). Factor Xa, in the presence of PZ, is responsible for the consumption of ZPI in tissue factor–induced coagulation. Factor XIa also contributes, however, when coagulation is initiated by direct contact activation (e.g., kaolin) and relatively large concentrations of factor XIa are generated (4).

# PROTEIN Z/PROTEIN Z–DEPENDENT PROTEASE INHIBITOR AND CLINICAL COAGULATION

## Protein Z and Hemorrhage

It has been suggested that PZ deficiency is associated with a hemorrhagic disorder, perhaps related to capillary fragility (35). Thirty-six individuals with bleeding disorders of unknown etiology were studied. Many of these individuals had a positive Rumpel-Leede test (83%) and a prolonged bleeding time (43%). The mean PZ level in the patients was 54% (range 22% to 112%). In additional studies, prothrombin complex concentrates, which contain PZ, have been used to prevent perioperative hemorrhage in individuals with a bleeding history and perceived PZ deficiency (36,37). Two subsequent studies, however, have failed to detect a relation between PZ deficiency and a bleeding tendency (38,39), and it should be noted that 10% of apparently healthy individuals (Red Cross blood donors) have PZ levels of less than 50% (14). Further, PZ-null mice have normal bleeding times and do not have a hemorrhagic phenotype (30,40). Therefore, a clear relation between low levels of PZ and a hemorrhagic diathesis remains to be established.

## Protein Z and Thrombosis

Unchallenged, PZ knockout mice do not express an obvious phenotype. When combined with the homozygous factor $V_{Leiden}$ ($FV^{\lambda/\lambda}$) genotype, however, the $PZ^{-/-}$ genotype causes intrauterine and perinatal thrombosis and an apparent consumptive coagulopathy that leads to near absolute mortality (30). The genetic combinations $FV^{\lambda/\lambda}/PZ^{+/-}$ and $FV^{\lambda/+}/PZ^{-/-}$ also reduce the survival of mice by greater than 50%. It should be noted that the factor $V_{Leiden}$ genotype appears to produce a more severe thrombotic phenotype in mice than the factor $V_{Leiden}$ genotype in humans. Nevertheless, the results of the murine $PZ \times FV_{Leiden}$ crosses strongly suggest that PZ deficiency is a prothrombotic trait and are consistent with human data showing that a combination of prothrombotic traits significantly increases the risk of thrombosis.

Studies exploring the association between PZ levels and ischemic stroke have produced conflicting results (13,41–45). In a group of 169 young patients (mean age 33 years) without hypertension or dyslipidemia, Vasse et al. found that low convalescent PZ levels (<15th percentile) were associated with a fourfold increased risk of stroke (41). Heeb et al. studying 154 older individuals (median age 58 years), reported that low PZ (<15th percentile) was associated with an increased risk of stroke in men [odds ratio (OR), 3.6; 95% confidence intervals (CI), 1.5 to 4.3] and those aged above 58 years (OR, 2.6; 95% CI, 1.4 to 4.9) (43). They (Heeb et al.) found that the risk of stroke associated with a low PZ was most apparent in individuals without diabetes, hypertension, or hypercholesterolemia, and other risk factors for stroke.

In contrast, Kobelt et al. reported an association of high PZ levels with stroke in a group of 125 patients (mean age 40 years) without a history of venous thrombosis (42). After adjusting for possible confounders (age, sex, hypertension, diabetes, smoking, body mass index, hyperlipidemia, and fibrinogen), the risk of stroke in individuals with PZ in the highest quartile (>150%) versus the lowest quartile (<76%) was 2.5-fold (95% CI, 1.05 to 5.72). Lichy et al. analyzed the PZ intron F g79a polymorphism in a group of 200 patients with stroke and found that the presence of at least one "a" allele is associated with a reduced risk of stroke (OR, 0.6; 95% CI, 0.4 to 0.95) after adjusting for age, sex, hypertension, hypercholesterolemia, and family history (13). They also noted a significant relation between the "a" allele and reduced PZ plasma levels in healthy individuals, implying that lower levels of PZ may protect against stroke. In this study of individuals from southwest Germany, the genotypes of 30% (60/200) of the stroke cases and 41% (81/199) of the healthy controls contained at least one "a." Interestingly, the prevalence of the intron F "a" allele in an Italian population is 37%, whereas in an English population it appears to be much lower, 20% (11,12). Because the intron F g79a polymorphism is unlikely to directly affect PZ expression, its association with PZ levels may reflect the effect of a separate polymorphism with which it is in a high degree of linkage disequilibrium.

Two additional studies detected no relation between stroke and convalescent PZ levels (44,45). McQuillan et al. however, reported that significantly higher PZ levels were found in plasma samples from patients with stroke, taken within 7 days of the acute event (45). In contrast, Fedi et al. found an association between low PZ levels (<15th percentile) and the acute coronary syndrome (OR, 3.3; 95% CI, 1.1 to 9.7) that was increased further by concomitant smoking (OR, 9.5; 95% CI, 2.4 to 37.2) (46). Low plasma concentrations of PZ have also been reported in ischemic colitis (47).

In regard to venous thrombosis, one study did not find a relation with low levels of PZ in a small cohort of patients (41), and another study, in which PZ levels were not determined, failed to detect a relation with polymorphisms within the PZ gene (11). A report (48) that low PZ affects the age of onset and the severity of thrombosis in patients with the factor $V_{Leiden}$ mutation was not confirmed in a later study (18). Recent results from the Leiden Thrombophilia Study (LETS) showed a modestly increased risk of venous thrombosis with low PZ (<10th percentile) in men (OR, 2.4; 95% CI, 1.2 to 4.9) and older individuals (>55 years, OR, 3.3; 95% CI, 1.2 to 8.7) on subgroup analysis (18). These same groups, men and older individuals, are those in which Heeb et al. found an association between low PZ (<15th percentile) and ischemic stroke (43). A mechanism, however, to explain why younger women may be protected from the thrombotic risk associated with low levels of PZ is lacking. In LETS, neither high nor low concentrations of ZPI were related to venous thrombosis (43).

Low levels (<5th percentile) of PZ are common in individuals with antiphospholipid antibodies and are associated with the thrombotic complications and fetal wastage of the antiphospholipid syndrome (OR, 6.6; 95% CI, 2.3 to 19.4) (49–51). Reduced levels of PZ (<15th percentile) are also associated with early miscarriage in the absence of antiphospholipid antibodies (OR, 6.7; 95% CI, 3.1 to 14.8) and maternal anti-PZ antibodies are reportedly related to early fetal death and other pregnancy complications (52–54).

In sum, available clinical data provide a conflicting picture of the role of PZ (and ZPI) in thrombotic disease. That PZ and ZPI produce potent inhibition of factor Xa suggests that deficiencies of these proteins could be associated with a procoagulant state, and the results of the studies in $PZ^{-/-} \times$ factor $V_{Leiden}$ mice appear to confirm this notion (2,30). On the other hand, certain clinical studies report that high levels of PZ predispose to stroke or that low levels of PZ may protect from stroke (13,42). The biologic foundation for these latter results is not readily apparent. The frequently offered explanation of effect of bovine PZ on the binding of inactive thrombin to phospholipids does not hold for active thrombin or human PZ (13,24–26,35,42). Finally, it must be noted that the very broad range of the plasma levels of PZ

and ZPI implies that their plasma concentrations need not be maintained near their population means for a critical physiologic purpose. This suggests that isolated low or high plasma levels of these proteins are unlikely to produce a dramatic pathologic effect and/or, alternatively, that the physiologically important roles of PZ and ZPI occur outside the plasma milieu. Only additional investigation will clarify these issues.

## References

1. Prowse C, Esnouf M. The isolation of a new warfarin-sensitive protein from bovine plasma. *Biochem Soc Trans* 1977;5:255–256.
2. Han X, Fiehler R, Broze G Jr. Isolation of a protein Z-dependent plasma protease inhibitor. *Proc Natl Acad Sci U S A* 1998;97:6734–6738.
3. Han X, Huang Z-F, Fiehler R, et al. The protein Z-dependent protease inhibitor is a serpin. *Biochemistry* 1999;38:11073–11078.
4. Han X, Fiehler R, Broze G Jr. Characterization of protein Z-dependent protease inhibitor. *Blood* 2000;96:3049–3055.
5. Broze G Jr, Miletich J. Human protein Z. *J Clin Invest* 1984;73:933–938.
6. Sejima H, Hayashi T, Deyashiki Y, et al. Primary structure of vitamin K-dependent human protein Z. *Biochem Biophys Res Commun* 1990;171:661–668.
7. Ichinose A, Takeya H, Espling E, et al. Amino acid sequence of human protein Z, a vitamin K-dependent plasma glycoprotein. *Biochem Biophys Res Commun* 1990;172:1139–1144.
8. Nishimura H, Kawabata S, Kisiel W, et al. Identification of a disaccharide (Xyl-Glc) and a trisaccharide (Xyl2-Glc) O-glycosidically linked to a serine residue in the first epidermal growth factor–like domain of human factors VII and IX and human protein Z and bovine protein Z. *J Biol Chem* 1989;264:20320–20325.
9. Hojrup P, Jensen M, Petersen T. Amino acid sequence of bovine protein Z. A vitamin K-dependent serine protease homologue. *FEBS Lett* 1985;184:333–338.
10. Fujimaki K, Yamzaki T, Masafumi T, et al. The gene for human protein Z is localized to chromosome 13 at band q34 and is coded by eight regular exons and one alternative exon. *Biochemistry* 1998;37:6838–6846.
11. Rice G, Futers S, Grant P. Identification of novel polymorphisms within the protein Z gene, haplotype distribution and linkage analysis. *Thromb Haemost* 2001;85:1023–1024.
12. Santacroce R, Cappucci F, Di Perna P, et al. Protein Z gene polymorphisms are associated with protein Z plasma levels. *J Thromb Haemost* 2004;2:1197–1199.
13. Lichy C, Sropp S, Song-Si T, et al. A common polymorphism of the protein Z gene is associated with protein Z plasma levels and with risk of cerebral ischemia in the young. *Stroke* 2003;35:40–45.
14. Miletich J, Broze G Jr. Human plasma protein Z antigen: range in normal subjects and effect of warfarin therapy. *Blood* 1987;69:1580–1586.
15. Vossen C, Hasstedt S, Rosendaal F, et al. Heritability of plasma concentrations of clotting factors and measures of a prethrombotic state in a protein C–deficient family. *J Thromb Haemost* 2004;2:242–247.
16. Kemkes-Matthes B, Matthes K. Protein Z, a new haemostatic factor, in liver disease. *Haemostasis* 1995;25:312–316.
17. Yurdakok M, Gurakan B, Ozbag E, et al. Plasma protein Z levels in healthy newborn infants. *Am J Hematol* 1995;48:206–207.
18. Al-Shanqeeti A, van Hycklama A, Berntorp E, et al. Protein Z and protein Z–dependent protease inhibitor: determinants of levels and risk of venous thrombosis. *Thromb Haemost* 2005;93:411–413.
19. Usalan C, Erdem Y, Altun B, et al. Protein Z levels in haemodialysis patients. *Int Urol Nephrol* 1999;31:541–545.
20. Malyszko J, Malyszko S, Mysliwiec M. Markers of endothelial cell injury and thrombin activatable fibrinolysis inhibitor in nephrotic syndrome. *Blood Coagul Fibrinolysis* 2002;13:615–621.
21. Vasse M, Denoyelle C, Legrand E, et al. Weak regulation of protein Z biosynthesis by inflammatory cytokines. *Thromb Haemost* 2002;87:350–351.
22. Greten J, Kreis I, Liliensiek B, et al. Localisation of protein Z in vascular lesions of patients with atherosclerosis. *Vasa* 1998;27:144–148.
23. McDonald J, Shah A, Schwalbe R, et al. Comparison of naturally occurring vitamin K–dependent proteins: correlation of amino acid sequences and membrane binding properties suggests a membrane contact site. *Biochemistry* 1997;36:5120–5127.
24. Hogg P, Stenflo J. Interaction of vitamin K–dependent protein Z with thrombin. *J Biol Chem* 1990;266:10953–10958.
25. Hogg P, Stenflo J. Interaction of human protein Z with thrombin: evaluation of the species difference in the interaction between bovine and human protein Z and thrombin. *Biochem Biophys Res Commun* 1991;178:801–807.
26. Morita T, Kaetsu H, Mizuguchi J, et al. A characteristic property of vitamin K–dependent plasma protein Z. *J Biochem* 1988;104:368–374.
27. Ichinose A, Davie E. The blood coagulation factors: their cDNAs, genes, and expression. In: Colman R, Hirsh J, Marder V, et al., eds. *Hemostasis and thrombosis: basic principles and clinical practice.* Philadelphia, PA: JB Lippincott Co, 1994:19–54.

28. New L, Liu K, Kamali V, et al. cDNA cloning of rasp-1, a novel gene encoding a plasma protein associated with liver regeneration. *Biochem Biophys Res Commun* 1996;223:404–412.
29. Tabatabai A, Fiehler R, Broze G Jr. Protein Z circulates in plasma in a complex with protein Z–dependent protease inhibitor. *Thromb Haemost* 2001;85:655–660.
30. Yin Z-F, Huang Z-F, Cui J, et al. Prothrombotic phenotype of protein Z deficiency. *Proc Natl Acad Sci U S A* 2000;97:6734–6738.
31. Rezaie A, Copper S, Church F, et al. Protein C inhibitor is a potent inhibitor of the thrombin-thrombomodulin complex. *J Biol Chem* 1995;270:25336–25339.
32. Ehrlich H, Gebbink R, Keijer J, et al. Alteration of serpin specificity by a protein cofactor: vitronectin endows plasminogen activator with thrombin inhibitory properties. *J Biol Chem* 1990;265:13029–13035.
33. Broze G Jr. Protein Z and thrombosis. *Lancet* 2001;357:900–901.
34. Danielsson A, Bjork I. Properties of antithrombin-thrombin complex formed in the presence and absence of heparin. *Biochem J* 1983;213:345–353.
35. Kemkes-Matthes B, Matthes K. Protein Z deficiency: a new cause of bleeding tendency. *Thromb Res* 1995;79:49–55.
36. Greten J, Kemkes-Matthes B, Nawroth P. Prothrombin complex concentrate contains protein Z and prevents bleeding in a patient with protein Z deficiency. *Thromb Haemost* 1995;74:992–993.
37. Kemkes-Matthes B, Matthes K. Protein Z. *Semin Thromb Hemost* 2001;27:551–556.
38. Gamba G, Bertolino G, Montani N, et al. Bleeding tendency of unknown origin and protein Z levels. *Thromb Res* 1998;90:291–295.
39. Ravi S, Mauron T, Lammle B, et al. Protein Z in healthy human individuals and in patients with a bleeding tendency. *Br J Haematol* 1998;102:1219–1223.
40. Broze G Jr, Yin Z-F, Lasky N. A tail vein bleeding time model and delayed bleeding in hemophiliac mice. *Thromb Haemost* 2001;85:747–748.
41. Vasse M, Guegan-Massardier E, Borg J-Y, et al. High frequency of protein Z deficiency in patients with ischemic stroke. *Lancet* 2001;357:933–934.
42. Kobelt K, Biasiutti F, Mattle H, et al. Protein Z in ischaemic stroke. *Br J Haematol* 2001;114:169–173.
43. Heeb M, Paganini-Hill A, Griffin J, et al. Low protein Z levels and risk of ischemic stroke: differences by diabetic status and gender. *Blood Cells Mol Dis* 2002;29:139–144.
44. Lopaciuk S, Bykowska K, Kwiecinski H, et al. Protein Z in young survivors of ischemic stroke. *Thromb Haemost* 2002;88:436.
45. McQuillan A, Eikelboom J, Hankey G, et al. Protein Z in ischemic stroke and its etiologic subtypes. *Stroke* 2003;34:2415–2419.
46. Fedi S, Sofi F, Brogi D, et al. Low protein Z plasma levels are independently associated with acute coronary syndromes. *Thromb Haemost* 2003;90:1173–1178.
47. Koutroubakis I, Theodoropoulou A, Sfiridaki A, et al. Low plasma protein Z levels in patients with ischemic colitis. *Dig Dis Sci* 2003;48:1673–1676.
48. Kemkes-Matthes B, Matzdorff A, Matthes K. Protein Z influences the prothrombotic phenotype of factor V Leiden in humans. *Thromb Res* 2002;106:183–185.
49. Steffano B, Forastiero R, Marinuzzo M, et al. Low plasma protein Z levels in patients with antiphospholipid antibodies. *Blood Coagul Fibrinolysis* 2001;12:411–412.
50. McColl M, Deans A, Maclean P, et al. Plasma protein Z deficiency is common in women with antiphospholipid antibodies. *Br J Haematol* 2003;120:907–915.
51. Forastiero R, Matinuzzo M, Broze G Jr. Autoimmune antiphospholipid antibodies impair the inhibition of activated factor X by protein Z/protein Z-dependent protease inhibitor. *J Thromb Haemost* 2003;1:1754–1770.
52. Gris J-C, Quere I, Dechaud H, et al. High frequency of protein Z deficiency in patients with unexplained early fetal loss. *Blood* 2002;99:2606–2608.
53. Gris J-C, Amadio C, Mercier E, et al. Anti–protein Z antibodies in women with pathologic pregnancies. *Blood* 2003;101:4850–4852.
54. Gris J-C, Mercier E, Quere I, et al. Low-molecular-weight heparin versus low-dose aspirin in women with one fetal loss and a constitutional thrombophilic disorder. *Blood* 2004;103:3695–3699.

# CHAPTER 12 ■ FACTOR XI

PETER N. WALSH AND DAVID GAILANI

Coagulation factor XI, previously known as plasma thromboplastin antecedent (PTA), was first identified by Rosenthal et al. (1) as a deficiency in the plasma of patients with abnormal bleeding and, subsequently, was found to be particularly common in patients of Ashkenazi Jewish descent (2,3). Factor XI is present in human plasma at a concentration of 4 to 6 $\mu$g per mL (approximately 30 nM) and was first purified from bovine (4) and human (5) plasma as a 160-kDa homodimeric protein that participates in interactions with coagulation proteins of the contact phase of blood coagulation (6–9). Factor XI is the zymogen of a trypsinlike serine protease that is activated by factor XIIa and by both thrombin and factor XIa (10,11), and it can then recognize factor IX as its normal macromolecular substrate in plasma (12–14).

## GENE STRUCTURE AND REGULATION

The factor XI gene, 23 kb, is located on the distal end of the long arm of chromosome 4 (4q35) (15,16). The gene contains 15 exons with 14 introns, the first exon coding for the 5' untranslated region and the second exon coding for a signal peptide (see Fig. 12-1). The complementary deoxyribonucleic acid (cDNA) for human factor XI was originally isolated from a $\lambda$gt11 expression library from human liver, demonstrating that the messenger RNA (mRNA) consists of 2,097 nucleotides (17). Factor XI is synthesized as a polypeptide chain with a typical leader sequence of 18 amino acids. The mature protein consists of 607 amino acids encoded by 13 exons, the first 8 of which (exons III to X) encode four tandem repeat sequences termed *apple domains*, whereas the remaining 5 exons (exons XI to XV) encode the trypsinlike catalytic domain. The introns are located at a similar position within each of the four apple domains; the last four introns are located in the same positions as those in the genes for human tissue plasminogen activator and human urokinase (15). The cDNA for factor XI contains a stop codon (TGA) and a potential polyadenylation sequence located 21 nucleotides upstream from the poly(A) tail within the 166 nucleotides that constitute the 3' noncoding sequence of the mRNA. In addition, there are five potential N-glycosylation sites found in each of the two identical chains of factor XI. The cDNA sequence of factor XI is highly homologous (58% identity) with human plasma prekallikrein (17), which, like factor XI, contains four apple domains that have considerable structural homology with the N-terminal domains of plasminogen, hepatocyte growth factor, and numerous nematode proteins, referred to as the PAN module, as well as with a microneme protein from *Eimeria tenella* (18–20). Nonetheless, a recent examination of the puffer fish genome found orthologs for 21 of 26 different proteins involved in coagulation and fibrinolysis, with the exception of genes for the "contact system" proteins (i.e., factor XI, factor XII, and prekallikrein), suggesting that the gene duplication leading to factor XI and prekallikrein must be a very recent event in evolution (21).

This suggestion is particularly intriguing in the context of the observation that the presence of a tyrosine or phenylalanine at position 225 (chymotrypsin numbering system), which correlates with the presence of an AGY codon for serine 195, confers the property of Na$^+$-induced allosteric regulation of catalytic activity in serine proteases, such as thrombin and factors VIIa, IXa, and Xa, which apparently evolved from a thrombinlike ancestor. On the other hand, the presence of a proline at position 225, which correlates with the presence of an TCN codon for serine 195, precludes Na$^+$-induced allosteric regulation of catalytic activity in serine proteases, such as factors XIa, XIIa, and plasma kallikrein, which apparently evolved from a trypsinlike ancestor (22). The human factor XI gene promoter has recently been cloned and characterized (23). A binding site for the transcription factor hepatocyte nuclear factor-4$\alpha$ (HNF-4$\alpha$) appears to be required for hepatocyte-specific expression of factor XI (23). A full-length cDNA for murine factor XI also has been cloned from a murine liver cDNA library. The 2.8-kb murine cDNA codes for a protein of 624 amino acids with 78% homology to human factor XI (24). The recent molecular cloning and biochemical characterization of rabbit factor XI (25) discloses a protein with 87% identity with human factor XI (91% within the catalytic domain) in which a His residue replaces the Cys321 that forms an interchain disulfide linkage in human factor XI, thereby explaining why rabbit factor XI migrates by sodium dodecyl sulfate-polyacrylamide gel electrophoresis (SDS-PAGE) as monomer (26). In contrast, rabbit factor XI exists in plasma as a noncovalent homodimer and is functionally identical to human factor XI (25).

Although little is known about the details of processing and posttranslational modifications that factor XI undergoes during its biosynthesis, it is clearly found to undergo glycosylation at N72, N108, N432, and N473, but not at N335, another potential glycosylation site (17). In addition, it appears that not only does dimer formation (mediated by the A4 domain of factor XI) occur during intracellular processing but dimerization also is required for normal biosynthesis (27–29). Therefore, type III mutation of factor XI (see section, "Molecular Genetics of Factor XI Deficiency"), in which F283 in the fourth apple domain is substituted by L (27), is characterized by impaired dimerization and secretion, as demonstrated (28). Subsequent studies, in which the A4 domain of factor XI was substituted by that of tissue plasminogen activator (tPA), demonstrated dimerization that was specific to the A4 domain and that was required for normal secretion of the protein. Therefore, the A4 domain of factor XI contains residues that initially mediate noncovalent dimerization of the two subunits, which are then stabilized by the formation of the interchain disulfide bond involving C321. These events appear to be essential for dimer formation and secretion.

The normal site of synthesis of plasma factor XI is thought to be the liver because factor XI levels decrease in liver disease and a patient with previously normal hemostasis is found to develop factor XI deficiency after receiving a liver transplant from a factor XI–deficient donor (30). Furthermore, Northern

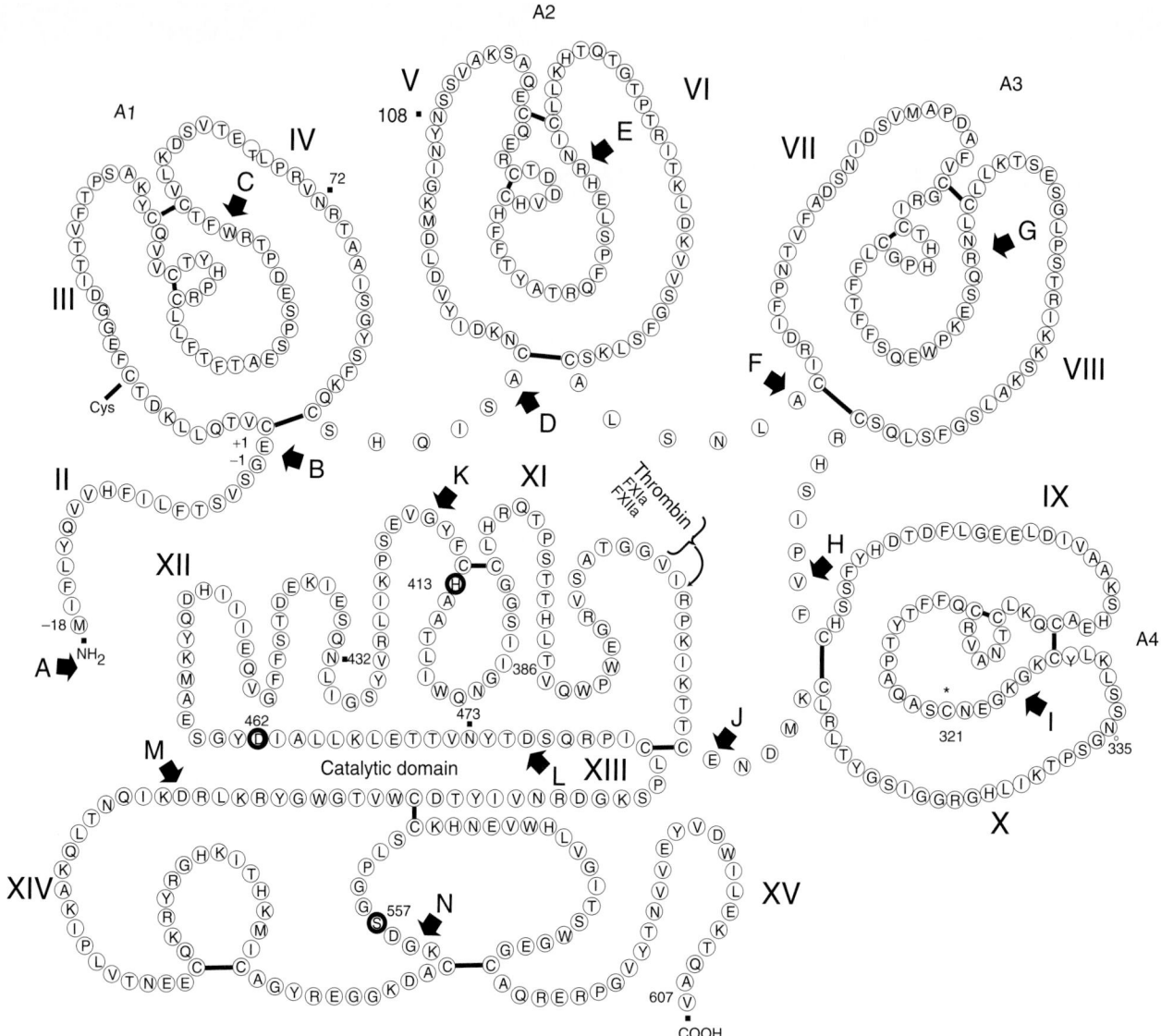

**FIGURE 12-1.** Amino acid sequence and primary structure of human factor XI. The signal sequence (numbered ×18 to ×1) is removed during biosynthesis by signal peptidase by the cleavage of the G–E bond between −1 and −2. Factor XI circulates in plasma as a homodimer connected by a single disulfide bond linking C321 in both of the fourth apple domains. The 14 introns (A to N) are shown by *solid arrows*. The exons are denoted by II–XV amino- to carboxy-terminus, with exon II representing the propeptide and exon I (not shown) representing the 5′ untranslated region. The four apple domains (consisting of 90 to 91 amino acids) are labeled as A1, A2, A3, and A4. The site of cleavage catalyzed by thrombin, factor XIa, or factor XIIa during the conversion of factor XI to factor XIa is shown with a *small, curved arrow*. The three members of the catalytic triad (H413, D462, and S557) are circled in *bold*. The four N-linked carbohydrate chains (i.e., N72, N108, N432, and N473) are shown by solid squares. (Figure redrawn and modified from McMullen BA, Fujikawa K, Davie EW. Location of the disulfide bonds in human coagulation factor XI: the presence of tandem apple domains. *Biochemistry* 1991;30:2056–2060.)

blot analyses of mRNA from various tissues show that murine factor XI message is expressed exclusively in the liver, whereas mRNA for human factor XI was identified in liver, pancreas, and kidney (24).

## PROTEIN STRUCTURE

Human factor XI is a disulfide-linked homodimer containing approximately 5% carbohydrate (i.e., 0.6% hexose, 2.7% N-acetylhexosamine, and 1.7% N-acetylneuraminic acid), with a molecular weight ($M_r$) ratio of approximately 143,000. Factor XI is present in human plasma at a concentration of 4 to 6 μg per mL (approximately 30 nM) in the form of a zymogen that requires proteolytic activation to develop serine protease activity (5,8,31–33). The zymogen form of the protein is unique among coagulation factors because it is a disulfide-linked homodimer consisting of two identical polypeptide chains. Each factor XI polypeptide contains 607 amino acids; each can be proteolytically activated by factor XIIa at an internal R369–I370 bond to yield a heavy chain (i.e., 369 amino acids) and a light chain (i.e., 238 amino acids) that contain a typical trypsinlike catalytic triad, consisting of H413, D464, and S557, with a typical trypsinlike substrate-binding pocket (17,34). After cleavage at R369–I360 bond, the catalytic domain contains an amino-terminal sequence of I-V-G-G characteristic of most serine proteases. The $M_r$ of the homodimer is 135,979 without carbohydrate, and 143,000 with four carbohydrate chains at N72 and N108 within the heavy chain and at N432 and N473 within the catalytic domain, whereas no carbohydrate is present on N335, another potential *N*-glycosylation site (17).

The primary sequence and domain structure of factor XI, including its disulfide linkages, are shown in Figure 12-1. The amino-terminal 369 residues of each factor XI monomer after propeptide cleavage comprises the heavy-chain region of factor XIa, which consists of four tandem repeat sequences of 90 to 91 amino acids, each containing six or seven cysteine residues that form three internal disulfide bonds. Each repeat sequence, or apple domain, contains an amino acid sequence that is 23% to 34% identical to the other apple domains of factor XI and that is 58% identical to the corresponding apple domains of plasma prekallikrein. In both plasma factor XI (17,34) and plasma prekallikrein, a characteristic disulfide-bonding pattern links the first and sixth, second and fifth, and third and fourth cysteines in each of the four apple domains (34). An additional cysteine is present at position 11 in the A1 domain of factor XI and forms a disulfide bond with another cysteine residue, whereas C321 in the A4 domain is disulfide-linked to the corresponding C321 to form the homodimer (34).

# PLATELET FACTOR XI

Platelet factor XI coagulant activity and antigen are present in well-washed platelet suspensions and constitute approximately 0.5% of the factor XI activity in normal plasma (35–39), from which it can be concluded that there are approximately 300 molecules of platelet factor XI per platelet. Platelet factor XI migrates on SDS-PAGE with an apparent $M_r$ of approximately 220,000, which decreases to approximately 55,000 after reduction, compared to plasma factor XI that has an $M_r$ of approximately 160,000 and a subunit $M_r$ of approximately 80,000 (35–37,40). From these facts, it has been suggested that platelet factor XI could represent a disulfide-linked tetramer of four identical 55,000-$M_r$ subunits, each being a truncated form of plasma factor XI lacking exon V, or, alternatively, it could represent a 55,000-$M_r$ protein disulfide linked to a platelet membrane protein (36,41,42). A possible candidate for this putative platelet factor XI–binding membrane protein on the platelet surface is glycoprotein Ib (GP Ib) ($M_r$ approximately 170,000). This possibility is supported by studies demonstrating that platelets from patients with the hereditary giant platelet (Bernard-Soulier) syndrome who lacked GP Ib contained no detectable factor XI activity in washed platelet suspensions (43). It is not known whether platelet factor XI is the product of an alternatively spliced mRNA lacking exon V in megakaryocytes (41) or that of a full-length factor XI mRNA in megakaryocytes or liver (44), and whether the protein undergoes posttranslational modifications. By using reverse-transcriptase polymerase chain reaction (RT-PCR), 12 of the 13 exons (excluding exon V) coding mature plasma factor XI were amplified from human platelet mRNA. A factor XI mRNA transcript of approximately 1.9 kb was detected by Northern hybridization in megakaryocytic cells, compared with approximately 2.1 kb in liver cells. Factor XI cDNA was cloned from a megakaryocytic library, and the sequence was found to be identical to that of plasma factor XI, with the exception of the absence of exon V. The splicing of exon IV to exon VI maintained the open reading frame without altering the amino acid sequence, except for deletion of amino acids A91–R144 within the amino-terminal portion of the apple 2 (A2) domain. These observations have led to the suggestion that platelet factor XI is either an alternative splicing product of the factor XI gene or the product of a separate gene lacking exon 5 and is localized to platelets and megakaryocytes but absent from other blood cells (41). In contrast, recent studies have confirmed the presence of factor XI mRNA amplified by RT-PCR from platelets and megakaryocytes that constituted only a full-length message that is identical to mRNA from liver (44).

# STRUCTURE–FUNCTION RELATIONSHIPS

## Factor XI Activation

Plasma factor XI circulates as a zymogen in human plasma as a complex with high-molecular-weight kininogen (HK) (7), which is required for binding of factor XI to negatively charged surfaces (45) (see Chapter 6). Factor XI can be activated by three biologically relevant proteases: factor XIIa, factor XIa, and thrombin (5,10,11). It can participate in the contact phase of blood coagulation in a reaction that requires the presence of anionic surfaces for optimal surface-mediated *in vitro* activation by factor XIIa (6,7,45–47). However, because deficiencies of factor XII, prekallikrein, and HK are not associated with hemostatic abnormalities but deficiency of factor XI produces abnormal bleeding complications in at least 50% of affected individuals (2,3,48–50), it has been suggested that the more relevant *in vivo* pathway for activation of plasma factor XI might be by the feedback activation by thrombin or, possibly, by autoactivation by factor XIa (10,11, 51). A recent study that requires confirmation suggests that $\beta_2$-glycoprotein I binds factor XI and inhibits its activation by thrombin and factor XIIa, whereas cleaved $\beta_2$-glycoprotein I binds factor XI but fails to inhibit activation of factor XI (52). All three proteases (i.e., thrombin, factor XIIa, and factor XIa) cleave each monomer of factor XI at the R369–I370 bond, generating the new amino-terminal sequence of the catalytic domain, I-V-G-G, which then activates the catalytic triad of the serine protease. It has been postulated that on anionic surfaces, such as in extracorporeal circulation, a ternary complex is formed when factor XI, in stoichiometric complex with HK in plasma, is adsorbed to the negatively charged surface, where factor XIIa recognizes it as a substrate (6,7,45–47,53–56). The factor XI homodimer is thereby cleaved to generate two disulfide-linked heavy chains ($M_r$ 45,000 to 50,000) and two active-site–containing light chains ($M_r$ 30,000 to 35,000) (5,8).

## Functional Domains of Factor XI

Specific three-dimensional information on structure is not available for either plasma factor XI or platelet factor XI. Although reasonable predictions can be made about the structure of the catalytic domain of factor XIa by homology modeling on the basis of the known structures of serine proteases such as trypsin, no such information is available about the apple domains of factor XI or about the only other known protein with high homology (58%) to factor XI (i.e., prekallikrein) (17). However, molecular models of all four apple domains have been published (57–61) on the basis of energy minimization calculations and the known disulfide linkages within the apple domains (34). From these molecular models and on the basis of the use of monoclonal antibodies, conformationally constrained synthetic peptides, and recombinant proteins (62) with site-directed mutations, the binding sites within factor XI or factor XIa for a number of physiologically relevant plasma or cellular ligands have been identified and characterized. This information is summarized in Table 12-1.

**TABLE 12-1**

STRUCTURAL BIOLOGY OF FACTOR XI AND FACTOR XI INTERACTIONS

| | Function | Domain | Subdomain | Residues | Reference |
|---|---|---|---|---|---|
| FXI/HK Domain 6 | Complex with HK in presence of $Zn^{2+}$ promotes FXI binding to platelets and FXI activation by FXIa or thrombin | A1 (E1–S90) A2 (A95–L180) A4 (F272–E361) | F56–S86 | V64, I77 | 57,59,64, 66,67 |
| FXI/Prothrombin kringle 2 domain | Complex with prothrombin in presence of $Ca^{2+}$ promotes FXI binding to platelets and FXI activation by thrombin | A1 (E1–S90) | A45–S86 | ? | 51,64,68 |
| FXI/Thrombin | Activation of FXI by thrombin on GP Ibα expressed on platelets | A1 (E1–S90) | A45–R70 | D51, E66 | 63–65 |
| FXI/Platelet GP Ibα | Membrane binding for FXI activation | A3 (A181–V271) | N235–R266 | N248, R250, K255, F260, Q263 | 61,69–76 |
| FXI/Heparin | ? Binding to glycosaminoglycans | A3 (A181–V271) | T249–F260 | K252, K253, ? K255 | 77,78 |
| FXI/FXI | Dimerization of FXI | A4 (F272–E361) | ? | C321, F283 | 28,29, 79–83 |
| FXI/FXIIa | Activation of FXI by FXIIa | A4 (F272–E361) | A317–G350 | ? | 60,69 |
| FXIa/FIX | Substrate-binding site | A2 (A95–L180) A3 (A181–V271) | A134–L172 I183–V191 S195–I197 F260–S265 | ? ? | 14,58,84 85,86 |
| FXIa/Platelets | Membrane binding of FXIa for FIX activation | Catalytic Domain (I370–V607) | C527–C542 | ? | 87–89 |
| FXIa/Heparin | ? Binding of FXIa to glycosaminoglycans | Catalytic Domain (I370–V607) | C527–R532 | K529, R530, R532 | 90,91 |
| FXIa/Protease Nexin-2 | Inhibition of FXIa; Binding of Kunitz protease inhibitor domain of PN2 to catalytic domain of FXIa | Catalytic Domain (I370–V607) | ? | ? | |

FXI, factor XI; FXIa, factor XIa; ?, specific information not available.

Thrombin (3–65), HK (57,59,64,66,67), and the kringle 2 domain of prothrombin (51,64,68) have all been shown to bind to contiguous subdomains within the carboxy-terminal half of the A1 domain (E1–S90). Molecular modeling of the three-dimensional structure of the A1 domain demonstrates the possibility that three surface-exposed loop structures are present, each consisting of antiparallel β-strands connected by β-turns. Although these structures may not conform precisely to the actual structure of factor XI once it is determined from nuclear magnetic resonance or x-ray crystallography, the models have been used to predict the amino acid side chains that might mediate various ligand interactions and to design experiments using conformationally constrained synthetic peptides and recombinant A1 domain constructs. Thereby, it has been determined that HK binds to a subdomain within the A1 domain comprising residues F56–S86, whereas thrombin binds to a partially overlapping and contiguous site comprising subdomain A45–R70. Different amino acid side chains appear to be essential for these interactions because E51 and E66 are important for thrombin interactions with factor XI but not for

HK binding, whereas V64 and I77 are important for HK binding but not for thrombin binding (66). The kringle 2 domain of prothrombin can bind to a subdomain comprising residues A45–S86, but fine mapping of this site has not yet been accomplished (51,68). Occupancy of these sites by their respective ligands is likely to be important in promoting the binding of factor XI to platelets either in the presence of HK and $Zn^{2+}$ ions or prothrombin and $Ca^{2+}$ ions, leading to the preferential activation of factor XI by thrombin (and also by factor XIIa) on the GP Ibα subunit of the GP Ib/IX/V complex on the platelet surface (51,64,65).

The A3 domain of factor XI also has been identified as the locus of binding sites for both platelets (61,69–76) and heparin (77,78). Therefore, activated platelets expose specific reversible, high-affinity binding sites for factor XI that requires the presence of HK and $ZnCl_2$ (92), or prothrombin and $CaCl_2$ (51). Binding of factor XI to activated platelets through the A3 domain (61) is required for optimal rates of factor XI activation by factor XIIa (93) or by thrombin (51). The sequence of residues within the A3 domain of factor XI (i.e., N235–R266) that comprises a contact surface for interaction with a platelet receptor consisting of the GP Ibα subunit of the GP Ib/IX/V complex (73,74) contains amino acids that mediate this binding, including N248, R250, K255, F260, and Q263 (70,72). The A3 domain of factor XI also contains all the binding energy required for interaction of factor XI with heparin in a heparin-binding consensus sequence (i.e., T249–F260) that contains amino acids K252 and K253, and possibly K255, which at least in part mediate the binding of factor XI to heparin (77,78).

A major role of the A4 domain of factor XI is to mediate dimer formation between the two identical polypeptide chains comprising factor XI through disulfide bond formation at C321 (17,28,29,34,79,80). The functional significance of the event has been postulated to facilitate efficient activation of factor IX by dimeric factor XIa on the platelet surface (81), where factor XIa is protected from inactivation by protease nexin-2 (PN2)(87,90,94). It has been clearly demonstrated that the A4 domain mediates noncovalent interactions between the two identical subunits and that the dimer is stabilized by covalent linkage between two cysteine residues in each monomer at position 321 (17,28,29,34,79,80,82,83). Furthermore, a natural mutation in factor XI resulting in diminished intracellular dimerization and secretion of the protein involves mutation of F283L, which implies that F283 is important for noncovalent dimer formation (28). In addition, a sequence of residues (i.e., A317–G350) within the A4 domain of factor XI appears to contain three peptide structures, possibly consisting of three antiparallel $\beta$-strands that together comprise a contact surface for interaction with factor XIIa. This site may participate in the activation of factor XI by factor XIIa (60,69).

# CELLULAR INTERACTIONS

Early observations suggesting that platelets participate in the contact phase of blood coagulation (95–99) were subsequently confirmed by the evidence that isolated human platelets activated with either adenosine diphosphate or collagen could promote the proteolytic activation of factor XII by kallikrein and, subsequently, the activation of factor XI by factor XIIa in the presence of HK (38,93,100,101). The mechanism underlying the role of activated platelets in the activation of factor XI involves the generation of high-affinity (dissociation constant, $K_d$, approximately 10 nM), specific, saturable binding sites (approximately 1,500 sites per platelet) on the surface of activated platelets that require the presence of HK and $Zn^{2+}$ ions (92). The observation that HK also binds to platelets under similar conditions originally suggested that the two proteins bind to the platelet surface as a complex (102,103). However, it has subsequently been shown that HK interacts with factor XI through a surface-exposed site encompassing residues F56–S86 within the A1 domain (57,59,104), resulting in the exposure of a platelet binding site encompassing residues N235–R266 within the A3 domain of factor XI (61). Perhaps most importantly, it has been demonstrated that prothrombin can substitute for HK as a cofactor for the binding of factor XI to the surface of activated platelets and for platelet-mediated factor XI activation by thrombin (51). In this way, prothrombin appears to bind to a site in the A1 domain of factor XI contiguous to the site used by HK for binding to the A1 domain (51). Occupancy of this site results in the exposure of a surface in the A3 domain of factor XI that binds with high affinity and specificity to the surface of activated platelets, resulting in an approximately 5,000- to 10,000-fold acceleration of rates of factor XI activation by thrombin (51), as shown in schematic form in Figure 12-2. The platelet receptor that binds factor XI and colocalizes it with thrombin for efficient activation has

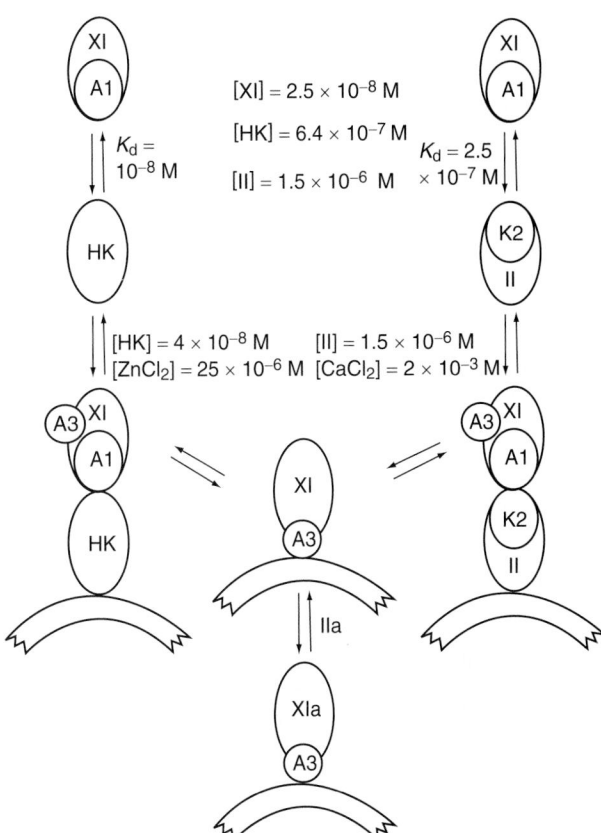

**FIGURE 12-2.** Schematic diagram of the role of prothrombin and high-molecular-weight kininogen in factor XI binding to activated platelets and thrombin-mediated factor XI activation. The crescentic figure represents the activated platelet surface. A1, apple 1 domain; A3, apple 3 domain; II, prothrombin; XI, factor XI; XIa, factor XIa; HK, high-molecular-weight kininogen; K2, kringle 2 domain of prothrombin.

recently been shown to consist of the GP Ibα subunit of the GP Ib/IX/V complex that is localized within platelet membrane microdomains referred to as *lipid rafts* (73,74). This interaction of factor XI with surface membranes of activated platelets has been shown to be mediated by binding of residues (i.e., R250, K252, K253, K255, F260, and Q263) within the A3 domain of factor XI (75) to the leucine-rich repeat motifs of GP Ibα (76). Finally, it has recently been demonstrated that activation of factor XI by thrombin on activated platelets requires the interaction of factor XI and platelet GP Ibα with thrombin anion-binding exosites I and II, respectively (65,105,106).

Endothelial cells can expose specific, saturable, high-affinity binding sites for both factor XI and HK, which raises the possibility that endothelium as well as platelets can participate in the activation of factor XI by factor XIIa (107–113). However, it has recently been shown that what was interpreted as a specific interaction of factor XI with the endothelial cell surface is an artifact of binding to microtiter plates. Activated platelets, but not endothelial cells, participate in the initiation of the consolidation phase of blood coagulation. Moreover, the interaction of factor XIa with activated platelets, but not with endothelial cells, promotes the activation of factor IX (87,114). Therefore, the endothelial cell surface is generally regarded as anticoagulant and nonthrombogenic (see Chapter 45), and it has been suggested that the binding of HK to endothelial cells may be more important for the regulation of bradykinin production (115–117) and for the activation of prourokinase (118) and plasminogen (115,118) than for the procoagulant functions promoted by factor XI (87,114,116,117).

## Factor XIa Enzymatic Activity

After activation on artificial surfaces, factor XIa remains surface bound and recognizes factor IX as its normal macromolecular substrate (12–14,119). In the presence of calcium ions, factor XIa cleaves factor IX, a single-chain 57,000-$M_r$ glycoprotein with 17% carbohydrate, at an internal R145–A146 bond, forming an intermediate that is subsequently hydrolyzed at an R180–V181 bond to generate active factor IXa and to form a 10,000-$M_r$ activation peptide, 50% of which is composed of carbohydrate (12–14,119–124). The light chain of factor XIa or catalytic domain (i.e., C362–V607) contains a typical trypsinlike catalytic triad comprising residues H413, D462, and S557, which are activated when factor XI is cleaved at R369–I370 bond to expose a new amino-terminal tetrapeptide, I-V-G-G, typical of trypsinlike serine proteases. The serine protease active site of factor XIa can cleave and activate two major macromolecular substrates, including factor IX (12–14) and factor XI (10,11). In addition, factor XIa (and plasma kallikrein) has recently been shown to activate prohepatocyte growth factor, raising the possibility that they may regulate processes that involve the HGF/c-Met pathway, such as tissue repair and angiogenesis (125).

The interaction of factor XIa with its preferred macromolecular substrate, factor IX, involves $Ca^{2+}$-dependent binding of factor IX to a substrate-binding site within the heavy chain of factor XIa (14,84,126). The location and characterization of this substrate-binding site have been studied in two laboratories with conflicting results (58,85,86). One of these studies used molecular modeling and conformationally constrained synthetic peptides to identify a sequence of residues (i.e., A134–L172) within the A2 domain of factor XIa that contains three antiparallel β-strands connected by β-turns that have the characteristics of a substrate-binding site for factor IX because they act as competitive inhibitors of factor IX activation by factor XIa (58). In contrast, recombinant factor XI proteins, in which each of the four apple domains is individually replaced with the corresponding domain from the homologous but functionally distinct protein prekallikrein, revealed that when the A3 domain of prekallikrein was inserted into factor XIa, the Michaelis constant ($K_m$) for activation of factor IX was 35-fold higher than the $K_m$ for activation by wild-type factor XIa or by the other factor XI/PK chimeras (85,86). Mapping of the A3 domain of factor XIa by alanine-scanning mutagenesis has identified residues in the N-terminus (i.e., I183–V191, and possibly S195–I197) and the C-terminus (i.e., F260–S265) of the A3 domain that are required for factor IX activation (86). Recent evidence indicates that the interaction of factor XIa with factor IX is dependent on the γ-carboxyglutamic acid domain of factor IX (127). Therefore, the putative substrate-binding site for factor IX resides either within the A2 domain or within the A3 domain of factor XIa. A possible resolution of these two apparently conflicting studies is that intimate interdomainal interactions between A2 and A3 may be required for maintaining an intact substrate-binding site that interacts with the Gla domain of factor IX.

## Cellular Interactions and Regulation of Factor XIa

The regulation of factor XIa depends on its localization (i.e., whether it appears on the platelet surface, in the proximity of endothelium, or in the plasmatic compartment of the blood). Within the plasma, four separate serine protease inhibitors (serpins) have been demonstrated to inactivate factor XIa: antithrombin III, $\alpha_1$-protease inhibitor, C1 inhibitor, and $\alpha_2$-antiplasmin (8,31,128–137). It has recently been shown that another serpin, protease nexin 1, which is not present at physiologically significant concentrations in plasma but which is secreted in low concentrations from platelet α-granules, inhibits factor XIa in the presence of heparin with potency greater than that of C1 inhibitor (138). Factor XIa also has been reported to be inhibited by plasminogen activator inhibitor 1 (139) and protein C inhibitor (140). The inhibition of factor XIa within the plasma compartment has been postulated to occur predominantly through the action of $\alpha_1$-protease inhibitor (130), although studies on the modulation of contact system proteases by glycosaminoglycans indicate a selective enhancement of the inhibition of factor XIa by C1 inhibitor (141) and by protease nexin 1 (138).

Because factor XIa can be formed on the platelet surface (38,92,93,101) and it can bind to high-affinity ($K_d$ approximately 800 pM), specific, saturable receptors (130 to 500 sites per platelet) on activated platelets in the presence of HK, the binding being mediated by the catalytic domain of the enzyme and distinct from those for factor XI (87–89), it has been suggested that factor IX activation by factor XIa might also occur on the platelet surface (142). Although the binding of factor XIa to platelets does not appear to enhance rates of factor IX activation (81,87,142), both factor XIa (87,88) and factor IX (143) can bind to high-affinity, saturable receptors on activated platelets. Within the environment of activated platelets, factor XIa is regulated by different mechanisms from those operative in plasma because platelet-bound factor XIa is protected from inactivation by $\alpha_1$-protease inhibitor (132). In addition, platelets are known to secrete inhibitors of factor XIa (144–148) including PN2, a truncated form of the transmembrane Alzheimer β-amyloid protein precursor that contains a Kunitz-type serine protease inhibitor domain. PN2 is a potent inhibitor of factor XIa (inhibition constant, $K_i$ 2.9 to $4.5 \times 10^{-10}$ M) that has considerably enhanced inhibitory activity in the presence of heparin ($K_i$ 2.5 to $4.5 \times 10^{-11}$ M) (90,91,94,146–150), which provides a template for the assembly of factor XIa/PN2 complexes (90). Although the release of PN2 from activated platelets inhibits plasma factor XIa activity in the environment of the hemostatic thrombus, platelet-bound dimeric (but not monomeric) factor XIa is protected from inactivation by PN2 (81,87,94). In contrast, endothelial cells have no such protective effect, suggesting that whereas factor XIa is protected from inactivation by PN2 when bound to the platelet surface, inactivation of factor XIa by PN2 might be enhanced on the surface of endothelial cells that contain heparan sulfate glycosaminoglycans. Therefore, it has been suggested that the colocalization of dimeric factor XIa and factor IX to the activated platelet surface may serve to localize the factor IX activation and subsequent coagulation reactions to the activated platelet surface that contains specific, high-affinity, saturable binding sites for the enzyme factor IXa. In the presence of factor VIII, the occupancy of these sites can increase the catalytic efficiency ($k_{cat}/K_m$) of factor X activation by more than 20 million–fold (143,151–153).

# MOLECULAR GENETICS OF FACTOR XI DEFICIENCY

Hereditary deficiency of factor XI is an autosomal disorder characterized by trauma- and surgery-related hemorrhage, and only rarely by the "spontaneous" soft tissue and joint bleeding that is typical of factor VIII or factor IX deficiency (154–157).

Clinical manifestations and treatment of factor XI deficiency are discussed elsewhere (see Chapters 58 and 59). Bleeding is highly variable, although it tends to be more prevalent in patients with severe reductions in plasma factor XI (<0.2 U per mL) (49,154,158). Patients with milder factor XI deficiency (0.2 to 0.5 U per mL) can experience bleeding complications and those with very severe deficiency (<0.05 U per mL) may not bleed excessively (2,3,49,154,158,159). This situation has contributed to difficulties in establishing patterns of inheritance. First described by Rosenthal in 1953 (1), factor XI deficiency was initially considered a dominant disorder with variable penetrance (48,160,161). This contrasts with other inherited coagulation protease deficiencies that are usually symptomatic in the homozygous or compound heterozygous state. Hypothetically, the dimeric structure of factor XI could explain some cases of apparent dominant transmission (5) because heterozygosity for a factor XI gene mutation could result in formation of defective heterodimers with normal factor XI (see following text). In contrast, Rapaport et al. suggested that factor XI deficiency exists in major (i.e., factor XI level <1% to 20%) and minor (i.e., level 30% to 65%) forms, which is most consistent with a recessive or intermediate mode of inheritance (2). A recessive inheritance pattern is generally accepted for the more common forms of the disorder caused by the type II and type III mutations (see subsequent text) (3,156,162).

Although factor XI deficiency is rare in general, it is common in the Ashkenazi Jewish population, in whom the abnormal allele frequency is estimated to be 5% to 11%

(154,163,164). More than 90% of abnormal factor XI alleles in the Jewish population are caused by two-point mutations of roughly equal prevalence, E117 Stop and F283L (154,164). E117 Stop (type II mutation) truncates the factor XI polypeptide within the A2 domain and is essentially a null allele (27). Homozygotes for E117 Stop, therefore, lack plasma factor XI antigen or activity. F283L (type III mutation) is located in the A4 domain (27,154), an area that is critical for dimer formation (29). F283L causes a partial defect in dimerization (28,165). Because dimerization is a prerequisite for factor XI secretion, the F283L mutation causes retention of monomeric factor XI within cells (28,165). Homozygotes for F283L have plasma factor XI levels that are approximately 10% of normal (154) and the factor XI–F283L in plasma is dimeric and functions normally (28). Heterozygotes for E117 Stop and F283L have plasma factor XI levels of $52 \pm 18\%$ and $67 \pm 24\%$ of normal, respectively, (154), and exhibit relatively few bleeding symptoms, consistent with a recessive mode of inheritance.

More than 80 mutations in the factor XI gene associated with factor XI deficiency have been reported since the original description of the type II and type III mutations (http://www.med.unc.edu/isth/mutations-databases/Factor_XI.htm). A partial list of those associated with single amino acid substitutions is shown in Table 12-2. Most cases are characterized by commensurate decreases in plasma factor XI activity and antigen (49,50,158, 166–168), consistent with the fact that nearly all mutations that give rise to factor XI deficiency reduce

## TABLE 12-2

### MUTATIONS ASSOCIATED WITH FACTOR XI (FXI) DEFICIENCY

| Exon | cDNA | Mutation | Domain | Defect | Reference |
|---|---|---|---|---|---|
| 3 | 143G → C | D16H | Apple 1 | Reduced secretion | 170 |
| 3 | 209T → C | C38R | Apple 1 | Reduced secretion | 183 |
| 5 | 408G → A | G104D | Apple 2 | Unknown | 185 |
| 5 | 446G → T | E117X | Apple 2 | Premature termination | 27,154 |
| 6 | 561G → A | G155E | Apple 2 | Unknown | 185 |
| 7 | 781G → C | W228C | Apple 3 | Reduced secretion | 187 |
| 8 | 807G → A | C237Y | Apple 3 | Reduced secretion | 183 |
| 8 | 840G → A | S248N | Apple 3 | CRM+ platelet binding defect | 72,174 |
| 9 | 944T → C | F283L | Apple 4 | Reduced secretion—dimerization defect | 27,28 |
| 9 | 1002T → C | L302P | Apple 4 | Reduced secretion | 170 |
| 9 | 1008C → T | T304I | Apple 4 | Reduced secretion | 170 |
| 9 | 1019C → T | R308C | Apple 4 | Reduced secretion | 187 |
| 9 | 1064G → A | E323K | Apple 4 | Reduced secretion | 170 |
| 10 | 1103G → A | G336R | Apple 4 | CRM+ | 182 |
| 10 | 1146G → A | G350E | Apple 4 | Reduced secretion—dimerization defect | 28,165 |
| 10 | 1146G → C | G350A | Apple 4 | CRM+ | 182 |
| 11 | 1254C → A | T386N | Catalytic | Reduced secretion | 173 |
| 11 | 1290G → A | C398Y | Catalytic | Reduced secretion | 188 |
| 11 | 1296G → T | G400V | Catalytic | Reduced secretion dominant negative | 165 |
| 11 | 1332C → T | A412V | Catalytic | Reduced secretion | 187 |
| 12 | 1421T → G | F442V | Catalytic | Reduced secretion | 171 |
| 12 | 1475G → A | G460R | Catalytic | Unknown | 185 |
| 12 | 1521C → T | T475I | Catalytic | Reduced secretion | 187 |
| 13 | 1574T → C | Y493H | Catalytic | Reduced secretion | 183 |
| 14 | 1651G → C | K518N | Catalytic | Reduced secretion | 175 |
| 14 | 1656C → T | P520L | Catalytic | CRM+ mild defect in factor IX activation | 188 |
| 15 | 1761G → A | G555E | Catalytic | CRM+ defect in factor IX activation | 189 |
| 15 | 1803G → C | W569S | Catalytic | Reduced secretion dominant negative | 165 |
| 15 | 1821C → T | T575M | Catalytic | CRM+ | 182 |
| 15 | 1825C → A | S576R | Catalytic | Reduced secretion | 187 |

CRM+, cross-reactive material positive.
Base pair refers to position in the human factor XI cDNA (17).

protein secretion [cross-reactive material negative (CRM–) deficiency] (27,154,169–175). Gene mutations that result in CRM–factor XI deficiency appear to fall into three mechanistic categories (a) mutations that interfere with or prevent the synthesis of the factor XI polypeptide, which include premature stop codons, such as E117 Stop (27,171,176–182), frame shifts (175,179,183), deletions (184), intronic splicing defects (170,172,175,183,185), and, probably, amino acid substitutions that cause protein instability or severe structural perturbations (perhaps most of the mutations in Table 12-2); (b) mutations that interfere with protein dimer formation (i.e., F283L and G350E) (28,165), resulting in retention of factor XI monomer in the cell; and, (c) mutations that result in a poorly secreted polypeptide that can form homodimers or heterodimers with normal factor XI polypeptide, effectively trapping a portion of the normal factor XI polypeptide in the cell (G400V and W569S) (165). This third mechanism may account for families in which factor XI deficiency is inherited as an autosomal dominant condition (160,165,186). Experiments in fibroblasts demonstrate that cotransfection of factor XI–G400V or W569S with wild-type factor XI reduces wild-type protein secretion (dominant negative effect) (165). The negative effect on factor XI release is not seen during the cotransfection of wild-type factor XI with the type II or type III mutations, which is consistent with the apparent recessive mode of inheritance for these mutations (165).

A few factor XI mutations are associated with dysfunctional protein in plasma (CRM+ deficiency) or with protein secreted by transfected cells in culture. Factor XI–Q226R and factor XI–S248N were identified in a compound heterozygous individual with recurrent epistaxis that caused iron deficiency anemia (174). Factor XI–Q226R does not appear to have a considerable functional abnormality (174) and is probably a polymorphism (190). Factor XI–S248N has activity similar to that of the wild-type factor XI in plasma clotting assays (174) but is defective in platelet binding and is activated poorly by thrombin on the surface of activated platelets *in vitro* (72). Because thrombin-mediated activation of factor XI on platelets is a likely physiologic mechanism for factor XI activation *in vivo* (51,81,191), the defective interaction with platelets may explain the bleeding symptoms in the patient and his family members. Zivelin et al. (189) identified a patient who was homozygous for a G555E substitution in the catalytic domain, with normal factor XI antigen level and very low factor XI activity (<0.01 U per mL). This mutation interferes with interactions of factor XIa with factor IX and that of factor XIa with the serpin inhibitor antithrombin III (189). Heterozygosity for a P520L substitution was identified in a child with mild bleeding symptoms (188). Although it is not known if the patient is CRM+, factor XI–P520L is expressed by transfected fibroblast in culture and has a mild defect in factor IX activation. Finally, E350A and T575M are associated with discrepant antigen and activity levels (182); however, the functional consequences of these mutations have not been reported.

# PHYSIOLOGY AND PATHOPHYSIOLOGY OF FACTOR XI

A great deal of information has been acquired on the physiologic role of factor XI through the study of patients with factor XI deficiency and through the definition of the associated genetic defects. However, in many patients, the reported lack of correlation between the plasma level of factor XI and the severity of clinical bleeding manifestations (2,3,42,49,154, 158,159) emphasizes the incomplete nature of the understanding of how factor XI participates in hemostasis. The molecular

characterization of platelet factor XI [either as an alternative splicing product of the factor XI gene lacking exon V and expressed exclusively in megakaryocytes (41) or as the product of a full-length message that is identical to mRNA from liver (44)] and the demonstration that a small number of selected patients with severe plasma factor XI deficiency and minimal or absent hemostatic defects have platelet factor XI by flow cytometry (42) support the suggestion that platelet factor XI can participate in hemostasis and may even substitute for plasma factor XI (35,36,42,43,49). However, future studies are required to determine the biochemical relation between plasma factor XI and platelet factor XI, including the mechanisms and enzymes that activate these two proteins and the substrate specificity of each of the activated proteases.

An important tool to facilitate investigations of the physiologic roles of plasma factor XI (and possibly of platelet factor XI) is the development of a murine model of severe plasma factor XI deficiency using the technique of homologous recombination in embryonic stem cells (192). In this model, the murine factor XI gene (24) was disrupted by the introduction of a neomycin phosphotransferase gene into exon V, resulting in the absence of factor XI activity in plasma and of factor XI mRNA from liver. No evidence of hemostatic deficiency was detected in homozygous null mice, and the genotypes of progeny from mating of mice heterozygous for the factor XI null allele showed the expected Mendelian ratio of wild-type, heterozygous, and homozygous null animals, suggesting that increased intrauterine mortality did not result from severe factor XI deficiency. It is not known whether normal murine platelets contain platelet factor XI, but if they do, it is possible that disruption of exon V with a neomycin phosphotransferase gene would not prevent the expression of platelet factor XI that lacks exon V. Future studies with murine factor XI knockout models may provide important insights into the relative contributions of plasma factor XI and platelet factor XI to physiologic and pathologic processes.

The details of the clinical manifestations and management of factor XI deficiency are presented in Chapters 58 and 59. However, insights into normal physiologic function can be gleaned from certain clinical facts. For example, responses to the infusion of plasma in patients with factor XI deficiency provide evidence that the recovery of factor XI is greater than 90% after infusion and that the half-life of the plasma protein is $52 \pm 22$ (mean $\pm$ SD) hours (193,194). Another clinical fact worthy of note is that patients with severe plasma factor XI deficiency are especially at risk for bleeding from tissues with high local fibrinolytic activity, including the urinary tract, the nose, the oral cavity, and the tonsils (154,195). Moreover, factor XI can be activated by thrombin (10,11,51) and appears to play a role in the protection of fibrin clots against fibrinolysis (196). These facts suggest that factor XI, in addition to its procoagulant activity, has an antifibrinolytic activity. This factor XI–dependent downregulation of the activation of fibrinolysis (196) has been postulated to occur as a consequence of a factor XI–dependent burst in thrombin generation, resulting in the activation of thrombin-activatable fibrinolysis inhibitor (TAFI) or procarboxypeptidase B (197–200), which inhibits the activation of plasminogen by removing carboxy-terminal lysines from fibrin that are essential for plasminogen binding and activation (199–201).

In addition to its demonstrable role in hemostasis, recent evidence has focused attention on the possible contributions of high levels of factor XI as a risk factor for venous thrombosis (202) and cardiovascular disease in women (203), although inherited factor XI deficiency apparently confers no protection against acute myocardial infarction (204). One recent study followed 600 patients with a first episode of venous thromboembolism and found an increased risk of recurrence, especially among those with increased levels of TAFI and factor

XI (205), whereas another study showed that increased levels of TAFI, but not factor XI, increased the risk of venous thromboembolism in patients with factor $V_{Leiden}$ carrier status (206). These studies are consistent with the results of an investigation in rabbits demonstrating increase in rabbit jugular vein thrombolysis by antibody neutralization of factor XI because of diminished indirect activation of TAFI (207). Two recent studies in mice with targeted factor XI gene deletion, either alone (208) or in combination with targeted deficiency of protein C (209), showed protection from $FeCl_3$-induced carotid thrombosis (208) or from early lethality caused by thrombosis in protein-C–deficient animals (209). Another study reported the dependence of surface- and tissue-factor–initiated thrombus propagation on factor XI in primates (210). Therefore, factor XI levels may comprise a significant risk factor for thrombosis, and the factor XI molecule may constitute a reasonable target for the development of antithrombotic drugs.

The physiologic pathways by which plasma factor XI and platelet factor XI are activated and the mechanisms by which they participate in normal blood coagulation and hemostasis are important aspects of a revised theory of blood coagulation that focuses on the assembly of coagulation protein complexes on the platelet surface. The original theories of blood coagulation (211,212) envisioned a series of enzymatic reactions initiated by activation of intrinsic blood coagulation by the assembly of the contact proteins on a foreign surface. However, the absence of bleeding complications in patients with deficiencies of factor XII, prekallikrein, and HK, and the presence of hemostatic defects in patients with factor XI deficiency, has led to a search for alternative pathways of factor XI activation. Although the demonstration (213,214) that the tissue factor–factor VIIa complex can directly activate not only factor X but also factor IX has been used to suggest an explanation for the absence of bleeding manifestations in patients with contact phase deficiencies (215); this observation does not account for the presence of abnormal bleeding in some patients with factor XI deficiency. Nonetheless, evidence exists that the initiation of blood coagulation *in vivo* is a consequence of the formation of the catalytic complex that occurs when factor VII or factor VIIa is assembled on the transmembrane protein tissue factor found in many cell types (216). Furthermore, the discovery of the tissue factor pathway inhibitor (TFPI) and the elucidation of its mechanism of action provides some of the information necessary to understand why both factor XI and factor VII appear to be necessary for normal hemostasis (217–223). The complex of tissue factor and factor VIIa is almost immediately inhibited when a complex is formed between factor Xa and TFPI (224,225). Therefore, the generation of factor Xa results in the immediate inactivation of the enzyme complex that initially forms it (i.e., tissue factor–factor VIIa). Furthermore, it has been observed that the formation of thrombin through the extrinsic pathway is transient and that the continuous generation of thrombin by the intrinsic pathway is required to assure normal hemostasis (225). All of these observations suggest that factor XI is required for normal functioning of the intrinsic pathway and that an alternative mechanism for the activation of factor XI exists independent of the contact proteins.

A schematic model of the mechanism of factor XI activation and the expression of factor XIa enzymatic activity on the platelet surface is presented in Figure 12-2. Both Naito and Fujikawa (10) and Gailani and Broze (11) have independently demonstrated that human factor XI can be activated either by thrombin or by factor XIa (i.e., autoactivation of factor XI). Although the kinetics of factor XI activation by thrombin in solution are quite unfavorable, the presence of dextran sulfate as a negatively charged surface enhances the rate of activation of factor XI by thrombin by approximately 2,000-fold (10, 11,226). However, the presence of either HK (10,11,227) or fibrinogen (227) have major inhibitory effects on the autoactivation and the thrombin-mediated activation of factor XI in the presence of dextran sulfate. On the other hand, activated platelets have been shown to promote factor XI activation by thrombin at initial rates that are two- to fivefold greater than that promoted by dextran sulfate and 5,000- to 10,000-fold greater than that in solution in the presence of either HK and $ZnCl_2$ or in the presence of prothrombin (or prothrombin fragment 1) and $CaCl_2$ (51). On the activated platelet surface, thrombin has been shown to be the preferred activator, compared with factor XIIa or factor XIa (64), and the platelet receptor that binds factor XI and thrombin for efficient activation is the GP Ib/IX/V complex (73), within membrane microdomains referred to as lipid rafts (74). The factor XIa thereby generated then binds to a separate, unknown, high-affinity, low-capacity receptor through the catalytic domain (in contrast to factor XI, which binds to GP Ibα via the apple 3 domain) to promote factor IX activation by dimeric factor XIa, which is protected from inactivation by the platelet-secreted Kunitz inhibitor, PN2, a potent inhibitor of unbound factor XIa (81,94,87–89).

# ACKNOWLEDGMENTS

This study was supported by research grants from the National Institutes of Health: HL46213, HL70683, PO1 HL74124, and PO1 HL64943 to PNW and HL58837 to DG. DG is an established investigator of the American Heart Association. We are grateful to Patricia Pileggi for assistance in chapter preparation.

## *References*

1. Rosenthal RL, Dreskin OH, Rosenthal N. New hemophilia-like disease caused by deficiency of a third plasma thromboplastin factor. *Proc Soc Exp Biol Med* 1953;82:171–174.
2. Rapaport SI, Proctor RR, Patch MJ, et al. The mode of inheritance of PTA deficiency: evidence for the existence of a major PTA deficiency and a minor PTA deficiency. *Blood* 1961;18:149–155.
3. Leiba H, Ramot B, Many A. Hereditary and coagulation studies in ten families with factor XI (plasma thromboplastin antecedent) deficiency. *Br J Haematol* 1965;11:654–665.
4. Koide T, Kato H, Davie EW. Isolation and characterization of bovine factor XI (plasma thromboplastin antecedent). *Biochemistry* 1977;16:2279–2286.
5. Bouma BN, Griffin JH. Human blood coagulation factor XI. Purification, properties, and mechanism of activation by activated factor XII. *J Biol Chem* 1977;252:6432–6437.
6. Ratnoff OD, Davie EW, Mallett DL. Studies on the action of Hageman factor: evidence that activated Hageman factor in turn activates plasma thromboplastin antecedent. *J Clin Invest* 1961;40:803–819.
7. Thompson RE, Mandle R, Kaplan AP Jr. Association of factor XI and high molecular weight kininogen in human plasma. *J Clin Invest* 1977;60:1376–1380.
8. Kurachi K, Davie EW. Activation of human factor XI (plasma thromboplastin antecedent) by factor XIIa (activated Hageman factor). *Biochemistry* 1977;16:5831–5839.
9. Kurachi K, Fujikawa K, Davie EW. Mechanism of activation of bovine factor XI by factor XII and factor XIIa. *Biochemistry* 1980;19: 1330–1338.
10. Naito K, Fujikawa K. Activation of human blood coagulation factor XI independent of factor XII. Factor XI is activated by thrombin and factor XIa in the presence of negatively charged surfaces. *J Biol Chem* 1991;266:7353–7358.
11. Gailani D, Broze GJ Jr. Factor XI activation in a revised model of blood coagulation. *Science* 1991;253:909–912.
12. Fujikawa K, Legaz ME, Kato H, et al. The mechanism of activation of bovine factor IX (Christmas factor) by bovine factor XIa (activated plasma thromboplastin antecedent). *Biochemistry* 1974;13:4508–4516.
13. Di Scipio RG, Kurachi K, Davie EW. Activation of human factor IX (Christmas factor). *J Clin Invest* 1978;61:1528–1538.
14. Sinha D, Seaman FS, Walsh PN. Role of calcium ions and the heavy chain of factor XIa in the activation of human coagulation factor IX. *Biochemistry* 1987;26:3768–3775.
15. Asakai R, Davie EW, Chung DW. Organization of the gene for human factor XI. *Biochemistry* 1987;26:7221–7228.

16. Kato A, Asakai R, Davie EW, et al. Factor XI gene (F11) is located on the distal end of the long arm of human chromosome 4. *Cytogenet Cell Genet* 1989;52:77–78.

17. Fujikawa K, Chung DW, Hendrickson LE, et al. Amino acid sequence of human factor XI, a blood coagulation factor with four tandem repeats that are highly homologous with plasma prekallikrein. *Biochemistry* 1986;25:2417–2424.

18. Tordai H, Banyai L, Patthy L. The PAN module: the N-terminal domains of plasminogen and hepatocyte growth factor are homologous with the apple domains of the prekallikrein family and with a novel domain found in numerous nematode proteins. *FEBS Lett* 1999;461:63–67.

19. Brown PJ, Billington KJ, Bumstead JM, et al. A microneme protein from Eimeria tenella with homology to the Apple domains of coagulation factor XI and plasma pre-kallikrein. *Mol Biochem Parasitol* 2000;107:91–102.

20. Brown PJ, Gill AC, Nugent PG, et al. Domains of invasion organelle proteins from apicomplexan parasites are homologous with the Apple domains of blood coagulation factor XI and plasma pre-kallikrein and are members of the PAN module superfamily. *FEBS Lett* 2001;497:31–38.

21. Jiang Y, Doolittle RF. The evolution of vertebrate blood coagulation as viewed from a comparison of puffer fish and sea squirt genomes. *Proc Natl Acad Sci U S A* 2003;100:7527–7532. *Epub 2003 Jun 7513.*

22. Dang QD, Di Cera E. Residue 225 determines the Na(+)-induced allosteric regulation of catalytic activity in serine proteases. *Proc Natl Acad Sci U S A* 1996;93:10653–10656.

23. Tarumi T, Kravtsov DV, Zhao M, et al. Cloning and characterization of the human factor XI gene promoter. transcription factor hepatocyte nuclear factor 4alpha (HNF-4alpha) is required for hepatocyte-specific expression of factor XI. *J Biol Chem* 2002;277:18510–18516.

24. Gailani D, Sun MF, Sun Y. A comparison of murine and human factor XI. *Blood* 1997;90:1055–1064.

25. Sinha D, Marcinkiewicz M, Gailani D, et al. Molecular cloning and biochemical characterization of rabbit factor XI. *Biochem J* 2002;367:49–56.

26. Wiggins RC, Cochrane CG, Griffin JH. Rabbit blood coagulation factor XI. Purification and properties. *Thromb Res* 1979;15:475–486.

27. Asakai R, Chung DW, Ratnoff OD, et al. Factor XI (plasma thromboplastin antecedent) deficiency in Ashkenazi Jews is a bleeding disorder that can result from three types of point mutations. *Proc Natl Acad Sci U S A* 1989;86:7667–7671.

28. Meijers JC, Davie EW, Chung DW. Expression of human blood coagulation factor XI: characterization of the defect in factor XI type III deficiency. *Blood* 1992;79:1435–1440.

29. Meijers JC, Mulvihill ER, Davie EW, et al. Apple four in human blood coagulation factor XI mediates dimer formation. *Biochemistry* 1992;31:4680–4684.

30. Clarkson K, Rosenfeld B, Fair J, et al. Factor XI deficiency acquired by liver transplantation. *Ann Intern Med* 1991;115:877–879.

31. Heck LW, Kaplan AP. Substrates of Hageman factor. I. Isolation and characterization of human factor XI (PTA) and inhibition of the activated enzyme by alpha 1-antitrypsin. *J Exp Med* 1974;140:1615–1630.

32. Movat HZ, Ozge-Anwar AH. The contact phase of blood coagulation: clotting factors XI and XII, their isolation and interaction. *J Lab Clin Med* 1974;84:861–878.

33. Saito H, Goldsmith GH Jr. Plasma thromboplastin antecedent (PTA, factor XI): a specific and sensitive radioimmunoassay. *Blood* 1977;50:377–385.

34. McMullen BA, Fujikawa K, Davie EW. Location of the disulfide bonds in human coagulation factor XI: the presence of tandem apple domains. *Biochemistry* 1991;30:2056–2060.

35. Lipscomb MS, Walsh PN. Human platelets and factor XI. Localization in platelet membranes of factor XI-like activity and its functional distinction from plasma factor XI. *J Clin Invest* 1979;63:1006–1014.

36. Tuszynski GP, Bevacqua SJ, Schmaier AH, et al. Factor XI antigen and activity in human platelets. *Blood* 1982;59:1148–1156.

37. Schiffman S, Yeh CH. Purification and characterization of platelet factor XI. *Thromb Res* 1990;60:87–97.

38. Walsh PN. The effects of collagen and kaolin on the intrinsic coagulant activity of platelets. Evidence for an alternative pathway in intrinsic coagulation not requiring factor XII. *Br J Haematol* 1972;22:393–405.

39. Schiffman S, Rapaport SI, Chong MM. Platelets and initiation of intrinsic clotting. *Br J Haematol* 1973;24:633–642.

40. Komiyama Y, Nomura S, Murakami T, et al. Purification and characterization of platelet-type factor XI from human platelets. *Thromb Haemost* 1993;69:1238. (Abstract)

41. Hsu TC, Shore SK, Seshsmma T, et al. Molecular cloning of platelet factor XI, an alternative splicing product of the plasma factor XI gene. *J Biol Chem* 1998;273:13787–13793.

42. Hu CJ, Baglia FA, Mills DC, et al. Tissue-specific expression of functional platelet factor XI is independent of plasma factor XI expression. *Blood* 1998;91:3800–3807.

43. Walsh PN, Mills DC, Pareti FI, et al. Hereditary giant platelet syndrome. Absence of collagen-induced coagulant activity and deficiency of factor-XI binding to platelets. *Br J Haematol* 1975;29:639–655.

44. Martincic D, Kravtsov V, Gailani D. Factor XI messenger RNA in human platelets. *Blood* 1999;94:3397–3404.

45. Wiggins RC, Bouma BN, Cochrane CG, et al. Role of high-molecular-weight kininogen in surface-binding and activation of coagulation Factor XI and prekallikrein. *Proc Natl Acad Sci U S A* 1977;74:4636–4640.

46. Griffin JH, Cochrane CG. Mechanisms for the involvement of high molecular weight kininogen in surface-dependent reactions of Hageman factor. *Proc Natl Acad Sci U S A* 1976;73:2554–2558.

47. Meier HL, Pierce JV, Colman RW, et al. Activation and function of human Hageman factor. The role of high molecular weight kininogen and prekallikrein. *J Clin Invest* 1977;60:18–31.

48. Rosenthal RL, Dreskin OH, Rosenthal N. Plasma thromboplastin antecedent (PTA) deficiency: clinical coagulation, therapeutic and hereditary aspects of a new hemophilia-like disease. *Blood* 1955;10:120–131.

49. Ragni MV, Sinha D, Seaman F, et al. Comparison of bleeding tendency, factor XI coagulant activity, and factor XI antigen in 25 factor XI-deficient kindreds. *Blood* 1985;65:719–724.

50. Rimon A, Schiffman S, Feinstein DI, et al. Factor XI activity and factor XI antigen in homozygous and heterozygous factor XI deficiency. *Blood* 1976;48:165–174.

51. Baglia FA, Walsh PN. Prothrombin is a cofactor for the binding of factor XI to the platelet surface and for platelet-mediated factor XI activation by thrombin. *Biochemistry* 1998;37:2271–2281.

52. Shi T, Iverson GM, Qi JC, et al. Beta-2-glycoprotein I binds factor XI and inhibits its activation by thrombin and factor XIIa: loss of inhibition by clipped beta-2-glycoprotein I. *Proc Natl Acad Sci U S A* 2004;101:3939–3944.

53. Liu CY, Scott CF, Bagdasarian A, et al. Potentiation of the function of Hageman factor fragments by high molecular weight kininogen. *J Clin Invest* 1977;60:7–17.

54. Saito H, Ratnoff OD, Marshall JS, et al. Partial purification of plasma thromboplastin antecedent (factor XI) and its activation by trypsin. *J Clin Invest* 1973;52:850–861.

55. Schiffman S, Lee P. Preparation, characterization, and activation of a highly purified factor XI: evidence that a hitherto unrecognized plasma activity participates in the interaction of factors XI and XII. *Br J Haematol* 1974;27:101–114.

56. Schiffman S, Markland FS Jr. Effect of intermediates of extrinsic clotting on purified factor XI: factor VII and/or thromboplastin. *Thromb Res* 1975;6:273–279.

57. Baglia FA, Jameson BA, Walsh PN. Localization of the high molecular weight kininogen binding site in the heavy chain of human factor XI to amino acids phenylalanine 56 through serine 86. *J Biol Chem* 1990;265:4149–4154.

58. Baglia FA, Jameson BA, Walsh PN. Identification and chemical synthesis of a substrate-binding site for factor IX on coagulation factor XIa. *J Biol Chem* 1991;266:24190–24197.

59. Baglia FA, Jameson BA, Walsh PN. Fine mapping of the high molecular weight kininogen binding site on blood coagulation factor XI through the use of rationally designed synthetic analogs. *J Biol Chem* 1992;267:4247–4252.

60. Baglia FA, Jameson BA, Walsh PN. Identification and characterization of a binding site for factor XIIa in the Apple 4 domain of coagulation factor XI. *J Biol Chem* 1993;268:3838–3844.

61. Baglia FA, Jameson BA, Walsh PN. Identification and characterization of a binding site for platelets in the Apple 3 domain of coagulation factor XI. *J Biol Chem* 1995;270:6734–6740.

62. Walsh PN, Baglia FA, Jameson BA. Factor XI: structure-function relationships utilizing monoclonal antibodies protein modification, computational chemistry, and rational synthetic peptide design. *Meth Enzymol* 1993;222:65–96.

63. Baglia FA, Walsh PN. A binding site for thrombin in the apple 1 domain of factor XI. *J Biol Chem* 1996;271:3652–3658.

64. Baglia FA, Walsh PN. Thrombin-mediated feedback activation of factor XI on the activated platelet surface is preferred over contact activation by factor XIIa or factor XIa. *J Biol Chem* 2000;275:20514–20519.

65. Yun TH, Baglia FA, Myles T, et al. Thrombin activation of Factor XI on activated platelets requires the interaction of factor XI and platelet glycoprotein Ib{alpha} with thrombin anion-binding exosites I and II, respectively. *J Biol Chem* 2003;278:48112–48119.

66. Seaman FS, Baglia FA, Gurr JA, et al. Binding of high-molecular-mass kininogen to the Apple 1 domain of factor XI is mediated in part by Val64 and Ile77. *Biochem J* 1994;304:715–721.

67. Renne T, Gailani D, Meijers JC, et al. Characterization of the H-kininogen-binding site on factor XI: a comparison of factor XI and plasma prekallikrein. *J Biol Chem* 2002;277:4892–4899.

68. Baglia FA, Badellino KO, Ho DH, et al. A binding site for the kringle II domain of prothrombin in the apple 1 domain of factor XI. *J Biol Chem* 2000;275:31954–31962.

69. Baglia FA, Seaman FS, Walsh PN. The Apple 1 and Apple 4 domains of factor XI act synergistically to promote the surface-mediated activation of factor XI by factor XIIa. *Blood* 1995;85:2078–2083.

70. Ho DH, Baglia FA, Walsh PN. Factor XI binding to activated platelets is mediated by residues R(250), K(255), F(260), and Q(263) within the Apple 3 domain. *Biochemistry* 2000;39:316–323.

71. Ho DH, Badellino K, Baglia FA, et al. The role of high molecular weight kininogen and prothrombin as cofactors in the binding of factor XI A3 domain to the platelet surface. *J Biol Chem* 2000;275:25139–25145.

72. Sun MF, Baglia FA, Ho D, et al. Defective binding of factor XI-N248 to activated human platelets. *Blood* 2001;98:125–129.

73. Baglia FA, Badellino KO, Li CQ, et al. Factor XI binding to the platelet glycoprotein Ib-IX-V complex promotes factor XI activation by thrombin. *J Biol Chem* 2002;277:1662–1668.

74. Baglia FA, Shrimpton CN, Lopez JA, et al. The glycoprotein Ib-IX-V complex mediates localization of factor XI to lipid rafts on the platelet membrane. *J Biol Chem* 2003;278:21744–21750.

75. Baglia FA, Lopez JA, Walsh PN. Identification of a binding site for glycoprotein Ib alpha in the Apple 3 domain of factor XI. *J Thromb Haemost* 2003;1:P1097.

76. Baglia FA, Shrimpton CN, Emsley J, et al. Factor XI interacts with the leucine-rich repeats of glycoprotein Ibalpha on the activated platelet. *Blood* 2003;102:129a.

77. Ho DH, Badellino K, Baglia FA, et al. A binding site for heparin in the apple 3 domain of factor XI. *J Biol Chem* 1998;273:16382–16390.

78. Zhao M, Abdel-Razek T, Sun MF, et al. Characterization of a heparin binding site on the heavy chain of factor XI. *J Biol Chem* 1998;273:31153–31159.

79. Cheng Q, Sun MF, Kravtsov DV, et al. Factor XI apple domains and protein dimerization. *J Thromb Haemost* 2003;1:2340–2347.

80. Dorfman R, Walsh PN. Noncovalent interactions of the Apple 4 domain that mediate coagulation factor XI homodimerization. *J Biol Chem* 2001;276:6429–6438.

81. Gailani D, Ho D, Sun MF, et al. Model for a factor IX activation complex on blood platelets: dimeric conformation of factor XIa is essential. *Blood* 2001;97:3117–3122.

82. Riley PW, Chong PL-G, Roder H, et al. Fluorescence anisotropy and circular dichroism studies of the monomer-dimer equilibrium and the associated unfolding states of coagulation factor XI Apple 4 domain. *Blood* 2003;102:302a.

83. Yang X, Chang Y-J, Lin S-W, et al. Identification of residues Asn 89, Ile 90 and Val 107 of the factor IXa second epidermal growth factor domain that are essential for the assembly of the factor-X activating complex on activated platelets. *Blood* 2003;102:304a.

84. Sinha D, Koshy A, Seaman FS, et al. Functional characterization of human blood coagulation factor XIa using hybridoma antibodies. *J Biol Chem* 1985;260:10714–10719.

85. Sun Y, Gailani D. Identification of a factor IX binding site on the third apple domain of activated factor XI. *J Biol Chem* 1996;271:29023–29028.

86. Sun MF, Zhao M, Gailani D. Identification of amino acids in the factor XI apple 3 domain required for activation of factor IX. *J Biol Chem* 1999;274:36373–36378.

87. Baird TR, Walsh PN. The interaction of factor XIa with activated platelets but not endothelial cells promotes the activation of factor IX in the consolidation phase of blood coagulation. *J Biol Chem* 2002;277:38462–38467.

88. Sinha D, Seaman FS, Koshy A, et al. Blood coagulation factor XIa binds specifically to a site on activated human platelets distinct from that for factor XI. *J Clin Invest* 1984;73:1550–1556.

89. Miller TN, Baird TR, Baglia FA, et al. The catalytic domain of the enzyme (factor XIa) mediates Zn2+-dependent binding to a site on activated platelets distinct from the binding site for zymogen (factor XI). *Blood* 2002;100:489a. (Abstract)

90. Zhang Y, Scandura JM, Van Nostrand WE, et al. The mechanism by which heparin promotes the inhibition of coagulation factor XIa by protease nexin-2. *J Biol Chem* 1997;272:26139–26144.

91. Badellino KO, Walsh PN. Localization of a heparin binding site in the catalytic domain of factor XIa. *Biochemistry* 2001;40:7569–7580.

92. Greengard JS, Heeb MJ, Ersdal E, et al. Binding of coagulation factor XI to washed human platelets. *Biochemistry* 1986;25:3884–3890.

93. Walsh PN, Griffin JH. Contributions of human platelets to the proteolytic activation of blood coagulation factors XII and XI. *Blood* 1981;57:106–118.

94. Scandura JM, Zhang Y, Van Nostrand WE, et al. Progress curve analysis of the kinetics with which blood coagulation factor XIa is inhibited by protease nexin-2. *Biochemistry* 1997;36:412–420.

95. Castaldi PA, Larrieu MJ, Caen J. Availability of platelet Factor 3 and activation of factor XII in thrombasthenia. *Nature* 1965;207:422–424.

96. Mustard JF, Hegardt B, Roswell HC, et al. Effect of adenosine nucleotides on platelet aggregation and clotting time. *J Lab Clin Med* 1964;65:548–559.

97. Mustard JF, Rowsell HC, Lotz F, et al. The effect of adenine nucleotides on thrombus formation, platelet count, and blood coagulation. *Exp Mol Pathol* 1966;5:43–60.

98. Pizzuto J, Giorgio AJ, Didisheim P. [The effect of "ADP" in coagulation]. *Rev Invest Clin* 1966;18:297–305.

99. Weiss HJ, Kochwa S. Studies of platelet function and proteins in 3 patients with Glanzmann's thrombasthenia. *J Lab Clin Med* 1968;71:153–165.

100. Walsh PN. Albumin density gradient separation and washing of platelets and the study of platelet coagulant activities. *Br J Haematol* 1972;22:205–217.

101. Walsh PN. The role of platelets in the contact phase of blood coagulation. *Br J Haematol* 1972;22:237–254.

102. Greengard JS, Griffin JH. Receptors for high molecular weight kininogen on stimulated washed human platelets. *Biochemistry* 1984;23:6863–6869.

103. Gustafson EJ, Schutsky D, Knight LC, et al. High molecular weight kininogen binds to unstimulated platelets. *J Clin Invest* 1986;78:310–318.

104. Baglia FA, Sinha D, Walsh PN. Functional domains in the heavy-chain region of factor XI: a high molecular weight kininogen-binding site and a substrate-binding site for factor IX. *Blood* 1989;74:244–251.

105. Celikel R, McClintock RA, Roberts JR, et al. Modulation of alpha-thrombin function by distinct interactions with platelet glycoprotein Ibalpha. *Science* 2003;301:218–221.

106. Dumas JJ, Kumar R, Seehra J, et al. Crystal structure of the GpIbalpha-thrombin complex essential for platelet aggregation. *Science* 2003;301:222–226.

107. Stern DM, Drillings M, Kisiel W, et al. Activation of factor IX bound to cultured bovine aortic endothelial cells. *Proc Natl Acad Sci U S A* 1984;81:913–917.

108. Stern DM, Drillings M, Nossel HL, et al. Binding of factors IX and IXa to cultured vascular endothelial cells. *Proc Natl Acad Sci U S A* 1983;80:4119–4123.

109. Stern DM, Nawroth PP, Kisiel W, et al. A coagulation pathway on bovine aortic segments leading to generation of Factor Xa and thrombin. *J Clin Invest* 1984;74:1910–1921.

110. Berrettini M, Schleef RR, Heeb MJ, et al. Assembly and expression of an intrinsic factor IX activator complex on the surface of cultured human endothelial cells. *J Biol Chem* 1992;267:19833–19839.

111. Schmaier AH, Kuo A, Lundberg D, et al. The expression of high molecular weight kininogen on human umbilical vein endothelial cells. *J Biol Chem* 1988;263:16327–16333.

112. Hasan AA, Cines DB, Herwald H, et al. Mapping the cell binding site on high molecular weight kininogen domain 5. *J Biol Chem* 1995;270:19256–19261.

113. Herwald H, Hasan AA, Godovac-Zimmermann J, et al. Identification of an endothelial cell binding site on kininogen domain D3. *J Biol Chem* 1995;270:14634–14642.

114. Baird TR, Walsh PN. Activated platelets but not endothelial cells participate in the initiation of the consolidation phase of blood coagulation. *J Biol Chem* 2002;277:28498–28503.

115. Motta G, Rojkjaer R, Hasan AA, et al. High molecular weight kininogen regulates prekallikrein assembly and activation on endothelial cells: a novel mechanism for contact activation. *Blood* 1998;91:516–528.

116. Baird TR, Walsh PN. Factor XI, but not prekallikrein, blocks high molecular weight kininogen binding to human umbilical vein endothelial cells. *J Biol Chem* 2003;278:20618–20623.

117. Mahdi F, Shariat-Madar Z, Schmaier AH. The relative priority of prekallikrein and factors XI/XIa assembly on cultured endothelial cells. *J Biol Chem* 2003;278:43983–43990. *Epub 42003 Aug 43927.*

118. Lin Y, Harris RB, Yan W, et al. High molecular weight kininogen peptides inhibit the formation of kallikrein on endothelial cell surfaces and subsequent urokinase-dependent plasmin formation. *Blood* 1997;90:690–697.

119. Osterud B, Bouma BN, Griffin JH. Human blood coagulation factor IX. Purification, properties, and mechanism of activation by activated factor XI. *J Biol Chem* 1978;253:5946–5951.

120. Anson DS, Choo KH, Rees DJ, et al. The gene structure of human antihaemophilic factor IX. *EMBO J* 1984;3:1053–1060.

121. Jaye M, de la Salle H, Schamber F, et al. Isolation of a human antihaemophilic factor IX cDNA clone using a unique 52-base synthetic oligonucleotide probe deduced from the amino acid sequence of bovine factor IX. *Nucleic Acids Res* 1983;11:2325–2335.

122. Jagadeeswaran P, Lavelle DE, Kaul R, et al. Isolation and characterization of human factor IX cDNA: identification of Taq I polymorphism and regional assignment. *Somat Cell Mol Genet* 1984;10:465–473.

123. Kurachi K, Davie EW. Isolation and characterization of a cDNA coding for human factor IX. *Proc Natl Acad Sci U S A* 1982;79:6461–6464.

124. Yoshitake S, Schach BG, Foster DC, et al. Nucleotide sequence of the gene for human factor IX (antihemophilic factor B). *Biochemistry* 1985;24:3736–3750.

125. Peek M, Moran P, Mendoza N, et al. Unusual proteolytic activation of pro-hepatocyte growth factor by plasma kallikrein and coagulation factor XIa. *J Biol Chem* 2002;277:47804–47809.

126. van der Graaf F, Greengard JS, Bouma BN, et al. Isolation and functional characterization of the active light chain of activated human blood coagulation factor XI. *J Biol Chem* 1983;258:9669–9675.

127. Aktimur A, Gabriel MA, Gailani D. The factor IX gamma-carboxyglutamic acid (Gla) domain is involved in interactions between factor IX and factor XIa. *J Biol Chem* 2003;278:7981–7987. *2002 Epub Dec 7920.*

128. Beeler DL, Marcum JA, Schiffman S, et al. Interaction of factor XIa and antithrombin in the presence and absence of heparin. *Blood* 1986;67:1488–1492.

129. Scott CF, Schapira M, Colman RW. Effect of heparin on the inactivation rate of human factor XIa by antithrombin-III. *Blood* 1982;60:940–947.

130. Scott CF, Schapira M, James HL, et al. Inactivation of factor XIa by plasma protease inhibitors: predominant role of alpha 1-protease inhibitor and protective effect of high molecular weight kininogen. *J Clin Invest* 1982;69:844–852.

131. Forbes CD, Pensky J, Ratnoff OD. Inhibition of activated Hageman factor and activated plasma thromboplastin antecedent by purified serum C1 inactivator. *J Lab Clin Med* 1970;76:809–815.

132. Walsh PN, Sinha D, Kueppers F, et al. Regulation of factor XIa activity by platelets and alpha 1-protease inhibitor. *J Clin Invest* 1987;80:1578–1586.

133. Damus PS, Hicks M, Rosenberg RD. Anticoagulant action of heparin. *Nature* 1973;246:355–357.

134. Soons H, Janssen-Claessen T, Tans G, et al. Inhibition of factor XIa by antithrombin III. *Biochemistry* 1987;26:4624–4629.

135. Meijers JC, Vlooswijk RA, Bouma BN. Inhibition of human blood coagulation factor XIa by C-1 inhibitor. *Biochemistry* 1988;27:959–963.

136. Saito H, Goldsmith GH, Moroi M, et al. Inhibitory spectrum of alpha 2-plasmin inhibitor. *Proc Natl Acad Sci U S A* 1979;76:2013–2017.

137. Scott CF, Colman RW. Factors influencing the acceleration of human factor XIa inactivation by antithrombin III. *Blood* 1989;73:1873–1879.

138. Knauer DJ, Majumdar D, Fong PC, et al. SERPIN regulation of factor XIa. The novel observation that protease nexin 1 in the presence of heparin is a more potent inhibitor of factor XIa than C1 inhibitor. *J Biol Chem* 2000;275:37340–37346.

139. Berrettini M, Schleef RR, Espana F, et al. Interaction of type 1 plasminogen activator inhibitor with the enzymes of the contact activation system. *J Biol Chem* 1989;264:11738–11743.

140. Espana F, Berrettini M, Griffin JH. Purification and characterization of plasma protein C inhibitor. *Thromb Res* 1989;55:369–384.

141. Wuillemin WA, Eldering E, Citarella F, et al. Modulation of contact system proteases by glycosaminoglycans. Selective enhancement of the inhibition of factor XIa. *J Biol Chem* 1996;271:12913–12918.

142. Walsh PN, Sinha D, Koshy A, et al. Functional characterization of platelet-bound factor XIa: retention of factor XIa activity on the platelet surface. *Blood* 1986;68:225–230.

143. Ahmad SS, Rawala-Sheikh R, Walsh PN. Comparative interactions of factor IX and factor IXa with human platelets. *J Biol Chem* 1989;264:3244–3251.

144. Soons H, Janssen-Claessen T, Hemker HC, et al. The effect of platelets in the activation of human blood coagulation factor IX by factor XIa. *Blood* 1986;68:140–148.

145. Cronlund AL, Walsh PN. A low molecular weight platelet inhibitor of factor XIa: purification, characterization, and possible role in blood coagulation. *Biochemistry* 1992;31:1685–1694.

146. Bush AI, Martins RN, Rumble B, et al. The amyloid precursor protein of Alzheimer's disease is released by human platelets. *J Biol Chem* 1990;265:15977–15983.

147. Smith RP, Higuchi DA, Broze GJ. Jr. Platelet coagulation factor XIa-inhibitor, a form of Alzheimer amyloid precursor protein. *Science* 1990;248:1126–1128.

148. Van Nostrand WE, Schmaier AH, Farrow JS, et al. Protease nexin-II (amyloid beta-protein precursor): a platelet alpha-granule protein. *Science* 1990;248:745–748.

149. Badellino KO, Walsh PN. Protease nexin II interactions with coagulation factor XIa are contained within the Kunitz protease inhibitor domain of protease nexin II and the factor XIa catalytic domain. *Biochemistry* 2000;39:4769–4777.

150. Navaneetham D, Jin L, Babine RE, et al. Molecular interactions between the Kunitz protease inhibitory domain of protease nexin 2 and the catalytic subunit of factor XIa revealed by x-ray crystallography and mutational analysis. *Blood* 2003;102:127a.

151. Ahmad SS, Rawala-Sheikh R, Walsh PN. Platelet receptor occupancy with factor IXa promotes factor X activation. *J Biol Chem* 1989;264:20012–20016.

152. Ahmad SS, Rawala-Sheikh R, Ashby B, et al. Platelet receptor-mediated factor X activation by factor IXa. High-affinity factor IXa receptors induced by factor VIII are deficient on platelets in Scott syndrome. *J Clin Invest* 1989;84:824–828.

153. Rawala-Sheikh R, Ahmad SS, Ashby B, et al. Kinetics of coagulation factor X activation by platelet-bound factor IXa. *Biochemistry* 1990;29:2606–2611.

154. Asakai R, Chung DW, Davie EW, et al. Factor XI deficiency in Ashkenazi Jews in Israel. *N Engl J Med* 1991;325:153–158.

155. Kitchens CS. Factor XI: a review of its biochemistry and deficiency. *Semin Thromb Hemost* 1991;17:55–72.

156. Seligsohn U. Factor XI deficiency. *Thromb Haemost* 1993;70:68–71.

157. Gailani D. Advances and dilemmas in factor XI. *Current Opin Hematol* 1994;1:347–353.

158. Bolton-Maggs PH, Young Wan-Yin B, McCraw AH, et al. Inheritance and bleeding in factor XI deficiency. *Br J Haematol* 1988;69:521–528.

159. Sidi A, Seligsohn U, Jonas P, et al. Factor XI deficiency: detection and management during urologic surgery. *J Urol* 1978;119:528–530.

160. Campbell EW, Mednicoff IB, Dameshek MD. Plasma thromboplastin antecedent (PTA) deficiency. *AMA Arch Int Med* 1957;100:232–240.

161. Cavins JA, Wall RL. Clinical and laboratory studies of plasma thromboplastin antecedent deficiency (PTA). *Am J Med* 1960;29:444–448.

162. Seligsohn U, Griffin JH. Contact activation and factor XI. In: Scriver CR, Beaudet AL, Sly WS, et al, eds. *Metabolic and molecular basis of inherited disease*, 7th ed. New York: McGraw-Hill, 1995:3285–3311.

163. Seligsohn U. High gene frequency of factor XI (PTA) deficiency in Ashkenazi Jews. *Blood* 1978;51:1223–1228.

164. Peretz H, Mulai A, Usher S, et al. The two common mutations causing factor XI deficiency in Jews stem from distinct founders: one of ancient Middle Eastern origin and another of more recent European origin. *Blood* 1997;90:2654–2659.

165. Kravtsov DV, Wu W, Meijers JC, et al. Dominant factor XI deficiency caused by mutations in the factor XI catalytic domain. *Blood* 2004;16:16.

166. Forbes CD, Ratnoff OD. Studies on plasma thromboplastin antecedent (factor XI), PTA deficiency and inhibition of PTA by plasma: pharmacologic inhibitors and specific antiserum. *J Lab Clin Med* 1972;79:113–127.

167. Saito H, Ratnoff OD, Bouma BN, et al. Failure to detect variant (CRM+) plasma thromboplastin antecedent (factor XI) molecules in hereditary plasma thromboplastin antecedent deficiency: a study of 125 patients of several ethnic backgrounds. *J Lab Clin Med* 1985;106:718–722.

168. Mannhalter C, Hellstern P, Deutsch E. Identification of a defective factor XI cross-reacting material in a factor XI-deficient patient. *Blood* 1987;70:31–37.

169. Hancock JF, Wieland K, Pugh RE, et al. A molecular genetic study of factor XI deficiency. *Blood* 1991;77:1942–1948.

170. Pugh RE, McVey JH, Tuddenham EG, et al. Six point mutations that cause factor XI deficiency. *Blood* 1995;85:1509–1516.

171. Imanaka Y, Lal K, Nishimura T, et al. Identification of two novel mutations in non-Jewish factor XI deficiency. *Br J Haematol* 1995;90:916–920.

172. Peretz H, Zivelin A, Usher S, et al. A 14-bp deletion (codon 554 del AAG-gtaacagagtg) at exon 14/intron N junction of the coagulation factor XI gene disrupts splicing and causes severe factor XI deficiency. *Hum Mutat* 1996;8:77–78.

173. Wistinghausen B, Reischer A, Oddoux C, et al. Severe factor XI deficiency in an Arab family associated with a novel mutation in exon 11. *Br J Haematol* 1997;99:575–577.

174. Martincic D, Zimmerman SA, Ware RE, et al. Identification of mutations and polymorphisms in factor XI genes of an African-American family by dideoxyfingerprinting. *Blood* 1998;92:3309–3317.

175. Ventura C, Santos AI, Tavares A, et al. Molecular genetic analysis of factor XI deficiency: identification of five novel gene alterations and the origin of type II mutation in Portuguese families. *Thromb Haemost* 2000;84:833–840.

176. Iijima K, Udagawa A, Kawasaki H, et al. A factor XI deficiency associated with a nonsense mutation (Trp501stop) in the catalytic domain. *Br J Haematol* 2000;111:556–558.

177. Dossenbach-Glaninger A, Krugluger W, Schrattbauer K, et al. Severe factor XI deficiency caused by compound heterozygosity for the type III mutation and a novel insertion in exon 9 (codons 324/325 +G). *Br J Haematol* 2001;114:875–877.

178. Kawaguchi T, Koga S, Hongo H, et al. A novel type of factor XI deficiency showing compound genetic abnormalities: a nonsense mutation and an impaired transcription. *Int J Hematol* 2000;71:84–89.

179. Au WY, Cheung JW, Lam CC, et al. Two factor XI mutations in a Chinese family with factor XI deficiency. *Am J Hematol* 2003;74:136–138.

180. Wu WM, Wang HL, Wang XF, et al. [Identification of two novel factor XI non-sense mutation Trp228stop and Trp383stop in a Chinese pedigree of congenital factor XI deficiency]. *Zhonghua Xue Ye Xue Za Zhi* 2003;24:126–128.

181. Bolton-Maggs P, Butler R, Mountford R, et al. Eleven novel mutations in non-Jewish factor XI deficient kindred detected by SSCP with heteroduplex analysis followed by sequencing. *J Thromb Haemost* 2003;1(Suppl. 1):P1687.

182. Quelin F, Trossaert M, Sigaud M, et al. Molecular basis of severe factor XI deficiency in seven families from the west of France. Seven novel mutations, including an ancient Q88X mutation. *J Thromb Haemost* 2004;2:71–76.

183. Zivelin A, Bauduer F, Ducout L, et al. Factor XI deficiency in French Basques is caused predominantly by an ancestral Cys38Arg mutation in the factor XI gene. *Blood* 2002;99:2448–2454.

184. Mitchell MJ, Harrington P, Cutler J, et al. An alu-mediated 31.5 kb deletion as the cause of factor XI deficiency in two unrelated patients. *Blood* 2003;102:444 (Abstract).

185. Mitchell M, Harrington P, Cutler J, et al. Eighteen unrelated patients with factor XI deficiency, four novel mutations and a 100% detection rate by denaturing high-performance liquid chromatography. *Br J Haematol* 2003;121:500–502.

186. Litz CE, Swaim WR, Dalmasso AP. Factor XI deficiency: genetic and clinical studies of a single kindred. *Am J Hematol* 1988;28:8–12.

187. Mitchell M, Cutler J, Thompson S, et al. Heterozygous factor XI deficiency associated with three novel mutations. *Br J Haematol* 1999;107:763–765.

188. Gailani D, Bolton-Maggs PHB, Blinder M, et al. Amino acid substitutions in the factor XI catalytic domain associated with factor XI deficiency. *Thromb Haemost* 2001;P1112.

189. Zivelin A, Ogawa S, Bulvik S, et al. Severe factor XI deficiency caused by a Gly555 to Glu mutation (factor XI-Glu555): a cross-reactive material positive variant defective in factor IX activation. *J Thromb Haemost* 2004;2:1782–1789.

190. Cargill M, Altshuler D, Ireland J, et al. Characterization of single-nucleotide polymorphisms in coding regions of human genes. *Nat Genet* 1999;22:231–238.

191. Walsh PN. Roles of platelets and factor XI in the initiation of blood coagulation by thrombin. *Thromb Haemost* 2001;86:75–82.

192. Gailani D, Lasky NM, Broze GJ. Jr. A murine model of factor XI deficiency. *Blood Coagul Fibrin* 1997;8:134–144.

193. Nossel HL, Niemetz J, Sawitsky A. Blood PTA (factor XI) levels following plasma infusion. *Proc Soc Exp Biol Med* 1964;115:896–897.

194. Bolton-Maggs PH, Wensley RT, Kernoff PB, et al. Production and therapeutic use of a factor XI concentrate from plasma. *Thromb Haemost* 1992;67:314–319.

195. Berliner S, Horowitz I, Martinowitz U, et al. Dental surgery in patients with severe factor XI deficiency without plasma replacement. *Blood Coagul Fibrin* 1992;3:465–468.

196. von dem Borne PA, Meijers JC, Bouma BN. Feedback activation of factor XI by thrombin in plasma results in additional formation of thrombin that protects fibrin clots from fibrinolysis. *Blood* 1995;86:3035–3042.

197. Wang W, Hendriks D, Scharpe S. Carboxypeptidase U, a plasma carboxypeptidase with high affinity for plasminogen. *J Biol Chem* 1994;269: 15937–15944.

198. Hendriks D, Scharpe S, Van Sande M, et al. Characterization of a carboxypeptidase in human serum distinct from carboxypeptidase. *Clin Chem Clin Biochem* 1989;27:277–285.

199. Tan AK, Eaton DL. Activation and characterization of procarboxypeptidase B from human plasma. *Biochemistry* 1995;34:5811–5816.

200. Bajzar L, Manuel R, Nesheim ME. Purification and characterization of TAFI, a thrombin-activatable fibrinolysis inhibitor. *J Biol Chem* 1995; 270:14477–14484.

201. Redlitz A, Tan AK, Eaton DL, et al. Plasma carboxypeptidases as regulators of the plasminogen system. *J Clin Invest* 1995;96:2534–2538.

202. Meijers JC, Tekelenburg WL, Bouma BN, et al. High levels of coagulation factor XI as a risk factor for venous thrombosis. *N Engl J Med* 2000;342: 696–701.

203. Berliner JI, Rybicki AC, Kaplan RC, et al. Elevated levels of Factor XI are associated with cardiovascular disease in women. *Thromb Res* 2002;107: 55–60.

204. Salomon O, Steinberg DM, Dardik R, et al. Inherited factor XI deficiency confers no protection against acute myocardial infarction. *J Thromb Haemost* 2003;1:658–661.

205. Eichinger S, Schoenauer V, Weltermann A, et al. Thrombin activatable fibrinolysis inhibitor (TAFI) and the risk of recurrent venous thromboembolism. *Blood* 2004;22:22.

206. Libourel EJ, Bank I, Meinardi JR, et al. Co-segregation of thrombophilic disorders in factor V Leiden carriers; the contributions of factor VIII, factor XI, thrombin activatable fibrinolysis inhibitor and lipoprotein(a) to the absolute risk of venous thromboembolism. *Haematologica* 2002;87: 1068–1073.

207. Minnema MC, Friederich PW, Levi M, et al. Enhancement of rabbit jugular vein thrombolysis by neutralization of factor XI. *In vivo* evidence for a role of factor XI as an anti-fibrinolytic factor. *J Clin Invest* 1998;101:10–14.

208. Rosen ED, Gailani D, Castellino FJ. FXI is essential for thrombus formation following FeCl3-induced injury of the carotid artery in the mouse. *Thromb Haemost* 2002;87:774–776.

209. Chan JC, Ganopolsky JG, Cornelissen I, et al. The characterization of mice with a targeted combined deficiency of protein c and factor XI. *Am J Pathol* 2001;158:469–479.

210. Gruber A, Hanson SR. Factor XI-dependence of surface- and tissue-factor–initiated thrombus propagation in primates. *Blood* 2003;102:953–955. *Epub 2003 Apr 2010.*

211. Davie EW, Ratnoff OD. Waterfall sequence for intrinsic blood clotting. *Science* 1964;145:1310–1312.

212. MacFarlane RG. An enzyme cascade in the blood clotting mechanism, and its function as a biochemical amplifier. *Nature* 1964;202:498–499.

213. Zur M, Nemerson Y. Kinetics of factor IX activation via the extrinsic pathway dependence of Km on tissue factor. *J Biol Chem* 1980;255: 5703–5707.

214. Jesty J, Silverberg SA. Kinetics of the tissue factor-dependent activation of coagulation factors IX and X in a bovine plasma system. *J. Biol Chem* 1979;254:12337–12345.

215. Marlar RA, Kleiss AJ, Griffin JH. An alternative extrinsic pathway of human blood coagulation. *Blood* 1982;60:1353–1358.

216. Steinberg M, Nemerson Y. Activation of factor X. In: Colman RW, Hirsh J, Marder VJ, et al, eds. *Hemostasis and Thrombosis. Basic Principles and Clinical Practice*, 2nd. Philadelphia: J.B. Lippincott, 1987:112–119.

217. Morrison SA, Jesty J. Tissue factor-dependent activation of tritium labeled factor IX and factor X in human plasma. *Blood* 1984;63:1338–1347.

218. Sanders NL, Bajaj SP, Zivelin A, et al. Inhibition of tissue factor/factor VIIa activity in plasma requires factor X and an additional plasma component. *Blood* 1985;66:204–212.

219. Hubbard AR, Jennings CA. Inhibition of tissue thromboplastin-mediated blood coagulation. *Thromb Res* 1986;42:489–498.

220. Rao LVM, Rapaport SI. Studies on the mechanisms of inactivation of the extrinsic pathway of coagulation. *Blood* 1987;69:645–651.

221. Broze GJJ, Miletich JP. Characterization of the inhibition of tissue factor in serum. *Blood* 1987;69:150–155.

222. Broze GJJ, Miletich JP. Isolation of the tissue factor inhibitor produced by HepG2 hepatoma cells. *Proc Natl Acad Sci U S A* 1987;84:1886–1890.

223. Hubbard AR, Jennings CA. Inhibition of the tissue factor-factor VII complex: involvement of factor Xa and lipoproteins. *Thromb Res* 1987;46: 527–537.

224. Broze GJ Jr, Warren LA, Novotny WF, et al. The lipoprotein-associated coagulation inhibitor that inhibits the factor VII-tissue factor complex also inhibits factor Xa: insight into its possible mechanism of activation. *Blood* 1988;71:335–343.

225. Broze GJ, Girard TJ, Novotny WF. Jr. Regulation of coagulation by a multivalent Kunitz-type inhibitor. *Biochemistry* 1990;29:7539–7546.

226. Gailani D, Broze GJ. Jr. Factor XII-independent activation of factor XI in plasma: effects of sulfatides on tissue factor-induced coagulation. *Blood* 1993;82:813–819.

227. Scott CF, Colman RW. Fibrinogen blocks the autoactivation and thrombin-mediated activation of factor XI on dextran sulfate. *Proc Natl Acad Sci U S A* 1992;89:11189–11193.

# CHAPTER 13 ■ ANTITHROMBIN III AND HEPARIN COFACTOR II

SUSAN C. BOCK

## ANTITHROMBIN III

### Overview

Antithrombin III (ATIII) is a plasma proteinase inhibitor that inactivates thrombin and the enzymes responsible for the generation of thrombin. This combination of properties makes ATIII a very powerful and important endogenous anticoagulant molecule and explains why patients with even modest ATIII deficiencies experience clinical thrombosis. The anticoagulant activity of pharmaceutical heparin derives from their ability to potentiate the inhibitory activity of ATIII by mechanisms that are similar to physiologic activation of ATIII by vessel-wall heparan sulfate proteoglycans (HSPGs). In addition to its well-known anticoagulant activity, ATIII also has antiinflammatory, antiproliferative, antiangiogenic, and antiviral properties that are related to its ability to block noncoagulant as well as coagulant functions of thrombin and to its ability to assume a variety of protein conformations.

### Biochemistry

The plasma concentration of human ATIII (1) is about 2.4 $\mu$M (i.e., 140 $\mu$g per mL) (2). It circulates as two glycoforms: The predominant ATIII-$\alpha$ glycoform accounts for more than 90% of the ATIII in plasma, whereas the minor ATIII-$\beta$ variant represents less than 10% of ATIII concentration (3). Both isoforms have an identical polypeptide backbone, for which the complete amino acid sequence is known (4,5). Disulfide bonds link cysteines 8 with 128, 21 with 95, and 247 with 430 (4). The major $\alpha$-ATIII isoform is modified with four identical sialylated, biantennary complex oligosaccharides on asparagines 96, 135, 155, and 192 (6,7), and these account for 15% of the total mass of 58,000 Da. The minor $\beta$-ATIII isoform is not glycosylated on asparagine135, and some of its properties are distinct from those of the $\alpha$-isoform, as discussed in the section on $\beta$-antithrombin. Both ATIII isoforms adopt several different protein conformations, which have distinct physical and functional properties. Crystal structures are available for several conformations and have considerably advanced the understanding of ATIII mechanism and regulation (8–13).

The enzymes that are targets of ATIII inhibitory activity mediate blood coagulation, platelet activation, protease-activated receptor (PAR) signaling, and cell proliferation (see Fig. 13-1). The name "antithrombin" is somewhat misleading because it suggests that ATIII is primarily an inhibitor of thrombin, when in fact, it has broad inhibitory activity for many different factors in the coagulation cascade. ATIII serves as an important regulator of hemostasis and thrombosis at several levels by blocking: (a) thrombin-mediated fibrin clot formation, (b) common pathway factor Xa- (FXa)-mediated thrombin generation, and (c) coagulation factors that are higher up in the intrinsic and extrinsic pathways [factors IXa, XIa, XIIa (and its fragments), and plasma kallikrein (high-molecular-weight kininogen) and factor VIIa–TF]. ATIII inhibition of thrombin also serves to regulate its noncoagulant functions that mediate platelet activation and vascular cell signaling and proliferation (Fig. 13-1).

### Serpin Inhibition Mechanism

ATIII exhibits sequential, structural, and functional homology to members of the serpin (*serine proteinase inhibitor*) gene family (4,14). Many different serpins are present in blood and contribute to the regulation of coagulation (i.e., ATIII and HcII), complement (C1 inhibitor), fibrinolytic [i.e., plasminogen activator inhibitor-1 (PAI-1) and $\alpha_2$-antiplasmin], and inflammatory [i.e., $\alpha_1$-antitrypsin ($\alpha_1$-proteinase inhibitor)] pathways. Serpins inhibit their target enzymes by using a suicide-substrate inhibition mechanism that requires full function of the target proteinase catalytic apparatus and the formation of a covalent complex between the enzyme active site serine and the serpin (15). Serpins are globular molecules with protruding reactive center loops (RCLs) containing substratelike sequences that serve as "bait" for their target enzymes. Inhibitory complex formation begins when a target enzyme cleaves the scissile P1–P1' bond [nomenclature of Schechter and Berger, (16)] of the RCL substratelike sequence. This generates an acyl–enzyme complex in which the P1 residue is covalently linked to the target proteinase active site serine, and in which the polypeptides generated by reactive loop cleavage become mobile and get rearranged (17,18). The P1-containing polypeptide incorporates as an additional strand in the central $\beta$-sheet of the serpin, translocating the covalently bound target enzyme approximately 70 Å to the opposite pole of the serpin (19). The crystallographic structure of the $\alpha_1$-antitrypsin–trypsin (see Fig. 13-2) shows that inhibitory complex formation results in significant protein conformational changes in the inhibitor and the target enzyme (20). The serpin is converted from a stressed, 5-stranded A-sheet metastable conformation to a relaxed and hyperstable, 6-stranded A-sheet conformation. Physical deformation by crushing of the translocated target enzyme molecule against the hyperstable serpin molecule prevents regeneration of active proteinase by distorting catalytic triad geometry and preventing deacylation, and by facilitating efficient proteolysis of structurally disordered regions.

235

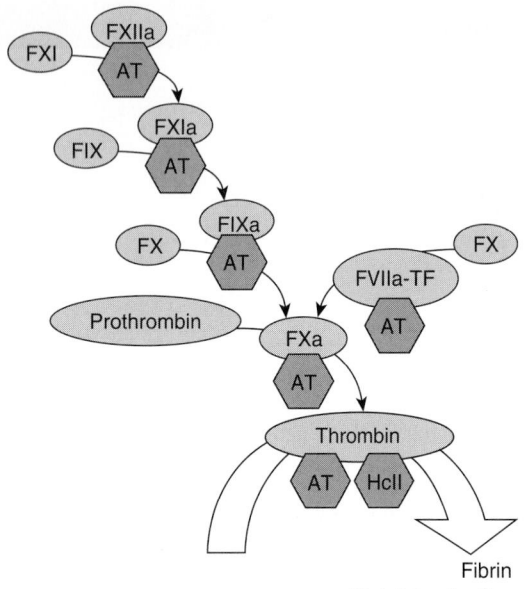

**FIGURE 13-1.** Antithrombin III (ATIII) and heparin cofactor II (HcII) target enzymes. ATIII inhibits coagulation factors in the intrinsic, extrinsic, and common pathways. ATIII and HcII inhibit thrombin, which has coagulant and noncoagulant functions. SMC, smooth muscle cell; EC NO, endothelial cell nitric oxide.

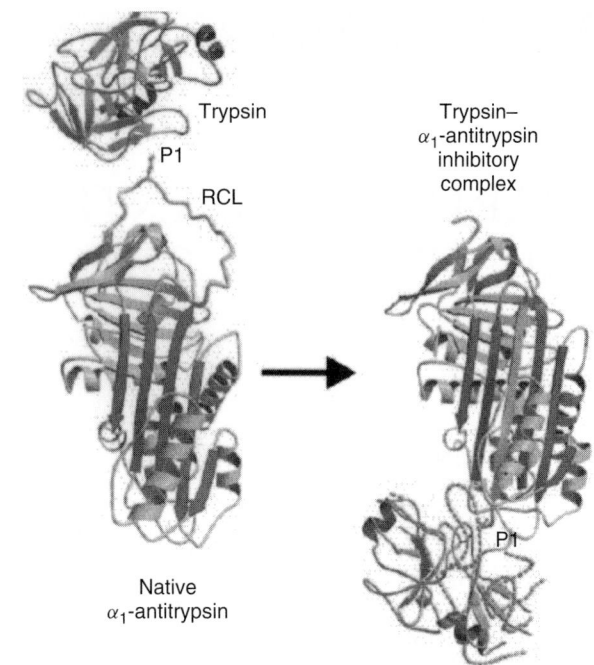

**FIGURE 13-2.** Serpin inhibition mechanism. **Left:** The native $\alpha_1$-antitrypsin molecule contains a 5-stranded central $\beta$-sheet (*red*) and an intact and fully exposed reactive center loop (RCL) (*yellow*) that is recognized as a substrate by target enzymes, including trypsin. **Right:** Formation of an inhibitory complex between $\alpha_1$-antitrypsin and trypsin involves: (a) trypsin recognition and cleavage of the P1–P1' peptide bond in the RCL polypeptide, (b) formation of a covalent acyl linkage between the serpin P1 residue and the enzyme active site serine, (c) expansion of the serpin central $\beta$-sheet by incorporation of the cleaved RCL polypeptide as a sixth strand, (d) translocation of the P1 residue and covalently bound enzyme from the north pole to the south pole of the serpin molecule, and (e) deformation of the translocated trypsin molecule. Target enzyme deformation in the inhibitory complex alters active-site geometry, which prevents deacylation and facilitates proteolytic destruction of disordered regions (interrupted coils) (see Color Fig. 13-2). (From Huntington J, Read R, Carrell R. Structure of a serpin-protease complex shows inhibition by deformation. *Nature* 2000;407:923–926, with permission.)

## Heparin Cofactor Binding to and Activation of Antithrombin III

ATIII exhibits the general serpin structural and mechanical features described in the preceding section, but it is somewhat unusual in being a considerably less efficient inhibitor than typical members of this family. Whereas rate constants for target proteinase inhibition by most serpins are in the $10^6$ to $10^7$ $M^{-1}$ $sec^{-1}$, the values for ATIII inhibition of thrombin and FXa are approximately three orders of magnitude lower. As illustrated in Figure 13-3, the limited reactivity of ATIII with its target enzymes is caused by a structural idiosyncrasy.

In contrast with other serpins that have fully exposed reactive loops (Fig. 13-3A), native ATIII circulates as a self-constrained molecule (Fig. 13-3B) in which the amino-terminal end of its reactive loop (*blue*) is partially inserted into its central $\beta$-sheet (9–11). This limits target enzyme access to the P1–P1' scissile bond (*purple*) of the reactive loop (21). However, ATIII can be activated fully for thrombin and for FXa inhibition by the binding of a cofactor molecule containing a specific heparin pentasaccharide sequence. Pentasaccharide binding to a site that is approximately 30 Å from the reactive loop allosterically induces its full exposure (Fig. 13-3C), which is accompanied by a 300-fold increase in the FXa inhibition rate.

The specific pentasaccharide sequence (22,23) required for high-affinity binding and activation of ATIII has the structure illustrated in Figure 13-4. This pentasaccharide is present in the approximately 30% of pharmaceutical heparin molecules having anticoagulant activity (24) and in the vascular wall and matrix HSPGs, which are endogenous ATIII receptors and activators (25,26).

ATIII-mediated thrombin, FXa, and FIXa inhibition rates are accelerated up to several 1,000-fold by a combination of heparin-dependent conformational change and bridging mechanisms. The relative importance of these mechanisms varies

with the target proteinase. The bridging effect is the most important factor in the activation of thrombin inhibition. Thrombin inhibition is accelerated just twofold in the presence of pentasaccharide, whereas pentasaccharide-containing heparin chains of greater than 18 sugar units in length accelerate the rate of inhibitory complex formation by more than 1000-fold (27). In contrast, an allosteric conformational change mechanism plays a large role in the acceleration of antithrombin III, FXa, and FIXa inhibition by heparin. Pentasaccharide alone accelerates rates of FXa and FIXa inhibitory complex formation by approximately 300 times (24,28,29). In the presence of $Ca^{2+}$, full-length heparin produces further 10- to 1,000-fold increases in rates of FXa and FIXa inhibition (28–30). An exosite, including strand 3C under the reactive center loop of ATIII, is exposed by heparin binding and contributes to cofactor acceleration of FXa and FIXa inhibition rates (31).

The ATIII pentasaccharide binding site is located on the surface of the inhibitor molecule at the junction of its N-terminal polypeptide and A and D helices (Fig. 13-3C and Fig. 13-5 for long-range and close-up views, respectively). The crystal structure of the AT*H complex (11,12) allowed direct identification of ATIII surface residues that contact the cofactor and largely confirmed heparin binding site residue assignments previously made on the basis of early chemical modification studies and

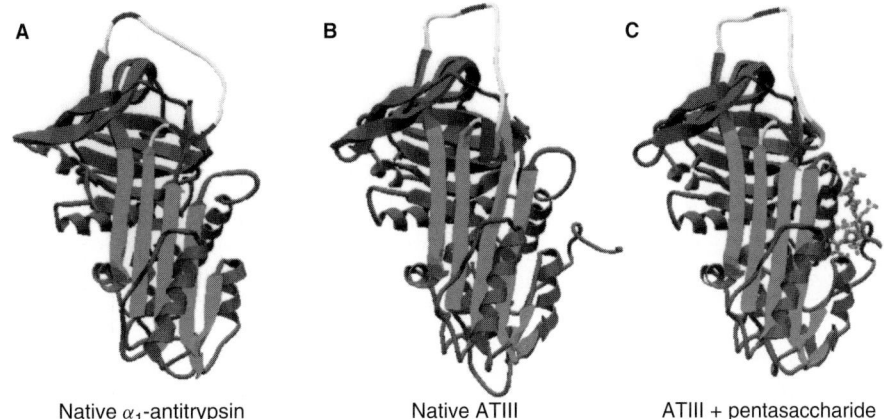

A    Native α₁-antitrypsin    B    Native ATIII    C    ATIII + pentasaccharide

**FIGURE 13-3.** Structural basis for limited reactivity of native ATIII, and ATIII allosteric activation by heparin pentasaccharide. Serpin–reactive center loop (RCL) polypeptides are drawn in *yellow*, with the P1–P1′ scissile bonds marked in *purple* and the P14 residues marked in *blue*. Central A β-sheets are *orange*. **A:** RCL loops of most serpins, such as α₁-antitrypsin, are fully exposed and unconstrained by A-sheet insertion, and they inhibit their target enzymes rates of approximately $10^6 \, M^{-1} \, sec^{-1}$. **B:** The RCL loop of native ATIII is constrained by insertion of its P14 residue into β-sheet-A, which reduces rates of native ATIII target enzyme inhibition to approximately $10^3 \, M^{-1} \, sec^{-1}$. **C:** Heparin pentasaccharide binding to ATIII allosterically expels the RCL loop and restores FXa inhibition rates into the approximately $10^6 \, M^{-1} \, sec^{-1}$ range. Figures are drawn using 1QLP.pbd for α₁-antitrypsin, 1E05.pbd for native ATIII, and 1E03.pbd for ATIII pentasaccharide (see Color Fig. 13-3).

the analysis of naturally occurring antithrombin mutants with heparin-binding defects. Detailed information about the roles of specific residues and their quantitative contributions to the binding of the cofactor and to the stabilization of the high-affinity AT*H complex have more recently become available from investigations of recombinant mutant ATIIIs.

Heparin binding to and activation of ATIII occurs according to the two-step mechanism illustrated in Figure 13-6 (32). An initial weak binding complex, AT–H, forms first; then, in a second step, a protein conformational change converts the AT–H intermediate to the activated, high-affinity AT*H complex that is competent for rapid FXa and FIXa inhibition. The overall affinity ($K_d$) of antithrombin for heparin results from the combined effects of the $K_1$ binding and $k_{+2}$ and $k_{-2}$ rate constants defined in the two-step mechanism. $K_1$ represents the dissociation equilibrium constant for formation of the initial weak binding complex, AT–H. $k_{+2}$ measures the rate for conformational conversion of initial weak AT–H complex to the high-affinity AT*H complex. Finally, $k_{-2}$ represents the reverse rate of the conformational change (i.e., the stability of the AT*H complex). The extent to which individual ATIII residues and pentasaccharide components contribute to each of the previously described processes was determined by measuring the binding equilibrium and kinetic constant values for

ATIII mutants and truncated pentasaccharides and by comparing them to those of ATIII and pentasaccharide controls.

$K_1$ analysis shows that initial recognition and low-affinity binding of the pentasaccharide to native ATIII is mediated by its DEF nonreducing end, which interacts with (a) K125 from helix D, (b) K114 in polypeptide that will become helix P, and (c) K11 in the N-terminal polypeptide. The basic residues that participate in the initial interaction with the pentasaccharide cofactor are circled in the native structure of Figure 13-5A (33–37).

The weak binding interaction of the first step leads to conformational adjustments in both the pentasaccharide and the antithrombin molecules. Pentasaccharide DEF complementarity with ATIII is enhanced and creates a complementary secondary site for binding a preferred conformer of the GH disaccharide (33,34). On the antithrombin side, the protein conformational change converting AT–H to AT*H requires K114, K125, and F122 (35,36,38), which make the largest contributions to $k_{+2}$ and mediate the formation of a new helix P in the activated inhibitor. (Compare *purple* polypeptide backbone in Figs. 13-5A and 13-5B.) The activated AT*H complex that forms is stabilized by interactions requiring F122, R129, and, especially, K114, as evidenced by large increases in $k_{-2}$ when these residues are mutated (36,38,39).

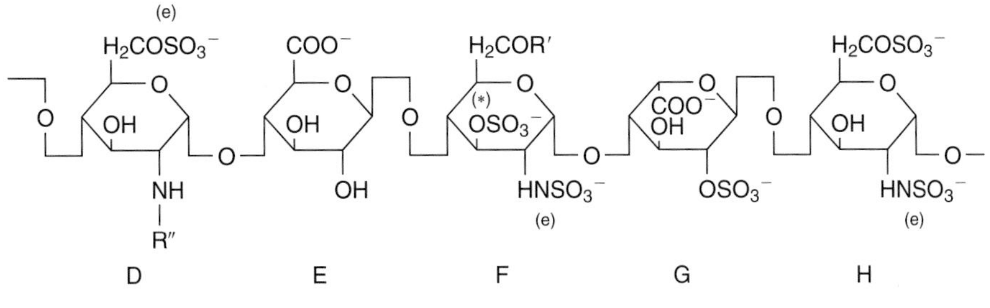

(e)
H₂COSO₃⁻    COO⁻    H₂COR′    H₂COSO₃⁻

D    E    F    G    H

**FIGURE 13-4.** Structure of the heparin pentasaccharide that binds ATIII with high affinity and activates it for efficient target proteinase inhibition. Structural variants are indicated by R′ ($-H$ or $-SO_3^-$) and R″ ($-SO_3^-$ and $-COCH_3$). The 3-O-sulfate group marked by an asterisk is unique to the antithrombin-binding region of the heparin molecule. In addition, the three sulfate groups indicated by (e) are essential to the high-affinity binding of antithrombin. (From Lindahl U, Feingold DS, Roden L. Biosynthesis of heparin. *TIBS* 1986;11:221, with permission.)

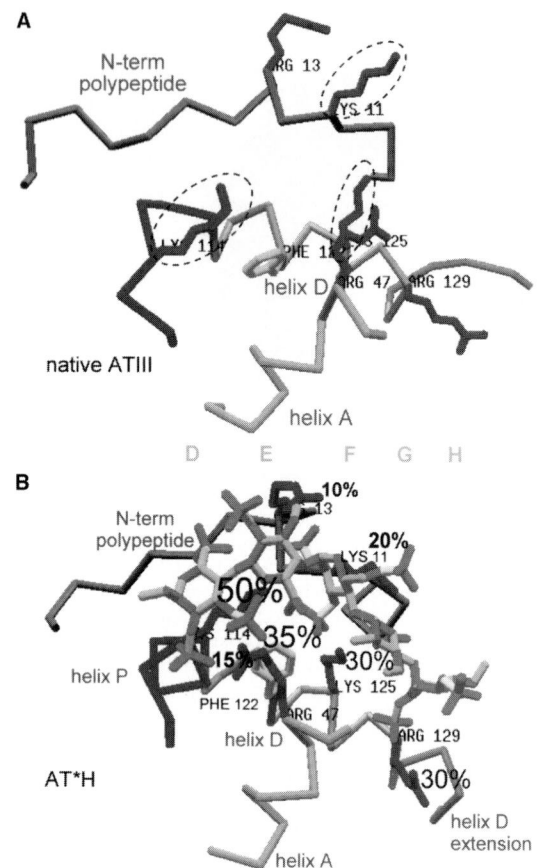

$$AT + H \xrightarrow{K_1} AT - H \underset{k_{-2}}{\overset{k_{+2}}{\rightleftharpoons}} AT * H$$

**FIGURE 13-6.** Two-step mechanism for heparin binding to and the activation of antithrombin III (ATIII). AT, antithrombin III; H, heparin; AT–H, initial weak antithrombin–heparin intermediate; $K_1$, dissociation equilibrium constant for AT–H formation; AT*H, high-affinity antithrombin–heparin complex that is competent for rapid FXa inhibition; $k_{+2}$ rate of conformational conversion of the weak AT-H intermediate to the high-affinity AT*H complex; $k_{-2}$ reverse rate of the conformational change.

**FIGURE 13-5.** Pentasaccharide occupancy of the heparin binding site on ATIII induces a protein conformational change that leads to high-affinity binding of the cofactor, reactive center loop expulsion, and acceleration of FXa inhibition. (**A**) and (**B**) show pentasaccharide binding surfaces of native ATIII (1E05.pdb) and of AT*H (1E03.pdb), respectively. Side chains of the basic residues of heparin binding site are *blue*, and that of phenylalanine122 is *green*. **A:** Circled lysine125, 114, and 11 residues of native ATIII (**A**) participate in cofactor recognition and in the formation of the initial weak AT–H intermediate. **B:** Pentasaccharide atoms are drawn in *aqua* (carbon), *red* (oxygen), and *yellow* (sulfur), and the D–H sugar labels are in *aqua*. Numbers indicate the percentage of pentasaccharide-free energy of binding that is lost upon mutation of indicated residues. Conformational changes induced by pentasaccharide binding can be visualized by comparing the main-chain polypeptide backbones of key structural elements in native (**A**) and AT*H (**B**) molecules. *Orange* shows elongation of helical region at arginine47 end of helix A; *purple* shows formation of helix P at the amino-terminal end of helix D (*light blue*), and *pink* shows elongation of helix D at its carboxy terminus (see Color Fig. 13-5).

As mentioned in the preceding text, the $K_1$ binding and $k_{+2}$ and $k_{-2}$ rate constants from the two-step mechanism of Figure 13-6 together determine the overall affinity of the ATIII–pentasaccharide interaction. At physiologic pH and at ionic strength, the $K_d$ for binding of the major α-ATIII isoform of human plasma to pentasaccharide and longer chain high-affinity (i.e., pentasaccharide-containing) heparin molecules are approximately 50 nM and 20 nM, respectively, as determined by both binding equilibrium and binding kinetic measurements (40). Numbers in Figure 13-5B show percentage losses in the free energy of binding with pentasaccharide for mutants of key heparin-binding-site residues. Therefore, lysine114 and phenylalanine122 make the greatest contributions to the binding energy (36,38). Lysine125 and arginine129 also make significant contributions (35,39), whereas lysine11 and arginines13 and 47 make only small contributions (37,41). Analysis of binding energy losses across the mutant series also indicates

that cooperative interactions between combinations of the previously described residues contribute to high-affinity cofactor binding (42).

The binding of pentasaccharide and ATIII is mediated by ionic as well as nonionic interactions. From the salt dependence of the $K_d$, it has been determined that ionic interactions of the pentasaccharide and the six basic residues on ATIII are responsible for approximately 40% of the free energy of binding (24,27,35–37,39,41). Nonionic interactions (i.e., hydrogen bonds and van der Waals and hydrophobic interactions) contribute an approximately 60% greater portion of the binding free energy, with centrally located phenylalanine122 (*green* in Fig. 13-5B) being responsible for a substantial share by positioning R47 and K114 for extensive contact with the cofactor and with bridging structural elements being involved in forming and stabilizing the high-affinity conformation (38).

Pentasaccharide binding–dependent ATIII conformational changes are integral to development of the high-affinity AT*H complex that has its distal reactive center loop expelled and is activated for efficient FXa inhibition. Structural elements of the pentasaccharide binding region that exhibit cofactor binding–dependent conformational changes and that are thought to contribute to the propagation of conformational change toward the reactive loop are marked in Figure 13-5. By comparing the polypeptide backbones for the purple, orange, and pink segments of the native ATIII (Fig. 13-5A) and AT*H (Fig. 13-5B) molecules, pentasaccharide binding can be observed to induce helix-P formation and helix-A and helix-D elongation. As previously discussed, lysine114- and phenylalanine122-mediated helix-P formation (*purple*) is crucial for stabilizing the high-affinity AT*H complex (38). Helix-D elongation (*pink*) also appears to be a requirement for tight heparin binding and for activation of inhibition. ATIII mutants in which the elongation of hD helix was inhibited by deletion(s) (43) or by proline introduction (44) exhibited decreased pentasaccharide and heparin binding affinities and could not be fully activated for FXa inhibition. The process of conformational change propagation between the initial site of cofactor binding and the site of target proteinase recognition has received less experimental attention and is less well understood than the initial binding interaction. However, it is inferred from analyses of crystal structures for native-, intermediate-, and pentasaccharide-bound antithrombins that conformational change transmission and RCL expulsion involve the rearrangement of bonding networks formed by residues in the A-sheet, the hF arm, and the reactive loop polypeptide (13,45). The longer length of the ATIII-reactive center loop compared with the RCLs of other serpins also contributes to the reduction of the native inhibition rate, and the deletion of two RCL residues partially (10-fold) activates ATIII anti-fXa inhibition (46).

In summary, the constrained reactive loop of six-stranded native ATIII is responsible for its poor performance as a proteinase inhibitor. Pentasaccharide cofactor binding converts native ATIII to a five-stranded, reactive, loop-expelled conformation resembling the five-stranded native structures of other serpins and fully activates ATIII proteinase inhibitory activity.

## Endogenous Activation of Antithrombin III

Because of the structural constraints discussed in the preceding text, ATIII molecules circulating in the blood have limited inhibitory activity. They become activated, however, upon binding to vessel wall HSPG$^{act}$ molecules (3-O-sulfated pentasaccharide-bearing anticoagulantly active heparan sulfate proteoglycan). HSPG$^{act}$ is present on vascular endothelium and in the underlying matrix and serves to localize and concentrate activated antithrombin on and in the vessel wall. It is generally believed that activated ATIII molecules bound to vascular surface HSPG$^{act}$ receptors contribute substantively to the anticoagulant and antithrombotic properties of the endothelium by inhibiting free thrombin, FXa, and other activated coagulation-factor molecules that are generated by membrane-bound activation complexes, and released into the diffusion layer at the blood vessel–wall interface.

Physiologic activation of ATIII by a vascular component was initially investigated in a rat hindlimb quarters model perfused with ATII and thrombin. A tightly bound, heparinase-sensitive component accelerated the rate of thrombin–antithrombin complex formation 15- to 19-fold (25). Further studies with normal versus mast cell–deficient mice established that the accelerating vascular component was HSPG$^{act}$ rather than a mast cell–derived heparin species (47). This anticoagulantly active HSPG$^{act}$ species constitutes about 5% of the total HSPG associated with rat microvascular endothelial cells (48). The integral membrane proteins ryudocan and syndecan serve as core proteins for both HSPG$^{act}$ and HSPG$^{inact}$ (anticoagulantly inactive HSPG) (49). Ryudocan and syndecan have, respectively, three and five extracellular serine attachment sites that are posttranslationally modified with glycosaminoglycans (GAGs) composed of alternating N-acetylglucosamine and glucuronic acid/iduronic acid residues. The copolymer is further modified by multiple sulfation reactions to generate heparan sulfate chains with regions of varying structure. The presence of chains bearing pentasaccharide sequence(s) with essential 3-O-sulfation on a small portion (see Fig. 13-4) confers HSPG$^{act}$ status on a subset of HSPG molecules.

The anatomic localization of HSPG$^{act}$ has been studied using immunohistochemistry and radiolabeled ATIII perfusion techniques. ATIII localization was investigated using immunohistochemistry techniques in biopsies of normal human hearts before transplantation (50). Venous endothelium, but not capillary endothelium, stained positively for ATIII. ATIII was also present around smooth muscle cells and around intima of small arteries and arterioles, but not around large arteries, in apparent contradiction to the results of subsequent studies in which normal rat aorta was perfused with $^{125}$I-labeled ATIII. The perfusion studies (26) demonstrated the presence of ATIII-binding HSPG$^{act}$ on and under the aortic endothelium. Small amounts of HSPG$^{act}$ (1%) were observed on the luminal side of aortic endothelial cells, whereas the subendothelial basement membrane and extracellular matrix on the abluminal side of the endothelium contained much greater amounts of ATIII-binding HSPG$^{act}$. This distribution suggests that luminal HSPG$^{act}$ may provide a basal level of activated ATIII for scavenger inhibition of activated coagulation enzymes exposed to the endothelium and that these basal levels may be dramatically increased in injured regions following endothelial damage and liberation of the larger pool of abluminal HSPG$^{act}$ and its associated bound and activated ATIII.

The physiologic importance of ATIII binding to endogenous vascular surface HSPG$^{act}$ is supported by the occurrence of lethal thrombosis in mice homozygous for an ATIII mutation that reduces binding to heparin/HSPG (51). Similarly, thrombosis was prevented in stents coated with the high-affinity, pentasaccharide-containing fraction of heparin (which binds antithrombin) but not in stents coated with low-affinity, pentasaccharide-depleted heparin (which does not support ATIII binding) (52). Therefore, antithrombin–HSPG interactions play a crucial role in maintaining circulatory system patency. A previous contrary report based on the nonthrombotic phenotype of mice deficient for 3-OST-1 (53) may reflect redundancy of enzymes that mediate 3-O-sulfation of the pentasaccharide sequence of HSPG (54,55).

Finally, in addition to vascular HSPGs, the endothelial cell thrombin receptor thrombomodulin can bind ATIII and enhance its inhibition of receptor bound thrombin by a factor of approximately eight (56). This thrombin-specific effect is mediated by a highly sulfated chondroitin sulfate chain on thrombomodulin (57,58), which interacts with both thrombin [at exosite II, (59)] and with ATIII. Chondroitin sulfate occupancy of exosite II of anticoagulant thrombin (i.e., thrombomodulin-bound thrombin) blocks heparin binding to the enzyme and precludes heparin/ATIII inhibition at the very rapid rates observed for procoagulant thrombin (60).

## Pharmacologic Activation of Antithrombin III

The clinical use of heparin as an anticoagulant began more than 60 years ago (61). The name heparin derives from the fact that the anticoagulant was originally extracted from liver; however, commercial preparations are now usually obtained from pig intestinal mucosa or bovine lung, which are good sources of mast cells. Mast cell heparin proteoglycan is composed of a serglycin core protein modified with 60 to 100,000 Da heparin sulfate glycosaminoglycan chains (62). The heparin proteoglycan polysaccharide chains are intracellularly cleaved to form smaller fragments (7,000 to 25,000 Da) that are present in pharmaceutical heparin. Standard pharmaceutical heparin is a heterogeneous mixture of polysaccharide molecules (average 15,000 to 18,000 Da). In addition to a high degree of size/length heterogeneity, there is also a significant amount of compositional heterogeneity. Typically, only one third of the molecules in a standard pharmaceutical heparin preparation bear the ATIII-binding pentasaccharide sequence and exhibit anticoagulant activity.

Unfractionated heparin is used widely in clinical settings. It is given to prevent and treat venous thrombosis and for the management of arterial disease. Intravenous administration of heparin doses that prolong the aPTT (activated partial thromboplastin time) to 1.5 to 2.5 times control values is highly effective for the prevention and treatment of venous thrombosis (63). Heparin is also widely utilized in extracorporeal circulation, for flushing indwelling catheters, for coating biomaterials and medical devices, and in many other hospital procedures. However, there are major drawbacks associated with the use of unfractionated heparin, including increased risk of hemorrhage and thrombocytopenia, variable patient response, and prolonged hospitalization because of the need for anticoagulant monitoring and dosing adjustments. In addition to inhibiting clotting enzyme function, heparin also interferes with platelet function, which contributes to its hemorrhagic side effects. On the basis of studies with size-fractionated heparins, which indicated that the high-molecular-weight fraction (average 20,000 Da) was considerably more active at inducing platelet aggregation than was the low-molecular-weight fraction (average 7,000 Da) (64), low-molecular-weight heparins (LMWHs) were suggested as a potentially advantageous alternative to standard heparin (65).

Several LMWHs have been developed and evaluated in clinical trials and are now frequently used in hospital and outpatient settings. LMWHs are derived from unfractionated heparin by enzymatic or chemical cleavage. Their range of fragment size is from 1,800 to 12,000 Da, with an average of around 5,000 Da. As a result of their small fragment size and the cleavage into smaller pieces of most chains that were long enough (>18 sugars) to approximate (bridge) ATIII and thrombin, LMWHs preferentially inhibit factor Xa and have antifactor Xa to antithrombin ratios of 2:1 to 4:1 (vs. 1:1 for standard heparin). Compared with standard heparin, LMWHs have decreased affinity for endothelial cells (66,67) and exhibit reduced nonspecific binding to heparin-binding proteins (68). These properties improve bioavailability and produce a more predictable dose response. The improved pharmacokinetic profile permits LMWHs to be administered subcutaneously once or twice daily on a weight-adjusted basis without laboratory monitoring. These attributes are an important advantage over standard heparin, which has a highly variable patient response that necessitates frequent laboratory monitoring, dose adjustment, and prolonged hospitalization. Clinical trials have established that for eligible patients with deep vein thrombosis, outpatient, unmonitored, subcutaneous, weight-adjusted LMWH is as effective and as safe as inpatient treatment with intravenous, unfractionated heparin and affords considerable cost reductions (69).

A synthetic pentasaccharide, fondaparinux, has also been developed as an anticoagulant pharmaceutical (70). Fondaparinux accelerates ATIII inhibition of FXa but has no activity against thrombin. It is believed that this profile of inhibition is advantageous because amplification steps resulting in the generation of large numbers of thrombin molecules through the common and intrinsic pathways are downregulated, while still permitting the trace thrombin that does form to facilitate hemostasis. The half-life of fondaparinux is approximately 17 hours and is dose independent, which allows for once daily subcutaneous administration without monitoring of coagulation parameters. Fondaparinux has been approved for thromboprophylaxis after major orthopedic surgery.

Other efforts to develop pharmaceuticals that activate ATIII without the side effects of standard heparin have led to the chemical synthesis of a heparin mimetic that potentiates factor Xa *and thrombin* inhibition but has reduced interactions with platelet factor 4 (PF4) and, therefore, a decreased tendency to induce thrombocytopenia (71). This heparin mimetic has a pentasaccharide domain for ATIII binding and a sulfated hexasaccharide domain for thrombin binding. These are joined by a neutral hexasaccharide linker that allows approximation of a thrombin molecule bound to the thrombin-binding domain, with an ATIII molecule bound to the pentasaccharide domain. The judicious use of neutral saccharides in the linker region eliminates binding of the mimetic to PF4 by limiting the extent of the charged domains to fewer than eight sugars long, which is the length required for interaction with PF4.

## Antithrombin III Inhibition of Target Enzymes Associated with Activating Complexes and Fibrin Clots

Freely circulating and purified thrombin and factor Xa are readily inhibited by ATIII and ATIII/heparin. However, when associated with the surface-activating complexes that generated the thrombin and FXa or with platelets or with fibrin clots, these target enzymes are resistant to ATIII and ATIII/heparin inhibition. Factor Xa in prothrombinase complexes formed by its addition to platelets or reconstitution with factor V, phospholipid, and calcium is blocked from inhibition by ATIII (72–75). Meizothrombin, a fragment 2–containing, fibrinogen-clotting intermediate in the generation of thrombin from prothrombin, is less susceptible to inhibition by ATIII and heparin than is thrombin. This effect is mediated by fragment-2 of prothrombin (76), which interacts with the heparin binding

site of thrombin. The gradient of fragment 2 around a clot contributes to the reduction in ATIII inhibition of thrombin in the immediate vicinity of the clot and allows for more rapid thrombin inhibition at greater distances from the site of injury where fragment 2 concentrations are reduced (76). Platelet-bound thrombin is protected from inactivation by ATIII/heparin by platelet GP Ibα occupancy of its exosite 2 heparin binding site (77).

Clot-bound thrombin and thrombin bound to soluble fibrin degradation peptides generated by tPA-induced clot lysis are refractive to inhibition by ATIII/heparin (78,79). Fibrin blocks ATIII/heparin thrombin inhibition by prior formation of ternary thrombin–fibrin–heparin complexes in which thrombin exosite 1 interacts with fibrin, and thrombin exosite 2 binds the heparin molecule of the ternary complex (which is also connected to the ternary complex through the heparin binding site of fibrin). Therefore, thrombin in the ternary complex is resistant to ATIII/heparin inhibition because the ATIII/heparin cannot access exosite 2, which is occupied by the heparin molecule from the ternary complex (80). Clot-associated factor Xa is also resistant to inhibition by ATIII/heparin (81). Therefore, coagulation is difficult to regulate in the immediate microenvironment of a clot because clot-bound factor Xa is able to generate thrombin (and fragment 2—see the preceding discussion) from prothrombin, and, by binding to fibrin, the newly formed thrombin may also evade inactivation by ATIII/heparin. In contrast to ATIII inhibition of factor Xa and thrombin, which is attenuated in activation complexes, ATIII inhibition of kallikrein and factor VIIa (FVIIa) is potentiated by the association of these intrinsic and extrinsic enzymes with activating surface-bound proteins.

In contrast to ATIII inhibition of factor Xa and thrombin, which is attenuated in activation complexes, ATIII inhibition of kallikrein and factor VIIa (FVIIa) is potentiated by the association of these intrinsic and extrinsic enzymes with activating surface-bound proteins. In the case of kallikrein, binding of high-molecular-weight kininogen promotes inhibition by ATIII/heparin through a bridging mechanism that involves binding of ATIII and kallikrein–kininogen to the same heparin molecule (82). FVIIa also becomes more sensitive to ATIII inhibition when bound to its activating cofactor, tissue factor (83,84). In this case, increased reactivity of FVIIa with ATIII has been attributed to a conformational change in the enzyme active site that is induced by tissue factor binding.

## Antithrombin III as a Scavenger

As discussed in preceding text, native ATIII, HSPG^act-bound ATIII, and ATIII/heparin that are formed by administration of the pharmaceutical inhibit "free" factor Xa and "free" thrombin more efficiently than they inhibit factor Xa and thrombin located on activation surfaces and in fibrin clots. Hence, these forms of ATIII may serve as scavengers in the blood and on vascular surfaces and may neutralize thrombin and factor Xa molecules that have escaped from activation complexes and clots. In this capacity, ATIII would serve an important role in blocking coagulation and thrombin non-coagulant functions in uninjured areas, where they are less necessary.

ATIII may also play a role in regulating the low-level coagulation activation that occurs normally in the unperturbed circulation. ATIII regulation of tissue factor–induced coagulation has been studied from several angles, and these investigations collectively suggest that there are multiple points at which ATIII may contribute to the control of coagulation initiation. ATIII inhibits FVIIa–TF complexes formed on OC2008 cells (which express TF and cell surface GAGs constitutively) in the presence, as well as in the absence, of heparin (84). ATIII in combination with tissue factor pathway inhibitor (TFPI) was also able to prevent the formation of prothrombinase activity in a model system containing FVIIa–TF, FVIII, FV, FIX, FX, and prothrombin reconstituted on phosphatidyl choline and phosphatidyl serine (PCPS) vesicles. This model procoagulant system contained physiologic concentrations of the listed components, but no heparin or HSPG. TFPI potentiated the action of ATIII by decreasing the rate of prothrombinase formation and by enabling ATIII to effectively scavenge the limited amounts of FIXa and FXa formed in the presence of TFPI (85). Studies in a different model system reconstituted with zymogen FVII and human brain thromboplastin suggest that ATIII may also contribute to regulation of tissue factor–induced coagulation through its ability, in the presence of heparin, to inhibit the activation of plasma FVII by FXa, thrombin, FIXa, and other proteinases (86). Therefore, ATIII (in combination with TFPI) appears to play a crucial role in controlling low-level basal activation of the coagulation system that occurs in the normal circulation.

## Antithrombin III Clearance

Different conformations and complexes of ATIII are cleared from the circulation by different pathways. High-affinity binding of the native conformation to vessel wall HSPG$^{act}$ mediates its clearance from plasma into noncirculating vascular-associated and extravascular pools (87,88). As will be discussed in the next section, the β-ATIII isoform clears from plasma 2.5 times faster than the α-ATIII isoform (89). Thrombin–ATIII (TAT) inhibitory complexes (and, presumably, inhibitory complexes of ATIII with other target enzymes) are rapidly cleared from the circulation by the liver (90). This clearance mechanism is specific for complexed ATIII, with TAT complexes being eliminated from the plasma many times more rapidly than native and cleaved ATIII (91). Furthermore, clearance of ATIII inhibitory complexes exhibits competition with the clearance of other serpin complexes, indicating that serpin–enzyme complexes utilize a common clearance pathway (90–92). The primary receptor for clearance of serpin–enzyme complexes is LRP (low density lipoprotein receptor–related protein) (92). LRP is expressed by many tissues and cell types and is a prominent receptor in the liver. It interacts with numerous ligands, including serpin–enzyme complexes, and plays a key role in proteinase regulation and lipoprotein metabolism.

## β-Antithrombin III

β-ATIII is a naturally occurring glycoform of ATIII that binds to heparin and HSPGs with higher affinity than the predominant ATIII isoform, α-ATIII (3,89). β-ATIII synthesis is the result of inefficient utilization of the N-X-S type consensus sequence specifying N-glycosylation of asparagine135 (93). Because of partial glycosylation at this site, plasma contains two ATIII glycoforms: α-ATIII, which is glycosylated at all four consensus sequences, and β-ATIII, which is glycosylated at only three consensus sequences [the asparagine135 N-X-S remains unmodified (94)].

β-ATIII binds heparin and pentasaccharide, respectively, six times and three times more tightly than does α-ATIII because of elimination of asparagine135 oligosaccharide effects on the formation of the initial AT–H intermediate and on its conformational conversion to activated AT*H and the stabilization of this complex (40). The enhanced affinity of the β isoform for heparin and its more rapid clearance from the circulation compared with α-ATIII suggest that β-ATIII, although a minor species in the plasma, may play an important role on the vessel wall (89). β-ATIII associates 30% to 50% faster with uninjured aorta, and three times faster with deendothelialized

aorta, than does α-ATIII, and approximately five times more β-ATIII than α-ATIII was recovered in detergent extracts of intima media from uninjured rabbit aortas (95). Compared to plasma, a higher proportion of the ATIII in extracts of human organs is β-ATIII (96). β-ATIII is also more effective than α-ATIII at inhibiting thrombin appearance on the wall of injured aorta (97). Because it is believed that antithrombin molecules that are bound in an activated conformation to vessel wall HSPGs are crucial for efficient scavenging of activated thrombin and other coagulation factors, β-ATIII may represent a functionally important component in the physiologic regulation of coagulation enzyme activity, despite the fact that it is only a minor component in blood. Furthermore, according to this hypothesis, the apparently low content of β-ATIII (<10%) compared with α-ATIII (>90%) in plasma may actually reflect its increased binding and physiologic consumption on vascular surfaces.

## Inherited Antithrombin III Deficiencies and Their Treatment

ATIII is an essential physiologic anticoagulant (98). Its complete absence is incompatible with life, and its partial deficiency in mice (99) and humans increases the individual's risk for thrombosis. The prevalence of genetic ATIII deficiency in humans is approximately 0.02 to 0.05% [reviewed in (100)]. However, this increases to approximately 5% for patients with a history of thromboembolic disease (101).

The ATIII gene is composed of 7 exons and 6 introns and spans 13,477 base pairs of genomic DNA (102) in the q23-q25 region of chromosome 1 (103). Genetic ATIII deficiencies, therefore, exhibit an autosomal dominant pattern of inheritance, with functional activity levels of the affected heterozygotes usually ranging from 40% to 60% of normal, and antigen levels varying according to the type of deficiency. Type I ATIII deficiencies result from failure of ATIII synthesis or from defective secretion of ATIII from hepatocytes, and exhibit parallel reduction of functional activity and antigen levels to approximately 50% of normal values. Type I deficiencies are caused by a wide variety of mutations, including insertions and deletions, missense mutations, nonsense mutations, and the introduction of cryptic splice sites. Type II ATIII deficiencies are caused by missense mutations and N-glycosylation consensus sequence mutations that lead to the production of variant antithrombins with altered functional properties. ATIII antigen levels generally exceed ATIII functional levels in patients with type II deficiencies, and the characterization of numerous type II variant proteins has provided extensive ATIII structure–function information [reviewed in (100,104)].

There is great variability in the occurrence and severity of symptomatic thrombosis in individuals with genetic ATIII deficiencies. The onset of thrombotic episodes most often occurs in the third decade, but a considerable number of affected individuals reach old age without thrombotic problems, whereas some infants and children develop thrombosis early in life. Disease severity and age of onset are influenced by properties of the specific defective ATIII allele that is inherited, and by other factors that can decrease or enhance the thrombotic tendency caused by genetic ATIII deficiency. For example, protein C resistance secondary to the factor V$_{Leiden}$ mutation (FV R506Q) has been shown to influence the expression of thrombosis in patients with genetic ATIII deficiencies. In a study of six families that segregated type I and type II ATIII defects and factor V$_{Leiden}$, the coinheritance of the factor V$_{Leiden}$ allele with the ATIII alleles reduced the age of onset and increased the clinical severity of thrombosis (105).

Thrombotic episodes in individuals with genetic ATIII deficiencies are mainly confined to the venous system. Common problems include recurrent episodes of deep vein thrombosis, mesenteric thrombosis, and/or pulmonary emboli. Similar to venous thrombosis occurring in persons without ATIII deficiency, precipitating factors in patients with ATIII deficiency include pregnancy, surgery, trauma, and infection. However, many episodes of thrombosis in genetically deficient persons appear to occur spontaneously, without a precipitating event. Pregnancy is a time of increased thrombotic risk in women with genetic ATIII deficiency. In a retrospective study, the incidence of thromboembolic complications during pregnancy in women with congenital ATIII deficiency has been estimated at about 70%. Prophylactic subcutaneous administration of heparin may be considered as soon as the pregnancy has been diagnosed, and supplementation with ATIII concentrates to normalize antithrombin levels during delivery and postpartum is also recommended (106). As with any genetic disease, patient education is important because it enables the patient to avoid stimuli that are likely to induce thrombosis and to effectively recognize and to seek prompt treatment for thrombotic symptoms when they do occur.

Episodes of acute venous thromboembolism in patients who have ATIII deficiency have been successfully managed by heparin alone or heparin in combination with antithrombin concentrates. Administration of ATIII concentrates together with heparin is considered the treatment of choice for patients with known hereditary ATIII deficiency and who present with massive and potentially life-threatening thromboembolic disease (107). By increasing the plasma antithrombin concentration, it is believed that potential "heparin resistance" secondary to genetically low levels of ATIII can be overcome more readily, and clinical benefit can be achieved more rapidly. However, a retrospective study of Swedish patients with ATIII–deficiency suggested that heparin resistance may not actually represent a substantial problem for most of these individuals because administration of heparin alone produced a more than 1.5 times prolongation of the aPTT in at least 90% of patients (108).

Individuals with ATIII deficiency are at a high risk for postoperative and posttraumatic thrombosis, as well as thromboembolism during pregnancy and after delivery, and antithrombin concentrates have been used in combination with heparin for prophylaxis during surgery, delivery, and postpartum (109–111). Although there are no randomized clinical trials establishing the efficacy of this approach, the preponderance of favorable outcomes reported in the literature suggests that prophylactic treatment with ATIII concentrates and heparin is helpful. Prophylactic anticoagulation with vitamin K antagonists is sometimes prescribed for genetically deficient persons who have experienced recurring episodes of thrombosis. In contrast, prophylactic anticoagulation of asymptomatic carriers of ATIII deficiency genes is regarded as unnecessary and is not recommended (112).

Estrogen-containing contraceptives and postmenopausal replacement therapies should be avoided by women with genetic ATIII deficiencies because estrogen usage has been associated with the development of thrombosis in normal women, as well as in ATIII deficient females (113,114). Progestogen-containing contraceptives, on the other hand, do not appear to lower ATIII levels (115).

## Acquired Antithrombin III Deficiencies

Acquired antithrombin deficiencies are encountered more frequently than genetic ATIII deficiencies. Acquired ATIII deficiencies occur in association with many conditions and procedures, including severe sepsis, trauma, burns, malignancies, extracorporeal circulation, and surgery. These disorders have consumptive coagulation and acute inflammatory components. Antithrombin levels decline because of stoichiometric consumption of ATIII during neutralization of activated coagulation enzymes. Additionally, in inflammatory settings, activated leukocytes release neutrophil elastase and matrix metalloproteinases that cleave the reactive loop of ATIII (116–118) and induce a functional activity deficiency.

Data from several studies suggest that a decrease in plasma ATIII concentration to below 60% to 70% of normal represents a crucial point in the pathogenesis of venous thrombosis. A study of patients with nephrotic syndrome reported that eight of 11 patients with antithrombin concentrations of less than 70% developed thrombosis, whereas only one of 37 patients with ATIII concentrations of greater than 70% experienced thrombosis (119). Finally, in trials of antithrombin concentrate in patients undergoing hip or knee replacement, all patients with nadir ATIII concentrations of less than 60% developed thrombosis (120).

ATIII levels decrease profoundly during cardiopulmonary bypass to 40% to 50% of preoperative levels and remain low even after protamine neutralization (121). Several factors contribute to the development of ATIII deficiency during bypass including: (a) hemodilution, (b) ATIII consumption by the formation of inhibitory complexes, and (c) increased systemic neutrophil elastase concentrations and the heparin-mediated elastase inactivation of ATIII (122).

ATIII deficiency also develops in response to high-dose chemotherapy regimens used to prepare patients with hematopoietic malignancies for bone marrow transplantation (BMT). ATIII levels decline in parallel with albumin and prealbumin levels, suggesting that impaired hepatic synthesis and/or extravascular redistribution contribute to ATIII deficiency in BMT. Nadir ATIII levels typically occur at 2 to 3 weeks following the start of the preparative regimen and are correlated with the development of vascular occlusive disease of the liver, pulmonary dysfunction, and central nervous system dysfunction. Patients who developed multiorgan failure had lower ATIII levels than those who did not develop organ failure or who experienced single organ failure (123,124).

Localized ATIII deficiency has been observed in unstable cardiac allografts (50). Immunohistologic studies on serial biopsies from donor and transplanted organs (for periods of up to a decade) have shown that clinically stable grafts maintain a normal pattern of vascular ATIII reactivity in contrast to grafts that fail. Interestingly, a proportion of late unstable allografts, which have progressed to the stage of losing normal venous and arterial ATIII reactivity and showing evidence of fibrin deposition, may go on to subsequently develop a system of ATIII-reactive capillaries. Appearance of these ATIII-reactive capillaries shifts the prognosis for graft survival from bad to good.

## Antithrombin III Concentrates

ATIII concentrates have been produced by the blood plasma fractionation industry since the mid-1970s using heparin affinity chromatography methods (125). The manufacturing process also includes a heat treatment step to inactivate viral pathogens. ATIII concentrates are considered safe, and the transmission of HIV, hepatitis B, or non-A non-B hepatitis has not been reported in patient follow-up studies [reviewed in (110,126)]. However, the pasteurization step used to inactivate viruses induces formation of aggregated protein and latent ATIII molecules, which are devoid of anticoagulant activity because of uptake of the reactive center loop as a central sixth strand in β-sheet A. Sixteen percent to 40% of the ATIII in five extensively analyzed batches of one antithrombin concentrate existed as inactive, latent molecules (127). Another study of 23 lots of four different ATIII concentrates produced by four different manufacturers demonstrated the presence of denatured antithrombin in all preparations except in those that had received additional solvent/detergent treatment and further purification steps (128). This study also found levels of TAT and cleaved antithrombin to be substantially elevated in concentrates relative to normal plasma. TAT increased 20- to 1,600-fold, whereas cleaved ATIII increased 50- to 230-fold. Therefore, elevated TAT and cleaved ATIII levels in patients who have received ATIII concentrates should be interpreted with caution.

In the United States, ATIII concentrates are mainly utilized for patients with genetic ATIII deficiencies, as discussed in a previous section. However, in some European countries and in Japan, ATIII concentrates are additionally administered to patients with acquired antithrombin deficiencies [e.g., disseminated intravascular coagulation (DIC), sepsis, trauma, hematopoietic malignancy] and to patients undergoing BMT, orthopedic surgery, and cardiopulmonary bypass and to obstetrics patients. Although ATIII supplementation improved hemostatic parameters and survival in several animal models of sepsis [reviewed in (129)], the large double-blind, placebo-controlled, multicenter phase III Kybersept trial of human plasma-derived high-dose ATIII for patients with severe sepsis failed to show any benefit with respect to 28-day all-cause mortality (130).

## Antiinflammatory Properties of Antithrombin III

ATIII exhibits antiinflammatory properties that are both independent of, and related to, its ability to inhibit thrombin. Work in endotoxemia and ischemia/reperfusion models attributed ATIII antiinflammatory effects on leukocyte accumulation, vascular permeability, and TNF-$\alpha$ and iNOS induction to endothelial prostacyclin release (131–133). Prostacyclin administration mimicked the ATIII-mediated antiinflammatory effects, whereas indomethacin pretreatment antagonized these responses to ATIII. Antiinflammatory effects were lost in experiments using a chemically modified ATIII with reduced affinity for heparin, suggesting that prostacyclin-mediated antiinflammatory effects require ATIII interaction with cell surface HSPGs. ATIII has also been demonstrated to block thrombin-mediated, neutrophil-dependent ischemia-reperfusion damage. Postreperfusion treatment with ATIII attenuated the P selectin mediated leukocyte recruitment response, and similar results were also observed in an *in vitro* model using human blood neutrophils and cultured endothelial cells (134).

Direct ATIII effects on inflammatory responses of peripheral blood cells have also been demonstrated. ATIII inhibits chemokine-induced migration of neutrophils, lymphocytes, and monocytes, and, in the absence of chemokines, stimulates their migration (135–137). In monocytes and endothelial cells, ATIII potently blocks activation of nuclear factor kappa beta (NF$\kappa$B), a transcription factor involved in immediate early gene activation during inflammation (138). ATIII-mediated NF$\kappa$B downregulation also involves binding of ATIII to cell surface HSPGs, and this interaction has been proposed to interfere with signal transduction leading to NF$\kappa$B activation.

Therefore, on the basis of the recently described antiinflammatory and the well-established anticoagulant properties of ATIII, ATIII supplementation has been proposed for clinical reversal of microvascular dysfunction in acute inflammatory disorders such as sepsis. High-dose ATIII failed to improve overall 28-day survival in severe sepsis patients of the Kybersept trial; however, decreased mortality was noted for patients who did not receive heparin (130). It has been suggested that clinical benefit was observed in this subgroup because

concomitant systemic heparin did not block the antiinflammatory effects of ATIII (137).

## Antithrombin III—Antiproliferative, Antiangiogenic, and Antiviral Activities

Independent of its anticoagulant and antiinflammatory properties, ATIII also has antiproliferative, antiangiogenic, and antiviral activities. ATIII inhibits thrombin-induced proliferation of human arterial smooth muscle cells and human mesangial cells *in vitro* (139,140) and is also reported to inhibit rat spleen T-cell proliferation in a thrombin-independent manner (141).

Several conformations of ATIII lack anticoagulant activity but exhibit antiangiogenic and antitumor growth properties that are of potential physiologic and therapeutic importance. These activities are not present in the native, inhibitory conformation of antithrombin but are acquired after the protein undergoes structural conversion to cleaved and latent forms, which feature incorporation of the reactive loop polypeptide as strand 4 of the central A $\beta$-sheet. The antiangiogenic antithrombins (142,143) exert their effects through downregulation in endothelial cells of the proangiogenic heparan sulfate proteoglycan, perlecan (144), and disrupt cell–matrix interactions through uncoupling of focal adhesion kinase (145). A "prelatent" conformation of ATIII, which has undergone only limited conformational change and is still able to bind heparin and inhibit thrombin, also exhibits potent antiangiogenic and tumor inhibition activities (146).

Finally, antiviral activity has been reported for several ATIII conformations (147). Native, cleaved, and prelatent conformations of ATIII inhibit human immunodeficiency virus (HIV)-1 replication, but latent ATIII does not. Activated $CD8^+$ T cells from HIV-1-seropositive individuals modified serum ATIII into an HIV inhibitory factor, suggesting that ATIII may play a role in the progression of HIV infection.

# HEPARIN COFACTOR II

## Overview

HcII is a plasma serpin with 30% homology to ATIII. Compared with ATIII, there are similarities as well as differences in HcII interactions with coagulation enzymes and GAGs. Like ATIII, HcII inactivates thrombin; but unlike ATIII, it is not a broad-spectrum inhibitor of coagulation enzymes and does not inhibit factor Xa or other clotting factors. The circulating form of HcII, like the circulating form of ATIII, is an inefficient inhibitor of thrombin. Both are activated more than three orders of magnitude by heparin; however, the structural mechanisms for heparin activation of HcII and ATIII are distinct. Dermatan sulfate, which only minimally activates ATIII, is an efficient activator of HcII. Proposed physiologic roles of HcII include extravascular thrombin inhibition, inflammatory signaling, and thrombin regulation during pregnancy. In contrast to ATIII, HcII deficiency is not strongly associated with venous thrombosis but may contribute to the prevention of arterial thrombosis.

## Biochemistry and Molecular Genetics

HcII (also known as leuserpin 2) is a 66-kDa glycoprotein with a pI of 4.95 to 5.15 (148). HcII contains approximately 10% carbohydrate, two sulfated tyrosine residues (149), and three free sulfhydryls. The plasma concentration and plasma half-life of HcII are, respectively, approximately 1.2 $\mu$M (approximately 80 $\mu$g per mL) and approximately 2.5 days (150,151). The complete amino acid sequence of the 480-residue mature protein is known from complementary deoxyribonucleic acid (cDNA) analysis (152,153). The serpin domain is approximately 30% homologous to ATIII and other serpins, uses leucine as its P1 residue, and is preceded by an *N*-terminal polypeptide sequence that contains two highly acidic hirudin-like repeats. In contrast to ATIII, which is a broad-spectrum inhibitor of thrombin, factor Xa, and other intrinsic and extrinsic pathway coagulation enzymes, HcII inhibition of clotting pathway enzymes is limited to thrombin (Fig. 13-1). However, HcII also inhibits cathepsin G (154) and chymotrypsin (155) in accordance with its P1 leucine residue. HcII inhibition of thrombin, but not of chymotrypsin, is potentiated by heparin and dermatan sulfate (155). HcII–thrombin inhibitory complexes are rapidly cleared by low density lipoprotein receptor–related protein (LRP) (92), which also clears ATIII inhibitory complexes. The HcII gene spans 14 kb of DNA in the q11 region of chromosome 22 and has 5 exons and 4 introns (156).

## Target Enzyme Specificity and Mechanism of Glycosaminoglycan Activation

The leucine P1 residue of HcII confers primary specificity for inhibition of cathepsin G and chymotrypsin, which prefer medium-sized nonpolar residues, but not for thrombin, FXa, or related coagulation factors, which cleave arginine-containing substrate sequences. HcII inhibits thrombin exclusively among clotting enzymes, and this specificity is conferred by a GAG cofactor binding–dependent interaction between two negatively charged hirudin-like sequences in the amino-terminal domain of HcII and thrombin's anion-binding exosite I.

Figure 13-7A shows the 2.35-Å structure of native HcII (157). As in native ATIII (Fig. 13-3B), target enzyme access to the reactive center loop is reduced by its partial insertion into central $\beta$-sheet A. Binding sites for heparin and dermatan sulfate occupy overlapping areas in the helix-D region, and most of the positively charged HcII residues that interact with these GAGs are located in homologous positions to basic residues of the ATIII heparin binding site (Fig. 13-5). As a result of perturbations caused by intermolecular contacts in the dimeric native

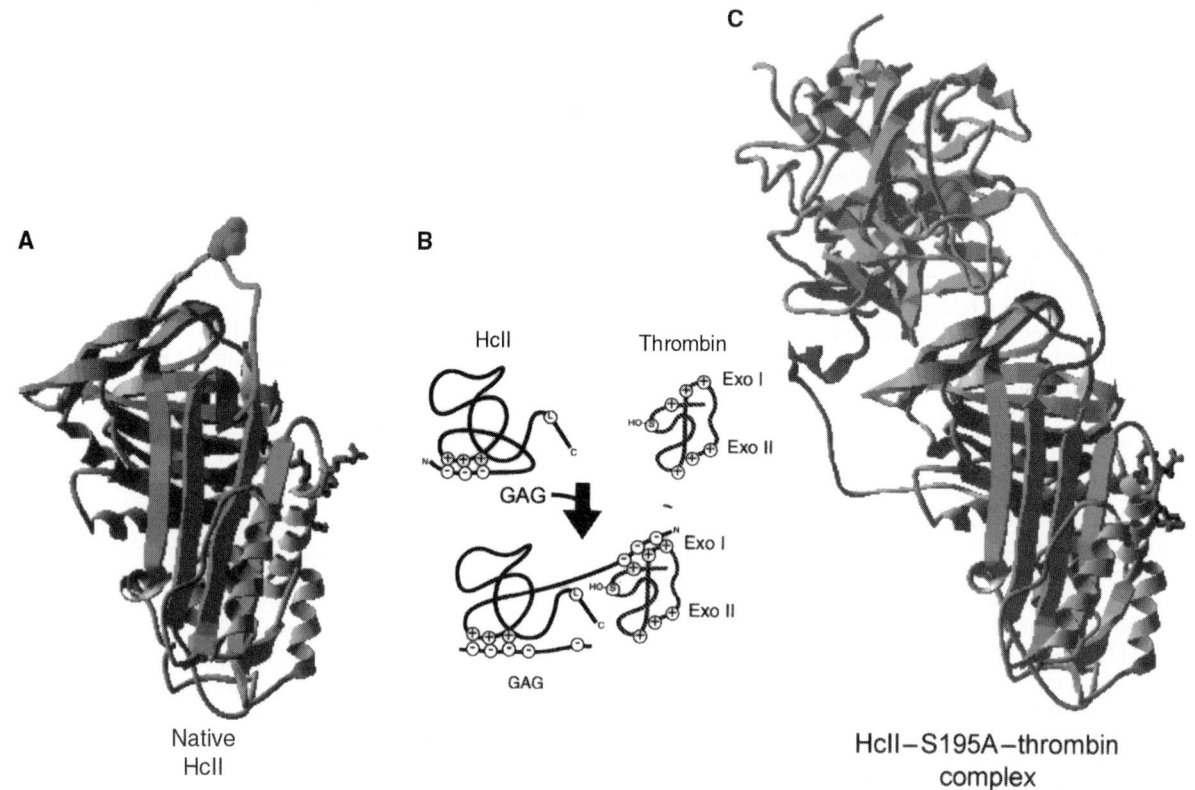

FIGURE 13-7. Heparin cofactor II (HcII) inhibition of thrombin. **A:** Native HcII. The reactive center loop (*orange and purple*) of native HcII is constrained because of incorporation of its C-terminal end (*purple*) into $\beta$-sheet-A (*pink*). The leucine P1 residue of the reactive center loop is shown as a *red* van der Waals surface, and side chains of positively charged residues in the GAG-binding site are drawn in *aqua*. The *N*-terminal hirudin-like polypeptide of HcII was not visible in this structure because perturbations caused by intermolecular contacts in the dimeric native HcII crystal structure largely prevented assignment of its location. **B:** Cartoon model of native HcII shows intramolecular binding of its *N*-terminal, negatively charged hirudin-like and positively charged GAG-binding domains, as inferred from mutagenesis studies. Activation occurs when cofactor heparin or dermatan sulfate molecules bind HcII and competitively displace its *N*-terminal domain from its GAG-binding site. This uncoupling leads to: (a) allosteric HcII conformational changes and (b) HcII *N*-terminal domain binding to the thrombin anion-binding exosite I, which together increase the specificity, rate, and strength of the inhibitory complex formation. **C:** S195A-thrombin–HcII Michaelis complex. In this structure, the *N*-terminal anionic binding site (*dark blue ribbon*) interacts with exosite I on thrombin (*green*), and the allosteric change leading to expulsion of the reactive center loop (*purple* and *orange*) from the A $\beta$-sheet has occurred (see Color Fig. 13-7). (**A** and **C:** From Protein Data Bank structures 1JMJ and 1JMO, respectively. **B:** From Tollefsen D. Heparin cofactor II. *Adv Exp Med Biol* 1997;425:35–44, with permission.)

HcII crystal structure, the location of the anionic hirudin-like N-terminal domain of HcII could not be assigned for the most part. However, from functional studies with HcII N-terminal anionic and helix-D GAG-binding region mutants, it is inferred that in native HcII, in the absence of GAG cofactors, there is intramolecular binding of the hirudin-like repeats with the positively charged GAG-binding region, as is schematically depicted in Figure 13-7B (158–160). Upon addition of heparin or dermatan sulfate, cofactor binding and occupancy of the GAG-binding site makes dual contributions to activating HcII for more efficient thrombin inhibition. First, GAG binding competitively displaces the anionic amino-terminal polypeptide from the GAG-binding site, freeing it to interact with thrombin exosite I (161), as illustrated in the Figure 13-7B cartoon. This association is observed in the 2.2-Å crystal structure of the HcII–S195A–thrombin complex (Fig. 13-7C) (157) and improves the specificity, rate, and strength of the interaction. Secondly, by analogy to the mechanism for heparin activation of ATIII (Fig. 13-5), the release of the binding interaction between the N-terminal "hirudin" domain and the helix-D GAG-binding domain through mutation (160,162), or cofactor binding, is inferred to induce a long-range protein conformational change, which expels the reactive center loop from sheet A and improves reactivity with thrombin (157). The binding sites for heparin and dermatan sulfate on HcII overlap, but are not identical [reviewed in (163)], and distinct protein conformational changes are induced by the GAGs (162). In contrast to heparin cofactor inhibition of thrombin by ATIII, both heparin and dermatan sulfate primarily utilize an allosteric mechanism, rather than a template mechanism, to accelerate thrombin inactivation (164). In the presence of heparin, large decreases in rates of HcII and ATIII inhibition of fibrin clot-bound thrombin occur as a result of the formation of thrombin–fibrin–heparin ternary complexes, which reduce the access of heparin–serpin complexes to the enzyme (80). However, in the presence of dermatan sulfate, HcII inhibition of clot-bound thrombin remains almost as efficient as its inhibition of free thrombin because of the lack of dermatan sulfate—fibrin cross-linking in the DS–thrombin–fibrin complex that is formed (165).

## Biologic Roles of Heparin Cofactor II

On the basis of their distinct patterns of target proteinase specificity and cofactor activation as discussed in preceding text, it is expected that HcII and ATIII evolved to fulfill distinct biologic roles. HcII contributes to thrombin inhibition in the body as indicated by the presence of low levels of thrombin–HcII inhibitory complexes in normal plasma samples (166) and human organ extracts (96). However, in contrast to ATIII deficiency, HcII deficiency is not strongly associated with thrombosis and contributes only to thrombotic risk in combination with other deficiencies [reviewed in (167)]. Approximately 1% of apparently healthy individuals (no history of thrombosis) have HcII levels of less than 60% (168), and the frequency of HcII deficiency is similar in the general population and thrombosis patients. Furthermore, in contrast to ATIII-null mice, HcII-null mice are fully viable and do not exhibit spontaneous thrombosis (169). However, complete HcII deficiency in mice was associated with more rapid vessel occlusion after carotid artery injury and was prevented by previous infusion of purified HcII (169). These findings are consistent with the proposed role of HcII as an extravascular thrombin inhibitor that is activated by fibroblast and smooth muscle cell dermatan sulfate proteoglycans (170). Administration of porcine skin dermatan sulfate prolonged arterial occlusion times in HcII wild-type mice but not in HcII-null mice (171). Therefore, HcII in conjunction with physiologic or pharmaceutical dermatan sulfates may contribute to the protection against arterial thrombosis. A recent report of reduced rates of in-stent restenosis in patients with high plasma HcII levels is consistent with this view (172).

Several kinds of evidence suggest that HcII may play a role in protection from thrombosis during pregnancy. Dermatan sulfate proteoglycans (presumably of placental origin) increase in the maternal and fetal circulations during pregnancy (173) and thrombin-HcII complexes are prominent in placental extracts (96). Elevated HcII has been reported in pregnant women, with levels increasing to three times normal at term (174,175). HcII levels have also been observed to decrease in preeclampsia patients (176). However, recent transgenic mouse investigations indicate that despite the previously noted associations, HcII is not essential during pregnancy or for normal development because HcII-null mice are born at the expected Mendelian frequency and do not exhibit abnormalities (169).

Finally, a role for HcII in inflammation, wound healing, and tissue repair has also been proposed, on the basis of the ability of proteolytically derived N-terminal peptides of HcII to act as leukocyte chemoattractants (177).

## References

1. Rosenberg R, Damus P. Purification and mechanism of action of human antithrombin-heparin cofactor. *J Biol Chem* 1973;248:6490–6505.
2. Murano G, Williams L, Miller-Anderson M, et al. Some properties of antithrombin III and its concentration in human plasma. *Thromb Res* 1980;18:259–262.
3. Peterson C, Blackburn M. Isolation and characterization of an antithrombin III variant with reduced carbohydrate content and enhanced heparin binding. *J Biol Chem* 1985;260:610–615.
4. Petersen T, Dudek-Wojciechowska G, Sottrup-Jensen L, et al. Primary structure of antithrombin-III (heparin cofactor). Partial homology between α1-antitrypsin and antithrombin-III. In: Collen DD, Wiman B, Verstraete M, eds. *The physiological inhibitors of coagulation and fibrinolysis.* Amsterdam; Elsevier 1979:43–54.
5. Bock S, Wion K, Vehar G, et al. Cloning and expression of the cDNA for human antithrombin III. *Nucl Acids Res* 1982;10:8113–8125.
6. Franzen L-F, Svensson S, Larm O. Structural studies on the carbohydrate portion of antithrombin III. *J Biol Chem* 1980;255:5090–5093.
7. Mizuochi T, Fujii J, Kurachi K, et al. Structural studies of the carbohydrate moiety of human antithrombin III. *Arch Biochem Biophys* 1980;203:458–465.
8. Mourey L, Samama J, Delarue M, et al. Crystal structure of cleaved bovine antithrombin III at 3.2A resolution. *J Mol Biol* 1993;232:223–241.
9. Schreuder H, deBoer B, Dijkema R, et al. The intact and cleaved human antithrombin III complex as a model for serpin-proteinase interactions. *Struct Biol* 1994;1:48–54.
10. Skinner R, Abrahams J, Whisstock J, et al. The 2.6A structure of antithrombin indicates a conformational change at the heparin binding site. *J Mol Biol* 1997;266:601–609.
11. Jin L, Abrahams J, Skinner R, et al. The anticoagulant activation of antithrombin by heparin. *Proc Natl Acad Sci U S A* 1997;94:14683–14688.
12. McCoy A, Pei X, Skinner R, et al. Structure of beta-antithrombin and the effect of glycosylation on antithrombin's heparin affinity and activity. *J Mol Biol* 2003;326:823–833.
13. Johnson D, Huntington J. Crystal structure of antithrombin in a heparin-bound intermediate state. *Biochemistry* 2003;42:8712–8719.
14. Huber R, Carrell R. Implications of the three-dimensional structure of alpha1-antitrypsin for structure and function of serpins. *Biochem* 1989;28:8951–8965.
15. Olson S, Bock P, Kvassman J, et al. Role of the catalytic serine in the interactions of serine proteinases with protein inhibitors of the serpin family. Contribution of a covalent interaction to the binding energy of serpin-proteinase complexes. *J Biol Chem* 1995;270:30007–30017.
16. Schechter I, Berger A. On the size of the active site in proteases. I. Papain. *Biochem Biophys Res Comm* 1967;27:157–162.
17. Lawrence D, Ginsburg D, Day D, et al. Serpin-protease complexes are trapped as stable acyl-enzyme intermediates. *J Biol Chem* 1995;270:25309–25312.
18. Wilczynska M, Fa M, Ohlsson P-I, et al. The inhibition mechanism of serpins. Evidence that the mobile reactive center loop is cleaved in the native protease-inhibitor complex. *J Biol Chem* 1995;270:29652–29655.
19. Wright H, Scarsdale J. Structural basis of serpin inhibitor activity. *Proteins: Struct Funct Genet* 1995;22:210–225.

20. Huntington J, Read R, Carrell R. Structure of a serpin-protease complex shows inhibition by deformation. *Nature* 2000;407:923–926.

21. Pike R, Potempa J, Skinner R, et al. Heparin-dependent modification of the reactive center arginine of antithrombin and consequent increase in heparin binding affinity. *J Biol Chem* 1997;272:19652–19655.

22. Lindahl U, Backstrom G, Thunberg L, et al. Evidence for a 3-O-sulfated D-glucosamine residue in the antithrombin-binding sequence of heparin. *Proc Natl Acad Sci U S A* 1980;77:6551–6555.

23. Choay J, Petitou M, Lormeau J, et al. Structure-activity relationship in heparin: a synthetic pentasaccharide with high affinity for antithrombin III and eliciting high anti-factor Xa activity. *Biochem Biophys Res Comm* 1983;116:492–499.

24. Olson ST, Bjork I, Sheffer R, et al. Role of the antithrombin-binding pentasaccharide in heparin acceleration of antithrombin-proteinase reactions. *J Biol Chem* 1992;267:12528–12538.

25. Marcum J, McKenney J, Rosenberg R. The acceleration of thrombin-antithrombin complex formation in rat hind-limb quarters via naturally occurring heparin-like molecules bound to the endothelium. *J Clin Invest* 1984;74:341–350.

26. deAgostini A, Watkins S, Slayter H, et al. Localization of anticoagulantly active heparan sulfate proteoglycans in vascular endothelium: antithrombin binding on cultured endothelial cells and perfused rat aorta. *J Cell Biol* 1990;111:1293–1304.

27. Olson S, Bjork I. Predominant contribution of surface approximation to the mechanism of heparin acceleration of the antithrombin-thrombin reaction. Elucidation from salt concentration effects. *J Biol Chem* 1991; 266:6353–6364.

28. Bedsted T, Swanson R, Chuang Y, et al. Heparin and calcium ions dramatically enhance antithrombin reactivity with factor IXa by generating new interaction exosites. *Biochemistry* 2003;42:8143–8152.

29. Wiebe E, Stafford A, Fredenburgh J, et al. Mechanism of catalysis of inhibition of factor IXa by antithrombin in the presence of heparin or pentasaccharide. *J Biol Chem* 2003;278:35767–35774.

30. Rezaie A. Calcium enhances heparin catalysis of the antithrombin-factor Xa reaction by a template mechanism. Evidence that calcium alleviates Gla domain antagonism of heparin binding to factor Xa. *J Biol Chem* 1998;273:16824–16827.

31. Izaguirre G, Zhang W, Swanson R, et al. Localization of an antithrombin exosite that promotes rapid inhibition of factors Xa and IXa dependent on heparin activation of the serpin. *J Biol Chem* 2003;278:51433–51440.

32. Olson S, Shore J. Demonstration of a two-step reaction mechanism for inhibition of alpha-thrombin by antithrombin III and identification of the step affected by heparin. *J Biol Chem* 1982;257:14891–14895.

33. Desai U, Petitou M, Bjork I, et al. Mechanism of heparin activation of antithrombin. Role of individual residues of the pentasaccharide activating sequence in the recognition of native and activated states of antithrombin. *J Biol Chem* 1998;273:7478–7487.

34. Desai U, Petitou M, Bjork I, et al. Mechanism of heparin activation of antithrombin: evidence for an induced-fit model of allosteric activation involving two interaction subsites. *Biochemistry* 1998;37:13033–13041.

35. Schedin-Weiss S, Desai U, Bock S, et al. Importance of lysine 125 for heparin binding and activation of antithrombin. *Biochemistry* 2002;41: 4779–4788.

36. Arocas V, Bock S, Raja S, et al. Lysine 114 of antithrombin is of crucial importance for the affinity and kinetics of heparin pentasaccharide binding. *J Biol Chem* 2001;276:43809–43817.

37. Schedin-Weiss S, Desai U, Bock S, et al. Roles of N-terminal region residues Lys11, Arg12 and Arg24 of antithrombin in heparin recognition and in promotion and stabilization of the heparin-induced conformational change. *Biochemistry* 2004;43:675–683.

38. Jairajpuri M, Lu A, Desai U, et al. Antithrombin III phenylalanines 122 and 121 contribute to its high affinity for heparin and its conformational activation. *J Biol Chem* 2003;278:15941–15950.

39. Desai U, Swanson R, Bock S, et al. Role of arginine 129 in heparin binding and activation of antithrombin. *J Biol Chem* 2000;275:18967–18984.

40. Turk B, Brieditis I, Bock S, et al. The oligosaccharide side chain on Asn-135 of alpha-antithrombin, absent in beta-antithrombin, decreases the affinity of the inhibitor by affecting the heparin-induced conformational change. *Biochemistry* 1997;36:6682–6691.

41. Arocas V, Bock S, Olson S, et al. The role of Arg46 and Arg47 of antithrombin in heparin binding. *Biochemistry* 1999;38:10196–10204.

42. Olson S, Bjork I, Bock S. Identification of critical molecular interactions mediating heparin activation of antithrombin. Implications for the design of improved heparin anticoagulants. *Trends Cardiovasc Med* 2002;12: 198–205.

43. Meagher J, Olson S, Gettins P. Critical role of the linker region between helix D and strand 2A in heparin activation of antithrombin. *J Biol Chem* 2000;275:2698–2704.

44. Belzar K, Zhou A, Carrell R, et al. Helix D elongation and allosteric activation of antithrombin. *J Biol Chem* 2002;277:8551–8558.

45. Whisstock J, Pike R, Jin L, et al. Conformational changes in serpins: II. The mechanism of activation of antithrombin by heparin. *J Mol Biol* 2000;301:1287–1306.

46. Rezaie A. Partial activation of antithrombin without heparin through deletion of a unique sequence on the reactive site loop of the serpin. *J Biol Chem* 2002;277:1235–1239.

47. Marcum J, McKenney J, Galli S, et al. Anticoagulantly active heparin-like molecules from mast cell-deficient mice. *Am J Physiol* 1986;250: H879–H888.

48. Kojima T, Leone C, Marchildon G, et al. Isolation and characterization of heparan sulfate proteoglycan core proteins produced by cloned rat microvascular endothelial cells. *J Biol Chem* 1992;267:4859–4869.

49. Kojima T, Shworak N, Rosenberg R. Molecular cloning and expression of two distinct cDNA encoding heparan sulfate proteoglycan core proteins from a rat endothelial cell line. *J Biol Chem* 1992;267:4870–4877.

50. Faulk W, Labarrere C. Modulation of vascular antithrombin III in human cardiac allografts. *Haemostasis* 1993;23(Suppl. 1):194–201.

51. Dewerchin M, Hérault J-P, Wallays G, et al. Life-threatening thrombosis in mice with targeted Arg48-to-Cys mutation of the heparin-binding domain of antithrombin. *Circ Res* 2003;93:1120–1126.

52. Kocsis J, Llanos G, Holmer E. Heparin-coated stents. *J Long-Term Eff Med* 2000;10:19–45.

53. HajMohammadi S, Enjyoji K, Princivalle M, et al. Normal levels of anticoagulant heparan sulfate are not essential for normal hemostasis. *J Clin Invest* 2003;111:989–999.

54. Weitz J. Heparan sulfate: antithrombotic or not?. *J Clin Invest* 2003;111: 952–954.

55. Duncan M, Chen J, Krise J, et al. The biosynthesis of anticoagulant heparan sulfate by heparan sulfate 3-O-sulfotransferase isoform 5. *Biochim Biophys Acta* 2004;1671:34–43.

56. Preissner K, Delvos U, Muller-Berghaus G. Binding of thrombin to thrombomodulin accelerates inhibition of the enzyme by antithrombin III. Evidence for a heparin-independent mechanism. *Biochemistry* 1987; 26:2521–2528.

57. Bourin M-C, Lundgren-Akerlund E, Lindahl U. Isolation and characterization of the glycosaminoglycan component of rabbit thrombomodulin proteoglycan. *J Biol Chem* 1990;265:15424–15431.

58. Preissner K, Koyama T, Muller D, et al. Domain structure of the endothelial cell receptor thrombomodulin as deduced from modulation of its anticoagulant functions. Evidence for a glycosaminoglycan-dependent secondary binding site for thrombin. *J Biol Chem* 1990;265:4915–4922.

59. Ye J, Rezaie A, Esmon C. Glycosaminoglycan contributions to both protein C activation and thrombin inhibition involve a common arginine-rich site in thrombin that includes residues arginine 93, 97 and 101. *J Biol Chem* 1994;269:17965–17970.

60. Bourin M-C. Effect of rabbit thrombomodulin on thrombin inhibition by antithrombin in the presence of heparin. *Thromb Res* 1989;54:27–39.

61. Best C. Preparation of heparin and its use in the first clinical cases. *Circulation* 1959;19:79–86.

62. Robinson H, Horner A, Hook M, et al. A proteoglycan form of heparin and its degradation to single chain molecules. *J Biol Chem* 1978;253: 6687–6693.

63. Basu D, Gallus A, Hirsh J, et al. A prospective study of the value of monitoring heparin treatment with the activated partial thromboplastin time. *N Engl J Med* 1972;287:324–327.

64. Salzman E, Rosenberg R, Smith M, et al. Effect of heparin and heparin fractions on platelet aggregation. *J Clin Invest* 1980;65:64–73.

65. Hirsh J, Ofosu F, Buchanan M. Rationale behind the development of low molecular weight heparin derivatives. *Semin Thromb Hemost* 1985;11: 13–16.

66. Hirsh J, Levine M. Low molecular weight heparin. *Blood* 1992;79:1–17.

67. Barzu T, Molho P, Tobelem G, et al. Binding of heparin and low molecular weight heparin fragments to human vascular endothelial cells in culture. *Nouv Rev Fr Hematol* 1984;26:243–247.

68. Young E, Cosmi B, Weitz J, et al. Comparison of the non-specific binding of unfractionated heparin and low molecular weight heparin (Enoxaparin) to plasma proteins. *Thromb Haemost* 1993;70:625–630.

69. Hirsh J, Crowther M. Low molecular weight heparin for the out-of-hospital treatment of venous thrombosis: rationale and clinical results. *Thromb Haemost* 1997;78:689–692.

70. Bauer K. New pentasaccharides for prophylaxis of deep vein thrombosis. *Pharmacology Chest* 2003;124:364S–370S.

71. Petitou M, Herault J-P, Bernat A, et al. Synthesis of thrombin-inhibiting heparin mimetics without side effects. *Nature* 1999;398:417–422.

72. Marciniak E. Factor-Xa inactivation by antithrombin III: evidence for biological stabilization of factor Xa by factor V-phospholipid complex. *Brit J Haematol* 1973;24:391–400.

73. Miletich J, Jackson C, Majerus P. Properties of the factor Xa binding site on human platelets. *J Biol Chem* 1978;253:6908–6916.

74. Teitel J, Rosenberg R. Protection of factor Xa from neutralization by the heparin-antithrombin complex. *J Clin Invest* 1983;71:1383–1391.

75. Lindhout T, Baruch D, Schoen P, et al. Thrombin generation and inactivation in the presence of antithrombin III and heparin. *Biochemistry* 1986; 25:5962–5969.

76. Walker F, Esmon C. The effect of prothrombin fragment 2 on the inhibition of thrombin by antithrombin. *J Biol Chem* 1979;254:5618–5622.

77. DeCristofaro R, DeCandia E, Rutella S, et al. The Asp272-Glu282 region of platelet glycoprotein Ib alpha interacts with the heparin-binding site of alpha-thrombin and protects the enzyme from the heparin-catalyzed inhibition by antithrombin III. *J Biol Chem* 2000;275:3887–3895.

78. Weitz J, Hudoba M, Massel D, et al. Clot bound thrombin is protected from inhibition by heparin-antithrombin III but susceptible to inactivation

by antithrombin III-independent inhibitors. *J Clin Invest* 1990;86: 385–391.

79. Weitz J, Leslie B, Hudoba M. Thrombin binds to soluble fibrin degradation products where it is protected from inhibition by heparin-antithrombin by susceptible to inactivation by antithrombin-independent inhibitors. *Circulation* 1998;97:544–552.

80. Becker D, Fredenburgh J, Stafford A, et al. Exosites 1 and 2 are essential for protection of fibrin-bound thrombin from heparin-catalyzed inhibition by antithrombin and heparin cofactor II. *J Biol Chem* 1999;274: 6226–6233.

81. Eisenberg P, Siegel J, Abendschein D, et al. Importance of factor Xa in determining the procoagulant activity of whole-blood clots. *J Clin Invest* 1993;91:1877–1883.

82. Olson S, Francis A, Sheffer R, et al. Parallel mechanisms of high molecular weight kininogen action as a cofactor in kallikrein inactivation and prekallikrein activation reactions. *Biochemistry* 1993;32:12148–12159.

83. Lawson JH, Butenas S, Ribarik N, et al. Complex-dependent inhibition of factor VIIa by antithrombin III and heparin. *J Biol Chem* 1993;268: 767–770.

84. Rao LVM, Rappaport SI, Hoang AD. Binding of factor VIIa to tissue factor permits rapid antithrombin III/heparin inhibition of factor VIIa. *Blood* 1993;81:2600–2607.

85. van'tVeer C, Mann KG. Regulation of tissue factor initiated thrombin generation by the stoichiometric inhibitors tissue factor pathway inhibitor, antithrombin-III, and heparin cofactor II. *J Biol Chem* 1997;272:4367–4377.

86. Broze GJ, Kikert K, Higuchi D. Inhibition of factor VIIa/tissue factor by antithrombin III and tissue factor pathway inhibitor. *Blood* 1993;82: 1679–1680.

87. Carlson T, Atencio A, Simon T. *In vivo* behavior of radioiodinated rabbit antithrombin III. Demonstration of a noncirculating vascular compartment. *J Clin Invest* 1984;74:191–199.

88. Carlson T, Simon T, Atencio A. *In vivo* behavior of human radioiodinated antithrombin III: distribution among three physiologic pools. *Blood* 1985; 66:13–19.

89. Carlson T, Atencio A, Simon T. Comparison of the behavior *in vivo* of two molecular forms of antithrombin III. *Biochem J* 1985;225:557–564.

90. Fuchs H, Shiffman M, Pizzo S. *In vivo* catabolism of alpha1-proteinase inhibitor-trypsin, antithrombin III-thrombin and alpha2 macroglobulin-methylamine. *Biochim Biophys Acta* 1982;716:151–157.

91. Mast A, Enghild J, Pizzo S, et al. Analysis of the plasma elimination kinetics and conformational stabilities of native, proteinase-complexed, and reactive site cleaved serpins: comparison of alpha1-proteinase inhibitor, alpha1-antichymotrypsin, antithrombin III, alpha2 antiplasmin, angiotensinogen and ovalbumin. *Biochemistry* 1991;30:1723–1730.

92. Kounnas M, Church F, Argraves W, et al. Cellular internalization and degradation of antithrombin III-thrombin, heparin cofactor II-thrombin, and alpha1-antitrypsin complexes is mediated by the low density lipoprotein receptor-related protein. *J Biol Chem* 1996;271:6523–6529.

93. Picard V, Ersdal-Badju E, Bock S. Partial glycosylation of antithrombin III asparagine135 is caused by the serine in the third position of its N-glycosylation consensus sequence and is responsible for production of beta-antithrombin III isoform with enhanced heparin affinity. *Biochemistry* 1995; 34:8433–8440.

94. Brennan S, George P, Jordan R. Physiological variant of antithrombin-III lacks carbohydrate sidechain at Asn 135. *FEBS Lett* 1987;219:431–436.

95. Witmer M, Hatton M. Antithrombin III-beta associates more readily than antithrombin III-alpha with uninjured and de-endothelialized aortic wall *in vitro* and *in vivo*. *Arterioscler Thromb* 1991;11:530–539.

96. Kamp P-B, Strathmann A, Ragg H. Heparin cofactor II, antithrombin-beta and their complexes with thrombin in human tissues. *Thromb Res* 2001; 101:483–491.

97. Frebelius S, Isaksson S, Swedenborg J. Thrombin inhibition by antithrombin III on the subendothelium is explained by the isoform AT-beta. *Thromb Vasc Biol* 1996;16:1292–1297.

98. Ishiguro K, Kojima T, Kadomatsu K, et al. Complete antithrombin deficiency in mice results in embryonic lethality. *J Clin Invest* 2000;106: 873–878.

99. Yanada M, Kojima T, Ishiguro K, et al. Impact of antithrombin deficiency in thrombogenesis: lipopolysaccharide and stress-induced thrombus formation in heterozygous antithrombin-deficient mice. *Blood* 2002;99: 2455–2458.

100. Perry D, Carrell R. Molecular genetics of human antithrombin III deficiency. *Hum Mutat* 1996;7:7–22.

101. Harper P, Luddington R, Daly M, et al. The incidence of dysfunctional antithrombin variants: four cases in 210 patients with thromboembolic disease. *Br J Haematol* 1991;77:360–364.

102. Olds R, Lane D, Chowdhuri V, et al. Complete nucleotide sequence of the antithrombin gene. Evidence for homologous recombination causing thrombophilia. *Biochemistry* 1993;32:4216–4224.

103. Bock S, Harris J, Balazs I, et al. Assignment of the human antithrombin III gene to chromosome 1q23-25. *Cytogenet Cell Genet* 1985;39:67–69.

104. vanBoven H, Lane D. Antithrombin III and its inherited deficiency states. *Semin Hematol* 1997;34:188–204.

105. vanBoven H, Reitsma P, Rosendaal F, et al. Factor V Leiden (FV R506Q) in families with inherited antithrombin deficiency. *Thromb and Haemost* 1996;75:417–421.

106. Hellgren M, Tengborn L, Abildgaard U. Pregnancy in women with congenital antithrombin III deficiency: experience of treatment with heparin and antithrombin. *Gynecol Obstet Invest* 1982;14:127–141.

107. Lechner K, Kyrle P. Antithrombin III concentrates—are they clinically useful? *Thromb Haemost* 1995;73:340–348.

108. Schulman S, Tengborn L. Treatment of venous thromboembolism in patients with congenital deficiency of antithrombin. *Thromb Haemost* 1992; 68:634–636.

109. Jackson M, Olsen S, Gomez E, et al. Use of antithrombin III concentrates to correct antithrombin III deficiency during vascular surgery. *J Vasc Surg* 1995;22:804–807.

110. Menache D, O'Malley J, Schorr J, et al. Evaluation of the safety, recovery, half-life, and clinical efficacy of antithrombin III (human) in patients with hereditary antithrombin III deficiency. *Blood* 1990;75:33–39.

111. Schwartz R, Bauer K, Rosenberg R, et al. Clinical experience with antithrombin III concentrate in treatment of congenital and acquired deficiency of antithrombin. *Am J Med* 1989;87(suppl. 3B):3B, 53S–3B,60S.

112. Rosendaal F, Heijboer H, Briet E, et al. Mortality in hereditary antithrombin-III deficiency—1830-1989. *Lancet* 1991;337:260–262.

113. Fagerhol M, Abildgaard U, Bergsjo P, et al. Oral contraceptives and low antithrombin III concentration. *Lancet* 1970;I:1175.

114. Pabinger I, Schneider B, The GTH Study Group on Natural Inhibitors. Thrombotic risk of women with hereditary antithrombin III-, protein C- and protein S-deficiency taking oral contraceptive medication. *Thromb Haemost* 1994;71:548–552.

115. Bergsjo P, Fagerhol M, Abildgaard U. Antithrombin III concentration in women using low dose progestogen for contraception. *Am J Obstet Gynecol* 1972;112:938–940.

116. Jochum M, Lander S, Heimburger N, et al. Effect of human granulocytic elastase on isolated human antithrombin III. *Hoppe-Seyler's Z Physiol Chem* 1981;362:103–112.

117. Jordan R, Kilpatrick J, Nelson R. Heparin promotes the inactivation of antithrombin by neutrophil elastase. *Science* 1987;237:777–779.

118. Mast A, Enghild J, Nagase H, et al. Kinetics and physiological relevance of the inactivation of alpha1-proteinase inhibitor, alpha1-antichymotrypsin and antithrombin III by matrix metalloproteinases-1 (tissue collagenase), -2 (72 kDa gelatinase/type IV collagenase) and -3 (stromelysin). *J Biol Chem* 1991;266:15810–15816.

119. Kauffmann R, Veltkamp J, VanTilburg N, et al. Acquired antithrombin III deficiency and thrombosis in the nephrotic syndrome. *Am J Med* 1978; 65:607–613.

120. Francis C, Pellegrini V, Harris C, et al. Prophylaxis of venous thrombosis following total hip and total knee replacement using antithrombin III and heparin. *Semin in Hematol* 1991;28:39–45.

121. Hashimoto K, Yamagishi M, Sasaki T, et al. Heparin and antithrombin III levels during cardiopulmonary bypass: correlation with subclinical plasma coagulation. *Ann Thorac Surg* 1994;58:799–805.

122. Cohen J, Tenenbaum N, Sarfati I, et al. *In vivo* inactivation of antithrombin III is promoted by heparin during cardiopulmonary bypass. *J Invest Surg* 1992;5:45–49.

123. Gordon B, Haire W, Kessinger A. High frequency of antithrombin III and protein C deficiency following autologous bone marrow transplantation for lymphoma. *Bone Marrow Transpl* 1991;8:497–502.

124. Haire W. Antithrombin deficiency in special clinical syndromes—Part II: hematologic malignancies and bone marrow transplantation. *Semin Hematol* 1995;32:56–60.

125. Miller-Andersson M, Borg H, Andersson L. Purification of antithrombin III by affinity chromatography. *Thromb Res* 1974;5:439–452.

126. Nunez H, Drohan W. Purification of antithrombin III (human). *Semin Hematol* 1991;28:24–30.

127. Harper P, Park G, Carrell R. The plasma turnover of transfused antithrombin concentrate in patients with acquired antithrombin deficiency. *Transfusion Med* 1996;6:45–50.

128. Hellstern P, Moberg U, Ekblad M, et al. *In vitro* characterization of antithrombin III concentrates—a single-blind study. *Haemostasis* 1995;25: 193–201.

129. Emerson T, Fournel M, Redens T, et al. Efficacy of antithrombin III supplementation in animal models of fulminant *Escherichia coli* endotoxemia or bacteremia. *Am J of Med* 1989;87(Suppl. 38):27S–33S.

130. Warren B, Eid A, Singer P, et al. High-dose antithrombin III in severe sepsis: a randomized controlled trial. *JAMA* 2001;286:1869–1878.

131. Uchiba M, Okajima K, Murakami K, et al. Attenuation of endotoxin-induced pulmonary vascular injury by antithrombin III. *Am J Physiol* 1996; 270:L921–L930.

132. Mizutani A, Okajima K, Uchiba M, et al. Antithrombin reduces ischemia/reperfusion-induced renal injury in rats by inhibiting leukocyte activation through promotion of prostacyclin production. *Blood* 2003;101: 3029–3036.

133. Isobe H, Okajima K, Uchiba M, et al. Antithrombin prevents endotoxin-induced hypotension by inhibiting the induction of nitric oxide synthase in rats. *Blood* 2002;99:1638–1645.

134. Ostrovsky L, Woodman R, Payne D, et al. Antithrombin III prevents and rapidly reverses leukocyte recruitment in ischemia/reperfusion. *Circulation* 1997;96:2302–2310.

135. Dunzendorfer S, Kaneider N, Rabensteiner A, et al. Cell-surface heparan sulfate proteoglycan-mediated regulation of human neutrophil migration by the serpin antithrombin III. *Blood* 2001;97:1079–1085.

136. Kaneider N, Reinisch C, Dunsendorfer S, et al. Syndecan-4 mediates antithrombin-induced chemotaxis of human peripheral blood lymphocytes and monocytes. *J Cell Sci* 2002;115:227–236.

137. Kaneider N, Forster E, Moshelmer B, et al. Syndecan-4-dependent signaling in the inhibition of endotoxin-induced endothelial adherence of neutrophils by antithrombin. *Thromb Haemost* 2003;90:1150–1157.

138. Oelschlager C, Romisch J, Staubitz A, et al. Antithrombin III inhibits nuclear factor kappa B activation in human monocytes and vascular endothelial cells. *Blood* 2002;99:4015–4020.

139. Hedin U, Frebelius S, Sanchez J, et al. Antithrombin III inhibits thrombin-induced proliferation in human arterial smooth muscle cells. *Arterioscler Thromb* 1994;14:254–260.

140. Pahl M, Vaziri N, Oveisi F, et al. Antithrombin III inhibits mesangial cell proliferation. *J Am Soc Nephrol* 1996;7:2249–2253.

141. Okada Y, Zuo X, Marchevsky A, et al. Antithrombin III treatment improves parameters of acute inflammation in a highly histoincompatible model of rat lung allograft rejection. *Transplantation* 1999;67:526–528.

142. O'Reilly M, Pirie-Shepherd S, Lane W, et al. Antiangiogenic activity of the cleaved conformation of the serpin antithrombin. *Science* 1999;285:1926–1928.

143. Kisker O, Onizuka S, Banyard J, et al. Generation of multiple angiogenesis inhibitors by human pancreatic cancer. *Cancer Res* 2001;61:7298–7304.

144. Zhang W, Chuang Y, Swanson R, et al. Antiangiogenic antithrombin down-regulates the expression of the proangiogenic heparan sulfate proteoglycan, perlecan, in endothelial cells. *Blood* 2004;103:1185–1191.

145. Larsson H, Sjoblom T, Dixelius J, et al. Antiangiogenic effects of latent antithrombin through perturbed cell-matrix interactions and apoptosis of endothelial cells. *Cancer Res* 2000;60:6723–6729.

146. Larsson H, Akerud P, Nordling K, et al. A novel anti-angiogenic form of antithrombin with retained proteinase binding ability and heparin affinity. *J Biol Chem* 2001;276:11996–12002.

147. Geiben-Lynn R, Brown N, Walker B, et al. Purification of a modified form of bovine antithrombin III as an HIV-1 CD8+ T-cell antiviral factor. *J Biol Chem* 2002;277:42352–42357.

148. Tollefsen D, Majerus D, Blank M. Heparin cofactor II. Purification and properties of a heparin-dependent inhibitor of thrombin in human plasma. *J Biol Chem* 1982;257:2162–2169.

149. Hortin G, Tollefsen D, Strauss A. Identification of two sites of sulfation of human heparin cofactor II. *J Biol Chem* 1986;261:15827–15830.

150. Tollefsen D, Petska C. Heparin cofactor II activity in patients with disseminated intravascular coagulation and hepatic failure. *Blood* 1985;66:769–774.

151. Sie P, Dupouy D, Pichon J, et al. Turnover study of heparin cofactor III in healthy man. *Thromb Haemost* 1985;54:635–638.

152. Ragg H. A new member of the plasma protease inhibitor family. *Nucl Acids Res* 1988;14:1073–1088.

153. Blinder M, Marasa J, Reynolds C, et al. Heparin cofactor II: cDNA sequence, chromosome localization, restriction fragment length polymorphism, and expression in E. coli. *Biochem* 1988;27:752–759.

154. Parker K, Tollefsen D. The protease specificity of heparin cofactor II. Inhibition of thrombin generated during coagulation. *J Biol Chem* 1985;260:3501–3505.

155. Church F, Noyes C, Griffith M. Inhibition of chymotrypsin by heparin cofactor II. *Proc Natl Acad Sci U S A* 1985;82:6431–6434.

156. Herzog R, Lutz S, Blin N, et al. Complete nucleotide sequence of the gene for human heparin cofactor II and mapping to chromosomal band 22q11. *Biochemistry* 1991;30:1350–1357.

157. Baglin T, Carrell R, Church F, et al. Crystal structures of native and thrombin-complexed heparin cofactor II reveal a multistep allosteric mechanism. *Proc Natl Acad Sci U S A* 2002;99:11079–11084.

158. Ragg H, Ulshofer T, Gerewitz J. On the activation of human leuserpin-2, a thrombin inhibitor, by glycosaminoglycans. *J Biol Chem* 1990;265:5211–5218.

159. VanDeerlin V, Tollefsen D. The N-terminal acidic domain of heparin cofactor II mediates the inhibition of alpha-thrombin in the presence of glycosaminoglycans. *J Biol Chem* 1991;266:20223–20231.

160. Mitchell J, Church F. Aspartic acid residues 72 and 75 and tyrosine-sulfate 73 of heparin cofactor II promote intramolecular interactions during glycosaminoglycan binding and thrombin inhibition. *J Biol Chem* 2002;277:19823–19830.

161. Sheehan J, Wu Q, Tollefsen D, et al. Mutagenesis of thrombin selectively modulates inhibition by serpins heparin cofactor II and antithrombin III. Interaction with the anion-binding exosite determines heparin cofactor II specificity. *J Biol Chem* 1993;268:3639–3645.

162. Liaw P, Austin R, Fredenburgh J, et al. Comparison of heparin- and dermatan sulfate-mediated catalysis of thrombin inactivation by heparin cofactor II. *J Biol Chem* 1999;274:27597–27604.

163. Tollefsen D. Heparin cofactor II. *Adv Exp Med Biol* 1997;425:35–44.

164. Sheehan J, Tollefsen D, Sadler J. Heparin cofactor II is regulated allosterically and not primarily by template effects. Studies with mutant thrombins and glycosaminoglycans. *J Biol Chem* 1994;269:32747–32751.

165. Liaw P, Becker D, Stafford A, et al. Molecular basis for the susceptibility of fibrin-bound thrombin to inactivation for heparin cofactor II in the presence of dermatan sulfate, but not heparin. *J Biol Chem* 2001;276:20959–20965.

166. Andersson T, Sie P, Pelzer H, et al. Elevated levels of thrombin-heparin cofactor II complex in plasma from patients with disseminated intravascular coagulation. *Thromb Res* 1992;66:591–598.

167. Tollefsen D. Heparin cofactor II deficiency. *Arch Pathol Lab Med* 2002;126:1394–1400.

168. Andersson T, Larsen M, Handeland G, et al. Heparin cofactor II activity in plasma: application of an automated assay method to study the normal adult population. *Scand J Hematol* 1986;36:96–102.

169. He L, Vincente C, Westrick R, et al. Heparin cofactor II inhibits arterial thrombosis after arterial injury. *J Clin Invest* 2002;109:213–219.

170. McGuire E, Tollefsen D. Activation of heparin cofactor II by fibroblasts and vascular smooth muscle cells. *J Biol Chem* 1987;262:169–175.

171. Vincente C, He L, Pavao M, et al. Antithrombotic activity of dermatan sulfate in heparin cofactor II deficient mice. *Blood* 2004;104:3965–3970.

172. Takamori N, Azuma H, Kato M, et al. High plasma heparin cofactor II activity is associated with reduced incidence of in-stent restenosis after percutaneous coronary intervention. *Circulation* 2004;109:213–219.

173. Andrew M, Mitchell L, Berry L, et al. An anticoagulant dermatan sulfate proteoglycan circulates in the pregnant woman and her fetus. *J Clin Invest* 1992;89:321–326.

174. Massouh M, Jatoi A, Gordon E, et al. Heparin cofactor II activity in plasma during pregnancy and oral contraceptive use. *J Lab Clin Med* 1989;114:697–699.

175. Liu L, Dewar L, Song Y, et al. Inhibition of thrombin by antithrombin III and heparin cofactor II *in vivo*. *Thromb Haemost* 1995;73:405–412.

176. Sandset P, Hellgren M, Uvebrandt M, et al. Extrinsic coagulation pathway inhibitor and heparin cofactor II during normal and hypotensive pregnancy. *Thromb Res* 1989;55:665–670.

177. Church F, Pratt C, Hoffman M. Leukocyte chemoattractant peptides from the serpin heparin cofactor II. *J Biol Chem* 1991;266:704–709.

# CHAPTER 14 ■ PROTEIN C, PROTEIN S, AND THROMBOMODULIN

CHARLES T. ESMON

The protein C anticoagulant pathway has become the focus of intense interest recently. The pathway serves as an "on demand" anticoagulant system that can be regulated by inflammatory mediators. Abnormal function of the pathway is relatively common and associated with an increased risk of venous and probably arterial thrombosis. Several lines of evidence suggest that protein C consumption contributes to the pathogenesis of some forms of septic shock. This chapter focuses on our current understanding of the mechanisms by which the pathway functions, the interactions and mediators that control the function of the system, and the biochemistry of the proteins. Several reviews are available on the biochemistry (1–10), physiology, and clinical impact (11–25) of the protein C pathway.

Our current understanding of the protein C pathway is represented schematically in Figure 14-1. Thrombin binds to thrombomodulin (TM) [$K_d$ approximately 0.5 to 5 nM, depending on reaction conditions (26,27) and whether the TM is covalently modified with chondroitin sulfate (27)] on the surface of the endothelial cell. Thrombin binding to TM increases the rate of protein C activation dramatically (28). An endothelial cell protein C receptor (EPCR) has also been identified (29) and shown to augment protein C activation (30). In vivo, protein C binding increases the rate of thrombin-dependent protein C activation between 10- and 20-fold (31). EPCR binds to both protein C and activated protein C (APC) with similar affinities ($K_d$ approximately 30 nM), but APC bound to EPCR does not appear to be able to inactivate factor Va (32). Presumably, APC dissociates from EPCR and interacts with protein S, probably on endothelial (33,34) or activated platelet surfaces (35–38), where the complex inactivates factors Va (39) or VIIIa (40). In both cases, the activated forms of the cofactors are the preferred substrate for APC (41,42). The inactivation of these cofactors prevents effective thrombin generation. The early suggestion that combined factor V and VIII deficiency were due to lack of protein C inhibitor (PCI) was subsequently shown to be incorrect (43,44). Thrombin bound to TM can be inhibited more rapidly by PCI (45,46) and antithrombin (47) than can free thrombin. APC is neutralized by $\alpha_1$-antiproteinase inhibitor, PCI, and $\alpha_2$ macroglobulin (48–56). The estimated half-life for inactivation of the thrombin–TM complex is approximately 2 to 3 seconds (45) compared to 15 minutes or more for APC inhibition (57). The half-life of protein C is also rather short, approximately 10 hours (58,59).

In addition to activating protein C and catalyzing the inactivation of thrombin, TM in complex with thrombin can promote the activation of a procarboxypeptidase B, often referred to as thrombin activatable fibrinolysis inhibitor or TAFI (60). TM accelerates thrombin activation of TAFI and protein C comparably (61). Suppression of thrombin generation by APC and the subsequent prevention of thrombin activation of TAFI appear to

be responsible for the profibrinolytic activity of APC in plasma clots (60,62). This carboxypeptidase results in partial inhibition of fibrin degradation presumably by removing carboxy-terminal lysine residues. TM also accelerates the proteolytic inactivation of prourokinase by thrombin (63,64). These apparent clot stabilization functions of TM would seem to oppose its many anticoagulant functions. This carboxypeptidase appears to have other functions near the vessel wall. In particular, many vasoactive substances, such as C5a, are inactivated by removal of their carboxy-terminal Arg. In many in vivo experiments, infusion of soluble TM has resulted in a net antithrombotic and/or antiinflammatory effect (65–74). Recently, TAFI has been shown to effectively inactivate C5a and bradykinin (75,76). Whether the main function of TAFI is to inhibit fibrinolysis or to dampen vasoactive substance functions remains in some doubt. Perhaps its main physiologic functions may be dependent on the setting. It seems likely that inhibition of the vasoactive peptides might predominate in the microcirculation where TM concentrations are high and transit is rapid.

## IDENTIFICATION OF PROTEIN C, PROTEIN S, THROMBOMODULIN, AND ENDOTHELIAL CELL PROTEIN C RECEPTOR

### Protein C

In 1960, Mammen et al. identified an anticoagulant activity that arose spontaneously upon incubation of their prothrombin preparation (77). They referred to this anticoagulant as autoprothrombin II-A. The initial work suggested that this inhibitor functioned as a competitive inhibitor of prothrombin activation. The authors subsequently isolated the inhibitor (78). Perhaps because our understanding of coagulation was rather incomplete at that time, and therefore detailed interpretation of the function of the inhibitor was precluded, these pioneering observations did not garner the attention that they deserved. Later, Stenflo isolated bovine protein C (79), which was named protein C because it was the third peak to elute from the DEAE column. Interest in the protein was sparked by the demonstration that this was a vitamin K–dependent protein (79) and a precursor to a membrane-binding serine esterase that was immunochemically distinct from the known plasma clotting factors (80). Now there were at least five vitamin K–dependent plasma factors. By exchanging reagents, Seegers was able to show that the "new" protein C was the precursor of autoprothrombin II-A [see (78) for review of the early work of Dr. Seegers on this protein]. Subsequently, human protein C was isolated, and a slow release of a 12-residue

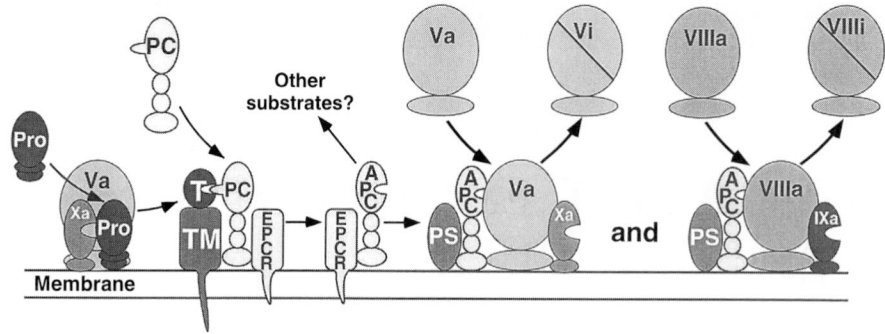

**FIGURE 14-1.** Model of the function of the protein C anticoagulant pathway. Thrombin (T) is generated from prothrombin (Pro) by the factor Va–factor Xa complex. T then binds to thrombomodulin (TM) to form the protein C activation complex. Protein C binds to the endothelial cell protein C receptor (EPCR), if present, and this complex is activated by the T–TM complex. Activated protein C (APC) can remain bound to EPCR, but this complex does not seem to be capable of inactivating factor Va, presumably an indication that it is targeted to as yet unidentified alternative substrates. When APC dissociates from EPCR, it can then bind to protein S (PS). This complex inactivates factor Va or factor VIIIa, thereby shutting down T formation and preventing blood clot extension. [Modified figure reprinted with permission from Stearns-Kurosawa DJ, et al. The endothelial cell protein C receptor augments protein C activation by the thrombin-thrombomodulin complex. *Proc Natl Acad Sci U S A* 93:10212–10216, figure 6, copyright 1996 National Academy of Sciences, U S A, and from Esmon CT, The protein C anticoagulant pathway. *Arterioscl Thromb* 12(2):135–145, Figure 1, copyright 1992 Waverly.]

peptide by thrombin was demonstrated to activate human protein C (81).

Purified preparations of bovine factor V and factor Va became available, and it was shown that APC could inactivate factor V slowly (82), and that APC inactivated factor Va much more rapidly than factor V (41). APC inactivation involved a selective cleavage in the heavy chain of factor Va (41). This inactivation process was attenuated by factor Xa (41).

## Protein S

Protein S was initially identified by DiScipio and Davie (83) as a sixth vitamin K–dependent plasma protein, which they isolated from bovine and human plasma. No function was ascribed to protein S. Walker, searching for a cofactor for APC, demonstrated that protein S could facilitate APC inactivation of factor Va and augmented the plasma anticoagulant response to APC (84). These studies indicated that the two new vitamin K–dependent proteins were both part of an anticoagulant system, further elevating interest in the potential physiologic and clinical contributions of the system.

## Thrombomodulin

Thrombin activation of protein C in the presence of physiologic $Ca^{2+}$ is extremely slow (85). Esmon and Owen (28,86) reasoned that if protein C were to be able to function as a physiologic activator, there must be a mechanism to enhance the activation rate. This mechanism did not seem to be present in blood or plasma because almost all of the protein C can be isolated from serum as the zymogen (87) and inhibition or removal of protein C from plasma does not influence standard clotting assays (80). Because thrombin could activate protein C slowly, one possible mechanism for protein C activation would be for thrombin to bind to a cofactor, thereby increasing the protein C activation rate. The endothelium, with its well-established antithrombotic potential, was a logical cell type to test. Due to the very high surface area of endothelium exposed to blood in the microcirculation (88), the perfused rabbit coronary microcirculation was chosen as the

test system to explore the possible existence of an endothelial cell cofactor for thrombin-dependent protein C activation (28). Perfusion of the coronary microcirculation with thrombin plus protein C elicited potent anticoagulant activity, whereas thrombin or protein C perfusion alone did not. Protein C activation was blocked by active site-inhibited thrombin, consistent with a cofactor-mediated process. Human endothelial cells in culture were also shown to have thrombin-dependent protein C activation potential (28,89). TM was subsequently isolated from rabbit (90), rat (91), bovine (92), and human (93) tissue(s).

## Endothelial Cell Protein C Receptor

Early studies of endothelial cell protein C activation demonstrated that some cell lines showed a distinct preference for activating protein C containing the Gla domain, whereas other cell lines failed to distinguish between intact protein C and protein C lacking the Gla domain (residues 1 to 44) (94). This, coupled with the incompletely understood antiinflammatory activities of APC (see subsequent text), prompted Fukudome and Esmon (29) to search for cell-specific binding sites for protein C/APC. Such binding sites were identified on endothelium (29,95) and shown to be downregulated by tumor necrosis factor α (TNF-α) (29), indicating a high probability that binding was dependent on a cell surface protein. EPCR was subsequently identified by an expression cloning strategy (29). The expressed soluble form of the receptor was shown to bind to protein C selectively and with comparable affinities for protein C and APC (96).

## Schematic Structures of the Members of the Protein C Anticoagulant Pathway

The schematic structure of protein C, protein S, TM, and EPCR are shown in Figure 14-2. Protein C and protein S are vitamin K–dependent proteins; hence, their biosynthesis is blocked by oral anticoagulants (see Table 14-1). In contrast, TM and EPCR are integral membrane proteins.

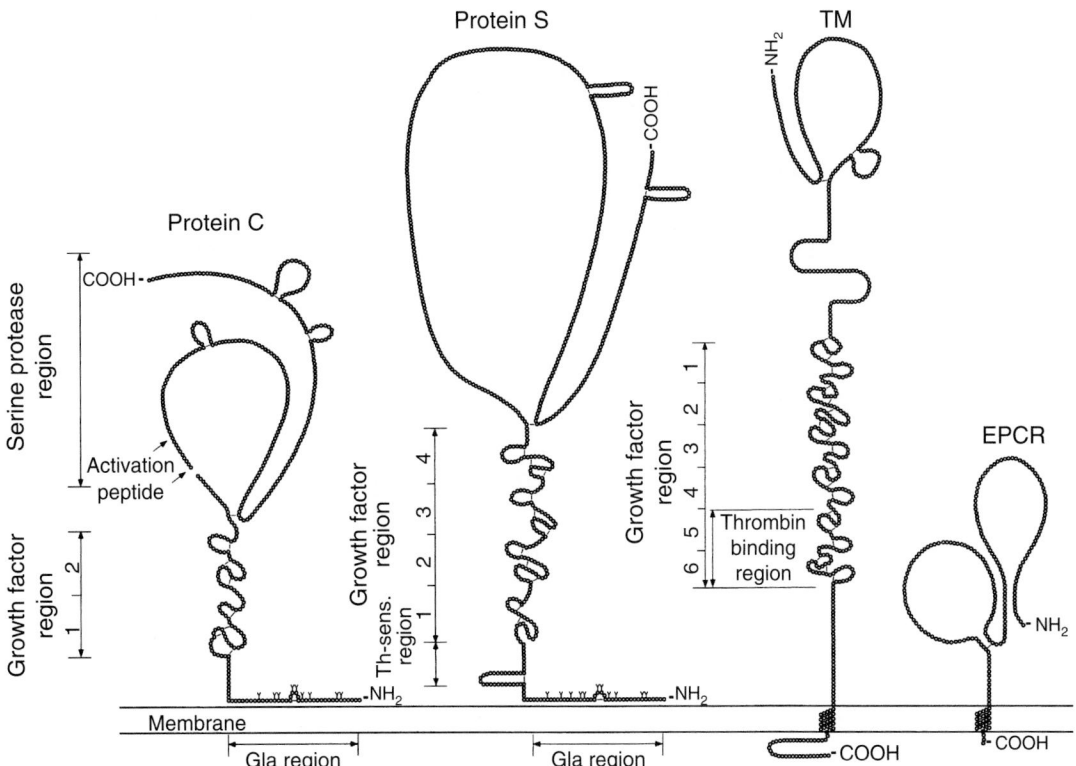

**FIGURE 14-2.** Schematic representation of protein C, protein S, thrombomodulin, and endothelial cell protein C receptor (EPCR). Specific domains of each protein are identified. Gla, γ-carboxyglutamic acids; Th-sens., thrombin-sensitive; TM, thrombomodulin. (Modified figure reprinted with permission from *J Biol Chem* 1989;264:4743, copyright the American Society of Biochemistry and Molecular Biology, Inc., 1989.)

# PROTEIN C STRUCTURE AND FUNCTION

Protein C is synthesized with a leader peptide and a propeptide involved in the carboxylation of protein C, which are removed proteolytically during maturation (97–100). The sequence of human protein C is shown in Figure 14-3. The mature protein C molecule consists of an amino-terminal Gla domain, a hydrophobic stack region that connects the Gla domain to the two epidermal growth factor (EGF) domains, and a protease domain with homology to trypsin. In general, at the gene level, these domains are separated by introns [(101); also see Chapter 2]. Human protein C circulates primarily as a two-chain zymogen, but approximately 10% of the protein C circulates as a single chain (102). Human protein C activation occurs by cleavage of

**TABLE 14-1**

### PROPERTIES OF THE COMPONENTS OF THE PROTEIN C PATHWAY

| | Chains | AA Residues | Vitamin K–dependent (Gla) | Integral membrane | Function |
|---|---|---|---|---|---|
| TM | 1 | 557(184) | No | Yes | Cofactor |
| EPCR | 1 | 220(29) | No | Yes | Cofactor |
| Thrombin | 2 | 295(422)[b] | Yes[d] | No | Enzyme |
| Protein C | 2[a] | 461(143)[c] | Yes | No | Substrate |
| APC | 2 | 447(81) | Yes | No | Enzyme |
| Protein S | 1 | 635(151) | Yes | No | Cofactor |

AA, amino acid; Gla, gamma-carboxyglutamic acid; TM, thrombomodulin; EPCR, endothelial cell protein C receptor; APC, activated protein C.
[a]Approximately 5% to 10% of protein C circulates as single chain.
[b]This reference describes the crystal structure of thrombin and the chymotrypsinogen numbering system for thrombin used throughout this chapter.
[c]Number of residues in single-chain protein C.
[d]Prothrombin is vitamin K–dependent. The vitamin K–dependent region is released from thrombin during activation.

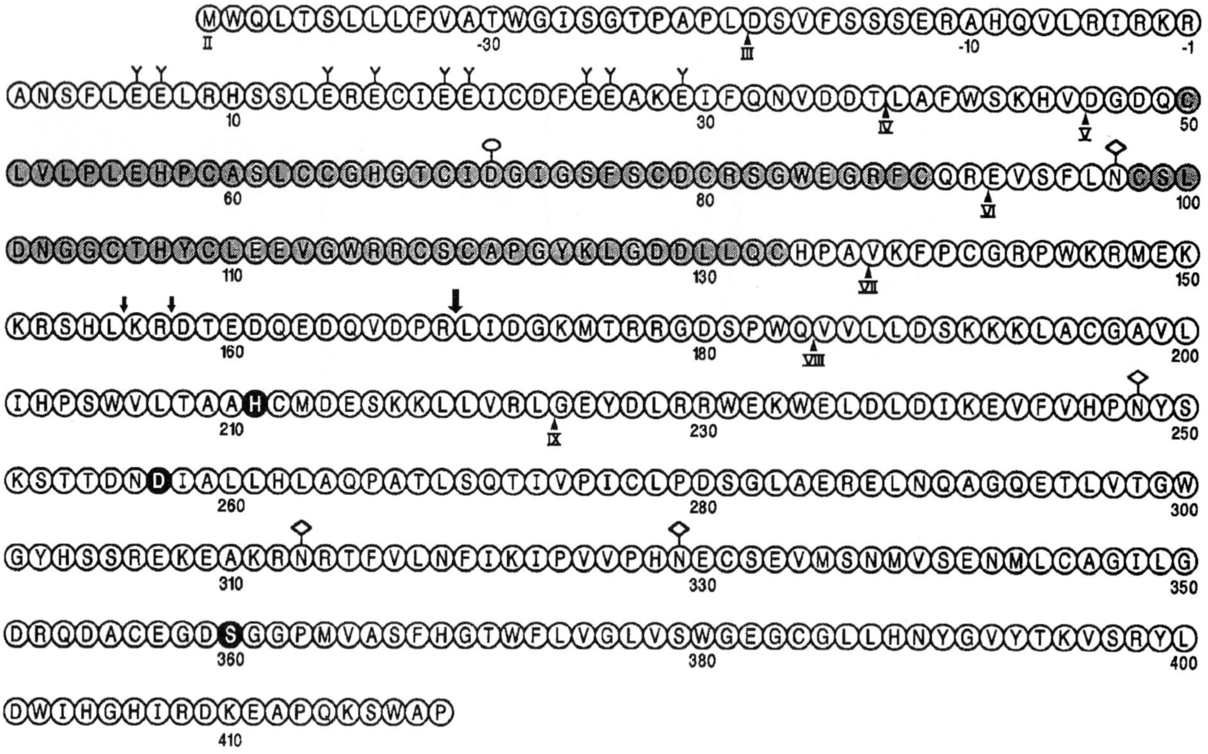

**FIGURE 14-3.** Amino acid sequence of human protein C. Amino acids are numbered from the amino-terminus of the mature protein. *Y* depicts γ-carboxylation, and an *oval* depicts hydroxylation of an amino acid. *Diamonds* represent sites of N-linked glycosylation. Residues within the two EGF-like domains are *shaded*. The serine, aspartic acid, and histidine residues that constitute the active catalytic site are identified in *black*. ▲ denotes the location of an intron in the protein C gene, and the *roman numeral* identifies the following exon. The dipeptide proteolytically removed during the posttranslational processing of most protein C molecules is marked by the *small arrows*. The site of proteolytic cleavage during protein C activation is identified by the *large arrow*.

DPRLID sequence (Asp-Pro-Arg-Leu-Ile-Asp) at Arg169, releasing a 12 residue peptide (81). In the single-chain protein C, no peptide is released during activation. The thrombin–TM complex is the major physiologic activator (103). There are $Ca^{2+}$ binding sites located in the Gla domain (1), the first EGF domain (6,104,105), and the protease domain of protein C (106). The metal binding sites in the Gla domain are required for binding to phospholipid (1) and to EPCR (107). Mutational studies of the Gla domain suggest that the *N*-terminal half of the domain is critical for membrane interaction (1). Mutations of Gla residues 7, 20, 26, and 29 result in nearly complete loss of APC anticoagulant activity. Mutation of Gla25 decreases activity 75%, but Gla6, 14, and 19 do not appear to be critical for APC functions tested to date [(108–111); and reviewed in (1)]. Mutation of the hydrophobic residues near the *N*-terminus also disrupt phospholipid binding, particularly Leu5 (112). Arg15, which is highly conserved in the vitamin K–dependent clotting factors, also appears to be important in $Ca^{2+}$ binding (113). The disulfide bond in the Gla domain is also important for function (1). His10 in human protein C has been shown to be largely responsible for the 10-fold higher membrane binding affinity over bovine protein C, which has a Pro at this position (114). Methods for expression and isolation of protein C mutants have been reviewed recently (115).

APC functions much better on phospholipid vesicles containing phosphatidylethanolamine (116,117), and protein C activation proceeds more rapidly on these vesicles (118). APC function is also enhanced significantly by glucosylceramides (119), and low levels of these lipids in the circulation appear to correlate with an increased risk of thrombosis. In contrast, the

prothrombin activation complex demonstrates a lower phosphatidylethanolamine dependence. Chimeric protein C in which the Gla domain (first 46 residues) is replaced with that of prothrombin lack the phosphatidylethanolamine-dependence characteristic of the wild type (117). Plasma anticoagulant activity of this chimera is also protein S–independent. Further analysis revealed that it is the carboxy-terminal 24 residues that are responsible for the phosphatidylethanolamine dependence (117). This same region is necessary for protein S–dependent enhancement of factor Va inactivation and for the participation of protein S as an anticoagulant in plasma.

When the Gla domain of protein C is exchanged for that of prothrombin, all detectable interaction with EPCR (107) is lost, although the anticoagulant activity of the resultant APC mutant is increased approximately fourfold (117). Undercarboxylation, by as little as one Gla residue, reduces the affinity for EPCR approximately 10-fold (107).

The $Ca^{2+}$ binding site in the first EGF domain is probably important to aid in the appropriate folding of the $Ca^{2+}$ stabilized conformation of the protein C Gla domain (120,121). This site is not critical for activation by the thrombin–TM complex in solution (122). Protein C also contains a β hydroxy aspartic acid residue (123) in this domain. Mutation of this residue to Glu (124) or Ala (125) impairs APC $Ca^{2+}$ binding and anticoagulant activity. A synthetic peptide corresponding to the Gla domain of protein C (residues 1 to 48) can bind $Ca^{2+}$ and phospholipid similarly to intact protein C (126).

Protein C activation exhibits a very strong dependence on $Ca^{2+}$, which inhibits activation of protein C by thrombin (85). This inhibition is not dependent on the Gla (127) or EGF1 domains (122). In contrast, activation by the thrombin–TM complex depends on the presence of $Ca^{2+}$ (127). The site responsible for these $Ca^{2+}$ effects is located in the protease domain of the protein C molecule (106) and is structurally similar to the $Ca^{2+}$ binding site in trypsin (106,128).

The structure of APC lacking the Gla domain has been determined to 2.8 Å (see Fig. 14-4) (128), and a molecular model of APC has been published (129). Regions of APC thought to be functionally important are discussed in the context of the APC structures in these two papers. APC shows several unique properties that may contribute to its unusual specificity. Like thrombin, APC has an extended groove that could engage P′ residues of substrates. The groove is located almost exactly where anion-binding exosite 1 in thrombin is located. In APC, the groove terminates near the $Ca^{2+}$ binding site, which is located on almost the opposite side of the protease domain of protein C from the active site. By analogy with thrombin, this groove may be able to elicit conformational changes and/or interact with receptors. Support for this conclusion comes from mutagenesis studies, which show that residues in this region do play an important role in factor Va inactivation (130). In thrombin, anion-binding exosite 1 is the docking site for TM (131,132), the protease activated thrombin receptor 1 (133–137), fibrinogen (138–140), factor V, and factor VIII (141). Of interest, factors V and VIII have highly conserved sequences on the P′ side near Arg506 (142), a major APC cleavage site in factors Va and VIIIa. These sequences are rich in acidic and hydrophobic residues similar to the corresponding domain in the thrombin receptor (134).

The active site of APC is relatively open compared to that of thrombin. The S2 and S3/S4 pockets are more hydrophilic and somewhat larger than those of thrombin or factor Xa. This may contribute to the resistance of APC to inhibition by plasma proteinase inhibitors. The second EGF domain makes extensive contact with the protease domain of APC. The first EGF domain is unusual in that it contains an "extra" disulfide bridge (143,144) that forms a loop within one of the loops (128). There is a rather large peptide region between the first and second EGF domains that is likely to allow considerable flexibility between the two domains. Flexibility in the APC molecule may contribute to the observed topographical changes in APC, which are observed following interaction with protein S, discussed in subsequent text (145). In the crystal structures, the two EGF domains of protein C and factor IXa are located in quite different positions (145,146). Whether the opposite bends in the EGF domains reflect real differences in the structures of the two proteins, different flexible conformers in the molecules, or are due to crystal packing influences, is uncertain.

Highly variable posttranslational modification makes human protein C particularly complex at the biochemical level. It circulates at approximately 65 nM in both single- and two-chain forms, and each of these forms has several glycosylation variants with 4, 3, and to a lesser extent, 2 N-linked carbohydrate chains (102). The variants separate on gel electrophoresis, giving rise to very complex patterns for purified protein C. All forms can be activated, but glycosylation variants seem to have differing anticoagulant activities and rates of activation (147). Glycosylation at Asn329 is probably responsible for the highest molecular weight ($\alpha$) form of protein C. Elimination of all glycosylation sites increases APC anticoagulant activity two- to threefold, and elimination of the glycosylation site at 313 results in a 2.5-fold increase in activation rate due to a corresponding reduction in the $K_m$. Expression of protein C in human kidney 293 cells leads to decreased sialic acid and an increase in GalNAc and fucose (148) compared to plasma protein C. A polylactosamine on protein C also has been implicated in inhibiting cell adhesion through E selectin (149), a potential antiinflammatory function of protein C.

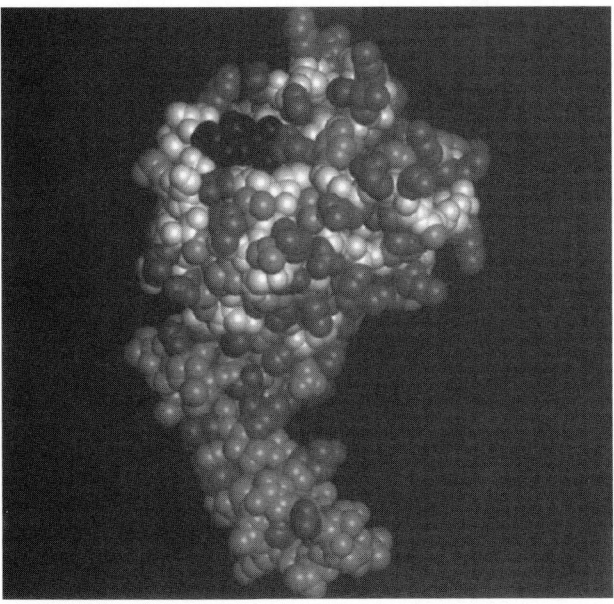

**FIGURE 14-4.** Space-filling model of the activated protein C crystal. The model is based on the previously determined structure of activated protein C lacking the Gla domain (128). The active site inhibitor is shown in *black*. Basic residues are in *blue*, acidic residues are *red*, and hydrophobic residues are *gold*. Other residues in the protease domain are *white*. The acidic, basic, and hydrophobic residues of the EGF domains follow the same convention, but the other residues are in *green* to set off the EGF domains from the protease domain. The three basic residues critical for activation by the thrombin–TM complex are at the top of the figure. The exosite runs just underneath these residues. The $Ca^{2+}$ binding site is to the far right of the protease domain near the acidic (*red*) residue that is almost completely hidden by the basic (*blue*) residues (see Color Fig. 14-4).

# PROTEIN S STRUCTURE AND FUNCTION

Protein S is synthesized with a leader and a propeptide involved in carboxylation, which are released proteolytically during expression (150–152). The sequence of protein S is shown in Figure 14-5. In the mature protein, the vitamin K–dependent Gla domain is followed by an aromatic stack, a unique 29-residue thrombin-sensitive domain encoded by exon IV (150,152), four EGF-like domains, and a terminal domain homologous to the sex hormone–binding globulin and androgen-binding protein (153,154). Cleavage at Arg49, 60, or 70 in the thrombin-sensitive region destroys protein S-cofactor function (155–158), as shown by the mutation of these three sites to generate a thrombin-resistant form of protein S (155). Like protein C, physiologic levels of $Ca^{2+}$ inhibit thrombin proteolysis of protein S (159). Activated platelets (160) and neutrophils (161) contain proteases that can cleave protein S in this region and inactivate the protein. The first EGF domain contains a $\beta$-hydroxylated aspartic acid residue; the remaining three EGF domains contain $\beta$ hydroxylated asparagine residues. Hydroxylation of these residues is incomplete, however, in human protein S (162,163). The EGF domains function cooperatively to bind a $Ca^{2+}$ (163), the combination of EGF domains binding $Ca^{2+}$ up to 10,000 times tighter than the isolated domains (163). The N-terminal EGF domain is critical for the cofactor function (164). Antibodies directed toward the EGF domains of protein S inhibit cofactor activity (165).

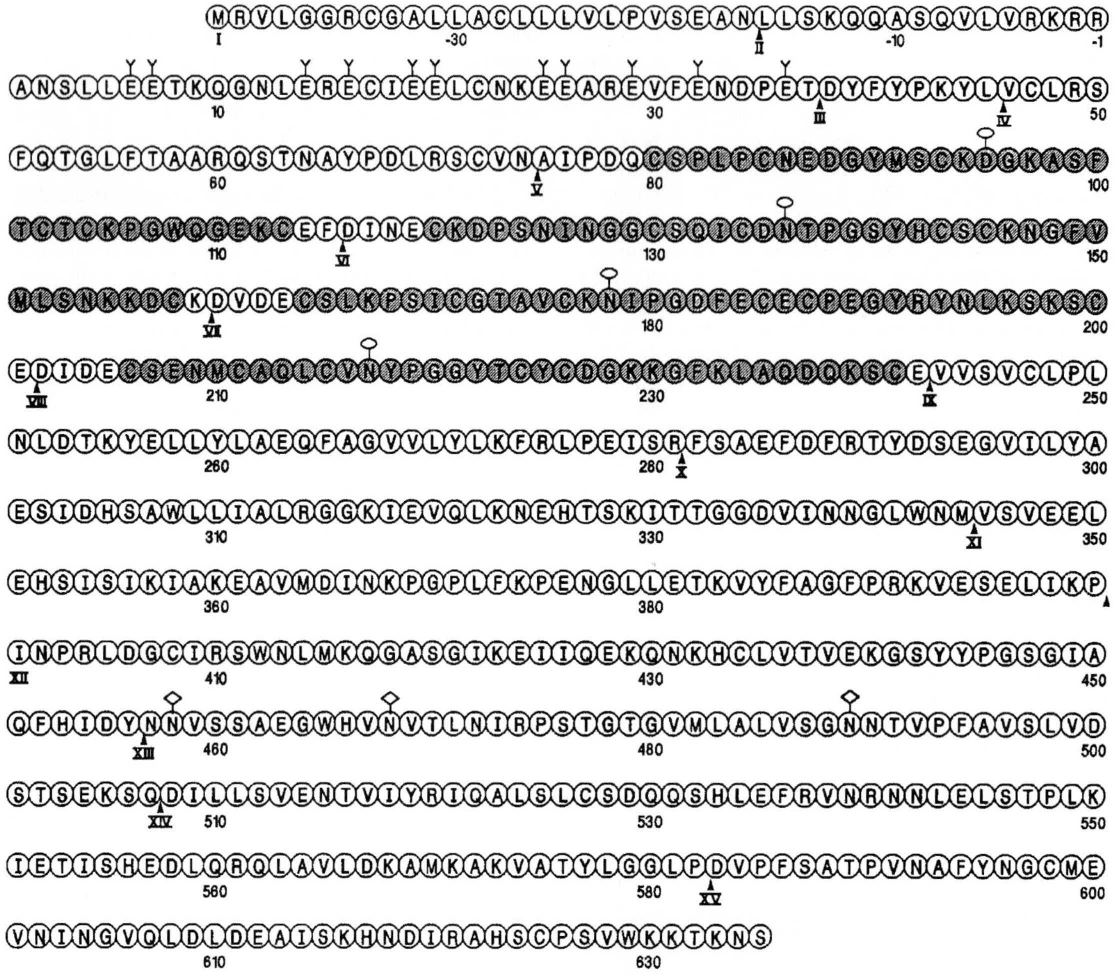

FIGURE 14-5. Amino acid sequence of human protein S. Amino acids are numbered from the amino-terminus of the mature protein. Y depicts γ-carboxylation, and an *oval* depicts potential hydroxylation of an amino acid. *Diamonds* represent potential sites of N-linked glycosylation. Residues within the four EGF-like domains are *shaded*. ˅ denotes the location of an intron in the protein S-gene, and the *roman numeral* identifies the following exon. The amino acid sequence is that reported by Schmidel et al. (152).

The steroid hormone–binding globulin domain is not required for protein S–cofactor activity (166). Protein S is a complicated protein, however, and early work demonstrated that C4BP, a regulatory protein of the complement system, binds to protein S (167) with approximately 60% of the protein S in this complex. This interaction is important because the protein S–C4BP complex lacks cofactor activity for APC in plasma anticoagulant assays (168,169). C4BP and protein S interact reversibly and with very high affinity in plasma, an interaction that is tightened substantially by the presence of $Ca^{2+}$ (170,171). The sex hormone–binding globulin domain appears to be required and sufficient for this binding (172). Deletion of the domain eliminates detectable C4BP interaction (166), a deletion mutant involving the carboxy-terminal residues 583 to 635, and exhibits a 1,000-fold reduction for C4BP. Peptides corresponding to 420 to 434 (173) and 414 to 433 (174) have been implicated in C4BP interaction.

C4BP exists as a large protein (540 kDa) containing six or seven identical α chains approximately 70 kDa each (175). By electron microscopy, C4BP appears as a spiderlike structure with long arms corresponding to the α chains (175,176). Protein S sits at the base of the α chains and interacts with the single β chain that forms the protein S–binding site (175,177). Most, but not all, circulating C4BP molecules have a covalently linked

β chain (2,178). C4BP is an acute-phase reactant, but only the C4BP α chains seem to be elevated in the acute-phase response (179). Although both bovine and human protein S can interact with human C4BP, bovine C4BP does not interact with either protein S-molecule (168). Both types of chains are composed of short consensus repeats. Truncation studies of the β chain revealed that the protein S–binding site is located in the first three repeats (180) and subsequently in the N-terminal repeat (177). Bovine C4BP, which apparently does not bind to protein S, lacks the N-terminal repeat (181,182).

# THROMBOMODULIN STRUCTURE AND FUNCTION

Thrombomodulin is a type 1 transmembrane protein. It is synthesized with a leader peptide. The mature human TM molecule is 559 residues in length, as deduced from the cDNA sequence (183–186), and a single copy of the gene is localized to 20p-12 cen (184,187). The sequence of the mature protein is shown in Figure 14-6. The gene is without introns (183,186); hence, unlike the other members of the family, the different domains cannot be separated or inferred from exon–intron

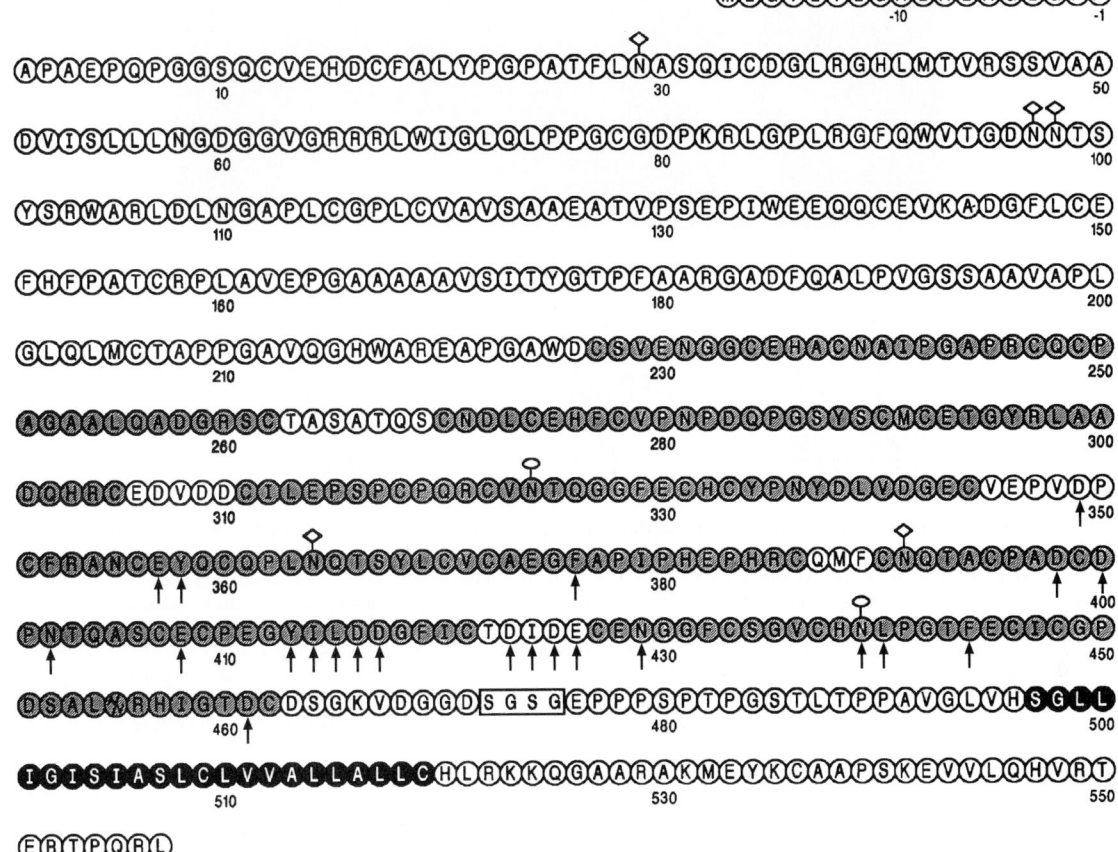

**FIGURE 14-6.** Amino acid sequence of human thrombomodulin. Amino acids are numbered from the amino-terminus of the mature protein. *Ovals* depict sites of potential hydroxylation, and *diamonds* represent potential sites of N-linked glycosylation. Residues within the six EGF-like domains are *shaded*. Residues in the putative transmembrane domain are shown in *black*. The consensus sequence for the possible attachment of a glycosaminoglycan is *boxed*. A/V denotes a genetic polymorphism. *Arrows* point to the 22 residues thought to be critical for cofactor activity within EGF domains 4 to 6 (199).

boundaries. The amino-terminal domain (226 residues) has weak homology (approximately 20%) with the lectins, such as the asialoglycoprotein receptor (188). Recently, this domain, whether free or attached to TM, has been shown to dampen endothelial cell inflammatory responses (mitogen-activated kinase and nuclear factor κB activation). By so doing, the presence of the *N*-terminal domain limits endothelial cell activation that promotes leukocyte adhesion (189). TM, and specifically the lectin domain of TM, has been shown to participate in cell adhesion (190). Cells transfected with full-length TM formed clusters that could be disrupted by chondroitin sulfate or mannose. No comparable clumping was observed when the cells were transfected with TM lacking the lectin domain.

The lectin domain is followed by six EGF-like domains (236 residues). EGF domains 5 and 6 are responsible for most of the thrombin-binding affinity (191), but this fragment cannot support protein C activation. Good rates of protein C activation require the linker region between EGF3 and EGF repeats 4 to 6 (192–195), or less effectively, repeats 4 to 5 (196). EGF 3 is required for rapid thrombin–dependent TAFI activation (197). Many point mutations within EGF 4, 5, and 6 have been identified that reduce thrombin affinity or protein C activation rates (198,199). Using relative affinities to select conformers of EGF 5 from a yeast expression system, White et al. suggested that EGF 5 of TM does not have the canonical disulfide bonding pattern (200). Recent crystal structure determination of the TM 4 to 6 bound to thrombin confirmed this proposal (201)

(see Fig. 14-7). Indeed, unlike the usual disulfide pairing for EGF domains (1–3, 2–4, and 5–6), in EGF 5 the disulfides are paired 1 to 2, 3 to 4, 5 to 6, resulting in an elongated domain that shifts the overall conformation considerably. EGF 4, a domain known to have many residues required for protein C activation, is pointed away from thrombin. The crystal structure did not reveal a significant change in thrombin's conformation. However, despite the lack of a visible change in thrombin conformation, mutational and spectral data indicate that thrombin conformation(s) can be altered by TM [see Rezaie and Yang (130) for a recent update].

Following the EGF domains is a 34-residue region rich in Ser and Thr, corresponding to potential O-linked glycosylation sites. The region also contains two sites of potential addition of chondroitin sulfate. Mutational analysis has shown that Ser474 and 472 are potential sites of chondroitin sulfate addition (202). The sequence of this attachment site is Ser(472)-Gly-Ser(474)-Gly-Glu-Pro. Which Ser is modified depends on the cell line in which the TM is expressed. In the same study, evidence was presented that placental TM can contain chondroitin sulfate(s). This was an issue because isolated human TM preparations (93) did not display the characteristic high molecular weight and diffuse electrophoretic pattern observed with rabbit TM (9,47,90,203–205). It is unclear whether the human TM has less chondroitin sulfate addition *in vivo* or the chondroitin containing material is lost differentially during preparation. However, TM containing chondroitin sulfate can be isolated

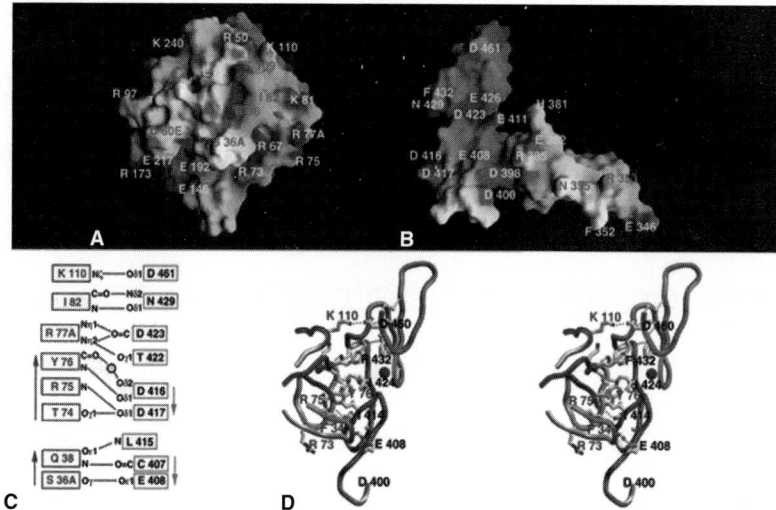

**FIGURE 14-7.** The thrombin–thrombomodulin interaction interface is dominated by hydrophobic contacts. Graphical representation and analysis of surface properties (GRASP) (425) electrostatic surface potentials of α-thrombin (**A**) and TME456 (**B**). Both moieties have been slightly rotated around the *y* axis to present their interaction interfaces to the viewer. Note the overall complementarity of electrostatic potentials. **C:** Major hydrogen–bonding interactions (*dotted lines*) between thrombin and TM. **D:** Detail of the interaction interface, highlighting its primary hydrophobic character. Selected hydrogen bonds are indicated as *green spheres*. Note that single, solvent-exposed salt bridge forms between thrombin and TM (Lys110 Nζ-Asp461 Oδ2). For clarity, only residues Asp400-Cys462 of TM and thrombin loops of the contact interface are shown (see Color Fig. 14-7). (Reprinted with permission from Fuentes-Prior P, et al. *Nature* 2000;404:518–525, copyright 2000.)

from human tissues (202,206). The issue is important because the presence of chondroitin sulfate (a) tightens thrombin affinity more than 10-fold (207); (b) increases the ability of TM to block fibrinogen clotting and platelet activation (9,47); (c) stimulates inhibition by antithrombin (9,208) and PCI (45); and (d) modulates the $Ca^{2+}$ dependence of protein C activation (207,208). In addition, the chondroitin sulfate has been shown to facilitate plasmodium falciparum infected erythrocytes (209), probably playing a role in disease progression. Lack of chondroitin sulfate probably accounts for the relatively ineffective direct anticoagulant activity observed with human TM preparations (210). Recombinant soluble TM can have chondroitin sulfate attached with relatively high fidelity (211,212).

Following the O-linked sugar region is a 23-residue hydrophobic region that corresponds to the transmembrane region. This region is highly conserved among species (213,214), suggesting a potentially important and selective function for the domain. The cytoplasmic tail is 38 residues in length, contains one tyrosine, one serine, and two threonine residues that are potential sites of phosphorylation. Phosphorylation of serine has been observed following stimulation with phorbol myristate acetate (213). There is also a Cys residue in this domain. No consensus sequence for internalization by coated pit–mediated endocytosis is present. Nevertheless, coated and noncoated pit–mediated endocytosis has been observed with TM (215). The constitutive internalization instead seems to be a property of the N-terminal lectinlike domain (216). Recently, TM has been localized to caveolae (217), which probably accounts for the constitutive internalization. Whether localization to caveolae is dependent on the lectin domain remains to be determined.

# ENDOTHELIAL CELL PROTEIN C RECEPTOR STRUCTURE AND FUNCTION

EPCR is a type 1 transmembrane protein (29). It is homologous to the MHC class 1 family of molecules. The N-terminal region

has only two of the three domains normally present in this family and is missing the domain that is thought to be primarily responsible for interaction with β2 microglobulin. The sequence of mature EPCR is shown in Figure 14-8. The α- and β-domains of EPCR interact intimately, making a rather compact structure, with a deep groove between the two domains (218) (see Fig. 14-9). A β-pleated sheet is located below the two helical domains. A phospholipid, mostly phosphatidylcholine, is bound in the groove. It is positioned in almost the identical location as peptide and glycolipid antigens bound in the MHC class 1 family members. Between the α- and β-domains and the membrane is a short region with several potential O-linked glycosylation sites. The 25-residue transmembrane region is somewhat unusual in that it contains two Gly–Gly sequences that are not normally favorable for α-helix formation. The cytoplasmic domain is very short and quite conserved among species, consisting of an Arg-Arg-Cys sequence in human (29) and murine (219) EPCR and Arg-Arg-Arg-Cys in bovine EPCR (219). Human EPCR appears to be palmitoylated on the terminal Cys (220,221).

The EPCR gene has both a thrombin response element (222) and multiple Sp1 (223) binding sites that modulate EPCR expression. These have been identified in the genomic sequences of both murine (224) and human (225) EPCR. There are also several haplotypes of the EPCR gene, one of which results in a different coding sequence that leads to increased circulating EPCR and is associated with an increased risk of thrombosis (226).

Interruption of the murine EPCR gene leads to early embryonic lethality with thrombosis around the embryonically derived trophoblast giant cells (227). In a partial deletion resulting in approximately a 10-fold decrease in EPCR, the mice are viable (228).

# PROTEIN C ACTIVATION

The thrombin–TM complex is almost certainly the major physiologic activator of protein C (103). However, other activators have been described. Plasmin has also been reported to activate

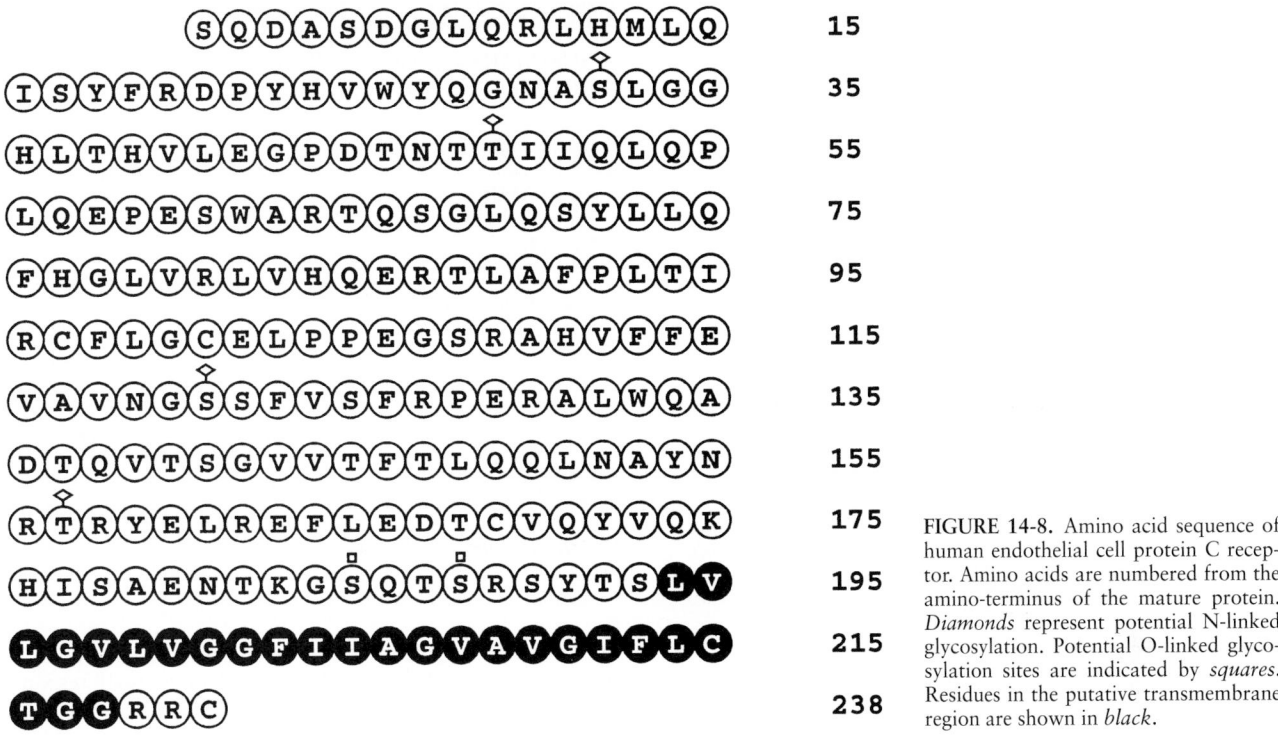

FIGURE 14-8. Amino acid sequence of human endothelial cell protein C receptor. Amino acids are numbered from the amino-terminus of the mature protein. *Diamonds* represent potential N-linked glycosylation. Potential O-linked glycosylation sites are indicated by *squares*. Residues in the putative transmembrane region are shown in *black*.

and then degrade protein C (229,230). Copperhead snake venom contains a protein C activator that is useful in coagulation assays (231). Activation of protein C by the factor Xa–TM complex has been reported (232), and TM has been reported to inhibit factor Xa activation of prothrombin (233). Several laboratories, including our own, have failed to confirm protein C activation by this complex (234) or binding to TM (235). If TM does bind to factor Xa, it must utilize a completely different mechanism because factor Xa lacks an equivalent to anion-binding exosite 1 in thrombin that is the major TM binding site. Meizothrombin can also interact with TM to efficiently activate protein C (236,237). In the presence of negatively charged phospholipid, the activation by meizothrombin is more efficient than that of thrombin (237). The ability of TM to interact with meizothrombin or meizothrombin des fragment 1 (236) is consistent with the observation that anion-binding exosite 1 is formed in the meizothrombin des fragment 1 structure (238).

## Protein C Activation on Endothelial Cells

Endothelial cells maintain antithrombotic properties that would be compromised if negatively charged phospholipid were constitutively expressed on their surface. Nevertheless, protein C is a vitamin K–dependent protein and, by analogy with other vitamin K–dependent proteins, activation should be enhanced if protein C were bound to the surface. EPCR can substitute for negatively charged phospholipid in promoting protein C activation. EPCR binds directly to protein C through the Gla domain. Binding requires nearly complete $\gamma$ carboxylation (29,107). Binding to EPCR promotes protein C activation primarily by decreasing the $K_m$ (30,239). Soluble EPCR inhibits protein C activation by blocking protein C binding to the cellular EPCR (240). EPCR involvement in protein C activation presumably varies in different vascular beds. EPCR is expressed at high levels in large vessels, particularly arteries, and at low to undetectable levels in the capillaries (241). Consistent with direct staining of the large vessels for EPCR, protein C can be stained immunohistochemically only on vessels that are positive for EPCR staining (241). Therefore, the effective affinity for protein C can be anticipated to differ dramatically among vessels. In addition to EPCR, human, but not bovine (242), factor Va can augment protein C activation on endothelium (243). Unlike EPCR, human factor Va can also accelerate protein C activation in solution (244). The factor Va light chain is responsible for this activity (242,245).

In solution, EGF domains 4 to 6 of TM are sufficient for protein C activation. On cell surfaces, however, the O-linked sugar region is necessary, possibly to elevate thrombin to the appropriate height from the membrane surface (246). Consistent with this observation, the distance from the surface of phospholipid-TM vesicles to the active site of thrombin bound to TM is approximately 65 Å (247). This indicates that the O-linked sugar region of TM must be rather extended and rigid. It apparently rises approximately perpendicular to the membrane surface.

Cellular modulation of TM expression and function can be controlled by a large number of factors, which are summarized in Table 14-2. For instance, platelet factor 4 can enhance protein C activation by the thrombin–TM complex both *in vivo* (248) and *in vitro*, increasing the rate of activation more than 10-fold at low protein C concentrations (249,250). The influence on activation rate involves primarily a decrease in the $K_m$ for protein C from 8.3 $\mu$M to 0.27 $\mu$M (250,251). These changes in protein C activation rates were almost completely lost when the Gla domain of protein C was removed.

Not all cationic proteins enhance protein C activation. The major basic protein from eosinophils inhibits protein C activation by the thrombin–TM complex in a concentration-dependent fashion (252). Inhibition is dependent on the presence of the chondroitin sulfate on TM. Inhibition was observed on human aortic and umbilical vein endothelial cells. Once major basic protein was incubated with the endothelial cell surface and the cells were subsequently washed, it required more than 5 hours to regain most of the protein C activating activity of the cell surface. Inhibition by this eosinophil protein could conceivably contribute to hypereosinophilic heart disease (252).

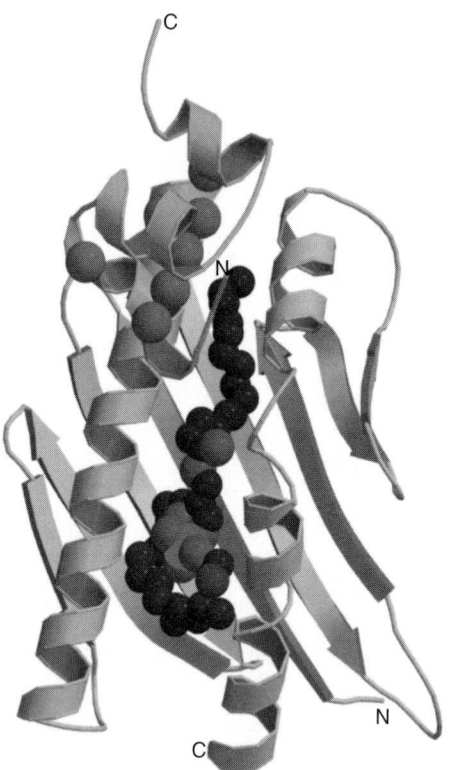

FIGURE 14-9. The rs-endothelial cell protein C receptor (EPCR) molecule with a portion of the protein C Gla domain and a lipid molecule. In EPCR (*yellow ribbon*), two $\alpha$-helices and an eight-stranded $\beta$-sheet create a groove that is filled with phospholipid (the space-filling balls in the center). Binding of $Ca^{2+}$ ions (*spheres in magenta*) to the protein C Gla domain (*green ribbon*) exposes the N-terminal "omega" loop, which in the absence of EPCR interacts with the phospholipid surfaces on the membrane. There do not appear to be direct interactions between the protein C Gla domain and the lipid molecule located in the groove of rsEPCR. The model of the complex consists of residues 7 to 177 of rsEPCR and the first 33 residues of the protein C Gla domain (422–424) (see Color Fig. 14-9). [Reprinted with permission from Oganesyan et al., *The J Biol Chem* 2002;277(28):24851–24854, copyright 2002.]

Although it is extremely unlikely that significant negatively charged phospholipid is present on the cell surface of quiescent endothelium cells, activation can lead to exposure of these lipids. In addition to phosphatidylserine, cell activation exposes phosphatidylethanolamine. This phospholipid exerts approximately a fourfold enhancement on protein C activation (118). The phospatidylethanolamine effect was dependent on the unsaturated fatty acids at both positions. This is commonly found in naturally occurring phosphatidylethanolamine (253).

Many agents, particularly those involved in inflammation, can downregulate protein C activation on cultured endothelial cells. These include endotoxin (254), interleukin 1 $\beta$ (255–257), transforming growth factor $\beta$ (258), and TNF-$\alpha$ (257,259–263). In the last case, the mechanism of TM downregulation is primarily at the level of transcriptional control (257,260–263) with even a transient exposure of endothelium to TNF-$\alpha$ leading to a prolonged inhibition of TM transcription. The TNF-$\alpha$ responsive region of the gene has been mapped to a region starting at $-51$ and containing the TATA box sequence (263). Agents that elevate cyclic adenosine monophosphate (AMP) (256,262,264) and retinoic acid (265–268) can decrease this downregulation. Retinoic acid response elements have been identified in the 5'

## TABLE 14-2

### A SUMMARY OF MOLECULAR MODULATORS OF THROMBOMODULIN EXPRESSION AND FUNCTION

| Upregulation | Downregulation |
|---|---|
| Cyclic AMP | Tumor necrosis factor $\alpha$ |
| Retinoic acid | Interleukin 1 |
| Thrombin | Endotoxin |
| Heat shock | Eosinophil major basic protein |
| Vascular endothelial cell growth factor | Shear stress |
| Platelet factor 4 | Transforming growth factor $\beta$ |
| | Homocysteine |
| | Hypoxia |
| | Neutrophil activation (elastase and oxidation) |
| | Glucose modified proteins |

AMP, adenosine monophosphate.

untranslated region of the TM gene that seem to be responsible for this regulatory behavior (266,267). A cyclic AMP response element responsible for the elevation in TM level is located in the 3' region (264).

Homocysteine is another mediator that downregulates TM expression on the endothelium *in vitro* (269,270). In this case, the impact seems to be on the protein rather than on transcription, since the mRNA levels were elevated slightly in response to homocysteine (270). For a recent review of the homocysteine regulation of the pathway, see reference (271). Hypoxia can also downregulate TM surface expression and mRNA (272). Expression can also be downregulated by glucose-modified albumin (273), possibly linking diabetic thrombotic complications to TM downregulation. TM, but not EPCR, is also downregulated in rat models of diabetes (274).

In rabbit models, when veins, but not arteries, are used to bypass the coronary artery, there is a rapid and profound downregulation of TM expression that appears to be associated with increased thrombosis and leukocyte infiltration (275). Consistent with these findings, Waugh et al. (276,277) have found that overexpression of TM on vessels subjected to deep arterial injury resulted in inhibition of thrombosis, leukocyte infiltration, and reduced neointimal formation.

Atherosclerosis also appears to regulate TM and EPCR expression (278). Both proteins are reduced on the endothelium overlying the lesions. The mechanisms responsible for the downregulation are uncertain, but inflammatory cytokines are likely contributors. Of potential clinical interest, statins have been shown to prevent the TM downregulation at least in cell culture (279,280).

Cultured endothelial cell TM expression is sensitive to shear stress (281). TM mRNA and protein expression dropped to approximately 37% of the control levels after a 36-hour exposure to a laminar sheer stress of 15 dynes per $cm^2$. The cells recover normal mRNA levels within 6 hours after removing the shear stress.

Thrombin effects on TM regulation are somewhat controversial. TM–dependent thrombin internalization has been described (282), and this internalization is blocked by protein C (283). Thrombin and TM internalization and endothelial cell transcytosis have been observed by electron microscopy (284). In contrast, the thrombin–TM complex appeared to be stable in the perfused heart (28) or cultured endothelial cells (285) except when anti-TM antibodies are present (286). Thrombin treatment of endothelial cells can upregulate TM mRNA levels (287–289) through activation of the thrombin receptor (290). This is probably a reflection of protein kinase C activation, because phorbol esters will also increase TM mRNA levels (287,288).

TM can also be downregulated by proteolytic release from the cell surface. The major protease implicated to date is neutrophil elastase (291,292). TNF-$\alpha$ works synergistically to facilitate neutrophil-mediated release of TM from endothelial cells (291). The neutrophils can also cause oxidative damage to TM. There is a methionine in TM that is particularly sensitive to oxidation (293). This oxidation results in severe decreases in TM activity. Particularly interesting in this regard is the observation that the soluble TM degradation products, consisting of the EGF domain repeats, are mitogenic for Swiss 3T3 cells (a fibroblast cell line) (294), suggesting a possible role in wound healing or proliferative responses to inflammatory injury.

Downregulation of TM on cell surfaces may not only limit protein C activation, but can apparently poise the cell for activation by thrombin through the thrombin receptor. As an example, expression of TM on smooth muscle cells, which normally lack TM, leads to a lowered sensitivity of the smooth muscle cells to thrombin by shifting the thrombin dose–response curve to the right (295). The extent of the shift increased with increasing TM expression levels. This observation may be physiologically relevant. Smooth muscle cells have the capacity to synthesize TM, at least in cell culture (296), raising the possibility that TM expression on these cells, in response to trauma, may limit the ability of thrombin to serve as a mitogen. Blocking thrombin binding to TM with a monoclonal antibody increased the mitogenic response of endothelial cells to thrombin (297). On the basis of recent studies by Conway et al. (189), this could be due to the signaling mechanisms initiated by the lectin domain of TM. A similar function for TM appears to occur on endothelial cells. Perhaps TM and the thrombin receptor on endothelium are colocalized, and the TM effect is therefore localized to specific regions of the cell surface.

In contrast to these injury/inflammation–mediated downregulation events, heat shock can induce a sustained elevation in TM mRNA (298). The upregulation is delayed and remains high for a prolonged period after heat shock. Vascular endothelial cell growth factor can also upregulate TM expression and mRNA (approximately twofold) on cultured endothelium (299).

TM is also found on keratinocytes and is upregulated during epidermal development (300). TM is also found at very high levels in the neural crest during embryonic development in the mouse. The protein in the neural crest, which was originally termed fetomodulin (301,302), is subject to upregulation by cyclic AMP and retinoic acid in fetal F9 cells (265). Studies in which a TM gene was replaced (knocked in) with a 2.4-kb reporter gene construct revealed tissue-specific expression within the parietal endoderm (303).

The TM gene has been deleted by homologous recombination. The deletion causes embryonic lethality on day 8.5 (304). This is before the development of a functional cardiovascular system and may imply that TM has functions in addition to its role in the anticoagulant and fibrinolytic processes described previously. Replacement of TM with a mutant form, which has reduced activity, creates a mouse with an organ-specific hypercoagulable state (103). Selective deletion of TM in the developing embryo (as opposed to the placenta) delays, but does not prevent, embryonic death (305). In addition, replacing the normal TM gene with a mutant with much less protein C activation capability results in a viable mouse with a hypercoagulable state (306). Lack of TM in the trophoblast giant cells results in impaired proliferation and increased apoptosis (307).

## The Biochemistry of Protein C Activation by the Thrombin–TM Complex

TM accelerates protein C activation in solution, as well as on membrane surfaces. TM decreases the $K_m$ from approximately 60 to 2 to 6 $\mu$M (127) and increases $k_{cat}$ from approximately 1 mol per minute to 250 mol per minute (127). Several models have been presented to explain this enhancement. Thrombin–TM interaction is mediated, in large part, by anion-binding exosite 1 on thrombin. Sadler et al. were the first to show that point mutations within this region, which bind both fibrinogen and TM, could disrupt fibrinogen clotting or protein C activation by the thrombin–TM complex differentially (10,308). This research led to the concept that thrombin mutants could be generated that are primarily protein C activators with little residual fibrinogen clotting activity. There are Glu residues at positions 192 (309) and 39 (310) in thrombin that appear to make unfavorable interactions with the Asp residues in the P3 and P3′ (311–313) positions of protein C. These unfavorable interactions are largely overcome by TM. Increasing the P3-binding energetics by mutation of Glu217 to Lys in thrombin resulted in considerably enhanced protein C activation rates (312,314) and converted thrombin into an anticoagulant protein.

There is also an Na$^+$ binding site in thrombin (196,315,316). When sodium is bound in this site, it enhances fibrinogen clotting activity approximately eightfold (317,318) and decreases protein C activation rates by the thrombin–TM complex approximately 30% [reviewed in (319)]. Mutation of this site has been utilized to generate thrombin mutants with increased anticoagulant to fibrinogen clotting activity (316). On the basis of detailed kinetic analysis, residues Glu39, Glu192, and Trp60D are among several residues that are linked to the Na$^{2+}$ transition (320), consistent with the earlier mutagenesis studies described previously. From a kinetic analysis of the influence of TM and TM fragments on synthetic substrate specificity, it has been concluded that the TM effect is due to protein C interaction (196). This conclusion is consistent with the observation that mutation of Asp349 to Ala resulted in an altered Ca$^{2+}$ dependence for protein C activation (195). Furthermore, it is possible to mutate protein C to selectively inhibit activation by the thrombin–TM complex (321). Specifically, mutation of Lys37 to 39 to acidic or neutral residues had no influence on the activation rates of protein C by thrombin or the Ca$^{2+}$–dependent inhibition of this process. In contrast, the mutants were activated at least 10-fold slower by the thrombin–TM complex at all Ca$^{2+}$ concentrations tested (321).

It seems highly unlikely, however, that all of the TM influence on protein C activation is mediated by TM interaction with protein C. Many lines of evidence suggest that TM mediates conformational changes in the thrombin. These include changes in fluorescence of covalently attached dyes (131,322,323), selective changes in the electron spin resonance of covalently attached probes (324), and changes in synthetic substrate hydrolysis (131,196,325).

With the covalent fluorescent dyes, differences in the conformational changes in thrombin can be detected between inactive TM fragments (EGF 5 to 6) and active fragments (TM EGF 4 to 6 or 1 to 6) (323). Also consistent with thrombin conformational changes playing a significant role in increased protein C activation, a low-molecular-weight agent has been identified that binds to thrombin and increases protein C activation while reducing fibrinogen clotting activity (326,327). Furthermore, the natural substrate and inhibitor specificity is changed markedly. As described earlier, protein C, thrombin-activatable fibrinolytic inhibitor, prourokinase, and PCI all interact much better with the thrombin–TM complex than with free thrombin. It seems unlikely that TM would make direct protein–protein contacts with such diverse substrates and inhibitors. However, because these are all natural substrates, this possibility cannot be excluded. To gain an insight into molecular rearrangements in the active center of thrombin, the Kunitz inhibitor bovine pancreatic trypsin inhibitor (BPTI) has been employed. BPTI reacts very poorly with thrombin. Reaction is restricted in large part by Trp60D, which sits over the active site pocket (328). When Glu192 in thrombin is mutated to Gln, the thrombin–BPTI complex is tightened (329) sufficiently to allow structural studies of the complex (328). In the complex, Trp60D is shifted approximately 8 Å from its normal position, consistent with previous modeling studies (330). Interestingly, all of the insertion loops in thrombin, even those not contacting BPTI, are displaced significantly in the BPTI-thrombin E192Q crystal. These loops bear many of the residues thought to be involved in TM-mediated effects. If the conformational changes associated with BPTI docking resemble those induced by TM, then TM interaction with thrombin should enhance the on rate of BPTI interaction. Kinetic analysis showed that TM does increase the on rate approximately 10-fold (331). The inactive TM fragment, containing only EGF domains 5 to 6 molecule, did not enhance BPTI interaction (331). These studies suggest that TM does induce considerable conformational changes in thrombin that are, at least partially, responsible for the altered substrate and inhibitor specificity.

Because of the interest in protein C as a potential antithrombotic agent, other approaches have been used to favor protein C activation. In particular, mutation of both the P3 and P3' residues of protein C augment protein C activation (311,332) and can increase the rate of thrombin activation sufficiently to allow protein C to serve as a plasma anticoagulant *in vitro* (333).

## Assembly of the Factor VIIIa and Va Inactivation Complexes

Factor Va and VIIIa are inactivated rapidly on the surface of negatively charged phospholipids (8,39,40,334–340). von Willebrand factor protects factor VIIIa from inactivation (337,341). Factor IXa and factor Xa protect factors VIIIa and Va, respectively, from inactivation by APC, an effect that is largely eliminated by protein S (38,40,342,343). Factor Va inactivation involves cleavage at Arg506 and Arg306 (39,334, 335,343,344). Arg679 is also cleaved by APC, but this does not appear to inactivate factor Va (39). Cleavage of Arg306 is almost totally dependent on phospholipid (336,345). Arg306 cleavage is the only one enhanced by protein S. Protein S interaction with APC moves the active site of APC approximately 10 Å closer to the membrane surface, from 94 to 84 Å (145). This molecular motion is likely to explain the alteration in bond cleavage preference.

APC interaction with its substrates involves binding interactions distal from the active site of APC or the cleavage sites in the substrates. Specifically, APC can interact with the factor Va light chain (346,347) and factor VIIIa light chain (347). After cleavage at Arg306 in factor Va, the A2 domain dissociates, resulting in total loss of activity (336). Cleavage of Arg506 results in partial loss of activity. The amount of inactivation observed is strongly dependent on the factor Xa concentration employed in the assay (39). Inactivation of factor VIIIa can be accomplished by cleavage of either Arg336 or 562 because both sites have to be mutated to yield a resistant form of factor VIIIa (348). Inactivation of factor VIIIa is stimulated significantly by factor V (349,350), but the factor V$_{Leiden}$ (Arg506 replaced with Gln) does not stimulate factor VIIIa inactivation (350). This may account for the original observation that the

APC-resistant phenotype could be corrected by factor V and that assays involving factor VIII are more sensitive to the factor V mutation than those that monitor only factor V inactivation (351,352).

Plasma studies have been performed to explore the proteolytic inactivation of factor V and factor V$_{Leiden}$ by APC (353). In these studies, the factor V$_{Leiden}$ heavy chain of factor Va remained relatively resistant to proteolytic inactivation. The anticoagulant effects of APC in plasma are synergistic with heparin because of selective stimulation of factor V (not factor Va) inactivation (354). Plasma anticoagulant activity of APC and rates of factor Va inactivation are potently stimulated by the presence of phosphatidylethanolamine in the membrane (116). This enhancement is due, in part, to a synergistic increase in membrane-binding affinity that is dependent on phosphatidylethanolamine, protein S, and factor Va (117).

## Species Specificity

APC anticoagulant activity is very species-specific (355–357). Much of this species specificity is due to protein S (357–359). Because of this species specificity, *in vivo* studies with protein C/APC, which are not within the same species, may miss contributions of protein C/APC to anticoagulant or antiinflammatory events.

# OTHER ACTIVITIES OF PROTEIN S

Protein S has been reported to serve as a direct anticoagulant. Binding of protein S to factor Xa (360), factor VIII (361), and factor Va (362) has been described. These binding interactions can inhibit prothrombin activation *in vitro* (34). The C4BP-protein S complex can also inhibit the factor X activation complex (363). *In vivo*, the influence of increasing C4BP levels is to generate a hypercoagulable state that can be corrected by further supplementation with protein S (364,365). The significance of these inhibitory activities, however, is unclear because inhibition or removal of protein S from plasma has little effect on clotting activity or thrombin generation (366). The direct protein S–anticoagulant activity may depend on blood flow. Recently, protein S removal has been shown to increase thrombin generation in flowing plasma (367).

Bovine protein S has also been shown to bind to Tyro3, a protein kinase (368). Subsequent studies showed that human protein S did not interact with the human receptor, but a closely related vitamin K–dependent protein (369), gas6, did (370,371). The significance of these observations is not known at this time.

# SITES OF SYNTHESIS OF THROMBOMODULIN, PROTEIN C, PROTEIN S, AND ENDOTHELIAL CELL PROTEIN C RECEPTOR

TM expression has been observed in (a) mesothelial cells (372); (b) pulmonary andenocarcinoma (373); (c) neutrophils, where it is cryptic and seems to be incapable of accelerating protein C activation (374); (d) synovial fluid cells (375); (e) in the developing neural crest (301); (f) keratinocytes (376,377); (g) mouse brain astrocytes (378); (h) platelets (379); (i) monocytes (380,381); (j) macrophages (381); and (k) syncytiotrophoblasts (382). Of these cells, the skin and endothelium stain most intensely for TM (241). TM is expressed at very low levels in the human brain microcirculation (383) and at low levels in the liver sinusoidal endothelium (241).

Protein S is expressed in liver hepatocytes (384), osteoclasts (385), Leydig cells (386), and endothelial cells (387–389) and is found in platelets (390). It is also expressed in lymphoid cells, primarily T cells, following stimulation with Il-4 (391). Cross-linking protein S on the T cells promotes aggregation and inhibits proliferation (392), suggesting a potential role in the regulation of inflammatory processes. A detailed survey of rabbit tissue indicates that protein S is synthesized in interstitial cells of the ovary, epithelial cells of the epididymis, the endometrium, bronchial epithelial cells, alveolar macrophages, and several cell types within the central nervous system (393).

Protein C is expressed in liver (58,144) and in endothelium (394). The liver is probably the major site of synthesis because protein C levels drop very significantly in liver disease (58).

EPCR is expressed primarily on endothelial cells of large blood vessels (241). It is also expressed at very low levels on monocytes (395).

# THE PROTEIN C PATHWAY IN SEPTIC SHOCK AND STROKE

The protein C pathway appears to be one of the major mechanisms controlling inflammation-initiated coagulation events (396). Part of the mechanism clearly involves the capacity of the pathway to regulate thrombin production and hence to dampen the ability of thrombin to initiate inflammatory functions such as leukocyte adhesion and activation (134). A large body of *in vivo* studies, and some *in vitro* studies, have suggested that the pathway serves antiinflammatory functions in addition to inhibition of thrombin formation (397). APC alters gene expression profiles in cultured human endothelial cells (398). The net effect was antiapoptotic and antiinflammatory. Some of this signaling appears to be mediated by APC bound to EPCR-cleaving protease activated receptors, particularly protease activated receptor 1 (PAR-1) (399). The physiologic importance of these observations is illustrated by the finding that APC infusion can block p53-mediated apoptosis in endothelium and is also neuroprotective in mouse models (400–402). This may be particularly important because this pathway appears to be impaired in infection-associated strokes (403). The combination of antiinflammatory, anticoagulant, and antiapoptotic activities of APC appears to contribute to the effectiveness in treating both experimental models of sepsis (404) and severe sepsis in humans (405). In patients with severe sepsis, APC infusion decreased the relative risk of death 19.4%, with the greatest impact in patients who are most severely ill (405).

One common hypothesis is that the anticoagulant activity of APC is its primary physiologic protective function in severe sepsis. Both experiments in mice and analysis of the APC treated patients with severe sepsis argue against this proposal. Mice heterozygous for the factor $V_{Leiden}$ mutation (APC resistant) actually have a better survival profile than wild-type mice (406). Furthermore, patients with severe sepsis and factor $V_{Leiden}$ exhibited a benefit from APC treatment comparable to that of patients without factor $V_{Leiden}$ (406).

One of the first indications that the protein C system might be involved in preventing endotoxin-mediated shock came from studies in which thrombin was infused before a challenge with $LD_{100}$ levels of *Escherichia coli*. All thrombin-treated animals survived (99). This result was surprising because thrombin causes the disseminated intravascular coagulation that probably contributes to the vascular injury and organ failure. Thrombin infusion had previously been shown to lead to formation of a net anticoagulant response (407) due to the formation of APC (408), making APC a candidate for the protective effects mediated by thrombin. Subsequently, APC was shown to block the septic response initiated by *E. coli* in primates (409) and rats (410). Blocking the protein C anticoagulant pathway, either by inhibiting protein C activation or by blocking protein S function with C4BP, exacerbated the response to a Gram-negative bacterial challenge, converting the response from sublethal to lethal (365,409).

The lung is a major organ impacted in septic shock. Recent studies have shown that APC has protective effects on models of lung injury (411,412). The protection involves, among other things, reducing TGF-$\beta$ levels. Protection is also EPCR dependent. APC can be instilled into the lung to achieve protection.

Inhibition of the protein C pathway increases neutrophil activation in response to low-level endotoxin challenge, suggesting that the pathway plays a role in modulating neutrophil activation and probably diminishes adherence that would lead to loss of microvascular integrity (413). In addition to facilitating the coagulation response, inhibition of the protein C pathway increased inflammatory cytokine levels (TNF-$\alpha$ in particular). In rats, APC dampens the TNF-$\alpha$ response to endotoxin (410) and can block TNF-$\alpha$ formation in tissues following compression-induced spinal cord injury (414). This may be due to a direct effect of APC on monocytes because the enzyme and protein S functioned synergistically to block endotoxin-induced cytokine production by more than 90% (410). APC did not block production of reactive oxygen intermediates, upregulation of MHC class II, ICAM-1 or IL-2 receptor, or downregulation of CD59, suggesting that adhesion, phagocytosis, and bacteria-killing activities remain intact (415).

Monocytes appear to have specific binding sites for APC (416) that are functionally and structurally distinct from EPCR (417). The engagement of APC receptors on monocytes has been reported to block the ability of agonists such as interferon $\gamma$ (IFN $\gamma$) to elevate intracellular $Ca^{2+}$ levels (416). This receptor remains to be characterized biochemically; the exact mechanisms of its antiinflammatory activity therefore remain unknown. Monocytes can synthesize TM (380,381, 418), but unlike endothelial cells, endotoxin enhances TM expression. Therefore, at inflammatory sites involved in organ rejection, TM levels are low to absent on the endothelium but readily apparent on the intragraft macrophages (419). This may provide a mechanism for generating APC to perform the antiinflammatory functions even when TM has been downregulated on endothelium.

In severe sepsis, the protein C activation mechanisms can be downregulated (420). The inhibition of protein C activation appears to vary quite widely among patients (421). Whether the extent of downregulation is predictive of patient survival remains to be determined.

# SUMMARY

This chapter outlines some of the key areas in this rapidly emerging protein C anticoagulant pathway. This is a very powerful pathway and one in which there are many unresolved issues. In the near future, one can anticipate an ever-increasing level of sophistication in our understanding of the biochemical, cellular, and genetic regulation of this system.

# ACKNOWLEDGMENTS

I would like to thank Dr. Naomi Esmon for her helpful editorial comments and Nici Kobzdej for final preparation of the manuscript. Dr. Charles Esmon is an investigator for the Howard Hughes Medical Institute.

# References

1. Castellino FJ. Human protein C and activated protein C. *Trends Cardiovasc Med* 1995;5:55–62.
2. Dahlbäck B. Protein S and C4b-binding protein: components involved in the regulation of the protein C anticoagulant system. *Thromb Haemost* 1991;66:49–61.
3. Davie EW, Fujikawa K, Kisiel W. The coagulation cascade: initiation, maintenance and regulation. *Biochemistry* 1991;30:10363–10370.
4. Esmon CT. The roles of protein C and thrombomodulin in the regulation of blood coagulation. *J Biol Chem* 1989;264:4743–4746.
5. Esmon CT. Thrombomodulin as a model of molecular mechanisms that modulate protease specificity and function at the vessel surface. *FASEB J* 1995;9:946–955.
6. Stenflo J. Structure-function relationships of epidermal growth factor modules in vitamin K-dependent clotting factors. *Blood* 1991;78:1637–1651.
7. Preissner KT. Biological relevance of the protein C system and laboratory diagnosis of protein C and protein S deficiencies. *Clin Sci* 1990;78:351–364.
8. Walker FJ, Fay PJ. Regulation of blood coagulation by the protein C system. *FASEB J* 1992;6:2561–2567.
9. Bourin MC, Lindahl U. Glycosaminoglycans and the regulation of blood coagulation. *Biochem J* 1993;289:313–330.
10. Sadler JE, Lentz SR, Sheehan JP, et al. Structure-function relationships of the thrombin-thrombomodulin interaction. *Haemostasis* 1993;23:183–193.
11. Aiach M, Borgel D, Gaussem P, et al. Protein C and protein S deficiencies. *Semin Hematol* 1997;34:205–217.
12. Alving BM, Comp PC. Recent advances in understanding clotting and evaluating patients with recurrent thrombosis. *Am J Obstet Gynecol* 1992;167:1184–1191.
13. Esmon CT, Schwarz HP. An update on clinical and basic aspects of the protein C anticoagulant pathway. *Trends Cardiovasc Med* 1995;5:141–148.
14. Florell SR, Rodgers GM. Inherited thrombotic disorders: an update. *Am J Hematol* 1997;54:53–60.
15. Gladson CL, Groncy P, Griffin JH. Coumarin necrosis, neonatal purpura fulminans, and protein C deficiency. *Arch Dermatol* 1987;123:1701a–1706a.
16. Lane DA, Mannucci PM, Bauer KA, et al. Inherited thrombophilia: part 2. *Thromb Haemost* 1996;76:824–834.
17. Marlar RA, Neumann A. Neonatal purpura fulminans due to homozygous protein C or protein S deficiencies. *Semin Thromb Hemost* 1990;16:299–309.
18. Reitsma PH, Poort SR, Bernardi F, et al. Protein C deficiency: a database of mutations. For the protein C & S subcommittee of the scientific and standardization committee of the International Society on Thrombosis and Haemostasis. *Thromb Haemost* 1993;69:77–84.
19. Reitsma PH, Bernardi F, Doig RG, et al. Protein C deficiency: a database of mutations, 1995 update. *Thromb Haemost* 1995;73(5):876–879.
20. Lane DA, Mannucci PM, Bauer KA, et al. Inherited thrombophilia: part 1. *Thromb Haemost* 1996;76:651–662.
21. Gandrille S, Borgel D, Ireland H, et al. Protein S deficiency: a database of mutations. For the plasma coagulation inhibitors subcommittee of the scientific and standardization committee of the International Society on Thrombosis and Haemostasis. *Thromb Haemost* 1997;77:1201–1214.
22. Bertina RM. Factor V Leiden and other coagulation factor mutations affecting thrombotic risk. *Clin Chem* 1997;43:1678–1683.
23. Dahlbäck B. Physiological anticoagulation. Resistance to activated protein C and venous thromboembolism. *J Clin Invest* 1994;94:923–927.
24. Pabinger I, Brucker S, Kyrle PA, et al. Hereditary deficiency of antithrombin III, protein C and protein S: prevalence in patients with a history of venous thrombosis and criteria for rational patient screening. *Blood Coagul Fibrinolysis* 1992;3:547–553.
25. Kemkes-Matthes B. Acquired protein S deficiency. *Clin Investig* 1992;70:529–534.
26. Hofsteenge J, Taguchi H, Stone SR. Effect of thrombomodulin on the kinetics of the interaction of thrombin with substrates and inhibitors. *Biochem J* 1986;237:243–251.
27. Parkinson JF, Garcia JGN, Bang NU. Decreased thrombin affinity of cell-surface thrombomodulin following treatment of cultured endothelial cells with β-D-xyloside. *Biochem Biophys Res Commun* 1990;169:177–183.
28. Esmon CT, Owen WG. Identification of an endothelial cell cofactor for thrombin-catalyzed activation of protein C. *Proc Natl Acad Sci U S A* 1981;78:2249–2252.
29. Fukudome K, Esmon CT. Identification, cloning and regulation of a novel endothelial cell protein C/activated protein C receptor. *J Biol Chem* 1994;269:26486–26491.
30. Stearns-Kurosawa DJ, Kurosawa S, Mollica JS, et al. The endothelial cell protein C receptor augments protein C activation by the thrombin-thrombomodulin complex. *Proc Natl Acad Sci U S A* 1996;93:10212–10216.
31. Taylor FB Jr, Peer GT, Lockhart MS, et al. EPCR plays an important role in protein C activation *in vivo. Blood* 2001;97:1685–1688.
32. Regan LM, Stearns-Kurosawa DJ, Kurosawa S, et al. The endothelial cell protein C receptor: inhibition of activated protein C anticoagulant function without modulation of reaction with proteinase inhibitors. *J Biol Chem* 1996;271:17499–17503.
33. Stern DM, Nawroth PP, Harris K, et al. Cultured bovine aortic endothelial cells promote activated protein C-protein S-mediated inactivation of factor Va. *J Biol Chem* 1986;261:713–718.

34. Hackeng TM, Hessing M, van't Veer C, et al. Protein S binding to human endothelial cells is required for expression of cofactor activity for activated protein C. *J Biol Chem* 1993;268:3993–4000.
35. Tans G, Rosing J, Thomassen MCLGD, et al. Comparison of anticoagulant and procoagulant activities of stimulated platelets and platelet-derived microparticles. *Blood* 1991;77:2641–2648.
36. Harris KW, Esmon CT. Protein S is required for bovine platelets to support activated protein C binding and activity. *J Biol Chem* 1985;260:2007–2010.
37. Dahlbäck B, Wiedmer T, Sims PJ. Binding of anticoagulant vitamin K-dependent protein S to platelet-derived microparticles. *Biochemistry* 1992;31:12769–12777.
38. Solymoss S, Tucker MM, Tracy PB. Kinetics of inactivation of membrane-bound factor Va by activated protein C. *J Biol Chem* 1988;263:14884–14890.
39. Egan JO, Kalafatis M, Mann KG. The effect of Arg306 ≥ Ala and Arg506 ≥ Gln substitutions in the inactivation of recombinant human factor Va by activated protein C and protein S. *Protein Sci* 1997;6:2016–2027.
40. Regan LM, Lamphear BJ, Huggins CF, et al. Factor IXa protects factor VIIIa from activated protein C. *J Biol Chem* 1994;269:9445–9452.
41. Walker FJ, Sexton PW, Esmon CT. Inhibition of blood coagulation by activated protein C through selective inactivation of activated factor V. *Biochim Biophys Acta* 1979;571:333–342.
42. Vehar GA, Davie EW. Preparation and properties of bovine factor VIII (antihemophilic factor). *Biochemistry* 1980;19:401–410.
43. Canfield WM, Kisiel W. Evidence of normal functional levels of activated protein C inhibitor in combined factor V/VIII deficiency disease. *J Clin Invest* 1982;70:1260–1272.
44. Nichols WC, Seligsohn U, Zivelin A, et al. Mutations in the ER-Golgi intermediate compartment protein ERGIC-53 cause combined deficiency of coagulation factors V and VIII. *Cell* 1998;93:61–70.
45. Rezaie AR, Cooper ST, Church FC, et al. Protein C inhibitor is a potent inhibitor of the thrombin-thrombomodulin complex. *J Biol Chem* 1995;270:25336–25339.
46. Elisen MGLM, Borne PAK, Bouma BN, et al. Protein C inhibitor acts as a procoagulant by inhibiting the thrombomodulin-induced activation of protein C in human plasma. *Blood* 1998;91:1542–1547.
47. Bourin M-C, Öhlin A-K, Lane DA, et al. Relationship between anticoagulant activities and polyanionic properties of rabbit thrombomodulin. *J Biol Chem* 1988;263:8044–8052.
48. Heeb MJ, Mosher D, Griffin JH. Activation and complexation of protein C and cleavage and decrease of protein S in plasma of patients with intravascular coagulation. *Blood* 1989;73:455–461.
49. Scully MF, Toh CH, Hoogendoorn H, et al. Activation of protein C and its distribution between its inhibitors, protein C inhibitor, α1−antitrypsin and α2−macroglobulin, in patients with disseminated intravascular coagulation. *Thromb Haemost* 1993;69:448–453.
50. España F, Griffin JH. Determination of functional and antigenic protein C inhibitor and its complexes with activated protein C in plasma by ELISA's. *Thromb Res* 1989;55:671–682.
51. España F, Gilabert J, Aznar J, et al. Complexes of activated protein C with α1-antitrypsin in normal pregnancy and in severe preeclampsia. *Am J Obstet Gynecol* 1991;164:1310–1316.
52. España F, Gruber A, Heeb MJ, et al. *In vivo* and *in vitro* complexes of activated protein C with two inhibitors in baboons. *Blood* 1991;77:1754–1760.
53. Heeb MJ, España F, Geiger M, et al. Immunological identity of heparin-dependent plasma and urinary protein C inhibitor and plasminogen activator inhibitor-3. *J Biol Chem* 1987;262:15813–15816.
54. Heeb MJ, España F. Physiologic inhibition of human activated protein C by alpha-1-antitrypsin. *J Biol Chem* 1988;263:11613–11616.
55. Heeb MJ, España F, Griffin JH. Inhibition and complexation of activated protein C by two major inhibitors in plasma. *Blood* 1989;73:446–454.
56. Heeb MJ, Gruber A, Griffin JH. Identification of divalent metal ion-dependent inhibition of activated protein C by alpha2-macroglobulin and alpha2-antiplasmin in blood and comparisons to inhibition of factor Xa, thrombin, and plasmin. *J Biol Chem* 1991;266:17606–17612.
57. Okajima K, Koga S, Kaji M, et al. Effect of protein C and activated protein C on coagulation and fibrinolysis in normal human subjects. *Thromb Haemost* 1990;63:48–53.
58. D'Angelo SV, Comp PC, Esmon CT, et al. Relationship between protein C antigen and anticoagulant activity during oral anticoagulation and in selected disease states. *J Clin Invest* 1986;77:416–425.
59. Dreyfus M, Masterson M, David M, et al. Replacement therapy with a monoclonal antibody purified protein C concentrate in newborns with severe congenital protein C deficiency. *Semin Thromb Hemost* 1995;21:371–381.
60. Bajzar L, Manuel R, Nesheim ME. Purification and characterization of TAFI, a thrombin-activable fibrinolysis inhibitor. *J Biol Chem* 1995;270:14477–14484.
61. Bajzar L, Morser J, Nesheim M. TAFI, or plasma procarboxypeptidase B, couples the coagulation and fibrinolytic cascades through the thrombin-thrombomodulin complex. *J Biol Chem* 1996;271:16603–16608.
62. Bajzar L, Nesheim M. The effect of activated protein C on fibrinolysis in cell-free plasma can be attributed specifically to attenuation of prothrombin activation. *J Biol Chem* 1993;268:8608–8616.

63. de Munk GAW, Groeneveld E, Rijken DC. Acceleration of the thrombin inactivation of single chain urokinase-type plasminogen activator (pro-urokinase) by thrombomodulin. *J Clin Invest* 1991;88:1680–1684.

64. Molinari A, Giogetti C, Lansen J, et al. Thrombomodulin is a cofactor for thrombin degradation of recombinant single-chain urokinase plasminogen activator *in vitro* and in a perfused rabbit heart model. *Thromb Haemost* 1992;67:226–232.

65. Gomi K, Zushi M, Honda G, et al. Antithrombotic effect of recombinant human thrombomodulin on thrombin-induced thromboembolism in mice. *Blood* 1990;75:1396–1399.

66. Uchiba M, Okajima K, Murakami K, et al. Recombinant human soluble thrombomodulin reduces endotoxin-induced pulmonary vascular injury via protein C activation in rats. *Thromb Haemost* 1995;74:1265–1270.

67. Mohri M, Oka M, Aoki Y, et al. Intravenous extended infusion of recombinant human soluble thrombomodulin prevented tissue factor-induced disseminated intravascular coagulation in rats. *Am J Hematol* 1994;45:298–303.

68. Ono M, Nawa K, Marumoto Y. Antithrombotic effects of recombinant human soluble thrombomodulin in a rat model of vascular shunt thrombosis. *Thromb Haemost* 1994;72:421–425.

69. Gonda Y, Hirata S, Saitoh K-I, et al. Antithrombotic effect of recombinant human soluble thrombomodulin on endotoxin-induced disseminated intravascular coagulation in rats. *Thromb Res* 1993;71:325–335.

70. Aoki Y, Takei R, Mohri M, et al. Antithrombotic effects of recombinant human soluble thrombomodulin (rhs-TM) on arteriovenous shunt thrombosis in rats. *Am J Hematol* 1994;47:162–166.

71. Solis MM, Vitti M, Cook J, et al. Recombinant soluble human thrombomodulin: a randomized, blinded assessment of prevention of venous thrombosis and effects on hemostatic parameters in a rat model. *Thromb Res* 1994;73:385–394.

72. Hasegawa N, Kandra TG, Husari AW, et al. The effects of recombinant human thrombomodulin on endotoxin-induced multiple-system organ failure in rats. *Am J Respir Crit Care Med* 1996;153:1831–1837.

73. Uchiba M, Okajima K, Murakami K, et al. Recombinant thrombomodulin prevents endotoxin-induced lung injury in rats by inhibiting leukocyte activation. *Am J Physiol* 1996;271:L470–L475.

74. Uchiba M, Okajima K, Murakami K, et al. rhs-TM prevents ET-induced increase in pulmonary vascular permeability through protein C activation. *Am J Physiol* 1997;273:L889–L894.

75. Myles T, Nishimura T, Yun TH, et al. Thrombin activatable fibrinolysis inhibitor: a potential regulator of vascular inflammation. *J Biol Chem* 2003;278:51059–51067.

76. Campbell WD, Lazoura E, Okada N, et al. Inactivation of C3a and C5a octapeptides by carboxypeptidase R and carboxypeptidase N. *Microbiol Immunol* 2002;46:131–134.

77. Mammen EF, Thomas WR, Seegers WH. Activation of purified prothrombin to autoprothrombin I or autoprothrombin II (platelet cofactor II) or autoprothrombin II-A. *Thromb Diath Haemorrh* 1960;5:218–250.

78. Seegers WH. Protein C and autoprothrombin II-A. *Semin Thromb Hemost* 1981;7:257–262.

79. Stenflo J. A new vitamin K-dependent protein: purification from bovine plasma and preliminary characterization. *J Biol Chem* 1976;251:355–363.

80. Esmon CT, Stenflo J, Suttie JW, et al. A new vitamin K dependent protein: a phospholipid binding zymogen of a serine esterase. *J Biol Chem* 1976;251:2770–2776.

81. Kisiel W. Human plasma protein C: isolation, characterization and mechanism of activation by α-thrombin. *J Clin Invest* 1979;64:761–769.

82. Kisiel W, Canfield WM, Ericsson LH, et al. Anticoagulant properties of bovine plasma protein C following activation by thrombin. *Biochemistry* 1977;16:5824–5831.

83. DiScipio RG, Davie EW. Characterization of protein S, a gamma-carboxyglutamic acid containing protein from bovine and human plasma. *Biochemistry* 1979;18:899–904.

84. Walker FJ. Regulation of activated protein C by a new protein: a role for bovine protein S. *J Biol Chem* 1980;255:5521–5524.

85. Amphlett GW, Kisiel W, Castellino FJ. Interaction of calcium with bovine plasma protein C. *Biochemistry* 1981;20:2156–2161.

86. Esmon CT, Owen WG. The discovery of thrombomodulin. *J Thromb Haemost* 2004;2:209–213.

87. Kisiel W, Ericsson LH, Davie EW. Proteolytic activation of protein C from bovine plasma. *Biochemistry* 1976;15:4893–4900.

88. Busch C, Cancilla P, DeBault L, et al. Use of endothelium cultured on microcarriers as a model for the microcirculation. *Lab Invest* 1982;47:498–504.

89. Owen WG, Esmon CT. Functional properties of an endothelial cell cofactor for thrombin-catalyzed activation of protein C. *J Biol Chem* 1981;256:5532–5535.

90. Esmon NL, Owen WG, Esmon CT. Isolation of a membrane-bound cofactor for thrombin-catalyzed activation of protein C. *J Biol Chem* 1982;257:859–864.

91. Esmon CT, Esmon NL, Saugstad J. Activation of protein C by a complex between thrombin and an endothelial cell surface protein. In: Nossel HL, Vogel HJ, eds. *Pathobiology of the endothelial cell.* New York: Academic Press, 1982:121–136.

92. Jakubowski HV, Kline MD, Owen WG. The effect of bovine thrombomodulin on the specificity of bovine thrombin. *J Biol Chem* 1986;261:3876–3882.

93. Salem HH, Maruyama I, Ishii H, et al. Isolation and characterization of thrombomodulin from human placenta. *J Biol Chem* 1984;259:12246–12251.

94. Esmon NL, Esmon CT. Protein C and the endothelium. *Semin Thromb Hemost* 1988;14:210–215.

95. Bangalore N, Drohan WN, Orthner CL. High affinity binding sites for activated protein C and protein C on cultured human umbilical vein endothelial cells independent of protein S and distinct from known ligands. *Thromb Haemost* 1994;72(3):465–474.

96. Fukudome K, Kurosawa S, Stearns-Kurosawa DJ, et al. The endothelial cell protein C receptor: cell surface expression and direct ligand binding by the soluble receptor. *J Biol Chem* 1996;271:17491–17498.

97. Furie B, Furie BC. The molecular basis of blood coagulation. *Cell* 1988;53:505–518.

98. Grinnell BW, Walls JD, Gerlitz B, et al. Native and modified recombinant human protein C: function, secretion, and posttranslational modifications. In: Bruley DF, Drohan WN, eds. *Protein C and related anticoagulants, Advances in applied biotechnology series.* Vol. 11. Houston, TX: Gulf Publishing Co, 1991:29–63.

99. Taylor FB Jr, Chang A, Hinshaw LB, et al. A model for thrombin protection against endotoxin. *Thromb Res* 1984;36:177–185.

100. Comp PC. Hereditary disorders predisposing to thrombosis. *Prog Hemost Thromb* 1986;8:71–102.

101. Plutzky J, Hoskins J, Long GL, et al. Evolution and organization of the human protein C gene. *Proc Natl Acad Sci U S A* 1986;83:546–550.

102. Miletich JP, Broze GJ Jr. β Protein C is not glycosylated at asparagine 329: the rate of translation may influence the frequency of usage at asparagine-X-cysteine sites. *J Biol Chem* 1990;265:11397–11404.

103. Weiler-Guettler H, Christie PD, Beeler DL, et al. A targeted point mutation in thrombomodulin generates viable mice with a prethrombotic state. *J Clin Invest* 1998;101:1983–1991.

104. Öhlin A-K, Stenflo J. Calcium-dependent interaction between the EGF region of human protein C and a monoclonal antibody. *J Biol Chem* 1987;262:13798–13804.

105. Öhlin A-K, Linse S, Stenflo J. Calcium binding to the epidermal growth factor homology region of bovine protein C. *J Biol Chem* 1988;263:7411–7417.

106. Rezaie AR, Mather T, Sussman F, et al. Mutation of Glu 80 [to] Lys results in a protein C mutant that no longer requires $Ca^{2+}$ for rapid activation by the thrombin-thrombomodulin complex. *J Biol Chem* 1994;269:3151–3154.

107. Regan LM, Mollica JS, Rezaie AR, et al. The interaction between the endothelial cell protein C receptor and protein C is dictated by the Gla domain of protein C. *J Biol Chem* 1997;272:26279–26284.

108. Christiansen WT, Tulinsky A, Castellino FJ. Functions of individual gamma-carboxyglutamic acid (Gla) residues of human protein C. Determination of functionally nonessential Gla residues and correlations with their mode of binding of calcium. *Biochemistry* 1994;33:14993–15000.

109. Colpitts TL, Prorok M, Castellino FJ. Binding of calcium to individual gamma-carboxyglutamic acid residues of human protein C. *Biochemistry* 1995;34:2424–2430.

110. Jhingan A, Zhang L, Christiansen WT, et al. The activities of recombinant gamma-carboxyglutamic-acid-deficient mutants of activated human protein C toward human coagulation factor Va and factor VIII in purified systems and in plasma. *Biochemistry* 1994;33:1869–1875.

111. Zhang L, Jhingan A, Castellino FJ. Role of individual gamma-carboxyglutamic acid residues of activated human protein C in defining its *in vitro* anticoagulant activity. *Blood* 1992;80:942–952.

112. Zhang L, Castellino FJ. The binding energy of human coagulation protein C to acidic phospholipid vesicles contains a major contribution from leucine 5 in the gamma-carboxyglutamic acid domain. *J Biol Chem* 1994;269:3590–3595.

113. Thariath A, Castellino FJ. Highly conserved residue arginine-15 is required for the Ca2+-dependent properties of the gamma-carboxyglutamic acid domain of human anticoagulation protein C and activated protein C. *Biochem J* 1997;322:309–315.

114. Shen L, Shah AM, Dahlbäck B, et al. Enhancing the activity of protein C by mutagenesis to improve the membrane-binding site: studies related to proline-10. *Biochemistry* 1997;36:16025–16031.

115. Castellino FJ, Geng J-P. Expression of human anticoagulation protein C and gamma-carboxyglutamic acid mutants in mammalian cell cultures. *Methods Enzymol* 1997;282:369–385.

116. Smirnov MD, Esmon CT. Phosphatidylethanolamine incorporation into vesicles selectively enhances factor Va inactivation by activated protein C. *J Biol Chem* 1994;269:816–819.

117. Smirnov MD, Safa O, Regan L, et al. A chimeric protein C containing the prothrombin Gla domain exhibits increased anticoagulant activity and altered phospholipid specificity. *J Biol Chem* 1998;273:9031–9040.

118. Horie S, Ishii H, Hara H, et al. Enhancement of thrombin-thrombomodulin-catalysed protein C activation by phosphatidylethanolamine containing unsaturated fatty acids: possible physiological significance of phosphatidylethanolamine in anticoagulant activity of thrombomodulin. *Biochem J* 1994;301:683–691.

119. Deguchi H, Fernández JA, Pabinger I, et al. Plasma glucosylceramide deficiency as potential risk factor for venous thrombosis and modulator of anticoagulatn protein C pathway. *Blood* 2001;97:1907–1914.

120. Sunnerhagen M, Forsén S, Hoffrén A-M, et al. Structure of the Ca²⁺-free GLA domain sheds light on membrane binding of blood coagulation proteins. Nat Struct Biol 1995;2:504–509.
121. Öhlin A-K, Bjork I, Stenflo J. Proteolytic formation and properties of a fragment of protein C containing the gamma-carboxyglutamic acid rich domain and the EGF-like region. Biochemistry 1990;29:644–651.
122. Rezaie AR, Esmon NL, Esmon CT. The high affinity calcium-binding site involved in protein C activation is outside the first epidermal growth factor homology domain. J Biol Chem 1992;267:11701–11704.
123. Drakenberg T, Fernlund P, Roepstorff P, et al. Beta-hydroxyaspartic acid in vitamin K-dependent protein C. Proc Natl Acad Sci U S A 1983;80:1802–1806.
124. Öhlin A-K, Landes G, Bourdon P, et al. Beta-hydroxyaspartic acid in the first epidermal growth factor–like domain of protein C: its role in Ca²⁺ binding and biological activity. J Biol Chem 1988;263:19240–19248.
125. Cheng C-H, Geng J-P, Castellino FJ. The functions of the first epidermal growth factor homology region of human protein C as revealed by a charge-to-alanine scanning mutagenesis investigation. Biol Chem 1997;378:1491–1500.
126. Colpitts TL, Castellino FJ. Calcium and phospholipid binding properties of synthetic gamma-carboxyglutamic acid-containing peptides with sequence counterparts in human protein C. Biochemistry 1994;33:3501–3508.
127. Esmon NL, DeBault LE, Esmon CT. Proteolytic formation and properties of gamma-carboxyglutamic acid-domainless protein C. J Biol Chem 1983;258:5548–5553.
128. Mather T, Oganessyan V, Hof P, et al. The 2.8 Å crystal structure of Gla-domainless activated protein C. EMBO J 1996;15:6822–6831.
129. Fisher CL, Greengard JS, Griffin JH. Models of the serine protease domain of the human antithrombotic plasma factor activated protein C and its zymogen. Protein Sci 1994;3:588–599.
130. Rezaie AR, Yang L. Thrombomodulin allosterically modulates the activity of the anticoagulant thrombin. Proc Natl Acad Sci U S A 2003;100:12051–12056.
131. Ye J, Liu L-W, Esmon CT, et al. The fifth and sixth growth factor–like domains of thrombomodulin bind to the anion exosite of thrombin and alter its specificity. J Biol Chem 1992;267:11023–11028.
132. Mathews II, Padmanabhan KP, Tulinsky A, et al. Structure of a nonadecapeptide of the fifth EGF domain of thrombomodulin complexed with thrombin. Biochemistry 1994;33:13547–13552.
133. Mathews II, Padmanabhan KP, Ganesh V, et al. Crystallographic structures of thrombin complexed with thrombin receptor peptides: existence of expected and novel binding modes. Biochemistry 1994;33:3266–3279.
134. Coughlin SR. Thrombin receptor function and cardiovascular disease. Trends Cardiovasc Med 1994;4:77–83.
135. Liu L-W, Vu T-KH, Esmon CT, et al. The region of the thrombin receptor resembling hirudin binds to thrombin and alters enzyme specificity. J Biol Chem 1991;266:16977–16980.
136. Vu T-KH, Wheaton VI, Hung DT, et al. Domains specifying thrombin-receptor interaction. Nature 1991;353:674–677.
137. Vu T-KH, Hung DT, Wheaton VI, et al. Molecular cloning of a functional thrombin receptor reveals a novel proteolytic mechanism of receptor activation. Cell 1991;64:1057–1068.
138. Stubbs MT, Oschkinat H, Mayr I, et al. The interaction of thrombin with fibrinogen. A structural basis for its specificity. Eur J Biochem 1992;206:187–195.
139. Martin P, Robertson W, Turk D, et al. The structure of residues 7-16 of the A-alpha-chain of human fibrinogen bound to bovine thrombin at 2.3-Å resolution. J Biol Chem 1992;267:7911–7920.
140. Naski MC, Fenton JW II, Maraganore JM, et al. The COOH-terminal domain of hirudin: an exosite-directed competitive inhibitor of the action of alpha-thrombin on fibrinogen. J Biol Chem 1990;265:13484–13489.
141. Esmon CT, Lollar P. Involvement of thrombin anion-binding exosites 1 and 2 in the activation of factor V and factor VIII. J Biol Chem 1996;271:13882–13887.
142. Kane WH, Davie EW. Blood coagulation factors V and VIII: structural and functional similarities and their relationship to hemorrhagic and thrombotic disorders. Blood 1988;71:539–555.
143. Beckmann RJ, Schmidt RJ, Santerre RF, et al. The structure and evolution of a 461 amino acid human protein C precursor and its messenger RNA, based upon the DNA sequence of cloned human liver cDNAs. Nucleic Acids Res 1985;13:5233–5247.
144. Foster DC, Davie EW. Characterization of a cDNA coding for human protein C. Proc Natl Acad Sci U S A 1984;81:4766–4770.
145. Yegneswaran S, Wood GM, Esmon CT, et al. Protein S alters the active site location of activated protein C above the membrane surface. J Biol Chem 1997;272:25013–25021.
146. Le Tonqueze M, Dueymes M, Giovangrandi Y, et al. The relationship of anti-endothelial cell antibodies to anti-phospholipid antibodies in patients with giant cell arteritis and/or polymyalgia rheumatica. Autoimmunity 1995;20:59–66.
147. Grinnell BW, Walls JD, Gerlitz B. Glycosylation of human protein C affects its secretion, processing, functional activities, and activation by thrombin. J Biol Chem 1991;226:9778–9785.
148. Yan SB, Chao YB, van Halbeek H. Novel Asn-linked oligosaccharides terminating in GalNAcβ(1 to 4)[Fucα(1 to 3)]GlcNAcβ(1 to·) are present in recombinant human protein C expressed in human kidney 293 cells. Glycobiology 1993;3:597–608.
149. Grinnell BW, Hermann RB, Yan SB. Human protein C inhibits selectin-mediated cell adhesion: role of unique fucosylated oligosaccharide. Glycobiology 1994;4:221–226.
150. Edenbrandt C-M, Lundwall A, Wydro R, et al. Molecular analysis of the gene for vitamin K-dependent protein S and its pseudogene. Cloning and partial gene organization. Biochemistry 1990;29:7861–7868.
151. Lundwall A, Dackowski W, Cohen E, et al. Isolation and sequence of the cDNA for human protein S, a regulator of blood coagulation. Proc Natl Acad Sci U S A 1986;83:6716–6720.
152. Schmidel DK, Tatro AV, Phelps LG, et al. Organization of the human protein S genes. Biochemistry 1990;29:7845–7852.
153. Joseph DR, Baker ME. Sex hormone-binding globulin, androgen-binding protein, and vitamin K-dependent protein S are homologous to laminin A, merosin, and drosophila crumbs protein. FASEB J 1992;6:2477–2481.
154. Gershagen S, Fernlund P, Edenbrandt C-M. The genes for SHBG/ABP and the SHBG-like region of vitamin K- dependent protein S have evolved from a common ancestral gene. J Steroid Biochem Mol Biol 1991;40:763–769.
155. Chang GTG, Aaldering L, Hackeng TM, et al. Construction and characterization of thrombin-resistant variants of recombinant human protein S. Thromb Haemost 1994;72(5):693–697.
156. Dahlbäck B. Purification of human vitamin K-dependent protein S and its limited proteolysis by thrombin. Biochem J 1983;209:837–846.
157. Walker FJ. Regulation of vitamin K-dependent protein S. Inactivation by thrombin. J Biol Chem 1984;259:10335–10339.
158. Suzuki K, Nishioka J, Hashimoto S. Regulation of activated protein C by thrombin-modified protein S. J Biochem (Tokyo) 1983;94:699–705.
159. Sugo T, Dahlbäck B, Holmgren A, et al. Calcium binding of bovine protein S. Effect of thrombin cleavage and removal of the gamma-carboxyglutamic acid-containing region. J Biol Chem 1986;261:5116–5120.
160. Mitchell CA, Salem HH. Cleavage of protein S by a platelet membrane protease. J Clin Invest 1987;79:374–379.
161. Oates AM, Salem HH. The binding and regulation of protein S by neutrophils. Blood Coagul Fibrinolysis 1991;2:601–607.
162. Stenflo J, Lundwall A, Dahlbäck B. β-Hydroxyasparagine in domains homologous to the epidermal growth factor precursor in vitamin K-dependent protein S. Proc Natl Acad Sci U S A 1987;84:368–372.
163. Stenberg Y, Linse S, Drakenberg T, et al. The high affinity calcium-binding sites in the epidermal growth factor module region of vitamin K-dependent protein S. J Biol Chem 1997;272:23255–23260.
164. Stenberg Y, Drakenberg T, Dahlbäck B, et al. Characterization of recombinant epidermal growth factor (EGF)-like modules from vitamin K-dependent protein S expressed in Spodoptera cells. The cofactor activity depends on the N-terminal EGF module in human protein S. Eur J Biochem 1998;251(558):564.
165. Dahlbäck B, Hildebrand B, Malm J. Characterization of functionally important domains in human vitamin K-dependent protein S using monoclonal antibodies. J Biol Chem 1990;265(14):8127–8135.
166. van Wijnen M, Stam JG, Chang GTG, et al. Characterization of mini-protein S, a recombinant variant of protein S that lacks the sex hormone binding globulin-like domain. Biochem J 1998;330:389–396.
167. Dahlbäck B, Stenflo J. High molecular weight complex in human plasma between vitamin K-dependent protein S and complement component C4b-binding protein. Proc Natl Acad Sci U S A 1981;78:2512–2516.
168. Dahlbäck B. Inhibition of protein Ca cofactor function of human and bovine protein S by C4b-binding protein. J Biol Chem 1986;261:12022–12027.
169. Comp PC, Nixon RR, Cooper MR, et al. Familial protein S deficiency is associated with recurrent thrombosis. J Clin Invest 1984;74:2082–2088.
170. Dahlbäck B, Frohm B, Nelsestuen G. High affinity interaction between C4b-binding protein and vitamin K-dependent protein S in the presence of calcium. J Biol Chem 1990;265:16082–16087.
171. Griffin JH, Gruber A, Fernandez JA. Reevaluation of total, free, and bound protein S and C4b-binding protein levels in plasma anticoagulated with citrate or hirudin. Blood 1992;79:3203–3211.
172. He X, Shen L, Malmborg A-C, et al. Binding site for C4b-binding protein in vitamin K-dependent protein S fully contained in carboxy-terminal laminin-G-type repeats. A study using recombinant factor IX-protein S chimeras and surface plasmon resonance. Biochemistry 1997;36:3745–3754.
173. Greengard JS, Fernandez JA, Radtke K-P, et al. Identification of candidate residues for interaction of protein S with C4b binding protein and activated protein C. Biochem J 1995;305:397–403.
174. Fernandez JA, Heeb MJ, Griffin JH. Identification of residues 413-433 of plasma protein S as essential for binding to C4b-binding protein. J Biol Chem 1993;268:16788–16794.
175. Dahlbäck B, Smith CA, Muller-Eberhard HJ. Visualization of human C4b-binding protein and its complexes with vitamin K-dependent protein S and complement protein C4b. Proc Natl Acad Sci U S A 1983;80:3461–3465.
176. Dahlbäck B, Muller-Eberhard HJ. Ultrastructure of C4b-binding protein fragments formed by limited proteolysis using chymotrypsin. J Biol Chem 1984;259:11631–11634.
177. Härdig Y, Dahlbäck B. The amino-terminal module of the C4b-binding protein β-chain contains the protein S-binding site. J Biol Chem 1996;271:20861–20867.
178. Hillarp A, Dahlbäck B. Novel subunit in C4b-binding protein required for protein S binding. J Biol Chem 1988;263:12759–12764.
179. Garcia de Frutos P, Alim RIM, Hardig Y, et al. Differential regulation of α and beta chains of C4b-binding protein during acute-phase response

resulting in stable plasma levels of free anticoagulant protein S. *Blood* 1994;84:815–822.

180. Härdig Y, Rezaie A, Dahlbäck B. High affinity binding of human vitamin K-dependent protein S to a truncated recombinant β-chain of C4b-binding protein expressed in *Escherichia coli*. *J Biol Chem* 1993;268:3033–3036.

181. Hillarp A, Pardo-Manuel F, Ruiz RR, et al. The human C4b-binding protein β-chain gene. *J Biol Chem* 1993;268:15017–15023.

182. Hillarp A, Thern A, Dahlbäck B. Bovine C4b binding protein. Molecular cloning of the α- and β-chains provides structural background for lack of complex formation with protein S. *J Immunol* 1994;153:4190–4199.

183. Jackman RW, Beeler DL, Fritze L, et al. Human thrombomodulin gene is intron depleted: nucleic acid sequences of the cDNA and gene predict protein structure and suggest sites of regulatory control. *Proc Natl Acad Sci U S A* 1987;84:6425–6429.

184. Wen D, Dittman WA, Ye RD, et al. Human thrombomodulin: complete cDNA sequence and chromosome localization of the gene. *Biochemistry* 1987;26:4350–4357.

185. Suzuki K, Kusumoto H, Deyashiki Y, et al. Structure and expression of human thrombomodulin, a thrombin receptor on endothelium acting as a cofactor for protein C activation. *EMBO J* 1987;6:1891–1897.

186. Shirai T, Shiojiri S, Ito H, et al. Gene structure of human thrombomodulin, a cofactor for thrombin-catalyzed activation of protein C. *J Biochem (Tokyo)* 1988;103:281–285.

187. Espinosa RI, Sadler JE, LeBeau MM. Regional localization of the human thrombomodulin gene to 20p12-cen. *Genomics* 1989;5:649–650.

188. Petersen TE. The amino-terminal domain of thrombomodulin and pancreatic stone protein are homologous with lectins. *FEBS Lett* 1988;231:51–53.

189. Conway EM, Van de Wouwer M, Pollefeyt S, et al. The lectin-like domain of thrombomodulin confers protection from neutrophil-mediated tissue damage by suppressing adhesion molecule expression via nuclear factor kappaB and mitogen-activated protein kinase pathways. *J Exp Med* 2002;196:565–577.

190. Huang H-C, Shi G-Y, Jiang S-J, et al. Thrombomodulin-mediated cell adhesion: involvement of its lectin-like domain. *J Biol Chem* 2003;278:46750–46759.

191. Kurosawa S, Stearns DJ, Jackson KW, et al. A 10-kDa cyanogen bromide fragment from the epidermal growth factor homology domain of rabbit thrombomodulin contains the primary thrombin binding site. *J Biol Chem* 1988;263:5993–5996.

192. Stearns DJ, Kurosawa S, Esmon CT. Micro-thrombomodulin: residues 310–486 from the epidermal growth factor precursor homology domain of thrombomodulin will accelerate protein C activation. *J Biol Chem* 1989;264:3352–3356.

193. Suzuki K, Hayashi T, Nishioka J, et al. A domain composed of epidermal growth factor–like structures of human thrombomodulin is essential for thrombin binding and for protein C activation. *J Biol Chem* 1989;264:4872–4876.

194. Zushi M, Gomi K, Yamamoto S, et al. The last three consecutive epidermal growth factor–like structures of human thrombomodulin comprise the minimum functional domain for protein C-activating cofactor activity and anticoagulant activity. *J Biol Chem* 1989;264:10351–10353.

195. Zushi M, Gomi K, Honda G, et al. Aspartic acid 349 in the fourth epidermal growth factor–like structure of human thrombomodulin plays a role in its $Ca^{2+}$-mediated binding to protein C. *J Biol Chem* 1991;266:19886–19889.

196. Vindigni A, White CE, Komives EA, et al. Energetics of thrombin-thrombomodulin interaction. *Biochemistry* 1997;36:6674–6681.

197. Wang W, Nagashima M, Schneider M, et al. Elements of the primary structure of thrombomodulin required for efficient thrombin-activable fibrinolysis inhibitor activation. *J Biol Chem* 2000;275:22942–22947.

198. Lentz SR, Chen Y, Sadler JE. Sequences required for thrombomodulin cofactor activity within the fourth epidermal growth factor–like domain of human thrombomodulin. *J Biol Chem* 1993;268:15312–15317.

199. Nagashima M, Lundh E, Leonard JC, et al. Alanine-scanning mutagenesis of the epidermal growth factor–like domains of human thrombomodulin identifies critical residues for its cofactor activity. *J Biol Chem* 1993;268:2888–2892.

200. White CE, Hunter MJ, Meininger DP, et al. The fifth epidermal growth factor–like domain of thrombomodulin does not have an epidermal growth factor–like disulfide bonding pattern. *Proc Natl Acad Sci U S A* 1996;93:10177–10182.

201. Fuentes-Prior P, Iwanaga Y, Huber R, et al. Structural basis for the anticoagulant activity of the thrombin-thrombomodulin complex. *Nature* 2000;404:518–525.

202. Lin J-H, McLean K, Morser J, et al. Modulation of glycosaminoglycan addition in naturally expressed and recombinant human thrombomodulin. *J Biol Chem* 1994;269(40):25021–25030.

203. Bourin M, Boffa M, Bjork I, et al. Functional domains of rabbit thrombomodulin. *Proc Natl Acad Sci U S A* 1986;83:5924–5928.

204. Bourin MC, Lundgren-Åkerlund E, Lindahl U. Isolation and characterization of the glycosaminoglycan component of rabbit thrombomodulin proteoglycan. *J Biol Chem* 1990;265:15424–15431.

205. Bourin M-C. Effect of rabbit thrombomodulin on thrombin inhibition by antithrombin in the presence of heparin. *Thromb Res* 1989;54:27–39.

206. Xu J, Esmon NL, Esmon CT. Reconstitution of the human endothelial cell protein C receptor with thrombomodulin in phosphatidylcholine vesicles enhances protein C activation. *J Biol Chem* 1999;274:6704–6710.

207. Ye J, Rezaie AR, Esmon CT. Glycosaminoglycan contributions to both protein C activation and thrombin inhibition involve a common arginine-rich site in thrombin that includes residues arginine 93, 97, and 101. *J Biol Chem* 1994;269:17965–17970.

208. He X, Ye J, Esmon CT, et al. Influence of arginines 93, 97, and 101 of thrombin to its functional specificity. *Biochemistry* 1997;36:8969–8976.

209. Gysin J, Pouvelle B, Le Tonquèze M, et al. Chondroitin sulfate of thrombomodulin is an adhesion receptor for plasmodium falciparum-infected erythrocytes. *Mol Biochem Parasitol* 1997;88:267–271.

210. Maruyama I, Salem HH, Ishii H, et al. Human thrombomodulin is not an efficient inhibitor of procoagulant activity of thrombin. *J Clin Invest* 1985;75:987–991.

211. Parkinson JF, Vlahos CJ, Yan SCB, et al. Recombinant human thrombomodulin: regulation of cofactor activity and anticoagulant function by a glycosaminoglycan side chain. *Biochem J* 1992;283:151–157.

212. Parkinson JF, Koyama T, Bang NU, et al. Thrombomodulin: an anticoagulant cell surface proteoglycan with physiologically relevant glycosaminoglycan moiety. *Adv Exp Med Biol* 1992;313:177–188.

213. Dittman WA, Kumada T, Sadler JE, et al. The structure and function of mouse thrombomodulin. Phorbol myristate acetate stimulates degradation and synthesis of thrombomodulin without affecting mRNA levels in hemangioma cells. *J Biol Chem* 1988;263:15815–15822.

214. Jackman RW, Beeler DL, VanDeWater L, et al. Characterization of a thrombomodulin cDNA reveals structural similarity to the low density lipoprotein receptor. *Proc Natl Acad Sci U S A* 1986;83:8834–8838.

215. Conway EM, Boffa M-C, Nowakowski B, et al. An ultrastructural study of thrombomodulin endocytosis: internalization occurs via clathrin-coated and non-coated pits. *J Cell Physiol* 1992;151:604–612.

216. Conway EM, Pollefeyt S, Collen D, et al. The amino terminal lectin-like domain of thrombomodulin is required for constitutive endocytosis. *Blood* 1997;89:652–661.

217. Mulder AB, Smit JW, Bom VJJ, et al. Association of endothelial tissue factor and thrombomodulin with caveolae. *Blood* 1996;88:3667–3670.

218. Oganesyan V, Oganesyan N, Terzyan S, et al. The crystal structure of the endothelial protein C receptor and a bound phospholipid. *J Biol Chem* 2002;277:24851–24854.

219. Fukudome K, Esmon CT. Molecular cloning and expression of murine and bovine endothelial cell protein C/activated protein C receptor (EPCR). The structural and functional conservation in human, bovine, and murine EPCR. *J Biol Chem* 1995;270:5571–5577.

220. Xu J, Qu D, Esmon CT. Characterization of endothelial protein C receptor. Book of Abstracts, *Vascular Biology '98 Scientific Conference of American Heart Association and North American Vascular Biology Organization*, 61, 1998, Abstract.

221. Xu J, Qu D, Esmon CT. Thrombin enhanced release of soluble EPCR mediated by metalloproteinases associated with caveolae. Book of Abstracts, *Vascular Biology '98 Scientific Conference of American Heart Association and North American Vascular Biology Organization*, 62, 1998, Abstract.

222. Gu JM, Fukudome K, Esmon CT. Characterization and regulation of the 5′-flanking region of the murine endothelial protein C receptor gene. *J Biol Chem* 2000;275:12481–12488.

223. Rance JB, Follows GA, Cockerill PN, et al. Regulation of the human endothelial cell protein C receptor gene promoter by multiple Sp1 binding sites. *Blood* 2003;101:4393–4401.

224. Liang Z, Rosen ED, Castellino FJ. Nucleotide structure and characterization of the murine gene encoding the endothelial cell protein C receptor. *Thromb Haemost* 1999;81:585–588.

225. Simmonds RE, Lane DA. Structural and functional implications of the intron/exon organization of the human endothelial protein C/activated protein C receptor (EPCR) gene: comparison with the structure of CD1/major histocompatibility complex α1 and α2 domains. *Blood* 1999;94:632–641.

226. Saposnik B, Reny HL, Gaussem P, et al. A haplotype of the EPCR gene is associated with increased plasma levels of sEPCR and is a candidate risk factor for thrombosis. *Blood* 2003;103:1311–1318.

227. Gu J-M, Crawley JTB, Ferrell G, et al. Disruption of the endothelial cell protein C receptor gene in mice causes placental thrombosis and early embryonic lethality. *J Biol Chem* 2002;277:43335–43343.

228. Castellino FJ, Liang Z, Volkir SP, et al. Mice with a severe deficiency of the endothelial protein C receptor gene develop, survive, and reproduce normally, and do not present with enhanced arterial thrombosis after challenge. *Thromb Haemost* 2002;88:462–472.

229. Varadi K, Philapitsch A, Santa T, et al. Activation and inactivation of human protein C by plasmin. *Thromb Haemost* 1994;71:615–621.

230. Epstein DJ, Begum PW, Bajaj SP, et al. Radioimmunoassays for protein C and factor X. Plasma antigen levels in abnormal hemostatic states. *Am J Clin Pathol* 1984;82:573–581.

231. Klein JD, Walker FJ. Purification of a protein C activator from the venom of the southern copperhead snake (*Agkistrodon contortrix contortrix*). *Biochemistry* 1986;25:4175–4179.

232. Haley PE, Doyle MF, Mann KG. The activation of bovine protein C by factor Xa. *J Biol Chem* 1989;264:16303–16310.

233. Thompson EA, Salem HH. Inhibition by human thrombomodulin of factor Xa-mediated cleavage of prothrombin. *J Clin Invest* 1986;78:13–17.

234. Thompson EA, Salem HH. Factors $IX_a$, $X_a$, $XI_a$ and activated protein C do not have protein C activating ability in the presence of thrombomodulin. *Thromb Haemost* 1988;59:339.

235. Wu Q, Tsiang M, Lentz SR, et al. Ligand specificity of human thrombomodulin: equilibrium binding of human thrombin, meizothrombin, and factor Xa to recombinant thrombomodulin. *J Biol Chem* 1992;267:7083–7088.

236. Doyle MF, Mann KG. Multiple active forms of thrombin. IV. Relative activities of meizothrombins. *J Biol Chem* 1990;265:10693–10701.

237. Cote HCF, Bajzar L, Stevens WK, et al. Functional characterization of recombinant human meizothrombin and meizothrombin(desF1). Thrombomodulin-dependent activation of protein C and thrombin-activable fibrinolysis inhibitor (TAFI), platelet aggregation, antithrombin-III inhibition. *J Biol Chem* 1997;272:6194–6200.

238. Martin PD, Malkowski MG, Box J, et al. New insights into the regulation of the blood clotting cascade derived from the X-ray crystal structure of bovine meizothrombin des F1 in complex with PPACK. *Structure* 1997; 5:1681–1693.

239. Fukudome K, Ye X, Tsuneyoshi N, et al. Activation mechanism of anticoagulant protein C in large blood vessels involving the endothelial cell protein C receptor. *J Exp Med* 1998;187:1029–1035.

240. Kurosawa S, Stearns-Kurosawa DJ, Hidari N, et al. Identification of functional endothelial protein C receptor in human plasma. *J Clin Invest* 1997;100:411–418.

241. Laszik Z, Mitro A, Taylor FB Jr, et al. Human protein C receptor is present primarily on endothelium of large blood vessels: implications for the control of the protein C pathway. *Circulation* 1997;96:3633–3640.

242. Salem HH, Esmon NL, Esmon CT, et al. Effects of thrombomodulin and coagulation factor Va-light chain on protein C activation *in vitro*. *J Clin Invest* 1984;73:968–972.

243. Maruyama I, Salem H, Majerus P. Coagulation factor Va binds to human umbilical vein endothelial cells and accelerates protein C activation. *J Clin Invest* 1984;74:224–230.

244. Salem H, Broze G, Miletich J, et al. Human coagulation factor Va is a cofactor for the activation of protein C. *Proc Natl Acad Sci U S A* 1983;80:1584–1588.

245. Salem H, Broze G, Miletich J, et al. The light chain of factor Va contains the activity of factor Va that accelerates protein C activation by thrombin. *J Biol Chem* 1983;258:8531–8534.

246. Tsiang M, Lentz S, Sadler JE. Functional domains of membrane-bound human thrombomodulin. EGF- like domains four to six and the serine/threonine-rich domain are required for cofactor activity. *J Biol Chem* 1992; 267:6164–6170.

247. Lu R, Esmon NL, Esmon CT, et al. The active site of the thrombin-thrombomodulin complex: a fluorescence energy transfer measurement of its distance above the membrane surface. *J Biol Chem* 1989;264:12956–12962.

248. Slungaard A, Fernandez JA, Griffin JH, et al. Platelet factor 4 enhances generation of activated protein C *in vitro* and *in vivo*. *Blood* 2003;102: 146–151.

249. Mannucci PM, Vigano S. Deficiencies of protein C, an inhibitor of blood coagulation. *Lancet* 1982;2:463–467.

250. Dudek AZ, Pennell CA, Decker TD, et al. Platelet factor 4 binds to glycanated forms of thrombomodulin and to protein C. A potential mechanism for enhancing generation of activated protein C. *J Biol Chem* 1997; 272:31785–31792.

251. Slungaard A, Key NS. Platelet factor 4 stimulates thrombomodulin protein C-activating cofactor activity. A structure-function analysis. *J Biol Chem* 1994;269(41):25549–25556.

252. Slungaard A, Vercellotti GM, Tran T, et al. Eosinophil cationic granule proteins impair thrombomodulin function. A potential mechanism for thromboembolism in hypereosinophilic heart disease. *J Clin Invest* 1993; 91:1721–1730.

253. Ford DA, Gross RW. Lipobiology. In: Bittar EE, Bittar N, eds. *Cell chemistry and physiology*. Part I. Greenwich, CT: JAI Press, 1995:335–361.

254. Moore KL, Andreoli SP, Esmon NL, et al. Endotoxin enhances tissue factor and suppresses thrombomodulin expression of human vascular endothelium *in vitro*. *J Clin Invest* 1987;79:124–130.

255. Nawroth PP, Handley DA, Esmon CT, et al. Interleukin-1 induces endothelial cell procoagulant while suppressing cell surface anticoagulant activity. *Proc Natl Acad Sci U S A* 1986;83:3460–3464.

256. Hirokawa K, Aoki N. Regulatory mechanisms for thrombomodulin expression in human umbilical vein endothelial cells *in vitro*. *J Cell Physiol* 1991;147:157–165.

257. Maruyama I, Soejima Y, Osame M, et al. Increased expression of thrombomodulin on the cultured human umbilical vein endothelial cells and mouse hemangioma cells by cyclic AMP. *Thromb Res* 1991;61:301–310.

258. Ohji T, Urano H, Shirahata A, et al. Transforming growth factor beta1 and beta2 induce down-modulation of thrombomodulin in human umbilical vein endothelial cells. *Thromb Haemost* 1995;73:812–818.

259. Moore KL, Esmon CT, Esmon NL. Tumor necrosis factor leads to internalization and degradation of thrombomodulin from the surface of bovine aortic endothelial cells in culture. *Blood* 1989;73:159–165.

260. Conway EM, Rosenberg RD. Tumor necrosis factor suppresses transcription of the thrombomodulin gene in endothelial cells. *Mol Cell Biol* 1988; 8:5588–5592.

261. Lentz SR, Tsiang M, Sadler JE. Regulation of thrombomodulin by tumor necrosis factor-α: comparison of transcriptional and posttranscriptional mechanisms. *Blood* 1991;77:543–550.

262. Ohdama S, Takano S, Ohashi K, et al. Pentoxifylline prevents tumor necrosis factor-induced suppression of endothelial cell surface thrombomodulin. *Thromb Res* 1991;62:745–755.

263. Yu K, Morioka H, Fritze LMS, et al. Transcriptional regulation of the thrombomodulin gene. *J Biol Chem* 1992;267:23237–23247.

264. Tazawa R, Yamamoto K, Suzuki K, et al. Presence of functional cyclic AMP responsive element in the 3'-untranslated region of the human thrombomodulin gene. *Biochem Biophys Res Commun* 1994;200:1391–1397.

265. Weiler-Guettler H, Yu K, Soff G, et al. Thrombomodulin gene regulation by cAMP and retinoic acid in F9 embryonal carcinoma cells. *Proc Natl Acad Sci U S A* 1992;89:2155–2159.

266. Ishii H, Horie S, Kizaki K, et al. Retinoic acid counteracts both the downregulation of thrombomodulin and the induction of tissue factor in cultured human endothelial cells exposed to tumor necrosis factor. *Blood* 1992;80:2556–2562.

267. Dittman WA, Nelson SC, Greer PK, et al. Characterization of thrombomodulin expression in response to retinoic acid and identification of a retinoic acid response element in the human thrombomodulin gene. *J Biol Chem* 1994;269:16925–16932.

268. Koyama T, Hirosawa S, Kawamata N, et al. All-trans retinoic acid upregulates thrombomodulin and down regulates tissue-factor expression in acute promyelocytic leukemia cells: distinct expression of thrombomodulin and tissue factor in human leukemic cells. *Blood* 1994;84(9):3001–3009.

269. Hayashi T, Honda G, Suzuki K. An atherogenic stimulus homocysteine inhibits cofactor activity of thrombomodulin and enhances thrombomodulin expression in human umbilical vein endothelial cells. *Blood* 1992;79: 2930–2936.

270. Lentz SR, Sadler JE. Inhibition of thrombomodulin surface expression and protein C activation by the thrombogenic agent homocysteine. *J Clin Invest* 1991;88:1906–1914.

271. Lentz SR. Homocysteine and vascular dysfunction. *Life Sci* 1997;61: 1205–1215.

272. Ogawa S, Gerlach H, Esposito C, et al. Hypoxia modulates the barrier and coagulant function of cultured bovine endothelium: increased monolayer permeability and induction of procoagulant properties. *J Clin Invest* 1990;85:1090–1098.

273. Esposito C, Gerlach H, Brett J, et al. Endothelial receptor-mediated binding of glucose-modified albumin is associated with increased monolayer permeability and modulation of cell surface coagulant properties. *J Exp Med* 1989;170:1387–1407.

274. Laszik ZG, Zhou XJ, Silva FG, et al. Thrombomodulin (TM) but not endothelial cell protein C receptor (EPCR) mRNA is downregulated in streptozotocin-induced diabetic rat kidneys Abstract. *Mod Pathol* 2003; 16(1218):267A.

275. Kim AY, Walinsky PL, Kolodgie FD, et al. Early loss of thrombomodulin expression impairs vein graft thromboresistance: implications for vein graft failure. *Circ Res* 2002;90:205–212.

276. Waugh JM, Yuksel E, Li J, et al. Local overexpression of thrombomodulin for *in vivo* prevention of arterial thrombosis in a rabbit model. *Circ Res* 1999;84:84–92.

277. Waugh JM, Li-Hawkins J, Yuksel E, et al. Thrombomodulin overexpression to limit neointima formation. *Circulation* 2000;102:332–337.

278. Laszik ZG, Zhou XJ, Ferrell GL, et al. Down-regulation of endothelial expression of endothelial cell protein C receptor and thrombomodulin in coronary atherosclerosis. *Am J Pathol* 2001;159:797–802.

279. Masamura K, Oida K, Kanehara H, et al. Pitavastatin-induced thrombomodulin expression by endothelial cells acts via inhibition of small G proteins of the Rho family. *Arterioscler Thromb Vasc Biol* 2003;23:512–517.

280. Shi J, Wang J, Zheng H, et al. Statins increase thrombomodulin expression and function in human endothelial cells by a nitric oxide-dependent mechanism and counteract tumor necrosis factor alpha-induced thrombomodulin downregulation. *Blood Coagul Fibrinolysis* 2003;14:575–585.

281. Malek AM, Jackman R, Rosenberg RD, et al. Endothelial expression of thrombomodulin is reversibly regulated by fluid shear stress. *Circ Res* 1994;74:852–860.

282. Maruyama I, Majerus PW. The turnover of thrombin-thrombomodulin complex in cultured human umbilical vein endothelial cells and A549 lung cancer cells: endocytosis and degradation of thrombin. *J Biol Chem* 1985; 260:15432–15438.

283. Maruyama I, Majerus PW. Protein C inhibits endocytosis of thrombin-thrombomodulin complexes in A549 lung cancer cells and human umbilical vein endothelial cells. *Blood* 1987;69:1481–1484.

284. Horvat R, Palade GE. Thrombomodulin and thrombin localization on the vascular endothelium; their internalization and transcytosis by plasmalemma vesicles. *Eur J Cell Biol* 1993;61:299–313.

285. Beretz A, Freyssinet J-M, Gauchy J, et al. Stability of the thrombin-thrombomodulin complex on the surface of endothelial cells from human saphenous vein or from the cell line EA.hy 926. *Biochem J* 1989;259: 35–40.

286. Brisson C, Archipoff G, Hartmann M-L, et al. Antibodies to thrombomodulin induce receptor-mediated endocytosis in human saphenous vein endothelial cells. *Thromb Haemost* 1992;68:737–743.

287. Hirokawa K, Aoki N. Up-regulation of thrombomodulin in human umbilical vein endothelial cells *in vitro*. *J Biochem (Tokyo)* 1990;108:839–845.

288. Bartha K, Brisson C, Archipoff G, et al. Thrombin regulates tissue factor and thrombomodulin mRNA levels and activates in human saphenous vein endothelial cells by distinct mechanisms. *J Biol Chem* 1993;268:421–429.

289. Dittman WA, Kumada T, Majerus PW. Transcription of thrombomodulin mRNA in mouse hemangioma cells is increased by cycloheximide and thrombin. *Proc Natl Acad Sci U S A* 1989;86:7179–7182.

290. Ma S-F, Garcia JGN, Reuning U, et al. Thrombin induces thrombomodulin mRNA expression via the proteolytically activated thrombin receptor in cultured bovine smooth muscle cells. *J Lab Clin Med* 1997;129:611–619.

291. Boehme MWJ, Deng Y, Raeth U, et al. Release of thrombomodulin from endothelial cells by concerted action of TNF-α and neutrophils: *in vivo* and *in vitro* studies. *Immunol* 1996;87:134–140.

292. Takano S, Kimura S, Ohdama S, et al. Plasma thrombomodulin in health and diseases. *Blood* 1990;76:2024–2029.

293. Glaser CB, Morser J, Clarke JH, et al. Oxidation of a specific methionine in thrombomodulin by activated neutrophil products blocks cofactor activity. *J Clin Invest* 1992;90:2565–2573.

294. Hamada H, Ishii H, Sakyo K, et al. The epidermal growth factor–like domain of recombinant human thrombomodulin exhibits mitogenic activity for Swiss 3T3 cells. *Blood* 1995;86(1):225–233.

295. Grinnell BW, Berg DT. Surface thrombomodulin modulates thrombin receptor responses on vascular smooth muscle cells. *Am J Physiol* 1996;270:H603–H609.

296. Soff GA, Jackman RW, Rosenberg RD. Expression of thrombomodulin by smooth muscle cells in culture: different effects of tumor necrosis factor and cyclic adenosine monophosphate on thrombomodulin expression by endothelial cells and smooth muscle cells in culture. *Blood* 1991;77:515–518.

297. Lafay M, Laguna R, Le Bonniec BF, et al. Thrombomodulin modulates the mitogenic response to thrombin of human umbilical vein endothelial cells. *Thromb Haemost* 1998;79:848–852.

298. Conway EM, Liu L, Nowakowski B, et al. Heat shock of vascular endothelial cells induces an up-regulatory transcriptional response of the thrombomodulin gene that is delayed in onset and does not attenuate. *J Biol Chem* 1994;269(36):22804–22810.

299. Calnek DS, Grinnell BW. Thrombomodulin-dependent anticoagulant activity is regulated by vascular endothelial growth factor. *Exp Cell Res* 1998;238:294–298.

300. Raife TJ, Lager DJ, Madison KC, et al. Thrombomodulin expression by human keratinocytes. Induction of cofactor activity during epidermal differentiation. *J Clin Invest* 1994;93:1846–1851.

301. Imada S, Yamaguchi H, Nagumo M, et al. Identification of fetomodulin, a surface marker protein of fetal development, as thrombomodulin by gene cloning and functional assays. *Dev Biol* 1990;140:113–122.

302. Imada M, Imada S, Iwasaki H, et al. Fetomodulin: marker surface protein of fetal development which is modulatable by cyclic AMP. *Dev Biol* 1987;122:483–491.

303. Weiler-Guettler H, Aird WC, Rayburn H, et al. Developmentally regulated gene expression of thrombomodulin in postimplantation mouse embryos. *Development* 1996;122:2271–2281.

304. Healy AM, Rayburn HB, Rosenberg RD, et al. Absence of the blood-clotting regulator thrombomodulin causes embryonic lethality in mice before development of a functional cardiovascular system. *Proc Natl Acad Sci U S A* 1995;92:850–854.

305. Isermann B, Hendrickson SB, Hutley K, et al. Tissue-restricted expression of thrombomodulin in the placenta rescues thrombomodulin-deficient mice from early lethality and reveals a secondary developmental block. *Development* 2001;128(6):827–838.

306. Weiler H, Lindner V, Kerlin B, et al. Characterization of a mouse model for thrombomodulin deficiency. *Arterioscler Thromb Vasc Biol* 2001; 21(9):1531–1537.

307. Weiler H, Isermann H. Thrombomodulin. *J Thromb Haemost* 2003;1: 1515–1524.

308. Wu Q, Sheehan JP, Tsiang M, et al. Single amino acid substitutions dissociate fibrinogen-clotting and thrombomodulin-binding activities of human thrombin. *Proc Natl Acad Sci U S A* 1991;88:6775–6779.

309. Le Bonniec BF, Esmon CT. Glu-192 [to] Gln substitution in thrombin mimics the catalytic switch induced by thrombomodulin. *Proc Natl Acad Sci U S A* 1991;88:7371–7375.

310. Le Bonniec BF, MacGillivray RTA, Esmon CT. Thrombin Glu-39 restricts the P′3 specificity to nonacidic residues. *J Biol Chem* 1991;266: 13796–13803.

311. Rezaie AR, Esmon CT. The function of calcium in protein C activation by thrombin and the thrombin-thrombomodulin complex can be distinguished by mutational analysis of protein C derivatives. *J Biol Chem* 1992; 267:26104–26109.

312. Tsiang M, Jain AK, Dunn KE, et al. Functional mapping of the surface residues of human thrombin. *J Biol Chem* 1995;270(28):16854–16863.

313. Friedrich U, Potzsch B, Preissner KT, et al. Calcium-dependent activation of protein C by thrombin/thrombomudulin: role of negatively charged amino acids within the activation peptide of protein C. *Thromb Haemost* 1994;72(4):567–572.

314. Gibbs CS, Coutré SE, Tsiang M, et al. Conversion of thrombin into an anticoagulant by protein engineering. *Nature* 1995;378:413–416.

315. Di Cera E, Guinto ER, Vindigni A, et al. The Na+ binding site of thrombin. *J Biol Chem* 1995;270:22089–22092.

316. Dang QD, Guinto ER, Di Cera E. Rational engineering of activity and specificity in a serine protease. *Nat Biotechnol* 1997;15:146–149.

317. Dang QD, Vindigni A, Di Cera E. An allosteric switch controls the procoagulant and anticoagulant activities of thrombin. *Proc Natl Acad Sci U S A* 1995;92:5977–5981.

318. Wells CM, Di Cera E. Thrombin is a Na+-activated enzyme. *Biochemistry* 1992;31:11721–11730.

319. Di Cera E, Dang QD, Ayala YM. Molecular mechanisms of thrombin function. *Cell Mol Life Sci* 1997;53:701–730.

320. Guinto ER, Vindigni A, Ayala YM, et al. Identification of residues linked to the slow [to] fast transition of thrombin. *Proc Natl Acad Sci U S A* 1995;92:11185–11189.

321. Gerlitz B, Grinnell BW. Mutation of protease domain residues Lys[37–39] in human protein C inhibits activation by the thrombomodulin-thrombin complex without affecting activation by free thrombin. *J Biol Chem* 1996; 271:22285–22288.

322. Ye J, Esmon CT, Johnson AE. The chondroitin sulfate moiety of thrombomodulin binds a second molecule of thrombin. *J Biol Chem* 1993;268: 2373–2379.

323. Ye J, Esmon NL, Esmon CT, et al. The active site of thrombin is altered upon binding to thrombomodulin: two distinct structural changes are detected by fluorescence, but only one correlates with protein C activation. *J Biol Chem* 1991;266:23016–23021.

324. Musci G, Berliner LJ, Esmon CT. Evidence for multiple conformational changes in the active center of thrombin induced by complex formation with thrombomodulin: an analysis employing nitroxide spin labels. *Biochemistry* 1988;27:769–773.

325. Liu L-W, Rezaie AR, Carson CW, et al. Occupancy of anion binding exosite 2 on thrombin determines Ca2+ dependence of protein C activation. *J Biol Chem* 1994;269:11807–11812.

326. Berg DT, Wiley MR, Grinnell BW. Enhanced protein C activation and inhibition of fibrinogen cleavage by a thrombin modulator. *Science* 1996; 273:1389–1391.

327. Grinnell BW. Tipping the balance of blood coagulation. *Nat Biotechnol* 1997;15:124–125.

328. van de Locht A, Bode W, Huber R, et al. The thrombin E192Q-BPTI complex reveals gross structural rearrangements: implications for the interaction with antithrombin and thrombomodulin. *EMBO J* 1997;16:2977–2984.

329. Guinto ER, Ye J, Le Bonniec BF, et al. Glu[192] [to] Gln substitution in thrombin yields an enzyme that is effectively inhibited by bovine pancreatic trypsin inhibitor and tissue factor pathway inhibitor. *J Biol Chem* 1994;269:18395–18400.

330. Bode W, Turk D, Karshikov A. The refined 1.9-Å X-ray crystal structure of D-Phe-Pro-Arg chloromethylketone-inhibited human alpha-thrombin: structure analysis, overall structure, electrostatic properties, detailed active-site geometry, and structure-function relationships. *Protein Sci* 1992; 1:426–471.

331. Rezaie AR, He X, Esmon CT. Thrombomodulin increases the rate of thrombin inhibition by BPTI. *Biochemistry* 1998;37:693–699.

332. Ehrlich HJ, Grinnell BW, Jaskunas SR, et al. Recombinant human protein C derivatives: altered response to calcium resulting in enhanced activation by thrombin. *EMBO J* 1990;9:2367–2373.

333. Richardson MA, Gerlitz B, Grinnell BW. Enhancing protein C interaction with thrombin results in a clot-activated anticoagulant. *Nature* 1992; 360:261–264.

334. Kalafatis M, Rand MD, Mann KG. The mechanism of inactivation of human factor V and human factor Va by activated protein C. *J Biol Chem* 1994;269:31869–31880.

335. Kalafatis M, Bertina RM, Rand MD, et al. Characterization of the molecular defect in factor V[R506Q]. *J Biol Chem* 1995;270(8):4053–4057.

336. Mann KG, Hockin MF, Begin KJ, et al. Activated protein C cleavage of factor V leads to dissociation of the A2 domain. *J Biol Chem* 1997;272: 20678–20683.

337. Fay PJ, Coumans J-V, Walker FJ. von Willebrand factor mediates protection of factor VIII from activated protein C-catalyzed inactivation. *J Biol Chem* 1991;266:2172–2177.

338. Fay PJ, Smudzin TM, Walker FJ. Activated protein C-catalyzed inactivation of human factor VIII and factor VIII[a]. *J Biol Chem* 1991;266: 20139–20145.

339. Koedam JA, Meijers JCM, Sixma JJ, et al. Inactivation of human factor VIII by activated protein C. Cofactor activity of protein S and protective effect of von Willebrand factor. *J Clin Invest* 1988;82:1236–1243.

340. Bakker HM, Tans G, Janssen-Claessen T, et al. The effect of phospholipids, calcium ions, and protein S on rate constants of human factor Va inactivation by activated human protein C. *Eur J Biochem* 1992;208: 171–178.

341. Koppelman SJ, van Hoeij M, Vink T, et al. Requirements of von Willebrand factor to protect factor VIII from inactivation by activated protein C. *Blood* 1996;87:2292–2300.

342. Nicolaes GAF, Tans G, Thomassen MCLGD, et al. Peptide bond cleavages and loss of functional activity during inactivation of factor Va and factor Va[R506Q] by activated protein C. *J Biol Chem* 1995;270:21158–21166.

343. Rosing J, Hoekema L, Nicolaes GAF, et al. Effects of protein S and factor Xa on peptide bond cleavages during inactivation of factor Va and factor Va[R506Q] by activated protein C. *J Biol Chem* 1995;270:27852–27858.

344. Heeb MJ, Kojima Y, Greengard JS, et al. Activated protein C resistance: molecular mechanisms based on studies using purified Gln506-factor V. *Blood* 1995;85:3405–3411.

345. Kalafatis M, Mann KG. Role of the membrane in the inactivation of factor Va by activated protein C. *J Biol Chem* 1993;268:27246–27257.

346. Krishnaswamy S, Williams EB, Mann KG. The binding of activated protein C to factors V and Va. *J Biol Chem* 1986;261:9684–9693.

347. Walker FJ, Scandella D, Fay PJ. Identification of the binding site for activated protein C on the light chain of factors V and VIII. *J Biol Chem* 1990;265:1484–1489.

348. Amano K, Michnick DA, Moussalli M, et al. Mutation at either Arg336 or Arg562 in factor VIII is insufficient for complete resistance to activated protein C (APC)-mediated inactivation: implications for the APC resistance test. *Thromb Haemost* 1998;79:557–563.

349. Shen L, Dahlbäck B. Factor V and protein S as synergistic cofactors to activated protein C in degradation of factor VIIIa. *J Biol Chem* 1994;269: 18735–18738.

350. Varadi K, Rosing J, Tans G, et al. Factor V enhances the cofactor function of protein S in the APC-mediated inactivation of factor VIII: influence of the factor V$^{R506Q}$ mutation. *Thromb Haemost* 1996;76:208–214.

351. Dahlbäck B, Hildebrand B. Inherited resistance to activated protein C is corrected by anticoagulant cofactor activity found to be a property of factor V. *Proc Natl Acad Sci U S A* 1994;91:1396–1400.

352. Dahlbäck B, Carlsson M, Svensson PJ. Familial thrombophilia due to a previously unrecognized mechanism characterized by poor anticoagulant response to activated protein C: prediction of a cofactor to activated protein C. *Proc Natl Acad Sci U S A* 1993;90:1004–1008.

353. Kalafatis M, Haley PE, Lu D, et al. Proteolytic events that regulate factor V activity in whole plasma from normal and activated protein C (APC)-resistant individuals during clotting: an insight into the APC-resistance assay. *Blood* 1996;87:4695–4707.

354. Petaja J, Fernandez JA, Gruber A, et al. Anticoagulant synergism of heparin and activated protein C *in vitro*. *J Clin Invest* 1997;99(11):2655–2663.

355. Marciniak E. Coagulation inhibitor elicited by thrombin. *Science* 1970; 170:452–453.

356. Marciniak E. Inhibitor of human blood coagulation elicited by thrombin. *J Lab Clin Med* 1972;79:924–934.

357. Walker FJ. Regulation of bovine activated protein C by protein S: the role of the cofactor protein in species specificity. *Thromb Res* 1981;22:321–327.

358. Shen L, He X, Dahlbäck B. Synergistic Cofactor function of factor V and protein S to activated protein C in the inactivation of the factor VIIIa-factor IXa complex. *Thromb Haemost* 1997;78:1030–1036.

359. He X, Shen L, Dahlbäck B. Expression and functional characterization of chimeras between human and bovine vitamin-K-dependent protein-S-defining modules important for the species specificity of the activated protein C cofactor activity. *Eur J Biochem* 1995;227:443–440.

360. Heeb MJ, Rosing J, Bakker HM, et al. Protein S binds to and inhibits factor Xa. *Proc Natl Acad Sci U S A* 1994;91:2728–2732.

361. Koppelman SJ, Hackeng TM, Sixma JJ, et al. Inhibition of the intrinsic factor X activating complex by protein S: evidence for a specific binding of protein S to factor VIII. *Blood* 1995;86:1062–1071.

362. Heeb MJ, Mesters RM, Tans G, et al. Binding of protein S to factor Va associated with inhibition of prothrombinase that is independent of activated protein C. *J Biol Chem* 1993;268:2872–2877.

363. Koppelman SJ, van't Veer C, Sixma JJ, et al. Synergistic inhibition of the intrinsic factor X activation by protein S and C4b-binding protein. *Blood* 1995;86:2653–2660.

364. Taylor FB Jr, Dahlbäck B, Chang ACK, et al. Role of free protein S and C4b binding protein in regulating the coagulant reponse to *Escherichia coli*. *Blood* 1995;86:2642–2652.

365. Taylor F, Chang A, Ferrell G, et al. C4b-binding protein exacerbates the host response to *Escherichia coli*. *Blood* 1991;78:357–363.

366. Duchemin J, Pittet J-L, Tartary M, et al. A new assay based on thrombin generation inhibition to detect both protein C and protein S deficiencies in plasma. *Thromb Haemost* 1994;71:331–338.

367. van't Veer C, Hackeng TM, Biesbroeck D, et al. Increased prothrombin activation in protein S-deficient plasma under flow conditions on endothelial cell matrix: an independent anticoagulant function of protein S in plasma. *Blood* 1995;85:1815–1821.

368. Stitt TN, Conn G, Gore M, et al. The anticoagulation factor protein S and its relative, Gas6, are ligands for the tyro 3/Axl family of receptor tyrosine kinases. *Cell* 1995;80:661–670.

369. Manfioletti G, Brancolini C, Avanzi G, et al. The protein encoded by a growth arrest-specific gene (gas6) is a new member of the vitamin K-dependent proteins related to protein S, a negative coregulator in the blood coagulation cascade. *Mol Cell Biol* 1993;13(8):4976–4985.

370. Godowski PJ, Mark MR, Chen J, et al. Reevaluation of the roles of protein S and Gas6 as ligands for the receptor tyrosine kinase Rse/Tyro 3. *Cell* 1995;82:355–358.

371. Nyberg P, He X, Härdig Y, et al. Stimulation of Sky tyrosine phosphorylation by bovine protein S: domains involved in the receptor-ligand interaction. *Eur J Biochem* 1997;246:147–154.

372. Collins CL, Fink LM, Hsu S-M, et al. Thrombomodulin staining of mesothelioma cells. *Hum Pathol* 1992;23:966.

373. Collins CL, Ordonez NG, Schaefer R, et al. Thrombomodulin expression in malignant pleural mesothelioma and pulmonary adenocarcinoma. *Am J Pathol* 1992;141:827–833.

374. Conway EM, Nowakowski B, Steiner-Mosonyi M. Human neutrophils synthesize thrombomodulin that does not promote thrombin-dependent protein C activation. *Blood* 1992;80:1254–1263.

375. Conway EM, Nowakowski B. Biologically active thrombomodulin is synthesized by adherent synovial fluid cells and is elevated in synovial fluid of patients with rheumatoid arthritis. *Blood* 1993;81:726–733.

376. Mizutani H, Hayashi T, Nouchi N, et al. Functional and immunoreactive thrombomodulin expressed by keratinocytes. *J Invest Dermatol* 1994; 103:825–828.

377. Jackson DE, Mitchell CA, Bird P, et al. Immunohistochemical localization of thrombomodulin in normal human skin and skin tumours. *J Pathol* 1995;175:421–432.

378. Pindon A, Hantai D, Jandrot-Perrus M, et al. Novel expression and localization of active thrombomodulin on the surface of mouse brain astrocytes. *Glia* 1997;19:259–268.

379. Suzuki K, Nishioka J, Hayashi T, et al. Functionally active thrombomodulin is present in human platelets. *J Biochem (Tokyo)* 1988;104:628–632.

380. Satta N, Freyssinet J-M, Toti F. The significance of human monocyte thrombomodulin during membrane vesiculation and after stimulation by lipopolysaccharide. *Br J Haematol* 1997;96:534–542.

381. McCachren SS, Diggs J, Weinberg JB, et al. Thrombomodulin expression by human blood monocytes and by human synovial tissue lining macrophages. *Blood* 1991;78:3128–3132.

382. Maruyama I, Bell CE, Majerus PW. Thrombomodulin is found on endothelium of arteries, veins, capillaries, lymphatics, and on syncytiotrophoblast of human placenta. *J Cell Biol* 1985;101:363–371.

383. Ishii H, Salem HH, Bell CE, et al. Thrombomodulin, an endothelial anticoagulant protein, is absent from the human brain. *Blood* 1986;67:362–365.

384. Hoskins J, Norman DK, Beckmann RJ, et al. Cloning and characterization of human liver cDNA encoding a protein S precursor. *Proc Natl Acad Sci U S A* 1987;84:349–353.

385. Maillard C, Berruyer M, Serre CM, et al. Protein-S, a vitamin K-dependent protein, is a bone matrix component synthesized and secreted by osteoblasts. *Endocrinology* 1992;130:1599–1604.

386. Malm J, He X, Bjartell A, et al. Vitamin K-dependent protein S in Leydig cells of human testis. *Biochem J* 1994;302:845–850.

387. Fair DS, Marlar RA, Levin EG. Human endothelial cells synthesize protein S. *Blood* 1986;67:68–71.

388. Stern DM, Brett J, Harris K, et al. Participation of endothelial cells in the protein C-protein S anticoagulant pathway: the synthesis and release of protein S. *J Cell Biol* 1986;102:1971–1978.

389. Hooper WC, Phillips DJ, Ribeiro MJA, et al. Tumor necrosis factor -α downregulates protein S secretion in human microvascular and umbilical vein endothelial cells but not in the HepG-2 hepatoma cell line. *Blood* 1994;84:483–489.

390. Schwarz HP, Heeb MJ, Wencel-Drake JD, et al. Identification and quantitation of protein S in human platelets. *Blood* 1985;66:1452–1455.

391. Smiley ST, Boyer SN, Heeb MJ, et al. Protein S is inducible by interleukin 4 in T cells and inhibits lymphoid cell procoagulant activity. *Proc Natl Acad Sci U S A* 1997;94:11484–11489.

392. Smiley ST, Stitt TN, Grusby MJ. Cross-linking of protein S bound to lymphocytes promotes aggregation and inhibits proliferation. *Cell Immunol* 1997;181:120–126.

393. He X, Shen L, Bjartell A, et al. The gene encoding vitamin K-dependent anticoagulant protein S is expressed in multiple rabbit organs as demonstrated by northern blotting, in situ hybridization, and immunohistochemistry. *J Histochem Cytochem* 1995;43(1):85–96.

394. Tanabe S, Sugo T, Matsuda M. Synthesis of protein C in human umbilical vein endothelial cells. *J Biochem (Tokyo)* 1991;109:924–928.

395. Ginsberg JS, Wells P, Brill-Edwards P, et al. Antiphospholipid antibodies and venous thromboembolism. *Blood* 1995;86:3685–3691.

396. Esmon CT. Inflammation and thrombosis: mutual regulation linked through the protein C anticoagulant pathway. *Immunologist* 1998;6:84–89.

397. Okajima K. Regulation of inflammatory responses by natural anticoagulants. *Immunol Rev* 2001;184:258–274.

398. Joyce DE, Gelbert L, Ciaccia A, et al. Gene expression profile of antithrombotic protein C defines new mechanisms modulating inflammation and apoptosis. *J Biol Chem* 2001;276:11199–11203.

399. Riewald M, Petrovan RJ, Donner A, et al. Activation of endothelial cell protease activated receptor 1 by the protein C pathway. *Science* 2002;296: 1880–1882.

400. Cheng T, Liu D, Griffin JH, et al. Activated protein C blocks p53-mediated apoptosis in ischemic human brain endothelium and is neuroprotective. *Nat Med* 2003;9:338–342.

401. Shibata M, Kumar SR, Amar A, et al. Anti-inflammatory, antithrombotic, and neuroprotective effects of activated protein C in a murine model of focal ischemic stroke. *Circulation* 2001;103:1799–1805.

402. Malyszko J, Skrzydlewska E, Malyszko S, et al. Protein Z, a vitamin K-dependent protein in patients with renal failure. *J Thromb Haemost* 2003;1:195–196.

403. Macko RF, Ameriso SF, Gruber A, et al. Impairments of the protein C system and fibrinolysis in infection-associated stroke. *Stroke* 1996;27:2005–2011.

404. Ettingshausen CE, Halimeh S, Kurnik K, et al. Symptomatic onset of severe hemophilia A in childhood is dependent on the presence of prothrombotic risk factors. *Thromb Haemost* 2001;85:218–220.

405. Bernard GR, Vincent JL, Laterre PF, et al. Efficacy and safety of recombinant human activated protein C for severe sepsis. *N Engl J Med* 2001; 344:699–709.

406. Kerlin BA, Yan SB, Isermann BH, et al. Survival advantage associated with heterozygous factor V Leiden mutation in patients with severe sepsis and in mouse endotoxemia. *Blood* 2003;102:3085–3092.

407. Hyde E, Wetmore H, Gurewich V. Isolation and characterization of an *in vivo* thrombin-induced anticoagulant activity. *Scand J Haematol* 1974; 13:121.

408. Comp PC, Jacocks RM, Ferrell GL, et al. Activation of protein C *in vivo*. *J Clin Invest* 1982;70:127–134.

409. Taylor FB Jr, Chang A, Esmon CT. Protein C prevents the coagulopathic and lethal effects of *E. coli* infusion in the baboon. *J Clin Invest* 1987;79: 918–925.

410. Hancock WW, Tsuchida A, Hau H, et al. The anticoagulants protein C and protein S display potent anti-inflammatory and immunosuppressive effects relevant to transplant biology and therapy. *Transplant Proc* 1992; 24:2302–2303.

411. Hataji O, Taguchi O, Gabazza EC, et al. Activation of protein C pathway in the airways. *Lung* 2002;180:47–59.

412. Yasui H, Gabazza EC, Tamaki S, et al. Intratracheal administration of activated protein C inhibits bleomycin-induced lung fibrosis in the mouse. *Am J Respir Crit Care Med* 2001;163:1660–1668.

413. Esmon CT, Taylor FB Jr, Snow TR. Inflammation and coagulation: linked processes potentially regulated through a common pathway mediated by protein C. *Thromb Haemost* 1991;66:160–165.

414. Taoka Y, Okajima K, Uchiba M, et al. Activated protein C reduces the severity of compression-induced spinal cord injury in rats by inhibiting activation of leukocytes. *J Neurosci* 1998;18:1393–1398.

415. Grey ST, Tsuchida A, Hau H, et al. Selective inhibitory effects of the anticoagulant activated protein C on the responses of human mononuclear phagocytes to LPS, IFN-gamma, or phorbol ester. *J Immunol* 1994;153: 3664–3672.

416. Hancock WW, Grey ST, Hau L, et al. Binding of activated protein C to a specific receptor on human mononuclear phagocytes inhibits intracellular calcium signaling and monocyte-dependent proliferative responses. *Transplantation* 1995;60:1525–1532.

417. Ahmad MF, Bach FH, Esmon CT, et al. Cloning and *in vitro* analysis of the endothelial protein C receptor (EPCR) on human monocytes show that monocyte EPCR does not mediate the anti-inflammatory effects of activated protein C. Abstract. *Blood* 1997;90:32a.

418. Oida K, Tohda G, Ishii H, et al. Effect of oxidized low density lipoprotein on thrombomodulin expression by THP-1 cells. *Thromb Haemost* 1997; 78:1228–1233.

419. Grey ST, Hancock WW. A physiologic anti-inflammatory pathway based on thrombomodulin expression and generation of activated protein C by human mononuclear phagocytes. *J Immunol* 1996;156:2256–2263.

420. Faust SN, Levin M, Harrison OB, et al. Dysfunction of endothelial protein C activation in severe meningococcal sepsis. *N Engl J Med* 2001; 345:408–416.

421. Liaw PCY, Ferrell G, Esmon CT. A monoclonal antibody against activated protein C allows rapid detection of activated protein C in plasma and reveals a calcium ion dependent epitope involved in factor Va inactivation. *J Thromb Haemost* 2003;1:662–670.

422. Bode W, Mayr I, Baumann U, et al. The refined 1.9 Å crystal structure of human α-thrombin: interaction with D-Phe-Pro-Arg chlorometheylketone and significance of the Tyr-Pro-Pro-Trp insertion segment. *EMBO J* 1989; 8:3467–3475.

423. Bacon DJ, Anderson WF. A fast algorithm for rendering spacefilling molecule pictures. *J Mol Graph Model* 1988;6:219–220.

424. Kraulis PJ. Molscript: a program to produce both detailed and schematic plots of protein structures. *J Appl Cryst* 1991;24:946–950.

425. Nicholls A, Bharadwaj R, Honig B. GRASP-graphical representation and analysis of surface properties. *Biophys J* 1993;64:A166.

# CHAPTER 15 ■ HEPARIN AND VASCULAR PROTEOGLYCANS

DOUGLAS M. TOLLEFSEN AND LIJUAN ZHANG

Heparin is a sulfated glycosaminoglycan isolated from mammalian tissues that are rich in mast cells. When administered intravenously, heparin binds to the plasma protein antithrombin (previously known as antithrombin III), causing it to rapidly inhibit proteases of the intrinsic and common coagulation pathways. This interaction produces a potent anticoagulant effect. Endogenous heparinlike molecules appear to be involved in the inhibition of coagulation within normal blood vessels and may have a variety of other biologic functions. Although heparin is an effective agent for the treatment of venous thromboembolic disease, unstable angina, and acute myocardial infarction, it occasionally produces life-threatening bleeding or triggers an immune reaction, causing thrombocytopenia associated with venous and arterial thrombosis.

## HISTORICAL OVERVIEW

The term *heparin* was used by Howell in 1923 to describe an aqueous extract of canine liver that inhibited coagulation of blood *in vitro* (1). These extracts later were shown to consist of mixtures of sulfated polysaccharides containing uronic acid and glucosamine (2). The suggestion that heparin might be used to treat thromboembolism was initially greeted with skepticism because of the fear that patients given heparin would bleed to death. According to Jaques (3), this fear was allayed by a dramatic demonstration conducted by Charles Best at the University of Toronto in 1937:

> Best asked me [Jaques] to anesthetize a dog, prepare it for laparotomy, and inject heparin intravenously. When the most illustrious surgeons in the world arrived, Best explained what I had done (a blood sample which I had taken was incoagulable). Best then picked up a scalpel and handed it to Dr. Balfour with the request that he make a midline incision. The surgeons, properly dressed in their morning suits, jumped back, whereupon Best made the incision and I applied haemostats to two tiny bleeding points and showed a clean dry incision. Within months of this demonstration, surgeons all over the world took up heparin enthusiastically.

Canadian and Swedish investigators reported success in the use of heparin to treat recurrent thrombosis and pulmonary embolism in 1939 (2,4). The indications for heparin were soon expanded to include vascular surgical procedures, extracorporeal circulation, and prophylaxis of thromboembolism.

Despite the ensuing widespread clinical use of heparin, its mechanism of action remained obscure for several decades. As early as 1895, "thrombin" had been observed to lose activity gradually when added to defibrinated plasma or serum (5); this inhibitory potential became known as the progressive antithrombin activity. In 1939, Brinkhous et al. showed that heparin was effective as an anticoagulant only in the presence of a nondialyzable plasma component that they termed *heparin cofactor* (6). These early observations were linked in 1968, when Abildgaard reported that a single protein

(i.e., antithrombin) isolated from human plasma possessed both progressive antithrombin and heparin cofactor activity (7). Rosenberg and Damus purified larger quantities of antithrombin, enabling a more detailed physicochemical characterization of the protein (8). Subsequently, a second protein with heparin cofactor activity was purified from plasma by Tollefsen et al. and termed *heparin cofactor II* (HCII) (9).

In the sections that follow, we discuss the structure, biosynthesis, and isolation of heparin and heparan sulfate (HS); the synthesis of anticoagulantly active heparan sulfate proteoglycans (HSPGs) by endothelial cells; the physiologic role of the heparin–antithrombin system; some of the nonanticoagulant actions of heparin; the synthesis of anticoagulant heparin analogs; and the interaction of HCII with glycosaminoglycans. A discussion of the structures and mechanisms of action of antithrombin and HCII is presented in Chapter 13.

## STRUCTURE, BIOSYNTHESIS, AND ISOLATION OF HEPARIN AND HEPARAN SULFATE

Heparin is a highly sulfated polymer built on a backbone of alternating D-glucuronic acid and N-acetyl-D-glucosamine residues (10,11) that is widely distributed in the animal kingdom, being found in both vertebrates and invertebrates (12). In mammals, heparin is initially synthesized in mast cells as a heparin proteoglycan in which multiple heparin chains, each containing 100 to 150 disaccharide units, are covalently linked to a core protein called *serglycin* (13,14). Once generated, the heparin proteoglycan is degraded by three different types of lysosomal enzymes: (i) proteases that cleave the polypeptide chain; (ii) endoglycosidases that cut the heparin chain between glucuronic acid and glucosamine residues; and (iii) exoglycosidases that remove monosaccharide units from the nonreducing ends of heparin oligosaccharides (15). The degraded products are then stored in the secretory granules of mast cells, which are widely distributed in a variety of organs, including the liver, heart, lungs, kidneys, and intestine.

Pharmaceutical grade heparin is usually isolated from mammalian tissues such as the lung or intestinal mucosa. Preparation of the polysaccharide involves homogenization of tissues; treatment of the resultant material with proteolytic enzymes, such as papain, or extraction at elevated pH and temperature; differential precipitation of complex sugars with quaternary ammonium salts such as cetylpyridinium chloride; and chromatography of the substances on anion exchange resins such as QAE-Sephadex (16). The purified products behave as single glycosaminoglycan chains with molecular weights varying from approximately 3,000 to 35,000, with a mean of approximately 12,000. If oxidizing agents have been avoided during the purification procedure, approximately 15% to 30% of the polysaccharide chains remain covalently linked to fragments of the core protein. The remainder have free uronic acid or glucosamine reducing groups. This suggests that the polysaccharide species are generated by cleavage of the larger individual polysaccharide chains of the heparin proteoglycan at three to five separate sites. In most commercial preparations of heparin, oxidizing agents are used late in the isolation procedure to "bleach" the polysaccharide. This treatment appears to be responsible for the absence of protein linkage regions within these preparations.

Mammalian cells also synthesize HSPGs that consist of core proteins with covalently attached HS chains of 50 to 150 disaccharide units (17). Both heparin and HS chains exhibit structural diversity, which arises from various patterns of N-sulfation, N-acetylation, and O-sulfation of the disaccharide units. The distinction between heparin proteoglycan and HSPGs is based on (i) the structure of the core protein; (ii) the location of the glycoconjugate within the cell; and (iii) the relative amounts of N-acetylglucosamine and glucuronic acid present in the carbohydrate chains. In particular, the heparin core protein is small and relatively simple in structure with extended runs of Ser-Gly attachment sites (13,14,18), whereas HS core proteins are large and more diverse in structure (19) with short runs of Ser-Gly or closely spaced Ser-Gly attachment sites (20); heparin proteoglycan is found within mast cell granules, whereas HSPGs are located on cell surfaces or in the surrounding matrix (21); and heparin contains larger amounts of N-sulfate, O-sulfate, and iduronic acid, whereas HS is less extensively modified.

Biosynthesis of a heparin or HS proteoglycan occurs in the Golgi apparatus and is initiated by attachment of a linkage region tetrasaccharide containing one xylose, two galactose, and one glucuronic acid to the serine hydroxyl group of a Ser-Gly (or Ala) dipeptide in the core protein (10,11). The formation of heparin/HS chains depends on nearby acidic or hydrophobic residues or close spacing of Ser-Gly sites (20–22). In humans, the heparin core protein serglycin contains an extended run of eight Ser-Gly repeats, in which virtually all of the Ser residues

become modified with the linkage region tetrasaccharide. The tetrasaccharide is synthesized by the sequential action of four glycosyltransferases (xylosyltransferase, galactosyltransferase I, galactosyltransferase II, and glucuronyltransferase I) that use uridine diphosphate (UDP) sugars as their substrates. The structures of serglycin and its linkage region are depicted in Figure 15-1.

Immediately after formation of the linkage region tetrasaccharide, α-N-acetylglucosaminyltransferase I adds an N-acetylglucosamine residue and thereby commits the nascent chain to the heparin/HS biosynthetic pathway (see Fig. 15-2) (11). Linkage region tetrasaccharides on other core proteins can be modified at this stage by β-N-acetylgalactosaminyltransferase I, resulting in biosynthesis of chondroitin sulfate or dermatan sulfate chains (21). The heparin/HS chain is assembled by the alternate incorporation of glucuronic acid and N-acetylglucosamine from the corresponding UDP sugars. This is accomplished through the action of copolymerases that are members of the *EXT* gene family having β-glucosaminyltransferase II and α-N-acetyl-glucosaminyltransferase II activities. Thereafter, this simple copolymer is modified by a concerted process that leads to different modifications in various regions of the glycosaminoglycan chain.

First, glucosamine residues are partially N-deacetylated, and the exposed amino groups serve as acceptors of sulfate groups in a transfer reaction with 3'-phosphoadenosine-5'-phosphosulfate (PAPS). These two reactions are carried out by a bifunctional enzyme, N-acetylglucosamine N-deacetylase/N-sulfotransferase (NDST), which is composed of a single polypeptide chain. Four isoforms of human NDST (NDST-1, -2, -3, and -4) have been identified, differing in their expression in various tissues and in their relative N-deacetylase and N-sulfotransferase activities (23). Mice that lack NDST-2 do not synthesize mast cell heparin but produce HS (24,25), whereas mice that lack NDST-1 produce undersulfated HS and die at birth of lung failure (26,27). At this stage of biosynthesis, the nascent heparin or HS polymer contains stretches of N-sulfoglucosamine interspersed with unmodified N-acetylglucosamine residues.

**A** 1     MMQKLLKCSR LVLALALILV LESSVQGYPT QRARYQWVRC NPDSNSANCL EEKGPMFELL

    61     PGESNKIPRL RTDLFPKTRI QDLNRIFPLS EDY⎡SGSG⎤FG⎡S GSGSGSGSGS G⎤FLTEMEQDY

  121    QLVDESDAFH DNLRSLDRNL PSDSQDLGQH GLEEDFML

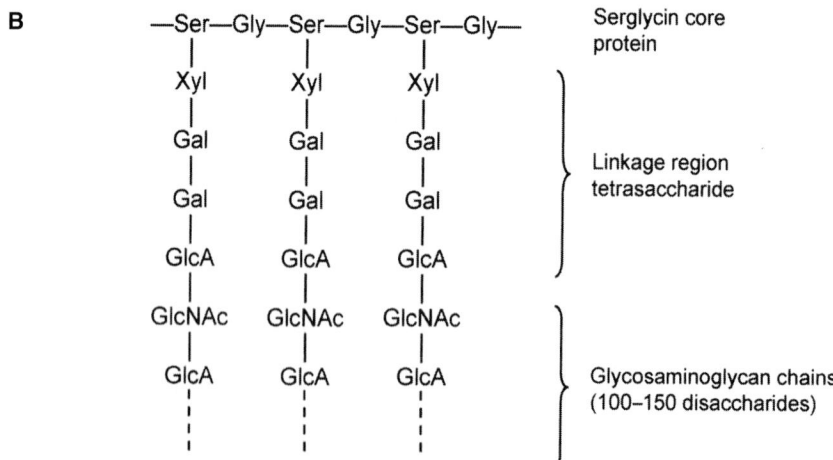

**FIGURE 15-1.** Heparin proteoglycan structure. **A:** Amino acid sequence of the human serglycin core protein. The boxed residues comprise the glycosaminoglycan attachment sites. **B:** Structure of the linkage region. Ser, serine; Gly, glycine; Xyl, xylose; Gal, galactose; GlcA, glucuronic acid; GlcNAc, N-acetyl-glucosamine.

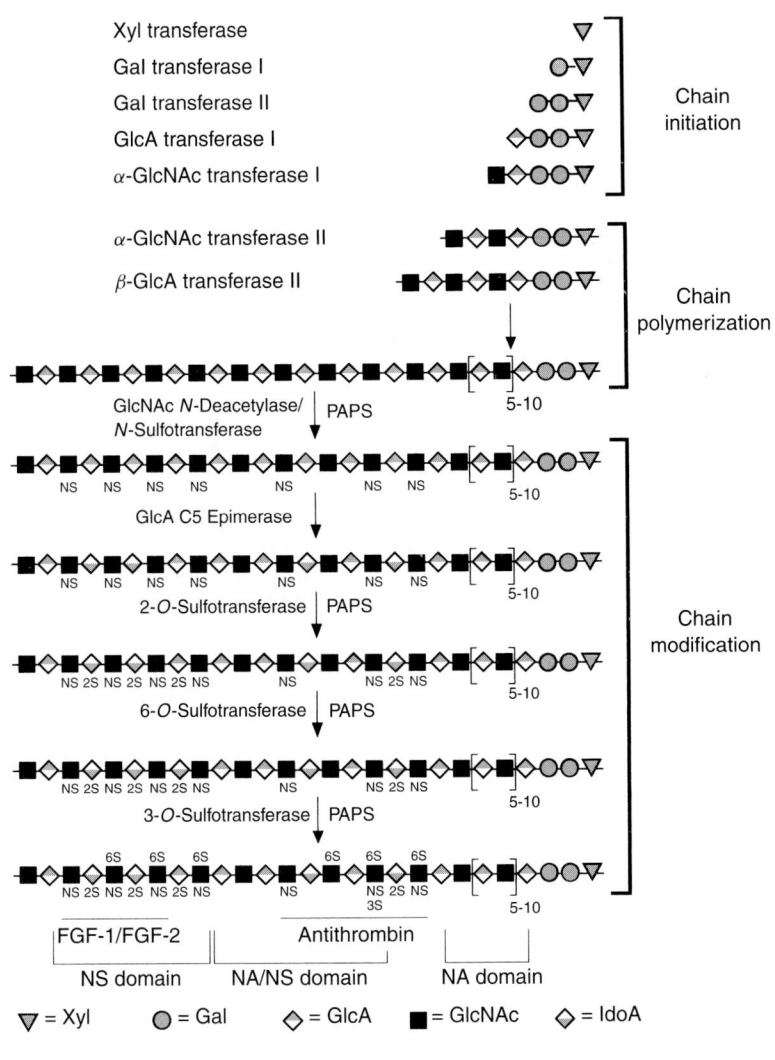

**FIGURE 15-2.** Heparin/heparan sulfate biosynthesis. The symbols are defined by the structures shown below the scheme. Representative tracts of contiguous N-acetylated disaccharide units (NA domains), contiguous N-sulfated sequences of variable length (NS domains), and alternating N-acetylated and N-sulfated units (NA/NS domains) in HS are indicated. Heparin is predominantly composed of a single, extended NS domain. Regions that have been implicated in binding of fibroblast growth factors FGF-1/ FGF-2 and antithrombin are shown. IdoA, iduronic acid; PAPS, 3'-phosphoadenosine-5'-phosphosulfate. Other abbreviations are defined in the legend to Figure 15-1. (Reprinted from Esko JD, Lindahl U. Molecular diversity of heparan sulfate. *J Clin Invest* 2001;108:169–173, with permission.)

Next, glucuronic acid residues are variably epimerized to iduronic acid by glucuronyl C5-epimerase. Then the iduronic acid residues and, to a lesser extent, glucuronic acid residues are partially O-sulfated at the C2-position. Finally, the glucosamine moieties are O-sulfated to a variable extent at the C6 and the C3-positions. Epimerization and O-sulfation occur only in regions of the polymer that contain N-sulfoglucosamine, but these modifications are incomplete. As a result, a wide variety of oligosaccharide structures can be formed, each having the ability to interact with a different protein (e.g., antithrombin) or class of proteins (e.g., fibroblast growth factors or viral capsid proteins) (10). One HS 2-O-sulfotransferase, three HS

6-O-sulfotransferases, and six HS 3-O-sulfotransferases have been identified in humans (23). Multiple isoforms make possible tissue-specific and developmentally regulated expression of the corresponding enzyme activities. Because the enzymatic properties of the isoforms may differ in subtle ways, their selective expression may be responsible for unique oligosaccharide sequences found in heparin/HS in different tissues and different animals. For example, 3-O-sulfotransferase-1 is primarily responsible for sulfation of the C3-position of glucosamine in the sequence GlcA-GlcNS, which gives rise to the high-affinity antithrombin-binding site (discussed in the subsequent text).

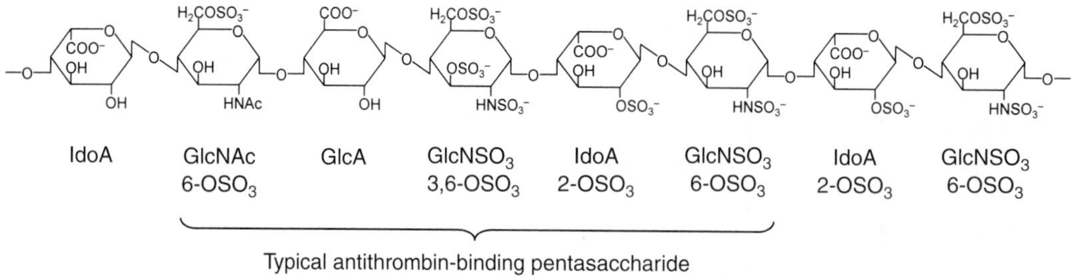

**FIGURE 15-3.** Representative region of a heparin chain containing a typical antithrombin-binding sequence. IdoA, iduronic acid; GlcA, glucuronic acid; GrcNAc, N-acetyl-glucosamine.

# ANTITHROMBIN-BINDING SEQUENCES IN HEPARIN

A segment of a heparin chain containing an antithrombin-binding site is depicted in Figure 15-3. It is important to emphasize that this sequence is only one of many possible arrangements of uronic acid and glucosamine moieties found elsewhere in the polymer. As progress was being made in defining various aspects of the biosynthesis, linear sequence, and three-dimensional configuration of heparin and HS, it was tacitly assumed that heparin may exhibit numerous alternative structures equally capable of interacting with antithrombin (28). This assumption was shown to be incorrect in 1976, when several groups demonstrated that only approximately 30% of commercial heparin is able to bind to antithrombin but that the bound fraction is responsible for virtually all of the anticoagulant activity (29–31).

These findings led to investigations designed to determine the structural differences between high-affinity (active) and low-affinity (inactive) heparin species (28). Briefly, Rosenberg et al. showed that oligosaccharides produced from high-affinity heparin were enriched in a tetrasaccharide sequence that contained glucuronic acid and N-acetylglucosamine (32). Leder isolated an enzyme that removes sulfate from the 3-O position of glucosamine (33), and Lindahl et al. showed that this substituent is critical for high-affinity binding of heparin to antithrombin (34). These observations were confirmed and extended by Choay et al. who synthesized a series of pentasaccharides that are able to catalyze the factor Xa–antithrombin reaction (35, 36). The contributions of individual substituents within the antithrombin-binding pentasaccharide have been evaluated by comparing the avidity of synthetic oligosaccharides for antithrombin (37). On the basis of these data, the relative importance of individual residues is shown in Figure 15-4. The presence of an N-sulfate in place of the N-acetyl group on the first glucosamine residue increases the affinity for antithrombin approximately twofold. Similarly, the 2-O-sulfate and 6-O-sulfate groups on the fourth and fifth residues of the pentasaccharide increase the affinity but are not absolutely required for high-affinity binding. Therefore, some variability in the structure of heparin at these sites is compatible with antithrombin binding and anticoagulant activity. In contrast, certain structures are critical for antithrombin binding, including the presence and orientation of carboxylate groups on the two uronic acid residues, the 6-O-sulfate on the first glucosamine, the 3-O-sulfate and N-sulfate on the middle glucosamine, and the N-sulfate on the last glucosamine of the pentasaccharide.

Although synthetic heparin pentasaccharides that bind to antithrombin with high affinity accelerate the factor Xa–antithrombin interaction, they do not significantly increase the rate of neutralization of thrombin or other hemostatic enzymes. Isolation of oligosaccharides derived from partial chemical depolymerization of heparin revealed that molecules at least 16 monosaccharide units in length are required to accelerate both the thrombin–antithrombin and factor Xa–antithrombin interactions (38). For inhibition of factor Xa to occur, it is sufficient to form a binary complex between heparin and antithrombin that leads to a conformational change in the reactive site loop of the inhibitor. To facilitate thrombin inhibition, however, longer heparin chains must bind simultaneously to thrombin

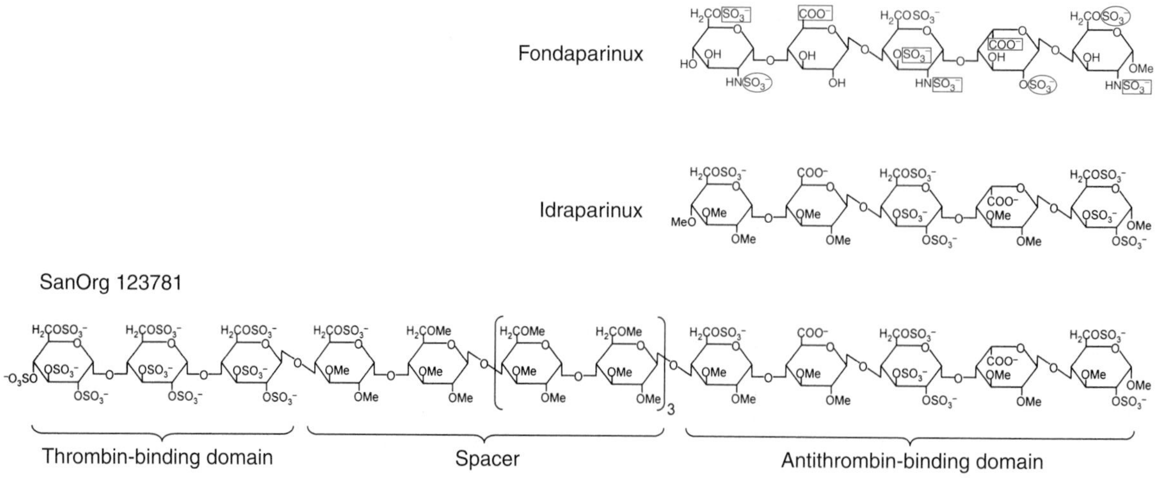

**FIGURE 15-4.** Synthetic heparinlike oligosaccharides. Sulfate and carboxylate groups required for high-affinity binding to antithrombin are indicated by *boxes* in the structure of fondaparinux. Sulfate groups that are not essential but that contribute to high-affinity binding are *circled*.

and antithrombin to form a ternary thrombin–heparin–antithrombin complex. These differences in mechanism of inhibition explain why smaller heparin molecules can inhibit factor Xa while failing to inhibit thrombin. The inhibitory mechanism of antithrombin is discussed in more detail in Chapter 13.

# SYNTHESIS OF ANTICOAGULANTLY ACTIVE HEPARAN SULFATE PROTEOGLYCANS BY ENDOTHELIAL CELLS

Mast cells were once thought to be the only site of synthesis of anticoagulantly active heparin. These cells are located beneath the endothelium and sequester heparin within their secretory granules (39), where it forms crystalline arrays with cationic molecules such as histamine and neutral proteases. Ordinarily, heparin is not released from mast cells into the circulation; one exception may be patients with systemic mastocytosis, in whom small amounts of heparin can appear in the bloodstream and slightly prolong the activated partial thromboplastin time (40). Therefore, mast cell heparin is unlikely to affect hemostasis under normal circumstances. These considerations led to the suggestion that endothelial cells might synthesize HSPGs endowed with the critical oligosaccharide structure required to bind and activate antithrombin (41). In parallel investigations of the structure of anticoagulantly active mast cell heparin, HSPGs synthesized by endothelial cells were shown to contain a small subpopulation (approximately 1%) of HS (HS$^{act}$) that binds antithrombin with high affinity and accelerates inhibition of thrombin and factor Xa by antithrombin in vitro (42). As discussed in the following section, these studies suggested that HS$^{act}$ might be a major physiologic modulator of hemostasis.

Early investigations revealed that HS is present in the aorta and other vessels and exhibits trace amounts of anticoagulant activity (43,44). It proved difficult, however, to rule out the possibility that mast cells were the source of this material. Direct evidence that endothelial cells are able to generate anticoagulantly active HSPGs was eventually obtained by Marcum and Rosenberg, who studied cloned microvascular endothelial cells isolated from the rat epididymal fat pad (45). They showed that polysaccharides extracted from these cells possessed antithrombin accelerating activity that could be completely eliminated by treatment with purified Flavobacterium heparinase. Virtually all of the heparinlike material could be harvested by a brief exposure of the endothelial cells to dilute trypsin, which suggested that these components are located on the cell surface. Furthermore, metabolic labeling of the polysaccharides with [$^{35}$S]sulfate, followed by affinity fractionation with antithrombin and structural analysis, revealed the presence of oligosaccharide structures typically found in anticoagulantly active commercial heparin. Similar studies conducted with cloned bovine aortic endothelial cells gave virtually identical results and indicated that the level of anticoagulantly active HS species present would correspond to approximately 50,000 antithrombin-binding sites per endothelial cell (46). This estimate of surface-bound anticoagulantly active polysaccharide was in excellent agreement with the data generated by characterization of the interactions of antithrombin with bovine aortic tissue sections.

Two major endothelial cell core proteins that are endowed with anticoagulantly active HS chains have been characterized. Kojima et al. isolated intact HSPGs from rat microvascular endothelial cells using a combination of ion-exchange chromatography, affinity fractionation with antithrombin, and gel filtration in denaturing solvents (47). The anticoagulantly active HSPGs

bound to antithrombin constituted approximately 5% the of total HSPGs and were endowed almost entirely with anticoagulantly active HS chains, whereas the anticoagulantly inactive HSPGs that did not interact with antithrombin represented approximately 95% of the total HSPGs. The two types of HS chains had the same molecular mass of approximately 25 to 30 kDa, and the anticoagulantly active HS chains possessed a single antithrombin-binding region. The core proteins of the anticoagulantly active and inactive HSPGs (HSPG$^{act}$ and HSPG$^{inact}$) were isolated after treatment with Flavobacterium heparitinase and purification by ion-exchange chromatography. Peptide mapping studies suggested that HSPG$^{act}$ and HSPG$^{inact}$ contained the same two major core proteins with molecular masses of 50 kDa and 30 kDa.

The primary sequences of internal peptides derived from the HSPG core proteins were used to molecularly clone two cDNAs from a rat microvascular endothelial cell library (48). The first cDNA constituted a previously unidentified species, termed syndecan-4 (ryudocan), whereas the second cDNA represented the rat ortholog of syndecan-1. The latter molecule was a known proteoglycan that was originally thought to be limited in its distribution to epithelial cells. The two cDNAs encode integral membrane proteins of 202 amino acids (syndecan-4) and 313 amino acids (syndecan-1), respectively, which have extraordinarily homologous transmembrane and intracellular domains but very distinct extracellular regions. Syndecan-4 has three potential glycosaminoglycan attachment sites in its extracellular domain, whereas syndecan-1 has five. Both molecules are expressed at high levels (0.1% to 0.5% of total mRNA) in primary endothelial cells, primary smooth muscle cells, and primary fibroblasts. The possibility that slightly different core proteins direct the synthesis of HSPG$^{act}$ and HSPG$^{inact}$ was excluded by stably expressing an epitope-tagged syndecan-4 in cells that synthesize anticoagulantly active and anticoagulantly inactive HS chains; after isolation of the proteoglycan with a specific antibody against the epitope, both HS$^{act}$ and HS$^{inact}$ were found to be present (49). This finding suggested that the presence of HS biosynthetic enzymes rather than expression of specific core proteins determine the fine structure of the HS chains. Further studies suggested that in addition to syndecan-1 and syndecan-4, glypican-1 (50) and perlecan (51) synthesized by endothelial cells also bear anticoagulantly active HS chains.

The HS biosynthetic pathway generates limiting amounts of anticoagulant HSPGs with regions of defined structure that contain the antithrombin-binding site; this pathway also produces the more abundant nonanticoagulant HSPGs with regions of varying structure that carry out other biologic functions. Analyses of cell mutants, created by overexpression of the syndecan-4 core protein or by chemical mutagenesis, revealed that anticoagulant HS generation requires a component present in limiting amounts (52,53). To identify this component, a cell-free system was developed by Shworak et al. in which wild-type microsomes were incubated with radiolabeled HSPG precursor extracted from mutant cells blocked during anticoagulant HSPG generation (54); coincubation of these two extracts resulted in the production of large amounts of anticoagulant HSPG. Furthermore, in many different cell types the concentration of this "microsomal conversion activity" correlated with the cell's ability to generate anticoagulant HSPG. Treatment of microsomal and cell surface HSPGs from wild-type cells with excess microsomal conversion activity transformed up to 35% of total HSPGs into anticoagulant HSPG. This extent of conversion was much greater than the normal levels of cell surface anticoagulant HSPGs, which average approximately 1% to 5% of total HSPGs (54). These investigations provided evidence that a microsomal component limits transformation of small amounts of a HSPG precursor population into anticoagulant HSPGs.

The assay described in the preceding text was then used to isolate the limiting component, which proved to be the long-sought glucosaminyl 3-O-sulfotransferase-1 (3-OST-1) (55,56). This enzyme usually is present in trace amounts as compared to other HS biosynthetic enzymes. When 3-OST-1 is no longer limiting, the cell's capacity to generate HS[act] is determined by the abundance of HS[act] precursors (57). In vitro 3-O-sulfation with purified 3-OST-1 was used to tag the regions of the HS[act] precursors destined to become antithrombin-binding sites and allow the HS[act] precursors to be captured. The tagged regions were then structurally examined (58). It was shown that six 3-O-sulfation sites existed per HS[act] precursor chain. At least five out of the six 3-O-sulfate-tagged oligosaccharides in HS[act] precursors bound antithrombin, whereas none of 3-O-sulfate-tagged oligosaccharides from HS[inact] precursors bound antithrombin. When treated with low pH nitrous acid or heparitinase, 3-O-sulfate-tagged HS[act] and HS[inact] precursors exhibited clearly different structural features: they had different uronic acid epimerization and O-sulfation patterns around the 3-O-sulfate acceptor sites. 3-O-sulfate-tagged HS[act] hexasaccharides were antithrombin affinity purified, sequenced by chemical and enzymatic degradation, and shown to have structures compatible with the antithrombin-binding sequence illustrated in Figure 15-3. The differences in structure surrounding potential 3-O-sulfate acceptor sites in HS[act] and HS[inact] precursors suggested that these precursors might be generated by different concerted assembly mechanisms in the same cell (58).

## ANATOMIC LOCATION OF ANTICOAGULANTLY ACTIVE HEPARAN SULFATE PROTEOGLYCANS

The anatomic location of HSPG[act] was investigated by de Agostini et al., who perfused normal rat aorta for short periods of time with [125]I-antithrombin and observed that the labeled protein was bound to the aortic subendothelium (see Fig. 15-5) (59). Quantitation of the data revealed that only approximately 1% of the bound [125]I-antithrombin was associated with the luminal surface of the endothelium and that only small amounts were associated with smooth muscle cells or connective tissue deeper in the vessel wall. The labeled antithrombin was also noted to bind to regions around capillaries, especially in the subendothelium associated with the basal lamina/basement membrane. Perfusion of the aorta with [125]I-antithrombin-labeled bovine serum albumin produced no detectable binding, which indicated that the binding of [125]I-antithrombin within the aorta was not due to nonspecific interactions or trapping of the labeled protein. To demonstrate that the [125]I-antithrombin specifically interacted with HS chains, the vasculature was perfused with Flavobacterium heparinase before perfusion with labeled

antithrombin. This treatment effectively prevented any binding of [125]I-antithrombin to all regions, including the subendothelium, while leaving the endothelial layer intact.

These data were consistent with the known synthesis of HSPG[act] by endothelial cells and suggested that the proteoglycans are released from these cells and accumulate predominantly in the basement membrane. This observation suggested two possible ways in which coagulation system activity could be regulated by blood vessel wall HSPG[act]. On the one hand, the small amounts of luminal HSPG[act] could be in a critical position to bind and activate antithrombin and thereby regulate hemostatic activity at the blood–vessel wall interface. The much larger quantities of abluminal HSPG[act] could serve as a potential reservoir that could be brought into play with extensive damage to the overlying endothelium. On the other hand, plasma antithrombin may have relatively free access to the much greater amounts of HSPG[act] that accumulate on the abluminal surface of the endothelial cells, as suggested by studies that document the permeability of the endothelial cell layer (60). Indeed, the presence of [125]I-antithrombin bound to subendothelium after ex vivo perfusion suggests that this region is readily accessible to antithrombin. The accessibility of subendothelial HSPG[act] would also explain kinetic tracer data, which suggest that 10% to 20% of antithrombin partitions to an extravascular compartment (61). These observations imply that coagulation proteases might be inhibited by antithrombin bound to HSPG[act] in the subendothelium.

Marcum et al. obtained evidence that intact blood vessels possess HSPGs that stimulate the activity of plasma antithrombin (62). In their experiments, rat hindlimb preparations were perfused with purified thrombin at a constant level, and purified antithrombin was infused at several different concentrations. The amount of thrombin–antithrombin complex formed within the vasculature was estimated by a specific radioimmunoassay for the interaction product. The rate of complex formation was enhanced 19-fold in the animal with respect to the uncatalyzed rate in vitro. The antithrombin stimulating activity detected in the hindlimb vasculature appeared to be due to an HSPG, because the rate of thrombin–antithrombin complex formation was reduced to the uncatalyzed rate by pre-infusion of the vasculature with Flavobacterium heparinase. Furthermore, when the hindlimb preparation was perfused with antithrombin chemically modified at Trp49 to decrease its affinity for HS, complex formation also occurred at the uncatalyzed rate. Finally, when purified human platelet factor 4 (PF4) was added to the perfusion stream along with antithrombin, thrombin inhibition occurred at the uncatalyzed rate. These data suggested that PF4, after being released from activated platelets, may play a role in thrombogenesis by neutralizing anticoagulantly active vascular HSPGs. Similar results were obtained with mice genetically deficient in mast cells, strongly suggesting that mast cell heparin plays little or no role in this phenomenon (63).

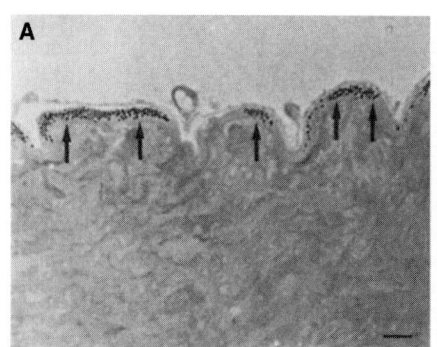
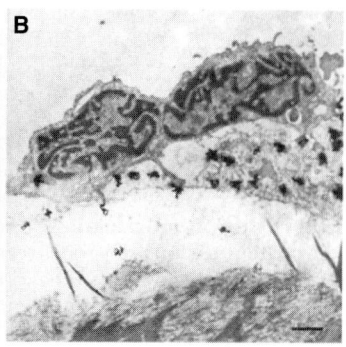

FIGURE 15-5. Autoradiography of normal rat aortas perfused with [125]I-antithrombin. A: Light microscopic autoradiograph. Intense labeling is present in the basement membrane beneath the endothelial cells (arrows). Bar, 10 μm. B: Electron microscopic autoradiograph. Labeling is again evident beneath the endothelium. Bar, 1.0 μm. (Reprinted from de Agostini AI, Watkins SC, Slayter HS, et al. Localization of anticoagulantly active heparan sulfate proteoglycans in vascular endothelium: antithrombin binding on cultured endothelial cells and perfused rat aorta. J Cell Biol 1990;111:1293–1304, with permission.)

In summary, it appeared likely that a small fraction of plasma antithrombin is normally bound to HSPG$^{act}$ associated with endothelial cells of the blood vessel wall. It was unclear whether the functionally important HSPGs are primarily the small amounts present on the luminal surface of the endothelium or the much larger quantities located in the subendothelial region, or both. In either case, the endothelial HSPGs could interact with antithrombin to produce an antithrombotic effect at blood–surface interfaces where coagulation proteases are commonly generated. Therefore, antithrombin would be in a position to protect surfaces lined by normal endothelium against thrombus formation. Furthermore, the catalytic nature of anticoagulantly active HS species would ensure the continual regeneration of the nonthrombogenic properties of the endothelial cell layer.

# THE PHENOTYPE OF 3-O-SULFOTRANSFERASE-1-DEFICIENT MICE

As discussed in the preceding section, a critical limiting factor in the biosynthesis of HS$^{act}$ is the presence of 3-OST-1, which creates the high-affinity antithrombin-binding motif by modification of selected regions within the HS polymer (55,56). 3-OST-5 can also generate HS$^{act}$, although much less efficiently than 3-OST-1 (64). Therefore, 3-OST-1 is likely to be the major enzyme responsible for generation of HS$^{act}$ in vivo. Mice lacking the gene that encodes 3-OST-1 (Hs3st1) were generated by HajMohammadi et al. to evaluate the biologic role of HS$^{act}$ (65). The absence of 3-OST-1 enzyme caused large reductions (75% to 98%) in HS$^{act}$ levels in most tissues as determined by the ability of HS purified from these tissues to accelerate inhibition of factor Xa by antithrombin. Unexpectedly, removal of most HS$^{act}$ did not alter the basal rate of fibrin generation in 3-OST-1–deficient mice, nor did it lead to enhanced fibrin deposition in the lungs under hypoxemic conditions known to produce a strong procoagulant stimulus. To evaluate the possibility that HS$^{act}$ plays a role only after endothelial injury, which might allow direct contact of the blood with the subendothelial matrix, mice were investigated in a carotid arterial injury model in which application of ferric chloride to the adventitia rapidly induces endothelial denudation leading to thrombosis. However, Hs3st1$^{-/-}$ and Hs3st1$^{+/+}$ mice had similar thrombotic occlusion times and equivalent postinjury levels of thrombin–antithrombin complexes, despite the virtual absence of HS$^{act}$ in the uninjured carotid artery of the Hs3st1$^{-/-}$ mice as determined by $^{125}$I-antithrombin binding.

Because 3-OST-1–deficient mice lack an obvious procoagulant phenotype, hemostatic balance does not appear to be tightly correlated with HS$^{act}$ levels. Whereas Hs3st1$^{-/-}$ mice appeared normal on a mixed C57BL/6 × 129S4/SvJae genetic background, intrauterine growth retardation and early postnatal lethality were observed in Hs3st1$^{-/-}$ mice backcrossed into the C57BL/6 background. Although the cause of neonatal mortality in these mice is unclear, histologic examination did not reveal evidence of focal thrombosis as seen in antithrombin-deficient embryos (66), which further suggests a lack of association between 3-OST-1 and antithrombin activity. The unexplained phenotype of Hs3st1$^{-/-}$ mice raises the possibility that HS$^{act}$ participates in a novel biologic function(s). Indeed, recent analyses of Drosophila deficient in the orthologous enzyme, 3-O-sulfotransferase-B, suggest a critical role in Notch signaling pathways (67). Novel functions might even occur outside of the vascular system, because 3-OST-1–derived HS$^{act}$ is produced in several nonendothelial cell types (57, 68,69).

The lack of a prothrombotic phenotype in 3-OST-1 knockout mice challenges the concept that HS$^{act}$ plays a major role in hemostasis. However, unprovoked thrombosis occurs in humans or mice homozygous for antithrombin mutations that reduce the inhibitor's affinity for HS (70,71). These findings suggest that HS binding is required for proper antithrombin function in vivo. How, then, could one explain the 3-OST-1 knockout data?

First, the residual 2% to 20% anticoagulant HS activity in the 3-OST-1–deficient mice likely reflects 3-O-sulfation by 3-O-sulfotransferase isoforms other than 3-OST-1. As indicated in the preceding text, 3-OST-5 might play an important role if hemostatic balance requires only low levels of HS$^{act}$ (64). Because the plasma antithrombin concentration (2 $\mu$M to 5 $\mu$M) greatly exceeds the dissociation constant of antithrombin for HS$^{act}$ (approximately 15 nM), small amounts of HS$^{act}$ might always be saturated with antithrombin and thereby exert a basal anticoagulant tone. Assessment of this possibility will require deletion of the gene for 3-OST-5, and perhaps other isoforms that may be responsible for synthesis of the HS$^{act}$ present in Hs3st$^{-/-}$ mice.

Second, HS$^{act}$ may not be responsible for the anticoagulant properties of HS in vivo. Scully et al. reported that HS, which failed to bind to a column of immobilized antithrombin (generally defined as HS$^{inact}$), accelerated the factor Xa-antithrombin reaction by 1,100-fold, although much higher concentrations were required in comparison with high-affinity HS (HS$^{act}$) (72). They proposed that the nonthrombogenic property of blood vessels is due to acceleration of the factor Xa–antithrombin interaction by the greater mass of vascular HS$^{inact}$ rather than by the much smaller proportion of HS$^{act}$ molecules. If this hypothesis is true, one would predict that defective HS synthesis would lead to a procoagulant phenotype. To complicate matters, HS interacts with a great variety of proteins other than antithrombin, and multiple functions have been attributed to HS throughout embryonic development, including interactions with the fibroblast growth factor (FGF), Wnt, TGF-$\beta$, and hedgehog (Hh) signaling pathways (73). Targeted disruption of EXT1, one of the genes responsible for HS chain polymerization, resulted in loss of HS, disruption of gastrulation, and embryonic lethality before embryonic day 8.5 (74). Conditional knockouts of EXT1 or other HS biosynthetic genes in vascular tissue at later stages of development could be more informative with regard to the hemostatic properties of HS but have not yet been achieved. Knockout of the syndecan-4 gene (Synd4) suggests that HS might be involved in anticoagulation of the placenta (75). Syndecan-4, a transmembrane protein bearing both HS$^{act}$ and HS$^{inact}$ chains, was detected in the fetal vessels of the placenta by in situ hybridization and immunohistochemical staining. During late gestation, degeneration of fetal vessels in the placental labyrinth was more extensive in Synd4$^{-/-}$ embryos than in wild-type controls and was associated with deposition of fibrin(ogen). These findings suggest that absence of syndecan-4 produces a deficit in placental anticoagulation.

Third, chondroitin sulfate or dermatan sulfate in the vessel wall might compensate for the reduction in anticoagulant HS activity in the 3-OST-1 knockout mouse. For example, the chondroitin sulfate moiety on thrombomodulin enhances the reactivity of thrombomodulin-bound thrombin with antithrombin (76,77), and dermatan sulfate may promote inhibition of thrombin by HCII in the carotid arterial injury model, as discussed in the subsequent text (78).

Fourth, HS$^{act}$ synthesized by 3-OST-1 might serve an anticoagulant role in a distinct subset of tissues or under pathologic conditions not yet examined (65).

Fifth, unmasking of an overt procoagulant effect might require a second genetic defect in addition to 3-OST-1 deficiency. For example, the combination of factor V$_{Leiden}$ and protein Z deficiency produces a much greater procoagulant phenotype than does either of the two deficiencies alone (79).

# SYNTHETIC HEPARINLIKE ANTICOAGULANT DRUGS

In the early 1980s, the total chemical synthesis of a pentasaccharide related to the antithrombin-binding domain in heparin was achieved in more than 60 individual steps by chemists at Sanofi and Organon (37). Extensive structure-activity studies using a variety of other synthetic oligosaccharides, as well as nuclear magnetic resonance (NMR) and x-ray crystallography were subsequently performed (80). On the basis of these studies, a concerted drug development effort was undertaken to develop the synthetic pentasaccharide fondaparinux, which has proven effective in human trials and is now used clinically as an anticoagulant drug (81) (Fig. 15-4). Fondaparinux mediates factor Xa inhibition by antithrombin but does not cause thrombin inhibition because of its short polymer length. In fact, fondaparinux has a stronger affinity for antithrombin and a higher anti-Xa activity in comparison with the most common antithrombin-binding pentasaccharide structure in porcine heparin. These differences have been attributed to the first glucosamine residue in fondaparinux being N-sulfated, whereas that of porcine heparin is N-acetylated. Fondaparinux does not interact significantly with platelets or with plasma proteins other than antithrombin and therefore has predictable pharmacokinetic behavior. Because it does not interact with PF4, fondaparinux is unlikely to trigger heparin-induced thrombocytopenia. A more highly sulfated derivative (idraparinux) with a longer half-life than fondaparinux is also being evaluated in clinical trials (82) (Fig. 15-4).

A careful analysis of heparin indicates that a synthetic polymer that could mimic heparin's full anticoagulant activity (i.e., inhibition of both thrombin and factor Xa) would need to have both an antithrombin-binding domain and a thrombin-binding domain. Thrombin binds nonspecifically to highly sulfated heparin oligosaccharides and to other anionic polymers. Therefore, heparin analogs have been synthesized to contain a highly sulfated oligosaccharide linked to the nonreducing end of an antithrombin-binding pentasaccharide through a neutral spacer region (83). In these compounds, N-sulfate groups were replaced by O-sulfates, and hydroxyl groups were alkylated, thereby greatly simplifying the synthetic process. The resulting compounds, one of which is depicted in Figure 15-4, catalyzed inhibition of thrombin by antithrombin and were fivefold to 10-fold more potent than standard heparin in in vivo models. This is probably because these compounds interact much less avidly with basic plasma proteins including PF4, thereby leaving more molecules available for binding to thrombin and antithrombin. More importantly, these compounds seem to have little effect on platelets; they do not activate platelets in the presence of plasma from patients with heparin-induced thrombocytopenia and do not affect the bleeding time of rats while still inhibiting thrombosis.

Enzymatic and chemoenzymatic methods have also been employed to synthesize heparinlike anticoagulants. Rosenberg's group has synthesized a series of potent anticoagulant heparin analogs by using a capsular bacterial polysaccharide (heparosan) obtained from Escherichia coli K5 and different mammalian-expressed HS sulfotransferases and epimerase with yields in the microgram range (84–86). This approach is currently limited by the high cost of the enzymes and the low yield compared to commercial heparin production.

Lindahl et al. have been able to generate gram amounts of "neoheparin" with antifactor Xa and antithrombin activities similar to those of heparin using chemoenzymatic modifications of heparosan (87). However, it is unknown whether the significant amounts of nonnaturally occurring 3-O-sulfated GlcA and IdoA residues in the neoheparin molecule might create undesirable side effects in vivo.

# NONANTICOAGULANT ACTIONS OF HEPARIN AND HEPARAN SULFATE

Heparin and HS have a wide variety of biologic actions that are independent of its anticoagulant effects. As one of the most acidic biopolymers found in nature, heparin interacts with hundreds of proteins such as growth factors, cytokines, chemokines, extracellular matrix components, protease inhibitors, proteases, and lipases (88). HS has been implicated in the control of many processes in multicellular organisms, including cell division, adhesion, spreading, migration, chemoattraction, inflammation, axon guidance, matrix assembly, lipoprotein uptake, extracellular proteolysis, tumor metastasis, angiogenesis, body size, body weight, and uptake of bacteria and viruses (10,19,73,89–96). In this section, we briefly consider a few examples of the nonanticoagulant effects of heparin and HS.

## Effects on Platelets

Heparin administration commonly produces an immediate, mild reduction in the platelet count, which is thought to result from enhanced platelet aggregation (97). This phenomenon, termed *nonimmune heparin-associated thrombocytopenia*, probably results from direct interactions between heparin and platelets (98). Heparin binds in a saturable and specific manner to approximately 2,500 sites on the platelet surface (99,100). The affinity of heparin for platelets increases with the size and charge density of the polymer. Dissociation constants of 1.3 $\mu$M and 0.3 $\mu$M have been determined for heparin molecules having molecular weights of approximately 3,000 and approximately 15,000, respectively (101). Although it has been reported that the $\alpha_{IIb}\beta_3$ integrin (fibrinogen receptor) interacts with heparin (102), the binding sites for heparin on platelets have not been identified with certainty.

When added to citrate-anticoagulated platelet-rich plasma, heparin alone weakly stimulates platelet aggregation and potentiates platelet activation induced by adenosine 5′-diphosphate (ADP) or other agonists (103–107). These effects are probably not artifacts of decreased ionized calcium produced by the citrate anticoagulant, because heparin also enhances platelet aggregation induced by collagen in hirudin-anticoagulated whole blood (108). Low-molecular-weight heparin is less able to stimulate platelet aggregation than is unfractionated heparin (98,103,105–107,109–111), consistent with the relative binding affinities of these polymers (101). Furthermore, heparin species with low affinity for antithrombin or fibronectin are more active, presumably because these proteins competitively inhibit binding of heparin to platelets (98,110). The mechanism by which heparin enhances platelet function is unknown, in part, because inconsistent effects of heparin on aggregation of washed platelets have been observed (98,109, 110,112,113). Nevertheless, it is clear that the mechanism is distinct from that of heparin-induced thrombocytopenia, which is triggered by antibodies that bind to neoepitopes on PF4–heparin complexes and activate platelets by their Fc receptors (114).

Heparin may also interfere with platelet function and thereby contribute to the hemorrhagic side effects of the drug. In the presence of antithrombin, heparin blocks activation of platelets induced by thrombin (109,115). Heparin also inhibits binding of von Willebrand factor to platelets, reducing adhesion of platelets to the subendothelium of an injured vessel (116,117). These effects may cause prolongation of the bleeding time in patients receiving heparin (118,119).

## Inhibition of Selectins

The selectins (L, P, and E selectin) are integral membrane proteins involved in cell adhesion interactions, including lymphocyte homing, inflammation, and tumor metastasis (120). L selectin is expressed constitutively on leukocytes, whereas P-selectin is rapidly translocated from secretory granules to the cell surface upon activation of platelets or endothelial cells. E-selectin expression is induced more slowly in endothelial cells by proinflammatory agonists. Selectins bind to carbohydrate structures related to the sialyl-Lewis$^x$ tetrasaccharide; these structures are components of glycoproteins found on the surface of leukocytes, activated endothelium, and mucinous adenocarcinoma cells. Heparin and HS also interact with L selectin and P selectin (but not E selectin) and inhibit binding of these proteins to sialyl-Lewis$^x$ at concentrations less than those typically used for anticoagulation (121). In mouse models, heparin produces a potent antiinflammatory effect, which appears to be caused by blockade of L and P selectins; modified heparins that lack anticoagulant activity are also effective in these models (122).

Experimental studies suggest that heparin inhibits tumor cell proliferation, migration across the endothelial barrier, invasion of tissues, and angiogenesis (123). Furthermore, some clinical studies have documented a survival benefit for patients with cancer receiving heparin (124). In most cases, the mechanisms responsible for these effects are unknown. Recent studies indicate that adhesion of activated platelets expressing P selectin to mucin-bearing tumor cells is blocked by heparin (125). In a mouse model in which human colon adenocarcinoma cells were injected intravenously, tumor cell–platelet aggregates accumulated rapidly in the pulmonary vasculature, and tumor foci were detectable in the lungs 6 weeks later. A single dose of heparin administered 30 minutes before injection of the tumor cells markedly decreased the number of metastatic foci at 6 weeks (125).

Selectin-mucin interactions also may trigger migratory thrombophlebitis (Trousseau syndrome) in patients with mucinous adenocarcinomas (126). In wild-type mice, injection of mucins extracted from human colon carcinoma cells led to formation of platelet-rich microthrombi in the lungs. Thrombus formation was inhibited by heparin but not by hirudin and therefore appeared to be independent of thrombin generation. Furthermore, thrombus formation was largely absent in mice deficient in either P selectin or L selectin. Although the mucins did not activate platelets suspended in buffer or plasma, platelet activation occurred when mucins were added to whole blood. Platelet activation by mucins *in vitro* was inhibited by heparin and did not occur in blood from L selectin–deficient mice. These observations are consistent with a model in which soluble carcinoma mucins first bind to L selectin on leukocytes, stimulating release of an unidentified platelet agonist. The activated platelets then bind to mucins via P selectin and become cross-linked to form aggregates or bind to P selectin glycoprotein ligand-1 on neutrophils or monocytes to signal production of thromboxane $A_2$ or tissue factor. Heparin could block some or all of these selectin interactions. This mechanism may explain the clinical observation that heparin is generally more effective than vitamin K antagonists for treatment of Trousseau syndrome.

## Complement, Antiphospholipid Antibodies, and Fetal Loss

Heparin is used to prevent fetal loss in patients with the antiphospholipid syndrome (127). Injection of pregnant mice with human IgG containing antiphospholipid antibodies caused fetal resorption at a rate of more than 40%; in comparison, approximately 10% of fetuses were absorbed in mice given normal human IgG. Experiments with gene-targeted mice showed that activation of both the classical and alternative complement pathways is necessary to produce fetal loss in this model (128). Fetal loss was prevented by treatment with unfractionated or low-molecular-weight heparin but not by fondaparinux or hirudin (129). *In vivo* and *in vitro* experiments showed that heparin inhibited activation of complement factor C3, as well as deposition of C3b on the surface of placental trophoblasts. Therefore, the ability of heparin to inhibit complement may explain its beneficial effect in pregnant patients with antiphospholipid antibodies; heparin may also inhibit the inflammatory response that normally follows complement activation by blockade of P- and L selectins, as described in the preceding section.

## Microbial Adherence and Invasion

A wide variety of bacteria, parasites, and viruses adhere to HSPGs on cultured cells *in vitro* and are displaced from the cell surface by soluble heparin (93). In some cases, binding of the microbe to an HSPG is thought to mediate internalization or tissue tropism. Although some of these interactions may be nonspecific, specific adhesion molecules that bind to heparin have been identified on the surfaces of pathogens such as *Plasmodium falciparum*, *Trypanosoma cruzi*, *Bordetella pertussis*, human immunodeficiency virus (HIV), and herpes simplex virus (HSV). One of the best-studied examples is HSV-1. This virus contains two envelope glycoproteins, gB and gC, that are responsible for reversible adhesion of the virus to HSPGs on target cells. A third viral glycoprotein, gD, then interacts with one of several other cellular proteins to mediate fusion of the viral envelope with the cell membrane, resulting in entry of the viral nucleocapsid into the cytoplasm. Although the first proteins found to interact with gD did not have attached glycosaminoglycan chains, HSPGs with HS chains modified by a specific 3-O-sulfotransferase (3-OST-3) also bind to gD (95). Therefore, HSPGs may be sufficient for adhesion and entry of HSV-1 into susceptible cells.

## Growth Factor Signaling

HSPGs serve as coreceptors for a variety of soluble ligands, including FGFs, vascular endothelial growth factors (VEGFs), transforming growth factors-$\beta$, CC and CXC chemokines, and various cytokines (130). An example that has been well studied is the interaction of FGF2 with the receptor tyrosine kinase FGFR1. Efficient signal transduction by FGFR1 does not occur in cells that are unable to synthesize HS or cells treated with enzymes that degrade HS (131,132), but addition of soluble heparin to these cells restores the signaling pathway. Heparin or an HS chain of syndecan or glypican on the cell surface appears to facilitate formation of a complex containing two FGF monomers and two FGF receptors, which leads to receptor dimerization and signaling. Although crystallographic studies have identified potential heparin-binding sites in both FGF and its receptor, the precise orientation of heparin in the signaling complex is unknown. Heparin oligosaccharides with a minimum of 12 sugar residues are required for FGF signaling. Binding to FGF requires N-sulfation of glucosamine and iduronic acid 2-O-sulfate, whereas binding to the receptor also requires 6-O-sulfation of glucosamine (Fig. 15-2) (133).

These studies suggest that regulation of HS biosynthesis plays a critical role in development.

## Functions of Heparan Sulfate in Development

Direct evidence implicating proteoglycans in development was obtained initially from studies with *Drosophila*, in which mutations at the *dally* (*division abnormally delayed*) locus cause morphologic abnormalities in the wings, eyes, antennae, and other tissues (73,94). The *dally* gene and its homolog *dlp* (*dally-like protein*) encode HSPG core proteins homologous to vertebrate glypicans, which are attached to the plasma membrane by glycosyl phosphatidylinositol linkers. Subsequent studies revealed that *dally* or *dlp* mutations affect signaling pathways that involve known HS-binding growth factors, including decapentaplegic (Dpp), hedgehog, and wingless (Wg) (134). Mutations that affect development in *Drosophila* have also been discovered in genes involved in glycosaminoglycan biosynthesis. These genes include *sugarless*, which encodes a UDP-glucose dehydrogenase homolog required for synthesis of UDP-glucuronic acid; *sulfateless*, which encodes an *N*-deacetylase/*N*-sulfotransferase homolog; and *tout-velu*, which encodes an HS-specific copolymerase homologous to EXT1. Mutations in these genes appear to affect pathways involving the growth factors Dpp, Hh, Wg, and FGF. Enzymes that determine specific sulfation patterns in HS are also important in development. For example, downregulation of *Drosophila* 3-*O*-sulfotransferase-B by RNA interference causes neural abnormalities due to defects in Notch signaling pathways (67). The mechanisms by which HSPGs affect these growth factors are not entirely clear. HSPGs may serve as coreceptors that facilitate activation of signaling receptors on the cell surface as in the case of FGF, they may control diffusion of growth factors from their sites of production and thereby assist in formation of morphogenic gradients in tissues, or they may be involved in stabilization or clearance of the growth factors or their receptors.

Mutations that affect vertebrate HSPGs also cause developmental abnormalities (94). For example, Simpson-Golabi-Behmel syndrome is a human disorder caused by mutations in glypican-3. This syndrome is characterized by overgrowth of many somatic tissues, including heart, kidneys, and bone, as well as increased susceptibility to Wilms tumors and neuroblastoma. A murine knockout of glypican-3 produced a similar phenotype. Other examples include mutations in the HS copolymerase genes *EXT1* and *EXT2*, which cause familial exostoses (cartilaginous tumors of the growth plates of bones), and targeted mutations in the murine HS 2-*O*-sulfotransferase gene, which lead to renal agenesis as well as eye and skeletal defects.

## Lipoprotein Metabolism

HSPGs bind to lipoprotein lipase and anchor this enzyme to the luminal surface of endothelial cells, where it hydrolyzes triglycerides in circulating lipoprotein particles (19). The lipoprotein particles also interact with endothelial HSPGs through their apolipoprotein B or E components. Interestingly, lipoprotein lipase is synthesized by myocytes and adipocytes, and transport of the enzyme from the basal to the luminal side of the endothelial cell appears to require HSPGs on the basal surface of the cell (135). Intravenous administration of unfractionated or low-molecular-weight heparin displaces lipoprotein lipase from the endothelium into the circulation, from which the enzyme is cleared by hepatic receptors (136). By this mechanism, repeated exposure to heparin may contribute to the elevated serum triglyceride levels observed in patients undergoing hemodialysis and play a role in the development of atherosclerosis.

# ACTIVATION OF HEPARIN COFACTOR II BY DERMATAN SULFATE AND OTHER POLYANIONS

The rate of inhibition of thrombin by HCII increases more than 1,000-fold in the presence of heparin, HS, or dermatan sulfate (137). HCII is unique in its ability to be stimulated by dermatan sulfate and binds to a minor subpopulation of dermatan sulfate oligosaccharides (138). The high-affinity binding site for HCII in porcine skin dermatan sulfate is a tandem repeat of three iduronic acid 2-*O*-sulfate → *N*-acetylgalactosamine 4-*O*-sulfate disaccharide subunits (see Fig. 15-6). The HCII-binding site in dermatan sulfate from tissues other than porcine skin may also include iduronic acid → *N*-acetylgalactosamine 4,6-*O*-disulfate subunits (139,140). Unlike antithrombin, HCII binds nonspecifically to heparin oligosaccharides at least 4 monosaccharide units in length (141).

The hexasaccharide sequence with high affinity for HCII is present at low abundance in dermatan sulfates of mammalian origin (138). Dermatan sulfates with the same backbone structure but with different patterns of sulfation are present in ascidians (marine invertebrates commonly known as sea squirts). All of the ascidian dermatan sulfates isolated so far have a high content of iduronic acid 2-*O*-sulfate residues, but they differ in the pattern of sulfation of the *N*-acetylgalactosamine units. For example, the *N*-acetylgalactosamine residues of *Halocynthia pyriformis* are predominantly 4-*O*-sulfated (142), whereas those of *Ascidia nigra* are quantitatively 6-*O*-sulfated (143). These dermatan sulfates stimulate thrombin inhibition by HCII with the following $IC_{50}$s: *H. pyriformis*, 0.3 $\mu$g per mL; mammalian, 3.0 $\mu$g per mL; and *A. nigra*, 300 $\mu$g per mL (142,143). These results indicate that the ability of dermatan sulfate to activate HCII is not simply a function of the overall charge density of the polymer, because the total sulfate contents of the ascidian dermatan sulfates are similar; instead, activity appears to require the presence of *N*-acetylgalactosamine 4-*O*-sulfate residues.

A variety of sulfated polyanions in addition to heparin and dermatan sulfate stimulate the HCII-thrombin reaction, and many of these polyanions have been studied as potential antithrombotic agents. They include naturally occurring compounds such as chondroitin sulfate E from mast cell granules (144) and fucoidan from seaweed (145), as well as semisynthetic polyanions such as dextran sulfate (146), pentosan polysulfate (147,148), and sulfated bis-lactobionic acid amide (149).

Mice with targeted deletion of the gene for HCII develop normally and have no evidence of spontaneous thrombosis (78). However, the time of formation of an occlusive thrombus in the carotid artery following photochemically induced endothelial injury is significantly shorter in HCII-deficient mice than in wild-type controls. The antithrombotic effect of HCII may result from activation of the inhibitor by dermatan sulfate in the wall of the injured artery. To test this hypothesis, HCII-deficient mice were injected before arterial injury with recombinant native HCII or with HCII mutants with decreased affinity for either heparin or dermatan sulfate (150). Both native HCII and the mutant with defective heparin binding restored the thrombotic occlusion time to normal, whereas the mutant with defective

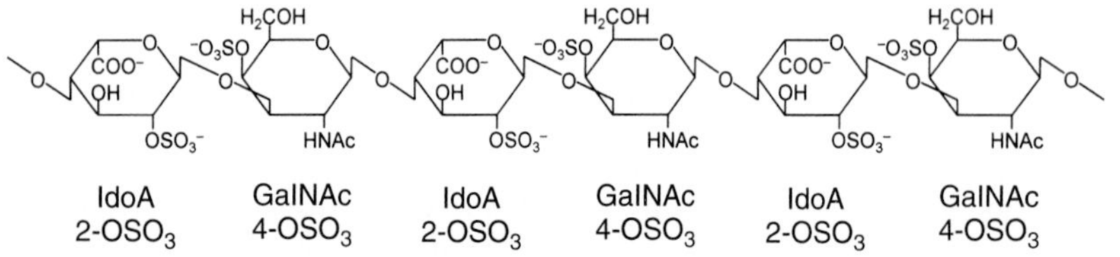

**FIGURE 15-6.** Structure of a dermatan sulfate hexasaccharide with high affinity for heparin cofactor II. IdoA, iduronic acid; GalNAc, *N*-acetylgalactosamine.

dermatan sulfate binding did not (He L, Vincent CP, Tollefsen DM, 2005, unpublished observations). These results provide evidence for a physiologic interaction between HCII and dermatan sulfate present in the arterial wall.

## References

1. Howell WH. Heparin as an anticoagulant. *Am J Physiol* 1923;63: 434–435.
2. Jorpes E. *Heparin: its chemistry, physiology, and application in medicine.* London: Oxford University Press, 1939.
3. Jaques LB. The Howell theory of blood coagulation: a record of the pernicious effects of a false theory. *Can Bull Med Hist* 1988;5:143–165.
4. Murray DWG. Heparin in thrombosis and embolism. *Br J Surg* 1939;27: 567–598.
5. Contejean C. Recherches sur les injections intraveineuses de peptone et leaur influence sur la coagulabilite du sang chez le chien. *Arch Physiol Norm Pathol* 1895;7:45.
6. Brinkhous KM, Smith HP, Warner ED, et al. The inhibition of blood clotting: an unidentified substance which acts in conjunction with heparin to prevent the conversion of prothrombin to thrombin. *Am J Physiol* 1939; 125:683–687.
7. Abildgaard U. Highly purified antithrombin III with heparin cofactor activity prepared by disc electrophoresis. *Scand J Clin Lab Invest* 1968; 21:89–91.
8. Rosenberg RD, Damus PS. The purification and mechanism of action of human antithrombin-heparin cofactor. *J Biol Chem* 1973;248:6490–6505.
9. Tollefsen DM, Majerus DW, Blank MK. Heparin cofactor II. Purification and properties of a heparin-dependent inhibitor of thrombin in human plasma. *J Biol Chem* 1982;257:2162–2169.
10. Esko JD, Lindahl U. Molecular diversity of heparan sulfate. *J Clin Invest* 2001;108:169–173.
11. Sugahara K, Kitagawa H. Heparin and heparan sulfate biosynthesis. *IUBMB Life* 2002;54:163–175.
12. Medeiros GF, Mendes A, Castro RA, et al. Distribution of sulfated glycosaminoglycans in the animal kingdom: widespread occurrence of heparin-like compounds in invertebrates. *Biochim Biophys Acta* 2000;1475: 287– 294.
13. Stevens RL, Avraham S, Gartner MC, et al. Isolation and characterization of a cDNA that encodes the peptide core of the secretory granule proteoglycan of human promyelocytic leukemia HL-60 cells. *J Biol Chem* 1988; 263:7287–7291.
14. Avraham S, Stevens RL, Nicodemus CF, et al. Molecular cloning of a cDNA that encodes the peptide core of a mouse mast cell secretory granule proteoglycan and comparison with the analogous rat and human cDNA. *Proc Natl Acad Sci U S A* 1989;86:3763–3767.
15. Jacobsson KG, Lindahl U. Degradation of heparin proteoglycan in cultured mouse mastocytoma cells. *Biochem J* 1987;246:409–415.
16. Linhardt RJ, Gunay NS. Production and chemical processing of low molecular weight heparins. *Semin Thromb Hemost* 1999;25(Suppl. 3):5–16.
17. Bernfield M, Gotte M, Park PW, et al. Functions of cell surface heparan sulfate proteoglycans. *Annu Rev Biochem* 1999;68:729–777.
18. Bourdon MA, Oldberg A, Pierschbacher M, et al. Molecular cloning and sequence analysis of a chondroitin sulfate proteoglycan cDNA. *Proc Natl Acad Sci U S A* 1985;82:1321–1325.
19. Rosenberg RD, Shworak NW, Liu J, et al. Heparan sulfate proteoglycans of the cardiovascular system. Specific structures emerge but how is synthesis regulated? *J Clin Invest* 1997;99:2062–2070.
20. Zhang L, David G, Esko JD. Repetitive Ser-Gly sequences enhance heparan sulfate assembly in proteoglycans. *J Biol Chem* 1995;270:27127–27135.
21. Esko JD, Zhang L. Influence of core protein sequence on glycosaminoglycan assembly. *Curr Opin Struct Biol* 1996;6:663–670.
22. Zhang L, Esko JD. Amino acid determinants that drive heparan sulfate assembly in a proteoglycan. *J Biol Chem* 1994;269:19295–19299.
23. Kusche-Gullberg M, Kjellen L. Sulfotransferases in glycosaminoglycan biosynthesis. *Curr Opin Struct Biol* 2003;13:605–611.
24. Forsberg E, Pejler G, Ringvall M, et al. Abnormal mast cells in mice deficient in a heparin-synthesizing enzyme. *Nature* 1999;400:773–776.
25. Humphries DE, Wong GW, Friend DS, et al. Heparin is essential for the storage of specific granule proteases in mast cells. *Nature* 1999;400:769–772.
26. Fan G, Xiao L, Cheng L, et al. Targeted disruption of NDST-1 gene leads to pulmonary hypoplasia and neonatal respiratory distress in mice. *FEBS Lett* 2000;467:7–11.
27. Ringvall M, Ledin J, Holmborn K, et al. Defective heparan sulfate biosynthesis and neonatal lethality in mice lacking N-deacetylase/N-sulfotransferase-1. *J Biol Chem* 2000;275:25926–25930.
28. Petitou M, Casu B, Lindahl U. 1976-1983, a critical period in the history of heparin: the discovery of the antithrombin binding site. *Biochimie* 2003;85:83–89.
29. Lam LH, Silbert JE, Rosenberg RD. The separation of active and inactive forms of heparin. *Biochem Biophys Res Commun* 1976;69:570–577.
30. Hook M, Bjork I, Hopwood J, et al. Anticoagulant activity of heparin: separation of high-activity and low-activity heparin species by affinity chromotography on immobilized antithrombin. *FEBS Lett* 1976;66:90–93.
31. Andersson LO, Barrowcliffe TW, Holmer E, et al. Anticoagulant properties of heparin fractionated by affinity chromotography on matrix-bound antithrombin III and by gel filtration. *Thromb Res* 1976;9:575–583.
32. Rosenberg RD, Armand G, Lam L. Structure-function relationships of heparin species. *Proc Natl Acad Sci U S A* 1978;75:3065–3069.
33. Leder IG. A novel 3-O sulfatase from human urine acting on methyl-2-deoxy-2-sulfamino-alphs-D-glucopyranoside 3-sulfate. *Biochem Biophys Res Commun* 1980;94:1183–1189.
34. Lindahl U, Backstrom G, Thunberg L, et al. Evidence for a 3-O-sulfated D-glucosamine residue in the antithrombin-binding sequence of heparin. *Proc Natl Acad Sci U S A* 1980;77:6551–6555.
35. Choay J, Lormeau JC, Petitou M, et al. Anti-Xa active heparin oligosaccharides. *Thromb Res* 1980;18:573–578.
36. Choay J, Petitou M, Lormeau JC, et al. Structure-activity relationship in heparin: a synthetic pentasaccharide with high affinity for antithrombin III and eliciting high anti-factor Xa activity. *Biochem Biophys Res Commun* 1983;116:492–499.
37. Petitou M, van Boeckel CA. A synthetic antithrombin III binding pentasaccharide is now a drug! What comes next? *Angew Chem Int Ed Engl* 2004;43:3118–3133.
38. Oosta GM, Gardner WT, Beeler DL, et al. Multiple functional domains of the heparin molecule. *Proc Natl Acad Sci U S A* 1981;78:829–833.
39. Caulfield JP, Lewis RA, Hein A, et al. Secretion in dissociated human pulmonary mast cells. Evidence for solubilization of granule contents before discharge. *J Cell Biol* 1980;85:299–312.
40. Nenci GG, Berrettini M, Parise P, et al. Persistent spontaneous heparinaemia in systemic mastocytosis. *Folia Haematol Int Mag Klin Morphol Blutforsch* 1982;109:453–463.
41. Damus PS, Hicks M, Rosenberg RD. Anticoagulant action of heparin. *Nature* 1973;246:355–357.
42. Marcum JA, Atha DH, Fritze LM, et al. Cloned bovine aortic endothelial cells synthesize anticoagulantly active heparan sulfate proteoglycan. *J Biol Chem* 1986;261:7507–7517.
43. Teien AN, Abildgaard U, Hook M. The anticoagulant effect of heparan sulfate and dermatan sulfate. *Thromb Res* 1976;8:859–867.
44. Thomas DP, Merton RE, Barrowcliffe TW, et al. Anti-factor Xa activity of heparan sulphate. *Thromb Res* 1979;14:501–506.
45. Marcum JA, Rosenberg RD. Heparinlike molecules with anticoagulant activity are synthesized by cultured endothelial cells. *Biochem Biophys Res Commun* 1985;126:365–372.
46. Stern D, Nawroth P, Marcum J, et al. Interaction of antithrombin III with bovine aortic segments. Role of heparin in binding and enhanced anticoagulant activity. *J Clin Invest* 1985;75:272–279.
47. Kojima T, Leone CW, Marchildon GA, et al. Isolation and characterization of heparan sulfate proteoglycans produced by cloned rat microvascular endothelial cells. *J Biol Chem* 1992;267:4859–4869.
48. Kojima T, Shworak NW, Rosenberg RD. Molecular cloning and expression of two distinct cDNA-encoding heparan sulfate proteoglycan core proteins from a rat endothelial cell line. *J Biol Chem* 1992; 267:4870–4877.
49. Shworak NW, Shirakawa M, Mulligan RC, et al. Characterization of ryudocan glycosaminoglycan acceptor sites. *J Biol Chem* 1994;269: 21204–21214.
50. Weksberg R, Squire JA, Templeton DM. Glypicans: a growing trend. *Nat Genet* 1996;12:225–227.
51. Murdoch AD, Liu B, Schwarting R, et al. Widespread expression of perlecan proteoglycan in basement membranes and extracellular matrices of human tissues as detected by a novel monoclonal antibody against domain III and by in situ hybridization. *J Histochem Cytochem* 1994;42: 239–247.
52. Shworak NW, Shirakawa M, Colliec-Jouault S, et al. Pathway-specific regulation of the synthesis of anticoagulantly active heparan sulfate. *J Biol Chem* 1994;269:24941–24952.
53. Colliec-Jouault S, Shworak NW, Liu J, et al. Characterization of a cell mutant specifically defective in the synthesis of anticoagulantly active heparan sulfate. *J Biol Chem* 1994;269:24953–24958.
54. Shworak NW, Fritze LM, Liu J, et al. Cell-free synthesis of anticoagulant heparan sulfate reveals a limiting converting activity that modifies an excess precursor pool. *J Biol Chem* 1996;271:27063–27071.
55. Liu J, Shworak NW, Fritze LM, et al. Purification of heparan sulfate D-glucosaminyl 3-O-sulfotransferase. *J Biol Chem* 1996;271:27072– 27082.
56. Shworak NW, Liu J, Fritze LM, et al. Molecular cloning and expression of mouse and human cDNAs encoding heparan sulfate D-glucosaminyl 3-O-sulfotransferase. *J Biol Chem* 1997;272:28008–28019.
57. Zhang L, Schwartz JJ, Miller J, et al. The retinoic acid and cAMP-dependent up-regulation of 3-O-sulfotransferase-1 leads to a dramatic augmentation of anticoagulantly active heparan sulfate biosynthesis in F9 embryonal carcinoma cells. *J Biol Chem* 1998;273:27998–28003.
58. Zhang L, Yoshida K, Liu J, et al. Anticoagulant heparan sulfate precursor structures in F9 embryonal carcinoma cells. *J Biol Chem* 1999;274: 5681–5691.
59. de Agostini AI, Watkins SC, Slayter HS, et al. Localization of anticoagulantly active heparan sulfate proteoglycans in vascular endothelium: antithrombin binding on cultured endothelial cells and perfused rat aorta. *J Cell Biol* 1990;111:1293–1304.
60. Simionescu N. Cellular aspects of transcapillary exchange. *Physiol Rev* 1983;63:1536–1579.

61. Carlson TH, Simon TL, Atencio AC. *In vivo* behavior of human radio-iodinated antithrombin III: distribution among three physiologic pools. *Blood* 1985;66:13–19.

62. Marcum JA, McKenney JB, Rosenberg RD. Acceleration of thrombin-antithrombin complex formation in rat hindquarters by heparinlike molecules bound to the endothelium. *J Clin Invest* 1984;74:341–350.

63. Marcum JA, McKenney JB, Galli SJ, et al. Anticoagulantly active heparin-like molecules from mast cell-deficient mice. *Am J Physiol* 1986;250: H879–H888.

64. Xia G, Chen J, Tiwari V, et al. Heparan sulfate 3-O-sulfotransferase isoform 5 generates both an antithrombin-binding site and an entry receptor for herpes simplex virus, type 1. *J Biol Chem* 2002;277:37912–37919.

65. HajMohammadi S, Enjyoji K, Princivalle M, et al. Normal levels of anticoagulant heparan sulfate are not essential for normal hemostasis. *J Clin Invest* 2003;111:989–999.

66. Ishiguro K, Kojima T, Kadomatsu K, et al. Complete antithrombin deficiency in mice results in embryonic lethality. *J Clin Invest* 2000;106:873–878.

67. Kamimura K, Rhodes JM, Ueda R, et al. Regulation of Notch signaling by Drosophila heparan sulfate 3-O sulfotransferase. *J Cell Biol* 2004;166: 1069–1079.

68. de Agostini AI, Ramus MA, Rosenberg RD. Differential partition of anticoagulant heparan sulfate proteoglycans synthesized by endothelial and fibroblastic cell lines. *J Cell Biochem* 1994;54:174–185.

69. Hosseini G, Liu J, de Agostini AI. Characterization and hormonal modulation of anticoagulant heparan sulfate proteoglycans synthesized by rat ovarian granulosa cells. *J Biol Chem* 1996;271:22090–22099.

70. van Boven HH, Lane DA. Antithrombin and its inherited deficiency states. *Semin Hematol* 1997;34:188–204.

71. Dewerchin M, Herault JP, Wallays G, et al. Life-threatening thrombosis in mice with targeted Arg48-to-Cys mutation of the heparin-binding domain of antithrombin. *Circ Res* 2003;93:1120–1126.

72. Scully MF, Ellis V, Kakkar VV. Heparan sulphate with no affinity for antithrombin III and the control of haemostasis. *FEBS Lett* 1988;241:11–14.

73. Lin X. Functions of heparan sulfate proteoglycans in cell signaling during development. *Development* 2004;131:6009–6021.

74. Lin X, Wei G, Shi Z, et al. Disruption of gastrulation and heparan sulfate biosynthesis in EXT1-deficient mice. *Dev Biol* 2000;224:299–311.

75. Ishiguro K, Kadomatsu K, Kojima T, et al. Syndecan-4 deficiency impairs the fetal vessels in the placental labyrinth. *Dev Dyn* 2000;219: 539–544.

76. Preissner KT, Delvos U, Muller-Berghaus G. Binding of thrombin to thrombomodulin accelerates inhibition of the enzyme by antithrombin III. Evidence for a heparin-independent mechanism. *Biochemistry* 1987;26: 2521–2528.

77. Bourin MC, Lundgren-Akerlund E, Lindahl U. Isolation and characterization of the glycosaminoglycan component of rabbit thrombomodulin proteoglycan. *J Biol Chem* 1990;265:15424–15431.

78. He L, Vicente CP, Westrick RJ, et al. Heparin cofactor II inhibits arterial thrombosis after endothelial injury. *J Clin Invest* 2002;109:213–219.

79. Yin ZF, Huang ZF, Cui J, et al. Prothrombotic phenotype of protein Z deficiency. *Proc Natl Acad Sci U S A* 2000;97:6734–6738.

80. Hricovini M, Guerrini M, Bisio A, et al. Conformation of heparin pentasaccharide bound to antithrombin III. *Biochem J* 2001;359:265–272.

81. Bauer KA. Fondaparinux: a new synthetic and selective inhibitor of Factor Xa. *Best Pract Res Clin Haematol* 2004;17:89–104.

82. Ma Q, Fareed J. Idraparinux sodium. Sanofi-Aventis. *IDrugs* 2004;7: 1028–1034.

83. Petitou M, Herault JP, Bernat A, et al. Synthesis of thrombin-inhibiting heparin mimetics without side effects. *Nature* 1999;398:417–422.

84. Kuberan B, Beeler DL, Lawrence R, et al. Rapid two-step synthesis of mitrin from heparosan: a replacement for heparin. *J Am Chem Soc* 2003; 125:12424–12425.

85. Kuberan B, Beeler DL, Lech M, et al. Chemoenzymatic synthesis of classical and non-classical anticoagulant heparan sulfate polysaccharides. *J Biol Chem* 2003;278:52613–52621.

86. Kuberan B, Lech MZ, Beeler DL, et al. Enzymatic synthesis of antithrombin III-binding heparan sulfate pentasaccharide. *Nat Biotechnol* 2003;21: 1343–1346.

87. Lindahl U, Li JP, Kusche-Gullberg M, et al. Generation of "neoheparin" from E. coli K5 capsular polysaccharide. *J Med Chem* 2005;48:349–352.

88. Conrad HE. *Heparin-binding proteins*. San Diego, CA: Academic Press, 1998.

89. Iozzo RV, San Antonio JD. Heparan sulfate proteoglycans: heavy hitters in the angiogenesis arena. *J Clin Invest* 2001;108:349–355.

90. Lander AD, Selleck SB. The elusive functions of proteoglycans: *in vivo* veritas. *J Cell Biol* 2000;148:227–232.

91. Lindahl U. What else can 'heparin' do? *Haemostasis* 1999;29(Suppl. S1): 38–47.

92. Reizes O, Lincecum J, Wang Z, et al. Transgenic expression of syndecan-1 uncovers a physiological control of feeding behavior by syndecan-3. *Cell* 2001;106:105–116.

93. Rostand KS, Esko JD. Microbial adherence to and invasion through proteoglycans. *Infect Immun* 1997;65:1–8.

94. Selleck SB. Proteoglycans and pattern formation: sugar biochemistry meets developmental genetics. *Trends Genet* 2000;16:206–212.

95. Shukla D, Liu J, Blaiklock P, et al. A novel role for 3-O-sulfated heparan sulfate in herpes simplex virus 1 entry. *Cell* 1999;99:13–22.

96. Vlodavsky I, Friedmann Y. Molecular properties and involvement of heparanase in cancer metastasis and angiogenesis. *J Clin Invest* 2001;108: 341–347.

97. Horne MK, 3rd. Nonimmune heparin-platelet interactions: implications for the pathogenesis of heparin-induced thrombocytopenia. In: Warkentin TE, Greinacher A, eds. *Heparin-induced thrombocytopenia*, 3rd ed. New York: Marcel Dekker Inc, 2004:149–163.

98. Salzman EW, Rosenberg RD, Smith MH, et al. Effect of heparin and heparin fractions on platelet aggregation. *J Clin Invest* 1980;65:64–73.

99. Sobel M, Adelman B. Characterization of platelet binding of heparins and other glycosaminoglycans. *Thromb Res* 1988;50:815–826.

100. Horne MK 3rd, Chao ES. Heparin binding to resting and activated platelets. *Blood* 1989;74:238–243.

101. Horne MK 3rd, Chao ES. The effect of molecular weight on heparin binding to platelets. *Br J Haematol* 1990;74:306–312.

102. Sobel M, Fish WR, Toma N, et al. Heparin modulates integrin function in human platelets. *J Vasc Surg* 2001;33:587–594.

103. Holmer E, Lindahl U, Backstrom G, et al. Anticoagulant activities and effects on platelets of a heparin fragment with high affinity for antithrombin. *Thromb Res* 1980;18:861–869.

104. Chen J, Sylven C. Heparin potentiation of collagen-induced platelet aggregation is related to the GPIIb/GPIIIa receptor and not to the GPIb receptor, as tested by whole blood aggregometry. *Thromb Res* 1992;66:111–120.

105. Xiao Z, Theroux P. Platelet activation with unfractionated heparin at therapeutic concentrations and comparisons with a low-molecular-weight heparin and with a direct thrombin inhibitor. *Circulation* 1998;97:251–256.

106. Aggarwal A, Sobel BE, Schneider DJ. Decreased platelet reactivity in blood anticoagulated with bivalirudin or enoxaparin compared with unfractionated heparin: implications for coronary intervention. *J Thromb Thrombolysis* 2002;13:161–165.

107. Klein B, Faridi A, von Tempelhoff GF, et al. A whole blood flow cytometric determination of platelet activation by unfractionated and low molecular weight heparin *in vitro*. *Thromb Res* 2002;108:291–296.

108. Chen J, Karlberg KE, Sylven C. Heparin enhances platelet aggregation irrespective of anticoagulation with citrate or with hirudin. *Thromb Res* 1992;67:253–262.

109. Westwick J, Scully MF, Poll C, et al. Comparison of the effects of low molecular weight heparin and unfractionated heparin on activation of human platelets *in vitro*. *Thromb Res* 1986;42:435–447.

110. Chong BH, Ismail F. The mechanism of heparin-induced platelet aggregation. *Eur J Haematol* 1989;43:245–251.

111. Brace LD, Fareed J. Heparin-induced platelet aggregation. II. Dose/response relationships for two low molecular weight heparin fractions (CY 216 and CY 222). *Thromb Res* 1990;59:1–14.

112. Eika C. The platelet aggregating effect of eight commercial heparins. *Scand J Haematol* 1972;9:480–482.

113. Saba HI, Saba SR, Morelli GA. Effect of heparin on platelet aggregation. *Am J Hematol* 1984;17:295–306.

114. Visentin GP, Liu CY, Aster RH. Molecular immunopathogenesis of heparin-induced thrombocytopenia. In: Warkentin TE, Greinacher A, eds. *Heparin-induced thrombocytopenia*, 3rd ed. New York: Marcel Dekker Inc; 2004: 179–196.

115. Cofrancesco E, Colombi M, Manfreda M, et al. Effect of heparin and related glycosaminoglycans (GAGs) on thrombin-induced platelet aggregation and release. *Haematologica* 1988;73:471–475.

116. Sobel M, McNeill PM, Carlson PL, et al. Heparin inhibition of von Willebrand factor-dependent platelet function *in vitro* and *in vivo*. *J Clin Invest* 1991;87:1787–1793.

117. Sobel M, Soler DF, Kermode JC, et al. Localization and characterization of a heparin binding domain peptide of human von Willebrand factor. *J Biol Chem* 1992;267:8857–8862.

118. Hjort PF, Borchgrevink CF, Iverson OH, et al. The effect of heparin on the bleeding time. *Thromb Diath Haemorrh* 1960;4:389–399.

119. Heiden D, Mielke CH Jr, Rodvien R. Impairment by heparin of primary haemostasis and platelet [14C]5-hydroxytryptamine release. *Br J Haematol* 1977;36:427–436.

120. Kansas GS. Selectins and their ligands: current concepts and controversies. *Blood* 1996;88:3259–3287.

121. Koenig A, Norgard-Sumnicht K, Linhardt R, et al. Differential interactions of heparin and heparan sulfate glycosaminoglycans with the selectins. Implications for the use of unfractionated and low molecular weight heparins as therapeutic agents. *J Clin Invest* 1998;101:877–889.

122. Wang L, Brown JR, Varki A, et al. Heparin's anti-inflammatory effects require glucosamine 6-O-sulfation and are mediated by blockade of L- and P-selectins. *J Clin Invest* 2002;110:127–136.

123. Smorenburg SM, Van Noorden CJ. The complex effects of heparins on cancer progression and metastasis in experimental studies. *Pharmacol Rev* 2001;53:93–105.

124. Cosgrove RH, Zacharski LR, Racine E, et al. Improved cancer mortality with low-molecular-weight heparin treatment: a review of the evidence. *Semin Thromb Hemost* 2002;28:79–87.

125. Borsig L, Wong R, Feramisco J, et al. Heparin and cancer revisited: mechanistic connections involving platelets, P-selectin, carcinoma mucins, and tumor metastasis. *Proc Natl Acad Sci U S A* 2001;98:3352–3357.

126. Wahrenbrock M, Borsig L, Le D, et al. Selectin-mucin interactions as a probable molecular explanation for the association of Trousseau syndrome with mucinous adenocarcinomas. *J Clin Invest* 2003;112:853–862.

127. Derksen RH, Khamashta MA, Branch DW. Management of the obstetric antiphospholipid syndrome. *Arthritis Rheum* 2004;50:1028–1039.

128. Girardi G, Berman J, Redecha P, et al. Complement C5a receptors and neutrophils mediate fetal injury in the antiphospholipid syndrome. *J Clin Invest* 2003;112:1644–1654.

129. Girardi G, Redecha P, Salmon JE. Heparin prevents antiphospholipid antibody-induced fetal loss by inhibiting complement activation. *Nat Med* 2004;10:1222–1226.

130. Park PW, Reizes O, Bernfield M. Cell surface heparan sulfate proteoglycans: selective regulators of ligand-receptor encounters. *J Biol Chem* 2000; 275:29923–29926.

131. Rapraeger AC, Krufka A, Olwin BB. Requirement of heparan sulfate for bFGF-mediated fibroblast growth and myoblast differentiation. *Science* 1991;252:1705–1708.

132. Yayon A, Klagsbrun M, Esko JD, et al. Cell surface, heparin-like molecules are required for binding of basic fibroblast growth factor to its high affinity receptor. *Cell* 1991;64:841–848.

133. Esko JD, Selleck SB. Order out of chaos: assembly of ligand binding sites in heparan sulfate. *Annu Rev Biochem* 2002;71:435–471.

134. Han C, Yan D, Belenkaya TY, et al. Drosophila glypicans dally and dally-like shape the extracellular Wingless morphogen gradient in the wing disc. *Development* 2005;132:667–679.

135. Saxena U, Klein MG, Goldberg IJ. Transport of lipoprotein lipase across endothelial cells. *Proc Natl Acad Sci U S A* 1991;88:2254–2258.

136. Nasstrom B, Stegmayr B, Gupta J, et al. A single bolus of a low molecular weight heparin to patients on haemodialysis depletes lipoprotein lipase stores and retards triglyceride clearing. *Nephrol Dial Transplant* 2005;20: 1172–1179.

137. Tollefsen DM, Pestka CA, Monafo WJ. Activation of heparin cofactor II by dermatan sulfate. *J Biol Chem* 1983;258:6713–6716.

138. Maimone MM, Tollefsen DM. Structure of a dermatan sulfate hexasaccharide that binds to heparin cofactor II with high affinity. *J Biol Chem* 1990; 265:18263–18271.

139. Mascellani G, Liverani L, Bianchini P, et al. Structure and contribution to the heparin cofactor II-mediated inhibition of thrombin of naturally oversulphated sequences of dermatan sulphate. *Biochem J* 1993;296:639–648.

140. Mascellani G, Liverani L, Prete A, et al. Relative influence of different disulphate disaccharide clusters on the HCII-mediated inhibition of thrombin by dermatan sulphates of different origins. *Thromb Res* 1994;74:605–615.

141. Tollefsen DM. The interaction of glycosaminoglycans with heparin cofactor II: structure and activity of a high-affinity dermatan sulfate hexasaccharide. *Adv Exp Med Biol* 1992;313:167–176.

142. Pavao MSG, Aiello KRM, Werneck CC, et al. Highly sulfated dermatan sulfates from ascidians: structure versus anticoagulant activity of these glycosaminoglycans. *J Biol Chem* 1998;273:27848–27857.

143. Pavao MSG, Mourao PAS, Mulloy B, et al. A unique dermatan sulfate-like glycosaminoglycan from ascidian: its structure and the effect of its unusual sulfation pattern on anticoagulant activity. *J Biol Chem* 1995;270: 31027–31036.

144. Scully MF, Ellis V, Seno N, et al. The anticoagulant properties of mast cell product, chondroitin sulphate E. *Biochem Biophys Res Commun* 1986; 137:15–22.

145. Church FC, Meade JB, Treanor RE, et al. Antithrombin activity of fucoidan. The interaction of fucoidan with heparin cofactor II, antithrombin III, and thrombin. *J Biol Chem* 1989;264:3618–3623.

146. Yamagishi R, Niwa M, Kondo S, et al. Purification and biological property of heparin cofactor II: activation of heparin cofactor II and antithrombin III by dextran sulfate and various glycosaminoglycans. *Thromb Res* 1984; 36:633–642.

147. Sie P, Fernandez F, Caranobe C, et al. Inhibition of thrombin-induced platelet aggregation and serotonin release by antithrombin III and heparin cofactor II in the presence of standard heparin, dermatan sulfate and pentosan polysulfate. *Thromb Res* 1984;35:231–236.

148. Scully MF, Kakkar VV. Identification of heparin cofactor II as the principal plasma cofactor for the antithrombin activity of pentosan polysulphate (SP54). *Thromb Res* 1984;36:187–194.

149. Klauser RJ. Interaction of the sulfated lactobionic acid amide LW 10082 with thrombin and its endogenous inhibitors. *Thromb Res* 1991;62: 557–565.

150. Colwell NS, Grupe MJ, Tollefsen DM. Amino acid residues of heparin cofactor II required for stimulation of thrombin inhibition by sulphated polyanions. *Biochim Biophys Acta* 1999;1431:148–156.

# CHAPTER 16 ■ FIBRINOGEN STRUCTURE AND PHYSIOLOGY

ROY R. HANTGAN AND SUSAN T. LORD

Fibrinogen, an adhesive protein whose structure and function have roots dating 450 million years ago in the Paleozoic Era (1,2), has come of age in the new millennium. Recent advances in structural biology now enable us to visualize fibrinogen's molecular makeup at atomic resolution (3–10), confirming and extending clotting factor I's trinodular architecture first revealed by electron microscopy in 1959 (11). Parallel studies have focused on thrombin binding to fibrinogen's central domain, where it cleaves small peptides, enabling the previously soluble 340,000-Da protein to form a highly interconnected network of insoluble strands termed fibrin. We can now understand fibrin structure in terms of the bricks (fibrinogen) and mortar (subunit interactions, noncovalent, and crosslinked) that stabilize both a hemostatic plug and an occlusive thrombus. Investigators have demonstrated how the structure, stability, and lifetime of fibrin are controlled by a complex interplay with other molecular/cellular components of the hemostatic system. These components include factor XIIIa, which crosslinks fibrin to itself and to other adhesive proteins; integrin receptors that link fibrin tightly to cell surfaces; and the components of the fibrinolytic system, which assemble on the fibrin matrix, poised to dissolve the clot when its function has been fulfilled. Remarkable growth in the field of molecular genetics continues to expand our understanding of the biosynthesis of fibrinogen, especially the regulation of this process by control of gene expression. Each of these topics is explored in the sections that follow.

## AMINO ACID SEQUENCE AND DISULFIDE BONDING

The fibrinogen molecule is a dimer (12) consisting of three pairs of disulfide-bonded polypeptide chains, designated A$\alpha$, B$\beta$, and $\gamma$, as illustrated schematically in Figure 16-1. The length of each bar in the figure is proportional to the size of the polypeptide chain, and the sequences have been aligned so that the positions of disulfide bonds linking the three chains are in register (13,14). The nomenclature of the chains derives from the fact that relatively small polypeptides, called fibrinopeptides A and B, which constitute only approximately 2% of the total protein content, are released from A$\alpha$ and B$\beta$ chains by thrombin (15,16). Molecules devoid of fibrinopeptides A and/or B are referred to as *fibrin monomers*.

The entire amino acid sequence of human fibrinogen, a total of 1,482 residues in each set of three polypeptide chains, has been determined by classic protein chemistry techniques (17,18). In addition, the amino acid sequence has been deduced from the nucleotide sequence of the cDNAs coding for the A$\alpha$, B$\beta$, and $\gamma$ chains (17–23). There are 610, 461, and 411 amino acid residues in the common forms of the A$\alpha$, B$\beta$, and $\gamma$ chains,

respectively (17,18). The computed respective molecular weights are 66,500, 52,000, and 46,500, for a total molecular weight of approximately 330,000 for two copies of each chain (18). Less common structural variants exist, with the most frequent one (<10%) being a variant of the $\gamma$ chain in which residues 408 to 411 have been replaced with a 20-residue sequence ending in leucine at position 427 (24–28). Similarly, a less common variant of the A$\alpha$ chain, designated A$\alpha$E, has an additional 236 amino acids at the carboxyl terminal (29). All three chains contain carbohydrate, each of molecular weight 2,500, attached covalently at residues B$\beta$364, $\gamma$52, and A$\alpha$E 667 (30–33). Therefore, the computed molecular weight of the common form of fibrinogen is approximately 340,000, confirming the results obtained by physical chemical measurements (34).

The amino acid sequences of the A$\alpha$, B$\beta$, and $\gamma$ chains are homologous, indicating that they have evolved from a common ancestor (13). However, there are important differences in sequence among the three chains, which is the root of their functional differences. Fibrinopeptide A (16 residues) and fibrinopeptide B (14 residues) are present at the N-termini of the A$\alpha$ and B$\beta$ chains (35). After thrombin cleavage, the N-terminal residues of the A$\alpha$ and B$\beta$ chains are converted from alanine and pyroglutamic acid, respectively, to glycine (35). Factor XIIIa–susceptible crosslink sites are present on the A$\alpha$ and $\gamma$ chains but not on the B$\beta$ chain (36,37). A single pair of glutamine and lysine are located close to the carboxyl terminal of the $\gamma$ chain (38); two glutamine sites and perhaps as many as five lysine sites on the A$\alpha$ chain are located approximately 200 residues apart on the long polar region (39). This region, which is peculiar to this chain, is a highly exposed portion of the molecule, readily cleaved by proteolytic enzymes (13). Liberation of part or all of this 403-residue sequence from fibrinogen is the first cleavage step by plasmin and is the major change that converts fibrinogen to fragment X (40). Another critical plasmin cleavage site involves all three of the chains and is located approximately midway between the proximal and distal disulfide rings of the coiled-coils (Figure 16-1) (40,41).

The disulfide bonds between the six chains have also been located by studies of the disulfide-rich cyanogen bromide fragments. There are 8, 11, and 10 cysteine residues on the A$\alpha$, B$\beta$, and $\gamma$ chains, respectively; all of the 58 cysteine residues in the molecule participate in 29 disulfide bonds (42,43). As illustrated in Figure 16-1, the N-termini of all six chains are held together by 11 disulfide bonds in a region termed the central domain or N-disulfide knot (N-DSK) (44,45). Five interchain disulfide bonds tie the two halves of the dimeric molecule together in this region (including one that links the A$\alpha$ chains, two that link the $\gamma$ chains, and two that link the A$\alpha$ and B$\beta$ chains) (46). The $\gamma$ chains are joined by disulfide bonds in an antiparallel manner, which implies that the two halves of the molecule are also joined in this same

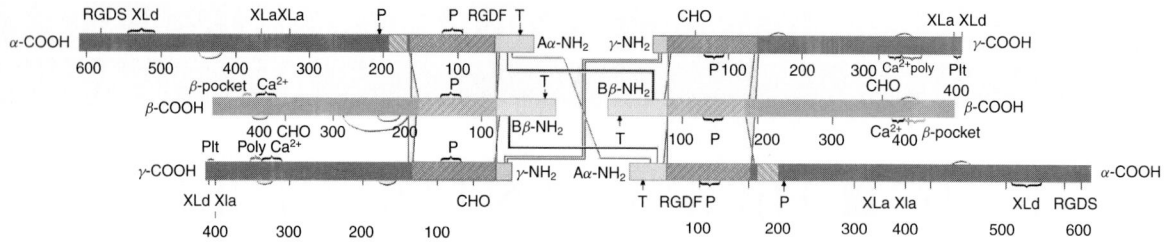

**FIGURE 16-1.** Schematic diagram of the six polypeptide chains of fibrinogen: The Aα, Bβ, and γ chains of human fibrinogen are represented by bars (*blue, green,* and *red,* respectively) that are proportional to the number of residues of each chain; the numbers beneath the rectangles define the sequence number. Note the three disulfide bonds (*yellow lines*) that connect the two halves of the molecule in an antiparallel arrangement; a twofold symmetry axis passes through the center of this region, perpendicular to the plane of the page. The seven pairs of interchain disulfide bonds are represented by *straight yellow lines* and the six pairs of intrachain disulfide bonds by *curved, yellow lines.* Thrombin cleavage sites on the Aα and Bβ chains are indicated by a *T* and an *arrow. Brackets* define the plasmin-sensitive regions within the coiled-coil regions; the *single arrow* with a P indicates the plasmin cleavage that releases the polar portion of the carboxyl terminal of the α chain. The positions of lysine and glutamine residues, which have been identified as crosslink electron donor and acceptor sites, are indicated by XLd and XLa, respectively; regions of the α chain that contain lysine donor sites are identified by brackets. Regions of the β and γ chains involved in calcium binding are marked with brackets and Ca²⁺. Sequences on the γ chain that interact with GPRP, thereby defining a polymerization site involved in fibrin assembly, are indicated by poly (*red brackets*), and those involved in platelet binding by Plt. Regions on the β chain that interact with GHRP are denoted by β-pocket (*green brackets*). Sites of carbohydrate attachment are indicated by CHO. The different shadings and colors within each rectangle indicate the portions of the polypeptide chain that define the central domain (*dotted*), the coiled-coil region (*right diagonals*), the outer domains (β-domain, *solid green*; γ-domain, *solid red*), and in the case of the Aα chain, the polar region (*solid blue*). The *small, blue, left-diagonal region* on the α chain denotes its "hairpin helix" (see Color Fig. 16-1).
Complete details of the sequences of each polypeptide can be found in electronic databases with the following identifiers:
FIBRINOGEN ALPHA/ALPHA-E CHAIN PRECURSOR. (GENE: FGA) FIBA_HUMAN
Primary accession number: P02671
FIBRINOGEN BETA CHAIN PRECURSOR. (GENE: FGB) FIBB_HUMAN
Primary accession number: P02675
FIBRINOGEN GAMMA-A CHAIN PRECURSOR. (GENE: FGG) FIBG_HUMAN
Primary accession number: P02679.

antiparallel arrangement (Fig. 16-1) (12). A set of three cystine linkages that tie the three polypeptide chains together completes the N-DSK (44,45). A similar triplet of interchain disulfide bridges occurs in a region 111 to 112 residues toward the carboxyl terminal of the molecule (44,45,47,48). The remainder of the Aα chain contains one intrachain disulfide (44,45), whereas three such connections are found in the Bβ chain and two in the γ chain (43–45,47,48).

## STRUCTURAL INSIGHTS FROM LIMITED PROTEOLYSIS OF FIBRINOGEN

Enzymatic fragmentation of fibrinogen by plasmin and trypsin indicates that regions of extreme susceptibility exist and that large-core fragments can easily be produced by such degradation (40,49,50). Plasmin cleavage of fibrinogen initially yields derivatives that contain not only the central and/or terminal cores but also portions of the connector regions as part of fragments Y, D, and E (51–54). The plasmin degradation product, fragment E, shares much of its primary sequence with N-DSK. The terminal domains, which correspond essentially to fragment D, contain mostly the carboxyl, two thirds of the Bβ and γ chains, and only a short sequence of the Aα chain, which emerges from this domain as a long polar region containing one disulfide bond and the crosslink sites (Fig. 16-1). The asymmetric scheme of fragmentation (see Chapter 23) (55–57) accounts for all of the enzyme-sensitive intermediates and enzyme-resistant final degradation products and is entirely compatible with the trinodular electron-microscopic picture. According to this scheme, fibrinogen is first converted to a clottable derivative, fragment X ($M_r$ 240,000 to 260,000), which is then split asymmetrically into a fragment Y ($M_r$ 150,000) and a fragment D ($M_r$ 100,000). Fragment Y is subsequently split into a second fragment D and a fragment E ($M_r$

50,000). This sequence correlates with the trinodular model: Fragment X is composed of all three nodules minus the polar appendage of the Aα chain; fragment Y is composed of the smaller central nodule (fragment E) connected to either larger lateral nodule (fragment D). Fragment E and the second fragment D are liberated separately when the coiled-coil of fragment Y is degraded.

A critical confirmation of this asymmetric cleavage pattern was provided by Budzynski et al. who demonstrated that the component polypeptide chains of fragment Y were of two distinct groups (58). The three large chains extended from the *N*-terminal ends in the central (fragment E) domain to the lateral (fragment D) domains, whereas the three small-chain remnants were limited to the other half of the central domain. A direct visual demonstration of these predicted structures has been provided by shadow-cast electron micrographs of purified fragments (59). The difference in structure between the central and terminal domains was demonstrated by immunologic studies that showed distinct antigenic determinants for fragments D (terminal) and E (central) (60). The fact that both nodules contribute to fragment Y and fragment X structure was demonstrated by the existence of both D and E determinants in purified fragments X and Y, tested against appropriately absorbed antisera (56). The locations of fragments D and E and N-DSK within the multinodular fibrinogen structure have been confirmed by immunoelectron-microscopy (61–63).

## THREE-DIMENSIONAL STRUCTURE

### Molecular Architecture

Fibrinogen, the first biologic macromolecule visualized by electron microscopy, was described in 1959 in an elegant publication by Hall and Slayter (11) as a trinodular particle with an overall length of 475 Å, comprised of two roughly spherical nodules of 65 Å in diameter connected by thin threads of 8 Å to 15 Å in diameter to a central nodule 50 Å in diameter (11). The validity of the trinodular model was subsequently confirmed in both shadowed and negatively stained specimens of human fibrinogen, such as those presented in Figure 16-2. The resolution of the outer D-domains into two ellipsoidal regions, and the overall S-shaped arrangement of the multinodular fibrinogen molecules (64), can be seen in these micrographs. Recent progress in defining the structure of fibrinogen *at atomic resolution* can be appreciated by comparing these images to the structure of (chicken) fibrinogen determined at 2.7 Å resolution by x-ray diffraction crystallography in 2001 (4). Figure 16-2 includes a color-coded ribbon drawing of fibrinogen's three-dimensional structure and a surface representation, designed to facilitate comparison to the images obtained by electron microscopy. Chicken fibrinogen displays a strong sequence homology with its human counterpart, but fortunately it lacks the flexible carboxyl-terminal segment of the α chains that hindered crystallization of vertebrate fibrinogen molecules (3,65–68).

There is a striking agreement between the dimensions (460 Å × 65 Å), and overall sigmoid shape of the crystallographically determined fibrinogen structure, and the features deduced from electron microscopy. For example, note how two sets of three-stranded coiled-coils link the central domain to the outer β and γ globular domains. The x-ray structure of chicken fibrinogen also provided many details that were not seen by microscopy, including the "fourth helix" (4) formed by a segment of the α chain that folds back on the classical three-stranded coil-coil for approximately 60 residues. This structure confirmed the presence of a pair of *disulfide swivels* comprised of covalently crosslinked cysteine residues β76-α49, α45-γ23, and γ19-β80 that initiate the helical regions of the *three-stranded rope* motif,

as predicted by Doolittle (71). This structure also confirmed the presence of a small interruption in the coiled-coils in a protease-sensitive region (41) approximately 100 Å from the center of the molecule (4,72). Similar structural features were observed, albeit at a lower resolution (approximately 4 Å), in a crystallographic study of proteolytically modified bovine fibrinogen (3). Both structures displayed a twofold symmetry axis, pointing upward from the central domain in the top panel of Figure 16-2, which places key polymerization sites on the upper face of the elongated, dimeric fibrinogen molecule (3,4).

Segmental flexibility was recognized as an important feature that contributes to fibrinogen's hemostatic functions by facilitating contacts between polymerizing molecules and cell surface receptors (3,4,65). However, molecular motions have so far precluded precise determination of certain features of fibrinogen's three-dimensional structure. Although the positions of approximately 70% of the 2,728 residues present in each chicken fibrinogen molecule were determined in its 2.7 Å resolution structure, considerable segments of the αC domains, 96 residues in the central domain, and 16 in the γ-chain carboxyl terminal, yielded too little electron density to be mapped (4). Likewise, the carboxyl-terminal α-chain 170 residues were not visible in the crystal structure of the 285-kDa (modified) bovine fibrinogen structure (3). Fortunately, x-ray diffraction crystallography has provided additional insights into fibrinogen structure by examining the molecular morphology of several individual domains of this multinodular protein (65).

## Central Domain Organization

The *N*-terminal regions of all six chains in a dimeric fibrinogen molecule are tightly folded into an approximately globular

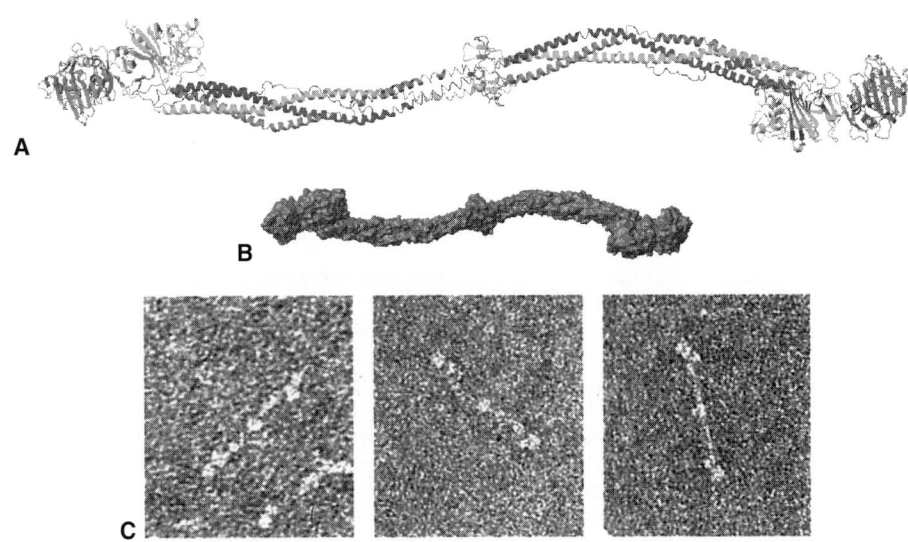

**FIGURE 16-2.** Fibrinogen structure determined by x-ray diffraction crystallography and electron microscopy. The **top** image depicts a color-coded chain-tracing of fibrinogen structure based on the crystal structure chicken fibrinogen reported by Yang et al. 2001 (4). The color scheme used in Figure 16-1 to represent the intact fibrinogen molecule, namely α chain (*blue*), β chain (*green*), and γ chain (*red*), is used here to represent the path of each main chain in fibrinogen. α-helices are shown as *ribbons* and β-strands as *wide arrows*. Starting with the small globular central domain, coiled-coil regions formed by the entwined α, β, and γ chains extend to both the right and left, then they connect to the carboxyl-terminal β and γ segments that fold into independent globular domains. The α chain folds back on itself to form a "hairpin helix"; however, the chicken fibrinogen molecule lacks the long carboxyl-terminal segment found on human fibrinogen. This figure was prepared using the molecular graphics software MOLMOL (69) and is patterned after Figure 1 of Yang Z, Kollman JM, Pandi L, et al. Crystal structure of native chicken fibrinogen at 2.7 A resolution. *Biochemistry* 2001;40:12515–12523. (Coordinates are available from the Protein Data Bank as entry 1JFE.PDB.) The middle panel depicts a surface representation of the fibrinogen molecule at approximately twofold smaller scale than the color-coded structural diagram. The **bottom** panel depicts images of fibrinogen obtained by electron microscopy reported by Fowler and Erickson, 1983 (70). These images are at approximately fivefold smaller scale than the color-coded fibrinogen structural diagram (see Color Fig. 16-2).

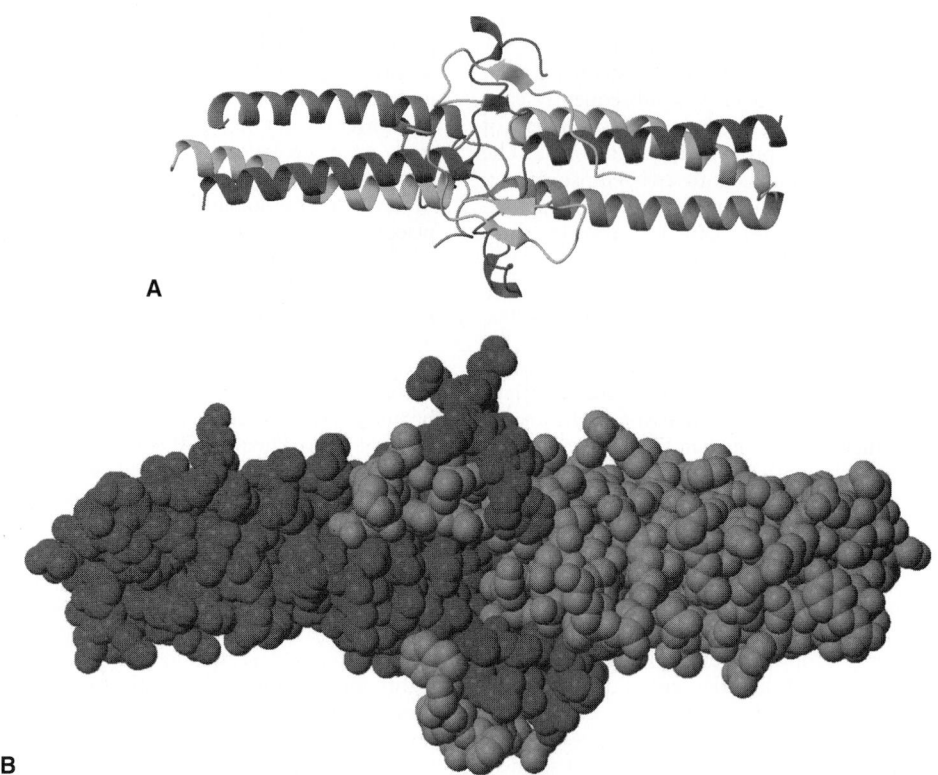

**FIGURE 16-3. A:** Structural diagram of the constituent polypeptide chains of fragment E (bovine). The color scheme used in Figure 16-1 to represent the intact fibrinogen molecule, namely $\alpha$ chain (*blue*), $\beta$ chain (*green*), and $\gamma$ chain (*red*), is used here to represent the path of each main chain in the dimeric fragment $E_5$. $\alpha$-helices are shown as *ribbons* and $\beta$-strands as *wide arrows*. This 35-kDa fragment contains the N-terminal disulfide knot and portions of the coiled-coils from the $\alpha$, $\beta$, and $\gamma$ chains but not the fibrinopeptides. Crystal structure of the central region of bovine fibrinogen (E5 fragment) at 1.4 Å resolution (coordinates are available from the Protein Data Bank as entry 1JY2.PDB). **B:** Space-filling diagram of the structure of fragment $E_5$. Note how the two halves (*red* and *blue*) of this dimeric central domain fragment form a "handshake" interface (see Color Fig. 16-3). This figure was prepared using the molecular graphics software MOLMOL (69) and is patterned after Figure 2 of Madrazo J, Brown JH, Litvinovich S, et al. Crystal structure of the central region of bovine fibrinogen (E5 fragment) at 1.4 Å resolution. *Proc Nat'l Acad Sci* 2001;98:11867–11972. (Coordinates are available from the Protein Data Bank as entry 1JY2.PDB.)

dimeric central domain that is stabilized by disulfide bonds and contains fibrinopeptides A and B (61). Key features of this region, illustrated schematically in Figure 16-3A, have been revealed in a high-resolution (1.4 Å) structure for a 35-kDa E-domain fragment of bovine fibrinogen (5). The remarkable thermal stability (73) of this "handshake" interface (Fig. 16-3B) between the segments of the dimeric fibrinogen molecule can now be understood in terms of its extensive noncovalent contacts and network of reciprocal disulfide crosslinks. In fact, the approximately 2,500 Å² contact area is probably sufficient, on its own, to promote dimer formation (5). Indeed, only the A$\alpha$ to B$\beta$ disulfides are required to assemble the fibrinogen dimer (46,74). Molecular flexibility prevented visualization of the fibrinopeptides, although we revisit this issue later in the chapter when thrombin binding is considered.

## Fragment-D Structure

The structure of fragment D, isolated as an 86-kDa tryptic fragment of human fibrinogen, was first solved in 1997 by Spraggon et al. (8), who employed x-ray diffraction crystallography to obtain data at sufficient resolution (2.9 Å) to define

not only the paths of each constituent polypeptide chain but also the location of several interchain disulfide bridges and the positions of critical side chain atoms. The 734 residues of this fragment D, which include $\alpha$-chain residues 111 to 197, $\beta$-chain residues 134 to 461 and $\gamma$-chain residues 88 to 406, account for approximately 50% of the entire mass of the 340-kDa fibrinogen molecule (8). The structure of the main chain of plasma fragment D is shown in Figure 16-4 as a set of color-coded lines to specify the paths of the polypeptide chains: $\alpha$ (*blue*), $\beta$ (*green*), and $\gamma$ chains (*red*).

Described by the Spraggon et al. (8) as "plough-shaped," fragment D contains a three-stranded "remnant coiled-coil" comprised of roughly half the residues present in the intact connector region, with about equal representations from the $\alpha$, $\beta$, and $\gamma$ chains. Consistent with protein packing principles and the predictions of R. Doolittle (75), most nonpolar residues in this truncated rope point inward to form a hydrophobic core. However, additional $\alpha$ chain residues form a fourth, amphipathic helix that folds back and packs against the three-stranded coiled-coil itself. Carboxyl-terminal residues of the $\beta$ and $\gamma$ chains depart to form separate globular domains, with the $\beta$-domain closest to the central domain, displaced by an approximately 130-degree angle from the distal

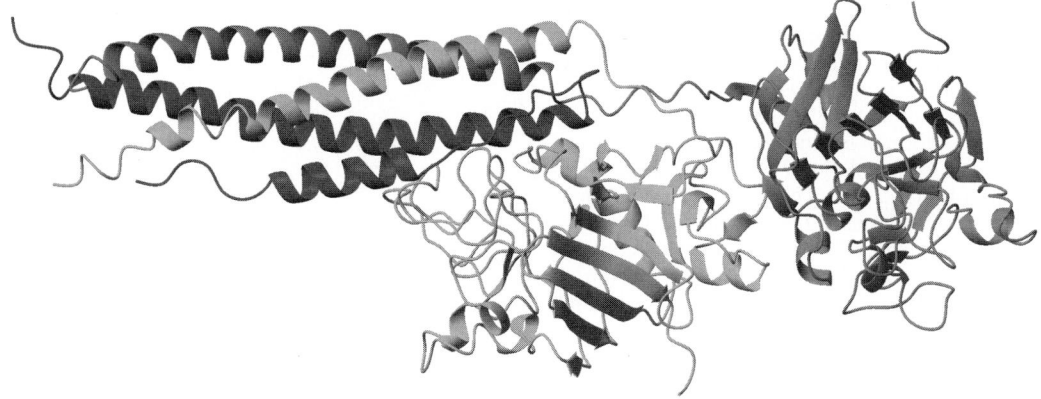

**FIGURE 16-4.** Structural diagram of the constituent polypeptide chains of fragment D. The color scheme used in Figure 16-1 to represent the intact fibrinogen molecule, namely α chain (*blue*), β chain (*green*), and γ chain (*red*), is used here to represent the path of each main chain in fragment D. α-helices are shown as *ribbons* and β-strands as *wide arrows*. Note the coiled-coil regions formed by the entwined α, β, and γ chains, and how the carboxyl-terminal β and γ segments fold into independent globular domains. In contrast, the α chain folds back on itself to form the "hairpin helix" (see Color Fig. 16-4). This figure has been prepared using MOLMOL, molecular graphics software (69) and is patterned after Figure 2a of Spraggon G, Everse SJ, Doolittle RF: Crystal structures of fragment D from human fibrinogen and its crosslinked counterpart from fibrin. *Nature* 1997;389:455–462. (Coordinates are available from the Protein Data Bank as entry 1FZA.PDB.)

γ-domain. This point may be best appreciated by comparing the structure of isolated fragment D (Fig. 16-4) to the distal domains in the structural diagram of the intact fibrinogen molecule (Fig. 16-2).

Subsequently, Kostelansky et al. (10) reported a 2.8-Å resolution structure for a 79-kDa recombinant fragment D construct. The positions of residues α126 to α190, β161 to β458, and γ96 to γ394 were determined in that study. Although the structures of the plasma and recombinant proteins are nearly superimposable, differing on average by about the radius of a single carbon atom, there are differences in the loop regions, the positions of which are somewhat better determined in the recombinant fragment-D structure (10). These advances in structural and molecular biology complement the view of fibrinogen's molecular morphology determined by electron microscopy (11,64,67,70) and provide new insights into the form and function of the "outer nodules" of fibrinogen first described by Hall and Slayter nearly 50 years ago!

## Structures of the Homologous βC and γC Domains

Structural studies (6–8) have also confirmed predictions, based on amino acid homology (75), that the β and γ chains would form carboxyl-terminal domains with similar folded structures. Yee et al. (6) first reported that the 30-kDa globular γC domain is characterized by a "unique fold," structurally distinct from any of the more than 6,000 structures (or approximately 200 independently folded domains) then reported in the Protein Data Bank (see Fig. 16-5). This image is color-coded to identify secondary structural features: α-helices are *red*, β-strands are *blue*, and *loops* are *gray*. Subsequently, Spraggon et al. noted remarkably similar structures for both the globular βC and γC domains, and pointed out that each domain can be further divided into three subdomains, with each subdomain containing a distinctive mix of α-helical and β-stranded structures (8,76). Conformational changes in the βC and γC domains in response to ligand and calcium ion binding are explored in subsequent sections.

## Structure of the αC Domain

The hydrophilic carboxyl-terminal portions of each α chain depart from the terminal domains of the β and γ chains to

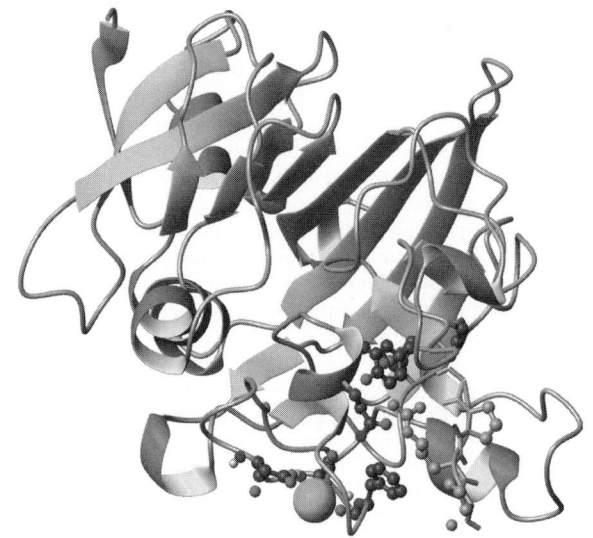

**FIGURE 16-5.** Structural diagram of the γ-chain carboxyl-terminal domain. The path of the main chain is represented by a tube, color-coded according to secondary structure such that *red* denotes α–helical regions, *blue* indicating regions of β-structure, and *yellow* indicates non-repetitive structural elements. Residues that bind a calcium ion (*green*) are shown in *ball and stick* representation with *red* indicating oxygen, *blue* indicating nitrogen, and *gray* indicating carbon atoms. The same format is used to highlight residues that bind the polymerization inhibitor GPRP (*orange*) (see Color Fig. 16-5). This figure has been prepared using MOLMOL molecular graphics software (69), and is patterned after Figure 4 of Pratt KP, Cote HCF, Chung DW, et al. The primary fibrin polymerization pocket: Three-dimensional structure of a 30-kDa C-terminal γ chain fragment complexed with the peptide Gly-Pro-Arg-Pro, *Proc Natl Acad Sci U S A* 1997;94:7176–7181. (Coordinates are available from the Protein Data Bank as entry 2FIB.PDB.)

form a structure termed the "alpha-C domain" (77) that was first visualized by electron microscopy (61,70,78) and characterized as an independent folding unit by calorimetry (79). No high-resolution structural data are available for the αC domain, as the carboxyl-terminal third of the Aα chain is missing on the proteolytically modified form of bovine fibrinogen whose structure has been solved at 4-Å resolution (3), and is disordered in chicken fibrinogen, solved to 2.7 Å (4). However, spectroscopic and calorimetric characterizations of the thermal unfolding patterns of recombinant αC domain fragments support secondary structure predictions that the αC domain contains a compact globular segment (Aα392–610) followed by an N-terminal connector (Aα221–391) with a left-handed polyproline helix (80,81).

## Structure of the AαE Domain

The crystal structure of recombinant human fibrinogen AαE carboxyl-terminal domain has been determined at a resolution of 2.1 Å (30). Unlike the carboxyl terminal of the common form of the Aα chain, the AαEC domain shows significant homology to the globular domains of the β and γ chain C-termini (82). A comparison of the crystal structure of AαEC domain with the structures of the carboxyl-terminal domains of human fibrinogen β and γ chains revealed a binding cleft that is essentially neutral. Therefore, this binding pocket is thought not to bind Gly-Pro-Arg or Gly-His-Arg peptides, suggesting that the AαE domain does not participate directly in fibrin polymerization. Nonetheless, it has been proposed that the binding cleft of AαEC binds a carbohydrate-containing ligand such as sialic acid (30).

# FIBRIN FORMATION

The dramatic conversion of soluble fibrinogen into an insoluble polymer can be considered in three steps: (a) Cleavage of fibrinopeptides by thrombin, resulting in the formation of fibrin monomer, (b) a three-step noncovalent assembly process, and (c) covalent stabilization of fibrin by factor XIIIa–catalyzed crosslinking. Each of these events is discussed in detail in the sections that follow. These steps are illustrated schematically in Figure 16-6; corresponding images obtained by electron microscopy during the time course of fibrin assembly are depicted in Figure 16-7. The latter figure includes images of fibrinogen obtained by negative staining (panel A) and rotary shadowing (panel B).

## Fibrinopeptide Release

When thrombin acts on fibrinogen, specific Arg–Gly bonds of the Aα and Bβ chains are hydrolyzed (Fig. 16-1), and 2 mol each of fibrinopeptides A and B are released (83). These peptides constitute less than 2% of the mass of fibrinogen, but their removal has profound consequences, that result in formation of a fibrin clot.

The mechanism governing thrombin's ability to initiate fibrin gelation by selectively catalyzing the hydrolysis of only two particular Arg–Gly bonds on the Aα or Bβ chains of fibrinogen continues to be a subject of active investigation. The substrate specificity arises in part from a set of hydrophobic residues present on fibrinopeptide A that bind to a complementary apolar region on thrombin, positioning the Arg16–Gly17 peptide bond in the catalytic site (84–90). The three-dimensional structure of fibrinopeptide A, shown by solution nuclear magnetic resonance (NMR) and x-ray crystallography data to contain a

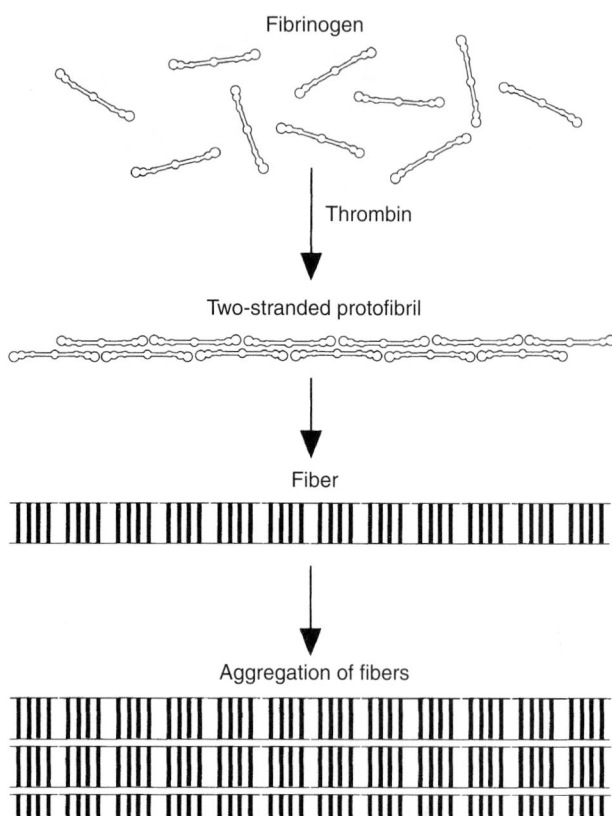

**FIGURE 16-6.** Schematic of the three-step noncovalent fibrin assembly process. Thrombin-catalyzed fibrinopeptide release leads to formation of two-stranded fibrin protofibrils, which are stabilized by the A–a and B–b contacts as described in the text. Next, a fiber is formed by lateral association of long protofibrils; the repetitive band pattern results from the half-staggered overlap configuration of the protofibrils that form the fiber. In the third step, fibers composed of 14 to 22 protofibrils aggregate laterally to form thick bundles of fibrin. Crossbanded fibers in varying stages of lateral aggregation can be seen in the electron micrograph of Figure 16-7E. However, note that the network branch points that characterize the fibrin clot have been omitted from this schematic. (From Weisel JW. Fibrin assembly. Lateral aggregation and the role of the two pairs of fibrinopeptides. *Biophys J* 1986;50:1079, with permission.)

short turn of α helix at its midsection that follows a region of multiple chain reversals (87,89,91,92), also contributes to thrombin–fibrinogen interactions. Studies with genetically engineered fibrinogen Aα-fusion proteins have shown that single-site substitutions within the fibrinopeptide A sequence have different effects on catalysis and binding (93), supporting the postulate that these functions map to distinct regions of both the fibrinogen and thrombin molecules.

## Thrombin: Fragment-E Structure

In addition to its active site, thrombin contains a cluster of positively charged residues termed the "anion-binding exosite" (94), which binds via ionic interactions (94–96) to a region contained within the central domain of fibrinogen (97,98). These interactions can now be visualized at atomic resolution, thanks to the recently published 3.65 Å resolution crystal structure of a complex formed between thrombin and human fibrinogen fragment E$_{ht}$ (99). Figure 16-8A presents a

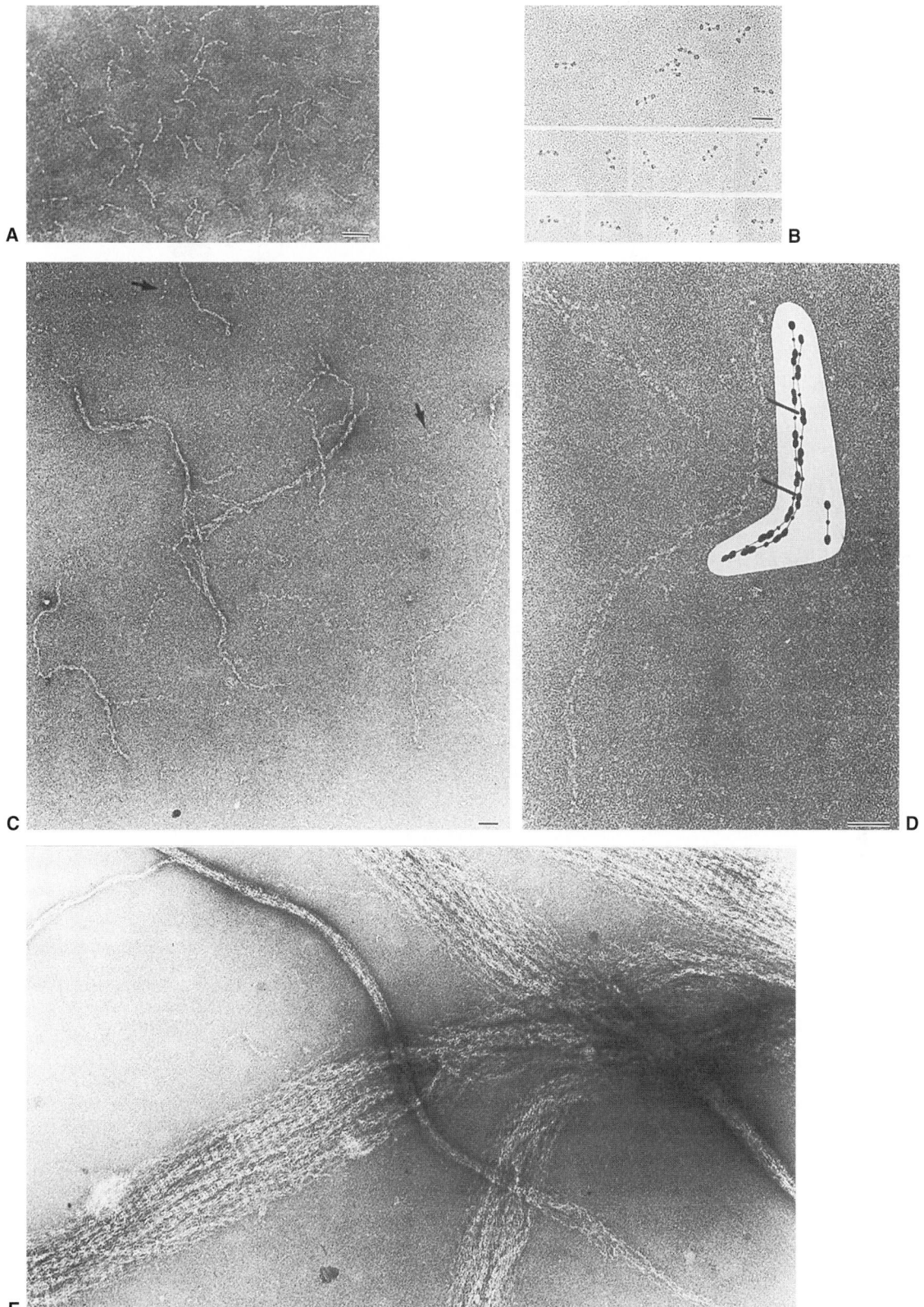

FIGURE 16-7. Electron micrographs of fibrinogen and fibrin. (A) and (B) depict fibrinogen that has been visualized by negative staining and shadowing, respectively. The multidomainal structure with an overall length of 450 Å can clearly be seen in both micrographs. The subdivision of the outer domain into two distinct nodules and the domain formed by the ends of the α chains are most evident in the negatively stained and shadowed specimens, respectively. Negatively stained protofibrils, obtained shortly after addition of thrombin to fibrinogen in buffered normal saline, are shown in (C) (*arrows*) and at higher magnification in (D). Note the half-staggered overlap arrangement of the individual fibrin monomer units in (D) (*illustrated schematically in the inset*). (E) depicts thick fibers (just before the gel point) that have been assembled by the lateral association of as many as 50 protofibrils. Interfiber connections are formed after protofibrils bridge between two thicker strands of fibrin. *Bars* represent 450 Å (length of the fibrinogen molecule) in (A) through (E). (A and B: From Erickson HP, Fowler WE. Electron microscopy of fibrinogen and its plasmin fragments and small polymers. *Ann N Y Acad Sci* 1983;408:146; C to E: From Hantgan RR, Fowler RW, Erickson HP, et al. Fibrin assembly: a comparison of electron microscopic and light scattering results. *Thromb Haemost* 1980;44:119, with permission.)

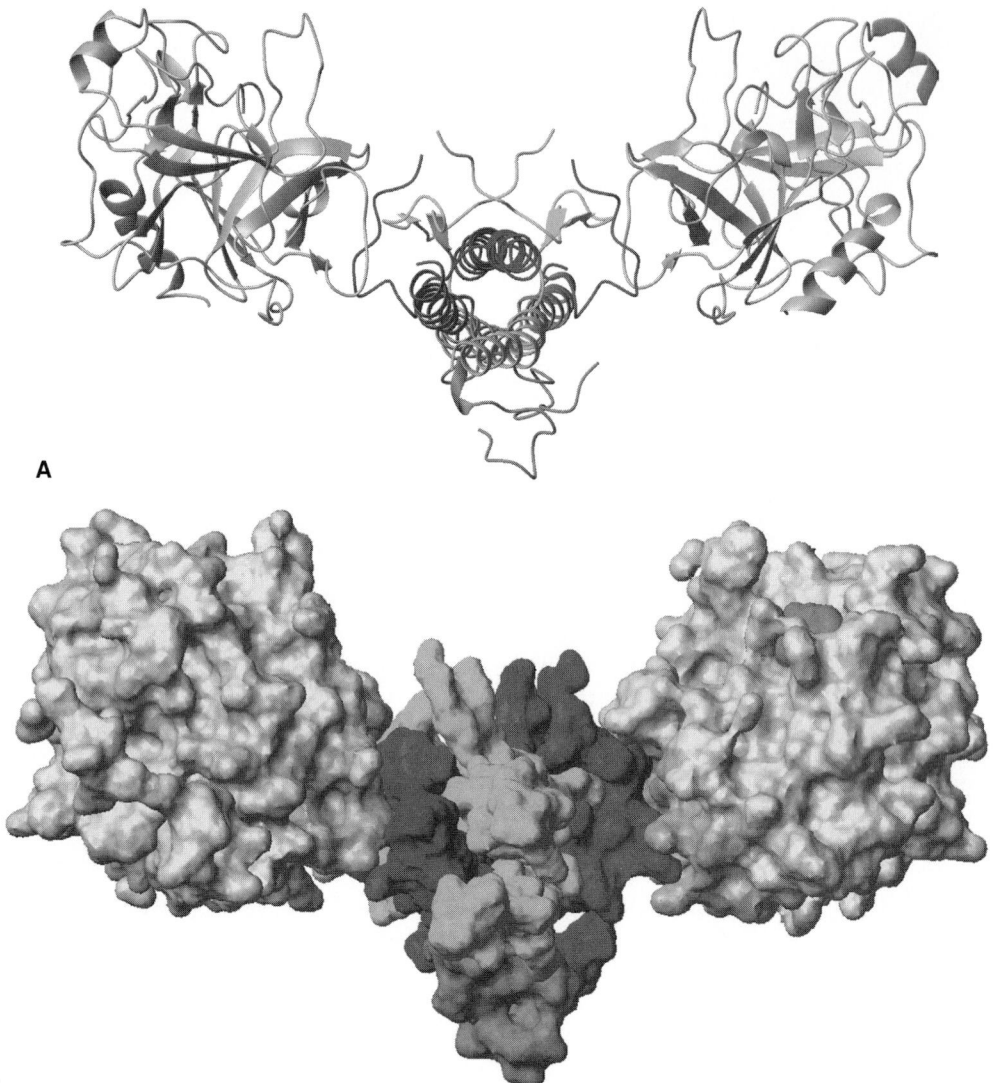

**FIGURE 16-8. A:** Structural diagram of the constituent polypeptide chains of the complex formed between fragment E and two thrombin molecules. The color scheme used in Figure 16-3 to represent the fragment E, namely α chain (*blue*), β chain (*green*), and γ chain (*red*), is also used here. The polypeptide chains of each thrombin molecule are represented by *gold lines*, with α-helices shown as *ribbons* and β-strands as *wide arrows*. This figure has been prepared using the molecular graphics software MOL-MOL (69), and is patterned after Figure 1.C. of Pechik I, Madrazo J, Mosesson MW, et al. Crystal structure of the complex formed between thrombin and the central "E" region of fibrin. *Proc Nat'l Acad Sci* 2004;101:2718–2723. (Coordinates are available from the Protein Data Bank as entry 1QVH.PDB.) **B:** Space-filling diagram of the structure of the thrombin: fragment-E complex. The color-coding follows that in panel (**A**), except that the hydrophobic core of fragment E is shown in *gray*, the sites on thrombin where the inhibitor PPACK binds are shown in *magenta*, and thrombin's exosites is shown in *orange*. Note that only a portion of the exosites makes direct contact with fragment E (see Color Fig. 16-8).

chain-tracing of this V-shaped complex, looking directly into the core of fibrinogen's central domain (imagine rotating the fragment-E structure in Fig. 16-3A by 90 degrees so that the coiled-coils point out of the page; the color-coding for fragment-E is the same in both figures). Figure 16-8B shows the same thrombin: fragment E structure in space-filling mode (99). The γN domain (*red*) of fragment E sits at the bottom of the figure with the α (*blue*) and β (*green*) chains straddling the coiled-coils (*dark gray*). Two thrombin molecules are bound, each by their exosites (*orange*); the inhibitor PPACK occupies each active site (*magenta*). Because both fibrinopeptides are absent in fragment E$_{ht}$, we may only imagine the paths between

these flexible substrates and the catalytic sites on thrombin. Each facet of this tight noncovalent complex is stabilized by a hydrophobic interior (each thrombin molecule buries 1,200 Å$^2$ of surface area) complemented by a network of three hydrogen bonds and three salt bridges (99).

## Fibrinopeptide Release Rates

Following the early observation that fibrinopeptide A is released more rapidly than fibrinopeptide B from fibrinogen (15,100), investigators have debated whether prior release of fibrinopeptide A is a prerequisite for removal of fibrinopeptide B (101–107). Both peptides can be released simultaneously from fibrinogen, but the B peptide is cleaved so slowly that its release may appear to follow that of the A peptide (102,105). A sequential model has been proposed in which fibrinopeptide B is released at a statistically significant rate only from molecules lacking fibrinopeptide A (106,107). Studies with recombinant fibrinogen variants suggest, however, that the ordered release of fibrinopeptides is dictated by the specificity of thrombin for its substrates (108). Studies of the temperature-dependence and salt concentration–dependence of fibrinopeptide release provide strong support for the sequential mechanism and further indicate that electrostatic interactions enable thrombin to bind rapidly, that is, at a diffusion controlled rate, to fibrinogen and fibrin (109–111). Once bound, hydrophobic interactions cause a conformational change in thrombin, which is an inherently allosteric enzyme (112), converting it to a faster form with increased catalytic efficiency (109). As polymerization to protofibrils proceeds, the rate of fibrinopeptide B release increases approximately sevenfold (102,105,106), consistent with the hypothesis that either this peptide is preferentially removed from soluble fibrin polymers (113) or that polymerization-induced conformational changes facilitate its release (102,105). A recent detailed kinetic study demonstrated that the rates of FPA and FPB release exhibited differential sensitivity to both ionic strength and calcium ion concentrations, perhaps indicative of calcium-linked conformational changes in fibrinogen's AαC domains (114).

# FIBRIN ASSEMBLY

## First Steps

The thrombin-catalyzed release of the fibrinopeptides from fibrinogen results in the formation of an intermediate, termed fibrin monomer, with an overall structure indistinguishable from that of the parent molecule (64,66,115,116). Removal of fibrinopeptide A by either the physiologic enzyme, thrombin, or batroxobin, a protease derived from the venom of *Bothrops atrox*, exposes new binding sites, termed *A knobs*, on the central, E-domain of fibrin monomer, which can interact with complementary sites, termed *γC holes*, which are always present on the γC domain of another fibrin molecule monomer (117–119). Similarly, removal of fibrinopeptide B by either thrombin or venzyme, isolated from the venom of Agkistrodon contortrix, exposes a *B knob* on the central domain, which can form a noncovalent association with a *βC hole* present on the βC domain (8,76,117). Release of either set of fibrinopeptides initially leads to the formation of a fibrin dimer, which is characterized by a half-staggered overlap structure and is stabilized by noncovalent interactions between complementary polymerization sites present on the central and outer domains of fibrin (66,116,120).

## Protofibril Growth

Continuing thrombin-catalyzed cleavage of the fibrinopeptides leads to the formation of two-stranded polymers of fibrin, termed protofibrils, in a rapid bimolecular polymerization process (see Fig. 16-9) (101,113,115). The central role of the protofibril in fibrin assembly was first proposed by Ferry some four decades ago (121). Protofibrils have been extensively studied in inhibited clotting systems (116,122–127) and have been shown to be obligatory intermediates on the fibrin assembly pathway (113,128). The protofibrils shown in the high-resolution negatively stained electron micrographs in

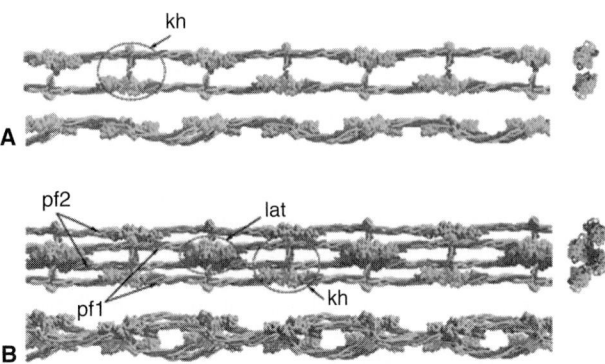

**FIGURE 16-9. A:** schematic of fibrin protofibril structure. Individual fibrin monomer molecules with the two-stranded protofibrils are shown in space-filling mode with α chains in *magenta*, β chains in *blue*, and γ chains in *green*. The *red oval* outlines the knob-hole (kh) noncovalent contacts that stabilize each protofibril. The views are presented: top, side, and end-on. **B:** Schematic of two protofibrils (pf1, pf2) laterally associated as the first step in formation of a thick fibrin fiber. Note that the lateral contacts between these aligned protofibrils (lat) are distinct from the knob-hole interaction that stabilizes the individual protofibrils (see Color Fig. 16-9). (From Yang Z, Mochalkin I, Doolittle RF. A model of fibrin formation based on crystal structures of fibrinogen and fibrin fragments complexed with synthetic peptides. *Proc Natl Acad Sci U S A* 2000;97:14156, with permission.)

Figure 16-7, panels C and D, were prepared from samples in the early stages of fibrin assembly (115,128). The structure of the protofibril is illustrated schematically in Figure 16-9. Protofibrils are stabilized by the same "A–a" and "B–b" *knob/hole* noncovalent contacts that stabilize the fibrin dimer (116,120, 129,130) and additional stability is provided by noncovalent interactions between the distal D-domains of fibrin molecules aligned end to end in the same strand of each protofibril (116).

## Protofibril Stability

Recent advances in structural biology have led to a new understanding of the noncovalent interactions between the *A knobs* on the central E-domain of one fibrin monomer and the corresponding γC *holes* on the outer D-domain of another fibrin subunit. The *A knob* on the central E-domain has been shown to involve residues that are newly exposed on the α chain following the release of fibrinopeptide A (6–8,76). Early evidence supporting this concept came from the observation that short peptides containing the sequence Gly-Pro-Arg, the three *N*-terminal α-chain residues, bind to fibrinogen and are effective polymerization inhibitors (119). Crystallographic data reported independently by different groups (6–8) has defined, at the molecular level, details of these *knob-hole* contacts.

Yee et al. reported the crystal structure of a 30-kDa carboxyl-terminal fragment of the γ chain, purified from a yeast expression system (6), and Pratt et al. solved the structure of the complex formed between this γ-domain and the polymerization inhibitor Gly-Pro-Arg-Pro (GPRP) (7). This high-resolution (2.0 Å) structure is presented in Figure 16-5, although it is important to emphasize that Spraggon et al. (8) reported a very similar structure for the γ-domain–GPRP complex isolated from a proteolytic digest of crosslinked human fibrin. Comparison to the unliganded γ-domain structure reveals that only subtle conformational rearrangements accompany binding of GPRP, which is held in place largely by electrostatic interactions with residues present on loops in the P-domain (7). Residues in direct contact with the positively charged GPRP ligand are annotated on Figure 16-5 and include Gln329,

Asp330, His340, and Asp364. Tyr363, shown by photoaffinity labeling to participate in polymerization (131), is indeed present in the binding pocket, but its interaction with GPRP is mediated through a bridging water molecule (7). The residues contacting the single tightly bound calcium ion in the γ-domain structure are in quite distinct locations from the GPRP binding pocket (Fig. 16-5) (7,132).

Structural studies with a larger proteolytic fragment of crosslinked fibrin, which contained both the γ- and β-domains, led Spraggon et al. to similar conclusions, namely, that ligand binding sites for GPRP are present on three extended loops that form a cavity on the γ-domain in an area that is rich in negatively charged side chains and contains Tyr363 (7). Everse et al. subsequently described the crystal structure of crosslinked D-dimer (DD), complexed with both GPR and GHR peptides bound to separate locations on the γ and β chains, respectively (76). Additional crystallographic studies from this group have demonstrated that a major conformational change accompanies binding of Gly-His-Arg-Pro-Amide (GHRPam), a peptide mimetic of the *B knob*, to the βC domain; in particular, two carboxylate anions (BβGlu397 and BβAsp398) rotate inward to complete formation of the β-chain pocket in the liganded structure (9). Combining protein engineering and x-ray diffraction crystallography, Kostelansky et al. recently demonstrated a critical role for BβAsp398 in binding GHRPam to the βC *hole* (133). They also demonstrated that mutating BβGlu397 and BβAsp398 to alanine residues impaired protofibril formation and lateral association, whereas mutating BβAsp432 had no effect. The latter result was unexpected, as previous crystallographic studied described a key role for BβAsp432 in the *B knob*–βC interactions (76).

## Protofibril Structure

The wealth of structural data now available has enabled Doolittle et al. (65,117,134) to propose a detailed model for the assembly and molecular architecture of fibrin protofibrils. Key to this understanding is the complementary yet asymmetric interface formed between γ-chain residues 270 to 310 that abut in the DD structure: Arg275 in one γC domain contacts Tyr280 of the second molecule whereas Arg275 of the second points toward Ser300 of the first (117). During protofibril growth, these end-to-end contacts are reinforced by electrostatic knob–hole interactions with the A and B knobs provided by a third fibrin molecule that sits atop these two, as illustrated in Figure 16-10. Although flexibility within the segments harboring the knobs has precluded their precise location, knowledge of the hole locations on DD has fixed the distance between the two aligned strands of a protofibril at approximately 80 Å, in good agreement with observations by electron microscopy (116,128). Replicating these contacts yields two-molecule thick polymers with the second strand offset from the first by half the length of single fibrin molecule, yielding the characteristic 225-Å band pattern seen in electron micrographs, such as Figure 16-7E.

## Thick Fiber Formation

Light scattering kinetic data, combined with electron-microscopic observations, demonstrate that the second step in fibrin assembly is the lateral association of long protofibrils into thicker fibrin fibers (113,116,128) (Fig. 16-7). Lateral association of protofibrils into fibrin strands takes place at an appreciable rate only when the oligomers reach a sufficient length, in the range of 600 to 800 nm. The requirement for a critical length suggests that the contacts that enable protofibrils to associate into bundles, thereby forming thicker fibers,

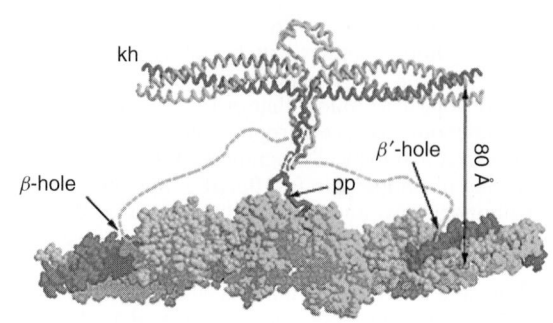

**FIGURE 16-10.** Schematic of the knob–hole interactions that stabilize a fibrin protofibril. The color-coding follows that in Figure 16-8. The upper molecule, the central domain of a fibrin monomer, is shown in polypeptide backbone mode with *dashed lines* corresponding to the flexible segments of the α and β chains that have not been visualized in crystal structures. The lower molecule, separated by 80 Å, is a fragment DD shown in space-filling mode. "*pp*" denotes the binding sites for the A-knob mimetic peptide Gly-Pro-Arg-Pro-amide (see Color Fig. 16-10). (From Yang Z, Mochalkin I, Doolittle RF. A model of fibrin formation based on crystal structures of fibrinogen and fibrin fragments complexed with synthetic peptides. *Proc Natl Acad Sci U S A* 2000;97:14156, with permission.)

are relatively weak, and a large number of these contacts must form to stabilize the fibrin strands (101,113,128–130). Structural considerations indicate that interactions between D-domains in laterally aligned protofibrils are likely to be responsible for this aspect of fiber growth (116,124,129,130). Recently, Doolittle et al. have proposed that noncovalent interactions between the γC domains of laterally aligned protofibrils, especially those that shield residues γ350 to γ360 and γ370 to γ380 from water, stabilize bundles of protofibrils (117). These intraprotofibril contacts are labeled "lat" in Figure 16-9 and are quite distinct from the "kh" contacts that stabilize individual double-stranded polymers.

## Effects of Fibrinopeptides on Fibrin Assembly

A subject that remained controversial for many years is the impact of fibrinopeptide A versus fibrinopeptide B release in determining the rate and extent of lateral association and the overall impact on the structure of fibrin. Some investigators have interpreted turbidity data to mean that removal of fibrinopeptide A alone leads only to formation of fine clots composed of protofibrils and thin fibers, whereas release of fibrinopeptide B was thought to be required for assembly of a coarse network composed of thick fibrin fibers (101,135–137). On the other hand, both light scattering and electron-microscopic data support the view that release of fibrinopeptide A alone is sufficient to initiate the entire fibrin assembly process, although the stability of the protofibrils and the rate of thick fiber formation are enhanced by fibrinopeptide B removal (113,128,138). Biophysical studies demonstrate that fibrin can also be formed by removing fibrinopeptide B alone, although only at low temperatures (139,140); electron microscopy revealed a heterogeneous mixture of thick fibers with frequent interconnecting thin strands under these conditions (141).

This issue has been resolved by J. Weisel, who performed extensive electron-microscopic analyses and found a remarkably invariant fiber diameter of 85 ± 13 nm, whether fibrinogen was clotted with thrombin, batroxobin, or venzyme to form αβ-fibrin, α-fibrin, or β-fibrin, respectively (120). Furthermore, the complex pattern of light and dark bands seen in electron micrographs of negatively stained specimens (such as those in Fig. 16-7E) was also present under all of these conditions.

Computer modeling showed that there is a unique molecular packing that gives rise to this band pattern. Fibrin fibers are formed by the lateral association of protofibrils (approximately 14 to 22 across), and each protofibril is composed of two strands of fibrin arranged in a half-staggered overlap pattern (66,67,120,142). Electron microscopy of shadowed specimens reveals that fibrin fibers are similar in width and also display a twist (115,141,143,144). Weisel et al. have proposed that each additional protofibril added to such a twisted fiber must be stretched slightly to remain in register. When the energy required to achieve this deformation exceeds that gained from additional noncovalent bond formation, fiber growth ceases, limiting fiber diameters to less than 100 nm (144). It is the last step in fibrin formation (namely, lateral aggregation of 85-nm fibers into larger bundles, illustrated schematically in Fig. 16-9) that is primarily responsible for the difference between coarse and fine clots (113,120,123). In particular, thicker bundles of fibrin are formed upon removal of both sets of fibrinopeptides (120). Contacts between $\beta$C domain residues 330–375 in adjacent protofibrils, interactions that follow a conformational change linked to knob/hole interactions that follow release of fibrinopeptides B, have been proposed to provide a subsidiary source of stability that can explain these observations (117). We will revisit this issue when the effects of calcium ions on fibrin assembly are considered, in a subsequent section.

## Fibrin Network Branchpoints

The net result of the fibrin assembly process is the formation of a highly interconnected network of fibrin fibers, which has sufficient mechanical stability to serve as a hemostatic plug. Protofibrils and thin fibers may be connected to more than one thick fibrin strand by the same lateral contacts that promote the association of protofibrils into fibers (Fig. 16-7E) (129,130). In addition to these bridging strands, a recent report has described a new structure, termed the trimolecular branch point, in which one double-stranded protofibril forms a junction with two separate double-stranded protofibrils (145). Other investigators have proposed models in which the formation of network branch points involves a different type of interfiber contact (135–137). In addition, electron-microscopic examination of the structure of fibrin formed from fragment X revealed a near-complete absence of branching, indicating that the carboxyl-terminal two thirds of the $\alpha$ chain plays a major role in formation of a stable, three-dimensional fibrin network (146). Immunoelectron-microscopy demonstrated that the full-length $\alpha$ chains interact to form a globular domain, termed the $\alpha$C domain, that associates with the central domain of fibrinogen at neutral, but not at acidic, pH (77). Concomitant with fibrinopeptide release and/or polymerization, the $\alpha$C domain is displaced from the central domain, allowing the individual $\alpha$ chains to participate in fibrin assembly (77). Additional studies with fragment X preparations that lacked one or both $\alpha$-chain carboxyl-terminal segments showed the resultant fibrin clots to exhibit substantial branching, comparable to that observed with intact fibrin. However, differences in fiber bundling were noted with fragment X fibrin, leading to the conclusion that the $\alpha$C domain does participate in fiber growth/branchpoint formation (147). Carbohydrate residues also influence both lateral association and branch point formation, because complete deglycosylation of fibrinogen has been shown to result in a more porous clot composed of thicker fibers with fewer network branch points (148).

## Fibrin Structure

Investigators have conducted a search for lateral order in fibrin, such as that proposed by Hermans (149), to explain the observation that only 20% of the volume of a fiber is protein, with the remainder being solvent (150). Electron-microscopic examination of thin sections of clots revealed essentially no regular pattern of fiber packing; rather, 10- to 30-nm channels were observed between regions of tightly packed protofibrils (143). Protofibrils are held together by a limited number of lateral contacts, and this lack of lateral order actually favors network branch point formation (143). X-ray diffraction and electron-microscopic data indicate a longitudinal repeat of 22.5 nm, half the length of fibrinogen, which has been attributed to the half-staggered overlap arrangement of the fibrin molecules within the protofibrils (145,151–153), but extensive optical diffraction studies of electron micrographs of fibrin also demonstrated only limited lateral order in fibrin fibers. In contrast, very thick fibers formed under the orienting influence of a strong magnetic field did display evidence of lateral order (154,155). Doolittle et al. have recently proposed a fibrin packing model where each strand of a protofibril interacts with another protofibril, related by a half-staggered overlap to avoid steric clashes; the dimensions of this model precisely replicate data obtained by neutron diffraction with magnetically oriented fibrin (117,154).

## Fibrin Assembly in Plasma and Whole Blood

In addition to the sequential fibrin assembly mechanism described in the preceding text, fibrinogen–fibrin complexes are likely to be important in certain pathologic situations in which the thrombin concentration is low and fibrin polymer growth is limited by incomplete removal of fibrinopeptide A (156, 157). For example, thrombus growth *in vivo* could be restricted by unactivated fibrinogen molecules or fibrin degradation products such as DD, which can cap the polymerization sites normally available at the ends of each protofibril (157). Furthermore, fibrin assembly kinetics measured with purified proteins differs from results obtained in plasma. Using changes in magnetic birefringence to monitor fiber growth, Torbet showed that even the addition of albumin promotes the rapid formation of thick fibrin fibers in a model system (158). Furthermore, results obtained in citrated plasma showed evidence of inhibited gelation due to antithrombin III, whereas in $Ca^{2+}$-containing plasma, fiber growth increased linearly with time, then reached an abrupt plateau (158). However, the effects of albumin on fibrin assembly remain controversial; albumin either promotes rapid fiber growth (159), favors formation of thin fibrils (160), or has no considerable effect on either the kinetics or extent of fiber growth (112). Recent studies of the activation of the extrinsic, tissue-factor mediated coagulation system in whole blood have shown rapid release of fibrinopeptide A in parallel with activation of factor XIII, leading to substantial fibrin formation and $\gamma$-chain crosslinking prior to release of fibrinopeptide B (161,162).

## Alternative Polymerization Models

The central role of the two-stranded fibrin protofibril in fibrin assembly is not universally accepted. Biophysical measurements and electron micrographs support a distinct interlocked single-strand model of fibrin network formation (163–165). This model stresses the importance of linear, single-stranded polymers of fibrin stabilized by noncovalent interactions involving a D:E:D trinodular unit under conditions in which polymerization is limited by low thrombin concentrations, and partially activated fibrin molecules (with only one fibrinopeptide A removed) block further elongation. Subsequent fibrinopeptide release favors a highly branched fibrin network, with lateral association promoted by D-domain contacts between nearby single-stranded polymers (165). Evidence for the importance of single-stranded fibrin polymers in the early stages of the assembly process has also been obtained by stopped-flow, multiangle laser light scattering, a technique well suited to detecting transient intermediates (166,167).

# FACTOR XIIIA–CATALYZED CROSSLINKING OF FIBRIN

In parallel with its fibrinopeptide-liberating action on fibrinogen, thrombin converts the inactive $\alpha$ chains in plasma factor XIII (168–170) to a calcium-dependent transglutaminase (171) that links the side chains of lysine and glutamine residues by isopeptide bonds. As many as six crosslinks can form between one fibrin monomer and its neighbors (172,173), in a process that renders the fibrin clot mechanically stronger (174,175) and more resistant to chemical (6 M urea) and enzymatic (plasmin) lysis (176–180).

In the early stages of the fibrin assembly process, protofibrils are stabilized by the factor XIIIa–catalyzed formation of crosslinks between the $\gamma$ chains of the assembling fibrin molecules (36). The lysine and glutamine residues involved in this reciprocal crosslink formation are both located near the carboxyl-terminal of the $\gamma$ chains of individual fibrin molecules (38), themselves held in close proximity by noncovalent interactions that determine the structure of the fibrin protofibril. Evidence supporting this concept comes from the observation that the ability of factor XIIIa to promote crosslinking of isolated D-domain fragments was enhanced by fragment E and that this effect was abolished by the tetrapeptide GPRP (181).

## $\gamma$-Chain Crosslink Locations

Although most investigators would agree that structural biology has resolved an ongoing controversy about the location of the covalent crosslinks between $\gamma$Gln398 and $\gamma$Lys406 chains within fibrin protofibrils in favor of the longitudinal model, the debate continues as evidenced by a recent exchange between Mosessson and Weisel (182,183). Early electron-microscopic examination of crosslinked fibrinogen dimers and dimer–fibrin monomer complexes indicated that these isopeptide bonds are formed between the D-domains of fibrin molecules adjacent in the same strand of a protofibril, termed longitudinal or end-to-end crosslinks (184). These findings were confirmed and extended to fibrin by further electron-microscopic examination of soluble, crosslinked fibrin fragments produced by the sequential actions of thrombin, factor XIIIa, and plasmin on the parent fibrinogen molecule (185). Under native conditions, these fragments were double-stranded, consistent with the known topology of fibrin protofibrils. In contrast, dissociation of all noncovalent interactions with dilute acetic acid yielded exclusively single-stranded oligomers that were taken as evidence for the end-to-end crosslinking pattern (185). Conversely, other investigators have presented evidence from electron-microscopic and immunologic studies indicating that transverse crosslinks were formed between the D-domains of molecules related by a half-staggered overlap within the protofibrils (145,186–189). Recently, Siebenlist et al. (190) reported autoradiography data obtained with fibrinogen-fibrin mixtures containing $\gamma_A$ and $\gamma'$ splice variants indicating a preponderance of transverse crosslinks.

The structure of crosslinked fragment D, isolated and crystallized from a plasmin digest of factor XIIIa–ligated fibrin, has been solved at 2.9 Å resolution, which is, sufficient detail

to show that the crosslinks are indeed end to end (longitudinal), as shown in Figure 16-11A, B. The upper panel shows a space-filling structure (8); the lower panel shows polypeptide chain tracings, color-coded for secondary structure. The authors were careful to point out that flexibility in this region precluded direct observation of the residues involved in the electron density map, but distance constraints were only consistent with longitudinal crosslinks (8). A reciprocal crosslink has been visualized in the crystal structure of lamprey crosslinked fragment D (191). Although the lamprey DD interface differed from that typically observed in human DD structures, due to flexibility inherent in fibrin structure, this crosslink was not consistent with the transverse model proposed by Mosesson et al. (182).

## $\alpha$-Chain Crosslinking

After pairing of virtually all of the $\gamma$ chains in the fibrin clot, a slower process of multiple crosslink formation between $\alpha$ chains proceeds. Because each $\alpha$ chain has two glutamyl acceptor sites (in positions 328 and 366) and five potential lysine donor sites (between positions 518 and 584) (39), a highly intricate crosslink network may result. Studies with a recombinant 45-kDa $\alpha$-chain fragment have demonstrated the ability of factor XIIIa to catalyzed crosslinks between glutamine residues at $\alpha$-chain positions 221, 237, and 328 and lysine residues at positions 539, 556, 580, and 601. However, it is unclear if all three glutamyl acceptors sites are reactive in intact fibrin (192). These interwoven $\alpha$-chain bonds are probably more critical for clot lysis resistance (179,180,193,194) than is the limited geometry of the $\gamma$–$\gamma$ crosslinks. Additional resistance to plasmin digestion comes from the slow formation of higher order $\gamma$-chain multimers (195). Crosslinked clots formed from a minor fibrinogen variant with a 20-residue carboxyl-terminal $\gamma$-chain extension also exhibit increased lytic resistance, probably due to their increased affinity for factor XIIIa (196,197).

# PLASMIN DIGESTION OF CROSSLINKED FIBRIN

Because of their unique presence in stabilized fibrin, the crosslink bonds are responsible for the liberation of specific degradation products during plasmin proteolysis (198). These degradation products bear strong resemblance to those of fibrinogen or noncrosslinked fibrin, but their unique structure provides information regarding fibrin polymerization and crosslinking and is also an important consideration for clinical assays of circulating derivatives. The unique characteristics of these degradation products result from prior crosslinking of fibrin, not from an alteration in proteolytic attack by plasmin. The sites of plasmin action attack and the sequence of cleavages are remarkably similar for fibrinogen and crosslinked fibrin. Following liberation of the "protective" covering of multiple crosslinked $\alpha$ chains, the thin portion of the coiled-coils between the D- and E-domains is exposed and then cleaved, leading to the liberation of solubilized derivatives from particulate fibrin.

Initial structural studies of crosslinked fibrin degradation products considered those derivatives present in a terminal lysate, prepared by prolonged *in vitro* exposure to plasmin. A unique fragment, termed DD (199–201), consists of fragment D moieties of two adjacent fibrin monomers covalently bound by the crosslinks between their $\gamma$-chain remnants. Fragment E was identified, as was a noncovalent complex of DD with

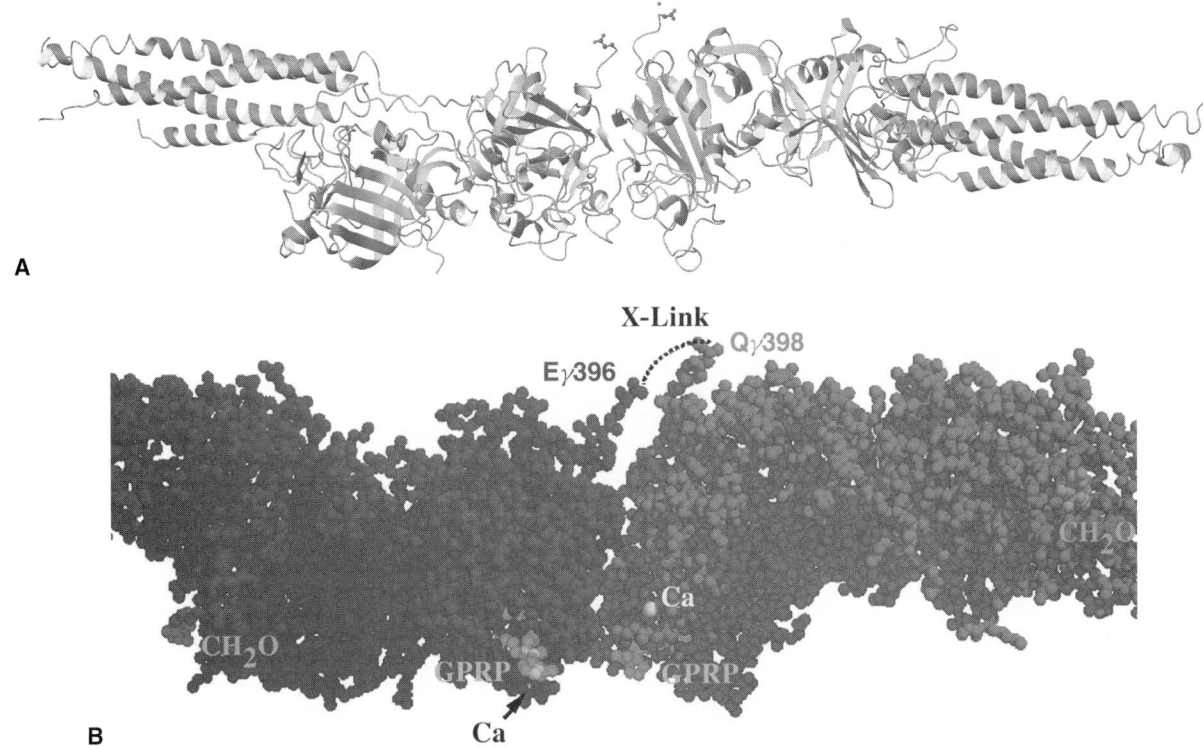

**FIGURE 16-11. A:** Structural diagram of cross-linked fragment D-Dimer. The path of each of the six constituent polypeptide chains is represented by a tube, color-coded according to secondary structure such that *red* denotes α-helical regions, *blue* indicates regions of β-structure, and *yellow* indicates nonrepetitive structural elements. Note how the γ-domains are aligned end to end in crosslinked fragment D. This figure was prepared using MOLMOL molecular graphics software (69) and is patterned after Figure 6 of Spraggon G, Everse SJ, Doolittle RF: Crystal structures of fragment D from human fibrinogen and its crosslinked counterpart from fibrin. *Nature* 1997;389:455–462. (Coordinates are available from the Protein Data Bank as entry 1FZB.PDB.) **B:** Space-filling representation of a portion of the crosslinked fragment D-Dimer shown in panel (**A**). The last carboxyl-terminal residue in each γ-chain that could be visualized in the crystal structure, γGLU396 and γGLN398 are annotated, and a *dotted line* denotes the putative path of the cross-linking site (see Color Fig. 16-11). (From Figure 6 of Spraggon G, Everse SJ, Doolittle RF: Crystal structures of fragment D from human fibrinogen and its crosslinked counterpart from fibrin. *Nature* 1997;389:455–462.)

fragment E (202,203). The derivation of the complex can be readily envisioned from the half-overlap model. The noncovalent forces between the central and terminal domains that led to fibrin monomer attraction and protofibril formation continue to operate after fibrinolysis and result in the liberation of the overlapping E and DD moieties still attached by lateral and longitudinal contacts. Once the α chains are cleaved, the critical cleavages leading to liberation of such fibrin products are between the appropriate D- and E-domains.

The structure of four large complexes, including their covalently bound component parts, has been elucidated and their origin within the fibrin matrix proposed (see Chapter 23) (204,205). This series of noncovalently bound derivatives is the simplest series of complexes that could logically arise from two-stranded, half-staggered overlap fibrin, primarily as a result of interdomainal cleavages in the thin portion of the coils between the D- and E-domains. Each complex is composed of elements from two adjacent fibrin strands, with the same interstrand noncovalent bonding between the D- and E-domains as that proposed for DD/E. Larger complexes contain subunits as large as DY (YD would be the antiparallel form), YY, DXD, and YXD (or DXY). These complexes can be separated into component fragments and identified electrophoretically, and they have been identified in the blood of patients with various thrombotic or thrombolytic disorders (see Chapter 23).

# ROLE OF CALCIUM IN FIBRINOGEN STRUCTURE AND FUNCTION

## Calcium Ion Binding Sites

Divalent calcium ions play a major role in maintaining the structure and stability of fibrinogen. Equilibrium dialysis experiments have demonstrated the existence of three high-affinity $Ca^{2+}$ binding sites on human fibrinogen (206). Detailed structural data from x-ray diffraction crystallography first identified a $Ca^{2+}$ binding site on a loop in the carboxyl-terminal P subdomain of the γ-domain of fibrinogen (6). Subsequent structural studies with plasma fragment D (9) and recombinant fragment D (10) defined three calcium binding sites, one on the γC domain and two on the βC domain. These sites and their network of oxygen-rich calcium-coordinating residues are shown in Figure 16-12. One area that remains unsettled is the extent to which the conformational change in BβAsp398, which occurs upon occupancy of the βC hole by the b-knob mimetic GHRPam, influences calcium binding. Kostelansky et al. (10), who studied recombinant fragment D, concluded that under

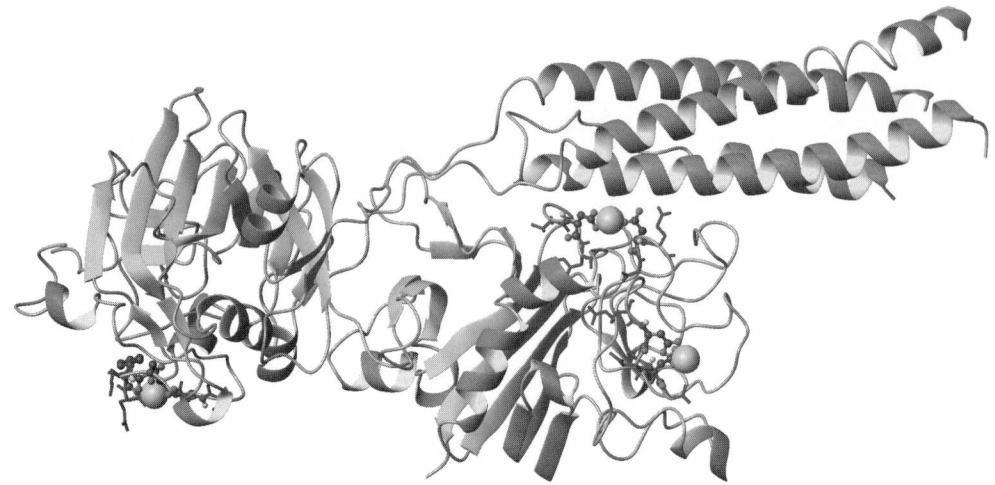

**FIGURE 16-12.** Structural diagram of (recombinant) fragment D. The path of the main chain is represented by a tube, color-coded according to secondary structure such that *red* denotes α–helical regions, *blue* indicates regions of β-structure and *yellow* indicates nonrepetitive structural elements. Residues that bind a calcium ion (*green*) are shown in *ball and stick* representation in which *red* indicates oxygen, *blue* indicates nitrogen, and *gray* indicates carbon atoms (see Color Fig. 16-12). This figure has been prepared using MOLMOL molecular graphics software (69) and is patterned after Figure 3 of Kostelansky MS, Betts L, Gorkun OV, et al. 2.8 Å crystal structures of recombinant fragment D with and without two peptide ligands: GHRP binding to the "b" site disrupts its nearby calcium-binding site. *Biochemistry* 2002;41:12124–12132. (Coordinates are available from the Protein Data Bank as entry 1LTJ.PDB.)

physiologic conditions occupancy of the b-site would displace the nearby calcium ion, whereas Everse et al. observed calcium bound in the presence of the a-knob mimetic GR-PRam, which can also bind to the b-hole (9).

## Calcium Ion Binding Affinities

Because the $K_d$ for $Ca^{2+}$ binding to these sites on human fibrinogen (206) (19 μM) is well below the free $Ca^{2+}$ concentration in plasma (1.5 mM), they will be fully occupied in circulating fibrinogen. Low-affinity binding sites, which would not be fully saturated under these conditions and could play a regulatory role, are found in bovine (207) and rat (206) species; evidence indicates that sialic residues in human fibrinogen provide low-affinity $Ca^{2+}$ binding sites that may fulfill this function (208). Millimolar calcium concentrations limit the extent of plasmin digestion of both fibrinogen and fibrin and protect fibrinogen against denaturation by heat and high pH (209,210). Calcium chloride (20 mM) limits the extent of disulfide bond reduction (211).

## Calcium Ion Effects on Fibrin Assembly

Calcium does not enhance thrombin-catalyzed fibrinopeptide release but does accelerate the rate of at least one of the subsequent assembly events (101,212–214). Because the calcium binding site on the γC domain is physically distinct from the polymerization pocket, it would appear unlikely that calcium binding has a direct effect on the first step in fibrin assembly, protofibril growth (6–8). However, engineered fibrinogen variants with single-site mutations at key calcium-binding residues in the γC domain (γD318A and γD320A) exhibited defective polymerization with thrombin and no detectable polymerization with batroxobin (215). These observations

indicate that protofibril formation, at least with γD318A and γD320A fibrinogen, requires B–b interactions (215).

Calcium enhances the rate and extent of lateral fiber growth when clotting is initiated by low concentrations of thrombin, batroxobin (216,217), or an enzyme isolated from the venom of Agkistrodon contortrix, which preferentially releases fibrinopeptide B (218). These effects are consistent with the earlier observation that the mechanical strength of clots formed in the presence of millimolar $Ca^{2+}$ concentrations is considerably greater than that formed in its absence (174). Calorimetric studies have provided evidence for a calcium-dependent conformational change in fibrin during the latter stages of the assembly process and have correlated this effect with the removal of fibrinopeptide B (218,219). Furthermore, measurements of $Ca^{2+}$ binding to fibrin during fibrin assembly show that approximately two $Ca^{2+}$ binding sites shift from low to high affinity, that this effect is closely tied to release of fibrinopeptide B, and that it proceeds at the same rate as the calcium-dependent conformational change (220). As noted earlier, calcium-dependent conformational changes in the βC domain that follow occupancy of its βC holes may explain some of these observations (10,117).

Additional evidence for a complex interplay among calcium binding, fibrinopeptide B release, and fibrin assembly comes from the observation that Gly-His-Arg-Pro (the terminal tetrapeptide of the β chain of fibrin) binds 10-fold more tightly to fibrinogen in the presence of 2-mM $Ca^{2+}$ than it does in its absence; the binding of the α-chain terminal tripeptide Gly-Pro-Arg is not influenced by calcium (221). The β-domain, to which Gly-His-Arg-Pro binds, does have a functional, albeit low affinity, calcium-binding site (76). Further mechanistic insights come from the engineered fibrinogen variant γE132A, which contains a mutation in one of the βC domain calcium-binding sites. At physiologic calcium concentrations, this variant exhibited increased lateral association, consistent with a role for B-b interactions in protofibril bundling (222).

# INTERACTION OF FIBRIN WITH OTHER PLASMA PROTEINS

## Thrombin

Following the early report by Seegers et al. that fibrin exhibited anticoagulant activity (223), considerable progress has been made in characterizing the affinity of thrombin for the fibrin clot. Binding to the fibrin network has been characterized by two classes of sites, one with a dissociation constant in the micromolar range and the second approximately 10-fold weaker (224). In addition to its catalytic site, thrombin binds to fibrin through two physically distinct positively charged locations termed exosites I and II. Solution of the three-dimensional structure of thrombin by x-ray diffraction crystallography has shown that exosite I resides on a loop structure on the surface of the molecule, near the rim of the deep cleft that forms the primary substrate binding pocket. Thrombin binds to the central domain of fibrin through exosite I (94,95,97–99). Exosite II, which is found near the carboxyl-terminal B-chain helix (225), may be primarily responsible for high-affinity fibrin binding. Exosite II recognizes sulfated tyrosine residues at positions 418 and 427 of the $\gamma'$ chain (226,227). However, recent evidence indicates that optimum high-affinity interactions with fibrin require the participation of both thrombin exosites (228).

Studies with fibrinogen fragments initially identified residues that contribute to the nonsubstrate, thrombin-binding site on the E-domain on its $\gamma$-chain sequence (97,98) and A$\alpha$ 17 to A$\alpha$50 (229,230) and $\beta$15 to $\beta$42 (231). Thanks to the recently published crystal structure of a complex with two thrombin molecules bound to fragment E (99), we can visualize these interactions at atomic resolution (Fig. 16-8). This study has defined the fibrinogen residues that contact thrombin's exosite I to include A$\alpha$ Trp33, Phe35, Asp38 and Glu39, B$\beta$ Ala68 and Asp69, and $\gamma$ Asp27 and Ser30 (99). In addition, four hydrophobic residues on each thrombin molecule contact complementary nonpolar residues on fragment E. Additional stability comes from a network of hydrogen bonds and salt bridges. Additional insights into thrombin–fibrinogen interactions are presented in a recent, richly detailed three-dimensional model (232).

When bound through both the catalytic site and exosite I, fibrin-bound thrombin efficiently catalyzes the release of fibrinopeptide B. Thrombin bound through exosite I alone can activate factor XIII, and it can be inhibited by antithrombin III (233). Thrombin bound through exosite I can also serve as a cofactor that accelerates fibrin assembly (234). Francis et al. have shown that thrombin bound to insoluble fibrin or associated with plasmin fibrin derivatives retains its enzymatic activity (235). Small amounts of active thrombin are bound to fibrin in pathologic clots, suggesting that it may play a role in propagation of thrombosis (235). Indeed the complex formed between thrombin bound to fragment E, the one recently visualized by x-ray diffraction crystallography, may well represent this catalytically active form of thrombin (99).

## Factor XIII

Interactions among factor XIII, Ca$^{2+}$, thrombin, and fibrin(ogen) are also critical in generating the active transglutaminase at physiologically significant rates [see (236,237) for comprehensive reviews]. This activation process involves thrombin cleavage of the a$_2$b$_2$ zymogen form of factor XIII, followed by a calcium-dependent dissociation that releases the active a$_2$ subunits. Fibrinogen lowers the calcium concentration required for the dissociation step to that found in plasma (1.5 mM); fragments derived from the midrange of the $\alpha$ chains of fibrinogen

have been implicated in this process (238). Factor XIII binds to fibrinogen with a dissociation constant (10 nM) tight enough to ensure that nearly all of the zymogen will circulate as a noncovalent complex with fibrinogen (239). Sedimentation equilibrium data demonstrate that factor XIII interacts cooperatively with fibrinogen to form a 2:1 complex (240). factor XIII binds approximately 20-fold more tightly to $\gamma'$ fibrinogen, implying a special role for the anionic carboxyl-terminal segment of the $\gamma'$ chain in localizing transglutaminase activity to a fibrin clot (240). When fibrinogen and factor XIII are present in dilute solution at equal concentrations, thrombin first removes fibrinopeptide A from fibrinogen, then the activation peptide from factor XIII; fibrinopeptide B release lags behind both of these proteolytic events (241). Fibrinopeptide A is released at a rate some 40-fold faster than that of factor XIII activation; this difference may reflect the nearly 30-fold difference in concentrations of the two thrombin substrates (242).

The ability of thrombin to catalyze activation of factor XIII and to initiate fibrin assembly raises the possibility that interactions between fibrin, thrombin, and factor XIII(a) play a role in the regulation of hemostatic plug formation (239,243,244). Considerable evidence demonstrates that fibrin polymers (as distinct from fibrin monomer or the crosslinked fibrin clot) are responsible for the fibrin(ogen)-dependent acceleration of factor XIII activation (242–247). The mechanism for this effect involves formation of a tight ternary complex between fibrin, thrombin, and factor XIII in which thrombin releases the activation peptide from factor XIII nearly 100-fold faster than from free factor XIII (248). However, recent results indicate that only fibrinopeptide release is required to observe factor XIII activation enhancement and that $\gamma'$ fibrino(gen) is especially effective in this regard (249).

Structural studies support the concept that fibrin binding to factor XIII induces a large conformational change that exposes the buried active site (250). In addition, fibrin-bound thrombin retains the ability to remove fibrinopeptide B from $\alpha$-fibrin and to activate factor XIII (248). The products of these reactions, namely $\alpha\beta$ fibrin and factor XIIIa, remain bound through interactions that are distinct from the active site of factor XIIIa (251), a region centered on the catalytic triad of residues Cys314-His373-Asp396 (250). Binding of fibrin to the catalytically active A2* subunits of factor XIIIa can be blocked by an antibody that does not inhibit the enzyme's active site (252). Likewise, factor XIIIa activity can be blocked by synthetic peptides corresponding to residues encoded by exons 3 and 5 of factor XIII, Asn72–Asp97 and Asp190–230, respectively, that are distinct from the active site, which is encoded by exon 7 (253,254). These observations suggest that factor XIIIa, like thrombin, has an *exosite* (251). Regions within the fibrin carboxyl-terminal region, A$\alpha$ 389–402 and A$\alpha$ 241–476, have been implicated in the binding interaction between fibrin and factor XIIIa (255), whereas blocking a site contained within $\gamma$-chain residues 402 to 411 with a monoclonal antibody has been shown to inhibit $\gamma$-chain crosslinking (256).

These observations are consistent with a mechanism proposed by Hornyak and Shafer (251) in which a reorientation occurs following the initial binding event that enables factor XIIIa to efficiently catalyze the formation of covalent crosslinks within the developing fibrin fibers. However, kinetic studies performed in the presence of physiologic fibrinogen and calcium concentrations have shown that the ability of fibrin polymers to accelerate release of the factor XIII activation peptide is lost when $\gamma$–$\gamma$ dimer formation reaches 40% completion (244). This mechanism could ensure that factor XIIIa activity will be targeted to the growing fibrin protofibrils, without excessive crosslinking of the fully assembled fibrin clot (244).

Investigators have reached somewhat different conclusions about the role of the noncatalytic b subunits of factor XIII in the fibrin-dependent activation mechanism. Greenberg et al. found that fibrin did not enhance the rate of thrombin activation of the platelet factor XIII $a_2$ molecule but did affect the appearance of activity in the presence of purified b chains; they concluded that the $a_2b_2$ tetramer binds to fibrin in a conformation that facilitates its activation by thrombin (257). Hornyak et al. found similar kinetic parameters for the thrombin-catalyzed release of the activation peptide from platelet and plasma factor XIII and concluded that the b subunits do not inhibit this step in the activation pathway (258). Only the active $a_2$ subunits of factor XIII remain bound to fibrin (259,260), which leaves open the possibility that slow dissociation of the b subunits limits the appearance of cross-linking activity. All of these events are correlated, so active factor XIIIa becomes available only when it is needed to crosslink the $\gamma$ and $\alpha$ chains of the assembling fibrin clot (241,243).

## Fibronectin

Fibronectin is a 520,000-Da heterodimeric glycoprotein that circulates in plasma at a concentration approximately 10-fold lower than that of fibrinogen (261,262). The serum concentration is less than half that in plasma, indicating some involvement of fibronectin in coagulation. Analysis of the primary structure of fibronectin reveals that each subunit is composed of three types of repeated homologous sequences (263–265). Functional characterization of fragments obtained by protease digestions has identified binding sites for fibrin on the type I repeats (also called finger domains), which are clustered as a group of five motifs on the N-terminal region of fibronectin and three on its carboxyl-terminal domain (266, 267). The solution structure of a pair of these N-terminal fibronectin type 1 modules (denoted 4F1 and 5F1) has been determined by two-dimensional NMR spectroscopy (268,269). Each module displays a type 1 consensus structure composed of a double-stranded $\beta$-sheet folded onto a triple-stranded $\beta$-sheet with additional stabilization provided by two disulfide bonds. Hydrophobic interactions between pairs of $\beta$-sheets stabilize the elongated structure formed by the combined 4F1 and 5F1 subunits (269). Although the 4F1.5F1 pair exhibits substantial fibrin-binding activity, higher activity was found on a proteolytic fragment with all five finger domains (270). Conversely, studies with recombinant domains indicated that only fingers 4 and 5 were capable of binding to immobilized fibrin (271). A high-affinity site has also been localized to the carboxyl-terminal region of fibronectin, subunits 10F1–12F1, although maximum affinity was observed with full-length fibronectin (272). Recently, a cryptic high-affinity binding site for fibronectin has been localized to residues 221–391 of the $\alpha$C domain of fibrinogen (273).

In addition to these relatively weak noncovalent interactions, factor XIIIa can catalyze the formation of a covalent crosslink between the $\alpha$-chains of fibrin(ogen) and a glutamine residue located at position 3, near the N-terminus of fibronectin (274–277). High-resolution structural studies have shown that this glutamine resides on an extended, flexible 18-residue segment that makes it available for crosslinking (278). Electron micrographs of fibronectin–fibrinogen complexes have shown fibronectin molecules that appear to have been crosslinked to either the central or outer domains of fibrinogen, although this may be due to the flexible conformation of the $\alpha$ chains of fibrinogen (70,279).

Evidence for the role of fibronectin in fibrin assembly has been somewhat contradictory. Fibronectin prolongs the clotting time in plasma and decreases the turbidity (an index of fiber thickness) in a purified system (280). On the other hand, there is a substantial increase in the turbidity of fibrin clots formed in the presence of relatively high fibronectin concentrations, in

which approximately 1 mol of fibronectin was covalently crosslinked per mole of fibrin by factor XIIIa (281). Fibronectin alone does not affect fibrin structure, but both fiber size and density are increased when factor XIII is present, and fibronectin becomes covalently incorporated into the developing clot (282). Studies in a purified system, under near physiologic buffer conditions, have also demonstrated a more than twofold increase in clot strength due to fibronectin ligation to fibrin by factor XIIIa (283). In addition, the extent of fibronectin incorporation into a developing fibrin clot is strongly dependent on the factor XIIIa activity present. Clots with a fibronectin–fibrin mole ratio of 1:20 were obtained with normal plasma, while this value was increased to 1:2 in a purified system containing a 10-fold higher factor XIIIa concentration (284). Despite incorporation of fibronectin into fibrin, studies with plasma clots have shown only minimal effects of fibronectin on the mechanical properties of clots (285).

## Thrombospondin

Thrombospondin is a 540,000-Da glycoprotein released from the $\alpha$-granules of stimulated platelets, which plays a role in platelet aggregation by stabilizing the initially reversible platelet–fibrinogen interaction (286–288). Thrombospondin forms a reversible, noncovalent complex with fibrinogen (287, 289). The resultant fibrinogen-thrombosponin-fibrinogen crossbridges help to stabilize platelet–platelet contacts at physiologic shear rates (290). The 120- and 140-kDa fragments derived from thrombospondin by thermolysin digestion retain the ability to bind to fibrinogen (291). Initial immunologic studies implicated residues 241 to 476 of the fibrinogen $\alpha$ chain as being involved in thrombospondin binding (289), whereas later investigations using fibrinogen fragments and synthetic peptides localized binding sites to A$\alpha$-chain residues 113 to 126 and B$\beta$-chain residues 243 to 252 (288,292,293). Thrombospondin is also incorporated into the fibrin clot during its assembly in a manner described as copolymerization, because the process did not show evidence of saturation and was nearly complete prior to the gel point (294). Factor XIIIa crosslinking was not required for this incorporation, which resulted in faster fibrin polymerization and a significant decrease in fiber thickness, as indicated by turbidity measurements and electron-microscopic observations (294–296). These results indicate that platelet–fibrin interactions *in vivo* may be influenced by thrombospondin (294–296).

## von Willebrand Factor

von Willebrand factor (VWF) is a glycoprotein that circulates in plasma in the form of multimers ranging from 500- to 20,000-kDa and is present at a concentration approximately 200-fold lower than that of fibrinogen. VWF plays an important role in hemostasis by promoting the adhesion of platelets to sites of vascular damage (297,298). The observation that the VWF concentration in serum obtained from slowly clotting plasma (i.e., from patients with hemophilia A or normal plasma in the presence of a thrombin inhibitor) had reduced VWF concentrations suggested an association between VWF and fibrin(ogen) (299,300). Recent work indicates that interactions between fibrin and platelets, mediated by VWF and glycoprotein Ib, enhance the rate of thrombin generation in platelet-rich plasma (301). Other studies have demonstrated that factor XIIIa can crosslink VWF to fibrin in a slow process with VWF providing the requisite glutamine acceptor residues (302). Additional evidence supports a role for VWF in formation of a platelet–fibrin thrombus (303,304) through a noncovalent association of VWF with fibrin, which is characterized by a dissociation constant of approximately 15 $\mu$g per mL, comparable to the plasma VWF concentration (303). A high-affinity fibrin binding site has been localized to the carboxyl-terminal region of VWF, in the C1C2 domains that are distinct from its RGD site (305). Further support for a noncovalent VWF–fibrin association comes from the demonstration that high-molecular-weight multimers of VWF, released from cultured endothelial cells, bind to both crosslinked and non-crosslinked fibrin (306). Adhesive interactions between VWF and fibrin have also been shown to play a major role in anchoring platelets to fibrin in rapidly flowing blood (307,308).

## Fibulin

The fibulins are an emerging family of extracellular matrix and blood proteins presently having several members, two of which, fibulin-1 and fibulin-2, have been most characterized (309,310) Fibulin-1 is the predominant fibulin in blood, present at a concentration of 30 to 40 $\mu$g per mL, approximately 1,000-fold higher than fibulin-2. Purified fibulin-1 binds to fibrinogen and fibrin with a dissociation constant ($K_d$) of 2.9 ± 1.6 $\mu$M. Proteolytic fragments of fibrinogen containing the carboxyl-terminal region of the B$\beta$ chain (residues 216-468) bind to fibulin-1. Fibulin-1 is able to incorporate into fibrin clots formed *in vitro* and is detected within newly formed fibrin-containing thrombi associated with human atherectomy specimens (310). In perfusion chamber assays, platelets in whole blood under flow conditions attach and spread on surfaces coated with fibulin-1. It was shown that fibulin-1 supports platelet adhesion via a bridge of fibrinogen to the platelet integrin $\alpha_{IIb}\beta_3$. Platelet adherence to fibroblast monolayers containing extracellular matrix-incorporated fibulin-1 also required the presence of fibrinogen (311).

## Fibroblast Growth Factor-2

Fibrin formed at sites of tissue injury provides the temporary matrix needed to support the initial endothelial cell responses for vessel repair. Fibroblast growth factor-2 (FGF-2/bFGF) also acts at sites of injury and stimulates similar vascular cell responses. Binding studies demonstrated specific and saturable binding of FGF-2 to fibrinogen and fibrin, with maximum molar binding ratios of FGF-2 to fibrinogen between 2.0 and 4.0 (312). Scatchard analysis indicated two classes of binding sites for FGF-2 to fibrinogen and fibrin with the high-affinity sites showing $K_d$ values of approximately 1 nM and the lower affinity sites showing $K_d$ values approximately 100-fold weaker (312). A high-affinity binding site for fibrin has recently been localized to a set of five residues present in two nearby clusters near the carboxyl-terminal of FGF-2 (313). These residues are absent on FGF-1, a structurally similar molecule that does not bind fibrinogen (314). Proteolytic digestion experiments indicate the carboxyl-terminal region of fragment D that contains the binding site for FGF-2 (315). The binding of FGF-2 to fibrin(ogen) as a component of the provisional matrix may serve to localize and concentrate the growth factor at sites of tissue injury where it is most needed to facilitate wound repair and angiogenesis.

# INTERACTIONS OF FIBRIN WITH PROTEINS OF THE FIBRINOLYTIC SYSTEM

According to the model proposed by Wiman and Collen, dissolution of fibrin clots under physiologic conditions requires binding of the circulating zymogen plasminogen to the clot, conversion of plasminogen to the active protease plasmin by tissue-type plasminogen activator, proteolysis of the clot, and, finally, inactivation of released plasmin by circulating antiplasmin (316) (see also Chapters 18 and 69). A central feature of both naturally occurring is fibrin selectivity: the targeted generation of plasmin activity at the clot surface (317,318).

## Plasminogen–Fibrin(ogen) Binding

The ability of the fibrinolytic system to specifically degrade fibrin and not fibrinogen is largely due to the increased affinity of both plasminogen and tissue-type plasminogen activator for fibrin, compared to fibrinogen (319). However, somewhat divergent reports have appeared concerning the association of fibrinogen with plasminogen: Lucas et al. found no detectable interaction between glu-plasminogen and fibrinogen (320), whereas Lewis et al. reported cooperative binding characterized by four sites with dissociation constants ranging from 0.9 nmol to 47 $\mu$mol (321). Likewise, dissociation constants ranging from greater than 25 $\mu$mol per L (320–322) to 1 $\mu$M (323–325) have been reported for glu-plasminogen binding to fibrin, with differences perhaps attributable to the type of fibrin surface employed.

## tPA–Fibrin Complexes

Kinetic studies have shown that fibrin formation is accompanied by a dramatic increase in the efficiency of plasminogen activation by tissue-type plasminogen activator (tPA) (326,327), whereas blocking fibrin assembly with the tetrapeptide inhibitor Gly-Pro-Arg-Pro largely abolishes this stimulatory effect (328). Fibrin protofibrils have been identified as the smallest molecular species required for enhanced tPA generation, with increased activity associated with limited proteolysis that yields fragment X polymers (329,330). Both kinetic and direct-binding studies indicate a positive feedback mechanism in which early clot lysis exposes new high-affinity binding sites on fibrin for plasminogen (327,331–334). These high-affinity sites probably correspond to the zwitterionic carboxyl-terminal lysine residues exposed by plasmin cleavage of fibrin, and they most likely interact with complementary "lysine binding sites" present on kringles 1 to 4 of plasminogen; additional regions of plasminogen, termed "aminohexyl sites," appear to recognize the positively charged side chains of intrachain lysines present on intact fibrin (317,319,335). Fibrinogen fragments D and E bind to immobilized lys-plasminogen (336,337); the sequence B$\beta$ Leu121-Lys122 of the coiled-coil region of fragment E appears to be especially important for fibrin–plasminogen interactions (338).

## Plasmin(ogen)–Tissue-Type Plasminogen Activator–Fibrin Complexes

Efficient, targeted generation of fibrinolytic activity requires formation of a ternary complex composed of tPA–plasminogen–fibrin (339,340). Although early studies were interpreted in terms of an ordered, sequential binding mechanism in which tPA binds first to fibrin followed by plasminogen (326), recent work supports a steady-state template model in which tPA and plasminogen interact independently with distinct molecular recognition sites on intact fibrin to form the catalytically active ternary complex that generates plasmin (341). Considerable progress has been made in identifying the regions of fibrin that mediate tPA binding. Carboxyl-terminal fragments of fibrinogen prepared by digestion with either plasmin (fragment D) or cyanogen bromide (residues A$\alpha$ 148–160 of FCB-2 and residues $\gamma$ 312–324 of FCB-5) retain the ability to bind to immobilized tPA and accelerate plasminogen activation by tPA, whereas fragment E lacks these properties (337,342–345). In fact, both FCB-2 and FCB-5 bind tPA with an affinity comparable to fibrin itself, which exhibits a $K_d$ approximately 1 nM for tPA (346).

Additional studies have identified A$\alpha$ 154 to A$\alpha$ 159, which contains a critical lysine at position 157, as the minimal $\alpha$ chain sequence that retains the ability to accelerate tPA catalysis of plasminogen activation (343,347). Although sites A$\alpha$ 148 to A$\alpha$ 160 and $\gamma$ 312 to $\gamma$ 324 are not functional on fibrinogen, conformational changes associated with either fibrinogen aggregation or fibrin polymerization expose these tPA binding sites (346,348,349). Structural studies have shown that A$\alpha$ 154 to A$\alpha$ 159 is present on a solvent-inaccessible region of the coiled-coils in fragment D (8). Recent studies demonstrate that epitopes corresponding to both the A$\alpha$ 148 and A$\alpha$ 160 and $\gamma$ 312 to $\gamma$ 324 sites become exposed upon proteolytic digestion of the $\beta$C and $\gamma$C domains on fragment D, and that both epitopes are available in a noncovalent DD–fragment E complex (350). Independent high-affinity binding sites for plasminogen and tPA are also present on the compact carboxyl-terminal regions of the $\alpha$C domains (residues A$\alpha$ 392–610) (351). These "cryptic" sites (352) become available upon fibrin formation, probably as a result of the switch between intramolecular and intermolecular interactions between the aC domains that accompanies fibrin polymerization (340,353).

Analysis of the primary structure of tPA shows that it is composed of five distinct structural regions: a N-terminal "finger" domain, an epidermal growth factor–like domain, two kringles with sequence similarity to plasminogen, and a carboxyl-terminal catalytic domain typical of serine proteases (354,355). Studies of deletion-mutant proteins lacking specific tPA domains have shown that both kringle 2, which contains a lysine binding site, and the finger domain, which is similar to the fibrin-recognition region of fibronectin, are involved in fibrin binding (356–360).

The following mechanism has been proposed, which incorporates many of the kinetic and structural aspects of the tPA–plasminogen–fibrin interaction (356). Initially, a weak ternary complex with minimal catalytic activity is formed as tPA binds to fibrin by the tPA finger domain and plasminogen binds to fibrin through the plasminogen aminohexyl site. Photo affinity labeling coupled with electron microscopy has shown that plasminogen binds to the ends of fibrin strands and spans regions where two D-domains are aligned end to end in a fibrin protofibril, thereby placing the nascent protease in an optimum position to cleave any nearby fibrin molecules (361). The resultant plasmin generated at the fibrin surface then cleaves fibrin, exposing new carboxyl-terminal lysine residues that enable more tPA and plasminogen to bind through lysine binding sites present on specific kringles on the activator and its substrate. This positive feedback mechanism can regulate fibrinolysis, ensuring that plasmin activity is initially generated at a slow pace and is targeted to the fully assembled fibrin clot (356). This process is also regulated by a proteolytic enzyme termed thrombin-activatable fibrinolysis inhibitor (TAFI), that is activated by the thrombin–thrombomodulin system (362). TAFI, through its carboxypeptidase activity, cleaves the carboxyl-terminal lysine residues formed on fibrin although plasmin digestion, thereby limiting positive feedback mechanism that converts glu-plasminogen to lys-plasminogen (363).

## $\alpha_2$-Antiplasmin and Fibrin

Interactions between fibrin, plasminogen, and $\alpha_2$-antiplasmin also play a major role in regulation of the fibrinolytic process. $\alpha_2$-antiplasmin rapidly inactivates plasmin, interferes with plasminogen binding to fibrin, and is crosslinked to fibrin by factor XIIIa (364–366). However, the relative contributions of plasma and platelet factorXIIIa in promoting $\alpha_2$-antiplasmin crosslinking to fibrin remains an area of active investigation (367–369). The carboxyl-terminal region of $\alpha_2$-antiplasmin is rich in lysine residues that can bind to the lysine binding sites present on the kringles of plasminogen, thereby blocking the association of plasminogen with fibrin (370–372). In addition, $\alpha_2$-antiplasmin has a glutamine residue adjacent to its amino-terminus that is covalently coupled to a lysine residue at position 303 of the fibrin(ogen) $\alpha$ chain in a rapid reaction, catalyzed by factor XIIIa at a rate faster than ligation of the fibrin $\gamma$ chains (364,373,374). When crosslinked to fibrin, $\alpha_2$-plasmin inhibitor retains its ability to inactivate plasmin, and this process has physiologic significance in preventing early clot lysis (375–377). Additional antifibrinolytic activity comes from the covalent crosslinking of plasminogen activator inhibitor 2 (PAI-2) to fibrin, a process mediated both by tissue transglutaminase and factor XIIIa. The lysine residues on the A$\alpha$ chain to which PAI-2 becomes crosslinked are distinct from the ligation sites for $\alpha_2$-plasmin inhibitor, enabling the simultaneous incorporation of both inhibitors into a developing fibrin clot (378,379).

## Plasminogen Activator Inhibitor 1 and Fibrin

The thrombolytic process is also regulated by plasminogen activator inhibitor 1 (PAI-1), a 50-kDa serine protease inhibitor that is present in plasma and is released in an active conformation from both platelets and endothelial cells in response to pathophysiologic stimuli (380,381). Active PAI-1 binds reversibly to fibrin through a small number of high-affinity sites ($K_d$ <1nM) and a larger number of low-affinity sites ($K_d$ approximately 4 $\mu$M) (382). Because PAI-1 bound to fibrin retains its ability to inhibit tissue plasminogen activator (383,384), this constitutes an important pathway for limiting fibrinolysis, especially at sites of interaction between platelets and endothelial cells, such as platelet-rich thrombi (385–387). Vitronectin also modulates the interactions between PAI-1 and fibrin, enhancing its affinity for fibrin and protecting it from rapid inactivation (388).

## Lipoprotein (a) and Fibrin

Additional regulation of the fibrinolytic process may be provided by lipoprotein (a) [Lp(a)], a plasma particle composed of a lipid core and an apolipoprotein B-100 subunit disulfide-bonded to apolipoprotein (a) [apo(a)] subunit (389,390). The primary structure of apo(a) is strikingly similar to that of plasminogen in that it contains 37 copies of kringle 4, one copy of kringle 5, and an (inert) serine protease-like domain (391,392). Lp(a) has functional similarities to plasminogen in that it binds tightly to immobilized fibrin(ogen) (393,394). Partial disulfide bond reduction by sulfhydryl reagents such as homocysteine, cysteine, and glutathione increases the affinity of Lp(a) for fibrin (395). Limited plasmin digestion of fibrin(ogen) exposes new lysine binding sites for Lp(a) located on both the D- and E-domains (393). Recently, a binding site for Lp(a) has been localized to fibrinogen's $\alpha$C domain (residues 392–610) (396). Proteolytic cleavage of apo(a) yields a 170-kDa carboxyl-terminal fragment that contains fibrin binding sites and an N-terminal domain of variable size that lacks these sites (397).

However, the functional consequences of these Lp(a)–fibrin interactions remain unresolved. Some investigators have reported *in vitro* studies indicating that Lp(a) competes with plasminogen for binding to fibrin (394,398), inhibits its activation by tPA (393,394,399,400) and causes a modest inhibition of lysis of plasma clots (393). Conversely, others have observed that purified Lp(a) increased the binding of plasminogen to fibrin (401) and that this fibrin-bound Lp(a) increased the rate of tPA catalyzed plasmin generation, especially at physiologic salt and plasminogen concentrations (402). The presence of multiple isoforms of apoliprotein (a) has further complicated interpretation of the potential physiologic effects of Lp(a) on the human fibrinolytic system (403,404). However, a recent study has demonstrated that human Lp(a) and a 17-kringle recombinant apo(a) construct strongly inhibited fibrin-mediated plasminogen activation (405).

# INTERACTIONS OF FIBRIN WITH PLATELET, ENDOTHELIAL CELL, AND LEUKOCYTE INTEGRINS

## $\alpha_{IIb}\beta_3$

Platelet membrane glycoproteins IIb and IIIa form a $Ca^{2+}$-dependent, noncovalent complex originally termed GP IIb/IIIa that functions as a receptor for the adhesive proteins fibrinogen, fibronectin, and VWF (406). Analysis of the primary structures of the individual subunits (deduced from their cDNA sequences) (407–409) has shown GP IIb/IIIa to be a member of the integrin family of cell adhesion receptors, now termed $\alpha_{IIb}\beta_3$ (410,411). Although no three-dimensional structure is available for integrin $\alpha_{IIb}\beta_3$, it shares a common subunit with integrin $\alpha_V\beta_3$, whose ectodomain structure has recently been solved by x-ray diffraction crystallography (412,413). The 36% identity/54% similarity of the $\alpha_{IIb}$ and $\alpha_V$ subunits have enabled investigators to build models of $\alpha_{IIb}\beta_3$ (414), with special emphasis on characterizing the ligand recognition regions on its large extracellular region (415,416). Fibrinogen binds to stimulated platelets in a specific, saturable manner (417,418), although details of the number of bound molecules, the rate of binding, and the question of reversibility remain controversial, as discussed in a comprehensive review by Peerschke (419). Identification of $\alpha_{IIb}\beta_3$ as the fibrinogen receptor has been obtained by direct-binding experiments (417–419), studies of Glanzmann thrombasthenic platelets, immunologic studies employing monoclonal antibodies directed against these proteins (420,421), and by purification and reconstitution studies (422–424). Human cell lines tandemly transfected with plamids expressing the individual $\alpha_{IIb}$ and $\beta_3$ subunits exhibit functional integrin receptors capable of specifically binding fibrinogen, VWF, and vitronectin (425).

Each $\gamma C$ domain of fibrinogen contains at least two integrin recognition regions: the primary binding site at carboxyl-terminal residues 400 to 411 (HHLGGAKQAGDV) of the $\gamma C$ domain (426–431), and an auxiliary site localized to residues 370 to 383 (432). Both these regions are near to, but distinct from, the $\gamma C$ fibrin polymerization site and the site of $\gamma$-chain crosslinking (427). Furthermore, mutations or deletions in the $\gamma 316$ to $\gamma 322$ segment result in defective platelet aggregation and platelet adhesion to immobilized fibrinogen (215,433,434). Electron-microscopic images of complexes formed between isolated $\alpha_{IIb}\beta_3$ and fibrinogen show a specific interaction between the distal domains of trinodular fibrinogen molecules and the integrin globular head region (435). This orientation is consistent with a dominant role for the fibrinogen $\gamma$ chain carboxyl-terminal sequence in binding to $\alpha_{IIb}\beta_3$.

Two additional receptor-recognition regions, which share a common RGD sequence, have been identified on the A$\alpha$ chain (429–431,436–439). The RGDS sequence, present at positions 572 to 575 of fibrinogen (and on the other adhesive ligands–VWF and fibronectin), has been implicated in integrin–fibrinogen interactions (429,438). However, several lines of evidence indicate that the $\gamma$-chain carboxyl-terminal sequences, rather than the RGD sequences, provide the primary sites for $\alpha_{IIb}\beta_3$–fibrin(ogen) interactions (440). Recombinant fibrinogens engineered to contain RGE sequences, rather than the native RGD sequence at positions $\alpha 97$ or $\alpha 574$, supported platelet aggregation (441). In contrast, a genetically engineered $\gamma$-chain variant in which carboxyl-terminal residues 408 to 411 were replaced by a 20-residue insert, did not function normally in platelet aggregation assays (441); this variant also exhibited decreased binding to the GP IIb/IIIa complex (442). Gene-targeting technology has been used in mice to truncate the carboxyl-terminal sequence QAGDV from fibrinogen; mice homozygous for this $\gamma\Delta 5$-fibrinogen variant had normal fibrinogen levels, clotting times, and fibrin crosslinking. However, platelet function studies yielded the paradoxical result of defective platelet aggregation but normal clot retraction (443). Recombinant human fibrinogen molecules lacking the carboxyl-terminal AGDV sequence also failed to support platelet aggregation but exhibited normal platelet-mediated clot retraction (444). These observations indicate that different receptors and/or different receptor-recognition sequences on fibrin(ogen) are required for platelet aggregation and clot retraction.

## $\alpha_V\beta_3$, $\alpha_5\beta_1$, and $\alpha_M\beta_2$

Integrins $\alpha_V\beta_3$ and $\alpha_5\beta_1$, present on platelets and endothelial cells, bind fibrinogen in part through the RGD sequence near the carboxyl-terminal of the A$\alpha$ chain residues 572 to 574 (445–451), which may become covalently crosslinked through the A$\alpha$ chains, possibly by endothelial cell transglutaminase (452). Additional binding sites for $\alpha_V\beta_3$ have been localized to residues $\gamma 190$ to $\gamma 202$ and $\gamma 346$ to $\gamma 358$, segments that although distant in sequence are adjacent on the three-dimensional structure of fibrinogen's $\gamma C$ domain (453,454). The $\gamma C$ domain also harbors a binding site for $\alpha_5\beta_1$, recently localized to residues 370 to 383 (432). Fibrinogen also binds to the leukocyte integrin $\alpha_M\beta_2$, and its homolog $\alpha_X\beta_2$ (455) through binding sites present on both the $\gamma C$ domain (456–458) and the A$\alpha$EC domain (459). Residues $\gamma 383$ to $\gamma 395$ were initially identified as a "cryptic" binding site for $\alpha_M\beta_2$ (456,458), one that became accessible through limited proteolysis of fibrinogen's D-domain. A subsequent report narrowed the $\alpha_M\beta_2$-recognition site to $\gamma 390$ to $\gamma 395$ (457). Integrins $\beta 1$ and $\beta 3$ in human smooth muscle cells interact with fibrin in vitro and mediate adhesion to and contraction of fibrin clots (460).

# BIOSYNTHESIS AND METABOLISM

## Gene Regulation

Human fibrinogen is the product of three closely linked genes, FGA, FGB, and FGG, specifying the amino acid sequences of the A$\alpha$, B$\beta$, and $\gamma$ polypeptide chains, respectively [reviewed in (23,461,462)]. The three genes are clustered in a 50-kb region on chromosome 4q28 (463–467), in the order FGG, FGA, and FGB, with six, eight, and 10 exons, respectively (441,461,462,464,468–474). FGG and FGA are transcribed from one strand, whereas FGB is transcribed from opposite strand (463). Therefore, the upstream regulatory regions of FGG and FGB border the fibrinogen gene cluster. The cDNAs that encode the three chains are similar to each other (20–22), and to the cDNAs encoding the rat fibrinogen polypeptides (475–477). This homology extends to the genomic sequences, with two intron/exon boundaries conserved in all three genes and a third junction common to FGB and FGG (467,475). This evidence indicates the three genes evolved from a common ancestral gene through a series of duplications and inversions that began approximately 1 billion years ago (13,17,18,27,471–474,478–482). It is hypothesized that this ancestral gene duplicated to form FGA and a preFGG. The preFGG then duplicated approximately 500 million years ago into FGG and FGB. Similar, "fibrinogen-like" sequences have been found, including the genes encoding scabrous of the developing Drosophila eye (483,484), fibroleukin, formerly identified as protein pT49 from cytotoxic T lymphocytes (480,485,486), and the tenascin family of extracellular matrix proteins (487–491), reviewed in (14, 23,82,492–494).

The fibrinogen genes share a common regulatory mechanism, likely mediated by common transcriptional regulatory molecules that recognize sequence motifs in the immediate 5'-flanking regions of each gene (23,461,462). Significant regions of homology immediately upstream from the sites of transcription initiation contain cis-acting regulatory elements that control expression of these genes (469,471,481,495–500). Expression is coordinated (471,501), such that, at least in hepatocytes, the relative proportion of each mRNA is nearly equal (462). Coordinated expression was seen first in rats following defibrination with Malayan pit viper venom. Here the onset, rate, and maximal accumulation of mRNAs coding for the A$\alpha$, B$\beta$, and $\gamma$ chains were nearly the same, each mRNA increasing approximately 12-fold (501). Under normal, that is, basal, conditions the mRNAs of the three fibrinogen genes are constitutively expressed in the liver (462,495,502–506). FGG, but not FGA and FGB, is also expressed in a variety of extrahepatic epithelial cells *in vitro* (499) and tissues *in vivo* (507,508). The mechanisms regulating the more ubiquitous expression of FGG have not been determined, although reporter gene studies with the 5'-flanking region from human FGG have confirmed that the TATA-like sequence (−20 to −23 bp), a CAAT-like sequence (−54 to −57 bp), and an USF binding site (−66 to −77 bp) constitute a minimal promoter that mediates liver-specific expression (481). In contrast, the tissue-specific expression of the FGA and FGB is controlled by liver-specific transcription factors including hepatocyte-specific nuclear factor-1 (HNF-1) (497,503–506,509). HNF-1, a 92-kDa nuclear protein, binds to an upstream sequence, ATTAAC, common to the promoter regions of several liver-specific genes, including those for $\alpha_1$-antitrypsin, albumin, $\alpha$-fetoprotein, and transthyretin (505), and FGA and FGB, but not FGG (506).

Fibrinogen is one of several hepatic proteins whose plasma levels increase in response to injury (462,510–512). This acute-phase response is characterized by the production of cytokines, which act on tissues and cells resulting in multiple responses including fever, proliferation of immune cells, and changes in expression of several liver-specific proteins known collectively as the acute-phase proteins. The acute-phase response is conserved across species, with plasma levels of fibrinogen increased twofold to 10-fold, whereas albumin concentrations decrease by approximately 50%. This upregulation of fibrinogen expression in liver is mediated by interleukin 6 (IL-6) through type II-IL-6 response elements in the 5'-flanking region of all three fibrinogen genes (481,495,498,500,513). When hepatocytes are incubated in the presence of IL-6, the three fibrinogen mRNAs increase simultaneously and equally, with a concomitant increase

in secreted fibrinogen (496,499,514,515). Indeed fibrin(ogen) degradation products may have a specific role in a feedback regulation of fibrinogen synthesis as these fragments stimulate peripheral blood monocytes/macrophages to produce IL-6 and consequently increase fibrinogen synthesis (516–520). The tumor promoter 12-0-tetradecanolyphorbol-13-acetate and synthetic diacylglycerol also upregulate fibrinogen expression in a rat hepatoma cell line, which responds similarly to IL-6 (496). These results suggest that the extracellular mediator IL-6 activates an intracellular signaling mechanism involving protein kinase C to stimulate the production of the mRNAs for fibrinogen (496) and other class II acute-phase proteins (495,498,499, 510–512,515,521,522). A glucocorticoid response element, identified in the 5'-flanking region of the B$\beta$- and $\gamma$-chain genes, also mediates upregulation of fibrinogen expression (498,521).

In addition to these cis-acting response elements, regions in the 5'-flanking sequences have been identified as negative regulators of transcription. A negative element with sequence homology to several silencer elements was identified in the region −348 to −390 bp of human FGG (481), although the mechanism that reduces fibrinogen gene expression has not been elucidated. The antiinflammatory cytokines IL-4, IL-10, and IL-13 alone or in combination downregulate fibrinogen gene expression and protein production in hepatocarcinoma cells (523). Paradoxically, the proinflammatory cytokine, IL-1$\beta$, which induces expression of class I acute-phase proteins, has no effect (524) or an inhibitory effect (525) on hepatocyte synthesis of fibrinogen. In addition, transforming growth factor-$\beta$ (TGF-$\beta$) induces a decrease in the basal level of fibrinogen mRNAs in cultured hepatocytes (526). Furthermore, TFG-$\beta$ efficiently antagonizes the IL-6 induction of fibrinogen mRNA at late (12 to 48 hours) but not early (6 hours) times after IL-6 treatment. The early stimulatory and late inhibitory effects exerted by IL-6 and TGF-$\beta$, respectively, may coordinate to regulate fibrinogen synthesis during inflammation (526).

Each of the fibrinogen mRNAs is initiated at a single site. Multiple mRNAs exist for each gene (462), arising from polyadenylation site selection in all three genes, and alternative processing of the A$\alpha$ and $\gamma$ chain transcripts (26,27,82, 137,461,462,472–474,477,507,508,527–529). The predominant $\gamma$-chain mRNA results from splicing all 10 exons in FGG and encodes the 411 residue $\gamma$ chain, also designated $\gamma$50 or $\gamma$Val-411 (530). The minor form of the mRNA results from retention of the last intron as an exon and alternative polyadenylation site selection and encodes the 427 residue $\gamma'$ chain, also designated $\gamma$57.5 or $\gamma$Leu-427 (468,508,530,531). Similarly, mRNA processing results in two A$\alpha$-chain variants, the predominant 610 residue A$\alpha$ polypeptide and a minor, longer 847 residue polypeptide called A$\alpha$E (472). The A$\alpha$E polypeptide is translated from an alternatively spliced mRNA that incorporates a sixth exon (532). Therefore, the two forms are identical through residue Val610, which is followed by Arg611, encoded in exon V, and 236 residues encoded by exon VI. These residues fold into a globular domain that is homologous to the globular carboxyl-terminal domains of the B$\beta$ and $\gamma$ chains (472). Interestingly, the mature mRNA for the predominant A$\alpha$ chain encodes a 625 residue polypeptide (22,473). Apparently, proteolytic cleavage of the longer A$\alpha$ chain removes the carboxyl-terminal 15 amino acids as a normal processing event during the maturation of the nascent polypeptide (533). Expression of the alternative mRNAs is less efficient, such that in plasma fibrinogen $\gamma'$ and A$\alpha$E are 10% and 2% of their counterparts, $\gamma$ and A$\alpha$, respectively (28,472,474,527–529,534, 535). In contrast, in rat hepatocytes approximately 30% of the $\gamma$-chain transcripts are specific for the longer polypeptide, called $\gamma$A (462); the reason for this species difference remains unknown.

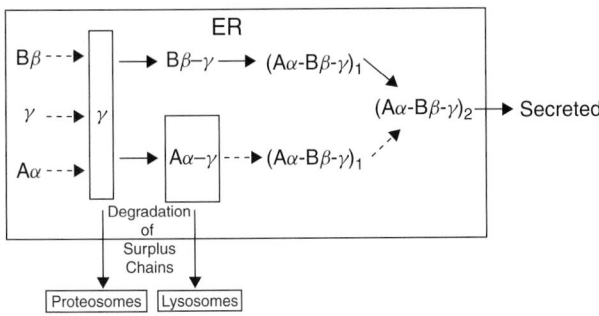

**FIGURE 16-13.** Schematic of the steps in the assembly and secretion of fibrinogen. The three chains are synthesized on separate polysomes, with each chain cotranslationally directed into the edoplasmic reticulum, represented by the *large box* labeled ER. Studies with cultured human hepatoma cells, HepG2, demonstrate both $\gamma$ chains and A$\alpha$–$\gamma$ complexes accumulated as intracellular pools, indicated by the *smaller boxes.* The principal pathway for assembly is indicated by the *solid arrows;* an alternate pathway is indicated by the *dashed arrows.* Pulse-chase experiments demonstrate a precursor-product relation from B$\beta$–$\gamma$ to (A$\alpha$-B$\beta$-$\gamma$)$_1$ to (A$\alpha$-B$\beta$-$\gamma$)$_2$. The fibrinogen dimer transits from the ER into the Golgi for further posttranslational processing prior to secretion from the cell. Surplus fibrinogen chains are degraded either by proteosomes or by lysosomes. Studies with specific inhibitors indicate that A$\alpha$–$\gamma$ complexes are degraded by hydolases in lysosomes, whereas $\gamma$ chains are retrotranslocated from the ER by proteosomes and degraded following ubiquitin conjugation.

## Synthesis and Secretion

The six polypeptides of fibrinogen are assembled in the rough endoplasmic reticulum (ER) in an ordered pattern elucidated by Redman et al. in studies with cultured human hepatocellular carcinoma cells, called HepG2, as illustrated in Figure 16-13 (536). Pulse-chase experiments have shown that $\gamma$ chains and A$\alpha$–$\gamma$ chain complexes accumulate in intracellular pools, whereas B$\beta$ chains are quickly incorporated into first B$\beta$–$\gamma$ complexes, then half-fibrinogen molecules and lastly fibrinogen (A$\alpha$B$\beta\gamma$)$_2$. Contrasting results have been obtained with cultured rat hepatocytes, where the rate-limiting step appears to be synthesis of the A$\alpha$ chain (537). Cultured chicken hepatocytes also exhibit nonstoichiometric synthesis of the fibrinogen subunits, with notably lower levels of A$\alpha$ chain synthesis (538,539). Studies with stably transfected COS, BHK, or CHO cells expressing each of the chains, combinations of chains, or all three chains have provided evidence for these assembly intermediates and other two-chain complexes, that is, A$\alpha$–$\gamma$, and further, have shown that secretion of individual polypeptide chains or pairs of chains is minimal relative to secretion of the fully assembled fibrinogen molecule (46,540–550). Because essentially normal fibrinogen is assembled and secreted when all three chains are expressed in these cell lines, assembly is clearly not hepatocyte specific.

Studies with HepG2 cells and stably transfected COS cells provide insight into the mechanisms that regulate this assembly pathway (536,551). Using N-linked glycosylation to identify chains in the ER, MG132 to inhibit degradation by proteosomes, and sequential immunoprecipitation, these studies examined the association of fibrinogen with Sec61$\beta$, a component of the translocon, and Hsp70, a cytosolic chaperone. The data show that glycosylated B$\beta$ chains associate with Sec61$\beta$ in COS cells that express only the B$\beta$ chain. In HepG2 cells, all the chains associate with Sec61$\beta$, although the association with B$\beta$ precedes the association with both A$\alpha$ and $\gamma$ chains. All chains in HepG2 cells also associate with Hsp70, but more A$\alpha$ and $\gamma$ chains are bound than were B$\beta$ chains.

Taken together these data suggest that B$\beta$ chains do not accumulate in the ER because they are rapidly retrotranslocated, as indicated by their rapid association with to Sec61$\beta$. The lower association of B$\beta$ chains with Hsp70 is consistent with this chain being more rapidly degraded. The slower association of A$\alpha$ and $\gamma$ chains with Sec61$\beta$ is consistent with the accumulation of these chains in HepG2 cells. Further studies are clearly needed to comprehend the mechanisms by which these and perhaps other chaperones coordinate the steps in chain assembly in the ER. Studies are also needed to determine the mechanisms that regulate transit of assembled chains through the Golgi and secretion from the cell.

The fibrinogen chains are linked by 29 inter- and intra-chain disulfide bonds, originally determined by peptide chemistry studies (23). Subsequent analyses utilizing expression of variant fibrinogens in transfected cells have demonstrated that five pairs of disulfide bonds link the two half-molecules and determined which of these disulfides are essential for assembly and secretion of the dimeric molecule (46,74). Surprisingly, the two asymmetric disulfides, between A$\alpha$Cys36 and B$\beta$Cys65, by themselves are sufficient for synthesis of the fibrinogen dimer. Extensive studies of expressed variants with substitutions or deletions have demonstrated that the N-terminal domains of each chain, including the N-terminal half of the coiled-coil regions and the N-terminal disulfide ring, are critical for dimer assembly, that the C-terminal half of the coiled-coil and intrachain disulfides proximate to the coiled-coil in the B$\beta$ and $\gamma$ chains are critical for formation of the initial two-chain complexes, that the C-terminal disulfide ring is essential for all chain assembly, that the C-terminal intrachain disulfide in the $\gamma$ chain is critical for secretion but not intracellular assembly, and that the C-terminal intrachain disulfides in the A$\alpha$ and B$\beta$ chains are not critical for either assembly or secretion (536). Recent studies with truncated variants indicate that residues near the C-terminus of the $\gamma$ chain, in particular $\gamma$Ile387, are also critical for formation of the initial two-chain complexes (552).

The recent identification of mutations that cause afibrinogenemia and hypofibrinogenemia provide an increased understanding of the primary structures required for fibrinogen synthesis and secretion *in vivo.* These mutations are described in Chapter 62. Many of these mutations are large deletions, nonsense or frameshift mutations that would eliminate substantial portions of the encoded chains. Because liver biopsies are unusual, it is unknown whether these mutations alter synthesis, assembly, or secretion. Interestingly, single residue substitutions have only been identified in FGB. These encode the B$\beta$ chain substitutions L383R, G430D and G444S. To assess whether these substitutions could cause afibrinogenemia, transient expression of the mutant fibrinogens was examined in COS cells. These experiments demonstrated that B$\beta$ chains were synthesized and fibrinogen molecules were assembled in the cells, but not secreted into the medium (553,554). These cases suggest that the B$\beta$ chain in the distal D nodule of fibrinogen has a critical role in secretion.

## TISSUE-SPECIFIC SYNTHESIS

Plasma fibrinogen is synthesized in the liver, with a steady-state rate of 1.7 to 5.0 g per day (555,556). The synthetic reserve is large, and up to 20-fold increases in production rates have been found in patients with peripheral consumption of fibrinogen (557). Approximately 75% of fibrinogen is found in the plasma (556), with much of the remainder distributed in interstitial fluid and in lymph. The plasma half-life is 3 to 5 days (558,559). Although there is evidence that thrombin and plasmin may play a role in the normal catabolism of fibrinogen, their overall contribution appears to account for only 2%

to 3% of fibrinogen breakdown (560,561). The mechanism and location of the major catabolic pathway therefore remain unknown.

Circulating fibrinogen exists not only in the plasma but also within the α-granules in platelets (see Chapter 38). Intraplatelet fibrinogen is structurally distinct from plasma fibrinogen, as the γ′ chain is not found in platelets, suggesting the fibrinogen is differentially expressed in platelets (527,562–564). Nevertheless, most studies show that fibrinogen in megakaryocytes and platelets originates from receptor-mediated endocytosis of plasma fibrinogen, with its subsequent storage in α-granules (565–572). The implicated receptor is the integrin $\alpha_{IIb}\beta_3$, which also mediates platelet aggregation through interactions that depend on the C-terminal residues of the predominant γ chain. The origin of platelet fibrinogen is currently thought to arise from $\alpha_{IIb}\beta_3$-mediated endocytosis, such that only fibrinogen with two γ chains, and no γ′ chain, is present. This conclusion is entirely consistent with studies of mice expressing fibrinogen that lacks the C-terminal 5 residues of the γ chain, FgγΔ5 (573). Immunoblot analysis of lysed platelets showed markedly reduced amounts of fibrinogen in platelets isolated from mice expressing FgγΔ5 compared to platelets isolated from normal mice. Interestingly, platelets for the FgγΔ5 mice contained elevated levels of fibronectin, indicating that the interaction between $\alpha_{IIb}\beta_3$ and fibrinogen controls the fibronectin content of platelets.

Extrahepatic synthesis of relatively lower amounts of fibrinogen has been reported. These studies suggest a fibrinogen function, independent of hemostasis, in cellular adhesion or the structural integrity of tissues. Only FGG expression has been demonstrated in normal extrahepatic tissue *in vivo*, including brain, lung, and marrow (507,508,574). In contrast, *in vitro* expression of all three genes and secretion of fibrinogen chains has been demonstrated in nonhepatic epithelial cells, in response to appropriate physiologic stimuli (575). Following estrogen stimulation of ovarian granulosa cells, Bβ and γ chains were secreted (576). Epithelial cells from human intestine (Caco-2) respond to IL-6 induction by a modest increase in synthesis and secretion of fibrinogen (577). In addition, the synthesis and secretion of fully assembled fibrinogen by a lung alveolar epithelial cell line (A549) has been demonstrated (578). Although little constitutive fibrinogen expression occurs in the lung cells, transcription was upregulated 5- to 10-fold after induction with dexamethasone and IL-6 (510, 578,579). Secretion of fibrinogen from lung epithelial cells occurs in a polarized manner toward the basolateral face of the plasma membrane by a microtubule-dependent mechanism. These data suggest that lung epithelium may incorporate fully assembled fibrinogen into its extracellular matrix during inflammation, and cultured lung alveolar epithelial cells do indeed incorporate newly synthesized fibrinogen into the extracellular matrix (580). Furthermore, on deposition of fibrinogen into the matrix, its conformation is altered to display the β15-21 epitope thought to be exposed only on thrombin-generated fibrin (580). FGA and FGB expression does not occur in epithelial cells of normal lung *in vivo*, but inducible expression of all three genes is clearly evident during *Pneumocystis carinii* pneumonia (581). The dramatic upregulation of fibrinogen expression in response to inflammatory stimuli suggests that fibrinogen may contribute to the pathogenesis of fibrotic lung disease (90,582,583). As an extracellular matrix protein, fibrinogen may be important in normal physiology and in disease pathogenesis. Recent studies have shown that fibrinogen in cultured cell medium incorporates into the extracellular matrix during the active secretion and assembly of fibronectin from fibroblasts (584). Subsequent studies demonstrated that matrix fibrinogen enhances both cell proliferation and cell migration following scrape-wounding of cultured dermal fibroblasts (585). These data indicate that fibrinogen, as opposed to fibrin, is an important matrix constituent that enhances wound repair. Therefore, fibrinogen joins the list of adhesive glycoproteins, including fibronectin, thrombospondin, vitronectin, VWF, and fibulin, that function as both plasma and matrix proteins (586–596).

## A Risk Factor in Cardiovascular Disease

Multiple epidemiologic studies have demonstrated that elevated levels of fibrinogen are predictive for cardiovascular disease. Three recent reviews with metaanalyses that combined multiple prospective studies have clearly confirmed the association between high fibrinogen and increased risk of cardiovascular disease (597–599). Nevertheless, because fibrinogen is an acute-phase protein, it remains unclear whether elevated levels of fibrinogen makes a causal contribution to disease pathogenesis or elevated fibrinogen level is a marker for early stage, clinically silent disease. This dilemma is complicated by studies that examined the associations between fibrinogen levels and genetic polymorphisms. One analysis of multiple studies concluded that there is an association between a polymorphism in the promoter region of the β chain, −455G/A, and the level of circulating fibrinogen, but not between this polymorphism and cardiovascular disease (600). These authors note, however, that based on the established level of risk with increased fibrinogen levels, a study with more than 10,000 individuals with the less common allele would be needed to provide sufficient power to detect an association between the polymorphism and disease. Another review concludes that the −455A allele within a specific haplotype is associated with atherothrombotic disease (601). A recent study indicates that a polymorphism in the β3 integrin gene, is associated with increased risk of cardiovascular disease only in the presence of elevated fibrinogen levels (602). This finding suggests that genetic polymorphisms outside the fibrinogen locus in association with elevated fibrinogen may provide a more reliable prognostic indicator.

Multiple studies also show that environmental factors influence fibrinogen levels. Indeed, estimates from segregation analysis suggest that significantly less than half of the plasma fibrinogen level is genetically determined (603). Fibrinogen levels are known to increase with natural life events such as age, pregnancy, and menopause. Fibrinogen levels also increase with other disease risk factors, such as smoking, hypertension, diabetes, infection, and obesity. Interestingly, fibrinogen levels decrease with moderate alcohol consumption (604). In her thoughtful review, de Maat has summarized and appraised studies that examined the effects of diet and drugs on fibrinogen levels. She concluded that plasma levels of fibrinogen are likely regulated by a complex interplay between environmental and genetic factors (605). Iacoviello et al. also concluded that gene–environment interactions are likely to make a statistically significant contribution to plasma fibrinogen levels (600). Two specific examples substantiate this conclusion. First, individuals with *Helobacter pylori* infection who carry the B2 allele within FGG show an additional increase in fibrinogen levels and in the risk of myocardial infarction compared to infected individuals who carry the B1 allele (606). Second, fibrinogen levels were increased following strenuous physical exercise, but the extent of increase was dependent on the FGB allele, with higher levels in −455A carriers relative to −455G carriers (607).

Elevated fibrinogen clearly compounds the risk for cardiovascular disease in patients with diabetes. Recent studies suggest an increased rate of fibrinogen synthesis is correlated with obesity and type 2 diabetes. In a small study with six healthy postpubertal obese girls and six age-matched lean control girls, the synthesis rate of fibrinogen was measured by mass spectroscopy following infusion of L-[$^{13}$C]leucine (608). The data showed the fractional synthesis rate of fibrinogen in obese girls was twice that of lean girls. Although the mechanism that associates the synthesis rate with obesity remains unknown, these studies suggest that elevated levels of fibrinogen in obese individuals is a consequence of an increased rate of fibrinogen synthesis. Using a similar experimental protocol, Barazzoni et al. measured the fractional and absolute synthesis rates of fibrinogen in seven middle-aged men with type 2 diabetes and matched nondiabetic controls (609). These studies showed both basal fibrinogen concentration and absolute synthesis rates of fibrinogen were greater in diabetics.

# References

1. Xu X, Doolittle RF. Presence of a vertebrate fibrinogen-like sequence in an echinoderm. *Proc Natl Acad Sci U S A* 1990;87:2097.
2. Davidson CJ, Tuddenham EG, McVey JH. 450 million years of hemostasis. *J Thromb Haemost* 2003;1:1487.
3. Brown JH, Volkmann N, Jun G, et al. The crystal structure of modified bovine fibrinogen. *Proc Natl Acad Sci U S A* 2000;97:85.
4. Yang Z, Kollman JM, Pandi L, et al. Crystal structure of native chicken fibrinogen at 2.7 A resolution. *Biochemistry* 2001;40:12515.
5. Madrazo J, Brown JH, Litvinovich S, et al. Crystal structure of the central region of bovine fibrinogen (E5 fragment) at 1.4-A resolution. *Proc Natl Acad Sci U S A* 2001;98:11967.
6. Yee VC, Pratt KP, Côté HCF, et al. Crystal structure of a 30 kDa C-terminal fragment from the gamma chain of human fibrinogen. *Structure* 1997;5:125.
7. Pratt KP, Côté HCF, Chung DW, et al. The primary fibrin polymerization pocket: three-dimensional structure of a 30-kDa C-terminal gamma chain fragment complexed with the peptide Gly-Pro-Arg-Pro. *Proc Natl Acad Sci U S A* 1997;94:7176.
8. Spraggon G, Everse SJ, Doolittle RF. Crystal structures of fragment D from human fibrinogen and its crosslinked counterpart from fibrin. *Nature* 1997;389:455.
9. Everse SJ, Spraggon G, Veerapandian L, et al. Conformational changes in fragments D and double-D from human fibrin(ogen) upon binding the peptide ligand Gly-His-Arg-Pro-amide. *Biochemistry* 1999;38:2941.
10. Kostelansky MS, Betts L, Gorkun OV, et al. 2.8 A crystal structures of recombinant fragment D with and without two peptide ligands: GHRP binding to the "b" site disrupts its nearby calcium binding site. *Biochemistry* 2002;41:12124.
11. Hall CE, Slayter HS. The fibrinogen molecule: its size, shape and mode of polymerization. *J Biophys Biochem Cytol* 1959;5:11.
12. Hoeprich PD, Doolittle RF. Dimeric half-molecules of human fibrinogen are joined through disulfide bonds in an antiparallel orientation. *Biochemistry* 1983;22:2049.
13. Doolittle RF. The amino acid sequence of the alpha-chain of human fibrinogen. *Nature* 1979;280:464.
14. Henschen A. On the structure of functional sites in fibrinogen. *Thromb Res* 1983;(Suppl. 5):27.
15. Bailey K, Bettelheim FR, Lorand L, et al. Action of thrombin in the clotting of fibrinogen. *Nature* 1951;167:233.
16. Blomback B, Blomback M. The molecular structure of fibrinogen. *Ann N Y Acad Sci* 1972;202:77.
17. Henschen A, Lottspeich F, Kehl M, et al. Covalent structure of fibrinogen. *Ann N Y Acad Sci* 1983;408:28.
18. Doolittle RF. The structure and evolution of vertebrate fibrinogen. *Ann N Y Acad Sci* 1983;408:13.
19. Rixon MW, Chan WY, Davie EW, et al. Characterization of a complementary deoxyribonucleic acid coding for the alpha chain of human fibrinogen. *Biochemistry* 1983;22:3237.
20. Chung DW, Que BGF, Rixon MW, et al. Characterization of complementary deoxyribonucleic and genomic deoxyribonucleic acid for the beta chain of human fibrinogen. *Biochemistry* 1983;22:3244.
21. Chung DW, Chan WY, Davie EW. Characterization of a complementary deoxyribonucleic acid coding for the gamma chain of human fibrinogen. *Biochemistry* 1983;22:3250.
22. Kant JA, Lord ST, Crabtree GR. Partial mRNA sequences for human A alpha, B beta, and gamma fibrinogen chains: evolutionary and functional implications. *Proc Natl Acad Sci U S A* 1983;80:3953.
23. Doolittle RF. Fibrinogen and fibrin. *Annu Rev Biochem* 1984;53:195.
24. Francis CW, Marder VJ, Martin SE. Demonstration of a large molecular weight variant of the gamma chain of normal human plasma fibrinogen. *J Biol Chem* 1980;255:5599.
25. Wolfenstein-Todel C, Moesson MW. Human plasma fiabrinogen heterogeneity: evidence for an extended carboxylterminal sequence in a normal gamma chain variant. *Proc Natl Acad Sci U S A* 1980;77:5069.
26. Chung DW, Davie EW. gamma and gamma' chains of human fibrinogen are produced by alternative mRNA processing. *Biochemistry* 1984;23:4232.
27. Fornace AJ Jr, Cummings DE, Comeau CM, et al. Structure of the human gamma-fibrinogen gene. Alternate mRNA splicing near the 3' end of the gene produces gamma A and gamma B forms of gamma-fibrinogen. *J Biol Chem* 1984;259:12826.
28. Francis CW, Muller E, Henschen A, et al. Carboxyl-terminal amino acid sequences of two variant forms of the gamma chain of human plasma fibrinogen. *Proc Natl Acad Sci U S A* 1988;85:3358.
29. Fu Y, Grieninger G. Fib$_{420}$: a normal human variant of fibrinogen with two extended a chains. *Proc Natl Acad Sci U S A* 1994;91:2625.
30. Spraggon G, Applegate D, Everse SJ, et al. Crystal structure of a recombinant alphaEC domain from human fibrinogen-420. *Proc Natl Acad Sci U S A* 1998;95:9099.
31. Mills DA, Triantaphyllopoulos DC. Distribution of carbohydrate among the polypeptide chains and plasmin digest products of human fibrinogen. *Arch Biochem Biophys* 1969;135:28.
32. Blomback B, Grondahl NJ, Hessel B. Primary structure of human fibrinogen and fibrin. II. Structural studies on NH2-terminal part of chain. *J Biol Chem* 1973;248:5806.
33. Topfer-Peterson E, Lottspeich F, Henschen A. Carbohydrate linkage site in the beta chain of human fibrin. *Hoppe Seylers Z Physiol Chem* 1976;357:1509.
34. Scheraga HA, Laskowski M Jr. The fibrinogen-fibriin conversion. *Adv Protein Chem* 1957;12:1.
35. Blomback B, Yamashina I. On the N-terminal amino acids in fibrinogen and fibrin. *Arkiv Kemi* 1958;12:299.
36. Chen R, Doolittle RF. Identification of the polypeptide chains involved in the cross-linking of fibrin. *Proc Natl Acad Sci U S A* 1969;63:420.
37. McKee PA, Mattock P, Hill RL. Subunit structure of human fibrinogen, soluble fibrin, and cross-linked insoluble fibrin. *Proc Natl Acad Sci U S A* 1970;66:738.
38. Chen R, Doolittle RF. Gamma-gamma crosslinking sites in human and bovine fibrinogen. *Biochemistry* 1971;10:4486.
39. Cottrell BA, Strong DD, Watt KWK, et al. Amino acid sequence studies of the alpha chain of human fibrinogen: exact location of Crosslinking acceptor sites. *Biochemistry* 1979;18:5405.
40. Nussenzweig V, Seligmann M, Pelmont U, et al. Les produits de degradation du fibrinogene humain par la plasmine. I. Separation et proprietes physico-chimiques. *Ann Inst Pasteur* 1961;100:377.
41. Takagi T, Doolittle RF. Amino acid sequence studies on plasmin-derived fragments of human fibrinogen: N-terminal sequences of intermediate and terminal fragments. *Biochemistry* 1975;14:940.
42. Henschen A. Number and reactivity of disulfide bonds in fibrinogen and fibrin. *Arkiv Kemi* 1964;22:355.
43. Garlund B, Hessel B, Marguerie G, et al. Primary structure of human fibrinogen: characterization of disulfide-containing cyanogen-bromide fragments. *Eur J Biochem* 1977;77:595.
44. Blomback B, Blomback M, Henschen A, et al. N-terminal disulphide knot of human fibrinogen. *Nature* 1968;218:130.
45. Blomback B, Hessel B, Hogg D. Disulfide bridges in NH2-terminal part of human fibrinogen. *Thromb Res* 1976;8:639.
46. Zhang J-Z, Kudryk B, Redman CM. Symmetrical disulfide bonds are not necessary for assembly and secretion of human fibrinogen. *J Biol Chem* 1993;268:11278.
47. Bouma H, Takagi T, Doolittle RF. The arrangement of disulfide bonds in fragment D from human fibrinogen. *Thromb Res* 1978;13:557.
48. Henschen A. Disulfide bridges in the middle part of human fibrinogen. *Hoppe Seylers Z Physiol Chem* 1979;359:1757.
49. Nussenzweig V, Seligmann M. Analyse, par des methodes immunochimiques de la degradation par la plasmine du fibrinogene humain et de la fibrine, a differents stades. *Rev Hematol* 1960;15:451.
50. Mihalyi E, Godfrey JE. Digestion of fibrinogen by trypsin. II. Characterization of the large fragment obtained. *Biochim Biophys Acta* 1963;67:90.
51. Kowalska-Loth B, Garlund B, Egberg N, et al. Plasmic degradation products of human fibrinogen. II. Chemical and immunological relation between fragment E and N-DSK. *Thromb Res* 1973;2:423.
52. Garlund B, Kowalska-Loth B, Grondahl NH, et al. Plasmic degradation products of human fibrinogen. I. Isolation and characterization of fragments E and D and their relation to "disulfide knots". *Thromb Res* 1972;1:371.
53. Marder VJ, Budzynski AZ, James HL. High molecular weight derivatives of human fibrinogen produced by plasmin. III. Their NH2-terminal amino acids and comparison with the NH2-terminal disulfide knot. *J Biol Chem* 1972;247:4775.
54. Marder VJ. Identification and purification of fibrinogen degradation products produced by plamsin: considerations on the structure of fibrinogen. *Scand J Haematol Suppl*, 1971;13:21.
55. Marder VJ, Shulman NR, Carroll WR. The importance of intermediate degradation products of fibrinogen in fibrinolytic hemorrhage. *Trans Assoc Am Physicians* 1987;80:156.
56. Marder VJ, Shulman NR, Carroll WR. High molecular weight derivatives of human fibrinogen produced by plasmin. I. Physiochemical and immunological characterization. *J Biol Chem* 1969;244:2111.
57. Francis CW, Marder VJ. A molecular model of plasmic degradation of crosslinked fibrin. *Semin Thromb Hemost* 1982;8:25.
58. Budzynski AZ, Marder VJ, Shainoff JR. Structure of plasmic degrdation products of human fibrinogen. *J Biol Chem* 1974;249:2294.

59. Fowler WE, Fretto LJ, Erickson HP, et al. Electron microscopy of plasmic fragments of human fibrinogen as related to trinodular structure of the intact molecule. *J Clin Invest* 1980;66:50.

60. Nussenzweig V, Seligmann M, Grabar P. Les produits de degradation du fibrinogene humain par la plasmine. II. Etude immunologique: mise en evidence d'anticorps antifibrinogene natif possedant des specificites differentes. *Ann Inst Pasteur* 1961;100:490.

61. Telford JN, Nagy JA, Hatcher PA, et al. Location of peptide fragments in the fibrinogen molecule by immunoelectron microscopy. *Proc Natl Acad Sci U S A* 1980;77:2372.

62. Price TM, Strong DD, Rudee ML, et al. Shadow-cast electron microscopy of fibrinogen with antibody fragments bound to specific regions. *Proc Natl Acad Sci U S A* 1981;78:200.

63. Norton PA, Slayter HS. Immune labeling of the D and E regions of human fibrinogen by electron microscopy. *Proc Natl Acad Sci U S A* 1981; 78:1661.

64. Williams RC. Morphology of bovine fibrinogen monomers and fibrin oligomers. *J Mol Biol* 1981;150:399.

65. Doolittle RF. Structural basis of the fibrinogen-fibrin transformation: contributions from X-ray crystallography. *Blood Rev* 2003;17:33.

66. Weisel JW, Phillips GN, Cohen C. A model from electron microscopy for the molecular structure of fibrinogen and fibrin. *Nature* 1981;289:263.

67. Weisel J, Stauffacher CV, Bullitt E, et al. A model for fibrinogen:domains and sequence. *Science* 1985;230:1388.

68. Rao SP, Poojary MD, Elliott BW Jr, et al. Fibrinogen structure in projection at 18 a resolution. Electron density by co-ordinated cryo-electron microscopy and X-ray crystallography. *J Mol Biol* 1991;222:89.

69. Koradi R, Billeter M, Wuthrich K. MOLMOL: a program for display and analysis of macromolecular structures. *J Mol Graph* 1996;14:51.

70. Erickson HP, Fowler WE. Electron microscopy of fibrinogen and its plasmic fragments and small polymers. *Ann N Y Acad Sci* 1983;408:146.

71. Doolittle RF, Goldbaum DM, Doolittle LR. Designation of sequences involved in the "coiled-coil" interdomainal connections in fibrinogen: construction of an atomic scale model. *J Mol Biol* 1978;120:311.

72. Rao SPS, Poojary MD, Elliott BW Jr, et al. Fibrinogen structure in projection at 18 Å resolution. Electron density by co-ordinated cryo-electron microscopy and x-ray crystallography. *J Mol Biol* 1991;222:89.

73. Donovan JW, Mihalyi E. Conformation of fibrinogen: caloriemtric evidence for a three-nodule structure. *Proc Natl Acad Sci U S A* 1974;71:4125.

74. Huang S, Cao Z, Davie EW. The role of N-terminal disulfide bonds in the structure and assembly of human fibrinogen. *Biochem Biophys Res Commun* 1993;190:488.

75. Doolittle RF. A detailed consideration of a principal domain of vertebrate fibrinogen and its relatives. *Prot Sci* 1992;1:1563.

76. Everse SJ, Spraggon G, Veerapandian L, et al. Crystal structure of fragment double-D from human fibrin with two different bound ligands. *Biochemistry* 1998;37:8637.

77. Veklich YI, Gorkun OV, Medved LV, et al. Carboxyl-terminal portions of the a chains of fibrinogen and fibrin. Localization by electron microscopy and the effects of isolated aC fragments on polymerization. *J Biol Chem* 1993;268:13577.

78. Mosesson MW, Hainfeld J, Haschemeyer RH, et al. Identification and mass analysis of human fibrinogen molecules and their domains by scanning transmission electron microscopy. *J Mol Biol* 1981;153:695.

79. Medved LV, Gorkun OV, Privalov PL. Structural organization of C-terminal parts of fibrinogen A alpha chains. *FEBS Lett* 1983;160:291.

80. Weisel JW, Medved L. The structure and function of the alpha C domains of fibrinogen. *Ann N Y Acad Sci* 2001;936:312.

81. Tsurupa G, Tsonev L, Medved L. Structural organization of the fibrin(ogen) alpha C-domain. *Biochemistry* 2002;41:6449.

82. Fu YP, Cao Y, Hertzberg KM, et al. Fibrinogen a genes: conservation of bipartite transcripts and carboxy-terminal-extended a subunits in vertebrates. *Genomics* 1995;30:71.

83. Blomback B. Studies on the action of thrombotic enzymes on bovine fibrinogen as measured by N-terminal analysis. *Arkiv Kemi* 1958;12:321.

84. Marsh HC, Meinwald YC, Thannhauser TW, et al. Mechanism of action of thrombin on fibrinogen: kinetic evidence for involvement of aspartic acid at position P10. *Biochemistry* 1983;22:4170.

85. Nagy JA, Meinwald YC, Scheraga HA. Immunochemical determination of conformational equilibria for fragments of the A-alpha chain of fibrinogen. *Biochemistry* 1982;21:1794.

86. Marsh HC Jr, Meinwald YC, Lee S, et al. Mechanism of action of thrombin on fibrinogen: NMR evidence for a beta-bend at or near fibrinogen A alpha Gly(P5)-Gly(P4). *Biochemistry* 1985;24:2806.

87. Ni F, Scheraga HA, Lord ST. High-resolution NMR studies of fibrinogen-like peptides in solution: resonance assignments and conformational analysis of residues 1-23 of the A alpha chain of human fibrinogen. *Biochemistry* 1988;27:4481.

88. Ni F, Konishi Y, Frazier RB, et al. High-resolution NMR studies of fibrinogen-like peptides in solution: interaction of thrombin with residues 1-23 of the A alpha chain of human fibrinogen. *Biochemistry* 1989;28:3082.

89. Ni F, Meinwald YC, Vásquez M, et al. High-resolution NMR studies of fibrinogen-like peptides in solution: structure of a thrombin-bound peptide corresponding to residues 7-16 of the A alpha chain of human fibrinogen. *Biochemistry* 1989;28:3094.

90. Lord ST, Fowlkes DM. Expression of a fibrinogen fusion peptide in Escherichia coli: a model thrombin substrate for structure/function analysis. *Blood* 1989;73:166.

91. Stubbs MT, Oschkinat H, Mayr I, et al. The interaction of thrombin with fibrinogen—a structural basis for its specificity. *Eur J Biochem* 1992; 206:187.

92. Martin PD, Robertson W, Turk D, et al. The structure of residues 7-16 of the Aa-chain of human fibrinogen bound to bovine thrombin at 2.3-Å resolution. *J Biol Chem* 1992;267:7911.

93. Lord ST, Byrd PA, Hede KL, et al. Analysis of fibrinogen Aa-fusion proteins. Mutants which inhibit thrombin equivalently are not equally good substrates. *J Biol Chem* 1990;265:838.

94. Fenton JW, Olson TA, Zabinski MP, et al. Anion-binding exosite of human alpha-thrombin and fibrin(ogen) recognition. *Biochemistry* 1988; 27:7106.

95. Berliner LJ, Sugawara Y. Human alpha-thrombin binding to nonpolymerized fibrin-agarose: evidence for an anionic binding region. *Biochemistry* 1985;24:7005.

96. Kaminski M, McDonagh J. Inhibited thrombins. Interactions with fibrinogen and fibrin. *Biochem J* 1987;242:881.

97. Vali Z, Scheraga HA. Localization of the binding site on fibrin for the secondary binding site of thrombin. *Biochemistry* 1988;27:1956.

98. Kaczmarek E, McDonagh J. Thrombin binding to the A alpha-, B beta-, and gamma-chains of fibrinogen and to their remnants contained in fragment E. *J Biol Chem* 1988;263:13896.

99. Pechik I, Madrazo J, Mosesson MW, et al. Crystal structure of the complex between thrombin and the central "E" region of fibrin. *Proc Natl Acad Sci U S A* 2004;101:2718.

100. Blomback B, Vestermark A. Isolation of fibrinopeptides by chromatography. *Arkiv Kemi* 1958;12:173.

101. Blomback B, Hessel B, Hogg D, et al. A two-step fibrinogen-fibrin transition in blood coagulation. *Nature* 1978;275:501.

102. Martinelli RA, Scheraga HA. Steady-state kinetic study of the bovine thrombin-fibrinogen interaction. *Biochemistry* 1980;19:2343.

103. Hurlet-Jensen A, Cummins HZ, Nossel HL, et al. Fibrin-polymerization and release of fibrinopeptide B by thrombin. *Thromb Res* 1982;27:419.

104. Higgins DL, Lewis SD, Shafer JA. Steady state kinetic parameters for the thrombin-catalyzed conversion of human fibrinogen to fibrin. *J Biol Chem* 1982;258:9276.

105. Hanna LS, Scheraga HA, Francis CW, et al. Comparison of structures of various fibrinogens and a derivative thereof by a study of the kinetics of release of fibrinopeptides. *Biochemistry* 1984;23:4681.

106. Lewis SD, Shields PP, Shafer JA. Characterization of the kinetic pathway for liberation of fibrinopeptides during assembly of fibrin. *J Biol Chem* 1985;260:10192.

107. Mihalyi E. Clotting of bovine fibrinogen. Kinetic analysis of the release of the fibrinopeptides by thrombin and of the calcium uptake upon clotting at high fibrinogen concentrations. *Biochemistry* 1988;27:976.

108. Mullin JL, Gorkun OV, Binnie CG, et al. Recombinant fibrinogen studies reveal that thrombin specificity dictates order of fibrinopeptide release. *J Biol Chem* 2000;275:25239.

109. Vindigni A, Di Cera E. Release of fibrinopeptides by the slow and fast forms of thrombin. *Biochemistry* 1996;35:4417.

110. De Cristofaro R, Di Cera E. Modulation of thrombin-fibrinogen interaction by specific ion effects. *Biochemistry* 1992;31:257.

111. Hopfner K-P, Di Cera E. Energetics of thrombin-fibrinogen interaction. *Biochemistry* 1992;31:11567.

112. Carr ME. Turbidimetric evaluation of the impact of albumin on the structure of thrombin-mediated fibrin gelation. *Haemostasis* 1987;17:189.

113. Hantgan RR, Hermans J. Assembly of fibrin: a light scattering study. *J Biol Chem* 1979;254:11272.

114. Profumo A, Turci M, Damonte G, et al. Kinetics of fibrinopeptide release by thrombin as a function of CaCl2 concentration: different susceptibility of FPA and FPB and evidence for a fibrinogen isoform-specific effect at physiological Ca2+ concentration. *Biochemistry* 2003;42:12335.

115. Krakow W, Endres GF, Siegel BM, et al. An electron microscopic investigation of the polymerization of bovine fibrin monomer. *J Mol Biol* 1972;71:95.

116. Fowler WE, Hantgan RR, Hermans J, et al. Structure of the fibrin protofibril. *Proc Natl Acad Sci U S A* 1981;78:4872.

117. Yang Z, Mochalkin I, Doolittle RF. A model of fibrin formation based on crystal structures of fibrinogen and fibrin fragments complexed with synthetic peptides. *Proc Natl Acad Sci U S A* 2000;97:14156.

118. Olexa SA, Budzynski AZ. Evidence for four different polymerization sites involved in human fibrin formation. *Proc Natl Acad Sci U S A* 1980;77:1374.

119. Laudano AP, Doolittle RF. Studies on synthetic peptides that bind fibrinogen and present fibrin polymerization. *Proc Natl Acad Sci U S A* 1978;75:3085.

120. Weisel JW. Fibrin assembly. Lateral aggregation and the role of the two pairs of fibrinopeptides. *Biophys J* 1986;50:1079.

121. Ferry JD. The mechanism of polymerization of fibrin. *Proc Natl Acad Sci U S A* 1952;38:566.

122. Fowler WR, Erickson HP. Trinodular structure of fibrinogen: confirmation by both shadowing and negative-stain electron microscopy. *J Mol Biol* 1979;134:241.

123. Ferry JD, Morrison PR. Preparation and properties of serum and plasma proteins. VIII. The conversion of human fibrinogen to fibrin under various conditions. *J Am Chem Soc* 1947;69:388.

124. Siegel BM, Mernan JP, Scheraga HP. The configuration of native and partially polymerized fibrinogen. *Biochim Biophys Acta* 1953;11:329.

125. Nelb GW, Kamykowski GW, Ferry JD. Kinetics of ligation of fibrin oligomers. *J Biol Chem* 1980;255:6398.

126. Bale MD, Janmey PA, Ferry JD. Kinetics of formation of fibrin oligomers. II. Size distribution of ligated oligomers. *Biopolymers* 1982;21:2265.

127. Janmey PA, Erdile L, Bale MD, et al. Kinetics of fibrin oligomer formation observed by electron microscopy. *Biochemistry* 1983;22:4336.

128. Hantgan RR, Fowler RW, Erickson HP, et al. Fibrin assembly: a comparison of electron microscopic and light scattering results. *Thromb Haemost* 1980;44:119.

129. Hermans J, McDonagh J. Fibrin: structure and interactions. *Semin Thromb Hemost* 1982;8:11.

130. Hantgan RR, McDonagh J, Hermans J. Fibrin assembly. *Ann N Y Acad Sci* 1983;408:344.

131. Yamazumi K, Doolittle RF. Photoaffinity labeling of the primary fibrin polymerization site: localization of the label to gamma-chain Tyr-363. *Proc Natl Acad Sci U S A* 1992;89:2893.

132. Côté HCF, Pratt KP, Davie EW, et al. The polymerization pocket "a" within the carboxyl-terminal region of the gamma chain of human fibrinogen is adjacent to but independent from the calcium-binding site. *J Biol Chem* 1997;272:23792.

133. Kostelansky MS, Bolliger-Stucki B, Betts L, et al. BbetaGlu397 and BbetaAsp398 but not BbetaAsp432 are required for "B:b" interactions. *Biochemistry* 2004;43:2465.

134. Doolittle RF. X-ray crystallographic studies on fibrinogen and fibrin. *J Thromb Haemost* 2003;1:1559.

135. Wiltzius P, Deitler G, Kanzig W, et al. Fibrin aggregation before sol-gel transition. *Biophys J* 1982;38:123.

136. Mueller M, Burchard W. Fibrinogen-fibrin transformations characterized during the course of reaction by their intermediate structures: a light scattering study in dilute solution under physiological conditions. *Biochim Biophys Acta* 1978;537:208.

137. Muller MF, Ris H, Ferry JD. Electron microscopy of fine fibrin clots and fine and coarse fibrin films: observations of fibers in cross-section and in deformed states. *J Mol Biol* 1984;174:369.

138. Shen LL, Hermans J, McDonagh J, et al. Role of fibrinopeptide B release: comparison of fibrins produced by thrombin and Ancrod. *Am J Physiol* 1977;232:H629.

139. Shainoff JR, Dardik BN. Fibrinopeptide B and aggregation of fibrinogen. *Science* 1979;204:200.

140. Shimzu A, Schindlauer G, Ferry JD. Interaction of fibrinogen-binding tetrapeptide Gly-Pro-Arg-Pro with fine clots and oligomers of alpha fibrin; comparisons with ALBE-fibrin. *Biopolymers* 1988;27:775.

141. Mosesson MW, DiOrio JP, Muller MF, et al. Studies on the ultrastructure of fibrin lacking fibrinopeptide B (beta-fibrin). *Blood* 1987;69:1073.

142. Weisel JW, Phillips GN, Cohen C. The structure of fibrinogen and fibrin. II. Architecture of the fibrin clot. *Ann NY Acad Sci* 1983;408:367.

143. Voter WA, Lucaveche C, Blaurock AE, et al. Lateral packing of protofibrils in fibrin fibers and fibrinogen polymers. *Biopolymers* 1986;25:2359.

144. Weisel JW, Nagaswami C, Makowski L. Twisting of fibrin fibers limits their radial growth. *Proc Natl Acad Sci U S A* 1987;84:8991.

145. Mosesson MW, Siebenlist KR, Amrani DL, et al. Identification of covalently linked trimeric and tetrameric D domains in crosslinked fibrin. *Proc Natl Acad Sci U S A* 1989;86:1113.

146. Weisel JW, Papsun DM. Involvement of the COOH-terminal portion of the alpha-chain of fibrin in the branching of fibers to form a clot. *Thromb Res* 1987;47:155.

147. Gorkun OV, Veklich YI, Medved LV, et al. Role of the alpha C domains in clot formation. *Biochemistry* 1994;33:6986.

148. Langer BG, Weisel JW, Dinauer PA, et al. Deglycosylation of fibrinogen accelerates polymerization and increases lateral aggregation of fibrin fibers. *J Biol Chem* 1988;263:15056.

149. Hermans J. Models of fibrin. *Proc Natl Acad Sci U S A* 1979;76:1189.

150. Carr ME, Hermans J. Size and density of fibrin fibers from turbidity. *Macromolecules* 1978;11:46.

151. Cohen C, Weisel JW, Phillips GN, et al. The structure of fibrinogen and fibrin. I. Electron microscopy and x-ray crystallography of fibrinogen. *Ann N Y Acad Sci* 1983;408:194.

152. Stryer L, Cohen C, Langridge R. Axial period of fibrinogen and fibrin. *Nature* 1963;197:793.

153. Gollwitzer R, Bode W, Schramm H-J, et al. Laser diffraction of oriented fibrinogen. *Ann N Y Acad Sci* 1983;408:214.

154. Torbet J, Freyssinet J-M, Hudry-Clergeon G. Oriented fibrin gels formed by polymerization in strong magnetic fields. *Nature* 1981;289:91.

155. Freyssinet J-M, Torbet J, Hudry-Clergeon G, et al. Fibrinogen and fibrin structure and fibrin formation measured by using magnetic orientation. *Proc Natl Acad Sci U S A* 1983;80:1616.

156. Wilf J, Minton AP. Soluble fibrin-fibrinogen complexes as intermediates in fibrin gel formation. *Biochemistry* 1986;25:3124.

157. Husain SS, Weisel JW, Budzynski AZ. Interaction of fibrinogen and its derivatives with fibrin. *J Biol Chem* 1989;264:11414.

158. Torbet J. Fibrin assembly in human plasma and fibrinogen/albumin mixtures. *Biochemistry* 1986;25:5309.

159. Wilf J, Gladner JA, Minton AP. Acceleration of fibrin gel formation by unrelated proteins. *Thromb Res* 1985;37:681.

160. Galanakis DK, Lane BP, Simon SR. Albumin modulates lateral assembly of fibrin polymers: evidence of enhanced fine fibril formation and of unique synergism with fibrinogen. *Biochemistry* 1987;26:2389.

161. Brummel KE, Butenas S, Mann KG. An integrated study of fibrinogen during blood coagulation. *J Biol Chem* 1999;274:22862.

162. Mann KG, Brummel K, Butenas S. What is all that thrombin for? *J Thromb Haemost* 2003;1:1504.

163. Dietler G, Kanzig W, Haberli A, et al. Experimental tests of a geometrical abstraction of fibrin polymerization. *Biopolymers* 1986;25:905.

164. Hunziker EB, Straub PW, Haeberji A. Molecular morphology of fibrin monomers and early oligomers during fibrin polymerization. *J Ultrastruct Mol Struct Res* 1988;98:60.

165. Hunziker EB, Straub PW, Haeberli A. A new concept of fibrin formation based upon the linear growth of interlacing and branching polymers and molecular alignment into interlocked single-stranded segments. *J Biol Chem* 1990;265:7455.

166. Rocco M, Bernocco S, Turci M, et al. Early events in the polymerization of fibrin. *Ann N Y Acad Sci* 2001;936:167.

167. Bernocco S, Ferri F, Profumo A, et al. Polymerization of rod-like macromolecular monomers studied by stopped-flow, multiangle light scattering: set-up, data processing, and application to fibrin formation. *Biophys J* 2000;79:561.

168. Schwartz ML, Pizzo SV, Hill RL, et al. Human factor XIII from plasma and platelets. *J Biol Chem* 1973;248:1395.

169. Lorand L, Konishi K. Activation of the fibrin stabilizing factor of plasma by thrombin. *Arch Biochem Biophys* 1964;105:58.

170. Loewy AG, Dunathan K, Kriel R, et al. Fibrinase. I. Purification of substrate and enzyme. *J Biol Chem* 1961;236:2625.

171. Folk JE, Chung SI. Molecular and catalytic properties of transglutaminases. *Adv Enzymol* 1973;38:109.

172. Folk JE, Finlayson JS. The epsilon-(gamma-glutamyl)lysine crosslink and the catalytic role of transglutaminases. *Adv Protein Chem* 1977;31:1.

173. Pisano JJ, Finlayson JS, Peyton MP. Crosslink in fibrin polymerized by factor XIII: epsilon-(gamma-glutamyl)lysine. *Science* 1968;160:892.

174. Shen LL, Hermans J, McDonash J, et al. Effects of calcium ion and covalent crosslinking on formation an delasticity of fibrin gels. *Thromb Res* 1975;6:255.

175. Gerth C, Roberts WW, Ferry JD. Rheology of fibrin clots. II. Linear viscoelastic behavior in shear creep. *Biophys Chem* 1974;2:208.

176. Robbins KC. A study on the conversion of fibrinogen to fibrin. *Am J Physiol* 1944;142:581.

177. Laki K, Lorand L. On the solubility of fibrin clots. *Science* 1948;108:280.

178. McDonagh RP, McDonagh J, Duckert F Jr. The influence of fibrin crosslinking on the kinetics of urokinase-induced clot lysis. *Br J Haematol* 1971;21:323.

179. Shen LL, McDonagh RP, McDonagh J, et al. Early events in the plasmin digestion of fibrinogen and fibrin: effects on fibrin polymerization. *J Biol Chem* 1977;252:6184.

180. Francis CW, Marder VJ. Increased resistance to plasmic degradation of fibrin with highly crosslinked alpha-polymer chains formed at high factor XIII concentrations. *Blood* 1988;71:1361.

181. Samokhin GP, Lorand L. Contact with the N termini in the central E domain enhances the reactivities of the distal D domains of fibrin to factor XIIIa. *J Biol Chem* 1995;270:21827.

182. Mosesson MW. Cross-linked gamma-chains in fibrin fibrils bridge 'transversely' between strands: yes. *J Thromb Haemost* 2004;2:388.

183. Weisel JW. Cross-linked gamma-chains in fibrin fibrils bridge transversely between strands: no. *J Thromb Haemost* 2004;2:394.

184. Fowler WE, Erickson HP, Hantgan RR, et al. Cross-linked fibrinogen dimers demonstrate a feature of the molecular packing in fibrin fibers. *Science* 1981;211:287.

185. Weisel JW, Francis CW, Nagaswami C, et al. Determination of the topology of factor XIIIa-induced fibrin gamma-chain cross-links by electron microscopy of ligated fragments. *J Biol Chem* 1993;268:26618.

186. Mosesson MW. Thrombin interactions with fibrinogen and fibrin. *Semin Thromb Hemost* 1993;19:361.

187. Siebenlist KR, Meh DA, Wall JS, et al. Orientation of the carboxy-terminal regions of fibrin gamma chain dimers determined from the crosslinked products formed in mixtures of fibrin, fragment D, and factor XIIIa. *Thromb Haemost* 1995;74:1113.

188. Mosesson MW, Siebenlist KR, Hainfeld JF, et al. The covalent structure of factor XIIIa crosslinked fibrinogen fibrils. *J Struct Biol* 1995;115:88.

189. Mosesson MW. Fibrinogen and fibrin polymerization: appraisal of the binding events that accompany fibrin generation and fibrin clot assembly. *Blood Coagul Fibrinolysis* 1997;8:257.

190. Siebenlist KR, Meh DA, Mosesson MW. Position of gamma-chain carboxy-terminal regions in fibrinogen/fibrin cross-linking mixtures. *Biochemistry* 2000;39:14171.

191. Yang Z, Pandi L, Doolittle RF. The crystal structure of fragment double-D from cross-linked lamprey fibrin reveals isopeptide linkages across an unexpected D-D interface. *Biochemistry* 2002;41:15610.

192. Matsuka YV, Medved LV, Migliorini MM, et al. Factor XIIIa-catalyzed cross-linking of recombinant alpha C fragments of human fibrinogen. *Biochemistry* 1996;35:5810.

193. Schwartz ML, Pizzo SV, Hill RL, et al. The effect of fibrin stabilizing factor on the subunit structure of human fibrin. *J Clin Invest* 1971;50:1506.

194. Gaffney PJ, Whitaker AN. Fibrin cross-links and lysis rates. *Thromb Res* 1979;14:85.

195. Siebenlist KR, Mosesson MW. Progressive cross-linking of fibrin gamma chains increases resistance to fibrinolysis. *J Biol Chem* 1994;269:28414.

196. Falls LA, Farrell DH. Resistance of gammaA/gamma' fibrin clots to fibrinolysis. *J Biol Chem* 1997;272:14251.

197. Siebenlist KR, Meh DA, Mosesson MW. Plasma factor XIII binds specifically to fibrinogen molecules containing gamma chains. *Biochemistry* 1996;35:10448.

198. Marder VJ, Budzynski AZ. Degradation products of fibrinogen and crosslinked fibrin: projected clinical applications. *Thromb Diath Haemorrh* 1974;32:49.

199. Kopec M, Teisseyre E, Dudek-Wojciechowska G. Studies on "double D" fragment from stabilized bovine fibrin. *Thromb Res* 1973;2:283.

200. Gaffney PJ, Brasher M. Subunit structure of the plasmin-induced degradation products of cross-linked fibrin. *Biochim Biophys Acta* 1973;295:308.

201. Pizzo SV, Taylor LM, Schwartz ML Jr. Subunit structure of fragment D from fibrinogen and cross-linked fibrin. *J Biol Chem* 1973;248:4584.

202. Hudry-Clergeon G, Paturel L, Suscillon M. Identification d'un complexe (D-D) ... E dans les produits de degradation de la fibrine bovine stabilisee par le facteur XIII. *Pathol Biol* 1974;(Suppl. 22):47.

203. Gaffney PJ, Lane DA, Kakkar VV, et al. Characterization of a soluble D dimer-E complex in cross-linked fibrin digests. *Thromb Res* 1975;7:89.

204. Francis CW, Marder VJ, Barlow GH. Plasmic degradation of crosslinked fibrin: characterization of new macromolecular soluble complexes and a model of their structure. *J Clin Invest* 1980;66:1033.

205. Francis CW, Marder VJ, Martin SE. Plasmic degradation of crosslinked fibrin. I. Structural analysis of the particulate clot and identification of new macromolecular-soluble complexes. *Blood* 1980;56:456.

206. Nieuwenhuizen W, van Ruijven-Vermeer IAM, Nooijen WJ, et al. Recalculation of calcium-binding properties of human and rat fibrin(ogen) and their degradation products. *Thromb Res* 1981;22:653.

207. Marguerie G, Chagniel G, Suscillon M. The binding of calcium to bovine fibrinogen. *Biochim Biophys Acta* 1977;490:94.

208. Dang CV, Shin CK, Bell WR, et al. Fibrinogen sialic acid residues are low affinity calcium- binding sites that influence fibrin assembly. *J Biol Chem* 1989;264:15104.

209. Ly B, Godal HC. Denaturation of fibrinogen: the protective effect of calcium. *Haemostasis* 1973;1:204.

210. Odrljin TM, Rybarczyk BJ, Francis CW, et al. Calcium modulates plasmin cleavage of the fibrinogen D fragment gamma chain N-terminus: mapping of monoclonal antibody J88B to a plasmin sensitive domain of the gamma chain. *Biochim Biophys Acta* 1996;1298:69.

211. Procyk R, Blombäck B. Disulfide bond reduction in fibrinogen: calcium protection and effect on clottability. *Biochemistry* 1990;29:1501.

212. Endres GF, Scheraga HA. Equilibria in the fibrinogen-fibrin conversion. IX. Effects of calcium ions on the reversible polymerization of fibrin monomer. *Arch Biochem Biophys* 1977;153:266.

213. Boyer MH, Shainoff JR, Ratnoff OD. Acceleration of fibrin polymerization by calcium ions. *Blood* 1972;39:382.

214. Brass EP, Forman WB, Edwards RV, et al. Fibrin formation: effect of calcium ions. *Blood* 1978;52:564.

215. Lounes KC, Ping L, Gorkun OV, et al. Analysis of engineered fibrinogen variants suggests that an additional site mediates platelet aggregation and that "B-b" interactions have a role in protofibril formation. *Biochemistry* 2002;41:5291.

216. Hardy JJ, Carrell NA, McDonagh J. Calcium ion functions in fibrinogen conversion to fibrin. *Ann N Y Acad Sci* 1983;408:279.

217. Carr ME, Gabriel DA, McDonagh J. Influence of Ca2+ on the structure of reptilase-derived and thrombin-derived fibrin gels. *Biochem J* 1990;239:513.

218. Dyr JE, Blomback B, Hessel B, et al. Conversion of fibrinogen to fibrin induced by preferential release of fibrinopeptide B. *Biochim Biophys Acta* 1989;990:18.

219. Donovan JW, Mihalyi E. Clotting of fibrinogen. 1. Scanning calorimetric study of the effect of calcium. *Biochemistry* 1985;24:3434.

220. Mihalyi E. Clotting of bovine fibrinogen. Calcium binding to fibrin during clotting and its dependence on release of fibrinopeptide B. *Biochemistry* 1988;27:967.

221. Yamazumi K, Doolittle RF. The synthetic peptide Gly-Pro-Arg-Pro-amide limits the plasmic digestion of fibrinogen in the same fashion as calcium ion. *Protein Sci* 1992;1:1719.

222. Kostelansky MS, Lounes KC, Ping LF, et al. Calcium-binding site beta2, adjacent to the "b" polymerization site, modulates lateral aggregation of protofibrils during fibrin polymerization. *Biochemistry* 2004;43:2475.

223. Seegers WH, Nieft M, Loomis EC. Note on the adsorption of thrombin on fibrin. *Science* 1945;101:520.

224. Liu CY, Nossel HL, Kaplan KL. The binding of thrombin by fibrin. *J Biol Chem* 1979;254:10421.

225. Bode W, Turk D, Karshikov A. The refined 1.9 A X-ray crystal structure of D-Phe-Pro-Arg chloromethylketone-inhibited human alpha-thrombin. *Protein Sci* 1992;1:426.

226. Meh DA, Siebenlist KR, Brennan SO, et al. The amino acid sequence in fibrin responsible for high affinity thrombin binding. *Thromb Haemost* 2001;85:470.

227. Lovely RS, Moaddel M, Farrell DH. Fibrinogen gamma' chain binds thrombin exosite II. *J Thromb Haemost* 2003;1:124.

228. Pospisil CH, Stafford AR, Fredenburgh JC, et al. Evidence that both exosites on thrombin participate in its high affinity interaction with fibrin. *J Biol Chem* 2003;278:21584.

229. Hsieh KH. Thrombin interaction with fibrin polymerization sites. *Thromb Res* 1997;86:301.

230. Binnie CG, Lord ST. A synthetic analog of fibrinogen alpha 27-50 is an inhibitor of thrombin. *Thromb Res* 1991;65:165.

231. Siebenlist KR, DiOrio JP, Budzynski AZ, et al. The polymerization and thrombin-binding properties of des- (Bb1-42)-fibrin. *J Biol Chem* 1990;265:18650.

232. Rose T, Di Cera E. Three-dimensional modeling of thrombin-fibrinogen interaction. *J Biol Chem* 2002;277:18875.

233. Naski MC, Shafer JA. αα-Thrombin-catalyzed hydrolysis of fibrin I. Alternative binding modes and the accessibility of the active site in fibrin I-bound αα-thrombin. *J Biol Chem* 1990;265:1401.

234. Kaminski M, Siebenlist KR, Mosesson MW. Evidence for thrombin enhancement of fibrin polymerization that is independent of its catalytic activity. *J Lab Clin Med* 1991;117:218.

235. Francis CW, Markham RE Jr, Barlow GH, et al. Thrombin activity of fibrin thombi and soluble plasmic derivatives. *J Lab Clin Med* 1983;102:220.

236. Muszbek L, Yee VC, Hevessy Z. Blood coagulation factor XIII: structure and function. *Thromb Res* 1999;94:271.

237. Lorand L. Factor XIII: structure, activation, and interactions with fibrinogen and fibrin. *Ann N Y Acad Sci* 2001;936:291.

238. Credo BR, Curtis CG, Lorand L. Alpha chain domain of fibrinogen controls generation of fibrinoligase (coagulation factor XIIIa): calcium ion regulatory aspects. *Biochemistry* 1981;20:3770.

239. Greenberg CS, Shuman MA. The zymogen forms of blood coagulation factor XIII bind specifically to fibrinogen. *J Biol Chem* 1982;257:6096.

240. Moaddel M, Farrell DH, Daugherty MA, et al. Interactions of human fibrinogens with factor XIII: roles of calcium and the gamma' peptide. *Biochemistry* 2000;39:6698.

241. Janus TJ, Lewis SD, Lorand L, et al. Promotion of thrombin-catalyzed activation of factor XIII by fibrinogen. *Biochemistry* 1983;22:6269.

242. Greenberg CS, Miraglia CC, Rickles FR, et al. Cleavage of blood coagulation. Factor XIII and fibrinogen by thrombin during in vitro clotting. *J Clin Invest* 1985;75:1453.

243. Greenberg CS, Dobson JV, Miraglia CC. Regulation of plasma factor XIII binding to fibrin in vitro. *Blood* 1985;66:1028.

244. Lewis SD, Janus TJ, Lorand L, et al. Regulation of formation of factor XIIIa by its fibrin substrates. *Biochemistry* 1985;24:6772.

245. Greenberg CS, Miraglia CC. The effect of fibrin polymers of thrombin-catalyzed plasma factor XIIIa formation. *Blood* 1985;66:466.

246. Greenberg CS, Achyuthan KE, Miraglia CC. Thrombin binding to fibrin is necessary for fibrin polymers to enhance factor XIIIa formation. *Semin Thromb Hemost* 1986;12:226.

247. Greenberg CS, Achyuthan KE, Rajagopalan S, et al. Characterization of the fibrin polymer structure that accelerates thrombin cleavage of plasma factor XIII. *Arch Biochem Biophys* 1988;262:142.

248. Naski MC, Lorand L, Shafer JA. Characterization of the kinetic pathway for fibrin promotion of a-thrombin-catalyzed activation of plasma factor XIII. *Biochemistry* 1991;30:934.

249. Moaddel M, Falls LA, Farrell DH. The role of gamma A/gamma ' fibrinogen in plasma factor XIII activation. *J Biol Chem* 2000;275:32135.

250. Yee VC, Le TI, Bishop PD, et al. Structure and function studies of factor XIIIa by x-ray crystallography. *Semin Thromb Hemost* 1996;22:377.

251. Hornyak TJ, Shafer JA. Interactions of factor XIII with fibrin as substrate and cofactor. *Biochemistry* 1992;31:423. Jan 21.

252. McDonagh J, Fukue H. Determinants of substrate specificity for factor XIII. *Semin Thromb Hemost* 1996;22:369.

253. Achyuthan KE, Slaughter TF, Santiago MA, et al. Factor XIIIa-derived peptides inhibit transglutaminase activity. Localization of substrate recognition sites. *J Biol Chem* 1993;268:21284.

254. Hettasch JM, Peoples KA, Greenberg CS. Analysis of factor XIII substrate specificity using recombinant human factor XIII and tissue transglutaminase chimeras. *J Biol Chem* 1997;272:25149.

255. Procyk R, Bishop PD, Kudryk B. Fibrin—recombinant human factor XIII a-subunit association. *Thromb Res* 1993;71:127.

256. Taubenfeld SM, Song Y, Sheng D, et al. A monoclonal antibody against a peptide sequence of fibrinogen gamma chain acts as an inhibitor of factor XIII-mediated crosslinking of human fibrin. *Thromb Haemost* 1995;74:923.

257. Greenberg CS, Achyuthan KE, Fenton JW. Factor XIIIa formation promoted by complexing of alpha-thrombin, fibrin, and factor XZIII. *Blood* 1987;69:867.

258. Hornyak TJ, Bishop PD, Shafer JA. Alpha-thrombin-catalyzed activation of human platelet factor XIII: relationship between proteolysis and factor XIIIa activity. *Biochemistry* 1989;28:7326.

259. Ikematsu SR, McDonagh RP, Reisner HM, et al. Immunochemical studies of human factor XIII radioimmunoassay of the carrier subunit of the zymogen. *J Lab Clin Med* 1981;97:662.

260. Skrzynia C, Reisner HM, McDonah J. Characterization of the catalytic subunit of factor XIII by radioimmunoassay. *Blood* 1982;60:1089.

261. Rocco M, Infusini E, Daga MG, et al. Models of fibronectin. *EMBO J* 1987;6:2343.

262. Sjobert B, Pap S, Osterlund E, et al. Solution structure of human plasma fibronectin using small-angle x-ray and neutron scattering at physiological pH and ionic strength. *Arch Biochem Biophys* 1987;255:347.

263. Petersen TE, Skorstengaard K. Primary structure. In: McDonagh J, ed. *Plasma fibronectin. Structure and function.* New York: Marcel Dekker Inc, 1985.

264. Petersen TE, Skorstengaard K, Vibe-Pedersen K. Primary structure of fibronectin. In: Mosher DF, ed. *Fibronectin.* San Diego, CA: Academic Press, 1989.

265. Hynes R. Molecular biology of fibronectin. *Annu Rev Cell Biol* 1985; 1:67.

266. Hormann H. Interaction with fibrinogen and fibrin. In: McDonagh J, ed. *Plasma fibronectin. Structure and function.* New York: Marcel Dekker Inc, 1985.

267. Yamada KM. Fibronectin domains and receptors. In: Mosher DF, ed. *Fibronectin.* San Diego, CA: Academic Press, 1989.

268. Potts JR, Campbell ID. Structure and function of fibronectin modules. *Matrix Biol* 1996;15:313.

269. Williams MJ, Phan I, Harvey TS, et al. Solution structure of a pair of fibronectin type 1 modules with fibrin binding activity. *J Mol Biol* 1994;235:1302.

270. Rostagno A, Williams MJ, Baron M, et al. Further characterization of the NH2-terminal fibrin-binding site on fibronectin. *J Biol Chem* 1994;269:31938.

271. Matsuka YV, Medved LV, Brew SA, et al. The NH2-terminal fibrin-binding site of fibronectin is formed by interacting fourth and fifth finger domains. Studies with recombinant finger fragments expressed in Escherichia coli. *J Biol Chem* 1994;269:9539.

272. Rostagno AA, Schwarzbauer JE, Gold LI. Comparison of the fibrin-binding activities in the N- and C-termini of fibronectin. *Biochem J* 1999;338:375.

273. Makogonenko E, Tsurupa G, Ingham K, et al. Interaction of fibrin(ogen) with fibronectin: further characterization and localization of the fibronectin-binding site. *Biochemistry* 2002;41:7907.

274. McDonaagh RP, McDonagh J, Petersen TE, et al. Amino acid sequence of the factor XIIIa acceptor site in bovine plasma fibronectin. *FEBS Lett* 1981;127:1374.

275. Mosher DF. Action of fibrin-stabilizing factor on cold-insoluble globulin and alpha 2 macroglobulin in clotting plasma. *J Biol Chem* 1975;250:6614.

276. Ehrlich PH, Sobel JH, Moustafa ZA, et al. Monoclonal antibodies to alpha-chain regions of human fibrinogen that participate in polymer formation. *Biochemistry* 1983;22:4184.

277. Procyk R, Blomback B. Factor XIII-induced crosslinking in solutions of fibrinogen and fibronectin. *Biochim Biophys Acta* 1988;967:304.

278. Potts JR, Phan I, Williams MJ, et al. High-resolution structural studies of the factor XIIIa crosslinking site and the first type 1 module of fibronectin [letter]. *Nat Struct Biol* 1995;2:946.

279. Erickson HP, Carrell N, McDonagh J. Fibronectin molecule visualized in electron microscopy: a long, thin flexible strand. *J Cell Biol* 1981;91:673.

280. Niewiarowska J, Cierniewski CS. Inhibitory effect of fibronectin on the fibrin gel structure. *Thromb Res* 1982;27:611.

281. Okada M, Blomback B, Chang MD, et al. Fibronectin and fibrin gel structure. *J Biol Chem* 1985;260:1811.

282. Carr ME, Gabriel DA, McDonagh J. Influence of factor XIII and fibronectin on fiber size and density in thrombin-induced fibrin gels. *J Lab Clin Med* 1987;110:747.

283. Kamykowski GW, Mosher DF, Lorand L, et al. Modification of sheer modulus and creep compliance of fibrin clots by fibronectin. *Biophys Chem* 1981;13:25.

284. McDonagh J, Hada M, Kaminski M. Plasma fibronectin and fibrin formation. In: McDonagh J, ed. *Plasma fibronectin. Structure and function.* New York: Marcel Dekker Inc, 1985.

285. Chow TW, McIntire LV, Peterson DM. Importance of plasma fibronectin in determining PFP and PRP mechanical properties. *Thromb Res* 1983;29:243.

286. Leung LL. The role of thrombospondin in platelet aggregation. *J Clin Invest* 1984;74:1764.

287. Leung LKL, Nachman RL. Complex formation of platelet thrombospondin with fibrinogen. *J Clin Invest* 1982;70:542.

288. Bacon-Baguley T, Kudryk BJ, Walz DA. Thrombospondin interaction with fibrinogen. Evidence for binding to the A alpha- and B beta-chains of fibrinogen. *J Biol Chem* 1987;262:1927.

289. Tuszynski GP, Srivastava S, Switalska HI, et al. The interaction of human platelet thrombospondin with fibrinogen. Thrombospondin purification and specificity of interaction. *J Biol Chem* 1985;260:12240.

290. Bonnefoy A, Hantgan R, Legrand C, et al. A model of platelet aggregation involving multiple interactions of thrombospondin-1, fibrinogen, and GPIIbIIIa receptor. *J Biol Chem* 2001;276:5605.

291. Dixit VM, Grant GA, Frazier WA, et al. Isolation of the fibrinogen-binding region of platelet thrombospondin. *Biophys Res Commun* 1983;119:1075.

292. Bacon-Baguley T, Ogilvie ML, Gartner TK, et al. Thrombospondin binding to specific sequences within the Aa- and Bb-chains of fibrinogen. *J Biol Chem* 1990;265:2317.

293. Walz DA, Bacon-Baguley T, Kendra-Franczak S, et al. Binding of thrombospondin to immobilized ligands: specific interaction with fibrinogen, plasminogen, histidine-rich glycoprotein, and fibronectin. *Semin Thromb Hemost* 1987;13:317.

294. Bale MD, Westrick LG, Mosher DF. Incorporation of thrombospondin into fibrin clots. *J Biol Chem* 1985;260:7502.

295. Bale MD, Mosher DF. Effects of thrombospondin on fibrin polymerization and structure. *J Biol Chem* 1986;261:862.

296. Bale MD. Noncovalent and covalent interactions of thrombospondin with polymerizing fibrin. *Semin Thromb Hemost* 1987;13:326.

297. Girma J-P, Meyer D, Verweij CL, et al. Structure-function relationship of human von Willebrand factor. *Blood* 1987;70:605.

298. Ruggeri ZM, Zimmerman TS. von Willebrand factor and von Willebrand disease. *Blood* 1987;70:895.

299. Ballard JO, Sanders JC, Easter ME. Altered serum factor VIII-related antigen (VII:AGN)/von Willebrand factor (VIII:vWf) in haemophiliacs with inhibitors to factor VIII procoagulant activity (VIII:C). *Thromb Haemost* 1981;45:68.

300. Hada M, Kato M, Ikematsu S, et al. Possible cross-linking of factor VIII related antigen to fibrin by factor XIII in delayed coagulation process. *Thromb Res* 1982;25:163.

301. Beguin S, Kumar R. Thrombin, fibrin and platelets: a resonance loop in which von Willebrand factor is a necessary link. *Thromb Haemost* 1997;78:590.

302. Hada M, Kaminski M, Bockenstedt P, et al. Covalent crosslinking of von Willebrand factor to fibrin. *Blood* 1986;68:95.

303. Loscalzo J, Inbal A, Handin RI. von Willebrnad factor facilitates platelet incorporation in polymerizing fibrin. *J Clin Invest* 1986;78:1112.

304. Parker RI, Gralnick HR. Fibrin monomer induces binding of endogenous platelet von Willebrand factor to the glycocalicin portion of platelet glycoprotein Ib. *Blood* 1987;70:1589.

305. Keuren JF, Baruch D, Legendre P, et al. von Willebrand factor C1C2 domain is involved in platelet adhesion to polymerized fibrin at high shear rate. *Blood* 2004;103:1741.

306. Ribes JA, Francis CW. Multimer size dependence of von Willebrand factor binding to crosslinked or noncrosslinked fibrin. *Blood* 1990;75:1460.

307. Endenburg SC, Hantgan RR, Lindeboom-Blokzijl L, et al. On the role of von Willebrand factor in promoting platelet adhesion to fibrin in flowing blood. *Blood* 1995;86:4158.

308. Hantgan RR, Hindriks G, Taylor RG, et al. Glycoprotein Ib, von Willebrand factor, and glycoprotein IIb:IIIa are all involved in platelet adhesion to fibrin in flowing whole blood. *Blood* 1990;76:345.

309. Tran H, Mattei M, Godyna S, et al. Human fibulin-1D: molecular cloning, expression and similarity with S1-5 protein, a new member of the fibulin gene family. *Matrix Biol* 1997;15:479.

310. Tran H, Tanaka A, Litvinovich SV, et al. The interaction of fibulin-1 with fibrinogen. A potential role in hemostasis and thrombosis. *J Biol Chem* 1995;270:19458.

311. Godyna S, Diaz-Ricart M, Argraves WS. Fibulin-1 mediates platelet adhesion via a bridge of fibrinogen. *Blood* 1996;88:2569.

312. Sahni A, Odrljin T, Francis CW. Binding of basic fibroblast growth factor to fibrinogen and fibrin. *J Biol Chem* 1998;273:7554.

313. Peng H, Sahni A, Fay P, et al. Identification of a binding site on human FGF-2 for fibrinogen. *Blood* 2004;103:2114.

314. Sahni A, Altland OD, Francis CW. FGF-2 but not FGF-1 binds fibrin and supports prolonged endothelial cell growth. *J Thromb Haemost* 2003;1:1304.

315. Sahni A, Francis CW. Plasmic degradation modulates activity of fibrinogen-bound fibroblast growth factor-2. *J Thromb Haemost* 2003;1:1271.

316. Wiman B, Collen D. Molecular mechanism of physiological fibrinolysis. *Nature* 1978;272:549.

317. Collen D. Fibrin-specific thrombolytic therapy. *Thromb Res* 1988;VIII:3.

318. Marder VJ, Sherry S. Thrombolytic therapy: current status. *N Engl J Med* 1988;318:1512.

319. Nieuwenhuizen W. Fibrinogen and its induced specific sites for modulation of t-PA induced fibrinolysis. In: Kluft C, ed. *Tissue-type plasminogen activator (t-PA): physiological and clinical aspects.* Boca Raton, FL: CRC Press, 1988:171.

320. Lucas MA, Fretto LJ, McKee PA. The binding of human plasminogen to fibrin and fibrinogen. *J Biol Chem* 1983;258:4249.

321. Lewis MS, Carmassi F, Chung SI. Cooperative association of plasminogen with fibrinogen. *Biochemistry* 1984;23:3874.

322. Park K, Mosher DF, Cooper SL. Acute surface-induced thrombosis in the canine *ex vivo* model: importance of protein composition of the initial monolayer and platelet activation. *J Biomed Mater Res* 1986;20:589.

323. Fleury V, Angles-Cano E. Characterization of the binding of plasminogen to fibrin surfaces: the role of carboxy-terminal lysines. *Biochemistry* 1991;30:7630.

324. Fleury V, Loyau S, Lijnen HR, et al. Molecular assembly of plasminogen and tissue-type plasminogen activator on an evolving fibrin surface. *Eur J Biochem* 1993;216:549.

325. Nesheim M, Fredenburgh JC, Larsen GR. The dissociation constants and stoichiometries of the interactions of Lys-plasminogen and chloromethyl ketone derivatives of tissue plasminogen activator and the variant delta FEIX with intact fibrin. *J Biol Chem* 1990;265:21541.

326. Hoylaerts M, Rijken DC, Lijnen HR, et al. Kinetics of the activation of plasminogen by human tissue plasminogen activator. Role of fibrin. *J Biol Chem* 1982;257:2912.

327. Norman B, Wallen P, Ranby M. Fibrinolysis mediated by tissue plasminogen ativator. *Eur J Biochem* 1985;149:193.

328. Kaczmarek E, Lee MH, McDonagh J. Initial interaction between fibrin and tissue plasminogen activator (t-PA). The Gly-Pro-Arg-Pro binding site on fibrin(ogen) is important for t-PA activity. *J Biol Chem* 1993;268:2474.

329. Suenson E, Bjerrum P, Holm A, et al. The role of fragment X polymers in the fibrin enhancement of tissue plasminogen activator-catalyzed plasmin formation. *J Biol Chem* 1990;265:22228.

330. Bauer R, Hansen SL, Jones G, et al. Fibrin structures during tissue-type plasminogen activator-mediated fibrinolysis studied by laser light scattering: relation to fibrin enhancement of plasminogen activation. *Eur Biophys J* 1994;23:239.

331. Suenson E, Lutzen O, Thorsen S. Initial plasmin degradation of fibrin as the basis for a positive feedback mechanism for fibrinolysis. *Eur J Biochem* 1984;140:513.

332. Harpel PC, Chang T-S, Verderber E. Tissue plasminogen activator and urokinase mediate the binding of glu-plasminogen to plasma fibrin I. *J Biol Chem* 1985;260:4432.

333. Tran-Thang C, Kruithof EKO, Atkinson J. High affinity binding sites for glu-plasminogen unveiled by limited plasmic degradation of human fibrin. *Eur J Biochem* 1986;160:599.

334. Suenson E, Peterson LC. Fibrin and plasminogen structures essential to stimulation of plasmin formation by tissue-type plasminogen activator. *Biochim Biophys Acta* 1986;870:510.

335. Castellino FJ. Structure/function relationships of human plasminogen and plasmin. In: Kluft C, ed. *Tissue-type palsminogen activator (t-PA): physiological and clinical aspects.* Boca Raton, FL: CRC Press, 1988:145.

336. Varadi A, Patthy L. Location of plasminogen-binding sites in human fibrin(ogen). *Biochemistry* 1983;22:2440.

337. Bosma PJ, Rijken DC, Nieuwenhuizen W. Binding of tissue-type plasminogen activator to fibrin fragments. *Eur J Biochem* 1988;172:399.

338. Varadi A, Patthy L. Beta (Leu 121-Lys 122) segment of fibrinogen is in a region essential for plasminogen binding by fibrin fragment E. *Biochemistry* 1984;23:2108.

339. Hoylaerts M, Rijken DC, Lijnen HR, et al. Kinetics of the activation of plasminogen by human tissue plasminogen activator. Role of fibrin. *J Biol Chem* 1982;257:2912.

340. Medved L, Nieuwenhuizen W. Molecular mechanisms of initiation of fibrinolysis by fibrin. *Thromb Haemost* 2003;89:409.

341. Horrevoets AJG, Pannekoek H, Nesheim ME. A steady-state template model that describes the kinetics of fibrin-stimulated [Glu$^1$]- and [Lys$^{78}$] plasminogen activation by native tissue-type plasminogen activator and variants that lack either the finger or kringle-2 domain. *J Biol Chem* 1997;272:2183.

342. Nieuwenhuizen W, Vermond A, Voskuilen M, et al. Identification of a site in fibrin(ogen) which is involved in the acceleration of plasminogen activation by tissue-type plasminogen activator. *Biochim Biophys Acta* 1983;748:86.

343. Nieuwenhuizen W, Schielen WJG, Yonekawa O, et al. Studies on the localization and accessibility of sites in fibrin which are involved in the acceleration of the activation of plasminogen by tissue-type plasminogen activator. *Adv Exp Med Biol* 1990;281:83.

344. Schielen WJG, Adams HPHM, Van Leuven K, et al. The sequence gamma-(312-324) is a fibrin-specific epitope. *Blood* 1991;77:2169.

345. Yonekawa O, Voskuilen M, Nieuwenhuizen W. Localization in the fibrinogen gamma-chain of a new site that is involved in the acceleration of the tissue-type plasminogen activator-catalysed activation of plasminogen. *Biochem J* 1992;283:187.

346. Grailhe P, Nieuwenhuizen W, Anglés-Cano E. Study of tissue-type plasminogen activator binding sites on fibrin using distinct fragments of fibrinogen. *Eur J Biochem* 1994;219:961.

347. Schielen WJG, Adams HPHM, Voskuilen M, et al. Structural requirements of position Aa-157 in fibrinogen for the fibrin-induced rate enhancement of the activation of plasminogen by tissue-type plasminogen activator. *Biochem J* 1991;276:655.

348. Voskuilen M, Vermond A, Veeneman GH, et al. Fibrinogen lysine residue A-alpha 157 plays a cruical role in the fibrin-induced acceleration of plasminogen activation, catalyzed by tissue-type plasminogen activator. *J Biol Chem* 1987;262:5944.

349. Haddeland U, Sletten K, Bennick A, et al. Aggregated, conformationally changed fibrinogen exposes the stimulating sites for t-PA-catalysed plasminogen activation. *Thromb Haemost* 1996;75:326.

350. Yakovlev S, Makogonenko E, Kurochkina N, et al. Conversion of fibrinogen to fibrin: mechanism of exposure of tPA- and plasminogen-binding sites. *Biochemistry* 2000;39:15730.

351. Tsurupa G, Medved L. Identification and characterization of novel tPA- and plasminogen-binding sites within fibrin(ogen) alpha C-domains. *Biochemistry* 2001;40:801.

352. Tsurupa G, Medved L. Fibrinogen alpha C domains contain cryptic plasminogen and tPA binding sites. *Ann N Y Acad Sci* 2001;936:328.

353. Nieuwenhuizen W. Fibrin-mediated plasminogen activation. *Ann N Y Acad Sci* 2001;936:237.

354. Pennica D, Holmes WE, Kohr WJ. Cloning and expression of human tissue-type plasminogen activator cDNA in E. coli. *Nature* 1983;301:214.

355. Banyai L, Varadi A, Patthy L. Common evolutionary origin of the fibrin-binding structures of fibronectin and tissue-type plasminogen activator. *FEBS Lett* 1983;163:37.

356. van Zonneveld AJ, Veerman H, Pannekoek H. On the interaction of the finger and the kringle-2 domain of tissue-type plasminogen activator with fibrin: inhibition of kringle-2 binding by epsilon-amino caproic acid. *J Biol Chem* 1986;261:14214.

357. Larsen GR, Henson K, Blue Y. Variants of human tissue-type plasminogen activator. Fibrin binding, fibrinolytic, and fibrinogenolytic characterization of genetic variants lacking the fibronectin finger-like and/or the epidermal growth factor domains. *J Biol Chem* 1988;263:1023.

358. De Munk GAW, Caspers MPM, Chang GTG, et al. Binding of tissue-type plasminogen activator to lysine, lysine analogues, and fibrin fragments. *Biochemistry* 1989;28:7318.

359. Burck PJ, Berg DH, Warrick MW, et al. Characterization of a modified human tissue plasminogen activator comprising a kringle-2 and a protease domain. *J Biol Chem* 1990;265:5170.

360. Linjen HR, Nelles L, Van Hoef B, et al. Biochemical and functional characterization of human tissue-type plasminogen activator variants obtained by deletion and/or duplication of structural/functional domains. *J Biol Chem* 1990;265:5677.

361. Weisel JW, Nagaswami C, Korsholm B, et al. Interactions of plasminogen with polymerizing fibrin and its derivatives, monitored with a photoaffinity cross-linker and electron microscopy. *J Mol Biol* 1994;235:1117.

362. Nesheim M, Walker J, Wang W, et al. Modulation of fibrin cofactor activity in plasminogen activation. *Ann N Y Acad Sci* 2001;936:247.

363. Wang W, Boffa MB, Bajzar L, et al. A study of the mechanism of inhibition of fibrinolysis by activated thrombin-activable fibrinolysis inhibitor. *J Biol Chem* 1998;273:27176.

364. Aoki N, Harpel PC. Inhibitors of the fibrinolytic system. *Semin Thromb Hemost* 1984;10:24.

365. Aoki N. Fibrinolysis: its initiation and regulation. *J Protein Chem* 1986;5:269.

366. Saito H. Alpha2-plasmin inhibitor and its deficiency states. *J Lab Clin Med* 1988;112:671.

367. Azhar A, Ausat FS, Ahmad F, et al. Snake venoms as probes to study the kinetics of formation and architecture of fibrin network structure. *Adv Exp Med Biol* 1996;391:417.

368. Devine DV, Bishop PD. Platelet-associated factor XIII in platelet activation, adhesion, and clot stabilization. *Semin Thromb Hemost* 1996;22:409.

369. Reed GL, Matsueda GR, Haber E. Platelet factor XIII increases the fibrinolytic resistance of platelet-rich clots by accelerating the crosslinking of alpha 2-antiplasmin to fibrin. *Thromb Haemost* 1992;68:315.

370. Sasaki T, Morita T, Iwanaga S. Identification of the plasminogen-binding site of human alpha2-plasmin inhibitor. *J Biochem* 1986;99:1699.

371. sugiyama N, Sasaki T, Iwamoto M, et al. Binding site of alpha2-plasmin inhibitor to plasminogen. *Biochim Biophys Acta* 1988;952:1.

372. Hortin GL, Trimpe BL, Fok KF. Plasmin's peptide-binding specificity: characterization of ligand sites in alpha2-antiplasmin. *Thromb Res* 1989;54:621.

373. Tamaki T, Aoki N. Cross-linking of alpha 2-plasmin inhibitor to fibrin catalyzed by activated fibrin-stabilizing factor. *J Biol Chem* 1982;257:14767.

374. Kimura S, Aoki N. Cross-linking site in fibrinogen for alpha 2-plasmin inhibitor. *J Biol Chem* 1986;261:15591.

375. Sakata Y, Aoki N. Cross-linking of a2-plasmin inhibitor to fibrin by fibrin stabilizing factor. *J Clin Invest* 1980;65:290.

376. Sakata Y, Aoki N. Significance of cross-linking of alpha 2 plasmin inhibitor to fibrin in inhibition of fibrinolysis and in hemostasis. *J Clin Invest* 1982;69:536.

377. Aoki N, Sakata Y, Ichinose A. Fibrin-associated plasminogen activation in alpha2-plasmin inhibitor deficiency. *Blood* 1983;62:1118.

378. Ritchie H, Lawrie LC, Mosesson MW, et al. Characterization of crosslinking sites in fibrinogen for plasminogen activator inhibitor 2 (PAI-2). *Ann N Y Acad Sci* 2001;936:215.

379. Ritchie H, Lawrie LC, Crombie PW, et al. Cross-linking of plasminogen activator inhibitor 2 and alpha 2-antiplasmin to fibrin(ogen). *J Biol Chem* 2000;275:24915.

380. Krishnamurti C, Alving BM. Plasminogen activator inhibitor type 1: biochemistry and evidence for modulation of fibrinolysis *in vivo*. *Semin Thromb Hemost* 1992;18:67.

381. Wiman B. Plasminogen activator inhibitor 1 (PAI-1) in plasma: its role in thrombotic disease. *Thromb Haemost* 1995;74:71.

382. Reilly CF, Hutzelmann JE. Plasminogen activator inhibitor-1 binds to fibrin and inhibits tissue plasminogen activator-mediated fibrin dissolution. *J Biol Chem* 1992;267:17128.

383. Keijer J, Linders M, Van Zonneveld A-J, et al. The interaction of plasminogen activator inhibitor 1 with plasminogen activators (tissue-type and urokinase-type) and fibrin: localization of interaction sites and physiologic relevance. *Blood* 1991;78:401.

384. Stringer HAR, Pannekoek H. The significance of fibrin binding by plasminogen activator inhibitor 1 for the mechanism of tissue-type plasminogen activator-mediated fibrinolysis. *J Biol Chem* 1995;270:11205.

385. Braaten JV, Handt S, Jerome WG, et al. Regulation of fibrinolysis by platelet-released plasminogen activator inhibitor 1 (PAI-1): light scattering and ultrastructural examination of a model platelet-fibrin thrombus. *Blood* 1993;81:1290.

386. Handt S, Jerome WG, Tietze L, et al. PAI-1 secretion by endothelial cellls increases fibrinolytic resistance of an *in vitro* fibrin clot: evidence for a key role of endothelial cells in thrombolytic resistance. *Blood* 1996;87:4204–4213.

387. Hantgan RR, Jerome WG, Handt S. Platelets and endothelial cells act in concert to delay thrombolysis. Evidence from an *in vitro* model of the human occlusive thrombus. *Thromb Haemost* 1998;79:620-628.

388. Podor TJ, Peterson CB, Lawrence DA, et al. Type 1 plasminogen activator inhibitor binds to fibrin via vitronectin. *J Biol Chem* 2000;275: 19788.

389. Brown MS, Goldstein JL. Plasma lipoproteins. *Nature* 1987;330:113.

390. Scanu AM. Lipoprotein(a). *Arch Pathol Lab Med* 1988;112:1045.

391. McLean JW, Tomlinson JE, Kuang W, et al. cDNA sequence of human apolipoprotein(a) is homologous to plasminogen. *Nature* 1987;330:132.

392. Eaton DL, Fless GM, Kohr WJ. Partial amino acid sequence of apoprotein(a) shows that it is homologous to plasminogen. *Proc Natl Acad Sci U S A* 1987;84:3224.

393. Harpel PC, Gordon BR, Parker TS. Plasmin catalyzes binding of lipoprotein (a) to immobilized fibrinogen and fibrin. *Proc Natl Acad Sci U S A* 1989;86:3847.

394. Loscalzo J, Weinfeld M, Fless GM, et al. Lipoprotein(a), fibrin binding, and plasminogen activation. *Arteriosclerosis* 1990;10:240.

395. Harpel PC, Chang VT, Borth W. Homocysteine and other sulfhydryl compounds enhance the binding of lipoprotein(a) to fibrin: a potential biochemical link between thrombosis, atherogenesis, and sulfhydryl compound metabolism. *Proc Natl Acad Sci U S A* 1992;89:10193.

396. Tsurupa G, Ho-Tin-Noe B, Angles-Cano E, et al. Identification and characterization of novel lysine-independent apolipoprotein(a)-binding sites in fibrin(ogen) alphaC-domains. *J Biol Chem* 2003;278:37154.

397. Huby T, Schröder W, Doucet C, et al. Characterization of the N-terminal and C-terminal domains of human apolipoprotein(a): relevance to fibrin binding. *Biochemistry* 1995;34:7385.

398. Rouy D, Laplaud PM, Saboureau M, et al. Hedgehog lipoprotein(a) is a modulator of activation of plasminogen at the fibrin surface: an *in vitro* study. *Arterioscler Thromb* 1992;12:146.

399. Edelberg JM, Gonzalez-Gronow M, Pizzo SV. Lipoprotein(a) inhibition of plasminogen activation by tissue-type plasminogen activator. *Thromb Res* 1990;57:155.

400. Anglés-Cano E, Hervio L, Rouy D, et al. Effects of lipoprotein(a) on the binding of plasminogen to fibrin and its activation by fibrin-bound tissue-type plasminogen activator. *Chem Phys Lipids* 1994;67-68:369.

401. Liu J, Harpel PC, Pannell R, et al. Lipoprotein(a): a kinetic study of its influence on fibrin-dependent plasminogen activation by prourokinase or tissue plasminogen activator. *Biochemistry* 1993;32:9694.

402. Liu J, Harpel PC, Gurewich V. Fibrin-bound lipoprotein(a) promotes plasminogen binding but inhibits fibrin degradation by plasmin. *Biochemistry* 1994;33:2554.

403. Hervio L, Durlach V, Girard-globa A, et al. Multiple binding with identical linkage: a mechanism that explains the effect of lipoprotein(a) on fibrinolysis. *Biochemistry* 1995;34:13353.

404. Fless GM, Snyder ML. Polymorphic forms of Lp(a) with different structural and functional properties: cold-induced self-association and binding to fibrin and lysine-Sepharose. *Chem Phys Lipids* 1994;67-68:69.

405. Hancock MA, Boffa MB, Marcovina SM, et al. Inhibition of plasminogen activation by lipoprotein(a): critical domains in apolipoprotein(a) and mechanism of inhibition on fibrin and degraded fibrin surfaces. *J Biol Chem* 2003;278:23260.

406. Phillips DR, Charo IF, Parise LV, et al. The platelet membrane glycoprotein IIb-IIIa complex. *Blood* 1988;71:831.

407. Poncz M, Eisman R, Heidenreich R, et al. Structure of the platelet membrane glycoprotein IIb. Homology to the A subunits of the vitronectin and fibronectin membrane receptors. *J Biol Chem* 1987;262:8476.

408. Fitzgerald LA, Steiner B, Rall SC, et al. Protein sequence of endothelial glycoprotein IIIa derived from a cDNA clone. *J Biol Chem* 1987;262: 3936.

409. Zimrin AB, Eisman R, Vilaire G, et al. Structure of platelet glycoprotein IIIa. *J Clin Invest* 1988;81:1470.

410. Shattil SJ, Kashiwagi H, Pampori N. Integrin signaling: the platelet paradigm. *Blood* 1998;91:2645.

411. Shattil SJ, Ginsberg MH. Integrin signaling in vascular biology. *J Clin Invest* 1997;100:S91–S95.

412. Xiong JP, Stehle T, Diefenbach B, et al. Crystal structure of the extracellular segment of integrin alpha Vbeta3. *Science* 2001;294:339.

413. Xiong JP, Stehle T, Zhang R, et al. Crystal structure of the extracellular segment of integrin alpha Vbeta3 in complex with an Arg-Gly-Asp ligand. *Science* 2002;296:151.

414. Hantgan RR, Lyles DS, Mallett TC, et al. Ligand binding promotes the entropy-driven oligomerization of integrin AIIbB3. *J Biol Chem* 2003;278: 3417.

415. Feuston BP, Culberson JC, Hartman GD. Molecular model of the alpha(IIb)beta(3) integrin. *J Med Chem* 2003;46:5316.

416. Filizola M, Hassan SA, Artoni A, et al. Mechanistic insights from a refined three-dimensional model of integrin aIIbb3. *J Biol Chem* 2004;279: 24624–24630.

417. Marguerie GA, Plow EF, Edgington TS. Human platelet possess an inducible and saturable receptor specific for fibrinogen. *J Biol Chem* 1979;254:5357.

418. Mustard JF, Packham MA, Kinlough-Rathbone RL, et al. Fibrinogen and ADP-induced platelet aggregation. *Blood* 1978;52:453.

419. Peerschke EIB. The platelet fibrinogen receptor. *Semin Hematol* 1985; 22:241.

420. Bennett JS, Hoxie JA, Leitman SF, et al. Inhibition of fibrinogen binding to stimulated human platelets by a monoclonal antibody. *Proc Natl Acad Sci U S A* 1983;80:2417.

421. Pidard D, Montgomery RR, Bennett JS, et al. Interaction of AP-2, a monoclonal antibody specific for the human platelet glycoprotein IIb-IIIa complex, with intact platelets. *J Biol Chem* 1983;258:12582.

422. Nachman RL, Leung LKL. Complex formation of platelet membrane glycoproteins IIb and IIIa with fibrinogen. *J Clin Invest* 1982;69:263.

423. Jennings LK, Phillips DR. Purification of glycoproteins IIb and IIIa from human blood platelet plasma membranes and characterization of a calcium-dependent glycoprotein IIb-IIIa complex. *J Biol Chem* 1982;257: 10458.

424. Parise LV, Phillips DR. Reconstitution of the purified platelet fibrinogen receptor. *J Biol Chem* 1985;260:10698.

425. Bodary SC, Napier MA, McLean JW. Expression of recombinant platelet glycoprotein IIbIIIa results in a functional fibrinogen-binding complex. *J Biol Chem* 1989;264:18859.

426. Hawiger J, Timmons S, Kloczewiak M, et al. Gamma and alpha chains of human fibrinogen possess sites reactive with human platelet receptors. *Proc Natl Acad Sci U S A* 1982;79:2068.

427. Kloczewiak M, Timmons S, Hawiger J. Recognition site for the platelet receptor is present on the 15-residue carboxy-terminal fragment of the gamma chain of human fibrinogen and is not involved in the fibrin polymerization reaction. *Thromb Res* 1983;29:249.

428. Kloczewiak M, Timmons S, Lukas TJ, et al. Platelet receptor recognition site on human fibrinogen. synthesis and structure-function relationships of peptides corresponding to the carboxy-terminal segment of the gamma chain. *Biochemistry* 1984;23:1767.

429. Lam SCT, Plow EF, Smith MA, et al. Evidence that arginyl-glycyl-aspartate peptides and fibrinogen gamma chain peptides share a common binding site on platelets. *J Biol Chem* 1987;262:947.

430. Kloczewiak M, Timmons S, Bednarek MA, et al. Platelet receptor recognition domain on the gamma chain of human fibrinogen and its synthetic peptide analogues. *Biochemistry* 1989;28:2915.

431. Andrieux A, Hudry-Clergeon G, Ryckewaert J-J, et al. Amino acid sequences in fibrinogen mediating its interaction with its platelet receptor, GPIIbIIIa. *J Biol Chem* 1989;264:9258.

432. Podolnikova NP, Yakubenko VP, Volkov GL, et al. Identification of a novel binding site for platelet integrins alpha IIbbeta 3 (GPIIbIIIa) and alpha 5beta 1 in the gamma C-domain of fibrinogen. *J Biol Chem* 2003; 278:32251–32258.

433. Hogan KA, Gorkun OV, Lounes KC, et al. Recombinant fibrinogen Vlissingen/Frankfurt IV. The deletion of residues 319 and 320 from the gamma chain of firbinogen alters calcium binding, fibrin polymerization, cross-linking, and platelet aggregation. *J Biol Chem* 2000;275:17778.

434. Remijn JA, IJsseldijk MJ, van Hemel BM, et al. Reduced platelet adhesion in flowing blood to fibrinogen by alterations in segment gamma316-322, part of the fibrin-specific region. *Br J Haematol* 2002;117:650.

435. Weisel JW, Nagaswami C, Vilaire G, et al. Examination of the platelet membrane glycoprotein IIb-IIIa complex and its interaction with fibrinogen and other ligands by electron microscopy. *J Biol Chem* 1992;267:16637.

436. Marguerie GA, Thomas-Maison N, Ginsberg MH, et al. The platelet-fibrinogen interaction: evidence for proximity of the A alpha chain of fibrinogen to platelet membrane glycoproteins IIb/III. *Eur J Biochem* 1984; 139:5.

437. Plow EF, Srouji AH, Meyer D, et al. Evidence that three adhesive proteins interact with a common recognition site on activated platelets. *J Biol Chem* 1984;259:5388.

438. Gartner TK, Bennett JS. The tetrapeptide analogue of the cell attachment site of fibronectin inhibits platelet aggregation and fibrinogen binding to activated platelets. *J Biol Chem* 1985;260:11891.

439. Hawiger J, Kloczewiak M, Bednarek MA, et al. Platelet receptor recognition domains on the alpha chain of human fibrinogen: structure-function analysis. *Biochemistry* 1989;28:2909.

440. Hawiger J. Adhesive ends of fibrinogen and its antiadhesive peptides: the end of a saga. *Semin Hematol* 1995;32:99.

441. Farrell DH, Thiagarajan P, Chung DW, et al. Role of fibrinogen a and gamma chain sites in platelet aggregation. *Proc Natl Acad Sci U S A* 1992;89:10729.

442. Farrell DH, Thiagarajan P. Binding of recombinant fibrinogen mutants to platelets. *J Biol Chem* 1994;269:226.

443. Holmbäck K, Danton MJS, Suh TT, et al. Impaired platelet aggregation and sustained bleeding in mice lacking the fibrinogen motif bound by integrin $a_{IIb}b_3$. *EMBO J* 1996;15:5760.

444. Rooney MM, Parise LV, Lord ST. Dissecting clot retraction and platelet aggregation–clot retraction does not require an intact fibrinogen gamma chain C terminus. *J Biol Chem* 1996;271:8553.

445. Cheresh DA, Berliner SA, Vicente V, et al. Recognition of distinct adhesive sites on fibrinogen by related integrins on platelets and endothelial cells. *Cell* 1989;58:945.

446. Dejana E, Languino LR, Colella S, et al. The localization of a platelet GpIIb-IIIa-related protein in endothelial cell adhesion structures. *Blood* 1988;71:566.

447. Suehiro K, Gailit J, Plow EF. Fibrinogen is a ligand for integrin $a_5b_1$ on endothelial cells. *J Biol Chem* 1997;272:5360.

448. Suehiro K, Plow EF. Ligand recognition by beta 3 integrins. *Keio J Med* 1997;46:111.

449. Suehiro K, Smith JW, Plow EF. The ligand recognition specificity of b3 integrins. *J Biol Chem* 1996;271:10365.

450. Tranqui L, Andrieux A, Hudry-Clergeon G, et al. Differential structural requirements for fibrinogen binding to platelets and to endothelial cells. *J Cell Biol* 1989;108:2519.

451. Francis CW, Bunce LA, Sporn LA. Endothelial cell responses to fibrin mediated by FPB cleavage and the amino terminus of the b chain. *Blood Cells* 1993;19:291.

452. Martinez J, Rich E, Barsigian C. Transglutaminase-mediated cross-linking of fibrinogen by human umbilical vein endothelial cells. *J Biol Chem* 1989;264:20502.

453. Yokoyama K, Erickson HP, Ikeda Y, et al. Identification of amino acid sequences in fibrinogen gamma -chain and tenascin C C-terminal domains critical for binding to integrin alpha vbeta 3. *J Biol Chem* 2000;275:16891.

454. Plow EF, Haas TA, Zhang L, et al. Ligand binding to integrins. *J Biol Chem* 2000;275:21785.

455. Ugarova TP, Yakubenko VP. Recognition of fibrinogen by leukocyte integrins. *Ann N Y Acad Sci* 2001;936:368.

456. Yakubenko VP, Solovjov DA, Zhang L, et al. Identification of the binding site for fibrinogen recognition peptide gamma 383–395 within the alpha(M)I-domain of integrin alpha(M)beta2. *J Biol Chem* 2001;276:13995.

457. Ugarova TP, Lishko VK, Podolnikova NP, et al. Sequence gamma 377–395(P2), but not gamma 190–202(P1), is the binding site for the alpha MI-domain of integrin alpha M beta 2 in the gamma C-domain of fibrinogen. *Biochemistry* 2003;42:9365.

458. Lishko VK, Kudryk B, Yakubenko VP, et al. Regulated unmasking of the cryptic binding site for integrin alpha M beta 2 in the gamma C-domain of fibrinogen. *Biochemistry* 2002;41:12942.

459. Lishko VK, Yakubenko VP, Hertzberg KM, et al. The alternatively spliced alpha(E)C domain of human fibrinogen-420 is a novel ligand for leukocyte integrins alpha(M)beta(2) and alpha(X)beta(2). *Blood* 2001;98:2448.

460. Yee KO, Rooney MM, Giachelli CM, et al. Role of beta-1 and beta-3 integrins in human smooth muscle cell adhesion to and contraction of fibrin clots *in vitro*. *Circ Res* 1998;83:241.

461. Chung DW, Harris JE, Davie EW. Nucleotide sequences of the three genes coding for human fibrinogen. *Adv Exp Med Biol* 1990;281:39.

462. Crabtree GR. The molecular biology of fibrinogen. In: Stamatoyannopoulos G, Nienhuis AW, Leder P et al., eds. *The molecular basis of blood diseases*. Philadelphia, PA: WB Saunders, 1987:631–661.

463. Kant JA, Fornace AJ Jr, Saxe D, et al. Evolution and organization of the fibrinogen locus on chromosome 4: gene duplication accompanied by transposition and inversion. *Proc Natl Acad Sci U S A* 1989;82:2344.

464. Kant JA, Crabtree GR. The rat fibrinogen genes. Linkage of the A alpha and gamma chain genes. *J Biol Chem* 1983;258:4666.

465. Olaisen B, Teisberg P, Gedde Dahl T Jr. Fibrinogen gamma chain locus is on chromosome 4 in man. *Hum Genet* 1982;61:24.

466. Henry I, Uzan G, Weil D, et al. The genes coding for A alpha-, B beta-, and gamma-chains of fibrinogen map to 4q2. *Am J Hum Genet* 1984;36:760.

467. Kant JA, Fornace AJJ, Saxe D, et al. Evolution and organization of the fibrinogen locus on chromosome 4: gene duplication accompanied by transposition and inversion. *Proc Natl Acad Sci U S A* 1985;82:2344.

468. Crabtree GR, Kant JA. Organization of the rat gamma-fibrinogen gene: alternative mRNA splice patterns produce the gamma A and gamma B (gamma ') chains of fibrinogen. *Cell* 1982;31:159.

469. Crabtree GR, Kant JA, Fornace AJ Jr, et al. Regulation and characterization of the mRNAs for the A alpha, B beta and gamma chains of fibrinogen. *Ann N Y Acad Sci* 1983;408:457.

470. Fornace AJ Jr, Cummings DE, Comeau CM, et al. Single-copy inverted repeats associated with regional genetic duplications in gamma fibrinogen and immunoglobulin genes. *Science* 1984;224:161.

471. Fowlkes DM, Mullis NT, Comeau CM, et al. Potential basis for regulation of the coordinately expressed fibrinogen genes: homology in the 5' flanking regions. *Proc Natl Acad Sci U S A* 1984;81:2313.

472. Fu Y, Weissbach L, Plant PW, et al. Carboxy-terminal-extended variant of the human fibrinogen a subunit: a novel exon conferring marked homology to b and gamma subunits. *Biochemistry* 1992;31:11968.

473. Rixon MW, Chan W-Y, Davie EW. Nucleotide sequence of the gene for the gamma chain of human fibrinogen. *Biochemistry* 1983;22:3244.

474. Weissbach L, Grieninger G. Bipartite mRNA for chicken alpha-fibrinogen potentially encodes an amino acid sequence homologous to beta- and gamma-fibrinogens. *Proc Natl Acad Sci U S A* 1990;87:5198.

475. Crabtree GR, Comeau CM, Fowlkes DM, et al. Evolution and structure of the fibrinogen genes. Random insertion of introns or selective loss? *J Mol Biol* 1985;185:1.

476. Eastman EM, Gilula NB. Cloning and characterization of a cDNA for the B beta chain of rat fibrinogen: evolutionary conservation of translated and 3'-untranslated sequences. *Gene* 1989;79:151.

477. Morgan JG, Holbrook NJ, Crabtree GR. Nucleotide sequence of the gamma chain gene of rat fibrinogen: conserved intronic sequences. *Nucleic Acids Res* 1987;15:2774.

478. Strong DD, Moore M, Cottrell BA, et al. Lamprey fibrinogen gamma chain: cloning, cDNA sequencing, and general characterization. *Biochemistry* 1985;24:92.

479. Doolittle RF, Cottrell BA, Riley M. Amino acid compositions of the subunit chains of lamprey fibrinogen. Evolutionary significance of some structural anomalies. *Biochim Biophys Acta* 1976;453:439.

480. Koyama T, Hall LR, Haser WG, et al. Structure of a cytotoxic T-lymphocyte-specific gene shows a strong homology to fibrinogen beta and gamma chains. *Proc Natl Acad Sci U S A* 1987;84:1609.

481. Mizuguchi J, Hu CH, Cao Z, et al. Characterization of the 5'-flanking region of the gene for the gamma chain of human fibrinogen. *J Biol Chem* 1995;270:28350.

482. Takagi T, Doolittle RF. Amino acid sequence of the carboxy-terminal cyanogen bromide peptide of the human fibrinogen beta-chain: homology with the corresponding gamma-chain peptide and presence in fragment D. *Biochim Biophys Acta* 1975;386:617.

483. Baker NE, Mlodzik M, Rubin GM. Spacing differentiation in the developing Drosophila eye: a fibrinogen-related lateral inhibitor encoded by scabrous. *Science* 1990;250:1370.

484. Lee EC, Hu X, Yu SY, et al. The scabrous gene encodes a secreted glycoprotein dimer and regulates proneural development in Drosophila eyes. *Mol Cell Biol* 1996;16:1179.

485. Marazzi S, Blum S, Hartmann R, et al. Characterization of human fibroleukin, a fibrinogen-like protein secreted by T lymphocytes. *J Immunol* 1998;161:138.

486. Ruegg C, Pytela R. Sequence of a human transcript expressed in T-lymphocytes and encoding a fibrinogen-like protein. *Gene* 1995;160:257.

487. Clark RA, Erickson HP, Springer TA. Tenascin supports lymphocyte rolling. *J Cell Biol* 1997;137:755.

488. Copertino DW, Jenkinson S, Jones FS, et al. Structural and functional similarities between the promoters for mouse tenascin and chicken cytotactin. *Proc Natl Acad Sci U S A* 1995;92:2131.

489. Jones FS, Burgoon MP, Hoffman S, et al. A cDNA clone for cytotactin contains sequences similar to epidermal growth factor–like repeats and segments of fibronectin and fibrinogen. *Proc Natl Acad Sci U S A* 1988;85:2186.

490. Van Eyken P, Sciot R, Desmet VJ. Expression of the novel extracellular matrix component tenascin in normal and diseased human liver. An immunohistochemical study. *J Hepatol* 1990;11:43.

491. Vrucinic-Filipi N, Chiquet-Ehrismann R. Tenascin function and regulation of expression. *Symp Soc Exp Biol* 1993;47:155.

492. Doolittle RF. The evolution of vertebrate blood coagulation: a case of Yin and Yang. *Thromb Haemost* 1993;70:24.

493. Doolittle RF, Everse SJ, Spraggon G. Human fibrinogen: anticipating a 3-dimensional structure. *FASEB J* 1996;10:1464.

494. Doolittle RF, Spraggon G, Everse SJ. Evolution of vertebrate fibrin formation and the process of its dissolution. *Ciba Found Symp* 1997;212:4.

495. Dalmon J, Laurent M, Courtois G. The human beta fibrinogen promoter contains a hepatocyte nuclear factor 1-dependent interleukin-6-responsive element. *Mol Cell Biol* 1993;13:1183.

496. Evans E, Courtois GM, Kilian PL, et al. Induction of fibrinogen and a subset of acute phase response genes involves a novel monokine which is mimicked by phorbol esters. *J Biol Chem* 1987;262:10850.

497. Hu CH, Harris JE, Davie EW, et al. Characterization of the 5'-flanking region of the gene for the a chain of human fibrinogen. *J Biol Chem* 1995;270:28342.

498. Huber P, Laurent M, Dalmon J. Human b-fibrinogen gene expression. Upstream sequences involved in its tissue specific expression and its dexamethasone and interleukin 6 stimulation. *J Biol Chem* 1990;265:5695.

499. Simpson-Haidaris PJ. Induction of fibrinogen biosynthesis and secretion from cultured pulmonary epithelial cells. *Blood* 1997;89:873.

500. Zhang Z, Fuentes NL, Fuller GM. Characterization of the IL-6 responsive elements in the gamma fibrinogen gene promoter. *J Biol Chem* 1995;270:24287.

501. Crabtree GR, Kant JA. Coordinate accumulation of the mRNAs for the alpha, beta, and gamma chains of rat fibrinogen following defibrination. *J Biol Chem* 1982;257:7277.

502. Grieninger G, Plant PW, Liang TJ, et al. Hormonal regulation of fibrinogen synthesis in cultured hepatocytes. *Ann N Y Acad Sci* 1983;408:469.

503. Baumhueter S, Courtois G, Morgan JG. The role of HNF-1 in liver-specific gene expression. *Ann N Y Acad Sci* 1989;557:272.

504. Baumhueter S, Mendel DB, Conley PB, et al. HNF-1 shares three sequence motifs with the POU domain proteins and is identical to LF-B1 and APF. *Genes Dev* 1990;4:372.

505. Courtois G, Baumhueter S, Crabtree GR. Purified hepatocyte nuclear factor 1 interacts with a family of hepatocyte-specific promoters. *Proc Natl Acad Sci U S A* 1988;85:7937.

506. Courtois G, Morgan JG, Campbell LA, et al. Interaction of a liver-specific nuclear factor with the fibrinogen and alpha 1-antitrypsin promoters. *Science* 1987;238:688.

507. Haidaris PJ, Courtney MA. Tissue-specific and ubiquitous expression of fibrinogen gamma-chain mRNA. *Blood Coagul Fibrinolysis* 1990;1:433.

508. Haidaris PJ, Courtney MA. Liver-specific RNA processing of the ubiquitously transcribed rat fibrinogen gamma-chain gene. *Blood* 1992;79:1218.

509. Baumhueter S, Courtois G, Crabtree GR. A variant nuclear protein in dedifferentiated hepatoma cells binds to the same functional sequences in the beta fibrinogen gene promoter as HNF-1. *EMBO J* 1988;7:2485.

510. Dowton SB, Colten HR. Acute phase reactants in inflammation and infection. *Semin Hematol* 1988;25:84.

511. Castell JV, Gomez-Lechon MJ, David M, et al. Acute-phase response of human hepatocytes: regulation of acute-phase protein synthesis by interleukin-6. *Hepatology* 1990;12:1179.

512. Weber J. Interleukin-6: multifunctional cytokine. *Biol Ther Cancer Updat* 1993;3:1.

513. Anderson GM, Shaw AR, Shafer JA. Functional characterization of promoter elements involved in regulation of human B beta-fibrinogen expression. Evidence for binding of novel activator and repressor proteins. *J Biol Chem* 1993;268:22650.

514. Fuller GM, Otto JM, Woloski BM, et al. The effects of hepatocyte stimulating factor on fibrinogen biosynthesis in hepatocyte monolayers. *J Cell Biol* 1985;101:1481.

515. Otto JM, Grenett HE, Fuller GM. The coordinated regulation of fibrinogen gene transcription by hepatocyte-stimulating factor and dexamethasone. *J Cell Biol* 1987;105:1067.

516. Ritchie DG, Levy BA, Adams MA, et al. Regulation of fibrinogen synthesis by plasmin-derived fragments of fibrinogen and fibrin: an indirect feedback pathway. *Proc Natl Acad Sci U S A* 1982;79:1530.

517. Kessler CM, Bell WR. The effect of homologous thrombin and fibrinogen degradation products on fibrinogen synthesis in rabbits. *J Lab Clin Med* 1979;93:768.

518. Barnhart MI, Cress DC, Noonan SM, et al. Influence of fibrinolytic products on hepatic release and synthesis of fibrinogen. *Thromb Diath Haemorrh* 1970;39:143.

519. Princen HM, Moshage HJ, Emeis JJ, et al. Fibrinogen fragments X, Y, D and E increase levels of plasma fibrinogen and liver mRNAs coding for fibrinogen polypeptides in rats. *Thromb Haemost* 1985;53:212.

520. Nham S-U, Fuller GM. Effect of fibrinogen degradation products on production of hepatocyte stimulating factor by a macrohage cell line (P388D1). *Thromb Res* 1986;44:467.

521. Asselta R, Duga S, Modugno M, et al. Identification of a glucocorticoid response element in the human γ chain fibrinogen promoter. *Thromb Haemost* 1998;79:1144.

522. Princen HM, Moshage HJ, de Haard HJ, et al. The influence of glucocorticoid on the fibrinogen messenger RNA content of rat liver *in vivo* and in hepatocyte suspension culture. *Biochem J* 1984;220:631.

523. Vasse M, Paysant I, Soria J, et al. Down-regulation of fibrinogen biosynthesis by IL-4, IL-10 and IL-13. *Br J Haematol* 1996;93:955.

524. Amrani DL. Regulation of fibrinogen biosynthesis: glucocorticoid and interleukin-6 control. *Blood Coagul Fibrinolysis* 1990;1:443.

525. Conti P, Bartle L, Barbacane RC, et al. The down-regulation of IL-6-stimulated fibrinogen steady state mRNA and protein levels by human recombinant IL-1 is not PGE2-dependent: effects of IL-1 receptor antagonist (IL-1RA). *Mol Cell Biochem* 1995;142:171.

526. Hassan JH, Chelucci C, Peschle C, et al. Transforming growth factor beta (TGF-beta) inhibits expression of fibrinogen and factor VII in a hepatoma cell line. *Thromb Haemost* 1992;67:478.

527. Haidaris PJ, Francis CW, Sporn LA, et al. Megakaryocyte and hepatocyte origins of human fibrinogen biosynthesis exhibit hepatocyte-specific expression of gamma chain-variant polypeptides. *Blood* 1989;74:743.

528. Homandberg GA, Williams JE, Evans DB, et al. Evidence that rat platelet fibrinogen molecules lack the gamma' chain variant found in plasma fibrinogen molecules. *Thromb Res* 1985;39:203.

529. Wolfenstein-Todel C, Mosesson MW. Carboxy-terminal amino acid sequence of a human fibrinogen gamma-chain variant (gamma'). *Biochemistry* 1981;20:6146.

530. Francis CW, Mosesson MW. Terminology for fibrinogen gamma-chains differing in carboxyl terminal amino acid sequence. *Thromb Haemost* 1989;62:813.

531. Chung DW, Chan WY, Davie EW. Characterization of a complementary deoxyribonucleic acid coding for the gamma chain of human fibrinogen. *Biochemistry* 1983;22:3250.

532. Grieninger G. Contribution of the alpha EC domain to the structure and function of fibrinogen-420. *Ann N Y Acad Sci* 2001;936:44.

533. Farrell DH, Huang S, Davie EW. Processing of the carboxyl 15-amino acid extension in the α-chain of fibrinogen. *J Biol Chem* 1993;268:10351.

534. Homandberg GA, Evans DB, Kane CM, et al. Amino acid sequences of the carboxyl-terminal regions of rat plasma fibrinogen gamma A and gamma' chains. *Thromb Res* 1985;39:263.

535. Lawrence SO, Wright TW, Francis CW, et al. Purification and functional characterization of homodimeric gammaB-gammaB fibrinogen from rat plasma. *Blood* 1993;82:2406.

536. Redman CM, Xia H. Fibrinogen biosynthesis. Assembly, intracellular degradation, and association with lipid synthesis and secretion. *Ann N Y Acad Sci* 2001;936:480.

537. Hirose S, Oda K, Ikehara Y. Biosynthesis, assembly and secretion of fibrinogen in cultured rat hepatocytes. *Biochem J* 1988;251:373.

538. Grieninger G, Plant PW, Chiasson MA. Fibrinogen precursors: order of assembly of fibrinogen chains. *J Biol Chem* 1984;259:10574.

539. Plant PW, Grieninger G. Noncoordinate synthesis of the fibrinogen subunits in hepatocytes cultured under hormone-deficient conditions. *J Biol Chem* 1986;261:2331.

540. Farrell DH, Mulvihill ER, Huang S, et al. Recombinant human fibrinogen and sulfation of the gamma' chain. *Biochemistry* 1991;30:9414.

541. Huang SM, Cao ZY, Chung DW, et al. The role of β–γ and α–γ complexes in the assembly of human fibrinogen. *J Biol Chem* 1996;271:27942.

542. Huang S, Mulvihill ER, Farrell DH, et al. Biosynthesis of human fibrinogen. Subunit interactions and potential intermediates in the assembly. *J Biol Chem* 1993;268:8919.

543. Roy S, Overton O, Redman C. Overexpression of any fibrinogen chain by Hep G2 cells specifically elevates the expression of the other two chains. *J Biol Chem* 1994;269:691.

544. Roy S, Sun A, Redman C. *In vitro* assembly of the component chains of fibrinogen requires endoplasmic reticulum factors. *J Biol Chem* 1996;271:24544.

545. Roy S, Yu S, Banerjee D, et al. Assembly and secretion of fibrinogen. Degradation of individual chains. *J Biol Chem* 1992;267:23151.

546. Zhang JZ, Redman C. Fibrinogen assembly and secretion. Role of intrachain disulfide loops. *J Biol Chem* 1996;271:30083.

547. Zhang JZ, Redman CM. Identification of B beta chain domains involved in human fibrinogen assembly. *J Biol Chem* 1992;267:21727.

548. Zhang J-Z, Redman CM. Role of interchain disulfide bonds on the assembly and secretion of human fibrinogen. *J Biol Chem* 1994;269:652.

549. Zhang JZ, Redman CM. Assembly and secretion of fibrinogen. Involvement of N-terminal domains in dimer formation. *J Biol Chem* 1996;271:12674.

550. Binnie CG, Hettasch JM, Strickland E, et al. Characterization of purified recombinant fibrinogen: partial phosphorylation of fibrinopeptide A. *Biochemistry* 1993;32:107.

551. Xia H, Redman CM. Differential degradation of the three fibrinogen chains by proteasomes: involvement of Sec61p and cytosolic Hsp70. *Arch Biochem Biophys* 2001;390:137.

552. Okumura N, Terasawa F, Tanaka H, et al. Analysis of fibrinogen gamma-chain truncations shows the C-terminus, particularly gammaIle387, is essential for assembly and secretion of this multichain protein. *Blood* 2002;99:3654.

553. Duga S, Asselta R, Santagostino E, et al. Missense mutations in the human beta fibrinogen gene cause congenital afibrinogenemia by impairing fibrinogen secretion. *Blood* 2000;95:1336.

554. Vu D, Bolton-Maggs PH, Parr JR, et al. Congenital afibrinogenemia: identification and expression of a missense mutation in FGB impairing fibrinogen secretion. *Blood* 2003;102:4413.

555. Straub PW. A study of fibrinogen production by human liver slices *in vitro* by immunoprecipitation method. *J Clin Invest* 1963;42:130.

556. Takeda Y. Studies of the metabolism and distribution of fibrinogen in healthy men with autologous 125I-labeled fibrinogen. *J Clin Invest* 1966;45:103.

557. Reeve EB, Franks JJ. Fibrinogen synthesis, distribution and degradation. *Semin Thromb Hemost* 1974;1:129.

558. Collen D, Tytgat GN, Claeys H, et al. Metabolism and distribution of fibrinogen. I. Fibrinogen turnover in physiological conditions in humans. *Br J Haematol* 1972;22:681.

559. Rausen AA, Cruchaud A, McMillan CW, et al. A study of fibrinogen turnover in classical hemophilia and congenital afibrinogenemia. *Blood* 1961;18:710.

560. Nossel HL. Radioimmunoassay of fibrinopeptides in relation to intravascular coagulation and thrombosis. *N Engl J Med* 1976;295:428.

561. Sherman LA, Fletcher AP, Sherry S. *In vitro* transformation between fibrinogen varying ethanol solubilities: a pathway of fibrinogen catabolism. *J Lab Clin Med* 1969;73:574.

562. Francis CW, Nachman RL, Marder VJ. Plasma and platelet fibrinogen differ in gamma chain content. *Thromb Haemost* 1984;51:84.

563. Mosesson MW, Homandberg GA, Amrani DL. Human platelet fibrinogen gamma chain structure. *Blood* 1984;63:990.

564. Francis CW, Kraus DH, Marder VJ. Structural and chromatographic heterogeneity of normal plasma fibrinogen associated with the presence of three gamma-chain types with distinct molecular weights. *Biochim Biophys Acta* 1983;744:155.

565. Cramer EM, Debili N, Martin JF, et al. Uncoordinated expression of fibrinogen compared with thrombospondin and von Willebrand factor in maturing human megakaryocytes. *Blood* 1989;73:1123.

566. Cramer EM, Harrison P, Savidge GF, et al. Uncoordinated expression of alpha-granule proteins in human megakaryocytes. *Prog Clin Biol Res* 1990;356:131.

567. Handagama PJ, Amrani DL, Shuman MA. Endocytosis of fibrinogen into hamster megakaryocyte a granules is dependent on a dimeric gamma$_A$ configuration. *Blood* 1995;85:1790.

568. Handagama PJ, Shuman MA, Bainton DF. Incorporation of intravenously injected albumin, immunoglobulin G, and fibrinogen in guinea pig megakaryocyte granules. *J Clin Invest* 1989;84:73.

569. Handagama PJ, Shuman MA, Bainton DF. *In vivo* defibrination results in markedly decreased amounts of fibrinogen in rat megakaryocytes and platelets. *Am J Pathol* 1990;137:1393.

570. Handagama PJ, Shuman MA, Bainton DF. The origin of platelet alpha-granule proteins. *Prog Clin Biol Res* 1990;356:119.

571. Harrison P, Wilbourn B, Debili N, et al. Uptake of plasma fibrinogen into the alpha granules of human megakaryocytes and platelets. *J Clin Invest* 1989;84:1320.

572. Louache F, Debili N, Cramer E, et al. Fibrinogen is not synthesized by human megakaryocytes. *Blood* 1991;77:311.

573. Ni H, Papalia JM, Degen JL, et al. Control of thrombus embolization and fibronectin internalization by integrin alpha IIb beta 3 engagement of the fibrinogen gamma chain. *Blood* 2003;102:3609.

574. Courtney MA, Stoler MH, Marder VJ, et al. Developmental expression of mRNAs encoding platelet proteins in rat megakaryocytes. *Blood* 1991;77:560.

575. Lee SY, Lee KP, Lim JW. Identification and biosynthesis of fibrinogen in human uterine cervix carcinoma cells. *Thromb Haemost* 1996;75:466.

576. McDonagh J, Fukue H. Determinants of substrate specificity for factor XIII. *Semin Thromb Hemost* 1996;22:369.

577. Molmenti EP, Ziambaras T, Perlmutter DH. Evidence for an acute phase response in human intestinal epithelial cells. *J Biol Chem* 1993;268:14116.

578. Haidaris PJ. Induction of fibrinogen biosynthesis and secretion from cultured pulmonary epithelial cells. *Blood* 1997;89:873.

579. Castell JV, Gomez-Lechon MJ, David M, et al. Interleukin-6 is the major regulator of acute phase protein synthesis in adult human hepatocytes. *FEBS Lett* 1989;242:237.

580. Guadiz G, Sporn LA, Simpson-Haidaris PJ. Thrombin cleavage-independent deposition of fibrinogen in extracellular matrices. *Blood* 1997;90:2644.

581. Simpson-Haidaris PJ, Courtney MA, Wright TW, et al. Induction of fibrinogen expression in lung epithelium during Pneumocystis carinii pneumonia. *Infect Immun* 1998;66:4431–4439.

582. De Moerloose P, De Benedetti E, Nicod L, et al. Procoagulant activity in bronchoalveolar fluids: no relationship with tissue factor pathway inhibitor activity. *Thromb Res* 1992;65:507.

583. Jacobson W, Park GR, Saich T, et al. Surfactant and adult respiratory distress syndrome. *Br J Anaesth* 1993;70:522.

584. Pereira M, Rybarczyk BJ, Odrljin TM, et al. The incorporation of fibrinogen into extracellular matrix is dependent on active assembly of a fibronectin matrix. *J Cell Sci* 2002;115:609.

585. Rybarczyk BJ, Lawrence SO, Simpson-Haidaris PJ. Matrix-fibrinogen enhances wound closure by increasing both cell proliferation and migration. *Blood* 2003;102:4035.

586. Asch AS, Tepler J, Silbiger S, et al. Cellular attachment to thrombospondin. Cooperative interactions between receptor systems. *J Biol Chem* 1991;266:1740.

587. Clark RA. Fibronectin matrix deposition and fibronectin receptor expression in healing and normal skin. *J Invest Dermatol* 1990;94:128S.

588. Epperlein HH, Halfter W, Tucker RP. The distribution of fibronectin and tenascin along migratory pathways of the neural crest in the trunk of amphibian embryos. *Development* 1988;103:743.

589. Godyna S, Mann DM, Argraves WS. A quantitative analysis of the incorporation of fibulin-1 into extracellular matrix indicates that fibronectin assembly is required. *Matrix Biol* 1995;14:467.

590. Grant DS, Kleinman HK. Regulation of capillary formation by laminin and other components of the extracellular matrix. *EXS* 1997;79:317.

591. Hiscott P, Larkin G, Robey HL, et al. Thrombospondin as a component of the extracellular matrix of epiretinal membranes: comparisons with cellular fibronectin. *Eye* 1992;6:566.

592. Labat-Robert J, Bihari-Varga M, Robert L. Extracellular matrix. *FEBS Lett* 1990;268:386.

593. Mounier F, Foidart JM, Gubler MC. Distribution of extracellular matrix glycoproteins during normal development of human kidney. An immuno-histochemical study. *Lab Invest* 1986;54:394.

594. Peters JH, Hynes RO. Fibronectin isoform distribution in the mouse. I. The alternatively spliced EIIIB, EIIIA, and V segments show widespread codistribution in the developing mouse embryo. *Cell Adhes Commun* 1996;4:103.

595. Roman J, McDonald JA. Fibulin's organization into the extracellular matrix of fetal lung fibroblasts is dependent on fibronectin matrix assembly. *Am J Respir Cell Mol Biol* 1993;8:538.

596. Tuckett F, Morriss-Kay GM. The distribution of fibronectin, laminin and entactin in the neurulating rat embryo studied by indirect immunofluorescence. *J Embryol Exp Morphol* 1986;94:95.

597. Maresca G, Di Blasio A, Marchioli R, et al. Measuring plasma fibrinogen to predict stroke and myocardial infarction: an update. *Arterioscler Thromb Vasc Biol* 1999;19:1368.

598. Danesh J, Collins R, Appleby P, et al. Association of fibrinogen, C-reactive protein, albumin, or leukocyte count with coronary heart disease: meta-analyses of prospective studies. *JAMA* 1998;279:1477.

599. Folsom AR, Wu KK, Shahar E et al, The Atherosclerosis Risk in Communities (ARIC) Study Investigators. Association of hemostatic variables with prevalent cardiovascular disease and asymptomatic carotid artery atherosclerosis. *Arterioscler Thromb* 1993;13:1829.

600. Iacoviello L, Vischetti M, Zito F, et al. Genes encoding fibrinogen and cardiovascular risk. *Hypertension* 2001;38:1199.

601. Green FR. Fibrinogen polymorphisms and atherothrombotic disease. *Ann N Y Acad Sci* 2001;936:549.

602. Boekholdt SM, Peters RJ, de Maat MP, et al. Interaction between a genetic variant of the platelet fibrinogen receptor and fibrinogen levels in determining the risk of cardiovascular events. *Am Heart J* 2004;147:181.

603. Pankow JS, Folsom AR, Province MA, et al. Segregation analysis of plasminogen activator inhibitor-1 and fibrinogen levels in the NHLBI family heart study. *Arterioscler Thromb Vasc Biol* 1998;18:1559.

604. Sierksma A, van der Gaag MS, Kluft C, et al. Moderate alcohol consumption reduces plasma C-reactive protein and fibrinogen levels; a randomized, diet-controlled intervention study. *Eur J Clin Nutr* 2002;56:1130.

605. de Maat MP. Effects of diet, drugs, and genes on plasma fibrinogen levels. *Ann N Y Acad Sci* 2001;936:509.

606. Zito F, Di Castelnuovo A, Amore C, et al. Bcl I polymorphism in the fibrinogen beta-chain gene is associated with the risk of familial myocardial infarction by increasing plasma fibrinogen levels. A case-control study in a sample of GISSI-2 patients. *Arterioscler Thromb Vasc Biol* 1997;17:3489.

607. Brull DJ, Dhamrait S, Moulding R, et al. The effect of fibrinogen genotype on fibrinogen levels after strenuous physical exercise. *Thromb Haemost* 2002;87:37.

608. Balagopal P, Sweeten S, Mauras N. Increased synthesis rate of fibrinogen as a basis for its elevated plasma levels in obese female adolescents. *Am J Physiol Endocrinol Metab* 2002;282:E899–E904.

609. Barazzoni R, Kiwanuka E, Zanetti M, et al. Insulin acutely increases fibrinogen production in individuals with type 2 diabetes but not in individuals without diabetes. *Diabetes* 2003;52:1851.

# CHAPTER 17 ■ FACTOR XIII AND FIBRIN STABILIZATION

CHARLES S. GREENBERG, DAVID C. SANE, AND THUNG-SHEN LAI

Fibrin is a complex three-dimensional biological structure that requires covalent modification by factor XIIIa to function effectively during hemostasis and wound healing. The reactions that factor XIIIa catalyze are often called cross-linking reactions, but they are more accurately defined as the covalent ligation of molecules through formation of intramolecular and intermolecular isopeptide bonds. Factor XIIIa covalently ligates fibrin molecules to each other and cross-links $\alpha_2$-antiplasmin inhibitor ($\alpha_2$-AP) and other molecules to fibrin to regulate fibrinolysis. Covalent modification of fibrin by factor XIIIa transforms it into a mechanically resilient and protease-resistant barrier to blood loss. Factor XIIIa also stabilizes the bond between adhesion molecules in the extracellular matrix (ECM). In this chapter, the structure, function, and regulation of factor XIIIa are reviewed. The diagnosis and treatment of inherited and acquired deficiencies of factor XIII are also presented. Although factor XIII deficiency causes hemorrhage, thrombosis may result when intravascular fibrin formation and stabilization are not regulated. The roles of factor XIII in modifying thrombotic risks are summarized, and therapeutic applications of factor XIII are reviewed.

## IDENTIFYING FIBRIN STABILIZING ENZYME AND CLINICAL SIGNIFICANCE

Biochemical studies first identified a calcium-dependent factor that causes fibrin to resist solubilization in alkaline solutions, to resist protease degradation, and to exhibit greater tensile strength (1–3). The factor was subsequently identified as a thrombin-dependent protein and purified from plasma (1,2,4).

Factor XIIIa was ultimately characterized as a transglutaminase enzyme that catalyzes displacement of ammonia at the $\gamma$-position in glutamine (Q) residues and replaces it with another amine, usually an $\varepsilon$-amino group from a lysine residue (5). A covalent isopeptide bond between the $\gamma$-carboxylamide and $\varepsilon$-amino groups of protein-bound glutamine and lysine residues in adjacent fibrin molecules was discovered to produce fibrin stabilization (see Fig. 17-1). The enzyme is designated as endo-$\gamma$-glutamine:epsilon-lysine transferase (EC 2.3.2.13). Factor XIIIa uses a free sulfhydryl to catalyze a reaction that is similar to the reverse reaction of a calcium-dependent protease (6).

The protein was first identified as a component of the coagulation system and designated as factor XIII before the first patient deficient in fibrin stabilizing activity was identified in 1960 (7). The patient had extensive bleeding, validating the clinical significance of factor XIII in hemostasis (7). Patients were subsequently discovered with either congenital or acquired deficiencies in factor XIII (8). Recent advances in molecular biology and protein biochemistry have provided further insights regarding the structure and function of factor XIII in hemostasis and thrombosis (9–11). Detailed studies of the molecular defects produced by inherited mutations and the production of a mouse model in which the factor XIII gene has been inactivated provided valuable new information on the structure and function of this protein (12–14). This information has led to a better understanding of factor XIII deficiency, development of factor XIIIa inhibitors, and the discovery that factor XIIIa plays a role in fibrinolysis, ECM biology, and thrombosis.

## PLASMA FACTOR XIII STRUCTURE

The plasma factor XIII molecule is a 320-kDa heteroteramer, $A_2B_2$, which is the product of two separate genes coding for A and B chains. The A chain is composed of 730 amino acids, 83 kDa, and dimerizes forming a nonglycosylated globular molecule that remains intracellular and is also secreted into plasma (15). The A chain has nine free sulfhydryl groups, including the active site at Cys314 (15,16). The $A_2$ molecule contains the activation peptide, catalytic triad, calcium-binding site, and fibrin-binding and substrate-recognition domains (17). Free A chains are not detected in plasma (18). The B chains are secreted by hepatocytes and complex rapidly with the $A_2$-subunit and also circulate in monomeric form (13,18,19). How and when the $A_2B_2$ complex is assembled remains poorly defined because the components are synthesized by different cells and must form a complex in plasma. The plasma–$A_2B_2$ complex circulates at a concentration of 14 to 28 mg per liter according to data from enzyme-linked immunosorbent assay (ELISA) (18,20).

### The Structure of the Factor XIII $A_2$-Subunit

Recombinant DNA technology was used to express the A chains in yeast and methods were developed to purify and crystallize the $A_2$-subunit (17,21,22). The results of these studies have identified critical domains and residues that regulate enzyme function and protein stability. Molecular analysis of mutant molecules identified in patients with factor XIII deficiency has confirmed the importance of various residues to *in vivo* function (see subsequent text). Factor XIII A chains have been expressed and purified from mammalian cells, *Escherichia coli*, and plants.

The $A_2$-zymogen crystal revealed that the A chains were folded into four distinct domains (see Fig. 17-2). The N-terminus contains activation peptides (numbers 1 to 37) followed by a $\beta$-sandwich domain (numbers 38 to 184), the catalytic core (numbers 185 to 515), and then two $\beta$-barrels (barrel 1: numbers 516 to 628; barrel 2: 629 to 730) domains. The dimer folds to form a hexagonal globular molecule with the $\beta$-barrel

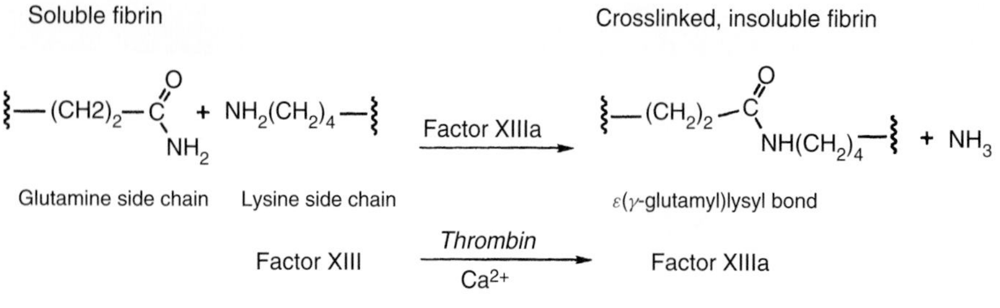

Soluble fibrin                                        Crosslinked, insoluble fibrin

**FIGURE 17-1.** The reaction catalyzed by the enzyme factor XIIIa, bringing about the covalent ligating of fibrin with Nε-(γ-glutamyl) lysine bonds. The zymogen factor XIII is converted by thrombin and $Ca^{2+}$ into the active enzyme.

domains arranged around the sides. The protein remains inactive until the active site cysteine, which is buried at the base of a depression in the molecule, is exposed by movement of the activation peptide and β-barrel domains. The activation peptide crosses the dimer interface to prevent substrates reacting with the Cys314 residues located in the active site pocket of the other chain (23). The activation peptide may not move until after the glutamine substrate binds to the protein because there are no major changes in the x-ray–crystal structure of the thrombin-cleaved $A_2$-subunit or the thrombin-cleaved $A_2$-subunit in the presence of calcium ions (24). It is possible that the packing of the $A_2$ molecules in the crystals may prevent the thrombin-cleaved protein from adopting the active conformation (23).

There are *cis*-peptide bonds located at Gly410 to Pro411, Arg310 to Tyr311, and Gln425 to Phe426 (25,26). The *cis*-peptide bonds could change to the transorientation and produce a substantial conformational change that promotes catalysis (26). Additional studies are needed to visualize the enzyme–substrate complex to further define the structure of the enzyme.

## The Structure of the Factor XIII $B_2$-Subunit

The B chain is a glycosylated protein that is secreted through the *Golgi* and is 77 kDa, with 661 amino acids containing 10 disulfide bonded repeats, called *sushi domains*, with two disulfide bonds in each sushi domain (19). The B chains are flexible, rod-shaped molecules, which bind to surface-exposed residues on the $A_2$-subunit. That patients deficient in the B chain also have lower plasma A chain levels suggests that the B chain may help regulate the survival of the A chain in plasma (13). The location of the B chain's binding sites on the $A_2$-subunit and how they modulate plasma factor XIII half-life and activation remain poorly defined. B chains dissociate from the fibrin clot, whereas factor XIIIa remains bound (27). The B chains rapidly dissociate from A chains during hemostasis and may bind to other proteins, cell surfaces, or non–cross-linked γ′ chains, a variant of γ chain, in the fibrin clot (28,29). The B chains in the $A_2B_2$ complex binds to the γ′ chain in a select population of fibrinogen molecules (30).

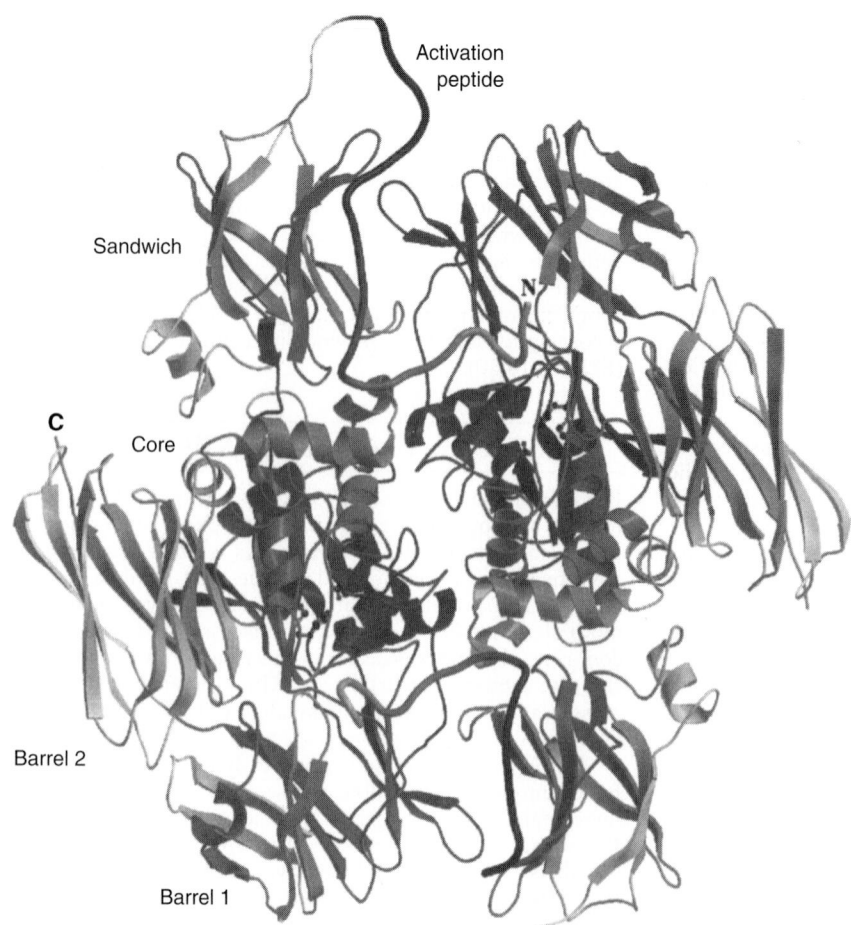

**FIGURE 17-2.** X-ray crystal structure of the factor XIII $A_2$-zymogen, shown in ribbon representation. The labeled structural domains are colored separately, with the colors ramped from less intense at the N-terminus to more intense at the C-terminus. Side-chain groups of the catalytic triad residues in the core domain are shown as space-filling structures (see Color Fig. 17-2). (Figure scaled to approximately 11 cm × 11 cm.)

The binding of the B chains to the γ′ chain accounts for the association of plasma factor XIII with fibrinogen (30,31).

The B chains must dissociate to fully activate the plasma factor XIII molecule after thrombin cleavage (32). The calcium concentration required to dissociate the B chains is higher than the physiologic plasma concentration. However, when fibrinogen is present, the calcium ion requirement is lowered to physiologic levels (33). It is unknown whether the B chains bind in a well-defined manner or if they associate at multiple sites to impede thrombin cleavage of plasma factor XIII (34). Thrombin cleavage may not be an absolute requirement for plasma factor XIII activation because the plasma zymogen expresses fibrin cross-linking activity when it interacts with fibrin polymers in the presence calcium ions (35). The B chains are not readily degraded by proteases and prevent the proteolytic inactivation of the $A_2$-subunit (34). The B chains enable the $A_2$-subunit to bind to fibrinogen, and this reaction is critical for localization of plasma factor XIII to sites where fibrin polymers and thrombin assemble a reaction that also accelerates thrombin cleavage of the $A_2B_2$ complex before a fibrin gels forms (29,30,36).

# FACTOR XIII ACTIVATION

Thrombin cleavage of the A chains releasing activation peptide is necessary to activate the plasma tetramer and the dimeric platelet factor XIII molecules, called factor XIIIa (37,38). However, because other serine proteases can also attack Arg–X bonds, activation of factor XIII by cleavage of the Arg37-Gly38 peptide bond can occur by other serine proteases as well as thrombin. Both endogenous platelet acid protease and calpain have been reported to activate factor XIII (39,40). In fact, the rate of thrombin cleavage of the protein is too slow for it to be activated in a physiologically appropriate timeframe.

Fibrin polymers serve as an important cofactor to generate factor XIIIa (41–43). A complex between thrombin, fibrin polymers, and plasma factor XIII forms and accelerates the cleavage of the A chain. The rate-enhancing effects of fibrin polymers has some important implications for hemostasis. Factor XIIIa will not form until a critical mass of fibrin polymerizes. This delay in factor XIIIa formation ensures that the hemostatic plug has a supply of factor XIIIa as it is forming. The generation of factor XIIIa in plasma can be triggered when as little as 1% to 2% of fibrinogen is converted to fibrin polymers. However, because a fibrin gel requires at least 20% of the fibrinogen to be cleaved to fibrin before a visible clot can be seen, factor XIIIa must begin stabilizing fibrin polymers before a visible thrombus appears. The plasma concentrations of the factor XIII $A_2$-subunit and fibrinogen are approximately 15 μg per mL and 3 mg per mL, respectively. Therefore, the molar ratio of factor XIII to fibrinogen in plasma is 1:100. This excess of fibrinogen supports the efficient mechanism for accelerating the conversion of factor XIII to factor XIIIa by fibrin polymers (23,41,44).

Platelet factor XIII is rapidly activated by thrombin. In contrast, there is a significant lag phase between thrombin cleavage and expression of the active plasma factor XIII. This lag phase, in activation, represents the time it takes for the B chains to dissociate from plasma factor XIIIa (16). Dissociation of the B chains from the A chains is also necessary to expose the active site cysteine 314 (32). There are no B chains bound to the fibrin clot, suggesting that the B chains dissociate as fibrin gels (45,46). The dissociation of the B chains from thrombin-cleaved plasma factor XIII can be regulated by either a domain in the central region of the Aα chain of fibrinogen, defined by residues 242 to 424, or by polymerizing fibrin (47). In contrast to the B chains, more than 90% of the A chains remain bound to fibrin (45,48).

## Catalytic Triad

The catalytic triad involving Cys314-His373-Asp396 is present in the central core catalytic domain (see Fig. 17-3) and has a configuration similar to the cysteine protease, papain (6,17). Site-directed mutagenesis of either Cys314, His373, or Asp396 produces an inactive protein and confirms the importance of these residues in catalysis. Site-directed mutagenesis and x-ray crystallography established that factor XIIIa uses a reverse proteolytic mechanism to catalyze the covalent isopeptide (49). There are other conserved residues within the active site pocket, including His342, Asp343, Glu434, Trp279, and Tyr560 (13,23). Site-directed mutagenesis has established that Trp279 is also important for stabilizing the oxyanion intermediate during catalysis (49,50). Because the active site Cys314 residue is hydrogen bonded with Tyr560 in the β-barrel domain (Fig. 17-3), a conformational change is needed to allow entry of the glutamine-containing substrate (17,23,24,51–53). The lysine substrate may gain entry after the salt bridge between Arg11 and Asp343 if the other chain is disrupted (23). In addition, the His342, which is hydrogen bonded to Glu434 (Fig. 17-3), could function to either align the lysine residue with the glutamine substrate or reduce the positive charge in lysine to promote catalysis. When His342 is mutated to alanine, the protein loses 85% of it transglutaminase activity (54). Development of specific inhibitors to factor XIIIa that can interact with the active site Cys314-SH have been developed and could be effective to promote thrombolysis (55).

## Calcium-Binding Site

Calcium ions are required for the $A_2$-subunit to display transglutaminase activity (56–58), a function to promote the interaction between the glutamine substrate and active sites (59–62), and promote the dissociation of the B chains from the A chains (63). Calcium ions bind to the A chains within an acidic binding domain with amino acids Asp435, Glu485, and Glu490 (58). The carbonyl group in Ala457 is also involved in the binding (23). There are additional weaker sites that can bind calcium at high concentrations (23). A terbium-binding site at the dimer interface, near residues Asp270 and Glu272, may disrupt the dimeric structure and lead to inhibition of factor XIIIa (23). The terbium-binding site (Asp270 to Glu272) is only five residues away from Trp279, which is important for catalysis (23) and could also explain how terbium inhibits the factor XIIIa (64). Pharmaceutical agents that could bind to specific domains in factor XIII could theoretically be developed to inhibit the intracellular activation and the extracellular function of factor XIIIa (55,65–68).

The mechanism by which calcium promotes catalysis could be related to the location of the binding site and its effect on controlling conformational change that is needed for catalysis (6,23). The calcium-binding site is only 10 Å from barrel 1, which blocks entry to the active site by interacting with Tyr560 (69). Calcium ions may induce a conformational change in barrel 1, which then exposes the active site and allows entry of the glutamine substrate (23). At high calcium ion levels, the $A_2$-subunit is activated in the absence of thrombin cleavage of the activation peptide (6,70). The calcium-binding site also forms close contacts with the active site in the other monomer, and this may stabilize the protein structure during catalysis (71). Allosteric interaction between the calcium-binding site of one monomer and the active site in the other chain may enable reciprocal catalysis at the fibrin D-dimer interface (11,13,72,73).

Calcium ions also make factor XIIIa resistant to degradation by serine proteases, including plasmin, thrombin, and trypsin (2,14). The second thrombin cleavage site (K513–Ser514) is in

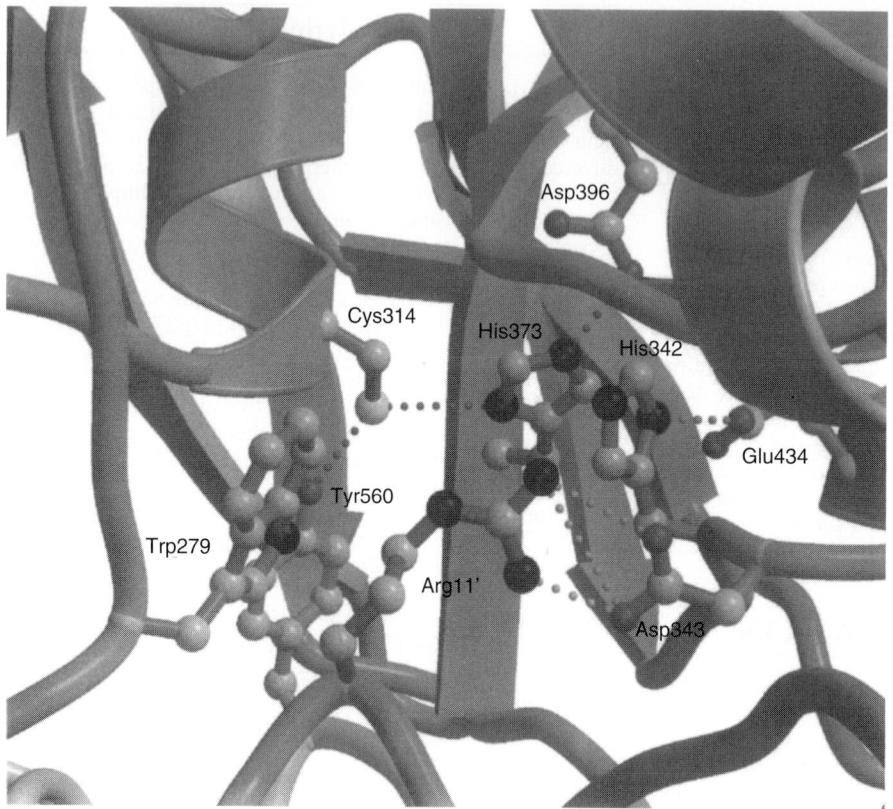

**FIGURE 17-3.** Close-up view of the factor XIII active site in the crystal structure of the zymogen. Side-chain groups of the Cys314-His373-Asp396 catalytic triad and of other conserved residues in the region are shown. Hydrogen-bonding interactions are represented by *dotted lines* (see Color Fig. 17-3). (Figure scaled to approximately 11 cm wide × 9.8 cm long.)

the C-terminus, which is more protease-sensitive in the absence of calcium ions (2,14). Once the C-terminus is removed from the protein, additional sites for proteolytic degradation are exposed. When the C-terminal β-barrels are removed by proteolysis, the dimer is destabilized and has lower transglutaminase activity (14). In summary, calcium plays a critical role in allowing the enzyme to adopt the proper conformation that promotes catalysis and resist proteolytic degradation (14).

## Active Site Pocket

When fibrinogen and fibrin bind to the thrombin-cleaved A chains, a conformational change in the A$_2$-subunit must occur to allow the substrates to enter the active site pocket, which is not solvent exposed (51,53). Once a substrate is inside the active site pocket, it must fit directly into a highly conserved region surrounding Cys314. The amino acids surrounding the active site Cys314 are highly conserved among the different transglutaminases (13), which place major constraints on the enzyme for effective catalysis. This is demonstrated in alanine mutagenesis of the amino acids flanking the active site Cys314, including Arg310 to Phe317 (49). Of the eight mutations, only one, Gly312-Ala, retains activity (49).

The ability of factor XIIIa to recognize the cross-linking site in the fibrin γ chain and rapidly catalyze two covalent bonds between each D-domain is a remarkable process that is not fully explained. To determine to what extent the primary amino acid sequence within the active site pocket defines substrate specificity, active site pocket (exon 7) was replaced with the corresponding exon of tissue transglutaminase (TTG) (74). Two other exons (3 and 5), previously identified as important domains for substrate recognition, were also replaced (74). The exon 3 chimera (residue 43–105, β-sandwich domain) was inactive (74). In contrast, the exon 5 chimera

molecule (190–229 in the catalytic core) had reduced activity but still retained preference for formation of cross-linked γ–γ dimers (74). The exon 7 chimera had normal transglutaminase activity, but the substrate specificity was changed to cross-link fibrin to Aα-γ complexes, a pattern similar to the cross-linking by TTG (74). These studies demonstrate that the residues close to the active site Cys314 help control access of the α and γ chains to the active site in factor XIIIa and modulate substrate specificity (74).

## Glutamine Substrate Recognition

There is a growing list of molecules that serve as substrates for factor XIIIa. Factor XIIIa substrates exist within the fibrin clot, in plasma, within the ECM, on cell surfaces, and inside cells. Fibrinogen, fibrin, fibronectin, and α$_2$-AP are the major substrates that interact with factor XIIIa in the clot and in plasma (38).

The first step in the enzymatic process is the interaction between factor XIIIa and a protein-bound glutamine (5). The ability for this reaction to occur depends on both the three-dimensional geometry in the enzyme and substrate. There still remains a limited understanding of this process, and further research is needed. However, during substrate recognition, there are changes in the enzyme conformation that facilitate the interaction with the active cysteine located deep in the active site pocket.

In the case of proteins substrates, the glutamine must be surface exposed and not hindered from reacting with factor XIIIa's active site (51). One-dimensional proton line-broadening and two-dimensional transferred–nuclear overhauser enhancement spectroscopy (NOESY) studies reveal that the glutamines and residues located C-terminally come in direct contact with the enzyme and adopt an extended conformation. Substrates with sequences similar to $\alpha_2$-AP (1 to 15) are proposed to bind both at the catalytic site and at a neighboring apolar region (51).

There are also regions in factor XIIIa that are remote from the active process cysteine that may bind substrates or undergo conformational changes that effect catalysis. Synthetic peptides from factor XIIIa were studied for whether they could alter substrate recognition and cross-linking (75). There were two peptides, Asn72-Asp97 and Asp190-Phe230, that modified cross-linking. Kinetic analysis revealed these peptides altered the first step in the catalytic reaction (75). When the peptide inhibitor was expressed in cells, it interfered with factor XIIIa cross-linking of the angiotensin II receptor in cells and inhibited atherosclerosis (76). Factor XIIIa cross-linked angiotensin II receptors are associated with hypertension (69,76).

These peptides could function also by binding to the glutamine substrates and thereby interfere with entry of the enzyme into the active site pocket. Identifying domains in factor XIIIa that undergo changes in conformation during the activation process has provided some insight into what portions of the molecule are undergoing changes during activation by thrombin and calcium ions. Labeling the cysteine and lysine side chains of factor XIIIa before and after activation of factor XIII demonstrated that there was acetylation of Lys73 and Lys221after activation. These lysine residues are within regions identified as potential sites that could bind to the glutamine substrates (77). The active site Cys314 and Cys409, located near the dimer interface, were also alkylated during activation. The $\beta$-barrel 2 domain at Cys695 also was alkylated, and Lys (677 or 678) is no longer acetylated in the activated enzyme, suggesting a substantial conformation change in this part of the molecule when activated (77).

Hydrogen–deuterium exchange experiments were conducted on recombinant factor XIII $A_2$-subunits after being exposed to thrombin and/or calcium (51). A conformation in the catalytic core (residue numbers 220 to 230) was detected when the protein was activated by thrombin. A change in conformation of this site was dependent upon the calcium concentration. In addition, a portion of the $\beta$-sandwich domain (residue numbers 98 to 104) changed when exposed to calcium alone. Changes in the $\beta$-barrel 1 domain at amino acids 526 to 546 occurred with calcium but did not change with thrombin alone. In conclusion, there are clearly domains in the $A_2$-subunit that can differentially change in response to thrombin and calcium ions (51) and are important for substrate recognition and catalysis.

Factor XIIIa must recognize the substrate, bind and fit into the active site to react with the glutamine (Glu398–399), and then react with a closely aligned lysine (Lys411) (30,78) in the $\gamma$ chain of an adjacent fibrin molecule aligned by fibrin polymerization (29,79). The enzyme must then be released to react with other sites and perform this reaction rapidly and with specificity.

The active site of one A chain appears to interact with the active site in the other A chain, and they may collaborate to catalyze the two isopeptide bonds that exist at the D-dimer interface (79). Each A chain may function independently and not simultaneously during intermolecular $\gamma$ chain cross-linking reaction (73). The reaction of other glutamine substrates in $\alpha_2$ antiplasmin and fibronectin does not involve two glutamines and two lysines aligned on different proteins (80,81). Therefore, only one active-site cysteine may be used to catalyze these reactions. It is possible that cleavage of one activation peptide is sufficient to promote a plasma factor XIII activation.

The primary amino sequence surrounding the glutamine substrate has an effect on XIIIa catalysis (82). Variations in specificity observed with factor XIIIa for peptides containing single and multiple substitutions in peptide sequence have demonstrated that several important features control substrate recognition (82). Amino acid residues at several locations in proximity to the glutamine are important determinants for the specificities of human plasma factor XIIIa (82). Peptides do not have the same reactivity as the native protein, suggesting there are other macromolecular structural domains that regulate substrate specificity (82).

## Lysine Substrate Recognition

The transglutaminase reaction is less selective toward lysine residues than toward glutamine residues. The nature of the amino acids immediately before the lysine influences the catalytic process (83). The presence of amino acids with either uncharged, basic polar residues or small aliphatic residues can enhance transglutaminase reactivity, whereas the presence of aspartic acid, glycine, proline, and histidine residues will inhibit the reaction (61,83). Steric hindrance could also contribute to the inability of some lysine residues to interact with factor XIIIa (61,83).

## Fibrinogen Binding

Fibrinogen plays an important role in controlling where and how plasma factor XIII functions during blood coagulation. In plasma, the $A_2B_2$ complex is bound to a select population of fibrinogen molecules that contain the C-terminal $\gamma'$ extension (28,31). This C-terminal $\gamma'$ extension is formed by alternate splicing of the $\gamma$ chain gene (30,78,84). The B chains that surround the $A_2$-subunit direct the B chains to the D-domain of the fibrinogen molecules that contain this unique sequence, which exists in approximately 15% of the plasma fibrinogen molecules (28,31). When fibrinogen is polymerized by thrombin or other agents, plasma factor XIII remains bound as the $A_2B_2$ complex (45). The only requirement to get plasma factor XIII into the clot is polymerization of fibrinogen (45). Fibrinogen binding provides a mechanism for localization of plasma factor XIII to sites of fibrin polymerization, which align the molecules for intermolecular ligation (31,41). In addition, fibrin polymerization may bring plasma factor XIII into contact with thrombin bound to fibrin (29).

The fibrin polymerization site on the D-domain of fibrinogen is always available and will react with the complimentary site in the E-domain after thrombin cleavage (78). Thrombin binds fibrin or fibrinogen at sites on fragment E or the $\gamma'$ chain (29). The thrombin concentration required to cleave plasma factor XIII is lowered to levels achieved during blood coagulation in order to promote thrombin-dependent activation of plasma factor XIII (41,43,85).

Thrombin appears to recognize a domain on plasma factor XIII that gets exposed by interaction of plasma factor XIII with fibrin polymers. These sites may be initially unavailable when the B chain is bound to the $A_2B_2$ complex. The B chain will dissociate more readily from the thrombin-cleaved A chains after the fibrinogen $\alpha$ chain binds to the protein (32,47). The calcium ion concentration required to activate the molecule is reduced to physiologic levels by the interaction with the $\alpha$ chain of fibrinogen (32). This site on fibrinogen is sufficiently large to have multiple points of contact with plasma factor XIII during fibrin polymerization (78).

## Fibrin Binding

Once a fibrin clot forms, the B chains appear free in the serum, but the thrombin-cleaved $A_2$-subunits do not readily dissociate (27,45). The fibrin-binding site for factor XIIIa appears to be different from the site for plasma factor XIII binding (86). Once factor XIIIa covalently modifies fibrin, it does not serve as an effective surface to promote thrombin cleavage or dissociate the B chains (87). The B chains may remain bound to the nonpolymerized γ chains of fibrinogen, which could help to mark regions of the clot that need further ligation. Factor XIIIa does not remain active for long within the clot, and there may exist some *in vivo* mechanism to inactivate it (88). Nitric oxide production by endothelial cells or other forms of oxidative stress could inactivate the cysteine residue in the active site (89). Proteolysis by plasmin, thrombin, or other proteases released by cells that infiltrate fibrin could regulate the function of the enzyme within the clot (90).

## Time Course of Factor XIIIa Formation

The time course of thrombin cleavage of plasma factor XIII has been studied in purified systems, blood and in plasma and there is agreement that plasma factor XIII cleavage by thrombin occurs soon after thrombin cleaves fibrinogen as soluble fibrin polymers assemble and before the appearance of a fibrin gel (41,91). This finding has important clinical implications for hemostasis and thrombosis.

Factor XIIIa begins to generate soluble cross-linked complexes that contain the D-dimer antigen (41,92) before a fibrin gel obstructs a vessel. The D-dimer antigen is exposed after plasmin cleaves cross-linked soluble complexes (92,93). Therefore, D-dimer antigen measurements are not solely measurements of the D-dimer released from an insoluble fibrin clot (92,94,95). D-dimer antigen measurements can be considered a marker of ongoing intravascular fibrin formation and fibrinolysis in the absence of complete vessel obstruction. The absence of D-dimer in the blood can exclude the presence of an intravascular thrombotic process, and this fact has been applied to diagnosis of deep vein thrombosis (92). Because many inflammatory states and other forms of tissue injury can trigger intravascular fibrin formation and fibrinolytic activation, elevated plasma D-dimer antigen levels may exist without thrombosis (92).

## The Nature of Covalent Intermolecular γ Chain Ligation

The C-terminus of the γ chain is a critical site for several reactions that promote hemostasis (29). The γ and γ′ chains can regulate plasma factor XIII binding, incorporation of factor XIII into the fibrin clot, thrombin binding, fibrin polymerization, and platelet aggregation (29,30). A monoclonal antibody directed at this site displays many different antithrombotic activities due to its antiplatelet and profibrinolytic functions, confirming the importance of this domain in normal hemostasis and providing a potential target for development of antithrombotic agents (96). Dysfibrinogens and specific fibrinogen mutants that disrupt the γ chain site have been shown to interfere with fibrin polymerization, cross-linking, and platelet function (29,30,97,98).

There is substantial flexibility in the C-terminus of the γ chain at the cross-linking site, which may facilitate entry into the active site pocket of factor XIIIa (99). The A₂-subunit is not a small molecule, and binding to this site, which is composed of two D-domains in adjacent fibrin molecules, requires exquisite specificity (23). X-ray crystallography of cross-linked D-dimers reveals that there is excellent alignment at the D-dimer interface to promote catalysis between fibrin molecules (100). Because there are two active sites in the A₂-dimer and these are oriented in different directions, they must bind to different γ chains at the D-dimer interface. The possibility that each A chain reacts independently and not simultaneously was proposed on the basis of kinetic data of factor XIII function (73) and would be feasible on the basis of the alignment of the molecules.

Ligation of γ chains between aligned chains at glutamine at position 398 or 399 of one γ chain and lysine at position 406 of another produces γ-dimers (101). At each D-dimer interface, only one of the two potential bonds is necessary for intermolecular fibrin dimers to form. The ligation between α chains creates very large oligomers, and this reaction occurs more slowly than γ chain dimer formation. There is also a minor amount of cross-linking between α chains and γ chains. Factor XIIIa can also cross-link α chains to γ chain dimers (102).

There are also higher forms of γ chain ligation producing γ-trimers and γ-tetramers (103,105). These must form because not all of the γ-dimers contain two isopeptide bonds. These cross-links may form at branch points or between fibrin fibers to produce covalent bonds between the fibrils (106). The γ chain multimers form slowly compared to α chain polymers at normal plasma factor XIII levels (104); however, γ chain multimers can form more rapidly when factor XIIIa levels are increased. The extent of resistance to fibrinolysis can be controlled by the degree of γ chain multimerization (105). In addition, the rheologic properties of fibrin can be modified by ligation reactions other than γ-dimer formation (107,108).

The rate at which fibrinogen and fibrin are cross-linked by factor XIIIa is regulated in part by the requirement to have D-domains aligned to allow the A₂-subunit to interact with two different fibrin molecules. The reaction that regulates the thrombin-dependent exposure of the fibrin polymerization on the fragment E then becomes the rate-controlling step. Directly adding thrombin-cleaved fragment E or a bivalent synthetic peptide that contains the fibrin polymerization sites causes the rate of fibrinogen ligation to increase to the same rate as fibrin polymers (54,101). Kinetic analysis of the cross-linking of γ chain and α chain cross-linking rates suggests that the reaction favors the γ chains when the molecules are aligned (109). Because the first step of the reaction involves reaction with the glutamine followed by a productive interaction with the lysine residue, there is a substantial barrier to this specific reaction that is overcome by fibrin polymerization and the binding of the plasma factor XIII to the γ′ chain of fibrinogen. Recently, the ability of the plasma factor XIII zymogen to cross-link was demonstrated, and this reaction is controlled by the binding of plasma factor XIII to the γ′ chain (35). These results suggest that the binding of plasma factor XIII to fibrin polymers is sufficient to induce catalysis. This reaction may be important when thrombin concentration is limited and a low amount of fibrin needs to be stabilized.

When the time course of factor XIIIa formation fibrin formation and covalent ligation are measured in plasma or blood, there is evidence that thrombin initially releases the fibrinopeptide A, then factor XIIIa is formed by thrombin and rapidly starts to cross-link the soluble fibrin polymer complexes (54). Whether thrombin-cleaved plasma factor XIIIa or the plasma zymogen initiates the initial cross-linking or the cross-linking occurs later, after more fibrin polymers assemble, is not well established. However, infusion of ancrod, which generates fibrin polymers, actually generates cross-linked fibrin complexes both *in vivo* and *in vitro*, confirming that in the presence of calcium and fibrin polymers, the zymogen form of plasma factor XIII can cross-link soluble fibrin polymers (110).

The ability of plasma factor XIII to cross-link γ chains early during the assembly of the fibrin polymers may also change the nature of the final fibrin fiber network (41). Changes in the size of fibrin fibers, the fiber thickness, and fibrin porosity could be altered by the timing of factor XIIIa formation (41,111).

One area of controversy regarding factor XIIIa cross-linking is whether the γ chains are cross-linked in a *cis* and/or *trans*-orientation (112,113). The fact that the cross-linking domain in the C-terminus domain of fibrin is flexible would argue that both types could exist within a fibrin gel (100), and evidence supports this argument (100). Biochemical and structural evidence supporting a *trans*-pattern has also been presented and confirmed by others (100).

## Multivalent α Chain Cross-linking

As the clot matures after fibrin gelation, fibrin α chain is modified by factor XIIIa very slowly. This may be because the α chains are mobile and infrequently interact with factor XIIIa. The glutamine substrates in the Aα chains are located in the midportion of the chain at Gln328 and Gln366. The lysine residues that are involved in forming α-chain multimers were initially located at Lys508 and at 556 or 562. Lys303 was determined as the position where α$_2$-AP is covalently attached (114). When the N-terminal synthetic peptide of α$_2$-AP was incubated with factor XIIIa and fibrin, 12 of 23 lysine residues between residues 208 and 610 in the Aα chain were covalently modified. Lys556 and Lys580 represented 50% of the cross-linking, and the other 50% was distributed between other lysyl residues (115). There are multiple sites in the Aα chain that can participate in multimer formation (115). The rate at which the α chain gets cross-linked to itself, to γ chain multimers, and to α$_2$-AP inhibitor plays a major role in regulating the susceptibility of fibrin to degradation (105,116–118). The isopeptide bond does not have any known specific protease to allow fibrin fibers to be degraded. Therefore, once extensive intermolecular isopeptide bond formation has occurred, serine proteases must degrade multiple sites in the fibrin molecule and fibrin fiber to promote disruption of the clot. The multivalent nature of the α chain lysines interacting with substrates in plasma, fibrin, and extracellular matrix provides additional sites to stabilize a fibrin clot *in vivo*.

There is evidence that a low concentration of circulating plasma fibrinogen (1% to 2%) has intramolecular cross-link formation between the α and γ chains (119). Intramolecular α-γ dimers interferes with thrombin-dependent fibrin polymerization (120). However, the formation of this intramolecular bond is catalyzed by the tissue TG molecule rather than factor XIIIa (120).

## Disrupting the Covalent Isopeptide Bond

The isopeptide bond is not susceptible to proteases that exist in human plasma or tissue (121). However, evidence suggests that factor XIIIa itself may reverse the isopeptide bond once it forms (44). Synthetic substrates to quantitate this reaction documented a relatively low $K_m$ (0.01 to 0.1 μM), suggesting this reaction could occur within the fibrin clot (121,122). The entire ligation process in fibrin may be more dynamic that previously suspected. The best evidence that the factor XIIIa–dependent reaction may be reversible was reported for the ligation of α$_2$-AP to fibrin (81,123). Additional studies are needed to determine the physiologic significance of reversing the isopeptide bond. To date, efforts to isolate a specific isopeptidase remain inconclusive (124). However, should an enzyme be discovered that could disrupt the isopeptide bond, it could potentially promote fibrinolysis.

## Fibrinolytic Inhibitors are Factor XIIIa Substrates

The cross-linking of protease inhibitors to the fibrin is another mechanism for factor XIIIa–mediated fibrin stabilization.

α$_2$-AP is the major fast-acting inhibitor of plasmin that circulates at a concentration of 1 μM in plasma. Patients congenitally deficient in α$_2$-AP experience a serious hemorrhagic disorder that has clinical features of factor XIII deficiency (81,125). Approximately 30% of α$_2$-AP is absent from serum and was found to bind covalently to fibrin. Factor XIIIa cross-links α$_2$-AP to fibrin's α chain (126). Early studies reported that Glutamine-2 is the major cross-linking site in α$_2$-AP and Lys 303 in the α chain site (127,128). Fibrin-bound α$_2$-AP can bind and inactivate plasmin when plasmin is present at low concentrations (128).

Two forms of α$_2$-AP circulate in human plasma: A 464-residue protein with methionine as the amino-terminus (Met–α$_2$-AP) and an N-terminally shortened 452-residue form with asparagine as the amino-terminus (Asn–α$_2$-AP) (129,130). Human plasma contains approximately 30% Met–α$_2$-AP and approximately 70% Asn–α$_2$-AP (129). The major form (Asn–α$_2$-AP) is more rapidly cross-linked to fibrin than the other form (129). Both plasma and fibrin cross-linked α$_2$-AP play a role in controlling the rate at which fibrin is degraded (125,131). A plasma protease that controls the conversion of the Met form to the Asn form of α$_2$-AP was recently isolated (129). This enzyme could play a vital role in regulating the antifibrinolytic function with the clot (129).

In recent studies, the contribution of factor XIIIa–mediated fibrin–fibrin cross-linking and α$_2$-AP–fibrin cross-linking to the fibrinolytic resistance of experimental pulmonary emboli were studied. These studies reveal that both forms of cross-linking can play a role in regulating clot lysis rates (118). Also apparent is the importance of platelets retracting and releasing α$_2$-AP (132) or other substances in making platelet-rich thrombi resistant to degradation (133–136).

Plasminogen activator inhibitor 2 (PAI-2), an inhibitor of plasmin formation, is also cross-linked to fibrin by factor XIIIa (137). Bound to fibrin, PAI-2 remains active and inhibits urokinase and tissue-type plasminogen activator (137). The glutamines in PAI-2 that serve as substrates were identified as residues 83 and 86, and are in a 33-residue loop that is separated from the active site of PAI-2 (137). Factor XIIIa ligates PAI-2 to Lys148, 230, and/or 413 in the α chain of fibrin. Because α$_2$-AP is ligated to a distinct residue (Lys303), there is no interference with PAI-2 coupling. The ability of the clot to localize agents that inhibit plasmin formation may augment fibrin stabilization (118,136,138). PAI-2 does not circulate in plasma until pregnancy (139). However, PAI-2 is secreted into the matrix, and it could function to modify fibrinolysis during tissue repair (140).

Recently, the plasma procarboxypeptidase B called thrombin activatable fibrinolysis inhibitor (TAFI) was discovered to be a factor XIIIa substrate (141). TAFI functions to connect thrombin formation with inhibition of fibrinolysis. TAFI is activated by the thrombin–thrombomodulin complex and cleaves carboxy-terminal lysine residues from fibrin (141). Once the lysine residues are removed by TAFI, plasminogen and plasmin binding to fibrin are reduced and fibrinolysis inhibited. This reaction provides yet another mechanism for rendering fibrin resistant to degradation. Localizing this protein to the fibrin clot surface could further promote fibrin stabilization (141).

The trappin genes are an interesting group of proteins that have an N-terminal sequence with a consensus sequence for cross-linking by transglutaminases and a disulfide-bonded domain that has protease inhibitor activity. These protease inhibitors are expressed in response to injury and are attached to ECM molecules, where they may limit tissue damage by elastase and other proteases that are released during inflammation. The relative importance of factor XIIIa (142) versus the TTG (143) in mediating the biologic action of these genes needs further investigation.

## Extracellular Matrix Molecules and Adhesive Glycoproteins Substrates: Fibronectin

Two distinct types of fibronectin (plasma and cellular) can interact with factor XIIIa and function as substrates (144,145). Plasma fibronectin (cold-insoluble globulin) is a 520,000-Da (144) heterodimer that circulates in plasma at a concentration that is 10% of fibrinogen (144). Fibronectin is covalently cross-linked to itself and to fibrin(ogen) by factor XIIIa. The cross-linked products of fibronectin may play a role in cell migration, attachment of fibrin to the ECM, and wound healing. Fibronectin is the second-most prevalent (4%) protein in the fibrin gel (145). The glutamines in fibronectin serving as factor XIIIa substrates were localized to the amino-terminus in both chains and at the carboxy-terminal domain in the longer protein (146). Glutamine 3 is involved in the cross-linking of fibronectin to fibrin (147). When fibrinogen and fibronectin are in solution, factor XIIIa catalyzes the formation of two cross-linked products. There are hybrid oligomers consisting of equimolar amounts of fibrinogen and fibronectin and fibrinogen oligomers. The size of these complexes grows and then are cross-linked to each other to form a gel (148). Although fibronectin alone has no impact on soluble fibrin assembly, when factor XIIIa is present, it becomes incorporated into fibrin. The resulting fibrin fibers are larger and denser, which increase the tensile strength of the clot. This reaction could play a role in modulating clot architecture and susceptibility of the fibrin to degradation. Plasma fibronectin is cross-linked by factor XIIIa to several ECM molecules in different tissues (146,149,150). The migration and adhesion of cells on factor XIII cross-linked fibronectin matrices is increased (151–155).

Factor XIIIa is associated with a number of processes in the adhesion of cells and in the ECM, including tissue repair (153,156), collagen synthesis (156), and reducing susceptibility of collagen precursors to proteolysis (157). The cross-linking of fibronectin to collagen may participate in anchoring the blood clot to the vessel wall. The fibronectin–collagen cross-linking reaction occurs for types I, II, III, and V collagen, but not for type IV (158). Other cross-linking reactions initiated by factor XIIIa have so far been identified such as fibrin–vinculin (159,160), fibronectin–von Willebrand protein (161), fibrin–von Willebrand protein (162), collagen–von Willebrand protein (161), laminin–von Willebrand protein (163), vitronectin–vitronectin (164), and fibrin–factor V (165,166). Osteopontin, an extracellular glycoprotein with multiple roles including bone homeostasis, tumor growth and metastasis, and angiogenesis, is a factor XIIIa substrate (167). Several ECM substrates of TTG, such as osteonectin (SPARC) (142), nidogen, and fibrillin (168), might also be factor XIIIa substrates, but further studies are needed in this area.

Factor XIIIa is a proangiogenic molecule, an effect mediated by the down regulation of thrombospondin (TSP)-1 expression and by enhancement of formation of $\alpha_V\beta_3$/vascular endothelial growth factor receptor (VEGFR)-2 complex. These complexes have a downstream influence on tyrosine phosphorylation and activation of VEGFR-2, which leads to upregulation of c-Jun and Egr-1, with the subsequent downregulation of TSP-1 by c-Jun through WT-1 pathway (169). In addition, there is a potential impact of factor XIIIa on atherosclerosis by localizing lipoprotein [Lp(a)] to fibrin (170). Immunohistochemical studies revealed that factor XIII antigen is colocalized with Lp(a) in atherosclerotic plaques (171). The accumulation of Lp(a) within the vessel by factor XIIIa could promote atherosclerosis. A monoclonal antibody to $\varepsilon$ ($\gamma$-glutamyl) lysine isopeptide bonds demonstrates transglutaminase activity within the atherosclerotic plaque. However, much of this activity may be attributable to tissue TG (171,172).

## Intracellular Substrates for Factor XIIIa

The interaction of factor XIIIa with intracellular cytoskeletal proteins may control the force generated by clot retraction and could also play a role in modulating actin polymerization if the enzyme functions to deaminate the glutamine in Rho which controls polymerization events. It has been established that when transglutaminases do not have a reactive lysine they may convert glutamines to glutamic acid by a hydrolytic process that uses water molecules (5).

Cross-linking of actin to fibrin by factor XIIIa has been demonstrated and Glu-Lys cross-links are generated by factor XIIIa during actin polymerization (173). The cross-linking of platelet and skeletal muscle myosin by factor XIIIa has also been reported (174,175). TSP and gelsolin are other platelet proteins that have been crosslinked to themselves (176,177) and to the fibrin clots (178). Local control of TSP concentrations can play a role in regulating angiogenesis (169).

## Factor XIII and Fibrin Rheology

Fibrin stabilization by factor XIIIa produces a substantial effect on the mechanical properties of fibrin gels. Covalent bonds catalyzed by factor XIIIa enhance the mechanical stiffness of fibrin fivefold compared to the ionic-bonded gel (179–181).

The placement of covalent bonds within fibrin gels prevents the rearrangement of fibrin fibers in the clot structure as detected when strain is applied to the clot (3) factor XIIIa, induces a slight decrease in fiber diameter and an increase in fiber length that can be detected. Recent evidence suggests that $\gamma$ chain dimer formation alone does not modify clot rheology when examined at low strain. However, the formation of high-molecular-weight covalent complexes between $\alpha$ and $\gamma$ chain multimers promotes optimal clot rigidity.

In plasma the nature of the fibrin gel is altered to some extent by other proteins (fibronectin, vitronectin, TSP) which are bound to fibrin and provide addition covalent ligations that could have a significant rheologic impact *vivo* (107,182).

## Platelets and Factor XIII

Platelet contains 50% of the fibrin stabilizing activity in whole blood (11). Platelet factor XIII serves as a catalyst that can enhance fibrin cross-linking and ligating of $\alpha_2$-AP to fibrin (134). There is a unique set of platelets that retain procoagulant and adhesive molecules called collagen- and thrombin-activated (COAT) platelets that are formed by factor XIIIa (183). Platelets need to be stimulated by thrombin and collagen to produce this modification. Factor XIIIa cross-links serotonin to several molecules derived from the platelet $\alpha$-granules. These serotonylated molecules are specifically bound to fibrinogen and TSP that remain bound to their cell surface membrane receptors (183). The fact that drugs that disrupt integrin receptor function on platelets *enhance* formation of the COAT platelets could explain why some of these agents cause a paradoxical increase in thrombosis.

The major platelet binding site for plasma factor XIII has been identified as the integrin $\alpha_{IIb}\beta_3$ (184). Plasma factor XIIIa also binds to thrombin activated platelets and the binding of factor XIIIa is inhibited by plasmin (185). Excess plasmin formation could destroy this binding and contribute to platelet dysfunction during disseminated intravascular coagulation (DIC) and thrombolytic therapy. Factor XIIIa binding to activated platelets is mediated through activation of glycoprotein (GP) IIb/IIIa. In addition, factor XIII binds to fibrinogen which is associated with activated platelets. High local concentration of factor XIIIa at the platelet surface could be important to promote clot stability during tissue repair.

Kulcarni and Jackson (186) demonstrated an important role for platelet factor XIII in regulating $\alpha_{IIb}\beta_3$ adhesive function. Platelet factor XIII and calpain were found to have important roles in limiting platelet recruitment and developing aggregates thereby limiting thrombus formation. These authors demonstrated that platelets undergoing a high level of cytosolic calcium flux exhibit factor XIII and calpain-dependent morphological changes that are associated with downregulation of the adhesive functions of the fibrinogen receptor. Although the mechanism for this activity is unclear, it is possible that factor XIII mediated covalent cross-linking of one or more of the ligands for $\alpha_{IIb}\beta_3$ (such as fibronectin, TSP, fibrinogen, vitronectin, and von Willebrand factor) or possibly the fibrinogen receptor itself may contribute to the ability of factor XIII to downregulate platelet adhesive activity.

The role of intracytoplasmic factor XIII is still poorly defined. Intracytoplasmic platelet factor XIII can be activated without releasing the activation peptide (40,160). Intracellular factor XIII also cross-links platelet cytoskeletal components including vinculin and filamin following platelet activation (160). This reaction may play a role during clot retraction or during platelet adhesion to enhance the stability of platelets when they are exposed to sheer forces in flowing blood.

Plasma factor XIII can also enhance the interaction of platelets with endothelial cells by binding to the endothelial $\alpha_V\beta_3$ and platelet GP IIb/IIIa integrins (187). Sustained elevation of calcium after platelets are activated by collagen can activate platelet factor XIII which then modifies platelet membrane $\alpha_{IIb}\beta_3$ adhesive function and limits thrombus growth (186). Flow cytometry was used to detect platelet-associated factor XIII which could serve as a marker of platelet activation in patients with peripheral vascular disease (188). Further studies are needed to ascertain how platelet factor XIII can modulate hemostatic and thrombotic processes

After activation of human platelets with thrombin, thymosin $\beta_4$ is released and cross-linked to fibrin in a time- and calcium-dependent manner (189,190). This provides a mechanism to increase the local concentration of thymosin where it may contribute to wound healing, angiogenesis, and inflammation. Efforts to bioengineer fibrin matrices with different cytokines attached by factor XIIIa are in progress to aid wound healing (191).

## Utilizing Factor XIIIa Activity to Image Acute Thrombus Formation

The cross-linking of $\alpha_2$-AP into thrombi occurs early after thrombus formation. Recently, Jaffer et al. (192) have synthesized a peptide based on the amino-terminus of $\alpha_2$-AP and coupled this to a near infrared fluorescent compound. The near infrared fluorescence (NIRF) agent (designated A15) demonstrated enhancement of thrombus imaging both *in vitro* and in a murine model. A15 was shown to be covalently bound to fibrin. This agent would be useful in detecting acute thrombi but not aged (>24 hours) thrombi because of the known decline in factor XIIIa activity over time.

## Factor XIII Gene Structure and Regulation

The A chain gene located on chromosome six at position 6p24–25 is more than 160 kb (193,194). It contains 15 exons producing a 3.9-kb messenger RNA (mRNA), with an 84-base pair 5′ untranslated region, a 2.2-kb open reading frame, and a long 1.6-kb 3′ untranslated region. The coding regions and splice junctions were sequenced and large introns remains uncharacterized (13).

The B chain gene is located on a different chromosome, at the 1q31–32.1 position (195). The 28-kb gene was sequenced and has 12 exons encoding a 2-kb messenger RNA (mRNA) (196). The mRNA contains a leader sequence characteristic for proteins that are secreted, an open reading frame coding for 641 amino acids, and a poly-A tail. Exons 2 to 11 code for homologous domains called sushi domains, which may have evolved through exon shuffling. Each sushi domain contains approximately 60 amino acids and is stabilized by two disulfide bonds. This disulfide-bonded sushi motif exists in other proteins, including the six complement control proteins factor H, C4 binding protein (C4bp), CR1, CR1 and decay accelerating factor (DAF), and the membrane cofactor proteins (MCP) (19,196,197).

The regulation of factor XIII A- and B chain gene expression is not thoroughly understood. The A chain is expressed mostly in bone marrow cells, including megakaryocytes, and carried by platelets (198) as well as the monocyte–macrophage lineage (199). The A chain can be detected in monocytes as they undergo differentiation at all stages of development (200) and remains expressed after leukemic transformation (201). Although the liver is not the major site of synthesis for the A chain (202), small quantities of $A_2$ chain are transcribed and translated in the liver (203). Furthermore, *in situ* hybridization reveals that the A-subunit mRNA was expressed in three different cell types in the liver, including histiocytes, Kupffer cells, and hepatocytes (203). Bone marrow and liver transplantation studies demonstrates the that $A_2$-subunit originates predominantly from bone marrow cells, although in some patients, additional extrahematopoietic synthetic sites probably contribute to a lesser extent (202). The cell-specific expression of the factor XIII A chains in monocytoid and megakaryocytoid cell lines has been studied and the promoter region analyzed. The binding of myeloid transcription factors GATA-1, Ets-1, and myeloid zinc finger-1 (MZF-1) (198), and transcription factors SP-1 and NF-1 in the factor XIII A chain promoter play a role in modifying gene expression. The regulation of the expression of the B-subunit has not been reported, but it is known to be expressed predominantly in the liver (198).

# FACTOR XIII DEFICIENCY

Factor XIII deficiency is inherited as an autosomal recessive disorder that can afflict individuals of all races and sexes. A wide variety of mutations and molecular genetic mechanism can produce this disorder (204). The frequency of factor XIII deficiency has been generally estimated at one per 2 million (204, 205). Factor XIII deficiency is typically associated with the absence of cross-linking of plasma fibrin as well as $\alpha_2$-AP and leads to a bleeding tendency of varying severity.

Initially, the disease was classified as type I and type II deficiencies. The genetic defect in type I deficiency is the absence of the B chain (206). However, the intracellular A chain is present and functional. In type II deficiency, there is a genetic defect in the A chain, although lower levels of the B chain circulate (206).

## Genetic Defects Causing Factor XIII Deficiency

Molecular genetic analysis has demonstrated that factor XIII deficiency is a highly heterogenous disorder (205). Substitutions that produce missense, nonsense mutations, or splice defects are scattered throughout the factor XIII A chain gene. Deletions and/or insertions are increased around exons 2, 3, and 11. There have been no reported mutations in exons 13 and 15 or residues within the catalytic triad (Cys314, His373, Asp396). Missense mutations represent approximately 50% of the abnormalities (205). Nonsense mutations, splice-site defects, small insertions, and small deletions have also been reported (205).

The structural consequences of these missense mutations have been predicted using the experimentally determined crystal structure of the factor XIII A2 zymogen as a starting scaffold for computer molecular modeling (207–211). In Figure 17-4, the distribution of the changes in the A chain structure is shown. Although none of the active site residues is altered, most of the affected amino acids are located in the catalytic core domain. The amino acid residues affected by the missense mutations are involved in interatomic interactions that are important for protein folding and stability (208).

When cases were studied, mRNA levels were normal, whereas intracellular antigen levels were not detectable, suggesting the proteins are not stable enough to survive intracellularly (208,211,212). Expression of mutant molecules in mammalian cells also demonstrated that the intracellular half-lives of these mutant molecules were substantially reduced (197,208).

The molecular genetics of factor XIII B chain deficiency has been reported to be due to a Cys430Phe substitution that destroyed a disulfide bond in the seventh sushi domain, impairing intracellular transport, and in another case, an insertion within the codon for exon 3 caused a stop codon at Tyr80 in the second sushi domain (213–216).

## Severity of Congenital Factor XIII Deficiency

Patients deficient in factor XIII lack plasma and platelet factor XIII, although some experience only a mild bleeding tendency

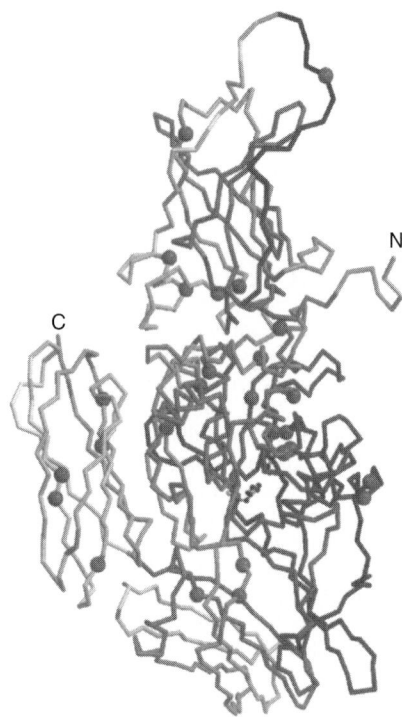

**FIGURE 17-4.** Distribution of the 21 amino acid residues altered by factor XIII–deficiency missense mutations. The factor XIII–A-subunit structure is shown as a backbone carbon trace colored by domain, similar to that shown in Color Figure 17-2 with labeled *N*- and *C*-termini. The 21 residues affected by deficiency mutations are represented by *red* carbon spheres; four polymorphism sites appear as *blue* carbon spheres. The side-chain groups of the Cys314, His373, Asp396 catalytic triad residues are drawn as *ball-and-stick* structures (see Fig. 17-3) (see Color Fig. 17-4).

(204). It has been recognized for many years that low plasma factor XIII levels (<5% of normal) are sufficient to control bleeding. In one case, there was a low-level expression of a normal factor XIII transcript despite a splice-site mutation. In another patient, homozygous Val414Phe missense mutation was associated with the homozygous Leu34 allele, which may have increased activity of the mutant molecule. The Leu34 allele produces molecules with higher specific activity compared to the Val34 variant. There is a correlation between other single nucleotide polymorphisms (SNPs) (codons 204, 564, 650, and 651) and the level of factor XIII activity in plasma.

B chains are required for the survival of the A chain in plasma. A patient with inherited isolated B deficiency had very low levels of A chain in plasma, and the half-life of A chain infusions was reduced. Ideally, these patients need therapy that contains a source of B chains (e.g., plasma).

## Clinical Findings in Inherited Factor XIII Deficiency

The bleeding diathesis in inherited factor XIII deficiency is usually severe. Bleeding a few days after birth at the umbilical cord site occurs in approximately 80% of cases. Bleeding after circumcision and a family history of fatal intracranial bleeding immediately after delivery has been reported (204,217). Bleeding into the skin and subcutaneous tissues can cause extensive bruises, and patients may be mistaken for "battered" children (218). Bleeding into muscles and around joints but not into the joint space can cause giant hematomas and prolonged hospitalizations (204).

A few patients experience a very mild bleeding syndrome that comes to light only when they present with a bleeding complication (e.g., after a surgical operation). Wound-healing problems described in a small proportion of the reported cases (approximately 14%) are not usually reported and may relate to replacement therapy having been used (204). Women who are factor XIII deficient require replacement because stabilization of fibrin at the maternal fetal interface is required to maintain pregnancy (204). The factor XIII gene–deficient mouse displayed a similar phenotype (14).

## Diagnosis of Factor XIII Deficiency

Routine laboratory tests of blood coagulation, including PT, activated partial thromboplastin time (aPTT), thrombin time, and fibrinogen level, are normal in factor XIII deficiency. Laboratory diagnosis still relies on the standard clot solubility test. A plasma clot from a patient deficient in factor XIII is easily disrupted by urea, acids, and bases (8,204,217). A small volume of plasma is incubated at room temperature with thrombin and calcium for 1 hour and then suspended in a solution of 5M urea. If there is no factor XIII activity, the clot will dissolve within 60 minutes. This is a qualitative test in which 1% to 3% of normal factor XIII activity can make a clot insoluble (7). If clot solubility is found, mixing experiments with normal plasma are required to be sure the deficiency is not due to an inhibitor. Factor XIII deficiency should be confirmed by a quantitative assay (219,220). In addition, the concentrations of the A- and B-subunits should then be determined by immunological techniques (18,220–222).

## Treatment of Inherited Factor XIII Deficiency

Fresh frozen plasma and cryoprecipitate have been used as sources of factor XIII because low levels of factor XIII in plasma can control bleeding. The *in vivo* half-life of factor XIII after infusion of plasma or factor XIII concentrates is from 11 to 14 days (204,217). It is therefore possible to infuse a nonconcentrated solution of factor XIII to prevent bleeding. Patients managed for over 30 years are reported to have their quality of life improved dramatically by replacement therapy. The plasma-derived Fibrogammin P is given as 1,000 U of the concentrate every 6 weeks. This therapy raises levels to 30% to 35%, and after 6 weeks (three half-lives), levels are 3% to 5%. A dose of 1,000 U is also given before any minor surgical procedures or invasive investigations or minor trauma to prevent bleeding. A recent survey revealed that only 68% of patients were on a regular replacement regimen (223). All patients need replacement because intracranial bleeding is unpredictable and can cause death or serious morbidity.

# ROLE OF FACTOR XIIIa IN HEMOSTASIS

It is not possible to isolate one biochemical or biologic reaction involving factor XIIIa as the most important for effective hemostasis. The unique property of the isopeptide bond allows factor XIIIa to confer hemostatic properties to fibrin through multiple pathways, including intermolecular cross-linking of fibrin molecules to each other, ligation of $\alpha_2$-AP to fibrin, and alteration of the mechanical properties of fibrin.

The mechanical strength of the fibrin gel is important to impede blood loss when exposed to sheer forces in the circulation. There is a shift in the equilibrium between formation of soluble fibrin polymers and assembly of insoluble fibrin fibers (107). Factor XIIIa lowers the fibrin concentration needed for an insoluble clot to form.

Factor XIII activity confers a relative increase in resistance to lysis of the fibrin gel by plasmin (81,116,136,224). Resistance of factor XIIIa–modified fibrin gels to plasmin degradation can be detected using either purified proteins, plasma, or blood. When normal plasma is clotted in the presence of calcium, the resulting clot is composed of cross-linked fibrin, $\alpha_2$-AP, and fibronectin (225). The possibility also exists that other plasma proteins may become cross-linked to fibrin and could also contribute to hemostatic properties of fibrin *in vivo* (11,41). von Willebrand protein is cross-linked to fibrin if the rate of blood coagulation is slowed (226). The multivalent potential of the lysine residues in the $\alpha$ chain and proteins that contain glutamine substrates suggest that there are many different cross-linked complexes that make fibrin a more effective hemostatic agent (41,227).

# ACQUIRED FACTOR XIII INHIBITORS

Whenever a patient presents with a bleeding disorder and routine coagulation tests, including aPTT, prothrombin time (PT), thrombin time, and fibrinogen level, are normal, either a deficiency in factor XIII or a defect in fibrinolysis should be considered. The urea clot solubility test should be performed, and mixing studies can be conducted rapidly to monitor for the presence of an inhibitor. Antibodies (IgG antibodies) to plasma factor XIII are acquired in several patient populations. Patients deficient in factor XIII can develop antibodies after they are exposed to the antigen by replacement therapy. In addition, antibody inhibitors can develop after exposure to certain drugs, including phenytoin (228,229), isoniazid (INH) (230), penicillin (231,232), and valproate (233,234).

The immunoglobulin (IgG) inhibitors have specific antigenic targets that react with both the plasma factor XIII molecule

$A_2B_2$ and platelet zymogen $A_2$, or just one form of the zymogen (235–237). Inhibitors were directed against various activated forms of factor XIII, and one appeared to be directed toward the fibrin-binding and cross-linking site (235,238). Antibodies directed toward the B chain have not been reported.

There are also certain clinical disorders associated with acquired deficiency of factor XIII including acute leukemia (239,240), chronic leukemia (231,241), prematurity (242), plasmacytoma (243), surgery, disseminated intravascular coagulation, sepsis, inflammatory bowel disease, and Henoch-Shönlein purpura. However, levels in these conditions are not as low, and the patients may not experience any adverse effects (231). Nevertheless, there is growing evidence that supplementing plasma factor XIII levels in some patient populations in which there are hemostatic defects as a consequence of surgery or other medical condition could reduce blood loss and improve wound healing (244–248).

Treatment for patients with factor XIII inhibitor is a medical emergency. Patients with an acquired factor XIII inhibitor need to have bleeding controlled by increasing the plasma level of factor XIII and/or by removing the inhibitor. Increasing the level of factor XIII requires administering a blood product that has concentrated levels of factor XIII. Cryoprecipitate or pasteurized factor XIII from human placenta (Fibrogammin P) has been used (249). Recombinant factor XIII may also become available for use in the future and has been shown to be safe when infused into human volunteers. The frequent infusion of high doses of factor XIII are required to overcome an inhibitor, especially if the titer of the antibody is high. Control of hemorrhage has been achieved with factor XIII infusions ranging from 50 to 150 U per kg. Because most of the antibodies are of the IgG class, they can bind to staphylococcus A columns, and this treatment has been used in several patients (250,251). One patient was reportedly treated with intravenous $\gamma$-globulins and responded within several days. Patients could also be treated with antifibrinolytic therapy, including e-aminocaproic acid (EACA) tranexamic acid or aprotinin, because the noncross-linked clots are very prone to fibrinolysis (231). Most patients reported on the literature also received immunosuppressive therapy with prednisone or cyclophosphamide (236,252–254). The use of Rituximab to deplete the B cells that are producing the antibody has not been reported but could be helpful because it has some utility in acquired factor VIII inhibitors. The response to therapy is variable, and more than 50% of the patients have fatal outcomes. The aggressive use of immunoadsorption, intravenous $\gamma$-globulin, immunosuppressive therapy, antifibrinolytic agent, and replacement therapy in this life-threatening condition may lead to improved clinical outcomes. However, very careful follow-up and treatment is needed to prevent recurrent life-threatening bleeding in this disorder.

# NEW APPROACHES TO DEVELOP THERAPEUTIC FACTOR XIIIa INHIBITORS

The caterpillar *Lonomia achelous* causes a severe hemorrhagic diathesis in humans that is associated with a deficiency of factor XIII (255). Lonomia V is a highly specific protease that degrades both the A and B chains of factor XIII (256). The crude salivary gland extract of the giant Amazon leech *Haementeria ghilianii* contains an inhibitor of plasma and platelet factor XIIIa called tridegin, which has been purified to homogeneity, yielding a single band on sodium dodecyl sulfate polyacrylamide gel electrophoresis (SDS/PAGE) with an apparent molecular mass of 7.3 kDa. Microsequencing has shown tridegin to be a peptide of 66 amino acids. Tridegin is the most potent inhibitor of factor XIII yet described (257). Finally, derivatives of 2-[(2-oxopropy1) thio] are a novel class of highly specific inactivators of factor XIIIa and human erythrocyte transglutaminase (65).

# EMERGING CLINICAL USES OF FACTOR XIII

The safety, distribution, and immunogenicity of a single dose of recombinant factor XIII was studied after administration to healthy volunteers. Recombinant factor XIII was well tolerated at dosages of up to 50 U/kg/second and may enter clinical trials for congenital deficiency and other acquired deficiency states. A number of gastrointestinal disorders associated with bleeding and low factor XIII levels, including ulcerative colitis (258), are reported to respond to factor XIII–supplementation therapy. In drug-induced hemorrhagic cystitis, low levels of factor XIII have been reported, and the administration of factor XIII concentrates appears to promote hemostasis (259).

## Factor XIII and Intraoperative and Postoperative Bleeding

Factor XIII influences bleeding after coronary surgery and was found to reduce the need for blood transfusions. In patients with prolonged diffuse bleeding, there is growing interest in using factor XIII replacement therapy (260). Low factor XIII levels were associated with increased blood loss after coronary artery bypass grafting, as measured by chest tube drainage (247).

Factor XIIIA and clot strength after cardiopulmonary bypass (CPB) were recently examined (247). Baseline factor XIII A chain antigen levels dropped to 64%, and clot strength was reduced to 77% after 45 minutes of surgery. These values remained abnormal postoperatively (247). Clot strength was correlated with platelet count and fibrinogen levels (247). Postoperative bleeding at 2 hours was inversely correlated with platelet count, factor XIII A chain antigen levels, and clot strength measured at the end of CPB. Maintenance of adequate platelet counts and factor XIIIA levels at the end of CPB may play a role in maintaining clot strength and reducing blood loss.

After major noncardiac surgery, plasma factor XIII levels are decreased, and the minimum levels occur precisely when increased fibroblast growth should be greatest. Moreover, infusion of factor XIII concentrates into patients enhances the stability of surgical wounds (248). Decreased factor XIII levels and reduction of clot firmness were found to be associated with unexplained intraoperative bleeding in 226 consecutive elective surgical patients (248,261). Fibrinogen and factor XIII were more rapidly consumed in bleeders, and computerized thromboelastography showed a significant reduction in clot firmness (248). There is a need to examine in a prospective trial whether rheologic properties can be used to identify patients at increase risk for bleeding. An increased risk for postoperative hemorrhage after neurosurgery was reported in patients with decreased factor XIII activity (261). Postoperative intracranial hematomas that required surgical evacuation was increased 6.4-fold in patients with postoperative factor XIII less than 60%. The risk was further increased 12-fold in patients who had fibrinogen levels less than 1.5 g per L and increased ninefold in patients with platelet counts less than $150 \times 10^9$ per L and low factor XIII levels (<60%).

## Fibrin Sealants and Factor XIII

Fibrin sealant, or fibrin "glue," is a biologic surgical hemostatic agent material that is used with growing frequency in a variety of surgical situations. This is a is a two-component system that has a concentrated fibrinogen and factor XIII solution combined with a solution of thrombin and calcium that forms a covalently modified fibrin gel after the solutions are mixed. Some commercial preparations also contain antifibrinolytic agents to further reduce fibrinolysis. Commercially prepared fibrin sealants are used extensively in Europe. The Food and Drug Administration (FDA) approved the first commercial fibrin sealant in 1998 and subsequent use in the United States has increased (262).

Virtually every surgical discipline has found an application for fibrin sealant, although most widespread applications and acceptance appear in the cardiovascular and neurosurgical areas. Topical application of factor XIII to patients with chronic, nonhealing leg ulcers (263); with liver and spleen lacerations (264); with dental extractions in hemophilia (265); at cannulation sites in ECMO (extracorporeal circulating membrane oxygenation) (266); direct application to gastric ulcers (267); vascular grafts; and replacement for nasal packing in endonasal operations (268) showed clinical improvement in a few weeks. Applications to aid adhesion and tissue repair include (269) sealing of dural leaks (270); promoting union of middle ear bones (271); skin grafting after burn injuries (272); reconstructive urologic surgery (273); sealing bronchopleural fistulas (274); alternative suturing in plastic surgery (275); and providing a matrix for the repair of bony defects (245).

Patients with liver disease and other coagulation abnormalities often need surgery, and local hemostasis could be a problem. A clinical trial using fibrin glue showed that it could be effective in preventing local hemorrhagic complications after inguinal hernia repair in patients with concurrent coagulation disorders (264).

Prevention of bleeding at sites where vascular grafts were inserted was examined in an animal model using porcine vascular grafts (276). Fibrin sealants that contained factor XIII reduced blood loss compared to absorbable gelatin sponges coated with thrombin (277).

Intracranial hemorrhages (ICHs) are a serious problem in premature infants. As for administration of supplemental factor XIII in cases of extremely premature infants (weighing <1,000 g), survival without craniotomy was achieved (242). In a randomized trial, premature infants were randomly divided into a treated group with a factor XIII concentrate and a nontreated group. Bleeding occurred in only 15.4% compared to (75.0%) in the nontreated group. Factor XIII replacement could become an effective agent to prevent intraventricular hemorrhage (IVH) in premature infants, although additional studies are needed (242).

The binding of fibrin sealant to collagen was recently found to be dependent on whether cross-linked fibrinogen–fibronectin complexes were present in the preparation. Fibrin must maintain a firm attachment to collagen in the ECM (278).

Serious gastrointestinal bleeding often develops in Henoch-Schönlein purpura (279). Low factor XIII levels have been reported, and bleeding has been successfully managed by factor XIII replacement (279). Clinical evaluation of a pasteurized factor XIII concentrate administration was conducted in a group of patients with moderately severe Henoch-Schönlein purpura. Symptoms improved in 3 days as factor XIII level increased (279).

Activated factor XIII reduced in vitro and prevented the loss of endothelial barrier function when endothelium was energy depleted (endothelial permeability). An effect on the paracellular passageways in endothelial monolayers was considered as the potential mechanism (280). On the basis of these studies, factor XIII was found to prevent the development of myocardial edema in children during cardiac surgery for congenital heart disease (281).

Direct application of factor XIII to chronic wounds improved wound healing in most patients by 3 weeks. The therapy reduced bleeding and secretions from the wound surface (282).

Factor XIII infusions enhanced the healing of bone defects in diabetic rats (245). The administration of factor XIII also accelerated mucosal healing of gastric stress ulcers in a rat model (283).

## Role of Factor XIII in Hypertension and Atherosclerosis

Recently, the ATI receptor in the monocytes from patients with essential hypertension were discovered to be dimeric and cross-linked by factor XIII (76). Site-directed mutagenesis established that a glutamine residue at position 315 (Gln315) in the carboxy terminus of the AT1 receptor was a substrate (76). The dimeric AT1 receptors were hypersensitive to angiotensin II (76). Treatment with angiotensin-converting enzyme (ACE) inhibitors changed the receptors to a monomeric form and reduced their responsiveness to angiotensin II (76). Inhibition of factor XIIIa in apo-E–deficient mice inhibited formation of AT1 dimers and prevented monocytes from infiltrating vascular tissue and causing atherosclerosis (284).

# POLYMORPHISMS OF THE FACTOR XIIIa-SUBUNIT GENE

There are five relatively common polymorphisms in the protein expressed by the A chain gene (285,286). There is a G to T change that leads to the replacement of valine with a leucine (41,285). There is also a tyrosine to phenylamine at amino acid 204, which is present in 1% to 3% of the population (41) and was associated with an increased risk of recurrent miscarriage (41). There is also proline to leucine change at amino acid 564 in the first β-barrel domain, a Val650 to isoleucine and a Glu651 to glutamine in barrel 2 that changes to migration of plasma factor XIII when analyzed by isoelectric focusing (41,287).

There are also two polymorphisms in the promoter of the A chain, which is in proximity to the SP-1– and MZF-1–binding sites that may regulate tissue-specific expression (9). The other is a four-nucleotide repeat, AAAG, that exists approximately 860 bp upstream of the transcription start site near GATA-1 binding site (12). This site was used for the prenatal diagnosis of factor XIII deficiency (288).

## The Activation Peptide Polymorphisms: Factor XIII Val34Leu

The activation peptide of XIII Val34Leu polymorphisms is located just three amino acids from the thrombin cleavage site Arg37-Gly39. The Leu allele is relatively common and levels vary between populations (41). Thirty percent of whites express the Leu allele, whereas only 1% of Japanese have the Leu allele. The highest levels are in the Pima Indians (41). Thrombin-dependent activation of the Leu34 molecule is more rapid than that of the Val34 variant either in the presence or in the absence of the B chains (111). Kinetic analysis reveals that the catalytic efficiency is increased 2.5-fold for the Leu34 molecule (111). The interaction between thrombin and a synthetic XIII activation peptide from residues 28 to 37 has been documented by x-ray crystallography (289). Analysis of the three-dimensional structure suggested that that a bulkier side-chain at residue 34 would alter the substrate peptide conformation. Furthermore, the main interaction between thrombin and factor XIII resides in the P4-P1 (Val/Leu34-Arg37) segment of the activation peptide (289).

When the kinetics of this reaction were analyzed in the presence of fibrin polymers, the activation of factor XIII Leu34 remained faster than that of Val34, with a catalytic efficiency of 4.8 compared with 2.2 $\mu$M.

The cleavage of the Leu34 activation peptide occurs at the same rate at fibrinopeptide A (111). In contrast, the rate of Val34 peptide cleavage is delayed and appears as the fibrinopeptide B is cleaved. These data suggest that factor XIII Leu34 is activated at the time of des-A fibrin formation, whereas the Val34 variant is activated when des-AB fibrin is formed. One could postulate that the rapidly formed factor XIIIa generated by the Leu34 allele would function to restrict lateral aggregation by making the protofibril more rigid. Fibrin clots formed with the Leu34 protein were thinner, with smaller pores, and alter permeation properties compared to the Val34 variant (111).

### The Leu34 Allele and Coronary Artery Disease

Studies concerning the effect of the Leu34 allele on carriership of the risk for myocardial infarction (MI) are quite variable (290). In the initial study involving a Caucasian patient population, the Leu34 allele provided a protective effect against MI. The other common polymorphisms, Pro564Leu, Val650Ile, and Glu651Gln, were associated with protection against coronary artery disease (41). A protective effect of the 34Leu allele was confirmed by studies from Finland (291), Brazil, and Italy. In contrast, studies in southern France, Spain, and Italy did not find any effect of the Leu34 allele on the risk of MI (9). The Atherosclerosis Risk in Communities (ARIC) study from a Newfoundland population found that failure to protect by the Leu34 allele was not limited to Mediterranean populations (292). In addition, the combination of factor XIII Leu34 and prothrombin 20210A alleles caused a 12-fold higher MI risk (292). The Leu34 allele did not protect young women and even reduced the efficiency of thrombolytic therapy (293). However, there may be other genetic and environmental factors that could modify the effect of the Leu34 allele. In obese young women, the Leu34 allele provided protection against MI, whereas in nonobese subjects, it had no influence (293). The Leu34 allele reduced risk of MI in women receiving postmenopausal estrogen therapy and a polymorphism in the B chain, His95Arg, reduced the risk further (294).

### The Leu34 Allele and Cerebrovascular Disease

The first study of cerebrovascular disease demonstrated a higher prevalence of the Leu34 allele in subjects with primary ICH and no association with ischemic stroke. The largest case–control study of cerebral infarction reported a major protective effect of Leu34. The effect was strong enough to reduce the high risk associated with smoking. A smaller study from Spain reported no association between the Leu34 allele and ischemic stroke. However, a large, well-matched case–control study of cerebral infarction reported a major protective effect of Leu34, with interactions with smoking that modified risk of stroke. These findings were supported by a smaller study from Italy (9,41).

However, a recent study from the United States did not find a protective effect of Leu34 in a small group of young women with cerebral infarction but found that the Phe204 allele was associated with a mildly increased risk of ischemic stroke. The Phe204 and Leu564 alleles were associated with an increased risk of hemorrhagic stroke (41).

Individuals homozygous for the Leu34 allele had an increased risk of retinal artery occlusion (295). Clearly, there is no consensus regarding whether bleeding and thrombosis in the cerebral circulation and other genetic or environmental factors could contribute to the variability of results.

### The Leu34 Allele and Venous Thrombotic Disorders

Several studies have investigated the relation between the Leu34 allele and venous thrombosis (41). Some studies found a protective effect similar to that described for MI, whereas others found no association. The interactions between the Leu34 allele and factor $V_{Leiden}$ did not show any increased risk of thrombosis (296). A common polymorphism in the A$\alpha$ chain (Thr312Ala) of fibrinogen and the factor XIII Leu34 allele negates the protective effect of the Leu34 allele (9,41). Amino acid 312 in the fibrinogen $\alpha$ chain is close to the factor XIII cross-linking and $\alpha_2$-AP incorporation sites and could have an interaction with factor XIIIa function.

# POLYMORPHISMS OF THE FACTOR XIIIb-SUBUNIT GENE

There are three known alleles of the factor XIII $\beta$ chain that can be identified by isoelectric focusing (297,298). However the molecular basis of these $\beta$ chain alleles is not established. There is a replacement of histidine with arginine in the second sushi domain that occurs in 10% of the Caucasian population. There is also an Alu insertion in the noncoding region of the $\beta$ chain gene.

## References

1. Loewy AG. Some thoughts on the state in nature, biosynthetic origin, and function of factor XIII. *Ann N Y Acad Sci* 1972;202:41–58.
2. Lorand L. Fibrinoligase: the fibrin-stabilizing factor system of blood plasma. *Ann N Y Acad Sci* 1972;202:6–30.
3. Roberts WW, Kramer O, Rosser RW, et al. Rheology of fibrin clots. I. Dynamic viscoelastic properties and fluid permeation. *Biophys Chem* 1974;1:152–160.
4. Schwartz ML, Pizzo SV, Hill RL, et al. Purification and subunit structure of human plasma and platelet fibrin-stabilizing factor. *J Lab Clin Med* 1971;78:848.
5. Folk JE, Chung SI. Transglutaminases. *Methods Enzymol* 1985;113:358–375.
6. Pedersen LC, Yee VC, Bishop PD, et al. Transglutaminase factor XIII uses proteinase-like catalytic triad to crosslink macromolecules. *Protein Sci* 1994;3:1131–1135.
7. Duckert F. Documentation of the plasma factor XIII deficiency in man. *Ann N Y Acad Sci* 1972;202:190–199.
8. Kitchens CS, Newcomb TF. Factor XIII. *Medicine* 1979;58:413–429.
9. Bereczky Z, Katona E, Muszbek L. Fibrin stabilization (factor XIII), fibrin structure and thrombosis. *Pathophysiol Haemost Thromb* 2003;33:430–437.
10. Muszbek L, Yee VC, Hevessy Z. Blood coagulation factor XIII: structure and function. *Thromb Res* 1999;94:271–305.
11. Lorand L. Factor XIII: structure, activation, and interactions with fibrinogen and fibrin. *Ann N Y Acad Sci* 2001;936:291–311.
12. Aslam S, Standen GR. Molecular analysis in factor XIIIA deficiency. *Thromb Haemost* 1995;73:895.
13. Ichinose A. Physiopathology and regulation of factor XIII. *Thromb Haemost* 2001;86:57–65.
14. Lauer P, Metzner HJ, Zettlmeissl G, et al. Targeted inactivation of the mouse locus encoding coagulation factor XIII-A: hemostatic abnormalities in mutant mice and characterization of the coagulation deficit. *Thromb Haemost* 2002;88:967–974.
15. Ichinose A, Hendrickson LE, Fujikawa K, et al. Amino acid sequence of the a subunit of human factor XIII. *Biochemistry* 1986a;25:6900–6906.
16. Curtis CG, Brown KL, Credo RB, et al. Calcium-dependent unmasking of active center cysteine during activation of fibrin stabilizing factor. *Biochemistry* 1974;13:3774–3780.
17. Yee VC, Pedersen LC, Le Trong I, et al. Three-dimensional structure of a transglutaminase: human blood coagulation factor XIII. *Proc Natl Acad Sci U S A* 1994;91:7296–7300.
18. Yorifuji H, Anderson K, Lynch GW, et al. B protein of factor XIII: differentiation between free B and complexed B. *Blood* 1988;72:1645–1650.
19. Ichinose A, McMullen BA, Fujikawa K, et al. Amino acid sequence of the b subunit of human factor XIII, a protein composed of ten repetitive segments. *Biochemistry* 1986b;25:4633–4638.
20. Murdock PJ, Owens DL, Chitolie A, et al. Development and evaluation of ELISAs for factor XIIIA and XIIIB subunits in plasma. *Thromb Res* 1992;67:73–79.
21. Bishop PD, Teller DC, Smith RA, et al. Expression, purification, and characterization of human factor XIII in *Saccharomyces cerevisiae*. *Biochemistry* 1990b;29:1861–1869.
22. Bishop PD, Lasser GW, Le Trong I, et al. Human recombinant factor XIII from *Saccharomyces cerevisiae*. Crystallization and preliminary x-ray data. *J Biol Chem* 1990a;265:13888–13889.
23. Yee VC, Le Trong I, Bishop PD, et al. Structure and function studies of factor XIIIa by x-ray crystallography. *Semin Thromb Hemost* 1996;22:377–384.
24. Yee VC, Pedersen LC, Bishop PD, et al. Structural evidence that the activation peptide is not released upon thrombin cleavage of factor XIII. *Thromb Res* 1995;78:389–397.
25. Jabs A, Weiss MS, Hilgenfeld R. Non-proline cis peptide bonds in proteins. *J Mol Biol* 1999;286:291–304.
26. Weiss MS, Metzner HJ, Hilgenfeld R. Two non-proline cis peptide bonds may be important for factor XIII function. *FEBS Lett* 1998;423:291–296.
27. Greenberg CS, Miraglia CC, Rickles FR, et al. Cleavage of blood coagulation factor XIII and fibrinogen by thrombin during *in vitro* clotting. *J Clin Invest* 1985b;75:1463–1470.
28. Mosesson MW. Fibrinogen gamma chain functions. *J Thromb Haemost* 2003;1:231–238.
29. Moaddel M, Farrell DH, Daugherty MA, et al. Interactions of human fibrinogens with factor XIII: roles of calcium and the gamma' peptide. *Biochemistry* 2000b;39:6698–6705.
30. Farrell DH. Pathophysiologic roles of the fibrinogen gamma chain. *Curr Opin Hematol* 2004;11:151–155.
31. Siebenlist KR, Meh DA, Mosesson MW. Plasma factor XIII binds specifically to fibrinogen molecules containing gamma chains. *Biochemistry* 1996;35:10448–10453.
32. Credo RB, Curtis CG, Lorand L. Ca2+-related regulatory function of fibrinogen. *Proc Natl Acad Sci U S A* 1978;75:4234–4237.
33. Curtis CG, Janus TJ, Credo RB, et al. Regulation of factor XIIIa generation by fibrinogen. *Ann N Y Acad Sci* 1983;408:567–576.
34. Mary A, Achyuthan KE, Greenberg CS. b-chains prevent the proteolytic inactivation of the a-chains of plasma factor XIII. *Biochim Biophys Acta* 1988a;966:328–335.
35. Siebenlist KR, Meh DA, Mosesson MW. Protransglutaminase (factor XIII) mediated crosslinking of fibrinogen and fibrin. [See comment]. *Thromb Haemost* 2001;86:1221–1228.
36. Moaddel M, Falls LA, Farrell DH. The role of gamma A/gamma' fibrinogen in plasma factor XIII activation. *J Biol Chem* 2000a;275:32135–32140.
37. Muszbek L, Adany R, Mikkola H. Novel aspects of blood coagulation factor XIII. I. Structure, distribution, activation, and function. *Crit Rev Clin Lab Sci* 1996;33:357–421.
38. Lorand L. Activation of blood coagulation factor XIII. *Ann N Y Acad Sci*, 1986;485:144–158.
39. Ando Y, Imamura S, Yamagata Y, et al. Platelet factor XIII is activated by calpain. *Biochem Biophys Res Commun* 1987;144:484–490.
40. Muszbek L, Polgar J, Boda Z. Platelet factor XIII becomes active without the release of activation peptide during platelet activation. *Thromb Haemost* 1993;69:282–285.
41. Greenberg CS, Miraglia CC. The effect of fibrin polymers on thrombin-catalyzed plasma factor XIIIa formation. *Blood* 1985;66:466–469.
42. Greenberg CS, Achyuthan KE, Fenton JW III. Factor XIIIa formation promoted by complexing of alpha-thrombin, fibrin, and plasma factor XIII. *Blood* 1987;69:867–871.
43. Ariens RA, Lai TS, Weisel JW, et al. Role of factor XIII in fibrin clot formation and effects of genetic polymorphisms. *Blood* 2002;100:743–754.
44. Makarova KS, Aravind L, Koonin EV. A superfamily of archaeal, bacterial, and eukaryotic proteins homologous to animal transglutaminases. *Protein Sci* 1999;8:1714–1719.
45. Triantaphyllopoulos DC. Factor XIII consumption as an indicator of thrombin generation. *J Lab Clin Med* 1974;84:74–80.
46. Greenberg CS, Dobson JV, Miraglia CC. Regulation of plasma factor XIII binding to fibrin *in vitro*. *Blood* 1985a;66:1028–1034.
47. Credo RB, Curtis CG, Lorand L. Alpha-chain domain of fibrinogen controls generation of fibrinoligase (coagulation factor XIIIa). Calcium ion regulatory aspects. *Biochemistry* 1981;20:3770–3778.
48. Greenberg CS, Enghild JJ, Mary A, et al. Isolation of a fibrin-binding fragment from blood coagulation factor XIII capable of cross-linking fibrin(ogen). *Biochem J* 1988;256:1013–1019.
49. Hettasch JM, Greenberg CS. Analysis of the catalytic activity of human factor XIIIa by site-directed mutagenesis. *J Biol Chem* 1994;269:28309–28313.
50. Iwata Y, Tago K, Kiho T, et al. Conformational analysis and docking study of potent factor XIIIa inhibitors having a cyclopropenone ring. *J Mol Graph Model* 2000;18:591–599.
51. Marinescu A, Cleary DB, Littlefield TR, et al. Structural features associated with the binding of glutamine-containing peptides to factor XIII. *Arch Biochem Biophys* 2002;406:9–20.
52. Turner BT Jr, Maurer MC. Evaluating the roles of thrombin and calcium in the activation of coagulation factor XIII using H/D exchange and MALDI-TOF MS. *Biochemistry* 2002;41:7947–7954.
53. Mitkevich OV, Shainoff JR, DiBello PM, et al. Coagulation factor XIIIa undergoes a conformational change evoked by glutamine substrate. Studies on kinetics of inhibition and binding of XIIIA by a cross-reacting antifibrinogen antibody. *J Biol Chem* 1998;273:14387–14391.

54. Lorand L, Parameswaran KN, Murthy SN. A double-headed Gly-Pro-Arg-Pro ligand mimics the functions of the E domain of fibrin for promoting the end-to-end crosslinking of gamma chains by factor XIIIa. *Proc Natl Acad Sci U S A* 1998;95:537–541.

55. Shebuski RJ, Sitko GR, Claremon DA, et al. Inhibition of factor XIIIa in a canine model of coronary thrombosis: effect on reperfusion and acute re-occlusion after recombinant tissue-type plasminogen activator. *Blood* 1990; 75:1455–1459.

56. Curtis CG, Stenberg P, Chou CH, et al. Titration and subunit localization of active center cysteine in fibrinoligase (thrombin-activated fibrin stabilizing fector). *Biochem Biophys Res Commun* 1973;52:51–56.

57. Hornyak TJ, Shafer JA. Role of calcium ion in the generation of factor XIII activity. *Biochemistry* 1991;30:6175–6182.

58. Lai TS, Slaughter TF, Peoples KA, et al. Site-directed mutagenesis of the calcium-binding site of blood coagulation factor XIIIa. *J Biol Chem* 1999; 274:24953–24958.

59. Chung SI, Folk JE. Kinetic studies with transglutaminases. The human blood enzymes (activated coagulation factor 13) and the guinea pig hair follicle enzyme. *J Biol Chem* 1972;247:2798–2807.

60. Cooke RD, Pestell TC, Holbrook JJ. Calcium and thiol reactivity of human plasma clotting factor XIII. *Biochem J* 1974;141:675–682.

61. Stenberg P, Curtis CG, Wing D, et al. Transamidase kinetics. Amide formation in the enzymic reactions of thiol esters with amines. *Biochem J* 1975;147:153–163.

62. Folk JE. Mechanism and basis for specificity of transglutaminase-catalyzed epsilon-(gamma-glutamyl) lysine bond formation. *Adv Enzymol Relat Areas Mol Biol* 1983;54:1–56.

63. Lorand L, Gray AJ, Brown K, et al. Dissociation of the subunit structure of fibrin stabilizing factor during activation of the zymogen. *Biochem Biophys Res Commun* 1974;56:914–922.

64. Achyuthan KE, Mary A, Greenberg CS. Tb(III)-ion-binding-induced conformational changes in platelet factor XIII. *Biochem J* 1989;257:331–338.

65. Seale L, Finney S, Sawyer RT, et al. Tridegin, a novel peptidic inhibitor of factor XIIIa from the leech, *Haementeria ghilianii*, enhances fibrinolysis *in vitro*. *Thromb Haemost* 1997;77:959–963.

66. Leidy EM, Stern AM, Friedman PA, et al. Enhanced thrombolysis by a factor XIIIa inhibitor in a rabbit model of femoral artery thrombosis. *Thromb Res* 1990;59:15–26.

67. Freund KF, Doshi KP, Gaul SL, et al. Transglutaminase inhibition by 2-[(2-oxopropyl)thio]imidazolium derivatives: mechanism of factor XIIIa inactivation. *Biochemistry* 1994;33:10109–10119.

68. Nilsson JL, Hoffmann KJ, Ljunggren C, et al. Fibrin-stabilizing factor inhibitors. 8. Pyridine derivatives as charge-transfer complex acceptors. *Acta Pharm Suec* 1973;10:209–214.

70. Cooke RD. Calcium-induced dissociation of human plasma factor XIII and the appearance of catalytic activity. *Biochem J* 1974;141:683–691.

71. Fox BA, Yee VC, Pedersen LC, et al. Identification of the calcium binding site and a novel ytterbium site in blood coagulation factor XIII by x-ray crystallography. *J Biol Chem* 1999;274:4917–4923.

72. Hornyak TJ, Bishop PD, Shafer JA. Alpha-thrombin-catalyzed activation of human platelet factor XIII: relationship between proteolysis and factor XIIIa activity. *Biochemistry* 1989;28:7326–7332.

73. Seelig GF, Folk JE. Half-of-the-sites and all-of-the-sites reactivity in human plasma blood coagulation factor XIIIa. *J Biol Chem* 1980;255: 9589–9593.

74. Hettasch JM, Peoples KA, Greenberg CS. Analysis of factor XIII substrate specificity using recombinant human factor XIII and tissue transglutaminase chimeras. *J Biol Chem* 1997;272:25149–25156.

75. Achyuthan KE, Slaughter TF, Santiago MA, et al. Factor XIIIa-derived peptides inhibit transglutaminase activity. Localization of substrate recognition sites. *J Biol Chem* 1993;268:21284–21292.

76. AbdAlla S, Lother H, Langer A, et al. Factor XIIIA transglutaminase crosslinks AT1 receptor dimers of monocytes at the onset of atherosclerosis. [See comment]. *Cell* 2004;119:343–354.

69. Thomas WG. Double trouble for type 1 angiotensin receptors in atherosclerosis. *N Engl J Med* 2005;352:506–508.

77. Turner BT Jr, Sabo TM, Wilding D, et al. Mapping of factor XIII solvent accessibility as a function of activation state using chemical modification methods. *Biochemistry* 2004;43:9755–9765.

78. Mosesson MW, Siebenlist KR, Meh DA. The structure and biological features of fibrinogen and fibrin. *Ann N Y Acad Sci* 2001;936:11–30.

79. Samokhin GP, Lorand L. Contact with the N termini in the central E domain enhances the reactivities of the distal D domains of fibrin to factor XIIIa. *J Biol Chem* 1995;270:21827–21832.

80. Sakata Y, Aoki N. Cross-linking of alpha 2-plasmin inhibitor to fibrin by fibrin-stabilizing factor. *J Clin Invest* 1980;65:290–297.

81. Mosher DF, Johnson RB. Specificity of fibronectin—fibrin cross-linking. *Ann N Y Acad Sci* 1983;408:583–594.

82. Gorman JJ, Folk JE. Structural features of glutamine substrates for human plasma factor XIIIa (activated blood coagulation factor XIII). *J Biol Chem* 1980;255:419–427.

83. Grootjans JJ, Groenen PJ, de Jong WW. Substrate requirements for transglutaminases. Influence of the amino acid residue preceding the amine donor lysine in a native protein. *J Biol Chem* 1995;270:22855–22858.

84. Wolfenstein-Todel C, Mosesson MW. Human plasma fibrinogen heterogeneity: evidence for an extended carboxyl-terminal sequence in a normal gamma chain variant (gamma'). *Proc Natl Acad Sci U S A* 1980;77:5069–5073.

85. Janus TJ, Lewis SD, Lorand L, et al. Promotion of thrombin-catalyzed activation of factor XIII by fibrinogen. *Biochemistry* 1983;22:6269–6272.

86. Hornyak TJ, Shafer JA. Interactions of factor XIII with fibrin as substrate and cofactor. *Biochemistry* 1992;31:423–429.

87. Lewis SD, Janus TJ, Lorand L, et al. Regulation of formation of factor XIIIa by its fibrin substrates. *Biochemistry* 1985;24:6772–6777.

88. Robinson BR, Houng AK, Reed GL. Catalytic life of activated factor XIII in thrombi. Implications for fibrinolytic resistance and thrombus aging. *Circulation* 2000;102:1151–1157.

89. Catani MV, Bernassola F, Rossi A, et al. Inhibition of clotting factor XIII activity by nitric oxide. *Biochem Biophys Res Commun* 1998;249:275–278.

90. Mary A, Achyuthan KE, Greenberg CS. The binding of divalent metal ions to platelet factor XIII modulates its proteolysis by trypsin and thrombin. *Arch Biochem Biophys* 1988b;261:112–121.

91. Undas A, Brummel K, Musial J, et al. Blood coagulation at the site of microvascular injury: effects of low-dose aspirin. *Blood* 2001;98:2423–2431.

92. Dempfle CE. Use of D-dimer assays in the diagnosis of venous thrombosis. *Semin Thromb Hemost* 2000;26:631–641.

93. Pfitzner SA, Dempfle CE, Matsuda M, et al. Fibrin detected in plasma of patients with disseminated intravascular coagulation by fibrin-specific antibodies consists primarily of high molecular weight factor XIIIa-crosslinked and plasmin-modified complexes partially containing fibrinopeptide A. *Thromb Haemost* 1997;78:1069–1078.

94. Merskey C, Johnson AJ, Harris JU, et al. Isolation of fibrinogen-fibrin related antigen from human plasma by immuno-affinity chromatography: its characterization in normal subjects and in defibrinating patients with *abruptio placentae* and disseminated cancer. *Br J Haematol* 1980;44:655–670.

95. Elms MJ, Bunce IH, Bundesen PG, et al. Rapid detection of cross-linked fibrin degradation products in plasma using monoclonal antibody-coated latex particles. *Am J Clin Pathol* 1986;85:360–364.

96. Jirouskova M, Smyth SS, Kudryk B, et al. A hamster antibody to the mouse fibrinogen gamma chain inhibits platelet-fibrinogen interactions and FXIIIa-mediated fibrin cross-linking, and facilitates thrombolysis. *Thromb Haemost* 2001;86:1047–1056.

97. Okumura N, Gorkun OV, Terasawa F, et al. Substitution of the gamma-chain Asn308 disturbs the D:D interface affecting fibrin polymerization, fibrinopeptide B release, and FXIIIa-catalyzed cross-linking. *Blood* 2004; 103:4157–4163.

98. Mosesson MW. Dysfibrinogenemia and thrombosis. *Semin Thromb Hemost* 1999;25:311–319.

99. Yee VC, Pratt KP, Cote HC, et al. Crystal structure of a 30 kDa C-terminal fragment from the gamma chain of human fibrinogen. *Structure* 1997; 5:125–138.

100. Yang Z, Pandi L, Doolittle RF. The crystal structure of fragment double-D from cross-linked lamprey fibrin reveals isopeptide linkages across an unexpected D-D interface. *Biochemistry* 2002;41:15610–15617.

101. Mosesson MW, Siebenlist KR, Hernandez I, et al. Fibrinogen assembly and crosslinking on a fibrin fragment E template. *Thromb Haemost* 2002; 87:651–658.

102. Shainoff JR, Urbanic DA. Multicolour immuno-staining of fibrinogen polypeptide chains for identification of their derivatives in electrophoregrams. *Blood Coagul Fibrinolysis* 1990;1:479–484.

103. Shainoff JR, Urbanic DA, DiBello PM. Immunoelectrophoretic characterizations of the cross-linking of fibrinogen and fibrin by factor XIIIa and tissue transglutaminase. Identification of a rapid mode of hybrid alpha-/gamma-chain cross-linking that is promoted by the gamma-chain cross-linking. *J Biol Chem* 1991;266:6429–6437.

104. Siebenlist KR, Mosesson MW. Progressive cross-linking of fibrin gamma chains increases resistance to fibrinolysis. *J Biol Chem* 1994;269: 28414–28419.

105. Siebenlist KR, Mosesson MW. Factors affecting gamma-chain multimer formation in cross-linked fibrin. *Biochemistry* 1992;31:936–941.

106. Mosesson MW, Siebenlist KR, Amrani DL, et al. Identification of covalently linked trimeric and tetrameric D domains in crosslinked fibrin. *Proc Natl Acad Sci U S A* 1989;86:1113–1117.

107. Carr ME Jr, Gabriel DA, McDonagh J. Influence of factor XIII and fibronectin on fiber size and density in thrombin-induced fibrin gels. *J Lab Clin Med* 1987;110:747–752.

108. Lim BC, Ariens RA, Carter AM, et al. Genetic regulation of fibrin structure and function: complex gene-environment interactions may modulate vascular risk. [Erratum appears in *Lancet* 2003;361:2250]. *Lancet* 2003; 361:1424–1431.

109. Lewis KB, Teller DC, Fry J, et al. Crosslinking kinetics of the human transglutaminase, factor XIII[A2], acting on fibrin gels and gamma-chain peptides. *Biochemistry* 1997;36:995–1002.

110. Dempfle CE, Argiriou S, Alesci S, et al. Fibrin formation and proteolysis during ancrod treatment. Evidence for des-A-profibrin formation and thrombin independent factor XIII activity. *Ann N Y Acad Sci* 2001;936:210–214.

111. Ariens RA, Philippou H, Nagaswami C, et al. The factor XIII V34L polymorphism accelerates thrombin activation of factor XIII and affects cross-linked fibrin structure. *Blood* 2000;96:988–995.

112. Weisel JW, Francis CW, Nagaswami C, et al. Determination of the topology of factor XIIIa-induced fibrin gamma-chain cross-links by electron microscopy of ligated fragments. *J Biol Chem* 1993;268:26618–26624.

113. Mosesson MW, Siebenlist KR, Meh DA, et al. The location of the carboxy-terminal region of gamma chains in fibrinogen and fibrin D domains. *Proc Natl Acad Sci U S A* 1998;95:10511–10516.

114. Kimura S, Aoki N. Cross-linking site in fibrinogen for alpha 2-plasmin inhibitor. *J Biol Chem* 1986;261:15591–15595.

115. Sobel JH, Gawinowicz MA. Identification of the alpha chain lysine donor sites involved in factor XIIIa fibrin cross-linking. *J Biol Chem* 1996;271: 19288–19297.

116. Reed GL, Houng AK. The contribution of activated factor XIII to fibrinolytic resistance in experimental pulmonary embolism. [See comment]. *Circulation* 1999;99:299–304.

117. Francis CW, Marder VJ. Increased resistance to plasmic degradation of fibrin with highly crosslinked alpha-polymer chains formed at high factor XIII concentrations. *Blood* 1988;71:1361–1365.

118. McDonagh RP Jr, McDonagh J, Duckert F. The influence of fibrin crosslinking on the kinetics of urokinase-induced clot lysis. *Br J Haematol* 1971;21:323–332.

119. Siebenlist KR, Mosesson MW. Evidence of intramolecular cross-linked A alpha.gamma chain heterodimers in plasma fibrinogen. *Biochemistry* 1996;35:5817–5821.

120. Murthy SN, Lorand L. Cross-linked A alpha.gamma chain hybrids serve as unique markers for fibrinogen polymerized by tissue transglutaminase. *Proc Natl Acad Sci U S A* 1990;87:9679–9682.

121. Parameswaran KN, Cheng XF, Chen EC, et al. Hydrolysis of gamma:epsilon isopeptides by cytosolic transglutaminases and by coagulation factor XIIIa. *J Biol Chem* 1997;272:10311–10317.

122. Loewy AG, Blodgett JK, Blase FR, et al. Synthesis and use of a substrate for the detection of isopeptidase activity. *Anal Biochem* 1997;246:111–117.

123. Kimura S, Tamaki T, Aoki N. Acceleration of fibrinolysis by the N-terminal peptide of alpha 2-plasmin inhibitor. *Blood* 1985;66:157–160.

124. Zavalova L, Lukyanov S, Baskova I, et al. Genes from the medicinal leech (*Hirudo medicinalis*) coding for unusual enzymes that specifically cleave endo-epsilon (gamma-Glu)-Lys isopeptide bonds and help to dissolve blood clots. *Mol Gen Genet* 1996;253:20–25.

125. Kluft C, Vellenga E, Brommer EJ, et al. A familial hemorrhagic diathesis in a Dutch family: an inherited deficiency of alpha 2-antiplasmin. *Blood* 1982;59:1169–1180.

126. Sakata Y, Aoki N. Significance of cross-linking of alpha 2-plasmin inhibitor to fibrin in inhibition of fibrinolysis and in hemostasis. *J Clin Invest* 1982; 69:536–542.

127. Ichinose A, Tamaki T, Aoki N. Factor XIII-mediated cross-linking of NH2-terminal peptide of alpha 2-plasmin inhibitor to fibrin. *FEBS Lett* 1983;153:369–371.

128. Lee KN, Jackson KW, Christiansen VJ, et al. Alpha2-antiplasmin: potential therapeutic roles in fibrin survival and removal. *Curr Med Chem Cardiovasc Hematol Agents* 2004a;2:303–310.

129. Lee KN, Jackson KW, Christiansen VJ, et al. A novel plasma proteinase potentiates alpha2-antiplasmin inhibition of fibrin digestion. *Blood* 2004b; 103:3783–3788.

130. Lee KN, Lee CS, Tae WC, et al. Crosslinking of alpha 2-antiplasmin to fibrin. *Ann N Y Acad Sci* 2001;936:335–339.

131. Tamaki T, Aoki N. Cross-linking of alpha 2-plasmin inhibitor to fibrin catalyzed by activated fibrin-stabilizing factor. *J Biol Chem* 1982;257: 14767–14772.

132. Aoki N. Clot retraction increases clot resistance to fibrinolysis by condensing alpha 2-plasmin inhibitor crosslinked to fibrin. [Comment]. *Thromb Haemost* 1993;70:376.

133. Hevessy Z, Haramura G, Boda Z, et al. Promotion of the crosslinking of fibrin and alpha 2-antiplasmin by platelets. *Thromb Haemost* 1996;75: 161–167.

134. Devine DV, Bishop PD. Platelet-associated factor XIII in platelet activation, adhesion, and clot stabilization. *Semin Thromb Hemost* 1996;22:409–413.

135. Reed GL, Matsueda GR, Haber E. Platelet factor XIII increases the fibrinolytic resistance of platelet-rich clots by accelerating the crosslinking of alpha 2-antiplasmin to fibrin. [See comment]. *Thromb Haemost* 1992;68: 315–320.

136. Reed GL, Matsueda GR, Haber E. Fibrin-fibrin and alpha 2-antiplasmin-fibrin cross-linking by platelet factor XIII increases the resistance of platelet clots to fibrinolysis. *Trans Assoc Am Physicians* 1991;104:21–28.

137. Ritchie H, Lawrie LC, Mosesson MW, et al. Characterization of crosslinking sites in fibrinogen for plasminogen activator inhibitor 2 (PAI-2). *Ann N Y Acad Sci* 2001;936:215–218.

138. Ritchie H, Lawrie LC, Crombie PW, et al. Cross-linking of plasminogen activator inhibitor 2 and alpha 2-antiplasmin to fibrin(ogen). *J Biol Chem* 2000;275:24915–24920.

139. Ritchie H, Robbie LA, Kinghorn S, et al. Monocyte plasminogen activator inhibitor 2 (PAI-2) inhibits u-PA-mediated fibrin clot lysis and is cross-linked to fibrin. *Thromb Haemost* 1999;81:96–103.

140. Jensen PH, Lorand L, Ebbesen P, et al. Type-2 plasminogen-activator inhibitor is a substrate for trophoblast transglutaminase and factor XIIIa. Transglutaminase-catalyzed cross-linking to cellular and extracellular structures. *Eur J Biochem* 1993;214:141–146.

141. Valnickova Z, Enghild JJ. Human procarboxypeptidase U, or thrombin-activable fibrinolysis inhibitor, is a substrate for transglutaminases. Evidence for transglutaminase-catalyzed cross-linking to fibrin. *J Biol Chem* 1998;273:27220–27224.

142. Aeschlimann D, Mosher D, Paulsson M. Tissue transglutaminase and factor XIII in cartilage and bone remodeling. *Semin Thromb Hemost* 1996; 22:437–443.

143. Greenberg CS, Birckbichler PJ, Rice RH. Transglutaminases: multifunctional cross-linking enzymes that stabilize tissues. *FASEB J* 1991;5: 3071–3077.

144. Mosher DF. Fibronectin. *Prog Hemost Thromb* 1980;5:111–151.

145. Hynes RO, Yamada KM. Fibronectins: multifunctional modular glycoproteins. *J Cell Biol* 1982;95:369–377.

146. Mosher DF, Fogerty FJ, Chernousov MA, et al. Assembly of fibronectin into extracellular matrix. *Ann N Y Acad Sci* 1991;614:167–180.

147. Mosher DF, Schad PE, Vann JM. Cross-linking of collagen and fibronectin by factor XIIIa. Localization of participating glutaminyl residues to a tryptic fragment of fibronectin. *J Biol Chem* 1980;255:1181–1188.

148. Procyk R, Blomback B. Factor XIII-induced crosslinking in solutions of fibrinogen and fibronectin. *Biochim Biophys Acta* 1988;967:304–313.

149. Mosher DF. Cross-linking of fibronectin to collagenous proteins. *Mol Cell Biochem* 1984;58:63–68.

150. Zhang Q, Mosher DF. Cross-linking of the NH2-terminal region of fibronectin to molecules of large apparent molecular mass. Characterization of fibronectin assembly sites induced by the treatment of fibroblasts with lysophosphatidic acid. *J Biol Chem* 1996;271:33284–33292.

151. Corbett SA, Lee L, Wilson CL, et al. Covalent cross-linking of fibronectin to fibrin is required for maximal cell adhesion to a fibronectin-fibrin matrix. *J Biol Chem* 1997;272:24999–25005.

152. Brown LF, Lanir N, McDonagh J, et al. Fibroblast migration in fibrin gel matrices. *Am J Pathol* 1993;142:273–283.

153. Lanir N, Ciano PS, Van de Water L, et al. Macrophage migration in fibrin gel matrices. II. Effects of clotting factor XIII, fibronectin, and glycosaminoglycan content on cell migration. *J Immunol* 1988;140:2340–2349.

154. Grinnell F. Fibronectin and wound healing. *J Cell Biochem* 1984;26: 107–116.

155. Naito M, Nomura H, Iguchi A, et al. Effect of crosslinking by factor XIIIa on the migration of vascular smooth muscle cells into fibrin gels. *Thromb Res* 1998;90:111–116.

156. Paye M, Nusgens BV, Lapiere CM. Factor XIII of blood coagulation modulates collagen biosynthesis by fibroblasts *in vitro*. *Haemostasis* 1989;19: 274–283.

157. Paye M, Nusgens B, Lapiere CM. Factor XIII of blood coagulation decreases the susceptibility of collagen precursors to proteolysis. *Biochim Biophys Acta* 1991;1073:437–441.

158. Mosher DF, Schad PE. Cross-linking of fibronectin to collagen by blood coagulation Factor XIIIa. *J Clin Invest* 1979;64:781–787.

159. Serrano K, Devine DV. Intracellular factor XIII crosslinks platelet cytoskeletal elements upon platelet activation. *Thromb Haemost* 2002;88: 315–320.

160. Asijee GM, Muszbek L, Kappelmayer J, et al. Platelet vinculin: a substrate of activated factor XIII. *Biochim Biophys Acta* 1988;954:303–308.

161. Bockenstedt P, McDonagh J, Handin RI. Binding and covalent cross-linking of purified von Willebrand factor to native monomeric collagen. *J Clin Invest* 1986;78:551–556.

162. Hada M, Kaminski M, Bockenstedt P, et al. Covalent crosslinking of von Willebrand factor to fibrin. *Blood* 1986;68:95–101.

163. Usui T, Takagi J, Saito Y. Propolypeptide of von Willebrand factor serves as a substrate for factor XIIIa and is cross-linked to laminin. *J Biol Chem* 1993;268:12311–12316.

164. Sane DC, Moser TL, Pippen AM, et al. Vitronectin is a substrate for transglutaminases. *Biochem Biophys Res Commun* 1988;157:115–120.

165. Francis RT, McDonagh J, Mann KG. Factor V is a substrate for the transamidase factor XIIIa. *J Biol Chem* 1986;261:9787–9792.

166. Wang DL, Annamalai AE, Ghosh S, et al. Human platelet factor V is crosslinked to actin by FXIIIa during platelet activation by thrombin. *Thromb Res* 1990;57:39–57.

167. Prince CW, Dickie D, Krumdieck CL. Osteopontin, a substrate for transglutaminase and factor XIII activity. *Biochem Biophys Res Commun* 1991; 177:1205–1210.

168. Raghunath M, Cankay R, Kubitscheck U, et al. Transglutaminase activity in the eye: cross-linking in epithelia and connective tissue structures. *Invest Ophthalmol Vis Sci* 1999;40:2780–2787.

169. Dardik R, Solomon A, Loscalzo J, et al. Novel proangiogenic effect of factor XIII associated with suppression of thrombospondin 1 expression. *Arterioscler Thromb Vasc Biol* 2003;23:1472–1477.

170. Borth W, Chang V, Bishop P, et al. Lipoprotein (a) is a substrate for factor XIIIa and tissue transglutaminase. *J Biol Chem* 1991;266:18149–18153.

171. Romanic AM, Arleth AJ, Willette RN, et al. Factor XIIIa cross-links lipoprotein(a) with fibrinogen and is present in human atherosclerotic lesions. *Circ Res* 1998;83:264–269.

172. Valenzuela R, Shainoff JR, DiBello PM, et al. Immunoelectrophoretic and immunohistochemical characterizations of fibrinogen derivatives in atherosclerotic aortic intimas and vascular prosthesis pseudo-intimas. *Am J Pathol* 1992;141:861–880.

173. Cohen I, Blankenberg TA, Borden D, et al. Factor XIIIa-catalyzed cross-linking of platelet and muscle actin. Regulation by nucleotides. *Biochim Biophys Acta* 1980;628:365–375.

174. Cohen I, Young-Bandala L, Blankenberg TA, et al. Fibrinoligase-catalyzed cross-linking of myosin from platelet and skeletal muscle. *Arch Biochem Biophys* 1979;192:100–111.

175. Kahn DR, Cohen I. Factor XIIIa-catalyzed coupling of structural proteins. *Biochim Biophys Acta* 1981;668:490–494.

176. Nurminskaya M, Linsenmayer TF. Identification and characterization of up-regulated genes during chondrocyte hypertrophy. *Dev Dyn* 1996;206: 260–271.
177. Karlsson C, Korayem AM, Scherfer C, et al. Proteomic analysis of the Drosophila larval hemolymph clot. *J Biol Chem* 2004;279:52033–52041.
178. Bale MD, Mosher DF. Thrombospondin is a substrate for blood coagulation factor XIIIa. *Biochemistry* 1986;25:5667–5673.
179. Bale MD, Ferry JD. Strain enhancement of elastic modulus in fine fibrin clots. *Thromb Res* 1988;52:565–572.
180. Mockros LF, Roberts WW, Lorand L. Viscoelastic properties of ligation-inhibited fibrin clots. *Biophys Chem* 1974;2:164–169.
181. Nielsen VG, Gurley WQ Jr, Burch TM. The impact of factor XIII on coagulation kinetics and clot strength determined by thrombelastography. *Anesth Analg* 2004;99:120–123.
182. Carr ME Jr. Turbidimetric evaluation of the impact of albumin on the structure of thrombin-mediated fibrin gelation. *Haemostasis* 1987;17:189–194.
183. Dale GL, Friese P, Batar P, et al. Stimulated platelets use serotonin to enhance their retention of procoagulant proteins on the cell surface. *Nature* 2002;415:175–179.
184. Cox AD, Devine DV. Factor XIIIa binding to activated platelets is mediated through activation of glycoprotein IIb-IIIa. *Blood* 1994;83:1006–1016.
185. Kreager JA, Devine DV, Greenberg CS. Cytofluorometric identification of plasmin-sensitive factor XIIIa binding to platelets. *Thromb Haemost* 1988; 60:88–93.
186. Kulkarni S, Jackson SP. Platelet factor XIII and calpain negatively regulate integrin alphaIIbbeta3 adhesive function and thrombus growth. *J Biol Chem* 2004;279:30697–30706.
187. Dardik R, Shenkman B, Tamarin I, et al. Factor XIII mediates adhesion of platelets to endothelial cells through alpha(v)beta(3) and glycoprotein IIb/IIIa integrins. *Thromb Res* 2002;105:317–323.
188. Devine DV, Andestad G, Nugent D, et al. Platelet-associated factor XIII as a marker of platelet activation in patients with peripheral vascular disease. *Arterioscler Thromb* 1993;13:857–862.
189. Huff T, Otto AM, Muller CS, et al. Thymosin beta4 is released from human blood platelets and attached by factor XIIIa (transglutaminase) to fibrin and collagen. *FASEB J* 2002;16:691–696.
190. Makogonenko E, Goldstein AL, Bishop PD, et al. Factor XIIIa incorporates thymosin beta4 preferentially into the fibrin(ogen) alphaC-domains. *Biochemistry* 2004;43:10748–10756.
191. Zisch AH, Schenk U, Schense JC, et al. Covalently conjugated VEG—fibrin matrices for endothelialization. *J Control Release* 2001;72:101–113.
192. Jaffer FA, Tung CH, Wykrzykowska JJ, et al. Molecular imaging of factor XIIIa activity in thrombosis using a novel, near-infrared fluorescent contrast agent that covalently links to thrombi. *Circulation* 2004;110: 170–176.
193. Ichinose A, Davie EW. Characterization of the gene for a subunit of human factor XIII (plasma transglutaminase), a blood coagulation factor. *Proc Natl Acad Sci U S A* 1988;85:5829–5833.
194. Board PG, Webb GC, McKee J, et al. Localization of the coagulation factor XIII A subunit gene (F13A) to chromosome bands 6p24–p25. *Cytogenet Cell Genet* 1988;48:25–27.
195. Griffiths LR, Board PG, Zwi MB, et al. The B subunit of coagulation factor XIII is linked to renin and the Duffy blood group to alpha-spectrin on human chromosome 1. *Hum Hered* 1989;39:107–109.
196. Bottenus RE, Ichinose A, Davie EW. Nucleotide sequence of the gene for the b subunit of human factor XIII. *Biochemistry* 1990;29:11195–11209.
197. Ichinose A, Kaetsu H. Molecular approach to structure-function relationship of human coagulation factor XIII. *Methods Enzymol* 1993;222:36–51.
198. Kida M, Souri M, Yamamoto M, et al. Transcriptional regulation of cell type-specific expression of the TATA-less A subunit gene for human coagulation factor XIII. *J Biol Chem* 1999;274:6138–6147.
199. Henriksson P, Becker S, Lynch G, et al. Identification of intracellular factor XIII in human monocytes and macrophages. *J Clin Invest* 1985; 76:528–534.
200. Conkling PR, Achyuthan KE, Greenberg CS, et al. Human mononuclear phagocyte transglutaminase activity cross-links fibrin. *Thromb Res* 1989; 55:57–68.
201. Invernizzi R, De Fazio P, Iannone AM, et al. Immunocytochemical detection of factor XIII A—subunit in acute leukemia. *Leuk Res* 1992;16:829–836.
202. Poon MC, Russell JA, Low S, et al. Hemopoietic origin of factor XIII A subunits in platelets, monocytes, and plasma. Evidence from bone marrow transplantation studies. *J Clin Invest* 1989;84:787–792.
203. Adany R, Antal M. Three different cell types can synthesize factor XIII subunit A in the human liver. *Thromb Haemost* 1996;76:74–79.
204. Anwar R, Miloszewski KJ. Factor XIII deficiency. *Br J Haematol* 1999; 107:468–484.
205. Anwar R, Stewart AD, Miloszewski KJ, et al. Molecular basis of inherited factor XIII deficiency: identification of multiple mutations provides insights into protein function. *Br J Haematol* 1995;91:728–735.
206. Girolami A, Cappellato MG, Vicarioto MA. Congenital factor XIII deficiency: type I and type II disease. *Br J Haematol* 1985;60:375–377.
207. Aslam S, Yee VC, Narayanan S, et al. Structural analysis of a missense mutation (Val414Phe) in the catalytic core domain of the factor XIII(A) subunit. *Br J Haematol* 1997;98:346–352.
208. Ichinose A, Souri M, Izumi T, et al. Molecular and genetic mechanisms of factor XIII A subunit deficiency. *Semin Thromb Hemost* 2000;26:5–10.
209. Kangsadalampai S, Chelvanayagam G, Baker R, et al. Identification and characterization of two missense mutations causing factor XIIIA deficiency. *Br J Haematol* 1999;104:37–43.
210. Kangsadalampai S, Yenchitsomanus P, Chelvanayagam G, et al. Identification of a new mutation (Gly420Ser), distal to the active site, that leads to factor XIII deficiency. *Eur J Haematol* 2000;65:279–284.
211. Mikkola H, Muszbek L, Haramura G, et al. Molecular mechanisms of mutations in factor XIII A-subunit deficiency: *in vitro* expression in COS-cells demonstrates intracellular degradation of the mutant proteins. *Thromb Haemost* 1997;77:1068–1072.
212. Mikkola H, Palotie A. Gene defects in congenital factor XIII deficiency. *Semin Thromb Hemost* 1996;22:393–398.
213. Koseki S, Souri M, Koga S, et al. Truncated mutant B subunit for factor XIII causes its deficiency due to impaired intracellular transportation. [Erratum appears in *Blood* 2001;97:3712 Note: Shitishima T (corrected to Shichishima T)]. *Blood* 2001;97:2667–2672.
214. Souri M, Izumi T, Higashi Y, et al. A founder effect is proposed for factor XIII B subunit deficiency caused by the insertion of triplet AAC in exon III encoding the second Sushi domain. *Thromb Haemost* 1998;80:211–213.
215. Izumi T, Hashiguchi T, Castaman G, et al. Type I factor XIII deficiency is caused by a genetic defect of its b subunit: insertion of triplet AAC in exon III leads to premature termination in the second sushi domain. *Blood* 1996; 87:2769–2774.
216. Hashiguchi T, Ichinose A. Molecular and cellular basis of deficiency of the b subunit for factor XIII secondary to a Cys430-Phe mutation in the seventh sushi domain. *J Clin Invest* 1995;95:1002–1008.
217. Losowsky MS, Miloszewski KJ. Factor XIII. *Br J Haematol* 1977;37:1–5.
218. Newman RS, Jalili M, Kolls BJ, et al. Factor XIII deficiency mistaken for battered child syndrome: case of "correct" test ordering negated by a commonly accepted qualitative test with limited negative predictive value. *Am J Hematol* 2002;71:328–330.
219. Al-Sharif FZ, Aljurf MD, Al-Momen AM, et al. Clinical and laboratory features of congenital factor XIII deficiency. *Saudi Med J* 2002;23: 552–554.
220. Francis JL. The detection and measurement of factor XIII activity: a review. *Med Lab Sci* 1980;37:137–147.
221. Francis JL, Todd PJ. Factor XIII deficiency. A family study by measurement of factor XIII subunits A and S. *Acta Haematol* 1979;62:167–172.
222. Katona EE, Ajzner E, Toth K, et al. Enzyme-linked immunosorbent assay for the determination of blood coagulation factor XIII A-subunit in plasma and in cell lysates. *J Immunol Methods* 2001;258:127–135.
223. Seitz R, Duckert F, Lopaciuk S, et al. Study Group. ETRO Working Party on Factor XIII questionnaire on congenital factor XIII deficiency in Europe: status and perspectives. *Semin Thromb Hemost* 1996;22:415–418.
224. Rampling MW. Factor XIII cross-linking and the rate of fibrinolysis induced by streptokinase and urokinase. *Thromb Res* 1978;12:287–295.
225. Mosher DF. Action of fibrin-stabilizing factor on cold-insoluble globulin and alpha2-macroglobulin in clotting plasma. *J Biol Chem* 1976;251: 1639–1645.
226. Hada M, Kato M, Ikematsu S, et al. Possible cross-linking of factor VIII related antigen to fibrin by factor XIII in delayed coagulation process. *Thromb Res* 1982;25:163–168.
227. Lorand L, Credo RB, Janus TJ. Factor XIII (fibrin-stabilizing factor). *Methods Enzymol* 1981;80(Pt C):333–341.
228. Board PG, Losowsky MS, Miloszewski KJ. Factor XIII: inherited and acquired deficiency. *Blood Rev* 1993;7:229–242.
229. Lechner K. Acquired inhibitors in nonhemophilic patients. *Haemostasis* 1974;3:65–93.
230. Otis PT, Feinstein DI, Rapaport SI, et al. An acquired inhibitor of fibrin stabilization associated with isoniazid therapy: clinical and biochemical observations. *Blood* 1974;44:771–781.
231. Tosetto A, Castaman G, Rodeghiero F. Acquired plasma factor XIII deficiencies. *Haematologica* 1993;78:5–10.
232. Bidwell E. Acquired inhibitors of coagulants. *Annu Rev Med* 1969;20:63–74.
233. Pohlmann-Eden B, Peters CN, Wennberg R, et al. Valproate induces reversible factor XIII deficiency with risk of perioperative bleeding. *Acta Neurol Scand* 2003;108:142–145.
234. Teich M, Longin E, Dempfle CE, et al. Factor XIII deficiency associated with valproate treatment. *Epilepsia* 2004;45:187–189.
235. Lorand L, Velasco PT, Hill JM, et al. Intracranial hemorrhage in systemic lupus erythematosus associated with an autoantibody against actor XIII. *Thromb Haemost* 2002;88:919–923.
236. Nilsson JL, Stenberg P, Ljunggren C, et al. Fibrin-stabilizing factor inhibitors. *Ann N Y Acad Sci* 1972;202:286–296.
237. Lorand L, Velasco PT, Rinne JR, et al. Autoimmune antibody (IgG Kansas) against the fibrin stabilizing factor (factor XIII) system. *Proc Natl Acad Sci U S A* 1988;85:232–236.
238. Fukue H, Anderson K, McPhedran P, et al. A unique factor XIII inhibitor to a fibrin-binding site on factor XIIIA. *Blood* 1992;79:65–74.
239. Barbui T, Rodeghiero F, Dini E. Factor-XIII subunits-A and -S in congenital deficiency and in acute myeloblastic leukemia. *Haematologica* 1974;59: 458–466.
240. Rodeghiero F, Barbui T, Dal Belin-Peruffo A, et al. Defective fibrin crosslinking in acute leukemia. *Thromb Haemost* 1984;52:343–346.
241. Petri M, Ellman L, Carey R. Acquired factor XIII deficiency with chronic myelomonocytic leukemia. *Ann Intern Med* 1983;99:638–639.

242. Shirahata A, Nakamura T, Shimono M, et al. Blood coagulation findings and the efficacy of factor XIII concentrate in premature infants with intracranial hemorrhages. *Thromb Res* 1990;57:755–763.

243. Eipe J, Yakulis V, Costea N. Factor XIII deficiency in BALB/c mice with plasmacytoma. *Cancer Res* 1977;37:3551–3555.

244. Zamboni P, De Mattei M, Ongaro A, et al. Factor XIII contrasts the effects of metalloproteinases in human dermal fibroblast cultured cells. *Vasc Endovasc Surg* 2004;38:431–438.

245. el-Hakim IE. The effect of fibrin stabilizing factor (F.XIII) on healing of bone defects in normal and uncontrolled diabetic rats. *Int J Oral Maxillofac Surg* 1999;28:304–308.

246. Cario E, Goebell H, Dignass AU. Factor XIII modulates intestinal epithelial wound healing *in vitro. Scand J Gastroenterol* 1999;34:485–490.

247. Chandler WL, Patel MA, Gravelle L, et al. Factor XIIIA and clot strength after cardiopulmonary bypass. *Blood Coagul Fibrinolysis* 2001;12:101–108.

248. Menzebach A, Cassens U, Van Aken H, et al. Strategies to reduce perioperative blood loss related to non-surgical bleeding. *Eur J Anaesthesiol* 2003; 20:764–770.

249. Gootenberg JE. Factor concentrates for the treatment of factor XIII deficiency. *Curr Opin Hematol* 1998;5:372–375.

250. Rivard GE, St Louis J, Lacroix S, et al. Immunoadsorption for coagulation factor inhibitors: a retrospective critical appraisal of 10 consecutive cases from a single institution. *Haemophilia* 2003;9:711–716.

251. Gailani D. An IgG inhibitor against coagulation factor XIII: resolution of bleeding after plasma immunoadsorption with staphylococcal protein A. *Am J Med* 1992;92:110–112.

252. Tosetto A, Rodeghiero F, Gatto E, et al. An acquired hemorrhagic disorder of fibrin crosslinking due to IgG antibodies to FXIII, successfully treated with FXIII replacement and cyclophosphamide. *Am J Hematol* 1995;48: 34–39.

253. Lewis JH, Szeto IL, Ellis LD, et al. An acquired inhibitor to coagulation factor 13. *Johns Hopkins Med J* 1967;120:401–407.

254. Fear JD, Miloszewski KJ, Losowsky MS. An acquired inhibitor of factor XIII with a qualitative abnormality of fibrin cross-linking. *Acta Haematol* 1984;71:304–309.

255. Guerrero Guerrero BA, Arocha-Pinango CL, Gil San Juan A. *Lonomia achelous* caterpillar venom (LACV) selectively inactivates blood clotting factor XIII. *Thromb Res* 1997;87:83–93.

256. Guerrero BA, Arocha-Pinango CL, Gil San Juan A. Degradation of human factor XIII by lonomin V, a purified fraction of *Lonomia achelous* caterpillar venom. *Thromb Res* 1997;87:171–181.

257. Finney S, Seale L, Sawyer RT, et al. Tridegin, a new peptidic inhibitor of factor XIIIa, from the blood-sucking leech *Haementeria ghilianii. Biochem J* 1997;324:797–805.

258. Chamouard P, Grunebaum L, Wiesel ML, et al. Significance of diminished factor XIII in Crohn's disease. *Am J Gastroenterol* 1998;93:610–614.

259. Demesmay K, Tissot E, Bulabois CE, et al. Factor XIII replacement in stem-cell transplant recipients with severe hemorrhagic cystitis: a report of four cases. *Transplantation* 2002;74:1190–1192.

260. Godje O, Haushofer M, Lamm P, et al. The effect of factor XIII on bleeding in coronary surgery. *Thorac Cardiovasc Surg* 1998;46:263–267.

261. Gerlach R, Raabe A, Zimmermann M, et al. Factor XIII deficiency and postoperative hemorrhage after neurosurgical procedures. *Surg Neurol* 2000;54:260–264; discussion 264–265.

262. Albala DM. Fibrin sealants in clinical practice. *Cardiovasc Surg* 2003; 11(Suppl. 1):5–11.

263. Hildenbrand T, Idzko M, Panther E, et al. Treatment of nonhealing leg ulcers with fibrin-stabilizing factor XIII: a case report. *Dermatol Surg* 2002;28:1098–1099.

264. Canonico S. The use of human fibrin glue in the surgical operations. *Acta Bio Medica* 2003;74(Suppl. 2):21–25.

265. Dunn CJ, Goa KL. Fibrin sealant: a review of its use in surgery and endoscopy. *Drugs* 1999;58:863–886.

266. Moront MG, Katz NM, O'Connell J, et al. The use of topical fibrin glue at cannulation sites in neonates. *Surg Gynecol Obstet* 1988;166: 358–359.

267. Groitl H, Scheele J. Initial experience with the endoscopic application of fibrin tissue adhesive in the upper gastrointestinal tract. *Surg Endosc* 1987; 1:93–97.

268. Hayward PJ, Mackay IS. Fibrin glue in nasal septal surgery. *J Laryngol Otol* 1987;101:133–138.

269. Bergsland J, Kalmbach T, Balu D, et al. Fibrin seal—an alternative to suture repair in experimental pulmonary surgery. *J Surg Res* 1986;40:340–345.

270. Cain JE Jr, Dryer RF, Barton BR. Evaluation of dural closure techniques. Suture methods, fibrin adhesive sealant, and cyanoacrylate polymer. *Spine* 1988;13:720–725.

271. Epstein GH, Weisman RA, Zwillenberg S, et al. A new autologous fibrinogen-based adhesive for otologic surgery. *Ann Otol Rhinol Laryngol* 1986;95:40–45.

272. Lilius P. Fibrin adhesive: its use in selected skin grafting. Practical note. *Scand J Plast Reconstr Surg Hand Surg* 1987;21:245–248.

273. Miyake K, Gotoh M, Sai S. Clinical application of a new fibrin adhesive (Tisseel) in urologic surgery. *Hinyokika Kiyo* 1985;31:357–364.

274. Regel G, Sturm JA, Neumann C, et al. Occlusion of bronchopleural fistula after lung injury—a new treatment by bronchoscopy. *J Trauma Injury Infect Crit Care* 1989;29:223–226.

275. Pers M. Plastic surgery for pressure sores. *Paraplegia* 1987;25:275–278.

276. Dickneite G, Metzner H, Nicolay U. Prevention of suture hole bleeding using fibrin sealant: benefits of factor XIII. *J Surg Res* 2000;93:201–205.

277. Gundry SR, Behrendt DM. A quantitative and qualitative comparison of fibrin glue, albumin, and blood as agents to pretreat porous vascular grafts. *J Surg Res* 1987;43:75–77.

278. Marx G, Mou X. Characterizing fibrin glue performance as modulated by heparin, aprotinin, and factor XIII. *J Lab Clin Med* 2002;140:152–160.

279. Kamitsuji H, Tani K, Yasui M, et al. Activity of blood coagulation factor XIII as a prognostic indicator in patients with Henoch-Schonlein purpura. Efficacy of factor XIII substitution. *Eur J Pediatr* 1987;146:519–523.

280. Noll T, Wozniak G, McCarson K, et al. Effect of factor XIII on endothelial barrier function. *J Exp Med* 1999;189:1373–1382.

281. Wozniak G, Noll T, Akinturk H, et al. Factor XIII prevents development of myocardial edema in children undergoing surgery for congenital heart disease. *Ann N Y Acad Sci* 2001;936:617–620.

282. Wozniak G, Noll T, Brunner U, et al. Topical treatment of venous ulcer with fibrin stabilizing factor: experimental investigation of effects on vascular permeability. *Vasa* 1999;28:160–163.

283. D'Argenio G, Iovino P, Cosenza V, et al. Factor XIII improves gastric stress lesions in rats. *Digestion* 2001;63:220–228.

284. Ogawa S, Glass CK. Factor XIIIA (cross)links AT1 receptors to atherosclerosis. [Comment]. *Cell* 2004;119:313–314.

285. Suzuki K, Iwata M, Ito S, et al. Molecular basis for subtypic differences of the "a" subunit of coagulation factor XIII with description of the genesis of the subtypes. *Hum Genet* 1994;94:129–135.

286. Suzuki K, Henke J, Iwata M, et al. Novel polymorphisms and haplotypes in the human coagulation factor XIII A-subunit gene. *Hum Genet* 1996; 98:393–395.

287. Anwar R, Gallivan L, Edmonds SD, et al. Genotype/phenotype correlations for coagulation factor XIII: specific normal polymorphisms are associated with high or low factor XIII specific activity. *Blood* 1999;93:897–905.

288. Killick CJ, Barton CJ, Aslam S, et al. Prenatal diagnosis in factor XIII-A deficiency. *Arch Dis Child Fetal Neonatal Ed* 1999;80:F238–F239.

289. Sadasivan C, Yee VC. Interaction of the factor XIII activation peptide with alpha-thrombin. Crystal structure of its enzyme-substrate analog complex. *J Biol Chem* 2000;275:36942–36948.

297. Board PG. Genetic heterogeneity of the B subunit of coagulation factor XIII: resolution of type 2. *Ann Hum Genet* 1984;48:223–228.

298. Komatsu N, Kido A, Kimura Y, et al. Polymorphism of coagulation factor XIII B subunit: further occurrence of FXIIIB*15 in Japanese and phenotyping in bloodstains. *Int J Legal Med* 1992;104:317–319.

290. Balogh I, Szoke G, Karpati L, et al. Val34Leu polymorphism of plasma factor XIII: biochemistry and epidemiology in familial thrombophilia. *Blood* 2000;96:2479–2486.

291. Wartiovaara U, Perola M, Mikkola H, et al. Association of FXIII Val34Leu with decreased risk of myocardial infarction in Finnish males. *Atherosclerosis* 1999;142:295–300.

292. Butt C, Zheng H, Randell E, et al. Combined carrier status of prothrombin 20210A and factor XIII-A Leu34 alleles as a strong risk factor for myocardial infarction: evidence of a gene-gene interaction. [See comment]. *Blood* 2003;101:3037–3041.

293. Marin F, Gonzalez-Conejero R, Lee KW, et al. A pharmacogenetic effect of factor XIII valine 34 leucine polymorphism on fibrinolytic therapy for acute myocardial infarction. *J Am Coll Cardiol* 2005;45:25–29.

294. Reiner AP, Heckbert SR, Vos HL, et al. Genetic variants of coagulation factor XIII, postmenopausal estrogen therapy, and risk of nonfatal myocardial infarction. *Blood* 2003;102:25–30.

295. Weger M, Renner W, Stanger O, et al. Role of factor XIII Val34Leu polymorphism in retinal artery occlusion. *Stroke* 2001;32:2759–2761.

296. Morange PE, Henry M, Brunet D, et al. Factor XIIIV34L is not an additional genetic risk for venous thrombosis in factor V Leiden carriers. *Blood* 2001;97:1894–1895.

# CHAPTER 18 ■ PLASMINOGEN–PLASMIN SYSTEM

NUALA A. BOOTH AND FEDOR BACHMANN

Hemostasis requires mechanisms both to stop bleeding by formation of a hemostatic plug and to limit the plug's development, allowing reestablishment of normal blood flow. The latter function is largely accomplished by localized activation of the plasminogen–plasmin enzyme system, also called the *fibrinolytic system*. The system is finely tuned, as it has to be to accomplish healing of a vascular lesion without compromising the early stability of the hemostatic plug and to limit activity to the injured area. There is a dynamic balance between coagulant and fibrinolytic activities, each of which represents a further balance between proteolytic and inhibitory proteins. Excessive local or systemic fibrinolytic activity can result in bleeding, often occurring after a delay, as the weakened plug is dissolved. Conversely, an inadequate fibrinolytic response may retard lysis of a thrombus and contribute to its extension.

Plasmin is the main fibrinolytic enzyme. It is a trypsinlike serine protease that degrades fibrin, and it is generated by activation of the zymogen, plasminogen. The central players dictating the activity of the system are the plasminogen activators (PAs) and the inhibitors of both the activation stage and of plasmin activity. The two major PAs that occur in the circulating blood, tissue-type plasminogen activator (tPA) and urinary-type plasminogen activator (uPA), also called *urokinase* or UK, are also serine proteases. Inhibitors, most of which are of the serine protease inhibitor (serpin) family, regulate the proteases. These are PA inhibitors, plasminogen activator inhibitor 1 (PAI-1; see Chapter 19) and PAI-2, and $\alpha_2$-antiplasmin, the principal inhibitor of plasmin. Receptors and binding proteins for plasminogen and the PAs on endothelial cells (see Chapter 22), platelets and leucocytes regulate local generation of plasmin. The best characterized of these receptors is the urinary-type plasminogen activator receptor (uPAR). Tables 18-1 and 18-2 list several of the properties of the genes, messenger ribonucleic acids (mRNAs), and proteins of the components of the fibrinolytic system, together with modulating factors. These include factor XII and the contact phase of coagulation, in which interactions with prekallikrein and kininogen also promote plasminogen activation. They also include apolipoprotein (a), cytokines, growth factors and hormones (see Chapter 6), the PAI-1–binding protein vitronectin, the thrombin-activatable fibrinolytic inhibitor (TAFI) (see Chapter 20), the low density lipoprotein receptor–related protein (LRP, identical to the $\alpha_2$-macroglobulin receptor), the mannose receptor, annexin II, and several other inhibitors that affect the physiology of fibrinolysis (see Chapter 23).

Like the serine proteases of blood coagulation, fibrinolytic proteases generally exist in a zymogen form, a single-chain form of the molecule that is activated by cleavage of a single peptide bond. All the active serine proteases cleave arginine and/or lysine bonds and originated from a simple trypsinlike ancestor protease (1,2). In the case of the fibrinolytic proteases, the products are all in a two-chain form held together by one or more disulfide bonds. An exception to this rule is tPA, which is an active protease in its single-chain form; tPA can be considered to be at one end of the scale of zymogenicity, with plasminogen as a totally inactive example at the other (3).

The typical structure of these proteases (Fig. 18-1) is that they have an N-terminal A chain containing several independently folded modules or domains, which have particular binding properties, and a C-terminal B chain, which is the protease domain. The kringle domain—named after a Danish pastry—is approximately 80 residues long and is held together by three internal disulfide bonds. The finger domains are homologous to type I and type II fibronectin regions. Type I finger domains are approximately 50 residues long, contain two internal disulfide bonds, and may play a role in fibrin binding. The epidermal growth factor (EGF) domains, which are homologous with a module in the EGF precursor, contain 53 residues and three internal disulfide bonds. In several proteins, these domains bind to specific cell-surface receptors or binding proteins. The apple domain has been found only in prekallikrein and factor XI, in which it occurs as a quadruple repeat of 90 residues in the N-terminal portion of these molecules. Like the kringle domains, it contains three internal disulfide bonds. The protease domain contains the catalytic triad, Ser195, His57, and Asp102 (chymotrypsin numbering), and the domain comprises approximately 250 amino acid residues and four disulfide bonds. The protease domain is well conserved, with particularly high sequence identity in the vicinity of the three active site residues and at the N-terminus.

The components of the fibrinolytic system are discussed next, beginning with the central enzyme, plasmin, and its precursor, plasminogen, then considering in turn plasminogen activators, the different inhibitors of plasmin, and plasmin generation, with a final summary on the balance of the system.

## PLASMINOGEN

Human plasminogen (PLG) is the zymogen form of the main fibrinolytic protease, plasmin (EC 3.4.21.7). PLG is a single-chain glycoprotein of 92 kDa, consisting of 791 amino acid residues and approximately 2% carbohydrate (Table 18-1). In the human adult, the plasma concentration of PLG is approximately 200 mg per L, which corresponds to 2 $\mu$M (Table 18-2). The half-life ($t_{1/2}$) of native PLG, which has a glutamic acid residue at its N-terminus (Glu–PLG), is approximately 2.2 days; the slightly degraded Lys–PLG (see subsequent section, "Activation of Plasminogen to Plasmin") has a much shorter $t_{1/2}$ of 0.8 days (4). The principal production site for PLG is the liver, but PLG is present in the extravascular space of most tissues, and some, such as eosinophils, the kidney, and the cornea, may be capable of synthesizing it (5–8).

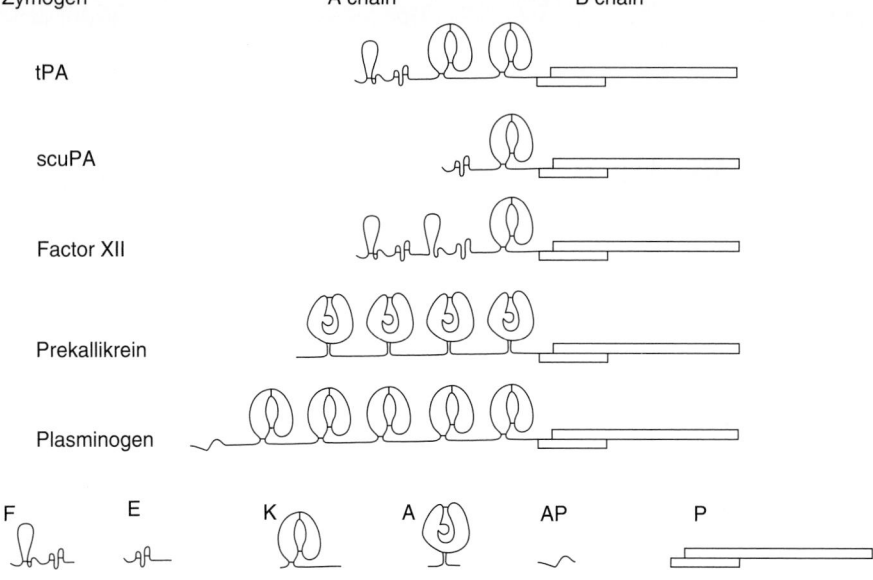

**FIGURE 18-1.** Structural elements of some serine proteases. A, apple domain (approximately 80 residues); AP, activation peptide; E, epidermal growth factor domain (approximately 32 residues); F, fibronectin finger (approximately 40 residues); K, kringle (approximately 90 residues); P, protease domain (B chain) (approximately 250 residues); scuPA, single-chain urokinase; tPA, tissue-type plasminogen activator.

## TABLE 18-1

### CHROMOSOME LOCATION AND GENE ORGANIZATION IN CONSTITUENTS OF THE PLASMINOGEN-PLASMIN SYSTEM

| Factor | Symbol | Chromosome | Gene (kb) | mRNA (kb) | Exons |
|---|---|---|---|---|---|
| Plasminogen | *PLG* | 6q26-q27 | 52.5 | 2.9 | 19 |
| tPA | *PLAT* | 8p12-p11 | 32.7 | 2.7 | 14 |
| uPA | *PLAU* | 10q24 | 6.4 | 2.4 | 11 |
| PAI-1 | *PLANH1* | 7q21.3-q22 | 12.2 | 2.4/3.2 | 9 |
| PAI-2 | *PLANH2* | 18q22.1 | 16.5 | 1.9 | 8 |
| Factor XII | *F12* | 5q33-qter | 12 | 2.6 | 14 |
| Prekallikrein | *KLK3* | 4q34-q35 | 22 | 2.4 | 15 |
| HMW kininogen | *KNG* | 3q27 | 27 | 3.2 | 11 |
| Vitronectin | *VTN* | 17q11 | 4.5 | 1.6 | 8 |
| C1-inhibitor | *C1NH* | 11q12-q13.1 | 17 | 1.8 | 8 |
| $\alpha_2$-Antiplasmin | *PLI* | 17p13 | 16 | 2.2 | 10 |
| $\alpha_2$-Macroglobulin | *A2M* | 12p13.3-p12.3 | 48 | 4.6 | 36 |
| Histidine-rich glycoprotein | *HRG* | 3q27 | 15.5 | 2.1 | 7 |
| Tetranectin, monomer | *TNA* | 3p22-p21.3 | 12 | 0.9 | 3 |
| Apolipoprotein (a) | *APOAL2.1* | 6q26-27 | [b] | [b] | [b] |
| TAFI | *CPB* | 13q14.11 | 48 | 1.8 | 11 |
| uPAR | *PLAUR* | 19q13.1-q13.2 | 23 | 1.4 | 7 |
| Annexin II[a] | *ANX2* | 15q21-q22 | — | 1.3 | — |
| LRP ($\alpha_2$-MR) | *LRP1* | 12q13-q13.3 | 92 | 15 | 89 |
| $\alpha$-Enolase | *ENO1* | 1pter-1p36.13 | >18 | 1.7 | 12 |
| Mannose-receptor | *MRC1* | 10p13 | — | 5.1 | — |

mRNA, messenger ribonucleic acid; tPA, tissue-type plasminogen activator; uPA, urinary-type plasminogen activator; PAI-1, plasminogen activator inhibitor 1; PAI-2, plasminogen activator inhibitor 2; HMW, high-molecular-weight; C1-inhibitor, complement component 1 esterase inhibitor; TAFI, thrombin-activatable fibrinolysis inhibitor; uPAR, urinary-type plasminogen activator receptor; LRP, low density lipoprotein receptor–related protein; MR, macroglobulin receptor.
[a]Heavy chain of tetramer.
[b]Variable, depending on the number of kringle 4 inserts.

## TABLE 18-2

### PROPERTIES OF PROTEIN CONSTITUENTS OF THE PLASMINOGEN-PLASMIN SYSTEM

| Factor | $M_r$ (kDa) | Amino acid residues | Concentration (mg/L) | Molar concentration | Carbohydrates (%) | $t_{1/2}$ | Function |
|---|---|---|---|---|---|---|---|
| Plasminogen | 92 | 791 | 200 | 2 $\mu$M | 2 | 2.2 d | z |
| tPA | 68 | 530 | 0.005 | 70 pM | 7/13 | 4 min | p |
| uPA | 54 | 411 | 0.002 | 40 pM | 7 | 7 min | z |
| PAI-1 | 52 | 379 | 0.01 | 200 pM | 5 | 8 min | i |
| PAI-2 | 46/70 | 393 | <0.005 | <70 pM | 0/35 | — | i |
| Factor XII | 80 | 596 | 30 | 0.375 $\mu$M | 17 | 2–3 d | z |
| Prekallikrein | 88 | 619 | 40 | 0.45 $\mu$M | 15 | — | z |
| HMW kininogen | 110 | 626 | 70 | 0.60 $\mu$M | 54[a] | 9 h | c |
| Vitronectin | 78 | 459 | 350 | 4.5 $\mu$M | 44[a] | — | c |
| C1-inhibitor | 105 | 478 | 180 | 1.7 $\mu$M | 49 | 70 h | i |
| $\alpha_2$-Antiplasmin | 70 | 452 | 70 | 1 $\mu$M | 13 | 3 d | i |
| $\alpha_2$-Macroglobulin | 725 | 1,451 | 2,500 | 3 $\mu$M | 8 | — | i |
| Histidine-rich glycoprotein | 75 | 507 | 100 | 1.5 $\mu$M | 14 | 3 d | i |
| Tetranectin, monomer[b, c] | 22.5 | 181 | 10 | 0.5 mM | 0 | 3 d | c |
| Apolipoprotein(a)[d] | 300–800 | — | <7 | — | 29 | — | m |
| TAFI (pro-CpU) | 60 | 401 | 5 | 75 nM | 23[a] | 10 min[e] | z, i |
| uPAR | 55 | 313 | — | — | 57[a] | — | r |
| Annexin II[b, f] | 38 | 338 | — | — | — | — | r |
| LRP ($\alpha_2$-MR) | 600 | 4,525 | — | — | 15[a] | — | r, i |
| $\alpha$-Enolase | 54 | 433 | — | — | 15[a] | — | r |
| Mannose receptor | 175 | 1,437 | — | — | 8[a] | — | r |

z, protease zymogen; tPA, tissue-type plasminogen activator; p, protease; uPA, urinary-type plasminogen activator; PAI-1, plasminogen activator inhibitor 1; i, inhibitor; PAI-2, plasminogen activator inhibitor 2; HMW, high-molecular-weight; c, cofactor; C1-inhibitor, complement component 1 esterase inhibitor; m, modulator; TAFI, thrombin-activatable fibrinolysis inhibitor; uPAR, urinary-type plasminogen activator receptor; LRP, low density lipoprotein receptor–related protein; MR, macroglobulin receptor; r, receptor.
$M_r$ of mature proteins is listed.
[a]Estimated value, calculated from difference of molecular weight determined by SDS-PAGE and weight of sum of amino acids derived from complementary DNA.
[b]$M_r$ of nonglycosylated form as listed in Swiss protein base ExPASy.
[c]Heavy chain of homotrimer.
[d]Many isoforms due to 13 up to 37 type 4 kringle motifs.
[e]Activated form.
[f]Heavy chain of heterotetramer (formed by two heavy and two 10-kDa light chains).

## Structural Organization

The PLG gene is 52.5 kb, the largest among the fibrinolytic proteins. It is located on chromosome 6q26-q27 (9), close to two genes for apolipoprotein (a) and for the PLG-related genes A and B (10,11). Amino acid sequence analysis showed the structural features of N-terminal activation peptide, five kringles, and the protease domain (12). Subsequent isolation of mRNA, and later of the gene, confirmed the original sequence, except for an additional isoleucine residue at position 67 (13).

The 19 exons of the *PLG* gene are separated by 18 introns that follow the general GT-AG rule found in other eukaryotic genes. The first exon encodes the signal sequence, with two exons encoding the activation peptide and each kringle; the remaining six exons code for the intervening sequence and the protease domain (see Fig. 18-2). Each of the five kringles consists of 78 to 80 residues, and they are well-conserved between species (14). Functionally, the kringles give PLG the ability to bind to exposed lysyl residues in fibrin (15,16), $\alpha_2$-antiplasmin (17), tetranectin (18), histidine-rich glycoprotein (19), collagen (20), high-molecular-weight (HMW) and low-molecular-weight (LMW) kininogen (21), thrombospondin (22), and cell surface receptors. The affinity of the kringles for lysyl residues is also exploited to isolate it from human plasma by affinity chromatography (23).

The kringle structure is shaped by a characteristic 1–6, 2–4, 3–5 disulfide bond pattern involving six conserved Cys residues

in positions 1, 22, 51, 63, 75, and 80 (kringle 5 numbering). A single nonconserved Cys in position 4 of kringle 2 forms an interkringle disulfide bond with Cys43 in kringle 3 (not shown on Fig. 18-2) and thereby restricts the mobility of kringles 2 and 3. Solution structures have been determined for kringle 1 (24), kringle 2 (25), kringle 2 + 3 (26), and kringle 4 (27). Crystallographic structures have been solved for kringle 1 (28,29), kringle 4 (30), and kringle 5 (31). The human PLG kringles have different affinities and specificities for $\omega$-amino acid ligands. The tightest binding site for $\varepsilon$-aminocaproic acid ($\varepsilon$ACA) is provided by kringle 1 [dissociation constant ($K_d$) of 9 $\mu$M] (32,33) followed by kringle 4 (32,34,35) and kringle 5 (34,35). Kringle 2 displays only a weak interaction with $\varepsilon$ACA, probably not of functional significance, whereas kringle 3 shows no interaction (36).

Experimentally, kringle 4 can be isolated from PLG by digestion with elastase, which cleaves after small amino acids and at relatively frequent Val–Val sequences. Therefore, digestion with elastase typically yields three major components: a fragment containing kringles 1 through 3, isolated kringle 4, and kringle 5 attached to the protease portion of PLG (12). The latter fragment, also called *mini-PLG*, can be activated to plasmin by PAs (37–39). Although it has some affinity for fibrin (16,40), it does not bind to lysine–Sepharose and therefore is separated from kringles 1–3 and kringle 4, which do bind lysine (12,32). Kringle 1 can be obtained from kringles 1–3 by further digestion with other enzymes, such as *Staphylococcus aureus* V8 protease (41).

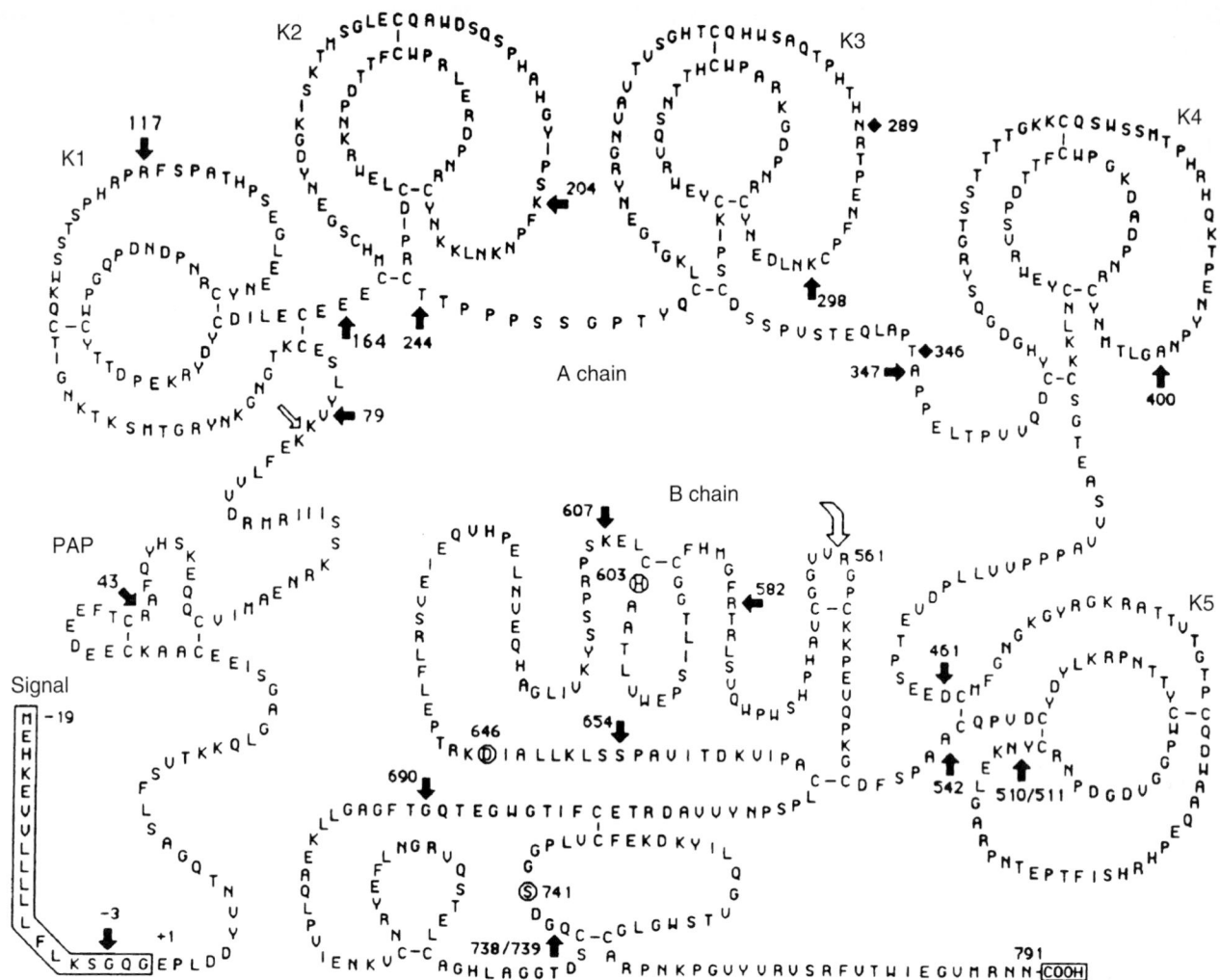

**FIGURE 18-2.** Sequence of the human plasminogen molecule. Positions of the 18 introns are indicated by *solid arrows* at (for type 1 and 2 introns) or in between (for type 0 introns) residues. The 19-residue signal peptide (shown in a box with *negative numbers*) is cleaved by signal peptidase at the Gly–Glu peptide bond. Conversion of plasminogen to plasmin occurs after the peptide bond Arg561–Val562 (shown by an *open, curved arrow*) is cleaved by plasminogen activators. PAP refers to the preactivation peptide generated by the action of plasmin on Glu–plasminogen; primary (but not sole) cleavage site is Lys77–Lys78 bond (shown by an *open, straight arrow*). K1–K5, kringles, located in the A chain; the B chain remains attached to the A chain after cleavage of the 561–562 bond via the disulfide bonds Cys548–Cys666 and Cys558–Cys566. Carbohydrate attachment sites (Asn289 and Thr346) are shown by *diamonds*. (From Petersen TE, Martzen MR, Ichinose A, et al. Characterization of the gene for human plasminogen, a key proenzyme in the fibrinolytic system. *J Biol Chem* 1990;265:6104, with permission.)

Crystallography has revealed that the kringle 4 structure is highly stabilized by an internal hydrophobic core and an extensive hydrogen bonding network. The lysine binding site (LBS) on the surface of kringle 4 is an open, elongated, shallow trough, formed by the hydrophobic residues Trp62, Phe64, and Trp72, surrounded by the positively charged Lys35 and Arg71 on one side and, at a distance of approximately 7 Å, the negatively charged side chains of Asp55 and Asp57 (see Fig. 18-3) (30). This structure provides for ideal docking of zwitterions such as lysine or εACA, whose opposite charges also are approximately 7 Å apart. The interaction between binding site and ligand is enhanced further by the close van der Waals contacts between the methylene carbons of ligand and the aromatic residues of the amino acids in the center of the binding site (30). The binding sites in kringles 1 and 5 are similarly constructed. In kringle 1, Arg34 takes the place of Lys35 in kringle 4 (30,42); in kringle 5, Leu71 is substituted for Arg71 in kringle 4 (31).

The catalytic domain of PLG (B chain) is made up of 230 residues and is homologous with the trypsin family of serine proteases. In the active site, it contains three amino acids: His603, Asp646, and Ser741. Two groups of investigators have elucidated the crystal structure of micro-PLG mutants. The main observations, a deformed catalytic triad and a blocked S1 specificity pocket, are similar in the two crystal structures (43,44). This unusual structural feature has only been observed in the crystal structure of factor D of the complement system, in contrast to the preformed catalytic triad observed in other trypsinlike structures.

## Activation of Plasminogen to Plasmin

All known PAs cleave the Arg561–Val562 bond in PLG (see Fig. 18-4). The B chain of the resulting two-chain Glu–plasmin

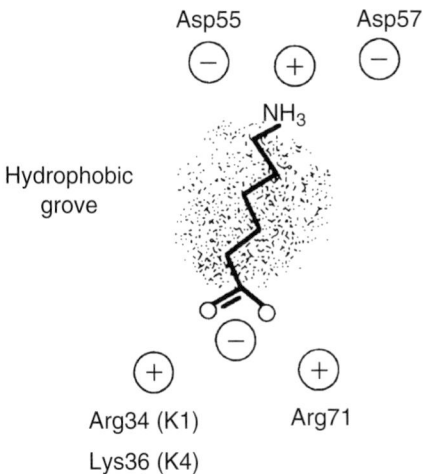

**FIGURE 18-3.** Model of the interaction site of plasminogen kringles 1 and 4 with ε-aminocaproic acid (depicted in *heavy lines*), a lysine analog. A hydrophobic core on the surface of an elongated shallow trough is surrounded by two clusters of positively and negatively charged amino acids.

molecule remains attached to the A chain by two disulfide bonds. When these PAs are added to Glu–PLG *in vitro*, the generation of trace amounts of plasmin results in cleavage of the *N*-terminus by hydrolysis of one or several of the following bonds: Arg68–Met69, Lys77–Lys78, or Lys78– Val79 (45,46). The final product obtained is Lys–plasmin (Fig. 18-4). Under physiologic conditions, the plasmin-mediated conversion to Lys–PLG probably does not occur in circulating blood (47) because free

plasmin is inactivated rapidly by $\alpha_2$-antiplasmin. Studies with monoclonal antibodies that recognize Lys–PLG but not Glu–PLG revealed no free Lys–PLG nor bound Lys–plasmin in normal human plasma and only minimal increases of these forms in patients who received thrombolytic therapy (48).

Several ω-aminocarboxylic acids, such as 6-aminohexanoic acid (εACA, 6-AHA), *p*-aminomethyl benzoic acid (*p*-AMBA), and *trans*-4-amino-methyl-cyclohexane-carboxylic acid (*trans*-AMCA, also known as tranexamic acid), inhibit the functional activity of plasmin *in vitro* and *in vivo* by binding to the LBS of plasmin(ogen), thereby inhibiting the binding of plasmin(ogen) to fibrin (49,50). These compounds are therefore termed *antifibrinolytic*. It should be noted that their effects depend strongly on the concentration used; at micromolar to low millimolar concentrations, these compounds actually increase the activation rate. They do this by inducing a conformational change, making Glu–PLG adopt a structure similar to that of Lys–PLG, which is more easily activated to plasmin. The change reflects the loss of interaction of the *N*-terminal preactivation peptide with LBS on the kringles (51,52). It causes a marked decrease in the Michaelis constant ($K_M$) for activation with tPA or uPA, by approximately one order of magnitude, down to the range of the physiologic concentration of PLG in human plasma (53,54). In Glu–PLG, Lys50 binds to LBSs on kringles (51,52), making these LBS less available for binding to C-terminal lysine in fibrin, PLG receptors, and other proteins. Therefore Lys–PLG binds with higher affinity to fibrin than does Glu–PLG.

Conformational differences between Glu– and Lys–PLG have been revealed by small-angle neutron scattering. Glu–PLG goes from having a radius of gyration of 39 Å to 56 Å in the presence of εACA (55). The closed form, in which the five kringle domains and the catalytic domain interact to produce an ellipsoid shape, is less activatable than the open form (see Fig. 18-5),

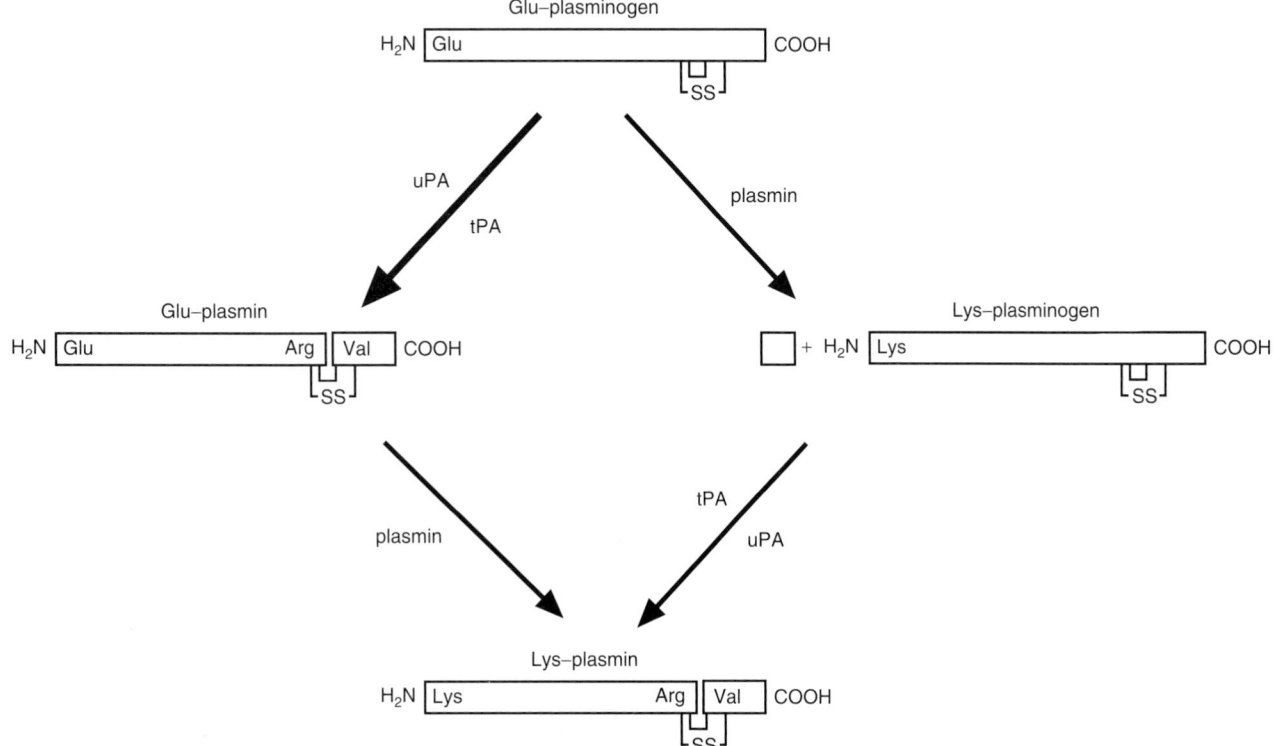

**FIGURE 18-4.** Activation of native Glu–plasminogen. In the absence of plasmin inhibitors, tissue plasminogen activator (tPA) or urinary plasminogen activator (uPA) converts Glu–plasminogen to Glu–plasmin; the latter then converts Glu–plasmin(ogen) to Lys–plasmin(ogen).

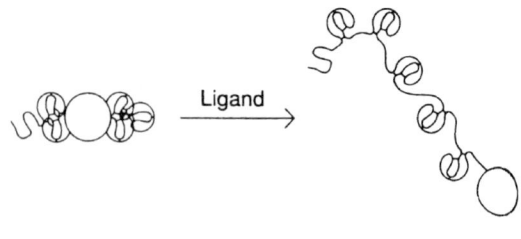

**Closed form**            **Open form**

FIGURE 18-5. A sketch of the conformational change in plasminogen induced on occupation of a weak lysine binding site by the ligand ε-aminocaproic acid. In the absence of ligand, the domains in plasminogen interact to form a molecule with the overall shape of a prolate ellipsoid. Binding of the ligand converts this into an extended flexible structure in which the interaction between the domains is abolished. The closed and open forms are drawn to scale. (From Mangel WF, Lin B, Ramakrishnan V. Characterization of an extremely large, ligand-induced conformational change in plasminogen. *Science* 1990;248:69, with permission.)

whose increased flexibility facilitates the binding of PAs, leading to approximately a 10-fold decrease of $K_M$. Furthermore, the open form, taken up by PLG after binding to fibrin, enables the proteolytic domain to sweep over a larger area and therefore be more efficient in the digestion of fibrin than a closed form with restricted mobility. Activatability of Glu–PLG by PAs is dependent on other factors as well, such as the presence of anions, which in the human plasma are mainly chloride ions, and of the divalent cations $Ca^{2+}$, $Mg^{2+}$, and $Mn^{2+}$. All these ions counteract the effect of εACA and stabilize PLG in the Glu-form, which is poorly activatable by PAs (54,56).

Many modulators increase or decrease the rate of PLG activation; the most important of these is fibrin. PLG binds to fibrin, directing the process of clot lysis to its target, binding that is competed by ω-amino carboxylic acids (57). Identification of the binding sites was achieved by examining the products of elastase digestion of PLG. Kringle 1–3 and miniplasminogen bound to fibrin, but kringle 4 did not (15,16,58,59). Notably, there is no close correlation between the affinities of kringles for fibrin and lysine/εACA (see Table 18-3).

Partial degradation of fibrin by plasmin creates a positive feedback mechanism, whereby native Glu–PLG is bound to newly created C-terminal lysines on the fibrin molecules, particularly on the C-terminal portion of the α chain (60–64). A few studies support the concept that PLG might bridge adjoining fibrin molecules and that probably both kringle 5 and kringle 1

## TABLE 18-3

AFFINITIES OF PLASMINOGEN KRINGLES FOR $ε_2$-AMINOCAPROIC ACID AND FOR NATIVE FIBRIN

| Kringle number(s) | Affinity for εACA | Affinity for native fibrin |
|---|---|---|
| 1–3 | High | Moderate |
| 4 | Moderate | Very low[a] |
| 5 | Low | High |

[a]A nuclear magnetic resonance imaging study has shown that kringle 4 can bind to partially digested fibrin, which has many C-terminal lysyl sites exposed (58). This binding was abolished by ε-aminocaproic acid (εACA).

bind to fibrin, albeit not at the same binding site (59,65,66). There is little consensus on the values of the dissociation constants and number of binding sites for the binding of PLG, particularly of Glu–PLG to fibrin. Taking all reported figures together, it appears that an average $K_d$ for the binding of Glu–PLG to native fibrin is approximately 5 $μM$ and that of Lys–PLG, roughly one order of magnitude lower. In the presence of partially digested fibrin, the $K_d$ for the binding of Glu–PLG approaches that of Lys–PLG for native fibrin (0.5 $μM$) (63,64). This probably means that Glu–PLG, after binding to fibrin, takes on the open configuration (Fig. 18-5) and functionally behaves like Lys–PLG.

Recombinant microplasminogen, consisting of residues 542–791, can be activated to microplasmin by all four common PAs: tPA, uPA, streptokinase (SK), and staphylokinase (SAK) (39). Autocatalytically produced microplasmin consisting of the last 31 amino acid residues of the A chain and B chain exhibited a similar affinity for fibrin as regular plasmin but a markedly lower catalytic rate constant ($k_{cat}$ = 0.0076 per second vs. 0.064 per second for plasmin) (38).

## Cell Binding of Plasminogen

PLG binds to different cell types and a number of binding proteins have been identified on human and other cells (67), α-enolase (68) and annexin II (69) being the most studied. All are abundant proteins, and generally the binding occurs through Lys residues. Interestingly, PLG binding to the prion protein PrPsc distinguishes between the normal and misfolded conformers (70). The association of PLG with the various binding proteins is not always of high affinity, and the fact that so many proteins can serve this function precludes their being viewed strictly as PLG receptors. The abundance of such binding sites does make it likely that this phenomenon indeed potentiates local plasmin generation (71).

## Angiostatins

Many primary tumors have been found to suppress the growth of their remote metastases or of a second and different tumor. At least in part, this effect is due to angiostatin, originally described as a 38-kDa protein and identified as an internal proteolytic fragment of PLG comprising kringles 1–4 (72). It appears that tumor-mediated proteolysis is responsible for the generation of angiostatin, through uPA-induced PLG activation and the opening up the inter-kringle and other disulfide bonds by plasmin reductases (73,74), which include known PLG-binding proteins that act as plasmin reductases (67,75,76). Similarly, proteolytic cleavage of PLG by macrophage elastase (MMP-12), or stromelysin-1 (MMP-3), or a 24-kDa endopeptidase from a *Chrysobacterium* species generated angiostatinlike fragments (77,78).

The antiproliferative effect of PLG fragments is not restricted to the originally described kringle 1–4 or 1–5 fragments. Recombinant fragments containing kringles 1–3 (79–81), or even isolated kringles 1, 2, 3, or 5, but not kringle 4, had antiproliferative activity similar to the originally described larger fragments (79,82,83). On the other hand, isolated kringle 4 was potent in inhibiting endothelial cell migration (84). Endothelial cell proliferation assays revealed that angiostatin induces apoptosis (85) and also appears to have a role in the prevention of atherosclerosis, in that it inhibits smooth muscle cell proliferation and migration *in vitro* (86). In all of these assays, intact PLG was inactive. The sum of these data suggests that various internal fragments of PLG exert powerful biological effects and that fragments of HMW kininogen (87) and of apolipoprotein (a) (88) have similar effects.

## Variants of Plasminogen

The PLG molecule is subject to considerable variation in the normal population. In addition to the limited proteolysis and activation processes already discussed, the two important sources of variation are glycosylation and genetic polymorphism.

### Glycosylation

Human Glu–PLG occurs in two variants that differ in glycosylation. PLG variant 1 is diglycosylated, with N-linked carbohydrate moiety of the mannose type with 10 to 11 monosaccharide units on Asn289, and an O-linked moiety of three to four residues on Thr346 (89). PLG 2, which accounts for a little more than half of the PLG molecules, contains only the carbohydrate group at Thr346 (90). Both of these forms exhibit, on isoelectric focusing, additional heterogeneity with respect to their sialic acid content (45,46,91,92). Therefore, each of the two variants produces six additional isoforms with pIs between 6.1 and 6.6. All 12 molecular forms are present in plasma from single donors (4).

In the absence of fibrin, PLG 1 appears to be more easily activated to plasmin than is PLG 2, but this difference is not observed in the presence of fibrin. Variant 1 changes its conformation more easily in the presence of fibrin or tranexamic acid than does variant 2 (93). Variant 2 was cleared more rapidly than variant 1 and bound five times faster to a deendothelialized vessel surface (94–96). A novel glycosylation site containing a trisaccharide on Ser249 has been described (97), and another may exist at Ser339 (98); a further serine residue, Ser578, can be phosphorylated (99).

### Polymorphism

Isoelectric focusing of neuraminidase-treated plasma (which removes sialic acid) revealed several bands of activatable PLG, representing the genetic polymorphism of PLG alleles. The nomenclature, adopted in 1984 (100), is that the two most commonly observed variants found in all races are called *PLG A* (A for acidic pI) and *PLG B* (B for basic pI). Recently, the molecular basis of these common polymorphisms was reported: PLG A have Asp453, and PLG B have Asn453 (101). Variants with intermediate pI are designated as PLG M. Variants with more acidic pI than PLG A receive, in addition to the letter A, a numerical suffix that increases with decreasing pI of the variant. The variants with more basic pI than PLG B receive a numerical suffix that increases with increasing pI of the variant. Alleles are designated with an asterisk (e.g., PLG*A3), and silent (null) PLG alleles are designated PLG*Q0, with Q0 standing for quantitatively zero or nonexpressed. The frequency of the alleles in 1,330 unrelated West Germans was 70.1% for PLG*A, 27.7% for PLG*B, 1.5% for PLG*A3, 0.6% for PLG*R (R: the sum of all other rare PLG alleles), and 0.35% for PLG*Q0 (100). In the Japanese population, the frequency of the allele PLG*A is considerably higher (95%) than in the Western population (102).

Since the first report in 1978 of a hereditary molecular abnormality in PLG in a patient with recurrent thrombosis (103), several hundred cases have been described with a deficiency of PLG antigen and activity (type I), or a normal level of antigen but reduced activity (type II, dysplasminogenemia). In most instances, a thromboembolic event or the presence of ligneous conjunctivitis has been the starting point for family studies. Only those cases in which the molecular defect has been identified are listed in Table 18-4 (101–114); updates can be found

## TABLE 18-4

### CONGENITAL PLASMINOGEN MUTATIONS

| Residue | Mutation | References | Type | Other names | Clinical manifestations |
|---------|----------|------------|------|-------------|-------------------------|
| 9 | Thr to Asn | 106 | I | — | — |
| 19 | Lys to Glu | 106 | I | — | — |
| 128 | Lys to Pro | 101 | I | — | — |
| 133 | Cys to stop | 104 | I | — | — |
| 134 | Arg to Lys | 101 | I | — | — |
| 212 | Lys deletion | 106 | I | — | — |
| 216 | Arg toHis | 105 | I | — | Ligneous conjunctivitis |
| 355 | Val to Phe | 107 | II | Nagoya | Thrombophilia |
| 374 | Val to Phe | 107 | — | Nagoya-I | Thrombophilia |
| 453 | Asp to Asn | 101 | — | — | — |
| 460 | Glu to stop | 108 | I | — | — |
| 513 | Arg to His | 106 | I | — | — |
| 572 | Ser to Pro | 108 | I | — | Thrombophilia (secretion defect) |
| 597 | Trp to Cys | 105,106 | I | — | Ligneous conjunctivitis |
| 597 | Trp to stop | 104 | I | — | Ligneous conjunctivitis |
| 601 | Ala to Thr | 107,112 | II | Tochigi, Osaska II | Thrombophilia |
| 620 | Ala to Thr | 107 | I | Nagoya-II, Tochigi, Kagoshima | Thrombophilia |
| 675 | Ala to Thr | 109,111 | I | | Thrombophilia? |
| 676 | Asp to Asn | 112,113 | II | Osaka-II, III | None |
| 693 | Gly to Arg | 101 | II | — | — |
| 732 | Gly to Arg | 114 | II | Kanagawa-I | — |

on the OMIM (Online Mendelian Inheritance in Man) Web site. The sum of all data does not prove conclusively that the heterozygous presence of one mutant PLG gene results in an increased incidence of thromboembolism (115,116). In healthy subjects, the Ala601Thr mutation is found in 2.2% and 2.9%, respectively, of the Japanese and Chinese Han populations (107,112). Similarly, Lys19 to Glu occurs relatively frequently in association with hypoplasminogenemia (104,117), and there is controversy over whether it should be regarded as a polymorphism (118). Homozygous deficiencies, however, are clearly associated with ligneous conjunctivitis, caused primarily by Arg216 to His or Trp597 to stop mutations (106), and replacement therapy with PLG is effective (108).

It is not yet clear why some mutations cause ligneous conjunctivitis and why very low functional PLG levels can be tolerated in some individuals, without thrombosis occurring (106).

PLG-deficient mice, depending on genetic background, also develop ligneous conjunctivitis (119). These mice are predisposed to severe thrombosis and deposit intravascular and extravascular fibrin in many tissues (120,121). Growth is retarded, rectal prolapse is frequent, and Plg$^{-/-}$ mice die prematurely, but ovulation, embryonic development, and reproduction are normal (122). Wound healing and tissue remodeling are impaired (123,124), and response to an inflammatory stimulus is diminished (125). After electric injury to the femoral artery, wound healing, removal of necrotic debris, leukocyte infiltration, smooth muscle cell immigration, and arterial neointima formation were greatly delayed in Plg$^{-/-}$ mice (126), suggesting that PLG deficiency might reduce the development of atherosclerosis. However, in Plg$^{-/-}$ mice crossed with apolipoprotein E–deficient mice prone to develop early atherosclerotic lesions, the spontaneous development of intimal lesions was greatly accelerated (127). Plg$^{-/-}$ mice crossed with fibrinogen$^{-/-}$ mice were restored to normality in many of these cases, demonstrating the causative role of intravascular and extravascular fibrin deposition (128,129).

## Regulation of Expression

Plasma levels of PLG are generally rather stable, as discussed further in the section, "Balance of the System", but there is an increase in the acute-phase response (130). Two sequence elements of CTGGGA common to acute-phase reactant genes are at position 76 to 81 and −553 to −558 (13). Three interleukin-6 (IL-6)–responsive elements are at positions −830, −518, and +117 in the 5′-flanking region (131).

The PLG gene has a TATA-like sequence, TGTAA, at position −16 rather than a canonical TATA box. This sequence corresponds exactly to the TATAA box of the homologous apo(a) gene, located 31 bp upstream from its transcription start site. Accordingly, the TGTAA sequence is probably involved in the expression of the TATA-less promoter in the PLG gene (131). Two main regions conferring liver specificity of expression to the PLG gene were found in the cis-acting element, AAAAATA, at −2194 to −2188 and +48 to +61 (132). Several other putative regulatory transcription elements are present in the 5′-flanking region (reviewed in 131). On the 3′-flanking region, the location of the consensus polyadenylation sequence AATAAA and of potential CAYTG signals suggests the presence of three polyadenylation sites (13).

## PLASMINOGEN ACTIVATORS

There are two physiologic PAs, tPA (tissue-type) and uPA (urinary-type, UK), named after the original sources of purified proteins. A further activation system, which is dependent on factor XII, prekallikrein, and HMW kininogen, is known as the contact PA pathway. There are also PAs from bacteria and the vampire bat, which are included here because of their therapeutic use in thrombolysis; they are also of mechanistic interest. The two human proteases, tPA and uPA, are also implicated respectively in neurobiology (133) and tumor biology (134). These aspects are not considered further in this chapter, which focuses on PAs in hemostasis.

## TISSUE-TYPE PLASMINOGEN ACTIVATOR

tPA, a serine protease of 68 kDa (EC 3.4.21.68), also known as vascular PA or extrinsic activator, is a glycoprotein of 527 residues. It exerts its effect primarily in the vascular system, because it is produced and secreted by endothelial cells (135); many other cells in culture also synthesize tPA. In normal plasma, the antigen concentration of tPA is approximately 5 μg per L, which corresponds to approximately 70 pM (136). Most of the tPA is present in a complex with its primary inhibitor, PAI-1 (137,138).

### Structural Organization

The gene for tPA comprises 32.7 kb and is located on bands p12-p11 on chromosome 8 (139), containing 14 exons (140) (Table 18-1). The mature protein exists in two forms of different length. The N-terminus of Bowes melanoma cell tPA can be either glycine or serine (141), but serine is nearly always the N-terminus of recombinant tPA (142). In this chapter, the numbering is based on the Ser-terminus of recombinant tPA because of the extensive literature that exists on structure-function in this form of tPA. In this numbering, glycine −3 probably represents the real N-terminus of tPA.

The structure of tPA (Fig. 18-1) shows a finger and EGF domain, and two kringle domains in the A chain, whereas the protease domain is the B chain. The finger domain extends from residues 6 to 43 and is 34% identical to the first finger of bovine fibronectin. It is involved in the binding of tPA to fibrin, as shown by mutants lacking kringle domains, which still bound to fibrin (143). Consistent with this, a degraded form of tPA that had lost the N-terminal 12 kDa bound less well to fibrin than wild-type tPA (144). The binding of the finger domain is independent of LBS, in that it cannot be blocked by εACA (145). Structurally, the finger domain is very similar to the seventh type 1 repeat of human fibronectin (146).

The epidermal growth factor domain (residues 44–92) is structurally similar to other EGF structures, as shown by nuclear magnetic resonance (NMR) (147). There is some evidence from deletion mutagenesis that the EGF domain binds to the mannose receptor and is involved in tPA clearance. Kringle 2 has affinity for lysine, ω-amino acids such as εACA, and fibrin, whereas no function has yet been ascribed to kringle 1 (143). The affinity for the binding of εACA (a model for C-terminal lysine residues) and of N-acetyllysine methyl ester (a model for intrachain lysine residues) is approximately equal, suggesting that tPA does not prefer C-terminal lysine residues (as PLG does) for binding. Intact tPA and a variant consisting only of kringle 2 and the protease domains were found to bind to the cyanogen bromide (CNBr) fibrinogen fragment FCB-2, which also binds PLG and acts as a stimulator of tPA-catalyzed PLG activation. In both cases, binding was completely inhibited by εACA, pointing to the involvement of LBS in this interaction (143).

The structure–function relations among kringle 2 and ω-amino acids and lysine have been studied in detail, using

NMR (148), microcalorimetry (149), crystallography (150), and site-directed mutagenesis (42,149,151). The crystal structure of kringle 2 resembles that of PLG kringle 4; there are, however, differences in the lysine-binding pocket. The core of kringle 2 is formed by a hydrophobic cluster of three tryptophan residues in positions 25, 63, and 74, surrounded by aromatic and hydrophobic side chains that form, at the surface of the kringle, a hydrophobic grove. Ligand binding appears to rely mostly on the integrity of Trp63 and Trp74, and an aromatic residue at position 76, which is normally Tyr (152). Mutation of the critical amino acids Lys33, Asp55, Asp57, or Trp72 markedly diminished binding to lysine–Sepharose, or interaction with εACA, or both (153).

The catalytic domain of tPA is typical of other serine proteases, with the catalytic triad His322, Asp371, and Ser478. The 2.3-Å crystal structure of the protease domain revealed strong structural similarity with other trypsinlike serine proteases, thrombin in particular (154). The active site cleft is shaped and narrowed by four surface loops. The loop around Arg299 exhibits five additional residues, Arg298-Arg-Ser-Pro-Gly302, compared with chymotrypsin. It projects out of the molecular surface as a β-hairpin and is of fundamental importance for the interaction with PAI-1 (3). The 60-loop around Arg327 is similar to but shorter than the corresponding loop in thrombin. Further loops are found around Ser381 and Gly465. The fully solvent-exposed hydrophobic region, comprising amino acids 420 to 423 of tPA, which forms a surface loop near one edge of the active site of tPA, constitutes an important secondary site for the interaction of tPA with PLG in the absence of fibrin.

tPA is secreted as a single-chain molecule (sctPA) but can easily be converted to the two-chain form (tctPA) by plasmin, which cleaves the Arg275–Ile276 peptide bond. Surprisingly, the single-chain form is not a zymogen but a protease which, in the presence of fibrin, is nearly as active as the two-chain form (155). The nonzymogenicity of tPA has been explored in a series of comparisons, with confirmatory mutagenesis studies (3,156). It emerges that other zymogens have a triad Asp194, His40 and Ser32 (chymotrypsin numbering), the His and Ser of which are replaced in tPA by Phe305 and Ala292, respectively. The constructed double mutant Phe305His and Ala292Ser was more zymogenic (156).

## Enzymatic Properties of Tissue-Type Plasminogen Activator

tPA is unusually specific; its major substrate is PLG, in which it cleaves the Arg561–Val562 bond. It is an inefficient activator of PLG in the absence of fibrin, but in its presence the activation of PLG is greatly potentiated (157). Since Thorsen et al.'s original observation that fibrin binds tPA but not urokinase (158), this phenomenon has been much studied. Binding of sctPA and tPA is roughly comparable, although the single-chain form may bind slightly better (159). The $K_d$ for binding of tPA to fibrin clots in the absence of PLG ranges from 140 nM to 400 nM (155,159,160). In the presence of PLG, the affinity of tPA to fibrin increases approximately 20-fold ($K_d$ 20 nM) (161). These observations are explained by formation of a ternary complex comprising tPA, PLG, and fibrin or binding of tPA to PLG, which, on binding to fibrin, has taken on an open conformation. The isolated A chain of tPA was indeed shown to bind to Glu- and mini-PLG with a $K_d$ of 100 nM (162).

The kinetic parameters reported for the activation of PLG by tPA show great variation. This is due to many potential experimental variables, different tPA and PLG preparations, different substrate concentrations, and, for studies using fibrin or fibrin derivatives, the nature of the fibrin stimulator used. In the absence of fibrin, $K_M$ values for the activation of Glu–PLG by tPA range from 9 μM to slightly more than 100 μM (155,163,164). In general, $K_M$ is three to four times lower with tPA than with sctPA when the activation of Glu–PLG is investigated in the absence of fibrin. This difference disappears when fibrin is present and $K_M$ values typically are two orders of magnitude smaller, with only moderate increases of $k_{cat}$. Values for $K_M$ in the presence of fibrin range from 0.16 μM to 1.1 μM PLG, and $k_{cat}$ values from 0.1 per second to 1.1 per second (155,164). Several authors found nonlinear enzyme kinetics (162,163,165), and there appear to be two phases in the activation of Glu–PLG by tPA in the presence of fibrin, with an initial $K_M$ of 1.05 μM and $k_{cat}$ 0.15 per second. Later in the process, as new high-affinity binding sites for PLG and tPA are exposed in partially digested fibrin (61–63,166, 167), $K_M$ decreased to 0.07 μM, whereas the $k_{cat}$ was unchanged (165). The important message from these studies is that PLG is not activated by tPA in the presence of fibrin, because it is only in the presence of fibrin that the $K_M$ for the reaction is consistent with the circulating concentration of 2 μM.

Distinct sites in the fibrin molecule have been identified as accelerating PLG activation; notably they are not available for binding in fibrinogen but become exposed in fibrin (168). The D-region of fibrin binds both PLG and tPA in a region that encompasses the sequence Aα148–160, and tPA alone, in a site including γ312–324. Both these associations are of low affinity and in the circulation the Aα148–160 site would bind PLG, which is present in much higher concentrations than tPA. Another binding in the D-region encompasses γ311–336 and γ337–379, which are linked by a disulfide bond (169). Antibodies have revealed that there is a tPA binding site that includes γ312–324 (170). Higher affinity sites for binding tPA and PLG are in the C-terminus of the α chain, within the region Aα392–610 (171). The conformational changes that occur on fibrinogen cleavage and fibrin assembly (172) reveal new sites for binding of tPA and PLG, and for enhancement of PLG activation.

Huge numbers of mutations have been engineered into tPA to change its characteristics, with the aim of making it an even more effective therapeutic agent. The most striking of these is the series of mutations to make tPA resistant to PAI-1. Madison et al. identified the importance of interactions between the positively charged tPA sequence 298–302 and the negatively charged PAI-1 sequence 350–355 (173). Mutagenesis of Arg298, 299, and 304 resulted in a mutant that was inhibited 120,000 times less rapidly by PAI-1 than wild-type tPA (174). These observations led, in part, to the development of the new tPA mutant tenecteplase (TNK–tPA), in which the sequence 296–299 (Lys-His-Arg-Arg) is replaced by four alanines (175). This variant also exhibits slower clearance, by virtue of its changed glycosylation, and its enhancement of PLG activation is more selective for fibrin above fibrinogen and the fibrin fragment DDE (176).

## Tissue-Type Plasminogen Activator Receptors and Binding Proteins

A number of structurally unrelated components that bind tPA have been described. Some have the potential to localize tPA on a surface to which PLG also binds, and therefore to potentiate activation. Many of the proteins in this group contain a C-terminal lysyl group and therefore also are receptors for PLG, as already discussed (69). This group includes 42-kDa annexin II (69,177), 45-kDa actin (178), heparan sulfate and chondroitin sulfate–like proteoglycans (179), cytokeratin 8 and 18 (180), and tubulin (181). Overexpression of the tPA receptor annexin II, as it occurs in patients with promyelocytic leukemia exhibiting the t(15;17) translocation in the leukemic cells, is associated with a hyperfibrinolytic state. The abnormally high levels of annexin II bind PLG and tPA and generate plasmin, with consumption of $\alpha_2$-antiplasmin, leading to bleeding (182). Interestingly, other studies show that such patients also have abnormally high fibrinolytic activity that is clearly due to uPA (183).

Several as yet poorly defined tPA receptors have been identified on endothelial cells, and it is not clear yet whether some of these are identical with each other (184). In addition to actin, human umbilical vein endothelial cells (HUVEC) express two further 37-kDa and 45-kDa tPA–binding proteins (178), whereas another study found a 20-kDa tPA binding protein, which was characterized and purified (185). This protein did not interact with PLG, but binding was inhibited by $\omega$-amino acids, suggesting that the lysine-binding site of tPA is involved, but the purified protein was not recognized by antibodies to annexin II or $\alpha$-enolase. In the presence of this receptor, PLG activation by tPA was enhanced 90-fold. A receptor that interacts with the B chain of tPA and potentiates PLG activation approximately 100-fold has been described on vascular smooth muscle cells (186). It has now been defined as type-II transmembrane protein p63 (CKAP4) (187).

## Glycosylation of Tissue-Type Plasminogen Activator

tPA has four potential glycosylation sites, of which three are occupied in type I (Asn117, Asn184, and Asn448) and two in type II tPA (Asn117 and Asn448), making it 3 kDa smaller (163). Residue 117 is predominantly N-glycosylated with oligomannose-type structures, whatever the source. Residues 184 and 448 are predominantly associated with complex-type structures in recombinant tPA and in tPA isolated from fibroblast cell lines, but with both complex- and oligomannose-type structures when isolated from melanoma cells (188). Glycosylation at residue 184 influences the biological properties of tPA. The type II form has a higher affinity for lysine (and fibrin) and a higher fibrinolytic activity (189). tPA, like uPA, has an O-linked fucose on Thr61 in the EGF domain (190) and this affects binding to HepG2 cells and may be relevant to clearance (191).

## Polymorphisms

The best-studied polymorphism is an Alu insertion/deletion polymorphism. Most clinical studies including a large prospective study (192), found no correlation with acute myocardial infarction or stroke, but one case–control study found that homozygotes for the insertion had twice as many cases of acute myocardial infarction as homozygotes for the deletion (193). The homozygous insertion polymorphism is also associated with a high rate of release of tPA in response to stress (194). Further study of the promoter identified additional polymorphisms, one of which ($-7351C > T$) has been shown to be functional at the level of transcription, with decreased release of tPA in individuals carrying the T allele (195).

## Synthesis, Release, and Clearance of Tissue-Type Plasminogen Activator

tPA is produced by many different cell types in culture, and its synthesis can be upregulated by diverse agents. Endothelial cells are a principal source and, in these cells, release rather than synthesis is also important in controlling local tPA. Finally, tPA is very rapidly cleared from the circulation. These three aspects are now reviewed briefly.

### Synthesis

tPA expression in cultured cells can be stimulated through multiple intracellular signaling pathways. Vasoactive substances, such as thrombin and histamine, increase tPA synthesis in HUVEC, acting through their G-coupled receptors and the protein kinase C (PKC) pathway (196–198). Steroid hormones (199,200) and retinoids can increase synthesis of tPA (201,202). It is important to note that not all endothelial cells synthesize tPA *in vivo* and that expression is restricted to small vessels (203–205).

The tPA gene contains common transcription elements, with three TATA boxes; a CAAT box is present at position $-112$ to $-116$. DNase I protection analysis of the tPA gene promoter in human endothelial- and phorbol-stimulated HeLa cells revealed several protected regions. A cytotoxic factor/nephritic factor-1–like element is at $-92$ to $-77$; three Sp1 binding sites are at positions $-72$ to $-66$, $-48$ to $-39$, and $+60$ to $+74$; a cyclic adenosine monophosphate–responsive element CRE-like/tetradecanoyl phorbolacetate–responsive element TRE-like element is between $-102$ and $-115$; and three GC/GT boxes are between $-43$ and $+68$ (196,206,207). Several of these *cis*-acting elements have been shown to be involved in constitutive and phorbol ester–induced expression of tPA mRNA. Between $-2,288$ to $-2,129$ and $-2,390$ to $-2,289$ are two further regulatory elements necessary for constitutive expression of the tPA gene in Bowes melanoma cells (208). Far upstream at $-7.3$ kb is located a functional retinoic acid response element consisting of a direct repeat of the GGGTCA motif spaced by five nucleotides (209). The region $-7,145$ to $-9,758$ comprises a multihormone-responsive enhancer that is activated by glucocorticoids, progesterone, androgens, mineralocorticoids, and 1,25-dihydroxyvitamin $D_3$, but not by estrogens (199,200). A nuclear factor NF1 site, 600 bp upstream from the transcription start site, acts as a repressor of tPA expression and confers cell specificity to tPA expression (205).

### Release

Acute release of tPA is established from early studies on venous occlusion for 10 or 20 minutes, a procedure widely used in patients (210–212). During venous stasis, at midway between systolic and diastolic blood pressure, venous outflow from the occluded segment decreases more than the (diminished) arterial inflow and represents approximately one third of remaining arterial inflow (210). Much of the locally produced tPA therefore remains in the occluded limb and is not cleared. Young patients with a history of recurrent venous thromboembolism exhibited an abnormal response to venous occlusion and this could be attributed either to subnormal tPA release or, more often, to elevated PAI-1 (137,211,212). In isolated cases with severe forms of von Willebrand disease, a complete lack of response to venous stasis and the infusion of 1-deamino-8-D-arginine vasopressin (DDAVP) was found (213). These patients may have a functional or structural defect in their endothelial cells. It should be noted, however, that release of von Willebrand factor (VWF) and tPA occur by different mechanisms (214). Lower PA activity is found in leg veins than in proximal veins. It has been estimated that the synthesis and release rate of tPA during forearm occlusion ranges between 0.5 to 1.1 ng per mL of blood, but only 0.08 to 0.11 ng per mL in an occluded leg (210). Increased hydrostatic pressure in the leg veins may be responsible for the diminished production of tPA. Applying a 20-minute venous occlusion test, patients who were immobilized were found to release considerably more tPA from leg veins after 12 to 33 days of recumbency than at the beginning of immobilization (215). The low content of tPA in human calf veins therefore may be one etiologic factor for development of deep venous thrombosis.

There is evidence that continuous release of tPA from the vasculature can diminish a thrombotic response. The human tPA gene was cloned into an adenoviral vector under the control of the Rous sarcoma virus (RSV) promoter and the construct was tested in an *in vivo* model of arterial thrombosis. All animals developed obstructive thrombosis except those treated with the viral vector; this was actually more effective than tPA therapeutic regime (216). This echoes two independent studies in the 1980s of patients who had consistently raised tPA activity as the cause of a hereditary lifelong hemorrhagic disorder (217,218). One of these (217) had a total absence of fibrin deposits or thrombi, despite widespread arterial disease; he died of cerebral bleeding. The underlying cause was not a deficiency of PAI-1 or any other known inhibitor. No further cases have been reported, despite an intensive search in many laboratories.

The mechanism of release has been studied in cultured endothelial cells, from which much of the tPA is released continuously, but there is an additional regulated pathway, where tPA is stored in specialized storage vesicles (219–222). Extracellular stimuli then trigger the release of stored tPA to the cell surface. The amount of tPA stored in storage vesicles in various cells, such as endothelial, neuroendocrine, and adrenal chromaffin cells, is large (220,222). In rats, the tissue stores of tPA were calculated to be sufficient to maintain a steady-state plasma level of tPA for 2 days in the absence of protein synthesis (223). Compounds that triggered release within a few minutes include bradykinin, histamine, eledoisin, acetylcholine, $\beta$-adrenergic agents, platelet-activating factor, endothelin, calcium ionophore A-23187, and acidosis (224,225). These compounds induce calcium influx into the endothelial cell and activate G-protein–coupled receptors (226). Some interventions that cause elevated tPA act through decreased clearance, as discussed in the next section. Among these are exercise and $\alpha$-adrenergic agents (227). In all situations in which epinephrine levels are increased, such as stress, anxiety, and exercise, tPA antigen levels increase (138,228).

DDAVP was widely used in the 1980s to study the release potential for tPA in patients with idiopathic or recurrent thrombosis (215,229–231). Earlier observations had suggested that DDAVP acts through a release of a pituitary PA–releasing hormone (229). Comparison of the effects of DDAVP and sodium nitroprusside showed that nitroprusside produced an even greater increase of forearm blood flow but no increase of tPA, but that DDAVP indeed stimulated tPA release from the vascular bed (232). The increase of circulating tPA levels after intraarterial infusion of acetylcholine and methacholine was shown to be mediated by muscarinic receptors (232–234). Bradykinin and substance P both induced tPA release after being infused into the forearm of volunteers (235,236), and the releasable pool of tPA, rather than the availability of PAI-1 to inhibit it, was the key factor (237).

## Clearance

Free tPA and tPA in complex with inhibitors are rapidly removed from the circulation and bound to receptors on endothelial cells and hepatocytes. In normal individuals, the $t_{1/2}$ of tPA is approximately 3 minutes (238,239). Studies on isolated rat hepatocytes suggested that the complex was cleared more rapidly than free tPA (240) but, *in vivo* in humans, clearance of tPA was calculated to be faster in subjects with low PAI-1 (3.5 minutes) versus high PAI-1 (5.3 minutes; $P = 0.006$), consistent with $t_{1/2}$ of 2.4 minutes for free tPA and $t_{1/2}$ of 5.0 minutes for tPA/PAI-1 complexes ($P = 0.006$) (241). Because of its clearance by the liver and the dependence of clearance on liver blood flow (242–244), the $t_{1/2}$ may be considerably prolonged in patients with hepatic cirrhosis (239,245).

Early studies showed that the uptake of tPA by liver endothelial and by Kupffer cells was inhibited by ovalbumin, leading to the identification of the mannose receptor as a major tPA receptor (246). Binding of ligands to the mannose receptor is pH sensitive and dependent on $Ca^{2+}$ ions. Binding is inhibited by mannose-albumin, mannan, D-mannose, and L-fucose, and particularly by cluster mannosides of the composition $M_6L_5$ (246–248). tPA has a high affinity ($K_d$ 1 to 4 nM) for the mannose receptor compared to other glycoproteins, the $K_d$ for most being 60 to 600 nM (248). In mice, the administration of estradiol leads to increased expression of the mannose receptor and increased clearance of tPA (249). Mutants of tPA have been engineered for slower clearance by replacement of Asn117, which is normally glycosylated, with Gln. Such mutants, including TNK–tPA, are cleared more slowly than wild-type tPA. It is not known whether the fucose residue at Thr61 in the EGF domain also binds to the mannose receptor or to the previously described fucose receptor (250).

The other major pathway for tPA clearance involves the LRP/$\alpha_2$-macroglobulin receptor (251,252). The 600-kDa LRP, the largest plasma membrane protein described, comprises 4,525 residues. It mediates the clearance of apolipoprotein E–enriched chylomicron remnants, toxins, cytokines, complexes of $\alpha_2$-macroglobulin with proteases from all subclasses, and free tPA and tPA/PAI-1 and uPA/PAI-1 complexes. Complex formation of tPA with PAI-1 increases the rate of clearance by LRP by at least one order of magnitude compared with that of free tPA (253). The binding sites for tPA/PAI-1 and for uPA/PAI-1 complexes are situated in the second complement-type domain cluster of LRP (254–256). The receptor-associated protein (RAP) inhibits endocytosis of most ligands to LRP (251,254,257).

Other LRP-like multiligand receptors, such as glycoprotein 330 and the 130-kDa very low density lipoprotein (VLDL) receptor, also can mediate the clearance of free and PAI-1 complexed tPA (258–260). For efficient uptake and clearance of several ligands, LRP works in cooperative fashion with coreceptors, for instance uPAR for the LRP-mediated degradation of uPA/PAI-1 complexes (261,262). Some monocytelike cell lines that expressed LRP on the cell surface were unable to degrade tPA, leading to the idea that a coreceptor was necessary for efficient degradation of tPA by LRP (263).

## Deficiency

Congenital deficiencies of tPA or uPA have not been described in humans and were assumed to constitute a lethal condition, until these genes were successfully deleted in mice (264). Unexpectedly, mice with a disrupted tPA gene developed normally. Microscopic examination revealed mild glomerulonephritis. In a plasma clot lysis assay, fibrinolytic activity was lower than in wild-type animals. After endotoxin-induced thrombogenic stimulation, tPA$^{-/-}$ mice had more extended thrombotic lesions than tPA$^{+/+}$ mice. The abnormalities found were rather mild, but mice with a double deficiency of tPA and uPA had severe spontaneous thrombosis and exhibited impaired health, reduced survival, and diminished fertility (264,265). It can be concluded that, in mice, there is some redundancy of biological functions with respect to PAs. On the other hand, it is obvious that a complete knockout of the fibrinolytic activators leads to severe disease. It is not known to what extent these results apply to human pathophysiology. The double knockout has a similar phenotype to the PLG knockout, consistent with tPA and uPA being the major mammalian activators of PLG. These mice have had a profound impact on understanding other functions of tPA, in areas as diverse as reproduction (266), neuronal development (133,267) and learning (133,268).

# URINARY-TYPE PLASMINOGEN ACTIVATOR

The urinary-type PA (EC 3.4.2.73; urokinase, uPA) is found in urine at 40 to 80 $\mu g$ per L (269) and is synthesized by several cell types, particularly cells with a fibroblastlike morphology, but also by epithelial cells (270) and monocytes and macrophages (271,272). Stimulation by endotoxin or tumor necrosis factor causes cultured endothelial cells to produce uPA, and synthesis has also been demonstrated by the human endothelium *in vivo* (273,274). uPA activates PLG by the cleavage of Arg561–Val562, as does tPA, but importantly can do so in the absence of fibrin. This characteristic has generated the view that tPA functions in fibrinolysis in the vasculature, whereas uPA's primary role is in processes such as degradation of extracellular matrix and cell migration, with consequences for wound healing, inflammation, embryogenesis, and invasion of tumor cells and metastasis (275,276). These clear functions of the uPA system do not argue against its importance in fibrin degradation, functions that have emerged from both human and animal studies, as discussed in subsequent text.

## Structural Organization

The complete primary amino acid sequence of uPA was determined in 1982 (277). The cDNA and the genomic DNA of uPA have been isolated and their nucleotide sequences established (278,279). The human uPA gene is 6.4 kb and on chromosome 10q24 (280). It contains 11 exons, and the intron–exon organization of the uPA gene closely resembles that of the tPA gene. uPA is produced as a 54-kDa, single-chain glycoprotein, 411 residues long and containing three domains: an epidermal growth factor domain, a kringle, and a protease domain (Fig. 18-1). The EGF domain interacts with the uPAR found on many cells, as discussed in subsequent text. The kringle domain has no affinity for fibrin, and its function has been unclear; a recent report shows that it stabilizes the interaction of uPA with uPAR (281). The protease domain has the residues His204, Asp255, and Ser356 as the catalytic triad, and sequence identity with tPA is approximately 40% (140). uPA is normally glycosylated at Asn302, whereas a covalently attached single monosaccharide, fucose to Thr18 (282), appears to affect the mitogenicity of uPA (283). There are two phosphorylation sites on Ser138 and Ser303. The phosphorylated form diminishes uPA's interaction with cells and PAI-1 (284).

Activation of single-chain urinary plasminogen activator (scuPA, also called *proUK*) to the active enzyme, uPA (UK), is by cleavage of Lys158–Ile159 (285). Many enzymes can cleave this bond but the most important to hemostasis are plasmin (286), factor XIIa, and kallikrein (287). The activation of scuPA in PLG-deficient mice was characterized as being due to kallikrein (288). Cleavage close to this site results in inactive uPA. Thrombin cleaves Arg156–Phe157 in scuPA (287,289, 290) and the inactive product can be activated by release of the N-terminal dipeptide of its B chain by cathepsin C or, albeit slowly, by plasmin (285,291). Granulocyte elastase and cathepsin G cleave the Ile159–Ile160 peptide bond; again, the resulting two-chain urinary-type plasminogen activator (tcuPA) is inactive (292).

uPA was originally characterized as having two active forms: HMW-UK and LMW-UK (293). These are, respectively, full-length active uPA and a processed form, cleaved at Lys135–Lys136 to yield the amino-terminal fragment (ATF), which interacts with uPAR, leaving 21 residues of the A chain and an intact B chain. Cleavage within the uPAR binding region (e.g., of the Lys23–Tyr24 bond) abolishes uPA receptor binding and therefore modulates cell surface uPA activity (294,295).

The conformation of uPA and of its domains has been studied by NMR (296,297). Essentially, the domains are similar to those in other serine proteases (Fig. 18-1) with few considerable differences. The crystal structure of the catalytic domain of recombinant, nonglycosylated human uPA has been solved at a resolution of 2.5 Å (298). At six positions, insertions of extra residues in loop regions create unique surface areas. The interaction of Lys300 with Asp335 in the flexible loop region 297–313 stabilizes the conformation of scuPA (299). The positively charged residues 179–184 in a surface loop interact with PAI-1 (297). A number of modified uPA molecules have been crystallized and used as a basis for drug design (300,301).

## Enzymatic Properties of Urinary-Type Plasminogen Activator and Single-Chain Urinary Plasminogen Activator

The question of whether scuPA is a true zymogen was hotly debated for several years, a controversy that was fueled by the problem of trace plasmin or uPA contamination, with reciprocal activation of scuPA and PLG (302). The issue has been resolved by studies on mutant forms of the proteins and by examining scuPA in the absence of PLG. For instance, the Lys158Glu mutant of scuPA, which cannot be cleaved by plasmin into uPA, still converted PLG to plasmin (303). The emerging consensus is that scuPA has approximately 0.4% of the activity of uPA (304–307). Therefore, scuPA lies on the spectrum between PLG, a true zymogen, and tPA, which is almost fully active in its single-chain form. Lys300 and Asp355 are key structural elements of scuPA's enzymatic activity. Lys300, situated in the flexible loop region 297–313, forms a weak interaction with Asp355 adjacent to the active site Ser356 and pulls Ser356 close to the position found in a fully active protease. Site-directed mutagenesis of Lys300 to Ala resulted in a 40-fold lower activity than in wild-type scuPA (308). Likewise, a mutation of Asp355 to Asn resulted in a 270-fold reduction of scuPA activity (299). When the flexibility of the 297–313 loop was enhanced, intrinsic catalytic activity was reduced. By contrast, when the loop was made less flexible, intrinsic catalytic activity increased (309).

## Urinary-Type Plasminogen Activator Receptor

A cellular receptor for uPA (uPAR; CD87) was first demonstrated on freshly collected human monocytes (310) but is expressed on several cell types. The gene for uPAR (gene code PLAUR) is on chromosome 19 and consists of seven exons and six introns extending over 23 kb (311,312). Constitutive expression of the uPAR gene is dependent on the $-141$ to $-61$ region (313), and expression can be increased by tumor promoters, growth factors, cytokines, and hormones. Interestingly, it can be upregulated by one of the plasmin reductases, phosphoglycerate kinase (75,314). The 1.4-kb mRNA encodes a signal peptide of 22 and a protein of 313 residues, with a glycosylphosphatidyl inositol (GPI) anchor, by which the receptor is attached to cell surface phospholipids (see Fig. 18-6). The receptor consists of three homologous domains, and high-affinity binding of uPA to the receptor is mediated by region 1, but region 2 and 3 enhance this binding (315–317).

scuPA and uPA bind to uPAR receptor by the ATF (315). The binding is of high affinity ($K_d$ $10^{-9}$ to $10^{-11}$, depending on the cell type) (318) and can localize and enhance uPA–mediated PLG activation on cell surfaces (71). The mechanism is a colocalization of scuPA and PLG; uPAR does not play a catalytic role

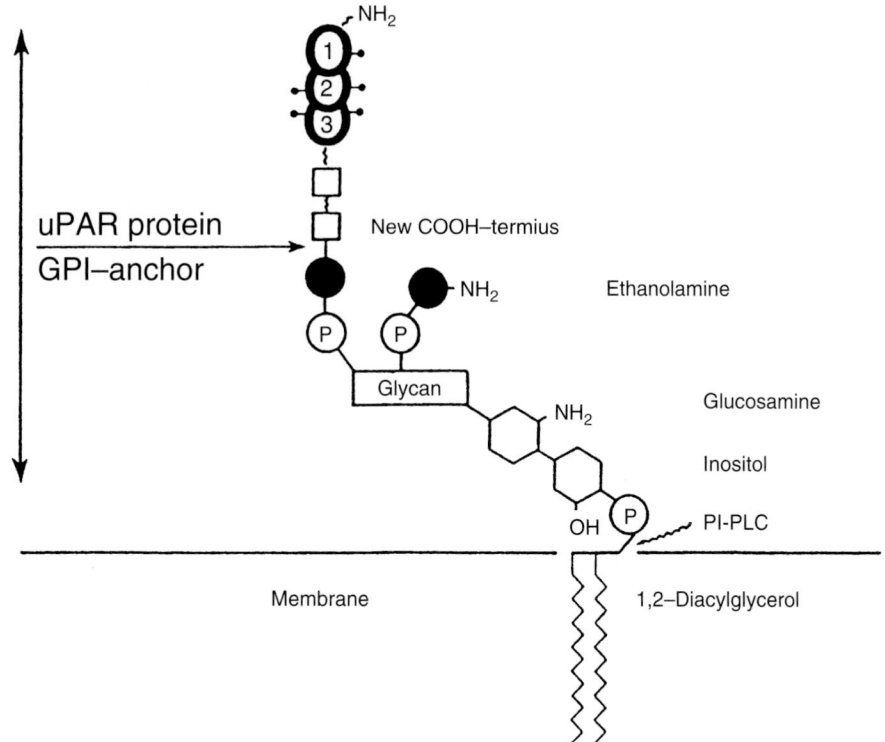

**FIGURE 18-6.** A simplified diagram of the domain structure of urinary-type plasminogen activator receptor (uPAR) and its attachment to the cell-surface glycosylphosphatidylinositol (GPI) membrane anchor. The N-terminal portion of the uPAR is composed of three domains. Potential glycosylation sites are indicated by •–. The C-terminal amino acids are depicted by *squares*. The linkage between the protein and the glycolipid is through a phosphoethanolamine that forms an amide bond with the a-carboxyl group of the protein and a phosphodiester bond with the glycan portion of the glycolipid. (PI-PLC, phosphatidylinositol-specific phospholipase C.) (From Ploug M, Behrendt N, Løber D, et al. Protein structure and membrane anchorage of the cellular receptor for urokinase-type plasminogen activator. *Semin Thromb Hemost* 1991;17:183–193, with permission.)

(319). Binding can also elicit a number of intracellular signaling responses, acting through the extracellular regulated kinase (ERK)/mitogen activated protein kinase (MAPK) pathway (320). Because uPAR is not a transmembrane protein, other components must participate to transmit a signal to the intracellular compartment. Several proteins are known to bind uPAR, including vitronectin and integrins in complex with caveolin (321). Such interactions regulate cell adhesion and are discussed further in the context of PAI-1 in Chapter 19. On some cells, the complex uPA/uPAR is associated with Endo 180, also known as uPAR-associated protein (uPARAP) (322), and is involved in collagen IV internalization (323). Receptor-bound uPA still is susceptible to inactivation by PAI-1, but the inhibition is somewhat less efficient than in free solution (319). The uPA/PAI-1 enzyme/inhibitor complexes are internalized, and the uPAR is recycled to the surface. This process requires the cooperation of LRP (262,324).

## Urinary-Type Plasminogen Activator in the Circulation

scuPA is found in plasma in concentrations of 2 to 4 ng per mL (325,326), which seem to remain fairly stable. In contrast with tPA and PAI-1, there is little circadian fluctuation in plasma uPA (327). Venous occlusion did not increase uPA antigen once values were corrected for the increase of hematocrit (136), but there are reports of increases of uPA antigen after venous stasis

(326), DDAVP infusion (328), and strenuous physical exercise (329). The activation of scuPA in plasma has not been studied in any detail, and uPA activity is not normally detected in plasma, but both leukocyte-associated and free scuPA are elevated in leukemia (183) and other disorders, including liver disease (330). Plasma uPA is cleared quickly, with a $t_{1/2}$ of approximately 7 minutes, in a manner that depends on hepatic blood flow (331). The LRP system binds and internalizes scuPA and uPA-PAI-1 complexes (251,261,262). The asialoglycoprotein receptor, located exclusively on parenchymal liver cells, also removes nonsialated uPA from the circulation (331).

The activity of scuPA is increased by two orders of magnitude when it is bound to uPAR on the surface of monocytes (332,333), which is now understood to reflect colocalization with PLG rather than a direct catalytic effect of uPAR (319). This local activity is relevant to thrombus stability, into which monocytes migrate (334) and express fibrinolytic activity (335). In freshly formed model thrombi, there is considerable spontaneous generation of fibrinolytic activity, most of which can be inhibited by antibodies to uPA (336). Polymorphonuclear cells, primarily neutrophils, generate this local uPA activity, apparently on uPAR (337); plasma $\alpha_1$-antitrypsin is crucial in protecting the activity from neutrophil elastase (338). The integrin $\alpha_M\beta_2$ is important in the generation of such local activity (339). When scuPA is present on uPAR, for instance on monocytes, it can associate with PAI-1 and other serpins, not in a classic covalent complex but in a reversible manner (340). This has given rise to the ideas that receptor-bound scuPA initiates proteolytic activity and that conversion to uPA is primarily a way of achieving inhibition by PAI-1 and other inhibitors and thereby regulating the activity (341). Platelets also contain uPAR (342) and a further 70-kDa protein, distinct from uPAR bound uPA in resting platelets with a $K_d$ of 43 nM (343). On other cells, too, cell-associated PLG activation by uPA is not mediated exclusively by uPAR and other receptors may come into play (344).

Although it does not bind to fibrin, scuPA has some fibrin specificity in that it degrades fibrin with less systemic degradation of fibrinogen and other plasma proteins than does uPA. It therefore is a more potent thrombolytic agent than uPA (306,345). The explanations for this include the different but complementary mechanisms by which tPA and scuPA induce fibrinolysis (346). tPA activates Glu–PLG, which is bound to an internal lysine, probably A$\alpha$ Lys157, which is exposed in nondegraded fibrin. As soon as some fibrin is digested by plasmin, new C-terminal lysyl residues are generated, increasing the binding of Glu–PLG (61,63) to fibrin. scuPA binds with high affinity to PLG ($K_d$ approximately 65 nM) and appears to activate selectively Glu–PLG, which is bound to C-terminal lysines in partially degraded fibrin (347,348). The generation of small amounts of fibrin-bound plasmin also converts scuPA to uPA, explaining the typical lag phase observed for fibrinolysis by scuPA. Efficient scuPA-mediated lysis occurs after some fibrin has been degraded by tPA. Therefore, sequential administration of tPA followed by scuPA resulted in increased thrombolysis in a rabbit jugular vein thrombosis model; the reverse order was less effective (349).

During coagulation, there is activation of the contact system generating kallikrein also. Because kallikrein is an efficient activator of scuPA (287,350), it is likely that scuPA is activated wherever activation of the contact phase of coagulation has occurred. This process also takes place in the absence of PLG. In a plasma milieu, clot lysis by scuPA is enhanced approximately 20-fold after dextran sulphate mediated activation of the contact phase (350). It is not entirely clear if this *in vitro* generated activity of kallikrein fully explains the contact system of PLG activation (351). Part of the dextran sulfate mediated activation may also be due to factor XII activity. Factor XIIa is a poor activator of PLG but is present at high concentrations in plasma (352).

## Regulation of Expression

The expression of scuPA has been reviewed in detail (353). The gene is regulated by several elements, with a typical TATA box 25 bp upstream of the transcription initiation site. A region of 500 bp contains potential binding sites for the transcription factor Sp1. Two putative AP-2 binding sites close to the transcription initiation site are responsible for protein kinase A–dependent induction of uPA expression. Two NF-$\kappa$B elements occur at −1,580 and −1,865 bp. The latter site acts as a repressor, as do two further negative regulatory sites, one situated between −1,824 and −1,572 bp, the other involving an enhancer-dependent cell-specific silencer region between −660 and −536 bp. The promoter is strongly enhanced by a region approximately 2,000 bp upstream of the transcription initiation site. This enhancer consists of an upstream PEA/AP-1A site and a downstream AP-1B site. All three sites are required for induction of uPA gene transcription by a variety of extracellular stimuli, such as phorbol ester, EGF, okadaic acid, and cytoskeleton disruption (354). Synergism between PEA/AP-1 and AP-1B depends on the integrity of an intervening cooperation mediator site that contains several sequences for binding of urokinase enhancer factors (355,356). In the 3' untranslated region UTR stretching from bp 1,368 to 2,260 of the human uPA gene, fragments were identified that exerted a positive or negative influence on chimeric reporter genes. Fragments

1,999 to 2,190 behaved like transcriptional enhancers, whereas fragments 1,532 to 1,723 had an inhibitory effect on the expression of uPA (357). At least three elements were found in the 5' UTR that confer instability to the uPA mRNA (358).

## Urinary-Type Plasminogen Activator/Urinary-Type Plasminogen Activator Receptor Deficiency

There are no known deficiencies of uPA or uPAR in humans, but mice with these disrupted genes reveal a number of interesting insights. uPA$^{-/-}$ mice, like tPA$^{-/-}$ mice, developed some fibrin deposits but did not spontaneously clot; challenge with endotoxin led to more venous thrombosis than in uPA$^{+/+}$ mice (264,265). Lysis of plasma clots was normal (264), but monocyte-dependent lysis was greatly decreased by the absence of uPA (359). This is consistent with the earlier findings that fibrin resolution was affected in mice deficient in uPA but not by deficiency in tPA or uPAR (360). Much lower plasmin generation, and hence matrix metalloproteinase activation, was observed in mice with combined apoE and uPA deficiency, so that they were protected from the atherosclerotic lesions that were induced in apoE$^{-/-}$ mice (361). Wound healing in uPA$^{-/-}$ mice is greatly disturbed and, after injury-induced depletion of vascular smooth muscle cells, repopulation of the injured area with smooth muscle cells was slow in uPA$^{-/-}$ mice (362). Perhaps surprisingly, the healing process does not involve binding to uPAR (363), and there are several other reports on uPAR-independent but uPA-dependent phenomena (364) as well as some in which both uPA and uPAR deficiency produce related effects (365). Some aspects of uPAR biology, such as the delayed clearance of platelets in uPAR$^{-/-}$ mice (366), macrophage infiltration into the vessel wall (367), and cancer cell growth and invasion (368), are independent of uPA. Studies on mice are helping to unravel which effects of uPA and uPAR operate independently of each other and which effects require their common functions.

# OTHER PLASMINOGEN ACTIVATORS

## Streptokinase

In 1933, it was shown that hemolytic streptococci produced an extracellular protein that could induce lysis of human plasma clots (369), and it has been a useful thrombolytic drug over several decades. Streptokinase and other bacterial activators have presumably evolved for the purpose of invasion of the mammalian host (370). SK is not an enzyme; rather, it acts by forming a 1:1 complex with PLG, which undergoes a change of conformation to expose an active site in the altered PLG molecule (371). The modified PLG in the equimolar complex (SK-PLG') autocatalytically converts to plasmin, and the activated complex is a potent PA (372). It retains the fibrin binding of the PLG moiety with consequent relative protection from inhibition by $\alpha_2$-antiplasmin (373). The C-terminus of SK regulates the PLG binding and activation, and mutational studies have revealed the essential features (374).

SK is a 47-kDa protein, containing no cysteines. NMR and crystallographic studies revealed a three-domain structure (375,376). The binding site for a kringle in PLG is located at the tip of a fully exposed hairpin loop in the $\beta$-domain of SK (377,378). The physicochemical properties of SK and the methods for its assay are reviewed (379); a new reference method that allows direct comparison with other PA has been developed (380).

SK is highly antigenic. Most apparently healthy persons have anti-SK antibodies in their blood, owing presumably to previous infections with $\beta$-hemolytic streptococci, and anti-SK titers may rise several hundredfold after administration to humans (381,382). After intravenous injection of SK into humans, dogs, or mice, SK is cleared from the circulation with a $t_{1/2}$ of 15 to 30 minutes (383). Clearance mostly takes place in the liver, primarily by the liver $\alpha_2$-macroglobulin receptor (383), now known to be identical to LRP (251).

## Anisoylated Plasminogen–Streptokinase Activator Complex

Plasmin generated in whole blood or plasma is immediately inactivated, but plasmin bound via its high-affinity LBS to fibrin is inactivated at a much lower rate by $\alpha_2$-antiplasmin. In the search for more efficient thrombolytic agents, researchers acylated the active site center of plasmin and of the SK–Plg' activator complex, in which a conformational change also exposes the active plasmin(ogen) site. Coupling of $p$-anisoyl to the active site serine of the PLG portion of SK–Plg' led to the development of the anisoylated PLG–SK activator complex (APSAC, Eminase). Its catalytic site is blocked, but its affinity to fibrin via the LBS is preserved. APSAC deacylates with a $t_{1/2}$ of approximately 40 minutes at 37°C (384). As it binds to fibrin, it is feasible to administer this drug in the form of a bolus injection. Evaluation in experimental animal models showed that APSAC had better clot specificity than SK, in that it caused less fibrinogenolysis and consumption of PLG and $\alpha_2$-antiplasmin and had a lesser hypotensive effect *in vivo* (385). Clinical studies showed that APSAC is an effective thrombolytic agent, but the systemic effects are comparable with SK.

## Staphylokinase

Staphylokinase (SAK) a protein with an $M_r$ of 15,000, produced by *Staphylococcus aureus*, has been known for more than 40 years to have thrombolytic properties (386,387). As recombinant techniques made production possible in larger quantities, there was renewed interest in its thrombolytic efficacy (388). Like SK, SAK is not an enzyme but forms a stable stoichiometric complex with PLG (372). In the absence of fibrin, it does not activate PLG. Trace amounts of plasmin, such as may be found on the surface of a thrombus, convert the SAK–PLG complex to SAK–plasmin complex that is a highly fibrin-specific PA. The complex binds to fibrin via the LBS of PLG, and the bound activator complex is somewhat protected from inactivation by $\alpha_2$-antiplasmin. The molecule is quite antigenic, and extensive mutagenesis has been undertaken to decrease this property (389). Coupling of SAK mutants to polyethylene glycol of $M_r$ 20,000 was shown to increase the $t_{1/2}$ of the complex severalfold, which would permit single bolus thrombolytic therapy in humans (390). Several clinical studies with SAK have been reported. In peripheral arterial occlusions and in patients with myocardial infarction, SAK compared favorably with tPA (391,392).

## Vampire Bat Plasminogen Activator

Many hematophagous animals, such as leeches, hookworms, mosquitoes, and the vampire bat, produce substances that interfere with the clotting or fibrinolysis mechanisms. In the 1960s, a potent PA was found in the saliva of the common vampire *Desmodus rotundus* (393). The bat lives exclusively on blood and uses the enzyme in its saliva to keep blood in a fluid state. The *D. rotundus* salivary plasminogen activator (DSPA) was cloned independently by two research groups and shows more than 70% identity with human tPA (394,395). Three major forms were identified: DSPA-$\alpha$, which contains a finger, EGF, kringle, and protease domain; DSPA-$\beta$, which lacks the finger domain; and DSPA-$\gamma$, which has just a kringle and a protease domain.

DSPA-$\alpha$ comprises 441 residues and, like SAK, has higher fibrin specificity than tPA (396). In the absence of fibrin, hardly any PLG activation occurs (397,398). PLG activation by DSPA is barely stimulated by D-dimer or the DDE complex, whereas these fibrin fragments strongly enhance tPA activity (399). The crystal structure of the catalytic domain of DSPA-$\alpha_1$ has been solved at 2.9 Å resolution (400) and shows strong similarity to tPA, which is also active in the single-chain form. Experiments in animals revealed that the thrombolytic potential of DSPA was at least equal to, and the clearance rate approximately 10 times slower than, that of tPA (401–403). The hope that high fibrin specificity would result in lesser bleeding at comparable thrombolytic potential was not fully realized (401), but this agent has several promising features, long clearance time, and fibrin specificity, which permits bolus administration and may be useful in stroke as well as acute myocardial infarction (404).

# INHIBITORS OF THE FIBRINOLYTIC SYSTEM

Several inhibitors control and modulate the expression of fibrinolytic activity. These act at the PLG activation step or on plasmin (see Fig. 18-7), and they prevent excessive systemic fibrinolytic activity. The principal inhibitor of tPA and uPA is PAI-1 (see Chapter 19), whereas $\alpha_2$-antiplasmin inhibits plasmin. Both are members of the serpin family, which also includes antithrombin and heparin cofactor (see Chapter 13). The serpins all function in the same way: They present to the target protease a reactive center loop, the P1-P1' of which mimics a substrate. A stable inactive 1:1 complex is formed between protease and serpin, lowering the effective protease concentration. Dissociation of the covalent complex, which occurs at different rates for different protease–serpin pairs, results in a cleaved form of the serpin, which lacks the short peptide from P1' to the original C-terminus. The serpins have marked specificity for particular proteases, but the specificity is not absolute, so that other inhibitors present at high concentration provide a back-up inhibitory system.

## $\alpha_2$-Antiplasmin

$\alpha_2$-Antiplasmin, also called *plasmin inhibitor*, is the primary fast-acting inhibitor of plasmin (405). It is a single-chain molecule of $M_r$ of 70,000, comprising 452 residues, the additional mass accounted for by approximately 13% carbohydrates on four potential asparagine glycosylation sites. The plasma concentration of $\alpha_2$-antiplasmin is 70 mg per L (i.e., 1 $\mu$M), approximately half the concentration of PLG on a molar basis. It is synthesized in the liver and consequently decreased in patients with advanced impairment of hepatic function. The $t_{1/2}$ of the native inhibitor is approximately 3 days, whereas the plasmin/$\alpha_2$-antiplasmin complex is cleared with a $t_{1/2}$ of approximately 0.5 days (406). The cDNA has been cloned (407), the organization of the gene determined (408), and the amino acid sequence derived. The gene for $\alpha_2$-antiplasmin (gene symbol PLI) has been localized to chromosome 17p13 (409). The inhibitory activity of $\alpha_2$-antiplasmin resides in its reactive center loop, in which the P1-P1' is Arg-Met (see Fig. 18-8); as with

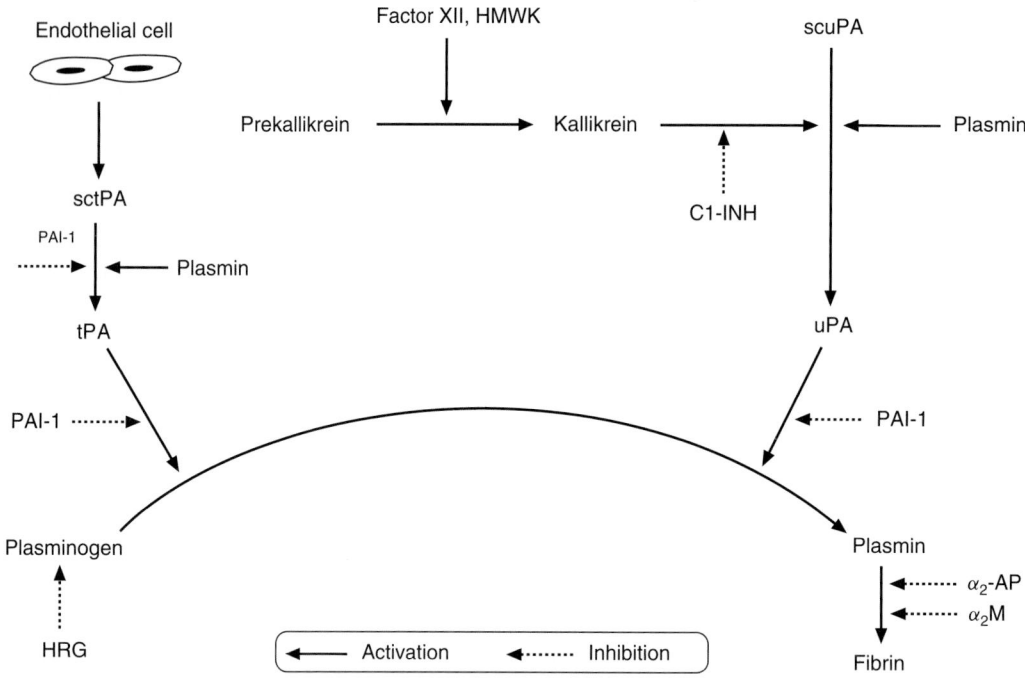

**FIGURE 18-7.** Activators and inhibitors of the blood fibrinolytic system. scuPA, single-chain urinary plasminogen activator; sctPA, single-chain tissue plasminogen activator; HMWK, high-molecular-weight kininogen; $\alpha_2$-AP, $\alpha_2$-antiplasmin; $\alpha_2$M, $\alpha_2$-macroglobulin; C1-INH, complement C1 esterase inhibitor; HRG, histidine-rich glycoprotein; PAI-1, plasminogen activator inhibitor 1.

other serpins, mutation of Arg to Ala destroys inhibitory function (410). The rate of interaction of wild-type $\alpha_2$-antiplasmin with plasmin is very fast, with a rate constant of $4 \times 10^7$ per M per second (411), comparable with the interaction of tPA and PAI-1.

Plasma $\alpha_2$-antiplasmin can occur in four different forms, depending on limited proteolysis at N- and C-termini. This processing appears not to affect the inhibitory capacity of $\alpha_2$-antiplasmin, which resides in the core of the protein. The N-terminus of $\alpha_2$-antiplasmin was originally identified as Asn (407), but it was later recognized that there is also a proform with an additional 12 residues at the N-terminus (412). Plasma $\alpha_2$-antiplasmin was shown to have about equal amounts of the two forms (413), whereas HepG2 cells produced the Met-form, which, after addition to plasma, was cleaved to the Asn form (414). An enzyme that removes the 12 residue N-terminal fragment has been purified and characterized (415). The importance of the N-terminal processing lies in the accessibility of Gln (at position 2 in the processed form); the proform terminus blocks access to the cross-linking site (412). Gln2 in $\alpha_2$-antiplasmin is cross-linked by factor XIIIa to the A$\alpha$ chain of fibrinogen or fibrin, at Lys303 (416,417). Fibrin with bound $\alpha_2$-antiplasmin is markedly more resistant to lysis than fibrin alone, and this observation was the basis of discovering the first deficiency of $\alpha_2$-antiplasmin (416). The cross-linking site can be saturated, as elegantly shown by studies with wild-type $\alpha_2$-antiplasmin and an active site Arg to Ala mutant (418). Antibodies specific for cross-linked $\alpha_2$-AP greatly stimulated lysis of fibrin (419).

Other studies focused on the C-terminus of $\alpha_2$-antiplasmin, which is extended relative to other serpins by approximately 50 residues (407). Two forms are detectable in normal human plasma (420). The native, full-length form binds PLG, whereas a processed form retains inhibitory capacity but cannot bind PLG (421). The two forms were distinguished by two-dimensional immunoelectrophoresis, with PLG incorporated in the gel in the first dimension (422). The ratio of the PLG

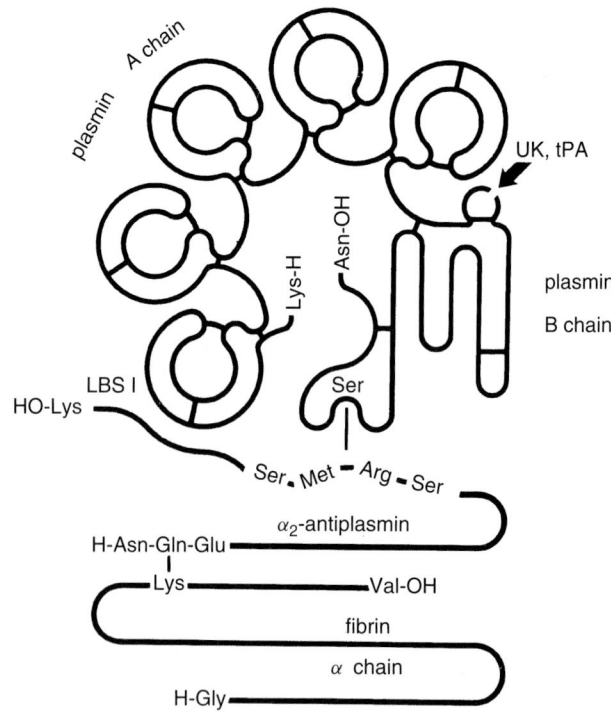

**FIGURE 18-8.** Interaction of $\alpha_2$-antiplasmin with plasmin and with the $\alpha$ chain of fibrinogen. For Lys–plasmin, only the high-affinity lysine binding site (LBS) 1 is indicated. H- denotes the N-termini and -OH the C-termini of the three proteins depicted. Lys residues in the C-terminus of $\alpha_2$-antiplasmin interacts with the LBS 1 of plasmin, and the N-terminal Gln2 is covalently cross-linked to Lys303 in the $\alpha$ chain of fibrin by factor XIIIa. tPA, tissue-type plasminogen activator; UK, urokinase. (From Bachmann F. Fibrinolysis. In: Verstraete M Vermylen J, Lijnen HR, et al., eds. *Thrombosis and haemostasis.* Leuven: Leuven University Press, 1987:227, with permission.)

binding to nonbinding form remains relatively constant in plasma samples, at approximately 65:35, even in patients with advanced liver cirrhosis (330).

The ability of $\alpha_2$-antiplasmin to bind PLG interferes with the fibrin-PLG interaction, because both involve LBS-1, as illustrated in Figure 18-8. It is also crucial to the fate of plasmin formed on the fibrin surface, to which both tPA and PLG bind by virtue of their lysine-binding sites. Plasmin formed on fibrin is therefore relatively protected from the action of $\alpha_2$-antiplasmin (423). This concept arose from experiments using lysine analogues, where $\alpha_2$-AP was shown to be approximately 100 times less effective toward plasmin in the presence of lysine analogues (424). The exact Lys residues responsible for binding the C-terminal region of $\alpha_2$-antiplasmin to LBS-1 in PLG are not yet defined. Binding of recombinant C-terminal peptide (55 residues) showed that binding to isolated kringles was most affected by mutation of Lys452 but that other internal Lys residues "tether" the kringles (425). A different study, in which each Lys from position 429 to the C-terminal Lys452 was separately mutated, indicated that Lys436 had the greatest effect; their modeling suggested that Lys452 is too close to Phe448 for it to be able to interact with the LBS (426).

The importance of $\alpha_2$-AP in stabilizing fibrin has been revealed in several *in vitro* systems, including clot lysis (427,428). A mutant of tPA that is relatively resistant to $\alpha_2$-AP was very efficient in lysing both clots and model thrombi (429). Deficiency of $\alpha_2$-AP results in delayed bleeding, but initial hemostasis is normal, and this is characteristic of fibrinolytic defects (217). Inheritance was autosomal recessive in a well-characterized Japanese family (430,431). An interesting defect in $\alpha_2$-AP Enschede was explained by the abnormal protein behaving as a substrate for plasmin rather than as an inhibitor (432), as a result of the extended (by one Ala residue) reactive center loop (433). Mice deficient in $\alpha_2$-AP were essentially normal in many respects, but they did show enhanced endogenous fibrinolytic activity without overt bleeding (434). In experimental models, the lack of $\alpha_2$-AP had effects on liver regeneration (435), platelet aggregation (436), and pulmonary heart failure (437).

## $\alpha_2$-Macroglobulin

$\alpha_2$-Macroglobulin is a major inhibitor of wide specificity and is the backup inhibitor of several proteases, including plasmin (438). It comes into play when the fibrinolytic system is fully activated and when the capacity of $\alpha_2$-antiplasmin is exhausted; it also forms complexes with tPA and uPA (183). $\alpha_2$-Macroglobulin is a glycoprotein of $M_r$ 725,000 that consists of four identical chains of $M_r$ 160,000 and contains approximately 8% carbohydrate (Table 18-1). Its plasma concentration is 2.5 g per L (3 $\mu$M). The tetramer is arranged as a pair of dimers, each consisting of two monomers linked together via a disulfide bond. The complete sequence of this 1,451-residue molecule has been established and the gene locus (gene symbol A2M) attributed to chromosome 12p13.3-p12.3 (439,440). The inhibitor contains two reactive sites. The sequence Arg-Val-Gly-Phe-Tyr-Glu (681–686) acts as a bait region that contains sites for proteases of different specificities (441). Cleavage results in a conformational change and activates the thioester site at positions 949–952. Electron microscopic studies showed that the catalytic domain of the rod-shaped plasmin molecule is entrapped inside the $\alpha_2$-macroglobulin cavity, whereas its N-terminal kringle domains protrude outside one end between the two armlike features of the transformed $\alpha_2$-macroglobulin structure (442). It is noteworthy that proteases inhibited by $\alpha_2$-macroglobulin can still act on small peptide substrates, but their position in the inhibitor cavity makes larger targets nonaccessible.

# PLASMINOGEN ACTIVATOR INHIBITOR 1

This is the principal inhibitor of both tPA and uPA and is discussed in detail in Chapter 19; the emphasis in this chapter is therefore to place it in the context of regulation of the PLG/plasmin system in the vasculature. In addition to its inhibition of tPA and uPA, PAI-1 has a role in regulating cell adhesion processes relevant to tissue remodeling, mediated by its binding to the adhesive glycoprotein vitronectin, rather than by proteinase inhibition (443).

The 52-kDa glycoprotein consists of 379 residues. It is unusual among the serpins in its tendency to lose activity through spontaneous insertion of the reactive center loop into the body of the molecule, forming an extra strand of $\beta$-sheet A. This form was termed *latent* because, after denaturation and refolding, activity was regained (444); there are no physiologic conditions under which this can occur. The noncovalent binding of vitronectin stabilizes the active form of PAI-1 (445), which is present in plasma at low concentrations, approximately 20 ng per mL (446–448). Because it has a $t_{1/2}$ of less than 10 minutes, its rate of synthesis must be high. The variation between normal individuals is rather high, ranging from 1 to 40 ng per mL, corresponding to 1 to 40 U per mL, the unit being the activity that neutralizes one unit of tPA in 10 minutes.

PAI-1 is produced by most cultured cells, and early publications identified it as a platelet protein (449), a product of megakaryocytes (450), endothelial cells (451), or hepatocytes (452); more recently, the production by adipocytes has been stressed (453–455). The source of resting plasma PAI-1 is not certain. Studies showing that normal endothelium or hepatocytes do not express PAI-1 (456) point to adipocytes as the normal source, whereas elevations in the acute-phase are likely to result from hepatocytes (457). Platelets constitute the major pool of circulating PAI-1. Although it is less active than plasma PAI-1, platelet PAI-1 accounts for about half the circulating PAI-1 activity, by virtue of the abundance of the protein in platelets (447). Large amounts of platelet PAI-1 accumulate in thrombi (458,459), and this directly correlates with their lysability (459).

PAI-1 inhibits tPA (tc and sc) and uPA (460). It does not inhibit scuPA, which is largely inactive, but it does associate with scuPA noncovalently, as discussed in the section on uPA (340). PAI-1 in plasma is in excess over tPA; therefore, most of the tPA is present in a complex with PAI-1. The second-order rate constants for the interaction with tPA and uPA are greater than $10^7$ $M^{-1}$ $S^{-1}$, a little lower for sctPA (see Table 18-5).

Hereditary deficiency of PAI-1 in humans is quite rare but leads to a lifelong bleeding disorder, presumably caused by premature lysis of hemostatic plugs at sites of vascular trauma, and consistent with this, bleeding occurs after a delay (461–464). The oral administration of fibrinolytic inhibitors such as AMCA has been effective in normalizing hemostatic function (463,464).

Mice with a disrupted *PAI-1* gene demonstrate normal development, fertility, and survival. The lack of inhibitor activity induces a mild hyperfibrinolytic state and confers a greater resistance to the prothrombotic effect of endotoxin injected into the footpad (465). After arterial injury, wound healing in PAI$^{-/-}$ mice was accelerated with rapid migration of smooth muscle cells from the uninjured tissue (466). In an arterial thrombosis model, time to development of an occlusive thrombus was approximately twice as long in PAI-1$^{-/-}$ than in PAI-1$^{+/+}$ mice (467). In another model of carotid artery injury, platelet-rich thrombi were generated and residual thrombi evaluated 24 hours later. Partially or completely occlusive thrombi were found in 34% of PAI$^{-/-}$ mice and 65% of PAI$^{+/+}$ mice (468).

SECOND-ORDER RATE CONSTANTS FOR THE INHIBITION OF TISSUE-TYPE PLASMINOGEN ACTIVATOR AND URINARY-TYPE PLASMINOGEN ACTIVATOR BY SERPINS

| | Second-order rate constant of inhibition/ M/s | | |
|---|---|---|---|
| | sctPA | tctPA | uPA |
| PAI-1 | $10^7$ | $3 \times 10^7$ | $5 \times 10^7$ |
| PAI-2 | $10^3$ | $2 \times 10^5$ | $10^6$ |
| Protease nexin | $1.5 \cdot 10^3$ | $3 \times 10^4$ | $1.5 \times 10^6$ |
| Protein C inhibitor | $10^3$ | $10^3$ | |
| C1-inhibitor | 1.3 | 5 | |
| $\alpha_2$-Antiplasmin | 13 | $\approx 10^2$ | $\approx 10^2$ |

sctPA, single-chain tissue-type plasminogen activator; tctPA, two-chain tissue-type plasminogen activator; uPA, urinary-type plasminogen activator; PAI-1, plasminogen activator inhibitor-1; PAI-2, plasminogen activator inhibitor-2; C1-inhibitor, complement 1 esterase inhibitor.
From Kruithof EKO. Inhibitors of plasminogen activators. In: Kluft C, ed. *Tissue-type plasminogen activator (tPA). Physiological and clinical aspects*, Vol I. Boca Raton, FL: CRC Press, 1988:189–210; Lobov S, Wilczynska M, Bergstrom F, et al. Structural bases of the redox-dependent conformational switch in the serpin PAI-2. *J Mol Biol* 2004;344:1359–1368; Huisman LGM, Van Griensven JMT, Kluft C. On the role of C1-inhibitor as inhibitor of tissue-type plasminogen activator in human plasma. *Thromb Haemost* 1995;73:466–471, with permission.

The opposite phenomenon, high plasma PAI-1, has been the subject of many studies that examined potential links with thrombosis. Mice overexpressing human PAI-1 in endothelium are subject to age-dependent development of arterial thrombosis (469). In humans, high circulating PAI-1 is clearly associated with a variety of pathologies, including cardiovascular disease (470–472) and cancer (473). Many studies have been conducted to investigate causal significance, and it appears that high PAI-1 does not independently predict disease, once other factors like obesity, diabetes, and elevated triglycerides are taken into account (474). A guanine insertion/deletion polymorphism at position 675 in the PAI-1 promoter (475) is associated with differences in circulating PAI-l (476). Despite promising early findings (477), the current view is that the predictive power of studying this polymorphism is low (474,478). In contrast to these studies on subtle variation in plasma PAI-1, Gram-negative septicemic patients have plasma PAI-1 concentraions that are sometimes raised as much as 50-fold over normal, and this is associated with high mortality (479).

## Chemical Inhibitors of Plasminogen Activator Inhibitor 1

Compounds that inhibit the synthesis or action of PAI-1 have been sought because of the relation between elevated PAI-1 and disease. They might be useful for enhancement of constitutive fibrinolytic activity or as adjuvant drugs in the thrombolytic treatment of thrombotic disorders. Gemfibrozil and clofibric acid act at the level of PAI-1 synthesis, decreasing it by approximately 40% (480). Also acting at the level of PAI-1 synthesis, a butadiene derivative T-686, administered to mice for 8 days before an injection of lipopolysaccharide, protected mice from its lethal effect in a dose-dependent fashion (481). In a rat thrombosis model, it limited thrombus growth (482)

and also attenuated development of atherosclerotic lesions in rabbits subjected to a high-cholesterol diet (483).

A 14–amino acid peptide, corresponding to the PAI-1 reactive center loop (residues 333 to 346), rapidly inhibited PAI-1 function and prevented the formation of a complex between tPA and PAI-1. It also enhanced considerably *in vitro* lysis of platelet-rich clots (484). Sideroxylonal C, a phloroglucinol dimer isolated from the flowers of *Eucalyptus albens*, inhibited PAI-1 in an *in vitro* assay without having a considerable effect on tPA (485). AR-H029953XX is a derivative of flufenamic acid, known to inhibit the C1-inhibitor. It prevents complex formation of tPA with PAI-1 through binding to Arg76 or Arg118, or both (486). A series of diketopiperazine-based inhibitors of PAI-1, XR334, XR1853, and XR5082, inhibited the action of PAI-1 on tPA and tcuPA ($IC_{50}$: 5 to 80 $\mu$M) and slowed the time to blood vessel occlusion in a rat carotid artery injury model (487). XR5118 binds to a region in PAI-1 (residues 110 to 145) known to interact with tPA, and it stimulated endogenous lysis of rabbit jugular vein thrombi and diminished thrombus growth (488). XR5118 binds to PAI-1 at $\beta$-sheet A, which causes an inactivating conformational change (489).

## Plasminogen Activator Inhibitor 2

The gene for PAI-2 (gene symbol *PLANH2*) spans 16.5 kb and is located on chromosome 18q22.1 (490). The cDNA of 1.9 kb encodes a protein of 415 residues. A segment of more than 5 kb has been sequenced in the 5′-flanking region and contains many regulatory elements important for constitutive and for stimulated gene expression (491,492).

PAI-2 was initially identified as a urokinase inhibitor in human placenta (493); it later was purified from human placenta and from the monocytoid cell line U-937 (494,495). PAI-2 is the predominant PA inhibitor of squamous epithelia in epidermis, esophagus, cornea, oral mucosa, tongue, and vagina (496). It is incorporated into the cornified envelope during terminal differentiation of the keratinocyte via transglutaminase-catalyzed crosslinks (497). Monocytes are an important source of PAI-2 (498) and may increase fibrin stability on migration into thrombi, especially because the PAI-2 is cross-linked to fibrin (499).

PAI-2 belongs to a subgroup of serpins called the *ovalbumin-related serpin family* (ov-serpins). Members of this subgroup lack a cleavable N-terminal signal sequence (490), and accordingly much of the protein is intracellular. In addition to this nonglycosylated form of apparent mass 47 kDa, some secreted, glycosylated 60-kDa PAI-2 is found in cultured U937 cells (500). All of the potential glycosylation sites on Asn75, Asn115, and Asn339 appear to be used. Peripheral blood monocytes also secrete some nonglycosylated PAI-2 by a mechanism distinct from the secretion system for interleukin 1$\beta$ and other nonclassically secreted proteins (499,501). PAI-2 exhibits an unusually long sequence between helices C and D, 33 residues that probably protrude from the molecule. The crystal structure for PAI-2 is of a form from which this loop was deleted (502). The loop contains three glutamines in positions 83, 84, and 86 that are essential for transglutaminase-mediated cross-linking of PAI-2 to trophoblast membranes, the cornified envelope of epidermis (503), and fibrin (499,504). Residues between 66 and 98 act as a protein-binding domain, which binds annexins I, II, IV, and V, among others (505). Purified PAI-2 polymerizes spontaneously at room temperature by inserting the reactive center loop into the A-sheet of another molecule, a loop-sheet polymerization that has some similarity to that which occurs in the Z-mutant of $\alpha_1$-antitrypsin (506). This polymerization depends on disulfide bond formation between Cys residues 37 (in the C-D loop) and 161, which can occur as a result of the mobility of the C-D loop (507). Alternatively, monomeric PAI-2, with a reduced Cys37, can form disulfide bonds with other molecules such as vitronectin (508).

PAI-2 is an efficient inhibitor of tcuPA, with a second-order rate constant of $10^6$ $M^{-1}$ $S^{-1}$; it reacts approximately five times more slowly with tctPA and quite poorly with sctPA (Table 18-5) (460,495). In normal plasma, there are no measurable levels of PAI-2, but high levels are found in pregnancy, with a steady rise until approximately 33 weeks, to reach approximately 250 ng per mL (509). Lesser increases during pregnancy were observed during intrauterine growth retardation (510–512). PAI-2 might therefore be a marker for decreased placental function (511,512). Different forms of PAI-2 occur in plasma in pregnancy (513), and it is not clear whether these represent PAI-2 disulfide-bonded or cross-linked to other proteins.

PAI-2 is also found in the plasma of patients with acute myeloblastic leukemia of the $M_4$ and the $M_5$ type (514), and in patients with sepsis, in whom PAI-1 is also increased (515). Speculation remains on the real function of PAI-2. Its intracellular location suggests roles other than inhibition of PA, and it was found to protect cells from the rapid cytopathic effects of alphavirus infection (516). It also acts intracellularly as a retinoblastoma protein (Rb)-binding protein (517). Its local activity appears to be relevant to a number of cancers (518,519). Mice with a disrupted PAI-2 gene did not present any phenotypic abnormalities (520); it will be interesting to see if appropriate inflammatory challenges reveal a phenotype.

## C1-Inhibitor

C1-inhibitor is a highly glycosylated 105-kDa serpin, consisting of 478 residues (Tables 18-1 and 18-2). The 16 kb gene is located on chromosome 11q12-q13.1 (521–523). It inhibits the activated subcomponents, C1r and C1s, of complement C1, and factors XIIa and XIa, plasma kallikrein, and plasmin. Its high plasma concentration (1.7 $\mu$M) gives it the capacity to inhibit tPA when it is present in excess over PAI-1 (138,330, 524). By virtue of its inhibitory effect on components of the contact system, it probably plays a role in controlling contact phase–dependent fibrinolysis and the conversion of scuPA to uPA.

## Histidine-Rich Glycoprotein

Histidine-rich glycoprotein (HRG) is named for the region between residues 330 and 389, which are similar to the histidine-rich regions in human and bovine kininogen (525). The 75-kDa protein has 507 residues and approximately 14% of carbohydrate. HRG competitively inhibits PLG associations by binding LBS-1 of PLG ($K_d$ 1 $\mu$M). It is suggested, on the basis of their relative concentrations, that PLG (2 $\mu$M) and HRG (1.5 $\mu$M) would circulate predominantly in a 1:1 reversible complex (526), which would decrease the PLG available for binding to fibrin. However, $\alpha_2$-antiplasmin had a greater effect than HRG on binding of PLG to fibrin (527). It has recently been proposed that HRG tethers PLG to the cell surface, which would enhance the cells' migratory potential (528). Only one family with congenital heterozygous HRG deficiency has been described. The proband, but none of the other five family members with low HRG levels, had thrombotic disease (529).

## Thrombin-Activatable Fibrinolysis Inhibitor

The generation of $C$-terminal lysyl residues is an important feedback mechanism for the binding of PLG to fibrin and the enhancement of fibrinolysis. These residues can be removed by TAFIa (EC 3.4.17.20; synonyms: carboxypeptidase B, U, or R), further regulating fibrinolysis (530), as discussed fully in Chapter 20. The zymogen TAFI is activated by thrombin/thrombomodulin and functionally connects the fibrinolytic and coagulant pathways (531).

TAFI is primarily produced by the liver and circulates at approximately 75 nM, but the normal variation is wide (530, 532). The more important variable is the circulating active enzyme, which has a very short $t_{1/2}$ and only a small proportion has to be activated for full function (533). The function of TAFIa was shown originally in clot lysis assays; potato tuber carboxypeptidase inhibitor relieves the inhibition (531,534). The effect of TAFIa has also been shown in model thrombi made from whole blood (535) and in animal studies, where TAFIa activity increased the time taken to restore blood flow in a canine coronary artery thrombosis model (536). Inhibitors of TAFIa enhanced endogenous fibrinolysis and also thrombolysis by tPA (537,538). The homozygous-deficient mouse shows enhanced plasma clot lysis but is comparable to wild-type mouse in many thrombus models, mostly those in which time taken to occlusion rather than thrombus resolution is assessed (539).

There are some reports of elevated TAFI as a mild risk factor for thrombosis, and it is elevated in inflammation, correlating with other acute-phase markers (540). Several polymorphisms in the TAFI gene have been reported. These seem to explain the wide normal range of concentrations but do not correlate strongly with disease (541). Some methods show bias toward particular polymorphic variants of TAFI (542,543); associations with disease therefore need to be interpreted with caution.

TAFIa activity appears to be the reason for increased fibrinolysis in hemophilia, where thrombin generation may be sufficient for fibrin formation but suboptimal for TAFI activation. Most thrombin is formed after clot formation, mainly via the intrinsic pathway by activation of factor XI by thrombin. This leads to a positive feedback mechanism and optimal activation of pro-TAFI (544). Factor IX–deficient plasma clots lysed prematurely, but the defect could be reversed by the addition of factor IX or of thrombomodulin to the plasma (545). Similarly, addition of TAFI, thrombomodulin, or factor VIII to hemophilia A plasma restored normal fibrinolysis (546). Consistent with this, incorporation of anti–factor XI antibodies or inhibition of TAFI in a rabbit model resulted in an almost twofold increase of endogenous thrombolytic activity (547).

## Lipoprotein (a)

Apolipoprotein (a), a component of lipoprotein (a) [Lp(a)], is linked by a disulfide bond to apolipoprotein B-100. Apo(a) has a wide size distribution, which depends on the number of kringle repeats; these are similar to kringle 4 of PLG (548). The total mass of Lp(a) therefore varies between 800 and 1,300 kDa. There is also a wide range of plasma Lp(a) concentrations, from 10 to 1,000 mg per L, and a skewed distribution, median value 50 mg per L. Besides apo(a), a gene cluster on chromosome 6q26-27 also contains PLG and two apo(a)-related genes (11,549,550).

Lp(a) binds to fibrin, extracellular matrix, platelets, and cells by its kringles; predictably, binding is inhibited by lysine and εACA. Lp(a) therefore competes with PLG and tPA for binding to fibrin and may thus exert an antifibrinolytic effect (551–553). PLG binding and activation on platelets (554) as well as on fibrin (555–558) is attenuated by Lp(a). Transgenic mice expressing the human apo(a) gene resolved experimental thrombi poorly when treated with tPA (559). These observations are consistent with the association of high Lp(a) with coronary artery disease (560–562). It is now clear that Lp(a) size is a key factor; only the smaller forms bind with high affinity to fibrin (563–565). Individuals with the combination of high Lp(a) levels and predominance of the small isoform showed the lowest fibrinolytic activity (565).

# BALANCE OF THE SYSTEM

The fibrinolytic system is normally kept quiescent as a result of two factors: the relative abundance of inhibitors over proteases and the requirement for fibrin or cell surfaces for initiation of activity. In normal individuals, steady-state levels of PLG in plasma are rather stable, whereas both the PA and their inhibitors are subject to change, suggesting that regulation of fibrinolytic activity occurs mainly via up- and down-regulation of the expression of the PA and their inhibitors. This general statement relates both to the relative concentrations of PA, many orders of magnitude lower than the PLG concentration, and to the very short half-lives of PA compared to PLG, minutes rather than days (Table 18-2).

The fibrinolytic system is geared to remove fibrin from the circulation in a controlled way, and therefore to prevent excessive fibrin accumulation. Circulating PLG is not normally converted to plasmin, which would cause generalized proteolysis and degradation of clotting factors, particularly factor V, factor VIII, VWF, and platelet glycoproteins. Instead, fibrin acts as a focus for the generation of activity, which is relatively protected from inhibitors. Although fibrin deposition plays an important role in hemostasis, wound healing, and inflammatory processes, fibrin formation must always be limited in time, and fibrin should be removed once it has fulfilled its role. The primary role of the PLG–plasmin system is not to lyse large formed blood clots, but to prevent excessive build-up of fibrin formation. That said, the system has been harnessed usefully for therapy, mainly by administering activators. Recently there has been a resurgence of interest in therapeutic use of plasmin (566).

Fibrin acts to assemble the fibrinolytic components, which is central to the control of the system. At the earliest stages of fibrin formation, tPA and PLG bind to the forming fibrin strands. Once small amounts of tPA and PLG are bound to fibrin in the form of a ternary complex, the catalytic efficiency of tPA for PLG is several hundred times higher than it is in the absence of fibrin. Plasmin generation causes proteolytic cleavage of fibrin that starts at the C-terminal portion of the $\alpha$ chain of fibrin and produces new C-terminal lysyl residues. Partially digested fibrin binds up to 10 times more Glu–PLG than undegraded fibrin. scuPA binds to and appears to activate selectively Glu–PLG bound to C-terminal lysines in the partially degraded fibrin. Trace amounts of plasmin also activate scuPA to uPA, and there is reciprocal activation of PLG to plasmin.

In healthy individuals, there is a molar excess of active PAI-1 in plasma over tPA (Table 18-2). Consequently, most of the tPA in plasma is in the form of an inactive complex with PAI-1 (241). Small amounts of free tPA occur in the circulation as a result of the high synthetic rate of both proteins and the finite time it takes for complex formation to occur. Even though PAI-1 in plasma is kept in its active conformation by its interaction with vitronectin, its tendency to lose activity does increase the possibility of plasma tPA expressing some of its activity. Normally, tPA activity is detectable at approximately 0.1 to 0.5 U per mL of plasma, even when blood is collected in an acidified anticoagulant to prevent complexing of any free tPA by PAI-1 (567). The maximum activity normally seen is equivalent to 1 $\mu$g per L; tPA has a specific activity of 500,000 to 700,000 U per mg (568). This low tPA activity is generally close to the borderline for detection, which is why procedures like euglobulin preparation, which removes most plasma inhibitors, but notably only about half the PAI-1 (447), are used. Even after the levels of free tPA increase severalfold, after strenuous exercise, venous occlusion, or intravenous injection of DDAVP to healthy volunteers, no circulating plasmin forms because PLG activation does not occur at these still physiologic tPA concentrations. This does not apply during the treatment of acute myocardial infarction with recombinant tPA, during which circulating plasma concentrations of tPA are achieved that are up to 1,000-fold higher than those observed in normal plasma.

Changes in the balance of tPA and PAI-1 are a clear example of how fibrinolytic activity can be initiated. Indeed, these components of the system fluctuate remarkably during a 24-hour period (569). tPA activity is lowest at night and in the early morning and then increases up to threefold during the day. PAI-1 antigen and activity are highest in the early morning hours and then gradually decline during the day, reaching their lowest level in the early afternoon. Consequently, if a drug (or placebo) is given at 8 AM, the activity of the fibrinolytic system invariably is higher a few hours later, and only trials in which a comparison to placebo is made are valid. Various factors may interfere with the normal circadian rhythm (327).

There is a large literature on the predictive value of tPA antigen and PAI-1 as risk factors for acute myocardial infarction, stroke, and peripheral vascular disease (472,477,478, 570). High tPA antigen is found to be associated with disease in a number of studies, and this probably reflects the tPA/PAI-1 complex (241,571).

It is generally assumed that PLG, present in plasma at approximately 2 $\mu$M, is not rate-limiting for fibrinolysis. Even though the concentration is so much higher than the activators (Table 18-2), it is indeed possible for it to become a limiting factor. The need to consider local PLG concentration, especially when the activators are used therapeutically, has been clearly shown (572). The effect on variation in available PLG is highlighted in studies on TAFIa (573). The effect of TAFIa on tPA-initiated lysis is usually stressed, in line with tPA's known fibrin dependence, but TAFIa also has strong effects on uPA and scuPA-induced lysis, pointing to its primary effect being on PLG binding (535).

Global circulating (a rare observation, unless thrombolytic agents are administered to patients at high doses) and local fibrinolytic activity are modulated by serpins. tPA and uPA are efficiently inhibited by PAI-1. More than 90% of blood PAI-1 is located in the platelets and promptly released on platelet activation. Although most of the platelet PAI-1 is inactive, there is still enough active PAI-1 in platelets to stabilize platelet-rich thrombi, as occur in the arterial circulation in which the blood pressure is high and premature lysis of a hemostatic plug is undesirable. Plasmin bound to fibrin is partly protected from inactivation by $\alpha_2$-antiplasmin. This assures that fibrinolysis proceeds on the surface of a clot. However, free plasmin that spills over into the general circulation is rapidly inactivated by $\alpha_2$-antiplasmin. After massive activation of the fibrinolytic system has taken place, such as in thrombolytic therapy, the amount of $\alpha_2$-antiplasmin does not suffice to inhibit all circulating plasmin, and $\alpha_2$-macroglobulin acts as a scavenger protease inhibitor.

The fibrinolytic system is a highly modulated enzyme system, and nature has taken many steps to limit its action in time and space but has also provided the necessary feedback loops that enhance the fibrinolytic system on the local level.

## References

1. Davidson CJ, Tuddenham EG, McVey JH. 450 million years of hemostasis. *J Thromb Haemost* 2003;1:1487–1494.
2. Patthy L. Evolutionary assembly of blood coagulation proteins. *Semin Thromb Hemost* 1990;16:245–259.

3. Madison EL. Probing structure-function relationships of tissue-type plasminogen activator by site-specific mutagenesis. *Fibrinolysis* 1994;8(Suppl. 1):221–236.

4. Collen D, De Maeyer L. Molecular biology of human plasminogen. I. Physicochemical properties and microheterogeneity. *Thromb Diath Haemorrh* 1975;34:396–402.

5. Raum D, Marcus D, Alper CA, et al. Synthesis of human plasminogen by the liver. *Science* 1980;208:1036–1037.

6. Highsmith RF, Kline DL. Kidney: primary source of plasminogen after acute depletion in the cat. *Science* 1971;174:141–142.

7. Twining SS, Wilson PM, Ngamkitidechakul C. Extrahepatic synthesis of plasminogen in the human cornea is up-regulated by interleukins-1α and −1β. *Biochem J* 1999;339:705–712.

8. Zhang L, Seiffert D, Fowler BJ, et al. Plasminogen has a broad extrahepatic distribution. *Thromb Haemost* 2002;87:493–501.

9. Murray JC, Buetow KH, Donovan M, et al. Linkage disequilibrium of plasminogen polymorphism and assignment of the gene to human chromosome 6q26-6q27. *Am J Hum Genet* 1987;40:338–350.

10. Frank SL, Klisak I, Sparkes RS, et al. A gene homologous to plasminogen located on human chromosome 2q11-p11. *Genomics* 1989;4:449–451.

11. Ichinose A. Multiple members of the plasminogen-apolipoprotein(a) gene family associated with thrombosis. *Biochemistry* 1992;31:3113–3118.

12. Sottrup-Jensen L, Claeys H, Zajdel M, et al. The primary structure of human plasminogen: isolation of two lysine-binding fragments and one "mini"-plasminogen (MW 38,000) by elastase-catalyzed-specific limited proteolysis. In: Davidson JF, Rowan RM, Samama MM et al., eds. *Progress in chemical fibrinolysis and thrombolysis*, Vol. 3. New York: Raven Press, 1978: 191–209.

13. Petersen TE, Martzen MR, Ichinose A, et al. Characterization of the gene for human plasminogen, a key proenzyme in the fibrinolytic system. *J Biol Chem* 1990;265:6104–6111.

14. Degen SJF, Bell SM, Schaefer LA, et al. Characterization of the cDNA coding for mouse plasminogen and localization of the gene to mouse chromosome 17. *Genomics* 1990;8:49–61.

15. Wiman B, Wallén P. The specific interaction between plasminogen and fibrin. A physiological role of the lysine binding site in plasminogen. *Thromb Res* 1977;10:213–222.

16. Thorsen S, Clemmensen I, Sottrup-Jensen L, et al. Adsorption to fibrin of native fragments of known primary structure from human plasminogen. *Biochim Biophys Acta* 1981;668:377–387.

17. Wiman B, Lijnen HR, Collen D. On the specific interaction between the lysine-binding sites in plasmin and complementary sites in α₂-antiplasmin and in fibrinogen. *Biochim Biophys Acta* 1979;579:142–154.

18. Clemmensen I, Petersen LC, Kluft C. Purification and characterization of a novel, oligomeric, plasminogen kringle 4 binding protein from human plasma: tetranectin. *Eur J Biochem* 1986;156:327–333.

19. Lijnen HR, Hoylaerts M, Collen D. Isolation and characterization of a human plasma protein with affinity for the lysine binding sites in plasminogen. *J Biol Chem* 1980;255:10214–10222.

20. Kelm RJ Jr, Swords NA, Orfeo T, et al. Osteonectin in matrix remodeling. A plasminogen-osteonectin-collagen complex. *J Biol Chem* 1994;269: 30147–30153.

21. Selim TE, Ghoneim HR, Uknis AB, et al. High-molecular-mass and low-molecular-mass kininogens block plasmin-induced platelet aggregation by forming a complex with kringle 5 of plasminogen/plasmin. *Eur J Biochem* 1997;250:532–538.

22. Silverstein RL, Leung LLK, Harpel PC, et al. Complex formation of platelet thrombospondin with plasminogen: modulation of activation by tissue activator. *J Clin Invest* 1984;74:1625–1633.

23. Deutsch DG, Mertz ET. Plasminogen: purification from human plasma by affinity chromatography. *Science* 1970;170:1095–1096.

24. Rejante MR, Llinás M. Solution structure of the ε-aminohexanoic acid complex of human plasminogen kringle 1. *Eur J Biochem* 1994;221:939–949.

25. Marti DN, Schaller J, Llinás M. Solution structure and dynamics of the plasminogen kringle 2-AMCHA complex: 3₁-helix in homologous domains. *Biochemistry* 1999;38:15741–15755.

26. Söhndel S, Hu CK, Marti D, et al. Recombinant gene expression and ¹H-NMR characteristics of the kringle (2 + 3) supermodule: spectroscopic functional individuality of plasminogen kringle domains. *Biochemistry* 1996;35:2357–2364.

27. Atkinson RA, Williams RJP. Solution structure of the kringle 4 domain from human plasminogen by ¹H nuclear magnetic resonance spectroscopy and distance geometry. *J Mol Biol* 1990;212:541–552.

28. Wu T-P, Padmanabhan KP, Tulinsky A. The structure of recombinant plasminogen kringle 1 and the fibrin binding site. *Blood Coagul Fibrinolysis* 1994;5:157–166.

29. Mathews II, Vanderhoff-Hanaver P, Castellino FJ, et al. Crystal structures of the recombinant kringle 1 domain of human plasminogen in complexes with the ligands ε-aminocaproic acid and *trans*-4-(aminomethyl)cyclohexane-1-carboxylic acid. *Biochemistry* 1996;35:2567–2576.

30. Wu T-P, Padmanabhan K, Tulinsky A, et al. The refined structure of the ε-aminocaproic acid complex of human plasminogen kringle 4. *Biochemistry* 1991;30:10589–10594.

31. Chang Y, Mochalkin I, McCance SG, et al. Structure and ligand binding determinants of the recombinant kringle 5 domain of human plasminogen. *Biochemistry* 1998;37:3258–3271.

32. Lerch PG, Rickli EE, Lergier W, et al. Localization of individual lysine-binding regions in human plasminogen and investigations on their complex-forming properties. *Eur J Biochem* 1980;107:7–13.

33. Menhart N, Sehl LC, Kelley RF, et al. Construction, expression, and purification of recombinant kringle 1 of human plasminogen and analysis of its interaction with omega-amino acids. *Biochemistry* 1991;30:1948–1957.

34. Novokhatny VV, Matsuka YV, Kudinov SA. Analysis of ligand binding to kringles 4 and 5 fragments from human plasminogen. *Thromb Res* 1989; 53:243–252.

35. McCance SG, Menhart N, Castellino FJ. Amino acid residues of the kringle-4 and kringle-5 domains of human plasminogen that stabilize their interactions with ω-amino acid ligands. *J Biol Chem* 1994;269:32405–32410.

36. Marti D, Schaller J, Ochensberger B, et al. Expression, purification and characterization of the recombinant kringle 2 and kringle 3 domains of human plasminogen and analysis of their binding affinity for ω-aminocarboxylic acids. *Eur J Biochem* 1994;219:455–462.

37. Christensen U, Sottrup-Jensen L, Magnusson S, et al. Enzymic properties of the neo-plasmin-val-442 (miniplasmin). *Biochim Biophys Acta* 1979; 567:472–481.

38. Komorowicz E, Kolev K, Machovich R. Fibrinolysis with des-kringle derivatives of plasmin and its modulation by plasma protease inhibitors. *Biochemistry* 1998;37:9112–9118.

39. Lasters I, Van Herzeele N, Lijnen HR, et al. Enzymatic properties of phage-displayed fragments of human plasminogen. *Eur J Biochem* 1997; 244:946–952.

40. Thewes T, Constantine K, Byeon IL, et al. Ligand interactions with the kringle 5 domain of plasminogen. A study by ¹H NMR spectroscopy. *J Biol Chem* 1990;265:3906–3915.

41. Motta A, Laursen RA, Llinás M, et al. Complete assignment of the aromatic magnetic resonance spectrum of the kringle 1 domain from human plasminogen: structure of the ligand-binding site. *Biochemistry* 1987;26: 3827–3836.

42. Tulinsky A. The structures of domains of blood proteins. *Thromb Haemost* 1991;66:16–31.

43. Peisach E, Wang J, de los Santos T, et al. Crystal structure of the proenzyme domain of plasminogen. *Biochemistry* 1999;38:11180–11188.

44. Wang X, Terzyan S, Tang J, et al. Human plasminogen catalytic domain undergoes an unusual conformational change upon activation. *J Mol Biol* 2000;295:903–914.

45. Wallén P, Wiman B. Characterization of human plasminogen. I. On the relationship between different molecular forms of plasminogen demonstrated in plasma and found in purified preparations. *Biochim Biophys Acta* 1970;221:20–30.

46. Wallén P, Wiman B. Characterization of human plasminogen. II. Separation and partial characterization of different molecular forms of human plasminogen. *Biochim Biophys Acta* 1972;257:122–134.

47. Violand BN, Castellino FJ. Mechanism of the urokinase-catalysed activation of human plasminogen. *J Biol Chem* 1976;251:3906–3912.

48. Holvoet P, Lijnen HR, Collen D. A monoclonal antibody specific for Lys-plasminogen. Application to the study of the activation pathways of plasminogen *in vivo*. *J Biol Chem* 1985;260:12106–12111.

49. Violand BN, Byrne R, Castellino FJ. The effect of α-, ω-amino acids on human plasminogen structure and activation. *J Biol Chem* 1978;253: 5395–5401.

50. Urano T, Chibber BAK, Castellino FJ. The reciprocal effects of ω-aminohexanoic acid and chloride ion on the activation of human [Glu¹] plasminogen by human urokinase. *Proc Natl Acad Sci U S A* 1987;84: 4031–4036.

51. An SSA, Carreño C, Marti DN, et al. Lysine-50 is a likely site for anchoring the plasminogen N-terminal peptide to lysine-binding kringles. *Protein Sci* 1998;7:1960–1969.

52. Cockell CS, Marshall JM, Dawson KM, et al. Evidence that the conformation of unliganded human plasminogen is maintained via an intramolecular interaction between the lysine-binding site of kringle 5 and the N-terminal peptide. *Biochem J* 1998;333:99–105.

53. Sjöholm I, Wiman B, Wallén P. Studies on the conformational changes of plasminogen induced during activation to plasmin by 6-aminohexanoic acid. *Eur J Biochem* 1973;39:471–479.

54. Castellino FJ. Biochemistry of human plasminogen. *Semin Thromb Hemost* 1984;10:18–23.

55. Mangel WF, Lin B, Ramakrishnan V. Characterization of an extremely large, ligand-induced conformational change in plasminogen. *Science* 1990; 248:69–73.

56. Stack S, Gonzales-Gronow M, Pizzo SV. The effect of divalent cations of the conformation and function of human plasminogen. *Arch Biochem Biophys* 1991;284:58–62.

57. Thorsen S. Differences in the binding to fibrin of native plasminogen and plasminogen modified by proteolytic degradation. Influence of ε-amino carboxylic acids. *Biochim Biophys Acta* 1972;393:55–65.

58. Rejante M, Elliott BW Jr, Llinás M. A ¹H-NMR study of plasminogen kringle 4 interactions with intact and partially digested fibrinogen. *Fibrinolysis* 1991;5:87–92.

59. Wu HL, Chang BI, Wu DH, et al. Interaction of plasminogen and fibrin in plasminogen activation. *J Biol Chem* 1990;265:19658–19664.

60. Lucas MA, Fretto LJ, McKee PA. The binding of human plasminogen to fibrin and fibrinogen. *J Biol Chem* 1983;258:4249–4256.

61. Suenson E, Lützen O, Thorsen S. Initial plasmin-degradation of fibrin as the basis of a positive feedback mechanism in fibrinolysis. *Eur J Biochem* 1984;140:513–522.

62. Harpel PC, Chang T, Verderber E. Tissue plasminogen activator and urokinase mediate the binding of Glu-plasminogen to plasma fibrin I. Evidence for new binding sites in plasmin-degraded fibrin I. *J Biol Chem* 1985;260:4432–4440.

63. Tran-Thang Ch, Kruithof EKO, Atkinson J, et al. High-affinity binding sites for human Glu-plasminogen unveiled by limited plasmic degradation of human fibrin. *Eur J Biochem* 1986;160:599–604.

64. Fleury V, Anglés-Cano E. Characterization of the binding of plasminogen to fibrin surfaces: the role of carboxy-terminal lysines. *Biochemistry* 1991;30:7630–7638.

65. Garman AM, Smith RAG. The binding of plasminogen to fibrin: evidence for plasminogen-bridging. *Thromb Res* 1982;27:311–320.

66. Petersen LC, Suenson E. Effect of plasminogen and tissue-type plasminogen activator on fibrin gel structure. *Fibrinolysis* 1990;5:51–59.

67. Crowe JD, Sievwright IK, Auld GC, et al. *Candida albicans* binds human plasminogen: identification of eight plasminogen-binding proteins. *Mol Microbiol* 2003;47:1637–1651.

68. Miles LA, Dahlberg CM, Plescia J, et al. Role of cell-surface lysines in plasminogen binding to cells: identification of α-enolase as a candidate plasminogen receptor. *Biochemistry* 1991;30:1682–1691.

69. Cesarman GM, Guevara CA, Hajjar KA. An endothelial cell receptor for plasminogen/tissue plasminogen activator (t-PA). Annexin II-mediated enhancement of t-PA-dependent plasminogen activation. *J Biol Chem* 1994;269:21198–21203.

70. Fischer MB, Roeckl C, Parizek P, et al. Binding of disease-associated prion protein to plasminogen. *Nature* 2000;408:479–483.

71. Ellis V. Plasminogen activation at the cell surface. *Curr Top Dev Biol* 2003;54:263–312.

72. O'Reilly MS, Holmgren L, Shing Y, et al. Angiostatin: a novel angiogenesis inhibitor that mediates the suppression of metastases by a Lewis lung carcinoma. *Cell* 1994;79:315–328.

73. Stathakis P, Fitzgerald M, Matthias LJ, et al. Generation of angiostatin by reduction and proteolysis of plasmin. Catalysis by a plasmin reductase secreted by cultured cells. *J Biol Chem* 1997;272:20641–20645.

74. Gately S, Twardowski P, Stack MS, et al. The mechanism of cancer-mediated conversion of plasminogen to the angiogenesis inhibitor angiostatin. *Proc Natl Acad Sci U S A* 1997;94:10868–10872.

75. Lay AJ, Jiang XM, Kisker O, et al. Phosphoglycerate kinase acts in tumour angiogenesis as a disulphide reductase. *Nature* 2000;408:869–873.

76. Kwon M, Caplan JF, Filipenko NR, et al. Identification of annexin II heterotetramer as a plasmin reductase. *J Biol Chem* 2002;277:10903–10911.

77. Cornelius LA, Nehring LC, Harding E, et al. Matrix metalloproteinases generate angiostatin: effects on neovascularization. *J Immunol* 1998;161:6845–6852.

78. Lijnen HR, Van Hoef B, Ugwu F, et al. Specific proteolysis of human plasminogen by a 24 kDa endopeptidase from a novel *Chryseobacterium* sp. *Biochemistry* 2000;39:479–488.

79. Cao YH, Ji RW, Davidson D, et al. Kringle domains of human angiostatin. Characterization of the anti-proliferative activity on endothelial cells. *J Biol Chem* 1996;271:29461–29467.

80. Joe Y-A, Hong Y-K, Chung D-S, et al. Inhibition of human malignant glioma growth *in vivo* by human recombinant plasminogen kringles 1-3. *Int J Cancer* 1999;82:694–699.

81. MacDonald NJ, Murad AC, Fogler WE, et al. The tumor-suppressing activity of angiostatin protein resides within kringles 1 to 3. *Biochem Biophys Res Commun* 1999;264:469–477.

82. Barendsz-Janson AF, Griffioen AW, Muller AD, et al. *In vitro* tumor angiogenesis assays: plasminogen lysine binding site 1 inhibits *in vitro* tumor-induced angiogenesis. *J Vasc Res* 1998;35:109–114.

83. Ji W-R, Barrientos LG, Llinás M, et al. Selective inhibition by kringle 5 of human plasminogen on endothelial cell migration, an important process in angiogenesis. *Biochem Biophys Res Commun* 1998;247:414–419.

84. Ji W-R, Castellino FJ, Chang Y, et al. Characterization of kringle domains of angiostatin as antagonists of endothelial cell migration, an important process in angiogenesis. *FASEB J* 1998;12:1731–1738.

85. Lucas R, Holmgren L, Garcia I, et al. Multiple forms of angiostatin induce apoptosis in endothelial cells. *Blood* 1998;92:4730–4741.

86. Walter JJ, Sane DC. Angiostatin binds to smooth muscle cells in the coronary artery and inhibits smooth muscle cell proliferation and migration *in vitro*. *Arterioscler Thromb Vasc Biol* 1999;19:2041–2048.

87. Colman RW. The contact system and angiogenesis: potential for therapeutic control of malignancy. *Semin Thromb Hemost* 2004;30:45–61.

88. Kim JS, Chang JH, Yu HK, et al. Inhibition of angiogenesis and angiogenesis-dependent tumor growth by the cryptic kringle fragments of human apolipoprotein(a). *J Biol Chem* 2003;278:29000–29008.

89. Hayes ML, Castellino FJ. Carbohydrate of the human plasminogen variants. III. Structure of the O-glycosidically linked oligosaccharide unit. *J Biol Chem* 1979;254:8777–8780.

90. Hayes ML, Castellino FJ. Carbohydrate of the human plasminogen variants. I. Carbohydrate composition, glycopeptide isolation, and characterization. *J Biol Chem* 1979;254:8768–8771.

91. Summaria L, Arzadon L, Bernabe P, et al. Studies on the isolation of the multiple molecular forms of human plasminogen and plasmin by isoelectric focusing methods. *J Biol Chem* 1972;247:4691–4702.

92. Pirie-Shepherd SR, Jett EA, Andon NL, et al. Sialic acid content of plasminogen 2 glycoforms as a regulator of fibrinolytic activity. Isolation, carbohydrate analysis, and kinetic characterization of six glycoforms of plasminogen 2. *J Biol Chem* 1995;270:5877–5881.

93. Mølgaard L, Ponting CP, Christensen U. Glycosylation at Asn-289 facilitates the ligand-induced conformational changes of human Glu-plasminogen. *FEBS Lett* 1997;405:363–368.

94. Gonzalez-Gronow M, Grenett HE, Fuller GM, et al. The role of carbohydrate in the function of human plasminogen: comparison of the protein obtained from molecular cloning and expression in *Escherichia coli* and COS cells. *Biochim Biophys Acta* 1990;1039:269–276.

95. Hatton MWC, Southward S, Ross-Ouellet B. Catabolism of plasminogen glycoforms I and II in rabbits: relationship to plasminogen synthesis by the rabbit liver *in vitro*. *Metabolism* 1994;43:1430–1437.

96. Hatton MW, Day S, Ross B, et al. Plasminogen II accumulates five times faster than plasminogen I at the site of a balloon de-endothelializing injury *in vivo* to the rabbit aorta: comparison with other hemostatic proteins. *J Lab Clin Med* 1999;134:260–266.

97. Pirie-Shepherd SR, Stevens RD, Andon NL, et al. Evidence for a novel O-linked sialylated trisaccharide on Ser-248 of human plasminogen 2. *J Biol Chem* 1997;272:7408–7411.

98. Hortin GL. Isolation of glycopeptides containing O-linked oligosaccharides by lectin affinity chromatography on jacalin-agarose. *Anal Biochem* 1990;191:262–267.

99. Wang H, Prorok M, Bretthauer RK, et al. Serine-578 is a major phosphorylation locus in human plasma plasminogen. *Biochemistry* 1997;36:8100–8106.

100. Skoda U, Bertrams J, Dykes D, et al. Proposal for the nomenclature of human plasminogen (PLG) polymorphism. *Vox Sang* 1986;51:244–248.

101. Tefs K, Georgieva M, Seregard S, et al. Characterization of plasminogen variants in healthy subjects and plasminogen mutants in patients with inherited plasminogen deficiency by isoelectric focusing gel electrophoresis. *Thromb Haemost* 2004;92:352–357.

102. Yamaguchi M, Doi S, Yoshimura M. Plasminogen phenotypes in a Japanese population. Four new variants including one with a functional defect. *Hum Hered* 1989;39:356–360.

103. Aoki N, Moroi M, Sakata Y. Abnormal plasminogen: a hereditary molecular abnormality found in a patient with recurrent thrombosis. *J Clin Invest* 1978;61:1186.

104. Schuster V, Zeitler P, Seregard S, et al. Homozygous and compound-heterozygous type I plasminogen deficiency is a common cause of ligneous conjunctivitis. *Thromb Haemost* 2001;85:1004–1010.

105. Schuster V, Mingers AM, Seidenspinner S, et al. Homozygous mutations in the plasminogen gene of two unrelated girls with ligneous conjunctivitis. *Blood* 1997;90:958–966.

106. Schuster V, Seidenspinner S, Zeitler P, et al. Compound-heterozygous mutations in the plasminogen gene predispose to the development of ligneous conjunctivitis. *Blood* 1999;93:3457–3466.

107. Ichinose A, Espling ES, Takamatsu J, et al. Two types of abnormal genes for plasminogen in families with a predisposition for thrombosis. *Proc Natl Acad Sci U S A* 1991;88:115–119; and correction *Proc Natl Acad Sci U S A* 1991;88:2967.

108. Schott D, Dempfle C-E, Beck P, et al. Therapy with a purified plasminogen concentrate in an infant with ligneous conjunctivitis and homozygous plasminogen deficiency. *N Engl J Med* 1998;339:1679–1686.

109. Azuma H, Uno Y, Shigekiyo T, et al. Congenital plasminogen deficiency caused by a Ser$^{572}$ to Pro mutation. *Blood* 1993;82:475–480.

110. Takeda-Shitaka M, Umeyama H. Elucidation of the cause for reduced activity of abnormal human plasmin containing an Ala$^{55}$-Thr mutation: importance of highly conserved Ala$^{55}$ in serine proteases. *FEBS Lett* 1998;425:448–452.

111. Mima N, Azuma H, Shigekiyo T, et al. A novel missense mutation in two families with congenital plasminogen deficiency—identification of an Ala(675) to Thr(675) substitution. *Thromb Haemost* 1996;75:96–100.

112. Tsutsumi S, Saito T, Sakata T, et al. Genetic diagnosis of dysplasminogenemia: detection of an Ala601-Thr mutation in 118 out of 125 families and identification of a new Asp676-Asn mutation. *Thromb Haemost* 1996;76:135–138.

113. Yamaguchi M, Sugiyama S, Noda H, et al. A novel missense mutation D676N in the plasminogen gene causes loss of functional activity. *Hum Hered* 1997;47:234–236.

114. Higuchi Y, Furihata K, Ueno I, et al. Plasminogen Kanagawa-I, a novel missense mutation, is caused by the amino acid substitution G732R. *Br J Haematol* 1998;103:867–870.

115. Tait RC, Walker ID, Conkie JA, et al. Isolated familial plasminogen deficiency may not be a risk factor for thrombosis. *Thromb Haemost* 1996;76:1004–1008.

116. Demarmels Biasiutti F, Sulzer I, Stucki B, et al. Is plasminogen deficiency a thrombotic risk factor? A study of 23 thrombophilic patients and their family members. *Thromb Haemost* 1998;80:167–170.

117. Sartori TM, Saggiorato G, Pellati D, et al. Contraceptive pills induce an improvement in congenital hypoplasminogenemia in two unrelated patients with ligneous conjunctivitis. *Thromb Haemost* 2003;90:86–91.

118. Tefs K, Ziegler M, Georgieva M, et al. A nucleic acid exchange in Intron F (Intron F-14T > G) in the human plasminogen gene is only a common polymorphism and not a true mutation. *Thromb Haemost* 2004;91:830–831.

119. Drew AF, Kaufman AH, Kombrinck KW, et al. Ligneous conjunctivitis in plasminogen-deficient mice. *Blood* 1998;91:1616–1624.

120. Ploplis VA, Carmeliet P, Vazizadeh S, et al. Effects of disruption of the plasminogen gene on thrombosis, growth, and health in mice. *Circulation* 1995;92:2585–2593.

121. Bugge TH, Flick MJ, Daugherty CC, et al. Plasminogen deficiency causes severe thrombosis but is compatible with development and reproduction. *Genes Dev* 1995;9:794–807.

122. Ny A, Leonardsson G, Hägglund A-C, et al. Ovulation in plasminogen-deficient mice. *Endocrinology* 1999;140:5030–5035.

123. Rømer J, Bugge TH, Pyke C, et al. Impaired wound healing in mice with a disrupted plasminogen gene. *Nat Med* 1996;2:287–292.

124. Bezerra JA, Bugge TH, Melin-Aldana H, et al. Plasminogen deficiency leads to impaired remodeling after a toxic injury to the liver. *Proc Natl Acad Sci U S A* 1999;96:15143–15148.

125. Ploplis VA, French EL, Carmeliet P, et al. Plasminogen deficiency differentially affects recruitment of inflammatory cell populations in mice. *Blood* 1998;91:2005–2009.

126. Carmeliet P, Moons L, Ploplis V, et al. Impaired arterial neointima formation in mice with disruption of the plasminogen gene. *J Clin Invest* 1997;99:200–208.

127. Xiao Q, Danton MJ, Witte DP, et al. Plasminogen deficiency accelerates vessel wall disease in mice predisposed to atherosclerosis. *Proc Natl Acad Sci U S A* 1997;94:10335–10340.

128. Bugge TH, Kombrinck KW, Flick MJ, et al. Loss of fibrinogen rescues mice from the pleiotropic effects of plasminogen deficiency. *Cell* 1996;87:709–719.

129. Palumbo JS, Talmage KE, Liu H, et al. Plasminogen supports tumor growth through a fibrinogen-dependent mechanism linked to vascular patency. *Blood* 2003;102:2819–2827.

130. Bannach FG, Gutierrez A, Fowler BJ, et al. Localization of regulatory elements mediating constitutive and cytokine-stimulated plasminogen gene expression. *J Biol Chem* 2002;277:38579–38588.

131. Kida M, Wakabayashi S, Ichinose A. Expression and induction by IL-6 of the normal and variant genes for human plasminogen. *Biochem Biophys Res Commun* 1997;230:129–132.

132. Meroni G, Buraggi G, Mantovani R, et al. Motifs resembling hepatocyte nuclear factor 1 and activator protein 3 mediate the tissue specificity of the human plasminogen gene. *Eur J Biochem* 1996;236:373–382.

133. Strickland S. Tissue plasminogen activator in nervous system function and dysfunction. *Thromb Haemost* 2001;86:138–143.

134. Rosenberg S. The urokinase-type plasminogen activator system in cancer and other pathological conditions: introduction and perspective. *Curr Pharm Des* 2003;9:4p.

135. Levin EG, Loskutoff DJ. Cultured bovine endothelial cells produce both urokinase and tissue-type plasminogen activators. *J Cell Biol* 1982;94:631–636.

136. Nicoloso G, Hauert J, Kruithof EKO, et al. Fibrinolysis in normal subjects—comparison between plasminogen activator inhibitor and other components of the fibrinolytic system. *Thromb Haemost* 1988;59:299–303.

137. Stalder M, Hauert J, Kruithof EKO, et al. Release of vascular plasminogen activator (vPA) after venous stasis: electrophoretic-zymographic analysis of free and complexed vPA. *Br J Haematol* 1985;61:169–176.

138. Booth NA, Walker E, Maughan R, et al. Plasminogen activator in normal subjects after exercise and venous occlusion: tPA circulates as complexes with C1 inhibitor and PAI-1. *Blood* 1987;69:1354–1362.

139. Benham FJ, Spurr N, Povey S, et al. Assignment of tissue-type plasminogen activator to chromosome 8 in man and identification of a common restriction length polymorphism within the gene. *Mol Biol Med* 1984;2:251–259.

140. Degen SJF, Rajput B, Reich E. The human tissue plasminogen activator gene. *J Biol Chem* 1986;261:6972–6985.

141. Jörnvall H, Pohl G, Bergsdorf N, et al. Differential proteolysis and evidence for a residue exchange in tissue plasminogen activator suggest possible association between two types of protein microheterogeneity. *FEBS Lett* 1983;156:47–50.

142. Pennica D, Holmes WE, Kohr WJ, et al. Cloning and expression of human tissue-type plasminogen activator cDNA in *E. coli*. *Nature* 1983;301:214–221.

143. Van Zonneveld A-J, Veerman H, Pannekoek H. On the interaction of the finger- and kringle 2-domain of tissue-type plasminogen activator with fibrin. Inhibition of kringle-2 binding to fibrin by ε-aminocaproic acid. *J Biol Chem* 1986;261:14214–14218.

144. Bányai L, Váradi A, Patthy L. Common evolutionary origin of the fibrin-binding structures of fibronectin and tissue-type plasminogen activator. *FEBS Lett* 1983;163:37–41.

145. de Munk GAW, Caspers MPM, Chang GTG, et al. Binding of tissue-type plasminogen activator to lysine, lysine analogues, and fibrin fragments. *Biochemistry* 1989;28:7318–7325.

146. Downing AK, Driscoll PC, Harvey TS, et al. Solution structure of the fibrin binding finger domain of tissue-type plasminogen activator determined by ¹H nuclear magnetic resonance. *J Mol Biol* 1992;225:821–833.

147. Smith BO, Downing AK, Dudgeon TJ, et al. Secondary structure of fibronectin type 1 and epidermal growth factor modules from tissue-type plasminogen activator by nuclear magnetic resonance. *Biochemistry* 1994;33:2422–2429.

148. Byeon I-JL, Kelley RF, Mulkerrin MG, et al. Ligand binding to the tissue-type plasminogen activator kringle 2 domain: structural characterization by ¹H-NMR. *Biochemistry* 1995;34:2739–2750.

149. Kelley RF, DeVos AM, Cleary S. Thermodynamics of ligand binding and denaturation for His64 mutants of tissue plasminogen activator kringle-2 domain. *Proteins: Struct Funct Genet* 1991;11:35–44.

150. de Vos AM, Ultsch MH, Kelley RF, et al. Crystal structure of the kringle 2 domain of tissue plasminogen activator at 2.4-Å resolution. *Biochemistry* 1992;31:270–279.

151. Collen D, Lijnen HR, Bulens F, et al. Biochemical and functional characterization of human tissue-type plasminogen activator variants with mutagenized kringle domains. *J Biol Chem* 1990;265:12184–12191.

152. Chang Y, Nilsen SL, Castellino FJ. Functional and structural consequences of aromatic residue substitutions within the kringle-2 domain of tissue-type plasminogen activator. *J Pept Res* 1999;53:656–664.

153. de Serrano VS, Sehl LC, Castellino FJ. Direct identification of lysine-33 as the principal cationic center of the ω-amino acid binding site of the recombinant kringle 2 domain of tissue-type plasminogen activator. *Arch Biochem Biophys* 1992;292:206–212.

154. Lamba D, Bauer M, Huber R, et al. The 2.3 Å crystal structure of the catalytic domain of recombinant two-chain human tissue-type plasminogen activator. *J Mol Biol* 1996;258:117–135.

155. Rijken DC, Hoylaerts M, Collen D. Fibrinolytic properties of one-chain and two-chain human extrinsic (tissue-type) plasminogen activator. *J Biol Chem* 1982;257:2920–2925.

156. Tachias K, Madison EL. Converting tissue-type plasminogen activator into a zymogen. *J Biol Chem* 1996;271:28749–28752.

157. Camiolo SM, Thorsen S, Astrup T. Fibrinogenolysis and fibrinolysis with tissue plasminogen activator, urokinase, streptokinase-activated human globulin, and plasmin. *Proc Soc Exp Biol Med* 1971;138:277–280.

158. Thorsen S, Glas-Greenwalt P, Astrup T. Differences in the binding to fibrin of urokinase and tissue plasminogen activator. *Thromb Diath Haemorrh* 1972;28:65–74.

159. Higgins D, Vehar GA. Interaction of one-chain and two-chain tissue plasminogen activator with intact and plasmin-degraded fibrin. *Biochemistry* 1987;26:7786–7791.

160. Larsen GR, Henson H, Blue Y. Variants of human tissue-type plasminogen activator. Fibrin binding, fibrinolytic, and fibrinogenolytic characterization of genetic variants lacking the fibronectin finger-like and/or the epidermal growth factor domains. *J Biol Chem* 1988;263:1023–1029.

161. Rånby M, Bergsdorf N, Nilsson T. Enzymatic properties of the one- and two-chain form of tissue plasminogen activator. *Thromb Res* 1982;27:175–183.

162. Geppert AG, Binder BR. Allosteric regulation of tPA-mediated plasminogen activation by a modifier mechanism: evidence for a binding site for plasminogen on the tPA A-chain. *Arch Biochem Biophys* 1992;297:205–212.

163. Rånby M. Studies on the kinetics of plasminogen activation by tissue plasminogen activator. *Biochim Biophys Acta* 1982;704:461–469.

164. Hoylaerts M, Rijken DC, Lijnen HR, et al. Kinetics of the activation of plasminogen by human tissue plasminogen activator. Role of fibrin. *J Biol Chem* 1982;257:2912–2919.

165. Norrman B, Wallén P, Rånby M. Fibrinolysis mediated by tissue plasminogen activator. Disclosure of a kinetic transition. *Eur J Biochem* 1985;149:193–200.

166. Rijken DC, Wijngaards G, Zaal De Jong M, et al. Purification and partial characterization of plasminogen activator from human uterine tissue. *Biochim Biophys Acta* 1979;580:140–153.

167. De Vries C, Veerman H, Koornneef E, et al. Tissue-type plasminogen activator and its substrate Glu-plasminogen share common binding sites in limited plasmin-digested fibrin. *J Biol Chem* 1990;265:13547–13552.

168. Medved L, Nieuwenhuizen W. Molecular mechanisms of initiation of fibrinolysis by fibrin. *Thromb Haemost* 2003;89:409–419.

169. Yonekawa O, Voskuilen M, Nieuwenhuizen W. Localization in the fibrinogen γ-chain of a new site that is involved in the acceleration of the tissue-type plasminogen activator-catalysed activation of plasminogen. *Biochem J* 1992;283:187–191.

170. Schielen WJG, Adams HPHM, van Leuven K, et al. The sequence γ-(312-324) is a fibrin-specific epitope. *Blood* 1991;77:2169–2173.

171. Tsurupa G, Medved L. Identification and characterization of novel tPA- and plasminogen-binding sites within fibrin(ogen) αC-domains. *Biochemistry* 2001;40:801–808.

172. Mosesson MW, Siebenlist KR, Voskuilen M, et al. Evaluation of the factors contributing to fibrin-dependent plasminogen activation. *Thromb Haemost* 1998;79:796–801.

173. Madison EL, Goldsmith FJ, Gerard RD, et al. Serpin-resistant mutants of human tissue-type plasminogen activator. *Nature* 1989;339:721–724.

174. Madison EL, Goldsmith EJ, Gerard RD, et al. Amino acid residue that affect interaction of tissue-type plasminogen activator with plasminogen activator inhibitor 1. *Proc Natl Acad Sci U S A* 1990;87:3530–3533.

175. Paoni NF, Keyt BA, Refino CJ, et al. A slow clearing, fibrin-specific, PAI-1 resistant variant of tPA (T103N, KHRR 296-299 AAAA). *Thromb Haemost* 1993;70:307–312.

176. Stewart RJ, Fredenburgh JC, Leslie BA, et al. Identification of the mechanism responsible for the increased fibrin specificity of TNK-tissue plasminogen activator relative to tissue plasminogen activator. *J Biol Chem* 2000;275:10112–10120.

177. Hajjar KA, Krishnan S. Annexin II: a mediator of the plasmin/plasminogen activator system. *Trends Cardiovasc Med* 1999;9:128–138.

178. Dudani AK, Ganz PR. Endothelial cell surface actin serves as a binding site for plasminogen, tissue plasminogen activator and lipoprotein(a). *Br J Haematol* 1996;95:168–178.

179. Bohm T, Geiger M, Binder BR. Isolation and characterization of tissue-type plasminogen activator-binding proteoglycans from human umbilical vein endothelial cells. *Arterioscler Thromb Vasc Biol* 1996;16:665–672.

180. Hembrough TA, Kralovich KR, Li L, et al. Cytokeratin 8 released by breast carcinoma cells *in vitro* binds plasminogen and tissue-type plasminogen activator and promotes plasminogen activation. *Biochem J* 1996;317:763–769.

181. Beebe DP, Wood LL, Moos M. Characterization of tissue plasminogen activator binding proteins isolated from endothelial cells and other cell types. *Thromb Res* 1990;59:339–350.

182. Menell JS, Cesarman GM, Jacovina AT, et al. Annexin II and bleeding in acute promyelocytic leukemia. *N Engl J Med* 1999;340:994–1004.

183. Bennett B, Booth NA, Croll A, et al. The bleeding disorder in acute promyelocytic leukaemia: fibrinolysis due to uPA rather than defibrination. *Br J Haematol* 1989;71:511–517.

184. Redlitz A, Plow EF. Receptors for plasminogen and tPA: an update. *Baillieres Clin Haematol* 1995;8:313–327.

185. Fukao H, Matsuo O. Analysis of tissue-type plasminogen activator receptor (tPAR) in human endothelial cells. *Semin Thromb Hemost* 1998;24:269–273.

186. Werner F, Razzaq TM, Ellis V. Tissue plasminogen activator binds to human vascular smooth muscle cells by a novel mechanism. Evidence for a reciprocal linkage between inhibition of catalytic activity and cellular binding. *J Biol Chem* 1999;274:21555–21561.

187. Razzaq TM, Bass R, Vines DJ, et al. Functional regulation of tissue plasminogen activator on the surface of vascular smooth muscle cells by the type-II transmembrane protein p63 (CKAP4). *J Biol Chem* 2003;278:42679–42685.

188. Parekh RB, Dwek RA, Thomas JR, et al. Cell-type-specific and site-specific N-glycosylation of type I and type II human tissue plasminogen activator. *Biochemistry* 1989;28:7644–7662.

189. Dwek RA. Glycobiology: "Towards understanding the function of sugars." *Biochem Soc Trans* 1995;23:1–25.

190. Harris RJ, Leonard CK, Guzzetta AW, et al. Tissue plasminogen activator has an O-linked fucose attached to threonine-61 in the epidermal growth factor domain. *Biochemistry* 1991;30:2311–2314.

191. Hajjar KA, Reynolds CM. α-Fucose-mediated binding and degradation of tissue-type plasminogen activator by HepG2 cells. *J Clin Invest* 1994;93:703–710.

192. Ridker PM, Baker MT, Hennekens CH, et al. Alu-repeat polymorphism in the gene coding for tissue-type plasminogen activator (tPA) and risks of myocardial infarction among middle-aged men. *Arterioscler Thromb Vasc Biol* 1997;17:1687–1690.

193. van der Bom JG, de Knijff P, Haverkate F et al. The Rotterdam Study. Tissue plasminogen activator and risk of myocardial infarction. *Circulation* 1997;95:2623–2627.

194. Jern C, Ladenvall P, Wall U, et al. Gene polymorphism of t-PA is associated with forearm vascular release rate of t-PA. *Arterioscler Thromb Vasc Biol* 1999;19:454–459.

195. Tjarnlund-Wolf A, Medcalf RL, Jern C. The t-PA −7,351C > T enhancer polymorphism decreases Sp1 and Sp3 protein binding affinity and transcriptional responsiveness to retinoic acid. *Blood* 2005;105:1060–1067.

196. Arts J, Herr I, Lansink M, et al. Cell-type specific DNA-protein interactions at the tissue-type plasminogen activator promoter in human endothelial and Hela cells *in vivo* and *in vitro*. *Nucleic Acids Res* 1997;25:311–317.

197. Levin EG, Santell L. Stimulation and desensitization of tissue plasminogen activator release from human endothelial cells. *J Biol Chem* 1988;263:9360–9365.

198. Levin EG, Marotti KR, Santell L. Protein kinase C and the stimulation of tissue plasminogen activator release from human endothelial cells: dependence on the elevation of messenger RNA. *J Biol Chem* 1989;264:16030–16036.

199. Bulens F, Merchiers P, Ibañez-Tallon I, et al. Identification of a multihormone responsive enhancer far upstream from the human tissue-type plasminogen activator gene. *J Biol Chem* 1997;272:663–671.

200. Merchiers P, Bulens F, Stockmans I, et al. 1,25-Dihydroxyvitamin D$_3$ induction of the tissue-type plasminogen activator gene is mediated through its multihormone-responsive enhancer. *FEBS Lett* 1999;460:289–296.

201. Kooistra T, Opdenberg JP, Toet K, et al. Stimulation of tissue-type plasminogen activator synthesis by retinoids in cultured human endothelial cells and rat tissues *in vivo*. *Thromb Haemost* 1991;65:565–572.

202. Medh RD, Santell L, Levin EG. Stimulation of tissue plasminogen activator production by retinoic acid: synergistic effect on protein kinase C-mediated activation. *Blood* 1992;80:981–987.

203. Levin EG, del Zoppo GJ. Localization of tissue plasminogen activator in the endothelium of a limited number of vessels. *Am J Pathol* 1994;144:855–861.

204. Levin EG, Santell L, Osborn KG. The expression of tissue plasminogen activator *in vivo*: a function defined by vessel size and anatomic location. *J Cell Sci* 1997;110:139–148.

205. Pham NL, Franzen A, Levin EG. NF1 regulatory element functions as a repressor of tissue plasminogen activator expression. *Arterioscler Thromb Vasc Biol* 2004;24:982–987.

206. Costa M, Shen Y, Maurer F, et al. Transcriptional regulation of the tissue-type plasminogen-activator gene in human endothelial cells: identification of nuclear factors that recognise functional elements in the tissue-type plasminogen-activator gene promoter. *Eur J Biochem* 1998;258:123–131.

207. Medcalf RL, Rüegg M, Schleuning WD. A DNA motif related to the cAMP-responsive element and an exon-located activator protein-2 binding site in the human tissue-type plasminogen activator gene promoter cooperate in basal expression and convey activation by phorbol ester and cAMP. *J Biol Chem* 1990;265:14618–14626.

208. Fujiwara J, Kimura T, Ayusawa D, et al. A novel regulatory sequence affecting the constitutive expression of tissue plasminogen activator (tPA) gene in human melanoma (Bowes) cells. *J Biol Chem* 1994;269:18558–18562.

209. Bulens F, Ibañez-Tallon I, van Acker P, et al. Retinoic acid induction of human tissue-type plasminogen activator gene expression via a direct repeat element (DR5) located at −7 kilobases. *J Biol Chem* 1995;270:7167–7175.

210. Keber D, Blinc A, Fettich J. Increase of tissue plasminogen activator in limbs during venous occlusion: a simple haemodynamic model. *Thromb Haemost* 1990;64:433–437.

211. Juhan-Vague I, Valadier J, Alessi MC, et al. Deficient tPA release and elevated PA inhibitor levels in patients with spontaneous or recurrent deep venous thrombosis. *Thromb Haemost* 1987;57:67–72.

212. Nguyen G, Horellou MH, Kruithof EKO, et al. Residual plasminogen activator inhibitor activity after venous stasis as criterion for hypofibrinolysis: a study in 83 patients with confirmed deep vein thrombosis. *Blood* 1988;72:601–605.

213. Jeanneau C, Bachouchi NO, Gorin I, et al. Absence of functional activity of tissue plasminogen activator in patients with severe forms of von Willebrand's disease. *Br J Haematol* 1987;56:79–88.

214. Knop M, Aareskjold E, Bode G, et al. Rab3D and annexin A2 play a role in regulated secretion of VWF, but not tPA, from endothelial cells. *EMBO J* 2004;23:2982–2992.

215. Keber D, Stegnar M, Kluft C. Different tissue plasminogen activator release in the arm and leg during venous occlusion is equalized after DDAVP infusion. *Thromb Haemost* 1990;63:72–75.

216. Waugh JM, Kattash M, Li J, et al. Gene therapy to promote thromboresistance: local overexpression of tissue plasminogen activator to prevent arterial thrombosis in an *in vivo* rabbit model. *Proc Natl Acad Sci U S A* 1999;96:1065–1070.

217. Booth NA, Bennett B, Wijngaards G, et al. A new life-long hemorrhagic disorder due to excess plasminogen activator. *Blood* 1983;61:267–275.

218. Aznar J, Estellés A, Vila V, et al. Inherited fibrinolytic disorder due to an enhanced plasminogen activator level. *Thromb Haemost* 1984;52:196–200.

219. Emeis JJ, van den Eijnden-Schrauwen Y, Van den Hoogen CM, et al. An endothelial storage granule for tissue-type plasminogen activator. *J Cell Biol* 1997;139:245–256.

220. Parmer RJ, Mahata M, Mahata S, et al. Tissue plasminogen activator (tPA) is targeted to the regulated secretory pathway. Catecholamine storage vesicles as a reservoir for the rapid release of tPA. *J Biol Chem* 1997;272:1976–1982.

221. Rosnoblet C, Vischer UM, Gerard RD, et al. Storage of tissue-type plasminogen activator in Weibel-Palade bodies of human endothelial cells. *Arterioscler Thromb Vasc Biol* 1999;19:1796–1803.

222. Santell L, Marotti KR, Levin EG. Targeting of tissue plasminogen activator into the regulated secretory pathway of neuroendocrine cells. *Brain Res* 1999;816:258–265.

223. Padró T, Van den Hoogen CM, Emeis JJ. Distribution of tissue-type plasminogen activator (activity and antigen) in rat tissues. *Blood Coagul Fibrinolysis* 1990;1:601–608.

224. Tappy L, Hauert J, Bachmann F. Effects of hypoxia and acidosis on vascular plasminogen activator release in the pig ear perfusion system. *Thromb Res* 1984;33:117–124.

225. Vaughan DE. The renin-angiotensin system and fibrinolysis. *Am J Cardiol* 1997;79:12–16.

226. van den Eijnden-Schrauen Y, Atsma DE, Lupu F, et al. Involvement of calcium and G proteins in the acute release of tissue-type plasminogen activator and von Willebrand factor from cultured human endothelial cells. *Arterioscler Thromb Vasc Biol* 1997;17:2177–2187.

227. Chandler WL, Levy WC, Stratton JR. The circulatory regulation of TPA and UPA secretion, clearance, and inhibition during exercise and during the infusion of isoproterenol and phenylephrine. *Circulation* 1995;92:2984–2994.

228. Jern C, Selin L, Jern S. *In vivo* release of tissue-type plasminogen activator across the human forearm during mental stress. *Thromb Haemost* 1994;72:285–291.

229. Cash JD. Control mechanisms of activator release. In: Davidson JF, Rowan RM, Samama MM et al., eds. *Progress in chemical fibrinolysis and thrombolysis*, Vol. 3. New York: Raven Press, 1978:65–75.

230. Mannucci PM, Rota L. Plasminogen activator response after DDAVP: a clinico-pharmacological study. *Thromb Res* 1980;20:69–76.

231. Brommer EJP, Barrett-Bergshoeff MM, Allen RA, et al. The use of desmopressin acetate (DDAVP) as a test of fibrinolytic capacity of patients—analysis of responders and non-responders. *Thromb Haemost* 1982;48:156–161.

232. Wall U, Jern S, Tengborn L, et al. Evidence of a local mechanism for desmopressin-induced tissue-type plasminogen activator release in human forearm. *Blood* 1998;91:529–537.

233. Stein CM, Brown N, Vaughan DE, et al. Regulation of local tissue-type plasminogen activator release by endothelium-dependent and endothelium-independent agonists in human vasculature. *J Am Coll Cardiol* 1998;32:117–122.

234. Dell'Omo G, Ferrini L, Morale M, et al. Acetylcholine-mediated vasodilatation and tissue-type plasminogen activator release in normal and hypertensive men. *Angiology* 1999;50:273–282.

235. Brown NJ, Gainer JV, Stein CM, et al. Bradykinin stimulates tissue plasminogen activator release in human vasculature. *Hypertension* 1999;33:1431–1435.

236. Newby DE, Wright RA, Ludlam CA, et al. An *in vivo* model for the assessment of acute fibrinolytic capacity of the endothelium. *Thromb Haemost* 1997;78:1242–1248.

237. Hrafnkelsdottir T, Gudnason T, Wall U, et al. Regulation of local availability of active tissue-type plasminogen activator *in vivo* in man. *J Thromb Haemost* 2004;2:1960–1968.

238. Tanswell P, Seifried E, Su PCAF, et al. Pharmacokinetics and systemic effects of tissue-type plasminogen activator in normal subjects. *Clin Pharmacol Ther* 1989;46:155–162.

239. Huber K, Kirchheimer JC, Korninger C, et al. Hepatic synthesis and clearance of components of the fibrinolytic system in healthy volunteers and in patients with different stages of liver cirrhosis. *Thromb Res* 1991;62:491–500.

240. Wing LR, Hawksworth GM, Bennett B, et al. Clearance of t-PA, PAI-1, and t-PA-PAI-1 complex in an isolated perfused rat liver system. *J Lab Clin Med* 1991;117:109–114.

241. Chandler WL, Alessi MC, Aillaud MF, et al. Clearance of tissue plasminogen activator (TPA) and TPA/plasminogen activator inhibitor type 1 (PAI-1) complex: relationship to elevated TPA antigen in patients with high PAI-1 activity levels. *Circulation* 1997;96:761–768.

242. Bounameaux H, Stassen JM, Seghers C, et al. Influence of fibrin and liver blood flow on the turnover and the systemic fibrinogenolytic effects of recombinant human tissue-type plasminogen activator in rabbits. *Blood* 1986;67:1493–1497.

243. de Boer A, Kluft C, Kroon JM, et al. Liver blood flow as a major determinant of the clearance of recombinant human tissue-type plasminogen activator. *Thromb Haemost* 1992;67:83–87.

244. Van Griensven JMT, Huisman LGM, Stuurman T, et al. Effects of increased liver blood flow on the kinetics and dynamics of recombinant tissue-type plasminogen activator. *Clin Pharmacol Ther* 1996;60:504–511.

245. Fletcher AP, Biederman O, Moore D, et al. Abnormal plasminogen-plasmin system activity (fibrinolysis) in patients with hepatic cirrhosis: its cause and consequences. *J Clin Invest* 1964;43:681–695.

246. Otter M, Barrett-Bergshoeff MM, Rijken DC. Binding of tissue-type plasminogen activator by the mannose receptor. *J Biol Chem* 1991;266:13931–13935.

247. Biessen EAL, van Teijlingen M, Vietsch H, et al. Antagonists of the mannose receptor and the LDL receptor-related protein dramatically delay the clearance of tissue plasminogen activator. *Circulation* 1997;95:46–52.

248. Noorman F, Barrett-Bergshoeff MM, Rijken DC. Role of carbohydrate and protein in the binding of tissue-type plasminogen activator to the human mannose receptor. *Eur J Biochem* 1998;251:107–113.

249. Lansink M, Jong M, Bijsterbosch M, et al. Increased clearance explains lower plasma levels of tissue-type plasminogen activator by estradiol: evidence for potently enhanced mannose receptor expression in mice. *Blood* 1999;94:1330–1336.

250. Lehrman MA, Hill RL. The binding of fucose-containing glycoproteins by hepatic lectins. *J Biol Chem* 1986;261:7419–7474.

251. Strickland DK, Ranganathan S. Diverse role of LDL receptor-related protein in the clearance of proteases and in signaling. *J Thromb Haemost* 2003;1:1663–1670.

252. Narita M, Bu G, Herz J, et al. Two receptor systems are involved in the plasma clearance of tissue-type plasminogen activator (tPA) *in vivo*. *J Clin Invest* 1995;96:1164–1168.

253. Camani C, Bachmann F, Kruithof EKO. The role of plasminogen activator inhibitor type 1 in the clearance of tissue-type plasminogen activator by rat hepatoma cells. *J Biol Chem* 1994;269:5770–5775.

254. Moestrup SK, Holtet TL, Etzerodt M, et al. $\alpha_2$-Macroglobulin-proteinase complexes, plasminogen activator inhibitor type-1-plasminogen activator complexes, and receptor-associated protein bind to a region of the $\alpha_2$-macroglobulin receptor containing a cluster of eight complement-type repeats. *J Biol Chem* 1993;268:13691–13696.

255. Willnow TE, Orth K, Herz J. Molecular dissection of ligand binding sites on the low density lipoprotein receptor-related protein. *J Biol Chem* 1994;269:15827–15832.

256. Horn IR, Van den Berg BMM, van der Meijden PZ, et al. Molecular analysis of ligand binding to the second cluster of complement-type repeats of the low density lipoprotein receptor-related protein. Evidence for an allosteric component in receptor-associated protein-mediated inhibition of ligand binding. *J Biol Chem* 1997;272:13608–13613.

257. Herz J, Goldstein JL, Strickland DK, et al. 39-kDa protein modulates binding of ligands to low density lipoprotein receptor-related protein/$\alpha_2$-macroglobulin receptor. *J Biol Chem* 1991;266:21232–21238.

258. Andreasen PA, Sottrup-Jensen L, Kjøller L, et al. Receptor-mediated endocytosis of plasminogen activators and activator/inhibitor complexes. *FEBS Lett* 1994;338:239–245.

259. Moestrup SK. The $\alpha_2$-macroglobulin receptor and epithelial glycoprotein-330: two giant receptors mediating endocytosis of multiple ligands. *Biochim Biophys Acta* 1994;1197:197–213.

260. Kasza A, Petersen HH, Heegaard CW, et al. Specificity of serine proteinase/serpin complex binding to very-low-density lipoprotein receptor and $\alpha_2$-macroglobulin receptor/low-density-lipoprotein-receptor-related protein. *Eur J Biochem* 1997;248:270–281.

261. Kounnas MZ, Henkin J, Argraves WS, et al. Low density lipoprotein receptor-related protein/$\alpha_2$-macroglobulin receptor mediates cellular uptake of pro-urokinase. *J Biol Chem* 1993;268:21862–21867.

262. Nykjaer A, Kjøller L, Cohen RL, et al. Regions involved in binding of urokinase-type-1 inhibitor complex and pro-urokinase to the endocytic $\alpha_2$-macroglobulin receptor/low density lipoprotein receptor-related protein. Evidence that the urokinase receptor protects pro-urokinase against binding to the endocytic receptor. *J Biol Chem* 1994;269:25668–25676.

263. Camani C, Gavin O, Kruithof EKO. Cellular degradation of free and inhibitor-bound tissue-type plasminogen activator. Requirement for a co-receptor? *Thromb Haemost* 2000;83:290–296.

264. Carmeliet P, Schoonjans L, Kieckens L, et al. Physiological consequences of loss of plasminogen activator gene function in mice. *Nature* 1994;368:419–424.

265. Carmeliet P, Collen D. Targeted gene manipulation and transfer of the plasminogen and coagulation systems in mice. *Fibrinolysis* 1996;10:195–213.

266. Leonardsson G, Peng X-R, Liu K, et al. Ovulation efficiency is reduced in mice that lack plasminogen activator gene function: functional redundancy among physiological plasminogen activators. *Proc Natl Acad Sci U S A* 1995;92:12446–12450.

267. Seeds NW, Basham ME, Haffke SP. Neuronal migration is retarded in mice lacking the tissue plasminogen activator gene. *Proc Natl Acad Sci U S A* 1999;96:14118–14123.

268. Baranes D, Lederfein D, Huang Y-Y, et al. Tissue plasminogen activator contributes to the late phase of LTP and to synaptic growth in the hippocampal mossy fiber pathway. *Neuron* 1998;21:813–825.

269. Husain SS, Gurewich V, Lipinski B. Purification and partial characterization of a single-chain molecular weight form of urokinase from human urine. *Arch Biochem Biophys* 1983;220:31–38.

270. Larsson L, Skriver L, Nielsen LS, et al. Distribution of urokinase-type plasminogen activator immunoreactivity in the mouse. *J Cell Biol* 1984;98:894–903.

271. Grau E, Moroz LA. Fibrinolytic activity of normal human blood monocytes. *Thromb Res* 1989;53:145–162.

272. Manchanda N, Schwartz BS. Lipopolysaccharide-induced modulation of human monocyte urokinase production and activity. *J Immunol* 1990;145:4174–4180.

273. Van Hinsbergh VWM, Kooistra T, van den Berg EA, et al. Tumor necrosis factor increases the production of plasminogen activator inhibitor in human endothelial cells *in vitro* and in rats *in vivo*. *Blood* 1988;72:1467–1473.

274. Camoin L, Pannell R, Anfosso F, et al. Evidence for the expression of urokinase-type plasminogen activator by human venous endothelial cells *in vivo*. *Thromb Haemost* 1998;80:961–967.

275. Danø K, Andreasen PA, Grøndahl-Hansen J, et al. Plasminogen activators, tissue degradation, and cancer. *Adv Cancer Res* 1985;44:139–266.

276. Duffy MJ. The urokinase plasminogen activator system: role in malignancy. *Curr Pharm Des* 2004;10:39–49.

277. Steffens GJ, Günzler WA, Ötting F, et al. The complete amino acid sequence of low molecular mass urokinase from human urine. *Hoppe Seylers Z Physiol Chem* 1982;363:1043–1058.

278. Holmes WE, Pennica D, Blaber M, et al. Cloning and expression of the gene for pro-urokinase in *Escherichia coli*. *Biotechnology* 1985;3:923–929.

279. Riccio A, Grimaldi G, Verde P, et al. The human urokinase plasminogen activator gene and its promoter. *Nucleic Acids Res* 1985;13:2753–2771.

280. Triputti P, Blasi F, Verde P, et al. Human urokinase gene is located on the long arm of chromosome 10. *Proc Natl Acad Sci U S A* 1985;82:4448–4452.

281. Bdeir K, Kuo A, Sachais BS, et al. The kringle stabilizes urokinase binding to the urokinase receptor. *Blood* 2003;102:3600–3608.

282. Buko AM, Kentzer EJ, Petros A, et al. Characterization of a posttranslational fucosylation in the growth factor domain of urinary plasminogen activator. *Proc Natl Acad Sci U S A* 1991;88:3992–3996.

283. Rabbani SA, Mazar AP, Bernier SM, et al. Structural requirements for the growth factor activity of the amino-terminal domain of urokinase. *J Biol Chem* 1992;267:14151–14156.

284. Franco P, Iaccarino C, Chiaradonna F, et al. Phosphorylation of human pro-urokinase on Ser138/303 impairs its receptor-dependent ability to promote myelomonocytic adherence and motility. *J Cell Biol* 1997;137:779–791.

285. Lijnen HR, Van Hoef B, Collen D. Activation with plasmin of two-chain urokinase-type plasminogen activator derived from single-chain urokinase-type plasminogen activator by treatment with thrombin. *Eur J Biochem* 1987;169:359–364.

286. Bernik MB, Oller EP. Increased plasminogen activator (urokinase) in tissue culture after fibrin deposition. *J Clin Invest* 1973;42:823–834.

287. Ichinose A, Fujikawa K, Suyama T. The activation of pro-urokinase by plasma kallikrein and its inactivation by thrombin. *J Biol Chem* 1986; 261:3486–3489.

288. List K, Jensen ON, Bugge TH, et al. Plasminogen-independent initiation of the pro-urokinase activation cascade *in vivo*. Activation of pro-urokinase by glandular kallikrein (mGK-6) in plasminogen-deficient mice. *Biochemistry* 2000;39:508–515.

289. Gurewich V, Pannell R. Inactivation of single-chain urokinase (pro-urokinase) by thrombin and thrombin-like enzymes: relevance of the findings to the interpretation of fibrin-binding experiments. *Blood* 1987;69:769–772.

290. Braat EAM, Levi M, Bos R, et al. Inactivation of single-chain urokinase-type plasminogen activator by thrombin in human subjects. *J Lab Clin Med* 1999;134:161–167.

291. Nauland U, Rijken DC. Activation of thrombin-inactivated single-chain urokinase-type plasminogen activator by dipeptidyl peptidase I (cathepsin C). *Eur J Biochem* 1994;223:497–501.

292. Schmitt M, Kanayama N, Henschen A, et al. Elastase released from human granulocytes stimulated with N-formyl-chemotactic peptide prevents activation of tumor cell prourokinase (pro-uPA). *FEBS Lett* 1989; 255:83–88.

293. Günzler WA, Steffens GJ, Ötting F, et al. Structural relationship between human high and low molecular mass urokinase. *Hoppe Seylers Z Physiol Chem* 1982;363:133–141.

294. Learmonth MP, Li W, Namiranian S, et al. Modulation of the cell binding property of single chain urokinase-type plasminogen activator by neutrophil cathepsin G. *Fibrinolysis* 1992;6(Suppl. 4):113–116.

295. Marcotte PA, Henkin J, Credo RB, et al. A-chain isozymes of recombinant and natural urokinases: preparation, characterization, and their biochemical and fibrinolytic properties. *Fibrinolysis* 1992;6:69–78.

296. Li X, Bokman AM, Llinás M, et al. Solution structure of the kringle domain from urokinase-type plasminogen activator. *J Mol Biol* 1994;235: 1548–1559.

297. Hansen AP, Petros AM, Meadows RP, et al. Solution structure of the amino-terminal fragment of urokinase-type plasminogen activator. *Biochemistry* 1994;33:4847–4864.

298. Spraggon G, Phillips C, Nowak UK, et al. The crystal structure of the catalytic domain of human urokinase-type plasminogen activator. *Structure* 1995;3:681–691.

299. Sun Z, Liu BF, Chen Y, et al. Analysis of the forces which stabilize the active conformation of urokinase-type plasminogen activator. *Biochemistry* 1998;37:2935–2940.

300. Zeslawska E, Schweinitz A, Karcher A, et al. Crystals of the urokinase type plasminogen activator variant β(c)-uPA in complex with small molecule inhibitors open the way towards structure-based drug design. *J Mol Biol* 2000;301:465–475.

301. Schweinitz A, Steinmetzer T, Banke IJ, et al. Design of novel and selective inhibitors of urokinase-type plasminogen activator with improved pharmacokinetic properties for use as antimetastatic agents. *J Biol Chem* 2004;279:33613–33622.

302. Petersen LC. Kinetics of reciprocal pro-urokinase/plasminogen activation. Stimulation by a template formed by the urokinase receptor bound to poly(D-lysine). *Eur J Biochem* 1997;245:316–323.

303. Lijnen HR, Van Hoef B, Nelles L, et al. Plasminogen activation with single-chain urokinase-type plasminogen activator scuPA. Studies with active site mutagenized plasminogen (Ser[740]Ala) and plasmin-resistant scuPA (Lys[158]Glu). *J Biol Chem* 1990;265:5232–5236.

304. Pannell R, Gurewich V. Activation of plasminogen by single-chain urokinase or by two-chain urokinase—a demonstration that single-chain urokinase has a low catalytic activity (pro-urokinase). *Blood* 1987;69:22–26.

305. Lijnen HR, Van Hoef B, De Cock F, et al. The mechanism of plasminogen activation and fibrin dissolution by single chain urokinase-type plasminogen activator in a plasma milieu *in vitro*. *Blood* 1989;73:1864–1872.

306. Gurewich V, Pannell R, Louie S, et al. Effective and fibrin-specific clot lysis by a zymogen precursor form of urokinase (pro-urokinase): a study *in vitro* and in two animal species. *J Clin Invest* 1984;73:1731–1739.

307. Ellis V, Scully MF, Kakkar VV. Plasminogen activation by single-chain urokinase in functional isolation. *J Biol Chem* 1987;262:14998–15003.

308. Liu J-N, Tang W, Sun Z-Y, et al. A site-directed mutagenesis of pro-urokinase which substantially reduces its intrinsic activity. *Biochemistry* 1996;35:14070–14076.

309. Sun Z, Jiang Y, Ma Z, et al. Identification of a flexible loop region (297-313) of urokinase-type plasminogen activator, which helps determine its catalytic activity. *J Biol Chem* 1997;272:23818–23823.

310. Vassalli J, Baccino D, Belin D. A cellular binding site for the $M_r$ 55,000 form of the human plasminogen activator, urokinase. *J Cell Biol* 1985; 100:86–92.

311. Børglum AD, Byskov A, Ragno P, et al. Assignment of the urokinase-type plasminogen activator receptor gene (PLAUR) to chromosome 19q13.1-q 13.2. *Am J Hum Genet* 1992;50:492–497.

312. Casey JR, Petranka JG, Kottra J, et al. The structure of the urokinase-type plasminogen activator receptor gene. *Blood* 1994;84:1151–1156.

313. Dang J, Boyd D, Wang H, et al. A region between −141 and −61 bp containing a proximal AP-1 is essential for constitutive expression of urokinase-type plasminogen activator receptor. *Eur J Biochem* 1999;264:92–99.

314. Shetty S, Muniyappa H, Haldy PK, et al. Regulation of urokinase receptor expression by phosphoglycerate kinase. *Am J Respir Cell Mol Biol* 2004; 31:100–106.

315. Ploug M. Identification of specific sites involved in ligand binding by photoaffinity labeling of the receptor for the urokinase-type plasminogen activator. Residues located at equivalent positions in uPAR domains I and III participate in the assembly of a composite ligand-binding site. *Biochemistry* 1998;37:16494–16505.

316. Oda M, Shiraishi A, Hasegawa M. Analysis of the ternary complex formation of human urokinase with the separated two domains of its receptor. *Eur J Biochem* 1998;256:411–418.

317. Gårdsvoll H, Danø K, Ploug M. Mapping part of the functional epitope for ligand binding on the receptor for urokinase-type plasminogen activator by site-directed mutagenesis. *J Biol Chem* 1999;274:37995–38003.

318. Behrendt N, Rønne E, Danø K. The structure and function of the urokinase receptor, a membrane protein governing plasminogen activation on the cell surface. *Biol Chem Hoppe Seyler* 1995;376:269–279.

319. Ellis V. Functional analysis of the cellular receptor for urokinase in plasminogen activation. Receptor binding has no influence on the zymogenic nature of pro-urokinase. *J Biol Chem* 1996;271:14779–14784.

320. Webb DJ, Nguyen DH, Gonias SL. Extracellular signal-regulated kinase functions in the urokinase receptor-dependent pathway by which neutralization of low density lipoprotein receptor-related protein promotes fibrosarcoma cell migration and matrigel invasion. *J Cell Sci* 2000;113: 123–134.

321. Wei Y, Yang X, Liu Q, et al. A role for caveolin and the urokinase receptor in integrin-mediated adhesion and signaling. *J Cell Biol* 1999;144:1285–1294.

322. Wienke D, MacFadyen JR, Isacke CM. Identification and characterization of the endocytic transmembrane glycoprotein Endo180 as a novel collagen receptor. *Mol Biol Cell* 2003;14:3592–3604.

323. Kjoller L, Engelholm LH, Høyer-Hansen M, et al. uPARAP/endo180 directs lysosomal delivery and degradation of collagen IV. *Exp Cell Res* 2004;293:106–116.

324. Nykjaer A, Conese M, Christensen EI, et al. Recycling of the urokinase receptor upon internalization of the uPA:serpin complexes. *EMBO J* 1997; 16:2610–2620.

325. Wun TC, Schleuning D, Reich E. Isolation and characterization of urokinase from human plasma. *J Biol Chem* 1982;257:3276–3283.

326. Darras V, Thienpont M, Stump DC, et al. Measurement of urokinase-type plasminogen activator (uPA) with an enzyme-linked immunosorbent assay (ELISA) based on three murine monoclonal antibodies. *Thromb Haemost* 1986;56:411–414.

327. Andreotti F, Kluft C. Circadian variation of fibrinolytic activity in blood. *Chronobiol Int* 1991;8:336–351.

328. Levi M, ten Cate JW, Dooijewaard G, et al. DDAVP induces systemic release of urokinase-type plasminogen activator. *Thromb Haemost* 1989;62: 686–689.

329. Dooijewaard G, de Boer A, Turion PNC, et al. Physical exercise induces enhancement of urokinase-type plasminogen activator (uPA) levels in plasma. *Thromb Haemost* 1991;65:82–86.

330. Booth NA, Anderson JA, Bennett B. Plasminogen activators in alcoholic cirrhosis: demonstration of increased tissue type and urokinase type activator. *J Clin Pathol* 1984;37:772–777.

331. van der Kaaden ME, Rijken DC, Van Berkel TJC, et al. Plasma clearance of urokinase-type plasminogen activator. *Fibrinolysis and Proteolysis* 1998; 12:251–258.

332. Ellis V, Scully MF, Kakkar VV. Plasminogen activation initiated by single-chain urokinase-type plasminogen activator. Potentiation by U937 monocytes. *J Biol Chem* 1989;264:2185–2188.

333. Manchanda N, Schwartz BS. Single chain urokinase. Augmentation of enzymatic activity upon binding to monocytes. *J Biol Chem* 1991;266: 14580–14584.

334. McGuinness CL, Humphries J, Waltham M, et al. Recruitment of labelled monocytes by experimental venous thrombi. *Thromb Haemost* 2001;85: 1018–1024.

335. Grau E, Moroz LA. Fibrinolytic activity of normal human blood monocytes. *Thromb Res* 1989;53:145–162.

336. Mutch NJ, Moir E, Robbie LA, et al. Localization and identification of thrombin and plasminogen activator activities in model human thrombi by *in situ* zymography. *Thromb Haemost* 2002;88:996–1002.

337. Moir E, Booth NA, Bennett B, et al. Polymorphonuclear leucocytes mediate endogenous thrombus lysis via a u-PA-dependent mechanism. *Br J Haematol* 2001;113:72–80.

338. Moir E, Robbie LA, Bennett B, et al. Polymorphonuclear leucocytes have two opposing roles in fibrinolysis. *Thromb Haemost* 2002;87: 1006–1010.

339. Pluskota E, Soloviev DA, Bdeir K, et al. Integrin $\alpha_M\beta_2$ orchestrates and accelerates plasminogen activation and fibrinolysis by neutrophils. *J Biol Chem* 2004;279:18063–18072.

340. Manchanda N, Schwartz BS. Interaction of single-chain urokinase and plasminogen activator inhibitor type 1. *J Biol Chem* 1995;270:20032–20035.

341. Schwartz BS, España F. Two distinct urokinase-serpin interactions regulate the initiation of cell surface-associated plasminogen activation. *J Biol Chem* 1999;274:15278–15283.

342. Piguet PF, Vesin C, Donati Y, et al. Urokinase receptor (uPAR, CD87) is a platelet receptor important for kinetics and TNF-induced endothelial adhesion in mice. *Circulation* 1999;99:3315–3321.

343. Jiang YP, Pannell R, Liu JN, et al. Evidence for a novel binding protein to urokinase-type plasminogen activator in platelet membranes. *Blood* 1996; 87:2775–2781.

344. Longstaff C, Merton RE, Fabregas P, et al. Characterization of cell-associated plasminogen activation catalyzed by urokinase-type plasminogen activator, but independent of urokinase receptor (uPAR, CD87). *Blood* 1999;93:3839–3846.

345. Stump DC, Stassen JM, Demarsin E, et al. Comparative thrombolytic properties of single-chain forms of urokinase-type plasminogen activator. *Blood* 1987;69:592–596.

346. Pannell R, Black J, Gurewich V. Complementary modes of action of tissue-type plasminogen activator and pro-urokinase by which their synergistic effect on clot lysis may be explained. *J Clin Invest* 1988;81:853–859.

347. Longstaff C, Clough AM, Gaffney PJ. Kinetics of plasmin activation of single chain urinary-type plasminogen activator (scuPA) and demonstration of a high affinity interaction between scuPA and plasminogen. *J Biol Chem* 1992;267:173–179.

348. Lenich C, Pannell R, Gurewich V. The effect of the carboxy-terminal lysine of urokinase on the catalysis of plasminogen activation. *Thromb Res* 1991;64:69–80.

349. Collen D, Stassen J-M, De Cock F. Synergistic effect of thrombolysis of sequential infusion of tissue-type plasminogen activator (tPA), single chain urokinase-type plasminogen activator (scuPA) and urokinase in the rabbit jugular vein thrombosis model. *Thromb Haemost* 1987;58:943–946.

350. Hauert J, Nicoloso G, Schleuning WD, et al. Plasminogen activators in dextran sulfate-activated euglobulin fractions: a molecular analysis of factor XII- and prekallikrein-dependent fibrinolysis. *Blood* 1989;73:994–999.

351. Binnema DJ, Dooijewaard G, Iersel JJL, et al. The contact-system dependent plasminogen activator from human plasma: identification and characterization. *Thromb Haemost* 1990;64:390–397.

352. Schousboe I, Feddersen K, Rojkjaer R. Factor XIIa is a kinetically favorable plasminogen activator. *Thromb Haemost* 1999;82:1041–1046.

353. Besser D, Verde P, Nagamine Y, et al. Signal transduction and the uPA/uPAR system. *Fibrinolysis* 1997;10:215–237.

354. Irigoyen JP, Nagamine Y. Cytoskeletal reorganization leads to induction of the urokinase-type plasminogen activator gene by activating FAK and Src and subsequently the Ras/Erk signaling pathway. *Biochem Biophys Res Commun* 1999;262:666–670.

355. D'Orazio D, Besser D, Marksitzer R, et al. Cooperation of two PEA3/AP1 sites in uPA gene induction by TPA and FGF-2. *Gene* 1997;201:179–187.

356. De Cesare D, Palazzolo M, Berthelsen J, et al. Characterization of UEF-4, a DNA-binding protein required for transcriptional synergism between two AP-1 sites in the human urokinase enhancer. *J Biol Chem* 1997;272: 23921–23929.

357. Smicun Y, Kopf E, Miskin R. The 3′-untranslated region of the urokinase gene enhances the expression of chimeric genes in cultured cells and correlates with specific brain expression in transgenic mice. *Eur J Biochem* 1998;251:704–715.

358. Nanbu R, Menoud PA, Nagamine Y. Multiple instability-regulating sites in the 3′ untranslated region of the urokinase-type plasminogen activator mRNA. *Mol Cell Biol* 1994;14:4920–4928.

359. Singh I, Burnand KG, Collins M, et al. Failure of thrombus to resolve in urokinase-type plasminogen activator gene-knockout mice: rescue by normal bone marrow-derived cells. *Circulation* 2003;107:869–875.

360. Bugge TH, Flick MJ, Danton MJ, et al. Urokinase-type plasminogen activator is effective in fibrin clearance in the absence of its receptor or tissue-type plasminogen activator. *Proc Natl Acad Sci U S A* 1996;93:5899–5904.

361. Carmeliet P, Moons L, Lijnen R, et al. Urokinase-generated plasmin activates matrix metalloproteinases during aneurysm formation. *Nat Genet* 1997;17:439–444.

362. Carmeliet P, Moons L, Herbert J-M, et al. Urokinase but not tissue type plasminogen activator mediates arterial neointima formation in mice. *Circ Res* 1997;81:829–839.

363. Carmeliet P, Moons L, Dewerchin M, et al. Receptor-independent role of urokinase-type plasminogen activator in pericellular plasmin and matrix metalloproteinase proteolysis during vascular wound healing in mice. *J Cell Biol* 1998;140:233–245.

364. Deindl E, Ziegelhoffer T, Kanse SM, et al. Receptor-independent role of the urokinase-type plasminogen activator during arteriogenesis. *FASEB J* 2003;17:1174–1176.

365. Gyetko MR, Aizenberg D, Mayo-Bond L. Urokinase-deficient and urokinase receptor-deficient mice have impaired neutrophil antimicrobial activation *in vitro*. *J Leukoc Biol* 2004;76:648–356.

366. Piguet PF, Vesin C, Donati Y, et al. Urokinase receptor (uPAR, CD87) is a platelet receptor important for kinetics and TNF-induced endothelial adhesion in mice. *Circulation* 1999;99:3315–3321.

367. Gu JM, Johns A, Morser J, et al. Urokinase plasminogen activator receptor promotes macrophage infiltration into the vascular wall of ApoE deficient mice. *J Cell Physiol* 2005; 204:73–82.

368. Jo M, Thomas KS, Wu L, et al. Soluble urokinase-type plasminogen activator receptor inhibits cancer cell growth and invasion by direct urokinase-independent effects on cell signaling. *J Biol Chem* 2003;278:46692–46698.

369. Tillett WS, Garner RL. The fibrinolytic activity of hemolytic streptococci. *J Exp Med* 1933;68:485–502.

370. Gladysheva IP, Turner RB, Sazonova IY, et al. Coevolutionary patterns in plasminogen activation. *Proc Natl Acad Sci U S A* 2003;100:9168–9172.

371. Wohl RC, Summaria L, Arzadon L, et al. Steady state kinetics of activation of human and bovine plasminogens by streptokinase and its equimolar complexes with various activated forms of human plasminogen. *J Biol Chem* 1978;253:1402–1407.

372. Parry MA, Zhang XC, Bode I. Molecular mechanisms of plasminogen activation: bacterial cofactors provide clues. *Trends Biochem Sci* 2000;25: 53–59.

373. Cederholm-Williams SA, De Cock F, Lijnen HR, et al. Kinetics of the reaction between streptokinase, plasmin and $\alpha_2$-antiplasmin. *Eur J Biochem* 1979;100:125–132.

374. Mundada LV, Prorok M, DeFord ME, et al. Structure-function analysis of the streptokinase amino terminus (residues 1–59). *J Biol Chem* 2003;278: 24421–24427.

375. Conejerolara F, Parrado J, Azuaga AI, et al. Thermal stability of the three domains of streptokinase studied by circular dichroism and nuclear magnetic resonance. *Protein Sci* 1996;5:2583–2591.

376. Wang X, Lin X, Loy JA, et al. Crystal structure of the catalytic domain of human plasmin complexed with streptokinase. *Science* 1998;281: 1662–1665.

377. Wang X, Tang J, Hunter B, et al. Crystal structure of streptokinase β-domain. *FEBS Lett* 1999;459:85–89.

378. Chaudhary A, Vasudha S, Rajagopal K, et al. Function of the central domain of streptokinase in substrate plasminogen docking and processing revealed by site-directed mutagenesis. *Protein Sci* 1999;8:2791–2805.

379. Reddy KNN. Streptokinase: biochemistry and clinical application. *Enzyme* 1988;40:79–89.

380. Longstaff C, Whitton CM. A proposed reference method for plasminogen activators that enables calculation of enzyme activities in SI units. *J Thromb Haemost* 2004;2:1416–1421.

381. Bachmann F. Development of antibodies against perorally and rectally administered streptokinase in man. *J Lab Clin Med* 1968;72:228–238.

382. Ojalvo AG, Pozo L, Labarta V, et al. Prevalence of circulating antibodies against a streptokinase C-terminal peptide in normal blood donors. *Biochem Biophys Res Commun* 1999;263:454–459.

383. Gonias SL, Einarsson M, Pizzo SV. Catabolic pathways for streptokinase, plasmin and streptokinase activator complex in mice: *in vivo* reaction of plasminogen activator with $\alpha_2$-macroglobulin. *J Clin Invest* 1982; 7:412–423.

384. Hibbs MJ, Fears R, Ferres H, et al. Determination of the deacetylation rate of p-anisoyl plasminogen streptokinase activator complex (APSAC, EMINASE) in human plasma, blood and plasma clots. *Fibrinolysis* 1989;3:235–240.

385. Fears R. Development of anisoylated plasminogen-streptokinase activator complex from the acyl enzyme concept. *Semin Thromb Hemost* 1989;15: 129–139.

386. Lack CH. Staphylokinase: an activator of plasma protease. *Nature* 1948; 161:559–560.

387. Lewis JH, Ferguson JH. A proteolytic enzyme sytem of the blood. III. Activation of dog serum profibrinolysin by staphylokinase. *Am J Physiol* 1951;166:594–603.

388. Collen D. Staphylokinase: a potent, uniquely fibrin-selective thrombolytic agent. *Nat Med* 1998;4:279–284.

389. Laroche Y, Heymans S, Capaert S, et al. Recombinant staphylokinase variants with reduced antigenicity due to elimination of B-lymphocyte epitopes. *Blood* 2000;96:1425–1432.

390. Vanwetswinkel S, Plaisance S, Zhi-Yong Z, et al. Pharmacokinetic and thrombolytic properties of cysteine-linked polyethylene glycol derivatives of staphylokinase. *Blood* 2000;95:936–942.

391. Vanderschueren S, Barrios L, Kerdsinchai P et al, The STAR Trial Group. A randomized trial of recombinant staphylokinase versus alteplase for coronary artery patency in acute myocardial infarction. *Circulation* 1995; 92:2044–2049.

392. Heymans S, Vanderschueren S, Verhaeghe R, et al. Outcome and one year follow-up of intra-arterial staphylokinase in 191 patients with peripheral arterial occlusion. *Thromb Haemost* 2000;83:666–671.

393. Hawkey C. Plasminogen activator in the saliva of the vampire bat *Desmodus rotundus*. *Nature* 1966;211:434–435.

394. Gardell SJ, Duong LT, Diehl RE, et al. Isolation, characterization and cDNA cloning of a vampire bat salivary plasminogen activator. *J Biol Chem* 1989;264:17947–17952.

395. Krätzschmar J, Haendler B, Langer G, et al. The plasminogen activator family from the salivary gland of the vampire bat *Desmodus rotundus*: cloning and expression. *Gene* 1991;105:229–237.

396. Schleuning W-D, Donner P. *Desmodus rotundus* (common vampire bat) salivary plasminogen activator. In: Bachmann F, ed. *Fibrinolytics and antifibrinolytics, handbook of experimental pharmacology.* Heidelberg: Springer, 2000:447–468.

397. Bergum PW, Gardell SJ. Vampire bat salivary plasminogen activator exhibits a strict and fastidious requirement for polymeric fibrin as its cofactor, unlike human tissue-type plasminogen activator. A kinetic analysis. *J Biol Chem* 1992;267:17726–17731.

398. Bringmann P, Gruber D, Liese A, et al. Structural features mediating fibrin selectivity of vampire bat plasminogen activators. *J Biol Chem* 1995;270: 25596–25603.

399. Stewart RJ, Fredenburgh JC, Weitz JI. Characterization of the interactions of plasminogen and tissue and vampire bat plasminogen activators with fibrinogen, fibrin, and the complex of D-dimer noncovalently linked to fragment E. *J Biol Chem* 1998;273:18292–18299.

400. Renatus M, Stubbs MT, Huber R, et al. Catalytic domain structure of vampire bat plasminogen activator: a molecular paradigm for proteolysis without activation cleavage. *Biochemistry* 1997;36:13483–13493.

401. Montoney M, Gardell SJ, Marder VJ. Comparison of the bleeding potential of vampire bat salivary plasminogen activator versus tissue plasminogen activator in an experimental rabbit model. *Circulation* 1995;91: 1540–1544.

402. Witt W, Maass B, Baldus B, et al. Coronary thrombolysis with *Desmodus* salivary plasminogen activator in dogs. Fast and persistent recanalization by intravenous bolus administration. *Circulation* 1994;90:421–426.

403. Hildebrand M, Bhargava AS, Bringmann P, et al. Pharmacokinetics of the novel plasminogen activator *Desmodus rotundus* plasminogen activator in animals and extrapolation to man. *Fibrinolysis* 1996;10:269–276.

404. Liberatore GT, Samson A, Bladin C, et al. Vampire bat salivary plasminogen activator (desmoteplase): a unique fibrinolytic enzyme that does not promote neurodegeneration. *Stroke* 2003;34:537–543.

405. Collen D, Wiman B. Fast-acting plasmin inhibitor in human plasma. *Blood* 1978;51:563–569.

406. Mast AE, Enghild JJ, Pizzo SV, et al. Analysis of the plasma elimination kinetics and conformational stabilities of native, proteinase-complexed, and reactive site cleaved serpins: comparison of $\alpha_1$-proteinase inhibitor, $\alpha_1$-antichymotrypsin, antithrombin III, $\alpha_2$-antiplasmin, angiotensinogen, and ovalbumin. *Biochemistry* 1991;30:1723–1730.

407. Holmes WE, Nelles L, Lijnen HR, et al. Primary structure of human $\alpha_2$-antiplasmin, a serine protease inhibitor (serpin). *J Biol Chem* 1987;262: 1659–1664.

408. Hirosawa S, Nakamura Y, Miura O, et al. Organization of the human $\alpha_2$-plasmin inhibitor gene. *Proc Natl Acad Sci U S A* 1988;85:6836–6840.

409. Kato A, Hirosawa S, Toyota S, et al. Localization of the human $\alpha_2$-plasmin inhibitor gene (PLI) to 17p13. *Cytogenet Cell Genet* 1993;62: 190–191.

410. Lee KN, Tae W-C, Jackson KW, et al. Characterization of wild-type and mutant $\alpha_2$-antiplasmins: fibrinolysis enhancement by reactive site mutant. *Blood* 1999;94:164–171.

411. Wiman B, Boman L, Collen D. On the kinetics of the reaction between human antiplasmin and a low-molecular-weight form of plasmin. *Eur J Biochem* 1978;87:143–146.

412. Sumi Y, Ichikawa Y, Nakamura Y, et al. Expression and characterization of pro $\alpha_2$-plasmin inhibitor. *J Biochem* 1989;106:703–707.

413. Bangert K, Johnsen AH, Christensen U et al. Different *N*-terminal forms of $\alpha_2$-plasmin inhibitor in human plasma. *Biochem J* 1993;291:523–625.

414. Koyama T, Koike Y, Toyota S, et al. Different NH$_2$-terminal form with 12 additional residues of $\alpha_2$-plasmin inhibitor from human plasma and culture media of Hep G2 cells. *Biochem Biophys Res Commun* 1994;200: 417–422.

415. Lee KN, Jackson KW, Christiansen VJ, et al. A novel plasma proteinase potentiates $\alpha_2$-antiplasmin inhibition of fibrin digestion. *Blood* 2004;103: 3783–3788.

416. Kimura S, Aoki N. Cross-linking site in fibrinogen for $\alpha_2$-plasmin inhibitor. *J Biol Chem* 1986;261:15591–15595.

417. Booth NA. Regulation of fibrinolytic activity by localization of inhibitors to fibrin(ogen). *Fibrinolysis Proteolysis* 2000;14:206–213.

418. Lee KN, Tae W-C, Jackson KW, et al. Characterization of wild-type and mutant $\alpha_2$-antiplasmins: fibrinolysis enhancement by reactive site mutant. *Blood* 1999;94:164–171.

419. Reed GL, Matsueda GR, Haber E. Synergistic fibrinolysis: combined effects of plasminogen activators and an antibody that inhibits $\alpha_2$-antiplasmin. *Proc Natl Acad Sci U S A* 1990;87:1114–1118.

420. Clemmensen I, Thorsen S, Müllertz S, et al. Properties of three different molecular forms of $\alpha_2$-plasmin inhibitor. *Eur J Biochem* 1981;120: 105–122.

421. Sasaki T, Morita T, Iwanaga S. Identification of the plasminogen-binding site of human $\alpha_2$-plasmin inhibitor. *J Biochem* 1986;99:1696–1705.

422. Kluft C, Los N. Demonstration of two forms of $\alpha_2$-antiplasmin in plasma by modified crossed immunoelectrophoresis. *Thromb Res* 1981;21: 65–71.

423. Collen D. On the regulation and control of fibrinolysis. *Thromb Haemost* 1980;43:77–89.

424. Wiman B, Collen D. On the kinetics of the reaction between human antiplasmin and plasmin. *Eur J Biochem* 1978;84:573–578.

425. Frank PS, Douglas JT, Locher M, et al. Structural/functional characterization of the $\alpha_2$-plasmin inhibitor C-terminal peptide. *Biochemistry* 2003;42: 1078–1085.

426. Wang H, Yu A, Wiman B, et al. Identification of amino acids in antiplasmin involved in its noncovalent 'lysine-binding site'-dependent interaction with plasmin. *Eur J Biochem* 2003;270:2023–2029.

427. Paramo JA, Gascoine PS, Pring JB, et al. The relative inhibition by $\alpha_2$-antiplasmin and plasminogen activator inhibitor-1 of clot lysis *in vitro*. *Fibrinolysis* 1990;4:169–175.

428. Robbie LA, Booth NA, Croll AM, et al. The roles of $\alpha_2$-antiplasmin and plasminogen activator inhibitor 1 (PAI-1) in the inhibition of clot lysis. *Thromb Haemost* 1993;70:301–306.

429. Robbie LA, Bennett B, Keyt BA, et al. Effective lysis of model thrombi by a t-PA mutant (A473S) that is resistant to $\alpha_2$-antiplasmin. *Br J Haematol* 2000;111:517–523.

430. Koie K, Kamiya T, Ogata K, et al. $\alpha_2$-Plasmin-inhibitor deficiency (Miyasato disease). *Lancet* 1978;2:1334–1336.

431. Aoki N, Saito H, Kamiya T, et al. Congenital deficiency of $\alpha_2$-plasmin inhibitor associated with severe hemorrhagic tendency. *J Clin Invest* 1979; 63:877–884.

432. Rijken DC, Groeneveld E, Kluft C, et al. $\alpha_2$-Antiplasmin Enschede is not an inhibitor, but a substrate, of plasmin. *Biochem J* 1988;255:609–615.

433. Holmes WE, Lijnen HR, Nelles L, et al. $\alpha_2$-Antiplasmin Enschede: alanine insertion and abolition of plasmin inhibitory activity. *Science* 1987;238: 209–211.

434. Lijnen HR, Okada K, Matsuo O, et al. $\alpha_2$-Antiplasmin gene deficiency in mice is associated with enhanced fibrinolytic potential without overt bleeding. *Blood* 1999;93:2274–2281.

435. Okada K, Ueshima S, Imano M, et al. The regulation of liver regeneration by the plasmin/$\alpha_2$-antiplasmin system. *J Hepatol* 2004;40:110–116.

436. Takei M, Matsuno H, Okada K, et al. Lack of $\alpha_2$-antiplasmin enhances ADP induced platelet micro-aggregation through the presence of excess active plasmin in mice. *J Thromb Thrombolysis* 2002;14:205–211.

437. Matsuno H, Kozawa O, Yoshimi N, et al. Lack of $\alpha_2$-antiplasmin promotes pulmonary heart failure via overrelease of VEGF after acute myocardial infarction. *Blood* 2002;100:2487–2493.

438. Sakurai Y, Takahashi T, Arakawa H, et al. Trypsin-like endopeptidase(s) naturally entrapped in human blood $\alpha_2$-macroglobulin. *Biomed Res* 1996; 17:347–350.

439. Sottrup-Jensen L, Stepanik TM, Kristensen T, et al. Primary structure of human $\alpha_2$-macroglobulin. V. The complete structure. *J Biol Chem* 1984; 259:8318–8327.

440. Kan CC, Solomon E, Belt KT, et al. Nucleotide sequence of cDNA encoding human $\alpha_2$-macroglobulin and assignment of the chromosomal locus. *Proc Natl Acad Sci U S A* 1985;82:2282–2286.

441. Travis J, Salvesen GS. Human plasma proteinase inhibitors. *Annu Rev Biochem* 1983;52:655–709.

442. Kolodziej SJ, Klueppelberg HU, Nolasco N, et al. Three-dimensional structure of the human plasmin $\alpha_2$-macroglobulin complex. *J Struct Biol* 1998;123:124–133.

443. Czekay RP, Aertgeerts K, Curriden SA, et al. Plasminogen activator inhibitor-1 detaches cells from extracellular matrices by inactivating integrins. *J Cell Biol* 2003;160:781–791.

444. Hekman CM, Loskutoff DJ. Endothelial cells produce a latent inhibitor of plasminogen activators that can be activated by denaturants. *J Biol Chem* 1985;260:11581–11587.

445. Declerck PJ, De Mol M, Alessi M-C, et al. Purification and characterization of a plasminogen activator inhibitor 1 binding protein from human plasma. Identification as a multimeric form of S protein (vitronectin). *J Biol Chem* 1988;263:15454–15461.

446. Kruithof EKO, Gudinchet A, Bachmann F. Plasminogen activator inhibitor 1 and plasminogen activator inhibitor 2 in various disease states. *Thromb Haemost* 1988;59:7–12.

447. Booth NA, Simpson AJ, Croll A, et al. Plasminogen activator inhibitor (PAI-1) in plasma and platelets. *Br J Haematol* 1988;70:327–333.

448. Declerck PJ, Alessi M-C, Verstreken MV, et al. Measurement of plasminogen activator inhibitor 1 in biologic fluids with a murine monoclonal antibody-based enzyme-linked immunosorbent assay. *Blood* 1988;71:220–225.

449. Johnson SA, Schneider CL. The existence of antifibrinolysin activity in platelets. *Science* 1953;117:229–230.

450. Konkle BA, Schick PK, He X, et al. Plasminogen activator inhibitor-1 mRNA is expressed in platelets and megakaryocytes and the megakaryoblastic cell line CHRF-288. *Arterioscler Thromb* 1993;13:669–674.

451. van Mourik JA, Lawrence DA, Loskutoff DJ. Purification of an inhibitor of plasminogen activator (antiactivator) synthesized by endothelial cells. *J Biol Chem* 1984;259:14914–14921.

452. Cwikel BJ, Barouski-Miller PA, Coleman PL, et al. Dexamethasone induction of an inhibitor of plasminogen activator in HTC hepatoma cells. *J Biol Chem* 1984;259:6847–6851.

453. Morange PE, Alessi MC, Verdier M, et al. PAI-1 produced *ex vivo* by human adipose tissue is relevant to PAI-1 blood level. *Arterioscler Thromb Vasc Biol* 1999;19:1361–1365.

454. Loskutoff DJ, Samad F. The adipocyte and hemostatic balance in obesity: studies of PAI-1. *Arterioscler Thromb Vasc Biol* 1998;18:1–6.

455. Crandall DL, Quinet EM, Morgan GA, et al. Synthesis and secretion of plasminogen activator inhibitor-1 by human preadipocytes. *J Clin Endocrinol Metab* 1999;84:3222–3227.

456. Loskutoff DJ. Regulation of PAI-1 gene expression. *Fibrinolysis* 1991;5: 197–206.

457. Booth NA. The natural inhibitors of fibrinolysis. In: Bloom AL, Forbes CD, Thomas DP, et al., eds. *Haemostasis and thrombosis*, 3rd ed. Edinburgh: Churchill Livingstone, 1994:699–717.

458. Robbie LA, Bennett B, Croll AM, et al. Proteins of the fibrinolytic system in human thrombi. *Thromb Haemost* 1996;75:127–133.

459. Potter van Loon BJ, Rijken DC, Brommer EJP, et al. The amount of plasminogen, tissue-type plasminogen activator and plasminogen activator inhibitor type 1 in human thrombin and relation to *ex vivo* lysability. *Thromb Haemost* 1992;67:101–105.

460. Kruithof EKO. The inhibitors of the fibrinolytic system. In: Bachmann F, ed. *Fibrinolytics and antifibrinolytics. Handbook of experimental pharmacology.* Vol 146. Berlin, Springer, 2001:113–139.

461. Diéval J, Nguyen G, Gross S, et al. A lifelong bleeding disorder associated with a deficiency of plasminogen activator inhibitor type 1. *Blood* 1991; 77:528–532.

462. Fay WP, Shapiro AD, Shih JL, et al. Complete deficiency of plasminogen-activator inhibitor type 1 due to a frame-shift mutation. *N Engl J Med* 1992;327:1729–1733.

463. Lee MH, Vosburgh E, Anderson K, et al. Deficiency of plasma plasminogen activator inhibitor 1 results in hyperfibrinolytic bleeding. *Blood* 1993; 81:2357–2362.

464. Fay WP, Parker AC, Condrey LR, et al. Human plasminogen activator inhibitor-1 (PAI-1) deficiency: characterization of a large kindred with a null mutation in the PAI-1 gene. *Blood* 1997;90:204–208.

465. Carmeliet P, Stassen JM, Schoonjans L, et al. Plasminogen activator inhibitor-1 gene-deficient mice. II. Effects on hemostasis, thrombosis and thrombolysis. *J Clin Invest* 1993;92:1756–2760.

466. Carmeliet P, Moons L, Lijnen R, et al. Inhibitory role of plasminogen activator inhibitor-1 in arterial wound healing and neointima formation. A gene targeting and gene transfer study in mice. *Circulation* 1997;96: 3180–3191.

467. Eitzman DT, Westrick RJ, Nabel EG, et al. Plasminogen activator inhibitor-1 and vitronectin promote vascular thrombosis in mice. *Blood* 2000;95:577–580.

468. Farrehi PM, Ozaki CK, Carmeliet P, et al. Regulation of arterial thrombolysis by plasminogen activator inhibitor-1 in mice. *Circulation* 1998;97: 1002–1008.

469. Eren M, Painter CA, Atkinson JB, et al. Age-dependent spontaneous coronary arterial thrombosis in transgenic mice that express a stable form of human plasminogen activator inhibitor-1. *Circulation* 2002;106:491–496.

470. Bachmann F. The role of plasminogen activator inhibitor type 1 (PAI-1) in the clinical setting, including deep vein thrombosis. In: Glas-Greenwalt P, ed. *Fibrinolysis in disease. Molecular and hemovascular aspects of fibrinolysis.* Boca Raton, FL: CRC Press, 1995:79–86.

471. Vaughan DE. Plasminogen activator inhibitor-1: a common denominator in cardiovascular disease. *J Investig Med* 1998;46:370–376.

472. Juhan-Vague I, Pyke SDM, Alessi MC, et al. Fibrinolytic factors and the risk of myocardial infarction or sudden death in patients with angina pectoris. *Circulation* 1996;94:2057–2063.

473. Carroll VA, Binder BR. The role of the plasminogen activation system in cancer. *Semin Thromb Hemost* 1999;25:183–197.

474. Scarabin P-Y, Aillaud M-F, Amouyel P et al, The PRIME Study. Associations of fibrinogen, factor VII and PAI-1 with baseline findings among 10,500 male participants in a prospective study of myocardial infarction. *Thromb Haemost* 1998;80:749–756.

475. Dawson S, Hamsten A, Wiman B, et al. Genetic variation at the plasminogen activator inhibitor-1 locus is associated with altered levels of plasma plasminogen activator inhibitor-1 activity. *Arterioscler Thromb* 1991;11: 183–190.

476. Eriksson P, Kallin B, Van'T Hooft FM, et al. Allele-specific increase in basal transcription of the plasminogen-activator inhibitor 1 gene is associated with myocardial infarction. *Proc Natl Acad Sci U S A* 1995;92: 1851–1855.

477. Wiman B, Hamsten A. Impaired fibrinolysis and risk of thromboembolism. *Prog Cardiovasc Dis* 1991;34:179–192.

478. Lowe GDO, Yarnell JWG, Sweetnam PM, et al. Fibrin D-dimer, tissue plasminogen activator, plasminogen activator inhibitor, and the risk of major ischaemic heart disease in the Caerphilly study. *Thromb Haemost* 1998;79:129–133.

479. Pralong G, Calandra T, Glauser MP, et al. Plasminogen activator inhibitor 1: a new prognostic marker in septic shock. *Thromb Haemost* 1989;61: 459–462.

480. Arts J, Kockx M, Princen HMG, et al. Studies on the mechanism of fibrate-inhibited expression of plasminogen activator inhibitor-1 in cultured hepatocytes from cynomolgus monkey. *Arterioscler Thromb Vasc Biol* 1997;17:26–32.

481. Murakami J, Ohtani A, Murata S. Protective effect of T-686, an inhibitor of plasminogen activator inhibitor-1 production, against the lethal effect of lipopolysaccharide in mice. *Jpn J Pharmacol* 1997;75:291–294.

482. Ohtani A, Murakami J, Hirano-Wakimoto A. T-686, a novel inhibitor of plasminogen activator inhibitor-1, inhibits thrombosis without impairment of hemostasis in rats. *Eur J Pharmacol* 1997;330:151–156.

483. Vinogradsky B, Bell SP, Woodcock-Mitchell J, et al. A new butadiene derivative, T-686, inhibits plasminogen activator inhibitor type-1 production *in vitro* by cultured human vascular endothelial cells and development of atherosclerotic lesions *in vivo* in rabbits. *Thromb Res* 1997;85:305–314.

484. Eitzman DT, Fay WP, Lawrence DA, et al. Peptide-mediated inactivation of recombinant and platelet plasminogen activator inhibitor-1 *in vitro*. *J Clin Invest* 1995;95:2416–2420.

485. Neve J, Leone PA, Carroll AR, et al. Sideroxylonal C, a new inhibitor of human plasminogen activator inhibitor type-1, from the flowers of *Eucalyptus albens*. *J Nat Prod* 1999;62:324–326.

486. Björquist P, Ehnebom J, Inghardt T, et al. Identification of the binding site for a low-molecular-weight inhibitor of plasminogen activator inhibitor type 1 by site-directed mutagenesis. *Biochemistry* 1998;37:1227–1234.

487. Charlton PA, Faint RW, Bent F, et al. Evaluation of a low molecular weight modulator of human plasminogen activator inhibitor-1 activity. *Thromb Haemost* 1996;75:808–815.

488. Friederich PW, Levi M, Biemond BJ, et al. Novel low-molecular-weight inhibitor of PAI-1 (XR5118) promotes endogenous fibrinolysis and reduces postthrombolysis thrombus growth in rabbits. *Circulation* 1997;96: 916–921.

489. Einholm AP, Pedersen KE, Wind T, et al. Biochemical mechanism of action of a diketopiperazine inactivator of plasminogen activator inhibitor-1. *Biochem J* 2003;373:723–732.

490. Ye RD, Ahern SM, Le Beau MM, et al. Structure of the gene for human plasminogen activator inhibitor-2. The nearest mammalian homologue of chicken ovalbumin. *J Biol Chem* 1989;264:5495–5502.

491. Bachmann F. The enigma PAI-2. Gene expression, evolutionary and functional aspects. *Thromb Haemost* 1995;74:172–179.

492. Kruithof EK, Baker MS, Bunn CL. Biological and clinical aspects of plasminogen activator inhibitor type 2. *Blood* 1995;86:4007–4024.

493. Kawano T, Morimoto K, Uemura Y. Partial purification and properties of urokinase inhibitor from human placenta. *J Biochem (Tokyo)* 1970;67: 333–342.

494. Åstedt B, Lecander I, Brodin T, et al. Purification of a specific placental plasminogen activator inhibitor by monoclonal antibody and its complex formation with plasminogen activation. *Thromb Haemost* 1985;53:122–125.

495. Kruithof EKO, Vassalli J-D, Schleuning W-D, et al. Purification and characterization of a plasminogen activator inhibitor from the histiocytic lymphoma cell line U-937. *J Biol Chem* 1986;261:11207–11213.

496. Risse BC, Brown H, Lavker RM, et al. Differentiating cells of murine stratified squamous epithelia constitutively express plasminogen activator inhibitor type 2 (PAI-2). *Histochem Cell Biol* 1998;110:559–569.

497. Jensen PH, Lorand L, Ebbesen P, et al. Type-2 plasminogen-activator inhibitor is a substrate for trophoblast transglutaminase and factor XIII$_a$. Transglutaminase-catalyzed cross-linking to cellular and extracellular structures. *Eur J Biochem* 1993;214:141–146.

498. Schwartz BS, Bradshaw JD. Differential regulation of tissue factor and plasminogen activator inhibitor by human mononuclear cells. *Blood* 1989; 74:1644–1650.

499. Ritchie H, Robbie LA, Kinghorn S, et al. Monocyte plasminogen activator inhibitor 2 (PAI-2) inhibits u-PA-mediated fibrinolysis and is cross-linked to fibrin. *Thromb Haemost* 1999;81:96–103.

500. Genton C, Kruithof EK, Schleuning WD. Phorbol ester induces the biosynthesis of glycosylated and nonglycosylated plasminogen activator inhibitor 2 in high excess over urokinase-type plasminogen activator in human U-937 lymphoma cells. *J Cell Biol* 1987;104:705–712.

501. Ritchie H, Booth NA. Secretion of plasminogen activator inhibitor 2 by human peripheral blood monocytes occurs via an endoplasmic reticulum-golgi-independent pathway. *Exp Cell Res* 1998;242:439–450.

502. Harrop SJ, Jankova L, Coles M, et al. The crystal structure of plasminogen activator inhibitor 2 at 2.0 Å resolution: implications for serpin function. *Structure Fold Des* 1999;7:43–54.

503. Jensen PH, Schüler E, Woodrow G, et al. A unique interhelical insertion in plasminogen activator inhibitor-2 contains three glutamines, Gln$^{83}$, Gln$^{84}$, Gln$^{86}$, essential for transglutaminase-mediated cross-linking. *J Biol Chem* 1994;269:15394–15398.

504. Ritchie H, Lawrie LC, Crombie PW, et al. Cross-linking of plasminogen activator inhibitor 2 and α$_2$-antiplasmin to fibrin(ogen). *J Biol Chem* 2000; 275:24915–24920.

505. Jensen PH, Jensen TG, Laug WE, et al. The exon 3 encoded sequence of the intracellular serine proteinase inhibitor plasminogen activator inhibitor 2 is a protein binding domain. *J Biol Chem* 1996;271:26892–26899.

506. Mikus P, Urano T, Liljeström P, et al. Plasminogen-activator inhibitor type 2 (PAI-2) is a spontaneously polymerising SERPIN—biochemical characterisation of the recombinant intracellular and extracellular forms. *Eur J Biochem* 1993;218:1071–1082.

507. Wilczynska M, Lobov S, Ohlsson PI, et al. A redox-sensitive loop regulates plasminogen activator inhibitor type 2 (PAI-2) polymerization. *EMBO J* 2003;22:1753–1761.

508. Lobov S, Wilczynska M, Bergstrom F, et al. Structural bases of the redox-dependent conformational switch in the serpin PAI-2. *J Mol Biol* 2004; 344:1359–1368.

509. Kruithof EKO, Tran-Thang C, Gudinchet A, et al. Fibrinolysis in pregnancy: a study of plasminogen activator inhibitors. *Blood* 1987;69:460–466.

510. Bonnar J, Daly L, Sheppard BL. Changes in the fibrinolytic system during pregnancy. *Sem Thromb Hemostas* 1990;16:221–229.

511. Reith A, Booth NA, Moore NR, et al. Plasminogen activator inhibitors (PAI-1 and PAI-2) in normal pregnancies, pre-eclampsia and hydatidiform mole. *Br J Obstet Gynaecol* 1993;100:370–374.

512. Grancha S, Estellés A, Gilabert J, et al. Decreased expression of PAI-2 mRNA and protein in pregnancies complicated with intrauterine fetal growth retardation. *Thromb Haemost* 1996;76:761–767.

513. Booth NA, Reith A, Bennett B. A plasminogen activator inhibitor (PAI-2) circulates in two molecular forms during pregnancy. *Thromb Haemost* 1988;59:77–79.

514. Scherrer A, Kruithof EKO, Grob J-P. Plasminogen activator inhibitor-2 in patients with monocytic leukemia. *Leukemia* 1991;5:479–486.

515. Robbie LA, Dummer S, Booth NA, et al. Plasminogen activator inhibitor 2 and urokinase-type plasminogen activator in plasma and leucocytes in patients with severe sepsis. *Br J Haematol* 2000;109:342–348.

516. Antalis TM, La Linn M, Donnan K, et al. The serine proteinase inhibitor (serpin) plasminogen activation inhibitor type 2 protects against viral cytopathic effects by constitutive interferon α/β priming. *J Exp Med* 1998; 187:1799–1811.

517. Darnell GA, Antalis TM, Johnstone RW, et al. Inhibition of retinoblastoma protein degradation by interaction with the serpin plasminogen activator inhibitor 2 via a novel consensus motif. *Mol Cell Biol* 2003;23:6520–6532.

518. Mueller BM, Yu YB, Laug WE. Overexpression of plasminogen activator inhibitor 2 in human melanoma cells inhibits spontaneous metastasis in scid/scid mice. *Proc Natl Acad Sci U S A* 1995;92:205–209.

519. Varro A, Noble PJ, Pritchard DM, et al. Helicobacter pylori induces plasminogen activator inhibitor 2 in gastric epithelial cells through nuclear factor-kappaB and RhoA: implications for invasion and apoptosis. *Cancer Res* 2004;64:1695–1702.

520. Dougherty KM, Pearson JM, Yang AY, et al. The plasminogen activator inhibitor-2 gene is not required for normal murine development or survival. *Proc Natl Acad Sci U S A* 1999;96:686–691.

521. Salvesen GS, Catanese JJ, Kress LF, et al. Primary structure of the reactive site of human C1-inhibitor. *J Biol Chem* 1985;260:2432–2436.

522. Tosi M, Duponchel C, Bourgarel P, et al. Molecular cloning of human C1 inhibitor: sequence homologies with $\alpha_1$-antitrypsin and other members of the serpins superfamily. *Gene* 1986;42:265–272.

523. Bock SC, Skriver K, Nielsen E, et al. Human C1 inhibitor: primary structure, cDNA cloning, and chromosomal localization. *Biochemistry* 1986;25:4292–4301.

524. Huisman LGM, Van Griensven JMT, Kluft C. On the role of C1-inhibitor as inhibitor of tissue-type plasminogen activator in human plasma. *Thromb Haemost* 1995;73:466–471.

525. Koide T, Foster D, Yoshitake S, et al. Amino acid sequence of human histidine-rich glycoprotein derived from the nucleotide sequence of its cDNA. *Biochemistry* 1986;25:2220–2225.

526. Lijnen HR, Hoylaerts M, Collen D. Isolation and characterization of a human plasma protein with affinity for the lysine binding sites in plasminogen. *J Biol Chem* 1980;255:10214–10222.

527. Ichinose A, Mimuro J, Koide T, et al. Histidine-rich glycoprotein and $\alpha_2$-plasmin inhibitor in inhibition of plasminogen binding to fibrin. *Thromb Res* 1984;33:401–407.

528. Jones AL, Hulett MD, Altin JG, et al. Plasminogen is tethered with high affinity to the cells surface by the plasma protein, histidine-rich glycoprotein. *J Biol Chem* 2004;279:38267–38276.

529. Shigekiyo T, Ohshima T, Oka H, et al. Congenital histidine-rich glycoprotein deficiency. *Thromb Haemost* 1993;70:263–265.

530. Nesheim M. Fibrinolysis and the plasma carboxypeptidase. *Curr Opin Hematol* 1998;5:309–313.

531. Bajzar L, Nesheim M, Morser J, et al. Both cellular and soluble forms of thrombomodulin inhibit fibrinolysis by potentiating the activation of thrombin-activable fibrinolysis inhibitor. *J Biol Chem* 1998;273:2792–2798.

532. Bouma BN, Marx PF, Mosnier LO, et al. Thrombin-activatable fibrinolysis inhibitor (TAFI, plasma procarboxypeptidase B, procarboxypeptidase R, procarboxypeptidase U). *Thromb Res* 2001;101:329–354.

533. Bajzar L, Morser J, Nesheim M. TAFI, or plasma procarboxypeptidase B, couples the coagulation and fibrinolytic cascades through the thrombin-thrombomodulin complex. *J Biol Chem* 1996;271:16603–16608.

534. Leurs J, Wissing BM, Nerme V, et al. Different mechanisms contribute to the biphasic pattern of carboxypeptidase U (TAFIa) generation during *in vitro* clot lysis in human plasma. *Thromb Haemost* 2003;89:264–271.

535. Mutch NJ, Moore NR, Wang E, et al. Thrombus lysis by uPA, scuPA and tPA is regulated by plasma TAFI. *J Thromb Haemost* 2003;1:2000–2007.

536. Redlitz A, Nicolini FA, Malycky JL, et al. Inducible carboxypeptidase activity. A role in clot lysis *in vivo*. *Circulation* 1996;93:1328–1330.

537. Nagashima M, Werner M, Wang M, et al. An inhibitor of activated thrombin-activatable fibrinolysis inhibitor potentiates tissue-type plasminogen activator-induced thrombolysis in a rabbit jugular vein thrombolysis model. *Thromb Res* 2000;98:333–342.

538. Klement P, Liao P, Bajzar L. A novel approach to arterial thrombolysis. *Blood* 1999;94:2735–2743.

539. Nagashima M, Yin ZF, Zhao L, et al. Thrombin-activatable fibrinolysis inhibitor (TAFI) deficiency is compatible with murine life. *J Clin Invest* 2002;109:101–110.

540. Silveira A, Schatteman K, Goossens F, et al. Plasma procarboxypeptidase U in men with symptomatic coronary artery disease. *Thromb Haemost* 2000;84:364–368.

541. Morange PE, Aillaud MF, Nicaud V, et al. Ala147Thr and C+1542G polymorphisms in the TAFI gene are not associated with a higher risk of venous thrombosis in FV Leiden carriers. *Thromb Haemost* 2001;86:1583–1584.

542. Gils A, Alessi MC, Brouwers E, et al. Development of a genotype 325-specific proCPU/TAFI ELISA. *Arterioscler Thromb Vasc Biol* 2003;23:1122–1127.

543. Guimaraes AH, van Tilburg NH, Vos HL, et al. Association between thrombin activatable fibrinolysis inhibitor genotype and levels in plasma: comparison of different assays. *Br J Haematol* 2004;124:659–665.

544. Bouma BN, Meijers JCM. Fibrinolysis and the contact system: a role for factor XI in the down-regulation of fibrinolysis. *Thromb Haemost* 1999;82:243–250.

545. Broze GJ, Higuchi DA. Coagulation-dependent inhibition of fibrinolysis-role of carboxypeptidase-U and the premature lysis of clots from hemophilic plasma. *Blood* 1996;88:3815–3823.

546. Mosnier LO, Lisman T, van den Berg HM, et al. The defective down regulation of fibrinolysis in haemophilia A can be restored by increasing the TAFI plasma concentration. *Thromb Haemost* 2001;86:1035–1039.

547. Minnema MC, Friederich PW, Levi M, et al. Enhancement of rabbit jugular vein thrombolysis by neutralization of factor XI. *In vivo* evidence for a role of factor XI as an anti-fibrinolytic factor. *J Clin Invest* 1998;101:10–14.

548. Scanu AM, Edelstein C. Kringle-dependent structural and functional polymorphism of apolipoprotein(a). *Biochim Biophys Acta* 1995;1256:1–12.

549. Lindahl G, Gersdorf E, Menzel HJ, et al. The gene for the Lp(a)-specific glycoprotein is closely linked to the gene for plasminogen on chromosome 6. *Hum Genet* 1989;81:149–152.

550. Byrne CD, Schwartz K, Meer K, et al. The human apolipoprotein(a)/plasminogen gene cluster contains a novel homologue transcribed in liver. *Arterioscler Thromb* 1994;14:534–541.

551. Miles LA, Fles GM, Levin EG, et al. A potential basis for the thrombotic risks associated with lipoprotein(a). *Nature* 1989;339:301–303.

552. Hajjar KA, Gavish D, Breslow JL, et al. Lipoprotein(a) modulation of endothelial cell surface fibrinolysis and its potential role in atherosclerosis. *Nature* 1989;339:303–305.

553. Gonzalez-Gronow M, Edelberg JM, Pizzo SV. Further characterization of the cellular plasminogen binding site: evidence that plasminogen 2 and lipoprotein(a) compete for the same site. *Biochemistry* 1989;28:2374–2377.

554. Ezratty A, Simon DI, Loscalzo J. Lipoprotein(a) binds to human platelets and attenuates plasminogen binding and activation. *Biochemistry* 1993;32:4628–4633.

555. Plow EF, Herren T, Redlitz A, et al. The cell biology of the plasminogen system. *FASEB J* 1995;9:939–945.

556. Sangrar W, Gabel BR, Boffa MB, et al. The solution phase interaction between apolipoprotein(a) and plasminogen inhibits the binding of plasminogen to a plasmin-modified fibrinogen surface. *Biochemistry* 1997;36:10353–10363.

557. Angles-Cano E, Rojas G. Apolipoprotein(a): structure-function relationship at the lysine-binding site and plasminogen activator cleavage site. *Biol Chem* 2002;383:93–99.

558. Tsurupa G, Ho-Tin-Noe B, Angles-Cano E, et al. Identification and characterization of novel lysine-independent apolipoprotein(a)-binding sites in fibrin(ogen) $\alpha$C-domains. *J Biol Chem* 2003;278:37154–37159.

559. Palabrica TM, Liu AC, Aronovitz MJ, et al. Antifibrinolytic activity of apolipoprotein(a) *in vivo*: human apolipoprotein(a) transgenic mice are resistant to tissue plasminogen activator-mediated thrombolysis. *Nat Med* 1995;1:256–259.

560. Mooser V, Mancini FP, Bopp S, et al. Sequence polymorphisms in the apo(a) gene associated with specific levels of Lp(a) in plasma. *Hum Mol Genet* 1995;4:173–181.

561. Dahlén GH. Lipoprotein(a), atherosclerosis and thrombosis. *Prog Lipid Res* 1991;30:189–194.

562. Longenecker JC, Klag MJ, Marcovina SM, et al. Small apolipoprotein(a) size predicts mortality in end-stage renal disease: the CHOICE study. *Circulation* 2002;106:2812–2818.

563. Hervio L, Durlach V, Girard-Globa A, et al. Multiple binding with identical linkage: a mechanism that explains the effect of lipoprotein(a) on fibrinolysis. *Biochemistry* 1995;34:13353–13358.

564. Angles-Cano E, de la Pena Diaz A, Loyau S. Inhibition of fibrinolysis by lipoprotein(a). *Ann N Y Acad Sci* 2001;936:261–275.

565. Falcó C, Estellés A, Dalmau J, et al. Influence of lipoprotein (a) levels and isoforms on fibrinolytic activity—study in families with high lipoprotein (a) levels. *Thromb Haemost* 1998;79:818–823.

566. Novokhatny VV, Jesmok GJ, Landskroner KA, et al. Locally delivered plasmin: why should it be superior to plasminogen activators for direct thrombolysis? *Trends Pharmacol Sci* 2004;25:72–75.

567. Nilsson TK, Mellbring G. Impact of immediate acidification of blood on measurement of plasma tissue plasminogen activator (tPA) activity in surgical patients. *Clin Chem* 1989;35:1999.

568. Gaffney PJ, Curtis AD. A collaborative study to establish the second international standard for tissue plasminogen activator (tPA). *Thromb Haemost* 1987;59:1085–1087.

569. Grimaudo V, Hauert J, Bachmann F, et al. Diurnal variation of the fibrinolytic system. *Thromb Haemost* 1988;59:495–499.

570. Ridker PM, Vaughan DE, Stampfer MJ, et al. Endogenous tissue-type plasminogen activator and risk of myocardial infarction. *Lancet* 1993;341:1165–1168.

571. Nordenhem A, Wiman B. Tissue plasminogen activator (tPA) antigen in plasma: correlation with different tPA/inhibitor complexes. *Scand J Clin Lab Invest* 1998;58:475–483.

572. Rijken DC, Sakharov DV. Basic principles in thrombolysis: regulatory role of plasminogen. *Thromb Res* 2001;103(Suppl. 1):S41–S49.

573. Sakharov DV, Plow EF, Rijken DC. On the mechanism of the antifibrinolytic activity of plasma carboxypeptidase B. *J Biol Chem* 1997;272:14477–14482.

# CHAPTER 19 ■ PLASMINOGEN ACTIVATOR INHIBITOR-1

MANUEL YEPES, DAVID J. LOSKUTOFF, AND DANIEL A. LAWRENCE

Plasminogen activators (PAs) are specific serine proteinases that activate the proenzyme plasminogen, by cleavage of a single Arg-Val peptide bond, to the broad-specificity enzyme plasmin. Plasminogen activation provides an important source of localized proteolytic activity during a number of physiologic and pathologic processes such as fibrinolysis, ovulation, cell migration, epithelial differentiation, vascular disease, and cancer (1–3). Therefore, accurate regulation of PAs constitutes a critical feature of many physiologic and pathologic events. Two PAs are found in mammals: tissue-type PA (tPA) and urokinase-type PA (uPA) (4). The regulation of PAs is a complex process that involves regulation of gene expression by factors such as hormones, growth factors, and cytokines (1,4), as well as regulation of enzyme activity through interactions with fibrin (5) or with specific receptors for uPA (6), tPA (7), and plasminogen (8). PA activity is also regulated by specific inhibitors termed *plasminogen activator inhibitors* (PAIs) (9). However, of the five different PAIs [i.e., PAI-1 (10); PAI-2 (11); PAI-3, also called the *activated protein C inhibitor* (APCI) (12); protease nexin-1 (13); and neuroserpin (14)], only PAI-1, which is the most kinetically efficient, appears to play a significant role in regulating PA activity in blood and most tissues. The exception to this may be in the central nervous system (CNS), where neuroserpin is an important regulator of tPA activity (15,16). This chapter focuses on the biochemical, genetic, physiologic, and pathologic properties of PAI-1. The basic properties of PAI-1 are analyzed in the first part, whereas the second half examines the evidence linking PAI-1 to the pathogenesis of human disease.

## BASIC PROPERTIES OF PLASMINOGEN ACTIVATOR INHIBITOR-1

### Protein Structure and Function

Formerly known as the *endothelial cell PAI* (10,17–19), the *"fast-acting" inhibitor of tPA in plasma* (20), and the β-*migrating PAI* (21–23), PAI-1 is a single-chain glycoprotein having an $M_r$ of approximately 50,000 and was first identified in the year 1983 (10,24,25). PAI-1 has three potential N-linked glycosylation sites and contains between 15% and 20% carbohydrate (19,23). It belongs to the serine proteinase inhibitors superfamily (serpins), which is a gene family that includes many of the proteinase inhibitors found in blood, as well as other proteins with unrelated or unknown functions (26) (see Chapter 13). The serpins share a tertiary structure (27) and have evolved from a common ancestor (28,29). They act as "suicide inhibitors" [i.e., they react only once with their target protease to form sodium dodecyl sulfate (SDS)–stable complexes (30–33)]. The interaction between the

serpin and its target protease occurs at an amino acid residue located in the reactive center loop (RCL) of the serpin, which is known as a "bait" residue. This "bait" residue is thought to mimic the normal substrate of the enzyme and to associate by its side-chain atoms with the specificity crevice (S1 site) of the enzyme (34–37). The "bait" amino acid is called the P1 residue, with the amino acids toward the amino-terminal side of the scissile RCL bond being labeled in the order P1, P2, P3, and so on, and the amino acids on the carboxyl side being labeled P1′, P2′, P3′, and so on (38). Upon cleavage of the "bait" amino acid by a target proteinase, there is a large conformational change in the serpin that involves the rapid insertion of the RCL into the major structural element of the serpin, the β-sheet A (33,39–41). This results in a tight docking of the enzyme to the serpin surface and in a large increase in the structural stability of the serpin. This leads to distortion of the enzyme structure, including the active site, which traps the proteinase in an acyl–enzyme complex with the serpin (42–44).

The PAI-1 complementary deoxyribonucleic acid (cDNA) encodes a protein of 402 amino acids that includes a typical secretion signal sequence (23,45–47). Mature human PAI-1 is composed of two variants in approximately equal proportions (i.e., 381 and 379 amino acids), which likely arise from alternative cleavage of the secretion signal sequence and generate proteins with overlapping amino-terminal sequences of Ser-Ala-Val-His-His and Val-His-His-Pro-Pro (45,48). The latter sequence does not contain cysteines because the single cysteine residue present in the signal peptide is removed during membrane translocation (46,47). This property facilitates the efficient expression and isolation of recombinant PAI-1 from *Escherichia coli* (48–52), which, in contrast to PAI-1 purified from mammalian cell culture, is predominantly produced in the active form (48).

### Reactive Center Loop

The P1 "bait" amino acid of PAI-1 (Arg346) is contained within the RCL near the carboxyl terminus of the molecule and serves as a pseudosubstrate for the target serine proteinase (33,37). Either arginine or lysine at P1 is essential for PAI-1 to function as an effective inhibitor of uPA (36,37), and the residues surrounding P1 can modulate PAI-1 inhibitory activity by up to two orders of magnitude and can also alter the target–protease specificity (42,53,54). In the case of tPA other P1 residues are tolerated, and this is most likely due to tighter exosite interactions between PAI-1 and tPA (53,55–57).

### Plasminogen Activator Inhibitor-1 Conformations

Native PAI-1 exists in at least two distinct conformations: an active form that is produced by cells and is secreted and an inactive

## PAI-1 structure

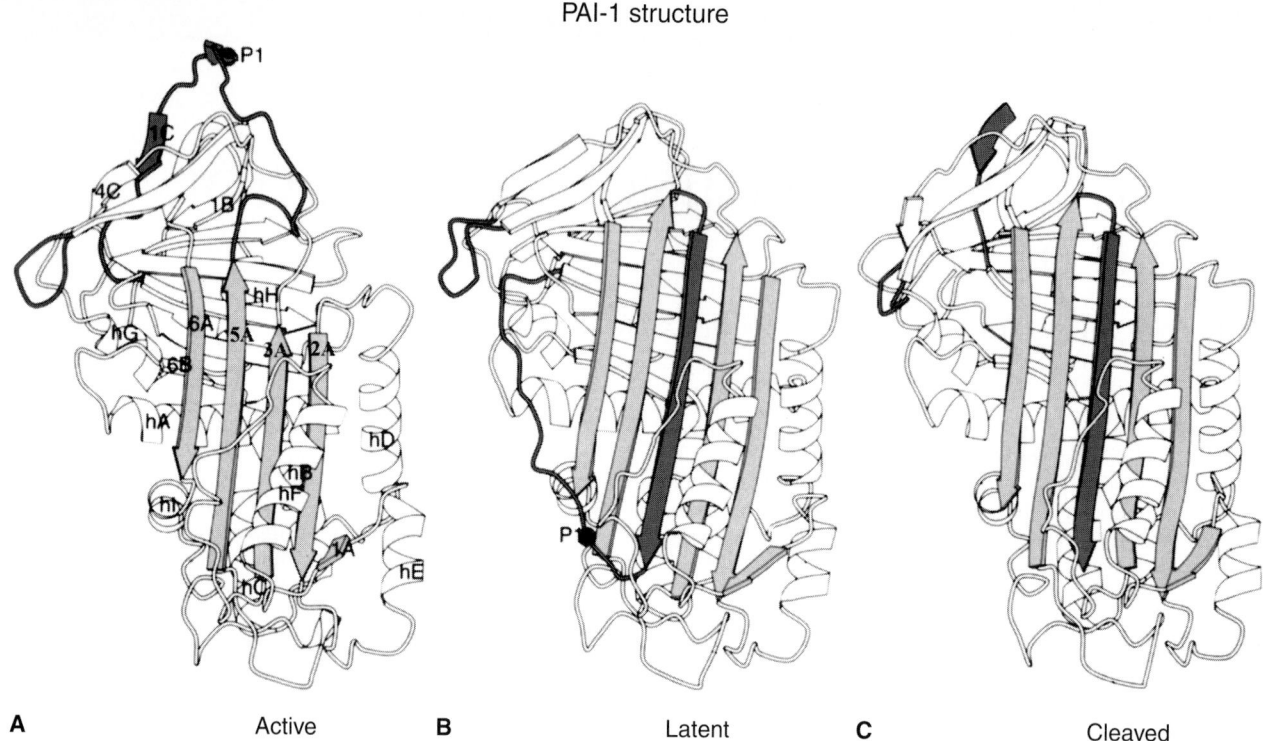

**A**    Active    **B**    Latent    **C**    Cleaved

**FIGURE 19-1.** Schematic illustration of the three conformations of plasminogen activator inhibitor-1 (PAI-1). The major β-sheet (β-sheet A) is highlighted in *light gray*, and the reactive center loop (RCL) is in *dark gray*. **A:** The active conformation of a stable mutant of PAI-1 (61). **B:** The latent conformation of PAI-1 (60). **C:** The cleaved conformation of PAI-1 (287). In both the latent and cleaved forms of PAI-1, the RCL is inserted into β-sheet A to form a new β-strand, (strand 4A) (see Color Fig. 19-1). (From Sharp AM, Stein PE, Pannu NS, et al. The active conformation of plasminogen activator inhibitor 1, a target for drugs to control fibrinolysis and cell adhesion. *Structure Fold Des* 1999;7:111–118, with permission.)

or latent form that accumulates in cell culture medium over time (58–60) (see Fig. 19-1). In blood and tissues, most of the PAI-1 is in the active form; however, in platelets both the active and the latent PAI-1 are found (21). In the active form of PAI-1, the RCL is part of an exposed loop on the surface of the molecule (61). Upon reaction with a proteinase, this RCL cleaves and integrates into the center of its own β-sheet A (33,61). In the latent form, the RCL is intact, but instead of being exposed, the entire amino-terminal side of the RCL is inserted as the central strand into the β-sheet A (60). This insertion accounts for the increased stability of latent PAI as well as for its lack of inhibitory activity (58,62,63). The active form spontaneously converts to the latent form with a half-life of about 1 to 2 hours at 37°C at neutral or slightly alkaline pH (48,59,64–66). The latent form can also be converted into the active form by treatment with denaturants or negatively charged phospholipids, or can be converted very slowly in the presence of the protein vitronectin (58,66,67). This spontaneous reversible interconversion between the active and latent structures is unique for PAI-1 and distinguishes it from other serpins.

Other inactive forms of PAI-1 have also been identified. The first form results from the oxidation of one or more critical methionine residues within active PAI-1 (68,69). This form differs from latent PAI-1 in that it can be partially reactivated by treatment with an enzyme that specifically reduces oxidized methionine residues (68). Oxidative inactivation of PAI-1 may be an additional mechanism for the regulation of the PA system. Oxygen radicals produced locally by neutrophils or other cells could inactivate PAI-1 and thereby facilitate the generation of plasmin activity at sites of infections

or in areas of tissue remodeling (70). A fourth conformational form of PAI-1 has also been identified. This is a noninhibitory substrate form that can be induced by the addition of SDS and can be converted back to the active or latent forms by treatment with 4 M guanidine HCl (71,72). The significance of this form and whether it exists *in vivo* is not known. PAI-1 can also exist in two different cleaved forms. As noted previously, PAI-1 that is complexed with a proteinase is cleaved at the P1–P1′ site, and PAI-1 can also be found not in complex with a proteinase but with its RCL cleaved. This can arise from dissociation of the PAI-1–PA complex or from the cleavage of the RCL by a nontarget proteinase at a site other than the P1–P1′ (63,73). None of these forms of PAI-1 is able to inhibit proteinase activity; however, they may interact with other nonproteinase substrates.

## Biochemical Properties

### Interaction with Tissue-Type Plasminogen Activator, Urokinase-Type Plasminogen Activator, and Plasmin

Inhibition of PAs by PAI-1 occurs in a rapid and stoichiometric manner, resulting in the formation of a covalent bond between the two molecules. Several studies indicate that PAI-1 is cleaved during this reaction and that the amino-terminal end of the RCL inserts as an antiparallel strand into β-sheet A (74,75). The inhibitor is consumed in the process, giving rise to the discussed term *suicide inhibitor*.

Kinetic studies demonstrate that PAI-1 inhibits the naturally occurring single-chain form of tPA with a second-order rate constant of approximately $10^6 \, M^{-1} S^{-1}$, a value that is at least 1,000 times higher than those for the interactions of PAI-2, PAI-3, and protease nexin-1 with single-chain tPA (9,42). Moreover, approximately 70% of the total tPA in carefully collected normal human plasma is detected in complex with PAI-1, suggesting that the inhibition of tPA by PAI-1 is a normal, ongoing process. PAI-1 is also an important uPA inhibitor because the second-order rate constant for its interaction with uPA is also at least two orders of magnitude higher than that of other PAIs (9,42,76). PAI-1 can also efficiently and directly inhibit plasmin (64,77). Therefore, PAI-1 is the chief regulator of plasmin generation *in vivo*, and, as such, it appears to play an important role in both fibrinolytic and thrombotic diseases (3,78–80).

## Interaction with Vitronectin and Members of the Low Density Lipoprotein Receptor Family (LDL-Rs)

Most of the active PAI-1 in blood circulates in the form of a complex with the glycoprotein vitronectin. The binding site of vitronectin to PAI-1 has been identified in a region centered around residues 101 to 123 of the three-dimensional structure (81–84), whereas the binding site to members of the LDL-R family has been less well characterized and appears to be located in a region associated with $\alpha$ helix D containing residues Arg76 and Lys69 (85,86). Vitronectin is present in plasma and in the extracellular matrix (87,88), mainly at sites of injury or remodeling. Vitronectin is also specifically incorporated into fibrin clots (89). Vitronectin may be considered a cofactor for PAI-1 because it stabilizes PAI-1 in its active conformation, thereby increasing its biologic half-life. In turn, PAI-1 converts vitronectin from its native, plasma form, which does not support cell adhesion, to an "activated" form that is able to bind ligands such as integrins (90). Vitronectin also increases the inhibitory efficiency of PAI-1 for thrombin approximately 300-fold, making it a more efficient inhibitor of thrombin than antithrombin III in the absence of heparin (91,92) (see Fig. 19-2).

Upon complex formation with a proteinase, the conformational change in PAI-1 associated with RCL insertion results in a loss in high affinity binding to vitronectin but in a gain in high affinity binding to the clearance receptors of the (LDL-R) family (85,93). This is a result of a conformational change in PAI-1 that disrupts the vitronectin binding site, exposing, at the same time, a cryptic receptor binding site that is revealed only when PAI-1 is in an active conformation complex with a proteinase (54,61,85). This results in an approximately 1,000,000-fold shift in the relative affinity of PAI-1 from vitronectin to a member of the LDL-R family, which leads to a rapid clearance of PAI-1 by internalization through the LDL-R family members (85).

The uPA receptor (uPAR) (6) is a glycosyl phosphatidyl inositol (GPI)–anchored protein that localizes uPA on the cell surface, frequently at the invading edge of cells (94). Receptor occupancy has been shown to activate intracellular signaling pathways. Like PAI-1, uPAR also binds to vitronectin with high affinity as well as to various integrins (95–98), and the binding of uPAR to vitronectin is inhibited by PAI-1. The fact that uPAR and integrins also may bind to vitronectin raises the possibility that, as discussed later in this chapter, PAI-1 could regulate cell adhesion and migration.

## Binding to Heparin and Fibrin

PAI-1 also binds to heparin with high affinity (48,99). This binding does not affect the interaction of PAI-1 with uPA or tPA but, in contrast, enhances the interaction of PAI-1 with thrombin (91,100). The heparin binding domain on PAI-1 has been mapped to a region homologous to the heparin binding domain of antithrombin III on and around $\alpha$ helix D (101). Critical residues appear to include lysines 65, 69, 80, and 88, and arginine 76. It has also been reported that PAI-1 binds to fibrin *in vitro* with a $K_d$ of 3.8 $\mu$M, and, while bound, remains capable of inhibiting uPA and tPA (102–105). However, more recent data suggest that most of the PAI-1 localized to fibrin clots is vitronectin dependent (106,107).

# Structure and Regulation of the Plasminogen Activator Inhibitor-1 Gene

The human gene for PAI-1 is located on chromosome 7q21.3-22 (108). It is 12.3 kb in length, composed of 9 exons and 8 introns, and is similar in structure to that of protease nexin I and neuroserpin (109–115). The promoter contains a typical TATA box but no CAAT sequence. Segments of PAI-1 promoter containing as little as 187 bp of upstream sequence have shown to direct transcription in several mammalian cell types (111,116,117). Comparison of the rat and human PAI-1 promoter sequences shows a striking region of conservation in

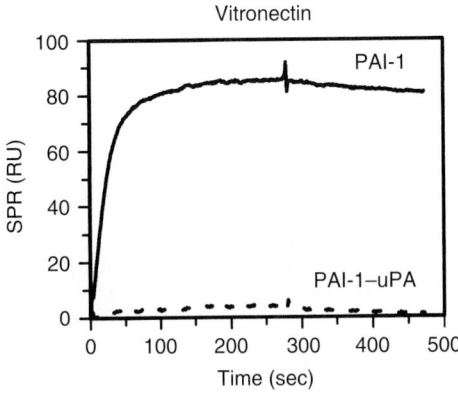
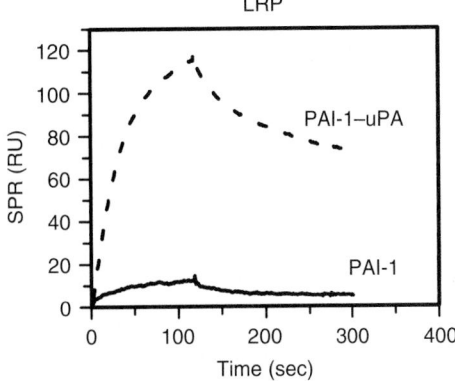

**FIGURE 19-2.** Plasminogen activator inhibitor-1 (PAI-1) association with vitronectin and low density lipoprotein receptors (LDL-Rs) is conformationally controlled. Surface plasmin resonance analysis of PAI-1 or PAI-1–uPA complexes binding to either vitronectin or the LDL-R family member LRP. The *solid lines* in each panel are PAI-1 only and the *dashed lines* in each panel are the PAI-1–uPA covalent complex. (From Natalia Gorlatova and Daniel A. Lawrence.)

the proximal promoter (from the TATA box to −90) and a distal sequence of −510 to −753 of the rat sequence. Changes in plasma PAI-1 levels can be correlated with variations in the structure of the PAI-1 gene. To date, three polymorphic variations in the gene have been reported: a single nucleotide insertion per deletion (4G/5G) polymorphism in the promoter region, an allelic variation at a (C–A)$_n$ dinucleotide repeat polymorphism in intron 3, and a HindIII restriction fragment length polymorphism (RFLP) due to a base change at the 3′ flanking region of the gene (118). However, no link between PAI-1 polymorphism and human disease has been consistently demonstrated. Relative to the HindIII RFLP polymorphism, three genotypes—1/1, 1/2, and 2/2—have been described, on the basis of the presence ("2" allele) or the absence ("1" allele) of the HindIII polymorphic site. Interestingly, genotype 1/1 exhibits higher plasma PAI-1 activity than genotype 2/2 (119). Two sizes of PAI-1 messenger ribonucleic acid (mRNA) are observed in human cells, approximately 3 kb and 2 kb in length, respectively. This difference has been shown to be because of alternative polyadenylation, with both mRNAs encoding the same protein, but with an additional 1 kb of 3′ untranslated region present in the larger message (109–112). The additional 3′ untranslated region in the larger message contains a 75-base pair AT-rich sequence that has been postulated to play a role in PAI-1 gene regulation by a posttranscriptional mechanism (47,120–123).

Although PAI-1 is present at low concentrations in plasma, its relatively short half-life in blood (i.e., 10 minutes) suggests a high biosynthetic rate (124). Moreover, its concentration rapidly increases in response to a variety of agents or changes in physiologic state, indicating that the amount of PAI-1 in plasma is subject to dynamic regulation. For example, the concentration of plasma PAI-1 increases dramatically during endotoxemia (125). Endotoxin [lipopolysaccharide (LPS)] induces PAI-1 mRNA in virtually all tissues of the mouse (126), suggesting that plasma PAI-1 may originate from multiple tissues during sepsis. In situ hybridization analysis reveals that endotoxin induces PAI-1 mRNA in endothelial cells at all levels of the vasculature, including larger arteries, veins, and capillaries. PAI-1 gene expression is also induced in hepatocytes and in adipocytes (127,128).

Many of the effects of endotoxin are mediated through the release of cytokines from inflammatory cells [e.g., tumor necrosis factor-α (TNF-α) and interleukin-1 (IL-1)]. Indeed, a variety of studies have shown that most of the same tissues of the mouse that produce PAI-1 in response to endotoxin (i.e., liver, heart, and lung) also produce it in response to TNF-α (126) Therefore, endotoxin and TNF-α upregulate PAI-1 expression primarily in endothelial cells in most mouse tissues and induces it in vitro in various bovine and human endothelial cells. Growth modulators such as transforming growth factor-β (TGF-β) also induce plasma PAI-1 antigen and tissue PAI-1 mRNA in several animal models (126). In murine models, TGF-β induces PAI-1 mRNA in vascular and nonvascular smooth muscle cells, in adipocytes, and in cells in the myocardium and kidney (126). Although TGF-β induces PAI-1 in cultured bovine endothelial cells (129), it does not appear to induce it in murine endothelium in vivo. Whether this apparent inconsistency reflects differences between in vitro and in vivo systems or between species remains to be determined.

Several studies have identified DNA sequence elements in the first 1.3 kb of the promoter/5′-upstream flanking region of the PAI-1 gene that mediate cytokine responsiveness in transfected cells (130). However, little is known about the role of these sequences in PAI-1 promoter function in vivo. PAI-1 mRNA levels are determined by both transcriptional and posttranscriptional mechanisms. Factors that have been shown to increase the rate of PAI-1 mRNA transcription in different cell types are glucocorticoids, TNF-α, insulin, and IL-1 (130). In HepG2 cells, IGF-1 (insulinlike growth factor-1) and insulin are also able to induce PAI-1 synthesis by increasing mRNA stability (131). Moreover, it has been suggested that PAI-1 gene regulation is of even greater complexity because it also could depend on genetic polymorphisms.

Expression of PAI-1 has been observed in a wide range of cell types including adipocytes, fibrosarcoma, hepatoma, and ovarian and endothelial cells. However, studies in transgenic mice carrying the PAI-1 promoter linked to an indicator gene suggest that PAI-1 expression may be much more limited in vivo (126). Although the hepatoma cells produce large amounts of PAI-1 in vitro and have been used as a model to study its regulation, it is known that hepatocytes do not normally synthesize PAI-1 in vivo (132,133). Nevertheless, these hepatocytes and the endothelial cells can be induced by endotoxin to produce PAI-1 in vivo (133). These observations raise important concerns about the validity of in vitro tissue culture as a model for the regulation of fibrinolysis in vivo.

# PLASMINOGEN ACTIVATOR INHIBITOR-1 IN PATHOLOGIC CONDITIONS

In healthy individuals, PAI-1 is expressed primarily in megakaryocytes, smooth muscle cells, and adipocytes (128, 130,134,135). However, as noted in the preceding text, its expression can be rapidly and markedly induced in many cell types by stress, or injury, or by growth factors and cytokines (133,136,137). The last part of this chapter analyzes the link between PAI-1 and different pathologic events such as cancer, obesity, atherosclerosis, and vascular, pulmonary, and renal diseases (see Fig. 19-3).

## Cancer

The existence of a link between fibrinolysis and tumor growth was first suggested by the observations that patients with malignant tumors have increased fibrinolytic activity and that tumor tissues can degrade fibrin clots (1,138–140). Therefore, it was quite unexpected when high PAI-1 levels were found to be strongly correlated with a poor prognosis in patients with many different neoplasias, including gastric and breast carcinomas, as well as with brain, ovarian, and lung tumors and with metastatic lesions from renal cell carcinoma, melanoma,

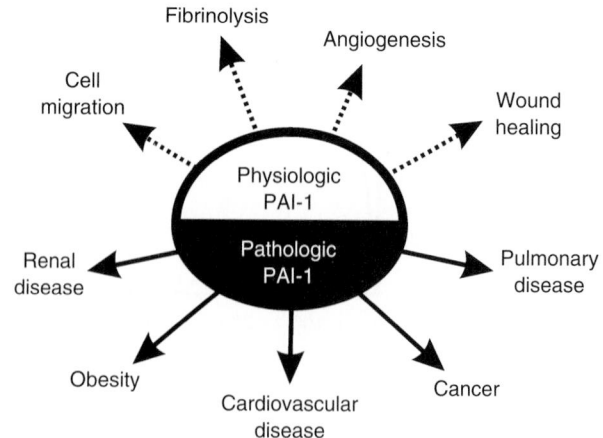

**FIGURE 19-3.** Plasminogen activator inhibitor-1 (PAI-1) association with normal and pathologic physiology.

and colorectal cancer (141–146). Analysis of human colon carcinomas has demonstrated the presence of PAI-1 mRNA in vascular endothelial cells, in the stroma surrounding the invasive tumor, in granulation tissue, and in some capillaries within the tumor (147). Strong staining for PAI-1 antigen has also been observed in proliferative vessels in intracranial tumors such as high-grade gliomas and metastatic tumors, as well as in blood vessels near the necrotic center of tumors (147,148). In these studies, PAI-1 was localized to the vascular basement membrane and perivascular connective tissue, whereas endothelial cells themselves showed only weak reactivity. In contrast, an immunochemical study on Lewis lung carcinoma transplanted in mice showed PAI-1 protein in the tumor cells themselves (149). Like PAI-1, uPA and its receptor, uPAR, have also been correlated with a poor prognosis in cancer (150,151). In this section of the chapter, the role of PAI-1 in cancer has been addressed from two perspectives: cell migration and tumor angiogenesis.

## Cell Migration

Although uPA has been associated with physiologic events that involve cell migration such as wound healing, vascular remodeling (152–154), neural cell migration (155), and monocyte invasiveness (156), its precise role in these processes is not clear. Increased uPA levels have been reported in many transformed cells including myeloid leukemic cells (157), hepatomas (158), gliomas (159), and carcinomas (160), and inhibitors of uPA have been shown to reduce cell migration and metastasis (161–164). The long-established explanation of these data was that the main role of uPA was to activate plasmin, which directly, and indirectly through the activation of matrix metalloproteases (MMPs), degrades the basement membrane and clears a path for cells to migrate (165,166) (see Fig. 19-4A). However, by the 1990s, this "matrix barrier model" of proteases and cell migration started to be challenged. For example, it was shown that uPA and plasmin as well as other proteases could produce a "limited proteolysis" that preserved the architecture of the basement membrane but exposed cryptic sites within the matrix that could enhance cell adhesion and or migration (167–171). Plasmin could also promote cell proliferation and migration through the activation of growth factors such as TGF-$\beta$ (172,173) or through the release of "sequestered" growth factors from the matrix such as fibroblast growth factor (FGF) and vascular endothelial growth factor (VEGF) (174–177). More recent studies have expanded on these observations and have begun to suggest that the role of uPA and, in particular, PAI-1 in cell migration may be far more subtle and elegant than previously thought and may involve interactions on the cell surface with a number of receptors including uPAR, integrins, and members of the LDL-R family.

Cell surface uPA and uPAR were originally shown to localize at the focal contacts (178,179) and at the leading edge of migrating cells (180). As already noted, uPAR not only serves as a receptor for uPA but also binds to vitronectin in the matrix, and, through this binding, can mediate cell adhesion directly (181). uPAR can also associate either directly or indirectly with integrins, and this association can affect both cell signaling and migration (95–98,182,183). In vitro studies have demonstrated that both PAI-1 and uPAR bind to the somatomedin B-domain of vitronectin, although uPAR binds with significantly lower affinity (184,185). Therefore, PAI-1 competes with uPAR for binding to vitronectin and may inhibit uPAR-mediated cell attachment (185–187). PAI-1, uPA, and uPAR can also modulate integrin-mediated cell adhesion (167,168,188). For example, the integrin $\alpha_V\beta_3$ binding site on vitronectin overlaps the PAI-1 binding site, resulting in a potential competition between $\alpha_V\beta_3$ and PAI-1 for vitronectin binding (167,184). Therefore, in smooth muscle cells where vitronectin promotes cell migration, the inhibition of $\alpha_V\beta_3$ binding to vitronectin by the addition of PAI-1 results in an inhibition of cell migration (167). Exogenous PAI-1 also inhibits the migration of stimulated endothelial, human amnion WISH and epidermal carcinoma cells, as well as the invasion of human monocytes (167,168,189,190). However, the effects of PAI-1 on cell adhesion and migration are fully reversible by PAs because, as discussed at the beginning of this chapter, upon complex formation with a protease, PAI-1 undergoes a conformational change that alters the PAI-1 vitronectin binding site and renders the PA–PAI-1 complex unable to bind to vitronectin. Therefore, the relative concentrations of uPA (or tPA) and active PAI-1 at the cell matrix interface are able to regulate cell-matrix interactions mediated through vitronectin.

In addition to blocking cell-matrix interactions and cell migration, PAI-1 can also promote cell migration under some conditions. In the studies discussed in the preceding text, high concentrations of exogenous PAI-1 were used to block migration. However, recent work by Palmieri et al. has established that the stable expression of PAI-1 can actually stimulate adhesion and migration on several different matrix proteins (191). And although this activity required the inhibition of uPA, it did not specifically require PAI-1, because another uPA inhibitor, PAI-3, could also stimulate this activity. The inhibition of uPA by either PAI-1 or PAI-3 also increased the surface expression of several integrin subunits. Czekay et al. demonstrated that the binding of uPA to uPAR promotes the association of the uPA–uPAR complex with the integrins $\alpha_V\beta_3$ or $\alpha_V\beta_5$, and showed that by adding PAI-1 to this complex, they could induce the cells to detach from the matrix by stimulating endocytosis of the integrin–uPAR–uPA–PAI-1 complex by a member of the LDL-R family (188). The endocytosed integrins could then recycle back to the cell surface, where, upon activation, they could reengage the matrix. These studies have lead to the hypothesis that the inhibition of uPA by PAI-1 could promote the type of cycled attachment–detachment–reattachment required for cell migration (166,188). Importantly, this activity appears to be independent of the matrix composition, suggesting that it may represent a general mechanism in which inhibition of uPA promotes cell migration (Fig. 19-4B). This model is consistent with much of the literature examining the roles of uPA and PAI-1 in cell migration. It provides a compelling explanation as to why both uPA and its inhibitor PAI-1 are strongly correlated with a poor prognosis in cancer patients because both molecules are needed for the maximal enhancement of cell migration. In this context, it is also interesting to note that PAI-1 differs from other serpins in that it is a trace protein in plasma and tissues, with a relatively short half-life (approximately 10 minutes). Moreover, it is an immediate early gene and has been shown to accumulate at focal points of adhesion (192). Finally, its biosynthesis is stimulated rapidly by a variety of inflammatory mediators, growth factors, and hormones (130,136). The short half-life and ability to be rapidly and dramatically unregulated are the expected properties of molecules with the potential to rapidly initiate or terminate biologic processes (i.e., molecular switches) (80,185). Therefore, by regulating the production rate or activity of PAI-1, cells may be able to control their adhesiveness and movement.

Finally, PAI-1 can also regulate cell motility by effecting uPA-dependent cell signaling by phosphorylation of the extracellular signal-regulated kinase (ERK). This signaling requires uPA binding to uPAR and requires endocytosis of the PAI-1–uPA–uPAR complex by the VLDLR and recycling of uPAR back to the cell surface (193). The effect of PAI-1 inhibition of

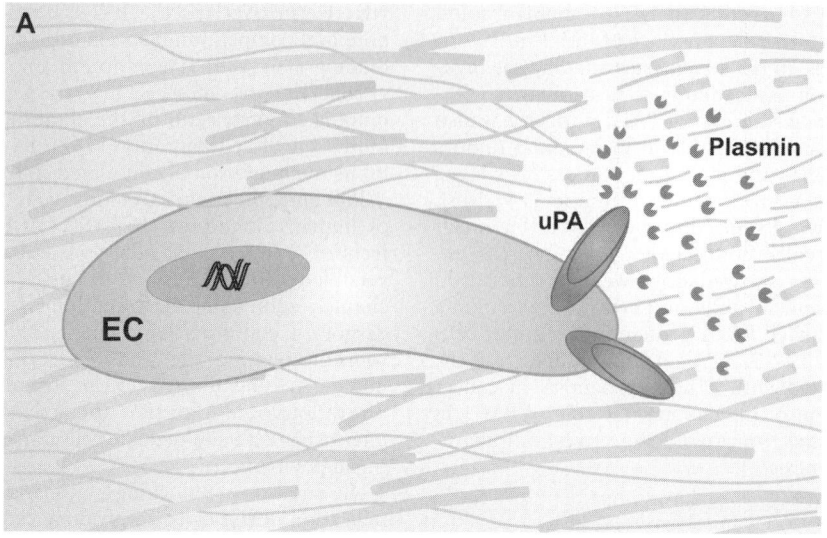

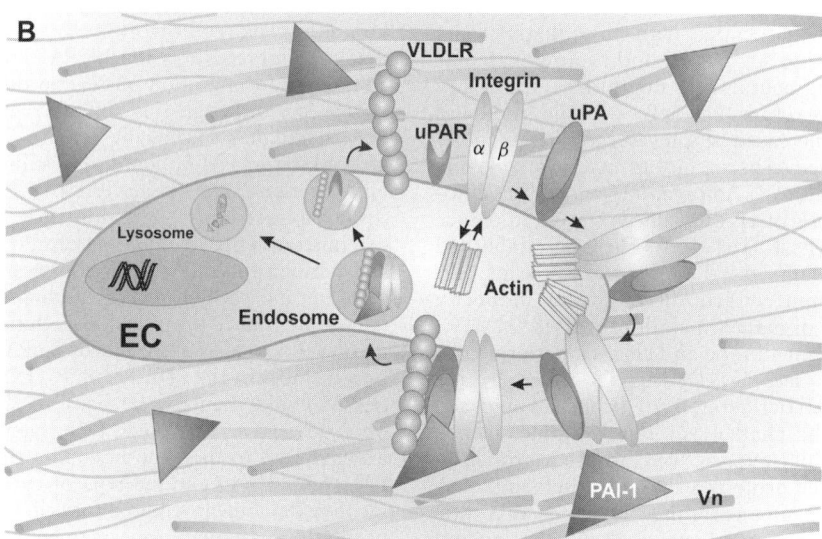

**FIGURE 19-4.** The evolution of our understanding of the role of plasminogen activator inhibitor-1 (PAI-1) in cell migration. **A:** Before the multiple actions of urokinase PA (uPA), urokinase-type plasminogen activator receptor (uPAR), and PAIs were fully understood, the simplest model for the function of uPA in cell migration was based solely on its ability to activate plasmin. Plasmin in turn degraded extracellular matrix (ECM) proteins, which allowed the cell to escape its matrix barrier and migrate. **B:** A model of the potential role of PAI-1 in cell migration that assumes that the cell surface receptors uPAR, integrins, and low density lipoprotein receptor (LDL-R) family, such as the very low density lipoprotein receptor (VLDLR), are expressed by the cell. The integrin may or may not be attached to the matrix and connected to the cytoskeleton, and uPA may be expressed by the same cell or by a nearby cell. Binding of the secreted uPA to uPAR may enhance the association of uPAR with an integrin, which may also promote adhesion. If there is also PAI in the surrounding milieu, it can then bind to the uPA present in the ternary complex. This PAI would most likely be PAI-1 because its expression is stimulated by conditions associated with cell migration and because it will specifically localize to the matrix through binding to vitronectin. The binding of PAI-1 to uPA induces the conformational change in PAI-1 that simultaneously reduces its affinity for the matrix while enhancing its affinity for the clearance receptor (Fig. 19-2). This association also promotes integrin disengagement from the matrix, and very likely from the cytoskeleton as well, and binding to the clearance receptor (VLDLR). Whether the integrin first disengages from the matrix and then binds to the clearance receptor or whether it is the association of the quaternary complex with the clearance receptor that induces the integrin to disengage is not yet clear. Regardless of the exact sequence of events, the quaternary complex is then endocytosed, and, in the endosome, the PAI–uPA complex separates from the three receptors and is targeted to the lysosome for degradation. The LDL-R, uPAR, and the integrin are then recycled back to the cell surface where the process can be repeated. This cycled attachment–detachment–reattachment of integrins is necessary for cell migration. This figure does not indicate the many potential intracellular signaling events that each one of these interactions could generate, but each one of these receptor interactions could signal the cell. The downstream consequences of these events undoubtedly also modulate cell adhesion and migration through other pathways (see Color Fig. 19-4). (From Stefansson S, Lawrence DA. Old dogs and new tricks, proteases, inhibitors, and cell migration. *Sci STKE* 2003;e24, with permission.)

uPA and endocytosis of the complex is unclear: It was shown to inhibit uPA-induced chemotaxis in one study (194), whereas in another report, PAI-1–uPA complexes increased cell migration and proliferation in a process that required association with the LDL-R family and was dependent upon uPAR recycling (193).

## Tumor Angiogenesis

Angiogenesis is an important factor for tumor growth and metastasis. It has been proposed that extracellular matrix remodeling is necessary to allow invasion of the newly forming blood vessels, which would explain why uPA and its receptor are elevated in several types of cancers. However, it is the spatial relationship between uPA and PAI-1 that seems to be critical for the tumorigenic response. Immunohistochemical staining and *in situ* hybridization of aortic explants and cocultures of endothelial cells and fibroblasts have shown uPA to be predominantly located in the sprouting endothelium, whereas PAI-1 expression is strong in the population of stromal fibroblasts that are directly in contact with the migrating endothelial cells (195). These findings have also been described in breast carcinomas, where PAI-1 expression is found primarily in fibroblasts, and this expression is associated with an increased incidence of tumor invasion (196,197).

The effects of PAI-1 on tumor growth and angiogenesis in ectopic or transplant tumor models are variable and are sometimes opposed (77,198–206). A potential explanation for these differences is that PAI-1, *in vivo*, normally plays a regulatory role to either enhance or reduce cell migration and/or angiogenesis during wound healing. This system then may also play a role in tumor growth, and the potential importance of this regulation is likely to be very context specific. For example, in transplant tumor models, small differences in the initial conditions of either the tumor or the recipient of the transplant may have very large effects on early events such as the number of transplanted cells that survive or the adhesion and engraftment of the tissue, and it may be these very early events that are largely determining the final outcome of the experiments. Nevertheless, the potential for PAI-1 to regulate angiogenesis has been shown in several nontumor models, where PAI-1 has been found to be a potent regulator of angiogenesis (204). The inhibitory effect of PAI-1 on angiogenesis in this model can be explained by the ability of PAI-1 to inhibit both integrin access to vitronectin and proteinase activity (77).

A dual role for PAI-1 in tumor growth and angiogenesis has been demonstrated by the finding that physiologic levels of PAI-1 promote the growth of M21 human melanoma tumors in nude mice, whereas pharmacologic levels of PAI-1 are inhibitory (204). This pattern of growth is mirrored in the extent of angiogenesis, with the treatment of tumors with low doses of PAI-1 increasing the density of vessel branching, whereas substantially fewer branches are observed upon treatment with higher doses (80,204). This dose-response curve has also been observed in Matrigel implants in mice (204) (see Fig. 19-5) and in an *ex vivo* aortic ring explant assay (205). Therefore, PAI-1 concentrations at or near to the normal physiologic range appear to promote angiogenesis, whereas pharmacologic levels of PAI-1 appear to inhibit angiogenesis. These data yield a classic bell-shaped curve for the effects of PAI-1 on angiogenesis, consistent with its potential role as a regulator of angiogenesis *in vivo*.

### Clinical Implications

As noted previously, high tumor levels of PAI-1 are one of the most informative markers of poor prognosis in several types of cancers (141–146). This would suggest that, despite the various results obtained in different *in vivo* and *in vitro* models of tumor growth and angiogenesis, PAI-1 might be used as a prognostic marker in patients with cancer, as well as a predictive factor for therapy response. Moreover, these results also suggest that therapeutic modulation of PAI-1 levels might be a potential target for anticancer treatment.

---

## Plasminogen Activator Inhibitor-1 in Vascular Disease

In addition to tumor growth and angiogenesis, PAI-1 is also important in vascular disease. In this section, the role of PAI-1 in vascular disease is addressed from four different perspectives: vascular fibrinolysis, vascular wound healing, atherosclerosis, and cardiovascular and cerebrovascular disease.

### Vascular Fibrinolysis

The coagulation cascade is a stepwise activation and amplification of plasma proteinases resulting in the conversion of prothrombin to thrombin, with the generation of the fibrin clot. The coagulation cascade also leads to platelet activation

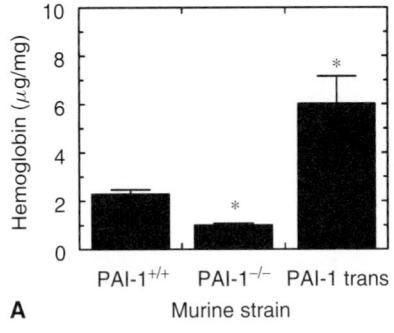
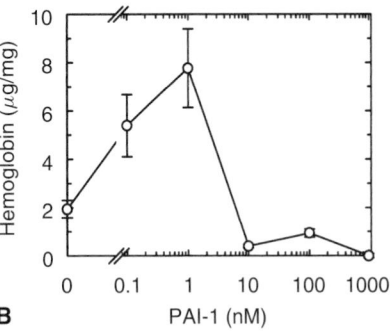

**FIGURE 19-5.** Quantitative analysis of angiogenesis in Matrigel implants. Wild-type, plasminogen activator inhibitor (PAI)-1–deficient or PAI-1–transgenic C57/B6J mice were injected subcutaneously with Matrigel alone or with Matrigel containing fibroblast growth factor (FGF)-2 and heparin at a final concentration of 250 ng per mL of FGF-2 and 0.0025 U per mL of heparin. Wild-type mice were also injected with FGF-2/heparin and with increasing concentrations of PAI-1. After 5 to 7 days, the Matrigel implant was harvested and solubilized in 0.1% Triton X-100 and then centrifuged to remove particulates. The concentration of hemoglobin in the supernatant was then determined directly by measuring the absorbance at 405 nm and by comparing to a standard curve for purified hemoglobin. **A:** Hemoglobin content from implants containing FGF-2 in wild-type, PAI-1–deficient (*, P <0.05), or PAI-1–transgenic mice (*, P <0.05). **B:** Hemoglobin content in implants containing FGF-2 with increasing concentrations of fully active PAI-1. In both panels, n ≥4 for each condition, and the mean ± SE (standard error) are shown. As a control for background, the hemoglobin levels from implants without FGF-2 was subtracted form each sample. (From McMahon GA, Petitclerc E, Stefansson S, et al. Plasminogen activator inhibitor-1 regulates tumor growth and angiogenesis. *J Biol Chem* 2001;276:33964–33968, with permission.)

by a proteinase-activated receptor (207). Activated platelets then release their granular content into the clot, which includes PAI-1 and vitronectin. The dissolution of the fibrin clot is primarily mediated by tPA, which is synthesized and stored within endothelial cells. tPA binds fibrin and is incorporated into the clot along with its substrate plasminogen, which also binds fibrin. PAI-1 released from platelets is also localized within the thrombus, where it is associated with vitronectin (107). In humans most of the PAI-1 in platelets is latent (21,208–210). However, there is enough active PAI-1 in platelets to ensure that the initial fibrin matrix is not prematurely lysed by tPA activation of plasminogen (211). PAI-1 deficiency in humans results in a hyperfibrinolytic state (212), and complete absence of PAI-1 results in posttraumatic bleeding without other manifestations (212–214).

## Vascular Wound Healing and Restenosis

Abnormal expression of the fibrinolytic system may also promote the development of luminal stenosis resulting from arterial neointima formation after vascular injury. As with tumor growth and angiogenesis, studies analyzing the role of PAI-1 in neointima formation and restenosis are variable and are frequently contradictory. A role for PAI-1 in vascular restenosis was first suggested by studies where an electrical injury to the femoral artery was induced in mice genetically deficient in tPA, uPA, or PAI-1 (215,216). These studies demonstrated that in this model, neointima formation was primarily the result of smooth muscle cell migration and proliferation, which, compared to wild-type animals, was enhanced in the PAI-1$^{-/-}$, reduced in uPA$^{-/-}$, and unchanged in tPA$^{-/-}$ mice. These results were similar to those obtained in *in vitro* cell migration assays, showing that PAI-1 can inhibit smooth muscle cell migration by obscuring the cell adhesion site to vitronectin (167,217). However, work by other groups using different vascular injury models has yielded opposite conclusions about the role of PAI-1 in neointima formation. In studies using either copper-induced (218,219) oxidative vascular injury (220,221) or carotid ligation (221), PAI-1 was found to inhibit neointima formation. Consistent with these reports, PAI-1 overexpression by adenovirus transgene transduction was found to increase vascular stenosis after balloon injury in a rat (222).

The binding of PAI-1 to vitronectin has also been shown to alter smooth muscle cell migration in different experimental models (167). Studies with vitronectin$^{-/-}$ mice (221) have shown that vitronectin deficiency results in a smaller neointima formation following vascular injury. Likewise, there is no difference between the smooth muscle cell proliferation in the vitronectin-null mice compared to wild-type mice, suggesting that vitronectin could promote neointima formation by enhancing smooth muscle cell migration. These results raise the possibility that, because vitronectin can bind simultaneously to fibrin and PAI-1, it can also promote the inhibition of fibrinolysis by targeting PAI-1 to the fibrin surface. Therefore, vitronectin may support neointima formation both by stabilizing fibrin in a PAI-1-dependent manner and by enhancing the interaction between the provisional matrix and the smooth muscle cells through integrins.

## Atherosclerosis

Although most patients with generalized arterial atherosclerosis exhibit normal plasma fibrinolytic profiles, the local fibrinolytic balance in these patients may be severely disturbed. Intravascular or mural thrombosis is a frequent histologic feature of atherosclerotic lesions and appears to play a role in the intimal

thickening and fibrosis characteristic of advanced lesions (223). To determine whether localized alterations in fibrinolytic activity could influence this process, PAI-1 mRNA expression was evaluated in segments of severely diseased and relatively normal human arteries obtained from patients undergoing reconstructive surgery for aortic occlusive or aneurysmal disease (224) (see Fig. 19-6). Compared with normal or mildly affected arteries, PAI-1 mRNA levels in severely atherosclerotic vessels that were analyzed by Northern blot were considerably increased. In most cases, the level of PAI-1 gene expression correlated with the degree of atherosclerosis. Analysis by *in situ* hybridization demonstrated an abundance of PAI-1 mRNA-positive cells within the thickened intima of atherosclerotic arteries, mainly around the base of the plaque, and in cells scattered within the necrotic material. In contrast to these results, PAI-1 mRNA was detected primarily within the luminal endothelial cells of normal-appearing aortic tissues (224). These observations have been confirmed and extended (225) in studies showing that both endothelial cells and smooth muscle cells of apparently normal arteries were positive for PAI-1 antigen and mRNA. In advanced atherosclerotic lesions, increased expression of PAI-1 was seen in the smooth muscle cells within the fibrous cap of the necrotic core. In addition, large quantities of PAI-1 were present in the extracellular matrix in close association with elastic lamina and collagen bundles.

PAI-1 has also been found to increase considerably during the progression from normal vessels to fatty streaks to the developed atherosclerotic plaque (226). Staining for PAI-1 is strongly positive, particularly in the areas adjacent to the plaque, whereas tPA shows the opposite trend, being lowest in lesions with plaque (226). Therefore, higher concentrations of PAI-1, together with lower levels of tPA, are characteristic of advanced atheromatous lesions and alterations in the balance of the fibrinolytic system that favor its inhibition appear to be a component of the atherosclerotic process and its common clinical complications.

The role of PAI-1 in the development of atherosclerotic lesions was also studied in mice lacking either apolipoprotein E (apoE$^{-/-}$) or the LDL-R$^{-/-}$. These mice develop atheroscleroticlike lesions when fed a high fat diet. Studies where apoE$^{-/-}$ or LDL-R$^{-/-}$ mice were crossed with either transgenic mice overexpressing PAI-1 or mice deficient in PAI-1 have indicated that, contrary to observations made in human autopsy specimens (226), PAI-1 expression levels have no effect on the progression of the disease in the region of the aortic arch (227). In contrast, a different study, where apoE$^{-/-}$ mice and animals deficient in both apoE and PAI-1 were compared, showed a statistically significant protection from the development of atherosclerosis at the carotid artery bifurcation in mice lacking PAI-1 (228).

## Cardiovascular and Cerebrovascular Disease

A role for PAI-1 in thrombotic events has been studied in animals and humans. PAI-1–transgenic mice develop age-dependent coronary artery thrombosis (229), and PAI-1$^{-/-}$ mice exhibit accelerated clot-lysis time (230). There is a statistically significant increase in the PAI-1 expression in mice as a result of stress (231). The importance of PAI-1 in human vascular disease is suggested by the finding that human plasma concentrations of PAI-1 increase by almost 10-fold at the site of injury when platelets are activated (232). Likewise, a link between increased PAI-1 levels, decreased fibrinolytic activity, and cardiovascular disease has been suggested by several studies (233–235), and, as was discussed earlier, increased PAI-1 levels constitute the link between obesity, insulin resistance, and the resultant increase in the risk of cardiovascular disease (135,236,237).

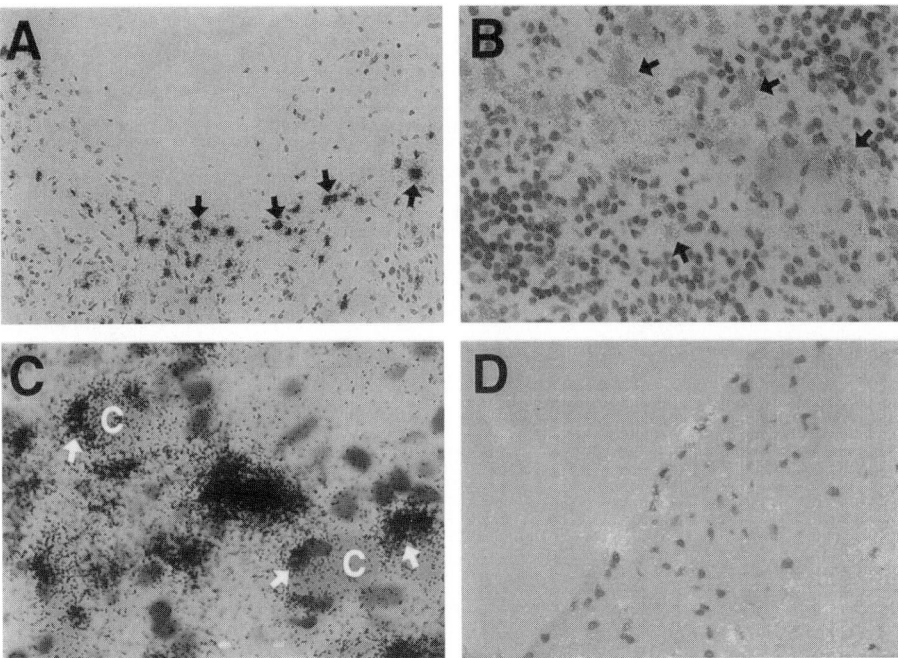

**FIGURE 19-6.** Plasminogen activator inhibitor-1 (PAI-1) gene expression in the abdominal aortic aneurysm wall. Tissue samples were analyzed for the expression of PAI-1 mRNA (messenger ribonucleic acid) by *in situ* hybridization. **A:** Atherosclerotic aneurysm wall. The PAI-1 transcript is expressed in cells (*arrows*) aligned at the base of the necrotic atheroma core, ×200, bright field. **B:** Atherosclerotic aneurysm wall. Macrophagelike cells expressing PAI-l mRNA (*arrows*) within the inflammatory infiltrate, ×400, epiluminescence. **C:** Atherosclerotic aneurysm wall. PAI-l mRNA expression in circumferentially arranged cells (*arrows*), which depict a cross-section of ringlike structures that are assumed to be small caliber capillaries (C) within an inflammatory infiltrate, ×1,000, bright field. **D:** Normal aorta. PAI-1 mRNA signal is detected in luminal endothelium and in a few subintimal cells, ×400, epiluminescence (see Color Fig. 19-6). (From Schneiderman J, Bordin GM, Engelberg I, et al. Expression of fibrinolytic genes in atherosclerotic abdominal aortic aneurysm wall. A possible mechanism for aneurysm expansion. *J Clin Invest* 1995;96:639–645, with permission.)

A number of sequence variations in the promoter region of the *PAI-1* gene have been described. One of them, referred to as the 4G/5G polymorphism, is the guanosine deletion/insertion 675 bp upstream from start of transcription. Although some *in vitro* studies have suggested that the 4G allele is associated with higher PAI-1 activity compared to the 5G allele (238), no association between PAI-1 genotype (4G/5G polymorphism) and arterial or venous thrombosis has been found (239), except in patients with combined protein S deficiency (240). Therefore, there is no reason to include the study of PAI-1 4G/5G polymorphism as part of the diagnostic process in patients with cerebrovascular or cardiovascular disease. Nevertheless, some studies with human subjects have suggested that patients with 4G/5G polymorphism and insulin resistance syndrome or sepsis have an increased risk of myocardial infarction (240) and vascular complications during systemic infections (118).

The role for PAI-1 in cerebral ischemia is less well characterized. In animal models, PAI-1 mRNA substantially increases in the ischemic area early after the onset of cerebral ischemia (241,242), and inactivation of the PAI-1 gene results in a considerable increase in the volume of the ischemic area following middle cerebral artery occlusion (243). However, studies in nonhuman primates have failed to show any link between PAI-1 levels and neuronal death following cerebral ischemia (242). Likewise, as with cardiovascular disease, no link has been demonstrated between 4G/5G polymorphism and increased risk of ischemic stroke (244).

## Obesity

PAI-1 synthesis has been reported in murine adipocyte cell lines (128,245–248), human adipose tissue explants (236,245,249), and primary cultures of human adipocytes (250,251) (see Fig. 19-7). There is a considerable correlation between the amount of visceral fat and plasma levels of PAI-1 in humans (236,252–254) and mice (255,256). Adipose tissue PAI-1 mRNA levels are enhanced in obese individuals (128), and a potential role for PAI-1 in obesity has been suggested by the finding that genetically obese and diabetic (ob/ob) mice crossed into a PAI-1-deficient background had considerably reduced body weight and had improved metabolic profiles compared to lean mice (237). Likewise, nutritionally induced obesity and insulin resistance were dramatically attenuated in wild-type mice lacking PAI-1 (257). The improved adiposity and insulin resistance may be related to the observation that PAI-1-deficient mice fed a high fat diet had increased metabolic rates and total energy expenditure compared to wild-type mice and that peroxisome proliferator-activated receptor γ (PPARγ) and adiponectin were maintained (257). These observations suggest that PAI-1 has a direct role in obesity and insulin resistance.

PAI-1 is dramatically upregulated in obesity, and it is now clear that accelerated atherosclerosis, increased risk for fatal myocardial infarction, hypertension, insulin resistance, and type 2 diabetes also frequently accompany this disorder. The possibility that adipose tissue itself may directly contribute to

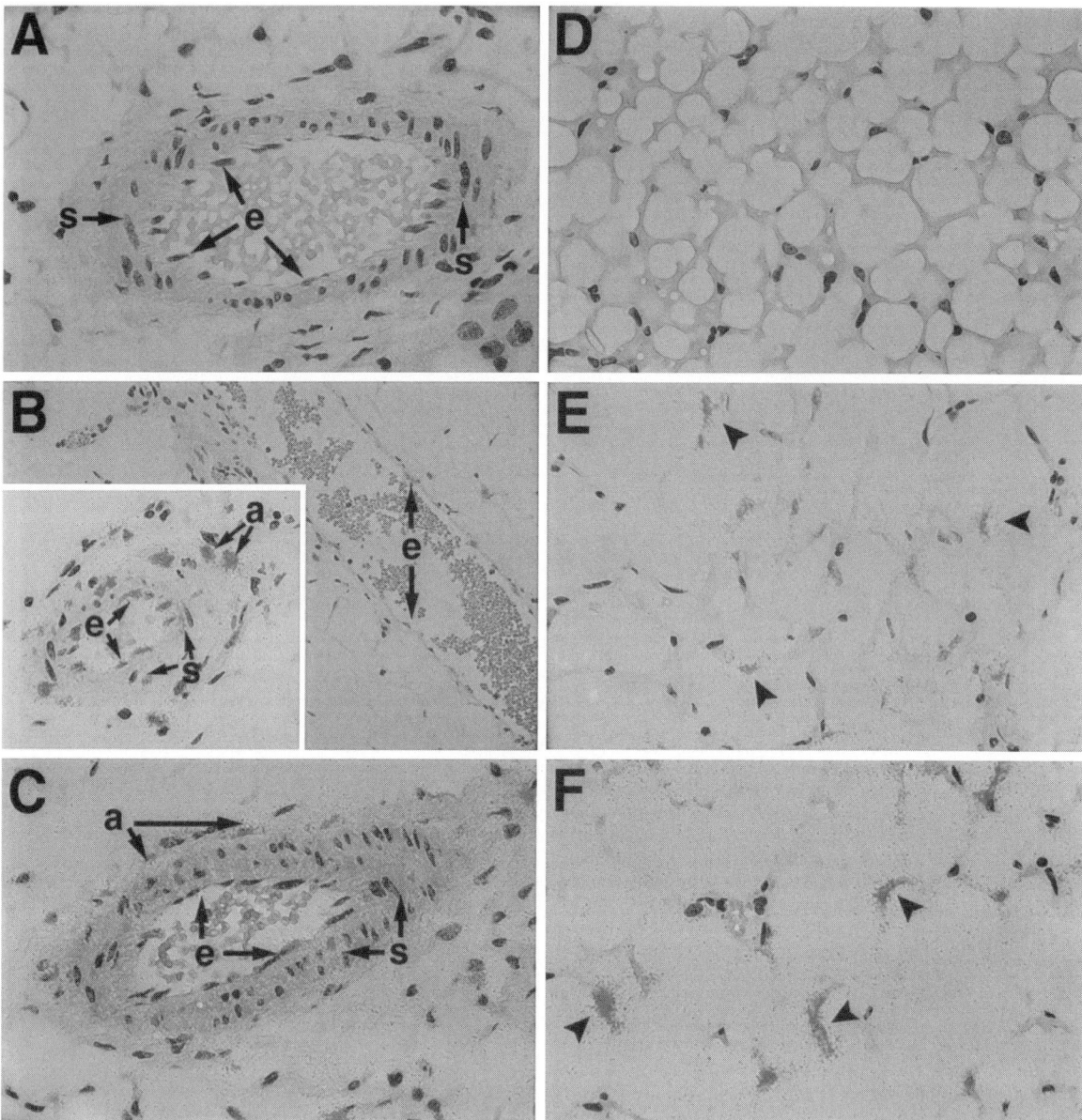

**FIGURE 19-7.** Localization of plasminogen activator inhibitor-1 (PAI-1) messenger ribonucleic acid (mRNA) in the adipose tissue of CB6 mice after lipopolysaccharide (LPS) or tumor necrosis factor (TNF)-α treatment. *In situ* hybridization of paraffin sections showing vasculature from epididymal fat pads of untreated mice (**A**) or from mice treated with LPS (**B**) or with TNF-α (**C**) for 3 hours. *e*, endothelial cells; *a*, adventitial cells; *s*, cells within smooth muscle layers. *In situ* hybridization on sections of epididymal fat pad–containing adipocytes and microvascular endothelial cells from untreated mice (**D**) or from mice treated with LPS (**E**) or TNF-α (**F**) for 3 hours. Some positive cells are indicated by *arrowheads*. Slides were exposed for 8 weeks at 4°C and were stained with hematoxylin and eosin (see Color Fig. 19-7). Original magnification, ×400. (From Samad F, Yamamoto K, Loskutoff DJ. Distribution and regulation of plasminogen activator inhibitor-1 in murine adipose tissue *in vivo*. Induction by tumor necrosis factor-alpha and lipopolysaccharide. *J Clin Invest* 1996;97:37–46, with permission.)

the elevated expression of PAI-1 in obesity has gained considerable attention. Initial clues for such a hypothesis came from the observation that the adipose tissue of mice contains relatively high levels of PAI-1 mRNA (126). Moreover, clinical studies demonstrated that weight loss due to surgical treatment, diet, and so on, considerably reduced plasma PAI-1 levels in obese humans (258). These findings were noteworthy because, in obesity, the size and number of adipocytes and, therefore, the amount of adipose tissue mass typically increase severalfold. Therefore, in obesity, the PAI-1 biosynthetic capacity of adipose tissue may approach or even exceed that of other tissues.

These initial observations have been extended considerably by studies in genetically obese (ob/ob) mice (128,255). Plasma PAI-1 activity is approximately fivefold higher in these mice than in their lean counterparts, and this elevation increases further with age (255). Moreover, studies with genetically obese and diabetic mice (ob/ob) lacking the *PAI-1* gene (PAI-1$^{-/-}$) have demonstrated that elevated PAI-1 is associated with hyperglycemia, hyperinsulinemia, and insulin resistance syndrome (237).

A variety of observations implicate specific hormones or cytokines in the increased expression of PAI-1 by adipose tissue in obesity. For example, the observations that TNF-$\alpha$, TNF-$\beta$, and insulin are elevated in obesity and induce PAI-1 in the plasma and adipose tissue of lean mice (135) certainly suggest the involvement of these mediators in the regulation of PAI-1 in obesity. The observation that inhibiting TNF-$\alpha$ in obese mice considerably decreases plasma PAI-1 antigen and adipose tissue PAI-1 mRNA (259) strongly supports this hypothesis. Triglycerides and free fatty acids also may be involved because they stimulate PAI-1 gene expression in adipocytes. These studies of PAI-1 suggest that these mediators may promote the increased risk for cardiovascular disease in obesity or type 2 diabetes.

## Renal Disease

Although PAI-1 is essentially undetectable in normal kidneys, PAI-1 mRNA and PAI-1 protein levels have been found to be increased in several renal diseases (260–263). A role for PAI-1 has been described in acute renal disorders such as proliferative glomerulonephritis, renal vasculitis, thrombotic microangiopathy, and membranous nephropathy, as well as in chronic progressive renal disease.

**PAI-1 in Acute Renal Disease.** PAI-1 mRNA has been detected in human and animal models of proliferative glomerulonephritis, particularly in those cases associated with fibrin deposition (264). Moreover, it has been observed that inhibition of plasminogen activators results in a considerable worsening in the severity of the glomerular injury. PAI-1 reduces glomerular mesangial turnover by inhibiting plasminogen activators, thereby decreasing plasmin generation and plasmin-mediated matrix degradation. Because fibrin accumulation is an important mediator of acute glomerular injury, strategies designed to enhance fibrinolysis by blocking PAI-1, or to prevent fibrin formation, might be therapeutic in patients with glomerulosclerosis. Although the role of PAI-1 in renal vasculitis is less clear, PAI-1 protein has been identified together with fibrin deposits in renal biopsy specimens from patients with focal necrotizing glomerulonephritis due to systemic lupus erythematosus (265).

In thrombotic microangiopathy, which is a condition that typically involves fibrin deposition in glomerular capillaries and extraglomerular arterioles, PAI-1 plays an active role in the generation of the fibrin thrombi that are formed in response to glomerular endothelial cell injury. PAI-1 deposition has been identified in the kidneys of patients with this disorder (266). Likewise, elevated plasma PAI-1 levels have been associated with disease outcome in several studies of patients with hemolytic uremic syndrome (267). Finally, in membranous nephropathy, PAI-1 transcripts have been found to be abundant (265), and PAI-1 protein colocalizes with vitronectin within the transmembranous deposits (268).

**PAI-1 in Progressive Chronic Renal Disease.** In this disease, there is a pathologic accumulation of extracellular matrix (269,270). PAI-1 mediates several effects that may facilitate matrix accumulation through the impairment of matrix turnover. Likewise, TGF-$\beta$, which is a critical mediator of renal fibrosis, is a powerful inducer of PAI-1 expression (271), and several studies have demonstrated a link between the renin–angiotensin–aldosterone cascade, TGF-$\beta$, and PAI-1 in the pathophysiology of glomerulosclerosis (269). Angiotensin II stimulates PAI-1 production (272), and the renoprotective effects of pharmacologic inhibition of angiotensin II are mediated, at least in part, by a reduction in PAI-1 expression (273). Likewise, recent studies using a rat model of mesangioproliferative nephritis, known as anti–Thy-1 nephritis, demonstrated that treatment with a dominant-negative human mutant PAI-1 that binds to matrix vitronectin but does not inhibit plasminogen activators enhances plasmin generation, increases matrix turnover, and decreases matrix accumulation in experimental glomerulonephritis (274–276).

## Lung Disease

PAI-1 has been identified as a major deleterious mediator in many acute and chronic inflammatory lung disorders. Adult respiratory distress syndrome (ARDS) (277,278), idiopathic pulmonary fibrosis (IPF) (279,280), sarcoidosis (281), hyperoxic lung injury (282), and bronchopulmonary dysplasia (283) are all associated with prominent intraalveolar fibrin deposition and development of pulmonary fibrosis. Fibrin turnover is tightly regulated by the concerted action of proteases and antiproteases, and inhibition of plasmin-mediated proteolysis could account for fibrin accumulation in lung alveoli. The fibrinolytic activity in bronchoalveolar lavage (BAL) supernatant fluids obtained from patients with these diseases has been found to be suppressed (282,283). Moreover, PAI-1 levels in BAL fluids from patients with ARDS and IPF are considerably elevated, and it was shown that this PAI-1 upregulation impairs the fibrinolytic capacity of the fluid (277,278). Bleomycin administration has been used extensively to study the pathogenesis of pulmonary fibrosis in a variety of animal models (284). Bleomycin causes a pneumonitis that progresses to fibrosis in a dose-dependent manner within 2 weeks, while simultaneously suppressing the fibrinolytic activity of BAL fluid in a pattern similar to that seen in human inflammatory lung disease (284). In mice, it was demonstrated that PAI-1 is upregulated after bleomycin administration and that the PAI-1 expression localizes to areas of fibrin-rich fibroproliferative lesions (285).

Transgenic mice that either overexpress PAI-1 or are genetically deficient in PAI-1 have been used to determine whether a cause-and-effect relation exists between PAI-1 expression and the development of pulmonary fibrosis. The results of one study demonstrated a strong relation between PAI-1 gene expression and the degree of pulmonary fibrosis that followed bleomycin administration (286). In another study, it was shown that the lungs of mice exposed to hyperoxia overproduced PAI-1 and that PAI-1 upregulation impaired fibrinolytic activity in the alveolar compartment (282). It was found that mice genetically deficient in PAI-1 did not develop intraalveolar fibrin deposits in response to hyperoxia. These findings suggest that alterations in the fibrinolytic environment during inflammatory injury influence the subsequent development of pulmonary fibrosis and provide evidence for the pathologic contribution of PAI-1 in this event.

In conclusion, there is a strong link between PAI-1 and human disease. Currently, there are several ongoing clinical trials testing the effects of the modification of human PAI-1 in different diseases. Results of these studies will provide new and definitive insight into the role of PAI-1 in the pathologic and physiologic processes.

## References

1. Dano K, Andreasen PA, Grondahl-Hansen J, et al. Plasminogen activators, tissue degradation, and cancer. *Adv Cancer Res* 1985;44:139–266.
2. Vassalli J-D, Sappino A-P, Belin D. The plasminogen activator/plasmin system. *J Clin Invest* 1991;88:1067–1072.
3. Kohler HP, Grant PJ. Plasminogen-activator inhibitor type 1 and coronary artery disease. *N Engl J Med* 2000;342:1792–1801.
4. Saksela O, Rifkin DB. Cell-associated plasminogen activation: regulation and physiological functions. *Annu Rev Cell Biol* 1988;4:93–126.
5. Hoylaerts M, Rijken DC, Lijnen HR, et al. Kinetics of the activation of plasminogen by human tissue plasminogen activator. *J Biol Chem* 1982; 257:2912–2919.
6. Ellis V, Dano K. Plasminogen activation by receptor-bound urokinase. *Semin Thromb Hemost* 1991;17:194–200.
7. Hajjar KA, Hamel NM, Harpel PC, et al. Binding of tissue plasminogen activator to cultured human endothelial cells. *J Clin Invest* 1987;80:1712–1719.
8. Plow EF, Felez J, Miles LA. Cellular regulation of fibrinolysis. *Thromb Haemost* 1991;66:32–36.
9. Lawrence DA, Ginsburg D. Plasminogen activator inhibitors. In: High KA, Roberts HR, eds. *Molecular basis of thrombosis and hemostasis*, New York: Marcel Dekker, 1995:517–543.

10. Loskutoff DJ, van Mourik JA, Erickson LA, et al. Detection of an unusually stable fibrinolytic inhibitor produced by bovine endothelial cells. *Proc Natl Acad Sci U S A* 1983;80:2956–2960.

11. Astedt B, Lecander I, Ny T. The placental type plasminogen activator PAI-2. *Fibrinolysis* 1987;1:203–208.

12. Geiger M. Protein C inhibitor/plasminogen activator inhibitor 3. *Fibrinolysis* 1988;2:183–188.

13. Scott RW, Bergman BL, Bajpai A, et al. Protease nexin. Properties and a modified purification procedure. *J Biol Chem* 1985;260:7029–7034.

14. Osterwalder T, Contartese J, Stoeckli ET, et al. Neuroserpin, an axonally secreted serine protease inhibitor. *EMBO J* 1996;15:2944–2953.

15. Hastings GA, Coleman TA, Haudenschild CC, et al. Neuroserpin, a brain-associated inhibitor of tissue plasminogen activator is localized primarily in neurons. Implications for the regulation of motor learning and neuronal survival. *J Biol Chem* 1997;272:33062–33067.

16. Yepes M, Lawrence DA. Neuroserpin: a selective inhibitor of tissue-type plasminogen activator in the central nervous system. *Thromb Haemost* 2004;91:457–464.

17. Emeis JJ, van Hinsbergh VWM, Verheijen JH, et al. Inhibition of tissue-type plasminogen activator by conditioned medium from cultured human and porcine vascular endothelial cells. *Biochem Biophys Res Commun* 1983;110:392–398.

18. Philips M, Juul AG, Thorsen S. Human endothelial cells produce a plasminogen activator inhibitor and a tissue-type plasminogen activator-inhibitor complex. *Biochim Biophys Acta* 1984;802:99–110.

19. van Mourik JA, Lawrence DA, Loskutoff DJ. Purification of an inhibitor plasminogen activator (antiactivator) synthesized by endothelial cells. *J Biol Chem* 1984;259:14914–14921.

20. Kruithof EKO, Tran-Thang C, Ransijn A, et al. Demonstration of a fast-acting inhibitor of plasminogen activators in human plasma. *Blood* 1984;64:907–913.

21. Erickson LA, Ginsberg MH, Loskutoff DJ. Detection and partial characterization of an inhibitor of plasminogen activator in human platelets. *J Clin Invest* 1984;74:1465–1472.

22. Erickson LA, Hekman CM, Loskutoff DJ. Denaturant-induced stimulation of the beta-migrating plasminogen activator inhibitor in endothelial cells and serum. *Blood* 1986;68:1298–1305.

23. Ny T, Sawdey M, Lawrence D, et al. Cloning and sequence of a cDNA coding for the human beta-migrating endothelial-cell-type plasminogen activator inhibitor. *Proc Natl Acad Sci U S A* 1986;83:6776–6780.

24. Chmielewska J, Rånby M, Wiman B. Evidence for a rapid inhibitor to tissue plasminogen activator in plasma. *Thromb Res* 1983;31:427–436.

25. Kruithof EKO, Ransijn A, Bachmann F. Inhibition of tissue plasminogen activator by human plasma. In: Davidson JF, Bachmann F, Bouvier CA, et al, eds. *Progress in Fibrinolysis Volume VI*, Edinburgh: Churchill Livingstone, 1983:365–369.

26. Gettins PGW, Patston PA, Olson ST. *Serpins: structure, function and biology*. Austin, Texas: R.G. Landes Company, 1996.

27. Doolittle RF. Angiotensinogen is related to the antitrypsin-antithrombin-ovalbumin family. *Science* 1983;222:417–419.

28. Irving JA, Pike RN, Lesk AM, et al. Phylogeny of the serpin superfamily: implications of patterns of amino acid conservation for structure and function. *Genome Res* 2000;10:1845–1864.

29. Irving JA, Steenbakkers PJ, Lesk AM, et al. Serpins in prokaryotes. *Mol Biol Evol* 2002;19:1881–1890.

30. Cohen AB, Gruenke LD, Craig JC, et al. Specific lysine labeling by [18]OH- during alkaline cleavage of the α-1-antitrypsin-trypsin complex. *Proc Natl Acad Sci U S A* 1977;74:4311–4314.

31. Wiman B, Collen D. On the mechanism of the reaction between human alpha 2-antiplasmin and plasmin. *J Biol Chem* 1979;254:9291–9297.

32. Levin EG. Latent tissue plasminogen activator produced by human endothelial cells in culture: evidence for an enzyme-inhibitor complex. *Proc Natl Acad Sci U S A* 1983;80:6804–6808.

33. Lawrence DA, Ginsburg D, Day DE, et al. Serpin-protease complexes are trapped as stable acyl-enzyme intermediates. *J Biol Chem* 1995;270:25309–25312.

34. Huber R, Carrell RW. Implications of the three-dimensional structure of alpha 1-antitrypsin for structure and function of serpins. *Biochem* 1989;28:8951–8966.

35. Shubeita HE, Cottey TL, Franke AE, et al. Mutational and immunochemical analysis of plasminogen activator inhibitor 1. *J Biol Chem* 1990;265:18379–18385.

36. York JD, Li P, Gardell SJ. Combinatorial mutagenesis of the reactive site region in plasminogen activator inhibitor I. *J Biol Chem* 1991;266:8495–8500.

37. Sherman PM, Lawrence DA, Yang AY, et al. Saturation mutagenesis of the plasminogen activator inhibitor-1 reactive center. *J Biol Chem* 1992;267:7588–7595.

38. Schechter I, Berger A. On the size of the active site in proteases. I. Papain. *Biochem Biophys Res Commun* 1967;27:157–162.

39. Wilczynska M, Fa M, Ohlsson PI, et al. The inhibition mechanism of serpins: evidence that the mobile reactive center loop is cleaved in the native protease-inhibitor complex. *J Biol Chem* 1995;270:29652–29655.

40. Lawrence DA, Olson ST, Muhammad S, et al. Partitioning of serpin-proteinase reactions between stable inhibition and substrate cleavage is regulated by the rate of serpin reactive center loop insertion into beta-sheet A. *J Biol Chem* 2000;275:5839–5844.

41. Hagglof P, Bergstrom F, Wilczynska M, et al. The reactive-center loop of active PAI-1 is folded close to the protein core and can be partially inserted. *J Mol Biol* 2004;335:823–832.

42. Lawrence DA, Strandberg L, Ericson J, et al. Structure-function studies of the SERPIN plasminogen activator inhibitor type 1: analysis of chimeric strained loop mutants. *J Biol Chem* 1990;265:20293–20301.

43. Huntington JA, Read RJ, Carrell RW. Structure of a serpin-protease complex shows inhibition by deformation. *Nature* 2000;407:923–926.

44. Huntington JA, Carrell RW. The serpins: nature's molecular mousetraps. *Sci Prog* 2001;84:125–136.

45. Andreasen PA, Riccio A, Welinder KG, et al. Plasminogen activator inhibitor type-1: reactive center and amino-terminal heterogeneity determined by protein and cDNA sequencing. *FEBS Lett* 1986;209:213–218.

46. Pannekoek H, Veerman H, Lambers H, et al. Endothelial plasminogen activator inhibitor (PAI): a new member of the Serpin gene family. *EMBO J* 1986;5:2539–2544.

47. Ginsburg D, Zeheb R, Yang AY, et al. cDNA cloning of human plasminogen activator-inhibitor from endothelial cells. *J Clin Invest* 1986;78:1673–1680.

48. Lawrence D, Strandberg L, Grundström T, et al. Purification of active human plasminogen activator inhibitor 1 from *Escherichia coli*. Comparison with natural and recombinant forms purified from eucaryotic cells. *Eur J Biochem* 1989;186:523–533.

49. Franke AE, Danley DE, Kaczmarek FS, et al. Expression of human plasminogen activator inhibitor type-1 (PAI-1) in Escherichia coli as a soluble protein comprised of active and latent forms. Isolation and crystallization of latent PAI-1. *Biochim Biophys Acta* 1990;1037:16–23.

50. Reilly TM, Seetharam R, Duke JL, et al. Purification and characterization of recombinant plasminogen activator inhibitor-1 from Escherichia coli. *J Biol Chem* 1990;265:9570–9574.

51. Keijer J, Ehrlich HJ, Linders M, et al. Vitronectin governs the interaction between plasminogen activator inhibitor 1 and tissue-type plasminogen activator. *J Biol Chem* 1991;266:10700–10707.

52. Seetharam R, Dwivedi AM, Duke JL, et al. Purification and characterization of active and latent forms of recombinant plasminogen activator inhibitor 1 produced in Escherichia coli. *Biochem* 1992;31:9877–9882.

53. Sherman PM, Lawrence DA, Verhamme IM, et al. Identification of tPA-specific plasminogen activator inhibitor-1 mutants: evidence that second sites of interaction contribute to target specificity. *J Biol Chem* 1995;270:9301–9306.

54. Stefansson S, Yepes M, Gorlatova N, et al. Mutants of plasminogen activator inhibitor-1 designed to inhibit neutrophil elastase and cathepsin G are more effective *in vivo* than their endogenous inhibitors. *J Biol Chem* 2004;279:29981–29987.

55. Kvassman JO, Verhamme I, Shore JD. Inhibitory mechanism of serpins: loop insertion forces acylation of plasminogen activator by plasminogen activator inhibitor-1. *Biochem* 1998;37:15491–15502.

56. Olson ST, Swanson R, Day D, et al. Resolution of Michaelis complex, acylation, and conformational change steps in the reactions of the serpin, plasminogen activator inhibitor- 1, with tissue plasminogen activator and trypsin. *Biochem* 2001;40:11742–11756.

57. Ibarra CA, Blouse GE, Christian TD, et al. The contribution of the exosite residues of plasminogen activator inhibitor-1 to proteinase inhibition. *J Biol Chem* 2004;279:3643–3650.

58. Hekman CM, Loskutoff DJ. Endothelial cells produce a latent inhibitor of plasminogen activators that can be activated by denaturants. *J Biol Chem* 1985;260:11581–11587.

59. Levin EG, Santell L. Conversion of the active to latent plasminogen activator inhibitor from human endothelial cells. *Blood* 1987;70:1090–1098.

60. Mottonen J, Strand A, Symersky J, et al. Structural basis of latency in plasminogen activator inhibitor-1. *Nature* 1992;355:270–273.

61. Sharp AM, Stein PE, Pannu NS, et al. The active conformation of plasminogen activator inhibitor 1, a target for drugs to control fibrinolysis and cell adhesion. *Structure Fold Des* 1999;7:111–118.

62. Lawrence DA, Olson ST, Palaniappan S, et al. Engineering plasminogen activator inhibitor-1 (PAI-1) mutants with increased functional stability. *Biochem* 1994;33:3643–3648.

63. Lawrence DA, Olson ST, Palaniappan S, et al. Serpin reactive-center loop mobility is required for inhibitor function but not for enzyme recognition. *J Biol Chem* 1994;269:27657–27662.

64. Hekman CM, Loskutoff DJ. Bovine plasminogen activator inhibitor 1: specificity determinations and comparison of the active, latent, and guanidine-activated forms. *Biochem* 1988;27:2911–2918.

65. Lindahl TL, Sigurdardóttir O, Wiman B. Stability of plasminogen activator inhibitor 1 (PAI-1). *Thromb Haemost* 1989;62:748–751.

66. Lambers JW, Cammenga M, Konig BW, et al. Activation of human endothelial cell-type plasminogen activator inhibitor (PAI-1) by negatively charged phospholipids. *J Biol Chem* 1987;262:17492–17496.

67. Wun T-C, Palmier MO, Siegel NR, et al. Affinity purification of active plasminogen activator inhibitor- 1 (PAI-1) using immobilized anhydrourokinase. *J Biol Chem* 1989;264:7862–7868.

68. Lawrence DA, Loskutoff DJ. Inactivation of plasminogen activator inhibitor by oxidants. *Biochem* 1986;25:6351–6355.

69. Strandberg L, Lawrence DA, Johansson LB-A, et al. The oxidative inactivation of plasminogen activator inhibitor type 1 results from a conformational change in the molecule and does not require the involvement of the P1′ methionine. *J Biol Chem* 1991;266:13852–13858.

70. Weiss SJ, Regiani S. Neutrophils degrade subendothelial matrices in the presence of alpha-1-proteinase inhibitor. Cooperative use of lysosomal proteinases and oxygen metabolites. *J Clin Invest* 1984;73: 1297–1303.

71. Declerck PJ, De Mol M, Vaughan DE, et al. Identification of a conformationally distinct form of plasminogen activator inhibitor-1, acting as a noninhibitory substrate for tissue-type plasminogen activator. *J Biol Chem* 1992;267:11693–11696.

72. Urano T, Strandberg L, Johansson LB, et al. A substrate-like form of plasminogen-activator-inhibitor type 1—conversions between different forms by sodium dodecyl sulphate. *Eur J Biochem* 1992;209:985–992.

73. Wu K, Urano T, Ihara H, et al. The cleavage and inactivation of plasminogen activator inhibitor type 1 by neutrophil elastase: the evaluation of its physiologic relevance in fibrinolysis. *Blood* 1995;86:1056–1061.

74. Lawrence DA. The serpin-proteinase complex revealed. *Nat Struct Biol* 1997;4:339–341.

75. Wilczynska M, Fa M, Karolin J, et al. New structural insights into native serpin-protease complexes reveal the inhibitory mechanism of serpins. *Nat Struct Biol* 1997;4:354–357.

76. Sprengers ED, Kluft C. Plasminogen activator inhibitors. *Blood* 1987;69: 381–387.

77. Stefansson S, Petitclerc E, Wong MK, et al. Inhibition of Angiogenesis *in vivo* by Plasminogen activator inhibitor-1. *J Biol Chem* 2001;276:8135–8141.

78. Booth NA. Fibrinolysis and thrombosis. *Baillieres Best Pract Res Clin Haematol* 1999;12:423–433.

79. Huber K. Plasminogen activator inhibitor type-1 (part one): basic mechanisms, regulation, and role for thromboembolic disease. *J Thromb Thrombolysis* 2001;11:183–193.

80. Stefansson S, McMahon GA, Petitclerc E, et al. Plasminogen activator inhibitor-1 in tumor growth, angiogenesis and vascular remodeling. *Curr Pharma Design* 2003;9:1545–1564.

81. Lawrence DA, Berkenpas MB, Palaniappan S, et al. Localization of vitronectin binding domain in plasminogen activator inhibitor-1. *J Biol Chem* 1994;269:15223–15228.

82. Xu Z, Balsara RD, Gorlatova NV, et al. Conservation of critical functional domains in murine plasminogen activator inhibitor-1. *J Biol Chem* 2004; 279:17914–17920.

83. Jensen JK, Wind T, Andreasen PA. The vitronectin binding area of plasminogen activator inhibitor-1, mapped by mutagenesis and protection against an inactivating organochemical ligand. *FEBS Lett* 2002;521:91–94.

84. Zhou A, Huntington JA, Pannu NS, et al. How vitronectin binds PAI-1 to modulate fibrinolysis and cell migration. *Nat Struct Biol* 2003;10:541–544.

85. Stefansson S, Muhammad S, Cheng XF, et al. Plasminogen activator inhibitor-1 contains a cryptic high affinity binding site for the low density lipoprotein receptor-related protein. *J Biol Chem* 1998;273:6358–6366.

86. Horn IR, van den Berg BM, Moestrup SK, et al. Plasminogen activator inhibitor 1 contains a cryptic high affinity receptor binding site that is exposed upon complex formation with tissue-type plasminogen activator. *Thromb Haemost* 1998;80:822–828.

87. Tomasini BR, Mosher DF. Vitronectin. *Prog Hemost Thromb* 1991;10: 269–305.

88. Seiffert D. Constitutive and regulated expression of vitronectin. *Histol Histopathol* 1997;12:787–797.

89. Podor TJ, Campbell S, Chindemi P, et al. Incorporation of vitronectin into fibrin clots. Evidence for a binding interaction between vitronectin and gamma A/gamma' fibrinogen. *J Biol Chem* 2002;277:7520–7528.

90. Seiffert D, Smith JW. The cell adhesion domain in plasma vitronectin is cryptic. *J Biol Chem* 1997;272:13705–13710.

91. Keijer J, Linders M, Wegman JJ, et al. On the target specificity of plasminogen activator inhibitor 1: the role of heparin, vitronectin, and the reactive site. *Blood* 1991;78:1254–1261.

92. Naski MC, Lawrence DA, Mosher DF, et al. Kinetics of inactivation of α-thrombin by plasminogen activator inhibitor-1: comparison of the effects of native and urea-treated forms of vitronectin. *J Biol Chem* 1993; 268:12367–12372.

93. Lawrence DA, Palaniappan S, Stefansson S, et al. Characterization of the binding of different conformational forms of plasminogen activator inhibitor-1 to vitronectin: implications for the regulation of pericellular proteolysis. *J Biol Chem* 1997;272:7676–7680.

94. Grondahl-Hansen J, Lund LR, Ralfkiær E, et al. Urokinase-tissue-type plasminogen activators in keratinocytes during wound reepithelialization. *J Invest Dermatol* 1988;90:790–795.

95. Yebra M, Parry GCN, Stromblad S, et al. Requirement of receptor-bound urokinase-type plasminogen activator for integrin $\alpha_v \beta_5$-directed cell migration. *J Biol Chem* 1996;271:29393–29399.

96. Carriero MV, Del Vecchio S, Capozzoli M, et al. Urokinase receptor interacts with alpha(v)beta5 vitronectin receptor, promoting urokinase-dependent cell migration in breast cancer. *Cancer Res* 1999;59:5307–5314.

97. Tarui T, Mazar AP, Cines DB, et al. Urokinase-type plasminogen activator receptor (cd87) is a ligand for integrins and mediates cell-cell interaction. *J Biol Chem* 2001;276:3983–3990.

98. Chapman HA, Wei Y. Protease crosstalk with integrins: the urokinase receptor paradigm. *Thromb Haemost* 2001;86:124–129.

99. Lindahl T, Wiman B. Purification of high and low molecular weight plasminogen activator inhibitor 1 from fibrosarcoma cell-line HT 1080 conditioned medium. *Biochim Biophys Acta* 1989;994:253–257.

100. Ehrlich HJ, Keijer J, Preissner KT, et al. Functional interaction of plasminogen activator inhibitor type 1 (PAI-1) and heparin. *Biochem* 1991;30: 1021–1028.

101. Ehrlich HJ, Gebbink RK, Keijer J, et al. Elucidation of structural requirements on plasminogen activator inhibitor 1 for binding to heparin. *J Biol Chem* 1992;267:11606–11611.

102. Braaten JV, Handt S, Jerome WG, et al. Regulation of fibrinolysis by platelet-released plasminogen activator inhibitor 1: light scattering and ultrastructural examination of lysis of a model platelet-fibrin thrombus. *Blood* 1993;81:1290–1299.

103. Wagner OF, de Vries C, Hohmann C, et al. Interaction between plasminogen activator inhibitor type 1 (PAI- 1) bound to fibrin and either tissue-type plasminogen activator (t-PA) or urokinase-type plasminogen activator (u-PA). *J Clin Invest* 1989;84:647–655.

104. Keijer J, Linders M, van Zonneveld A-J, et al. The interaction of plasminogen activator inhibitor 1 with plasminogen activators (tissue-type and urokinase-type) and fibrin: localization of interaction sites and physiologic relevance. *Blood* 1991;78:401–409.

105. Reilly CF, Hutzelmann JE. Plasminogen activator inhibitor-1 binds to fibrin and inhibits tissue-type plasminogen activator-mediated fibrin dissolution. *J Biol Chem* 1992;267:17128–17135.

106. Podor TJ, Shaughnessy SG, Blackburn MN, et al. New insights into the size and stoichiometry of the plasminogen activator inhibitor type-1. vitronectin complex. *J Biol Chem* 2000;275:25402–25410.

107. Podor TJ, Peterson CB, Lawrence DA, et al. Type 1 plasminogen activator inhibitor binds to fibrin via vitronectin. *J Biol Chem* 2000;275: 19788–19794.

108. Klinger KW, Winqvist R, Riccio A, et al. Plasminogen activator inhibitor type 1 gene is located at region q21.3-q22 of chromosome 7 and genetically linked with cystic fibrosis. *Proc Natl Acad Sci U S A* 1987;84: 8548–8552.

109. Loskutoff DJ, Linders M, Keijer J, et al. Structure of the human plasminogen activator inhibitor 1 gene: nonrandom distribution of introns. *Biochem* 1987;26:3763–3768.

110. Strandberg L, Lawrence D, Ny T. The organization of the human plasminogen-activator-inhibitor 1 gene. *Eur J Biochem* 1988;176:609–616.

111. Follo M, Ginsburg D. Structure and expression of the human gene encoding plasminogen activator inhibitor, PAI-1. *Gene* 1989;84:447–453.

112. Bosma PJ, van den Berg EA, Kooistra T, et al. Human plasminogen activator inhibitor-1 gene: promoter and structural gene nucleotide sequences. *J Biol Chem* 1988;263:9129–9141.

113. McGrogan M, Kennedy J, Golini F. Structure of the human protease nexin gene and expression of recombinant forms of PN-1. In: Festoff BW, ed. *Serine proteases and their serpin inhibitors in the nervous system.* New York: Plenum Press, 1990:147–161.

114. Bosma PJ, Kooistra T, Siemieniak DR, et al. Further characterization of the 5′-flanking DNA of the gene encoding human plasminogen activator inhibitor-1. *Gene* 1991;100:261–266.

115. Berger P, Kozlov SV, Krueger SR, et al. Structure of the mouse gene for the serine protease inhibitor neuroserpin (PI12). *Gene* 1998;214:25–33.

116. van Zonneveld A-J, Curriden SA, Loskutoff DJ. Type 1 plasminogen activator inhibitor gene: functional analysis and glucocorticoid regulation of its promoter. *Proc Natl Acad Sci U S A* 1988;85:5525–5529.

117. Riccio A, Lund LR, Sartorio R, et al. The regulatory region of the human plasminogen activator inhibitor type-1 (PAI-1) gene. *Nucleic Acids Res* 1988;16:2805–2824.

118. Dawson SJ, Wiman B, Hamsten A, et al. The two allele sequences of a common polymorphism in the promoter of the plasminogen activator inhibitor-1 (PAI-1) gene respond differently to interleukin-1 in HepG2 cells. *J Biol Chem* 1993;268:10739–10745.

119. Dawson SJ, Hamsten A, Wiman B, et al. Genetic variation at the plasminogen activator inhibitor-1 locus is associated with altered levels of plasma plasminogen activator inhibitor-1 activity. *Arterioscler Thromb* 1991;11:183–190.

120. van den Berg EA, Sprengers ED, Jaye M, et al. Regulation of plasminogen activator inhibitor-1 mRNA in human endothelial cells. *Thromb Haemost* 1988;60:63–67.

121. Konkle BA, Ginsburg D. The addition of endothelial cell growth factor and heparin to human umbilical vein endothelial cell cultures decreases plasminogen activator inhibitor-1 expression. *J Clin Invest* 1988;82:579–585.

122. Irigoyen JP, Munoz-Canoves P, Montero L, et al. The plasminogen activator system: biology and regulation. *Cell Mol Life Sci* 1999;56:104–132.

123. Heaton JH, Dlakic WM, Gelehrter TD. Posttranscriptional regulation of PAI-1 gene expression. *Thromb Haemost* 2003;89:959–966.

124. Kruithof EKO, Gudinchet A, Bachmann F. Plasminogen activator inhibitor 1 and plasminogen activator inhibitor 2 in various disease states. *Thromb Haemost* 1988;59:7–12.

125. Colucci M, Paramo JA, Collen D. Generation in plasma of a fast-acting inhibitor of plasminogen activator in response to endotoxin stimulation. *J Clin Invest* 1985;75:818–824.

126. Sawdey MS, Loskutoff DJ. Regulation of murine type 1 plasminogen activator inhibitor gene expression *in vivo*. Tissue specificity and induction by lipopolysaccharide, tumor necrosis factor-α, and transforming growth factor-β. *J Clin Invest* 1991;88:1346–1353.

127. Fearns C, Loskutoff DJ. Induction of plasminogen activator inhibitor 1 gene expression in murine liver by lipopolysaccharide. Cellular localization and

role of endogenous tumor necrosis factor-alpha. *Am J Pathol* 1997;150: 579–590.

128. Samad F, Yamamoto K, Loskutoff DJ. Distribution and regulation of plasminogen activator inhibitor-1 in murine adipose tissue *in vivo*. Induction by tumor necrosis factor-alpha and lipopolysaccharide. *J Clin Invest* 1996;97:37–46.

129. Sawdey M, Podor TJ, Loskutoff DJ. Regulation of type 1 plasminogen activator inhibitor gene expression in cultured bovine aortic endothelial cells. *J Biol Chem* 1989;264:10396–10401.

130. Loskutoff DJ. Regulation of PAI-1 gene expression. *Fibrinolysis* 1991; 5:197–206.

131. Fattal PG, Schneider DJ, Sobel BE, et al. Post-transcriptional regulation of expression of plasminogen activator inhibitor type 1 on mRNA by insulin and insulin-like growth factor 1. *J Biol Chem* 1992;267:12412–12415.

132. Konkle BA, Schuster SJ, Kelly MD, et al. Plasminogen activator inhibitor-1 messenger RNA expression is induced in rat hepatocytes *in vivo* by dexamethasone. *Blood* 1992;79:2636–2642.

133. Loskutoff DJ, Sawdey M, Keeton M, et al. Regulation of PAI-1 gene expression *in vivo*. *Thromb Haemost* 1993;70:135–137.

134. Simpson AJ, Booth NA, Moore NR, et al. Distribution of plasminogen activator inhibitor (PAI-1) in tissues. *J Clin Pathol* 1991;44:139–143.

135. Loskutoff DJ, Samad F. The adipocyte and hemostatic balance in obesity: studies of PAI-1. *Arterioscler Thromb Vasc Biol* 1998;18:1–6.

136. Lawrence DA, Ginsburg D. Gene expression and function of plasminogen activator inhibitor-1. In: Glas-Greenwalt P, ed. *Fibrinolysis in disease: molecular and Hhemovascular aspects of fibrinolysis*, Boca Raton: CRC Press, 1995;21–29.

137. Mutch NJ, Wilson HM, Booth NA. Plasminogen activator inhibitor-1 and haemostasis in obesity. *Proc Nutr Soc* 2001;60:341–347.

138. Unkeless J, Dano K, Kellerman GM, et al. Fibrinolysis associated with oncogenic transformation. Partial purification and characterization of the cell factor, a plasminogen activator. *J Biol Chem* 1974;249:4295–4305.

139. Astrup T. Cell-induced fibrinolysis: a fundamental process. In: Reich E, Rifkin DB, Shaw E, eds. *Proteases and Biological Control*, Cold Spring Harbor: Cold Spring Harbor Laboratory, 1975:343–355.

140. Duffy MJ. Plasminogen activators and cancer. *Blood Coagul Fibrinolysis* 1990;1:681–687.

141. Schmitt M, Wilhelm O, Janicke F, et al. Urokinase-type plasminogen activator (uPA) and its receptor (CD87): a new target in tumor invasion and metastasis. *J Obstet Gynaecol* 1995;21:151–165.

142. Hofmann R, Lehmer A, Buresch M, et al. Clinical relevance of urokinase plasminogen activator, its receptor, and its inhibitor in patients with renal cell carcinoma. *Cancer* 1996;78:487–492.

143. Quax PH, van Muijen GN, Weening-Verhoeff EJ, et al. Metastatic behavior of human melanoma cell lines in nude mice correlates with urokinase-type plasminogen activator, its type 1 inhibitor, and urokinase-mediated matrix degradation. *J Cell Biol* 1991;115:191–199.

144. Sier CF, Vloedgraven HJ, Ganesh S, et al. Inactive urokinase and increased levels of its inhibitor type 1 in colorectal cancer liver metastasis. *Gastroenterology* 1994;107:1449–1456.

145. Pedersen H, Brunner N, Francis D, et al. Prognostic impact of urokinase, urokinase receptor, and type 1 plasminogen activator inhibitor in squamous and large cell lung cancer tissue. *Cancer Res* 1994;54:4671–4675.

146. Nekarda H, Siewert JR, Schmitt M, et al. Tumour-associated proteolytic factors uPA and PAI-1 and survival in totally resected gastric cancer. *Lancet* 1994;343:117.

147. Pyke C, Kristensen P, Ralfkiaer E, et al. The plasminogen activation system in human colon cancer: messenger RNA for the inhibitor PAI-1 is located in endothelial cells in the tumor stroma. *Cancer Res* 1991;51: 4067–4071.

148. Pyke C, Kristensen P, Ralfkiaer E, et al. Urokinase-type plasminogen activator is expressed in stromal cells and its receptor in cancer cells at invasive foci in human colon adenocarcinomas. *Am J Pathol* 1991;138:1059–1067.

149. Kristensen P, Pyke C, Lund LR, et al. Plasminogen activator inhibitor-type 1 in Lewis lung carcinoma. *Histochemistry* 1990;93:559–566.

150. Rabbani SA, Xing RH. Role of urokinase (uPA) and its receptor (uPAR) in invasion and metastasis of hormone-dependent malignancies. *Int J Oncol* 1998;12:911–920.

151. Konno H, Baba M, Shoji T, et al. Cyclooxygenase-2 expression correlates with uPAR levels and is responsible for poor prognosis of colorectal cancer. *Clin Exp Metastasis* 2002;19:527–534.

152. Pepper MS, Montesano R. Proteolytic balance and capillary morphogenesis. *Cell Differ Dev* 1990;32:319–327.

153. Romer J, Lund LR, Eriksen J, et al. Differential expression of urokinase-type plasminogen activator and its type-1 inhibitor during healing of mouse skin wounds. *J Invest Dermatol* 1991;97:803–811.

154. Lang IM, Moser KM, Schleef RR. Elevated expression of urokinase-like plasminogen activator and plasminogen activator inhibitor type 1 during the vascular remodeling associated with pulmonary thromboembolism. *Arterioscler Thromb Vasc Biol* 1998;18:808–815.

155. Erickson CA, Isseroff RR. Plasminogen activator activity is associated with neural crest cell motility in tissue culture. *J Exp Zool* 1989;251: 123–133.

156. Kirchheimer JC, Remold HG. Endogenous receptor-bound urokinase mediates tissue invasion of human monocytes. *J Immunol* 1989;143: 2634–2639.

157. Wilson EL, Jacobs P, Dowdle EB. The secretion of plasminogen activators by human myeloid leukemic cells *in vitro*. *Blood* 1983;61:568–574.

158. Levin EG, Fair DS, Loskutoff DJ. Human hepatoma cell line plasminogen activator. *J Lab Clin Med* 1983;102:500–508.

159. Hsu DW, Efird JT, Hedley-Whyte ET. Prognostic role of urokinase-type plasminogen activator in human gliomas. *Am J Pathol* 1995;147:114–123.

160. Ossowski L. Invasion of connective tissue by human carcinoma cell lines: requirement for urokinase, urokinase receptor, and interstitial collagenase. *Cancer Res* 1992;52:6754–6760.

161. Coen D, Bottazzi B, Bini A, et al. Plasminogen activator activity of metastatic variants from a murine fibrosarcoma: effect of thrombin *in vitro*. *Int J Cancer* 1983;32:67–70.

162. Yu HR, Schultz RM. Relationship between secreted urokinase plasminogen activator activity and metastatic potential in murine B16 cells transfected with human urokinase sense and antisense genes. *Cancer Res* 1990;50:7623–7633.

163. Hearing VJ, Law LW, Corti A, et al. Modulation of metastatic potential by cell surface urokinase of murine melanoma cells. *Cancer Res* 1988;48: 1270–1278.

164. Ossowski L. Plasminogen activator dependent pathways in the dissemination of human tumor cells in the chick embryo. *Cell* 1988;52:321–328.

165. Mignatti P, Robbins E, Rifkin DB. Tumor invasion through the human amniotic membrane: requirement for a proteinase cascade. *Cell* 1986;47: 487–498.

166. Stefansson S, Lawrence DA. Old dogs and new tricks, proteases, inhibitors, and cell migration. *Sci STKE* 2003;189;pe24.

167. Stefansson S, Lawrence DA. The serpin PAI-1 inhibits cell migration by blocking integrin $\alpha_v \beta_3$ binding to vitronectin. *Nature* 1996;383:441–443.

168. Kjoller L, Kanse SM, Kirkegaard T, et al. Plasminogen activator inhibitor-1 represses integrin- and vitronectin-mediated cell migration independently of its function as an inhibitor of plasminogen activation. *Exp Cell Res* 1997;232:420–429.

169. Giannelli G, Falk-Marzillier J, Schiraldi O, et al. Induction of cell migration by matrix metalloprotease-2 cleavage of laminin-5. *Science* 1997;277: 225–228.

170. Xu J, Rodriguez D, Petitclerc E, et al. Proteolytic exposure of a cryptic site within collagen type IV is required for angiogenesis and tumor growth *in vivo*. *J Cell Biol* 2001;154:1069–1079.

171. Hangai M, Kitaya N, Xu J, et al. Matrix metalloproteinase-9-dependent exposure of a cryptic migratory control site in collagen is required before retinal angiogenesis. *Am J Pathol* 2002;161:1429–1437.

172. Sato Y, Tsuboi R, Lyons R, et al. Characterization of the activation of latent TGF-beta by co-cultures of endothelial cells and pericytes or smooth muscle cells: a self-regulating system. *J Cell Biol* 1990;111:757–763.

173. Lyons RM, Gentry LE, Purchio AF, et al. Mechanism of activation of latent recombinant transforming growth factor beta 1 by plasmin. *J Cell Biol* 1990;110:1361–1367.

174. Saksela O, Rifkin DB. Release of basic fibroblast growth factor-heparan sulfate complexes from endothelial cells by plasminogen activator-mediated proteolytic activity. *J Cell Biol* 1990;110:767–775.

175. Ribatti D, Leali D, Vacca A, et al. *In vivo* angiogenic activity of urokinase: role of endogenous fibroblast growth factor-2. *J Cell Sci* 1999;112(Pt 23):4213–4221.

176. Houck KA, Leung DW, Rowland AM, et al. Dual regulation of vascular endothelial growth factor bioavailability by genetic and proteolytic mechanisms. *J Biol Chem* 1992;267:26031–26037.

177. Matsuno H, Kozawa O, Yoshimi N, et al. Lack of alpha2-antiplasmin promotes pulmonary heart failure via overrelease of VEGF after acute myocardial infarction. *Blood* 2002;100:2487–2493.

178. Pöllänen J, Hedman K, Nielsen LS, et al. Ultrastructural localization of plasma membrane-associated urokinase-type plasminogen activator at focal contacts. *J Cell Biol* 1988;106:87–95.

179. Hebert CA, Baker JB. Linkage of extracellular plasminogen activator to the fibroblast cytoskeleton: colocalization of cell surface urokinase with vinculin. *J Cell Biol* 1988;106:1241–1247.

180. Bastholm L, Nielsen MH, De Mey J, et al. Confocal fluorescence microscopy of urokinase plasminogen activator receptor and cathepsin D in human MDA-MB-231 breast cancer cells migrating in reconstituted basement membrane. *Biotech Histochem* 1994;69:61–67.

181. Wei Y, Waltz DA, Rao N, et al. Identification of the urokinase receptor as an adhesion receptor for vitronectin. *J Biol Chem* 1994;269:32380–32388.

182. Wei Y, Eble JA, Wang Z, et al. Urokinase receptors promote beta1 integrin function through interactions with integrin alpha3beta1. *Mol Biol Cell* 2001;12:2975–2986.

183. Simon DI, Rao NK, Xu H, et al. Mac-1 (CD11b/CD18) and the urokinase receptor (CD87) form a functional unit on monocytic cells. *Blood* 1996;88:3185–3194.

184. Okumura Y, Kamikubo Y, Curriden SA, et al. Kinetic analysis of the interaction between vitronectin and the urokinase receptor. *J Biol Chem* 2002;277:9395–9404.

185. Deng G, Curriden SA, Wang S, et al. Is plasminogen activator inhibitor-1 the molecular switch that governs urokinase receptor-mediated cell adhesion and release? *J Cell Biol* 1996;134:1563–1571.

186. Kanse SM, Kost C, Wilhelm OG, et al. The urokinase receptor is a major vitronectin-binding protein on endothelial cells. *Exp Cell Res* 1996;224: 344–353.

187. Waltz DA, Natkin LR, Fujita RM, et al. Plasmin and plasminogen activator inhibitor type 1 promote cellular motility by regulating the interaction between the urokinase receptor and vitronectin. *J Clin Invest* 1997;100:58–67.

188. Czekay RP, Aertgeerts K, Curriden SA, et al. Plasminogen activator inhibitor-1 detaches cells from extracellular matrices by inactivating integrins. *J Cell Biol* 2003;160:781–791.

189. Inyang AL, Tobelem G. Tissue-plasminogen activator stimulates endothelial cell migration in wound assays. *Biochem Biophys Res Commun* 1990;171:1326–1332.

190. Kirchheimer JC, Binder BR, Remold HG. Matrix-bound plasminogen activator inhibitor type 1 inhibits the invasion of human monocytes into interstitial tissue. *J Immunol* 1990;145:1518–1522.

191. Palmieri D, Lee JW, Juliano RL, et al. Plasminogen activator inhibitor-1 and -3 increase cell adhesion and motility of MDA-MB-435 breast cancer cells. *J Biol Chem* 2002;277:40950–40957.

192. Ciambrone GJ, McKeown-Longo PJ. Plasminogen activator inhibitor type I stabilizes vitronectin- dependent adhesions in HT-1080 cells. *J Cell Biol* 1990;111:2183–2195.

193. Webb DJ, Thomas KS, Gonias SL. Plasminogen activator inhibitor 1 functions as a urokinase response modifier at the level of cell signaling and thereby promotes MCF-7 cell growth. *J Cell Biol* 2001;152:741–752.

194. Degryse B, Sier CF, Resnati M, et al. PAI-1 inhibits urokinase-induced chemotaxis by internalizing the urokinase receptor. *FEBS Lett* 2001;505:249–254.

195. Bacharach E, Itin A, Keshet E. Apposition-dependent induction of plasminogen activator inhibitor type 1 expression: a mechanism for balancing pericellular proteolysis during angiogenesis. *Blood* 1998;92:939–945.

196. Dublin E, Hanby A, Patel NK, et al. Immunohistochemical expression of uPA, uPAR, and PAI-1 in breast carcinoma. Fibroblastic expression has strong associations with tumor pathology. *Am J Pathol* 2000;157:1219–1227.

197. Pedersen AN, Christensen IJ, Stephens RW, et al. The complex between urokinase and its type-1 inhibitor in primary breast cancer: relation to survival. *Cancer Res* 2000;60:6927–6934.

198. Soff GA, Sanderowitz J, Gately S, et al. Expression of plasminogen activator inhibitor type I by human prostate carcinoma cells inhibits primary tumor growth, tumor-associated angiogenesis, and metastasis to lung and liver in any athymic mouse model. *J Clin Invest* 1995;96:2593–2600.

199. Eitzman DT, Krauss JC, Shen T, et al. Lack of plasminogen activator inhibitor-1 effect in a transgenic mouse model of metastatic melanoma. *Blood* 1996;87:4718–4722.

200. Jankun J, Keck RW, Skrzypczak-Jankun E, et al. Inhibitors of urokinase reduce size of prostate cancer xenografts in severe combined immunodeficient mice. *Cancer Res* 1997;57:559–563.

201. Bajou K, Noel A, Gerard RD, et al. Absence of host plasminogen activator inhibitor 1 prevents cancer invasion and vascularization. *Nat Med* 1998;4:923–928.

202. Gutierrez LS, Schulman A, Brito-Robinson T, et al. Tumor development is retarded in mice lacking the gene for urokinase- type plasminogen activator or its inhibitor, plasminogen activator inhibitor-1. *Cancer Res* 2000;60:5839–5847.

203. Bajou K, Masson V, Gerard RD, et al. The plasminogen activator PAI-1 controls *in vivo* tumor vascularization by interaction with proteases, not vitronectin. Implications for antiangiogenic strategies. *J Cell Biol* 2001;152:777–784.

204. McMahon GA, Petitclerc E, Stefansson S, et al. Plasminogen activator inhibitor-1 regulates tumor growth and angiogenesis. *J Biol Chem* 2001;276:33964–33968.

205. Devy L, Blacher S, Grignet-Debrus C, et al. The pro- or antiangiogenic effect of plasminogen activator inhibitor 1 is dose dependent. *FASEB J* 2002;16:147–154.

206. Curino A, Mitola DJ, Aaronson H, et al. Plasminogen promotes sarcoma growth and suppresses the accumulation of tumor-infiltrating macrophages. *Oncogene* 2002;21:8830–8842.

207. Vu TH, Hung DT, Wheaton VI, et al. Molecular cloning of a functional thrombin receptor reveals a novel proteolytic mechanism of receptor activation. *Cell* 1991;64:1057–1068.

208. Erickson LA, Hekman CM, Loskutoff DJ. The primary plasminogen-activator inhibitors in endothelial cells, platelets, serum, and plasma are immunologically related. *Proc Natl Acad Sci U S A* 1985;82:8710–8714.

209. Booth NA, Simpson AJ, Croll A, et al. Plasminogen activator inhibitor (PAI-1) in plasma and platelets. *Br J Haematol* 1988;70:327–333.

210. Declerck PJ, Verstreken M, Kruithof EKO, et al. Measurement of plasminogen activator inhibitor 1 in biologic fluids with a murine monoclonal antibody-based enzyme-linked immunoabsorbent assay. *Blood* 1988;71:220–225.

211. Fay WP, Eitzman DT, Shapiro AD, et al. Platelets inhibit fibrinolysis *in vitro* by both plasminogen activator inhibitor-1 dependent and independent mechanisms. *Blood* 1994;83:351–356.

212. Fay WP, Parker AC, Condrey LR, et al. Human plasminogen activator inhibitor-1 (PAI-1) deficiency: characterization of a large kindred with a null mutation in the PAI-1 gene. *Blood* 1997;90:204–208.

213. Fay WP, Shapiro AD, Shih JL, et al. Complete deficiency of plasminogen-activator inhibitor type 1 due to a frame-shift mutation. *N Engl J Med* 1992;327:1729–1733.

214. Minowa H, Takahashi Y, Tanaka T, et al. Four cases of bleeding diathesis in children due to congenital plasminogen activator inhibitor-1 deficiency. *Haemostasis* 1999;29:286–291.

215. Carmeliet P, Moons L, Lijnen R, et al. Inhibitory role of plasminogen activator inhibitor-1 in arterial wound healing and neointima formation: a gene targeting and gene transfer study in mice. *Circulation* 1997;96:3180–3191.

216. Carmeliet P, Moons L, Herbert JM, et al. Urokinase but not tissue plasminogen activator mediates arterial neointima formation in mice. *Circ Res* 1997;81:829–839.

217. Redmond EM, Cullen JP, Cahill PA, et al. Endothelial cells inhibit flow-induced smooth muscle cell migration: role of plasminogen activator inhibitor-1. *Circulation* 2001;103:597–603.

218. Ploplis VA, Cornelissen I, Sandoval-Cooper MJ, et al. Remodeling of the vessel wall after copper-induced injury is highly attenuated in mice with a total deficiency of plasminogen activator inhibitor-1. *Am J Pathol* 2001;158:107–117.

219. Ploplis VA, Castellino FJ. Attenuation of neointima formation following arterial injury in PAI-1 deficient mice. *Ann NY Acad Sci* 2001;936:466–468.

220. Zhu Y, Farrehi PM, Fay WP. Plasminogen activator inhibitor type 1 enhances neointima formation after oxidative vascular injury in atherosclerosis-prone mice. *Circulation* 2001;103:3105–3110.

221. Peng L, Bhatia N, Parker AC, et al. Endogenous vitronectin and plasminogen activator inhibitor-1 promote neointima formation in murine carotid arteries. *Arterioscler Thromb Vasc Biol* 2002;22:934–939.

222. DeYoung MB, Tom C, Dichek DA. Plasminogen activator inhibitor type 1 increases neointima formation in balloon-injured rat carotid arteries. *Circulation* 2001;104:1972–1971.

223. Juhan-Vague I, Collen D. On the role of coagulation and fibrinolysis in atherosclerosis. *Ann Epidemiol* 1992;2:427–438.

224. Schneiderman J, Sawdey MS, Keeton MR, et al. Increased type 1 plasminogen activator inhibitor gene expression in atherosclerotic human arteries. *Proc Natl Acad Sci U S A* 1992;89:6998–7002.

225. Lupu F, Bergonzelli GE, Heim DA, et al. Localization and production of plasminogen activator inhibitor-1 in human healthy and atherosclerotic arteries. *Arterioscler Thromb* 1993;13:1090–1100.

226. Robbie LA, Booth NA, Brown AJ, et al. Inhibitors of fibrinolysis are elevated in atherosclerotic plaque. *Arterioscler Thromb Vasc Biol* 1996;16:539–545.

227. Sjoland H, Eitzman DT, Gordon D, et al. Atherosclerosis progression in LDL receptor-deficient and apolipoprotein E-deficient mice is independent of genetic alterations in plasminogen activator inhibitor-1. *Arterioscler Thromb Vasc Biol* 2000;20:846–852.

228. Eitzman DT, Westrick RJ, Xu Z, et al. Plasminogen activator inhibitor-1 deficiency protects against atherosclerosis progression in the mouse carotid artery. *Blood* 2000;96:4212–4215.

229. Eren M, Painter CA, Atkinson JB, et al. Age-dependent spontaneous coronary arterial thrombosis in transgenic mice that express a stable form of human plasminogen activator inhibitor-1. *Circulation* 2002;106:491–496.

230. Carmeliet P, Kieckens L, Schoonjans L, et al. Plasminogen activator inhibitor-1 gene-deficient mice. I. Generation by homologous recombination and characterization. *J Clin Invest* 1993;92:2746–2755.

231. Yamamoto K, Takeshita K, Shimokawa T, et al. Plasminogen activator inhibitor-1 is a major stress-regulated gene: implications for stress-induced thrombosis in aged individuals. *Proc Natl Acad Sci U S A* 2002;99:890–895.

232. Juhan-Vague I, Moerman B, De Cock F, et al. Plasma levels of a specific inhibitor of tissue-type plasminogen activator (and urokinase) in normal and pathological conditions. *Thromb Res* 1984;33:523–530.

233. Meade TW, Ruddock V, Stirling Y, et al. Fibrinolytic activity, clotting factors, and long-term incidence of ischaemic heart disease in the Northwick Park Heart Study. *Lancet* 1993;342:1076–1079.

234. Thompson SG, Kienast J, Pyke SD, et al. Hemostatic factors and the risk of myocardial infarction or sudden death in patients with angina pectoris. European concerted action on thrombosis and disabilities angina pectoris study group. *N Engl J Med* 1995;332:635–641.

235. Folsom AR, Aleksic N, Park E, et al. Prospective study of fibrinolytic factors and incident coronary heart disease: the Atherosclerosis Risk in Communities (ARIC) study. *Arterioscler Thromb Vasc Biol* 2001;21:611–617.

236. Alessi MC, Peiretti F, Morange P, et al. Production of plasminogen activator inhibitor 1 by human adipose tissue: possible link between visceral fat accumulation and vascular disease. *Diabetes* 1997;46:860–867.

237. Schafer K, Fujisawa K, Konstantinides S, et al. Disruption of the plasminogen activator inhibitor 1 gene reduces the adiposity and improves the metabolic profile of genetically obese and diabetic ob/ob mice. *FASEB J* 2001;15:1840–1842.

238. Eriksson P, Kallin B, 't Hooft FM, et al. Allele-specific increase in basal transcription of the plasminogen-activator inhibitor 1 gene is associated with myocardial infarction. *Proc Natl Acad Sci U S A* 1995;92:1851–1855.

239. Ridker PM, Hennekens CH, Lindpaintner K, et al. Arterial and venous thrombosis is not associated with the 4G/5G polymorphism in the promoter of the plasminogen activator inhibitor gene in a large cohort of US men. *Circulation* 1997;95:59–62.

240. Zoller B, Garcia dF, Dahlback B. A common 4G allele in the promoter of the plasminogen activator inhibitor-1 (PAI-1) gene as a risk factor for pulmonary embolism and arterial thrombosis in hereditary protein S deficiency. *Thromb Haemost* 1998;79:802–807.

241. Zhang ZG, Chopp M, Goussev A, et al. Cerebral microvascular obstruction by fibrin is associated with upregulation of PAI-1 acutely after onset of focal embolic ischemia in rats. *J Neurosci* 1999;19:10898–10907.

242. Hosomi N, Lucero J, Heo JH, et al. Rapid differential endogenous plasminogen activator expression after acute middle cerebral artery occlusion. *Stroke* 2001;32:1341–1348.

243. Nagai N, De Mol M, Lijnen HR, et al. Role of plasminogen system components in focal cerebral infarction: a gene targeting and gene transfer study in mice. *Circulation* 1999;99:2440–2444.

244. Chen CH, Eng HL, Chang CJ, et al. 4G/5G promoter polymorphism of plasminogen activator inhibitor-1, lipid profiles, and ischemic stroke. *J Lab Clin Med* 2003;142:100–105.

245. Morange PE, Aubert J, Peiretti F, et al. Glucocorticoids and insulin promote plasminogen activator inhibitor 1 production by human adipose tissue. *Diabetes* 1999;48:890–895.

246. Sakamoto T, Woodcock-Mitchell J, Marutsuka K, et al. TNF-alpha and insulin, alone and synergistically, induce plasminogen activator inhibitor-1 expression in adipocytes. *Am J Physiol* 1999;276:C1391–C1397.

247. Samad F, Schneiderman J, Loskutoff D. Expression of fibrinolytic genes in tissues from human atherosclerotic aneurysms and from obese mice. *Ann NY Acad Sci* 1997;811:350–358.

248. Lundgren CH, Brown SL, Nordt TK, et al. Elaboration of type-1 plasminogen activator inhibitor from adipocytes. A potential pathogenetic link between obesity and cardiovascular disease. *Circulation* 1996;93:106–110.

249. Cigolini M, Tonoli M, Borgato L, et al. Expression of plasminogen activator inhibitor-1 in human adipose tissue: a role for TNF-alpha? *Atherosclerosis* 1999;143:81–90.

250. Crandall DL, Groeling TM, Busler DE, et al. Release of PAI-1 by human preadipocytes and adipocytes independent of insulin and IGF-1. *Biochem Biophys Res Commun* 2000;279:984–988.

251. Gottschling-Zeller H, Rohrig K, Hauner H. Troglitazone reduces plasminogen activator inhibitor-1 expression and secretion in cultured human adipocytes. *Diabetologia* 2000;43:377–383.

252. Vague P, Juhan-Vague I, Aillaud MF, et al. Correlation between blood fibrinolytic activity, plasminogen activator inhibitor level, plasma insulin level, and relative body weight in normal and obese subjects. *Metabolism* 1986;35:250–253.

253. Mavri A, Stegnar M, Krebs M, et al. Impact of adipose tissue on plasma plasminogen activator inhibitor-1 in dieting obese women. *Arterioscler Thromb Vasc Biol* 1999;19:1582–1587.

254. Giltay EJ, Elbers JM, Gooren LJ, et al. Visceral fat accumulation is an important determinant of PAI-1 levels in young, nonobese men and women: modulation by cross-sex hormone administration. *Arterioscler Thromb Vasc Biol* 1998;18:1716–1722.

255. Samad F, Loskutoff DJ. Tissue distribution and regulation of plasminogen activator inhibitor-1 in obese mice. *Mol Med* 1996;2:568–582.

256. Shimomura I, Funahashi T, Takahashi M, et al. Enhanced expression of PAI-1 in visceral fat: possible contributor to vascular disease in obesity. *Nat Med* 1996;2:800–803.

257. Ma LJ, Mao SL, Taylor KL, et al. Prevention of obesity and insulin resistance in mice lacking plasminogen activator inhibitor 1. *Diabetes* 2004; 53:336–346.

258. Calles-Escandon J, Ballor D, Harvey-Berino J, et al. Amelioration of the inhibition of fibrinolysis in elderly, obese subjects by moderate energy intake restriction. *Am J Clin Nutr* 1996;64:7–11.

259. Samad F, Uysal KT, Wiesbrock SM, et al. Tumor necrosis factor alpha is a key component in the obesity-linked elevation of plasminogen activator inhibitor 1. *Proc Natl Acad Sci U S A* 1999;96:6902–6907.

260. Duymelinck C, Dauwe SE, De Greef KE, et al. TIMP-1 gene expression and PAI-1 antigen after unilateral ureteral obstruction in the adult male rat. *Kidney Int* 2000;58:1186–1201.

261. Eddy AA, Giachelli CM. Renal expression of genes that promote interstitial inflammation and fibrosis in rats with protein-overload proteinuria. *Kidney Int* 1995;47:1546–1557.

262. Brown NJ, Nakamura S, Ma L, et al. Aldosterone modulates plasminogen activator inhibitor-1 and glomerulosclerosis *in vivo*. *Kidney Int* 2000; 58:1219–1227.

263. Keeton M, Ahn C, Eguchi Y, et al. Expression of type 1 plasminogen activator inhibitor in renal tissue in murine lupus nephritis. *Kidney Int* 1995; 47:148–157.

264. Rerolle JP, Hertig A, Nguyen G, et al. Plasminogen activator inhibitor type 1 is a potential target in renal fibrogenesis. *Kidney Int* 2000;58:1841–1850.

265. Hamano K, Iwano M, Akai Y, et al. Expression of glomerular plasminogen activator inhibitor type 1 in glomerulonephritis. *Am J Kidney Dis* 2002;39:695–705.

266. Xu Y, Hagege J, Mougenot B, et al. Different expression of the plasminogen activation system in renal thrombotic microangiopathy and the normal human kidney. *Kidney Int* 1996;50:2011–2019.

267. Bergstein JM, Riley M, Bang NU. Role of plasminogen-activator inhibitor type 1 in the pathogenesis and outcome of the hemolytic uremic syndrome. *N Engl J Med* 1992;327:755–759.

268. Nakamura T, Tanaka N, Higuma N, et al. The localization of plasminogen activator inhibitor-1 in glomerular subepithelial deposits in membranous nephropathy. *J Am Soc Nephrol* 1996;7:2434–2444.

269. Border WA, Noble NA. Transforming growth factor beta in tissue fibrosis. *N Engl J Med* 1994;331:1286–1292.

270. Border WA, Okuda S, Nakamura T. Extracellular matrix and glomerular disease. *Semin Nephrol* 1989;9:307–317.

271. Lund LR, Riccio A, Andreasen PA, et al. Transforming growth factor-beta is a strong and fast acting positive regulator of the level of type-1 plasminogen activator inhibitor mRNA in WI-38 human lung fibroblasts. *EMBO J* 1987;6:1281–1286.

272. Kerins DM, Hao Q, Vaughan DE. Angiotensin induction of PAI-1 expression in endothelial cells is mediated by the hexapeptide angiotensin IV. *J Clin Invest* 1995;96:2515–2520.

273. Oikawa T, Freeman M, Lo W, et al. Modulation of plasminogen activator inhibitor-1 *in vivo*: a new mechanism for the anti-fibrotic effect of renin-angiotensin inhibition. *Kidney Int* 1997;51:164–172.

274. Huang Y, Haraguchi M, Lawrence DA, et al. A mutant, noninhibitory plasminogen activator inhibitor type 1 decreases matrix accumulation in experimental glomerulonephritis. *J Clin Invest* 2003;112:379–388.

275. Fogo AB. Renal fibrosis: not just PAI-1 in the sky. *J Clin Invest* 2003; 112:326–328.

276. Ingelfinger JR. Forestalling fibrosis. *N Engl J Med* 2003;349:2265–2266.

277. Bertozzi P, Astedt B, Zenzius L, et al. Depressed bronchoalveolar urokinase activity in patients with adult respiratory distress syndrome. *N Engl J Med* 1990;322:890–897.

278. Idell S, Peters J, James KK, et al. Local abnormalities of coagulation and fibrinolytic pathways that promote alveolar fibrin deposition in the lungs of baboons with diffuse alveolar damage. *J Clin Invest* 1989;84:181–193.

279. Chapman HA, Allen CL, Stone OL. Abnormalities in pathways of alveolar fibrin turnover among patients with interstitial lung disease. *Am Rev Respir Dis* 1986;133:437–443.

280. Kotani I, Sato A, Hayakawa H, et al. Increased procoagulant and antifibrinolytic activities in the lungs with idiopathic pulmonary fibrosis. *Thromb Res* 1995;77:493–504.

281. Hasday JD, Bachwich PR, Lynch JP, et al. III. Procoagulant and plasminogen activator activities of bronchoalveolar fluid in patients with pulmonary sarcoidosis. *Exp Lung Res* 1988;14:261–278.

282. Barazzone C, Belin D, Piguet PF, et al. Plasminogen activator inhibitor-1 in acute hyperoxic mouse lung injury. *J Clin Invest* 1996;98:2666–2673.

283. Viscardi RM, Broderick K, Sun CC, et al. Disordered pathways of fibrin turnover in lung lavage of premature infants with respiratory distress syndrome. *Am Rev Respir Dis* 1992;146:492–499.

284. Idell S, Gonzalez K, Bradford H, et al. Procoagulant activity in bronchoalveolar lavage in the adult respiratory distress syndrome. Contribution of tissue factor associated with factor VII. *Am Rev Respir Dis* 1987; 136:1466–1474.

285. Olman MA, Mackman N, Gladson CL, et al. Changes in procoagulant and fibrinolytic gene expression during bleomycin-induced lung injury in the mouse. *J Clin Invest* 1995;96:1621–1630.

286. Eitzman DT, McCoy RD, Zheng X, et al. Bleomycin-induced pulmonary fibrosis in transgenic mice that either lack or overexpress the murine plasminogen activator inhibitor-1 gene. *J Clin Invest* 1996;97:232–237.

287. Aertgeerts K, De Bondt HL, De Ranter CJ, et al. Mechanisms contributing to the conformational and functional flexibility of plasminogen activator inhibitor-1. *Nat Struct Biol* 1995;2:891–897.

# CHAPTER 20 ■ THROMBIN-ACTIVATABLE FIBRINOLYSIS INHIBITOR AKA PROCARBOXYPEPTIDASE U

MICHAEL E. NESHEIM, JUDITH LEURS, AND DIRK F. HENDRIKS

Thrombin-activatable fibrinolysis inhibitor (TAFI) is a plasma glycoprotein of 401 amino acids that circulates at a concentration of approximately 5.0 $\mu$g per mL (1,2). It is the precursor of zinc ion–dependent, carboxypeptidase B–like enzyme, designated TAFIa, that suppresses fibrinolysis. It is activated by proteolysis at the Arg92–Ala93 bond. The amino-terminal portion is an activation fragment, and the carboxy-terminal portion is the enzyme TAFIa. Thrombin and plasmin are capable of activating TAFI, but they are relatively inefficient in doing so. The physiologic activator is thought to be the thrombin–thrombomodulin complex (3). The gene for TAFI is located on chromosome 13 (4). It contains 11 exons and spans approximately 48 kb of genomic DNA and is expressed in the liver (5).

As is the case with many complex biologic molecules, TAFI made its existence known in several laboratories through independent and unrelated investigations, each of which resulted in a new name for the previously unknown entity. As a consequence, the protein has acquired several monikers, each of which, as learned in retrospect, refers to the same entity. Among its names are procarboxypeptidase U (6,7), plasma procarboxypeptidase B (1,8), procarboxypeptidase R (9), and TAFI (2). The name procarboxypeptidase U was assigned because the protein is the precursor of an unstable carboxypeptidase B–like enzyme found in serum. It was named plasma procarboxypeptidase B because it is the precursor of carboxypeptidase B–like enzyme homologous to the carboxypeptidase B precursor found in the pancreas. It was called procarboxypeptidase R because it has a preference for removal of arginine, as apposed to lysine, from the carboxy terminus of proteins and peptides. This distinguishes the enzyme from the other carboxypeptidase B–like enzyme of plasma, known as carboxypeptidase N (6). It was named TAFI because it was discovered in a search for an entity that gives rise to an inhibitor of fibrinolysis in response to prothrombin activation.

This chapter provides information regarding the presumed balance between the deposition and removal of fibrin and the role of the TAFI pathway in it; the activation of TAFI; the mechanisms by which TAFIa suppresses fibrinolysis; TAFI and the factor XI–dependent pathway of coagulation; assays for TAFI and TAFIa; the physiologic and pathophysiologic roles of the TAFI pathway; and an update on the epidemiology of TAFI. Several recent reviews on TAFI are available (10–26).

## THE BALANCE BETWEEN FIBRIN DEPOSITION AND REMOVAL

The vasculature system has within it two powerful, well-regulated systems that operate to both stop blood flow at the site of an injury and to maintain blood fluidity elsewhere. These systems are known, respectively, as the coagulation and fibrinolytic cascades. These systems involve plasma proteins, formed elements of blood, particularly platelets, and cells lining the blood vessel wall. They are latent, and therefore their potential is not obvious without overt stimulation. When triggered, however, they can be very potent. This point has been demonstrated, for example, in chimpanzees that were injected over a 30-second period with trace quantities of a combination of blood coagulation factor Xa and procoagulant phospholipid vesicles (27). Within 1 minute, all of the plasma fibrinogen had been converted to fibrin, and the platelet count had dropped to zero. This startling and dramatic coagulation response, which might be expected to be fatal, had no long-term effects on the animals because it was immediately followed by an equally potent fibrinolytic response. Within a minute or two, the circulating level of tissue-type plasminogen activator (tPA) had risen approximately 800-fold, and all of the fibrin that had been deposited within the vascular system was solubilized to fibrin degradation products. These experiments demonstrated, in the systemic circulation, events that presumably can happen locally when required to prevent local blood loss or remove inappropriately deposited fibrin.

A further appreciation of the potential of the coagulation system can be gained by considering that thrombin added to plasma at 1 NIH U per mL will provide a clot in approximately 15 seconds. The plasma, however, has in it sufficient prothrombin to generate approximately 150 NIH U of thrombin per mL if fully activated. Therefore, were the coagulation system to be fully activated instantaneously, the blood would be fully gelled within 1 or 2 seconds, and the rate-limiting step would be the polymerization of fibrin. Likewise, plasmin sustained at a level of approximately 2 nM will lyse a fibrin clot within approximately 30 minutes. Plasma has plasminogen in it at a level of approximately 2,000 nM. Therefore, if the plasminogen were instantly turned to plasmin, a clot could be expected to be fully solubilized in approximately 2 seconds. These considerations suggest that the coagulation and fibrinolytic systems are potentially extremely powerful. They also tend to rationalize the many levels of control that exist in these systems so that they can perform their respective functions without doing untoward damage to the host.

The balance between fibrin deposition and removal is depicted in Figure 20-1. In response to vascular injury, the coagulation cascade is upregulated to convert prothrombin to thrombin, which then converts fibrinogen to fibrin, thereby producing the familiar blood clot. In response to fibrin, the fibrinolytic cascade can be upregulated to convert plasminogen to plasmin, which then digests fibrin into soluble fibrin

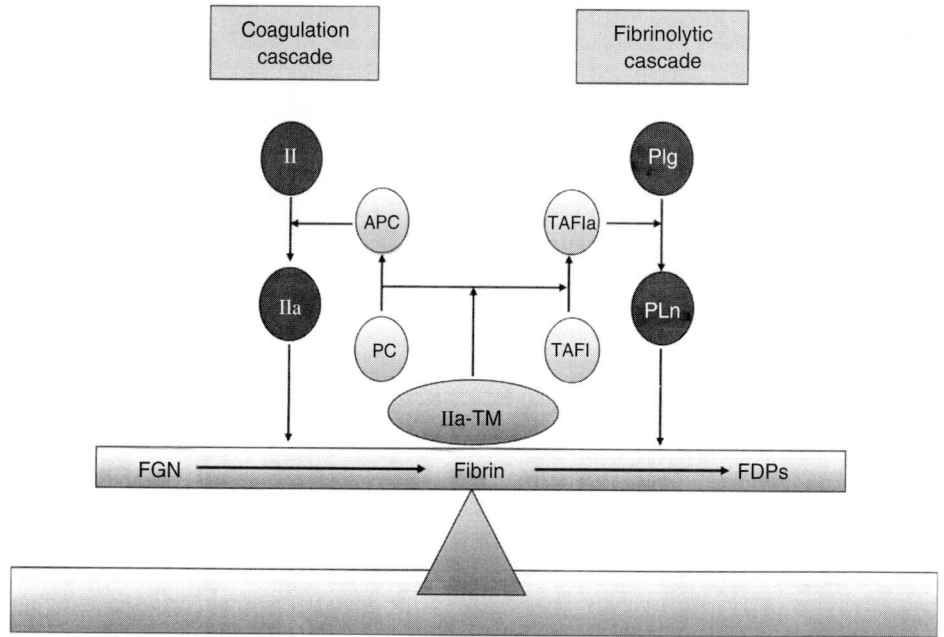

**FIGURE 20-1.** The balance between fibrin deposition and removal. Prothrombin (II) is activated to thrombin (IIa) by the coagulation cascade, and fibrin deposition occurs. Subsequently, plasminogen (Plg) is activated to plasmin (PLn) by the fibrinolytic cascade, and fibrin is removed. The thrombin–thrombomodulin complex (IIa-TM) activates protein C (PC) and thrombin-activatable fibrinolysis inhibitor (TAFI) to the enzymes-activated protein C (APC) and TAFIa, which respectively downregulate the coagulation and fibrinolytic cascades. The TAFI pathway provides a regulatory link between the two cascades such that activation of coagulation suppresses fibrinolysis. FGN, fibrinogen; FDP; fibrin degradation products.

degradation products. When these processes are properly balanced, the physiologic roles of these systems are realized. When they are unbalanced, however, bleeding or thrombosis can occur. The systems are regulated at many levels, most of which are not depicted in the figure. One very important mode for the regulation of coagulation, however, is indicated. It involves the protein C pathway, whereby the thrombin–thrombomodulin complex converts the zymogen protein C to the enzyme, activated protein C (APC), which, through a negative feedback loop, downregulates thrombin formation (28). Studies with TAFI have shown that a similar feedback loop exists on fibrinolytic side of the balance (2,3). In this case, the thrombin–thrombomodulin complex activates the zymogen TAFI to the enzyme, TAFIa, which suppresses the fibrinolytic cascade. Because TAFI is activated by the thrombin–thrombomodulin complex, the TAFI pathway provides an explicit molecular connection between the coagulation and fibrinolytic cascades, such that activation of the former can suppress the activation of the latter.

The importance of the protein C pathway in the regulation of the coagulation cascade has been demonstrated by the existence of severe thrombosis in the congenital absence of protein C (28,29) and the elevated risk of thrombosis in the condition known as activation protein C resistance, associated with factor $V_{Leiden}$ (30). Whether defects in TAFI exist and to what extent they might be associated with hemostatic abnormalities is not known as yet.

# THE ACTIVATION OF THROMBIN-ACTIVATABLE FIBRINOLYSIS INHIBITOR

TAFI is activated by proteolytic cleavage at the Arg92–Ala93 bond (1,2). The enzyme TAFIa is composed of amino acids 93 through

401 (1). Enzymes known to catalyze this cleavage are thrombin, plasmin, and trypsin (1,2). The reactions catalyzed by thrombin and plasmin are very inefficient compared to many other reactions catalyzed by these enzymes. The efficiency of the reaction catalyzed by thrombin, however, is stimulated by a factor of 1,250 by thrombomodulin (3). This magnitude of increase accomplished by thrombomodulin is similar to that obtained in protein C activation (31). Heparin stimulates the activation of TAFI by plasmin, but not to the same extent as thrombomodulin stimulates the thrombin-catalyzed reaction (32). Because thrombomodulin so potently stimulates TAFI activation by thrombin, the thrombin–thrombomodulin complex is thought to be the physiologic activator.

The activation of TAFI is calcium ion–dependent (33). It shows a monophasic dependence on the calcium ion concentration with a half maximal effect at a concentration of approximately 0.25 mM. This is in sharp contrast to the calcium ion concentration dependence of protein C activation, which is biphasic with a peak at a calcium ion concentration of approximately 0.25 mM (33,34).

The kinetics of TAFI activation are consistent with what has been referred to as an enzyme-central, parallel assembly model (3,35). According to this model, as shown in Figure 20-2, the enzyme thrombin can bind to either TAFI or thrombomodulin to form the corresponding binary complexes. These can interact further to bind the third component (either TAFI or thrombomodulin) to form the ternary thrombin–thrombomodulin–TAFI complex, from which the enzyme TAFIa is generated. Three parameters are associated with this model: the dissociation constant for the thrombin–thrombomodulin interaction, the $K_m$ for thrombin TAFI interaction, and the $k_{cat}$, or turnover number, of the ternary complex. The three respective parameters were evaluated to be 10 nM, 1 $\mu$M, and 1 per second, respectively (3). The $K_m$ number is high relative to the plasma concentration of TAFI, as is the case with protein C activation (31). This implies that the rate of TAFI activation *in vivo* would be proportional to

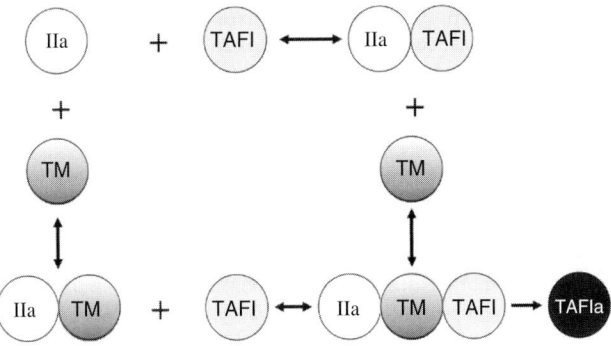

**FIGURE 20-2.** A model of the mechanism of activation of thrombin-activatable fibrinolysis inhibitor (TAFI) by thrombin plus thrombomodulin. This is an enzyme-central, parallel assembly model whereby thrombin (IIa) interacts with either TAFI or thrombomodulin (TM) to form the corresponding binary complexes. These then interact further to form the ternary thrombin–thrombomodulin–TAFI complex from which TAFIa is generated. Thrombin alone will catalyze activation of TAFI, but thrombomodulin increases the efficiency of the process by a factor of 1,250.

the plasma concentration, which has in fact been demonstrated (36,37). In addition, the relatively low plasma levels of both protein C and TAFI, compared to their $K_m$ values, indicates that they would not compete appreciably with each other for the thrombin–thrombomodulin complex, and activation of both would occur simultaneously with little if any interference from each other. The activation of TAFI has been demonstrated not only with soluble thrombomodulin but also with the thrombomodulin found in endothelial cells (38,39). Consistent with a relative lack of interference with each other, competition for protein C activation by TAFI on endothelial cells, although present, was only modest even at concentrations of TAFI several times its plasma concentration (39). The same was observed regarding the inhibition of TAFI activation by protein C (38).

Thrombomodulin has five recognized domains (40). In order, from the amino-terminus, they are a lectinlike domain, six tandem epidermal growth factor (EGF)-like domains, a chondroitin sulfate rich domain, a transmembrane domain, and an intracellular domain. The minimal structure required for protein C activation comprises the fourth, fifth, and sixth EGF-like domains, plus the small peptide that connects epidermal growth factor domains three and four (41). This same structure is necessary, but not sufficient, for TAFI activation (33,42). In addition, the thirteen residues comprising the third disulfide loop of the third epidermal growth factor domain are required. Therefore, although the elements of thrombomodulin structure required for efficient activation of TAFI and protein C are similar, they are not identical. Two amino acid residues are particularly intriguing. One is Met388, which is found in the small peptide that connects the fourth and fifth epidermal growth factor domains. This residue is essential for protein C activation, but not for TAFI activation (42). In addition, it can be oxidized in the presence of neutrophils (43). When this occurs, activity with respect to protein C activation is lost, but activity in TAFI activation is retained (33). This, in turn, suggests that in an inflammatory milieu, a strong shift in the balance between fibrin deposition and removal could occur in favor of thrombosis, because the anticoagulant pathway through protein C would be severely attenuated, but the antifibrinolytic pathway through TAFI would not. The other residue that stands out is Phe376, which is in the fourth epidermal growth factor domain. When this residue is replaced with alanine, activity in TAFI activation is retained, but activity in protein C activation is lost; therefore, Phe376 appears very important for protein C, but not for TAFI activation (33). Because of the differences in elements of structure of

thrombomodulin required for the two reactions, the potential exists to create recombinant forms of thrombomodulin that are specific for either protein C or TAFI activation.

The elements of thrombin structure required for the two reactions are overlapping, but not identical. Alanine-scanning mutagenesis of thrombin showed that the activation of both TAFI and protein C depends on residues of thrombin that map to exosite I, where thrombomodulin is known to bind (44). Other residues, however, were identified that are selectively needed for one or the other of the two reactions. Therefore, a region "below" the active site was found to be necessary specifically for protein C activation, whereas another region "above" the active site was found to be necessary specifically for TAFI activation. In addition, mutagenesis studies in which key tryptophan residues of thrombin were exchanged for phenylalanine showed that Trp215 of the active site of thrombin is very important in protein C, but not TAFI, activation, whereas the opposite is true for Trp60d (45).

The elements of structure of TAFI that confer thrombomodulin dependence upon its activation have not been identified to date. They, however, apparently do not map to amino acids comprising the P6 to P3′ positions around the activation cleavage site. Mutagenesis studies of this region showed that even when several of these residues were replaced with those found around the thrombin cleavage site in the $\beta$ chain of fibrinogen, full thrombomodulin dependence of TAFI activation was retained, and no catalytic efficiency was lost (46). Remarkably, when the residues of TAFI around the cleavage site were replaced with those around the cleavage site of protein C, the mutant TAFI did not express well, and its activation by thrombin–thrombomodulin was very inefficient.

## MECHANISMS BY WHICH ACTIVE THROMBIN-ACTIVATABLE FIBRINOLYSIS INHIBITOR SUPPRESSES FIBRINOLYSIS

TAFIa is a carboxypeptidase B–like enzyme; that is, it catalyzes removal of basic (arginine and lysine) residues from the carboxy termini of selected peptides or proteins. This property confers upon TAFIa its ability to suppress fibrinolysis. When thrombin catalyzes the removal of fibrinopeptides A and B from the amino-termini of the A$\alpha$ and B$\beta$ chains of fibrinogen E-domains, the cleaved fibrinogen monomers associate noncovalently with the D-domains of neighboring molecules and the fibrin polymer is formed, thereby providing the major proteinaceous component of the familiar blood clot (47). The fibrin polymer is further stabilized by covalent isopeptide bonds formed between the D-domains of adjacent fibrin protomers in the clot. These bonds are formed through the action of factor XIIIa.

In response to fibrin, the vasculature is capable of releasing tPA, a serine protease enzyme (48). This enzyme then catalyzes activation of glu plasminogen through a single proteolytic cleavage to form glu plasmin, also a serine protease. The activation of glu plasminogen is stimulated by a factor of approximately 500 by fibrin (49,50), an effect that presumably keeps plasminogen activation localized to the site of a clot. This stimulation occurs through a mechanism in which fibrin acts as a template to bind both glu plasminogen and tPA (50). Once formed, plasmin begins to digest the clot by catalyzing cleavages after selected arginine and lysine residues in the $\alpha$, $\beta$, and $\gamma$ chains in regions connecting the D- and E-domains of the fibrin protomers (47,51). These cleavages expose carboxy-terminal lysine residues in the fibrin mesh that provide additional binding sites, especially for glu plasminogen. As a consequence, the cofactor activity of fibrin in glu plasminogen activation increases by a factor of approximately 3, and glu plasminogen activation is accelerated

(52,53). In addition, the partially cleaved fibrin serves as a cofactor for a reaction in which a peptide comprising the first 77 amino acids of glu plasminogen and glu plasmin are liberated by a cleavage catalyzed by plasmin. These reactions produce species known as lys plasminogen and lys plasmin, respectively. Lys plasminogen is a much better substrate for tPA than glu plasminogen (approximately 20-fold) (49,50,54). Therefore, (lys) plasmin formation is further accelerated. These two phenomena (upregulation of the cofactor activity of fibrin and generation of lys plasminogen) comprise potent positive feedback steps in the process of plasminogen activation. TAFIa interferes with this positive feedback by removing the newly exposed carboxy-terminal arginine and lysine residues as they appear in fibrin (53). It therefore eliminates the positive feedback steps in plasminogen activation and slows down the process of fibrinolysis.

TAFIa also functions by modulating the inhibition of plasmin by antiplasmin. Both glu and lys plasmin are very rapidly inhibited by antiplasmin, such that free plasmin in plasma has a half-life of approximately 0.1 second (55). Fibrin, however, attenuates this effect somewhat, such that the rate constant for inhibition of plasmin by antiplasmin is reduced approximately threefold by intact fibrin. As the fibrin is modified by plasmin, the magnitude of this effect increases an additional 10- to 15-fold, such that the rate constant for inhibition of plasmin in the presence of plasmin-modified fibrin is only approximately 2% to 3% of the value found in the absence of fibrin (56–58). As a consequence, plasmin is highly protected from the inhibitor in the presence of fibrin, especially when it has newly exposed carboxy-terminal lysine and arginine residues. The net effect of this is to substantially raise the steady-state level of plasmin during the fibrinolytic process, thereby promoting the rate at which the clot is dissolved (57). TAFIa, by removing the carboxy-terminal lysine and arginine residues, eliminates most of this protective effect. Therefore, in the presence of TAFIa, the steady state level of plasmin is considerably lower than it is in the absence of TAFIa, and the process of fibrinolysis is prolonged (57).

Another more subtle effect likely occurs directly in the digestion of fibrin by plasmin. Fibrin is solubilized when the $\alpha$, $\beta$, and $\gamma$ chains of adjacent protomers within the polymer are cleaved. For adjacent D- and E-domains on neighboring protomers to be separated, six cleavages must occur at the same location. Exhaustive digestion, which includes all such connections, is not necessary for complete solubilization, because fibrin degradation products can be released as a family of molecules of various molecular weights, the larger ones having many D, E connections not severed completely (59,60). Therefore, fibrin can be completely solubilized with only a fraction of all D, E connections cleaved through. The cleavages made by plasmin do not occur randomly, presumably because the new carboxy-terminal lysine and or arginine residues that result from cleavage at one of the $\alpha$, $\beta$, or $\gamma$ chains tends to bind plasmin and localize it so that the other chains are cleaved at the same D, E site (60). As a consequence, relatively few cleavages are needed to completely solubilize the fibrin. In the presence of TAFIa, however, this retention of plasmin does not occur to the same extent, and more cleavages are required to completely dissolve the fibrin because they occur randomly throughout the fibrin network. This also can prolong the process of fibrinolysis.

Most of the enzymes of coagulation and fibrinolysis can be downregulated by protease inhibitors, especially by antithrombin, antiplasmin, and plasminogen activator inhibitor-1 (PAI-1). TAFIa is exceptional in this regard in that, to date, no physiologic inhibitor of it has been reported. Instead, TAFIa spontaneously loses activity, an effect that presumably represents the means by which it is physiologically downregulated (6,61). The rate of decay is highly dependent on temperature, such that at body temperature the TAFIa half-life is approximately

10 minutes, but at room temperature it is approximately 2 hours, and at ice temperature it is indefinitely stable (61). Because TAFIa is unstable, it suppresses fibrinolysis only transiently, an effect that in part determines the potency of TAFIa as an antifibrinolytic agent (62). The loss of activity occurs in the absence of proteolysis, but once TAFIa loses activity, it is susceptible to proteolysis by thrombin or plasmin at Arg302 (61,63). Mutagenesis studies have identified a region of TAFIa comprising residues 302 to 330 to which the tendency to decay can be attributed (61,63). A naturally occurring polymorphism is found within this region at residue 325, which comprises either a threonine or an isoleucine residue (62,64). The latter variant of TAFIa has a half-life that is double that of the former; in addition, it is approximately 60% more potent as an antifibrinolytic agent (62). Approximately 10% of the population is homozygous for the more stable variant and 40% for the less stable one (64). Whether pathologic tendencies correlate with one or the other is currently under investigation.

When the time to lyze a clot is measured *in vitro* at various input concentrations of TAFIa, it increases at low concentrations and eventually appears to reach a plateau (2,3,61,62). Typically, the time to lyze in the plateau is three to four times that observed in the absence of TAFIa. The concentration needed to obtain a half-maximal prolongation is typically approximately 1 nM, a concentration which is only approximately 1% of the plasma concentration of the zymogen TAFI. Therefore, although TAFIa does not appear to completely eliminate fibrinolysis, even at relatively high levels, it is very potent in that only a small fraction of available TAFI needs to be activated to have an appreciable effect. The magnitude of the maximal prolongation obtained with TAFIa is directly proportional to its stability. Variants with a relatively short half-life therefore show only a small maximal increase, whereas those with a long half-life show the opposite. In fact, mutagenesis studies have shown that the maximal prolongation is directly proportional to the half-life of the variant (61,62). An example is shown in Figure 20-3. This observation had proven difficult to rationalize, because the expectation is that a relatively short half-life could be offset with an elevated TAFIa concentration. Further studies, however, provided an explanation for this and disclosed a curious property of the fibrinolytic system and its regulation by TAFIa (65,66). The studies showed that the TAFIa concentration dependence of lysis prolongation is not best represented by a saturating function, but rather by relation, whereby the lysis time increases linearly with respect to the TAFIa concentration up to some critical value, and then logarithmically thereafter. Therefore, the lysis time *versus* TAFIa concentration relation does not show a true plateau; it gives only a superficial impression of a plateau because of the linear-to-logarithmic switch in the relation. The explanation for this switch is based on the proposition that so long as TAFIa is present at or above some key threshold value, fibrin degradation essentially ceases, only to begin again once TAFIa decays to a level below the threshold value. The time interval over which the TAFIa level stays above the threshold is determined by both the initial input concentration of TAFIa and its half-life for first-order decay. Therefore, although TAFIa might, in principle, totally suppress fibrinolysis, it does not appear to do so because it decays. A stable carboxypeptidase (pancreatic carboxypeptidase B), however, can virtually stop fibrinolysis if present at a sufficiently high level (66). If TAFIa were to be generated acutely, and then decay, the effect would be to delay, but not eliminate, eventual fibrinolysis. If it were to be generated chronically, however, such that it were replenished over time, a situation might exist whereby fibrinolysis would be eliminated so long as the coagulant stimulus were present. Whether this can or does occur *in vivo* is not known, however. This raises the intriguing possibility, although, that under some conditions, TAFIa might function as an absolute inhibitor of fibrinolysis.

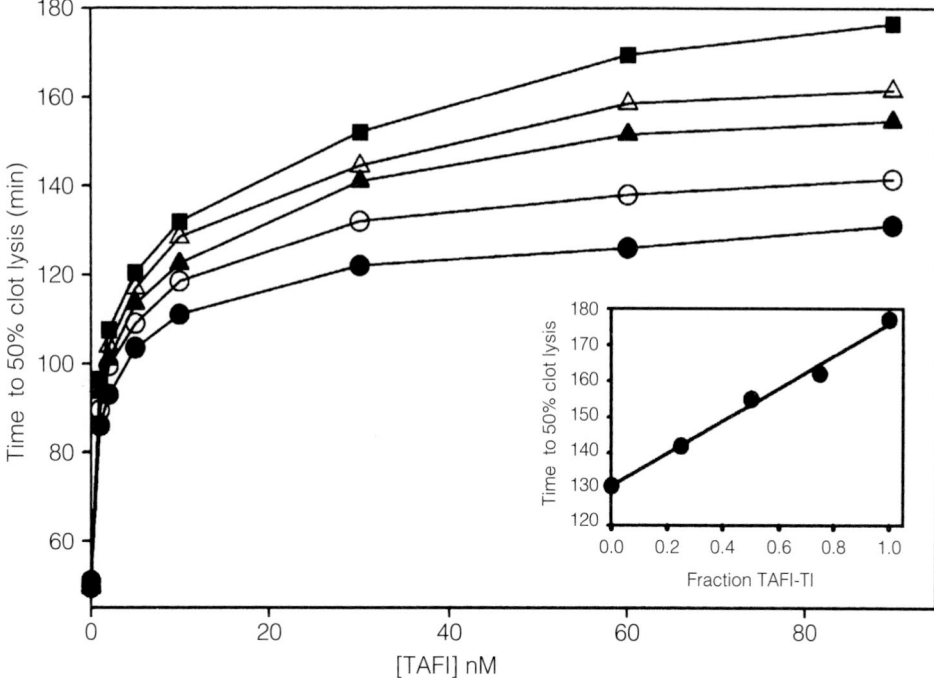

**FIGURE 20-3.** Prolongation of fibrinolysis by variants of thrombin-activatable fibrinolysis inhibitor (TAFI) with different half-lives. The time to lyze a clot is prolonged when TAFIa is included. Pseudosaturation occurs in the relation between the lysis time and the TAFIa concentration. The maximum prolongation depends on the half-life of the TAFIa. The data shown in *solid circles* was obtained with a TAFIa variant having threonine at position 325 and a half-life of 10 minutes. The data shown in *solid squares* were obtained with a TAFIa variant having isoleucine at position 325 and a 20-minute half-life. The other data were obtained mixtures of the two. They gave maximal lysis times between the extremes, as indicated in the *insert*, where TAFI-TI is the proportion of the sample consisting of the Ile325 variant. [From Schneider M, Boffa M, Stewart R, et al. Two naturally occurring variants of TAFI (Thr-325 and Il-325) differ substantially with respect to thermal stability and antifibrinolytic activity of the enzyme. *J Biol Chem* 2002;277(2):1021–1030.]

The combination of pseudosaturation in the relation between the time to lyze a clot and the TAFIa concentration, and a tendency for reversible inhibitors of TAFIa to stabilize it, gives rise to a complex relation between effects on fibrinolysis and the concentration of such inhibitors. Therefore, when reversible inhibitors of TAFIa were examined *in vitro* for their effects on the time to lyze a clot, they both prolonged and promoted lysis, depending on the dose (67,68). Typically, at relatively low concentrations, such inhibitors actually retard fibrinolysis, sometimes by a considerable margin, because they stabilize the TAFIa population but do not completely inhibit all the TAFIa molecules. Only at relatively high concentrations are they able to sufficiently inhibit the whole population to overcome the stabilizing effect.

# THROMBIN-ACTIVATABLE FIBRINOLYSIS INHIBITOR AND THE FACTOR XI–DEPENDENT PATHWAY OF COAGULATION

When clotting is triggered in whole blood or plasma, a series of events occur that collectively have been designated, in sequence, the initiation, propagation, and termination phases (69). In the initiation phase, events such as platelet activation, factor V and factor VIII activation, and prothrombin activation at a low level occur. At the end of the initiation phase, clotting occurs. At this point, approximately 1% or 2% of the prothrombin has been activated. This is followed by the propagation phase in which the factor XI–dependent (intrinsic) pathway is triggered, presumably through activation of factor XI by thrombin (70), and massive prothrombin activation occurs within the clot. This is followed by the termination phase in which the reactions of the coagulation cascade subside and thrombin is consumed by antithrombin. Samples of plasma with defects in the factor XI–dependent pathway, such as those with severe hemophilia A or B, display the initiation phase (69,71), but not the intense thrombin formation of the propagation phase.

Several investigators noted early on that when clotting and subsequent fibrinolysis were induced by adding tPA and thrombin to normal plasmas, or those with defects in the factor XI–dependent pathway, fibrinolysis occurred early in the defective plasmas (72–74). For example, clots made in normal plasma would lyze under the extant condition in 2 hours, and those made in the deficient plasmas would lyze in approximately 30 minutes. The phenomenon was designated "premature lysis" (72). The mechanism for this subsequently was shown to be dependent on the TAFI pathway, in that normal plasma showed premature lysis when TAFIa was inhibited, and normal lysis could be restored in hemophilia plasma by promoting TAFI activation (72,74). These and other studies showed that the massive level of thrombin transiently formed after clotting in normal plasma is sufficient, even in the absence of thrombomodulin, to activate enough of the TAFI pool to subsequently suppress fibrinolysis (71–75). This suggests the concept that a role of the factor

XI–dependent pathway of coagulation is to suppress fibrinolysis through the activation of TAFI, thereby stabilizing the newly formed clot. The concept of premature lysis has also led to the hypothesis that bleeding in hemophiliacs is caused as much by a failure to trigger the TAFI pathway and therefore suppress fibrinolysis as it is by the formation of a clot in the first place. This hypothesis, although very plausible, has yet to be tested in a systematic way.

# ASSAYS FOR THROMBIN-ACTIVATABLE FIBRINOLYSIS INHIBITOR AND ACTIVE THROMBIN-ACTIVATABLE FIBRINOLYSIS INHIBITOR

Numerous assays for TAFI and TAFIa have been described, and some are available commercially. The assays for TAFI are either immunologic assays based on measurements of antigen or functional assays based on measurements of the activity of TAFIa following the complete activation of TAFI by thrombin–thrombomodulin. Some of the immunologic assays are compromised somewhat because they respond differentially to various forms of the antigen that can arise because of proteolysis of it (76,77). In addition, some assays have been shown to respond very differently to the Ile325/Thr325 isoforms of TAFI (78). Such assays have been applied to the determination of the average TAFI concentration and its distribution about the average in several large populations. Substantial difference in the averages have been reported by several groups, but all report a fairly broad concentration distribution (77,79). The individual variations have been reported to be determined mostly by genetics, as opposed to by environment (80). The difference in average values reported by different groups may reflect differences in concentrations assigned to assay standards rather than real differences between the populations studied.

Assays for the enzyme TAFIa are based on measuring its carboxypeptidase B–like function with a variety of substrates. These assays are complicated by the existence at relatively high levels of the constitutively active carboxypeptidase B–like enzyme, known as carboxypeptidase N, in plasma. Its concentration is approximately 100 nM, which is about 100 times the level at which TAFIa would have a significant effect on fibrinolysis. Therefore, detecting TAFIa at levels in the range of 1 nM, for example, requires a substrate that is highly selective for TAFIa or an inhibitor that is highly specific for carboxypeptidase N. No synthetic substances with absolute specificity have been described to date, but the judicious use of partially selective substrates has indicated that the endogenous basal level of TAFIa is less than 100 pM (81,82). Another assay has been described for TAFIa that is on the basis of its ability to downregulate plasminogen activation (83). In this assay, high-molecular-weight soluble fibrin degradation products are incubated for a designated period with the plasmin sample containing TAFIa. Following this, the residual cofactor activity of the fibrin degradation products is measured in cleavage of a fluorescent plasminogen derivative by the vampire bat plasminogen activator. This assay is very specific for TAFIa, as opposed to carboxypeptidase N, and it responds to TAFIa in the sample at levels ranging from 5 to 200 pM. Therefore, it is both very specific and highly sensitive. The application of it to five freshly drawn plasma samples from apparently healthy volunteers showed the basal level of plasma TAFIa to be 11 pM. This is only approximately 0.01% of the TAFI level in plasma, suggesting very little systemic activation of the TAFI pathway under basal conditions.

# ACTIVATION OF THROMBIN-ACTIVATABLE FIBRINOLYSIS INHIBITOR *IN VITRO* AND *IN VIVO*

Indirect evidence for the activation of TAFI upon clotting *in vitro* is provided by the timing of subsequent fibrinolysis when a plasminogen activator is included in the experiments. The time to achieve lysis after clotting is considerably reduced when a carboxypeptidase B inhibitor is included. Quantitatively similar results are obtained if a monoclonal antibody directed at TAFI that prevents its activation is included. From such observations, the conclusion is reached that TAFI activation occurs following clotting in plasma. Studies to directly measure TAFIa over time, when a clot is formed through the coagulation cascade and subsequently lyzed because of included tPA, have shown that TAFIa is formed shortly after clotting. Its concentration exhibits a transient peak that decays with a half-life of approximately 10 minutes. The activator is presumably thrombin, formed after the clot is made. Some time later, fibrinolysis occurs, and this is accompanied by a second transient burst of TAFIa activity; in this case, the activator is presumably plasmin (81). TAFIa generated in the first peak appears to delay fibrinolysis, but that which occurs in the second peak does not because it is likely formed too late in the sequence of events. Evidence for activation of TAFI in spontaneously clotting whole blood is provided by the transient increase in carboxypeptidase B–like activity in serum. This activity is unstable and therefore appears only transiently (6). Its appearance, in retrospect, provided the first clue to the existence of TAFI. Studies in thrombolysis models in animals indirectly indicate that TAFI can be activated *in vivo* and that TAFIa can retard fibrinolysis (76,84,85). A particularly revealing study (76) within an arterial thrombolysis model in the rabbit showed that a TAFIa inhibitor included along with tPA could increase the apparent potency of the activator by approximately threefold. It could also reduce the time to reperfusion and markedly enhance patency, with no appreciable increase in bleeding. A similar study in a dog model showed directly that TAFI is activated during thrombolysis and that this could be diminished or eliminated with a reversible synthetic thrombin inhibitor (86). All of these studies together show that TAFI is activated postclotting *in vitro* and that it can be activated *in vivo*. However, the scope of conditions under which it is activated *in vivo*, the extent to which it is activated, and the duration are not yet known in detail.

# PHYSIOLOGIC AND PATHOPHYSIOLOGIC ROLES OF THE THROMBIN-ACTIVATABLE FIBRINOLYSIS INHIBITOR PATHWAY

Studies *in vivo* and in selected animal models indicate that the TAFI pathway suppresses the activity of the fibrinolytic cascade when coagulation is triggered. This observation strongly suggests that it contributes to the balance between fibrin deposition and removal. Because the plasma level of TAFI is considerably lower than the $K_m$ value for its activation by thrombin–thrombomodulin, its rate of activation, all other things being equal, would be expected to be proportional to its plasma concentration. Therefore, the impact on fibrinolysis could be expected to vary with the plasma concentration, and this expectation has been confirmed experimentally (87). Theoretically, therefore, variations in plasma levels would associate with tendencies to bleed or thrombose. Whether this occurs has been examined in numerous epidemiologic studies (88–136), results of which are summarized in Table 20-1. Among the

**TABLE 20-1**

OVERVIEW OF STUDIES OF proCPU (THROMBIN-ACTIVATABLE FIBRINOLYSIS INHIBITOR)
AS A RISK FACTOR FOR CARDIOVASCULAR DISEASE

| Authors | Results | Assay method[a] | Reference |
|---|---|---|---|
| **VENOUS THROMBOEMBOLISM** | | | |
| Libourel et al. | Factor $V_{Leiden}$ carriers with venous thromboembolism have higher proCPU plasma concentrations than their first-degree relatives (also factor $V_{Leiden}$ carriers); 115% (76,88–146), $n = 17$ versus 103% (76–83,85,86,88–193), $n = 136$, $P = 0.009$ (median and range) | 1 | 88 |
| Schroeder et al. | No difference in proCPU plasma antigen levels between patients with acute pulmonary embolism (PE) and patients with suspected but excluded pulmonary embolism (121.9% ± 30%, $n = 71$ vs. 114.9 ± 42.9, $n = 49$); in patients was PE, proCPU was higher in patients with high occlusion rate (occlusion rate 95%–100%, proCPU: 134.8% ± 52% vs. occlusion rate <50%, proCPU: 107.8 ± 30.4, $P = 0.033$) | 2 | 89 |
| van Tilburg et al. | No difference in proCPU plasma levels between patients with venous thrombosis and control subjects (107 ± 14 U/dL, $n = 474$ and 107 ± 12 U/dL, $n = 474$ patients and controls respectively), but more patients than controls with high proCPU levels (>90th percentile); OR, 1.7 (95% CI, 1.1–2.5) | 3 | 90 |
| **ARTERIAL DISEASE** | | | |
| Brouwers et al. | Higher proCPU levels in patients with nonrefractory unstable angina pectoris than in refractory patients; 114.4 (109.0–120.2) U/dL, $n = 133$ versus 105.6 (99.0–111.6) U/dL, $n = 76$, $P = 0.042$ (median and 95% CI) | 4 | 91 |
| Juhan-Vague et al. | No difference in proCPU plasma concentration in men who subsequently had myocardial infarction or coronary death when compared with their controls in France or in Northern Ireland (France: 119% ± 3%, $n = 94$ vs. 113% ± 4%, $n = ?$ $P = 0.21$, Northern Ireland: 115% ± 4%, $n = 65$ vs. 119% ± 5% $n = ?$, $P = 0.58$) (mean ± SEM) | 2 | 93 |
| Lau et al. | Higher preprocedural proCPU plasma levels in patients with restenosis (108% ± 33% vs. 94% ± 30%, $P = 0.011$) and pro CPU plasma levels correlated with 6 mo % diameter stenosis after percutaneous coronary intervention ($n = 159$, $r = 0.21$, $P = 0.013$) | 5 | 94 |
| Leurs et al. | No difference in proCPU plasma concentration between patients who had myocardial infarction and their controls; (570.3 ± 84:4 U/L, $n = 283$ vs. 578.2 U/L, $n = 291$, $P > 0.05$) | 1 | 95 |
| Montaner et al. | Higher proCPU plasma levels determined in samples drawn within the first 24 h after onset of symptoms in patients with ischemic stroke, but before treatment was started compared to the levels found in healthy controls (158.4% ± 53.2%, $n = 30$ vs. 105.6% ± 30.2%, $n = 30$, $P > 0.01$) | 6 | 96 |
| Morange et al. | In France, mean levels of proCPU were significantly higher in men who subsequently developed angina pectoris than in their controls (mean ± SD: 119% ± 5%, $n = 81$ vs. 107% ± 3%, $n = 81$, $P = 0.02$), whereas no difference was observed in Northern Ireland (124% ± 6%, $n = 62$ vs. 121% ± 4% $n = 124$, $P > 0.05$) (mean ± *SEM*) | 2 | 97 |
| Salomon et al. | No difference in proCPU plasma levels in patients with factor XI deficiency with or without a history of myocardial infarction (121.2% ± 30.7%, $n = 16$ vs. 134.3% ± 47.2%, $n = 79$, $P = 0.23$) | 4 | 98 |
| Santamaria et al. | Higher proCPU plasma levels in patients with ischemic stroke than in healthy controls (113.7% ± 25 %, $n = 114$ vs. 102% ± 19%, $n = 150$, $P > 0.05$) | 7 | 99 |
| Schroeder et al. | No difference in the proCPU concentration determined in venous plasma of patients with coronary arterial disease (defined as the presence of at least one stenosis of >20% in a major coronary artery or in one of the branches) compared to controls, but higher levels in the intracoronary plasma samples [venous: 115 (110.9–119.2)%, $n = 362$ vs. 109.0 (102.7–115.4)%, $n = 134$, $P = 0.158$; intracoronary: 110.2 (105.6–114.8)% vs. 101.4 (95.0–107.8)%, $P = 0.044$]; no difference in proCPU levels determined in venous intracoronary plasma when CAD was defined as more than 50% stenosis (standard cutoff value median and 95% CI) | 2 | 100 |

*(continued)*

## TABLE 20-1

CONTINUED

| Authors | Results | Assay method[a] | Reference |
|---------|---------|-----------------|-----------|
| Silveira et al. | Higher proCPU plasma concentration in men requiring coronary artery bypass grafting because of stable angina pectoris than in control (1,029 ± 154 U/L, $n = 110$, vs. 974 ± 140 U/L, $n = 56$, $P > 0.05$) | 1 | 101 |
| Zorio et al. | Young patients with myocardial infarction compared with controls had higher proCPU plasma levels when measured with an activity assay, but lower when antigen was determined (activity-based: 11.6 ± 1.23 μg/mL, $n = 96$ vs. 10.39 ± 1.42 μg/mL, $n = 99$, $P > 0.001$; antigen: 94.09% ± 29.80% vs. 103.78 ± 28.25 $P > 0.05$) | 8,9 | 102 |
| Colucci et al. | ProCPU plasma concentration measured with ELISA and activity assay is reduced in patients with cirrhosis compared to healthy subjects [proCPU measured with a functional assay: 8.7 (5.6–12.3) μg/mL, $n = 30$ vs. 21.7 (16.6–26.7) μg/mL, $n = 30$, $P > 0.05$] | 8,9 | 103 |
| Guo et al. | No difference in proCPU antigen levels in plasma in patients with rheumatoid arthritis ($n = 50$) in comparison with controls ($n = 80$), whereas severe hepatitis ($n = 11$) was associated with lower proCPU plasma concentrations | 10 | 104 |
| Lisman et al. | Low proCPU plasma levels in plasma in patients with mild, moderate, and severe cirrhosis compared to controls (66% ± 13%, $n = 19$; 55% ± 22%, $n = 20$; 47% ± 18%, $n = 25$ vs. 103% ± 20%, $n = 20$, $P > 0.001$) in all three cases | 11 | 105 |
| van Gorp et al. | ProCPU plasma concentrations measured with ELISA and an activity-based assay are reduced in patients with dengue hemorrhagic fever in comparison to pooled plasma from 150 controls. Antigen 31.8% $n = 50$; activity, 46% proCPU plasma levels were lower in nonsurvivors than in survivors. Antigen: 33.5%, $n = 13$ versus 48.7%, $n = 37$ and activity: 20.1% versus 34% (median) | 7,11 | 106 |
| van Thiel et al. | Lower proCPU plasma concentration in patients with liver disease than in controls; range of mean proCPU concentration in different types of liver diseases 1.0–2.2 μg/mL, controls: 6.3 ± 1 μg/mL (mean ± SEM) | 8 | 107 |
| Watanabe et al. | Lower proCPU plasma concentrations in patients with DIC than in non-DIC and healthy subjects (antigen: 106.9% ± 16.1% $n = 36$, 127.8% ± 15.1%, $n = 15$ and 122.8% ± 10.2%, $n = 17$, activity-based: 1.97 ± 1.41 μg/mL, 3.37 ± 1.21 μg/mL, 3.52 ± 0.33 μg/mL, respectively) | 8,11 | 108 |

### COAGULATION AND HEMATOLOGICAL DISORDERS

| Authors | Results | Assay method[a] | Reference |
|---------|---------|-----------------|-----------|
| Antovic et al. | Lower proCPU plasma concentration in patients with hemophilia A than in age-matched controls when proCPU is measured with an activity-based assay, but not when antigen is measured (activity-based: 13.09 ± 3.81 μg/mL, $n = 17$ vs. 17.85 ± 4.62 μg/mL, $n = 13$, $P = 0.01$; antigen: 83.02% ± 34.49% vs. 98.87% ± 37.4% $P = 0.28$) | 8 | 109 |
| Meijers et al. | Patients with acute promyelocytic leukemia have lower plasma proCPU levels than their controls when measured with an activity-based assay, but not when measured with ELISA; proCPU plasma levels determined with an activity-based assay: 37% ± 39% versus 107 ± 41, $P < 0.0001$ and proCPU antigen levels: 97% ± 21%, versus 97% ± 21%, $P > 0.05$, $n = 15$ and 20, patients and controls, respectively. | 7,11 | 110 |

### KIDNEY TRANSPLANTATION, NEPHROTIC SYNDROME, AND DIALYSIS

| Authors | Results | Assay method[a] | Reference |
|---------|---------|-----------------|-----------|
| Brzosko et al. | No correlation between proCPU plasma antigen levels and intima media thickness of the common carotid artery, which relates to coronary and arterial disease in patients with a kidney transplant ($n = 33$) | 4 | 111 |
| Hryszko et al. | Higher proCPU plasma levels in patients undergoing peritoneal dialysis than in controls (proCPU antigen 227.1% ± 143.5% $n = 14$ | 4,8 | 112 |

*(continued)*

## TABLE 20-1

CONTINUED

| Authors | Results | Assay method[a] | Reference |
|---|---|---|---|
| | vs. 106.1% ± 58%; $n = 18$ $P < 0.05$; proCPU determined with the activity-based assay: $0.7 \pm 0.2$ $\mu$g/mL vs. $0.3 \pm 0.2$ $\mu$g/mL $P < 0.0001$); no difference in proCPU plasma levels in patients undergoing hemodialysis compared to controls (proCPU antigen: 125.9% ± 85.2%, $n = 21$ vs. 106.1% ± 58.8%, $n = 18$, proCPU measured with activity-based assay: $0.5 \pm 0.4$ $\mu$g/mL vs. $0.3 \pm 0.2$ $\mu$g/mL) | | |
| Hryszko et al. | Higher proCPU plasma antigen levels in nondiabetic patients with a kidney transplant than in age- and sex-matched controls (128.8% ± 58.7%, $n = 29$ vs. 53.1% ± 29.4%, $n = 18$) | 4 | 113 |
| Malyszko et al. | Higher proCPU plasma levels in patients with kidney transplant and with hypercholesterolemia than in patients having normal serum lipids (antigen 283% ± 123% vs. 234% ± 98%, $P < 0.05$; proCPU determined with the activity-based assay: 1.9 $\mu$g/mL vs. 1.26 $\mu$g/mL $P < 0.05$; $n = 26$ and 20, respectively) | 4,8 | 114 |
| Malyszko et al. | Higher proCPU levels in patients with nephrotic syndrome than in controls; proCPU antigen: 162% ± 70.8% versus 110.6% ± 44.2%, $P < 0.05$; proCPU determined with an activity-based assay: $4.16 \pm 3.41$ $\mu$g/mL versus $0.78 \pm 0.31$ $\mu$g/mL, $P < 0.01$, $n = 22$ and 21, patient and controls, respectively | 4,8 | 115 |
| Malyszko et al. | Recombinant human erythropoietin does not influence proCPU levels in patients on continuous ambulatory peritoneal dialysis; proCPU before and after 3 mo treatment; antigen 302% ± 208% versus 204% ± 141%, $P = 0.07$, functional: 1.25% ± 0.66 $\mu$g/mL versus $0.98 \pm 0.61$ $\mu$g/mL $P = 0.06$, $n = 17$ | 4,8 | 116 |
| Malyszko et al. | In patients on continuous ambulatory peritoneal dialysis, plasma levels of proCPU decreased after 6 mo of simvastatin treatment reaching values comparable to controls (baseline: 122.99% ± 50.89%, after 6 mo treatment: 80.72% ± 30.67%, $P < 0.02$, controls 53.06% ± 29.37%) 6 mo after simvastatin withdrawal proCPU plasma levels were not different from the baseline value (118.76% ± 56.43%, $P > 0.05$) $n = 7$ | 4 | 117 |
| Malyszko et al. | Azathioprine does not influence proCPU plasma concentration in kidney transplant recipients on cyclosporine and prednisone (proCPU antigen: 268.8% ± 138.9%, $n = 14$, vs. 246.0% ± 114.8% $n = 31$; proCPU determined with activity-based assay: 0.82 $\mu$g/mL ± 0.28 vs. $0.76 \pm 0.33$ $\mu$g/mL, treatment with azathioprine and without, respectively) | 4,8 | 118 |
| **DIABETES AND OBESITY** | | | |
| Antovic et al. | No difference in proCPU plasma levels in patients with type I diabetes mellitus with or without microvascular complications compared to healthy subjects; proCPU antigen: 59.7% ± 7.2%, 73.4% ± 8.9% versus 91.9% ± 12.2%; functional levels $18.6 \pm 1.3$ $\mu$g/mL, $17.4 \pm 1.1$ $\mu$g/mL and $17.3 \pm 0.6$ $\mu$g/mL in diabetic with ($n = 18$) and without ($n = 20$) microvascular complications and controls ($n = 20$) $P > 0.05$ | 4,8 | 119 |
| Aubert et al. | Higher proCPU plasma antigen levels in obese than in lean subjects; ELISA 1: 107 (82,83,81,85,86,76,88–116) versus 89 (78–83,85,86,76, 88–104), $P < 0.001$ ELISA 2:114 (95–137) versus 88 (77–83,85,86,76, 88–105), $P < 0.001$ $n = 89$ and 64, respectively (median and 25 and 75 percentile) | 2,10 | 120 |
| Hori et al. | Higher proCPU plasma concentrations determined with ELISA and activity-based assay in type 2 DM patients versus controls (antigen: 143% vs. 115%, $P < 0.05$; activity 39% vs. 21%, $P < 0.05$ $n = 57$ and 30, respectively) Higher proCPU plasma levels in obese patients with DM than in nonobese patients with DM Higher proCPU plasma antigen levels in obese nondiabetic persons | 7,12 | 121 |

*(continued)*

**TABLE 20-1**

CONTINUED

| Authors | Results | Assay method[a] | Reference |
|---|---|---|---|
| | than in nonobese (142.1%, $n = 10$ vs. 100.8%, $n = 20$, $P < 0.05$) whereas no difference was detected withan activity-based assay (mean $\pm$ SEM) | | |
| Schatteman et al. | Higher proCPU level in patients with type 2 diabetes than in controls; proCPU: 1,080 $\pm$ 152 U/L, $n = 50$ versus 996 $\pm$ 181 U/L, $n = 50$, $P = 0.013$ | 1 | 122 |
| Yano et al. | Higher proCPU plasma levels in patients with diabetes than in controls (147.4% $\pm$ 11.6%, $n = 39$ vs. 99.5% $\pm$ 4.9%, $n = 20$, $P < 0.05$) Higher plasma levels of proCPU in patients with diabetes and microalbuminuria than in diabetics without microalbuminuria (194% $\pm$ 24.5%, $n = 12$ vs. 128.8 $\pm$ 12.3, $n = 27$, $P < 0.05$) | 12 | 123 |
| **HORMONE THERAPY AND PREGNANCY** | | | |
| Antovic et al. | Preeclampsia with or without fetal growth retardation is associated with decreased proCPU plasma concentrations in comparison to normal pregnancies (48.89% $\pm$ 26.83%, $n = 46$ vs. 116.30% $\pm$ 74.1%, $n = 16$, $P < 0.0001$) | 4 | 124 |
| Bladbjerg et al. | 5–6 yr of hormone replacement (oestradiol alone or combined with noretisterone acetate) had no effect on plasma concentrations of proCPU in postmenopausal women (treatment: 132.9% $\pm$ 39.3%, $n = 187$, no treatment: 132.1% $\pm$ 41.6%, $n = 249$, $P = 0.86$) | 10 | 125 |
| Juhan-Vague et al. | The use of OC did not influence the plasma concentration of proCPU, whereas hormone replacement therapy (HRT) reduced the proCPU plasma concentration (women using HRT 103% $\pm$ 41%, $n = 43$ vs. 111% $\pm$ 35%, $n = 108$, $P < 0.01$) | 2 | 126 |
| Kemmeren et al. | Second- (30 $\mu$g ethinyloestradiol/150 $\mu$g levonorgestrel) and third-generation (30 $\mu$g ethinyloestradiol/150 $\mu$g desogestrel) OC increased plasma levels of proCPU, whereas no change in proCPU plasma concentration was observed when levonorgestrel or desogestrel were given alone; mean difference (95% CI) levonorgestrel containing OC versus levonorgestrel only: 7.3 (2.7–11.9) %, $n = 24$, desogestrel containing OC versus desogestrel only: 11.8 (1.7–2.2)%, $n = 27$; second- and third-generation OC increased proCPU levels in carriers of factor$V_{Leiden}$; desogestrel given alone reduced the proCPU plasma concentration, whereas levonorgestrel had no effect; mean difference (95% CI) levonorgestrel OC versus levonorgestrel only 9.8 (2.3–17.3)%, $n = 19$; desogestrel containing OC versus desogestrel only: 20.1 (14.1–26.0)%, $n = 16$ | 11 | 127 |
| Libourel et al. | Higher proCPU plasma levels in female factor $V_{Leiden}$ carriers using OC than in nonusers younger than 50 yr of age; 111%, $n = 25$ versus 101%, $n = 20$, $P = 0.02$ (median) | 1 | 88 |
| Meijers et al. | ProCPU antigen levels increased on second-generation OC (30 $\mu$g ethinyloestradiol, 150 $\mu$g levonorgestrel) and on third-generation OC (30 $\mu$g ethinyloestradiol, 150 $\mu$g desogestrel); percentage change from baseline: second-generation OC 8.4% $\pm$ 8.2%, $n = 28$; third-generation OC 12.7% $\pm$ 9.1%, $n = 28$ | 11 | 128 |
| Post et al. | Oestradiol combined with trimegestone reduced the proCPU plasma concentration; mean (95% CI) percentage change from baseline versus placebo was −8.4% (−15.7 to −1.1) after 4 wk and −5.9% (−11.7 to −0.1) after 12 wk, placebo $n = 16$, treatment $n = 14$; oestradiol alone or combined with dydrogesterone had no effect | 13 | 129 |
| Stromqvist et al. | Higher proCPU plasma levels in women receiving hormone therapy than in nonusers (14.0 $\pm$ 2.3 $\mu$g/mL, $n = 127$) versus (12.7 $\pm$ 2.5 $\mu$g/mL, $n = 141$, $P < 0.0001$) | 10 | 130 |
| Schatteman et al. | Higher proCPU plasma concentrations in women receiving hormone therapy than in nonusers (1,006 $\pm$ 152 U/L, $n = 130$) versus (930 $\pm$ 156 U/L, $n = 144$, $P < 0.0001$) | 1 | 131 |
| Vogelvang et al. | Raloxifene reduced proCPU plasma concentrations, whereas equine oestradiol combined with medroxyprogesterone acetate had no effect; | 13 | 132 |

*(continued)*

## TABLE 20-1

CONTINUED

| Authors | Results | Assay method[a] | Reference |
|---------|---------|-----------------|-----------|
| | mean percentage (95% CI) change from baseline versus placebo ($n = 23$) after 24 mo of treatment was $-4.3\%$ ($-8.5$ to $-0.2$) and $-4.0\%$ ($-10.0$ to $2.0$), treatment with raloxifene 60 mg ($n = 23$) and 150 mg ($n = 20$), respectively | | |
| Mousa et al. | proCPU levels increased during pregnancies from $6.6 \pm 1.2$ $\mu$g/mL at booking to $9.6 \pm 1.2$ $\mu$g/mL at 35–39 wk of gestation ($P < 0.001$), then dropped to $7.2 \pm 1.1$ $\mu$g/mL 24 h after delivery; *in vitro* clot lysis times followed the same trend and a negative correlation with APC resistance phenotype was found | 4 | 133 |
| Alacagioglu et al. | proCPU antigen levels measured in 30 healthy and 30 preeclamptic pregnant women; $12.6 \pm 1.9$ $\mu$g/mL in healthy, $12.3 \pm 3.0$ $\mu$g/mL preeclampsia ($P > 0.05$) | 4 | 134 |
| **ACUTE CORONARY DISEASE AND RESTENOSIS** | | | |
| Santamaria et al. | Case–control study (174 cases, 211 controls) of TAFI levels in acute CAD; no significant differences overall; however, adjusted odds ratio for CAD in highest proCPU quartile ($>126\%$) was 3.5 (95% CI, 1.3–8.7) | 7 | 135 |
| Lau et al. | Restenosis investigated in 159 patients with stable angina who had angioplasty or stenting; a significant positive correlation found between preprocedural proCPU level and 6 mo % diameter stenosis ($r = 0.21$, $P = 0.013$) | 4 | 136 |

CI, confidence interval; CAD, coronary artery disease; ELISA, enzyme-linked immunosorbent assay; DIC, disseminated intravascular coagulation; DM, diabetes mellitus; HRT, hormone replacement therapy; OC, oral contraceptives; APC, activated protein C.
[a]Assay methods: 1, activity-based assay for TAFI (133); 2, ELISA (Milan Analytica); 3, in-rocket immunoelectrophoresis; 4, ELISA (Affinity Biologicals); 5, ELISA (American Diagnostica); 6, ELISA (Hyphen Biomed); 7, Activity-based assay for TAFI (89); 8, Activity-based assay for TAFI (American Diagnostica); 9, ELISA (Chromagenix, Milan Italy); 10, ELISA in-house methods; 11, ELISA (89); 12, ELISA (Kordia Laboratory Supply); 13, Activity-based assay for TAFI (95).

findings are the following: (a) elevated levels of plasma TAFI are found in patients with stroke; (b) men requiring coronary artery bypass grafting because of stable angina pectoris had a higher plasma TAFI level than age-matched controls; (c) the restenosis rate 6 months after percutaneous coronary intervention correlated with the plasma TAFI level; (d) increased plasma TAFI correlates with an increased incidence of angina pectoris in France but not in Northern Ireland; (e) no difference is observed between plasma levels of TAFI in those who have a myocardial infarction or coronary death compared to controls, but fewer patients than controls had a TAFI concentration above the 90th percentile; (f) oral contraceptives or hormone replacement therapy are variously associated with changes in plasma TAFI levels; (g) plasma TAFI is low in patients with liver cirrhosis or dengue hemorrhagic fever; and (h) in promyeolocytic leukemia, plasma TAFI measured as antigen is normal but measured as activity is low. Studies to date generally suggest association of the TAFI pathway with various thrombotic pathologies, but no definitive mechanistic connections have yet been identified.

The TAFI knockout mouse is viable and has no obvious thrombotic or bleeding phenotype (137). When crossed with a heterozygous plasminogen knockout, however, a TAFI-deficient phenotype is clearly evident in models involving both clot lysis and leukocyte migration in peritoneal inflammation (138). Therefore, in the context of the partially plasminogen-deficient mouse, the observed phenotypes with respect to TAFIa deficiency are consistent with the conclusion that the TAFI pathway modulates fibrinolysis *in vivo*. The TAFI knockout mouse has been demonstrated to have readily measured deficiencies in wound healing (139,140). This, too, could be a consequence of

deregulated fibrinolysis, but it also might be a consequence of other actions of the TAFI pathway.

# OTHER POTENTIAL FUNCTIONS OF THE ACTIVE THROMBIN-ACTIVATABLE FIBRINOLYSIS INHIBITOR PATHWAY

That the TAFI pathway might have functions other than modulation of fibrinolysis is plausible because TAFIa is able to target molecules other than partially degraded fibrin. Therefore, it might function, like many other members of the carboxypeptidase family of enzymes, as modulators of other processes.

Targets of TAFIa other than plasmin-modified fibrin have been identified. It is very active toward bradykinin and some encephalins, for example (8). It also effectively catalyzes removal of carboxy-terminal arginine or lysine residues from peptides associated with inflammation, such as the anaphylatoxins C5a, and C3a, and thrombin-cleaved osteopontin, which has adhesive and cell-signaling functions thought to be important in inflammatory responses (141–143). A study by Myles et al. (142) suggested that the enzyme TAFIa is considerably more efficient than the constitutively active plasma enzyme carboxypeptidase N in catalyzing cleavage of peptides with sequences based on anaphylatoxins, osteopontin, and bradykinin. They also provided data that indicated in their experimental animal model that TAFIa was more potent than carboxypeptidase N in preventing a hypotensive response to bradykinin. They also suggested that thrombin could upregulate the proinflammatory properties of osteopontin and that subsequent action of TAFIa could down-regulate them.

Clinical evidence for a potential role of the TAFI pathway comes from a recent study by Hovinga et al. on the association between a functional single-nucleotide dimorphism in the coding region of the TAFI gene and outcome (survival or death) in meningococcal disease (144). The dimorphism codes for either threonine or isoleucine at amino acid 325 in the TAFI protein. The Ile325 variant of TAFIa is twice as stable and 60% more potent as an antifibrinolytic than the Thr325 variant. The genotype of survivors and many of their relatives were determined, as were the genotypes of relatives of the nonsurvivors. The analysis indicated that patients whose parents were carriers of the TAFIa Ile325 genotype had a 1.6-fold [confidence interval (CI), 0.7 to 3.7] higher risk of contracting meningococcal disease and a 3.1-fold (CI, 1.0 to 9.5) increased risk of dying from the disease compared with all other genotypes. The mechanistic basis for this can only be speculated upon at this point, but the observations suggest that the TAFI pathway might be significant in the response to sepsis. Two recent reviews have been published on the potential connections between the TAFI pathway and inflammation (145,146). In them, evidence suggesting that TAFI participates in crosstalk between coagulation or fibrinolysis and inflammation is discussed. However, a definitive understanding of these linkages remains to be gathered.

## References

1. Eaton DL, Malloy BE, Tsai SP, et al. Isolation, molecular cloning, and partial characterization of a novel carboxypeptidase B from human plasma. *J Biol Chem* 1991;266:21833–21838.
2. Bajzar L, Manuel R, Nesheim ME. Purification and characterization of TAFI, a thrombin activatable fibrinolysis inhibitor. *J Biol Chem* 1995;270:14477–14484.
3. Bajzar L, Morser J, Nesheim M. TAFI, or plasma procarboxypeptidase B, couples the coagulation and fibrinolytic cascades through the thrombin-thrombomodulin complex. *J Biol Chem* 1996;271:16603–16608.
4. Vanhoof G, Wauters J, Schatteman K, et al. The gene for human carboxypeptidase U (CPU)—a proposed novel regulator of plasminogen activation—maps to 13q14.11. *Genomics* 1996;38:454–455.
5. Boffa MB, Reid TS, Joo E, et al. Characterization of the gene encoding human TAFI (thrombin-activable fibrinolysis inhibitor; plasma procarboxypeptidase B). *Biochemistry* 1999;38(20):6547–6558.
6. Hendriks D, Scharpe S, van Sande M, et al. Characterization of a carboxypeptidase in human serum distinct from carboxypeptidase N. *J Clin Chem Clin Biochem* 1989;27:277–285.
7. Wang W, Hendriks DF, Scharpe SS. Carboxypeptidase U, a plasma carboxypeptidase with high affinity for plasminogen. *J Biol Chem* 1994;269:15937–15944.
8. Tan AK, Eaton DL. Activation and characterization of procarboxypeptidase B from human plasma. *Biochemistry* 1995;34:5811–5816.
9. Campbell W, Okada H. An arginine specific carboxypeptidase generated in blood during coagulation or inflammation which is unrelated to carboxypeptidase N or its subunits. *Biochem Biophys Res Commun* 1989;162:933–939.
10. Nesheim M, Wang W, Boffa M, et al. Thrombomodulin and TAFI in the molecular link between coagulation and fibrinolysis. *Thromb Haemost* 1997;78:386–391.
11. Bouma BN, Meijers JC. Role of blood coagulation factor XI in downregulation of fibrinolysis. *Curr Opin Hematol* 2000;7(5):266–272.
12. Bajzar L. Thrombin activatable fibrinolysis inhibitor and an antifibrinolytic pathway. *Arterioscler Thromb Vasc Biol* 2000;20(12):2511–2518.
13. Booth NA. TAFI meets the sticky ends. *Thromb Haemost* 2001;85(1):1–2.
14. Wu KK, Matijevic-Aleksic N. Thrombomodulin: a linker of coagulation and fibrinolysis and predictor of risk of arterial thrombosis. *Ann Med* 2000;32 (Suppl. 1):73–77.
15. Schatteman K, Goossens F, Leurs J, et al. Carboxypeptidase U at the interface between coagulation and fibrinolysis. *Clin Appl Thromb Hemost* 2001;7(2):93–101.
16. Bouma BN, Marx PF, Mosnier LO, et al. Thrombin-activatable fibrinolysis inhibitor (TAFI, plasma procarboxypeptidase B, procarboxypeptidase R, procarboxypeptidase U). *Thromb Res* 2001;101(5):329–354.
17. Nesheim M. Myocardial infarction and the balance between fibrin deposition and removal. *Ital Heart J* 2001;2(9):641–645.
18. Nagashima M, Yin ZF, Broze GJ Jr, et al. Thrombin-activatable fibrinolysis inhibitor (TAFI) deficient mice. *Front Biosci* 2002;7:556–568.
19. Boffa MB, Nesheim ME, Koschinsky ML. Thrombin activable fibrinolysis inhibitor (TAFI): molecular genetics of an emerging potential risk factor for thrombotic disorders. *Curr Drug Targets Cardiovasc Haematol Disord* 2001; 1(2):59–74.
20. Bouma BN, Meijers JC. Thrombin-activatable fibrinolysis inhibitor (TAFI, plasma procarboxypeptidase B, procarboxypeptidase R, procarboxypeptidase U). *J Thromb Haemost* 2003;1(7):1566–1574.
21. Nesheim M. Thrombin and fibrinolysis. *Chest* 2003;124(Suppl. 3):33S–39S.
22. Antovic JP. Thrombin activatable fibrinolysis inhibitor. A link between coagulation and fibrinolysis. *Clin Lab* 2003;49(9-10):475–486.
23. Bouma BN, Meijers JC. New insights into factors affecting clot stability: a role for thrombin activatable fibrinolysis inhibitor (TAFI; plasma procarboxypeptidase U, procarboxypeptidase R). *Semin Hematol* 2004;41(1 Suppl. 1):13–19.
24. Van de Wouwer M, Conway EM. Novel functions of thrombomodulin in inflammation. *Crit Care Med* 2004;32(Suppl. 5):S254–S261.
25. Bajzar L, Jain N, Wang P, et al. Thrombin activatable fibrinolysis inhibitor: not just an inhibitor of fibrinolysis. *Crit Care Med* 2004; 32 (Suppl. 5): S320–S324.
26. Marx PF. Thrombin-activatable fibrinolysis inhibitor. *Curr Med Chem* 2004; 11(17):2335–2348.
27. Giles AR, Nesheim ME, Herring SW, et al. The fibrinolytic potential of the normal primate following the generation of thrombin *in vivo*. *Thromb Haemost* 1990;63(3):476–481.
28. Esmon CT. Regulation of blood coagulation. *Biochem Biophys Acta Protein Struct Mol Enzymol* 2000;1477(1-2):349–360.
29. Nizzi FA Jr, Kaplan HS. Protein C and S deficiency. *Semin Thromb Hemost* 1999;25(3):265–272.
30. Nicolaes GA, Dahlback B. Activated protein C resistance (FV(Leiden)) and thrombosis: factor V mutations causing hypercoagulable states. *Hematol Oncol Clin North Am* 2003;17(1):37–61.
31. Le Bonniec BF, MacGillivray RTA, Esmon CT. Thrombin Glu-39 restricts the P'3 specificity to nonacidic residues. *J Biol Chem* 1991;266:13796–13803.
32. Mao SS, Cooper CM, Wood T, et al. Characterization of plasmin-mediated activation of plasma procarboxypeptidase B. Modulation by glycosaminoglycans. *J Biol Chem* 1999;274(49):35046–35052.
33. Wang W, Nagashima M, Schneider M, et al. Elements of the primary structure of thrombomodulin required for efficient thrombin-activable fibrinolysis inhibitor activation. *J Biol Chem* 2000;275:22942–22947.
34. Esmon CT, Esmon NL. Protein C activation. *Semin Thromb Hemost* 1984; 10:122–130.
35. Boskovic DS, Giles AR, Nesheim ME. Studies of the role of factor Va in the factor Xa-catalyzed activation of prothrombin, fragment 1.2-prethrombin-2 and dansyl-L-glutamyl-glycyl-L-arginine-meizothrombin in the absence of phospholipid. *J Biol Chem* 1990;265:10497–10505.
36. Mosnier LO, von dem Borne PAKr, Meijers JCM, et al. Plasma TAFI levels influence the clot lysis time in healthy individuals in the presence of an intact intrinsic pathway of coagulation. *Thromb Haemost* 1998;80:829–839.
37. Strömqvist M, Schatteman K, Leurs J, et al. Immunological assay for the determination of procarboxypeptidase U antigen levels in human plasma. *Thromb Haemost* 2001;85:12–17.
38. Bajzar L, Nesheim ME, Morser J, et al. Both cellular and soluble forms of thrombomodulin inhibit fibrinolysis by potentiating the activation of thrombin-activable fibrinolysis inhibitor. *J Biol Chem* 1998;273:2792–2798.
39. Kokame K, Zheng X, Sadler JE. Activation of thrombin activable fibrinolysis inhibitor requires epidermal growth factor-like domain 3 of thrombomodulin and is inhibited competitively by protein C. *J Biol Chem* 1998; 273(20):12135–12139.
40. Sadler JE. Thrombomodulin structure and function. *Thromb Haemost* 1997;78(1):392–395.
41. Clarke JH, Light DR, Blasko E, et al. The short loop between epidermal growth factor-like domains 4 and 5 is critical for human thrombomodulin function. *J Biol Chem* 1993;268:6309–6315.
42. Wang W, Nagashima M, Morser J, et al. Comparison of the structures of thrombomodulin required for the activation of protein C and TAFI. *Fibrinolysis and Proteolysis* 1998;12:11–26.
43. Glaser CB, Morser J, Clarke JH, et al. Oxidation of a specific methionine in thrombomodulin by activated neutrophil products blocks cofactor activity. A potential rapid mechanism for modulation of coagulation. *J Clin Invest* 1992;90:2565–2573.
44. Hall SC, Nagashima M, Zhao L, et al. Thrombin interacts with thrombomodulin, protein C and thrombin activable fibrinolysis inhibitor via specific and distinct domains. *J Biol Chem* 1999;274(36):25510–25516.
45. Bell R, Stevens WK, Jia ZC, et al. Fluorescence properties and functional roles of tryptophan residues 60d, 96, 148, 207, and 215 of thrombin. *J Biol Chem* 2000;275(38):29513–29520.
46. Schneider M, Nagashima M, Knappe S, et al. Amino acid residues in the P6-P'3 region of thrombin-activable fibrinolysis inhibitor (TAFI) do not determine the thrombomodulin dependence of TAFI activation. *J Biol Chem* 2002;277(12):9944–9951.
47. Doolittle RF. Fibrinogen and fibrin. *Ann Rev Biochem* 1984;53:195–229.
48. Wall U, Jern C, Jern S. High capacity for tissue-type plasminogen activator release from vascular endothelium *in vivo*. *J Hypertens* 1997;15:1641–1647.
49. Hoylaerts M, Rijken DC, Lijnen HR, et al. Kinetics of the activation of plasminogen by human tissue plasminogen activator role of fibrin. *J Biol Chem* 1982;257:2912–2919.

50. Horrevoets AJG, Pannekoek H, Nesheim ME. A steady-state template model that describes the kinetics of fibrin-stimulated Glu1– and Lys78- plasminogen activation by native tissue type plasminogen activator and variants that lack either the finger or kringle 2 domain. *J Biol Chem* 1997;272:2183–2191.

51. Castellino FJ. Recent advances in the chemistry of the fibrinolytic system. *Chem Rev* 1981;81:431–446.

52. Suenson E, Lutzen O, Thorsen S. Initial plasmin-degradation of fibrin as the basis of a positive feed-back mechanism in fibrinolysis. *Eur J Biochem* 1984; 140:513–522.

53. Wang W, Boffa MB, Bajzar L, et al. A study of the mechanism of inhibition of fibrinolysis by activated thrombin-activable fibrinolysis inhibitor. *J Biol Chem* 1998;273(42):27176–27181.

54. Collen D, Lijnen HR. Basic and clinical aspects of fibrinolysis and thrombolysis. *Blood* 1991;78:3114–3124

55. Lijnen HR, Collen D. Alpha 2-antiplasmin. In: Barrett AJ, Salvesen G, eds. *Proteinase inhibitors*. New York: Elsevier Science Publishers BV, 1986:457–476.

56. Lee AYY, Fredenburgh JC, Stewart RJ, et al. Like fibrin, (DD)E, the major degradation product of crosslinked fibrin, protects plasmin from inhibition by $\alpha_2$-antiplasmin. *Thromb Haemost* 2001;85(3):502–508.

57. Schneider M, Nesheim M. A study of the protection of plasmin from antiplasmin inhibition within an intact fibrin clot during the course of clot lysis. *J Biol Chem* 2004;279(14):13333–13339.

58. Schneider M, Brufatto N, Neill E, et al. Activated thrombin-activatable fibrinolysis inhibitor reduces the ability of high molecular weight fibrin degradation products to protect plasmin from antiplasmin. *J Biol Chem* 2004;279(14):13340–13345.

59. Francis CW, Marder VJ. A molecular model of plasmic degradation of crosslinked fibrin. *Semin Thromb Haemost* 1982;8:25–35.

60. Walker JB, Nesheim ME. The molecular weights, mass distribution, chain composition, and structure of soluble fibrin degradation products released from a fibrin clot perfused with plasmin. *J Biol Chem* 1999;274(8):5201–5212.

61. Boffa MB, Bell R, Stevens WK, et al. Roles of thermal instability and proteolytic cleavage in regulation of activated thrombin activable fibrinolysis inhibitor. *J Biol Chem* 2000;275(17):12868–12878.

62. Schneider M, Boffa M, Stewart R, et al. Two naturally occurring variants of TAFI (Thr-325 and Il-325) differ substantially with respect to thermal stability and antifibrinolytic activity of the enzyme. *J Biol Chem* 2002;277(2):1021–1030.

63. Marx PF, Hackeng TM, Dawson PE, et al. Inactivation of active thrombin-activable fibrinolysis inhibitor takes place by a process that involves conformational instability rather than proteolytic cleavage. *J Biol Chem* 2000;275 (17):12410–12415.

64. Brouwers GJ, Vos HL, Leebeek FWG, et al. A novel, possibly functional, single nucleotide polymorphism in the coding region of the *Thrombin-activatable Fibrinolysis Inhibitor (TAFI)* gene is also associated with TAFI levels. *Blood* 2001;98(6):1992–1993.

65. Leurs J, Nerme V, Sim Y, et al. Carboxypeptidase U (TAFIa) prevents lysis from proceeding into the propagation phase through a threshold-dependent mechanism. *J Thromb Haemost* 2004;2(3):416–423.

66. Walker JB, Bajzar L. The intrinsic threshold of the fibrinolytic system is modulated by basic carboxypeptidases, but the magnitude of the antifibrinolytic effect of activated thrombin-activatable fibrinolysis inhibitor is masked by its instability. *J Biol Chem* 2004;279(27):27896–27904.

67. Walker JB, Hughes B, James I, et al. Stabilization *versus* inhibition of TAFIa by competitive inhibitors *in vitro*. *J Biol Chem* 2003;278(11):8913–8921.

68. Schneider M, Nesheim M. Reversible inhibitors of TAFIa can both promote and inhibit fibrinolysis. *J Thromb Haemost* 2003;1(1):147–154.

69. Brummel KE, Paradis SG, Butenas S, et al. Thrombin functions during tissue factor-induced blood coagulation. *Blood* 2002;100(1):148–152.

70. Broze GJ Jr, Gailani D. The role of factor XI in coagulation. *Thromb Haemost* 1993;70:72–74.

71. Mann KG, Butenas S, Brummel K. The dynamics of thrombin formation. *Arterioscler Thromb Vasc Biol* 2003;23(1):17–25.

72. Broze GJ Jr, Higuchi DA. Coagulation-dependent inhibition of fibrinolysis: role of carboxypeptidase-U and the premature lysis of clots from hemophilic plasma. *Blood* 1996;88:3815–3823.

73. von dem Borne PAKr, Meijers JCM, Bouma BN. Feedback activation of factor XI by thrombin in plasma results in additional formation of thrombin that protects fibrin clots from fibrinolysis. *Blood* 1995;86:3035–3042.

74. von dem Borne PAKr, Bajzar L, Meijers JCM, et al. Thrombin mediated activation of factor XI results in a thrombin-activatable fibrinolysis inhibitor-dependent inhibition of fibrinolysis. *J Clin Invest* 1997;99(10): 2323–2327.

75. Bajzar L, Nesheim ME, Tracy PB. The profibrinolytic effect of activated protein C in clots formed from plasma is TAFI-dependent. *Blood* 1996;88: 2093–2100.

76. Klement P, Liao P, Bajzar L. A novel approach to arterial thrombolysis. *Blood* 1999;94(8):2735–2743.

77. Guimaraes AH, van Tilburg NH, Vos HL, et al. Association between thrombin activatable fibrinolysis inhibitor genotype and levels in plasma: comparison of different assays. *Br J Haematol* 2004;124(5):659–665.

78. Gils A, Alessi MC, Brouwers E, et al. Development of a genotype 325-specific proCPU/TAFI ELISA. *Arterioscler Thromb Vasc Biol* 2003; 23:1122–1127.

79. Chetaille P, Alessi MC, Kouassi D, et al. Plasma TAFI antigen variations in healthy subjects. *Thromb Haemost* 2000;83(6):902–905.

80. Henry M, Aubert H, Morange PE, et al. Identification of polymorphisms in the promoter and the 3′ region of the TAFI gene: evidence that plasma TAFI antigen levels are strongly genetically controlled. *Blood* 2001;97(7): 2053–2058.

81. Leurs J, Wissing BM, Nerme V, et al. Different mechanisms contribute to the biphasic pattern of carboxypeptidase U (TAFIa) generation during in vitro clot lysis in human plasma. *Thromb Haemost* 2003;89(2):264–271.

82. Mao SS, Colussi D, Bailey CM, et al. Electrochemiluminescence assay for basic carboxypeptidases: inhibition of basic carboxypeptidases and activation of thrombin-activatable fibrinolysis inhibitor. *Anal Biochem* 2003;319(1): 159–170.

83. Neill EK, Stewart RJ, Schneider MM, et al. A functional assay for measuring activated thrombin-activatable fibrinolysis inhibitor in plasma. *Anal Biochem* 2004;330(2):332–341.

84. Redlitz A, Nicolini FA, Malycky JL, et al. Inducible carboxypeptidase activity. A role in clot lysis in vivo. *Circulation* 1996;93:1328–1330.

85. Refino CJ, DeGuzman L, Schmitt D, et al. Consequences of inhibition of plasma carboxypeptidase B on in vivo thrombolysis, thrombosis and hemostasis. *Fibrinolysis and Proteolysis* 2000;14(5):305–314.

86. Mattsson C, Bjorkman JA, Abrahamsson T, et al. Local proCPU (TAFI) activation during thrombolytic treatment in a dog model of coronary artery thrombosis can be inhibited with a direct, small molecule thrombin inhibitor (melagatran). *Thromb Haemost* 2002;(4):557–562.

87. Mosnier LO, von dem Borne PAKr, Meijers JCM, et al. Plasma TAFI levels influence the clot lysis time in healthy individuals in the presence of an intact intrinsic pathway of coagulation. *Thromb Haemost* 1998;80:829–839.

88. Libourel E, Bank I, Meinardi J, et al. Co-segregation of thrombophilic disorders in factor V leiden carriers; the contributions of factor VIII, factor XI, thrombin activatable fibrinolysis inhibitor and lipoprotein(a) to the absolute risk of venous thromboembolism. *Haematologica* 2002;87:1068–1073.

89. Schroeder V, Kucher N, Kohler HP. Role of thrombin activatable fibrinolysis inhibitor (TAFI) in patients with acute pulmonary embolism. *J Thromb Haemost* 2003;1:492–493.

90. van Tilburg NH, Rosendaal FR, Bertina RM. Thrombin activatable fibrinolysis inhibitor and the risk for deep vein thrombosis. *Blood* 2000;95:2855–2859.

91. Brouwers GJ, Leebeek F, Tanck M, et al. Association between thrombinactivatable fibrinolysis inhibitor (TAFI) and clinical outcome in patients with unstable angina pectoris. *Thromb Haemost* 2003;90:92–100.

92. Juhan-Vague I, Morange PE, Aubert H, et al. Plasma thrombin-activatable fibrinolysis inhibitor antigen concentration and genotype in relation to myocardial infarction in the north and south of Europe. *Arterioscler Thromb Vasc Biol* 2002;22:867–873.

93. Juhan-Vague I, Morange PE. Very high TAFI antigen levels are associated with a lower risk of hard coronary events: the PRIME Study. *J Thromb Haemost* 2003;1:2243–2244.

94. Lau HK, Segev A, Hegele RA, et al. Thrombin-activatable fibrinolysis inhibitor (TAFI): a novel predictor of angiographic coronary restenosis. *Thromb Haemost* 2003;90:1187–1191.

95. Schatteman K, Goossens F, Leurs J, et al. Fast homogeneous assay for plasma procarboxypeptidase U. *Clin Chem Lab Med* 2001;39:806–810.

96. Montaner J, Ribo M, Monasterio J, et al. Thrombin-activatable fibrinolysis inhibitor levels in the acute phase of ischemic stroke. *Stroke* 2003;34:1038–1040.

97. Morange PE, Juhan-Vague I, Scarabin PY, et al. Association between TAFI antigen and ala 147Thr polymorphism of the TAFI gene and the angina pectoris incidence—the PRIME Study. *Thromb Haemost* 2003;89:554–560.

98. Salomon O, Steinberg DM, Dardik R, et al. Inherited factor XI deficiency confers no protection against acute myocardial infarction. *J Thromb Haemost* 2003;1:658–661.

99. Santamaria A, Oliver A, Borrell M, et al. Risk of ischemic stroke associated with functional thrombin-activatable fibrinolysis inhibitor plasma levels. *Stroke* 2003;34:2387–2391.

100. Schroeder V, Chatterjee T, Mehta H, et al. Thrombin activatable fibrinolysis inhibitor (TAFI) levels in patients with coronary artery disease investigated by angiography. *Thromb Haemost* 2002;88:1020–1025.

101. Silveira A, Schatteman K, Goossens F, et al. Plasma procarboxypeptidase U in men with symptomatic coronary artery disease. *Thromb Haemost* 2000; 84:364.

102. Zorio E, Castello R, Falcb C, et al. Thrombin-activatable fibrinolysis inhibitor in young patients with myocardial infarction and its relationship with the fibrinolytic function and the protein C system. *Br J Haematol* 2003;122: 958–965.

103. Colucci M, Binetti BM, Branca MG, et al. Deficiency of thrombin activatable fibrinolysis inhibitor in cirrhosis is associated with increased plasma fibrinolysis. *Hepatology* 2003;38:230–237.

104. Guo X, Morioka A, Kaneko Y, et al. Arginine carboxypeptidase (CPR) in human plasma determined with sandwich ELISA. *Microbiol Immunol* 1999; 43:691–698.

105. Lisman T, Leebeek F, Mosnier L, et al. Thrombin-activatable fibrinolysis inhibitor deficiency in cirrhosis is not associated with increased plasma fibrinolysis. *Gastroenterology* 2001;121:131–139.

106. van Gorp E, Minnema M, Suharti C, et al. Activation of coagulation factor XI, without detectable contact activation in dengue haemorrhagic fever. *Br J Haematol* 2001;113:94–99.

107. van Thiel DH, George M, Fareed J. Low levels of thrombin activatable fibrinolysis inhibitor (TAFI) in patients with chronic liver disease. *Thromb Haemost* 2001;85:667–670.

108. Watanabe R, Wada H, Watanabe Y, et al. Activity and antigen levels of thrombin-activatable fibrinolysis inhibitor in plasma of patients with disseminated intravascular coagulation. *Thromb Res* 2001;104:1–6.

109. Antovic J, Schulman S, Eelde A, et al. Total thrombin-activatable fibrinolysis inhibitor (TAFI) antigen and pro-TAFI in patients with haemophilia A. *Haemophilia* 2001;7:557–560.

110. Meijers JC, Oudijk EJ, Mosnier LO, et al. Reduced activity of TAFI (thrombin-activatable fibrinolysis inhibitor) in acute promyelocytic leukaemia. *Br J Haematol* 2000;108:518–523.

111. Brzosko S, Hryszko T, Lebkowska U, et al. Plasma tissue-type plasminogen activator, fibrinogen, and time on dialysis prior to transplantation are related to carotid intima media thickness in renal transplant recipients. *Transplant Proc* 2003;35:2931–2934.

112. Hryszko T, Malyszko J, Malyszko JS, et al. Patients on peritoneal dialysis but not on hemodialysis have elevated concentration and activity of thrombin-activatable fibrinolysis inhibitor. *Thromb Res* 2001;104:233–238.

113. Hryszko T, Malyszko J, Malyszko JS, et al. A possible role of thrombinactivatable fibrinolysis inhibitor in disturbances of fibrinolytic system in renal transplant recipients. *Nephrol Dial Transplant* 2001;16:1692–1696.

114. Malyszko J, Malyszko JS, Hryszko T, et al. Thrombin-activatable fibrinolysis inhibitor in kidney transplant recipient with dyslipidemia. *Transplant Proc* 2003;35:2219–2221.

115. Malyszko J, Malyszko JS, Mysliwiec M. Markers of endothelial cell injury and thrombin activatable fibrinolysis inhibitor in nephrotic syndrome. *Blood Coagul Fibrinolysis* 2002;13:615–621.

116. Malyszko J, Suchowierska E, Malyszko JS, et al. Some aspects of haemostasis in CAPD patients treated with erythropoietin. *Kidney Blood Press Res* 2002;25:240–244.

117. Malyszko J, Malyszko JS, Hryszko T, et al. Simvastatin affects TAFI and thrombomodulin in CAPD patients. *Thromb Haemost* 2001;86:930–931.

118. Malyszko J, Malyszko JS, Hryszko T, et al. Some aspects of haemostasis in kidney transplant recipients maintained on cyclosporine, azathioprine, and prednisone in comparison to patients treated with cyclosporine and prednisone. *Transplant Proc* 2003;35:2940–2942.

119. Antovic JP, Yngen M, Ostenson CG, et al. Thrombin activatable fibrinolysis inhibitor and hemostatic changes in patients with type I diabetes mellitus with and without microvascular complications. *Blood Coagul Fibrinolysis* 2003;14:551–556.

120. Aubert H, Frere C, Aillaud MF, et al. Weak and non-independent association between plasma TAFI antigen levels and the insulin resistance syndrome. *J Thromb Haemost* 2003;1:791–797.

121. Hori Y, Gabazza EC, Yano Y, et al. Insulin resistance is associated with increased circulating level of thrombin-activatable fibrinolysis inhibitor in type 2 diabetic patients. *J Clin Endocrinol Metab* 2002;87:660–665.

122. Schatteman K, Van Gaal L, Goossens F, et al. Increased procarboxypeptidase U levels in type II diabetes may reflect decreased firbinolytic rate. *Fibrinolysis and Proteolysis* 2000;14:69.

123. Yano Y, Kitagawa N, Gabazza EC, et al. Increased plasma thrombin-activatable fibrinolysis inhibitor levels in normotensive type 2 diabetic patients with microalbuminuria. *J Clin Endocrinol Metab* 2003;88:736–741.

124. Antovic JP, Rafik HR, Antovic A, et al. Does thrombin activatable fibrinolysis inhibitor (TAFI) contribute to impairment of fibrinolysis in patients with preeclampsia and/or intrauterine fetal growth retardation? *Thromb Haemost* 2002;88:644–647.

125. Bladbjerg EM, Madsen JS, Kristensen SR, et al. Effect of long-term hormone replacement therapy on tissue factor pathway inhibitor and thrombin activatable fibrinolysis inhibitor in healthy postmenopausal women: a randomized controlled study. *J Thromb Haemost* 2003;1:1208–1214.

126. Juhan-Vague I, Renucci JF, Grimaux M, et al. Thrombinactivatable fibrinolysis inhibitor antigen levels and cardiovascular risk factors. *Arterioscler Thromb Vasc Biol* 2000;20:2156–2161.

127. Kemmeren JM, Algra A, Meijers JC, et al. Effect of second- and third- generation oral contraceptives on fibrinolysis in the absence and presence of the factor V leiden mutation. *Blood Coagul Fibrinolysis* 2002;13:373–381.

128. Meijers J, Middeldorp S, Tekelenburg W, et al. Increased fibrinolytic activity during use of oral contraceptives is counteracted by an enhanced factor XI-independent down regulation of fibrinolysis: a randomized cross-over study of two low-dose oral contraceptives. *Thromb Haemost* 2000;84:9–14.

129. Post MS, Hendriks DF, Van Der Mooren MJ, et al. Oral oestradiol/trimegestone replacement reduces procarboxypeptidase U (TAFI): a randomized, placebo-controlled, 12-week study in early postmenopausal women. *J Intern Med* 2002;251:245–251.

130. Stromqvist M, Schatteman K, Leurs J, et al. Immunological assay for the determination of procarboxypeptidase U antigen levels in human plasma. *Thromb Haemost* 2001;85:12–17.

131. Schatteman K, Goossens F, Scharpe S, et al. Assay of procarboxypeptidase U, a novel determinant of the fibrinolytic cascade, in human plasma. *Clin Chem* 1999;45:807–813.

132. Vogelvang T, Leurs J, van der Mooren MJ, et al. Raloxifene reduces procarboxypeptidase U, an antifibrinolytic marker. A 2-year randomised, placebo-controlled study in healthy early postmenopausal women. *Menopause* 2004; 11:110–115.

133. Mousa HA, Downey C, Alfirevic Z, et al. Thrombin activatable fibrinolysis inhibitor and its fibrinolytic effect in normal pregnancy. *Thromb Haemost* 2004;92(5):1025–1031.

134. Alacacioglu I, Ozcan MA, Alacacioglu A, et al. Plasma levels of thrombin activatable fibrinolysis inhibitor in normal and preeclamptic pregnant women. *Thromb Res* 2004;114:155–159.

135. Santamaria A, Martinez-Rubio A, Borrell M, et al. Risk of acute coronary artery disease associated with functional thrombin activatable fibrinolysis inhibitor plasma level. *Haematologica* 2004;89:880–881.

136. Lau HK, Segev A, Hegele RA, et al. Thrombin-activatable fibrinolysis inhibitor (TAFI): a novel predictor of angiographic coronary restenosis. *Thromb Haemost* 2003;90(6):1187–1191.

137. Nagashima M, Yin ZF, Zhao L, et al. Thrombin-activatable fibrinolysis inhibitor (TAFI) deficiency is compatible with murine life. *J Clin Invest* 2002; 109(1):101–110.

138. Swaisgood CM, Schmitt D, Eaton D, et al. *In vivo* regulation of plasminogen function by plasma carboxypeptidase B. *J Clin Invest* 2002;110(9): 1275–1282.

139. Te Velde EA, Wagenaar GT, Reijerkerk A, et al. Impaired healing of cutaneous wounds and colonic anastomoses in mice lacking thrombin-activatable fibrinolysis inhibitor. *J Thromb Haemost* 2003;1(10):2087–2096.

140. Boffa MB. TAFI and wound healing: closing a knowledge gap. *J Thromb Haemost* 2003;1(10):2075–2077.

141. Denhardt DT, Noda M, O'Regan AW, et al. Osteopontin as a means to cope with environmental insults: regulatin of inflammation, tissue remodeling, and cell survival. *J Clin Invest* 2001;107:1055–1061.

142. Myles T, Nishimura T, Yun TH, et al. Thrombin activatable fibrinolysis inhibitor, a potential regulator of vascular inflammation. *J Biol Chem* 2003; 278(51):51059–51067.

143. Campbell WD, Lazoura E, Okada N, et al. Inactivation of C3a and C5a octapeptides by carboxypeptidase R and carboxypeptidase N. *Microbiol Immunol* 2002; 46(2):131–134.

144. Hovinga JAK, Franco RF, Zago MA, et al. A functional single nucleotide polymorphism in the thrombin-activatable fibrinolysis inhibitor (TAFI) gene associates with outcome of meningococcal disease. *J Thromb Haemost* 2004;2:54–57.

145. Bajzar L, Jain N, Wang P, et al. Thrombin activatable fibrinolysis inhibitor: not just an inhibitor of fibrinolysis. *Crit Care Med* 2004;32:S320–S324.

146. Van de Wouwer M, Conway EM. Novel functions of thrombinomodulin in inflammation. *Crit Care Med* 2004;32:S254–S261.

# CHAPTER 21 ■ α-MACROGLOBULINS AND KUNINS

JUSTIN P. HART AND SALVATORE V. PIZZO

Proteinases play a wide variety of roles in biologic systems, such as in the clotting and fibrinolytic pathways, activation of zymogens in the digestive system, cleavage of signaling molecule precursors, and initiation and execution of apoptotic cascades; they also provide immune defense against invasion by foreign organisms. Given the diversity of proteinase functions, it is not surprising that a complex system of proteinase inhibitors has evolved to maintain the exquisite balance between proteolytic activation and inhibition.

Because proteinases are the main proteins involved in the clotting and fibrinolytic cascade, the objective of this chapter is to review our current understanding of the structure, mechanism, and biologic functions of the proteinase inhibitors that regulate coagulation and fibrinolysis. In particular, two classes of proteinase inhibitors—the α-macroglobulins and the kunins—are discussed in detail. A third, and the largest, class of inhibitors of the coagulation and fibrinolytic cascades, the serine proteinase inhibitors, or serpins, is discussed in Chapter 13.

Historically, research in the field of proteinase and proteinase inhibitors has been driven by the concept of specificity (i.e., a unique pairing of one proteinase with a particular cognate proteinase inhibitor). This method of investigation has led to the identification of many useful proteinase–proteinase inhibitor pairs that have both high affinity and specificity *in vitro*; however, this conceptual simplification often results in poor explanation of *in vivo* phenomena when tested in complex biologic systems. This is particularly the case with α-macroglobulins and kunins because they are often considered "backup" inhibitors, either because of their broad specificity, as in the case of α-macroglobulins, or because of their lack of high-affinity targets, as in the case of kunins.

The interaction between proteinase and proteinase inhibitor does not end with the inhibition of a target proteinase by its selective inhibitor. The complexes must be rapidly cleared from circulation to prevent dissociation, leading to regeneration of proteolytic activity. Moreover, some proteinase inhibitors, or proteinase–proteinase inhibitor complexes, act either directly as biologic effectors *in vivo* or indirectly by regulating the biologic activity of other signaling molecules. It is possible that these effects may be the true physiologic functions of α-macroglobulins and kunins. In addition to a detailed review of the proteinase inhibitory mechanisms of α-macroglobulins and kunins, we also consider: (a) the receptor-mediated clearance and signal transduction of α-macroglobulin–proteinase complexes, (b) the mechanism by which α-macroglobulin–proteinase complexes facilitate enhanced adaptive immune responses against specific antigens, and (c) the regulation of cytokines and growth factors by α-macroglobulin and α-macroglobulin–proteinase complexes. Moreover, the roles of α-macroglobulin and kunins in biologic fluids are discussed because, during inflammation, these proteinase inhibitors are often extravasated into tissues and extracellular fluids in which significant proteolysis occurs.

## PROTEINASES

A wide variety of proteinases are involved in many different biologic processes. Despite their specificity for particular substrates, most, if not all, of them can be categorized on the basis of one of the four mechanistic classes of substrate hydrolysis—serine, cysteine, aspartic acid, and metalloproteinases (1). Of these four classes, the largest group is the serine proteinases. This group includes many digestive enzymes, such as trypsin and chymotrypsin; all the coagulation and fibrinolytic proteinases; proteinases involved in the complement and contact system; and some of the cellular inflammatory proteinases, such as neutrophil elastase and mast cell tryptase. Most of the mammalian serine proteinases can be placed in a single large family referred to as the *chymotrypsin superfamily* (2). The importance of the active-site serine and histidine is highlighted by the effectiveness of diisopropyl fluorophosphate (DFP), which irreversibly interacts with serine, and of chloromethyl ketone, which reacts with histidine, in abolishing the activity of these proteinases. All the proteinases involved in the pathways of coagulation and fibrinolysis are serine proteinases of the chymotrypsin superfamily.

## INHIBITORS

The importance of proteinase inhibition is reflected in the abundance of proteinase inhibitors in human plasma. If albumin, fibrinogen, and the immunoglobulins are excluded, approximately 20% of all remaining proteins in plasma are proteinase inhibitors. Whereas cysteine and metalloproteinase inhibitors are present constitutively at low levels in the plasma and extracellular fluids (2), serine proteinase inhibitors are extremely abundant. This finding is not surprising, given the predominance of serine proteinases in many biologic processes.

Proteinases that activate the coagulation and fibrinolytic cascades have very limited substrate specificity. They serve primarily to activate the zymogen precursors of one or, at the most, two components of the pathway, usually by a single peptide bond cleavage. Given the strict conformational requirement for clotting and fibrinolytic factor cleavage, it is not surprising that few specific inhibitors of these cascades have been identified. Because the coagulation and fibrinolytic systems are enzyme-amplified cascades, one molecule of initiator (e.g., factor XIIa or tissue plasminogen activator) would theoretically lead to the rapid consumption of all circulating components. This, however, does not occur because of the abundance of coagulation-specific inhibitors that restrict proteolytic activities such as antithrombin III (ATIII) and activated protein C (APC); fibrinolysis-specific inhibitors such as plasminogen activator inhibitors (PAIs) and $\alpha_2$-antiplasmin ($\alpha_2$AP); and broad-specificity inhibitors such as $\alpha_2$-macroglobulin ($\alpha_2$M). The bulk of the clotting and fibrinolytic cascade inhibition does not involve shutting down the pathways at critical points, as might be inferred from the presence of specific inhibitors of these pathways. Rather, they involve a generalized inhibition of all the activated clotting and fibrinolytic factors by $\alpha_2$M and other proteinase inhibitors, resulting in a limited activation that is localized only to the site where this process is initiated.

The remainder of this chapter focuses on two classes of inhibitors: the $\alpha$-macroglobulins and kunins. $\alpha_2$M is biologically unique in that it is the only known proteinase inhibitor that reacts with all four mechanistic classes of proteinases. Although a few patients have been described with somewhat decreased $\alpha_2$M levels, no major deficiency of this protein has been reported in the literature. It is possible that such a deficiency is incompatible with survival. By contrast, there are well-known deficiency diseases of several serpins.

The kunins are a group of less well-known plasma serine proteinase inhibitors. However, this group includes tissue factor pathway inhibitor (TFPI) [also known as *lipoprotein-associated coagulation inhibitor* (LACI)], which binds to the blood coagulation protein factor Xa and inhibits its function.

## $\alpha_2$-Macroglobulin

### General Considerations

$\alpha_2$M is present in human plasma at concentrations ranging from 2 to 5 $\mu$M. It is also present in extravascular fluids at concentrations of approximately 70% of this level. A variety of cells produce $\alpha_2$M, including hepatocytes, fibroblasts, and macrophages (3–5). The half-life of native $\alpha_2$M in humans is approximately 5 to 6 days (6). From these data and from the known plasma concentration of $\alpha_2$M, it can be estimated that 1.0 to 2.5 g of $\alpha_2$M must be eliminated every day. Because the only known mechanism for plasma $\alpha_2$M elimination requires proteinase attack (5,7–11), it is reasonable to speculate that a large fraction of the $\alpha_2$M pool is constantly being eliminated as a result of proteinase scavenging. $\alpha$-Macroglobulins are an ancient class of proteins that have existed for more than 600 million years. The protein is present in the hemolymph of the horseshoe crab, *Limulus polyphemus*, as well as in other invertebrates, and is found in the plasma of all vertebrate species (3–5,12). An interesting feature of this protein family is that multiple forms may be found in various species. One or more of these forms may be constitutive, whereas some forms may appear only during acute-phase reactions or even during pregnancy (3–5).

In general, the protein is composed either of two or four identical subunits of 180 kDa (3,4,13,14). The invertebrate and fish proteins appear to be dimeric forms, whereas the protein present in reptiles, birds, and mammals is a tetrameric form consisting of two pairs of disulfide-bonded subunits (3–5,7,8,12–14). Amphibian plasma contains both a dimeric and a tetrameric protein (7,14). During human pregnancy, in addition to the tetrameric $\alpha_2$M, a dimeric form called *pregnancy zone protein* (PZP) appears in the plasma (4,15,16). This protein reaches peak levels during the last trimester.

An exception to the rule that $\alpha$-macroglobulins are multimeric proteins has been found in mice, rats, and guinea pigs (17–19). These species possess a 180-kDa subunit inhibitor as well as a normally circulating tetrameric protein. The mechanism of proteinase inhibition by this monomeric protein shares some features common to the mechanism of the multimeric inhibitors (20), but it also shows certain distinct properties. Because this form of the inhibitor does not occur in humans, it is not considered in any detail in this chapter. A tetrameric $\alpha$-macroglobulin has been found in tropical snail *Biomphalaria glabrata*, suggesting that invertebrates may also possess multimeric forms of $\alpha$-macroglobulin (21).

The complete amino acid sequence of human $\alpha_2$M has been determined by protein sequencing (22), and studies demonstrate that human $\alpha_2$M is part of a superfamily that includes not only the monomeric, dimeric, and tetrameric proteinase inhibitors but also the complement components C3, C4, and C5 (22,23).

### Mechanism of Proteinase Inhibition by $\alpha_2$-Macroglobulin

$\alpha$-Macroglobulins are unique in their ability to inhibit proteinases from each of the four mechanistic classes (3–5,24,25). The mechanism by which human $\alpha_2$M achieves this broad specificity is also unique. Most of the early work establishing this mechanism was the result of studies performed by Barrett, and their terminology is used to describe the events leading to proteinase inhibition (1,2).

An essential feature of the mechanism by which $\alpha_2$M "inhibits" proteinases is that the active site of the proteinase is not involved in a complex with the inhibitor. Therefore, Ganrot was able to show that the $\alpha_2$M–proteinase complex preserves the ability to cleave small substrates, although it shows little or no proteolytic activity against most macromolecular substrates (26). The initial step in the reaction of $\alpha_2$M with a proteinase involves limited proteolysis on a region of the $\alpha_2$M molecule termed the *bait region* (25) (see Fig. 21-1). The bait

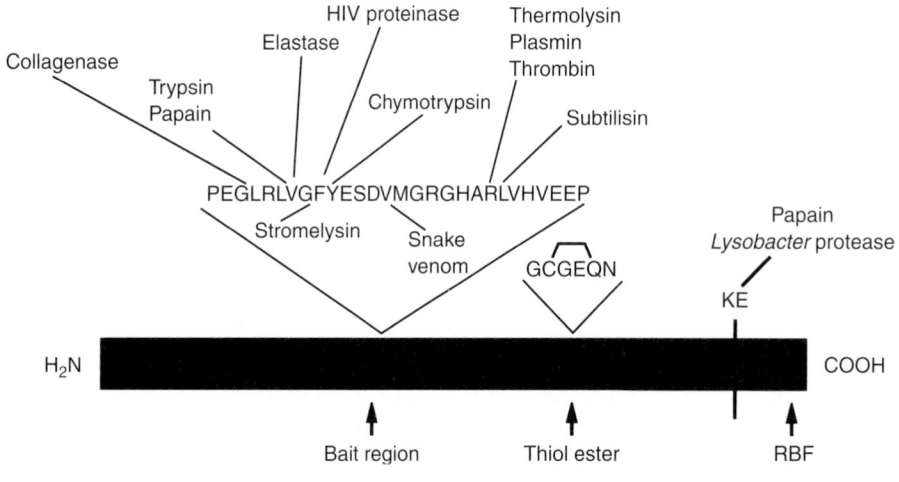

FIGURE 21-1. Subunit structure of the $\alpha_2$-macroglobulin ($\alpha_2$M) monomer. The linear structure of monomeric $\alpha_2$M is shown in this figure. The bait region, thiol ester region, and receptor-binding fragment (*RBF*) are indicated by their respective *arrows*. The cleavage sites for various different proteinases are shown above. The amino acid sequence representing the intrasubunit $\gamma$-glutamyl-$\beta$-cysteinyl thioester bond is shown above the *bar* for the thiol ester region. HIV, human immunodeficiency virus. (From Chu CT, Pizzo SV. Alpha 2-macroglobulin, complement, and biologic defense: antigens, growth factors, microbial proteases, and receptor ligation. *Lab Invest* 1994;71: 792–812, with permission.)

region consists of a sequence of approximately 25 amino acids that corresponds to the different specifications of many proteases and is located approximately halfway down the length of each $\alpha_2$M subunit (27,28). Unless a proteinase cleaves the bait region, it cannot be inhibited by $\alpha_2$M. Studies using recombinant $\alpha_2$M that contain bait region variants show that, in addition to its role as a proteinase cleavage site, the bait region is involved in the noncovalent association of $\alpha_2$M dimers into functional tetramers (29,30). Mutation in this site not only alters the specificity of proteinase cleavage but also prohibits association between $\alpha_2$M dimers. After the initial bait region cleavage, the inhibitor undergoes a large-scale conformational change that entraps the proteinase inside the $\alpha_2$M molecule (24,25,31). This conformational change can be observed as a change in the ultraviolet (UV) and circular dichroic spectra of the protein (31), in migration when electrophoresed under nondenaturing conditions (24,25), or in the sedimentation rate when studied in the ultracentrifuge (31). Because the inhibitor migrates faster after reaction with proteinase when electrophoresed in nondenaturing polyacrylamide gels, Barrett (24) and Barrett and Starkey (25) termed the *conformational* change "slow to fast" transition. Ultracentrifuge studies demonstrated a dramatic change in sedimentation, with the $S_{20,w}$ increasing from 18.5 to 20.3 after proteinase reaction (31). This change is indicative of an approximately 10% compaction of the $\alpha_2$M molecule when it reacts with a proteinase, and it explains the slow to fast change in gel migration (24,25) (Fig. 21-1).

Another important feature of $\alpha_2$M is the presence of a $\gamma$-glutamyl-$\beta$-cysteinyl thiol ester that is composed of the side chains of two residues located at approximately two thirds of the distance from the amino-terminal of each subunit, a feature that is also present in the homologous complement proteins C3 and C4 (32–35) (Fig. 21-1). These thiol esters may react directly with small nucleophiles such as ammonia or methylamine (34,36–38). In human $\alpha_2$M, reaction with methylamine triggers a conformational change similar to that seen after proteinase attack on the bait region (31,39). The conformational change that occurs in methylamine-treated human $\alpha_2$M also prevents proteinases from binding to the inhibitor.

Shortly after proteolytic cleavage of the bait region of native $\alpha_2$M (40), the thiol esters become more highly reactive to nucleophilic attack (41,42). The resultant short-lived intermediate, termed *nascent* $\alpha_2$M (42), has a thiol ester that is susceptible to nucleophilic attack not only by ammonia or small amines, but also by water or the surface lysine residues of the trapped proteinase. Reaction with the lysine $\varepsilon$-amino group generates a $\gamma$-glutamyl-$\varepsilon$-lysyl cross-link, which releases a free cysteine thiol group (33).

A major question raised by these observations is the role of the thiol ester in proteinase inhibition. The tetrameric $\alpha$-macroglobulin from hens' eggs, ovostatin, lacks a thiol ester; however, it is still an effective proteinase inhibitor that functions by a similar trap mechanism (43,44). In fact, it can be demonstrated that human $\alpha_2$M inhibits proteinases just as effectively without forming a covalent cross-link (41,45). In these situations, the inhibition still occurs by a trapping mechanism of the type already described, in which the conformational change is crucial to the mechanism of proteinase inhibition.

What, then, is the function of the thiol ester? A possible hint to its role derives from the study of the $\alpha_2$M homologues PZP and rat $\alpha$-1-inhibitor-3 ($\alpha$1I3). For these proteins to function as inhibitors, the covalent cross-linking of the proteinase seems to be essential (16,20). Proteinases that do not form such a bond are able to degrade $\alpha$1I3. It can possibly be speculated that in the earliest forms of $\alpha$-macroglobulin, the thiol ester played a role similar to that seen in rat $\alpha$1I3. Therefore, the thiol ester may be viewed as an evolutionary remnant. However, some studies using site-directed mutagenesis demonstrate that

the thiol ester may be required for proper folding and maintenance of the native $\alpha_2$M structure, suggesting that the function of the thiol ester may extend beyond its role in trap closure and proteinase inhibition (46,47).

## Structural Model of $\alpha_2$-Macroglobulin

One of the unusual features of human $\alpha_2$M is that this protein of four identical subunits binds either one or two molecules of a proteinase (3–5). The stoichiometry, moreover, depends on the size of the proteinase and on the rate of inhibition. Small proteinases, such as trypsin, maximally form 2:1 complexes with $\alpha_2$M, whereas large proteinases, such as plasmin and kallikrein, form 1:1 complexes.

When human $\alpha_2$M is mildly reduced and carboxamidomethylated to block the free cysteines, it is possible to separate the two halves of the molecule (48,49). Each of these "half-molecules" can be shown to bind a molecule of either a small or large proteinase. The data suggest that two potential traps exist in each $\alpha_2$M molecule. But why does only one plasmin bind to the native molecule, which can accommodate two molecules of a smaller proteinase?

In addition to these data, electron microscopic and small-angle x-ray scatter studies are available for human $\alpha_2$M. These various observations, as well as the symmetry considerations, suggest a three-dimensional structure for human $\alpha_2$M (50,51) (see Fig. 21-2). The model in the figure has the appearance of a hollow cylinder organized into two separate units. Each unit has a pocket large enough to trap one proteinase molecule if this molecule is no more than approximately 6 nm in diameter. A molecule as large as plasmin barely fits into a pocket of each unit. Moreover, plasmin is an extremely asymmetric molecule, with a very high axial ratio that causes it to project into the second binding pocket (52). The structure shown in Figure 21-2 suggests an obvious mechanism for trapping proteinases. Proteinases are envisioned as entering the traps, where they cleave the bait regions. Subsequently, the long arms undergo a large-scale movement to close the traps around the proteinase. On the basis of previous data and theoretical considerations (50–53), the thiol esters were placed at the base of each long arm, whereas the bait regions were placed at the base of each short arm. Such a placement fits well with the data described in the preceding text (i.e., that direct methylamine attack on the thiol esters can trigger a conformational change similar to that caused by a proteinase attack) (24,25,31). A wealth of data supports the basic concepts proposed in this model. To cite a few examples, (a) kinetic studies suggest that each half-molecule can function independently when proteinases attack $\alpha_2$M (40); (b) studies with monoclonal antibodies that probe the topology of plasmin suggest that the proteinase active site must be deep inside the molecule, whereas the back end of the plasmin molecule actually protrudes beyond the distal ends of the trap arms (54); (c) nuclear magnetic resonance studies indicate that the thiol esters and bait regions in each half-molecule are coplanar. During the large-scale conformational change that closes each trap, they remain coplanar (55), an essential prediction that follows from the proposed symmetry (53) (Fig. 21-2).

When human $\alpha_2$M is attacked by either proteinases or methylamine, a similar conformational change is triggered in the inhibitor (24,27,31). Herein lies a paradox; ovostatin lacks a thiol ester yet traps proteinases by the same mechanism as seen with human $\alpha_2$M. Moreover, rat plasma contains a tetrameric $\alpha$-macroglobulin ($\alpha_1$M), the thiol esters of which react with methylamine, but the inhibitor does not show any conformational change until the bait regions are attacked by a proteinase (5). Clearly, the bait region cleavage is the major driving force for conformational change and trap

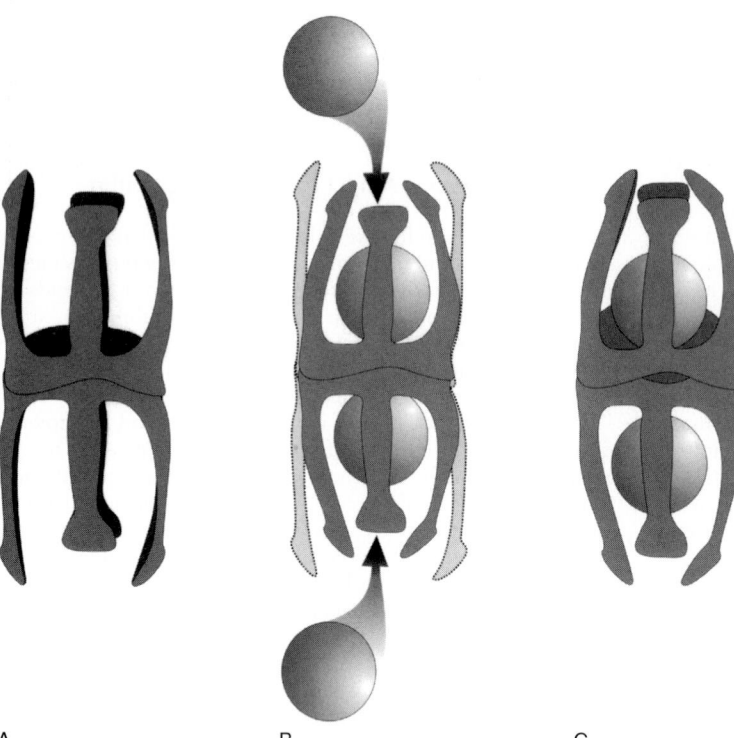

FIGURE 21-2. Structural model of human $\alpha_2$-macroglobulin ($\alpha_2$M). **A:** A form of $\alpha_2$M before binding of proteinase. **B:** The "slow to fast" transition of $\alpha_2$M during proteinase incorporation. **C:** The fully closed form after binding of a small proteinase such as trypsin.

A                    B                    C

closure. Presumably, in some α-macroglobulins such as human $\alpha_2$M, the thiol ester bond cleavage is a sufficient condition to trigger movement of the long arms of each half-molecule, subsequently producing a compacted molecule with empty traps; however, in other α-macroglobulins, thiol ester cleavage is insufficient to cause conformational change.

Numerous electron microscopic studies support the basic assumptions of the structural model of $\alpha_2$M. More recent electron microscopic data suggests that $\alpha_2$M undergoes a significant conformational change during its activation, which includes rotation of the molecule along its major axis (56). Although the functional division of the $\alpha_2$M molecule lies on its minor axis (50,57), Qazi et al. suggest that the $\alpha_2$M dimers are arranged on the major axis of this molecule (56). Analysis of a half-transformed $\alpha_2$M complex suggests that the dimers rotate 45 degrees during this transition. This untwisting of the molecule results in a doubling of the size of the openings within $\alpha_2$M, allowing for the entrapment of molecules up to approximately 50 Å. Indeed, we have observed incorporation of proteins as large as 120 kDa within the $\alpha_2$M complex (Cianciolo G and Pizzo SV, unpublished observations). Following this transformation, the $\alpha_2$M dimers retwist and enclose the entrapped proteinase. The resulting $\alpha_2$M* demonstrates a 90-degree rotation of the receptor-binding domain (RBD) about the major axis. Therefore, the COOH-terminal tips of the long arm, containing the RBD, swing outward in the $\alpha_2$M* structure.

These data provide an intriguing model for $\alpha_2$M* structure and function. However, more work is needed to better define the localization of the proteolytic bait region within the native and activated forms of $\alpha_2$M. Additionally, the observation that the COOH-termini of the subunits are further separated in the $\alpha_2$M* conformation than in the native $\alpha_2$M seems to contradict the previous demonstration that $\alpha_2$M* is considerably more compact in structure than $\alpha_2$M is. These issues will be addressed when higher resolution structures of the dynamic molecule are studied.

## Receptors for $\alpha_2$-Macroglobulin

When $\alpha_2$M–proteinase complexes are injected into the circulatory system of animals or humans, they have a half-life of only 2 to 5 minutes and are eliminated soon (5,9). *In vitro* binding studies have identified specific, saturable, high-affinity receptors for $\alpha_2$M–proteinase complexes on many cell types, including fibroblasts, adipocytes, hepatocytes, and reticuloendothelial cells ranging from monocytes to tissue macrophages (5,9,58–61). In all of these cell types, the affinity is very high, with a dissociation constant ($K_d$) of approximately 0.5 nM, irrespective of the cell type studied or the proteinase that is bound to human $\alpha_2$M (7–11,58–62). The murine or human receptor recognizes proteinase complexes of α-macroglobulins from humans, rodents, birds, and amphibians with a similar affinity (7–11,58–62). This receptor represents one of the most highly conserved complex-recognition systems in all of evolution.

Considerable efforts were made in the 1990s to identify the receptor responsible for plasma clearance and receptor-mediated endocytosis of $\alpha_2$M. The search concluded with the identification of the low density lipoprotein receptor–related protein (LRP), a 600-kDa member of the low density lipoprotein (LDL) receptor family, as the receptor for $\alpha_2$M (63). LRP is a multiligand receptor that binds to a number of unrelated ligands, including LDL, apolipoprotein E (apoE)–enriched very low density lipoprotein (VLDL), lipoprotein lipase, tissue plasminogen activator–plasminogen activator inhibitor complexes, *Pseudomonas* exotoxin A, lactoferrin, and RAP that was copurified with LRP and was later determined to serve as an intracellular molecular chaperone for LRP (64). $\alpha_2$M–proteinase complexes bind to the extracellular 515-kDa portion of LRP and become internalized through the noncovalently associated 85-kDa transmembrane portion of the receptor (63). After internalization, $\alpha_2$M is dissociated from the receptor and becomes degraded within the phagolysosome. It is generally believed that LRP binding represents an end-metabolic pathway for $\alpha_2$M.

A second receptor for $\alpha_2$M was originally characterized in 1994, and, more recently, this $\alpha_2$M* signaling receptor has been identified as GRP78 (65). Prior to this positive identification of GRP78, several lines of evidence suggested the presence of a second $\alpha_2$M* receptor. The addition of $\alpha_2$M* results in a transient hyperpolarization in the membrane potential of rat osteosarcoma cells (66). When murine peritoneal macrophages, human trabecular meshwork cells, and hepatocyte cell lines are treated with $\alpha_2$M–methylamine or $\alpha_2$M–proteinase complexes, a transient elevation of inositol triphosphate and intracellular calcium levels occurs, as well as activation of adenylate cyclase, leading to increase in cyclic adenosine monophosphate (cAMP) (67–71). This effect is not inhibited by RAP, which abolishes the binding of all known ligands to LRP, and the affinity of $\alpha_2$M* binding to the signaling receptor is approximately 10 times greater than the affinity for binding to LRP ($K_d$ approximately 50 pM vs. 0.5 nM) (72,73). The $\alpha_2$M* signaling receptor is expressed in very low numbers relative to the number of LRP on the cell surface (i.e., 1,500 vs. 35,000 per cell), making the isolation and purification of this receptor difficult. Despite this low level of expression, GRP78 was identified as a cell surface protein capable of binding to $\alpha_2$M*. Further studies demonstrated that GRP78, but not LRP, was responsible for inducing $\alpha_2$M*-mediated cellular signaling. The identification of GRP78 has resolved many long-standing questions about the nature of $\alpha_2$M*-mediated cellular signal transduction. Currently, it is believed that GRP78 may serve as a coreceptor with LRP for $\alpha_2$M* in a manner that is analogous to the uPAR/LRP coreceptor for urokinase (uPA).

Considerable progress has also been made in locating the receptor-recognition site on the $\alpha_2$M molecule, which is present at the tips of the molecule's four long arms (62) (Fig. 21-2). When the long arms swing inward to trap proteinases, a conformational change occurs at the tips of the long arms that exposes this site. The conformational change that occurs after reaction of the thiol esters with methylamine also exposes the receptor-recognition sites (10,11). Structural studies have located the receptor-recognition site in a 40-kDa COOH-terminal fragment that ends at the last residue of the polypeptide chain (74–79). At least two epitopes have been identified within the receptor-recognition site in this 40-kDa fragment. One is present in the distal 20-kDa segment of the COOH-terminal, whereas the second is in the adjacent 20-kDa region (77). Moreover, it is known that the receptor-recognition sequence present in the proximal region of the 40-kDa COOH-terminal fragment is susceptible to oxidation and binds the antitumor agent cis-dichlorodiammine-platinum (II) (cis-DDP) (76,77,80). On the basis of the available chemical data, it appears that the target of oxidants or cis-DDP in human $\alpha_2$M may be either a methionine or a lysine residue. An antiidiotypic antibody to the cis-DDP-sensitive site has been obtained, which binds to LRP with extremely high affinity ($K_d$ 0.2 nM) (79).

These studies are all consistent with the hypothesis that the proximal 20-kDa region of $\alpha_2$M COOH-terminal 40-kDa fragment contains the receptor-recognition site to the LRP receptor. When the distal 20-kDa region of the $\alpha_2$M COOH-terminus was cloned and expressed, it was found that this fragment also binds to the LRP receptor (81). Moreover, this ligand can induce intracellular signaling to the same, if not greater, extent as the whole molecule (69). A detailed analysis of the amino acid residues in the COOH-terminal 20-kDa fragment using site-directed mutagenesis shows that lysine at position 1,370 is crucial for binding to LRP (72), whereas lysine at 1,374 is essential for binding to the signaling receptor. Structural prediction of the receptor-binding fragment (RBF) using the profile-fed neural network system from Heidelberg (PHD) demonstrates that residues 1,372 to 1,376 form a surface-exposed $\alpha$-helix flanked by two loops (72). Given these

findings, we propose that the RBD of $\alpha_2$M to LRP is composed of residues starting at 40 kDa upstream of the COOH-terminal and ending at residue 1,370, whereas the RBD to the signaling receptor begins from residue 1,374 and ends at the COOH-terminal.

## Biologic Role of $\alpha_2$-Macroglobulin

**Proteinase Inhibition.** The structure, function, and receptor biology of $\alpha_2$M have been extensively studied, but a major question remains to be answered: What does $\alpha_2$M actually do *in vivo*? As noted earlier (see the section, "Inhibitors"), lack of $\alpha_2$M may be incompatible with human life. In 1971, it was shown that when the circulatory system of a dog was infused with sufficient trypsin to deplete $\alpha_2$M, it produced shock and hypercoagulability, followed by activation of the fibrinolytic system (82). Depletion of even 30% to 50% of plasma $\alpha_2$M was followed by death within 15 minutes to 6 hours (82). However, $\alpha_2$M does not appear to be the primary inhibitor of any of the proteinases that could potentially be generated in plasma. Rather, $\alpha_2$M appears to function in a backup capacity. For example, during streptokinase infusion, large-scale generation of plasmin depletes its specific inhibitor $\alpha_2$-antiplasmin, and $\alpha_2$M becomes the major antiplasmin (83,84). Studies have suggested that $\alpha_2$M might be the primary inhibitor of blood coagulation factor Xa (85), but this appears to be a species-specific effect that is not seen in humans (86). Therefore, it seems inconsistent that, given the primary role of $\alpha_2$M as a backup proteinase inhibitor in the circulation, no complete deficiency has been found in humans, despite the large number (>150,000) of plasma samples screened.

To better understand the biologic function of $\alpha_2$M, the transgenic mouse technology was used to produce homozygous deletion of the mouse $\alpha_2$M gene (87). This study showed that $\alpha_2$M-deficient mice were viable, with normal-sized litters and with no obvious hematologic or thrombotic disorders. Compared to wild-type mice, however, the expression of murinoglobulin (a structural and functional homolog of $\alpha_2$M found only in mice) was increased 3.5-fold during pregnancy, suggesting that the redundancy in the $\alpha$-macroglobulin family of proteins may compensate for specific $\alpha_2$M deletion. It remains to be seen whether the absence of human $\alpha_2$M is compatible with life because no other $\alpha$-macroglobulin is available to serve as a backup. Given the data summarized in the preceding text, $\alpha_2$M appears to function during pathophysiologic states, such as disseminated intravascular coagulation or acute pancreatitis, when large amounts of proteinases are released into the circulation and during normal physiologic states, such as pregnancy and wound repair, when proteinases are secreted into the tissues to help support growth and development.

Although $\alpha_2$M may function as a secondary or "fail-safe" inhibitor of serine proteinases in the plasma compartment, it probably is a major inhibitor of metalloproteinases in tissues. In rheumatoid arthritis, $\alpha_2$M–collagenase complexes can be found in the synovial fluid (88). In addition, kinetic studies of $\alpha_2$M interactions with collagenase suggest that $\alpha_2$M is as good a metalloproteinase inhibitor as some of the tissue inhibitors of metalloproteinases (TIMPs) (89,90). $\alpha_2$M may play an important role in regulating the degree of tissue damage during inflammation by minimizing the proteinase-mediated degradation of extracellular matrix proteins.

**Regulation of the Adaptive Immune System by $\alpha_2$-Macroglobulin.** In addition to functioning as a proteinase inhibitor, more recent studies indicate that $\alpha_2$M* also facilitates the activation of the adaptive immune response. Evidence suggests that $\alpha_2$M* functions as a molecular transporter that is capable of enhancing the delivery of antigens found at sites of inflammation directly to antigen-presenting cells that express LRP.

Following proteolytic cleavage within the bait region of $\alpha_2$M*, the large arms of each monomer fold inward, effectively trapping proteinases within a molecular cage (Fig. 21-2). Numerous studies have demonstrated that in addition to proteinases, a wide range of protein antigens can also be trapped within the activated form of $\alpha_2$M (91–94). As discussed previously, this activated form of $\alpha_2$M is recognized and rapidly internalized by cells expressing the scavenger receptor LRP. Recent studies have demonstrated that this receptor is expressed on a number of important cells within the immune system, such as antigen-presenting cells, including lin-CD11c$^+$ blood dendritic cells, Langerhans cells, monocytes, and macrophages (94–96). Dendritic cells are the most potent antigen-presenting cells, and they function by internalizing, processing, and presenting antigens within major histocompatibility complexes for recognition by antigen-specific T cells. The interaction between T cells and properly loaded antigen-presenting cells induces the activation of antigen-specific T cells and of the adaptive immune response during infection. The LRP$^+$ APC discussed earlier is distributed throughout the body and readily internalizes $\alpha_2$M*–antigen complexes that are formed at sites of tissue damage or infection. This receptor targeting of antigens within $\alpha_2$M* results in markedly enhanced antigen uptake within antigen-presenting cell when compared to soluble antigen alone. Furthermore, this enhanced uptake induces increased stimulation of antigen-specific T cells.

Because increased levels of proteolysis are associated with both infection and inflammation, the proteolytically activated form of $\alpha_2$M may play an important role in delivering antigens present at sites of tissue damage to LRP$^+$ APC. In doing so, $\alpha_2$M* would efficiently target foreign antigens to the cells most capable of inducing antigen-specific immune responses. This cotrapping and delivery of antigens by $\alpha_2$M* is unique in that $\alpha_2$M* is able to incorporate a wide range of unrelated antigens. Therefore, the $\alpha_2$M*/LRP axis can target a diverse array of antigens to APC. In the absence of receptor-mediated delivery, the uptake of antigens by APC is less efficient. The uptake of antigens by receptor-mediated endocytosis has gained increasing attention on the basis of the demonstration that the stimulation of T cells is directly related to the amount of antigen internalized by these APC (97,98). $\alpha_2$M* may play an important role in initiating the adaptive immune system during infection, in which case, antigens are believed to be present at very low concentrations.

**Regulation of Cytokines and Growth Factors.** Evidence has accumulated about the role of $\alpha_2$M in modulating the biologic activity of various plasma and extracellular fluid cytokines and growth factors. $\alpha_2$M has been shown to bind specifically to tumor necrosis factor-$\alpha$ (TNF-$\alpha$), interleukin-1$\beta$ (IL-1$\beta$), IL-2, IL-6, IL-8, platelet-derived growth factor (PDGF), nerve growth factor (NGF), transforming growth factor-$\beta$ (TGF-$\beta$), basic fibroblast growth factor (bFGF), vascular endothelial growth factor (VEGF), and others (99–101). As one might expect with the multiple unrelated cytokines binding to the same protein, many different binding mechanisms exist (102).

Most cytokines (except TGF-$\beta$ type 1 and bFGF) do not cross-compete for PDGF binding to $\alpha_2$M (103). This suggests that different binding sites are present on $\alpha_2$M as well. Previously described mechanisms of cytokine binding to $\alpha_2$M include (a) noncovalent attachment to the protein, (b) covalent binding by disulfide exchange, and (c) covalent binding to the $\gamma$-glutamate of the thiol ester during the "nascent" state, as was demonstrated for insulin (92). It is unknown whether a direct attack of cytokine on the thiol ester during the "nascent" state can occur in vivo; however, this process is extremely useful in vitro for making covalent adducts of $\alpha_2$M with an array of proteins and peptides. Investigation by Crookston et al. (104) showed that approximately 70% of TGF-$\beta$ type 1 binding to $\alpha_2$M is noncovalent. Three fourths of the remaining

30% can be released by disulfide exchange with dithiothreitol (DTT). Because covalent binding through disulfide exchange requires exposure of free sulfhydryl groups (one per $\alpha_2$M subunit), this may explain why $\alpha_2$M–methylamine and $\alpha_2$M–proteinase have slightly higher binding affinity to most cytokines than native $\alpha_2$M does (104–107). The only exception known is TGF-$\beta$ type 2, which has equal affinity to both $\alpha_2$M and $\alpha_2$M–methylamine. The $K_d$ values for $\alpha_2$M–cytokine interactions range from 13 nM for TGF-$\beta$ type 2 to greater than 1.3 $\mu$M for TNF-$\alpha$ (104).

The precise role of $\alpha_2$M in the regulation of cytokines is unknown. Some studies have suggested that serum $\alpha_2$M serves as a storage pool of a latent form of TGF-$\beta$ (99,108,109); it also regulates growth factor–mediated cell proliferation (110–112). On fibroblasts, PDGF-BB and $\alpha_2$M appear to synergistically enhance cell growth (110). In this case, $\alpha_2$M is thought to be responsible for delivering cytokines to the cell surface, thereby increasing the local concentration of cytokines for binding to their receptors. Other studies have hypothesized that cytokine binding to $\alpha_2$M is an important cytokine clearance mechanism in the plasma and in extracellular space (112–115). Once cytokine-bound $\alpha_2$M reacts with a proteinase, it becomes receptor-recognized and can carry cytokine into cells. As a potential regulator of the autocrine feedback loop, $\alpha_2$M can bind to TGF-$\beta$ that is secreted by macrophages and can decrease TGF-$\beta$–mediated inhibition of nitric oxide production by the same cells (116). $\alpha_2$M appears to inhibit the interaction between TGF-$\beta$ and its cell surface receptors in this case. Additional studies comparing $\alpha_2$M-deficient plasma versus normal mouse plasma in regulating TGF-$\beta$ activity showed that $\alpha_2$M deficiency resulted in increased TGF-$\beta$ binding to cells.

The mechanism by which $\alpha_2$M regulates cytokine and growth factor functions in vivo is currently unknown. Several studies have shed new light on the potential role of $\alpha_2$M in regulating cytokines. Recent evidence suggests that the clearance of $\alpha_2$M*–cytokine complexes may be altered by the presence of a soluble form of LRP (117). This soluble form of LRP may play a role in reducing cytokine clearance and in augmenting inflammatory responses in specific types of tissue injury (118). Although the full extent to which $\alpha_2$M regulates cytokine and growth factors in vivo remains unknown, recent studies demonstrate links between $\alpha_2$M and the pathogenesis of infection and sepsis. Waghabi et al. demonstrated that $\alpha_2$M reduced the cardiac parasite load in a mouse model of *Trypanosoma cruzi* (119). It is important to point out that these authors employed a murine $\alpha_2$M/murine murinoglobulin double knockout, thereby eliminating all of the murine $\alpha$-macroglobulins. Further, $\alpha_2$M* altered trypomastigote morphology and motility and impaired *T. cruzi* invasion of cardiomyocytes. Increased levels of TGF-$\beta$, correlating with increased fibrosis and infection, were also observed in the $\alpha$-macroglobulin-deficient mice. These data demonstrate a clear role for $\alpha$-macroglobulins in limiting the extent of infection and in regulating the subsequent cytokine- and growth-factor–mediated tissue response to inflammation.

# Kunins

## General Considerations

The kunins, a superfamily of proteins homologous to aprotinin, are also known as *pancreatic trypsin inhibitor (Kunitz)* or, under a common trade name, *Trasylol*. The term originated from "bikunin," a contraction of *bis Kunitz inhibitor* (120), which is the tandemly repeated two-domain Kunitz-type proteinase inhibitor human plasma inter-$\alpha$-trypsin inhibitor (ITI)

(121). Because proteins containing one, two, or three Kunitz-type domains are known, the term *kunin* was introduced to encompass these types of proteins (122,123).

Contrary to a previous report (124), kunins are now known to occur only in animals. The soybean trypsin inhibitor family of proteinase inhibitors and the aprotinin family have been designated "Kunitz" inhibitors after their discoverer (125). The common nomenclature, therefore, is a historic accident, and we stress that the term *kunin* should be applied only to homologs of aprotinin.

## Structure and Mechanism

A kunin domain consists of approximately 58–amino acid residues, much smaller than the serpins. The overall amino acid identities between kunins are low, and may even be as low as 20%. The property that makes proteins recognizable as kunins is the absolute conservation of cysteine residues. Unlike serpins, the structure of which does not depend on disulfide bonds, kunins are likely to be dependent on the correct formation of three disulfide bonds per domain. Indeed, the archetypal kunin, aprotinin, is an intensely studied protein, and much is known of its folding and structural requirements (126). Some kunin-containing proteins do not function as proteinase inhibitors, the best known being β-bungarotoxin B subunit (127).

Mammalian kunins often are embedded in other proteins, sometimes undergoing apparently complex posttranslational proteolytic processing. Some of the most commonly studied mammalian kunins are listed in Figure 21-3. Increasing evidence suggests that three of these kunins, namely, trypstatin; TFPI, also known as LACI; and protease nexin-2 (PN-2), are involved in regulating coagulation and fibrinolysis (see Figs. 21-3 and 21-4).

## Inter-α-Trypsin Inhibitor

The kunin family of proteinase inhibitors includes trypstatin (rat), bikunin (human), inter-α-trypsin inhibitor (ITI), PαI, and other structural variants such as inter-α-like inhibitor and ITI family heavy-chain–related protein (129). These mature polypeptides are derived from extensive posttranslational processing of five major gene products: α₁-microglobulin/bikunin precursor (AMPB) and four heavy-chain precursors, H1, H2,

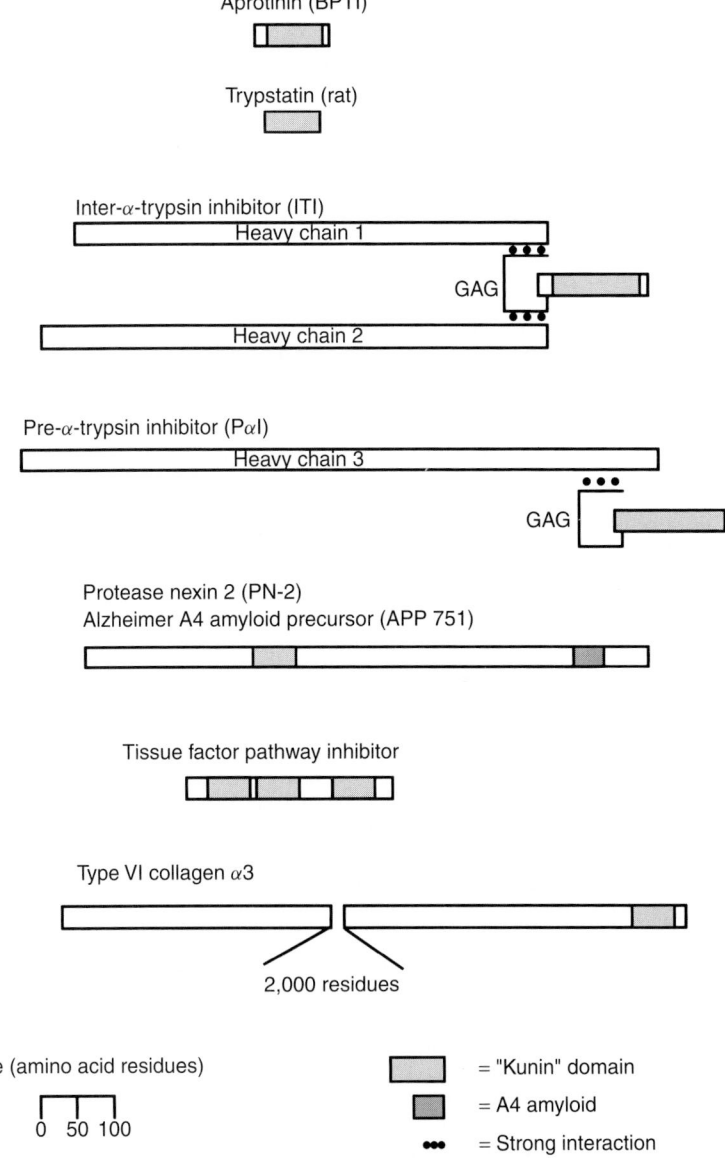

FIGURE 21-3. Proteins containing kunin domains. The prototypic kunin, bovine aprotinin, contains a single domain (*hatched boxes*) with short peptide extensions (*open boxes*) at the N- and C-terminals (128). Trypstatin is the aprotinin homolog in rat. The inter-α-inhibitor (ITI) family is represented here by bikunin, ITI, and pre-α-inhibitor (PαI). Bikunin contains two adjacent kunin domains, as the name suggests. ITI is composed of two distinct heavy chains attached to the bikunin domains, probably by a glycosaminoglycan (GAG) link (*thin line*) (129). PαI is composed of one heavy chain, different from the two ITI heavy chains, attached to the bikunin by an equivalent GAG-like link (129). The *dots* between the GAG chain and the protein chain represent the strong forces that help assemble the complexes; in the case of PαI, the link between GAG and heavy chain 3 is covalent (130). Most Alzheimer peptide precursors (APPs) contain a single kunin domain and a membrane-spanning domain close to the A4 amyloid segment. Secreted forms of APPs (lacking the membrane-spanning domain) are known as protease nexin-2 (PN-2) (see text). TFPI contains three consecutive kunin domains and is therefore a "trikunin." The domains are separated by short connecting peptides. Human type VI collagen α3 chain contains almost 2,000 residues (131), so its structure is abbreviated in the figure.

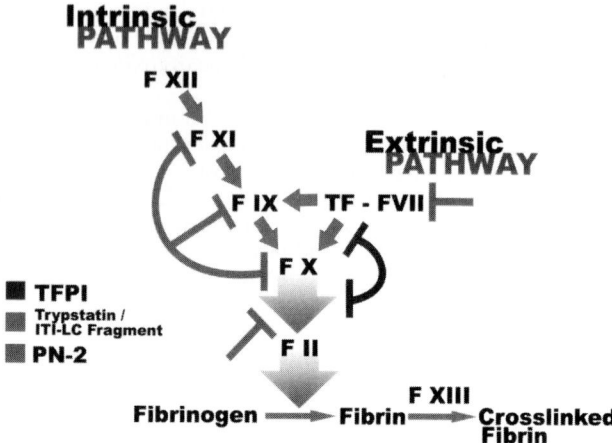

**FIGURE 21-4.** Kunin inhibitors and the coagulation cascade. Increasing evidence suggests that the kunins protease nexin-2 (PN-2), trypstatin/inter-α-trypsin inhibitor light chain (ITI-LC) fragment, and tissue factor pathway inhibitor (TFPI) are capable of regulating a number of factors within both the intrinsic and extrinsic coagulation pathway. Activated coagulation factors and factors V and VIII have been omitted in order to simplify this schematic (see Color Fig. 21-4).

H3, and H4. The polypeptide precursors undergo sequential $NH_2$- and COOH-terminal cleavages followed by covalent protein–glycosaminoglycan–protein modification to generate the final products (129,132).

The highest level of expression occurs in the liver and is driven by a series of liver-specific transcription factors called *hepatocyte nuclear factors* (HNFs). Secondary expression occurs in the brain, but this appears to be restricted only to the heavy-chain genes (129). Although members of the kunin family are generally considered proteinase inhibitors, some also regulate cell functions (133,134). Indeed, during the preovulatory period, the participation of ITI family members is required for preventing the loss of cumulus cells by stabilizing pericellular hyaluronan (135). This effect does not appear to be related to the proteinase inhibitory properties of the bikunin. Because no evidence exists that any member of this family other than trypstatin is a physiologic regulator of plasma proteinases, despite their appreciable presence in blood, we limit our discussion of the ITI protein family to trypstatin and its human homolog, inter-α-trypsin inhibitor light chain (ITI-LC) (20,121,129,136).

### Trypstatin/Inter-α-Trypsin Inhibitor Light Chain

Trypstatin is found in rat mast cells at the same cellular location as aprotinin in cows (137). Indeed, aprotinin may be the bovine analog of trypstatin. Following its identification, rat trypstatin was found to be genetically identical to rat ITI-LC, also known as bikunin (136). Interestingly, rat mast cells which contained trypstatin/ITI-LC lack messenger ribonucleic acid (mRNA) for this protein, leading these authors to suggest that mast cells have incorporated plasma ITI-LC and have proteolytically processed it into trypstatin (136). Although the role of trypstatin/ITI-LC is still unclear, Kido et al. have postulated an intriguing role for it as a regulator of coagulation. The inhibitor is located in the granules of mast cells, where it may exist as a preformed complex with tryptase, a mast cell proteinase with trypsinlike specificity (138). Tryptase converts prothrombin to thrombin with a similar range of $k_{cat}/K_m$ values as factor Xa, leading to the proposal that it may be involved in mast cell–mediated coagulation events (139). However, trypstatin/ITI-LC binds to factor Xa almost as tightly as

it binds to tryptase [inhibition constant ($K_i$) in the $10^{-10}$ M range (138)], leading to the additional proposal that the inhibitor may act as an anticoagulant around venules upon degranulation of mast cells (138). This effect would be apparent only in the immediate vicinity of the degranulating cells because diffusion would rapidly decrease the trypstatin/ITI-LC concentration below its $K_i$ to a level at which it would no longer form complexes with tryptase or factor Xa.

This proposed scheme may further apply to humans because human mast cells also contain ITI-LC (140). Studies demonstrating this point were performed by immunohistochemistry, suggesting that human mast cells contain ITI-LC or some fragment of this molecule. As noted previously, rat mast cells contain a portion of ITI-LC also known as trypstatin. Although full-length ITI-LC does not inhibit any coagulation proteinases, a fragment of human ITI-LC containing the second kunin domain (identical to trypstatin) does inhibit factor Xa in a concentration-dependent and competitive manner. The addition of this cleaved form of human ITI-LC considerably prolongs the plasma-based activated partial thromboplastin time (aPTT) (141). Together, these findings suggest that human mast cells contain a fragment of ITI-LC, which, like trypstatin, is capable of inhibiting factor Xa. Therefore, degranulating mast cells may play a role in maintaining vascular homeostasis by releasing kunins with anticoagulant activities. These mast cell anticoagulants may be essential for maintaining blood flow following the upregulation of procoagulant factors found within inflamed tissue.

### Tissue Factor Pathway Inhibitor

TFPI is a trikunin present at very low levels in the human circulation (approximately 2.5 nM). It was originally identified as a plasma lipoprotein–associated protein and was given the name *LACI*. This name is quite misleading, however, because LDL–associated TFPI has no proteinase inhibitory activity (142). The nature of this association is unclear, but TFPI is released from its complex with lipoproteins by treatment with disulfide-reducing reagents, which suggests that stabilization of the complex involves disulfide bonds between TFPI and lipoproteins (124).

TFPI exhibits tight binding (in the nM $K_d$ range) to factor Xa and trypsin, but much weaker binding to other coagulation proteinases (124). Inhibition of factor Xa is enhanced in the presence of heparin, which may serve to increase the frequency of productive binding of the initial encounter complex between the proteinase and the inhibitor. Detailed studies on the effects of glycosaminoglycan GAG on the interactions between TFPI and factor Xa show that high–molecular-weight heparin (>10 kDa) is more effective in binding to TFPI than low–molecular-weight heparin (143).

Much of the early work on characterization of TFPI centered on its ability to inhibit the extrinsic pathway of coagulation by inhibition of the factor VIIa/tissue factor (TF) activator complex (144,145). The factor VIIa/TF activator complex is not inhibited by TFPI alone; it also requires the presence of factor Xa. Experiments in which the P1 residues of the first or second domain were varied by site-directed mutagenesis indicated that factor Xa inhibition was accomplished by the second domain and the factor VIIa/TF inhibition by the first domain (146). The emerging view from these studies is that TFPI binds factor Xa by the second kunin domain, endowing this binary complex with the ability to bind factor VIIa/TF by the first kunin domain (146). Although no proteolytic inhibitory function has been assigned to the third domain of TFPI, studies have demonstrated that this domain is recognized by the VLDL receptor (147). Through this association, TFPI inhibits endothelial cell proliferation in response to bFGF. The fact that the major pool of TFPI is the endothelial cell–associated form is noteworthy, suggesting that this kunin may be an important regulator of angiogenesis (148). Indeed, recent studies demonstrate that TFPI blocks tumor growth, and this was attributed in part to inhibition of angiogenesis (149).

In addition to the VLDL receptor, the search for cell surface–binding proteins of TFPI has led to the discovery of an interesting convergence between $\alpha$-macroglobulin and kunins. TFPI was initially shown to bind to two classes of cell surface receptors. The high-affinity receptor ($K_d$, approximately 2.3 nM; 41,000 sites per cell) was subsequently identified as LRP/$\alpha_2$-macroglobulin receptor (150), and the low-affinity receptor ($K_d$, approximately 40 nM; $2 \times 10^6$ sites per cell) was found to be a cell surface glycosylphosphatidylinositol-anchored proteoglycan, glypican-3 (151).

Whether the role of TFPI as a regulator of the intrinsic pathway by combined inhibition of factor Xa and factor VIIa/TF represents its physiologic role is difficult to ascertain because no human deficiency has been identified, and homozygous deletion of the mouse TFPI gene results in mice that are lethal *in utero* (152). These mice exhibit signs of hemorrhage of yolk sac, central nervous system, and tail because of intravascular thrombi formation consequent to consumptive coagulopathy. The central role of TFPI in hemostasis is further supported by the ability of factor VII deficiency to "rescue" mice with complete TFPI deficiency (153). Broze et al. have noted that the plasma concentration of the inhibitor is below the $K_i$ of its encounter complex with factor Xa (124), indicating that plasma TFPI would not be an effective inhibitor. However, as is the case with other inhibitors that may bind to cell surfaces or connective tissue components, its efficacy may be enhanced in these local environments.

TFPI has also attracted attention as a potential therapeutic agent for the prevention of thrombosis. During vascular injury, the initiation of thrombosis induces the expression of adhesion molecules, leukocyte activation, and migration of smooth muscle cells. A number of studies have demonstrated that administration of TFPI successfully reduces thrombosis and restenosis after arterial injury (148,154–159). On the basis of the successful reduction of restenosis in animal models, further studies are required to determine whether TFPI will successfully reduce restenosis in human patients with atherosclerosis. TFPI is also being tested as an antithrombotic for treatment of sepsis. Low doses of TFPI have effectively reduced mortality in a rabbit model of septic shock (160). However, a recent phase III trial examining the effect of TFPI on patients with severe sepsis demonstrated reduced mortality only among a small subset of severely septic patients whose international normalized ratio (INR) was less than 1.2 (161).

## Protease Nexin-2

PN-2 is the extracellular form of the protein known as alzheimer peptide precursors (APP). Although PN-2 was identified before APP, most of the characterization of the protein was based on work deriving from the cloning of the precursor of the A4, or $\beta$, peptide associated with senile plaques characteristic of Alzheimer disease. The discovery that PN-2 and APP shared the same polypeptide precursor (162,163) integrated these separate research areas and has led to several hypotheses of the role played by this kunin. The primary transcript of the APP gene undergoes a variety of alternate messenger RNA splicing events that lead to one of several species (164–169). APPs also undergo a number of processing events after synthesis, including N-glycosylation at two to three sites, O-glycosylation, and Tyr-sulfation (170). After synthesis in cell lines and in cell lines transformed with APP-containing vectors, characteristic proteins in the range of 90 to 130 kDa are detected by APP antisera. Most of the alternative

APPs translated from the single gene are transmembrane proteins, and a consensus of work on the processing of APPs in various lines shows the following kinetics: The precursors are synthesized as proteins of 90 to 110 kDa that undergo glycosylation into 110- to 130-kDa species (170,171). Although secretion is thought to occur after removal of the transmembrane domain, no evidence of this has yet been presented, other than the lack of reaction of COOH-terminal antisera with secreted APPs (170,171). The structure of A4 amyloid does not establish the site of cleavage because the $NH_2$-terminal is ragged and highly likely to have been proteolyzed (172). It is now apparent, however, that proteolytic release of the extracellular portion of APPs normally takes place by cleavage within the A4 amyloid domain (173,174). This is presumed to prevent deposition of the A4 amyloid because, under normal circumstances, constitutive proteolytic processing cannot generate the peptide. It is speculated that amyloid deposition occurs as a result of aberrant cleavage of APPs in the absence of normal proteolytic processing (173,174). Because the secreted form of the first APP to be discovered, APP695, does not contain a Kunitz domain (165), it cannot be called PN-2. Those forms that do contain the domain can be called PN-2s, and the remainder of this section uses this terminology to indicate this fact.

Because PN-2 is a kunin, it should obey the standard mechanism of inhibition similar to other serpins, and its kinetics of reaction with several proteinases have been analyzed. PN-2 is somewhat broader than TFPI in the range of proteinases it inhibits. It shows moderate affinity for chymotrypsin ($K_i$ in the nM range) but very little affinity for other proteinases with chymotrypsinlike specificity (163,175,176). PN-2 has been implicated in the regulation of coagulation through inhibition of the intrinsic pathway proteinase factor XIa, which it inhibits with $K_i$ in the range of 300 to 650 pM (176,177). Further studies demonstrate that PN-2 is an inhibitor of factor VIIa and factor VIIa–TF complex (178). Because PN-2 is present in the free circulation at very low levels, it is unlikely that substantial inhibition of factor XIa occurs here. However, PN-2 is highly enriched in platelets and lymphocytes, and, when released, it can achieve local concentrations of 30 nM (179). Because heparin potentiates the binding of factor XIa by PN-2 by 4- to 15-fold (176,177), its inhibitory efficiency may be enhanced in these local environments, which is reminiscent of the hypothesized role of TFPI in regulating the initiation of the extrinsic pathway. An analysis of the mechanism of the enhancement of factor XIa inhibition by PN-2 shows that only heparin molecules containing at least 32 saccharide units (approximately 10 kDa) are able to mediate this enhancement, which supports this hypothesis (180), suggesting that heparin may serve as a platform on which factor XIa and PN-2 complexes are assembled. Additional investigation into the role of PN-2 in coagulation showed that PN-2 can also inhibit factors IXa and Xa in the prothrombinase complex, either alone or in the presence of phospholipid vesicles. Together, these observations support the previously stated hypothesis that PN-2 may function in regulating the clotting process at sites of vascular injury (181).

Despite compelling hypotheses implicating the Kunitz domain in the development of Alzheimer senile plaques (182), PN-2 is almost certainly released before the A4 peptide is laid down, limiting the likelihood of its direct participation in the formation of plaques. Some data indicate that PN-2 may play an indirect role in plaque development. PN-2 binds to a high-affinity cell surface receptor also identified as the LRP (183). This binding is mediated by the Kunitz domain in the molecule. Because the $\varepsilon$4 allele of apoE has been established as a risk factor for late-onset Alzheimer disease (184) and because LRP is a major cell surface receptor for apoE, this finding should generate renewed interest in the role of PN-2 in the pathogenesis of Alzheimer disease. Further, studies suggest that PN-2 binds to fibrillar deposits in cerebral vessels and induces localized anticoagulation that may contribute to the cerebral hemorrhage associated with severe cases of cerebral amyloid angiopathy (185).

# UNRESOLVED ISSUES

Overall, the evidence that proteinase inhibitors, as a group, play a major role in regulating coagulation and fibrinolysis is quite strong. The extent to which α-macroglobulins and kunins are directly involved in normal hemostasis or in pathologic episodes remains an area of ongoing investigation. With several of the serpins, the discovery of deficiency states has led to identification of their roles. One would expect that the same would be true for the macroglobulins and kunins, although none has been described.

The results from a wide range of disciplines continue to expand our understanding of $\alpha_2M$ and the multiple functions of this serum protein. With the identification of the $\alpha_2$MSR, GRP78, further studies are under way to more clearly characterize cellular responses, within both lymphocytes and tumor cells, following exposure to $\alpha_2M^*$. The identification of an LRP$^+$ DC suggests that $\alpha_2M^*$ plays an important role in the development of antigen-specific immune responses. Further studies are needed to examine the extent of LRP expression on additional DC subsets in order to determine how the $\alpha_2M^*$-LRP axis augments adaptive immunity *in vivo*. Considerable advances in our understanding of the role of $\alpha_2M$ in response to infection have been made through the use of double knockout mice deficient in murine $\alpha_2M$/murine murinoglobulin. The availability of these mice will allow for further characterization of the role of the α-macroglobulins in models of microbial infection and pathogenesis. In addition, these double knockout mice provide a valuable resource for determining the biologic importance of the cytokine- and growth-factor–binding properties of $\alpha_2M$ *in vivo*.

Despite the lack of a unique physiologic target for kunins, increasing experimental evidence suggests that these proteins play a role in regulating thrombosis. Following the identification of a human homolog of trypstatin, ITI-LC, further studies are needed to more closely examine the effects of mast cell degranulation on vascular hemostasis, particularly in sites of inflammation. On the basis of the initial success of TFPI in preventing restenosis in several animal models, further studies are needed to test the ability of TFPI to reduce restenosis in the clinical setting. Preliminary studies suggest that TFPI may inhibit restenosis by blocking thrombosis as well as neointimal proliferation. Additionally, administration of TFPI was found to inhibit tumor growth, an effect believed to be in part due to the inhibition of tumor angiogenesis. These antitumor effects of TFPI require further characterization and could lead clinical trials designed to examine the therapeutic benefit of TFPI in human malignancy.

## References

1. Barrett AJ. Introduction: the classification of proteinases. Paper presented at: Ciba Found Symposium, 1980;Basel, Switzerland.
2. Barrett AJ. An introduction to the proteinases. In: Salvesen G, ed. *Proteinase inhibitors*. New York: Elsevier Science, 1986:3–15.
3. Travis J, Salvesen GS. Human plasma proteinase inhibitors. *Annu Rev Biochem* 1983;52:655–709.
4. Sottrup-Jensen L. α2-Macroglobulin and related thiol ester plasma proteins. In: FW Putnam ed. *The plasma proteins*, 2nd ed., Vol. 5. Orlando, FL: Academic Press, 1987:191–287.
5. Pizzo SV, Gonias SL. Receptor-mediated protease degradation. In: Conn PM, ed. *The receptors*, Vol. 1. Orlando, FL: Academic Press, 1984:177–206.
6. Blatrix C, Amouch P, Drouet J, et al. Study on the plasmatic elimination of the alpha2-macroglobulin-proteinase complexes. *Pathol Biol (Paris)* 1973;21(Suppl):11–14.

7. Feldman SR, Pizzo SV. Comparison of the binding of chicken alpha-macroglobulin and ovomacroglobulin to the mammalian alpha 2-macroglobulin receptor. *Arch Biochem Biophys* 1984;235(1):267–275.
8. Feldman SR, Pizzo SV. Purification and characterization of frog alpha-macroglobulin: receptor recognition of an amphibian glycoprotein. *Biochemistry* 1985;24(10):2569–2575.
9. Gonias SL, Pizzo SV. Chemical and structural modifications of alpha 2-macroglobulin: effects on receptor binding and endocytosis studied in an *in vivo* model. *Ann N Y Acad Sci* 1983;421:457–471.
10. Imber MJ, Pizzo SV. Clearance and binding of two electrophoretic "fast" forms of human alpha 2-macroglobulin. *J Biol Chem* 1981;256(15):8134–8139.
11. Kaplan J, Ray FA, Keogh EA. Recognition of nucleophile-treated alpha 2-macroglobulin by the alveolar macrophage alpha-macroglobulin protease complex receptor. *J Biol Chem* 1981;256(15):7705–7707.
12. Starkey PM, Barrett AJ. Evolution of alpha 2-macroglobulin. The structure of a protein homologous with human alpha 2-macroglobulin from plaice (Pleuronectes platessa L.) plasma. *Biochem J* 1982;205(1):105–115.
13. Quigley JP, Armstrong PB. An endopeptidase inhibitor found in Limulus plasma: an ancient form of alpha 2-macroglobulin. *Ann N Y Acad Sci* 1983;421:119–124.
14. Feldman SR, Pizzo SV. Purification and characterization of a "half-molecule" alpha 2-macroglobulin from the southern grass frog: absence of binding to the mammalian alpha 2-macroglobulin receptor. *Biochemistry* 1986;25(3):721–727.
15. Carlsson-Bosted L, Moestrup SK, Gliemann J, et al. Three different conformational states of pregnancy zone protein identified by monoclonal antibodies. *J Biol Chem* 1988;263(14):6738–6741.
16. Christensen U, Simonsen M, Harrit N, et al. Pregnancy zone protein, a proteinase-binding macroglobulin. Interactions with proteinases and methylamine. *Biochemistry* 1989;28(24):9324–9331.
17. Saito A, Sinohara H. Murinoglobulin, a novel protease inhibitor from murine plasma. Isolation, characterization, and comparison with murine alpha-macroglobulin and human alpha-2-macroglobulin. *J Biol Chem* 1985;260(2):775–781.
18. Saito A, Sinohara H. Rat plasma murinoglobulin: isolation, characterization, and comparison with rat alpha-1- and alpha-2-macroglobulins. *J Biochem (Tokyo)* 1985;98(2):501–516.
19. Suzuki Y, Sinohara H. Guinea pig plasma murinoglobulin. Purification and some properties. *Biol Chem Hoppe Seyler* 1986;367(7):579–589.
20. Enghild JJ, Salvesen G, Thogersen IB, et al. Proteinase binding and inhibition by the monomeric alpha-macroglobulin rat alpha 1-inhibitor-3. *J Biol Chem* 1989;264(19):11428–11435.
21. Bender RC, Bayne CJ. Purification and characterization of a tetrameric alpha-macroglobulin proteinase inhibitor from the gastropod mollusc Biomphalaria glabrata. *Biochem J* 1996;316(Pt 3):893–900.
22. Sottrup-Jensen L, Stepanik TM, Kristensen T, et al. Primary structure of human alpha 2-macroglobulin. V. The complete structure. *J Biol Chem* 1984;259(13):8318–8327.
23. Sottrup-Jensen L, Stepanik TM, Kristensen T, et al. Common evolutionary origin of alpha 2-macroglobulin and complement components C3 and C4. *Proc Natl Acad Sci U S A* 1985;82(1):9–13.
24. Barrett AJ. Alpha 2-macroglobulin. *Methods Enzymol* 1981;80(Pt C):737–754.
25. Barrett AJ, Starkey PM. The interaction of alpha 2-macroglobulin with proteinases. Characteristics and specificity of the reaction, and a hypothesis concerning its molecular mechanism. *Biochem J* 1973;133(4):709–724.
26. Ganrot PO. Inhibition of plasmin activity by alpha-2-macroglobulin. *Clin Chim Acta* 1967;16(2):328–329.
27. Harpel PC. Studies on human plasma alpha 2-macroglobulin-enzyme interactions. Evidence for proteolytic modification of the subunit chain structure. *J Exp Med* 1973;138(3):508–521.
28. Mortensen SB, Sottrup-Jensen L, Hansen HF, et al. Primary and secondary cleavage sites in the bait region of alpha 2-macroglobulin. *FEBS Lett* 1981;135(2):295–300.
29. Gettins PG, Hahn KH, Crews BC. Alpha 2-macroglobulin bait region variants. A role for the bait region in tetramer formation. *J Biol Chem* 1995;270(23):14160–14167.
30. Bowen ME, Gettins PG. Bait region involvement in the dimer-dimer interface of human alpha 2-macroglobulin and in mediating gross conformational change. Evidence from cysteine variants that form interdimer disulfides. *J Biol Chem* 1998;273(3):1825–1831.
31. Gonias SL, Reynolds JA, Pizzo SV. Physical properties of human alpha 2-macroglobulin following reaction with methylamine and trypsin. *Biochim Biophys Acta* 1982;705(3):306–314.
32. Tack BF, Harrison RA, Janatova J, et al. Evidence for presence of an internal thiolester bond in third component of human complement. *Proc Natl Acad Sci U S A* 1980;77(10):5764–5768.
33. Sottrup-Jensen L, Petersen TE, Magnusson S. A thiol-ester in alpha 2-macroglobulin cleaved during proteinase complex formation. *FEBS Lett* 1980;121(2):275–279.
34. Howard JB. Reactive site in human alpha 2-macroglobulin: circumstantial evidence for a thiolester. *Proc Natl Acad Sci U S A* 1981;78(4):2235–2239.
35. Harrison RA, Thomas ML, Tack BF. Sequence determination of the thiolester site of the fourth component of human complement. *Proc Natl Acad Sci U S A* 1981;78(12):7388–7392.

36. Howard JB. Methylamine reaction and denaturation-dependent fragmentation of complement component 3. Comparison with alpha2-macroglobulin. *J Biol Chem* 1980;255(15):7082–7084.

37. Gorski JP, Howard JB. Effect of methylamine on the structure and function of the fourth component of human complement, C4. *J Biol Chem* 1980;255(21):10025–10028.

38. Swenson RP, Howard JB. Characterization of alkylamine-sensitive site in alpha 2-macroglobulin. *Proc Natl Acad Sci U S A* 1979;76(9):4313–4316.

39. Barrett AJ, Brown MA, Sayers CA. The electrophoretically 'slow' and 'fast' forms of the alpha 2-macroglobulin molecule. *Biochem J* 1979;181(2):401–418.

40. Strickland DK, Bhattacharya P, Olson ST. Kinetics of the conformational alterations associated with nucleophilic modification of alpha 2-macroglobulin. *Biochemistry* 1984;23(14):3115–3124.

41. Salvesen GS, Sayers CA, Barrett AJ. Further characterization of the covalent linking reaction of alpha 2-macroglobulin. *Biochem J* 1981;195(2):453–461.

42. Sottrup-Jensen L, Petersen TE, Magnusson S. Trypsin-induced activation of the thiol esters in alpha 2-macroglobulin generates a short-lived intermediate ('nascent' alpha 2-M) that can react rapidly to incorporate not only methylamine or putrescine but also proteins lacking proteinase activity. *FEBS Lett* 1981;128(1):123–126.

43. Nagase H, Harris ED Jr, Woessner JF Jr, et al. Ovostatin: a novel proteinase inhibitor from chicken egg white. I. Purification, physicochemical properties, and tissue distribution of ovostatin. *J Biol Chem* 1983;258(12):7481–7489.

44. Nagase H, Harris ED Jr. Ovostatin: a novel proteinase inhibitor from chicken egg white. II. Mechanism of inhibition studied with collagenase and thermolysin. *J Biol Chem* 1983;258(12):7490–7498.

45. Van Leuven F, Cassiman JJ, Van den Berghe H. Functional modifications of alpha 2-macroglobulin by primary amines. II. Inhibition of covalent binding of trypsin to alpha 2 M by methylamine and other primary amines. *J Biol Chem* 1981;256(17):9023–9027.

46. Gettins PG, Boel E, Crews BC. Thiol ester role in correct folding and conformation of human alpha 2-macroglobulin. Properties of recombinant C949S variant. *FEBS Lett* 1994;339(3):276–280.

47. Gettins PG. Thiol ester cleavage-dependent conformational change in human alpha 2-macroglobulin. Influence of attacking nucleophile and of Cys949 modification. *Biochemistry* 1995;34(38):12233–12240.

48. Gonias SL, Pizzo SV. Characterization of functional human alpha 2-macroglobulin half-molecules isolated by limited reduction with dithiothreitol. *Biochemistry* 1983;22(3):536–546.

49. Gonias SL, Pizzo SV. Reaction of human alpha 2-macroglobulin half-molecules with plasmin as a probe of protease binding site structure. *Biochemistry* 1983;22(21):4933–4940.

50. Feldman SR, Gonias SL, Pizzo SV. Model of alpha 2-macroglobulin structure and function. *Proc Natl Acad Sci U S A* 1985;82(17):5700–5704.

51. Feldman SR, Pizzo SV. A three-dimensional model of a unique proteinase inhibitor: alpha 2-macroglobulin. *Semin Thromb Hemost* 1986;12(3):223–225.

52. Pochon F, Favaudon V, Tourbez-Perrin M, et al. Localization of the two protease binding sites in human alpha 2-macroglobulin. *J Biol Chem* 1981;256(2):547–550.

53. Gettins P, Cunningham LW. A unique pair of zinc binding sites in the human alpha 2-macroglobulin tetramer. A 35Cl and 37Cl NMR study. *Biochemistry* 1986;25(18):5004–5010.

54. Cummings HS, Castellino FJ. Interaction of human plasmin with human alpha 2-macroglobulin. *Biochemistry* 1984;23(1):105–111.

55. Ruben GC, Harris ED Jr, Nagase H. Electron microscopic studies of free and proteinase-bound duck ovostatins (ovomacroglobulins). Model of ovostatin structure and its transformation upon proteolysis. *J Biol Chem* 1988;263(6):2861–2869.

56. Qazi U, Gettins PG, Strickland DK, et al. Structural details of proteinase entrapment by human alpha2-macroglobulin emerge from three-dimensional reconstructions of Fab labeled native, half-transformed, and transformed molecules. *J Biol Chem* 1999;274(12):8137–8142.

57. Roche PA, Salvesen GS, Pizzo SV. Symmetry of the inhibitory unit of human alpha 2-macroglobulin. *Biochemistry* 1988;27(20):7876–7881.

58. Van Leuven F, Cassiman JJ, Van den Berghe H. Uptake and degradation of alpha2-macroglobulin-protease complexes in human cells in culture. *Exp Cell Res* 1978;117(2):273–282.

59. Feldman SR, Ney KA, Gonias SL, et al. In vitro binding and in vivo clearance of human alpha 2-macroglobulin after reaction with endoproteases from four different classes. *Biochem Biophys Res Commun* 1983;114(2):757–762.

60. Ney KA, Gidwitz S, Pizzo SV. Changes in the binding of "fast"-form alpha 2-macroglobulin to 3T3-L1 cells after differentiation to adipocytes. *Biochemistry* 1984;23(15):3395–3403.

61. Van Leuven F, Cassiman JJ, Van Den Berghe H. Demonstration of an alpha2-macroglobulin receptor in human fibroblasts, absent in tumor-derived cell lines. *J Biol Chem* 1979;254(12):5155–5160.

62. Delain E, Barray M, Tapon-Bretaudiere J, et al. The molecular organization of human alpha 2-macroglobulin. An immunoelectron microscopic study with monoclonal antibodies. *J Biol Chem* 1988;263(6):2981–2989.

63. Krieger M, Herz J. Structures and functions of multiligand lipoprotein receptors: macrophage scavenger receptors and LDL receptor-related protein (LRP). *Annu Rev Biochem* 1994;63:601–637.

64. Willnow TE, Rohlmann A, Horton J, et al. RAP, a specialized chaperone, prevents ligand-induced ER retention and degradation of LDL receptor-related endocytic receptors. *Embo J* 1996;15(11):2632–2639.

65. Misra UK, Gonzalez-Gronow M, Gawdi G, et al. The role of Grp 78 in alpha 2-macroglobulin-induced signal transduction. Evidence from RNA interference that the low density lipoprotein receptor-related protein is associated with, but necessary for, GRP 78-mediated signal transduction. *J Biol Chem* 2002;277(44):42082–42087.

66. Dixon SJ, Aubin JE. Serum and alpha 2-macroglobulin induce transient hyperpolarizations in the membrane potential of an osteoblastlike clone. *J Cell Physiol* 1987;132(2):215–225.

67. Misra UK, Chu CT, Rubenstein DS, et al. Receptor-recognized alpha 2-macroglobulin-methylamine elevates intracellular calcium, inositol phosphates and cyclic AMP in murine peritoneal macrophages. *Biochem J* 1993;290(Pt 3):885–891.

68. Misra UK, Chu CT, Gawdi G, et al. Evidence for a second alpha 2-macroglobulin receptor. *J Biol Chem* 1994;269(17):12541–12547.

69. Misra UK, Chu CT, Gawdi G, et al. The relationship between low density lipoprotein-related protein/alpha 2-macroglobulin (alpha 2M) receptors and the newly described alpha 2M signaling receptor. *J Biol Chem* 1994;269(28):18303–18306.

70. Misra UK, Gawdi G, Pizzo SV. Ligation of the alpha 2-macroglobulin signalling receptor on macrophages induces protein phosphorylation and an increase in cytosolic pH. *Biochem J* 1995;309(Pt 1):151–158.

71. Howard GC, Roberts BC, Epstein DL, et al. Characterization of alpha 2-macroglobulin binding to human trabecular meshwork cells: presence of the alpha 2-macroglobulin signaling receptor. *Arch Biochem Biophys* 1996;333(1):19–26.

72. Howard GC, Yamaguchi Y, Misra UK, et al. Selective mutations in cloned and expressed alpha-macroglobulin receptor binding fragment alter binding to either the alpha2-macroglobulin signaling receptor or the low density lipoprotein receptor-related protein/alpha2-macroglobulin receptor. *J Biol Chem* 1996;271(24):14105–14111.

73. Wu SM, Boyer CM, Pizzo SV. The binding of receptor-recognized alpha2-macroglobulin to the low density lipoprotein receptor-related protein and the alpha2M signaling receptor is decoupled by oxidation. *J Biol Chem* 1997;272(33):20627–20635.

74. Sottrup-Jensen L, Gliemann J, Van Leuven F. Domain structure of human alpha 2-macroglobulin. Characterization of a receptor-binding domain obtained by digestion with papain. *FEBS Lett* 1986;205(1):20–24.

75. Van Leuven F, Marynen P, Sottrup-Jensen L, et al. The receptor-binding domain of human alpha 2-macroglobulin. Isolation after limited proteolysis with a bacterial proteinase. *J Biol Chem* 1986;261(24):11369–11373.

76. Roche PA, Strickland DK, Enghild JJ, et al. Evidence that the platinum-reactive methionyl residue of the alpha 2-macroglobulin receptor recognition site is not in the carboxyl-terminal receptor binding domain. *J Biol Chem* 1988;263(14):6715–6721.

77. Enghild JJ, Thogersen IB, Roche PA, et al. A conserved region in alpha-macroglobulins participates in binding to the mammalian alpha-macroglobulin receptor. *Biochemistry* 1989;28(3):1406–1412.

78. Pizzo SV, Roche PA, Feldman SR, et al. Further characterization of the platinum-reactive component of the alpha 2-macroglobulin-receptor recognition site. *Biochem J* 1986;238(1):217–225.

79. Isaacs IJ, Steiner JP, Roche PA, et al. Use of anti-idiotypic antibodies to establish that monoclonal antibody 7H11D6 binds to the alpha 2-macroglobulin receptor recognition site. *J Biol Chem* 1988;263(14):6709–6714.

80. Gonias SL, Pizzo SV. Altered clearance of human alpha 2-macroglobulin complexes following reaction with cis-dichlorodiammineplatinum(II). *Biochim Biophys Acta* 1981;678(2):268–274.

81. Salvesen G, Quan LT, Enghild JJ, et al. Expression of a functional alpha-macroglobulin receptor binding domain in Escherichia coli. *FEBS Lett* 1992;313(2):198–202.

82. Ohlsson K, Ganrot PO, Laurell CB. In vivo interaction between trypsin and some plasma proteins in relation to tolerance to intravenous infusion of trypsin in dog. *Acta Chir Scand* 1971;137(2):113–121.

83. Nilehn JE, Robertson B. On the degradation products of fibrinogen or fibrin after infusion of streptokinase in patients with venous thrombosis. *Scand J Haematol* 1965;2(4):267–276.

84. Gonias SL, Einarsson M, Pizzo SV. Catabolic pathways for streptokinase, plasmin, and streptokinase activator complex in mice. In vivo reaction of plasminogen activator with alpha 2-macroglobulin. *J Clin Invest* 1982;70(2):412–423.

85. Fuchs HE, Pizzo SV. Regulation of factor Xa in vitro in human and mouse plasma and in vivo in mouse. Role of the endothelium and plasma proteinase inhibitors. *J Clin Invest* 1983;72(6):2041–2049.

86. Friedberg RC, Hagen PO, Pizzo SV. The role of endothelium in factor Xa regulation: the effect of plasma proteinase inhibitors and hirudin. *Blood* 1988;71(5):1321–1328.

87. Umans L, Serneels L, Overbergh L, et al. Targeted inactivation of the mouse alpha 2-macroglobulin gene. *J Biol Chem* 1995;270(34):19778–19785.

88. Abe S, Nagai Y. Evidence for the presence of a complex of collagenase with alpha2-macroglobulin in human rheumatoid synovial fluid: a possible regulatory mechanism of collagenase activity in vivo. *J Biochem (Tokyo)* 1973;73(4):897–900.

89. Sottrup-Jensen L, Birkedal-Hansen H. Human fibroblast collagenase-alpha-macroglobulin interactions. Localization of cleavage sites in the bait regions of five mammalian alpha-macroglobulins. *J Biol Chem* 1989; 264(1):393–401.

90. Enghild JJ, Salvesen G, Brew K, et al. Interaction of human rheumatoid synovial collagenase (matrix metalloproteinase 1) and stromelysin (matrix metalloproteinase 3) with human alpha 2-macroglobulin and chicken ovostatin. Binding kinetics and identification of matrix metalloproteinase cleavage sites. *J Biol Chem* 1989;264(15):8779–8785.

91. Cianciolo GJ, Enghild JJ, Pizzo SV. Covalent complexes of antigen and alpha(2)-macroglobulin: evidence for dramatically-increased immunogenicity. *Vaccine* 2001;20(3-4):554–562.

92. Chu CT, Rubenstein DS, Enghild JJ, et al. Mechanism of insulin incorporation into alpha 2-macroglobulin: implications for the study of peptide and growth factor binding. *Biochemistry* 1991;30(6):1551–1560.

93. Adlakha CL, Hart JP, Pizzo SV. Kinetics of nonproteolytic incorporation of a protein ligand into thermally activated alpha 2-macroglobulin: evidence for a novel nascent state. *J Biol Chem* 2001;276(45):41547–41552.

94. Hart JP, Gunn MD, Pizzo SV. A CD91-positive subset of CD11c+ blood dendritic cells: characterization of the APC that functions to enhance adaptive immune responses against CD91-targeted antigens. *J Immunol* 2004;172(1):70–78.

95. Moestrup SK. The alpha 2-macroglobulin receptor and epithelial glycoprotein-330: two giant receptors mediating endocytosis of multiple ligands. *Biochim Biophys Acta* 1994;1197(2):197–213.

96. Moestrup SK, Gliemann J, Pallesen G. Distribution of the alpha 2-macroglobulin receptor/low density lipoprotein receptor-related protein in human tissues. *Cell Tissue Res* 1992;269(3):375–382.

97. Lanzavecchia A, Reid PA, Watts C. Irreversible association of peptides with class II MHC molecules in living cells. *Nature* 1992;357(6375): 249–252.

98. Nelson CA, Petzold SJ, Unanue ER. Peptides determine the lifespan of MHC class II molecules in the antigen-presenting cell. *Nature* 1994; 371(6494):250–252.

99. LaMarre J, Wollenberg GK, Gonias SL, et al. Cytokine binding and clearance properties of proteinase-activated alpha 2-macroglobulins. *Lab Invest* 1991;65(1):3–14.

100. Bonner JC, Brody AR. Cytokine-binding proteins in the lung. *Am J Physiol* 1995;268(6 Pt 1):L869–L878.

101. Kurdowska A, Carr FK, Stevens MD, et al. Studies on the interaction of IL-8 with human plasma alpha 2-macroglobulin: evidence for the presence of IL-8 complexed to alpha 2-macroglobulin in lung fluids of patients with adult respiratory distress syndrome. *J Immunol* 1997;158(4):1930–1940.

102. Gonias SL. Alpha 2-macroglobulin: a protein at the interface of fibrinolysis and cellular growth regulation. *Exp Hematol* 1992;20(3):302–311.

103. Bonner JC, Goodell AL, Lasky JA, et al. Reversible binding of platelet-derived growth factor-AA, -AB, and -BB isoforms to a similar site on the "slow" and "fast" conformations of alpha 2-macroglobulin. *J Biol Chem* 1992;267(18):12837–12844.

104. Crookston KP, Webb DJ, Wolf BB, et al. Classification of alpha 2-macroglobulin-cytokine interactions based on affinity of noncovalent association in solution under apparent equilibrium conditions. *J Biol Chem* 1994;269(2):1533–1540.

105. Dennis PA, Saksela O, Harpel P, et al. Alpha 2-macroglobulin is a binding protein for basic fibroblast growth factor. *J Biol Chem* 1989;264(13): 7210–7216.

106. Borth W, Luger TA. Identification of alpha 2-macroglobulin as a cytokine binding plasma protein. Binding of interleukin-1 beta to "F" alpha 2-macroglobulin. *J Biol Chem* 1989;264(10):5818–5825.

107. Webb DJ, Crookston KP, Figler NL, et al. Differences in the binding of transforming growth factor beta 1 to the acute-phase reactant and constitutively synthesized alpha-macroglobulins of rat. *Biochem J* 1995;312 (Pt 2):579–586.

108. O'Connor-McCourt MD, Wakefield LM. Latent transforming growth factor-beta in serum. A specific complex with alpha 2-macroglobulin. *J Biol Chem* 1987;262(29):14090–14099.

109. Huang SS, O'Grady P, Huang JS. Human transforming growth factor beta. alpha 2-macroglobulin complex is a latent form of transforming growth factor beta. *J Biol Chem* 1988;263(3):1535–1541.

110. Bonner JC, Badgett A, Osornio-Vargas AR, et al. PDGF-stimulated fibroblast proliferation is enhanced synergistically by receptor-recognized alpha 2-macroglobulin. *J Cell Physiol* 1990;145(1):1–8.

111. Stouffer GA, LaMarre J, Gonias SL, et al. Activated alpha 2-macroglobulin and transforming growth factor-beta 1 induce a synergistic smooth muscle cell proliferative response. *J Biol Chem* 1993;268(24):18340–18344.

112. Bonner JC, Badgett A, Hoffman M, et al. Inhibition of platelet-derived growth factor-BB-induced fibroblast proliferation by plasmin-activated alpha 2-macroglobulin is mediated via an alpha 2-macroglobulin receptor/low density lipoprotein receptor-related protein-dependent mechanism. *J Biol Chem* 1995;270(11):6389–6395.

113. Danielpour D, Sporn MB. Differential inhibition of transforming growth factor beta 1 and beta 2 activity by alpha 2-macroglobulin. *J Biol Chem* 1990;265(12):6973–6977.

114. Wollenberg GK, LaMarre J, Rosendal S, et al. Binding of tumor necrosis factor alpha to activated forms of human plasma alpha 2 macroglobulin. *Am J Pathol* 1991;138(2):265–272.

115. LaMarre J, Hayes MA, Wollenberg GK, et al. An alpha 2-macroglobulin receptor-dependent mechanism for the plasma clearance of transforming growth factor-beta 1 in mice. *J Clin Invest* 1991;87(1):39–44.

116. Lysiak JJ, Hussaini IM, Webb DJ, et al. Alpha 2-macroglobulin functions as a cytokine carrier to induce nitric oxide synthesis and cause nitric oxide-dependent cytotoxicity in the RAW 264.7 macrophage cell line. *J Biol Chem* 1995;270(37):21919–21927.

117. Quinn KA, Grimsley PG, Dai YP, et al. Soluble low density lipoprotein receptor-related protein (LRP) circulates in human plasma. *J Biol Chem* 1997;272(38):23946–23951.

118. Williams EA, Ing RJ, Hart HP, et al. Soluble $\alpha_2$-macroglobulin receptor is increased in endotracheal aspirates from infants and children after cardiopulmonary bypass. *J Thorac Cardiovasc Surg* 2005;129:1098–1103.

119. Waghabi MC, Coutinho CM, Soeiro MN, et al. Increased Trypanosoma cruzi invasion and heart fibrosis associated with high transforming growth factor beta levels in mice deficient in alpha(2)-macroglobulin. *Infect Immun* 2002;70(9):5115–5123.

120. Gebhard W, Schreitmuller T, Hochstrasser K, et al. Two out of the three kinds of subunits of inter-alpha-trypsin inhibitor are structurally related. *Eur J Biochem* 1989;181(3):571–576.

121. Gebhard W, Hochstrasser K. Inter-α-trypsin inhibitor and its close relatives. In: Salvesen G, ed. *Proteinase inhibitors*. New York: Academic Press, 1986:389.

122. Enghild J, Thogersen IB, Pizzo SV. Polypeptide chain structure of inter-α-trypsin inhibitor and per-α-trypsin inhibitor: evidence for chain assembly by glycan and comparison with other "kunin" containing proteins. In: Festoff B, ed. *Serine proteases and serpins in the nervous system*. New York: Plenum Publishing, 1990:79.

123. Gebhard W, Hochstrasser K, Fritz H, et al. Structure of inter-alpha-inhibitor (inter-alpha-trypsin inhibitor) and pre-alpha-inhibitor: current state and proposition of a new terminology. *Biol Chem Hoppe Seyler* 1990;371(Suppl):13–22.

124. Broze GJ Jr, Girard TJ, Novotny WF. Regulation of coagulation by a multivalent Kunitz-type inhibitor. *Biochemistry* 1990;29(33):7539–7546.

125. Laskowski M Jr, Kato I. Protein inhibitors of proteinases. *Annu Rev Biochem* 1980;49:593–626.

126. Creighton TE. Understanding protein folding pathways and mechanisms. In: King J, ed. *Protein folding*. Washington, DC: American Association for the Advancement of Science, 1989:157.

127. Kondo K, Toda H, Narita K, et al. Amino acid sequence of beta 2-bungarotoxin from Bungarus multicinctus venom. The amino acid substitutions in the B chains. *J Biochem (Tokyo)* 1982;91(5):1519–1530.

128. Jourdain M, Carrette O, Tournoys A, et al. Effects of inter-alpha-inhibitor in experimental endotoxic shock and disseminated intravascular coagulation. *Am J Respir Crit Care Med* 1997;156(6):1825–1833.

129. Salier JP, Rouet P, Raguenez G, et al. The inter-alpha-inhibitor family: from structure to regulation. *Biochem J* 1996;315(Pt 1):1–9.

130. Creighton TE, Charles IG. Sequences of the genes and polypeptide precursors for two bovine protease inhibitors. *J Mol Biol* 1987;194(1):11–22.

131. Enghild JJ, Salvesen G, Hefta SA, et al. Chondroitin 4-sulfate covalently cross-links the chains of the human blood protein pre-alpha-inhibitor. *J Biol Chem* 1991;266(2):747–751.

132. Thogersen IB, Enghild JJ. Biosynthesis of bikunin proteins in the human carcinoma cell line HepG2 and in primary human hepatocytes. Polypeptide assembly by glycosaminoglycan. *J Biol Chem* 1995;270(31):18700–18709.

133. Kanayama N, Halim A, Maehara K, et al. Kunitz-type trypsin inhibitor prevents LPS-induced increase of cytosolic free Ca2+ in human neutrophils and HUVEC cells. *Biochem Biophys Res Commun* 1995;207(1):324–330.

134. Blom A, Pertoft H, Fries E. Inter-alpha-inhibitor is required for the formation of the hyaluronan-containing coat on fibroblasts and mesothelial cells. *J Biol Chem* 1995;270(17):9698–9701.

135. Chen L, Zhang H, Powers RW, et al. Covalent linkage between proteins of the inter-alpha-inhibitor family and hyaluronic acid is mediated by a factor produced by granulosa cells. *J Biol Chem* 1996;271(32):19409–19414.

136. Itoh H, Ide H, Ishikawa N, et al. Mast cell protease inhibitor, trypstatin, is a fragment of inter-alpha-trypsin inhibitor light chain. *J Biol Chem* 1994; 269(5):3818–3822.

137. Fritz H, Kruck J, Russe I, et al. Immunofluorescence studies indicate that the basic trypsin-kallikrein-inhibitor of bovine organs (Trasylol) originates from mast cells. *Hoppe Seylers Z Physiol Chem* 1979;360(3):437–444.

138. Kido H, Yokogoshi Y, Katunuma N. Kunitz-type protease inhibitor found in rat mast cells. Purification, properties, and amino acid sequence. *J Biol Chem* 1988;263(34):18104–18107.

139. Kido H, Fukusen N, Katunuma N, et al. Tryptase from rat mast cells converts bovine prothrombin to thrombin. *Biochem Biophys Res Commun* 1985;132(2):613–619.

140. Ide H, Itoh H, Yoshida E, et al. Immunohistochemical demonstration of inter-alpha-trypsin inhibitor light chain (bikunin) in human mast cells. *Cell Tissue Res* 1999;297(1):149–154.

141. Morishita H, Yamakawa T, Matsusue T, et al. Novel factor Xa and plasma kallikrein inhibitory-activities of the second Kunitz-type inhibitory domain of urinary trypsin inhibitor. *Thromb Res* 1994;73(3-4):193–204.

142. Hansen JB, Huseby KR, Huseby NE, et al. Tissue factor pathway inhibitor in complex with low density lipoprotein isolated from human plasma does not possess anticoagulant function in tissue factor-induced coagulation *in vitro*. *Thromb Res* 1997;85(5):413–425.

143. Valentin S, Larnkjer A, Ostergaard P, et al. Characterization of the binding between tissue factor pathway inhibitor and glycosaminoglycans. *Thromb Res* 1994;75(2):173–183.

144. Novotny WF, Girard TJ, Miletich JP et al. Purification and characterization of the lipoprotein-associated coagulation inhibitor from human plasma. *J Biol Chem* 1989;264(31):18832–18837.

145. Rao LV, Rapaport SI. Studies of a mechanism inhibiting the initiation of the extrinsic pathway of coagulation. *Blood* 1987;69(2):645–651.

146. Girard TJ, Warren LA, Novotny WF, et al. Functional significance of the Kunitz-type inhibitory domains of lipoprotein-associated coagulation inhibitor. *Nature* 1989;338(6215):518–520.

147. Hembrough TA, Ruiz JF, Papathanassiu AE, et al. Tissue factor pathway inhibitor inhibits endothelial cell proliferation via association with the very low density lipoprotein receptor. *J Biol Chem* 2001;276(15):12241–12248.

148. Kato H. Regulation of functions of vascular wall cells by tissue factor pathway inhibitor: basic and clinical aspects. *Arterioscler Thromb Vasc Biol* 2002;22(4):539–548.

149. Hembrough TA, Swartz GM, Papathanassiu A, et al. Tissue factor/factor VIIa inhibitors block angiogenesis and tumor growth through a nonhemostatic mechanism. *Cancer Res* 2003;63(11):2997–3000.

150. Warshawsky I, Broze GJ Jr, Schwartz AL. The low density lipoprotein receptor-related protein mediates the cellular degradation of tissue factor pathway inhibitor. *Proc Natl Acad Sci U S A* 1994;91(14):6664–6668.

151. Mast AE, Higuchi DA, Huang ZF, et al. Glypican-3 is a binding protein on the HepG2 cell surface for tissue factor pathway inhibitor. *Biochem J* 1997;327(Pt 2):577–583.

152. Huang ZF, Higuchi D, Lasky N, et al. Tissue factor pathway inhibitor gene disruption produces intrauterine lethality in mice. *Blood* 1997;90(3):944–951.

153. Chan JC, Carmeliet P, Moons L, et al. Factor VII deficiency rescues the intrauterine lethality in mice associated with a tissue factor pathway inhibitor deficit. *J Clin Invest* 1999;103(4):475–482.

154. Jang Y, Guzman LA, Lincoff AM, et al. Influence of blockade at specific levels of the coagulation cascade on restenosis in a rabbit atherosclerotic femoral artery injury model. *Circulation* 1995;92(10):3041–3050.

155. Park CT, Creasey AA, Wright SD. Tissue factor pathway inhibitor blocks cellular effects of endotoxin by binding to endotoxin and interfering with transfer to CD14. *Blood* 1997;89(12):4268–4274.

156. Kamikubo Y, Hamuro T, Matsuda J, et al. Antithrombotic effect of human recombinant tissue factor pathway inhibitor on endotoxin-induced intravascular coagulation in rats: concerted effect with antithrombin. *Thromb Haemostasis* 1996;76(4):621–626.

157. Chen D, Riesbeck K, McVey JH, et al. Regulated inhibition of coagulation by porcine endothelial cells expressing P-selectin-tagged hirudin and tissue factor pathway inhibitor fusion proteins. *Transplantation* 1999;68(6):832–839.

158. Chen D, Riesbeck K, Kemball-Cook G, et al. Inhibition of tissue factor-dependent and -independent coagulation by cell surface expression of novel anticoagulant fusion proteins. *Transplantation* 1999;67(3):467–474.

159. Sato Y, Asada Y, Marutsuka K, et al. Tissue factor pathway inhibitor inhibits aortic smooth muscle cell migration induced by tissue factor/factor VIIa complex. *Thromb Haemostasis* 1997;78(3):1138–1141.

160. Matyal R, Vin Y, Delude RL, et al. Extremely low doses of tissue factor pathway inhibitor decrease mortality in a rabbit model of septic shock. *Intensive Care Med* 2001;27(8):1274–1280.

161. Abraham E, Reinhart K, Opal S, et al. Efficacy and safety of tifacogin (recombinant tissue factor pathway inhibitor) in severe sepsis: a randomized controlled trial. *Jama* 2003;290(2):238–247.

162. Oltersdorf T, Fritz LC, Schenk DB, et al. The secreted form of the Alzheimer's amyloid precursor protein with the Kunitz domain is protease nexin-II. *Nature* 1989;341(6238):144–147.

163. Van Nostrand WE, Wagner SL, Suzuki M, et al. Protease nexin-II, a potent antichymotrypsin, shows identity to amyloid beta-protein precursor. *Nature* 1989;341(6242):546–549.

164. Kitaguchi N, Takahashi Y, Tokushima Y, et al. Novel precursor of Alzheimer's disease amyloid protein shows protease inhibitory activity. *Nature* 1988;331(6156):530–532.

165. Kang J, Lemaire HG, Unterbeck A, et al. The precursor of Alzheimer's disease amyloid A4 protein resembles a cell-surface receptor. *Nature* 1987;325(6106):733–736.

166. Ponte P, Gonzalez-DeWhitt P, Schilling J, et al. A new A4 amyloid mRNA contains a domain homologous to serine proteinase inhibitors. *Nature* 1988;331(6156):525–527.

167. Tanzi RE, McClatchey AI, Lamperti ED, et al. Protease inhibitor domain encoded by an amyloid protein precursor mRNA associated with Alzheimer's disease. *Nature* 1988;331(6156):528–530.

168. de Sauvage F, Octave JN. A novel mRNA of the A4 amyloid precursor gene coding for a possibly secreted protein. *Science* 1989;245(4918):651–653.

169. Palmert MR, Podlisny MB, Witker DS, et al. The beta-amyloid protein precursor of Alzheimer disease has soluble derivatives found in human brain and cerebrospinal fluid. *Proc Natl Acad Sci U S A* 1989;86(16):6338–6342.

170. Selkoe DJ, Podlisny MB, Joachim CL, et al. Beta-amyloid precursor protein of Alzheimer disease occurs as 110- to 135-kilodalton membrane-associated proteins in neural and nonneural tissues. *Proc Natl Acad Sci U S A* 1988;85(19):7341–7345.

171. Weidemann A, Konig G, Bunke D, et al. Identification, biogenesis, and localization of precursors of Alzheimer's disease A4 amyloid protein. *Cell* 1989;57(1):115–126.

172. Anderton BH. Alzheimer's disease. Progress in molecular pathology. *Nature*, 19–25 1987;325(6106):658–659.

173. Sisodia SS, Koo EH, Beyreuther K, et al. Evidence that beta-amyloid protein in Alzheimer's disease is not derived by normal processing. *Science* 1990;248(4954):492–495.

174. Esch FS, Keim PS, Beattie EC, et al. Cleavage of amyloid beta peptide during constitutive processing of its precursor. *Science* 1990;248(4959):1122–1124.

175. Sinha S, Dovey HF, Seubert P, et al. The protease inhibitory properties of the Alzheimer's beta-amyloid precursor protein. *J Biol Chem* 1990;265(16):8983–8985.

176. Van Nostrand WE, Wagner SL, Farrow JS, et al. Immunopurification and protease inhibitory properties of protease nexin-2/amyloid beta-protein precursor. *J Biol Chem* 1990;265(17):9591–9594.

177. Smith RP, Higuchi DA, Broze GJ Jr. Platelet coagulation factor XIa-inhibitor, a form of Alzheimer amyloid precursor protein. *Science* 1990;248(4959):1126–1128.

178. Mahdi F, Rehemtulla A, Van Nostrand WE, et al. Protease nexin-2/Amyloid beta-protein precursor regulates factor VIIa and the factor VIIa-tissue factor complex. *Thromb Res* 2000;99(3):267–276.

179. Van Nostrand WE, Schmaier AH, Farrow JS, et al. Protease nexin-2/amyloid beta-protein precursor in blood is a platelet-specific protein. *Biochem Biophys Res Commun* 1991;175(1):15–21.

180. Schmaier AH, Dahl LD, Hasan AA, et al. Factor IXa inhibition by protease nexin-2/amyloid beta-protein precursor on phospholipid vesicles and cell membranes. *Biochemistry* 1995;34(4):1171–1178.

181. Van Nostrand WE, Schmaier AH, Farrow JS, et al. Protease nexin-II (amyloid beta-protein precursor): a platelet alpha-granule protein. *Science* 1990;248(4956):745–748.

182. Selkoe DJ. Aging, amyloid, and Alzheimer's disease. *N Engl J Med* 1989;320(22):1484–1487.

183. Kounnas MZ, Moir RD, Rebeck GW, et al. LDL receptor-related protein, a multifunctional ApoE receptor, binds secreted beta-amyloid precursor protein and mediates its degradation. *Cell* 1995;82(2):331–340.

184. Strittmatter WJ, Saunders AM, Schmechel D, et al. Apolipoprotein E: high-avidity binding to beta-amyloid and increased frequency of type 4 allele in late-onset familial Alzheimer disease. *Proc Natl Acad Sci U S A* 1993;90(5):1977–1981.

185. Wagner MR, Keane DM, Melchor JP, et al. Fibrillar amyloid beta-protein binds protease nexin-2/amyloid beta-protein precursor: stimulation of its inhibition of coagulation factor XIa. *Biochemistry* 2000;39(25):7420–7427.

# CHAPTER 22 ■ HUMAN ENDOTHELIAL CELL PLASMIN–GENERATING SYSTEM

KATHERINE A. HAJJAR AND RALPH L. NACHMAN

## THE ENDOTHELIUM

Endothelial cells form the lining of all blood vessels, thereby creating a conduit for delivery of nutrients, oxygen, and macromolecules, as well as a barrier against toxins, drugs, and infectious agents (1–3). The close association of endothelial cells with flowing blood endows this 1-kg, 1-trillion cell organ with the ability to regulate blood pressure, vascular tone, immune responses, platelet reactivity, vascular repair and remodeling, hemostasis, and angiogenesis (4). The endothelial cell surface, comprising about 7 m² in the adult, is the target of an array of stimuli ranging from fluid dynamic forces and soluble mediators to infectious agents and adhesion events involving many other cell types. Among the systems that respond to these influences is the endothelial plasminogen–generating system.

## THE FIBRINOLYTIC SYSTEM

Fibrinolysis is a physiologic response to the deposition of intra- or extravascular fibrin (5). Formed upon hydrolysis of the Arg560–Val561 peptide bond of plasminogen, plasmin cleaves a series of fibrin-specific peptide bonds, culminating in the release of soluble degradation products. The generation of plasmin on a fibrin surface, which classically involves the formation of a ternary complex of plasminogen, tissue plasminogen activator (tPA), and fibrin, may serve as a prototype for understanding its generation in other biologic contexts.

The endothelial cell plays a central role in the control of plasmin generation through its expression of plasminogen activators, activator inhibitors, and cofactor/receptors (6). In this chapter, we consider the role of the endothelial cell, uniquely situated at the blood–vessel interface, in the regulation of plasmin generation. In addition, we examine the possible roles that cell-surface–fibrinolytic systems may play in maintaining the patency of blood vessels, in mediating vascular remodeling and in promoting angiogenesis.

## ENDOTHELIAL CELL SYNTHESIS, SECRETION, AND ASSEMBLY OF FIBRINOLYTIC PROTEINS

### Plasminogen

N-terminal glutamic acid plasminogen (Glu-PLG), the $M_r$ 93,000 zymogen precursor of plasmin, is synthesized by the liver and circulates in plasma at a concentration of approximately 1.5 μM (5,6). Plasminogen can be activated by either urokinase (uPA) or tissue plasminogen activator (tPA), both of which hydrolyze the Arg560–Val561 peptide bond,

yielding the two-chain, active serine protease, plasmin (see Table 22-1). Plasminogen activation by tPA is enhanced several hundred–fold on surfaces that contain fibrin because of increases in enzyme–substrate affinity (i.e., decreased Michaelis constant, $K_m$) (7,8).

Human plasminogen deficiency was first described in a 30-year-old man with a history of repeated episodes of thrombophlebitis, intracranial and mesenteric venous thrombosis, and pulmonary embolism (23). Reduced plasminogen activity (i.e., 50% of normal) in the patient's plasma was traced to an Ala601Thr point mutation, and since then several more patients with this defect or related substitutions that resulted in a predisposition to thrombosis have been described (24). However, there is now another group of patients with plasminogen deficiency who appear to be free of thrombotic disease but who have fibrin deposition within mucous membranes—the so-called ligneous conjunctivitis (25,26). The factors that govern fibrin deposition in intravascular versus extravascular locations are presently unknown.

The biologic role of plasmin as a fibrinolytic agent has been further confirmed through analysis of plasminogen "knock-out" mice (see Table 22-2). Plasminogen-null mice undergo normal embryogenesis and development, are fertile, and survive to adulthood (27,28). In addition to runting and ligneous conjunctivitis (29), these animals display a predisposition to thrombosis with spontaneous thrombi in liver, stomach, colon, rectum, lung, and pancreas; fibrin deposition in liver; and ulcerative lesions in the gastrointestinal tract and rectum. These results suggest that plasminogen is not strictly required for normal development but does play a crucial role in postnatal intra- and extravascular fibrinolysis. Bolus administration of plasminogen restores thrombolytic potential in these animals (30).

Many studies have demonstrated equilibrium binding of plasminogen to a wide variety of cell types, including cultured endothelial cells (54–57). Plasminogen binds rapidly, reversibly, and with high affinity [dissociation constant ($K_d$) 310 nM] and capacity ($B_{max}$ 1,400,000 sites per cell) to cultured human umbilical vein endothelial cells (see Fig. 22-1) (58). This interaction is lysine binding site (LBS)–specific, thereby implicating the disulfide-linked "kringle" structures of plasminogen. Interaction of Glu-PLG with the cell surface results in a 12.7-fold enhancement in the efficiency of plasmin generation by tPA because of a logarithmic increase in apparent enzyme–substrate affinity (58,59). During this process, the circulating form of plasminogen, Glu-PLG, is converted to a more efficiently activated, plasmin-modified form called *N-terminal lysine plasminogen* (Lys-PLG) (60,61).

### Tissue Plasminogen Activator

For the last four decades, focal plasminogen activator activity has been recognized to be associated with the walls of blood

**TABLE 22-1**

SOME ACTIONS OF PLASMIN

| Action | Reference |
|---|---|
| **FIBRINOLYTIC PROTEIN MODIFICATION** | |
| N-terminal Glu-plasminogen | 8–10 |
| Single-chain tissue plasminogen activator | 11 |
| Single-chain urokinase | 12 |
| **INACTIVATION OF COAGULATION FACTORS** | |
| Factor Va | 13 |
| Factor VIIIa | 14 |
| **MATRIX PROTEIN MODIFICATION** | |
| Laminin | 15 |
| Fibrinogen | 16 |
| **PROTEASE ACTIVATION** | |
| MMP-1 | 17 |
| MMP-3 | 18,19 |
| **GROWTH AND DIFFERENTIATION FACTOR ACTIVATION** | |
| Transforming growth factor-β | 20,21 |
| Brain-derived neurotrophic factor | 22 |

MMP, matrix metalloproteinase.

vessels (62,63). tPA expression *in vivo* appears to be highly restricted to smaller vessels in specific anatomic locations, a pattern that likely reflects the vast heterogeneity of endothelial cells because they respond to a myriad of tissue-specific cues (2). In the baboon, for example, tPA antigen and messenger RNA (mRNA) were readily detected in 7- to 30-$\mu$m diameter precapillary arterioles, postcapillary venules, and vasa vasora but not in femoral artery, femoral vein, carotid artery, or aorta (64). In the mouse lung, similarly, bronchial blood vessels displayed endothelial cell–associated tPA antigen, especially at branch points, whereas pulmonary blood vessels were uniformly negative for the antigen (65,66).

The endothelium appears to be the principal source of tPA in blood (67). Because the *in vivo* circulating half-life of tPA is only about 5 minutes, acute changes in its release from the endothelium could have profound functional effects. The infusion of DDAVP (desmopressin), bradykinin, platelet activating factor, endothelin, and thrombin stimulates the release of tPA within minutes (67). In addition, hyperoxia leads to a 4.5-fold upregulation of tPA mRNA in small vessel endothelial cells in the mouse lung (65). In humans, the infusion of tumor necrosis factor (TNF) into patients with malignancy is associated with an increase in tPA (68). Decreased release of tPA in response to venous occlusion in humans has been associated with deep venous thrombotic vascular disease (69), as well as with atrophie blanche and other cutaneous vasculitides (70).

Although tPA functions efficiently on a fibrin surface, it is also associated with the membrane of endothelial cells (Fig. 22-1) (71–73). tPA binding to endothelial cells is a specific, reversible, high-affinity interaction (73) that involves a major binding site [$K_d$ 18 nM; binding maximum ($B_{max}$) 815,000 sites per cell] now known to be annexin 2. This interaction is independent of the lysine binding site and is inhibited by a peptide derived from the N-terminal domain of tPA (58). Once localized on the surface of the endothelial cell, tPA appears to be protected from its physiologic inhibitor, plasminogen activator inhibitor-1 (PAI-1) (73).

Complete deficiency of tPA appears to have no effect on embryonic mouse development, viability, fertility, or lifespan (Table 22-2) (38). When challenged, however, tPA knockouts

exhibit reduced *in vivo* lysis of a fibrin clot and an increased rate of endotoxin-induced thrombosis. These data indicate that tPA plays a fundamental role in both thrombolysis and fibrinolytic surveillance. Finally, combined tPA/uPA deficiency results in a phenotype characterized by cachexia; reduced fertility and lifespan; fibrin deposition in liver, lungs, and gonads; ulceration of gastrointestinal tract and skin; and rectal prolapse (38). These data suggest substantial overlap in physiologic function of tPA and uPA.

## Annexin 2

Isolated endothelial cell membranes bind both tPA and plasminogen at a single saturable high-affinity binding site ($K_d$ 30 nM and 114 nM, respectively) (74,75). In ligand blotting experiments, both tPA and plasminogen interacted specifically with an $M_r$ 36,000 membrane protein, which was distinct from the uPAR and PAI-1 (71,74,76). Internal peptide sequencing of the purified coreceptor revealed its identity with the calcium-regulated, phospholipid-binding protein annexin 2 (see Fig. 22-2) (77). Receptor identity was confirmed when both polyclonal antibodies and antisense oligonucleotides blocked ligand binding to endothelial cells. In addition, human embryonic kidney (HEK 293) cells that were transfected with the annexin 2 complementary deoxyribonucleic acid (DNA) acquired the ability to bind both tPA and plasminogen. Annexin 2 is expressed abundantly on tumor cells (78–80), myeloid cells (81), monocyte/macrophages (82,83), and endothelial cells (84–86).

Kinetic analysis of purified native human annexin 2 revealed its ability to stimulate tPA-dependent plasminogen activation in a purified protein system (88). Lineweaver–Burk plots indicated a 60-fold increase in the catalytic efficiency of tPA-mediated activation of plasminogen, an effect that was completely dependent upon basic carboxy-terminal amino acids. These data suggest that annexin 2 possesses the fibrinlike property of stimulating tPA-dependent plasminogen activation in a lysine-binding site–dependent manner. Corroborating studies suggest that the annexin 2 heterotetramer (Fig. 22-2), composed of two annexin monomers and two p11 (S100A10) subunits, may have even greater stimulatory effects on tPA-dependent plasmin generation at the endothelial cell surface (85).

Annexin 2 is an outer face, peripheral membrane protein, although it lacks a classic signal peptide. It is translocated to the endothelial cell surface by both constitutive and regulated pathways (89). Within minutes to hours of stress-related stimuli such as heat shock, the translocation of annexin 2 from a cytoplasmic pool to the extracytoplasmic plasma membrane face occurs both *in vitro* and *in vivo* (Fig. 22-2) (90). Although the details of the translocation pathway are currently unknown, the process clearly depends upon coexpression of protein p11. In addition, translocation requires phosphorylation of annexin 2 at tyrosine 23 by an src-like kinase. This phosphorylation "switch" dramatically increases the fibrinolytic potential and may represent a novel stress-induced pathway of protein secretion.

Several pieces of evidence indicate that annexin 2 is crucial for maintaining fibrinolytic balance *in vivo*. In rats, pretreatment of the carotid artery with wild-type annexin 2—but not a mutant form of the protein—prevents vessel thrombosis in response to oxidative injury with ferric chloride (91). In addition, overexpression of annexin 2 on leukemic blast cells from humans with acute promyelocytic leukemia is associated with dysregulated plasmin generation and a hyperfibrinolytic, hemorrhagic state (81). Finally, homozygous annexin 2–null mice display considerable defects in fibrin homeostasis (Table 22-2) (46). These mice deposit fibrin within microvessels and are unable to completely clear injury-induced arterial thrombi. Although these animals demonstrated normal lysis of a fibrin-containing plasma clot, tPA-dependent plasmin generation at

**TABLE 22-2**

GENETIC MOUSE MODELS RELEVANT TO ENDOTHELIAL CELL FIBRINOLYSIS

| Genotype | Phenotype | Reference |
|---|---|---|
| **GENE DEFICIENCY MODELS** | | |
| Plasminogen: | | |
| PLG$^{-/-}$ | Spontaneous thrombosis, runting, premature death | 27,31 |
| | Fibrin in liver, lungs, stomach; gastric ulcers | 27,31 |
| | Impaired wound healing; ligneous conjunctivitis | 29,32 |
| | Impaired monocyte recruitment | 33 |
| | Impaired neointima formation after electrical injury | 34 |
| | Impaired dissemination of *Borrelia burgdorferi* | 35 |
| | Reduced excitotoxic neuronal cell death in brain | 15 |
| | Reduced transplantation arteriosclerosis | 36 |
| | Increased atherogenesis | 37 |
| **PLASMINOGEN ACTIVATORS** | | |
| tPA$^{-/-}$ | Reduced lysis of fibrin clot | 38 |
| | Increased endotoxin-induced thrombosis | 38 |
| uPA$^{-/-}$ | Occasional fibrin in liver/intestine | 38 |
| | Rectal prolapse, ulcers of eyelids, face, and ears | 38 |
| | Reduced macrophage degradation of fibrin | 38 |
| | Increased endotoxin-induced thrombosis | 38 |
| | Reduced aortic and ventricular aneurysm | 39,40 |
| uPA$^{-/-}$/tPA$^{-/-}$ | Reduced growth, fertility, and lifespan; cachexia | 38 |
| | Fibrin deposits in liver, gonads, and lungs | 38 |
| | Ulcers in intestine, skin, and ears; rectal prolapse | 38 |
| | Impaired clot lysis | 38 |
| **INHIBITORS** | | |
| PAI-1$^{-/-}$ | Mildly increased lysis of fibrin clot | 41 |
| | Resistance to endotoxin-induced thrombosis | 42 |
| **RECEPTORS** | | |
| LRP$^{-/-}$ | Embryonic lethal day 13.5 after conception | 43,44 |
| uPAR$^{-/-}$ | Essentially normal | 45 |
| | Reduced macrophage PLG activation *in vitro* | 45 |
| | Normal matrix degradation | 45 |
| Annexin 2$^{-/-}$ | Mild runting, fibrin deposition in microvasculature | 46 |
| | Impaired clearance of arterial thrombi | 46 |
| | Impaired postnatal neoangiogenesis | 46 |
| **OVEREXPRESSION MODELS** | | |
| Apo(a)$^{+/+}$ | Atherosclerotic lesions with high-fat diet | 47 |
| | Reduced cell-associated plasmin and activation of TGF-$\beta$ | 48 |
| | Resistance to tPA-mediated clot lysis | 49 |
| Apo(a)$\Delta$LBS$^{+/+}$ | Reduced lipid deposition | 50 |
| PAI-1$^{+++/+++}$ | Venous thrombosis | 51 |
| | Tail necrosis, hindfoot edema | |
| uPA$^{+++/+++}$ | Fatal neonatal hemorrhage | 52 |
| | Impaired learning | 53 |

PLG, plasminogen; tPA, tissue-type plasminogen activator; uPA, urokinase plasminogen activator; PAI-1, plasminogen activator inhibitor-1; LRP, lipoprotein receptor related protein; uPAR, urokinase receptor; Apo(a), apolipoprotein (a); TGF-$\beta$, transforming growth factor-$\beta$.

the surface of isolated endothelial cells was markedly reduced. Directed migration of annexin 2–null endothelial cells through fibrin and collagen lattices *in vitro* was also reduced.

## Urokinase

Under resting conditions, renal tubular epithelium, rather than endothelium, appears to be the major source of *in vivo* uPA (92,93). However, the expression of uPA is strongly induced in endothelium during wound repair and physiologic angiogenesis, such as in the ovarian follicle (94). The association of uPA with the blood vessel wall appears to reflect its association with the uPAR.

Although uPA has been regarded as the major extravascular plasminogen activator, uPA-deficient mice display a surprisingly mild phenotype (Table 22-2). They exhibit normal development, viability, fertility, and lifespan (38). Macroscopic findings are limited to occasional rectal prolapse and ulcerations of the face, ears, and eyelids. Microscopically, fibrin

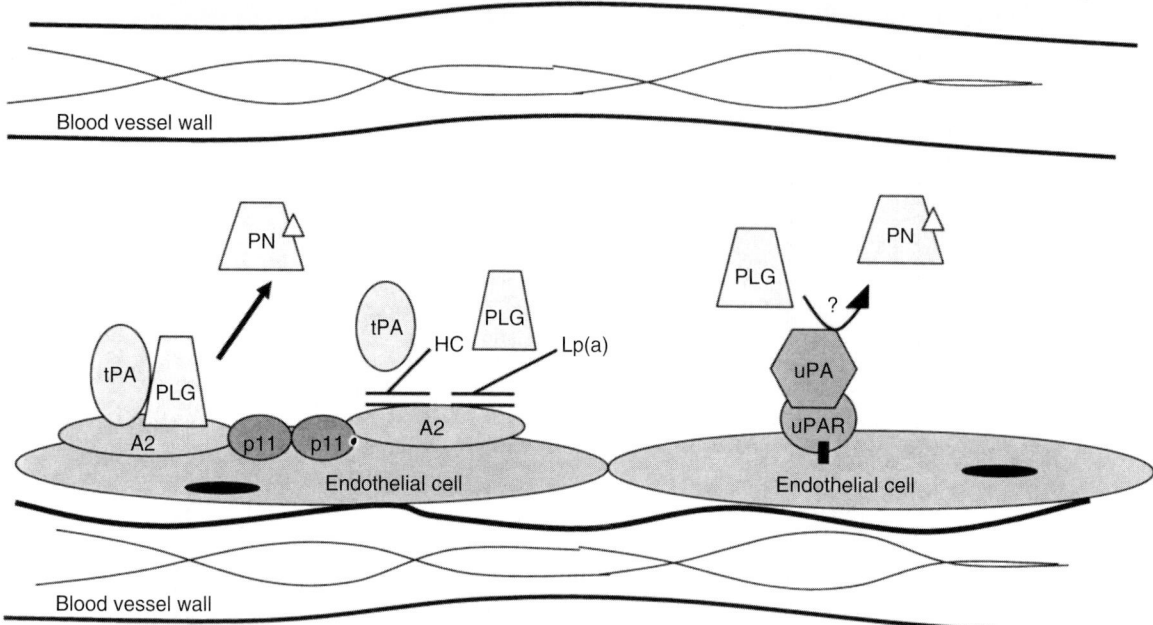

**FIGURE 22-1.** Fibrinolytic assembly on endothelial cells. Annexin 2 (*A2*), in heterotetrameric complex with protein *p11*, is expressed on the surface of vascular endothelial cells. *tPA*, produced by the endothelial cell, as well as circulating plasminogen (*PLG*), bind to annexin 2 at independent sites, giving rise to efficient generation of plasmin (*PN*). tPA binding is blocked by homocysteine (*HC*), which derivatizes the tPA binding site. Lipoprotein (a) [*Lp(a)*] competes with plasminogen for its binding site on annexin 2. On interaction with its receptor, urokinase receptor (*uPAR*), uPA may also accelerate the generation of plasminogen.

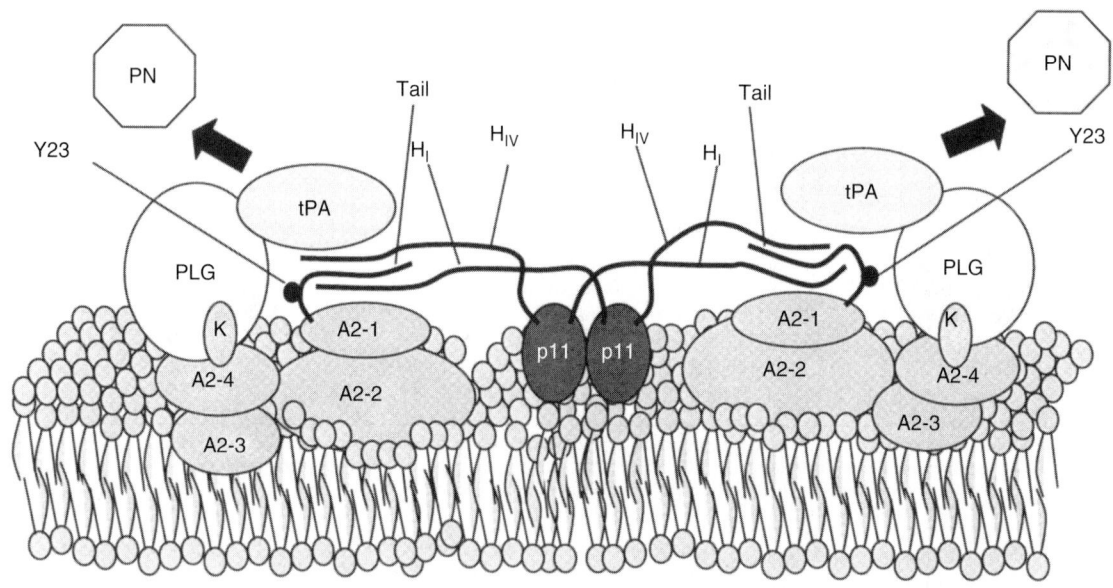

**FIGURE 22-2.** Schematic model of the annexin 2 tetramer complex with associated plasminogen (*PLG*) and tissue plasminogen activator (*tPA*). Annexin 2 binds PLG by a lysine residue (*K*) within core domain 4 (*A2-4*). tPA binding requires a linear amino acid sequence within the tail domain. The four core domains of annexin 2 (*A2-1* through *A2-4*) maintain its close association with membrane phospholipid. Twin p11 molecules bind the *N*-terminal tail of annexin 2 through hydrophobic interactions with helix 1 ($H_I$) of one p11 and helix 4 ($H_{IV}$) of the second p11, thereby imparting increased membrane affinity to the complex (87). The tyrosine phosphorylation site (*Y23*) of annexin 2 is necessary for its transport to the cell surface. Assembly of zymogen and activator greatly favors the catalytic efficiency of activation of plasminogen and generation of plasmin (*PN*).

deposits are sometimes seen in hepatic sinusoids and intestine. uPA$^{-/-}$ macrophages show reduced capacity to degrade fibrin *in vitro*, and uPA-null mice are more susceptible to endotoxin-induced thrombosis than littermate controls are.

## Urokinase Receptor

The interaction of uPA with many cell types, including human umbilical vein endothelial cells, requires the high-affinity ($K_d$ 0.5 nM; $M_r$ 55,000 to 60,000) uPAR (Fig. 22-1) (95–108). This glycosyl–phosphatidylinositol–anchored protein accepts high-molecular-weight uPA, prouPA, and the amino-terminal fragment (ATF) of uPA, but not low-molecular-weight uPA or tissue plasminogen activator (97,99,109,110). uPA associated with this receptor maintains its susceptibility to its physiologic inhibitor PAI-1, suggesting a possible clearance function (111,112). The uPA receptor possesses three structural domains, the first of which interacts with uPA (113).

In the adult mouse, uPAR mRNA, which is not normally detected in resting endothelial cells, appears in endothelial cells of multiple organs following exposure to endotoxin (114); the same stimulus reduces its expression in the renal tubules (93). Recent evidence, furthermore, indicates that uPAR-associated uPA may fulfill mainly nonproteolytic functions including directed cell migration, cellular adhesion, differentiation, and proliferation (115).

uPAR may fulfill nonproteolytic functions ranging from directed cell migration to cellular adhesion, differentiation, and regulation of integrin function (115,116). uPAR binds the adhesive glycoprotein vitronectin at a site distinct from the uPA binding domain (117,118). uPAR-transfected 293 cells acquire enhanced adhesion to vitronectin, but lose their adhesion to fibronectin (119). uPAR, furthermore, colocalizes with integrins in focal contacts at the leading edge of migrating cells (119,120). In endothelial cells, uPAR also associates with caveolae, structures that appear to coordinate a variety of signaling events (121).

uPAR–deficient mice, interestingly, have an essentially normal phenotype (Table 22-2) (45). Although their macrophages show a reduced rate of uPA-dependent plasminogen activation, *in vitro* matrix degradation is normal. In addition, simultaneous deletion of both uPAR and tPA does not impair development, fertility, or wound repair capability (122). Histologic analysis of these animals revealed only occasional fibrin deposits in hepatic sinusoids. Therefore, the role of uPAR in fibrinolytic surveillance seems tenuous.

# OTHER FIBRINOLYSIS-RELATED ACTIONS OF PLASMIN

## Activation of Fibrinolytic Proteins

With respect to the fibrinolytic system, plasmin may amplify its own generation in several ways (Table 22-1). *In vitro*, plasmin can convert the circulating form of its parent zymogen, plasminogen (Glu-PLG) to a truncated form 10 to 20 times more readily activated by either tPA or uPA (8–10). This modified molecule, *N*-terminal lysine plasminogen (lysplasminogen), does not circulate under normal conditions (61), but can be found on cell surfaces, particularly the endothelial cell (60), where it may serve as a preferred substrate for plasminogen activators.

*In vitro*, plasmin can convert single-chain forms of both major plasminogen activators (single-chain tPA and prourokinase) to two-chain molecules that possess enhanced plasmin

generating activity. tPA is synthesized by endothelial cells as a single-chain polypeptide ($M_r$ 72,000) that can be cleaved to its two-chain homolog by plasmin, tissue kallikrein, and factor Xa (123). Two-chain tPA is more active than one-chain tPA plasminogen activation, except in the presence of fibrin (124). Therefore, conversion of tPA to its two-chain form may have special relevance to fibrin-free systems, such as cell surfaces.

uPA, secreted in single-chain form by a variety of cultured cell types including the endothelial cell is also converted to two-chain form on exposure to plasmin (12,125–127). Although one series of studies describes prourokinase as a zymogen devoid of intrinsic plasminogen activating activity (12, 125,126), others have elucidated the ability of single-chain uPA to bind to fibrin (128) and activate plasminogen (129, 130). Although uPA may gain catalytic activity upon conversion to the two-chain form, it also loses its fibrin binding specificity (98). Therefore, its conversion to the two-chain form may be important at the cell surface, and in locations that are relatively devoid of fibrin.

## Inactivation of Procoagulant Proteins

Further *in vitro* studies suggest that plasmin can modify cofactors important in the thrombin-generating coagulation cascade (Table 22-1). Plasmin has been shown to inactivate bovine factor Va *in vitro* by cleaving both the heavy and light chains of this protein ($M_r$ 168,000) (13). This lipid-dependent inactivation results in a series of plasmin-specific cleavages that are distinct from those produced by activated protein C (131). The inactivation of human factor V by plasmin may be preceded by transient generation of procoagulant fragments that are subsequently degraded to inactive form (132). Plasmin also can inactivate factor VIIIa, another procoagulant cofactor that is structurally homologous to factor Va (14).

## Modification of Platelet Function

The effects of plasmin on *in vitro* platelet function are complex and probably depend on the dose and duration of plasmin treatment. Exposure of platelets to plasmin *in vitro* has been associated with platelet activation (133,134), platelet inhibition (135), and platelet disaggregation (136). Early in the thrombotic process, platelet fibrinogen is converted to fibrin by thrombin in parallel with enhanced plasminogen–platelet interaction (137). However, plasmin generated on the platelet surface could degrade platelet glycoproteins IIb/IIIa and Ib, receptors for fibrinogen and von Willebrand factor, respectively, leading to impaired platelet adhesion and aggregation (138,139). Indeed, prolonged bleeding times were found in patients 90 minutes after tPA infusion for thrombolysis, suggesting early impairment of platelet function upon plasmin generation (140). Finally, platelets may play a late role in thrombotic reocclusion after successful thrombolytic therapy (141).

# NONFIBRINOLYTIC FUNCTIONS OF PLASMIN

Within the blood vessel, it is likely that plasmin fulfills roles beyond the degradation of fibrin. Nonfibrin substrates suggested by *in vivo* studies include promatrix metalloproteinases-1 and -3 (18), laminin within the central nervous system (15), and proBDNF in the mouse hippocampus (22) (Table 22-1). Therefore, with the development of new transgenic and null deletion mouse models, expanding roles are emerging for the fibrinolytic system in tissue remodeling (1).

## Wound Healing

A number of transgenic mouse models of vascular disease have elucidated a complex role for the fibrinolytic system in wound healing (Table 22-2). Plasminogen-deficient mice display impaired healing of cutaneous wounds because of impaired keratinocyte migration (32). This abnormality is not seen in the simultaneous absence of fibrinogen, suggesting that the fibrinolytic activity of plasmin is required for normal wound healing in the skin (142).

## Inflammation

In the peritoneal cavity, recruitment of inflammatory cells is profoundly inhibited in the absence of plasminogen (33). Plasmin may promote invasion of leukocytes into inflammatory lesions such as the advanced or evolving atherosclerotic plaque (143). In transplant-associated arteriosclerosis, similarly, the extent of disease is considerably reduced in plasminogen-deficient mice, reflecting, at least in part, the reduced influx of macrophages, with attenuated medial necrosis, fragmentation of elastic laminae and remodeling of the adventitia (Table 22-2) (36).

In other studies, PAI-1 is likely to function as a major regulator of endothelial cell plasmin generation, especially in inflammatory settings. Although quiescent endothelial cells express little or no PAI-1 *in vivo*, inflammatory cytokines are powerful inducers of PAI-1. In both rats and humans with active malignancy, injecting TNF results in a striking increase in plasma concentrations of PAI-1 (67,68). In addition, endothelial expression of PAI-1 is detected in the ovary near neovascular sprouts that also express uPA (94). Elevated levels of circulating PAI-1 have been linked epidemiologically with risk of myocardial infarction (69).

## Atherogenesis

On the basis of observations that inflammatory cell migration is impaired in plasminogen deficiency, one might predict that atherosclerotic plaque formation would be impaired in mice that are doubly deficient in plasminogen and apolipoprotein E (ApoE). However, such mice showed an *increased* predisposition to atherosclerosis compared with animals deficient in ApoE alone (Table 22-2) (37). Mice with ApoE deficiency combined with either uPA or tPA deficiency showed no increase in fatty streak or advanced plaque formation, suggesting that elimination of both uPA and tPA may be necessary to accelerate atherogenesis (39). Therefore, rather than mediating inflammatory and smooth muscle cell invasion during plaque initiation, the dominant role for plasmin may be in degrading fibrin and other matrix constituents after the lesion has begun to form. Clearly, more studies are needed to resolve these issues.

In humans, the atherogenic, prothrombotic amino acid, homocysteine (HC), accumulates in association with nutritional deficiency of vitamin $B_6$, vitamin $B_{12}$, or folic acid, or in inherited deficiencies of cystathionine $\beta$-synthase, methylenetetrahydrofolate reductase, or methionine synthase (144). Elevated levels of HC are highly associated with atherosclerosis, venous thromboembolism, and cardiovascular death (145,146). *In vitro* studies indicate that HC may promote vascular compromise by blocking tPA binding to its endothelial cell receptor, annexin 2. HC directly disables the tPA-binding "tail" domain of annexin 2 by forming a covalent disulfide adduction product with cysteine 9 within the LCKLSL sequence (147). Mutation of C9 within the tPA binding sequence results in severely impaired tPA interaction (148). HC-treated cultured endothelial cells bind approximately 50% less tPA than untreated cells do and also activate approximately 50% less plasminogen, thereby possibly impairing fibrin clearance prior to plaque formation (148).

Lipoprotein (a) [Lp(a)] is a low density lipoprotein (LDL)–like particle that is an independent risk factor for atherosclerosis (149–152). In addition to apolipoprotein B-100, Lp(a) contains a disulfide-linked moiety called *apolipoprotein (a)* [apo(a)]. Apo(a) shares a remarkable degree of homology with plasminogen, including multiple tandem repeats of domains similar to kringle 4, a single region resembling kringle 5, and a pseudoprotease segment (153). Plasminogen and apo(a), furthermore, are genetically linked on chromosome 6 and may have arisen from a common ancestral gene (154). The disulfide-linked kringle 37 of the originally cloned apo(a) resembles kringle 4 of plasminogen in that it possesses amino acids corresponding to three of the four key LBS residues (i.e., Asp55, Asp57, and Arg71) (155). Lp(a) binds to plasmin-treated fibrin (156) and colocalizes with fibrin in atheromatous tissue, possibly displacing plasminogen (157,158).

Both Lp(a) and apo(a) inhibit Lys–PLG binding to both endothelial cells (median inhibitory dose, is more than 36-fold) (158) and U937 cells (159). Lp(a) also binds to annexin 2 *in vitro* and can inhibit 95% of plasminogen activation by tPA at the endothelial cell surface (89). The estimated dissociation constants for apo(a) and plasminogen with respect to the endothelial cell surface are comparable, suggesting that receptor occupancy *in vivo* is largely determined by the ambient level of Lp(a) because plasminogen concentrations do not appear to change considerably (158–160).

Because Lp(a) levels are, at best, only transiently responsive to diet (161,162), heredity may play a more important role in regulating fibrinolytic potential at the endothelial cell surface (163–165). In general, plasma Lp(a) concentrations appear to correlate inversely with the ratio of kringle 4 to kringle 5 encoding domains within the apo(a) gene (166,167). Therefore, the larger the apo(a) gene product, reflected in a greater number of kringle 4 domains, the lower the concentration of apo(a) in plasma. In addition, Lp(a) appears to represent an acute-phase reactant in the postsurgical and postmyocardial infarction setting (163) and in patients with cancer (165), suggesting a role for soluble inflammatory mediators in regulating its synthesis or assembly.

Cell-associated plasmin activity is reduced *in vivo* when apo(a) is overexpressed (48). Similarly, apo(a)-overexpressing transgenic mice are resistant to lysis of an artificial thrombus by tPA (Table 22-2) (49). Lp(a) may exert an antifibrinolytic effect by enhancing functional, antigenic, and transcript levels of PAI-1 (168). Alternatively, Lp(a) may act as an inhibitor of plasminogen activators (169) by directly competing with plasminogen for binding to streptokinase (170), by competitively inhibiting tPA in the presence of fibrinogen (171) or by uncompetitively inhibiting the fibrin-dependent enhancement of tPA-induced plasmin generation (172).

When Lp(a) was overexpressed in mice receiving a high-fat diet, atherosclerotic lesions containing both lipid and anti-apo(a) cross-reactive material were observed (47). On the other hand, the deposition of both lipid and apo(a) was reduced in mice expressing apo(a) in which LBSs had been mutated (50). These data indicate that LBSs of apo(a) are crucial to its atherogenicity.

## Aneurysm

Plasmin may play a central role in aneurysm formation and progression (Table 22-2). uPA, but not tPA, deficiency is associated with reduced medial destruction and reduced activation of downstream plasmin-dependent matrix metalloproteinases in a murine model of aortic aneurysm (39). Similarly, uPA-deficient, but not tPA-deficient, mice appear to be protected from cardiac rupture secondary to ventricular aneurysm, and treatment with PAI-1 or the general matrix metalloproteinase inhibitor, TIMP-1, seems to protect wild-type mice from aortic rupture (173).

## Restenosis

Arterial restenosis reflects neointima formation following vascular injury, usually secondary to an acute therapeutic intervention. Because restenosis involves leukocyte invasion, proliferation and migration of smooth muscle cells, deposition of extracellular matrix, and reendothelialization, plasmin activity may be required at any of several steps. Neointima formation in models involving severe electrical or mechanical arterial injury requires intact expression of plasminogen and uPA, but not tPA (34,174,175) or uPAR (176). PAI-1, furthermore, appears to substantially temper the neointimal/stenotic response (177). Because such injury models are not associated with severe thrombosis, it is thought that fibrinolytic activity is required for migration of smooth muscle cells and leukocytes within the arterial wall rather than for thrombolysis (178). On the other hand, when jugular vein segments were surgically grafted into the carotid artery, neointima formed even in the complete absence of host plasminogen; these data suggest that although proteolytic activity is required to overcome barriers to cell migration in the arterial wall, it may be less important in the vein wall (179).

Early thrombosis may play a much more prominent role in the overall response to injury with ferric chloride, Rose Bengal, or the copper cuff. In these models, the loss of uPA accelerates thrombotic occlusion (180), whereas deficiency of PAI-1 attenuates thrombosis (181,182). Absence of PAI-1 was also associated with reduced vascular stenosis regardless of whether ApoE was also absent (183,184) or present (185). Finally, in balloon-injured rat carotid arteries transduction of a PAI-1-expressing gene led to increased restenosis of the vessel, again suggesting that clearance of the initial thrombus may have long-term effects on vessel patency and neointima formation (186). Therefore, in these systems, plasmin may function to clear an initial thrombus, thereby eliminating the scaffold for later restenosis.

Plasmin appears to be an important modulator of growth factor activity and processing (Table 22-1). Plasma transforming growth factor-$\beta$ (TGF-$\beta$), which can serve as a survival factor for smooth muscle cells or as an inhibitor of endothelial cell proliferation, is reduced in atherosclerosis, possibly because of impaired activation by plasmin (187,188). In addition, the *in vitro* mitogenic and chemotactic effects of basic fibroblast growth factor (bFGF) and platelet-derived growth factor depend upon uPA and tPA, respectively (189).

## Angiogenesis

The endothelial cell fibrinolytic system may play a complex role in regulating the development of new blood vessels during wound healing or in response to tumor growth. uPA, uPAR, and PAI-1 are all expressed by endothelial cells during angiogenesis, and all are induced by the angiogenic growth factors' vascular endothelial cell growth factor (VEGF) and bFGF *in vivo* (190–192). On the other hand, developmental angiogenesis and vasculogenesis appear to be unimpeded in plasminogen-deficient mice.

Annexin 2 appears to be an important component of the endothelial cell's angiogenic repertoire (46). An annexin 2 peptide, which mimics sequences necessary for tPA binding, blocked endothelial cell invasion of Matrigel implants in wild-type mice. In addition, annexin 2–deficient mice displayed markedly diminished neovascularization of the FGF-stimulated cornea and of the oxygen-primed neonatal retina (Table 22-2). Capillary sprouting from annexin 2–deficient aortic ring explants was markedly reduced in association with severe impairment of activation of metalloproteinase-9 and -13. These data establish annexin 2 as a regulator of cell surface plasmin generation and show, additionally, that impaired endothelial cell fibrinolytic activity constitutes a barrier to effective neoangiogenesis.

Angiostatin is a circulating inhibitor of angiogenesis that was originally isolated from the urine of Lewis lung carcinoma–bearing mice (193). This protein ($M_r$ 38,000), which bears complete homology to kringles 1 through 4 of plasminogen, inhibits bFGF-stimulated endothelial cell proliferation *in vitro* and blocks formation of new blood vessels in both the chick chorioallantoic membrane and mouse cornea assays. In several experimental animal models, exogenous angiostatin induced tumor dormancy by initiation of apoptosis rather than by direct inhibition of the cell cycle (194). Blockade of primary and metastatic tumor growth is also seen on implantation of tumor cells that are stably transfected with an angiostatin gene in a murine fibrosarcoma model (195). The cellular target or receptor for angiostatin is unknown. Formation of angiostatin may involve cleavage of plasmin(ogen) by a tumor-associated metalloelastase (196), a plasmin reductase (197), or by matrix metalloproteinases-7 and -9 (198).

## References

1. Hajjar KA, Esmon NL, Marcus AJ. Vascular function in hemostasis. In: Lichtman MA, Beutler E, Kipps TJ, et al., eds. *Williams hematology*, New York: McGraw-Hill, 2005.
2. Augustin HG, Kozian DH, Johnson RC. Differentiation of endothelial cells: analysis of the constitutive and activated endothelial cell phenotypes. *BioEssays* 1994;16:901–906.
3. Cines DB, Pollak ES, Buck CA, et al. Endothelial cells in physiology and in the pathophysiology of vascular disorders. *Blood* 1998;91:3527–3561.
4. Hajjar KA. *The endothelium in health and disease*, High KA et al., eds., 2006. McGraw-Hill, New York (*in press*).
5. Hajjar KA. The molecular basis of fibrinolysis. In: Nathan DG, Orkin SH, Ginsburg D, et al., eds. *Hematology of infancy and childhood.*, Philadelphia, PA: WB Saunders, 2003:1497–1514.
6. Hajjar KA. Molecular mechanisms of fibrinolysis. In: Lichtman MA, Beutler E, Kipps TJ et al., eds. *Williams hematology.*, New York: McGraw-Hill, 2005.
7. Ranby M. Studies on the kinetics of plasminogen activation by tissue plasminogen activator. *Biochem Biophys Acta* 1982;704:461–469.
8. Hoylaerts M, Rijken DC, Lijnen HR, et al. Kinetics of the activation of plasminogen by human tissue plasminogen activator: role of fibrin. *J Biol Chem* 1982;257:2912–2929.
9. Markus G, Evers JL, Hobika GH. Comparison of some properties of native (glu) and modified (lys) human plasminogen. *J Biol Chem* 1978;253:733–739.
10. Markus G, Priore RL, Wissler FC. The binding of tranexamic acid to native (glu) and modified (lys) human plasminogen and its effect on conformation. *J Biol Chem* 1979;254:1211–1216.
11. Ichinose A, Takio K, Fujikawa K. Localization of the binding site of tissue-type plasminogen activator to fibrin. *J Clin Invest* 1986;78:163–169.
12. Kasai S, Arimura H, Nishida M, et al. Primary structure of single-chain pro-urokinase. *J Biol Chem* 1985;260:12382–12389.
13. Omar MN, Mann KG. Inactivation of factor Va by plasmin. *J Biol Chem* 1987;262:9750–9755.
14. McKee PA, Anderson JC, Switzer ME. Molecular structural studies of human factor VIII. *Ann N Y Acad Sci* 1975;240:8–33.
15. Chen ZL, Strickland SE. Neuronal death in the hippocampus is promoted by plasmin-catalyzed degradation of laminin. *Cell* 1997;91:917–925.
16. Marder VJ, Sherry S. Thrombolytic therapy: current status. *N Engl J Med* 1988;318:1512–1520.
17. Netzel-Arnett S, Mitola DJ, Yamada SS, et al. Collagen dissolution by keratinocytes requires cell surface plasminogen activation and matrix metalloproteinase activity. *J Biol Chem* 2002;277:45154–45161.
18. Loskutoff DJ, Quigley JP. PAI-1, fibrosis, and the elusive provisional fibrin matrix. *J Clin Invest* 2000;106:1441–1443.
19. Ramos-DeSimone N, Hahn-Dantona E, Sipley J, et al. Activation of matrix metalloproteinase-9 (MMP-9) via a converging plasmin/stromelysin-1 cascade enhances tumor cell invasion. *J Biol Chem* 1999;274:13066–13076.

20. Lyons RM, Gentry LE, Purchio AF, et al. Mechanism of activation of latent recombinant transforming growth factor beta1 by plasmin. *J Cell Biol* 1990;110:1361–1367.

21. Sporn MB, Roberts AB, Wakefield LM, et al. Transforming growth factor-beta: biological function and chemical structure. *Science* 1986;233:532–534.

22. Pang PT, Teng HK, Zaitsev E, et al. Cleavage of proBDNF by tPA/plasmin is essential for long-term hippocampal plasticity. *Science* 2004;306:487–491.

23. Aoki N, Moroi M, Sakata Y, et al. Abnormal plasminogen: a hereditary molecular abnormality found in a patient with recurrent thrombosis. *J Clin Invest* 1978;61:1186–1195.

24. Ichinose A, Espling ES, Takamatsu J, et al. Two types of abnormal genes for plasminogen in families with a predisposition for thrombosis. *Proc Natl Acad Sci U S A* 1991;88:115–119.

25. Schott D, Dempfle CE, Beck P, et al. Therapy with a purified plasminogen concentrate in an infant with ligneous conjunctivitis and homozygous plasminogen deficiency. *N Engl J Med* 1998;339:1679–1686.

26. Schuster V, Seregard S. Ligneous conjunctivitis. *Surv Ophthalmol* 2003; 48:369–388.

27. Bugge TH, Flick MJ, Daugherty CC, et al. Plasminogen deficiency causes severe thrombosis but is compatible with development and reproduction. *Genes Dev* 1995;9:794–807.

28. Carmeliet P, Collen D. Gene targeting and gene transfer studies of the plasminogen/plasmin system: implications in thrombosis, hemostasis, neointima formation, and atherosclerosis. *FASEB J* 1995;9:934–938.

29. Drew AF, Kaufman AH, Kombrinck KW, et al. Ligneous conjunctivitis in plasminogen-deficient mice. *Blood* 1998;91:1616–1624.

30. Lijnen HR, Carmeliet P, Bouche A, et al. Restoration of thrombolytic potential in plasminogen-deficient mice by bolus administration of plasminogen. *Blood* 1996;88:870–876.

31. Ploplis VA, Carmeliet P, Vazirzadeh S, et al. Effects of disruption of the plasminogen gene on thrombosis, growth, and health in mice. *Circulation* 1995;92:2585–2593.

32. Romer J, Bugge TH, Pyke C, et al. Impaired wound healing in mice with a disrupted plasminogen gene. *Nature Med* 1996;2:287–292.

33. Ploplis VA, French EL, Carmeliet P, et al. Plasminogen deficiency differentially affects recruitment of inflammatory cell populations in mice. *Blood* 1998;91:2005–2009.

34. Carmeliet P, Moons L, Ploplis VA, et al. Impaired arterial neointima formation in mice with disruption of the plasminogen gene. *J Clin Invest* 1997;99:200–208.

35. Coleman JL, Gebbia JA, Piesman J, et al. Plasminogen is required for efficient dissemination of B. burgdorferi in ticks and for enhancement of spirochetemia in mice. *Cell* 1997;89:1111–1119.

36. Moons L, Wi C, Ploplis V, et al. Reduced transplant arteriosclerosis in plasminogen-deficient mice. *J Clin Invest* 1998;102:1788–1797.

37. Xiao Q, Danton MJS, Witte DP, et al. Plasminogen deficiency accelerates vessel wall disease in mice predisposed to atherosclerosis. *Proc Natl Acad Sci U S A* 1997;94:10335–10340.

38. Carmeliet P, Schoonjans L, Kieckens L, et al. Physiological consequences of loss of plasminogen activator gene function in mice. *Nature* 1994; 368:419–424.

39. Carmeliet P, Moons L, Lijnen R, et al. Urokinase-generated plasmin activates matrix metalloproteinases during aneurysm formation. *Nat Genet* 1997;17:439–444.

40. Heymans S, Luttun AND, Theilmeier G, et al. Inhibition of plasminogen activators or matrix metalloproteinases prevents cardiac rupture but impairs therapeutic angiogenesis and causes cardiac failure. *Nat Med* 1999; 5:1135–1142.

41. Carmeliet P, Kieckens L, Schoonjans L, et al. Plasminogen activator inhibitor-1 gene-deficient mice: I. Generation by homologous recombination and characterization. *J Clin Invest* 1993;92:2746–2755.

42. Carmeliet P, Stassen JM, Schoonjans L, et al. Plasminogen activator inhibitor-1 gene-deficient mice: II. Effects on hemostasis, thrombosis, and thrombolysis. *J Clin Invest* 1993;92:2756–2760.

43. Herz J, Clouthier DE, Hammer RE. LDL receptor-related protein internalizes and degrades uPA-PAI-1 complexes and is essential for embryo implantation. *Cell* 1992;71:411–421.

44. Herz J, Clouthier DE, Hammer RE. Correction: LDL receptor-related protein internalizes and degrades uPA-PAI-1 complexes and is essential for embryo implantation. *Cell* 1993;73:428.

45. Dewerchin M, Van Nuffelen A, Wallays G, et al. Generation and characterization of urokinase receptor-deficient mice. *J Clin Invest* 1996;97:870–878.

46. Ling Q, Jacovina AT, Deora AB, et al. Annexin II is a key regulator of fibrin homeostasis and neoangiogenesis. *J Clin Invest* 2004;113:38–48.

47. Lawn RM, Wade DP, Hammer RE. Atherogenesis in transgenic mice expressing human apolipoprotein(a). *Nature* 1992;360:670–672.

48. Grainger DJ, Kemp PR, Liu AC, et al. Activation of transforming growth factor-beta is inhibited in transgenic apolipoprotein(a) mice. *Nature* 1994; 370:460–462.

49. Palabrica TM, Liu AC, Aronovitz MJ, et al. Antifibrinolytic activity of apolipoprotein(a) *in vivo*: human apolipoprotein(a) transgenic mice are resistant to tissue plasminogen activator-mediated thrombolysis. *Nat Med* 1995;1:256–259.

50. Boonmark NW, Lou XJ, Schwartz K, et al. Modification of apolipoprotein(a) lysine binding site reduces atherosclerosis in transgenic mice. *J Clin Invest* 1997;100:558–564.

51. Erickson LA, Fici GJ, Lund JE, et al. Development of venous occlusions in transgenic mice for the plasminogen activator inhibitor-1 gene. *Nature* 1990;346:74–76.

52. Heckel JL, Sandgren EP, Degen JL, et al. Neonatal bleeding in transgenic mice expressing urokinase-type plasminogen activator. *Cell* 1990;62: 447–456.

53. Meiri N, Masos T, Rosenblum K, et al. Overexpression of urokinase-type plasminogen activator in transgenic mice is correlated with impaired learning. *Proc Natl Acad Sci U S A* 1994;91:3196–3200.

54. Hajjar KA. Cellular receptors in the regulation of plasmin generation. *Thromb Haemostasis* 1995;74:294–301.

55. Burtin P, Chavanel G, Andre J. The plasmin system in human colonic tumors: an immunofluorescent study. *Int J Cancer* 1985;35:307–314.

56. Burtin P, Chavanel G, Andre-Bougaran J, et al. The plasmin system in human adenocarcinomas and their metastases. A comparative immunofluorescence study. *Int J Cancer* 1987;39:170–178.

57. Clavel C, Chavanel G, Birembaut P. Detection of the plasmin system in human mammary pathology using immunofluorescence. *Cancer Res* 1986;46:5743–5747.

58. Hajjar KA, Harpel PC, Jaffe EA, et al. Binding of plasminogen to cultured human endothelial cells. *J Biol Chem* 1986;261:11656–11662.

59. Schafer A, Rodriguez R, Loscalzo J, et al. Inhibition of vascular endothelial cell prostacyclin synthesis by plasmin. *Blood* 1989;74:1015–1020.

60. Hajjar KA, Nachman RL. Endothelial cell-mediated conversion of glu-plasminogen to lys-plasminogen: further evidence for assembly of the fibrinolytic system on the endothelial cell surface. *J Clin Invest* 1988;82: 1769–1778.

61. Holvoet P, Lijnen HR, Collen D. A monoclonal antibody specific for lys-plasminogen. *J Biol Chem* 1985;260:12106–12111.

62. Todd AS. Fibrinolysis autographs. *Nature* 1958;181:495–496.

63. Todd AS. Localization of fibrinolytic activity in tissues. *Br Med Bull* 1964;20:210–212.

64. Levin EG, del Zoppo GJ. Localization of tissue plasminogen activator in the endothelium of a limited number of vessels. *Am J Pathol* 1994;144: 855–861.

65. Levin EG, Santell L, Osborn KG. The expression of endothelial tissue plasminogen activator *in vivo*: a function defined by vessel size and anatomic location. *J Cell Sci* 1997;110:139–148.

66. Levin EG, Osborn KG, Schleuning WD. Vessel-specific gene expression in the lung: tissue plasmingen activator is limited to bronchial arteries and pulmonary vessels of discrete size. *Chest* 1998;114:68S.

67. Van Hinsbergh VWM, Kooistra T, Emeis JJ, et al. Regulation of plasminogen activator production by endothelial cells: role in fibrinolysis and local proteolysis. *Int J Radiat Biol* 1991;60:261–272.

68. Van Hinsbergh VWM, Bauer KA, Kooistra T, et al. Progress of fibrinolysis during tumor necrosis factor infusions in humans. Concomitant increase in tissue-type plasminogen activator, plasminogen activator inhibitor type-1, and fibrin(ogen) degradation products. *Blood* 1990;76: 2284–2289.

69. Hamsten A, Wiman B, De Faire U, et al. Increased plasma levels of a rapid inhibitor of tissue plasminogen activator in young survivors of myocardial infarction. *N Engl J Med* 1985;313:1557–1563.

70. Pizzo SV, Murray JC, Gonias SL. Atrophie blanche: a disorder associated with defective release of tissue plasminogen activator. *Arch Pathol Lab Med* 1986;110:517–519.

71. Barnathan ES, Kuo A, Van der Keyl H, et al. Tissue-type plasminogen activator binding to human endothelial cells: evidence for two distinct binding sites. *J Biol Chem* 1988;263:7792–7799.

72. Beebe DB. Binding of tissue plasminogen activator to human umbilical vein endothelial cells. *Thromb Res* 1987;46:241–254.

73. Hajjar KA, Hamel NM, Harpel PC, et al. Binding of tissue plasminogen activator to cultured human endothelial cells. *J Clin Invest* 1987;80: 1712–1719.

74. Hajjar KA, Hamel NM. Identification and characterization of human endothelial cell membrane binding sites for tissue plasminogen activator and urokinase. *J Biol Chem* 1990;265:2908–2916.

75. Hajjar KA. The endothelial cell tissue plasminogen activator receptor: specific interaction with plasminogen. *J Biol Chem* 1991;266:21962–21970.

76. Sakata Y, Okada M, Noro A, et al. Interaction of tissue-type plasminogen activator inhibitor-1 on the surface of endothelial cells. *J Biol Chem* 1988;263:1960–1969.

77. Hajjar KA, Jacovina AT, Chacko J. An endothelial cell receptor for plasminogen and tissue plasminogen activator: I. Identity with annexin II. *J Biol Chem* 1994;269:21191–21197.

78. Tressler RJ, Nicolson GL. Butanol-extractable and detergent-solubilized cell surface components from murine large cell lymphoma cells associated with adhesion to organ microvessel endothelial cells. *J Cell Biochem* 1992;48:162–171.

79. Tressler RJ, Updyke TV, Yeatman TJ, et al. Extracellular annexin is associated with divalent cation-dependent tumor cell adhesion of metastatic RAW 117 large-cell lymphoma cells. *J Cell Biochem* 1993;53:265–276.

80. Yeatman TJ, Updyke TV, Kaetzel MA, et al. Expression of annexins on the surfaces of non-metastatic human and rodent tumor cells. *Clin Exp Metastasis* 1993;11:37–44.

81. Menell JS, Cesarman GM, Jacovina AT, et al. Annexin II and bleeding in acute promyelocytic leukemia. *N Engl J Med* 1999;340:994–1004.

82. Brownstein C, Deora AB, Jacovina AT, et al. Annexin II mediates plasminogen-dependent matrix invasion by human monocytes: enhanced expression by macrophages. *Blood* 2004;103:317–324.

83. Falcone DJ, Borth W, Faisal Khan KM, et al. Plasminogen-mediated matrix invasion and degradation by macrophages is dependent on surface expression of annexin II. *Blood* 2001;97:777–784.

84. Chung CY, Erickson HP. Cell surface annexin II is a high affinity receptor for the alternatively spliced segment of tenascin-C. *J Cell Biol* 1994;126:539–548.

85. Kassam G, Choi KS, Ghuman J, et al. The role of annexin II tetramer in the activation of plasminogen. *J Biol Chem* 1998;273:4790–4799.

86. Wright JF, Kurosky A, Wasi S. An endothelial cell-surface form of annexin II binds human cytomegalovirus. *Biochem Biophys Res Commun* 1994;198:983–989.

87. Rety S, Sopkova J, Renouard M, et al. The crystal structure of a complex of p11 with the annexin II N-terminal peptide. *Nat Struct Biol* 1999;6:85–89.

88. Cesarman GM, Guevara CA, Hajjar KA. An endothelial cell receptor for plasminogen/tissue plasminogen activator: II. Annexin II-mediated enhancement of t-PA-dependent plasminogen activation. *J Biol Chem* 1994;269:21198–21203.

89. Hajjar KA, Guevara CA, Lev E, et al. Interaction of the fibrinolytic receptor, annexin II, with the endothelial cell surface: essential role of endonexin repeat 2. *J Biol Chem* 1996;271:21652–21659.

90. Deora AB, Kreitzer G, Jacovina AT, et al. An annexin 2 phosphorylation switch mediates its p11-dependent translocation to the cell surface. *J Biol Chem* 2004;279:43411–43418.

91. Ishii H, Yoshida M, Hiraoka M, et al. Recombinant annexin II modulates impaired fibrinolytic activity *in vitro* and in rat carotid artery. *Circ Res* 2001;89:1240–1245.

92. Kristensen P, Larson LI, Nielsen LS, et al. Human endothelial cells contain one type of plasminogen activator. *FEBS Lett* 1984;168:33–37.

93. Yamamoto K, Loskutoff DJ. Fibrin deposition in tissues from endotoxin-treated mice correlates with decreases in the expression of urokinase-type but not tissue-type plasminogen activator. *J Clin Invest* 1996;97:2440–2451.

94. Bacharach E, Itin A, Keshet E. *In vivo* patterns of expression of urokinase and its inhibitor PAI-1 suggest a concerted role in regulating physiological angiogenesis. *Proc Natl Acad Sci U S A* 1992;89:10686–10690.

95. Blasi F, Conese M, Moller LB, et al. The urokinase receptor: structure, regulation and inhibitor-mediated internalization. *Fibrinolysis* 1994;8:182–188.

96. Appella E, Robinson A, Ullrich SJ, et al. The receptor-binding sequence of urokinase. *J Biol Chem* 1987;262:4437–4440.

97. Cubellis MV, Nolli ML, Cassani G, et al. Binding of single chain prourokinase to the urokinase receptor of human U937 cells. *J Biol Chem* 1986;261:15819–15822.

98. Stoppelli MP, Corti A, Soffientini A, et al. Differentiation-enhanced binding of the amino-terminal fragment of human urokinase plasminogen activator to a specific receptor on U937 monocytes. *Proc Natl Acad Sci U S A* 1985;82:4939–4943.

99. Vassalli JD, Baccino D, Belin D. A cellular binding site for the Mr 55,000 form of the human plasminogen activator, urokinase. *J Cell Biol* 1985;100:86–92.

100. Fibbi G, Dini G, Pasquali F, et al. The Mr 17500 region of the A chain of urokinase is required for interaction with a specific receptor in A431 cells. *Biochim Biophys Acta* 1986;885:301–308.

101. Stoppelli MP, Tacchetti C, Cubellis MV, et al. Autocrine saturation of pro-urokinase receptors on human A431 cells. *Cell* 1986;45:675–684.

102. Bajpai A, Baker JB. Cryptic urokinase binding sites on human foreskin fibroblasts. *Biochem Biophys Res Commun* 1985;133:994–1000.

103. Bajpai A, Baker JB. Urokinase binding sites on human foreskin cells. Evidence for occupancy with endogenous urokinase. *Biochem Biophys Res Commun* 1985;133:475–482.

104. Del Rosso M, Dini G, Fibbi G. Receptors for plasminogen activator, urokinase, in normal and Rous sarcoma virus-transformed mouse fibroblasts. *Cancer Res* 1985;45:630–636.

105. Huarte J, Belin D, Bosco D, et al. Plasminogen activator and mouse spermatozoa: urokinase synthesis in the male genital tract and binding of the enzyme to the sperm cell surface. *J Cell Biol* 1987;104:1281–1289.

106. Del Rosso M, Pucci M, Fibbi G, et al. Interaction of urokinase with specific receptors abolishes the time of commitment to terminal differentiation of murine erythroleukemia cells. *Br J Haematol* 1987;66:289–294.

107. Shuman MA, Merkel CH. Urokinase binding to bovine corneal endothelial cells. *Exp Eye Res* 1985;41:371–382.

108. Barnathan E, Kuo A, Rosenfeld L, et al. Interaction of single-chain urokinase-type plasminogen activator with human endothelial cells. *J Biol Chem* 1990;265:2865–2872.

109. Nielsen LS, Kellerman GM, Behrendt N, et al. A 55,000–60,000 Mr receptor protein for urokinase-type plasminogen activator. *J Biol Chem* 1988;263:2358–2363.

110. Ploug M, Ronne E, Behrendt N, et al. Cellular receptor for urokinase plasminogen activator. Carboxyl-terminal processing and membrane anchoring by glycosylphosphatidylinositol. *J Biol Chem* 1991;266:1926–1933.

111. Cubellis MV, Andreasson P, Ragno P, et al. Accessibility of receptor-bound urokinase to type-1 plasminogen activator inhibitor. *Proc Natl Acad Sci U S A* 1989;86:4828–4832.

112. Ellis V, Wun TC, Behrendt N, et al. Inhibition of receptor-bound urokinase by plasminogen activator inhibitor. *J Biol Chem* 1990;265:9904–9908.

113. Dano K, Behrendt N, Brunner N, et al. The urokinase receptor: protein structure and role in plasminogen activation and cancer invasion. *Fibrinolysis* 1994;8:189–203.

114. Almus-Jacobs F, Varki N, Sawdey MS, et al. Endotoxin stimulates expression of the murine urokinase receptor gene *in vivo*. *Am J Pathol* 1995;147:688–698.

115. Blasi F, Carmeliet P. uPAR: a versatile signalling orchestrator. *Nat Rev Mol Cell Biol* 2002;3:932–943.

116. Chapman HA. Plasminogen activators, integrins, and the coordinated regulation of cell adhesion and migration. *Curr Opin Cell Biol* 1997;9:714–724.

117. Waltz DA, Chapman HA. Reversible cellular adhesion to vitronectin linked to urokinase receptor occupancy. *J Biol Chem* 1994;269:14746–14750.

118. Wei Y, Waltz DA, Rao N, et al. Identification of the urokinase receptor as an adhesion receptor for vitronectin. *J Biol Chem* 1994;269:32380–32388.

119. Wei Y, Lukashev M, Simon DI, et al. Regulation of integrin function by the urokinase receptor. *Science* 1996;273:1551–1555.

120. Xue W, Kindzelskii AL, Todd RF, et al. Physical association of complement receptor type 3 and urokinase-type plasminogen activator in neutrophil membranes. *J Immunol* 1994;152:4630–4640.

121. Stahl A, Mueller BM. The urokinase-type plasminogen activator receptor, a GPI-linked protein, is localized in caveolae. *J Cell Biol* 1995;129:335–344.

122. Bugge TH, Flick MJ, Danton MJS, et al. Urokinase-type plasminogen activator is effective in fibrin clearance in the absence of its receptor or tissue-type plasminogen activator. *Proc Natl Acad Sci U S A* 1996;93:5899–5904.

123. Ichinose A, Kisiel W, Fujikawa K. Proteolytic activation of tissue plasminogen activator by plasma and tissue enzymes. *FEBS Lett* 1984;175:412–418.

124. Tate KM, Higgins DL, Holmes WE, et al. Functional role of proteolytic cleavage at arginine-275 of human tissue plasminogen activator as assessed by site-directed mutagenesis. *Biochemistry* 1987;26:338–343.

125. Nielsen LS, Hansen JG, Skriver L, et al. Purification of zymogen to plasminogen activator from human glioblastoma cells by affinity chromatography with monoclonal antibody. *Biochemistry* 1982;21:6410–6415.

126. Wun TC, Ossowski L, Reich E. A proenzyme form of human urokinase. *J Biol Chem* 1982;257:7262–7268.

127. Booyse FM, Scheinbuks J, Radek J, et al. Immunologic identification and comparison of plasminogen activator forms in cultured normal human endothelial cells and smooth muscle cells. *Thromb Res* 1981;24:495–504.

128. Pannell R, Gurewich V. Pro-urokinase: a study of its stability in plasma and of a mechanism for its selective fibrinolytic effect. *Blood* 1986;67:1215–1223.

129. Collen D, Zamarron C, Lijnen HR, et al. Activation of plasminogen by pro-urokinase. *J Biol Chem* 1986;261:1259–1266.

130. Lijnen HR, Zamarron C, Blaber M, et al. Activation of plasminogen by pro-urokinase. *J Biol Chem* 1986;261:1253–1258.

131. Esmon CT. Regulation of blood coagulation. *Biochim Biophys Acta* 2000;1477:349–360.

132. Lee CD, Mann KG. Activation/inactivation of human factor V by plasmin. *Blood* 1989;73:185–190.

133. Puri RN, Zhou FX, Colman RF, et al. Plasmin-induced platelet aggregation is accompanied by cleavage of aggregin and indirectly mediated by calpain. *Am J Physiol* 1990;259:C862–C868.

134. Schafer AI, Adelman B. Plasmin inhibition of platelet function and of arachidonate metabolism. *J Clin Invest* 1985;75:456–461.

135. Schafer AI, Maas AK, Ware JA, et al. Platelet protein phosphorylation, elevation of cytosolic calcium, and inositol phospholipid breakdown in platelet activation induced by plasmin. *J Clin Invest* 1986;78:73–79.

136. Loscalzo J, Vaughan DE. Tissue plasminogen activator promotes platelet disaggregation. *J Clin Invest* 1986;79:1749–1755.

137. Miles LA, Ginsberg MA, White JG, et al. Plasminogen interacts with platelets through two distinct mechanisms. *J Clin Invest* 1986;77:2001–2009.

138. Adelman B, Michelson AD, Loscalzo J, et al. Plasmin effect on platelet glycoprotein Ib-von Willebrand factor interactions. *Blood* 1985;65:32–40.

139. Stricker RB, Wong D, Shiu DT, et al. Activation of plasminogen by tissue plasminogen activator on normal and thrombasthenic platelets: effects on surface proteins and platelet aggregation. *Blood* 1986;68:275–280.

140. Gimple LW, Gold HK, Leinbach RC, et al. Correlation between template bleeding times and spontaneous bleeding during treatment of acute myocardial infarction with recombinant issue type plasminogen activator. *Blood* 1989;80:581–588.

141. Coller BS. Platelets and thrombolytic therapy. *N Engl J Med* 1990;322:33–42.

142. Bugge TH, Kombrinck KW, Flick MJ, et al. Loss of fibrinogen rescues mice from the pleiotropic effects of plasminogen deficiency. *Cell* 1996;87:709–719.

143. Plow EF, Ploplis VA, Busuttil S, et al. A role of plasminogen in atherosclerosis and restenosis models in mice. *Thromb Haemost* 1999;82(Suppl. 1):4–7.

144. Kraus JP. Molecular basis of phenotype expression in homocystinuria. *J Inher Metab Dis* 1994;17:383–390.

145. Boushey CJ, Beresford SAA, Omenn GS, et al. A quantitative assessment of plasma homocysteine as a risk factor for vascular disease. *JAMA* 1995;274:1049–1057.

146. Refsum H, Ueland PM, Nygard O, et al. Homocysteine and cardiovascular disease. *Ann Rev Med* 1998;49:31–62.

147. Hajjar KA, Mauri L, Jacovina AT, et al. Tissue plasminogen activator binding to the annexin II tail domain: direct modulation by homocysteine. *J Biol Chem* 1998;273:9987–9993.

148. Hajjar KA. Homocysteine-induced modulation of tissue plasminogen activator binding to its endothelial cell membrane receptor. *J Clin Invest* 1993;91:2873–2879.

149. Hajjar KA, Nachman RL. The role of lipoprotein(a) in atherogenesis and thrombosis. *Annu Rev Med* 1996;47:423–442.

150. Loscalzo J. Lipoprotein(a), a unique risk factor for atherothrombotic disease. *Arteriosclerosis* 1990;10:672–679.

151. Scanu AM, Fless GM. Lipoprotein(a) heterogeneity and biologic relevance. *J Clin Invest* 1990;85:1709–1715.

152. Utermann G. The mysteries of lipoprotein(a). *Science* 1989;246:904–910.

153. McLean JW, Tomlinson JE, Kuang WJ, et al. cDNA sequence of human apolipoprotein(a) is homologous to plasminogen. *Nature* 1987;330:132–137.

154. Weitkamp LR, Guttormsen SA, Schultz JS. Linkage between the loci for the Lp(a) lipoprotein (Lp) and plasminogen (PLG). *Hum Genet* 1988;79:80–82.

155. Armstrong VW, Harrach B, Robenek H, et al. Heterogeneity of human lipoprotein Lp(a): cytochemical and biochemical studies on the interaction of two Lp(a) species with the LDL receptor. *J Lipid Res* 1990;31:429–441.

156. Harpel PC, Gordon BR, Parker TS. Plasmin catalyzes binding of lipoprotein(a) to immobilized fibrinogen and fibrin. *Proc Natl Acad Sci U S A* 1989;56:3847–3851.

157. Wolf K, Rith M, Niendorf A, et al. Thrombosis: cellular elements of the vasculature. *Circulation* 1989;80:522.

158. Hajjar KA, Gavish D, Breslow J, et al. Lipoprotein(a) modulation of endothelial cell surface fibrinolysis and its potential role in atherosclerosis. *Nature* 1989;339:303–305.

159. Miles LA, Fless GM, Levin EG, et al. A potential basis for the thrombotic risks associated with lipoprotein(a). *Nature* 1989;339:301–303.

160. Gonzales-Gronow M, Edelberg JM, Pizzo SV. Further characterization of the cellular plasminogen binding site: evidence that plasminogen 2 and lipoprotein a compete for the same site. *Biochemistry* 1989;28:2374–2377.

161. Neven L, Khalil A, Pfaffinger D, et al. Rhesus monkey model of familial hypercholesterolemia: relation between plasma Lp(a) levels, apo(a) isoforms and LDL-receptor function. *J Lipid Res* 1990;31:633–643.

162. Pfaffinger D, Schuelke J, Kim C, et al. Relationship between apo(a) isoforms and Lp(a) density in subjects with different apo(a) phenotype: a study before and after a fatty meal. *J Lipid Res* 1991;32:679–683.

163. Maeda S, Abe A, Seishima M, et al. Transient changes of serum lipoprotein(a) as an acute phase protein. *Atherosclerosis* 1989;78:145–150.

164. Utermann G, Menzel HJ, Kraft HG, et al. Lp(a) glycoprotein phenotypes. *J Clin Invest* 1987;80:458–465.

165. Wright LC, Sullivan DR, Muller M, et al. Elevated apolipoprotein(a) levels in cancer patients. *Int J Cancer* 1989;43:241–244.

166. Gavish D, Azrolan N, Breslow JL. Fish oil reduces plasma Lp(a) levels and affects post-prandial association of apo(a) with triglyceride rich lipoproteins. *J Clin Invest* 1989;84:2021–2027.

167. Koschinsky ML, Beisiegel U, Henne-Bruns D, et al. Apolipoprotein(a) size heterogeneity is related to variable number of repeat sequences in its mRNA. *Biochemistry* 1990;29:640–644.

168. Etingin OR, Hajjar DP, Hajjar KA, et al. Lipoprotein(a) regulates plasminogen activator inhibitor-1 expression in endothelial cells. *J Biol Chem* 1990;266:2459–2465.

169. Karadi I, Kostner GM, Gries A, et al. Lipoprotein(a) and plasminogen are immunochemically related. *Biochim Biophys Acta* 1988;960:91–97.

170. Edelberg JM, Gonzales-Gronow M, Pizzo SV. Lipoprotein(a) inhibits streptokinase-mediated activation of human plasminogen. *Biochemistry* 1989;28:2370–2374.

171. Edelberg JM, Gonzales-Gronow M, Pizzo SV. Lipoprotein(a) inhibition of plasminogen activation by tissue-type plasminogen activator. *Thromb Res* 1990;57:155–162.

172. Loscalzo J, Weinfeld M, Fless G, et al. Lipoprotein(a), fibrin binding, and plasminogen activation. *Arteriosclerosis* 1990;10:240–245.

173. Heymans S, Luttun A, Nuyens D, et al. Inhibition of plasminogen activators or matrix metalloproteinases prevents cardiac rupture but impairs therapeutic angiogenesis and causes cardiac failure. *Nat Med* 2003;5:1135–1142.

174. Lijnen HR, Van Hoef B, Lupu F, et al. Function of the plasminogen/plasmin and matrix metalloproteinase systems after vascular injury in mice with targeted inactivation of fibrinolytic system genes. *Arterioscler Thromb Vasc Biol* 1998;18:1035–1045.

175. Carmeliet P, Moons L, Herbert Jm, et al. Urokinase but not tissue plasminogen activator mediates arterial neointima formation in mice. *Circ Res* 1997;81:829–839.

176. Carmeliet P, Moons L, Dewerchin M, et al. Receptor-independent role of urokinase-type plasminogen activator in pericellular plasmin and matrix metalloproteinase proteolysis during vascular wound healing in mice. *J Cell Biol* 1998;140:233–245.

177. Carmeliet P, Moons L, Lijnen R, et al. Inhibitory role of plasminogen activator inhibitor-1 in arterial wound healing and neointima formation. *Circulation* 1997;96:3180–3191.

178. Konstantinides S, Schafer K, Loskutoff DJ. Do PAI-1 and vitronectin promote or inhibit neointima formation? *Arterioscler Thromb Vasc Biol* 2002;22:1943–1945.

179. Shi C, Patel A, Zhang D, et al. Plasminogen is not required for neointima formation in a mouse model of vein graft stenosis. *Circ Res* 1999;84:883–890.

180. Schafer K, Konstantinides S, Riedel C, et al. Different mechanisms of increased luminal stenosis after arterial injury in mice deficient for urokinase- or tissue-type plasminogen activator. *Circulation* 2002;106:1847–1852.

181. Eitzman DT, Westrick RJ, Nabel EG, et al. Plasminogen activator inhibitor-1 and vitronectin promote vascular thrombosis in mice. *Blood* 2000;95:577–580.

182. Konstantinides S, Schafer K, Thinnes T, et al. Plasminogen activator inhibitor-1 and its cofactor vitronectin stabilize arterial thrombi following vascular injury in mice. *Circulation* 2001;103:576–583.

183. Schafer K, Muller K, Hecker A, et al. Enhanced thrombosis in atherosclerosis-prone mice is associated with increased arterial expression of plasmingen activator. *Arterioscler Thromb Vasc Biol* 2003;23:2097–2103.

184. Zhu Y, Farrehi PM, Fay WP. Plasminogen activator inhibitor type 1 enhances neointima formation after oxidative vascular injury in atherosclerosis-prone mice. *Circulation* 2001;103:3105–3110.

185. Ploplis VA, Cornelissen I, Sandoval-cooper MJ, et al. Remodeling of the vessel wall after copper-induced injury is highly attenuated in mice with a total deficiency of plasminogen activator inhibitor-1. *Am J Pathol* 2001;158:107–117.

186. DeYoung MB, Tom C, Dichek DA. Plasminogen activator inhibitor type 1 increases neointima formation in balloon-injured rat carotid arteries. *Circulation* 2001;104:1972–1981.

187. Grainger DJ, Kemp PR, Metcalfe JC, et al. The serum concentration of active transforming growth factor-β is severely depressed in advanced atherosclerosis. *Nat Med* 1995;1:74–79.

188. Herbert JM, Carmeliet P. Involvement of u-PA in the antiapoptotic activity of TGF beta for vascular smooth muscle cells. *FEBS Lett* 1997;413:401–404.

189. Herbert JM, Lamarche I, Carmeliet P. Urokinase and tissue-type plasminogen activator are required for the mitogenic and chemotactic effects of bovine fibroblast growth factor and platelet-derived growth factor-BB for vascular smooth muscle cells. *J Biol Chem* 1997;272:23585–23591.

190. Mignatti P, Rifkin DB. Plasminogen activators and matrix metalloproteinases in angiogenesis. *Enzyme Protein* 1996;49:117–137.

191. Pepper MS, Montesano R, Mandriota S, et al. Angiogenesis: a paradigm for balanced extracellular proteolysis during cell migration and morphogenesis. *Enzyme Protein* 1996;49:138–162.

192. Pepper MS. Manipulating angiogenesis: from basic science to the bedside. *Arterioscler Thromb Vasc Biol* 1997;17:605–619.

193. O'Reilly MS, Holmgren L, Shing Y, et al. Angiostatin: a novel angiogenesis inhibitor that mediates the suppression of metastases by a Lewis lung carcinoma. *Cell* 1995;79:315–328.

194. O'Reilly MS, Holmgren L, Chen C, et al. Angiostatin induces and sustains dormancy of human primary tumors in mice. *Nat Med* 1996;2:689–692.

195. Cao Y, O'Reilly MS, Marshall B, et al. Expression of angiostatin cDNA in a murine fibrosarcoma suppresses primary tumor growth and produces long-term dormancy of metastases. *J Clin Invest* 1998;101:1055–1063.

196. Dong Z, Kumar R, Yang X, et al. Macrophage-derived metallo-elastase is responsible for the generation of angiostatin in Lewis lung carcinoma. *Cell* 1997;88:801–810.

197. Stathakis P, Fitzgerald M, Matthias LJ, et al. Generation of angiostatin by reduction and proteolysis of plasmin: catalysis by a plasmin reductase secreted by cultured cells. *J Biol Chem* 1997;272:20641–20645.

198. Patterson BC, Sang QXA. Angiostatin-converting enzyme activities of human matrilysin (MMP-7) and gelatinase B/type IV collagenase (MMP-9). *J Biol Chem* 1997;272:28823–28825.

# CHAPTER 23 ■ PHYSIOLOGIC REGULATION OF FIBRINOLYSIS

VICTOR J. MARDER AND CHARLES W. FRANCIS

The fibrinolytic system is the principal effector of clot removal and controls the enzymatic degradation of fibrin. Its action is coordinated through the interaction of activators, zymogens, enzymes, inhibitors, and receptors to provide local activation at sites of fibrin deposition. This chapter focuses on physiologic regulation of fibrinolysis that clears intravascular fibrin locally while preventing systemic derangements that could result in pathologic conditions of excessive activation. Basic aspects of fibrinolysis are described in Chapters 18 and 23, and clinical aspects are included in Chapter 69, and as part of other chapters in the sections, "Therapy, New Directions, and Complications in Thrombotic Disorders" and "Therapy of Bleeding Disorders."

## FIBRINOLYTIC BALANCE: THROMBOSIS VERSUS BLEEDING

Physiologic coagulation and fibrinolysis are highly coordinated physiologically, providing for prompt control of bleeding with eventual resolution and healing. Disruption of control of fibrinolysis can shift the balance of clot formation and dissolution and lead to bleeding if there is excessive fibrinolysis or to thrombosis if there is inappropriate fibrinolytic inhibition (1,2). Figure 23-1 shows this complex interaction. For example, bleeding caused by an excess of a fibrinolytic stimulus can be corrected by administration of a fibrinolytic inhibitor. However, if the patient is predisposed to venous thrombosis or disseminated intravascular coagulation (DIC), clinical thrombosis could occur. On the other hand, stimulation of fibrinolysis through therapeutic administration of plasminogen activator for treatment of thrombosis may result in successful thrombolysis, but may also result in a bleeding complication in a susceptible patient. Pathologic abnormalities of the fibrinolytic system that may result in thrombosis or bleeding are described in Chapter 69.

## MOLECULAR COMPONENTS

A detailed description of the structure, genetic control, and biochemistry of the substrates, activators, and inhibitors that constitute the plasminogen–plasmin enzyme system is described in detail in Chapters 18 and 23.

### Plasminogen

Plasminogen is the zymogen form of the active fibrinolytic enzyme plasmin, synthesized in the liver and present in plasma at a concentration of 2.4 $\mu$M (see Table 23-1). In its intact form, plasminogen is a 791–amino acid, single-chain molecule of $M_r$ 88,000. Activators convert plasminogen to the two-chain plasmin molecule by cleaving the Arg561–Val bond at the junction of the heavy (A) and light (B) chains (see Fig. 23-2).

The initial amino-terminal 77 residues, called the *activation peptide*, can be liberated by plasmin to produce a smaller molecule with an amino-terminal lysine (Lys-plasminogen) (3–7). Lys-plasminogen has a higher affinity for binding to fibrin and greater reactivity with plasminogen activators (8–13). Its formation therefore tends to accelerate and improve the efficiency of plasmin formation and fibrin degradation. The heavy chain contains five homologous structures termed *kringles* that contribute to fibrin binding and to interactions with antiplasmin and cell surfaces (14–16). Binding to fibrin is mediated by *lysine binding sites*, so named because of their interaction with lysine or with lysine analogues such as ε-aminocaproic acid (EACA), which inhibits plasmin by competitive binding with lysine sites on fibrin (see Chapter 79) (17,18). The activity of the principal physiologic fibrinolytic inhibitor, $\alpha_2$-plasmin inhibitor, is mediated in part by binding to lysine binding sites in addition to the catalytic site (19–21).

### Activators

Contact activation of Hageman factor (factor XII) results in the generation of fibrinolytic activity (22–24), and prekallikrein activation can occur on endothelial cells (see Chapter 22) (25). The physiologic importance of contact activation is uncertain, but it is of interest that the original patient with Hageman factor deficiency died of a pulmonary embolus and that thrombotic events have occurred in patients deficient in prekallikrein and kininogen (26). Physiologic plasminogen activators (PA) can be divided into two types: Tissue-type plasminogen activator (tPA) and urokinase-type plasminogen activator (uPA), both of which are serine proteases with a high specific activity for converting plasminogen to plasmin. Single-chain tPA with an $M_r$ of 72,000 is synthesized and secreted by endothelial cells and can be converted into a two-chain molecule by cleavage of the Arg275-Ile bond by kallikrein, plasmin, or factor Xa (27–31). The amino-terminal heavy chain contains a domain similar to the finger region of fibronectin, a domain partially homologous to epidermal growth factor and disulfide-bonded kringle structures that are closely homologous to those of plasminogen (32–34). tPA binds avidly to fibrin, a property mediated by sites located on the finger and second kringle regions and possibly also the first kringle (30,35–40), and expresses greater enzymatic activity in the presence of fibrin (30,41,42), enhancement of which is mediated by a cyclic ternary complex composed of tPA, plasminogen, and fibrin (42). The site on fibrin that interacts with tPA is on the A$\alpha$ chain part of the coiled-coil (see Chapter 16) (43–45).

Urokinase (UK) is the PA responsible for the fibrinolytic activity of urine (46). It is synthesized by kidney and endothelial cells as a single-chain molecule that is converted to the two-chain form (47–49). uPA differs from tPA in regard to the fibronectinlike finger domain, immunologic reactivity, lack of high-affinity binding for fibrin, and lack of increased PA activity in the presence of fibrin (33,36,37,50,51). A single-chain

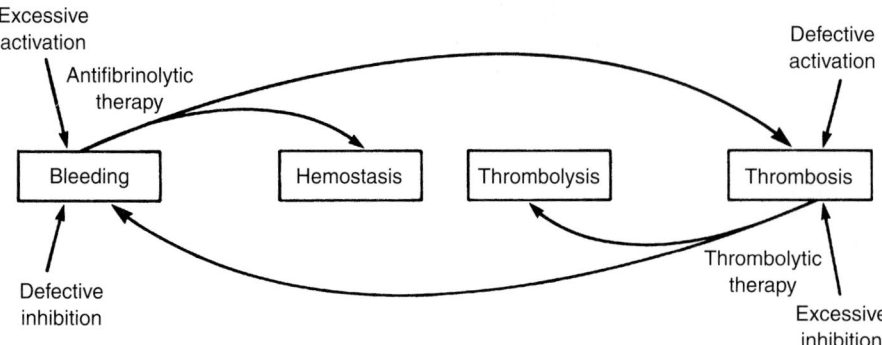

**FIGURE 23-1.** Disruption of the balance between the opposing forces of fibrinolysis and antifibrinolysis, leading to bleeding or thrombotic manifestations. Bleeding may result from defective inhibition of excessive activation of fibrinolysis. Conversely, defective activation or excess inhibition of fibrinolysis may result in thrombosis. Therapy with fibrinolytic agents may dissolve a thrombus, but bleeding may complicate the clinical management. Bleeding caused by excess fibrinolysis may be improved by antifibrinolytic therapy or result in a thrombotic complication.

form of uPA, single-chain urokinase plasminogen activator (scuPA), has been isolated from urine and plasma and has been produced by recombinant DNA technology (52–57). Plasmin and kallikrein cleave the Lys158–Ile bond in scuPA, converting it to tcuPA, whereas thrombin cleaves the Arg156–Phe bond, resulting in an inactive two-chain derivative (58–60). scuPA has low enzymatic activity in the absence of fibrin; in the presence of fibrin, scuPA converts plasminogen to plasmin, which in turn converts scuPA to tcuPA (61–63). Exposure of fibrin to plasmin renders it more susceptible to lysis as a result of increased binding of plasminogen to newly exposed lysine residues (64).

The first exogenous "therapeutic" activators were purified from human urine, from the culture medium of human embryonic kidney cells (UK), and from culture of α-hemolytic streptococci, streptokinase (SK). Fibrinolytic agents with improved

## TABLE 23-1

### MOLECULAR COMPONENTS OF THE PLASMIN FIBRINOLYTIC SYSTEM

| | $M_r$ | Plasma concentration | Plasma half-life | Selected functional properties |
|---|---|---|---|---|
| **SUBSTRATE/ENZYME** | | | | |
| Plasminogen | 88,000 (Glu1) | 2.4 $\mu$M (210 mg/L) | 2.2 d | Zymogen; lysine binding sites for fibrin on |
| | 83,000 (Lys77) | | 0.8 d | the kringle portions; activator-sensitive site at Arg561–Val562 |
| Plasmin | 88,000 (Glu1) | 0 | <1 min | Serine protease; active site on the light chain |
| | 83,000 (Lys77) | | | ($M_r$ 26,000); variable heavy chain containing |
| | 38,000 (Val442) | | | kringle structures |
| **PLASMINOGEN ACTIVATORS** | | | | |
| Endogenous | | | | |
| tPA | 72,000 | 70 pM (0.005 $\mu$g/L) | 5 min | Single-chain form converted to two-chain form by plasmin, increased activity in the presence of fibrin |
| scuPA | 54,000 | 40 pM (0.002 mg/L) | 7 min | Low intrinsic activity, plasmin converts to a two-chain active enzyme (urokinase) |
| Exogenous | | | | |
| SK | 48,000 | NA | 30 min | Inactive by itself; forms active equimolar complex with plasminogen |
| Reteplase | 40,000 | NA | 15 min | Mutant deletion of tPA, retains kringle 2 and protease domains |
| Tenecteplase | 72,000 | NA | 20 min | Substituted amino acids of tPA at three sites, long half-life |
| **INHIBITORS** | | | | |
| $\alpha_2$-plasmin inhibitor | 69,000 | 1 $\mu$M (69 mg/L) | 2.6 d | Binds to fibrin by XIIIa; inhibits plasmin by forming irreversible complex with catalytic site; prevents plasmin binding to fibrin |
| PAI-1 | 50,000 | 0.2 nM (0.01 $\mu$g/L) | 8 min | Interacts with catalytic site of UK or tPA to form an inactive complex, occurs in active and latent forms |

tPA, tissue-type plasminogen activator; scuPA, single-chain urokinase plasminogen activator (prourokinase); SK, streptokinase; NA, not applicable; PAI-1, plasminogen activator inhibitor-1; UK, urokinase.

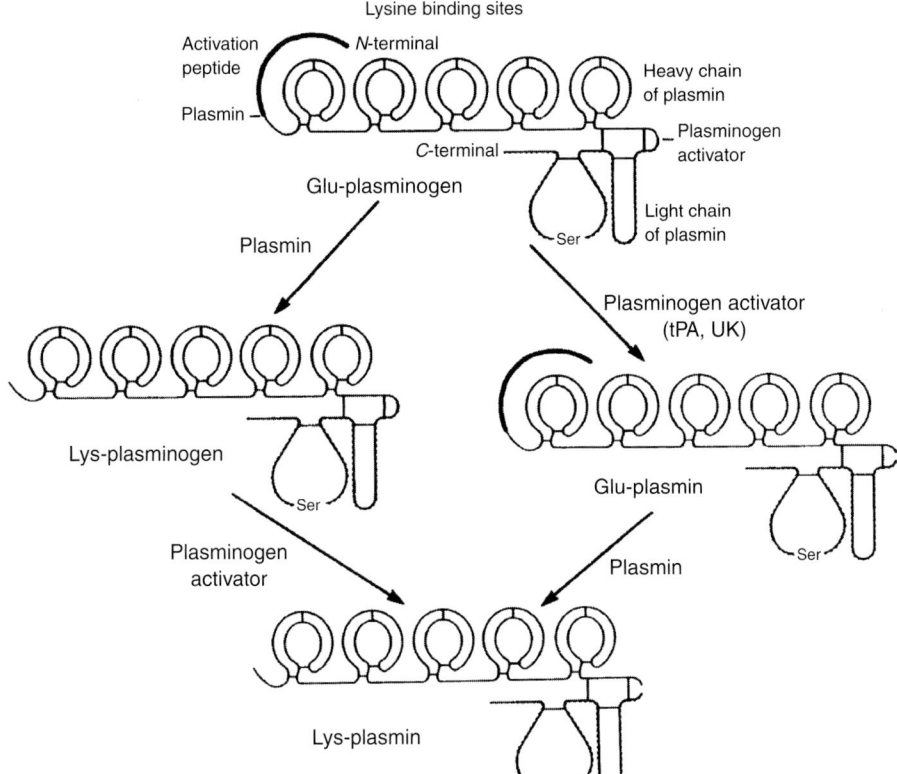

**FIGURE 23-2.** Activation of plasminogen by plasminogen activator, showing two pathways leading to plasmin. Plasminogen activator cleaves at Arg560–Val, separating the protein into light (catalytic site) and heavy (kringle domains) chains. The Glu-plasminogen and Glu-plasmin forms both contain the amino-terminal activation peptide. Plasmin has the potential to cleave this activation peptide (*left side*), producing Lys-plasminogen, an intermediate form that binds better to fibrin and is more sensitive to plasminogen activator, properties that accelerate activation to plasmin. Plasmin also can cleave the activation peptide from Glu-plasmin, leading as well to Lys-plasmin (*right side*). The activation peptide extends from the Glu1 residue to Lys76. The five kringle structures of the heavy chain are involved in fibrin binding, with the first four kringles containing a single high-affinity site, as well as several low-affinity lysine binding sites. The catalytic center contains the typical serine-histidine-aspartic acid residues and is the major site of interaction with the inhibitor, $\alpha_2$-antiplasmin.

pharmacologic properties led to the development of several newer plasminogen activators, including recombinant tPA, scuPA, staphylokinase, Bat PA derived ultimately from vampire bat salivary gland, and mutant forms of tPA [reteplase, tenectoplase (TNK–tPA), lanetoplase]. SK has no intrinsic plasminogen activator activity, but in complex with plasminogen it acquires PA activity (65,66). Both SK and UK have low affinity for fibrin, so their therapeutic use usually results in proteolytic degradation of plasma fibrinogen (the lytic state). tPA has high affinity for fibrin and low enzymatic activity in the absence of fibrin, properties that make it a relatively "fibrin-specific" agent, producing less fibrinogen degradation than occurs with SK or UK (67,68). Bleeding complications are equally common with tPA and SK (69) and intracranial hemorrhages are more common with tPA (70), indicating that fibrin specificity does not protect against hemorrhagic events.

Reteplase lacks the finger and epidermal growth factor domains, as well as the kringle 1 domain, retaining only the kringle 2 domain and the protease site of tPA (71). The resultant molecule has less fibrin-binding capacity, but a clearly longer half-life than tPA (15 vs. 4 minutes) (72), allowing it to be administered as an intravenous bolus injection. TNK–tPA retains the domain structure of tPA but incorporates site-directed mutagenesis to produce amino acid substitutions at three sites (73), resulting in longer half-life, greater resistance to plasminogen activator inhibitor (PAI)-1, and less effect on plasma fibrinogen than is exhibited by tPA (74). The unifying feature of these tPA variants is their longer half-life and, consequently, their potential for bolus administration (75,76), similar to that previously achieved by acylated derivatives of plasminogen activator complexes (77,78). Staphylokinase is similar to SK in that its complex with plasminogen is capable of converting plasminogen to plasmin (79).

## Plasmin

Cleavage of the Arg561–Val bond in plasminogen by any of the plasminogen activators converts plasminogen to a protease (80,81). The three principal molecular forms of plasmin are the Glu-1 type, which consists of the intact molecule with only the Arg561–Val bond cleaved; the Lys78 form, which lacks the amino-terminal 77-residue activation peptide; and the Val442 form, which contains an intact light chain, but only one kringle structure, and lacks all of the lysine binding sites (82). All forms of plasmin are endopeptidases that hydrolyze susceptible arginine and lysine bonds in proteins at neutral pH and act on most synthetic substrates and proteins susceptible to trypsin (83). In addition to fibrinogen and fibrin, plasmin hydrolyzes coagulation factors V and VIII, complement, adrenocorticotropic hormone, growth hormone, and glucagon, and also cleaves the activation peptide from plasminogen (4–7,84). This latter action serves to accelerate plasminogen conversion to plasmin, because the Lys form is more susceptible to activator cleavage than is intact Glu-plasminogen (Fig. 23-2) (10–13).

## Inhibitors

The principal physiologic inhibitor of plasmin is $\alpha_2$-antiplasmin, which is synthesized in the liver and present in plasma at a concentration of 1 $\mu$M, as well as in platelets (85–88). The plasmin–antiplasmin interaction is central to the physiologic control of fibrinolysis, which must provide for intermittent activation at sites of fibrin deposition without initiating a systemic proteolytic state (see Fig. 23-3). In plasma, $\alpha_2$-antiplasmin reacts quickly with plasmin, irreversibly inhibiting the enzyme by forming a stable bimolecular complex with catalytic site serine (19,20,89). In the process, $\alpha_2$-antiplasmin is itself

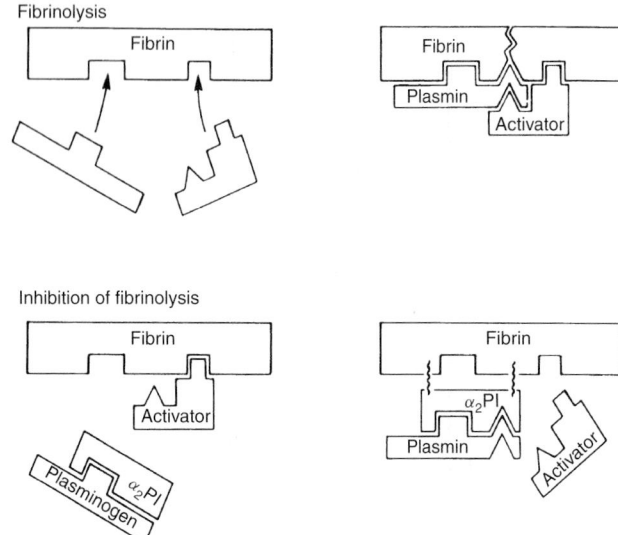

**FIGURE 23-3.** Schematic representation of the interaction of surface-oriented plasminogen activator with plasminogen and fibrin. In solution, $\alpha_2$-antiplasmin prevents binding of plasminogen or plasmin to fibrin. $\alpha_2$-Antiplasmin may cross-link with fibrin, in which case the inhibitor not only prevents plasmin from binding to its fibrin substrate, but also neutralizes the serine catalytic site of plasmin.

partially degraded by plasmin (89). As the lysine binding sites of free plasmin are accessible to the inhibitor in solution, free plasmin is more readily inactivated than is fibrin-bound plasmin. $\alpha_2$-plasmin inhibitor is present in blood in two forms, differing in their ability to bind plasminogen (19,20,90); approximately 70% is in the plasminogen-binding form (91–93). Factor XIIIa cross-links $\alpha_2$-antiplasmin to the $\alpha$-chains of fibrin, making the fibrin more resistant to plasmic degradation and contributing to the increased resistance of cross-linked fibrin clots to lysis (94–97).

$\alpha_2$-Plasmin inhibitor is the most important plasma antiplasmin, but other inhibitors such as $\alpha_2$-macroglobulin may exert a limited role, particularly if the capacity of $\alpha_2$-plasmin inhibitor is exceeded by a high concentration of free plasmin (85,87). Although the plasma concentration of $\alpha_2$-macroglobulin is high (3 $\mu$M), its inhibitory capacity may be limited, and complexes may retain residual protease activity on some protein substrates (98,99) (see Chapter 18). Other plasma protease inhibitors, such as antithrombin III, $\alpha_1$-antitrypsin, and $C_1$ inactivator have some antiplasmin activity *in vitro* but exert a minimal physiologic effect in the blood (99).

Inhibitors of PA (PAI-1, PAI-2, PAI-3, and protease nexin) also play an important role in the regulation of fibrinolysis. It is unlikely that PAI-3 and protease nexin are physiologically significant inhibitors, mostly because of slow kinetics of interaction. PAI-2 (100,101) is present in placenta, monocytes, macrophages, some tumor cells, and the plasma of pregnant women (102,103), but an important role in regulation of fibrinolysis has not been established. PAI-1 ($M_r$ 52,000) is homologous with other serpin inhibitors and is the primary inhibitor of PA in plasma, with a second-order rate constant of inhibition of both tPA and uPA greater than $10^{-7}$ mol/L/second (104–107). Synthesis by endothelial cells and hepatocytes (108–112) is stimulated by endotoxin, thrombin, interleukin-1, tumor necrosis factor, fibroblast growth factor-2, angiotensin II, and lipoproteins (113–115). Secreted PAI-1 is active, but spontaneously decays to a "latent" form in which it cannot inactivate uPA or tPA, but can be reactivated by sodium dodecyl sulfate or urea and possibly *in vivo* (116–119). In plasma, PAI-1 bound to vitronectin is stabilized in the active conformation (120–122). In

the subendothelial matrix, PAI-1 is protected from inactivation and may function to inhibit local proteolysis (123,124). Fibrin-bound PAI-1 inhibits uPA and tPA, thereby localizing its inhibitory activity at sites of fibrin deposition (125).

# PHYSIOLOGIC CONTROL OF THROMBOLYSIS

The physiologic response to the formation of a hemostatic plug or thrombus requires localized activation of fibrinolysis for removing fibrin without systemic plasminemia. Thrombolysis is regulated (see Table 23-2) by the concentration of plasminogen, activators, and inhibitors at the site of fibrin formation and by binding of fibrinolytic reactants to fibrin, cells, and matrix components of the thrombus (see Fig. 23-4).

Plasminogen binds to fibrin as it polymerizes and is incorporated throughout the thrombus, with binding mediated through lysine binding sites on kringle domains. Activation of bound plasminogen is facilitated by binding of tPA to fibrin and by the increased activity of both tPA and scuPA in the presence of fibrin (30,36,37,41,63,64). Fast-acting inhibitors such as $\alpha_2$-antiplasmin and PAI-1 are efficient at inhibiting free plasmin or tPA, but not fibrin-bound enzyme (19,20,126), thereby allowing localized plasmin proteolysis of fibrin while preventing systemic effect. Secretion of tPA by endothelial cells may be stimulated by fibrin, by thrombin bound to the thrombus, or by the effects of vessel occlusion, thereby increasing the local concentration of PA (127–131). Fibrin also may inhibit endothelial cell secretion of PAI-1, preventing inactivation of tPA (132). Fibrinolysis is regulated by the platelet content of thrombi. Platelets can bind both plasminogen (15) and tPA (133), increasing plasmin formation, but also they may limit fibrinolysis through secretion of PAI-1 and $\alpha_2$-antiplasmin stored in $\alpha$-granules (134–136).

The initial action of plasmin on the thrombus accelerates fibrinolysis through several positive feedback mechanisms. Plasmin converts Glu- to Lys-plasminogen, which has greater fibrin affinity (8,9) converts single-chain tPA to the two-chain form, which increases its binding to fibrin, and plasmic cleavages expose new plasminogen and tPA lysine binding sites (137,138). Several properties of the thrombus serve to limit dissolution, an effect that is more important for hemostasis and protection of hemostatic plugs. The small surface area of endothelium adjacent to a large thrombus limits effective tPA content. On the contrary, the increased ratio of endothelial cell surface to clot volume in microvascular clots, for example, those of DIC, may result in more rapid and complete clot lysis.

Thrombus dissolution also is limited by fibrinolytic inhibitors. PAI-1 bound to fibrin inhibits both tPA and uPA, and in complex with tPA, competes with free tPA for fibrin-binding sites (125), and factor XIIIa cross-links $\alpha_2$-plasmin inhibitor to fibrin $\alpha$-polymer chains (94,95). Therefore, inhibitors of both tPA and plasmin are specifically localized to the thrombus to downregulate fibrinolysis. The slow cross-linking of fibrin $\alpha$-chains into large polymers by factor XIIIa renders the fibrin more resistant to plasmic degradation, contributing to the relative resistance of older thrombi to fibrinolysis (139,140). Additionally, thrombin-activatable fibrinolysis inhibitor (TAFI) cleaves newly exposed lysine binding sites to decrease binding of tPA and plasminogen (141–143).

Endothelial cells interact with the fibrinolytic system to modulate activity (see Fig. 23-5) (see Chapter 22). Endothelial cells possess binding sites for plasminogen, plasmin, and PA; cell-bound PA retains activity (16,144–148); and Glu-plasminogen is rapidly converted to the more active Lys-plasminogen form, all of which serves to localize and enhance fibrinolytic activity at the vessel wall–thrombus interface (144). These processes are

## TABLE 23-2

### PHYSIOLOGIC FACTORS THAT INFLUENCE THROMBOLYSIS

| Promotes thrombolysis | Limits thrombolysis |
| --- | --- |
| Local release of tPA by endothelial cells | Local release of PAI-1 and $\alpha_2$-antiplasmin by platelets |
| Plasminogen and tPA incorporation into thrombus | Finite amount of plasminogen available |
| Plasmin formation | Fibrin cross-linking by factor XIIIa increases resistance to plasmin-induced thrombolysis |
| Exposure of new lysine residues by plasmin proteolysis promotes further plasminogen and tPA binding | TAFI-induced cleavage of lysine residues eliminates binding sites for plasminogen and tPA |
| Bound plasmin is resistant to inhibition by free $\alpha_2$-antiplasmin | Prior presence of fibrin-bound $\alpha_2$-antiplasmin and PAI-1 |

tPA, tissue-type plasminogen activator; TAFI, thrombin-activatable fibrinolysis inhibitor; PAI-1, plasminogen activator inhibitor-1.

important in maintaining the nonthrombogenic properties and vascular patency of intact vessels by generating a fibrinolytic response to nascent fibrin deposits. PAI-1 bound to subendothelial matrix prevents plasminogen activation at sites of vascular injury, maintains hemostatic plug integrity, and protects the matrix from proteolytic degradation (149,150). Lipoprotein (a) [Lp(a)] is a low density lipoprotein–like particle with kringle structural homology with plasminogen, competing for its endothelial cell receptor and reducing cell-associated plasmin generation (151,152). The increased risk of atherosclerosis associated with elevated plasma concentrations of lipoprotein (a) may be related in part to decreased endothelial cell fibrinolytic potential.

Plasma normally has a low concentration of PA activity (53,153–156), but tPA activity can rapidly increase with stimuli such as exercise, epinephrine, desmopressin [1-deamino-8-D-arginine vasopressin (DDAVP)], nicotine, histamine, and venous occlusion, suggesting release from storage sites in endothelial cells. Net plasma fibrinolytic activity also reflects the level of PAI-1, whose release from endothelial cells can be induced by steroids, endotoxin, thrombin, interleukin-1, and tissue necrosis factor (112–115,157). These effects may be important in the thrombotic tendency of inflammatory states (114,158); for example, elevated PAI-1 during septicemia resulting from endotoxin stimulation may contribute to complex hemostatic changes (111).

An entirely distinct mechanism of fibrinolytic regulation relates to plasma carboxypeptidase B (159,160), an enzyme that exists as a precursor protein that can be activated by thrombin (161). It has been purified and named TAFI (141),

and its activity explains the effect of thrombin to decrease fibrinolysis induced by tPA (162) and the effect of activated protein C (APC) to increase fibrinolysis by limiting thrombin generation (163). The endothelial surface effects this "coupling of the coagulation and fibrinolytic cascades" (142) by virtue of thrombin–thrombomodulin complex formation as the likely modality for TAFI activation (142,164,165).

The ultimate mechanism of action of TAFI is by liberation of C-terminal lysine residues from degrading fibrin or from cell surfaces (166,167). Because these lysine residues serve as tPA and plasminogen binding sites (168), TAFI inhibits lysis by preventing attachment of plasminogen and limiting further plasmin action on fibrin. The prothrombotic potential of APC resistance or factor $V_{Leiden}$ derives in great measure by absent feedback inhibition of thrombin production, leading to pathologic fibrin formation (169,170). However, this failure to inhibit thrombin generation also results in increased thrombin-generated TAFI and, therefore, an accumulation of plasmin-resistant fibrin in the thrombus (171).

In contrast, diminished thrombin formation in hemophiliacs results in less TAFI activation and less inhibition of clot lysis (172). Therefore, bleeding in patients with absent factor VIII or factor IX results not only from decreased fibrin formation, but also from the absence of an important antifibrinolytic mechanism provided by TAFI. In addition, TAFI is affected by factor XIII, which cross-links TAFI to fibrin (94,173), and by activated factor XI, leading to amplification of the clotting cascade and even more TAFI activation (174). Because thrombomodulin promotes thrombin-induced APC formation (a mechanism of decreasing coagulation), as well as thrombin-induced

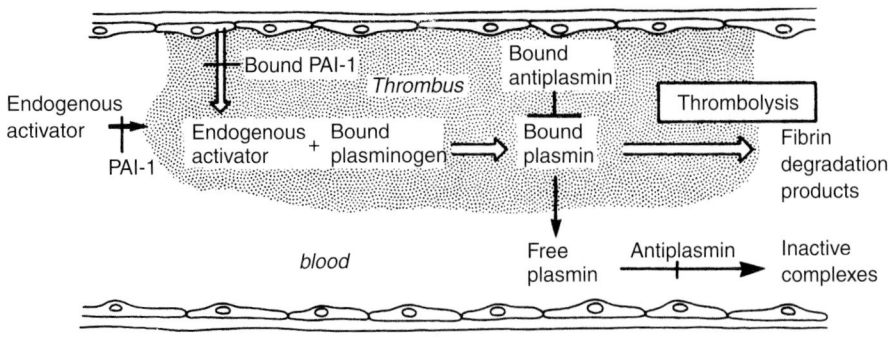

FIGURE 23-4. Schematic representation of physiologic fibrinolysis. In response to the formation of an intravascular thrombus, endothelial cells release endogenous activator tissue-type plasminogen activator (tPA) and initiate thrombolysis that is efficient for small thrombi or hemostatic plugs, less so for large thrombi in major vessels. Small amounts of plasmin released into the blood are rapidly neutralized by antiplasmin, preventing degradation of plasma proteins. Plasmic degradation of the thrombus results in formation of fibrin degradation products, especially D-dimer. PAI-1, plasminogen activator inhibitor-1.

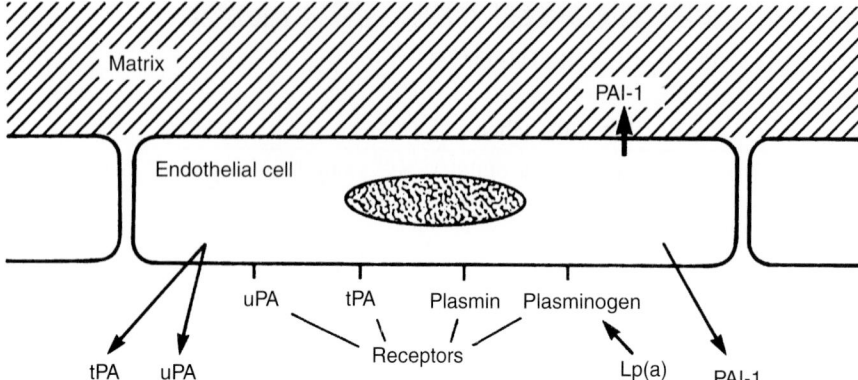

**FIGURE 23-5.** Endothelial cell participation in fibrinolysis. Endothelial cell secretion of tPA and uPA is modulated by cytokines, drugs, vascular occlusion, and local hemostasis. PAI-1 is secreted into the blood and onto subendothelial matrix. Surface receptors for plasminogen, plasmin, and PA promote localized fibrinolysis. LP(a) may limit local activation of fibrinolysis by competing for the endothelial cell plasminogen receptor. tPA, tissue-type plasminogen activator; uPA, urokinase-type plasminogen activator; LP(a), lipoprotein (a); PAI-1, plasminogen activator inhibitor-1.

TAFI formation (a mechanism of promoting clot stability) (175), it would seem that these endothelial cell surface–mediated reactions work at cross purposes. One possible explanation for this seeming discrepancy is that TAFI binding to thrombomodulin inhibits protein C activation by thrombomodulin (175), suggesting a competitive advantage to thrombomodulin-mediated reactions that promote rather than inhibit clot formation.

## GENETICALLY MODIFIED MICE

Genetic manipulations of embryonic cells that result in transgenic overexpression of proteins or "knockout" recombinations resulting in loss of functional protein expression have been applied to assess the fibrinolytic balance (176–181) (see Table 23-3). Several synopses summarize the varied effects of plasmin in addition to its obvious role in fibrin lysis, including extracellular matrix degradation, tissue and vascular remodeling, cell migration, angiogenesis, and tumor biology. Still, Bugge et al. conclude that the "critical physiologic role of the plasminogen-activating system is fibrinolysis" (177). Hypothetically, animals deficient in a plasminogen activator, plasminogen, or urokinase plasminogen activator receptor or with increased levels of PAI-1 should have an increased predilection to vascular thrombotic events or increased fibrin deposition in organs. In fact, mice without tPA or uPA survive gestation, mature into adults, and reproduce (176,177,182–188). However, animals that lack uPA may demonstrate fibrin deposition in the gastrointestinal tract, and the combination of tPA and uPA deficiency exaggerates the thrombotic effect. Although plasminogen deficiency still allows animals to survive to adulthood, the effects are similar to those that occur for the uPA plus tPA knockout combination, including gastrointestinal and skin ulcerations, thrombotic organ damage, wasting, decreased healing, and early mortality (177). The additional knockout of PAI-1 (189,190) reduced this thrombotic tendency, although the fibrinolytic response per se was not improved (189).

Increased production of PAI-1 in transgenic animals curtails a physiologic response to vascular injury. Although these mice do not have thrombotic problems *in utero*, spontaneous venous occlusions and ischemic necrosis of the tail and the digits occurs at birth (191,192). Animals with increased apolipoprotein (a) activity (193) have decreased thrombolytic response to tPA, but they manifest lesions of early atherosclerosis (fatty streaks) rather than the venous occlusions of the PAI-1 transgenics.

Mouse models that promote coagulation by removing natural coagulation inhibitors seem to induce a greater threat than disruption of single components of the fibrinolytic system. For example, lack of tissue factor pathway inhibitor (TFPI) or protein C causes death *in utero* (194–197), suggesting that there is a limited capacity of natural fibrinolytic responses to respond to uncontrolled hypercoagulation.

Animals with a deficiency of a fibrinolytic inhibitor such as PAI-1 or $\alpha_2$-plasmin, or with increased amounts of uPA, could manifest a hemorrhagic tendency. The results in animals are interesting in that a deficiency of inhibitor induced biochemical effects of heightened fibrin lysis, as well as an improved thrombolytic response to artificial clots (197–201), but did not manifest the spontaneous bleeding that occurs in humans with hereditary deficiency of inhibitor. Knockout of the antifibrinolytic component TAFI does not cause increased bleeding or attenuation in thrombotic models (202), although such a deficiency impairs skin wound repair and colonic anastomotic closure (203).

Total lack of fibrinogen induces a potential for hemorrhagic events in adult mice (177). The fibrinogen-deficient animals are not dissimilar from the human condition of hereditary hypofibrinogenemia, which can be relatively asymptomatic in the absence of major trauma. Interestingly, although such fibrinogen deficiency prevents the thrombotic and fibrin-deposition manifestations of plasminogen deficiency, the latter does not modify the hemorrhagic potential in animals that lack fibrinogen (177,192). The severest effect on hemostasis is induced in transgenic animals that overproduce uPA; such mice manifest severe hemorrhagic complications at birth in half of the subjects. Perhaps the high uPA levels in mice resemble human subjects with increased hemorrhagic potential after administration of therapeutic plasminogen activators.

## ABERRANT FIBRINOLYTIC MECHANISMS

Aberrations of physiologic fibrinolysis may result in clinical bleeding or thrombotic disorders (see Table 23-4), as described in Chapter 69. In general, heightened activity or diminished inhibition of fibrinolysis can predispose to hemorrhage, whereas the opposite tendencies of decreased fibrinolysis and increased fibrinolytic inhibition may cause thrombotic disease. The latter association is not a proven association, although a recent report suggests that a prolonged tPA-induced clot lysis time is associated with predisposition to deep vein thrombosis (DVT) (204).

### Excessive Fibrinolysis

The normal plasma concentration of $\alpha_2$-plasmin inhibitor is approximately 1 $\mu$M, less than half that of plasminogen. Although $\alpha_2$-macroglobulin complexes with excess plasmin, the amount of plasmin generated exceeds the neutralizing capacity of inhibitors, resulting in *hyperfibrino(geno)lysis* (Fig. 23-6).

## TABLE 23-3

### EFFECT OF SELECTED KNOCKOUTS AND TRANSGENICS ON THE FIBRINOLYTIC BALANCE

| Knockout(s) | Transgenic | Observed effects |
|---|---|---|
| **A. ANTIFIBRINOLYTIC (PROTHROMBOTIC)** | | |
| tPA | — | Normal development |
| uPA | — | Essentially normal development, but may have fibrin deposition in organs |
| uPAR | — | Similar to uPA deficiency |
| tPA + uPA | — | Fibrin deposition and ischemic changes in organs |
| Plasminogen | — | Develop to maturity, but may demonstrate wasting, skin and gastrointestinal ulcerations, thrombotic organ damage |
| | PAI-1 | Thrombotic venous occlusion and ischemic necrosis of tail and digits at birth |
| | Lp(a) | Fatty streaks (atherosclerosis), decreased thrombolytic response to administered tPA |
| **B. PROFIBRINOLYTIC (HEMORRHAGE)** | | |
| | uPA | Severe and fatal hemorrhagic complications in newborns |
| PAI-1 or $\alpha_2$-antiplasmin | — | No spontaneous hemorrhage, but improved experimental clot-lysis response |
| Fibrinogen | — | Hemorrhagic manifestations in adults |
| TAFI | — | Impaired wound healing, anastomotic repair |
| **C. COMBINED PRO- AND ANTIFIBRINOLYTIC** | | |
| tPA + uPA + PAI-1 | — | PAI-1 decreases the thrombotic phenotype of tPA + uPA |
| Plasminogen + *fibrinogen* | — | Absence of fibrinogen alleviates thrombosis of plasminogen deficiency, but absence of plasminogen does not correct the bleeding potential of afibrinogenemia |

Lp(a), lipoprotein a; PAI-1, plasminogen activator inhibitor 1; tPA, tissue-type plasminogen activator; uPA, urokinase-type plasminogen activator; uPAR, urokinase-type plasminogen activator receptor; TAFI, thrombin-activatable fibrinolysis inhibitor.

Therapeutic administration of PA for treatment of thrombosis usually induces a plasma lytic state, marked by degradation of fibrinogen and fibrin and coagulation factors V and VIII, more so with SK or UK than with tPA or scuPA. The risk of bleeding is increased, but this is caused by lysis of hemostatic plugs more than by the lytic state.

Physiologic stimuli such as stress and exhaustive exercise induces release of PA from endothelial cells, but not in amounts that exceed the neutralizing capacity of PAI-1. Excessive release may occur with hypotension, surgical trauma, tumors, heatstroke, and other pathologic influences (see Chapter 69) and may result in primary hyperfibrinolysis and bleeding (205). Accelerated fibrinolysis is common in patients with severe liver disease. Such patients may have elevated levels of plasminogen activator and PAI-1 with decreased $\alpha_2$-plasmin inhibitor (206–210), disrupting an already complex hemorrhagic state, and contribute to major bleeding events. Pathologic fibrinolysis also may contribute to severe hemorrhage in orthotopic liver transplantation, especially during the anhepatic phase (211), due to reduced hepatic clearance of tPA, a situation which improves after revascularization of the transplant. Hepatic ischemia and dysfunction also may cause primary fibrinolysis upon supraceliac clamping of the aorta during aneurysm repair (212).

Congenital hemorrhagic states due to heightened systemic fibrinolysis occurs as increased PA synthesis (213,214), or decreased $\alpha_2$-antiplasmin (215–220) or PAI-1 (221,222). In patients with increased PA levels or decreased PAI-1, tests show shortened clot lysis times, low fibrinogen, and increased plasma tPA levels, as opposed to preserved fibrinogen concentrations in patients with $\alpha_2$-antiplasmin deficiency. All of these patients may have a life-long hemorrhagic diathesis, but with $\alpha_2$-antiplasmin deficiency, bleeding is caused by premature lysis of hemostatic plugs rather than by systemic plasminemia. Treatment with antifibrinolytic agents corrects abnormal laboratory parameters and controls or prevents bleeding in all of these hereditary conditions (see Chapter 79).

The fibrinolytic activation of DIC typically is quite a different process, representing local microvascular responses to thrombotic occlusion rather than a systemic lytic state, and serves an important function in restoring small vessel patency. Tissues differ in their fibrinolytic potential, with the renal pelvis, endometrium, and prostate being especially rich in PA (223). Hemorrhage occurring after prostatectomy may reflect such excessive local fibrinolysis, and treatment with EACA often decreases blood loss (224,225). Local fibrinolysis is part of the physiology of menstruation; in patients with menorrhagia, local fibrinolysis may contribute to pathologic bleeding and be responsive to antifibrinolytic therapy (226) (see Chapter 79).

**TABLE 23-4**

PATHOLOGIC ABERRATIONS OF THE FIBRINOLYTIC BALANCE THAT MAY
CAUSE THROMBOSIS OR BLEEDING

| Imbalance | Pathologic cause(s) | Selected disorder(s) |
|---|---|---|
| **BLEEDING** | | |
| Excessive activation of fibrinolysis | Excessive release of circulating vascular tPA | Primary hyperfibrinolysis |
| | Iatrogenic | Administration of exogenous activator |
| | Defective clearance of activator | Hepatic cirrhosis |
| | Localized excess activator | Menorrhagia, postprostatectomy |
| Defective inhibition of fibrinolysis | Molecular defect of plasma protein | Hereditary deficiency of antiplasmin or PAI-1 |
| **THROMBOSIS** | | |
| Defective activation of fibrinolysis | Inadequate release of tPA | Endothelial cell defect or injury |
| | Molecular defect of a plasma protein | Hereditary defect or deficiency of plasminogen or fibrinogen |
| Excessive inhibition of fibrinolysis | Iatrogenic | Administration of antifibrinolytic agent (EACA) |
| | Elevated blood level of tPA inhibitor | Hereditary, transgenic mouse |
| | Global prolongation of lysis time | No specific component identified |

EACA, ε-aminocaproic acid; PAI-1, plasminogen activator inhibitor 1; tPA, tissue-type plasminogen activator.

## Decreased Fibrinolysis

Predisposition to thrombosis can result from an excessive procoagulant tendency that overwhelms a physiologic fibrinolytic response or from an inadequate fibrinolytic response to an otherwise benign thrombophilic processes. Thrombotic disease caused by defective fibrinolysis, secondary to either decreased plasminogen activation or increased inhibition, is difficult to evaluate because fibrinolytic assays are less sensitive to decreased activity than to increased activity.

Congenital defects in the fibrinolytic system have been associated with thrombosis, specifically due to abnormalities of fibrinogen and plasminogen. Aoki et al. described a patient with recurrent venous thrombotic disease who had a normal plasminogen antigen concentration, but 50% functional activity (227), the result of an amino acid substitution near the active

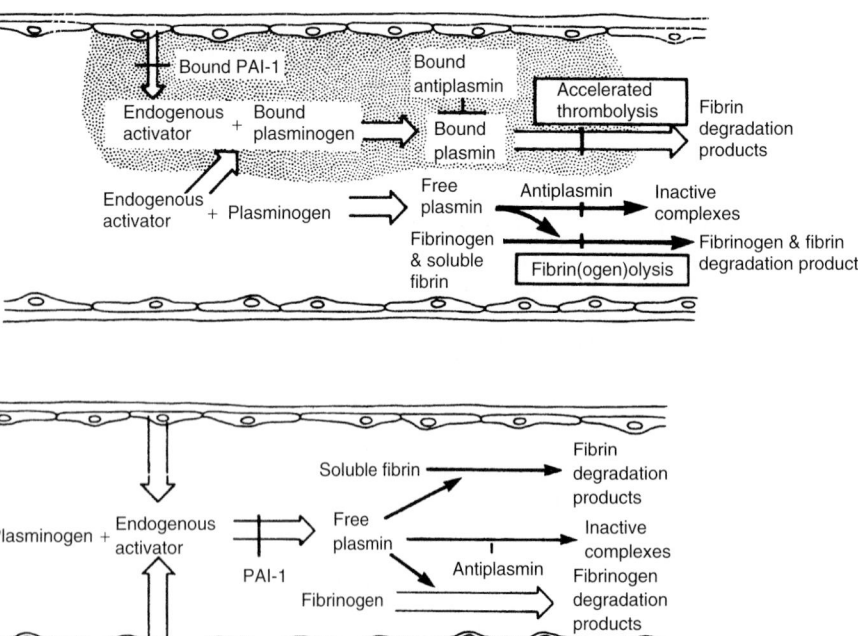

FIGURE 23-6. Schematic representation of excess fibrinolytic activation. (**Top**) Plasminogen activator therapy for thrombotic disease. With the administration of an excess of plasminogen activator, plasminogen activation in the thrombus is accelerated to a clinically relevant speed. Abundant free plasmin is formed in the blood, and this exceeds the capacity of plasma $\alpha_2$-antiplasmin to neutralize protease activity. The result is degradation of fibrinogen and other plasmin-susceptible substrates, producing the so-called plasma proteolytic state. (**Bottom**) Excess release of tissue-type plasminogen activator (tPA) from endothelial cells. In response to an extreme stimulus, large amounts of tPA are released into the blood from endothelial cells, mimicking the therapeutic administration of plasminogen activator, except that thrombus is not present. Free plasmin degrades fibrinogen and soluble fibrin, resulting in fibrinogen and fibrin degradation products in the blood. PAI-1, plasminogen activator inhibitor-1.

site histidine (228). The same defect has been found in two additional cases (229). Because no other family members, including one homozygous individual, experienced clinical disease, the contribution of the plasminogen variant to the thrombosis is problematic. Furthermore, a review of the literature suggests that the risk of thrombosis is no higher in individuals who are plasminogen deficient than in those who are not, and that plasminogen deficiency occurs equally in persons with or without thrombosis (230). Therefore, the correlation of venous thrombotic disease with homozygous plasminogen deficiency has been called into question (230–232), especially in view of the absence of ischemic venous occlusion in plasminogen knockouts and the neonatal clinical entity of ligneous conjunctivitis (233,234), lesions of which contain fibrin without plasminogen and can be reversed by plasminogen infusion (234).

Dysfibrinogenemia is usually asymptomatic, but a subset of patients have bleeding or thrombosis (see Chapter 62). Several mechanisms may explain the thrombotic tendency in some families, including abnormalities in the interaction of fibrinogen with tPA, plasminogen, or plasmin (235). For example, fibrinogen Chapel Hill III, identified in a patient with recurrent venous thrombosis (236), exhibited defective polymerization, abnormally rigid fibrin gels, and resistance to plasmic degradation, as also noted for fibrinogen Tampere (237) and fibrinogen Dusard (238). Fibrinogen New York I, which shows defective plasminogen activation by tPA (239), contains a Bβ–chain deletion that pinpoints the sequence that interacts with tPA (240).

Familial thrombotic disease also has been associated with defective fibrinolytic response to stimulation by venous occlusion or DDAVP infusion (241–243). Vessel wall fibrinolytic activity was histochemically normal, suggesting that the defect is a decreased release of plasminogen activator. One family also showed a subnormal increase in von Willebrand factor, suggesting a more global endothelial cell defect in processing or storage of proteins (243). Interestingly, increased fibrinolytic activity associated with postoperative external pneumatic compression has been cited as a mediator of DVT prophylaxis (244–246), perhaps lending credence to the physiologic role of endothelial cell release of PA.

About the importance of increased levels of fibrinolytic inhibitors in causing DVT, information is available from several clinical conditions. Surgical trauma results in a postoperative increase in PAI-1 and a corresponding reduction of global fibrinolytic activity (212,247–249), although any association with DVT is not strong enough to be clinically reliable for predicting events (247–252).

Pregnancy is associated with a marked decrease in plasma euglobulin fibrinolytic activity (253,254). Although increases in PA occur during pregnancy, these are overwhelmed by greater increases in PAI-1 and PAI-2 (255–257). PAI-1 decreases rapidly after delivery, whereas PAI-2 remains elevated for several days (255). Preeclampsia is associated with elevated inhibitor levels, which correlate with the severity of placental damage (257–262).

Patients with coronary artery disease have elevated PAI-1 (263,264), which may be a risk factor for reinfarction in young survivors of myocardial infarction (MI) (265). Elevated blood concentrations of PAI-1, tPA, or both have been linked with increased risk of acute MI or ischemic stroke, and because tPA circulates mostly in complex with PAI-1, it is not surprising that both parameters of fibrinolysis are elevated in the same subjects. There is a significant correlation of tPA antigen concentration with acute MI, relative risk of 2.8 in the highest quintile (266), and of tPA and PAI-1 for subsequent MI or sudden coronary death in patients with angina (267). The PAI-1 predictive relation usually is eliminated after correcting for insulin resistance or other risk factors (267–269), but the tPA relation with subsequent MI or stroke has usually (268–272),

but not uniformly (273), been independent of known cardiovascular risk factors. A prospective trial (274) showed no predictive quality of PAI-1 concentration in post-MI blood for a subsequent coronary event. There is no prospective correlation of venous thromboembolic disease with PAI-1 or tPA levels (275).

Reports have described higher PAI-1 and the 4G/5G polymorphism as risk factors for MI (276), as concomitant events in patients with a history of coronary thrombosis (277), or in association with a shorter time course for development of acute coronary syndromes (278), but other reports show a relation of PAI-1 concentration but not the 4G/5G polymorphism in relation to stroke (279), or an association of PAI-1 with the 4G/5G polymorphism but not with an increased risk of MI (280). The Physician's Health Study group showed no relation of the PAI-1 polymorphism with development of arterial or venous thrombotic disease (281).

Thrombosis due to excessive fibrinolytic inhibition could result from administration of an antifibrinolytic agent to predisposed patients, especially those with ongoing severe DIC or mucin-secreting adenocarcinoma (see Chapter 79). Intravascular coagulation normally leads to activation of compensatory fibrinolysis, presumably, in part, because of stimulation of plasminogen activator release from endothelial cells. This response contributes to the maintenance of vascular patency, and inhibition of fibrinolysis may exacerbate the thrombotic process (282–284). Because EACA is excreted in the urine, ureteral obstruction may develop in patients who have urinary tract bleeding; therefore, antifibrinolytic therapy must be used with caution in patients with hematuria. Elevated PAI-1 levels have been noted in patients with DVT (285,286), but there is no clear association between elevated PAI-1 and thrombosis.

A recent retrospective assessment of global fibrinolysis suggests that patients at the 90th percentile prolongation were at double the risk of DVT, although no insight was possible as to the individual protein that caused such lysis time prolongation (204). Further studies are required to determine whether this laboratory result is causal or the consequence of venous thromboembolic disease, and whether a specific factor can account for the data.

# FIBRINOGEN AND FIBRIN DEGRADATION PRODUCTS

## Fibrinogen

Plasmin has trypsinlike specificity, with an affinity for the hydrolysis of lysyl and arginyl bonds, although only 50 to 60 of the potential 362 lysine and arginine residues of fibrinogen are cleaved, 10% rapidly and the remainder more slowly (287). Degraded fibrinogen can be separated by ion-exchange chromatography into five fractions (A, B, C, D, and E), of which fragments D and E are the major end products of the original molecule (288). The identification and characterization of the intermediate fragments X and Y (289,290) provided the insight for the asymmetric scheme of fibrinogen degradation (291) (see Fig. 23-7, left). The initial cleavages liberate the carboxy-terminal appendage of the Aα chain and a peptide from the N-terminal portion of the Bβ chain, producing fragment X. Cleavages of all three polypeptide chains along one coiled-coil connecting the central (E) and terminal (D) domains of fragment X split it asymmetrically. The result is one fragment D molecule that consists of carboxy-terminal portions of the three chains and a fragment Y moiety consisting of central and terminal domains still connected by a coiled-coil. At the same time, a 42-residue fragment (Bβ1–42) containing fibrinopeptide B is split from the amino-terminal end of the

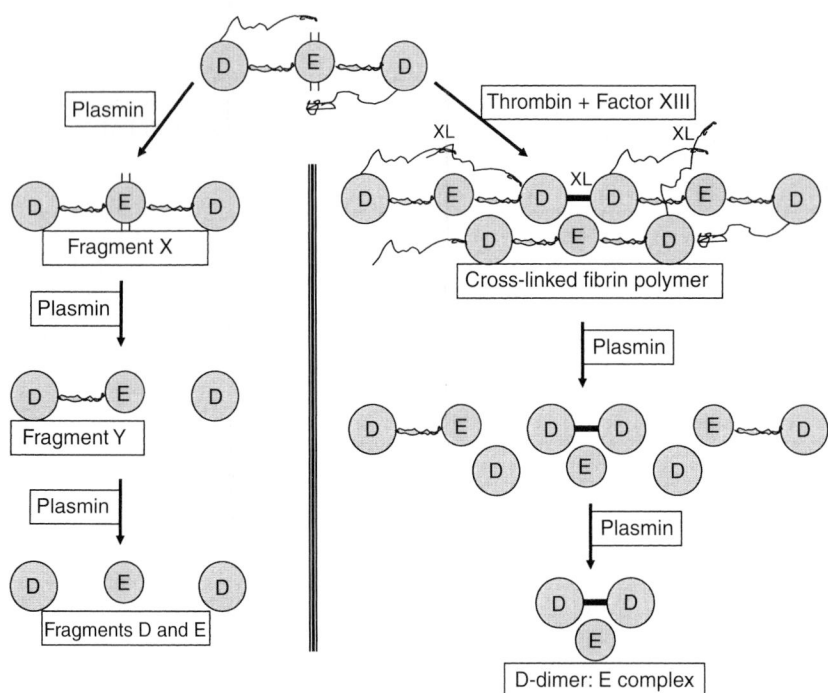

**FIGURE 23-7.** Plasmic degradation of fibrinogen and of cross-linked fibrin by plasmin. The principal structures of fibrinogen (**top**) are three globular domains from which degradation fragments D and E derive, the $\alpha$-helical coiled-coils that connect them, and A$\alpha$-chain extensions from the carboxy-terminal region of the D-domains. Shown on the left, fibrinogen is degraded asymmetrically (291) by cleavage of the coiled-coils. Intermediate degradation fragment X consists of all three domains connected by coiled-coils, but lacks the A$\alpha$-chain extensions and the B$\beta$1-42 sequence. Fragment Y consists of the central E-domain connected by a coiled-coil to a fragment D-domain. Formation of cross-linked fibrin from fibrinogen is shown schematically on the right, by enzymatic actions of thrombin and factor XIII. Thrombin liberates fibrinopeptides from the E-domain, and factor XIII cross-links (XL) fibrin longitudinally between D-domains and in a less well-defined manner, between the $\alpha$-chain extensions (see Chapter 16). Plasmic cleavage of the two-stranded protofibrils removes the cross-linked $\alpha$ chains first, then cleaves the coiled-coils to liberate a series of complexes, the smallest of which is DD/E. Complexes that are larger than DD/E (such as DY/YD) also are liberated from cross-linked fibrin, but they are subsequently degraded to the DD/E moiety.

B$\beta$ chain. Subsequent cleavage of the coiled-coil of fragment Y produces a second fragment D and fragment E. Fragment X is slowly coagulable by thrombin, but fragments Y and D have potent antipolymerizing effects, mostly a result of disruption of the proper alignment of fibrin protofibrils (290,292,293). Fragment E contains the amino-terminal portion of all six polypeptide chains (290).

In the presence of physiologic concentrations of calcium (294–296), the molecular weight of fragments D and E vary from $M_r$ 85,000 to 100,000 and $M_r$ 35,000 to 50,000, respectively (291,297–299). Under denaturing conditions (300) or with limited calcium content, fragment D can be further degraded to $M_r$ 46,000. The late cleavages of fragment E disrupt binding sites involved in fibrin monomer polymerization, bonds that are probably critical for complex formation with D-dimer (DD) as well (301,302) (Fig. 23-7, right).

## Cross-Linked Fibrin

Plasmic degradation of non–cross-linked fibrin is identical to that of fibrinogen, supporting the view that there is little structural change during polymerization (303,304). On the other hand, cross-linked fibrin is degraded by plasmin more slowly, and the factor XIIIa–mediated cross-link (XL) isopeptide bonds result in significantly different degradation products (305–307). Prolonged exposure of fibrin to plasmin *in vitro* produces a unique fragment (D-dimer), consisting of two fragment D moieties from adjacent fibrin monomers, covalently bound by cross-links between their $\gamma$-chain remnants (308–310) (Fig. 23-7, right). Fragment E exists in both free and noncovalent complex with D-dimer (DD/E complex) (311,312). The derivation of this complex from degraded fibrin can be envisioned on the basis of the two-stranded, half-staggered overlap structure of the fibrin protofibril (see Chapter 16), and these structures have been confirmed by electron microscopic studies (313). A variety of large degradation products are released by plasmin from cross-linked fibrin (305,306,314–317). These noncovalently bound complexes represent ever-longer stretches of the two-stranded, half-staggered fibrin protofibril (306), each of which is held in apposition with the same

noncovalent bonds that influenced fibrin polymer formation. The smallest complex is DD/E, with larger forms being longitudinal strings of the DD/E complex held together by uncleaved coiled-coils (306).

## Assays for Fibrinogen and Fibrin Derivatives

At a site of tissue injury, physiologic local thrombin action produces an insoluble fibrin network, but fibrin monomers remain soluble and circulate in complex with fibrinogen, degradation products, and other fibrin monomers (318–322). Quantitation of fibrinopeptides, fibrin monomers, and polymers and degradation products of fibrin in plasma may be useful in assessing hypercoagulability, ongoing thrombosis, pathologic fibrinolysis, and response to therapy.

Properties of soluble fibrin that are useful for assay include low solubility, tendency to polymerize, large molecular size, neoantigens, and ability to accelerate tPA activity. The paracoagulation reaction uses ethanol, protamine sulfate, or cooling to 4°C to precipitate fibrin polymers from plasma (323–326). Although positive in pathologic thrombosis or intravascular coagulation, these assays show inadequate specificity and sensitivity for diagnostic utility. Because fibrin polymers in complexes have a molecular weight greater than that of fibrinogen, they can be identified by their early elution from gel-filtration columns. Abnormal results have been reported in patients with venous thrombosis and arterial occlusive disease, but are most clearly positive in patients with DIC (327–329). Fibrin monomer binds to fibrinogen and may be quantitated after affinity chromatography using fibrinogen bound to agarose beads (330), and elevated levels have been found in patients with thrombotic disease or DIC (331).

Thrombin-induced cleavage of fibrinopeptides from fibrinogen exposes new antigenic sites, and fibrin neoepitopes result from conformational changes after polymerization, providing foundation for enzyme-linked immunosorbent assays (ELISA) that recognize fibrin monomer or polymer, but not fibrinogen (332–334). Another method for measuring soluble fibrin is based on the principle that fibrin stimulates the activation of plasminogen by tPA (335), allowing for detection of increased fibrin monomer in the presence of fibrin(ogen) degradation products (335,336).

Interpretation of results for soluble fibrin assay is hindered by the variation in normal plasma concentration, from 0.1% of plasma fibrinogen by chromogenic assay to 7.7% by gel-filtration chromatography (329,335), probably reflecting the different molecular species that are identified (337,338). Soluble fibrin levels are sensitive in the diagnosis of DIC (339,340) and venous thromboembolic disease (341–343) and have also been elevated in acute MI (344–346) and obstetric complications (347).

The development of sensitive radioimmunoassays for the fibrinopeptides, especially fibrinopeptide A, has allowed accurate measurements of the kinetics of thrombin action, particularly in thrombotic states and as altered by anticoagulant therapy (348–351). The assays are technically demanding and are sensitive to thrombin generation *in vitro* or during venipuncture. Plasmin cleaves the amino-terminus of the Bβ chain, which includes fibrinopeptide B, so either thrombin (hypercoagulability) or plasmin (increased fibrinolysis) action could produce elevated levels (352). In healthy subjects, the mean plasma fibrinopeptide A concentration is less than 2 nmol per L, and the plasma half-life is 3 minutes (350). Because fibrinopeptide A is a specific marker of thrombin action, the finding of even low concentrations in healthy subjects implies that there is a baseline level of thrombin action that accounts for up to 3% of fibrinogen catabolism. Elevated levels have been found in patients with both thrombotic and inflammatory diseases, thereby limiting diagnostic specificity (353–355). Heparin infusion into patients with venous thromboembolic disease rapidly decreases the fibrinopeptide A concentration, indicating an effective inhibition of the thrombotic process (348).

Activated factor XIII rapidly forms covalent isopeptide cross-links between pairs of γ chains (356), more slowly between α chains, each of which may cross-link with two other α chains (357). Large α-chain polymers (358–360) also include covalently cross-linked fibronectin and $α_2$-plasmin inhibitor (94,357,361). By electrophoresis of plasma extracts, a low concentration of cross-linked fibrin polymer has been demonstrated in normal plasma (344), with increased amounts in patients with acute MI in whom 4% of total fibrinogen exists as fibrin dimers (344).

Most immunologic techniques for the detection of fibrinogen degradation products also react with fibrinogen (362,363), thereby precluding their use in plasma or in incompletely clotted blood due to the presence of heparin (364). More specific assays for plasmic derivatives of fibrinogen include an ELISA that uses a "capture" monoclonal antibody that reacts with degradation products of both fibrinogen and fibrin, and a second monoclonal antibody that reacts with a thrombin-sensitive site on the Aα chain, so the combination detects plasmic derivatives of fibrinogen, but not fibrin (365). Comparison of plasma levels of β15–42 and Bβ1–42 may be interpreted as reflecting the ratio of plasmic degradation of fibrin to fibrinogen (366,367).

## Clinical Relevance of Degradation Products

An assay that detects unique plasmic derivatives of fibrin in plasma would have important clinical use. Because *in vivo* thrombi are cross-linked (368,369), one approach has been to measure the unique factor XIII–cross-linked plasmin degradation products. A technique that relies on electrophoresis of plasma is useful for characterizing the extent of fibrinolysis and fibrinogenolysis during fibrinolytic therapy and in patients with liver disease, but it is time consuming and technically demanding, making it unsuitable for routine clinical use (370–372). The current standard for fibrin derivative

measurement is the DD assay (373–377), which, because of low cross-reactivity with fibrinogen, can be applied in assays of plasma.

DD levels are elevated in nearly all patients with DIC, making the assay a sensitive marker for this pathology (377–381). However, the assay is not as specific as it is sensitive, because positive results occur in many other conditions (382,383). As an example, one survey found an elevated DD level in 28% of random plasma samples from hospitalized patients (384). Plasma levels of fibrin and fibrinogen degradation products have been measured in patients receiving fibrinolytic therapy, with a goal of noninvasively assessing thrombolysis. In the treatment of acute MI, fibrinogen degradation as measured by plasma levels of $Bβ_{1-42}$ is greater with SK than with tPA, and with 150 mg of tPA compared with 100 mg of tPA, findings that are consistent with the decrease in plasma fibrinogen during such treatment (385,386). Levels of plasma cross-linked fibrin degradation products, measured as DD, also increase to high levels early during fibrinolytic therapy, but the degree of elevation during treatment of acute MI, pulmonary embolism (PE) or DVT does not correlate with reperfusion success (387–391).

A possible explanation for this unexpected discrepancy concerns the effect of PA on plasma soluble fibrin (Fig. 23-7) (391). Although the amount of plasma soluble fibrin is small compared to the concentration of fibrinogen, the amount of plasma soluble fibrin is large compared to the fibrin of a coronary artery thrombus or even of deep leg vein thrombus. Consequently, the limited correlation of DD levels with thrombolysis can be explained by the derivation of circulating fibrin degradation products from plasma soluble fibrin rather than from the pathologic thrombus. In patients receiving fibrinolytic therapy for DVT, correction of DD levels for the contribution from soluble fibrin allows for good correlation between plasma DD levels and angiographically documented clot lysis (392).

Before therapy, patients diagnosed with DVT or PE have increased plasma DD levels, reflecting background physiologic lysis of thrombus (387,388,393–399). Therefore, a normal level in such a patient would be unexpected and could be of value in ruling out the diagnosis. A substantial effort has been devoted to this issue, because noninvasive approaches to documenting DVT or PE would have considerable implication for initial management (400). A number of immunologic DD assays have been developed, and comparisons have pointed to general equivalence of the assays (401) or to the superiority of the ELISA over turbidometric approaches (402). Literature reviews generally support the contention that DD assays are sufficiently reliable to allow the physician to defer invasive (or noninvasive) studies for documenting new or recurrent venous thromboembolic disease (402–406). Not all analyses agree with the conclusion that a DD assay can be applied as a "standalone test" (407). Also, certain caveats do exist; for example, a negative DD value did not exclude thrombotic disease early (4 days) after trauma (408) and did not predict DVT in critically ill patients (409) or in patients after traumatic brain injury (410). However, DD has been used as a marker for an ongoing hypercoagulable state, with higher levels correlating with subsequent DVT after total hip replacement surgery (411).

These observations illustrate the complexity of fibrinogen and fibrin degradation products, but also the potential for reasoned application of such assays in the understanding and management of pathologic thrombotic states.

## References

1. Astrup T. The haemostatic balance. *Thromb Diath Haemorrh* 1958;2:347.
2. Nossel H. Relative proteolysis of the fibrinogen Bβ chain by thrombin and plasmin as a determinant of thrombosis. *Nature* 1981;291:165.

3. Walther PJ, Steinmann HM, Hill RL, et al. Activation of human plasminogen by urokinase: partial characterization of a preactivation peptide. *J Biol Chem* 1970;249:1173.

4. Wallen P, Wiman B. Characterization of human plasminogen. I: on the relationship between different molecular forms of plasminogen demonstrated in plasma and found in purified preparations. *Biochim Biophys Acta* 1970;221:20.

5. Rickli EE, Cuendet PA. Isolation of plasmin-free human plasminogen with N-terminal glutamic acid. *Biochim Biophys Acta* 1971;250:447.

6. Wallen P, Wiman B. Characterization of different molecular forms of human plasminogen. *Biochim Biophys Acta* 1972;257:122.

7. Summaria L, Arzadon L, Bernabe P, et al. Characterization of the NH₂-terminal glutamic acid and NH₂-terminal lysine forms of human plasminogen isolated by affinity chromatography and isoelectric focusing methods. *J Biol Chem* 1973;248:2984.

8. Thorsen S. Differences in the binding to fibrin of native plasminogen and plasminogen modified by proteolytic degradation influence of ε-aminocarboxylic acids. *Biochim Biophys Acta* 1975;393:55.

9. Lucas MA, Fretto LJ, McKee PA. The binding of human plasminogen to fibrin and fibrinogen. *J Biol Chem* 1983;258:4249.

10. Claeys H, Vermylen J. Physico-chemical and proenzyme properties of NH₂-terminal lysine human plasminogen: influence of 6-aminohexanoic acid. *Biochim Biophys Acta* 1974;342:351.

11. Thorsen S, Kok P, Astrup T. Reversible and irreversible alterations of human plasminogen indicated by changes in susceptibility to plasminogen activator and in response to epsilon-aminocaproic acid. *Thromb Diath Haemorrh* 1974;32:325.

12. Hoylaerts M, Rijken DC, Lijnen HR, et al. Kinetics of the activation of plasminogen by human tissue plasminogen activator. Role of fibrin. *J Biol Chem* 1982;257:2912.

13. Lijnen HR, Zamarron C, Collen D. Characterization of the high-affinity interaction between human plasminogen and pro-urokinase. *Eur J Biochem* 1985;150:141.

14. Markus G, DePasquale JL, Wissler FC. Quantitative determination of the binding of epsilon-aminocaproic acid to native plasminogen. *J Biol Chem* 1978;253:727.

15. Miles LA, Plow EF. Binding and activation of plasminogen on the platelet surface. *J Biol Chem* 1985;260:4303.

16. Bauer PI, Machovich R, Buki KG, et al. Interaction of plasmin with endothelial cells. *Biochem J* 1984;218:119.

17. Abiko Y, Iwamoto M, Tomikawa M. Plasminogen-plasmin system. V: as stoichiometric equilibrium complex of plasminogen and a synthetic inhibitor. *Biochim Biophys Acta* 1969;185:424.

18. Brockway WJ, Castellino FJ. The mechanisms of the inhibition of plasmin activity by ε-aminocaproic acid. *J Biol Chem* 1969;246:424.

19. Christensen U, Clemmensen I. Kinetic properties of the primary inhibitor of plasmin from human plasma. *Biochem J* 1977;163:389.

20. Wiman B, Collen D. On the kinetics of the reaction between human antiplasmin and plasmin. *Eur J Biochem* 1978;84:573.

21. Moroi M, Aoki N. Inhibition of plasminogen binding to fibrin by α₂-plasmin inhibitor. *Thromb Res* 1977;10:581.

22. Kaplan AP, Silverberg M. The coagulation-kinin pathway of human plasma. *Blood* 1987;70:1.

23. Colman RW, Schmaier AH. Contact system: a vascular biology modulator with anticoagulant, profibrinolytic, and proinflammatory attributes. *Blood* 1997;90:3819.

24. Bouma BN, Meijers JCM. Fibrinolysis and the contact system: a role for factor XI in the down regulation of fibrinolysis. *Thromb Haemost* 1999;82:243.

25. Motta G, Røjkjaer R, Hasan AAK, et al. High molecular weight kininogen regulates prekallikrein assembly and activation on endothelial cells: a novel mechanism for contact activation. *Blood* 1998;91:516.

26. Ratnoff OD, Busce FJ, Sheon RP. The demise of John Hageman. *N Engl J Med* 1968;279:760.

27. Ichinose A, Kisiel W, Fujikawa K. Proteolytic activator of tissue plasminogen activator by plasmin and tissue enzymes. *FEBS Lett* 1984;175:412.

28. Binder BR, Spragg J, Austen KF. Purification and characterization of human vascular plasminogen activator derived from blood vessel perfusates. *J Biol Chem* 1979;244:1998.

29. Wallen P, Ranby M, Bergsdorf N. Purification and characterization of tissue plasminogen activator: on the occurrence of two different forms and their enzymatic properties. In: Davidson JF, Nilsson IM, Astedt B, eds. *Progress in fibrinolysis*, Vol. 5. Edinburgh: Churchill Livingstone, 1981.

30. Rijken DC, Hoylaerts M, Collen D. Fibrinolytic properties of one-chain human extrinsic (tissue-type) plasminogen activator. *J Biol Chem* 1982;257:2920.

31. Ranby M, Bergsdorf N, Nilsson T. Enzymatic properties of the one- and two-chain form of tissue plasminogen activator. *Thromb Res* 1982;27:175.

32. Pennica D, Holmes WE, Kohn WJ, et al. Cloning and expression of human tissue-type plasminogen activator cDNA in *E. coli*. *Nature* 1983;301:214.

33. Banyai L, Varadi A, Patthy L. Common evolutionary origin of the fibrin-binding structures of fibronectin and tissue-type plasminogen activator. *FEBS Lett* 1983;163:37.

34. Sottrup-Jensen L, Claeys H, Zajdel M, et al. The primary structure of human plasminogen: isolation of two lysine-binding fragments and one "mini"-plasminogen (MW, 38,000) by elastase-catalyzed specific limited proteolysis. In: Davidson JF, Rowan RM, Samama MM, et al., eds. *Progress in chemical fibrinolysis and thrombolysis*, Vol. 3. New York: Raven Press, 1978.

35. Camiolo SM, Thorsen S, Astrup T. Fibrinogenolysis and fibrinolysis with tissue plasminogen activator, urokinase, streptokinase-activated human globulin, and plasmin. *Proc Soc Exp Biol Med* 1971;138:277.

36. Thorsen S, Glas-Greenwalt P, Astrup T. Differences in the binding to fibrin of urokinase and tissue plasminogen activator. *Thromb Diath Haemorrh* 1972;28:65.

37. Thorsen S. Human urokinase and porcine tissue plasminogen activator. *Dan Med Bull* 1977;24:189.

38. Ichinose A, Takio K, Fujikawa K. Localization of the binding site of tissue-type plasminogen activator to fibrin. *J Clin Invest* 1986;78:163.

39. van Zonneveld A-J, Veerman H, Pannekoek H. On the interaction of the finger and kringle-2 domains of tissue-type plasminogen activator with fibrin. *J Biol Chem* 1986;261:14214.

40. Gething M-J, Adler B, Boose J-A, et al. Variants of human tissue-type plasminogen activator that lack specific structural domains of the heavy chain. *EMBO J* 1988;7:2731.

41. Ranby M. Studies on the kinetics of plasminogen activation by tissue plasminogen activator. *Biochim Biophys Acta* 1982;704:461.

42. Hoylaerts M, Rijken DC, Lijnen HR, et al. Kinetics of the activation of plasminogen by human tissue plasminogen activator: role of fibrin. *J Biol Chem* 1982;257:2912.

43. Bosma PJ, Rijken DC, Nieuwenhuizen W. Binding of tissue-type plasminogen activator to fibrinogen fragments. *Eur J Biochem* 1988;172:399.

44. Nieuwenhuizen W, Vermond A, Voskuilen M, et al. Identification of a site in fibrin(ogen) which is involved in the acceleration of plasminogen activation by tissue-type plasminogen activator. *Biochim Biophys Acta* 1983;748:86.

45. Voskuilen M, Vermond A, Veenenman GH, et al. Fibrinogen lysine residue A-alpha 157 plays a crucial role in the fibrin-induced acceleration of plasminogen activation, catalyzed by tissue-type plasminogen activator. *J Biol Chem* 1987;262:5944.

46. Williams JRB. The fibrinolytic activity of urine. *Br J Exp Pathol* 1951;32:530.

47. Bernik MB, Kwaan HC. Origin of fibrinolytic activity in cultures of human kidney. *J Lab Clin Med* 1967;70:650.

48. White WF, Barlow GH, Mozen MM. The isolation and characterization of plasminogen activators (urokinase) from human urine. *Biochemistry* 1966;5:2160.

49. Barlow GH, Francis CW, Marder VJ. On the conversion of high-molecular-weight urokinase to the low-molecular-weight form by plasmin. *Thromb Res* 1981;23:541.

50. Rijken DC, Wijngaards G, Zaal DeJong M, et al. Purification and partial characterization of plasminogen activator from human uterine tissue. *Biochim Biophys Acta* 1979;580:140.

51. Wiman B, Wallen P. The specific interaction between plasminogen and fibrin: a physiological role of the lysine binding site in plasminogen. *Thromb Res* 1977;10:213.

52. Husain SS, Gurewich V, Lipinski B. Purification and partial characterization of a single-chain high-molecular-weight form of urokinase from human urine. *Arch Biochem Biophys* 1983;220:31.

53. Wun TC, Schleuning WD, Reich E. Isolation and characterization of urokinase from human plasma. *J Biol Chem* 1982;257:3276.

54. Wun TC, Ossowski L, Reich E. A proenzyme form of human urokinase. *J Biol Chem* 1982;257:7262.

55. Stump DC, Lijnen HR, Collen D. Purification and characterization of single-chain urokinase-type plasminogen activator (scu-PA) from human cell cultures. *J Biol Chem* 1986;261:1274.

56. Holmes WE, Pennica D, Blaber M, et al. Cloning and expression of the gene for pro-urokinase in *Escherichia coli*. *Biotechnology* 1985;3:923.

57. Winkler ME, Blaber M, Bennett GL, et al. Purification and characterization of recombinant urokinase from *E. coli*. *Biotechnology* 1985;3:990.

58. Gurewich V, Pannell R, Louie S, et al. Effective and fibrin-specific clot lysis by a zymogen precursor form of urokinase (pro-urokinase). A study *in vitro* and in two animal species. *J Clin Invest* 1984;73:1731.

59. Zamarron C, Lijnen HR, Van Hoef B, et al. Biological and thrombolytic properties of proenzyme and active forms of urokinase. I: fibrinolytic and fibrinogenolytic properties in human plasma *in vitro* of urokinases obtained from human urine or by recombinant DNA technology. *Thromb Haemost* 1984;52:19.

60. Gurewich V, Pannell R. Inactivation of single-chain urokinase (pro-urokinase) by thrombin and thrombin-like enzymes: relevance of the findings to the interpretation of fibrin-binding experiments. *Blood* 1987;69:769.

61. Pannell R, Gurewich V. Pro-urokinase: a study of its stability in plasma and of a mechanism for its selective fibrinolytic effect. *Blood* 1986;67:1215.

62. Collen D, Zamarron C, Lijnen HR, et al. Activation of plasminogen by pro-urokinase, II: kinetics. *J Biol Chem* 1986;261:1259.

63. Lijnen HR, Van Hoef B, DeCock F, et al. The mechanism of plasminogen activation and fibrin dissolution by single-chain urokinase-type plasminogen activator in a plasma milieu *in vitro*. *Blood* 1989;73:1846.

64. Pannell R, Black J, Gurewich V. Complementary modes of action of tissue-type plasminogen activator and pro-urokinase by which their synergistic effect on clot lysis may be explained. *J Clin Invest* 1988;81:853.

65. Wohl RC, Summaria L, Arzadon L, et al. Steady-state kinetics of activation of human and bovine plasminogens by streptokinase and its equimolar complexes with various activated forms of human plasminogen. *J Biol Chem* 1978;253:1402.

66. Castellino FJ, Violand BN. The fibrinolytic system—basic considerations. *Prog Cardiovasc Dis* 1979;21:241.

67. Topol EJ, Bell WR, Weisfeldt ML. Coronary thrombolysis with recombinant tissue-type plasminogen activator. *Ann Intern Med* 1985;103:837.

68. Verstraete M, Bory M, Collen D, et al. Randomised trial of intravenous recombinant tissue-type plasminogen activator versus intravenous streptokinase in acute myocardial infarction. *Lancet* 1985;1:842.

69. Rao AK, Pratt C, Berke A, et al. Thrombolysis in myocardial infarction trial, hemorrhagic manifestations and changes in plasma fibrinogen and the fibrinolytic system in patients treated with recombinant tissue plasminogen activator and streptokinase. *J Am Coll Cardiol* 1988;11:1.

70. Marder VJ, Stewart D. Towards safer thrombolytic therapy. *Semin Hematol* 2002;39:206.

71. Kohnert U, Rudolph R, Verheijen JH, et al. Biochemical properties of the kringle 2 and protease domains are maintained in the refolded t-PA deletion variant BM 06.022. *Protein Eng* 1992;5:93.

72. Martin U, Bader R, Bohm C, et al. BM 06.022: a novel recombinant plasminogen activator. *Cardiovasc Drugs Ther* 1993;11:299.

73. Keyt BA, Paoni NF, Refino CJ, et al. A faster-acting and more potent form of tissue plasminogen activator. *Proc Natl Acad Sci U S A* 1994;91:3670.

74. Paoni NF, Keyt BA, Refino CJ, et al. A slow clearing fibrin specific PAI-1 resistant of t-PA (T103N, KHRR 296-299 AAAA). *Thromb Haemost* 1993;70:307.

75. Verstraete M. Newer thrombolytic agents. *Ann Acad Med Singapore* 1999;28:424.

76. White HD, Van de Werf FJ. Thrombolysis for acute myocardial infarction. *Circulation* 1998;97:1632.

77. Smith RAG, Dupe RJ, English PD, et al. Fibrinolysis with acylenzymes: a new approach to thrombolytic therapy. *Nature* 1981;290:505.

78. Marder VJ, Rothbard RL, Fitzpatrick PG, et al. Rapid lysis of coronary artery thrombi by a (2-4 minute) bolus intravenous injection of APSAC (anisoylated plasminogen:streptokinase activator). *Ann Intern Med* 1986;104:304.

79. Collen D, Zhao ZA, Holvoet P, et al. Primary structure and gene structure of staphylokinase. *Fibrinolysis* 1992;6:226.

80. Robbins KC, Summaria L, Hsieh B, et al. The peptide chains of human plasmin: mechanism of activation of human plasminogen to plasmin. *J Biol Chem* 1967;242:2333.

81. Summaria L, Hsieh B, Robbins KC. The specific mechanism of activation of human plasminogen to plasmin. *J Biol Chem* 1967;242:4279.

82. Christensen U, Sottrup-Jensen L, Magnusson S, et al. Enzymic properties of the neo-plasmin-Val442 (miniplasmin). *Biochim Biophys Acta* 1979;567:472.

83. Weinstein MJ, Doolittle RF. Differential specificities of thrombin, plasmin, trypsin with regard to synthetic and natural substrates and inhibitors. *Biochim Biophys Acta* 1972;258:577.

84. Violand BN, Castellino FJ. Mechanism of the urokinase-catalyzed activation of human plasminogen. *J Biol Chem* 1976;251:3906.

85. Collen D. Identification and some properties of a new fast-reacting plasmin inhibitor in human plasma. *Eur J Biochem* 1976;69:209.

86. Moroi M, Aoki N. Isolation and characterization of alpha-2-plasmin inhibitor from human plasma: a novel proteinase inhibitor which inhibits activator-induced clot lysis. *J Biol Chem* 1976;251:5956.

87. Müllertz S, Clemmensen I. The primary inhibitor of plasmin in human plasma. *Biochem J* 1976;159:545.

88. Plow EF, Collen D. The presence and release of $\alpha_2$-antiplasmin from human platelets. *Blood* 1981;58:69.

89. Wiman B, Collen D. On the mechanism of the reaction between human $\alpha_2$-antiplasmin and plasmin. *J Biol Chem* 1979;254:9291.

90. Clemmensen I. Different molecular forms of alpha-2-antiplasmin. In: Collen D, Wiman B, Verstraete M, eds. *The physiological inhibitors of coagulation and fibrinolysis.* Amsterdam: Elsevier/North-Holland, 1979.

91. Kluft C, Los N. Demonstration of two forms of $\alpha_2$-antiplasmin in plasma by modified crossed immunoelectrophoresis. *Thromb Res* 1981;21:65.

92. Clemmensen I, Thorsen S, Müllertz S, et al. Properties of three different molecular forms of the $\alpha_2$-plasmin inhibitor. *Eur J Biochem* 1981;120:105.

93. Kluft C, Los P, Jie AFH, et al. The mutual relationship between the two molecular forms of the major fibrinolysis inhibitor alpha-2-antiplasmin in blood. *Blood* 1986;67:105.

94. Sakata Y, Aoki N. Crosslinking of $\alpha_2$-plasmin inhibitor to fibrin by fibrin-stabilizing factor. *J Clin Invest* 1980;65:290.

95. Sakata Y, Aoki N. Significance of crosslinking of $\alpha_2$-plasmin inhibitor to fibrin in inhibition of fibrinolysis and in hemostasis. *J Clin Invest* 1982;69: 536.

96. Gormsen J, Fletcher A, Alkjaersig N, et al. Enzymic lysis of plasma clots: the influence of fibrin stabilization on lysis rates. *Arch Biochem Biophys* 1967;120:654.

97. Gaffney PJ, Whitaker AN. Fibrin crosslinks and lysis rates. *Thromb Res* 1979;14:85.

98. Harpel PC, Mosesson MW. Degradation of human fibrinogen by plasma $\alpha_2$-macroglobulin-enzyme complexes. *J Clin Invest* 1973;52:2175.

99. Aoki N, Harpel PC. Inhibitors of the fibrinolytic enzyme system. *Semin Thromb Hemost* 1984;10:24.

100. Astedt B, Haegerstrand I, Lecander I. Cellular localization in placenta of placental type plasminogen activator inhibitor. *Thromb Haemost* 1986;56:63.

101. Wohlwend A, Belin D, Vassalli JD. Plasminogen activator-specific inhibitors produced by human monocytes/macrophages. *J Exp Med* 1987; 165:320.

102. Kawano T, Morimoto K, Uemura Y. Urokinase inhibitor in human placenta. *Nature* 1968;217:253.

103. Lecander I, Astedt B. Isolation of a new specific plasminogen activator from pregnancy plasma. *Br J Haematol* 1986;62:221.

104. Kruithof KEO, Tran-Thang C, Ransijn A, et al. Demonstration of a fast-acting inhibitor of plasminogen activators in human plasma. *Blood* 1984;64:907.

105. Thorsen S, Philips M. Isolation of tissue-type plasminogen activator-inhibitor complexes from human plasma. Evidence for a rapid plasminogen activator inhibitor. *Biochim Biophys Acta* 1984;802:111.

106. Colucci M, Paramo JA, Collen DA. Inhibition of one-chain and two-chain forms of human tissue-type plasminogen activator by the fast-acting inhibitor of plasminogen activator *in vitro* and *in vivo*. *J Lab Clin Med* 1986;108:53.

107. Kruithof EKO, Tran-Thang C, Bachmann F. The fast-acting inhibitor of tissue-type plasminogen activator in plasma is also the primary plasma inhibitor of urokinase. *Thromb Haemost* 1986;55:65.

108. Loskutoff DJ, Edgington TS. Synthesis of a fibrinolytic activator and inhibitor by endothelial cells. *Proc Natl Acad Sci U S A* 1977;74:3903.

109. Loskutoff DJ, Edgington TS. An inhibitor of plasminogen activator in rabbit endothelial cells. *J Biol Chem* 1981;256:4142.

110. Philips M, Juul AG, Thorsen S. Human endothelial cells produce a plasminogen activator inhibitor and a tissue-type plasminogen activator-inhibitor complex. *Biochim Biophys Acta* 1984;802:99.

111. van Mourik JA, Lawrence DA, Loskutoff DJ. Purification of an inhibitor of plasminogen activator (antiactivator) synthesized by endothelial cells. *J Biol Chem* 1984;259:14914.

112. Ginsburg D, Zeheb R, Yang AY, et al. cDNA cloning of human plasminogen activator-inhibitor from endothelial cells. *J Clin Invest* 1986;78:1673.

113. Bevilacqua MP, Schleef RR, Gimbrone MA Jr, et al. Regulation of the fibrinolytic system of cultured human vascular endothelium by interleukin-1. *J Clin Invest* 1986;78:587.

114. Emeis JJ, Kooistra T. Interleukin-1 and lipopolysaccharide induce an inhibitor of tissue-type plasminogen activator *in vivo* and in cultured endothelial cells. *J Exp Med* 1986;163:1260.

115. Schleef RR, Bevilacqua MP, Sawdey M, et al. Cytokine activation of vascular endothelium: effects on tissue-type plasminogen activator and type 1 plasminogen activator inhibitor. *J Biol Chem* 1988;263:5797.

116. Sprengers ED, Verheijen JH, Van Hinsbergh VWM, et al. Evidence for the presence of two different fibrinolytic inhibitors in human endothelial cell conditioned medium. *Biochim Biophys Acta* 1984;801:163.

117. Hekman CM, Loskutoff DJ. Endothelial cells produce a latent inhibitor of plasminogen activators that can be activated by denaturants. *J Biol Chem* 1985;260:11581.

118. Levin EG, Santell L. Conversion of the active to latent plasminogen activator inhibitor from human endothelial cells. *Blood* 1987;70:1090.

119. Vaughan DE, Deckercj PJ, Van Houtte E, et al. Studies of recombinant plasminogen activator inhibitor-1 in rabbits: pharmacokinetics and evidence for reactivation of latent plasminogen activator inhibitor-1 *in vivo*. *Circ Res* 1986;67:1281.

120. Declerck PJ, De Mol M, Alessi M-C, et al. Purification and characterization of a plasminogen activator inhibitor 1 binding protein from human plasma. Identification as a multimeric form of S protein (vitronectin). *J Biol Chem* 1988;263:15454.

121. Mimuro J, Loskutoff DJ. Purification of a protein from bovine plasma that binds to type 1 plasminogen activator inhibitor and prevents its interaction with extracellular matrix. *J Biol Chem* 1989;264:936.

122. Salonen E-M, Vaheri A, Pöllänen J, et al. Interaction of plasminogen activator inhibitor (PAI-1) with vitronectin. *J Biol Chem* 1989;264:6339.

123. Levin EG, Santell L. Association of plasminogen activator inhibitor with the growth substratum and membrane of human endothelial cells. *J Cell Biol* 1987;105:2543.

124. Mimuro J, Schleef RR, Luskutoff DJ. Extracellular matrix of cultured bovine aortic endothelial cells contains functionally active type I plasminogen activator inhibitor. *Blood* 1987;70:721.

125. Wagner OF, de Vries C, Hohmann C, et al. Interaction between plasminogen activator inhibitor type 1 bound to fibrin and either tissue-type plasminogen activator or urokinase-type plasminogen activator. Binding of t-PA/PAI-1 complexes to fibrin mediated by both the finger and the kringle-1 domain of t-PA. *J Clin Invest* 1989;84:647.

126. Tran-Thang C, Kruithof EKO, Bachmann F. The mechanism of *in vitro* clot lysis induced by vascular plasminogen activator. *Blood* 1984;63:1331.

127. Kaplan KL, Mather T, DeMarco L, et al. Effect of fibrin on endothelial cell production of prostacyclin and tissue plasminogen activator. *Arteriosclerosis* 1989;9:43.

128. Levin EG, Marzec U, Anderson J, et al. Thrombin stimulates tissue plasminogen activator release from cultured human endothelial cells. *J Clin Invest* 1984;74:1988.

129. Hanss M, Collen D. Secretion of tissue-type plasminogen activator and plasminogen activator inhibitor by cultured human endothelial cells: modulation by thrombin, endotoxin, and histamine. *J Lab Clin Med* 1987;109:97.

130. Amery A, Vermylen J, Maes H, et al. Enhancing the fibrinolytic activity in human blood by occlusion of blood vessels. *Thromb Diath Haemorrh* 1962; 7:70.

131. Wiman B, Mellbring G. Plasminogen activator release during venous stasis and exercise as determined by a new specific assay. *Clin Chim Acta* 1983; 127:279.

132. Fukao H, Ueshima S, Tanaka N, et al. Suppression of plasminogen activator inhibitor I release by fibrin from human umbilical vein endothelial cells. *Thromb Res Suppl* 1990;10:11.

133. Vaughan DE, Mendelsohn ME, Declerck P, et al. Characterization of the binding of human tissue-type plasminogen activator to platelets. *J Biol Chem* 1989;264:15869.

134. Braaten JV, Handt S, Jerome WG, et al. Regulation of fibrinolysis by platelet-released plasminogen activator inhibitor 1: light scattering and ultrastructural examination of lysis of a model platelet-fibrin thrombus. *Blood* 1993;81:1290.

135. Kruithof EKO, Tran-Thang C, Backmann F. Studies on the release of plasminogen activator inhibitor by human platelets. *Thromb Haemost* 1986; 55:201.

136. Cogstad GO, Stormorken H, Solum NO. Platelet alpha-2-antiplasmin is isolated in the platelet alpha-granules. *Thromb Res* 1983;31:387.

137. Suenson E, Lützen O, Thorsen S. Initial plasmin-degradation of fibrin as the basis of a positive feedback mechanism in fibrinolysis. *Eur J Biochem* 1984;140:513.

138. Tran-Thang C, Kruithof EKO, Atkinson J, et al. High-affinity binding sites for human Glu-plasminogen unveiled by limited plasmic degradation of human fibrin. *Eur J Biochem* 1986;160:599.

139. Francis CW, Marder VJ. Rapid formation of large-molecular-weight α-polymers in crosslinked fibrin induced by high factor XIII concentrations. *J Clin Invest* 1987;80:1459.

140. Francis CW, Marder VJ. Increased resistance to plasmic degradation of fibrin with highly crosslinked α-polymer chains formed at high Factor XIII concentrations. *Blood* 1988;70:1361.

141. Bajzar L, Manuel R, Nesheim ME. Purification and characterization of TAFI, a thrombin activatable fibrinolysis inhibitor. *J Biol Chem* 1995; 270:14477.

142. Bajzar L, Morser J, Nesheim M. TAFI, or plasma procarboxypeptidase B couples the coagulation and fibrinolytic cascades through the thrombin-thrombomodulin complex. *J Biol Chem* 1996;271:16603.

143. Nesheim M, Wang W, Boffa M, et al. Thrombin, thrombomodulin and TAFI in the molecular link between coagulation and fibrinolysis. *Thromb Haemost* 1997;78:386.

144. Hajjar K, Harpel P, Jaffe E, et al. Binding of plasminogen to cultured human endothelial cells. *J Biol Chem* 1986;261:11656.

145. Miles LA, Levin EG, Plescia J, et al. Plasminogen receptors, urokinase receptors, and their modulation on human endothelial cells. *Blood* 1988; 72:628.

146. Hajjar KA, Hamel NM, Harpel PC, et al. Binding of tissue plasminogen activator to cultured human endothelial cells. *J Clin Invest* 1987;80:1712.

147. Hajjar KA, Nachman RL. Endothelial cell-mediated conversion of Glu-plasminogen to Lys-plasminogen. Further evidence for assembly of the fibrinolytic system on the endothelial cell surface. *J Clin Invest* 1988;82:1769.

148. Lijnen HR, Collen D. Endothelium in hemostasis and thrombosis. *Prog Cardiovasc Dis* 1997;39:343.

149. Mimuro J, Loskutoff DJ. Binding of type 1 plasminogen activator inhibitor to the extracellular matrix of cultured bovine endothelial cells. *J Biol Chem* 1989;264:5058.

150. Mimuro J, Schleef RR, Luskutoff DJ. Extracellular matrix of cultured bovine aortic endothelial cells contains functionally active type 1 plasminogen activator inhibitor. *Blood* 1987;70:721.

151. Hajjar KA, Gavish D, Breslow JL, et al. Lipoprotein(a) modulation of endothelial cell surface fibrinolysis and its potential role in atherosclerosis. *Nature* 1989;339:303.

152. Miles LA, Fless GM, Levin EG, et al. A potential basis for the thrombotic risks associated with lipoprotein(a). *Nature* 1989;339:301.

153. Daras V, Thienpont M, Stump DC, et al. Measurement of urokinase-type plasminogen activator with an enzyme-linked immunosorbent assay based on three murine monoclonal antibodies. *Thromb Haemost* 1986;56:411.

154. Rijken DC, Juhan-Vague I, DeCock F, et al. Measurement of human tissue-type plasminogen activator by a two-site immunoradiometric assay. *J Lab Clin Med* 1983;101:274.

155. Bergsdorf N, Nilsson T, Wallén P. An ELISA for determination of tissue plasminogen activator applied to patients with thromboembolic disease. *Thromb Haemost* 1983;50:740.

156. Holvoet P, Boes J, Collen D. Measurement of free, one-chain tissue-type plasminogen activator in human plasma with an enzyme-linked immunosorbent assay based on an active site-specific murine monoclonal antibody. *Blood* 1987;69:284.

157. Levin EG, Loskutoff DJ. Regulation of plasminogen activator production by cultured endothelial cells. *Ann N Y Acad Sci* 1982;401:184.

158. Bevilacqua MP, Prober JS, Majeau GR, et al. Recombinant tumor necrosis factor induced procoagulant activity in cultured human vascular endothelium: characterization and comparison with the actions of interleukin. *Proc Natl Acad Sci U S A* 1986;83:4533.

159. Redlitz A, Tan AK, Eaton DL, et al. Plasma carboxypeptidases as regulators of the plasminogen system. *J Clin Invest* 1995;96:2534.

160. Loskutoff DJ. Carboxypeptidases: new regulators of plasminogen activation *in vivo*. *J Clin Invest* 1995;96:2104.

161. Tan AK, Eaton DL. Activation and characterization of carboxypeptidase B from human plasma. *Biochemistry* 1995;34:5811.

162. Bajzar L, Nesheim ME. The effect of activated protein C on fibrinolysis on cell-free plasma can be attributed specifically to attenuation of prothrombin activation. *J Biol Chem* 1993;268:8608.

163. Fredenburgh JC, Nesheim ME. Lys-plasminogen is a significant intermediate in the activation of Glu-plasminogen during fibrinolysis *in vitro*. *J Biol Chem* 1992;267:26150.

164. Bajzar L, Nesheim M, Morser J, et al. Both cellular and soluble forms of thrombomodulin inhibit fibrinolysis by potentiating the activation of thrombin-activable fibrinolysis inhibitor. *J Biol Chem* 1998;273:2792.

165. Hosaka Y, Takahashi Y, Ishii H. Thrombomodulin in human plasma contributes to inhibit fibrinolysis through acceleration of thrombin-dependent activation of plasma procarboxypeptidase B. *Thromb Haemost* 1998; 79:371.

166. Odrljin TM, Rybarczyk BJ, Francis CW, et al. Calcium modulates plasmin cleavage of the fibrinogen D fragment γ chain N-terminus: mapping of monoclonal antibody J88B to plasmin sensitive domain of the γ chain. *Biochim Biophys Acta* 1996;1298:69.

167. Sakharov DV, Plow EF, Rijken DC. On the mechanism of the antifibrinolytic activity of plasma carboxypeptidase B. *J Biol Chem* 1997;272:14477.

168. Collen D, Lijnen R. Basic and clinical aspects of fibrinolysis and thrombolysis. *Blood* 1992;78:23114.

169. Dahlbäck B, Carlsson M, Svensson PJ. Familial thrombophilia due to a previously unrecognized mechanism characterized by poor anticoagulant response to activated protein C: prediction of a cofactor to activated protein C. *Proc Natl Acad Sci U S A* 1993;90:1004.

170. Bertina RM, Koeleman RPC, Koster T, et al. Mutation in blood coagulation factor V associated with resistance to activated protein C. *Nature* 1994;369:64.

171. Bajzar L, Kalafatis M, Simioni P, et al. An antifibrinolytic mechanism describing the prothrombotic effect associated with factor V Leiden. *J Biol Chem* 1996;271:22949.

172. Broze GJ Jr, Higuchi DA. Coagulation-dependent inhibition of fibrinolysis: role of carboxypeptidase-U and the premature lysis of clots from hemophilic patients. *Blood* 1996;88:3815.

173. Valnickova Z, Enghild JJ. Human procarboxypeptidase U, or thrombin-activable fibrinolysis inhibitor, is a substrate for transglutaminases. Evidence for transglutaminase-catalyzed cross-linking to fibrin. *J Biol Chem* 1998;273:27220.

174. Von dem Borne PA, Bajzar L, Meijers JC, et al. Thrombin-mediated activation of factor XI results in a thrombin-activatable fibrinolysis inhibitor-dependent inhibition of fibrinolysis. *J Clin Invest* 1997;99:2323.

175. Kokame K, Zheng X, Sadlerl JE. Activation of thrombin-activable fibrinolysis inhibitor requires epidermal growth factor-like domain 3 of thrombomodulin and is inhibited competitively by protein C. *J Biol Chem* 1995; 273:12135.

176. Carmeliet P, Collen D. Gene targeting and gene transfer studies of the biological role of the plasminogen/plasmin system. *Thromb Haemost* 1995; 74:429.

177. Bugge TH, Kombrinck KW, Flick MJ, et al. Loss of fibrinogen rescues mice from the pleiotropic effects of plasminogen deficiency. *Cell* 1996;87:709.

178. Brodsky SV. Coagulation, fibrinolysis and angiogenesis: new insights from knockout mice. *Exp Nephrol* 2002;10:299.

179. Ploplis VA, Castellino FJ. Gene targeting of components of the fibrinolytic system. *Thromb Haemost* 2002;87:22.

180. Degen JL, Drew AF, Palumbo JS, et al. Genetic manipulation of fibrinogen and fibrinolysis in mice. *Ann N Y Acad Sci* 2001;936:276.

181. Drew AF, Tucker HL, Kombrinck KW, et al. Plasminogen is a critical determinant of vascular remodeling in mice. *Circ Res* 2000;87:133.

182. Carmeliet P, Schoonjans L, Kieckens L, et al. Physiological consequences of loss of plasminogen activator gene function in mice. *Nature* 1994; 368: 419.

183. Dewerchin M, Nuffelen AV, Wallays G, et al. Generation and characterization of urokinase receptor-deficient mice. *J Clin Invest* 1996;97:870.

184. Bugge TH, Flick MJ, Danton MJS, et al. Urokinase plasminogen activator is effective in fibrin clearance in the absence of its receptor or tissue-type plasminogen activator. *Proc Natl Acad Sci U S A* 1996;93:5899.

185. Bugge TH, Flick MJ, Daugherty CC, et al. Plasminogen deficiency causes severe thrombosis but is compatible with development and reproduction. *Genes Dev* 1995;9:794.

186. Ploplis VA, Carmeliet P, Vazizadeh S, et al. Effects of disruption of the plasminogen gene on thrombosis, growth, and health in mice. *Circ Res* 1995; 92:2585.

187. Romer J, Bugge TH, Pyke C, et al. Impaired wound healing in mice with a disrupted plasminogen gene. *Nat Med* 1996;2:287.

188. Carmeliet P, Moons L, Ploplis V, et al. Impaired arterial neointima formation in mice with disruption of the plasminogen gene. *J Clin Invest* 1997; 99:200.

189. Lijnen HR, Moons L, Beelen V, et al. Biological effects of combined inactivation of plasminogen activator and plasminogen activator inhibitor-1 gene function in mice. *Thromb Haemost* 1995;74:1126.

190. Pinsky DJ, Liao H, Lawson CA, et al. Coordinated induction of plasminogen activator inhibitor-1 (PAI-1) and inhibition of plasminogen activator

gene expression by hypoxia promotes pulmonary vascular fibrin deposition. *J Clin Invest* 1998;102:919.

191. Erickson LA, Fici GJ, Lund JE, et al. Development of venous occlusions in mice transgenic for the plasminogen activator inhibitor-1 gene. *Nature* 1990;346:74.

192. Carmeliet P, Stassen JM, Van Vlaenderen I, et al. Adenovirus-mediated transfer of tissue-type plasminogen activator augments thrombolysis in tissue-type plasminogen activator-deficient and plasminogen activator inhibitor-1-overexpressing mice. *Blood* 1997;90:1527.

193. Palabrica TM, Liu AC, Aronovitz MJ, et al. Antifibrinolytic activity of apolipoprotein(a) *in vivo*: human apolipoprotein(a) transgenic mice are resistant to tissue plasminogen activator-mediated thrombolysis. *Nat Med* 1995;1:256.

194. Huang Z-F, Higuchi D, Lasky N, et al. Tissue factor pathway inhibitor gene disruption produces intrauterine lethality in mice. *Blood* 1997;90:944.

195. Chan JCY, Carmeliet P, Moons L, et al. Factor VII deficiency rescues the intrauterine lethality in mice associated with tissue factor pathway inhibitor deficit. *J Clin Invest* 1999;103:475.

196. Jalbert LR, Rosen ED, Moons L, et al. Inactivation of the gene for anticoagulant protein C causes lethal perinatal consumptive coagulopathy in mice. *J Clin Invest* 1998;102:1481.

197. Carmeliet P, Kieckens L, Schoonjans L, et al. Plasminogen activator inhibitor-1 gene-deficient mice. I: Generation by homologous recombination and characterization. *J Clin Invest* 1993;92:2746.

198. Carmeliet P, Stassen JM, Schoonjans L, et al. Plasminogen activator inhibitor-1 gene-deficient mice. II: Effects on hemostasis, thrombosis and thrombolysis. *J Clin Invest* 1993;92:2756.

199. Lijnen HR, Okada K, Matsuo O, et al. Alpha2-antiplasmin gene deficiency in mice is associated with enhanced fibrinolytic potential without overt bleeding. *Blood* 1999;93:2274.

200. Lijnen HR, Carmeliet P, Bouche A, et al. Restoration of thrombolytic potential in plasminogen-deficient mice by bolus administration of plasminogen. *Blood* 1996;88:870.

201. Heckel JL, Sandgren EP, Degen JL, et al. Neonatal bleeding in transgenic mice expressing urokinase-type plasminogen activator. *Cell* 1990;62:447.

202. Nagashima M, Yin ZF, Broze GJ Jr., et al. Thrombin-activatable fibrinolysis inhibitor (TAFI) deficient mice. *Front Biosci* 2002;7:d556.

203. te Velde EA, Wagenaar GT, Reijerkerk A, et al. Impaired healing of cutaneous wounds and colonic anastomoses in mice lacking thrombin-activatable fibrinolysis inhibitor. *J Thromb Haemost* 2003;1:2087.

204. Lisman T, de Groot PG, Joost CM, et al. Reduced plasma fibrinolytic potential is a risk factor for venous thrombosis. *Blood* 2005;105:1102.

205. Meikle AW, Graybill JF. Fibrinolysis and hemorrhage in a fatal case of heat stroke. *N Engl J Med* 1967;276:911.

206. Comp PC, Jacocks RM, Rubenstein C, et al. A lysine-adsorbable plasminogen activator is elevated in conditions associated with increased fibrinolytic activity. *J Lab Clin Med* 1981;97:637.

207. Booth NA, Anderson JA, Bennett B. Plasminogen activators in alcoholic cirrhosis: demonstration of increased tissue-type and urokinase-type activator. *J Clin Pathol* 1984;37:772.

208. Hersch SL, Kunelis T, Francis RB Jr. The pathogenesis of accelerated fibrinolysis in liver cirrhosis: a critical role for tissue plasminogen activator inhibitor. *Blood* 1987;69:1315.

209. Tran-Thang C, Fasel-Felley J, Pralong G, et al. Plasminogen activators and plasminogen activator inhibitors in liver deficiencies caused by chronic alcoholism or infectious hepatitis. *Thromb Haemost* 1989;62:651.

210. Aoki N, Yamanaka T. The alpha-2 plasmin inhibitor levels in liver disease. *Clin Chim Acta* 1978;84:99.

211. Bohmig HJ. The coagulation disorder of orthotopic hepatic transplantation. *Semin Thromb Hemost* 1977;4:57.

212. Illig KA, Green RM, Ouriel K, et al. Primary fibrinolysis during supraceliac aortic clamping. *J Vasc Surg* 1997;25:244.

213. Booth NA, Bennett B, Wijngaards G, et al. A new life-long hemorrhagic disorder due to excess plasminogen activator. *Blood* 1983;61:267.

214. Aznar J, Estellés A, Vila V, et al. Inherited fibrinolytic disorder due to an enhanced plasminogen activator level. *Thromb Haemost* 1984;52:196.

215. Koie E, Kamiya T, Ogata K, et al. $\alpha_2$-plasmin-inhibitor deficiency 7 (Miyasato disease). *Lancet* 1978;2:1334.

216. Aoki N, Saito H, Kamiya T, et al. Congenital deficiency of $\alpha_2$-plasmin inhibitor associated with severe hemorrhagic tendency. *J Clin Invest* 1979;63:877.

217. Kluft C, Vellenga E, Brommer EJP. Homozygous alpha-2-antiplasmin deficiency. *Lancet* 1979;2:206.

218. Miles LA, Plow EF, Donnelly J, et al. A bleeding disorder due to deficiency of alpha-1-antiplasmin. *Blood* 1982;59:1246.

219. Saito H. $\alpha_2$-Plasmin inhibitor and its deficiency states. *J Lab Clin Med* 1988;112:671.

220. Kluft C, Nieuwenhuis HK, Rijken DC, et al. Alpha-2-antiplasmin Enschede: a dysfunctional alpha-2-antiplasmin molecule, associated with an autosomal recessive hemorrhagic disorder. *J Clin Invest* 1987;80:1391.

221. Schleef RR, Higgins DL, Pillemer E, et al. Bleeding diathesis due to decreased functional activity of type 1 plasminogen activator inhibitor. *J Clin Invest* 1989;83:1747.

222. Diéval J, Nguyen G, Gross S, et al. A lifelong bleeding disorder associated with a deficiency of plasminogen activator inhibitor type I. *Blood* 1991;77:528.

223. Astrup T. Tissue activators of plasminogen. *Fed Proc* 1966;25:42.

224. Sack E, Spaet TH, Gentile RL, et al. Reduction of postprostatectomy bleeding by epsilon-aminocaproic acid. *N Engl J Med* 1962;266:541.

225. Vinnicombe J, Shuttleworth KED. Aminocaproic acid in the control of haemorrhage after prostatectomy: a controlled trial. *Lancet* 1966;1:230.

226. Nilsson L, Rybo G. Treatment of menorrhagia with epsilon-aminocaproic acid: a double-blind investigation. *Acta Obstet Gynecol Scand* 1965;44:467.

227. Aoki NB, Moroi M, Sakata Y, et al. Abnormal plasminogen: a hereditary molecular abnormality found in a patient with recurrent thrombosis. *J Clin Invest* 1978;61:1186.

228. Miyata T, Iwanaga S, Sakata Y, et al. Plasminogen Tochigi: inactive plasmin resulting from replacement of alanine-600 by threonine in the active site. *Proc Natl Acad Sci U S A* 1982;79:6132.

229. Miyata T, Iwanaga S, Sakata Y, et al. Plasminogens Tochigi II and Nagoya: two additional molecular defects with Ala-600 Thr replacement found in plasmin light chain variants. *J Biochem* 1984;96:277.

230. Prins MH, Hirsh J. A critical review of the evidence supporting a relationship between impaired fibrinolysis and venous thromboembolism. *Arch Intern Med* 1991;151:1721.

231. Ploplis VA, Carmeliet P, Vazirzadeh S, et al. Effects of disruption of the plasminogen gene on thrombosis, growth, and health in mice. *Circulation* 1995;92:2585.

232. Tait RC, Walker ID, Conkie JA, et al. Isolated familial plasminogen deficiency may not be a risk factor for thrombosis. *Thromb Haemost* 1996;76:1004.

233. Mingers AM, Heimburger N, Zeitler P, et al. Homozygous type I plasminogen deficiency. *Semin Thromb Hemost* 1997;23:259.

234. Schuster V, Mingers AM, Seidenspinner S, et al. Homozygous mutations in the plasminogen gene of two unrelated girls with ligneous conjunctivitis. *Blood* 1997;90:958.

235. Haverkate F, Samama M. Familial dysfibrinogenemia and thrombophilia. Report on a study of the SSC Subcommittee on Fibrinigen. *Thromb Haemost* 1995;73:151.

236. Carrell N, Gabriel DA, Blatt PM, et al. Hereditary dysfibrinogenemia in a patient with thrombotic disease. *Blood* 1983;62:439.

237. Hessel B, Silveira AM, Carlsson K, et al. Fibrinogenemia Tampere—a dysfibrinogenemia with defective gelation and thromboembolic disease. *Thromb Res* 1995;78:323.

238. Soria J, Soria C, Caen JP. A new type of congenital dysfibrinogenaemia with defective fibrin lysis—Dusard syndrome: possible relation to thrombosis. *Br J Haematol* 1983;53:575.

239. Al-Mondhiry HAB, Bilezikian SB, Nossel HL. Fibrinogen "New York"—an abnormal fibrinogen associated with thromboembolism: functional evaluation. *Blood* 1975;45:607.

240. Liu CY, Koehn JA, Morgan FJ. Characterization of fibrinogen New York 1. A dysfunctional fibrinogen with a deletion of B$\beta$ (9-72) corresponding exactly to exon 2 of the gene. *J Biol Chem* 1985;260:4390.

241. Johansson L, Hedner U, Nilsson IM. A family with thromboembolic disease associated with deficient fibrinolytic activity in vessel wall. *Acta Med Scand* 1978;203:477.

242. Jorgensen M, Mortensen JZ, Madsen AG, et al. A family with reduced plasminogen activator activity in blood associated with recurrent venous thrombosis. *Scand J Haematol* 1982;29:217.

243. Stead NW, Bauer KA, Kinney TR, et al. Venous thrombosis in a family with defective release of vascular plasminogen activator and elevated plasma Factor VIII/von Willebrand's factor. *Am J Med* 1983;74:33.

244. Allenby F, Pflug JJ, Boardman L, et al. Effects of external pneumatic intermittent compression on fibrinolysis in man. *Lancet* 1973;2:1412.

245. Tarnay TJ, Rohr PR, Davidson AG, et al. Pneumatic calf compression, fibrinolysis, and the prevention of deep venous thrombosis. *Surgery* 1980;88:489.

246. Comerota AJ, Chouhan V, Harada RN, et al. The fibrinolytic effects of intermittent pneumatic compression: mechanism of enhanced fibrinolysis. *Ann Surg* 1997;226:306.

247. Knight MTN, Dawson R, Melrose DG. Fibrinolytic response to surgery. Labile and stable patterns and their relevance to postoperative deep venous thrombosis. *Lancet* 1977;2:370.

248. Páramo JA, Alfaro MJ, Rocha E. Postoperative changes in the plasmatic level of tissue-type plasminogen activator and its fast-acting inhibitor relationship to deep vein thrombosis and influence of prophylaxis. *Thromb Haemost* 1985;54:713.

249. Eriksson BI, Eriksson E, Gyzander E, et al. Thrombosis after hip replacement. Relationship to the fibrinolytic system. *Acta Orthop Scand* 1989;60:159.

250. Clayton JK, Anderson JA, McNicol GP. Preoperative prediction of postoperative deep vein thrombosis. *BMJ* 1976;2:910.

251. Rakoczi I, Chamone D, Collen D, et al. Prediction of postoperative legvein thrombosis in gynaecological patients. *Lancet* 1978;1:509.

252. Gordon-Smith IC, Hickman JA, Le Quesne LP. Postoperative fibrinolytic activity and deep vein thrombosis. *Br J Surg* 1974;61:213.

253. Bonnar J, McNicol GP, Douglas AS. Coagulation and fibrinolytic mechanisms during and after normal childbirth. *BMJ* 1970;2:200.

254. Walker JE, Gow L, Campbell DM, et al. The inhibition by plasma of urokinase and tissue activator-induced fibrinolysis in pregnancy and the puerperium. *Thromb Haemost* 1983;49:21.

255. Kruithof EKO, Tran-Thang C, Gudinchet A, et al. Fibrinolysis in pregnancy: a study of plasminogen activator inhibitors. *Blood* 1987;69:460.

256. Gore M, Eldon S, Trofatter KF, et al. Pregnancy-induced changes in the fibrinolytic balance: evidence for defective release of tissue plasminogen activator and increased levels of the fast-acting tissue plasminogen activator inhibitor. *Am J Obstet Gynecol* 1987;156:674.

257. Estellés A, Gilabert J, Aznar J, et al. Changes in the plasma levels of type 1 and type 2 plasminogen activator inhibitors in normal pregnancy and in patients with severe preeclampsia. *Blood* 1989;74:1332.

258. Bellart J, Gilabert R, Fontcuberta J, et al. Coagulation and fibrinolytic parameters in normal pregnancy and in pregnancy complicated by intrauterine growth retardation. *Am J Perinatol* 1998;15:81.

259. Gris J, Ripart-Neveu S, Maugard C, et al. Respective evaluation of the prevalence of haemostasis abnormalities in unexplained primary early recurrent miscarriages, The Nimes Obstetricians and Haematologists (NOHA) Study. *Thromb Haemost* 1997;77:1096.

260. Schjetlein R, Haugen G, Wisloff F. Markers of intravascular coagulation and fibrinolysis in preeclampsia: association with intrauterine growth retardation. *Acta Obstet Gynecol Scand* 1997;76:541.

261. Nakashima A, Kobayashi T, Terao T. Fibrinolysis during normal pregnancy and severe preeclampsia relationships between plasma levels of plasminogen activators and inhibitors. *Gynecol Obstet Invest* 1996;42:95.

262. Kanfer A, Bruch JF, Nguyen G, et al. Increased placental antifibrinolytic potential and fibrin deposits in pregnancy-induced hypertension and preeclampsia. *Lab Invest* 1996;74:253.

263. Hamsten A, Wiman B, DeFaire U, et al. Increased plasma levels of a rapid inhibitor of tissue plasminogen activator in young survivors of myocardial infarction. *N Engl J Med* 1985;313:1557.

264. Paramo JA, Colucci M, Collen D, et al. Plasminogen activator inhibitor in the blood of patients with coronary artery disease. *BMJ* 1985;291:573.

265. Hamsten A, Walldius G, Szamosi A, et al. Plasminogen activator inhibitor in plasma: risk factor for recurrent myocardial infarction. *Lancet* 1987;2:3.

266. Ridker PM, Vaughan DE, Stampfer MJ, et al. Endogenous tissue-type plasminogen activator and risk of myocardial infarction. *Lancet* 1993; 341:1165.

267. Juhan-Vague I, Pyke SDM, Alessi MC, et al. Fibrinolytic factors and the risk of myocardial infarction or sudden death in patients with angina pectoris. *Circulation* 1996;94:2057.

268. Thögersen AM, Jansson J-H, Boman K, et al. High plasminogen activator inhibitor and tissue plasminogen activator levels in plasma precede a first acute myocardial infarction in both men and women. Evidence for the fibrinolytic system as an independent primary risk factor. *Circulation* 1998; 98:2241.

269. Juhan-Vague I, Alessi MC. PAI-1, obesity, insulin resistance and risk of cardiovascular events. *Thromb Haemost* 1997;78:656.

270. Smith FB, Lee AJ, Fowkes FG, et al. Hemostatic factors as predictors of ischemic heart disease and stroke in the Edinburgh Artery Study. *Arterioscler Thromb Vasc Biol* 1997;17:3321.

271. Carter AM, Catto AJ, Grant PJ. Determinants of tPA antigen and associations with coronary artery disease and acute cerebrovascular disease. *Thromb Haemost* 1998;80:632.

272. Macko RF, Kittner SJ, Epstein A, et al. Elevated tissue plasminogen activator antigen and stroke risk: the Stroke Prevention in Young Women Study. *Stroke* 1999;30:7.

273. Van der Bom JG, de Knijff P, Haverkate F, et al. Tissue plasminogen activator and risk of myocardial infarction. The Rotterdam Study. *Circulation* 1997;95:2623.

274. Moss AJ, Goldstein RE, Marder VJ, et al. THROMBO Research Group. Thrombogenic factor and recurrent coronary events after myocardial infarction. *Circulation* 1999;99:2517.

275. Ridker PM, Vaughan DE, Stampfer MJ, et al. Baseline fibrinolytic state and the risk of future venous thrombosis. A prospective study of endogenous tissue-type plasminogen activator and plasminogen activator inhibitor. *Circulation* 1992;85:1822.

276. Gray RP, Yudkin JS, Patterson DL. Plasminogen activator inhibitor: a risk factor for myocardial infarction in diabetic patients. *Br Heart J* 1993;69: 228.

277. Ossei-Gerning N, Mansfield MW, Stickland MH, et al. Plasminogen activator inhibitor-1 promoter 4G/5G genotype and plasma levels in relation to a history of myocardial infarction in patients characterized by coronary angiography. *Arterioscler Thromb Vasc Biol* 1997;17:33.

278. Iwai N, Shimoike H, Nakamura Y, et al. The 4G/5G polymorphism of the plasminogen activator inhibitor gene is associated with the time course of progression to acute coronary syndromes. *Atherosclerosis* 1998;136:109.

279. Catto AJ, Carter AM, Stickland M, et al. Plasminogen activator inhibitor-1 (PAI-1) 4G/5G promoter polymorphism and levels in subjects with cerebrovascular disease. *Thromb Haemost* 1997;77:730.

280. Ye S, Green FR, Scarabin PY, et al. The 4G/5G genetic polymorphism in the promoter of the plasminogen activator inhibitor-1 (PAI-1) gene is associated with differences in plasma PAI-1 activity but not with risk of myocardial infarction in the ECTIM study: Etude CasTemoins de l'infarctus du Mycocarde. *Thromb Haemost* 1995;74:837.

281. Ridker PM, Hennekens CH, Lindpaintner K, et al. Arterial and venous thrombosis is not associated with the 4G/5G polymorphism in the promoter of the plasminogen activator inhibitor gene in a large cohort of US men. *Circulation* 1997;95:59.

282. Gralnick HR, Greipp P. Thrombosis with epsilon-aminocaproic acid therapy. *Am J Clin Pathol* 1971;56:151.

283. Naeye RL. Thrombotic state after a hemorrhagic diathesis: a possible complication of therapy with epsilon-aminocaproic acid. *Blood* 1962;19:694.

284. Charytan C, Purtilo D. Glomerular capillary thrombosis and acute renal failure after epsilon-aminocaproic acid therapy. *N Engl J Med* 1969;280: 1102.

285. Engesser L, Brommer EJP, Kluft C, et al. Elevated plasminogen activator inhibitor, a cause of thrombophilia—a study in 203 patients with familial or sporadic venous thrombophilia. *Thromb Haemost* 1989;62:673.

286. Angles CE, Gris JC, Loyau S, et al. Familial association of high levels of histidine-rich glycoprotein and plasminogen activator inhibitor-1 with venous thromboembolism. *J Lab Clin Med* 1993;121:646.

287. Mihalyi E, Weinberg RM, Towne DW, et al. Proteolytic fragmentation of fibrinogen. I: comparison of the fragmentation of human and bovine fibrinogen by trypsin or plasmin. *Biochemistry* 1976;15:5372.

288. Nussenzweig V, Seligmann M, Pelmont U, et al. Les produits de degradation du fibrinogene humain par la plasmine. I: separation et proprietes physicochimiques. *Ann Inst Pasteur* 1961;100:377.

289. Marder VJ, Shulman NR, Carroll WR. The importance of intermediate degradation products of fibrinogen in fibrinolytic hemorrhage. *Trans Assoc Am Physicians* 1967;80:156.

290. Marder VJ, Shulman NR, Carroll WR. High-molecular-weight derivatives of human fibrinogen produced by plasmin. I: Physicochemical and immunological characterization. *J Biol Chem* 1969;244:2111.

291. Marder VJ, Budzynski AZ. The structure of the fibrinogen degradation products. *Prog Hemost Thromb* 1974;2:141.

292. Marder VJ. Identification and purification of fibrinogen degradation products produced by plasmin. Considerations on the structure of fibrinogen. *Scand J Haematol Suppl* 1971;13:21.

293. Marder VJ, Shulman NR. High-molecular-weight derivatives of human fibrinogen produced by plasmin. II: mechanism of their anticoagulant activity. *J Biol Chem* 1969;244:2120.

294. Haverkate F, Timan G. Protective effect of calcium in the plasmin degradation of fibrinogen and fibrin products D. *Thromb Res* 1977;10:803.

295. Nieuwenhuizen W, Vermond A, Haverkate F. Factors influencing the structure of terminal plasmin degradation products of human fibrinogen and fibrin. *Biochim Biophys Acta* 1981;667:321.

296. Dang CV, Ebert RF, Bell WR. Localization of a fibrinogen calcium binding site between $\gamma$ subunit positions 311 and 336 by terbium fluorescence. *J Biol Chem* 1985;260:9713.

297. Furlan M, Beck EA. Plasmic degradation of human fibrinogen. I: structural characterization of degradation products. *Biochim Biophys Acta* 1972; 263:631.

298. Furlan M, Beck EA. Plasmic degradation of human fibrinogen. II: further characterization of Fragment D. *Biochim Biophys Acta* 1973;310:205.

299. Southan C, Thompson E, Panico M, et al. Characterization of peptides cleaved by plasmin from the C-terminal polymerization domain of human fibrinogen. *J Biol Chem* 1985;260:13095.

300. Furlan M, Kemp G, Beck EA. Plasmic degradation of human fibrinogen. III: molecular model of the plasmin-resistant disulfide knot in monomeric fragment D. *Biochim Biophys Acta* 1970;400:95.

301. Olexa SA, Budzynski AZ. Effects of fibrinopeptide cleavage on the plasmic degradation pathways of human crosslinked fibrin. *Biochemistry* 1980; 19:647.

302. Olexa SA, Budzynski AZ. Binding phenomena of isolated unique plasmic degradation products of human crosslinked fibrin. *J Biol Chem* 1979;254: 4925.

303. Dudek GA, Kloczewiak M, Budzynski AZ, et al. Characterization and comparison of macromolecular end products of fibrinogen and fibrin proteolysis by plasmin. *Biochim Biophys Acta* 1970;214:44.

304. Pizzo SV, Schwartz ML, Hill RL, et al. The effect of plasmin on the subunit structure of human fibrin. *J Biol Chem* 1973;248:4574.

305. Francis CW, Marder VJ, Martin SE. Plasmic degradation of crosslinked fibrin. I: Structural analysis of the particulate clot and identification of new macromolecular soluble complexes. *Blood* 1980;56:456.

306. Francis CW, Marder VJ, Barlow GH. Plasmic degradation of crosslinked fibrin: characterization of new macromolecular soluble complexes and a model of their structure. *J Clin Invest* 1980;66:1033.

307. Francis CW, Marder VJ. A molecular model of plasmic degradation of crosslinked fibrin. *Semin Thromb Hemost* 1982;8:25.

308. Kopec M, Teisseyre E, Dudek-Wojciechowska G, et al. Studies on "double D" fragment from stabilized bovine fibrin. *Thromb Res* 1973;2:283.

309. Gaffney PJ, Brasher M. Subunit structure of the plasmin-induced degradation products of crosslinked fibrin. *Biochim Biophys Acta* 1973;295:308.

310. Pizzo SV, Taylor LM Jr, Schwartz ML, et al. Subunit structure of fragment D from fibrinogen and crosslinked fibrin. *J Biol Chem* 1973;248:4584.

311. Hudry-Clergeon G, Paturel L, Suscillon M, et al. Identification d'un complexe (D-D) ... E dans les produits de degradation de la fibrine bovine stabilisee par la. *Pathol Biol (Paris)* 1974;(Suppl. 22):47.

312. Gaffney PJ, Lane DA, Kakkar VV, et al. Characterization of a soluble D dimer-E complex in crosslinked fibrin digests. *Thromb Res* 1975;7:89.

313. Veklich Y, Francis CW, White J, et al. Structural studies of fibrinolysis by electron microscopy. *Blood* 1998;92:4721.

314. Blomback B, Hessel B, Hogg D, et al. A two-step fibrinogen-fibrin transition in blood coagulation. *Nature* 1978;275:501.

315. Olexa SA, Budzynski AZ. Evidence for four different polymerization sites involved in human fibrin formation. *Proc Natl Acad Sci U S A* 1980; 77: 1374.

316. Olexa SA, Budzynski AZ. Localization of a fibrin polymerization site. *J Biol Chem* 1981;256:3544.

317. Reganon E, Vila V, Aznar J. Identification of high-molecular-weight derivatives of plasmic digests of crosslinked human fibrin. *Thromb Haemost* 1978;40:368.

318. Sasaki T, Page IH, Shainoff JR. Soluble complex of fibrinogen and fibrin. *Science* 1966;152:1069.

319. von Hugo R, Hafter R, Stein B, et al. Incorporation of 125I-fibrinogen in circulating soluble fibrin monomer complexes during hypercoagulability. *Thromb Res* 1977;10:703.

320. Jakobsen E, Ly B, Kierulf P. Incorporation of fibrinogen into soluble fibrin complexes. *Thromb Res* 1974;4:499.

321. Williams JE, Hjantgan RR, Hermans J, et al. Characterization of the inhibition of fibrin assembly by fibrinogen fragment D. *Biochem J* 1981;197:661.

322. Alkjaersig N, Fletcher AP. Formation of soluble fibrin oligomers in purified systems and in plasma. *Biochem J* 1983;213:75.

323. Kopec M, Kowalski E, Stachurska J. Studies on paracoagulation: role of antithrombin VI. *Thromb Diath Haemorrh* 1960;5:285.

324. Godal HC, Abildgaard U. Gelation of soluble fibrin in plasma by ethanol. *Scand J Haematol* 1966;3:342.

325. Breen FA Jr, Tullis JL. Ethanol gelation: a rapid screening test for intravascular coagulation. *Ann Intern Med* 1968;69:1197.

326. Niewiarowski S, Gurewich V. Laboratory identification of intravascular coagulation: the serial dilution protamine sulfate test for the detection of fibrin monomer and fibrin degradation products. *J Lab Clin Med* 1971; 77:665.

327. Fletcher AP, Alkjaersig N, O'Brien J, et al. Blood hypercoagulability and thrombosis. *Trans Assoc Am Physicians* 1970;83:159.

328. Vermylen J, Donati MB, Verstraete M. The identification of fibrinogen derivatives in plasma and serum by agarose gel filtration. *Scand J Haematol Suppl* 1972;13:219.

329. Fletcher AP, Alkjaersig NK, Ghani FM, et al. Blood coagulation system pathophysiology in acute myocardial infarction: the influence of anticoagulant treatment on laboratory findings. *J Lab Clin Med* 1979;93:1054.

330. Heene DL, Matthias FR. Adsorption of fibrinogen derivatives on insolubilized fibrinogen and fibrin. *Thromb Res* 1973;2:137.

331. Matthias FR, Reinicke R, Heene DL. Affinity chromatography and quantitation of soluble fibrin from plasma. *Thromb Res* 1977;10:365.

332. Scheefers-Borchel U, Muller-Berghaus G, Fuhge P, et al. Discrimination between fibrin and fibrinogen by a monoclonal antibody against a synthetic peptide. *Proc Natl Acad Sci U S A* 1985;82:7091.

333. Dempfle CE, Doll M, Lill H, et al. Binding of a new monoclonal antibody against N-terminal heptapeptide of fibrin α-chain to fibrin polymerization site 'A': effects of fibrinogen and fibrinogen derivatives, and pretreatment of samples with NaSCN. *Blood Coagul Fibrinolysis* 1993;4:79.

334. Soe G, Jihno I, Inuzuka K, et al. A monoclonal antibody that recognizes a neo-antigen in the E domain of fibrin monomer complexes with fibrinogen or its derivatives: its application to the measurement of soluble fibrin in plasma. *Blood* 1996;88:2109.

335. Wiman B, Radanby M. Determination of soluble fibrin in plasma by a rapid and quantitative spectrophotometric assay. *Thromb Haemost* 1986; 55:189.

336. Bredbacka S, Blombäck M, Wiman B. Soluble fibrin: a predictor for the development and outcome of multiple organ failure. *Am J Hematol* 1994; 46:289.

337. Halvorsen S, Skjonsberg OH, Ruyter R, et al. Comparison of methods for detecting soluble fibrin in plasma, an *in vitro* study. *Thromb Res* 1990; 57:489.

338. McCarron BI, Marader VJ, Francis CW. Reactivity of soluble fibrin assays with plasmic degradation products of fibrin and in patients receiving fibrinolytic therapy. *Thromb Haemost* 1999;82:1722.

339. Bredbacka S, Blombäck M, Wiman B, et al. Laboratory methods for detecting disseminated intravascular coagulation (DIC): new aspects. *Acta Anaesthesiol Scand* 1993;37:125.

340. Wada H, Wakita Y, Nakae T, et al. Increased plasma-soluble fibrin monomer levels in patients with disseminated intravascular coagulation. *Am J Hematol* 1996;51:255.

341. Ginsberg JS, Siragusa S, Douketis J, et al. Evaluation of a soluble fibrin assay in patients with suspected deep vein thrombosis. *Thromb Haemost* 1995;74:833.

342. Vogel G, Dempfle C-E, Spannagl M, et al. The value of quantitative fibrin monomer determination in the early diagnosis of postoperative deep vein thrombosis. *Thromb Res* 1996;81:241.

343. Ginsberg JS, Siragusa S, Douketis J, et al. Evaluation of a soluble fibrin assay in patients with suspected pulmonary embolism. *Thromb Haemost* 1996;75:551.

344. Francis CW, Connaghan DG, Scott WL, et al. Increased plasma concentration of crosslinked fibrin polymers in acute myocardial infarction. *Circulation* 1987;75:1170.

345. Lee LV, Ewald GA, McKenzie CR, et al. The relationship of soluble fibrin and crosslinked fibrin degradation products to the clinical course of myocardial infarction. *Arterioscler Thromb Vasc Biol* 1997;17:628.

346. Terres W, Kümmel P, Sudrow A, et al. Enhanced coagulation activation in troponin T-positive unstable angina pectoris. *Am Heart J* 1998;135:281.

347. Östlund E, Bremme K, Wiman B. Soluble fibrin in plasma as a sign of activated coagulation in patients with pregnancy complications. *Acta Obstet Gynecol Scand* 1998;77:165.

348. Nossel HL, Younger LR, Wilner GD, et al. Radioimmunoassay of human fibrinopeptide A. *Proc Natl Acad Sci U S A* 1971;68:2350.

349. Budzynski AZ, Marder VJ, Sherry S. Reaction of plasmic degradation products of fibrinogen in the radioimmunoassay of human fibrinopeptide A. *Blood* 1975;45:757.

350. Nossel HL, Yudelman I, Canfield RE, et al. Measurement of fibrinopeptide A in human blood. *J Clin Invest* 1974;54:43.

351. Bilezikian SB, Nossel HL, Butler VP Jr, et al. Radioimmunoassay of human fibrinopeptide B and kinetics of fibrinopeptide cleavage by different enzymes. *J Clin Invest* 1975;56:438.

352. Butler VP Jr, Weber DA, Nossel HL, et al. Immunochemical studies of antisera to human fibrinopeptide-B. *Blood* 1982;59:1006.

353. Nossel HL, Wasser J, Kaplan KL, et al. Sequence of fibrinogen proteolysis and platelet release after intrauterine infusion of hypertonic saline. *J Clin Invest* 1979;64:1371.

354. Cronlund M, Hardin J, Burton J, et al. Fibrinopeptide A in plasma of normal subjects and patients with disseminated intravascular coagulation and systemic lupus erythematosus. *J Clin Invest* 1976;58:142.

355. Nossel HL. Radioimmunoassay of fibrinopeptides in relation to intravascular coagulation and thrombosis. *N Engl J Med* 1976;295:428.

356. Chen R, Doolittle RF. γ-γ crosslinking sites in human and bovine fibrin. *Biochemistry* 1971;10:4486.

357. Schwartz ML, Pizzo SV, Hill RI, et al. The effect of fibrin-stabilizing factor on the subunit structure of human fibrin. *J Clin Invest* 1971;50:1506.

358. Ly B, Kierulf P, Jakobsen E. Stabilization of soluble fibrin/fibrinogen complexes by fibrin stabilizing factor. *Thromb Res* 1974;4:509.

359. Nelb GW, Kamykowski GW, Perry JD. Kinetics of ligation of fibrin oligomers. *J Biol Chem* 1980;255:6398.

360. Selmayr E, Mahn I, Muller-Berghaus G. Crosslinking of soluble fibrin and fibrinogen. *Thromb Res* 1985;39:467.

361. Mosher DF. Action of fibrin-stabilizing factor on cold-insoluble globulin and α₂-macroglobulin in clotting plasma. *J Biol Chem* 1976;251:1639.

362. Merskey C, Lalezari P, Johnson AJ. A rapid, simple, sensitive method for measuring fibrinolytic split products in human serum. *Proc Soc Exp Biol Med* 1969;131:871.

363. Marder VJ, Cruz GO, Schumer BR. Evaluation of a new antifibrinogen-coated latex particle agglutination test in the measurement of serum fibrin degradation products. *Thromb Haemost* 1977;37:183.

364. Connaghan DG, Francis CW, Ryan DH, et al. Prevalence and clinical implications of heparin-associated false-positive tests for serum firbin(ogen) degradation products. *Am J Clin Pathol* 1986;86:304.

365. Koppert PW, Kuipers W, Hoegee-de Nobel B. et al. A quantitative enzyme immunoassay for primary fibrinogenolysis products in plasma. *Thromb Haemost* 1987;57:25.

366. Weitz JI, Koehn JA, Canfield RE, et al. Development of a radioimmunoassay for the fibrinogen-derived peptide Bβ1-42. *Blood* 1986;67:1014.

367. Kudryk B, Robinson D, Netre C, et al. Measurement in human blood of fibrinogen/fibrin fragments containing the Bβ 15-42 sequence. *Thromb Res* 1982;25:277.

368. Gaffney PJ, Brasher M, Lord K, et al. Fibrin subunits in venous and arterial thromboembolism. *Cardiovasc Res* 1976;10:421.

369. Francis CW, Markham RE Jr, Marder VJ. Demonstration of in situ fibrin degradation in pathologic thrombi. *Blood* 1984;63:1216.

370. Connaghan DG, Francis CW, Lane DA, et al. Specific identification of fibrin polymers, fibrinogen degradation products, and crosslinked fibrin degradation products in plasma and serum with a new sensitive technique. *Blood* 1985;65:589.

371. Francis CW, Doughney K, Brenner B, et al. Increased immunoreactivity of plasma after fibrinolytic activation in an anti-DD ELISA system. Role of soluble crosslinked fibrin polymers. *Circulation* 1989;79:666.

372. Van De Water L, Carr JM, Aronson D, et al. Analysis of elevated fibrin(ogen) degradation product levels in patients with liver disease. *Blood* 1986;67: 1468.

373. Rylatt DB, Blake AS, Cottis LE, et al. An immunoassay for human D-dimer using monoclonal antibodies. *Thromb Res* 1983;31:767.

374. Whitaker AN, Elms MJ, Masci PP, et al. Measurement of crosslinked fibrin derivatives in plasma: an immunoassay using monoclonal antibodies. *J Clin Pathol* 1984;37:882.

375. Brenner B, Francis CW, Marder VJ. The role of soluble crosslinked fibrin in D dimer immunoreactivity of plasmic digests. *J Lab Clin Med* 1989; 113:682.

376. Koppert PW, Koopman J, Haverkate F, et al. Production and characterization of a monoclonal antibody reactive with a specific neoantigenic determinant (comprising Bβ 54-118) in degradation products of fibrin and fibrinogen. *Blood* 1986;68:437.

377. Koopman J, Haverkate F, Koppert PW, et al. New enzyme immunoassay of fibrin-fibrinogen degradation products in plasma using a monoclonal antibody. *J Lab Clin Med* 1987;109:75.

378. Gaffney PJ, Creighton LJ, Perry MJ, et al. Monoclonal antibodies to crosslinked fibrin degradation products, II: Further evaluation in a variety of clinical states. *Br J Haematol* 1988;68:91.

379. Carr JM, McKinney M, McDonagh J. Diagnosis of disseminated intravascular coagulation. Role of D-dimer. *Am J Clin Pathol* 1989;91:280.

380. Wilde JT, Kitchen S, Kinsey S, et al. Plasma D-dimer levels and their relationship to serum fibrinogen/fibrin degradation products in hypercoagulable states. *Br J Haematol* 1989;71:65.

381. Prisco D, Paniccia R, Bonechi F, et al. Evaluation of new methods for the selective measurement of fibrin and fibrinogen degradation products. *Thromb Res* 1989;56:547.

382. Bounameaux H, de Moerloose P, Perrier A, et al. Plasma measurement of D-dimer as diagnostic aid in suspected venous thromboembolism: an overview. *Thromb Haemost* 1994;71:1.

383. Brill-Edwards E, Lee A. D-dimer testing in the diagnosis of acute venous thromboembolism. *Thromb Haemost* 1999;82:688.

384. Greenberg CS, Devine DV, McCrae KM. Measurement of plasma fibrin D-dimer levels with the use of a monoclonal antibody coupled to latex beads. *Am J Clin Pathol* 1987;87:94.

385. Owen J, Friedman KD, Grossman BA, et al. Quantitation of fragment X formation during thrombolytic therapy with streptokinase and tissue plasminogen activator. *J Clin Invest* 1987;79:1642.

386. Eisenberg PR, Sobel BE, Jaffe AS. Characterization *in vivo* of the fibrin specificity of activators of the fibrinolytic system. *Circulation* 1988;78:592.

387. Vaughan DE, Goldhaber SZ, Kim H, et al. Recombinant tissue plasminogen activator in patients with pulmonary embolism: correlation of fibrinolytic specificity and efficacy. *Circulation* 1987;75:1200.

388. Faivre R, Mirshahi M, Ducellier D, et al. Evolution of plasma specific fibrin degradation products during thrombolytic therapy in patients with thromboembolism. *Thromb Res* 1988;50:583.

389. Lew AS, Berberian L, Cercek B, et al. Elevated serum D-dimer: a degradation product of crosslinked fibrin (XDP) after intravenous streptokinase during acute myocardial infarction. *J Am Coll Cardiol* 1986;7:1320.

390. Eisenberg PR, Sherman LA, Tiefenbrunn AJ, et al. Sustained fibrinolysis after administration of t-PA despite its short half-life in the circulation. *Thromb Haemost* 1987;57:35.

391. Francis CW, Connaghan DG, Marder VJ. Assessment of fibrin degradation products during fibrinolytic therapy for acute myocardial infarction. *Circulation* 1986;74:1027.

392. Brenner B, Francis CW, Totterman S, et al. Quantitation of venous clot lysis with the D-dimer immunoassay during fibrinolytic therapy requires correction for soluble fibrin degradation products. *Circulation* 1990;81:1818.

393. Koppert PW, Hoegee-de Nobel E. A monoclonal antibody-based enzyme immunoassay for fibrin degradation products in plasma. *Thromb Haemost* 1988;59:310.

394. Declerck PJ, Mombaerts P, Holvoet P, et al. Fibrinolytic response and fibrin fragment D-dimer levels in patients with deep vein thrombosis. *Thromb Haemost* 1987;58:1024.

395. Rowbotham BJ, Carroll P, Whitaker AN, et al. Measurement of crosslinked fibrin derivatives—use in the diagnosis of venous thrombosis. *Thromb Haemost* 1987;57:59.

396. Mirshahi M, Soria C, Soria J, et al. Changes in plasma fibrin degradation products as a marker of thrombus evolution in patients with deep vein thrombosis. *Thromb Res* 1988;51:295.

397. Goldhaber SZ, Vaughan DE, Tumeh SS, et al. Utility of crosslinked fibrin degradation products in the diagnosis of pulmonary embolism. *Am Heart J* 1988;116:505.

398. Tardy B, Tardy-Poncet B, Viallon A, et al. Evaluation of D-dimer ELISA test in elderly patients with suspected pulmonary embolism. *Thromb Haemost* 1998;79:38.

399. Freyburger G, Trillaud H, Labrouche S, et al. D-dimer strategy in thrombosis exclusion. A gold standard study in 100 patients suspected of deep venous thrombosis or pulmonary embolism: 8 DD methods compared. *Thromb Haemost* 1998;79:32.

400. Bounameaux H, Perrier A, Wells PS. Cinical and laboratory diagnosis of deep vein thrombosis: new cost-effective strategies. *Semin Vasc Med* 2001;1:39.

401. Gosselin RC, Owings JT, Kehoe J, et al. Comparison of six D-dimer methods in patients suspected of deep vein thrombosis. *Blood Coagul Fibrinolysis* 2003;14:545.

402. Stein PD, Hull RD, Patel KC, et al. D-dimer for the exclusion of acute venous thrombosis and pulmonary embolism: a systematic review. *Ann Intern Med* 2004;140:589.

403. Bates SM, Kearon C, Crowther M, et al. A diagnostic strategy involving a quantitative latex D-dimer assay reliably excludes deep venous thrombosis. *Ann Intern Med* 2003;138:787.

404. Siragusa S, Anastasio R, Porta C, et al. Deferment of objective assessment of deep vein thrombosis and pulmonary embolism without increased risk of thrombosis: a practical approach based on the pretest clinical model, D-dimer testing, and the use of low-molecular-weight heparins. *Arch Intern Med* 2004;164:2477.

405. Rathbun SW, Whitsett TL, Raskob GE. Negative D-dimer result to exclude recurrent deep venous thrombosis: a management trial. *Ann Intern Med* 2004;141:839.

406. ten Wolde M, Kraaijenhagen RA, Prins MH, et al. The clinical usefulness of D-dimer testing in cancer patients with suspected deep venous thrombosis. *Arch Intern Med* 2002;162:1880.

407. Heim SW, Schectman JM, Siadaty MS, et al. D-dimer testing for deep venous thrombosis: a metaanalysis. *Clin Chem* 2004;50:1136.

408. Wahl WL, Ahrns KS, Zajkowski PJ, et al. Normal D-dimer levels do not exclude thrombotic complications in trauma patients. *Surgery* 2003;134:529.

409. Crowther MA, Cook DJ, Griffith LE, et al. Neither baseline tests of molecular hypercoagulability nor D-dimer levels predict deep venous thrombosis in critically ill medical-surgical patients. *Intensive Care Med* 2005;31:48.

410. Meythaler JM, Fisher WS, Rue LW, et al. Screening for venous thromboembolism in traumatic brain injury: limitations of D-dimer assay. *Arch Phys Med Rehabil* 2003;84:285.

411. Arnesen H, Dahl OE, Aspelin T, et al. Sustained prothrombotic profile after hip replacement surgery: the influence of prolonged prophylaxis with dalteparin. *J Thromb Haemost* 2003;1:971.

# CHAPTER 24 ■ OVERVIEW OF PLATELET STRUCTURE AND FUNCTION

JAMES N. GEORGE AND ROBERT W. COLMAN

Platelets have a unique origin, being fragments of megakaryocyte cytoplasm, yet they contain many structural, metabolic, and signaling components of nucleated cells. Because platelets participate in many physiologic functions and because of their accessibility, they have been models for advances in cell biology. Platelets have been important for the initial discovery of actin in nonmuscle cells (1), the initial description of the structure of the integrin family of receptors (2) and their role in disease (3), the initial description of the structure and function of the selectin family of receptors (4), and the discovery of protease-activated receptors (5). Platelets are essential for normal hemostasis (6) and are also important contributors to thrombotic disorders (7). Understanding their role in thrombosis has led to important therapies for cardiovascular disease (8–10).

## PLATELET PRODUCTION

The development of megakaryocytes and the production of platelets are unique phenomena. Megakaryocyte maturation is endomitotic, with repeated cycles of nuclear duplication without cell division until a modal DNA level of 16N or greater is reached. This process results in giant cells, 40 to 50 $\mu$m in diameter, with vast cytoplasm. Cytoplasmic organelles become organized into domains representing nascent platelets, demarcated by a network of invaginated membrane channels derived from the plasma membrane (11). Megakaryocytes develop within the marrow hematopoietic extravascular compartment, in which they are localized along the albuminal face of the sinusoidal endothelium, frequently in clusters (12). This position facilitates the exit of segments of cytoplasm, termed *proplatelets*, into the circulation (13). The final fragmentation of megakaryocyte cytoplasm into individual platelets has similarities to apoptosis (14) and perhaps results from the shear forces of circulating blood in the pulmonary circulation (15). The liberation of new, individual platelets from the pseudopods of megakaryocyte cytoplasm is facilitated by alignment of the demarcation membranes, dilatation of their channels, and microtubule reorganization (13,16).

Thrombopoietin is the dominant cytokine regulating both megakaryocyte proliferation and differentiation (17). But multiple cytokines and hormones, including interleukin (IL)-3, IL-6, IL-11, and stem cell factor, also participate (17,18). Hematopoietic lineage-specific transcription factors, GATA-1 (19), Tal-1 (20), p45-NF-E2 (21), RUNX1 (22), and the Ets family of transcription factors (23) are required for megakaryocyte growth and platelet development. Mice genetically deficient in c-mpl (the thrombopoietin receptor) (24), GATA-1 (19), or p45-NF-E2 (21) are profoundly thrombocytopenic. However, maintenance of circulating platelet levels that are 5% to 15% of normal in these mice is consistent with the activity of multiple cytokines and transcription factors regulating platelet production (17–23).

## PLATELET STRUCTURE

The ultrastructure of inactivated and activated platelets is shown in Figure 24-1. The process of activation, triggered by diverse soluble agonists, such as thrombin and adenosine diphosphate (ADP), or insoluble vessel wall matrix proteins, such as collagen or von Willebrand factor (VWF), results in dramatic reorganization of the platelet membrane, cytoskeleton, and cytoplasm organelles. These three components of platelet structure are considered separately.

### Platelet Membranes

Although circulating platelets maintain a compact disc shape, their surrounding plasma membrane is complex. Invaginated channels, termed the *surface-connected canalicular system*, form a membrane network throughout the interior of the platelet, providing an enormous expansion of available surface area. Further expansion of the plasma membrane occurs with fusion of $\alpha$-granule membranes with the plasma membrane during activation and secretion. A distinct internal membrane system is the dense tubular system, derived from megakaryocyte endoplasmic reticulum. The dense tubular system concentrates a storage pool of calcium, analogous to sarcoplasmic reticulum of muscle, and is the site of prostaglandin synthesis (25).

Receptor glycoproteins (GPs) are anchored in the plasma membrane, both on the platelet surface and within the open canalicular system, as well as on the $\alpha$-granule membranes. The location of these receptors is dynamic on platelet activation—GP IIb/IIIa is translocated from within the platelet to the surface, whereas GP Ib/IX/V is withdrawn from the surface into the interior. Table 24-1 provides a summary of the structural and functional features of these two principal platelet membrane GPs.

GP IIb/IIIa is a member of the integrin family of membrane receptors, named so because the integrins integrate extracellular ligands with the intracellular cytoskeleton (26). In the integrin nomenclature, GP IIb is the $\alpha_{IIb}$ subunit, and GP IIIa is the $\beta_3$ subunit. GP IIb synthesis is restricted to megakaryocytes and platelets; GP IIIa synthesis also occurs in endothelial cells and in many other cells as the $\beta_3$ subunit of the vitronectin receptor. GP IIb/IIIa is the most abundant GP on the cell surface membrane; it is also abundant on platelet $\alpha$-granule membranes. Therefore, the surface density of functional GP IIb/IIIa receptors can increase by 30% to 50% after activation and secretion, from approximately 40,000 available molecules per platelet to approximately 80,000 (27). Active shuttling of GP IIb/IIIa between the cell surface and $\alpha$-granules is the proposed mechanism for $\alpha$-granule acquisition of fibrinogen (28,29). GP IIb/IIIb in resting platelets has low affinity for fibrinogen and other soluble ligands. Platelet activation results in inside-out signaling, from the cytoplasmic domain of

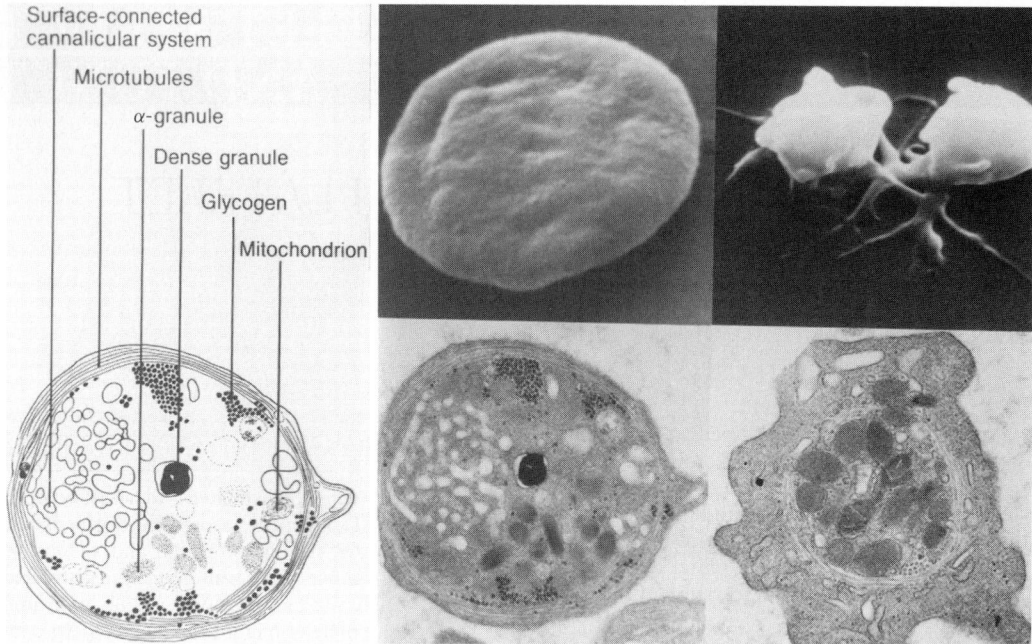

**FIGURE 24-1.** Electron micrograph of resting and activated platelets. The **top** photographs are scanning electron micrographs demonstrating the disc shape of normal circulating platelets (**left**, magnification ×20,000) and the more spherical form of activated platelets with many long pseudopodia (**right**, magnification ×10,000). The **bottom left** photograph is a transmission electron micrograph of the cross section of a resting platelet (magnification ×21,000) with a matched drawing (**far left**) labeling the normal subcellular structures. In the **bottom right** photograph (magnification ×30,000) of an activated platelet, the constriction of the microtubular ring around the centralized granules and the formation of pseudopodia can be seen. (Electron micrographs courtesy James G. White, M.D., and Marcy Krumwiede, University of Minnesota; remaining from George JN. Hemostasis and fibrinolysis. In: Stein JH. *Internal medicine*, 5th ed. Mosby: St. Louis, 1998:534–540, with permission.)

## TABLE 24-1

### STRUCTURE AND FUNCTION OF THE MAJOR PLATELET MEMBRANE GLYCOPROTEIN RECEPTORS, GP IIB/IIIA AND GP IB/IX/V

|  | GP IIb/IIIa | GP Ib/IX/V |
|---|---|---|
| Structure | Integrin family of receptors with two trans-membrane subunits; covalent heterodimer of αIIb (GP IIb) and β3 (GP IIIa) required for cell surface expression | Four transmembrane subunits (Ibα, Ibβ, IX, V), each a member of the leucine-rich repeat superfamily; covalent heterodimer of Ibα-Ibβ, and 1:1 noncovalent association of Ib with IX required for cell surface expression; noncovalent 2:1 association of Ib/IX with V |
| Synthesis | IIb: chromosome 17, megakaryocyte-specific IIIa: chromosome 17, many cell types | All principally expressed in megakaryocytes; limited expression in endothelium<br>Ibα: chromosome 17<br>Ibβ: chromosome 22<br>IX: chromosome 3<br>V: chromosome 3 |
| Location and density | Surface plasma membrane, surface-connected canalicular system and, α-granule membrane; surface density increases from 40,000 to 80,000 molecules/platelet with activation | Surface plasma membrane; surface density decreases with activation by translocation to surface-connected canalicular system; GP Ib/IX: 25,000 molecules/platelet; GP V: 12,500 molecules/platelet |
| Ligands | Principally fibrinogen; also fibrin, VWF, fibronectin, vitronectin, thrombospondin; receptor function requires platelet activation | Principally VWF; constitutive receptor function for matrix-bound VWF |
| Mutations with loss of function | Glanzmann thrombasthenia | Bernard-Soulier syndrome |
| Mutations with gain of function | None | Platelet-type von Willebrand disease |
| Antithrombotic agents | Fibrinogen-receptor antagonists | None |

GP, glycoprotein; VWF, von Willebrand factor.

GP IIb/IIIa to its extracellular ligand recognition sites, causing a conformational change that markedly enhances ligand binding affinity (30). The major ligand for GP IIb/IIIa is fibrinogen, a principal mediator of platelet aggregation (31), but GP IIb/IIIa also can bind fibrin, VWF, fibronectin, vitronectin, and thrombospondin. These proteins also can bind to other platelet receptors. This feature of multiple ligands binding to one receptor and each ligand being able to bind to multiple receptors provides a redundancy that protects patients with congenital defects from continual, severe bleeding (32).

GP Ib/IX/V is a complex of four gene products; the complex is a covalent heterodimer of Iba-Ibb and is in noncovalent association with GP IX and GP V. There are approximately 12,000 copies of GP Ib/IX/V on the platelet surface, each with two copies of GP Ib/IX associated with a single copy of GP V (33). In contrast to GP IIb/IIIa, GP Ib/IX/V exists principally on the platelet surface with negligible concentration on internal and α-granule membranes. Also in contrast to GP IIb/IIIa, the surface concentration of GP Ib/IX/V decreases during platelet activation with translocation into the surface-connected canalicular system (34,35). GP Ib/IX/V is the principal platelet receptor for VWF; therefore, it is principally responsible for platelet adhesion to subendothelium as the initial event of hemostasis (36). GP Ib/IX/V binding of VWF is also involved in platelet aggregation, both directly (31) and by activation of GP IIb/IIIa (37). GP Ib/IX/V, unlike GP IIb/IIIa, has greater specificity for VWF as a ligand; its interactions with other ligands are less important.

## Platelet Cytoskeleton

Platelet disc shape is maintained by a circumferential coil of microtubules (38). During activation (Fig. 24-1), the microtubule coil constricts, allowing the platelet to become spherical and directing movement of the secretory granules toward the cell center, where they are close to membrane channels leading to the surface.

Platelet disc shape also is maintained by a membrane cytoskeleton composed of actin, spectrin, and associated proteins located immediately underneath the plasma membrane. The cytoskeleton further serves to anchor the cytoplasmic portion of transmembrane receptor proteins and to transmit signals from the platelet interior to the ligand receptor sites on the plasma surface (inside-out signaling).

Most of the platelet actin and cytoskeletal-associated proteins and filaments are distributed throughout the platelet cytoplasm. No ordered structure is apparent because most of the actin is soluble rather than assembled into filaments, but these cytoskeletal proteins are assumed to direct the traffic of organelles, proteins, and intracellular signaling molecules. These proteins, particularly actin and myosin, also are rapidly assembled into microfilaments on platelet activation, providing the contractile force for the dramatic shape change and pseudopod formation (Fig. 24-1).

## Platelet Granules

α-Granules are the principal platelet secretory granules and are also the most numerous and prominent platelet organelles. Their ultrastructure is characteristic (Fig. 24-1) (39). A dense nucleoid region contains proteoglycans and the associated platelet-specific basic proteins, platelet factor 4 and β-thromboglobulin. A lighter zone contains tubular structures that are high-molecular-weight multimers of VWF. A zone between these regions contains fibrinogen, albumin, and, presumably, other acquired proteins.

The variety of proteins contained within granules is vast and includes many proteins, such as fibrinogen and VWF, that are essential components for the platelet-mediated initial reactions of hemostasis. α-Granule proteins are acquired by several mechanisms (28): (i) endogenous synthesis (e.g., VWF and platelet factor 4), (ii) receptor-mediated endocytosis (e.g., fibrinogen) (29), and (iii) fluid-phase pinocytosis (e.g., albumin and IgG, for which the platelet concentration mirrors the plasma concentration) (28).

The number of dense granules in the platelets is less than the number of α-granules, but they are readily recognizable by their dense core surrounded by a clear halo (Fig. 24-1). Dense granules are the storage and secretory organelles for small molecules—serotonin, nonmetabolic ADP and adenosine triphosphate (ATP), catecholamines, $Ca^{2+}$, and $Mg^{2+}$—rather than for proteins. However, similar to α-granules, their contents are important components for platelet hemostatic function.

Lysosomes are few, and their function is unclear because there is not the requirement for catabolism as in more metabolically active cells. It is assumed that secreted lysosomal enzymes have a role in digestion of clot and vessel matrix components as part of wound healing.

## PLATELET FUNCTION

Platelets provide for the initial arrest of bleeding and, with small wounds, can provide definitive hemostasis. This is apparent from the experience of patients with hemophilia, who have no excessive bleeding from small cuts but a delayed onset of prolonged and potentially severe bleeding from larger wounds. With larger wounds, the platelet aggregate is not sufficiently stable without fibrin stabilization.

The complementary role of platelets and coagulation in hemostasis is well illustrated by the bleeding time. Bleeding times are prolonged in patients with severe thrombocytopenia or platelet function disorders, but they are normal, or almost normal, in patients with hemophilia. Aspirin, which causes partial impairment of platelet function, causes a modest increase of the bleeding time in some healthy subjects. However, after patients with severe hemophilia were given aspirin, the combination of impaired platelet function and deficient fibrin formation caused extremely prolonged bleeding even from these small wounds; several patients ultimately required factor VIII infusions to stop the bleeding (40).

Initial platelet adhesion to exposed subendothelial tissue is primarily mediated by collagen and VWF. Platelet GP Ia/IIa and GP VI are receptors for collagen (41), and GP Ib/IX/V is the constitutively active receptor for VWF. These membrane proteins act in concert because VWF reactivity with platelets is enhanced by its binding to collagen. Platelet adhesion initiates the reactions of platelet shape change, secretion, and activation of GP IIb/IIIa ligand-binding sites. These reactions result in the formation of platelet–platelet interactions, leading to the formation of the hemostatic platelet aggregate. Platelet aggregate formation requires the synergistic interaction of both major platelet receptors, GP IIb/IIIa and GP Ib/IX/V, and both of their principal ligands, fibrinogen and VWF (31).

## PLATELET RECEPTORS FOR SMALL AGONISTS AND ANTAGONISTS

Activation of GP IIb/IIIa ligand binding sites also is achieved through signaling by a number of agonists that bind to G protein–coupled seven-transmembrane receptors (STRs). Some of these small molecules come from the platelet itself: serotonin, which stimulates platelets through a 5-HT-2 subtype of serotonin receptor (42); thromboxane $A_2$, the product of cyclooxygenase-catalyzed synthesis that binds to a specific thromboxane receptor (43); and ADP, which is released from the dense granules and binds principally to two receptors, P2Y$_1$ and P2Y$_{12}$ (44). Other agonists for STRs are hormones released from other tissues, including epinephrine, which binds to platelet $\alpha_2$-adrenergic receptors (45), and vasopressin, arising from the posterior pituitary gland. Finally, thrombin uniquely activates its STR by cleaving it to allow a new N-terminal peptide to bind to a more C-terminal portion of the receptor (5,46). Most of these agonists mainly cause activation of GP IIb/IIIa, but thrombin can directly cause platelet secretion. One must also consider the receptors for inhibitory agonists such as prostacyclin (PGI$_2$), prostaglandin E$_2$, and prostaglandin D$_2$. There are at least four families of receptors with multiple isotypes (47). All are STRs, and most act by stimulating adenylate cyclase through coupling to Gs. Because PGI$_2$ is a major inhibitor derived from activated endothelial cells and prostaglandin D$_2$ is synthesized in platelets, all of these receptors operate to modulate platelet activation.

## PLATELET INTRACELLULAR SIGNALING

The heterodimer G proteins, which are coupled to STRs (48), are frequently but not always the inhibitors of cell signaling. One of the earliest responses dependent on G proteins is the activation of PLC-$\beta$ (49). This enzyme is responsible for phosphoinositol hydrolysis yielding diacylglycerol, which activates protein kinase C, leading to protein phosphorylation, granule secretion, and fibrinogen receptor expression (50). The other product of hydrolysis by PLC is inositol-phosphate, which binds to dense tubule receptors to release sequential Ca$^{2+}$ (51). A kinase that phosphorylates phosphatidylinositol in the D-3 portion of the inositol ring (PI3K) is important in regulating activation of the integrin $\alpha_{IIb}\beta_3$ (52).

The second major pathway, in addition to phosphatidylinositol hydrolysis, is the eicosanoid pathway, initiated by phospholipase A$_2$, which reduces arachidonate from membrane phospholipids (53). Arachidonate release is the rate-limiting step for synthesis of prostanoids and leukotrienes.

An increase in intracellular calcium is a constant accompaniment of platelet activation and is mediated by IP3. A variety of enzymes involved in platelet signaling require Ca$^{2+}$, including PLA$_2$, PLC, and myosin light chain kinase. In addition, potent proteases, calpains I and II, are activated and digest cytoskeleton proteins (54) and translocate PLC.

## CONGENITAL DISORDERS OF PLATELET FUNCTION

Defective platelet function or thrombocytopenia must be severe for clinically important bleeding to occur, and even with severe abnormalities, bleeding may be intermittent and unpredictable. For example, the congenital absence of GP IIb/IIIa in Glanzmann thrombasthenia has a profound effect on the laboratory assessment of platelet function, yet these patients may have only intermittent and minor bleeding (32). The normal platelet number, 150,000 to 350,000 per $\mu$L, far exceeds the number that is essential for hemostasis; spontaneous major bleeding does not occur until the platelet count is less than 10,000 per $\mu$L, and even then it is uncommon. Hereditary disorders of common platelet membrane receptors such as Glanzmann thrombasthenia and Bernard-Soulier syndrome (32) are rare, as are abnormalities of platelet granules such as storage pool deficiency.

Primary secretion defects, as a group, are a common but mild disorder and are extremely heterogeneous. They are best conceptualized as defects in the signal transduction pathway, which comprises receptors, G proteins, and intracellular effectors. Receptor defects have been documented for thromboxane A$_2$ receptors (55) and collagen receptors, including GP Ia/IIa (56) and GP VI (57). A defect in one of the ADP receptors, P2Y$_{12}$ (58), has also been reported as the cause of a mild hemorrhagic disorder. Defects have been reported in arachidonate liberation secondary to defective Ca$^{2+}$ mobilization, leading to decreased phospholipase A$_2$ levels. Cyclooxygenase deficiency has been reported and may be due to a quantitative or qualitative abnormality in the enzyme. Finally, the defect in Wiskott-Aldrich syndrome has been identified as a mutation in WASP, a gene on the X chromosome whose product regulates cytoskeletal function (59).

## ACQUIRED PLATELET FUNCTION DEFECTS

Acquired platelet function defects secondary to drugs are mild and ubiquitous, considering, for example, the number of individuals who take aspirin regularly and who therefore have impaired platelet function caused by irreversible inhibition of cyclooxygenase-dependent thromboxane formation. In addition to aspirin, more than 100 other medications, food, spices, and vitamins have been reported to impair platelet function (60). For almost all agents, the data are limited to descriptions of abnormal *in vitro* platelet aggregation tests or a prolonged bleeding time, which may have no clinical importance. The low risk for major bleeding in patients with hereditary and acquired disorders of platelet function has been exploited in the use of aspirin, thienopyridines, and platelet GP IIb/IIIa blockers as antithrombotic agents.

Other than pharmacologic agents, certain pathologic conditions are also frequently associated with platelet dysfunction and clinical bleeding. These conditions include the myeloproliferative disorders, in which abnormal platelets are produced (61); uremia, in which small toxic compounds such as guanidinosuccinic acid accumulate in the plasma; and cardiopulmonary bypass, in which platelets are exposed to artificial surfaces, resulting in activation and depletion of granula contents and antibodies. Both hemorrhage and thrombosis have been reported in myeloproliferative disorders, with a wide range of clinical laboratory abnormalities. Dysproteinemias are associated with qualitative platelet defects.

## PHARMACOLOGIC INHIBITION OF PLATELET FUNCTION TO PREVENT THROMBOSIS

With the demonstration that aspirin is effective in the primary prevention of myocardial infarction (8), it has become a standard treatment for patients with cardiovascular and cerebrovascular diseases. However, the use of angioplasty and stent placement to open obstructed coronary arteries has required more effective antithrombotic agents to prevent restenosis. Clopidogrel, which blocks the platelet ADP receptor, is a standard agent for patients with coronary artery stents, and ticlopidine has demonstrated greater efficacy than aspirin for prevention of recurrent stroke (9). The most effective antithrombotic agents for coronary artery disease are drugs that block the platelet fibrinogen receptor GP IIb/IIIa (10).

### References

1. Bettex-Galland M, Luscher EF. Thrombosthenin—a contractile protein from thrombocytes. Its extraction from human blood platelets and some of its properties. *Biochim Biophys Acta* 1961;49:536.

2. Kunicki TJ, Pidard D, Rosa JP, et al. The formation of calcium-dependent complexes of platelet membrane glycoproteins IIb and IIIa in solution as determined by crossed immunoelectrophoresis. *Blood* 1981;58:268–276.

3. Nurden AT, Caen JP. An abnormal platelet glycoprotein pattern in three cases of Glanzmann's thrombasthenia. *Br J Haematol* 1974;28:253–260.

4. McEver RP. Selectins: novel receptors that mediate leukocyte adhesion during inflammation. *Thromb Haemost* 1991;65:223–228.

5. Coughlin SR. Thrombin signalling and protease-activated receptors. *Nature* 2000;407:258–264.

6. George JN. Platelets. *Lancet* 2000;355:1531–1539.

7. Ruggeri ZM. Platelets in atherothrombosis. *Nat Med* 2002;8:1227–1234.

8. Steering Committee of the Physicians' Health Study Research Group. Final report of the aspirin component of the ongoing Physicians' Health Study. *N Engl J Med* 1989;321:129–135.

9. Sharis PJ, Cannon CP, Loscalzo J. The antiplatelet effects of ticlopidine and clopidogrel. *Ann Intern Med* 1998;129:394–405.

10. Topol EJ, Byzova TV, Plow EF. Platelet GP IIb-IIIa blockers. *Lancet* 1999; 353:227–231.

11. Behnke O. An electron microscope study of megakaryocytes of rat bone marrow. I. The development of the demarcation membrane system and the platelet surface coat. *J Ultrastruct Res* 1968;24:412–433.

12. Lichtman MA, Chamberlain JK, Simon W, et al. Parasinusoidal location of megakaryocytes in marrow: a determinant of platelet release. *Am J Hematol* 1978;4:303–312.

13. Cramer EM, Norol F, Guichard J, et al. Ultrastructure of platelet formation by human megakaryocytes cultured with the Mpl ligand. *Blood* 1997;89: 2336–2346.

14. De Botten S, Sabri S, Daugas E, et al. Platelet formation is the consequence of caspase activation within megakaryocytes. *Blood* 2003;100:1310–1317.

15. Behnke O, Forer A. From megakaryocytes to platelets: platelet morphogenesis takes place in the bloodstream. *Eur J Haematol* 1998;60:3–23.

16. Hartwig JH, Italiano J. The birth of the platelet. *J Thromb Haemost* 2003;1: 1580–1586.

17. Kaushansky K. Thrombopoietin. *N Engl J Med* 1998;339:746–754.

18. Norol F, Vitrat N, Cramer E, et al. Effects of cytokines on platelet production from blood and marrow CD34+ cells. *Blood* 1998;91:830–843.

19. Shivdasani RA, Fujiwara Y, McDevit M, et al. A lineage-selective knockout establishes the critical role of transcription factor GATA-1 in megakaryocyte growth and platelet development. *EMBO J* 1997;16:3965–3973.

20. Mikkola HK, Klintman J, Yang H, et al. Haematopoietic stem cells retain long-term repopulating activity and multipotency in the absence of stem-cell leukemia SCL/Tal-1 gene. *Nature* 2003;421:547–551.

21. Levin J, Peng J, Baker GR, et al. Pathophysiology of thrombocytopenia and anemia in mice lacking transcription factor NF-E2. *Blood* 1999;94: 3037–3047.

22. Ichikawa M, Asai T, Saito T, et al. AML-1 is required for megakaryocytic maturation and lymphocytic differentiation, but not for maintenance of hematopoietic stem cells in adult hematopoiesis. *Nat Med* 2004;10: 299–304.

23. Hart A, Melet F, Grossfeld P, et al. Fli-1 is required for murine vascular and megakaryocytic development and is hemizygously deleted in patients with thrombocytopenia. *Immunity* 2000;13:167–177.

24. Gurney AL, Carver-Moore K, De Sauvage FJ, et al. Thrombocytopenia in c-*mpl*-deficient mice. *Science* 1994;265:1445–1447.

25. Gerrard JM, White JG, Rao GH. Localization of platelet prostaglandin production in the platelet dense tubular system. *Am J Pathol* 1976;83:283–298.

26. Hynes RO. Integrins: bidirectional, allosteric signaling machines. *Cell* 2002; 110:673–687.

27. Wagner CL, Mascelli MA, Neblock DS, et al. Analysis of GP IIb/IIIa receptor number by quantification of 7E3 binding to human platelets. *Blood* 1996;88:907–914.

28. George JN. Platelet immunoglobulin G: Its significance for the evaluation of thrombocytopenia and for understanding the origin of alpha-granule proteins. *Blood* 1990;76(5):859–870.

29. Handagama P, Scarborough RM, Shuman MA, et al. Endocytosis of fibrinogen into megakaryocyte and platelet α-granules is mediated by $\alpha_{IIb}\beta_3$ (glycoprotein IIb-IIIa). *Blood* 1993;82:135–138.

30. Shattil SJ, Kashiwagi H, Pampori N. Integrin signaling: the platelet paradigm. *Blood* 1998;91:2645–2657.

31. Ruggeri ZM, Dent JA, Saldivar E. Contribution of distinct adhesive interactions to platelet aggregation in flowing blood. *Blood* 1999;94:172–178.

32. George JN, Caen JP, Nurden AT. Glanzmann's thrombasthenia: the spectrum of clinical disease. *Blood* 1990;75:1383–1395.

33. Lopez JA, Andrews RK, Afshar-Kharghan V, et al. Bernard-Soulier syndrome. *Blood* 1998;91:4397–4418.

34. Hourdille P, Heilmann E, Combrié R, et al. Thrombin induces a rapid redistribution of glycoprotein Ib-IX complexes within the membrane systems of activated human platelets. *Blood* 1990;76:1503–1513.

35. Cramer EM, Lu H, Caen JP, et al. Differential redistribution of platelet glycoproteins Ib and IIb-IIIa after plasmin stimulation. *Blood* 1991;77: 694–699.

36. Savage B, Sixma JJ, Ruggeri ZM. Functional self-association of von Willebrand factor during platelet adhesion under flow. *Proc Natl Acad Sci U S A* 2002;99:425–430.

37. Kasirer-Friede A, Cozzi MR, Mazzuczto M, et al. Signaling through GP Ib-IX-V activates alphaIIb-beta3 independently of other receptors. *Blood* 2004;103:3403–3411.

38. White JG, Rao GH. Microtubule coils versus the surface membrane cytoskeleton in maintenance and restoration of platelet discoid shape. *Am J Pathol* 1998;152:597–609.

39. Harrison P, Cramer EM. Platelet α-granules. *Blood Rev* 1993;7:52–62.

40. Kaneshiro MM, Mielke CH Jr, Kasper CK, et al. Bleeding time after aspirin in disorders of intrinsic clotting. *N Engl J Med* 1969;281:1039–1042.

41. Nieswandt B, Watson SP. Platelet-collagen interaction: is GP VI the central receptor? *Blood* 2003;102:449–461.

42. Julius D, Huang KN, Livelli TJ, et al. The 5HT2 receptor defines a family of structurally distinct but functionally conserved serotonin receptors. *Proc Natl Acad Sci U S A* 1990;87:928–932.

43. Hirata M, Hayashi Y, Shikubi F, et al. Cloning and expression of cDNA for a human thromboxane A2 receptor. *Nature* 1991;349:617–620.

44. Jin J, Quinton TM, Zhang J, et al. Adenosine diphosphate (ADP)-induced thromboxane A2 generation in human platelets requires coordinated signaling through integrin alpha(IIb)beta(3) and ADP receptors. *Blood* 2002; 99:193–198.

45. Regan JW, Nakata H, DeMarinis RM, et al. Purification and characterization of the human platelet alpha 2-adrenergic receptor. *J Biol Chem* 1986; 261:3894–3900.

46. Vu TK, Hung DT, Wheaton VI, et al. Molecular cloning of a functional thrombin receptor reveals a novel proteolytic mechanism of receptor activation. *Cell* 1991;64:1057–1068.

47. Coleman RA, Smith WL, Narumiya S. International union of pharmacology classification of prostanoid receptors: properties, distribution, and structure of the receptors and their subtypes. *Pharmacol Rev* 1994;46:205–229.

48. Hamm HE. How activated receptors couple to G proteins. *Proc Natl Acad Sci U S A* 2001;98:4819–4821.

49. Cockcroft S, Thomas GM. Inositol-lipid specific phospholipase C isoenzymes and their differential regulation by receptors. *Biochem J* 1992;288: 1–14.

50. Shattil SJ, Brass LF. Induction of the fibrinogen receptor on human platelets by intracellular mediators. *J Biol Chem* 1987;262:992–1000.

51. Brass LF, Joseph SK. A role for inositol triphosphate in intracellular Ca2+ mobilization and granule secretion in platelets. *J Biol Chem* 1985;260: 15172–15179.

52. Kucera GL, Rittenhouse SE. Human platelets form 3-phosphorylated phosphoinositides in response to alpha-thrombin, U46619, or GTP gamma S. *J Biol Chem* 1990;265:5345–5348.

53. Leslie CC. Properties and regulation of cytosolic phospholipase A2. *J Biol Chem* 1997;272:16709–16712.

54. Tsujinaka T, Sakon M, Kambayashi J, et al. Cleavage of cytoskeletal proteins by two forms of Ca2+ activated neutral proteases in human platelets. *Thromb Res* 1982;28:149–156.

55. Hirata T, Kakizuka A, Ushikubi F, et al. Arg60 to Leu mutation of the human thromboxane A2 receptor in a dominantly inherited bleeding disorder. *J Clin Invest* 1994;94:1662–1667.

56. Nieuwenhuis HK, Sakariassen KS, Houdijk WPM, et al. Deficiency of platelet membrane glycoprotein Ia associated with a decreased platelet adhesion to subendothelium: a defect in platelet spreading. *Blood* 1986;68: 692–695.

57. Moroi M, Jung SM, Okuma M, et al. A patient with platelets deficient in glycoprotein VI that lack both collagen-induced aggregation and adhesion. *J Clin Invest* 1989;84:1440–1445.

58. Cattaneo M, Zighetti ML, Lombardi R, et al. Molecular bases of defective signal transduction in the platelet P2Y12 recpetor of a patient with congenital bleeding. *Proc Natl Acad Sci U S A* 2003;100:1978–1983.

59. Zhu QL, Watanabe C, Liu T, et al. Wiskott-Aldrich syndrome/X-linked thrombocytopenia: WASP gene mutations, protein expression, and phenotype. *Blood* 1997;90:2680–2689.

60. George JN, Shattil SJ. The clinical importance of acquired abnormalities of platelet function. *N Engl J Med* 1991;324:27–39.

61. Schafer AI. Bleeding and thrombosis in the myeloproliferative disorders. *Blood* 1984;64:1–12.

# CHAPTER 25 ■ PLATELET PRODUCTION: CELLULAR AND MOLECULAR REGULATION

ELISABETH M. CRAMER AND WILLIAM VAINCHENKER

Platelets are derived from the cytoplasm fragmentation of giant bone marrow cells, the megakaryocytes (MK; they are the largest cells of the marrow—up to 35 $\mu$m), which are characterized by a single polylobulated nucleus and represent less than 0.05% of marrow cells. MK arise and mature in the bone marrow along with the other blood cell precursors (e.g., granulocytes and erythroblasts). Given the normal platelet count (i.e., 150 to $400 \times 10^9$ per L) and platelet life time (i.e., 10 days), an average of $15 \times 10^{10}$ platelets must be produced every day to maintain blood platelet level.

MK are unique cells in the human body in that they display a single polyploid nucleus and grow by undergoing an unparalleled phenomenon called *endomitosis*, during which the nucleus multiplies its deoxyribonucleic acid (DNA) content without dividing, and the cytoplasmic mass grows and develops considerably, proportional to and under the control of the ploidy classes. After achieving the full maturation state, MK deform and their internal membrane system spreads out to form long extensions. Platelets eventually detach and are shed in the peripheral blood from the tips of the extensions as well as from their length. Although their large size causes them to appear prominent, MK are actually relatively rare in normal bone marrow. MK study is difficult because bone marrow samples are required and because of the general low number of these cells (i.e., <1% of marrow cells), but scientific advances and techniques have helped to improve our understanding of MK maturation and platelet formation. The development of *in vitro* MK culture systems, which is the study of specific and early markers that made possible the immunologic detection of MK and their precursors that were not recognizable by classical light microscopy, has made MK study much more feasible by making possible the isolation and purification of those cells. Finally, the identification, purification, and cloning of thrombopoietin (TPO), a specific regulator of platelet production, and the availability of its recombinant form for experimental purposes have facilitated the preparation of large enriched populations of MK. In this chapter we focus on the cellular and molecular aspects of MK differentiation with the exception of TPO and its receptor: c-mpl.

## MICROENVIRONMENT AND MEGAKARYOCYTE LOCALIZATION IN THE BONE MARROW

Normal human MK are located primarily in the bone marrow. They are often gathered into small groups, usually up to three, which consist of different cells of various size, ploidy, and maturation stages. They are often located in proximity to a vascular sinusoid (1) (see Fig. 25-1). This is important because MK and endothelial cells cross-talk by many potential pathways:

MK express mitogenic factors for endothelial cells, for example, vascular endothelial growth factor (VEGF) (2,3), whereas endothelial cells express receptors and adhesion molecules that can potentially retain MK close to the bloodstream where future platelets could be shed (4). Their accumulation near the sinusoids represents a potential physical barrier for other marrow cells migrating into the circulation. However, foreign cells are able to penetrate the MK through the open channels of the demarcation membranes and transmigrate across the entire volume of MK without any serious damage to either cell. This natural phenomenon, termed "emperipolesis," is occasionally observed within normal bone marrow but is distinct from phagocytosis (5). Nevertheless, in pathologic conditions, for example, myeloproliferative syndromes with myelofibrosis, the frequency of emperipolesis is not only increased but also becomes pathogenic to both cell types with disastrous consequences to the immediate cellular environment (6). In animal species such as mice and rats, but not humans, maturing MK are distributed equally in the bone marrow and the spleen, and to a lesser extent in the liver (7). In addition, MK are observed within the pulmonary circulation of both human and animals.

Remarkably, mature bone marrow MK are extremely deformable and not only can adhere to the sinusoidal endothelial barrier but can also transmigrate across the barrier to enter the circulation. The first capillary bed that the MK encounter is the pulmonary microcirculation in which they can be easily entrapped. Intact, fully mature, large MK have definitely been recovered in the lung circulation, and large MK naked nuclei can be found downstream from the lungs, in the aorta (8). These observations, which implicate the lung as a major site of platelet production, are discussed in detail in the section, "Platelet Shedding" in this chapter.

## CELLULAR ASPECTS OF MEGAKAROCYTOPOIESIS

### Megakaryocytic Cells

MK differentiation is a branch of hematopoietic cell lineage. Platelet production derives from the differentiation of a multipotent hematopoietic stem cell (HSC) into MK. HSCs are the only long-life cells of the hematopoietic system and are capable of regenerating all the hematopoietic tissue by their self-renewal capacities. HSCs commit to MK differentiation and in the meantime lose self-renewal capacities and multipotent properties. These committed cells are called *hematopoietic* progenitors. The loss of potential appears through precise developmental stages. In a first step, the HSC gives rise to a common myeloid progenitor and a common lymphoid progenitor. The common myeloid progenitors subsequently commit toward specific lineages. However, the erythroid and MK lineage derive from a

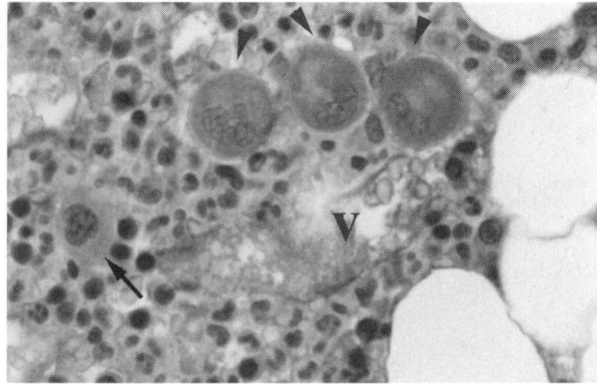

**A**

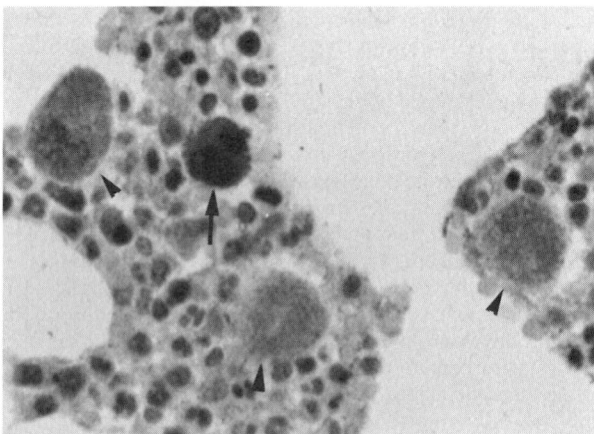

**B**

FIGURE 25-1. Human normal bone marrow biopsy immunostained for fibrinogen (**A**) and von Willebrand factor (VWF) (**B**) by the alkaline phosphatase–anti-alkaline phosphatase (APAAP) technique. **A:** Megakaryocytes (MK) are frequently located along a vascular sinusoid (*V*). Fibrinogen displays a centrifugal staining pattern typical of an α-granule protein endocytosed from the extracellular medium. The staining intensity is weak in the small immature MK (*arrow*) even as it is maximal in large, mature MK (*arrowheads*). **B:** VWF displays a centripetal staining pattern (*arrowheads*) with a stronger expression in the paranuclear region in large, mature MK. The staining intensity is maximal in the small MK (*arrow*).

common progenitor called either *E/MK* progenitor or BFU-E/MK (9–11). This bipotent progenitor has been characterized both in mouse and in humans and gives rise to colonies containing mostly erythroblasts and a few MK. The phenotype of this progenitor has been clearly assessed in the mouse, whereas in humans it has the same phenotype as other primitive progenitors (CD34$^+$ CD38$^{low}$).

The MK lineage becomes restricted to MK at the subsequent developmental stage where the progenitor is only committed toward the MK lineage. The subsequent differentiation stages are divided into three main developmental stages. The MK progenitor cells are capable of proliferation and of giving rise *in vitro* to MK colonies. MK progenitor cell further differentiates through a variable number of mitoses to a transitional cell [promegakaryoblast (PMKB)] that enters an endomitotic process with an average of three DNA cycles of duplication (modal ploidy of 16N). These cells correspond to MK that have begun to synthesize the main platelet proteins and are already morphologically identifiable. The cytoplasm maturation subsequently accelerates to yield a typical MK. Finally, the

mature MK sheds platelets in the circulation outside the marrow territory itself.

## Megakaryocytic Progenitors

Several clonal assays have made it possible to distinguish three main types of MK progenitors (12). This hierarchical classification of MK progenitors is essentially based on their proliferative capacities: The bigger the colony size or the longer the period required for the colonies to develop, the more primitive the progenitor. However, other criteria may also be important, such as ploidy of MK composing an individual colony (13,14), physical properties of MK progenitors, and immunologic phenotype of these progenitors (see subsequent text).

**BFU-MK.** BFU-MK are the most primitive MK-committed progenitors, which produce colonies composed of more than 50 cells organized into subcolonies. BFU-MK follow the same model as BFU-E–derived colonies: They mature in 12 days in mice (15) and in 21 days in humans (16). These progenitors are found both in the bone marrow and less frequently in the blood.

**CFU-MK.** CFU-MK progenitor cells differ from the BFU-MK by lower capacities of proliferation: They give rise to colonies comprising three to 50 cells in 5 days in mice (10,17) and in 12 days in humans (9,18). Unlike BFU-MK that are in the G0/G1 phase of the cell cycle, CFU-MK have a high $^3$H-thymidine suicide rate and are destroyed by chemical agents such as 5-fluorouracil. BFU-MK and CFU-MK are also found in fetal tissues, especially in fetal and neonatal blood (19,20).

**Low Density CFU-MK (LD-CFU-MK).** LD-CFU-MK have been identified in the mouse as an MK progenitor with a density less than 1,050 mg per mL. In 2 to 3 days, they give rise to colonies composed of a few MK with a high ploidy (21). The developmental stage of these last progenitors is extremely close to that of the transitional cell, which has switched toward an endomitotic process. The use of differentiation markers has allowed more precise delineation of the compartments of MK progenitors and transitional cells.

## Megakaryocyte Diploid Precursors

As the size of a diploid precursor is that of a small lymphocyte, with no characteristic morphologic features, it can be identified as such only because of the presence of specific immunologic markers on its surface (22). Electron microscopy is also a sensitive tool that can cytochemically detect the presence of platelet peroxidase (23). This enzymatic activity, which reflects the capacity of the cell to synthesize prostaglandins (24), is characteristic for this cell line. Platelet peroxidase was first demonstrated in certain leukemia cells, where it was remarkable both for its chemical properties and subcellular distribution. This enzymatic activity is labile and is quite sensitive to fixation; it is present in the perinuclear cistern and the lumen of the endoplasmic reticulum (ER) and is absent from the Golgi complex (except for an occasional cistern) and secretion granules. It persists during all stages of maturation of the MK lineage (see Fig. 25-2A). Its presence has been further demonstrated in early erythroid precursors, but the cytochemical activity is generally less pronounced than in MK precursors and soon disappears with maturation.

## Megakaryocytes

**Classification of Megakaryocyte Maturation Stages.** MK differentiation is a continuous process, but for the sake of clarity it has been classified into three distinct maturation stages (see Fig. 25-3) (25). Megakaryocytic differentiation

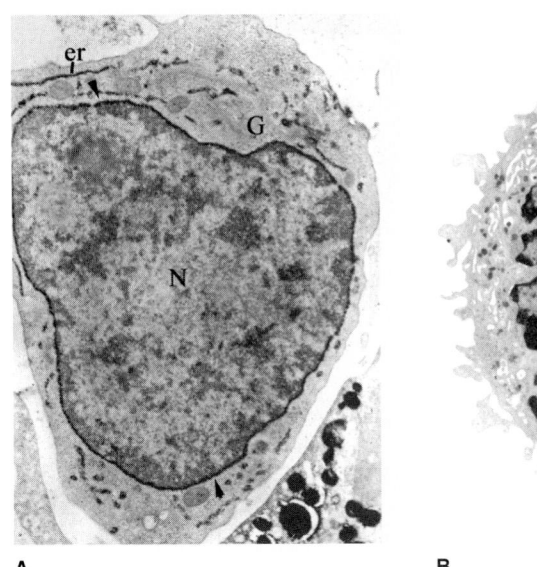
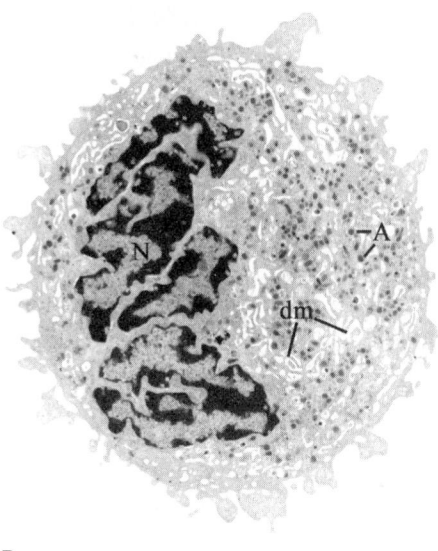

**FIGURE 25-2. A:** The diploid megakaryocyte (MK) precursor lacks distinctive morphologic features but can be identified on the basis of its content of peroxidase activity, which is revealed by a cytochemical reaction that opacifies structures in which it is contained: the perinuclear cisternae (*arrowheads*) and endoplasmic reticulum (*er*). Golgi complex (*G*) (apart from an occasional cisternae) and the rare secretion granules are consistently negative N, nucleus; (magnification ×10,000). **B:** Mature MK is characterized by its large size and multilobed nucleus. It contains specific organelles [i.e., numerous α-granules (*A*)] and a well-developed demarcation membrane system (*dm*) regularly scattered throughout the cytoplasm. This system is formed by invagination of the plasma membrane; it develops rapidly and is the precursor of the platelet membrane system (i.e., plasma membrane and surface-connected canalicular system) (magnification ×5,940).

becomes morphologically identifiable as such after the nuclear ploidy becomes a multiple of 2N. The type I stage immature MK (Fig. 25-3A) has a basophilic cytoplasm and can be distinguished from the diploid hemoblast only because of its large polyploid nucleus, frequent cytoplasm blebs, and relatively large cell volume (i.e., >14 μm in diameter). At this stage, no additional cell division occurs, and the cells undergo only endomitosis. The nuclear to cytoplasm ratio (N/C) is high, the chromatin is thin, and the cytoplasm is basophilic and without azurophilic granules. The type II MK of intermediate maturation (Fig. 25-3B) is larger (i.e., 15 to 40 μm), with a polylobulated nucleus and a cytoplasm that is deep blue because of the richness in ribonucleic acid (RNA). This intense basophilia coincides with the high number of free ribosomes in the cytoplasm and a well-developed rough ER, attesting to the active protein synthesis. Sometimes, an azurophilic area is visible near the cell center where granule formation begins. As the cell matures, the N/C ratio decreases and the amount of cytoplasm dramatically increases and becomes azurophilic, whereas the nuclear lobes become more distinct and the chromatin condenses. The mature MK type III (Fig. 25-3C) has a low N/C ratio. The nucleus is dark purple, with a dense chromatin texture and clearly distinct nuclear lobes. The cytoplasm is vast and is uniformly granular and azurophilic. At this stage, the MK is ready to fragment and liberate its platelets. It has been estimated that each MK can produce from 400 to 8,000 platelets (26).

### Cytoplasm Differentiation.

*Demarcation membrane system.* During the maturation process, the demarcation membrane system (DMS), a network of smooth membrane channels, is formed and is located initially near the plasma membrane. These channels derive from multiple invaginations of the MK plasma membrane (27) (Fig. 25-2B). The DMSs are always in contact with the extracellular medium, as demonstrated by the penetration of electron dense tracers, such as horseradish peroxidase. This membrane system grows rapidly and becomes widespread within the whole cytoplasm volume, expanding by more than 700% within 72 hours. Although some differences between the protein components of the two membrane systems have

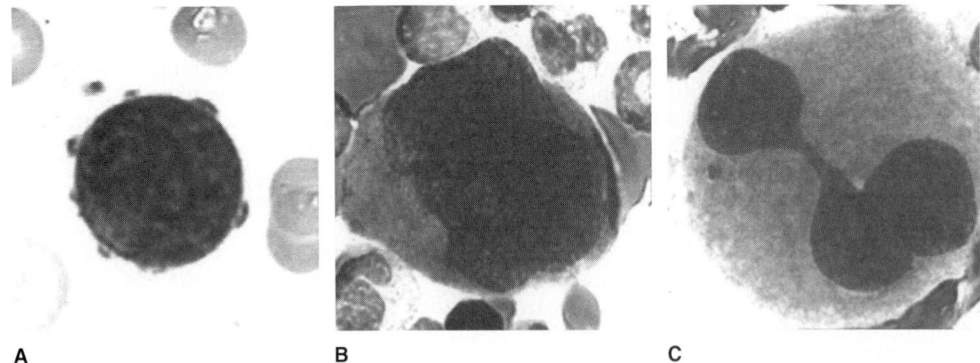

**FIGURE 25-3.** Light microscopic appearance of the three different maturation stages of megakaryocytes (MK) from a bone marrow smear stained by the Romanovski technique. **A:** Immature MK or megakaryoblast (type I): The relatively large size of this otherwise poorly differentiated hemoblast [high nucleus/cytoplasm (N/C) ratio, thin chromatin, and basophilic cytoplasm] allows it to be assigned to the MK lineage. **B:** MK of intermediate maturation (type II): This stage is characterized by large size, convoluted polyploid large nucleus, which is surrounded by a uniformly basophilic cytoplasm; some azurophilic granules appear toward the cell center. **C:** Mature MK (type III): In this stage, the MK appears as a large cell with a polylobulated nucleus and a uniformly granular and azurophilic cytoplasm.

been pointed out by freeze fracture studies (28), the main platelet surface (glycoprotein) GP receptors expressed on the plasma membrane are found equally on DMS (29).

The role of the DMS is clearly related to the delimitation of future platelet territories, and several theories concerning the mechanism of platelet shedding are described in the section, "Platelet Shedding" in this chapter.

*Golgi complexes and centrioles.* Several Golgi complexes within a single MK appear to follow the migration of centrioles. The localization of centrioles within the cell is at random, as are the Golgi complexes. The latter are found more frequently near the cell center, however, in the paranuclear region. Their number would, therefore, be proportional to ploidy. Proteins stored in the granules, which are endogenously synthesized by MK, can be immunodetected initially in the trans-Golgi network (TGN), where they undergo glycosylation, concentration, and precipitation. Proteins endocytosed from the extracellular medium are not immunodetected in the TGN (30). Membrane GPs also transit through the Golgi complex. It is noteworthy that the immunolabeling for the GP Ib/IX/V complex is weak, whereas GP IIb/IIIa and P selectin, which are major components of the α-granule membrane, are more prominently seen (31).

*Endoplasmic reticulum.* Rough ER and free ribosomes are abundant in immature MK and are responsible for the intense basophilia observed with panoptic dyes. The smooth ER that derives from the rough ER after loss of ribosomes remains abundant until the end of the maturation process, and is closely associated with the DMS. It contains some enzymes, including NADH–cytochrome $c$ reductase, cyclooxygenase, thromboxane synthase, and $Ca^{2+}$ $Mg^{2+}$ adenosine triphosphatase (ATPase). In humans, platelet peroxidase cytochemical activity is located in the ER and reflects the content of cyclooxygenase, an early marker of the cell line (Fig. 25-1A), the presence of which demonstrates that the ER gives rise to the dense tubular system of platelets (23). In rodents, acetylcholinesterase (AchE), a marker absent from mature human MK, is also specifically located in the ER.

*Formation and packaging of cytoplasm granules.* Four different types of platelet storage granules are formed during MK maturation: α-granules, dense granules, lysosomes, and peroxisomes. Their content is detailed in Table 25-1; the following sections focus on their mechanism of formation.

**α-Granules.** α-Granules appear early during MK maturation, concomitantly with the initial development of demarcation membranes (32). They arise from the TGN, where a dark nucleoid is rapidly visible within the budding vesicles. α-Granules are unique organelles in that they acquire their protein content by two distinct mechanisms: (a) biosynthesis, predominantly taking place in the MK (33,34); and (b) endocytosis of plasma proteins, either receptor-mediated or through a fluid phase (35,36), that occurs in both MK and platelets (37–39). The cytoplasmic markers are initially immunodetected in a diffuse staining pattern when located in the cisterns of synthesis and later in a granular pattern when packaged in granules. Two interesting types of information are provided by immunolabeling observations of α-granules proteins: Endocytosed proteins (e.g., fibrinogen and immunoglobulins) appear later in the MK than endogenously synthesized proteins [e.g., von Willebrand factor (VWF)] (30), and their distribution patterns within the maturing MK cytoplasm are distinct (i.e., centrifugal and maximal at the cell periphery for the former but centripetal and predominant in the juxtanuclear area for the latter) (40). VWF multimers are apparent in the form of 20-nm tubular structures, first appearing in the TGN and in the α-granules (41). As detailed in the section, "Platelet Shedding," the α-granule membrane contains numerous receptors that

## TABLE 25-1

### α-GRANULE PROTEINS

| Matrix | Membrane |
|---|---|
| **PRESENT IN PLASMA** | α-**GRANULE MEMBRANE** |
| (Endocytosed) | **RESTRICTED** |
| Fibrinogen | P selectin |
| Albumin | GMP33 |
| Fibronectin | Osteonectin |
| IgG, IgA, IgM | |
| (MK synthesized) | α-**GRANULE MEMBRANE** |
| VWF | **AND PLASMA MEMBRANE** |
| Coagulation factor V | GP IIb/IIIa (alphaIIb/beta3) |
| Thrombospondin | GP IV |
| | CD9 |
| **ABSENT FROM PLASMA** | PECAM1 |
| (Platelet specific) | GP Ib/IX/V |
| Multimerin | rap1b |
| β-Thromboglobulin | |
| Platelet factor 4 | |
| PDGF | |
| EGF | |
| TGF-β | |
| VEGF/VPF | |

Ig, immunoglobulin; MK, megakaryocyte; VWF, von Willebrand factor; PDGF, platelet-derived growth factor; EGF, endothelial growth factor; TGF-β, transforming growth factor-β; GP, glycoprotein; PECAM1, Platelet/endothelial cell adhesion molecule-1; VEGF/VPF, vascular endothelial growth factor/vascular permeability factor.

appear during MK maturation: P selectin, GP IIb/IIIa, CD36, CD9, and PE CAM1 (31,42). Some are detectable in the Golgi apparatus and seem to be transported directly to α-granules, but many seem to transit by the plasma membrane and are subsequently internalized. Evidence based on intracellular trafficking suggests that GP IIb/IIIa present in the α-granule originates directly from the internalized plasma membrane pool (43). Multivesicular bodies, present in MK and only occasionally in platelets, have been identified as a sorting compartment, intermediately between TGN and α-granules and dense granules (44,45). Evidently, and in contrast to numerous secretory cells such as endothelial cells, virtually no constitutive secretion occurs in MK and the quasi-totality of secretion proteins follow the regulated pathway and are packaged within secretory granules (46).

*Dense granules.* Dense granules are the final marker of cytoplasm maturation at the ultrastructural level (47). Indeed, they acquire their dense appearance quite late, but their limiting membrane and intrinsic receptors (48) are probably formed earlier. They arise from TGN, and their components are sorted from the α-granule components in multivesicular bodies (45).

*Lysosomes and peroxisomes.* Lysosomes and peroxisomes can be detected cytochemically within maturing MK because of their specific enzymatic content, acid hydrolases (49), and catalase, respectively.

**Nucleus.** The nucleus displays several sparse rounded lobes with abundant euchromatin and conspicuous nucleoli (type I) (Fig. 25-1A). Its maturation is characterized by constant size increase and segmentation and by chromatin clumping (type II) (Fig. 25-1B). Although the number of nuclear lobes is not strictly equivalent to ploidy, it is proportional to ploidy. Through a unique process known as *endomitosis*, nuclear lobulation and ploidy are increased without any division, with the

DNA duplicating until a level ranging from 4N to 64N (rarely 128N) is reached (see section, "The Endomitotic Process"). The first study on the number of nuclear lobes was performed on squash preparations. The study demonstrated this number always to be a multiple of two, the most common form being the 8-lobed cell, one fourth with 4 lobes, and one fourth with 16 lobes. This pattern reflects the ploidy measurements made by later analysis of DNA content. Finally, the nucleus has terminated its growth after the main events of the synthesis of cytoplasm organelles have occurred. Close to the final maturation stage of MK, the nucleus changes texture and aspect (type III). The nuclear lobes tend to elongate and gather, the chromatin becomes coarser, and long clefts of cytoplasm extend between each lobe. The structural changes of nucleus shape and chromatin texture announce the start of proplatelet formation and platelet shedding steps. Because constitutive formation of the proplatelet-bearing MK was recently reported to be caspase

dependent, involving mitochondrial release of cytochrome *c*, a known proapoptogenic factor, it is therefore tempting to correlate the ultrastructural nuclear changes to an apoptotic event. In immunologic thrombocytopenic purpura (ITP), unusual aspects of MK chromatin have been described as paraapoptotic (50).

**Megakaryocyte Activation.** In the presence of appropriate agonists, such as adenosine diphosphate (ADP) and thrombin, MK, like platelets, react by striking morphologic changes (see Fig. 25-4). The plasma membrane becomes bristled and emits numerous and thin pseudopods, the nucleus becomes eccentric, and the cytoplasm organelles become centralized and surrounded by a dense meshwork of microtubules and microfilaments. The cisterns of DMS widen, and secretion granules fuse with the membrane of the DMS, into the lumen of which they discharge their contents (51). This phenomenon, which leads to inappropriate secretion of granule contents, including growth factors, might be implicated in pathologic

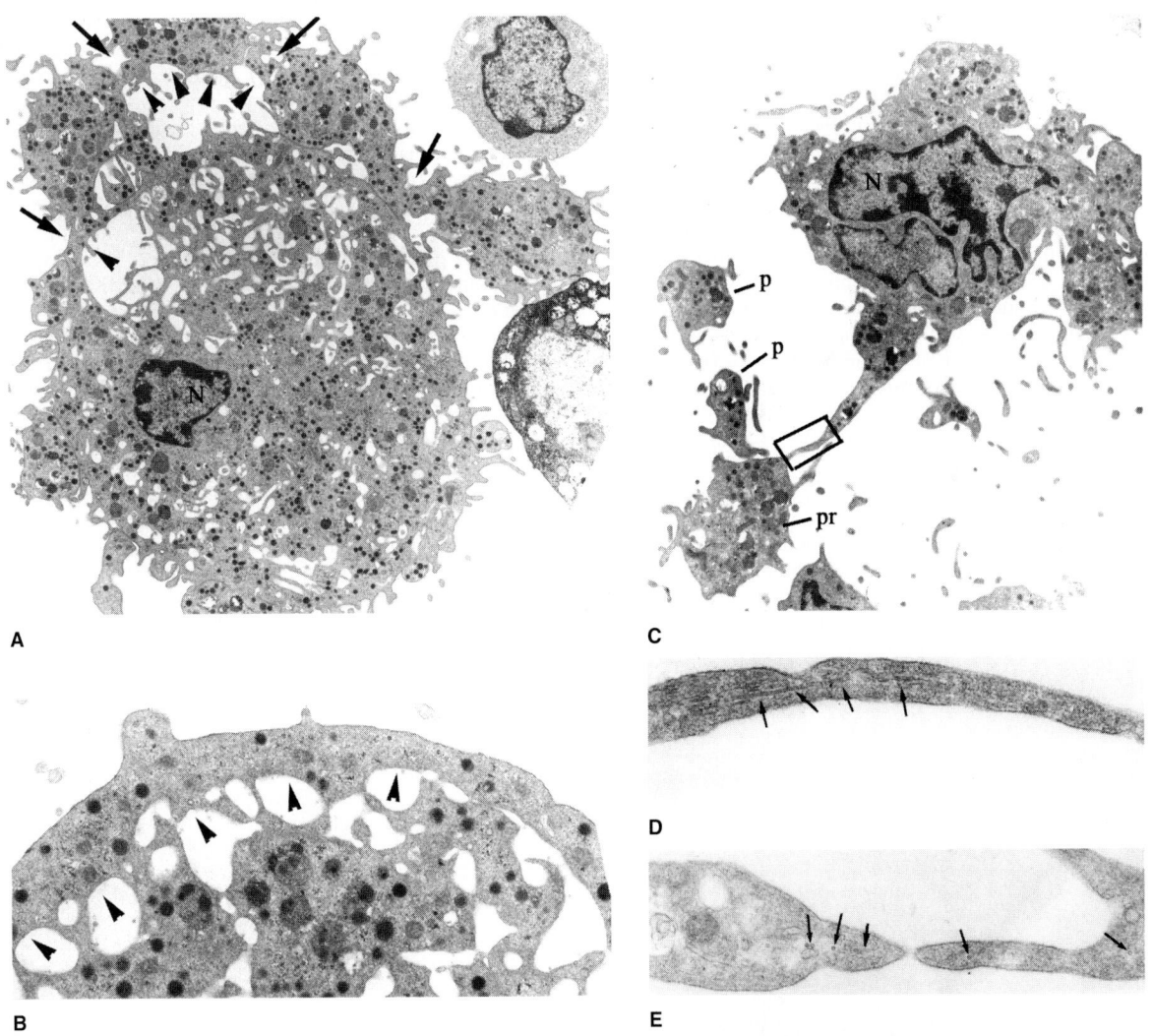

**FIGURE 25-4.** **A** and **B**: After reaching full maturation, megakaryocytes (MK) display the alignment and dilatation of some peripheral demarcation membranes (*arrowheads*), creating an outer ring of cytoplasm. The peripheral sheet of cytoplasm unfolds from the cell core, forming an elongated proplatelet process. Constriction zones are regularly disposed along this cytoplasmic extension (*arrows*), delimiting future platelet territories (*N*, nucleus) [magnification (**A**), ×3,520; (**B**), ×9,560]. **C**: Cytoplasm extends away (*box*) from the core of the mother cell, forming a proplatelet (*pr*). Some platelets (*p*) have detached from its tip (*N*, nucleus). **D**: A high magnification of the constriction zone shows some elongated parallel microtubules stretching along the long axis of the proplatelet (*arrow*) (magnification ×36,650). **E**: At places of constriction along the proplatelets, transverse microtubules appear (*arrows*) that might help increase local fragility, leading to breakage and liberation of a newly formed platelet (magnification ×35,650).

states such as fibroblast activation and myelofibrosis development (52).

## The Endomitotic Process

At the end of the proliferative phase, 2N MK precursors become polyploid. Polyploidization of MK is unique among mammalian cells in that multiples of 2N chromosomes are enclosed in a single nucleus and are surrounded by a single nuclear membrane. To achieve this, MK undergo endomitosis, during which DNA duplicates without nuclear and cytoplasmic division but is followed by nuclear segmentation. Designation of this process as endomitosis may not be totally appropriate, and some investigators have described this phenomenon as endoreplication (53,54).

### Description

MK are the only cells that become polyploid during their normal differentiation, whereas other cells become polyploid after stress. Polyploidy is a manner of increasing platelet production because the cytoplasm volume of MK increases in parallel with ploidy. An increase in MK ploidy is one of the first events occurring after the induction of an acute severe thrombocytopenia in mice: as early as 24 hours after the modal ploidy increases from 16N to 32N. These changes are maximal at 48 hours and return at 120 hours to basal values.

In a first step, MK increase their ploidy and can stop DNA duplication at any stage between 2N and 64N, rarely going up to 128N. In humans, as well as in most mammals, the modal ploidy is 16N (for about 50% of the MK). However, in some mouse species such as C3H mice, the modal MK ploidy is higher (32N) (55). During human ontogenesis, MK increase their ploidy, and in culture most fetal MK are only 2N or 4N (56). Low ploidy MK [i.e., micromegakaryocytes (2N and 4N)] have been shown to be able to shed platelets both *in vitro* as well as in human malignant pathologies. This suggests that the regulation of polyploidization may be independent of the cytoplasm maturation leading to platelet shedding.

MK endomitoses are rare events that remain difficult to observe. Originally, the term endomitosis was given to the mechanisms of polyploidization because it was suggested that the mitotic process occurs without rupture of the nuclear envelope.

However, some ultrastructural studies have described the endomitotic process. The first steps of endomitosis are identical to those of mitosis. They begin by chromosome condensation and by disappearance of the nuclear membrane (57). Several mitotic spindles are subsequently formed with two centrosomes by the tetraploid nucleus (58,59). Each of these centrosomes is active and participates in the mitotic spindle elongation. At the metaphase, chromosomes are aligned at the equator and have sizes similar to those of mitotic cells (57).

By using *in vitro* cultures in the presence of TPO, it easier to precisely describe the endomitotic process, with use of immunolabeling of the various proteins of the mitotic apparatus. An endomitosis corresponds to a mitosis that has skipped anaphase B and cytokinesis. The beginning of endomitosis is identical to normal mitosis: duplication of the centrosome, development of a mitotic spindle, condensation of chromosome (prophase), rupture of the nuclear envelope, alignment of the chromosomes on the equatorial plate (metaphase), and separation of the sister chromatids (anaphase). The main differences between mitosis and endomitosis lie at the level of the mitotic spindle. After the beginning of the anaphase, the spindle in polyploidizing MK remains short and does not elongate as in normal mitosis. Therefore, chromatids move toward each pole and appear as a round mass around each pole at anaphase, but each DNA mass remains tight as a consequence of the absence of spindle elongation. There is no development of a midzone in anaphase. Subsequently, decondensation of the chromosome and reformation of the nuclear membrane occurs. There is no karyokinesis or cytokinesis. At the end of endomitosis an MK contains a single nucleus with a single nuclear membrane. Each nuclear lobe corresponds to each pole of the multipolar spindle and their number is directly reflects the ploidy (60). When the MK is polyploid, the spindle is multipolar with a number of poles corresponding to the ploidy level. However, each pole does not correspond to 2N chromosome because segregation of chromatids is asymmetrical during endomitosis (60) (see Fig. 25-5).

Therefore, the cell cycle of an MK undergoing polyploidization is very similar to a mitotic process. There is clearly the succession of a G1, an S, a G2, and an M phase, but the M phase is incomplete. After the M phase, the cell reenters in G1 to undergo a subsequent cell cycle to duplicate DNA. However, the molecular mechanisms responsible for the switch from a mitotic to an endomitotic cycle, as well as the mechanism that stops this process at the end, are abnormal.

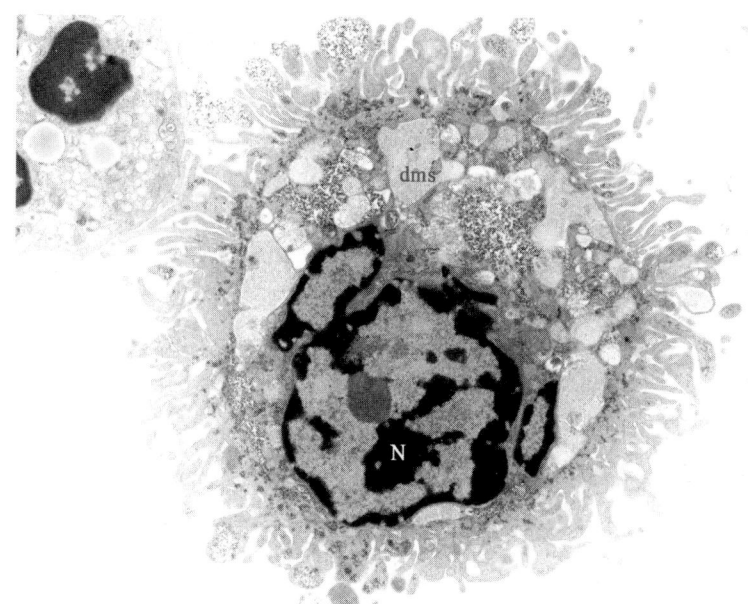

**FIGURE 25-5.** Like platelets, megakaryocytes can become activated. Thrombin induces shape change, pseudopod emission, organelle centralization, and granule secretion into the dilated channels of the demarcation membrane system (*dms*). The nucleus (*N*) is pushed to the cell periphery (magnification ×7,260).

## Regulation

■ The main mitosis regulators are effective during the endomitotic process:

– Cyclin D3, cyclin E, and A are normally expressed during G, E, and G2/M phases, respectively.

– The presence of cyclin B1 during the endomitotic process has been a subject of debate. There is now a large body of evidence indicating that cyclin B1 is expressed during the endomitotic cycle and degraded in anaphase. The presence of cyclin B1 is absolutely necessary for an entry in mitosis because the cdc2 (CDK1) kinase activity is indispensable for rupture of the nuclear envelope and chromatid condensation.

– The APC (anaphase-promoting complex), a proteasome complex that regulates the end of mitosis by successive degradation of mitotic regulator, is globally functional in the MK, and this is true both for the p55cdc20 subunit and cdh1 because cyclin B1, p55cdc20, and Aurora B are destroyed during the endomitotic process.

– Some CDK inhibitors such as p21 and p27 are expressed at high levels in polyploid MK and are not involved directly in the endomitotic process. These inhibitors could contribute to the mitotic arrest—although the ploidy of MK is normal in p21$^{-/-}$ and p27$^{-/-}$ mice (61).

■ However, some differences from a normal cell cycle are observed:

– The level of cyclin D3 is extremely high in MK, and an increase in cyclin D is capable of increasing MK ploidy (62).

– Cyclin E may also play an important role because cyclin E$^{-/-}$ mice have a marked defect in MK ploidization (63). In contrast, a proliferation defect is not observed in the other mitotic cells.

Whatever the molecular mechanisms involved, the cell cycle of the endomitotic MK presents two main abnormalities:

(a) One occurs at the end of mitosis, which remains to be understood, and leads to insufficient spindle elongation and cytokinesis. This may be related to a dysregulation of anaphase actors, possibly by inadequate protein degradation by the proteasome.

(b) The second abnormality is at the G1/S transition. Indeed, a normal cell cannot become polyploid because an unknown sensor detects the level of ploidy and blocks the subsequent reentry in S phase. This checkpoint is mainly regulated by p53 (64).

■ The advantages of polyploidization on the platelet formation are have been unclear until now. Theoretically, an endomitotic cycle could be shorter than a mitotic cycle because late phases of the cell cycle are abrogated. However, the time for DNA duplication seems identical for both processes (65). During terminal differentiation, MK must synthesize a high quantity of membranes to produce platelets. The endomitotic process could result in considerable economy of nuclear and plasma membrane synthesis, which may be helpful to produce platelets more efficiently. Finally polyploidization may be a method to markedly increase protein synthesis and to allow a much higher protein synthesis. Recently, it has been shown that during polyploidization, all the alleles of a gene remain functional; therefore, polyploidization is a true gene amplification (66). How polyploidization may also modify protein synthesis and gene expression remains to be determined. It has been reported that a linear correlation between messenger RNA (mRNA) or protein expression and ploidy is observed. However, at high ploidy, the expression may reach a plateau. For a long time, the issue of whether platelets arising from MK of different ploidy have similar or different size and function has been a matter of debate. After induction of an acute or severe thrombocytopenia, the mean platelet volume increases with ploidy. In addition, these young platelets are hyperfunctional. However, there is no direct evidence that high ploidy MK shed bigger and more functional platelets. In C3H mice, the platelet size is normal despite a 32N modal MK ploidy and changes in the mean platelet volume precede ploidy alterations after thrombocytopenia induction (67). In addition, there is currently no evidence that high ploidy MK have higher or different capacities for protein synthesis. Therefore, the altered platelet volume and function may be related either to the release of young platelets or to the effects of cytokines involved in platelet homeostasis on MK and platelet functions. In the same direction, TPO, which increases ploidy, enhances MK traduction machinery (68).

## Platelet Shedding

It is important to emphasize that the morphologic changes accompanying platelet production have not yet been observed *in vivo* in the bone marrow biopsy of a healthy subject, human or animal. The observations have only been made *in vitro* either on culture MK or on bone marrow MK placed on a glass slide. Although TPO is not necessary for platelet production, it is only since its discovery and use in culture dishes that images of platelet producing MK have been consistently observed. A noteworthy development is that definite structural differences have been identified between murine and human proplatelet formation by MK (7).

### Description

The mechanisms of platelet shedding have been better understood recently thanks to culture systems in the presence of TPO. Given that the precursor action is performed on bone marrow MK incubated *in vitro*, it is known that the formation of long cytoplasm extensions (proplatelet formation) are required, which are quite different from the cytoplasm blebs observed in PMKBs, for example (see Fig. 25-6) The development of these cytoplasm extensions gives to platelet shedding MK the typical morphologic appearance of an octopus (69,70).

The following events leading to platelet formation are sequentially observed *in vitro*: Demarcation membranes tend to open and widen, creating a furrow that individualizes an external band of cytoplasm forming a long process (Fig. 25-6A). This process elongates and extends off the cell, guided by a bundle of microtubules, forming the so-called proplatelet. The proplatelet bends, and branches, and bends again, each elbow being surrounded by a circular microtubule belt. The future platelet is able to detach from this extremity. The formation of proplatelet is accompanied with trafficking of an alignment of organelles, mainly granules, and mitochondria, moving in both directions, forward and backward, until they reach the tip of the proplatelet where they are immobilized, unable to go backward again. It could be the circular microtubule that stops them from going backward again (71).

The following summarizes the sequential subcellular events of platelet production:

(a) Peripheral redistribution and alignment of demarcation membranes; dilatation of the demarcation membranes (Fig. 25-6A, B)

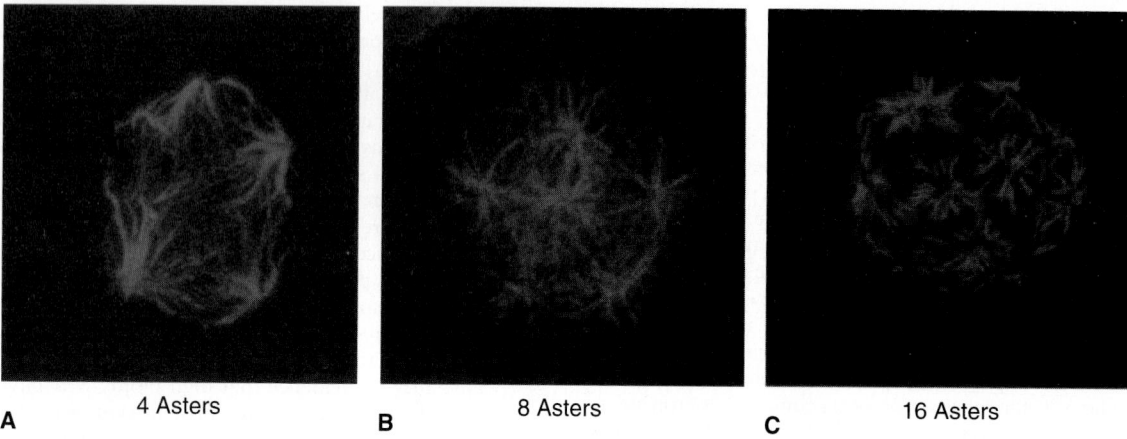

**FIGURE 25-6.** Immunofluorescent labeling of α and β tubulin in megakaryocytes (MK) undergoing endomitosis. These images of promet aphasis of endomitosis from 4N to 8N, 8N to 16N, and 16N to 32N show the structure and assymmetry of the multipolar mitotic spindles.

(b) Extension of a proplatelet displaying an axial bundle of microtubules and regular constriction zones (Fig. 25-6B, C) (Microcinema shows that proplatelets are mobile and reversible structures and that the future platelet organelles freely move along its long axis) (72,73)

(c) Appearance of constriction areas along the proplatelet located at the distal tip of the proplatelet extension

(d) Curving of the proplatelet forming an elbow, which thereby displays a circular belt of microtubule at its extremity

(e) Breakage of a distal constriction area and liberation of a newly formed platelet.

In the above model, only platelets detached from the tip of the proplatelet display a circular loop of microtubules, formed through the curling of this extremity (74). In order to explain the presence of the circular microtubule belt in platelets, it has also been suggested that newly formed platelets that still bear a longitudinal bundle of microtubules in the circulation, bend, curl, and form a loop with a central vacuole even as both its extremities fuse together, then the vacuole shrinks and the circumferential belt of microtubule is formed.

### Organelles Involved

The following platelet organelles play a key role in platelet shedding:

**Demarcation Membranes.** Mature MK evaginate the channels of demarcation membranes to their surface, which elongate to take a filamentous aspect and form long proplatelet extensions. Therefore, demarcation membranes do not delineate platelet territories in MK cytoplasm. However, the number and size of platelets released by individual MK are directly dependent of their development (75,76).

### Cytoskeleton

*Microtubules.* Pharmacologic inhibitors of microtubule formation prevent proplatelet extensions (73,77,78). Microtubules that are longitudinally oriented are present in these cytoplasm extensions. Microtubules are oriented along these processes, and constrictions occur that delineate the future platelets. It has been suggested that microtubules in each proplatelet are derived from one centriole enabling the existence of a direct relation between platelet shedding and ploidy (75). Proplatelet elongation is under the control of microtubules, which appear to be oriented in opposite directions within the same bundle, and they are able to slide back and forth along each other, thereby ensuring changes in the proplatelet length (79,80).

*Microfilaments.* Paradoxically, the process of proplatelet formation is enhanced by actin cytoskeleton disruption, showing that the filamentous network is not involved in proplatelet extension (73,78). However, and importantly, it is implicated in the bending and branching of these extensions that determine the size and number of shed platelets (71).

**Platelet Volume.** The final size of the shed platelet is critical in view of the fact that large platelets are functionally more active than small platelets. The subcellular structures just described are involved in determining platelet volume: The main regulatory element is the microfilament network. Indeed, the ability of proplatelet bending and kinking seems to be critical for platelet territory formation (71). Actin filaments are linked to the plasma membrane receptor GP Ib/V/IX through actin binding protein (ABP) or filamin, and abnormalities of one of these proteins are able to generate abnormally large platelets, which are then produced in decreased number: A typical example is Bernard-Soulier syndrome (81). Other congenital macrothrombocytopenia, mainly May-Hegglin, Sebastian, and Fechner syndromes, now united under the name of MYH9-related disorders, are autosomal dominant syndromes, variably affecting platelet formation. These results follow from mutations in the human nonmuscle myosin-IIA heavy chain gene, another component of the microfilament network (82). In ITP, platelet volume increases and this can be compared to the effect on red blood cells in hemolytic anemia, where accelerated production increases cell size. Accelerated platelet production leads to a quasi-immediate increase in platelet size, and this can be attributed to the repartition of the constriction zones, which, when closer to the MK core along the proplatelet, delimit larger territories (72,74,75). Finally, pathologic states like myelodysplasia are often characterized by an increased mean platelet volume. Given that acquired mutations of the transcription factor GATA1 that accompany some preleukemic states may also lead to macrothrombocytopenia (83), the increased platelet volume of myelodysplasia probably originates from a complex combination of cellular and molecular abnormalities.

### Apoptosis and Platelet Production

Cell apoptosis is characterized by cell fragmentation; platelet formation by MK, which is characterized by cytoplasm fragmentation, therefore, is similar to the apoptotic process. Moreover, terminal differentiation associated with loss of the nucleus (as it occurs in keratinocytes or during erythropoiesis) can be regulated by caspases, a class of proteases usually activated during apoptosis. It was demonstrated that caspase inhibition *in vitro* blocks proplatelet formation and causes thrombocytopenia in the animal model. A major effect was obtained with the pan-caspase inhibitor Z-VAD.fMk and to a lesser extent with caspase 9 and caspase 3 inhibitors (84). Bcl2 superexpression also blocks proplatelet formation.

### Embryonic Stem Cells and Platelet Production

By differentiating murine embryonic stem (ES) cells in coculture with stromal cells, Fujimoto et al. (85) succeeded in producing functional platelets able to spread, aggregate, bind fibrinogen, and express P selectin. The model promises to be extremely useful because these cells are able to closely mimic culture MK, including proplatelet and platelet production. Further production of gene-transferred platelets has been made possible by differentiating ES cells that were transfected with genes of interest.

### Localization

**Megakaryocyte Chemotaxis.** MK express the chemokine receptor CXCR4. The action of its ligand, the chemokine stromal cell–derived factor-1 (SDF-1) was found to induce MK chemotaxis, that is, migration toward a chemotactic gradient (86). The experiment was conducted in a modified Boyden chamber, showing that whole intact mature MK oriented themselves with the formation of a unilateral cytoplasmic pseudopod, the nuclear lobes being gathered at the opposite pole, and such MK can migrate through a transwell of bone marrow endothelial cells. MK are also able to react to agonists in a manner similar to that of platelets (51) (Fig. 25-5); therefore, their presence in the circulation might be pathogenic in some situations such as lung diseases. Thrombin induces dramatic morphologic changes as early as the megakaryoblastic stage, showing that the protease-activated receptor (PAR) is expressed early on this cell line. Two other groups carried out comparable studies and also observed that CXCR4 expression increases with MK maturation, but mature MK as well as platelets do not respond to SDF-1, suggesting that the signaling induced by SDF-1 is not operating: These results were interpreted as a potential mechanism for retaining immature MK in the marrow, whereas mature MK can migrate into the blood (87,88).

In normal individuals, platelet shedding does not seem to occur in the marrow but directly in the circulation. In the marrow, MK are located in the subendothelial region, in close contact with endothelial cells that may be involved in their terminal differentiation (89). Long cytoplasm pseudopods may pass through the endothelial barrier and enter into the marrow sinusoids (1,90–92). Alternatively, mature MK can also migrate through this blood barrier (91), and they are actually detected in the circulating blood. Several authors have pointed out that MK are present in considerable numbers in the small vessels of the lung and are trapped in the pulmonary capillary beds where they release platelets (93). Platelet release occurs by breaking off the long proplatelet extension at the level of the constrictions, and this rupture may be due only to the mechanic power induced by the blood flow pressure. Initially, proplatelets are released with a longitudinal orientation of the microtubules and their tip is elongated (like a teardrop) (94,95); subsequently, in the circulation, a rearrangement of microtubules occurs, giving a marginal microtubule coil, and platelets acquire their definitive discoid shape. The elegant model of Italiano et al. (74) argues against the theory of delayed formation of the circular microtubule belt: Indeed, the model shows its formation when the proplatelet extremity curves, allowing a new platelet to be formed; however, the model fails to show any platelet detachment in the culture system (71).

# MEGAKARYOCYTE DIFFERENTIATION STAGE-SPECIFIC MARKERS

## Megakaryocyte Progenitors

Initially, it was suggested that MK progenitors do not express platelet-specific proteins. In humans, MK progenitors have been characterized by differentiation markers, which are also present in other hematopoietic progenitors such as the CD34, CD31, and the AC133 antigens. Because of the expression of HLA-DR, one can distinguish between BFU-MK (HLA-DR$^{low}$) and CFU-MK (HLA-DR$^{high}$) (see Fig. 25-7) (16). In the mouse, it has been possible to purify MK progenitors close to homogeneity, on the basis of the expression of several antigens. The expression of the CD9 on MK progenitors helps distinguish them from erythroid progenitors.

## Megakaryocyte Precursors

Different platelet markers have been identified at later stages of differentiation. Initial studies have been undertaken by using a cytochemical marker, AchE, in the mouse (96,97). AchE staining, which is easily detected with light microscopy, is a very convenient marker for investigating murine megakaryocytopoiesis *in vitro*. In humans, AchE predominates in the erythroid lineage and cannot be used to identify megakaryocytic cells.

Studies in the mouse have shown the presence in the marrow of a compartment of small AchE-positive cells (SACHE) with a 2N ploidy. These cells are the direct precursors of MK and differentiate into polyploid MK in a few days (97–99). Most of these 2N cells have no proliferate capacities and subsequently undergo endoreplication cycles. Their number is greatly increased or reduced in induced thrombocytopenia or thrombocytosis, respectively. A very similar type of cells has been identified in normal human bone marrow using the platelet peroxidase marker at the ultrastructural level and has been called PMKB (22,23). Platelet peroxidase reflects cyclogenase activity. It is located in the perinuclear cistern and ER and is absent from Golgi complex and secretion granules.

## Platelet Markers on Megakaryocytes

More recent studies have used monoclonal antibodies directed against platelet proteins and have allowed a better understanding of MK differentiation. Most studies have focused on the main platelet glycoproteins, the GP IIb/IIIa (i.e., $\alpha_2\beta_3$ integrin or CD41b) and the GP Ib complex (i.e., GP Iba, GP Ibb, GP IX, and GP V or CD42a, b, c, and d).

CD41, or $\alpha_{IIb}$-$\beta_3$ integrin, is composed of CD41a or GP IIb and CD61 or GP IIIa or $\beta_3$ integrin. CD61 is not specific to the MK because, as a $\beta$ integrin, it can associate with a different chain than CD41a and especially with the vitronectin receptor ($\alpha v$). Therefore, CD61 can be detected on nonmegakaryocytic cells such as endothelial cells, activated macrophages, and osteoclasts. In contrast, CD41a (GP IIb) or CD41b (GP IIb/IIIa complex) appears specific for the MK lineage, especially in adults. In the marrow, a very tiny compartment (0.8 to $2.5 \times 10^4$ marrow cells) of small cells expressing platelet proteins can be detected by an anti–GP IIb antibody (100–103). During *in vitro* CFU-MK culture, a large number of these small cells are present just before the development of recognizable MK colonies (around day 6) (103,104).

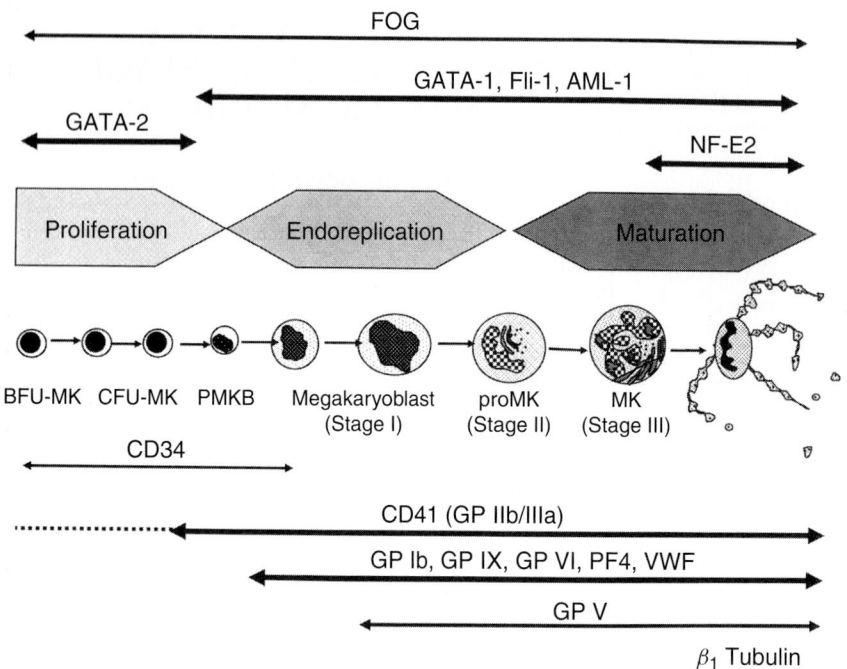

FIGURE 25-7. MK maturation markers. FOG, friend of GATA; BFU, burst-forming unit; CFU, colony-forming unit; GP, glycoprotein; PMKB, promegakaryoblast; PF4, platelet factor 4; VWF, von Willebrand factor.

However, CD41 was also detected on CD34$^+$ cells. Most of the CD34$^+$ CD41$^+$ cells in the adult correspond to late MK progenitors capable of giving rise to clusters of MK (from one to 10 cells) in 5 days (105) and to typical CFU-MK. But other experiments based on the use of the thymidine kinase gene under the GP IIb promoter, in transgenic or knockin mice, have shown that, after ganciclovir treatment, most of the hematopoietic progenitors as well as some HSCs were killed (106,107).

More recently, it has been shown that CD41 was an ontogenic marker of hematopoiesis. It is the first marker of definitive hematopoiesis in ES cells as well as in the embryo (108,109). During later development, CD41 becomes restricted to the megakaryocytic lineage in the adult (108,110). In humans, CD41 is not restricted to the megakaryocytic lineage in the neonate, where it is detected on hematopoietic progenitors, especially on the bipotent erythroid/MK progenitors, lymphoid progenitors, and some HSCs capable of reconstituting hematopoiesis in immunodeficient animals (SCID-RC) (111). It is noteworthy that the expression of Mpl, the receptor of TPO, mimics the expression of CD41 in certain ways. It is expressed at a low level on HSCs and all types of hematopoietic progenitors. Its expression markedly increases after commitment toward the MK lineage (112).

CD41 expression precedes the detection of other major platelet proteins (104). The CD42 antigen is detected slightly later on a cell that expresses the CD34 and CD41 antigens. These cells are capable of giving rise to a single MK or a cluster of less than four MK. The proliferation capacities of these cells are quite similar to those of the human CFU-MK defined in agar medium (113,114). The CD41$^+$ and CD42$^+$ cells have also been called *transitional* cells because these cells can switch from a mitotic stage to an endomitotic stage. In contrast to the CD41, CD42 is mainly restricted to the MK lineage, although some late erythroid progenitors may express this marker. The CD42 is a complex of four proteins. However, to detect the CD42 antigen on the surface, the GP Ibα (CD42b), GP Ibβ (CD42c), and GP IX (CD42a) must be expressed together. In contrast, GP V (CD42d) is not necessary and may be synthesized later than the other proteins (115).

Expression of CD42 corresponds to a later differentiation that is correlated with a marked increase in the expression of Mpl, GP VI (the collagen receptor), the α2β1 integrin, and CD36 and in the detection of proteins contained in the α-granules such as platelet factor 4 (PF4) and VWF. The next expression of these different proteins definitely increases in parallel, whereas the CD34 antigen disappears during the endomitotic process.

## CD4

Immature MK express the CD4 molecule, which may be relevant for the mechanisms of thrombocytopenia in HIV infection (116,117).

Finally, expression of some markers such as thromboxane synthase may increase at the end of maturation. β1-tubulin may be expressed only at the stage of proplatelet formation (results are summarized in Fig. 25-7.)

# MOLECULAR REGULATION OF MEGAKARYOCYTOPOIESIS

Investigations of molecular regulation of megakaryocytopoiesis have permitted large progresses in the understanding of normal MK differentiation, especially the association between erythroid and megakaryocytic differentiation and platelet shedding, as well as congenital and acquired MK pathologies.

Three main approaches have allowed this understanding:

- Studies of the promoters of MK-specific genes
- Knockout and knockin of transcription factor genes
- Studies of MK pathologies

## GATA Family and Partners

Sequencing of the promoter of MK-specific genes such as GP IIb, PF4, GP Ibα, β-thromboglobulin, GP IX, or GP V has shown the presence of consensus binding sequences (WGATAR) for transcription factors of the GATA family (118–122) already observed in erythroid-specific genes (123,124). MK-specific gene promoters also possess DNA consensus sequence for the Ets family (GGA/T), some of them being in tandem with the GATA motifs (125). Mutations that impair Ets binding reduce 60% of the activity of the MK promoters (125). Therefore, GATA and Ets binding sites are equally important for the activity of MK gene promoters. Ets binding sites are not found in erythroid-specific genes, whereas CGCC or CACC motifs are associated with GATA binding sites (124,126,127).

Among the GATA proteins, the GATA-1 protein was first described as a specific regulator of erythroid-specific genes (128) but was later detected in MK (129,130). GATA-1 knockout transgenic mice have lethal anemia in the embryo (131). But when a knockout of GATA-1 restrained to the MK lineage was obtained in mice, the animals were viable but presented profound macrothrombocytopenia with an excess of small immature MK in the marrow (132,133). These cells exhibit an increased proliferation capacity. In addition, synthesis of all the main platelet glycoproteins is markedly decreased.

GATA-1 protein is associated with several other transcription factors. One of its partners, called FOG-1 (Friend of GATA-1), was subsequently identified by a double hybrid approach. The knockout of FOG-1 gave a phenotype similar to that of GATA-1 in the erythroid lineage but with profound additional abnormalities in the megakaryocytic lineage (i.e., absence of MK progenitors), suggesting that FOG-1 may have another partner in the early stage of the megakaryocytic lineage. There is much evidence now to show that this partner is GATA-2, another member of the GATA family.

The importance of GATA-1 and FOG-1 was demonstrated in studies of human pathologies. First, some congenital thrombocytopenia with X chromosome transmission, with very large-sized platelets (macroplatelets) and moderate dyserythropoiesis, were related to mutations in the GATA-1 gene in positions 205 and 218 at the site of interaction of GATA-1 with FOG-1 (134). More recently, it has been shown that megakaryoblastic leukemia (AML-M7) of the Down syndrome is associated with mutations in the second exon of GATA-1 (135). These mutations lead to a shorter form of GATA-1 in its N-terminus, which has less transcriptional activity than the long form of GATA-1. These mutations are already detected in the transient myeloproliferative syndrome of the Down syndrome (136), suggesting that (a) these mutations occur in utero and (b) that a second genetic event is necessary for the development of an acute leukemia.

This mutation of GATA-1 in AML-M7 is observed only in the leukemia of trisomy 21: GATA-1 may, therefore, cooperate with a gene located on the chromosome 21 and thereby become overexpressed.

## Tal-1

The transcription factor Tal-1 is also associated with GATA-1 in a large complex involved in the regulation of erythroid genes. Tal-1 is also expressed in MK (137). Tal-1 knockout is lethal in the embryo because of the absence of HSC and, consequently, of hematopoiesis (138). Therefore, from this approach, it was difficult to assess the precise role of Tal-1 in the MK differentiation. An inducible knockout of Tal-1 surprisingly demonstrated that Tal-1 is not necessary for stem cell properties of hematopoietic cells but is a master gene in the commitment of a mesenchymatous cell toward hematopoiesis (109). In addition, Tal-1 is indispensable for the development of the erythroid and megakaryocytic lineages (109). The target genes of Tal-1 during megakaryocytopoiesis are currently unknown.

## AML-1

In cases of familial thrombocytopenia with propensity to develop AML, it has been demonstrated that the presence of a mutation in one allele of AML-1 usually leads to an inactive allele (139). Therefore, the thrombocytopenia may be related to this haploinsufficiency (139). AML-1, now called RUNX1, is one of the three constituents of the core binding factor-α and has been identified in the fusion transcript of AML-M2 with the t (8;21) translocation. Point mutations of AML-1 have been described in sporadic leukemia. Its role in megakaryocytopoiesis was unknown and could not be predicted from the phenotype of constitutive knockout mice. Recently, it has been shown that AML-1 may cooperate with GATA-1 (140). Inducible AML-1 knockout mice in the adult show a defect in MK maturation (141).

## Ets Family

The Ets family of transcription factors includes more than 13 different proteins. Two possible candidate genes are Ets-1 and Fli-1, which are both expressed in MK cell lines and in MK and are able to transactivate MK-specific genes (142). Ets-1 knockout mice have a marked defect in lymphoid lineages, but normal megakaryocytopoiesis. In contrast, the Fli-1 knockout is lethal in the embryo on account of a defect in vascular development and in megakaryocytopoiesis (143). There is a marked thrombocytopenia, with an excess of small immature MK undergoing apoptosis. These abnormalities are related to those observed in the Paris-Trousseau syndrome thrombocytopenia, or in the Jacobsen syndrome. These syndromes correspond to a deletion in 11q23 involving both Ets-1 and Fli-1. Recently, it has been shown that the in vitro defect in megakaryocytopoiesis observed in this syndrome can be corrected by Fli-1 expression. Therefore, it appears now that Fli-1 is the member of the Ets family that is involved in regulation of megakaryocytic genes. Fli-1 cooperates with GATA-1 to activate the transcription of GP IX and GP Ib (144). In addition, in contrast to GATA-1 and to the other transcription factors involved in the regulation of megakaryocytic genes, Fli-1 is not detected at a remarkable level in the erythroid lineage. Furthermore, its overexpression in the murine erythroid lineage may lead to an erythroleukemia. Therefore, Fli-1 may be involved in the commitment towards the megakaryocytic lineage.

## p45$^{NF-E2}$

p45$^{NF-E2}$ is a bZip (basic-leucine zipper) protein transcription factor. It forms a heterodimer with proteins of the maf family to form an active NF-E2 transcription factor. p45$^{NF-E2}$ has been identified in erythroid cells, where it regulates genes involved in heme synthesis. Surprisingly, p45$^{NF-E2}$ knockout mice die at birth from a severe thrombocytopenia with no defect in the erythroid lineage. In these p45$^{NF-E2-/-}$ mice, there is an increased MK number with marked maturation defects, especially in the development of demarcation membranes and in the distribution of α-granules (145). More interestingly, p45$^{NF-E2-/-}$ MK are unable to form proplatelets in vitro, and this correlates with acute thrombocytopenia (145,146). The partner of p45$^{NF-E2}$ in MK is essentially MafG and, to a lesser extent, MafK (147). The double knockout mice, MafG$^{-/-}$ MafK$^{-/-}$, have thrombocytopenia similar to that of p45$^{NF-E2-/-}$ mice. Therefore, discovery of the target genes of p45$^{NF-E2}$ was an avenue to characterize the genes involved in proplatelet formation.

Three genes are effectively involved in the process of proplatelet formation. β1-Tubulin was first identified (148); it is restricted to the megakaryocytic lineage and is expressed at late stages of differentiation. $\beta$1-tubulin knockout mice have a thrombocytopenia with abnormal-shaped platelets (i.e., absence of a discoid shape) (149). In contrast, reexpression of $\beta$1-tubulin in p45$^{NF-E2-/-}$ MK did not restore proplatelet formation (148) More recently, it has been shown that the three $\beta$- HSD genes involved in estrogen synthesis were regulated by NF-E2 (150). Normal murine MK synthesize estradiol, which regulates proplatelet formation in an autocrine or paracrine manner. Reexpression of the 3$\beta$-HSD in p45$^{NF-E2-/-}$ MK partially restores their capacity to form proplatelets (150). Reexpression of $\beta$1-tubulin and 3$\beta$-HSD completely corrects proplatelet formation from p45$^{NF-E2-/-}$ MK (150). It has also been shown that Rab27b, a small G protein involved in granule trafficking is a target gene of p45$^{NF-E2}$ and may also play a role in proplatelet formation (151). In contrast, thromboxane synthase, also a target gene of p45$^{NF-E2}$, has no role in proplatelet formation (152,153).

## Others

More recently, knockout of transcription factors or study of acute megakaryoblastic leukemia (AML-M7) has suggested that other transcription factors were involved in MK development.

GFI-1b is a transcription factor with a SNAG domain and is considered to be a transcriptional repressor (154). It is mainly expressed during the erythroid and megakaryocytic differentiation (155). Its knockout is lethal in the embryo, where major abnormalities in the erythroid and megakaryocytic differentiation lead to fatal anemia and thrombocytopenia (155). Its target genes responsible for this phenotype as well as its partners are unknown.

Neonate AML-M7 are usually associated with a t (1;22) translocation, which leads to a fusion protein between two ubiquitous transcription factors OTT and MAL1 (156). MAL1 may be an important transcription factor for MK development because it is a coactivator of the serum responsive factor (SRF), which is regulated by Rho signaling pathway. MAL-1 is associated with G-actin in the cytoplasm of nonactivated cell. When the Rho pathway is activated, G-actin is sequestered and MAL-1 is translocated to the nucleus. In combination with SRF, it

then activates target genes that are compounds of the cytoskeleton (157).

# REGULATION OF MEGAKARYOCYTOPOIESIS

Studies on the regulation of megakaryocytopoiesis (see Fig. 25-8) have largely been dominated by two concepts: (a) a humoral regulation by a late differentiation factor called TPO (158–160), which would be the equivalent of erythropoietin for the MK lineage and (b) a sequential dual regulation corresponding to different developmental stages: one being early in differentiation, by proliferative factors called MK-CSF, and the second being late, by differentiation factors also called potentiators or synergistic factors (161). In fact, the identification of TPO, the humoral factor regulating platelet production, has demonstrated that this hypothesis was actually true because TPO acts both on early and late stages of megakaryopoiesis. However, in contrast to erythropoietin (Epo), TPO is not the only growth factor that acts on late stages of megakaryocytopoiesis; in particular, it does not regulate proplatelet formation. Indeed, c-mpl$^{-/-}$ and TPO$^{-/-}$ mice have thrombocytopenia corresponding to about one tenth of the normal platelet number, less severe than expected, thereby suggesting that other growth factors may regulate platelet production in homeostatic conditions. In addition, a negative regulation by feedback may also influence platelet production.

## Stimulating Factors

### Steel Factor or Stem Cell Factor or Kit Ligand

Stem cell factor (SCF) is one of the most important cytokines, which acts as a synergistic factor with most hematopoietic growth factors. It is synthesized by marrow stromal cells. Its effect predominates on the erythroid lineage as a costimulator with Epo and in the early stages of hematopoiesis. SCF also seems to play an important physiologic role in megakaryocytopoiesis.

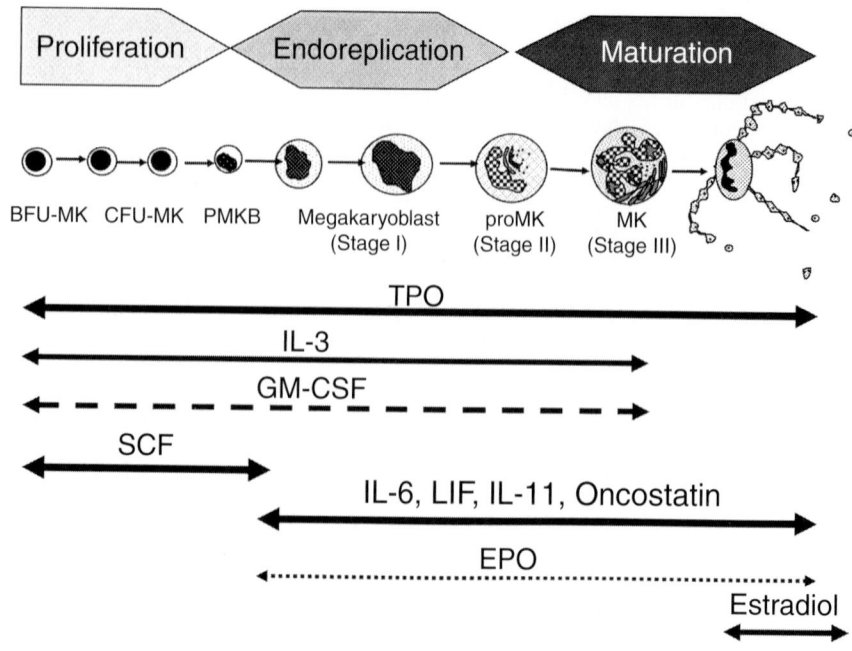

**FIGURE 25-8.** Cytokine regulation of megakaryocytopoiesis. BFU, burst-forming unit; CFU, colony-forming unit; PMKB, promegakaryoblast; MK, megakaryocytes; TPO, thrombopoietin; GM-CSF, granulocyte-macrophage colony-stimulating factor; SCF, stem cell factor; EPO, erythropoietin.

W/W$^v$ mice (deficient in the c-kit receptor) or Steel mice (deficient in SCF) have abnormal megakaryocytopoiesis, exhibiting a decrease in MK number but an increase in MK size, leading to normal platelet count (162–164). Furthermore, Steel mice have no rebound thrombocytosis after 5-fluorouracil treatment (165). When Steel mice are treated with SCF, they are able to undergo rebound thrombocytosis, like their wild-type litter mates (166). *In vitro*, SCF greatly potentiates the effects of other cytokines (including TPO) on the growth of MK progenitors, increasing both the cloning efficiency and the size of MK colonies (167–169). Surprisingly, SCF not only has a proliferative activity in early stages on megakaryocytopoiesis (170) but also acts in late stages (167,169,171). On purified MK, SCF slightly increases the ³H-thymidine incorporation (167), probably inducing their polyploidization. It increases MK adherence to fibroblasts (167). It also has a slight effect on the proliferation of transitional cells and favors the development of demarcation membranes in association with IL-3 (interleukin-3) and IL-6 (169,171).

*In vivo*, injection of SCF accelerates platelet recovery after myelosuppression. In addition, SCF mobilizes efficiently hematopoietic progenitors as well as MK progenitors. However, its use in clinical situations is impaired by its toxicity.

### Interleukin-3 and Granulocyte-Macrophage Colony-Stimulating Factor

IL-3 and granulocyte-macrophage colony-stimulating factor (GM-CSF) are two cytokines, which have many similarities in their action as well as in their receptor structure. IL-3 is a 14- to 22-kDa glycoprotein synthesized essentially by T cells but not by stromal cells. GM-CSF is a 22-kDa glycoprotein, which is synthesized by a larger number of cells such as T cells, monocyte/macrophages, and stromal cells. Both cytokines directly act on CFU-MK, IL-3 having a much higher activity (172–178). With the exception of TPO, IL-3 is the only cytokine that is able to induce MK colony formation alone. The effects of these two cytokines predominate in the early stages of megakaryocytopoiesis. It has even been suggested that IL-3 may impair MK terminal differentiation.

IL-3$^{-/-}$ and GM-CSF$^{-/-}$ mice have no thrombocytopenia. In addition, these two cytokines are not responsible for the remaining platelet production in TPO$^{-/-}$ mice.

Preclinical trials of IL-3 or a fusion protein between IL-3 and GM-CSF were promising because their injection enhanced platelet production (179) or platelet recovery in primates. In contrast, clinical trials were disappointing, with minimum effect on platelet counts and with considerable toxicity (180).

### Erythropoietin

Epo is synthesized by the kidneys and regulates erythropoiesis. The Epo receptor is present on MK and platelets. Although it was initially thought that Epo could induce MK colony formation by itself (9,10,181,182), there are now strong indications that Epo is essentially a maturation cytokine (172,183). Therefore, it acts more effectively as a costimulator with other cytokines and is able to favor terminal differentiation. Epo may also potentiate proplatelet formation by purified murine MK (184).

*In vivo* Epo does not appear as a major regulator of platelet production but may increase platelet functions. In humans, chronic administration of Epo may slightly increase platelet production (185–187). Epo has been observed to increase platelet number in one case of congenital thrombocytopenia, the thrombocytopenia with absence of radius (TAR syndrome).

**Interleukin-6, Interleukin-11, Leukemia Inhibitory Factor, and Oncostatin M.** Several cytokines [IL-6, lleukemia inhibitory factor (LIF), IL-11, oncostatin M, and ciliary neurotrophic factor (CNTF)] have pleiotropic effects on numerous cell types (188). The redundancy of these cytokines is explained by the molecular biology of their receptors. All these cytokines utilize a common signal transducing chain (GP130). They are essentially mediators of the inflammatory response.

IL-6 was the first molecule of this family to be studied on megakaryocytopoiesis. It is a 21- to 26-kDa glycoprotein, which is synthesized by a large number of cells, especially monocyte/macrophages, T cells, and stromal cells (189). It may also be an autocrine mediator and was initially considered as an interferon ($\beta$2-interferon). MK also synthesize IL-6 (190). The main role of IL-6 in hematopoiesis focuses on B-cell regulation.

IL-6 has a minimal effect on MK colony formation, especially in humans, but acts in synergy with IL-3 and SCF (191,192). In humans and *in vitro*, the combination of SCF, IL-3, and IL-6 has a similar efficiency as TPO alone. Studies on the effects of IL-6 on MK have shown that *in vitro* this cytokine induces an enhancement of (a) MK size, (b) MK ploidy (193,194), (c) cytoplasmic maturation including synthesis of platelet proteins (193,195), and (d) number (196). IL-6 also induces proplatelet formation by isolated MK (184).

However, IL-6 is not a physiologic regulator of thrombopoiesis and its level is not increased by thrombocytopenia. In addition, IL-6$^{-/-}$ mice have no quantitative or qualitative defects of platelets, and IL-6 is not responsible for the basal platelet number in TPO$^{-/-}$ or c-mpl$^{-/-}$ mice (197). IL-6 and IL-11 are probably responsible for the increase in platelet production in inflammatory diseases although this effect might be indirect and related to an increased synthesis of TPO.

Effects of IL-6 on platelet production have been studied in several animal models. IL-6 was able to increase the platelet count in a dose-dependent manner, with differences between species: In mice and primates, IL-6 has a major effect on MK ploidy where the modal ploidy increases from 16N to 64N (198,199), whereas no noticeable effect on ploidy is observed in dogs (200). IL-6 leads to marked enhancement of thrombocytopoiesis in dogs, with the release of large platelets with altered function. At higher dose, it increases platelet counts, MK, and CFU-MK numbers. A synergistic effect between IL-3 and IL-6 on platelet production has been described *in vivo* (201).

Clinical trials on the effects of IL-6 on platelet recovery have shown some effect on the platelet count but also some toxicity.

In the mouse, LIF potentiates the effects of IL-3 on MK colony formation (202); its injection induces thrombocytosis (203). However, in humans, its effect on *in vitro* megakaryocytopoiesis is less pronounced than that of IL-6 (169,204). LIF knockout mice have normal platelet count (205).

*Oncostatin M has similar effects on thrombopoiesis as leukemia inhibitory factor.* The effects of IL-11 on thrombocytopoiesis both *in vivo* and *in vitro* have been the subject of much study. IL-11 has marked effects on thrombocytopoiesis: *In vitro* IL-11 alone has no MK-stimulating activity alone but acts in synergy with IL-3 to stimulate murine and human colony formation (206,207). IL-11 acts on the late differentiation by increasing MK size and ploidy in humans (206). IL-11 injection in mice results in 1.25-fold increase in platelet counts that is caused by an increase in 32N MK, but not in MK numbers. In addition, the number of CFU-MK is increased in the spleen, but IL-11 effects on platelet counts are not abrogated by splenectomy (208). Mice have been hematologically reconstituted, with marrow cells expressing high levels of IL-11 after retroviral gene transfer (209). A sustained rise in platelet count is constantly seen without change in the number of leukocytes and of red blood cells. However, numerous systemic effects of IL-11 are observed including acute-phase protein reaction and behavioral changes.

IL-11 has been extensively studied in clinical trials. It accelerates platelet recovery by increasing the number of marrow CFU-MK and MK. It only has weak reversible toxicity, including anemia, and an elevation of inflammation markers (i.e., fibrinogen and C-reactive protein) (210).

The use of IL-11 has been approved in the United States in the treatment of chemotherapy-induced thrombocytopenia.

## Stromal Cell–Derived Factor 1

SDF-1, also called *pre–B-cell growth stimulating factor*, is a CXC chemokine. It binds a unique receptor, CXCR4, which is a seven transmembrane receptor coupled to G proteins. CXCR4 is also a coreceptor for HIV (211). SDF-1 is synthesized by stromal cells, bone marrow, endothelial, and dendritic cells. Gene disruption of CXCR4 and SDF-1 in the mouse has shown that these molecules play an essential function in different tissues: Mice die at birth from numerous developmental abnormalities including cerebellar and cardiac abnormalities and abnormal blood vessel formation. CXCR4 and SDF-1 play a major role in hematopoiesis, namely in B-cell development and in bone marrow colonization from fetal liver by HSC during ontogenesis. Indeed, SDF-1$^{-/-}$ embryos have a marked defect in marrow myelopoiesis, whereas fetal liver myelopoiesis is normal (212,213). SDF-1 is a chemoattractant for human CD34$^+$ hematopoietic progenitors, and CXCR4 may be involved in the bone marrow homing of HSC (214,215). There is increasing evidence that SDF-1/CXCR4 plays a major role in the retention of hematopoietic cells in the marrow (216). Therefore, SDF-1 is absolutely required for prolonged establishment of HSC in the marrow. In addition, mobilization of hematopoietic progenitors in blood is related to down-regulation of CXCR4 membrane expression, either related to a proteolysis by neutrophil proteases or by receptor endocytosis (215,217). SDF-1/CXCR4 is also involved in the marrow exit of hematopoietic precursors.

In addition, SDF-1 behaves as a growth factor. It regulates HSC, although with controversial results (218,219). MK progenitors and MK express the CXCR4 receptor, the expression of which increases with maturation (220). However, there is evidence that despite this increase in expression, mature MK are poorly responsive to SDF-1, at least in chemotactic assays (87,88). SDF-1 has a synergetic effect with growth factors such as TPO on MK colony formation. SDF-1 can directly affect MK polyploidization and maturation, increasing proplatelet formation (221). High SDF-1 or fibroblast growth factor (FGF)-4 expression can restore a normal platelet production in TPO$^{-/-}$ and c-mpl$^{-/-}$ mice (222). But this effect is not direct and is related to the chemo attraction of MK precursors toward a hematopoietic vascular niche that is permissive to MK maturation (222). Therefore, it seems likely that TPO-independent platelet production is not directly related to a specific cytokine but rather to the interaction of megakaryocytic cells with the bone marrow environment and endothelial cells.

## Other Hematopoietic Growth Factors

Several other characterized cytokines may also act *in vivo* or *in vitro* on megakaryocytopoiesis. One of the most studied cytokines is IL-1 $\alpha$ or $\beta$. These two cytokines have a positive effect on megakaryocytopoiesis (173,223), but most effects, if not all, seem indirect by the induction of numerous cytokines such as IL-6, GM-CSF, or SCF. IL-1 injected in both animals and humans shows an increase in platelet production. IL-1 has major toxic effects that reduce its interest as a therapeutic agent.

G-CSF also has a synergistic effect with IL-3 on the growth of MK progenitors; it has been shown recently that platelets are able to bind G-CSF and to functionally respond to this cytokine (224). *In vivo* injection of G-CSF has no effect on platelet recovery in humans.

IL-9 has been isolated for its proliferative activity on a factor-dependent megakaryoblastic cell line (MO-7E). This cytokine may favor MK maturation in synergy with TPO (225).

## Nonhematopoietic Growth Factors

Basic fibroblast growth factor (bFGF), a nonhematopoietic growth factor, acts on megakaryocytopoiesis, probably by both direct and indirect effects (226). The bFGF effects are suppressed by antibodies against IL-6 (227). Notably, MK expresses bFGF and synthesizes its receptor (228) and bFGF increases the number of CFU-MK generated in *ex vivo* expansion protocols (229).

---

# Inhibitory Factors

As soon as the MK colony assay was available, it was evident that it was different from the erythroid or granulocytic lineages because MK colony formation was partially inhibited by serum in a dose-dependent manner. In contrast, plasma or serum derived from platelet-poor plasma had no inhibitory effect (230–232). These results strongly indicated that platelets store and secrete one or several molecules inhibiting megakaryocytopoiesis.

It has been subsequently demonstrated that these inhibitory proteins are present inside platelets, especially in $\alpha$-granules. Five different proteins may be involved in this inhibition: TGF-$\beta$, PF4 associated peptides, $\beta$-thromboglobulin, and connective tissue activating peptide (CTAP-III) (227,233–236) as well as an incompletely characterized glycoprotein (237).

The inhibitory effects of TGF-$\beta$ on megakaryocytopoiesis are extremely potent (227,238–240). The inhibitory effect of TGF-$\beta$ is in no way specific for megakaryocytopoiesis as all primitive hematopoietic progenitors including HSCs are also inhibited by TGF-$\beta$ (241,242). However, the effects of TGF-$\beta$ on the MK lineage differ from those observed in other cell lines: TGF-$\beta$ not only inhibits the growth of MK progenitors but also inhibits the endomitotic process and the cytoplasmic maturation (239,243), thereby acting on late stages of differentiation. This inhibitory effect may be related to an inhibition of TPO signaling (244). Treatment of mice for 7 to 14 days with TGF-$\beta$1 induces a 95% reduction in the platelet count as well as an anemia and an increase in granulopoiesis (245).

PF4, $\beta$-thromboglobulin, and CTAP-III belong to the same family of cytokines (chemokines) and they are also able to bind heparin. Their inhibitory effects may be related to a common dodecapeptide, Asn–Gly–Arg–Lys–Ile–Cys–Leu–Asp–Leu–Glu–Ala–Pro, present in the sequence of theses cytokines (236). *In vivo* injection of PF4 in mice induces a thrombocytopenia. PF4 inhibits MK progenitor proliferation, MK polyploidization, and proplatelet formation (246). However, the inhibitory effect of PF4 on megakaryocytopoiesis is nonspecific. Similar to other members of this family such as MIP-1$\alpha$ (247), PF4 acts on primitive hematopoietic cells and may also inhibit angiogenesis. Thrombospondin 1 may also inhibit MK *in vitro* through the CD36 molecule (248).

Outside these platelet molecules, other cytokines such as interferons and TNF-$\alpha$ also inhibit megakaryocytopoiesis *in vitro* (249,250).

The effects of IL-4 on megakaryocytopoiesis remain controversial and may differ among different species. However, more recent evidence suggests that IL-4 inhibits MK colony formation by a direct effect in MK progenitor. This IL-4 inhibitory effect is not affected by neutralizing antibodies against TGF-$\beta$, interferons, and TNF-$\alpha$ (251).

The physiologic relevance of platelet inhibitory molecules on platelet production is currently unknown. These molecules could play a role in a feedback regulation process and could be involved in the mechanisms that render platelet production dependent on the platelet mass.

# CONCLUSION

Megakaryopoiesis, the cellular process responsible for platelet production, is part of the general hematopoietic proliferation and differentiation process that takes place in the bone marrow. It takes an average of 1 week for an undifferentiated bone marrow stem cell to give birth to mature platelets. Megakaryopoiesis has numerous specificities compared to the other hematopoietic cell lines:

- Proximity to the erythroid lineage during the early steps of differentiation.
- A switch during differentiation from a proliferative mitotic (DNA duplication followed by cytokinesis) to an endomitotic process (DNA duplication without cytokinesis), which leads to a polyploid cell with a single polylobulated nucleus. This process is quasi-obligatory during differentiation, in contrast to many other cell systems where polyploidization is a stress response.
- At the end of differentiation, platelets are born from the cytoplasmic fragmentation of MK by a regulated and dynamic process called *proplatelet* formation. Thus the number of platelets formed is not the direct reflection of MK number but of the MK mass. However, the precise site into which platelets are released from mature MK still remains to be established.

## *References*

1. Lichtman MA, Chamberlain JK, Simon W, et al. Parasinusoidal location of megakaryocytes in marrow: a determinant of platelet release. *Am J Hematol* 1978;4:303–312.
2. Mohle R, Green D, Moore MA, et al. Constitutive production and thrombin-induced release of vascular endothelial growth factor by human megakaryocytes and platelets. *PNAS U S A* 1997;94:663–668.
3. Mohle R, Green D, Moore MA, et al. Constitutive production and thrombin-induced release of vascular endothelial growth factor by human megakaryocytes and platelets. *Proc Natl Acad Sci U S A* 1997;94:663–668.
4. Almeida-Porada G, Ascensao JL. Isolation, characterization, and biologic features of bone marrow endothelial cells. *J Lab Clin Med* 1996;128:399–407.
5. Breton-Gorius J. On the alleged phagocytosis by megakaryocytes. *Br J Haematol* 1981;47:635–636.
6. Schmitt A, Jouault H, Guichard J, et al. Pathologic interaction between megakaryocytes and polymorphonuclear leukocytes in myelofibrosis. *Blood* 2000;96:1342–1347.
7. Schmitt A, Guichard J, Masse JM, et al. Of mice and men: comparison of the ultrastructure of megakaryocytes and platelets. *Exp Hematol* 2001;29:1295–1302.
8. Levine RF, Eldor A, Shoff PK, et al. Circulating megakaryocytes: delivery of large numbers of intact, mature megakaryocytes to the lungs. *Eur J Haematol* 1993;51:233–246.
9. Vainchenker W, Bouget J, Guichard J, et al. Megakaryocyte colony formation from human bone marrow precursors. *Blood* 1979;54:940–947.
10. McLeod DL, Shreeve MM, Axelrad AA. Induction of megakaryocyte colonies with platelet formation *in vitro*. *Nature* 1976;261:492–494.
11. Debili N, Coulombel L, Croisille L, et al. Characterization of a bipotent erythro-megakaryocytic progenitor in human bone marrow. *Blood* 1996;88:1284–1296.
12. Hoffman R. Regulation of megakaryocytopoiesis. *Blood* 1989;74:1196–1212.
13. Levin J, Levin FC, Penington DG, et al. Measurement of ploidy distribution in megakaryocyte colonies obtained from culture with studies of the effects of thrombocytopenia. *Blood* 1981;57:287–297.
14. Paulus J-M, Prenant M, Deschamps J-F, et al. Polyploid megakaryocytes develop randomly from a multicompartmental system of committed progenitors. *Proc Natl Acad Sci U S A* 1982;79:4410–4414.
15. Long MW, Gragowski LL, Heffner CH, et al. Phorbol diesters stimulate the development of an early murine progenitor cell: The burst forming unit-megakaryocyte. *J Clin Invest* 1985;76:431–438.

16. Briddell RA, Brandt JE, Straneva JE, et al. Characterization of the human burst-forming unit-megakaryocyte. *Blood* 1989;74:145–151.
17. Metcalf D, McDonald HR, Odartchenko N, et al. Growth of mouse megakaryocyte colonies *in vitro*. *Proc Natl Acad Sci U S A* 1975;72:1744–1748.
18. Mazur EM, Hoffman R, Chasis J, et al. Immunofluorescent identification of human megakaryocyte colonies using an antiplatelet glycoprotein antiserum. *Blood* 1981;57:277–286.
19. Vainchenker W, Guichard J, Breton-Gorius J. Growth of human megakaryocyte colonies in culture from fetal, neonatal and adult peripheral blood cells. Ultrastructural analysis. *Blood Cells* 1979;5:25–39.
20. Zauli G, Valvassori L, Capitani S. Presence and characteristics of circulating megakaryocyte progenitor cells in human fetal blood. *Blood* 1993;81:385–390.
21. Chatelain C, Debast M, Symann M. Identification of a light density murine megakaryocyte progenitor (LD-CFU-M). *Blood* 1988;72:1187–1192.
22. Breton-Gorius J, Vainchenker W. Expression of platelet proteins during the *in vitro* and *in vivo* differentiation of megakaryocytes and morphological aspects of their maturation. *Sem Hematol* 1986;28:43–67.
23. Breton-Gorius J, Guichard J. Ultrastructural localization of peroxidase activity in human platelets and megakaryocytes. *Am J Pathol* 1972;66:277–286.
24. Gerrard JM, White JG, Rao GH, et al. Localization of platelet prostaglandin production in the platelet dense tubular system. *Am J Pathol* 1976;83:283–298.
25. Williams N, Levine RF. The origin, development and regulation of megakaryocytes. *Br J Haematol* 1982;52:173–180.
26. Stenberg PE, Levin J. Mechanisms of platelet production. *Blood Cells* 1989;15:23–47.
27. Behnke O. An electron microscope study of megakaryocytes of rat bone marrow. I. The development of the demarcation membrane system and the platelet surface coat. *J Ultrastruct Res* 1968;24:412–433.
28. Zucker-Franklin D, Petursson J. Thrombocytopoiesis: analysis by membrane tracer and freeze fracture studies on fresh human and cultured human megakaryocytes. *J Cell Biol* 1984;99:390–402.
29. Debili N, Kieffer N, Nakazawa M, et al. Expression of platelet glycoprotein Ib by cultured human megakaryocytes: ultrastructural localization and biosynthesis. *Blood* 1990;76:368–376.
30. Cramer EM, Debili N, Martin JF, et al. Uncoordinated expression of fibrinogen compared with thrombospondin and von Willebrand factor in maturing human megakaryocytes. *Blood* 1989;73:1123–1129.
31. Cramer EM, Savidge GF, Vainchenker W, et al. Alpha-granule pool of glycoprotein IIb-IIIa in normal and pathologic platelets and megakaryocytes. *Blood* 1990;75:1220–1227.
32. Heijnen HFG, Debili N, Vainchenker W, et al. Multivesicular bodies are an intermediate stage in the formation of platelet α-granules. *Blood* 1998;91:2313–2325.
33. Cramer E, Vainchenker W, Vinci G, et al. Gray platelet syndrome: immunoelectron microscopic localization of fibrinogen and von Willebrand factor in platelets and megakaryocytes. *Blood* 1985;66:1309–1316.
34. Cramer EM, Harrison P, Savidge GF, et al. Uncoordinated expression of alpha-granule proteins in human megakaryocytes. *Prog Clin Biol Res* 1990;356:131–142.
35. Handagama P, Bainton DF, Jacques Y, et al. Kistrin, an integrin antagonist, blocks endocytosis of fibrinogen into guinea pig megakaryocyte and platelet alpha-granules. *JCI* 1993;91:193–200.
36. George JN. Platelet immunoglobulin G: its significance for the evaluation of thrombocytopenia and for understanding the origin of α-granule proteins. *Blood* 1990;76:895–870.
37. Handagama PJ, Shuman MA, Bainton DF. Incorporation of intravenously injected albumin, immunoglobulin G, and fibrinogen in guinea pig megakaryocyte granules. *JCI* 1989;84:73–82.
38. Handagama P, Rappolee DA, Werb Z, et al. Platelet alpha-granule fibrinogen, albumin, and immunoglobulin G are not synthesized by rat and mouse megakaryocytes. *JCI* 1990;86:1364–1368.
39. Harrison P, Wilbourn B, Debili N, et al. Uptake of plasma fibrinogen into the alpha granules of human megakaryocytes and platelets. *J Clin Invest* 1989;84:1320–1324.
40. de Larouziere V, Brouland JP, Souni F, et al. Inverse immunostaining pattern for synthesized versus endocytosed alpha-granule proteins in human bone marrow megakaryocytes. *Br J Haematol* 1998;101:618–625.
41. Cramer EM, Breton-Gorius J, Beesley JE, et al. Ultrastructural demonstration of tubular inclusions coinciding with von Willebrand factor in pig megakaryocytes. *Blood* 1988;71:1533–1538.
42. Berger G, Caen J-P, Berndt MC, et al. Ultrastructural demonstration of CD36 in the α-granule membrane of human platelets and megakaryocytes. *Blood* 1993;82:3034–3044.
43. Masse JM, Perlemuter K, Debili N, et al. Intracellular trafficking of the ααIIbβ3 receptor antagonist, abciximab, in normal and Glanzmann's disease megakaryocytes. *Br J Haematol* 1999;107:720–730.
44. Heijnen HF, Schiel AE, Fijnheer R, et al. Activated platelets release two types of membrane vesicles: microvesicles by surface shedding and exosomes derived from exocytosis of multivesicular bodies and alpha-granules. *Blood* 1999;94:3791–3799.
45. Youssefian T, Cramer EM. Megakaryocyte dense granule components are sorted in multivesicular bodies. *Blood* 2000;95:4004–4007.

46. Veljkovic DK, Cramer EM, Alimardani G, et al. Studies of alpha-granule proteins in cultured human megakaryocytes. *Thromb Haemost* 2003;90: 844–852.

47. Youssefian T, Masse J-M, Rendu F, et al. Platelet dense granule membrane contains glycoproteins Ib and IIb-IIIa. *Blood* 1997;89:4047–4057.

48. Israels SJ, Gerrard JM, Jacques YV, et al. Platelet dense granule membranes contain both granulophysin and P-selectin (GMP-140). *Blood* 1992;80:143–152.

49. Bentfeld-Barker ME, Bainton DF. Identification of primary lysosomes in human megakaryocytes and platelets. *Blood* 1982;59:472–481.

50. Houwerzijl EJ, Blom NR, van der Want JJ, et al. Ultrastructural study shows morphologic features of apoptosis and para-apoptosis in megakaryocytes from patients with idiopathic thrombocytopenic purpura. *Blood* 2004;103:500–506.

51. Cramer EM, Massé J-M, Caen J-P, et al. Effect of thrombin on maturing human megakaryocytes. *Am J Pathol* 1993;143:1498–1508.

52. Villeval J, Cohen-Solal K, Tulliez M, et al. High thrombopoietin production by hematopoietic cells induces a fatal myeloproliferative syndrome in mice. *Blood* 1997;90:4369–4383.

53. Nagata Y, Muro Y, Todokoro K. Thrombopoietin-induced polyploidization of bone marrow megakaryocytes is due to a unique regulatory mechanism in late mitosis. *J Cell Biol* 1997;139:449–457.

54. Vitrat N, Cohen-Solal K, Pique C, et al. Endomitosis of human megakaryocytes are due to abortive mitosis. *Blood* 1998;91:3711–3723.

55. Jackson CW, Steward SA, Chenaille PJ, et al. An analysis of megakaryocytopoiesis in the C3H mouse: an animal model whose megakaryocytes have 32N as the modal DNA class. *Blood* 1990;76:690–696.

56. Hegyi E, Nakazawa M, Debili N, et al. Developmental changes in human megakaryocyte ploidy. *Exp Hematol* 1991;19:87–94.

57. Radley JM. Ultrastructure of endomitosis in megakaryocytes. *Nouv Rev Fr Hematol* 1989;31:232a.

58. Goyanes-Villaescuca V. Cycles of reduplication in megakaryocyte nuclei. *Cell Tissue Kinet* 1969;2:165–168.

59. Moskwin-Taerkhanov MI, Onishenko GE. Centrioles in megakaryocytes of mouse bone marrow. *Tsilogiia* 1978;20:1436–1438.

60. Roy L, Coullin P, Vitrat N, et al. Asymmetrical segregation of chromosomes with a normal metaphase:anaphase checkpoint in polyploid megakaryocytes. *Blood* 2001;97:2238–2247.

61. Baccini V, Roy L, Vitrat N, et al. Role of p21Cip1/Waf1 in cell cycle exit of endomitotic megakaryocytes. *Blood* 2001;98:3274–3282.

62. Wang Z, Zhang Y, Kamen D, et al. Cyclin D3 is essential for megakaryocytopoiesis. *Blood* 1995;86:3783–3788.

63. Geng Y, Yu Q, Sicinska E, et al. Cyclin E ablation in the mouse. *Cell* 2003; 114:431–443.

64. Meraldi P, Honda R, Nigg EA. Aurora-A overexpression reveals tetraploidization as a major route to centrosome amplification in p53$^{-/-}$ cells. *EMBO J* 2002;21:483–492.

65. Odell TTJ, Jackson CW. Generation cycle of rat megakaryocytes. *Exp Cell Res* 1968;53:321–328.

66. Raslova H, Roy L, Vourc'h C, et al. Megakaryocyte polyploidization is associated with a functional gene amplification. *Blood* 2003;101:541–544.

67. Corash L, Chen HY, Levin J. Regulation of thrombopoiesis: effects of the degree of thrombocytopenia on megakaryocyte ploidy and platelet volume. *Blood* 1987;70:177–185.

68. Caron S, Charon M, Cramer E, et al. Selective modification of eukaryotic initiation factor 4F (eIF4F) at the onset of cell differentiation: recruitment of eIF4GII and long-lasting phosphorylation of eIF4E. *Mol Cell Biol* 2004;24:4920–4928.

69. Thiery JB, Bessis M. La genèse des plaquettes à partir des mégacaryocytes observés sur la cellule vivante. *C R Acad Sci* 1956;242:290–292.

70. Thiery JB, Bessis M. Mécanisme de la plaquettogenèse. Etude *in vitro* par la microcinématographie. *Rev Hemat* 1956;II:162–176.

71. Italiano JE Jr, Lecine P, Shivdasani RA, et al. Blood platelets are assembled principally at the ends of proplatelet processes produced by differentiated megakaryocytes. *J Cell Biol* 1999;147:1299–1312.

72. Cramer EM, Norol F, Guichard J, et al. Ultrastructure of platelet formation by human megakaryocytes cultured with the Mpl ligand. *Blood* 1997;89:2336–2346.

73. Tablin F, Castro M, Leven RM. Blood platelet formation *in vitro*: the role of the cytoskeleton in megakaryocyte fragmentation. *J Cell Sci* 1990;97: 59–70.

74. Hartwig J, Italiano J Jr. The birth of the platelet. *J Thromb Haemost* 2003;1:1580–1586.

75. Radley JM, Scurfield G. The mechanism of platelet release. *Blood* 1980; 56:996–999.

76. Radley JM, Haller CJ. The demarcation membrane system of the megakaryocyte: a misnomer? *Blood* 1982;60:213–219.

77. Handagama PJ, Feldman BF, Jain BC, et al. *In vitro* platelet release by rat megakaryocytes: effect of metabolic inhibitors and cytoskeletal disrupting agents. *Am J Vet Res* 1987;48:1142–1146.

78. Leven RM, Yee MK. Megakaryocyte morphogenesis stimulated *in vitro* by whole and partially fractionated thrombocytopenic plasma: a model system for the study of platelet formation. *Blood* 1987;69:1046–1052.

79. Hartwig J, Italiano J Jr. The birth of the platelet. *J Thromb Haemost* 2003;1:1580–1586.

80. Italiano JE Jr, Shivdasani RA. Megakaryocytes and beyond: the birth of platelets. *J Thromb Haemost* 2003;1:1174–1182.

81. Rao AK, Jalagadugula G, Sun L. Inherited defects in platelet signaling mechanisms. *Semin Thromb Hemost* 2004;30:525–535.

82. Balduini CL. Giant platelet syndromes and the MYH9 mutations. *Lab Hematol* 2004;10:187–188.

83. Gurbuxani S, Vyas P, Crispino JD. Recent insights into the mechanisms of myeloid leukemogenesis in Down syndrome. *Blood* 2004;103:399–406.

84. De Botton S, Sabri S, Daugas E, et al. Platelet formation is the consequence of caspase activation within megakaryocytes. *Blood* 2002;100: 1310–1317.

85. Fujimoto TT, Kohata S, Suzuki H, et al. Production of functional platelets by differentiated embryonic stem (ES) cells *in vitro*. *Blood* 2003;102: 4044–4051.

86. Hamada T, Mohle R, Hesselgesser J, et al. Transendothelial migration of megakaryocytes in response to stromal cell-derived factor 1 (SDF-1) enhances platelet formation. *J Exp Med* 1998;188:539–548.

87. Kowalska MA, Ratajczak J, Hoxie J, et al. Megakaryocyte precursors, megakaryocytes and platelets express the HIV co-receptor CXCR4 on their surface: determination of response to stromal-derived factor-1 by megakaryocytes and platelets. *Br J Haematol* 1999;104:220–229.

88. Riviere C, Subra F, Cohen-Solal K, et al. Phenotypic and functional evidence for the expression of CXCR4 receptor during megakaryocytopoiesis. *Blood* 1999;93:1511–1523.

89. Avraham H, Cowley S, Chi SY, et al. Characterization of adhesive interactions between human endothelial cells and megakaryocytes. *J Clin Invest* 1993;91:2378–2384.

90. Behnke O. An electron microscope study of the rat megakaryocyte. II. Some aspects of platelet release and microtubules. *J Ultrastruct Res* 1969; 26:111–129.

91. Tavassoli M, Aoki M. Migration of entire megakaryocyte through the marrow-barrier. *B J Hematol* 1981;48:25–29.

92. Zucker-Francklin D, Petursson S. Thrombocytopoiesis: analysis by membrane tracer and freeze-fracture on fresh human and cultured mouse megakaryocytes. *J Cell Biol* 1984;99:390–402.

93. Trowbridge EA, Martin JF, Slater DN. Evidence for a theory of physical fragmentation of megakaryocytes implying that all platelets are produced in the pulmonary circulation. *Thromb Res* 1982;28:461–475.

94. Radley JM, Hartshorn MA. Megakaryocyte fragments and the microtubule coil. *Blood Cells* 1987;12:603–610.

95. Becker RP, De Bruyn PP. The transmural passage of blood cells into myeloid sinusoids and the entry of platelets into the sinusoidal circulation: a scanning electron microscopic investigation. *Am J Anat* 1976;145:183–205.

96. Zajicek J. Studies on the histogenesis of blood platelets. I. Histochemical investigations of the acetylcholinesterase activity of megakaryocytes and platelets in different animal species. *Acta Haematol* 1954;12: 238–244.

97. Jackson CN. Cholinesterase as a possible marker for early cells of the megakaryocytic series. *Blood* 1973;42:413–421.

98. Long MW, Williams N. Differences in the regulation of megakaryocytopoiesis in the murine bone marrow and spleen. *Leukoc Res* 1982;6: 721–728.

99. Long MW, Williams N. Immature megakaryocytes in the mouse: *in vitro* relationship to megakaryocyte progenitor cells and mature megakaryocytes. *J Cell Physiol* 1982;112:339–344.

100. Ishibashi T, Ruggeri ZM, Harker LA, et al. Separation of human megakaryocytes by state of differentiation on continuous gradients of Percoll: size and ploidy analysis of cells identified by monoclonal antibody to glycoprotein IIb/IIIa. *Blood* 1986;67:1286–1292.

101. Rabellino EM, Nachman RL, Williams N, et al. Human megakaryocytes. I. Characterization of the membrane and cytoplasmic components of isolated marrow megakaryocytes. *J Exp Med* 1979;149:1273–1287.

102. Rabellino EM, Levene RB, Leung LLK, et al. Human megakaryocytes. II. Expression of platelet proteins in early marrow megakaryocytes. *J Exp Med* 1981;154:85–100.

103. Vainchenker W, Deschamps JF, Bastin JM, et al. Two monoclonal antiplatelet antibodies as markers of human megakaryocyte maturation: immunofluorescent staining and platelet peroxidase detection in megakaryocyte colonies and *in vivo* cells from normal and leukemic patients. *Blood* 1982;59:514–521.

104. Vinci G, Tabilio A, Deschamps J-F, et al. Immunological study of *in vitro* maturation of human megakaryocytes. *Br J Haematol* 1984;56:589–605.

105. Debili N, Issaad C, Massé J-M, et al. Expression of CD34 and platelet glycoproteins during human megakaryocytic differentiation. *Blood* 1992;80: 3022–3035.

106. Tronik-Le Roux D, Roullot V, Schweitzer A, et al. Suppression of erythromegakaryocytopoiesis and the induction of reversible thrombocytopenia in mice transgenic for the thymidine kinase gene targeted by the platelet glycoprotein αIIb promoter. *J Exp Med* 1995;181:2141–2151.

107. Tropel P, Roullot V, Vernet M, et al. A 2.7-kb portion of the 5′flanking region of the murine glycoproteinIIb is transcriptionally active in primitive hematopoietic progenitor cells. *Blood* 1997;90:2995.

108. Mitjavila-Garcia MT, Cailleret M, Godin I, et al. Expression of CD41 on hematopoietic progenitors derived from embryonic hematopoietic cells. *Development* 2002;129:2003–2013.

109. Mikkola HK, Klintman J, Yang H, et al. Haematopoietic stem cells retain long-term repopulating activity and multipotency in the absence of stem-cell leukaemia SCL/tal-1 gene. *Nature* 2003;421:547–551.

110. Emambokus NR, Frampton J. The glycoprotein IIb molecule is expressed on early murine hematopoietic progenitors and regulates their numbers in sites of hematopoiesis. *Immunity* 2003;19:33–45.

111. Debili N, Robin C, Schiavon V, et al. Different expression of CD41 on human lymphoid and myeloid progenitors from adults and neonates. *Blood* 2001;97:2023–2030.

112. Debili N, Wendling F, Cosman D, et al. The Mpl receptor is expressed in the megakaryocytic lineage from late progenitors to platelets. *Blood* 1995;85:391–401.

113. Levene RB, Williams NT, Lamazierre J-MD, et al. Human megakaryocyte IV growth and characterization of clonable megakaryocyte progenitors in agar. *Exp Hematol* 1987;15:181–189.

114. Levene RB, Daniel Lemaziere JM, Broxmeyer HE, et al. Human megakaryocytes. V. Changes in the phenotypic profile of differentiating megakaryocytes. *J Exp Med* 1985;161:457–474.

115. Lepage A, Leboeuf M, Cazenave JP, et al. The αaIIbβ3 integrin and GPIb-V-IX complex identify distinct stages in the maturation of CD34(+) cord blood cells to megakaryocytes. *Blood* 2000;96:4169–4177.

116. Gewirtz AM, Boghosian-Sell L, Catani L, et al. Expression of FcγRII and CD4 receptors by normal human megakaryocytes. *Exp Hematol* 1992;20:512–516.

117. Kouri YH, Borkowsky W, Nardi M, et al. Human megakaryocytes have a CD4 molecule capable of binding human immunodeficiency virus-1. *Blood* 1993;81:2664–2670.

118. Hickey MJ, Roth GJ. Characterization of the gene encoding human platelet glycoprotein IX. *J Biol Chem* 1993;268:3438–3443.

119. Majumdar S, Gonder D, Koutis B, et al. Characterization of the human β-thromboglobulin gene. *J Biol Chem* 1991;266:5785–5789.

120. Prandini MH, Uzan G, Martin F, et al. Characterization of a specific erythromegakaryocytic enhancer within the glycoprotein IIb promoter. *J Biol Chem* 1992;267:10370–10374.

121. Ravid K, Doi T, Beeler L, et al. Transcriptional regulation of the rat platelet factor 4 gene: interaction between an enhancer/silencer domain and the GATA-1 site. *Mol Cell Biol* 1991;11:6116–6127.

122. Wenger RH, Kieffer N, Wicki AN, et al. Structure of the human blood platelet membrane glycoprotein Ibα gene. *Biochem Biophys Res Commun* 1988;156:389–395.

123. Orkin SH. GATA-binding transcription factors in hematopoietic cells. *Blood* 1992;80:575–581.

124. Raich N, Roméo PH. Erythroid regulatory elements. *Stem Cells* 1993;11:95–104.

125. Lemarchandel V, Ghysdael J, Mignotte V, et al. Gata and Ets *cis*-acting sequence mediate megakaryocyte-specific expression. *Mol Cell Biol* 1993;13:668–676.

126. Audit I, Eléouet JF, Roméo P-H. Transcriptional regulation of the pyruvate kinase erythroid specific promoter. *J Biol Chem* 1993;268:5431–5437.

127. Eléouet JF, Roméo PH. CCACC or Sp1 binding proteins cooperate with hGATA-1 to direct erythroid-specific transcription and to mediate 5′ HS-2 sensitivity of a TATA-less promoter. *Eur J Biochem* 1993;212:763–770.

128. Tsai S-F, Martin DI, Zon LI, et al. Cloning of the cDNA for the major DNA-binding protein of the erythroid lineage through expression in mammalian cells. *Nature* 1989;339:446–451.

129. Martin DIK, Zon LI, Mutter G, et al. Expression of an erythroid transcription factor in megakaryocytic and mast cell lineages. *Nature* 1990;344:444–447.

130. Roméo P-H, Prandini MH, Joulin V, et al. Megakaryocytic and erythrocytic lineages share specific transcription factors. *Nature* 1990;344:447–449.

131. Pevny L, Simon MC, Roberston E, et al. Erythroid differentiation in chimeric mice blocked by a targeted mutation in the gene for transcription factor GATA-1. *Nature.* 1991;349:257–261.

132. Shivdasani R, Fujiwara Y, McDevit M, et al. A lineage-selective knockout establishes the critical role of transcription factor GATA-1 in megakaryocyte growth and platelet development. *EMBO J* 1997;16:3965–3973.

133. Vyas P, Ault K, Jackson CW, et al. Consequences of GATA-1 deficiency in megakaryocytes and platelets. *Blood* 1999;93:2867–2875.

134. Nichols KE, Crispino JD, Poncz M, et al. Familial dyserythropoietic anaemia and thrombocytopenia due to an inherited mutation in *GATA1*. *Nat Genet* 2000;24:266–270.

135. Wechsler J, Greene M, McDevitt MA, et al. Acquired mutations in GATA1 in the megakaryoblastic leukemia of Down syndrome. *Nat Genet* 2002;32:148–152.

136. Groet J, McElwaine S, Spinelli M, et al. Acquired mutations in GATA1 in neonates with Down's syndrome with transient myeloid disorder. *Lancet* 2003;361:1617–1620.

137. Mouthon MA, Bernard O, Mitjavila MT, et al. Expression of tal-1 and GATA-binding proteins during human hematopoiesis. *Blood* 1993;81:647–655.

138. Shivdasani RA, Mayer E, Orkin SH. Absence of blood formation in mice lacking the T-cell leukaemia oncoprotein tal-1/SCL. *Nature* 1995;373:432–434

139. Song WJ, Sullivan MG, Legare RD, et al. Haploin sufficiency of CBFA2 causes familial thrombocytopenia with propensity to develop acute myelogenous leukaemia. *Nat Genet* 1999;23:166–175.

140. Elagib KE, Racke FK, Mogass M, et al. RUNX1 and GATA-1 coexpression and cooperation in megakaryocytic differentiation. *Blood* 2003;101:4333–4341.

141. Ichikawa M, Asai T, Saito T, et al. AML-1 is required for megakaryocytic maturation and lymphocytic differentiation, but not for maintenance of hematopoietic stem cells in adult hematopoiesis. *Nat Med* 2004;10:299–304.

142. Zhang L, Lemarchandel V, Romeo PH, et al. The Fli-1 proto-oncogene, involved in erythroleukemia and Ewing's sarcoma, encodes a transcriptional activator with DNA-binding specificities distinct from other Ets family members. *Oncogene* 1993;8:1621–1630.

143. Hart A, Melet F, Grossfeld P, et al. Fli-1 is required for murine vascular and megakaryocytic development and is hemizygously deleted in patients with thrombocytopenia. *Immunity* 2000;13:167–177.

144. Wang X, Crispino JD, Letting DL, et al. Control of megakaryocyte-specific gene expression by GATA-1 and FOG-1: role of Ets transcription factors. *EMBO J* 2002;21:5225–5234.

145. Shivdasani RA, Rosenblatt MF, Zucker-Franklin D, et al. Transcription factor NF-E2 is required for platelet formation independent of the actions of thrombopoietin/MGDF in megakaryocyte development. *Cell* 1995;81:695–704.

146. Lecine P, Villeval JL, Vyas P, et al. Mice lacking transcription factor NF-E2 provide *in vivo* validation of the proplatelet model of thrombocytopoiesis and show a platelet production defect that is intrinsic to megakaryocytes. *Blood* 1998;92:1608–1616.

147. Shavit JA, Motohashi H, Onodera K, et al. Impaired megakaryopoiesis and behavioral defects in mafG-null mutant mice. *Genes Dev* 1998;12:2164–2174.

148. Lecine P, Italiano JEJ, Kim SW, et al. Hematopoietic-specific beta 1 tubulin participates in a pathway of platelet biogenesis dependent on the transcription factor NF-E2. *Blood* 2000;96:1366–1373.

149. Schwer HD, Lecine P, Tiwari S, et al. A lineage-restricted and divergent beta-tubulin isoform is essential for the biogenesis, structure and function of blood platelets. *Curr Biol* 2001;11:579–586.

150. Nagata Y, Yoshikawa J, Hashimoto A, et al. Proplatelet formation of megakaryocytes is triggered by autocrine-synthesized estradiol. *Genes Dev* 2003;17:2864–2869.

151. Tiwari S, Italiano JEJ, Barral DC, et al. A role for Rab27b in NF-E2-dependent pathways of platelet formation. *Blood* 2003;102:3970–3979.

152. Deveaux S, Cohen-Kaminsky S, Shivdasani R, et al. p45 NF-E2 Regulates expression of thromboxane synthase in megakaryocytes. *EMBO J* 1997;16:5654–5661.

153. Vitrat N, Letestu R, Masse A, et al. Thromboxane synthase has the same pattern of expression as platelet specific glycoproteins during human megakaryocyte differentiation. *Thromb Haemost* 2000;83:759–768.

154. Tong B, Grimes HL, Yang TY, et al. The Gfi-1B proto-oncoprotein represses p21WAF1 and inhibits myeloid cell differentiation. *Mol Cell Biol* 1998;18:2462–2473.

155. Saleque S, Cameron S, Orkin SH. The zinc-finger proto-oncogene Gfi-1b is essential for development of the erythroid and megakaryocytic lineages. *Genes Dev* 2002;16:301–306.

156. Mercher T, Coniat MB, Monni R, et al. Involvement of a human gene related to the Drosophila spen gene in the recurrent t(1;22) translocation of acute megakaryocytic leukemia. *Proc Natl Acad Sci U S A* 2001;98:5776–5779.

157. Miralles F, Posern G, Zaromytidou AI, et al. Actin dynamics control SRF activity by regulation of its coactivator MAL. *Cell* 2003;113:329–342.

158. Ebbe S, Stohlman FJ, Donovan J, et al. Megakaryocytic maturation rate in thrombocytopenic rats. *Blood* 1968;32:787–795.

159. Levin J, Evatt BL. Humoral control of thrombopoiesis. *Blood Cells* 1979;5:105–121.

160. McDonald TP. Thrombopoietin: its biology, purification, and characterization. *Exp Hematol* 1988;16:201–205.

161. Williams N, Eger RR, Jackson HM, et al. Two-factor requirement for murine megakaryocyte colony formation. *J Cell Physiol* 1982;110:101–104.

162. Ebbe S, Phalen E, Stohlman FJ. Abnormalities of megakaryocytes in $Sl/Sl^d$ mice. *Blood* 1973;42:865–869.

163. Ebbe S, Phalen E, Stohlman FJ. Abnormalities of megakaryocytes in $W/W^v$ mice. *Blood* 1973;42:857–862.

164. Ebbe S, Carpenter D, Yee T. Megakaryocytopenia in $W/W^v$ mice is accompanied by an increase in size within ploidy groups and acceleration of maturation. *Blood* 1989;74:94–98.

165. Ebbe S, Phalen E. Regulation of megakaryocytes in $W/W^v$ mice. *J Cell Physiol* 1978;96:73–79.

166. Hunt P, Zsebo KM, Hokom MM, et al. Evidence that stem cell factor is involved in the rebound thrombocytosis that follows 5-Fluorouracil treatment. *Blood* 1992;80:904–911.

167. Avraham H, Vannier E, Cowley S, et al. Effects of the stem cell factor, c-kit ligand, on human megakaryocytic cells. *Blood* 1992;79:365–371.

168. Briddell RA, Bruno E, Cooper RJ, et al. Effect of c-kit ligand on *in vitro* human megakaryocytopoiesis. *Blood* 1991;78:2854–2859.

169. Debili N, Massé J, Katz A, et al. Effects of recombinant hematopoietic growth factors (IL-3, IL6, SCF, LIF) on the megakaryocyte differentiation of CD34 positive cells. *Blood* 1993;82:84–95.

170. Tanaka R, Koike K, Imai T, et al. Stem cell factor enhances proliferation, but not maturation, of murine megakaryocytic progenitors in serum-free culture. *Blood* 1992;80:1743–1749.

171. Debili N, Breton-Gorius J. Hemopoietic growth factors and human megakaryocyte differentiation. *Bone Marrow Transpl* 1992;9(Suppl. 1): 11–15.

172. Bruno E, Briddell R, Hoffman R. Effect of recombinant and purified hematopoietic growth factors on human megakaryocyte colony formation. *Exp Hematol* 1988;16:371–377.

173. Lu L, Briddell RA, Graham CD, et al. Effect of recombinant and purified human haematopoietic growth factors on *in vitro* colony formation by enriched populations of human megakaryocyte progenitor cells. *Br J Haematol* 1988;70:149–156.

174. Mazur EM, Cohen JL, Bogart L, et al. Recombinant gibbon interleukin-3 stimulates megakaryocyte colony growth *in vitro* from human peripheral blood progenitor cells. *J Cell Physiol* 1988;136:439–446.

175. Sieff C, Niemeyer CM, Nathan DG, et al. Stimulation of human hematopoietic colony formation by recombinant gibbon multi-colony-stimulating factor or interleukin 3. *J Clin Invest* 1987;80:818–823.

176. Messner HA, Yarnasky K, Jama N, et al. Growth of human hemopoietic colonies in response to recombinant gibbon interleukin 3. Comparison with human recombinant granulocyte and granulocyte-macrophage colony stimulating factor. *Proc Natl Acad Sci U S A* 1987;84:6765–6769.

177. Quesenberry PJ, McGrath HE, Williams ME, et al. Multifactor stimulation of megakaryocytopoiesis: effect of interleukin 6. *Exp Hematol* 1991;19:35–41.

178. Mazur EM, Cohen JE, Wong CG, et al. Modest stimulating effect of recombinant human GM-CSF on colony growth from peripheral blood human megakaryocyte progenitor cells. *Exp Hematol* 1987;15:1128–1133.

179. Farese AM, Williams DE, Seiler FR, et al. Combination protocols of cytokine therapy with interleukin-3 and granulocyte-macrophage colony-stimulating factor in a primate model of radiation-induced marrow aplasia. *Blood* 1993;82:3012–3018.

180. Brown JR, Demetri GD. Challenges in the development of platelet growth factors: low expectations for low counts. *Curr Hematol Rep* 2002;1: 110–118.

181. Sakaguchi M, Kawakita M, Matsushita J, et al. Human erythropoietin stimulates murine megakaryocytopoiesis in serum free culture. *Exp Hematol* 1987;15:1028–1034.

182. Williams N, Jackson H, Iscove NN, et al. The role of erythropoietin, thrombopoietic stimulating factor, and myeloid colony-stimulating factors. *Exp Hematol* 1984;12:734–744.

183. Dessypris EN, Gleaton JH, Armstrong OL. Effect of human recombinant erythropoietin on human marrow megakaryocyte colony formation *in vitro*. *Br J Haematol* 1987;67:265–269.

184. An E, Ogata K, Kuriya S, et al. Interleukin-6 and erythropoietin act as direct potentiators and inducers of *in vitro* cytoplasmic process formation on purified mouse megakaryocytes. *Exp Hematol* 1994;22:149–156.

185. Dessypris EN, Graber SE, Krantz SB, et al. Effects of recombinant erythropoietin on the concentration and cycling status of human marrow hematopoietic progenitor cells *in vivo*. *Blood* 1988;72:2060–2062.

186. Eschbach JW, Abdlhadi MH, Browne JK, et al. Recombinant human erythropoietin in anemic patients with end-stage renal disease. *Ann Intern Med* 1989;111:992–1000.

187. Stone WJ, Graber SE, Krantz SB, et al. Treatment of the anemia of predialysis patients with recombinant human erythropoietin: a randomized placebo-controlled trial. *Am J Med Sci* 1988;296:171–179.

188. Kishimoto T, Taga T, Akira S. Cytokine signal transduction. *Cell* 1994;76: 253–262.

189. Kishimoto T. The biology of interleukin-6. *Blood* 1989;74:1–10.

190. Navarro S, Debili N, Le Couedic J-P, et al. Interleukin-6 and its receptor are expressed by human megakaryocytes. *In vitro* effects on proliferation and endoreplication. *Blood* 1991;77:461–471.

191. Leary AG, Zeng HQ, Clark SC, et al. Growth factor requirements for survival in G₀ and entry into the cell cycle of primitive human hemopoietic progenitors. *Proc Natl Acad Sci U S A* 1992;89:4013–4017.

192. Ikebuchi K, Wong GG, Clark SC, et al. Interleukin 6 enhancement of interleukin 3-dependent proliferation of multipotential hemopoietic progenitors. *Proc Natl Acad Sci U S A* 1987;84:9035–9039.

193. Ishibashi T, Kimura H, Uchida T, et al. Human interleukin 6 is a direct promoter of maturation of megakaryocytes *in vitro*. *Proc Natl Acad Sci U S A* 1989;86:5953–5957.

194. Kimura H, Ishibashi T, Shikama Y, et al. Interleukin-1 beta (IL-1β) induces thrombocytosis in mice: possible implication of IL-6. *Blood* 1990; 76:2493–2500.

195. Kimura H, Ishibashi T, Uchida T, et al. Interleukin 6 is a differentiation factor for human megakaryocytes *in vitro*. *Eur J Immunol* 1990;20:1927–1931.

196. Navarro S, Mitjavila M-T, Katz A, et al. Expression of Interleukin 6 and its specific receptor by untreated and PMA-stimulated human erythroid and megakaryocytic cell lines. *Exp Hematol* 1991;19:11–17.

197. Gainsford T, Nandurkar H, Metcalf D, et al. The residual megakaryocyte and platelet production in c-mpl-deficient mice is not dependent on the actions of interleukin-6, interleukin-11, or leukemia inhibitory factor. *Blood* 2000;95:528–534.

198. Hill RJ, Warren MK, Stenberg P, et al. Stimulation of megakaryocytopoiesis in mice by human recombinant interleukin-6. *Blood* 1991;77:42–48.

199. Stahl CP, Zucker-Franklin D, Evatt BL, et al. Effects of human interleukin-6 on megakaryocyte development and thrombocytopoiesis in primates. *Blood* 1991;78:1467–1475.

200. Burstein S, Mei R-L, Henthorn J, et al. Leukemia inhibitory factor and interleukin-11 promote maturation of murine and human megakaryocytes *in vitro*. *J Cell Physiol* 1992;153:305–312.

201. Geissler K, Valent P, Bettelheim P, et al. *In vivo* synergism of recombinant human interleukin-3 and recombinant human interleukin-6 on thrombopoiesis in primates. *Blood* 1992;79:1155–1160.

202. Metcalf D, Hilton D, Nicola NA. Leukemia inhibitory factor can potentiate murine megakaryocyte production *in vitro*. *Blood* 1991;77:2150–2153.

203. Metcalf D, Nicola NA, Gearing DP. Effects of injected leukemia inhibitory factor in hematopoietic and other tissues in mice. *Blood* 1990;76: 50–56.

204. Burstein SA, Downs T, Friese P, et al. Thrombocytopoiesis in normal and sublethally irradiated dogs: response to human interleukin-6. *Blood* 1992;80:420–428.

205. Escary JL, Perreau J, Dumenil D, et al. Leukaemia inhibitory factor is necessary for maintenance of haematopoietic stem cells and thymocyte stimulation. *Nature* 1993;63:361–364.

206. Teramura M, Kobayashi S, Hoshino S, et al. Interleukin-11 enhances human megakaryocytopoiesis *in vitro*. *Blood* 1992;79:327–331.

207. Bruno E, Briddell RA, Cooper J, et al. Effects of recombinant interleukin 11 on human megakaryocyte progenitor cells. *Exp Hematol* 1991;19: 378–381.

208. Neben TY, Loebelenz J, Hayes L, et al. Recombinant human interleukin-11 stimulates megakaryocytopoiesis and increases peripheral platelets in normal andd splenectomized mice. *Blood* 1993;81:901–908.

209. Hawley RG, Fong AZC, Ngan Y, et al. Progenitor cell hyperplasia with rare development of myeloid leukemia in interleukin 11 bone marrow chimeras. *J Exp Med* 1993;178:1175–1188.

210. Reynolds C. Clinical efficacy of rhIL-11. *Oncology (Huntingt)* 2000;14: 32–40.

211. Nagasawa T, Tachibana K, Kishimoto T. A novel CXC chemokine PBSF/SDF-1 and its receptor CXCR4: their functions in development, hematopoiesis and HIV infection. *Semin Immunol* 1998;10:179–185.

212. Nagasawa T, Hirota S, Tachibana K, et al. Defects of B-cell lymphopoiesis and bone-marrow myelopoiesis in mice lacking the CXC chemokine PBSF/SDF-1. *Nature* 1996;382(6592):635–638.

213. Zou YR, Kottmann AH, Kuroda M, et al. Function of the chemokine receptor CXCR4 in haematopoiesis and in cerebellar development. *Nature* 1998;393:595–599.

214. Peled A, Petit I, Kollet O, et al. Dependence of human stem cell engraftment and repopulation of NOD/SCID mice on CXCR4. *Science* 1999; 283:845–848.

215. Lapidot T, Kollet O. The essential roles of the chemokine SDF-1 and its receptor CXCR4 in human stem cell homing and repopulation of transplanted immune-deficient NOD/SCID and NOD/SCID/B2m(null) mice. *Leukemia* 2002;16:1992–2003.

216. Ma Q, Jones D, Springer TA. The chemokine receptor CXCR4 is required for the retention of B lineage and granulocytic precursors within the bone marrow microenvironment. *Immunity* 1999;10:463–471.

217. Levesque JP, Hendy J, Takamatsu Y, et al. Disruption of the CXCR4/CXCL12 chemotactic interaction during hematopoietic stem cell mobilization induced by GCSF or cyclophosphamide. *J Clin Invest* 2003; 111:187–196.

218. Lataillade JJ, Clay D, Bourin P, et al. Stromal cell-derived factor 1 regulates primitive hematopoiesis by suppressing apoptosis and by promoting G(0)/G(1) transition in CD34(+) cells: evidence for an autocrine/paracrine mechanism. *Blood* 2002;99:1117–1129.

219. Cashman J, Clark-Lewis I, Eaves A, et al. Stromal-derived factor 1 inhibits the cycling of very primitive human hematopoietic cells *in vitro* and in NOD/SCID mice. *Blood* 2002;99:792–799.

220. Wang JF, Liu ZY, Groopman JE. The alpha-chemokine receptor CXCR4 is expressed on the megakaryocytic lineage from progenitor to platelets and modulates migration and adhesion. *Blood* 1998;92:756–764.

221. Guerriero R, Mattia G, Testa U, et al. Stromal cell-derived factor 1alpha increases polyploidization of megakaryocytes generated by human hematopoietic progenitor cells. *Blood* 2001;97:2587–2595.

222. Avecilla ST, Hattori K, Heissig B, et al. Chemokine-mediated interaction of hematopoietic progenitors with the bone marrow vascular niche is required for thrombopoiesis. *Nat Med* 2004;10:64–71.

223. Briddell RA, Brandt JE, Leemhuiss TB, et al. Role of cytokines in sustaining long-term human megakaryocytopoiesis *in vitro*. *Blood* 1992;79: 332–337.

224. Shimoda K, Okamura S, Harada N, et al. Identification of a functional receptor for granulocyte colony-stimulating factor on platelets. *J Clin Invest* 1993;91:1310–1313.

225. Fujiki H, Kimura T, Minamiguchi H, et al. Role of human interleukin-9 as a megakaryocyte potentiator in culture. *Exp Hematol* 2002;30: 1373–1380.

226. Bruno E, Cooper RJ, Wilson EL, et al. Basic fibroblast growth factor promotes the proliferation of human megakaryocyte progenitor cells. *Blood* 1993;82:430–435.

227. Han ZC, Bellucci S, Wan HY, et al. New insights into the regulation of megakaryocytopoiesis by haematopoietic and fibroblastic growth factors and transforming growth factor β1. *Br J Haematol* 1992;81:1–5.

228. Bikfavi A, Han ZC, Fuhrmann G. Interaction of fibroblast growth factor (FGF) with megakaryocytopoiesis and demonstration of FGF receptor

expression in megakaryocytes and megakaryocyte-like cells. *Blood* 1992; 80:1905–1913.

229. Kashiwakura I, Takahashi TA. Basic fibroblast growth factor-stimulated *ex vivo* expansion of haematopoietic progenitor cells from human placental and umbilical cord blood. *Br J Haematol* 2003;122:479–488.

230. Vainchenker W, Chapman J, Deschamps JF, et al. Normal human serum contains a factor(s) capable of inhibiting megakaryocyte colony formation. *Exp Hematol* 1982;10:650–660.

231. Kimura H, Burstein SA, Thorming SA, et al. Human megakaryocytic progenitors (CFU-M) assaying in methylcellulose: physical characteristics and requirements for growth. *J Cell Physiol* 1984;118:87–96.

232. Messner HA, Jamal N, Izaguirre CA. The growth of large megakaryocyte colonies from human bone marrow. *J Cell Physiol* 1982;1(Suppl. 1):45–51.

233. Abgrall J, Han Z, Sensebe L, et al. Inhibitory effect of highly purified human platelet beta-thromboglobulin on *in vitro* human megakaryocyte colony formation. *Exp Hematol* 1991;19:202–205.

234. Gewirtz AM, Calabretta B, Rucinski B, et al. Inhibition of human megakaryocytopoiesis by platelet factor 4 (PF4) and a synthetic C-terminal PF4 peptide. *J Clin Invest* 1989;83:1477–1486.

235. Han ZC, Bellucci S, Walz A, et al. Negative regulation of human megakaryocytopoiesis by human platelet factor 4 (PF4) and connective tissue-activating peptide III (CTAP-III). *Int J Cell Cloning* 1990;8:253–259.

236. Caen J-P, Han ZC. Contrôle du développement du megacaryocyte: des données fondamentales aux résultats cliniques. *C R Acad Sci Paris* 1993;316:925–930.

237. Dessypris EN, Gleaton JH, Sawyer ST, et al. Suppression of maturation of megakaryocyte colony forming unit *in vitro* by a platelet released glycoprotein. *J Cell Physiol* 1987;130:361–368.

238. Ishibashi T, Miller SL, Burstein SA. Type beta transforming growth factor is a potent inhibitor of murine megakaryocytopoiesis *in vitro*. *Blood* 1987;69:1737–1741.

239. Mitjavila MT, Vinci G, Villeval JL, et al. Human platelet alpha granules contain a non specific inhibitor of megakaryocyte colony formation: its relationship to type $\beta$ transforming growth factor (TGF-$\beta$). *J Cell Physiol* 1988;134:93–100.

240. Solberg LA, Tucker RF, Grant MN, et al. Transforming growth factor-$\beta$ inhibits colony formation from megakaryocytic, erythroid and multipotent stem cells. In: Najman A, Guigon M, eds. *The inhibitors of hematopoiesis*, Vol. 162. Paris: Colloque INSERM, John Libbey Eurotext, 1987:111–121.

241. Cashman JD, Eaves AC, Raines EW, et al. Mechanisms that regulate the cell cycle status of very primitive hematopoietic cells in long-term human marrow cultures. I. Stimulatory role of a variety of mesenchymal cell activators and inhibitory role of TGF-$\beta$. *Blood* 1990;75:96–101.

242. Keller JS, McNIece IK, Sill KT, et al. Transforming growth factor $\beta$ directly regulates primitive murine hematopoietic cell proliferation. *Blood* 1990; 75:596–602.

243. Kuter DJ, Gminski DM, Rosenberg RD. Transforming growth factor $\beta$ inhibits megakaryocyte growth and endomitosis. *Blood* 1992;79:619–626.

244. Kalina U, Koschmieder S, Hofmann WK, et al. Transforming growth factor-beta1 interferes with thrombopoietin-induced signal transduction in megakaryoblastic and erythroleukemic cells. *Exp Hematol* 2001;29:602–608.

245. Carlino JA, Higley HR, Creson JR, et al. Transforming growth factor $\beta$1 systemically modulates granuloid, erythroid, lymphoid, and thrombocytic cells in mice. *Exp Hematol* 1992;20:943–950.

246. Oda M, Kurasawa Y, Todokoro K, et al. Thrombopoietin-induced CXC chemokines, NAP-2 and PF4, suppress polyploidization and proplatelet formation during megakaryocyte maturation. *Genes Cells* 2003;8:9–15.

247. Graham GJ, Wright EG, Hewick R, et al. Identification and characterization of an inhibitor of haematopoietic stem cell proliferation. *Nature* 1990;344:442–444.

248. Yang M, Li K, Ng MH, et al. Thrombospondin-1 inhibits *in vitro* megakaryocytopoiesis via CD36. *Thromb Res* 2003;109:47–54.

249. Carlo-Stella C, Cazzola M, Ganser A, et al. Synergistic antiproliferative effect of recombinant interferon-$\gamma$ with recombinant interferon-$\alpha$ on chronic myelogenous leukemia hematopoietic progenitor cells (CFU-GEMM, CFU-MK, BFU-E, and CFU-GM). *Blood* 1988;72:1293–1299.

250. Ganser A, Carlo-Stella C, Greher J, et al. Effects of recombinant interferon alpha and gamma on human bone marrow-derived megakaryocytic progenitor cells. *Blood* 1987;70:1173–1178.

251. Sonoda Y, Kuzuyama Y, Tanaka S, et al. Human interleukin-4 inhibits proliferation of megakaryocyte progenitor cells in culture. *Blood* 1993; 81:624–630.

# CHAPTER 26 ■ PLATELETS: STRUCTURE RELATED TO FUNCTION

ELISABETH M. CRAMER AND MICHAËLA FONTENAY

Platelets are small, anucleated cells that circulate in the blood at an average concentration of 150 to $400 \times 10^9$ per L. Platelets constitute a primary defense against bleeding. As a consequence, in the absence of bleeding, they circulate in a basal resting state with minimal interaction with the other blood components and vessel wall (1). Their smooth, regular, and discoid shape is ideally designed to help them behave this way. On appropriate demand and stimulation, platelets flatten and spread on the denuded endothelium; then they recruit all of their diverse artillery of anatomic and functional capacities, becoming rough and sticky, to build a hemostatic plug and, secondary to their content in growth factors, to eventually contribute to wound healing. They are also involved in the generation of thrombotic disorders under pathologic circumstances. This chapter presents the structural tools involved in adapting the state of the platelet to the need of its environment.

## GENERALITY ON THE STRUCTURE OF RESTING PLATELETS

Circulating platelets are lentil (biconvex lens)-shaped (see Fig. 26-1). This shape is well preserved by citrate anticoagulant, but it is artifactually rounded up by ethylenediaminetetraacetic acid (EDTA). Human platelets have axes with mean lengths of 2.5 versus 0.5 $\mu$M and a volume ranging from 7 to 9 fL. They display striking heterogeneity among themselves. They are anucleated cells, produced by the fragmentation of the cytoplasm of a mother cell, the megakaryocyte (MK). The precise mechanisms that regulate this fragmentation are not yet fully clear (i.e., what subcellular events lead to the delimitation of the future platelet territories, determining their size and organelle content). Nevertheless, the surface glycoproteins (GPs), such as the GP Ib/IX/V complex, and the cytoskeleton, microtubules, and actin filaments play major roles, as evidenced by the association of pathologic disorders involving these structures with abnormal platelet volume.

The platelet volume histogram has the characteristic of a log–normal distribution (2). The same pattern is found in platelet populations with an increased number of newly born platelets. This observation has been considered evidence that platelet heterogeneity is established at platelet birth and is not a consequence of aging. It coincides with the ultrastructural aspects of proplatelet budding and constriction zones and with a decrease in size of the future platelet territories along the proplatelet length: the smaller, the more distal; and the larger, the closer to the cell core (3). Platelet size and density also are under the control of MK size and ploidy (e.g., high ploidy MKs give rise to platelets rich in canalicular membranes, thereby with a low density) (4,5).

## LIGHT MICROSCOPIC EXAMINATION OF PLATELETS

On blood smeared from the fingertip, platelets tend to form aggregates. In the presence of anticoagulant, they appear as relatively sparse, tiny cellular elements spaced on the smear. After Wright stain and panoptic stains, two main zones are evident: the hyalomere, a peripheral transparent or slightly basophilic zone formed by the peripheral membrane and cytoskeleton elements, and the centrally located granulomere, containing azurophilic granulations corresponding to the cytoplasmic organelles, mainly secretory granules, and mitochondria. The most numerous are $\alpha$-granules, characterized by their dense core, rich in proteoglycans, which are responsible for azurophilia. Indeed, pathologic platelets deprived of this dense nucleoid appear colorless on Wright stain. Moreover, gray platelets (e.g., from the gray platelet syndrome), which lack morphologically recognizable $\alpha$-granules, also look gray on Wright and Romanowsky stain. Apart from appreciating the number, size, and tinctorial affinity, light microscopic examination of platelets is quite limited.

## ULTRASTRUCTURE

For the sake of clarity, platelet ultrastructure (see Fig. 26-2) is subdivided into three topographical parts related to function.

- The platelet membranes/intracellular and extracellular interactions
- The granules and intracytoplasmic organelles/platelet secretion
- The cytoskeleton/motor proteins

### Plasma Membrane

The first aim of platelet function is to maintain vascular integrity and to stop bleeding. To ensure this function, the platelet surface plays a crucial role of contact, first ensuring adhesion to the exposed subendothelium components, and then aggregation of platelets to build the platelet plug. It is difficult and artificial to describe sequential physiologic events that lead to eventual control of hemorrhage by looking at isolated platelets in suspension. Nevertheless, analysis of sequential physiologic changes in the protein organization of the platelet surface during *in vitro* activation helps clarify the puzzle of building the platelet plug.

The platelet is surrounded by the plasma membrane that extends through multiple channels of the *surface-connected canalicular system* (SCCS). Through the electron microscope, the platelet membrane, like most biological membranes, appears

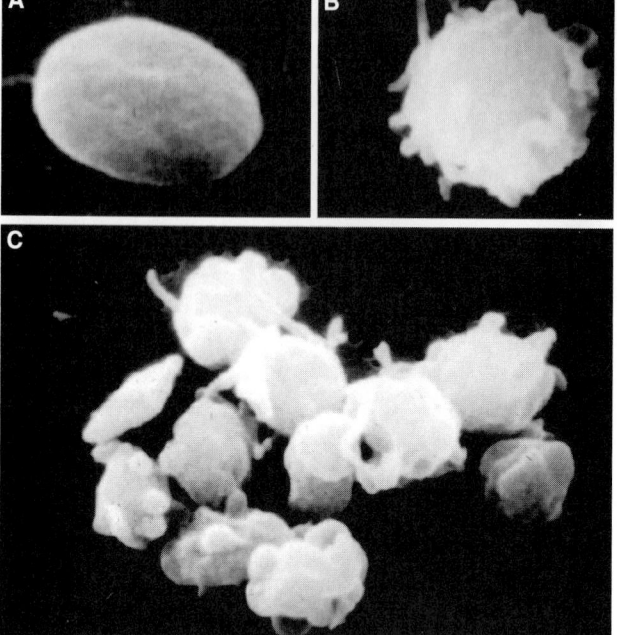

**FIGURE 26-1.** Scanning electron microscopic view of human platelets undergoing activation. **A:** Smooth, lentil-shaped platelets tend to round up and become spheroid, whereas short filopods extend from the surface. **B:** The platelet surface becomes rough and ruffled. **C:** Platelets develop contacts among each other through their filopods.

as a trilaminar unit membrane made of two dense leaflets separated by a constant space, the overall structure being 20 nm thick. The plasma membrane plays the fundamental role of maintaining cytoplasmic integrity because it is the surface of external interaction between vascular and plasma proteins and platelets, and of intracellular interaction with cytoskeletal elements. Therefore, it is the main mediator for the platelet functions of adhesion, secretion, aggregation, and final contraction.

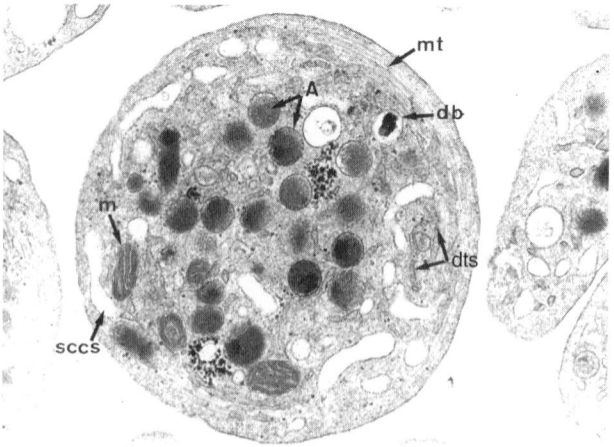

**FIGURE 26-2.** Electron microscopic view of a platelet section shows the various intracellular compartments. A ring of microtubules (*mt*) circles the cell periphery. The plasma membrane (pm) invaginates at several points to form the surface-connected canalicular system (*SCCS*). This system is closely associated with the dense tubular system (*dts*), a residual of the smooth endoplasmic reticulum. Secretion granules, among which the most numerous are the α-granules (*A*), are recognizable because of a dense nucleoid (*arrowhead*). Dense bodies or granules (*db*) display natural electron density of their core. Mitochondria (*m*) and glycogen are scattered in the cytoplasm (magnification, ×40,000).

Platelet membranes do not differ from other biologic membranes and are composed of proteins and lipids. The major membrane lipids are phospholipids and cholesterol. Phospholipids are arranged as a bilayer, with their polar heads oriented to the external and internal aqueous milieu and their long acyl chains positioned perpendicular to the plane of the membrane, forming a hydrophobic chain. They are deployed asymmetrically within the bilayer: Neutral phospholipids are located predominantly at the outer layer, and anionic phospholipids are placed mainly in the inner layer. Cholesterol molecules intercalated between phospholipid molecules are solubilized by phospholipids, and variations in cholesterol–phospholipid ratios modulate the fluidity of the lipid bilayer.

The plasma membrane determines permeability properties, is sensitive to surface-active agents, and supplies lipid activators to coagulation. Receptor GPs are anchored in the lipid bilayer, their glycosylated receptor component turned toward the plasmatic side. The glycocalix or cell coat appears as a fuzzy layer, 20 to 30 nm thick, lining the entire cell surface when observed by negative stain (6). The cell coat is made up of the oligosaccharide side chains of glycolipids and integral membrane GPs and the polysaccharide chains of integral membrane proteoglycans. In addition, adsorbed proteins, such as albumin and fibrinogen, and adsorbed plasma proteoglycans, contribute to the glycocalyx. The membrane-associated pool of plasma proteins constitutes the first line of interaction of the platelet with its environment and participates in the process of plasma protein endocytosis and further storage into secretion granules. Antigens, GP receptors, and several enzymes are embedded in the coat material. The exterior coat provides platelets with their potential adhesive properties. This anatomic entity is more prominent than on any other circulating blood cell, red or white, and reflects the close and permanent interaction of the platelet with its extracellular medium, namely plasma proteins. The old-fashioned concept of a periplatelet atmosphere, if too vague in its molecular definition, is nevertheless a good illustration of the fact that platelets carry their functional environment within themselves. The glycocalix also is responsible for the strong negative charge of the platelet surface, which repels undesired interactions with other cellular elements of the vascular wall and circulating blood. Several glycosylphosphatidyl inositol (GPI)-anchored proteins are found at the platelet surface, including the prion protein PrP (7).

The platelet membrane invaginates to give rise to a system of channels and canalicules that forms a network within the entire cytoplasmic volume, the SCCS (see Fig. 26-3). Within the invaginated surface membrane domain, the glycocalix seems to be less developed: It is noteworthy that immunolabeling for GP Ib shows, as an example, that this GP is preferentially located around the cell surface and that labeling within the SCCS is only minimal. Moreover, the glycosylated tails of the molecules appear to constitute an obturation at the opening of the canalicular system, possibly forming a filter to control the entry of plasma proteins. These openings widen after platelets become activated and actin polymerizes, and in parallel, GP Ib redistributes to the surface of the canalicular system.

This chapter concentrates on the data provided by morphologic examinations, mainly ultrastructural. On the resting platelet surface, several GPs that play a role during the first steps of platelet activation can be immunolabeled by specific antibodies, showing that they display an even and regular distribution. The complementary data provided by electron microscopic examination gives details about the distribution of the intracellular pools of the major functional platelet membrane GPs.

(a) The adhesion receptor formed with the complex of three types of GPs (GP Ib, GP IX, and GP V) is the receptor for surface-bound subendothelial von Willebrand factor (VWF) and also binds thrombin. The *GP Ib/IX/V complex*

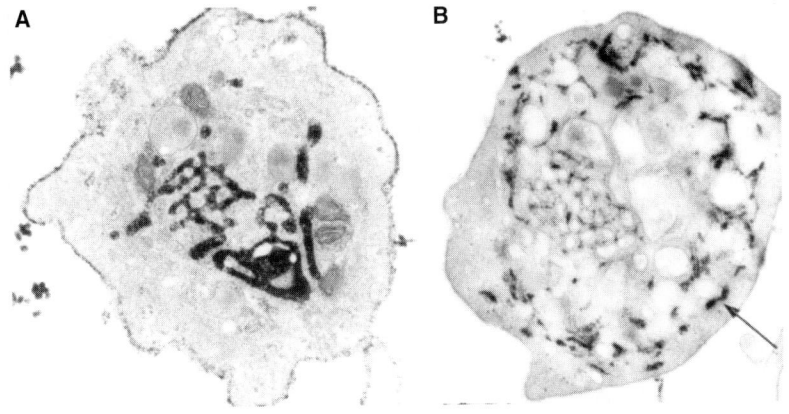

**FIGURE 26-3. A:** Within the platelet intracellular space extends a vast surface-connected canalicular system (SCCS) connected to the surface membrane. This surface connection is demonstrated by the penetration of extracellular electron-dense tracers; here, horseradish peroxidase (magnification, ×27,300). **B:** Close to the SCCS is the dense tubular system (*arrow*). It originates from the endoplasmic reticulum of megakaryocytes and is specifically visualized by electron microscopy (EM) because of its content of cyclooxygenase, here cytochemically detected by its peroxidase activity (*arrow*) (magnification, ×26,730).

is the paradigm of receptors implicated in platelet adhesion (8,9). Correlated with this function, immunogold labeling for the three components shows that this GP complex is present along the cell surface of resting platelets. However, the channels of the SCCS display only occasional and weak labeling for the complex. In addition, between 5% and 10% of the total platelet labeling is also present on the granule membrane, where it is colocalized with its stored ligand, VWF (10). Because of the connection of the GP Ib/IX/V complex with the network of submembranous actin through actin-binding protein (ABP) (11), it is possible that the differential distribution of GP Ib/IX/V along the membrane reflects the architecture of the actin meshwork, preferentially underlining the platelet surface. The attachment of this GP complex to the contractile proteins is particularly important in the modulation of platelet adhesive property after activation.

(b) *GP VI*, the major activating receptor for collagen, is also involved in the early events of platelet function. It plays a crucial role in collagen-induced activation and aggregation.

(c) *GP IIb/IIIa* ($\alpha_{IIB}\beta_3$) is the principal aggregation receptor, and its main function is to bind fibrinogen (12); it also binds VWF at high shear rates. This GP complex is typical of the aggregative step. GP IIb/IIIa is homogeneously distributed on the cell surface. The same uniform pattern of distribution is present on the SCCS membrane. Furthermore, immunogold labeling performed on platelet sections allows the recognition of a consistent pool of GP IIb/IIIa at the limiting membrane of $\alpha$-granules (13), with the receptor site oriented toward the inside of the granule. This pool seems to account for as much as 30% of the total platelet pool of GP IIb/IIIa. The incorporation of plasma fibrinogen and its storage in the $\alpha$-granules has been demonstrated to be dependent on and regulated by the $\alpha$-granule pool of GP IIb/IIIa (14).

(d) *GP IV* (CD36) is involved in both the adhesive and aggregative properties of platelets. It functions as a receptor for collagen II and thrombospondin and is involved in signal transduction (15). Electron microscopic examination detected GP IV on the entire platelet surface and the canalicular system; it also showed its presence on the $\alpha$-granule membrane, accounting for approximately 20% of the total immunolabeling (16). A relation between granule GP IV and its stored ligand thrombospondin is not yet demonstrated.

(e) *GP Ia/IIa* ($\alpha_2\beta_1$) binds collagen, whereas GP Ic/IIa and GP Ic*/IIa ($\alpha_5\beta_1$, $\alpha_6\beta_1$) bind laminin and fibronectin, respectively; and the $\alpha_V\beta_3$ receptor, a minor component

present only in 100 copies per platelet, binds adhesive proteins such as fibrinogen, fibronectin, and VWF (17).

(f) *CD9 and platelet–endothelial cell adhesion molecule-1 (PECAM 1)* are components of the plasma and SCCS membranes. CD9 is a tetraspan protein demonstrated to be closely related to GP IIb/IIIa in platelet activation. It also may serve as a fibronectin receptor and may be involved in a receptor function for growth factors (18). PECAM 1 is an adhesion molecule associated with the cytoskeleton of activated platelets and also is expressed on endothelial cells (19). Immunogold studies of both proteins have allowed the recognition of a pool of these GPs located in the $\alpha$-granule membrane (25% of total cell immunolabeling) (13).

## Activated Platelet Membrane

After activation, constituents of the plasma membrane become reorganized and exposed to serve as a catalytic surface for plasma proteins: Anionic phospholipids asymmetrically located in the plasma membrane are repositioned from the inside to the outside layer after thrombin activation to promote clotting.

Contraction of the platelet cytoskeleton leads to the liberation and undulation of peripheral membranes and contributes to pseudopod formation (see Figs. 26-1 and 26-4). However, this is strictly controlled by the linkage of the plasma membrane proteins to elements of the platelet cytoskeleton located on the cytoplasmic side of the plasma membrane, particularly with the filamentous form of actin (20). Indeed, a network of crisscrossing and overlapping filaments lies just beneath the plasma membrane. On activation, major changes in the organization of the components of the plasma membrane occur. First, GP Ib is rapidly cleared from the cell surface and is translocated into the superficial channels of the SCCS (see Fig. 26-5). This was shown with a variety of agonists such as adenosine 5'-diphosphate (ADP), thrombin, and plasmin at low concentration (21,22). The unavailability of GP Ib on the platelet surface is evidenced *in vitro* by the parallel functional decrease in ristocetin agglutinability: This process is reversible and is not caused by receptor degradation, as shown by a constant GP Ib platelet content measured in cell lysate. At this stage, the inactivation of the agonists by a specific inhibitor leads to a complete restoration of platelet function and of ristocetin-induced agglutination (23). Glycocalicin, the glycosylated part of GP Ib, which is highly sensitive to enzymatic degradation, can be cleaved from the GP Ib molecule by thrombin and plasmin, showing that platelet coat and surface charge can be modified on activation; translocation to the intracellular compartments may be a way to protect the receptors from enzymatic degradation. As the GP complex is attached to the ABP, it is possible that its internalization is caused by

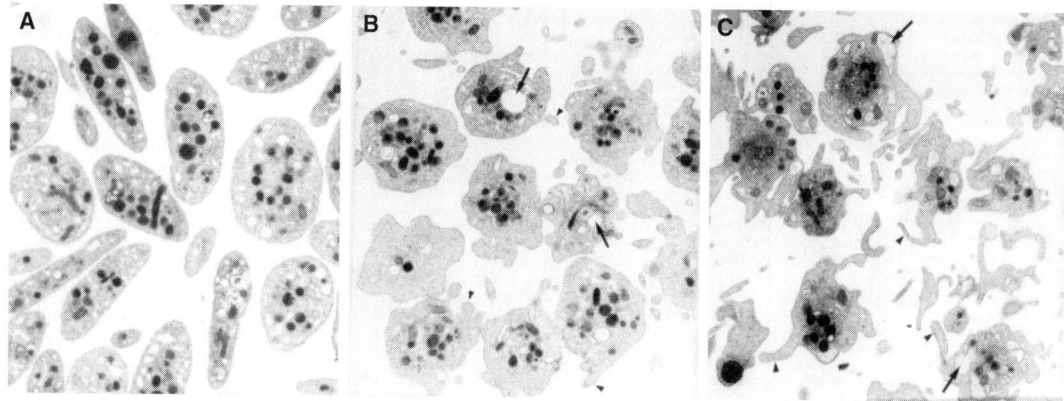

**FIGURE 26-4. A:** Electron microscopic view of a normal platelet population isolated from human blood. A striking feature is the heterogeneity among platelets: In spite of a generally regular discoid shape and smooth surface, platelets differ among themselves because of their size, content of secretion granules, and richness in surface canalicular system (magnification, ×13,400). **B:** When activated, platelets change shape, become spherical, and emit pseudopods (*arrowheads*). The microtubule ring contracts and cytoplasmic organelles tend to centralize. Initially, when aggregation is reversible, no secretion of α-granules occur, α-granules remain in the cell center, and the cisternae of the surface-connected canalicular system (SCCS) remain empty (*arrows*) (magnification, ×12,200). **C:** On stronger or more prolonged activation, platelets react as described in (**B**) but, in addition, α-granules that have been compressed toward the cell center fuse with the membrane limiting the SCCS and release their content in the lumen (*arrows*). Platelets are transformed into a sticky skeleton with a ball of microfilaments remaining in the cell center; long pseudopods (*arrowheads*) bristle the platelet surface.

actin contraction pulling GP Ib toward the inside of the cell in conjunction with contraction. Cytochalasin D completely blocks GP Ib internalization, showing the involvement of actin polymerization in this phenomenon. In parallel, clustering of the fibrinogen receptors (GP IIb/IIIa) occurs immediately after platelet activation (24), reflecting the necessity of cross-linking of the receptor for it to become functional (25).

The second event, which may or may not follow shape change, is the fusion of α-granules with the limiting membrane of the SCCS followed by secretion of their contents. The small G protein rap1b, which is expressed within platelets, is associated with membranes, including the SCCS and α-granule membranes, which suggests that it may be implicated in the secretion step (26). In addition, several cytoskeleton-signaling molecules have been identified in association with intracytoplasmic clathrin-coated vesicles responsible for the endocytic-exocytic transport (27). Finally, after secretion has occurred, the internalization of the GP Ib/IX complex from the plasma membrane into the SCCS is no longer fully reversible by specific inhibitors of platelet activation (28). After activation, the plasma membrane GP Ib decreases, whereas the level of expression of the other aggregative receptors, such as GP IIb/IIIa (Fig. 26-5B) and CD36, increases (10,29,30). These observations correlate with the passage of the platelet from an adhesive to an aggregative state.

Furthermore, during the early phase of platelet secretion, the immunoelectron observation of the localization of soluble proteins, such as fibrinogen, thrombospondin, and VWF, shows that these proteins redistribute from the matrix to the periphery of the α-granules and stick to the wall of the SCCS (31). This finding emphasizes the function of the α-granule associated receptors, which contribute to the presentation and concentration of adhesive-aggregative proteins on the platelet surface, leading to their optimal function.

## Dense Tubular System

The dense tubular system originates from the MK endoplasmic reticulum, of which it is the residue, and is composed of channels closely placed beside the SCCS cisternae. It is the site where calcium, important for triggering contraction of actomyosin, is sequestered, and resembles the sarcoplasmic reticulum of muscle cells. It contains several enzymatic activities, $Ca^{2+}$ adenosine triphosphate (ATP)ases, and cyclooxygenase II, which is cytochemically detectable by its characteristic platelet peroxidase activity and is involved in prostaglandin synthesis (32,33) (Fig. 26-3B). In diverse pathologies, both membrane systems may be in close apposition, forming a so-called membrane complex.

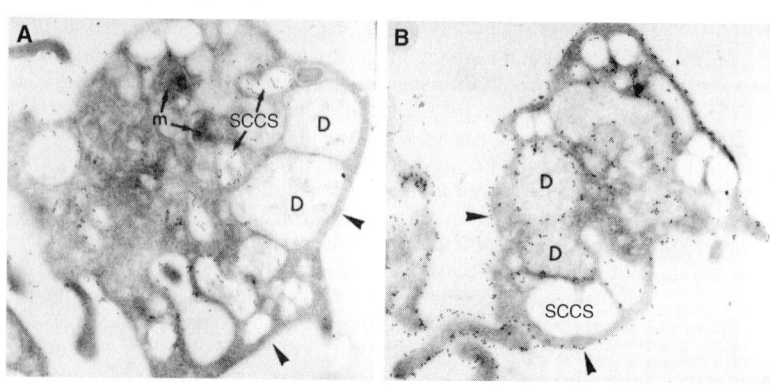

**FIGURE 26-5.** After platelets become activated, surface glycoproteins (GPs) move within the lipidic bilayer and segregate in different locations. **A:** GP Ib is cleared from the cell surface (*arrrowheads*) and translocates to the internal membranes of the surface-connected canalicular system (*SCCS*). Some dilated cisterns (*D*) of the canalicular system are filled with granule secretion products (magnification, ×24,800). **B:** In parallel, GP IIbIIIa is still strongly expressed at the platelet surface (*arrowheads*), its plasma membrane expression having been enhanced by the fusion of the plasma membrane with the α-granule membrane (*D*, dilated SCCS cisterns) (magnification, ×24,800).

## Secretory Granules

Platelets contain four main types of cytoplasmic granules classified according to their respective ultrastructures, densities, and content: the granules, the dense bodies (or dense granules), the lysosomes, and the peroxisomes.

### α-Granules

α-Granules are the most prominent and numerous population of storage granules, with a mean number of 50 to 80 α-granules per platelet. They are formed during early MK maturation and arise from the trans-Golgi network (TGN) in the form of small vesicles and immature granules that transit through multivesicular bodies, then progressively enlarge and increase in density until they reach a definitive size (34).

**Morphology.** Mature granules are generally round or ovoid, with diameters ranging from 200 to 500 nm, each enclosed within a unit membrane. They sometimes display an elongated shape when platelets are fixed in whole blood without anticoagulant. This demonstrates that granules are able to deform according to the physicochemical state of their subcellular environment.

Their ultrastructure is characteristic (see Fig. 26-6). The matrix can be divided into three distinct zones with different densities under the electron microscope (35). A dark nucleoid is apparent early, when the granules are still small and the rest of the matrix electron lucent. Although mature MK granules appear identical to those within platelets, there is evidence that they can continue to acquire some of their content during platelet life, at least by endocytosis. The electron-dense nucleoid is the most characteristic region and has been shown to colocalize with proteoglycans and the platelet-specific proteins, β-thromboglobulin and platelet factor 4 (PF4). The light zone, located at the periphery and opposite the dense nucleoid, contains a group of one to five tubular structures, regularly spaced and aligned, and measuring 20 to 25 nm (36). They colocalize with VWF immunostaining and represent the coiled VWF. They are missing from platelets with type 3 von Willebrand disease that lack VWF (37). Their close resemblance with the tubules found in the Weibel-Palade bodies, which are VWF storage organelles in endothelial cells, shows that they correspond to VWF in its high-molecular-weight multimeric form (38). The intermediate zone is situated between the nucleoid and the light zone and is associated with labeling for fibrinogen, thrombospondin, and albumin, as well as growth factors. The unit membrane of the granules also contains membrane-associated receptors whose receptor sites are oriented toward the inner side of the membrane.

**Content.** α-granules contain a multifunctional array of adhesive proteins, coagulation factors, growth factors, protease inhibitors, and proteoglycans, as well as immunoglobulins. The α-granular proteins can be broadly subdivided into two classes: (i) Platelet-specific proteins absent from the plasma and synthesized within the MK (e.g., β-thromboglobulin and PF4) and (ii) proteins identical to those in the plasma, some of which are not synthesized by MK, such as fibrinogen, albumin, and fibronectin, and others that are synthesized in the MK, such as VWF, VWF AgII, coagulation factor V, thrombospondin, fibronectin, platelet-derived growth factor, transforming growth factor-β, vascular endothelial growth factor/vascular permeability factor, protein C inhibitor, protease-nexin-2 (amyloid protein precursor), high-molecular-weight kininogen, plasminogen, plasminogen activator inhibitor, platelet-derived collagenase inhibitor proteins, $α_2$-macroglobulin, $α_1$-antitrypsin, $α_2$-antiplasmin, and multimerin (P155) (39). This list continues to grow and is not exhaustive (see Table 25-1 in Chapter 25).

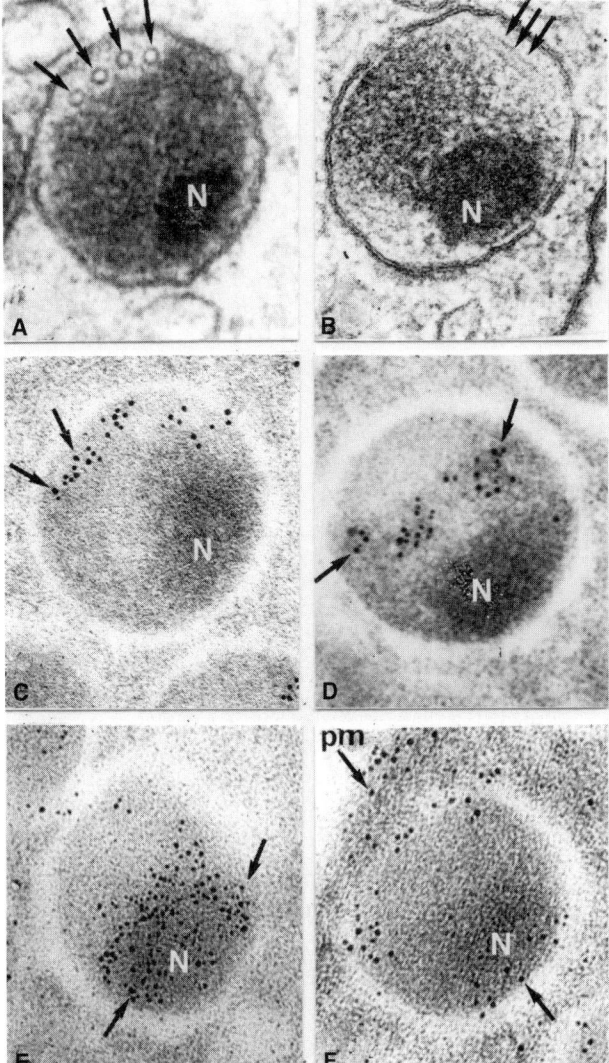

**FIGURE 26-6.** Compartmentalization within α-granules. When observed by transmission EM, α-granules exhibit evidence of compartmentalization of the various stored proteins into four distinct zones. **A:** An electron-dense nucleoid (N), opposite to it an electron lucent zone, and in between a zone of intermediary electron density. The granule is surrounded by a limiting membrane. In the electron lucent zone, tubular structures (here transversely sectioned) in groups of up to five can be seen (arrows); they represent the high-molecular-weight multimers of von Willebrand factor (VWF). **B:** On this section, the tubular structure is longitudinally sectioned (arrows) and is similar to the structures found in the Weibel-Palade bodies of endothelial cells that contain large VWF multimers. **C:** Immunogold labeling for VWF is restricted to the electron lucent zone (arrows) and colocalized with these tubules. **D:** In the intermediary zone, other proteins such as fibrinogen (arrows), albumin, and growth factors can be immunodetected. **E:** The dense nucleoid (N) of α-granules composed of proteoglycans and of platelet-specific proteins such as platelet factor 4 and β-thromboglobulin (arrows). **F:** The limiting membrane contains several types of receptors, either specific to the α-granule (e.g., P selectin) or shared with the plasma membrane (pm) (e.g., GP IIb/IIIa, shown here) (magnification, ×120,000).

The α-granule–limiting membrane has been shown to contain a number of different receptor molecules. Some are specific to the α-granule membrane. This is the case for P selectin (40), osteonectin, and GMP33; they are absent from the plasma membrane of resting platelets, and P selectin in particular becomes a marker of activation when expressed at the cell surface (see Fig. 26-7). The same reasoning can be applied to soluble

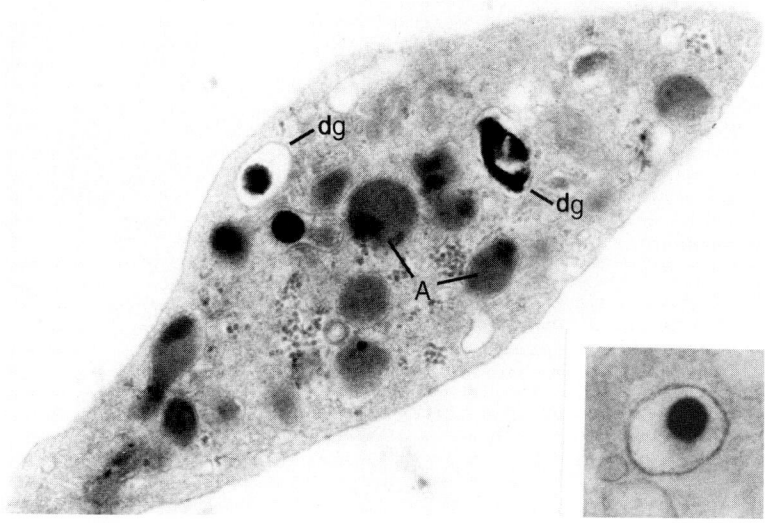

**FIGURE 26-7.** Dense granules (*dg*). Their natural electron density can be enhanced by specific cytochemical reactions. Several dense granule profiles often can be seen on the same platelet section. Wholemount preparations typically demonstrate an average number of two to seven dense granules per platelet. With the technique of White, dense granules can be distinguished from other granules by their enhanced density (magnification, ×27,300). *A*, α-granules **Inset:** The technique of Richards and Da Prada opacifies the dense granule limiting membrane as well (magnification, ×54,380).

platelet-specific granule proteins (β-thromboglobulin and PF4), which, when detected in the plasma, are accurate markers of platelet secretion and therefore of activation. Other receptors are present both on the α-granule membrane and on the plasma membrane of the resting platelets. This is the case for most plasma membrane proteins to different extents, the most striking example being GP IIb/IIIa (29), which is abundantly represented on α-granules. Other plasma membrane receptors [e.g., CD9, PECAM 1, and CD36 (GP IV) (13,16)] are found in the granule membrane at intermediary rates (10% to 30% of total), and the GP Ib/IX/V complex, although present, is only detected in trace amounts. The regulatory mechanism that leads certain plasma membrane receptors, such as GP IIb/IIIa, to be massively retained in the granule membrane, and others, such as the GP Ib/V/IX complex, to be only minimally internalized (about 10% of total platelet content in granules) is not known. But the EM observations are only static and cannot recognize constant compartment exchanges and receptor recycling. The study of a rare congenital disease, the gray platelet syndrome, helps the understanding of the role of α-granules in platelet physiology. In this syndrome, platelets contain abnormal empty α-granules that possess the α-granule membrane but no soluble contents (41). The origin of this abnormality is found in MK in which endogenously synthesized granule matricidal proteins are released in large amounts into the extracellular space within the lumen of the demarcation membrane system (42,43). Platelets of these patients appear gray after Romanowsky staining and exhibit a decreased aggregation response to ADP, collagen, and thrombin *in vitro* and therefore are a good model for studying the role of α-granules in hemostasis.

### Dense Granules (Dense Bodies)

Dense granules owe their name to their natural opacity to electrons in osmium-stained platelets and their capacity to be seen under the electron microscope on unstained preparations. There are between two and seven dense granules per platelet, and they measure approximately 200 to 300 nm in diameter. Under the electron microscope, they have a characteristic morphology distinct from the other cytoplasmic granules. They exhibit a dense core surrounded by a clear halo. Because of their low number, they are not observed on every platelet section by EM. Two cytochemical techniques have been used to enhance their natural electron density (Fig. 26-7): The technique of White (44) opacifies the serotonin content, and the technique of Richards and Da Prada (45) uses uranyl acetate to stain ADP and adenosine triphosphate (ATP). This technique

has the advantage of visualizing not only dense granule content but also its membrane, making detection more sensitive. Dense granules can also be visualized by fluorescent optical microscopy because of their ability to uptake a fluorescent dye derived from quinidine, mepacrine. This property also allows quantitative measurements to be made by flow cytometry (46).

Dense granules are the storage organelles for serotonin of powerful vasoconstrictive effect (90% of circulating serotonin is bound to platelets), catecholamines, divalent cations, $Ca^{2+}$ and $Mg^{2+}$, and the nonmetabolic pool of ADP and ATP. Finally, receptors have been identified in their limiting membrane, either specific such as granulophysin (CD63), whose function is unknown, or similar to the ones found in the granule membrane, for example, P selectin and GP IIb/IIIa (16,47). This raises the question of parenthood between these two types of granules, α-granules and dense granules. After activation, the dense granule content is directly secreted by fusion with the plasma membrane, unlike α-granules, which are centripetally secreted through the SCCS. The membrane proteins are translocated to the plasma membrane.

### Lysosomes

Lysosomes are granules smaller than 300 nm in diameter and homogeneous in structure. Only a few are present per platelet, and they can be visualized with specific, enzymatic cytochemical stains such as acid phosphatase, arylsulfatase, and β-glucuronidase. Using a sensitive ultrastructural technique for the detection of acid phosphatase based on cerium as the electron opaque agent, Behnke demonstrated the frequency of autophagic vacuoles and secondary lysosomes in platelets (48,49). The role of lysosomal enzymes during platelet activation seems to be related to their interaction with the vessel wall and digestion of matrix components. They also have a role inside the platelet, eliminating the autophagic debris. Several GPs, lysosome-associated membrane protein (LAMP)-1, LAMP-2, and CD63, are present in the lysosome membrane and redistribute to the cell surface after strong activation.

### Peroxisomes

In addition to the preceding three categories of secretory granules, a cytochemical technique that detects the peroxidase activity of catalase makes it possible to demonstrate that some of the small granules in platelets stain for catalase and are similar to peroxisomes found in many other tissues (50).

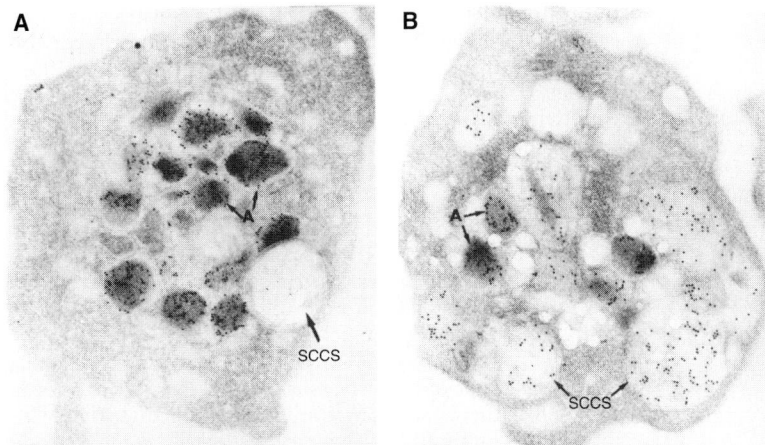

**FIGURE 26-8.** Immunogold labeling for fibrinogen in activated platelets. **A:** Initially, α-granules (*A*) that contain fibrinogen centralize and get close to the surface-connected canalicular system (*SCCS*) but do not secrete, and the lumen of the SCCS remains clear (*arrow*) (magnification, ×25,000). **B:** In the later stage, α-granules disappear from the cytoplasm, and their fibrinogen content is secreted into the dilated channels of the SCCS (magnification, ×25,000).

## Secretory Granules and Platelet Activation

Initially, when activation is reversible, α-granules centralize (see Figs. 26-4B and 26-8A), encompassed between the tightening microtubule belt. They come close to the cisternae of the SCCS but do not fuse with it. At the second stage, after activation is maintained or stronger agonists are used (thrombin, collagen, or ADP 20 μmol per L), the limiting membrane of the centralized granules fuse with that of the canalicular system and their contents are released into the channel lumen and disappear from the cytoplasm (Figs. 26-4C and 26-8B). The protein components of the granule membrane incorporated into the SCCS membrane, including P selectin, diffuse freely within the lipid bilayer and redistribute to the plasma membrane, where they are expressed (see Fig. 26-9). GP IIb/IIIa receptors that have undergone early activation bind their ligand fibrinogen early during secretion. Therefore, α-granule fibrinogen rather than plasma fibrinogen is preferentially linked to the α-granule receptor and appears to play a definite role in building the platelet aggregate (see Fig. 26-10). Fusion of α-granules, directly with the platelet plasma membrane or between themselves, is only seldom observed and seems to be a minor phenomenon (30,51).

The mode of secretion of dense granules is classically different, because they are able to migrate toward the cell periphery, where they are often located in the resting cell, and fuse with the plasma membrane, releasing their dense content directly into the extracellular medium. Studies performed on bovine platelets that lack SCCS have helped to describe this phenomenon.

The fate of lysosomes is comparable but not similar to that of α-granules and dense granules during activation. Indeed, their content is released into the extracellular medium, but secretion of dense granules can occur, whereas lysosomes remain in the cytoplasm, depending on the nature and dose of the agonist. In the intact platelet, the dose-response curve for lysosomal secretion lies to the right of that for amine storage secretion. The sequence of secretion for α-granules versus dense granules is not as well correlated, and some agonists seem to be able to induce dense granule secretion preferentially, whereas activation inhibitors such as aspirin preferentially block α-granule secretion, leaving intact dense granule release (52).

## Stress Platelets and Reticulated Platelets

Platelets produced during recovery from acute thrombocytopenia show a striking increase in volume, with large and even giant forms apparent on the smear as early as 4 hours after the induction of thrombocytopenia. These stress platelets look spheric in EDTA and, when harvested with citrated anticoagulant, display an elongated shape, often beaded in appearance, strongly resembling MK proplatelets (53). Reticulated platelets are young platelets that contain some free ribosomes and sparse cisternae of rough endoplasmic reticulum (ER), responsible for a residual RNA content rapidly degraded after platelet release in the circulation. By analogy to reticulocytes, they are called *reticulated platelets*. This property makes them colorable by fluorochromes and supravital dyes, particularly by thiazole orange (54), and is used for the quantitative evaluation of platelet production (55). However, thiazole orange can be actively taken up by dense granules in the same way as dense granules can take up the fluorescent dye mepacrine (see preceding text), and this would interfere with the reticulated platelet count, falsely increasing it. Thus it is important to perform the staining reaction on paraformaldehyde lightly fixed platelets.

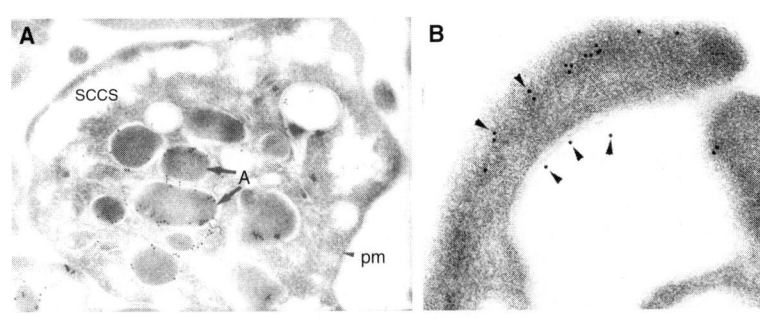

**FIGURE 26-9. A:** Immunogold labeling for P selectin shows that this receptor is located at the periphery of α-granules (*A*) in resting platelets and is absent from the plasma membrane (*pm*) and surface-connected canalicular system (*SCCS*) (magnification, ×22,000) **B:** After fully activated platelets undergo secretion, P selectin, the α-granule membrane marker, redistributes to the plasma membrane and pseudopod surface (*arrowheads*) (magnification, ×70,000).

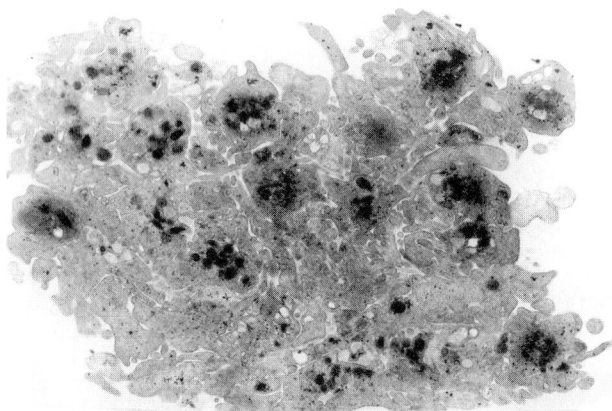

**FIGURE 26-10.** After adhering to a wounded surface and forming a monolayer, platelets build an aggregate by sticking to each other (magnification, ×13,000).

# PLATELET CYTOSKELETON

## Cytoskeleton in Resting Platelets

The cytoplasm is spatially organized by a network of structural proteins called the *cytoskeleton*. It mainly contains tubulin and actin polymers (11). The cytoskeleton has a dual function, static and dynamic (11); the circulating unactivated platelets have a discoid shape. After activation, they undergo a dynamic shape change in order to ensure their hemostatic function. They become spheric, extend filopodia, and spread on a surface by forming lamellipodia. Therefore, cell shape is critical first, to maintain a hemodynamic smooth and circular form in resting circulating platelets, and second, to contribute to platelet aggregative function by becoming ecchinocytic upon activation. The cytoskeleton and bound signaling molecules play a critical role in mediating these shape changes.

The platelet cytoskeleton consists of two main structures: a microtubule coil near the membrane and a dense network of actin filaments (56,57).

### Microtubules

**Description.** A thick annular bundle of microtubules underlies the cell membrane at its greater circumference, forming a solid loop that sustains the discoid cell shape. When sectioned parallel to the plane of the disc, the microtubule bundle underlies the cell membrane and is not in contact with the plasma membrane. Forty percent of platelet tubulin forms a coil that consists of a single microtubule wound 10 times just under the plasma membrane. Cross section of a circular microtubule shows that it measures approximately 25 nm in diameter and appears on transversal EM sections as round, hollow figures, typically surrounded by a clear halo that makes them easily distinguishable from other filamentous cytoplasmic structures; each microtubule is formed by a ring of 12 to 15 protofilaments arrayed in parallel and often depicting a central filament. Microtubules are composed of tubulin molecules, which are heterodimers of two closely related globular polypeptides, the α-tubulin and β-tubulin. In addition to tubulin, submembranous microtubules are composed of the tubulin associated motor proteins, kinesin and dynein. Microtubules are able to dissociate partially or in totality into subunits. The mode of formation of the platelet circular microtubule by MK has not been clearly visualized yet. The origin of this structure in platelets has been hypothesized by Behnke, who showed, in the rat species, that newly formed platelets freshly detached from the proplatelet through breakage of the constriction zones are spindle shaped and crossed in their long axis by a parallel bundle of microtubules (58). Subsequently, the fusiform platelet transforms into a circular shape by curving into a ring, which closes by fusion at the tips. It is presumed that the curving of the fusiform platelet is mediated by curving of its contained bundle of microtubules, which becomes the marginal bundle of the disc-shaped platelet. More recently, Italiano et al. showed that the coil may be formed in the mature MK at the extremity of the proplatelet: Repetitive kinking of the proplatelets allows new extremities to be formed, allowing shedding from the newly formed elbows of newborn platelets with already formed circumferential microtubule coil (59).

**Function.** The microtubule coil is involved in maintaining the discoid shape of the resting platelet (60). It also provides the compliance that is necessary during activation after the microtubule coil contracts, enabling the platelet to become spheroid. During shape change, the microtubule belt constricts, clasping toward the cell center the secretion granules and cytoplasmic organelles. This also concentrates the secretion granules close to the channels of the canalicular system. In parallel, fragments of microtubules appear at the cell periphery, subtending the cytoplasmic extensions and pseudopods (61,62).

The relation between platelet discoid shape and microtubules is shown by experiments performed by lowering the temperature or with agents known to depolymerize microtubules, such as colchicine, vinblastine, and vincristine. At low temperature or in the presence of these chemical agents, platelets lose their discoid form and become relatively spherical and regular. This is accompanied by the disappearance of the circumferential band of microtubules. This phenomenon is reversible, and reformation of the microtubule coil leads to recovery of the discoid shape.

Their various roles in platelet function have been confirmed by the use of taxol, an agent that prevents disassembly of preexisting microtubules. Indeed, in the presence of taxol, shape change and secretory functions of platelets are unaltered, and this observation establishes that microtubule disassembly is not required for any step of the physiologic response of platelet to activation and is not responsible for microtubule topographic redistribution in stimulated cells. The association of the circumferential microtubules with submembrane and intracytoplasmic filaments 5 nm across is established, and stabilization of the tubules results from this connection.

Apart from maintaining resting platelets in discoid shape, microtubules regulate the assembly of integrin-induced cytoskeletal complexes through a connection with the cytoplasmic domain of integrins (57,63,64).

The integrity of the microtubule coil is essential for platelet function. Microtubule disruption occurs through the physical forces exerted by the contracting associated filaments, rather than through depolymerization. Granule extrusion, pseudopod retraction, and even clot retraction are also under the control of microtubules. The microtubule coil disruption after treatment with major depolymerizing agents such as vinca alkaloids prevents platelet aggregation and secretion. However, platelet shape change and secretion are still observed when the microtubules are only tightly disorganized by a chemical agent such as paclitaxel. Approximately 90% of the β-tubulin in platelets is β1-tubulin. β1-null mice have reduced proplatelet formation, thrombocytopenia, and platelet spherocytosis. In the absence of β1-tubulin, the marginal band of microtubules that maintains platelet discoid shape is broken. However, platelets function normally under physiologic shear conditions (59). The defective organization of microtubules in β1-null mice is the same as that observed in GATA-1–null mice. These abnormalities may result from a limiting amount of microtubule polymers in these platelets. Therefore, the discoid shape of platelets is apparently dispensable for many aspects of platelet functions such as their life span, dense granule secretion, aggregation in response to various stimuli, and hemostasis in injured arterioles.

## Actin Network

**Description.** The actin filament-based cytoskeleton can be subdivided in two components: the submembranous skeleton and the cytoplasmic filaments.

*Submembrane cytoskeleton.* The area lying just under the unit membrane of the platelet surface is occupied by a continuous layer of filamentous elements that prevents contact of any cytoplasmic organelles with the plasma membrane (11,65). The submembranous filaments are located peripheral to the circumferential band of microtubules in the discoid cell. Biochemical and ultrastructural investigations have shown that they are short, actin filaments that are associated with detergent-insoluble components of the plasma membrane. The assembly of submembrane actin filaments is inhibited by cytochalasin B. When dissecting morphologic changes during activation, it is important to discriminate between the adherence and spreading of platelets on a surface, and activation of platelets in suspension. After being activated in suspension by agonists such as ADP, thrombin, epinephrine, and collagen, discoid platelets become spheroid, and their membrane emits irregular protrusions with thin pseudopodia. Therefore, the initial morphologic event induced is a change in cell shape. The agent responsible for microtubule fragmentation is actin contraction; constraints on the resting membrane skeleton before fragmentation are imposed by connections running between the side of actin filaments underlying the plasma membrane and GP Ib/IX/V. Microtubule fragmentation is followed by the dispatching of the fragments at the cell periphery, in the cytoplasmic extensions and pseudopods.

*Cytoplasmic intermediate and actin filaments.* Intermediate filaments are strong, ropelike polymers of fibrous polypeptides that resist stretch and play a structural and tension-bearing role in the cells. In platelets, desmin and vimentin are the principal constituents. They are called intermediate because in EM their apparent diameter (8 to 12 nm) is between that of the thin actin filaments and the thick microtubules. After cells are treated with concentrated salt solutions and nonionic detergents, the intermediate filaments remain, whereas most of the cytoskeleton is lost.

Intermediate and actin filaments fill the cytoplasm and mediate contractile events of the platelets. Their observation is obscured by the other elements of the cytoplasmic background ultrastructure. Several methods have been used to study the filament cytoskeleton, including negative stains, detergent extraction, quick-freeze deep etching (66), high-voltage transmission, and scanning EM.

Resting platelets are apparently devoid of assembled actin, the cytoplasm having an amorphous aspect and being poorly dense to electrons. Because cellular actin is maintained in an equilibrium between unpolymerized and filamentous actin, the cytoplasmic space has been called the sol–gel zone. The sol–gel zone contains both motor and chassis components. Gels of actin are formed of microfilaments 5 nm across connected to microtubules (67).

## Biochemistry of the Actin Network

In addition to the microtubules, actin is the other major component of platelet cytoskeleton. It represents 20% of the total platelet proteins. It is distributed in two forms: first, monomers of globular actin (G-actin), and second, filamentous actin (F-actin). In resting platelets, 40% of actin is in filamentous form and assembled into 2,000 to 5,000 filaments. Actin filaments are polarized structures with pointed (minus) ends and barbed (plus) ends. The barbed ends represent the site of active assembly reaction. Several proteins and glycoproteins (GPs) are closely associated to actin filaments; they can also be distinguished in two pools accompanying the two main compartments of the actin cytoskeleton: Transmembrane GP associated to the membrane cytoskeleton and proteins associated with the cytoplasmic network of actin. These are the filamin A (ABP-280), talin, $\alpha$-actinin, and myosins II and I bearing ATPase activities (68,69).

### Structural Proteins Regulating the Stability of the Actin Network

In circulating and nonactivated platelets, actin is prevented from polymerizing by two mechanisms. The first mechanism is the trapping of actin monomers by carrier proteins: In resting platelets, monomers of actin are sequestered by thymosin $\beta 4$ and profilin (70). The second one is the presence of capping proteins located at the barbed ends of actin filaments that prevent the addition of actin monomers. As an example, the calcium-dependent protein gelsolin binds to barbed ends, forms a cap on the exposed plus end of the filament, and breaks up the cross-linked network of actin filament (71). However, in gelsolin$^{-/-}$ mice, the actin filament content of unstimulated platelets is only slightly higher than normal, indicating that gelsolin is not the only capping protein in platelets (72). Other candidates for efficient inhibition of actin filament elongation are the $Ca^{2+}$-insensitive capping proteins CapZ and CapG (73,74). They regulate the number and accessibility of actin filament barbed ends. These capping proteins are more important than initially suggested, because they determine the choice between the formation of lamellipodia or filopodia. Indeed, depletion of capping proteins by using short hairpin RNAs causes the loss of lamellipodia and the explosive formation of filopodia. Therefore, the selective formation of lamellipodia versus filopodia depends on the presence of capping proteins at the actin barbed ends, that are negative regulators of filopodia (74) (see Fig. 26-11).

### Structural Proteins Associated with Actin in the Membrane Cytoskeleton

Proteins interacting with actin filaments are involved (i) in the stabilization of membrane skeleton network in resting platelets, as is the case for the filamin A (ABP-280), and spectrin; and (ii) in the cross-linking of membrane proteins with this network, as is the case for talin, moesin, vinculin, and skelemin (see Table 26-1).

The membrane skeleton is connected to the membrane receptors GP Ib/IX/V and $\alpha_{IIb}\beta_3$, to the tyrosine kinases (pp60$^{c-src}$, pp62$^{c-yes}$, pp72$^{syk}$) and the phosphatase SHP-1, to the scaffold protein 14-3-3$\zeta$, and to the $Ca^{2+}$-dependent protease calpain (65,75,76) (see Table 26-1).

**ABP-280.** The most important protein of the platelet membrane skeleton network is filamin A (ABP-280). It belongs to the ABP family of proteins, which consists of dimers that associate head to head. ABP monomer has a C-terminal dimerization domain and a N-terminal actin-binding site (77). In resting platelets, ABP binds actin filaments and participates in the organization of filaments in parallel by interacting with $\alpha$-actinin. This creates a strong network in the cytoplasm and under the plasma membrane. ABP associates with the cytoplasmic domain of GP Ib$\alpha$ and also with tissue factor, Fc$\gamma$ receptor, and $\beta_1$ integrin (63,77–79). The lack of GP Ib$\alpha$–ABP complex in platelets of patients with a Bernard-Soulier syndrome may decrease the strength of the interactions between the plasma membrane and the cytoskeleton, and this could account for the abnormal size of these platelets. ABP can bind members of the Ras superfamily of the low-molecular-weight (LMW) G proteins, Cdc42, Rac, and RalA (80), the latter being an upstream regulator of ABP, which induces the formation of filopodia. Upon platelet activation, ABP is phosphorylated and cleaved by calpain. After cleavage, it loses its ability to bind GP Ib/IX/V and subsequently loses its cross-linking function.

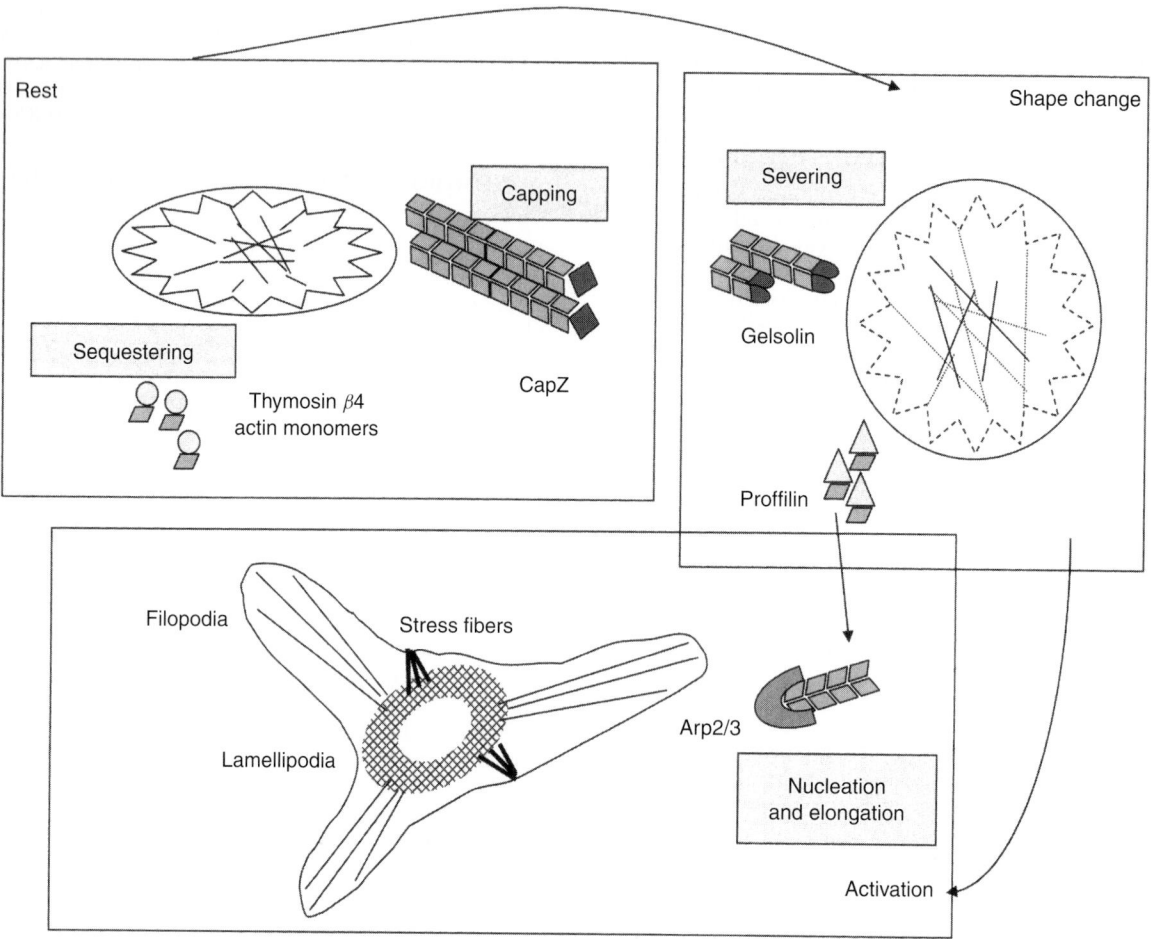

**FIGURE 26-11.** Schematic representation of different steps of the regulation of actin polymerization in platelets at rest, during platelet shape change and after full activation. In resting platelets, actin monomers are sequestered by thymosin $\beta4$ and actin filaments elongation is prevented by capping protein, CapZ. During shape change, actin filaments are severed by gelsolin, and new monomers are transported by profilin to the barbed ends of shortened filaments. Actin polymerization for lamellipodia, filopodia, and stress fibers formation is orchestrated by the Arp2/3 complex located at the nucleation sites.

**Spectrin.** Platelet spectrin consists of dimers that associate head to head to form tetramers of approximately 180 nm in length. It forms complexes with $\alpha_{IIb}\beta_3$ and binds actin filament ends. Spectrin is located at the cytoplasmic side of the plasma membrane and cross-links actin filaments to the membrane. In the red blood cell, the spectrin tetramers are linked to the plasma membrane by ankyrin and protein 4.1, both identified in platelets (81). The interaction of $\alpha_{IIb}\beta_3$ with spectrin may regulate the ability of $\alpha_{IIb}\beta_3$ to become activated (82). Cleavage of spectrin by calpain during platelet aggregation results in dissociation of the tetramer and loss of the ability to cross-link actin (83). Spectrin also contains (i) a pleckstrin homology (PH) domain that mediates its interaction with the plasma membrane, (ii) a Src homology (SH) domain allowing the recruitment of signaling molecules, and (iii) a $Ca^{2+}$/calmodulin-binding regulatory domain that binds actin. These domains are implicated in the location of spectrin in focal adhesion regions along with integrin $\alpha_{IIb}\beta_3$ during platelet activation.

**Moesin and Talin.** Moesin and talin serve as bridges between membrane receptors and actin filaments. These bridges are formed through the direct binding of integrin, at least for talin (84,85). Both moesin and talin are regulated by phosphorylation (86,87). Moesin is the only member of the ERM (Ezrin/Radixin/Moesin) family of proteins present in platelets.

This family of proteins consists of closely related proteins whose C-terminal domain interacts with actin.

The N-terminal domain of talin in platelets has a high degree of homology to the N-terminal region of ERM proteins, through which it directly binds the cytoplasmic domain of $\beta_1$ and $\beta_3$ integrins (85). The C-terminal end of talin binds to actin, focal adhesion protein, and vinculin by a mechanism that depends on the generation of phosphatidylinositol 4,5-bisphosphate [PI (4,5)$P_2$] during platelet activation. Talin is released from its binding with $\beta$ integrins by calpain-dependent proteolysis.

Structural proteins that ensure the stability of the actin cytoskeleton in platelets also bear posttranslational modifications upon platelet activation. This suggests that they are implicated in the stabilization of the cytoskeleton in activated platelets.

## Reorganization of the Cytoskeleton in Activated Platelets

### From Platelet Shape Change to Platelet Aggregation

**Morphology.** When activation is initiated following an injury of the vessel wall, or after adhesion on a substratum,

**TABLE 26-1**

PLATELET PROTEINS IMPLICATED IN CYTOSKELETON MAINTENANCE
IN RESTING PLATELETS AND IN CYTOSKELETON REORGANIZATION
IN ACTIVATED PLATELETS

| Cytoskeletal proteins | Cytoskeleton-associated proteins | Membrane receptors | Signaling proteins: Kinases Phosphatases Proteases | Regulators of actin polymerization |
|---|---|---|---|---|
| Actin | Filamin A (ABP-280) | GP Ib/IX | pp60$^{c\text{-}src}$ | Cdc42, Rac1, RhoA |
| Myosin | Spectrin | GP IIbIIIa | pp62$^{c\text{-}yes}$ | WASp, WAVE |
| α-actinin | Talin | GP VI | pp72$^{Syk}$ | Cortactin |
| | Vinculin | | *ras*GAP | Arp2/3 |
| | Ankyrin | | PI 3-K | Gelsolin, CapZ, CapG |
| | Protein 4.1 | | PI 5-K | Thymosin beta4 |
| | Moesin | | SHP-1 | Profilin |
| | Skelemin | | MLCK | Cofilin |
| | | | ROCK | |
| | | | PAK | |
| | | | Calpain | |

ABP, actin-binding protein; WASp, Wiskott-Aldrich syndrome protein; WAVE, WASp family, Verproline homologous proteins; MLCK, myosin–light chain kinase; ROCK, Rho kinase; PAK, p21-activated kinases.

platelets undergo a series of sequential morphologic changes: round shape, spreading with short filopodia, spindle shape, spreading with long filopodia, spreading with lamellipodia, and finally, full spreading (88). Platelet spreading is the initial step that pastes the vascular wound. Extrusion of the lamellipod is made possible by the rearrangement of the resting platelet cytoskeleton and a massive actin assembly reaction with fragmentation of the peripheral actin network by pleckstrin. Lamellipodia, or spreading veils, contain orthogonally arranged actin networks at the platelet periphery, which allow an outward flow of the membrane. Lamellipodia extend from the plasma membrane–actin filament interface, where the resultant actin filament fragments are linked to the membrane by the ABP–GP Ib/IX/V connections.

In addition to the extension of large lamellipodia, activated platelets assemble surface filopodia. Filopodia allow platelets to firmly attach to each other and thereby build a solid aggregate. These projections are cored by bundles of long actin filaments that originate in the cell center, resembling stress fibers. The actin assembly that drives the formation of filopodia based on spatial rearrangement of filaments is different from that which generates lamellipodia. It requires lengthening of actin filaments with coordinated uncapping, whereas lamellipod formation depends on filament fragmentation. Filopodia are long, thin extensions containing bundles of actin filaments that terminate at the filopodial tips, whereas lamellipodia are flat cytoplasmic veils. These different structures play important distinct roles in the adhesive process: Lamellipodia arrest vascular leakage by adhering to the wounded surface, and filopodia bind to fibrin and other platelets to form a three-dimensional clot (see Fig. 26-12).

Platelet shape change proceeds through four recognizable steps:

First, platelets spread active lamellipodia between the two banks of the wounded vessel that will close down during further platelet contact. This platelet monolayer contributes to seal the gap. In parallel to these changes, the microtubule coil depolymerizes, and the amount of F-actin increases. Initially, actin filaments form a circle toward the platelet center, and short filaments are created at the periphery. Later, the central circle disappears, and bundles of filaments radiate from the center to the cell periphery, causing a limited number of filopodia. This leads to plasma membrane ruffling, and lamellipodia are formed.

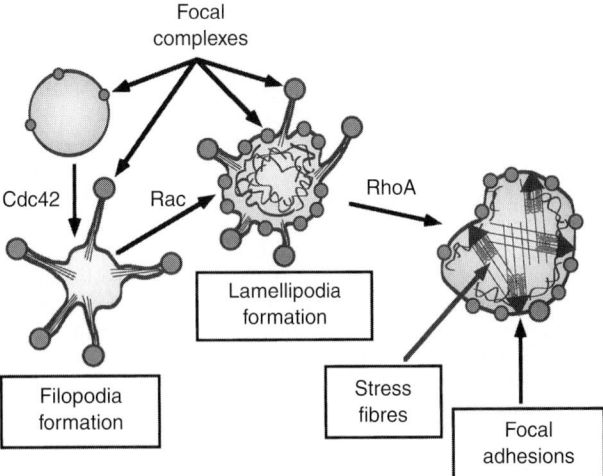

**FIGURE 26-12.** Schematic representation of different stages in cell spreading shows the involvement of Rho family members. After cells spread on an integrin substrate, Cdc42, Rac, and RhoA are activated. Cdc42 induces the formation of filopodia; Rac, the formation of submembranous actin filament networks and lamellipodia extension; and RhoA, the formation of stress fibers and focal adhesions.

Second, additional platelets are recruited to consolidate the initial sealing platelet monolayer. They are activated through heterotrimeric G-coupled receptors engagement: the thrombin receptor, protease activated receptor 1 (PAR-1). This results in the activation of the integrin $\alpha_{IIb}\beta_3$ (inside-out signaling). In turn, activated integrin $\alpha_{IIb}\beta_3$ binds fibrinogen (outside-in signaling) and transduces signals leading to the polymerization of the submembranous actin filament network. By extending numerous short filopodia, platelets aggregate and fit between themselves like small bricks to form a thick platelet plug.

Third, platelet contraction seals the two banks of the wounded vessel wall through the formation of actin ropes, anchored in focal adhesion zones, also called stress fibers. They are linked to the strings of fibrin, which they pull and retract during platelet contraction. Contraction results in platelet secretion of procoagulant molecules and growth factors (platelet-derived growth factor, transforming growth factor-$\beta$) that contribute to achieve the wound healing repair. Platelet shedding of procoagulant microparticles also disseminates a procoagulant signal to recruit more platelets at the site of injury.

Fourth, after secretion, exhausted platelets passively spread in the aggregate. The $\alpha$-granular glycoprotein, P selectin, expressed at the surface of platelets during activation, serves as an attractant for polymorphonuclear cells and monocytes/macrophages. Both phagocytic cell types express the P selectin glycoprotein ligand-1 (PSLG-1). This terminal step cleans the zone from platelet leftovers and fibrin debris (89).

**Integrin Signaling and Reorganization of Actin Filaments.** As platelets are activated, interactions between the plasma membrane and the submembranous skeleton have to be broken. Integrin-dependent signaling mechanisms include (i) the tyrosine phosphorylation of the $\beta_3$-integrin subunit, (ii) the association of myosin–light chain with phosphorylated integrin, and (iii) the cleavage of the $\beta_3$-subunit, spectrin, talin, and filamin A (ABP-280) by calpain (65,83,90) (see Table 26-1). Therefore, the $Ca^{2+}$-dependent protease calpain, activated after stimulation of platelets and signaling across activated GP IIbIIIa, plays a major role in regulating shape change and aggregation. Inhibition of calpain correlates with inhibition of platelet spreading, secretion, and aggregation in thrombin-treated platelets. Calpain is also required for procoagulant membrane blebbing after platelet adhesion to collagen through GP VI (91,92).

To achieve shape changes, it is necessary that GP IIbIIIa interacts with three other cytoskeletal proteins: $\alpha$-actinin, skelemin, and vinculin. $\alpha$-actinin, a protein present in the network of cytoplasmic actin filaments, also interacts with the Gp Ib/IX/V complex at high shear stress, downstream of the binding of VWF to its receptor (93,94). In focal complexes, $\alpha_{IIb}\beta_3$ binds skelemin, an $M_r$ approximately 210 kDa cytoskeletal protein. The membrane-proximal region of the cytoplasmic domain of $\beta_1$- and $\beta_3$ integrin subunits is implicated in this interaction that supports early platelet spreading induced by integrin activation (95). Vinculin-containing complexes, with actin and talin, are also present in focal adhesions that form at the extremity of stress fibers during platelet aggregation.

**Lipid Rafts.** Lipid rafts are cholesterol-enriched membrane microdomains. Their importance in platelet activation has been recently emphasized. Although their involvement in platelet signaling and shape change is unclear, it is known that the GP Ib/IX/V complexes are concentrated into lipid rafts, mostly along filopodia (96). Early steps of platelet activation, by the collagen receptor GP VI (97) and by Fc$\gamma$ RIIa, preferentially occur in these microdomains. In addition, lipid rafts contribute to platelet activation via heterotrimeric G protein–coupled receptors, leading

to a local generation of the second messenger phosphatidylinositol 3,4,5-trisphosphate (98). Lipid rafts microdomains maintain membrane receptors and signaling molecules in close vicinity, a state that could facilitate signal transduction.

**Posttranslational Regulation of Actin-Binding Proteins by Tyrosine or Serine/Threonine Kinases.** Numerous kinases become phosphorylated during platelet activation; however, many of their function remain unclear. Among them, protein-tyrosine kinases, including members of the Src family (pp60$^{c-src}$, pp60$^{c-fyn}$, pp62$^{c-yes}$, pp54/58$^{c-yes}$, $pp72^{syk}$) could be activated after signaling through the thrombin receptor and through $\alpha_{IIb}\beta_3$ integrin. The main substrate of tyrosine kinases pp60$^{c-src}$ and pp72$^{syk}$ is cortactin (99). Cortactin is a SH3-containing protein that cross-links actin filaments. It colocalizes with actin in platelet lamellipodia. Whether the tyrosine phosphorylation of cortactin enhances or diminishes its ability to bind F-actin is still a matter of debate. The activation of the focal adhesion kinase (FAK) is strictly dependent on integrin GP IIb/IIIa. Interestingly, $\alpha$-actinin is phosphorylated on its actin-binding site by FAK, and this tyrosine phosphorylation reduces the amount of $\alpha$-actinin that binds actin filaments (100). In this case, the tyrosine phosphorylation of $\alpha$-actinin negatively regulates its actin-binding activity. Therefore, ABPs are tightly regulated by tyrosine phosphorylation.

Among the serine/threonine kinases, protein kinase C (PKC) and the mitogen-activated protein (MAP) kinases have been well studied in platelets. Members of the MAP kinases, ERK1/2, enhance platelet secretion (101). Recently, evidence has been provided that a serine/threonine kinase, named integrin-linked kinase (ILK), associates with and phosphorylates integrin $\beta_3$. It also phosphorylates a subunit of the myosin phosphatase at an inhibitory site (102,103). This indicates that ILK is a key player in outside-in signaling induced by the binding of fibrinogen to the $\alpha_{IIb}\beta_3$ integrin and regulates the interaction between the GP IIb/IIIa integrin and the cytoskeleton.

Downstream of the complex integrin, src and FAK coupled to talin, skelemin, and $\alpha$-actinin, actin movements are regulated by other serine/threonine kinases: the myosin–light chain kinase (MLCK) and the Rho kinase (ROCK) (104). ROCK is an $M_r$ approximately 160 kDa recruited to the platelet membrane by active Rho. Both MLCK and ROCK phosphorylate the myosin–light chain and myosin phosphatase. This results in an increased phosphorylation of myosin–light chain, association of myosin with actin filaments, and the formation of stress fibers. An alternative pathway implicates the tyrosine phosphorylation of the proto-oncogene Vav by Syk. In turn, Vav activates Rac1, leading to an increase in membrane ruffling due the lamellipodia formation (see Fig. 26-13). Finally, phosphorylation is a key event to control ABPs and their upstream regulators.

**Rho Family Members and Their Effectors.** Members of the Rho subfamily of the LMW G proteins include Rac1, Cdc42, and RhoA. Studies in which constitutively active forms of Rho family members have been microinjected into cultured cells have shown that each family member has a dramatically different effect (105,106):

- Cdc42 induces the formation of short filopodia;
- Rac then induces the formation of lamellipodia; and
- RhoA induces the formation of stress fibers and long filopodia, and regulates the contractility of stress fibers anchored in focal adhesions (107) (Fig. 26-12).

Rho proteins are activated in guanosine triphosphate (GTP)–bound and inactivated in guanosine diphosphate (GDP)–bound states. Several GTP exchange factors (GEFs) allow GTP binding and the conversion of LMW G proteins to an active state. GEFs can be activated either indirectly by interactions of their pleckstrin homology domains with phospholipid substrates of the phosphatidylinositol 3-kinase (PI 3-K) or

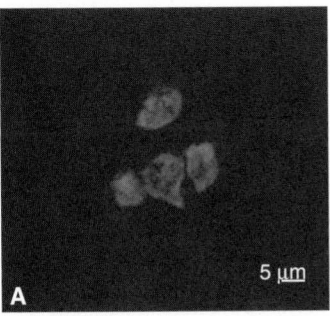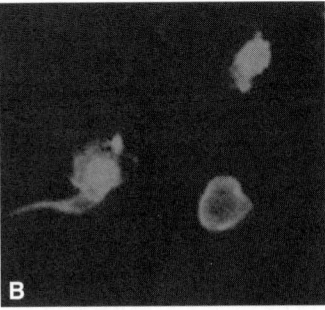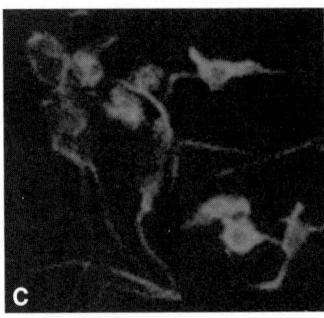

**FIGURE 26-13.** Immunofluorescence images of actin filaments in resting platelets (**A**), in platelets spreading on collagen and exhibiting lamellipodia (**B**), and in platelets in suspension treated with ionomycin that induced the protrusion of thin and long filopodia (**C**). Actin filaments were stained with fluorescently labeled phalloidin. Bar = 5 μm.

directly by tyrosine phosphorylation (108–110). For instance, the proto-oncogene Vav is an exchange factor that becomes tyrosine-phosphorylated during platelet activation and can induce activation of both Rac and Rho (111). In a similar way, RhoA, Rac, and Cdc42 are activated after platelet stimulation by thrombin; RhoA and Rac1 are also activated, in a PI 3-K–dependent manner, after signaling through integrin GP IIb/IIIa (112–115) (Fig. 26-13).

Conversely, targets for Cdc42, Rac and Rho include phosphatidylinositol-kinases (PIK) such as PI 3-K and PI 5-K (113,116,117). The engagement of the thrombin receptor and/or of $\alpha_{IIb}\beta_3$ integrin leads to the activation of PI 3-K, which becomes associated with the cytoskeleton. Downstream of Rac, Cdc42, or RhoA, PI 3-K is activated and induces the generation of PI $(3,4,5)P_3$ and PI $(3,4)P_2$ (110,117–119). After stimulation of platelets by thrombin, activation of PI 5-K by Cdc42, Rac and Rho induce the generation of PI $(4,5)P_2$ and initiate actin polymerization (113). Indeed, PI $(4,5)P_2$ is the major phosphatidylinositide involved in cytoskeletal reorganizations and is mainly implicated in regulating the interactions between talin and vinculin at the focal adhesion points (120).

Rac and Cdc42 bind and activate a family of serine/threonine kinases of $M_r$ approximately 65 kDa, the p21-activated kinases (PAK) (121). $p65^{PAK}$ becomes phosphorylated during platelet activation, and it has been implicated in the regulation of cytoskeletal reorganizations (122). Several PAK substrates or binding partners have been implicated in the effects of PAK, including the filamin A, myosin, and the LIM kinase. In resting platelets, the isoform PAK1 is associated with the cortical-ABP cortactin. Cortactin dissociates from PAK1 upon stimulation by thrombin and this coincides with its relocalization to the cytoskeleton, in a Rac1-dependent manner (123). Cortactin may be a downstream effector of Rac1 during the formation of lamellipodia (see Fig. 26-14). PAK and ABP interact by the C-terminal domain of filamin A and by the domain of PAK that interact with Cdc42 and Rac1. Binding of filamin A has been shown to activate PAK. The LIM kinase is activated by phosphorylation by both PAK and ROCK. In turn, LIM kinase phosphorylates and inactivates cofilin, a protein that promotes depolymerization of F-actin. The result of this cascade is the stabilization of the actin network in lamellae. Formation of stress fibers is thought to be regulated after activation of Rho through the activation of the

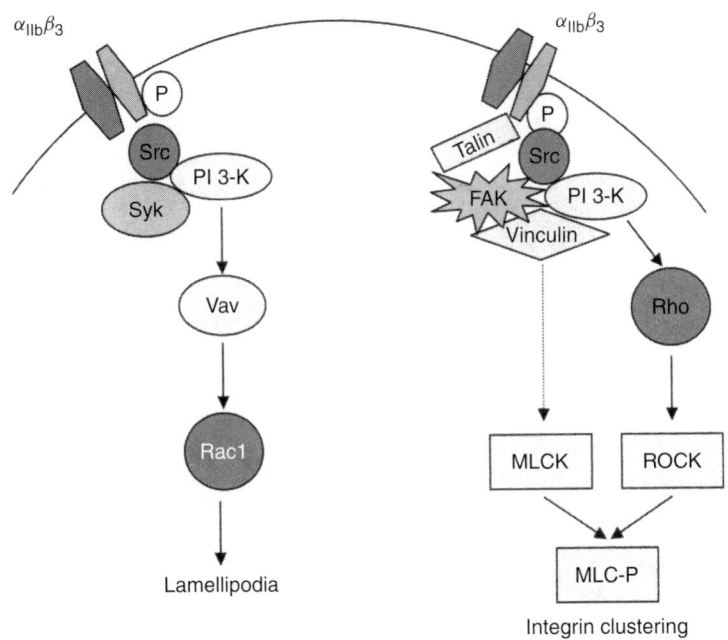

**FIGURE 26-14.** Integrin-dependent pathways of actin remodeling GP IIbIIIa activates Rac through a Src/Syk/PI 3-K–dependent pathway to induce lamellipodia formation. GP IIbIIIa also recruits the tyrosine kinase FAK (focal adhesion kinase) to directly activate myosin–light chain kinase (MLCK) or to indirectly activate the Rho kinase (ROCK) through Rho. Both result in the phosphorylation of the myosin–light chain (MLC), which allows the clustering of integrin and stress fiber formation.

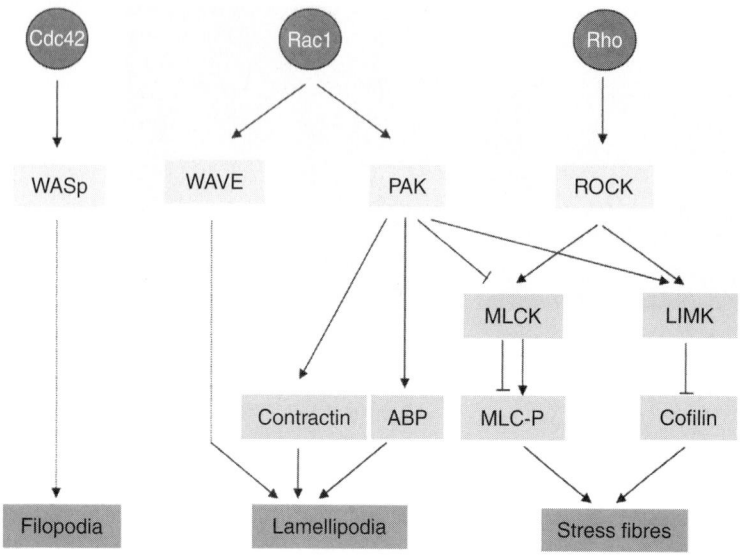

**FIGURE 26-15.** Small G proteins and downstream regulators of actin remodeling. Different stages in cell spreading show the involvement of Rho family members. After cells spread on an integrin substrate, Cdc42, Rac, and RhoA are activated. Cdc42 induces the formation of filopodia through Wiskott-Aldrich syndrome protein (WASp); Rac regulates the formation of submembranous actin filament networks and lamellipodia extension through the activation of WASp family Verproline homologous proteins (WAVE) and p21-activated kinases (PAK), which controls the ABP-280 and cortactin. RhoA and its effector, the Rho kinase (ROCK), activates the kinases LIMK and MLCK to govern the formation of stress fibers and focal adhesions. MLCK, myosin-light chain kinase.

Rho kinase ROCK. Targets of ROCK are (i) the MLCK that activate myosin through the phosphorylation of MLC and (ii) the LIM kinase that inhibits cofilin (see Fig. 26-15).

IQGAP2 is another GTP-dependent effector of Rac1 recently identified in platelets. In response to thrombin, it binds Rac1-GTP and the complex Arp2/3 that regulates actin polymerization (124). The Wiskott-Aldrich syndrome protein (WASp) is an $M_r$ approximately 62 kDa proline-rich protein and is a direct target for Cdc42. This protein is defective in the Wiskott-Aldrich syndrome, a bleeding disorder characterized by thrombocytopenia and lymphopenia. Platelets are small and can generate only few filopodia (125). Because WASp is thought to be necessary for regulating actin depolymerization, it clearly appears that platelet morphology and shape change depend on a tight equilibrium between actin depolymerization and polymerization (see subsequent text).

### Contraction and Secretion

Platelet secretion of procoagulant granule products allows the recruitment of naive platelets. Secretion is ensured by the contraction of actin filaments and requires the conversion of myosin to a form that is able to interact with cytoplasmic actin filaments (126). The association of myosin with actin filaments depends on the phosphorylation of myosin–light chains, which are targets for MLCK. Upon thrombin stimulation, activation of MLCK occurs, which is enhanced by $Ca^{2+}$/calmodulin. This allows the contractile force required for secretion to occur. In addition, a calmodulin-independent and RhoA-dependent mechanism induces myosin phosphorylation (127). Myosin-associated actin filaments contract in a ring around α-granules, forcing them toward the platelet center, where they release their content into the SCCS. Myosin phosphorylation is regulated by phosphatases and kinases that are activated by Rho family proteins (128,129). Secretion is an active, energy-dependent process.

### Clot Retraction

Physiologically, clot retraction follows platelet aggregation; it occurs through the binding of integrins $\alpha_{IIb}\beta_3$ to a network of fibrin. Little is known about signaling that occurs through the integrin when it binds fibrin. A consequence of outside-in signaling in a platelet aggregate is that the occupied integrin becomes incorporated into actin–myosin complexes that represent the contractile component of the cytoskeleton. The complexes formed in aggregating platelets contain the proteins that are involved in the integrin–membrane skeleton complexes and other signaling molecules, including PKC, p85/PI 3-K, FAK, PTP-1C/SH-PTP1/SHP-1, Cdc42Hs, RhoA, Rap1B, phospholipase C, and diglyceride kinase (82,130–133). Furthermore, the calcium-dependent protease calpain is recruited to focal adhesion points close to integrin $\alpha_{IIb}\beta_3$. When activated by phospholipids, calpain contacts and hydrolyzes its substrates: talin, filamin, spectrin, α-actinin, vinculin, src, and cortactin. Therefore, calpain participates in the relaxation of the fibrin clot retraction through the disruption of the connection between these focal proteins and the fibrin network. Finally, fibrin clot retraction is associated with dephosphorylation of tyrosine-phosphorylated substrates in an $\alpha_{IIb}\beta_3$- and actin cytoskeleton–dependent manner. This suggests that dephosphorylation regulates the forces required for full contraction of the fibrin network (134).

### Microparticle Shedding

The final step of platelet activation reflecting full activation is the shedding of microparticles (MP). Platelet dust is an anatomic concept first described by Wolf in 1967 (135), defining the platelet-related coagulant activity of the whole cell-free plasma and serum. Later, it was shown by Crawford (136) that these MP were formed by *in vivo* fracture of membrane buds detached from extended platelet pseudopods induced by calpain (137). Physiologically, microparticles are located at the periphery of platelet aggregates. EM examination revealed the presence of fibrin-associated MP, close to the thrombus formed on fibrillar collagen. Flow cytometry studies have also detected plasma membrane vesicles released from activated platelets. MP express integrin GP Ib and $\alpha_{IIb}\beta_3$ at their surface and also have a high density of prothrombotic proteins on their surface, including the adhesive receptor P selectin (138). However, it is possible that, depending on the state of activation after they are shed, their composition varies. They may functionally change from hemostatic to prothrombotic, according to their content of GP Ib and IIb/IIIa and to the extent of platelet secretion. MP adhere to platelets via integrin $\alpha_{IIb}\beta_3$, and also to neutrophils or monocytes via P selectin. Their prothrombotic effect is magnified by their ability to induce tissue factor synthesis when adhering to monocytes (139). Both activated platelets and MP express the aminophospholipid phosphatidylserine, thereby providing an essential procoagulant surface that supports the formation of activated clotting enzymes (i.e., Xase and prothrombinase complex) on membranes. Phosphatidylserine expression is responsible for the characteristic annexin V–binding property of microparticles (140). MP shed from other cell types, such as endothelial cells or monocytes, amplify the recruitment of platelets at the site of aggregation. For example, monocyte-derived MP that contain membrane phospholipids activate platelets through the generation of lysophosphatidic acid, resulting from hydrolysis of phospholipids by soluble phospholipase A2 (141). Therefore, in addition to procoagulant membrane dissemination, MP also facilitate the coagulation process through the transport of procoagulant membrane-soluble mediators.

Microparticles should be distinguished from platelet exosomes, released from multivesicular bodies, and α-granules, the function of which is still unknown (142). Microparticle shedding was found to accompany in vitro platelet production (3). This may be an auxiliary mechanism to provide a quick response to control hemorrhage induced by thrombocytopenia.

In vivo, extrinsic signals, such as endothelial wall injury and high levels of circulating factor VIIa, induce the activation of platelets expressing membrane tissue factor transferred from monocytes and subsequent release of MP. MP also can be produced in pathologic clinical conditions such as cardiopulmonary bypass, idiopathic thrombocytopenic purpura, and heparin-induced thrombocytopenia. In vitro, MP are generated by platelets incubated with the serum of patients with heparin-induced thrombocytopenia, with the complex C5b-9 of complement, and/or at high shear rates. Several reports have established that MP formation depends on the rise of intracellular calcium concentrations, because calcium ionophores are potent activators of MP formation. MP shedding depends on actin rearrangement because the inhibition of actin polymerization by cytochalasin D decreases the shedding of procoagulant MP (143,144). The main intracellular events observed during MP shedding are the activation of calpain, the increase of protein tyrosine phosphatase (PTP) activity, and the decrease of tyrosine phosphorylation (144,145). The activation of the calcium-dependent cysteine proteases, calpain or cathepsin L, could play a major role in breaking membrane–cytoskeleton interactions (146). Indeed, numerous structural and regulatory proteins, such as the cortical-ABP or cortactin, and Src, are proteolyzed during MP shedding. The Wiskott-Aldrich protein WASp accumulates in MP generated during MK differentiation initiated upon phorbol ester. Antisens oligonucleotides anti-WASp abolish this microvesiculation, suggesting a crucial role of this regulator of actin polymerization in MP shedding (147). In addition to calpain activity that is constantly detected, the activation of the p38 mitogen–activated protein kinase could be necessary (92). However, whether the engagement of integrin $\alpha_{IIb}\beta_3$ is required for shedding is still a matter of debate. MP shedding does not seem to require G protein–dependent actin reorganization, nor to follow classical pathways of cell activation.

## Regulation of Actin Polymerization and Depolymerization in Platelets

Filamentous actin represents approximately 40% of the total actin in resting platelets. After activation, the amount of F-actin increases to 60%–70%. However, actin reorganization is a dynamic process that includes both polymerization and depolymerization steps.

### Actin Polymerization in Activated Platelets

Following platelet activation, the generation of free barbed ends, which are hot spots of actin nucleation, is a necessary step before polymerization occurs. Increase in cytoplasmic calcium, which is a common feature of cell activation, activates the capping protein gelsolin, allowing it to sever actin filaments. Gelsolin remains bound to the new barbed ends of actin, unless PI (3,4)P$_2$

is generated. PI (3,4)P$_2$ increases as a result of Rac activation upon the stimulation of platelets with thrombin (that activates PI 3-K downstream of Rac1) (113). The generation of PI (3,4)P$_2$ induces the release of gelsolin and subsequently an increased number of free barbed ends available for the addition of monomeric actin and filament growth. The fluorescence resonance energy transfer (FRET)-based reporter protein, used to measure the dissociation of gelsolin, demonstrates that uncapping occurs in cells at sites of active actin assembly (148). Gelsolin-dependent severing is an upstream event that precedes the beginning of actin polymerization. When gelsolin, or its homolog CapG, dissociates from the barbed ends of actin filaments, the complex of proteins Arp2/3, required for actin polymerization, is activated (74,149). The assembly of a branched network of actin filaments requires a core set of proteins including monomers of actin bound to ATP, the Arp2/3 complex, profilin, capping proteins, and cofilin.

Arp2/3 is an acceptor for actin monomers that both amplifies actin nucleation and initiates new filaments, as branches on preexisting filaments. In vitro, the Arp2/3 nucleates actin filament assembly: It possesses at least two binding sites for actin, one that binds to the sides of actin filaments and one that binds to the pointed ends of actin monomers, nucleating barbed-end elongation (74). Indeed, antibodies to the p34 subunit of Arp2/3 inhibits the incorporation of actin monomers in platelet extracts. In addition, activation of platelets by thrombin receptor activating peptide induces the localization of Arp2/3 to the lamellipodia, where filaments branch, and to the filopodia, and it stimulates the polymerization of actin (74,150).

The activation of the Arp2/3 complex is regulated by two pathways: the WASp and the WAVE, also called Scar proteins. Little is known about the WAVE/Scar pathway, even if all three isoforms, WAVE1, WAVE2, and WAVE3, are expressed in platelets (151). The WASp pathway is better characterized. Unstimulated WASp holds in an autoinhibited, inactive conformation. It becomes active upon stimulation by the following signaling molecules: the small G protein Cdc42, the phosphatidylinositol 4,5-bisphosphate PIP$_2$ (152), and the recently characterized protein Toca-1 (transducer of Cdc42-dependent actin assembly). N-WASp, in neuronal cells, was initially reported as an inducer of filopodia (153). A recent paper, using FRET, shows that N-WASp is activated in response to inside cell stimulation extending filopodia. It also regulates membrane ruffling downstream PIP$_2$ and Cdc42 (154). The upstream activator Toca-1 binds both N-WASp and Cdc42 and activates N-WASp to promote actin nucleation (155).

Activated WASp is an upstream regulator of Arp2/3. The A-motif of WASp contains a cluster of acidic residues that mediates the interaction of WASp with Arp2/3 (152). The C-terminal domain of N-WASp, which sequesters Arp2/3 complex, inhibits by half the actin nucleation capacity in normal permeabilized platelets (152). WASp could localize to the membrane through its EVH domain and, after stimulation, recruit actin monomers to sites containing Arp2/3. Monomers of actin are transported by profilin that interacts with WASp. Profilin then releases the monomers of actin at the sites of nucleation and accelerates the polymerization of actin (156). Finally, WASp and N-WASp accelerate the actin nucleation activity to induce filopodia formation downstream Cdc42. By contrast, WAVE/Scar and cortactin orchestrate lamellae spreading downstream of Rac1 (157–160). Activation of Rac1 induced the relocalization of cortactin to the membrane cytoskeleton, where cortactin directly interacts with Arp2/3, and may contribute to lamellipodia formation (158). A positive regulatory role for cortactin in the activation of Arp2/3 has been demonstrated (159).

Although WASp is a direct target for Cdc42, the vasodilator-stimulated phosphoprotein (VASP), a protein related to WASp, may be important in regulating actin polymerization in response to Rho activation (161,162). VASP is a polypeptide of

$M_r$ approximately 40 kDa, which exists *in vivo* as a tetramer. VASP contains a proline-rich sequence for the binding of profilin, an EVH domain that interacts with zyxin and vinculin at focal adhesion points. It does not bind Arp2/3. In platelets, VASP is a substrate of cyclic adenosine monophosphate (cAMP)–dependent and cyclic guanosine monophosphate (cGMP)–dependent protein kinases. The serine/threonine phosphorylation of VASP inhibits platelet aggregation (163). These findings are consistent with a role for VASP in regulating actin polymerization in focal adhesions.

Finally, the molecular mechanisms for actin reorganization in filopodia and lamellae have been better understood since the role of Arp2/3 was elucidated. However, the fine regulation of actin polymerization at focal adhesion points remains to be precisely understood.

### Actin Depolymerization in Activated Platelets

After growth, capping proteins terminate the filament elongation. When filaments have aged by hydrolysis of their bound ATP, cofilin promotes debranching and depolymerization. Cofilin severs actin filaments and accelerates monomer release at the pointed ends (164). A bifunctional capping protein, CAP1, also facilitates depolymerization: CAP1 both accelerates F-actin depolymerization at the pointed ends and facilitates its elongation at barbed ends (165). Regeneration of easily polymerizable G-actin depends on the exchange of ADP to ATP. The ABP profilin catalyzes the exchange of ADP to ATP, thereby refilling the pool of ATP-actin monomers.

# CONCLUSION

Finally, the dynamic reorganization of cellular cytoskeleton aims to ensure cell motility, and also cell–cell contact, for instance platelet aggregation (166). Platelet shape is mainly controlled at rest by the microtubule circle. In the case of activated platelets, an assembly of a branched network of actin filaments allows the protrusion of lamellipodia. This network is broken when platelets extend filopodia and capping proteins control these two major events. However, to reach an irreversible stage of activation such as full aggregation and MP shedding, actin movements escape from control and stop. The dynamic cytoskeleton enters a steady state for physiologic functions such as clotting.

## References

1. Frenette PS, Moyna C, Hartwell DW, et al. Platelet-endothelial interactions in inflamed mesenteric venules. *Blood* 1998;91:1318–1324.
2. Paulus JM. Platelet size in man. *Blood* 1975;46:321–336.
3. Cramer EM, Norol F, Guichard J, et al. Ultrastructure of platelet formation by human megakaryocytes cultured with the Mpl ligand. *Blood* 1997;89:2336–2346.
4. Corash L, Chen HY, Levin J. Regulation of thrombopoiesis: effects of the degree of thrombocytopenia on megakaryocyte ploidy and platelet volume. *Blood* 1987;70:177–185.
5. Corash L, Levin J. The relationship between megakaryocyte ploidy and platelet volume in normal and thrombocytopenic C3H mice. *Exp Hematol* 1990;18:985–989.
6. Behnke O. Electron microscopical observations on the surface coating of human blood platelets. *J Ultrastruct Res* 1968;24:412–420.
7. Perini F, Frangione B, Prelli F. Prion protein released by platelets. *Lancet* 1996;347:1635–1636.
8. Ruggeri ZM. Mechanisms initiating platelet thrombus formation. *Thromb Haemost* 1997;78:611–616.
9. Lopez JA, Dong JF. Structure and function of the glycoprotein Ib-IX-V complex. *Curr Opin Hematol* 1997;4:3232–3329.
10. Berger G, Massé J-M, Cramer EM. Alpha-granule membrane mirrors the platelet plasma membrane and contains the glycoproteins I, IX and V. *Blood* 1996;87:1385–1395.
11. Fox JE. The platelet cytoskeleton. *Thromb Haemost* 1993;70:884–893.
12. Hoffman R. Control of thrombocytopoiesis: current state of the art. *Cancer Treat Res* 1995;80:25–49.
13. Cramer EM, Berger G, Berndt MC. Platelet α-granule and plasma membrane share two new components: CD9 and PECAMI. *Blood* 1994;84:1722–1730.
14. Handagama P, Bainton DF, Jacques Y, et al. Kistrin, an integrin antagonist, blocks endocytosis of fibrinogen into guinea pig megakaryocyte and platelet alpha-granules. *J Clin Invest* 1993;91:193–200.
15. Greenwalt DE, Lipsky RH, Ockenhouse CF, et al. Membrane glycoprotein CD36: a review of its roles in adherence, signal transduction, and transfusion medicine. *Blood* 1992;80:1105–1115.
16. Berger G, Caen J-P, Berndt MC, et al. Ultrastructural demonstration of CD36 in the α granule membrane of human platelets and megakaryocytes. *Blood* 1993;82:3034–3044.
17. Coller BS, Seligsohn U, West SM, et al. Platelet fibrinogen and vitronectin in glanzmann thrombasthenia: evidence consistent with specific roles for glycoprotein IIb/IIIa and α v β 3 integrins in platelet protein trafficking. *Blood* 1991;78:2603–2610.
18. Lagaudrière-Gesbert C, Le Naour F, Lebel-Binay S, et al. Functional analysis of four tetraspans, CD9, CD53, CD81, and CD82, suggests a common role in costimulation, cell adhesion, and migration: only CD9 upregulates HB-EGF activity. *Cell Immunol* 1997;182:105–112.
19. Newman PJ, Hillery CA, Albrecht R, et al. Activation-dependent changes in human platelet PECAM-1: phosphorylation, cytoskeletal association, and surface membrane redistribution. *J Cell Biol* 1992;119:239–246.
20. Fox JEB, Austin CD, Boyles JK, et al. Role of membrane skeleton in preventing the shedding of procoagulant-rich microvesicles from the platelet plasma membrane. *J Cell Biol* 1990;111:483–493.
21. Hourdillé P, Heilmann E, Combrie R, et al. Thrombin induces a rapid redistribution of glycoprotein Ib-IX complexes within the membrane systems of activated human platelets. *Blood* 1990;76:1503–1513.
22. Cramer E, Lu H, Caen JP, et al. Differential redistribution of platelet glycoproteins Ib and IIb-IIIa after plasmin stimulation. *Blood* 1991;77:694–699.
23. Lu H, Soria C, Soria J, et al. Reversible translocation of glycoprotein Ib in plasmin-treated platelets: consequences for platelet function. *Eur J Clin Invest* 1993;23:785–793.
24. Isenberg WM, McEver RP, Phillips DR. The platelet fibrinogen receptor: an immunogold-surface replica study of agonist-induced ligand binding and receptor clustering. *J Cell Biol* 1987;104:1655–1663.
25. Sims PJ, Ginsberg MH, Plow EF, et al. Effect of platelet activation on the conformation of the plasma membrane glycoprotein IIb-IIIa complex. *J Biol Chem* 1991;266:7345–7352.
26. Berger G, Quarck R, Tenza D, et al. Ultrastructural localization of the small GTP-binding protein Rap1 in human platelets and megakaryocytes. *Br J Haematol* 1994;88:372–382.
27. Stenberg PE, Pestina TI, Barrie RJ, et al. The Src family kinases, Fgr, Fyn, Lck, and Lyn, colocalize with coated membranes in platelets. *Blood* 1997;89:2384–2393.
28. Lu H, Menashi S, Garcia I, et al. Reversibility of thrombin-induced decrease in platelet glycoprotein Ib function. *Br J Haematol* 1993;85:116–123.
29. Cramer EM, Savidge GF, Vainchenker W, et al. Alpha granule pool of glycoprotein IIb-IIIa in normal and pathologic platelets and megakaryocytes. *Blood* 1990;75:1220–1227.
30. Kieffer N, Guichard J, Breton-Gorius J. Dynamic redistribution of major surface receptors after contact-induced platelet activation and spreading: an immunoelectron microscopic study. *Am J Pathol* 1992;40:57–73.
31. Suzuki H, Kinlough-Rathbone RL, Packham MA, et al. Immunocytochemical localization of fibrinogen during thrombin-induced aggregation of washed human platelets. *Blood* 1988;71:1310–1320.
32. Breton-Gorius J, Guichard J. Ultrastructural localization of peroxidase activity in human platelets and megakaryocytes. *Am J Pathol* 1972;66:277–286.
33. Gerrard JM, White JG, Rao GH, et al. Localization of platelet prostaglandin production in the platelet dense tubular system. *Am J Pathol* 1976;83:283–298.
34. Heijnen HFG, Debili N, Vainchenker W, et al. Multivesicular bodies are an intermediate stage in the formation of platelet α-granules. *Blood* 1998;91:2313–2325.
35. Harrison P, Cramer EM. Platelet α-granules. *Blood Rev* 1993;7:52–62.
36. Cramer EM, Meyer D, Le Menn R, et al. Eccentric localization of von Willebrand factor in an internal structure of platelet α-granule resembling that of Weibel-Palade bodies. *Blood* 1985;66:710–713.
37. Cramer EM, Caen JP, Drouet L, et al. Absence of tubular structures and immunolabeling for von Willebrand factor in the platelet alpha-granules from porcine von Willebrand disease. *Blood* 1986;68:774–778.
38. Harrison P, Wilbourn B, Lawrie A, et al. Porcine platelets contain an increased quantity of ultra-high molecular weight von Willebrand factor and numerous alpha-granular tubular structures. *Br J Haematol* 1993;83:608–615.
39. Hayward CP, Bainton DF, Smith JW, et al. Multimerin is found in the alpha-granules of resting platelets and is synthesized by a megakaryocytic cell line. *J Clin Invest* 1993;91:2630–2639.
40. Stenberg PE, McEver RP, Shuman MA, et al. A platelet alpha-granule membrane protein (GMP-140) is expressed on the plasma membrane after activation. *J Cell Biol* 1985;101:880–886.
41. Rosa JP, George JN, Bainton DF, et al. Gray platelet syndrome. Demonstration of alpha granule membranes that can fuse with the cell surface. *J Clin Invest* 1987;80:1138–1146.

42. Cramer E, Vainchenker W, Vinci G, et al. Gray platelet syndrome: immunoelectron microscopic localization of fibrinogen and von Willebrand factor in platelets and megakaryocytes. *Blood* 1985;66:1309–1316.

43. Breton-Gorius J, Vainchenker W, Nurdent A, et al. Defective alpha-granule production in megakaryocytes from gray platelet syndrome: ultrastructural studies of bone marrow cells and megakaryocytes growing in culture from blood precursors. *Am J Pathol* 1981;102:10–19.

44. White JG. The dense bodies of human platelets: Inherent electron opacity of the serotonin storage particles. *Blood* 1969;33:598–606.

45. Richards JG, Da Prada M. Uranaffin reaction: a new cytochemical technique for the localization of adenine nucleotides in organelles storing biogenic amines. *J Histochem Cytochem* 1977;25:1322–1326.

46. Wall J, Buijs-Wilts M, Arnold J, et al. A flow cytometric assay using mepacrine for study of uptake and release of platelet dense granule contents. *Br J Haematol* 1995;89:380–385.

47. Israels S, Gerrard J, Jacques Y, et al. Platelet dense granule membrane contains both granulophysin and P-selectin (GMP-140). *Blood* 1992;80:143.

48. Behnke O, Forer A. Blood platelet heterogeneity: evidence for two classes of platelets in man and rat. *Br J Haematol* 1993;84:686–693.

49. Menard M, Meyers KM, Prieur DJ. Demonstration of secondary lysosomes in bovine megakaryocytes and platelets using acid phosphatase cytochemistry with cerium as a trapping agent. *Thromb Haemost* 1990;63:127–132.

50. Breton-Gorius J, Vainchenker W. Expression of platelet proteins during the *in vitro* and *in vivo* differentiation of megakaryocytes and morphological aspects of their maturation. *Semin Hematol* 1986;28:43–67.

51. Stenberg PE, Shuman MA, Levine SP, et al. Redistribution of alpha-granules and their contents in thrombin-stimulated platelets. *J Cell Biol* 1984;98:748–760.

52. Rinder CS, Student LA, Bonan JL, et al. Aspirin does not inhibit adenosine diphosphate–induced platelet alpha-granule release. *Blood* 1993;82:505–512.

53. Tong M, Seth P, Penington DG. Proplatelets and stress platelets. *Blood* 1987;69:522–528.

54. Kienast J, Schmitz G. Flow cytometric analysis of thiazole orange uptake by platelets: a diagnostic aid in the evaluation of thrombocytopenic disorders. *Blood* 1990;75:116–121.

55. Robinson MS, Harrison C, Mackie IJ, et al. Reticulated platelets in primary and reactive thrombocytosis. *Br J Haematol* 1998;101:388–389.

56. White JG. Arrangements of actin filaments in the cytoskeleton of human platelets. *Am J Pathol* 1984;117:207–217.

57. White JG, Sauk JJ. Microtubule coils in spread blood platelets. *Blood* 1984;64:470–478.

58. Behnke O, Forer A. From megakaryocytes to platelets: platelet morphogenesis takes place in the bloodstream. *Eur J Haematol Suppl* 1998;61:3–23.

59. Italiano JJ, Bergmeier W, Tiwari S, et al. Mechanisms and implications of platelet discoid shape. *Blood* 2003;101:4789–4796.

60. White JG, Rao GH. Microtubule coils versus the surface membrane cytoskeleton in maintenance and restoration of platelet discoid shape. *Am J Pathol* 1998;152:597–609.

61. Steiner M, Ikada Y. Quantitative assessment of polymerized and depolymerized platelet microtubules. Changes caused by agregating agents. *J Clin Invest* 1979;63:443–448.

62. Steiner M. Fluorescence studies of platelet tubulin. *Biochemistry* 1980;19:4492–4499.

63. Andrews RK, Fox JE. Identification of a region in the cytoplasmic domain of the platelet membrane glycoprotein Ib-IX complex that binds to purified actin-binding protein. *J Biol Chem* 1992;267:18605–18611.

64. Kaverina I, Rottner K, Small JV. Targeting, capture, and stabilization of microtubules at early focal adhesions. *J Cell Biol* 1998;142:181–190.

65. Hartwig JH, DeSisto M. The cytoskeleton of the resting human blood platelet: structure of the membrane skeleton and its attachment to actin filaments. *J Cell Biol* 1991;112:407–425.

66. Hartwig J. Mechanism of actin rearrangements mediating platelet activation. *J Cell Biol* 1992;118:1421–1442.

67. Fox JE. Platelet activation: new aspects. *Haemostasis* 1996;26:102–131.

68. Fox JE, Boyles JK, Berndt MC, et al. Identification of a membrane skeleton in platelets. *J Cell Biol* 1988;106:1525–1538.

69. Fox JE, Lipfert L, Clark EA, et al. On the role of the platelet membrane skeleton in mediating signal transduction. Association of GP IIb-IIIa, pp60c-src, pp62c-yes, and the p21ras GTPase-activating protein with the membrane skeleton. *J Biol Chem* 1993;268:25973–25984.

70. Weber A, Nachmias VT, Pennise CR, et al. Interaction of thymosin $\beta$ 4 with muscle and platelet actin: implications for actin sequestration in resting platelets. *Biochemistry* 1992;31:6179–6185.

71. Hartwig JH, Chambers KA, Stossel TP. Association of gelsolin with actin filaments and cell membranes of macrophages and platelets. *J Cell Biol* 1989;108:467–479.

72. Witke W, Sharpe AH, Hartwig JH, et al. Hemostatic, inflammatory, and fibroblast responses are blunted in mice lacking gelsolin. *Cell* 1995;81:41–51.

73. Barkalow KL, Falet H, Italiano JE Jr., et al. Role for phosphoinositide 3-kinase in Fc gamma RIIA-induced platelet shape change. *Am J Physiol Cell Physiol* 2003;285:C797–C805.

74. Falet H, Hoffmeister KM, Neujahr R, et al. Importance of free actin filament barbed ends for Arp2/3 complex function in platelets and fibroblasts. *Proc Natl Acad Sci U S A* 2002;99:16782–16787.

75. Calverley DC, Kavanagh TJ, Roth GJ. Human signaling protein 14-3-3zeta interacts with platelet glycoprotein Ib subunits Ib$\alpha$ and Ib$\beta$. *Blood* 1998;91:1295–1303.

76. Xu W, Xie Z, Chung DW, et al. A novel human actin-binding protein homologue that binds to platelet glycoprotein Ib$\alpha$. *Blood* 1998;92:1268–1276.

77. Loo DT, Kanner SB, Aruffo A. Filamin binds to the cytoplasmic domain of the $\beta$1-integrin. Identification of amino acids responsible for this interaction. *J Biol Chem* 1998;273:23304–23312.

78. Ott I, Fischer EG, Miyagi Y, et al. A role for tissue factor in cell adhesion and migration mediated by interaction with actin-binding protein 280. *J Cell Biol* 1998;140:1241–1253.

79. Ohta Y, Stossel TP, Hartwig JH. Ligand-sensitive binding of actin-binding protein to immunoglobulin G Fc receptor I (Fc gamma RI). *Cell* 1991;67:275–282.

80. Ohta Y, Suzuki N, Nakamura S, et al. The small GTPase RalA targets filamin to induce filopodia. *Proc Natl Acad Sci U S A* 1999;96:2122–2128.

81. Davies GE, Cohen CM. Platelets contain proteins immunologically related to red cell spectrin and protein 4.1. *Blood* 1985;65:52–59.

82. Fox JE, Shattil SJ, Kinlough-Rathbone RL, et al. The platelet cytoskeleton stabilizes the interaction between $\alpha$IIb$\beta$3 and its ligand and induces selective movements of ligand-occupied integrin. *J Biol Chem* 1996;271:7004–7011.

83. Fox JE, Reynolds CC, Morrow JS, et al. Spectrin is associated with membrane-bound actin filaments in platelets and is hydrolyzed by the Ca2+-dependent protease during platelet activation. *Blood* 1987;69:537–545.

84. Tsukita S, Yonemura S. ERM (ezrin/radixin/moesin) family: from cytoskeleton to signal transduction. *Curr Opin Cell Biol* 1997;9:70–75.

85. Horwitz A, Duggan K, Buck C, et al. Interaction of plasma membrane fibronectin receptor with talin–a transmembrane linkage. *Nature* 1986;320:531–533.

86. Nakamura F, Amieva MR, Furthmayr H. Phosphorylation of threonine 558 in the carboxyl-terminal actin-binding domain of moesin by thrombin activation of human platelets. *J Biol Chem* 1995;270:31377–31385.

87. Bertagnolli ME, Locke SJ, Hensler ME, et al. Talin distribution and phosphorylation in thrombin-activated platelets. *J Cell Sci* 1993;106(Pt 4):1189–1199.

88. Stenberg PE, Barrie RJ, Pestina TI, et al. Prolonged bleeding time with defective platelet filpodia formation in the Wistar Furth rat. *Blood* 1998;91:1599–1608.

89. de Gaetano G, Cerletti C, Evangelista V. Recent advances in platelet-polymorphonuclear leukocyte interaction. *Haemostasis* 1999;29:41–49.

90. Du X, Saido TC, Tsubuki S, et al. Calpain cleavage of the cytoplasmic domain of the integrin $\beta$ 3 subunit. *J Biol Chem* 1995;270:26146–26151.

91. Croce K, Flaumenhaft R, Rivers M, et al. Inhibition of calpain blocks platelet secretion, aggregation, and spreading. *J Biol Chem* 1999;274:36321–36327.

92. Siljander P, Farndale RW, Feijge MA, et al. Platelet adhesion enhances the glycoprotein VI-dependent procoagulant response: involvement of p38 MAP kinase and calpain. *Arterioscler Thromb Vasc Biol* 2001;21:618–627.

93. Jenkins AL, Nannizzi-Alaimo L, Silver D, et al. Tyrosine phosphorylation of the $\beta$3 cytoplasmic domain mediates integrin-cytoskeletal interactions. *J Biol Chem* 1998;273:13878–13885.

94. Resendiz JC, Feng S, Ji G, et al. von Willebrand factor binding to platelet glycoprotein Ib-IX-V stimulates the assembly of an $\alpha$-actinin–based signaling complex. *J Thromb Haemost* 2004;2:161–169.

95. Reddy KB, Bialkowska K, Fox JE. Dynamic modulation of cytoskeletal proteins linking integrins to signaling complexes in spreading cells. Role of skelemin in initial integrin-induced spreading. *J Biol Chem* 2001;276:28300–28308.

96. Heijnen HF, Van Lier M, Waaijenborg S, et al. Concentration of rafts in platelet filopodia correlates with recruitment of c-Src and CD63 to these domains. *J Thromb Haemost* 2003;1:1161–1173.

97. Locke D, Chen H, Liu Y, et al. Lipid rafts orchestrate signaling by the platelet receptor glycoprotein VI. *J Biol Chem* 2002;277:18801–18809.

98. Bodin S, Giuriato S, Ragab J, et al. Production of phosphatidylinositol 3,4,5-trisphosphate and phosphatidic acid in platelet rafts: evidence for a critical role of cholesterol-enriched domains in human platelet activation. *Biochemistry* 2001;40:15290–15299.

99. Lopez I, Duprez V, Melle J, et al. Thrombopoietin stimulates cortactin translocation to the cytoskeleton independently of tyrosine phosphorylation. *Biochem J* 2001;356:875–881.

100. Izaguirre G, Aguirre L, Hu YP, et al. The cytoskeletal/non-muscle isoform of $\alpha$-actinin is phosphorylated on its actin-binding domain by the focal adhesion kinase. *J Biol Chem* 2001;276:28676–28685.

101. Toth-Zsamboki E, Oury C, Cornelissen H, et al. P2X1-mediated ERK2 activation amplifies the collagen-induced platelet secretion by enhancing myosin light chain kinase activation. *J Biol Chem* 2003;278:46661–46667.

102. Pasquet JM, Noury M, Nurden AT. Evidence that the platelet integrin $\alpha$IIb $\beta$3 is regulated by the thrombin-linked kinase, ILK, in a PI3-kinase dependent pathway. *Thromb Haemost* 2002;88:115–122.

103. Kiss E, Muranyi A, Csortos C, et al. Integrin-linked kinase phosphorylates the myosin phosphatase target subunit at the inhibitory site in platelet cytoskeleton. *Biochem J* 2002;365:79–87.

104. Amano M, Chihara K, Kimura K, et al. Formation of actin stress fibers and focal adhesions enhanced by Rho-kinase. *Science* 1997;275:1308–1311.

105. Hall A. Rho GTPases and the actin cytoskeleton. *Science* 1998;279: 509–514.

106. Nobes CD, Hall A. Rho, rac, and cdc42 GTPases regulate the assembly of multimolecular focal complexes associated with actin stress fibers, lamellipodia, and filopodia. *Cell* 1995;81:53–62.

107. Chrzanowska-Wodnicka M, Burridge K. Rho-stimulated contractility drives the formation of stress fibers and focal adhesions. *J Cell Biol* 1996; 133:1403–1415.

108. Crespo P, Schuebel KE, Ostrom AA, et al. Phosphotyrosine-dependent activation of Rac-1 GDP/GTP exchange by the vav proto-oncogene product. *Nature* 1997;385:169–172.

109. Ma AD, Metjian A, Bagrodia S, et al. Cytoskeletal reorganization by G protein-coupled receptors is dependent on phosphoinositide 3-kinase gamma, a Rac guanosine exchange factor, and Rac. *Mol Cell Biol* 1998; 18:4744–4751.

110. Han J, Luby-Phelps K, Das B, et al. Role of substrates and products of PI 3-kinase in regulating activation of Rac-related guanosine triphosphatases by Vav. *Science* 1998;279:558–560.

111. Cichowski K, Brugge JS, Brass LF. Thrombin receptor activation and integrin engagement stimulate tyrosine phosphorylation of the proto-oncogene product, p95vav, in platelets. *J Biol Chem* 1996;271: 7544–7550.

112. Leng L, Kashiwagi H, Ren XD, et al. RhoA and the function of platelet integrin αIIbβ3. *Blood* 1998;91:4206–4215.

113. Hartwig JH, Bokoch GM, Carpenter CL, et al. Thrombin receptor ligation and activated Rac uncap actin filament barbed ends through phosphoinositide synthesis in permeabilized human platelets. *Cell* 1995; 82:643–653.

114. Azim AC, Barkalow K, Chou J, et al. Activation of the small GTPases, rac and cdc42, after ligation of the platelet PAR-1 receptor. *Blood* 2000; 95:959–964.

115. Clark EA, King WG, Brugge JS, et al. Integrin-mediated signals regulated by members of the rho family of GTPases. *J Cell Biol* 1998;142:573–586.

116. Tolias KF, Cantley LC, Carpenter CL. Rho family GTPases bind to phosphoinositide kinases. *J Biol Chem* 1995;270:17656–17659.

117. Zheng Y, Bagrodia S, Cerione RA. Activation of phosphoinositide 3-kinase activity by Cdc42Hs binding to p85. *J Biol Chem* 1994;269:18727–18730.

118. Zhang J, King WG, Dillon S, et al. Activation of platelet phosphatidylinositide 3-kinase requires the small GTP-binding protein Rho. *J Biol Chem* 1993;268:22251–22254.

119. Guinebault C, Payrastre B, Racaud-Sultan C, et al. Integrin-dependent translocation of phosphoinositide 3-kinase to the cytoskeleton of thrombin-activated platelets involves specific interactions of p85 α with actin filaments and focal adhesion kinase. *J Cell Biol* 1995;129:831–842.

120. Chong LD, Traynor-Kaplan A, Bokoch GM, et al. The small GTP-binding protein Rho regulates a phosphatidylinositol 4-phosphate 5-kinase in mammalian cells. *Cell* 1994;79:507–513.

121. Manser E, Leung T, Salihuddin H, et al. A brain serine/threonine protein kinase activated by Cdc42 and Rac1. *Nature* 1994;367:40–46.

122. Teo M, Manser E, Lim L. Identification and molecular cloning of a p21cdc42/rac1-activated serine/threonine kinase that is rapidly activated by thrombin in platelets. *J Biol Chem* 1995;270:26690–26697.

123. Vidal C, Geny B, Melle J, et al. Cdc42/Rac1-dependent activation of the p21-activated kinase (PAK) regulates human platelet lamellipodia spreading: implication of the cortical-actin binding protein cortactin. *Blood* 2002;100:4462–4469.

124. Schmidt VA, Scudder L, Devoe CE, et al. IQGAP2 functions as a GTP-dependent effector protein in thrombin-induced platelet cytoskeletal reorganization. *Blood* 2003;101:3021–3028.

125. Symons M, Derry JM, Karlak B, et al. Wiskott-Aldrich syndrome protein, a novel effector for the GTPase CDC42Hs, is implicated in actin polymerization. *Cell* 1996;84:723–734.

126. Fox JE, Phillips DR. Role of phosphorylation in mediating the association of myosin with the cytoskeletal structures of human platelets. *J Biol Chem* 1982;257:4120–4126.

127. Paul BZ, Daniel JL, Kunapuli SP. Platelet shape change is mediated by both calcium-dependent and -independent signaling pathways. Role of p160 Rho-associated coiled-coil-containing protein kinase in platelet shape change. *J Biol Chem* 1999;274:28293–28300.

128. Bauer M, Retzer M, Wilde JI, et al. Dichotomous regulation of myosin phosphorylation and shape change by Rho-kinase and calcium in intact human platelets. *Blood* 1999;94:1665–1672.

129. Suzuki Y, Yamamoto M, Wada H, et al. Agonist-induced regulation of myosin phosphatase activity in human platelets through activation of Rho-kinase. *Blood* 1999;93:3408–3417.

130. Zhang J, Banfic H, Straforini F, et al. A type II phosphoinositide 3-kinase is stimulated via activated integrin in platelets. A source of phosphatidylinositol 3-phosphate. *J Biol Chem* 1998;273:14081–14084.

131. Lipfert L, Haimovich B, Schaller MD, et al. Integrin-dependent phosphorylation and activation of the protein tyrosine kinase pp125FAK in platelets. *J Cell Biol* 1992;119:905–912.

132. Falet H, Ramos-Morales F, Bachelot C, et al. Association of the protein tyrosine phosphatase PTP1C with the protein tyrosine kinase c-Src in human platelets. *FEBS Lett* 1996;383:165–169.

133. Dash D, Aepfelbacher M, Siess W. The association of pp125FAK, pp60Src, CDC42Hs and Rap1B with the cytoskeleton of aggregated platelets is a reversible process regulated by calcium. *FEBS Lett* 1995;363:231–234.

134. Osdoit S, Rosa JP. Fibrin clot retraction by human platelets correlates with α(IIb)β(3) integrin-dependent protein tyrosine dephosphorylation. *J Biol Chem* 2001;276:6703–6710.

135. Wolf P. The nature and significance of platelet products in human plasma. *Br J Haematol* 1967;13:269–288.

136. Crawford N. The presence of contractile proteins in platelet microparticles isolated from human and animal platelet-free plasma. *Br J Haematol* 1971;21:53–69.

137. Wiedmer T, Shattil SJ, Cunningham M, et al. Role of calcium and calpain in complement-induced vesiculation of the platelet plasma membrane and in the exposure of the platelet factor Va receptor. *Biochemistry* 1990; 29:623–632.

138. Hughes M, Hayward CPM, Warkentin TE, et al. Morphological analysis of microparticles generation in heparin-induced thrombocytopenia. *Blood* 2000;96:188–194.

139. Tans G, Rosing J, Thomassen MC, et al. Comparison of anticoagulant and procoagulant activities of stimulated platelets and platelet-derived microparticles. *Blood* 1991;77:2641–2648.

140. Dachary-Prigent J, Freyssinet JM, Pasquet JM, et al. Annexin V as a probe of aminophospholipid exposure and platelet membrane vesiculation: a flow cytometry study showing a role for free sulfhydryl groups. *Blood* 1993;81:2554–2565.

141. Fourcade O, Simon MF, Viode C, et al. Secretory phospholipase A2 generates the novel lipid mediator lysophosphatidic acid in membrane microvesicles shed from activated cells. *Cell* 1995;80:919–927.

142. Heijnen HF, Schiel AE, Fijnheer R, et al. Activated platelets release two types of membrane vesicles: microvesicles by surface shedding and exosomes derived from exocytosis of multivesicular bodies and alpha-granules. *Blood* 1999;94:3791–3799.

143. Fox JE, Austin CD, Reynolds CC, et al. Evidence that agonist-induced activation of calpain causes the shedding of procoagulant-containing microvesicles from the membrane of aggregating platelets. *J Biol Chem* 1991;266:13289–13295.

144. Pasquet JM, Dachary-Prigent J, Nurden AT. Microvesicle release is associated with extensive protein tyrosine dephosphorylation in platelets stimulated by A23187 or a mixture of thrombin and collagen. *Biochem J* 1998; 333(Pt 3):591–599.

145. Yano Y, Kambayashi J, Shiba E, et al. The role of protein phosphorylation and cytoskeletal reorganization in microparticle formation from the platelet plasma membrane. *Biochem J* 1994;299(Pt 1):303–308.

146. Schoenwaelder SM, Yuan Y, Cooray P, et al. Calpain cleavage of focal adhesion proteins regulates the cytoskeletal attachment of integrin αIIbβ3 (platelet glycoprotein IIb/IIIa) and the cellular retraction of fibrin clots. *J Biol Chem* 1997;272:1694–1702.

147. Miki H, Nonoyama S, Zhu Q, et al. Tyrosine kinase signaling regulates Wiskott-Aldrich syndrome protein function, which is essential for megakaryocyte differentiation. *Cell Growth Differ* 1997;8:195–202.

148. Allen PG. Actin filament uncapping localizes to ruffling lamellae and rocketing vesicles. *Nat Cell Biol* 2003;5:972–979.

149. Li Z, Kim ES, Bearer EL. Arp2/3 complex is required for actin polymerization during platelet shape change. *Blood* 2002;99:4466–4474.

150. Falet H, Hoffmeister KM, Neujahr R, et al. Normal Arp2/3 complex activation in platelets lacking WASp. *Blood* 2002;100:2113–2122.

151. Oda A, Miki H, Wada I, et al. WAVE/Scars in Platelets. *Blood* 2005;105: 3141–3148.

152. Rohatgi R, Ma L, Miki H, et al. The interaction between N-WASp and the Arp2/3 complex links Cdc42-dependent signals to actin assembly. *Cell* 1999;97:221–231.

153. Miki H, Sasaki T, Takai Y, et al. Induction of filopodium formation by a WASp-related actin-depolymerizing protein N-WASp. *Nature* 1998;391: 93–96.

154. Ward ME, Wu JY, Rao Y. Visualization of spatially and temporally regulated N-WASP activity during cytoskeletal reorganization in living cells. *Proc Natl Acad Sci U S A* 2004;101:970–974.

155. Ho HY, Rohatgi R, Lebensohn AM, et al. Toca-1 mediates Cdc42-dependent actin nucleation by activating the N-WASP-WIP complex. *Cell* 2004;118:203–216.

156. Suetsugu S, Miki H, Takenawa T. The essential role of profilin in the assembly of actin for microspike formation. *EMBO J* 1998;17:6516–6526.

157. Miki H, Suetsugu S, Takenawa T. WAVE, a novel WASP-family protein involved in actin reorganization induced by Rac. *EMBO J* 1998;17: 6932–6941.

158. Weed SA, Karginov AV, Schafer DA, et al. Cortactin localization to sites of actin assembly in lamellipodia requires interactions with F-actin and the Arp2/3 complex. *J Cell Biol* 2000;151:29–40.

159. Uruno T, Liu J, Zhang P, et al. Activation of Arp2/3 complex-mediated actin polymerization by cortactin. *Nat Cell Biol* 2001;3:259–266.

160. Head JA, Jiang D, Li M, et al. Cortactin tyrosine phosphorylation requires Rac1 activity and association with the cortical actin cytoskeleton. *Mol Biol Cell* 2003;14:3216–3229.

161. Reinhard M, Giehl K, Abel K, et al. The proline-rich focal adhesion and microfilament protein VASP is a ligand for profilins. *EMBO J* 1995;14: 1583–1589.

162. Prehoda KE, Lee DJ, Lim WA. Structure of the enabled/VASP homology 1 domain-peptide complex: a key component in the spatial control of actin assembly. *Cell* 1999;97:471–480.

163. Aszodi A, Pfeifer A, Ahmad M, et al. The vasodilator-stimulated phosphoprotein (VASP) is involved in cGMP- and cAMP-mediated inhibition of agonist-induced platelet aggregation, but is dispensable for smooth muscle function. *EMBO J* 1999;18:37–48.

164. Moriyama K, Yahara I. Two activities of cofilin, severing and accelerating directional depolymerization of actin filaments, are affected differentially by mutations around the actin-binding helix. *EMBO J* 1999;18:6752–6761.

165. Moriyama K, Yahara I. Human CAP1 is a key factor in the recycling of cofilin and actin for rapid actin turnover. *J Cell Sci* 2002;115:1591–1601.

166. Pollard TD, Borisy GG. Cellular motility driven by assembly and disassembly of actin filaments. *Cell* 2003;112:453–465.

# CHAPTER 27 ■ THROMBOPOIETIN

KENNETH KAUSHANSKY

## HISTORY

The term erythropoietin (EPO) was coined at the turn of the 20th century to describe the humoral substance responsible for red blood cell production. At that time, blood platelets were barely distinguishable in the best microscopes, prompting their dismissal as the "dust of the blood." However, the pioneering work of Carnot and of Wright and others in the early 20th century defined the crucial role of blood platelets in coagulation and their origin from the marrow megakaryocytes, ultimately prompting the Hungarian physician Keleman to coin the term *thrombopoietin* (TPO) to describe the humoral substance responsible for the recovery of platelet levels following thrombocytopenia (1).

In the mid 1960s, several groups set out to purify TPO from the plasma of thrombocytopenic animals. At the time, the only reliable assay on which to base a purification strategy was the $^{35}$S uptake assay into the peripheral blood platelets of mice or rats injected with the assay fraction. This *in vivo* assay proved cumbersome; the assay was too insensitive, costly, and time-consuming to be practical, and little progress was made. With the availability of *in vitro* megakaryocyte differentiation assays in the 1980s, additional purifications were attempted; nevertheless, although the availability of what was thought to be partially purified TPO helped to define its expected biological properties (2–4), none of the initial purification efforts led to amino acid determination or to the cloning of the molecule.

Occasionally in science, a finding from one field, although important in itself, can have a profound, catalytic effect on a seemingly unrelated area of research. The discovery and characterization of the murine myeloproliferative leukemia virus (MPLV) had such an influence on the search for TPO. This virus causes an acute myeloproliferative syndrome in infected mice (5). In 1990, the responsible oncogene was cloned, and the protooncogene was obtained 2 years later (6,7). On the basis of the predicted presence of four spatially conserved cysteine residues, and a juxtamembrane pentapeptide sequence (Trp–Ser–Naa–Trp–Ser), it was immediately evident that the cellular gene was a member of the hematopoietic cytokine receptor family (8), which includes the receptors for EPO; the granulopoietic factors interleukin-3 (IL-3), granulocyte colony-stimulating factor (G-CSF), and granulocyte macrophage colony-stimulating factor (GM-CSF); and multiple lymphokines. However, in 1992, the receptor's ligand was unknown; *c-mpl* encoded an orphan receptor. On the basis of the origin of the Mpl complementary deoxyribonucleic acid (cDNA), the bipotent erythroid/MK cell line HEL (9), and the antisense *c-mpl* knockout experiments that demonstrated a significant reduction in megakaryocytes (10), many groups postulated that the *mpl* ligand might be identical to TPO.

## THE CLONING OF THROMBOPOIETIN

Although progress in understanding megakaryocyte biology and in purifying TPO was being made using the c-Mpl receptor, others had developed improved bioassays for TPO and continued to make efforts using conventional purification strategies. Using a modified *in vivo* assay in which the polyploidy of marrow megakaryocytes from injected rats was examined, Kuter et al. performed an 11-step purification of ovine TPO (11), although the publication of this work did not report the cloning of the corresponding cDNA. In contrast, using an *in vitro* megakaryocyte assay, the scientists at Kirin Pharmaceuticals, in a 12-step conventional purification scheme, obtained sufficient plasma TPO from thrombocytopenic rats to obtain the amino acid sequence and cloned the cDNA for rat and then for multiple species of the protein, including the human hormone (12).

By using the *c-Mpl* protooncogene product coupled to affinity matrices, scientists at Genentech and at Amgen obtained microgram quantities of porcine and canine TPO, respectively, allowing their amino acid sequencing and cDNA cloning (13). In contrast to the biochemical purifications utilized by these four groups, an expression cloning strategy was used by Lok et al. to obtain cDNA for murine and then human TPO (14). In this approach, a hematopoietic cell line, BaF3, which requires IL-3 for survival and proliferation was engineered to express the *c-Mpl* protooncogene. In this way, if the c-Mpl ligand was present in the culture, the cells might remain viable and potentially proliferate after withdrawal of IL-3. The BaF3/mpl cells were chemically mutated, and autonomously growing sublines were obtained; although most such sublines were producing their own IL-3, others were producing the c-Mpl ligand. This subline was used as the source for cDNA library construction and as an additional functional cloning strategy. Remarkably, the cDNA obtained from the previously described four groups, three cloned simultaneously, but all encoded the same polypeptide (except for species differences). Initial *in vitro* experiments using the corresponding recombinant proteins demonstrated the effect of each of these substances on megakaryocyte maturation, and injections into normal mice resulted in impressive increases in peripheral blood platelet counts and marrow megakaryopoiesis. With these efforts, TPO was finally cloned.

## STRUCTURE OF THROMBOPOIETIN

The cloned human TPO cDNA encodes a polypeptide of 353 amino acids, including the 21–amino acid secretory leader sequence (15). The mature protein can be conveniently divided into two domains: The amino-terminal 154 residues bear a striking sequence homology to that of erythropoietin (EPO) and bind to the c-Mpl receptor; the carboxyl-terminal domain bears no resemblance to any known proteins but contains multiple sites of both N- and O-linked carbohydrate. This latter feature accounts for the large discrepancy between the predicted and actual molecular weight of the protein; approximately 50% of the 70-kDa TPO molecule is carbohydrate.

On the basis of its amino acid sequence, and like its closest homolog EPO, TPO is predicted to fold into a four-helix bundle protein. This prediction was recently confirmed with the determination of the tertiary structure of the receptor-binding domain of TPO in complex with an anti-TPO monoclonal antibody (16). Comparisons of the two proteins reveal striking similarities, but also some critical differences, likely accounting for the failure of the two hormones to cross-react with the receptors for the other hormone (17).

As noted, TPO can be conveniently divided into two domains on the basis of homology to EPO; expression of a truncated version that represents the domain most homologous to EPO revealed that this amino-terminal half of the molecule is responsible for binding to the Mpl receptor (18). However, the circulatory half-life of the isolated amino-terminal fragment is substantially shorter than the full-length molecule, unless it is modified with polyethylene glycol (19). A second biologic property recently assigned to the carboxyl-terminal domain of TPO is to enhance secretory efficiency of the protein; the level at which the isolated amino-terminal fragment is expressed from cells that normally produce TPO is reduced about five- to 10-fold compared with the secretory level of the full-length molecule (20–22). Whether this is due to enhanced folding of the polypeptide, protection from intracellular proteolysis, or other mechanisms is presently under study.

Several investigators have attempted to ascertain the sites on TPO responsible for binding to its receptor. By using site-directed alanine-scanning mutagenesis to study the functional activities of 40 solvent-exposed residues of the protein, monoclonal antibody epitope mapping and a phage display binding assay system, Pearce et al. determined that, the residues vital for hormone binding to c-Mpl are located in the first and fourth predicted $\alpha$-helices of the molecule and the segment connecting the first and second helices (23), locations previously shown to be important for functional interactions in several other cytokine/receptor systems (24). Subsequently, Jagerschmidt produced 20 TPO mutants and compared the mutants' ability to induce the proliferation of a c-Mpl–expressing cell line, M-O7e, with that of wild-type TPO (25). Among the mutations that substantially reduced biologic activity, three were found located in the A helix of the protein (Arg10, Lys14 and Arg17) and four in helix D (His133, Gln132, Lys138, and Phe141). Moreover, they found that Arg10 and Arg17 seem to be specific determinants for TPO/c-Mpl recognition, although Pearce et al. failed to find any reduction in binding affinity of an Arg10 to Ala mutation. Because these residues in EPO are Arg and Leu, respectively, the latter residue could help explain the failure of the two cytokines to cross-react in receptor-binding assays (17).

# THE REGULATION OF THROMBOPOIETIN EXPRESSION

As would be expected for the physiologic regulator of platelet production, plasma concentrations of TPO vary inversely with the platelet count in patients with marrow failure (26). Northern blot analyses of multiple organs reveal that TPO is widely expressed, with messenger ribonucleic acid (mRNA) being present at highest levels in the liver of normal animals, but the kidney, smooth muscle, and a number of other organs also express transcripts for the hormone (13,14,18). On the basis of the capacity of platelets to adsorb TPO from its surroundings, and internalize and destroy it, Kuter and Rosenberg (27) and other investigators (28) have proposed that the regulation of TPO levels in plasma is dependent entirely on platelet numbers; in the presence of thrombocytosis, the steady state level of hormone production is overwhelmed by platelet-mediated TPO removal and levels of TPO are low; in states of thrombocytopenia, little of the same amount of TPO produced is adsorbed, allowing the levels of TPO to rise. Initial findings of relatively low TPO levels in patients with immune thrombocytopenia were addressed by further postulating that the megakaryocytic hyperplasia seen in such states accounts for the increased TPO adsorption. Ancillary data for this assertion come from the *tpo* hemizygous mouse (29): Loss of one allele of *tpo* leads to a 40% reduction in platelet counts; if active regulation of TPO exists, then increased expression from the second, normal allele should have corrected the reduction in hormone levels and should have reestablished a normal platelet count, much like what occurs in the EPO system.

These arguments not withstanding, a growing body of evidence suggests that additional mechanisms operate to affect TPO expression. At baseline, it is very difficult to detect specific mRNA in marrow cells. However, transcript levels can be substantially induced in marrow stromal cells in response to thrombocytopenia (30–33), although at platelet levels less than the 60% found in the *tpo* hemizygous mice. In addition, a number of inflammatory states are associated with TPO levels greater than those expected for the platelet count (34–36), although this finding has not been universal (37). Recently, it has been shown that IL-6, a well known inflammatory response mediator, increases TPO production both *in vitro* and *in vivo* (38–40), potentially helping to explain the enhanced levels seen in inflammatory and possibly other pathologic states.

The mechanism by which TPO production is regulated is coming under increased investigation. By using platelet granule proteins, Sungaran et al. determined that the platelet $\alpha$ granule proteins PDGF-BB and FGF2 stimulated, and that platelet factor 4, thrombospondin, and TGF-$\beta$ inhibited TPO production from cultures of marrow stromal cells (41); on balance, whole platelet extracts suppressed TPO production. More recently, on the basis of their initial finding that all-*trans*-retinoic acid (ATRA) treatment of patients with acute promyelocytic leukemia led to increased levels of TPO, Kinjo et al. showed that treatment of the marrow stromal cell line KM101 with ATRA increased hormone production by twofold to threefold at both the mRNA and protein levels, that a retinoic acid response element (RARE) is present in the 5′-flanking region of the *Tpo* gene, and that this region binds stromal cell nuclear proteins in mobility shift assays and mediates a 2.6-fold increase in reporter gene activity in the KM101 cells (42). Therefore, accumulating evidence indicates that marrow stromal cells can be induced by exogenous stimuli to produce TPO and can help explain the response to inflammatory stimuli.

The *Tpo* gene displays an unusual 5′ untranslated region structure. Unlike most genes that initiate translation with the first ATG codon present in the mRNA, TPO translation initiates at the eighth ATG codon in the transcript, located in the third exon of a full-length mRNA (there are two transcription initiation sites that differ because of alternate splicing of the first exon) (43). Because the eighth ATG is out of frame with, but embedded in, the short open-reading frame of the seventh ATG, translation initiation is inefficient (44). Therefore, under normal circumstances, little TPO protein is produced for any given amount of mRNA. Although it is not yet certain whether this molecular arrangement has physiologic consequences (i.e., it can be differentially regulated), it is now clear from patients with familial essential thrombocythemia that mutation of the *Tpo* gene in noncoding sequences can lead to enhanced translation efficiency and thrombocytosis. Four cases of autosomal dominant familial thrombocytosis have been linked to mutations in the region surrounding the initiation codon. In two families, a single mutation in different nucleotides of the intron 3 splice donor sequence resulted in alternate splicing of the primary transcript, eliminating the seventh and eighth ATG codons, and creating a new amino-terminus by fusing of the fifth open-reading frame (ORF) with the hormone coding sequence. This novel *Tpo* mRNA is efficiently translated, resulting in supraphysiologic levels of hormone production and nonclonal expansion of thrombopoiesis (45,46). In another mutant *Tpo* allele, deletion of a single nucleotide within the seventh ORF leads to its fusion with the TPO coding sequence and now enhanced translation of TPO from the seventh ATG codon (47). Finally, another mutation within the seventh ORF leads to its premature termination, preventing its interference with translation initiation from the usual eighth initiation codon (48) and again enhancing protein production. The molecular mechanisms of diseases of mRNA translation have been recently summarized (49).

## MEGAKARYOPOIETIC ACTIVITIES OF THROMBOPOIETIN *IN VITRO*

As initially defined, TPO was thought to be a potent megakaryocyte differentiation factor but was not thought to influence cellular proliferation. However, as soon as recombinant protein was available, it was established that in contrast to the partially purified samples thought to contain the hormone, TPO clearly acts to induce proliferation of megakaryocytic progenitor cells (50) and, in synergy with other cytokines, to support the proliferation of multiple types of immature hematopoietic progenitor cells (51–54). It has been clear from the initial studies of its biologic properties that TPO is a potent megakaryocyte colony-stimulating factor. Approximately 75% of the maximal number of megakaryocyte colony-forming cells can be induced to grow by using optimal levels of TPO alone (50,55). A number of other cytokines and hormones, including IL-3, kit ligand, EPO, and IL-11, also act in synergy with lower levels of TPO to promote megakaryocyte colony formation (56). However, the hormone appears to exert its proliferative effect primarily on progenitors of limited developmental potential. The number of megakaryocytes present in each colony is greater for those that form in the presence of IL-3 or kit ligand, either alone or together with TPO, than those that form in the presence of TPO alone. However, in the absence of the hormone, IL-3– or kit ligand–induced megakaryocyte formation is aborted; the cells display low ploidy values and poor cytoplasmic maturation (55).

Serum-free suspension culture systems have been the most useful for demonstrating the differentiative effects of the hormone on megakaryocytes. By using the recombinant protein, several groups have established that TPO increases megakaryocyte cell size, shifts the cells to much higher ploidy classes, and enhances the expression of the lineage specific markers glycoprotein (GP) Ib and GP IIb/IIIa (50,57–59). When examined under the electron microscope, TPO-induced megakaryocytes display prominent membrane production and numerous platelet-specific granules, and the cytoplasm demarcates into regions destined to fragment into mature platelets (50,55,57). When cultured slightly longer, especially in the presence of plasma, the cells form "proplatelet processes," and fragment into platelets, which appear to function normally

upon exposure to classic platelet agonists (60). Moreover, this final process appears to be independent of TPO, instead being more dependent on a substance in normal plasma. One report suggests that the activity in plasma responsible for platelet formation is a complex of thrombin and antithrombin III (61). At present, this report remains unconfirmed, so that the nature of a (regulatable) stimulus (if there is one) for the final stage of platelet formation is presently unclear.

One relatively consistent property of hematopoietic growth factors has been that the cytokine or cytokines that stimulate the production of a given cell lineage also activate or "prime" the resulting mature blood cells for activation in response to other signals (62–64). Similar to that for IL-3, GM-CSF, and G-CSF, *in vitro* studies indicate that although incubation in the hormone leads to the priming of platelets to respond to an otherwise subthreshold level of classical platelet agonists (65–67), TPO does not lead to frank platelet reactivation.

## THROMBOPOIETIN AND THE HEMATOPOIETIC STEM CELL

Analogous to the lineage-specific characteristics of EPO, the biologic properties of TPO were initially thought to be restricted to cells of the megakaryocyte lineage. Nevertheless, early studies of the biologic activities of the hormone included the stimulation of sorted CD34+ cells (57). Because this population of cells includes megakaryocytic progenitors, it remained formally possible that the hormone was lineage restricted until two groups demonstrated that sorted marrow cells that were highly enriched in hematopoietic stem cells also survived in the presence of TPO alone and proliferated in synergy with IL-3 or kit ligand (53,54). Shortly after these *in vitro* findings were reported, the genetic elimination of the TPO receptor, *c-Mpl*, was found to result in a considerable reduction in the number of hematopoietic progenitors of all lineages (68), and then, using competitive repopulation, Solar et al. demonstrated that the number of hematopoietic stem cells were reduced sevenfold to eightfold in *c-Mpl*–null mice (69). More recently, as it came to be appreciated that the congenital form of amegakaryocytic thrombocytopenia is due to a homozygous or mixed heterozygous mutation in the c-Mpl receptor locus, the role of TPO on stem cells has been extended to humans because nearly all such children develop aplastic anemia on account of dwindling numbers of stem cells within the first 2 to 5 years of life (70–73). Consistent with this notion, we recently demonstrated that the self-renewal/expansion of hematopoietic stem cells is also vitally dependent on TPO, as transplantation of normal stem cells into *Tpo* null mice results in a 15- to 20-fold reduction in the level of stem cell expansion (74).

Therefore, it is now clear that TPO joins kit ligand and flt ligand as the only cytokines demonstrated to play a nonredundant role in stem cell survival, self-renewal, and proliferation.

## *IN VIVO* ACTIVITIES OF THROMBOPOIETIN

The effects of exogenous TPO on the kinetics of platelet production have been studied extensively. As would be expected from its megakaryopoietic effects *in vitro*, when TPO is administered to animals or to humans, the platelet count begins to rise after 3 to 5 days, depending on the dose and the recipient species (13,14,18,75–80). These results indicate that TPO does not cause the immediate release of platelets from megakaryocytes, consistent with its failure to accelerate fragmentation of proplatelet processes, the long exvaginations of megakaryocyte cytoplasm felt to represent the most immediate platelet precursor (60). Instead, TPO stimulates the development and maturation of new megakaryocytes. Once the size and numbers of megakaryocytes increase, the platelet count begins to rise until a new steady state level is reached, the height of which depends on a log-linear relationship with the administered dose (19). Because of a prolonged biologic effect (the result of its slow plasma clearance and action on both primitive and mature hematopoietic cells), enhanced platelet production resulting from parenteral administration of TPO occurs 6 to 16 days after a steady state level of the hormone is achieved (80,81).

Given the pan-hematopoietic effects of TPO *in vitro*, careful attention was paid to all of hematopoiesis in animals administered with the recombinant hormone; the *in vivo* effects of TPO were found to correlate with its *in vitro* properties. Administration of the hormone to either normal or myelosuppressed animals increased the numbers of all types of hematopoietic progenitor cells (82), and genetic elimination of *Tpo* or its receptor caused a 65% to 95% reduction in number of transplantable stem cells and hematopoietic precursors of multiple lineages (68). Therefore, TPO should be thought of as a lineage-dominant pan-hematopoietic cytokine that plays multiple roles in blood cell production.

As noted in the preceding text, a large body of evidence indicates that cytokines that stimulate hematopoietic cell production also activate the corresponding mature cell type. If this were also true for TPO, platelet activation and thrombosis could result. *In vitro* studies have indicated that the hormone primes platelets to aggregate in the presence of classical agonists but does not, by itself, lead to platelet activation (66). Studies performed *in vivo* are consistent with this conclusion; the administration of TPO to nonhuman primates (19) or humans did not result in *de novo* platelet activation (79), and an excess of thrombotic complications has not been seen in multiple clinical trials of two forms of the hormone (see subsequent text). Nevertheless, these clinical trials have all avoided enrolling individuals with any history of pathologic thrombosis, forcing a careful examination of this question in unselected patients administered with the hormone once it or a corresponding small molecule agonist gains U.S. Food and Drug Administration (FDA) approval as a thrombopoietic agent.

Despite this increased understanding of the vital role of TPO on thrombopoiesis, a remaining major question is what is responsible for the approximately 10% residual platelet formation present in mice and humans in which *Tpo* or its receptor are genetically altered. On the basis of the megakaryopoietic activities of IL-3, IL-6, IL-11, GM-CSF, and leukemia inhibitory factor, both *in vitro* and *in vivo*, in an attempt to identify the cytokine(s) responsible for residual platelet production in *Mpl*$^{-/-}$ mice, mice genetically deficient in IL-3, IL-6-R, IL-11-R, or the combined signaling subunit of the IL-3, GM-CSF, and IL-5 receptors ($\beta_C$) were crossed to *c-Mpl*–null animals; none of these double-to-quadruple cytokine/cytokine-receptor–deficient mice displayed more severe thrombocytopenia than found in the *c-Mpl*$^{-/-}$ mouse (83–86). Whether another known (or possibly unknown) cytokine is responsible for the residual platelet production in the absence of TPO function is unknown. However, it was recently suggested that the chemokine SDF-1, which displays a synergistic action on megakaryocyte growth (87), and endothelial cells (88), might be responsible for residual thrombopoiesis in *c-Mpl* mice.

## THE Mpl RECEPTOR AND MOLECULAR MECHANISMS OF THROMBOPOIETIN ACTION

The initial step in hematopoietic growth factor action is the binding to its specific cell-surface receptor. Recent studies of the response of many of these receptors have begun to provide molecular insights into cytokine-induced signaling. It is clear that the protein tyrosine phosphorylation of the receptor itself, and of several substrates, is an integral part of the cellular response to hematopoietic growth factor stimulation because protein tyrosine kinase inhibitors block the growth induced by many hematopoietic cytokines, whereas phosphatase inhibitors have the opposite effect (89,90). However, the TPO receptor does not display any enzymatic activity; rather, cytokine receptors recruit cytoplasmic kinases to activate signaling molecules. The EPO receptor was the first member of the hematopoietic cytokine receptor family shown to recruit and activate a member of the Janus family of cytoplasmic tyrosine kinases (JAKs). Subsequent work has shown that JAKs mediate much of the secondary protein tyrosine phosphorylation triggered by the binding of hematopoietic growth factors to their corresponding receptors (91,92). The role of other cytoplasmic kinases, such as src and the src-related kinases, in growth factor–induced signaling is also under active investigation (93,94). Although many of the signals involved in thrombopoietic cytokine action are rapidly being identified, major challenges lie ahead in deciphering the molecular basis of signal specificity. For example, the cellular response generated upon TPO binding is distinct from that originating at the IL-3 receptor, but many of the same molecules are activated by both receptors; a thorough analysis of the specific patterns of signaling intermediates activated by each of the cytokines that act directly on megakaryocytes will be required to more fully understand the role played by each during thrombopoiesis.

Progress has been rapid in deciphering the signaling pathways employed by TPO, although only recently cloned. Initial studies of TPO signal transduction concentrated on the JAK and STAT families of proteins because of the former's homology with EPO and that between c-Mpl and the rest of the cytokine receptor family. The first reports focused on leukemic cell lines that naturally express the c-Mpl receptor, or the ones engineered to do so. These studies identified JAK2 and TYK2 as the immediate kinases that bind to c-Mpl and become activated on exposure to TPO (95–103). Other proteins reported in various megakaryocytic cell lines to be phosphorylated in response to TPO include STAT3 and STAT5 (95,96,101,104,105); the adapter proteins Grb2 (101,102), Cbl (102), and SOS (102); Shc and its related phosphatase SHIP (96,101,102,106); phosphoinositol-3-kinase (PI 3-K) and its downstream kinase Akt (65,107, 108); an inhibitory transcription factor downstream of Akt, FKHRL-1 (109); the Raf-1/MAP kinase (101,110,111); and hematopoietic cytokine receptor-related phosphatases such as SHPTP-2 (109).

In addition to determining the intracellular signaling pathways activated by TPO, much work has been done to identify the site of the c-Mpl receptor from which each signal originates. For example, Tyr112 (numbering beginning with the first intracytoplasmic domain residue) in murine c-Mpl is phosphorylated in response to the hormone binding and serves to initiate both Shc and STAT3 activation (97,112). Truncation of the c-Mpl receptor 69 residues from the transmembrane domain eliminated both Shc and STAT3 activation; however, it only reduced activation of STAT5, PI 3-K, and ERK1/2, leaving a receptor that was still capable of supporting cell growth—conclusions that were verified *in vivo* when a similarly truncated *c-mpl* cDNA was knocked in to the *c-mpl* locus in mice (113). The resting platelet count of these mice was normal; however, platelet recovery following cytotoxic therapy–induced thrombocytopenia was considerably delayed, indicating that the proximal part of the Mpl receptor includes all signals required for baseline MK proliferation and maturation but that the additional signal intensity of STAT, ERK, and PI 3-K, and/or the distinct signals initiated from the distal part of the receptor are important for high-level thrombopoiesis. Similar conclusions that STAT responses serve an amplification role in cytokine signaling are derived from studies of STAT5a/STAT5b double knockout mice (96).

The nature of TPO signaling in mature platelets has also been explored (114–117) and reveals that the hormone stimulates the phosphorylation and activation of JAK2, STAT3, and STAT5. Because the hormone has been shown to prime platelets for an enhanced response to classical platelet agonists, additional studies now focus on determining how these signaling intermediates might participate in platelet activation.

# THE THERAPEUTIC POTENTIAL OF THROMBOPOIETIN

The toxicity and therapeutic efficacy of TPO have been tested in many animal species, from mice to man. In all studies, administration of any form of the hormone was safe; there were no signs of hepatic, renal, or pulmonary toxicity; capillary leak; coagulopathy; or hematopoietic toxicity, and no evidence of an acute-phase response that is characteristic of other cytokines known to affect megakaryocyte development. When tested in animals treated with nonablative doses of either chemotherapy or radiation or both, the administration of exogenous TPO resulted in higher nadir platelet counts and accelerated platelet recovery (75,82,118–122). Thrombopoietin administration also promoted improved recovery of the erythrocyte and granulocyte lineages in these animals, which was consistent with its *in vitro* stimulatory effects on cells of multiple hematopoietic lineages (53,54,82). In one study using rhesus monkeys, the administration of TPO after sublethal irradiation resulted in functional iron deficiency, confirming its effect on erythropoiesis and arguing for the study of prophylactic administration of iron in patients receiving the recombinant protein (122). Together, these results suggest that the therapeutic efficacy of the hormone might be greater than initially anticipated.

In contrast to the near-universal success of the hormone in ameliorating the thrombocytopenia and, in many studies, the pancytopenia associated with myelosuppressive therapy, its effectiveness in accelerating platelet recovery after myeloablative therapy and stem cell transplantation has been less impressive. The administration of TPO to lethally irradiated mice receiving bone marrow cells accelerated platelet recovery by 2 to 4 days in two studies (78,123) but did not augment hematopoietic recovery when fewer bone marrow cells were given (124). In mice receiving peripheral blood stem cell transplants, TPO accelerated platelet recovery by only 1 or 2 days as compared with mice receiving transplants but no exogenous hormone (123). Thrombopoietin also did not facilitate hematopoietic reconstitution in nonhuman primates undergoing autologous bone marrow transplantation or peripheral blood stem cell transplantation (125). For the most part, the preclinical studies of TPO have accurately predicted the response of patients administered with the hormone for reasons of myelosuppression. The results of many clinical trials of TPO therapy given for up to 10 days have now been published (79,81,126–132). In all studies the administration of either recombinant human TPO or pegylated recombinant human megakaryocyte growth and development factor to cancer patients was safe. Specifically, there were no significant changes in vital signs or weight and the frequency of symptoms or signs of bone pain, organ dysfunction, superficial or deep venous thrombosis, or platelet activation were similar in the treatment and placebo groups. It must be noted, however, that patients with a history of cardiac, pulmonary, vascular, or thrombotic disease were excluded from all of the studies. Only a single patient in any of these clinical trials developed antibodies to TPO (80). However, very few patients have been given more than a single course of treatment in the initial clinical trials, making any conclusions on the immunogenicity of the two products premature.

The efficacy of TPO in clinical trials has been mixed. Results from three studies using pegylated recombinant human megakaryocyte growth and development factor or recombinant human TPO in a total of 101 patients with cancer treated with carboplatinum-based chemotherapeutic regimens have been reported (126–128). In all three studies, platelet counts returned to baseline significantly faster, and, in two of the three studies, nadir platelet counts were higher in the patients given TPO, as compared with either those given placebo or the same patients during their first cycle of chemotherapy. However, the chemotherapeutic regimens administered in these two trials induced only modest thrombocytopenia (mean nadir platelet counts in the placebo groups being 60,000 per $mm^3$ to 111,000 per $mm^3$); in neither study was hospital discharge delayed because of thrombocytopenia nor were substantial numbers of platelet transfusions required. In the third study (128), compared with a first cycle of carboplatin-based therapy without the hormone, the nadir platelet values and the number of days with fewer than 20,000 platelets per $mm^3$ were both considerably improved by the administration of a single dose of TPO following the second cycle of chemotherapy ($P < 0.001$). Moreover, 59% of the patients enrolled in this study required platelet transfusions after their first cycle of chemotherapy, but only 26% needed them following the cycle of chemotherapy augmented with TPO ($P = 0.02$).

Several additional indications for TPO therapy have been envisioned. Thrombopoietin increases the number of megakaryocytic and other hematopoietic progenitors *in vitro* and *in vivo* (53,54), and it mobilizes stem and progenitor cells from the marrow into the circulation (80,123,129), properties that might benefit patients receiving stem cell transplants. In 75 patients with breast cancer who were undergoing autologous bone marrow transplantation, administration of pegylated recombinant human megakaryocyte growth and development factor led to a 5 to 6 day earlier rise in platelet count to 20,000 per $mm^3$ and a halving of the use of platelet transfusions as compared with placebo (130). However, when tested in 64 patients in a phase III trial, the drug failed to accelerate platelet recovery. Likewise, the recombinant hormone was administered to 38 patients with delayed platelet recovery after peripheral blood stem cell or bone marrow transplantation; the use of recombinant human TPO led to platelet transfusion independence in only two individuals (132).

More recently, TPO was tested as an aid in mobilizing stem cells for subsequent autologous transplantation. Somlo et al. found that compared to a group of autologous transplantation patients in whom stem cells were mobilized with G-CSF alone, the addition of TPO to the mobilization phase led to a reduction from a mean of three to a mean of one apheresis procedure necessary to collect the requisite number of $CD34^+$ cells, and, upon infusion, the patients who received cells mobilized with G-CSF and TPO demonstrated accelerated red blood cell and platelet recovery and required a small, but reduced number of platelet transfusions that was statistically significant compared with patients who received G-CSF mobilized stem cells (133).

Another potential indication for the hormone is in increasing platelet yields in normal individuals who donate platelets by apheresis. At present, a 2- to 3-hour apheresis of normal donors yields approximately $3 \times 10^{11}$ platelets, which, when transfused into a single donor results in a 10 to 40 $\times 10^9$ per L increment in platelet levels. By increasing the platelet count in a donor, the number of platelets recovered should increase, potentially increasing the mean platelet increment when the cells are subsequently infused into a single recipient; alternately, such enhanced platelet collections could allow a single donor a pheresis to be used for multiple recipients. A study by Kuter et al. addressed the former possibility (134); normal donors were administered a single subcutaneous injection of a truncated, pegylated form of TPO produced in bacteria and then underwent apheresis several days later at the height of their thrombocytosis. In this study, three times the number of platelets were derived from the TPO-injected donors as controls (mean platelet count at time of apheresis was $599 \times 10^9$ per L), and the recipients of the increased platelet numbers displayed a fourfold greater platelet increment. Most of these donors continued to receive intermittent injections and donated platelets. Unfortunately, several donors developed antibodies to the altered, recombinant form of the hormone used in the study, which negated its effectiveness in augmenting the platelet level prior to apheresis, and, even worse, in many of these normal platelet donors the antibodies cross-reacted with their native hormone, resulting in severe thrombocytopenia. As a result of this study, the manufacturer of that form of the hormone stopped all clinical trials of the agent.

Another potential indication for the administration of TPO is immune thrombocytopenia (ITP). Although the typical bone marrow examination of a patient with classic ITP demonstrates impressive megakaryopoiesis, it remains possible that the levels of the hormone attainable physiologically are less than necessary for maximal megakaryopoiesis and that levels attainable pharmacologically could further increase platelet levels in this disorder. At present, the literature contains only a single report on four patients so treated; one experienced an adverse, nonhematologic reaction after the first dose and was taken off the trial, the other three patients all demonstrated increased levels of new platelet production (135). Overall, the clinical performance of recombinant TPO has been mixed, and additional studies will be required to identify the precise settings in which therapeutic benefit will be significant.

# ROLE OF THROMBOPOIETIN AND ITS RECEPTOR IN PATHOLOGY

Other than the remarkable insights into the pathogenesis of chronic myelogenous leukemia afforded by the t(9;22) translocation, little is known about the pathogenesis of the chronic myeloproliferative disorders (MPDs), polycythemia vera (PV), essential thrombocythemia (ET), and idiopathic myelofibrosis (IMF). Evidence is now accumulating, however, that the cellular response to hematopoietic growth factors, or dysregulation of the growth factors themselves, might contribute to the etiology of these disorders. The concept of autocrine secretion of peptide growth factors by tumor cells dates to the work of Sporn and Todaro (136). Later work suggested that hematopoietic growth factors and their receptors might play an important role in the malignant transformation of marrow cells.

Myeloproliferative disorders share a common origin in a pluripotent hematopoietic progenitor cell. Consequently, if growth factors or their receptors play a role in these disorders, then that cytokine receptor must be expressed in hematopoietic stem cells. As illustrated previously, c-Mpl is present on the repopulating hematopoietic stem cell and genetic elimination of *Tpo* or *c-Mpl* leads to the conclusion that it plays a crucial, nonredundant role in these cells.

Several lines of evidence support the notion that TPO and/or its receptor play a role in myeloproliferative disorders. First, mutations of Mpl can lead to autonomous cell growth and leukemogenicity in mice. Perhaps the best example of this is the mutant form of *c-Mpl* that led to its discovery, the *v-Mpl*

oncogene (6). Following the characterization of a constitutively active mutant of the EPO receptor, Alexander et al. engineered constitutively active receptor mutants of c-Mpl by substituting cysteine residues into the dimer interface domain of the receptor. Factor-dependent hematopoietic cells transduced with the mutant receptor displayed constitutive phosphorylation of both Mpl and the signal transduction molecules implicated in Mpl function, suggesting a potential for contributing to the tumorigenicity of the mutant cells (137). Onishi et al. identified an activating mutation in the transmembrane domain of c-Mpl by using a combination of retrovirus-mediated gene transfer and polymerase chain reaction–driven random mutagenesis. This mutation resulted in the abrogation of factor dependency in all IL-3–dependent cell lines tested. One IL-3–dependent murine cell line that expressed only the mutated form of Mpl induced autocrine growth and leukemogenesis when transduced into syngeneic mice, apparently by constitutive activation of two distinct intracellular signaling pathways (138). Finally, our group has demonstrated that truncation of the membrane-distal part of the extracellular domain of c-Mpl induces autocrine growth in factor-dependent cell lines (139). These studies appear to confirm that certain mutations of the TPO receptor may contribute to the malignant transformation of some hematopoietic progenitors *in vivo*, at least in the mouse. Second, expression of normal c-Mpl in all marrow cells, or TPO in hematopoietic cells leads to myeloproliferative disorders. For example, Cocault et al. demonstrated that a retrovirus containing natural murine Mpl cDNA is erythroleukemogenic *in vivo* when injected into adult mice (140). Several groups have observed that transgenic overexpression of *Tpo* in mice induces megakaryocyte proliferation in the spleen and massive marrow fibrosis, a disorder bearing strong resemblance to agnogenic myeloid metaplasia and myelofibrosis in humans (141–143). Third, as noted, one of the most characteristic finding in patients with myeloproliferative syndromes is "autonomous" colony growth, which in reality represents growth factor hyperresponsiveness. Hematopoietic progenitor cells taken from blood and bone marrow that normally die in culture without exogenous growth factors survive and proliferate in the presence of serum alone. Li et al. have demonstrated, for example, that with the introduction of an antisense oligonucleotide to Mpl, there is a reduction in spontaneous colony formation in serum-free assays and in plasma clot assays (144). Similar conclusions were drawn by Taksin et al. using an inhibitory, soluble form of the c-Mpl receptor (145). This outcome suggests that the TPO receptor may influence autonomous growth of these cells in culture. Fourth, TPO levels and c-Mpl expression is altered in patients with several of the MPDs. For example, Pitcher et al. have observed that circulating TPO levels are unexpectedly high in patients with ET (146), although this has not been a universal finding (147). Moreover, c-Mpl expression on megakaryocytes from patients with MPDs has been abnormal (148,149), and a signaling defect has been observed in cells derived from patients with PV (150). In addition to being of potential diagnostic benefit, these findings again point to an abnormality in the TPO/c-Mpl system in patients with MPDs. An important very recent observation has begun to make sense of some of these and other observations relating to abnormal signaling in ET and the other myeloproliferative disorders. A single site mutation of JAKZ, the kinase responsible for TPO, EPO, IL-3 and several other hematopoietic growth factors, has been identified in from 30–95% of patients with PV, ET and IMF in several series (reviewed in Kaushansky K. On the molecular origins of the chronic myeloproliferative disorders: it all makes sense. *Blood* 2005;105:4187–4190.)

Although there is no direct evidence yet that TPO or its receptor plays a primary pathogenic role in acquired myeloid disorders in humans, there now exists striking evidence that congenital abnormalities of both molecules cause human disease.

Familial ET is a rare disorder characterized by excessive thrombocytosis, in the absence of other hematologic manifestations of the acquired disorder, in extremely young individuals or in older persons with a familial history. In many such patients, overexpression of TPO is responsible. At present, at least four distinct mutations of the *Tpo* gene have been described, leading to its overproduction because of the enhanced translational efficiency of the mutant mRNA (45–47,151). The stage for such disorders is set by the poor translation efficiency of wild-type TPO mRNA, owing in large measure to the native initiation codon being embedded within the cistron of a short, upstream, out of frame (with respect to the normal TPO reading frame) ORF. In two cases, different mutations in the splice donor site within intron 3 leads to elimination of exon 3, resulting in translation of TPO protein from an upstream initiation codon, one that is not hampered by an overlapping ORF. In another case, a stop codon is introduced in the overlapping, out-of-frame, upstream cistron, reducing its influence on translation from the native site, and, in a fourth case, a one-nucleotide deletion puts the upstream overlapping reading frame in frame with the TPO-coding sequence, which allows its enhanced translation. Such disorders of protein translation are being increasingly recognized as a cause of human disease (49).

Recent studies have identified homozygous elimination of *c-MPL* as causing a large number of cases of congenital amegakaryocytic thrombocytopenia (CAMT) (70–73,152). Infants with this disorder usually present with excessive bleeding in the perinatal period, although occasionally the diagnosis is delayed for a short time. A diagnostic bone marrow aspiration and biopsy usually reveals normal cellularity, although only a few megakaryocytes are initially found and those present are unusually small and hypolobated. With the availability of plasma TPO measurements, nearly every such patient has been found to display very high levels of the hormone, which is biologically active. More recently, further study has demonstrated that many of these children fail to express c-Mpl on their platelet surfaces, usually because of the presence of nonsense or severe missense codons in the extracellular domain of the receptor. Although children with CAMT usually present with isolated thrombocytopenia, they typically develop pancytopenia within a few years of birth, presaged by declining numbers of marrow-derived hematopoietic progenitors of all types (73). At this point, their marrow morphology resembles that seen in aplastic anemia, and stem cell transplantation is the only curative option. Also of great interest in this regard is the recent observation that the development of anti-TPO antibodies can lead to pancytopenia (153). As noted earlier, TPO plays an important role in stem cell biology, perhaps helping to explain the stem cell failure that characterizes the latter stages of CAMT and the aplasia associated with accidentally neutralizing endogenous TPO in patients. However, this finding also raises an interesting research question; mice nullizygous for c-MPL or TPO display similarly low platelet counts but do not develop pancytopenia. Further study into the cause of this discrepancy is likely to reveal much about stem cell kinetics in mouse and man.

Although most patients with immune thrombocytopenic purpura display enhanced megakaryopoiesis secondary to peripheral immune destruction of platelets, usually because of an autoantibody to platelet GP IIb/IIIa or GP Ib, careful platelet turnover studies reveal that not all patients have rapid platelet elimination (154). In such patients, it is possible that reduced production of platelets might be caused by antibodies against TPO or its receptor. More recent study has borne out this possibility, both as *de novo* disease and in response to administration of a genetically modified form of TPO (155–157). In both of these situations, the clue to the unusual pathophysiology was reduced megakaryopoiesis in the marrow of the patients with presumed immune thrombocytopenic purpura.

Soon after the *c-Mpl* protooncogene was identified, it became clear that it was expressed on a sizable proportion of blast cells from patients with myeloid malignancies (158). Although there is little evidence that disorders of *c-Mpl* are involved in the generation of acute leukemia, a sizable body of evidence suggests that its expression on the surface of leukemic cells adversely affects the response characteristics of the cells and the overall survival of the patients who develop such leukemias (159,160). The same is true of patients with myelodysplastic syndromes; the presence of c-Mpl on the surface of the dysplastic cells predicted enhanced likelihood of evolution to acute leukemia (161). In contrast, however, the adverse prognosis of expression of c-Mpl did not extend to chronic myelogenous leukemia (162).

## References

1. Kelemen ECI, Tanos B. Demonstration and some properties of human thrombopoietin in thrombocythemic sera. *Acta Haematol (Basel)* 1958; 20:350–355.
2. McDonald TP, Andrews RB, Clift R, et al. Characterization of a thrombocytopoietic-stimulating factor from kidney cell culture medium. *Exp Hematol* 1981;9(3):288–296.
3. Carter CD, Schultz TW, McDonald TP. Thrombopoietin from human embryonic kidney cells stimulates an increase in megakaryocyte size of sublethally irradiated mice. *Radiat Res* 1993;135(1):32–39.
4. Erickson-Miller CL, Ji H, Parchment RE, et al. Megakaryocyte colony-stimulating factor (Meg-CSF) is a unique cytokine specific for the megakaryocyte lineage. *Br J Haematol* 1993;84(2):197–203.
5. Wendling F, Varlet P, Charon M, et al. MPLV: a retrovirus complex inducing an acute myeloproliferative leukemic disorder in adult mice. *Virology* 1986;149(2):242–246.
6. Souyri M, Vigon I, Penciolelli JF, et al. A putative truncated cytokine receptor gene transduced by the myeloproliferative leukemia virus immortalizes hematopoietic progenitors. *Cell* 1990;63(6):1137–1147.
7. Vigon I, Mornon JP, Cocault L, et al. Molecular cloning and characterization of MPL, the human homolog of the v-mpl oncogene: identification of a member of the hematopoietic growth factor receptor superfamily. *Proc Natl Acad Sci U S A* 1992;89(12):5640–5644.
8. Cosman D. The hematopoietin receptor superfamily. *Cytokine* 1993;5(2): 95–106.
9. Long MW, Heffner CH, Williams JL, et al. Regulation of megakaryocyte phenotype in human erythroleukemia cells. *J Clin Invest* 1990;85(4): 1072–1084.
10. Methia N, Louache F, Vainchenker W, et al. Oligodeoxynucleotides antisense to the proto-oncogene c-Mpl specifically inhibit *in vitro* megakaryocytopoiesis. *Blood* 1993;82(5):1395–1401.
11. Kuter DJ, Beeler DL, Rosenberg RD. The purification of megapoietin: a physiological regulator of megakaryocyte growth and platelet production. *Proc Natl Acad Sci U S A* 1994;91(23):11104–11108.
12. Sohma Y, Akahori H, Seki N, et al. Molecular cloning and chromosomal localization of the human thrombopoietin gene. *FEBS Lett* 1994;353(1): 57–61.
13. de Sauvage FJ, Hass PE, Spencer SD, et al. Stimulation of megakaryocytopoiesis and thrombopoiesis by the c-Mpl ligand. *Nature* 1994;369 (6481):533–538.
14. Lok S, Kaushansky K, Holly RD, et al. Cloning and expression of murine thrombopoietin cDNA and stimulation of platelet production *in vivo*. *Nature* 1994;369(6481):565–568.
15. Kaushansky K. Thrombopoietin. *N Engl J Med* 1998;339(11):746–754.
16. Feese MD, Tamada T, Kato Y, et al. Structure of the receptor-binding domain of human thrombopoietin determined by complexation with a neutralizing antibody fragment. *Proc Natl Acad Sci U S A* 2004;101(7): 1816–1821.
17. Broudy VC, Lin NL, Sabath DF, et al. Human platelets display high-affinity receptors for thrombopoietin. *Blood* 1997;89(6):1896–1904.
18. Bartley TD, Bogenberger J, Hunt P, et al. Identification and cloning of a megakaryocyte growth and development factor that is a ligand for the cytokine receptor Mpl. *Cell* 1994;77(7):1117–1124.
19. Harker LA, Marzec UM, Hunt P, et al. Dose-response effects of pegylated human megakaryocyte growth and development factor on platelet production and function in nonhuman primates. *Blood* 1996;88(2):511–521.
20. Linden HM, Kaushansky K. The glycan domain of thrombopoietin enhances its secretion. *Biochemistry* 2000;39(11):3044–3051.
21. Muto T, Feese MD, Shimada Y, et al. Functional analysis of the C-terminal region of recombinant human thrombopoietin. C-terminal region of thrombopoietin is a "shuttle" peptide to help secretion. *J Biol Chem* 2000; 275(16):12090–12094.
22. Linden HM, Kaushansky K. The glycan domain of thrombopoietin (TPO) acts in trans to enhance secretion of the hormone and other cytokines. *J Biol Chem* 2002;277(38):35240–35247.

23. Pearce KH Jr, Potts BJ, Presta LG, et al. Mutational analysis of thrombopoietin for identification of receptor and neutralizing antibody sites. *J Biol Chem* 1997;272(33):20595–20602.

24. Kaushansky K. Structure-function relationships of the hematopoietic growth factors. *Proteins* 1992;12(1):1–9.

25. Jagerschmidt A, Fleury V, Anger-Leroy M, et al. Human thrombopoietin structure-function relationships: identification of functionally important residues. *Biochem J* 1998;333:779–734.

26. Nichol JL, Hokom MM, Hornkohl A, et al. Megakaryocyte growth and development factor. Analyses of *in vitro* effects on human megakaryopoiesis and endogenous serum levels during chemotherapy-induced thrombocytopenia. *J Clin Invest* 1995;95(6):2973–2978.

27. Kuter DJ, Rosenberg RD. The reciprocal relationship of thrombopoietin (c-Mpl ligand) to changes in the platelet mass during busulfan-induced thrombocytopenia in the rabbit. *Blood* 1995;85(10):2720–2730.

28. Fielder PJ, Gurney AL, Stefanich E, et al. Regulation of thrombopoietin levels by c-Mpl-mediated binding to platelets. *Blood* 1996;87(6):2154–2161.

29. de Sauvage FJ, Carver-Moore K, Luoh SM, et al. Physiological regulation of early and late stages of megakaryocytopoiesis by thrombopoietin. *J Exp Med* 1996;183(2):651–656.

30. McCarty JM, Sprugel KH, Fox NE, et al. Murine thrombopoietin mRNA levels are modulated by platelet count. *Blood* 1995;86(10):3668–3675.

31. Sungaran R, Markovic B, Chong BH. Localization and regulation of thrombopoietin mRNAexpression in human kidney, liver, bone marrow, and spleen using in situ hybridization. *Blood* 1997;89(1):101–107.

32. Guerriero A, Worford L, Holland HK, et al. Thrombopoietin is synthesized by bone marrow stromal cells. *Blood* 1997;90(9):3444–3455.

33. Hirayama Y, Sakamaki S, Matsunaga T, et al. Concentrations of thrombopoietin in bone marrow in normal subjects and in patients with idiopathic thrombocytopenic purpura, aplastic anemia, and essential thrombocythemia correlate with its mRNA expression of bone marrow stromal cells. *Blood* 1998;92(1):46–52.

34. Cerutti A, Custodi P, Duranti M, et al. Thrombopoietin levels in patients with primary and reactive thrombocytosis. *Br J Haematol* 1997;99(2):281–284.

35. Schoffski P, Tacke F, Trautwein C, et al. Thrombopoietin serum levels are elevated in patients with hepatitis B/C infection compared to other causes of chronic liver disease. *Liver* 2002;22(2):114–120.

36. Tacke F, Trautwein C, Zhao S, et al. Quantification of hepatic thrombopoietin mRNA transcripts in patients with chronic liver diseases shows maintained gene expression in different etiologies of liver cirrhosis. *Liver* 2002;22(3):205–212.

37. Wang JC, Chen C, Novetsky AD, et al. Blood thrombopoietin levels in clonal thrombocytosis and reactive thrombocytosis. *Am J Med* 1998;104(5):451–455.

38. Wolber EM, Jelkmann W. Interleukin-6 increases thrombopoietin production in human hepatoma cells HepG2 and Hep3B. *J Interferon Cytokine Res* 2000;20(5):499–506.

39. Kaser A, Brandacher G, Steurer W, et al. Interleukin-6 stimulates thrombopoiesis through thrombopoietin: role in inflammatory thrombocytosis. *Blood* 2001;98(9):2720–2725.

40. Wolber EM, Fandrey J, Frackowski U, et al. Hepatic thrombopoietin mRNA is increased in acute inflammation. *Thromb Haemost* 2001;86(6):1421–1424.

41. Sungaran R, Chisholm OT, Markovic B, et al. The role of platelet alpha-granular proteins in the regulation of thrombopoietin messenger RNA expression in human bone marrow stromal cells. *Blood* 2000;95(10):3094–3101.

42. Kinjo KMY, Uchida H, Ikeda Y, et al. A novel mechanism for thrombopoietin (TPO) production induced by all-trans retinoic acid via transcriptional activation through putative retinoic acid responsive element in the promoter region of TPO gene. *Blood* 2001;98:83a.

43. Chang MS, McNinch J, Basu R, et al. Cloning and characterization of the human megakaryocyte growth and development factor (MGDF) gene. *J Biol Chem* 1995;270(2):511–514.

44. Morris DR. Cis-acting mRNA structures in gene-specific translational control. *mRNA metabolism and post-transcriptional gene regulation.* New York: Wiley-Liss, 1997:165–180.

45. Wiestner A, Schlemper RJ, van der Maas AP, et al. An activating splice donor mutation in the thrombopoietin gene causes hereditary thrombocythaemia. *Nat Genet* 1998;18(1):49–52.

46. Jorgensen MJ, Raskind WH, Wolff JF, et al. Familial thrombocytosis associated with overproduction due to a novel splice donor site mutation. *Blood* 1998;92(10):205a.

47. Kondo T, Okabe M, Sanada M, et al. Familial essential thrombocythemia associated with one-base deletion in the 5'-untranslated region of the thrombopoietin gene. *Blood* 1998;92(4):1091–1096.

48. Ghilardi N, Wiestner A, Kikuchi M, et al. Hereditary thrombocythaemia in a Japanese family is caused by a novel point mutation in the thrombopoietin gene. *Br J Haematol* 1999;107(2):310–316.

49. Cazzola M, Skoda RC. Translational pathophysiology: a novel molecular mechanism of human disease. *Blood* 2000;95(11):3280–3288.

50. Kaushansky K, Lok S, Holly RD, et al. Promotion of megakaryocyte progenitor expansion and differentiation by the c-Mpl ligand thrombopoietin. *Nature* 1994;369(6481):568–571.

51. Kaushansky K, Broudy VC, Grossmann A, et al. Thrombopoietin expands erythroid progenitors, increases red cell production, and enhances erythroid recovery after myelosuppressive therapy. *J Clin Invest* 1995;96(3):1683–1687.

52. Kobayashi M, Laver JH, Kato T, et al. Recombinant human thrombopoietin (Mpl ligand) enhances proliferation of erythroid progenitors. *Blood* 1995;86(7):2494–2499.

53. Ku H, Yonemura Y, Kaushansky K, et al. Thrombopoietin, the ligand for the Mpl receptor, synergizes with steel factor and other early acting cytokines in supporting proliferation of primitive hematopoietic progenitors of mice. *Blood* 1996;87(11):4544–4551.

54. Sitnicka E, Lin N, Priestley GV, et al. The effect of thrombopoietin on the proliferation and differentiation of murine hematopoietic stem cells. *Blood* 1996;87(12):4998–5005.

55. Kaushansky K, Broudy VC, Lin N, et al. Thrombopoietin, the Mpl ligand, is essential for full megakaryocyte development. *Proc Natl Acad Sci U S A* 1995;92(8):3234–3238.

56. Broudy VC, Lin NL, Kaushansky K. Thrombopoietin (c-Mpl ligand) acts synergistically with erythropoietin, stem cell factor, and interleukin-11 to enhance murine megakaryocyte colony growth and increases megakaryocyte ploidy *in vitro*. *Blood* 1995;85(7):1719–1726.

57. Zeigler FC, de Sauvage F, Widmer HR, et al. *In vitro* megakaryocytopoietic and thrombopoietic activity of c-Mpl ligand (TPO) on purified murine hematopoietic stem cells. *Blood* 1994;84(12):4045–4052.

58. Wendling F, Maraskovsky E, Debili N, et al. cMpl ligand is a humoral regulator of megakaryocytopoiesis. *Nature* 1994;369(6481):571–574.

59. Debili N, Wendling F, Katz A, et al. The Mpl-ligand or thrombopoietin or megakaryocyte growth and differentiative factor has both direct proliferative and differentiative activities on human megakaryocyte progenitors. *Blood* 1995;86(7):2516–2525.

60. Choi ES, Nichol JL, Hokom MM, et al. Platelets generated *in vitro* from proplatelet-displaying human megakaryocytes are functional. *Blood* 1995; 85(2):402–413.

61. Ishida Y, Yano K, Ito T, et al. Purification of proplatelet formation (PPF) stimulating factor: thrombin/antithrombin III complex stimulates PPF of megakaryocytes *in vitro* and platelet production *in vivo*. *Thromb Haemost* 2001;85(2):349–355.

62. Weisbart RH, Kwan L, Golde DW, et al. primes neutrophils for enhanced oxidative metabolism in response to the major physiological chemoattractants. *Blood* 1987;69(1):18–21.

63. Valent P, Besemer J, Muhm M, et al. Interleukin 3 activates human blood basophils via high-affinity binding sites. *Proc Natl Acad Sci U S A* 1989; 86(14):5542–5546.

64. Balazovich KJ, Almeida HI, Boxer LA. Recombinant human G-CSF and GM-CSF prime human neutrophils for superoxide production through different signal transduction mechanisms. *J Lab Clin Med* 1991;118(6):576–584.

65. Chen J, Herceg-Harjacek L, Groopman JE, et al. Regulation of platelet activation *in vitro* by the c-Mpl ligand, thrombopoietin. *Blood* 1995;86(11):4054–4062.

66. Ezumi Y, Nishida E, Uchiyama T, et al. Thrombopoietin potentiates agonist-stimulated activation of p38 mitogen-activated protein kinase in human platelets. *Biochem Biophys Res Commun* 1999;261(1):58–63.

67. Eilers M, Schulze H, Welte K, et al. Thrombopoietin acts synergistically on Ca(2+) mobilization in platelets caused by ADP or thrombin receptor agonist peptide. *Biochem Biophys Res Commun* 1999;263(1):230–238.

68. Alexander WS, Roberts AW, Nicola NA, et al. Deficiencies in progenitor cells of multiple hematopoietic lineages and defective megakaryocytopoiesis in mice lacking the thrombopoietic receptor c-Mpl. *Blood* 1996;87(6):2162–2170.

69. Solar GP, Kerr WG, Zeigler FC, et al. Role of c-Mpl in early hematopoiesis. *Blood* 1998;92(1):4–10.

70. Ihara K, Ishii E, Eguchi M, et al. Identification of mutations in the c-Mpl gene in congenital amegakaryocytic thrombocytopenia. *Proc Natl Acad Sci U S A* 1999;96(6):3132–3136.

71. van den Oudenrijn S, Bruin M, Folman CC, et al. Mutations in the thrombopoietin receptor, Mpl, in children with congenital amegakaryocytic thrombocytopenia. *Br J Haematol* 2000;110(2):441–448.

72. Tonelli R, Scardovi AL, Pession A, et al. Compound heterozygosity for two different amino-acid substitution mutations in the thrombopoietin receptor (c-mpl gene) in congenital amegakaryocytic thrombocytopenia CAMT. *Hum Genet* 2000;107(3):225–233.

73. Ballmaier M, Germeshausen M, Schulze H, et al. c-mpl mutations are the cause of congenital amegakaryocytic thrombocytopenia. *Blood* 2001;97(1):139–146.

74. Fox N, Priestley G, Papayannopoulou T, et al. Thrombopoietin expands hematopoietic stem cells after transplantation. *J Clin Invest* 2002;110(3):389–394.

75. Ulich TR, del Castillo J, Senaldi G, et al. Systemic hematologic effects of PEG-rHuMGDF-induced megakaryocyte hyperplasia in mice. *Blood* 1996;87(12):5006–5015.

76. Harker LA, Hunt P, Marzec UM, et al. Regulation of platelet production and function by megakaryocyte growth and development factor in nonhuman primates. *Blood* 1996;87(5):1833–1844.

77. Andrews RG, Winkler A, Myerson D, et al. Recombinant human ligand for MPL, megakaryocyte growth and development factor (MGDF), stimulates thrombopoiesis *in vivo* in normal and myelosuppressed baboons. *Stem Cells* 1996;14(6):661–677.

78. Kabaya K, Akahori H, Shibuya K, et al. *In vivo* effects of pegylated recombinant human megakaryocyte growth and development factor on hematopoiesis in normal mice. *Stem Cells* 1996;14(6):651–660.

79. O'Malley CJ, Rasko JE, Basser RL, et al. Administration of pegylated recombinant human megakaryocyte growth and development factor to humans stimulates the production of functional platelets that show no evidence of *in vivo* activation. *Blood* 1996;88(9):3288–3298.

80. Vadhan-Raj S, Murray LJ, Bueso-Ramos C, et al. Stimulation of megakaryocyte and platelet production by a single dose of recombinant human thrombopoietin in patients with cancer. *Ann Intern Med* 1997;126(9):673–681.

81. Basser RL, Rasko JE, Clarke K, et al. Thrombopoietic effects of pegylated recombinant human megakaryocyte growth and development factor (PEG-rHuMGDF) in patients with advanced cancer. *Lancet* 1996; 348 (9037):1279–1281.

82. Kaushansky K, Lin N, Grossmann A, et al. Thrombopoietin expands erythroid, granulocyte-macrophage, and megakaryocytic progenitor cells in normal and myelosuppressed mice. *Exp Hematol* 1996;24(2):265–269.

83. Gainsford T, Roberts AW, Kimura S, et al. Cytokine production and function in c-Mpl-deficient mice: no physiologic role for interleukin-3 in residual megakaryocyte and platelet production. *Blood* 1998;91(8):2745–2752.

84. Chen Q, Solar G, Eaton DL, et al. IL-3 does not contribute to platelet production in c-Mpl-deficient mice. *Stem Cells* 1998;16(Suppl. 2):31–36.

85. Gainsford T, Nandurkar H, Metcalf D, et al. The residual megakaryocyte and platelet production in c-mpl-deficient mice is not dependent on the actions of interleukin-6, interleukin-11, or leukemia inhibitory factor. *Blood* 2000;95(2):528–534.

86. Scott CL, Robb L, Mansfield R, et al. Granulocyte-macrophage colony-stimulating factor is not responsible for residual thrombopoiesis in mpl null mice. *Exp Hematol* 2000;28(9):1001–1007.

87. Hodohara K, Fujii N, Yamamoto N, et al. Stromal cell-derived factor-1 (SDF-1) acts together with thrombopoietin to enhance the development of megakaryocytic progenitor cells (CFU-MK). *Blood* 2000;95(3):769–775.

88. Avecilla ST, Hattori K, Heissig B, et al. Chemokine-mediated interaction of hematopoietic progenitors with the bone marrow vascular niche is required for thrombopoiesis. *Nat Med* 2004;10(1):64–71.

89. Tojo A, Kasuga M, Urabe A, et al. Vanadate can replace interleukin 3 for transient growth of factor-dependent cells. *Exp Cell Res* 1987;171(1):16–23.

90. Satoh T, Uehara Y, Kaziro Y. Inhibition of interleukin 3 and granulocyte-macrophage colony-stimulating factor stimulated increase of active ras.GTP by herbimycin A, a specific inhibitor of tyrosine kinases. *J Biol Chem* 1992;267(4):2537–2541.

91. Darnell JE Jr, Kerr IM, Stark GR. Jak-STAT pathways and transcriptional activation in response to IFNs and other extracellular signaling proteins. *Science* 1994;264(5164):1415–1421.

92. Ihle JN, Kerr IM. Jaks and Stats in signaling by the cytokine receptor superfamily. *Trends Genet* 1995;11(2):69–74.

93. Corey SJ, Burkhardt AL, Bolen JB, et al. Granulocyte colony-stimulating factor receptor signaling involves the formation of a three-component complex with Lyn and Syk protein-tyrosine kinases. *Proc Natl Acad Sci U S A* 1994;91(11):4683–4687.

94. Anderson SM, Jorgensen B. Activation of src-related tyrosine kinases by IL-3. *J Immunol* 1995;155(4):1660–1670.

95. Bacon CM, Tortolani PJ, Shimosaka A, et al. Thrombopoietin (TPO) induces tyrosine phosphorylation and activation of STAT5 and STAT3. *FEBS Lett* 1995;370(1-2):63–68.

96. Socolovsky M, Fallon AE, Wang S, et al. Fetal anemia and apoptosis of red cell progenitors in Stat5a-/-5b-/- mice: a direct role for Stat5 in Bcl-X(L) induction. *Cell* 1999;98(2):181–191.

97. Drachman JG, Griffin JD, Kaushansky K. The c-Mpl ligand (thrombopoietin) stimulates tyrosine phosphorylation of Jak2, Shc, and c-Mpl. *J Biol Chem* 1995;270(10):4979–4982.

98. Sattler M, Durstin MA, Frank DA, et al. The thrombopoietin receptor c-MPL activates JAK2 and TYK2 tyrosine kinases. *Exp Hematol* 1995; 23(9):1040–1048.

99. Tortolani PJ, Johnston JA, Bacon CM, et al. Thrombopoietin induces tyrosine phosphorylation and activation of the Janus kinase, JAK2. *Blood* 1995;85(12):3444–3451.

100. Morella KK, Bruno E, Kumaki S, et al. Signal transduction by the receptors for thrombopoietin (c-mpL) and interleukin-3 in hematopoietic and nonhematopoietic cells. *Blood* 1995;86(2):557–571.

101. Mu SX, Xia M, Elliott G, et al. Megakaryocyte growth and development factor and interleukin-3 induce patterns of protein-tyrosine phosphorylation that correlate with dominant differentiation over proliferation of mpl-transfected 32D cells. *Blood* 1995;86(12):4532–4543.

102. Sasaki K, Odai H, Hanazono Y, et al. TPO/c-mpl ligand induces tyrosine phosphorylation of multiple cellular proteins including proto-oncogene products, Vav and c-Cbl, and Ras signaling molecules. *Biochem Biophys Res Commun* 1995;216(1):338–347.

103. Drachman JG, Millett KM, Kaushansky K. Thrombopoietin signal transduction requires functional JAK2, not TYK2. *J Biol Chem* 1999;274(19): 13480–13484.

104. Drachman JG, Sabath DF, Fox NE, et al. Thrombopoietin signal transduction in purified murine megakaryocytes. *Blood* 1997;89(2):483–492.

105. Drachman JG, Kaushansky K. Dissecting the thrombopoietin receptor: functional elements of the Mpl cytoplasmic domain. *Proc Natl Acad Sci U S A* 1997;94(6):2350–2355.

106. Hill RJ, Zozulya S, Lu YL, et al. Differentiation induced by the c-Mpl cytokine receptor is blocked by mutant Shc adaptor protein. *Cell Growth Differ* 1996;7(9):1125–1134.

107. Sattler M, Salgia R, Durstin MA, et al. Thrombopoietin induces activation of the phosphatidylinositol-3' kinase pathway and formation of a complex containing p85PI3K and the protooncoprotein p120CBL. *J Cell Physiol* 1997;171(1):28–33.

108. Miyakawa Y, Rojnuckarin P, Habib T, et al. Thrombopoietin induces phosphoinositol 3-kinase activation through SHP2, Gab, and insulin receptor substrate proteins in BAF3 cells and primary murine megakaryocytes. *J Biol Chem* 2001;276(4):2494–2502.

109. Tanaka M, Kirito K, Kashii Y, et al. Forkhead family transcription factor FKHRL1 is expressed in human megakaryocytes. Regulation of cell cycling as a downstream molecule of thrombopoietin signaling. *J Biol Chem* 2001;276(18):15082–15089.

110. Nagata Y, Todokoro K. Thrombopoietin induces activation of at least two distinct signaling pathways. *FEBS Lett* 1995;377(3):497–501.

111. Yamada M, Komatsu N, Okada K, et al. Thrombopoietin induces tyrosine phosphorylation and activation of mitogen-activated protein kinases in a human thrombopoietin-dependent cell line. *Biochem Biophys Res Commun* 1995;217(1):230–237.

112. Alexander WS, Maurer AB, Novak U, et al. Tyrosine-599 of the c-Mpl receptor is required for Shc phosphorylation and the induction of cellular differentiation. *EMBO J* 1996;15(23):6531–6540. Dec 2

113. Luoh SM, Stefanich E, Solar G, et al. Role of the distal half of the c-Mpl intracellular domain in control of platelet production by thrombopoietin *in vivo*. *Mol Cell Biol* 2000;20(2):507–515.

114. Oda A, Miyakawa Y, Druker BJ, et al. Thrombopoietin primes human platelet aggregation induced by shear stress and by multiple agonists. *Blood* 1996;87(11):4664–4670.

115. Ezumi Y, Takayama H, Okuma M. Thrombopoietin, c-Mpl ligand, induces tyrosine phosphorylation of Tyk2, JAK2, and STAT3, and enhances agonists-induced aggregation in platelets *in vitro*. *FEBS Lett* 1995; 374(1):48–52.

116. Miyakawa Y, Oda A, Druker BJ, et al. Recombinant thrombopoietin induces rapid protein tyrosine phosphorylation of Janus kinase 2 and Shc in human blood platelets. *Blood* 1995;86(1):23–27.

117. Rodriguez-Linares B, Watson SP. Thrombopoietin potentiates activation of human platelets in association with JAK2 and TYK2 phosphorylation. *Biochem J* 1996;316(Pt 1):93–98.

118. Grossmann A, Lenox J, Ren HP, et al. Thrombopoietin accelerates platelet, red blood cell, and neutrophil recovery in myelosuppressed mice. *Exp Hematol* 1996;24(10):1238–1246.

119. Grossmann A, Lenox J, Deisher TA, et al. Synergistic effects of thrombopoietin and granulocyte colony-stimulating factor on neutrophil recovery in myelosuppressed mice. *Blood* 1996;88(9):3363–3370.

120. Akahori H, Shibuya K, Obuchi M, et al. Effect of recombinant human thrombopoietin in nonhuman primates with chemotherapy-induced thrombocytopenia. *Br J Haematol* 1996;94(4):722–728.

121. Harker LA, Marzec UM, Kelly AB, et al. Prevention of thrombocytopenia and neutropenia in a nonhuman primate model of marrow suppressive chemotherapy by combining pegylated recombinant human megakaryocyte growth and development factor and recombinant human granulocyte colony-stimulating factor. *Blood* 1997;89(1):155–165.

122. Neelis KJ, Qingliang L, Thomas GR, et al. Prevention of thrombocytopenia by thrombopoietin in myelosuppressed rhesus monkeys accompanied by prominent erythropoietic stimulation and iron depletion. *Blood* 1997; 90(1):58–63.

123. Molineux G, Hartley CA, McElroy P, et al. Megakaryocyte growth and development factor stimulates enhanced platelet recovery in mice after bone marrow transplantation. *Blood* 1996;88(4):1509–1514.

124. Fibbe WE, Heemskerk DP, Laterveer L, et al. Accelerated reconstitution of platelets and erythrocytes after syngeneic transplantation of bone marrow cells derived from thrombopoietin pretreated donor mice. *Blood* 1995; 86(9):3308–3313.

125. Neelis KJ, Dubbelman YD, Wognum AW, et al. Lack of efficacy of thrombopoietin and granulocyte colony-stimulating factor after high dose total-body irradiation and autologous stem cell or bone marrow transplantation in rhesus monkeys. *Exp Hematol* 1997;25(10):1094–1103.

126. Fanucchi M, Glaspy J, Crawford J, et al. Effects of polyethylene glycol-conjugated recombinant human megakaryocyte growth and development factor on platelet counts after chemotherapy for lung cancer. *N Engl J Med* 1997;336(6):404–409.

127. Basser RL, Rasko JE, Clarke K, et al. Randomized, blinded, placebo-controlled phase I trial of pegylated recombinant human megakaryocyte growth and development factor with filgrastim after dose-intensive chemotherapy in patients with advanced cancer. *Blood* 1997;89(9):3118–3128.

128. Vadhan-Raj S, Verschraegen CF, Bueso-Ramos C, et al. Recombinant human thrombopoietin attenuates carboplatin-induced severe thrombocytopenia and the need for platelet transfusions in patients with gynecologic cancer. *Ann Intern Med* 2000;132(5):364–368.

129. Geissler K, Kabrna E, Stengg S, et al. Recombinant human megakaryocyte growth and development factor increases levels of circulating haemopoietic

progenitor cells post chemotherapy in patients with acute myeloid leukaemia. *Br J Haematol* 1998;102(2):535–543.

130. Schuster MW, Beveridge R, Frei-Lahr D, et al. The effects of pegylated recombinant human megakaryocyte growth and development factor (PEG-rHuMGDF) on platelet recovery in breast cancer patients undergoing autologous bone marrow transplantation. *Exp Hematol* 2002;30(9): 1044–1050.

131. Bolwell B, Vredenburgh J, Overmoyer B, et al. Phase 1 study of pegylated recombinant human megakaryocyte growth and development factor (PEG-rHuMGDF) in breast cancer patients after autologous peripheral blood progenitor cell (PBPC) transplantation. *Bone Marrow Transplant* 2000; 26(2):141–145.

132. Nash RA, Kurzrock R, DiPersio J, et al. A phase I trial of recombinant human thrombopoietin in patients with delayed platelet recovery after hematopoietic stem cell transplantation. *Biol Blood Marrow Transplant* 2000;6(1):25–34.

133. Somlo G, Sniecinski I, ter Veer A, et al. Recombinant human thrombopoietin in combination with granulocyte colony-stimulating factor enhances mobilization of peripheral blood progenitor cells, increases peripheral blood platelet concentration, and accelerates hematopoietic recovery following high-dose chemotherapy. *Blood* 1999;93(9):2798–2806.

134. Kuter D, McCullough J, Romo J, et al. Treatment of platelet (PLT) donors with pegylated recombinant human megakaryocyte growth and development factor (PEG-rHuMGDF) increases circulating PLT counts (CTS) and PLT apheresis yields and increases platelet increments in recipients of PLT transfusions. *Blood* 1997;90(10):2579–2579.

135. Nomura S, Dan K, Hotta T, et al. Effects of pegylated recombinant human megakaryocyte growth and development factor in patients with idiopathic thrombocytopenic purpura. *Blood* 2002;100(2):728–730.

136. Sporn MB, Todaro GJ. Autocrine secretion and malignant transformation of cells. *N Engl J Med* 1980;303(15):878–880.

137. Alexander WS, Metcalf D, Dunn AR. Point mutations within a dimer interface homology domain of c-Mpl induce constitutive receptor activity and tumorigenicity. *EMBO J* 1995;14(22):5569–5578.

138. Onishi M, Kinoshita S, Morikawa Y, et al. Applications of retrovirus-mediated expression cloning. *Exp Hematol* 1996;24(2):324–329.

139. Sabath DF, Kaushansky K, Broudy VC. Deletion of the extracellular membrane-distal cytokine receptor homology module of Mpl results in constitutive cell growth and loss of thrombopoietin binding. *Blood* 1999;94(1): 365–367.

140. Cocault L, Bouscary D, Le Bousse Kerdiles C, et al. Ectopic expression of murine TPO receptor (c-Mpl) in mice is pathogenic and induces erythroblastic proliferation. *Blood* 1996;88(5):1656–1665.

141. Yan XQ, Lacey D, Hill D, et al. A model of myelofibrosis and osteosclerosis in mice induced by overexpressing thrombopoietin (mpl ligand): reversal of disease by bone marrow transplantation. *Blood* 1996; 88(2):402–409.

142. Frey BM, Rafii S, Teterson M, et al. Adenovector-mediated expression of human thrombopoietin cDNA in immune-compromised mice: insights into the pathophysiology of osteomyelofibrosis. *J Immunol* 1998;160(2): 691–699.

143. Villeval JL, Cohen-Solal K, Tulliez M, et al. High thrombopoietin production by hematopoietic cells induces a fatal myeloproliferative syndrome in mice. *Blood* 1997;90(11):4369–4383.

144. Li Y, Hetet G, Kiladjian JJ, et al. Proto-oncogene c-mpl is involved in spontaneous megakaryocytopoiesis in myeloproliferative disorders. *Br J Haematol* 1996;92(1):60–66.

145. Taksin AL, Couedic JP, Dusanter-Fourt I, et al. Autonomous megakaryocyte growth in essential thrombocythemia and idiopathic myelofibrosis is not related to a c-Mpl mutation or to an autocrine stimulation by Mpl-L. *Blood* 1999;93(1):125–139.

146. Pitcher L, Taylor K, Nichol J, et al. Thrombopoietin measurement in thrombocytosis: dysregulation and lack of feedback inhibition in essential thrombocythaemia. *Br J Haematol* 1997;99(4):929–932.

147. Li J, Xia Y, Kuter DJ. The platelet thrombopoietin receptor number and function are markedly decreased in patients with essential thrombocythaemia. *Br J Haematol* 2000;111(3):943–953.

148. Moliterno AR, Hankins WD, Spivak JL. Impaired expression of the thrombopoietin receptor by platelets from patients with polycythemia vera. *N Engl J Med* 1998;338(9):572–580.

149. Yoon SY, Li CY, Tefferi A. Megakaryocyte c-Mpl expression in chronic myeloproliferative disorders and the myelodysplastic syndrome: immunoperoxidase staining patterns and clinical correlates. *Eur J Haematol* 2000;65(3):170–174.

150. Moliterno AR, Siebel KE, Sun AY, et al. A novel thrombopoietin signaling defect in polycythemia vera platelets. *Stem Cells* 1998;16(Suppl. 2):185–192.

151. Ghilardi N, Skoda RC. A single-base deletion in the thrombopoietin (TPO) gene causes familial essential thrombocythemia through a mechanism of more efficient translation of TPO mRNA. *Blood* 1999;94(4): 1480–1482.

152. Muraoka K, Ishii E, Tsuji K, et al. Defective response to thrombopoietin and impaired expression of c-Mpl mRNA of bone marrow cells in congenital amegakaryocytic thrombocytopenia. *Br J Haematol* 1997;96(2): 287–292.

153. Basser RL, O'Flaherty E, Green M, et al. Development of pancytopenia with neutralizing antibodies to thrombopoietin after multicycle chemotherapy supported by megakaryocyte growth and development factor. *Blood* 2002;99(7):2599–2602.

154. Ballem PJ, Segal GM, Stratton JR, et al. Mechanisms of thrombocytopenia in chronic autoimmune thrombocytopenic purpura. Evidence of both impaired platelet production and increased platelet clearance. *J Clin Invest* 1987;80(1):33–40.

155. Li J, Yang C, Xia Y, et al. Thrombocytopenia caused by the development of antibodies to thrombopoietin. *Blood* 2001;98(12):3241–3248.

156. Katsumata Y, Suzuki T, Kuwana M, et al. Anti-c-Mpl (thrombopoietin receptor) autoantibody-induced amegakaryocytic thrombocytopenia in a patient with systemic sclerosis. *Arthritis Rheum* 2003;48(6):1647–1651.

157. Chang M, Nakagawa PA, Williams SA, et al. Immune thrombocytopenic purpura (ITP) plasma and purified ITP monoclonal autoantibodies inhibit megakaryocytopoiesis *in vitro*. *Blood* 2003;102(3):887–895.

158. Vigon I, Dreyfus F, Melle J, et al. Expression of the c-Mpl proto-oncogene in human hematologic malignancies. *Blood* 1993;82(3):877–883.

159. Wetzler M, Baer MR, Bernstein SH, et al. Expression of c-Mpl mRNA, the receptor for thrombopoietin, in acute myeloid leukemia blasts identifies a group of patients with poor response to intensive chemotherapy. *J Clin Oncol* 1997;15(6):2262–2268.

160. Schroder JK, Kolkenbrock S, Tins J, et al. Analysis of thrombopoietin receptor (c-Mpl) mRNA expression in de novo acute myeloid leukemia. *Leuk Res* 2000;24(5):401–409.

161. Bouscary D, Preudhomme C, Ribrag V, et al. Prognostic value of c-Mpl expression in myelodysplastic syndromes. *Leukemia* 1995;9(5):783–788.

162. Kaban K, Kantarjian H, Talpaz M, et al. Expression of thrombopoietin and its receptor (c-Mpl) in chronic myelogenous leukemia: correlation with disease progression and response to therapy. *Cancer* 2000;88(3):570–576.

# CHAPTER 28 ■ PLATELET GLYCOPROTEIN POLYMORPHISMS AND RELATIONSHIP TO FUNCTION, IMMUNOGENICITY, AND DISEASE

THOMAS J. KUNICKI

Platelet adhesion to extracellular matrix proteins and platelet cohesion (i.e., platelet aggregation) are necessary stages of normal hemostasis. Disruption of the integrity of the endothelial cell monolayer through physical trauma, plaque rupture, or inflammation can lead to exposure of collagens, retention of von Willebrand factor (VWF), and the attachment of platelets to the site of injury. This process involves the concerted participation of a handful of important membrane receptors.

Under flow conditions ranging from a low ($\leq$300 per second) to high shear ($\geq$1,500 per second), platelets will initially arrest transiently on exposed collagen. This requires VWF acting as a bridge between collagen and the platelet glycoprotein Ib (GP Ib) complex (1,2). The GP Ib complex is not usually considered a receptor for collagen; however, it does initiate the first adhesive platelet contact with the collagen-rich matrix. It is collagen that captures the VWF molecule by binding to its A3 domain, thereby localizing it and somehow altering its conformation to make it bind through its A1 domain with greater avidity to the GP Ib complex. This interaction is relatively weak and of short duration, resulting in a slowing of platelet motion and a tethering or rolling of the platelet across the thrombogenic collagen-rich surface. More importantly, engagement of the GP Ib complex leads to signal transduction, which activates other platelet receptors, particularly platelet glycoprotein VI (GP VI) and the integrins $\alpha_2\beta_1$ and $\alpha_{IIb}\beta_3$. If VWF binding to the GP Ib complex is inhibited, neither this initial contact nor the ensuing stable platelet monolayer formation and thrombus formation will occur.

Shortly after this initial engagement, two primary collagen receptors, the integrin $\alpha_2\beta_1$ and the platelet-specific receptor GP VI, mediate enhanced signal transduction and a more stable attachment of platelets to collagen. GP VI plays a dominant role in enhancing the transduction of signals leading to platelet activation that are otherwise initiated by the GP Ib complex. $\alpha_2\beta_1$ affords a more avid platelet attachment and contributes to signaling, resulting in a stable monolayer of activated platelets that serve as a nidus for prothrombin conversion and thrombus formation (3–5). Like other integrins, $\alpha_2\beta_1$ can undergo an activation-dependent increase in avidity for collagens (6). Platelet adhesion in flowing blood mediated by $\alpha_2\beta_1$ is supported by several collagen types, including types I, III, IV, and VI (7–11), and the rate of platelet monolayer formation is directly proportional to the platelet $\alpha_2\beta_1$ density (12).

A conformational change in a second integrin $\alpha_{IIb}\beta_3$ facilitates platelet aggregation through the binding of fibrinogen and/or VWF. Thrombin generated at the site of platelet aggregation then converts fibrinogen to fibrin, which enhances and stabilizes thrombus growth. Genetic differences that might alter surface expression of any of these receptors or ligands involved in thrombus initiation and growth have the potential to influence risk for adverse outcomes. Consequently, there is increasing interest in the association of genetic variation in platelet glycoproteins with risk for acute coronary disease, excessive bleeding syndromes, resistance to antiplatelet drugs, and heightened immunogenicity.

Additional platelet-derived agonists, such as arachidonate, thromboxane $A_2$ (Tx$A_2$), and adenosine diphosphate (ADP), can amplify platelet activation and accelerate the rate of thrombus formation. Genetic differences in the ADP receptor, P2Y$_{12}$, and the Tx$A_2$ receptor can therefore modulate the platelet response to these agonists.

Platelets synthesize and release Tx$A_2$ upon stimulation with a variety of agonists, including thrombin, collagen, and ADP. Tx$A_2$ is then released from platelets where it stimulates platelet Tx$A_2$ receptors, resulting in activation of phospholipase C (PLC) and an increase in cytosolic calcium. The increase in calcium then amplifies platelet aggregation and stimulates the synthesis of additional Tx$A_2$ and the release of ADP. In this manner, both Tx$A_2$ and ADP participate in a positive feedback loop that leads to irreversible platelet aggregation. The antiplatelet activity of aspirin is based primarily on its ability to irreversibly inhibit platelet cyclooxygenase-1 (COX-1) and thereby suppresses Tx$A_2$ synthesis (13).

Platelets express at least three purinergic receptors, two of which interact with ADP (14): The P2Y$_1$ receptor responsible for mobilization of ionized calcium from internal stores, which mediates shape change and initiates aggregation induced by ADP, and the P2Y$_{12}$ receptor coupled to adenylyl cyclase inhibition, essential for the full aggregation response to ADP (15). Clopidogrel is an effective inhibitor of ADP-induced platelet aggregation because it is a specific antagonist of the P2Y$_{12}$ purinergic receptor (13). Patients with abnormalities of platelet function due to a severe defect of P2Y$_{12}$ have been described but are rare (14,16,17). Each was characterized by a lifelong history of mucosal bleeding, easy bruising and/or excessive postoperative bleeding, mildly to severely prolonged bleeding times, slight and rapidly reversible primary wave of aggregation induced by ADP and abnormalities of platelet aggregation induced by collagen, arachidonate, and Tx$A_2$ analogs but normal aggregation induced by high concentrations of thrombin.

# SINGLE NUCLEOTIDE POLYMORPHISMS AND CANDIDATE GENE HAPLOTYPES

## Receptor Glycoprotein Gene Haplotypes

Single nucleotide polymorphisms (SNPs) in platelet glycoprotein receptor genes can give rise to differences in expression levels, activity, and/or immunogenicity. Those that influence the immunogenicity of the receptor can be defined serologically as antigens and are designated by the prefix human platelet antigen (HPA-) (18), as shown in Table 28-1. Seven genes relevant to a discussion of genetic differences in platelet function include the integrin $\alpha_2$ subunit gene *ITGA2*, the integrin $\alpha$IIb subunit gene *ITGA2B*, the integrin $\beta_3$ subunit gene *ITGB3*, the GP Ib$\alpha$ subunit gene *GP1BA*, the GP VI gene *GP6*, the P2Y$_{12}$ ADP receptor gene *P2Y$_{12}$*, and the TxA$_2$ receptor gene *TXA2R*.

*ITGA2.* Quantitative differences in platelet $\alpha_2\beta_1$ have been correlated with inheritance of three major *ITGA2* haplotypes (see Fig. 28-1), which can be defined by the SNPs C807T and G1648A. Haplotype 1 (**807T/1648G**) is associated with the highest levels of $\alpha_2\beta_1$, whereas haplotypes 2 (**807C/1648G**) and 3 (**807C/1648A**) are associated with the lowest and intermediate levels, respectively (12). The SNP C807T is a silent polymorphism within exon 7 of ITGA2 that correlates with expression levels, whereas the G1648 substitution within exon 13 gives rise to the amino acid replacement Glu505 $\rightarrow$ Lys505, defining the HPA-5 (Br) alloantigen system (37).

To readily distinguish each of the three major *ITGA2* haplotypes, two additional polymorphisms within intron 7 are convenient: The G65265A and A65986G dimorphisms (GenBank NT_025718) that define *Bgl* II and *Ase* I restriction sites, respectively (38). Haplotype 1 is *Bgl* II (pos) *Ase* I (neg); haplotype 2 is *Bgl* II (neg) *Ase* I (pos); and haplotype 3 is *Bgl* II (neg) *Ase* I (neg).

Two other polymorphisms in the *ITGA2* promoter, C-52T and C-92G, can further modulate transcription rates and affect the expression of the platelet integrin $\alpha_2\beta_1$. The substitution $-52$T disrupts an *Sp1* binding site spanning $-58$ to $-47$, attenuates transcription, and is associated with reduced expression of $\alpha_2\beta_1$ (39). The substitution $-92$G is adjacent to an *Sp1* binding site at position $-107$ to $-99$ and further decreases the rate of transcription (39). The presence of the $-92$G haplotype also correlates with reduced densities of platelet $\alpha_2\beta_1$. Interestingly, strain-related, twofold differences in expression of ITGA2 have also been reported in mice (40).

*ITGA2B.* Two major *ITGA2B* haplotypes are characterized by the substitution T10893G (Ile843 $\rightarrow$ Ser843) that defines the Bak (HPA-3) alloantigen system (see Fig. 28-2) (22). This polymorphism lies adjacent to the binding site of the murine monoclonal antibody PMI-1, which has been shown to inhibit platelet adhesion and spreading on certain substrata (41). ADP stimulation of platelets results in a fibrinogen-dependent increase in binding of the PMI-1 antibody, and peptides containing

## TABLE 28-1

### HUMAN PLATELET ALLOANTIGENS

| Antigen | Synonym | Glycoprotein location | Nucleotide | Amino acid | Reference |
|---------|---------|----------------------|------------|------------|-----------|
| HPA-1a | Pl[A1], Zw[a] | Integrin $\beta_3$ | T196 | Leu33 | 19,20 |
| HPA-1b | Pl[A2], Zw[b] | | C196 | Pro33 | |
| HPA-2a | Ko[b] | GP Ib$\alpha$ | C524 | Thr145 | 21 |
| HPA-2b | Ko[a], Sib[a] | | T524 | Met145 | |
| HPA-3a | Bak[a], Lek[a] | Integrin $\alpha_{IIb}$ | T2622 | Ile843 | 22 |
| HPA-3b | Bak[b] | | G2622 | Ser843 | |
| HPA-4a | Yuk[b], Pen[a] | Integrin $\beta_3$ | G526 | Arg143 | 23 |
| HPA-4b | Yuk[b], Pen[a] | | A526 | Gln143 | |
| HPA-5a | Br[b], Zav[b] | Integrin $\alpha_2$ | G1648 | Glu505 | 24 |
| HPA-5b | Br[a], Zav[a], Hc[a] | | A1648 | Lys505 | |
| HPA-6bW | Ca[a], Tu[a] | Integrin $\beta_3$ | A1564 | Gln489 | 25 |
| | | | G1564 | Arg489 | |
| HPA-7bW | Mo[a] | Integrin $\beta_3$ | G1317 | Ala407 | 26 |
| | | | C1317 | Pro407 | |
| HPA-8bW | Sr[a] | Integrin $\beta_3$ | T2004 | Cys636 | 27 |
| | | | C2004 | Arg636 | |
| HPA-9bW | Max[a] | Integrin $\alpha_{IIb}$ | A2603 | Met837 | 28 |
| | | | G2603 | Val837 | |
| HPA-10bW | La[a] | Integrin $\beta_3$ | A281 | Gln62 | 29 |
| | | | G281 | Arg62 | |
| HPA-11bW | Gro[a] | Integrin $\beta_3$ | A1996 | His633 | 30 |
| | | | G1996 | Arg633 | |
| HPA-12bW | Iy[a] | GP Ib$\beta$ | A141 | Glu15 | 31 |
| | | | G141 | Gly15 | |
| HPA-13bW | Sit[a] | Integrin $\alpha_2$ | T2531 | Met799 | 32 |
| | | | C2531 | Thr799 | |
| | Oe[a] | Integrin $\beta_3$ | | | 33 |
| | Va[a] | Integrin $\beta_3$ | | | 34 |
| | Pe[a] | GP Ib$\alpha$ | | | 35 |
| | Gov[a/b] | CD109 | | | 36 |

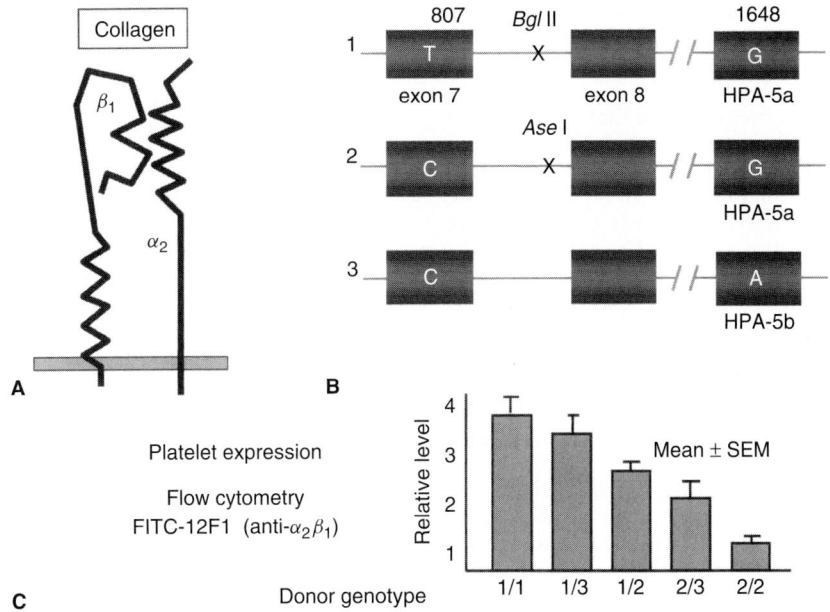

**FIGURE 28-1.** The integrin $\alpha_2$ (*ITGA2*) haplotypes. **A:** The platelet integrin $\alpha_2\beta_1$ is a collagen receptor composed of noncovalently associated $\alpha_2$ and $\beta_1$ subunits. **B:** There are three major haplotypes of the human $\alpha_2$ gene *ITGA2* that can be distinguished by a C807T substitution in exon 7, the presence or absence of unique *Bgl* II and *Ase* I restriction sites in intron 7, and a G1648A substitution in exon 13 that is responsible for the HPA-5a/5b diallelic alloantigen system. **C:** Platelet surface expression of integrin $\alpha_2\beta_1$, measured in flow cytometry by the binding of fluorescein isothiocynate (FITC) conjugated murine monoclonal antibody 12F1, varies up to fourfold and correlates with expression of haplotypes 1, 2, and 3. Haplotype 2 is associated with the lowest level of expression; haplotype 1, with the highest level; and haplotype 3, with intermediate levels. Bars represent the mean of greater than 10 determinations. Error bars represent one standard error of the mean.

Arginine-Glycine-Aspartate (RGD) also reversibly increase the binding of this antibody to cells and to purified glycoprotein $\alpha_{IIb}\beta_3$ (42). Therefore, the $\alpha_{IIb}$ region encompassing HPA-3 and PMI-1 epitopes may participate in adhesive functions through postreceptor occupancy events. The precise impact of the T10893G substitution on platelet function has not been characterized, but recent haplotype association studies in von Willebrand Disease (VWD) type 1 pedigrees have demonstrated that haplotype 10893T is associated with increased severity of bleeding (see subsequent text).

*ITGB3.* In the integrin $\beta_3$ subunit, the SNP T196C results in a Leu33 → Pro33 substitution defining the Pl^A1 (HPA-1a) and Pl^A2 (HPA-1b) haplotypes (see Fig. 28-3) (19,20). The influence of *ITGB3* Pl^A2 on platelet function has been vigorously debated. Several reports have provided evidence that Pl^A2 confers either enhanced function of $\alpha_{IIb}\beta_3$ or an increased resistance to inhibitors of platelet function. For example, it has been reported that Chinese hamster ovary (CHO) or human kidney 293 cells transfected with the Pl^A2 haplotype show increased adhesion to fibrinogen, but not fibronectin

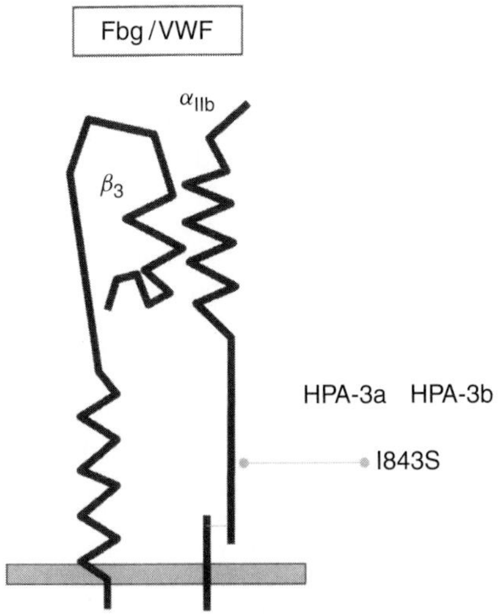

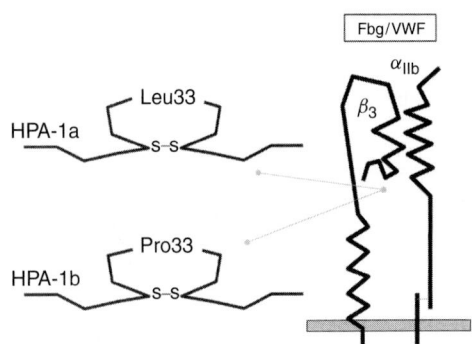

**FIGURE 28-2.** The integrin $\alpha_{IIb}$ (*ITGA2B*) haplotypes. The platelet integrin $\alpha_{IIb}\beta_3$ is a receptor for fibrinogen (Fbg) or von Willebrand Factor (VWF) composed of noncovalently associated $\alpha_{IIb}$ and $\beta_3$ subunits. The $\alpha_{IIb}$ subunit bears a prominent I843S substitution that creates two major haplotypes represented by the alloantigens HPA-3a and HPA-3b, respectively.

**FIGURE 28-3.** The integrin $\beta 3$ (*ITGB3*) haplotypes. The platelet integrin $\alpha_{IIb}\beta_3$ is a receptor for fibrinogen (Fbg) or von Willebrand Factor (VWF) composed of noncovalently associated $\alpha_{IIb}$ and $\beta_3$ subunits. The $\beta_3$ subunit bears a prominent L33P substitution within an amino-terminal loop that creates two major haplotypes represented by the alloantigens HPA-1a and HPA-1b, respectively.

(43), characterized by increased outside-in signaling through focal adhesion kinase (FAK) to mitogen activated protein kinase (MAPK) and greater actin reorganization (44), in a manner that is augmented by shear (45). It has also been reported that Pl$^{A2}$ enhances receptor function of $\beta_3$ in the context of both $\alpha_{IIb}\beta_3$ and $\alpha_V\beta_3$. Therefore, CHO cells transfected with Pl$^{A2}$ exhibited enhanced migration to fibrinogen or VWF, but not to fibronectin or vitronectin, whereas CHO cell lines expressing $\alpha_V\beta_3$ showed enhanced migration to vitronectin or osteopontin, but not to fibrinogen (46).

Pl$^{A2}$ enhancement has also been observed with endogenous platelet $\alpha_{IIb}\beta_3$. Compared to Pl$^{A1/A1}$ platelets, Pl$^{A2}$-positive platelets exhibit a gene dosage effect leading to significantly greater surface P selectin expression, $\alpha_{IIb}\beta_3$-bound fibrinogen, and activated $\alpha_{IIb}\beta_3$ in response to low-dose ADP (47). Upon adhesion to fibrinogen, human platelets and CHO cells expressing Pl$^{A2}$ exhibit enhanced activation of the ERK2 substrate myosin light chain kinase (MLCK). Platelets expressing Pl$^{A2}$ show greater alpha-granule release, clot retraction, and adhesion to fibrinogen under shear stress, all of which can be blocked completely by MLCK and MAPK kinase inhibition (44). These results suggest that the basis for the Pl$^{A2}$ difference lies in postintegrin occupancy signaling through MAPK and MLCK after $\alpha_{IIb}\beta_3$ cross-linking (44).

It should be noted that not all studies have observed an increased biologic activity associated with the Pl$^{A2}$ haplotype (48,49).

*GP1BA.* The GP Ib complex is a heptamer composed of four distinct gene products: two molecules of GP Ib$\alpha$, two of GP Ib$\beta$, two of GP IX, and one of GP V. VWF is directly bound by the GP Ib$\alpha$ subunits, each of which is disulfide-linked to a GP Ib$\beta$ subunit. Relevant polymorphisms have been associated with the gene *GP1BA* encoding the GP Ib$\alpha$ subunit (see Fig. 28-4), and two major haplotypes can be distinguished by a Thr145 → Met145 substitution within the ligand binding region that also defines the HPA-2 (Ko) alloantigen system (21,50).

The Met145/Thr145 SNP is in linkage disequilibrium (LD) with a variable number of tandem repeats (VNTR) polymorphism within the mucinlike macroglycopeptide region of GP Ib$\alpha$. This is reflected by the duplication of a 13–amino acid sequence either once (VNTR A), twice (VNTR B), thrice (VNTR C), or four times (VNTR D),

VNTR = Variable number of tandem repeats

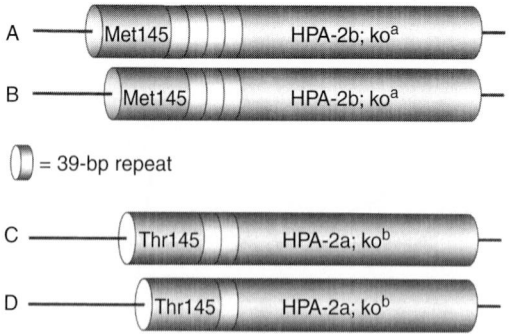

**FIGURE 28-4.** The glycoprotein Ib$\alpha$ (*GP1BA*) haplotypes. The Ib$\alpha$ gene is characterized by a major T145M substitution that creates the HPA-2a and HPA-2b alloantigens. A second polymorphism, represented by a variable number of tandem 39 base pair repeats is in linkage disequilibrium (LD) with T145M. Therefore, variable number of tandem repeats (VNTR) A and B (four and three repeats, respectively) is usually associated with M145 (HPA-2b), whereas VNTR C and D (two and one repeat, respectively) is normally associated with T145 (HPA-2a).

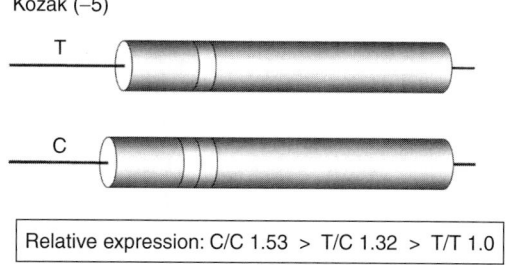

**FIGURE 28-5.** Additional glycoprotein Ib$\alpha$ (*GP1BA*) haplotypes. In addition to VNTR and T145M (Fig. 28-4), the Ib$\alpha$ gene is characterized by a T/C substitution in the 5′-untranslated region that is at position −5 relative to the start codon. This substitution is adjacent to a consensus Kozak sequence and influences the relative translation rate of the transcript. Thus, donors who are homozygous for a C at this position (C/C) express approximately 1.5 times as much GP Ib$\alpha$ as those donors who are homozygous for a T at this position (T/T).

and results in a polypeptide length of 610, 623, 636, or 649 amino acids, respectively (51,52). Because these repeats are rich in proline, serine, and threonine, they can be potentially glycosylated, and each repeat could add up to 32 Å to the length of the GP Ib$\alpha$ extracellular domain (51). In a simple model, this could extend the GP Ib$\alpha$ binding sites for VWF and thrombin further above the plane of the plasma membrane, increasing the avidity for these ligands and accounting for the observed increased risk for acute coronary artery disease associated with the longer variants, VNTR C and VNTR D, which are in LD with Met145 (53,54).

In addition, a T/C substitution in the region of the translation start site, at a position 5 nucleotides upstream (−5) from the initiator codon [antithymocyte globulin (ATG)] (see Fig. 28-5) (55,56), influences translation efficiency. The presence of the −5C haplotype increases the mean level of GP Ib$\alpha$ on the platelet plasma membrane (roughly, a 50% increase in homozygous individuals and a 33% increase in heterozygous individuals) (55). Interestingly, the −5C/T haplotypes and the Met145/Thr145 haplotypes are in complete linkage equilibrium (57).

*GP6.* The two major haplotypes of the human gene *GP6* are designated a and b and have frequencies in white non-Hispanics of 0.84 and 0.16, respectively (see Fig. 28-6). They are characterized by five–amino acid substitutions: a = 219S-237K-249T-317Q-322H and b = 219P-237E-249A-317L-322N. There is evidence that haplotype b attenuates GP VI function perhaps through an influence on its expression (58). Consistent with this biological evidence, inheritance of haplotype b is associated with increased bleeding severity in VWD type 1 (see subsequent text).

*P2Y$_{12}$.* Differences in platelet responses to ADP between normal donors may be associated with the recently described H1 and H2 haplotypes of P2Y$_{12}$ (59). As for the other platelet ADP receptors, P2X$_1$ and P2Y$_1$, heritable polymorphisms have not yet been identified, and it is not evident that platelet mRNA levels vary markedly between individuals (60).

*TXA2R.* The two isoforms of this receptor, TXR$\alpha$ and TXR$\beta$, exhibit similar ligand binding properties and PLC activation, but TXR$\alpha$ activates adenylyl cyclase, whereas TXR$\beta$ inhibits it. Both isoforms are present in platelets. Two major haplotypes are defined by T924C. Haplotype 2 (924C) has been positively associated with

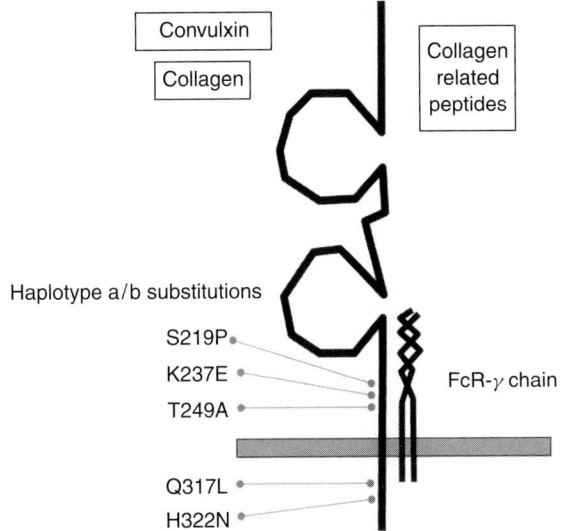

**FIGURE 28-6.** Glycoprotein VI (*GP6*) haplotypes. Platelet GP VI is a receptor specifically for collagens or the snake venom protein convulxin (CVX) that is also specifically recognized by collagen-related peptides (CRP). It associates noncovalently with the coreceptor FcR-γ chain. There are two major haplotypes of human GP VI, a and b, that bear substitutions at five positions, which are in linkage disequilibrium (LD). Haplotype a is represented by S219/K237/T249/ Q317/H322, whereas haplotype b is represented by P219/E237/ A249/L317/N322.

bronchial asthma (61) and may directly influence the rate of transcription or translation of *TXA2R*.

## Non–Receptor Gene Haplotypes

In addition to the aforementioned genetic differences in platelet glycoprotein receptor genes, there are heritable polymorphisms in glycoprotein ligand and/or cytokine genes that can influence the expression levels of these glycoproteins and thereby have an impact on platelet function or activity. These include the VWF gene *VWF*, the fibrinogen Bβ chain gene *FGB*, and the interleukin 6 gene *IL6*.

*VWF.* Two major haplotypes of the *VWF* gene have been defined that influence expression: haplotype 1 (−1793G/−1234C/ 1185A/−1015G) and haplotype 2(−1793G/−1234T/1185G/ −1051A) (62,63). Individuals homozygous for haplotype 1 have the highest mean VWF:Ag levels (mean = 0.962 U per mL); heterozygotes have intermediate levels (0.867 U per mL); and those homozygous for haplotype 2 have the lowest levels (0.776 U per mL) (63). Circulating levels of plasma VWF may be determined, in part, by this polymorphic variation in the promoter region of the *VWF* gene.

*FGB.* Elevated levels of fibrinogen are an independent risk factor for coronary vascular events among healthy individuals or those with coronary artery disease (64). An increase in as little as 0.1 mg per mL of plasma fibrinogen will increase cardiovascular risk by approximately 15% (65). Because production of the fibrinogen Bβ chain is the rate-limiting step in fibrinogen biosynthesis, the major *FGB* haplotypes defined by G-455A are directly linked to expression levels (64).

*IL6.* Inflammation is a key component of coronary heart disease, and genes coding for cytokines are candidates for predisposing to risk for coronary heart disease. Humphries et al. (66) showed that the −174C haplotype is associated with a significantly (*P* = 0.007) higher systolic blood pressure and increased risk for development of coronary heart disease.

## PLATELET GLYCOPROTEIN IMMUNOGENETICS

Our progress in understanding the biology of platelet membrane glycoprotein receptors was stimulated by the study of platelet immunogenicity, because these glycoproteins figure prominently as alloantigens, autoantigens, and targets of drug-dependent antibodies. The molecular nature of glycoprotein epitopes is therefore an appropriate focus of this review. Platelet membrane glycolipids and phospholipids also represent autoantigenic components, but much less is known about the structure and immunogenicity of these platelet constituents, and it is the intent of this review to highlight the immunogenetics of platelet glycoproteins.

Two clinically important syndromes, neonatal alloimmune thrombocytopenia (NATP) and posttransfusion purpura (PTP), can result from sensitization to platelet-specific alloantigens. The development of these alloantibodies can represent a major obstacle to platelet transfusion therapy in sensitized patients, such as those undergoing chemotherapy in conjunction with myelodysplastic syndromes or hematopoietic stem cell transplantation.

**Neonatal Alloimmune Thrombocytopenia (NATP).** NATP is caused by maternal sensitization to paternal alloantigens on fetal platelets, and human platelet antigen 1 (HPA-1) is the alloantigen system most often involved in patients in the United States. The response to HPA-1a among individuals homozygous for HPA-1b is HLA restricted (67–69), and responsive individuals are almost exclusively HLA DRB3*0101 (68) or DQB1*02 (70,71). For DRB3*0101, the calculated risk factor is 141, a risk level equivalent to that of HLA B27 in ankylosing spondylitis (71). On the other hand, the converse response of homozygous HPA-1a individuals to the more rare HPA-1b haplotype is not linked to HLA (71,72).

It is probable that T cells are responsible for the HLA restriction in this case, and Maslanka et al. (71) reported that in one case of NATP, T cells that share CDR3 motifs are stimulated by peptides that contain the same Leu33 substitution that is recognized by anti-HPA-1a alloantibodies. With respect to another platelet alloantigen, HPA-6b, there appears to be an association between responsiveness and the MHC genes HLA DRB1*1501, DQA1*0102 or DQB1*0602 (73).

**Posttransfusion Purpura (PTP).** PTP can result within 7 to 10 days after an immunogenic blood (platelet) transfusion and most often affects previously nontransfused, multiparous women. As with NATP, there is an increased risk to develop PTP among HLA-DR3–positive individuals, and HPA-1a is the antigen most often implicated in white populations (67,74).

## HAPLOTYPE FREQUENCIES IN DIFFERENT RACIAL/ETHNIC GROUPS

A substantial amount of information has been accumulated with respect to the relative frequency of the major alloantigen haplotypes among different racial and ethnic populations (see Table 28-2). The data for four of the most clinically prominent alloantigen haplotypes are depicted: HPA-1b, HPA-2b, HPA-3b, and HPA-5b (*ITGA2* haplotype 3). Each of these alloantigens represents one of a diallelic system. Therefore, while the frequencies of the immunogenic, less common alleles are depicted in Table 28-3, those of the more common alleles can be readily deduced.

HPA-1b has a relatively higher frequency among whites of European background, North Africans, African Americans, and Western Indians (≥0.08), and is much rarer among Asians,

## TABLE 28-2

### HAPLOTYPE FREQUENCIES IN DIFFERENT POPULATIONS

| Population | HPA-1b | HPA-2b | HPA-3b | HPA-5b | Reference |
|---|---|---|---|---|---|
| **BRAZIL** | | | | | |
| American Indians | 0 | 0.04 | 0.43 | 0 | 75,76 |
| | 0 | 0.04 | 0.29 | 0.04 | 77 |
| Blacks | 0.12 | 0.15 | 0.35 | 0.20 | 75,76 |
| | 0.10 | 0.19 | 0.33 | 0.12 | 78 |
| Whites | 0.11 | 0.10 | 0.50 | 0.03 | 75,76 |
| | 0.08 | 0.15 | 0.40 | 0.08 | 78 |
| Japanese | — | — | 0.45 | 0.03 | 76 |
| **EUROPE** | | | | | |
| Austrian | 0.15 | 0.08 | 0.39 | 0.11 | 79 |
| Danish | 0.17 | 0.08 | 0.37 | 0.08 | 80 |
| Dutch | 0.15 | 0.07 | 0.44 | 0.10 | 81 |
| Finnish | 0.14 | 0.09 | 0.41 | 0.05 | 82 |
| French | 0.15 | 0.08 | 0.38 | 0.13 | 83 |
| German | 0.18 | 0.08 | 0.37 | 0.10 | 84 |
| Italian (Milan) | 0.21 | 0.09 | 0.45 | 0.15 | 57 |
| Polish | 0.13 | 0.10 | 0.41 | 0.06 | 85 |
| Slovenian | 0.19 | 0.11 | 0.41 | 0.07 | 86 |
| Spanish | 0.15 | 0.11 | 0.27 | 0.16 | 87 |
| Welsh | 0.17 | 0.10 | 0.39 | 0.10 | 88 |
| **AFRICA** | | | | | |
| Moroccan Berber | 0.25 | 0.18 | 0.32 | 0.14 | 89 |
| Tunisian | 0.25 | — | 0.31 | 0.22 | 90 |
| **NORTH AMERICA** | | | | | |
| African American | 0.08 | 0.18 | 0.37 | 0.21 | 91 |
| | | | | 0.16 | 92 |
| White, Non-Hispanic | 0.17 | 0.08 | 0.41 | 0.09 | 57 |
| | — | 0.09 | — | 0.11 | 91 |
| | | | | 0.08 | 92 |
| Native American | — | 0.12 | — | 0.02 | 92 |
| **ASIA** | | | | | |
| Korean | 0.005 | — | — | — | 91 |
| | 0.012 | 0.08 | 0.44 | 0.02 | 93 |
| Japanese | 0.009 | 0.10 | | 0.03 | 94 |
| | 0.002 | — | — | — | 95 |
| | 0.002 | 0.10 | 0.41 | 0.04 | 78 |
| Thais Northeastern | 0.03 | 0.06 | 0.47 | 0.04 | 96 |
| Thais | 0.015 | 0.06 | 0.49 | 0.04 | 97,98 |
| Hong Kong Chinese | 0.005 | 0.02 | 0.47 | 0.03 | 99 |
| Chinese Han | 0.003 | 0.05 | 0.40 | 0.01 | 100 |
| Chinese Taiwan | 0.001 | 0.05 | 0.39 | 0.18 | 97,101 |
| Saisiat Taiwan | 0 | 0.04 | 0.55 | 0.03 | 102 |
| Bunun Taiwan | 0 | 0.01 | 0.58 | 0 | 102 |
| Tsou Taiwan | 0 | 0 | 0.75 | 0.02 | 102 |
| Puyuma Taiwan | 0 | 0.01 | 0.44 | 0.03 | 102 |
| Indonesian | 0.009 | 0.06 | 0.49 | 0.005 | 97,98 |
| | 0.009 | | 0.54 | 0.05 | 103 |
| Vietnamese Kinh | 0.014 | 0.05 | 0.51 | 0.03 | 104 |
| Filipino | — | — | 0.47 | — | 97 |
| Ma'ohis (Polynesian) | 0.025 | 0.09 | 0.40 | 0.02 | 104 |
| Indian, Western | 0.095 | — | — | — | 105 |
| **AUSTRALIA** | | | | | |
| Aboriginal | 0.008 | — | 0.06 | 0.15 | 106 |
| | 0.003 | 0 | 0.07 | 0.25 | 107 |
| White | 0.14 | 0.07 | 0.38 | 0.09 | 107 |

Native North Americans, and Aboriginals (≤0.03) (see Fig. 28-7). Not surprisingly, the most frequent antigen target in NATP in white populations is HPA-1a (estimated at 78%) (110). However, among Asians, anti-HPA-1a has never been shown to be involved in NATP (111).

HPA-2b has the highest frequencies among African Americans and North Africans (≥0.15) (see Fig. 28-8), but is also highly represented in whites (0.07 to 0.15) and one study of Native North Americans (0.12). It has a uniformly lower frequency in Native South Americans (American Indians) (0.04)

**TABLE 28-3**

PROTHROMBOTIC HAPLOTYPE FREQUENCIES
IN DIFFERENT POPULATIONS

| | *ITGA2* Haplotype 1 (807T) | *GP1BA* −5C | Reference |
|---|---|---|---|
| Whites | 0.38 | 0.13–0.14 | 57,108,109 |
| Whites, Hispanic | 0.51 | | 109 |
| Asian | 0.30 | | 91 |
| African American | 0.34 | 0.17 | 108,109 |
| Native North American | 0.54 | | 109 |
| American Indian | | 0.254 | 108 |

and is nonexistent among aboriginals. The reports of HPA-2b frequency among Asians have provided disparate values ranging from 0 to 0.1. HPA-2a has been implicated in NATP among both whites and Asians (112–115), but much more commonly among whites.

With one exception, HPA-3b seems to be prominently represented among all races, with frequencies ranging from 0.26 to 0.78 (see Fig. 28-9). The sole exception is aboriginals, among whom the frequency is 0.06 to 0.07. HPA-3a is a frequent target for alloimmunization in NATP and PTP among whites.

The highest frequencies of HPA-5b are found among North Africans (0.14 to 0.22), African Americans (0.12 to 0.21), and aboriginals (0.15 to 0.25) (see Fig. 28-10). The lowest frequencies are found among Asians (≤0.05), American Indians (≤0.04), and Native North Americans (0.02), whereas intermediate frequencies are characteristic of white populations (0.04 to 0.16).

Other nonimmunogenic haplotypes figure prominently in risk for thrombosis or bleeding, particularly *ITGA2* haplotype

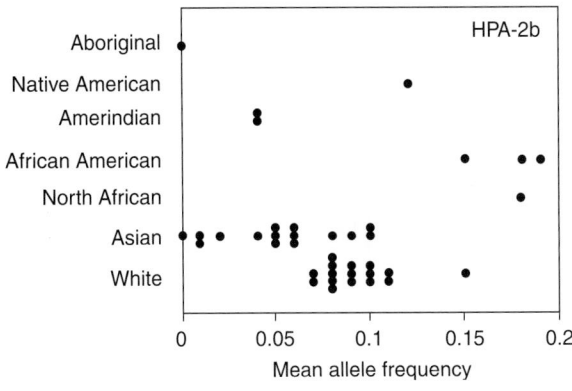

**FIGURE 28-8.** Mean allele frequencies of the Alloantigen HPA-2b in different populations. Depicted in this figure are the mean frequencies of the HPA-2b allele obtained in separate studies of diverse racial/ethnic populations. Each data point represents the mean value reported in a single published study. The individual studies are itemized in Table 28-2. The populations listed on the ordinate are (**top** to **bottom**): Aboriginal Australians; Native North Americans; South-American American Indians; African Americans; North Africans; Asians; and whites of European origin. The mean allele frequency is shown on the abscissa.

1(807T), *ITGA2* haplotype 2(807C), *GPIBA* −5C, and *GPIBA*–5T. Differences in frequencies of these haplotypes are important in understanding the demographics of disease (Table 28-3).

# CANDIDATE GENE HAPLOTYPES AND RESISTANCE TO ANTITHROMBOTIC DRUGS

The paradigm for genetic resistance to antiplatelet drugs is aspirin resistance (ASAR). The Antiplatelet Trialists Collaboration has concluded that low-dose aspirin (ASA) (75 to 150 mg daily) is an effective antiplatelet regimen for long-term use among patients with increased risk for occlusive vascular events (116). However, there are significant differences among

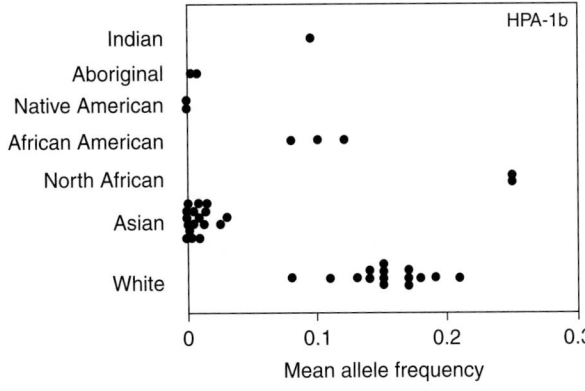

**FIGURE 28-7.** Mean allele frequencies of the alloantigen HPA-1b in different populations. Depicted in this figure are the mean frequencies of the HPA-1b allele obtained in separate studies of diverse racial/ethnic populations. Each data point represents the mean value reported in a single published study. The individual studies are itemized in Table 28-2. The populations listed on the ordinate are (**top** to **bottom**): Western Indians; Aboriginal Australians; Native North Americans; African Americans; North Africans; Asians; and whites of European origin. The mean allele frequency is shown on the abscissa.

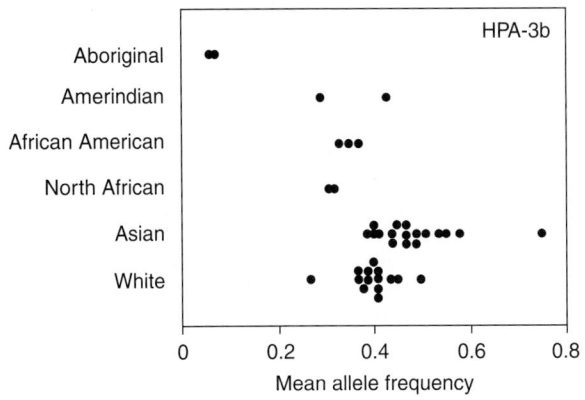

**FIGURE 28-9.** Mean allele frequencies of the alloantigen HPA-3b in different populations. Depicted in this figure are the mean frequencies of the HPA-3b allele obtained in separate studies of diverse racial/ethnic populations. Each data point represents the mean value reported in a single published study. The individual studies are itemized in Table 28-2. The populations listed on the ordinate are (**top** to **bottom**): Aboriginal Australians; South-American American Indians; African Americans; North Africans; Asians; and whites of European origin. The mean allele frequency is shown on the abscissa.

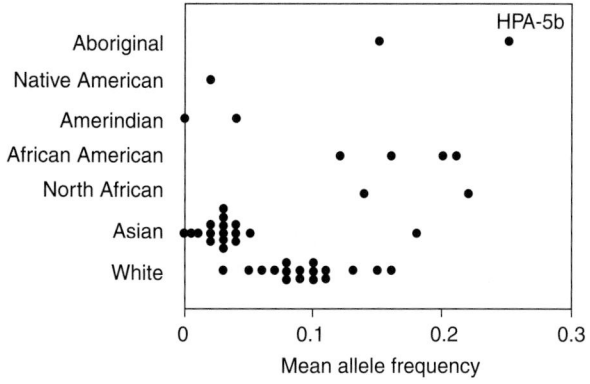

**FIGURE 28-10.** Mean allele frequencies of the alloantigen HPA-5b in different populations. Depicted in this figure are the mean frequencies of the HPA-5b allele obtained in separate studies of diverse racial/ethnic populations. Each data point represents the mean value reported in a single published study. The individual studies are itemized in Table 28-2. The populations listed on the ordinate are (**top to bottom**): Aboriginal Australians; Native North Americans; South-American American Indians; African Americans; North Africans; Asians; and whites of European origin. The mean allele frequency is shown on the abscissa.

patients or controls with respect to the extent to which ASA can inhibit platelet function. This variability influences the beneficial effect of low-dose ASA in prevention of stroke or acute cardiovascular events (117).

Those genetic differences that influence the rate and efficiency of platelet responses might also influence the ability of an inhibitor, such as ASA, to attenuate platelet function. Because ASA exerts its effect on platelet function through its inhibition of platelet COX-1, resulting in a significant decrease in $TxA_2$ production, one would suspect that aspirin resistance might be related to genetic variation in COX-1. However, although 14 variants of COX-1 were identified among ASA nonresponders with recurrence of ischemic stroke, carriers and noncarriers of these mutations behaved similarly when platelet aggregation was studied with collagen, ADP, or arachidonic acid (118). It would appear that the genetic differences responsible for resistance to ASA inhibition are more complex, involving any number of the receptor–ligand interactions that contribute to platelet adhesion and aggregation.

The report of Weber et al. (119) provides a basis for classification of ASAR that helps to distinguish "true" ASAR from the more common variability in responsiveness to ASA inhibition. In the more common type 1 ASAR (roughly 15% of normal donors or patients with ischemic coronary disease), platelet responsiveness to collagen and platelet $TxA_2$ formation are not inhibited by *in vivo* low-dose ASA (81 to 325 mg per day for ≥3 days), but subsequent addition of ASA to platelet-rich plasma or whole blood *in vitro* (100 $\mu$M) can completely block collagen-induced aggregation and significantly increase the PFA-100 CEPI-CT. In the less common type 2 ASAR (roughly 5% of donors), platelet function and $TxA_2$ formation are inhibited both *in vivo* and *in vitro*. It is the latter type that is more akin to true aspirin resistance.

The PFA-100 is one convenient method to analyze interdonor differences in responsiveness to ASA. This apparatus measures platelet thrombus formation under high shear in citrated whole blood initiated by exposure to collagen and activation with ADP or epinephrine. ASA prolongs the rate of thrombus formation (closure time; CT) of blood activated by epinephrine (CEPI-CT) (120). There is already substantial evidence that the PFA-100 may reliably substitute for the bleeding time as a platelet function–screening test in the clinical setting, producing fewer false-positive results (120–122). Homoncik et al. (123) convincingly showed that the PFA-100 is suitable for monitoring the extent of ASA-induced platelet dysfunction. They reported a dose-dependent prolongation of CEPI-CT that correlated well with basal values and was markedly influenced by VWF antigen (VWF:Ag) levels.

Several studies reviewed in the preceding text emphasized an increased sensitivity of the $Pl^{A2}$ haplotype to a variety of platelet agonists. Conversely, $Pl^{A2}$ may increase resistance to platelet inhibition (124). In one of the first studies of this nature, bleeding times before or after ASA ingestion were shown to be influenced by the $Pl^{A1}$ versus $Pl^{A2}$ haplotype. In 80 healthy men, aged 20 to 25 years, the bleeding time prior to ASA ingestion was shorter in carriers of the $Pl^{A2}$ haplotype than in those homozygous for the $Pl^{A1}$ haplotype. It was concluded that carriers of the $Pl^{A2}$ haplotype appear to be more resistant to the antithrombotic action of ASA (125).

# CANDIDATE GENE HAPLOTYPES AND RISK FOR THROMBOSIS IN ACUTE CORONARY AND CEREBROVASCULAR DISEASE

Ischemic heart disease and cerebrovascular disease are the leading causes of morbidity and mortality among both adult men and women in the developed western world (126–129). These diseases result from interactions between genetic susceptibility factors, chronic environmental influences (for example, hormonal imbalance, smoking, or obesity), and intercurrent disorders, such as diabetes, hypertension, dyslipidemia, or hyper-homocysteinemia. Acute myocardial infarction (MI), resulting from the formation of an occlusive thrombus at the site of a ruptured atherosclerotic plaque, is the most devastating outcome of these disorders, and the critical role of platelets in this process is now well accepted (130).

Not only the extent but also the rate of platelet activation influences these outcomes, controlled by heritable differences in the expression and avidity of key platelet receptors and their protein ligands.

There is correlation between *ITGA2* haplotype 1 (807T) (high receptor density) and risk for arterial thrombosis in younger men with a history of MI (131,132), women who are heavy smokers (133), patients with diabetic retinopathy (134), and younger patients with stroke (135).

A number of reports have found an association between the expression of *ITGB3* Pro33 ($Pl^{A2}$ alloantigen) and risk for thrombosis, particularly among young individuals (136,137), and a notable decrease in its frequency among young survivors of MI (138). A number of other studies on large patient cohorts have failed to find an association with risk for MI (139,140) or stroke (139). Interestingly, one recent metaanalysis concluded that there is no association between $Pl^{A2}$ and increased thrombotic risk (141), whereas a second recent metaanalysis (142) concluded that there is a weak but significant correlation.

Reiner et al. (143) found that homozygosity for haplotype 2 (10893G) is associated with an approximately fivefold increased risk of ischemic stroke among subgroups of women who carried a diagnosis of hypertension or diabetes [odds ratio (OR), 4.51; 95% confidence intervals (CI), 1.01 to 20.13] or had elevated plasma homocysteine levels (OR, 5.94; 95% CI, 1.53 to 23.05).

An association has been found between inheritance of the *GP1BA* Met145 haplotype and risk for coronary artery disease (53,54) or stroke (54,144) in younger individuals. The biologic effect of the Met145/Leu145 substitution remains to be determined but is thought to reflect a change in the avidity of the GP Ib complex for VWF. There is an indication of an association between the *GP1BA* −5C haplotype and the severity of negative outcomes following acute MI in younger individuals (≤62 years old) (145). Moreover, a recent study has documented a synergistic effect of −5C and Met145 that results in an increased risk for stroke in younger individuals (146).

Homozygosity for the *GP6* haplotype b (Pro219/Pro219) has been associated with risk for MI, particularly among older women (≥60 years old) who were smokers and carried the fibrinogen Bβ -455A haplotype (higher fibrinogen level).

Elevated levels of plasma fibrinogen are an independent risk factor for coronary vascular events among healthy individuals or those with coronary artery disease (64). An increase in as little as 0.1 mg per mL of plasma fibrinogen will increase cardiovascular risk by approximately 15% (65). Because production of the fibrinogen Bβ chain is the rate-limiting step in fibrinogen biosynthesis, it is not surprising that the promoter region SNP G-455A was shown to have a direct effect on transcription (64). In a recent study of 250 male army recruits undergoing basic training, fibrinogen levels (mg per mL) were significantly elevated over baseline levels 2, 48, and 96 hours after a strenuous 48 hour final military exercise (FME), representing increases of 15.7%, 3.4%, and 7.6%, respectively. Higher levels were attained in −455A haplotype carriers, relative to −455GG subjects: $3.17 \pm 0.05$ versus $2.94 \pm 0.05$ ($P <0.001$) at 2 hours post FME; $2.86 \pm 0.05$ versus $2.60 \pm 0.05$ ($P <0.0005$) at 48 hours; and $2.98 \pm 0.06$ versus $2.69 \pm 0.06$ ($P <0.0005$) at 96 hours. At the same time, there was no effect of a second SNP G-854A on fibrinogen levels. Therefore, the fibrinogen Bβ chain SNP G-455A influences fibrinogen levels following exercise.

Humphries et al. (66) examined the effect of the *IL6* −174 G → C substitution in the promoter of the IL-6 gene on risk of coronary heart disease, and on intermediate risk traits including fibrinogen and systolic blood pressure, in 2,751 middle-aged healthy UK men. The −174C haplotype (frequency 0.43) was associated with a significantly ($P = 0.007$) higher systolic blood pressure. Compared to men with genotype GG, those carrying the −174C haplotype had a relative risk of coronary heart disease of 1.54 ($P = 0.048$). This effect was exacerbated among heavy smokers (compared to GG nonsmokers, relative risk = 2.66). These effects remained statistically significant even after adjusting for classical risk factors, including blood pressure ($P = 0.04$). In a subset of the genotyped men ($n = 494$), carriers of the −174C haplotype had higher levels of C-reactive protein than noncarriers. These data confirm the importance of the inflammatory system in the development of coronary heart disease. They suggest that, at least in part, the effect of the IL-6 −174 (G/C) SNP on blood pressure is likely to be operating through inflammatory mechanisms. The molecular mechanisms underlying the effects of this genetically determined differences in plasma levels of IL-6 remain to be determined. However, the fact that IL-6 can influence the expression of other potential risk factors, such as fibrinogen and VWF, makes it an important target in a comprehensive study of the genetics of arterial thrombosis. For these reasons, the IL-6 −174 (G/C) SNP should be included in any list of candidate gene SNPs relevant to arterial thrombosis.

# CANDIDATE GENE HAPLOTYPES AND RISK FOR BLEEDING

Genetic variation in platelet glycoprotein receptors can have an impact on platelet function *in vivo*, particularly in mild forms of von Willebrand Disease (VWD) type 1, which account for at least 60% of all cases of VWD (147). The paradox of VWD type 1 is that bleeding risk does not correlate with plasma VWF levels (147).

Among normal donors, plasma VWF levels vary over a wide range, and 95% of all values fall within 50% and 200% of the mean. ABO blood type has a major influence on VWF levels such that the average level for persons who are blood type O is 25% to 35% lower than that of persons who are non-O (148). This accounts for approximately 30% of the genetic variance of VWF (149). The SNP G-1793C in the VWF promoter also correlates with small changes in mean VWF level. Among blood group O donors, mean VWF levels are 77% for genotype CC, 86% for genotype GC, and 93% for genotype GG (63). Because of the high haplotype frequency of −1793C (0.65), it can contribute to the variation in VWF levels.

In an initial case–control study (150), we showed that the 807C dimorphism of the integrin gene *ITGA2* is associated with diminished platelet responsiveness to collagen in a high shear environment, reflected by a prolongation of the PFA-100 (Dade-Behring International) collagen/epinephrine-closure time. That study preceded the finding that there are two major haplotypes that share the 807C allele: haplotype 3 (807C/1648A), which is associated with higher levels of the integrin, and haplotype 2 (807C/1648G), which is associated with markedly reduced levels of this receptor (12).

A subsequent study of the pedigrees of index cases of VWD type 1 provided additional insight into the genetic differences that influence bleeding severity and clarified the association between bleeding and *ITGA2* haplotypes 2 and 3 (57). In that study, a positive influence of −1793C on plasma VWF:Ag and VWF:RCo was confirmed, but the impact of VWF promoter haplotypes was not sufficiently important that they were directly associated with variation in bleeding phenotype. A bleeding severity score was derived from a detailed history and adjusted for age, providing a normal distribution of this quantitative trait. VWF:RCo levels, followed by VWF:Ag levels, had the strongest influence on bleeding severity score. *ITGA2* haplotype 2 contributes to increased bleeding severity score and increased risk, whereas haplotype 3 is protective. This study reinforced the need to distinguish the major haplotypes 2 and 3 of *ITGA2*, which share the 807C SNP, as each has a quantitatively and perhaps qualitatively opposite influence on the function of this integrin.

With regard to *GP6* haplotypes, a statistically significant, albeit weaker, association was found between haplotype b (Pro219) and risk for bleeding. Conversely, haplotype a (Ser219) was protective. These findings are not consistent with the observation of Croft et al. (151) that homozygosity for haplotype b would be associated with risk for acute MI, but are consistent with the observations of Joutsi-Korhonen et al. (58) that haplotype a confers increased reactivity to the receptor.

The involvement of *ITGA2* and *GP6* haplotypes in risk for bleeding in mild VWD is certainly not a coincidence. Although some have argued that one or the other of GP VI or integrin $\alpha_2\beta_1$ is the more important for platelet adhesion and signaling on collagens, it is more likely that the concerted activity of both is essential for optimum platelet function. Receptor cooperation is supported by several observations: Mice genetically deficient in GP VI exhibit a modest abnormality in hemostatic function (152) whereby platelet adhesion and thrombus formation persist, albeit with some loss of thrombus stability. At the same time, similar results occur with mice that are deficient in $\alpha_2\beta_1$ (153), where adhesion and thrombus formation are moderately impaired but not completely eliminated. Consistent with this theme, two receptor models of platelet adhesion to collagen and resultant platelet activation emphasize the integrated crosstalk between these two receptors. Last, mouse strain differences in platelet aggregability by collagen have been recently correlated with a difference in expression of integrin $\alpha_2\beta_1$, but not other prominent receptors, such as GP VI, GP Ibα or integrin $\alpha_{IIb}\beta_3$.

Reiner et al. (143) have reported that homozygosity for the *ITGA2B* haplotype 2 (HPA-3b allele) was associated with an approximately fivefold increased risk of ischemic stroke among subgroups of women who carried a diagnosis of hypertension or diabetes (OR, 4.51; 95% CI, 1.01 to 20.13) or had elevated plasma homocysteine levels (OR, 5.94; 95% CI, 1.53 to 23.05). This study is consistent with the hypothesis that *ITGA2B* haplotype 2 confers increased platelet cohesiveness. The results of the VWD type 1 association study (57) would support this hypothesis, because the complementary haplotype 1 would decrease the tendency to thrombosis and thereby increase risk for bleeding in VWD type 1.

We next analyzed the association of bleeding severity with candidate gene haplotypes within pedigrees of 12 index cases of VWD type 2 (six type 2M, three type 2A, and three type 2B) (154). In addition to the 12 index cases, these pedigrees included 58 affected and 55 unaffected relatives, as defined by plasma Ristocetin cofactor (VWF:RCo) levels. Once again, VWF:RCo levels, followed by VWF:Ag levels, had the strongest influence on bleeding severity score. *ITGA2* promoter haplotype −52T and *ITGA2B* haplotype 1 (Ile843) were each associated with an increase in bleeding severity score per age ($P = 0.026$ and $P = 0.016$, respectively). These associations remained statistically significant when the analysis was performed on only type 2A plus type 2M pedigrees ($P = 0.01$ and $P = 0.036$, respectively).

Despite its variability and poor heritability, the level of VWF, measured as antigen or ristocetin cofactor, remains the single most important parameter associated with bleeding severity and bleeding times in families of VWD type 1 or 2. In addition, *ITGA2*, *GP6*, and *ITGA2B* haplotypes are important modifiers of disease outcome, demonstrating that genetically controlled attenuation of certain adhesion receptors (whether through expression or activity) can influence risk for morbidity in clinical settings where hemostasis is compromised.

# SUMMARY

Platelet glycoprotein polymorphisms figure prominently in the efficiency of normal hemostasis, in the risk for pathologic outcome of thrombosis or bleeding, and in the immunogenicity of the platelet. The contribution of platelet glycoprotein polymorphisms as genetic risk factors for disease is a relatively new area of human genomics that is still evolving. Differences in the degree to which these are involved in risk for clinical thrombosis, bleeding syndromes, or resistance to antithrombotic drugs are largely attributable to clinical study design. Presently, there is substantial evidence that the integrin $\beta_3$ $Pl^{A2}$ haplotype, the GP Ibα Met145 haplotype, the GP Ibα −5C haplotype, and the integrin $\alpha_2$ haplotype 1 (807T) can each contribute to the risk for and morbidity of thrombotic disease. Likewise, the integrin $\beta_3$ $Pl^{A2}$ haplotype seems to impede the antithrombotic efficacy of ASA prophylaxis. At the same time, risk for bleeding in VWD type 1 is enhanced by inheritance of the integrin $\alpha_2$ haplotype 2 (807C), the GP VI haplotype b, or the integrin αIIb haplotype 1. These findings reinforce the notion that in future genetic and epidemiologic studies, the cumulative effects of multiple platelet and plasma glycoprotein gene haplotypes must be evaluated concurrently.

## References

1. Moroi M, Jung SM, Nomura S, et al. Analysis of the involvement of the von Willebrand factor-glycoprotein Ib interaction in platelet adhesion to a collagen-coated surface under flow conditions. *Blood* 1997;90(11):4413–4424.

2. Savage B, Almus-Jacobs F, Ruggeri ZM. Specific synergy of multiple substrate-receptor interactions in platelet thrombus formation under flow. *Cell* 1998;94:657–666.

3. Kamiguti AS, Theakston RD, Watson SP, et al. Distinct contributions of glycoprotein VI and alpha(2)beta(1) integrin to the induction of platelet protein tyrosine phosphorylation and aggregation. *Arch Biochem Biophys* 2000;374:356–362.

4. Kehrel B, Wierwille S, Clemetson KJ, et al. Glycoprotein VI is a major collagen receptor for platelet activation: it recognizes the platelet-activating quaternary structure of collagen, whereas CD36, glycoprotein IIb/IIIa, and von Willebrand factor do not. *Blood* 1998;91:491–499.

5. Ichinohe T, Takayama H, Ezumi Y, et al. Collagen-stimulated activation of Syk but not c-Src is severely compromised in human platelets lacking membrane glycoprotein VI. *J Biol Chem* 1997;272:63–68.

6. Jung SM, Moroi M. Platelets interact with soluble and insoluble collagens through characteristically different reactions. *J Biol Chem* 1998;273: 14827–14837.

7. Santoro SA, Rajpara SM, Staatz WD, et al. Isolation and characterization of a platelet surface collagen binding complex related to VLA-2. *Biochem Biophys Res Commun* 1988;153:217–223.

8. Kunicki TJ, Nugent DJ, Staats SJ, et al. The human fibroblast class II extracellular matrix receptor mediates platelet adhesion to collagen and is identical to the platelet glycoprotein Ia-IIa complex. *J Biol Chem* 1988;263:4516–4519.

9. Pischel KD, Bluestein HG, Woods VL. Platelet glycoprotein Ia,Ic, and IIa are physicochemically indistinguishable from the very late activation antigens adhesion- related proteins of lymphocytes and other cell types. *J Clin Invest* 1988;81:505–513.

10. Takada Y, Wayner EA, Carter WG, et al. Extracellular matrix receptors, ECMRII and ECMRI, for collagen and fibronectin correspond to VLA-2 and VLA-3 in the VLA family of heterodimers. *J Cell Biochem* 1988;37: 385–393.

11. Saelman EUM, Nieuwenhuis HK, Hese KM, et al. Platelet adhesion to collagen types I through VIII under conditions of stasis and flow is mediated by GPIa/IIa (alpha 2 beta 1 integrin). *Blood* 1994;83:1244–1250.

12. Kritzik M, Savage B, Nugent DJ, et al. Nucleotide polymorphisms in the alpha 2 gene define multiple alleles which are associated with differences in platelet alpha 2 beta 1. *Blood* 1998;92:2382–2388.

13. Clutton P, Folts JD, Freedman JE. Pharmacological control of platelet function. *Pharmacol Res* 2001;44:255–264.

14. Cattaneo M, Lecchi A, Randi AM. Identification of a new congenital defect of platelet function characterized by severe impairment of platelet responses to adenosine diphosphate. *Blood* 1992;80:2787–2796.

15. Hollopeter G, Jantzen HM, Vincent D, et al. Identification of the platelet ADP receptor targeted by antithrombotic drugs. *Nature* 2001;409:202–207.

16. Cattaneo M, Lecchi A, Lombardi R, et al. Platelets from a patient heterozygous for the defect of P2CYC receptors for ADP have a secretion defect despite normal thromboxane A2 production and normal granule stores: further evidence that some cases of platelet 'primary secretion defect' are heterozygous for a defect of P2CYC receptors. *Arterioscler Thromb Vasc Biol* 2000;20:E101–E106.

17. Nurden P, Savi P, Heilmann E, et al. An inherited bleeding disorder linked to a defective interaction between ADP and its receptor on platelets. Its influence on glycoprotein IIb-IIIa complex function. *J Clin Invest* 1995;95: 1612–1622.

18. von dem Borne AEGKr. Nomenclature of platelet antigen systems. *Br J Haematol* 1990;74:239–240.

19. Shulman NR, Aster RH, Leitner A, et al. Immunoreactions involving platelets: V. Post-transfusion purpura due to a complement-fixing antibody against a genetically controlled platelet antigen. A proposed mechanism for thrombocytopenia and its relevance in "autoimmunity.". *J Clin Invest* 1961;40:1597–1620.

20. Newman PJ, Derbes RS, Aster RH. The human platelet alloantigens, PLA1 and PLA2, are associated with a leucine33/proline33 amino acid polymorphism in membrane glycoprotein IIIa, and are distinguishable by DNA typing. *J Clin Invest* 1989;83:1778–1781.

21. Kuijpers RWAM, Faber NM, Cuypers HTM, et al. NH$_2$-terminal globular domain of human platelet glycoprotein Ibα has a methionine$^{145}$/threonine$^{145}$ amino acid polymorphism, which is associated with the HPA-2 (Ko) alloantigens. *J Clin Invest* 1992;89:381–384.

22. Lyman S, Aster RH, Visentin GP, et al. Polymorphism of human platelet membrane glycoprotein IIb associated with the Bak$^a$/Bak$^b$ alloantigen system. *Blood* 1990;75:2343–2348.

23. Wang R, Furihata K, McFarland JG, et al. An amino acid polymorphism within the RGD binding domain of platelet membrane glycoprotein IIIa is responsible for the formation of Pen$^a$/Pen$^b$ alloantigen system. *J Clin Invest* 1992;90:2038–2043.

24. Mellins E, Cameron P, Amaya M, et al. A mutant human histocompatibility leukocyte antigen DR molecule associated with invariant chain peptides. *J Exp Med* 1994;179:541–549.

25. Wang R, McFarland JG, Kekomaki R, et al. Amino acid 489 is encoded by a mutational "hot spot" on the beta 3 integrin chain: the CA/TU human platelet alloantigen system. *Blood* 1993;82(11):3386–3391.

26. Kuijpers RWAM, Simsek S, Faber NM, et al. Single point mutation in human glycoprotein IIIa is associated with a new platelet-specific alloantigen (Mo) involved in neonatal alloimmune thrombocytopenia. *Blood* 1993;81:70–76.

27. Santoso S, Kalb R, Kiefel V, et al. A point mutation leads to an unpaired cysteine residue and a molecular weight polymorphism of a functional platelet beta 3 integrin subunit. The Sra alloantigen system of GPIIIa. *J Biol Chem* 1994;269:8439–8444.

28. Noris P, Simsek S, De Bruijne-admiraal LG, et al. Max^a, a new low-frequency platelet-specific antigen localized on glycoprotein IIb, is associated with neonatal alloimmune thrombocytopenia. *Blood* 1995;86:1019–1026.

29. Peyruchaud O, Bourre F, Morel-Kopp M-C, et al. HPA-10w^b (La^a): genetic determination of a new platelet-specific alloantigen on glycoprotein IIIa and its expression in COS-7 cells. *Blood* 1997;89:2422–2428.

30. Simsek S, Folman C, Van der Schoot CE, et al. The Arg633His substitution responsible for the platelet antigen Gro^a unravelled by SSCP analysis and direct sequencing. *Br J Haematol* 1997;97:330–335.

31. Sachs UJH, Kiefel V, Bohringer M, et al. Single amino acid substitution in human platelet glycoprotein Ib beta is responsible for the formation of the platelet-specific alloantigen Iy^a. *Blood* 2000;95:1849–1855.

32. Santoso S, Amrhein J, Hofmann HA, et al. A point mutatin Thr$_{799}$Met on the alpha-2 integrin leads to the formation of new human platelet alloantigen Sit^a and affects collagen-induced aggregation. *Blood* 1999;94:4103–4111.

33. Santoso S, Pylipiw R, Wilke LG, et al. One amino acid deletion of the Pl^{A2} allelic form of GPIIIa leads to the formation of the new platelet alloantigen, Oe^a. *Blood* 1998;92:472a.

34. Kekomaki R, Raivio P, Kero P. A new low-frequency platelet alloantigen, Va^a, on glycoprotein IIb/IIIa associated with neonatal alloimmune thrombocytopenia. *Transf Med* 1992;2:27–33.

35. Kekomaki R, Partanen J, Pitkanen S, et al. Glycoprotein Ib/IX-specific alloimmunization in an HPA 2b-homozygous mother in association with neonatal thrombocytopenia. *Thromb Haemost* 1993;69:99.

36. Kelton JG, Smith JW, Horsewood P, et al. Gov^{a/b} alloantigen system on human platelets. *Blood*. 1990;75:2172–2176.

37. Santoso S, Kalb R, Walka V, et al. The human platelet alloantigens Br(a) and Br(b) are associated with a single amino acid polymorphism on glycoprotein Ia (integrin subunit α2). *J Clin Invest* 1993;92:2427–2432.

38. Jacquelin B, Tarantino M, Kritzik M, et al. Allele-dependent transcriptional regulation of the human integrin alpha 2 gene. *Blood* 2001;97:1721–1726.

39. Jacquelin B, Rozenshteyn D, Kanaji S, et al. Characterization of inherited differences in transcription of the human integrin alpha 2 gene. *J Biol Chem* 2001;276:23518–23524.

40. Li TT, Larrucea S, Souza S, et al. Genetic variation responsible for mouse strain differences in integrin {alpha}2 expression is associated with altered platelet responses to collagen. *Blood* 2004;103:3396–3402.

41. Shadle PJ, Ginsberg MH, Plow EF, et al. Platelet-collagen adhesion: inhibition by a monoclonal antibody that binds glycoprotein IIb. *J Cell Biol* 1984;99:2056–2060.

42. Frelinger AL III, Lam SC-T, Plow EF, et al. Occupancy of an adhesive glycoprotein receptor modulates expression of an antigenic site involved in cell adhesion. *J Biol Chem* 1988;263:12397–12402.

43. Vijayan KV, Goldschmidt-clermont PJ, Roos C, et al. The P1(A2) polymorphism of integrin beta(3) enhances outdie-in signaling and adhesive functions. *J Clin Invest* 2000;105:793–802.

44. Vijayan KV, Liu Y, Dong JF, et al. Enhanced activation of mitogen-activated protein kinase and myosin light chain kinase by the Pro33 polymorphism of integrin beta 3. *J Biol Chem* 2003;278:3860–3867.

45. Vijayan KV, Huang TC, Liu Y, et al. Shear stress augments the enhanced adhesive phenotype of cells expressing the Pro33 isoform of integrin beta3. *FEBS Lett* 2003;540:41–46.

46. Sajid M, Vijayan KV, Souza S, et al. PlA polymorphism of integrin beta 3 differentially modulates cellular migration on extracellular matrix proteins. *Arterioscler Thromb Vasc Biol* 2002;22:1984–1989.

47. Michelson AD, Furman MI, Goldschmidt-Clermont P, et al. Platelet GP IIIa PI(A) polymorphisms display different sensitivities to agonists. *Circulation* 2000;101:1013–1018.

48. Andrioli G, Minuz P, Solero P, et al. Defective platelet response to arachidonic acid and thromboxane A(2) in subjects with Pl(A2) polymorphism of beta(3) subunit (glycoprotein IIIa). *Br J Haematol* 2000;110:911–918.

49. Bennett JS, Catella-Lawson F, Rut AR, et al. Effect of the Pl(A2) alloantigen on the function of beta(3)-integrins in platelets. *Blood* 2001;97:3093–3099.

50. Murata M, Furihata K, Ishida F, et al. Genetic and structural characterization of an amino acid dimorphism in glycoprotein Ibα involved in platelet transfusion refractoriness. *Blood* 1992;79:3086–3090.

51. Lopez JA, Ludwig EH, McCarthy BJ. Polymorphism of human glycoprotein Ibα results from a variable number of tandem repeats of a 13-amino acid sequence in the mucin-like macroglycopeptide region. *J Biol Chem* 1992;267:10055–10061.

52. Ishida F, Furihata K, Ishida K, et al. The largest variant of platelet glycoprotein Ibα_has four tandem repeats of 13 amino acids in the macroglycopeptide region and a genetic linkage with Methionine$^{145}$. *Blood* 1995;86:1356–1360.

53. Murata M, Matsubara Y, Kawano K, et al. Coronary artery disease and polymorphisms in a receptor mediating shear stree-dependent platelet activation. *Circulation* 1997;96:3281–3286.

54. Gonzalez-Conejero R, Lozano ML, Rivera J, et al. Polymorphisms of platelet membrane glycoprotein Ib alpha associated with arterial thrombotic disease. *Blood* 1998;92:2771–2776.

55. Afshar-Kharghan V, Li CQ, Khoshnevis-Asl M, et al. Kozak sequence polymorphism of the glycoprotein (GP) Ibalpha gene is a major determinant of the plasma membrane levels of the platelet GP Ib- IX-V complex. *Blood* 1999;94:186–191.

56. Kaski S, Kekomaki R, Partanen J. Systematic screening for genetic polymorphism in human platelet glycoprotein Ib alpha. *Immunogenetics* 1996;44:170–176.

57. Kunicki TJ, Federici AB, Salomon DR, et al. An association of candidate gene haplotypes and bleeding severity in von Willebrand Disease (VWD) type 1 pedigrees. *Blood* 2004;104:2359–2367.

58. Joutsi-Korhonen L, Smethurst PA, Rankin A, et al. The low-frequency allele of the platelet collagen signaling receptor glycoprotein VI is associated with reduced functional responses and expression. *Blood* 2003;101:4372–4379.

59. Fontana P, Dupont A, Gandrille S, et al. Adenosine diphosphate-induced platelet aggregation is associated with P2Y12 gene sequence variations in healthy subjects. *Circulation* 2003;108:989–995.

60. Wang L, Ostberg O, Wihlborg AK, et al. Quantification of ADP and ATP receptor expression in human platelets. *J Thromb Haemost* 2003;1:330–336.

61. Unoki M, Furuta S, Onouchi Y, et al. Association studies of 33 single nucleotide polymorphisms (SNPs) in 29 candidate genes for bronchial asthma: positive association a T924C polymorphism in the thromboxane A2 receptor gene. *Hum Genet* 2000;106:440–446.

62. Harvey PJ, Keightley AM, Lam YM, et al. A single nucleotide polymorphism at nucleotide -1793 in the von Willebrand Factor (VWF) regulatory region is associated with plasma VWF:Ag levels. *Br J Haematol* 2000;109:349–353.

63. Keightley AM, Lam YM, Brady JN, et al. Variation at the von Willebrand Factor (vWF) gene locus is associated with plasma vWF: Ag levels: identification of three novel single nucleotide polymorphisms in the vWF gene promoter. *Blood* 1999;93:4277–4283.

64. Brull DJ, Dhamrait S, Moulding R, et al. The effect of fibrinogen genotype on fibrinogen levels after strenuous physical exercise. *Thromb Haemost* 2002;87:37–41.

65. Ernst E, Resch KL. Fibrinogen as a cardiovascular risk factor: a meta-analysis and review of the literature. *Ann Intern Med* 1993;118:956–963.

66. Humphries SE, Luong LA, Ogg MS, et al. The interleukin-6 -174 G/C promoter polymorphism is associated with risk of coronary heart disease and systolic blood pressure in healthy men. *Eur Heart J* 2001;22:2243–2252.

67. Reznikoff-Etievant MF, Dangu C, Lobet R. HLA-B8 antigen and anti-P1^{A1} alloimmunization. *Tissue Antigens* 1981;18:66–68.

68. Valentin N, Vergracht A, Bignon JD, et al. HLA-Drw52a is involved in alloimmunization against PL-A1 antigen. *Human Immunol* 1990;27:73–79.

69. Reznikoff-Etievant MF, Muller JY, Julien F, et al. An immune response gene linked to MHC in man. *Tissue Antigens* 1981;22:312.

70. L'Abbé D, Tremblay L, Filion M, et al. Alloimmunization to platelet antigen HPA-1a (PI^{A1}) is strongly associated with both HLA-DRB3*0101 and HLA-DQB1*0201. *Hum Immunol* 1992;34:107–114.

71. Maslanka K, Yassai M, Gorski J. Molecular identification of T cells that respond in a primary buk culture to a peptide derived from a platelet glycoprotein implicated in neonatal alloimmune thrombocytopenia. *J Clin Invest* 1996;98:1802–1808.

72. Kuijpers RWAM, von dem Borne AE, Kifel V, et al. Leucine 33-proline 33 substitution in human platelet glycoprotein IIIa determines HLA-DRw52a (Dw24) association of the immune response against HPA-1a (Zwa/PIA1) and HPA-1b (Zwb/PIA2). *Human Immunol* 1992;34(4):253–256.

73. Westman P, Hashemi-Tavoularis S, Blanchette V, et al. Material DRB1* 1501, DQA1*0102,DQB1*0602 haplotype in fetomaternal alloimmunization against human platelet alloantigen HPA-6b (GPIIIa-Gln489). *Tissue Antigens* 1997;50:113–118.

74. Mueller-Eckhardt C. HLA-B8 antigen and anti-P1^{A1} alloimmunization. *Tissue Antigens* 1982;19:154–158.

75. Covas DT, Delgado M, Zeitune MM, et al. Gene frequencies of the HPA-1 and HPA-2 platelet antigen alleles among the Amerindians. *Vox Sang* 1997;73:182–184.

76. Covas DT, Biscaro TA, Nasciutti DC, et al. Gene frequencies of the HPA-3 and HPA-5 platelet antigen alleles among the Amerindians. *Eur J Haematol* 2000;65:128–131.

77. Chiba AK, Bordin JO, Kuwano ST, et al. Platelet alloantigen frequencies in amazon indians and brazilian blood donors. *Transfus Med* 2000;10:207–212.

78. Castro V, Origa AF, Annichino-Bizzacchi JM, et al. Frequencies of platelet-specific alloantigen systems 1-5 in three distinct ethnic groups in Brazil. *Eur J Immunogenet* 1999;26:355–360.

79. Holensteiner A, Walchshofer S, Adler A, et al. Human platelet antigen gene frequencies in the Austrian population. *Haemostasis* 1995;25:133–136.

80. Steffensen R, Kaczan E, Varming K, et al. Frequency of platelet-specific alloantigens in a Danish population. *Tissue Antigens* 1996;48:93–96.

81. Simsek S, Faber NM, Bleeker PM, et al. Determination of human platelet antigen frequencies in the Dutch population by immunophenotyping and DNA (allele-specific restriction enzyme) analysis. *Blood* 1993;81:835–840.

82. Kekomaki S, Partanen J, Kekomaki R. Platelet alloantigens HPA-1, -2, -3, -5 and -6b in Finns. *Transfus Med* 1995;5:193–198.

83. Merieux Y, Debost M, Bernaud J, et al. Human platelet antigen frequencies of platelet donors in the French population determined by polymerase chain reaction with sequence-specific primers. *Pathol Biol (Paris)* 1997;45:697–700.

84. Chen DF, Pastucha LT, Chen HY, et al. Simultaneous genotyping of human platelet antigens by hot start sequence-specific polymerase chain reaction with DNA polymerase AmpliTaq Gold. *Vox Sang* 1997;72:192–196.

85. Drzewek K, Brojer E, Zupanska B. The frequency of human platelet antigen (HPA) genotypes in the polish population. *Transfus Med* 1998;8:339–342.

86. Rozman P, Drabbels J, Schipper RF, et al. Genotyping for human platelet-specific antigens HPA-1, -2, -3, -4 and -5 in the Slovenian population reveals a slightly increased frequency of HPA-1b and HPA-2b as compared to other European populations. *Eur J Immunogenet* 1999;26:265–269.

87. Nogues N, Subirana L, Garcia Manzano A, et al. Human platelet alloantigens in a Mexican population: a comparative gene frequency study [abstract]. *Vox Sang* 2000;78:P060.

88. Sellers J, Thompson J, Guttridge MG, et al. Human platelet antigens: typing by PCR using sequence-specific primers and their distribution in blood donors resident in Wales. *Eur J Immunogenet* 1999;26:393–397.

89. Ferrer G, Muniz-Diaz E, Aluja MP, et al. Analysis of human platelet antigen systems in a Moroccan Berber population. *Transfus Med* 2002;12:49–54.

90. Mojaat N, Halle L, Proulle V, et al. Gene frequencies of human platelet antigens in the Tunisian population. *Tissue Antigens* 1999;54:201–204.

91. Kim HO, Jin Y, Kickler TS, et al. Gene frequencies of the five major human platlet antigens in African American, white and Korean populations. *Transfusion* 1995;35:863–867.

92. Reiner AP, Aramaki KM, Teramura G, et al. Analysis of platelet glycoprotein Ia ($\alpha_2$ integrin) allele frequencies in three north american populations reveals genetic association between nucleotide 807C/T and amino acid 505 Glu/Lys (HPA-5) dimorphisms. *Thromb Haemost* 1998;80:449–456.

93. Seo DH, Park SS, Kim DW, et al. Gene frequencies of eight human platelet-specific antigens in Koreans. *Transfus Med* 1998;8:129–132.

94. Legler TJ, Kohler M, Mayr WR, et al. Genotyping of the human platelet antigen systems 1 through 5 by multiplex polymerase chain reaction and ligation-based typing. *Transfusion* 1996;36:426–431.

95. Tanaka S, Ohnoki S, Shibata H, et al. Gene frequencies of human platlet antigens on glycoprotein IIIa in Japanese. *Transfusion* 1996;36:813–817.

96. Romphruk AV, Akahat J, Srivanichrak P, et al. Genotyping of human platelet antigens in ethnic Northeastern Thais by the polymerase chain reaction-sequence specific primer technique. *J Med Assoc Thai* 2000;83:1333–1339.

97. Shih MC, Liu TC, Lin IL, et al. Gene frequencies of the HPA-1 to HPA-13, Oe and Gov platelet antigen alleles in Taiwanese, Indonesian, Filipino and Thai populations. *Int J Mol Med* 2003;12:609–614.

98. Liu TC, Shih MC, Lin CL, et al. Gene frequencies of the HPA-1 to HPA-8w platelet antigen alleles in Taiwanese, Indonesian, and Thai. *Ann Hematol* 2002;81:244–248.

99. Chang YW, Mytilineos J, Opelz G, et al. Distribution of human platelet antigens in a Chinese population. *Tissue Antigens* 1998;51:391–393.

100. Dazhuang L, Zhenyu L, Yuqin B, et al. Genotyping of human platelet antigens (HPA) and investigation of their gene frequencies [abstract]. *Chin J Blood Transfus* 2001;14:177.

101. Tsao KC, Sun CF, Lai NC. The phenotype and gene frequencies of human platelet specific antigens among Chinese in Taiwan. *Zhonghua Min Guo Wei Sheng Wu Ji Mian Yi Xue Za Zhi* 1992;25:48–55.

102. Chu CC, Lee HL, Chu TW, et al. The use of genotyping to predict the phenotypes of human platelet antigens 1 through 5 and of neutrophil antigens in Taiwan. *Transfusion* 2001;41:1553–1558.

103. Santoso S, Kiefel V, Masri R, et al. Frequency of platelet-specific antigens among Indonesians. *Transfusion* 1993;33:739–741.

104. Halle L, Bach KH, Martageix C, et al. Eleven human platelet systems studied in the Vietnamese and Ma'ohis Polynesian populations. *Tissue Antigens* 2004;63:34–40.

105. Kulkarni B, Mohanty D, Ghosh K, et al. Frequency distribution of antigens in the human platelet antigen-1 system in the western Indian population. *Transfusion* 2002;42:317–320.

106. Chen Z, Lester S, Boettcher B, et al. Platelet antigen allele frequencies in Australian aboriginal and Caucasian populations. *Pathology* 1997;29:392–398.

107. Bennett JA, Palmer LJ, Musk AW, et al. Gene frequencies of human platelet antigens 1-5 in indigenous Australians in Western Australia. *Transfus Med* 2002;12:199–203.

108. Ozelo MC, Costa DS, Siqueira LH, et al. Genetic variability of platelet glycoprotein Ibalpha gene. *Am J Hematol* 2004;77:107–116.

109. Dinauer DM, Friedman KD, Hessner MJ. Allelic distribution of the glycoprotein Ia (alpha2-integrin) C807T/G873A dimorphisms among caucasian venous thrombosis patients and six racial groups. *Br J Haematol* 1999;107:563–565.

110. Mueller-Eckhardt C, Kiefel V, Grubert A, et al. 348 cases of suspected neonatal alloimmune thrombocytopenia. *Lancet* 1989;1:363–366.

111. Shibata Y, Matsuda I, Miyaji T, et al. Yuk$^a$, a new platelet antigen involved in two cases of neonatal alloimmune thrombocytopenia. *Vox Sang* 1986;50:177–180.

112. von dem Borne A, von Riesz E, Verheugt F, et al. Bak$^a$, a new platelet-specific antigen involved in neonatal alloimmune thrombocytopenia. *Vox Sang* 1980;39:113–120.

113. McGrath K, Minchinton R, Cunningham I, et al. Platelet anti-Bak$^b$ antibody associated with neonatal alloimmune thrombocytopenia. *Vox Sang* 1989;57:182–184.

114. Mueller-Eckhardt C, Becker T, Weishet M, et al. Neonatal alloimmune thrombocytopenia due to fetomaternal Zw$^b$ in compatability. *Vox Sang* 1986;50:94–96.

115. Grenet P, Dausset J, Dugas M, et al. Purpura thrombopenique neonatal avec isoimmunisation foeto-maternelle anti-Ko$^a$. *Arch Fr Pediatr* 1965;22:1165–1174.

116. Antithrombotic Trialists' Collaboration. Collaborative meta-analysis of randomised trials of antiplatelet therapy for prevention of death, myocardial infarction, and stroke in high risk patients. *BMJ* 2002;324:71–86.

117. Gum PA, Kottke-Marchant K, Poggio ED, et al. Profile and prevalence of aspirin resistance in patients with cardiovascular disease. *Am J Cardiol* 2001;88:230–235.

118. Hillarp A, Palmqvist B, Lethagen S, et al. Mutations within the cyclooxygenase-1 gene in aspirin non-responders with recurrence of stroke. *Thromb Res* 2003;112:275–283.

119. Weber AA, Przytulski B, Schanz A, et al. Towards a definition of aspirin resistance: a typological approach. *Platelets* 2002;13:37–40.

120. Marshall PW, Williams AJ, Dixon RM, et al. A comparison of the effects of aspirin on bleeding time measured using the simplate method and closure time measured using the PFA-100, in healthy volunteers. *Br J Clin Pharmacol* 1997;44:151–155.

121. Fressinaud E, Veyradier A, Sigaud M, et al. Therapeutic monitoring of von Willebrand disease: interest and limits of a platelet function analyser at high shear rates. *Br J Haematol* 1999;106:777–783.

122. Francis JL. Platelet dysfunction detected at high shear in patients with heart valve disease. *Platelets* 2000;11:133–136.

123. Homoncik M, Jilma B, Hergovich N, et al. Monitoring of aspirin (ASA) pharmacodynamics with the platelet function analyzer PFA-100. *Thromb Haemost* 2000;83:316–321.

124. Cooke GE, Bray PF, Hamlington JD, et al. PIA2 polymorphism and efficacy of aspirin. *Lancet* 1998;351:1253.

125. Szczeklik A, Undas A, Sanak M, et al. Relationship between bleeding time, aspirin and the PlA1/A2 polymorphism of platelet glycoprotein IIIa. *Br J Haematol* 2000;110:965–967.

126. Centers for Disease Control and Prevention. Mortality from coronary heart disease and acute myocardial infarction—United States, 1998. *MMWR Morb Mortal Wkly Rep* 2001;50:90–93.

127. Bedinghaus J, Leshan L, Diehr S. Coronary artery disease prevention: what's different for women? *Am Fam Physician* 2001;63:1393–1396.

128. Brass LM. The impact of cerebrovascular disease. *Diabetes Obes Metab* 2000;2(Suppl. 2):S6–S10.

129. Pellicano R, Oliaro E, Gandolfo N, et al. Ischemic cardiovascular disease and helicobacter pylori. Where is the link? *J Cardiovasc Surg (Torino)* 2000;41:829–833.

130. Rauch U, Osende JI, Fuster V, et al. Thrombus formation on atherosclerotic plaques: pathogenesis and clinical consequences. *Ann Intern Med* 2001;134:224–238.

131. Moshfegh K, Wuillemin WA, Redondo M, et al. Association of two silent polymorphisms of platelet glycoprotein Ia/IIa receptor with risk of myocardial infarction: a case-control study. *Lancet* 1999;353:351–354.

132. Santoso S, Kunicki TJ, Kroll H, et al. Association of the platelet glycoprotein Ia $C_{807}$T gene polymorphism with myocardial infarction in younger patients. *Blood* 1999;93:2449–2453.

133. Roest M, Banga JD, Grobbee DE, et al. Homozygosity for 807 T polymorphism in alpha(2) subunit of platelet alpha(2)beta(1) is associated with increased risk of cardiovascular mortality in high-risk women. *Circulation* 2000;102:1645–1650.

134. Matsubara Y, Murata M, Maruyama T, et al. Association between diabetic retinopathy and genetic variations in alpha-2 beta-1 integrin, a platelet receptor for collagen. *Blood* 2000;95:1560–1564.

135. Carlsson LE, Santoso S, Spitzer C, et al. The alpha 2 gene coding sequences $T_{807}/A_{873}$ of the platelet collagen receptor integrin alpha2 beta1 might be a genetic risk factor for the development of stroke in younger patients. *Blood* 1999;93:3583–3586.

136. Carter AM, Ossei-Gerning N, Grant PJ. Platelet glycoprotein IIIa PIA polymorphism in young men with myocardial infarction. *Lancet* 1996;348:485–486.

137. Weiss EJ, Bray PF, Tayback M, et al. A polymorphism of a platelet glycoprotein receptor as an inherited risk factor for coronary thrombosis. *N Engl J Med* 1996;334:1090–1094.

138. Ardissino D, Mannucci PM, Merlini PA, et al. Prothrombotic genetic risk factors in young survivors of myocardial infarction. *Blood* 1999;94:46–51.

139. Ridker PM, Hennekens CH, Schmitz C, et al. Pl$^{A1/A2}$ polymorphism of platelet glycoprotein IIIa and risks of myocardial infarction, stroke, and venous thrombosis. *Lancet* 1997;349:385–388.

140. Herrmann SM, Poirier O, Marques-Vidal P, et al. The Leu$^{33}$/Pro polymorphism (Pl$^{A1}$/Pl$^{A2}$) of the glycoprotein IIIa (GPIIIa) receptor is not related to myocardial infarction in the ECTIM study. *Thromb Haemost* 1977;77:1179–1181.

141. Zhu MM, Weedon J, Clark LT. Meta-analysis of the association of platelet glycoprotein IIIa PlA1/A2 polymorphism with myocardial infarction. *Am J Cardiol* 2000;86:1000–1005.

142. Di Castelnuovo A, De Gaetano G, Donati MB, et al. Platelet glycoprotein receptor IIIa polymorphism PLA1/PLA2 and coronary risk: a meta-analysis. *Thromb Haemost* 2001;85:626–633.

143. Reiner AP, Kumar PN, Schwartz SM, et al. Genetic variants of platelet glycoprotein receptors and risk of stroke in young women. *Stroke* 2000;31:1628–1633.

144. Sonoda A, Murata M, Ito D, et al. Association between platelet glycoprotein Ib alpha genotype and ischemic cerebrovascular disease. *Stroke* 2000;31:493–497.

145. Santoso S, Zimmermann P, Sachs UJ, et al. The impact of the Kozak sequence polymorphism of the glycoprotein Ib alpha gene on the risk and extent of coronary heart disease. *Thromb Haemost* 2002;87:345–346.

146. Sonoda A, Murata M, Ikeda Y, et al. Stroke and platelet glycoprotein Ibα polymorphisms. *Thromb Haemost* 2001;85:573–574.

147. Sadler JE. Von Willebrand disease type 1: a diagnosis in search of a disease. *Blood* 2003;101:2089–2093.

148. Gill JC, Endres-Brooks J, Bauer PJ, et al. The effect of ABO blood group on the diagnosis of von Willebrand disease. *Blood* 1987;69:1691–1695.

149. Orstavik KH, Kornstad L, Reisner H, et al. Possible effect of secretor locus on plasma concentration of factor VIII and von Willebrand factor. *Blood* 1989;73:990–993.

150. Di Paola J, Federici AB, Sacchi E, et al. Low platelet alpha 2 beta 1 levels in type I von Willebrand disease correlate with impaired platelet function in a high shear stress system. *Blood* 1999;93:3578–3582.

151. Croft SA, Samani NJ, Teare MD, et al. Novel platelet membrane glycoprotein VI dimorphism is a risk factor for myocardial infarction. *Circulation* 2001;104:1459–1463.

152. Kato K, Kanaji T, Russell S, et al. The contribution of glycoprotein VI to stable platelet adhesion and thrombus formation illustrated by targeted gene deletion. *Blood* 2003;102:1701–1707.

153. Chen J, Diacovo TG, Grenache DG, et al. The alpha(2) integrin subunit-deficient mouse : a multifaceted phenotype including defects of branching morphogenesis and hemostasis. *Am J Pathol* 2002;161:337–344.

154. Kunicki TJ, Baronciani L, Canciani MT, et al. An association of candidate gene haplotypes and bleeding severity in von Willebrand Disease (VWD) type 2 pedigress 2004 Submitted.

# CHAPTER 29 ■ MOLECULAR MECHANISMS OF DRUG-INDUCED THROMBOCYTOPENIA

BENG H. CHONG AND JULIANA C. KWOK

Drug-induced thrombocytopenia is a relatively common and potentially serious adverse effect of a number of clinical agents (1–3). This condition is characterized by petechiae, purpuric lesions, and, occasionally, serious bleeding such as intracranial hemorrhage. The patient's platelet count usually decreases to values below $20 \times 10^9$ per L but recovers upon withdrawal of the offending drug (1,3,4). Drug-induced thrombocytopenia can be caused by inhibition of megakaryocyte proliferation and platelet production or by destruction of platelets in the peripheral circulation (2). Peripheral platelet destruction may occur by immune-mediated mechanisms (1,2), which cause antibodies to bind to platelets in the presence of the offending drug, resulting in enhanced platelet clearance by the reticuloendothelial system.

More than 200 drugs have been reported to cause thrombocytopenia (5–8). However, many of these case studies have not definitively proven a causal relation between the drug and thrombocytopenia (6,8). With an increasing number of drugs available for clinical use each year, the frequency of such case reports will also increase (9–14). Drugs most commonly associated with immune thrombocytopenia include quinine and its optical isomer, quinidine, sulfonamides, penicillins, and heparin. More recently, agents including mirtazapine (15), carbimazole (16), tiagabine (17), roxifiban (18,19), and abciximab (20) have been implicated in drug-induced thrombocytopenia.

This review focuses on immune drug-induced thrombocytopenia due to increased platelet destruction, of which quinine-induced thrombocytopenia is a prototype. Because the clinical presentation and pathogenesis of thrombocytopenia induced by heparin are quite different, this topic is discussed separately in Chapter 114.

## QUININE-TYPE DRUG-INDUCED THROMBOCYTOPENIA

### Historical Perspective

The pathogenesis of drug-induced immune thrombocytopenia has been the subject of much debate since Ackroyd first demonstrated drug-dependent antibodies against platelets in 1949 (21). In his work examining thrombocytopenia induced by the sedative sedormid, a series of *in vitro* studies demonstrated agglutination of normal human platelets in the presence of the drug and serum derived from patients with sedormid-induced thrombocytopenia. Addition of complement resulted in lysis of the platelets (22). From this work, Ackroyd proposed that the drug acts as a hapten, combining covalently with platelets to form a drug–platelet antigenic complex (see Fig. 29-1). This leads to the production of a drug-dependent antibody, which recognizes and binds this complex (Fig. 29-1A). The antibody-coated platelets are then prematurely cleared by the reticuloendothelial system, resulting in thrombocytopenia (22).

However, Ackroyd's hapten hypothesis was subsequently challenged by Miescher et al. (24,25) and Shulman (23,26,27). On the basis of his work on quinidine-induced thrombocytopenia, Shulman demonstrated that binding of the drug to platelets was weak and could be washed off the cells relatively easily. In addition, excess free drug did not inhibit binding of the antibody to platelets (23). His contention that the hapten theory was incorrect was supported by animal studies demonstrating that haptens did not bind firmly to macromolecules, were not immunogenic, and that excess hapten inhibits antibody binding (28). Therefore, Shulman proposed the immune complex or "innocent bystander" hypothesis (23).

In the innocent bystander mechanism, the drug binds tightly to a plasma protein and elicits an antibody response (Fig. 29-1B). Binding of the antibody to the drug–protein complex forms an immune complex that becomes nonspecifically absorbed by neighboring platelets via their Fc receptors (Fig. 29-1B), resulting in platelet destruction (23). However, recent work has provided evidence against this mechanism, including the observation that antibodies bind platelets via the Fab domain, not the Fc domain (29–32), and that antibodies recognize specific platelet glycoproteins (1,16,29,31, 33–45). In addition, when the drug-dependent antibodies affect more than one blood cell type (e.g., platelets and granulocytes), causing thrombocytopenia and neutropenia, two distinct antibodies reacting with two different platelet and granulocyte antigens have been demonstrated (29); the concomitant cytopenias were not due to the nonspecific deposition of drug–antibody complexes on both platelets and granulocytes, as previously believed.

### Pathogenesis

Current experimental data suggest that neither the hapten hypothesis proposed by Ackroyd nor the innocent bystander hypothesis proposed by Miescher and Shulman is the basis of immune thrombocytopenia caused by most drugs. One possible exception may be the thrombocytopenia caused by large doses of penicillin and related drugs. These drugs are capable of linking covalently to platelet membranes, and the hapten mechanism may account for the thrombocytopenia in this condition. Another exception is heparin-induced thrombocytopenia (HIT) in which heparin-platelet factor 4 (PF4)-antibody complexes bind to platelets by the FcγIIA receptors on platelets in a mechanism similar to the innocent bystander hypothesis. However, even in HIT, this mechanism accounts only for the initial steps in the drug–antibody–platelet interactions, as we have demonstrated that the HIT antibody also binds to platelets

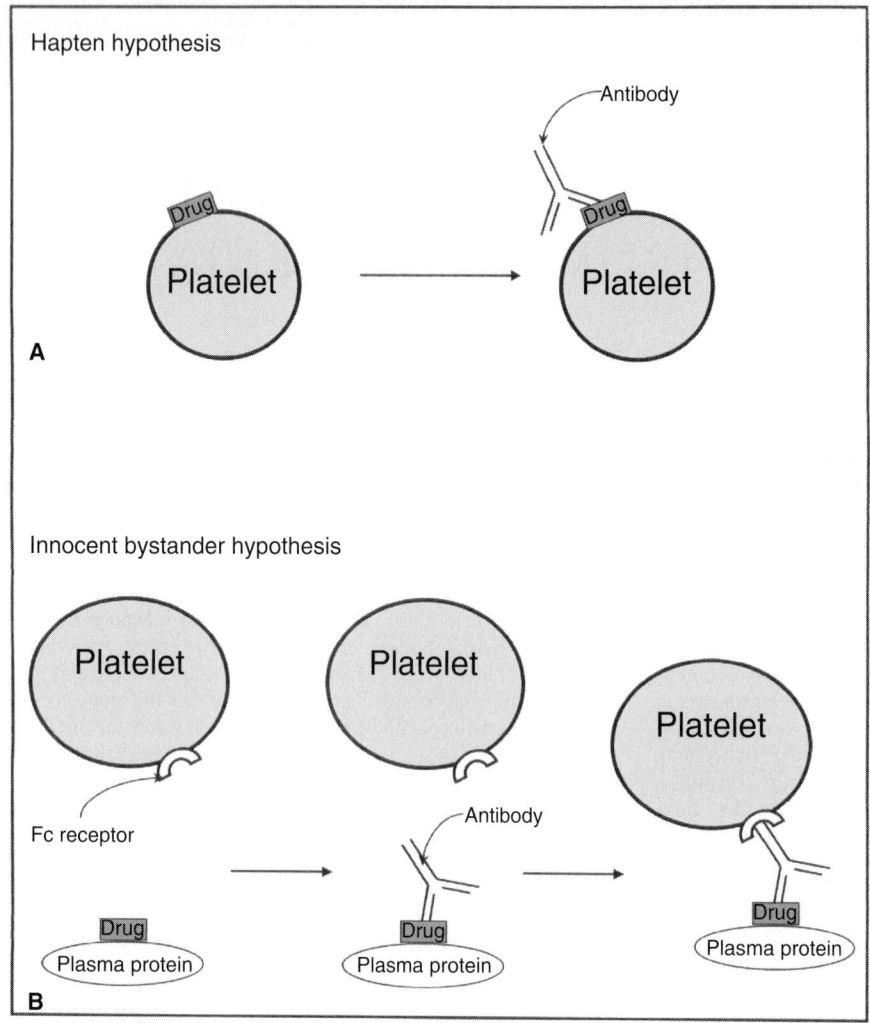

**FIGURE 29-1.** The hapten hypothesis (**A**) and the innocent bystander hypothesis (**B**) of drug-dependent antibodies. **A:** According to Ackroyd's hapten hypothesis, the drug acts as a hapten, binding covalently to platelets. The drug-dependent antibody recognizes and binds the drug–platelet antigenic complex. The antibody-coated platelets are then cleared prematurely by reticuloendothelial system (22). **B:** In the innocent bystander hypothesis, the drug binds tightly to a plasma protein and elicits an antibody response. The antibody binds to the drug–plasma protein complex, forming an immune complex. This is then nonspecifically adsorbed onto the surrounding platelets by their Fc receptors, resulting in platelet destruction (23).

via its Fab domain to PF4/heparin complexes on the platelet surface once platelets become activated (46).

Recent studies revealed that in most immune drug-induced thrombocytopenias, the antibody reacts with an epitope or epitopes formed by the interaction of the drug with one or more platelet glycoproteins, including GP Ib/IX, GP IIb/IIIa, GP V, and platelet/endothelial cell adhesion molecule-1 (PECAM-1) (see Fig. 29-2) (1,16,35–39,41,43–45). Binding of the drug-dependent antibody to platelets (Fig. 29-2) results in destruction of the opsonized platelets by macrophages in the reticuloendothelial system. The precise mechanism by which drug/platelet glycoprotein epitopes are formed is not fully known. However, it is likely that binding of the drug to the platelet glycoprotein causes a conformational change, exposing an otherwise cryptic domain of the glycoprotein that has not been previously seen by the cells of the immune system, thereby resulting in the formation of an autoantigen or neoantigen (1,43,47) (Fig. 29-2). It is also possible, but less likely, that close interaction of the drug and a peptide domain on the glycoprotein results in a compound epitope (1,43,48).

The earlier cases of drug-induced thrombocytopenia implicated quinine and its optic isomer, quinidine, as the causative agents (23,26,27,49,50). Quinine is used for the clinical treatment of malaria and muscle cramps and is also present in tonic water. Quinidine was previously used for the treatment of cardiac arrhythmia. Much effort has been dedicated to elucidating the mechanism of quinine- and quinidine-induced thrombocytopenia (29,31–34,36–39,42,44). These studies have

demonstrated that quinine induces antibodies that are specific to the platelet membrane glycoprotein, GP Ib/IX complex (38,41,44). Antibodies directed against other platelet glycoproteins such as GP IIb/IIIa (36–39,45), GP V (35) and PECAM-1 (16) have also been described. Binding of platelet glycoproteins by antibodies results in increased platelet clearance by the reticuloendothelial system, and hence, thrombocytopenia.

Recently, a number of other structurally unrelated drugs have also been reported to trigger thrombocytopenia through induction of antiplatelet antibodies. These agents include rifampicin (used for the treatment of tuberculosis) (51,52), ranitidine (histamine H2 receptor antagonist) (53), carbimazole (used for the treatment of hyperthyroidism) (16), and drug metabolites of naproxen and acetaminophen (54).

## GP Ib/IX Complex

GP Ib/IX is a major glycoprotein complex expressed on the platelet surface at approximately 25,000 copies per platelet (1). This complex consists of three polypeptides, GP Ibα, GP Ibβ, and GP IX, each encoded by a different gene (55,56). The GP Ibα subunit ($M_r$ = 143 kDa) is disulfide-linked to GP Ibβ ($M_r$ = 25 kDa), and these two subunits are noncovalently linked to GP IX ($M_r$ = 22 kDa) (56) (see Fig. 29-3). The three subunits are expressed in a 1:1:1 ratio (57). On the platelet membrane, GP Ib/IX is also noncovalently associated with GP V ($M_r$ = 82 kDa) (58) in a 2:1 ratio (57). All four subunits are

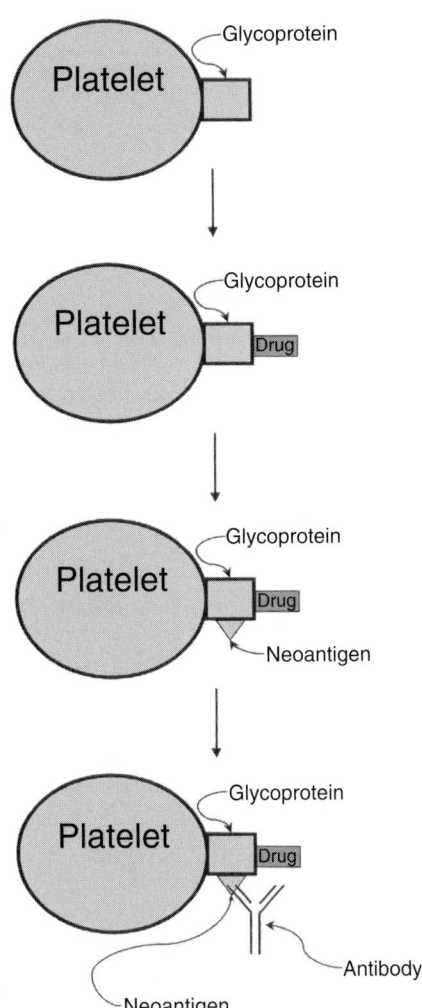

**FIGURE 29-2.** Immune-mediated drug-induced thrombocytopenia. The drug binds to a platelet membrane glycoprotein such as GP Ib/IX, GP IIb/IIIa, GP V, or platelet/endothelial cell adhesion molecule-1 (PECAM-1) (1,16,35–39,41,43–45), causing a conformational change. This induces the formation of a neoantigen that is recognized by drug-dependent antibodies. Binding of drug-dependent antibodies to platelets results in premature clearance of platelets by the reticuloendothelial system.

members of the leucine-rich motif (LRM) superfamily that are involved in diverse processes such as cell signaling, cell adhesion, and development (30,56,59). The extracellular region of GP Ibα contains an O-glycosylated region and an amino-terminal domain. The latter region contains eight LRMs (60,61) and is the binding site for von Willebrand factor (VWF) (62), P selectin, Mac-1, and thrombin (63) (Fig. 29-3). Binding of VWF to GP Ib/IX results in activation of platelets and its adhesion to the exposed subendothelium (57).

The first experimental evidence that drug-dependent antibodies react with the GP Ib/IX complex came from observations that platelets from patients with Bernard-Soulier syndrome (BSS) were not lysed by quinine-dependent antibodies (33). Patients with BSS lack GP Ib/IX, GP V, and a 100-kDa protein (64) and, as a result, have lifelong bleeding conditions characterized by giant platelets. This suggested that one or more of these deficient glycoproteins are the target antigen.

In 1983, we provided the first direct evidence that GP Ib/IX is the platelet autoantigen for quinine/quinidine-dependent antibodies (29). We observed that GP Ib and GP IX could be immunoprecipitated in a drug-dependent manner using serum from patients with quinidine-induced thrombocytopenia (29). This was subsequently confirmed by Devine and Rosse (65). Further studies have now shown that GP Ib/IX is the target antigen in most patients diagnosed with quinine/quinidine-induced thrombocytopenia (38–40,42,44).

Our recent work has focused on characterizing the binding site of quinine-dependent antibodies on the GP Ib/IX complex. Studies were performed using mouse L cells and Chinese hamster ovary (CHO) cells transfected with different combinations of the three subunits of GP Ib/IX: GP Ibα, GP Ibβ, and GP IX. This work demonstrated that quinine-dependent antibodies roughly fall into three categories: Approximately 50% of patients have antibodies that target GP IX alone, approximately 10% have antibodies that bind GP Ibα only, and approximately 40% have antibodies that bind both domains (42).

Because GP IX is a major target for quinine-dependent antibodies, we mapped the structural regions recognized by these antibodies (44). On the basis of the knowledge that quinine-dependent antibodies are species specific, reacting only with glycoproteins present on human or primate platelets but not those of other species (66), we generated four chimeric mouse/human GP IX constructs (see Fig. 29-4). In each construct, a fragment of human GP IX was replaced by the corresponding fragment of mouse GP IX (Fig. 29-4). These constructs were then stably transfected in CHO cells in association with GP Ibα and GP Ibβ (44). Using the monoclonal antibody SZ1 that has been shown to bind an epitope similar to, or very close to, the binding site for quinine-dependent antibodies (38,41), we demonstrated that SZ1 did not bind chimera 3 that contains a mouse sequence at the C-terminal extracellular region of GP IX between amino acids 64 and 135 (Fig. 29-4) (44). These results suggested that quinine-dependent antibodies bind at this C-terminal extracellular domain of human GP IX (Fig. 29-4). This was further supported by the lack of drug-dependent antibody-binding to chimera 3 using sera from six patients with quinine-induced thrombocytopenia (44). By aligning the human and mouse sequences of this C-terminal region from amino acids 64 to 135, we identified the nonconserved residues (Fig. 29-3). These residues were mutated by a single amino acid change and the GP IX mutants were stably expressed in CHO cells. These studies demonstrated that arginine 110 (R110) and glutamine 115 (Q115) are essential for binding by both SZ1 and the patients' antibodies (Fig. 29-3) (44). Hence, these two residues in the C-terminal region of GP IX (Fig. 29-3) play an important role in the binding of quinine-induced anti–GP IX antibodies (44).

Recently, using a similar approach involving transfected CHO cells, the drug-dependent antibodies from patients with thrombocytopenia caused by three other drugs, ranitidine (a histamine H2 receptor antagonist) (53), rifampicin (used for the treatment of tuberculosis) (51), and quinidine (38), were also found to target the GP IX subunit of GP Ib/IX. Similar to quinine-dependent antibodies, the binding of the ranitidine-, rifampicin-, and quinidine-dependent antibodies to platelets was blocked by the monoclonal antibody SZ1 (38,51–53). These results suggest that antibodies induced by the four drugs, ranitidine, rifampicin, quinidine, and quinine, bind either to the same or an adjacent site on GP IX. Hence, this region of GP IX may play a crucial role in epitope formation for drug-induced antibodies. Further studies of this region may be important for elucidating the mechanisms by which drugs induce immune-mediated thrombocytopenia.

Although less frequent, quinine-dependent antibodies also target the GP Ib subunit of the GP Ib/IX complex. Early experiments in 1981 demonstrated that antibody-platelet binding was competitively inhibited in the presence of an anti–GP Ib alloantibody or purified GP Ib (34), suggesting that this latter glycoprotein is the target for quinine-dependent antibodies. Subsequently, more detailed studies in 12 patients showed that

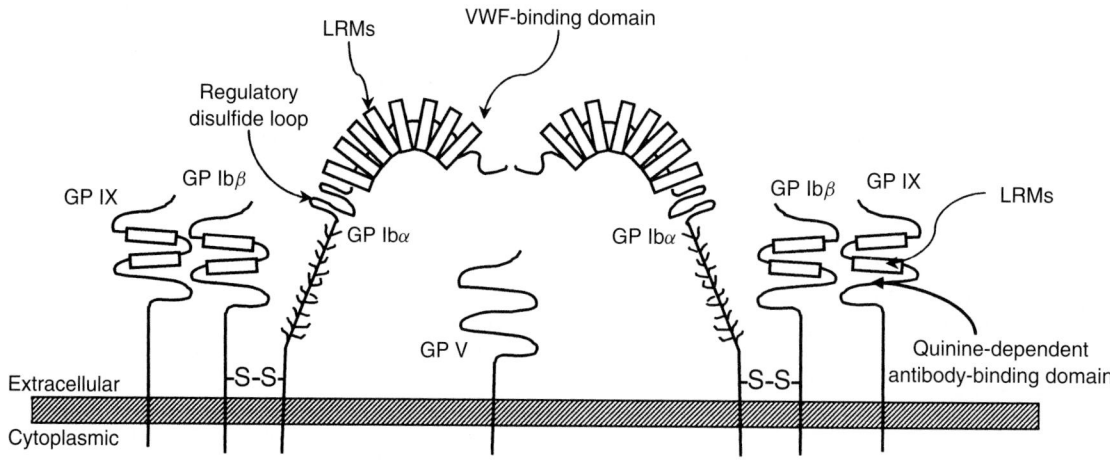

Quinine-dependent antibody-binding domain

64
**LDVTQNPWHCDCSLTYLRLWLEDRTPEALLQVRCAS**

**PSLAAHGPLGRLTGYQLGSCGWQLQASWVRPGVLWD**
135

**FIGURE 29-3.** Schematic illustration of the GP Ib/IX/V complex. This complex consists of four polypeptides: GP Ibα, GP Ibβ, GP IX, and GP V. The GP Ibα subunit is disulfide-linked to GP Ibβ, and these two subunits are noncovalently linked to GP IX (56). The GP Ib/IX complex is noncovalently associated with GP V (58). The four subunits are expressed in a 2:2:2:1 GP Ibα : GP Ibβ : GP IX : GP V ratio (57). The extracellular region of GP Ibα contains an O-glycosylated region and an amino-terminal domain. The latter region contains eight leucine-rich motifs (LRMs) (60,61) and is the binding site for von Willebrand factor (VWF) (62). GP IX contains a binding site for quinine-dependent antibodies between amino acids 64 and 135 (44). Nonconserved residues between human and mouse GP IX sequences (*bold*) were mutated by single–amino acid change. Stable expression of the mutant hGP IX in Chinese hamster ovary (CHO) cells demonstrated that SZ1 and quinine-dependent antibodies bind to arginine 110 (R110) and glutamine 115 (Q115) (*underlined*) (44). (From Andrews RK, Gardiner EE, Shen Y, et al. Glycoprotein Ib-IX-V. *Int J Biochem Cell Biol* 2003;35:1170–1174.)

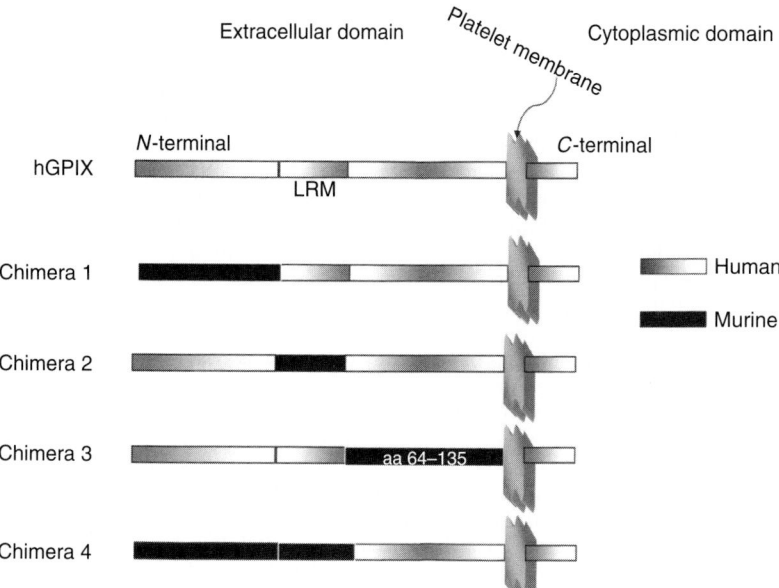

**FIGURE 29-4.** Schematic diagram of the chimeric mouse/human GP IX constructs. On the basis of the observation that quinine-dependent antibodies react only with glycoproteins present on human or primate platelets, but not those of other species (66), four chimeric GP IX constructs were generated. In each construct, a fragment of human GP IX was replaced by the corresponding fragment of mouse GP IX. The inability of the monoclonal antibody SZ1 to bind chimera 3, suggested that SZ1 and quinine-dependent antibodies target this region from amino acid 64 to 135 on human GP IX (44). LRM, leucine-rich motif.

the serum from one patient reacted with GP Ibα at the glyco-calicin N-terminal domain (38). This is in contrast to most drug-induced antiplatelet antibodies that predominantly recognize the membrane-associated region of the GP Ib/IX complex (38,39, 53,67). Further detailed studies involving enzymatic cleavage of GP Ibα at specific sites using mocarhagin and trypsin have mapped the target region on GP Ibα to be between amino acids 283 and 293 (42).

## Glycoprotein V

As mentioned in the previous text, GP Ib/IX is noncovalently associated with GP V, an 82-kDa membrane glycoprotein (58) (Fig. 29-3). The exact role of GP V is still unclear at present, but it is the major platelet membrane protein that acts as a substrate for thrombin (68,69). Hence, it was thought that GP V plays a role in thrombin activation. However, the observation that platelets from patients with Bernard-Soulier that lack GP V

can still be activated by thrombin (70) argues against this theory. Moreover, a thrombin receptor located on the surface of platelets and endothelial cells was recently identified (71) and found to be essential for thrombin-induced platelet activation (72). Cloning of this thrombin receptor demonstrated that it was distinct from GP V (71).

One study in 1986 documented binding of GP V by the sera of six patients with quinidine-induced thrombocytopenia (35). The antibodies did not react with GP Ib (35). However, this finding has not yet been duplicated by other investigators. Hence, it remains unclear whether GP V is a clinically relevant target in drug-induced thrombocytopenia.

## GP IIb/IIIa Complex

The GP IIb/IIIa complex is the most abundant integrin expressed on the surface of platelets at approximately 50,000 to 80,000 copies per platelet (73). The glycoprotein complex is a

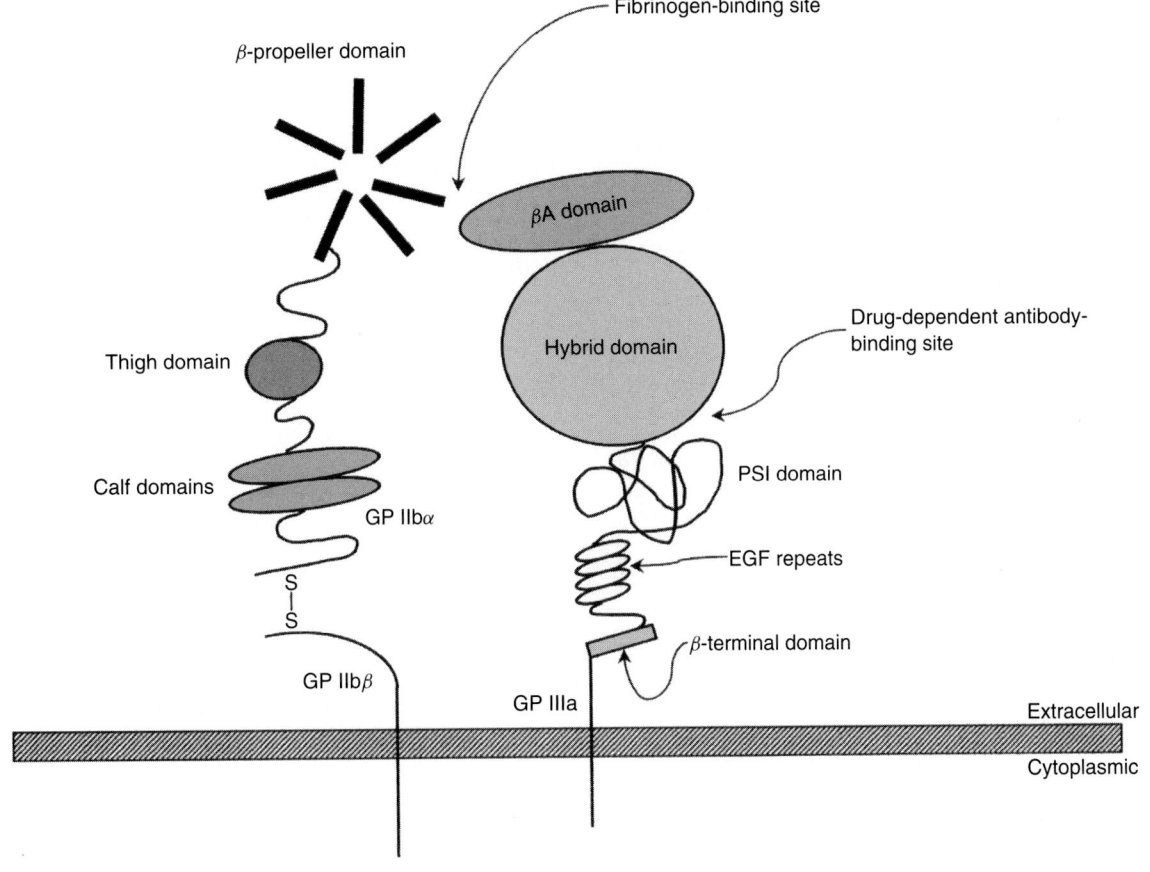

**FIGURE 29-5.** Schematic diagram of the GP IIb/IIIa complex. The glycoprotein complex is a heterodimer consisting of GP IIb and GP IIIa. The GP IIb subunit consists of an α and a β chain, linked by a disulfide bond. At the N-terminal of the GP IIbα subunit is a β-propeller structure. This domain consists of a series of amino acid repeats, arranged to form seven bladelike structures. The blades at the base of the β-propeller contain four divalent binding motifs. The N-terminal region of the GP IIIa subunit is not yet well defined, but a βA domain has been identified. This is followed by the hybrid and plexin, semaphorin, integrin (PSI) domains, linked to a series of four disulfide repeats, arranged in epidermal-growth factor (EGF)-like structures. The location of the PSI domain relative to the hybrid domain is not clear, because it could not be resolved by crystallographic studies. The binding site for fibrinogen is believed to lie somewhere between the β-propeller and βA domains (76). [From Quinn MJ, Byzova TV, Qin J, et al. Platelet activation and the formation of the platelet plug. *Arterioscler Thromb Vasc Biol* 2003;23:945–952; Peterson JA, Nyree CE, Newman PJ, et al. A site involving the "hybrid" and PSI homology domains of GP IIIa (β3-integrin subunit) is a common target for antibodies associated with quinine-induced immune thrombocytopenia. *Blood* 2003;101:937–942; Topol EJ, Byzova TV, Plow EF. Platelet GP IIb/IIIa blockers. *Lancet* 1999;353:227–231.]

heterodimer, consisting of GP IIb and GP IIIa, encoded by different genes (see Fig. 29-5) (74,75). The GP IIb subunit is synthesized as a single peptide and subsequently cleaved into α ($M_r$ = 132 kDa) and β ($M_r$ = 22 kDa) chains linked by a disulfide bond (Fig. 29-5) (75,76). GP IIIa is a single polypeptide, cross-linked by multiple intrachain disulfides (75). It has a molecular weight of 95 kDa in the nonreduced state and 114 kDa in the reduced state (75). Platelet activation results in conformational changes in the extracellular domain of the GP IIb/IIIa complex, allowing it to bind fibrinogen and VWF (Fig. 29-5), which subsequently leads to platelet aggregation and thrombus formation (1,76). Patients with Glanzman thrombasthenia lack GP IIb/IIIa (77), and their platelets fail to aggregate.

Although most quinine-dependent antibodies target the GP Ib/IX complex, some have been documented to target the GP IIb/IIIa complex (38,39,42). Quinine-dependent antibodies specific for GP IIb/IIIa were found to be conformation-dependent, with the intrachain disulfide bonds in GP IIIa playing an important role in maintaining the structural epitope (39). In fact, recent studies showed that quinine-induced antibodies from three patients were found to require only GP IIIa for binding (45). The site for antibody recognition on GP IIIa was initially determined to be close to the epitopes for the monoclonal antibodies, 22C4 and SZ22 (38). Further detailed characterization using chimera proteins of GP IIb/IIIa transiently expressed in HEK293T cells defined the antibody-binding site to be between residues 49 and 98 (45). These studies demonstrated that antibody binding to GP IIb/IIIa was lost when amino acids Ala50, Arg62, and Asp66 were mutated (45), suggesting that these residues play a crucial role. On the basis of crystal structure analysis (79), the target epitope on GP IIIa was determined to lie in the hybrid domain and the plexin, semaphorin, integrin (PSI) homology domain of the glycoprotein (Fig. 29-5).

In addition to quinine-dependent antibodies, GP IIb/IIIa has also been implicated as the target antigen for other drug-induced antibodies, including the antibodies that are related to drug metabolites of the nonsteroidal antiinflammatory drugs (NSAIDs), naproxen and acetaminophen (54) and the oral antidepressant mirtazapine (15). Further characterization of the epitopes recognized by drug-induced antibodies will increase our understanding of the molecular mechanisms whereby drugs promote immune-mediated destruction of platelets and other cell types.

## Platelet/Endothelial Cell Adhesion Molecule-1

PECAM-1 is a member of the immunoglobulin gene superfamily, expressed on the surface of platelets, leukocytes, and endothelial cells (at the intercellular junctions) (80). PECAM-1 consists of six extracellular immunoglobulinlike loops, a transmembrane region, and a variable cytoplasmic tail that is involved in cellular adhesion, migration, signal transduction, and vascular stability (81,82). Although the exact role of PECAM-1 on platelet is still unclear, PECAM-1 deficient platelets display enhanced aggregation and spreading, and form significantly larger thrombi under conditions of arterial flow (83,84). Hence, it is postulated that PECAM-1 plays a negative-regulatory role in platelet activation and thrombi formation (83–85).

Recently, five patients treated for hyperthyroidism using the thioamide carbimazole developed immune thrombocytopenia (16). Analysis of the sera from these patients revealed antibodies that were reactive against PECAM-1 on platelets and on endothelial cells (16). Detailed characterization using monoclonal antibodies against different epitopes and mutation studies demonstrated that the second extracellular domain was crucial for carbimazole-dependent antibody binding (16). This effect was specific for carbimazole, as the active metabolite, thiamazole, failed to induce reactivity in patient sera (86). Interestingly, sera from patients with quinine/quinidine-induced thrombocytopenia were also reactive with PECAM-1, although binding was not as strong as with GP Ib/IX and GP IIb/IIIa (16). These studies describe PECAM-1 as an important new target antigen for drug-induced antibodies (either alone or with other platelet antigens), and should be considered in addition to GP Ib/IX and GP IIb/IIIa in drug-induced thrombocytopenia.

# THROMBOCYTOPENIA INDUCED BY GP IIB/IIIA ANTAGONISTS

Because the GP IIb/IIIa receptor acts as the final common pathway for platelet aggregation, blocking the receptor will result in potent inhibition of platelet function and therefore thrombosis. This gave rise to the development of a new class of antithrombotic agents, the GP IIb/IIIa antagonists. By competitively blocking the binding of fibrinogen to GP IIb/IIIa, these agents inhibit platelet thrombi formation (78,87,88). Currently, three GP IIb/IIIa antagonists have been approved for clinical use in the United States: abciximab (87), tirofiban (89), and eptifibatide (90). These agents have been shown to be efficacious in the treatment of acute coronary thrombosis in a number of trials (91–93). However, these GP IIb/IIIa antagonists have also been associated with increased risk of severe or profound thrombocytopenia that can occur within hours after receiving the drug (94,95).

Unfortunately, the pathogenesis of GP IIb/IIIa antagonist-induced thrombocytopenia is still not fully understood. The current hypothesis is that binding of the drug to the GP IIb/IIIa receptor triggers an immune-mediated destruction of platelets, resulting in thrombocytopenia. However, whether the antigen is the drug itself, a neoepitope generated by binding of the antagonist to the receptor, or a compound antigen consisting of the drug and receptor complex is still unclear.

## Abciximab

Abciximab (also known as ReoPro) is a Fab fragment generated by the papain cleavage of a chimeric mouse/human IgG antibody. It contains a specificity-determining sequence from a murine monoclonal antibody (7E3) directed against the GP IIb/IIIa complex. Abciximab was the first fibrinogen receptor antagonist approved for clinical use (87). However, approximately 2.5% to 5.6% of patients treated with abciximab develop thrombocytopenia. In addition, approximately 0.5% to 1.0% of patients develop severe or profound life-threatening thrombocytopenia within a few hours of administration of abciximab (94,95). The incidence of severe and profound thrombocytopenia has been reported to increase with readministration (96).

Early studies identified the presence of anti-abciximab antibodies in drug-treated patients. The antibodies can be preexisting or induced upon drug exposure. In 1994, Christopoulos examined nine patients with unstable angina (97). The patients were treated with abciximab for 48 to 96 hours, and platelet-associated IgG (PA IgG) was measured. Within 24 hours of drug treatment, a significant rise in PA IgG was observed, lasting approximately 2 weeks (97). However, none of the patients developed thrombocytopenia (97). The rapid IgG response suggested the presence of preformed antibodies reactive with abciximab-coated platelets (97). An examination by Curtis et al. of the pretreatment sera of two patients with abciximab-induced thrombocytopenia also confirmed the presence of preexisting IgG reactive with abciximab-coated platelets (20).

Antibodies against abciximab could also be detected in healthy subjects with no prior exposure to abciximab. Christopoulos et al. examined 21 healthy subjects and found that in 15 (71%) sera contained antibodies against abciximab (97). Similarly, Curtis et al. examined sera from 104 healthy subjects and found IgG antibodies reactive with abciximab-coated platelets in 77 (74%) samples (20). Whether the presence of preexisting antibodies against abciximab in healthy subjects predisposes them to thrombocytopenia upon treatment with abciximab is not known.

The question as to which is the immunogenic portion of abciximab is unclear. In most cases, the antibodies target the human Fab fragment of the chimeric GP IIb/IIIa antagonists (97,98). However, in a small number of cases, the antibodies target the murine 7E3 fragment (97,98). Christopoulos et al. examined 21 healthy subjects and found 14 (67%) serum samples with antibodies specific for the human Fab portion of abciximab (97). Only one (4.8%) of the 21 subjects had antibodies specific for the mouse 7E3 segment (97). However, because these healthy subjects were not subsequently exposed to abciximab, no definitive association can be made between antibody specificity and occurrence of thrombocytopenia. Another study by Knight et al. showed that five of six (83%) patient sera had antibodies against human Fab, and only one patient (17%) had antibodies against mouse 7E3 (98). However, whether these antibodies are the cause of the thrombocytopenia in these patients is unclear, and further studies are required (98).

The apparent low incidence of antibodies specific for 7E3 of abciximab compared to antibodies specific for the human Fab portion coincides with the low incidence of patients developing severe thrombocytopenia upon first exposure to the drug (94,95). Hence, it is possible to speculate that severe thrombocytopenia is more likely to occur in patients with antibodies against 7E3. This suggestion is confirmed by a study that demonstrates two main differences between antibodies in normal subjects compared to patients with thrombocytopenia(20). First, Fab fragments prepared from normal IgG competitively inhibited reactivity against abciximab-coated platelets in 85% of healthy subjects compared to 36% of patients who developed thrombocytopenia (20). This strongly suggested that antibodies from healthy subjects target the human Fab fragment, whereas antibodies from patients target a different site on abciximab or GP IIb/IIIa (20). Second, sera from all patients with thrombocytopenia preferentially reacted with platelets sensitized to 7E3 compared to those sensitized with AP2 (murine monoclonal antibody specific for GP IIb/IIIa complex) or AP3 (murine monoclonal antibody specific for GP IIIa) (20). In contrast, sera from healthy subjects did not react with any of the monoclonal antibodies preferentially (20). These results suggested that sera from patients with thrombocytopenia contain antibodies specific for the 7E3 region on abciximab (20).

Collectively, these studies, while preliminary and limited, suggest that most of the healthy population have preexisting antibodies against the human Fab portion of abciximab, although this does not appear to play a major role in thrombocytopenia. Patients who develop severe thrombocytopenia upon exposure to the drug have antibodies specific for the murine 7E3 fragment. It presently remains unclear whether healthy subjects with preexisting antibodies specific for 7E3 are more susceptible to thrombocytopenia upon treatment with abciximab. In addition, the reason a healthy subject with no prior exposure to abciximab would have preexisting antibodies specific for 7E3 is not known. Further detailed studies are necessary to establish any correlation between antibody specificity and predisposition to abciximab-induced thrombocytopenia.

## Thrombocytopenia Caused by Other GP IIb/IIIa Antagonists

The two other clinically approved GP IIb/IIIa antagonists, tirofiban and eptifibatide, have also been reported to cause severe thrombocytopenia. Similar rates of thrombocytopenia have been found for these agents compared with abciximab (92,99,100). Tirofiban (also known as Aggrastat) is a nonpeptide mimetic and eptifibatide (also called Integrelin) is a synthetic peptide (101). Roxifiban is another GP IIb/IIIa antagonist, currently in phase II clinical trial that has been implicated in drug-induced thrombocytopenia. Although there have been few studies to date examining the mechanism of GP IIb/IIIa antagonist-induced thrombocytopenia, it has been suggested that the binding of these drugs to the GP IIb/IIIa receptor induces conformational changes in the glycoprotein. The changes result in the expression of new antigenic sites called ligand-induced binding sites (LIBS) (102), which then become the targets for antiplatelet antibodies.

These drug-related antiplatelet antibodies can also be preformed. Antibodies were detected in the pretreatment sera of patients with thrombocytopenia who were administered tirofiban (103), eptifibatide (103), and roxifiban (18,19), and in primates treated with ligand-mimetic drugs, L-738, 167-(A1-L), L-739, 758-(A2-L), and L-767, 679-(B) (104).

Generally, drug-induced antibodies did not appear to be present in the healthy population: Screening of 100 healthy subjects failed to show the presence of drug-dependent antibodies in the presence of tirofiban or eptifibatide (103). In a separate study, serum samples from 1,032 healthy human donors showed that only 1.7% had antibodies reactive with GP IIb/IIIa in the presence of ligand-mimetic drugs (104). Similar results were obtained in a study of 1,000 healthy human subjects and 41 chimpanzees tested in the presence of roxifiban (18). Unfortunately, in all these studies, the healthy subjects were not subsequently exposed to GP IIb/IIIa antagonists; therefore, it is not known whether they will develop thrombocytopenia. Hence, no correlation can be made between the presence of preexisting drug-dependent antibodies and the occurrence of thrombocytopenia. In addition, out of 23 patients treated with tirofiban or eptifibatide who did not develop thrombocytopenia, only two patients' sera reacted weakly in the presence of tirofiban (103). From these data, it can be speculated that ligand mimetic-induced antibodies are not present in the healthy population and generally exist only in the patients who develop drug-induced thrombocytopenia upon exposure to the agent. However, further studies are necessary to confirm the status of these drug-induced antibodies in the general population and in the patients.

A recent study of nine patients who developed tirofiban- or eptifibatide-induced thrombocytopenia demonstrated antibody reactivity with the GP IIb/IIIa complex (103). However, dissociation of the complex with ethylenediamine tetraacetic acid (EDTA) abolished reactivity, suggesting the importance of the intact glycoprotein structure (103). Binding of ligand mimetics to a single site in the fibrinogen-binding pocket of GP IIb/IIIa blocks binding of fibrinogen (105). In contrast, abciximab interferes with fibrinogen by occupying a site close to, but not identical to, the fibrinogen-binding site (106). Using this information, Bougie et al. (103) reasoned that drug-dependent antibodies recognizing a site close to the fibrinogen-binding site would be sterically inhibited by abciximab. Antibody binding was measured by reacting patient sera with platelets that were pretreated with tirofiban or eptifibatide, followed by saturating concentrations of abciximab. Reactivity could be divided into three groups: Antibody-binding from two out of nine patient sera was completely inhibited; binding in six patient sera was partially inhibited; and antibody-binding from the serum of one patient was relatively unaffected by the presence of saturating concentrations of abciximab (103). These results suggested that drug-dependent antibodies target three different epitopes on GP IIb/IIIa (103). One site is located very close to, or identical to, the binding site for abciximab and fibrinogen. A second site is in close proximity to, but not identical to, the abciximab specific epitope, thereby resulting in only partial inhibition of antibody-platelet reactivity. A third site is distal to the abciximab-binding site. However, whether these epitopes are a direct result of drug-induced glycoprotein conformational change, and whether they are specific targets for drug-induced antibodies, is still unclear.

In another study examining roxifiban, Billheimer et al. provided support for a LIBS-mediated immune mechanism (18). The sera from two patients with roxifiban-induced thrombocytopenia were found to be positive for drug-dependent antibodies (18). Antibody reactivity was lost in the presence of EDTA, implying the importance of GP IIb/IIIa structural conformation (18). Incubation of purified GP IIb/IIIa with roxifiban resulted in a supershift of the protein complex, as observed on SDS-PAGE gel under nonreducing conditions (18). Immunoblotting with patient sera showed antibody binding to the supershifted glycoprotein (18). Experiments using radiolabeled drug demonstrated that roxifiban did not remain associated with the supershifted glycoprotein under SDS-PAGE analysis (18), suggesting that the drug did not form part of the target epitope. From these results, Billheimer et al. suggested that roxifiban induced a conformation change in GP IIb/IIIa, resulting in electromobility shift of the protein. This conformational change resulted in the formation of LIBS, which were targeted by drug-induced antibodies (18).

Although the studies by Bougie et al. and Billheimer et al. lend support to the hypothesis that drug-induced antibodies recognize and bind to LIBS, whether these epitopes are a direct result of drug-induced glycoprotein conformational change is still uncertain. In addition, there is no strong evidence demonstrating the specific binding of drug-induced antibodies to the newly formed epitopes or LIBS. Further mapping of these antigenic target sites is required to definitively show drug-induced antibody binding to LIBS as the mechanism of GP IIb/IIIa antagonist-induced thrombocytopenia.

## Platelet Activation

An alternative antibody-independent mechanism for GP IIb/IIIa antagonist-induced thrombocytopenia is platelet activation by binding of the drug (3). In 1999, Peter et al. studied 26 patients treated with abciximab (107). One patient developed severe thrombocytopenia within 2 hours of the start of medication (107). Analysis of this patient's platelets revealed increased P selectin expression, indicative of increased platelet activation (107). Enhanced platelet P selectin expression could be reinduced, in vitro, in a concentration-dependent manner upon addition of abciximab to the patient's blood (107). In addition, the GP IIb/IIIa receptor was shown to be in a high-affinity state, as demonstrated by fibrinogen and PAC-1 binding at 10 minutes after commencement of abciximab treatment (107). Again, this high-affinity state could be reinduced in vitro, in the presence of the drug (107). This conformational change of GP IIb/IIIa from the low- to high-affinity state in the presence of abciximab results in fibrinogen binding and aggregation of platelets (108). The aggregated platelets are then cleared by the reticuloendothelial system. This study suggests abciximab-induced platelet activation resulting in platelet aggregation and clearance as an alternative mechanism of abciximab-induced thrombocytopenia. However, it is difficult to understand why fibrinogen binding can occur in the presence of abciximab, which should, in fact, block fibrinogen binding. Furthermore, because this is the

only documented case from a study of 26 patients, additional studies are essential to confirm the role of platelet activation in GP IIb/IIIa antagonist-induced thrombocytopenia.

## CONCLUSIONS

Drug-induced immune thrombocytopenia is a potentially life-threatening complication of a range of drugs. Because the number of agents available for clinical use increases each year, it is expected that reports of drug-induced thrombocytopenia will also increase. The condition is characterized by the presence of drug-dependent antibodies that target a particular epitope on the platelet surface or on the platelet-bound drug. This leads to enhanced clearance of platelets by the reticuloendothelial system, and hence to thrombocytopenia. Usually, the antibody target is a particular site on platelet glycoproteins such as GP Ib/IX, GP IIb/IIIa and PECAM-1. The antigenic site can also be on the offending drug itself, as is the case for abciximab. Understanding drug-induced antibody–platelet interactions may help in the identification of the patients at risk of developing thrombocytopenia. Several studies have mapped the amino acid sequences that are crucial for drug-dependent antibody binding to platelets. Future epitope mapping studies may reveal regions of homology in the antigenic glycoproteins on platelets and other target tissues. These studies will increase our understanding of the pathogenesis of drug-induced immune damage, not only to platelets, but also to other cells and tissue systems. This knowledge will contribute to the development of safer therapies with reduced risk of thrombocytopenia and other immune complications.

## ACKNOWLEDGMENTS

Some studies on quinine- and quinidine-induced thrombocytopenia described in this manuscript were supported by an NHMRC grant.

## References

1. Chong BH. Diagnosis, treatment and pathophysiology of autoimmune thrombocytopenias. Crit Rev Oncol Hematol 1995;20:271–296.
2. Aster RH. Drug-induced thrombocytopenia: an overview of pathogenesis. Semin Hematol 1999;36:2–6.
3. Greinacher A, Eichler P, Lubenow N, et al. Drug-induced and drug-dependent immune thrombocytopenias. Rev Clin Exp Hematol 2001;5:1 66–200.
4. Hackett T, Kelton JG, Powers P. Drug-induced platelet destruction. Semin Thromb Hemost 1982;8:116–137.
5. Pedersen-Bjergaard U, Andersen M, Hansen PB. Drug-induced thrombocytopenia: clinical data on 309 cases and the effect of corticosteroid therapy. Eur J Clin Pharmacol 1997;52:183–189.
6. George JN, Raskob GE, Shah SR, et al. Drug-induced thrombocytopenia: a systematic review of published case reports. Ann Intern Med 1998;129: 886–890.
7. Rizvi MA, Kojourni K, George JN. Drug-induced thrombocytopenia: an updated systematic review. Ann Intern Med 2001;134:346.
8. Hibbard AB, Medina PJ, Vesley SK. Reports of drug-induced thrombocytopenia. Ann Intern Med 2003;138:239.
9. Martin XD, Danese M. Dorzolamide-induced immune thrombocytopenia: a case report and literature review. Glaucoma 2001;10:133–135.
10. Bernstein WB, Trotta RF, Rector JT, et al. Mechanisms for linezolid-induced anemia and thrombocytopenia. Ann Pharmacother 2003;37:517–520.
11. Aljitawi OS, Krishnan K, Curtis BR, et al. Serologically documented loracarbef (Lorabid)-induced immune thrombocytopenia. Am J Hematol 2003;73:41–43.
12. Meyer O, Hoffmann T, Aslan T, et al. Diclofenac-induced antibodies against RBCs and platelets: two case reports and a concise review. Transfusion 2003;43:345–349.
13. D'Addario SF, Bryan ME, Stringer WA, et al. Minocycline-induced immune thrombocytopenia presenting as Schamberg's disease. J Drugs Dermatol 2003;2:320–323.
14. Garbe E, Meyer O, Andersohn F, et al. Amlodipine-induced immune thrombocytopenia. Vox Sang 2004;86:75–76.

15. Liu X, Sahud MA. Glycoprotein IIb/IIIa complex is the target in mirtaza-pine-induced immune thrombocytopenia. *Blood Cells Mol Dis* 2003;30:241–245.

16. Kroll H, Sun Q-H, Santoso S. Platelet endothelial cell adhesion molecule-1 (PECAM-1) is a target glycoprotein in drug-induced thrombocytopenia. *Blood* 2000;96:1409–1414.

17. Willert C, Englisch S, Schlesinger S, et al. Possible drug-induced thrombocytopenia secondary to tiagabine. *Neurology* 1999;52:889.

18. Billheimer JT, Dicker IB, Wynn R, et al. Evidence that thrombocytopenia observed in humans treated with orally bioavailable glycoprotein IIb/IIIa antagonists is immune mediated. *Blood* 2002;99:3540–3546.

19. Seiffert D, Stern AM, Ebling W, et al. Prospective testing for drug-dependent antibodies reduces the incidence of thrombocytopenia observed with the small molecule glycoprotein IIb/IIIa antagonist roxifiban: implications for the etiology of thrombocytopenia. *Blood* 2003;101:58–63.

20. Curtis BR, Swyers J, Divgi A, et al. Thrombocytopenia after second exposure to abciximab is caused by antibodies that recognize abciximab-coated platelets. *Blood* 2002;99:2054–2059.

21. Ackroyd JF. The pathogenesis of thrombocytopenic purpura due to hypersensitivity to sedermoid. *Clin Sci* 1949;7:248–249.

22. Ackroyd JF. The role of complement in sedormid purpura. *Clin Sci* 1951;10:185–205.

23. Shulman NR. Immunoreactions involving platelets. I. A steric and kinetic model for formation of a complex from a human antibody, quinidine as a hapten, and platelets; and for fixation of complement by the complex. *J Exp Med* 1958;107:665–690.

24. Miescher PA, Miescher A. Die sedormid-anaphylaxie. *Schweiz Med Wochenschr* 1952;82:1279.

25. Miescher P, Cooper N. The fixation of soluble antigen-antibody complexes upon thrombocytes. *Vox Sang* 1960:5:5138–5142.

26. Shulman NR. Immunoreactions involving platelets. IV. Studies on the pathogenesis of thrombocytopenia in drug purpura using test doses of quinidine in sensitized individuals: their implications in idiopathic thrombocytopenic purpura. *J Exp Med* 1958;117:711–729.

27. Shulman NR. Immunoreactions involving platelets. III. Quantitative aspects of platelet agglutination, inhibition of clot retraction, and other reactions caused by the antibody of quinidine purpura. *J Exp Med* 1958;107:697–710.

28. Green I, Paul W, Benacerraf B. The behaviour of hapten-poly-L-lysine conjugates as complete antigens in genetic responder and as haptens in non-responder guinea pigs. *J Exp Med* 1966;123:859–879.

29. Chong BH, Berndt MC, Koutts J, et al. Quinine-induced thrombocytopenia and leukopenia: demonstration and characterization of distinct antiplatelet and antileukocyte antibodies. *Blood* 1983;62:1218–1223.

30. Berndt MC, Gregory C, Kabral A, et al. Purification and preliminary characterization of the glycoprotein Ib complex im the human platelet membrane. *Eur J Biochem* 1985;151:637.

31. Christie DJ, Mullen PC, Aster RH. Fab-mediated binding of drug-dependent antibodies to platelets in quinidine- and quinine-induced thrombocytopenia. *J Clin Invest* 1985;75:310–314.

32. Smith ME, Reid DM, Jones CE, et al. Binding of quinine- and quinidine-dependent drug antibodies to platelets is mediated by the fab domain of the immunoglobulin G and is not Fc dependent. *J Clin Invest* 1987;79:912–917.

33. Kunicki TJ, Johnson MM, Aster RH. Absence of the platelet receptor for drug-dependent antibodies in the Bernard-Soulier syndrome. *J Clin Invest* 1978;62:716–719.

34. Kunicki TJ, Russell N, Nurden AT, et al. Further studies on the human platelet receptor for quinine- and quinidine-dependent antibodies. *J Immunol* 1981;126:398–402.

35. Stricker RB, Shuman MA. Quinidine purpura: evidence that glycoprotein V is a target platelet antigen. *Blood* 1986;67:1377–1381.

36. Christie DJ, Mullen PC, Aster RH. Quinine- and quinidine-platelet antibodies can react with GPIIb/IIIa. *Br J Haematol* 1987;67:213–219.

37. Pfueller SL, Bilston RA, Logan D, et al. Heterogeneity of drug-dependent platelet antigens and their antibodies in quinine- and quinidine-induced thrombocytopenia: involvement of glycoproteins Ib, IIIa and IX. *Blood* 1988;72:1155–1162.

38. Chong BH, Du X, Berndt MC, et al. Characterization of the binding domains on platelet glycoproteins Ib-IX and IIb/IIIa complexes for the quinine/quinidine-dependent antibodies. *Blood* 1991;77:2190–2199.

39. Visentin GP, Newman PJ, Aster RH. Characteristics of quinine- and quinidine-induced antibodies specific for platelet glycoproteins IIb and IIIa. *Blood* 1991;77:2668–2676.

40. Nieminen U, Kekomaki R. Quinidine-induced thrombocytopenia purpura: clinical presentation in relation to drug-dependent and drug-independent platelet antibodies. *Br J Haematol* 1992;80:77–82.

41. Lopez JA, Li CQ, Weisman S, et al. The glycoprotein Ib-IX complex-specific monoclonal antibody SZ1 binds to a conformational-sensitive epitope on glycoprotein IX: implications for the target antigen of quinine/quinidine-dependent autoantibodies. *Blood* 1995;85:1254–1258.

42. Burgess JK, Lopez JA, Berndt MC, et al. Quinine-dependent antibodies bind a restricted set of epitopes on the glycoprotein Ib-IX complex: characterization of the epitopes. *Blood* 1998;92:2366–2373.

43. Aster RH. Drug-induced thrombocytopenia. In: AD Michelson, ed. *Platelets*. Elsevier Science, San Diego & London. 2002:593–606.

44. Asvadi P, Ahmadi Z, Chong BH. Drug-induced thrombocytopenia: localization of the binding site of GPIX-specific quinine-dependent antibodies. *Blood* 2003;102:1670–1677.

45. Peterson JA, Nyree CE, Newman PJ, et al. A site involving the "hybrid" and PSI homology domains of GPIIIa (β3-integrin subunit) is a common target for antibodies associated with quinine-induced immune thrombocytopenia. *Blood* 2003;101:937–942.

46. Newman PM, Chong BH. Heparin-induced thrombocytopenia: new evidence for the dynamic binding of purified anti-PF4-heparin antibodies to platelets and the resultant platelet activation. *Blood* 2000;96:182–187.

47. Connellan JM, Deacon S, Thurlow PJ. Changes in platelet function and reactivity induced by quinine in relation to quinine (drug) induced immune thrombocytopenia. *Thromb Res* 1991;61:501–514.

48. Christie DJ, Aster RH. Drug-antibody-platelet interaction in quinine- and quinidine-induced thrombocytopenia. *J Clin Invest* 1982;70:989–998.

49. Steinkamp R, Moore CV, Doubek WG. Thrombocytopenic purpura caused by hypersensitivity to quinine. *J Lab Clin Med* 1955;45:18–29.

50. Bolton FG, Dameshek W. Thrombocytopenic purpura due to quinidine. I. Clinical studies. *Blood* 1956;11:527–546.

51. Burgess JK, Lopez JA, Gaudry LE, et al. Rifampicin-dependent antibodies bind a similar or identical epitope to glycoprotein IX-specific quinine-dependent antibodies. *Blood* 2000;95:1988–1992.

52. Pereira J, Hidalgo P, Ocqueteau M, et al. Glycoprotein Ib/IX complex is the target in rifampicin-induced immune thrombocytopenia. *Br J Haematol* 2000;110:907–910.

53. Gentilini G, Curtis BR, Aster RH. An antibody from a patient with ranitidine-induced thrombocytopenia recognizes a site on glycoprotein IX that is a favored target for drug-induced antibodies. *Blood* 1998;92:2359–2365.

54. Bougie D, Aster R. Immune thrombocytopenia resulting from sensitivity to metabolites of naproxen and acetaminophen. *Blood* 2001;97:3846–3850.

55. Hickey MJ, Deaven LL, Roth GJ. Human platelet glycoprotein IX characterization of cDNA and localization of the gene to chromosome 3. *FEBS Lett* 1990;274:189–192.

56. Lopez JA. The platelet glycoprotein Ib-IX complex. Blood coagulation and fibrinolysis. *Blood Coagul Fibrinolysis* 1994;5:97–119.

57. Andrews RK, Gardiner EE, Shen Y, et al. Glycoprotein Ib-IX-V. *Int J Biochem Cell Biol* 2003;35:1170–1174.

58. Modderman PW, Admiraal LG, Sonnenberg A, et al. Glycoproteins V and Ib-IX form a noncovalent complex in the platelet membrane. *J Biol Chem* 1992;267:364.

59. Kobe B, Deisenhofer J. The leucine-rich repeat: a versatile binding motif. *Trends Biochem Sci* 1994;19:415–421.

60. Huizinga EG, Tsuji S, Romjin RAP, et al. Structures of GPIbα and its complex with the vWF-A1 domain. *Science* 2002;297:1176–1179.

61. Uff S, Clemetson JM, Harrison T, et al. Crystal structure of the platelet GPIbα N-terminal domain reveals an unmasking mechanism for receptor activation. *J Biol Chem* 2002;277:35657–35663.

62. Handa M, Titani K, Holland LZ, et al. The von Willebrand factor-binding domain of platelet membrane glycoprotein Ib. Characterization by monoclonal antibodies and partial amino acid sequence analysis of proteolytic fragments. *J Biol Chem* 1986;261:12579–12585.

63. Harmon JT, Jamieson GA. The glycocalicin portion of platelet glycoprotein Ib expresses both high and moderate affinity receptor sites for thrombin. A soluble radioreceptor assay for the interaction of thrombin with platelets. *J Biol Chem* 1986;261:13224–13229.

64. Berndt MC, Gregory C, Chong BH, et al. Additional glycoprotein defects in Bernard-Soulier's syndrome: confirmation of genetic basis by parental analysis. *Blood* 1983;62:800–807.

65. Devine DV, Rosse WF. Identification of platelet proteins that bind alloantibodies and autoantibodies. *Blood* 1984;64:1240–1245.

66. Shulman NR, Reid DM. Mechanisms of drug-induced immunologically mediated cytopenias. *Transfus Med Rev* 1993;7:215–229.

67. Kekomaki R, Dawson B, McFarland JG, et al. Localization of human platelet autoantigens to the cystein-rich region of glycoprotein IIIa. *J Clin Invest* 1991;88:847–854.

68. Phillips DR, Agin PP. Platelet plasma membrane glycoproteins. Identification of a proteolytic substrate for thrombin. *Biochem Biophys Res Commun* 1977;75:940–947.

69. Mosher DF, Vaheri A, Choate JJ, et al. Action of thrombin on surface glycoproteins of human platelets. *Blood* 1979;53:437–445.

70. Jamieson GA, Okumura T. Reduced thrombin binding and aggregation in Bernard-Soulier platelets. *J Clin Invest* 1978;61:861–864.

71. Vu TK, Hung DT, Wheaton VI, et al. Molecular cloning of a functional thrombin receptor reveals a novel proteolytic mechanism of receptor activation. *Cell* 1991;64:1057–1068.

72. Hung DT, Vu TK, Wheaton VI, et al. Cloned platelet thrombin receptor is necessary for thrombin-induced platelet activation. *J Clin Invest* 1992;89:1350–1353.

73. Wagner CL, Mascelli MA, Neblock DS, et al. Analysis of GPIIb/IIIa receptor number by quantification of 7E3 binding to human platelets. *Blood* 1996;88:907–914.

74. Sosnoski DM, Emanuel BS, Hawkins AL, et al. Chromosomal localization of the genes for the vitronectin and fibronectin receptors α subunits and for platelet glycoproteins IIb and IIIa. *J Clin Invest* 1988;81:1993–1998.

75. Phillips DR, Charo IF, Scarborough RM. GPIIb-IIIa: the responsive integrin. *Cell* 1991;65:359–362.

76. Quinn MJ, Byzova TV, Qin J, et al. Platelet activation and the formation of the platelet plug. *Arterioscler Thromb Vasc Biol* 2003;23:945–952.

77. Phillips DR, Agin PP. Platelet membrane defects in Glanzmann's thrombasthenia: evidence for decreased amounts of two major glycoproteins. *J Clin Invest* 1977;60:535–545.

78. Topol EJ, Byzova TV, Plow EF. Platelet GPIIb/IIIa blockers. *Lancet* 1999;353:227–231.

79. Xiong JP, Stehle T, Diefenbach B, et al. Crystal structure of the extracellular segment of integrin $\alpha V\beta 3$. *Science* 2001;294:339–345.

80. Newman PJ, Berndt MC, Gorski J, et al. PECAM-1 (CD31) cloning and relation to adhesion molecules of the immunoglobulin gene superfamily. *Science* 1990;247:1219–1222.

81. Newman PJ. The role of PECAM-1 in vascular cell biology. *Ann N Y Acad Sci* 1994;714:165–174.

82. Newman PJ. The biology of PECAM-1. *J Clin Invest* 1997;99:3–8.

83. Rathore V, Stapleton MA, Hillery CA, et al. PECAM-1 negatively regulates GPIb/V/IX signaling in murine platelets. *Blood* 2003;102:3658–1664.

84. Jackson DE. The unfolding tale of PECAM-1. *FEBS Lett* 2003;540:7–14.

85. Thai le M, Ashman LK, Harbour SN, et al. Physical proximity and functional interplay of PECAM-1 with the Fc receptor Fc gamma RIIa on the platelet plasma membrane. *Blood* 2003;102:3637–3645.

86. Kroll H, Giptner A, Santoso S. Drug-dependent antibodies against the prodrug carbimazole do not react with the active metabolite thiamzole. *Blood* 2001;97:2186–2187.

87. Coller BS. Perspectives series: cell adhesion in vascular biology. Platelet GPIIb/IIIa antagonists: the first anti-integrin receptor therapeutics. *J Clin Invest* 1997;99:1467–1471.

88. Kereiakes DJ. Oral platelet glycoprotein IIb/IIIa inhibitors. *Coron Artery Dis* 1999;10:581–594.

89. Vickers S, Theohardies AD, Arison B, et al. *In vitro* and *in vivo* studies on the metabolism of tirofiban. *Drug Metab Dispos* 1999;27:1360–1366.

90. Phillips DR, Scarborough RM. Clinical pharmacology of eptifibatide. *Am J Cardiol* 1997;80:11B–20B.

91. The EPIC Investigators. Use of monoclonal antibody directed against the platelet glycoprotein IIb/IIIa receptor in high-risk coronary angioplasty. *N Engl J Med* 1994;330:956–961.

92. The RESTORE Investigators. Effects of platelet glycoprotein IIb/IIIa blockade with tirofiban on adverse cardiac events in patients with unstable angina or acute myocardial infarction undergoing coronary angioplasty. *Circulation* 1997;96:1445–1453.

93. The PURSUIT Investigators. Inhibition of the platelet glycoprotein IIb/IIIa with eptifibatide in patients with acute coronary syndromes without persistent ST-segment elevation. *N Engl J Med* 1998;339:436–443.

94. Jubelirer SJ, Koenig BA, Bates MC. Acute profound thrombocytopenia following C73 Fab (abciximab) therapy: case reports, review of the literature, and implications for therapy. *Am J Hematol* 1999;61:205–208.

95. Kereiakes DJ, Berkowitz SD, Lincoff AM, et al. Clinical correlates and course of thrombocytopenia during percutaneous coronary intervention in the era of abciximab platelet glycoprotein IIb/IIIa blockade. *Am Heart J* 2000;40:74–80.

96. Tcheng JE, Kereiakes DJ, Braden GA, et al. Readministration of abciximab: interim report of the ReoPro readministration registry. *Am Heart J* 1999;138:S33–S38.

97. Christopoulos C. Platelet surface IgG in patients receiving infusions of Fab chimeric monoclonal antibody to glycoprotein IIb/IIIa. *Clin Exp Immunol* 1994;98:6–11.

98. Knight DM, Wagner C, Jordan R, et al. The immunogenicity of the 7E3 murine monoclonal Fab antibody fragment variable region is dramatically reduced in humans by substitution of human for murine constant regions. *Mol Immunol* 1995;32:1271–1281.

99. Berkowitz SD, Sane DC, Sigmon KN, et al. Occurrence and clinical significance of thrombocytopenia in a population undergoing high-risk percutaneous coronary revascularization. Evaluation of c7E3 for the Prevention of Ischemic Complications (EPIC) study group. *J Am Coll Cardiol* 1998;32:311–319.

100. Hongo RH, Brent BN. Association of eptifibatide and acute profound thrombocyotpenia. *Am J Cardiol* 2001;88:428–431.

101. Giugliano RP. Drug-induced thrombocytopenia: is it a serious concern for glycoprotein IIb/IIIa receptor inhibitors? *J Thromb Thrombolysis* 1998;5:191–202.

102. Frelinger AL, Du XP, Plow EF, et al. Monoclonal antibodies to ligand-occupied conformers of integrin $\alpha IIb\beta 3$ (glycoprotein IIb-IIIa) alter receptor affinity, specificity, and function. *J Biol Chem* 1991;266:17106–17111.

103. Bougie DW, Wilker PR, Wuitschick ED, et al. Acute thrombocytopenia after treatment with tirofiban or eptifibatide is associated with antibodies specific for ligand-occupied GPIIb/IIIa. *Blood* 2002;100:2071–2076.

104. Bednar B, Cook JJ, Holahan MA, et al. Fibrinogen receptor antagonist-induced thrombocytopenia in chimpanzee and rhesus monkey associated with preexisting drug-dependent antibodies to platelet glycoprotein IIb/IIIa. *Blood* 1999;94:587–599.

105. Mousa SA, Bozarth JM, Naik UP, et al. Platelet GPIIb/IIIa binding characteristics of small molecule RGD mimetic: Distinct binding profile for roxifiban. *Br J Pharmacol* 2001;133:331–336.

106. Puzon-McLaughlin W, Kamata T, Takada Y. Multiple discontinuous ligand-mimetic antibody binding sites define a ligand-binding pocket in integrin $\alpha IIb\beta 3$. *J Biol Chem* 2000;275:7795–7802.

107. Peter K, Straub A, Kohler B, et al. Platelet activation as a potential mechanism of GP IIb/IIIa inhibitor-induced thrombocytopenia. *Am J Cardiol* 1999;84:519–524.

108. Peter K, Schwarz M, Ylanne J, et al. Induction of fibrinogen binding and platelet aggregation as a potential intrinsic property of various GP IIb/IIIa ($\alpha IIb\ \beta 3$) inhibitors. *Blood* 1998;92:3240–3249.

# CHAPTER 30 ■ INTEGRIN $\alpha_{IIb}\beta_3$ AND PLATELET AGGREGATION

ANA KASIRER-FRIEDE, JUN QIN, EDWARD F. PLOW, AND SANFORD J. SHATTIL

## PERSPECTIVE

Approximately 30 years ago, an important insight into the hemostatic function of platelets was established. In characterizing the membrane glycoproteins of platelets by gel electrophoresis, Phillips and Agin (1) noted that two major protein bands, which we now term $\alpha_{IIb}$ (GP IIb) and $\beta_3$ (GP IIIa), were missing from the platelets of patients with Glanzmann thrombasthenia, a rare inherited bleeding disorder associated with an absence of platelet aggregation. Nurden and Caen had earlier observed abnormal gel patterns of the membrane proteins of thrombasthenic platelets (2). These seminal observations triggered extensive investigations in many laboratories into the structure of $\alpha_{IIb}\beta_3$ (GP IIb/IIIa) and its functions in platelet adhesion, aggregation, and hemostasis. In the mid-1980s, another series of observations had a major impact on our understanding of the biology of $\alpha_{IIb}\beta_3$, culminating in the identification of $\alpha_{IIb}\beta_3$ as a member of a family of adhesion receptors called integrins, so called because they *integrated* their extracellular ligands with the intracellular cytoskeleton (3).

A second inherited defect, afibrinogenemia, provided additional key insights into the requirements for platelet aggregation. Platelets from patients with afibrinogenemia (4,5) or washed platelets suspended in defibrinated plasma (6) failed to aggregate, and addition of fibrinogen to the samples restored the response. In the late 1970s and early 1980s, the molecular basis for these observations was established when fibrinogen was found to associate with platelets (7), bind specifically to $\alpha_{IIb}\beta_3$ (8–10), and mediate platelet aggregation (10,11). Subsequently, molecular details of the interaction of fibrinogen with $\alpha_{IIb}\beta_3$ have been defined, and other ligands that interact with $\alpha_{IIb}\beta_3$ to influence platelet aggregation and adhesion have been identified. Work on $\alpha_{IIb}\beta_3$ and its ligands has culminated in the development of parenteral $\alpha_{IIb}\beta_3$ antagonists that have been found useful in the prevention and treatment of arterial thrombosis in specific clinical situations (12). Therefore, our knowledge of $\alpha_{IIb}\beta_3$ has evolved from bands on gels to a detailed understanding of its biology to its successful exploitation as a therapeutic target. Most recently, it has become apparent that integrins function not only as adhesion receptors but also as conduits for bidirectional communication; that is, integrins transmit both inside-out signals to regulate ligand binding and outside-in signals to regulate anchorage-dependent cellular responses, which in the platelet include full aggregation and granule secretion as well as clot retraction. This chapter focuses on $\alpha_{IIb}\beta_3$ and its role in platelet signaling and aggregation. Its relation to other integrin family members provides a backdrop of information that is relevant to its structure, function, and specificity as an adhesion receptor.

## EXPRESSION AND BIOSYNTHESIS OF $\alpha_{IIb}\beta_3$

The synthesis and expression of $\alpha_{IIb}\beta_3$ is restricted: It is primarily synthesized by megakaryocytes and is expressed by these cells and platelets. In addition, $\alpha_{IIb}$ expression has been noted in early murine hematopoietic progenitors and mast cells where its functions remain to be firmly established (13,14). Restricted expression is imposed by the $\alpha_{IIb}$ subunit, and its promoter has been used to target genes to megakaryocytes and platelets (15,16). This limitation is not the case for the $\beta_3$ subunit, because $\alpha_V\beta_3$ is expressed by many cell types, including platelets, endothelial cells, and smooth muscle cells. The genes for $\alpha_{IIb}$ and $\beta_3$ reside in close physical proximity on chromosome 17 (17). The two protein subunits must associate stoichiometrically into a 1:1 noncovalent complex for efficient cell-surface expression (18,19), and naturally occurring mutations that alter the biosynthesis of one subunit affect surface expression of the other (20–23). The subunit association required for surface expression occurs early in biosynthesis in the endoplasmic reticulum (21). Although $\alpha_{IIb}$ is synthesized as a single polypeptide chain, it is proteolytically processed into a heavy and a light chain. This processing is required for cell-surface expression and occurs after the subunits have complexed within the cell (19,24,25). $\alpha_{IIb}\beta_3$ is the most abundant cell-surface glycoprotein on platelets, present at approximately 40,000 to 80,000 copies per cell (18,26,27). In addition, an intracellular pool of $\alpha_{IIb}\beta_3$ is present in the membranes of $\alpha$-granules and can become surface-expressed upon agonist-induced platelet secretion, thereby increasing the number of functional $\alpha_{IIb}\beta_3$ receptors by approximately 30% to 50% (26,28–30). Rapid shuttling of $\alpha_{IIb}\beta_3$ between the cell surface and intracellular pools has been observed (31) and may be involved in the import of fibrinogen into platelet $\alpha$-granules (32).

## STRUCTURE OF $\alpha_{IIb}\beta_3$

$\alpha_{IIb}$ consists of 1,008 amino acids and $\beta_3$ of 762 amino acids (33,34). The extracellular domains of both subunits are glycosylated (24). As assessed by sodium dodecylsulfate polyacrylamide gel electrophoresis under nonreducing conditions, the apparent molecular weights of the $\alpha_{IIb}$ and $\beta_3$ subunits are approximately 130 kDa and approximately 95 kDa, respectively (18). Upon reduction, the $\alpha_{IIb}$ subunit separates into a heavy and light chain of 115 and 25 kDa, respectively. The light chain of $\alpha_{IIb}$ contains a 20–amino acid cytoplasmic tail, a transmembrane helix, and an extracellular segment that is disulfide-linked to the heavy chain. The $\beta_3$ subunit is relatively resistant to reducing conditions, which may reflect its extensive protected

517

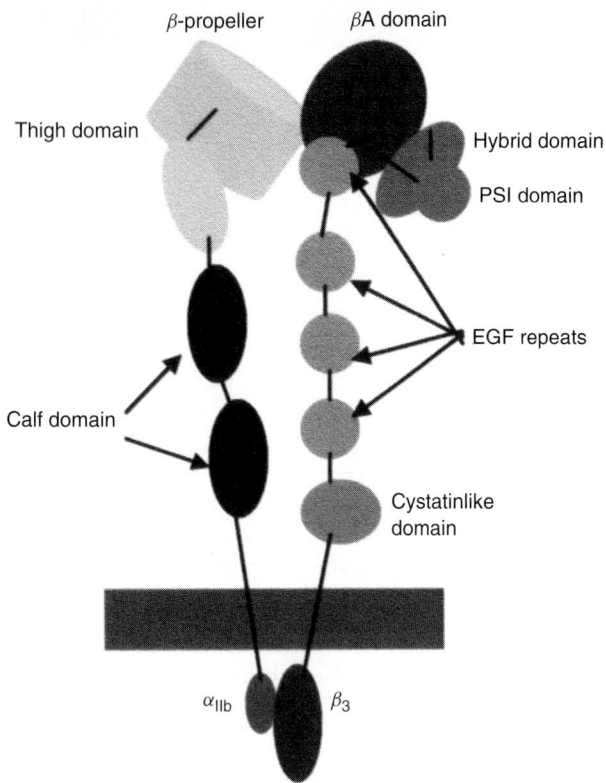

**FIGURE 30-1.** Schematic model showing the organization and structural domains of $\alpha_{IIb}\beta_3$. PSI, plexin-semaphorin-integrin; EGF, epidermal growth factor.

intrachain disulfide-bonding pattern (35). A schematic structural model of $\alpha_{IIb}\beta_3$ is shown in Figure 30-1. The overall shape depicted is based on a cryogenic electron micrographic image of the isolated receptor (36), crystal structures of the homologous $\alpha_V\beta_3$ extracellular domain (37,38), and nuclear magnetic resonance (NMR) analyses of the cytoplasmic face (39,40) and the transmembrane domains (41). In this model, $\alpha_{IIb}\beta_3$ is composed of a globular head resting on two extended

stalks. The head may be bent to approach the cell membrane in the resting state of the receptor and, as discussed in subsequent text, undergo switchblade extension upon activation of the receptor (42) (see Fig. 30-2). The two stalks interact with each other in the resting state and separate in the active state (39,41–45) (Fig. 30-2). Each extracellular subunit consists of a series of linked domains. At the N-terminal aspect of the $\alpha$ subunit is a $\beta$-propeller, a large domain composed of a series of approximately 60 amino acid repeats, which are arranged to form seven blades that extend out from a central core. At the base of the $\beta$-propeller in the $\alpha_{IIb}$ subunit are four divalent binding motifs in which oxygenated amino acids within short hairpin loops coordinate cations. The remainder of the $\alpha$-subunit consists of a thigh and two calf domains. Between the thigh and the first calf module is a "genu," a bend that allows the molecule to bend and compact. The transmembrane domain of the $\alpha_{IIb}$ is likely $\alpha$ helical (41,46) and extends into the cytoplasmic tail. The cytoplasmic helix terminates at a PP-containing turn that allows the acidic C-terminus to fold back to interact with the cytoplasmic helix (39,44). A cation-binding site is likely present and stabilizes the fold-back structure (44,47). The N-terminal aspect of $\beta_3$ was not present in the crystal structure of $\alpha_V\beta_3$ (37,38). Notable features of this region include Cys5, which forms a long disulfide loop to Cys435 (48), and position 33, the site of the PL(A1)/(A2) polymorphism, which has been linked to an increased risk of coronary artery disease in some studies (49). The first major identifiable domain in the $\beta_3$ subunit, the A-domain, is homologous to I-domains found within several integrin $\alpha$-subunits (50). The $\beta_3$A domain contains three divalent cation-binding sites, including a metal ion–dependent adhesion site (MIDAS) motif that is prominently involved in ligand binding. A hybrid and a plexin-semaphorin-integrin (PSI) domain connect the $\beta_3$A domain to a protease-resistant region in which a series of disulfide repeats are arranged into four EGF-like domains. Although these were not well resolved in the original crystal structure, they were later identified by NMR (51), and the PSI domain has since been built into the structure (52). These are followed by a cystatinlike domain (37). The final structural motif discerned in the crystal structure was the $\beta$TD. A transmembrane helix extends into the cytoplasmic tail (41). NMR studies revealed a membrane-proximal helix that interacts with $\alpha_{IIb}$ (39). The helix is followed by a long loop followed by an NPLY turn and another short helix (40).

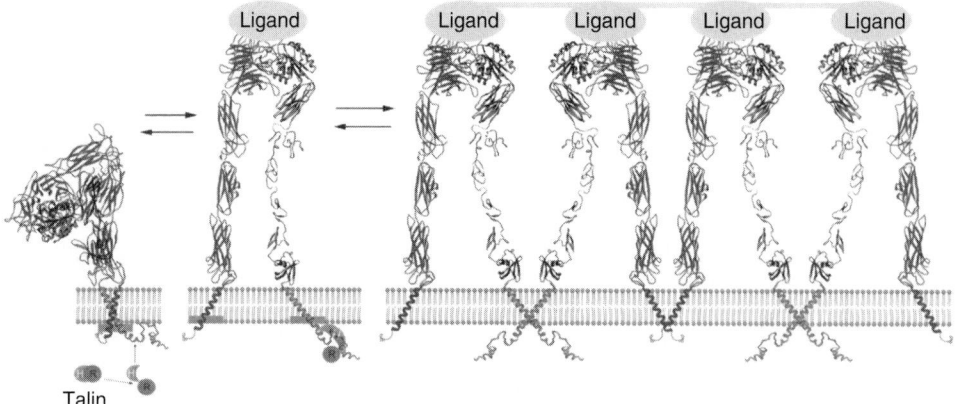

**FIGURE 30-2.** Model of a pathway for activation of $\alpha_{IIb}\beta_3$. Talin binding to the cytoplasmic tail of the $\beta_3$ subunit can lead to unclasping of integrin subunit tails and a membrane-associated structural change of the cytoplasmic face. This change may entail a transition from a bent conformation in its resting state to an extended conformation in which it becomes competent to bind soluble ligands. The receptors can also cluster, further enhancing their avidity for ligand. The $\alpha$-subunit is in *blue* and the $\beta$-subunit is in *red* (see Color Fig. 30-2). (Reproduced with permission from Qin J, Vinogradova O, Plow EF. Integrin bidirectional signaling: a molecular view. *PLoS Biol.* 2004;2:e169.)

The ligand-binding site with which fibrinogen and other adhesive ligands react resides within the globular head and is formed by both subunits (54). Point mutations within either $\alpha_{IIb}$ or $\beta_3$ can impair the capacity of the receptor to interact with ligand (55–59). Such analyses, together with the crystal structure of the homologous $\alpha_V\beta_3$ extracellular domain in complex with RGD peptide (also a ligand for $\alpha_{IIb}\beta_3$; see subsequent text) (38), studies of chemical cross-linking (60,61), synthetic peptides (62–64), and site-directed antibodies (65), have been used to implicate several specific sequences as ligand contact sites within $\alpha_{IIb}\beta_3$. These sequences indicate that the ligand-binding pocket is a complex three-dimensional structure formed by multiple discontinuous residues within each subunit (37).

# PLATELET AGGREGATION IS MEDIATED BY $\alpha_{IIb}\beta_3$

The primary function of $\alpha_{IIb}\beta_3$ is to serve as a receptor for macromolecular ligands (18). Engagement of these ligands bestows adhesive properties to platelets. Major adhesive ligands of $\alpha_{IIb}\beta_3$ include fibrinogen (8), fibrin (66), von Willebrand factor (VWF) (67), fibronectin (68), vitronectin (69), and thrombospondin (70). All of these ligands are constituents of extracellular matrices, and when presented in this format, their interactions with $\alpha_{IIb}\beta_3$ support platelet adhesion. Contributions of $\alpha_{IIb}\beta_3$ to platelet adhesion have been demonstrated with many of these ligands and under a variety of conditions (71–73). Each of these ligands can also interact with at least one additional receptor on platelets. For example, fibrinogen can bind to $\alpha_V\beta_3$ (74) and $\alpha_5\beta_1$ (75), VWF to GP Ib/IX/V (76), fibronectin to $\alpha_5\beta_1$ (77), vitronectin to $\alpha_V\beta_3$ (78), and thrombospondin to GP IV (CD36) (79,80).

Central to the function of $\alpha_{IIb}\beta_3$ on platelets is its capacity to mediate platelet aggregation. This response requires engagement of $\alpha_{IIb}\beta_3$ by soluble fibrinogen (8,10,11) or VWF (73). At high shear rates, such as those attained in stenosed arteries, VWF binding to $\alpha_{IIb}\beta_3$ is necessary for productive platelet aggregation (73,81–83). Key to $\alpha_{IIb}\beta_3$ function in platelet aggregation is its capacity to undergo a transformation from a *resting* low-affinity state to an *activated* high-affinity state (Fig. 30-2). As discussed in detail later, platelet agonists engage their receptors and induce intracellular responses, referred to as inside-out signaling, that converge on the cytoskeletal protein, talin. In turn, talin binds to the cytoplasmic tail of the $\beta_3$ subunit (84,85) and dissociates it from the $\alpha_{IIb}$ cytoplasmic tail (39). This triggers conformational changes that are transmitted through the transmembrane segments of the integrin to activate ligand binding to the extracellular domains. Transitions during integrin activation include a release of the receptor from the bent conformation in its resting state to an extended format in its activated state (42); local conformational changes within the $\beta_3$A domain (86); and changes in intermolecular interactions between the transmembrane domains that promote separation of those domains (87,88). In some cases, high-affinity ligand binding may occur in the absence of full extension of the head domain (89). Inside-out signaling may also promote the clustering of integrin heterodimers into oligomers (90), and clustering would be expected to increase receptor avidity or valency. However, conformational change and affinity modulation appear to be the dominant mechanism by which ligand binding to $\alpha_{IIb}\beta_3$ or $\alpha_V\beta_3$ is regulated (88,91).

## Ligand Recognition Specificity

Fibrinogen binding to activated $\alpha_{IIb}\beta_3$ is divalent cation-dependent, rapid, and initially reversible, with dissociation constant ($K_d$) approximately 300 nM (8,9,92,93). Stabilization then occurs, and the bound fibrinogen becomes essentially nondissociable (92–96). This transition stabilizes platelet aggregates and presumably depends upon the formation of additional molecular contacts between the ligand and $\alpha_{IIb}\beta_3$ (94,97). Stabilization may be promoted by multiple factors, including ligand-induced structural changes in the receptor (95,98), receptor clustering, cytoskeletal reinforcements (99), fibrinogen self-association or association of fibrinogen with other adhesive proteins, such as thrombospondin (100,101), and receptor internalization (102). Although the dimeric structure of fibrinogen and the multimeric structure of VWF may permit these ligands to bridge between receptors on adjacent platelets and thereby mediate aggregation (103), such cross-bridging may not be the only mechanism that determines the size of platelet aggregates (104,105). Postreceptor occupancy events occur upon binding of fibrinogen to $\alpha_{IIb}\beta_3$ (106) and are important for maximal aggregation. One direct manifestation of receptor occupancy is the induction of ligand-induced binding sites (LIBS), which serve as epitopes for monoclonal antibodies that react with the occupied but not with the resting or activated, unoccupied conformers of $\alpha_{IIb}\beta_3$ (107–109). Occupancy of $\alpha_{IIb}\beta_3$ also leads to a series of intracellular responses, referred to as *outside-in signaling* (see subsequent text) (104,110,111).

Two synthetic peptides of four to six amino acids define the recognition specificity of fibrinogen for $\alpha_{IIb}\beta_3$ (112). The first of these peptides corresponds to the extreme carboxy terminus of one of the three constituent chains of fibrinogen, the $\gamma$ chain (113, 114). The final six amino acids of the $\gamma$ chain are KQAGDV, and this peptide or variants thereof, referred to collectively as the $\gamma$ chain peptides, interacts with $\alpha_{IIb}\beta_3$ (115). The sequence is found in fibrinogen but not in other $\alpha_{IIb}\beta_3$ ligands. Nevertheless, the $\gamma$ chain peptide does inhibit the binding of other adhesive proteins to $\alpha_{IIb}\beta_3$ (105,116). A naturally occurring variant (the $\gamma'$ variant) of fibrinogen, in which an alternative sequence terminates the constituent chain, does not bind to $\alpha_{IIb}\beta_3$ and does not support platelet aggregation (117,118). Furthermore, mutational studies conducted *in vitro* (119) and *in vivo* (120) indicate that the $\gamma$ chain sequence is essential for productive interaction of fibrinogen with $\alpha_{IIb}\beta_3$. The second peptide, referred to as the RGD peptide, has Arg-Gly-Asp-X (where X is most amino acids) as its minimal sequence. Two RGD sequences reside in the A$\alpha$ chain of human fibrinogen, and RGD peptides inhibit fibrinogen binding to $\alpha_{IIb}\beta_3$ and platelet aggregation (121–123). Indeed, several of the $\alpha_{IIb}\beta_3$ therapeutic antagonists have been designed from the RGD sequence (12,124). However, mutation of either of these sequences does not alter fibrinogen recognition by the receptor (119). RGD sequences are present within and mediate the interaction of several other ligands with $\alpha_{IIb}\beta_3$. In particular, mutation of the RGD sequence in VWF (125) and vitronectin (126) prevents their interaction with $\alpha_{IIb}\beta_3$. Fibronectin contains an RGD sequence as well as several alternative sequences that interact with $\alpha_{IIb}\beta_3$ (127,128). Furthermore, RGD functions as a major recognition sequence for several other integrins, including $\alpha_V\beta_3$ (129). Secondary roles of the RGD or other sequences in stabilizing fibrinogen: $\alpha_{IIb}\beta_3$ interactions have not been excluded. Indeed, recent observations point to a role for still other sequences, unrelated to the RGD and $\gamma$ chain peptides, in $\alpha_{IIb}\beta_3$-dependent retraction of fibrin clots by platelets (130,131).

## $\alpha_{IIb}\beta_3$ Antagonists

Although platelet adhesion is mediated by many receptors and platelet aggregation can be induced by many agonists, aggregation itself is absolutely dependent upon $\alpha_{IIb}\beta_3$. This funneling of function onto $\alpha_{IIb}\beta_3$ provides a firm rationale for blockade of its ligand-binding activity as an antithrombotic strategy. This rationale has stimulated an intensive effort to develop specific and potent $\alpha_{IIb}\beta_3$ antagonists throughout the 1990s. In some respects, this effort was successful, but the hope that these drugs would provide both short-term and long-term protection against cardiovascular disease proved to be overly optimistic (131). Three $\alpha_{IIb}\beta_3$ antagonists, abciximab (ReoPro), eptifibatide (Integrilin), and tirofiban (Aggrastat), were approved by the FDA as antithrombotics for specific indications. These drugs are utilized widely to prevent acute coronary events in association with percutaneous coronary interventions (PCIs) and are very effective in this context (132). All three drugs are administered intravenously (PCI) and have similar mechanisms of action: blockade of ligand binding to $\alpha_{IIb}\beta_3$. Integrin antagonists may block function of the receptors by direct competition with ligand or by inducing allosteric changes in the integrin to perturb the ligand-binding site (45). The mechanism of action of the three FDA approved $\alpha_{IIb}\beta_3$ antagonists has not been firmly established, although they do not appear to react with a single site in the receptor (133). Abciximab, the first $\alpha_{IIb}\beta_3$ antagonist approved for human use, is a Fab fragment of a humanized mouse monoclonal antibody to $\alpha_{IIb}\beta_3$ (124,134,135). Abciximab also reacts with $\alpha_V\beta_3$ and $\alpha_M\beta_2$ and some of the positive effects of this drug may be attributable to this cross-reactivity (136). Integrilin is a cyclic peptide. Its origin is the snake venom disintegrin, barbourin, which was identified as a potent and specific inhibitor of $\alpha_{IIb}\beta_3$ and contains a K(Lys)GD within a structure rigidified within a disulfide loop (137). The RGD peptide was the starting point for the design of tirofiban, but this drug no longer has peptide bonds in its structure (138). Following on the early successes of these drugs in the setting of PCI, it was anticipated that they would also be efficacious in reducing acute coronary syndromes in general. However, clinical trials demonstrated only modest or no benefits, and they ultimately did not stack up well against more general platelet antagonists, such as clopidogrel, in terms of cost and efficacy. Also, there was great anticipation that orally active $\alpha_{IIb}\beta_3$ antagonists, which could be administered long-term, would reduce the risk of thrombotic events (139). In fact, several orally active and potent $\alpha_{IIb}\beta_3$ antagonists were developed and tested in clinical trials. These drugs were found in the best of cases to have little clinical benefit and, in the worst of cases, to be detrimental. Indeed, metaanalysis of the reported clinical trials suggested an increase in mortality in patients given oral $\alpha_{IIb}\beta_3$ antagonists (140). As a result, the development of oral $\alpha_{IIb}\beta_3$ antagonists has been largely abandoned. The basis for these negative results is not clear because the principle that blockade of the receptor should prevent thrombus formation is mechanistically sound. However, dosing is very complicated. Underdosing would be ineffective and overdosing could cause bleeding. The possibility that interaction of drug with $\alpha_{IIb}\beta_3$ may actually induce platelet activation received considerable attention in the literature but was not convincingly demonstrated. At this juncture, it appears that $\alpha_{IIb}\beta_3$ antagonists are useful but with limited indications (131).

# REGULATION OF THE LIGAND-BINDING FUNCTION OF $\alpha_{IIb}\beta_3$ (INSIDE-OUT SIGNALING)

The concentrations of VWF and fibrinogen in plasma are in excess of those needed to saturate $\alpha_{IIb}\beta_3$ receptors on the surface of platelets. Platelet aggregation and adhesion can also be supported by pools of $\alpha_{IIb}\beta_3$ normally shielded from the extracellular environment by virtue of their location in the membranes of $\alpha$-granules or the open canalicular system. In addition to inside-out activation of plasma membrane $\alpha_{IIb}\beta_3$, the functional contributions of these "internal" pools of receptors are dependent on signaling reactions that promote granule exocytosis and increased access of open canalicular

membranes to extracellular ligands. Interestingly, some of the $\alpha_{IIb}\beta_3$ within $\alpha$-granule membranes may already be complexed with fibrinogen stored within the granules (141).

Inside-out signaling can be triggered by the interaction of any one of a number of diverse agonists with their cognate receptors in the platelet plasma membrane (see Chapters 31 to 34). For example, thrombin, adenosine diphosphate (ADP), epinephrine, and thromboxane $A_2$ activate $\alpha_{IIb}\beta_3$ by binding to heptahelical, G protein–linked receptors (142–146); collagen interacts with integrin $\alpha_2\beta_1$ and GP VI (147); and VWF interacts with GP Ib/IX/V under conditions of high shear (72,148). Furthermore, ADP working through $P2Y_1$ and $P2Y_{12}$ receptors has been shown to constitute a significant component of the total platelet stimulus initiated through multiple other receptors (149,150). In pathologic situations, $\alpha_{IIb}\beta_3$ may also become activated by immune complexes through engagement of Fc$\gamma$RIIA receptors and by C5b-9, the membrane attack complex of complement (151). Studies conducted with selective inhibitors of various signaling molecules provide strong circumstantial evidence that a serine-threonine kinase; protein kinase C (PKC); and a lipid kinase, *phosphatidylinositide 3OH-kinase (PI 3-K)*, are important intermediates in a complicated network of biochemical reactions that lead to the activation of $\alpha_{IIb}\beta_3$ (see Fig. 30-3) (110). These networks involve various kinases, phosphatases, and adaptors, which together regulate the positive activation and negative downregulation of platelet functionality. However, critical gaps remain in our understanding of the reactions that link agonist or antagonist receptors to the ligand-binding function of $\alpha_{IIb}\beta_3$.

## Protein Kinase C

Platelets contain conventional ($\alpha$, $\beta I$, bII, $\gamma$), atypical ($\zeta$, $\iota/\lambda$) and novel ($\delta$I-III, $\theta$I-II, $\eta$) isoforms of PKC (152). The conventional isoforms are activated by diacylglycerol, a direct product of phospholipase C-mediated phosphoinositide hydrolysis, and by cytoplasmic free $Ca^{2+}$, levels of which are increased by IP3, the other product of phosphoinositide hydrolysis. PKC was first implicated in affinity modulation of $\alpha_{IIb}\beta_3$ by the effects of nonselective PKC inhibitors (153–155). Specific PKC isoforms may help to mediate inside-out signaling, whereas others may mediate outside-in signaling or granule secretion (156–163). At the present time, it has not been clearly established which PKC isoforms operate in inside-out signaling and what their relevant substrates are, although the RACK family of isozyme-selective membrane anchoring proteins, substrates for activated C-kinase (RACKs) (164), likely represent one basis for PKC isoform-specific functional selectivity (163,165).

Platelets contain at least five isoforms of phospholipase C, including phospholipases C$\beta$ and C$\gamma_2$ (166,167), which may all be activated by $Ca^{2+}$ *in vitro*. In addition, phospholipase C$\beta$ is activated directly by G$\alpha$q, which is coupled to several G protein–linked receptors in platelets (144,168). Phospholipase C$\gamma$2, however, may be activated by tyrosine phosphorylation in platelets stimulated with thrombin (169) or following tyrosine kinase–coupled receptor activation (170–173), and it is a known substrate for Src and Syk (174,175). Evidence that these or other tyrosine kinases are involved in inside-out signaling comes from studies using selective tyrosine kinase inhibitors, which partially block fibrinogen binding and platelet aggregation, and from studies using inhibitors of tyrosine phosphatases, which trigger platelet activation (174,176). Although mice deficient in PLC$\gamma$2 show weak collagen-induced activation of $\alpha_{IIb}\beta_3$, the intraperitoneal and gastrointestinal hemorrhaging described in these mice nevertheless allude to the importance of this phospholipase (177,178).

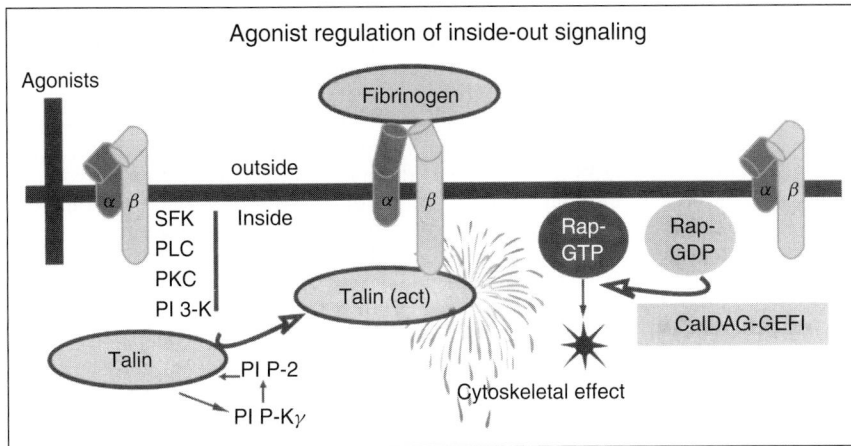

**FIGURE 30-3.** Model of a pathway for inside-out signaling to integrin $\alpha_{IIb}\beta_3$ in platelets. $\alpha_{IIb}\beta_3$ equilibrates between resting and activated states, the resting state predominating in unstimulated platelets and the activated state in stimulated platelets. Agonists induce activation of signaling intermediates, which leads to cytoskeletal changes, talin activation, affinity modulation of integrin $\alpha_{IIb}\beta_3$, and soluble ligand binding. The model depicted is incomplete and represents only some of the many molecules involved in this very complex process. Readers are referred to the text for a limited discussion. SFK, Src family kinase; PLC, phospholipase C; PKC, protein kinase C; PI 3-K, phosphatidylinositide 3OH-kinase; PI P-2, phosphatidylinositol-4'5'-biphosphate; PI P-K$\gamma$, phosphatidyl-inositol-phosphate kinase, gamma isoform.

## Phosphatidylinositide 3OH-Kinase

PI 3-K phosphorylates the 3OH group of phosphatidylinositols (PtdIns), including PtdIns(4)P and PtdIns(4,5)P2, to yield PtdIns(3,4)P2 and PtdIns(3,4,5)P3, respectively. At least four PI 3-K isoforms are present in platelets, including the two best characterized type I isoforms, p85/p110 and p110$\gamma$ (179–181). PtdIns(3,4)P2 and PtdIns(3,4,5)P3 are membrane-embedded and transduce signals in part by binding to specific PH and SH2 domains in relevant signaling proteins, thereby recruiting them to their locus of action at the membrane (182). Interestingly, 3-phosphorylated phosphoinositides can activate certain atypical and novel isoforms of PKC (182), suggesting one possible link between PI 3-K, PKC, and affinity modulation of $\alpha_{IIb}\beta_3$. Although 3-phosphorylated phosphoinositides produced in response to thrombin stimulation may function more to stabilize fibrinogen binding to $\alpha_{IIb}\beta_3$ rather than to initiate it (183), other studies suggest a more prominent role for PI 3-K in platelet activation: (i) ligation of GP Ib/IX/V induces the dissociation of PI 3-K from an $\alpha$-actinin/PtdIns(3,4)P2 complex (184) and its association with Src, an early upstream effector in the GP Ib/IX/V signaling pathway (185), (ii) mice deficient in Akt 1 and Akt 2 (important downstream effectors of PI 3-K) have impaired thrombin-induced fibrinogen binding (186), (iii) PI 3-K is necessary for $\alpha_{IIb}\beta_3$-independent Rac activation downstream of collagen (187), (iv) PI 3-K may amplify platelet secretion through an ADP-dependent feedback loop (188), and (v) a PI 3-K inhibitor greatly decreases binding of the ligand-mimetic antibody PAC-1 to $\alpha_{IIb}\beta_3$ in response to occupancy of GP Ib/IX/V by VWF (153).

## Ras Superfamily GTPases

Platelets contain members of the Ras [H-Ras, R-Ras, Rap1a, Rap2b (189), Rala (190), Rab] and Rho (cdc42, Rac1, RhoA) families of small GTPases (191,192). They may function as regulators of integrin affinity or of cytoskeletal organization and cell morphology. Ras family members are known primarily for their mitogenic effects and for activation of mitogen-activated protein (extracellular signal-regulated kinase) kinases in nucleated cells. However, in platelets, Ras and Erk may be activated independently of each other (193). Stimulation of the anucleate platelet by thrombin, convulxin, or thrombopoietin causes Ras GTP loading (194). Of note, when activated forms of H-Ras or Raf-1 are overexpressed in Chinese hamster ovary (CHO) cells, they *inhibit* the affinity/avidity state of $\alpha_{IIb}\beta_3$ (195). In contrast, expression of activated R-Ras *increases* integrin-mediated adhesion of cultured cells (196)

and of platelets (197) by sequences residing in the hypervariable C-terminal region (198).

Rap1, a small Ras-like GTPase, is activated in response to platelet agonists and upon adhesion to fibrinogen (199,200), and activation is dependent on increased cytoplasmic-free calcium (201) and PI 3-K (202). Rap1 associates with the actin cytoskeleton of activated platelets and is a substrate for protein kinase A (PKA) (203), although the effect of this phosphorylation is unknown. In mouse megakaryocytes activated through the Par-4 thrombin receptor, expression of Rap1b, the predominant isoform in platelets, has been shown to increase agonist-induced fibrinogen binding to $\alpha_{IIb}\beta_3$, an effect inhibited by blocking actin polymerization with cytochalasin D. Conversely, overexpression of Rap1-GTPase-activating protein (Rap1-GAP), which converts Rap1-GTP to Rap1-GDP, partially blocks agonist-induced fibrinogen binding (204). Therefore, Rap1b promotes, but is not sufficient for, inside-out signaling. Although some potential Rap1 regulators and effectors have recently been identified (205,206), the specific Rap effector(s) responsible for potentiating fibrinogen binding are unknown. The importance of Rap1 in platelet function is reflected by the defects found in mice lacking Cal-DAG, a GEFI for Rap1 (207). Mice show severe bleeding defects, decreased platelet aggregation, and thrombus formation (208). Furthermore, ablation of Rap1 itself is mostly embryonic lethal, with decreased platelet aggregation in survivors (209).

## Proximal Effectors of Inside-Out Signaling

Evidence implicating the transmembrane domains and cytoplasmic tails of $\alpha_{IIb}$ and/or $\beta_3$ in the process of affinity modulation comes from studies of naturally occurring and experimental integrin mutations, analyses of $\alpha_{IIb}\beta_3$ function in heterologous expression systems, and identification of integrin tail-binding proteins (87,88,110). These results suggest a working model in which the membrane-proximal portions and transmembrane domain of $\alpha_{IIb}$ interact with the corresponding portions of $\beta_3$; in particular, the cytoplasmic tails of $\alpha_{IIb}$ and $\beta_3$ interact through one or more salt bridges to form a "hinge" through which signals impacting on membrane-distal tail residues are propagated across the membrane to modulate receptor affinity. Certain membrane-proximal and transmembrane domain mutations or deletions can "break" this hinge, leaving the receptor in a permanent high-affinity state.

One $\beta_3$ tail interacting protein that has been strongly implicated in inside-out $\alpha_{IIb}\beta_3$ activation is talin. Talin is a highly flexible 270-kDa protein, which homodimerizes in an antiparallel fashion (210,211). Each subunit consists of an N-terminal 50-kDa FERM domain containing a head region and a 220-kDa carboxy-terminal rod region. Binding to $\beta$ integrins [$\beta_{1D}$, $\beta_2$, $\beta_3$ and $\beta_5$, and weakly to $\beta_7$ (212,213)], occurs primarily through the FERM domain in the head region, although an additional lower-affinity site resides in the tail (214). Talin is a good candidate to link integrin cytoplasmic domains to the actin cytoskeleton because there are multiple binding sites in the protein for vinculin and actin (215–219). Overexpression of a fragment of talin head domain, talin F2-F3, activates integrin $\alpha_{IIb}\beta_3$ by binding to $\beta_3$ cytoplasmic tails (39,213,220). Importantly, evidence suggesting that talin is a direct final inducer of $\alpha_{IIb}\beta_3$ activation has been accumulating: (a) NMR studies indicate that the normal interaction between the $\alpha_{IIb}$ and $\beta_3$ tails may be disrupted by talin, leading to integrin conformational changes (39,40,221); (b) a knockdown of talin in CHO cells expressing $\alpha_{IIb}\beta_3$, or in primary megakaryocytes, reduced energy-dependent $\beta_3$ integrin activation (85). Talin binding to integrin $\beta$ tails may be regulated by phosphorylation (222), calpain cleavage (223), PI P-2 (224), or competition for binding to talin head by phosphotidyl-inositol-phosphate kinase, gamma isoform (PI P-K$\gamma$) (225). In addition, binding of talin to PI P-K$\gamma$ activates the enzyme, further emphasizing talin's roles as a regulatory and structural protein of the cytoskeleton (226–228).

## Downregulation of Inside-Out Signaling

In addition to the aforementioned potential negative regulation of $\alpha_{IIb}\beta_3$ by H-Ras, ligand-binding to $\alpha_{IIb}\beta_3$ is suppressed by factors that increase platelet cyclic adenosine monophosphate (AMP) or cyclic guanosine 3'-5-monophosphate (GMP), such as PGI$_2$ and nitric oxide, respectively (229,230). A common substrate of cyclic AMP-dependent and cyclic GMP-dependent protein kinases is vasodilator-stimulated phospho-protein (VASP), a 50-kDa protein that binds to vinculin, localizes to focal adhesions, and regulates actin dynamics. Phosphorylation of VASP on specific serine residues by agents that increase cyclic AMP or cyclic GMP correlates with inhibition of platelet aggregation (229), whereas deletion of the VASP gene results in enhanced platelet aggregation (231). However, the role of VASP in $\alpha_{IIb}\beta_3$ function and the mechanisms by which cyclic nucleotides downregulate inside-out signaling remain to be determined. Surprisingly, mouse platelets lacking platelet/endothelial cell adhesion molecule-1 (PECAM-1) show similarly enhanced platelet aggregation (232). PECAM-1, an ITIM-containing inhibitory receptor, may counteract signal transduction pathways of ITAM-containing receptors through its ability to recruit and activate protein-tyrosine or inositol phosphatases, such as SHP2 (232). CD39, an ecto-ADPase on endothelial cells, may also downregulate platelet responses *in vivo* by removing the agonist, ADP, from the vascular milieu (233,234). As a corollary, all mechanisms that attenuate signaling prompted by direct or costimulatory agonists, newly generated or released, will also prevent continued activation.

# REGULATION OF PLATELET FUNCTION BY $\alpha_{IIb}\beta_3$ (OUTSIDE-IN SIGNALING)

Several platelet responses are dependent, in part, on the initial binding of fibrinogen or VWF to $\alpha_{IIb}\beta_3$. These include (a) firm adhesion under high shear conditions (73,235); (b) spreading on extracellular matrices containing fibrinogen or VWF (236); (c) secretion from platelet $\alpha$- and dense granules

in response to "weak" agonists, such as ADP or epinephrine; (d) conversion of small platelet aggregates into larger, more hemostatically effective ones; (e) fibrin clot retraction (237); and (f) development of platelet procoagulant activity and the generation of platelet microparticles in response to certain stimuli, for example, collagen, thrombin, C5b9 (238,239). Some of these responses may require only ligand binding to $\alpha_{IIb}\beta_3$ (adhesion, spreading), whereas others require platelet aggregation (secretion) or, under some experimental conditions, can be completely independent of $\alpha_{IIb}\beta_3$ (secretion, procoagulant activity). Of note, in a cell-free system, $\alpha_{IIb}\beta_3$ itself can evolve toward a conformational state minimizing dissociability of bound fibrinogen (97), and it may be from such a stabilized conformation that outside-in signals propagate. There is a temporal and spatial hierarchy to outside-in signaling in platelets that may be analogous to that observed in nucleated cells, although the details likely differ (240). Therefore, for physiologic function, platelets need to activate signaling pathways leading to cytoskeletal remodeling for platelet spreading, adhesion stabilization, and eventually clot retraction.

Ligation of $\alpha_{IIb}\beta_3$ by physiologic ligands initiates a cascade of outside-in signaling events (see Fig. 30-4) thought to begin with ligand occupancy and integrin oligomerization (91,241–243). Clustering may involve heterooligomerization of the integrin subunits as well as homooligomerization (244,245). A major early event following fibrinogen binding to $\alpha_{IIb}\beta_3$ is tyrosine phosphorylation of a number of platelet proteins triggered by Src family kinases. In resting platelets, c-Src is associated with the integrin $\beta_3$ tail (246), along with Csk, which phosphorylates Src Y529 and maintains Src in an autoinhibited state. Fibrinogen binding and $\alpha_{IIb}\beta_3$ clustering induce Csk dissociation from the $\alpha_{IIb}\beta_3$ complex, resulting in Y529 dephosphorylation and Src activation. At the same time, the Syk tyrosine kinase is recruited to the integrin complex and becomes activated. In the mouse, both Src family kinases and Syk are required for full platelet spreading on fibrinogen (243,246,247). This is because their localized activation results in the assembly of a larger signaling complex made up of additional enzymes, adapter molecules, and substrates, including Slp-76, Btk, Nck, and cdc 42, that promote actin polymerization and reorganization (110,248–250). c-Src-focal adhesion kinase (FAK) complexes form at later stages of adhesion to fibrinogen, or postthrombin-induced platelet aggregation (251), and are localized to focal complexes and focal adhesions (243). A homolog of FAK, phosphotyrosine kinase 2 (Pyk2) (252) is similarly phosphorylated following thrombin activation in aggregated platelets or platelets adherent to fibrinogen, but in contrast to FAK, it becomes activated soon after platelet stimulation by agonists, in a manner that is independent of adhesive ligand binding to $\alpha_{IIb}\beta_3$ (253).

Specific domains of $\beta_3$ serve to transduce signals subsequent to ligand binding. The region of $\beta_3$ encompassing residues 741 to 762, referred to as the ICY domain, contains two tyrosines (747:NpxY and 759:NITY) (254), which become phosphorylated following fibrinogen-dependent platelet aggregation induced by thrombin or LIBS antibodies (250,255,256). Tyrosine phosphorylation of these residues creates one or more docking sites for proteins important for cytoskeletal reorganization, including Shc, myosin, and possibly Pyk2 (255–257). Disruption of $\beta_3$ tyrosines (256) reduces spreading on fibrinogen and produces unstable platelet aggregates, without decreasing activation by ADP and thrombin (258–261). Tyrosine phosphorylation may also be regulated by sCD40L (262) and mu-calpain (263), and may, in turn, support the trafficking of additional signaling partners (256,264,265). In contrast to the proadhesive phenotype promoted by $\beta_3$ tyrosine phosphorylation, phosphorylation of threonine 753 appears to negatively regulate platelet adhesion and spreading on fibrinogen (264, 266,267). Changes in $\beta_3$ secondary structure, as noted in two

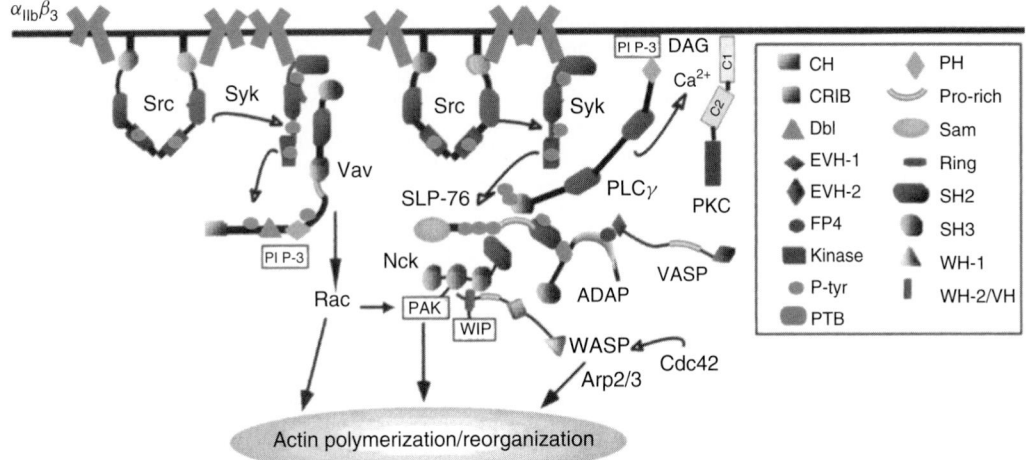

**FIGURE 30-4.** Cartoon depicting selected aspects of outside-in signaling in platelets. (1) Agonists induce affinity modulation, and ligand binding induces integrin clustering. (2) Ligated and clustered $\alpha_{IIb}\beta_3$ triggers early events, such as activation of Src and Syk, and (3) a cascade of signaling events lead to activation and recruitment of cytoskeletal proteins WIP, Wiskott-Aldrich syndrome protein (WASP), and Arp2/3, which can eventually nucleate actin filament growth and provoke cytoskeletal reorganization. The insert provides a key to some of the modules or domains within the proteins that mediate or regulate protein functions and/or interactions. Domain abbreviations: CH, calponin homology; P-tyr, phosphotyrosine; PTB, phosphotyrosine binding; PH, pleckstrin homology; WH, WASP homology; and VH, verprolin homology. WIP indicates WASP interacting protein; PLC$\gamma$, phospholipase C$\gamma$. No attempt is made to show all proteins involved or all interactions of a given protein (see Color Fig. 30-4). (Reproduced with permission from Shattil SJ, Newman PJ. Integrins: dynamic scaffolds for adhesion and signaling in platelets. *Blood* 2004; 104:1606–1615.)

polymorphisms [PL(A1) and PL(A2)], found in the N-terminal region (268), similarly alter $\beta_3$-mediated responses. In particular, the PL(A2) polymorphism enhances actin polymerization and cell spreading in a CHO cell model, while leaving soluble fibrinogen binding unaffected (269), although at present it is unclear how the modification in the extracellular domain can augment outside-in responses. Furthermore, still other integrin tail-binding proteins, for example, CIB, have the potential to modulate outside-in signaling, although their roles *in vivo* remain to be explored (270–272). Finally, outside-in signaling through $\alpha_{IIb}\beta_3$ may induce dense-granule secretion of ADP and generation of thromboxane A$_2$ (TxA$_2$) (273) for stabilization of adhesion under shear flow (248).

Because focal adhesions are dynamic structures, mechanisms must also exist to downregulate focal adhesion assembly. These may include the dephosphorylation of certain focal adhesion proteins by tyrosine phosphatases (274–276) and their cleavage by calpain and other proteases (237). In platelets, there are multiple layers of regulation: (a) beginning at the level of the integrin itself, the protein phosphatase 1 (PP1), which is associated with $\alpha_{IIb}$ cytoplasmic domain residues 989KVG992, dissociates and dephosphorylates myosin light chain following stimulation with thrombin (277); and certain Src family members, particularly Lyn, may attenuate outside-in signaling by phosphorylation of the inositol phosphatase, SHIP1 (278,279); and (b) farther downstream, dephosphorylation of FAK by PTEN also inhibits spreading and dephosphorylates products of PI 3-K in other cells, and likely in platelets (280–282).

## INTEGRIN $\alpha_V\beta_3$

Compared to the high expression of $\alpha_{IIb}\beta_3$, there are only a few hundred molecules of $\alpha_V\beta_3$ per platelet, and its physiologic significance in this cell is unclear. Nonetheless, this section provides a brief comparison of $\alpha_V\beta_3$ with $\alpha_{IIb}\beta_3$ to make several specific points. Reviews of $\alpha_V\beta_3$ should be consulted for more focused information on specific functions of this receptor (283–285). $\alpha_{IIb}\beta_3$ and $\alpha_V\beta_3$ share the same $\beta$ subunit, and the $\alpha$-subunits are approximately 40% identical in amino acid sequence. Among the most notable structural differences in $\alpha_{IIb}$ and $\alpha_V$, the cytoplasmic tail of $\alpha_V$ is longer than that of $\alpha_{IIb}$ (286). The two sister integrins bind many of the same ligands, including the two ligands that can mediate platelet aggregation, fibrinogen and VWF (287), but ligands that bind to one receptor but not the other have also been identified; for example, osteopontin (288) and adenovirus penton base (289) bind to $\alpha_V\beta_3$ but not to $\alpha_{IIb}\beta_3$, and barbourin binds to $\alpha_{IIb}\beta_3$ but not to $\alpha_V\beta_3$ (137). This pattern is recapitulated at the level of the fine recognition specificities of the two receptors; RGD peptides bind with much higher affinity to $\alpha_V\beta_3$ than to $\alpha_{IIb}\beta_3$, and $\gamma$ chain peptides bind with much higher affinity to $\alpha_{IIb}\beta_3$ than to $\alpha_V\beta_3$ (290). Drugs that react selectively with each receptor have been designed, although it remains to be determined if such specificity is any advantage among the $\alpha_{IIb}\beta_3$ antagonists. Like $\alpha_{IIb}\beta_3$, $\alpha_V\beta_3$ can undergo activation (91,291,292), even in platelets (293).

On adhesive cells such as osteoclasts, smooth muscle cells, or fibroblasts, $\alpha_V\beta_3$ localizes to podosomes or focal adhesions (294–296) and directly or indirectly mediates recruitment of signaling and cytoskeletal proteins into these structures. FAK, integrin-linked kinase (ILK), and Src kinases, several phosphatases, talin, vinculin, and actin, as well as other cytoskeletal-associated proteins, colocalize within these sites, which change dynamically over time (see preceding text). The breadth of the functions ascribed to $\alpha_V\beta_3$ has stimulated the development of specific $\alpha_V\beta_3$ antagonists, but data from clinical trials in humans are not yet available. In addition, $\alpha_V\beta_3$ is a cellular-binding site for adenoviruses, provides a route for cellular infectivity (297), and is a binding site for matrix metalloproteinase-2 (298), which may be important in the tissue remodeling associated with $\alpha_V\beta_3$-mediated cell migration.

Glanzmann thrombasthenia can arise from a defect in either the $\alpha_{IIb}$ or $\beta_3$ genes, with the latter giving rise to a deficiency of $\alpha_V$ as well as $\alpha_{IIb}$ (299). No distinct phenotype has been reported among individuals lacking one compared to both $\beta_3$ integrins. This lack of unique functions ascribable to $\alpha_V\beta_3$ in humans may be due to the existence of several other $\alpha_V$ integrins with overlapping functions (300). Knockout of the $\alpha_V$ gene in mice is lethal (301).

# References

1. Phillips DR, Agin PP. Platelet membrane defects in Glanzmann's thrombasthenia. Evidence for decreased amounts of two major glycoproteins. *J Clin Invest* 1977;60:535–545.
2. Nurden AT, Caen JP. An abnormal platelet glycoprotein pattern in three cases of Glanzmann's thrombasthenia. *Br J Haematol* 1974;28:253–260.
3. Hynes RO. Integrins: bidirectional, allosteric signaling machines. *Cell* 2002;110:673–687.
4. Inceman S, Caen J, Bernard J. Aggregation, adhesion, and viscous metamorphosis of platelets in congenital fibrinogen deficiencies. *J Lab Clin Med* 1966;68:21–32.
5. Weiss HJ, Rogers J. Fibrinogen and platelets in the primary arrest of bleeding. Studies in two patients with congenital afibrinogenemia. *N Engl J Med* 1971;285:369–374.
6. Solum NO, Stormorken H. Influence of fibrinogen on the aggregation of washed human blood platelets induced by adenosine diphosphate, thrombin, collagen, and adrenaline. *Scand J Clin Lab Invest* 1965;17 (Suppl. 84):170+.
7. Mustard JF, Packham MA, Kinlough-Rathbone RL, et al. Fibrinogen and ADP-induced platelet aggregation. *Blood* 1978;52:453–466.
8. Bennett JS, Vilaire G. Exposure of platelet fibrinogen receptors by ADP and epinephrine. *J Clin Invest* 1979;64:1393–1401.
9. Mustard JF, Kinlough-Rathbone RL, Packham MA, et al. Comparison of fibrinogen association with normal and thrombasthenic platelets on exposure to ADP or chymotrypsin. *Blood* 1979;54:987–993.
10. Marguerie GA, Plow EF, Edgington TS. Human platelets possess an inducible and saturable receptor specific for fibrinogen. *J Biol Chem* 1979;254:5357–5363.
11. Peerschke EI, Zucker MB, Grant RA, et al. Correlation between fibrinogen binding to human platelets and platelet aggregability. *Blood* 1980;55:841–847.
12. Bhatt DL, Topol EJ. Scientific and therapeutic advances in antiplatelet therapy. *Nat Rev Drug Discov* 2003;2:15–28.
13. Emambokus NR, Frampton J. The glycoprotein IIb molecule is expressed on early murine hematopoietic progenitors and regulates their numbers in sites of hematopoiesis. *Immunity* 2003;19:33–45.
14. Berlanga O, Emambokus N, Frampton J. GPIIb (CD41) integrin is expressed on mast cells and influences their adhesion properties. *Exp Hematol* 2005;33:403–412.
15. Uzan G, Prenant M, Prandini MH, et al. Tissue-specific expression of the platelet GPIIb gene. *J Biol Chem* 1991;266:8932–8939.
16. Tronik-Le Roux D, Roullot V, Schweitzer A, et al. Suppression of erythro-megakaryocytopoiesis and the induction of reversible thrombocytopenia in mice transgenic for the thymidine kinase gene targeted by the platelet glycoprotein alpha IIb promoter. *J Exp Med* 1995;181:2141–2151.
17. Sosnoski DM, Emanuel BS, Hawkins AL, et al. Chromosomal localization of the genes for the vitronectin and fibronectin receptors alpha subunits and for platelet glycoproteins IIb and IIIa. *J Clin Invest* 1988;81:1993–1998.
18. Phillips DR, Charo IF, Parise LV, et al. The platelet membrane glycoprotein IIb-IIIa complex. *Blood* 1988;71:831–843.
19. Duperray A, Troesch A, Berthier R, et al. Biosynthesis and assembly of platelet GPIIb-IIIa in human megakaryocytes: evidence that assembly between pro-GPIIb and GPIIIa is a prerequisite for expression of the complex on the cell surface. *Blood* 1989;74:1603–1611.
20. Coller BS, Seligsohn U, West SM, et al. Platelet fibrinogen and vitronectin in Glanzmann thrombasthenia: evidence consistent with specific roles for glycoprotein IIb/IIIA and alpha v beta 3 integrins in platelet protein trafficking. *Blood* 1991;78:2603–2610.
21. Bennett JS, Kolodziej MA, Vilaire G, et al. Determinants of the intracellular fate of truncated forms of the platelet glycoproteins IIb and IIIa. *J Biol Chem* 1993;268:3580–3585.
22. Poncz M, Rifat S, Coller BS, et al. Glanzmann thrombasthenia secondary to a Gly273 → Asp mutation adjacent to the first calcium-binding domain of platelet glycoprotein IIb. *J Clin Invest* 1994;93:172–179.
23. Wilcox DA, Paddock CM, Lyman S, et al. Glanzmann thrombasthenia resulting from a single amino acid substitution between the second and third calcium-binding domains of GPIIb. Role of the GPIIb amino terminus in integrin subunit association. *J Clin Invest* 1995;95:1553–1560.
24. Duperray A, Berthier R, Chagnon E, et al. Biosynthesis and processing of platelet GPIIb-IIIa in human megakaryocytes. *J Cell Biol* 1987;104:1665–1673.
25. Silver SM, McDonough MM, Vilaire G, et al. The *in vitro* synthesis of polypeptides for the platelet membrane glycoproteins IIb and IIIa. *Blood* 1987;69:1031–1037.
26. Niiya K, Hodson E, Bader R, et al. Increased surface expression of the membrane glycoprotein IIb/IIIa complex induced by platelet activation. Relationship to the binding of fibrinogen and platelet aggregation. *Blood* 1987;70:475–483.
27. Wagner CL, Mascelli MA, Neblock DS, et al. Analysis of GPIIb/IIIa receptor number by quantification of 7E3 binding to human platelets. *Blood* 1996;88:907–914.
28. Gogstad GO, Hagen I, Korsmo R, et al. Characterization of the proteins of isolated human platelet alpha-granules. Evidence for a separate alpha-granule-pool of the glycoproteins IIb and IIIa. *Biochim Biophys Acta* 1981;670:150–162.
29. Woods VL Jr, Wolff LE, Keller DM. Resting platelets contain a substantial centrally located pool of glycoprotein IIb-IIIa complex which may be accessible to some but not other extracellular proteins. *J Biol Chem* 1986;261:15242–15251.
30. Wencel-Drake JD, Dahlbäck B, White JG, et al. Ultrastructural localization of coagulation factor V in human platelets. *Blood* 1986;68:244–249.
31. Wencel-Drake JD. Plasma membrane GPIIb/IIIa. Evidence for a cycling receptor pool. *Am J Pathol* 1990;136:61–70.
32. Handagama P, Scarborough RM, Shuman MA, et al. Endocytosis of fibrinogen into megakaryocyte and platelet alpha-granules is mediated by alpha IIb beta 3 (glycoprotein IIb-IIIa). *Blood* 1993;82:135–138.
33. Fitzgerald LA, Poncz M, Steiner B, et al. Comparison of cDNA-derived protein sequences of the human fibronectin and vitronectin receptor alpha-subunits and platelet glycoprotein IIb. *Biochemistry* 1987;26:8158–8165.
34. Fitzgerald LA, Steiner B, Rall SC Jr, et al. Protein sequence of endothelial glycoprotein IIIa derived from a cDNA clone. Identity with platelet glycoprotein IIIa and similarity to "integrin." *J Biol Chem* 1987;262:3936–3939.
35. Jennings LK, Phillips DR. Purification of glycoproteins IIb and III from human platelet plasma membranes and characterization of a calcium-dependent glycoprotein IIb-III complex. *J Biol Chem* 1982;257:10458–10466.
36. Adair BD, Yeager M. Three-dimensional model of the human platelet integrin alphaIIbbeta3 based on electron cryomicroscopy and x-ray crystallography. *Proc Natl Acad Sci U S A* 2002;99:14059–14064.
37. Xiong JP, Stehle T, Diefenbach B, et al. Crystal structure of the extracellular segment of integrin alpha Vbeta3. *Science* 2001;294:339–345.
38. Xiong JP, Stehle T, Zhang R, et al. Crystal structure of the extracellular segment of integrin alpha Vbeta3 in complex with an Arg-Gly-Asp ligand. *Science* 2002;296:151–155.
39. Vinogradova O, Velyvis A, Velyviene A, et al. A structural mechanism of integrin alpha(IIb)beta(3) "inside-out" activation as regulated by its cytoplasmic face. *Cell* 2002;110:587–597.
40. Vinogradova O, Vaynberg J, Kong X, et al. Membrane-mediated structural transitions at the cytoplasmic face during integrin activation. *Proc Natl Acad Sci U S A* 2004;101:4094–4099.
41. Li R, Mitra N, Gratkowski H, et al. Activation of integrin alphaIIbbeta3 by modulation of transmembrane helix associations. *Science* 2003;300:795–798.
42. Takagi J, Petre BM, Walz T, et al. Global conformational rearrangements in integrin extracellular domains in outside-in and inside-out signaling. *Cell* 2002;110:599–511.
43. Kim M, Carman CV, Springer TA. Bidirectional transmembrane signaling by cytoplasmic domain separation in integrins. *Science* 2003;301:1720–1725.
44. Vinogradova O, Haas T, Plow EF, et al. A structural basis for integrin activation by the cytoplasmic tail of the alpha IIb-subunit. *Proc Natl Acad Sci U S A* 2000;97:1450–1455.
45. Lu C, Shimaoka M, Salas A, et al. The binding sites for competitive antagonistic, allosteric antagonistic, and agonistic antibodies to the I domain of integrin LFA-1. *J Immunol* 2004;173:3972–3978.
46. Luo BH, Springer TA, Takagi J. A specific interface between integrin transmembrane helices and affinity for ligand. *PLoS Biol* 2004;2:e153.
47. Haas TA, Plow EF. The cytoplasmic domain of alphaIIb beta3. A ternary complex of the integrin alpha and beta subunits and a divalent cation. *J Biol Chem* 1996;271:6017–6026.
48. Sun QH, Liu CY, Wang R, et al. Disruption of the long-range GPIIIa Cys(5)-Cys(435) disulfide bond results in the production of constitutively active GPIIb-IIIa (alpha(IIb)beta(3)) integrin complexes. *Blood* 2002;100:2094–2101.
49. Bray PF. Platelet glycoprotein polymorphisms as risk factors for thrombosis. *Curr Opin Hematol* 2000;7:284–289.
50. Leitinger B, Hogg N. Integrin I domains and their function. *Biochem Soc Trans* 1999;27:826–832.
51. Beglova N, Blacklow SC, Takagi J, et al. Cysteine-rich module structure reveals a fulcrum for integrin rearrangement upon activation. *Nat Struct Biol* 2002;9:282–287.
52. Xiong JP, Stehle T, Goodman SL, et al. A novel adaptation of the integrin PSI domain revealed from its crystal structure. *J Biol Chem* 2004;279:40252–40254.
53. Qin J, Vinogradova O, Plow EF. Integrin bidirectional signaling: a molecular view. *PLoS Biol* 2004;2:e169.

54. Weisel JW, Nagaswami C, Vilaire G, et al. Examination of the platelet membrane glycoprotein IIb-IIIa complex and its interaction with fibrinogen and other ligands by electron microscopy. *J Biol Chem* 1992;267:16637–16643.

55. Kamata T, Irie A, Tokuhira M, et al. Critical residues of integrin alphaIIb subunit for binding of alphaIIbbeta3 (glycoprotein IIb-IIIa) to fibrinogen and ligand-mimetic antibodies (PAC-1, OP-G2, and LJ-CP3). *J Biol Chem* 1996;271:18610–18615.

56. Kahn MJ, Kieber-Emmons T, Vilaire G, et al. Effect of mutagenesis of GPIIb amino acid 273 on the expression and conformation of the platelet integrin GPIIb-IIIa. *Biochemistry* 1996;35:14304–14311.

57. Loftus JC, O'Toole TE, Plow EF, et al. A beta 3 integrin mutation abolishes ligand binding and alters divalent cation-dependent conformation. *Science* 1990;249:915–918.

58. Bajt ML, Ginsberg MH, Frelinger AL III, et al. A spontaneous mutation of integrin alphaIIb beta 3 (platelet glycoprotein IIb-IIIa) helps define a ligand binding site. *J Biol Chem* 1992;267:3789–3794.

59. Chen YP, Djaffar I, Pidard D, et al. Ser-752 → Pro mutation in the cytoplasmic domain of integrin beta 3 subunit and defective activation of platelet integrin alpha IIb beta 3 (glycoprotein IIb-IIIa) in a variant of Glanzmann thrombasthenia. *Proc Natl Acad Sci U S A* 1992;89:10169–10173.

60. D'Souza SE. Chemical cross-linking of arginyl-glycyl-aspartic acid peptides to an adhesion receptor on platelets. *J Biol Chem* 1988;263:3943–3951.

61. D'Souza SE, Ginsberg MH, Burke TA, et al. The ligand binding site of the platelet integrin receptor GPIIb-IIIa is proximal to the second calcium binding domain of its alpha subunit. *J Biol Chem* 1990;265:3440–3446.

62. Santoro SA, Lawing WJ Jr. Competition for related but nonidentical binding sites on the glycoprotein IIb-IIIa complex by peptides derived from platelet adhesive proteins. *Cell* 1987;48:867–873.

63. Gartner TK, Taylor DB. The amino acid sequence Gly-Ala-Pro-Leu appears to be a fibrinogen binding site in the platelet integrin, glycoprotein IIb. *Thromb Res* 1990;60:291–309.

64. Lasz EC, McLane MA, Trybulec M, et al. Beta 3 integrin derived peptide 217-230 inhibits fibrinogen binding and platelet aggregation: significance of RGD sequences and fibrinogen A alpha-chain. *Biochem Biophys Res Commun* 1993;190:118–124.

65. Andrieux A, Hudry-Clergeon G, Ryckewaert JJ, et al. Amino acid sequences in fibrinogen mediating its interaction with its platelet receptor, GPIIbIIIa. *J Biol Chem* 1989;264:9258–9265.

66. Hantgan RR. Fibrin protofibril and fibrinogen binding to ADP-stimulated platelets: evidence for a common mechanism. *Biochim Biophys Acta* 1988;968:24–35.

67. Ruggeri ZM, Bader R, de Marco L. Glanzmann thrombasthenia: deficient binding of von Willebrand factor to thrombin-stimulated platelets. *Proc Natl Acad Sci U S A* 1982;79:6038–6041.

68. Ginsberg MH, Forsyth J, Lightsey A, et al. Reduced surface expression and binding of fibronectin by thrombin-stimulated thrombasthenic platelets. *J Clin Invest* 1983;71:619–624.

69. Thiagarajan P, Kelly KL. Exposure of binding sites for vitronectin on platelets following stimulation. *J Biol Chem* 1988;263:3035–3038.

70. Karczewski J, Knudsen KA, Smith L, et al. The interaction of thrombospondin with platelet glycoprotein GPIIb-IIIa. *J Biol Chem* 1989;264:21322–21326.

71. de Groot PG, Sixma JJ. Platelet adhesion. *Br J Haematol* 1990;75:308–312.

72. Savage B, Saldivar E, Ruggeri ZM. Initiation of platelet adhesion by arrest onto fibrinogen or translocation on von Willebrand factor. *Cell* 1996;84:289–297.

73. Savage B, Almus-Jacobs F, Ruggeri ZM. Specific synergy of multiple substrate-receptor interactions in platelet thrombus formation under flow. *Cell* 1998;94:657–666.

74. Smith JW, Ruggeri ZM, Kunicki TJ, et al. Interaction of integrins alpha v beta 3 and glycoprotein IIb-IIIa with fibrinogen. Differential peptide recognition accounts for distinct binding sites. *J Biol Chem* 1990;265:12267–12271.

75. Suehiro K, Gailit J, Plow EF. Fibrinogen is a ligand for integrin alpha5beta1 on endothelial cells. *J Biol Chem* 1997;272:5360–5366.

76. Ruggeri ZM. Von Willebrand factor, platelets and endothelial cell interactions. *J Thromb Haemost* 2003;1:1335–1342.

77. Pytela R, Pierschbacher MD, Ruoslahti E. Identification and isolation of a 140 kd cell surface glycoprotein with properties expected of a fibronectin receptor. *Cell* 1985;40:191–198.

78. Pytela R, Pierschbacher MD, Ruoslahti E. A 125/115-kDa cell surface receptor specific for vitronectin interacts with the arginine-glycine-aspartic acid adhesion sequence derived from fibronectin. *Proc Natl Acad Sci U S A* 1985;82:5766–5770.

79. Asch AS, Barnwell J, Silverstein RL, et al. Isolation of the thrombospondin membrane receptor. *J Clin Invest* 1987;79:1054–1061.

80. Dawson DW, Pearce SF, Zhong R, et al. CD36 mediates the *in vitro* inhibitory effects of thrombospondin-1 on endothelial cells. *J Cell Biol* 1997;138:707–717.

81. Weiss HJ, Hawiger J, Ruggeri ZM, et al. Fibrinogen-independent platelet adhesion and thrombus formation on subendothelium mediated by glycoprotein IIb-IIIa complex at high shear rate. *J Clin Invest* 1989;83:288–297.

82. Ikeda Y, Handa M, Kawano K, et al. The role of von Willebrand factor and fibrinogen in platelet aggregation under varying shear stress. *J Clin Invest* 1991;87:1234–1240.

83. Kulkarni S, Dopheide SM, Yap CL, et al. A revised model of platelet aggregation. *J Clin Invest* 2000;105:783–791.

84. Calderwood DA, Ginsberg MH. Talin forges the links between integrins and actin. *Nat Cell Biol* 2003;5:694–697.

85. Tadokoro S, Shattil SJ, Eto K, et al. Talin binding to integrin beta tails: a final common step in integrin activation. *Science* 2003;302:103–106.

86. Yang W, Shimaoka M, Chen J, et al. Activation of integrin beta-subunit I-like domains by one-turn C-terminal alpha-helix deletions. *Proc Natl Acad Sci U S A* 2004;101:2333–2338.

87. Partridge AW, Liu S, Kim S, et al. Transmembrane domain helix packing stabilizes integrin alphaIIbbeta3 in the low affinity state. *J Biol Chem* 2005;280:7294–7300.

88. Luo BH, Carman CV, Takagi J, et al. Disrupting integrin transmembrane domain heterodimerization increases ligand binding affinity, not valency or clustering. *Proc Natl Acad Sci U S A* 2005;102:3679–3684.

89. Adair BD, Xiong JP, Maddock C, et al. Three-dimensional EM structure of the ectodomain of integrin {alpha}V{beta}3 in a complex with fibronectin. *J Cell Biol* 2005;168:1109–1118.

90. Li W, Metcalf DG, Gorelik R, et al. A push-pull mechanism for regulating integrin function. *Proc Natl Acad Sci U S A* 2005;102:1424–1429.

91. Hato T, Pampori N, Shattil SJ. Complementary roles for receptor clustering and conformational change in the adhesive and signaling functions of integrin alphaIIb beta3. *J Cell Biol* 1998;141:1685–1695.

92. Marguerie GA, Edgington TS, Plow EF. Interaction of fibrinogen with its platelet receptor as part of a multistep reaction in ADP-induced platelet aggregation. *J Biol Chem* 1980;255:154–161.

93. Marguerie GA, Plow EF. Interaction of fibrinogen with its platelet receptor: kinetics and effect of pH and temperature. *Biochemistry* 1981;20:1074–1080.

94. Peerschke EI, Wainer JA. Examination of irreversible platelet-fibrinogen interactions. *Am J Physiol* 1985;248:C466–C472.

95. Muller B, Zerwes HG, Tangemann K, et al. Two-step binding mechanism of fibrinogen to alpha IIb beta 3 integrin reconstituted into planar lipid bilayers. *J Biol Chem* 1993;268:6800–6808.

96. Huber W, Hurst J, Schlatter D, et al. Determination of kinetic constants for the interaction between the platelet glycoprotein IIb-IIIa and fibrinogen by means of surface plasmon resonance. *Eur J Biochem* 1995;227:647–656.

97. Peerschke EI. Stabilization of platelet-fibrinogen interactions is an integral property of the glycoprotein IIb-IIIa complex. *J Lab Clin Med* 1994;124:439–446.

98. Peerschke EI. Regulation of platelet aggregation by post-fibrinogen binding events. Insights provided by dithiothreitol-treated platelets. *Thromb Haemost* 1995;73:862–867.

99. Torti M, Festetics ET, Bertoni A, et al. Agonist-induced actin polymerization is required for the irreversibility of platelet aggregation. *Thromb Haemost* 1996;76:444–449.

100. Simmons SR, Albrecht RM. Self-association of bound fibrinogen on platelet surfaces. *J Lab Clin Med* 1996;128:39–50.

101. Leung L, Nachman R. Molecular mechanisms of platelet aggregation. *Annu Rev Med* 1986;37:179–186.

102. Wencel-Drake JD, Boudignon-Proudhon C, Dieter MG, et al. Internalization of bound fibrinogen modulates platelet aggregation. *Blood* 1996;87:602–612.

103. Moon DG, Shainoff JR, Gonda SR. Electron microscopy of platelet interactions with heme-octapeptide-labeled fibrinogen. *Am J Physiol* 1990;259:C611–C618.

104. Prevost N, Woulfe D, Tanaka T, et al. Interactions between Eph kinases and ephrins provide a mechanism to support platelet aggregation once cell-to-cell contact has occurred. *Proc Natl Acad Sci U S A* 2002;99:9219–9224.

105. Plow EF, Srouji AH, Meyer D, et al. Evidence that three adhesive proteins interact with a common recognition site on activated platelets. *J Biol Chem* 1984;259:5388–5391.

106. Plow EF, D'Souza SE, Ginsberg MH. Ligand binding to GPIIb-IIIa: a status report. *Semin Thromb Hemost* 1992;18:324–332.

107. Frelinger AL III, Lam SC, Plow EF, et al. Occupancy of an adhesive glycoprotein receptor modulates expression of an antigenic site involved in cell adhesion. *J Biol Chem* 1988;263:12397–12402.

108. Frelinger AL III, Cohen I, Plow EF, et al. Selective inhibition of integrin function by antibodies specific for ligand-occupied receptor conformers. *J Biol Chem* 1990;265:6346–6352.

109. Plow EF, D'Souza SE, Ginsberg MH. Consequences of the interaction of platelet membrane glycoprotein GPIIb-IIIa (alpha IIb beta 3) and its ligands. *J Lab Clin Med* 1992;120:198–204.

110. Shattil SJ, Newman PJ. Integrins: dynamic scaffolds for adhesion and signaling in platelets. *Blood* 2004;104:1606–1615.

111. Brass LF, Stalker TJ, Zhu L, et al. Boundary events: contact-dependent and contact-facilitated signaling between platelets. *Semin Thromb Hemost* 2004;30:399–410.

112. Plow EF, Marguerie G, Ginsberg M. Fibrinogen, fibrinogen receptors, and the peptides that inhibit these interactions. *Biochem Pharmacol* 1987;36:4035–4040.

113. Kloczewiak M, Timmons S, Hawiger J. Recognition site for the platelet receptor is present on the 15-residue carboxy-terminal fragment of the

gamma chain of human fibrinogen and is not involved in the fibrin polymerization reaction. *Thromb Res* 1983;29:249–255.

114. Kloczewiak M, Timmons S, Lukas TJ, et al. Platelet receptor recognition site on human fibrinogen. Synthesis and structure-function relationship of peptides corresponding to the carboxy-terminal segment of the gamma chain. *Biochemistry* 1984;23:1767–1774.

115. Tranqui L, Andrieux A, Hudry-Clergeon G, et al. Differential structural requirements for fibrinogen binding to platelets and to endothelial cells. *J Cell Biol* 1989;108:2519–2527.

116. Timmons S, Kloczewiak M, Hawiger J. ADP-dependent common receptor mechanism for binding of von Willebrand factor and fibrinogen to human platelets. *Proc Natl Acad Sci U S A* 1984;81:4935–4939.

117. Kirschbaum NE, Mosesson MW, Amrani DL. Characterization of the gamma chain platelet binding site on fibrinogen fragment D. *Blood* 1992; 79:2643–2648.

118. Hettasch JM, Bolyard MG, Lord ST. The residues AGDV of recombinant gamma chains of human fibrinogen must be carboxy-terminal to support human platelet aggregation. *Thromb Haemost* 1992;68:701–706.

119. Farrell DH, Thiagarajan P, Chung DW, et al. Role of fibrinogen alpha and gamma chain sites in platelet aggregation. *Proc Natl Acad Sci U S A* 1992; 89:10729–10732.

120. Holmback K, Danton MJ, Suh TT, et al. Impaired platelet aggregation and sustained bleeding in mice lacking the fibrinogen motif bound by integrin alpha IIb beta 3. *EMBO J* 1996;15:5760–5771.

121. Plow EF, Pierschbacher MD, Ruoslahti E, et al. The effect of Arg-Gly-Asp-containing peptides on fibrinogen and von Willebrand factor binding to platelets. *Proc Natl Acad Sci U S A* 1985;82:8057–8061.

122. Gartner TK, Bennett JS. The tetrapeptide analogue of the cell attachment site of fibronectin inhibits platelet aggregation and fibrinogen binding to activated platelets. *J Biol Chem* 1985;260:11891–11894.

123. Hawiger J, Kloczewiak M, Bednarek MA, et al. Platelet receptor recognition domains on the alpha chain of human fibrinogen: structure-function analysis. *Biochemistry* 1989;28:2909–2914.

124. Coller BS. Anti-GPIIb/IIIa drugs: current strategies and future directions. *Thromb Haemost* 2001;86:427–443.

125. Beacham DA, Wise RJ, Turci SM, et al. Selective inactivation of the Arg-Gly-Asp-Ser (RGDS) binding site in von Willebrand factor by site-directed mutagenesis. *J Biol Chem* 1992;267:3409–3415.

126. Cherny RC, Honan MA, Thiagarajan P. Site-directed mutagenesis of the arginine-glycine-aspartic acid in vitronectin abolishes cell adhesion. *J Biol Chem* 1993;268:9725–9729.

127. Ginsberg M, Pierschbacher MD, Ruoslahti E, et al. Inhibition of fibronectin binding to platelets by proteolytic fragments and synthetic peptides which support fibroblast adhesion. *J Biol Chem* 1985;260:3931–3936.

128. Bowditch RD, Halloran CE, Aota S, et al. Integrin alpha IIb beta 3 (platelet GPIIb-IIIa) recognizes multiple sites in fibronectin. *J Biol Chem* 1991;266: 23323–23328.

129. Ruoslahti E. RGD and other recognition sequences for integrins. *Annu Rev Cell Dev Biol* 1996;12:697–715.

130. Rooney MM, Parise LV, Lord ST. Dissecting clot retraction and platelet aggregation. Clot retraction does not require an intact fibrinogen gamma chain C terminus. *J Biol Chem* 1996;271:8553–8555.

131. Quinn MJ, Plow EF, Topol EJ. Platelet glycoprotein IIb/IIIa inhibitors: recognition of a two-edged sword? *Circulation* 2002;106:379–385.

132. Topol EJ, Byzova TV, Plow EF. Platelet GPIIb-IIIa blockers. *Lancet* 1999; 353:227–231.

133. Nakada MT, Sassoli PM, Tam SH, et al. Abciximab pharmacodynamics are unaffected by antecedent therapy with other GPIIb/IIIa antagonists in non-human primates. *J Thromb Thrombolysis* 2002;14:15–24.

134. Coller BS. Antiplatelet agents in the prevention and therapy of thrombosis. *Annu Rev Med* 1992;43:171–180.

135. Jordan RE, Mascelli MA, Nakada MT. Pharmacology and clinical development of abciximab (c7E3 Fab, ReoPro): a monoclonal antibody inhibitor of GPIIb/IIIa and aVb3. In: Sasahara AA, Loscalzo J, eds. *New therapeutic agents in thrombosis and thrombolysis.* New York: Marcel Dekker, 1997:291–313.

136. Topol EJ, Califf RM, Weisman HF, et al. The EPIC investigators. Randomised trial of coronary intervention with antibody against platelet IIb/IIIa integrin for reduction of clinical restenosis: results at six months. *Lancet* 1994;343:881–886.

137. Scarborough RM, Rose JW, Hsu MA, et al. Barbourin. A GPIIb-IIIa-specific integrin antagonist from the venom of Sistrurus m. barbouri. *J Biol Chem* 1991;266:9359–9362.

138. Barrett JS, Murphy G, Peerlinck K, et al. Pharmacokinetics and pharmacodynamics of MK-383, a selective non-peptide platelet glycoprotein-IIb/IIIa receptor antagonist, in healthy men. *Clin Pharmacol Ther* 1994;56:377–388.

139. Agah R, Plow EF, Topol EJ. GPIIb-IIIa antagonists. In: Michelson A, ed. *Platelets.* Burlington: MAA Academic Press, 2002:769–785.

140. Chew DP, Bhatt DL, Sapp S, et al. Increased mortality with oral platelet glycoprotein IIb/IIIa antagonists: a meta-analysis of phase III multicenter randomized trials. *Circulation* 2001;103:201–206.

141. Nurden AT. Association of fibrinogen-bound glycoprotein IIb-IIIa complexes on the activated platelet surface. *J Lab Clin Med* 1996;128:7–8.

142. Hung DT, Vu TK, Wheaton VI, et al. Cloned platelet thrombin receptor is necessary for thrombin-induced platelet activation. *J Clin Invest* 1992;89: 1350–1353.

143. Daniel JL, Dangelmaier C, Jin J, et al. Molecular basis for ADP-induced platelet activation. I. Evidence for three distinct ADP receptors on human platelets. *J Biol Chem* 1998;273:2024–2029.

144. Brass LF, Manning DR, Cichowski K, et al. Signaling through G proteins in platelets: to the integrins and beyond. *Thromb Haemost* 1997;78:581–589.

145. Eckly A, Gendrault JL, Hechler B, et al. Differential involvement of the P2Y1 and P2YT receptors in the morphological changes of platelet aggregation. *Thromb Haemost* 2001;85:694–701.

146. Kauffenstein G, Bergmeier W, Eckly A, et al. The P2Y(12) receptor induces platelet aggregation through weak activation of the alpha(IIb)beta(3) integrin—a phosphoinositide 3-kinase-dependent mechanism. *FEBS Lett* 2001; 505:281–290.

147. Moroi M, Jung SM. Platelet receptors for collagen. *Thromb Haemost* 1997;78:439–444.

148. Siljander PR, Hamaia S, Peachey AR, et al. Integrin activation state determines selectivity for novel recognition sites in fibrillar collagens. *J Biol Chem* 2004;279:47763–47772.

149. Adam F, Bouton MC, Huisse MG, et al. Thrombin interaction with platelet membrane glycoprotein Ib alpha. *Trends Mol Med* 2003;9:461–464.

150. Li Z, Zhang G, Le Breton GC, et al. Two waves of platelet secretion induced by thromboxane A2 receptor and a critical role for phosphoinositide 3-kinases. *J Biol Chem* 2003;278:30725–30731.

151. Sims PJ, Wiedmer T. Induction of cellular procoagulant activity by the membrane attack complex of complement. *Semin Cell Biol* 1995;6:275–282.

152. Poole AW, Pula G, Hers I, et al. PKC-interacting proteins: from function to pharmacology. *Trends Pharmacol Sci* 2004;25:528–535.

153. Kasirer-Friede A, Cozzi MR, Mazzucato M, et al. Signaling through GP Ib-IX-V activates alpha IIb beta 3 independently of other receptors. *Blood* 2004;103:3403–3411.

154. Quinton TM, Kim S, Dangelmaier C, et al. Protein kinase C- and calcium-regulated pathways independently synergize with Gi pathways in agonist-induced fibrinogen receptor activation. *Biochem J* 2002;368:535–543.

155. Quinton TM, Ozdener F, Dangelmaier C, et al. Glycoprotein VI-mediated platelet fibrinogen receptor activation occurs through calcium-sensitive and PKC-sensitive pathways without a requirement for secreted ADP. *Blood* 2002;99:3228–3234.

156. Tabuchi A, Yoshioka A, Higashi T, et al. Direct demonstration of involvement of protein kinase Calpha in the Ca2+-induced platelet aggregation. *J Biol Chem* 2003;278:26374–26379.

157. Murugappan S, Tuluc F, Dorsam RT, et al. Differential role of protein kinase C delta isoform in agonist-induced dense granule secretion in human platelets. *J Biol Chem* 2004;279:2360–2367.

158. Crosby D, Poole AW. Physical and functional interaction between protein kinase C delta and Fyn tyrosine kinase in human platelets. *J Biol Chem* 2003;278:24533–24541.

159. Gilligan DM, Sarid R, Weese J. Adducin in platelets: activation-induced phosphorylation by PKC and proteolysis by calpain. *Blood* 2002;99:2418–2426.

160. Polanowska-Grabowska R, Gear AR. Activation of protein kinase C is required for the stable attachment of adherent platelets to collagen but is not needed for the initial rapid adhesion under flow conditions. *Arterioscler Thromb Vasc Biol* 1999;19:3044–3054.

161. Libersan D, Merhi Y. Platelet P-selectin expression: requirement for protein kinase C, but not protein tyrosine kinase or phosphoinositide 3-kinase. *Thromb Haemost* 2003;89:1016–1023.

162. Giuliano S, Nesbitt WS, Rooney M, et al. Bidirectional integrin alphaIIb-beta3 signalling regulating platelet adhesion under flow: contribution of protein kinase C. *Biochem J* 2003;372:163–172.

163. Buensuceso CS, Arias-Salgado EG, Shattil SJ. Protein-protein interactions in platelet alphaIIbbeta3 signaling. *Semin Thromb Hemost* 2004;30:427–439.

164. Chang BY, Chiang M, Cartwright CA. The interaction of Src and RACK1 is enhanced by activation of protein kinase C and tyrosine phosphorylation of RACK1. *J Biol Chem* 2001;276:20346–20356.

165. Schechtman D, Mochly-Rosen D. Adaptor proteins in protein kinase C-mediated signal transduction. *Oncogene* 2001;20:6339–6347.

166. Banno Y, Nakashima S, Ohzawa M, et al. Differential translocation of phospholipase C isozymes to integrin-mediated cytoskeletal complexes in thrombin-stimulated human platelets. *J Biol Chem* 1996;271:14989–14994.

167. Philip F, Guo Y, Scarlata S. Multiple roles of pleckstrin homology domains in phospholipase Cbeta function. *FEBS Lett* 2002;531:28–32.

168. Rhee SG, Bae YS. Regulation of phosphoinositide-specific phospholipase C isozymes. *J Biol Chem* 1997;272:15045–15048.

169. Tate BF, Rittenhouse SE. Thrombin activation of human platelets causes tyrosine phosphorylation of PLC-gamma 2. *Biochim Biophys Acta* 1993; 1178:281–285.

170. Suzuki-Inoue K, Wilde JI, Andrews RK, et al. Glycoproteins VI and Ib-IX-V stimulate tyrosine phosphorylation of tyrosine kinase Syk and phospholipase Cgamma2 at distinct sites. *Biochem J* 2004;378:1023–1029.

171. Chacko GW, Duchemin AM, Coggeshall KM, et al. Clustering of the platelet Fc gamma receptor induces noncovalent association with the tyrosine kinase p72syk. *J Biol Chem* 1994;269:32435–32440.

172. Ichinohe T, Takayama H, Ezumi Y, et al. Collagen-stimulated activation of Syk but not c-Src is severely compromised in human platelets lacking membrane glycoprotein VI. *J Biol Chem* 1997;272:63–68.

173. Poole A, Gibbins JM, Turner M, et al. The Fc receptor gamma-chain and the tyrosine kinase Syk are essential for activation of mouse platelets by collagen. *EMBO J* 1997;16:2333–2341.

174. Jackson SP, Schoenwaelder SM, Yuan Y, et al. Non-receptor protein tyrosine kinases and phosphatases in human platelets. *Thromb Haemost* 1996; 76:640–650.

175. Wilde JI, Watson SP. Regulation of phospholipase C gamma isoforms in haematopoietic cells: why one, not the other? *Cell Signal* 2001;13:691–701.

176. Lerea KM, Tonks NK, Krebs EG, et al. Vanadate and molybdate increase tyrosine phosphorylation in a 50-kilodalton protein and stimulate secretion in electropermeabilized platelets. *Biochemistry* 1989;28: 9286–9292.

177. Wang D, Feng J, Wen R, et al. Phospholipase Cgamma2 is essential in the functions of B cell and several Fc receptors. *Immunity* 2000;13:25–35.

178. Rathore V, Wang D, Newman DK, et al. Phospholipase Cgamma2 contributes to stable thrombus formation on VWF. *FEBS Lett* 2004;573:26–30.

179. Jackson SP, Yap CL, Anderson KE. Phosphoinositide 3-kinases and the regulation of platelet function. *Biochem Soc Trans* 2004;32:387–392.

180. Tang X, Downes CP. Purification and characterization of Gbetagamma-responsive phosphoinositide 3-kinases from pig platelet cytosol. *J Biol Chem* 1997;272:14193–14199.

181. Zhang J, Banfic H, Straforini F, et al. A type II phosphoinositide 3-kinase is stimulated via activated integrin in platelets. A source of phosphatidylinositol 3-phosphate. *J Biol Chem* 1998;273:14081–14084.

182. Toker A, Cantley LC. Signalling through the lipid products of phosphoinositide-3-OH kinase. *Nature* 1997;387:673–676.

183. Kovacsovics TJ, Bachelot C, Toker A, et al. Phosphoinositide 3-kinase inhibition spares actin assembly in activating platelets but reverses platelet aggregation. *J Biol Chem* 1995;270:11358–11366.

184. Resendiz JC, Feng S, Ji G, et al. von Willebrand factor binding to platelet glycoprotein Ib-IX-V stimulates the assembly of an alpha-actinin-based signaling complex. *J Thromb Haemost* 2004;2:161–169.

185. Wu Y, Asazuma N, Satoh K, et al. Interaction between von Willebrand factor and glycoprotein Ib activates Src kinase in human platelets: role of phosphoinositide 3-kinase. *Blood* 2003;101:3469–3476.

186. Woulfe D, Jiang H, Morgans A, et al. Defects in secretion, aggregation, and thrombus formation in platelets from mice lacking Akt2. *J Clin Invest* 2004;113:441–450.

187. Soulet C, Gendreau S, Missy K, et al. Characterisation of Rac activation in thrombin- and collagen-stimulated human blood platelets. *FEBS Lett* 2001;507:253–258.

188. Dangelmaier C, Jin J, Smith JB, et al. Potentiation of thromboxane A2-induced platelet secretion by Gi signaling through the phosphoinositide-3 kinase pathway. *Thromb Haemost* 2001;85:341–348.

189. Greco F, Sinigaglia F, Balduini C, et al. Activation of the small GTPase Rap2B in agonist-stimulated human platelets. *J Thromb Haemost* 2004;2: 2223–2230.

190. Clough RR, Sidhu RS, Bhullar RP. Calmodulin binds RalA and RalB and is required for the thrombin-induced activation of Ral in human platelets. *J Biol Chem* 2002;277:28972–28980.

191. Etienne-Manneville S, Hall A. Rho GTPases in cell biology. *Nature* 2002; 420:629–635.

192. Offermanns S. G-proteins as transducers in transmembrane signaling. *Prog Biophys Mol Biol* 2003;83:101–130.

193. Tulasne D, Bori T, Watson SP. Regulation of RAS in human platelets. Evidence that activation of RAS is not sufficient to lead to ERK1-2 phosphorylation. *Eur J Biochem* 2002;269:1511–1517.

194. Shock DD, He K, Wencel-Drake JD, et al. Ras activation in platelets after stimulation of the thrombin receptor, thromboxane A2 receptor or protein kinase C. *Biochem J* 1997;321(Pt 2):525–530.

195. Hughes PE, Renshaw MW, Pfaff M, et al. Suppression of integrin activation: a novel function of a Ras/Raf-initiated MAP kinase pathway. *Cell* 1997;88:521–530.

196. Zhang Z, Vuori K, Wang H, et al. Integrin activation by R-ras. *Cell* 1996; 85:61–69.

197. Sethi T, Ginsberg MH, Downward J, et al. The small GTP-binding protein R-Ras can influence integrin activation by antagonizing a Ras/Raf-initiated integrin suppression pathway. *Mol Biol Cell* 1999;10:1799–1809.

198. Hansen M, Prior IA, Hughes PE, et al. C-terminal sequences in R-Ras are involved in integrin regulation and in plasma membrane microdomain distribution. *Biochem Biophys Res Commun* 2003;311:829–838.

199. de Bruyn KM, Zwartkruis FJ, de Rooij J, et al. The small GTPase Rap1 is activated by turbulence and is involved in integrin [alpha]IIb[beta]3-mediated cell adhesion in human megakaryocytes. *J Biol Chem* 2003; 278:22412–22417.

200. Larson MK, Chen H, Kahn ML, et al. Identification of P2Y12-dependent and -independent mechanisms of glycoprotein VI-mediated Rap1 activation in platelets. *Blood* 2003;101:1409–1415.

201. Franke B, Akkerman JW, Bos JL. Rapid Ca2+-mediated activation of Rap1 in human platelets. *EMBO J* 1997;16:252–259.

202. Woulfe D, Jiang H, Mortensen R, et al. Activation of Rap1B by G(i) family members in platelets. *J Biol Chem* 2002;277:23382–23390.

203. Franke B, van Triest M, de Bruijn KM, et al. Sequential regulation of the small GTPase Rap1 in human platelets. *Mol Cell Biol* 2000;20:779–785.

204. Bertoni A, Tadokoro S, Eto K, et al. Relationships between Rap1b, affinity modulation of integrin alpha IIbbeta 3, and the actin cytoskeleton. *J Biol Chem* 2002;277:25715–25721.

205. Schultess J, Danielewski O, Smolenski AP. Rap1GAP2 is a new GTPase-activating protein of Rap1 expressed in human platelets. *Blood* 2005;105: 3185–3192.

206. Lafuente EM, van Puijenbroek AA, Krause M, et al. RIAM, an Ena/VASP and Profilin ligand, interacts with Rap1-GTP and mediates Rap1-induced adhesion. *Dev Cell* 2004;7:585–595.

207. Eto K, Murphy R, Kerrigan SW, et al. Megakaryocytes derived from embryonic stem cells implicate CalDAG-GEFI in integrin signaling. *Proc Natl Acad Sci U S A* 2002;99:12819–12824.

208. Crittenden JR, Bergmeier W, Zhang Y, et al. CalDAG-GEFI integrates signaling for platelet aggregation and thrombus formation. *Nat Med* 2004;10: 982–986.

209. Chrzanowska-Wodnicka M, Smyth SS, Schoenwaelder SM, et al. Rap1b is required for normal platelet function and hemostasis in mice. *J Clin Invest* 2005;115:680–687.

210. Goldmann WH, Bremer A, Haner M, et al. Native talin is a dumbbell-shaped homodimer when it interacts with actin. *J Struct Biol* 1994;112:3–10.

211. Winkler J, Lunsdorf H, Jockusch BM. Energy-filtered electron microscopy reveals that talin is a highly flexible protein composed of a series of globular domains. *Eur J Biochem* 1997;243:430–436.

212. Critchley DR. Focal adhesions - the cytoskeletal connection. *Curr Opin Cell Biol* 2000;12:133–139.

213. Calderwood DA, Zent R, Grant R, et al. The Talin head domain binds to integrin beta subunit cytoplasmic tails and regulates integrin activation. *J Biol Chem* 1999;274:28071–28074.

214. Xing B, Jedsadayanmata A, Lam SC. Localization of an integrin binding site to the C terminus of talin. *J Biol Chem* 2001;276:44373–44378.

215. Lee HS, Bellin RM, Walker DL, et al. Characterization of an actin-binding site within the talin FERM domain. *J Mol Biol* 2004;343:771–784.

216. Hemmings L, Rees DJ, Ohanian V, et al. Talin contains three actin-binding sites each of which is adjacent to a vinculin-binding site. *J Cell Sci* 1996; 109(Pt 11):2715–2726.

217. McCann RO, Craig SW. The I/LWEQ module: a conserved sequence that signifies F-actin binding in functionally diverse proteins from yeast to mammals. *Proc Natl Acad Sci U S A* 1997;94:5679–5684.

218. Papagrigoriou E, Gingras AR, Barsukov IL, et al. Activation of a vinculin-binding site in the talin rod involves rearrangement of a five-helix bundle. *EMBO J* 2004;23:2942–2951.

219. Fillingham I, Gingras AR, Papagrigoriou E, et al. A vinculin binding domain from the talin rod unfolds to form a complex with the vinculin head. *Structure (Camb)* 2005;13:65–74.

220. Calderwood DA, Yan B, de Pereda JM, et al. The phosphotyrosine binding-like domain of talin activates integrins. *J Biol Chem* 2002;277: 21749–21758.

221. Ulmer TS, Calderwood DA, Ginsberg MH, et al. Domain-specific interactions of talin with the membrane-proximal region of the integrin beta3 subunit. *Biochemistry* 2003;42:8307–8312.

222. Litchfield DW, Ball EH. Phosphorylation of the cytoskeletal protein talin by protein kinase C. *Biochem Biophys Res Commun* 1986;134:1276–1283.

223. Franco SJ, Rodgers MA, Perrin BJ, et al. Calpain-mediated proteolysis of talin regulates adhesion dynamics. *Nat Cell Biol* 2004;6:977–983.

224. Morgan JR, Di Paolo G, Werner H, et al. A role for talin in presynaptic function. *J Cell Biol* 2004;167:43–50.

225. Calderwood DA, Tai V, Di Paolo G, et al. Competition for talin results in trans-dominant inhibition of integrin activation. *J Biol Chem* 2004;279: 28889–28895.

226. de Pereda JM, Wegener K, Santelli E, et al. Structural bases for phosphatidylinositol phosphate kinase type I-gamma binding to talin at focal adhesions. *J Biol Chem* 2005;280:8381–8386.

227. Di Paolo G, Pellegrini L, Letinic K, et al. Recruitment and regulation of phosphatidylinositol phosphate kinase type 1 gamma by the FERM domain of talin. *Nature* 2002;420:85–89.

228. Ling K, Doughman RL, Firestone AJ, et al. Type I gamma phosphatidylinositol phosphate kinase targets and regulates focal adhesions. *Nature* 2002; 420:89–93.

229. Schwarz UR, Walter U, Eigenthaler M. Taming platelets with cyclic nucleotides. *Biochem Pharmacol* 2001;62:1153–1161.

230. Freedman JE, Loscalzo J, Benoit SE, et al. Decreased platelet inhibition by nitric oxide in two brothers with a history of arterial thrombosis. *J Clin Invest* 1996;97:979–987.

231. Massberg S, Gruner S, Konrad I, et al. Enhanced *in vivo* platelet adhesion in vasodilator-stimulated phosphoprotein (VASP)-deficient mice. *Blood* 2004;103:136–142.

232. Rathore V, Stapleton MA, Hillery CA, et al. PECAM-1 negatively regulates GPIb/V/IX signaling in murine platelets. *Blood* 2003;102:3658–3664.

233. Marcus AJ, Broekman MJ, Drosopoulos JH, et al. The endothelial cell ecto-ADPase responsible for inhibition of platelet function is CD39. *J Clin Invest* 1997;99:1351–1360.

234. Marcus AJ, Broekman MJ, Drosopoulos JH, et al. Heterologous cell-cell interactions: thromboregulation, cerebroprotection and cardioprotection by CD39 (NTPDase-1). *J Thromb Haemost* 2003;1:2497–2509.

235. Ruggeri ZM. Mechanisms initiating platelet thrombus formation. *Thromb Haemost* 1997;78:611–616.

236. Weiss HJ, Turitto VT, Baumgartner HR. Further evidence that glycoprotein IIb-IIIa mediates platelet spreading on subendothelium. *Thromb Haemost* 1991;65:202–205.

237. Schoenwaelder SM, Yuan Y, Cooray P, et al. Calpain cleavage of focal adhesion proteins regulates the cytoskeletal attachment of integrin alphaIIb-beta3 (platelet glycoprotein IIb/IIIa) and the cellular retraction of fibrin clots. *J Biol Chem* 1997;272:1694–1702.

238. VanWijk MJ, VanBavel E, Sturk A, et al. Microparticles in cardiovascular diseases. *Cardiovasc Res* 2003;59:277–287.

239. Chang CP, Zhao J, Wiedmer T, et al. Contribution of platelet microparticle formation and granule secretion to the transmembrane migration of phosphatidylserine. *J Biol Chem* 1993;268:7171–7178.

240. Miyamoto S, Teramoto H, Coso OA, et al. Integrin function: molecular hierarchies of cytoskeletal and signaling molecules. *J Cell Biol* 1995;131:791–805.

241. Hantgan RR, Stahle M, Del Gaizo V, et al. AlphaIIb's cytoplasmic domain is not required for ligand-induced clustering of integrin alphaIIbbeta3. *Biochim Biophys Acta* 2001;1540:82–95.

242. Buensuceso C, de Virgilio M, Shattil SJ. Detection of integrin alpha IIbbeta 3 clustering in living cells. *J Biol Chem* 2003;278:15217–15224.

243. de Virgilio M, Kiosses WB, Shattil SJ. Proximal, selective, and dynamic interactions between integrin alphaIIbbeta3 and protein tyrosine kinases in living cells. *J Cell Biol* 2004;165:305–311.

244. Li R, Babu CR, Lear JD, et al. Oligomerization of the integrin alphaIIbbeta3: roles of the transmembrane and cytoplasmic domains. *Proc Natl Acad Sci U S A* 2001;98:12462–12467.

245. Li R, Gorelik R, Nanda V, et al. Dimerization of the transmembrane domain of Integrin alphaIIb subunit in cell membranes. *J Biol Chem* 2004;279:26666–26673.

246. Obergfell A, Eto K, Mocsai A, et al. Coordinate interactions of Csk, Src, and Syk kinases with [alpha]IIb[beta]3 initiate integrin signaling to the cytoskeleton. *J Cell Biol* 2002;157:265–275.

247. Woodside DG, Obergfell A, Leng L, et al. Activation of Syk protein tyrosine kinase through interaction with integrin beta cytoplasmic domains. *Curr Biol* 2001;11:1799–1804.

248. Goncalves I, Hughan SC, Schoenwaelder SM, et al. Integrin alpha IIb beta 3-dependent calcium signals regulate platelet-fibrinogen interactions under flow. Involvement of phospholipase C gamma 2. *J Biol Chem* 2003;278:34812–34822.

249. Obergfell A, Judd BA, del Pozo MA, et al. The molecular adapter SLP-76 relays signals from platelet integrin alphaIIbbeta3 to the actin cytoskeleton. *J Biol Chem* 2001;276:5916–5923.

250. Wonerow P, Pearce AC, Vaux DJ, et al. A critical role for phospholipase Cgamma2 in alphaIIbbeta3-mediated platelet spreading. *J Biol Chem* 2003;278:37520–37529.

251. Ohmori T, Yatomi Y, Asazuma N, et al. Involvement of proline-rich tyrosine kinase 2 in platelet activation: tyrosine phosphorylation mostly dependent on alphaIIbbeta3 integrin and protein kinase C, translocation to the cytoskeleton and association with Shc through Grb2. *Biochem J* 2000;347:561–569.

252. Avraham H, Ellis MH, Jhun BH, et al. Tyrosine kinases in megakaryocytopoiesis. *Stem Cells* 1995;13:380–392.

253. Raja S, Avraham S, Avraham H. Tyrosine phosphorylation of the novel protein-tyrosine kinase RAFTK during an early phase of platelet activation by an integrin glycoprotein IIb-IIIa-independent mechanism. *J Biol Chem* 1997;272:10941–10947.

254. Iwashima M, Irving BA, van Oers NS, et al. Sequential interactions of the TCR with two distinct cytoplasmic tyrosine kinases. *Science* 1994;263:1136–1139.

255. Law DA, Nannizzi-Alaimo L, Phillips DR. Outside-in integrin signal transduction. Alpha IIb beta 3-(GP IIb IIIa) tyrosine phosphorylation induced by platelet aggregation. *J Biol Chem* 1996;271:10811–10815.

256. Jenkins AL, Nannizzi-Alaimo L, Silver D, et al. Tyrosine phosphorylation of the beta3 cytoplasmic domain mediates integrin-cytoskeletal interactions. *J Biol Chem* 1998;273:13878–13885.

257. Butler B, Blystone SD. Tyrosine phosphorylation of beta 3 integrin provides a binding site for Pyk2. *J Biol Chem* 2005;280:14556–14562.

258. Law DA, DeGuzman FR, Heiser P, et al. Integrin cytoplasmic tyrosine motif is required for outside-in alphaIIbbeta3 signalling and platelet function. *Nature* 1999;401:808–811.

259. Litjens PE, Gorter G, Ylanne J, et al. Involvement of the beta3 E749ATSTFTN756 region in stabilizing integrin alphaIIbbeta3-ligand interaction. *J Thromb Haemost* 2003;1:2216–2224.

260. Derrick JM, Shattil SJ, Poncz M, et al. Distinct domains of alphaIIbbeta3 support different aspects of outside-in signal transduction and platelet activation induced by LSARLAF, an alphaIIbbeta3 interacting peptide. *Thromb Haemost* 2001;86:894–901.

261. Schaffner-Reckinger E, Gouon V, Melchior C, et al. Distinct involvement of beta3 integrin cytoplasmic domain tyrosine residues 747 and 759 in integrin-mediated cytoskeletal assembly and phosphotyrosine signaling. *J Biol Chem* 1998;273:12623–12632.

262. Prasad KS, Andre P, He M, et al. Soluble CD40 ligand induces beta3 integrin tyrosine phosphorylation and triggers platelet activation by outside-in signaling. *Proc Natl Acad Sci U S A* 2003;100:12367–12371.

263. Azam M, Andrabi SS, Sahr KE, et al. Disruption of the mouse mu-calpain gene reveals an essential role in platelet function. *Mol Cell Biol* 2001;21:2213–2220.

264. Kirk RI, Sanderson MR, Lerea KM. Threonine phosphorylation of the beta 3 integrin cytoplasmic tail, at a site recognized by PDK1 and Akt/PKB in vitro, regulates Shc binding. *J Biol Chem* 2000;275:30901–30906.

265. Cowan KJ, Law DA, Phillips DR. Identification of shc as the primary protein binding to the tyrosine-phosphorylated beta 3 subunit of alpha IIb beta 3 during outside-in integrin platelet signaling. *J Biol Chem* 2000;275:36423–36429.

266. Roll RL, Bauman EM, Bennett JS, et al. Phosphorylated pleckstrin induces cell spreading via an integrin-dependent pathway. *J Cell Biol* 2000;150:1461–1466.

267. Lerea KM, Cordero KP, Sakariassen KS, et al. Phosphorylation sites in the integrin beta3 cytoplasmic domain in intact platelets. *J Biol Chem* 1999;274:1914–1919.

268. Newman PJ, Derbes RS, Aster RH. The human platelet alloantigens, PlA1 and PlA2, are associated with a leucine33/proline33 amino acid polymorphism in membrane glycoprotein IIIa, and are distinguishable by DNA typing. *J Clin Invest* 1989;83:1778–1781.

269. Vijayan KV, Goldschmidt-Clermont PJ, Roos C, et al. The Pl(A2) polymorphism of integrin beta(3) enhances outside-in signaling and adhesive functions. *J Clin Invest* 2000;105:793–802.

270. Naik UP, Naik MU. Association of CIB with GPIIb/IIIa during outside-in signaling is required for platelet spreading on fibrinogen. *Blood* 2003;102:1355–1362.

271. Lau LM, Wee JL, Wright MD, et al. The tetraspanin superfamily member, CD151 regulates outside-in integrin {alpha}IIb{beta}3 signalling and platelet function. *Blood* 2004;104:2368–2375.

272. Andre P, Prasad KS, Denis CV, et al. CD40L stabilizes arterial thrombi by a beta3 integrin–dependent mechanism. *Nat Med* 2002;8:247–252.

273. Jin J, Quinton TM, Zhang J, et al. Adenosine diphosphate (ADP)-induced thromboxane A(2) generation in human platelets requires coordinated signaling through integrin alpha(IIb)beta(3) and ADP receptors. *Blood* 2002;99:193–198.

274. Falet H, Ramos-Morales F, Bachelot C, et al. Association of the protein tyrosine phosphatase PTP1C with the protein tyrosine kinase c-Src in human platelets. *FEBS Lett* 1996;383:165–169.

275. Osdoit S, Rosa JP. Fibrin clot retraction by human platelets correlates with alpha(IIb)beta(3) integrin-dependent protein tyrosine dephosphorylation. *J Biol Chem* 2001;276:6703–6710.

276. Rigacci S, Rovida E, Sbarba PD, et al. Low Mr phosphotyrosine protein phosphatase associates and dephosphorylates p125 focal adhesion kinase, interfering with cell motility and spreading. *J Biol Chem* 2002;277:41631–41636.

277. Vijayan KV, Liu Y, Li TT, et al. Protein phosphatase 1 associates with the integrin alphaIIb subunit and regulates signaling. *J Biol Chem* 2004;279:33039–33042.

278. Giuriato S, Bodin S, Erneux C, et al. pp60c-src associates with the SH2-containing inositol-5-phosphatase SHIP1 and is involved in its tyrosine phosphorylation downstream of alphaIIbbeta3 integrin in human platelets. *Biochem J* 2000;348(Pt 1):107–112.

279. Maxwell MJ, Yuan Y, Anderson KE, et al. SHIP1 and Lyn kinase negatively regulate integrin alpha IIb beta 3 signaling in platelets. *J Biol Chem* 2004;279:32196–32204.

280. Gu J, Tamura M, Yamada KM. Tumor suppressor PTEN inhibits integrin- and growth factor–mediated mitogen-activated protein (MAP) kinase signaling pathways. *J Cell Biol* 1998;143:1375–1383.

281. Maehama T, Dixon JE. The tumor suppressor, PTEN/MMAC1, dephosphorylates the lipid second messenger, phosphatidylinositol 3,4,5-trisphosphate. *J Biol Chem* 1998;273:13375–13378.

282. Leslie NR, Gray A, Pass I, et al. Analysis of the cellular functions of PTEN using catalytic domain and C-terminal mutations: differential effects of C-terminal deletion on signalling pathways downstream of phosphoinositide 3-kinase. *Biochem J* 2000;346(Pt 3):827–833.

283. Felding-Habermann B, Cheresh DA. Vitronectin and its receptors. *Curr Opin Cell Biol* 1993;5:864–868.

284. Byzova TV, Rabbani R, D'Souza SE, et al. Role of integrin alpha(v)beta3 in vascular biology. *Thromb Haemost* 1998;80:726–734.

285. Eliceiri BP, Cheresh DA. Role of alpha v integrins during angiogenesis. *Cancer J* 2000;6(Suppl. 3):S245–S249.

286. Suzuki S, Argraves WS, Pytela R, et al. cDNA and amino acid sequences of the cell adhesion protein receptor recognizing vitronectin reveal a transmembrane domain and homologies with other adhesion protein receptors. *Proc Natl Acad Sci U S A* 1986;83:8614–8618.

287. Hafdi Z, Lesavre P, Tharaux PL, et al. Role of alpha v integrins in mesangial cell adhesion to vitronectin and von Willebrand factor. *Kidney Int* 1997;51:1900–1907.

288. Hu DD, Hoyer JR, Smith JW. Ca2+ suppresses cell adhesion to osteopontin by attenuating binding affinity for integrin alpha v beta 3. *J Biol Chem* 1995;270:9917–9925.

289. Pampori N, Hato T, Stupack DG, et al. Mechanisms and consequences of affinity modulation of integrin alpha(V)beta(3) detected with a novel patch-engineered monovalent ligand. *J Biol Chem* 1999;274:21609–21616.

290. Suehiro K, Smith JW, Plow EF. The ligand recognition specificity of beta3 integrins. *J Biol Chem* 1996;271:10365–10371.

291. Pelletier AJ, Kunicki T, Quaranta V. Activation of the integrin alpha v beta 3 involves a discrete cation-binding site that regulates conformation. *J Biol Chem* 1996;271:1364–1370.

292. Mehta RJ, Diefenbach B, Brown A, et al. Transmembrane-truncated alphavbeta3 integrin retains high affinity for ligand binding: evidence for an "inside-out" suppressor? *Biochem J* 1998;330(Pt 2):861–869.

293. Bennett JS, Chan C, Vilaire G, et al. Agonist-activated alphavbeta3 on platelets and lymphocytes binds to the matrix protein osteopontin. *J Biol Chem* 1997;272:8137–8140.

294. Dejana E, Languino LR, Colella S, et al. The localization of a platelet GpIIb-IIIa-related protein in endothelial cell adhesion structures. *Blood* 1988;71:566–572.

295. Wayner EA, Orlando RA, Cheresh DA. Integrins alpha v beta 3 and alpha v beta 5 contribute to cell attachment to vitronectin but differentially distribute on the cell surface. *J Cell Biol* 1991;113:919–929.

296. Linder S, Aepfelbacher M. Podosomes: adhesion hot-spots of invasive cells. *Trends Cell Biol* 2003;13:376–385.

297. Wickham TJ, Mathias P, Cheresh DA, et al. Integrins alpha v beta 3 and alpha v beta 5 promote adenovirus internalization but not virus attachment. *Cell* 1993;73:309–319.

298. Brooks PC, Stromblad S, Sanders LC, et al. Localization of matrix metalloproteinase MMP-2 to the surface of invasive cells by interaction with integrin alpha v beta 3. *Cell* 1996;85:683–693.

299. Coller BS, Cheresh DA, Asch E, et al. Platelet vitronectin receptor expression differentiates Iraqi-Jewish from Arab patients with Glanzmann thrombasthenia in Israel. *Blood* 1991;77:75–83.

300. Friedlander M, Brooks PC, Shaffer RW, et al. Definition of two angiogenic pathways by distinct alpha v integrins. *Science* 1995;270:1500–1502.

301. Bader BL, Rayburn H, Crowley D, et al. Extensive vasculogenesis, angiogenesis, and organogenesis precede lethality in mice lacking all alpha v integrins. *Cell* 1998;95:507–519.

# CHAPTER 31 ■ THE PLATELET GLYCOPROTEIN Ib/IX/V COMPLEX AND PLATELET ADHESION

ADAM DALLAS MUNDAY, JOSÉ ARON LÓPEZ, AND MICHAEL CLAUDE BERNDT

## MOLECULAR AND CELLULAR MECHANISMS OF PLATELET ADHESION

The complications of arterial thrombosis, which include unstable angina, acute myocardial infarction, and stroke, are the leading combined causes of death in the developed world and among the most frequent causes of death in less developed countries. The thrombi causing these complications are rich in platelets, and, indeed, the platelets themselves initiate the process. The platelets can do this in two ways. They may adhere to exposed thrombogenic materials when an atherosclerotic plaque ruptures, become activated, spread, release the contents of their storage organelles, and become cohesive toward circulating platelets, resulting in occlusive thrombus. This is essentially the same cascade of events that occurs during hemostasis. Alternately, in the fluid phase, platelets can be activated by the pathologically high shear stresses present at sites of arterial stenosis, again with the potential to produce an occlusive thrombus. At a molecular level, these events are mediated by two specific platelet adhesion receptors: the glycoprotein (GP) Ib/IX/V complex, which binds von Willebrand factor (VWF) to initiate platelet adhesion, and the GP IIb/IIIa complex (integrin $\alpha_{IIb}\beta_3$), which binds VWF, fibrinogen, or both to mediate platelet aggregation.

Vascular injury exposes the subendothelial matrix, of which collagen is a major component. The two principal receptors for collagen on platelets are GP VI and the integrin $\alpha_2\beta_1$ (1), but these receptors are able to mediate platelet attachment to collagen only at low shear rates (<200 per second). At higher shear stresses, which are found in small arteries and arterioles, the attachment of platelets to collagen surfaces is carried out by the GP Ib/IX/V/VWF interaction with VWF serving as an intermediary between the receptor and collagen. This interaction then decelerates the platelets and allows for their interaction with collagen via GP VI, integrin $\alpha_2\beta_1$, and possibly GP V.

The seminal work of Savage et al. (2) demonstrated that at arterial flow rates, where the shear stress is high (>600 per second), the initial adhesion of platelets to the subendothelium is mediated exclusively by engagement of VWF by the GP Ib/IX/V complex. A critical level of flow is required to initiate GP Ib/IX/VWF-mediated cell adhesion. Translocation rates of platelets over VWF increase relatively linearly up to a shear rate of 1,500 per second and remain constant up to 6,000 per second. The interaction of the platelets with the matrix is transitory in nature, with the platelets adhering, remaining stationary for a short time, detaching, and reattaching. This transitory platelet–matrix interaction results from a fast dissociation rate constant for the GP Ib$\alpha$/VWF interaction (3). However, as the platelets translocate, they come in contact with the matrix, and this allows for the interaction of other receptors with their ligands. Critically, cell arrest is mediated by the interaction of integrin $\alpha_{IIb}\beta_3$ with fibrinogen and VWF.

VWF is present in the plasma in a form that is unable to bind GP Ib. VWF binds to collagen types I, II, and III by its A3 domain and can be deposited onto the subendothelium at sites of injury under conditions of high shear stress. This collagen-bound form of VWF can interact with GP Ib to initiate platelet adhesion at the site of vascular injury. VWF multimers can also self-associate (4), although whether this occurs *in vivo* is as yet unclear. Additional sources of VWF are endothelial cells and the platelets themselves. Endothelial cells contain ultra-large von Willebrand factor (ULVWF) multimers within Weibel-Palade bodies (5). As opposed to soluble VWF, ULVWF can support platelet adhesion in the absence of high shear. Endothelial cells are the major source of ULVWF. When stimulated, they secrete ULVWF from their Weibel-Palade bodies, with a portion of the ULVWF multimer remaining tethered to the endothelial cell surface as long stringlike structures by P selectin (6). These strings of VWF are able to support platelet adhesion (7,8). In a plasma milieu, ULVWF is very rapidly processed to the normal circulating forms of VWF by the metalloproteinase ADAMSTS-13 (7). Interestingly, the bond strength between either the isolated GP Ib-binding A1 domain of VWF or ULVWF has been demonstrated to be 11.4 pN (9), suggesting that, in contrast to processed VWF, the A1 domain in ULVWF is an activated adhesive conformation capable of spontaneously binding GP Ib. In the absence of shear stress, the modulator ristocetin, which is thought to physiologically mimic the action of shear, is required to elicit binding of plasma VWF to GP Ib. The strength of the plasma VWF/GP Ib bond in the presence of ristocetin, however, is 6.5 pN. This suggests that in a physiologic setting platelets would adhere better to ULVWF than to plasma VWF that had been deposited on the subendothelial surface.

In 1995, Wagner et al. demonstrated that platelets not only could bind to subendothelial matrix but also could translocate on, and stably adhere to, activated endothelium *in vivo* (10). In their initial study, the mesenteric venules of mice were acutely activated by treatment with the calcium ionophore A23187. The platelet–endothelial interactions occurred under these conditions with both resting and activated platelets and was critically dependent on the expression of endothelial P selectin. At very low shear rates (80 to 100 per second), however, translocation and adhesion of resting platelets on A23187- or histamine-activated endothelium is independent of P selectin and dependent on endothelial expression of VWF and platelet GP Ib (8).

In mice, both resting and activated platelets can translocate and adhere to inflamed endothelium chronically activated *in vivo* by tumor necrosis factor-α (TNFα) (11). Here, resting platelet adhesion is dependent on both endothelial P and E selectin and selectin counter-receptors on platelets, GP Ib (12), and P selectin glycoprotein ligand (PSGL-1) (13). Similarly, in endotoxin-treated rats, immunoneutralization of either endothelial P selectin or platelet GP Ib abolishes platelet interactions with vein endothelium (14). In contrast, the adhesion of activated platelets to TNF-activated venules appears to involve a distinct mechanism independent of GP Ib and is mediated by platelet P selectin and an unknown TNF-inducible P selectin receptor on endothelium (11).

Recent studies by Kulkarni et al. (15) have demonstrated that thrombus growth is also critically dependent on the VWF/GP Ib interaction. Here, the source of the VWF is platelet α-granules. Upon platelet deposition, activation signals induce the exocytosis of granule contents. This allows for a pool of VWF to be concentrated on the surface of the growing thrombus and provides a substrate for the arrest of more platelets through GP Ib and $\alpha_{IIb}\beta_3$ and hence further thrombus growth.

# STRUCTURE OF THE GLYCOPROTEIN Ib/IX/V COMPLEX

The GP Ib/IX/V complex is a unique plasma membrane GP complex unrelated in structure to other membrane receptors, including those also involved in mediating cell adhesion (16–19). The important structural features of the GP Ib/IX/V complex are shown in Figure 31-1. The GP Ib/IX/V complex consists of four transmembrane subunits — GP Ibα, GP Ibβ, GP IX, and GP V—each of which is a member of the leucine-rich repeat (LRR) protein superfamily. Proteins in this family participate in a variety of cell functions, including cell signaling, cell adhesion, and development (16,20). In the GP Ib/IX/V complex, each subunit contains either one copy or tandem repeats of a leucine-rich motif of approximately 24 amino acids flanked by conserved disulfide loop structures (21–24) at both the N- and C-termini. GP Ibα is disulfide-linked to GP Ibβ by cysteinyl residues proximal to the extracellular face of the plasma

membrane (25). GP Ib is noncovalently associated with GP IX as a 1:1 complex that can be purified from platelet membranes in the presence of Triton X-100 (26,27). GP V also associates with the complex noncovalently, and based on monoclonal antibody binding data, there are only half as many copies of this polypeptide on the platelet surface as there are GP Ib/IX complexes (26–28). The full GP Ib/IX/V complex can be solubilized in intact form with mild detergents such as digitonin (28).

The structure shown for the GP Ib/IX/V complex in Figure 31-1 is based on this apparent stoichiometry. As a cautionary note, it should be emphasized that this stoichiometry is based on studies with only two anti–GP V monoclonal antibodies and that other structures for the GP Ib/IX/V complex are plausible, including aggregate structures. Nevertheless, a number of experimental findings are consistent with this model. Expression studies of partial complexes in Chinese hamster ovary (CHO) cells suggest that GP V associates with GP Ibα in formation of the GP Ib/IX/V complex (29). This result, together with the apparent stoichiometry, suggests that one important function of GP V may be to bring into proximity two GP Ibα chains, a structural feature that may be important for GP Ib/IX/V complex–dependent signaling (see section, "Signaling through the Glycoprotein Ib/IX/V Complex"). Expression studies of partial complexes in CHO cells also suggest that GP Ibβ is the critical subunit linking GP Ibα and GP IX (30). In contrast, antibody crossblocking studies suggest a close association between GP Ibα and GP IX (31). These two findings are clearly not mutually exclusive and are consistent with rotary shadowing data that GP Ibβ, GP IX, and the membrane spanning C-terminal end of GP Ibα form a globular domain with a diameter of approximately 16 nm (32).

GP Ibα is 610 amino acids long (21) and has an apparent molecular weight on sodium dodecyl sulfate-polyacrylamide gel electrophoresis (SDS-PAGE) of 135 kDa, indicating that it contains approximately 50% carbohydrate by weight. Rotary shadowing electron microscopy indicates that GP Ibα has an N-terminal globular domain approximately 9 nm in diameter (32). This domain contains seven tandem LRRs with conserved N- and C-terminal flanking sequences (21,33). X-ray crystallography suggests that the N-terminus of GP Ibα consists of an N-terminal β-hairpin (residues 1 to 18), seven LRRs (34 to 198), with an overhang at each end (giving eight repeat structures), a

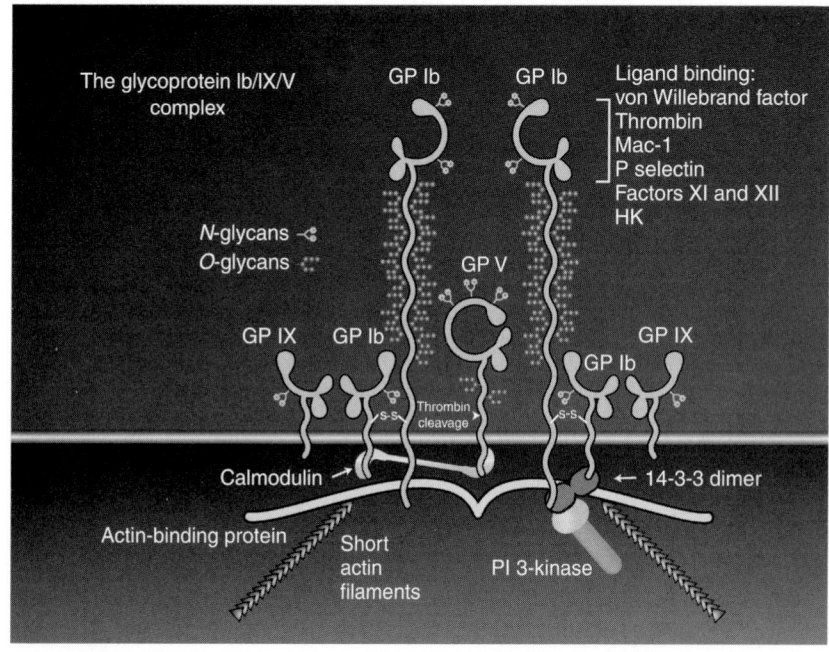

FIGURE 31-1. Schematic depiction of the glycoprotein (GP) Ib/IX/V complex and associated proteins. One possible arrangement of the GP Ib/IX/V complex is shown, with two GP Ib/IX complexes associated with one molecule of GP V. The actual complex may have a higher-order structure with the same stoichiometry. See the text for discussion. *Diamonds* on stalks depict N-linked carbohydrate chains; *circles* on stalks depict O-linked chains. S, sulfhydryl.

disulfide knot structure (amino acids 205 to 264), and a *C*-terminal anionic region (see Fig. 31-2). The *N*-terminal β-hairpin has two antiparallel strands with a disulfide bridge (C4 to C17) at its base. The seven LRRs fold into an arc shape, as seen in other LRR protein structures such as that of ribonuclease inhibitor. The GP Ibα *C*-terminal flanking sequence contains two disulfide bonds, C209 to C248 and C211 to C264, an α-helix (residues 214 to 223), and a loop (residues 227 to 242), which extends over the interior of the GP Ibα LRR concave face and which undergoes a dramatic change in conformation on binding VWF (see section, "Glycoprotein Ib/IX/V Complex as a von Willebrand Factor Receptor").

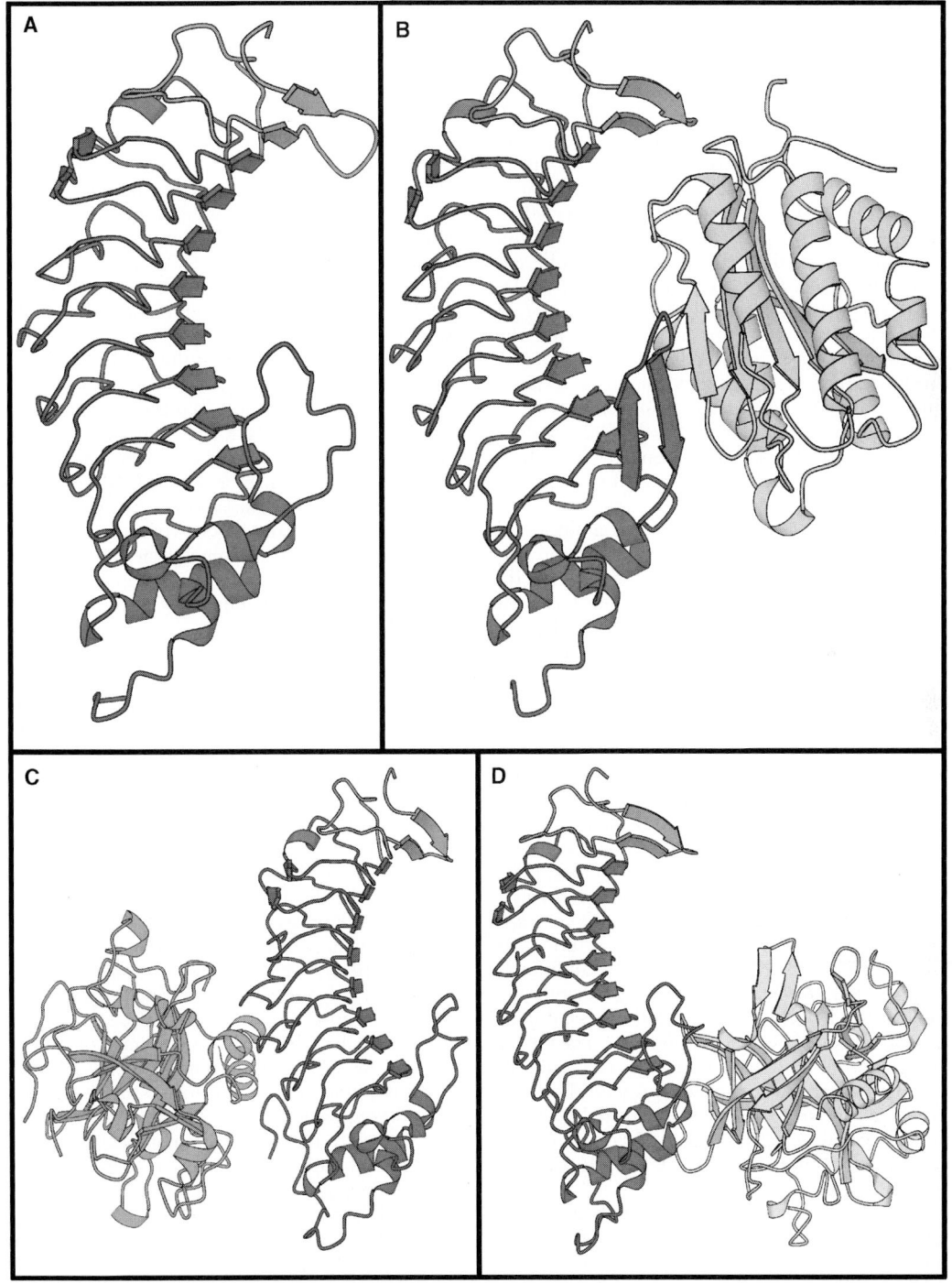

**FIGURE 31-2.** Summary of structural studies of glycoprotein (GP) Ibα and its binding partners. **A:** The 1.7-Å structure of the apo form of GP Ibα (pdb identifier 1P9A). The *N*-terminal "finger" is shown in *pink* and the *C*-terminal flank region in *magenta*. The eight tandem leucine-rich repeats are in *red*. **B:** The complex between GP Ibα [coloring as for part (A)] and von Willebrand factor A1 domain (*light green*) (pdb identifier 1SQ0). **C, D:** The crystal structure of GP Ibα [coloring as in (A)] in complex with thrombin reveals two possible binding sites. In panel (C), thrombin (*green*) is shown interacting with the sulfated tyrosine residues in the *C*-terminal tail of GP Ibα. In panel (D), thrombin (*yellow*) is interacting with the *C*-terminal flank (*magenta*) (see Color Fig. 31-2). (Celikel R, McClintock RA, Roberts JR, et al. Modulation of α-thrombin function by distinct interactions with platelet glycoprotein Ibα. *Science* 2003;301:218–221.)

The central region of GP Ibα consists of a sialomucin core rich in serine, threonine, and proline residues (21) that is heavily O-glycosylated (199). The major O-linked carbohydrate is a hexasaccharide containing sialic acid, galactose, N-acetylglucosamine, and N-acetylgalactosamine in a ratio of 2:2:1:1 (199, 200). Its structure has been determined to be NeuAc(α2-3)Gal (β1-3)[NeuAc(α2-3)Gal(β1-4)GalNAc(β1-6)]GalNAc-ol (34, 35,200). GP Ibα also contains four putative N-linked glycosylation sites (21), the saccharide structures of which have been partially determined (34). By rotary shadowing electron microscopy, the mucin core, or macroglycopeptide region, of GP Ibα is a linear structure approximately 35 nm long (32). The macroglycopeptide region of GP Ibα is polymorphic, with four variants, each specified by distinct alleles and varying in the number (1 to 4) of tandem repeats of a 13–amino acid sequence (36,37). On the basis of the similarity of this region to known mucin structures, each repeat would be expected to add approximately 2.5 nm to the overall length of GP Ibα (36). The structural and genetic implications of the different allelic forms, as well as their frequencies in different populations, are discussed in the section on polymorphisms.

Between the LRR C-terminal flanking sequence and the macroglycopeptide mucin core is a 19–amino acid sequence rich in negatively charged aspartate and glutamate residues (21). This sequence also contains three tyrosine residues within a sequence that favors their O-sulfation in the Golgi bodies. Sulfation of all three tyrosines has been confirmed, both in CHO cells expressing the GP Ib/IX complex (38) and in purified platelet GP Ibα (39).

The cytoplasmic tail of GP Ibα contains 96 amino acid residues (21) and binding sites for two proteins—filamin and 14-3-3ζ—implicated in regulating the function of the GP Ib/IX/V complex (40,41). The binding site for filamin has been localized to the internal sequence Thr536 to Leu554 (42), whereas the binding site for 14-3-3ζ has been localized to the C-terminus and involves phosphoserine residues at position Ser587, Ser590, and Ser609 (43–45).

GP Ibβ (25 kDa, 181 amino acids) and GP IX (22 kDa, 160 amino acids) both contain a single leucine-rich motif with conserved flanking sequences (22,23). The two polypeptides share sequence similarity throughout their extracellular and transmembrane regions, diverging significantly only in their cytoplasmic domains (16). GP Ibβ is disulfide-linked to GP Ibα immediately proximal to the platelet plasma membrane (22). The GP Ibβ cytoplasmic sequence of 34 amino acids contains a protein kinase A phosphorylation site at Ser166 (46) that appears to regulate platelet actin polymerization in response to agonist stimulation (47), as well as provides an additional 14-3-3ζ binding site (44,46–48). In addition, the membrane proximal region of the GP Ibβ cytoplasmic tail binds calmodulin, an association lost on platelet activation (49). The GP IX cytoplasmic tail comprises only five amino acids (23) with no known binding sites for complex-associated proteins. Both the GP Ibβ and GP IX cytoplasmic sequences can be palmitoylated at membrane proximal cysteinyl residues (50), a modification that is required for localization of the GP Ib/IX/V complex in lipid rafts (51).

GP V (82 kDa, 544 amino acids) has 15 LRRs and conserved N- and C-terminal flanking sequences. It has a short cytoplasmic tail of 16 amino acids (24,52), which also binds calmodulin. However, like GP Ibβ, this only occurs in resting platelets (49). Along with the seven-transmembrane-domain thrombin receptors, protease-activated receptor (PAR)-1 (53), PAR-3 (54), and PAR-4 (55,56), it is one of four potential thrombin receptors on the human platelet surface (57). Thrombin hydrolysis of GP V releases a large soluble fragment, GP Vf1, with an apparent molecular weight of 69.5 kDa (57).

# GENES, POLYMORPHISMS, AND EXPRESSION

Each of the polypeptides of the GP Ib/IX/V complex is encoded by its own gene. Each contains virtually the entire coding region within a single exon, with the exception of the gene for GP Ibβ, which has a small intron interrupting the region that encodes the signal peptide (58). All the genes also contain a small intron immediately 5′ to the translation start site. Therefore, the genes for the GP Ib/IX/V polypeptides each contain only one intron, except the GP Ibβ gene, which contains two. This paucity of introns confers a compact structure on the GP Ib/IX/V complex genes, with the largest, encoding GP Ibα, spanning only approximately 4 kb, including the upstream and downstream regulatory elements (59,60). Despite their similarities and the probability that they arose from a common ancestral gene, the genes are scattered throughout the human genome. The GP Ibα gene is located on chromosome 17 (17p12) (60), the GP Ibβ gene on chromosome 22 (22q11.2) (58,61), and the genes for GP IX and GP V on different regions of chromosome 3 (3q29 and 3q24, respectively) (62).

Transcription from all of the GP Ib/IX/V complex genes is controlled by a unique set of transcription factors that also control other genes whose expression is primarily restricted to the megakaryocyte. Each gene contains sequences for binding transcription factors of the GATA and Ets families, with GATA-1 being the member of the GATA family with the most important role in megakaryocyte gene expression (63). Another transcription factor, FOG-1 (friend of GATA-1) is a cofactor necessary for imparting some of the specificity of expression of these genes (64). Inducible expression of GP IX is similarly mediated through an Ets binding site involving the transcription factor Fli-1 (65,66).

Although most constitutive expression of the GP Ib/IX/V polypeptides is restricted to cells of the megakaryocytic lineage, considerable evidence exists that they are also expressed at lower levels in endothelial cells, particularly under cytokine stimulation. Two groups initially described the presence of an immunoreactive GP Ibα polypeptide in cultured human umbilical vein endothelium (67,68). It was later shown that it was possible to enhance expression of the GP Ibα messenger RNA by treating the cells with the inflammatory cytokines, interleukin-1 and TNF-α (69). The cloning of a complementary DNA for GP Ibα from an endothelial cell library further established the presence of this polypeptide in endothelial cells (70). Wu et al. (71) have provided evidence that all of the complex polypeptides can be found in endothelium.

Several polymorphisms affecting the genes and polypeptides of the GP Ib/IX/V complex have been described, primarily affecting GP Ibα These polymorphisms not only serve as useful markers for genetic studies but also may affect the expression, structure, function, or antigenicity of the affected polypeptide. In addition, evidence suggests that polymorphisms of GP Ibα may influence the risk of development of arterial thrombotic disease, although there is presently little agreement between different population studies (see Table 31-1).

In GP Ibα, two polymorphisms affect the structure of the polypeptide. One affects the length of the polypeptide, which can be 610, 623, 636, or 649 amino acid residues, depending on which of four alleles encodes it (the alleles and polypeptides are designated A, B, C, and D—from largest to smallest) (36,37). The difference is based on a variable number of tandem repeats (VNTR) polymorphism in the mucinlike macroglycopeptide region. A 13–amino acid sequence in this region has been exactly duplicated once, twice, or thrice, which accounts for the different lengths. Because each repeat is rich in threonine, serine, and proline residues, and because most of

**TABLE 31-1**

GP Ib POLYMORPHISMS AS PREDICTORS OF CARDIOVASCULAR AND DISEASE RISK

| Polymorphism | Risk factor (?) | Reference |
|---|---|---|
| GP Ibα | Met allele associated with CAD | 72 |
| HPA-2a/b | Met allele associated with CAD, CVD | 73 |
| | Met allele *not* associated with MI | 201 |
| | Met allele *not* associated with CAD | 202 |
| | Met allele associated with CAD | 203 |
| | Trend of Met allele association with stroke in women | 204 |
| | Met allele *not* associated with higher platelet activity in patients who have had a stroke | 205 |
| | Met allele associated with VNTR B and MI, sudden death | 206 |
| | Thr allele associated with higher affinity binding of VWF | 79 |
| GP Ibα | No association of increased VNTR (A or B) and stroke | 207 |
| VNTR A, B, C, D | VNTR A associated with CAD | 208 |
| | VNTR C/B associated with CHD and CVD | 73 |
| | No association of increased VNTR (A or B) and CAD | 202 |
| | VNTR C/D associated with increased platelet activity (PFA-100) in healthy subjects compared to VNTR C/C | 74 |
| | VNTR A or B associated with decreased age of CABG | 209 |
| | VNTR B associated with NAION | 210 |
| GP Ibα | C allele *not* associated with increased thrombosis | 211,212 |
| Kozak -5 T/C | C allele *not* associated with increased MI | 211 |
| | C allele *not* associated with increased MI or stroke in women | 213 |
| | C allele *not* associated with increased CAD | 214 |
| | C allele associated with ischemic stroke | 85 |
| | C allele associated with CAD | 215 |
| | T allele homozygote associated with CAD and MI | 216 |
| | C allele associated with MI | 217 |
| | T allele homozygote associated with increased platelet activity (PFA-100) in healthy subjects compared to T/C | 74 |
| | C allele associated with HIT-TEC in men | 218 |
| GP Ibβ | Glu15 substitution associated with neonatal alloimmune thrombocytopenia | 219 |
| Iyᵃ | | |

?, potential risk; HPA, human platelet antigens; CAD, coronary artery disease; CVD, cardiovascular disease; MI, myocardial infarction; VNTR, variable number of tandem repeats; CABG, coronary artery bypass grafting; NAION, non-arteritic ischemic optic neuropathy; HIT, heparin-induced thrombocytopenia.

the threonines and serines are likely to be glycosylated, each repeat could add up to 32 Å to the length of the GP Ibα extracellular domain (36). This may have important implications for the functions of the complex because each added repeat would position the ligand-binding domain farther above the platelet plasma membrane, thereby making it more accessible to ligands and possibly more susceptible to the influence of shear forces. Either or both of these effects could account for the demonstration in some studies of an increased risk for coronary artery disease (CAD) associated with the longer variants (72,73). However, VWF-dependent closure times on collagen-adrenaline using PFA-100 instrumentation are shorter in carriers of the C/D genotype than in those with the C/C genotype (74).

The VNTR polymorphism is also important for genetic studies. Heterozygosity for this marker ranges between 25% and 30% in all human populations tested, rendering it the most useful marker for the *GP Ibα* gene (75).

Another GP Ibα polymorphism of clinical importance is based on the presence of either Thr or Met at amino acid 145,

within the LRR region of the GP Ibα ligand-binding domain (76,77). This polymorphism is the basis of the human platelet antigens (HPA)-2 platelet alloantigen system. In Japanese and Caucasian populations, the allele frequencies for the Thr and Met alleles are approximately 90% and 10%, respectively (76,77). Heterozygous children of mothers homozygous for either allele are at risk for the development of alloimmune purpura caused by transplacental transfer of antibodies. Whether the HPA-2 polymorphism has functional consequences is presently unclear. Two recent studies found that VWF bound both the Thr and Met allelic forms of GP Ibα equally well (74,78), whereas a third study found that VWF bound with higher affinity to the Thr allelic form (79). The HPA-2 polymorphism has no effect on binding of thrombin to GP Ib as would be expected based on the GP Ib/thrombin crystal structures (Fig. 31-2C and D).

Kaski et al. found two other polymorphisms by sequencing random individuals in a Finnish population (80). One is a thymine (T)/cytosine (C) dimorphism at position −5 from the antithymocyte globulin (ATG) start codon, termed the Kozak polymorphism, and the second is an adenine/guanine dimorphism of the third base of the codon for Arg358, a silent change with no effect on the polypeptide sequence. The two rarer forms of these markers are both part of a mutant haplotype described in three unrelated patients with Bernard-Soulier syndrome (BSS) (81–83). The causative mutation in these patients is a deletion of the last two bases of the codon for Tyr492. Because it has been found in unrelated patients of northern European ancestry, this may represent a founder mutant haplotype that could account for a significant fraction of the alleles responsible for BSS in these populations.

The Kozak sequence polymorphism has been reported to be a major determinant of GP Ibα, and hence GP Ib/IX/V expression, on platelets due to more efficient translation of the −5C form of GP Ibα mRNA (84). Presence of one or both copies if the C allele has been reported as a risk marker of ischemic stroke (85,86).

# BIOSYNTHESIS OF THE GLYCOPROTEIN Ib/IX/V COMPLEX

On the platelet plasma membrane, the stoichiometry of the three GP Ib/IX polypeptides (GP Ibα, GP Ibβ, and GP IX) appears to be maintained tightly at equimolar levels (27). The number of GP V polypeptides in each complex is about one half that of the other polypeptides (28,71,87), although this ratio has not been examined closely enough to confidently state that it is a fixed requirement. Because the polypeptides of the complex are synthesized separately from individual mRNA species, this stoichiometry requires a mechanism either for their coordinate synthesis or for elimination of the uncomplexed polypeptides. Both of these mechanisms play a part in maintaining the stoichiometry, but the latter is predominant. In heterologous cells transfected with complementary DNA for the three polypeptides, a similar equimolar stoichiometry is achieved on the cell surface (88). In BSS heterozygotes, approximately one-half the normal levels of the complex appear on their platelets, whether the mutation affects GP Ibα, GP Ibβ, or GP IX (75). The stoichiometry is thereby maintained by the requirement of each polypeptide for the stability of the entire complex. In transfected cells, efficient expression of GP Ib on the cell surface requires all three of the polypeptides, with omission of either GP Ibβ or GP IX profoundly decreasing the surface levels of the complex (88). In partial complexes, GP Ibβ is able to independently associate with both GP Ibα and GP IX in the absence of the third subunit, but in the absence of GP Ibβ, GP Ibα does not associate with GP IX (30). Recent studies with Bernard-Soulier patient platelets also confirm the critical role of GP Ibβ in regulating both the processing and/or surface expression of GP Ibα and GP IX (89–91). The association of GP Ibβ and GP IX appears to be primarily regulated by the GP Ibβ N-terminal cysteine knot flanking sequence (92).

Like GP IX, GP V associates noncovalently with the complex (28). Unlike the other polypeptides of the complex, GP V appears on the plasma membrane of transfected cells when transfected alone, but its expression there is increased by the presence of the GP Ib/IX complex (29,93). GP V associates with the complex through a direct linkage with GP Ibα (29). This subunit is not required for efficient expression of the rest of the complex on the plasma membrane, although it may have a minor influence (29,93,94).

The polypeptide complex is assembled in the endoplasmic reticulum immediately after synthesis of its polypeptides and requires approximately 3 hours to complete the journey to the plasma membrane (95,96). On the way, the complex undergoes a large number of posttranslational modifications, including extensive N- and O-glycosylation, tyrosine sulfation, and fatty acylation. Each of these modifications is required for a fully functional complex and for expression on the cell surface (96). In cultured cells, complexes that lack GP IX are not as efficiently targeted to the plasma membrane and are degraded in the lysosome (95). This process is not influenced by the presence or absence of GP V.

# ROLE OF THE GLYCOPROTEIN Ib/IX/V COMPLEX IN PLATELET IMMUNOLOGY

Approximately 25,000 copies of the GP Ib/IX complex are found on platelets (26,27) and apparently one half as many copies of GP V (28,71). It is therefore not surprising that the GP Ib/IX/V complex plays a significant role in several important aspects of platelet immunology. The HPA-2 (Ko/Sib) alloantigen system (Thr or Met at residue 145) (76,77) has been associated with the pathogenesis of two clinical syndromes, neonatal alloimmune thrombocytopenia and refractoriness to platelet transfusion, in common with platelet alloantigens on other membrane glycoproteins such as $\alpha_{IIb}\beta_3$.

Early studies by Kunicki et al. (97,98) implicated the GP Ib/IX/V complex as the major platelet antigen involved in quinine/quinidine-induced thrombocytopenia. The thrombocytopenia is due to a Fab-mediated interaction with a neoepitope in the protein formed by binding of the drug. Binding of antibody to the drug-dependent epitope results in complement activation and subsequent platelet lysis. Studies with the monoclonal antibodies FMC25 and SZ1 implicate GP IX as the major binding site on the GP Ib/IX/V complex (99–101). Recently, the epitope has been mapped to GP IX subunit of the GP Ib/IX/V complex, specifically amino acids 64 to 135 (102). Another neoepitope is present within a 40-kDa polypeptide derived from the GP Ibα N-terminus (100). A more recent study indicates existence of at least three patterns of alloantiserum reactivity with the polypeptides of the GP Ib/IX/V complex (103). One group of alloantisera reacted with drug-dependent epitopes on both GP Ibα and GP IX, whereas the second and third groups of antisera reacted with epitopes on either GP IX or GP Ibα, respectively, but not with both polypeptides (103).

Rifampicin-dependent antibodies have been described that target the GP Ib/IX/V complex (104) and bind an epitope similar to the epitope recognized by quinine-dependent antibodies (105). Rifampicin is a drug used in the treatment of tuberculosis. The predominant target of antibodies isolated from patients with gold-induced autoimmune thrombocytopenia is GP V (106).

Although early studies suggested that only a small number of patients with chronic idiopathic thrombocytopenic purpura (ITP) had detectable anti–GP Ib/IX/V antibodies (107), a large number of studies using more sensitive techniques such as the monoclonal antibody immunoprecipitation assay have detected antibodies against the GP Ib/IX/V complex in 25% to 85% of patient sera (107–111). Autoantibodies against $\alpha_{IIb}\beta_3$ can also be detected in about one half of the patients with anti–GP Ib/IX/V antibodies (107–109). The autoantibodies are primarily IgG, with IgA and IgM antibodies occurring much less frequently (108,111), and they interact with the relevant platelet antigen through their Fab regions (112). In this regard, it is of interest that some studies suggest that the platelet Fc receptor, FcγRIIA, is in close proximity to the GP Ib/IX/V complex (113), a finding that may be relevant to the association of autoantibodies against GP Ib and a severe form of ITP (114). The epitopes on the GP Ib/IX/V complex recognized by autoantibodies in ITP have not been extensively characterized. In one study, three antibodies were localized to a disulfide-dependent epitope involving the plasma-membrane-proximal region of GP Ibα and GP Ibβ (107). Autoantibodies can also be detected against cytoplasmic regions of the GP Ib/IX/V complex, but these probably arise as a consequence of platelet destruction rather than being causative (108). Autoantibodies against the GP Ib/IX/V complex are also found in patients with thrombocytopenia and with primary biliary cirrhosis (115), systemic lupus erythematosus (116), and antiphospholipid antibodies (116,117). Antibodies against GP V have been detected in children with acute ITP after varicella zoster infection (118).

## GLYCOPROTEIN Ib/IX/V COMPLEX AS A VON WILLEBRAND FACTOR RECEPTOR

The binding or adhesion of VWF to the GP Ib/IX/V complex on platelets initiates the cascade of events that results in either hemostasis or thrombosis. In the normal circulation, this interaction is either absent or occurs with low affinity. Immobilization of VWF on a surface and high shear stresses are both believed to change the conformation of the A1 domain of VWF, making it a high-affinity ligand for the GP Ib/IX/V complex (119,120). Shear-dependent changes in the structure of the GP Ib/IX/V complex may also be important for increasing affinity for VWF (121). Treatment of VWF with modulators such as ristocetin and botrocetin, as well as its desialylation or proteolysis, also increases its affinity for the GP Ib/IX/V complex. The molecular mechanisms by which the antibiotic ristocetin and the snake venom proteins, botrocetin and bitiscetin, modulate VWF activity are yet to be fully defined. Nevertheless, the mechanism for VWF binding to GP Ib induced by ristocetin is much more similar to that which operates under shear than to the mechanism induced by botrocetin (122,123). Ristocetin binds proline-rich sequences in the N- and C-terminal flanking regions of the VWF A1 domain (124) and also binds one or more sites in GP Ibα (125,126). It has been proposed that ristocetin either binds VWF in proline-rich sequences proximal to the VWF A1 Cys509–Cys695 disulfide bond and alters the conformation of the A1 domain (124) or helps bridge the interaction between VWF and GP Ib (126,127). On the basis of botrocetin/A1 and bitiscetin cocrystal structures, botrocetin and bitiscetin bind distinct sites in the VWF A1 domain adjacent to the GP Ib–binding site. It has been proposed that both venom proteins stabilize VWF/GP Ib interaction by first binding VWF and then acting as bridge between ligand and receptor (128,129).

Sulfation of all three tyrosine residues in the negative charge cluster, Tyr276, Tyr278, and Tyr279, is necessary for optimal interaction of GP Ibα with VWF (130,131), particularly when induced by botrocetin. In this regard, an N-terminal GP Iα fragment comprising residues 1 to 275 is an order of magnitude worse as an inhibitor of botrocetin-dependent binding of VWF to platelets than a fragment comprising residues 1 to 282 (39). Finally, monoclonal antibodies that map into this region of GP Ibα selectively inhibit botrocetin-dependent, but not ristocetin-dependent, binding of VWF. In a similar manner, several anti–GP Ibα monoclonal antibodies have been reported that have the converse effect (123,132), suggesting that distinct regions of the GP Ib/IX/V complex can be used in VWF recognition.

It is now clearly established that the binding site for VWF is localized in the N-terminal globular region of the α chain of GP Ib, with the minimal fully functional sequence comprising residues His1 to Glu282 (39). Adhesion of VWF to GP Ibα involves electrostatic interactions between a negative patch within the LRRs of GP Ibα (within 59 and 128) and a complementary positive patch on the VWF-A1 domain (122,133). Residues N- and C-terminal to this region directly contact VWF in a cocrystal structure of a GP Ibα fragment (lacking N-linked glycosylation sites at Asn21 and Asn159) and a wild-type VWF-A1 fragment (residues 496–709) (Fig. 31-2B) (134). Gain-of-function point mutations within either GP Ibα (Met239/Val) or VWF-A1 (Arg543/Gln) alter the conformation of the affected protein and result in distinct mechanisms for their ligation involving different contact sites (134,135). In the case of VWF-A1, the mutation is greater than 15Å from a GP Ibα–contacting sequence, emphasizing the sensitivity of the interaction to conformational regulation (134). The VWF gain-of-function mutation at Arg543/Gln enhances affinity for GP Ibα by virtue of an approximately sixfold decrease in off-rate. On the other hand, the Met239/Val gain-of-function mutation of GP Ibα is within a β-hairpin structure in the C-terminal flank that is significantly altered when in complex with VWF-A1. This mutation stabilizes the β-hairpin and increases the affinity of VWF binding, also by approximately sixfold, but is associated with an increased on-rate and essentially unchanged off-rate (134). Together, these studies with isolated ligand and receptor fragments indicate how (shear stress-induced) conformational changes of native GP Ibα and VWF may regulate the affinity of the adhesive interaction and result in an on-rate/off-rate for platelet adhesion supporting either rolling or firm adhesion in flowing blood.

## PLATELET GP Ib/IX/V IS A UNIQUE RECEPTOR FOR THROMBIN

X-ray crystal structures published in 2003 have begun to explain many long-standing paradoxes of the thrombin–GP Ib/IX/V interaction (136–140), an interaction that is both literally and figuratively multifaceted. GP Ibα was identified as a high-affinity binding site for α-thrombin more than 20 years ago (138,139), but since then, establishing the functional consequences of this interaction has been problematic. Complications include the presence of other functional thrombin receptors on platelets, including protease-activated receptors PAR-1 and PAR-4; the undefined roles of other thrombin substrates, including GP V; the presence of multiple classes of thrombin-binding sites of different affinity (approximately 50 high-affinity binding sites on platelets compared with approximately 25,000 copies of GP Ib/IX); and the capacity of thrombin to activate platelets by different pathways, involving proteolytic or nonproteolytic mechanisms, at different doses (for example, the presence of GP Ib/IX/V facilitates the platelet response to low doses, but not high doses, of thrombin) (138–140). Recent analyses now suggest that GP Ibα promotes thrombin-dependent activation of PAR-1 (140,141); thrombin induces GP Ib–dependent signaling when GP V is absent (142); and GP Ibα mediates thrombin-dependent fibrin(ogen) cross-linking and regulation of clotting factor XI (143–145).

Thrombin associated with GP Ibα, therefore, has at least two potential roles: regulating clotting and activating platelets. The latter role has at least two potential mechanisms: GP Ibα serving as a cofactor for thrombin activation of PAR-1, and thrombin signaling directly by GP Ibα. The crystal structure of the thrombin–GP Ibα complex indicates that the molecules interact at the two sites, thrombin exosite I (which also binds fibrinogen) binding a region of GP Ibα within the C209 to C248 disulfide loop and thrombin exosite II binding the A/S region of GP Ibα [E268—two interactions, one involving the thrombin exosite I (that binds fibrinogen) and another exosite II (that binds heparin)] (136–140). How this pair of interactions with GP Ibα combine to regulate thrombin-dependent platelet activation and clot formation is one of the more intriguing recent advances in vascular biology.

One crystal structure used a GP Ibα fragment (N-terminal residues 1 to 290) and PPACK-inhibited thrombin (136); another used GP Ibα 1-279 (with N-linked glycosylation sites at Asn21 and Asn159 substituted by Glu) and DFP-thrombin (137). In brief, the thrombin exosite I interacted predominantly with 19 residues distributed within the C-terminal half of the fragment (residues 151 to 284) spanning the C-terminal 2–3 LRRs and anionic sulfated sequence; thrombin exosite II interacted mainly with residues 274, 275, and 277, and a region, 123–129, within the concave face of the canonical repeats; the sulfated tyrosine residues at 276, 278, and 279 interacted with both exosites (136,137). Thrombin binding minimally affects the structure of GP Ibα, except that of the anionic sequence (centered on 276 to 279), which is altered when thrombin binds by exosite II: surface-exposed GP Ibα Tyr276 and proximal acidic/sulfated residues, including Asp277, bind exosite II, which may then facilitate Tyr279 and associated residues contacting exosite I (136). These complexes reveal "striking charge complementarity between interacting surfaces of GP Ibα and thrombin" (137).

How do these interactions regulate the functions of thrombin or GP Ibα? Binding of thrombin by exosite II to GP Ibα opens the way for a second, sequential interaction of thrombin involving exosite I (stoichiometry of 2 thrombin: 1 GP Ibα)—this then inhibits thrombin-dependent fibrinogen cleavage (136). Thrombin bound to GP Ibα (by exosite II) accelerates PAR-1 cleavage and platelet activation: There is a sixfold to sevenfold increase in $k_{cat}/K_m$ for PAR-1 proteolysis on the platelet surface with intact GP Ibα (140,141). By an apparently analogous mechanism, thrombin associated with GP Ibα by exosite II is also ideally oriented for activation (by exosite I) of factor XI, potentially bound to a neighboring GP Ibα (145). Finally, two sites for thrombin on GP Ibα allow the former to cross-link two molecules of the latter, providing a mechanism for GP Ib-dependent platelet activation (in the absence of GP V) (142) and consistent with a receptor cross-linking mechanism for GP Ib/IX/V by other multivalent ligands (146,147). The pathophysiologic relevance of the thrombin/GP Ib/IX(/V) axis is at this stage speculative.

# GLYCOPROTEIN Ib/IX/V COMPLEX AS A RECEPTOR FOR OTHER LIGANDS

In addition to its functional role as a receptor for VWF and thrombin, the GP Ib/IX/V complex has been shown to be involved in other protein- and cell-binding interactions. This is consistent with the recent discovery that the lamprey utilizes LRR proteins as its equivalent to IgG for adaptive immune responses (148) and the finding that numerous molecules of the mammalian system of innate immunity, such as tolllike receptors (149), utilize LRRs as pattern recognition motifs capable of binding a diverse array of molecules. These observations suggest that, in general, LRR-containing proteins have the ability to bind a variety of different ligands.

A number of coagulation factors involved in initiation of the intrinsic pathway of coagulation bind GP Ib. It is known that kininogens inhibit binding of thrombin to platelets and thrombin-induced platelet aggregation. It has now been established that kininogen binds directly to the α chain of GP Ib at or near the binding site for α-thrombin (150). Factor XII zymogen is also able to bind GP Ibα (151). Upon binding, factor XII is converted to its active form (XIIa) by autolysis. This association also inhibits thrombin-induced platelet activation. This colocalization of both kininogen and factor XIIa to

GP Ibα may function to modulate the activity of thrombin at the platelet surface.

In addition, factor XI has been shown to bind GP Ib on activated platelets in a $Zn^{2+}$-dependent manner and preferentially binds raft-associated GP Ibα (152). Factor XI is a substrate for factor XIIa, and factor XI cleavage requires $Zn^{2+}$ and high molecular weight kininogen, the same prerequisite conditions as for factor XII association with platelets and its subsequent activation. Thrombin can also activate factor XI on the surface of activated platelets. This requires the formation of a trimolecular complex, including factor XI, GP Ibα, and thrombin. The binding of factor XI to thrombin exosites I and II is essential for thrombin-mediated activation of factor XI (145). The binding site on factor XI for GP Ib is within its apple 3 domain (153). These interactions therefore provide a mechanism whereby the platelet surface can provide the necessary environment for the initiation and maintenance of the coagulation cascade.

Fibrin monomer has been shown to modulate the binding of VWF to the GP Ib/IX/V complex, although the mechanism for this is unclear. Loscalzo et al. (154) found that VWF bound to fibrin monomer and that this interaction allowed subsequent binding to the GP Ib/IX/V complex. Similarly, in flowing blood, VWF must first bind to GP Ib to allow platelet adhesion to fibrin (155). In contrast, Parker and Gralnick (156) provided evidence that the initial step involved binding of fibrin monomer to the α chain of GP Ib.

Although the major ligand/receptor axis responsible for platelet adhesion is VWF binding to GP Ib/IX/V, other ligands have been demonstrated to participate in the adhesion of platelets by interacting with GP Ib/IX/V. These include P selectin, thrombospondin, and collagen. P selectin is expressed on the surface of platelets and activated endothelial cells. Recent work by Romo et al. (12) has demonstrated that P selectin can support platelet adhesion. Both immobilized P selectin and stimulated endothelial cells were able to support the binding and translocation (rolling) of GP Ib/IX expressing cells and washed platelets (12). Thrombospondin is also released on platelet activation (157) and is able to interact with numerous plasma proteins such as fibronectin and VWF. Agbanyo et al. (158) demonstrated that thrombospondin can support firm platelet adhesion at shear rates up to 4,000 per second. Onitsuka et al. (159) confirmed that platelets were able to adhere and roll on thrombospondin in a GP Ib–dependent manner, but showed that this relied on the initial deposition of VWF onto thrombospondin. More recently, however, Jurk et al. (160) provided evidence that GP Ib can directly support platelet adhesion to thrombospondin. Using platelets from patients who lack both plasma and platelet VWF, they demonstrated that VWF was not required as a bridge because platelets from these patients adhered to the same extent as platelets from normal controls. Because thrombospondin is secreted by activated platelets, the expression of thrombospondin on the platelet surface may play a facilitatory role to VWF in platelet capture and therefore in subsequent thrombus growth. In addition, atherosclerotic plaques are highly enriched in thrombospondin (161,162) and may provide a substrate for platelet adhesion upon plaque rupture.

Leukocytes have been demonstrated to be capable of attaching to and transmigrating through platelet thrombi. This process of transplatelet migration requires the leukocyte receptor Mac-1 (integrin $\alpha_M\beta_2$). Until recently, however, the ligand for Mac-1 remained elusive. Elegant studies performed by Simon et al. (163) demonstrated the ligand for Mac-1 on the platelet surface to be GP Ibα. Mac-1 binding to GP Ib has also been established as the mechanism of clearance of cold-treated platelets by phagocytic cells in the liver (164). Binding involves both the recognition of peptide sequence in the N-terminus of GP Ibα by the I-domain of Mac-1 (165) and the recognition of exposed β-N-acetylglucosamine residues of N-linked glycans on GP Ibα by a lectin-binding region of Mac-1 (166). In addition, maximal binding of Mac-1 to GP Ibα can be increased twofold by high molecular weight kininogen (167).

A large family of viper venom proteins structurally related to botrocetin also bind to the N-terminal region of GP Ibα [for a review, see Fujimura et al. (168)]. These proteins are disulfide-linked αβ heterodimers, approximately 25 to 30 kDa in molecular weight. The α and β chains display a high degree of sequence similarity and are related to the mammalian C-type lectin family. These proteins, however, do not require calcium ions for their GP Ib–binding activity. Members of this family of GP Ib–binding proteins include the various types of alboaggregin (169–171), echicetin (172), and CHH-A and CHH-B (171). Although all the GP Ib–binding proteins inhibit VWF binding, crossblocking studies with anti–GP Ib antibodies suggest that they bind to overlapping sites in the N-terminus, possibly in the LRRs (171). Interestingly, *Bothrops jararaca* venom contains not only botrocetins, which induce VWF binding to GP Ib, but also a protein called *jararaca GP Ib-BP*, which blocks the interaction (173).

Of the four GP Ib/IX/V polypeptides, GP V is the one least characterized functionally. GP V is cleaved by thrombin, which has been proposed to limit platelet activation by thrombin. Recently, however, Moog et al. (174) demonstrated that GP V plays a role in the adhesion and activation of platelets by collagen. Using GP V knockout mice and an intravital arterial thrombosis model, they showed that, in mice lacking GP V, platelet adhesion times were decreased and time to occlusion of the vessel was significantly increased. In addition, both the static adhesion of washed platelets and flow-based adhesion of platelets in whole blood to collagen type I were significantly reduced if GP V was absent.

Finally, a role for GP Ib/IX/V in infective endocarditis has been postulated. Infective endocarditis is a condition in which bacteria infect the heart valves. One common offending bacterium is *Streptococcus sanguis*, which has been shown to bind to and activate platelets (175,176) in a GP Ib–dependent manner (176). Therefore, platelets may be an initial contributing factor to infective endocarditis where injury of the valves or surrounding endothelium leads to the deposition of platelets and subsequent recruitment of bacteria via GP Ib interactions. This situation could be self-perpetuating whereby the bacteria cause localized platelet activation and thrombus formation.

# GLYCOPROTEIN Ib/IX/V COMPLEX ASSOCIATION WITH THE CYTOSKELETON

Solum and Olsen (177) first demonstrated that GP Ib was associated with the Triton X-100–insoluble fraction of platelet lysates, which is the operational definition of the cytoskeleton. Their study implied that the association was mediated by filamin because only disruption of this protein by a calcium-activated protease released the GP Ib/IX complex into the soluble fraction. This assumption was confirmed when two other groups directly demonstrated the association of GP Ib with filamin (40,178). The binding site for filamin was originally localized to a region in the middle of the GP Ibα cytoplasmic domain, between residues Thr536 and Phe568 (42), and more recently to residues 557 to 579 (179) and 557 to 575 (180). Association with the cytoskeleton has no effect on surface expression of the complex, but it does restrict its mobility on the cell surface and enables the complex to optimally bind VWF, at least when the interaction is induced by ristocetin (181, 182). Another process that may require the GP Ib/IX/V–filamin interaction is translocation of the complex from the platelet

exterior to an internal compartment (183–186). Redistribution requires participation of cytoskeletal structures because treatment of the platelets with cytochalasins inhibits the phenomenon. Whether this phenomenon actually occurs is controversial (187,188); if it does, it would provide a mechanism to facilitate platelet aggregation by reducing the electrostatic repulsion between platelets that is a consequence of the high negative charge imparted to the platelet surface by the dense coating of sialic acid residues within the macroglycopeptide of GP Ibα. Internalization of GP Ib/IX/V complexes after activation has also been proposed as a mechanism by which platelets might exert contractile tension on VWF bound to a matrix (189).

Association of the complex with the cytoskeleton may also be an essential factor in determining the size and shape of platelets and in decreasing the fluidity of their membranes. The platelets of patients with BSS are typically much larger than normal platelets (75), and their membranes deform much more easily (190). Recently, it has been shown that expression of a chimeric receptor IL-4Rα/GP Ibα cytoplasmic fusion protein in GP Ibα-deficient mice partially rescues the BSS-like phenotype with a doubling in circulating platelet count and a 50% reduction in platelet size when compared with platelets from the mouse model of the BSS. The chimeric receptor was confirmed to interact normally with filamin and 14-3-3ζ (191).

# SIGNALING THROUGH THE GLYCOPROTEIN Ib/IX/V COMPLEX

It is now well established that the interaction of GP Ib/IX/V with VWF elicits signals that potentiate the ability of the integrin $\alpha_{IIb}\beta_3$ to bind fibrinogen and VWF. The interaction of $\alpha_{IIb}\beta_3$ with either ligand induces stable platelet arrest and intracellular signals that result in irreversible platelet aggregation. The two integrin signaling phases are termed "inside-out" and "outside-in" signaling, respectively.

Many potential signaling pathways have been suggested to be involved in signaling from GP Ib/IX/V to $\alpha_{IIb}\beta_3$. These include gross physiologic changes in receptor localization on the platelet along with association with other receptors and/or costimulatory effects with other receptors. In addition, many intracellular signaling cascades have been suggested to be involved. However, to date little has been resolved as to what events are critical and which are peripheral to $\alpha_{IIb}\beta_3$ activation.

Several mechanisms have been proposed for GP Ib/IX/V signaling to $\alpha_{IIb}\beta_3$. Being a multimeric molecule, VWF may induce clustering of GP Ib/IX/V on the cell surface. Two groups have investigated whether clustering of GP Ib/IX/V induces activation of $\alpha_{IIb}\beta_3$. Chemical clustering of the GP Ib/IX/V complex in heterologous cells coexpressing $\alpha_{IIb}\beta_3$ did not result in an increase in the bond strength of $\alpha_{IIb}\beta_3$/fibrinogen (192) or induce PAC-1 binding (193). However, clustering of GP Ib/IX/V did result in both a decrease in the rolling velocity of the transfected CHO cells over VWF and an increase in stable adhesion under shear conditions. It appears, therefore, that while clustering of GP Ib/IX/V in suspension has no effect on the activation status of $\alpha_{IIb}\beta_3$, clustering of GP Ib/IX/V does result in intracellular signal generation. In this regard, Kasirer et al. (193) demonstrated that while clustering did not induce PAC-1 binding by $\alpha_{IIb}\beta_3$, protein tyrosine kinase activities were increased, evidenced by increased tyrosine phosphorylation of Syk.

Many groups have implied that other platelet receptors are absolutely required for GP Ib/IX/V-dependent signaling. Receptors implicated include the adenosine 5′-diphosphate (ADP) receptor P2Y$_{12}$, the FcR$\gamma$-chain, Fc$\gamma$RIIA, and the thromboxane A$_2$ receptor. Studies of shear-induced platelet aggregation have indicated that ADP, released from activated platelets, plays a costimulatory role in GP Ib/IX–dependent aggregation, because blockade of P2Y$_{12}$ leads to a decrease in platelet activation (194,195). The platelet Fc receptor Fc$\gamma$RIIA has been demonstrated to be physically and functionally associated with GP Ib (113) and, together with thromboxane A$_2$, plays a role in VWF/GP Ib/IX/V–dependent platelet activation (196). The FcR$\gamma$-chain has also been demonstrated to associate with GP Ib (197). FcR$\gamma$-chain has been shown to be required for full platelet activation because FcR$\gamma$-chain-deficient platelets show a blunted response to VWF-dependent shear-induced aggregation compared to normal platelets (198). Consistent with the notion that the ITAM-containing FcR$\gamma$-chain and/or Fc$\gamma$RIIA are involved in GP Ib–mediated platelet activation, Rathmore et al. (220) recently demonstrated that platelet endothelial cell adhesion molecule-1 (PECAM-1), which contains an immunoreceptor tyrosine-based inhibitory motif (ITIM), plays a negative regulatory role in GP Ib–dependent activation. This PECAM-1–mediated negative feedback loop has also been described for GP VI/FcR$\gamma$-chain signaling (221,222). Mice lacking PECAM-1 possess platelets that are hyperresponsive to VWF compared to control platelets.

GP Ib$\alpha$ associates with the cytoskeleton through interaction with filamin-1, and this linkage has been proposed to play a role in platelet activation. However, controversy surrounds the exact role of this cytoskeletal interaction. Cytochalasin D functions to depolymerise actin filaments and hence dissociate GP Ib/IX/V from the cytoskeleton. Several groups have used this approach and demonstrated that treatment of platelets with cytochalasin D enhances their aggregation response to VWF and shear (223,224). However, the use of a membrane permeable peptide directed against the filamin binding site of GP Ib$\alpha$ produced differing results (180). Incubation of the peptide with platelets resulted in dissociation of GP Ib$\alpha$ and filamin. In a dose-dependent manner, the peptide inhibited both ristocetin-induced and shear-induced platelet aggregation and reduced shear-induced protein tyrosine phosphorylation. Further clouding the issue are the conflicting results from heterologous cells expressing mutants of GP Ib$\alpha$. Several reports have demonstrated that removal of the filamin-1 binding site enhances VWF binding to GP Ib (224) and VWF-induced aggregation (223) under static and flow conditions (224). However, others found that disruption of the GP Ib–filamin association results in increased cell velocity (decreased VWF binding) (225) coupled with decreased attachment and even extraction of the receptor from the cell membrane under flow conditions (179).

In addition to its known association with filamin-1, GP Ib has been shown to associate with the scaffolding protein 14-3-3$\zeta$ (44,48,226–228). This association also regulates platelet activation. 14-3-3$\zeta$ binds to both GP Ib$\alpha$ and GP Ib$\beta$ in a phosphorylation-dependent manner (44,226,227) and plays a dual role in platelet activation; its association with GP Ib$\alpha$ is required for GP Ib/IX/V–mediated $\alpha_{IIb}\beta_3$ activation, and its association with GP Ib$\beta$ inhibits platelet activation. 14-3-3$\zeta$ binding to GP Ib$\beta$ requires phosphorylation of Ser166 within the cytoplasmic tail of the subunit. The kinase responsible is the cAMP-dependent protein kinase, protein kinase A (46). Cells expressing the GP Ib/IX complex, in which the GP Ib$\beta$ subunit has a mutation of Ser166, showed enhanced binding to VWF and platelets treated with a PKA inhibitor showed enhanced VWF binding (229). Feng et al. (227) demonstrated that a prerequisite for 14-3-3$\zeta$ association with GP Ib$\beta$ is that it first associate's with GP Ib$\alpha$. There are three known sites for 14-3-3$\zeta$ binding to GP Ib$\alpha$: Ser609 (230), Ser590, and Ser587 (45). Although deletion of either Ser609 (226) or Ser590, or to a lesser extent Ser587 (45), had no effect

on the GP Ib/IX–dependent adhesion of heterologous cells to VWF, GP Ib–dependent platelet spreading, which requires activated $\alpha_{IIb}\beta_3$, was significantly inhibited. The interaction of GP Ib with 14-3-3$\zeta$ has also been implicated in regulating megakaryocyte proliferation and ploidy (231).

Many signaling pathways have been proposed to play critical roles in GP Ib–mediated platelet activation. The particular pathway that predominates appears to depend on the method of investigation. Despite these controversies, it is apparent that intracellular calcium oscillations, phospholipase C (PLC), Src family kinases, and PI 3-kinase are required for inside-out signaling through GP Ib/IX/V and activation of $\alpha_{IIb}\beta_3$.

Intracellular calcium transients are perhaps the least controversial in terms of their requirement for platelet activation through GP Ib/IX/V. Initial studies demonstrated that under flow conditions, the interaction between GP Ib and VWF elicited a small rise in intracellular calcium, which was PI 3-kinase independent and due to release of calcium from internal stores (232,233). This rise in calcium was proposed to partially activate $\alpha_{IIb}\beta_3$ and induce stationary arrest of the platelets, subsequent $\alpha_{IIb}\beta_3$-mediated calcium responses, and firm adhesion. Subsequently, it has been shown that the calcium response is partially dependent on PLC$\gamma$2 but is independent of Fc$\gamma$RIIA and FcR$\gamma$-chain (234).

Src family kinases also appear to be indispensable for platelet activation induced by VWF binding to the GP Ib/IX/V complex. The pathway leading to calcium release appears to be initiated by Src activation. Although it is presently unclear whether Fc$\gamma$RIIA and FcR$\gamma$-chain (234) are directly involved in Src activation, several groups have demonstrated Src and Lyn association with FcR$\gamma$-chain (146,198) and/or GP Ib (197,235). It is thought that GP Ib-associated Src, through binding of either FcR$\gamma$-chain (146,198) or PI 3-kinase (235), becomes activated upon VWF binding. This leads to phosphorylation of FcR$\gamma$-chain, Syk, the adaptor molecules, linker for activation of T-cells (LAT) and Alzheimer disease associated protein (ADAP), and of protein kinase C (PKC) and PLC$\gamma$2. PLC$\gamma$2 hydrolyses phosphatidylinositol (PtdIns)(4,5)P$_2$ to form Ins(1,4,5)P$_3$, which is required for release of calcium from intracellular stores. Indeed, inhibition of Src with PP1 or PP2 abrogates all calcium responses and $\alpha_{IIb}\beta_3$ activation (146,234).

PI 3-kinase plays a significant role in the GP Ib/IX/V–mediated activation of $\alpha_{IIb}\beta_3$. It has been demonstrated that PI 3-kinase is associated with GP Ib (228,235) and that the PI 3-kinase–dependent production of PtdIns(3,4,5)P$_3$ and PtdIns(3,4)P$_2$ requires the interaction of VWF with GP Ib under conditions of shear (236,237). The use of PI 3-kinase inhibitors also demonstrates that PI 3-kinase is critically required for shear-dependent platelet adhesion, intracellular calcium mobilization, and spreading (237). Interestingly, under static conditions, PI 3-kinase is less important because its inhibition does not affect the intracellular calcium response but abrogates the activation of $\alpha_{IIb}\beta_3$ (146,237).

Finally, many other signaling enzymes/pathways have been implicated in VWF-GP Ib/IX/V–dependent activation of $\alpha_{IIb}\beta_3$. These include the kinases Lyn (197,235), Fyn (197), focal adhesion kinase (FAK) (238,239). and proline-rich tyrosine kinase 2 (239), as well as Src homology 2 domain-containing inositol 5-phosphatase (SHIP2) (240), mitogen-activating protein (MAP) kinase (241). and cGMP (242,243). The contributions of these signaling pathways remain to be fully elucidated.

## References

1. Nieswandt B, Watson SP. Platelet-collagen interaction: is GPVI the central receptor? *Blood* 2003;102:449–461.
2. Savage B, Saldivar E, Ruggeri ZM. Initiation of platelet adhesion by arrest onto fibrinogen or translocation on von Willebrand factor. *Cell* 1996;84: 289–297.

3. Doggett TA, Girdhar G, Lawshe A, et al. Selectin-like kinetics and biomechanics promote rapid platelet adhesion in flow: the GPIbα-vWF tether bond. *Biophys J* 2002; 83:194–205.

4. Savage B, Sixma JJ, Ruggeri ZM. Functional self-association of von Willebrand factor during platelet adhesion under flow. *Proc Natl Acad Sci U S A* 2002;99:425–430.

5. Sporn LA, Marder VJ, Wagner DD. Inducible secretion of large, biologically potent von Willebrand factor multimers. *Cell* 1986;46:185–190.

6. Padilla A, Moake JL, Bernardo A, et al. P-selectin anchors newly released ultralarge von Willebrand factor multimers to the endothelial cell surface. *Blood* 2004;103:2150–2156.

7. Dong JF, Moake JL, Nolasco L, et al. ADAMTS-13 rapidly cleaves newly secreted ultralarge von Willebrand factor multimers on the endothelial surface under flowing conditions. *Blood* 2002;100:4033–4039.

8. Andre P, Denis CV, Ware J, et al. Platelets adhere to and translocate on von Willebrand factor presented by endothelium in stimulated veins. *Blood* 2000;96:3322–3328.

9. Arya M, Anvari B, Romo GM, et al. Ultralarge multimers of von Willebrand factor form spontaneous high-strength bonds with the platelet glycoprotein Ib-IX complex: studies using optical tweezers. *Blood* 2002;99:3971–3977.

10. Frenette PS, Johnson RC, Hynes RO, et al. Platelets roll on stimulated endothelium *in vivo*: an interaction mediated by endothelial P-selectin. *Proc Natl Acad Sci U S A* 1995;92:7450–7454.

11. Frenette PS, Moyna C, Hartwell DW, et al. Platelet-endothelial interactions in inflamed mesenteric venules. *Blood* 1998;91:1318–1324.

12. Romo GM, Dong JF, Schade AJ, et al. The glycoprotein Ib-IX-V complex is a platelet counter-receptor for P-selectin. *J Exp Med* 1999;190:803–813.

13. Frenette PS, Denis CV, Weiss L, et al. P-Selectin glycoprotein ligand 1 (PSGL-1) is expressed on platelets and can mediate platelet-endothelial interactions *in vivo*. *J Exp Med* 2000;191:1413–1422.

14. Katayama T, Ikeda Y, Handa M, et al. Immunoneutralization of glycoprotein Ibα attenuates endotoxin-induced interactions of platelets and leukocytes with rat venular endothelium *in vivo*. *Circ Res* 2000;86:1031–1037.

15. Kulkarni S, Dopheide SM, Yap CL, et al. A revised model of platelet aggregation. *J Clin Invest* 2000;105:783–791.

16. López JA. The platelet glycoprotein Ib-IX complex. *Blood Coagul Fibrinolysis* 1994;5:97–119.

17. Clemetson KJ, Clemetson JM. Platelet GPIb-V-IX complex. Structure, function, physiology, and pathology. *Semin Thromb Hemost* 1995;21:130–136.

18. Andrews RK, López JA, Berndt MC. Molecular mechanisms of platelet adhesion and activation. *Int J Biochem Cell Biol* 1997;29:91–105.

19. López JA, Dong JF. Structure and function of the glycoprotein Ib-IX-V complex. *Curr Opin Hematol* 1997;4:323–329.

20. Kobe B, Deisenhofer J. The leucine-rich repeat: a versatile binding motif. *Trends Biochem Sci* 1994;19:415–421.

21. Lopez JA, Chung DW, Fujikawa K, et al. Cloning of the α chain of human platelet glycoprotein Ib: a transmembrane protein with homology to leucine-rich α2-glycoprotein. *Proc Natl Acad Sci U S A* 1987;84:5615–5619.

22. Lopez JA, Chung DW, Fujikawa K, et al. The α and β chains of human platelet glycoprotein Ib are both transmembrane proteins containing a leucine-rich amino acid sequence. *Proc Natl Acad Sci U S A* 1988;85:2135–2139.

23. Hickey MJ, Williams SA, Roth GJ. Human platelet glycoprotein IX: an adhesive prototype of leucine-rich glycoproteins with flank-center-flank structures. *Proc Natl Acad Sci U S A* 1989;86:6773–6777.

24. Hickey MJ, Hagen FS, Yagi M, et al. Human platelet glycoprotein V: characterization of the polypeptide and the related Ib-V-IX receptor system of adhesive, leucine-rich glycoproteins. *Proc Natl Acad Sci U S A* 1993;90:8327–8331.

25. Wicki AN, Clemetson KJ. The glycoprotein Ib complex of human blood platelets. *Eur J Biochem* 1987;163:43–50.

26. Berndt MC, Gregory C, Kabral A, et al. Purification and preliminary characterization of the glycoprotein Ib complex in the human platelet membrane. *Eur J Biochem* 1985;151:637–649.

27. Du X, Beutler L, Ruan C, et al. Glycoprotein Ib and glycoprotein IX are fully complexed in the intact platelet membrane. *Blood* 1987;69: 1524–1527.

28. Modderman PW, Admiraal LG, Sonnenberg A, et al. Glycoproteins V and Ib-IX form a noncovalent complex in the platelet membrane. *J Biol Chem* 1992;267:364–369.

29. Li CQ, Dong J-F, Lanza F, et al. Expression of platelet glycoprotein (GP) V in heterologous cells and evidence for its association with GP Ibα in forming a GP Ib-IX-V complex on the cell surface. *J Biol Chem* 1995;270:16302–16307.

30. López JA, Weisman S, Sanan DA, et al. Glycoprotein (GP) Ibβ is the critical subunit linking GP Ibα and GP IX in the GP Ib-IX complex. Analysis of partial complexes. *J Biol Chem* 1994;269:23716–23721.

31. Wu G, Meloni FJ, Shapiro SS. Platelet glycoprotein (Gp) IX associates with Gp Ibα in the platelet membrane GpIb complex. *Blood* 1996;87:2782–2787.

32. Fox JEB, Aggerbeck LP, Berndt MC. Structure of the glycoprotein Ib-IX complex from platelet membranes. *J Biol Chem* 1988;263:4882–4890.

33. Titani K, Takio K, Handa M, et al. Amino acid sequence of the von Willebrand factor-binding domain of platelet membrane glycoprotein Ib. *Proc Natl Acad Sci U S A* 1987;84:5610–5614.

34. Korrel SAM, Clemetson KJ, Van Halbeek H, et al. Structural studies on the O-linked carbohydrate chains of human platelet glycocalicin. *Eur J Biochem* 1984;140:571–576.

35. Tsuji T, Tsunehisa S, Watanabe Y, et al. The carbohydrate moiety of human platelet glycocalicin. The structure of the major ser/thr-linked chain. *J Biol Chem* 1983;258:6335–6339.

36. López JA, Ludwig EH, McCarthy BJ. Polymorphism of human glycoprotein Ibα results from a variable number of tandem repeats of a 13-amino acid sequence in the mucin-like macroglycopeptide region. Structure/function implications. *J Biol Chem* 1992;267:10055–10061.

37. Ishida F, Furihata K, Ishida K, et al. The largest variant of platelet glycoprotein Ibα has four tandem repeats of 13 amino acids in the macroglycopeptide region and a genetic linkage with methionine 145. *Blood* 1995;86:1357–1360.

38. Dong J-F, Li CQ, López JA. Tyrosine sulfation of the GP Ib-IX complex: identification of sulfated residues and effect on ligand binding. *Biochemistry* 1994;33:13946–13953.

39. Ward CM, Andrews RK, Smith AI, et al. Mocarhagin, a novel cobra venom metalloproteinase, cleaves the platelet von Willebrand factor receptor glycoprotein Ibα. Identification of the sulfated tyrosine/anionic sequence Tyr-276–Glu-282 of glycoprotein Ibα as a binding site for von Willebrand factor and α-thrombin. *Biochemistry* 1996;35:4929–4938.

40. Fox JEB. Linkage of a membrane skeleton to integral membrane glycoproteins in human platelets. Identification of one of the glycoproteins as glycoprotein Ib. *J Clin Invest* 1985;76:1673–1683.

41. Du X, Harris SJ, Tetaz TJ, et al. Association of a phospholipase A₂ (14-3-3 protein) with the platelet glycoprotein Ib-IX complex. *J Biol Chem* 1994;269:18287–18290.

42. Andrews RK, Fox JEB. Identification of a region in the cytoplasmic domain of the platelet membrane glycoprotein Ib-IX complex that binds to purified actin-binding protein. *J Biol Chem* 1992;267:18605–18611.

43. Du X, Fox JE, Pei S. Identification of a binding sequence for the 14-3-3 protein within the cytoplasmic domain of the adhesion receptor, platelet glycoprotein Ibα. *J Biol Chem* 1996;271:7362–7367.

44. Andrews RK, Harris SJ, McNally T, et al. Binding of purified 14-3-3ζ signaling protein to discrete amino acid sequences within the cytoplasmic domain of the platelet membrane glycoprotein Ib-IX-V complex. *Biochemistry* 1998;37:638–647.

45. Mangin P, David T, Lavaud V, et al. Identification of a novel 14-3-3ζ binding site within the cytoplasmic tail of platelet glycoprotein Ibα. *Blood* 2004;104:420–427.

46. Wardell MR, Reynolds CC, Berndt MC, et al. Platelet glycoprotein Ibβ is phosphorylated on serine 166 by cyclic AMP-dependent protein kinase. *J Biol Chem* 1989;264:15656–15661.

47. Fox JEB, Berndt MC. Cyclic AMP-dependent phosphorylation of glycoprotein Ib inhibits collagen-induced polymerization of actin in platelets. *J Biol Chem* 1989;264:9520–9526.

48. Calverley DC, Kavanagh TJ, Roth GJ. Human signaling protein 14-3-3ζ interacts with platelet glycoprotein Ib subunits Ibα and Ibβ. *Blood* 1998;91:1295–1303.

49. Andrews RK, Munday AD, Mitchell CA, et al. Interaction of calmodulin with the cytoplasmic domain of the platelet membrane glycoprotein Ib-IX-V complex. *Blood* 2001;98:681–687.

50. Muszbek L, Laposata M. Glycoprotein Ib and glycoprotein IX in human platelets are acylated with palmitic acid through thioester linkages. *J Biol Chem* 1989;264:9716–9719.

51. Shrimpton CN, Borthakur G, Larrucea S, et al. Localization of the adhesion receptor glycoprotein Ib-IX-V complex to lipid rafts is required for platelet adhesion and activation. *J Exp Med* 2002;196:1057–1066.

52. Lanza F, Morales M, de La Salle C, et al. Cloning and characterization of the gene encoding the human platelet glycoprotein V. A member of the leucine-rich glycoprotein family cleaved during thrombin-induced platelet activation. *J Biol Chem* 1993;268:20801–20807.

53. Vu T-KH, Hung DT, Wheaton VI, et al. Molecular cloning of a functional thrombin receptor reveals a novel proteolytic mechanism of receptor activation. *Cell* 1991;64:1057–1068.

54. Ishihara H, Connolly AJ, Zeng D, et al. Protease-activated receptor 3 is a second thrombin receptor in humans. *Nature* 1997;386:502–506.

55. Xu WF, Andersen H, Whitmore TE, et al. Cloning and characterization of human protease-activated receptor 4. *Proc Natl Acad Sci U S A* 1998;95:6642–6646.

56. Kahn ML, Zheng YW, Huang W, et al. A dual thrombin receptor system for platelet activation. *Nature* 1998;394:690–694.

57. Berndt MC, Phillips DR. Purification and preliminary physicochemical characterization of human platelet membrane glycoprotein V. *J Biol Chem* 1981;256:59–65.

58. Yagi M, Edelhoff S, Disteche CM, et al. Structural characterization and chromosomal location of the gene encoding human platelet glycoprotein Ibβ. *J Biol Chem* 1994;269:17424–17427.

59. Wenger RH, Kieffer N, Wicki AN, et al. Structure of the human blood platelet membrane glycoprotein Ibα gene. *Biochem Biophys Res Commun* 1988;156:389–395.

60. Wenger RH, Wicki AN, Kieffer N, et al. The 5′ flanking region and chromosomal localization of the gene encoding human platelet membrane glycoprotein Ibα. *Gene* 1989;85:517–524.

61. Kelly MD, Essex DW, Shapiro SS, et al. Complementary DNA cloning of the alternatively expressed endothelial cell glycoprotein Ibβ (GPIbβ) and localization of the GPIbβ gene to chromosome 22. *J Clin Invest* 1994; 93:2417–2424.

62. Yagi M, Edelhoff S, Disteche CM, et al. Human platelet glycoproteins V and IX: mapping of two leucine-rich glycoprotein genes to chromosome 3 and analysis of structures. *Biochemistry* 1995;34:16132–16137.

63. Shivdasani RA, Fujiwara Y, McDevitt MA, et al. A lineage-selective knock-out establishes the critical role of transcription factor GATA-1 in megakaryocyte growth and platelet development. *EMBO J* 1997;16: 3965–3973.

64. Tsang AP, Visvader JE, Turner CA, et al. FOG, a multiple zinc finger protein, acts as a cofactor for transcription factor GATA-1 in erythroid and megakaryocytic differentiation. *Cell* 1997;90:109–119.

65. Bastian LS, Kwiatkowski BA, Breininger J, et al. Regulation of the megakaryocytic glycoprotein IX promoter by the oncogenic Ets transcription factor Fli-1. *Blood* 1999;93:2637–2644.

66. Eisbacher M, Khachigian LM, Khin TH, et al. Inducible expression of the megakaryocyte-specific gene glycoprotein IX is mediated through an Ets binding site and involves upstream activation of extracellular signal-regulated kinase. *Cell Growth Differ* 2001;12:435–445.

67. Sprandio JD, Shapiro SS, Thiagarajan P, et al. Cultured human umbilical vein endothelial cells contain a membrane glycoprotein immunologically related to platelet glycoprotein Ib. *Blood* 1988;71:234–237.

68. Asch AS, Adelman B, Fujimoto M, et al. Identification and isolation of a platelet GPIb-like protein in human umbilical vein endothelial cells and bovine aortic smooth muscle cells. *J Clin Invest* 1988;81:1600–1607.

69. Konkle BA, Shapiro SS, Asch AS, et al. Cytokine-enhanced expression of glycoprotein Ibα in human endothelium. *J Biol Chem* 1990;265: 19833–19838.

70. Rajagopalan V, Essex DW, Shapiro SS, et al. Tumor necrosis factor–α modulation of glycoprotein Ibα expression in human endothelial and erythroleukemia cells. *Blood* 1992;80:153–161.

71. Wu G, Essex DW, Meloni FJ, et al. Human endothelial cells in culture and *in vivo* express on their surface all four components of the glycoprotein Ib/IX/V complex. *Blood* 1997;90:2660–2669.

72. Murata M, Matsubara Y, Kawano K, et al. Coronary artery disease and polymorphisms in a receptor mediating shear stress-dependent platelet activation. *Circulation* 1997;96:3281–3286.

73. Gonzalez-Conejero R, Lozano ML, Rivera J, et al. Polymorphisms of platelet membrane glycoprotein Ibα associated with arterial thrombotic disease. *Blood* 1998;92:2771–2776.

74. Jilma-Stohlawetz P, Homoncik M, Jilma B, et al. Glycoprotein Ib polymorphisms influence platelet plug formation under high shear rates. *Br J Haematol* 2003;120:652–655.

75. López JA, Andrews RK, Afshar-Kharghan V, et al. Bernard-Soulier syndrome. *Blood* 1998;91:4397–4418.

76. Murata M, Furihata K, Ishida F, et al. Genetic and structural characterization of an amino acid dimorphism in glycoprotein Ibα involved in platelet transfusion refractoriness. *Blood* 1992;79:3086–3090.

77. Kuijpers RWAM, Faber NM, Cuypers HTM, et al. NH2-terminal globular domain of human platelet glycoprotein Ibα has a methionine145/threonine145 amino acid polymorphism, which is associated with the HPA-2 (Ko) alloantigens. *J Clin Invest* 1992;89:381–384.

78. Li CQ, Garner SF, Davies J, et al. Threonine-145/Methionine-145 variants of baculovirus produced recombinant ligand binding domain of GPIbα express HPA-2 epitopes and show equal binding of von Willebrand factor. *Blood* 2000;95:205–211.

79. Ulrichts H, Vanhoorelbeke K, Cauwenberghs S, et al. Von Willebrand factor but not α-thrombin binding to platelet glycoprotein Ibα is influenced by the HPA-2 polymorphism. *Arterioscler Thromb Vasc Biol* 2003;23: 1302–1307.

80. Kaski S, Kekomäki R, Partanen J. Systematic screening for genetic polymorphism in human platelet glycoprotein Ibα. *Immunogenetics* 1996;44: 170–176.

81. Afshar-Kharghan V, López JA. Bernard-Soulier syndrome caused by a dinucleotide deletion and reading frameshift in the region encoding the glycoprotein Ibα transmembrane domain. *Blood* 1997;90:2634–2643.

82. Kenny D, Newman PJ, Morateck PA, et al. A dinucleotide deletion results in defective membrane anchoring and circulating soluble glycoprotein Ibα in a novel form of Bernard-Soulier syndrome. *Blood* 1997;90:2626–2633.

83. Kaski S, Partanen J, Salmi TT, et al. Different molecular origin of Bernard-Soulier syndrome (BSS) reflected in varying expression of platelet glycoprotein (GP) Ib/IX/V complex (Abstract). *Thromb Haemost* 1997;77:68.

84. Afshar-Kharghan V, Li CQ, Khoshnevis-Asl M, et al. Kozak sequence polymorphism of the glycoprotein (GP) Ibα gene is a major determinant of the plasma membrane levels of the platelet GP Ib-IX-V complex. *Blood* 1999;94:186–191.

85. Baker RI, Eikelboom J, Lofthouse E, et al. Platelet glycoprotein Ibα Kozak polymorphism is associated with an increased risk of ischemic stroke. *Blood* 2001;98:36–40.

86. Hsieh K, Funk M, Schillinger M, et al. Vienna stroke registry. Impact of the platelet glycoprotein Ib α Kozak polymorphism on the risk of ischemic cerebrovascular events: a case-control study. *Blood Coagul Fibrinolysis* 2004;15:469–473.

87. Michelson AD, Benoit SE, Furman MI, et al. The platelet surface expression of glycoprotein V is regulated by two independent mechanisms:

88. López JA, Leung B, Reynolds CC, et al. Efficient plasma membrane expression of a functional platelet glycoprotein Ib-IX complex requires the presence of its three subunits. *J Biol Chem* 1992;267:12851–12859.

89. Kenny D, Morateck PA, Gill JC, et al. The critical interaction of glycoprotein GP Ibβ with GPIX: a genetic cause of Bernard-Soulier syndrome. *Blood* 1999;93:2968–2975.

90. Moran N, Morateck PA, Deering A, et al. Surface expression of glycoprotein Ibα is dependent on glycoprotein Ibβ: evidence from a novel mutation causing Bernard-Soulier syndrome. *Blood* 2000;96:532–539.

91. Strassel C, Pasquet JM, Alessi MC, et al. A novel missense mutation shows that GPIbβ has a dual role in controlling the processing and stability of the platelet GPIb-IX adhesion receptor. *Biochemistry* 2003;42:4452–4462.

92. Kenny D, Morateck PA, Montgomery RR. The cysteine knot of platelet glycoprotein Ibβ (GPIbβ) is critical for the interaction of GPIbβ with GPIX. *Blood* 2002;99:4428–4433.

93. Meyer SC, Fox JE. Interaction of platelet glycoprotein V with glycoprotein Ib-IX regulates expression of the glycoprotein and binding of von Willebrand factor to glycoprotein Ib-IX in transfected cells. *J Biol Chem* 1995;270:14693–14699.

94. Calverley DC, Yagi M, Stray SM, et al. Human platelet glycoprotein V: its role in enhancing expression of the glycoprotein Ib receptor. *Blood* 1995; 86:1361–1367.

95. Dong JF, Gao S, López JA. Synthesis, assembly, and intracellular transport of the platelet glycoprotein Ib-IX-V complex. *J Biol Chem* 1998;273: 31449–31454.

96. Ulsemer P, Strassel C, Baas MJ, et al. Biosynthesis and intracellular posttranslational processing of normal and mutant platelet glycoprotein GP Ib-IX. *Biochem J* 2001;358:295–303.

97. Kunicki TJ, Johnson MM, Aster RH. Absence of the platelet receptor for drug-dependent antibodies in the Bernard-Soulier syndrome. *J Clin Invest* 1978;62:716–719.

98. Kunicki TJ, Russell N, Nurden AT, et al. Further studies of the human platelet receptor for quinine- and quinidine-dependent antibodies. *J Immunol* 1981;126:398–402.

99. Berndt MC, Chong BH, Bull HA, et al. Molecular characterization of quinine/quinidine drug-dependent antibody platelet interaction using monoclonal antibodies. *Blood* 1985;66:1292–1301.

100. Chong BH, Du X, Berndt MC, et al. Characterization of the binding domains on platelet glycoproteins Ib-IX and IIb/IIIa complexes for the quinine/quinidine-dependent antibodies. *Blood* 1991;77:2190–2199.

101. López JA, Li CQ, Weisman S, et al. The GP Ib-IX "complex-specific" monoclonal antibody SZ1 binds to a conformation-sensitive epitope on GP IX: implications for the target antigen of quinine/quinidine-dependent autoantibodies. *Blood* 1995;85:1254–1258.

102. Asvadi P, Ahmadi Z, Chong BH. Drug-induced thrombocytopenia: localization of the binding site of GPIX-specific quinine-dependent antibodies. *Blood* 2003;102:1670–1677.

103. Burgess JK, López JA, Berndt MC, et al. Quinine-dependent antibodies bind a restricted set of epitopes on the glycoprotein Ib-IX complex: characterization of the epitopes. *Blood* 1998;92:2366–2373.

104. Pereira J, Hidalgo P, Ocqueteau M, et al. Glycoprotein Ib/IX complex is the target in rifampicin-induced immune thrombocytopenia. *Br J Haematol* 2000;110:907–910.

105. Burgess JK, López JA, Gaudry LE, et al. Rifampicin-dependent antibodies bind a similar or identical epitope to glycoprotein IX-specific quinine-dependent antibodies. *Blood* 2000;95:1988–1992.

106. Garner SF, Campbell K, Metcalfe P, et al. Glycoprotein V: the predominant target antigen in gold-induced autoimmune thrombocytopenia. *Blood* 2002;100:344–346.

107. Kiefel V, Santoso S, Kaufmann E, et al. Autoantibodies against platelet glycoprotein Ib/IX: a frequent finding in autoimmune thrombocytopenic purpura. *Br J Haematol* 1991;79:256–262.

108. He R, Reid DM, Jones CE, et al. Spectrum of Ig classes, specificities, and titers of serum antiglycoproteins in chronic idiopathic thrombocytopenic purpura. *Blood* 1994;83:1024–1032.

109. Hou M, Stockelberg D, Kutti J, et al. Antibodies against platelet GPIb/IX, GPIIb/IIIa, and other platelet antigens in chronic idiopathic thrombocytopenic purpura. *Eur J Haematol* 1995;55:307–314.

110. Brighton TA, Evans S, Castaldi PA, et al. Prospective evaluation of the clinical usefulness of an antigen-specific assay (MAIPA) in idiopathic thrombocytopenic purpura and other immune thrombocytopenias. *Blood* 1996;88:194–201.

111. Kiefel V, Freitag E, Kroll H, et al. Platelet autoantibodies (IgG, IgM, IgA) against glycoproteins IIb/IIIa and Ib/IX in patients with thrombocytopenia. *Ann Hematol* 1996;72:280–285.

112. Hou M, Stockelberg D, Kutti J, et al. Fab-mediated binding of glycoprotein Ib/IX and IIb/IIIa specific antibodies in chronic idiopathic thrombocytopenic purpura. *Br J Haematol* 1995;91:944–950.

113. Sullam PM, Hyun WC, Szöllösi J, et al. Physical proximity and functional interplay of the glycoprotein Ib-IX-V complex and the Fc receptor FcγRIIA on the platelet plasma membrane. *J Biol Chem* 1998;273:5331–5336.

114. Hiraiwa A, Nugent DJ, Milner EC. Sequence analysis of monoclonal antibodies derived from a patient with idiopathic thrombocytopenic purpura. *Autoimmunity* 1990;8:107–113.

115. Feistauer SM, Penner E, Mayr WR, et al. Target platelet antigens of autoantibodies in patients with primary biliary cirrhosis. *Hepatology* 1997; 25:1343–1345.

116. Macchi L, Rispal P, Clofent-Sanchez G, et al. Anti-platelet antibodies in patients with systemic lupus erythematosus and the primary antiphospholipid antibody syndrome: their relationship with the observed thrombocytopenia. *Br J Haematol* 1997;98:336–341.

117. Galli M, Daldossi M, Barbui T. Anti-glycoprotein Ib/IX and IIb/IIIa antibodies in patients with antiphospholipid antibodies. *Thromb Haemost* 1994;71:571–575.

118. Mayer JL, Beardsley DS. Varicella-associated thrombocytopenia: autoantibodies against platelet surface glycoprotein V. *Pediatr Res* 1996; 40:615–619.

119. Miyata S, Goto S, Federici AB, et al. Conformational changes in the A1 domain of von Willebrand factor modulating the interaction with platelet glycoprotein Ibα. *J Biol Chem* 1996;271:9046–9053.

120. Siedlecki CA, Lestini BJ, Kottke-Marchant KK, et al. Shear-dependent changes in the three-dimensional structure of human von Willebrand factor. *Blood* 1996;88:2939–2950.

121. Peterson DM, Stathopoulos NA, Giorgio TD, et al. Shear-induced platelet aggregation requires von Willebrand factor and platelet membrane glycoproteins Ib and IIb-IIIa. *Blood* 1987;69:625–628.

122. Shen Y, Romo GM, Dong J, et al. Requirement of leucine-rich repeats of glycoprotein (GP) Ibα for shear-dependent and static binding of von Willebrand factor to the platelet membrane GP Ib-IX-V complex. *Blood* 2000;95:903–910.

123. Dong JF, Berndt MC, Schade A, et al. Ristocetin-dependent, but not botrocetin-dependent, binding of von Willebrand factor to the platelet glycoprotein Ib-IX-V complex correlates with shear-dependent interactions. *Blood* 2001;97:162–168.

124. Berndt MC, Ward CM, Booth WJ, et al. Identification of aspartic acid 514 through glutamic acid 542 as a glycoprotein Ib-IX complex receptor recognition sequence in von Willebrand factor. Mechanism of modulation of von Willebrand factor by ristocetin and botrocetin. *Biochemistry* 1992; 31:11144–11151.

125. Berndt MC, Du X, Booth WJ. Ristocetin-dependent reconstitution of binding of von Willebrand factor to purified human platelet membrane glycoprotein Ib-IX complex. *Biochemistry* 1988;27:633–640.

126. Scott JP, Montgomery RR, Retzinger GS. Dimeric ristocetin flocculates proteins, binds to platelets, and mediates von Willebrand factor-dependent agglutination of platelets. *J Biol Chem* 1991;266:8149–8155.

127. Hoylaerts MF, Nuyts K, Peerlinck K, et al. Promotion of binding of von Willebrand factor to platelet glycoprotein Ib by dimers of ristocetin. *Biochem J* 1995;306:453–463.

128. Fukuda K, Doggett TA, Bankston LA, et al. Structural basis of von Willebrand factor activation by the snake toxin botrocetin. *Structure (Camb)* 2002;10:943–950.

129. Maita N, Nishio K, Nishimoto E, et al. Crystal structure of von Willebrand factor A1 domain complexed with snake venom, bitiscetin: insight into glycoprotein Ibα binding mechanism induced by snake venom proteins. *J Biol Chem* 2003;278:37777–37781.

130. Dong J-F, Hyun W, López JA. Aggregation of mammalian cells expressing the platelet glycoprotein (GP) Ib-IX complex and the requirement for tyrosine sulfation of GP Ibα. *Blood* 1995;86:4175–4183.

131. Marchese P, Murata M, Mazzucato M, et al. Identification of three tyrosine residues of glycoprotein Ibα with distinct roles in von Willebrand factor and α-thrombin binding. *J Biol Chem* 1995;270:9571–9578.

132. Nishio K, Fujimura Y, Nishida S, et al. Antiplatelet glycoprotein Ib monoclonal antibody (OP-F1) totally abolishes ristocetin-induced von Willebrand factor binding, but has minimal effect on the botrocetin-induced binding. *Haemostasis* 1991;21:353–359.

133. Andrews RK, Gardiner EE, Shen Y, et al. Glycoprotein Ib-IX-V. *Int J Biochem Cell Biol* 2003;35:1170–1174.

134. Dumas JJ, Kumar R, McDonagh T, et al. Crystal structure of the wild-type von Willebrand factor A1-glycoprotein Ibα complex reveals conformation differences with a complex bearing von Willebrand disease mutations. *J Biol Chem* 2004;279:23327–23334.

135. Huizinga EG, Tsuji S, Romijn RA, et al. Structures of glycoprotein Ibα and its complex with von Willebrand factor A1 domain. *Science* 2002; 297:1176–1179.

136. Celikel R, McClintock RA, Roberts JR, et al. Modulation of α-thrombin function by distinct interactions with platelet glycoprotein Ibα. *Science* 2003;301:218–221.

137. Dumas JJ, Kumar R, Seehra J, et al. Crystal structure of the GpIbα-thrombin complex essential for platelet aggregation. *Science* 2003; 301:222–226.

138. Vanhoorelbeke K, Ulrichts H, Romijn RA, et al. The GPIbα-thrombin interaction: far from crystal clear. *Trends Mol Med* 2004;10:33–39.

139. Adam F, Bouton MC, Huisse MG, et al. Thrombin interaction with platelet membrane glycoprotein Ibα. *Trends Mol Med* 2003;9:461–464.

140. De Cristofaro R, De Candia E. Thrombin domains: structure, function and interaction with platelet receptors. *J Thromb Thrombolysis* 2003; 15: 151–163.

141. De Candia E, Hall SW, Rutella S, et al. Binding of thrombin to glycoprotein Ib accelerates the hydrolysis of Par-1 on intact platelets. *J Biol Chem* 2001;276:4692–4698.

142. Ramakrishnan V, DeGuzman F, Bao M, et al. A thrombin receptor function for platelet glycoprotein Ib-IX unmasked by cleavage of glycoprotein V. *Proc Natl Acad Sci U S A* 2001;98:1823–1828.

143. Beguin S, Keularts I, Al Dieri R, et al. Fibrin polymerization is crucial for thrombin generation in platelet-rich plasma in a VWF-GPIb-dependent process, defective in Bernard-Soulier syndrome. *J Thromb Haemost* 2004; 2:170–176.

144. Soslau G, Favero M. The GPIb-thrombin pathway: evidence for a novel role of fibrin in platelet aggregation. *J Thromb Haemost* 2004;2:522–524.

145. Yun TH, Baglia FA, Myles T, et al. Thrombin activation of factor XI on activated platelets requires the interaction of factor XI and platelet glycoprotein Ibα with thrombin anion-binding exosites I and II, respectively. *J Biol Chem* 2003;278:48112–48119.

146. Kasirer-Friede A, Cozzi MR, Mazzucato M, et al. Signaling through GP Ib-IX-V activates αIIβ3 independently of other receptors. *Blood* 2004; 103:3403–3411.

147. Andrews RK, Gardiner EE, Shen Y, et al. Platelet interactions in thrombosis. *IUBMB Life* 2004;56:13–18.

148. Pancer Z, Amemiya CT, Ehrhardt GR, et al. Somatic diversification of variable lymphocyte receptors in the agnathan sea lamprey. *Nature* 2004; 430:174–180.

149. Netea MG, van der Graaf C, Van der Meer JW, et al. Toll-like receptors and the host defense against microbial pathogens: bringing specificity to the innate-immune system. *J Leukoc Biol* 2004;75:749–755.

150. Bradford HN, Dela Cadena RA, Kunapuli SP, et al. Human kininogens regulate thrombin binding to platelets through the glycoprotein Ib-IX-V complex. *Blood* 1997;90:1508–1515.

151. Bradford HN, Pixley RA, Colman RW. Human factor XII binding to the glycoprotein Ib-IX-V complex inhibits thrombin-induced platelet aggregation. *J Biol Chem* 2000;275:22756–22763.

152. Baglia FA, Shrimpton CN, Lopez JA, et al. The glycoprotein Ib-IX-V complex mediates localization of factor XI to lipid rafts on the platelet membrane. *J Biol Chem* 2003;278:21744–21750.

153. Baglia FA, Badellino KO, Li CQ, et al. Factor XI binding to the platelet glycoprotein Ib-IX-V complex promotes factor XI activation by thrombin. *J Biol Chem* 2002;277:1662–1668.

154. Loscalzo J, Inbal A, Handin RI. von Willebrand protein facilitates platelet incorporation into polymerizing fibrin. *J Clin Invest* 1986;78: 1112–1119.

155. Endenburg SC, Hantgan RR, Lindeboom-Blokzijl L, et al. On the role of von Willebrand factor in promoting platelet adhesion to fibrin in flowing blood. *Blood* 1995;86:4158–4165.

156. Parker RI, Gralnick HR. Fibrin monomer induces binding of endogenous platelet von Willebrand factor to the glycocalicin portion of platelet glycoprotein Ib. *Blood* 1987;70:1589–1594.

157. Kehrel B, Flicker E, Wigbels B, et al. Thrombospondin measured in whole blood—an indicator of platelet activation. *Blood Coagul Fibrinolysis* 1996;7:202–205.

158. Agbanyo FR, Sixma JJ, de Groot PG, et al. Thrombospondin-platelet interactions. Role of divalent cations, wall shear rate, and platelet membrane glycoproteins. *J Clin Invest* 1993;92:288–296.

159. Onitsuka I, Jung SM, Ikeda H, et al. Real-time analysis of the interaction of platelets with immobilized thrombospondin under flow conditions. *Thromb Res* 2001;101:455–465.

160. Jurk K, Clemetson KJ, de Groot PG, et al. Thrombospondin-1 mediates platelet adhesion at high shear via glycoprotein Ib (GPIb): an alternative/backup mechanism to von Willebrand factor. *FASEB J* 2003;17: 1490–1492.

161. Wight TN, Raugi GJ, Mumby SM, et al. Light microscopic immunolocation of thrombospondin in human tissues. *J Histochem Cytochem* 1985; 33:295–302.

162. van Zanten GH, de Graaf S, Slootweg PJ, et al. Increased platelet deposition on atherosclerotic coronary arteries. *J Clin Invest* 1994;93:615–632.

163. Simon DI, Chen Z, Xu H, et al. Platelet glycoprotein Ibα is a counter-receptor for the leukocyte integrin Mac-1 (CD11b/CD18). *J Exp Med* 2000;192:193–204.

164. Hoffmeister KM, Felbinger TW, Falet H, et al. The clearance mechanism of chilled blood platelets. *Cell* 2003;112:87–97.

165. Ehlers R, Ustinov V, Chen Z, et al. Targeting platelet-leukocyte interactions: identification of the integrin Mac-1 binding site for the platelet counter receptor glycoprotein Ibα. *J Exp Med* 2003;198:1077–1088.

166. Hoffmeister KM, Josefsson EC, Isaac NA, et al. Glycosylation restores survival of chilled blood platelets. *Science* 2003;301:1531–1534.

167. Chavakis T, Santoso S, Clemetson KJ, et al. High molecular weight kininogen regulates platelet-leukocyte interactions by bridging Mac-1 and glycoprotein Ib. *J Biol Chem* 2003;278:45375–45381.

168. Fujimura Y, Kawasaki T, Titani K. Snake venom proteins modulating the interaction between von Willebrand factor and platelet glycoprotein Ib. *Thromb Haemost* 1996;76:633–639.

169. Peng M, Lu W, Kirby EP. Alboaggregin-B: a new platelet agonist that binds to platelet membrane glycoprotein Ib. *Biochemistry* 1991;30: 11529–11536.

170. Peng M, Lu W, Kirby EP. Characterization of three alboaggregins purified from *Trimeresurus albolabris* venom. *Thromb Haemost* 1992;67: 702–707.

171. Andrews RK, Kroll MH, Ward CM, et al. Binding of a novel 50-kDa alboaggregin from *Trimeresurus albolabris* and related viper venom proteins

to the platelet membrane glycoprotein Ib-IX-V complex. Effect on platelet aggregation and glycoprotein Ib-mediated platelet activation. *Biochemistry* 1996;35:12629–12639.

172. Peng M, Lu W, Beviglia L, et al. Echicetin: a snake venom protein that inhibits binding of von Willebrand factor and alboaggregins to platelet glycoprotein Ib. *Blood* 1993;81:2321–2328.

173. Kawasaki T, Fujimura Y, Usami Y, et al. Complete amino acid sequence and identification of the platelet glycoprotein Ib-binding site of jararaca GPIb-BP, a snake venom protein isolated from Bothrops jararaca. *J Biol Chem* 1996;271:10635–10639.

174. Moog S, Mangin P, Lenain N, et al. Platelet glycoprotein V binds to collagen and participates in platelet adhesion and aggregation. *Blood* 2001;98:1038–1046.

175. Sullam PM, Valone FH, Mills J. Mechanisms of platelet aggregation by viridans group streptococci. *Infect Immun* 1987;55:1743–1750.

176. Ford I, Douglas CW, Preston FE, et al. Mechanisms of platelet aggregation by Streptococcus sanguis, a causative organism in infective endocarditis. *Br J Haematol* 1993;84:95–100.

177. Solum NO, Olsen TM. Glycoprotein Ib in the Triton-insoluble (cytoskeletal) fraction of blood platelets. *Biochim Biophys Acta* 1984;799:209–220.

178. Okita JR, Pidard D, Newman PJ, et al. On the association of glycoprotein Ib and actin-binding protein in human platelets. *J Cell Biol* 1985;100:317–321.

179. Williamson D, Pikovski I, Cranmer SL, et al. Interaction between platelet glycoprotein Ibα and filamin-1 is essential for glycoprotein Ib/IX receptor anchorage at high shear. *J Biol Chem* 2002;277:2151–2159.

180. Feng S, Resendiz JC, Lu X, et al. Filamin A binding to the cytoplasmic tail of glycoprotein Ibalpha regulates von Willebrand factor-induced platelet activation. *Blood* 2003;102:2122–2129.

181. Dong J-F, Li CQ, Sae-Tung G, et al. The cytoplasmic domain of glycoprotein (GP) Ibα constrains the lateral diffusion of the GP Ib-IX complex and modulates von Willebrand factor binding. *Biochemistry* 1997;36:12421–12427.

182. Suzuki H, Yamamoto N, Tanoue K, et al. Glycoprotein Ib distribution on the surface of platelets in resting and activation states: an electron microscope study. *Histochem J* 1987;19:125–136.

183. George JN, Torres MM. Thrombin decreases von Willebrand factor binding to platelet glycoprotein Ib. *Blood* 1988;71:1253–1259.

184. Hourdillé P, Heilmann E, Combrié R, et al. Thrombin induces a rapid redistribution of glycoprotein Ib-IX complexes within the membrane systems of activated human platelets. *Blood* 1990;76:1503–1513.

185. Michelson AD, Ellis PA, Barnard MR, et al. Downregulation of the platelet surface glycoprotein Ib-IX complex in whole blood stimulated by thrombin, adenosine diphosphate, or an *in vivo* wound. *Blood* 1991; 77:770–779.

186. Cramer EM, Lu H, Caen JP, et al. Differential redistribution of platelet glycoproteins Ib and IIb-IIIa after plasmin stimulation. *Blood* 1991;77:694–699.

187. White JG, Krumwiede MD, Cocking-Johnson D, et al. Retention of glycoprotein Ib-IX receptors on external surfaces of thrombin-activated platelets in suspension. *Blood* 1995;86:3468–3478.

188. White JG, Escolar G. Fate of the GPIb/IX receptor complex following activation of human platelets. *Blood Coagul Fibrinolysis* 1996;7:262–265.

189. Kovacsovics TJ, Hartwig JH. Thrombin-induced GPIb-IX centralization on the platelet surface requires actin assembly and myosin II activation. *Blood* 1996;87:618–629.

190. White JG, Burris SM, Hasegawa D, et al. Micropipette aspiration of human blood platelets: a defect in Bernard-Soulier's syndrome. *Blood* 1984;63:1249–1252.

191. Kanaji T, Russell S, Ware J. Amelioration of the macrothrombocytopenia associated with the murine Bernard-Soulier syndrome. *Blood* 2002;100:2102–2107.

192. Arya M, López JA, Romo GM, et al. Glycoprotein Ib-IX-mediated activation of integrin $\alpha_{IIb}\beta_3$: effects of receptor clustering and von Willebrand factor adhesion. *J Thromb Haemost* 2003;1:1150–1157.

193. Kasirer-Friede A, Ware J, Leng L, et al. Lateral clustering of platelet GP Ib-IX complexes leads to up-regulation of the adhesive function of integrin αIIbβ3. *J Biol Chem* 2002;277:11949–11956.

194. Goto S, Tamura N, Eto K, et al. Functional significance of adenosine 5′-diphosphate receptor (P2Y12) in platelet activation initiated by binding of von Willebrand factor to platelet GP Ibα induced by conditions of high shear rate. *Circulation* 2002;105:2531–2536.

195. Resendiz JC, Feng S, Ji G, et al. Purinergic P2Y12 receptor blockade inhibits shear-induced platelet phosphatidylinositol 3-kinase activation. *Mol Pharmacol* 2003;63:639–645.

196. Canobbio I, Bertoni A, Lova P, et al. Platelet activation by von Willebrand factor requires coordinated signaling through thromboxane A2 and FcγIIA receptor. *J Biol Chem* 2001;276:26022–26029.

197. Falati S, Edmead CE, Poole AW. Glycoprotein Ib-V-IX, a receptor for von Willebrand factor, couples physically and functionally to the Fc receptor γ-Chain, fyn, and lyn to activate human platelets. *Blood* 1999;94:1648–1656.

198. Wu Y, Suzuki-Inoue K, Satoh K, et al. Role of Fc receptor γ-chain in platelet glycoprotein Ib-mediated signaling. *Blood* 2001;97:3836–3845.

199. Okumura T, Lombart C, Jamieson GA. Platelet glycocalicin. II. Purification and characterization. *J Biol Chem* 1976;251:5950–5955.

200. Judson PA, Anstee DJ, Clamp JR. Isolation and characterization of the major oligosaccharide of human platelet membrane glycoprotein GPIb. *Biochem J* 1982;205:81–90.

201. Ardissino D, Mannucci PM, Merlini PA, et al. Prothrombotic genetic risk factors in young survivors of myocardial infarction. *Blood* 1999;94: 46–51.

202. Ito T, Ishida F, Shimodaira S, et al. Polymorphisms of platelet membrane glycoprotein Ibα and plasma von Willebrand factor antigen in coronary artery disease. *Int J Hematol* 1999;70:47–51.

203. Sonoda A, Murata M, Ito D, et al. Association between platelet glycoprotein Ibα genotype and ischemic cerebrovascular disease. *Stroke* 2000; 31:493–497.

204. Reiner AP, Kumar PN, Schwartz SM, et al. Genetic variants of platelet glycoprotein receptors and risk of stroke in young women. *Stroke* 2000; 31:1628–1633.

205. Meiklejohn DJ, Vickers MA, Morrison ER, et al. *In vivo* platelet activation in atherothrombotic stroke is not determined by polymorphisms of human platelet glycoprotein IIIa or Ib. *Br J Haematol* 2001;112:621–631.

206. Mikkelsson J, Perola M, Penttila A, et al. Platelet glycoprotein Ibα HPA-2 Met/VNTR B haplotype as a genetic predictor of myocardial infarction and sudden cardiac death. *Circulation* 2001;104:876–880.

207. Carter AM, Catto AJ, Bamford JM, et al. Platelet GP IIIa PlA and GP Ib variable number tandem repeat polymorphisms and markers of platelet activation in acute stroke. *Arterioscler Thromb Vasc Biol* 1998;18: 1124–1131.

208. Murata M, Kawano K, Matsubara Y, et al. Genetic polymorphisms and risk of coronary artery disease. *Semin Thromb Hemost* 1998;24:245–250.

209. Donahue BS, Byrne DW, Gailani D, et al. Tissue factor and platelet glycoprotein Ib-α alleles are associated with age at first coronary bypass operation. *Anesthesiology* 2003;99:1287–1294.

210. Salomon O, Rosenberg N, Steinberg DM, et al. Nonarteritic anterior ischemic optic neuropathy is associated with a specific platelet polymorphism located on the glycoprotein Ibα gene. *Ophthalmology* 2004;111: 184–188.

211. Chevalier J, Nurden AT, Thiery JM, et al. Freeze-fracture studies on the plasma membranes of normal human, thrombasthenic, and Bernard-Soulier platelets. *J Lab Clin Med* 1979;94:232–245.

212. Croft SA, Hampton KK, Daly ME, et al. Kozak sequence polymorphism in the platelet GPIbα gene is not associated with risk of myocardial infarction. *Blood* 2000;95:2183–2184.

213. Frank MB, Reiner AP, Schwartz SM, et al. The Kozak sequence polymorphism of platelet glycoprotein Ibα and risk of nonfatal myocardial infarction and nonfatal stroke in young women. *Blood* 2001;97:875–879.

214. Ishida F, Ito T, Takei M, et al. Genetic linkage of Kozak sequence polymorphism of the platelet glycoprotein Ib α with human platelet antigen-2 and variable number of tandem repeats polymorphism, and its relationship with coronary artery disease. *Br J Haematol* 2000;111:1247–1249.

215. Meisel C, Afshar-Kharghan V, Cascorbi I, et al. Role of Kozak sequence polymorphism of platelet glycoprotein Ibα as a risk factor for coronary artery disease and catheter interventions. *J Am Coll Cardiol* 2001;38:1023–1027.

216. Douglas H, Michaelides K, Gorog DA, et al. Platelet membrane glycoprotein Ibα gene -5T/C Kozak sequence polymorphism as an independent risk factor for the occurrence of coronary thrombosis. *Heart* 2002;87:70–74.

217. Kenny D, Muckian C, Fitzgerald DJ, et al. Platelet glycoprotein Ibα receptor polymorphisms and recurrent ischaemic events in acute coronary syndrome patients. *J Thromb Thrombolysis* 2002;13:13–19.

218. Carlsson LE, Lubenow N, Blumentritt C, et al. Platelet receptor and clotting factor polymorphisms as genetic risk factors for thromboembolic complications in heparin-induced thrombocytopenia. *Pharmacogenetics* 2003;13:253–258.

219. Sachs UJ, Kiefel V, Bohringer M, et al. Single amino acid substitution in human platelet glycoprotein Ibβ is responsible for the formation of the platelet-specific alloantigen Iy(a). *Blood* 2000;95:1849–1855.

220. Rathore V, Stapleton MA, Hillery CA, et al. PECAM-1 negatively regulates GPIb/V/IX signaling in murine platelets. *Blood* 2003;102: 3658–3664.

221. Patil S, Newman DK, Newman PJ. Platelet endothelial cell adhesion molecule-1 serves as an inhibitory receptor that modulates platelet responses to collagen. *Blood* 2001;97:1727–1732.

222. Jones KL, Hughan SC, Dopheide SM, et al. Platelet endothelial cell adhesion molecule-1 is a negative regulator of platelet-collagen interactions. *Blood* 2001;98:1456–1463.

223. Mistry N, Cranmer SL, Yuan Y, et al. Cytoskeletal regulation of the platelet glycoprotein Ib/V/IX-von Willebrand factor interaction. *Blood* 2000;96:3480–3489.

224. Englund GD, Bodnar RJ, Li Z, et al. Regulation of von Willebrand factor binding to the platelet glycoprotein Ib-IX by a membrane skeleton-dependent inside-out signal. *J Biol Chem* 2001;276:16952–16959.

225. Schade AJ, Arya M, Gao S, et al. Cytoplasmic truncation of glycoprotein Ib α weakens its interaction with von Willebrand factor and impairs cell adhesion. *Biochemistry* 2003;42:2245–2251.

226. Gu M, Xi X, Englund GD, et al. Analysis of the roles of 14-3-3 in the platelet glycoprotein Ib-IX-mediated activation of integrin $\alpha_{IIb}\beta_3$ using a reconstituted mammalian cell expression model. *J Cell Biol* 1999;147:1085–1096.

227. Feng S, Christodoulides N, Resendiz JC, et al. Cytoplasmic domains of GpIbα and GpIbβ regulate 14-3-3ζ binding to GpIb/IX/V. *Blood* 2000; 95:551–557.

228. Munday AD, Berndt MC, Mitchell CA. Phosphoinositide 3-kinase forms a complex with platelet membrane glycoprotein Ib-IX-V complex and 14-3-3ζ. *Blood* 2000;96:577–584.

229. Bodnar RJ, Xi X, Li Z, et al. Regulation of glycoprotein Ib-IX-von Willebrand factor interaction by cAMP-dependent protein kinase-mediated

phosphorylation at Ser 166 of glycoprotein Ibβ. *J Biol Chem* 2002;277:47080–47087.

230. Bodnar RJ, Gu M, Li Z, et al. The cytoplasmic domain of the platelet glycoprotein Ibα is phosphorylated at serine 609. *J Biol Chem* 1999;274:33474–33479.

231. Kanaji T, Russell S, Cunningham J, et al. Megakaryocyte proliferation and ploidy regulated by the cytoplasmic tail of glycoprotein Ibα. *Blood* 2004;104:3161–3168 EPUB.

232. Nesbitt WS, Kulkarni S, Giuliano S, et al. Distinct glycoprotein Ib/V/IX and integrin α$_{IIb}$β$_3$-dependent calcium signals cooperatively regulate platelet adhesion under flow. *J Biol Chem* 2002;277:2965–2972.

233. Mazzucato M, Pradella P, Cozzi MR, et al. Sequential cytoplasmic calcium signals in a 2-stage platelet activation process induced by the glycoprotein Ibalpha mechanoreceptor. *Blood* 2002;100:2793–2800.

234. Mangin P, Yuan Y, Goncalves I, et al. Signaling role for phospholipase Cγ2 in platelet glycoprotein Ibα calcium flux and cytoskeletal reorganization. Involvement of a pathway distinct from FcRγ chain and FcγRIIA. *J Biol Chem* 2003;278:32880–32891.

235. Wu Y, Asazuma N, Satoh K, et al. Interaction between von Willebrand factor and glycoprotein Ib activates Src kinase in human platelets: role of phosphoinositide 3-kinase. *Blood* 2003;101:3469–3476.

236. Resendiz JC, Feng S, Ji G, et al. von Willebrand factor binding to platelet glycoprotein Ib-IX-V stimulates the assembly of an alpha-actinin-based signaling complex. *J Thromb Haemost* 2004;2:161–169.

237. Yap CL, Anderson KE, Hughan SC, et al. Essential role for phosphoinositide 3-kinase in shear-dependent signaling between platelet glycoprotein Ib/V/IX and integrin αIIbβ3. *Blood* 2002;99:151–158.

238. Mekrache M, Bachelot-Loza C, Ajzenberg N, et al. Activation of pp125FAK by type 2B recombinant von Willebrand factor binding to platelet GPIb at a high shear rate occurs independently of αIIbβ3 engagement. *Blood* 2003;101:4363–4371.

239. Canobbio I, Lova P, Sinigaglia F, et al. Proline-rich tyrosine kinase 2 and focal adhesion kinase are involved in different phases of platelet activation by vWF. *Thromb Haemost* 2002;87:509–517.

240. Dyson JM, Munday AD, Kong AM, et al. SHIP-2 forms a tetrameric complex with filamin, actin, and GPIb-IX-V: localization of SHIP-2 to the activated platelet actin cytoskeleton. *Blood* 2003;102:940–948.

241. Li BS, Ma W, Zhang L, et al. Activation of phosphatidylinositol-3 kinase (PI-3K) and extracellular regulated kinases (Erk1/2) is involved in muscarinic receptor-mediated DNA synthesis in neural progenitor cells. *J Neurosci* 2001;21:1569–1579.

242. Li Z, Xi X, Gu M, et al. A stimulatory role for cGMP-dependent protein kinase in platelet activation. *Cell* 2003;112:77–86.

243. Marshall SJ, Senis YA, Auger JM, et al. GPIb-dependent platelet activation is dependent on Src kinases but not MAP kinase or cGMP-dependent kinase. *Blood* 2004;103:2601–2609.

# CHAPTER 32 ■ PLATELET ADENOSINE 5′-DIPHOSPHATE RECEPTORS

SATYA P. KUNAPULI

Adenosine 5′-diphosphate (ADP) is the first low-molecular-weight platelet-activating agent to be identified (1). Along with adenosine 5′-triphosphate (ATP) and serotonin, ADP is stored in the dense granules of platelets and is released upon activation of platelets (2). The importance of ADP as a platelet-aggregating agent is substantiated by the observation that patients with storage-pool deficiencies or dysfunctional receptors have bleeding diatheses (3–9).

The cell surface receptors for nucleotides have been designated as P2 receptors and have been divided into two groups, P2X and P2Y receptors (10–12). The P2X receptors are ligand-gated channels, and molecular cloning has revealed seven subtypes of P2X receptors (11). The P2Y receptors are seven transmembrane receptors and elicit their effects through coupling to heterotrimeric G proteins. Nine distinct P2Y receptors are expressed in human tissues: $P2Y_1$, $P2Y_2$, $P2Y_4$, $P2Y_6$, $P2Y_{11}$, $P2Y_{12}$, $P2Y_{13}$, $P2Y_{14}$, and $P2Y_{15}$ (13–16) The ADP receptor on platelets were originally designated the P2T (thrombocyte P2) receptor (17).

## PHYSIOLOGIC EFFECTS OF ADENOSINE 5′-DIPHOSPHATE ON PLATELETS

Activation of platelets by ADP follows a defined sequence of events. The discoid-shaped resting platelet cells change shape when exposed to low concentrations of ADP (i.e., 0.1 to 0.5 $\mu$M) and are rapidly converted to spiculated spheres (18). Higher concentrations (i.e., 2 to 5 $\mu$M) of ADP cause platelet aggregation and granule secretion, which releases more ADP as well as many other substances including serotonin, ATP, and fibrinogen (2,18).

Platelet aggregation occurs because of the ability of ADP to expose the fibrinogen-binding site on the $\alpha_{IIb}\beta_3$ integrin [fibrinogen receptor; glycoprotein (GP) IIb/IIIa] (19). ADP causes primary aggregation, which is reversible under physiologic concentrations of extracellular calcium (20). ADP-induced release of arachidonic acid and the subsequently produced thromboxane A2, along with granule secretion, contribute to the irreversible secondary aggregation (21).

ADP causes the release of both $\alpha$-granules and dense granule contents (2,18) when the extracellular calcium concentration is low (22). The ADP-induced release of the contents of dense granules depends on thromboxane A2 because ADP fails to cause dense granule release in aspirin-treated and washed platelets (2). Whether ADP causes the release of the contents of $\alpha$-granules directly or indirectly through thromboxane A2 remains controversial. Several previous studies pointed to the direct role of ADP in the $\alpha$-granule release reaction (23–26), but other investigators have shown that ADP fails to expose P selectin (27) or $\beta$-thromboglobulin (28), both found in

$\alpha$-granules in aspirin-treated and washed platelets, suggesting that this event may require the generation of thromboxane A2.

## ADENOSINE 5′-DIPHOSPHATE–INDUCED PRIMARY INTRACELLULAR SIGNALING EVENTS IN PLATELETS

ADP, through its actions on cell surface receptors, modulates several second messenger systems in platelets (17,25,29). ADP inhibits platelet adenylyl cyclase through the stimulation of the $G\alpha_i$ protein and thereby decreases intracellular adenosine 3′,5′-cyclic monophosphate (cAMP) levels (30). Photoaffinity-labeling studies showed that this effect is mediated by $G\alpha_{i2}$ (31). ADP also causes rapid calcium influx when platelets are resuspended in physiologic calcium ion concentrations (32,33). ADP also induces inositol trisphosphate formation, which is well correlated with the mobilization of intracellular calcium stores in human platelets (34). Even in the absence of extracellular calcium, ADP causes an increase in intracellular calcium concentration through mobilization of intracellular calcium stores (35). In addition, ADP also causes the activation of phospholipase $A_2$ ($PLA_2$), resulting in the release of arachidonic acid from membrane phospholipids (21).

## THE THROMBOCYTE P2 RECEPTOR

All the physiologic and intracellular signaling events triggered by ADP in platelets were attributed initially to a single cell surface receptor. Because the molecular nature of this receptor was unknown, it was designated the P2T receptor. The historic studies and theories concerning P2T receptor have been dealt with in various review articles (17,25,29). The classic characteristics of the P2T receptor are the competitive antagonism by ATP and its presumably exclusive expression in platelets; at all other P2 receptors, ATP is an agonist. ADP and 2-methylthioADP (2MeSADP) are potent agonists of platelet aggregation, and ADP$\beta$S is a partial agonist, whereas ADP$\alpha$S is an antagonist. ATP derivatives that are substituted at the position 2 (e.g., 2MeSATP, 2ClATP, and 2MeS–AMP–PCP) are antagonists at this receptor. The ATP analogs ARL 66096 and ARL 67085 are antagonists at the P2T receptor and are a potential class of antithrombotic agents (36–38), which are currently in clinical trials. Other antithrombotic agents that interfere with the action of ADP on platelets are the thienopyridine derivatives, ticlopidine and clopidogrel, which prolong the bleeding time and are clinically effective antithrombotic agents (39–43).

Glycoprotein IIb (GP IIb), a component of the fibrinogen receptor, was proposed (44) to be the P2T receptor on the basis of binding studies with [$^3$H]-ADP on formalin-fixed platelets (45,46). However, platelets from patients with GP IIb deficiency respond normally to ADP and exhibit intracellular responses and shape change (47,48). Therefore, although the GP IIb may bind ADP (49), it does not appear to be a notable mediator of the functional effects of ADP.

A protein of approximately 100 kDa was identified by labeling with radiolabeled 5′-p-fluorosulfonylbenzoyl adenosine (FSBA) on platelets. This labeling was inhibited by ADP and by ATP (50–52). This protein was designated aggregin and was proposed to be the ADP receptor. FSBA inhibits ADP-induced platelet shape change and aggregation (50–52). FSBA has no effect on adenylyl cyclase in intact platelets nor does it inhibit the effect of ADP or interfere with the binding of 2MeSADP (53). Under conditions of covalent labeling of ADP binding sites, FSBA inhibits ADP-induced shape change but fails to block an increase in intracellular calcium or a decrease in cAMP levels (54). Further studies were carried out with ADP derivatives, which either stimulated or inhibited platelet aggregation at shorter incubation times and covalently modified the same 100-kDa aggregin at longer incubation times; these derivatives inhibited all ADP-induced platelet responses including the effect on adenylyl cyclase (55–58). Studies investigating whether aggregin is a platelet ADP receptor have been reviewed recently (25,58). However, these studies do not consider the possibility that the binding of FSBA or the ADP analogs to a nucleotide-binding protein or an ecto-ATPase can occur without physiologic implications and yet may exert their effects through the platelet ADP receptors. Considering the recent advances in the cloning and functional characterization of the platelet ADP receptors (discussed in subsequent part of text), aggregin may not be an ADP receptor.

# THE THREE-RECEPTOR MODEL FOR ADENOSINE 5′-DIPHOSPHATE–INDUCED PLATELET ACTIVATION

ARL 66096, a potent antagonist of ADP-induced platelet aggregation, and a P2X$_1$ receptor agonist, α,β-MeATP, were used to distinguish ADP-induced intracellular events (34). ARL 66096 blocked ADP-induced inhibition of adenylyl cyclase but failed to inhibit ADP-mediated intracellular calcium increases. Both ADP and 2-MeSADP caused a threefold increase in the inositol 1,4,5 trisphosphate and inositol 1,3,4 trisphosphate levels, which peaked in a similar fashion to the intracellular calcium increases. However, α,β-MeATP did not affect the formation of either forms of inositol trisphosphate. In addition, ARL 66096 failed to inhibit intracellular calcium mobilization, inositol trisphosphate formation, or shape change. On the basis of these observations, a three-receptor model was proposed (34). The first receptor is coupled for inhibition of adenylyl cyclase, designated P2T$_{AC}$ receptor; the second receptor is coupled for mobilization of calcium from intracellular stores through activation of phospholipase C (PLC) and inositol trisphosphate formation, designated P2T$_{PLC}$; the third receptor is an ionotropic P2X$_1$ receptor coupled for rapid calcium influx; A complementary deoxyribonucleic acid (DNA) clone encoding the P2Y$_1$ receptor was isolated from a human platelet cDNA library by homology screening and was shown to be the P2T$_{PLC}$ receptor (59). The Gαi-coupled P2T$_{AC}$ receptor has also been cloned recently and

designated the P2Y$_{12}$ receptor (60–63). Therefore, the concept of a single "P2T" receptor has been resolved into three P2 receptor subtypes (i.e., P2Y$_1$, P2Y$_{12}$, and P2X$_1$ receptors), each with distinct functions (see Fig. 32-1). Furthermore, other recent independent studies have also provided support for the three-receptor model by gene disruption approaches (64–66). A comparison of the properties of these three receptors is shown in Table 32-1.

## Function of the P2X$_1$ Receptor

MacKenzie et al. (33) demonstrated an ADP-gated channel on platelets, suggested to be the P2X$_1$ receptor, that could cause rapid calcium influx. A P2X$_1$ selective agonist, α,β-MeATP, causes an increase in intracellular calcium level through rapid calcium influx in the presence of 1-mM extracellular calcium (59). P2X$_1$ was found to be present in platelets initially by physiologic and pharmacologic means. Later, P2X$_1$ messenger ribonucleic acid (mRNA) was isolated from platelets (67), and the corresponding gene was subsequently isolated and cloned from human platelets and megakaryocytes (68,69).

It was initially thought that P2X$_1$ could be activated by both ATP and ADP (70). It was later shown that ADP was not an agonist for P2X$_1$ by using ADP that had been purified to remove contaminating amounts of ATP (71). In fact, purified ADP antagonizes α,β-MeATP-induced inward calcium currents in human platelets and prevents α,β-MeATP binding to the P2X$_1$ expressed in cultured cells (72). Furthermore, pyridoxine-α-4,5-monophosphate (MRS 2219) was found to be a selective agonist in rat P2X$_1$ receptors, whereas MRS 2220, the corresponding 6-azophenyl-2′, 5′-disulfonate derivative, was found to be a selective antagonist.

P2X$_1$-mediated, short-lived increases in intracellular calcium levels in platelets are sufficient for the onset of platelet shape change but not for platelet aggregation (73,74). Furthermore, P2X$_1$-mediated platelet shape change can occur under conditions in which fibrinogen receptor activation is prevented (74). P2X$_1$ activation may lead to the activation of extracellular signal–regulated kinase 2 (ERK2), with a resultant amplifying effect on the secretion of the platelet dense granule (75). In addition, costimulation of the P2X$_1$ and P2Y$_1$ receptors on human platelets by α,β-MeATP and ADP, respectively, potentiates an extent of calcium release that is faster and greater than the sum of the calcium releases from either agonist alone (76). However, platelets costimulated with α,β-MeATP and ADP in the presence of the P2Y$_1$ antagonist A3P5PS resulted only in shape change, indicating that no synergy exists between activation of the P2X$_1$ nd P2Y$_{12}$ receptors (77).

The possible involvement of P2X$_1$ in platelet activation was examined further in P2X$_1$ null mice and transgenic mice. The mice that were deficient in P2X$_1$ were healthy and did not appear to display any hemostatic defects (78). However, a 50% reduction in ADP-mediated inward calcium current was recently observed in P2X$_1$-deficient mice (76), possibly reflecting a role for secreted ATP in platelet activation. On the other hand, mice that overexpressed P2X$_1$ show an increase in collagen-mediated platelet secretion, aggregation, and ERK2 phosphorylation in comparison to wild-type mice (79).

*In vivo*, the functional role of P2X$_1$ was demonstrated in models of platelet-dependent thrombotic occlusion of small arteries (80). In a model of systemic thromboembolism, the mortality of P2X$_1^{-/-}$ mice, compared to wild-type mice, was reduced and the size of the mural thrombi formed after a laser-induced vessel wall injury was decreased, whereas the time for complete thrombus removal was shortened. Therefore, the P2X$_1$ receptor appears to contribute to the formation of platelet thrombi, particularly in small arteries in which shear forces are high (80).

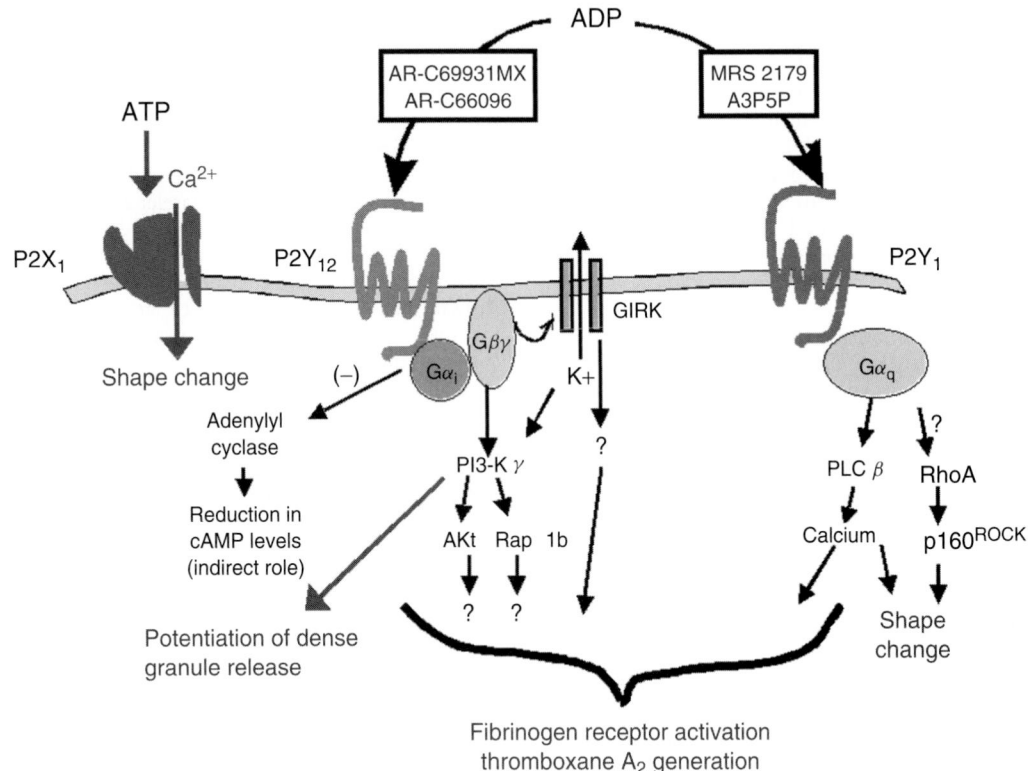

**FIGURE 32-1.** Functional roles of the platelet adenosine 5'-diphosphate (ADP) receptors (see Color Fig. 32-1). PLC, phospholipase C; GIRK, G protein–gated inwardly rectifying potassium; ATP, adenosine 5'-triphosphate; cAMP, adenosine 3',5'-cyclic monophosphate.

## Function of the P2Y₁ Receptor

The human P2Y$_1$ receptor was originally cloned from human erythroleukemia (HEL) cells (81) and endothelial cells (82). The platelet P2Y$_1$ receptor differs from the long and the short form of the HEL cell P2Y$_1$ receptors only in the length of the 3'-untranslated region because of utilization of the alternate polyadenylation site (59). The human P2Y$_1$ receptor is 373–amino acid long with seven putative hydrophobic transmembrane regions and is encoded by a single exon (83). The gene for the human P2Y$_1$ receptor has been localized to the chromosome 3q25 (83). The P2Y$_1$ receptor, when heterologously expressed in astrocytoma cells, has been shown to activate PLC through pertussis-toxin–insensitive G proteins of the Gq/11 class, resulting in inositol phosphate formation (84).

Although earlier studies had identified ATP as an agonist at this receptor (84–86), subsequently, Leon et al. (87)

### TABLE 32-1

**RESOLUTION OF THE THREE DISTINCT RECEPTORS BASED ON THE PHARMACOLOGIC PROPERTIES AND FUNCTION**

| | P2Y₁₂ receptor | P2Y₁ receptor | P2X₁ receptor |
|---|---|---|---|
| Agonists | ADP, 2MeSADP | ADP, 2MeSADP | ATP, $\alpha,\beta$-MeATP |
| Antagonists | AR-C69931MX | MRS2179 | ADP |
| | 2MeSAMP | A3P5P | MRS2159 |
| | ATP | ATP | |
| Rapid calcium influx | ? | ? | Yes |
| Mobilization of intracellular calcium stores | No | Yes | ? |
| Inhibition of adenylyl cyclase | Yes | No | No |
| Stimulation of IP₃ formation | No | Yes | No |
| Mediator of shape change | No | Yes | Yes |
| Essential for ADP-induced aggregation | Yes | Yes | No |
| Cloned in human platelets | Yes | Yes | Yes |
| Knockout mice developed | Yes | Yes | Yes |
| Prolonged bleeding times | Yes | Yes | No |

ADP, adenosine 5'-diphosphate; ATP, adenosine 5'-triphosphate.

demonstrated that ATP is a weak antagonist at the $P2Y_1$ receptor, with an estimated pKB of approximately 5. The $P2Y_1$ receptor is not coupled to adenylyl cyclase in platelets (59).

When activated by ADP, the platelet $P2Y_1$ receptor presumably couples to $G_q$ and causes intracellular calcium mobilization through the inositol trisphosphate pathway (88). Similar to the $P2Y_{12}$ receptor, the $P2Y_1$ receptor is also activated by ADP and by 2-substituted derivatives of ADP and is antagonized by ATP and by 2-substituted ATP analogs including ARL 66096 and ARL 67085. However, the potencies of these agonists and antagonists are different at the $P2Y_1$ and $P2Y_{12}$ receptors. For example, ADP is more potent at the $P2Y_1$ receptor ($EC_{50}$ approximately 0.3 $\mu$M) than at the $P2Y_{12}$ receptor ($EC_{50}$ approximately 2 $\mu$M). On the contrary, 2MeSADP is at least 100-fold more potent than ADP at the $P2Y_{12}$ receptor but only approximately fourfold more potent at the $P2Y_1$ receptor. These differences in potencies explain the distinct requirements for shape change and aggregation (as discussed in subsequent text). ATP appears to be an antagonist of similar potency at both the $P2Y_{12}$ and $P2Y_1$ receptors (pKB approximately 5) (87,89). ARL 66096 is a more potent antagonist at the $P2Y_{12}$ receptor than at the $P2Y_1$ receptor.

The $P2Y_1$ receptor selective antagonists (90), adenosine-3'-phosphate-5'-phosphosulfate (A3P5PS), adenosine-3'-phosphate-5'-phosphate (A3P5P), adenosine-2'-phosphate-5'-phosphate (A2P5P), and $N^6$-methyl 2'-deoxyadenosine 3',5'-bisphosphate (MRS2179), (91) inhibit ADP- or 2MeSADP-induced intracellular calcium mobilization and shape change in platelets in a concentration-dependent manner (59). These antagonists do not have any effect on the $P2Y_2$, $P2Y_4$, or the $P2Y_6$ receptors nor do they have any effect on the $P2Y_{12}$ receptor that mediates ADP-induced inhibition of adenylyl cyclase (92). The $EC_{50}$ for ADP at the cloned $P2Y_1$ receptor is approximately 0.3 $\mu$M(84), which is also the dose that is sufficient for platelet shape change (1). Studies with mice lacking $G\alpha_q$ revealed that signaling through Gq is essential for ADP-induced shape change (88). All the agents that cause platelet shape change, such as thrombin, thromboxane, and serotonin, also activate PLC (93). On the other hand, epinephrine, which does not activate PLC, fails to cause shape change in the absence of positive feedback activation mechanisms (94,95). These data therefore implicate PLC activation as the essential step in platelet shape change. Because the receptor mediating platelet shape change has been linked to the high-affinity ADP receptor on platelets (96), the $P2Y_1$ receptor is the high-affinity ADP receptor on platelets.

The $P2Y_1$ receptor causes platelet shape change through calcium-dependent and calcium-independent pathways (97,98). The calcium-dependent pathway is triggered by activation of PLC and by elevated intracellular calcium levels (98). The calcium-independent pathway involves activation of RhoA and $p160^{ROCK}$ (Rho kinase). In the $G\alpha_q$ null mice, ADP does not cause platelet shape change (88), suggesting that the RhoA pathway is downstream of Gq stimulation. However, it is not clear how Gq activates RhoA. Human platelets contain myosin phosphatase, which is phosphorylated and inactivated by the RhoA/$p160^{ROCK}$ pathway (99). A RhoA/Rho kinase–regulated pathway is required for the maintenance of a spherical platelet shape after agonist-dependent activation (97). Therefore, continued disruption of the cytoskeletal microtubule ring appears to be a Rho kinase–dependent event involved in the transformation of discoid platelets into spheres.

Pharmacologic approaches have also revealed the essential role of the $P2Y_1$ in ADP-induced platelet aggregation and in thromboxane A2 generation (100–102). ADP has been shown to cause the generation of a factor that can activate p38MAP kinase in non–aspirin-treated human platelets, and this response is mediated solely by the $P2Y_1$ receptor (103). Recently, it has been shown that the interactions of ADP with $P2Y_{12}$ and

with $P2Y_1$ are both essential for platelet adhesion on immobilized fibrinogen under physiologic flow conditions (104). In addition, the combined blocking of ADP receptors by both $P2Y_1$ and $P2Y_{12}$ has been shown to be effective in inhibiting direct shear-induced platelet aggregation (105).

Studies with mice that either lack the $P2Y_1$ or that overexpress the $P2Y_1$ receptor make it possible to determine the contributions of this receptor to platelet activation. Platelets from mice that lack $P2Y_1$ receptor neither change shape nor aggregate in response to ADP, with the exception of partial aggregation at very high concentrations of ADP (65,106). It was shown that $P2Y_1$-deficient mice are resistant to the acute thromboembolism induced by intravenous injection of ADP or collagen and adrenaline. In addition, these $P2Y_1$ receptor–null mice, as well as wild-type mice dosed with MRS2179, have also shown increased resistance to thromboembolism induced by tissue factor (107). On the other hand, overexpression of the $P2Y_1$ receptor, through transgene technology, led to a phenotype of platelet hyperreactivity in vitro, as evidenced by increased aggregation in response to lower concentrations of ADP and collagen than that required in wild-type mice (108). More interestingly, overexpression of the $P2Y_1$ receptor enabled ADP to induce dense granule secretion, which does not occur in wild-type platelets. This finding suggests that the level of $P2Y_1$ expression is critical for this event (108). Therefore, the $P2Y_1$ receptor plays an essential role in thrombotic states and represents a useful target in a wide range of thrombotic diseases. The potential of the $P2Y_1$ receptor as an antithrombotic agent target has been discussed in a recent review (109).

## Function of the $P2Y_{12}$ Receptor

The $P2Y_{12}$ receptor couples to $G\alpha_i$ and upon activation by ADP causes inhibition of $PGE_1$-stimulated adenylyl cyclase. ADP and 2-substituted derivatives of ADP are agonists at this receptor, whereas ATP and 2-substituted derivatives of ATP, including ARL 66096 and ARL 67085, are antagonists. Furthermore, clopidogrel and ticlopidine abolish ADP-induced adenylyl cyclase inhibition (110) by neutralizing the $P2Y_{12}$ receptor, through an active metabolite (111–113). In addition, two patients with congenitally defective ADP receptor function and aggregation (5,8) appear to have an abnormal $P2Y_{12}$ receptor (114,115).

2-{[(p-azidophenyl)-ethyl]-thio}-adenosine-5'-diphosphate (AzPET-ADP) inhibits adenylyl cyclase with a potency nearly 10-fold greater than that of ADP (116). On photolysis in the presence of human platelets, [$\beta$-$^{32}$P]-AzPET-ADP is predominantly incorporated into a protein of 43 kDa, and this labeling is inhibited by ADP, ATP, pCMBS (116), and ARL 66096 (late David C. B. Mills, personal communication). $\beta$-[$^{32}$P]-AzPET-ADP also labels a protein on platelets from rabbits, rats, and dogs that appears to be in the 43- to 50-kDa range (25). These studies suggest that the $P2Y_{12}$ receptor on human platelets is 43 kD.

Activation of the $P2Y_{12}$ receptor by ADP does not lead to PLC activation, intracellular calcium mobilization, or rapid calcium influx (59). $P2Y_{12}$ receptor does not play any significant role in ADP-induced platelet shape change (42,59) but is essential for ADP-induced platelet aggregation. Antagonists of this receptor have been shown to block both ADP-induced adenylyl cyclase inhibition (34,117) and platelet aggregation (38,117). Furthermore, a statistically significant correlation was found between pA2 (antagonist affinity constants) values for eight nucleotide analogs, as blockers of ADP-induced adenylyl cyclase inhibition and aggregation (89). The thienopyridines ticlopidine and clopidogrel when administered in vivo, negate ADP-induced inhibition of adenylyl cyclase and platelet aggregation (40,42,110). In two patients with defective ADP-induced platelet aggregation, adenylyl cyclase inhibition was also defective, suggesting that the receptor coupled to inhibition of adenylyl cyclase is essential for platelet aggregation (5,8).

The P2Y$_{12}$ receptor has been the target for antithrombotic thienopyridine compounds such as the aforementioned ticlopidine and clopidogrel (118), and CS747 (119). Even though these compounds have been effective in treating a variety of thrombotic diseases, they have been shown to cause the immune-mediated syndrome, thrombotic thrombocytopenic purpura (120). The P2Y$_{12}$ receptor was recently cloned by several groups, and P2Y$_{12}$ receptor knockout mice have been generated (66). Pharmacologic approaches have shown a role for the P2Y$_{12}$ receptor in ADP-induced platelet aggregation, thromboxane A2 generation, and potentiation of dense granule release and procoagulant activity (59,102,121–123). In response to ADP, platelets from mice lacking the P2Y$_{12}$ receptor aggregate poorly, fail to inhibit adenylyl cyclase, and do not respond to treatment with clopidogrel, but they retain P2Y$_1$-mediated shape change (66). A recent study shows the loss of inhibition of adenylyl cyclase and impaired platelet aggregation in response to ADP in platelets from G$\alpha_{i2}$-deficient mice, suggesting that G$\alpha_{i2}$ is associated with P2Y$_{12}$ responses and is important for ADP-induced inhibition of mouse platelet adenylyl cyclase *in vivo* (124). Of the four extracellular cysteines in the *N*-terminal region of P2Y$_{12}$, C17 and C270 were shown to be the targets of thiol reagents, suggesting that these could be the target of the active metabolites of the antiplatelet drugs clopidogrel and CS747 (113).

We have shown that agonist-induced fibrinogen receptor activation occurs in platelets through PKC-sensitive and calcium-sensitive pathways (125,126) and that the P2Y$_{12}$ receptor can independently synergize with either of these pathways (125). In addition, recent studies from Nieswandt et al. and from our lab have shown that concomitant signaling from the G12/13 activation and P2Y$_{12}$ receptor can cause fibrinogen receptor activation (127,128). Furthermore, the P2Y$_{12}$ receptor can synergize with the $\alpha_{2A}$-receptor, and costimulation of these two receptors leads to fibrinogen receptor activation and thromboxane A2 generation in an Src family kinase–dependent manner (129).

Yang et al. and we have shown that inhibition of adenylyl cyclase is not the signaling event that contributes to either P2Y$_{12}$-mediated ADP-induced fibrinogen receptor activation or potentiation of dense granule release reaction (122,130). The $\gamma$-isoform of phosphatidylinositol 3-kinase (PI 3-kinase) is activated by the $\beta\gamma$-regulatory subunits released from Gi proteins upon activation of the P2Y$_{12}$ receptor (131). Although mice lacking PI 3-kinase $\gamma$ are protected in a thromboembolic model, their platelets did not show significantly reduced aggregation in response to higher concentrations of ADP (132). We have shown that PI 3-kinase is an important signaling molecule in the P2Y$_{12}$ receptor-mediated potentiation of dense granule release reaction (122). The P2Y$_{12}$ receptor is able to induce partial aggregation of P2Y$_1$-deficient mouse platelets in response to a high concentration of ADP through the activation of PI 3-kinase (133). We have not only shown that the P2Y$_{12}$ stimulation leads to the production of PKB/Akt (another signaling molecule downstream of PI 3-kinase) but also demonstrated that P2Y$_{12}$ is important for thrombin-mediated Akt activation (134). Rap1b is a small GTPase that is activated in a PI 3-kinase $\gamma$–dependent mechanism following G$\alpha_i$/G$\alpha_z$-coupled receptor stimulation (135,136). It has been shown to play an important role in fibrinogen receptor activation in megakaryocytes (137). Recent studies have also shown that platelets from Rap1b knockout mice have a smaller extent of aggregation induced by ADP, compared to the wild-type mouse platelets (138). Therefore, Rap1b appears to be one of the functional effectors downstream of the P2Y$_{12}$ receptor. Platelets also express two isoforms of Akt (protein kinase

B) (139). Platelets from mice deficient in either isoform of Akt do not show significant abnormalities in agonist-induced platelet aggregation (139). Lack of both isoforms is embryonically lethal, suggesting their role in the early development (139). However, the fact that platelets from mice with three of the four alleles were knocked out show considerable deficiencies in aggregation (139). Because Rap1b and Akt are downstream of PI 3-kinase $\gamma$, these two effectors might be in the same functional effector pathway as PI 3-kinase $\gamma$ (Fig. 32-1). Recent studies from our lab have shown that G protein–gated inwardly rectifying potassium (GIRK) channels are important functional effectors of the P2Y$_{12}$ receptor in human platelets (140). Inhibitors of GIRK channels have been shown to block P2Y$_{12}$-mediated platelet aggregation, potentiation of dense granule release, and Akt activation, without affecting ADP-mediated inhibition of adenylyl cyclase, platelet shape change, or intracellular calcium increases (140). Other signaling molecules contributing to the P2Y$_{12}$-mediated platelet function remain to be elucidated.

Pharmacologic blockade of the P2Y$_{12}$ receptor in physiologic conditions of arterial flow revealed that this receptor is essential for platelet aggregation under shear conditions. Blood from a patient with a defective P2Y$_{12}$ receptor, or normal blood treated with AR-C69931MX, had a thrombus that was small and loosely packed, whereas healthy individuals formed large, densely packed thrombi under physiologic flow experiments (104).

Consistent with the central role of P2Y$_{12}$ receptor antagonists, these antagonists were found to reduce occlusive thrombosis in animal models. Patients and mice lacking functional P2Y$_{12}$ receptors have increased bleeding times (7,66). Clinical studies using clopidogrel demonstrated a reduced risk of peripheral artery disease, myocardial infarction, ischemic stroke, or vascular death, all in comparison to aspirin therapy (43). A combination therapy with aspirin has enhanced beneficial effects, as shown by the Clopidogrel in Unstable Angina to Prevent Recurrent Events (CURE) study, and has led to the approval of clopidogrel for the treatment of non–ST elevation acute coronary syndromes (141). An ongoing trial for the Management of Atherothrombosis with Clopidogrel in High-Risk Patients with Recent Transient Ischemic Attack or Ischemic Stroke (MATCH) is expected to test the effectiveness and safety of clopidogrel plus aspirin as against clopidogrel alone in patients who have experienced a transient ischemic attack or ischemic stroke (142). The results of this trial will further clarify the efficacy of combination therapy.

With the established role of the P2Y$_{12}$ receptor as the central point of thrombus formation, an *in vivo* analysis would clarify the mechanism by which the P2Y$_{12}$ receptor contributes to thrombus growth and stability. Andre et al. (143,144) recently demonstrated the role of the P2Y$_{12}$ receptor on *in vivo* thrombus formation using mice that are deficient in this receptor. The study showed that the P2Y$_{12}$ receptor, because of its effects on thrombus growth and stability *in vivo*, could be a target of antiplatelet agents that would be beneficial even in populations that do not respond to aspirin. In a complementary approach, van Gestel et al. (145) recently reported the effect of the P2Y$_{12}$ receptor antagonists (AR-C69931MX and clopidogrel) on *in vivo* thrombus growth and stability. They concluded that P2Y$_{12}$ receptor blockade (a) significantly reduces the total duration of embolization with fewer and smaller emboli being produced and (b) although the size of the initial thrombus is reduced, its stability was not affected (145). Contrary to this, Andre et al. concluded that the appearance of the first thrombus is delayed and that only small "unstable" thrombi formed in P2Y$_{12}^{-/-}$ mice (143,144). Contrary to the observations of van Gestel et al. (145), more embolization occurred in the P2Y$_{12}^{-/-}$ mice compared to wild-type or heterozygous mice. It is known that clopidogrel can be beneficial when only 50% of the $P2Y_{12}$ receptors is neutralized (118); therefore, an antagonist at the $P2Y_{12}$ receptor could be an effective therapeutic even with 50% of the $P2Y_{12}$ receptors being functional. However, the significant differences in embolization between homozygous and heterozygous mice in the study by Andre et al. (143,144) raise several important questions. Would a complete blockade of the $P2Y_{12}$ receptor formulate a better therapeutic goal and would it be more beneficial than clopidogrel because of abolished receptor function? Why are there differences between the studies with a $P2Y_{12}$ receptor antagonist and those with a $P2Y_{12}$ receptor knockout mice? Is the reason for increased bleeding time in the patients and in mice lacking the $P2Y_{12}$ receptor attributable to unstable thrombus formation or the small size of the thrombus? What are the reasons for differences in embolization in these two studies? Answers to these questions are important because, ultimately, the definition of the key role of the $P2Y_{12}$ receptor would translate into the development of a more effective antithrombotic agent, and the answers would affect the treatment modalities. Of course, the clinical data with humans will determine the effectiveness of such newer therapies.

# ACKNOWLEDGMENT

This work was supported by Research Grants HL60683, HL64943, and HL63933 from the National Institutes of Health.

## *References*

1. Gaarder A, Jonsen A, Laland S, et al. Adenosine diphosphate in red cells as a factor in the adhesiveness of human blood platelets. *Nature (London)* 1961;192:531–532.
2. Mills DCB, Robb IA, Roberts GCK. The release of nucleotides, 5-hydroxytryptamine and enzymes from human blood platelets during aggregation. *J Physiol* 1968;195:715–729.
3. Holmsen H, Weiss HJ. Hereditary defect in the platelet release reaction caused by a deficiency in the storage pool of platelet adenine nucleotides. *Br J Haematol* 1970;19:643–649.
4. Holmsen H, Weiss HJ. Secretable storage pools in platelets. *Ann Rev Med* 1979;30:119–134.
5. Cattaneo M, Lecchi A, Randi AM, et al. Identification of a new congenital defect of platelet aggregation characterized by severe impairment of platelet responses to adenosine 5'-diphosphate. *Blood* 1992;80:2787–2796.
6. Cattaneo M, Lombardi R, Zighetti ML, et al. Partial deficiency of [P-33]2mes-ADP binding sites on platelets from patients with congenital primary secretion defect—evidence that ADP potentiates platelet secretion independently of platelet aggregation and thromboxane A2 production. *Platelets* 1996;7:361.
7. Cattaneo M, Gachet C. ADP receptors and clinical bleeding disorders. *Arterioscler Thromb Vasc Biol* 1999;19:2281–2285.
8. Nurden P, Savi P, Heilmann E, et al. An inherited bleeding disorder linked to a defective interaction between ADP and its receptor on platelets. *J Clin Invest* 1995;95:1612–1622.
9. Nurden AT, Nurden P. Inherited defects of platelet function. *Rev Clin Exp Hematol* 2001;5:314–334.
10. Fredholm B, Abbracchio MP, Burnstock G, et al. Nomenclature and classification of purinoceptors. *Pharmacol Rev* 1994;46:143–156.
11. Fredholm BB, Abbracchio MP, Burnstock G, et al. Towards a revised nomenclature for P1 and P2 receptors. *Trends Pharmacol Sci* 1997;18: 79–82.
12. North RA, Barnard EA. Nucleotide receptors. *Curr Opin Neurobiol* 1997;7:346–357.
13. Inbe H, Watanabe S, Miyawaki M, et al. Identification and characterization of a cell-surface receptor, P2Y15, for AMP and adenosine. *J Biol Chem* 2004;279:19790–19799.
14. Burnstock G. Introduction: P2 receptors. *Curr Top Med Chem* 2004;4: 793–803.
15. Abbracchio MP, Boeynaems JM, Barnard EA, et al. Characterization of the UDP-glucose receptor (re-named here the P2Y14 receptor) adds diversity to the P2Y receptor family. *Trends Pharmacol Sci* 2003;24:52–55.
16. Dubyak GR. Knock-out mice reveal tissue-specific roles of P2Y receptor subtypes in different epithelia. *Mol Pharmacol* 2003;63:773–776.
17. Hourani SMO, Hall DA. Receptors for ADP on human platelets. *Trends Pharmacol Sci* 1994;15:103–108.
18. Born GVR. Aggregation of blood platelets by adenosine diphosphate and its reversal. *Nature (London)* 1962;194:927–929.
19. Macfarlane DE. Agonists and receptors: adenosine diphosphate. In: Holmsen H, ed. *Platelet responses and metabolism, Vol II: receptors and metabolism.* Boca Raton, FL: CRC Press, 1987:19–36.
20. Mustard JF, Perry DW, Kinlough-Rathbone RL, et al. Factors responsible for ADP induced release reaction of human platelets. *Am J Physiol* 1975; 228:1857–1865.
21. Macfarlane DE, Gardner S, Lipson C, et al. Malondialdehyde production by platelets during secondary aggregation. *Thromb Haemost* 1977;38: 1002–1009.
22. Packham MA, Bryant NL, Guccione MA, et al. Effect of concentration of Ca+2 in the suspending medium on the responses of human and rabbit platelets to aggregating agents. *Thromb Haemost* 1989;62:968–976.
23. Pengo V, Boschello A, Marzari A, et al. Adenosine diphosphate (ADP)-induced α-granules release from platelets of native whole blood is reduced by ticlopidine but not by aspirin or dipyridamole. *Thromb Haemost* 1986;56:147–150.
24. Rinder CS, Student LA, Bonan JL, et al. Aspirin does not inhibit adenosine diphosphate-induced platelet alpha-granule release. *Blood* 1993;82: 505–512.
25. Mills DCB. ADP receptor in platelets. *Thromb Haemost* 1996;76:835–856.
26. Quinton TM, Murugappan S, Kim S, et al. Different G protein-coupled signaling pathways involved in alpha granule release from human platelets. *J Thromb Haemost* 2004;2(6):978–984.
27. Rand ML, Perry DW, Packham MA, et al. Conditions influencing release of granule contents from human platelets in citrated plasma induced by ADP or the thrombin receptor activating peptide SFLLRN: direct measurement of percent release of b-thromboglobulin and assessment by flow cytometry of P-selectin expression. *Am J Hematol* 1996;52:288–294.
28. Kaplan KL, Broekman MJ, Chernoff A, et al. Platelet alpha-granule proteins: studies on release and subcellular localization. *Blood* 1979;53: 604–618.
29. Gachet C, Hechler B, Leon C, et al. Activation of ADP receptors and platelet function. *Thromb Haemost* 1997;77:271–275.
30. Cooper DMF, Rodbell M. ADP is a potent inhibitor of human platelet plasma membrane adenylate cyclase. *Nature* 1979;282:517–518.
31. Ohlmann P, Laugwitz KL, Nuernberg B, et al. The human platelet ADP receptor activates $G_{i2}$ proteins. *Biochem J* 1995;312:775–779.
32. Sage SO, Rink T. Kinetic differences between thrombin-induced and ADP-induced calcium influx and release from internal stores in fura-2-loaded human platelets. *Biochem Biophys Res Commun* 1986;136:1124–1129.
33. MacKenzie AB, Mahaut-Smith MP, Sage SO. Activation of receptor-operated cation channels via $P_{2X1}$ not $P_{2T}$ purinoceptors in human platelets. *J Biol Chem* 1996;271:2879–2881.
34. Daniel JL, Dangelmaier C, Jin J, et al. Molecular basis for ADP-induced platelet activation I: evidence for three distinct ADP receptors on platelets. *J Biol Chem* 1998;273:2024–2029.
35. Hallam TJ, Rink TJ. Response to adenosine diphosphate in human platelets loaded with the fluorescent calcium indicator quin 2. *J Physiol* 1985;368:131–146.
36. Humphries RG, Tomlinson W, Ingall AH, et al. FPL 66096: a novel, highly potent and selective antagonist at human platelet P2T-purinoceptors. *Br J Pharmacol* 1994;113:1057–1063.
37. Humphries RG, Tomlinson W, Clegg JA, et al. Pharmacological profile of the novel $P_{2T}$-purinergic receptor antagonist, FPL 67085 *in vitro* and in the anaesthetized rat *in vivo*. *Br J Pharmacol* 1995;115:1110–1116.
38. Humphries RG, Robertson MJ, Leff P. A novel series of $P_{2T}$ purinoceptor antagonists: definition of the role of ADP in arterial thrombosis. *Trends Pharmacol Sci* 1995;16:179–181.
39. Herbert JM, Frehel D, Vallee E, et al. Clopidogrel, a novel antiplatelet and antithrombotic agent. *Cardiovasc Drug Rev* 1993;11:180–198.
40. Gachet C, Cazenave J-P, Ohlmann P, et al. The thienopyridine ticlopidine selectively prevents the inhibitory effects of ADP but not of adrenaline on cAMP levels raised by stimulation of the adenylate cyclase of human platelets by $PGE_1$. *Biochem Pharmacol* 1990;40:2683–2687.
41. Gachet C, Stierle A, Cazenave J-P, et al. The thienopyridine PCR 4099 selectively inhibits ADP-induced platelet aggregation and fibrinogen binding without modifying the membrane glycoprotein IIb-IIIa complex in rat and in man. *Biochem Pharmacol* 1990;40:229–238.
42. Mills DCB, Puri RN, Hu C-J, et al. Clopidogrel inhibits the binding of ADP analogues to the receptor mediating inhibition of platelet adenylate cyclase. *Atheroscler Thromb* 1992;12:430–436.
43. Committee CS. A randomised, blinded, trial of clopidogrel versus aspirin in patients at risk of ischaemic events (CAPRIE). *Lancet* 1996;348: 1329–1339.
44. Greco NJ, Yamamoto N, Jackson BW, et al. Identification of a nucleotide-binding site on glycoprotein IIb. relationship to platelet activation. *J Biol Chem* 1991;266:13627–13633.
45. Agarwal AK, Tandon NN, Greco NJ, et al. Evaluation of the binding to fixed platelets of agonists and antagonists of ADP-induced platelet aggregation. *Thromb Haemost* 1989;62:1103–1106.
46. Greco NJ, Tandon NN, Jackson BW, et al. Low structural specificity for nucleoside triphosphates as antagonists of ADP-induced platelet activation. *J Biol Chem* 1992;267:2966–2970.
47. Mills DCB. Factors influencing the adenylate cyclase system in blood platelets. In: Sherry S, Scriabine A, eds. *Platelets and Thrombosis.* Baltimore, MD: University Park Press, 1974:45–67.

48. Powling MJ, Hardisty RM. Glycoprotein IIb-IIIa complex and Ca²⁺ influx into stimulated platelets. *Blood* 1985;66:731–734.

49. Mayinger P, Gawaz M. Photoaffinity labeling of integrin αIIβ₃ (glycoprotein IIb-IIIa) on intact platelets with 8-azido-[γ³²P]ATP. *Biochim Biophys Acta* 1992;1137:77–81.

50. Bennett JS, Colman RF, Colman RW. Identification of adenine nucleotide binding proteins in human platelet membranes by affinity labelling with 5-p-fluorosulfonylbenzoyl adenosine. *J Biol Chem* 1978;253:7346–7354.

51. Figures WR, Scearce L, Wachtfogel Y, et al. Platelet ADP receptor and α2-adrenoceptor interaction. evidence for an ADP requirement for epinephrine-induced platelet activation and an influence of epinephrine on ADP binding. *J Biol Chem* 1986;261:5981–5986.

52. Colman RW. Aggregin: a platelet ADP receptor that mediates aggregation. *FASEB J* 1990;3:1425–1435.

53. Mills DCB, Figures WR, Scearce LM, et al. Two mechanisms for inhibition of ADP-induced platelet shape change by 5′-p-fluorosulfonylbenzoyl adenosine: conversion to adenosine and covalent modification at an ADP binding site distinct from that which inhibits adenylate cyclase. *J Biol Chem* 1985;260:8078–8083.

54. Rao AK, Kowalska MA. ADP-induced platelet shape change and mobilization of cytoplasmic ionized calcium are mediated by distinct binding sites on platelets: 5′-p-fluorosulfonylbenzoyladenosine is a weak platelet agonist. *Blood* 1987;70:751–756.

55. Puri RN, Kumar A, Chen H, et al. Inhibition of ADP-induced platelet responses by covalent modification of aggregin, a putative ADP receptor, by 8-(4-bromo-2,3-dioxobutylthio)ADP. *J Biol Chem* 1995;270:24482–24488.

56. Puri RN, Colman RF, Colman RW. Platelet activation by 2-(4-bromo-2,3-dioxobutylthio)adenosine 5′diphosphate is mediated by its binding to a putative ADP receptor, aggregin. *Eur J Biochem* 1996;236:862–870.

57. Puri RN, Colman RW. Inhibition of ADP-induced platelet activation by 7-chloro-4-nitrobenz-2-oxa-1,3-diazole: covalent modification of aggregin, a putative ADP receptor. *J Cell Biochem* 1996;61:97–108.

58. Puri RN, Colman RW. ADP-induced platelet activation. *Crit Rev Biochem Mol Biol* 1997;3:437–502.

59. Jin J, Daniel JL, Kunapuli SP. Molecular basis for ADP-induced platelet activation II: The P2Y1 receptor mediates ADP-induced intracellular calcium mobilization and shape change in platelets. *J Biol Chem* 1998;273:2030–2034.

60. Takasaki J, Kamohara M, Saito T, et al. Molecular cloning of the platelet P2T(AC) ADP receptor: pharmacological comparison with another ADP receptor, the P2Y(1) receptor. *Mol Pharmacol* 2001;60:432–439.

61. Savi P, Labouret C, Delesque N, et al. P2y(12), a new platelet ADP receptor, target of clopidogrel. *Biochem Biophys Res Commun* 2001;283:379–383.

62. Zhang FL, Luo L, Gustafson E, et al. ADP is the cognate ligand for the orphan G-protein coupled receptor SP1999. *J Biol Chem* 2001;276:8608–8615.

63. Hollopeter J, Jantzen H-M, Vincent D, et al. Identification of the platelet ADP receptor targeted by antithrombotic drugs. *Nature* 2001;409:202–207.

64. Fabre JE, Nguyen M, Latour A, et al. Decreased platelet aggregation, increased bleeding time and resistance to thromboembolism in P2Y1-deficient mice. *Nat Med* 1999;5:1199–1202.

65. Leon C, Hechler B, Freund M, et al. Defective platelet aggregation and increased resistance to thrombosis in purinergic P2Y(1) receptor-null mice [see comments]. *J Clin Invest* 1999;104:1731–1737.

66. Foster CJ, Prosser DM, Agans JM, et al. Molecular identification and characterization of the platelet ADP receptor targeted by thienopyridine antithrombotic drugs. *J Clin Invest* 2001;107:1591–1598.

67. Vial C, Hechler B, Leon C, et al. Presence of P2X1 purinoceptors in human platelets and megakaryoblastic cell lines. *Thromb Haemost* 1997;78:1500–1504.

68. Scase TJ, Heath MF, Allen JM, et al. Identification of a P2X1 purinoceptor expressed on human platelets. *Biochem Biophys Res Commun* 1998;242:525–528.

69. Sun B, Li J, Okahara K, et al. P2X1 purinoceptor in human platelets. molecular cloning and functional characterization after heterologous expression. *J Biol Chem* 1998;273:11544–11547.

70. MacKenzie AB, Mahaut-Smith MP, Sage SO. Activation of receptor-operated cation channels via P2X1 not P2T purinoceptors in human platelets. *J Biol Chem* 1996;271:2879–2881.

71. Mahaut-Smith MP, Ennion SJ, Rolf MG, et al. ADP is not an agonist at P2X(1) receptors: evidence for separate receptors stimulated by ATP and ADP on human platelets. *Br J Pharmacol* 2000;131:108–114.

72. Oury C, Toth-Zsamboki E, Thys C, et al. The ATP-gated P2X1 ion channel acts as a positive regulator of platelet responses to collagen. *Thromb Haemost* 2001;86:1264–1271.

73. Takano S, Kimura J, Matsuoka I, et al. No requirement of P2X1 purinoceptors for platelet aggregation. *Eur J Pharmacol* 1999;372:305–309.

74. Rolf MG, Brearley CA, Mahaut-Smith MP. Platelet shape change evoked by selective activation of P2X1 purinoceptors with alpha, beta-methylene ATP. *Thromb Haemost* 2001;85:303–308.

75. Oury C, Toth-Zsamboki E, Vermylen J, et al. P2X(1)-mediated activation of extracellular signal-regulated kinase 2 contributes to platelet secretion and aggregation induced by collagen. *Blood* 2002;100:2499–2505.

76. Vial C, Rolf MG, Mahaut-Smith MP, et al. A study of P2X1 receptor function in murine megakaryocytes and human platelets reveals synergy with P2Y receptors. *Br J Pharmacol* 2002;135:363–372.

77. Rolf MG, Mahaut-Smith MP. Effects of enhanced P2X1 receptor Ca2+ influx on functional responses in human platelets. *Thromb Haemost* 2002;88:495–502.

78. Mulryan K, Gitterman DP, Lewis CJ, et al. Reduced vas deferens contraction and male infertility in mice lacking P2X1 receptors. *Nature* 2000;403:86–89.

79. Oury C, Kuijpers MJ, Toth-Zsamboki E, et al. Overexpression of the platelet P2X1 ion channel in transgenic mice generates a novel prothrombotic phenotype. *Blood* 2003;101:3969–3976.

80. Hechler B, Lenain N, Marchese P, et al. A role of the fast ATP-gated P2X1 cation channel in thrombosis of small arteries *in vivo*. *J Exp Med* 2003;198:661–667.

81. Ayyanathan K, Webb TE, Sandhu AK, et al. Cloning and chromosomal localization of human P2Y1 purinoceptor. *Biochem Biophys Res Commun* 1996;218:783–788.

82. Leon C, Vial C, Cazenave JP, et al. Cloning and sequencing of a human cdna encoding endothelial P2y(1) purinoceptor. *Gene* 1996;171:295–297.

83. Ayyanathan K, Naylor SL, Kunapuli SP. Structural characterization and fine chromosomal mapping of the human P2Y1 purinergic receptor gene (P2YR1). *Somat Cell Mol Genet* 1996;22:419–424.

84. Schachter JB, Li Q, Boyer JL, et al. Second messenger cascade specificity and pharmacological selectivity of the human P2y1-purinoceptor. *Br J Pharmacol* 1996;118:167–173.

85. Webb TE, Simon J, Krishek BJ, et al. Cloning and functional expression of a brain G-protein-coupled ATP receptor. *FEBS Lett* 1993;324:219–225.

86. Barnard EA, Simon J, Webb TE. Nucleotide receptors in the nervous system – an abundant component using diverse transduction mechanisms [Review]. *Mol Neurobiol* 1997;15:103–129.

87. Leon C, Hechler B, Vial C, et al. The P2Y(1) receptor is an ADP receptor antagonized by ATP and expressed in platelets and megakaryoblastic cells. *FEBS Lett* 1997;403:26–30.

88. Offermanns S, Toombs CF, Hu Y-H, et al. Defective platelet activation in G times q-deficient mice. *Nature* 1997;389:183–186.

89. Cusack NJ, Hourani SMO. Adenosine diphosphate antagonists and human platelets: no evidence that aggregation and inhibition of adenylate cyclase are mediated by different receptors. *Br J Pharmacol* 1982;76:221–227.

90. Boyer JL, Romeroavila T, Schachter JB, et al. Identification of competitive antagonists of the P2y(1) receptor. *Mol Pharmacol* 1996;50:1323–1329.

91. Boyer JL, Mohanram A, Camaioni E, et al. Competitive and selective antagonism of P2Y1 receptors by N6-methyl 2′-deoxyadenosine 3′,5′-bisphosphate. *Br J Pharmacol* 1998;124:1–3.

92. Eckly A, Gendrault JL, Hechler B, et al. Differential involvement of the P2Y1 and P2YT receptors in the morphological changes of platelet aggregation. *Thromb Haemost* 2001;85:694–701.

93. Hourani SMO, Cusack NJ. Pharmacological receptors on blood platelets. *Pharmacol Rev* 1991;43:243–298.

94. Lanza F, Stierle A, Gachet C, et al. Differential effects of extra-and intracellular calcium chelation on human platelet function and glycoprotein IIb-IIIa complex stability. *Nouv Rev Fr Hematol* 1992;34:123–131.

95. Steen VM, Holmsen H, Aarbakke G. The platelet-stimulating effect of adenaline through a 2-adrenergic receptors requires simultaneous activation by a true stimulatory platelet agonist. Evidence that adrenaline per se does not induce human platelet activation *in vitro*. *Thromb Haemost* 1993;70:506–513.

96. Savi P, Laplace MC, Herbert J-M. Evidence for the existence of two different ADP-binding sites on rat platelets. *Thromb Res* 1994;76:157–169.

97. Paul BZ, Kim S, Dangelmaier C, et al. Dynamic regulation of microtubule coils in ADP-induced platelet shape change by p160ROCK (Rho-kinase). *Platelets* 2003;14:159–169.

98. Paul BZ, Daniel JL, Kunapuli SP. Platelet shape change is mediated by both calcium-dependent and – independent signaling pathways. Role of p160 rho-associated coiled-coil-containing protein kinase in platelet shape change. *J Biol Chem* 1999;274:28293–28300.

99. Nemoto Y, Namba T, Teru-uchi T, et al. A rho gene product in human blood platelets. I. Identification of the platelet substrate for botulinum C3 ADP-ribosyltransferase as rhoA protein. *J Biol Chem* 1992;267:20916–20920.

100. Jin J, Daniel JL, Kunapuli SP. Molecular basis for ADP-induced platelet activation. II. The P2Y1 receptor mediates ADP-induced intracellular calcium mobilization and shape change in platelets. *J Biol Chem* 1998;273:2030–2034.

101. Jin J, Kunapuli SP. Coactivation of two different G protein-coupled receptors is essential for ADP-induced platelet aggregation. *Proc Natl Acad Sci U S A* 1998;95:8070–8074.

102. Jin J, Quinton TM, Zhang J, et al. Adenosine diphosphate (ADP)-induced thromboxane A(2) generation in human platelets requires coordinated signaling through integrin alpha(IIb)beta(3) and ADP receptors. *Blood* 2002;99:193–198.

103. Dangelmaier C, Jin J, Daniel JL, et al. The P2Y1 receptor mediates ADP-induced p38 kinase-activating factor generation in human platelets. *Eur J Biochem* 2000;267:2283–2289.

104. Remijn JA, Wu YP, Jeninga EH, et al. Role of ADP receptor P2Y(12) in platelet adhesion and thrombus formation in flowing blood. *Arterioscler Thromb Vasc Biol* 2002;22:686–691.

105. Turner NA, Moake JL, McIntire LV. Blockade of adenosine diphosphate receptors P2Y(12) and P2Y(1) is required to inhibit platelet aggregation in whole blood under flow. *Blood* 2001;98:3340–3345.

106. Fabre JE, Nguyen M, Latour A, et al. Decreased platelet aggregation, increased bleeding time and resistance to thromboembolism in P2Y1-deficient mice. *Nat Med* 1999;5:1199–1202.

107. Leon C, Freund M, Ravanat C, et al. Key role of the P2Y(1) receptor in tissue factor-induced thrombin- dependent acute thromboembolism: studies in P2Y(1)-knockout mice and mice treated with a P2Y(1) antagonist. *Circulation* 2001;103:718–723.

108. Hechler B, Zhang Y, Eckly A, et al. Lineage-specific overexpression of the P2Y1 receptor induces platelet hyper-reactivity in transgenic mice. *J Thromb Haemost* 2003;1:155–163.

109. Baurand A, Gachet C. The P2Y(1) receptor as a target for new antithrombotic drugs: a review of the P2Y(1) antagonist MRS-2179. *Cardiovasc Drug Rev* 2003;21:67–76.

110. Defreyn G, Gachet G, Savi P, et al. Ticlopidine and clopidogrel (SR25990C) selectively neutralize ADP inhibition of $PGE_1$-activated platelet adenylate cyclase in rats and rabbits. *Thromb Haemost* 1991;65:186–190.

111. Savi P, Herbert JM, Pflieger AM, et al. Importance of hepatic metabolism in the antiaggregating activity of the thienopyridine clopidogrel. *Biochem Pharmacol* 1992;44:527–532.

112. Savi P, Pereillo JM, Uzabiaga MF, et al. Identification and biological activity of the active metabolite of clopidogrel. *Thromb Haemost* 2000;84:891–896.

113. Ding Z, Kim S, Dorsam RT, et al. Inactivation of the human P2Y12 receptor by thiol reagents requires interaction with both extracellular cysteine residues, Cys17 and Cys270. *Blood* 2003;101:3908–3914.

114. Cattaneo M, Zighetti ML, Lombardi R, et al. Molecular bases of defective signal transduction in the platelet P2Y12 receptor of a patient with congenital bleeding. *Proc Natl Acad Sci U S A* 2003;100:1978–1983.

115. Hollopeter G, Jantzen HM, Vincent D, et al. Identification of the platelet ADP receptor targeted by antithrombotic drugs. *Nature* 2001;409:202–207.

116. Cristalli G, Mills DCB. Identification of a receptor for ADP on blood platelets by photoaffinity labelling. *Biochem J* 1993;291:875–881.

117. Macfarlane DE, Mills DCB. The effects of ATP on platelets: evidence against the central role of ADP in primary aggregation. *Blood* 1975;46:309–320.

118. Bennett JS. Novel platelet inhibitors. *Annu Rev Med* 2001;52:161–184.

119. Sugidachi A, Asai F, Yoneda K, et al. Antiplatelet action of R-99224, an active metabolite of a novel thienopyridine-type G(i)-linked P2T antagonist, CS-747. *Br J Pharmacol* 2001;132:47–54.

120. Bennett CL, Connors JM, Carwile JM, et al. Thrombotic thrombocytopenic purpura associated with clopidogrel. *N Engl J Med* 2000;342:1773–1777.

121. Jin J, Kunapuli SP. Co-activation of two different G protein-coupled receptors is essential for ADP-induced platelet aggregation. *Proc Natl Acad Sci U S A* 1998;95:8070–8074.

122. Dangelmaier C, Jin J, Smith JB, et al. Potentiation of thromboxane A2-induced platelet secretion by gi signaling through the phosphoinositide-3 kinase pathway. *Thromb Haemost* 2001;85:341–348.

123. Dorsam RT, Tuluc M, Kunapuli SP. Role of protease-activated and ADP receptor subtypes in thrombin generation on human platelets. *J Thromb Haemost* 2004;2:804–812.

124. Jantzen HM, Milstone DS, Gousset L, et al. Impaired activation of murine platelets lacking Galpha(i2). *J Clin Invest* 2001;108:477–483.

125. Quinton TM, Kim S, Dangelmaier C, et al. PKC-regulated and calcium-regulated pathways independently synergize with Gi pathways in agonist-induced fibrinogen receptor activation. *Biochem J* 2002;368:535–543.

126. Quinton TM, Ozdener F, Dangelmaier C, et al. Glycoprotein VI-mediated platelet fibrinogen receptor activation occurs through calcium-sensitive and PKC-sensitive pathways without a requirement for secreted ADP. *Blood* 2002;99:3228–3234.

127. Nieswandt B, Schulte V, Zywietz A, et al. Costimulation of gi-and G12/G13-mediated signaling pathways induces integrin alpha IIbbeta 3 activation in platelets. *J Biol Chem* 2002;277:39493–39498.

128. Dorsam RT, Kim S, Jin J, et al. Coordinated signaling through both G12/13 and G(i) pathways is sufficient to activate GPIIb/IIIa in human platelets. *J Biol Chem* 2002;277:47588–47595.

129. Dorsam RT, Kim S, Murugappan S, et al. Interplay of gi and gz signaling causes src family kinase-dependent GPIIb/IIIa activation and thromboxane A2 production in human platelets. 45th Annual American Society of Hematology, San Diego, CA, Blood; 2003:271.

130. Yang J, Wu J, Jiang H, et al. Signaling through gi family members in platelets. Redundancy and specificity in the regulation of adenylyl cyclase and other effectors. *J Biol Chem* 2002;277:46035–46042.

131. Abrams CS, Zhang J, Downes CP, et al. Phosphopleckstrin inhibits gbetagamma-activable platelet phosphatidylinositol-4,5-bisphosphate 3-kinase. *J Biol Chem* 1996;271:25192–25197.

132. Hirsch E, Bosco O, Tropel P, et al. Resistance to thromboembolism in PI3Kgamma-deficient mice. *FASEB J* 2001;15:2019–2021.

133. Kauffenstein G, Bergmeier W, Eckly A, et al. The P2Y(12) receptor induces platelet aggregation through weak activation of the alpha(IIb)beta(3) integrin—a phosphoinositide 3-kinase-dependent mechanism. *FEBS Lett* 2001;505:281–290.

134. Kim S, Jin J, Kunapuli SP. Akt activation in platelets depends on gi signaling pathways. *J Biol Chem* 2004;279:4186–4195.

135. Larson MK, Chen H, Kahn ML, et al. Critical role for the ADP receptor, P2Y12, in GPVI-mediated activation of RAP1b in platelets. *Blood* 2001;98;Abstract #3129.

136. Woulfe D, Jiang H, Mortensen R, et al. Activation of rap1B by G(i) family members in platelets. *J Biol Chem* 2002;277:23382–23390.

137. Bertoni A, Tadokoro S, Eto K, et al. Relationships between rap1b, affinity modulation of integrin alpha IIbbeta 3, and the actin cytoskeleton. *J Biol Chem* 2002;277:25715–25721.

138. Chrzanowska-Wodnicka M, Schoenwaelder S, White GC. II Rap1b regulates integrin IIb3 activity and platelet function - lessons from a knockout. Session type. *Blood* 2003;102.

139. Woulfe D, Jiang H, Morgans A, et al. Defects in secretion, aggregation, and thrombus formation in platelets from mice lacking akt2. *J Clin Invest* 2004;113:441–450.

140. Shankar H, Murugappan S, Kim S, et al. Role of G protein-gated inwardly-rectifying potassium channels in P2Y12 receptor-mediated platelet functional responses. *Blood* 2004;104(5)1335–1343.

141. Mitka M. Results of CURE trial for acute coronary syndrome. *JAMA* 2001;285:1828–1829.

142. Hacke W. From CURE to MATCH: ADP receptor antagonists as the treatment of choice for high-risk atherothrombotic patients. *Cerebrovasc Dis* 2002;13:22–26.

143. Andre P, LaRocca T, Delaney SM, et al. Anticoagulants (thrombin inhibitors) and aspirin synergize with P2Y12 receptor antagonism in thrombosis. *Circulation* 2003;108:2697–2703.

144. Andre P, Delaney SM, LaRocca T, et al. P2Y12 regulates platelet adhesion/activation, thrombus growth, and thrombus stability in injured arteries. *J Clin Invest* 2003;112:398–406.

145. van Gestel MA, Heemskerk JW, Slaaf DW, et al. *In vivo* blockade of platelet ADP receptor P2Y12 reduces embolus and thrombus formation but not thrombus stability. *Arterioscler Thromb Vasc Biol* 2003;23:518–523.

# CHAPTER 33 ■ PROTEASE-ACTIVATED RECEPTORS IN HEMOSTASIS, THROMBOSIS, AND VASCULAR BIOLOGY

SHAUN R. COUGHLIN, ERIC CAMERER, AND JUSTIN R. HAMILTON

In addition to cleaving soluble protein substrates, thrombin triggers a host of responses in platelets, endothelial cells, and other cells. This presents an intriguing question. How does thrombin, a protease, regulate the behavior of cells like a traditional hormone? Because of the central role played by thrombin and platelets in myocardial infarction and stroke, an understanding of thrombin signaling in platelets should suggest new strategies for the development of pharmaceuticals to prevent and to treat these and other thrombotic events. In addition, an understanding of thrombin signaling in other cell types should allow exploration of roles for coagulation beyond hemostasis and thrombosis.

Protease-activated receptors (PARs) provide an answer to the question of how thrombin signals. PARs are G protein–coupled receptors that utilize an intriguing mechanism to convert an extracellular proteolytic cleavage event into a transmembrane signal. As detailed in subsequent text, these receptors carry their own ligands, which remain silent until activated by receptor cleavage.

This chapter focuses on PAR activation by thrombin and on the roles of this system *in vivo*, with emphasis on platelets, hemostasis, and thrombosis. Recent advances in our understanding of PARs provide a working model for thrombin signaling in human platelets, and studies in mouse and primate models suggest that thrombin signaling in platelets is indeed important for hemostasis and thrombosis *in vivo*. Studies of PAR signaling in endothelial cells also evoke hypotheses about the roles of PARs in inflammation that can be tested in principle with knockout mouse models. Last, it is important to point out that PARs can mediate signaling to proteases other than thrombin and likely serve signaling functions in contexts outside of tissue injury. These issues are touched upon briefly.

Because PARs have been most intensely studied in the context of an effort to understand thrombin signaling, it is useful to consider when and where thrombin is generated as well as its known actions on cells.

## THROMBIN GENERATION

Thrombin is the main effector protease of the coagulation cascade—a series of zymogen conversions triggered when circulating coagulation factors contact tissue factor. Tissue factor, a type-I integral membrane protein, is an obligate cofactor for activation of zymogen factor X by factor VIIa. Factor Xa (with the assistance of cofactor factor Va) then converts zymogen prothrombin to active thrombin. Other zymogen conversions provide both amplification and negative feedback loops that regulate thrombin production. Importantly, thrombin generation occurs on the surface of cells, particularly on platelets, a situation that may favor thrombin's interaction with PARs nearby. Thrombin is short-lived in the circulation, and, in the context of a normal endothelium, thrombin acts to terminate its own production. Therefore, thrombin is thought to act near the site of its production (1).

Epithelial cells, macrophages, and other cell types that are normally segregated from blood constitutively express tissue factor (2). Classically, disruption of vascular integrity permits plasma coagulation factors to contact such extravascular tissue factor, thereby triggering thrombin generation. Circulating monocytes and vascular endothelial cells—cells that are normally bathed in coagulation factors—can be induced to express low levels of tissue factor by cytokines and other stimuli (3,4). Tethering of tissue factor–bearing monocytes and microparticles by activated platelets and endothelial cells may also recruit and concentrate tissue factor at sites of vascular injury, thereby contributing to activation of the coagulation cascade (5,6). The relative importance of circulating versus extravascular tissue factor for activation of coagulation in various settings remains to be determined. Regardless, both mechanisms link tissue injury and/or inflammation to the generation of coagulation proteases. Taken together, these considerations cast thrombin as a local mediator of responses to vascular injury or inflammation and suggest that thrombin's actions on cells should be considered in this context.

## CELLULAR RESPONSES TO THROMBIN

Thrombin has a host of direct actions on cells (7) (see Fig. 33-1). It is perhaps the most effective activator of platelets *ex vivo* (8). Thrombin provokes platelet shape change and release of the contents of platelet granules that contain adenosine 5'-diphosphate (ADP) and serotonin as well as chemokines and growth factors (9). Thrombin also triggers synthesis and release of thromboxane $A_2$ (10), mobilization of P selectin and CD40 ligand to the platelet surface (11,12), and activation of the integrin $\alpha_{IIb}/\beta_3$ (13). The latter binds fibrinogen and von Willebrand Factor (VWF) to mediate platelet aggregation (14). Thrombin causes expression of procoagulant activity on the platelet surface, which supports additional thrombin generation (15). In cultured endothelial cells, thrombin causes release of VWF (16), display of P selectin on the plasma membrane (16), and production of chemokines—actions that trigger binding of platelets and leukocytes to the endothelial surface *in vivo* (17,18). Endothelial cells change shape, and endothelial monolayers show increased permeability in response to thrombin (19) to promote local transudation of plasma proteins and edema (20). Thrombin can also regulate blood vessel diameter by endothelial-dependent vasodilatation (21–23); in

555

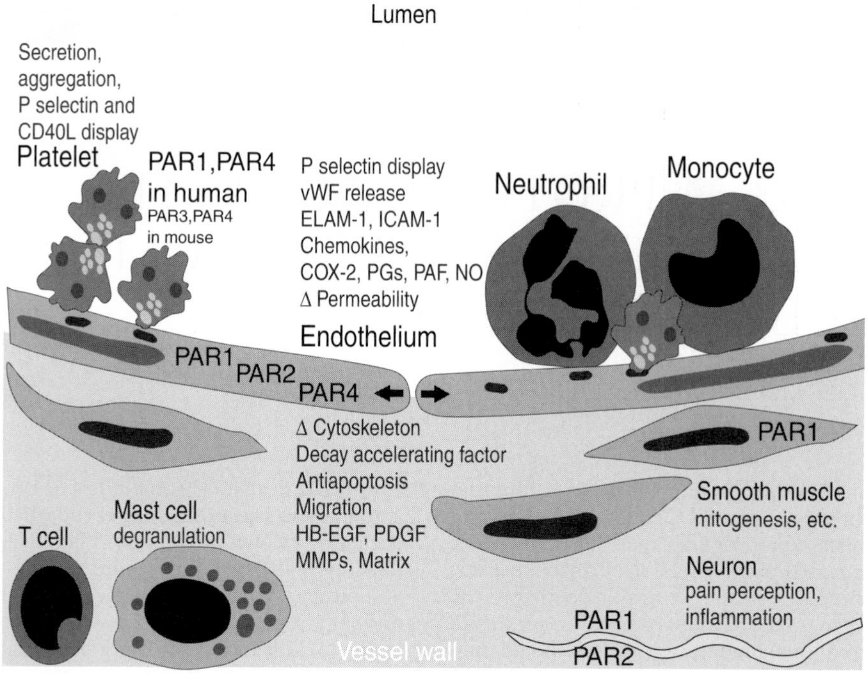

**FIGURE 33-1.** Thrombin's actions in the context of a blood vessel. Thrombin is a multifunctional serine protease generated at sites of vascular injury. It is arguably the most effective agonist for platelet activation. Thrombin also elicits a host of responses in the vascular endothelium, including shape and permeability changes, mobilization of adhesive molecules to the endothelial surface, and stimulation of autocoid and cytokine production. Many of the genes induced in endothelial cells encode proteins that promote inflammation, but others may be involved in protection against apoptosis. The latter might be important to prepare endothelial cells for an inflammatory environment rich in proapoptotic cytokines. Thrombin is also mitogenic for lymphocytes and mesenchymal cells. These actions of thrombin help orchestrate hemostatic and inflammatory responses to tissue injury. Possible roles in blood vessel development can also be readily envisioned. PAR, protease-activated receptor; VWF, von Willerband factor; ELAM, endothelial-leukocyte adhesion molecule; ICAM-1, intercellular adhesion molecule-1; COX, cyclooxygenase; PG, prostaglandin; PAF, platelet activating factor; NO, Nitric oxide; HB-EGF, heparin-binding EGF-like growth factor; PDGF, platelet-derived growth factor; MMP, matrix metalloprotease. (From Coughlin SR. Thrombin signalling and protease-activated receptors. *Nature* 2000;40(6801): 258–264, with permission.)

the absence of endothelium, the action of thrombin on smooth muscle cells evokes vasoconstriction (24). In fibroblast and vascular smooth muscle cell cultures, thrombin regulates cytokine production and is mitogenic, and thrombin triggers calcium signaling and other responses in T lymphocytes. Especially when taken in the context of thrombin being generated at sites of vascular injury, these cellular actions suggest that thrombin signaling connects tissue damage to responses involved in both hemostasis and inflammation. These and other responses to thrombin (7,25) also raise the possibility that regulation of endothelial and other cells by thrombin might play a role in contexts other than tissue injury (e.g., in leukocyte transmigration, vascular remodeling, and/or angiogenesis). Characterization of receptors that mediate thrombin signaling has provided opportunities to test these ideas.

## HOW CAN A PROTEASE ACT LIKE A HORMONE?

As noted in the introduction, thrombin signaling is mediated, at least in part, by a small family of G protein–coupled PARs (26). PAR1, the prototype for this family, is activated when thrombin cleaves its *N*-terminal exodomain at a specific site (27,28). This cleavage event unmasks a new *N*-terminus that then serves as a tethered ligand, binding intramolecularly to the body of the receptor to effect transmembrane signaling (see Fig. 33-2) (27). Intermolecular ligation of PARs can occur

but, not surprisingly, appears to be less efficient than intramolecular ligation (29,30). A synthetic hexapeptide of the sequence SFLLRN, which mimics the PAR1 tethered ligand, can activate the receptor independent of protease and receptor cleavage (27,31,32). In addition to providing evidence in support of the tethered ligand mechanism, such peptides have provided convenient pharmacologic tools for probing the effects of PAR activation in cells and tissues (33).

The role of thrombin in PAR1 activation appears to be simply to unmask the receptor's tethered ligand (7,26). PAR1–thrombin interactions are accounted for by the sequences surrounding the thrombin cleavage site within PAR1's *N*-terminal exodomain, and cleavage at that site is both necessary and sufficient for PAR1 activation by protease (29,34,35,37–39). Indeed, PAR1 mutants bearing enteropeptidase or trypsin cleavage sites in place of the thrombin cleavage site caused enteropeptidase or trypsin signaling, respectively, in heterologous expression systems (34,40). Therefore, PAR1 can be viewed as a peptide receptor that carries its own ligand. The latter remains silent until activated by cleavage of the receptor's *N*-terminal exodomain.

Some details are known about how PAR1's proteolytic switch works, that is, how the tethered ligand is kept silent in the uncleaved receptors and made active by cleavage. Receptor cleavage at the R41–S42 bond both removes amino-terminal sequence that sterically hinders ligand function and generates a new protonated amino group at the new *N*-terminus created by receptor cleavage. In the SFLLRN peptide, the cognate

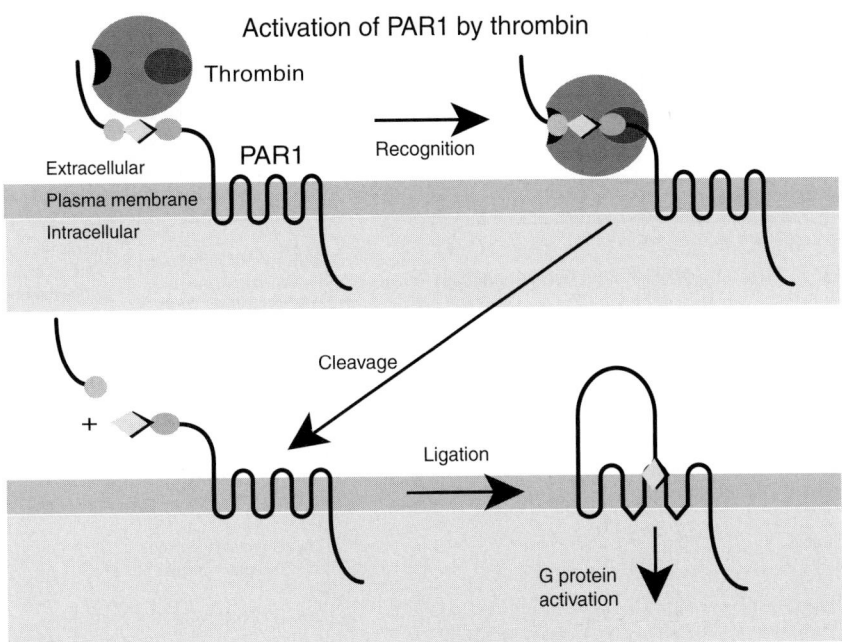

**FIGURE 33-2.** How a protease can act like a hormone: Mechanism of PAR1 activation. Thrombin (*large sphere*) recognizes the amino-terminal exodomain of the G protein–coupled thrombin receptor PAR1. This interaction utilizes sites both amino (P1–P4, *small sphere*) and the carboxyl terminal (P9′–P14′, *small oval*) of the thrombin cleavage site. The latter sequence resembles the carboxyl tail of the thrombin inhibitor hirudin and binds to thrombin's exosite 1 in an analogous manner (34–36). Thrombin severs the peptide bond between receptor residues Arg41 and Ser42. This cleavage event serves to unmask a new amino-terminus beginning with the sequence SFLLRN (*diamond*) that functions as a tethered ligand, docking intramolecularly to the body of the receptor to effect transmembrane signaling. A synthetic peptide having the sequence SFLLRN, which mimics the tethered ligand sequence, will function as an agonist for PAR1 independent of receptor cleavage. Therefore, PAR1 is, in essence, a peptide receptor that carries its own ligand, the latter being active only after receptor cleavage (27). PAR, protease-activated receptor. (From Coughlin SR. Thrombin signalling and protease-activated receptors. *Nature* 2000;407(6801):258–264, with permission.)

protonated amino group is critical for agonist activity (32,41). Parallels with zymogen activation in serine proteases are apparent (27,42). In conversion of trypsinogen to trypsin, the precise proteolytic cleavage generates a new amino-terminus that bears a new protonated amino group, which then docks intramolecularly to trap the protease in its active conformation (42).

The molecular details about how the exposed tethered ligand effects receptor activation remain unknown. Studies with receptor mutants and chimeras suggest that PAR1's extracellular loops and the exodomain just amino-terminal to the first transmembrane segment may interact to form a structure (43,44) that is an important determinant of the receptor's specificity for agonist peptides (45–48). Whether this structure serves as a kind of keyhole that determines access to a binding site within the heptahelical bundle or is by itself the site that binds the agonist and moves transmembrane domains so as to send information across the cell membrane remains to be determined.

Once ligated, PAR1 can bind and activate heterotrimeric G proteins of the G12/13, Gq, and Gi/z families and hence can activate a host of intracellular signaling pathways (see Fig. 33-3). Such pluripotent signaling fits well with the known effects of thrombin on platelets and on endothelial and other cells. For example, in mouse platelets, Gq is necessary for platelet secretion and aggregation in response to thrombin but is not necessary for thrombin-triggered shape change (49). G13 appears to contribute to platelet aggregation as well as shape change in response to low concentrations of thrombin but appears to be unnecessary at higher agonist concentrations; G12 appears to be dispensable for thrombin signaling in platelets (50). Gz, a Gi family member, is critical for epinephrine's ability to both

inhibit cAMP formation and increase the sensitivity of mouse platelets to be activated by other agonists (51). Therefore, PAR1 coupling to Gq, G13, and Gz may account for thrombin's remarkable efficacy as a platelet agonist.

# IRREVERSIBLE ACTIVATION AND DISPOSABLE RECEPTORS

The unusual mechanism by which PAR1 is activated raises important pharmacologic and cell biologic questions. Cleavage of the receptor is irreversible, and the "peptide agonist" that is unmasked by the cleavage remains tethered to the receptor. Given the irreversibility of the activation mechanism, how is PAR1 signaling terminated? Thrombin is an enzyme, implying that one thrombin molecule might cleave and activate several molecules of PAR1. If so, how does PAR1 mediate responses that depend on thrombin concentration? In addition, given the high effective local concentration of the tethered ligand, will it be possible to develop pharmaceuticals that block PAR1 signaling? There are hints of interesting answers (26).

Like other G protein–coupled receptors, PAR1 is rapidly uncoupled from signaling soon after activation and is then internalized by phosphorylation-dependent mechanisms (66–68). Interestingly, unlike the well-studied $\beta_2$-adrenergic receptor, PAR1 internalization appeared to be independent of $\beta$-arrestins (69). In addition, unlike $\beta_2$-adrenergic receptor, which recycles after internalization, internalized PAR1 is rapidly delivered to lysosomes and degraded (67,70–72). In addition to degradation in lysosomes, other mechanisms for terminating or regulating

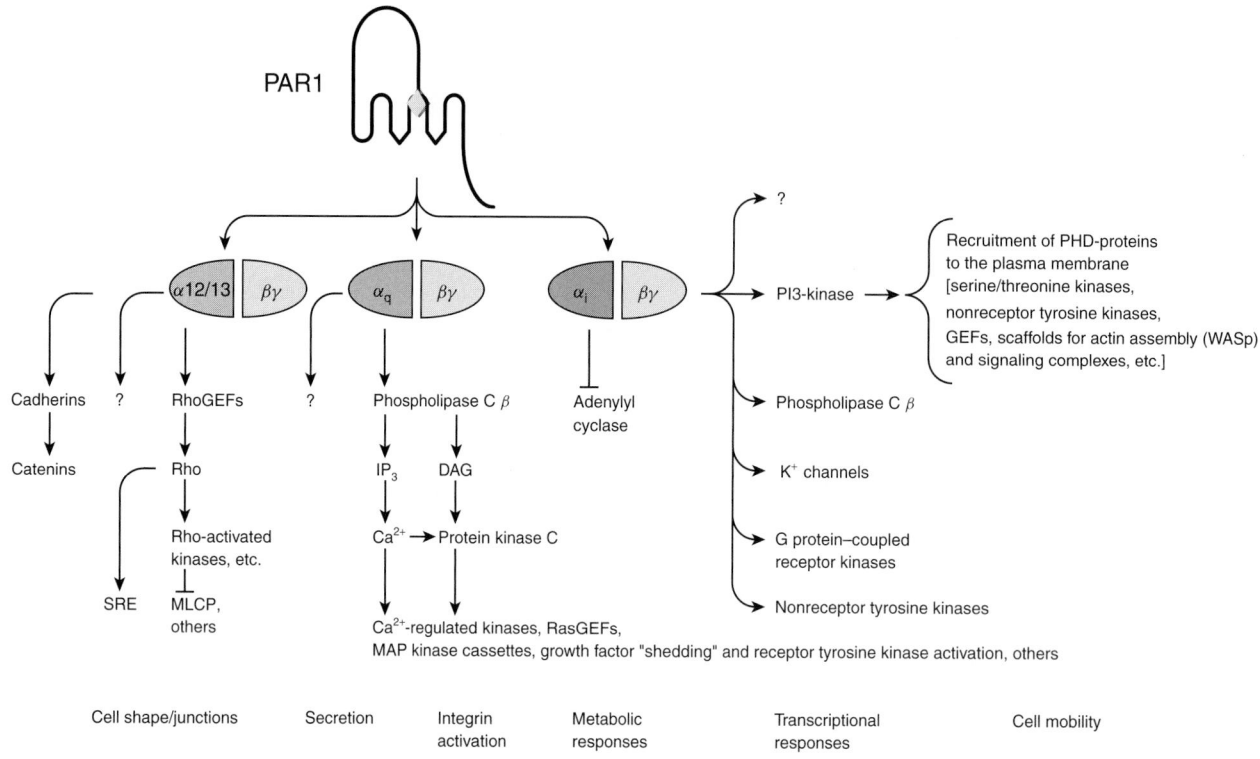

**FIGURE 33-3.** PAR1 signaling. PAR1 can couple to members of the G12/13, Gq, and Gi/z families (52–54) to impact a substantial network of signaling pathways. The α subunits of G12 and G13 bind RhoGEFs (guanine nucleotide exchange factors that activate small G proteins) (55–57), which in turn activate Rho and Rho-mediated cytoskeletal responses that may regulate shape in platelets (50,58) and permeability and migration in endothelial cells (59,60). Gα_q activates phospholipase CβI, thereby triggering phosphoinositide hydrolysis, calcium mobilization, and protein kinase C activation (61). This activation provides a path to calcium-regulated kinases and phosphatases, GEFs, MAP kinase cassettes, and other proteins that mediate cellular responses ranging from granule secretion, integrin activation, and aggregation in platelets (49) to transcriptional responses in endothelial and mesenchymal cells. Gα_i inhibits adenylyl cyclase, an action known to promote platelet responses. Gβγ subunits can activate phosphoinositide-3 kinase (62) and other lipid-modifying enzymes, protein kinases, and channels (63). Phosphoinositide-3 kinase modifies the inner leaflet of the plasma membrane to provide attachment sites for a host of signaling proteins (64). PAR1 activation can also activate cell surface "sheddases" that liberate ligands for receptor tyrosine kinases, providing a link between thrombin and receptor tyrosine kinases involved in cell growth and differentiation (65). The pleiotrophic effects of PAR1 activation are consistent with many of thrombin's diverse actions on cells. PAR, protease-activated receptor; GEF, guanine nucleotide exchange factor; WASp, Wiskott-Aldrich syndrome protein; IP3, inositol 1,4,5-trisphosphate; DAG, diacylglycerol; SRE, serum response element; MLC, myosin light chain phosphatase; MAP, mitogen-activating protein. [From Coughlin SR. Thrombin signalling and protease-activated receptors. *Nature* 2000;407(6801):258–264, with permission.]

PAR1 function seem to exist. Some PAR1 molecules that escape lysosomal degradation may return to the cell surface with the tethered ligand in an inactive state (40,73). Regulated metalloproteinase-dependent shedding of the PAR1 N-terminal exodomain has been recently described (74). Therefore, overall, PAR1 is used once and then discarded like other molecules that are activated by proteolytic mechanisms.

In fibroblasts and endothelial cells, responsiveness to thrombin is maintained by delivery of naive PAR1 to the cell surface from a preformed intracellular pool (70). By contrast, in human megakaryocytelike cell lines, recovery of PAR1 signaling requires synthesis of new protein (67,70). Perhaps, there is no need for a special resensitization mechanism in platelets. Once activated and incorporated into a clot, they are presumably not reused.

The rapid shutoff of activated PAR1 provides a plausible answer to how PAR1 mediates responses that are proportional to thrombin concentration (73). Each cleaved receptor is active for only a finite interval and, therefore, should elicit production of some average "unit" of second messenger (e.g., inositol trisphosphate) before shutting off. Because the second messenger is itself cleared, the level of second messenger achieved should be proportional to the rate at which receptors are cleaved and activated and hence to thrombin concentration.

Can an effective PAR1 inhibitor be developed? Antagonists that compete with the tethered ligand will likely need high affinity for PAR1 to effectively block ligand binding and receptor activation. However, because each activated PAR1 is rapidly shut off and because platelets in flowing blood or rolling on a nascent thrombus must presumably respond rapidly to contribute to a thrombus, it is conceivable that merely "slowing" thrombin receptor activation on platelets might have a therapeutic effect. Competitive antagonists structurally related to the PAR1-tethered ligand have been generated and have some use *in vivo* (see subsequent text) (75–78). In principle, noncompetitive antagonists may provide an alternative; the platelet ADP receptor blockers ticlopidine and clopidogrel provide an interesting precedent in this regard (79,80). Rationales for developing PAR1 antagonists as potential pharmaceuticals are discussed in subsequent text.

# A FAMILY OF PROTEASE-ACTIVATED RECEPTORS

Four PARs are known. Human PAR1 (27,28), PAR3 (81), and PAR4 (82,83) can be activated by thrombin. PAR2 can be activated by trypsin (84), tryptase (85), and coagulation factors VIIa and Xa (86–88) but not by thrombin. These receptors have a basic residue at P1 in the activating cleavage site, and, in principle, any protease capable of cleaving these sites can trigger PAR signaling. Therefore, it is certainly possible that these receptors mediate responses to other proteases *in vivo.* Moreover, cofactors that localize proteases to the cell surface and modulate their activity can help orchestrate PAR activation (87,89). Therefore, the full repertoire of proteases that signal through PARs remains to be defined.

Notably, the *N*-terminal exodomains of PAR1 and PAR3 have thrombin-interacting sequences *C*-terminal of the thrombin cleavage site (Fig. 33-2). In both cases, this sequence resembles the carboxyl tail of the leech anticoagulant hirudin and, like the latter, binds to the fibrinogen-binding exosite of thrombin; this interaction is important for receptor cleavage at low concentrations of thrombin (7,27,37,39,90,91). The presence of such extended thrombin-interacting sequences in PAR1 and PAR3 is consistent with the notion that these receptors evolved to mediate responses to thrombin versus other proteases. A hirudinlike sequence is not evident in PAR2 or PAR4. PAR2 cannot be cleaved by thrombin (92), and PAR4 requires higher thrombin concentrations for activation than PAR1 does (82,83).

# PROTEASE-ACTIVATED RECEPTORS AND PLATELET ACTIVATION

Available data provide a useful working model of thrombin signaling in human and mouse platelets at the receptor level and reveal both curious species differences and a variation on the paradigm for PAR activation (see Fig. 33-4). It is important to consider both species because general answers about the relative importance of PARs for thrombin signaling in platelets and for hemostasis and thrombosis *in vivo* can, at least in principle, be derived from studies of PAR knockout mice. The model casts PARs as necessary for activation of platelets by thrombin and frames important questions about the strategies for pharmaceutical development.

## Thrombin Receptors in Human Platelets

Human platelets express PAR1 and PAR4, and activation of either is sufficient to trigger platelet secretion and aggregation (27,82,83,93,94). Antibodies to the thrombin interaction site in PAR1 blocked receptor cleavage and platelet activation at low but not at high concentrations of thrombin (38,93,95). Similar results were obtained with a PAR1 antagonist (75,93). By contrast, PAR4-blocking antibodies by themselves had no effect on platelet activation by thrombin, but when these were combined with PAR1 blockade, platelet activation was markedly inhibited even at high concentrations of thrombin (93). These results suggest that PAR1 mediates activation of human platelets at low thrombin concentrations and that, in the absence of PAR1 function, PAR4 can mediate platelet activation but only at high thrombin concentrations (Fig. 33-4).

If PAR1 is sufficient to mediate platelet activation at low concentrations of thrombin, what does PAR4 contribute? It is possible that PAR4 simply provides some redundancy in an important system or that PAR1 and PAR4 interact. It is equally possible that PAR4, which lacks a thrombin-binding hirudin-like sequence, contributes responsiveness to proteases other than thrombin. In this regard, platelet activation by cathepsin G (96), a granzyme released by activated neutrophils, appears to be mediated by PAR4 (97); whether this phenomenon is important *in vivo* is unknown. An additional possibility is that qualitative differences in PAR1 versus PAR4 signaling make important contributions to platelet function. For example, PAR4 is activated and shutoff more slowly than PAR1, and the tempo of calcium signaling to thrombin in human platelets

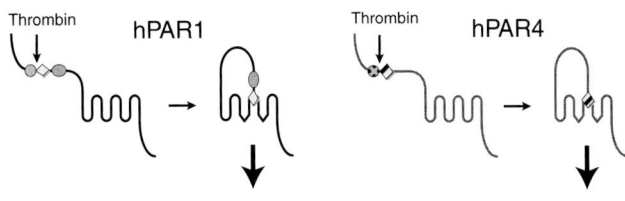

Thrombin signaling in human platelets

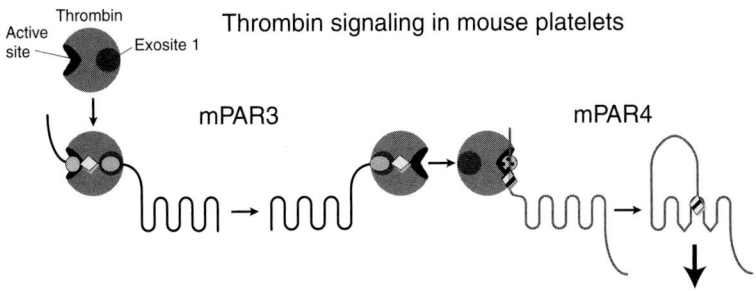

Thrombin signaling in mouse platelets

**FIGURE 33-4.** Thrombin receptors in human and mouse platelets. Human platelets express PAR1 and PAR4, and available data suggest that these receptors can independently mediate thrombin signaling—PAR1 is the main thrombin receptor and can mediate platelet activation by low concentrations of thrombin. In the absence of PAR1 function, PAR4 can trigger platelet activation but requires relatively high concentrations of thrombin to do so. In contrast, mouse platelets express PAR3 and PAR4, and, surprisingly, it appears that mouse PAR3, rather than mediating transmembrane signaling by itself, functions as a cofactor that supports cleavage and activation of PAR4 at low thrombin concentrations. As this model predicts, platelets from PAR3 knockout mice require more thrombin for activation than wild-type mice, and platelets from PAR4 knockout mice show no responses to even very high concentrations of thrombin. These mice provided an opportunity to assess the importance of thrombin signaling in hemostasis and thrombosis (see text). PAR, protease-activated receptor. [From Coughlin SR. Thrombin signalling and protease-activated receptors. *Nature* 2000;407(6801):258–264, with permission.]

appears to represent the sum of contributions from both receptors (98,99). Differences in G protein coupling also exist between PAR1 and PAR4 (at least for the human isoforms). Like hPAR1, hPAR4 activates Gq and probably G12/13 signaling, but, unlike hPAR1, hPAR4 does not appear to couple to Gi (82,83,93,100). The importance of such differences is not known for platelet function.

In addition to interacting with PARs, thrombin also binds to glycoprotein Ibα (GP Ibα) on the surface of human platelets (101). GP Ibα is part of a multifunctional protein complex that also binds VWF and P selectin (102). Platelets from patients with Bernard-Soulier syndrome lack surface GP Ibα and show decreased thrombin responsiveness, but such platelets are also structurally abnormal (103–106). However, antibodies that block thrombin binding to GP Ibα attenuate platelet activation by thrombin and decrease PAR1 cleavage (105,107,108). These and other observations (109) support the model that GP Ibα may serve as a cofactor that localizes thrombin to the platelet surface to support thrombin cleavage of PARs, which is analogous to the interaction between PAR3 and PAR4 in mouse platelets described in subsequent text (89). Attempts to directly demonstrate such activity by coexpressing the GP Ib complex with PARs have been unsuccessful (89), but the importance of such negative results is, of course, uncertain. Studies in mouse platelets (see subsequent text) also suggest a connection between the GP Ib complex and thrombin signaling, but the exact nature of that connection remains unclear.

The presence of PAR1 and PAR4 in human platelets raises an important question about the development of antithrombotic pharmaceuticals. Given that activation of PAR4 requires relatively high concentrations of thrombin for activation, will inhibition of PAR1 be sufficient to prevent thrombosis? Or will inhibition of both PAR1 and PAR4 be required? Preliminary answers are coming from studies in PAR-deficient mice and from primate models.

## Thrombin Receptors in Mouse Platelets

In contrast with human platelets, mouse platelets express PAR3 and PAR4 (83). Accordingly, PAR1-activating peptides that are fully active on both human and mouse PAR1 in heterologous expression systems (110) activate human but not mouse platelets (110–112). Moreover, knockout of mPAR1 had no effect on thrombin signaling in mouse platelets but ablated thrombin signaling in fibroblasts (110). These observations triggered a search for other thrombin receptors in mouse platelets and led to the identification of PAR3 (81). The expression of *human* PAR3 cDNA in COS cells or in *Xenopus* oocytes caused phosphoinositide hydrolysis in response to low concentrations of thrombin, and *in situ* hybridization using a mouse PAR3 probe detected mPAR3 mRNA in mouse megakaryocytes (81). Therefore, mouse PAR3 appeared to be a good candidate for the "missing" mouse platelet thrombin receptor, and, indeed, knockout mouse studies revealed that PAR3 is necessary for activation of mouse platelets at low but not at high concentrations of thrombin (83). Responses to high concentrations of thrombin in PAR3-deficient mouse platelets were attributable to mPAR4 (83). At face value, these data conjured a dual receptor model analogous to that described earlier for human platelets (Fig. 33-4)—but with PAR3 simply substituting for PAR1 as the "high-affinity" thrombin receptor in mouse platelets (83). However, subsequent characterization of the mouse homolog of PAR3 presented a paradox. Despite strong evidence that mPAR3 was necessary for mouse platelet responses to low concentrations of thrombin, expression of mPAR3 cDNA in heterologous expression systems

failed to result in thrombin signaling. Resolution of this paradox came in the form of an interesting variation on the mechanism of PAR activation (89). Although expression of mPAR3 in COS cells did not by itself produce thrombin signaling, coexpression of mPAR3 with mPAR4 reliably enhanced both mPAR4 cleavage and signaling at low concentrations of thrombin compared with that seen with mPAR4 alone. When tethered to the plasma membrane, the N-terminal exodomain of mPAR3 alone was sufficient for this activity, and the thrombin-interacting sequences within this domain were necessary. Therefore, it appears that mPAR3 does not by itself mediate transmembrane signaling but, instead, functions as a cofactor for the cleavage and activation of mPAR4 at low thrombin concentrations—a curious form of G protein–coupled receptor interaction in which one receptor acts as an accessory protein that aids "ligation" of another (Fig. 33-4) (89).

This model predicts that, in contrast with the case in human platelets, activation of mouse platelets by thrombin should be PAR4-dependent. Platelets from PAR4-deficient (*Par4*$^{-/-}$) mice are indeed unresponsive to even micromolar concentrations of thrombin despite the presence of PAR3 (113). This observation provides strong support for the model proposed in Figure 33-4. Available data do not support the notion that mPAR3 and mPAR4 form stable heterodimers (SRC and David Sulciner, 2000), and whether a ternary complex between PAR3, thrombin, and PAR4 ever exists is not known. Thrombin binding to PAR3 may simply increase the effective local concentration of thrombin at the surface of the mouse platelet.

Perhaps surprisingly, a similar cofactor relation between hPAR1 and hPAR4 or between GP Ibα and hPAR1 or hPAR4 could not be detected when these molecules were coexpressed in the same systems in which the mPAR3–mPAR4 interaction was readily demonstrated (89). It is certainly possible that such negative results were due to differences in absolute or relative expression levels achieved in these systems versus in platelets, or to other technical issues. Interestingly, mouse platelets that lack GP V, part of the GP Ib complex, have been reported to show enhanced responsiveness to thrombin (114) and to become responsive to active-site–inhibited thrombin preparations (115). Therefore, as in human platelets, there is evidence that the GP Ib complex contributes to thrombin responses in mouse platelets (114). However, the apparently absolute lack of thrombin responses in *Par4*$^{-/-}$ mouse platelets (113,116) suggests that the GP Ib complex is not sufficient to mediate platelet activation by thrombin. The observation that responses to high concentrations of active-site–inhibited thrombin preparations were also ablated in *Par4*$^{-/-}$ platelets (113) suggests the possibility that such responses may be triggered by active protease(s) in these preparations. The notion that GP Ib plays a cofactor role remains appealing.

## EVIDENCE FROM MOUSE AND PRIMATE MODELS THAT PROTEASE-ACTIVATED RECEPTORS ARE IMPORTANT IN HEMOSTASIS AND THROMBOSIS: IS PROTEASE-ACTIVATED RECEPTOR INHIBITION A RATIONAL STRATEGY FOR ANTITHROMBOTIC THERAPY?

Both thrombin and platelets play key roles in arterial thrombosis, and, given the remarkable effectiveness of thrombin as a platelet agonist, it is reasonable to postulate an important role for thrombin in platelet activation in this setting. However, multiple agonists present at sites of vascular injury can activate platelets (117,118), and thrombin itself has multiple actions, including mediating fibrin formation. Because platelets from $Par4^{-/-}$ mice were unresponsive to thrombin, such mice provided a long-awaited opportunity to assess the relative importance of platelet activation by thrombin among the many potentially redundant mechanisms that orchestrate hemostasis and thrombosis.

$Par4^{-/-}$ mice appear healthy, show no evidence of spontaneous bleeding, and are not anemic. Platelets are normal in number and morphology. Female mice that are $Par4^{-/-}$ can support pregnancies. However, $Par4^{-/-}$ mice do show markedly prolonged bleeding times when the challenge is sufficiently strong. [In this study, mice were anesthetized, the tail transected 0.5 cm from the tip so as to open tail artery and veins, the bleeding tip immersed in 37°C saline, and the time to cessation of flow was measured (113)]. In bone marrow reconstitution studies, this phenotype is fully attributable to PAR4 deficiency in cells of hematopoietic origin (116). These results provide strong genetic evidence that thrombin signaling in platelets is important for hemostasis.

The relatively mild hemostatic defect in $Par4^{-/-}$ mice indicated an interesting contrast between mice that lack the classic hemostatic effectors of thrombin—platelet activation and fibrin formation—and mice that lack thrombin itself. Like $Par4^{-/-}$ mice, mice that lack fibrinogen ($Fib^{-/-}$) have a relatively mild defect in hemostasis (119). Depending upon the strain, $Fib^{-/-}$ mice do exhibit some perinatal hemorrhage and pregnant female mice bleed at placentation, but $Fib^{-/-}$ mice regularly survive to "old age" without apparent problems. Neither $Par4^{-/-}$ nor $Fib^{-/-}$ mice have abnormal embryonic development. This observation is in contrast with mice that lack thrombin itself (prothrombin-deficient; $Pt^{-/-}$) (120,121). Approximately 50% of $Pt^{-/-}$ embryos die at midgestation with cardiovascular collapse, and virtually all that survive to birth exsanguinate in the perinatal period. This contrast raised the question of whether combined deficiency of PAR4 and fibrinogen might recapitulate the phenotypes associated with prothrombin deficiency. Combined deficiency of PAR4 and fibrinogen indeed recapitulated the severe hemostatic defect seen in prothrombin nulls: virtually all $Par4^{-/-}$ and $Fib^{-/-}$ pups exsanguinated at birth (122). Therefore, perhaps not surprisingly, platelet activation and fibrin formation together appear to account for the major hemostatic effects of thrombin. Interestingly, however, $Par4^{-/-}$ and $Fib^{-/-}$ mice showed no abnormality in embryonic development, consistent with the notion that thrombin has novel roles in the embryo beyond platelet activation and fibrin formation (110,122–124).

$Par4^{-/-}$ mice also displayed protection against thrombosis induced by a thrombin-dependent mechanism (i.e., thromboplastin-induced pulmonary embolism) and by a nonspecific vascular injury (i.e., ferric chloride-induced thrombosis of mesenteric arterioles) (113,125). Protection in the thromboplastin model could be attributed to PAR4 deficiency in bone marrow–derived cells (116) and was nearly as dramatic as that seen in NF-E2–deficient mice, which lack platelets (116,126). These results support the importance of platelet activation by thrombin in a thrombin-dependent model of thrombosis. Together, these studies provide strong genetic evidence that platelet activation by thrombin is important in hemostasis and thrombosis in mice despite the panoply of agonists and potentially redundant pathways involved in these processes. Whether the protection against thrombosis in $Par4^{-/-}$ mice is attributable to their lack of direct platelet activation by thrombin and/or to a consequent decrease in release of secondary mediators of platelet activation and/or to decreased platelet procoagulant activity and fibrin formation (15,127–129) remains to be determined.

The results described in preceding text were obtained in mice that appear to lack all thrombin signaling in platelets. It is unlikely that such complete ablation of thrombin signaling can be readily achieved using pharmaceuticals in humans because human platelets have two thrombin receptors, PAR1 and PAR4, that function independently. However, studies in mouse and primate models suggest that inhibition of PAR1 alone might be sufficient to achieve an antithrombotic effect.

The model in Figure 33-4 suggests that PAR3-deficient mouse platelets are analogous to PAR1-inhibited human platelets; both rely on PAR4 for thrombin signaling. Indeed, functionally, both show markedly decreased responses at low concentrations of thrombin and delayed responses at higher concentrations of thrombin (83,93). Perhaps surprisingly, PAR3-deficient mice showed a level of protection in thrombosis models that was similar to that seen in $Par4^{-/-}$ mice (125). How is it that PAR3-deficiency and PAR4-deficiency can have such similar effects? It is possible that the concentration of thrombin acting at the platelet surface is simply insufficient to activate platelets that lack PAR3's cofactor function and rely only on PAR4 for thrombin-mediated signaling. Alternatively, the local concentration of thrombin may be high enough to cleave PAR4, but not at a rate sufficient to activate platelets quickly enough for their incorporation into a thrombus. Regardless, the observation that PAR3-deficient mice have no spontaneous bleeding yet are protected in thrombosis models suggests that partial attenuation of thrombin signaling in mouse platelets can produce a useful antithrombotic effect. Several studies suggest that PAR1 inhibition in primates may yield similar results. Like human platelets, platelets in nonhuman primates express PAR1 and PAR4 (78). Polyclonal antibody directed against the thrombin-interacting sequences in attenuated platelet-dependent PAR1 decreases in blood flow in a carotid injury model in African green monkeys (130). More recent studies with a small molecule PAR1 antagonist yielded similar results in cynomolgus monkeys (78). Of note, PAR4 signaling was shown to be intact in this study. Therefore, PAR1 inhibition appears to be sufficient to achieve an antithrombotic effect in nonhuman primates, and PAR1 antagonists may have the potential utility to prevent and/or to treat thrombotic events in humans.

Why consider inhibition of platelet activation by thrombin instead of inhibition of thrombin itself? Inhibition of platelet activation by thrombin should leave other functions of thrombin including fibrin formation and protein C activation relatively intact (see Fig. 33-5). Excluding these important pathways might provide for a safer pharmaceutical and a higher therapeutic index when prevention or treatment of platelet-dependent arterial thrombosis is the goal.

# PROTEASE-ACTIVATED RECEPTORS IN INFLAMMATION

What functions do endothelial PARs serve? One might imagine the following scenario. Vascular injury, whether by trauma, infection, or metabolic or inflammatory mediators, triggers local generation of coagulation proteases and/or release of other proteases, which, via PARs, activate endothelial cells (see Fig. 33-6). The activated endothelial surface in turn promotes adhesion and rolling of platelets and leukocytes as well as access of plasma proteins to the extravascular space. Thrombin also triggers endothelial production of platelet-activating factor, a potent platelet and leukocyte activator (131), as well as IL-6 and IL-8 (132). Therefore, endothelial PARs may be part of a first response that helps link tissue

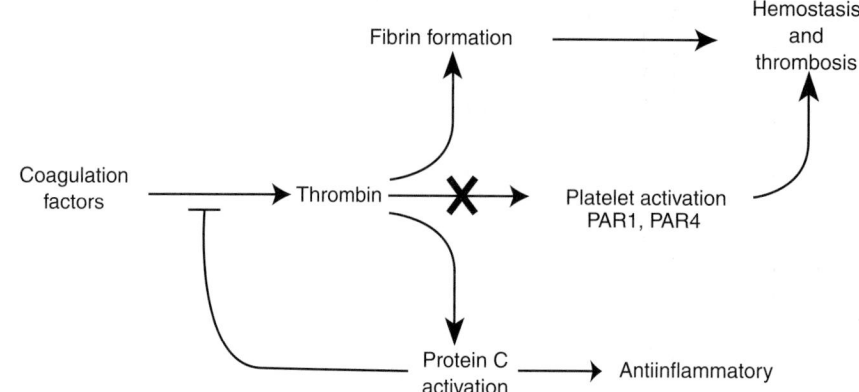

**FIGURE 33-5.** Why consider developing a protease-activated receptor 1 (PAR1) antagonist versus a direct thrombin inhibitor? In addition to activating PARs on platelets and other cells, thrombin mediates fibrin formation and protein C activation. PAR antagonists have the potential of blocking platelet activation by thrombin while sparing fibrin formation and protein C activation. Such a strategy might provide for a larger therapeutic index than might be achieved for thrombin inhibitors, particularly for prevention or treatment of thrombosis that is relatively platelet-dependent as in myocardial infarction and stroke. Use of anticoagulants in human suggests a relatively narrow therapeutic index, and mice that lack prothrombin exsanguinate at birth. By contrast, mice that lack all platelet responses to thrombin have virtually no spontaneous bleeding.

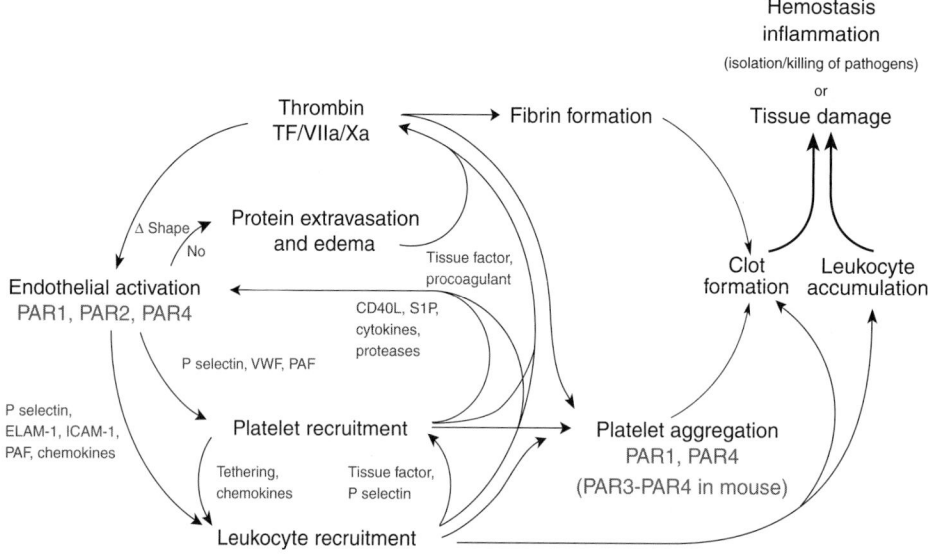

**FIGURE 33-6.** Possible interactions between coagulation and inflammation, and potential roles of protease-activated receptors (PARs). Thrombin activates endothelial PAR1. Factor Xa and/or tissue factor/factor VIIa complex (TF/VIIa) may activate endothelial PAR2 (87,88). PAR signaling upregulates adhesion molecules on the endothelial surface and triggers production of lipid mediators and chemokines (131,133–135). These events lead to adhesion, rolling, and, in some settings, attachment and activation of platelets and leukocytes at the endothelial surface. Recruitment of tissue factor–bearing leukocytes and microparticles (5,6) and platelet procoagulant activity (15) may promote further thrombin generation (136). Thrombin also increases endothelial permeability (137,138), and this too might promote additional thrombin generation because plasma coagulation factors contact extravascular tissue factor. Platelets and leukocytes can directly activate endothelial cells by presenting CD40L and other mediators, thereby upregulating not only adhesion molecules and cytokines (12) but also tissue factor and PAR2 (3,139). Leukocytes and platelets can themselves interact via P selectin (136), and neutrophils may activate platelets by release of the granzyme cathepsin G (97). Ultimately, leukocyte products may directly injure tissues, and thrombin may trigger fibrin formation, platelet aggregation, and microvascular thrombosis. When localized, such a system may be useful for isolating and destroying pathogens. Activation of endothelial PARs alone is sufficient to trigger platelet and leukocyte margination but not other sequelae. Therefore, it seems likely that endothelial PARs may help orchestrate "inspection" of sites of injury by platelets and leukocytes and that other stimuli are required for the more dramatic scenarios discussed above. Positive feedback between coagulation and inflammation is made more likely by cellular responses to endotoxin (140) and by genetic deficiencies in natural anticoagulant pathways (141), and, undamped, can be associated with hemorrhagic infarction of tissues. The relative importance of PARs in such settings remains to be determined (see text). TF, tissue factor; PAR, protease-activated receptor; S1P, sphingosine-1-phosphate; VWF, von Willebrand factor; PAF, platelet activating factor; ELAM, endothelial-leukocyte adhesion molecule; ICAM, intercellular adhesion module. [From Coughlin SR. Thrombin signaling and protease-activated receptors. *Nature* 2000;407(6801):258–264, with permission.]

injury to recruitment of platelets, leukocytes, and, by promoting transudation, immune effector proteins to "examine" the locale for damage and infection.

In mouse microvascular endothelial cell preparations, responses to thrombin are mediated primarily by PAR1 and, to a lesser extent, by PAR4 (142). PAR2 and, to a lesser extent, PAR1 appear to account for endothelial responses to the upstream coagulation proteases tissue factor/VIIa and Xa (143) (EC and SRC, 2003). Endothelial PARs may also act as receptors for activated protein C and for proteases released from leukocytes (25,85,97,144,145), but these appear to be weak agonists in our hands (EC and SRC, 2003).

On the basis of the observations in preceding text, PAR-deficient mice provide an opportunity to test the role of endothelial PARs in inflammatory responses. The species differences in PAR expression between mouse and human may be fortunate in this regard. PAR1 appears to be the major thrombin receptor in endothelial cells in both species. However, because PAR1 is not expressed in mouse platelets, PAR1-deficient mice offer an opportunity to ablate thrombin signaling in endothelial cells without perturbing platelet signaling, thereby defining the contribution of thrombin signaling in cells other than platelets in models of thrombosis and inflammation. PAR deficiency has been reported to be protective in various mouse models of pathologic inflammation (146). PAR1 deficiency provided protection against leukocyte infiltration and renal damage in a model of antibody-mediated glomerulonephritis (147), and both PAR1 deficiency (148) and PAR1 antagonists (149) reduced restenosis in arterial injury models. PAR2-deficient mice have reduced leukocyte rolling in exteriorized cremasteric preparations (150), and PAR2 deficiency has been reported to protect against inflammation in models of arthritis (151) and dermatitis (152,153). Both PAR1- and PAR2-deficient mice have been studied in mouse models of endotoxemia. Deficiency in either of the receptors alone failed to effect cytokine responses or lethality (154) (EC and SRC, unpublished). However, in the presence of the specific thrombin inhibitor hirudin, both PAR1 (155) and PAR2 (154) knockout animals showed decreased cytokine production compared with their identically treated wild-type littermates. Therefore, activation of multiple PARs by multiple coagulation proteases may contribute to inflammation in sepsis. Overall, evidence for a role for PARs in inflammation seems to be accumulating, but the effects reported are often small and variable, and important questions remain about cellular contributors and mechanisms of action. It has recently been reported that activation of PAR1 can prevent apoptosis in endothelial cells and neurons and that such an effect may mediate a protective effect of activated protein C in a mouse model of ischemic stroke (156,157). However, reports on whether PAR1 activation protects against or exacerbates cerebral ischemia–induced injury vary (157,158), and it is possible that dual roles for PAR activation—one antiapoptotic and protective and the other proinflammatory and deleterious—contribute to this complexity. More work is needed to determine whether PARs indeed play an important role in inflammation.

## PROTEASE-ACTIVATED RECEPTORS IN EMBRYONIC DEVELOPMENT

Coagulation proteases and PARs appear to play an important role in embryonic development that is unrelated to hemostasis in any usual sense, perhaps by contributing to normal blood vessel development. Approximately 50% of PAR1-deficient embryos die at midgestation with pericardial edema, bleeding, and delayed maturation of yolk sac vasculature (110,124). As emphasized above, PAR1 does not function in mouse platelets

(110–112), and mice that lack platelet responses to thrombin (113,122) as well as mice that lack the platelets (126) develop normally. Therefore, it is difficult to ascribe bleeding and death of PAR1-deficient embryos to a platelet function defect. At midgestation, PAR1 is expressed most abundantly in endocardial and endothelial cells, and a transgene in which the endothelial-specific Tie2 promoter drove PAR1 expression prevented death of PAR1-deficient embryos (124). Therefore, it appears that PAR1 signaling in endothelial cells (or perhaps in other Tie2-expressing cells) is necessary for proper blood vessel development. What does endothelial PAR1 sense biochemically in the developing embryo? Knockout of several coagulation factors causes variable degrees of embryonic loss at midgestation, which are in some cases associated with abnormal vascular development (120,121,123,159,160). Therefore, it is possible that PAR1 is sensing coagulation proteases in the embryo. If so, is this a system for sensing plasma—perhaps a mechanism for monitoring the leakiness of developing blood vessels or simply connectivity to the circulation? Which of the many endothelial cell responses to PAR1 activation are important in this context? Much work remains in this novel area.

## SUMMARY

The coagulation cascade and PAR together provide an elegant mechanism that links mechanical information in the form of tissue injury or vascular leak to cellular responses. In large part, these receptors appear to account for the cellular effects of thrombin, and an important role for PARs in hemostasis and thrombosis is well established in animal models. One might expect that the relative importance of PAR activation on platelets might vary according to the type of thrombus and to the extent to which it is dependent on thrombin, platelets or fibrin. Nonetheless, PAR inhibition remains an exciting area to explore for novel antithrombotic therapies. A complicated literature is emerging about the roles for PARs in inflammation. PAR activation on endothelial cells clearly can promote the recruitment of leukocytes and platelets and the transudation of plasma. However, a panoply of signaling systems and cell types orchestrates inflammatory responses, and efforts to define the relative contribution of PARs in endothelial cells and leukocytes in various inflammatory processes are just beginning. Last, unexpected roles for PARs in embryonic development are emerging, and whether these reflect new roles for the coagulation cascade and/or PAR signaling to other proteases remains to be explored.

## ACKNOWLEDGMENTS

Thanks to the members of my laboratory for helpful discussions. Figures 33-1 to 33-4 and 33-6 are from Coughlin SR. Thrombin signalling and protease-activated receptors. *Nature* 2000;407 (6801):258–264, and have been reproduced with permission from *Nature*.

## *References*

1. Colman R, Marder VJ, Clowes AW. Overview of coagulation and its regulation. In: Colman RW, Marder VJ, Clowes AW et al., eds. *Hemostasis and thrombosis: basic principles and clinical practice*, 5th ed. Philadelphia, PA: Lippincott Williams & Wilkins, 2005.
2. Drake TA, Morrissey JH, Edgington TS. Selective cellular expression of tissue factor in human tissues. Implications for disorders of hemostasis and thrombosis. *Am J Pathol* 1989;134(5):1087–1097.
3. Bevilacqua MP, Gimbrone MA Jr. Inducible endothelial functions in inflammation and coagulation. *Semin Thromb Hemost* 1987;13(4):425–433.
4. Camerer E, Kolstø AB, Prydz H. Cell biology of tissue factor, the principal initiator of blood coagulation. *Thromb Res* 1996;81:1–41.

5. Osterud B. Tissue factor expression by monocytes: regulation and patho-physiological roles. *Blood Coagul Fibrinolysis* 1998;9(6 Pt 2 Suppl. 1): S9–14.

6. Giesen PL, Rauch U, Bohrmann B, et al. Blood-borne tissue factor: another view of thrombosis. *Proc Natl Acad Sci U S A* 1999;96(5):2311–2315.

7. Coughlin SR. Sol Sherry lecture in thrombosis: how thrombin 'talks' to cells: molecular mechanisms and roles *in vivo*. *Arterioscler Thromb Vasc Biol* 1998;18(4):514–518.

8. Davey MG, Lüscher EF. Actions of thrombin and other coagulant and proteolytic enzymes on blood platelets. *Nature* 1967;216(118):857–858.

9. Brass LF, Manning DR, Cichowski K, et al. Signaling through G proteins in platelets: to the integrins and beyond. *Thromb Haemost* 1997;78(1): 581–589.

10. Hamberg M, Svensson J, Samuelsson B. Thromboxanes: a new group of biologically active compounds derived from prostaglandin endoperoxides. *Proc Natl Acad Sci U S A* 1975;72(8):2994–2998.

11. Stenberg PE, McEver RP, Shuman MA, et al. A platelet alpha-granule membrane protein (GMP-140) is expressed on the plasma membrane after activation. *J Cell Biol* 1985;101(3):880–886.

12. Henn V, Slupsky JR, Gräfe M, et al. CD40 ligand on activated platelets triggers an inflammatory reaction of endothelial cells. *Nature* 1998;391 (6667):591–594.

13. Hughes PE, Pfaff M. Integrin affinity modulation. *Trends Cell Biol* 1998; 8(9):359–364.

14. Colman RW, Marder VJ, Salzman EW. Overview of hemostasis. In: Colman RW, Marder VJ, Salzman EW et al., eds. *Hemostasis and thrombosis*, 3rd ed. Philadelphia, PA: JB Lippincott Co, 1994:3–18.

15. Sims PJ, Wiedmer T, Esmon CT, et al. Assembly of the platelet prothrombinase complex is linked to vesiculation of the platelet plasma membrane. *J Biol Chem* 1989;264:17049–17057.

16. Hattori R, Hamilton KK, Fugate RD, et al. Stimulated secretion of endothelial von willebrand factor is accompanied by rapid redistribution to the cell surface of the intracellular granule membrane protein GMP-140. *J Biol Chem* 1989;264(14):7768–7771.

17. Subramaniam M, Frenette PS, Saffaripour S, et al. Defects in hemostasis in P-selectin-deficient mice. *Blood* 1996;87(4):1238–1242.

18. Frenette PS, Mayadas TN, Rayburn H, et al. Susceptibility to infection and altered hematopoiesis in mice deficient in both P-and E-selectins. *Cell* 1996;84(4):563–574.

19. Lum H, Malik AB. Regulation of vascular endothelial barrier function. *Am J Physiol* 1994;267(3 Pt 1):L223–L241.

20. Cirino G, Cicala C, Bucci MR, et al. Thrombin functions as an inflammatory mediator through activation of its receptor. *J Exp Med* 1996;183(3): 821–827.

21. Tesfamariam B, Allen GT, Normandin D, et al. Involvement of the "tethered ligand" receptor in thrombin-induced endothelium-mediated relaxations. *Am J Physiol* 1993;265:H1744–H1749.

22. Hamilton JR, Frauman AG, Cocks TM. Increased expression of protease-activated receptor-2 (PAR2) and PAR4 in human coronary artery by inflammatory stimuli unveils endothelium-dependent relaxations to PAR2 and PAR4 agonists. *Circ Res* 2001;89(1):92–98.

23. Hamilton JR, Moffatt JD, Frauman AG, et al. Protease-activated receptor (PAR) 1 but not PAR2 or PAR4 mediates endothelium-dependent relaxation to thrombin and trypsin in human pulmonary arteries. *J Cardiovasc Pharmacol* 2001;V38(N1):108–119.

24. Ku DD, Zaleski JK. Receptor mechanism of thrombin-induced endothelium-dependent and endothelium-independent coronary vascular effects in dogs. *J Cardiovasc Pharmacol* 1993;22(4):609–616.

25. Riewald M, Petrovan RJ, Donner A, et al. Activation of endothelial cell protease activated receptor 1 by the protein C pathway. *Science* 2002; 296(5574):1880–1882.

26. Coughlin SR. How the protease thrombin talks to cells. *Proc Natl Acad Sci U S A* 1999;96:11023–11027.

27. Vu TK, Hung DT, Wheaton VI, et al. Molecular cloning of a functional thrombin receptor reveals a novel proteolytic mechanism of receptor activation. *Cell* 1991;64(6):1057–1068.

28. Rasmussen UB, Vouret-Craviari V, Jallat S, et al. cDNA cloning and expression of a hamster alpha-thrombin receptor coupled to Ca2+ mobilization. *FEBS Letts* 1991;288:123–128.

29. Chen J, Ishii M, Wang L, et al. Thrombin receptor activation: confirmation of the intramolecular tethered liganding hypothesis and discovery of an alternative intermolecular liganding mode. *J Biol Chem* 1994;269(23): 16041–16045.

30. O'Brien PJ, Prevost N, Molino M, et al. Thrombin responses in human endothelial cells. Contributions from receptors other than PAR1 include the transactivation of PAR2 by thrombin-cleaved PAR1. *J Biol Chem* 2000;275:13502–13509.

31. Vassallo RR Jr, Kieber-Emmons T, Cichowski K, et al. Structure-function relationships in the activation of platelet thrombin receptors by receptor-derived peptides. *J Biol Chem* 1992;267(9):6081–6085.

32. Scarborough RM, Naughton MA, Teng W, et al. Tethered ligand agonist peptides. Structural requirements for thrombin receptor activation reveal mechanism of proteolytic unmasking of agonist function. *J Biol Chem* 1992;267(19):13146–13149.

33. Hollenberg MD. Proteinase-mediated signaling: proteinase-activated receptors (PARs) and much more. *Life Sci* 2003;74(2-3):237–246.

34. Vu T-KH, Wheaton VI, Hung DT, et al. Domains specifying thrombin-receptor interaction. *Nature* 1991;353:674–677.

35. Liu L, Vu T-KH, Esmon CT, et al. The region of the thrombin receptor resembling hirudin binds to thrombin and alters enzyme specificity. *J Biol Chem* 1991;266:16977–16980.

36. Mathews II, Padmanabhan KP, Ganesh V, et al. Crystallographic structures of thrombin complexed with thrombin receptor peptides: existence of expected and novel binding modes. *Biochemistry* 1994;33(11):3266–3279.

37. Ishii K, Gerszten R, Zheng YW, et al. Determinants of thrombin receptor cleavage. Receptor domains involved, specificity, and role of the P3 aspartate. *J Biol Chem* 1995;270(27):16435–16440.

38. Hung DT, Vu TK, Wheaton VI, et al. Cloned platelet thrombin receptor is necessary for thrombin-induced platelet activation. *J Clin Invest* 1992; 89(4):1350–1353.

39. Mathews II, Padmanabhan KP, Ganesh V, et al. Crystallographic structures of thrombin complexed with thrombin receptor peptides: existence of expected and novel binding modes. *Biochemistry* 1994;33(11):3266–3279.

40. Hammes SR, Coughlin SR. Protease-activated receptor-1 can mediate responses to SFLLRN in thrombin-desensitized cells: evidence for a novel mechanism for preventing or terminating signaling by PAR1's tethered ligand. *Biochemistry* 1999;38(8):2486–2493.

41. Coller BS, Ward P, Ceruso M, et al. Thrombin receptor activating peptides: importance of the N-terminal serine and its ionization state as judged by pH dependence, NMR spectroscopy, and cleavage by aminopeptidase M. *Biochemistry* 1992;31:11713–11720.

42. Bode W, Schwager P, Huber R. The transition of bovine trypsinogen to a trypsin-like state upon strong ligand binding. *J Mol Biol* 1978;118:99–112.

43. Lerner DJ, Chen M, Tram T, et al. Agonist recognition by proteinase-activated receptor 2 and thrombin receptor. Importance of extracellular loop interactions for receptor function. *J Biol Chem* 1996;271(24):13943–13947.

44. Palczewski K, Kumasaka T, Hori T, et al. Crystal structure of rhodopsin: a G protein-coupled receptor. *Science* 2000;289(5480):739–745.

45. Gerszten RE, Chen J, Ishii M, et al. The thrombin receptor's specificity for agonist peptide is defined by its extracellular surface. *Nature* 1994;368: 648–651.

46. Nanevicz T, Ishii M, Wang L, et al. Mechanisms of thrombin receptor agonist specificity. Chimeric receptors and complementary mutations identify an agonist recognition site. *J Biol Chem* 1995;270(37):21619–21625.

47. Nanevicz T, Wang L, Chen M, et al. Thrombin receptor activating mutations. Alteration of an extracellular agonist recognition domain causes constitutive signaling. *J Biol Chem* 1996;271(2):702–706.

48. Bahou WF, Coller BS, Potter CL, et al. The thrombin receptor extracellular domain contains sites crucial for peptide-ligand induced activation. *J Clin Invest* 1993;91:1405–1413.

49. Offermanns S, Toombs CF, Hu YH, et al. Defective platelet activation in G alpha(q)-deficient mice. *Nature* 1997;389(6647):183–186.

50. Moers A, Nieswandt B, Massberg S, et al. G(13) is an essential mediator of platelet activation in hemostasis and thrombosis. *Nat Med* 2003; 9(11):1418–22.

51. Yang J, Wu J, Kowalska MA, et al. Loss of signaling through the G protein, Gz, results in abnormal platelet activation and altered responses to psychoactive drugs. *Proc Natl Acad Sci U S A* 2000;97(18):9984–9989.

52. Hung DT, Wong YH, Vu T-KH, et al. The cloned platelet thrombin receptor couples to at least two distinct effectors to stimulate both phosphoinositide hydrolysis and inhibit adenylyl cyclase. *J Biol Chem* 1992; 353:20831–20834.

53. Offermanns S, Laugwitz K-L, Spicher K, et al. G proteins of the G12 family are activated via thromboxane A2 and thrombin receptors in human platelets. *Proc Natl Acad Sci U S A* 1994;91:504–508.

54. Barr AJ, Brass LF, Manning DR. Reconstitution of receptors and GTP-binding regulatory proteins (G proteins) in Sf9 cells. A direct evaluation of selectivity in receptor.G protein coupling. *J Biol Chem* 1997;272(4):2223–2229.

55. Kozasa T, Jiang X, Hart MJ, et al. p115 RhoGEF, a GTPase activating protein for galpha12 and galpha13 [see comments]. *Science* 1998; 280(5372):2109–2111.

56. Hart MJ, Jiang X, Kozasa T, et al. Direct stimulation of the guanine nucleotide exchange activity of p115 RhoGEF by galpha13 [see comments]. *Science* 1998;280(5372):2112–2114.

57. Fukuhara S, Murga C, Zohar M, et al. A novel PDZ domain containing guanine nucleotide exchange factor links heterotrimeric G proteins to Rho. *J Biol Chem* 1999;274(9):5868–5879.

58. Klages B, Brandt U, Simon MI, et al. Activation of G12/G13 results in shape change and rho/rho kinase-mediated myosin light chain phosphorylation in mouse platelets. *J Cell Biol* 1999;144(4):745–754.

59. Vouret-Craviari V, Boquet P, Pouysségur J, et al. Regulation of the actin cytoskeleton by thrombin in human endothelial cells: role of Rho proteins in endothelial barrier function. *Mol Biol Cell* 1998;9(9):2639–2653.

60. Offermanns S, Mancino V, Revel J-P, et al. Vascular system defects and impaired cell chemokinesis as a result of G$\alpha_{13}$ deficiency. *Science* 1997; 275:533–536.

61. Taylor S, Chae H, Rhee S-G, et al. Activation of the B1 isozyme of phospholipase C by a subunits of the Gq class of G proteins. *Nature* 1991;350: 516–518.

62. Stoyanov B, Volinia S, Hanck T, et al. Cloning and characterization of a G protein-activated human phosphoinositide-3 kinase. *Science* 1995;269 (5224):690–693.

63. Clapham DE, Neer EJ. G protein beta gamma subunits. *Annu Rev Pharmacol Toxicol* 1997;37(2):167–203.

64. Leevers SJ, Vanhaesebroeck B, Waterfield MD. Signalling through phosphoinositide 3-kinases: the lipids take centre stage. *Curr Opin Cell Biol* 1999;11(2):219–225.

65. Prenzel N, Zwick E, Daub H, et al. EGF receptor transactivation by G-protein-coupled receptors requires metalloproteinase cleavage of proHB-EGF. *Nature* 1999;402(6764):884–888.

66. Lefkowitz RJ, Pitcher J, Krueger K, et al. Mechanisms of beta-adrenergic receptor desensitization and resensitization. *Adv Pharmacol* 1998;42(2):416–420.

67. Hoxie JA, Ahuja M, Belmonte E, et al. Internalization and recycling of activated thrombin receptors. *J Biol Chem* 1993;268(18):13756–13763.

68. Ishii K, Chen J, Ishii M, et al. Inhibition of thrombin receptor signaling by a G protein-coupled receptor kinase. Functional specificity among G protein-coupled receptor kinases. *J Biol Chem* 1994;269:1125–1130.

69. Paing MM, Stutts AB, Kohout TA, et al. beta – Arrestins regulate protease-activated receptor-1 desensitization but not internalization or downregulation. *J Biol Chem* 2002;277(2):1292–1300.

70. Hein L, Ishii K, Coughlin SR, et al. Intracellular targeting and trafficking of thrombin receptors: a novel mechanism for resensitization of a G protein-coupled receptor. *J Biol Chem* 1994;269:27719–27726.

71. Trejo J, Hammes SR, Coughlin SR. Termination of signaling by protease-activated receptor-1 is linked to lysosomal sorting. *Proc Natl Acad Sci U S A* 1998;95(23):13698–13702.

72. Trejo J, Coughlin SR. The cytoplasmic tails of protease-activated receptor-1 and substance P receptor specify sorting to lysosomes versus recycling. *J Biol Chem* 1999;274(4):2216–2224.

73. Ishii K, Hein L, Kobilka B, et al. Kinetics of thrombin receptor cleavage on intact cells. Relation to signaling. *J Biol Chem* 1993;268(13):9780–9786.

74. Ludeman MJ, Zheng YW, Ishii K, et al. Regulated shedding of PAR1 N-terminal exodomain from endothelial cells. *J Biol Chem* 2004;279(18):18592–18599.

75. Bernatowicz MS, Klimas CE, Hartl KS, et al. Development of potent thrombin receptor antagonist peptides. *J Med Chem* 1996;39(25):4879–4887.

76. Andrade-Gordon P, Maryanoff BE, Derian CK, et al. Design, synthesis, and biological characterization of a peptide-mimetic antagonist for a tethered-ligand receptor. *Proc Natl Acad Sci U S A* 1999;96(22):12257–12262.

77. Derian CK, Maryanoff BE, Zhang HC, et al. Therapeutic potential of protease-activated receptor-1 antagonists. *Expert Opin Drugs* 2003;12(2):209–221.

78. Derian CK, Damiano BP, Addo MF, et al. Blockade of the thrombin receptor protease-activated receptor-1 with a small-molecule antagonist prevents thrombus formation and vascular occlusion in nonhuman primates. *J Pharmacol Exp Ther* 2003;304(2):855–861.

79. Quinn MJ, Fitzgerald DJ. Ticlopidine and clopidogrel. *Circulation* 1999;100(15):1667–1672.

80. Savi P, Pereillo JM, Uzabiaga MF, et al. Identification and biological activity of the active metabolite of clopidogrel. *Thromb Haemost* 2000;84:891–896.

81. Ishihara H, Connolly AJ, Zeng D, et al. Protease-activated receptor 3 is a second thrombin receptor in humans. *Nature* 1997;386(6624):502–506.

82. Xu WF, Andersen H, Whitmore TE, et al. Cloning and characterization of human protease-activated receptor 4. *Proc Natl Acad Sci U S A* 1998;95(12):6642–6646.

83. Kahn ML, Zheng YW, Huang W, et al. A dual thrombin receptor system for platelet activation. *Nature* 1998;394(6694):690–694.

84. Nystedt S, Emilsson K, Wahlestedt C, et al. Molecular cloning of a potential proteinase activated receptor. *Proc Natl Acad Sci U S A* 1994;91(20):9208–9212.

85. Molino M, Barnathan ES, Numerof R, et al. Interactions of mast cell tryptase with thrombin receptors and PAR-2. *J Biol Chem* 1997;272(7):4043–4049.

86. Camerer E, Røttingen JA, Iversen JG, et al. Coagulation factors VII and X induce Ca2+ oscillations in Madin-Darby canine kidney cells only when proteolytically active. *J Biol Chem* 1996;271(46):29034–29042.

87. Camerer E, Huang W, Coughlin SR. Tissue factor-and factor X-dependent activation of protease-activated receptor 2 by factor VIIa. *Proc Natl Acad Sci U S A* 2000;97(10):5255–5260.

88. Riewald M, Ruf W. Mechanistic coupling of protease signaling and initiation of coagulation by tissue factor. *Proc Natl Acad Sci U S A* 2001;98(14):7742–7747.

89. Nakanishi-Matsui M, Zheng YW, Sulciner DJ, et al. PAR3 is a cofactor for PAR4 activation by thrombin. *Nature* 2000;404(6778):609–613.

90. Vu TK, Wheaton VI, Hung DT, et al. Domains specifying thrombin-receptor interaction. *Nature* 1991;353(6345):674–677.

91. Liu LW, Vu TK, Esmon CT, et al. The region of the thrombin receptor resembling hirudin binds to thrombin and alters enzyme specificity. *J Biol Chem* 1991;266(26):16977–16980.

92. Nystedt S, Emilsson K, Wahlestedt C, et al. Molecular cloning of a potential proteinase activated receptor [see comments]. *Proc Natl Acad Sci U S A* 1994;91(20):9208–9212.

93. Kahn ML, Nakanishi-Matsui M, Shapiro MJ, et al. Protease-activated receptors 1 and 4 mediate activation of human platelets by thrombin. *J Clin Invest* 1999;103(6):879–887.

94. Faruqi TR, Weiss EJ, Shapiro MJ, et al. Structure-function analysis of protease-activated receptor 4 tethered ligand peptides. Determinants of specificity and utility in assays of receptor function. *J Biol Chem* 2000;275(26):19728–19734.

95. Brass LF, Vassallo RJ, Belmonte E, et al. Structure and function of the human platelet thrombin receptor. Studies using monoclonal antibodies directed against a defined domain within the receptor N terminus. *J Biol Chem* 1992;267(20):13795–13798.

96. Selak MA, Chignard M, Smith JB. Cathepsin G is a strong platelet agonist released by neutrophils. *Biochem J* 1988;251(1):293–299.

97. Sambrano GR, Huang W, Faruqi T, et al. Cathepsin G activates protease-activated receptor-4 in human platelets. *J Biol Chem* 2000;275(10):6819–6823.

98. Shapiro MJ, Weiss EJ, Faruqi TR, et al. Protease-activated receptors 1 and 4 are shut off with distinct kinetics after activation by thrombin. *J Biol Chem* 2000;275(33):25216–25221.

99. Covic L, Gresser AL, Kuliopulos A. Biphasic kinetics of activation and signaling for PAR1 and PAR4 thrombin receptors in platelets. *Biochemistry* 2000;39(18):5458–5467.

100. Faruqi TR, Weiss EJ, Shapiro MJ, et al. Structure-function analysis of protease-activated receptor-4 tethered tigand peptides: determinants of specificity and utility in assays of receptor function. *J Biol Chem* 2000;275:19728–19734.

101. Okamura T, Hasitz M, Jamieson GA. Platelet glycocalicin: interaction with thrombin and role as thrombin receptor on the platelet surface. *J Biol Chem* 1978;253:3435–3443.

102. Andrews RK, Shen Y, Gardiner EE, et al. The glycoprotein Ib-IX-V complex in platelet adhesion and signaling. *Thromb Haemost* 1999;82(2):357–364.

103. Ware J, Russell SR, Vicente V, et al. Nonsense mutation in the glycoprotein Ib alpha coding sequence associated with bernard-soulier syndrome. *Proc Natl Acad Sci U S A* 1990;87(5):2026–2030.

104. De Marco L, Mazzucato M, Fabris F, et al. Variant bernard-soulier syndrome type bolzano. A congenital bleeding disorder due to a structural and functional abnormality of the platelet glycoprotein Ib-IX complex. *J Clin Invest* 1990;86(1):25–31.

105. De Marco L, Mazzucato M, Masotti A, et al. Function of glycoprotein Ib alpha in platelet activation induced by alpha-thrombin. *J Biol Chem* 1991;266(35):23776–23783.

106. Ruggeri ZM. The platelet glycoprotein Ib-IX complex. *Prog Hemost Thromb* 1991;10(7):35–68.

107. De Marco L, Mazzucato M, Masotti A, et al. Localization and characterization of an alpha-thrombin-binding site on platelet glycoprotein Ib alpha. *J Biol Chem* 1994;269(9):6478–6484.

108. De Candia E, Hall SW, Rutella S, et al. Binding of thrombin to glycoprotein Ib accelerates the hydrolysis of par-1 on intact platelets. *J Biol Chem* 2001;276(7):4692–4698. Epub 2000 Nov 4617.

109. Celikel R, McClintock RA, Roberts JR, et al. Modulation of alpha-thrombin function by distinct interactions with platelet glycoprotein Ibalpha. *Science* 2003;301(5630):218–221.

110. Connolly AJ, Ishihara H, Kahn ML, et al. Role of the thrombin receptor in development and evidence for a second receptor. *Nature* 1996;381(6582):516–519.

111. Connolly TM, Condra C, Feng DM, et al. Species variability in platelet and other cellular responsiveness to thrombin receptor-derived peptides. *Thromb Haemost* 1994;72(4):627–633.

112. Derian CK, Santulli RJ, Tomko KA, et al. Species differences in platelet responses to thrombin and SFLLRN. Receptor-mediated calcium mobilization and aggregation and regulation by protein kinases. *Thromb Res* 1995;6:505–519.

113. Sambrano GR, Weiss EJ, Zheng YW, et al. Role of thrombin signalling in platelets in haemostasis and thrombosis. [Comment in: nature. 2001 sep 6;413(6851):26-7 UI: 21429411]. *Nature* 2001;413(6851):74–78.

114. Ramakrishnan V, Reeves PS, DeGuzman F, et al. Increased thrombin responsiveness in platelets from mice lacking glycoprotein V. *Proc Natl Acad Sci U S A* 1999;V96(N23):13336–13341.

115. Ramakrishnan V, DeGuzman F, Bao M, et al. A thrombin receptor function for platelet glycoprotein Ib-IX unmasked by cleavage of glycoprotein V. *Proc Natl Acad Sci U S A* 2001;98(4):1823–1828.

116. Hamilton JR, Cornelissen I, Coughlin SR. Impaired hemostasis and protection against thrombosis in protease-activated receptor 4-deficient mice is due to lack of thrombin signaling in platelets. *J Thromb Haemostas* 2004;8:1429–1435.

117. Nieswandt B, Watson SP. Platelet-collagen interaction: is GPVI the central receptor? *Blood* 2003;102(2):449–461. Epub 2003 Mar 2020.

118. Kunapuli SP, Dorsam RT, Kim S, et al. Platelet purinergic receptors. *Curr Opin Pharmacol* 2003;3(2):175–180.

119. Suh TT, Holmback K, Jensen NJ, et al. Resolution of spontaneous bleeding events but failure of pregnancy in fibrinogen-deficient mice. *Genes Dev* 1995;9(16):2020–2033.

120. Sun WY, Witte DP, Degen JL, et al. Prothrombin deficiency results in embryonic and neonatal lethality in mice. *Proc Natl Acad Sci U S A* 1998;95(13):7597–7602.

121. Xue J, Wu Q, Westfield LA, et al. Incomplete embryonic lethality and fatal neonatal hemorrhage caused by prothrombin deficiency in mice. *Proc Natl Acad Sci U S A* 1998;95(13):7603–7607.

122. Camerer E, Duong DN, Hamilton JR, et al. Combined deficiency of protease-activated receptor-4 and fibrinogen recapitulates the hemostatic defect but not the embryonic lethality of prothrombin deficiency. *Blood* 2004;103(1):152–154.

123. Carmeliet P, Mackman N, Moons L, et al. Role of tissue factor in embryonic blood vessel development. *Nature* 1996;383(6595):73–75.

124. Griffin CT, Srinivasan Y, Zheng YW, et al. A role for thrombin receptor signaling in endothelial cells during embryonic development. [Comment in: science. 2001 aug 31;293(5535):1602-4 UI: 21425318]. *Science* 2001; 293(5535):1666–1670.

125. Weiss EJ, Hamilton JR, Lease KE, et al. Protection against thrombosis in mice lacking PAR3. *Blood* 2002;100(9):3240–3244.

126. Shivdasani RA, Rosenblatt MF, Zucker-Franklin D, et al. Transcription factor NF-E2 is required for platelet formation independent of the actions of thrombopoietin/MGDF in megakaryocyte development. *Cell* 1995; 81(5):695–704.

127. Mann KG. Biochemistry and physiology of blood coagulation. *Thromb Haemost* 1999;82:165–174.

128. Tracy PB. Regulation of thrombin generation at cell surfaces. *Semin Thromb Hemost* 1988;14(3):227–233.

129. Reverter JC, Beguin S, Kessels H, et al. Inhibition of platelet-mediated, tissue factor-induced thrombin generation by the mouse/human chimeric 7E3 antibody. Potential implications for the effect of c7E3 fab treatment on acute thrombosis and "clinical restenosis." *J Clin Invest* 1996;98(3):863–874.

130. Cook JJ, Sitko GR, Bednar B, et al. An antibody against the exosite of the cloned thrombin receptor inhibits experimental arterial thrombosis in the african green monkey. *Circulation* 1995;91(12):2961–2971.

131. Zimmerman GA, Elstad MR, Lorant DE, et al. Platelet-activating factor (PAF): signalling and adhesion in cell-cell interactions. Adv Exp Med Biol 1996;416(3):297–304.

132. Johnson K, Choi Y, DeGroot E, et al. Potential mechanisms for a proinflammatory vascular cytokine response to coagulation activation. *J Immunol* 1998;160(10):5130–5135.

133. Ali H, Tomhave ED, Richardson RM, et al. Thrombin primes responsiveness of selective chemoattractant receptors at a site distal to G protein activation. *J Biol Chem* 1996;271(6):3200–3206.

134. Colotta F, Sciacca FL, Sironi M, et al. Expression of monocyte chemotactic protein-1 by monocytes and endothelial cells exposed to thrombin. *Am J Pathol* 1994;144(5):975–985.

135. Ueno A, Murakami K, Yamanouchi K, et al. Thrombin stimulates production of interleukin-8 in human umbilical vein endothelial cells. *Immunology* 1996;88(1):76–81.

136. Palabrica T, Lobb R, Furie BC, et al. Leukocyte accumulation promoting fibrin deposition is mediated *in vivo* by P-selectin on adherent platelets. *Nature* 1992;359(6398):848–851.

137. Garcia JG, Siflinger-Birnboim A, Bizios R, et al. Thrombin-induced increase in albumin permeability across the endothelium. *J Cell Physiol* 1986;128(1):96–104.

138. Lum H, Andersen TT, Siflinger-Birnboim A, et al. Thrombin receptor peptide inhibits thrombin-induced increase in endothelial permeability by receptor desensitization. *J Cell Biol* 1993;120(6):1491–1499.

139. Nystedt S, Ramakrishnan V, Sundelin J. The proteinase-activated receptor 2 is induced by inflammatory mediators in human endothelial cells. Comparison with the thrombin receptor. *J Biol Chem* 1996;271(25):14910–14915.

140. Esmon CT. Introduction: are natural anticoagulants candidates for modulating the inflammatory response to endotoxin? *Blood* 2000;95(4):1113–1116.

141. Inbal A, Kenet G, Zivelin A, et al. Purpura fulminans induced by disseminated intravascular coagulation following infection in 2 unrelated children with double heterozygosity for factor V Leiden and protein S deficiency. *Thromb Haemost* 1997;77(6):1086–1089.

142. Kataoka H, Hamilton JR, McKemy DD, et al. Protease-activated receptors 1 and 4 mediate thrombin signaling in endothelial cells. *Blood* 2003; 102(9):3224–3231.

143. Camerer E, Kataoka H, Kahn M, et al. Genetic evidence that protease-activated receptors mediate factor Xa signaling in endothelial cells. *J Biol Chem* 2002;277(18):16081–16087.

144. Uehara A, Sugawara S, Muramoto K, et al. Activation of human oral epithelial cells by neutrophil proteinase 3 through protease-activated receptor-2. *J Immunol* 2002;169(8):4594–4603.

145. Uehara A, Muramoto K, Takada H, et al. Neutrophil serine proteinases activate human nonepithelial cells to produce inflammatory cytokines through protease-activated receptor 2. *J Immunol* 2003;170(11):5690–5696.

146. Coughlin SR, Camerer E. PARticipation in inflammation. *J Clin Invest* 2003;111(1):25–27.

147. Cunningham MA, Rondeau E, Chen X, et al. Protease-activated receptor 1 mediates thrombin-dependent, cell-mediated renal inflammation in crescentic glomerulonephritis. *J Exp Med* 2000;191(3):455–462.

148. Cheung WM, D'Andrea MR, Andrade-Gordon P, et al. Altered vascular injury responses in mice deficient in protease-activated receptor-1. *Arterioscler Thromb Vasc Biol* 1999;19(12):3014–3024.

149. Andrade-Gordon P, Derian CK, Maryanoff BE, et al. Administration of a potent antagonist of protease-activated receptor-1 (PAR-1) attenuates vascular restenosis following balloon angioplasty in rats. *J Pharmacol Exp Ther* 2001;298(1):34–42.

150. Lindner JR, Kahn ML, Coughlin SR, et al. Delayed onset of inflammation in protease-activated receptor-2-deficient mice. *J Immunol* 2000;165(11): 6504–6510.

151. Ferrell WR, Lockhart JC, Kelso EB, et al. Essential role for proteinase activated receptor-2 in arthritis. *J Clin Invest* 2003;III:35–41

152. Kawagoe J, Takizawa T, Matsumoto J, et al. Effect of protease-activated receptor-2 deficiency on allergic dermatitis in the mouse ear. *Jpn J Pharmacol* 2002;88(1):77–84.

153. Seeliger S, Derian CK, Vergnolle N, et al. Proinflammatory role of proteinase-activated receptor-2 in humans and mice during cutaneous inflammation *in vivo*. *FASEB J* 2003;17(13):1871–1885.

154. Pawlinski R, Pedersen B, Schabbauer G, et al. Role of tissue factor and protease activated receptors in a mouse model of endotoxemia. *Blood* 2003;23:23.

155. Pawlinski R, Mackman N. Tissue factor, coagulation proteases, and protease-activated receptors in endotoxemia and sepsis. *Crit Care Med* 2004; 32(Suppl. 5):S293–S297.

156. Cheng T, Liu D, Griffin JH, et al. Activated protein C blocks p53-mediated apoptosis in ischemic human brain endothelium and is neuroprotective. *Nat Med* 2003;3:3.

157. Guo H, Liu D, Gelbard H, et al. Activated protein C prevents neuronal apoptosis via protease activated receptors 1 and 3. *Neuron* 2004;41(4): 563–572.

158. Junge CE, Sugawara T, Mannaioni G, et al. The contribution of protease-activated receptor 1 to neuronal damage caused by transient focal cerebral ischemia. *Proc Natl Acad Sci U S A* 2003;100(22):13019–13024.

159. Bugge TH, Xiao Q, Kombrinck KW, et al. Fatal embryonic bleeding events in mice lacking tissue factor, the cell-associated initiator of blood coagulation. *Proc Natl Acad Sci U S A* 1996;93(13):6258–6263.

160. Cui J, O'Shea KS, Purkayastha A, et al. Fatal hemorrhage and incomplete block to embryogenesis in mice lacking coagulation factor V. *Nature* 1996;384(6604):66–68.

161. Coughlin SR. Thrombin signalling and protease-activated receptors. *Nature* 2000;407(6801):258–264.

# CHAPTER 34 ■ PLATELET–COLLAGEN RECEPTORS

MARY M. ZUTTER AND SAMUEL A. SANTORO

Platelets circulate throughout the vasculature as single, nonadhesive cellular elements. Platelet activation can be initiated by numerous agonists, including thrombin, adenosine 5'-diphosphate (ADP), and, as will be discussed in this chapter, interaction with collagen within the vessel wall that is exposed following injury (1–5). Vessel wall injury or atherosclerotic plaque rupture disrupts the vascular endothelium, allowing circulating platelets to contact components of the extracellular matrix in the subendothelium and to adhere to the vessel wall.

The fibrillar collagens have, for some time now, been recognized as the most thrombogenic macromolecular constituents of the blood vessel wall (6). The collagens serve not only as substrates for platelet adhesion but also as potent initiators of platelet activation. The molecular mechanisms by which platelets adhere to sites of vascular injury have been delineated by extensive studies over the past 10 to 15 years (3–5). The paradigm that defines the process of platelet adhesion and thrombus formation is thought to be remarkably similar to the paradigm that defines emigration of lymphocytes, neutrophils, and monocytes to sites of inflammation (7). The multistep process of platelet adhesion and thrombus formation requires the sequential engagement of several distinct adhesion molecules with their receptors, as diagrammed in Figure 34-1. In step one, platelet tethering and rolling on activated endothelium or exposed subendothelium requires von Willebrand factor (VWF) and its major platelet surface receptor, the glycoprotein (GP) Ib/IX/V complex (8). In step two, firm adhesion to the collagen-rich subendothelial matrix is mediated by the $\alpha_2\beta_1$ integrin. However, see discussion in subsequent text about an alternative model that invokes an early role for GP VI. In step three, platelet activation and granule release is mediated predominantly by the GP VI/$F_c$ receptor $\gamma$ ($F_cR\gamma$). In step four, platelet aggregation and clot formation is subsequently mediated by the $\alpha_{IIb}\beta_3$ integrin (GP IIb/IIIa) and its principal ligand, fibrinogen (3–5). Therefore, two primary platelet surface receptors for collagens, the $\alpha_2\beta_1$ integrin and GP VI, play complementary and perhaps synergistic roles in the complex process of platelet adhesion to vessel wall collagens and subsequent thrombus formation.

## THE $\alpha_2\beta_1$ INTEGRIN AND PLATELET FUNCTION

The $\alpha_2\beta_1$ integrin serves as a cell surface receptor on many cell types for collagens and/or laminin as well as for several other nonmatrix ligands (10–14). Interactions between the $\alpha_2\beta_1$ integrin and the extracellular matrix have been implicated in a number of biologic and pathobiologic processes (10,11,15).

As noted previously, interactions of platelets with subendothelial collagens following vascular injury are required for effective hemostasis. Several studies have indicated that the $\alpha_2\beta_1$ integrin is a critical mediator of platelet adhesion to collagen (10,11,16–18). Four complementary approaches underlie the observations and experimental basis of this important conclusion.

The initial suggestion that the $\alpha_2\beta_1$ integrin might serve as a platelet surface collagen receptor came from the description by Nieuwenhuis et al. of a patient with a bleeding disorder (19,20). The patient's platelets showed no response to collagen but exhibited normal responsiveness to other platelet agonists. Electrophoretic analysis of the platelets revealed the deficiency of GP Ia ($\alpha_2$ integrin subunit). In addition, other patients with either reduced levels of platelet expression of the $\alpha_2\beta_1$ integrin or the presence of autoantibodies to the integrin have been reported to exhibit impaired platelet activation by collagen but not by other agonists (21–24).

Second, purified human platelets adhere to collagens I to VIII via an $\alpha_2\beta_1$ integrin–dependent mechanism that requires $Mg^{2+}$ (25). Adhesion is inhibited by inhibitory monoclonal antibodies directed against the $\alpha_2\beta_1$ integrin (26,27). Effective inhibition of platelet deposition onto collagen substrates under both static and flow conditions in either platelet-rich plasma or whole blood demonstrates the importance of the $\alpha_2\beta_1$ integrin for platelet deposition onto collagen substrates under physiologic conditions (15).

Third, purified $\alpha_2\beta_1$ integrin incorporated into liposomes binds to collagen substrates in a $Mg^{2+}$-dependent manner and exhibits the same collagen-type specificity as intact platelets (17). The $\alpha_2\beta_1$ integrin–containing liposomes do not adhere to any other of several extracellular matrix proteins, confirming the specificity of collagen adhesion via the $\alpha_2\beta_1$ integrin platelet receptor.

Fourth, the development of mice deficient in the $\alpha_2\beta_1$ integrin (15,28) has extended and verified many of the concepts regarding $\alpha_2\beta_1$ integrin and platelet function but challenged others (29,30). As discussed in greater detail in subsequent text, we have reported that the integrin-deficient mice clearly exhibit impaired adhesion to collagen substrates, especially under conditions of shear, and reveal a marked decrement in thrombus formation *in vivo* following arterial injury (31). Somewhat surprisingly, the $\alpha_2\beta_1$ integrin–deficient mice exhibit only a modest defect in collagen-induced platelet aggregation in the aggregometer under the standard low/no shear conditions (15).

---

### Structure of the $\alpha_2\beta_1$ Integrin

The integrins are a family of heterodimeric adhesive receptors that play important roles in mediating the cell–substrate and cell–cell interactions of many different cell types, including platelets. Several excellent general reviews are available (32–35).

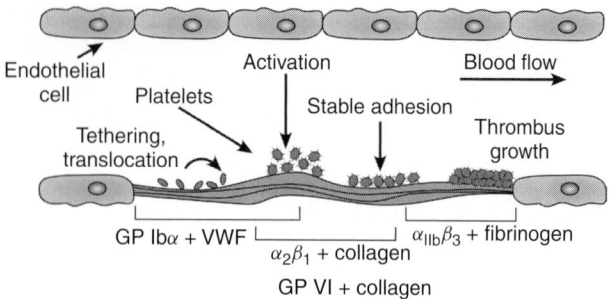

**FIGURE 34-1.** The multistep process of platelet adhesion to a collagenous substrate. Crucial steps include tethering, firm adhesion, activation, and thrombus formation. See text for details of the roles of the two collagen receptors, the $\alpha_2\beta_1$ integrin and glycoprotein (GP) VI (9). VWF, von Willebrand factor. (Adapted from McEver RP. P selectin/PSGL-1 and other interactions between platelets, leukocytes, and endothelium. In: Michelson AD, ed. *Platelets*. San Diego, CA: Academic Press, 2002:139–155.)

Structurally, integrins are composed of noncovalently associated, type I transmembrane $\alpha$ and $\beta$ subunits (36). At least 18 different $\alpha$ subunits and eight different $\beta$ subunits have been defined, resulting in the formation of at least 24 distinct heterodimers that have been identified in humans. Ligand specificity is a function of particular $\alpha/\beta$ combinations. Great redundancy is inherent in the system and other factors such as alternative splicing and the degree of integrin activation may contribute to ligand-binding specificity (36). The $\alpha_2\beta_1$ integrin is identical to the platelet membrane GP Ia/IIa complex, the very late activation antigen-2 (VLA-2) complex described on activated T cells, and the class II extracellular matrix receptor (ECMR II) defined on fibroblasts. It has also been designated CD49b/CD29 (37).

## The $\beta_1$ Subunit

The amino acid sequence of the $\beta_1$ subunit has been deduced from the corresponding cDNA sequence (38). The $\beta_1$ integrin subunit consists of a large extracellular domain, a transmembrane domain, and a short cytoplasmic domain. The large extracellular domain contains 56 conserved cysteine residues, 31 of which are clustered into four tandemly repeated segments, each of which is believed to contain a large number of internal disulfide bonds. The amino-terminal 45- to 50-kDa region contains within it several other regions of highly conserved sequence that are shared with other $\beta$ subunits. These regions, in association with the $\alpha$ subunit, may contribute to ligand-binding activity. The $\beta_1$ integrin hydrophobic transmembrane domain is of sufficient length to span the plasma membrane a single time. The $\beta_1$ subunit has a short cytoplasmic domain composed of the 40 or so most carboxy-terminal amino acid residues (38).

Takada et al. (39) have shown that mutation of the D130 residue in the extracellular domain of the $\beta_1$ integrin subunit results in loss of ligand binding of the $\alpha_2\beta_1$ integrin The D130 of the $\beta_1$ subunit is part of the sequence DXSXS that is conserved in all known integrin $\beta$ subunits. The DXSXS sequence is adjacent to the site of RGD cross-linking determined in $\beta_3$ integrins. Mutation of the homologous D119, S121, or S123 residues of the $\beta_3$ integrin subunit abolishes fibrinogen and RGD peptide binding to the $\alpha_{IIb}\beta_3$ integrin.

The extracellular domain of the $\beta_1$ subunit also contains the epitope recognized by activating monoclonal antibodies. Binding of activating antibodies to $\beta_1$ integrins enhances the ligand-binding activity of the integrin, presumably by either inducing or stabilizing as a consequence of antibody-binding changes in integrin conformation normally induced by inside-out signaling during the process of integrin and/or cellular activation. Somewhat surprisingly, the epitope recognized by these activating antibodies has been mapped to the same small region of the $\beta_1$ subunit, residues 207 to 218, recognized by monoclonal antibodies that inhibit ligand binding (40). The sequence is thought to exist as a bend structure lying between two sites implicated in ligand binding, residues 120 to 182 and 220 to 231. Takada and Puzon (40) have suggested that activating antibodies might fix the flexible turn in a conformation that facilitates ligand binding, whereas inhibitory antibodies fix the turn in a conformation that precludes ligand binding.

The $\beta_1$ cytoplasmic domain is subject to alternative splicing (41,42). One form of alternative splicing retains an intron located between the last two exons of the $\beta_1$ gene (41). The presence of a stop codon near the 5' end of this intron results in truncation of the $\beta_1$ cytoplasmic domain in this variant. Languino et al. (42) described a second alternatively spliced $\beta_1$ cytoplasmic domain. The variant, which they denoted as $\beta_{1s}$, is generated by the addition of a 116 base pair sequence between the two exons encoding the cytoplasmic domain. Although $\beta_{1s}$ mRNA represented only a minor fraction of total $\beta_1$ mRNA present, platelets were an exceptionally rich source of $\beta_{1s}$ mRNA. No data are yet available regarding the expression of $\beta_{1s}$ protein in platelets. The functional significance of the alternatively spliced $\beta_{1s}$ subunit cytoplasmic domain in platelet biology is, at present, unknown.

The cytoplasmic domain of the $\beta_1$ integrin subunit appears largely responsible for mediating the interactions of $\beta_1$-containing integrins with the actin cytoskeleton via interactions with other cytoskeletal components such as $\alpha$-actinin and talin (43). The regulation of integrin-cytoskeleton interactions is a focus of much current research. The extent of interaction of the $\alpha_2\beta_1$ integrin with the platelet cytoskeleton and the potential role of these cytoskeletal interactions in collagen-dependent signaling events are not clear. Kieffer et al. (44) concluded from their immunoelectron microscopic studies that platelet $\alpha_2\beta_1$ integrin was not associated with the cytoskeleton and did not cluster. This conclusion differs from the earlier report of Fox (45,46), who concluded that 50% of GP Ia (the $\alpha_2$ subunit) was associated with the platelet cytoskeleton. However, Fox's identification of the GP Ia subunit was based solely upon electrophoretic mobility. Subsequent studies by others have revealed that two polypeptides denoted Ia and Ia* exhibit identical electrophoretic mobilities (even in two-dimensional systems) and that Ia*, but not Ia, is associated with the cytoskeleton in activated platelets (47).

## The $\alpha_2$ Subunit

The amino acid sequence of the integrin $\alpha_2$ subunit has also been deduced from cDNA sequence (48). The $\alpha_2$ subunit exhibits molecular weights of 165 and 160 kDa under reducing and nonreducing conditions, respectively. The $\alpha_2$ chain and all other integrin $\alpha$ subunits share common structural features, including a large extracellular domain, a single hydrophobic membrane-spanning transmembrane domain, and a short cytoplasmic domain. Although some $\alpha$ subunits are cleaved posttranslationally to yield heavy- and light-chain components linked by a disulfide bond, the $\alpha_2$ subunit does not undergo such a posttranslational cleavage.

The $\alpha_2$ integrin subunit contains an additional segment of 191 amino acids inserted before the last five of the homologous repeats containing the divalent cation binding domains (48). Nine of the identified integrin $\alpha$ subunits have an inserted, or I-domain, near the amino-terminus of the protein. A variety of evidence, including mapping of function-blocking antibody epitopes, loss of function mutations, and expression of recombinant I-domains, have shown that I-domains are the major ligand-binding sites in integrins that contain I-domains (49–52). The I-domains are homologous to the collagen-binding A-domains of VWF and cartilage matrix protein and to domains within the complement factors B and C2 (53).

Binding of ligand to integrins requires divalent cations (49). The I-domains contain a metal-dependent adhesion site, or metal ion-dependent adhesion site (MIDAS) motif, that binds the divalent cation required for binding of ligand (49). Like the full-length integrin, recombinant I-domains bind to ligand in a divalent cation–dependent manner, and mutation of the MIDAS motif abolishes ligand binding (54). Cocrystal structures of the $\alpha_M$, $\alpha_L$, and $\alpha_2$ integrin I-domains with a ligand or ligand mimetic show that a negatively charged carboxylic oxygen in the ligand provides the final coordination site of the divalent cation bound to the MIDAS motif (50–52,55). Interestingly, although $Mg^{2+}$ and $Mn^{2+}$ have been shown to support the binding of ligand to both the integrin and the I-domain, $Ca^{2+}$ does not support the binding of the I-domain to ligand and, in fact, inhibits binding of full-length integrin to ligand but not the ligand to the I-domain (44).

The $\alpha_M$, $\alpha_L$, $\alpha_1$, and $\alpha_2$ integrin I-domains have been crystallized (50–52,55,56). The three-dimensional structures of these four I-domains are very similar. Each adopts the dinucleotide binding or Rossman fold, consisting of a core of largely parallel $\beta$-sheet structure surrounded by several $\alpha$ helices. All four contain the MIDAS motif in a crevice near the top of the $\beta$-sheet. Unique to the structure of the $\alpha_1$ and $\alpha_2$ integrin I-domains, however, is the addition of a short $\alpha C$ helix near the top of the domain in close proximity to the divalent cation-binding site (49–52). Sequence alignments indicate that the $\alpha C$ helix is also present in the $\alpha_{10}$ and $\alpha_{11}$ integrin I-domains, which are also collagen receptors, but is not found in the other $\alpha$ subunit integrin I-domains (49,57,58). Removal of the $\alpha C$ helix of the $\alpha_2$ integrin I-domain has been reported to increase nonspecific binding to collagen, which suggests that the $\alpha C$ helix evolved to minimize nonspecific binding to collagens (59).

Interestingly, both the $\alpha_2$ and $\alpha_M$ subunit I-domains have been crystallized in two conformations: the open conformation and the closed conformation (see Fig. 34-2) (50–52). The binding site is occupied in the $\alpha_2$ and $\alpha_M$ integrin I-domain open conformations, whereas the binding site is empty in the $\alpha_2$ and $\alpha_M$ integrin I-domain closed conformations. Therefore, it has been hypothesized that the open conformation represents the high-affinity, ligand-binding conformation and that the closed conformation represents the low-affinity, non–ligand-binding conformation. Recent experiments with the $\alpha_L$ integrin I-domain suggest that this hypothesis may be correct; mutant $\alpha_L$ integrin locked into the closed conformation had low affinity for ligand (60). In addition, computer modeling of the $\alpha_M$ integrin I-domain suggested that the closed conformation is the lower energy form, so that conversion to the high-affinity, open conformation requires an input of energy (61). It remains an open question whether this conformational change is induced by ligand binding or whether integrins can adopt the high-affinity, open conformation prior to ligand binding.

As mentioned earlier, cells can regulate the binding activity of integrins on the cell surface, and it has been hypothesized that a change in the integrin conformation could produce a change in affinity (62). Because the I-domain has been shown to be the ligand-binding site for integrins that contain them, integrin activation could result from a conformational change of the $\alpha_2$ integrin I-domain from the non–ligand-binding, closed conformation to the ligand-binding, open conformation. In the conformational change from closed to open, the $\alpha_2$ integrin I-domain makes three major movements: The chelation of the divalent cation in the MIDAS motif is altered, the $\alpha C$ helix is reorganized, and the $\alpha_7$ helix makes a large "slinking" motion as it rotates and drops down the body of the integrin (50–52). The changes that the $\alpha_M$ integrin I-domain makes in the conversion from the closed conformation to the open conformation are very similar to those of the $\alpha_2$ integrin I-domain; indeed, plotting the $\alpha C$ positions of these integrins demonstrates that the backbone of the I-domains are almost identical in both conformations (50). It has been hypothesized that the conversion from the closed to the open conformation promotes ligand binding by reorganizing MIDAS motif residues that chelate the divalent cation, making the $Mg^{2+}$ ion more electrophilic (50–52). The structural rearrangements of the MIDAS motif are coupled to backbone movements of the loops that bear the coordinating residues (50–52).

Although the amino acid residues just inside the plasma membrane (GFFKR) are highly conserved among all integrin $\alpha$ chains, the remainder of the cytoplasmic domains differ considerably in sequence. It has been shown that the cytoplasmic domain of the $\alpha_2$ integrin subunit makes significant contributions to postreceptor occupancy events such as collagen gel contraction and cell motility (63,64). In an analysis of chimeric integrin molecules created by replacing the cytoplasmic domain of the $\alpha_2$ integrin with cytoplasmic domains of the $\alpha_4$ and $\alpha_5$ integrins, Chan et al. (63) observed that integrins expressing each of the three cytoplasmic domains were expressed to similar extents in association with the $\beta_1$ subunit and effectively mediated cell attachment to collagen and laminin. The $\alpha_2$ and $\alpha_5$ cytoplasmic domains supported collagen gel contraction, whereas the $\alpha_4$ cytoplasmic domain conferred increased motility on collagen and laminin substrates. Truncation of the $\alpha_2$ cytoplasmic domain just beyond the conserved GFFKR motif resulted in complete loss of constitutive $\alpha_2\beta_1$ ligand-binding activity (65,66). Deletion of the cytoplasmic tail also eliminated activation of adhesive function in response to phorbol esters. Full activity could be restored by adding back five to seven amino acid residues beyond the GFFKR sequence. Despite these clues from studies of other cell types, the role of the $\alpha_2$ cytoplasmic domain in platelet biology is uncertain.

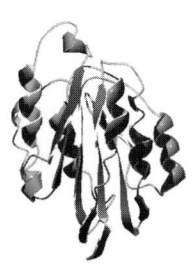
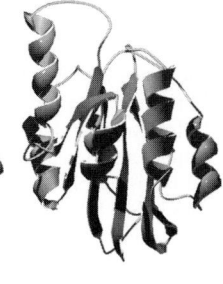

Closed         Open

**Movements**

1. Unwinding of $\alpha C$ into $\alpha_6$

2. Downward movement of $\alpha_7$

3. Movement of metal ion and associated loops

**FIGURE 34-2.** The transition from the closed, lower-affinity state to the open, higher-affinity state of the $\alpha_2$ integrin I-domain is illustrated.

# THE GP VI/F$_c$R$\gamma$ COMPLEX AND PLATELET FUNCTION

The GP VI/F$_c$R$\gamma$ complex constitutes the second major collagen receptor on platelets. GP VI was first identified on the surface of platelets in 1982 (67). A functional role for the receptor was initially indicated by a patient with autoimmune thrombocytopenia who presented with a defective response to collagen and who had autoantibodies to GP VI (68,69). Her antibodies were used to identify the target protein as GP VI on two-dimensional gel electrophoresis. The antibody has since been used to identify other patients lacking GP VI on their platelets (70). Patients lacking platelet GP VI present with a mild bleeding diathesis, moderately prolonged bleeding times, and defective collagen-induced platelet aggregation (68,69). Patients deficient in GP VI exhibit only modest defects in platelet adhesion to collagen. Severe bleeding complications due to deficiency of GP VI have not been reported. It is now apparent that GP VI is present on the platelet surface not as a single polypeptide but in complex with the F$_c$R$\gamma$ subunit (71,72).

## Structure of the GP VI/F$_c$R$\gamma$ Complex

GP VI, a 60- to 65-kDa platelet GP, is a member of the immunoglobulin Ig superfamily (73). The Ig superfamily represents a very large family of proteins with diverse function and one or more Ig-like domains as the basic building block (74). The relation of GP VI to other members of the Ig superfamily was established by Clemetson et al. by comparison with other amino acid sequences in the database (73). The GP VI sequence resembles most closely the sequence of the F$_c\alpha$ receptor and receptors on natural killer (NK) cells called *killer cell Ig-like receptors* (73,75,76). The extracellular domain consists of two Ig C2 domains connected by disulfide bridges that extend from the membrane by a mucinlike stalk rich in threonine and serine residues (73,75,76). The extracellular domain is followed by a transmembrane domain and a cytoplasmic tail that has no homology to other known Ig superfamily members. The transmembrane and cytoplasmic domains of GP VI are critical for its signaling role because these two domains mediate associations with adaptor molecules. Both the transmembrane domain and the cytoplasmic tail are required for the F$_c$R$\gamma$–GP VI interaction (77–80). GP VI noncovalently, but constitutively, associates with the F$_c$R$\gamma$ chain, forming a multimeric signaling complex (71,72). The F$_c$R$\gamma$ contains an immunoreceptor type activation motif (ITAM), which is phosphorylated by a Src family kinase, either Fyn or Lyn, following platelet adhesion to collagen. Phosphorylation and activation of the ITAM of the F$_c$R$\gamma$ following GP VI binding to collagens or collagen mimetics is required for platelet activation, granule release, and ultimate platelet aggregation (reviewed in reference 28).

# THE TWO-STEP, TWO-SITE MODEL OF COLLAGEN-INDUCED PLATELET ACTIVATION

We now understand that platelet adhesion to collagen is complex and that the process involves at least two collagen receptors on platelets. The results of a series of *in vitro* and *in vivo* studies have suggested a two-step, two-site model of collagen-induced platelet activation (27,81,82). In the original version of this model, first proposed by us, the $\alpha_2\beta_1$ integrin

supports the initial rapid platelet–collagen interaction that mediates platelet adhesion to the vessel wall under conditions of flow. This allows a second low-affinity signal transducing receptor to engage collagen and mediate collagen-induced platelet activation and aggregation. Studies by several groups indicate that the GP VI/F$_c$R$\gamma$ complex serves as the signal transducing coreceptor (73,82–85). In this model, the $\alpha_2\beta_1$ integrin mediates strong adhesion but does not contribute the necessary or sufficient signals to support platelet activation. Although this model has been of considerable utility in guiding studies since it was first proposed by us approximately 12 years ago, it may not be entirely correct. Recently, a somewhat revised version of the two-step, two-site model has been proposed. In the revised model, GP VI ligation precedes that of the integrin and is essential for activation of the integrin for stable adhesion (15,29).

The signaling pathways downstream of GP VI that lead to platelet activation have been extensively studied (29). GP VI is often activated by mimetics such as collagen-related peptide or snake venoms such as convulxin that bind GP VI but not the $\alpha_2\beta_1$ integrin (29,81). Ligation of GP VI with collagen, collagen-related peptide, or cross-linking by antibody signals activation (85). The ITAM domain of F$_c$R$\gamma$ is phosphorylated by a Src family kinase, either Fyn or Lyn, following platelet adhesion to collagen. Phosphorylation of the ITAM of the F$_c$R$\gamma$ stimulates recruitment and activation of Syk. Syk phosphorylation initiates a signaling cascade involving LAT-Gads-SLP-76 [Src homology 2 (SH2) domain–containing leukocyte protein of 76 kDa], leading to downstream activation of PI3K and phospholipase C$\gamma_2$ (PLC$\gamma_2$), and ultimate granule release, activation of the $\alpha_{IIb}\beta_3$ integrin via inside-out signaling, and platelet aggregation. Conclusions from some of these studies, at least those involving convulxin, have been confounded somewhat by the recent report that convulxin also binds and signals via the GP Ib/IX/V complex (86).

# DOES THE $\alpha_2\beta_1$ INTEGRIN PROVIDE A DISCRETE SUBSET OF SIGNALS FOLLOWING PLATELET ADHESION TO COLLAGEN?

Studies using intact collagen, snake venom, GP VI–deficient platelets, and/or inhibitory monoclonal antibodies suggest that the $\alpha_2\beta_1$ integrin may play a role independent of GP VI in mediating signals downstream of platelet adhesion to collagen. Collagen-induced phosphorylation of PLC$\gamma_2$ and Syk is inhibited by antibodies that block $\alpha_2\beta_1$ integrin–mediated platelet adhesion to collagen and by jararhagin, a snake venom that selectively cleaves the $\beta_1$ integrin subunit of the $\alpha_2\beta_1$ integrin (87,88). Furthermore, phosphorylation of PLC$\gamma_2$ and Syk is maintained in platelets from F$_c$R$\gamma$-deficient mice and patients with GP VI deficiency (84,89). In other studies, collagen-induced phosphorylation of c-Src is also maintained in GP VI–deficient human platelets (90). Recent studies using the snake venom rhodocytin demonstrate that Src and Lyn constitutively associate with the $\alpha_2\beta_1$ integrin and that Src kinase activity increases following rhodocytin stimulation of platelets (91). Src activation, presumably via the $\alpha_2\beta_1$ integrin, is accompanied by activation of the p130 Crk-associated substrate (Cas) (91). Additional signaling cascades are initiated via the $\alpha_2\beta_1$ integrin following platelet adhesion to collagen under flow conditions. Platelet adhesion to collagen under flow conditions results in rapid tyrosine phosphorylation of pp125 focal adhesion kinase (FAK) (92,93). Other evidence that the $\alpha_2\beta_1$ integrin mediates signals distinct from GP VI comes from a comparison of signals initiated by collagen or the GP VI mimetics. Platelet adhesion to intact collagen stimulates a different response than platelet adhesion to GP VI mimetics. It therefore appears that the $\alpha_2\beta_1$ integrin provides discreet signals independent of the GP VI/$F_cR\gamma$. Although the role that signals downstream of $\alpha_2\beta_1$ integrin ligation play in platelet aggregation remains controversial, signals downstream of $\alpha_2\beta_1$ integrin ligation have been well elucidated and shown to be of biologic significance in other cell types (10,11,65,66,94).

# PLATELET SURFACE COLLAGEN RECEPTORS AND VASCULAR DISEASE

Kunicki et al. (21,22) demonstrated that $\alpha_2\beta_1$ integrin density on the platelet surface varies among healthy individuals and correlates with platelet adhesiveness to Type I collagen (26). They went on to show that the level of platelet surface expression of the $\alpha_2\beta_1$ integrin is associated with the presence of several linked polymorphisms within the $\alpha_2$ integrin gene (21,95). The sequence variants include two silent polymorphisms at nucleotide 807 (T or C) and nucleotide 873 (A or G). The 807C/873G pair is associated with a lower level of $\alpha_2\beta_1$ integrin expression than is the 807T/873A pair. Several, but by no means all, epidemiologic studies suggest that high-level expression of the $\alpha_2\beta_1$ integrin on platelets is an independent risk factor for nonfatal myocardial infarction, the development of diabetic retinopathy in individuals with type II diabetes, and stroke in the young (<50 years) (96–101). The relative risk conveyed by high-level receptor expression for myocardial infarction appeared to be increased by the presence of obesity or a smoking history. Conversely, on the basis of experiments with the platelet function an alyzer-100 (PFA-100) surrogate bleeding time device, it has been suggested that lower levels of platelet surface $\alpha_2\beta_1$ integrin expression exacerbate the bleeding diathesis of mild von Willebrand disease (102). The potential cause-and-effect relation between the level of $\alpha_2\beta_1$ integrin expression and vascular diseases suggested by these intriguing findings needs to be validated and further explored by animal studies in order to definitively establish causality.

The clinically important HPA-5a/b (Zav$^b$, Br$^b$, Zav$^a$, Br$^a$, Hc$^a$) platelet alloantigen system resides on the $\alpha_2$ integrin subunit. Alloimmunization against these antigens has been implicated in refractoriness to platelet transfusion, neonatal alloimmune thrombocytopenia, and posttransfusion purpura (103–108). The gene frequencies for the HPA-5a and b alleles are 0.889 and 0.111, respectively, in the Caucasian population (109). The antigen system is a consequence of an A↔G polymorphism at base 1,648, which results in a lysine residue (AAG) in Br$^a$ human platelet antigens-5b (HPA-5b) or a glutamic acid residue glycosaminoglycan (GAG) in Br$^b$ (HPA-5a) at amino acid position 505 located between the first and second divalent cation–binding domains (110). Neither the polymorphism nor antibodies directed against it have been associated with altered $\alpha_2\beta_1$ function.

At least nine polymorphisms have been observed within the coding region of the human GP VI gene (111,112). Additional polymorphisms are also present within regions upstream of the translational start site. Unlike the situation described earlier for the $\alpha_2$ integrin polymorphisms, none of the GP VI gene polymorphisms has been associated with altered levels of GP VI expression (113). It is possible that one or more of the GP VI polymorphisms may exhibit an association with hemorrhagic, thrombotic, or other cardiovascular disease states (113,114). Some early data suggests an association of the GP VI 13,254 CC genotype with increased risk for myocardial infarction, particularly among older women (111,115).

# PLATELET RECEPTOR-DEFICIENT MOUSE MODELS

In recent years, genetic deletion in mice of many of the platelet and vascular cell integrin and nonintegrin receptor subunits has been accomplished (116,117). The resulting animal models have allowed the biology of the receptors to be explored experimentally, especially in the in vivo setting, in ways that are unapproachable with human material. This section discusses how studies with GP VI–null, $\alpha_2\beta_1$-null, and $F_cR\gamma$-null mice have defined the independent and cooperative roles of the $\alpha_2\beta_1$ integrin and the GP VI/$F_cR\gamma$ complex in platelet biology and addressed unresolved issues regarding the role of the two receptors in platelet adhesion, activation, signaling, and vascular pathobiology.

## $\alpha_2\beta_1$ Integrin-Deficient Mouse Models

The relative roles of the $\alpha_2\beta_1$ integrin and the GP VI/$F_cR\gamma$ chain complex, another platelet-collagen receptor, in platelet adhesion, platelet activation, and aggregation have been intensely debated (3–5,21,22,31). To better define the role of the $\alpha_2\beta_1$ integrin in vivo, we developed a genetically engineered mouse in which expression of the $\alpha_2\beta_1$ integrin was completely eliminated (15,28). Mice deficient in the $\alpha_2\beta_1$ integrin are viable and fertile and develop normally. The $\alpha_2$-deficient mice exhibit no obvious bleeding tendency (15,28). Platelets from $\alpha_2\beta_1$-deficient mice exhibit markedly impaired adhesion to collagen substrates under either static or flow conditions, yet they exhibit only mildly impaired collagen-induced platelet aggregation (4).

These results differed in some ways from those of Holtkotter et al. (28) Since their initial in vitro studies of platelet adhesion and aggregation using $\alpha_2\beta_1$-deficient platelets under flow conditions in whole blood failed to show a collagen-binding defect, they concluded that the $\alpha_2\beta_1$ integrin was not required for platelet adhesion to collagen under flow conditions (118). However, Kuijhers et al. (30) more recently reported that $\alpha_2\beta_1$-null platelets are, in fact, less adhesive to collagen and form loose platelet aggregates under flow conditions in vitro. All studies reported thus far are in accord that the $\alpha_2\beta_1$ integrin is not essential for platelet aggregation as measured in vitro.

Several factors likely contribute to the observed differences in the role of the $\alpha_2\beta_1$ integrin in the two models. First, it is likely that firm adhesion to collagen in the presence of shear requires the $\alpha_2\beta_1$ integrin. This role of the integrin would be analogous to the role of the leukocyte integrins in the leukocyte adhesion to the vascular endothelium under conditions of flow. Second, the unique signals identified by Inoue et al. (119) that are induced by ligation of the $\alpha_2\beta_1$ integrin with solid-phase collagen but not by fluid-phase collagen may be essential for the development of a thrombus resistant to shear at the blood vessel wall interface. Third, whereas some signals emanating from $\alpha_2\beta_1$ integrin ligation are independent of those emanating from the GP VI/$F_cR\gamma$ complex, others, such as the tyrosine phosphorylation of Src, Syk, and PLC$\gamma_2$, are derived from both receptors (89). It seems likely that stable thrombus formation at the blood vessel wall interface requires a more complete activation of these pathways that is dependent upon the presence and engagement of the $\alpha_2\beta_1$ integrin.

To explore the in vivo role of the $\alpha_2\beta_1$ integrin in acute thrombosis at the site of vascular injury, we utilized a model of carotid artery occlusion (31,120–122). Mice were subjected to photochemical injury (the rose bengal dye laser injury model) of the right common carotid artery. Carotid artery blood flow was monitored continuously throughout the experiment via a

Doppler flow probe. The length of time to complete arterial occlusion following injury was $47 \pm 9$ (mean $\pm$ SD) minutes in the wild-type littermates. In contrast, the time to arterial occlusion was $74 \pm 20$ minutes for the homozygous $\alpha_2$-deficient animals. The $\alpha_2$-deficient animals required almost twice the length of time to completely occlude the carotid artery following injury, a large and statistically significant difference.

This experimental result is consistent with the previously demonstrated correlation between high-level $\alpha_2\beta_1$ integrin expression and an increased risk for thrombosis involving coronary and cerebral vessels (21,95–97). On the basis of some epidemiologic data, we expected to observe a gene dosage effect in mice heterozygous for $\alpha_2\beta_1$ integrin deficiency. The time to occlusion was not different from the time to complete occlusion observed in the wild-type mice. Therefore, complete deficiency of the integrin was required for prolongation of the occlusion time following injury. Only homozygous deficient animals were protected. These results are in line with the studies of Moshfegh et al. They reported that homozygosity, but not heterozygosity, for the 807T/873A genotype was an independent risk factor for acute myocardial infarction (100). These findings suggest that if pharmacologic inhibition of the $\alpha_2\beta_1$ integrin is to be exploited clinically, a high degree of inhibition will be required for efficacy.

The role of the $\alpha_2\beta_1$ integrin was also evaluated in a mouse model in which pulmonary embolism was induced by the intravenous injection of collagen. Baseline platelet counts were similar in wild-type ($719 \pm 124 \times 103$ per $\mu L$) and $\alpha_2$ integrin–deficient ($735 \pm 144 \times 103$ per $\mu L$) mice. The jugular vein of wild-type or $\alpha_2$-null mice was injected with either saline or saline containing fibrillar collagen ($25\ \mu g$) and epinephrine ($1\ \mu g$). The absolute decrements in platelet count from baseline following injection of collagen (or saline) were similar between the $\alpha_2$-deficient mice and the wild-type littermate controls ($P > 0.05$). The numbers of intravascular thrombi in the lungs of wild-type and $\alpha_2$ integrin–deficient mice were not statistically different ($P > 0.5$) Although $\alpha_2\beta_1$ integrin deficiency did not protect mice from lethal pulmonary emboli, mice deficient in the $F_cR\gamma$ subunit of the GP VI/$F_cR\gamma$ were completely protected from collagen-induced formation of pulmonary emboli (31).

These studies suggest distinctly different roles for the $\alpha_2\beta_1$ integrin and GP VI/$F_cR\gamma$, the two platelet surface collagen receptors, in different models of *in vivo* thrombus formation. The carotid artery injury model in which the initial platelet–collagen interactions take place with collagen in the solid phase in the presence of shear forces at the flowing blood vessel wall interface revealed an obligatory role for the $\alpha_2\beta_1$ integrin. In contrast, in the model of pulmonary embolus formation following intravascular injection of collagen where the initial encounters of platelets with collagen occurred in suspension and in the absence of shear in a manner rather analogous to the conditions of collagen-induced platelet aggregation *in vitro*, no dependence upon the $\alpha_2\beta_1$ integrin was observed. As in the *in vitro* determination of collagen-induced platelet aggregation, GP VI was required. In the pulmonary embolism model, significant shear forces are encountered only after platelet aggregate formation is complete at the time thrombi lodge in the pulmonary vasculature.

Because the epidemiology data based on $\alpha_2$ integrin polymorphisms suggested an association between surface density of the $\alpha_2\beta_1$ integrin and the risk of thrombotic diseases such as myocardial infarction and stroke in the young, well-established complications of atherosclerosis, the contribution of the $\alpha_2\beta_1$ integrin to the development of atherosclerosis was tested using the well-defined mouse apoE model (123). After either 6 or 15 weeks on a high-cholesterol, atherogenic diet, there were no significant differences in the atherogenic lesions between the $\alpha_2$-null

animals and the wild-type animals (123). These results suggest that risk for arterial thrombotic disease associated with high-level $\alpha_2\beta_1$ integrin expression is not due to enhanced development of atherosclerosis *per se* but may rather be a consequence of thrombotic complications at the plaques.

## The GP VI–Deficient Mouse Models

The initial report of a mouse model involving deletion GP VI has only recently appeared (124). Mice deficient in GP VI are viable and fertile, and exhibit normal bleeding times, but GP VI–deficient platelets do not aggregate in response to collagen or GP VI mimetics (124). Interestingly, although the GP VI-deficient platelets did not form aggregates when perfused over a collagen surface under conditions of flow, they did form an adherent monolayer. Kato et al. (124) attributed the adhesion solely to VWF. However, that interpretation is not consistent with the marked impairment of monolayer formation that we observed with $\alpha_2\beta_1$–null platelets under flow. The relative roles of the two receptors are still to be clarified. Animals in which the common $\gamma$-chain subunit, a subunit of the $F_cR\gamma$ signaling GP VI coreceptor as well as a component of the high-affinity receptor for IgE, the low-affinity receptor for IgG and associated with the high-affinity receptor for IgG have been more extensively evaluated (84,85). These mice, which not only lack the GP VI/$F_cR\gamma$ coreceptor but also lack $F_c\varepsilon R\gamma I$, $F_c\gamma FIII$, and $F_c\gamma RI$, are immunodeficient with abnormalities in macrophage, NK cell, mast cell, and B cell function, but fail to manifest a bleeding diathesis. Abnormalities observed with $F_cR\gamma$-deficient platelets include defective secretion, platelet activation, and aggregation in response to collagen or GP VI mimetics. Bleeding and platelet function abnormalities are much less severe in $F_cR\gamma$-null mice than in mice lacking several of the downstream adaptor/signaling molecules such as SLP76 or PLC$\gamma$2. These data suggest that other collagen receptors in addition to GP VI/$F_cR\gamma$ also contribute to collagen-induced signals. We hypothesize that the other receptor contributing to signaling is the $\alpha_2\beta_1$ integrin (19).

## References

1. Shattil SJ, Ginsberg MH, Brugge JS. Adhesive signaling in platelets. *Curr Opin Cell Biol* 1994;6:695–704.
2. Shattil SJ, Newman PJ. Integrins: dynamic scaffolds for adhesion and signaling in platelets. *Blood* 2004;104:1606–1615.
3. Farndale RW, Siljander PR, Onley DJ, et al. Collagen-platelet interactions: recognition and signalling. *Biochem Soc Symp* 2003;70:81–94.
4. Prevost N, Woulfe D, Tognolini M, et al. Contact-dependent signaling during the late events of platelet activation. *J Thromb Haemost* 2003;1: 1613–1627.
5. Jackson SP, Nesbitt WS, Kulkarni S. Signaling events underlying thrombus formation. *J Thromb Haemost* 2003;1:1602–1612.
6. Baumgartner HR. Platelet interaction with collagen fibrils in flowing blood. I. Reaction of human platelets with alpha chymotrypsin-digested subendothelium. *Thromb Haemost* 1977;37:1–16.
7. Springer TA. Traffic signals for lymphocyte recirculation and leukocyte emigration: the multistep paradigm. *Cell* 1994;76:301–314.
8. Sadler JE. New concepts in Von Willebrand disease. *Annu Rev Med* 2005; 56:173–191.
9. McEver RP. P-selectin/PSGL-1 and other interactions between platelets, leukocytes, and endothelium. In: Michelson AD, ed. *Platelets*. San Diego, CA: Academic Press, 2002:139–155.
10. Santoro SA, Saelman E, Zutter MM. The alpha 2 beta1 integrin: structure, function, and regulation of a platelet surface collagen receptor. In: Lapetina EG, ed. *Advances in molecular and cell biology, the platelet*, Vol. 18. Greenwich, CT: Jai Press, 1997:109–128.
11. Zutter MM, Santoro SA. Function of the alpha 2 beta1 integrin. In: Gullberg D, ed. *I domains in integrins*. Georgetown, TX: Laudes Bioscience, 2003:42–58.
12. Staatz WD, Rajpara SM, Wayner EA, et al. The membrane glycoprotein Ia-IIa (VLA-2) complex mediates the $Mg^{++}$-dependent adhesion of platelets to collagen. *J Cell Biol* 1989;108:1917–1924.

13. Elices MJ, Hemler ME. The human integrin VLA-2 is a collagen receptor on some cells and a collagen/laminin receptor on others. *Proc Natl Acad Sci U S A* 1989;86:9906–9910.

14. Kirchhofer D, Languino LR, Ruoslahti E, et al. Alpha 2 beta 1 integrins from different cell types show different binding specificities. *J Biol Chem* 1990;265:615–618.

15. Chen J, Diacovo TG, Grenache DG, et al. The alpha(2) integrin subunit-deficient mouse: a multifaceted phenotype including defects of branching morphogenesis and hemostasis. *Am J Pathol* 2002;161:337–344.

16. Kehrel B. Platelet receptors for collagen. *Platelets* 1995;6:11.

17. Moroi M, Jung SM. Platelet receptors for collagen. *Thromb Haemost* 1997;78:439–444.

18. Sixma JJ, van Zanten GH, Huizinga EG, et al. Platelet adhesion to collagen: an update. *Thromb Haemost* 1997;78:434–438.

19. Nieuwenhuis HK, Akkerman JW, Houdijk WP, et al. Human blood platelets showing no response to collagen fail to express surface glycoprotein Ia. *Nature* 1985;318:470–472.

20. Nieuwenhuis HK, Sakariassen KS, Houdijk WP, et al. Deficiency of platelet membrane glycoprotein Ia associated with a decreased platelet adhesion to subendothelium: a defect in platelet spreading. *Blood* 1986;68:692–695.

21. Kunicki TJ, Kritzik M, Annis DS, et al. Hereditary variation in platelet integrin alpha 2 beta 1 density is associated with two silent polymorphisms in the alpha 2 gene coding sequence. *Blood* 1997;89:1939–1943.

22. Kunicki TJ. The influence of platelet collagen receptor polymorphisms in hemostasis and thrombotic disease. *Arterioscler Thromb Vasc Biol* 2002;22:14–20.

23. Kehrel B, Balleisen L, Kokott R, et al. Deficiency of intact thrombospondin and membrane glycoprotein Ia in platelets with defective collagen-induced aggregation and spontaneous loss of disorder. *Blood* 1988;71:1074–1076.

24. Kunicki TJ, Orchekowski R, Annis D, et al. Variability of integrin alpha 2 beta 1 activity on human platelets. *Blood* 1993;82:2693–2703.

25. Santoro SA. Identification of a 160,000 dalton platelet membrane protein that mediates the initial divalent cation-dependent adhesion of platelets to collagen. *Cell* 1986;46:913–920.

26. Staatz WD, Fok KF, Zutter MM, et al. Identification of a tetrapeptide recognition sequence for the alpha 2 beta 1 integrin in collagen. *J Biol Chem* 1991;266:7363–7367.

27. Santoro SA, Walsh JJ, Staatz WD, et al. Distinct determinants on collagen support alpha 2 beta 1 integrin-mediated platelet adhesion and platelet activation. *Cell Regul* 1991;2:905–913.

28. Holtkotter O, Nieswandt B, Smyth N, et al. Integrin alpha 2-deficient mice develop normally, are fertile, but display partially defective platelet interaction with collagen. *J Biol Chem* 2002;277:10789–10790.

29. Nieswandt B, Watson SP. Platelet-collagen interaction: is GP VI the central receptor? *Blood* 2003;102:449–461.

30. Kuijpers MJ, Schulte V, Bergmeier W, et al. Complementary roles of glycoprotein VI and alpha 2 beta 1 integrin in collagen-induced thrombus formation in flowing whole blood *ex vivo*. *FASEB J* 2003;17:685–687.

31. He L, Pappan LK, Grenache DG, et al. The contributions of the alpha 2 beta 1 integrin to vascular thrombosis *in vivo*. *Blood* 2003;102:3652–3657.

32. Giancotti FG. Complexity and specificity of integrin signaling. *Nat Cell Biol* 2000;2:E13–E14.

33. McDonald JA. Integrins minireview series. *J Biol Chem* 2000;275:21783.

34. Harris ES, McIntyre TM, Prescott SM, et al. The leukocyte integrins. *J Biol Chem* 2000;275:23409–23412.

35. Albelda SM. Role of integrins and other cell adhesion molecules in tumor progression and metastasis. *Lab Invest* 1993;68:4–17.

36. Hynes RO. Integrins: versatility, modulation, and signaling in cell adhesion. *Cell* 1992;69:11–25.

37. Hemler ME, Lobb RR. The leukocyte beta 1 integrins. *Curr Opin Hematol* 1995;2:61–67.

38. Argraves WS, Pytela R, Suzuki S, et al. cDNA sequences from the alpha subunit of the fibronectin receptor predict a transmembrane domain and a short cytoplasmic peptide. *J Biol Chem* 1986;261:12922–12924.

39. Takada Y, Huang C, Hemler ME. Fibronectin receptor structures in the VLA family of heterodimers. *Nature* 1987;326:607–609.

40. Takada Y, Puzon W. Identification of a regulatory region of integrin beta 1 subunit using activating and inhibiting antibodies. *Biol Chem* 1993;268:17597–17601.

41. Altruda F, Cervella P, Tarone G, et al. A human integrin beta 1 subunit with a unique cytoplasmic domain generated by alternative mRNA processing. *Gene* 1990;95:261–266.

42. Languino LR, Ruoslahti E. An alternative form of the integrin beta 1 subunit with a variant cytoplasmic domain. *J Biol Chem* 1992;267:7116–7120.

43. Liu S, Calderwood DA, Ginsberg MH. Integrin cytoplasmic domain-binding proteins. *J Cell Sci* 2000;113:3563–3571.

44. Kieffer N, Guichard J, Breton-Gorius J. Dynamic redistribution of major platelet surface receptors after contact-induced platelet activation and spreading. An immunoelectron microscopy study. *Am J Pathol* 1992;140:57–73.

45. Fox JE. The platelet cytoskeleton. *Thromb Haemost* 1993;70:884–893.

46. Fox JE, Boyles JK, Berndt MC, et al. Identification of a membrane skeleton in platelets. *J Cell Biol* 1988;106:1525–1538.

47. Fox JE. Cytoskeletal proteins and platelet signaling. *Thromb Haemost* 2001;86:198–213.

48. Takada Y, Hemler ME. The primary structure of the VLA-2/collagen receptor alpha 2 subunit (platelet GPIa): homology to other integrins and the presence of a possible collagen-binding domain. *J Cell Biol* 1989;109:397–407.

49. Dickeson SK, Santoro SA. Ligand recognition by the I domain-containing integrins. *Cell Mol Life Sci* 1998;54:556–566.

50. Emsley J, Knight CG, Farndale RW, et al. Structural basis of collagen recognition by integrin alpha 2 beta 1. *Cell* 2000;101:47–56.

51. Emsley J, King SL, Bergelson JM, et al. Crystal structure of the I domain from integrin alpha 2 beta 1. *J Biol Chem* 1997;272:28512–28517.

52. Lee JO, Rieu P, Arnaout MA, et al. Crystal structure of the A domain from the alpha subunit of integrin CR3 (CD11b/CD18). *Cell* 1995;80:631–638.

53. Whittaker CA, Hynes RO. Distribution and evolution of von Willebrand/integrin A domains: widely dispersed domains with roles in cell adhesion and elsewhere. *Mol Biol Cell* 2002;13:3369–3387.

54. Kamata T, Liddington RC, Takada Y. Interaction between collagen and the alpha(2) I-domain of integrin alpha(2) beta(1). Critical role of conserved residues in the metal ion-dependent adhesion site (MIDAS) region. *J Biol Chem* 1999;274:32108–32111.

55. Shimaoka M, Xiao T, Liu JH, et al. Structures of the alpha L I domain and its complex with ICAM-1 reveal a shape-shifting pathway for integrin regulation. *Cell* 2003;112:99–111.

56. Qu A, Leahy DJ. Crystal structure of the CD11a/CD18 (LFA-1, alpha L beta 2) integrin. *Proc Natl Acad Sci U S A* 1995;92:10277–10281.

57. Velling T, Kusche-Gullberg M, Sejersen T, et al. cDNA cloning and chromosomal localization of human alpha(11) integrin. A collagen-binding, I domain-containing, beta(1)-associated integrin alpha-chain present in muscle tissues. *J Biol Chem* 1999;274:25735–25742.

58. Camper L, Hellman U, Lundgren-Akerlund E. Isolation, cloning, and sequence analysis of the integrin subunit alpha10, a beta1-associated collagen binding integrin expressed on chondrocytes. *J Biol Chem* 1998;273:20383–20389.

59. Kapyla J, Ivaska J, Riikonen R, et al. Integrin alpha(2)I domain recognizes type I and type IV collagens by different mechanisms. *J Biol Chem* 2000;275:3348–3354.

60. Shimaoka M, Lu C, Palframan RT, et al. Reversibly locking a protein fold in an active conformation with a disulfide bond: integrin alphaL I domains with high affinity and antagonist activity *in vivo*. *Proc Natl Acad Sci U S A* 2001;98:6009–6014.

61. Shimaoka M, Shifman JM, Jing H, et al. Computational design of an integrin I domain stabilized in the open high affinity conformation. *Nat Struct Biol* 2000;7:674–678.

62. Liddington RC, Ginsberg MH. Integrin activation takes shape. *J Cell Biol* 2002;158:833–839.

63. Chan BM, Kassner PD, Schiro JA, et al. Distinct cellular functions mediated by different VLA integrin alpha subunit cytoplasmic domains. *Cell* 1992;68:1051–1060.

64. Hemler ME, Kassner PD, Chan BM. Functional roles for integrin alpha subunit cytoplasmic domains. *Cold Spring Harb Symp Quant Biol* 1992;57:213–220.

65. Klekotka PA, Santoro SA, Haochuan W, et al. Specific residues within the $\alpha_2$ integrin subunit cytoplasmic domain regulate migration and cell cycle progression via distinct MAPK pathways. *J Biol Chem* 2001;276:32353–32361.

66. Klekotka PA, Santoro SA, Zutter MM. $\alpha_2$ integrin subunit cytoplasmic domain-dependent cellular migration requires p38 MAPK. *J Biol Chem* 2001;276:9503–9511.

67. Clemetson KJ, McGregor JL, James E, et al. Characterization of the platelet membrane glycoprotein abnormalities in Bernard-Soulier syndrome and comparison with normal by surface-labeling techniques and high-resolution two-dimensional gel electrophoresis. *J Clin Invest* 1982; 70:304–311.

68. Sugiyama T, Okuma M, Ushikubi F, et al. novel platelet aggregating factor found in a patient with defective collagen-induced platelet aggregation and autoimmune thrombocytopenia. *Blood* 1987;69:1712–1720.

69. Moroi M, Jung SM, Okuma M, et al. A patient with platelets deficient in glycoprotein VI that lack both collagen-induced aggregation and adhesion. *J Clin Invest* 1989;84:1440–1445.

70. Arai M, Yamamoto N, Moroi M, et al. Platelets with 10% of the normal amount of glycoprotein VI have an impaired response to collagen that results in a mild bleeding tendency. *Br J Haematol* 1995;89:124–130.

71. Gibbins JM, Okuma M, Farndale R, et al. Glycoprotein VI is the collagen receptor in platelets which underlies tyrosine phosphorylation of the Fc receptor gamma-chain. *FEBS Lett* 1997;413:255–259.

72. Tsuji M, Ezumi Y, Arai M, et al. A novel association of Fc receptor gamma-chain with glycoprotein VI and their co-expression as a collagen receptor in human platelets. *J Biol Chem* 1997;272:23528–23531.

73. Clemetson JM, Polgar J, Magnenat E, et al. The platelet collagen receptor glycoprotein VI is a member of the immunoglobulin superfamily closely related to FcalphaR and the natural killer receptors. *J Biol Chem* 1999;274:29019–29024.

74. Frazer K, Capra JD. Immunoglobulins: structure and function. In: Paul WE, ed. *Fundamental immunology*, 4th ed. New York: Lippincott Williams & Wilkins, 1998.

75. Jandrot-Perrus M, Busfield S, Lagrue AH, et al. Cloning, characterization, and functional studies of human and mouse glycoprotein VI: a platelet-specific collagen receptor from the immunoglobulin superfamily. *Blood* 2000;96:1798–1807.

76. Ezumi Y, Uchiyama T, Takayama H. Molecular cloning, genomic structure, chromosomal localization, and alternative splice forms of the platelet collagen receptor glycoprotein VI. *Biochem Biophys Res Commun* 2000;277:27–36.

77. Berlanga O, Tulasne D, Bori T, et al. The Fc receptor gamma-chain is necessary and sufficient to initiate signalling through glycoprotein VI in transfected cells by the snake C-type lectin, convulxin. *Eur J Biochem* 2002;269:2951–2960.

78. Zheng YM, Liu C, Chen H, et al. Expression of the platelet receptor GP VI confers signaling via the Fc receptor gamma-chain in response to the snake venom convulxin but not to collagen. *J Biol Chem* 2001;276:12999–13006.

79. Suzuki-Inoue K, Tulasne D, Shen Y, et al. Association of Fyn and Lyn with the proline-rich domain of glycoprotein VI regulates intracellular signaling. *J Biol Chem* 2002;277:21561–21566.

80. Andrews RK, Suzuki-Inoue K, Shen Y, et al. Interaction of calmodulin with the cytoplasmic domain of platelet glycoprotein VI. *Blood* 2002;99:4219–4221.

81. Watson SP, Asazuma N, Atkinson B, et al. The role of ITAM- and ITIM-coupled receptors in platelet activation by collagen. *Thromb Haemost* 2001;86:276–288.

82. Clemetson KJ, Clemetson JM. Platelet collagen receptors. *Thromb Haemost* 2001;86:189–197.

83. Kehrel B, Wierwille S, Clemetson KJ, et al. Glycoprotein VI is a major collagen receptor for platelet activation: it recognizes the platelet-activating quaternary structure of collagen, whereas CD36, glycoprotein IIb/IIIa, and von Willebrand factor do not. *Blood* 1998;91:491–499.

84. Poole A, Gibbins JM, Turner M, et al. The Fc receptor gamma-chain and the tyrosine kinase Syk are essential for activation of mouse platelets by collagen. *EMBO J* 1997;16:2333–2341.

85. Watson SP, Gibbins J. Collagen receptor signalling in platelets: extending the role of the ITAM. *Immunol Today* 1998;19:260–264.

86. Kanaji S, Kanaji T, Furihata K, et al. Convulxin binds to native, human glycoprotein Ib alpha. *J Biol Chem* 2003;278:39452–39460.

87. Keely PJ, Parise LV. The alpha2beta1 integrin is a necessary co-receptor for collagen-stimulated activation of Syk and the subsequent phosphorylation of phospholipase Cgamma2 in platelets. *J Biol Chem* 1996;271:26668–26676.

88. Kamiguti AS, Markland FS, Zhou Q, et al. Proteolytic cleavage of the beta1 subunit of platelet alpha2beta1 integrin by the metalloproteinase jararhagin compromises collagen-stimulated phosphorylation of pp72. *J Biol Chem* 1997;272:32599–32605.

89. Inoue K, Ozaki Y, Satoh K, et al. Signal transduction pathways mediated by glycoprotein Ia/IIa in human platelets: comparison with those of glycoprotein VI. *Biochem Biophys Res Commun* 1999;256:114–120.

90. Ichinohe T, Takayama H, Ezumi Y, et al. Collagen-stimulated activation of Syk but not c-Src is severely compromised in human platelets lacking membrane glycoprotein VI. *J Biol Chem* 1997;272:63–68.

91. Suzuki-Inoue K, Ozaki Y, Kainoh M, et al. Rhodocytin induces platelet aggregation by interacting with glycoprotein Ia/IIa (GPIa/IIa, Integrin alpha 2beta 1). Involvement of GPIa/IIa-associated src and protein tyrosine phosphorylation. *J Biol Chem* 2001;276:1643–1652.

92. Polanowska-Grabowska R, Geanacopoulos M, Gear AR. Platelet adhesion to collagen via the alpha 2 beta 1 integrin under arterial flow conditions causes rapid tyrosine phosphorylation of pp125FAK. *Biochem J* 1993;296:543–547.

93. Polanowska-Grabowska R, Gibbins JM, Gear AR. Platelet adhesion to collagen and collagen-related peptide under flow: roles of the [alpha]2[beta]1 integrin, GPVI, and Src tyrosine kinases. *Arterioscler Thromb Vasc Biol* 2003;23:1934–1940.

94. Klekotka PA, Santoro SA, Ho A, et al. Mammary epithelial cell-cycle progression via the alpha(2)beta(1) integrin: unique and synergistic roles of the alpha(2) cytoplasmic domain. *Am J Pathol* 2001;159:983–992.

95. Kritzik M, Savage B, Nugent DJ, et al. Nucleotide polymorphisms in the alpha2 gene define multiple alleles that are associated with differences in platelet alpha2 beta1 density. *Blood* 1998;92:2382–2388.

96. Santoso S, Kunicki TJ, Kroll H, et al. Association of the platelet glycoprotein Ia C807T gene polymorphism with nonfatal myocardial infarction in younger patients. *Blood* 1999;93:2449–2453.

97. Matsubara Y, Murata M, Maruyama T, et al. Association between diabetic retinopathy and genetic variations in alpha2beta1 integrin, a platelet receptor for collagen. *Blood* 2000;95:1560–1564.

98. Benze G, Heinrich J, Schulte H, et al. Association of the GPIa C807T and GPIIIa PlA1/A2 polymorphisms with premature myocardial infarction in men. *Eur Heart J* 2002;23:325–330.

99. Furihata K, Nugent DJ, Kunicki TJ. Influence of platelet collagen receptor polymorphisms on risk for arterial thrombosis. *Arch Pathol Lab Med* 2002;126:305–309.

100. Moshfegh K, Wuillemin WA, Redondo M, et al. Association of two silent polymorphisms of platelet glycoprotein Ia/IIa receptor with risk of myocardial infarction: a case-control study. *Lancet* 1999;353:351–354.

101. Carlsson LE, Santoso S, Spitzer C, et al. The alpha2 gene coding sequence T807/A873 of the platelet collagen receptor integrin alpha2beta1 might be a genetic risk factor for the development of stroke in younger patients. *Blood* 1999;93:3583–3586.

102. Di Paola J, Federici AB, Mannucci PM, et al. Low platelet alpha2beta1 levels in type I von Willebrand disease correlate with impaired platelet function in a high shear stress system. *Blood* 1999;93:3578–3582.

103. Kaplan C, Morel-Kopp MC, Kroll H, et al. HPA-5b (Br(a)) neonatal alloimmune thrombocytopenia: clinical and immunological analysis of 39 cases. *Br J Haematol* 1991;78:425–429.

104. Kiefel V, Shechter Y, Atias D, et al. Neonatal alloimmune thrombocytopenia due to anti-Brb (HPA-5a). Report of three cases in two families. *Vox Sang* 1991;60:244–245.

105. Bettaieb A, Fromont P, Rodet M, et al. Brb, a platelet alloantigen involved in neonatal alloimmune thrombocytopenia. *Vox Sang* 1991;60:230–234.

106. Bierling P, Fromont P, Bettaieb A, et al. Anti-Bra antibodies in the French population. *Br J Haematol* 1989;73:428–429.

107. Christie DJ, Pulkrabek S, Putnam JL, et al. Posttransfusion purpura due to an alloantibody reactive with glycoprotein Ia/IIa (anti-HPA-5b). *Blood* 1991;77:2785–2789.

108. Warkentin TE, Smith JW, Hayward CP, et al. Thrombocytopenia caused by passive transfusion of anti-glycoprotein Ia/IIa alloantibody (anti-HPA-5b). *Blood* 1992;79:2480–2484.

109. Kiefel V, Santoso S, Katzmann B, et al. The Bra/Brb alloantigen system on human platelets. *Blood* 1989;73:2219–2223.

110. Santoso S, Kalb R, Walka M, et al. The human platelet alloantigens Br(a) and Brb are associated with a single amino acid polymorphism on glycoprotein Ia (integrin subunit alpha 2). *J Clin Invest* 1993;92:2427–2432.

111. Croft SA, Samani NJ, Teare MD, et al. Novel platelet membrane glycoprotein VI dimorphism is a risk factor for myocardial infarction. *Circulation* 2001;104:1459–1463.

112. Kunicki TJ, Head S, Salomon DR. Platelet receptor structures and polymorphisms. *Methods Mol Biol* 2004;273:455–478.

113. Best D, Senis YA, Jarvis GE, et al. GP VI levels in platelets: relationship to platelet function at high shear. *Blood* 2003;102:2811–2818.

114. Takagi S, Iwai N, Baba S, et al. A GP VI polymorphism is a risk factor for myocardial infarction in Japanese. *Atherosclerosis* 2002;165:397–398.

115. Kunicki TJ, Nugent DJ. The influence of platelet glycoprotein polymorphisms on receptor function and risk for thrombosis. *Vox Sang* 2002;83(Suppl. 1):85–90.

116. Hynes RO, Bader BL. Targeted mutations in integrins and their ligands: their implications for vascular biology. *Thromb Haemost* 1997;78:83–87.

117. Hynes RO. Targeted mutations in cell adhesion genes: what have we learned from them?. *Dev Biol* 1996;180:402–412.

118. Massberg S, Gawaz M, Gruner S, et al. A crucial role of glycoprotein VI for platelet recruitment to the injured arterial wall in vivo. *J Exp Med* 2003;197:41–49.

119. Inoue O, Suzuki-Inoue K, Dean WL, et al. Integrin alpha2beta1 mediates outside-in regulation of platelet spreading on collagen through activation of Src kinases and PLCgamma2. *J Cell Biol* 2003;160:769–780.

120. Fay WP, Parker AC, Ansari MN, et al. Vitronectin inhibits the thrombotic response to arterial injury in mice. *Blood* 1999;93:1825–1830.

121. Eitzman DT, Westrick RJ, Nabel EG, et al. Plasminogen activator inhibitor-1 and vitronectin promote vascular thrombosis in mice. *Blood* 2000;95:577–580.

122. Rosen ED, Raymond S, Zollman A, et al. Laser-induced noninvasive vascular injury models in mice generate platelet- and coagulation-dependent thrombi. *Am J Pathol* 2001;158:1613–1622.

123. Grenache DA, Coleman T, Semenkovich CF, et al. $\alpha_2\beta_1$ integrin and development of atherosclerosis in a mouse model – assessment of risk. *Arterioscler Thromb Vasc Biol* 2003;23:2104–2109.

124. Kato K, Kanaji T, Russell S, et al. The contribution of glycoprotein VI to stable platelet adhesion and thrombus formation illustrated by targeted gene deletion. *Blood* 2003;102:1701–1707.

# CHAPTER 35 ■ PLATELET PROSTANOID RECEPTORS

BARRIE ASHBY

Platelets can be stimulated to change shape and aggregate by potent activators such as thrombin. Platelet activation is augmented by secondary feedback through generation of thromboxane $A_2$ ($TxA_2$) by platelets themselves. Activation of platelets by thrombin or $TxA_2$ and other agonists is largely mediated by an elevation of intracellular calcium ($Ca^{2+}$) levels. Conversely, an increase in intracellular cyclic adenosine monophosphate (cAMP) level, either by stimulation of adenylyl cyclase or by inhibition of phosphodiesterase activity, inhibits platelet aggregation. Prostaglandins (PGs) such as prostacyclin ($PGI_2$), $PGE_1$ (generated by the vessel wall), and $PGD_2$ (produced by platelets) can stimulate platelet adenylyl cyclase and are potential antithrombotic agents. On the other hand, $PGE_2$ may act to inhibit adenylyl cyclase, modulating its effect on platelet inhibition.

This chapter discusses prostanoid receptors on the platelet surface that are involved in coupling to generation of second messengers, leading to activation or inhibition of platelets. All of the receptors belong to the G protein–coupled receptor superfamily.

## THROMBOXANE $A_2$ AND PROSTAGLANDINS

Thromboxane and PGs are members of a family of compounds called *eicosanoids*, which constitute a group of 20-carbon fatty acids derived from arachidonic acid (1). The eicosanoids exert profound effects on practically all cells and tissues. $TxA_2$ is produced by platelets themselves (2) following stimulation with other agonists such as thrombin and adenosine diphosphate (ADP). $PGD_2$ is also synthesized by platelets (3), whereas $PGI_2$ is produced by endothelial cells. In general, $TxA_2$ leads to vasoconstriction and stimulation of platelet activation, whereas PGs lead to vasodilation and inhibition of platelet activation.

PGs and $TxA_2$ are not stored, but produced *de novo* following stimulation; they act as autocrine or paracrine mediators, with their biological activities usually restricted to the cell or tissue where they are synthesized or to nearby cells. $TxA_2$ has a short chemical half-life, less than 1 minute at body temperature, whereas that of $PGI_2$ is approximately 5 minutes. $TxA_3$, produced from diets rich in eicosapentanoic acid (EPA) from fish oils, is less potent than $TxA_2$ relative to aggregation of platelets and constriction of blood vessels. $PGE_1$ resembles $PGI_2$ in its ability to inhibit platelet aggregation, a property not shared with $PGE_2$.

Aspirin is an important drug in blocking platelet activation because of its ability to prevent $TxA_2$ formation. Indeed, early work on platelets revealed that aspirin acts by selectively blocking prostanoid production (4).

## Synthesis of Prostaglandins and Other Eicosanoids

Platelet eicosanoid metabolism is discussed in detail in Chapter 36. The current short summary describes details relevant to a discussion of platelet prostanoid receptors. PGs are derived not only from essential fatty acids (usually arachidonic acid, C20:4) but also from EPA (C20:5), which is derived from cold water fish. Arachidonic acid and other fatty acids are released from membrane phospholipids by the action of phospholipase $A_2$ ($PLA_2$). There are three distinct $PLA_2$ enzymes designated cardiac $PLA_2$ ($cPLA_2$), cytosolic $PLA_2$, and secretory $PLA_2$. The last two are calcium-dependent enzymes, and they are mainly responsible for arachidonic acid release.

Once formed, arachidonic acid is converted into the precursor prostaglandin endoperoxides $PGG_2$ and $PGH_2$ by the action of cyclooxygenases (1). Cyclooxygenases are inhibited by nonsteroidal antiinflammatory drugs (NSAIDs) such as aspirin and ibuprofen, leading to inhibition of PG and thromboxane formation. Two distinct cyclooxygenases have been described (5), and they are designated COX-1 and COX-2. COX-1 is constitutively expressed, whereas COX-2 is inducible in response to inflammatory mediators such as cytokines and lipopolysaccharide. Selective COX-2 inhibitors such as celecoxib and refecoxib are useful in treating chronic inflammation because they cause less gastric disturbance than NSAIDs by allowing the formation of cytoprotective $PGE_2$ through COX-1.

Cyclooxygenase is abundant within the vasculature, although the principal products vary longitudinally along the vasculature and cross-sectionally within the blood vessel wall (e.g., endothelium vs. vascular smooth muscle). Within the coronary circulation, the larger blood vessels synthesize principally $PGI_2$, whereas $PGE_2$ predominates in microvessels.

## Mechanisms of Prostaglandin Action

PGs exert their effects by binding to specific cell surface receptors, all of which are members of the G protein–coupled receptor superfamily. The prostaglandin receptors differ in their potency toward different PGs and in the signal transduction system to which they are coupled. PGs may stimulate or inhibit adenylyl cyclase, or stimulate phospholipase C (PLC), leading to formation of diacylglycerol and inositol trisphosphate (which itself stimulates calcium mobilization) (6). The receptors are summarized in Table 35-1.

The receptors are classified according to their endogenous ligand. Hence, $PGD_2$ binds preferentially to the DP receptor, which couples to Gs to stimulate adenylyl cyclase. $PGI_2$ binds to the IP receptor, which also couples to Gs, leading to stimulation of adenylyl cyclase.

**TABLE 35-1**

CLASSIFICATION OF PROSTAGLANDIN RECEPTOR SUBTYPES

| Receptor type | Endogenous agonist | Rank order of potency | Signal transduction |
|---|---|---|---|
| DP | $PGD_2$ | D2 > E2, F2$\alpha$, I2, TxA$_2$ | cAMP ↑ |
| EP | $PGE_2$ | E2 > I2 ≥ F2$\alpha$ > D2 | |
| EP1 | | | PLC ↑ |
| EP2 | | | cAMP ↑ |
| EP3 (seven variants) | | | cAMP ↓ |
| EP4 | | | cAMP ↑ |
| FP | $PGF_{2\alpha}$ | F2$\alpha$ > D2 > E2 > I2 | PLC ↑ |
| IP | $PGI_2$ | I2 > D2, E2, F2$\alpha$, TxA$_2$ | cAMP ↑ |
| TP (two variants) | $TxA_2$ | TxA$_2$ > D2 > F2$\alpha$, I2, E2 | PLC ↑ |

PG, prostaglandin; cAMP, cyclic adenosine monophosphate; PLC, phospholipase C; TxA$_2$, thromboxane A$_2$; ↑, elevation; ↓, inhibition.

$PGF_{2\alpha}$ binds to the FP receptor, which couples to PLC. $TxA_2$ binds to the TP receptor, which couples to Gq to activate PLC and to $G_{13}$ to activate the small G proteins Rho and Rac. $PGE_2$ interacts with four distinct EP receptor subtypes that are the products of separate genes. EP1 couples to PLC, EP2 and EP4 couples to stimulate adenylyl cyclase, and EP3 couples to inhibit adenylyl cyclase.

In addition to the diversity of subtypes, several of the receptors exist as isoforms. The human EP3 receptor, for example, displays seven distinct carboxyl-terminal variants (7) and the TP receptor exists as two distinct carboxyl-terminal variants, TP$\alpha$ and TP$\beta$ (8). The variants differ in properties such as susceptibility to agonist-induced desensitization.

# ACTIONS OF PROSTAGLANDINS IN THE CARDIOVASCULAR SYSTEM

PGs have a variety of effects on the cardiovascular system ranging from blood flow regulation to control of kidney function (1). Effects on blood flow and platelet activation are discussed in subsequent text.

## Blood Flow Regulation

$PGE_1$, $PGE_2$, and $PGI_2$ are potent vasodilators, and endogenously produced $PGE_2$, and $PGI_2$ may be local regulators in many vascular beds. $PGI_2$ and its stable analogs are used to treat peripheral vascular disease; however, such use is restricted by the hypotension, headache, and flushing that result from IV infusion of these agents. $TxA_2$ is a potent constrictor of cerebral and coronary arteries, and $PGF_{2\alpha}$ constricts superficial veins in the hands. Prinzmetal angina, a vasoconstrictive problem in coronary arteries, may be partly caused by $TxA_2$ released from platelets.

## Platelet Aggregation

Platelets respond to PGs in a variety of ways and express several of the prostaglandin receptors (see Fig. 35-1). $TxA_2$ causes platelet activation, resulting in secretion and aggregation (acting through the TP receptor), whereas $PGI_2$, $PGE_1$, and $PGD_2$ inhibit platelet activation through stimulation of adenylyl cyclase and cAMP formation. In addition, platelets possess

a $PGE_2$ receptor linked to inhibition of adenylyl cyclase (EP3 receptor), limiting the amount of cAMP that can be generated and hence dampening the response to PGs (9,10).

The antiaggregatory vasodilator mediator $PGI_2$ is produced in the endothelial cells of the vessel wall, whereas the proaggregatory vasoconstrictor $TxA_2$ is produced by the platelet itself. The dynamic interplay at the platelet–endothelium interface between $TxA_2$ and $PGI_2$ is thought to affect thrombosis and ischemia. Interventions that favor $PGI_2$ production while decreasing the formation of $TxA_2$ have the greatest benefit. Aspirin inhibits cyclooxygenase irreversibly by covalent acetylation of a serine residue (11). Low-dose aspirin maximizes the effect on the cyclooxygenase on the platelet but has no effect on the cyclooxygenase on endothelial cells. Unlike the endothelium, platelets lack nuclei and cannot synthesize new cyclooxygenase to replace those that are inactivated by aspirin. The effects of aspirin therefore continue through the life of the platelet, or for more than 10 days. Hence, a deficiency in the production of $TxA_2$ by platelets cannot be corrected until new platelets form. In contrast, after being inhibited, vascular cyclooxygenase can be replaced by new cyclooxygenase. The use of low doses of aspirin limits the opportunity for aspirin to enter the systemic circulation to inhibit vascular cyclooxygenase but allows it to act on platelet cyclooxygenase in the portal circulation.

Differences in platelet aggregatory potency between the thromboxanes, $TxA_2$ and $TxA_3$, constitute part of the rationale for dietary supplementation with EPA, which is found primarily in cold water fish. The addition of EPA to the diet either in purified form or by consuming cold water fish has been suggested as a novel therapeutic strategy in the prevention of thrombosis (i.e., in the reduced formation of $TxA_2$).

A variety of studies, including functional studies, receptor binding studies, and receptor knockout studies in mice show that platelets contain the TP, IP, DP, and EP3 receptors. There is little evidence that the platelets contain EP1, EP2, EP4, or FP receptors.

Pathways involving prostanoid receptors on platelets are shown schematically in Figure 35-1.

# THROMBOXANE A$_2$ AND PLATELET ACTIVATION

## TP Receptor

$TxA_2$ is very unstable, with a half-life of only a few seconds in aqueous solution; however, acting through the TP receptor, it

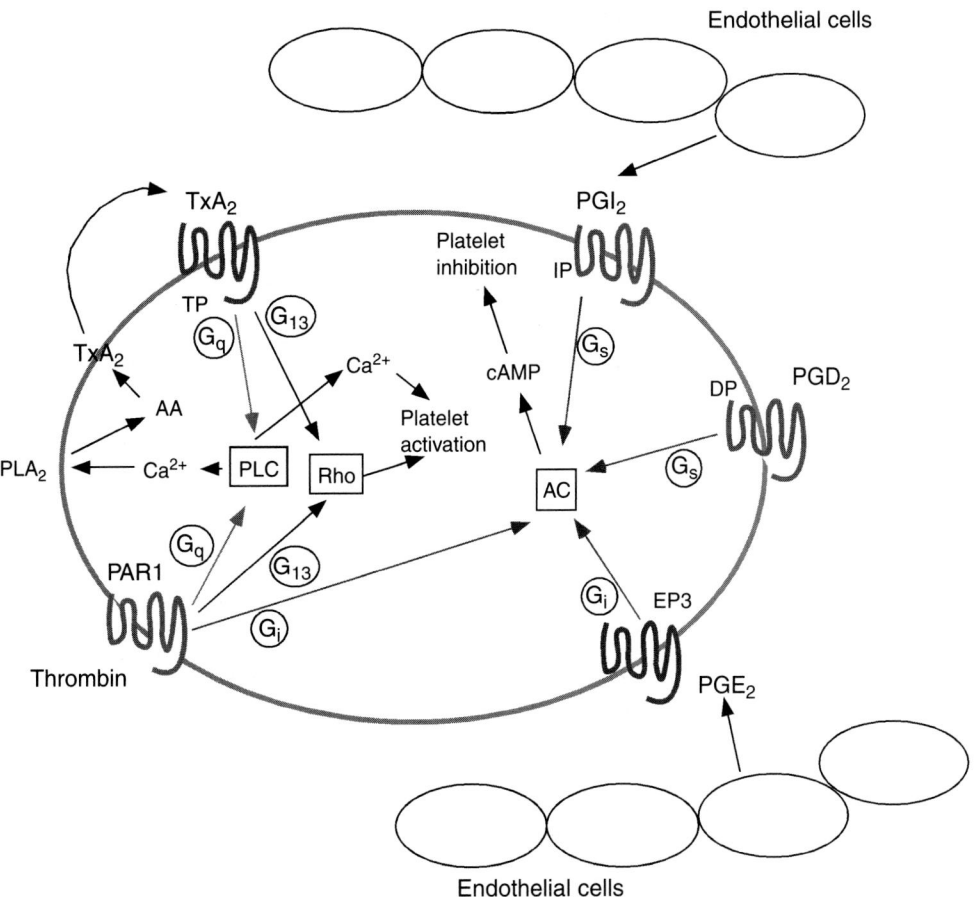

**FIGURE 35-1.** Platelet prostanoid receptors. G protein–coupled receptors, which all have seven transmembrane domains, are illustrated by the serpentine structures shown. Thrombin, acting through the PAR-1 receptor, activates phospholipase A$_2$ (PLA$_2$) and the arachidonic acid (AA) cascade, leading to formation of thromboxane A$_2$ (TxA$_2$). TxA$_2$ acts in a feedback loop to activate other platelets through the TP receptor. The TP receptor couples to G$_q$ and to G$_{13}$, leading to activation of phospholipase C and Rho, respectively, both of which contribute to shape change and aggregation. The IP receptor is activated by PGI$_2$ released from endothelial cells, leading to G$_s$-mediated activation of adenylyl cyclase (AC) and formation of cyclic adenosine monophosphate (cAMP). cAMP causes inhibition of platelet activation through a variety of mechanisms. PGD$_2$, acting through the DP receptor, also activates AC. In contrast, PGE$_2$ acts through the EP3 receptor and G$_i$ to inhibit AC.

is a potent stimulator of platelet aggregation and a constrictor of vascular and respiratory smooth muscles. Two stable synthetic analogs of PGH2, U44069 and U46619, are potent TP agonists. A number of synthetic antagonists of the TP receptor have been developed, including S-1456, which was used in the purification of the receptor. Other antagonists include SQ29546 and AH23848.

The TP receptor gene codes for two splice variants that give rise to two isoforms, TP$\alpha$ and TP$\beta$, that differ in their carboxyl tails. TP$\alpha$ is a protein of 343 amino acids (12,13), whereas TP$\beta$ is 64 amino acids longer than TP$\alpha$. The TP$\alpha$ isoform is the predominant form in platelets and is not expressed in endothelial cells, whereas TP$\beta$ is found in endothelial cells (14). TP receptors have also been found in bronchial smooth muscle and in mesangial cells of glomeruli. The prostaglandin endoperoxides PGG$_2$ and PGH$_2$ also bind to thromboxane receptors.

The role of the TP receptor in platelet activation was confirmed in mice genetically deficient in the receptor in which platelet activation is depressed (15).

In addition, a human genetic defect has been described in which arginine is replaced by leucine at residue 60 of the TP receptor (16). The mutant receptor binds ligands normally, but

exhibits impaired coupling to PLC and adenylyl cyclase. The defect appears to be related to an inherited bleeding disorder (16).

The major signal transduction pathway mediated by the TP receptor takes place through PLC and is mediated through the G protein Gq (17). The role of G$\alpha$q in platelet function was confirmed using gene knockout studies (18). Platelets from mice deficient in the $\alpha$ subunit of Gq are unresponsive to a variety of physiologic platelet activators including TxA$_2$, resulting in increased bleeding times.

The TP receptor also couples to the heterotrimeric G protein G13 and to the activation of the small G proteins Rho and Rac (19,20). Rho activation has been shown to depend on coupling of the TP receptor to a member of the G12/G13 family, rather than Gq, and to be independent of an increase in intracellular calcium level (19). Recent work (19) indicates that G13 is responsible for coupling of the TP receptor (and the thrombin and collagen receptors) to Rho and that G12 is not involved. Hence, G13 mediated signaling is required for normal hemostasis.

Myosin light chain kinase (MLCK) and p160 Rho-associated coiled-coil–containing protein kinase independently contribute to myosin light chain phosphorylation and platelet shape change, through Ca$^{2+}$-sensitive and Ca$^{2+}$-insensitive pathways, respectively (21). Rho activation leads to actin polymerization and phosphatidylinositol-4,5-bisphosphate formation, and to shape change. By contrast, Rac activation is dependent on an increase in intracellular calcium level that is mediated through TP receptor activation of Gq. However, Rac activation is through Gq and is not required for shape change.

In transfected cells, isoform TPα couples weakly to stimulate adenylyl cyclase, and TPβ couples weakly to inhibit adenylyl cyclase (22). In platelets, coupling of the TP receptor to adenylyl cyclase appears to have little role in modifying intracellular calcium mobilization and shape change. Rather, TxA$_2$-induced inhibition of adenylyl cyclase and platelet aggregation depends upon secretion of other agonists that stimulate Gi-coupled receptors (23).

Immunochemical studies show the localization of the TP receptor on platelets (24). Immunogold labeling with a polyclonal antibody to the C-terminal domain of TPα indicate that the receptor is present mainly at the platelet surface and is also present inside the platelet. Receptors were shown to be present in membranes of α-granules and in elements of the open-canalicular system. A similar distribution was found in megakaryocytes.

The significance of the TP receptor isoforms may lie in differences in their regulation. GPCRs frequently undergo agonist-induced desensitization that involves phosphorylation of certain serine or threonine residues in their carboxyl termini. Because TP agonists activate protein kinase C(PKC), it might be assumed that PKC phosphorylates the C-terminus, leading to selective desensitization of one or other of the isoforms. However, studies with transfected TPα and TPβ receptors (25) showed that whereas U46619, a TxA$_2$ mimetic, induced specific phosphorylation of both isoforms, inhibition of PKC had little effect on agonist-dependent phosphorylation of either isoform and failed to modulate homologous desensitization of agonist-induced stimulation of inositol phosphate formation. It therefore appears that although PKC phosphorylates both isoforms of TP, it contributes little to rapid agonist-induced phosphorylation of either isoform. Other studies showed that, although the number of TxA$_2$ binding sites decreased in TPα cells after prolonged stimulation with a TxA$_2$ mimetic, those in the TPβ cells increased markedly (26).

The isoprostane 8-epi-prostaglandin F2α (8-epiPGF$_{2α}$) is a compound with some of the properties of TxA$_2$. 8-epiPGF$_{2α}$ is a potent vasoconstrictor in lung and kidney and may be synthesized by platelets. However, 8-epiPGF$_{2α}$ is a weak platelet activator and induces shape change at concentrations of 1 or 10 μM and reversible, but not irreversible, aggregation at 100 μM (27). Studies support the idea that there is a distinct receptor for 8-epiPGF$_{2α}$ (28).

# PROSTAGLANDINS AND INHIBITION OF PLATELET AGGREGATION

PGI$_2$, PGE$_1$, and PGD$_2$ elevate cAMP levels in platelets and inhibit platelet function. Both PGI$_2$ and PGE$_1$ act through the IP receptor, whereas PGD$_2$ acts through the DP receptor. PGE$_2$ acts through the EP3 receptor to inhibit adenylyl cyclase, modulating the effects of cAMP on platelet function.

Elevation of cAMP level as a means to inhibit platelet activation also occurs through direct stimulation of adenylyl cyclase by use of the diterpene forskolin, a direct cell-permeable activator of the enzyme, and through use of cyclic nucleotide phosphodiesterase inhibitors.

The ways in which cAMP inhibits platelet activation are diverse and are not completely understood. An increase in intracellular cAMP level leads to a broad inhibition of platelet functions, including adhesion, secretion, and aggregation. The actions of cAMP are mainly mediated through cAMP-dependent protein kinase A (PKA), which acts at multiple points in platelet activation signaling cascades. PKA-mediated inhibition involves interference with steps in cytosolic Ca$^{2+}$ level elevation and effects on cytoskeleton-associated proteins including vasodilator-stimulated phosphoprotein (VASP), actin-binding protein (ABP), caldesmon, and MLCK that are involved in cytoskeletal reorganization.

Interference with calcium signaling includes inhibition of PLC activation, although direct inhibition of PLC has not been observed, and the mechanism probably involves a reduction in PIP2 synthesis (28). In addition, PKA phosphorylates IP3 receptors (29,30) that are responsible for the release of calcium stores from the dense tubular system, although the role of phosphorylation in the release of calcium stores is not clear. PKA may also phosphorylate the TxA$_2$ (TP) receptor, uncoupling it from interaction with Gq and PLC.

VASP, the protein located in focal adhesions and stress fibers of many cells, is phosphorylated by PKA. VASP is present in high concentrations in platelets (31). PKA-mediated phosphorylation of VASP reduces VASP binding to F-actin and inhibits actin polymerization (32). In VASP knockout mice, inhibition of platelet aggregation by cyclic nucleotides is impaired (33,34), suggesting that VASP phosphorylation may contribute to the inhibitory effects of cyclic nucleotides on platelet activation.

ABP cross-links and stabilizes actin filaments, and is cleaved by calpain during platelet activation, leading to loss of its ability to cross-link actin, which may allow reorganization of the cytoskeleton. Phosphorylation of ABP by PKA in platelets prevents proteolysis, so that the actin filament network is resistant to cytoskeletal reorganization (35).

The platelet protein caldesmon binds both actin and myosin, forming a complex that enhances translocation of actin filaments (36). Caldesmon is phosphorylated by PKA in platelets, and its phosphorylated form may stabilize the cytoskeleton and inhibit platelet activation (37).

PKA-mediated phosphorylation of MLCK reduces its affinity for calmodulin, thereby decreasing its phosphorylation by calcium-calmodulin kinase. MLCK is involved in myosin contractility and in the regulation of cytoskeletal reorganization during platelet shape change (38) so that this mechanism may contribute to inhibition of platelet activation. MLC phosphorylation may also be regulated through phosphorylation of the small G protein RhoA. RhoA stimulates Rho-kinase, leading to phosphorylation of myosin phosphatase and a decrease in its activity, which leads to increased MLC phosphorylation. In leukocytes, elevation of intracellular cAMP level inhibits RhoA activation and integrin-dependent adhesion (39).

The small G protein Rap1b is highly expressed in platelets, and it may be involved in cell adhesion processes. Rap1b is activated by both a PKC-independent Ca$^{2+}$-mediated mechanism and by a PKC-dependent mechanism (40). By contrast, PGI$_2$ treatment inhibits agonist-induced Rap1b activation (41–43), perhaps by effects on calcium mobilization.

PGs, acting through generation of cAMP, also inhibit cytoskeletal rearrangements involving glycoprotein Ib (GP Ib), a subunit of the GP Ib/V/IX complex. GP Ib is the platelet receptor for von Willebrand factor and mediates adhesion to the subendothelium. This complex is linked to actin filaments by ABP (44). PKA-mediated phosphorylation of GP Ib leads to inhibition of collagen-induced actin polymerization (45).

The rank order of potency of PGs as inhibitors of human platelet activation is PGI$_2$ > 6 keto-PGE$_1$ > PGE$_1$ > PGD$_2$ > 6-ketoPGF$_{2α}$ > PGE$_2$ > PGF$_{2α}$. The order reflects the importance of the prostacyclin (IP) receptor in mediating prostaglandin effects on platelet adenylyl cyclase.

## IP Receptor

PGI$_2$ (prostacyclin) is mainly synthesized in vascular endothelial cells, and it plays an important role in regulation of platelet aggregation and vascular tone. Prostacyclin has a half-life of approximately 3 minutes in aqueous solutions, so stable compounds have been developed as IP agonists. These compounds include iloprost and cicaprost, both of which are chemically stable. Both compounds have similar affinity for the IP receptor as native prostacyclin. No antagonists of the IP receptor are currently available.

The IP receptor, which is localized in platelets and vascular smooth muscle cells, mediates the action of PGI$_2$. In addition, PGE$_1$ binds to the IP receptor with relatively high affinity. The IP receptor is linked to stimulation of adenylyl cyclase through the G protein Gs. In heterologous expression systems, the receptor also couples to the mobilization of Ca$^{2+}$. The cloned human IP receptor codes for a protein of 386 amino acids (46,47). The messenger ribonucleic acid mRNA for the receptor is distributed most abundantly in kidney, with lesser amounts in lung and liver.

The IP receptor is desensitized by PKC but not by PKA (48). Studies on isolated platelets show that the IP receptor is also susceptible to downregulation (49–51).

PGI$_2$ plays a role in the cardiovascular response to TxA$_2$. Injury-induced vascular proliferation and platelet activation are enhanced in mice that are genetically deficient in the IP receptor but are depressed in mice that are genetically deficient in the TP or treated with a TP antagonist (15). The augmented response to vascular injury was abolished in mice deficient in both receptors. Therefore, PGI$_2$ modulates platelet-vascular interactions *in vivo* and specifically limits the response to TxA$_2$. This interplay may help explain the adverse cardiovascular effects associated with selective COX-2 inhibitors, which, unlike aspirin and NSAIDs, inhibit PGI$_2$ but not TxA$_2$.

## DP Receptor

PGD$_2$ inhibits platelet aggregation and relaxes vascular and non-vascular smooth muscle. The DP receptor is the only class of receptor identified to date that mediates the actions of PGD$_2$ (6). Selective DP agonists include 9-deoxy-D$^9$-PGD$_2$. Several DP receptor antagonists are available, including BWA868C, that demonstrate the presence of the DP receptor on platelets (52,53). PGD$_2$ exerts its effect by causing an increase in intracellular camp concentration. The DP receptor complementary deoxy ribonucleic acid (cDNA) codes for a protein of 359 amino acids and the recombinant receptor couples to stimulation of adenylyl cyclase (54).

## EP3 Receptor

PGE$_2$ acts through the EP3 receptor to mediate contraction of smooth muscle, inhibition of autonomic neurotransmitter release, and inhibition of gastric secretion (55). The receptor is also involved in inhibition of lipolysis and in inhibition of renal water reabsorption. Gene knockout studies indicate that the EP3 receptor is involved in temperature regulation in the preoptic nucleus and in the generation of fever (56).

The EP3 receptor is present on platelets, and PGE$_2$ acts to potentiate platelet aggregation; this action may be mediated through the EP3 receptor. The EP3 receptor couples to inhibition of adenylyl cyclase. Selective EP3 agonists include sulprostone, which also acts at the EP1 receptor, and enprostil. In addition, misoprostol, also a potent EP2 agonist, acts as an agonist at the EP3 receptor.

The human EP3 receptor has been cloned (57,58) and its gene structure has been determined (59). This receptor occurs as seven isoforms that are the product of alternative splicing of a single gene (7,60–62). The isoforms are identical over the first 369 amino acids but differ in carboxyl-terminal region, which varies in length from 6 to 65 amino acids following the seventh transmembrane helix.

Although all of the EP3 isoforms couple to inhibition of adenylyl cyclase, they differ in properties including susceptibility to desensitization and degree of constitutive activity. Some of the isoforms also couple to Ca$^{2+}$ mobilization. The short-tailed isoforms EP3III and EP3IV are markedly constitutively active, whereas isoforms EP3I and EP3II show little or no constitutive activity (63).

The EP3 receptor has been functionally demonstrated on platelets by the action of sulprostone in inhibiting adenylyl cyclase (64). Colocalization of the EP3 receptor on platelets with the IP receptor, which couples to stimulation of adenylyl cyclase, has led to the description of a novel mechanism of desensitization involving distinct stimulatory and inhibitory receptors (9,10). Hence, PGI$_2$ binds not only to the IP receptor with high affinity but also to the EP3 receptor with low affinity, causing stimulation of adenylyl cyclase at low concentration and inhibition of adenylyl cyclase at high concentration. Because PGs are local mediators, their concentration might be expected to vary as the autacoid is released and diffuses away from its site of action, so that the role of the inhibitory receptor may be to provide homeostatic control of cAMP level, buffering against rapid variations in agonist concentration.

Gene knockout studies of EP3 confirm its role in platelet activation (65). Low concentrations of PGE$_2$ enhanced platelet aggregation, whereas high PGE$_2$ levels inhibited aggregation. Activation of the EP3 receptor mediates the proaggregatory actions of PGE$_2$ at low concentration, whereas the IP receptor mediates the inhibitory effect of PGE$_2$ at higher concentrations. The relative activation of these two receptors, EP3 and IP, regulates the intracellular level of cAMP and, in this way, conditions the response of the platelet to aggregating agents. Consistent with these findings, loss of the EP3 receptor in a model of venous inflammation protects against formation of intravascular clots.

Other work on EP3 knockout mice suggests a similar role for the receptor (66). Mice lacking the EP3 receptor show an increased bleeding tendency and decreased susceptibility to thromboembolism, indicating this receptor in the augmentation of platelet responsiveness. In platelets from wild-type mice, EP3 agonists enhance platelet aggregation induced by the TP receptor agonist U46619. EP3 agonists alone do not induce aggregation but do lead to an increase in cytosolic Ca$^{2+}$ concentration and an inhibition of cAMP formation, suggesting Gi coupling to the EP3 receptor. The potentiating effects of PGE$_2$ on platelet aggregation and its effects on intracellular Ca$^{2+}$ and cAMP are absent in EP3 knockout mice, and the bleeding time was significantly prolonged. In addition, EP3 knockout mice were less susceptible than wild-type mice to mortality and to thrombus formation in the lung when given intravenous injections of arachidonic acid. The findings point to a mechanism in which PGE$_2$ potentiates TxA$_2$-induced platelet aggregation by acting through the EP3 receptor to increase intracellular Ca$^{2+}$ level or to decrease camp level, or both. The potentiating effect of the EP3 receptor appears to be involved in both physiologic and pathologic effects of PGE$_2$ *in vivo*.

Other works suggest that the EP3 receptor may act through other mechanisms to bring about cardioprotective effects (67, 68). Activation of the EP3 receptor by specific agonists has been shown to reduce myocardial infarct size in rodents. The reduction in infarct size was abolished by the protein kinase C inhibitors staurosporine and chelerythrine and by a selective inhibitor of adenosine triphosphate (ATP)-sensitive potassium channels, suggesting that the EP3 receptor reduces myocardial infarct size by mechanisms that involve protein kinase C and the opening of $K_{ATP}$ channels.

Other members of the EP receptor family (i.e., EP1, EP2, and EP4) and the FP receptor appear to have little, if any, role on platelets. These roles are described here briefly because they have effects that may impinge on the cardiovascular system.

## EP1 Receptor

The EP1 receptor mediates contraction of smooth muscle in various tissues (69). The EP1 receptor can be distinguished from other EP receptors by use of the antagonists, SC 19220 and AH 8609. 17-phenyl-w-trinor $PGE_2$ is a selective agonist at the EP1 receptor.

The EP1 receptor couples to mobilization of $Ca^{2+}$ through the phosphatidylinositol pathway. The human EP1 receptor cDNA has been cloned and codes for a protein of 402 amino acids (70). It is not clear whether the EP1 receptor is expressed on platelets.

## EP2 Receptor

The EP2 receptor was defined when relaxant and contractile effects of $PGE_2$ on guinea pig trachea smooth muscle were separated using the selective EP1 antagonists, SC 19220 and AH 8609 (71). The selective EP2 agonist butaprost has also proved useful in functional characterization of the receptor. Misoprostol, which also acts on the EP3 receptor, displays potent activity at the EP2 receptor.

The EP2 receptor couples to increase cAMP level. However, the EP4 receptor also couples to increase cAMP formation, so that some of the functions of $PGE_2$ attributed to EP2 may be mediated by EP4.

The human EP2 receptor cDNA codes for a protein of 358 amino acids (72). The recombinant receptor is resistant to agonist-induced short-term desensitization and internalization but undergoes downregulation in response to long-term desensitization (73,74). $PGE_2$ causes a small increase in cAMP levels in platelets, but it is not clear whether the effect is mediated through the EP2 or the EP4 receptors or by weak binding to the IP receptor.

## EP4 Receptor

The EP4 receptor couples to increase cAMP level, similar to the EP2 receptor. There are no selective agonists for the EP4 receptor; however, the EP2 selective agonist butaprost is not active at the EP4 receptor. Actions of $PGE_2$ at the EP4 receptor can be assigned by comparison of butaprost and other EP receptor agonists.

The human EP4 cDNA codes for a protein of 488 amino acids (75). The receptor has a long carboxyl-terminal domain containing numerous serine and threonine residues. The EP4 receptor is susceptible to agonist-induced short-term desensitization, which distinguishes it from the EP2 subtype. Truncation of the carboxyl-terminal domain abolishes short-term desensitization and internalization (74,76,77). The EP4 receptor also undergoes downregulation following long-term exposure to agonist (>12 hours), however, downregulation is also seen with the EP2 receptor. Abundant expression of the EP4 mRNA has been detected in the small intestine, thymus, lung, pancreas, spleen, leukocytes, uterus, and kidney.

The EP4 receptor has been suggested to mediate the actions of $PGE_2$ in remodeling the cardiovascular system in the newborn. PGs are necessary to maintain the ductus arteriosus in an open state. At birth, the ductus closes. Gene knockout of the EP4 receptor (78) in mice resulted in failure of closure of the ductus arteriosus, resulting in a left-to-right shunt of blood and subsequent death. The result indicates that the EP4 receptor is required for normal closure. However, approximately 5% of homozygous EP4 knockout mice survive, indicating that other genes can provide an alternative mechanism for ductus closure.

## FP Receptor

$PGF_{2\alpha}$ causes contraction of vascular and nonvascular smooth muscle, including bronchial and tracheal muscles. The FP receptor mediates the action of $PGF_{2\alpha}$. There are two selective FP receptor agonists, fluprostenol and cloprostenol, but no antagonists. The human FP receptor consists of 459 amino acids, and the expressed receptor couples to the G protein Gq to induce phosphatidyl inositol metabolism (79,80). Northern blot analysis shows that the receptor is abundantly expressed in the corpus luteum, kidney, heart, stomach, and lung.

## Platelet-Activating Factor

Platelet-activating factor (PAF) is a phospholipid (not an eicosanoid) produced from the phospholipid membrane after arachidonic acid is released. The proper name of PAF is 1-O-alkyl-2-acetyl-sn-glycero-3-phosphocholine; it is produced by inflammatory cells such as PMNs and mast cells and may act in complimentary fashion with the leukotrienes $LTC_4$ and $LTD_4$ to cause bronchoconstriction. Its properties include activation of platelets and neutrophils and increase of vascular permeability.

PAF induces platelet aggregation and secretion in a dose-dependent fashion. PAF has been hypothesized to induce platelet activation in rabbit platelets by a "third pathway" independent of $TxA_2$ and secreted ADP (81,82). However, this proposal has been controversial because studies present evidence both in favor of and against the proposal (83–87). Detailed studies on human platelets have shown that both aggregation and serotonin release were inhibited by aspirin and by ADP antagonists (88). Although PAF can mobilize arachidonic acid and stimulate $TxA_2$ synthesis, its effects on human platelets require close cell contact, $TxA_2$ synthesis, and ADP release. However, this requirement is in contrast to findings in rabbit and horse platelets (88). These findings are supported by the inability of platelets from patients with secretion defects to respond to PAF. The receptor for PAF has been cloned and sequenced and belongs to the G protein–coupled receptor superfamily (89). The deduced sequence indicates that the receptor consists of 342 amino acids.

## References

1. Campbell WB, Halushka PV. Lipid-derived autacoids: eicosanoids and platelet-activating factor. In: Hardman JG, Limbird LE, Molinoff PB, et al., eds. *Goodman & Gilman's the pharmacological basis of therapeutics.* 9th ed. New York: McGraw-Hill, 1996:601.
2. Hamberg M, Samuelsson B. Prostaglandin endoperoxides. Novel transformations of arachidonic acid in human platelets. *Proc Natl Acad Sci U S A* 1974;71:3400.
3. Oelz O, Oelz R, Knapp HR, et al. Biosynthesis of prostaglandin D2. 1. Formation of prostaglandin D2 by human platelets. *Prostaglandins* 1977;13:225.
4. Smith JB, Willis AL. Aspirin selectively inhibits prostaglandin production in human platelets. *Nat New Biol* 1971;231:235.
5. Needleman P, Isakson PC. The discovery and function of COX-2. *J Rheumatol Suppl* 1997;49:6.
6. Coleman RA, Smith WL, Narumiya S. International union of pharmacology classification of prostanoid receptors: properties, distribution, and structure of the receptors and their subtypes. *Pharmacol Rev* 1994;46:205.
7. Schmid A, Thierauch K-H, Schleuning W-D, et al. Splice variants of the human EP3 receptor for prostaglandin E2. *Eur J Biochem* 1995;228:23.

8. Yukawa M, Yokota R, Eberhardt RT, et al. Differential desensitization of thromboxane A2 receptor subtypes. *Circ Res* 1997;80:551.

9. Ashby B. Model of prostaglandin regulated cyclic AMP metabolism in platelets: examination of time-dependent effects on adenylate cyclase and phosphodiesterase activities. *Mol Pharmacol* 1989;36:866.

10. Ashby B. Novel mechanism of heterologous desensitization of adenylate cyclase: prostaglandins bind with different affinities to both stimulatory and inhibitory receptors on platelets. *Mol Pharmacol* 1990;38:46.

11. Roth GJ, Stanford N, Jacobs JW, et al. Acetylation of prostaglandin synthetase by aspirin. Purification and properties of the acetylated protein from sheep vesicular gland. *Biochemistry* 1977;16:4244.

12. Hirata M, Hayashi Y, Ushikubi F, et al. Cloning and expression of cDNA for a human thromboxane A2 receptor. *Nature* 1991;349:617.

13. Nusing RM, Hirata M, Kakizuka A, et al. Characterization and chromosomal mapping of the human thromboxane A2 receptor gene. *J Biol Chem* 1993;268:25252.

14. Raychowdury MK, Yukawa M, Collins LJ, et al. Alternative splicing produces a divergent cytoplasmic tail in the human endothelial cell thromboxane A2 receptor. *J Biol Chem* 1994;269:19255.

15. Cheng Y, Austin SC, Rocca B, et al. Role of prostacyclin in the cardiovascular response to thromboxane A2. *Science* 2002;296:539.

16. Hirata T, Kakizuka A, Ushikubi F, et al. Arg60 to Leu mutation of the human thromboxane A2 receptor in a dominantly inherited bleeding disorder. *J Clin Invest* 1994;194:1662.

17. Shenker A, Goldsmith P, Unson CG, et al. The G protein coupled to the thromboxane A2 receptor in human platelets is a member of the novel Gq family. *J Biol Chem* 1991;266:9309.

18. Offermanns S, Toombs CF, Hu Y-H, et al. Defective platelet activation in Gαq-deficient mice. *Nature* 1997;389:183.

19. Gratacap MP, Payrastre B, Nieswandt B, et al. Differential regulation of Rho and Rac through heterotrimeric G-proteins and cyclic nucleotides. *J Biol Chem* 2001;276:47906.

20. Moers A, Nieswandt B, Massberg S, et al. G13 is an essential mediator of platelet activation in hemostasis and thrombosis. *Nat Med* 2003;11:1418.

21. Paul BZ, Daniel JL, Kunapuli SP. Platelet shape change is mediated by both calcium-dependent and -independent signaling pathways. Role of p160 Rho-associated coiled-coil-containing protein kinase in platelet shape change. *J Biol Chem* 1999;274:28293.

22. Hirata T, Ushikubi F, Kakizuka A, et al. Two thromboxane A2 receptor isoforms in human platelets. Opposite coupling to adenylyl cyclase with different sensitivity to Arg60 to Leu mutation. *J Clin Invest* 1996;97:949.

23. Paul BZ, Jin J, Kunapuli SP. Molecular mechanism of thromboxane A2-induced platelet aggregation. Essential role for p2tac and alpha2a receptors. *J Biol Chem* 1999;274:29108.

24. Nurden P, Poujol C, Winckler J, et al. Immunolocalization of P2Y1 and TPalpha receptors in platelets showed a major pool associated with the membranes of alpha-granules and the open canalicular system. *Blood* 2003;101:1400.

25. Habib A, Vezza R, Creminon C, et al. Rapid, agonist-dependent phosphorylation *in vivo* of human thromboxane receptor isoforms—minimal involvement of protein kinase c. *J Biol Chem* 1997;272:7191.

26. Kinsella BT, O'Mahony DJ, Fitzgerald GA. The human thromboxane A2 receptor alpha isoform (TP-alpha) functionally couples to the G proteins Gq and G11 *in vivo* and is activated by the isoprostane 8-epi prostaglandin F2-alpha. *J Pharmacol Exp Ther* 1997;281:957.

27. Fukunaga M, Yura T, Grygorczyk R, et al. Evidence for the distinct nature of F2 isoprostane receptors from those of thromboxane A2. *Am J Physiol—Renal Fluid Electrolyte Physiol* 1997;41:F 477.

28. Ryningen A, Olav Jensen B, Holmsen H. Elevation of cyclic AMP decreases phosphoinositide turnover and inhibits thrombin-induced secretion in human platelets. *Biochim Biophys Acta* 1998;1394:235.

29. Cavallini L, Coassin M, Borean A, et al. Prostacyclin and sodium nitroprusside inhibit the activity of the platelet inositol 1,4,5-trisphosphate receptor and promote its phosphorylation. *J Biol Chem* 1996;271:5545.

30. El-Daher SS, Patel Y, Siddiqua A, et al. Distinct localization and function of 1,4,5 IP3 receptor subtypes and the 1,3,4,5 IP4 receptor GAP1IP4BP in highly purified human platelet membranes. *Blood* 2000;95:3412.

31. EigenthalerM M, Nolte C, Halbrügge M, et al. Concentration and regulation of cyclic nucleotides, cyclic-nucleotide-dependent protein kinases and one of their major substrates in human platelets. Estimating the rate of cAMP-regulated and cGMP-regulated protein phosphorylation in intact cells. *Eur J Biochem* 1992;205:471.

32. Reinhard M, Jarchau T, Walter U. Actin-based motility: stop and go with Ena/VASP proteins. *Trends Biochem Sci* 2001;26:243.

33. Aszodi A, Pfeifer A, Ahmad M, et al. The vasodilator-stimulated phosphoprotein (VASP) is involved in cGMP-and cAMP-mediated inhibition of agonist-induced platelet aggregation, but is dispensable for smooth muscle function. *EMBO J* 1999;18:37.

34. Hauser W, Knobeloch KP, Eigenthaler M, et al. Megakaryocyte hyperplasia and enhanced agonist-induced platelet activation in vasodilator-stimulated phosphoprotein knockout mice. *Proc Natl Acad Sci U S A* 1999;96:8120.

35. Chen M, Stracher A. *In situ* phosphorylation of platelet actin-binding protein by cAMP-dependent protein kinase stabilizes it against proteolysis by calpain. *J Biol Chem* 1989;264:14282.

36. Hemric ME, Tracy PB, Haeberle JR. Caldesmon enhances the binding of myosin to the cytoskeleton during platelet activation. *J Biol Chem* 1994;269:4125.

37. Hettasch JM, JSellers JR. Caldesmon phosphorylation in intact human platelets by cAMP-dependent protein kinase and protein kinase C. *J Biol Chem* 1991;266:11876.

38. Daniel JL, Molish IR, Rigmaiden M, et al. Evidence for a role of myosin phosphorylation in the initiation of the platelet shape change response. *J Biol Chem* 1984;259:9826.

39. Laudanna C, Campbell JJ, Butcher EC. Elevation of intracellular cAMP inhibits RhoA activation and integrin-dependent leukocyte adhesion induced by chemoattractants. *J Biol Chem* 1997;272:24141.

40. Franke B, van Triest M, de Bruijn KM, et al. Sequential regulation of the small GTPase Rap1 in human platelets. *Mol Cell Biol* 2000;20:779.

41. Siess W, Winegar DA, Lapetina EG. Rap1-B is phosphorylated by protein kinase A in intact human platelets. *Biochem Biophys Res Commun* 1990;170:944.

42. Lapetina EG, Lacal JC, Reep BR, et al. A ras-related protein is phosphorylated and translocated by agonists that increase cAMP levels in human platelets. *Proc Natl Acad Sci U S A* 1989;86:3131.

43. Reep BR, Lapetina EG. Nitric oxide stimulates the phosphorylation of rap1b in human platelets and acts synergistically with iloprost. *Biochem Biophys Res Commun* 1996;219:1.

44. Fox JEB. Identification of actin-binding protein as the protein linking the membrane skeleton to glycoproteins on platelet plasma membranes. *J Biol Chem* 1985;260:11970.

45. Fox JEB, Berndt MC. Cyclic AMP-dependent phosphorylation of glycoprotein Ib inhibits collagen-induced polymerization of actin in platelets. *J Biol Chem* 1989;264:9520.

46. Boie Y, Rushmore TH, Darmon-Goodwin A, et al. Cloning and expression of a cDNA the human prostanoid IP receptor. *J Biol Chem* 1994;269:12173.

47. Katsuyama M, Sugimoto Y, Namba T, et al. Cloning and expression of a cDNA for the human prostacyclin receptor. *FEBS Lett* 1994;344:74.

48. Smyth EM, Nestor PV, FitzGerald GA. Agonist-dependent phosphorylation of an-tagged human prostacyclin receptor. *J Biol Chem* 1996;271:33698.

49. Jaschonek K, Faul C, Schmidt H, et al. Desensitization of platelets to iloprost. Loss specific binding sites and heterologous desensitization of adenylate cyclase. *Eur J* 1988;147:187.

50. Alt U, Leigh PJ, Wilkins, AJ, et al. Desensitization of iloprost responsiveness in human platelets follows prolonged exposure to iloprost *in vitro*. *Br J Clin Pharmacol* 1986;22:118.

51. MacDermot J. Desensitization of prostacyclin responsiveness in platelets. *Biochem Pharmacol* 1986;35:2645.

52. Trist DG, Collins BA, Wood J, et al. The antagonism by BW A868C of PGD2 and BW245C activation of human platelet adenylate cyclase. *Br J Pharmacol* 1989;96:301.

53. Giles H, Leff P, Bolofo ML, et al. The classification of prostaglandin DP-receptors in platelets and vasculature using BW A868C, a novel, selective and potent competitive antagonist. *Br J Pharmacol* 1989;96:291.

54. Boie Y, Sawyer N, Slipetz DM, et al. Molecular cloning and characterization of the human prostanoid DP receptor. *J Biol Chem* 1995;270:18910.

55. Coleman RA, Humphrey PPA. In: Vane JR, O'Grady J, eds. *Prostanoid receptors: their function and classification in therapeutic applications of prostaglandins.* London: Edward Arnold, 1993:15.

56. Ushikubi F, Segi E, Sugimoto Y, et al. Impaired febrile response in mice lacking the prostaglandin E receptor subtype EP3. *Nature* 1998;395:281.

57. Kunapuli SP, Mao GF, Bastepe M, et al. Cloning and expression of a prostaglandin E receptor EP3 subtype from human erythroleukemia cells. *Biochem J* 1994;298:263.

58. Yang J, Xia M, Goetzl EJ, et al. Cloning and expression of the EP3 subtype of human receptors for prostaglandin E2. *Biochem Biophys Res Commun* 1994;198:999.

59. Kotani M, Tanaka I, Ogawa Y, et al. Structural organization of the human prostaglandin EP3 receptor subtype gene (PTGER3). *Genomics* 1997;40:424.

60. An S, Yang J, So SW, et al. Isoforms of the EP3 subtype of human prostaglandin E2 receptor transduce both intracellular calcium and cAMP signals. *Biochemistry* 1994;33:14496.

61. Regan JW, Bailey TJ, Donello JE, et al. Molecular cloning and expression of human EP3 receptors: evidence of three variants with differing carboxyl termini. *Br J Pharmacol* 1994;112:377.

62. Kotani M, Tanaka I, Ogawa Y, et al. Molecular cloning and expression of multiple isoforms of human prostaglandin E receptor EP3 subtype generated by alternative messenger RNA splicing: multiple second messenger systems and tissue specific distributions. *Mol Pharmacol* 1995;48:869.

63. Jin J-G, Mao G-F, Ashby B. Constitutive activity of human prostaglandin E receptor EP3 isoforms. *Br J Pharmacol* 1997;121:317.

64. Mao GF, Jin JG, Bastepe M, et al. Prostaglandin E2 both stimulates and inhibits adenyl cyclase on platelets: comparison of effects on cloned EP4 and EP3 prostaglandin receptor subtypes. *Prostaglandins* 1996;52:175.

65. Fabre JE, Nguyen M, Athirakul K, et al. Activation of the murine EP3 receptor for PGE2 inhibits cAMP production and promotes platelet aggregation. *J Clin Invest* 2001;107:603.

66. Ma H, Hara A, Xiao CY, et al. Increased bleeding tendency and decreased susceptibility to thromboembolism in mice lacking the prostaglandin E receptor subtype EP3. *Circulation* 2001;104:1176.

67. Zacharowski K, Olbrich A, Thiemermann C. Reduction of myocardial injury by the EP3 receptor agonist TEI-3356. Role of protein kinase C and of K(ATP)-channels. *Eur J Pharmacol* 1999;367:33.

68. Hide EJ, Thiemermann C. Sulprostone-induced reduction of myocardial infarct size in the rabbit by activation of ATP-sensitive potassium channels. *Br J Pharmacol* 1996;118:1409.

69. Coleman RA, Kennedy I, Humphrey PPA, et al. Neurotransmitter and autocoid receptors, prostanoid receptors. In: Hansch C, Sammes PG, Taylor JB et al., eds. *Comprehensive medicinal chemistry*. Oxford: Pergamon Press, 1990:643.

70. Funk CD, Furci L, FitzGerald GA, et al. Cloning and expression of a cDNA for the human prostaglandin E receptor EP1 subtype. *J Biol Chem* 1993;269:12173.

71. Coleman RA, Kennedy I, Sheldrick RL. New evidence with selective agonists and antagonists for the subclassification of PGE$_2$-sensitive (EP) receptors. *Adv Prostaglandin Thromboxane Leukot Res* 1987;17A:465.

72. Regan JW, Bailey TJ, Pepperl DJ, et al. Cloning of a novel human prostaglandin receptor with characteristics of the pharmacologically defined EP2 subtype. *Mol Pharmacol* 1994;46:213.

73. Nishigaki N, Negishi M, Ichikawa A. Two Gs-coupled prostaglandin E receptor subtypes, EP2 and EP4, differ in desensitization and sensitivity to the metabolic inactivation of the agonist. *Mol Pharmacol* 1996;50:1031.

74. Desai S, April H, Nwaneshiudu C, et al. Comparison of agonist-induced internalization of the human EP2 and EP4 prostaglandin receptors: role of the carboxyl terminus in EP4 receptor sequestration. *Mol Pharmacol* 2000;58:1279.

75. An S, Yang J, Xia M, et al. Cloning and expression of the EP2 subtype of human receptors for prostaglandin E2. *Biochem Biophys Res Commun* 1993;197:263.

76. Bastepe M, Ashby B. The long cytoplasmic carboxyl terminus of prostaglandin E receptor EP4 subtype is essential for agonist-induced desensitization. *Mol Pharmacol* 1997;51:343.

77. Desai S, Ashby B. Agonist-induced internalization and mitogen-activated protein kinase activation of the human prostaglandin EP4 receptor. *FEBS Lett* 2001;501:156.

78. Nguyen MT, Camenisch T, Snouwaert JN, et al. The prostaglandin receptor EP4 triggers remodelling of the cardiovascular system at birth. *Nature* 1997;390:78.

79. Abramovitz M, Boie Y, Nguyen T, et al. Cloning and expression of a cDNA for the human prostanoid FP receptor. *J Biol Chem* 1994;269:2632.

80. Cazenave JP, Benveniste J, Mustard JF. Aggregation of rabbit platelets by platelet-activator factor is independent of the release reaction and the arachidonate pathway and inhibited by membrane-active drugs. *Lab Invest* 1979;41:275.

81. Vargaftig BB, Chignard M, LeCouedic JP, et al. One, two, three, or more pathways for platelet aggregation. *Acta Med Scand* 1980;642:23.

82. McManus LM, Hanahan DJ, Pinckard RN. Human platelet stimulation by acetyl glyceryl ether phosphorylcholine. *J Clin Invest* 1981;67:903.

83. Chesney CM, Pifer DD, Byers LW, et al. Effect of platelet activating factor on human platelets. *Blood* 1982;59:582.

84. Marcus AJ, Safier LB, Ullman HL, et al. Effects of acetyl glyceryl ether phosphorylcholine on human platelet function *in vitro*. *Blood* 1981;58:1027.

85. Kloprogge E, DeHaas GH, Gorter G, et al. Stimulus-response coupling in human platelets: evidence against a role of PAF-acether in the "third pathway." *Thromb Res* 1983;30:107.

86. Rao GHR, Schmid HHO, Reddy KR, et al. Human platelet activation by an alkylacetyl analogue of phosphatidylcholine. *Biochim Biophys Acta* 1982;715:205.

87. Rao AK, Willis J, Hassel B, et al. Platelet-activating factor is a weak platelet agonist: evidence from normal human platelets and platelets with congenital secretion defects. *Am J Hematol* 1984;17:153.

88. Mauco G, Chap H, Douste-Blazy L. Platelet activating factor (PAF-acether) promotes an early degradation of phosphatidylinositol-4,5 biphosphate in rabbit platelets. *FEBS Lett* 1983;153:361.

89. Honda Z, Nakamura I, Miki I, et al. Cloning by functional expression of platelet activating receptor from guinea pig lung. *Science* 1991;349:342.

# CHAPTER 36 ■ PLATELET EICOSANOIDS

EMER M. SMYTH AND COLIN D. FUNK

Like most cells in the human body, platelets are capable of eicosanoid synthesis. Eicosanoids comprise a family of 20-carbon fatty acid derivatives that include prostaglandins, leukotrienes, hydroxy-eicosatetraenoic acids (HETEs), lipoxins, and other related molecules (1). In human platelets, the major eicosanoids, and the focus of this chapter, are thromboxane $A_2$ (Tx$A_2$) and 12-HETE. These lipid molecules are formed in response to platelet activation *in vitro* and *in vivo* (2) and are not stored preformed in dense granules or $\alpha$-granules but are synthesized *de novo* from the major precursor fatty acid arachidonic acid, which is released from membrane stores. The role of Tx$A_2$ in platelet and vascular biology has been understood to a large extent (see Table 36-1). Tx$A_2$ is a potent platelet proaggregatory substance, also capable of vasoconstriction in most vascular beds. On the other hand, the biological importance of 12-HETE formation has only been poorly understood.

Platelet activation plays an essential part in thromboembolic disorders (3). Clinicians and scientists worldwide recognize the importance of Tx$A_2$ synthesis by platelets. Therefore, aspirin, which blocks platelet Tx$A_2$ formation, is the current mainstay of preventive strategies against stroke and myocardial infarction. There are several other cellular sources of prostanoid biosynthesis that can alter platelet function. Prostacyclin (PG$I_2$), the major eicosanoid synthesized by the macrovascular endothelium, has potent actions that oppose Tx$A_2$ (Table 36-1). PG$I_2$ binds to specific platelet receptors, inhibits platelet aggregation, and even causes disaggregation of previously clumped platelets. High concentrations of PG$E_2$, released in response to major inflammatory mediators, also activate the PG$I_2$ receptor, known as IP, inhibiting platelet aggregation. In contrast, activation of one of the PG$E_2$ receptor subtypes (EP3), by low concentrations, leads to platelet aggregation (4). Prostacyclin also opposes the vascular actions of Tx$A_2$ because it is a potent vasodilatory compound. In this chapter, the eicosanoids generated by platelets are discussed.

## PLATELET EICOSANOID BIOSYNTHESIS AND METABOLISM

Two major pathways of eicosanoid production exist in platelets, and are often referred to as the cyclooxygenase (see Fig. 36-1) and the lipoxygenase (see Fig. 36-2) pathways. These pathways use the same substrate, arachidonic acid, but do not appear to compete directly for the same "pools" of substrate (i.e., the phospholipases that release the substrate are separately coupled to the downstream enzymes in different compartments of the platelet).

### Thromboxane $A_2$

Tx$A_2$ is formed when arachidonic acid is released from platelet membrane lipids by the sequential actions of phospholipase $A_2$,

PGH synthase, and thromboxane synthase (Fig. 36-1). Additional substrate may be delivered, as microparticles released from activated platelets, to adjacent platelets, thereby amplifying the generation of Tx$A_2$ (5). The reaction sequence is started when the C-13(S) hydrogen atom is abstracted from arachidonic acid by the cyclooxygenase activity of PGH synthase, followed by the insertion of two molecules of molecular oxygen, to form the unstable endoperoxide/hydroperoxide known as PG$G_2$ (6,7). The peroxidase activity of PGH synthase reduces the C-15 hydroperoxy moiety of PG$G_2$ to the corresponding alcohol group and yields PG$H_2$. Once synthesized, the PG$H_2$ intermediate is converted to Tx$A_2$ by thromboxane synthase (6,7). Both Tx$A_2$ and PG$H_2$ are unstable molecules with half-lives of approximately 30 seconds and 5 minutes *in vitro*, respectively. Because of its instability, Tx$A_2$ is rapidly converted nonenzymatically to thromboxane $B_2$ (Tx$B_2$).

Tx$A_2$ has an unusual oxetane chemical structure that is not commonly observed in biochemical reactions carried out in humans. It is formed by a free radical intermediate bound at the active site of thromboxane synthase by the C-9 oxygen of PG$H_2$ interacting with the heme iron (8). The intermediate also decomposes into malondialdehyde and 12-hydroxy-heptadecatrienoic acid (HHT). The HHT metabolite can be detected simultaneously with Tx$B_2$ in platelet incubations in an approximate 1:1 ratio (8).

### 12-Hydroxy-Eicosatetraenoic Acid

The 12-lipoxygenase pathway is initiated when arachidonic acid is liberated and bound by the enzyme for initial hydrogen atom abstraction at C-10, followed by stereospecific insertion of molecular oxygen at C-12 (7) (Fig. 36-2). This reaction results in the synthesis of a 12(S)-hydroperoxy-eicosatetraenoic acid [12(S)-HPETE] molecule. In the cellular environment, the hydroperoxy group of 12-HPETE gets rapidly reduced to the corresponding alcohol moiety to yield 12-HETE. This reduction is catalyzed to some extent by glutathione peroxidase, but also by other unknown factors, not by the 12-lipoxygenase itself (9–11).

## ENZYMES INVOLVED IN PLATELET EICOSANOID BIOSYNTHESIS

### Phospholipases

More than 95% of arachidonic acid is esterified in the *sn*-2 position of phospholipids in human platelets. Multiple types of phospholipase $A_2$ [e.g., group IIA secretory (sPL$A_2$), group IV cytosolic (cPL$A_2$), group V (sPL$A_2$), group VI calcium independent (iPL$A_2$), and group X (sPL$A_2$)] are classified into 12 groups and at least 19 PL$A_2$ enzymes have been cloned in

## TABLE 36-1

### BIOLOGICAL ROLES OF EICOSANOIDS ON PLATELETS AND VASCULATURE

| Eicosanoid | Platelet action | Vascular action |
|---|---|---|
| Thromboxane $A_2$ | Aggregation, amplification of aggregation in response to other agonists | Vasoconstriction |
| Prostacyclin | Inhibition of aggregation, disaggregation of previously clumped platelets | Vasodilation |
| Prostaglandin $D_2$ | Inhibition of aggregation | Variable |
| 12-Hydroxy-eicosatetraenoic acid | Modulation of aggregation in response to various agonists, modulation of platelet adhesion | Endothelial cell retraction |

mammals (12,13). The group IV 85-kDa $cPLA_2$ ($cPLA_2\alpha$) plays a critical role in $TxA_2$ formation, although alternative AA-releasing mechanisms, probably by other $PLA_2$s, produce enough $TxA_2$ to maintain platelet aggregation when $cPLA_2\alpha$ is absent (14). $cPLA_2$ has multiple phosphorylation sites that are rapidly regulated, and this facet of regulation is consistent with its role in immediate eicosanoid biosynthesis (15). The enzyme also requires micromolar calcium levels for activity/membrane interaction. On thrombin or collagen stimulation of platelets, 20% of total arachidonic acid from

all phospholipid classes (primarily phosphatidylinositol and phosphatidylcholine) is liberated. $cPLA_2$ appears to be a key initiating enzyme in 12-lipoxygenase product formation as well (14,16). Studies with inflammatory cell types (e.g., macrophages and mast cells) have provided some evidence for $sPLA_2$ action in eicosanoid biosynthesis under certain conditions, but a precise role in platelets has not been defined. An alternative mode of arachidonic acid release in platelets is the sequential action of phospholipase C and diglyceride lipase (17).

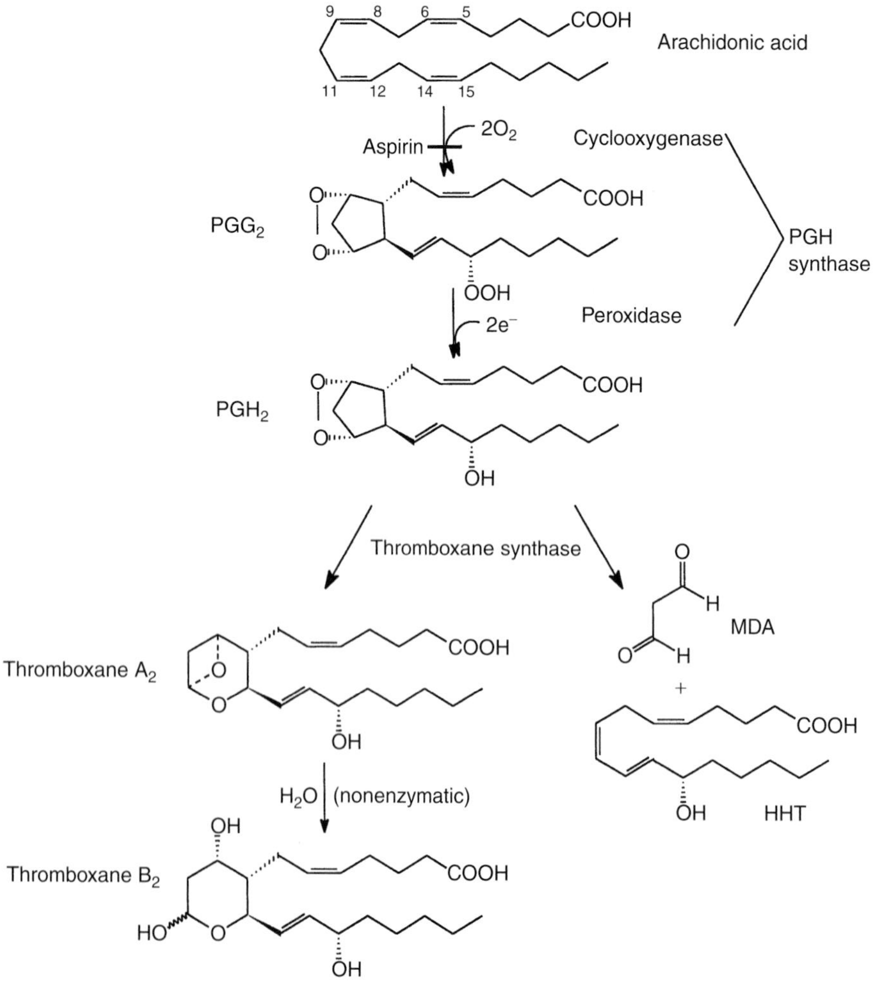

FIGURE 36-1. The cyclooxygenase pathway in human platelets. Arachidonic acid is released from membrane phospholipids by phospholipase $A_2$ enzyme action. The carboxyl group carbon is at position 1, and the four double bond positions are labeled. Two molecules of molecular oxygen are inserted into arachidonic acid, first at position 11 and then at position 15 by the cyclooxygenase activity of prostaglandin H (PGH) synthase. This is the aspirin-inhibitable step caused by acetylation of Ser529, which leads to blocked access of substrate in the active site. The prostaglandin $G_2$ ($PGG_2$) intermediate leaves the cyclooxygenase active site and is reduced by a distinct peroxidase site in PGH synthase to yield $PGH_2$. Thromboxane synthase forms unstable $TxA_2$ and two byproducts of $PGH_2$ transformation [malondialdehyde (MDA) and 12-hydroxy-5,8,10-heptadecatrienoic acid (HHT)]. No known platelet functions have been assigned to MDA and HHT. MDA is a highly reactive molecule that can cause protein cross-linking and is carcinogenic. $TxA_2$ undergoes nonenzymatic hydrolysis to form the inactive metabolite $TxB_2$.

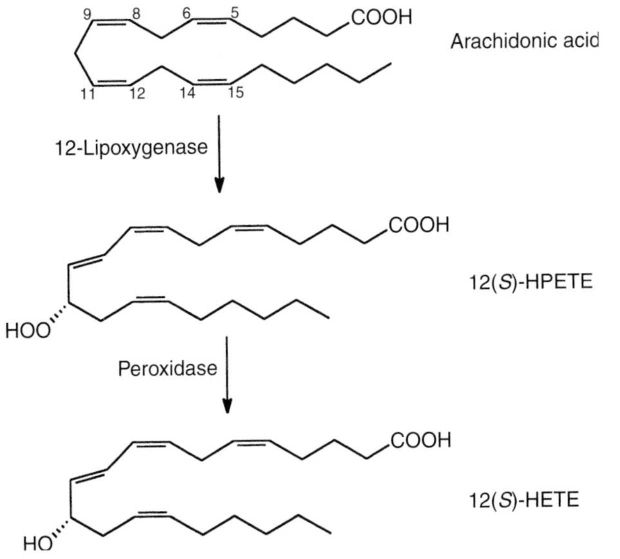

FIGURE 36-2. The platelet 12-lipoxygenase pathway. Arachidonic acid is the key substrate for platelet 12-lipoxygenase, as in the case of the cyclooxygenase pathway. The substrate "pool" for 12-lipoxygenase is distinct from the arachidonic acid metabolized by cyclooxygenase. 12-Lipoxygenase first abstracts a hydrogen atom from carbon 10, and molecular oxygen is inserted onto carbon 12 of the fatty acid radical to form 12(S)-hydroperoxy-eicosatetraenoic acid [12(S)-HPETE]. This molecule is rapidly metabolized by peroxidases in the platelet to 12-hydroxy-eicosatetraenoic acid (12-HETE). The synthesis of 12-HETE proceeds on a near-linear time course in activated platelets for many minutes, unlike the formation of $TxA_2$, which peaks rapidly within a minute because of PGH synthase "suicide" inactivation.

## Prostaglandin H Synthase

Two forms of PGH synthase (also referred to as PGHS-1, or COX-1, and PGHS-2, or COX-2) exist (18). It has long been thought that only PGHS-1 is expressed in human platelets, although it has become apparent that PGHS-2 is expressed in newly formed platelets (19,20). Under normal circumstances, therefore, less than 10% of circulating platelets express PGHS-2, and its major product, $PGE_2$, is produced in substantially less quantities than PGHS-1–derived $TxA_2$ (20). However, the levels of COX-2–positive platelets increase in settings of high platelet turnover, allowing generation of $PGE_2$ and $TxA_2$, with unknown vascular consequences. PGHS-1 is a 70-kDa, 599–amino acid, glycosylated membrane-bound heme protein. On the basis of the x-ray crystal structure of the ovine enzyme, it forms a homodimer and is placed in the membrane in such a way that it could efficiently acquire released arachidonic acid (21). The unique membrane-binding domain consists of four amphipathic helices embedded in only one leaflet of the lipid bilayer. The two subunits interact via a short epidermal growth factor–like motif near the N-terminus. PGHS-1 and PGHS-2 are essentially identical in their enzymatic activity and crystal structures but differ in the regulation and localization of their expression (18). Aspirin irreversibly acetylates a serine residue at position 529 of the human PGHS-1 enzyme (530 in ovine sequence) to block cyclooxygenase activity (18,22,23). This serine residue is not critical for enzyme activity; however, the acetylation process yields an enzyme whose active site is blocked from proper arachidonic acid access. Other nonsteroidal antiinflammatory drugs (NSAIDs) compete directly with arachidonate for binding to the cyclooxygenase site. A single amino acid difference between PGHS-1 and PGHS-2 allows for the development of PGHS-2 selective inhibitors. The valine found at position 523

in PGHS-2 is smaller than the isoleucine found in PGHS-1. This leaves a gap in the wall of the enzyme channel, giving access to a side-pocket, which is thought to be the site of binding of many selective drugs (24). Cyclooxygenase activity results in a rapid but transient burst in oxygen uptake, and the enzyme quickly undergoes suicide inactivation (18). The peroxidase activity is not inhibited by most NSAIDs, indicating that this site is spatially and functionally distinct from the cyclooxygenase active site.

## Thromboxane Synthase

Thromboxane synthase is a member of the cytochrome P-450 superfamily (8). This ferriheme-containing enzyme, based on complementary (cDNA) cloning, is a 61-kDa, 534-residue polypeptide (25). A shorter variant of 460 amino acids has also been deduced from cDNA cloning studies. Studies show that thromboxane synthase couples preferentially to PGHS-1, although PGHS-2–dependent $TxA_2$ generation has been reported (20). Like PGHS-1, thromboxane synthase also undergoes a mechanism-based suicide inactivation, and this may represent one factor for limiting $TxA_2$ biosynthesis by platelets. Numerous thromboxane synthase inhibitors have been developed with the anticipated promise of suppressing $TxA_2$ production while sparing vessel wall prostacyclin synthesis (3). This class of drugs has not resulted in useful clinical agents, perhaps because incidental ligands for the $TxA_2$ receptor (TP) such as prostaglandin endoperoxides and isoprostanes can still be generated.

## Platelet 12-Lipoxygenase

Several different isoforms of 12-lipoxygenase are classified according to their original site of isolation. Therefore, there are "platelet-type," "leukocyte-type," and "epidermal-type" 12-lipoxygenases (26,27). The human platelet 12-lipoxygenase is a 75-kDa, 663–amino acid, nonheme-iron–containing enzyme (28). It is a soluble enzyme but may be associated with membranes under various conditions and, presumably, for access to its substrate, arachidonic acid. Unlike the enzyme members of the cyclooxygenase pathway, the platelet 12-lipoxygenase does not undergo a rapid inactivation. Instead, 12-HPETE synthesis can continue in a near linear fashion for a sustained period (i.e., 20 to 60 minutes) (29). Therefore, this pathway may be involved in regulating longer-term processes rather than rapid platelet shape change, granule release, and aggregation. Indeed, 12-lipoxygenase studies have focused on its role in angiogenesis and cancer (30–32). A link between 12-lipoxygenase and integrin function has been reported (32). One of the difficulties in ascertaining functions of the platelet 12-lipoxygenase pathway has been the lack of specific inhibitors. Several nonspecific lipoxygenase inhibitors, including eicosatetraynoic acid, nordihydroguaiaretic acid, baicalein, esculetin, and phenidone, have yielded various results that indicate potential roles for the 12-lipoxygenase pathway in modulation of aggregation in response to different agonists [see (33), for example] or in modulation of platelet-adhesive events. A relatively new 12-HETE synthesis inhibitor OPC-29030 suppressed activation of the platelet glycoprotein (GP) IIb/IIIa in vitro and resulted in the inhibition of coronary thrombosis in vivo in dogs (34). Studies from platelet 12-lipoxygenase–deficient mice have indicated a role for this pathway in negatively modulating adenosine 5′-diphosphate (ADP)–induced aggregation (35). However, it should be noted that mouse platelets have a number of distinct properties compared to human platelets, including different expression profiles of thrombin (protease-activated) receptors (36).

# PLATELET EICOSANOID SIGNALING

## Thromboxane Receptors

The purification of the human platelet $TxA_2$ receptor (TP) was first accomplished in 1989 (37) using affinity chromatography with an immobilized antagonist [S-145; 5Z-7-(3-endo-phenylsulfonylamino-[2.2.1.]-bicyclohept-2-exo-yl)heptenoic acid]. Two years later, the cloning and expression of this receptor were reported from a placenta cDNA library (38). The TP receptor is a member of the seven transmembrane-spanning G protein–coupled receptor (GPCR) superfamily and consists of 343 amino acids. In 1994, it was determined that a second form of the TP receptor could be generated at the messenger RNA level in human endothelial cells (39). Therefore, the first form of the receptor has been designated the platelet/placenta or $TP\alpha$ receptor, and the second form, the endothelial or $TP\beta$ receptor. $TP\beta$ is identical to $TP\alpha$ for the first 328 amino acids. Only the carboxy terminus differentiates the two receptor forms because of alternative splicing of a single copy gene. Although the messenger RNA for both $TP\alpha$ and $TP\beta$ has been found in human platelets, only $TP\alpha$ protein is expressed in these cells (40).

Pharmacologic and radioligand-binding studies have concluded the presence of two subtypes of TP receptors on human platelets (41,42). $PGH_2$ binds to the same receptor as $TxA_2$ and its mimetics. Pharmacologic heterogeneity exists between the receptors that mediate vascular smooth muscle cell contraction and those that mediate platelet aggregation (43,44). On platelets, a high-affinity site for the $TxA_2$ mimetic known as I-BOP ([15- (1α,2β[5Z],3α-[1E,3S],4α)]-7-[3-(3-hydroxy-4-[p-iodophenoxy]-1-butenyl)-7-oxa-bicyclo[2.2.1]hept-2-yl]-5-heptenoic acid) or a reversible site for the antagonist GR32191 ([1r-(1α[Z],2β,3β,5α)]-(+)-7-[5-([(1,1′-biphenyl)-4-yl]methoxy) 3-hydroxy-2-(1-piperidinyl) cyclopentyl]-4-heptenoic acid hydrochloride) is associated with platelet shape change and increases in intracellular calcium (41,42). A low-affinity site for I-BOP or an irreversible binding site for GR32191 is linked to platelet aggregation, secretion, and phospholipase C activation. The molecular characterization of the two TP receptor subtypes cannot be explained in terms of $TP\alpha$ and $TP\beta$ forms because they show identical ligand binding properties but may be related to differential coupling to G proteins. $G_q$ is the main G protein interacting with TP in platelets (45). However, additional forms, such as $G\alpha_{11}$, $G\alpha_{12}$, $G\alpha_{13}$, and a high-molecular-weight G protein ($G_h$), may transduce $TxA_2$ actions (46,47). In transfected cell culture systems, both $TP\alpha$ and $TP\beta$ couple to phospholipase C activation, whereas the $TP\alpha$ form activates adenylate cyclase and $TP\beta$ inhibits it (48).

Exposure of human platelets to $TxA_2$ agonists results in rapid desensitization of biochemical and functional responses to interaction with its receptor, thereby limiting the potent amplifying effects of this eicosanoid. The pathways that govern desensitization of the $\alpha$ and $\beta$ isoforms vary, depending on whether they are natively expressed or transfected, and on the cell type used for expression studies, making it difficult to extrapolate these findings to native systems. Protein kinase C phosphorylation of the carboxy terminus of $TP\alpha$ appears to be the predominant regulatory pathway in platelets (49). Data consistent with TP downregulation in megakaryocytic cells have been presented (50). However, in transfection systems, $TP\alpha$, in contrast to $TP\beta$, undergoes neither constitutive nor agonist-induced internalization (51,52), leaving this phase of TP regulation in platelets as an open question. Therefore, the simplified signaling events for $TxA_2$ in platelets can be summarized as follows: (a) synthesis of $TxA_2$ and release from the

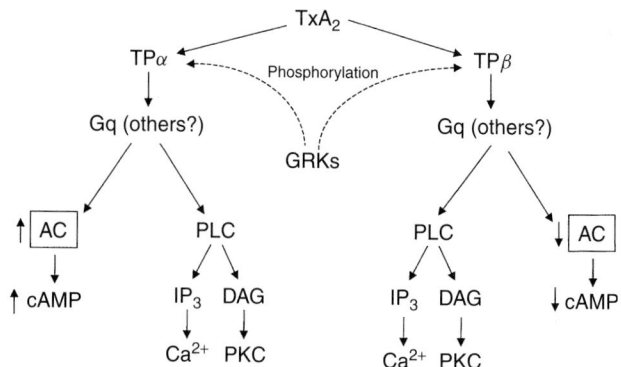

**FIGURE 36-3.** Thromboxane $A_2$ ($TxA_2$) signaling pathways. In human platelets, $TxA_2$ binds to the G protein–coupled receptor $TP\alpha$, which is coupled to the G protein Gq and others. This leads to activation of phospholipase C (PLC), formation of inositol trisphosphates ($IP_3$) and diacylglycerol (DAG), with ensuing elevation of intracellular calcium levels and activation of protein kinase C (PKC). In transfected cells, this receptor can also couple to the activation of adenylyl cyclase (AC), leading to the enhanced synthesis of adenosine 3′, 5′-cyclic monophosphate (cAMP). A similar pathway of activation via a thromboxane receptor variant $TP\beta$ exists in endothelial cells, but in transfected cells this pathway can inhibit AC. Desensitization of thromboxane receptor-mediated signaling is mediated by phosphorylation events by G protein receptor kinases (GRKs).

cell; (b) binding to a cell surface GPCR; (c) increase in intracellular calcium level and shape change; (d) phospholipase C activation, platelet secretion, and irreversible aggregation (see Fig. 36-3); and (e) PKC-dependent TP desensitization.

Isoprostanes, free radical-catalyzed products of arachidonic acid that are increased during vascular disease, may act as incidental ligands at the TP. Neither $TP\alpha$ nor $TP\beta$ ligate with $iPF_{2\alpha}III$, the most extensively studied isoprostane, when they are individually expressed (53). It is noteworthy that $TP\alpha$ can form heterodimers with $TP\beta$, leading to an increase in isoprostane signaling (54) and that membrane localization of $TP\beta$ is stabilized during exposure of $TP\beta$ overexpressing cells to oxidant stress (55). However, the relevance of these findings to platelet biology is not yet known. Therefore, it is worth considering that isoprostanes may propagate disease in syndromes where platelet activation and oxidant stress coincide.

It should be mentioned that human platelets have specific binding sites for other prostanoids. $PGI_2$, $PGE_2$, and $PGD_2$ interact with specific binding sites on platelets (see Fig. 36-4). Activation, at low concentrations, of the EP3 receptor for $PGE_2$, enhances platelet aggregation (4). In contrast, activation of the IP receptor (by $PGI_2$ or high concentrations of $PGE_2$) or the DP receptor antagonizes $TxA_2$ action by increases in adenosine 3′, 5′-cyclic monophosphate via Gs and adenylyl cyclase activation.

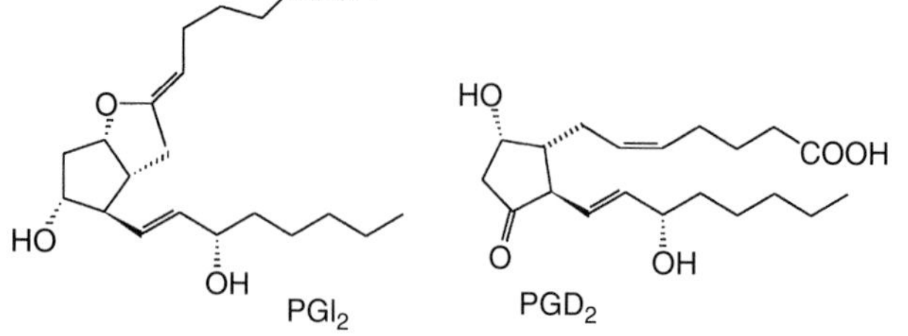

**FIGURE 36-4.** Platelet inhibitory eicosanoids. The structures of prostacyclin ($PGI_2$) and prostaglandin $D_2$ ($PGD_2$) are shown. These eicosanoids bind to prostacyclin (IP) and $PGD_2$ (DP) receptors, respectively, on human platelets and cause elevation of intracellular 3′, 5′-cyclic phosphate levels and inhibition of platelet aggregation.

## 12-Hydroxy-Eicosatetraenoic Acid Signaling

Even though the existence of the 12-lipoxygenase pathway in human platelets has been known since 1974, signaling through it is still clouded in mystery (7). 12-HETE, once formed, could exit the platelet and signal through a cell surface GPCR like other eicosanoids, but one has yet to be conclusively identified. There is evidence for this mode of binding in certain tumor cell lines that is linked to downstream protein kinase C activation (56). Data in support of an alternative mode of action indicate that 12-HETE binds to a large 650-kDa intracellular complex containing heat shock proteins in megakaryocytelike human erythroleukemia cells (57). Downstream signaling events are unknown. Alternatively, 12-HETE could be rapidly incorporated into platelet lipid membranes by acylases to influence membrane structure and various platelet biochemical parameters.

## CLINICAL IMPLICATIONS OF PLATELET EICOSANOIDS

Activated platelets release $TxA_2$, which induces aggregation in other platelets and constricts vascular smooth muscle. What is thromboxane's precise role in thrombosis and hemostasis? When platelet $TxA_2$ production is inhibited by aspirin ingestion, bleeding time is prolonged by 2 to 3 minutes. Nonetheless, such platelets still aggregate in response to thrombin or exposure to moderate doses of collagen (58,59). $TxA_2$ serves to amplify platelet responses to weak agonists like ADP and epinephrine. Taken together, these findings indicate a nonessential requirement of $TxA_2$ in hemostasis but a decreased ability of platelets to form a normal hemostatic plug if synthesis is blocked. $TxA_2$ synthesis is increased in a variety of cardiovascular diseases such as unstable angina pectoris, acute myocardial infarction, lupus nephritis, pregnancy-induced hypertension, and diabetes (60). Numerous studies have documented the efficacy of aspirin administration in reducing the risk of cardiovascular death, nonfatal myocardial infarction, transient ischemic attack, or stroke (61). At the doses used, most of the benefits are due to reduction in platelet thromboxane production through the PGHS-1 pathway. However, additional aspirin-evoked actions have been suggested and are possible. Recently, the phenomenon in which platelets are not fully inhibited by low-dose aspirin, termed "aspirin resistance," has been described [see (20) and references therein]. Indeed, low-dose, aspirin-insensitive $TxA_2$ production has been reported in patients with unstable coronary syndromes, and this may reflect PGHS-2–dependent $TxA_2$ biosynthesis, which is enhanced in clinical conditions associated with increased platelet regeneration. Traditional NSAIDs, which reversibly inhibit PGHS activity, do not afford the same cardiovascular protection as aspirin. On the contrary, at least one NSAID, ibuprofen, blocks the antiplatelet effects of aspirin when both drugs are used in combination (62).

Platelet activation in thromboembolic disorders is associated with episodic $TxA_2$ generation *in vivo*. Circulating and urinary thromboxane metabolites, such as 11-dehydro-$TxB_2$ and 2,3-dinor-$TxB_2$, can be measured as indices of platelet activation in these settings (63,64).

Cases of thromboxane deficiency and reduced 12-lipoxygenase product generation have been described in the medical literature (65,66). In these cases, no underlying genetic abnormalities have been found in the genes encoding PGHS, $TxA_2$ synthase, or 12-lipoxygenase. A genetic defect has been uncovered in the TP receptor in a dominantly inherited bleeding disorder characterized by a defect in platelet responsiveness to TP receptor agonists (65). An arginine-to-leucine codon mutation at residue 60, which

resides in the first intracellular loop, was found. This mutated receptor binds TP ligands normally but displays a diminished capacity to activate phospholipase C and adenylyl cyclase, on the basis of transfection studies. Therefore, this bleeding disorder could be caused by a genetic defect in an eicosanoid signaling pathway. More recently, genetic variations in the PGHS-1 gene have been described that could potentially influence the response to aspirin (67).

Prostacyclin synthesized by vascular endothelium is the most potent endogenous platelet antiaggregatory agent known (68). It inhibits aggregation in response to all known agonists, including thrombin. Prostacyclin production by the endothelium may be an important mechanism in preventing platelets from adhering to the vessel wall. When the vessel is damaged, the lack of synthesis in that region allows platelets to adhere to subendothelial collagen and subsequently aggregate, beginning the process of hemostatic plug formation. Recently, $PGI_2$ was shown to modulate platelet–vascular interactions *in vivo* and specifically limit the response to $TxA_2$ (69).

The benefit of aspirin in reducing thromboembolic events may be limited by two main factors. First, inhibition of PGHS is not tissue specific. Aspirin inhibits vascular production of prostacyclin, a potent platelet inhibitor, in addition to preventing platelet $TxA_2$ formation. Selective inhibition of platelet cyclooxygenase is not possible with currently available oral preparations. Doses as low as 80 mg per day may not inhibit basal $PGI_2$ synthesis but do prevent its increased formation after chemical or mechanical stimulation, such as during coronary angioplasty (70). However, platelet selectivity can be achieved by taking advantage of the pharmacokinetics and pharmacodynamics of the drug. Because platelets are unable to regenerate PGHS, after exposure to aspirin, the enzyme recovers with a half-life of 5 days, which is equivalent to the platelet half-life. Consequently, it is possible to achieve cumulative inhibition of this enzyme in the platelet with small, repetitive doses given orally. In contrast, the nucleated endothelial cell recovers enzyme activity and $PGI_2$ biosynthesis within hours. Alternatively, circulating platelets may be inhibited by slow, local administration of aspirin, without achieving high systemic levels of the drug. For example, continuous intraduodenal administration of low-dose aspirin inhibits circulating platelets, with little aspirin detected systemically (71). Platelets in the portal circulation are exposed to relatively high concentrations of aspirin. The inhibited platelets pass into the systemic circulation, whereas the aspirin is rapidly deacylated to salicylic acid by nonspecific esterases in plasma and in liver. A controlled-release formulation of aspirin (75 mg) has been shown to inhibit platelet $TxA_2$ selectively, without suppressing systemic $PGI_2$ synthesis (72).

Second, aspirin leads to irritation of the gastrointestinal mucosa. A subclass of NSAIDs, the PGHS-2 inhibitors or coxibs, cause fewer gastrointestinal complications (73). However, the PGHS-2 isozyme is the predominant source of $PGI_2$ generation *in vivo* (74), and at least one PGHS-2 inhibitor, rofecoxib, has been associated with increased risk of myocardial infarction (73).

Aside from aspirin, there are several other antithrombotic agents that influence platelet $TxA_2$ action. These agents include thromboxane synthase inhibitors, TP receptor antagonists, and dual-action synthase/TP receptor antagonists (see Fig. 36-5). The thromboxane synthase inhibitors offer the advantage over aspirin to redirect eicosanoid metabolism toward an increase in inhibitory prostacyclin or eicosanoids. However, thromboxane synthase inhibition yields an overproduction of the endoperoxide intermediate $PGH_2$ and does not decrease the generation of isoprostanes, both of which can activate TP receptors. Thromboxane synthase inhibitors have failed to reach the clinic because of their short duration of action, moderate potency, and disappointing effects in

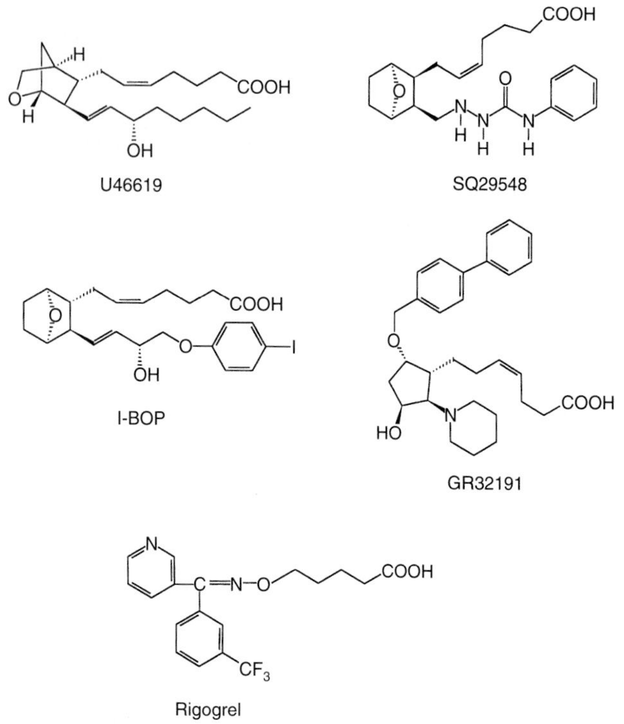

**FIGURE 36-5.** Drugs that influence thromboxane action or formation. U46619 and ([15-(1α,2β[5Z],3α-[1E,3S],4α)]-7-[3-(3-hydroxy-4-[*p*-iodophenoxy]-1-butenyl]-7-oxa-bicyclo (2.2.1) hept-2-yl]-5-heptenoic acid) (I-BOP) are two commonly used laboratory thromboxane mimetics. SQ29548 and GR32191 are frequently used *in vitro* thromboxane receptor antagonists. Ridogrel is a dual thromboxane synthase inhibitor/thromboxane receptor antagonist.

clinical trials of patients with coronary disease (3). Dual inhibitors would offer the best advantage because synthase inhibition would enhance inhibitory prostanoids at the expense of TxA$_2$, HHT, and malondialdehyde, whereas receptor antagonism would prevent PGH$_2$ action at the TP receptor. Ridogrel is a member of this class (Fig. 36-5).

Cases of platelet lipoxygenase deficiency in myeloproliferative disorders, characterized by frequent bleeding and thrombotic complications, have been detected (66). The platelets of some patients with the deficiency were able to synthesize elevated levels of thromboxane, and, paradoxically, episodes of hemorrhage were more prevalent than thrombosis in these patients. Bleeding complications occurred in significantly more patients with lipoxygenase deficiency than in patients with normal activity. In contrast, 13% of lipoxygenase-deficient patients, compared to 31% of patients with other myeloproliferative disorders, had thromboembolic complications. The mechanism for altered lipoxygenase expression affecting hemostasis and thrombosis awaits further research.

# ACKNOWLEDGMENTS

Supported in part by National Institutes of Health grant HL53558 and GM63130.

## References

1. Funk CD. Prostaglandins and leukotrienes: advances in eicosanoid biology. *Science* 2001;294:1871–1875.
2. Marcus AJ. Platelets and their disorders. In: Ratnoff OD, Forbes CD, eds. *Disorders of hemostasis*. Philadelphia: WB Saunders, 1996:79–137.
3. Verstraete M, Zoldhelyi P. Novel antithrombotic drugs in development. *Drugs* 1995;49:8566–8584.
4. Fabre JE, Nguyen M, Athirakul K, et al. Activation of the murine EP3 receptor for PGE$_2$ inhibits cAMP production and promotes platelet aggregation. *J Clin Invest* 2001;107:603–610.
5. Barry OP, Pratico D, Lawson JA, et al. Transcellular activation of platelets and endothelial cells by bioactive lipids in platelet microparticles. *J Clin Invest* 1997;99:2118–2127.
6. Needleman P, Turk J, Jakschik BA, et al. Arachidonic acid metabolism. *Annu Rev Biochem* 1986;55:69–102.
7. Hamberg M, Samuelsson B. Prostaglandin endoperoxides. Novel transformations of arachidonic acid in human platelets. *Proc Natl Acad Sci U S A* 1974;71:3400–3404.
8. Hecker M, Ullrich V. On the mechanism of prostacyclin and thromboxane A$_2$ biosynthesis. *J Biol Chem* 1989;264:141–150.
9. Siegel MI, McConnell RT, Porter NA, et al. Arachidonate metabolism via lipoxygenase and 12L-hydroperoxy-5,8,10,14-icosatetraenoic acid peroxidase sensitive to anti-inflammatory drugs. *Proc Natl Acad Sci U S A* 1980;77:308–312.
10. Ho YS, Magnenat JL, Bronson RT, et al. Mice deficient in cellular glutathione peroxidase develop normally and show no increased sensitivity to hyperoxia. *J Biol Chem* 1997;272:16644–16651.
11. Chen XS, Brash AR, Funk CD. Purification and characterization of recombinant histidine-tagged human platelet 12-lipoxygenase expressed in a baculovirus/insect cell system. *Eur J Biochem* 1993;214:845–852.
12. Six DA, Dennis EA. The expanding superfamily of phospholipase A(2) enzymes: classification and characterization. *Biochim Biophys Acta* 2000; 1488(1-2):1–19.
13. Kudo I, Murakami M. Phospholipase A$_2$ enzymes. *Prostaglandins Other Lipid Mediat* 2002; 68–69:3–58.
14. Wong DA, Kita Y, Uozumi N, et al. Discrete role for cytosolic phospholipase A(2)alpha in platelets: studies using single and double mutant mice of cytosolic and group IIA secretory phospholipase A(2). *J Exp Med* 2002; 196:349–357.
15. Clark JD, Schievella AR, Nalefski EA, et al. Cytosolic phospholipase A$_2$. *J Lipid Mediat Cell Signal* 1995;12:83–117.
16. Riendeau D, Guay J, Weech PK, et al. Arachidonyl trifluoromethyl ketone, a potent inhibitor of 85-kDa phospholipase A$_2$, blocks production of arachidonate and 12-hydroxyeicosatetraenoic acid by calcium ionophore–challenged platelets. *J Biol Chem* 1994;269:15619–15624.
17. Bell RL, Kennerly DA, Stanford N, et al. Diglyceride lipase: a pathway for arachidonate release from human platelets. *Proc Natl Acad Sci U S A* 1979;76:3238–3241.
18. Smith WL, Garavito RM, DeWitt DL. Prostaglandin endoperoxide H synthases (cyclooxygenases)-1 and -2. *J Biol Chem* 1996;271:33157–33160.
19. Weber AA, Zimmermann KC, Meyer-Kirchrath J, et al. Cyclooxygenase-2 in human platelets as a possible factor in aspirin resistance. *Lancet* 1999; 353:900.
20. Rocca B, Secchiero P, Ciabattoni G, et al. Cyclooxygenase-2 expression is induced during human megakaryopoiesis and characterizes newly formed platelets. *Proc Natl Acad Sci U S A* 2002;99:7634–7639.
21. Picot D, Loll PJ, Garavito RM. The x-ray crystal structure of the membrane protein prostaglandin H$_2$ synthase-1. *Nature* 1994;367:243–249.
22. Roth GJ, Stanford N, Jacobs JW, et al. Acetylation of prostaglandin synthetase by aspirin. Purification and properties of the acetylated protein from sheep vesicular gland. *Biochemistry* 1977;16:4244–4248.
23. Funk CD, Funk LB, Kennedy ME, et al. Human platelet/erythroleukemia cell prostaglandin G/H synthase: cDNA cloning, expression, and gene chromosomal assignment. *FASEB J* 1991;5:2304–2312.
24. Hawkey CJ. COX-2 inhibitors. *Lancet* 1999;353:307–314.
25. Ohashi K, Ruan KH, Kulmacz RJ, et al. Primary structure of human thromboxane synthase determined from the cDNA sequence. *J Biol Chem* 1992;267:789–793.
26. Yamamoto S, Suzuki H, Ueda N. Arachidonate 12-lipoxygenases. *Prog Lipid Res* 1997;36:23–41.
27. Funk CD. The molecular biology of mammalian lipoxygenases and the quest for eicosanoid functions using lipoxygenase-deficient mice. *Biochim Biophys Acta* 1996;1304:65–84.
28. Funk CD, Furci L, FitzGerald GA. Molecular cloning, primary structure, and expression of the human platelet/erythroleukemia cell 12-lipoxygenase. *Proc Natl Acad Sci U S A* 1990;87:5638–5642.
29. Nugteren DH. Arachidonate lipoxygenase. In: *Prostaglandins in hematology*. NY: Spectrum Publications, 1977:11–24.
30. Nie D, Tang K, Diglio C, et al. Eicosanoid regulation of angiogenesis: role of endothelial arachidonate 12-lipoxygenase. *Blood* 2000;95:2304–2311.
31. Virmani J, Johnson EN, Klein-Szanto AJ, et al. Role of 'platelet-type' 12-lipoxygenase in skin carcinogenesis. *Cancer Lett* 2001;162:161–165.
32. Pidgeon GP, Tang D, Cai YL, et al. Overexpression of platelet-type 12-lipoxygenase promotes tumor cell survival by enhancing alpha(v)beta(3) and alpha(v)beta(5) integrin expression. *Cancer Res* 2003;63:4258–4267.
33. Nyby MD, Sasaki M, Ideguchi Y, et al. Platelet lipoxygenase inhibitors attenuate thrombin- and thromboxane mimetic-induced intracellular calcium mobilization and platelet aggregation. *J Pharmacol Exp Ther* 1996; 278:503–509.
34. Katoh A, Ikeda H, Murohara T, et al. Platelet-derived 12-hydroxyeicosatetraenoic acid plays an important role in mediating canine coronary

thrombosis by regulating platelet glycoprotein IIb/IIIa activation. *Circulation* 1998;98:2891–2898.

35. Johnson EN, Brass LF, Funk CD. Increased platelet sensitivity to ADP in mice lacking platelet-type 12-lipoxygenase. *Proc Natl Acad Sci U S A* 1998;95:3100–3105.

36. Kahn ML, Zheng YW, Huang W, et al. A dual thrombin receptor system for platelet activation. *Nature* 1998;394:690–694.

37. Ushikubi F, Nakajima M, Hirata M, et al. Purification of the thromboxane $A_2$/prostaglandin $H_2$ receptor from human blood platelets. *J Biol Chem* 1989;264:16496–16501.

38. Hirata M, Hayashi Y, Ushikubi F, et al. Cloning and expression of cDNA for a human thromboxane $A_2$ receptor. *Nature* 1991;349:617–620.

39. Raychowdhury MK, Yukawa M, Collins LJ, et al. Alternative splicing produces a divergent cytoplasmic tail in the human endothelial thromboxane $A_2$ receptor. *J Biol Chem* 1994;269:19256–19261 [published erratum appears in *J Biol Chem* 1995;270: 7011].

40. Habib A, FitzGerald GA, Maclouf J. Phosphorylation of the thromboxane receptor a, the predominant isoform expressed in human platelets. *J Biol Chem* 1999;274:2645–2651.

41. Dorn GW II. Distinct platelet thromboxane $A_2$/prostaglandin $H_2$ subtypes. A radioligand binding study of human platelets. *J Clin Invest* 1989; 84:1883–1891.

42. Takahara K, Murray R, FitzGerald GA, et al. The response to thromboxane $A_2$ analogues in human platelets. Discrimination of two binding sites linked to distinct effector systems. *J Biol Chem* 1990;265:6836–6844.

43. Furci L, Fitzgerald DJ, FitzGerald GA. Heterogeneity of prostaglandin $H_2$/thromboxane $A_2$ receptors: distinct subtypes mediate vascular smooth muscle contraction and platelet aggregation. *J Pharmacol Exp Ther* 1991; 258:74–81.

44. Mais DE, Saussy DL Jr, Chaikhouni A, et al. Pharmacologic characterization of human and canine thromboxane $A_2$/prostaglandin $H_2$ receptors in platelets and blood vessels: evidence for different receptors. *J Pharmacol Exp Ther* 1985;233:418–424.

45. Shenker A, Goldsmith P, Unson CG, et al. The G protein coupled to the thromboxane $A_2$ receptor in human platelets is a member of the novel Gq family. *J Biol Chem* 1991;266:9309–9313.

46. Prevost N, Woulfe D, Tognolini M, et al. Contact-dependent signaling during the late events of platelet activation. *J Thromb Haemost* 2003;1: 1613–1627.

47. Vezza R, Habib A, FitzGerald GA. Differential signaling by the thromboxane receptor isoforms via the novel GTP-binding protein, Gh. *J Biol Chem* 1999;274:12774–12779.

48. Hirata T, Ushikubi F, Kakizuka A, et al. Two thromboxane $A_2$ receptor isoforms in human platelets. Opposite coupling to adenylyl cyclase with different sensitivity to Arg60 to Leu mutation. *J Clin Invest* 1996;97: 949–956.

49. Habib A, FitzGerald GA, Maclouf J. Phosphorylation of the thromboxane receptor alpha, the predominant isoform expressed in human platelets. *J Biol Chem* 1999;274:2645–2651.

50. Dorn GW II. Regulation of response to thromboxane $A_2$ in CHRF-288 megakaryocytic cells. *Am J Physiol* 1992;262(4 Pt 1):C991–C999.

51. Parent JL, Labrecque P, Orsini MJ, et al. Internalization of the $TxA_2$ receptor a and b isoforms. Role of the differentially spliced COOH terminus in agonist-promoted receptor internalization. *J Biol Chem* 1999;274: 8941–8948.

52. Parent JL, Labrecque P, Driss Rochdi M, et al. Role of the differentially spliced carboxyl terminus in thromboxane $A_2$ receptor trafficking: identification of a distinct motif for tonic internalization. *J Biol Chem* 2001; 276:7079–7085.

53. Pratico D, Smyth EM, Violi F, et al. Local amplification of platelet function by 8-Epi prostaglandin F2alpha is not mediated by thromboxane receptor isoforms. *J Biol Chem* 1996;271:14916–14924.

54. Huang AY, Kostetskaia E, McGinley K, et al. Interaction of human prostacyclin and thromboxane receptors. *Arterioscler Thromb Vasc Biol* 2003; 23(5):P324.

55. Valentin F, Field MC, Tippins JR. The mechanism of oxidative stress stabilization of the thromboxane receptor in COS-7 cells. *J Biol Chem* 2004; 279:8316–8324.

56. Liu B, Khan WA, Hannun YA, et al. 12(*S*)-hydroxyeicosatetraenoic acid and 13(*S*)-hydroxyoctadecadienoic acid regulation of protein kinase C–alpha in melanoma cells: role of receptor-mediated hydrolysis of inositol phospholipids. *Proc Natl Acad Sci U S A* 1995;92:9323–9327.

57. Herbertsson H, Kuhme T, Evertsson U, et al. Identification of subunits of the 650 kDa 12(*S*)-HETE binding complex in carcinoma cells. *J Lipid Res* 1998;39:237–244.

58. Zucker MB, Peterson J. Inhibition of adenosine diphosphate–induced secondary aggregation and other platelet functions by acetylsalicylic acid ingestion. *Proc Soc Exp Biol Med* 1967;127:547–552.

59. Zucker MB, Peterson J. Effect of acetylsalicylic acid, other nonsteroidal anti-inflammatory agents, and dipyridamole on human blood platelets. *J Lab Clin Med* 1970;76:66–71.

60. Fitzgerald DJ, Roy L, Catella F, et al. Platelet activation in unstable coronary disease. *N Engl J Med* 1986;315:983–989.

61. Catella-Lawson F, FitzGerald GA. Long-term aspirin in the prevention of cardiovascular disorders. Recent developments and variations on a theme. *Drug Saf* 1995;13:69–75.

62. Catella-Lawson F, Reilly MP, Kapoor SC, et al. Cyclooxygenase inhibitors and the antiplatelet effects of aspirin. *N Engl J Med* 2001;345:1809–1817.

63. Catella F, Healy D, Lawson JA, et al. 11-Dehydrothromboxane $B_2$: a quantitative index of thromboxane $A_2$ formation in the human circulation. *Proc Natl Acad Sci U S A* 1986;83:5861–5865.

64. Patrono C, Ciabattoni G, Davi G. Thromboxane biosynthesis in cardiovascular diseases. *Stroke* 1990;21(Suppl. 12):130–133.

65. Hirata T, Kakizuka A, Ushikubi F, et al. Arg60 to Leu mutation of the human thromboxane $A_2$ receptor in a dominantly inherited bleeding disorder. *J Clin Invest* 1994;94:1662–1667.

66. Schafer AI. Deficiency of platelet lipoxygenase activity in myeloproliferative disorders. *N Engl J Med* 1982;306:381–386.

67. Halushka MK, Walker LP, Halushka PV. Genetic variation in cyclooxygenase 1: effects on response to aspirin. *Clin Pharmacol Ther* 2003;73: 122–130.

68. Dusting GJ, MacDonald PS. Prostacyclin and vascular function: implications for hypertension and atherosclerosis. *Pharmacol Ther* 1990;48:323–344.

69. Cheng Y, Austin SC, Rocca B, et al. Role of prostacyclin in the cardiovascular response to thromboxane $A_2$. *Science* 2002;296:539–544.

70. Braden GA, Knapp HR, FitzGerald GA. Suppression of eicosanoid biosynthesis during coronary angioplasty by fish oil and aspirin. *Circulation* 1991;84:679–685.

71. FitzGerald GA, Lupinetti M, Charman SA, et al. Presystemic acetylation of platelets by aspirin: reduction in rate of drug delivery to improve biochemical selectivity for thromboxane $A_2$. *J Pharmacol Exp Ther* 1991; 259:1043–1049.

72. Clarke RJ, Mayo G, Price P, et al. Suppression of thromboxane $A_2$ but not of systemic prostacyclin by controlled-release aspirin. *N Engl J Med* 1991; 325:1137–1141.

73. Bombardier C, Laine L, Reicin A et al., VIGOR Study Group. Comparison of upper gastrointestinal toxicity of rofecoxib and naproxen in patients with rheumatoid arthritis. *N Engl J Med* 2000;343:1520–1528, 2 p following 1528.

74. McAdam BF, Catella-Lawson F, Mardini IA, et al. Systemic biosynthesis of prostacyclin by cyclooxygenase (COX)-2: the human pharmacology of a selective inhibitor of COX-2. *Proc Natl Acad Sci U S A* 1999;96: 272–277.

# CHAPTER 37 ■ PLATELET AND MEGAKARYOCYTE LIPIDS

PAUL K. SCHICK AND TRACEE S. PANETTI

Lipids in platelets are primarily membrane components and are integrally involved in platelet biologic activities such as membrane fluidity, platelet coagulant activities, the production of eicosanoids, and signaling pathways.

The lipid/protein ratios (w/w) in whole human platelets and platelet membranes are 0.28 and 0.58, respectively. Phospholipids are the most abundant class of lipids, constituting approximately 79% of total platelet lipids by weight. Five major phospholipids have been identified in human platelets: Phosphatidylcholine (PC) constitutes approximately 38% of total phospholipids; phosphatidylethanolamine (PE), 27%; sphingomyelin (SM), 17%; phosphatidylserine (PS), 10%; and phosphatidylinositol (PI), 5% (1) (see Table 37-1). Approximately 60% of PE is composed of plasmalogen PE, in which the acyl group at the C-1 position of the phospholipid is replaced by an alkenyl ether group. The importance of platelet plasmalogens is not known. However, it has been suggested that plasmalogens may protect platelet phospholipids against oxidative degradation (2). Platelet PC contains a subspecies of alkyl-PC, which may serve as a precursor for the formation of platelet activating factor (PAF) (3). Trace amounts of lysoPC, cardiolipin, and polyinositides have been detected in platelets.

Virtually all of the fatty acids in platelets are esterified in phospholipids, and only trace amounts of free fatty acids have been detected (1). The fatty acid composition of phospholipids would be expected to have a major influence on membrane-mediated platelet activities.

Cholesterol is the predominant neutral lipid in platelets and, like phospholipids, is an important structural and functional component of membranes (1). Glycolipids and ceramides have been detected in platelets, and these unique lipids may be important for platelet function, as well as for the maturation of megakaryocytes (MKs).

Platelets have a greater capacity for lipid metabolism than leukocytes and erythrocytes. For example, platelets are capable of de novo fatty acid and phospholipid synthesis (7,8). However, evidence suggests that lipid synthesis and uptake in MKs determine the content of certain platelet lipids such as cholesterol (9,10).

# PHOSPHOLIPIDS

## Organization of Phospholipids in Platelet Membranes

Cell membranes are highly organized structures with specific arrangements of proteins and lipids. The availability of lipids on the platelet surface is critical for platelet biology (1,11–16). The use of phospholipases and trinitrobenzene sulfonic acid (TNBS), a nonpenetrating membrane probe, has revealed that choline phospholipids (i.e., PC and SM) are primarily exposed on the platelet surface, whereas acidic phospholipids (i.e., PE, PS, and PI) are located in the inner leaflet of the platelet plasma membrane (1,4–6,11–20). This paradigm for the arrangement of phospholipids in platelet membrane also has been supported by studies using spin-labeled aminophospholipids (20) and annexin V, a protein that has a high affinity for aminophospholipids (12,21). In this respect, the distribution of phospholipids in platelet membranes is similar to that in erythrocytes and other cells. Phospholipases have been used to determine that 57% of total human platelet phospholipids are located in the plasma membrane (5,6) (see Fig. 37-1).

## Functional Aspects of Lipid Symmetry

Lipid asymmetry in platelet membranes has physiologic implications, because acidic phospholipids, particularly PS, are thought to promote platelet coagulant activities (see Chapter 38). Excessive thrombin formation on the platelet surface is less likely to occur because PS is not exposed on the surface of unstimulated platelets (22).

Evidence for the emergence of PS and PE on the surface of stimulated platelets has been provided by the use of thrombin (23), phospholipases (6,17), and with annexin V (12). Thrombin alone increased the exposure of PE but not PS on the platelet surface, as judged by labeling with TNBS (4). There were no differences in the fatty acid composition of PE that became exposed on the platelet surface in response to thrombin to that in PE that had not become expressed on the surface (24). Combinations of collagen and thrombin induced significant hydrolysis of PE and PS, but neither of these aggregating agents, when used alone, induced the hydrolysis of significant amounts of platelet lipids (5).

The extent of exteriorization of PS depends on the activator, and the most effective activator is $Ca^{2+}$ ionophore (6,22). The potency of physiologic activators decreases in the following order: Complement membrane attack complex (C5b-9), collagen plus thrombin, collagen, and thrombin.

The physiologic importance of exteriorization of PS in activated platelets is supported by a correlation with the extent of PS exposure and the development of platelet procoagulant activity. PS exposure on the platelet surface is reported to provide binding sites for prothrombin and factor IX that facilitate the assembly and activation of tenase and prothrombinase complexes (25). Patients with Scott syndrome provide further evidence of a role for PS. Patients with Scott syndrome have an isolated defect in platelet coagulant activity (impaired factor X and prothrombin activation) associated with a decrease in exposure of PS on the platelet surface (13). Patients with Scott syndrome have an isolated defect in platelet coagulant activity. The role of PS in platelet coagulant activity was supported by

591

DISTRIBUTION OF PLATELET PHOSPHOLIPIDS

| Platelet phospholipids | Percentage of total phospholipids | Percentage present on the surface (4–6) |
|---|---|---|
| Phosphatidylcholine | 38% | 60% |
| Phosphatidylethanolamine | 27% | 20% |
| Sphingomyelin | 17% | 90% |
| Phosphatidylserine | 10% | 0 to trace |
| Phosphatidylinositol | 5% | 0 to trace |

Approximately 79% of platelet lipids are phospholipids by weight.

evidence that the incubation of platelets with phospholipases [e.g., phospholipase A2 (PLA2)] that can attack PS inhibits platelet coagulant activities, whereas phospholipases that spare PS [e.g., phospholipase C (PLC) from *Clostridium perfringens* or sphingomyelinase] do not modify platelet prothrombinase activity (6).

PC present on the platelet surface may have a role in platelet aggregation and secretion. The hydrolysis of exposed PC by PLC from *C. perfringens* induces the release reaction in platelets, identical to that caused by thrombin (26). PC has also been implicated in platelet activation by the observation that naturally occurring myeloma anti-PC antibody can inhibit platelet aggregation (27).

The activation of platelets by calcium ionophore A23187, thrombin plus collagen, or complement proteins C5b-9 is associated with the shedding of small vesicles (microparticles) from the platelet surface that contain plasma membrane glycoproteins, P selectin, and cytoskeletal proteins (23,28–30). It has been proposed that the association of the membrane skeleton with the plasma membrane prevents the shedding of procoagulant-rich microvesicles from unstimulated platelets and that calpain-induced disruption of actin–membrane interactions may lead to the shedding of platelet microparticles (31). However, the inhibition of calpain activity with its inhibitor, MDL28170, did not prevent the formation of microparticles (32). It has been suggested that these microparticles are highly enriched with acidic phospholipids (12). However, the formation of platelet microparticles is important for the assembly of the prothrombin complex (13,23,28,29). The formation of microparticles was significantly decreased in platelets from a patient with Scott syndrome, an isolated defect in platelet procoagulant activity (23). The formation of microparticles may support platelet coagulant activity by increasing the availability of aminophospholipids for the assembly of the prothrombinase complex.

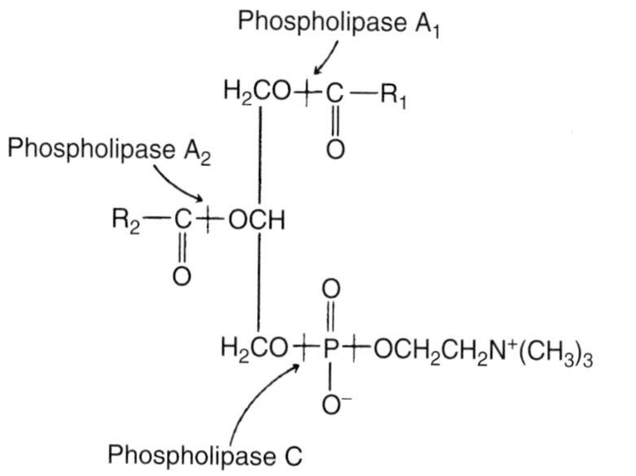

## Organization of Phospholipids in Membranes of Erythrocytes and Other Eukaryotic Cells

The understanding of erythrocyte membrane organization is relevant to understanding platelet coagulant activity. Intact erythrocytes in which PS is not exposed on the surface have no effect on coagulation. However, PS is exposed on the surface of thalassemic erythrocytes augment coagulant activity. This surface exposure may be responsible for the hypercoagulability in this disorder (33). *In vitro* studies in which PS is present on the surface of inside-out vesicles prepared from erythrocytes also support the role of the exposure of PS since these structures have prothrombinase activity (34).

Investigations of erythrocytes from patients with homozygous sickle cell anemia have provided new insights into transbilayer mobility of phospholipids. PS becomes exposed on the surface of irreversibly sickled erythrocytes and is associated with coagulant activity (35,36). In contrast, coagulant activity cannot be demonstrated in normal erythrocytes in which PS is not present on the cell surface. Several studies have indicated that sickling results in local uncoupling of the membrane lipid bilayer and cytoskeleton (37). It has been suggested that transbilayer movement of phospholipids and the exposure of PS are limited to these regions and that lipid organization is normal in the domains of the membrane in which membrane–cytoskeletal relationships are maintained (23,29).

There is evidence that in the Wiscott-Aldrich syndrome, the exposure of PS signals the premature removal of platelets by splenic macrophages (38).

In general, apoptosis occurs in nucleated cells and not in anucleated platelets. However, along with the expression of PS on platelet surfaces, platelets contain many of the components of the apoptotic mechanism (39). Whether or not classical apoptosis can be documented in platelets, the study of the role of PS exposure and platelet death is important for studying platelet removal and preservation.

MKs are nucleated cells. Apoptosis markers have been detected and are involved in MK scenescence (40). However, PS exposure has not been studied in MKs.

FIGURE 37-1. Effect of phospholipases on phospholipids. Phospholipases have been classified by their sites of hydrolysis as shown. Since they hydrolyze primarily exposed lipids, they have been used to study the lipid organization of platelet membranes.

## Regulation of Lipid Asymmetry

Several mechanisms for the control of the asymmetric organization of phospholipids in the surface membranes of eukaryocytic cells have been proposed. Fluorescent and spin-labeled lipid analogs, nucleotide-binding domain-PS (NBD-PS), and NBD-PC have been used to provide this information (14). Three activities have been described: (a) An inward-directed aminophospholipid translocase, (b) an outward-directed floppase, and (c) a bidirectional lipid scramblase.

An adenosine triphosphate (ATP)–dependent aminophospholipid translocase that rapidly transports PS and PE from the outer to the inner leaflet of plasma has been reported in platelet plasma membranes (14,32) and in other cells (41–43). The transporter is inhibited by micromolar $Ca^{2+}$ plasma concentrations (44). The identity of ATP-dependent floppase has not been determined, but the transporter appears to have biochemical properties similar to an ATP-dependent translocase in red blood cells (45). An ATP-dependent floppase is reported to slowly transport all phospholipids from the inner to the outer surface membrane (46). However, the predominance of choline phospholipids in the outer leaflet of plasma membranes may be due to passive translayer movement to compensate for the active maintenance of aminophospholipids in the inner leaflet (14). A lipid scramblase can induce rapid, random, bidirectional movement of all phospholipids in surface membranes and thereby the exposure of aminophospholipids on the cell surface. An increase in intracellular $Ca^{2+}$ levels is required to trigger lipid scrambling. This activity has been detected in a variety of cells but appears to be more pronounced in platelets (15). This rapid dissipation of phospholipid asymmetry is thought to enable platelets to generate coagulant activity. Decreased lipid scramblase activity (47,48) and disrupted floppase activity (49) are reported to be occur in Scott syndrome.

## Concluding Comments on the Phospholipid (Asymmetry in Platelets)

The studies using TNBS and phospholipases, as well as the use of annexin V (16) offer strong support for the concept that the exposure of aminophospholipids plays a role in platelet coagulant activity. However, the evidence for the change in aminophospholipid distribution on the surface of activated platelets is dependent on the absence of platelet lysis or increased permeability of the platelet, or both. Either circumstance would result in the hydrolysis of internally located aminophospholipids. The studies that demonstrate increased exposure of PS in thrombin- and collagen-treated platelets also provide evidence that approximately 10% platelet lysis occurred (6,17). Membrane perturbation can occur without evidence of overt lysis. Therefore, the agents used to activate platelets could conceivably have induced subtle changes in platelet plasma membrane permeability without evidence of lysis, which rendered aminophospholipids susceptible to hydrolysis by phospholipases. This possibility is relevant, because platelets exposed to diamide, A23187, and combinations of collagen and thrombin reacted readily with PLA2 from *Naja naja* alone. This PLA by itself had little action on resting platelets (5). This information indicates that the physical state of phospholipids, such as the packing of phospholipids, was altered in stimulated platelets and that significant membrane modification may have occurred.

The exposure of PE (50) and other membrane conformational changes also may have a role, along with PS, in triggering platelet coagulant activity under physiologic conditions. Thrombin induces little if any PS exposure, which may not be sufficient to support platelet coagulant activity (50). Evidence in experiments with reconstituted lipid vesicles indicates that the concomitant exposure of PE is necessary to support the binding of VIIIa to platelets (51). Changes in platelet aminophospholipid

orientation in platelet membranes may be associated with membrane conformation changes and the exposure of membrane proteins that, in conjunction with the exposure of PS, promote the generation of platelet coagulant activity.

# PHOSPHOINOSITIDES

Phosphoinositides (PPI) are involved in the activation of platelets and other mammalian cells. Specific aspects of the role of PPI in the activation of platelets are considered in Chapter 31.

PPI include PI and phosphatidylinositol phosphates—phosphatidylinositol 4-phosphate (PI 4-P), phosphatidylinositol 5-phosphate (PI 5-P), phosphatidylinositol 3-phosphate (PI 3-P), phosphatidylinositol-4,5-bisphosphate (PI 4,5-P2), phosphatidylinositol-3,4-bisphosphate (PI 3,4-P2), phosphatidylinositol-3,5-bisphosphate (PI 3,5-P2), and phosphatidylinositol-3,4,5-triphosphate (PI 3,4,5-P3), in which one, two, or three additional phosphate groups are present in the inositol ring (see Table 37-2). PI 3,4,5-P3; PI 3,4-P2; and PI 3,5-P2 are not present to any significant degree in unstimulated cells. PPI are present in small amounts in platelets and other cells. PI constitutes approximately 4% and PI 4-P plus PI 4,5-P2 fewer than 1% of total phospholipids present in human platelets.

Activation of platelets is associated with several interrelated changes in PPI and their metabolism. A fall in PI 4,5-P2 occurs early and transiently in activated platelets, as well as in other mammalian cells and tissues. It is regenerated by phosphorylation of PI and PI 4-P (52–58). In platelets, there is initially a diesteric cleavage of PI 4,5-P2 by inositol-specific PLC, which results in the production of 1,2-diacylglyceride (1,2-DG) and phosphatidylinositol-1,4,5-triphosphate (PI 1,4,5-P3). Subsequently, 1,2-DG can be deacylated to monoglyceride or phosphorylated to PA, which can be used for the resynthesis of PI (57). PA is also formed by phospholipase D acting on PC in activated platelets, but this contribution is minor (13%) compared to the contribution of inositol-specific PLC (58). These events constitute the PI cycle and are considered a major PI response during platelet stimulation (59).

Several of the enzymes necessary for the PI cycle have been demonstrated in human platelets. Platelet PLCs specific to PI mediate the diesteric hydrolysis of PI, PI 4,5-P2, and P I4-P *in vitro*, although PI 4,5-P2 is preferred (60,61). Platelets are capable of *de novo* synthesis of PI. DG kinase (for the PI cycle) is active in stimulated platelets. PA-cytidine monophosphate transferase, cytidine diphosphate diglyceride (CDP-diglyceride), and CDP-diglyceride myoinositol transferase, necessary for the use of PA for the resynthesis of PPI, also have been demonstrated in platelets (62,63).

Several potential physiologic roles of the PI response and the production of PA, diglyceride, and free arachidonate must be

## TABLE 37-2

### PLATELET PHOSPHOINOSITIDES

| | |
|---|---|
| Phosphatidylinositol | PI |
| Phosphatidylinositol 3-phosphate | PI 3-P |
| Phosphatidylinositol 4-phosphate | PI 4-P |
| Phosphatidylinositol 5-phosphate | PI 5-P |
| Phosphatidylinositol-3,4-bisphosphate | PI 3,4-P2 |
| Phosphatidylinositol-3,5-bisphosphate | PI 3,5-P2 |
| Phosphatidylinositol-4,5-bisphosphate | PI 4,5-P2 |
| Phosphatidylinositol-3,4,5-trisphosphate | PI 3,4,5-P3 |

PI is approximately 4% of platelet lipids, and PI 4-P plus PI 4,5-P2 are less than 1% of total phospholipids.

considered. 1,2-DG stimulates protein kinase C, probably by binding to the plasma membrane, which leads to the phosphorylation of the 47-kDa platelet protein (P47, pleckstrin) (64,65). The perturbation of platelet membranes by 1,2-DG also may promote the platelet release reaction.

The PI response stimulated by platelet agonists is thought to result in the production of free arachidonic acid (20:4). 1,2-DG (produced by the action of PLC) that is not phosphorylated to PA can be deacylated and serves as a potential source of free arachidonate by the action of diglyceride and monoglyceride lipases. These enzymes have been demonstrated in platelets (65–67). In addition, a PLA2 acting on PA has been found. However, it has been suggested that the PI response liberates only a fraction of the free 20:4 produced in thrombin-treated platelets (68). Other studies have indicated that the diglyceride/monoglyceride lipase pathway is not essential for the production of free 20:4 in activated platelets (69,70). PLA2 may be more important than PLC for the production of free 20:4 in activated platelets. PLA2 can liberate 20:4 by the deacylation of PE, PC, and other phospholipids apart from those in the PI cycle in activated platelets (71–73). When mass was measured, PC, rather than the other phospholipids, was the main source for free 20:4 in thrombin-treated platelets (74). 1,2-DG may promote the release of 20:4 by a PLA2-dependent pathway (75).

The conversion of PI 4,5-P2 to DG and inositol-1,4,5-trisphosphate is important for cellular activities, because the water-soluble PI 1,4,5-P3 is involved in the release of intracellular $Ca^{2+}$ (8,76). The phosphorylated PPI can be synthesized in platelets by the phosphorylation of PI by the action of kinases (59).

Most of these studies have been done with platelet lipids radiolabeled with $^{32}P$- or $^3H$-arachidonic acid (59). Because the incorporation of $^{32}P$ does not reflect endogenous distribution of PPI in platelets and the incorporation of $^3H$-arachidonic acid does not equilibrate with endogenous arachidonic acid, changes in the response of radiolabeled fatty acids may not provide reliable information about the metabolism of lipids and fatty acids in unlabeled pools (59–62,77). However, several studies have analyzed changes in lipid mass in activated platelets by chemical methods (68,77–81). This approach should provide more definitive information about phosphoinositide metabolism. One possible reason for the discrepancy between the distribution of radiolabeled 20:4 that had been incorporated into phospholipids after *in vitro* incubations, and the distribution of endogenous 20:4 is that MKs, but not platelets, may determine the content of all pools of lipids in platelets (15).

Several issues are unresolved concerning phosphoinositide metabolism in platelets (59,80). The relative roles of the PI and PPI cycles in activated platelets have not been defined. Although an extremely early fall in PI 4,5-P2 has been detected, it has been difficult to ascertain that this response is the initial event in platelet activation (59). Interestingly, there is evidence that phosphatidyl 4,5-biphosphate promotes PS exposure (82).

The relative roles of PI and other PPI in serving as sources for 1,2-DG in activated platelets have not been clarified (59, 83). It is unclear whether calcium has a primary or secondary role in the PI and PPI cycles (51). Further research may clarify the initial events in the lipid response to platelet activation and the role of the associated changes in cellular calcium and DG, PA, and inositol-1,4,5-trisphosphate in platelet activation.

Phosphatidylinositol 3-kinase (PI 3-K) is a heterodimer that has important roles in mitogenic signaling, cytoskeletal remodeling, and vesicular trafficking (84,85). The PI 3-K–dependent pathway may be responsible for signaling by collagen and in the priming action of thrombopoietin (86). The activation of $\alpha_{IIb}\beta_3$ in platelets induces the formation of PI 3-P, which is phosphorylated to PI 3,4-P2 and can activate protein kinase B/Akt. A C2 domain containing PI 3-K isoform (HsC2-PI3K) has been characterized in platelets and in a Children's Hospital Research

Foundation-288, a human cell line with MK features, and this PI 3-K isoform can induce the formation of PI3P. Therefore, Hs-PI 3-K may be an effector for integrin-dependent signaling in platelets (87).

# RECEPTOR-MEDIATED FUNCTIONS OF PLATELET LIPIDS

## Generation of Lysophospholipids

### Lysophosphatidic Acid

The Lysophosphatidic Acid (LPA) concentration in plasma is very low to undetectable (88–90). Serum LPA reaches concentrations of 1 to 5 $\mu$M and requires the presence of platelets (88,90) linking generation of LPA to platelet activation. LPA is generated enzymatically after platelet activation in a two-step process. Most LPA comes from an initial cleavage of PS, PC, or PE to lysolipids by phospholipases (88). Specifically, human platelets contain Group IIA secretory PLA2 and phosphatidylserine-specific phospholipase A1 (88). The PC, PS, PE may be derived from the plasma or the inner leaflet of the plasma membrane of the platelet (88,90). Subsequent exposure of the lysolipids to the plasma protein lyso phospholipase D (lysoPLD) promotes cleavage to generate LPA (88,90). Plasma lysoPLD and autotaxin, a cell surface lysoPLD that stimulates migration in tumor cells (91), are similar in their enzymatic activity, suggesting that plasma lysoPLD may be a secreted form of autotaxin. Lysolipids that are cleaved at the sn-1 position may require acyl migration from the sn-2 to the sn-1 position to be a substrate for lysoPLD and conversion to active LPA (90). An alternative source of lysophosphatidylcholine (LPC), a substrate of lysoPLD, in plasma may occur through conversion of PC to LPC by lecithin-cholesterol acyltransferase (LCAT). Patients deficient in LCAT have decreased generation of LPC and LPA in plasma (88). Mice deficient in the sPLA2-IIA have decreased LPA production, suggesting alternative mechanisms for the generation of LPA in serum (92). However, humans and rats express higher levels of sPLA2-IIA and may use the PLA2-IIA pathway preferentially (88). Therefore, sPLA2-IIa converts PS, PE, and PC from the platelet membrane to lysoPS, lysoPE, and lysoPC upon platelet activation, and subsequently lysoPLD converts the lysolipids to LPA in serum (see Fig. 37-2) (88,90).

### Sphingosine 1-phosphate

Sphingosine 1-phosphate (S1P) is synthesized from sphingosine by sphingosine kinase in platelets (89,93). S1P is stored by platelets and released into the extracellular fluid upon platelet activation in contrast to enzymatic generation of LPA (Fig. 37-2). Stable storage of S1P in platelets is most likely facilitated by the lack of a sphingosine lyase in platelets to rapidly degrade the S1P (93). The release of S1P from platelets occurs through a secretion mechanism that can be stimulated by thrombin in the presence of ethylene glycolbis (beta-aminoethyl ether tetraacetic acid (EGTA) or protein kinase C activation (90,93). The plasma concentration of S1P is approximately 200 nM, probably due to low-level secretion with a twofold increase in the serum concentration (400 nM) (89,90). Both LPA and S1P exist in plasma bound to the plasma protein albumin (89,90,94).

## Actions of Lysophospholipids on Platelets

Human platelets bind LPA and S1P through G protein–coupled receptors, specifically three LPA receptors—LPA1, LPA2, and

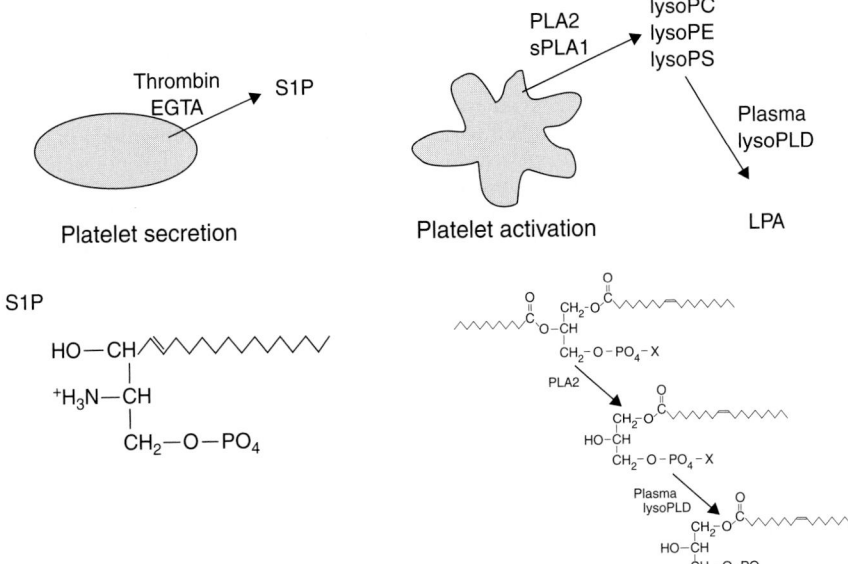

**FIGURE 37-2.** Schematic of sphingosine 1-phosphate (S1P) release from platelets with the chemical structure of S1P indicated underneath the platelet. A schematic of lysophosphatidic acid (LPA) generation from platelet lipids and serum enzymes with changes in the chemical structure indicated below the platelet.

LPA3—and a single S1P receptor, S1P4 (89,95). LPA and S1P promote $Ca^{2+}$ mobilization and reversible shape change in washed and aspirin-treated platelets, although LPA is more potent (92,95,96). In whole blood, LPA promotes platelet aggregation by stimulation of adenosine 5-diphosphate (ADP) secretion and activation of the $P2Y_{12}$ receptor to stimulate full aggregation (96).

# FATTY ACIDS

Developments in the understanding of the physiologic relevance of fatty acids and their metabolism in platelets are considered in this section. Chapter 36 is devoted exclusively to platelet arachidonate and eicosanoid metabolism.

Virtually all of the fatty acids in platelets are esterified and are primarily components of membrane phospholipids. Only trace amounts of free fatty acids have been detected in platelets (1). Because phospholipids are integral membrane components, their fatty acid content would be expected to have a marked influence on membrane fluidity, as well as on receptor-mediated and other membrane activities. For example, the experimental perturbation of platelet membranes with *cis*-unsaturated fatty acids had a marked inhibitory action on platelet function, emphasizing the importance of fatty acids (97). The manipulation of dietary fatty acids (e.g., fish oils, various unsaturated fatty acids, and saturated fatty acids) has resulted in modification of the fatty acid composition of platelets and has induced alterations in platelet reactivity and their ability to produce eicosanoids (97–104). The effects of diets enriched with ω-3 fatty acids on MK lipids have been described (105).

The orientation of fatty acids in membranes is relevant to platelet function. A specific arrangement of fatty acids in platelet membranes exists, because the fatty acid composition of each of the five major platelet phospholipids is distinct (1). For example, PI is composed primarily of stearoyl–arachidonyl species, PC consists of a variety of diacyl species, and SM contains a number of long-carbon-chain fatty acids (1). Various subspecies of phospholipids, defined by their acyl content, have been identified, and their importance in platelet physiologic activities is being investigated (77,106). In addition, there is an asymmetric distribution of phospholipids between the two leaflets of the platelet plasma membrane, and domains of phospholipids may be present in platelet membranes, as described in the previous section

(4,5,15). It would follow that there is a specific, nonrandom arrangement of fatty acids in platelet membranes. For example, it is thought that less than 10% of total platelet 20:4 is located on the platelet surface, whereas considerably greater amounts are present in the inner leaflet of the plasma membrane (5,24). A local increase in a given fatty acid (e.g., a diene or tetraene) would regulate fluidity in the membrane microenvironment and would influence platelet receptor and enzymatic activities.

Several metabolic processes that could influence the composition of fatty acids in platelet phospholipids and their arrangement in platelet membranes have been identified in human platelets. Platelets have the capacity for *de novo* fatty acid synthesis, for the elongation of fatty acids, for the uptake and exchange of fatty acids with plasma, and for the deacylation of membrane phospholipids (107–109).

Like all mammalian cells, platelets cannot synthesize essential fatty acids and must acquire linoleic acid by uptake from plasma. Platelets cannot desaturate linoleic acid or eicosatrienoic acid (20:3) for the synthesis of 20:4 (110). Eicosatrienoic acid and 20:4 are taken up to a considerably greater extent than are monoenes and dienes (i.e., oleic and linoleic acids) and saturated fatty acids (102).

The uptake of arachidonic acid has been extensively studied in human platelets, and approximately 70% of radiolabeled arachidonic acid is incorporated into platelet PC and PI. In contrast, only approximately 37% of total endogenous platelet arachidonic acid is present in these phospholipids. Half of endogenous arachidonic acid is present in PE, whereas only 20% of exogenously supplied radiolabeled arachidonic acid is taken up into PE (111). The basis for the discrepancy between the distribution of radioactive 20:4 incorporated into platelets, and the distribution of endogenous arachidonic acid in phospholipids is unclear (112). One explanation is that incorporation and exchange of unsaturated fatty acids occur primarily in phospholipids located on the platelet surface. It is thought that the arachidonic acid from PC, but not from PE or PS, exchanges with arachidonic acid in plasma (18,19). PC is located on the platelet surface and may be optimally located for rapid uptake and exchange of arachidonic acid and possibly other fatty acids. If this concept is valid, then the arachidonic acid content of acidic phospholipids located in the inner leaflet of the plasma membrane would have to be maintained by the transfer of arachidonic acid from PC to internally located PE, PS, and PI in circulating platelets. Experimental evidence exists that arachidonic acid can be transferred among endogenous phospholipids in resting and activated platelets (113).

Mammalian cells contain specific acyltransferases that can determine the fatty acid composition of phospholipids. Several acyltransferases for the acylation of lysophospholipids have been detected in platelets. Acyltransferases specific for the acylation of lysophospholipids (e.g., lysoPI and lysoPC) have been demonstrated in fractionated human platelets (114,115). These enzymes are highly specific for long-chain polyunsaturated fatty acids. An acyltransferase for the acylation of the C-2 position of glycerophosphate, an early phase of *de novo* phospholipid synthesis, has also been demonstrated in porcine platelets (114). This acyltransferase is selective but not entirely specific for saturated and monounsaturated fatty acids. Acyltransferases would be expected to be instrumental in establishing and maintaining the specific arrangement of fatty acids in individual phospholipids. Platelets can synthesize acylcoenzyme-As (CoAs), which serve as donors for acyltransferases, as acyl-CoA synthetase has been demonstrated and characterized in human platelets (116–118).

Transacylase activities for the transfer of 20:4 among endogenous phospholipids have been demonstrated in human platelets. A CoA-independent transacylase that mediates the transfer of 20:4 from PC to lysoplasmenylethanolamine and a CoA-dependent transacylase with specificity for the transfer of 20:4 from PC to lysoPS, lysoPE, and lysoPI have been demonstrated in platelets (119,120).

The uptake of unsaturated fatty acids into PC and their subsequent translocation to aminophospholipids could serve as a mechanism for establishing the 20:4 content of PE. However, this concept is dependent on platelets having extensive capacity for remodeling all pools of arachidonic acid. Exchange and turnover of 20:4 occur primarily in PC and do not occur to a significant extent in PE and PS (18,19). Undoubtedly, transacylation occurs in platelets. However, it is difficult to relate the rate and magnitude of transacylation noted in *in vivo* studies, because even optimal experimental conditions for *in vitro* experiments may be artifactual. Transacylase experiments have been performed in platelet membrane fractions or platelet lysates. Excessive concentrations of substrates needed for the assay may be higher than the critical micelle concentration, and using cell fractions can greatly overestimate or underestimate *in vivo* acylation. An example of this problem has been demonstrated by the investigation of CoA synthetase. The activity of this enzyme in *in vitro* studies in platelet fractions was found to be 200-fold greater than the activity measured in *in vivo* platelet studies (117).

Therefore, it would be premature to conclude that platelets have the capacity to remodel all pools of lipids. Conceptually, it would be inefficient for a cell specialized to respond rapidly to hemostatic injury to be involved in extensive renewal of structural membrane components. More likely, platelet acyltransferases and transacylases are involved in specific physiologic activities. For example, an acyltransferase and a CoA-independent transacylase specific for the acylation of PAF have been demonstrated in human platelets (121,122). These enzymes may serve to inactivate PAF and thereby regulate the amount of PAF in platelets. Platelets are known to contain a precursor of PAF and can synthesize PAF (123).

# NEUTRAL LIPIDS

Neutral lipids constitute approximately 28% of total platelet lipids, with free cholesterol being the predominant lipid. There also are small amounts of triacyl glycerol and monoacyl and diacyl glycerols and cholesterol esters in platelets (124). Cholesterol is a major component of platelet membranes and has

been shown to be present in platelet cytoskeletons (125). The sterol composition of platelets would be expected to influence the fluidity, organization, and physiologic activities of platelet membranes.

The synthesis, uptake, and regulation of cholesterol have been studied in guinea pig MKs and in both guinea pig and human platelets (126–128). MKs, but not platelets, can synthesize cholesterol. Platelets cannot take up cholesterol by receptor-mediated endocytosis of lipoproteins and do not have the capacity to accumulate cholesterol by net uptake from lipoproteins. The only mechanism for renewal of the cholesterol in platelets is exchange, which does not result in any net gain of cholesterol. The capacity for cholesterol exchange in MKs is considerably less than in platelets. It would appear that cholesterol synthesis in MKs is primarily responsible for establishing the sterol content of circulating platelets.

Type IIa hypercholesterolemia has been studied as a model for understanding the effects of altered platelet cholesterol (129–131). This genetic disease is associated with a propensity for thrombotic complications. An increase in the cholesterol to phospholipid ratio and association with increased platelet reactivity can be demonstrated in patients with this disease. Low density lipoproteins are increased in these patients and are reported to have a number effects on platelets and thereby alter platelet function (132,133). The incubation of normal human platelets with hypercholesterolemic plasma for up to 18 hours did not result in a change in the platelet cholesterol to phospholipid ratio. This is consistent with the observation that guinea pig platelets cannot take up cholesterol, and therefore an elevated plasma cholesterol level is not responsible for the development of the platelet abnormality. Also, normal platelets incubated with hypercholesterolemic plasma did not develop any abnormality in platelet function. These data indicate that the increased cholesterol content and platelet hypersensitivity in type IIa hypercholesterolemia is most likely not due to uptake of cholesterol from plasma.

Platelets can take up cholesterol from cholesterol-enriched liposomes but not from hypercholesterolemic plasma (134–136). However, there are most likely differences in the mechanisms for the accumulation of cholesterol in platelets from patients with type IIa hypercholesterolemia from those involved in the uptake of the sterol during the *in vitro* incubation of platelets with cholesterol-enriched liposomal dispersions. The ultrastructural distribution of the excess cholesterol in platelets from these patients differs from the sterol distribution in normal platelets that had been incubated with cholesterol-rich liposomes; in the former, excess cholesterol primarily is located in plasma membranes, whereas in the latter, cholesterol is present in both plasma membranes and organelles.

The information provided by this liposomal model is useful in understanding the effects of platelet cholesterol on platelet membrane fluidity and function. However, the process by which platelets take up cholesterol from liposomal dispersions obviously differs from that responsible for excess platelet cholesterol in type IIa hypercholesterolemia. Therefore, cholesterol-enriched liposomes do not appear to be an appropriate model system for the study of the congenital disorder.

The investigation of the consequences of diet-induced hypercholesterolemia in guinea pigs has further addressed this problem (128). The study showed that platelet cholesterol was increased in animals that had received these diets. As in the human studies, the cholesterol content of normal guinea pig platelets was not increased after incubation with hypercholesterolemic guinea pig plasma. MK size was noted to have increased, which indicates that hypercholesterolemia may induce a primary defect in MKs that results in the production of abnormal platelets (128).

# GLYCOLIPIDS AND CERAMIDES

Glycolipids are present in most mammalian cell membranes and are thought to be important for membrane physiology, cell adhesion, immune responses, and cellular maturation and differentiation. Therefore, glycolipids are likely to be important for MK maturation, platelet production, and platelet function.

Glycolipids are composed of three basic components: sphingosine, a fatty acid, and one or more carbohydrate moieties. Acidic glycolipids (gangliosides) are distinguished from neutral glycolipids by the presence of sialic acid. The backbone of a glycolipid or ganglioside is the ceramide moiety, which is composed of a fatty acid and a sphingosine base. The fatty acid and sphingosine portions of glycolipids are hydrophobic and are thought to be implanted in the lipid core of the membranes, whereas the carbohydrate moieties are hydrophilic and are exposed on the membrane surface (137).

The composition of glycolipids and ceramides has been established in human platelets. Neutral glycolipids, gangliosides, and ceramides constitute approximately 3.2% of platelet lipids on the basis of weight (138–140). Free ceramides are more abundant in platelets than in other blood cells and other mammalian cells (140,141). Ceramides have been shown to be actively synthesized in human platelets from radiolabeled acetate and palmitate (107).

Four neutral glycolipids have been identified in human platelets (138,140,142). Lactosyl ceramide is the most abundant glycolipid, constituting 64% of the total neutral glycolipids. Trihexosyl ceramide and globoside, and to a lesser extent glucosyl ceramide, are present in human platelets. More complex glycolipids have not been detected in platelets. Marcus et al. reported that there are three gangliosides and traces of two additional gangliosides in human platelets (139). Gangliosides account for approximately 0.5% of total platelet lipids and contain 6% of total platelet sialic acid. Ganglioside I has been identified as hematoside (GM3) and constitutes 92% of platelet gangliosides. Glycolipids are listed in Table 37-3.

Sulfatides have not been definitively identified in human platelets (138,139). Indirect evidence exists that platelet lipids, possibly sulfatides, can bind to human thrombospondin and von Willebrand factor (143,144). Sulfatides have been thought to provide a biologic surface for the binding of von Willebrand factor (144) and the activation of factor XII and prekallikrein (145–147).

Human platelets have been found to have the capacity to glycosylate ceramides for the production of glycosyl ceramide. Several hydrolytic enzymes that may be important for glycolipid metabolism have been detected in platelets. N-acetylhexosaminidase A and B, $\alpha$- and $\beta$-galactosidase, and, to a lesser extent, $\beta$-glucosidase have been found in human platelet $\alpha$-granules (142,148). Platelet hexosaminidase was decreased in platelets from patients with Sandhoff disease, and platelet $\alpha$-galactosidase A was decreased in Fabry disease (142). The estimation of platelet enzyme levels in homozygotes can serve as a means of diagnosing these disorders (142). The effects of these deficiencies on platelet function have not been studied.

The composition of two ceramides has been investigated in human platelets (140). The sphingosine content of the two ceramides (A and B) in human platelets differs. The sphingosine composition of ceramide A is similar to that of SM, whereas the composition of ceramide B is similar to that of glycolipids and gangliosides. This suggests that ceramide A serves as the precursor of SM and ceramide B as the source for glycolipids (140).

The participation of glycolipids in several important cellular activities has been attributed to their orientation in membranes. The hydrophilic carbohydrate moieties, exposed on the membrane surface, would be available for receptor and immunologically mediated activities. One study suggested that hematoside, globoside, and trihexosylceramide were exposed on the platelet surface, whereas lactosyl ceramide was not available (140).

The incubation of human platelets with thrombin caused marked changes in the availability of platelet glycolipids to external labeling agents. There was a 50% reduction in the exposure of trihexosyl ceramide and globoside, but a 100% increase in the availability of hematoside for this reaction (140). These observations indicate that the thrombin-platelet interaction results in the masking and unmasking of specific glycolipids on the platelet surface or, possibly, extensive reorganization of the platelet plasma membrane. The action of thrombin on the availability of glycolipids is considerably greater than on the exposure of platelet phospholipids (4). Platelet hematoside is a negatively charged molecule due to its content of sialic acid, and its exposure on the surface of thrombin-activated platelets could be important for platelet activation. In addition, there is evidence of an increase in the absolute amount of hematoside and a decrease in lactosyl ceramide in thrombin-treated platelets (138, 140). A recent study indicates that GD3 is rapidly formed from GM3 in activated platelets and is involved in platelet adhesion and spreading on subendothelium matrix (149).

Several studies indicate that gangliosides can bind serotonin (139,150). Marcus et al. have demonstrated significant irreversible binding of serotonin to platelet gangliosides (139). The binding was specific, as it occurred during incubation with hematoside (GM3) and a minor platelet ganglioside but did not occur with other glycolipids and phospholipids (139). Studies have verified that specific gangliosides (i.e., GM3 and GD3) can bind serotonin (150). There has been concern that only small amounts of serotonin were bound to ganglioside in these studies. A serotonin-binding protein has been isolated from several tissues, however, and gangliosides were shown to induce a fivefold increase in the binding of serotonin to this protein (150). A serotonin-binding protein has been isolated from platelets, but gangliosides did not increase the binding of serotonin to the serotonin-binding protein isolated from rat platelets (151,152). Therefore, the extent and relevance of the binding of serotonin to platelet gangliosides have not been determined.

GM1 ganglioside is thought to mediate cholera toxin binding to cellular GM1 ganglioside, which results in the stimulation of adenylate cyclase in intestinal mucosal cells and other vertebrate tissues (153). Cholera toxin has been shown to bind to platelets but does not lead to the alteration of cyclic nucleotide levels (154).

The concept that gangliosides serve as receptors has been challenged by several observations. For example, in most cells

## TABLE 37-3

### PLATELET GLYCOLIPIDS

| Platelet glycolipids (140) | nmol/109 platelets |
| --- | --- |
| Ceramides | 3.48 |
| Glucosylceramide | 0.022 |
| Lactosylceramide | 1.39 |
| Trihexosylceramide | 0.56 |
| Globoside | 0.42 |
| Hematoside | 0.63 |
| Ganglioside II | >0.03 |

Total glycolipids are less than 4% of total platelet lipids. Trihexosyl ceramide, globoside, and hematoside are exposed on the platelet surface.

and tissues, the binding of various bioactive substances to gangliosides has been of low affinity and specificity. On the other hand, there is growing evidence that gangliosides serve as cofactors, modulators, or auxiliary receptors for stimulus-response coupling (155,156). Gangliosides are thought to serve as modulators or auxiliary receptors for thyrotropin, interferon, and chorionic gonadotropin (157–159). It is possible that the exposure of hematoside on the surface of activated platelets facilitates the modulation and regulation of the platelet response to the agonist (140).

Glycolipids and phospholipids have been detected in human platelet cytoskeletons (125). Only two major platelet glycolipids are present in cytoskeletons prepared by Triton X-100 precipitation. Approximately 7% of total platelet trihexosyl ceramide and 2% of hematoside were detected. Although lactosyl ceramide is the predominant glycolipid in platelets, it was not detected in cytoskeletons. Two of the five major phospholipids, PC and SM, as well as cholesterol, were also detected in platelet cytoskeletons. The presence of lipids in cytoskeletons is not due to the trapping of lipids during the preparation of these structures, because radiolabeled cholesterol added just before the addition of Triton X-100 was not incorporated into the cytoskeletons. Glycolipids have been shown to be associated with cytoskeletal structures and microtubules in other cells. Cholera toxin was shown by immunohistologic methods to bind to Balb/c-3T3 cells, and the toxin was found to bind to the cytoskeletons of these cells (160). These experiments suggested that ganglioside GM1 was present in 3T3 cytoskeletons, as cholera toxin is known to recognize GM1. In another study, cholera toxin and an antiactinin affinity-purified antibody were used to show that capping GM1 in mouse lymphocytes was associated with the reorganization of the underlying cytoskeleton (161). Two other studies suggested that glycolipids are integral components of colchicine-sensitive microtubules in a number of cells and tissues (162,163).

Several implications for the presence of glycolipids in cytoskeletons in platelets, as well as in other cells and tissues exist. Glycolipids along with other lipids in cytoskeletons may provide structural support for cytoskeletons or possibly to mediate cytoskeletal physiologic activities (164).

Distinct differences in the composition of both neutral and acid glycolipids (gangliosides) have been reported to occur in immature versus mature tissues and cells (165,166). Also, the composition of glycolipids (i.e., fatty acid or carbohydrate components) may vary according to the stage of cellular maturation. The species of fatty acids, carbohydrates, and sphingosine bases in developing cells and tissues are most likely critical for maturation. Considerable evidence exists that glycolipids are involved in maturation and differentiation of various cells and tissues. Glycolipids appear to act as growth factors. Several studies have indicated that gangliosides are involved in the growth of neurites (167,168). It has been reported that glycolipids are involved in the maturation of erythroblasts. This study showed that ceramides and glycolipids with 24:0 (lignocerate) stimulated erythrocyte maturation, whereas those with 22:0 (behenate) were less effective (169). The basic mechanism for these observations has been suggested by a study that reported that GM1 and GM3 can modify cell growth by modulating platelet-derived growth factor receptor by affecting tyrosine phosphorylation (169).

The investigation of MKs revealed that glycolipid synthesis was greater in immature than in mature cells (170). Although platelets have the capacity for the synthesis of ceramides, the study indicated that ceramides and glycolipids are primarily synthesized in MKs. In addition, the glycosylation of free ceramides occurs almost exclusively in MKs rather than in platelets. These data indicate that MKs determine the composition of glycolipids in platelets and that there is considerable compartmentalization of glycolipid synthesis and membrane assembly at various stages of MK development.

# PROTEIN–LIPID INTERACTIONS AND PROTEIN ACYLATION

The covalent interaction of lipids with proteins represents a mechanism for the posttranslational modification of proteins. One example of this process is the interaction of glycosylphosphatidylinositol (GPI) with membrane proteins that results in the anchoring of the covalently bound protein (171,172). These GPI structures, which are attached to the C-terminal carboxyl group of a diverse group of proteins, consist of a complex oligoglycan linked to a PI molecule located in the lipid bilayer (172). The degradation of GPI by specific phospholipases leads to the release of the protein from the membrane. It has been suggested that proteins anchored by GPIs are easily released by appropriate stimuli and thereby influence biologic activities. For example, GPI anchors may be the source of intracellular mediators of the insulin reaction (171–173). Evidence suggests that a 150-kDa platelet glycoprotein is anchored by GPI (174). Deficiencies in GPI-anchored proteins have been detected in blood cells from patients with paroxysmal nocturnal hemoglobinuria (PNH) (175). Platelets from patients with PNH are deficient in GPI-anchored proteins CD55, CD59, and CD16 (176,177).

Protein acylation is another example of the ability of lipids to modify membrane proteins. Several cellular proteins have been found to be acylated—that is, they contain covalently bound fatty acids (178,179). Palmitic or myristic acids are the most common fatty acids covalently bound to proteins. Myristoylation of proteins is usually cotranslational, tightly coupled with protein synthesis, and can occur in cytosolic and in membrane proteins. Myristic acid is linked through an amide bond to N-terminal glycine. Palmitoylation of proteins is usually posttranslational, not associated with protein synthesis, and occurs primarily in proteins located in membranes. Palmitic acid is usually linked through a thioester bond to cysteine.

Several studies have demonstrated palmitoylation of platelet proteins. A 22-kDa platelet protein was found to be palmitoylated, and this protein was reported to be a leukocyte differentiation antigen, CD9 (180). Anti-CD9 antibody can activate platelets, and the antibody is thought to induce an association between CD9 and the platelet glycoprotein (GP) IIb/IIIa complex (181,182). In another study, the palmitoylation of 24- and 19-kDa proteins was detected, and these proteins were reported to be GP Ib/β and GP IX, respectively (183). Three platelet cytoskeletal proteins have been reported to be palmitoylated (184). Conflicting evidence exists as to whether GP IIb/IIIa is acylated in human platelets (184,185). The acylation of platelet membrane and cytoskeletal proteins may influence the anchorage of these proteins to the platelet surface. The acylation of platelet proteins occurs within minutes, and thrombin rapidly can alter the palmitoylation of platelet proteins (186). Rapid turnover of ankyrin acyl groups occurs in erythrocytes (187). These observations are consistent with the evidence that protein acylation and the turnover of acyl groups can be rapid, thereby dynamically modulating the orientation and function of membrane glycoproteins (188).

It has been proposed that acylated proteins are important for cell adhesion, anchoring proteins to membranes, cell–cell interactions, receptor-mediated activities, and cell maturation (175,176). Several proteins important for differentiation, such as lymphoma tyrosine protein kinase, and cyclic adenosine monophosphate–dependent protein kinase, are acylated (188, 189). Acylation may alter the orientation and anchorage of proteins in membranes and affect agonist–receptor interactions. Studies with the Rous sarcoma virus p60 protein provide evidence that acylation is essential for membrane localization (190). These studies show that the point mutation of the p60 protein resulted in a failure of myristoylation of the protein. In its nonacylated form, there was considerably less of the p60 protein present in the membrane than found in cells with the wild-type virus. On the other hand, the specificity in the lipid requirement for the functioning of ras p21 has been questioned (191). The anchoring of proteins by GPIs and protein acylation has been detected in several cells and tissues. However, the biologic significance of these lipid-induced modifications of membrane proteins should be better defined (178,179).

Protein acylation has been studied in guinea pig MKs (192). MKs, but not platelets, would be expected to be capable of myristoylating proteins, as protein synthesis occurs in MKs but not in platelets. The study found that GP IX was one of the major proteins to be myristoylated and that this event occurred during the later phases of the maturation of recognizable MKs. Myristoylation of GP IX was found to be cotranslational and amide-linked. An N-terminal lysine was the most likely site for myristoylation of GP IX in MKs, not an N-terminal glycine that generally is the site for myristoylation in most cells. GP Ib/β was primarily palmitoylated, and this event occurred during earlier phases of the maturation of MKs. Taken together, the study indicates that the myristoylation of GP IX has a role in the assembly and the expression of the GP Ib complex on the MK surface during the later phases of MK maturation and possibly in platelet shedding by MKs. MKs, but not platelets, can myristoylate GP IX, but both MKs and platelets can palmitoylate GP Ib/β. The palmitoylation of GP Ib/β occurs during the early phases of the maturation of recognizable MKs and may have a different role in the expression of the GP Ib complex than the myristoylation of GP IX. The palmityolation of GP Ib/β that persists in platelets may have a primary role in the localization of GP Ib in platelets.

## LIPID DOMAINS AND RAFTS

Lipid domains or clusters have been characterized in platelets and in other cells by several experimental approaches. Detergent-insoluble lipid domains (lipid rafts) have been characterized in platelets and other cells. These rafts are enriched with cholesterol and glycosphingolipids and therefore are also known as glycolipid enriched membrane domains (GEMs) (193). Transmission electron microscopy of the insoluble material revealed a heterogeneous population of vesicles ranging in size from 20 to 1,000 nm (194). Specific proteins are concentrated in lipid rafts: Stomatin, flotillin-1, flotillin-2, CD36, CD9, integrin $\alpha_{IIb}\beta_3$, and the glucose transporter GLUT-3. Stomatin, the flotillins, and CD36 were exclusively present in this lipid-raft fraction in platelets. Because stomatin is localized in α-granules, lipid rafts may be present in platelet α-granules (195). However, another study found that CD36 selectively partitioned while GPI-linked protein CD55 and $\alpha_{IIb}\beta_{3a}$ was not present in lipid rafts. This study also suggested that the inclusion of proteins is reversible and triggered by platelet activation (196).

Changes in proteins in platelet lipid rafts have been studied. In resting platelets, cholesterol was uniformly distributed on the cell surface and confined to distinct intracellular compartments (i.e., multivesicular bodies, dense granules, and the internal membranes of α-granules). Upon platelet activation, cholesterol accumulated at the tips of filopodia and at the leading edge of spreading cells. The adhesion-dependent raft aggregation was accompanied by concentration of the tyrosine kinase c-Src and the tetraspanin CD63 in these domains, whereas GP Ib was not selectively targeted to the raft clusters (197).

Although GP Ib was not found in platelet rafts in one study (197), other investigators have found factor XI is localized to GP Ib in membrane rafts and that this association is important for promoting the activation of factor XI by thrombin on the platelet surface. Interestingly, raft-associated GP Ib/IX/V was selectively palmitoylated in activated platelets, and the posttranslational modification may play a role in platelet adhesion and postadhesion signaling (198).

Lipid rafts appear to be important for the mediation and coordination of platelet activation. These domains are sites of early steps of platelet activation and can be enriched with signaling proteins. The Fc receptor γ chain (FcRγ) is constitutively present in rafts and orchestrates signaling by the platelet collagen receptor GP VI (199). Although lipid rafts or GEMs are important for the collagen receptor signaling, GEMs do not appear to play a role in fibrinogen receptor (Gp IIb/IIIa) signaling (192). Therefore, only GEMs mediate specific platelet activities.

Lipid rafts are sites of active phosphoinositide metabolism. G protein–coupled receptors mediate the production. They are sites where the PI metabolism is highly active. For example, heterotrimeric G protein–coupled receptors mediate the production of phosphatidic acid and phosphoinositide 3-kinase products. Thereby, lipid second messengers such as PI 3,4, 5-trisphosphate are generated (200).

Active Lyn protein tyrosine kinase has been found to be selectively enriched within membrane microdomains of resting platelets and plays a role in platelet survival (201). These findings suggest that lipid rafts are highly dynamic platelet membrane structures and play important roles in signaling mechanisms in activated platelets

The physiologic role of platelet lipid rafts has been investigated by state-of-the-art methods, including the use of lipophilic fluorescent dyes, cholesterol-binding cytolysin, and biotinylated BCθ that can be used to study lipid rafts in living cells and platelets. It was important to carry out these studies in resting and activated platelets (195,197,202,203). Some of the approaches, such as the depletion and repletion of cholesterol, would be expected to cause global effects on membrane organization and may provide misleading information. Nevertheless, lipid rafts undoubtedly have critical roles in platelet physiology, and the investigation of these domains most likely will clarify the basic mechanisms for platelet function.

Lipid–lipid and lipid–protein structural relations have also been studied in lipid domains with chemical cross-linking probes in erythrocyts and platelets (204–206). These studies suggested that PS is associated with other PS molecules in lipid domains in erythrocytes and in platelets (204–206). It was also shown that the organization of PS in platelet membranes differs from that in erythrocyte membranes. Although PS was associated with membrane proteins in erythrocyes, PS was not associated with proteins in platelets. The presence of lipid domains in platelet membranes conceivably could influence the availability of phospholipid arachidonate for the formation of eicosanoids, regulate membrane fluidity, and mediate receptor and enzyme activities.

## MEGAKARYOCYTE LIPIDS

The lipid content of guinea pig MKs has been determined (170,207). The content of neutral and phospholipid species is similar in MKs and platelets, but there is relatively more PI and less PS in MKs. The five major fatty acids in both cells were palmitic, stearic, oleic, linoleic, and arachidonic acids; the major difference was that there was half the arachidonic acid and a proportionate increase in oleic acid in MKs compared to platelets. The cholesterol to phospholipid ratio was 0.35 in MKs and 0.55 in platelets. This difference may be due to the presence of nuclei and endoplasmic reticulum in MKs with a low content of cholesterol relative to phospholipids.

To define lipid composition and metabolism during MK maturation, lipids were investigated in pure populations of MKs at different phases of maturation. The phospholipid and cholesterol contents were four times greater in mature MKs than in immature MKs, which paralleled the protein content and volume of mature and immature cells. The cholesterol-phospholipid ratio was similar, and there were no differences in phospholipid species in MKs at different stages of development (208).

Dramatic morphologic changes occur in MKs as they mature from progenitor cells to mature platelet-producing polyploid cells. From 1,000 to 4,000 platelets are thought to be produced in the cytoplasm of one MK; therefore, thrombopoiesis most likely is dependent on extensive membrane biogenesis and active lipid synthesis and metabolism in MKs, as lipids are integral membrane components.

MKs have a greater capacity for lipid synthesis and metabolism than platelets, and they determine the lipid composition of platelets (9,10,126,170,207,209). For example, only MKs, and not platelets, can synthesize cholesterol and glycosylate ceramides for the synthesis of glycolipids, and possess Δ-5 desaturase activity for the synthesis of arachidonic acid (126,170, 209). MKs may be responsible for determining the content of 20:4 and other fatty acids in PE and PS (209). A discrepancy exists between the distribution of eicosapentaenoic acid (20:5) in platelet phospholipids after the incubation of isolated platelets with the radiolabeled eicosapentaenoic acid and that after the oral intake of radiolabeled eicosapentaenoic acid (124). This information supports the contention that MKs play an important role in establishing the lipid content of platelets.

Lipid synthesis and metabolism have been studied in MKs at different phases of maturation (208,210). Most aspects of lipid synthesis and the uptake of arachidonic and palmitic acids occurred primarily in immature cells. Differences occurred in the acylation of phospholipid species with arachidonic acid in MKs at different stages of maturation, as the acylation of PC occurred primarily in immature MKs. These findings most likely are due to differences in MK arachidonyl acyltransferase and transacylase activities, because these enzymes play important roles in the organization of membrane lipids during MK maturation and platelet production.

In contrast, *de novo* synthesis of palmitic acid from radiolabeled acetate occurred predominantly in mature MKs (208). The enzymatic basis for this observation is that acetyl-CoA carboxylase, a key enzyme for *de novo* fatty acid synthesis, is expressed primarily in mature MKs (211). Acetyl-CoA carboxylase has been implicated in maturation. Acetyl-CoA carboxylase activity has been used as a measure of embryogenesis and may play a role in the differentiation of preadipocytes (212,213).

The delineation of lipid metabolism in MKs has provided the means to understand how the lipid content of platelets is established. The demonstration that there are distinct differences in the metabolism of fatty acids, ceramides and glycolipids, and other lipids in MKs at different phases of maturation indicates that lipids and their metabolism have important roles in MK maturation and the production of platelets.

# ACKNOWLEDGMENTS

Supported by grants from the National Institutes of Health (HL-25455, HL-26633, HL-14217, HL-39238, HL-51481) and the American Heart Association.

## *References*

1. Marcus AJ, Ullman HL, Safier LB. Lipid composition of subcellular particles of human blood platelets. *J Lipid Res* 1969;10:108.
2. Leray C, Cazenave JP, Gachet C. Platelet phospholipids are differentially protected against oxidative degradation by plasmalogens. *Lipids* 2002;37:285–290.
3. Mueller HW, Purdon AD, Smith JB, et al. 1-0-Alkyl-linked phosphoglycerides of human platelets: distribution of arachidonate and other acyl residues in the ether-linked and diacyl species. *Lipids* 1983;18:814.
4. Schick PK, Kurica KB, Chacko GK. Location of phosphatidylethanolamine and phosphatidylserine in human platelet plasma membranes. *J Clin Invest* 1976;57:1221.
5. Perret B, Chap HJ, Douste-Blazy L. Asymmetric distribution of arachidonic acid in the plasma membrane of human platelets: a determination using purified phospholipases and a rapid method for membrane isolation. *Biochim Biophys Acta* 1979;556:434.
6. Bevers EM, Comfurius P, Zwaal RF. Changes in membrane phospholipid distribution during platelet activation. *Biochim Biophys Acta* 1983;736:57.
7. Majerus PW, Smith MB, Clamon GH. Lipid metabolism in human platelets. I. Evidence for a complete fatty acid synthesizing system. *J Clin Invest* 1969;48:156.
8. Lewis N, Majerus PW. Lipid metabolism in human platelets. II. De novo phospholipid synthesis and the effect of thrombin on the pattern of synthesis. *J Clin Invest* 1969;48:2114.
9. Schick BP, Schick PK. Megakaryocyte biochemistry. *Semin Hematol* 1986;23:68.
10. Schick BP, Schick PK. The biochemistry of megakaryocytes. In: Levine RF, Levin J, Williams N, et al. eds. *Megakaryocytes: development and function.* New York: Alan R. Liss, 1986:265–279.
11. Rosing J, Rijn V, Bevers EM, et al. The role of activated human platelets in prothrombin and Factor X activation. *Blood* 1985;65:319.
12. Dachary-Prigent J, Freyssinet JM, Pasquet JM, et al. Annexin V as a probe of aminophospholipid exposure and platelet membrane vesiculation: a flow cytometry study showing a role for free sulfhydryl groups. *Blood* 1993;81:2554.
13. Rosing J, Bevers EM, Comfurius P, et al. Impaired factor X and prothrombin activation associated with decreased phospholipid exposure in platelets from a patient with a bleeding disorder. *Blood* 1985;65:1557.
14. Bevers EM, Comfurius P, Dekkers DW, et al. Transmembrane phospholipid distribution in blood cells: control mechanisms and pathophysiological significance. *J Biol Chem* 1998;379:973.
15. Zwaal RF, Comfurius P, Bevers EM. Mechanism and function of changes in membrane-phospholipid asymmetry in platelets and erythrocytes. *Biochem Soc Trans* 1993;21(2):248.
16. Thiagarajan P, Tait JF. Binding of annexin V/placental anticoagulant protein I to platelets. Evidence for phosphatidylserine exposure in the procoagulant response of activated platelets. *J Biol Chem* 1990;26:17420.
17. Bevers EM, Comfurius JP, van Rijn JL, et al. Generation of prothrombin-converting activity and the exposure of phosphatidylserine at the outer surface of platelets. *Eur J Biochem* 1982;122:429.
18. Bereziat G, Chambaz J, Trugman G, et al. Turnover of phospholipid linoleic and arachidonic acids in human platelets from plasma lecithins. *J Lipid Res* 1978;19:495.
19. Chambaz J, Wolf C, Pepin D, et al. Phospholipid and fatty acid exchange between human platelets and plasma. *Biol Cell* 1980;37:223.
20. Gaffet P, Basse F, Bienvenue A. Loss of phospholipid asymmetry in human platelet plasma membrane after 1–12 days of storage. An ESR study. *Eur J Biochem* 1994;222:1033.
21. van Engeland M, Nieland LJ, Ramaekers FC, et al. Annexin V-affinity assay: a review on an apoptosis detection system based on phosphatidylserine exposure. *Cytometry* 1998;31:1.
22. van Rijn J, Rosing J, van Dieijen G. Activity of human blood platelets in prothrombin and in factor X activation induced by ionophore A23187. *Eur J Biochem* 1983;133:1.
23. Sims PJ, Faioni EM, Wiedmer T, et al. Complement proteins C5b-9 cause release of membrane vesicles from the platelet surface that are enriched in the membrane receptor for coagulation factor Va and express prothrombinase activity. *J Biol Chem* 1988;263:18205.
24. Schick PK, Schick BP, Brandeis G, et al. Distribution of phosphatidylethanolamine arachidonic acid in platelet membranes. *Biochim Biophys Acta* 1981;643:659.
25. Heemskerk JW, Bevers EM, Lindhout T. Platelet activation and blood coagulation. *Thromb Haemost* 2002;88:186–193.
26. Schick PK, Yu BP. The role of platelet membrane phospholipids in the platelet release reaction. *J Clin Invest* 1974;54:1032.
27. Fiedel BA, Osmand AP, Gewurz H. Inhibition of platelet aggregation by a myeloma protein with anti-phosphocholine specificity. *Nature* 1976;263:687.
28. Bode AP, Sandberg H, Dombrose FA, et al. Association of factor V activity with membranous vesicles released from human platelets: requirement for platelet stimulation. *Thromb Res* 1985;39:49.
29. Sandberg H, Bode AP, Dombrose F, et al. Expression of coagulant activity in human platelets: release of membranous vesicles providing platelet factor 1 and platelet factor 3. *Thromb Res* 1985;39:63.
30. Sims PJ, Wiedmer T, Esmon CT, et al. Assembly of the platelet prothrombinase complex is linked to vesiculation of the platelet plasma membrane. *J Biol Chem* 1989;264:17049.
31. Fox JEB, Austin CD, Boyles JK, et al. Role of the membrane skeleton in preventing the shedding of procoagulant-rich microvesicles from the platelet plasma membrane. *J Cell Biol* 1990;111:483.
32. Comfurius P, Senden JMG, Tilly RHJ, et al. Loss of membrane phospholipid asymmetry in platelets and red cells may be associated with calcium-induced shedding of plasma membrane and inhibition of aminophospholipid translocase. *Biochim Biophys Acta* 1990;1026:153.
33. Kuypers FA, Yuan J, Lewis RA, et al. Membrane phospholipid asymmetry in human thalassemia. *Blood* 1998;91:3044.

34. Zwaal RF, Comfurius P, van Deenen LL. Membrane asymmetry and blood coagulation. *Nature* 1977;268:358.
35. Lubin B, Chiu D, Bastacky J, et al. Abnormalities in membrane phospholipid organization in sickled erythrocytes. *J Clin Invest* 1981;67:1643.
36. Franck PFH, Chiu DT-Y, Op den Kamp JAF, et al. Accelerated transbilayer movement of phosphatidylcholine in sickled erythrocytes: a reversible process. *J Biol Chem* 1983;258:18436.
37. Franck PFH, Bevers EM, Lubin BH, et al. Uncoupling of the membrane cytoskeleton from the lipid bilayer. *J Clin Invest* 1985;75:183.
38. Shcherbina A, Rosen FS, Remold-O'Donnell E. Pathological events in platelets of Wiskott-Aldrich syndrome patients. *Br J Haematol* 1999;106:875–883.
39. Li J, Xia Y, Bertino AM, et al. The mechanism of apoptosis in human platelets during storage. *Transfusion* 2000;40:1320–1329.
40. Zauli G, Vitale M, Falcieri E, et al. In vitro senescence and apoptotic cell death of human megakaryocytes. *Blood* 1997;90:2234–2243.
41. Daleke DL, Huestis WH. Incorporation and translocation of aminophospholipids in human erythrocytes. *Biochemistry* 1985;24:5406.
42. Connor J, Gillum K, Schroit AJ. Maintenance of lipid asymmetry in red blood cells and ghosts: effect of divalent cations and serum albumin on the transbilayer distribution of phosphatidylserine. *Biochim Biophys Acta* 1990;1025:82.
43. Connor J, Pak CH, Zwaal RF, et al. Bidirectional transbilayer movement of phospholipid analogs in human red blood cells. Evidence for an ATP-dependent and protein-mediated process. *J Biol Chem* 1992;267:19412.
44. Bitbol M, Fellmann P, Zachowski A, et al. Ion regulation of phosphatidylserine and phosphatidylethanolamine outside-inside translocation in human erythrocytes. *Biochim Biophys Acta* 1987;904:268.
45. Morrot G, Zachowski A, Devaux PF. Partial purification and characterization of the human erythrocyte Mg2(+)-ATPase. A candidate aminophospholipid translocase. *FEBS Lett* 1990;266(1–2):29.
46. Bettache N, Gaffet P, Allegre N, et al. Impaired redistribution of aminophospholipids with distinctive cell shape change during Ca²⁺-induced activation of platelets from a patient with Scott syndrome. *Br J Haematol* 1998;101:50.
47. Dachary-Prigent J, Pasquet JM, Fressinaud E, et al. Aminophospholipid exposure, microvesiculation and abnormal protein tyrosine phosphorylation in the platelets of a patient with Scott syndrome: a study using physiologic agonists and local anaesthetics. *Br J Haematol* 1997;99:959.
48. Dekkers DW, Comfurius P, Vuist WM, et al. Impaired Ca²⁺- induced tyrosine phosphorylation and defective lipid scrambling in erythrocytes from a patient with Scott syndrome: a study using an inhibitor for scramblase that mimics the defect in Scott syndrome. *Blood* 1998;9:2133.
49. Bettache N, Gaffet P, Allegre N, et al. Impaired redistribution of aminophospholipids with distinctive cell shape change during Ca²⁺-induced activation of platelets from a patient with Scott syndrome. *Br J Haematol* 1998;101:50–58.
50. Gilbert GE, Arena AA. Phosphatidylethanolamine induces high affinity binding sites for factor VIII on membranes containing phosphatidyl-L-serine. *J Biol Chem* 1995;270:18500.
51. Murer EH. The role of platelet calcium. *Semin Hematol* 1985;22:313.
52. Rittenhouse SE, Sasson JP. Measurement of IP3 mass as a monitor of phospholipase C activation in stimulated human platelets. *Nouv Rev Fr Hematol* 1985;27:239.
53. Agranoff BW, Murthy P, Seguin EB. Thrombin-induced phosphodiesteratic cleavage of phosphatidylinositol bisphosphate in human platelets. *J Biol Chem* 1983;258:2076.
54. Billah MM, Lapetina EG. Rapid decrease of phosphatidylinositol 4,5-bisphosphate in thrombin-stimulated platelets. *J Biol Chem* 1982;257:12705.
55. Watson SP, McConnell RT, Lapetina EG. The rapid formation of inositol phosphates in human platelets by thrombin is inhibited by prostacyclin. *J Biol Chem* 1984;259:13199.
56. Holmsen H, Dangelmaier CA, Rongved S. Tight coupling of thrombin-induced acid hydrolase secretion and phosphatidate synthesis to receptor occupancy in human platelets. *Biochem J* 1984;222:157.
57. Rittenhouse SE. Human platelets contain phospholipase C that hydrolyzes polyphosphoinositides. *Proc Natl Acad Sci U S A* 1983;80:5417.
58. Huang R, Kucera GL, Rittenhouse SE. Elevated cytosolic Ca⁺⁺ activates phospholipase D in human platelets. *J Biol Chem* 1991;266:1652.
59. Holmsen H. Platelet metabolism and activation. *Semin Hematol* 1985;22:219.
60. Low MG, Carroll RC, Weglicki WB. Multiple forms of phosphoinositide-specific phospholipase C of different relative molecular masses in animal tissues: evidence for modification of the platelet enzyme by Ca⁺⁺-dependent proteinase, *Biochem J* 1984;221:813.
61. Billah MM, Lapetina EG, Cuatrecasas P. Phospholipase A2 and phospholipase C activities of platelets: differential substrate specificity, Ca⁺⁺ requirement, pH dependence, and cellular localization. *J Biol Chem* 1980;255:10227.
62. Call FL II, Williams WJ. Biosynthesis of cytidine diphosphate diglyceride by human platelets. *J Clin Invest* 1970;49:392.
63. Lucas CT, Call FL II, Williams WJ. The biosynthesis of phosphatidylinositol in human platelets. *J Clin Invest* 1970;49:1949.
64. Kawahara Y, Takai Y, Minakuchi R, et al. Phospholipid turnover as a possible transmembrane signal for protein phosphorylation during human platelet activation by thrombin. *Biochem Biophys Res Commun* 1980;97:309.
65. Nishizuka Y. The role of protein kinase C in cell surface signal transduction and tumour promotion. *Nature* 1984;308:693.
66. Chau L-Y, Tai H-H. Release of arachidonate from diglyceride in human platelets requires the sequential action of a diglyceride lipase and a monoglyceride lipase. *Biochem Biophys Res Commun* 1981;100:1688.
67. Prescott SM, Majerus PW. Characterization of 1,2-diacylglycerol hydrolysis in human platelets: demonstration of an arachidonyl- monoacylglycerol intermediate. *J Biol Chem* 1983;258:764.
68. Mauco G, Dangelmaier CA, Smith JB. Inositol lipids, phosphatidate and diacylglycerol share stearoylarachidonoylglycerol as a common backbone in thrombin-stimulated human platelets. *Biochem J* 1984;224:933.
69. Chau L-Y, Tai H-H. Diglyceride/monoglyceride lipases pathway is not essential for arachidonate release in thrombin-activated human platelets. *Biochem Biophys Res Commun* 1983;113:241.
70. Imai A, Yano K, Kameyama Y, et al. Evidence for predominance of phospholipase A2 in release of arachidonic acid in thrombin-activated platelets: phosphatidylinositol-specific phospholipase C may play a minor role in arachidonate liberation. *Jpn J Exp Med* 1982;52:99.
71. Walenga RW, Opas EE, Feinstein MB. Differential effects of calmodulin antagonists on phospholipases A2 and C in thrombin- stimulated platelets. *J Biol Chem* 1981;256:12523.
72. Billah MM, Lapetina EG. Formation of lysophosphatidylinositol in platelets stimulated with thrombin or ionophore A23187. *J Biol Chem* 1982;257:5196.
73. Billah MM, Lapetina EG, Cuatrecasas P. Phospholipase A2 activity specific for phosphatidic acid: a possible mechanism of the production of arachidonic acid in platelets. *J Biol Chem* 1981;256:5399.
74. Purdon AD, Patelunas D, Smith JB. Evidence for the release of arachidonic acid through the selective action of phospholipase A2 in thrombin-stimulated human platelets. *Biochim Biophys Acta* 1987;920:205.
75. Halenda SP, Zavoico GB, Feinstein MB. Phorbol esters and oleoyl acetoyl glycerol enhance release of arachidonic acid in platelets stimulated by Ca⁺⁺ ionophore A23187. *J Biol Chem* 1985;260:12484.
76. Berridge MJ. Rapid accumulation of inositol triphosphate reveals that agonists hydrolyse polyphosphoinositides instead of phosphatidylinositol. *Biochem J* 1983;212:849.
77. Mahadevappa VG, Holub BJ. The molecular species composition of individual diacyl phospholipids in human platelets. *Biochim Biophys Acta* 1982;713:73.
78. Michell RH. Is phosphatidylinositol really out of the calcium gate? *Nature* 1982;296:492.
79. Bell RL, Majerus PW. Thrombin-induced hydrolysis of phosphatidylinositol in human platelets. *J Biol Chem* 1980;255:1790.
80. Perret BP, Plantavid M, Chap H, et al. Are polyphosphoinositides involved in platelet activation? *Biochem Biophys Res Commun* 1983;110:660.
81. Broekman MJ, Ward JW, Marcus AJ. Phospholipid metabolism in stimulated human platelets: changes in phosphatidylinositol, phosphatidic acid, and lysophospholipids. *J Clin Invest* 1980;66:275.
82. Bucki R, Janmey PA, Vegners R, et al. Involvement of phosphatidylinositol 4,5-bisphosphate in phosphatidylserine exposure in platelets: use of a permeant phosphoinositide-binding peptide. *Biochemistry* 2001;40:15752–15761.
83. Majerus PW, Wilson DB, Connolly TM, et al. Phosphoinositide turnover provides a link in stimulus-response coupling. *Trends Biochem Sci* 1985;10:168.
84. Geltz NR, Augustine JA. The p85 and p110 subunits of phosphatidylinositol 3-kinase-alpha are substrates, *in vitro*, for a constitutively associated protein tyrosine kinase in platelets. *Blood* 1998;91:930.
85. Wymann MP, Pirola L. Structure and function of phosphoinositide 3-kinase. *Boichem Biophys Acta* 1998;1436:127.
86. Pasquet JM, Gross BS, Gratacap MP, et al. Thrombopoietin potentiates collagen receptor signaling in platelets through a phosphatidylinositol 3-kinase-dependent pathway. *Blood* 2000;95:3429–3434.
87. Zhang J, Banfic H, Straforini F, et al. A type II phosphoinositide 3-kinase is stimulated via activated integrin. A source of phosphatidylinositol 3-phosphate. *J Biol Chem* 1998;273:14081.
88. Aoki J, Taira A, Takanezawa Y, et al. Serum lysophosphatidic acid is produced through diverse phospholipase pathways. *J Biol Chem* 2002;277:48737–48744.
89. Panetti TS. Differential effects of sphingosine 1-phosphate and lysophosphatidic acid on endothelial cells. *Biochim Biophys Acta* 2002;1582:190–196.
90. Sano T, Baker D, Virag T, et al. Multiple mechanisms linked to platelet activation result in lysophosphatidic acid and sphingosine 1-phosphate generation in blood. *J Biol Chem* 2002;277:21197–21206.
91. Umezu-Goto M, Kishi Y, Taira A, et al. Autotaxin has lysophospholipase D activity leading to tumor cell growth and motility by lysophosphatidic acid production. *J Cell Biol* 2002;158:227–233.
92. le Balle F, Simon MF, Meijer S, et al. Membrane sidedness of biosynthetic pathways involved in the production of lysophosphatidic acid. *Adv Enzyme Regul* 1999;39:275–284.
93. Yatomi Y, Yamamura S, Ruan F, et al. Sphingosine 1-phosphate induces platelet activation through an extracellular action and shares a platelet

surface receptor with lysophosphatidic acid. *J Biol Chem* 1997;272:5291–5297.

94. Yatomi Y, Ohmori T, Rile G, et al. Sphingosine 1-phosphate as a major bioactive lysophospholipid that is released from platelets and interacts with endothelial cells. *Blood* 2000;96:3431–3438.

95. Motohashi K, Shibata S, Ozaki Y, et al. Identification of lysophospholipid receptors in human platelets: the relations of two agonists, lysophosphatidic acid and sphingosine-1-phosphate. *FEBS Lett* 2000;468:189–193.

96. Haseruck N, Erl W, Pandey D, et al. The plaque lipid lysophosphatidic acid stimulates platelet activation and platelet-monocyte aggregate formation in whole blood: involvement of P2Y1 and P2Y12 receptors. *Blood* 2004;103:2585–2592.

97. MacIntyre DE, Hoover RL, Smith M, et al. Inhibition of platelet function by cis-unsaturated fatty acids. *Blood* 1984;63:848.

98. Galloway JH, Cartwright IJ, Woodcock BE, et al. Effects of dietary fish-oil supplementation on the fatty acid composition of the human platelet membrane: demonstration of selectivity in the incorporation of eicosapentaenoic acid into membrane phospholipid pools. *Clin Sci* 1985;68:449.

99. Thorngren M, Shafi S, Born GV. Delay in primary hemostasis produced by a fish diet without change in local thromboxane A2. *Br J Haematol* 1984;58:567.

100. Driss F, Vericel E, Lagarde M, et al. Inhibition of platelet aggregation and thromboxane synthesis after intake of small amount of icosapentaenoic acid. *Thromb Res* 1984;36:389.

101. Goodnight SH Jr, Harris WS, Conner WE. The effects of dietary omega-3 fatty acids on platelet composition and function in man: a prospective controlled study. *Blood* 1981;58:880.

102. Bruchner GG, German JB, Lokesh B, et al. Biosynthesis of prostanoids, tissue fatty acid composition and thrombotic parameters in rats fed diets enriched with docosahexaenoic (22:6n3) or eicosapentaenoic (20:5n3) acids. *Thromb Res* 1984;34:479.

103. Iritani N, Narita R. Changes of arachidonic acid and n-3 polyunsaturated fatty acids of phospholipid classes in liver, plasma and platelets during dietary fat manipulation. *Biochim Biophys Acta* 1984;793:441.

104. Norday A, Davenas E, Ciavatti M, et al. Effect of dietary (n-3) fatty acids on platelet function and lipid metabolism in rats. *Biochim Biophys Acta* 1985;835:491.

105. Schick PK, Menon S, Wojenski C. Effects of marine oil-enriched diets on guinea pig megakaryocyte and platelet lipids: effects on thromboxane synthesis and platelet function. *Biochim Biophys Acta* 1990;1022:49.

106. Mahadevappa VG, Holub BJ. The incorporation of (3H) glycerol and 1-(14C) acyl-sn-glycero-3-phosphocholine into different molecular species of phosphatidylcholine in human platelets. *Can J Biochem Cell Biol* 1984;62:827.

107. Deykin D, Desser RK. The incorporation of acetate and palmitate into lipids by human platelets. *J Clin Invest* 1968;47:1590.

108. Cohen P, Derksen A, van den Bosch H. Pathways of fatty acid metabolism in human platelets. *J Clin Invest* 1970;49:128.

109. Spector AA, Hoak JC, Warner ED, et al. Utilization of long-chain free fatty acids by human platelets. *J Clin Invest* 1970;49:1489.

110. Needleman SW, Spector AA, Hoak JC. Enrichment of human platelet phospholipids with linoleic acid diminishes thromboxane release. *Prostaglandins* 1982;24:607.

111. Bills TK, Smith JB, Silver MJ. Selective release of arachidonic acid from the phospholipids of human platelets in response to thrombin. *J Clin Invest* 1977;60:1.

112. Rittenhouse SE. Inositol lipid metabolism in the responses of stimulated platelets. *Cell Calcium* 1982;3:311.

113. Plantavid M, Perret BP, Chap H, et al. Asymmetry of arachidonic acid metabolism in the phospholipids of the human platelet membrane as studied with purified phospholipases. *Biochim Biophys Acta* 1982;693:451.

114. Iritani N, Ikeda Y, Kajitani H. Selectivities of 1-acylglycerophosphorylcholine acyltransferase and acyl-CoA synthetase for n-3 polyunsaturated fatty acids in platelets and liver microsomes. *Biochim Biophys Acta* 1984;793:416.

115. McKean ML, Smith JB, Silver MJ. Phospholipid biosynthesis in human platelets: formation of phosphatidylcholine from 1-acyl lysophosphatidylcholine by acyl-CoA. 1-acyl-sn-glycero-3-phosphocholine acyltransferase. *J Biol Chem* 1982;27:11278.

116. Wilson DB, Prescott SM, Majerus PW. Discovery of an arachidonyl coenzyme-A synthetase in human platelets. *J Biol Chem* 1982;257:3510.

117. Neufeld EJ, Wilson DB, Sprecher H, et al. High-affinity esterification of eicosanoid precursor fatty acids by platelets. *J Clin Invest* 1983;72:214.

118. Neufeld EJ, Sprecher H, Evans RW, et al. Fatty acid structural requirements for activity of arachidonyl-CoA synthetase. *J Lipid Res* 1984; 25:288.

119. Kramer RM, Deykin D. Arachidonyl transacylase in human platelets: coenzyme A-independent transfer of arachidonate from phosphatidylcholine to lysoplasmenylethanolamine. *J Biol Chem* 1983;258:13806.

120. Kramer RM, Pritzker CR, Deykin D. Coenzyme A-mediated arachidonic acid transacylation in human platelets. *J Biol Chem* 1984;259:2403.

121. McKean ML, Silver MJ. Phospholipid biosynthesis in human platelets: the acylation of lyso-platelet-activating factor. *Biochem J* 1985;225:723.

122. Kramer RM, Patton GM, Pritzker CR, et al. Metabolism of platelet activating factor in human platelets: transacylase-mediated synthesis of 1-O-alkyl-arachidonyl, sn-glycero-3 phosphocholine. *J Biol Chem* 1984;259:13316.

123. Blank ML, Lee TC, Cress EA, et al. Conversion of 1-alkyl-2 acetyl- sn-glycerols to platelet activating factor and related phospholipids by rabbit platelets. *Biochim Biophys Res Commun* 1984;124:156.

124. von Shacky C, Weber PC. Metabolism and effects on platelet function of the purified eicosapentaenoic and docosahexaenoic acids in humans. *J Clin Invest* 1985;76:2446.

125. Schick PK, Tuszynski GP, Vandervoort PW. Human platelet cytoskeletons: specific content of glycolipids and phospholipids. *Blood* 1983;61:163.

126. Schick BP, Schick PK. Cholesterol and phospholipid biosynthesis in guinea pig megakaryocytes. *Biochim Biophys Acta* 1981;663:249.

127. Schick BP, Schick PK. Cholesterol exchange in platelets, erythrocytes and megakaryocytes. *Biochim Biophys Acta* 1985;833:281.

128. Schick BP, Schick PK. The effect of hypercholesterolemia on guinea pig platelets, erythrocytes and megakaryocytes. *Biochim Biophys Acta* 1985;833:297.

129. Carvalho ACA, Colman RW, Lees RS. Platelet function in hyperbetalipoproteinemia. *N Engl J Med* 1974;290:434.

130. Shattil SJ, Bennett JS, Colman RW, et al. Abnormalities of cholesterol-phospholipid composition in platelets and low-density lipoproteins of human hyperbetalipoproteinemia. *J Lab Clin Med* 1977;89:341.

131. Tremoli E, Folco GC, Agradi E, et al. Platelet thromboxanes and serum cholesterol. *Lancet* 1979;1:107.

132. Dobner P, Engelmann B. Low-density lipoproteins supply phospholipid-bound arachidonic acid for platelet eicosanoid production. *Am J Physiol* 1998;275:E777–E784.

133. Relou IA, Hackeng CM, Akkerman JW, et al. Low-density lipoprotein and its effect on human blood platelets. *Cell Mol Life Sci* 2003;60:961–971.

134. Tandon N, Harmon JT, Rodbard D, et al. Thrombin receptors define responsiveness of cholesterol-modified platelets. *J Biol Chem* 1983;258:11840.

135. Stuart MJ, Gerrard JM, White JG. Effect of cholesterol on production of thromboxane b2 by platelets *in vitro*. *N Engl J Med* 1980;302:6.

136. Kramer RM, Jakubowski JA, Vaillancourt R, et al. Effect of membrane cholesterol on phospholipid metabolism in thrombin- stimulated human platelets: enhanced activation of platelet phospholipase(s) for liberation of arachidonic acid. *J Biol Chem* 1982;257:6844.

137. Zubay G. *Biochemistry*. Reading, MA: Addison-Wesley, 1983:527.

138. Tao RV, Sweeley CC, Jamieson GA. Sphingolipid composition of human platelets. *J Lipid Res* 1973;14:16.

139. Marcus AJ, Ullman HL, Safier LB. Studies on human platelet gangliosides. *J Clin Invest* 1972;51:2602.

140. Wang CT, Schick PK. The effect of thrombin on the organization of human platelet membrane glycosphingolipids: the sphingosine composition of platelet glycolipids and ceramides. *J Biol Chem* 1981;256:752.

141. Bouhours J-F, Bouhours D. Identification of free ceramide in human erythrocyte membrane. *J Lipid Res* 1984;25:613.

142. Snyder PD Jr, Desnick RJ, Krivit W. The glycosphingolipids and glycosyl hydrolases of human blood platelets. *Biochem Biophys Res Commun* 1972;46:1857.

143. Roberts DD, Haverstick DM, Dixit VM, et al. The platelet glycoprotein thrombospondin binds specifically to sulfated glycolipids. *J Biol Chem* 1985;260:9405.

144. Roberts DD, Williams SB, Gralnick HR, et al. von Willebrand factor binds specifically to sulfated glycolipids. *J Biol Chem* 1986;261:3306.

145. Shimada T, Sugo T, Kato H, et al. Activation of factor XII and prekallikrein with polysaccharide sulfates and sulfatides: comparison with kaolin-mediated activation. *J Biochem (Tokyo)* 1985;97:429.

146. Tans G, Rosing J, Griffin JH. Sulfatide-dependent autoactivation of human blood coagulation factor XII (Hageman factor). *J Biol Chem* 1983;258:8215.

147. Espana F, Ratnoff OD. Activation of Hageman factor (factor XII) by sulfatides and other agents in the absence of plasma proteases. *J Lab Clin Med* 1983;102:31.

148. Beutler E, Kuhl W. The diagnosis of the adult type Gaucher's disease and its carrier state by demonstration of deficiency of beta- glucosidase activity in peripheral blood leukocytes. *J Lab Clin Med* 1970;76:747.

149. Martini F, Riondino S, Pignatelli P, et al. Involvement of GD3 in platelet activation. A novel association with Fcgamma receptor. *Biochim Biophys Acta* 2002;1583:297–304.

150. Tamir H, Brunner W, et al. Enhancement by gangliosides of the binding of serotonin to serotonin binding protein. *J Neurochem* 1980;34:1719.

151. Pignatti PF, Cavalli-Sforza LL. Serotonin binding proteins from human blood platelets: an experimental model system for studies on properties of synaptic vesicles. *Neurobiology* 1975;5:65.

152. Tamir H, Gershon MD. Storage of serotonin and serotonin binding protein in synaptic vesicles. *J Neurochem* 1979;33:35.

153. Fishman PH. Role of membrane gangliosides in the binding and action of bacterial toxins. *J Membrane Biol* 1969;69:85.

154. Hughes RJ, Insel PA. Human platelets are defective in processing of cholera toxin. *Biochem J* 1983;212:669.

155. Bremer EG, Hakomori S-I. Gangliosides as receptor modulators. *Adv Exp Med Biol* 1984;174:381.

156. Dawson G, Berry-Kravis E. Gangliosides as modulators of the coupling of neurotransmitters to adenylate cyclase. *Adv Exp Med Biol* 1984;174:341.

157. Gardas A, Adler G, Lewartowska A, et al. Influence of antiganglioside antibodies on thyrotrophin binding and adenyl cyclase activity of thyroid plasma membranes. *Acta Endocrinol (Copenh)* 1983;104:333.

158. Vengris VE, Fernie BF, Pitha PM. The interaction between gangliosides and interferon. *Adv Exp Med Biol* 1980;125:479.

159. Lee G, Aloj SM, Brady RO, et al. The structure and function of glycoprotein hormone receptors: ganglioside interactions with human chorionic gonadotropin. *Biochem Biophys Res Commun* 1976;73:370.

160. Streuli CH, Patel B, Critchley DR. The cholera toxin receptor ganglioside GM1 remains associated with Triton-X-100 cytoskeletons of Balb/c-3T3 cells. *Exp Cell Res* 1981;136:247.

161. Kellie S, Patel B, Pierce EJ, et al. Capping of cholera toxin- ganglioside GM1 complexes on mouse lymphocytes is accompanied by co-capping of alpha-actinin. *J Cell Biol* 1983;97:447.

162. Nagai Y, Sakakibara K. Cytoskeleton-associated glycolipid (CAG) and its cell biological implication. *Adv Exp Med Biol* 1982;152:425.

163. Sakakibara K, Momoi T, Uchida T, et al. Evidence for association of glycosphingolipid with a colchicine-sensitive microtubule-like cytoskeleton structure of cultured cells. *Nature* 1981;293:76.

164. Tuszynski GP, Mauco GP, Koshy A, et al. The platelet cytoskeleton contains elements of the prothrombinase complex. *J Biol Chem* 1984;259:6947.

165. Fukuda MN, Levery SB. Glycolipids of fetal, newborn, and adult erythrocytes: glycolipid pattern and structural study of H3-glycolipid from newborn erythrocytes. *Biochemistry* 1983;22:5034.

166. Bouhours D, Bouhours JF. Developmental changes of hematoside of rat small intestine: postnatal hydroxylation of fatty acids and sialic acid. *J Biol Chem* 1983;258:299.

167. Ferrari G, Fabris M, Gorio A. Gangliosides enhance neurite outgrowth in PC12 cells. *Brain Res* 1983;284:215.

168. Schwartz M, Spirman N. Sprouting from chicken embryo dorsal root ganglia induced by nerve growth factor is specifically inhibited by affinity purified antiganglioside antibodies. *Proc Natl Acad Sci U S A* 1983;790:6080.

169. Bremer EG, Hakomori S, Bowen-Pope DF, et al. Ganglioside- mediated modulation of cell growth, growth factor binding, and receptor phosphorylation. *J Biol Chem* 1984;259:6818.

170. Schick PK, He X. Composition and synthesis of glycolipids in megakaryocytes and platelets: differences in synthesis in megakaryocytes at different stages of maturation. *J Lipid Res* 1990;31:1645.

171. Thomas JR, Dwek RA, Rademacher TW. Structure, biosynthesis, and function of glycosylphosphatidylinositols. *Biochemistry* 1990;29:5413.

172. Low MG. The glycosyl-phosphatidylinositol anchor of membrane proteins. *Biochim Biophys Acta* 1989;988:427.

173. Low MG, Saltiel AR. Structural and functional roles of glycosyl- phosphatidylinositol in membranes. *Science* 1988;239:268.

174. Dhar A, Shukla SD. Release of human platelet surface glycoprotein by phosphatidylinositol specific phospholipase(s) C. *J Cell Biol* 1988;107:559a.

175. Hall SE, Rosse WF. The use of monoclonal antibodies and flow cytometry in the diagnosis of paroxysmal nocturnal hemoglobinuria. *Blood* 1996;87:5332.

176. Maciejewski JP, Sloand EM, Sato T, et al. Impaired hematopoiesis in paroxysmal nocturnal hemoglobinuria/aplastic anemia is not associated with a selective proliferative defect in the glycosylphosphatidylinositol-anchored protein-deficient clone. *Blood* 1997;89:1173.

177. Bessler M, Hillmen P. Somatic mutation and clonal selection in the pathogenesis and in the control of paroxysmal nocturnal hemoglobinuria. *Semin Hematol* 1998;35:149–167.

178. Grand RJA. Acylation of viral and eukaryotic proteins. *Biochem J* 1989;258:625.

179. Schmidt MFG. Fatty acylation of proteins. *Biochim Biophys Acta* 1989;988:411.

180. Seehafer JG, Slupsky JR, Tang S-C, et al. The functional cell surface glycoprotein CD9 is distinguished by being the major fatty acid acylated and a major iodinated cell-surface component of the human platelet. *Biochim Biophys Acta* 1988;952:92.

181. Higashihara M, Maeda H, et al. A monoclonal anti-human platelet antibody: a new platelet aggregating substance. *Blood* 1985;65:382.

182. Slupsky JR, Seehafer JG, Tang S-C, et al. Evidence that monoclonal antibodies against CD9 antigen induce specific association between CD9 and the platelet glycoprotein IIb-IIIa complex. *J Biol Chem* 1989;264:12289.

183. Muszbek L, Laposata M. Glycoprotein Ib and glycoprotein IX in human platelets are acylated with palmitic acid through thioester linkages. *J Biol Chem* 1989;246:9716.

184. Muszbek L, Laposata M. Covalent modification of platelet proteins by palmitate. *Blood* 1989;74:1339.

185. Cierniewski CS, Kreslowska J, Pawlowska Z, et al. Palmitoylation of the glycoprotein IIb-IIIa complex in human blood platelets. *J Biol Chem* 1989;264:12158.

186. Huang EM. Agonist-enhanced palmitoylation of platelet proteins. *Biochim Biophys Acta* 1989;1011:134.

187. Aderem AA, Keum MM, Pure E, et al. Bacterial lipopolysaccharides, phorbol myristate acetate, and zymosan induce the myristoylation of specific macrophage proteins. *Proc Natl Acad Sci U S A* 1986;83:5817.

188. Marchildon GA, Casnellie JE, Walsh KA, et al. Covalently bound myristate in a lymphoma tyrosine protein kinase. *Proc Acad Natl Sci U S A* 1984;81:7679.

189. Carr SA, Biemann K, Shoji S, et al. n-Tetradecanoyl is the NH2- terminal blocking group of the catalytic subunit of cyclic AMP- dependent protein kinase from bovine cardiac muscle. *Proc Natl Acad Sci U S A* 1982;79:6128.

190. Buss JE, Kamps MP, Gould K, et al. The absence of myristic acid decreases membrane binding of p60src but does not affect tyrosine protein kinase activity. *J Virol* 1986;58:468.

191. Lacal PM, Pennington CY, Lacal JC. Transforming activity of ras proteins translocated to the plasma membrane by a myristoylation sequence from the src gene product. *Oncogene* 1988;2:533.

192. Schick PK, Walker J. The acylation of megakaryocyte proteins: glycoprotein IX is primarily myristoylated while glycoprotein Ib is palmitoylated. *Blood* 1996;87:1377.

193. Wonerow P, Obergfell A, Wilde JI, et al. Differential role of glycolipid-enriched membrane domains in glycoprotein VI- and integrin-mediated phospholipase Cgamma2 regulation in platelets. *Biochem J* 2002;364:755–765.

194. Dorahy DJ, Lincz LF, Meldrum CJ, et al. Biochemical isolation of a membrane microdomain from resting platelets highly enriched in the plasma membrane glycoprotein CD36. *Biochem J* 1996;319(Pt 1):67–72.

195. Mairhofer M, Steiner M, Mosgoeller W, et al. Stomatin is a major lipid-raft component of platelet alpha granules. *Blood* 2002;100:897–904.

196. Gousset K, Wolkers WF, Tsvetkova NM, et al. Evidence for a physiological role for membrane rafts in human platelets. *J Cell Physiol* 2002;190:117–128.

197. Heijnen HF, Van Lier M, Waaijenborg S, et al. Concentration of rafts in platelet filopodia correlates with recruitment of c-Src and CD63 to these domains. *J Thromb Haemost* 2003;1:1161–1173.

198. Shrimpton CN, Borthakur G, Larrucea S, et al. Localization of the adhesion receptor glycoprotein Ib-IX-V complex to lipid rafts is required for platelet adhesion and activation. *J Exp Med* 2002;196:1057–1066.

199. Locke D, Chen H, Liu Y, et al. Lipid rafts orchestrate signaling by the platelet receptor glycoprotein VI. *J Biol Chem* 2002;277:18801–18809.

200. Bodin S, Giuriato S, Ragab J, et al. Production of phosphatidylinositol 3,4,5-trisphosphate and phosphatidic acid in platelet rafts: evidence for a critical role of cholesterol-enriched domains in human platelet activation. *Biochemistry* 2001;40:15290–15299.

201. Dorahy DJ, Burns GF. Active Lyn protein tyrosine kinase is selectively enriched within membrane microdomains of resting platelets. *Biochem J* 1998;333(Pt 2):373–379.

202. Baglia FA, Shrimpton CN, Lopez JA, et al. The glycoprotein Ib-IX-V complex mediates localization of factor XI to lipid rafts on the platelet membrane. *J Biol Chem* 2003;278:21744–21750.

203. Waheed AA, Shimada Y, Heijnen HF, et al. Selective binding of perfringolysin O derivative to cholesterol-rich membrane microdomains (rafts). *Proc Natl Acad Sci U S A* 2001;98:4926–4931.

204. Marinetti GV, Love R. Differential reaction of cell membrane phospholipids and proteins with chemical probes. *Chem Phys Lipids* 1976;16:239.

205. Marinetti GV. Arrangement of phosphatidylserine and phosphatidylethanolamine in the erythrocyte membrane. *Biochim Biophys Acta* 1977;465:198.

206. Schick PK. The organization of aminophospholipids in human platelet membranes: selective changes induced by thrombin. *J Lab Clin Med* 1978;91:802.

207. Schick BP, Schick PK, Chase PR. Lipid composition of guinea pig platelets and megakaryocytes: the megakaryocyte as a probable source of platelet lipids. *Biochim Biophys Acta* 1981;663:239.

208. Schick PK, Williams-Gartner K, He X. Lipid composition and metabolism in megakaryocytes at different stages of maturation. *J Lipid Res* 1990;31:27.

209. Schick BP, Schick PK, Foster K, et al. Arachidonate synthesis and uptake in isolated guinea-pig megakaryocytes and platelets. *Biochim Biophys Acta* 1984;795:341.

210. Schick PK. Arachidonic acid is preferentially incorporated into immature megakaryocytes. *J Lab Clin Med* 1989;113:79.

211. He X, Schick PK, Wojenski C. The expression of acetyl-CoA carboxylase is related to megakaryocyte maturation. *J Lab Clin Med* 1995;126:178.

212. Turnham E, Northcote DH. The use of acetyl-CoA carboxylase activity and changes in wall composition as measures of embryogenesis in tissue cultures of oil palm. *Biochem J* 1982;208:323.

213. Pape E, Kim K-H. Effect of tumor necrosis factor on acetyl-coenzyme A carboxylase gene expression and preadipocyte differentiation. *Mol Endocrinol* 1988;2:395.

# CHAPTER 38 ■ ROLE OF PLATELETS IN BLOOD COAGULATION

PETER N. WALSH

The hemostatic response to vascular injury requires the initiation and propagation of blood coagulation, which consist of a series of proteolytic reactions that involve the assembly of enzymes, cofactors, and substrate molecules on cell surface receptors exposed on the plasma membranes of activated platelets and other intravascular cells including monocytes and neutrophils (1–4). The hemostatic mechanism has the remarkable capacity to maintain blood in a fluid state under normal physiologic conditions and to respond instantly when the integrity of the blood vessels is breached by the exposure of platelet and other cell membrane receptors. These proteins localize coagulation complex assembly within the hemostatic thrombus and prevent disseminated intravascular coagulation by protecting coagulation enzymes from inactivation by plasma and cellular inhibitors of serine proteases (1,3–8). The initial clear and comprehensive hypotheses on the normal coagulation mechanism, referred to as the *cascade* (9) and *waterfall* (10) *theories*, were proposed more than 40 years ago and have since been rather extensively revised (11–15). The purpose of this chapter is to present a postulated sequence of events that comprise the normal hemostatic mechanism, which localizes coagulant activity to the site of injury and dramatically amplifies the initiating stimulus by producing sufficient quantities of thrombin to cleave fibrinogen, thereby generating cross-linked fibrin that forms a physical barrier to extravasation of blood from the wound site. The contributions of other intravascular cells, such as leukocytes and monocytes, to coagulation complex assembly and the role of cell membrane receptors in the assembly of the anticoagulant complexes involving activated protein C, protein S, and thrombomodulin are not considered here because they are dealt with in other chapters (see Chapters 14 and 45, respectively). This chapter also does not consider in detail the role of artificial phospholipid membranes in the assembly of the factor X– and prothrombin-activating complexes that are dealt with elsewhere (see Chapter 10). Finally, the interactions of thrombin with platelets and other cells are considered in Chapter 13.

## SEQUENTIAL COAGULATION COMPLEX FORMATION

The cascade (9) and waterfall (10) theories of blood coagulation originally postulated a mechanism by which a minute initial stimulus was sequentially amplified through a series of enzymatic reactions to result in the local explosive generation of thrombin that is sufficient to convert fibrinogen to fibrin and to effect normal hemostasis. These hypotheses postulated two alternative pathways for the initiation of coagulation, each leading to the activation of factor X. One was termed the *intrinsic pathway*, by which the "contact factors" (i.e., factor XII, prekallikrein, high-molecular-weight kininogen,

and factor XI) were assembled on negatively charged surfaces (16), and the other was termed the *extrinsic pathway*, which was initiated by factor VIIa and by the exposure of tissue factor (TF) (14). It was subsequently shown that platelets make major contributions to each reaction step including alternative, platelet-dependent pathways for the activation of factor XI (2,17–21). However, these concepts required further revision because patients with deficiencies of factor XII, prekallikrein, and high-molecular-weight kininogen do not experience abnormal bleeding even after surgery or trauma (16), whereas patients with hemophilia A (i.e., factor VIII deficiency) and hemophilia B (i.e., factor IX deficiency) with severe, life-threatening, spontaneous, and posttraumatic bleeding (22,23), and patients with factor XI deficiency (24–31) and factor VII deficiency (14), although not usually subject to spontaneous hemorrhage, may bleed excessively after surgery or trauma. Therefore, it is clear that factors VIII and IX are essential for the activation of factor X. Because factor IX activation can be catalyzed not only by factor XIa (32–40) but also by factor VIIa tissue factor (41), it has been suggested that the TF pathway can initiate the intrinsic pathway directly and independently of the contact factor pathway. However, this suggestion does not account for the hemostatic defect observed in factor XI deficiency (24–31), indicating that factor XI activation is essential for activating factor IX and must proceed by a pathway independent of factor XII, prekallikrein, and high-molecular-weight kininogen. In 1991, an alternative mechanism for proteolytic activation of factor XI by thrombin (13,15) was demonstrated; this mechanism was subsequently shown to proceed at a 5,000- to 10,000-fold accelerated rate on the activated platelet surface (11,12, 42,43). The revised concept arising from these and other observations suggests that the initial event in hemostasis is the exposure of TF on cell membranes, resulting in the activation of factor X by factor VIIa tissue factor (14), and leading to the generation of only trace concentrations of thrombin because the TF pathway is rapidly shut down by TF pathway inhibitor (44–50). The initial traces of thrombin formed are insufficient to produce a hemostatic plug by converting fibrinogen to fibrin but are sufficient to activate platelets, factor XI, factor VIII, and factor V, which permit the consolidation (intrinsic) pathway of coagulation to generate sufficient quantities of thrombin to promote hemostasis (11–13,15,42,43,51–53). The consolidation pathway occurs on the surface membranes of activated platelets, which expose the specific plasma membrane receptors for factor XI (42,43,51–56), factor XIa (57–60), factor IX (61–64), factor IXa (61–73), factor VIII (60,74,75), factor VIIIa (60,74,75), factor X (75–77), factor Xa (78–90), factor V (78–90), factor Va (78–90), prothrombin (76,77), and thrombin (3,91). These platelet receptors promote the assembly of coagulation enzyme–cofactor–substrate complexes that, compared with solution-phase reactions, vastly accelerate the kinetics of factor

605

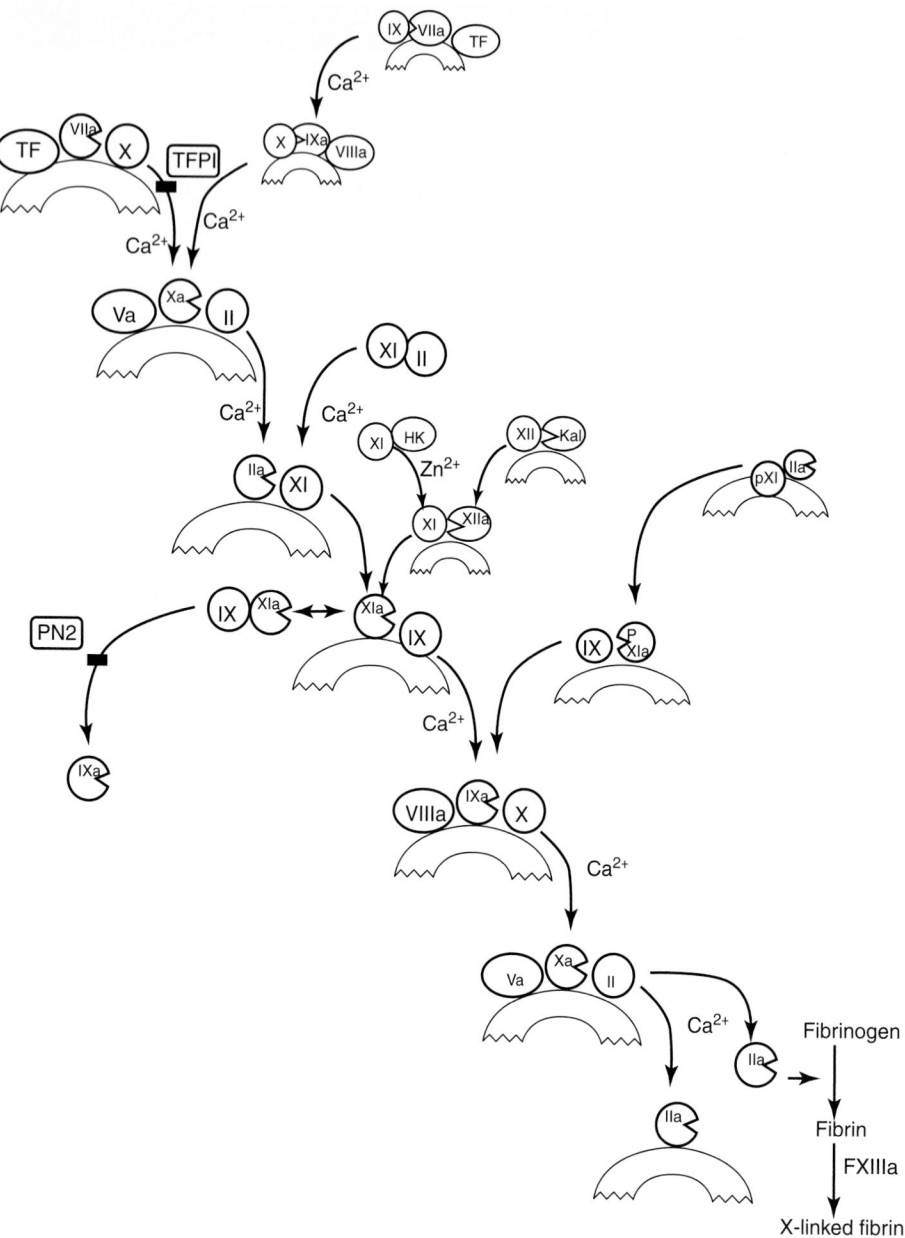

**FIGURE 38-1.** Schematic diagram representing a current hypothesis of the contribution of platelets to blood coagulation, and the postulated sequence of coagulation reactions that comprises the normal hemostatic mechanism. The crescentic forms represent the activated platelet membrane and the roman numerals represent the coagulation proteins including zymogens or substrates (*in circles*), cofactors (*in ellipses*), and enzymes (*in circles with segmental excisions*). TF, tissue factor; pXI, platelet factor XI; TFPI, tissue factor pathway inhibitor; PN2, protease nexin-2; the *arrows*, conversions from zymogen to enzyme; solid *black blocks* superimposed on arrow, the block imposed by the designated inhibitor. See text for detailed discussion and explanation (94). (From Walsh PN. Platelet coagulation-protein interactions. *Semin Thromb Hemost* 2004; 30:461–471, with permission.)

XI activation by factor XIIa (92) or by thrombin (11,12, 42,43,57), of factor X activation by factor IXa (61,62,66, 68–71,78–80,82–90,93), and of prothrombin activation by factor Xa (78–90). The assembly of these receptor-mediated coagulation complexes is presented in schematic form in Figure 38-1, which provides a point of reference for understanding the role of platelets and other cells in the initiation and consolidation pathways of blood coagulation.

## INITIATION PATHWAYS

The preponderance of evidence now supports the consensus that although the contact phase proteins can initiate intrinsic coagulation when foreign surfaces are introduced into the blood stream (16), the initiating event in hemostasis is the expression of the transmembrane protein, TF, on cell membranes exposed when the endothelial barrier is breached (14). The TF pathway is considered in detail in Chapter 5. Although a number of cell types, including monocytes and leukocytes and those underlying the endothelium, can synthesize and expose TF to plasma proteins, the specific cell type and mechanism of TF presentation has not been definitively identified (14). However, an intriguing possibility arising from a series of recent observations (95–101) is that tissue factor–bearing microparticles, derived from specialized membrane microdomains (i.e., lipid rafts) in monocytes, can fuse with platelet membranes utilizing adhesive receptors (i.e., P selectin on activated platelets and PSGL-1 on microparticles), thereby transferring TF by membrane fusion to platelets, which do not normally express it. Confirmation of this interesting and plausible hypothesis would provide a single locus (i.e., the activated platelet membrane) upon which all the enzyme–cofactor–substrate complexes of blood coagulation can be assembled, thereby avoiding the conundrum of requiring the initiation of blood coagulation on one cellular surface located in the subendothelium or upon monocytes, followed by the propagation of subsequent coagulation reactions on receptors exposed on activated platelets.

## Assembly and Regulation of the Tissue Factor Pathway

The initiating event in hemostasis is postulated to require the exposure of the transmembrane protein, TF, which binds factor VIIa, a vitamin K–dependent protease that has virtually no important activity as an enzyme in solution until bound to TF (14). A small amount of factor VIIa (i.e., <1% of the total factor VII in plasma) normally circulates in plasma (102) with a relatively long half-life for an active enzyme (i.e., approximately 2 hours) and is not susceptible to inactivation by plasma proteinase inhibitors (103). Factor VIIa then binds to TF exposed on cell membranes, where it can efficiently activate either factor IX or factor X, leading to the generation of a small quantity of factor Xa, which then facilitates the formation of a complex between TF pathway inhibitor, factor VIIa, factor Xa, and TF, resulting in the rapid and effective shutdown of any further formation of factor Xa (13,15,44–50). This initial assembly of the components of the TF pathway results in the assembly of the prothrombinase complex on platelet membranes (see subsequent text) and the generation of small quantities of thrombin that are insufficient to cleave fibrinogen or effect the formation of hemostatic thrombi but sufficient to activate platelets, factor XI, factor VIII, and factor V and to trigger the consolidation pathway of blood coagulation (1,4,8,104).

## Platelets and the Contact Activation Pathway

The biochemical mechanisms involved in the assembly and activation of the proteins constituting the contact phase of intrinsic coagulation (i.e., factor XII, prekallikrein, and high-molecular-weight kininogen) have been extensively studied and clearly elucidated (16,105–114) and are considered in detail in Chapter 6. It is clear that the reciprocal proteolytic activation of factor XII and prekallikrein on negatively charged surfaces in the presence of high-molecular-weight kininogen can lead to the limited proteolytic activation of factor XI (105–114) and the subsequent activation of intrinsic coagulation, leading to the generation of sufficient quantities of thrombin to cleave fibrinogen to fibrin. However, doubt has been cast upon the physiologic role of the contact-phase proteins in normal hemostasis because of the absence of hemostatic abnormalities in patients who are deficient in these proteins in contrast to the considerable bleeding complications that occur in some patients with factor XI deficiency (1,4,8,16,24–31,104). In fact, high-molecular-weight kininogen appears to downregulate the activation of platelets by interfering with the binding of thrombin to glycoprotein (GP) Ib/IX/V complex with platelet surface (see Chapter 6). Nonetheless, these observations do not exclude a possible role of the contact activation pathway either in normal hemostasis or in pathologic thrombus formation, especially in patients with prosthetic devices, such as artificial heart valves, implanted within the vasculature.

Following the presentation of early observations indicating that activated platelets participate in the assembly and activation of factor XII and factor XI and the subsequent assembly of the factor X–activating complex (2,17–21,92), it was demonstrated that isolated human platelets, activated by adenosine diphosphate (ADP) or by collagen, can promote the proteolytic activation of factor XII by kallikrein and the subsequent proteolytic activation of factor XI by factor XIIa (92), by exposing high-affinity ($K_d$ approximately 10 nM), specific, saturable binding sites (approximately 1,500 sites per platelet) that require the presence of either high-molecular-weight kininogen and zinc ions or prothrombin and calcium ions (11,12,51–53,55). Although subsequent evidence suggests that the activation of factor XI on the platelet surface by thrombin is preferred over factor XIIa–mediated factor XI activation (12), it remains a possibility that under certain physiologic or pathologic conditions, the assembly of contact pathway proteins on the activated platelet membrane can trigger the initiation of intrinsic coagulation by an alternative mechanism to the TF pathway.

# CONSOLIDATION PATHWAY

## Interactions of Activated Platelets with Factor XI

Factor XI is a unique, homodimeric coagulation protein that circulates in plasma as a zymogen in trace concentrations (approximately 30 nM) in complex with high-molecular-weight kininogen, which is required for the binding of factor XI to negatively charged surfaces and for efficient activation of factor XI by factor XIIa (105,113–118). The details concerning the biochemistry and physiology of factor XI can be found in Chapter 12. Each factor XI monomer contains 607 amino acids, consisting of four tandem repeat sequences, designated apple domains, followed by a typical trypsinlike, serine protease catalytic domain (119–122). The apple domains of factor XI contain binding sites for thrombin (123), high-molecular-weight kininogen (124–126), prothrombin (11,127), factor IX (39,128–131), platelets (51,53–55), heparin (132), and factor XIIa (54,133) and for homodimerization (134–136). Following the assembly of the TF pathway, minute quantities of thrombin, insufficient to generate a hemostatic thrombus, are produced in concentrations (0.05 to 1 nM) that are sufficient to activate platelet protease-activated receptors (PAR) and factor XI on the platelet surface (11–13,15,42,43). Optimal binding of factor XI, through its apple 3 (A3) domain, to the activated platelet surface requires the presence of either high-molecular-weight kininogen and zinc ions or prothrombin and calcium ions, each of which also promotes optimal rates of factor XI activation by thrombin on the platelet surface (11,12,51,53,55,123,127). The receptor on the activated platelet membrane that binds factor XI and thrombin is the GP Ib/IX/V complex, which colocalizes them in a productive enzyme– substrate complex within platelet membrane microdomains or lipid rafts (42,43). Therefore, the physiologic locus for the assembly of the thrombin–factor XI complex and for the initiation of the consolidation pathway of coagulation following the triggering events of the TF pathway appears to be the activated platelet membrane, whereas in contrast, neither quiescent nor activated endothelial cells appear to have a role in the initiation of the consolidation pathway of blood coagulation (57,137).

## Interactions of Factor XIa with Activated Platelets, Factor IX, and Protease Nexin-2

The fact that activated platelets accelerate factor XI activation by thrombin by 5,000- to 10,000-fold (11,12,51,53,55,123, 127) suggests that the enzyme, factor XIa, might also interact specifically with the activated platelet membrane for colocalization with and for efficient activation of its substrate, factor IX, which has also been shown to bind to specific, high-affinity ($K_d$ approximately 2.5 nM) binding sites (approximately 250 sites per platelet) on activated platelets (61). In fact, it has been demonstrated that factor XIa interacts with high affinity ($K_d$ approximately 1.7 nM) and specificity, with approximately 250 sites per activated platelet that are distinct from the lower-affinity ($K_d$ approximately 10 nM), higher-capacity (approximately 1,500 sites per platelet) binding sites for the zymogen, factor XI (57,59). Whereas factor XI binding to activated platelets requires the presence of high-molecular-weight kininogen and zinc ions and is mediated by the A3 domain of factor XI, factor XIa binding requires the presence of zinc ions but is unaffected by high-molecular-weight kininogen and is mediated by the catalytic domain of factor XIa (57). Interestingly, although both factor XIa (57,59) and factor IX (61) bind to activated platelets, the rate of factor IX activation by factor XIa is unaffected by the presence of activated platelets (57,138,139). However, factor XIa bound to the platelet surface is protected from inactivation by plasma proteinase inhibitors including $\alpha_1$-protease inhibitor (139).

Perhaps even more interesting and important is the potential role of protease nexin-2 (PN2) in the regulation of blood coagulation. PN2, a truncated form of the Alzheimer $\beta$-amyloid protein precursor that contains a Kunitz-type protease inhibitor domain, is a potent inhibitor of factor XIa ($K_i$ approximately 350 pM) that has substantially enhanced inhibitory activity ($K_i$ approximately 35 pM) in the presence of heparin (140–144). There is very little PN2 present (i.e., <60 pM) in normal human plasma (143), but the protein is present in sufficient amounts in platelet $\alpha$-granules to achieve a plasma concentration of 2 to 5 nM (141) and, possibly, even as high as approximately 30 nM (143) when platelets are stimulated to secrete their granule contents. These concentrations of PN2 are well above the $K_i$ value for factor XIa inhibition and have been shown to potently, rapidly, and completely inhibit factor XIa in solution, whereas factor XIa bound to its receptor on activated platelets is completely protected from inactivation by PN2 (57,141). In contrast, factor XIa bound to endothelial cells is not protected from inactivation by PN2 (57), suggesting that platelets, by secreting PN2 and by protecting factor XIa from inhibition, provide a nidus for localizing coagulation reactions to the platelet hemostatic thrombus, whereas the primary phenotype of endothelium is anticoagulant and nonthrombogenic (2,57,137,145).

## Platelet Factor XI

The biochemical nature and physiologic importance of the factor XI–like protein associated with the platelet plasma membrane are considered in detail in Chapter 12.

## Interactions of Activated Platelets with Factor IXa, Factor VIIIa, and Factor X

In 1972, it was shown that human platelets, activated with collagen but not with ADP, provide an activated membrane surface for the activation of factor X by factor IXa in the presence of factor VIII (17,21). These observations were subsequently confirmed, and it was shown that both activation of platelets by a variety of physiologic and nonphysiologic agonists and activation of factor VIII by thrombin were required for optimal rates of factor X activation by the factor IXa–factor VIIIa complex (146–150). A large body of work, reviewed elsewhere (see Chapters 7 and 8), has focused on the biochemical mechanisms of factor X activation in phospholipid model systems, supporting the view that aminophospholipids, exposed on the outer leaflet of activated platelets, participate in the assembly of the factor X–activating complex (151,152). A subsequent series of investigations designed to elucidate the mechanism by which platelets participate in the assembly of the factor X–activating complex (60–77,153–155) have given rise to the hypothesis that specific classes of receptors are exposed on the surface membranes of activated platelets and bind and colocalize factor IXa, factor VIIIa, and factor X for optimal factor X activation.

## Factor IXa Binding to Activated Platelets

Human factor IX is a single chain glycoprotein ($M_r$ approximately 57,000) present in plasma as a zymogen, containing a $\gamma$-carboxyglutamic acid (Gla) domain, two epidermal growth factor (EGF) domains, an activation peptide, and a serine protease catalytic domain, that is activated by limited proteolytic cleavage of two scissile bonds either by factor XIa or by factor VIIa to generate the active serine protease, factor IXa$\beta$, that recognizes factor X as its normal substrate (34,37,156–168). The initial evidence that supported platelet-receptor–mediated factor X activation was the observation that factor IXa binds to a discrete number (i.e., 500 to 600 sites per platelet) of high-affinity ($K_d$ approximately 2.5 nM), saturable receptors on activated platelets that are specific for the enzyme, about 50% (i.e., 250 to 300 sites per platelet) of which can also recognize the zymogen, factor IX, in the presence of calcium ions (61). The presence of the cofactor, factor VIIIa, and the substrate, factor X, increases the affinity ($K_d$ approximately 0.5 nM) of factor IXa binding by approximately fivefold, whereas they have no effect on the number or affinity of factor IX binding sites (61). The conclusion that these factor IXa binding sites are functionally active (62) is supported by fact that kinetic studies demonstrated that thrombin-activated platelets decrease the $K_m$ by greater than 200-fold and permit factor VIIIa to increase the $V_{max}$ by greater than 50,000-fold, resulting in the catalytic efficiency ($k_{cat}/K_m$) increasing by greater than $2 \times 10^8$-fold (70). These kinetic effects of platelets on the activation of factor X by factor IXa were almost identical to those of phospholipid (phosphatidylcholine/phosphatidylserine) vesicles (70,169) and were absolutely dependent on activation of platelets with thrombin or the thrombin receptor activation peptide (SFLLRN), whereas ADP had no capacity to expose factor IXa receptors on platelets (61,62, 76,77).

The observations that factor IXa binds to twice the number (i.e., approximately 500 sites per platelet) of receptors than the zymogen, factor IX (i.e., approximately 250 sites per platelet), with identical affinity ($K_d$ approximately 2.5 nM), and that factor IXa displaces all bound factor IX but factor IX displaces only 50% of the bound factor IXa (61) raise interesting questions concerning the functional and structural relations of these two binding sites. The structural determinants of factor IXa interactions with platelets have been investigated (discussed in subsequent text), leading to the conclusion that factor IX binding to activated platelets is mediated by the $\Omega$ loop (residues G4–Q11) within the Gla domain, whereas factor IXa binding to activated platelets is mediated by both the Gla domain $\Omega$ loop and the residues C88–C109 of the second EGF-2 domain (63,65,67,69, 71–73,155). Because factor IX would appear to displace factor IXa from its Gla-mediated binding site, it was surprising to observe that zymogen factor IX potentiates factor IXa–catalyzed factor X activation by substantially increasing the affinity of factor IXa for the intrinsic factor X–activating complex (64), possibly by displacing factor IXa from its shared factor IX/IXa binding site and by "feeding" it to its specific, high-affinity ($K_d$ approximately 0.5 nM) binding site (mediated by residues C88C109 of the EGF-2 domain) within the factor X–activating complex. Therefore, the sequence of functional events mediated by platelet receptors for factor IX/IXa is postulated to include: (a) the initial colocalization of factor XIa and factor IXa on their respective platelet receptors, where bound factor XIa is protected by PN2 from inactivation, for efficient factor XIa–catalyzed factor IX activation that is localized to the platelet hemostatic thrombus; (b) the progressive conversion of factor IX to factor IXa, both of which interact with the shared (Gla domain–mediated) factor IX/IXa binding site (approximately 250 sites per platelet; $K_d$ approximately 2.5 nM), from which factor IX can displace factor IXa; resulting in (c) the potentiation of high-affinity (approximately 250 sites per platelet; $K_d$ approximately 0.5 nM) binding of factor IXa to its specific platelet binding site (mediated by residues C88-C109 of the EGF-2 domain) for efficient factor X activation, the catalytic efficiency of which is more than $2 \times 10^8$-fold greater on the platelet surface than in solution.

## Structural Determinants of Factor IXa Interactions with Activated Platelets

A series of investigations that aimed at defining the structural requirements for factor IXa interactions with their receptors on activated platelets initially demonstrated that the active site of factor IXa is not involved in its high-affinity, factor VIIIa–dependent binding to activated platelets because active-site–blocked factor IXaβ competes with factor IXa for binding sites on activated platelets with a $K_i$ identical to the $K_d$ for factor IXa binding (62). Subsequent comparative platelet binding and kinetic studies with variant factor IXa molecules demonstrated that the presence of D47 is important for high-affinity, factor VIIIa–dependent factor IXa binding because the variant, factor IXa$_{Alabama}$ (D47 → G substitution), interacted with a normal number of binding sites (approximately 550 sites per platelet) with normal affinity ($K_d$ approximately 2.5 nM), but responded to the presence of factor VIIIa with a suboptimal decrease in $K_d$ (69). Moreover, the normal cleavage of factor IX at R145–A146 is essential for its specific, high-affinity interaction with factor IXa binding sites because the variant factor IXa$_{Chapel\ Hill}$ (D145 → H substitution), was found to interact only with the low-affinity ($K_d$ approximately 2.5 nM), low-capacity (approximately 250 sites per platelet) shared factor IXa binding sites (69). The first EGF-1 domain of factor IXa appears to have no role in the interactions of factor IXa with their receptors on activated platelets because a chimeric protein in which the EGF-1 of factor X replaces the corresponding residues in factor IX was shown to interact entirely normally with platelet receptors (68).

In contrast, a series of investigations utilizing chimeric and mutant proteins and synthetic peptides have implicated both the Ω loop (residues G4–Q11) within the Gla domain and residues C88–C109 within the EGF-2 domain in the interaction of factor IXa with platelet receptors (63,65,67,71–73, 155). Initially, it was shown that chemical modification of Gla residues or enzymatic removal of the entire Gla domain of factor IX resulted in factor IXa molecules that interacted with only 50% (approximately 250 sites per platelet) of the normal number of factor IXa binding sites with substantially reduced affinity ($K_d$ approximately 5 nM), compared with normal factor IXa binding (approximately 550 sites per platelet; $K_d$ approximately 0.5 nM) (71). Subsequently, very similar results were obtained with chimeric and mutant factor IXa molecules in which either factor VII or factor X residues were inserted into the factor IX Gla domain guided by molecular modeling (67). These studies implicated G4, K5, L6, F9, V10, and Q11 within the Ω loop (i.e., residues G4–Q11) of the Gla domain as important for factor IXa binding and for the assembly of the factor X–activating complex (67) and are entirely consistent with both functional and structural information definitively implicating the Gla domain Ω loop in binding to phospholipid membranes (170–173). However, it was subsequently found that although rationally designed, conformationally constrained synthetic peptides comprising residues G4–Q11 of the factor IX Gla domain were effective in displacing factor IXa molecules from 50% and factor IX from 100% of their respective binding sites with $K_i$ values identical to the $K_d$ values (approximately 3 nM), these peptides were relatively ineffective ($K_i$ approximately 165 μM) in inhibiting platelet-receptor–mediated activation of factor X by factor IXa. It was concluded that residues G4-Q11 of the factor IX Gla domain mediate factor IX/IXa binding to their shared platelet receptor, whereas the additional binding sites for the enzyme, factor IXa, that are functionally important in platelet-mediated factor X activation interact with some other region of the factor IXa molecule (63). A series of recent investigations utilized chimeric factor IX molecules with the EGF-2 domain or portions of it that are replaced with corresponding sequences from factor X or factor VII, are site-directed mutagenesis, and are conformationally constrained synthetic peptides. These studies have strongly implicated two disulfide-constrained loop structures, comprising residues C88–C109 within the EGF-2 domain in the high-affinity ($K_d$ approximately 0.5 nM in the presence of factor VIIIa, $K_d$ approximately 2.5 nM in the absence of factor VIII) binding site of the enzyme, factor IXa, but not the zymogen, factor IX to approximately 250 sites per platelet (65,72,73,155,174). When either the Ω loop (residues G4–Q11) within the Gla domain, or residues C88–C109 within the EGF-2 domain in factor IXa are mutated or replaced with residues from factor VII or factor X, deficient (i.e., low-affinity) binding to a reduced number (i.e., approximately 250 per platelet) of platelet sites is observed. In contrast, when both these domains are replaced or mutated, factor IXa fails entirely to bind to platelets or to promote factor X activation on the platelet surface. It can be concluded that the Ω loop (residues G4–Q11) within the Gla domain comprises the shared factor IXa platelet-binding site upon which factor IX is activated by factor XIa that provides a source of factor IXa. Factor IX then binds to the activated platelet membrane through the EGF-2 domain (residues C88–C109) for efficient assembly of the factor X–activating complex (65,72,73,155,174).

## Factor VIIIa Binding to Activated Platelets

Human factor VIII is a trace coagulation cofactor ($M_r$ approximately 280,000), bound in plasma to von Willebrand factor, with a domain structure consisting of A1-A2-B-A3-C1-C2. Factor VIII is cleaved by thrombin or factor Xa to generate a heterotrimeric active cofactor that participates nonenzymatically in the activation of factor X by factor IXa in the presence of activated platelets or phospholipids and calcium ions (152,175–187). Initially, it was shown by Nesheim et al. (188) that the pro-cofactor (factor VIII) interacts specifically with approximately 450 saturable, high-affinity ($K_d$ approximately 3.0 nM) sites per thrombin-activated platelet. These observations were subsequently confirmed and extended by the observation that the active cofactor (factor VIIIa) binds to an additional 300 to 500 sites per platelet with enhanced affinity ($K_d$ approximately 1.7 nM) and that in the presence of active-site–inhibited factor IXa and factor X, factor VIIIa binds to a total of approximately 1,200 sites per platelet with a $K_d$ of approximately 0.8 nM (74). Moreover, von Willebrand factor inhibits factor VIII binding but not factor VIIIa binding. Low concentrations of thrombin and the thrombin receptor activation peptide (SFLLRN) are potent agonists for factor VIIIa binding site expression, whereas ADP is inert. Further, factor Va does not compete with factor VIIIa for platelet binding, and annexin V is a potent inhibitor of factor VIIIa binding to activated platelets (74). Binding of factor VIIIa to thrombin-activated platelets is closely coupled to rates of factor X activation by factor IXa (74), it is mediated by the C2 domain of factor VIII (189–192), and it is facilitated by the presence of the A2 (and A1) domains (74). The importance of factor VIIIa binding to activated platelets and that of the assembly of the factor X–activating complex in maintaining normal hemostasis is underscored by the severe hemorrhagic diathesis observed in a patient with a platelet defect associated with impaired binding of both factor VIIIa and factor Va and with a deficiency in cell-surface exposure of phosphatidylserine (66,82,193).

## Factor X Binding to Activated Platelets

Factor X is a vitamin K–dependent plasma glycoprotein ($M_r$ approximately 59,000) containing an $N$-terminal light chain ($M_r$ approximately 16,000) and consisting of a Gla domain, followed by two EGF domains, and a typical trypsinlike serine protease catalytic domain ($M_r$ approximately 42,000) that is activated by either factor VIIa or factor IXa in a phospholipid-dependent reaction that requires the presence of calcium ions (33,151,157,159,194,195). Equilibrium binding studies have demonstrated the presence of a shared factor X per prothrombin binding site (approximately 16,000 sites per platelet; $K_d$ approximately 320 nM) on human platelets activated with either low concentrations of thrombin or the thrombin (or PAR-1) activation peptide (SFLLRN) but not with ADP (76,77). Detailed kinetic studies of factor IXa–catalyzed factor X activation in the presence of activated platelets demonstrate that factor X bound to the activated platelet surface is preferentially activated by platelet-bound factor IXa (77). Furthermore, the binding of factor VIIIa to the surface of activated platelets results in the generation of a lower capacity (approximately 1,000 sites per platelet), high-affinity ($K_d$ approximately 5 nM), specific factor X binding site that does not recognize prothrombin, occupancy of which is closely coupled to rates of factor X activation (74,75). Little is known about the molecular domains within factor X that mediate its interaction with the high-affinity, factor VIIIa–dependent binding site, but the binding of factor X and prothrombin to the low-affinity, high-capacity binding site (approximately 16,000 sites per platelet; $K_d$ approximately 320 nM) is mediated by the Gla domain presumably interacting with aminophospholipids on human platelets (76).

## Coordinate Binding of a Three-Receptor Complex

The hypothesis that emerges from the studies summarized in the preceding text requires that three classes of receptors be exposed on the surface membranes of activated platelets, including those that specifically bind factor IX/IXa$\beta$, factor VIII/VIIIa, and factor X. This hypothesis has recently been confirmed and extended by coordinate binding and kinetic factor Xa–generation studies (60,75) from which it can be concluded that the enzyme, factor IXa, generated from activation by factor XIa of platelet-bound factor IX binds to a specific, high-affinity (approximately 250 sites per platelet; $K_d$ approximately 0.5 nM) site on thrombin-activated platelets. The substrate, factor X, initially binds to a high-capacity, low-affinity (approximately 16,000 sites per platelet; $K_d$ approximately 320 nM) site on activated platelets that is shared with prothrombin, and the active cofactor, factor VIIIa, binds to a specific site (approximately 1,000 sites per platelet; $K_d$ approximately 0.8 nM) that binds factor X with high affinity and specificity (approximately 1,000 sites per platelet; $K_d$ approximately 5 nM) and presents it to the enzyme in a complex with an enzyme:cofactor:substrate stoichiometry of 1:4:4 for catalytic efficiency ($k_{cat}$ per $K_m$) that is greater than $10^8$-fold increased compared with solution-phase catalysis.

## Exposure of Platelet Receptors for Factor X Activation

Neither unactivated platelets nor platelets activated with supraphysiologic concentrations (i.e., 100 $\mu$M) of ADP bind to the components of the factor X–activating complex or promote rates of factor X activation, whereas low concentrations of thrombin, collagen, or the PAR-1 peptide, SFLLRN result in optimal rate enhancements and optimal binding of the components of the factor X–activating complex (3,21, 61,62,70,74,76,91,196). In contrast, the assembly of the prothrombin-activating complex requires concentrations of strong agonists (e.g., thrombin and collagen in combination) that are sufficiently high to result in maximal exposure of platelet membrane aminophospholipids (3,74,91,148,196–201). However, it seems reasonable to conclude that the exposure of negatively charged phospholipids on the external leaflet of the platelet plasma membrane is at least one prerequisite for platelet-mediated factor X activation because phospholipid vesicles containing phosphatidylserine promote factor X activation with kinetics similar to those obtained with activated platelets (70,150,153,169). Moreover, the calcium-dependent aminophospholipid-binding protein annexin V inhibits the binding of the components of the factor X–activating complex to the platelets, activation of factor X (74,76,153), and assembly of the prothrombinase complex (197–200,202–204). Similarly, in Scott syndrome, platelets with a genetic defect in aminophospholipid exposure following platelet activation manifest defective factor VIIIa binding, factor X activation, factor Va binding, and prothrombin activation (66,82,193). Nonetheless, it also seems reasonable to postulate that platelet proteins, in addition to aminophospholipids, exposed on the surface of activated platelets may play a role in the assembly of the factor X–activating complex because the affinity of factor IXa for activated platelets is approximately 30-fold higher than that for phospholipid vesicles because annexin V displays different inhibition kinetics on activated platelets and on phospholipid vesicles and because the kinetics of factor X activation in the presence of phospholipid vesicles is much more sensitive to variations in salt concentration than are the kinetics of factor X activation in the presence of activated platelets (153,154).

## Interactions of Activated Platelets with Factor Xa, Factor Va, and Prothrombin

A large body of early work beginning in 1964 (205) demonstrated that negatively charged aminophospholipids can provide a surface for assembly of the prothrombinase complex on which the vitamin K–dependent, Gla-containing enzyme (factor Xa) and substrate (prothrombin) can bind in a calcium-dependent manner and the cofactor (factor Va) can bind hydrophobically in a calcium-independent manner to phospholipid vesicles to accelerate the activation of prothrombin by approximately 300,000-fold compared with factor Xa–mediated prothrombin activation in solution (206–228). An extensive and elegant series of investigations has focused on the biochemical mechanisms of prothrombin activation in phospholipid model systems, supporting the view that aminophospholipids, exposed on the outer leaflet of activated platelets, participate in the assembly of the prothrombin-activating complex (198,229–237). These studies are reviewed in detail in Chapter 10 and elsewhere (151,152).

This chapter focuses on the mechanisms by which platelets promote prothrombin activation, which has been investigated utilizing enzyme kinetic measurements and equilibrium binding studies of the interaction of factor V, factor Va, and factor

Xa with both human (79–83,90,238) and bovine (78,85, 87–89) systems. It was initially shown that thrombin-activated human (80,81) and bovine (78) platelets bind factor Xa (approximately 250 binding sites per platelet; $K_d$ approximately 30 pM), and that platelet activation was required for this specific, high-affinity interaction, which was required to promote accelerated rates of prothrombin activation. Subsequent studies demonstrating reduced factor Xa binding to platelets from patients deficient in factor V (83), platelets studied in the presence of factor V alloantibodies (81), or platelets treated with activated protein C (239,240), which is a potent proteolytic inactivator of factor Va, were interpreted as providing evidence that factor Va is the receptor for factor Xa.

Biologically important differences between the bovine and human systems make direct comparisons somewhat problematic, but useful, complementary information has been derived from the study of both systems. In the bovine system it has been shown that factor Va binds to approximately 800 high-affinity ($K_d$ approximately 0.1 nM) and approximately 4,000 lower-affinity ($K_d$ approximately 1 nM) sites per platelet, whereas the procofactor, factor V, binds to approximately 800 low-affinity ($K_d$ approximately 1 nM) sites (87). Factor Va can displace all bound factor V, but factor V displaces only factor Va bound to low-affinity sites. The facts that platelet activation is not required for factor V/Va binding and that factor V is present in bovine plasma at a concentration of approximately $10^{-7}$ M means that factor V is always bound to the platelet surface (87). Coordinate binding studies in the bovine system have shown that approximately 2,500 factor Va–factor Xa complexes are platelet bound, of which only approximately 900 ($K_d$ approximately 0.2 nM) are functionally active in thrombin generation (85). These studies support the notion that in the bovine system, factor Va forms the receptor for factor Xa on the unactivated platelet surface and that a calcium-dependent, 1:1 stoichiometric factor Va–factor Xa complex ($K_d$ approximately 0.1 nM) comprises a high-affinity prothrombin-activating complex (85,87).

Coordinate factor Xa–factor Va binding studies have not been carried out in the human system in part because human platelet α-granules contain a large pool of factor V (i.e., 4,000 to 14,000 molecules per platelet) that is secreted upon platelet activation (241), thereby complicating the measurement of factor Va binding (which does not appear to require platelet activation), that is stimulated by the presence of factor Xa and prothrombin, and that is nonsaturable with as many as approximately 3,000 binding sites per platelet (79,238), in contrast to the approximately 250 sites per platelet that comprise the functional factor Xa binding sites important for prothrombin activation (80,81). However, analyses of kinetic measurements of prothrombin activation have been used to determine that a 1:1 stoichiometric complex of factor Va and factor Xa is colocalized on approximately 3,000 functional sites per platelet on thrombin-activated platelets with an apparent $K_d$ of approximately 0.1 nM and a $k_{cat}$ (i.e., number of moles of thrombin formed per mole of factor Xa bound) of approximately 30 per second (84,86). Nonetheless, the binding of factor Va to platelets, activated with concentrations of thrombin (0.05 to 1.0 nM) that are sufficient to effect maximal factor Va secretion from and binding to platelets, appears to be insufficient to support factor Xa binding (90). It was demonstrated that 50 nM thrombin is necessary to effect maximal factor Xa binding (approximately 6,000 sites per platelet), which depends both on the bound factor Va and on the expression of an additional binding site postulated to be mediated by effector cell protease receptor-1 (ECPR-1) (90), an integral membrane protein expressed by leukocytes (242), by pericytes derived from human brain microvessels (243), and by endothelial cells (244) that bind factor Xa in the absence of factor Va. Although this hypothesis is controversial (245), ECPR-1 has been identified in platelets and megakaryocytes in a platelet-activation–dependent form capable of binding factor Xa, and monoclonal antibodies specific for ECPR-1 have been reported to inhibit prothrombin activation by factor Va-Xa on activated platelets (90), giving rise to the suggestion that both ECPR-1 and membrane-bound factor Va are required for factor Xa binding and prothrombin-activating complex assembly on the activated platelet surface (90).

In addition to the postulated role of platelet proteins, such as ECPR-1 in the assembly of the prothrombin-activating complex, the exposure of anionic phospholipids (e.g., phosphatidylserine) in the outer leaflet of the activated platelet membrane has been correlated with the expression of prothrombinase complex formation, which (like the factor X–activating complex) is inhibited by the phospholipid-binding protein, annexin V (197–200,202–204). Because high concentrations of thrombin (>20 nM) or other "strong agonists" (e.g., the calcium ionophore A23187, mixtures of collagen and thrombin, or the complement protein lytic complex, C5b-9) are required to generate maximal factor Xa binding, functional prothrombinase complex assembly and aminophospholipid exposure, as well as platelet microparticle shedding, it has been suggested that the physiologic site for prothrombin-activation complex formation may consist of aminophospholipids exposed either on the outer leaflet of the platelet membrane or on platelet microparticles (80,204,246–250).

The facts that human platelet α-granules store and secrete a form of factor V that comprises 4,600 to 14,000 molecules per platelet, accounts for 20% to 25% of the total factor V in normal blood, and functions in the assembly of the prothrombinase complex are well established (241,251–259). Platelet factor V is stored in massive, disulfide-linked complexes with the α-granular protein, multimerin (253–256), and is secreted from platelets in a partially proteolyzed and activated form that can be further activated by factor Xa or thrombin to function in prothrombinase complex assembly (223,258,260–262). The origin of human platelet and megakaryocyte factor V (263–266) has not been definitively established. Two conflicting hypotheses have been advanced proposing either that platelet factor V is derived from plasma factor V that is endocytosed and packaged in α-granules by megakaryocytes and/or platelets (267–272) or that megakaryocytes synthesize factor V (263,264,273–275). The origin of platelet factor V notwithstanding, it appears to be a functionally distinct and physiologically unique protein because factor Xa activates platelet factor V 50- to 100-fold more effectively than thrombin (258), whereas the two proteases have equivalent activity in the activation of plasma factor V (276). In contrast to plasma factor V, the platelet protein is phosphorylated by a casein kinase II–like enzyme (277–279) and, when bound to platelet membranes, is much more resistant to inactivation by activated protein C (280,281). Furthermore, platelet factor V appears to play a preeminent role in hemostasis because patients with factor V$_{quebec}$, with severely deficient platelet factor V and near-normal levels of plasma factor V, have a severe bleeding diathesis (282–284), whereas no considerable bleeding was observed in a patient with normal platelet factor V but markedly reduced plasma factor V because of an anti–factor V autoantibody (261). The unique role of platelet factor V is emphasized by the substantially greater effectiveness of platelet transfusions over correction of plasma factor V in the management of hemorrhage associated with congenital factor V deficiency (285,286).

## CONCLUSIONS

The schematic diagram presented in Figure 38-1 summarizes a current view of the postulated sequence of biochemical events that comprise the normal hemostatic mechanism, emphasizing the intimate connections between the events of platelet activation, aggregation, and secretion on the one hand and blood coagulation on the other hand. The information summarized in this chapter demonstrates that the assembly of virtually all the coagulation enzyme–cofactor–substrate complexes that comprise the coagulation mechanism normally occur on the activated platelet surface (2). The platelet membrane comprises a surface for receptor-mediated catalytic complex assembly associated with major rate enhancements at each step in the reaction pathway (2,9,10). The activated platelet surface also provides a protective nidus, that is, the hemostatic thrombus, where binding of coagulation proteases protects them from inactivation by protease inhibitors, leading to the localization of coagulation reactions to the platelet surface, the prevention of disseminated intravascular coagulation, and the local explosive generation of thrombin at the site of vascular injury (2). Moreover, recent revisions in the theory of blood coagulation replace the view that the intrinsic and extrinsic mechanisms, initiated by contact activation and TF exposure, respectively, are separate and alternative pathways converging on the common pathway for factor X and prothrombin activation, with the revised hypothesis shown in Figure 38-1. Therefore, although blood coagulation can be triggered by exposure of the "contact factors" (factor XII, high-molecular-weight kininogen and prekallikrein) to negatively charged surfaces, the predominant mechanism for effecting normal hemostasis is initiated by TF exposure at sites of vascular injury resulting in the generation of minute quantities of thrombin, insufficient to convert fibrinogen to fibrin but sufficient to initiate the consolidation pathway by activating platelets, factor XI, factor VIII, and factor V, leading to factor IX activation, factor X activation, and prothrombin activation, with enormous amplification at each reaction step, to produce sufficient thrombin to form a consolidated platelet–fibrin thrombus.

# ACKNOWLEDGMENTS

Supported by research grants from the National Institute of Health (HL46213, HL64943, HL70683, and HL74124). We are grateful to Patricia Pileggi for assistance in chapter preparation.

## *References*

1. Walsh PN. Factor XI. In: Colman RW, Hirsh J, Marder VJ, et al., eds. *Hemostasis and thrombosis: basic principles and clinical practice*, 4th ed., Chap. 11. Philadelphia, PA: Lippincott Williams & Wilkins, 2001: 191–202.
2. Walsh PN. Platelet coagulant activities and hemostasis: a hypothesis. *Blood* 1974;43:597–605.
3. Tracy PB. Role of platelets and leukocytes in coagulation. In: Colman RW, Hirsh J, Marder VJ, et al., eds. *Hemostasis and thrombosis: basic principles and clinical practice*, 4th ed., Chap. 33. Philadelphia, PA: Lippincott Williams & Wilkins, 2001:575–596.
4. Ahmad SS, London FS, Walsh PN. The assembly of the factor X-activating complex on activated human platelets. *J Thromb Haemost* 2003;1: 48–59.
5. Bock SC. Antithrombin III and heparin cofactor II. In: Colman RW, Hirsh J, Marder VJ, et al., eds. *Hemostasis and thrombosis: basic principles and clinical practice*, 4th ed., Chap. 16 Philadelphia, PA: Lippincott Williams & Wilkins, 2001:321–365.
6. Esmon CT Protein C, protein S, and thrombomodulin. In: Colman RW, Hirsh J, Marder VJ, et al., eds. *Hemostasis and thrombosis: basic principles and clinical practice*, 4th ed., Chap. 17. Philadelphia, PA: Lippincott Williams & Wilkins, 2001:335–353.
7. Pizzo SV, Wu SM. Alpha-macroglobulins and kunins. In: Colman RW, Hirsh J, Marder VJ, et al., eds. *Hemostasis and thrombosis: basic principles and clinical practice*, 4th ed., Chap. 19. Philadelphia, PA: Lippincott Williams & Wilkins, 2001:367–379.
8. Walsh PN. Roles of factor XI, platelets and tissue factor-initiated blood coagulation. *J Thromb Haemost* 2003;1:2081–2086.
9. MacFarlane RG. An enzyme cascade in the blood clotting mechanism, and its function as a biochemical amplifier. *Nature* 1964;202:498–499.
10. Davie EW, Ratnoff OD. Waterfall sequence for intrinsic blood clotting. *Science* 1964;145:1310–1312.
11. Baglia FA, Walsh PN. Prothrombin is a cofactor for the binding of factor XI to the platelet surface and for platelet-mediated factor XI activation by thrombin. *Biochemistry* 1998;37:2271–2281.
12. Baglia FA, Walsh PN. Thrombin-mediated feedback activation of factor XI on the activated human platelet surface is preferred over contact activation by factor XIIa or factor XIa. *J Biol Chem* 2000;275:20514–20519.
13. Gailani D, Broze GJ Jr. Factor XI activation in a revised model of blood coagulation. *Science* 1991;253:909–912.
14. Morrissey JH. Tissue factor and factor VII initiation of coagulation. In: Colman RW, Hirsh J, Marder VJ, et al., eds. *Hemostasis and thrombosis: basic principles and clinical practice*, 4th ed., Chap. 5. Philadelphia, PA: Lippincott Williams & Wilkins, 2001:89–102
15. Naito K, Fujikawa K. Activation of human blood coagulation factor XI independent of factor XII. Factor XI is activated by thrombin and factor XIa in the presence of negatively charged surfaces. *J Biol Chem* 1991;266: 7353–7358.
16. Colman RW. Contact activation pathway: inflammatory, fibrinolytic, anticoagulant, antiadhesive and antiangiogenic activities. In: Colman RW, Hirsh J, Marder VJ, et al., eds. *Hemostasis and thrombosis: basic principles and clinical practice*, 4th ed., Chap. 6. Philadelphia, PA: Lippincott Williams & Wilkins, 2001:103–122.
17. Walsh PN. The effects of collagen and kaolin on the intrinsic coagulant activity of platelets. Evidence for an alternative pathway in intrinsic coagulation not requiring factor XII. *Br J Haematol* 1972;22:393–405.
18. Walsh PN. Albumin density gradient separation and washing of platelets and the study of platelet coagulant activities. *Br J Haematol* 1972;22:205–217.
19. Walsh PN. The role of platelets in the contact phase of blood coagulation. *Br J Haematol* 1972;22:237–254.
20. Walsh PN. The effect of dilution of plasma on coagulation. The significance of the dilution-activation phenomenon for the study of platelet coagulant activities. *Br J Haematol* 1972;22:219–236.
21. Walsh PN, Biggs R. The role of platelets in intrinsic factor-Xa formation. *Br J Haematol* 1972;22:743–760.
22. Kaufman RJ, Antonarakis SE, Fay PJ. Factor VIII and Hemophilia A. In: Colman RW, Hirsh J, Marder VJ, et al., eds. *Hemostasis and thrombosis: basic principles and clinical practice*, 4th ed., Chap. 8. Philadelphia, PA: Lippincott Williams & Wilkins, 2001:135–156.
23. Thompson AR. Molecular biology of factor IX. In: Colman RW, Hirsh J, Marder VJ, et al., eds. *Hemostasis and thrombosis: basic principles and clinical practice*, 4th ed., Chap. 7. Philadelphia, PA: Lippincott Williams & Wilkins, 2001:123–134.
24. Asakai R, Chung DW, Davie EW, et al. Factor XI deficiency in Ashkenazi Jews in Israel. *N Engl J Med* 1991;325:153–158.
25. Bolton-Maggs PH, Young Wan-Yin B, McCraw AH, et al. Inheritance and bleeding in factor XI deficiency. *Br J Haematol* 1988;69:521–528.
26. Hu CJ, Baglia FA, Mills DC, et al. Tissue-specific expression of functional platelet factor XI is independent of plasma factor XI expression. *Blood* 1998;91:3800–3807.
27. Leiba H, Ramot B, Many A. Hereditary and coagulation studies in ten families with factor XI (plasma thromboplastin antecedent) deficiency. *Br J Haematol* 1965;11:654–665.
28. Ragni MV, Sinha D, Seaman F, et al. Comparison of bleeding tendency, factor XI coagulant activity, and factor XI antigen in 25 factor XI-deficient kindreds. *Blood* 1985;65:719–724.
29. Rapaport SI, Proctor RR, Patch MJ, et al. The mode of inheritance of PTA deficiency: evidence for the existence of a major PTA deficiency and a minor PTA deficiency. *Blood* 1961;18:149–155.
30. Rosenthal RL, Dreskin OH, Rosenthal N. New hemophilia-like disease caused by deficiency of a third plasma thromboplastin factor. *Proc Soc Exp Biol Med* 1953;82:171–174.
31. Sidi A, Seligsohn U, Jonas P, et al. Factor XI deficiency: detection and management during urologic surgery. *J Urol* 1978;119:528–530.
32. Anson DS, Choo KH, Rees DJ, et al. The gene structure of human antihaemophilic factor IX. *EMBO J* 1984;3:1053–1060.
33. Di Scipio RG, Kurachi K, Davie EW. Activation of human factor IX (Christmas factor). *J Clin Invest* 1978;61:1528–1538.
34. Fujikawa K, Legaz ME, Kato H, et al. The mechanism of activation of bovine factor IX (Christmas factor) by bovine factor XIa (activated plasma thromboplastin antecedent). *Biochemistry* 1974;13:4508–4516.
35. Jagadeeswaran P, Lavelle DE, Kaul R, et al. Isolation and characterization of human factor IX cDNA: identification of Taq I polymorphism and regional assignment. *Somat Cell Mol Genet* 1984;10:465–473.
36. Jaye M, de la Salle H, Schamber F, et al. Isolation of a human antihaemophilic factor IX cDNA clone using a unique 52-base synthetic oligonucleotide probe deduced from the amino acid sequence of bovine factor IX. *Nucleic Acids Res* 1983;11:2325–2335.
37. Kurachi K, Davie EW. Isolation and characterization of a cDNA coding for human factor IX. *Proc Natl Acad Sci U S A* 1982;79:6461–6464.
38. Osterud B, Bouma BN, Griffin JH. Human blood coagulation factor IX. Purification, properties, and mechanism of activation by activated factor XI. *J Biol Chem* 1978;253:5946–5951.
39. Sinha D, Seaman FS, Walsh PN. Role of calcium ions and the heavy chain of factor XIa in the activation of human coagulation factor IX. *Biochemistry* 1987;26:3768–3775.

40. Yoshitake S, Schach BG, Foster DC, et al. Nucleotide sequence of the gene for human factor IX (antihemophilic factor B). *Biochemistry* 1985;24: 3736–3750.

41. Osterud B, Rapaport SI. Activation of factor IX by the reaction product of tissue factor and factor VII: additional pathway for initiating blood coagulation. *Proc Natl Acad Sci U S A* 1977;74:5260–5264.

42. Baglia FA, Badellino KO, Li CQ, et al. Factor XI binding to the platelet glycoprotein Ib-IX-V complex promotes factor XI activation by thrombin. *J Biol Chem* 2002;277:1662–1668.

43. Baglia FA, Shrimpton CN, Lopez JA, et al. The glycoprotein Ib-IX-V complex mediates localization of factor XI to lipid rafts on the platelet membrane. *J Biol Chem* 2003;278:21744–21750.

44. Broze GJJ, Miletich JP. Isolation of the tissue factor inhibitor produced by HepG2 hepatoma cells. *Proc Natl Acad Sci U S A* 1987;84:1886–1890.

45. Broze GJJ, Miletich JP. Characterization of the inhibition of tissue factor in serum. *Blood* 1987;69:150–155.

46. Hubbard AR, Jennings CA. Inhibition of tissue thromboplastin-mediated blood coagulation. *Thromb Res* 1986;42:489–498.

47. Hubbard AR, Jennings CA. Inhibition of the tissue factor-factor VII complex: involvement of factor Xa and lipoproteins. *Thromb Res* 1987;46: 527–537.

48. Morrison SA, Jesty J. Tissue factor-dependent activation of tritium labeled factor IX and factor X in human plasma. *Blood* 1984;63:1338–1347.

49. Rao LVM, Rapaport SI. Studies on the mechanisms of inactivation of the extrinsic pathway of coagulation. *Blood* 1987;69:645–651.

50. Sanders NL, Bajaj SP, Zivelin A, et al. Inhibition of tissue factor/factor VIIa activity in plasma requires factor X and an additional plasma component. *Blood* 1985;66:204–212.

51. Baglia FA, Jameson BA, Walsh PN. Identification and characterization of a binding site for platelets in the Apple 3 domain of coagulation factor XI. *J Biol Chem* 1995;270:6734–6740.

52. Greengard JS, Heeb MJ, Ersdal E, et al. Binding of coagulation factor XI to washed human platelets. *Biochemistry* 1986;25:3884–3890.

53. Ho DH, Baglia FA, Walsh PN. Factor XI binding to activated platelets is mediated by residues R(250), K(255), F(260), and Q(263) within the Apple 3 domain. *Biochemistry* 2000;39:316–323.

54. Baglia FA, Seaman FS, Walsh PN. The Apple 1 and Apple 4 domains of factor XI act synergistically to promote the surface-mediated activation of factor XI by factor XIIa. *Blood* 1995;85:2078–2083.

55. Ho DH, Badellino K, Baglia FA, et al. The role of high molecular weight kininogen and prothrombin as cofactors in the binding of factor XI A3 domain to the platelet surface. *J Biol Chem* 2000;275:25139–25145.

56. Sun MF, Baglia FA, Ho D, et al. Defective binding of factor XI-N248 to activated human platelets. *Blood* 2001;98:125–129.

57. Baird TR, Walsh PN. The interaction of factor XIa with activated platelets but not endothelial cells promotes the activation of factor IX in the consolidation phase of blood coagulation. *J Biol Chem* 2002;277:38462–38467.

58. Gailani D, Ho D, Sun MF, et al. Model for a factor IX activation complex on blood platelets: dimeric conformation of factor XIa is essential. *Blood* 2001;97:3117–3122.

59. Sinha D, Seaman FS, Koshy A, et al. Blood coagulation factor XIa binds specifically to a site on activated human platelets distinct from that for factor XI. *J Clin Invest* 1984;73:1550–1556.

60. Ahmad SS, London FS, Walsh PN. Binding studies of the enzyme (factor IXa) with the cofactor (factor VIII) in the assembly of factor-X activating complex on the activated platelet surface. *J Thromb Haemost* 2003;1: 2348–2355.

61. Ahmad SS, Rawala-Sheikh R, Walsh PN. Comparative interactions of factor IX and factor IXa with human platelets. *J Biol Chem* 1989;264:3244–3251.

62. Ahmad SS, Rawala-Sheikh R, Walsh PN. Platelet receptor occupancy with factor IXa promotes factor X activation. *J Biol Chem* 1989;264: 20012–20016.

63. Ahmad SS, Wong MY, Rawala R, et al. Coagulation factor IX residues G4-Q11 mediate its interaction with a shared factor IX/IXa binding site on activated platelets but not the assembly of the functional factor X activating complex. *Biochemistry* 1998;37:1671–1679.

64. London FS, Walsh PN. Zymogen factor IX potentiates factor IXa-catalyzed factor X activation. *Biochemistry* 2000;39:9850–9858.

65. Ahmad SS, Rawala R, Cheung WF, et al. The role of the second growth-factor domain of human factor IXa in binding to platelets and in factor-X activation. *Biochem J* 1995;310:427–431.

66. Ahmad SS, Rawala-Sheikh R, Ashby B, et al. Platelet receptor-mediated factor X activation by factor IXa. High-affinity factor IXa receptors induced by factor VIII are deficient on platelets in Scott syndrome. *J Clin Invest* 1989;84:824–828.

67. Ahmad SS, Rawala-Sheikh R, Cheung WF, et al. High-affinity, specific factor IXa binding to platelets is mediated in part by residues 3-11. *Biochemistry* 1994;33:12048–12055.

68. Ahmad SS, Rawala-Sheikh R, Cheung WF, et al. The role of the first growth factor domain of human factor IXa in binding to platelets and in factor X activation. *J Biol Chem* 1992;267:8571–8576.

69. Ahmad SS, Rawala-Sheikh R, Monroe DM, et al. Comparative platelet binding and kinetic studies with normal and variant factor IXa molecules. *J Biol Chem* 1990;265:20907–20911.

70. Rawala-Sheikh R, Ahmad SS, Ashby B, et al. Kinetics of coagulation factor X activation by platelet-bound factor IXa. *Biochemistry* 1990;29:2606–2611.

71. Rawala-Sheikh R, Ahmad SS, Monroe DM, et al. Role of gammacarboxyglutamic acid residues in the binding of factor IXa to platelets and in factor-X activation. *Blood* 1992;79:398–405.

72. Wilkinson FH, Ahmad SS, Walsh PN. The factor IXa second epidermal growth factor (EGF2) domain mediates platelet binding and assembly of the factor X activating complex. *J Biol Chem* 2002;277:5734–5741.

73. Wilkinson FH, London FS, Walsh PN. Residues 88-109 of factor IXa are important for assembly of the factor-X activating complex. *J Biol Chem* 2002;277:5725–5733.

74. Ahmad SS, Scandura JM, Walsh PN. Structural and functional characterization of platelet receptor-mediated factor VIII binding. *J Biol Chem* 2000;275:13071–13081.

75. Ahmad SS, Walsh PN. Coordinate binding studies of the substrate (factor X) with the cofactor (factor VIII) in the assembly of the factor X activating complex on the activated platelet surface. *Biochemistry* 2002;41: 11269–11276.

76. Scandura JM, Ahmad SS, Walsh PN. A binding site expressed on the surface of activated human platelets is shared by factor X and prothrombin. *Biochemistry* 1996;35:8890–8902.

77. Scandura JM, Walsh PN. Factor X bound to the surface of activated human platelets is preferentially activated by platelet-bound factor IXa. *Biochemistry* 1996;35:8903–8913.

78. Dahlback B, Stenflo J. Binding of bovine coagulation factor Xa to platelets. *Biochemistry* 1978;17:4938–4945.

79. Kane WH, Majerus PW. The interaction of human coagulation factor Va with platelets. *J Biol Chem* 1982;257:3963–3969.

80. Miletich JP, Jackson CM, Majerus PW. Interaction of coagulation factor Xa with human platelets. *Proc Natl Acad Sci U S A* 1977;74:4033–4036.

81. Miletich JP, Jackson CM, Majerus PW. Properties of the factor Xa binding site on human platelets. *J Biol Chem* 1978;253:6908–6916.

82. Miletich JP, Kane WH, Hofmann SL, et al. Deficiency of factor Xa factor Va binding sites on the platelets of a patient with a bleeding disorder. *Blood* 1979;54:1015–1022.

83. Miletich JP, Majerus DW, Majerus PW. Patients with congenital factor V deficiency have decreased factor Xa binding sites on their platelets. *J Clin Invest* 1978;62:824–831.

84. Tracy PB, Eide LL, Mann KG. Human prothrombinase complex assembly and function on isolated peripheral blood cell populations. *J Biol Chem* 1985;260:2119–2124.

85. Tracy PB, Nesheim ME, Mann KG. Coordinate binding of factor Va and factor Xa to the unstimulated platelet. *J Biol Chem* 1981;256:743–751.

86. Tracy PB, Nesheim ME, Mann KG. Platelet factor Xa receptor. *Methods Enzymol* 1992;215:329–360.

87. Tracy PB, Peterson JM, Nesheim ME, et al. Interaction of coagulation factor V and factor Va with platelets. *J Biol Chem* 1979;254:10354–10361.

88. Tracy PB, Mann KG. Prothrombinase complex assembly on the platelet surface is mediated through the 74,000-dalton component of factor Va. *Proc Natl Acad Sci U S A* 1983;80:2380–2384.

89. Tracy PB, Nesheim ME, Mann KG. Proteolytic alterations of factor Va bound to platelets. *J Biol Chem* 1983;258:662–669.

90. Bouchard BA, Catcher CS, Thrash BR, et al. Effector cell protease receptor1, a platelet activation-dependent membrane protein, regulates prothrombinase-catalyzed thrombin generation. *J Biol Chem* 1997;272: 9244–9251.

91. Walsh PN, Colman RW, Hirsh J, et al. Platelet-coagulant protein interactions. In: Colman RW, Hirsh J, Marder VJ, et al., eds. *Hemostasis and thrombosis: basic principles and clinical practice*, 3rd ed. Chap. 30. Philadelphia, PA: JB Lippincott Co, 1994: 629–651.

92. Walsh PN, Griffin JH. Contributions of human platelets to the proteolytic activation of blood coagulation factors XII and XI. *Blood* 1981;57: 106–118.

93. Berman CL, Yeo EL, Wencel-Drake JD, et al. A platelet alpha granule membrane protein that is associated with the plasma membrane after activation. Characterization and subcellular localization of platelet activation-dependent granule-external membrane protein. *J Clin Invest* 1986; 78:130–137.

94. Walsh PN. Platelet coagulation-protein interactions. *Semin Thromb Hemost* 2004;30:461–471.

95. Conde I, Shrimpton CN, Thiagarajan P, et al. Tissue factor-bearing microparticles arise from monocyte lipid rafts and can fuse with activated platelets, consolidating all of the membrane-bound coagulation reactions on the platelet surface. *J Thromb Haemost* 2003;1:OC146.

96. Falati S, Gross P, Merrill-Skoloff G, et al. Real-time *in vivo* imaging of platelets, tissue factor and fibrin during arterial thrombus formation in the mouse. *Nat Med* 2002;8:1175–1181.

97. Giesen PL, Rauch U, Bohrmann B, et al. Blood-borne tissue factor: another view of thrombosis. *Proc Natl Acad Sci U S A* 1999;96:2311–2315.

98. Himber J, Kling D, Fallon JT, et al. *In situ* localization of tissue factor in human thrombi. *Blood* 2002;99:4249–4250.

99. Morrissey JH. Tissue factor: in at the start … and the finish? *J Thromb Haemost* 2003;1:878–880.

100. Rauch U, Bonderman D, Bohrmann B, et al. Transfer of tissue factor from leukocytes to platelets is mediated by CD15 and tissue factor. *Blood* 2000;96:170–175.

101. Rauch U, Nemerson Y. Tissue factor, the blood, and the arterial wall. *Trends Cardiovasc Med* 2000;10:139–143.

102. Kondo S, Kisiel W. Regulation of factor VIIa activity in plasma: evidence that antithrombin III is the sole plasma protease inhibitor of human factor VIIa. *Thromb Res* 1987;46:325–335.

103. Seligsohn U, Kasper CK, Osterud B, et al. Activated factor VII: presence in factor IX concentrates and persistence in the circulation after infusion. *Blood* 1979;53:828–837.

104. Walsh PN. Roles of platelets and factor XI in the initiation of blood coagulation by thrombin. *Thromb Haemost* 2001;86:75–82.

105. Bouma BN, Griffin JH. Human blood coagulation factor XI. Purification, properties, and mechanism of activation by activated factor XII. *J Biol Chem* 1977;252:6432–6437.

106. Griffin JH, Cochrane CG. Mechanisms for the involvement of high molecular weight kininogen in surface-dependent reactions of Hageman factor. *Proc Natl Acad Sci U S A* 1976;73:2554–2558.

107. Liu CY, Scott CF, Bagdasarian A, et al. Potentiation of the function of Hageman factor fragments by high molecular weight kininogen. *J Clin Invest* 1977;60:7–17.

108. Meier HL, Pierce JV, Colman RW, et al. Activation and function of human Hageman factor. The role of high molecular weight kininogen and prekallikrein. *J Clin Invest* 1977;60:18–31.

109. Ratnoff OD, Davie EW, Mallett DL. Studies on the action of Hageman factor: evidence that activated Hageman factor in turn activates plasma thromboplastin antecedent. *J Clin Invest* 1961;40:803–819.

110. Saito H, Ratnoff OD, Marshall JS, et al. Partial purification of plasma thromboplastin antecedent (factor XI) and its activation by trypsin. *J Clin Invest* 1973;52:850–861.

111. Schiffman S, Lee P. Preparation, characterization, and activation of a highly purified factor XI: evidence that a hitherto unrecognized plasma activity participates in the interaction of factors XI and XII. *Br J Haematol* 1974;27:101–114.

112. Schiffman S, Markland FS Jr. Effect of intermediates of extrinsic clotting on purified factor XI: factor VII and/or thromboplastin. *Thromb Res* 1975;6:273–279.

113. Thompson RE, Mandle R Jr, Kaplan AP. Association of factor XI and high molecular weight kininogen in human plasma. *J Clin Invest* 1977;60:1376–1380.

114. Wiggins RC, Bouma BN, Cochrane CG, et al. Role of high-molecular-weight kininogen in surface-binding and activation of coagulation factor XI and prekallikrein. *Proc Natl Acad Sci U S A* 1977;74:4636–4640.

115. Heck LW, Kaplan AP. Substrates of Hageman factor. I. Isolation and characterization of human factor XI (PTA) and inhibition of the activated enzyme by alpha 1-antitrypsin. *J Exp Med* 1974;140:1615–1630.

116. Kurachi K, Davie EW. Activation of human factor XI (plasma thromboplastin antecedent) by factor XIIa (activated Hageman factor). *Biochemistry* 1977;16:5831–5839.

117. Movat HZ, Ozge-Anwar AH. The contact phase of blood coagulation: clotting factors XI and XII, their isolation and interaction. *J Lab Clin Med* 1974;84:861–878.

118. Saito H, Goldsmith GH Jr. Plasma thromboplastin antecedent (PTA, factor XI): a specific and sensitive radioimmunoassay. *Blood* 1977;50:377–385.

119. Asakai R, Davie EW, Chung DW. Organization of the gene for human factor XI. *Biochemistry* 1987;26:7221–7228.

120. Fujikawa K, Chung DW, Hendrickson LE, et al. Amino acid sequence of human factor XI, a blood coagulation factor with four tandem repeats that are highly homologous with plasma prekallikrein. *Biochemistry* 1986;25:2417–2424.

121. Kato A, Asakai R, Davie EW, et al. Factor XI gene (F11) is located on the distal end of the long arm of human chromosome 4. *Cytogenet Cell Genet* 1989;52:77–78.

122. McMullen BA, Fujikawa K, Davie EW. Location of the disulfide bonds in human coagulation factor XI: the presence of tandem Apple domains. *Biochemistry* 1991;30:2056–2060.

123. Baglia FA, Walsh PN. A binding site for thrombin in the Apple 1 domain of factor XI. *J Biol Chem* 1996;271:3652–3658.

124. Baglia FA, Jameson BA, Walsh PN. Localization of the high molecular weight kininogen binding site in the heavy chain of human factor XI to amino acids phenylalanine 56 through serine 86. *J Biol Chem* 1990;265:4149–4154.

125. Baglia FA, Jameson BA, Walsh PN. Fine mapping of the high molecular weight kininogen binding site on blood coagulation factor XI through the use of rationally designed synthetic analogs. *J Biol Chem* 1992;267:4247–4252.

126. Seaman FS, Baglia FA, Gurr JA, et al. Binding of high-molecular-mass kininogen to the Apple 1 domain of factor XI is mediated in part by Val64 and Ile77. *Biochem J* 1994;304:715–721.

127. Baglia FA, Badellino KO, Ho DH, et al. A binding site for the Kringle II domain of prothrombin in the Apple 1 domain of factor XI. *J Biol Chem* 2000;275:31954–31962.

128. Baglia FA, Jameson BA, Walsh PN. Identification and chemical synthesis of a substrate-binding site for factor IX on coagulation factor XIa. *J Biol Chem* 1991;266:24190–24197.

129. Sinha D, Koshy A, Seaman FS, et al. Functional characterization of human blood coagulation factor XIa using hybridoma antibodies. *J Biol Chem* 1985;260:10714–10719.

130. Sun Y, Gailani D. Identification of a factor IX binding site on the third Apple domain of activated factor XI. *J Biol Chem* 1996;271:29023–29028.

131. Sun MF, Zhao M, Gailani D. Identification of amino acids in the factor XI Apple 3 domain required for activation of factor IX. *J Biol Chem* 1999;274:36373–36378.

132. Ho DH, Badellino K, Baglia FA, et al. A binding site for heparin in the Apple 3 domain of factor XI. *J Biol Chem* 1998;273:16382–16390.

133. Baglia FA, Jameson BA, Walsh PN. Identification and characterization of a binding site for factor XIIa in the Apple 4 domain of coagulation factor XI. *J Biol Chem* 1993;268:3838–3844.

134. Meijers JC, Davie EW, Chung DW. Expression of human blood coagulation factor XI: characterization of the defect in factor XI type III deficiency. *Blood* 1992;79:1435–1440.

135. Meijers JC, Mulvihill ER, Davie EW, et al. Apple four in human blood coagulation factor XI mediates dimer formation. *Biochemistry* 1992;31:4680–4684.

136. Dorfman R, Walsh PN. Noncovalent interactions of the Apple 4 domain that mediate coagulation factor XI homodimerization. *J Biol Chem* 2001;276:6429–6438.

137. Baird TR, Walsh PN. Activated platelets but not endothelial cells participate in the initiation of the consolidation phase of blood coagulation. *J Biol Chem* 2002;277:28498–28503.

138. Walsh PN, Sinha D, Koshy A, et al. Functional characterization of platelet-bound factor XIa: retention of factor XIa activity on the platelet surface. *Blood* 1986;68:225–230.

139. Walsh PN, Sinha D, Kueppers F, et al. Regulation of factor XIa activity by platelets and alpha 1-protease inhibitor. *J Clin Invest* 1987;80:1578–1586.

140. Bush AI, Martins RN, Rumble B, et al. The amyloid precursor protein of Alzheimer's disease is released by human platelets. *J Biol Chem*. 1990;265:15977–15983

141. Scandura JM, Zhang Y, Van Nostrand WE, et al. Progress curve analysis of the kinetics with which blood coagulation factor XIa is inhibited by protease nexin-2. *Biochemistry* 1997;36:412–420.

142. Smith RP, Higuchi DA, Broze GJ Jr. Platelet coagulation factor XIa-inhibitor, a form of Alzheimer amyloid precursor protein. *Science* 1990;248:1126–1128.

143. Van Nostrand WE, Schmaier AH, Farrow JS, et al. Protease nexin-II (amyloid beta-protein precursor): a platelet alpha-granule protein. *Science* 1990;248:745–748.

144. Zhang Y, Scandura JM, Van Nostrand WE, et al. The mechanism by which heparin promotes the inhibition of coagulation factor XIa by protease nexin-2. *J Biol Chem* 1997;272:26139–26144.

145. Baird TR, Walsh PN. Factor XI, but not prekallikrein, blocks high molecular weight kininogen binding to human umbilical vein endothelial cells. *J Biol Chem* 2003;278:20618–20623.

146. Hultin MB. Role of human factor VIII in factor X activation. *J Clin Invest* 1982;69:950–958.

147. Neuenschwander P, Jesty J. A comparison of phospholipid and platelets in the activation of human factor VIII by thrombin and factor Xa, and in the activation of factor X. *Blood* 1988;72:1761–1770.

148. Rosing J, van Rijn JL, Bevers EM, et al. The role of activated human platelets in prothrombin and factor X activation. *Blood* 1985;65:319–332.

149. van Rijn J, Rosing J, van Dieijen G. Activity of human blood platelets in prothrombin and in factor X activation induced by ionophore A23187. *Eur J Biochem* 1983;133:1–10.

150. Walsh PN, Camp E, Dende D. Different requirements for intrinsic factor-Xa forming activity and platelet factor 3 activity and their relationship to platelet aggregation and secretion. *Br J Haematol* 1978;40:311–331.

151. Mann KG, Jenny RJ, Krishnaswamy S. Cofactor proteins in the assembly and expression of blood clotting enzyme complexes. *Annu Rev Biochem* 1988;57:915–956.

152. Mann KG, Nesheim ME, Church WR, et al. Surface-dependent reactions of the vitamin K-dependent enzyme complexes. *Blood* 1990;76:1–16.

153. London F, Ahmad SS, Walsh PN. Annexin V inhibition of factor IXa-catalyzed factor X activation on human platelets and on negatively-charged phospholipid vesicles. *Biochemistry* 1996;35:16886–16897.

154. London F, Walsh PN. The role of electrostatic interactions in the assembly of the factor X activating complex on both activated platelets and negatively-charged phospholipid vesicles. *Biochemistry* 1996;35:12146–12154.

155. Wong MY, Gurr JA, Walsh PN. The second epidermal growth factor–like domain of human factor IXa mediates factor IXa binding to platelets and assembly of the factor X activating complex. *Biochemistry* 1999;38:8948–8960.

156. Astermark J, Bjork I, Ohlin AK, et al. Structural requirements for $Ca^{2+}$ binding to the gamma-carboxyglutamic acid and epidermal growth factor–like regions of factor IX. Studies using intact domains isolated from controlled proteolytic digests of bovine factor IX. *J Biol Chem* 1991;266: 2430–2437.

157. Davie EW. The blood coagulation factors: their cDNA's, genes and expression. In: Colman RW, Hirsh J, Marder VJ, et al. eds. *Hemostasis and thrombosis: basic principles and clinical practice*, Vol. 3. Philadelphia, PA: JB Lippincott Co, 1987:242–267.

158. Davie EW, Fujikawa K, Kisiel W. The coagulation cascade: initiation, maintenance, and regulation. *Biochemistry* 1991;30:10363–10370.

159. Di Scipio RG, Hermodson MA, Yates SG, et al. A comparison of human prothrombin, factor IX (Christmas factor), factor X (Stuart factor), and protein S. *Biochemistry* 1977;16:698–706.

160. Fujikawa K, Legaz ME, Davie EW. Bovine factors X 1 and X 2 (Stuart factor). Isolation and characterization. *Biochemistry* 1972;11:4882–4891.

161. Handford PA, Baron M, Mayhew M, et al. The first EGF-like domain from human factor IX contains a high-affinity calcium binding site. *EMBO J* 1990;9:475–480.

162. Hedner U, Davie EW. Factor IX. In: Colman RW, Hirsh J, Marder VJ, et al., eds. *Hemostasis and thrombosis: basic principles and clinical practice*, Vol. 2. Philadelphia, PA: JB Lippincott Co, 1987:39–47.

163. Hultin MB, Jesty J. The activation and inactivation of human factor VIII by thrombin: effect of inhibitors of thrombin. *Blood* 1981;57:476–482.

164. Jesty J, Spencer AK, Nemerson Y. The mechanism of activation of factor X. Kinetic control of alternative pathways leading to the formation of activated factor X. *J Biol Chem* 1974;249:5614–5622.

165. Lollar P, Knutson GJ, Fass DN. Activation of porcine factor VIII:C by thrombin and factor Xa. *Biochemistry* 1985;24:8056–8064.

166. Ohlin AK, Linse S, Stenflo J. Calcium binding to the epidermal growth factor homology region of bovine protein C. *J Biol Chem* 1988;263:7411–7417.

167. Persson E, Selander M, Linse S, et al. Calcium binding to the isolated beta-hydroxyaspartic acid-containing epidermal growth factor–like domain of bovine factor X. *J Biol Chem* 1989;264:16897–16904.

168. Thompson AR. Structure, function, and molecular defects of factor IX. *Blood* 1986;67:565–572.

169. van Dieijen G, Tans G, Rosing J, et al. The role of phospholipid and factor VIIIa in the activation of bovine factor X. *J Biol Chem* 1981;256:3433–3442.

170. Toomey JR, Smith KJ, Roberts HR, et al. The endothelial cell binding determinant of human factor IX resides in the gamma-carboxyglutamic acid domain. *Biochemistry* 1992;31:1806–1808.

171. Freedman SJ, Blostein MD, Baleja JD, et al. Identification of the phospholipid binding site in the vitamin K-dependent blood coagulation protein factor IX. *J Biol Chem* 1996;271:16227–16236.

172. Morita T, Fukudome K, Miyata T, et al. gamma-carboxyglutamic acid (Gla)-domainless blood coagulation factor IXa species: preparation and properties. *J Biochem (Tokyo)* 1991;110:990–996.

173. Shikamoto Y, Morita T, Fujimoto Z, et al. Crystal structure of Mg$^{2+}$- and Ca$^{2+}$-bound Gla domain of factor IX complexed with binding protein. *J Biol Chem* 2003;278:24090–24094.

174. Yang X, Walsh PN. The omega-loop within the Gla domain (G4-Q11) and the EGF2 domain (C88-C124) of factor IXa are both essential for the assembly of the factor X activating complex on activated platelets. *J Thromb Haemost* 2003;1(Suppl.):OC198.

175. Chavin SI. Factor VIII: structure and function in blood clotting. *Am J Hematol* 1984;16:297–306.

176. Fay PJ. Subunit structure of thrombin-activated human factor VIIIa. *Biochim Biophys Acta* 1988;952:181–190.

177. Fay PJ, Smudzin TM, Walker FJ. Activated protein C-catalyzed inactivation of human factor VIII and factor VIIIa. Identification of cleavage sites and correlation of proteolysis with cofactor activity. *J Biol Chem* 1991;266:20139–20145.

178. Fulcher CA, Zimmerman TS. Characterization of the human factor VIII procoagulant protein with a heterologous precipitating antibody. *Proc Natl Acad Sci U S A* 1982;79:1648–1652.

179. Gitschier J, Wood WI, Goralka TM, et al. Characterization of the human factor VIII gene. *Nature* 1984;312:326–330.

180. Hoyer LW, Trabold NC. The effect of thrombin on human factor VIII. Cleavage of the factor VIII procoagulant protein during activation. *J Lab Clin Med* 1981;97:50–64.

181. Lollar P, Parker CG. Subunit structure of thrombin-activated porcine factor VIII. *Biochemistry* 1989;28:666–674.

182. Lollar P, Parker CG. pH-dependent denaturation of thrombin-activated porcine factor VIII. *J Biol Chem* 1990;265:1688–1692.

183. McKee PA, Andersen JC, Switzer ME. Molecular structural studies of human factor VIII. *Ann N Y Acad Sci* 1975;240:8–33.

184. Toole JJ, Knopf JL, Wozney JM, et al. Molecular cloning of a cDNA encoding human antihaemophilic factor. *Nature* 1984;312:342–347.

185. Vehar GA, Davie EW. Preparation and properties of bovine factor VIII (antihemophilic factor). *Biochemistry* 1980;19:401–410.

186. Weinstein MJ, Chute LE, Deykin D. Analysis of factor VIII coagulation antigen in normal, thrombin-related and hemophilic plasma. *Proc Natl Acad Sci U S A* 1981;78:5137–5142.

187. Wood WI, Capon DJ, Simonsen CC, et al. Expression of active human factor VIII from recombinant DNA clones. *Nature.* 1984;312:330–337.

188. Nesheim ME, Pittman DD, Wang JH, et al. The binding of 35S-labeled recombinant factor VIII to activated and unactivated human platelets. *J Biol Chem* 1988;263:16467–16470.

189. Foster PA, Fulcher CA, Houghten RA, et al. Synthetic factor VIII peptides with amino acid sequences contained within the C2 domain of factor VIII inhibit factor VIII binding to phosphatidylserine. *Blood* 1990;75:1999–2004.

190. Saenko EL, Scandella D. A mechanism for inhibition of factor VIII binding to phospholipid by von Willebrand factor. *J Biol Chem* 1995;270:13826–13833.

191. Pratt KP, Shen BW, Takeshima K, et al. Structure of the C2 domain of human factor VIII at 1.5 A resolution. *Nature* 1999;402:439–442.

192. Ahmad SS, Walsh PN. Lipid raft association of the factor VIII C2 domain mediates platelet membrane assembly of factor VIIIa into the factor-X-activating complex. *Blood* 2002;100:126a.

193. Bevers EM, Wiedmer T, Comfurius P, et al. Defective Ca(2+)-induced microvesiculation and deficient expression of procoagulant activity in erythrocytes from a patient with a bleeding disorder: a study of the red blood cells of Scott syndrome. *Blood* 1992;79:380–388.

194. Furie B, Furie BC. The molecular basis of blood coagulation. *Cell* 1988;53:505–518.

195. Jackson CM, Nemerson Y. Blood coagulation. *Annu Rev Biochem* 1980;49:765–811.

196. Walsh PN. Different requirements for intrinsic factor-Xa forming activity and platelet factor 3 activity and their relationship to platelet aggregation and secretion. *Br J Haematol* 1978;40:311–331.

197. Bevers EM, Comfurius P, Zwaal RF. Mechanisms involved in platelet procoagulant response. *Adv Exp Med Biol* 1993;344:195–207.

198. Bevers EM, Tilly RH, Senden JM, et al. Exposure of endogenous phosphatidylserine at the outer surface of stimulated platelets is reversed by restoration of aminophospholipid translocase activity. *Biochemistry* 1989;28:2382–2387.

199. Comfurius P, Senden JM, Tilly RH, et al. Loss of membrane phospholipid asymmetry in platelets and red cells may be associated with calcium-induced shedding of plasma membrane and inhibition of aminophospholipid translocase. *Biochim Biophys Acta* 1990;1026:153–160.

200. Thiagarajan P, Tait JF. Binding of annexin V/placental anticoagulant protein I to platelets. Evidence for phosphatidylserine exposure in the procoagulant response of activated platelets. *J Biol Chem* 1990;265:17420–17423.

201. Zwaal RF, Bevers EM, Comfurius P, et al. Loss of membrane phospholipid asymmetry during activation of blood platelets and sickled red cells; mechanisms and physiological significance. *Mol Cell Biochem* 1989;91:23–31.

202. Higgins DL, Callahan PJ, Prendergast FG, et al. Lipid mobility in the assembly and expression of the activity of the prothrombinase complex. *J Biol Chem* 1985;260:3604–3612.

203. Kung C, Hayes E, Mann KG. A membrane-mediated catalytic event in prothrombin activation. *J Biol Chem* 1994;269:25838–25848.

204. Thiagarajan P, Tait JF. Collagen-induced exposure of anionic phospholipid in platelets and platelet-derived microparticles. *J Biol Chem* 1991;266:24302–24307.

205. Milstone JH. Thrombokinase as prime activator of prothrombin: historical perspectives and present status. *Fed Proc* 1964;23:742–748.

206. Barton PG. Sequence theories of blood coagulation re-evaluated with reference to lipid-protein interactions. *Nature* 1967;215:1508–1509.

207. Barton PG, Hanahan DJ. Some lipid-protein interactions involved in prothrombin activation. *Biochim Biophys Acta* 1969;187:319–327.

208. Barton PG, Jackson CM, Hanahan DJ. Relationship between factor V and activated factor X in the generation of prothrombinase. *Nature* 1967;214:923–924.

209. Bull RK, Jevons S, Barton PG. Complexes of prothrombin with calcium ions and phospholipids. *J Biol Chem* 1972;247:2747–2754.

210. Cole ER, Koppel JL, Olwin JH. Interaction of bovine autoprothrombin C with phospholipids and divalent cations. *Can J Biochem Physiol* 1964;42:1595–1603.

211. Cole ER, Koppel JL, Olwin JH. Phospholipid-protein interactions in the formation of prothrombin activator. *Thromb Diath Haemorrh* 1965;14:431–444.

212. Esmon CT, Owen WG, Jackson CM. A plausible mechanism for prothrombin activation by factor Xa, factor Va, phospholipid, and calcium ions. *J Biol Chem* 1974;249:8045–8047.

213. Esmon CT, Suttie JW, Jackson CM. The functional significance of vitamin K action. Difference in phospholipid binding between normal and abnormal prothrombin. *J Biol Chem* 1975;250:4095–4099.

214. Esnouf MP, Jobin F. Lipids in prothrombin conversion. *Thromb Diath Haemorrh Suppl* 1965;17:103–110.

215. Gitel SN, Owen WG, Esmon CT, et al. A polypeptide region of bovine prothrombin specific for binding to phospholipids. *Proc Natl Acad Sci U S A* 1973;70:1344–1348.

216. Hemker HC, Esnouf MP, Hemker PW, et al. Formation of prothrombin converting activity. *Nature* 1967;215:248–251.

217. Hemker HC, Kahn MJ. Reaction sequence of blood coagulation. *Nature* 1967;215:1201–1202.

218. Hemker HC, Kahn MJ, Devilee PP. The adsorption of coagulation factors onto phospholipids. Its role in the reaction mechanism of blood coagulation. *Thromb Diath Haemorrh* 1970;24:214–223.

219. Kahn MJ, Hemker HC. Studies on blood coagulation factor V. I. The interaction of salts of fatty acids and coagulation factors. *Thromb Diath Haemorrh* 1969;22:417–430.

220. Lindhout T, Govers-Riemslag JW, van de Waart P, et al. Factor Va-factor Xa interaction. Effects of phospholipid vesicles of varying composition. *Biochemistry* 1982;21:5494–5502.

221. Nelsestuen GL, Suttie JW. The mode of action of vitamin K. Isolation of a peptide containing the vitamin K-dependent portion of prothrombin. *Proc Natl Acad Sci U S A* 1973;70:3366–3370.

222. Nesheim ME, Eid S, Mann KG. Assembly of the prothrombinase complex in the absence of prothrombin. *J Biol Chem* 1981;256:9874–9882.

223. Nesheim ME, Taswell JB, Mann KG. The contribution of bovine factor V and factor Va to the activity of prothrombinase. *J Biol Chem* 1979;254:10952–10962.

224. Papahadjopoulos D, Hanahan DJ. Observations on the interaction of phospholipids and certain clotting factors in prothrombin activator formation. *Biochim Biophys Acta* 1964;90:436–439.

225. Papahadjopoulos D, Yin ET, Hanahan DJ. Purification and properties of bovine factor X: molecular changes during activation. *Biochemistry* 1964; 19:1931–1939.

226. Rosing J, Tans G, Govers-Riemslag JW, et al. The role of phospholipids and factor Va in the prothrombinase complex. *J Biol Chem* 1980;255:274–283.

227. Stenflo J, Ganrot PO. Binding of Ca2+ to normal and dicoumarol-induced prothrombin. *Biochem Biophys Res Commun* 1973;50:98–104.

228. Stenflo J, Suttie JW. Vitamin K-dependent formation of gamma-carboxyglutamic acid. *Annu Rev Biochem* 1977;46:157–172.

229. Bevers EM, Comfurius P, van Rijn JL, et al. Generation of prothrombin-converting activity and the exposure of phosphatidylserine at the outer surface of platelets. *Eur J Biochem* 1982;122:429–436.

230. Bevers EM, Comfurius P, Zwaal RF. The nature of the binding for prothrombinase at the platelet surface as revealed by lipolytic enzymes. *Eur J Biochem* 1982;122:81–85.

231. Bevers EM, Comfurius P, Zwaal RF. Changes in membrane phospholipid distribution during platelet activation. *Biochim Biophys Acta* 1983;736:57–66.

232. Chap HJ, Zwaal RF, van Deenen LL. Action of highly purified phospholipases on blood platelets. Evidence for an asymmetric distribution of phospholipids in the surface membrane. *Biochim Biophys Acta* 1977;467:146–164.

233. Otnaess AB, Holm T. The effect of phospholipase C on human blood platelets. *J Clin Invest* 1976;57:1419–1425.

234. Schick PK. The organization of aminophospholipids in human platelet membranes: selective changes induced by thrombin. *J Lab Clin Med* 1978; 91:802–810.

235. Schick PK, Kurica KB, Chacko GK. Location of phosphatidylethanolamine and phosphatidylserine in the human platelet plasma membrane. *J Clin Invest* 1976;57:1221–1226.

236. Zwaal RF, Comfurius P, van Deenen LL. Membrane asymmetry and blood coagulation. *Nature* 1977;268:358–360.

237. Zwaal RFA, Rosing J, Tans G. Topological and kinetic aspects of phospholipids in blood coagulation. In: Mann KG, Taylor FB, eds. *Workshop on regulation of coagulation*. New York: Elsevier/North-Holland,1980.

238. Kane WH, Lindhout MJ, Jackson CM, et al. Factor Va-dependent binding of factor Xa to human platelets. *J Biol Chem* 1980;255:1170–1174.

239. Comp PC, Esmon CT. Activated protein C inhibits platelet prothrombin-converting activity. *Blood* 1979;54:1272–1281.

240. Dahlback B, Stenflo J. Inhibitory effect of activated protein C on activation of prothrombin by platelet-bound factor Xa. *Eur J Biochem* 1980; 107:331–335.

241. Tracy PB, Eide LL, Bowie EJ, et al. Radioimmunoassay of factor V in human plasma and platelets. *Blood* 1982;60:59–63.

242. Altieri DC, Edgington TS. Identification of effector cell protease receptor-1. A leukocyte-distributed receptor for the serine protease factor Xa. *J Immunol* 1990;145:246–253.

243. Bouchard BA, Shatos MA, Tracy PB. Human brain pericytes differentially regulate expression of procoagulant enzyme complexes comprising the extrinsic pathway of blood coagulation. *Arterioscler Thromb Vasc Biol* 1997; 17:1–9.

244. Nicholson AC, Nachman RL, Altieri DC, et al. Effector cell protease receptor-1 is a vascular receptor for coagulation factor Xa. *J Biol Chem* 1996;271:28407–28413.

245. Briede JJ, Heemskerk JW, van't Veer C, et al. Contribution of platelet-derived factor Va to thrombin generation on immobilized collagen- and fibrinogen-adherent platelets. *Thromb Haemost* 2001;85:509–513.

246. Sims PJ, Faioni EM, Wiedmer T, et al. Complement proteins C5b-9 cause release of membrane vesicles from the platelet surface that are enriched in the membrane receptor for coagulation factor Va and express prothrombinase activity. *J Biol Chem* 1988;263:18205–18212.

247. Sims PJ, Rollins SA, Wiedmer T. Regulatory control of complement on blood platelets. Modulation of platelet procoagulant responses by a membrane inhibitor of the C5b-9 complex. *J Biol Chem* 1989;264:19228–19235.

248. Sims PJ, Wiedmer T, Esmon CT, et al. Assembly of the platelet prothrombinase complex is linked to vesiculation of the platelet plasma membrane. Studies in Scott syndrome: an isolated defect in platelet procoagulant activity. *J Biol Chem* 1989;264:17049–17057.

249. Tans G, Rosing J, Thomassen MC, et al. Comparison of anticoagulant and procoagulant activities of stimulated platelets and platelet-derived microparticles. *Blood* 1991;77:2641–2648.

250. Weiss HJ, Lages B. Platelet prothrombinase activity and intracellular calcium responses in patients with storage pool deficiency, glycoprotein IIb-IIIa deficiency, or impaired platelet coagulant activity—a comparison with Scott syndrome. *Blood* 1997;89:1599–1611.

251. Chesney CM, Pifer D, Colman RW. Subcellular localization and secretion of factor V from human platelets. *Proc Natl Acad Sci U S A* 1981;78: 5180–5184.

252. Chesney CM, Pifer DD, Colman RW. The role of platelet factor V in prothrombin conversion. *Thromb Res* 1983;29:75–84.

253. Hayward CP, Bainton DF, Smith JW. et al. Multimerin is found in the alpha-granules of resting platelets and is synthesized by a megakaryocytic cell line. *J Clin Invest* 1993;91:2630–2639.

254. Hayward CP, Furmaniak-Kazmierczak E, Cieutat AM, et al. Factor V is complexed with multimerin in resting platelet lysates and colocalizes with multimerin in platelet alpha-granules. *J Biol Chem* 1995;270: 19217–19224.

255. Hayward CP, Kelton JG. Multimerin. *Curr Opin Hematol* 1995;2: 339–344.

256. Hayward CP, Warkentin TE, Horsewood P, et al. Multimerin: a series of large disulfide-linked multimeric proteins within platelets. *Blood* 1991; 77:2556–2560.

257. Mann FB, Hurn M, Magath TB. Observations on the conversion of prothrombin to thrombin. *Proc Soc Exp Biol Med* 1947;66:33–39.

258. Monkovic DD, Tracy PB. Functional characterization of human platelet-released factor V and its activation by factor Xa and thrombin. *J Biol Chem* 1990;265:17132–17140.

259. Ware AG, Fahey JL, Seegers WH. Platelet extracts, fibrin formation, and interaction of purified prothrombin and thromboplastin. *Am J Physiol* 1948;154:140–147.

260. Kalafatis M, Krishnaswamy S, Rand MD, et al. Proteolytic enzymes in coagulation, fibrinolysis, and complement activation. *Methods Enzymol* 1993;222:224–236.

261. Nesheim ME, Nichols WL, Cole TL, et al. Isolation and study of an acquired inhibitor of human coagulation factor V. *J Clin Invest* 1986;77:405–415.

262. Viskup RW, Tracy PB, Mann KG. The isolation of human platelet factor V. *Blood* 1987;69:1188–1195.

263. Gewirtz AM, Keefer M, Doshi K, et al. Biology of human megakaryocyte factor V. *Blood* 1986;67:1639–1648.

264. Gewirtz AM, Shapiro C, Shen YM, et al. Cellular and molecular regulation of factor V expression in human megakaryocytes. *J Cell Physiol* 1992; 153:277–287.

265. Nichols WL, Gastineau DA, Solberg LA Jr, et al. Identification of human megakaryocyte coagulation factor V. *Blood* 1985;65:1396–1406.

266. Wang DL, Annamalai AE, Ghosh S, et al. Human platelet factor V is crosslinked to actin by FXIIIa during platelet activation by thrombin. *Thromb Res* 1990;57:39–57.

267. Camire RM, Pollak ES, Kaushansky K, et al. Secretable human platelet-derived factor V originates from the plasma pool. *Blood* 1998;92:3035–3041.

268. Handagama P, Bainton DF, Jacques Y, et al. Kistrin, an integrin antagonist, blocks endocytosis of fibrinogen into guinea pig megakaryocyte and platelet alpha-granules. *J Clin Invest* 1993;91:193–200.

269. Handagama P, Rappolee DA, Werb Z, et al. Platelet alpha-granule fibrinogen, albumin, and immunoglobulin G are not synthesized by rat and mouse megakaryocytes. *J Clin Invest* 1990;86:1364–1368.

270. Handagama PJ, Shuman MA, Bainton DF. Incorporation of intravenously injected albumin, immunoglobulin G, and fibrinogen in guinea pig megakaryocyte granules. *J Clin Invest* 1989;84:73–82.

271. Harrison P, Wilbourn B, Debili N, et al. Uptake of plasma fibrinogen into the alpha granules of human megakaryocytes and platelets. *J Clin Invest* 1989;84:1320–1324.

272. Christella M, Thomassen LG, Castoldi E, et al. Endogenous factor V synthesis in megakaryocytes contributes negligibly to the platelet factor V pool. *Haematologica* 2003;88:1150–1156.

273. George JN. Platelet immunoglobulin G: its significance for the evaluation of thrombocytopenia and for understanding the origin of alpha-granule proteins. *Blood* 1990;76:859–870.

274. Chiu HC, Schick PK, Colman RW. Biosynthesis of factor V in isolated guinea pig megakaryocytes. *J Clin Invest* 1985;75:339–346.

275. Yang TL, Pipe SW, Yang A, et al. Biosynthetic origin and functional significance of murine platelet factor V. *Blood* 2003;102:2851–2855.

276. Monkovic DD, Tracy PB. Activation of human factor V by factor Xa and thrombin. *Biochemistry* 1990;29:1118–1128.

277. Kalafatis M. Identification and partial characterization of factor Va heavy chain kinase from human platelets. *J Biol Chem* 1998;273:8459–8466.

278. Kalafatis M, Rand MD, Jenny RJ, et al. Phosphorylation of factor Va and factor VIIIa by activated platelets. *Blood* 1993;81:704–719.

279. Rand MD, Kalafatis M, Mann KG. Platelet coagulation factor Va: the major secretory platelet phosphoprotein. *Blood* 1994;83:2180–2190.

280. Camire RM, Kalafatis M, Cushman M, et al. The mechanism of inactivation of human platelet factor Va from normal and activated protein C-resistant individuals. *J Biol Chem* 1995;270:20794–20800.

281. Camire RM, Kalafatis M, Simioni P, et al. Platelet-derived factor Va/Va Leiden cofactor activities are sustained on the surface of activated platelets despite the presence of activated protein C. *Blood* 1998;91:2818–2829.

282. Hayward CP, Cramer EM, Kane WH, et al. Studies of a second family with the Quebec platelet disorder: evidence that the degradation of the alpha-granule membrane and its soluble contents are not secondary to a defect in targeting proteins to alpha-granules. *Blood* 1997;89:1243–1253.

283. Janeway CM, Rivard GE, Tracy PB, et al. Factor V Quebec revisited. *Blood* 1996;87:3571–3578.

284. Tracy PB, Giles AR, Mann KG, et al. Factor V (Quebec): a bleeding diathesis associated with a qualitative platelet Factor V deficiency. *J Clin Invest* 1984;74:1221–1228.

285. Borchgrevink CF, Owren PA. The hemostatic effect of normal platelets in hemophilia and factor V deficiency. The importance of clotting factors adsorbed on platelets for normal hemostasis. *Acta Med Scand* 1961;170: 375–383.

286. Chediak J, Ashenhurst JB, Garlick I, et al. Successful management of bleeding in a patient with factor V inhibitor by platelet transfusions. *Blood* 1980;56:835–841.

# CHAPTER 39 ■ PLATELET SIGNAL TRANSDUCTION

CHARLES S. ABRAMS AND LAWRENCE F. BRASS

Platelets are activated when agonists such as collagen or thrombin bind to receptors on the platelet surface, initiating signaling-events within the platelet that eventually lead to the reorganization of the platelet cytoskeleton, aggregation, and granule secretion. This process can only occur when local barriers to platelet activation are exceeded or overwhelmed. Platelets are usually shielded from the connective tissue matrix within the vascular wall by a continuous barrier of endothelial cells, which physically separates platelets from molecules within the vessel wall that can cause platelet activation. When vascular injury occurs, platelets adhere to exposed collagen fibrils, forming a discontinuous carpet. *In vitro* adhesion to collagen can occur without the help of accessory molecules, but *in vivo* the shear forces and turbulence caused by flowing blood would strip platelets away from collagen were it not for the stabilizing effects of von Willebrand factor (VWF). A recently described metalloprotease, ADAMTS13, cleaves VWF, preventing the accumulation in plasma of ultra high-molecular-weight multimers that would otherwise cause spontaneous platelet clumping and arterial thrombosis (1–4). The binding of VWF to collagen by the A3 domain exposes binding sites on the VWF A1 and C1 domains for the platelet adhesion receptors, glycoprotein (GP) Ib/IX/V and $\alpha_{IIb}\beta_3$, respectively (5,6). These indirect interactions with collagen, combined with the activating signals produced when collagen binds directly to the $\alpha_2\beta_1$ integrin and GP VI on the platelet surface, platelets that have adhered to collagen change their shape, spreading along the fibrils and releasing thromboxane $A_2$ ($TxA_2$) and adenosine diphosphate (ADP) into the circulation.

The released $TxA_2$ and ADP recruit additional platelets, causing them to stick to each other and to the platelets directly adherent to collagen. The growing mound of activated platelets is eventually stabilized by a crosslinked fibrin clot. The critical contact between adjacent platelets depends on the binding of fibrinogen or fibrin to the integrin $\alpha_{IIb}\beta_3$ on the platelet surface, and this occurs only after platelets have been activated. Because fibrinogen is a symmetrical molecule, it can bind to two platelets. Repeated as many as 50,000 times per platelet, this binding allows platelets to stick to each other, a process that can be made to occur when platelets are in suspension, but usually this binding should occur only at a site of vascular injury. Like collagen, soluble platelet agonists cause platelets to change their shape, losing the discoid appearance that is characteristic of resting platelets and transforming them into an irregular sphere with pseudopodia. Underlying this change of shape is a rapid reorganization of the platelet cytoskeleton because actin filaments are uncapped, severed, and rebuilt in response to signals that involve changes in the cytosolic $Ca^{2+}$ concentration and the sequential activation of low-molecular-weight GTP-binding proteins such as Rac and Rho.

Collagen, ADP, and $TxA_2$ are not alone in their ability to activate platelets. Vascular injury and inflammation expose tissue factor, as well as collagen, and formation of the tissue factor/factor VIIa complex leads to the local generation of thrombin from prothrombin. Thrombin is a potent agonist, activating platelets at concentrations in the pM range by interacting with receptors on the platelet surface. Platelets facilitate this process by providing procoagulant phospholipids that accelerate thrombin generation. As a result, platelet activation and fibrin deposition are intimately linked, maximizing the growth and strength of the hemostatic plug. Human platelets express two G protein–coupled receptors (GPCR) that can be activated by thrombin. Cleavage of these receptors accounts for the long-established observation that only proteolytically active thrombin can activate platelets.

The process of transforming $\alpha_{IIb}\beta_3$ on the platelet surface into a competent receptor for fibrinogen is one of the most fascinating aspects of platelet biology. It is also the final common pathway in platelet responses to most agonists, making it a frequent target for drug development. Stated succinctly, the central issue is this: Although circulating platelets are surrounded by plasma proteins, they usually do not bind fibrinogen to their surface and stick to each other unless they have been activated. There are many reasons for this lack of binding, but this is ultimately due to the inability of fibrinogen or fibrin to bind to the resting conformation of $\alpha_{IIb}\beta_3$. Platelet activation alters the conformation of $\alpha_{IIb}\beta_3$ and exposes the fibrinogen-binding site. Usually, this should occur only at sites of vascular injury. However, even in the absence of substantial vascular injury, it is likely that the buffeting that the platelets withstand as they move through the circulation, perhaps encountering low concentrations of thrombin or being smashed against exposed atherosclerotic plaques, pushes them toward inappropriate activation.

Working against this tendency are a number of internal and external controls that dampen the intracellular signals that would otherwise promote platelet activation at sites that would lead to myocardial infarction or stroke. In addition to providing a physical barrier and a source of VWF, endothelial cells release prostacyclin ($PGI_2$) and nitric oxide (NO), two molecules that globally depress intracellular signaling in platelets by raising cyclic adenosine monophosphate (cAMP) and cyclic guanosine 3′-5-monophosphate (cGMP) levels (7–13). The ability of cyclic nucleotides to inhibit platelet activation has been exploited in the development of antiplatelet agents such as dipyridamole (Persantine), which raises cAMP levels inside platelets by inhibiting cAMP phosphodiesterase (14). cGMP also inhibits cAMP phosphodiesterase in platelets, contributing to the rise of cAMP levels. In turn, cAMP activates protein kinase A, which phosphorylates multiple platelet proteins including the $\beta$ chain of GP Ib (15,16), actin-binding protein (filamin) (17), myosin light chain (18,19), vasodilator-stimulated phosphoprotein (VASP) (20,21), and Rap1B (22). The net effect is a generalized inhibition of platelet activation. The importance of $PGI_2$ and NO as barriers to platelet activation is indicated not only by the effectiveness of molecules that mimic $PGI_2$ as antiplatelet agents, but also by the prothrombotic effects in mice of deleting the gene encoding the platelet $PGI_2$ receptor (IP) (23), and by the decrease in basal cAMP levels found in $IP^{-/-}$ platelets (24). In addition to releasing $PGI_2$ and NO, some endothelial cells express the *ecto*-ADPase, CD39, on their luminal surface. CD39 can hydrolyze small quantities of ADP released from damaged red cells and activated platelets, preventing the ADP from activating additional platelets (25,26). Other barriers to unwarranted platelet activation include the diluting effects of continued blood flow, the presence of natural anticoagulants that limit thrombin formation, and the short half-life of the platelet-derived agonist, $TxA_2$. Collectively, these provide a threshold that helps to prevent platelet activation at inappropriate times and places.

# THREE STAGES OF PLATELET PLUG FORMATION

As a starting point, one might consider the platelet surface as being crowded with receptors that support one or more of the phases of platelet plug formation. Those that are directly involved in binding to adhesive proteins such as collagen, VWF, and fibrinogen are present in greatest numbers. After recruitment of additional pools of receptors that are initially within the surface-connecting membrane system or in the membranes of $\alpha$-granules, there are approximately 80,000 copies of $\alpha_{IIb}\beta_3$ and 15,000 copies of GP Ib on the surface of human platelets. In contrast, receptors that primarily serve as signaling response elements for platelet agonists typically range from a few hundred to a few thousand per platelet (see Table 39-1). Although these numbers are not large in absolute terms, when placed in the context of the relatively small size of human platelets, the density is high. In cells other than platelets, it has been shown that some signaling molecules tend to be concentrated within or near cholesterol-enriched microdomains within the plasma membrane (27). There is growing evidence that this also occurs in platelets, increasing the efficiency of platelet activation (28–30).

The platelet monolayer that forms following the exposure of collagen and VWF initiates platelet plug formation, but is insufficient to prevent bleeding. The extension or recruitment phase of platelet plug formation occurs when additional activated platelets accumulate on top of the monolayer (50,51). Recruitment is mediated by the local accumulation of molecules that are released from platelets, such as ADP and $TxA_2$. Contacts between platelets are maintained by a variety of molecular interactions, of which the best-described and most critical is the binding of fibrinogen and VWF to activated $\alpha_{IIb}\beta_3$. Thrombin continues to participate in this phase of platelet activation and, in turn, activated platelets provide a procoagulant surface on which more thrombin can be generated by the assembly of the tenase and prothrombinase coagulation complexes. Circulating or locally secreted epinephrine causes vasoconstriction, and also potentiates the effects of other platelet agonists. In contrast to platelet activation by collagen, platelet activation by most of the agonists involved in extension of the platelet plug is very rapid, with some responses occurring within a fraction of a second. Teleologically, this makes sense because circulating platelets would not be expected to linger at a wound site long enough for a slower process to occur. Videos of thrombus formation at a site of focal injury show that initially most platelets move by the site of injury at speeds too rapid for activation to occur (50). As the thrombus develops, flow becomes more turbulent, slowing the forward movement of the platelets long enough for platelets to be activated by soluble agonists.

Formation of the platelet plug following vascular injury can be thought of as occurring in three stages: adhesion, activation, and secretion (see Fig. 39-1). Adhesion begins with the rolling, arrest, and activation of moving platelets by the collagen/VWF complex to form a platelet monolayer. Activation refers to the recruitment of additional platelets through the stimulation by fast-acting agonists such as thrombin, ADP, and $TxA_2$, all three of which activate platelets through GPCR on the platelet surface. This is arbitrarily separated into early stages initiated by the adhesion process itself, and later stages that result from activation of locally circulating agonists that predominantly stimulate the GPCR family. Finally, secretion of additional agonists and adhesive ligands perpetuates these events by recruiting additional platelets to participate in the formation of the platelet plug. These definitions are arbitrary,

## TABLE 39-1

### G PROTEIN–COUPLED RECEPTORS EXPRESSED ON HUMAN PLATELETS

| Agonist | Receptor | Approximate number of copies per platelet | G protein families | Reference |
|---|---|---|---|---|
| ADP | $P2Y_1$ | 150 | Impaired response to ADP; absent increase in cytosolic $Ca^{2+}$ and shape change in response to ADP | |
| | | | Normal inhibition of cAMP formation by ADP | 31,32 |
| | $P2Y_{12}$ | 600 | Greatly diminished aggregation in response to ADP; absent inhibition of adenylyl cyclase by ADP; increased bleeding time | 33 |
| Thrombin | PAR1 | 2,000 | Gq, G12, Gi (controversial) | 34–38 |
| | PAR4 | unknown | Gq, G12 | 39 |
| $TxA_2$ | TP$\alpha$ and TP$\beta$ | 1,000 | Gq, G12 | 40–45 |
| Epinephrine | $\alpha_{2A}$-adrenergic | 300 | Gi (particularly Gz) | 46–48 |
| $PGI_2$ | IP | unknown | Gs | 49 |

ADP, adenosine diphosphate; cAMP, cyclic adenosine monophosphate; PAR, protease-activated receptor; $TxA_2$, thromboxane $A_2$; $PGI_2$, prostacyclin.

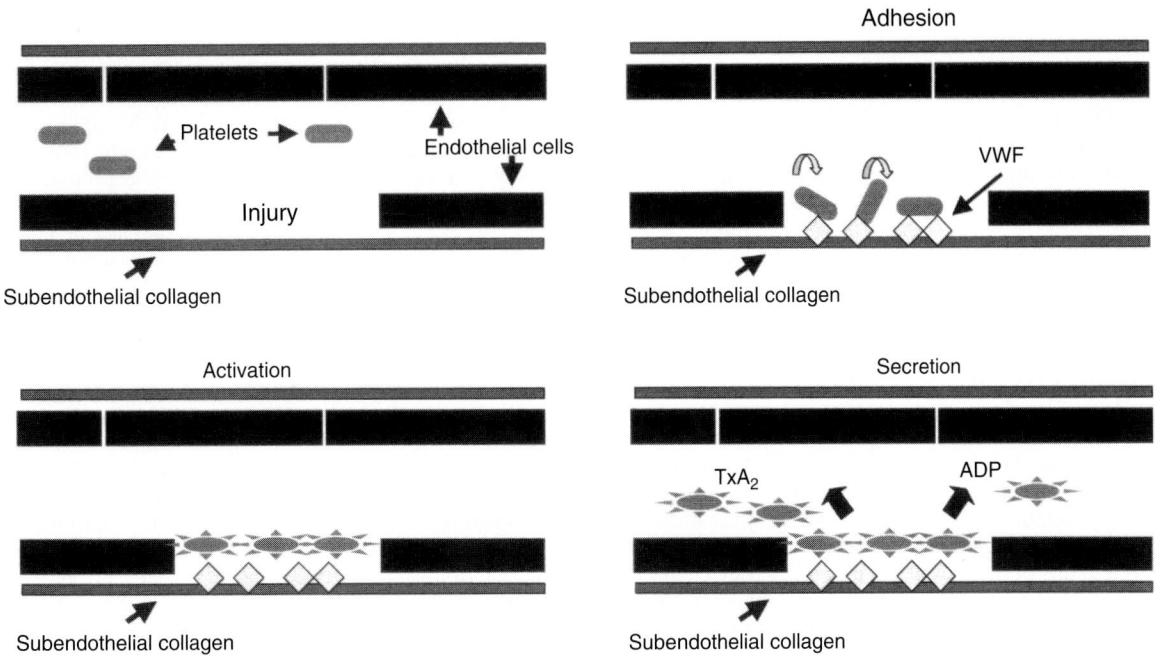

**FIGURE 39-1.** Stages in platelet plug formation. Before vascular injury, platelets are restrained from activation by the inability of plasma von Willebrand factor (VWF) to bind spontaneously to the platelet surface. The development of the platelet plug can be initiated by the exposure of collagen in the vessel wall or by the local generation of thrombin (or both). Rolling platelets adhere and spread on the collagen/VWF matrix, forming a monolayer of activated platelets that acts as a surface for subsequent recruitment of platelets by thrombin, adenosine diphosphate (ADP), and thromboxane (TxA₂).

because the adhesion of platelets to the collagen and VWF also initiates some of the early stages of activation.

## PLATELET ADHESION

The arrest and eventual activation of moving platelets by collagen is accomplished by receptors on the platelet surface that either bind directly to collagen (GP VI and the integrin $\alpha_2\beta_1$) or bind indirectly to collagen by VWF (the GP Ib/IX/V complex and the integrin $\alpha_{IIb}\beta_3$). The integrins require prior activation by intracellular "inside-out" signaling to engage collagen and VWF, after which they can contribute further platelet activation by generating outside-in signals. The presence of collagen and VWF

binding sites on GP VI and GP Ib allows platelets to slow down long enough to become activated and fully adherent. Platelet activation by collagen is summarized in Figure 39-2. Intracellular signaling in response to collagen is mediated by at least three receptors: GP VI, GP Ib, and, after integrin activation has occurred, $\alpha_2\beta_1$. The structure of GP VI places it in the immunoglobulin domain superfamily. Its ability to generate signals rests primarily on its constitutive association with a second molecule, the Fc receptor $\gamma$ chain (52). Platelets from mice that lack the $\gamma$ chain (53) have impaired responses to collagen. So do platelets from humans (54,55), but possibly not from mice (56), with reduced expression of $\alpha_2\beta_1$. Using blocking antibodies or a depletion strategy, Nieswandt et al. (56) concluded that GP VI is required for platelet responses to collagen.

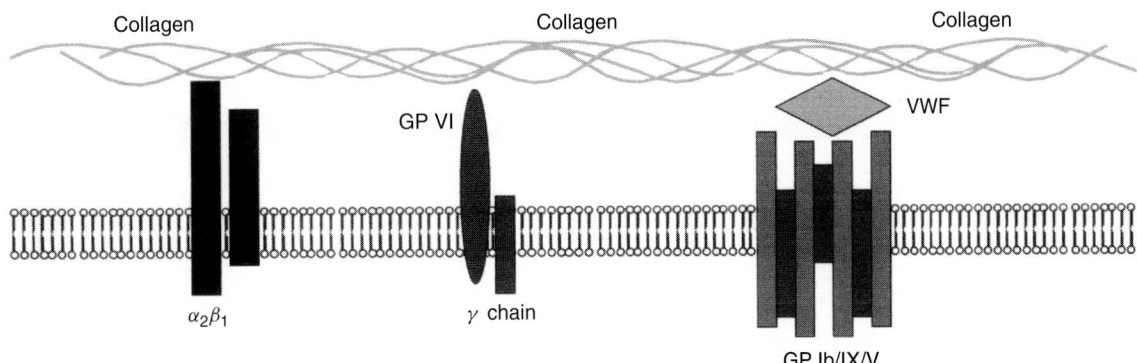

**FIGURE 39-2.** Platelet activation by collagen. Several distinct molecular complexes contribute platelet activation by collagen. These include: (1) The von Willebrand factor (VWF)–mediated binding of collagen to the glycoprotein (GP) Ib/IX/V complex, or direct interaction between collagen and either (2) the $\alpha_2\beta_1$ integrin, or (3) the GP VI/$\gamma$ chain complex. Ligation of these receptors induces signaling cascades that induce the secretion of adenosine diphosphate (ADP) and the production and release of thromboxane (TxA₂). ADP and TxA₂ bind to their own receptors in platelets, generating signals that support the more direct effects of collagen.

Signaling through GP VI can be studied in isolation with the snake venom protein, convulxin, or with synthetic "collagen-related" peptides (CRP). According to current models, collagen causes clustering of GP VI and its associated $\gamma$ chain. This promotes the phosphorylation of the $\gamma$ chain by nonreceptor tyrosine kinases in the Src family, creating a phosphotyrosine "ITAM" motif recognized by the tandem SH2 domains of Syk. Association of Syk with the GP VI/$\gamma$ chain complex activates Syk and leads to the phosphorylation and activation of phospholipase C (PLC)$\gamma$2. Loss of Syk impairs collagen responses (53). PLC$\gamma$ hydrolyzes membrane PI-4,5-P2 to form the second messengers 1,4,5-IP$_3$ and 1,2-diacylglycerol (DAG). Inositol 1,4,5-trisphosphate (IP$_3$) opens Ca$^{2+}$ channels in the platelet dense tubular system, raising the cytosolic Ca$^{2+}$ concentration and triggering Ca$^{2+}$ influx across the platelet plasma membrane. DAG and Ca$^{2+}$ activate the more common protein kinase C (PKC) isoforms that are expressed in platelets, making possible the regulatory serine/threonine phosphorylation events that are needed for platelet activation. At least one of those phosphorylation events regulates the exposure of fibrinogen-binding sites on $\alpha_{IIb}\beta_3$, but the full mechanism for activating $\alpha_{IIb}\beta_3$ remains obscure. The events triggered by GP VI lead to activation of $\alpha_2\beta_1$, as well as $\alpha_{IIb}\beta_3$. Engagement of the two integrins with their respective ligands initiates a further round of signaling that features some of the same molecules that are downstream of GP VI: Syk, SLP-76 and PLC$\gamma_2$ (57). This is a theme that repeats itself during platelet activation: different agonists with disparate receptors trigger signaling events that involve a common set of intermediates. Outside-in signaling is discussed at a greater length in the last section of this chapter.

Finally, GP Ib serves as both an anchor point for the platelet cytoskeleton, and as the focus for assembling signaling-complexes in platelets that have become bound to VWF (58–63). The cytoplasmic domain of GP Ib$\alpha$ can bind to filamin and to the scaffolding protein, 14-3-3$\zeta$. Src becomes associated with GP Ib following the binding of VWF. The p85 subunit of PI 3-kinase (PI 3-K) appears to mediate this association. In turn, Syk is activated. Therefore, signaling through GP Ib takes advantage of some of the same signaling molecules that are involved in GP VI– and integrin-dependent responses to collagen, with the same potential for causing protein tyrosine phosphorylation, PI-4,5-P2 hydrolysis, and recruitment of cytosolic proteins whose Pleckstrin homology (PH) domains can support associations with 3-phosphorylated phosphoinositides (64,65).

# PLATELET ACTIVATION

The agonists involved in the extension of the platelet plug typically cause platelet activation through GPCRs on the platelet surface. GPCRs are well suited for this task in a number of respects. First, most of these receptors bind ligands with high affinity. Second, GPCRs are composed of a single subunit that does not require oligomerization (although several recent studies have shown that some GPCR exist as homodimers or heterodimers even in the absence of their ligands) (66–68). Third, GPCRs are constitutively associated with G proteins, eliminating the time that would otherwise be required to recruit them into complexes (66). Fourth, because they act as guanine nucleotide exchange factors, each occupied receptor can activate multiple G proteins and, in some cases, more than one class of G proteins. This allows amplification of a signal that might begin with a relatively a small number of receptors. It also enables some receptors to signal through more than one effector pathway. Finally, because several generic mechanisms that can limit the activation of GPCR exist, platelet activation can be limited, a property that may be useful when platelet activation is inappropriate and needs to be contained (69,70).

GPCRs are composed of a single polypeptide chain with 7 transmembrane domains, an extracellular N-terminus, and an intracellular C-terminus. Binding sites for agonists can involve the N-terminus, the extracellular loops, or a pocket formed by the transmembrane domains (66). The G proteins that act as mediators for these receptors are heterotrimers composed of $\alpha$, $\beta$, and $\gamma$ subunits. Within this complex, the $\beta$ subunit forms a propellerlike structure that is tightly associated with the much smaller $\gamma$ subunit. The $\alpha$ subunit contains a guanine nucleotide–binding site that is usually occupied by guanosine diphosphate (GDP). Receptor activation causes the exchange of GTP for GDP, altering the conformation of the $\alpha$ subunit and exposing sites on both G$\alpha$ and G$\beta\gamma$ for interactions with downstream effectors (71–73). Hydrolysis of the GTP by the intrinsic GTPase activity of the $\alpha$ subunit restores the resting conformation of the heterotrimer, preparing it to undergo another round of activation and signaling (74). A family of GTPase activating proteins known as *regulators of G protein signaling* (RGS) proteins help accelerate the hydrolysis of GTP by G$\alpha$ (75). Prenylation of the $\gamma$ chain and acylation of the $\alpha$ subunit helps anchor the complete heterotrimer to the plasma membrane and continues to anchor G$\alpha$-GTP and G$\beta\gamma$ to the membrane when they dissociate from each other to expose effector binding sites. Platelets express 10 forms of G$\alpha$. There is little information about which types of G$\beta$ and G$\gamma$ are expressed (see Table 39-2). The best-described forms of G$\alpha$ fall into the Gs$\alpha$, Gi$\alpha$, Gq$\alpha$, and G12$\alpha$ families (74). Human platelets express at least one Gs$\alpha$ family member, four Gi$\alpha$ family members, three Gq$\alpha$ family members, and two G12$\alpha$ family members. On the basis of evidence from knockout and reconstitution studies, the abundance of G protein types in platelets appears to be necessary to support the actions of multiple dissimilar platelet agonists (24).

## TABLE 39-2

### G PROTEINS IN PLATELETS

| Family | G protein | Effectors | Function | Reference |
|--------|-----------|-----------|----------|-----------|
| Gq | Gq$\alpha$ | PLC | ↑ IP$_3$/DAG | 76,77 |
| | G11$\alpha$ | PLC | ↑ IP$_3$/DAG | 76,77 |
| | G16$\alpha$ G15$\alpha$ in mice | PLC | ↑ IP$_3$/DAG | 78–81 |
| G12 | G12$\alpha$, G13$\alpha$ | p115-RhoGEF? | Actin cytoskeleton | 77,82–84 |
| Gi | Gi2$\alpha$ > Gi3$\alpha$ ≫ Gi1$\alpha$ | Adenylyl cyclase, other effectors? | ↓ cAMP | 85 |
| | Gz$\alpha$ | Adenylyl cyclase, other effectors? | ↓ cAMP | 86–88 |
| | G$\beta\gamma$ from Gi family members | PLC$\beta$ PI 3-K($\gamma$) | ↑ IP$_3$/DAG ↑3-PPIs | |
| Gs | Gs$\alpha$ | Adenylyl cyclase | ↑ cAMP | 78 |

PLC, phospholipase C; IP$_3$, inositol 1,4,5-trisphosphate; DAG, diacylglycerol; cAMP, cyclic adenosine monophosphate; PPIs, phosphoinositides.

The structural features of GPCR that allow them to interact selectively with the various G proteins are not completely understood (66). Although the recent success in developing a crystallographic structure of rhodopsin has helped considerably, the completed structure of a receptor in its active state has not yet been elucidated. Mutagenesis studies have defined specific residues that may be important in any given receptor. These residues are typically located in the second or third intracellular loops of the receptor. Residues within the $\alpha$ subunit that help determine specificity are located at both ends of the $\alpha$ subunit. ADP-ribosylation of the C-terminus of three of the four Gi$\alpha$ family members in platelets (Gi1$\alpha$, Gi2$\alpha$ and Gi3$\alpha$) uncouples these G proteins from their associated receptors and prevents further signaling.

## G Protein–Coupled Receptors And Platelets

The GPCRs that respond to platelet agonists differ in their potency and their preferences for intracellular effector pathways. Some, such as the receptors for thrombin (PAR1 and PAR4), TxA$_2$ (TP) and ADP (P2Y$_{12}$) (see Fig. 39-3), cause phosphoinositide hydrolysis and raise the cytosolic Ca$^{2+}$ concentration by activating Gq (89). Others, such as the P2Y$_{12}$ receptor for ADP and the $\alpha_{2A}$-adrenergic receptor for epinephrine, are coupled by Gi2 and Gz, respectively, for inhibiting adenylyl cyclase and for activating PI 3-K and Rap1B (24,90–92). Optimal platelet activation by GPCRs is thought to require activation of both a Gq-coupled receptor and a Gi-coupled receptor (93). The ability of the four Gi family members that are expressed in platelets to inhibit adenylyl cyclase (which decreases cAMP formation) is most relevant when PGI$_2$ secreted by endothelial cells has inhibited platelet activation by raising platelet cAMP levels (24). Otherwise, it is probably other Gi effectors that account for the required activation of a Gi-coupled receptor during platelet activation. The biologic relevance of the Gi2-coupled P2Y$_{12}$ receptor for ADP is suggested by the phenotypes of the Gi2 and P2Y$_{12}$ knockout mice and by the well-established usefulness of the P2Y$_{12}$ antagonists ticlopidine and clopidogrel as antiplatelet agents (24,33,91,94,95). Thrombin and TxA$_2$ receptors can also cause the rearrangement of the actin cytoskeleton that underlies platelet shape change by coupling to guanine nucleotide exchange factors for Rho by G12 and G13 (82). In cells other than platelets, the link from G12 family members to Rho activation has been shown to be provided by proteins with RGS domains (for binding to G$\alpha$) and DBL-PH domains (for causing guanine nucleotide exchange on Rho family members)—proteins

such as p115 RhoGEF, LARG, and PDZ-RhoGEF (96). The role of these various proteins (if any) in platelets remains to be determined.

Platelet responses to agonists such as thrombin, ADP, TxA$_2$, and epinephrine can be mediated by a single class of receptors coupled to multiple different families of G proteins, by multiple classes of receptors, each coupled to a single family of G proteins, or by the cumulative effect of two or more agonists, each of which evokes only a subset of the necessary G-protein–mediated responses (97,98). The next section illustrates how this is thought to occur for several essential agonists, beginning with thrombin.

## Platelet Activation by Thrombin

Thrombin is able to activate platelets at concentrations as low as 0.1 nM (approximately 0.01 units per mL). Within seconds the cytosolic Ca$^{2+}$ concentration increases 10-fold to approximately 1 $\mu$M, triggering downstream Ca$^{2+}$-dependent events, including the activation of phospholipase A$_2$. Of these responses, aggregation, phosphoinositide hydrolysis, and the increase in cytosolic Ca$^{2+}$, but not shape change, have been shown to be abolished in platelets from mice lacking Gq$\alpha$ (89). Thrombin also activates Rac and Rho in platelets, leading to rearrangement of the actin cytoskeleton and shape change—presumably mediated by a combination of effector pathways coupled to G12 and Gq activation. Finally, thrombin is able to inhibit adenylyl cyclase activity in human platelets, either directly (by a Gi family member coupled to a thrombin receptor) (99) or indirectly by released ADP (100).

Thrombin activates platelets by GPCRs in the protease-activated receptor (PAR) family, the first member of which (PAR1) was identified in the Vu et al. (34) and Rasmussen et al. (101) laboratories [reviewed at greater length in (102)]. Prior work had shown that platelet responses to thrombin require the enzyme's proteolytic activity and are mediated by G proteins. Binding studies had identified high-affinity interactions with several sites on the platelet surface, including GP Ib$\alpha$, but efforts to establish any of these as a receptor in the signaling sense were not entirely successful. Substrates for thrombin were identified on the platelet surface, including GP V. However, cleavage of GP V did not appear to be required for platelet activation by thrombin.

Four PAR family members have been identified to date, three of which (PAR1, PAR3 and PAR4) are thrombin receptors. Studies on PAR1 established a paradigm that also applies to some of the other family members (see Fig. 39-4). PAR1 is usually activated when thrombin binds to the receptor N-terminus, cleaving it and exposing a new N-terminus that serves as a

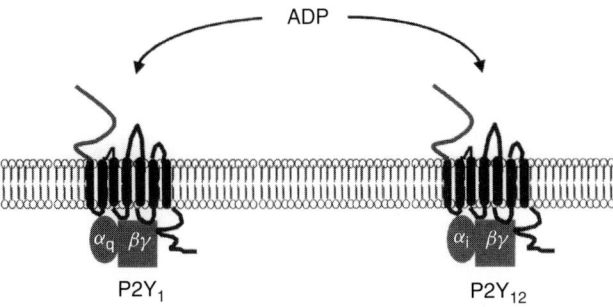

**FIGURE 39-3.** Platelet activation by adenosine diphosphate (ADP). Two receptors that can be activated by ADP have been identified in platelets. P2Y$_1$ and P2Y$_{12}$ are both G protein–coupled receptors but couple to different G protein families and, therefore, mediate different responses. Gq couples P2Y$_1$ receptors to the activation of phospholipase C (PLC)$\beta$. The Gi family member, Gi2, couples P2Y$_{12}$ to the inhibition of cyclic adenosine monophosphate (cAMP) formation (by Gi2$\alpha$) and to effector pathways that include PI 3-K and Rap1B (by G$\beta\gamma$).

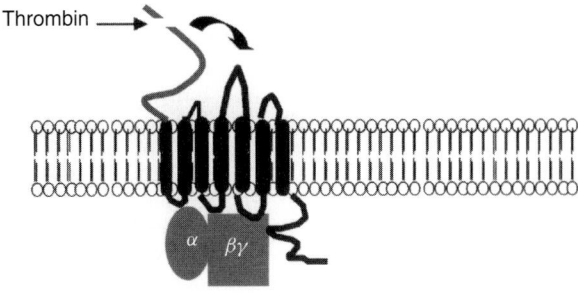

**FIGURE 39-4.** Platelet activation by thrombin. Human platelets express two protease activated receptor (PAR) family members, PAR1 and PAR4, which are coupled to effector pathways by Gq and G12. Cleavage of the receptors of PAR1 and PAR4 exposes a novel amino-terminus that serves as a tethered ligand that binds to the second extracellular loop of the receptor.

tethered ligand. Given sufficient substrate recognition, proteases other than thrombin can also activate PAR1 or, by cleaving in the "wrong" place, can render the receptor unresponsive to a subsequent addition of thrombin (103). The contact sites for the newly exposed tethered ligand have been localized to the membrane-proximal region of the N-terminus and parts of the second extracellular loop (104–106). Because the ligand is not free to diffuse away from the receptor, it is thought to effectively present a higher local concentration at the receptor and perhaps maintain signaling longer than would otherwise occur. Peptides corresponding to the tethered ligand domain (SFLLRN) can also activate PAR1, mimicking the effect of thrombin (34,107). The same is true for PAR2 and PAR4, but not for PAR3.

PAR1 was identified by expression cloning. The second PAR family member to be identified, PAR2, was cloned serendipitously. PAR2 is expressed by endothelial cells, but not by platelets. PAR2 can be cleaved and activated by trypsin, tryptase, TF/VIIa, and factor Xa (108,109), but not by thrombin (110,111). The third family member, PAR3, was identified after gene ablation studies showed that platelets from mice lacking PAR1 were still responsive to thrombin (112). PAR3 is a major regulator of thrombin responses in mouse platelets but appears to do so solely by facilitating cleavage of PAR4 (113,114). PAR4 is expressed on human and mouse platelets and accounts for the continued ability of platelets from PAR3 knockout mice to respond to thrombin (35,36). Simultaneous inhibition of human PAR1 and PAR4 with blocking antibodies or small-molecule antagonists completely abolishes platelet responses to thrombin (115), as does deletion of the gene encoding PAR4 in mice (116). Therefore, the four PAR family members have some features in common, but there are also differences among them. Two of the four family members, PAR1 and PAR3, have similar thrombin dose–response curves, whereas PAR4 requires 10- to 100-fold higher concentrations of thrombin, apparently because it lacks the hirudinlike sequences that can interact with thrombin's anion-binding exosite and facilitate receptor cleavage (35,36, 114,117). Loss of PAR3 expression on mouse platelets, shifts the thrombin dose–response curve to the right (35). Loss of PAR4 abolishes thrombin responses in mouse platelets (116).

Putting all of this together, current evidence suggests that thrombin activates human platelets by cleaving and activating PAR1 and PAR4 (Fig. 39-4). In turn, these receptors promote guanine nucleotide exchange on Gq, G12, and, perhaps, Gi family members, leading to the activation of PLCβ, PI 3-K, and the monomeric G proteins, Rho, Rac, and Rap1—and also

increasing in the cytosolic $Ca^{2+}$ concentration and inhibiting cAMP formation. This process is supported, particularly at suboptimal thrombin concentrations, by released ADP and $TxA_2$. Because cleavage of human PAR4 requires a higher concentration of thrombin than does cleavage of PAR1, it is likely that PAR1 is the predominant signaling receptor at low thrombin concentrations. Recent evidence suggests that once activated, PAR4 signals for a longer period than PAR1 (118,119). In contrast, mouse platelets express PAR3 and PAR4, but signaling appears to be mediated entirely by PAR4 with PAR3 serving solely to facilitate the cleavage of PAR4 at low thrombin concentrations (114,116).

One unresolved issue is the contribution of other thrombin receptors on platelets, particularly GP Ib. GP Ib is a heterodimer composed of an α and a β subunit that are disulfide-linked (120). There is a high-affinity binding site for thrombin at residues 268–287 on GP Ibα (121). Deletion of the extracellular domain of GP Ibα or blockade of the thrombin binding site decreases platelet responses to thrombin (122–125). In theory, the binding of thrombin to GP Ibα could facilitate the cleavage of a PAR family member on human platelets, much as the binding of thrombin to PAR3 is thought to facilitate cleavage of PAR4 on mouse platelets (125).

## Platelet Activation by Adenosine Diphosphate

ADP is stored in platelet dense granules and released upon platelet activation. It is also released from damaged red cells at sites of vascular injury. When added to platelets *in vitro*, ADP causes $TxA_2$ formation, protein phosphorylation, an increase in cytosolic $Ca^{2+}$, shape change, aggregation, and secretion. It also inhibits cAMP formation. These responses are half-maximal at approximately 1 μM concentration of ADP. However, ADP by itself is a weak activator of PLC in human platelets (126,127). According to current models, human platelets express two distinct GPCRs for ADP: $P2Y_1$ and $P2Y_{12}$. Both are members of the purinergic class of GPCRs (Table 39-1 and Fig. 39-3) (94,97,98,128,129). Optimal activation of platelets by ADP requires both $P2Y_1$ and $P2Y_{12}$. A third "ADP" receptor, $P2X_1$, has turned out to be an ATP-gated ion-channel that allow a transient influx of $Ca^{2+}$ before becoming desensitized (130–133). All three proteins have now been cloned and the genes for each have been deleted in mice (see Table 39-3) (31–33,134). In addition, $P2X_1$ has been overexpressed in mouse platelets by the

## TABLE 39-3

PLATELET PHENOTYPES OF G PROTEIN-COUPLED RECEPTOR KNOCKOUT MICE

| Agonist | Receptor | Phenotype | Reference |
|---------|----------|-----------|-----------|
| ADP | $P2Y_1$ and $P2Y_{12}$ | $P2Y_1$: Impaired response to ADP; no increase in cytosolic $Ca^{2+}$ concentration and shape change in response to ADP; normal inhibition of cAMP formation by ADP; greatly diminished aggregation in response to ADP; $P2Y_{12}$: No inhibition of adenylyl cyclase by ADP; increased bleeding time | 31–33 |
| Thrombin | PAR1 | None (not expressed on mouse platelets) | 112,136 |
| | PAR3 | Higher concentrations of thrombin required to elicit responses, presumably due to the loss of the normal contribution of PAR3 to PAR4 activation | 35 |
| | PAR4 | Complete loss of thrombin responsiveness | 116 |
| $TxA_2$ | TPα and TPβ | Prolonged bleeding time, absent aggregation in response to $TxA_2$ agonists, and delayed aggregation with collagen | 137 |
| $PGI_2$ | IP | Increased aggregation in response to ADP; increased thrombosis following vascular injury | 23 |

ADP, adenosine diphosphate; cAMP, cyclic adenosine monophosphate; PAR, protease-activated receptor; $TxA_2$, thromboxane $A_2$; $PGI_2$, prostacyclin.

introduction of a transgene driven by the GP IIb promoter (135). The phenotype of the transgenic mouse includes increased responsiveness to agonists and increased susceptibility to lethal thromboembolism upon injection with collagen plus epinephrine.

In the absence of P2Y$_1$, ADP is still able to inhibit cAMP formation in mouse platelets, but its ability to cause an increase in cytosolic Ca$^{2+}$, shape change, and aggregation is greatly impaired as was previously shown to be the case in platelets from mice that lack Gq$\alpha$ (89). P2Y$_1^{-/-}$ mice have a minimal bleeding time increase and are relatively resistant to disseminated thromboembolism following injection of ADP, but they show no predisposition to spontaneous hemorrhage. Primary responses to platelet agonists other than ADP are unaffected and when combined with serotonin, which is a weak stimulus for PLC in platelets, ADP causes the P2Y$_1^{-/-}$ platelets to aggregate. Therefore, the results with the P2Y$_1$ knockout agree with earlier studies using receptor antagonists (93,97). Taken together with observations made on Gq$\alpha^{-/-}$ mice, platelet P2Y$_1$ receptors are coupled to Gq and are responsible for activation of PLC. In view of the absence of ADP-induced shape change in Gq$\alpha$ knockout mouse platelets (89), it is thought that ADP receptors do not couple to G12 family members in platelets.

The second platelet ADP receptor, P2Y$_{12}$, is also a member of the large family of purinergic GPCRs (94,129). As predicted by inhibitor studies and by the phenotypes of individuals lacking functional P2Y$_{12}$ (138,139), platelets from P2Y$_{12}^{-/-}$ mice do not aggregate normally in response to ADP (139). They retain P2Y$_1$-associated responses, including shape change and PLC activation, but lack the ability to inhibit cAMP formation. The Gi family member associated with P2Y$_{12}$ responses appears to be primarily Gi2, because platelets from Gi2$\alpha^{-/-}$ mice have an impaired ability to aggregate, inhibit cAMP formation, and activate Rap1B in response to ADP, whereas those lacking Gi3$\alpha$ or Gz$\alpha$ respond normally (24,90–92).

The identification of the receptors that mediate platelet responses to ADP, the development of antagonists that target each of the known receptors, and the phenotypes observed in mice lacking the genes encoding P2Y$_1$, P2Y$_{12}$, Gq$\alpha$, or Gi2$\alpha$ have brought an increased appreciation of the contribution of ADP to platelet plug formation *in vivo*; so have studies performed *in vivo* with P2Y$_{12}^{-/-}$ mice in vascular injury and with disseminated thrombosis models. The absence of P2Y$_{12}$ produces a hemorrhagic phenotype in humans, although a relatively mild one (94,138,140) (Table 39-3). Deletion of either P2Y$_1$ or P2Y$_{12}$ prolongs the bleeding time and impairs platelet responses not only to ADP but also to thrombin and TxA$_2$, particularly at low concentrations (32,33,141). Because platelet TxA$_2$ receptors do not couple directly to Gi family members, platelet aggregation induced by TxA$_2$ requires the secretion of ADP to inhibit adenylyl cyclase (142). The identification of P2Y$_1$ and P2Y$_{12}$ has also made it possible to use the isolated receptors for the development of drugs to treat patients with cardiovascular and cerebrovascular disease. Two well-known thienopyridine compounds, ticlopidine and clopidogrel, produce metabolites that block P2Y$_{12}$ irreversibly.

## Platelet Activation by Epinephrine

In contrast to ADP and thrombin, epinephrine is a weak activator of human platelets and appears to serve primarily as a potentiator of platelet responses to other agonists. Nonetheless, there are reports of human families in which a mild bleeding disorder was associated with impaired epinephrine-induced aggregation and reduced numbers of $\alpha_2$-adrenergic receptors (143,144). Platelet responses to epinephrine are mediated by $\alpha_{2A}$-adrenergic receptors and are labile (Table 39-1) (46,47,145). The combination of epinephrine with a suboptimal concentration of ADP,

thrombin, or a TxA$_2$ analog is a stronger stimulus for platelet aggregation than any of these agonists alone. Potentiation has traditionally been attributed to the ability of epinephrine to inhibit cAMP formation, but it is now clear that other effector pathways are also involved, including pathways that lead to Rap1 activation (92). Epinephrine has no detectable direct effect on PLC in platelets and does not cause shape change (146). Taken together, these results suggest that platelet $\alpha_{2A}$-adrenergic receptors are coupled to Gi family members, but not to Gq or G12 family members. Identification of the Gi family member that is the preferred partner for $\alpha_{2A}$-adrenergic receptors in platelets has only recently become possible through studies on platelets lacking Gz$\alpha$.

Of the four Gi$\alpha$ family members in platelets, Gz$\alpha$ is most distinct. Where Gi1$\alpha$, Gi2$\alpha$, and Gi3$\alpha$ are more than 90% identical with each other, and ubiquitously expressed, Gz$\alpha$ is only 60% related to the others at the sequence level and has a restricted pattern of expression that includes some neurons and platelets. Gz$\alpha$ is also notable for having a relatively slow intrinsic rate of GTP hydrolysis (147) and for being a substrate for PKC (148) and p21-activated kinase (PAK) (149). One of the places that the sequence of Gz$\alpha$ diverges from the other Gi$\alpha$ family members is at the C-terminus, which is a domain that is crucial for receptor interactions. In particular, Gz$\alpha$ lacks the cysteine residue near the N-terminus that is the normal site for ADP-ribosylation by pertussis toxin. In reconstitution systems, overexpressed Gz will interact with a variety of receptors (99,150), but studies on platelets from Gz$\alpha^{-/-}$ mice suggest that Gz is the preferred partner for $\alpha_{2A}$-adrenergic receptors in platelets and that it does not contribute substantially to responses to agonists other than epinephrine (90). Aggregation in response to ADP or a PAR4 agonist peptide is normal, but the ability of epinephrine to potentiate responses to other agonists is absent at any concentration likely to be encountered *in vivo*. The diminished aggregation response is accompanied by a loss of epinephrine's normal ability to inhibit PGI$_2$-stimulated cAMP formation and by increased resistance to fatal thromboembolism following injection of epinephrine plus collagen, but not ADP plus collagen (90). Taking all of this together, these results suggest that epinephrine potentiates platelet activation by providing the type of Gi-dependent signaling that can also be seen with ADP but this is done by $\alpha_{2A}$-adrenergic receptors coupled to Gz, rather than by P2Y$_{12}$ receptors coupled to Gi2.

## Platelet Activation by Thromboxane A$_2$

TxA$_2$ is produced from arachidonate in platelets by the aspirin-sensitive cyclooxygenase pathway (see subsequent text). Once formed, TxA$_2$ can diffuse across the plasma membrane and can activate other platelets (Fig. 39-1) (151). Like ADP, this amplifies the initial stimulus for platelet activation and helps recruit additional platelets. This process is effective locally but is limited by the brief (approximately 30 seconds) half-life of TxA$_2$ in solution, helping to confine the spread of platelet activation to the original area of injury.

To date, only one gene encoding a TxA$_2$ receptor has been identified, but there are two splice variants (TP$\alpha$ and TP$\beta$) that differ in their cytoplasmic tails (Table 39-1) (40). Human platelets express both forms of the receptor. Biochemical studies have shown that platelet TxA$_2$ receptors can be physically associated with Gq$\alpha$ (41) and G13$\alpha$ (42) and are able to activate G12 family members (82), which is consistent with the observed ability of TxA$_2$ analogs to cause phosphoinositide hydrolysis and shape change in platelets. Loss of Gq$\alpha$ abolishes U46619-induced IP$_3$ formation and changes in cytosolic Ca$^{2+}$ but does not prevent platelet shape change (89) and U46619 continues to cause guanine nucleotide exchange on

G12$\alpha$/G13$\alpha$ in platelets from Gq$\alpha^{-/-}$ mice (83). Mice lacking G13$\alpha$ have a defect in shape change, aggregation, and thrombosis, whereas mice lacking G12$\alpha$ have no overt platelet phenotype (152). In cells other than platelets, TP has been shown to couple to pertussis toxin-sensitive Gi family members [e.g., see (153)]. However, in platelets, the inhibitory effects of U46619 on cAMP formation appear to be mediated by secreted ADP and are not observed when U46619 is added to platelet membranes (154). This suggests that platelet TP receptors are coupled to Gq and G12 family members, but not to Gi family members. Platelets from mice lacking the gene encoding TP have a prolonged bleeding time and are unable to aggregate in response to TxA$_2$ agonists (Table 39-3). They also show delayed aggregation with collagen, presumably reflecting the role of TxA$_2$ in platelet responses to collagen (137). A group of Japanese patients with impaired platelet responses to TxA$_2$ analogs, but normal ligand binding, have proved to be either homozygous or heterozygous for a missense mutation replacing Arg60 with Leu in the first cytoplasmic loop of TP (155), which presumably affects coupling, but not activation of the receptor.

# SECRETION

The secretory response results in the release of the contents of intracellular storage granules from within the platelet. Granule constituents include substances that can stimulate circulating platelets and cause them to acquire new adhesive properties. These stimulated platelets interact with one another, during platelet aggregation, to form an effective plug to seal the injured vessel wall and prevent excessive blood loss. Most of these substances that are actively and selectively secreted from platelets are packaged in preformed storage granules or are synthesized *de novo* from membrane phospholipids. Platelets contain three types of granules: (a) Dense granules that contain platelet agonists that serve to amplify platelet activation, (b) $\alpha$-granules that contain proteins that enhance the adhesive process, and (c) lysosomal granules that contain glycosidases and proteases that have an unclear function in platelet biology. Platelet secretion is triggered by a variety of strong agonists such as thrombin. Induction of secretion by weak agonists (e.g., ADP) occurs when the cells are brought into close contact such as occurs during aggregation (156,157). The latter secretory mechanism is clearly dependent on TxA$_2$ generated as a consequence of arachidonic acid release.

## Granule Exocytosis

As noted previously, the two morphologically prominent platelet storage granules, $\alpha$-granules and dense bodies, contain a variety of substances important in platelet function. Because these granules have a limiting membrane, it would seem likely that the final secretory event would involve exocytosis (158) (i.e., fusion of the secretory granule membrane with the plasma membrane). This has been observed in dense body secretion (159,160). Several families of proteins have been shown to be required for exocytosis in yeast and neuroendocrine cells. These include Rab GTPases and members of the soluble $N$-ethylmaleimide-sensitive-factor attachment protein receptor (SNARE)–SNAP complex (161–164).

Rab GTPases appear to be essential for both platelet $\alpha$ and dense granule release. The SNARE–SNAP complex has also been shown to be critical for platelet secretion. SNARE proteins are docking proteins that are present on the inner face of the cell membrane, as well as on the outer face of vesicular membranes. The fusion of the vesicular membrane with the cell membrane requires the formation of a core complex created by the binding of SNARE proteins on the opposing membranes. Soluble NSF-Attachment Proteins (SNAPs) facilitate this process. Platelets have been shown to contain numerous members of these families, and blocking antibodies directed against several SNAREs and SNAPs impair granule secretion in permeabilized platelets (162–164).

## Eicosanoids and Arachidonate

In addition to exocytosis of platelet granules, the passive release of TxA$_2$ from platelets is another mechanism to amplify platelet activation. Eicosanoids are formed from the arachidonate released from membrane phospholipids by phospholipase A$_2$ during platelet activation (165–167). Because the availability of arachidonate is the rate-limiting step in this process, phospholipase A$_2$ is tightly controlled. Platelet phospholipase A$_2$ is stimulated by the rise in the cytosolic Ca$^{2+}$ that accompanies platelet activation.

Once released from membrane phospholipids, arachidonate can be metabolized to TxA$_2$ by cyclooxygenase–1 (COX-1) (168). Aspirin acetylates COX-1 causing it to be irreversibly inactivated (169). Because platelets lack the ability to synthesize substantial amounts of protein, inactivation of COX-1 by aspirin blocks TxA$_2$ synthesis until new platelets are formed. Hence, aspirin is the most commonly used drug for antithrombotic therapy. However, there may be a subset of patients who are "aspirin resistant" although the molecular basis for this remains undetermined (170,171). Nonsteroidal antiinflammatory agents also inactivate COX-1, but without covalently modifying the enzyme (172).

Once formed, TxA$_2$ can diffuse across the plasma membrane and activate other platelets through signaling pathways (as described earlier in this chapter). Like ADP, TxA$_2$ amplifies the initial stimulus for platelet activation and helps to recruit additional platelets. This process is effective locally, but is limited by the short half-life of TxA$_2$ in solution, helping to confine the spread of platelet activation to the original area of injury.

# INTRACELLULAR SIGNALING EVENTS

After platelet activation by an agonist, intracellular signaling is needed for cytoskeletal reorganization, fibrinogen receptor exposure, and granule secretion. Two pathways that are central to platelet activation are the phosphoinositide hydrolysis pathway and the eicosanoid synthesis pathway. The phosphoinositide hydrolysis pathway begins when PLC cleaves membrane phosphatidylinositol 4,5-bisphosphate (PIP2) to form IP$_3$ and DAG, both of which serve as second messengers. The eicosanoid pathway begins when phospholipase A$_2$ releases arachidonate from membrane phospholipids to form TxA$_2$. As mentioned in the preceding text, most of the agonists that activate platelets do so by GPCRs, and it is the activation of G proteins that is the first step in the intracellular signaling pathway that leads to platelet second messenger formation.

## Inositol Signaling

### Phospholipase C and PI 3-kinases

One of the earliest responses of platelets to most agonists is the activation of PLC. Platelets contain $\beta$ and $\gamma$ forms of this enzyme. The $\beta$ forms are activated by G proteins, whereas the $\gamma$ forms (predominantly PLC$\gamma_2$) are regulated by tyrosine phosphorylation (173,174). PLC$\beta$ is thought to be primarily responsible for the rapid burst of phosphoinositide hydrolysis that occurs during platelet activation by agonists such as thrombin and TxA$_2$.

In general, PLC$\beta_1$ and PLC$\beta_3$ respond best to G$\alpha$, particularly members of the G$\alpha$q family, whereas PLC$\beta_2$ responds best to G $\beta$-$\gamma$. Coupling of specific heterotrimeric proteins to PLC has been discussed earlier in this chapter. Once activated, PLC hydrolyzes PI-4,5-P(2) to DAG plus IP(3) (175,176). DAG activates PKC and contributes to protein phosphorylation, and IP$_3$ binds to receptors in the dense tubular system and releases sequestered Ca$^{2+}$ (177,178). Additional discussion of these events is presented in the subsequent text.

PI 3-K are a group of enzymes that phosphorylate the D-3 position of the inositol ring of phosphatidylinositol to produce phosphatidylinositol 3-phosphate (PI 3-P), phosphatidylinositol 3,4-bisphosphates (PI 3,4-P2), and phosphatidylinositol 3,4,5-triphosphates (PI 3,4,5-P2 or PI P-3) (179). Four isoforms of PI 3-K that phosphorylate PI, PI 4-P and PIP2 have been described in humans, and are classified according to their catalytic subunit: p110$\alpha$, p110$\beta$, p110$\gamma$, and p110$\delta$.

Using pharmacologic inhibitors, and platelets obtained from genetically modified mice, investigators have begun to understand the role of different PI 3-K isoforms in platelets. Mice lacking the p110$\gamma$ catalytic subunit of PI 3-K have a defect in ADP-mediated platelet aggregation (180,181). Mice lacking the p85$\alpha$ regulatory subunit of PI 3-K have a defect in signaling events initiated by the platelet collagen receptor, GP VI, whereas there is no defect in platelet activation following stimulation by other platelet agonists such as ADP or thrombin (182). Together, the literature suggests that PI 3-K is involved in both the initial activation of GP IIb/IIIa and the subsequent stabilization of the GP IIb/IIIa/fibrinogen interaction that leads to irreversible platelet aggregation.

Cytosolic calcium ions Ca$^{2+}$ ions serve as intracellular second messengers, and like protein kinases, affect enzyme activity and protein–protein interactions. On the basis of studies with intracellular probes such as Fura-2, the cytosolic free Ca$^{2+}$ concentration in resting platelets is approximately 0.1 $\mu$M. Strong agonists, such as thrombin or collagen cause an increase to 1.0 $\mu$M. Weaker agonists, particularly epinephrine, may have little or no effect on cytosolic Ca$^{2+}$.

When platelets are activated, the cytosolic Ca$^{2+}$ concentration increases because of a combination of Ca$^{2+}$ release from the dense tubular system and Ca$^{2+}$ influx across the plasma membrane. The trigger for Ca$^{2+}$ release from the dense tubular system is 1,4,5-IP$_3$, and the trigger for the Ca$^{2+}$ influx may be secreted ATP binding to a gated ion-channel, the P(2X) purinergic receptor. The rise in cytosolic Ca$^{2+}$ concentration contributes to platelet activation by stimulating enzymes that are not optimally active at low Ca$^{2+}$ concentrations. Examples of these include cPLA(2), PLC, phosphorylase kinase, gelsolin, calpain, and myosin light chain kinase.

## Protein Kinase C

PKC isozymes are a family of serine/threonine kinases that play an essential role in the signal transduction mechanisms after activation of receptors. PKC has been identified as the cellular receptor for the lipid second messenger DAG, and it is therefore a key enzyme in the signaling events that follow activation of receptors coupled to PLC. PKC isozymes phosphorylate multiple cellular proteins on serine and threonine residues. Although some discrepancies between different studies on PKC isozyme expression exist, platelets probably express PKC $\alpha$, $\beta$, $\delta$, $\varepsilon$, $\eta$, $\theta$, and, perhaps, $\zeta$ and $\lambda$ (183).

Because of the limitations of platelets as a system for genetic studies, pharmacologic tools have been widely used in platelets. Consequently, both activation of PKC with phorbol esters (such as PMA or phorbol-12-myristate-13-acetate) and

pharmacologic inhibition with PKC have been the preferred approaches used to understand the involvement of PKC isozymes in platelet biology. PKC isozymes control a variety of functions, including aggregation, release of granular contents, mobilization of intracellular calcium, and regulation of cell shape. The $\delta$ and $\theta$ isoforms may be particularly important for these functions (184,185). PKC isozymes also play an important role in megakaryocyte differentiation.

## Other Protein Kinases

In addition to serine/threonine kinases such as PKC, platelets contain a large number of tyrosine kinases, some of which become active during platelet activation. Human platelets contain tyrosine kinases that are receptors for extracellular ligands, as well as large number of nonreceptor (cytoplasmic) tyrosine kinases, including Src, Fyn, Lyn, Hck, and Syk. Nonspecific inhibitors of tyrosine kinases, such as genistein or the tyrphostins, can inhibit platelet activation.

Inhibitors of phosphotyrosine phosphatases, such as vanadate, promote platelet activation. In general, tyrosine phosphorylation can serve two roles. It can have a regulatory effect on the phosphorylated protein, perhaps by causing a conformational change, or it can provide a binding site for modular domains located in other proteins, such as SH2 domains. Although studies of knockout mice have identified the role of some of these proteins in signaling pathways downstream of the GP VI collagen receptor, the function of most tyrosine kinases in platelets is still not completely understood (186).

## Cyclic Adenosine Monophosphate

Agents that raise the cAMP concentration in platelets inhibit platelet activation, but the mechanism by which this occurs is unclear. In general, the effects of cAMP are thought to be mediated by cAMP-dependent protein kinase, also known as protein kinase A.

Platelet substrates for this enzyme include the 24-kDa $\beta$ chain of GP Ib, actin-binding protein, and myosin light chain, VASP and Rap1B. Raising cAMP levels causes a number of specific changes in platelet function, including impaired phosphoinositide hydrolysis, a smaller increase in the cytosolic free Ca$^{2+}$ concentration in response to agonists, and an accelerated uptake of Ca$^{2+}$ into the dense tubular system.

PGI$_2$ released from activated endothelial cells elevates platelet cAMP levels by stimulating receptors on the platelet surface that are coupled to adenylyl cyclase by Gs. This results in an inhibition of platelet activation. Consequently, mice lacking the PGI$_2$ receptor show an increased risk of thrombosis (23). Most platelet agonists suppress cAMP formation by inhibiting adenylyl cyclase by one or more of the G$\alpha$i family members that are expressed in platelets.

The drug dipyridamole (Persantine) exerts antiplatelet effects by inhibiting cAMP phosphodiesterase, thereby raising cAMP levels within platelets (14). However, its efficacy has been debated. Sildenafil has phosphodiesterase activity and thereby decreases platelet cAMP levels. It has been speculated that this may contribute to the cardiovascular toxicity of this drug (187).

## Signals to and from $\alpha_{IIb}\beta_3$

One of the crucial unanswered questions in platelet biology, is the mechanism by which inside-out signaling pathways produce integrin activation. Activation of $\alpha_{IIb}\beta_3$ is required for fibrinogen to bind to the platelet surface and, therefore, for aggregation to occur. Human and mouse platelets that lack $\alpha_{IIb}\beta_3$ don't aggregate. Normal platelets incubated with $\alpha_{IIb}\beta_3$ blockers of many sorts also show reduced or absent aggregation. The intracellular events that link platelet agonists to integrin activation have proved to be elusive, in part because no single signaling pathways appears to be uniquely responsible. The early (receptor-proximal) events have been identified and the late (integrin-proximal) events are starting to be identified, but much that is in between remains *terra incognita*. In general terms, the early events include the activation of one or more PLC isoforms yielding a rise in the cytosolic $Ca^{2+}$ concentration and the activation of PKC. Late events include cytoskeletal proteins such as talin, which can bind to the cytoplasmic domain of $\beta_3$ (188). Rap1B and various guanine nucleotide exchange factor for Rap1B appear to be intermediates, but certainly are not the only ones (189–193).

In addition to the inside-out signaling events that lead to activation of GP IIb/IIIa, there are also outside-in signaling events that occur downstream of activated $\alpha_{IIb}\beta_3$ once fibrinogen binding has occurred. Fibrinogen binding to and clustering of $\alpha_{IIb}\beta_3$ stimulates rapid increases in the activities of integrin-associated Src family and Syk tyrosine kinases. Studies of platelets from mice lacking these kinases suggest that these events are required for the initiation of outside-in signaling and for full platelet spreading, irreversible aggregation, and clot retraction (194–197). Platelet aggregation results in the formation of large signaling and structural complexes that include $\alpha_{IIb}\beta_3$. One of the proteins in these complexes is the kinase, focal adhesion kinase (FAK), which, when phosphorylated, can provide a binding site for (among other proteins) Src and the p85 subunit of PI 3-K (198). Proteins capable of binding directly to the cytoplasmic domains of $\alpha_{IIb}\beta_3$ include $\beta_3$-endonexin (199), CIB (200,201), talin (188), Syk (202,203), myosin (204) and Shc (205). Shc binding requires phosphorylation of Y759 in the $\beta_3$ cytoplasmic domain (205). Myosin binding requires phosphorylation of both Y747 and Y759 (204). The binding of talin, $\beta_3$-endonexin, and CIB is thought to be independent of $\beta_3$ tyrosine phosphorylation. Some of the protein–protein interactions that involve the cytoplasmic domains of $\alpha_{IIb}\beta_3$ (including talin) help regulate integrin activation, others participate in outside-in signaling and clot retraction. Tyrosine phosphorylation of $\beta_3$ is thought to be integral to the latter two events.

Tyrosine residues 747 and 759 of $\beta_3$ become phosphorylated following the onset of platelet aggregation (204). Phosphorylation requires both activation of the integrin and its engagement with an adhesive protein. Inhibition of aggregation with an RGD-containing peptide or a peptidomimetic inhibits phosphorylation of $\beta_3$ (204). According to one model (195,196), platelet activation and aggregation leads to the activation of a Src family member and the subsequent phosphorylation of $\beta_3$. Consistent with this hypothesis, phosphorylation is diminished in Fyn$^{-/-}$ mouse platelets (196). Mutation of both Y747 and Y759 to phenylalanine produces mice whose platelets tend to disaggregate and that show reduced clot retraction and a tendency to rebleed from tail-bleeding time sites (206). Clot retraction refers to the decreased volume of a clot that occurs when embedded platelets pull on fibrin strands. Loss of clot retraction is a hallmark of $\alpha_{IIb}\beta_3$-deficient platelets from patients with Glanzmann thrombasthenia, reflecting the dependence of clot retraction on the interaction of $\alpha_{IIb}\beta_3$ with extracellular fibrin and with intracellular actin/myosin filaments. The diminished clot retraction in the Y747F/Y759F mice is consistent with a reduction in the binding of myosin to $\beta_3$. Failure to phosphorylate $\beta_3$ in the Y747F/Y759F mice would also prevent the binding of the adaptor protein Shc (205), abolishing any signaling pathways that lie downstream from that point.

## References

1. Moake JL. Thrombotic microangiopathies. *N Engl J Med* 2002;347: 589–600.
2. Dong J, Moake JL, Nolasco L, et al. ADAMTS13 rapidly cleaves newly secreted ultra-large von Willebrand factor multimers on the endothelial surface under flowing conditions. *Blood* 2002;100:4033–4039.
3. Chow TW, Turner NA, Chintagumpala M, et al. Increased von Willebrand factor binding to platelets in single episode and recurrent types of thrombotic thrombocytopenic purpura. *Am J Hematol* 1998;57:293–302.
4. Levy GG, Nichols WC, Lian EC. Mutations in a member of the ADAMTS gene family cause thrombotic thrombocytopenic purpura. *Nature* 2001;413:488–494.
5. Ruggeri ZM. Platelets in atherothrombosis. *Nat Med* 2002;8:1227–1234.
6. Huizinga EG, Tsuji S, Romijn RAP, et al. Structures of glycoprotein Ibalpha and its complex with von Willebrand factor A1 domain. *Science* 2002;297:1176–1179.
7. Moncada S, Ryglewski R, Bunting S, et al. An enzyme isolated from arteries transforms prostacglandin endoperoxides to an unstable substance that inhibits platelet aggregation. *Nature* 1976;263:663–665.
8. Miller OV, Gorman RR. Modulation of platelet cyclic nucleotide content by PGE1 and the prostaglandin endoperoxide PGG2. *J Cyclic Nucleotide Res* 1976;2:79–87.
9. Gorman RR, Fitzpatrick FA, Miller OV. Reciprocal regulation of human platelet cAMP levels by thromboxane A2 and prostacyclin. *Adv Cyclic Nucleotide Res* 1978;9:597–609.
10. Haslam RJ, Dickinson NT, Jang EK. Cyclic nucleotides and phosphodiesterases in platelets. *Thromb Haemost* 1999;82:412–423.
11. Mills DCB, Smith JB. The influence on platelet aggregation of drugs that affect the accumulation of adenosine 3′:5′ cyclic monophosphate in platelets. *Biochem J* 1971;121:185–196.
12. Eigenthaler M, Nolte C, Halbrugge M, et al. Concentration and regulation of cyclic nucleotides, cyclic-nucleotide-dependent protein kinases and one of their major substrates in human platelets. Estimating the rate of cAMP-regulated and cGMP-regulated protein phosphorylation in intact cells. *Eur J Biochem* 1992;205:471–481.
13. Keularts IMLW, Van Gorp RMA, Feijge MAH, et al. alpha2Aadrenergic receptor stimulation potentiates calcium release in platelets by modulating cAMP levels. *J Biol Chem* 2000;275:1763–1772.
14. Schwarz UR, Walter U, Eigenthaler M. Taming platelets with cyclic nucleotides. *Biochem Pharmacol* 2001;62:1153–1161.
15. Fox JEB, Reynolds CC, Johnson MM. Identification of glycoprotein Ibbeta as one of the major proteins phosphorylated during expsoure of intact platelets to agents that activate cAMP-dependent protein kinase. *J Biol Chem* 1987;262:12627–12631.
16. Wardell MR, Reynolds CC, Berndt MC, et al. Platelet glycoprotein Ibbeta is phosphorylated on serine 166 by cyclic AMP-dependent protein kinase. *J Biol Chem* 1989;264:15656–15661.
17. Wallach D, Davies PJA, Pastan I. Cyclic AMP-dependent phosphorylation of filamin in mammalian smooth muscle. *J Biol Chem* 1978;253:4739–4745.
18. Hathway DR, Adelstein RS. Human platelet myosin light chain kinase requires the calcium-binding protein calmodulin for activity. *Proc Natl Acad Sci U S A* 1979;76:1653–1657.
19. Hallam TJ, Daniel JL, Kendrick Jones J, et al. Relationship between cytoplasmic free calcium and myosin light chain phosphorylation in intact platelets. *Biochem J* 1985;232:373–377.
20. Halbrügge M, Walter U. Analysis, purification and properties of a 50 000-dalton membrane-associated phosphoprotein from human platelets. *J Chromatogr* 1990;521:335–343.
21. Nolte C, Eigenthaler M, Schanzenbacher P, et al. Comparison of vasodilatory prostaglandins with respect to cAMP-mediated phosphorylation of a target substrate in intact human platelets. *Biochem Pharmacol* 1991;42: 253–262.
22. Fischer TH, Gatling MN, Lacal J-C, et al. Rap1B, a cAMP-dependent protein kinase substrate, associates with the platelet cytoskeleton. *J Biol Chem* 1990;265:19405–19408.
23. Murata T, Ushikubi F, Matsuoka T, et al. Altered pain perception and inflammatory response in mice lacking prostacyclin receptor. *Nature* 1997; 388:678–682.
24. Yang J, Wu J, Jiang H, et al. Signaling through Gi family members in platelets: redundancy and specificity in the regulation of adenylyl cyclase and other effectors. *J Biol Chem* 2002;277:46035–46042.
25. Marcus AJ, Broekman MJ, Drosopoulos JHF, et al. The endothelial cell ecto-ADPase responsible for inhibition of platelet function is CD39. *J Clin Invest* 1997;99:1351–1360.
26. Gayle RB III, Maliszewski CR, Gimpel SD, et al. Inhibition of platelet function by recombinant soluble ecto-ADPase/CD39. *J Clin Invest* 1998; 101:1851–1859.
27. Simons K, Ikonen E. Functional rafts in cell membranes. *Nature* 1997; 387:569–572.
28. Locke D, Chen H, Liu Y, et al. Lipid rafts orchestrate signaling by the platelet receptor glycoprotein VI. *J Biol Chem* 2002;277:18801–18809.
29. Shrimpton CN, Borthakur G, Larrucea S, et al. Localization of the adhesion receptor glycoprotein Ib-IX-V complex to lipid rafts is required for platelet adhesion and activation. *J Exp Med* 2002;196:1057–1066.
30. Gousset K, Wolkers WF, Tsvetkova NM, et al. Evidence for a physiological role for membrane rafts in human platelets. *J Cell Physiol* 2002;190: 117–128.
31. Fabre J-E, Nguyen M, Latour A, et al. Decreased platelet aggregation, increased bleeding time and resistance to thromboembolism in P2Y1-deficient mice. *Nat Med* 1999;5:1199–1202.
32. Léon C, Hechler B, Freund M, et al. Defective platelet aggregation and increased resistance to thrombosis in purinergic P2Y1 receptor-null mice. *J Clin Invest* 1999;104:1731–1737.

33. Foster CJ. Molecular identification and characterization of the platelet ADP receptor targeted by thienopyridine drugs using P2Yac-null mice. *J Clin Invest* 2001;107:1591–1598.

34. Vu T-KH, Hung DT, Wheaton VI, et al. Molecular cloning of a functional thrombin receptor reveals a novel proteolytic mechanism of receptor activation. *Cell* 1991;64:1057–1068.

35. Kahn ML, Zheng YW, Huang W, et al. A dual thrombin receptor system for platelet activation. *Nature* 1998;394:690–694.

36. Xu W-F, Andersen H, Whitmore TE, et al. Cloning and characterization of human protease-activated receptor 4. *Proc Natl Acad Sci U S A* 1998; 95:6642–6646.

37. Brass LF, Vassallo RR Jr., Belmonte E, et al. Structure and function of the human platelet thrombin receptor: studies using monoclonal antibodies against a defined epitope within the receptor N-terminus. *J Biol Chem* 1992;267:13795–13798.

38. Ishihara H, Connolly AJ, Zeng D, et al. Protease-activated receptor 3 is a second thrombin receptor in humans. *Nature* 1997;386:502–506.

39. Faruqi TR, Weiss EJ, Shapiro MJ, et al. Structure-function analysis of protease-activated receptor 4 tethered ligand peptides -Determinants of specificity and utility in assays of receptor function. *J Biol Chem* 2000;275: 19728–19734.

40. Hirata T, Ushikubi F, Kakizuka A, et al. Two thromboxane A2 receptor isoforms in human platelets—Opposite coupling to adenylyl cyclase with different sensitivity to Arg60 to Leu mutation. *J Clin Invest* 1996;97:949–956.

41. Knezevic I, Borg C, Le Breton GC. Identification of Gq as one of the G-proteins which copurify with human platelet thromboxane A2/prostaglandin H2 receptors. *J Biol Chem* 1993;268:26011–26017.

42. Djellas Y, Manganello JM, Antonakis K, et al. Identification of Galpha13 as one of the G-proteins that couple to human platelet thromboxane A2 receptors. *J Biol Chem* 1999;274:14325–14330.

43. Hirata M, Hayashi Y, Ushikubi F, et al. Cloning and expression of cDNA for a human thromboxane A$_2$ receptor. *Nature* 1991;349:617–620.

44. Hanasaki K, Arita H. Characterization of thromboxane A$_2$/prostaglandin H$_2$(TXA$_2$/PGH$_2$) receptors of rat platelets and their interaction with TXA$_2$/PGH$_2$ receptor antagonists. *Biochem Pharmacol* 1988;37:3923–3929.

45. Furci L, Fitzgerald DJ, FitzGerald GA. Heterogeneity of prostaglandin H$_2$/thromboxane A$_2$ receptors: distinct subtypes mediate vascular smooth muscle contraction and platelet aggregation. *J Pharmacol Exp Ther* 1991; 258:74–81.

46. Kaywin P, McDonough M, Insel PA, et al. Platelet function in essential thrombocythemia: decreased epinephrine responsivenesss associated with a deficiency of platelet alpha-adrenergic receptors. *N Engl J Med* 1978; 299:505–509.

47. Motulsky HJ, Insel PA. [$^3$H]Dihydroergocryptine binding to alpha-adrenergic receptors of human platelets. A reassessment using the selective radioligands [$^3$H]prazosin, [$^3$H]yohimbine, and [$^3$H]rauwolscine. *Biochem Pharmacol* 1982;31:2591–2597.

48. Kobilka BK, Matsui H, Kobilka TS, et al. Cloning, sequencing, and expression of the gene coding for the human platelet $\alpha_2$-adrenergic receptor. *Science* 1987;238:650–656.

49. Vane JR, Botting RM. Pharmacodynamic profile of prostacyclin. *Am J Cardiol* 1995;75:3A–10A.

50. Falati S, Gross P, Merrill-Skoloff G, et al. Real-time *in vivo* imaging of platelets, tissue factor and fibrin during arterial thrombus formation in the mouse. *Nat Med* 2002;8:1175–1180.

51. Patel D, Vaananen H, Jirouskova M, et al. Dynamics of GP IIb/IIIa-mediated platelet-platelet interactions in platelet adhesion/thrombus formation on collagen *in vitro* as revealed by videomicroscopy. *Blood* 2003;101:929–936.

52. Clemetson JM, Polgar J, Magnenat E, et al. The platelet collagen receptor glycoprotein VI is a member of the immunoglobulin superfamily closely related to FcalphaR and the natural killer receptors. *J Biol Chem* 1999; 274:29019–29024.

53. Poole A, Gibbins JM, Turner M, et al. The Fc receptor gamma-chain and the tyrosine kinase Syk are essential for activation of mouse platelets by collagen. *EMBO J* 1997;16:2333–2341.

54. Nieuwenhuis HK, Akkerman JWN, Houdijk WPM, et al. Human blood platelets showing no response to collagen fail to express glycoprotein Ia. *Nature* 1985;318:470–472.

55. Sixma JJ, Van Zanten GH, Huizinga EG, et al. Platelet adhesion to collagen: an update. *Thromb Haemost* 1997;78:434–438.

56. Nieswandt B, Brakebusch C, Bergmeier W, et al. Glycoprotein VI but not alpha2beta1 integrin is essential for platelet interaction with collagen. *EMBO J* 2001;20:2120–2130.

57. Fujita H, Hashimoto Y, Russell S, et al. *In vivo* expression of murine platelet glycoprotein Ibalpha. *Blood* 1998;92:488–495.

58. Razdan K, Hellums JD, Kroll MH. Shear-stress-induced von Willebrand factor binding to platelets causes the activation of tyrosine kinase(s). *Biochem J* 1994;302:681–686.

59. Asazuma N, Ozaki Y, Satoh K, et al. Glycoprotein Ib von Willebrand factor interactions activate tyrosine kinases in human platelets. *Blood* 1997; 90:4789–4798.

60. Kasirer-Friede A, Ware J, Leng LJ, et al. Lateral clustering of platelet GP Ib-IX complexes leads to up-regulation of the adhesive function of integrin alphaIIbbeta3. *J Biol Chem* 2002;277:11949–11956.

61. Yap CL, Anderson KE, Hughan SC, et al. Essential role for phosphoinositide 3-kinase in shear-dependent signaling between platelet glycoprotein Ib/V/IX and integrin alphaIIbbeta3. *Blood* 2002;99:151–158.

62. Feng S, Resendiz JC, Lu X, et al. Filamin binding to the cytoplasmic tail of glycoprotein Ibalpha regulates von Willebrand factor-induced platelet activation. *Blood* 2003;102:2122–2129.

63. Wu Y, Asazuma N, Satoh K, et al. Interaction between von Willebrand factor and glycoprotein Ib activates Src kinases in human platelets: the role of phosphoinositide 3-kinase. *Blood* 2003;101:3469–3476.

64. Chow TW, Hellums DJ, Moake JL, et al. Shear stress-induced von Willebrand factor binding to platelet glycoprotein Ib initiates calcium influx associated with aggregation. *Blood* 1992;80:113–120.

65. Mazzucato M, Pradella P, Cozzi MR, et al. Sequential cytoplasmic calcium signals in a 2-stage platelet activation process induced by the glycoprotein Ibalpha mechanoreceptor. *Blood* 2002;100:2793–2800.

66. Hamm HE. How activated receptors couple to G proteins. *Proc Natl Acad Sci U S A* 2001;98:4819–4821.

67. Gomes I, Jordan BA, Gupta A, et al. G protein coupled receptor dimerization: implications in modulating receptor function. *J Mol Med* 2001;79: 226–242.

68. Jordan BA, Devi LA. G-protein-coupled receptor heterodimerization modulates receptor function. *Nature* 1999;399:697–700.

69. Bünemann M, Lee KB, Pals-Rylaarsdam R, et al. Desensitization of G-protein–coupled receptors in the cardiovascular system. *Annu Rev Physiol* 1999;61:169–192.

70. Penn RB, Pronin AN, Benovic JL. Regulation of G protein-coupled receptor kinases. *Trends Cardiovasc Med* 2000;10:81–89.

71. Lambright DG, Sondek J, Bohm A, et al. The 2.0 Å crystal structure of a heterotrimeric G protein. *Nature* 1996;379:311–319.

72. Ford CE, Skiba NP, Bae HS, et al. Molecular basis for interactions of G protein betagamma subunits with effectors. *Science* 1998;280:1271–1274.

73. Hamm HE. The many faces of G protein signaling. *J Biol Chem* 1998; 273:669–672.

74. Gilman AG. G proteins: transducers of receptor-generated signals. *Annu Rev Biochem* 1987;56:615–649.

75. Ross EM, Wilkie TM. GTPase-activating proteins for heterotrimeric G proteins: regulators of G protein signaling (RGS) and RGS-like proteins. *Annu Rev Biochem* 2000;69:795–827.

76. Shenker A, Goldsmith P, Unson CG, et al. The G protein coupled to the thromboxane A$_2$ receptor in human platelets is a member of the novel G$_q$ family. *J Biol Chem* 1991;266:9309–9313.

77. Brass LF, Hoxie JA, Manning DR. Signaling through G proteins and G protein-coupled receptors during platelet activation. *Thromb Haemost* 1993;70:217–223.

78. Van Willigen G, Donath J, Lapetina EG, et al. Identification of $\alpha$-subunits of trimeric GTP-binding proteins in human platelets by RT-PCR. *Biochem Biophys Res Commun* 1995;214:254–262.

79. Aragay AM, Quick MW. Functional regulation of Galpha16 by protein kinase C. *J Biol Chem* 1999;274:4807–4815.

80. Giesberts AN, Van Ginneken M, Gorter G, et al. Subcellular localization of alpha-subunits of trimeric G-proteins in human platelets. *Biochem Biophys Res Commun* 1997;234:439–444.

81. Tenailleau S, Corre J, Hermouet S. Specific expression of heterotrimeric G proteins G12 and G16 during human myeloid differentiation. *Exp Hematol* 1997;25:927–934.

82. Offermanns S, Laugwitz K-L, Spicher K, et al. G proteins of the G12 family are activated via thromboxane A2 and thrombin receptors in human platelets. *Proc Natl Acad Sci U S A* 1994;91:504–508.

83. Klages B, Brandt U, Simon MI, et al. Activation of G12/G13 results in shape change and Rho/Rho-kinase-mediated myosin light chain phosphorylation in mouse platelets. *J Cell Biol* 1999;144:745–754.

84. Offermanns S, Hu YH, Simon MI. Galpha12 and galpha13 are phosphorylated during platelet activation. *J Biol Chem* 1996;271:26044–26048.

85. Williams A, Woolkalis MJ, Poncz M, et al. Identification of the pertussis toxin-sensitive G proteins in platelets, megakaryocytes and HEL cells. *Blood* 1990;76:721–730.

86. Carlson K, Brass LF, Manning DR. Thrombin and phorbol esters cause the selective phosphorylation of a G protein other than G$_i$ in human platelets. *J Biol Chem* 1989;264:13298–13305.

87. Lounsbury KM, Brass LF, Manning DR. Phosphorylation of Gz$\alpha$ in human platelets: proximity to the amino-terminus of the subunit. *J Cell Biochem* 1990;111:334a.

88. Gagnon AW, Manning DR, Catani L, et al. Identification of Gz$\alpha$ as a pertussis toxin-insensitive G protein in human platelets and megakaryocytes. *Blood* 1991;78:1247–1253.

89. Offermanns S, Toombs CF, Hu YH, et al. Defective platelet activation in Galphaqdeficient mice. *Nature* 1997;389:183–186.

90. Yang J, Wu J, Kowalska MA, et al. Loss of signaling through the G protein, Gz, results in abnormal platelet activation and altered responses to psychoactive drugs. *Proc Natl Acad Sci U S A* 2000;97:9984–9989.

91. Jantzen H-M, Milstone DS, Gousset L, et al. Impaired activation of murine platelets lacking Galphai2. *J Clin Invest* 2001;108:477–483.

92. Woulfe D, Jiang H, Mortensen R, et al. Activation of Rap1B by Gi family members in platelets. *J Biol Chem* 2002;277:23382–23390.

93. Jin JG, Kunapuli SP. Coactivation of two different G protein–coupled receptors is essential for ADP-induced platelet aggregation. *Proc Natl Acad Sci U S A* 1998;95:8070–8074.

94. Hollopeter G, Jantzen HM, Vincent D, et al. Identification of the platelet ADP receptor targeted by antithrombotic drugs. *Nature* 2001;409: 202–207.

95. Gachet C. ADP receptors of platelets and their inhibition. *Thromb Haemost* 2001;86:222–232.

96. Fukuhara S, Chikumi H, Gutkind JS. RGS-containing RhoGEFs: the missing link between transforming G proteins and Rho? *Oncogene* 2001;20: 1661–1668.

97. Daniel JL, Dangelmaier C, Jin JG, et al. Molecular basis for ADP-induced platelet activation I. Evidence for three distinct ADP receptors on human platelets. *J Biol Chem* 1998;273:2024–2029.

98. Jin JG, Daniel JL, Kunapuli SP. Molecular basis for ADP-induced platelet activation II. The P2Y1 receptor mediates ADP-induced intracellular calcium mobilization and shape change in platelets. *J Biol Chem* 1998;273: 2030–2034.

99. Barr AJ, Brass LF, Manning DR. Reconstitution of receptors and GTP-binding regulatory proteins (G proteins) in Sf9 cells—A direct evaluation of selectivity in receptor. G protein coupling. *J Biol Chem* 1997; 272:2223–2229.

100. Kim S, Foster C, Lecchi A, et al. Protease-activated receptors 1 and 4 do not stimulate Gi signaling pathways in the absence of secreted ADP and cause human platelet aggregation independently of Gi signaling. *Blood* 2002;99:3629–3636.

101. Rasmussen UB, Vouret-Craviari V, Jallat S, et al. cDNA Cloning and expression of a hamster alpha-thrombin receptor coupled to Ca2+ mobilization. *FEBS Lett* 1991;288:123–128.

102. Brass LF. Thrombin and platelet activation. *Chest* 2003;124:18S–25S.

103. Molino M, Blanchard N, Belmonte E, et al. Proteolysis of the human platelet and endothelial cell thrombin receptor by neutrophil-derived cathepsin G. *J Biol Chem* 1995;270:11168–11175.

104. Bahou WF, Kutok JL, Wong A, et al. Identification of a novel thrombin receptor sequence required for activation-dependent responses. *Blood* 1994; 84:4195–4202.

105. Nanevicz T, Ishii M, Wang L, et al. Mechanisms of thrombin receptor agonist specificity -Chimeric receptors and complementary mutations identify an agonist recognition site. *J Biol Chem* 1995;270:21619–21625.

106. Gerszten RF, Chen J, Ishii M, et al. Specificity of the thrombin receptor for agonist peptide is defined by its extracellular surface. *Nature* 1994; 368:648–651.

107. Vassallo RR Jr, Kieber-Emmons T, Cichowski K, et al. Structure/function relationships in the activation of platelet thrombin receptors by receptor-derived peptides. *J Biol Chem* 1992;267:6081–6085.

108. Camerer E, Huang W, Coughlin SR. Tissue factor– and factor X–dependent activation of protease-activated receptor 2 by factor VIIa. *Proc Natl Acad Sci U S A* 2000;97:5255–5260.

109. Camerer E, Rottingen J-A, Gjernes E, et al. Coagulation factors VIIa and Xa induce cell signaling leading to up-regulation of the egr1 gene. *J Biol Chem* 1999;274:32225–32233.

110. Nystedt S, Emilsson K, Wahlestedt C, et al. Molecular cloning of a potential proteinase activated receptor. *Proc Natl Acad Sci U S A* 1994;91: 9208–9212.

111. Nystedt S, Emilsson K, Larsson AK, et al. Molecular cloning and functional expression of the gene encoding the human proteinase-activated receptor 2. *Eur J Biochem* 1995;232:84–89.

112. Connolly AJ, Ishihara H, Kahn ML, et al. Role of the thrombin receptor in development and evidence for a second receptor. *Nature* 1996;381: 516–519.

113. Ishihara H, Connolly AJ, Zeng D, et al. Protease-activated receptor 3 is a second thrombin receptor in humans. *Nature* 1997;386:502–508.

114. Nakanishi-Matsui M, Zheng YW, Sulciner DJ, et al. PAR3 is a cofactor for PAR4 activation by thrombin. *Nature* 2000;404:609–610.

115. Kahn ML, Nakanishi-Matsui M, Shapiro MJ, et al. Protease-activated receptors 1 and 4 mediate activation of human platelets by thrombin. *J Clin Invest* 1999;103:879–887.

116. Sambrano GR, Weiss EJ, Zheng Y-W, et al. Role of thrombin signaling in platelets in hemostasis and thrombosis. *Nature* 2001;413:74–78.

117. Ishii K, Gerszten R, Zheng YW, et al. Determinants of thrombin receptor cleavage. Receptor domains involved, specificity, and role of the P3 aspartate. *J Biol Chem* 1995;270:16435–16440.

118. Covic L, Gresser AL, Kuliopulos A. Biphasic kinetics of activation and signaling for PAR1 and PAR4 thrombin receptors in platelets. *Biochemistry* 2000;39:5458–5467.

119. Shapiro MJ, Weiss EJ, Faruqi TR, et al. Protease-activated receptors 1 and 4 are shut off with distinct kinetics after activation by thrombin. *J Biol Chem* 2000;275:25216–25221.

120. Lopez JA, Andrews RK, Afshar-Khargan V, et al. Bernard-Soulier syndrome. *Blood* 1998;91:4397–4418.

121. De Cristofaro R, De Candia E, Rutella S, et al. The Asp272-Glu282 region of platelet glycoprotein Ibalpha interacts with the heparin-binding site of alpha-thrombin and protects the enzyme from the heparin-catalyzed inhibition by antithrombin III. *J Biol Chem* 2000;275:3887–3895.

122. De Marco L, Mazzucato M, Masotti A, et al. Function of glycoprotein Ibalpha in platelet activation induced by alpha-thrombin. *J Biol Chem* 1991;266:23776–23783.

123. Harmon JT, Jamieson GA. Platelet activation by thrombin in the absence of the high affinity thrombin receptor. *Biochemistry* 1988;27:2151–2157.

124. Mazzucato M, De Marco L, Masotti A, et al. Characterization of the initial alpha-thrombin interaction with glycoprotein Ibalpha in relation to platelet activation. *J Biol Chem* 1998;273:1880–1887.

125. De Candia E, Hall SW, Rutella S, et al. Binding of thrombin to glycoprotein Ib accelerates hydrolysis of PAR1 on intact platelets. *J Biol Chem* 2001;276:4692–4698.

126. Fisher GJ, Bakshian S, Baldassare JJ. Activation of human platelets by ADP causes a rapid rise in cytosolic free calcium without hydrolysis of phosphatidylinositol-4,5-bisphosphate. *Biochem Biophys Res Commun* 1985;129:958–964.

127. Daniel JL, Dangelmaier CA, Selak M, et al. ADP stimulates IP3 formation in human platelets. *FEBS Lett* 1986;206:299–303.

128. Léon C, Hechler B, Vial C, et al. The P2Y1 receptor is an ADP receptor antagonized by ATP and expressed in platelets and megakaryoblastic cells. *FEBS Lett* 1997;403:26–30.

129. Zhang FL, Luo L, Gustafson E, et al. ADP is the cognate ligand for the orphan G protein-coupled receptor SP1999. *J Biol Chem* 2001;276:8608–8615.

130. McKenzie AB, Mahout-Smith MP, Sage SO. Activation of receptor-operated channels via P2X1 not P2T purinoreceptors in human platelets. *J Biol Chem* 1996;271:2879–2881.

131. Vial C, Hechler B, Léon C, et al. Presence of P2X1 purinoceptors in human platelets and megakaryoblastic cell lines. *Thromb Haemost* 1997;78: 1500–1504.

132. Sun B, Li J, Okahara K, et al. P2X1 purinoceptor in human platelets molecular cloning and functional characterization after heterologous expression. *J Biol Chem* 1998;273:11544–11547.

133. Mahaut-Smith MP, Ennion SJ, Rolf MG, et al. ADP is not an agonist at P2X1 receptors: evidence for separate receptors stimulated by ATP and ADP on human platelets. *Br J Pharmacol* 2000;131:108–114.

134. Mulryan K, Gitterman DP, Lewis CJ, et al. Reduced vas deferens contraction and male infertility in mice lacking P2X1 receptors. *Nature* 2000; 403:86–89.

135. Oury C, Kuijpers MJ, Toth-Zsamboki E, et al. Overexpression of the platelet P2X1 ion channel in transgenic mice generates a novel prothrombotic phenotype. *Blood* 2003;101:3969–3976.

136. Kawakami-Kimura N, Narita T, Ohmori K, et al. Involvement of hepatocyte growth factor in increased integrin expression on HepG2 cells triggered by adhesion to endothelial cells. *Br J Cancer* 1997;75:47–53.

137. Thomas DW, Mannon RB, Mannon PJ, et al. Coagulation defects and altered hemodynamic responses in mice lacking receptors for thromboxane A2. *J Clin Invest* 1998;102:1994–2001.

138. Nurden Pf, Savi P, Heilmann E, et al. An inherited bleeding disorder linked to a defective interaction between ADP and its receptor on platelets. Its influence on glycoprotein IIb-IIIa complex function. *J Clin Invest* 1995;95: 1612–1622.

139. Cattaneo M, Zighetti ML, Lombardi R, et al. Molecular bases of defective signal transduction in the platelet P2Y12 receptor of a patient with congenital bleeding. *Proc Natl Acad Sci U S A* 2003;100:1978–1983.

140. Cattaneo M, Gachet C. ADP receptors and clinical bleeding disorders. *Arterioscler Thromb Vasc Biol* 1999;19:2281–2285.

141. Fabre JE, Nguyen MT, Latour A, et al. Decreased platelet aggregation, increased bleeding time and resistance to thromboembolism in P2Y1-deficient mice. *Nat Med* 1999;5:1199–1202.

142. Paul BZS, Jin JG, Kunapuli SP. Molecular mechanism of thromboxane A2-induced platelet aggregation—Essential role for P2TAC and alpha2A receptors. *J Biol Chem* 1999;274:29108–29114.

143. Rao AK, Willis J, Kowalska MA, et al. Differential requirements for platelet aggregation and inhibition of adenylate cyclase by epinephrine. Studies of a familial platelet alpha2-adrenergic receptor defect. *Blood* 1988;71:494–501.

144. Tamponi G, Pannocchia A, Arduino C, et al. Congenital deficiency of alpha2-adrenoreceptors on human platelets: description of two cases. *Thromb Haemost* 1987;58:1012–1016.

145. Newman KD, Williams LT, Bishopric NH, et al. Identification of alpha-adrenergic receptors in human platelets by 3H-dihydroergocryptine binding. *J Clin Invest* 1978;61:395–402.

146. Siess W, Weber PC, Lapetina EG. Activation of phospholipase C is dissociated from arachidonate metabolism during platelet shape change induced by thrombin or platelet-activating factor. Epinephrine does not induce phospholipase C activation or platelet shape change. *J Biol Chem* 1984;259:8286–8292.

147. Casey PJ, Fong HKW, Simon MI, et al. Gz, a guanine nucleotide-binding protein with unique biochemical properties. *J Biol Chem* 1990;265:2383–2390.

148. Lounsbury KM, Casey PJ, Brass LF, et al. Phosphorylation of Gz in human platelets: selectivity and site of modification. *J Biol Chem* 1991;266: 22051–22056.

149. Wang J, Frost JA, Ross EM. Reciprocal signaling between heterotrimeric G proteins and the p21-stimulated protein kinase. *J Biol Chem* 1999;274: 31641–31647.

150. Ho MKC, Wong YH. Gz signaling: emerging divergence from Gi signaling. *Oncogene* 2001;20:1615–1625.

151. FitzGerald GA. Mechanisms of platelet activation: thromboxane A2 as an amplifying signal for other agonists. *Am J Cardiol* 1991;68:11B–15B.

152. Moers A, Nieswandt B, Massberg S, et al. G(13) is an essential mediator of platelet activation in hemostasis and thrombosis. *Nat Med* 2003;9:1418–1422.

153. Gao Y, Tang S, Zhou S, et al. The thromboxane A2 receptor activates mitogen-activated protein kinase via protein kinase C-dependent Gi coupling

and Src-dependent phosphorylation of the epidermal growth factor receptor. *J Pharmacol Exp Ther* 2001;296:426–433.

154. Brass LF, Woolkalis MJ, Manning DR. Interactions in platelets between G proteins and the agonists that stimulate phospholipase C and inhibit adenylyl cyclase. *J Biol Chem* 1988;263:5348–5355.

155. Higuchi W, Fuse I, Hattori A, et al. Mutations of the platelet thromboxane A2 (TXA2) receptor in patients characterized by the absence of TXA2-induced platelet aggregation despite normal TXA2 binding activity. *Thromb Haemost* 1999;82:1528–1531.

156. Charo IF, Feinman RD, Detwiler TC. Interrelations of platelet aggregation and secretion. *J Clin Invest* 1977;60:866–873.

157. Reed GL, Fitzgerald ML, Polgar J. Molecular mechanisms of platelet exocytosis: insights into the "secrete" life of thrombocytes. *Blood* 2000;96:3334–3342.

158. Palade G. Intracellular aspects of the process of protein synthesis. *Science* 1975;189:347–358.

159. Morgenstern E, Edelmann L, Reimers HJ, et al. Fibrinogen distribution on surfaces and in organelles of ADP stimulated human blood platelets. *Eur J Cell Biol* 1985;38:292–300.

160. Allen RD, Zacharski LR, Widirstky ST, et al. Transformation and motility of human platelets: details of the shape change and release reaction observed by optical and electron microscopy. *J Cell Biol* 1979;83:126–142.

161. Shirakawa R, Yoshioka A, Horiuchi H, et al. Small GTPase Rab4 regulates Ca2+-induced alpha-granule secretion in platelets. *J Biol Chem* 2000;275:33844–33849.

162. Feng D, Crane K, Rozenvayn N, et al. Subcellular distribution of 3 functional platelet SNARE proteins: human cellubrevin, SNAP-23, and syntaxin 2. *Blood* 2002;99:4006–4014.

163. Flaumenhaft R, Croce K, Chen E, et al. Proteins of the exocytotic core complex mediate platelet alpha-granule secretion. Roles of vesicle-associated membrane protein, SNAP-23, and syntaxin 4. *J Biol Chem* 1999;274:2492–2501.

164. Reed GL, Houng AK, Fitzgerald ML. Human platelets contain SNARE proteins and a Sec1p homologue that interacts with syntaxin 4 and is phosphorylated after thrombin activation: implications for platelet secretion. *Blood* 1999;93:2617–2626.

165. Takayama K, Kudo I, Kim DK, et al. Purification and characterization of human platelet phospholipase A$_2$ which preferentially hydrolyzes an arachidonoyl residue. *FEBS Lett* 1991;282:326–330.

166. Sharp JD, White DL, Chiou XG, et al. Molecular cloning and expression of human Ca(2+)-sensitive cytosolic phospholipase A2. *J Biol Chem* 1991;266:14850–14853.

167. Kramer RM, Roberts EF, Manetta J, et al. The Ca2(+)-sensitive cytosolic phospholipase A2 is a 100-kDa protein in human monoblast U937 cells. *J Biol Chem* 1991;266:5268–5272.

168. Vane JR. Biomedicine. Back to an aspirin a day? *Science* 2002;296:474–475.

169. Bunting S, Moncada S, Vane JR. The prostacyclin—thromboxane A2 balance: pathophysiological and therapeutic implications. *Br Med Bull* 1983;39:271–276.

170. Gum P, Kottke-Marchant K, Welch PA, et al. A prospective, blinded determination of the natural history of aspirin resistance among stable patients with caridovascular disease. *J Am Coll Cardiol* 2003;41:961–965.

171. Patrono C. Aspirin resistance: definition, mechanisms and clinical readouts. *J Thromb Haemost* 2003;1:1710–1713.

172. Stanford N, Roth GJ, Shen TY, et al. Lack of covalent modification of prostaglandin synthetase (cyclo-oxygenase) by indomethacin. *Prostaglandins* 1977;13:669–675.

173. Berridge MJ. Inositol trisphosphate and calcium signalling. *Nature* 1993;361:315–325.

174. Cockcroft S, Thomas GMH. Inositol-lipid–specific phospholipase C isoenzymes and their differential regulation by receptors. *Biochem J* 1992;288:1–14.

175. Lapetina EG, Billah MM, Cuatrecasas P. Lysophosphatidic acid potentiates the thrombin-induced production of arachidonate metabolites in platelets. *J Biol Chem* 1981;256:11984–11987.

176. Rittenhouse SE, Sasson JP. Mass changes in myoinositol trisphosphate in human platelets stimulated by thrombin. Inhibitory effects of phorbol ester. *J Biol Chem* 1985;260:8657–8660.

177. Kaibuchi K, Takai Y, Sawamura M, et al. Synergistic functions of protein phosphorylation and calcium mobilization in platelet activation. *J Biol Chem* 1983;258:6701–6704.

178. Brass LF, Joseph SK. A role for inositol triphosphate in intracellular Ca2+ mobilization and granule secretion in platelets. *J Biol Chem* 1985;260:15172–15179.

179. Cantley LC. The phosphoinositide 3-kinase pathway. *Science* 2002;296:1655–1657.

180. Hirsch E, Bosco O, Tropel P, et al. Resistance to thromboembolism in PI3Kgamma-deficient mice. *FASEB J* 2001;15:2019–2021.

181. Lian L, Wang Y, Draznin J, et al. The relative role of PLC{beta} and PI3K {gamma} in platelet activation. *Blood* 2005;106(1):110–117.

182. Watanabe N, Nakajima H, Suzuki H, et al. Functional phenotype of phosphoinositide 3kinase p85alpha-null platelets characterized by an impaired response to GP VI stimulation. *Blood* 2003;102:541–548.

183. Abrams CS, Kazanietz MG. Platelet signaling: protein kinase C. In: Gresele P, Page C, Fuster V et al, eds. *Platelets in thrombotic and non-thrombotic disorders*, Cambridge: Cambridge University Press, 2002.

184. Murugappan S, Tuluc F, Dorsam RT, et al. Differential role of protein kinase C delta isoform in agonist-induced dense granule secretion in human platelets. *J Biol Chem* 2004;279:2360–2367.

185. Sun L, Mao G, Rao AK. Association of CBFA2 mutation with decreased platelet PKC-theta and impaired receptor-mediated activation of GPIIb-IIIa and pleckstrin phosphorylation: proteins regulated by CBFA2 play a role in GPIIb-IIIa activation. *Blood* 2004;103:948–954.

186. Nieswandt B, Watson SP. Platelet-collagen interaction: is GPVI the central receptor? *Blood* 2003;102:449–461.

187. Li Z, Xi X, Gu M, et al. A stimulatory role for cGMP-dependent protein kinase in platelet activation. *Cell* 2003;112:77–86.

188. Calderwood DA, Zent R, Grant R, et al. The talin head domain binds to integrin beta subunit cytoplasmic tails and regulates integrin activation. *J Biol Chem* 1999;274:28071–28074.

199. Reedquist KA, Ross E, Koop EA, et al. The small GTPase, Rap1, mediates CD31-induced integrin adhesion. *J Cell Biol* 2000;148:1151–1158.

190. Tsukamato N, Hattori M, Yang H, et al. Rap1 GTPase activating protein SPA-1 negatively regulates cell adhesion. *J Biol Chem* 1999;274:18463–18469.

191. Katagiri K, Hattori M, Minato N, et al. Rap1 is a potent activation signal for leukocyte function-associated antigen 1 distinct from protein kinase C and phosphatidylinositol-3-OH kinase. *Mol Cell Biol* 2000;20:1956–1969.

192. Sebzda E, Bracke M, Tugal T, et al. Rap1A positively regulates T cells via integrin activation rather than inhibiting lymphocyte signaling. *Nat Immunol* 2002;3:251–258.

193. Bertoni A, Tadokoro S, Eto K, et al. Relationships between Rap1b, affinity modulation of integrin αIIbβ3, and the actin cytoskeleton. *J Biol Chem* 2002;277:25715–25721.

194. Payrastre B, Missy K, Trumel C, et al. The integrin alphaIIb/beta3 in human platelet signal transduction. *Biochem Pharmacol* 2000;60:1069–1074.

195. Philips DR, Prasad KSS, Manganello J, et al. Integrin tyrosine phosphorylation in platelet signaling. *Curr Opin Cell Biol* 2001;13:546–554.

196. Phillips DR, Nannizzi-Alaimo L, Prasad KSS. beta3 tyrosine phosphorylation in alphaIIbbeta3 (platelet membrane GP IIb-IIIa) outside-in integrin signaling. *Thromb Haemost* 2001;86:246–258.

197. Obergfell A, Eto K, Mocsai A, et al. Coordinate interactions of Csk, Src and Syk kinases with alphaIIbbeta3 initiate integrin signaling to the cytoskeleton. *J Cell Biol* 2002;157:265–275.

198. Guinebault C, Payrastre B, Racaud-Sultan C, et al. Integrin-dependent translocation of phosphoinositide 3-kinase to the cytoskeleton of thrombin-activated platelets involves specific interactions of p85alpha with actin filaments and focal adhesion kinase. *J Cell Biol* 1995;129:831–842.

199. Shattil SJ, O'Toole T, Eigenthaler M, et al. beta3-Endonexin, a novel polypeptide that interacts specificsally with the cytoplasmic tail of the integrin beta3 subunit. *J Cell Biol* 1995;131:807–816.

200. Naik UP, Patel PM, Parise LV. Identification of a novel calcium-binding protein that interacts with the integrin alphaIIb cytoplasmic domain. *J Biol Chem* 1997;272:4651–4654.

201. Shock DD, Naik UP, Brittain JE, et al. Calcium-dependent properties of CIB binding to the integrin alphaIIb cytoplasmic domain and translocation to the platelet cytoskeleton. *Biochem J* 1999;342:729–735.

202. Gao J, Zoller KE, Ginsberg MH, et al. Regulation of the pp72syk protein tyrosine kinase by platelet integrin alphaIIbbeta3. *EMBO J* 1997;16:6414–6425.

203. Woodside DG, Obergfell A, Leng L, et al. Activation of Syk protein tyrosine kinase through interaction with integrin beta cytoplasmic domains. *Curr Biol* 2001;11:1799–1804.

204. Jenkins AL, Nannizzi-Alaimo L, Silver D, et al. Tyrosine phosphorylation of the beta3 cytoplasmic domain mediates integrincytoskeletal interactions. *J Biol Chem* 1998;273:13878–13885.

205. Cowan KJ, Law DA, Phillips DR. Identification of Shc as the primary protein binding to the tyrosine-phosphorylated beta3 subunit of alphaIIbbeta3 during outside-in integrin platelet signaling. *J Biol Chem* 2000;275:36423–36429.

206. Law DA, DeGuzman FR, Heiser P, et al. Integrin cytoplasmic tyrosine motif is required for outside-in alphaIIbbeta3 signalling and platelet function. *Nature* 1999;401:808–811.

# CHAPTER 40 ■ OVERVIEW OF VASCULAR BIOLOGY, EMBRYOGENESIS, DEVELOPMENT, AND DISORDERS

MARK W. MAJESKY AND ALEXANDER W. CLOWES

The vascular system is remarkably dynamic and adaptive. From its inception in the embryo to its mature form in the adult, the circulatory network of arteries, veins, and lymphatic vessels continuously remodels. Although the first steps in vascular development are driven by pathways for angioblast self-assembly, all subsequent steps result from an intricate interplay of mechanical forces and cell–cell signaling interactions that act upon the vessel wall. Moreover, gene products that are crucial for the formation of blood and lymphatic vessels in the embryo reappear in adults during angiogenesis, adaptive growth and remodeling, wound repair, and vascular disease. This section on vascular biology (Section D) contains chapters illustrating these principles as they apply to processes that build and maintain a functioning vascular system.

Blood vessels are formed by the differentiation of angioblasts and by their subsequent assembly into a primitive vascular network. The nascent vascular plexus is patterned by a constant interplay of positive and negative signals for growth and survival that are encountered by endothelial cells in their local environment. Positive cues are provided by local growth factors, compatible matrix components, and relative tissue hypoxia, whereas negative cues result from repulsive signaling by an array of transmembrane plexins, semaphorins, and ephrins displayed on the endothelial cell surface. The fact that these repulsive signals for vascular patterning are the same as those that guide neurite extensions to their targets during nerve development illustrates the striking conservation of regulatory pathways that direct the formation of these two diverse networks. Newly formed blood vessels are fragile structures that require support cells to provide survival signals and to ensure mechanical stability. Endothelial cells recruit pericytes and smooth muscle cells (SMCs) to carry out these functions. Recent advances in genetic techniques for lineage mapping in mammalian embryos reveal a surprising diversity of origins for SMCs that interact with and stabilize newly formed vessels. These fate maps tell us that the vascular system is a mosaic structure in as much as it develops its smooth muscle coating in distinct segments, each with its own unique origins and developmental histories. The smooth muscle diversity revealed by these lineage maps suggests new ways of thinking about well-known variations in susceptibility to disease among different vessels in the same individual. Chapter 41 reviews our current understanding of the sequence of interdependent steps that are required to build a vascular system in the embryo.

Genetic analysis of vascular development also provides clear confirmation about the crucial roles played by short-range paracrine signaling factors in endothelial–smooth muscle communication. A chapter on nitric oxide as a mediator of endothelial cell signaling in the vessel wall (see Chapter 42) illustrates the diverse roles played by this essential short-range, diffusible substance for establishing and maintaining vascular structure and function. Through the production of nitric oxide, and the generation of labile and highly reactive oxygen radicals, endothelial cells can direct vasomotor responses by vascular smooth muscle, modulate platelet interactions with the luminal surface, and maintain a stable cell population in the vessel wall. Activation of the smooth muscle cyclic guanosine 3', 5'-monophosphate (GMP)-dependent protein kinases by endothelial cell–derived nitric oxide causes relaxation of resistance vessels, limits signaling from G protein–coupled cell surface receptors, and maintains a mature phenotype for vascular smooth muscle. A comparison of loss of function phenotypes for the three different nitric oxide synthase isoforms shows how precisely these gene products have evolved to respond to extracellular stimuli and to carry out the multiple roles of nitric oxide in the vasculature.

Vascular networks continuously monitor and adapt to changes in functional demand. This is seen as increases or decreases in capillary density, collateral reserve, and autoregulation of vascular tone. The endothelium has a primary role as both a sensor of chronic changes in blood flow rates and as a transducer for adaptive structural responses within the vessel wall. Mechanotransduction is a fundamental process by which cell–cell and cell–matrix contacts transmit information to the cell nucleus about physical forces acting upon the vessel wall. Genome-wide transcript profile analysis has provided much information about how changes in fluid shear stress imposed upon the endothelial surface modify patterns of endothelial gene expression. At the same time, the role of endothelial adhesion molecules as molecular "force transducers" that initiate intracellular signaling responses to changes in fluid shear stress is becoming more clear. Chapter 43 discusses the fundamental pathways by which vessel walls remodel in response to major changes in blood flow. Yet many challenges remain to extend these results, most of which are obtained with model systems *in vitro* and to living blood vessels *in vivo*. It will be important, for example, to identify pathways for compensatory outward remodeling in atherosclerotic arteries, a process that permits the growth of atheroma without impinging on the lumen, and to gain insights into factors that limit this response in individuals with more rapid disease progression. However, the fact that there are a large number of genes (>50 at present) whose mutant phenotypes result in failure of embryonic vascular remodeling precisely when blood flow rates begin their steady rise in early development suggests that the pathways for sensing changes in shear stress and transducing them into appropriate structural responses will be complex.

In addition to forming a branching network of arteries, veins, and lymphatic vessels, the maintenance of a functional circulatory system requires that these diverse elements of the circulation be kept separate and distinct. Great progress has been made in recent years to advance our understanding of the molecular basis of endothelial cell identity and diversity. From the initial discovery that arterial and venous endothelium can be distinguished even before the circulation has begun, by expression of ephrinB2 or EphB4, respectively, the number of markers for endothelial subtypes has progressively increased. Moreover, lymphatic vessels have been shown to express lymphatic endothelium-specific markers such as Prox-1 and LYVE-1. These markers provide new tools to enable investigators to study and modify the lymphatic vessel system independent of any effects on the systemic blood vascular system. These studies will continue to generate novel insights into how different parts of the vascular tree remain separate and distinct during development, and how new vessels are incorporated into existing vascular networks during adult angiogenesis. They will also lead to discoveries that will provide new avenues for therapeutic intervention in conditions such as lymphedema and tumor metastasis. The chapter on angiogenesis (see Chapter 44) covers this rapidly moving and exciting area of vascular biology.

Although adaptive structural remodeling is an ongoing process under normal conditions, blood vessels must also be able to repair vascular injuries while maintaining circulatory function. Vascular integrity can be readily restored after the small focal loss of endothelial cells by migration of surviving cells from the wound margins. Tissue homeostasis requires a dynamic endothelial surface that can respond to chemokines and inflammatory cytokines and that can appropriately modify interactions of platelets and monocytes with the vessel wall. A chapter on monocyte, platelet, and endothelial interactions (see Chapter 45) reviews the important classes of chemokines, chemokine receptors, and adhesion molecules that coordinate the recruitment and activation of these cell types. A separate chapter discusses the dynamics of platelet–vessel wall interactions in flowing blood (see Chapter 47). Repair of larger injuries to the vessel wall requires cooperative interactions among preexisting endothelial cells, platelets, neutrophils, monocytes, and circulating endothelial progenitor cells with the products of coagulation and inflammation. Under normal conditions, these repair processes are able to restore the vessel to its previous structure and functional capacity. If the injury stimulus is severe, however, a secondary set of responses is triggered that results in vessels with altered structure and function. Accumulation of macrophages, T lymphocytes, dedifferentiated smooth muscle cells, extracellular matrix (ECM) components, microthrombi, and cholesterol-rich lipid deposits can be found within the intima of chronically injured arteries, that produces disturbed blood flow, disrupts normal endothelial–smooth muscle communication, predisposes to thrombus formation, and alters the biomechanical properties of the vessel wall. These reactions of artery walls to chronic damage are reviewed in a chapter on vascular injury (see Chapter 50). Under most conditions, it is likely that such intimal lesions can persist for many years with no harmful outcome. Indeed, there is evidence to suggest that some lesions can even regress, particularly with dietary and lifestyle interventions. Under other conditions, however, degenerative changes within the intima continue to progress in ways that ultimately produce unstable plaques prone to hemorrhage, erosion or rupture, and thrombotic events. A great deal of information about the cellular and molecular pathways that underlie these degenerative

changes has been acquired in recent years, with a corresponding increase in the number of new therapeutic targets that have been brought to clinical trials as a result. The advent of coated stents for intervention in occlusive vascular diseases is one example of such an outcome. Yet many questions still remain about how the different cell types within the plaque interact with the products of coagulation and inflammation to stimulate lesion progression, and influence the outcome of chronic arterial disease processes. Chapter 53 reviews our current understanding of these complex interactions, and provides a framework for future work in this important area.

Although the pathogenesis of large vessel disease continues to demand our attention, advances in understanding basic pathways for vascular development have provided new tools and conceptual approaches to the problems of microvascular disease and tumor angiogenesis. Tumor vessels are highly variable in size, shape, and branching patterns, a reflection of the unusual environment of the growing tumor. They are often not organized in the conventional hierarchy of arteries, arterioles, capillaries, and venules and are frequently leaky, hemorrhagic, and defective in forming a well-defined pericyte covering. Many of the characteristic structural features of tumor vessels can be seen in the null phenotypes of genes involved in platelet-derived growth factor (PDGF) signaling during vascular development. Endothelial cells normally produce PDGF-BB, whereas smooth muscle cells and pericytes express its receptor, PDGF-R$\beta$. During normal microvessel formation, pericytes extend dendritic processes that intimately associate with the endothelial cell surface. Mice that lack the ability to produce PDGF-B or PDGF-R$\beta$ exhibit defects in recruitment and investment of pericytes and SMCs to the vessel wall, leading to leaky vessels that are prone to rupture. Moreover, deletion of the retention motif on PDGF-BB responsible for interaction with heparan sulfate proteoglycans (HSPG) resulted in a very similar defect in investment of pericytes around the microvessel wall. Likewise, forms of vascular endothelial growth factor (VEGF)-A that are unable to interact with HSPGs because of targeted deletion of long VEGF-A splice isoforms cannot support normal vascular development. Formation and degradation of the ECM is an important point of control for vascular wall formation, remodeling, regression, and disease. Cell–matrix contacts not only mediate adhesion, but also initiate intracellular signaling responses, and changes in the composition of the ECM produce corresponding changes in vascular cell phenotypes. The growing realization that adhesion receptors, growth factor receptors, and signaling proteins are organized in large multiprotein complexes, often coalesced in structured membrane subdomains called *lipid rafts*, illustrates how growth and survival signals can depend upon cell–cell and cell–matrix adhesion.

Finally, it is important to realize that the great wealth of information being acquired in the study of embryonic cardiovascular development using new approaches in genetics, genomics, and bioinformatics provides a rich potential source of new insights into vascular disease. Reactivation of embryonic programs of gene expression can be seen in response to vascular injury, thrombosis, and chronic inflammation in adult blood vessels. As our understanding of the composition and regulation of these embryonic gene sets improves, it can be anticipated that a corresponding enhancement in novel disease targets for atherothrombosis will be forthcoming. It is our hope that the chapters found in this section on vascular biology will serve to illustrate this principle.

# CHAPTER 41 ■ DEVELOPMENT OF THE VASCULAR SYSTEM

MARK W. MAJESKY, XIU-RONG DONG, AND SAN-PIN WU

Vascular development begins with the formation of angioblasts and with their differentiation into endothelial cells (ECs) (1,2). Nascent ECs self-assemble into a primary network of capillarylike vessels in the yolk sac and in the early embryo. The primary plexus then remodels to produce a series of large and small arteries, veins, and lymphatic vessels (3). At the onset of cardiac contraction, vascular ECs recruit a supporting layer of mesenchymal cells in response to increases in directional blood flow. Smooth muscle cell (SMC) differentiation occurs within these subendothelial cell clusters, followed by formation of a well-organized extracellular matrix (ECM) that supports and defines the vessel wall. Although these general features of vascular development have been known for many years, molecular pathways that control blood and lymphatic vessel formation have remained poorly understood. Recently, new genetic and cell transplantation methods have begun to identify genes that control the crucial steps in the formation and remodeling of the vascular system. As a result, new insights have been gained into the signaling pathways for endothelial–SMC interactions, arterial–venous identity, cross-talk between developing nerves and vessels, SMC recruitment and differentiation, and origins of intimal cell clusters that are forerunners of atherosclerotic plaques appearing later in life. This chapter reviews our current understanding of how blood and lymphatic vessels form in vertebrate embryos and illustrates how lessons learned from basic studies of vascular development can provide important insights into mechanisms that control vascular adaptation, repair, and disease processes in adult life.

# FORMATION OF THE TUNICA INTIMA

## Origins of Endothelial Cells

The first visible structures to appear in vascular development are clusters of hematopoietic cells surrounded by ECs; these structures are known as *blood islands* (4). The proximity of blood cells and ECs in blood islands led to the proposal of the presence of a common progenitor cell called the *hemangioblast* (5). Over the years, experimental support has accumulated for the existence of hemangioblasts. The monoclonal antibodies QH1 (6) and MB1 (7) recognize carbohydrate epitopes expressed on endothelial progenitors and on hematopoietic cells. QH1 immunostaining has been used to trace the emergence of the endothelial lineage in extraembryonic and splanchnic mesoderm (6,8). These studies identified the first angioblasts to appear in the embryo, revealed their robust migratory activity, and showed their coalescence into a primitive network of

vascular channels (6). Hemangioblasts are formed in limited numbers between embryonic days (EDs) 7.0 and 8.0 in the mouse and differentiate very quickly into ECs and blood cells (9). As a consequence, most ECs formed in the embryo probably do not arise from hemangioblasts but rather from angioblasts that lack hematopoietic potential. The process of vessel formation by the assembly of ECs that arise *de novo* is called *vasculogenesis* (10,11). Vasculogenesis is first observed in yolk sac blood islands and, shortly thereafter, within splanchnopleural mesoderm of the embryo itself. Although angioblast formation *per se* appears to be independent of endoderm signaling, subsequent endothelial cell differentiation and tube formation depends on an endoderm-derived factor. Vokes et al. reported that the secreted signaling protein sonic hedgehog (Shh) could restore vascular tube formation in endodermless embryos (12). Therefore, hedgehog signaling plays a crucial role in the early steps of vascular development that mediate lumen formation [for review see (13,14)].

Molecular genetic studies revealed that hemangioblast formation depends on the basic helix–loop–helix transcription factor stem cell leukemia (SCL)/Tal1 (15). SCL/Tal1 is coexpressed with both hematopoietic and endothelial markers in early mesoderm (15,16). Ectopic overexpression of SCL/Tal1 in zebrafish embryos disrupted vasculogenesis by overproduction of hemangioblasts (17). Deletion of SCL/Tal1 indicated its essential role in hematopoiesis, although vasculogenesis was not perturbed (18,19). Lack of effect on vasculogenesis is consistent with the concept that SCL/Tal1 directs early flk1$^+$ multipotential cells to a hemangioblast fate rather than remaining as committed angioblasts (20). These results suggest that SCL/Tal1 specifies hemangioblast formation and is required for hematopoietic differentiation in the mouse (14). Another recently identified marker for hemangioblasts in blood islands is the divergent homeobox gene Hex (21,22). Hex is also expressed in angioblasts throughout the embryo and is one of the earliest markers of endothelial lineage specification (23). Unlike other early endothelial markers, Hex is expressed only in endothelial precursors and becomes quickly downregulated on endothelial differentiation (22).

Once the major vessels have formed by vasculogenesis, extension of the vascular network occurs either by sprouting of new vessels from preexisting ones (angiogenesis), or by a process whereby a preexisting vessel splits into two daughter vessels by formation of transcapillary pillars (nonsprouting angiogenesis or intussusception) (24,25). Avascular regions of the developing central nervous system, lung, kidney, and limb bud become vascularized when sprouts of ECs originating from preexisting vessels invade these developing tissues. Angiogenesis requires a localized stimulus for the loss of endothelial cell–cell adhesion, gain of cell motility, increase in protease production, and synthesis of a specialized ECM (26). Multiple lines of evidence now show that a crucial mediator of angioblast formation and differentiation in the embryo is vascular endothelial growth factor (VEGF). Once the capillarylike primary vascular network has formed, remodeling of the vascular plexus into a circulatory tree of large and small vessels is shaped by a combination of local hypoxic, rheologic, and metabolic factors that act along with soluble signals produced by surrounding mesenchymal cells including angiopoietin-1 and TGF-$\beta$1 (see Fig. 41-1).

## Vascular Endothelial Growth Factor

The nutrient demands of the embryo shape the vascular development by the production of VEGF. Dvorak et al. discovered VEGF in the early 1980s as a factor that made blood vessels

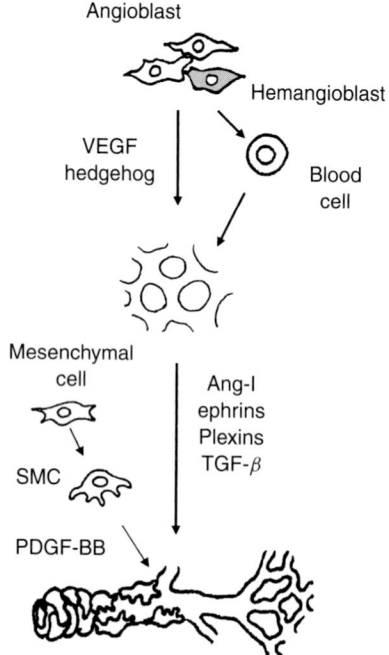

**FIGURE 41-1.** Development of the vessel wall. Formation of endothelial tubes and their assembly into a primitive vascular plexus is under control of vascular endothelial growth factor (VEGF) and hedgehog signaling. Remodeling of the initial network of capillarylike vessels into a system of large and small arteries, veins, and lymphatic vessels is the result of coordinated action by VEGFs, angiopoietins (Ang-1), ephrins, and plexins. Many of these vascular remodeling factors also function as guidance signals for nervous system development, reflecting the close interaction between developing nerves and vessels. Following initiation of blood flow, ECs recruit mesenchymal cells from multiple primary origins throughout the embryo to form a tunica media. Mesenchymal cells differentiate into pericytes and smooth muscle cells (SMCs) under the influence of transforming growth factor (TGF)-$\beta$ and platelet-derived growth factor (PDGF)-BB. In certain vascular beds, continued recruitment of SMCs occurs by migration of upstream SMCs along endothelial basement membranes to new downstream positions in response to chemoattractants such as PDGF-BB. This interaction is bidirectional because several SMC-derived factors (VEGF, Ang-1, TGF-$\beta$) are known to affect endothelial cell growth and survival. Differentiation of SMCs requires multiple signaling events that involve ECs, biomechanical forces, and extracellular matrix (ECM) interactions. Formation of a functionally mature vessel wall requires synthesis and assembly of appropriate ECM proteins [e.g., elastin (ELN), fibulins, fibrillins, and collagens] by medial SMCs to form a vasoactive and pressure-bearing blood vessel.

leaky; therefore, it was named *vascular permeability factor* (VPF) (27). Later, several groups of investigators showed that the same substance stimulated endothelial cell proliferation *in vitro* and was a potent angiogenic factor *in vivo*, therefore the name VEGF (28,29). VEGF/VPF is a heat-stable, 46-kDa dimeric protein with structural similarity and distant homology (18% to 20%, including all eight cysteines) to PDGF. Four different VEGF family members have been characterized to date (VEGF A–D) that display different binding selectivities for three VEGF receptor tyrosine kinases (see Fig. 41-2). VEGF-A can signal through VEGF-R1/flt1 or VEGF-R2/flk1/kinase insert domain receptor (KDR). VEGF-B and the related placenta growth factor (PlGF) signal through flt1/VEGF-R1, whereas VEGF-C and VEGF-D can use both VEGF-R2 and VEGF-R3 for signaling.

## Regulation of Vascular Endothelial Growth Factor Production by Hypoxia

VEGF is made by many different cell types, and its production is strongly upregulated by hypoxia. Indeed, a 28-bp enhancer element that mediates hypoxia-inducible transcription has been identified in the rat and human VEGF-A genes (30). Forsythe et al. cotransfected ECs with the hypoxia-inducible factors hypoxia inducible factor-1 (HIF-1)$\alpha$ and HIF-1$\beta$ [aryl hydrocarbon receptor nuclear translocator (ARNT)] and showed that these two DNA-binding proteins mediated strong upregulation of VEGF-A expression by hypoxia (31). Hypoxia also stabilizes VEGF-A mRNA by a 125-bp AU-rich sequence in the 3' untranslated region (3'UTR) (32,33). Targeted disruption of the HIF-1$\alpha$ gene in mice resulted in death by ED10.5 because of cardiovascular malformations and extensive mesenchymal cell apoptosis, particularly in cephalic mesenchyme (34,35). Vascular abnormalities in HIF-1$\alpha$ null embryos were evident by ED9.5 and included a loss of capillary profiles in head mesenchyme, severe hypoplasia of branchial arch vessels, and dilation of dorsal aortae and intersomatic arteries (34). HIF-1$\beta$/ARNT$^{-/-}$ mice also die around ED10.5 with defects in yolk sac vasculogenesis and branchial arch

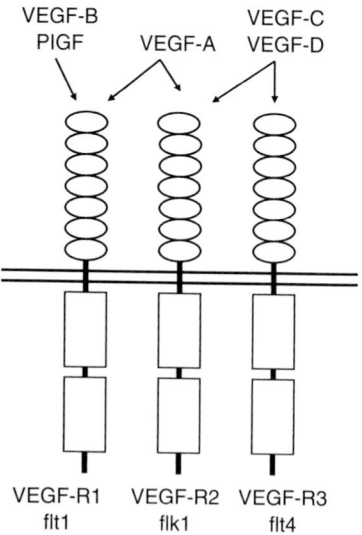

**FIGURE 41-2.** Vascular endothelial growth factor (VEGF) family members and VEGF receptors. The family of VEGF ligands interacts with the VEGF receptors as shown in the figure to mediate their effects on vascular development, angiogenesis, and lymphatic vessel formation.

arteries very similar to those observed in HIF-1$\alpha$ and VEGF-A–deficient mice (36). Quite surprisingly, VEGF mRNA levels exhibited normal developmental upregulation in HIF-1$\alpha$–null embryos (37). Careful analysis of HIF-1$\alpha^{-/-}$ embryos revealed that extensive mesenchymal cell death preceded overt vascular defects (37). Indeed, loss of mesenchymal cells resulted in failure to provide soluble factors and mechanical support needed for vascular development. The phenotype of HIF-1$\alpha$–null embryos suggests that control of glucose metabolism, rather than VEGF production, is a key function of HIF-1$\alpha$ in early vascular development. Consistent with this idea, HIF-1$\beta$/ARNT$^{-/-}$ ES cells failed to upregulate genes that are normally responsive to hypoglycemia, including the glucose transporter GLUT-1, phosphoglycerate kinase, and aldolase A (36). Therefore, the combined results from VEGF-A, HIF-1$\alpha$, and HIF-1$\beta$/ARNT knockouts suggest that rapid increases in tissue mass in the growing embryo produce local hypoglycemic and hypoxic conditions that act as strong stimuli for neovascularization by transcriptional upregulation of genes dependent on HIF-1$\alpha$ and HIF-1$\beta$/ARNT.

A second hypoxia-inducible transcription factor abundantly expressed in ECs is endothelial PAS protein–1 (EPAS-1) (also called HIF-2$\alpha$). HIF-1$\alpha$, ARNT, and EPAS-1 are members of the bHLH-PAS domain family of transcription factors that regulate genes involved in metabolic stress, detoxification of xenobiotics, control of circadian rhythm, and tissue patterning in embryonic development. EPAS-1 is 48% identical to HIF-1$\alpha$ at the amino acid level, and the two proteins have overlapping functional properties. Despite these similarities, expression patterns of the two genes are strikingly different. HIF-1$\alpha$ is expressed in SMCs that surround blood vessels,

whereas EPAS-1 is selectively expressed in ECs. EPAS-1-deficient embryos die beginning around ED12.5 because of circulatory failure (38) (see Table 41-1). Surprisingly, heart and blood vessels of EPAS-1$^{-/-}$ embryos develop normally with no structural defects evident by histology. The primary phenotype is circulatory failure secondary to profound bradycardia. The concentration of fetal circulating catecholamines are reduced to approximately 50% in EPAS-deficient mice, and administration of the catecholamine precursor dihydroxyphenylserine (DOPS) to pregnant female mice rescues the midgestational lethality of these embryos (38). The Organ of Zuckerkandl (OZ) is the primary oxygen-sensing organ in the embryo before the development of the carotid body and is a crucial site of EPAS-1 deficiency (38). Therefore, in the absence of EPAS-1, the OZ does not respond to hypoxia and fails to release catecholamines that would normally stimulate cardiac contraction and would maintain appropriate perfusion of the embryo. In adult models of wound healing in mice, introduction of adenovirus expressing EPAS-1 increased the expression of VEGF, flk1, flt1, and tie2; enhanced mural cell recruitment; and stimulated angiogenesis *in vivo* (39).

## Vascular Endothelial Growth Factor Receptors

The biological activities of VEGFs are mediated by three transmembrane receptor tyrosine kinases (Fig. 41-2). VEGF-R1/flt1 and VEGF-R2/flk1/KDR are expressed predominantly (but not exclusively) on vascular ECs and on their progenitors. By contrast, VEGF-R3/flt4 is expressed mostly on lymphatic ECs. VEGF-R1/flt1 has a higher affinity for VEGF-A (kDa = 15 to 30 pmol per L) than VEGF-R2/flk1/KDR (300 to 500

### TABLE 41-1

IMPORTANT GENES FOR VASCULAR DEVELOPMENT

| Gene | Expressed by | Phenotype | Time of death | References |
|------|--------------|-----------|---------------|------------|
| VEGF-A | ECs | Too few ECs | ED9.5 – ED10.5 | 47,48 |
| Ang-1 | ECs | Failure of EC remodeling | ED12.5 – ED13.5 | 76 |
| VEGF-R2/flk1 | ECs | No ECs, no blood vessels | ED8.5 – ED9.5 | 50 |
| VEGF-R1/flt1 | ECs | Failure of EC remodeling | ED8.5 – ED9.5 | 52 |
| Tie2 | ECs | Failure of EC remodeling | ED13.5 | 68,72 |
| EPAS-1 | ECs | Severe bradycardia | ED12.5 | 38 |
| HIF-1$\alpha$ | ECs | Multiple defects | ED11.5 | 34,35 |
| ARNT | ECs | Failure of EC remodeling | ED9.5 – ED10.5 | 36 |
| LKLF | ECs | SMC recruitment defects | ED12.5 – ED14.5 | 191 |
| TGF-$\beta$1 | Many cell types | Vasculogenesis defects | ED10.5 | 111 |
| Endoglin | ECs | Failure of EC remodeling | ED12.5 – ED13.5 | 192 |
| Smad2 | Many cell types | Multiple defects | ED9.5 | 130 |
| Smad5 | ECs | Failure of EC remodeling | ED9.5 – ED11.5 | 133 |
| VCAM-1 | ECs, myocardium | Coronary vessel defects | ED12.5 | 140 |
| $\alpha_4$- < integrin | ECs, PE | Coronary vessel defects | ED12.5 | 139 |
| Indian Hh | Yolk sac endoderm | Vasculogenesis defects | ED12.5 | 101,104 |
| Ephrin-B2 | ECs | Failure of EC remodeling | ED12.5 – ED14.5 | 85 |
| Eph-B4 | ECs | Failure of EC remodeling | ED12.5 – ED14.5 | 82 |
| PDGF-B | ECs | SMC recruitment defects | Birth | 175 |
| ELN | SMCs | Vascular occlusion | Birth | 196 |
| SRF | SMCs | Early gastrulation defects | ED9.5 | 230 |
| Myocardin | Myocardial cells | SMC recruitment defects | ED10.5 | 249 |

VEGF, vascular endothelial growth factor; ECs, endothelial cells; Ang-1, angiopoietin-1; EPAS, endothelial Per-ARNT-Sim domain protein-1 (also called HIF-2$\alpha$); HIF-1, hypoxia-inducible factor-1; ARNT, aryl hydrocarbon receptor nuclear transporter (also called HIF-1$\beta$); LKLF, lung Kruppel–like factor (also called KLF2); TGF-$\beta$1, transforming growth factor $\beta$1; VCAM-1, vascular cell adhesion molecule-1; ELN, elastin; SMCs, smooth muscle cells; Indian Hh, indian hedgehog; PDGF-B, platelet-derived growth factor-B; SRF, serum response factor; ED, embryonic days.

pmol per L). Hypoxia not only increases VEGF-A production, as discussed in the preceding text, but also strongly upregulates the expression of both VEGF-A receptor genes (40). Increased VEGF-R1/flt1 expression caused by hypoxia is mediated by a HIF-1 consensus binding site in the proximal promoter region of the flt1 gene (40). By contrast, upregulation of VEGF-R2/flk1 expression appears to be mediated indirectly by the production of paracrine factors by hypoxic target tissues (41). Therefore, a powerful forward amplifier system is built into developing vessels whereby hypoxia stimulates VEGF-A production in oxygen-starved tissues and simultaneously increases VEGF-A receptor expression in nearby ECs, resulting in a strong paracrine stimulus/response pathway for endothelial cell survival, proliferation, and angiogenesis.

## Isoforms of Vascular Endothelial Growth Factor-A

Four isoforms of VEGF-A are produced by alternative splicing. VEGF-120 and VEGF-165 are the major secreted, soluble forms of VEGF, whereas VEGF-189 and VEGF-221 are the membrane-bound forms. Different isoforms of VEGF-A play different roles in vascular development. For example, Carmeliet et al. produced mice that only make VEGF-120 by cre/loxP-mediated removal of VEGF exons 6 and 7. VEGF-120 alone was able to support complete vascular development *in utero* (42). However, approximately half of the VEGF$^{120/120}$ mice died within a few hours after birth because of hemorrhage in various tissues. The other half died from cardiac failure before postnatal day 12. Histologic analysis of hearts from VEGF$^{120/120}$ mice showed a reduced number of capillaries in myocardial tissue because of failure of postnatal angiogenesis to keep pace with normal cardiac growth. As a result, progressive ischemia developed in the myocardium, leading eventually to myocardial necrosis and cell death. Similar reductions in capillary density were found in kidney and skeletal muscle. These findings could mean that too little VEGF-120 is being made to maintain normal levels of total VEGF-A during tissue growth. Alternatively, different VEGF isoforms may have different biologic activities, and VEGF-120 cannot replace VEGF-165 or VEGF-189. In support of the latter possibility, Soker et al. found that VEGF-165, but not VEGF-120, specifically binds to neuropilin-1 (43). Binding to neuropilin-1 promotes activation of VEGF-R2/flk1 by VEGF-165 and enhances the chemotactic and mitogenic effects of VEGF-165 on ECs (43). Neuropilin-1 is a membrane protein that was first described in developing neurons in which it functions as a coreceptor for class 3 semaphorins, which are inhibitory axon guidance signals. Targeted inactivation of the neuropilin-1 gene in mice showed that neuropilin-1 regulates nerve fiber guidance in embryogenesis (44,45). Neuropilin-1 is also produced by ECs in developing blood vessels, and constitutive overexpression of neuropilin-1 in transgenic mice resulted in an excess of vascular profiles, dilation of blood vessels, malformed hearts, and lethality in midgestation embryos (46). Confirmation of the intriguing possibility that each VEGF isoform fulfills a unique functional requirement in angiogenesis awaits the production of mice expressing other isoform-specific variants of VEGF-A.

## Roles of Vascular Endothelial Growth Factor in Vasculogenesis

A critical role for VEGF-A in vasculogenesis has been established by gene deletion studies in mice (47–50). Embryos deficient in VEGF-R2/flk1 never develop a vascular system and die between ED8.5 and ED9.5, exhibiting reduced numbers of hemangioblasts and endothelial progenitor cells (50). Yolk sac blood islands are not formed, hematopoietic cells are severely reduced in number, and organized blood vessels could not be detected in the embryo or yolk sac in VEGF-R2/flk1$^{-/-}$ embryos. However, early endothelial marker genes were expressed

in VEGF-R2/flk1$^{-/-}$ embryos (50), suggesting that the role of VEGF may be to expand nascent endothelial cell pools rather than to direct angioblast differentiation *per se*. In agreement with this concept, Schuh et al. reported that early endothelial progenitors are in fact produced in the absence of flk1, lending support to the notion that VEGF acts primarily as a selective mitogen for primitive ECs in early vascular development (51). By contrast, disruption of the gene for VEGF-R1/flt1 is compatible with considerable early vascular development before failure occurs in remodeling of the primary vascular network. VEGF-R1/flt1–deficient embryos have thin-walled vessels that are frequently larger than normal diameter, exhibit hemorrhage and rupture, and die around ED9 to ED10 (49). Although VEGF-R1/flt1 binds VEGF-A with a higher affinity than flk-1, it has a much lower ligand-induced tyrosine kinase activity and may therefore effectively reduce local VEGF signaling. In support of this idea, Fong et al. reported that the primary defect in flt-1 knockout mice is an *increase* in the production of hemangioblasts, a response likely to be mediated by enhanced flk1 activation caused by the absence of a "VEGF trapping" effect of flt1 (52).

To determine the role played by the tyrosine kinase domain of VEGF-R1/flt1 in vascular development, Hiratsuka et al. produced mice that express a kinase-deleted form of the flt1 receptor (53). Remarkably, this flt1 ectodomain-only mutant mouse developed a normal vascular system and exhibited normal endothelial cell proliferation and permeability responses to VEGF-A. The only defect observed in these mice was not in the ECs at all but in the chemotactic responses of monocytes to VEGF. Therefore, the ligand-binding domain alone is sufficient to rescue the embryonic lethal phenotype of flt1 knockout mice. Possible explanations for these surprising results are (i) restoration of the proper distribution of VEGF between high- and low-affinity receptors, thereby producing the correct level of local flk1-dependent signaling and (ii) because VEGF is dimeric, it can initially bind to the high-affinity flt1 ectodomain and then recruit a low-affinity flk1 partner to the ligand–receptor complex, thereby activating signaling through the flk1 tyrosine kinase domain.

Mice with reduced capacity to produce the ligand VEGF-A by gene deletion also die at ED8.5 to ED9.5, with greatly reduced differentiation of ECs and with consequent impairment of both vasculogenesis and angiogenesis (47,48). Remarkably, VEGF-deficient embryos harboring only one inactivated VEGF-A allele exhibited a heterozygous lethal phenotype, suggesting a rigid requirement for threshold concentrations of VEGF-A to support normal development (47,48). It would seem that VEGF receptors are present in excess and that nascent ECs are extremely sensitive to variations in local concentrations of VEGF for new vessel formation. This prediction is borne out by the studies of Drake and Little who microinjected VEGF-165 into the normally avascular space between endoderm and splanchnic mesoderm in 5-somite quail embryos (54). These injections produced malformed vessels and excessive fusion of endothelial channels, leading to vessels with abnormally large lumens and altered branching patterns. Perhaps the most remarkable finding from the VEGF$^{+/-}$ mice is that other angiogenic factors produced in the embryo do not compensate for a reduction in amounts of VEGF-A at this stage of vascular development. Indeed, it is surprising that redundant and compensatory pathways do not appear to operate at such a crucial step in embryonic development to ensure that a vascular supply adequate to nourish the rapidly growing embryo is formed under conditions of reduced VEGF-A production. The studies of VEGF gene dosage effects indicate that the primary morphogens for early vascular development are those that control the production of VEGF, namely, hypoxia and hypoglycemia. Given the remarkable sensitivity for VEGF-A gene dosage during embryonic development, it is perhaps not surprising to find that small changes in local

VEGF concentrations in adult tissues appear to have profound effects on angiogenesis *in vivo* (55).

## Neuroprotective Effects of Vascular Endothelial Growth Factor

Although long considered a dedicated angiogenic factor, VEGF also has important neurotrophic effects (56). The first strong evidence for a neurotrophic function of VEGF came from analysis of mice that had low circulating levels of VEGF-A because of deletion of the hypoxia response element in the VEGF-A promoter, termed VEGF$^{\delta/\delta}$ (57). Unexpectedly, these VEGF hypomorphs developed symptoms of age-related motor neuron degeneration that was reminiscent of human amyotrophic lateral sclerosis (ALS) (Lou Gehrig disease). Laser Doppler studies showed that blood flow to spinal cord neurons was considerably reduced. Moreover, *in vitro* studies showed that VEGF-A had direct cell survival effects on cultured neurons, glial cells, and Schwann cells. Many patients with ALS are known to carry mutations in the Cu/Zn-superoxide dismutase-1 (SOD1) gene, and a mouse model of SOD1$^{G93A}$ develops ALS-like motor neuron degeneration (58). When SOD1$^{G93A}$ mice were intercrossed with VEGF$^{\delta/\delta}$ mice, the double transgenic offspring had more severe motor neuron defects than either single transgenic line alone (59). Taken together, these exciting results suggest a new role for VEGF-A as a neurotrophic factor, acting directly on neurons and glia, as well as indirectly by promoting adequate neuronal blood supply. These results raise the possibility that VEGF-A may have therapeutic applications for treatment of neurodegenerative disorders such as ALS/Lou Gehrig disease, Parkinson disease, Alzheimer disease, and stroke.

## Endocrine Gland–Derived Vascular Endothelial Growth Factor

A high-throughput screen for new angiogenesis factors identified a secreted protein named *endocrine gland–derived vascular endothelial growth factor* (EG-VEGF) (60). Despite its name, EG-VEGF is unrelated in sequence or structure to VEGFs A to D. Instead, EG-VEGF is a heparin-binding growth factor that acts by G protein–coupled receptors to produce chemoattractant and angiogenic effects for a remarkably narrow range of endothelial cell types. Bovine adrenal cortex capillary ECs respond strongly to EG-VEGF, whereas a wide variety of endothelial cell lines from other tissues were completely unresponsive. Steroidogenic tissues exhibited hypoxic upregulation of EG-VEGF production by a core HIF-1 response element. EG-VEGF can cooperate with VEGF-A to produce a highly permeable, fenestrated-type capillary endothelium characteristic of many endocrine glands. The discovery of EG-VEGF suggests the existence of a family of tissue-specific cofactors for VEGF-A signaling that may confer functional specialization on ECs in different organs and tissues.

## Development of Lymphatic Endothelium

The lymphatic system controls tissue fluid homeostasis, is a conduit for circulation of lymphocytes and antigen-presenting cells, and is a vehicle for dissemination of malignant cells during tumor metastasis. Lymphatic vessels originate as a specialized outgrowth of venous endothelium [for review see (61,62)]. Recent studies have identified transcription factors (Prox-1), growth factors (VEGF-C and VEGF-D), and cell surface markers (LYVE-1) that specifically identify lymphatic ECs in developing embryos (63).

VEGF-C is a ligand for VEGF-R3/flt4, a tyrosine kinase that is expressed primarily on lymphatic ECs. Indeed, VEGF-R3$^{-/-}$ mice are embryonically lethal. Surprisingly, the defects are in early blood vessel development before the appearance of lymphatic vessels. Yolk sac vasculature fails to undergo remodeling to form vitelline vessels in VEGF-R3$^{-/-}$ embryos, the dorsal aortae and cardinal veins are small or absent, and the pericardial cavity is greatly enlarged (64). The vessels that fail to develop strongly express VEGF-R3 in ECs at early stages of blood vessel formation when VEGF-C is expressed throughout the surrounding mesenchyme. The time at which embryonic development fails in VEGF-R3$^{-/-}$ mice is much later than that in flk-1/VEGF-R2–null mice, suggesting that VEGF-R3 has an important signaling function for vascular development that is distinct from that provided by flk-1/VEGF-R2. Consistent with this idea, VEGF-C/VEGF-R3 signaling cannot rescue the developmental defects produced by loss of only one copy of the VEGF-A gene (47,48).

Jeltsch et al. used a human keratin 14 promoter to drive VEGF-C expression in the dermis of adult mice (K14-VEGF-C) (65). These mice had hyperproliferative lymphatic ECs, leading to the formation of large, dilated lymphatic vessels and a swollen dermis (65). Although VEGF-C can stimulate VEGF-R2/flk-1, the capillary vessels of K14-VEGF-C transgenic mice had the same size, density, and leukocyte rolling responses as compared to wild-type mice. Therefore, the response to VEGF-C in adult tissues is specific to lymphatic ECs, a finding that suggests a therapeutic strategy to induce lymphangiogenesis *in vivo*.

Lymphatic vessels develop from specialized ECs in preexisting blood vessels, but the molecular signals that regulate this diversification and the ultimate separation of ECs into two distinct vascular networks are not known. Abtahian et al. recently reported that mice lacking the hematopoietic intracellular signaling protein SLP-76 (also called Syk) failed to separate emerging lymphatic vessels from their parent blood vessels (66). The aberrant formation of blood–lymphatic vascular connections led to severe embryonic hemorrhage and arteriovenous shunting. Expression of SLP-76 could not be detected in normal ECs. Moreover, blood-filled lymphatics also arose in wild-type mice reconstituted with SLP-76–deficient bone marrow, suggesting that the signaling function of SLP-76 is essential for the diversification of lymphatic vessels as a separate and distinct circulatory system (66).

Kaposi sarcoma is the most frequently occurring malignant tumor in individuals infected with human immunodeficiency virus (HIV). Kaposi sarcoma–associated herpesvirus (KSHV), also called *human herpesvirus-8*, is required for formation of Kaposi sarcoma tumors. Kaposi tumors are most often regarded as neoplasms of KSHV-infected lymphatic ECs. However, Hong et al. reported that infections of blood vascular ECs with KSHV led to a striking lymphatic reprogramming of these cells, including upregulation of Prox-1, LYVE-1, and connexin 37, together with downregulation of vascular endothelial markers, such as neuropilin-1, intercellular adhesion molecule-1 (ICAM-1), and placental growth factor (67). These findings suggest that KSHV infection of blood vascular ECs converts the cells to lymphatic endothelium with loss of vascular endothelial properties.

## Angiopoietins

A second family of receptor tyrosine kinases important for vascular development includes two proteins with immunoglobulin and epidermal growth factor–like ectodomains called tie1 and tie2/TEK (68–70). Ligands have thus far been identified only for the tie2/TEK receptor (71,72). Tie2-deficient embryos developed numerous incidences of hemorrhages, became edematous, and died by ED10.5 (68,72). Initial formation and patterning of early blood vessels were normal in Tie2-null embryos, but subsequent remodeling of initial vascular plexus into large and small vessels was defective. On histologic examination, most large vessels appeared normal, whereas the microvasculature exhibited disruption of vessel integrity, microaneurysms, and frequent ruptures. These defects result from a breakdown in cell–cell communication between ECs and surrounding mesenchymal cells leading to the failure of ECs to adhere properly to the underlying basement membrane and to each other.

## Angiopoietins—Ligands for tie2/Tek

Ligands for tie2/TEK were identified by expression cloning and were named *angiopoietins* (71). The angiopoietin family consists of four known members with the unique feature that two are receptor activators and two are receptor blockers (73). Therefore, turning off the tie2 receptor might prove to be just as important as turning it on for normal development and adult angiogenesis. The actions of angiopoietins on ECs are quite distinct from those of VEGF. Neither angiopoietin-1 (Ang1) nor angiopoietin-2 (Ang2) are mitogenic for ECs (71). Likewise, when administered alone, neither Ang1 nor Ang2 are angiogenic in a mouse corneal angiogenesis assay (74). However, when coadministered with VEGF, both Ang1 and Ang2 augmented the formation of new microvessels *in vivo* (74). Although both angiopoietins augment VEGF-dependent angiogenesis, they do so by different mechanisms. Ang1 promotes maturation and survival of new vessels, whereas Ang2 downregulates mature functions of preexisting vessels, thereby promoting endothelial detachment, migration, and angiogenesis (75).

A second prominent defect in mice lacking Ang1 or tie2 is a failure of heart development (76). In these embryos, the myocardium fails to trabeculate, and the endocardium appears detached from the myocardial layer. Because neuregulin-deficient mice exhibit a very similar failure in myocardial development (77), it remains possible that an endocardial-derived signal, namely neuregulin, controls production of Ang1 by the myocardium, which in turn acts on the endocardium by tie2 to promote normal endocardial–myocardial signaling. Therefore, interruption of endocardial–myocardial communication in mice deficient in tie2 signaling may underlie defects in heart development just as failure of endothelial–smooth muscle communication results in vascular defects. Transgenic mice overexpressing Ang1 in the dermis developed larger, more numerous, and more highly branched blood vessels than wild-type mice. Increased vascular density may result from the ability of Ang1 to promote vascular sprouting and branching (78) and/or from its ability to promote recruitment of pericytes and SMCs, thereby stabilizing new vessels from undergoing regression.

Factors that control the transcription of angiopoietins in vascular development are beginning to be identified. COUP-TFII is an orphan receptor of the steroid hormone family. Knockouts of COUP-TFII are embryonically lethal, with severe hemorrhage in the brain and pericardial sac (79). Endothelial cell differentiation initiates normally, and a primitive vascular plexus forms but does not remodel into large and small vessels. The role of COUP-TFII in vessel remodeling is especially evident in head mesenchyme where vessel rupture and hemorrhage are particularly obvious. Cranial vessel defects are accompanied by dilated dorsal aorta, regression of the sinus venosus, lack of branching of intersomatic arteries, and complete absence of posterior cardinal vein. These developmental defects resemble those seen in Ang1 knockouts, and reverse transcription–polymerase chain reaction (RT-PCR) analysis shows that Ang1 mRNA levels in the heart at ED9.5 are reduced eightfold to 10-fold in COUP-TFII–null mice. Therefore, one candidate transcription factor for control of Ang1 production in the development is COUP-TFII (79). Another is the MADS box factor Mef-2C (80). Mef-2C-null mice initiate vascular development normally but fail to remodel the primitive vascular plexus into a circulatory network

of large and small vessels (81). The vascular defects are probably due to a combination of direct effects on the vessel wall and indirect effects, due to defects in heart development. The cardiac defects include missing right ventricle, hypoplastic left ventricle, enlarged atria, and sinus venosus. By ED9.5, cardiac function is absent. Cranial vessels are greatly enlarged, possibly because of hypoxia-induced excess production of VEGF, and outflow arteries are hypoplastic because of loss blood flow after cardiac failure (80). RT-PCR analysis showed that levels of VEGF and Ang1 mRNAs are greatly decreased in the hearts of Mef2C$^{-/-}$ mice likely, resulting in the endocardial defects seen in these mice.

## Ephrins and Arterial–Venous Specification

The Eph receptor tyrosine kinases and their transmembrane ligands, the ephrins, mediate axon guidance, cell adhesion and migration, and patterning in the embryo [reviewed in (82)]. Ephrins control the migration of neural crest (NC) cells into branchial arches (83) and the patterning of the somites (84). Ephrins are also involved in control of blood vessel formation. The discovery that ephrin B2 and EphB4 are specifically expressed on arterial and venous ECs, respectively, before the initiation of blood flow introduced the concept of genetic determination of arterial and venous identity (85) [for review see (86)]. These pioneering studies suggested that the reciprocal and repulsive signaling between ephrinB2 and EphB4 was necessary to establish boundaries for arteries and veins, an essential step for normal vascular pattern formation (85). EphrinB1 promotes endothelial cell attachment and assembly into capillarylike structures *in vitro* (87). However, mouse embryos deficient in either ephrinB2 or EphB4 exhibit normal specification of arteries, veins, and lymphatics. Rather, a role for ephrinB2-EphB4 signaling seems to be evident at later stages of vascular remodeling, perhaps in the recruitment of mural cells (pericytes and SMCs) (88,89). EphrinA1 has been reported to mediate the angiogenic effects of tumor necrosis factor $\alpha$ (TNF-$\alpha$)–induced inflammatory responses (90).

Additional Eph/ephrin genes have been reported to be expressed in the developing cardiovascular system, indicating that Eph/ephrin interactions between ECs are not restricted to the boundaries between arteries and veins (91). Moreover, expression of ephrinB2 and EphB2 in mesenchyme surrounding early blood vessels suggests a role for Eph signaling in vascular SMC development. This idea is supported by the phenotype of EphB2/EphB3 double knockouts that had severe vascular defects including aortic arch artery malformations, delayed angiogenesis in cranial mesenchyme, abnormal cardinal veins, and extended pericardial sacs (91). These findings indicate that cell-to-cell signaling involving Eph/ephrin combinations is required for normal development and patterning of the vascular system. Additional important cues for arterial–venous fate determination are supplied by the notch signaling pathway, as demonstrated by gain and loss of function experiments in zebrafish (92,93) and in mice (94,95). Future studies will identify how important transcriptional controls for arterial–venous identity respond to environmental cues, including Shh and VEGF, to establish the correct vascular pattern before blood flow (92).

## Sonic Hedgehog

The vertebrate hedgehog (Hh) family consists of three known members: Shh, Indian hedgehog (Ihh), and desert hedgehog (Dhh). Hh proteins possess autocatalytic activity that cleaves a 413–amino acid precursor to release a 19-kDa *N*-terminal fragment with Hh signaling activity and a 28-kDa *C*-terminal peptide with cholesterol transferase activity. Shh normally contains palmitate at its *N*-terminus and cholesterol at its *C*-terminus (96). These lipid modifications enhance biological activity and reduce diffusion of Hh proteins from their source of synthesis. Hh proteins bind to 12-pass transmembrane proteins called patched (Ptc)-1 and Ptc-2. Ptc proteins do not signal. Rather, they control the activity of a 7-pass transmembrane protein called smoothened (Smo) (97,98). Smo transmits the Hh signal by a complex of proteins that associates with microtubules and controls the proteolytic processing of a family of Zn finger–containing transcription factors called gli-1, gli-2, and gli-3 (99,100).

Target genes whose expression is increased by activation of Smo signaling include ptc, gli-1, VEGF, Ang1, Ang2, fibroblast growth factor (FGF), bone morphogenetic proteins (BMPs), and Wnt proteins. A role for Hh signaling in vascular development was first suggested by the phenotype of Ihh knockout mice in which 50% of Ihh$^{-/-}$ embryos died at midgestation with severe yolk sac vascular defects (101). Formation of yolk sac blood vessels depends upon signaling from visceral endoderm to overlying mesoderm (2). Ihh is produced by visceral endoderm and is necessary and sufficient to direct yolk sac mesoderm to produce hematopoietic and endothelial cell lineages in explant culture systems (102,103). Embryonic stem cells isolated from Ihh-deficient mice are unable to form blood islands after conversion to embryoid bodies *in vitro* (104). Detailed analysis showed that Ihh$^{-/-}$ yolk sac blood vessels are smaller, fewer, and fail to undergo vascular remodeling when compared to wild-type. By contrast, Smo$^{-/-}$ yolk sac vessels arrest at an earlier stage of vascular development and do not undergo even the limited vascular remodeling observed in Ihh-null yolk sac.

A role for Hh signaling in adult angiogenesis has also been reported. Intramuscular injections of Shh following unilateral hindlimb ischemia stimulated angiogenesis and produced progressive increases in blood flow (105). When compared directly with VEGF-165 in a murine cornea angiogenesis model, both Shh and VEGF increased the number of blood vessels over a 6-day course. Shh produced a well-organized vascular network of dichotomous branching, large- and small-diameter vessels. By contrast, VEGF produced a halo of small, capillarylike vessels of uniform diameter. Similar experiments in Ptc-lacZ mice showed strong β-galactosidase staining that did not colocalize with endothelial or smooth muscle markers but rather was expressed by vimentin-positive interstitial fibroblasts (105). Administration of a Shh function–blocking monoclonal antibody (5E1) prevented upregulation of VEGF-A expression by resident fibroblasts in ischemic hind limbs and inhibited angiogenesis in this model (106). When tested *in vitro*, Shh had no direct effects on endothelial cell migration or proliferation and failed to activate Ptc gene expression. Instead, Shh strongly increased production of VEGF-A, Ang1, and Ang2 from a variety of cultured fibroblast cell lines. These findings suggest that Shh stimulates angiogenesis by a novel pathway that involves upregulation of two distinct families of angiogenic factors by mesenchymal cells in ischemic or injured tissues (105,106).

## Semaphorins

Semaphorins, similar to ephrins, are nerve-guiding and signaling molecules that are also implicated in vascular development and angiogenesis. The semaphorin family includes both transmembrane and secreted forms that bind to two different classes of receptors called *plexins* and *neuropilins* (107). It is currently thought that neuropilins provide a ligand-binding site for semaphorins, and plexins play a signaling role, although some semaphorins can bind directly to plexins (107). In vertebrates,

there are 19 semaphorins identified that are divided into five subgroups on the basis of structural features and on the basis of whether they are secreted or membrane bound (108). Binding of semaphorin 3A to neuropilin1 inhibits the motility of ECs *in vitro* and is thought to play a similar function in the developing embryo (44). The pexin D1 receptor on ECs was recently shown to be required for proper blood vessel pathfinding during the establishment of the initial vascular pattern of the major blood vessels in the zebrafish mutant out-of-bounds (109). Moreover, a loss of function mutation for pexin D1 in the mouse results in vascular patterning and outflow tract defects, including persistent truncus arteriosus, ectopic origin of coronary arteries, and, in some cases, right-sided aortic arch and absence of ductus arteriosus (110). These findings suggest an unexpected role of vascular endothelium in morphogenesis of the cardiac outflow tract.

## Transforming Growth Factor-β

The transforming growth factor-β (TGF-β) family of growth factors controls the development, adaptation, and repair of many tissues, including blood vessels. TGF-β binds to a receptor complex composed of two transmembrane serine–threonine kinases known as type I and type II TGF-β receptors (TβRI and TβRII). Binding of TGF-β to TβRII promotes the assembly of a heterotetrameric ligand–receptor complex that stimulates phosphorylation of TβRI by TβRII, thereby activating the serine–threonine kinase activity of TβRI. Activated TβRI phosphorylates receptor-bound proteins called *Smads*, thereby releasing them from binding sites on TβRI and leading to the association of phosphorylated receptor-Smads with the common coactivator, Smad4, followed by translocation of the Smad complex to the nucleus and stimulation of target gene transcription. Various studies, including genetic analyses in mice, indicate an important role for TGF-β signaling in vascular development.

### Transforming Growth Factor-βs 1-3

Mice deficient in TGF-β1 exhibit severe vascular developmental defects. Approximately 50% of TGF-β1$^{-/-}$ mice and 25% of TGF-β1$^{+/-}$ mice die around ED10.5 because of defects in yolk sac vasculogenesis and hematopoiesis (111). Embryos that survive this early lethality are viable at birth but die in the neonatal period from multifocal inflammatory disease (112). Embryonic lethality is correlated with defects in development of extraembryonic vasculature and disruption of chorioallantoic placental circulation (111). Blood islands appear and ECs differentiate normally in TGF-β1 mutant embryos, but later stages of vessel formation and/or survival are defective. At ED8.5, the number of ECs and yolk sac vessels was decreased in TGF-β1$^{-/-}$ mice compared to wild-type mice (111). It is curious that in two different studies, 50% of TGF-β1$^{-/-}$ mice exhibit early embryonic lethality with severe vascular defects, whereas 50% of embryos with the same mutant genotype do not display these developmental defects. The most likely explanation for this dichotomy is that because the null phenotype was examined on mixed genetic backgrounds, the differences between TGF-β1–deficient embryos that live or die *in utero* probably result from polymorphisms in modifier genes such as those involved in processing latent TGF-β1 to an active form or in elements of the receptor signaling pathway itself.

TGF-β2–deficient mice survive to term but die within minutes after birth after exhibiting cyanosis and respiratory failure (113). Multiple heart defects are found in TGF-β2$^{-/-}$ mice, including double outlet right ventricle, reduced myocardial trabeculation, and ventricular septal defects. The ascending aorta is hypocellular and thin-walled. Craniofacial defects are also present, consistent with a general deficiency in the migration or survival of cranial NC cells, which are the progenitors for SMCs in the aortic arch arteries (114,115). TGF-β3–null mice are born phenotypically normal but die within 8 to 24 hours because of difficulty in breathing and inability to suckle (116). These mice exhibit cleft palate because of failure of the palate edges to fuse along the midline. TGF-β3–deficient mice also have lung defects because of abnormal airway epithelial–mesenchymal interactions. The cardiovascular system in TGF-β3–null mice appears phenotypically normal.

### Activation of Latent Transforming Growth Factor-βs

TGF-βs are synthesized as inactive precursors. TGF-β1 is the C-terminal portion of a larger, 390–amino acid precursor that contains a latency-associated peptide (LAP) at the N-terminus. LAP is cleaved before secretion and remains noncovalently bound to TGF-β1 after secretion from the cell. This noncovalent complex is inactive and cannot bind to TGF-β receptors. The ability of LAP to bind and inactivate TGF-β1 is retained in its recombinant form, which can inhibit endogenous TGF-β1 when injected into mice (117). The latent TGF-β1 complex produced by most cells also contains a large secreted glycoprotein that is disulfide-linked to LAP known as *latent TGF-β binding protein* (LTBP). LTBP is composed of EGF-like repeats and cysteine-rich motifs that are structurally similar to domains found in fibrillin-1 and fibrillin-2. Moreover, LTBP forms fibrillar structures and undergoes transglutaminase-dependent cross-linking reminiscent of posttranslational modifications of fibrillins. The interaction of TGF-β1 with LAP and LTBP results in tight association of the growth factor, with the ECM in a latent or storage form.

Latent TGF-β1 can be activated *in vitro* by acid, heat, alkali, limited proteolysis, incubation with glycosidases, or binding to thrombospondin. The actual physiologic mechanisms for TGF-β1 activation *in vivo* are not known. ProTGF-β1 has an RHRR signal sequence for cleavage by mammalian convertase-type endoproteinases. Therefore, a candidate activator for latent TGF-β1 *in vivo* is the proprotein convertase furin. Purified furin efficiently converts proTGF-β1 into the mature 12.5-kDa form of TGF-β1 *in vitro* (118). Embryos that are deficient in furin because of a targeted gene deletion die between ED10.5 and ED11.5 from severe defects in yolk sac vasculogenesis and from arrest of cardiac looping (119). In the mutant yolk sacs, the appearance of blood islands and the timing of endothelial cell differentiation are not altered, but subsequent steps in vessel formation and maturation are defective. The phenotype of furin-deficient yolk sac vasculature is strikingly similar to that of TGF-β1–deficient yolk sacs (see preceding text) and lends support to the idea that furin and other members of the furinlike convertase family are physiologic activators of TGF-βs in the developing vascular system.

### Transforming Growth Factor-β Receptors

Any postulated role for TGF-βs in vascular development necessarily requires the presence of functional TβRI and TβRII. Consistent with an important role for TGF-β in blood vessel development, deficiencies in TβRII are embryonic lethal because of defects in yolk sac vasculogenesis and hematopoiesis (120). The phenotype of TβRII knockout mice is very similar to that of TGF-β1–deficient mice (111). More recently, a role for TβRIII in endocardial cell transformation in the heart was reported (121). TβRIII facilitates the binding of TGF-β2 to the TβRI-RII complex. Blocking antibodies to TβRIII inhibit endocardial to mesenchymal transformation, a crucial step in valve formation (121). Also, transfection of normally unresponsive ventricular endocardium with TβRIII enables these cells to undergo mesenchymal transformation when exposed to TGF-β2 (121). These experiments raise the possibility that TβRIII may either have an unsuspected signaling function or modify the TβRI–TβRII signaling complex to activate novel downstream factors.

### Smads

TβRI signals by phosphorylation of intracellular proteins called Smads (122). Vertebrate Smads were discovered by sequence homology to genes called MAD in *Drosophila* and sma in *Caenorhabditis elegans*, therefore the term Sma/Mad-related or Smad. By genetic analysis, MAD and sma act downstream of Dpp (a BMP/TGF-β homolog) and daf4 (a TGF-β receptor), respectively. Smads comprise a gene family of eight known members including the receptor-regulated Smads (Smads 1, 2, 3, 5, and 8), the common Smad (Smad 4), and the inhibitory Smads (Smads 6 and 7). Smads 1, 5, and 8 are substrates for BMPR-I and mediate BMP signals (123). Smads 2 and 3 are substrates for TβRI and ActRI and mediate TGF-β and activin signaling. All receptor-regulated Smads require dimerization with Smad4 to form complexes that translocate to the nucleus and activate target gene transcription either by direct DNA binding or by association with other DNA-binding proteins such as AP-1 (124) or Fast-1 (125). The inhibitory Smads were discovered by differential display cloning for genes whose expression is induced by laminar shear stress in ECs (126) and by screening of EST databases (127,128). Inhibitory Smads bind to the intracellular domain of type 1 signaling receptors but are not phosphorylated because they lack crucial C-terminal serine residues that are sites of phosphorylation in receptor-activated Smads (129). Bound inhibitory Smads block access of the signaling Smads to the type I receptor, thereby preventing their phosphorylation/activation. Smad6 preferentially inhibits BMP signaling and Smad7 inhibits both TGF-β and BMP signaling (123). Smad7 is induced by TGF-β1, suggesting an intracellular negative feedback loop that normally operates to regulate TGF-β signaling.

Smad2 is required for early mesoderm formation, anterior–posterior patterning, and normal craniofacial development (130). Although Smad2$^{-/-}$ mice die at ED9.5 from the generalized defects described in the preceding text, the early stages of vasculogenesis and hematopoiesis appear normal. Smad3-deficient mice are born viable and fertile, are smaller than wild-type littermates, and exhibit no overt defects in cardiovascular development (131,132). *In vitro* studies on embryonic fibroblasts isolated from Smad3-deficient mice suggest an important role for Smad3 in TGF-β1–mediated growth inhibition and transactivation of TGF-β1–responsive promoters (e.g., 3TP-lux, PAI-1, and c-jun). As expected from a common mediator of all Smad-dependent signaling, a null mutation introduced into the coactivator Smad4 produces an early embryonic lethality resulting from gastrulation defects, absence of mesoderm formation, and loss of normal anterior–posterior patterning of the embryo.

Although Smad5 is commonly regarded as a mediator of BMP signaling, Smad5-deficient mice have severe defects in vasculogenesis and hematopoiesis that strongly resemble the phenotype of TGF-β1–deficient mice (133,134). Yolk sac blood islands appear normally, ECs initiate differentiation and assemble a primitive vascular plexus at the correct time, but there is a defect in remodeling the primary network to a series of large/small vessels in Smad5-deficient mice. There is also a defect in hematopoiesis because the yolk sac is pale and anemic. Within the embryo, enlarged blood vessels were found to be surrounded by decreased numbers of vascular SMCs. Widespread apoptosis is detected throughout the mesenchyme, suggesting that the deficit in SMCs may be due to a reduced number of mesenchymal precursors. Therefore, Smad5 is essential for mesenchymal cell survival and for recruitment of SMCs during vascular development. The phenotype of Smad5-deficient mice resembles that of TGF-$\beta$1$^{-/-}$ mice and also of T$\beta$RII$^{-/-}$ mice, suggesting that Smad5 may be a physiologic mediator of TGF-$\beta$1 signaling in the developing embryo.

## Adhesion Molecules in Early Vessel Formation

Endothelial-specific cell–cell adhesion is required early in development to assemble vessel structures and then later to regulate transmural permeability and trafficking of leukocytes into surrounding tissues. ECs adhere to one another by tight junctions, gap junctions, and adherens junctions. The latter are formed by calcium-dependent adhesion molecules of the cadherin superfamily and include N-cadherin, which is expressed on many other cell types, and vascular-endothelial cadherin (VE-cadherin or cadherin-5), which is expressed exclusively on ECs (135). Consistent with an essential role for an endothelial-specific cadherin in vascular development, mice deficient in VE-cadherin do not survive beyond ED11.5 because of severe vascular defects (136,137). Absence of VE-cadherin did not disrupt hemangioblast formation, endothelial cell differentiation or early vessel formation. Remarkably, ECs lacking VE-cadherin exhibited normal cell adhesion and formed early capillarylike vessels despite the absence of a major endothelial-specific cell–cell adhesion molecule. By ED9.5, however, defects in remodeling and maturation of the primitive vascular plexus had become evident. Certain vessels had little or no lumen (thoracic aorta, anterior cardinal vein), whereas others had dilated vascular profiles. Increased endothelial cell apoptosis in VE-cadherin$^{-/-}$ embryos was found by terminal deoxynucleotidyl transferase biotin-dUTP nick end labeling (TUNEL), annexin V staining, and transmission electron microscopy (136). Endocardial cells detached from basal lamina, and embryonic vessels regressed, disintegrated, and collapsed, leading to progressive and widespread necrosis and finally to death of the embryo. Surprisingly, when examined by electron microscopy, ECs in blood islands had well-formed adherens junctions (137). If endothelial cell–cell adhesion is not defective in VE-cadherin$^{-/-}$ mice, what is the basis for the embryonic lethal phenotype? Carmeliet et al. showed that VE-cadherin and $\beta$-catenin could be coimmunoprecipitated with the VEGF receptor VEGF-R2/flk1 and Akt/protein kinase B in a large multiprotein complex that facilitates Akt-dependent survival signaling (136). Consistent with such a mechanism, the ability of VEGF-A to rescue ECs from apoptosis *in vitro* was found to require intact VE-cadherin. Physical interactions between VE-cadherin, $\beta$-catenin, and VEGF-R2/fkl1 are reminiscent of the finding that E-cadherin physically interacts with the EGF receptor (another receptor tyrosine kinase) by $\beta$-catenin (138). Therefore, VE-cadherin is not required for initial endothelial cell–cell adhesion but is required for formation of a continuous vascular network, for branching, and for VEGF-mediated cell survival during embryogenesis.

Endothelial cell interactions with the ECM are also crucial for vascular development. Indeed, defects in cell–matrix interactions may prove to be a major reason for failure of vessel maintenance in tie2- or Ang-1–deficient mice. $\alpha_4$-Integrins bind to both fibronectin and VCAM-1. Approximately half of the $\alpha_4$-integrin–deficient embryos exhibit early embryonic lethality because of defects in allantois fusion with the chorion (139). The remaining $\alpha_4$-integrin–deficient mice die between ED12.5 to ED13.5 from failure of the epicardium and lack of coronary vessel formation (139). VCAM-1, a counter-receptor for $\alpha_4$ integrin, is expressed by myocardial cells and appears to be the critical binding partner because VCAM-1 knockout mice exhibit very similar defects in placenta and coronary vessel formation (140). $\alpha_5$ Integrins appear to be crucial fibronectin receptors in early development because the severity of the $\alpha_5$-integrin–null phenotype more closely matches that of fibronectin null mice than other fibronectin-binding integrins (141).

$\alpha_V$-Containing integrins have been implicated in vascular development and angiogenesis. Drake et al. reported that $\alpha_V\beta_3$ antagonists disrupt vascular development and Friedlander et al. found that antagonists to $\alpha_V\beta_3$- and $\alpha_V\beta_5$-integrins blocked retinal neovascularization (142,143). Moreover, Brooks et al. showed that the anti-$\alpha_V\beta_3$ antibody LM609 inhibited tumor angiogenesis (144). It was therefore surprising to find that $\alpha_V$-integrin$^{-/-}$ mice exhibit normal vascular development up to ED12.5 when most embryos die from placental defects (256). Approximately 20% of $\alpha_V$-integrin–null mice survive until birth with a well-developed vascular system and then die in the perinatal period from vascular hemorrhage and rupture in cerebral and intestinal vessels. No vascular defects were found in other tissues of $\alpha_V$-integrin–deficient mice. Differences between findings with integrin antagonists and integrin-null mice may be due to overlapping functions and compensation by other integrins, species, or strain-specific differences in genetic background or due to transdominant inhibition of multiple integrins by interfering with one set of integrins following administration of a function-blocking antibody (145). Conditional $\alpha_V$-integrin alleles and chimeric mice will provide further insight into the specific role of $\alpha_V\beta_3$-integrins in vascular development and angiogenesis.

# FORMATION OF A TUNICA MEDIA

Once vascular remodeling has produced the basic pattern of large and small vessels, the next step in wall formation is the assembly of a tunica media to provide mechanical support, prevent hemorrhage and rupture, and to confer vasomotor and neurohumoral control of the circulation. Reciprocal signaling between ECs and mesenchymal cells is crucial to ensure endothelial cell survival and maturation, as well as for smooth muscle differentiation and matrix production. As with angiogenesis, the exchange of signals between ECs and SMCs that is initiated during vascular development continues throughout life to ensure that changing tissue demands for perfusion are coupled with corresponding adaptations in the structure and function of the tunica media.

## Origins of Vascular Smooth Muscle

Three pathways have been identified for investment of blood vessels with SMC: (i) recruitment from local mesenchyme, (ii) downstream extension from preexisting SMC, or (iii) differentiation of endotheliallike cells into SMCs. Most vascular SMCs are thought to arise by local recruitment of undifferentiated mesenchymal cells surrounding embryonic blood vessels (146,147). Although blood flow is not required for angioblasts to form capillarylike vessels in the early embryo, development of a tunica media is always associated with vessels through which blood flow can be demonstrated. As a result, it is assumed that crucial genes for SMC recruitment will exhibit flow-dependent upregulation in the embryonic endothelium. A second pathway for tunica media formation is by downstream extension of preexisting SMCs along the endothelial basement membranes of newly forming arterioles or venules (148,149). In this case, preexisting SMCs disassemble their cell–matrix and cell–cell connections to migrate along the outer surface of the nascent vessel and then reestablish a quiescent and differentiated phenotype at a new downstream location. This process may or may not be accompanied by cell division. Finally, evidence in gastrula-stage embryos or in embryoid bodies derived from mouse embryonic stem cells suggests that endothelial progenitor cells can differentiate either to ECs or to SMCs depending on environmental cues (9,20,150,151). Similarly, multipotential cells called *mesoangioblasts* can be isolated from the ED9.5 dorsal aorta that can differentiate directly into SMCs, ECs, blood cells, and skeletal muscle cells (152,153). De Ruiter et al. suggested that ECs in the dorsal aorta can undergo epithelial to mesenchymal transformation (EMT) and can transdifferentiate directly into SMCs (154). It is unlikely that mesenchymal transformation of aortic endothelium generates most of the aortic SMCs because we know that the bulk of the aortic media is made up of cardiac neural crest–derived SMCs (114). However, it is intriguing to consider that differentiation of an endothelial progenitor cell along a SMC pathway may produce a specialized subpopulation of SMCs within the intima or inner media that gives rise to diffuse intimal thickenings later in life. It will be important to determine whether this process can occur during angiogenesis, microvascular remodeling, or atherosclerotic plaque progression in adult vessels (155).

## Recruitment of Smooth Muscle Cells from Local Mesenchyme

Vascular SMC recruitment is initiated when diffusible factors released by ECs act on nearby mesenchymal cells to stimulate migration toward and clustering around developing blood vessels (156). Recruitment of SMCs from local mesenchyme is probably how most vessels acquire their smooth muscle coating. Vascular SMC differentiation can first be recognized when contractions of the tubular heart initiate the circulation. Embryonic blood vessels then acquire a tunica media to withstand the increasing blood pressure and flow rates that accompany the rapid growth of the embryo. Because SMCs are recruited locally and endothelial channels extend throughout

the embryo, it follows that vascular SMCs are recruited from many different sources of embryonic progenitors. Indeed, lineage mapping studies have provided evidence for at least four different origins of vascular SMCs in development (114,157,158) (see Fig. 41-3). One lineage produces SMCs that make up the wall of the proximal aorta, pulmonary artery, common carotid artery, innominate and subclavian arteries, and ductus arteriosus. These SMCs differentiate from cardiac neural crest–derived progenitors that migrate into the pharyngeal arches and are called *ectomesenchymal SMCs* (Ect SMCs) to denote their origin from ectoderm-derived NC cells. Lateral and splanchnopleural mesoderms comprise two additional origins for vascular SMCs and both sources give rise to cells called *mesenchymal SMCs* (Mes SMCs). In vessels where Ect and Mes SMCs coexist, the two SMC types are not equally distributed within the tunica media but exhibit sharp boundaries and transition zones (159). Ect SMCs are the predominant or exclusive type of SMC in the proximal segments of the major outflow vessels, whereas Mes SMCs are found in the distal segments of these vessels (114,115).

A third origin for vascular SMCs in the embryo was identified by lineage analysis studies employing retroviral markers, fluorescent tracers, or chick-quail chimeric embryos. Each of these approaches showed that progenitors for coronary SMCs originate from extracardiac coelomic mesothelium and reside within a transient structure called the *proepicardium* (PE) (160,161,162,163). The PE projects from the ventral body wall, contacts the looped heart tube, and migrates over the exposed surface of the heart to form the epicardial layer (162,163). Then, by a process of EMT, epicardial cells give rise to mesenchymal cells that enter the myocardium and migrate throughout the developing heart to form most of the nonmyocyte cell types in the heart (161). These epicardial-derived mesenchymal cells are progenitors for endothelial, smooth muscle, and adventitial cells of the coronary vessels, and a subset of valve mesenchymal cells. In addition, these cells are the source of instructive signals that direct competent myocardial

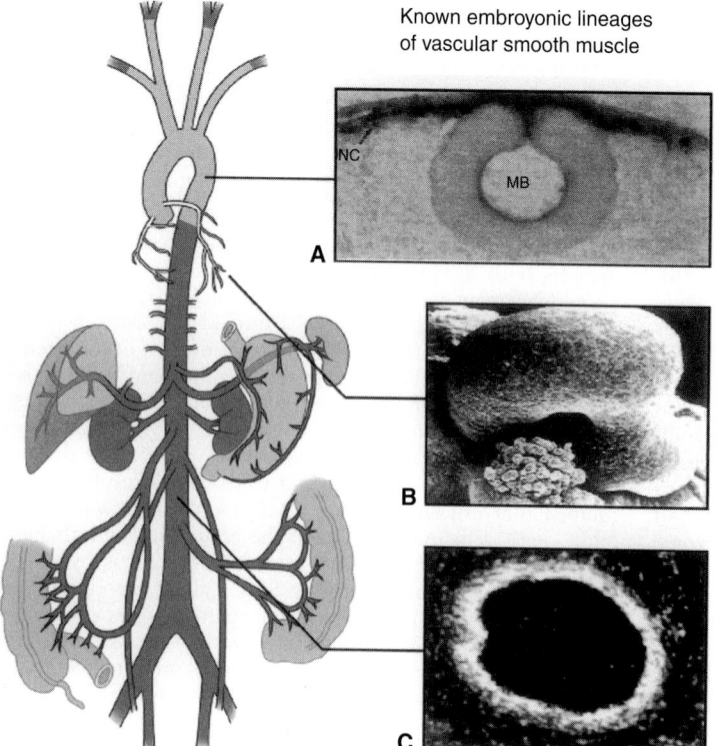

**Known embryonic lineages of vascular smooth muscle**

**FIGURE 41-3.** Vascular smooth muscle diversity. Fate mapping studies have identified at least three independent embryonic origins for vascular smooth muscle. **A:** Vessels that recruit smooth muscle cells (SMCs) from progenitors that originate in the cardiac neural crest (*NC*), here shown as migrating cells on the dorsal surface of the neural tube at the midbrain (*MB*) level that is positive for expression of the transcription factor slug. **B:** By contrast, coronary SMCs arise from mesothelial cells that line villuslike projections of the proepicardial organ, here shown just prior to contact with the looped heart tube. **C:** Vessels that recruit SMCs from local mesenchyme derived from splanchnic mesoderm.

cells to adopt a conduction tissue phenotype (164–166). Therefore, coronary SMCs are of a unique lineage that is distinct from that of any other type of SMC in the vascular system. It should also be pointed out that because coronary adventitial fibroblasts and coronary SMCs originate from the same progenitor cells and share an extensive developmental history in common, it may not be surprising to find that after injury to the coronary wall in adult hearts, adventitial cells can migrate into the damaged media and differentiate into coronary SMCs (167,168).

## Smooth Muscle Cell Recruitment by Extension of Preexisting Medial Cells

A morphologic hallmark of capillary arterialization in adult tissues is the acquisition of a pericyte coating. Pericytes are SMC-like cells that encircle the walls of precapillary and postcapillary arterioles and venules and adopt a contractile phenotype (169,170). ECs and pericytes make characteristic tight junction contacts and communicate directly through connexin-containing gap junctions (171,172). Formation of arterioles is essential for vascular development and adaptation; however, the mechanism of arteriolar wall formation has been unclear. Using antibodies directed against SMC-specific proteins, Price et al. showed an age-dependent increase in the number of terminal arterioles that were coimmunostained with anti–SM-MHC and anti-SMαActin in developing rat anterior gracilis muscle (173). They also found that new terminal arterioles exhibited SMαActin and SM-MHC labeling that was always continuous with upstream arterioles (149,173). These results implied that new arterioles were formed by pericyte extension from preexisting arteriolar medial cells (149). The findings of Price et al. (173) are reminiscent of those reported in the 1940s by the Clark and Clark who directly viewed the formation and regression of arterioles over many days in experimental chambers made in the skin of rabbit ears (174). They observed that upon delivery of a stimulus for increased blood flow, pericytes could be observed detaching from preexisting arterioles and migrating to more distal positions while maintaining close association with the precapillary vessel wall. Upon reduction in blood flow, pericytes were seen detaching from the arteriole, migrating away from the microvessel, and wandering into the interstitial matrix where they often underwent cell death. Taken together, these studies provide support for the idea that developing microvessels acquire a medial layer in response to increases in blood flow by extension of a preexisting population of SMCs through pericyte detachment and chemotaxis along the capillary endothelial cell basement membrane.

What are the signals that induce pericytes to detach from preexisting vessels and migrate downstream along capillary endothelium? Gene deletion studies in mice have shown that pericytes depend upon PDGF-B produced by capillary ECs for their development or survival (148,175) [for review see (176)]. PDGF-B expression by ECs in angiogenic sprouts is much greater than in quiescent stable microvessels. PDGF-β receptor–positive pericytes are normally found clustered around PDGF-B–expressing ECs and are recruited to migrate along sprouting capillary basement membranes by chemotaxis. In PDGF-B–deficient mice, capillary vessels are more tortuous, pericytes are frequently missing, and capillary walls are distended and exhibit numerous microaneurysms (175). PDGF-B–null mice also have a deficiency in pericytelike mesangial cells in renal glomeruli. Curiously, not all microvessels showed a requirement for PDGF-B signaling to support normal development. Vessels dependent upon PDGF-B were found in brain, heart, lung, and skeletal muscle, whereas vessels in the liver, gastrointestinal tract, adrenal gland, and perineural plexus were not affected by the absence of PDGF-B. A detailed study of PDGF-B/PDGF-β receptor signaling in

coronary development showed that subepicardial vessels in PDGF-deficient mice have fewer SMCs than those in wild-type hearts, whereas penetrating coronary arteries completely lack SMαActin-positive cells (148). These findings are consistent with the idea that penetrating coronary arteries acquire their media by downstream extension of SMCs from proximal sites along the main subepicardial coronary vessels in a PDGF-B-dependent manner. A similar mechanism may operate in brain vasculature where submeningeal arterioles contribute SMCs to downstream vessels that penetrate the brain by way of a PDGF-B–dependent downstream extension of preexisting SMCs. Although the normal appearance of the aorta and other large artery walls in PDGF-B–deficient mice suggests that they are independent of PDGF-B signaling for normal development, the possibility that compensatory mechanisms rescue large vessel defects in PDGF-B $^{-/-}$ mice should not be ruled out. Indeed, a study of chimeric mice composed of a mixture of wild-type and PDGF-β receptor–deficient cells showed that SMCs in large vessel walls normally respond to a PDGF-B signal for recruitment, proliferation, and/or survival during tunica media formation (177). Taken together, these studies suggest that for some vessels, PDGF-B is required for initial recruitment of SMCs or pericytes from surrounding mesenchyme. For most vessels, it appears that other factors provide the initial stimulus for SMC recruitment and PDGF-BB provides either a mitogenic/survival stimulus for expansion of the initial SMC pool or a chemotactic stimulus for downstream extension of preexisting SMCs.

Veins also acquire a SMC coating by an endothelial-dependent process. A point mutation in the angiopoietin-1 receptor gene *Tie2* is responsible for a human genetic deficiency called *venous malformation*. This mutation leads to an amino acid substitution that constitutively activates the receptor in a ligand-independent manner (178). Patients with venous malformation have thin-walled and dilated veins in specific locations under the skin. Venous dilation is associated with severe reduction in the number of venous SMCs. Because the tie2 receptor is not expressed in SMCs or their mesenchymal precursors, these data suggest that endothelial-dependent signals that are under the control of angiopoietin-1/tie2 signaling are required for recruitment of venous SMCs. As with arteries and veins, microvessels require ongoing bidirectional signaling between ECs and SMC/pericytes for formation and survival. One example of this interdependence is found in the postnatal development of the retinal vasculature. In this system, microvascular density is controlled primarily by the availability of oxygen. Hypoxia promotes new vessel formation, whereas hyperoxia promotes vascular regression. Careful analysis of the timing of hyperoxia-induced "vascular pruning" showed that it corresponds to a transient period characterized by the appearance of a pericyte-free neovascular plexus (179). Normally, retinal microvessels acquire a pericyte coating by migration of preexisting pericytes from upstream arterioles. In the absence of pericytes, new capillary vessels are labile and exhibit high rates of endothelial cell death. However, once the new vessels have acquired a pericyte cell layer, endothelial apoptosis rates drop sharply (179,180). VEGF is a known survival factor for ECs that is produced by pericytes and SMCs. Therefore, pericyte recruitment brings a source of VEGF in close contact with retinal capillary endothelium. Consistent with this idea, intraocular injection of VEGF accelerated pericyte coverage (179). Likewise, heparin-binding EGF (HB-EGF) was found to induce retinal neovascularization by stimulating VEGF production by SMCs/pericytes (181). By contrast, intraocular injection of PDGF-BB caused vascular regression because of detachment of PDGF β-receptor–positive pericytes from newly coated vessels while having no effect on already established vessels. Therefore, ECs and pericytes exchange crucial factors to ensure coordinated retinal microvascular formation and survival during postnatal development.

Lessons learned from embryonic vascular development can help us understand how angiogenesis is controlled in adult vessels. For example, using a rabbit cornea micropocket assay, Asahara et al. found that although VEGF alone induces angiogenesis, the process is enhanced by treatment with either angiopoietin-1 or angiopoietin-2 (74). Detailed morphometric analysis of vessel length, diameter, and density showed that angiopoietin-1 enhances VEGF-induced angiogenesis by promoting maturation of newly formed vessels, whereas angiopoietin-2 works to initiate endothelial sprouting by downregulating the stabilizing influence of angiopoietin-1. Therefore, the coordinated production of VEGF, angiopoietin-1, and angiopoietin-2 by pericytes and SMCs governs the ability of ECs to initiate angiogenesis and plays a major role in whether newly formed vessels regress or survive in adult tissues.

## Formation of Smooth Muscle Cells from Endothelial Cells

The notion that ECs can transdifferentiate into SMCs seems counterintuitive. However, it is not a new idea. In 1944, Altschul reported that histologic studies of human atherosclerosis showed that ECs could be observed to leave the surface lining, undergo a mesenchymal change, and become embedded in the aortic subendothelial matrix (182). He remarked that the number of endothelium-derived mesenchymal cells were "frequently great enough to produce a distinct thickening of the subendothelial space" (182). Arciniegas et al. reported that greater than 90% of bovine aortic ECs treated with TGF-β1 *in vitro* convert to spindle-shaped cells that coordinately gain SMαActin and lose factor VIII–related antigen expression (183). This phenotypic change became "irreversible" after 20 days of incubation in TGF-β1–containing medium. Sarkisov et al. observed capillary endothelial cell conversion into SMC-like myofibroblasts in granulation tissue during excisional wound repair (184). Moreover, Tuder et al. reported that ECs convert to myofibroblasts and SMCs in intimal thickenings associated with pulmonary hypertension (185). Finally, it should be pointed out that a very similar process of endothelial to mesenchymal transformation in heart development is well known (186). During cardiac valve formation, endocardial cells respond to factors produced by myocardium, transform into mesenchymal cells, invade cushion tissue ECM, and differentiate into valve interstitial cells (187). If endothelial to mesenchymal conversion occurs in endocardium during heart development, the possibility that a similar process occurs in vascular endothelium deserves careful consideration.

Two lines of experimental evidence support an origin of vascular SMCs from endotheliallike cells. First, DeRuiter et al. observed cells coexpressing markers for both ECs and SMCs directly beneath the endothelium in developing quail aorta (154). Furthermore, after injection of gold-labeled wheat germ agglutinin particles (Au-WGA) into the anterior vitelline vein, Au-WGA particles were detected both in surface lining ECs and in cells of the inner layer of the tunica media. The authors conclude that ECs endocytose Au-WGA particles at the luminal surface, undergo mesenchymal transformation, invade the subendothelial matrix, and acquire an SMC phenotype. Therefore, the subendothelial intima and inner media are seen as being built up of SMC-like cells that originate from the endothelial layer. Although this possibility awaits confirmation, a second line of evidence suggests that endotheliallike multipotential cells isolated from explants of ED9.5 to ED16 mouse embryo dorsal aorta (called mesoangioblasts) can produce cells capable of entering the myogenic lineage, expressing

MyoD, and participating in skeletal muscle fiber formation upon injection into adult muscle (188,189). At first glance, the finding that ECs could be a source of skeletal myoblasts seems remarkable. Yet it is important to note that somites and aortic endothelium are not so far removed from each other during early development. In fact, one source of angioblasts in the embryo is from somites, and the paired dorsal aortae are formed directly below, and in connection to, bilateral pairs of somites that differentiate from paraxial mesoderm (6). Moreover, when segments of quail or mouse embryo dorsal aorta known to contain mesoangioblasts were transplanted into host chick embryos, donor cells were found to differentiate not only into skeletal muscle but also into blood, cartilage, bone, smooth, and cardiac muscle (152). These findings suggest that mesoangioblasts are vessel-associated stem cells in the embryo and raise the intriguing possibility that these cells persist in adult vessels and participate in vascular repair and disease. In addition, multipotential cells in the ventral paraaortic region have been shown to produce both endothelial and hematopoietic cells (190). Similar kinds of multipotential vascular progenitor cells have been isolated from midgastrula stage embryos, from ES cell–derived embryoid bodies *in vitro*, and from the area of the dorsal aorta near the somites. These cells can differentiate into ECs or SMCs depending on the substrate and growth factors they are exposed to (9,20,150,151,153).

## Endothelial–Smooth Muscle Signaling in Tunica Media Formation

Vessel wall formation involves bidirectional signaling between ECs and SMCs. Differentiation and expansion of the initial endothelial cell pool is dependent upon VEGF produced by mesenchymal cells (47,48). Ang-1 is also produced by mesenchymal cells in close proximity to developing blood vessels and is required for normal vascular development (76). Ang-2 is a naturally occurring antagonist that blocks Ang-1 binding to tie2/tek. Knockouts of Ang-1 have severe defects in endothelial cell sprouting and vascular remodeling, and display embryonic lethality very similar to that of tie2 knockouts (76). Genetic evidence that ECs signal mesenchymal cells to form the tunica media is provided by the phenotypes of LKLF and endoglin knockout mice. LKLF (lung Kruppel–like factor, also called KLF2) is a Zn-finger transcription factor of the *Drosophila* Kruppel gene family that is selectively expressed in developing ECs (191). LKLF-null embryos die between ED12.5 and ED14.5 from vascular defects including hemorrhage and rupture. Vasculogenesis and primary network formation are normal in LKLF$^{-/-}$ mice, and SMαActin-positive cells appear in close apposition to vascular channels in LKLF knockout embryos. Therefore, LKLF is not required to specify either endothelial or smooth muscle lineages. However, the tunica media in LKLF null embryos is abnormally thin and disorganized, SMC differentiation is delayed, and ECM deposition is reduced (191). Absence of LKLF does not alter the expression of PDGF-B, tie2, tie1, flk1, HB-EGF, or TGF-β1 in ECs nor disrupt red cell, platelet, or myelomonocytic development. Because LKLF is not normally expressed by SMCs or their mesenchymal precursors, the phenotype of LKLF$^{-/-}$ mice strongly suggests that LKLF activity is required in ECs to control SMC recruitment, differentiation, or organization of the tunica media. Therefore, an important direction for future work will be to identify the crucial gene products for vessel wall formation controlled by LKLF in ECs.

Endoglin is a type III TGF-β receptor selectively expressed by ECs. Hypomorphic mutations in the endoglin locus cause human hereditary hemorrhagic telangectasia (HHT). In mice, endoglin gene deletion produces an embryonic lethal phenotype with severe vascular defects that resemble those in LKLF knockouts described in the preceding text (192). SMC recruitment and differentiation are defective causing failure of vascular development and early embryonic death. Again, vasculogenesis and early capillarylike vascular network formation are normal, endothelial differentiation markers are expressed normally, and blood cells are produced in endoglin $^{-/-}$ embryos at similar levels as that in wild-type mice. Vascular defects begin to appear around ED9.5 to ED10.5 and correlate with failure of SMC recruitment. Because endoglin is expressed by ECs and is absent in SMCs, the endoglin-null phenotype suggests that ECs respond to TGF-$\beta$1 and produce SMC recruitment factors. In this respect, it is noteworthy that approximately half of TGF-$\beta$1–deficient embryos exhibit failure of vascular development at point when endothelial–mesenchymal interactions are required (111).

## Differentiation and Maturation of the Tunica Media

The final steps in vessel wall development are growth, differentiation, maturation, and innervation of SMCs to form a mature and functional tunica media. Extensive studies of SMC differentiation over the years have identified a large number of contractile and cytoskeletal proteins whose expression can be correlated with maturation of the tunica media *in vivo*. Despite this progress, the crucial pathways that signal the transcriptional activation of these SMC-specific structural genes remain unclear. The following is a brief summary of SMC differentiation because it pertains to development of the tunica media. Emphasis is placed on identification of genes whose mutant phenotypes involve defects in formation of the tunica media. For more extensive coverage of the general topic of SMC differentiation, the reader is directed to several excellent recent reviews (147,193–195).

### The Role of Mechanical Forces and the Extracellular Matrix

As a general rule, the final thickness attained by the developing artery wall is proportional to wall stress, which, according to the law of Laplace, is a product of blood pressure and lumen diameter. Therefore, as lumen diameter increases, wall thickness correspondingly increases to normalize overall wall stress. Because blood flow is the primary determinant of lumen diameter, it follows that wall thickness is proportional to blood flow. Usually, the smooth muscle mass increases or decreases in tandem with that of ECM during wall remodeling, presumably as a result of signaling pathways activated by SMC-ECM adhesion receptors. The importance of this tightly coupled interaction for control of overall wall dimensions was revealed by the phenotype of the tropoelastin knockout mouse (196).

In large elastic arteries, tropoelastin is secreted into the extracellular space where it binds to scaffold proteins called *microfibril proteins* and then becomes cross-linked by lysyl oxidase into insoluble bands of ELN and microfibril proteins called *elastic lamellae*. Normally, inner and outer diameters of the aorta continue to increase throughout development in response to increases in cardiac output and blood flow. In mice unable to produce tropoelastin, pups are born but fail to survive beyond postnatal day 4.5 because of progressive obstruction of the major arteries (196). In elastin $^{-/-}$ mice, aortic diameters increase normally until around ED17.5 at which time the outer and inner diameters of the ascending aorta in mutant embryos start to become progressively smaller despite continued growth of the embryo. This change in wall structure was accompanied by progressive accumulation of SMCs in the subendothelium until the aortic lumen was obliterated (196).

No differences were found in endothelial cell injury, inflammation, or hemodynamics when aortas from ED16.5 elastin $^{-/-}$ versus wild-type embryos were compared. The process of subendothelial accumulation of SMCs was also found in systemic arteries of all sizes in ELN-null mice, including distributing arteries and even arterioles. It is interesting to note that the developmental age at which tropoelastin-null mice begin to show deviation from wild-type (ED17.5) is very close to the time that Majack et al. found aortic SMCs beginning to exit the cell cycle and normally become quiescent (197). These investigators further showed that exit from the cell cycle *in vivo* correlated with the loss of an autonomous growth phenotype characterized by the ability of SMCs cultured from embryonic rat aorta to proliferate in a defined serum-free medium without the addition of exogenous mitogens *in vitro* (197). Consistent with the idea that development of the elastic fiber is coupled to SMC cell cycle exit *in vivo*, proliferating cell nuclear antigen (PCNA) staining revealed that subendothelial SMC proliferation rates were much higher in elastin $^{-/-}$ mice than in wild-type mice (88% vs. 35%). In mice hemizygous for the tropoelastin gene, 35% increase in the number of elastic lamellae and SMC number was found (196). Examination of humans with hemizygosity for the *ELN* locus revealed a remarkable 2.5-fold increase in the number of elastic lamellae in the aortic wall (198). Unlike what was previously assumed, this work showed that the number of elastic lamellae is neither genetically fixed nor species specific. Rather, these studies revealed a remarkable sensitivity of arterial SMCs to proper formation of elastic fibers for normal vessel wall structure. However, adaptation to normalize wall stress by increasing the number of elastic lamellae only occurs early in development. After birth, the artery wall responds to increased wall tension by SMC hypertrophy and wall thickening but not by change in number of elastic lamellae. Therefore, development of large conduit arteries is extremely responsive to reductions in ELN content, with compensatory changes to normalize wall stress and elasticity being evidenced by an increase in SMC mass and in the number of rings of elastic fibers. These striking results suggest that acquisition of SMC quiescence and normal assembly of fibrillar collagen, proteoglycans, and elastic lamellae depend upon production of the correct amounts of tropoelastin within the tunica media during embryonic development. In addition, they raise the possibility that vascular injury, thrombosis, and inflammation later in life contribute to obstructive arterial disease by disrupting SMC–elastic fiber interactions. A similar argument can be made for fibrillar collagens in the artery wall. Koyama et al. reported that SMCs become arrested in the G1 phase of the cell cycle when plated on polymerized type I collagen fibrils as a result of increased levels of the cdk2 inhibitors p27-Kip1 and p21-Cip1/Waf1 (199). These effects on SMC cell cycle regulators were not seen if SMCs were plated on monomeric type I collagen (199).

Perhaps in retrospect, it should not be surprising to find that ECM components of the vessel wall play an active, instructive role in control of tunica media formation and SMC growth control (146,200). After all, vascular SMCs are surrounded by an extensively cross-linked ECM from the earliest times in their development (146). Moreover, the ECM is a rich depository for many different morphogens and growth factors. Cell–matrix interactions have been well documented as playing essential roles in the development and differentiation of many cell and tissue types (201), and the vessel wall is no exception (202,203). Moreover, matrix degradation and remodeling is essential for organogenesis in general and vessel wall formation in particular (3). Indeed, for large arteries at least, it could be argued that the main function of SMCs is to produce an ECM with an appropriate combination of elasticity and strength to function under high pulse pressures.

## Developmental Expression of Elastin, Fibulins, and Fibrillins

Transcription of the ELN gene begins just after the first recognizable SMCs appear in vascular development (204–206). ELN is the primary ECM molecule in large conduit arteries and serves a structural role in nearly all vessels (207). The arrangement of cross-linked elastic fibers differs significantly between vessels that contain neural crest–derived SMCs and those that contain mesoderm-derived SMCs (208). In addition to ELN itself, elastic fibers contain fibulin-1, fibulin-2, fibrillins, emelin, and nidogen-2. Fibulin-1 is a core component of microfibrils that provides a scaffold for elastic fiber formation. Fibulin-1 is among the first ECM proteins to be expressed as mesenchymal cells become committed to a SMC fate, and it functions first as a provisional matrix for assembly of the tunica media and later as a template for deposition of elastic fibers (209). Fibulins are well suited for a role as organizers of matrix formation because they can interact with many important ECM constituents including fibronectin, laminin, nidogen, aggrecan, versican, and tropoelastin (210). Moreover, in as much as fibulin-1 is strongly expressed at sites of epithelial to mesenchymal transformation throughout the embryo, it may also be important for transdifferentiation of ECs into SMCs, for transformation of endocardial cells into valve interstitial cells, and for conversion of epicardial cells into coronary SMCs (211).

Fibrillins 1 and 2 are additional microfibril components that play key roles in the development of the tunica media. Human mutations that map to fibrillin genes have been linked to connective tissue disorders with prominent vascular phenotypes. Marfan syndrome is caused by mutations in fibrillin-1 (212), and congenital contractural arachnodactyly maps to mutations in fibrillin-2 (213) [for review see (214)]. Studies of the developmental patterns of fibrillin gene expression during mammalian development led to the proposal that fibrillin-1 is primarily a load-bearing structural element in the vessel wall, whereas fibrillin-2 is largely involved with the control of elastic fiber assembly. Both fibrillin-1 and fibrillin-2 are expressed very early in vessel wall formation (210,215). Moreover, fibrillin-2 is an early marker of vascular SMC heterogeneity in developing avian embryo (209). Other important components of the elastic fiber include emilin, a 115-kDa protein that is particularly abundant at the elastin–microfibril interface and is thought to play a role in ELN fiber assembly (216), and microfibril-associated glycoprotein (MAGP), the major glycoprotein antigen of elastin-associated microfibrils.

## Smooth Muscle Differentiation

### Developmental Expression of Smooth Muscle Cell–Specific Contractile and Cytoskeletal Genes

Expression of SMαA is the earliest marker currently known for vascular SMC differentiation (147,217). The first cells to express SMαA during vascular development appear at the ventral surface of the dorsal aorta in apposition to the foregut endoderm (209). As development of the aortic wall proceeds, additional markers of the mature SMC phenotype appear in stages. Duband et al. reported that vascular SMC differentiation *in vivo* occurs in at least two steps, as defined by the timing of vascular SMC marker expression (218). For example, SMαA and desmin are representative early stage markers, whereas expression of calponin and SM22α signifies a later step in differentiation. Smooth muscle myosin heavy chain (SM-MHC) is a highly selective marker for developing SMCs that is not expressed in cardiac or skeletal muscle in the embryo (219). Smooth muscle–specific contractile and cytoskeletal proteins are produced not only by cell type–specific transcriptional controls but also by cell type–specific alternative splicing including α-tropomyosin, heavy caldesmon, metavinculin, SM1 and SM2 isoforms of SM-MHC, and smooth muscle α-actinin (220).

## Transcriptional Control of Smooth Muscle Cell Differentiation

In an effort to understand how transcription of SMC-specific contractile and cytoskeletal genes becomes activated in vascular development, the regulatory elements of several SMC-restricted marker genes have been studied, including SMαA (221), SM22α (222,223), SMγA (224,225), telokin (226), and SM-MHC (219,227). The objective of these studies was to identify cis-acting elements that mediate SMC-restricted gene expression. A common result was the identification of an evolutionarily conserved cis-regulatory element called the CArG box [5′-CC(AT)$_6$GG-3′] as a crucial element for SMC-specific transcription. CArG boxes form the core sequence of the serum response element (SRE), a DNA sequence that binds homodimers of the serum response factor (SRF) (194,228). Although regarded as a widely expressed transcription factor, SRF is most highly expressed in skeletal, cardiac, and smooth muscle–containing tissues in the developing embryo (229). Gene deletion studies have shown that SRF is required for very early stages of mesoderm formation, specification, and survival (230). No defect in cell proliferation was found in SRF$^{-/-}$ ES cells (230), which is consistent with the suggestion by Croissant et al. that an important role of SRF in developing embryos is the transcriptional control of muscle differentiation including skeletal, cardiac, and smooth muscle rather than cell proliferation *per se* (229).

### Role of Serum Response Factor

SRF is an evolutionarily conserved member of the MADS box family of DNA-binding proteins (194,231). It is composed of a central 60–amino acid MADS domain, responsible for DNA binding and dimerization, followed by a C-terminal transactivation domain (232). Many studies have shown that MADS box factors play important roles in muscle-specific gene transcription in vertebrates. A null mutation of the *Drosophila* MADS box factor DMef-2 resulted in failure of somatic, cardiac, and visceral muscle differentiation (233). A loss of function mutation in murine SRF was embryonic lethal at a very early stage of mesoderm formation resulting in the absence of smooth, skeletal, and cardiac muscle (230). A dependence upon SRF-binding CArG-elements for SMC-specific transcription has been reported for SMαA (234), SMγA (235), SM22α (236,240), SM-MHC (237), caldesmon (238), α$_1$ integrin (239), and telokin (226), among at least 33 known gene targets for SRF (194). Smooth muscle–restricted transcription of the SM22α promoter in transgenic mice was found to depend upon an upstream CArG box found within the first 280 bp of 5′ promoter sequence *in vivo* (240). Landerholm et al. used two different dominant-negative forms of SRF to show that coronary SMC differentiation from proepicardial cells requires transcriptionally active SRF (241). More recently, Miano et al. used a conditional knockout approach to remove SRF from vascular smooth and cardiac muscle only. They reported that SRF is required for initial SMC recruitment to the dorsal aorta at ED10.5 and for proper assembly of a contractile/cytoskeletal architecture in differentiating SMCs (242). This conclusion is consistent with loss of function studies for SRF in organisms, such as worms, flies, and frogs, which show that SRF has an ancient and evolutionarily conserved function to control the formation of a migration and contraction-competent cytoskeleton (242). Therefore, it seems likely that SRF is necessary for both activation of SMC-specific transcription during development (231,241) and maintenance of SMC-specific transcription in adult vessels (147,194,243).

### Importance of Serum Response Factor Coactivators for Smooth Muscle Myogenesis

SRF-CArG box interactions confer context-dependent and signal-responsive control of muscle-specific gene transcription. It is becoming increasingly clear that the physical association of SRF with cell-restricted and/or signal-dependent coactivators is crucial for coupling of SMC differentiation to environmental cues during vascular development. An important finding in this regard was the report by Sotiropoulos et al. showing that SRF activation was closely linked to the process of cytoplasmic actin treadmilling (244). In this model, stimulation of the rhoA/p160 Rho kinase pathway led to activation of LIM kinase–dependent phosphorylation of cofilin resulting in cytoplasmic actin stress fiber formation, focal adhesion assembly and activation of SRF-dependent transcription. Further, evidence for an important role of actin treadmilling in SRF-dependent SMC gene expression was provided by the discovery by Wang et al. of myocardin during an *in silico* screen for genes that are selectively expressed during early stages of cardiogenesis (245). Myocardin is a SAP domain–containing protein with conserved basic and polyglutamine-rich regions in the N-terminus and a strong transcriptional transactivation domain in the C-terminus (245). Myocardin is expressed in cardiac and smooth muscle lineages in developing embryos and is a potent transactivator of SRF-CArG box–dependent target genes (246–248). Myocardin$^{-/-}$ mice are reported to be embryonically lethal around ED10.5 with defects in vascular SMC recruitment and/or differentiation (249). In addition, two myocardin-related transcription factors (MRTFs) have been described that translocate from the cytoplasm to the nucleus when cytoplasmic G-actin pools are depleted by polymerization into F-actin and by assembly of F-actin into cytoskeletal structures (195,250–252). MRTF-A, also called MAL, is a strong SRF coactivator that contains two RPEL motifs that bind to unpolymerized actin. MRTF-A/MAL responds to rhoGTPase activation by dissociation from G-actin and accumulation in the nucleus (250). Another class of cytoskeletal-associated proteins that have SRF coactivator properties includes the cysteine-rich LIM-only proteins (Crp1 and Crp2) (253). Through N-terminal LIM domains, Crp1 and 2 can physically interact with the MADS domain of SRF and can then recruit GATA factors by Crp C-terminal LIM domains. This multiprotein complex assembled by Crp LIM domains strongly augments SRF-dependent transcription of SMC target genes (253). Both Crp1 and Crp2 were originally described as cytoskeletal proteins that bind to zyxin and α-actinin at cell–cell and cell–matrix attachment points. Chang et al. reported that Crp1/2 translocated from cytoskeletal complexes to the nucleus during the initial stages of coronary SMC differentiation from proepicardial cells and that dominant-negative Crp2 inhibited SRF-dependent SMC differentiation in this model (253). Therefore, cytoskeletal remodeling in response to rhoGTPase signaling allows for nuclear translocation of powerful SRF coactivators that couple extracellular cues for SMC differentiation to SRF-dependent gene transcription. Once SMC target genes are turned on, powerful feed forward pathways are activated to maintain the differentiated phenotype (194). The use of vertebrate models amenable to genetic analysis, coupled with high-throughput methods for analysis of gene expression and gene discovery, will accelerate the identification of essential genes involved in tunica media formation.

# SUMMARY

Lessons learned from basic studies of vascular development have led to important insights into adaptive and disease processes in adult blood vessels. Perhaps the greatest impact to date has been in the area of therapeutic angiogenesis where genetic analysis of early vascular development has clearly identified VEGFs, angiopoietins, neuropilins, ephrins, plexins, and semaphorins as crucial factors that play complementary roles in neovascularization, both in the embryonic and in the adult vasculature. Clinical trials are under way to test the efficacy of VEGF-A or angiopoietin-1 in therapeutic angiogenesis for myocardial infarction and peripheral vascular disease. It is anticipated that clinical applications will also be found for the use of multipotential stem cells, derived either from bone marrow or from mesenchymal tissues, in cardiovascular disease. Undoubtedly, therapeutic advances will result from a better understanding of the basic mechanisms of cell–cell signaling and molecular controls of cell differentiation underlying the normal development and fate of cardiac and vascular stem cells. Genetic analysis of endothelial and blood cell formation from hemangioblasts in the embryo will identify key molecules and pathways that will enable stem cells isolated from adult tissues to be directed along preselected cell lineages so as to enhance their ability to form specific cell types upon introduction into diseased adult tissues. Likewise, the production of artificial blood vessels and biomaterials will directly benefit from fundamental studies on how pressure-bearing ECM structures that make up to artery wall are formed during vascular development and on how they are coupled to SMC growth control.

A central principle of vessel wall formation in development is that lumen diameter and wall thickness are governed by the biomechanical forces exerted on vessel wall cells by the circulation. This is as true for developing embryonic vessels as it is for adaptive changes in the structure of adult vessels. Studies of genetically manipulable experimental models (e.g., mouse and zebrafish), as well as analysis of available human mutations, will continue to identify important and sometimes unanticipated gene products that convert these biomechanical stimuli into overall changes in vessel wall structure and function. These gene products will serve as important therapeutic targets for interventions in pathologic remodeling in diseased adult vessels including restenosis and vein graft failure. Recent studies of pathways that control formation and patterning of the skeleton in the embryo, for example, have led to important insights into molecular mechanisms for calcification of cardiac valves and artery walls in adult tissues.

Finally, lineage analysis studies of SMC origins in the embryo indicate that the vascular system is best viewed as a mosaic structure that is composed of unique parts that are pieced together from cells of different origins and developmental histories. When viewed in this way, the diversity in functional properties and disease propensities of different vessels is not so mysterious. The similarity in developmental origins between coronary SMC and adventitial fibroblast is a good example of how a better understanding of the ways in which the coronary vasculature develops can lead to more productive insights into how the coronary wall responds to injury and disease. It is almost axiomatic in pathology that disease recapitulates development. If that is so, then we can anticipate that further investigation of the basic mechanisms of vascular development in the embryo will continue to be a rich source of new insights and novel therapeutic targets for better understanding and prevention of vascular degeneration and disease in adults.

# ACKNOWLEDGMENTS

The author gratefully acknowledges helpful discussions with Robert J. Schwartz, Joseph Miano, Vicki Bautch, John Schwarz, Da-Zhi Wang, and Robert Tomanek. Work in the authors' laboratory was supported by grants from the National Institutes of Health (HL-19242, HL-07816), Astra-Zeneca Pharmaceuticals, and an Established Investigator Award from the American Heart Association.

## *References*

1. Carmeliet P. Mechanisms of angiogenesis and arteriogenesis. *Nat Med* 2000;6:389–395.
2. Rossant J, Howard L. Signaling pathways in vascular development. *Annu Rev Cell Dev Biol* 2002;18:541–573.
3. Carmeliet P, Collen D. Genetic analysis of blood vessel formation. *Trends Cardiovasc Med* 1997;7:271–281.
4. Gonzalez-Crussi F. Vasculogenesis in the chick embryo. An ultrastructural study. *Am J Anat* 1971;130:441–460.
5. Sabin F. Studies on the origin of blood-vessels and of red blood-corpuscles as seen in the living blastoderm of chicks during the second day of incubation. *Carnegie Inst Wash Contrib Embryol* 1920;9:213–262.
6. Pardanaud L, Altmann C, Kitos P, et al. Vasculogenesis in the early quail blastodisc as studied with a monoclonal antibody recognizing endothelial cells. *Development* 1987;100:339–349.
7. Labastie M, Poole T, Peault B, et al. MB1, a quail leukocyte endothelium antigen: partial characterization of the cell surface and secreted forms in cultured endothelial cells. *Proc Natl Acad Sci U S A* 1986;83:9016–9020.
8. Coffin J, Poole T. Embryonic vascular development: immunohistochemical identification of the origin and subsequent morphogenesis of the major vessel primordia in quail embryos. *Development* 1988;102:735–748.
9. Huber T, Kouskoff V, Fehling H, et al. Haemangioblast commitment is initiated in the primitive streak of the mouse embryo. *Nature* 2004;432:625–630.
10. Poole T, Coffin J. Vasculogenesis and angiogenesis: two distinct morphogenetic mechanisms establish embryonic vascular pattern. *J Exp Zool* 1989;251:224–231.
11. Risau W, Lemmon V. Changes in the vascular extracellular matrix during embryonic vasculogenesis and angiogenesis. *Dev Biol* 1988;125:441–450.
12. Vokes S, Yatskievych T, Heimark R, et al. Hedgehog signaling is essential for endothelial tube formation during vasculogenesis. *Development* 2004;131:4371–4380.
13. Risau W, Flamme I. Vasculogenesis. *Annu Rev Cell Biol* 1995;11:73–91.
14. Ema M, Rossant J. Cell fate decisions in early blood vessel formation. *Trends Cardiovasc Med* 2003;13:254–259.
15. Drake C, Brandt S, Trusk T, et al. TAL1/SCL is expressed in endothelial progenitor cells/angioblasts and defines a dorsal-to-ventral gradient of vasculogenesis. *Dev Biol* 1997;192:17–30.
16. Kallianpur A, Jordan J, Brandt S. The SCL/TAL-1 gene is expressed in progenitors of both the hematopoietic and vascular systems during embryogenesis. *Blood* 1994;83:1200–1208.
17. Gering M, Rodaway A, Gottgens B, et al. The SCL gene specifies haemangioblast development from early mesoderm. *EMBO J* 1998;17:4029–4045.
18. Robb L, Elwood N, Elefanty A, et al. The scl gene product is required for the generation of all hematopoietic lineages in the adult mouse. *EMBO J* 1996;15:4123–4129.
19. Shivdasani R, Mayer E, Orkin S. Absence of blood formation in mice lacking the T-cell leukaemia oncoprotein tal-1/SCL. *Nature* 1995;373:432–434.
20. Ema M, Faloon P, Zhang W, et al. Combinatorial effects of Flk1 and tal1 on vascular and hematopoietic development in the mouse. *Genes Dev* 2003;17:380–393.
21. Newman C, Chia F, Krieg P. The XHex homeobox gene is expressed during development of the vascular endothelium: overexpression leads to an increase in vascular endothelial cell number. *Mech Dev* 1997;66:83–93.
22. Thomas P, Brown A, Beddington R. Hex: a homeobox gene revealing peri-implantation asymmetry in the mouse embryo and an early transient marker of endothelial precursors. *Development* 1998;125:85–94.
23. Liao W, Ho C, Yan Y, et al. Hhex and Scl function in parallel to regulate early endothelial and blood differentiation in zebrafish. *Development* 2000;127:4303–4313.
24. Patan S, Haenni B, Burri P. Implementation of intussusceptive microvascular growth in the chicken chorioallantoic membrane. I. Pillar formation by folding of the capillary wall. *Microvasc Res* 1996;51:80–98.
25. Burri P, Hlushchuk R, Djonov V. Intussusceptive angiogenesis: its emergence, its characteristics, and its significance. *Dev Dyn* 2004;231:474–488.
26. Sage E, Bornstein P. Extracellular proteins that modulate cell-matrix interactions. *J Biol Chem* 1991;266:14831–14834.
27. Senger D, Galli S, Dvorak A, et al. Tumor cells secrete a vascular permeability factor that promotes accumulation of ascites fluid. *Science* 1983;219:983–985.
28. Connolly D, Heuvelman D, Nelson R, et al. Tumor vascular permeability factor stimulates endothelial cell growth and angiogenesis. *J Clin Invest* 1989;84:1470–1478.
29. Ferrara N, Henzel W. Pituitary follicular cells secrete a novel heparin-binding growth factor specific for vascular endothelial cells. *Biochem Biophys Res Commun* 1989;161:851–855.
30. Liu Y, Cox S, Morita T, et al. Hypoxia regulates vascular endothelial growth factor gene expression in endothelial cells. *Circ Res* 1995;77:638–643.
31. Forsythe J, Jiang B, Iyer N, et al. Activation of vascular endothelial growth factor gene transcription by hypoxia-inducible factor 1. *Mol Cell Biol* 1996;16:4604–4613.
32. Claffey K, Shih S, Mullen A, et al. Identification of a human VPF/VEGF 3' untranslated region mediating hypoxia-induced mRNA stability. *Mol Biol Cell* 1998;9:469–481.
33. Shih S, Claffey K. Regulation of human vascular endothelial growth factor mRNA stability in hypoxia by heterogeneous nuclear ribonucleoprotein L. *J Biol Chem* 1999;274:1359–1365.
34. Iyer N, Kotch L, Agani F, et al. Cellular and developmental control of O2 homeostasis by hypoxia-inducible factor 1 alpha. *Genes Dev* 1998;12:149–162.
35. Ryan H, Lo J, Johnson R. HIF-1 alpha is required for solid tumor formation and embryonic vascularization. *EMBO J* 1998;17:3005–3015.
36. Maltepe E, Schmidt J, Baunoch D, et al. Abnormal angiogenesis and responses to glucose and oxygen starvation in mice lacking the protein ARNT. *Nature* 1997;386:403–407.
37. Kotch L, Iyer N, Laughner E, et al. Defective vascularization of HIF-1α-null embryos is not associated with VEGF deficiency but with mesenchymal cell death. *Dev Biol* 1999;209:254–267.
38. Tian H, Hammer R, Matsumoto A, et al. The hypoxia-responsive transcription factor EPAS1 is essential for catecholamine homeostasis and protection against heart failure during embryonic development. *Genes Dev* 1998;12:3320–3324.
39. Takeda N, Maemura K, Imai Y, et al. Endothelial PAS domain protein 1 gene promotes angiogenesis through the transactivation of both vascular endothelial growth factor and its receptor, Flt-1. *Circ Res* 2004;95:146–153.
40. Gerber H, Condorelli F, Park J, et al. Differential transcriptional regulation of the two vascular endothelial growth factor receptor genes: flt-1, but not flk-1, is up-regulated by hypoxia. *J Biol Chem* 1997;272:23659–23667.
41. Brogi E, Schatteman G, Wu T, et al. Hypoxia-induced paracrine regulation of vascular endothelial growth factor receptor expression. *J Clin Invest* 1996;97:469–476.
42. Carmeliet P, Ng Y-S, Nuyens D, et al. Impaired myocardial angiogenesis and ischemic cardiomyopathy in mice lacking the vascular endothelial growth factor isoforms VEGF164 and VEGF188. *Nat Med* 1999;5:495–502.
43. Soker S, Takashima S, Miao H, et al. Neuropilin-1 is expressed by endothelial and tumor cells as an isoform-specific receptor for vascular endothelial growth factor. *Cell* 1998;92:735–745.
44. Miao H, Soker S, Feiner L, et al. Neuropilin-1 mediates collapsin-1/semaphorin III inhibition of endothelial cell motility: functional competition of collapsin-1 and vascular endothelial growth factor-165. *J Cell Biol* 1999;146:233–242.
45. Kawasaki T, Kitsukawa T, Bekku Y, et al. A requirement for neuropilin-1 in embryonic vessel formation. *Development* 1999;126:4895–4902.
46. Kitsukawa T, Shimono A, Kawakami A, et al. Overexpression of a membrane protein, neuropilin, in chimeric mice causes anomalies in the cardiovascular system, nervous system and limbs. *Development* 1995;121:4309–4318.
47. Carmeliet P, Ferreira V, Breier G, et al. Abnormal blood vessel development and lethality in embryos lacking a single VEGF allele. *Nature* 1996;380:435–439.
48. Ferrara N, Carver-Moore K, Chen H, et al. Heterozygous embryonic lethality induced by targeted inactivation of the VEGF gene. *Natue* 1996;380:439–442.
49. Fong G, Rossant J, Gertsenstein M, et al. Role of the Flt-1 receptor tyrosine kinase in regulating the assembly of vascular endothelium. *Nature* 1995;376:66–70.
50. Shalaby F, Rossant J, Yamaguchi T, et al. Failure of blood-island formation and vasculogenesis in Flk-1–deficient mice. *Nature* 1995;376:62–66.
51. Schuh A, Faloon P, Hu Q, et al. *In vitro* hematopoietic and endothelial potential of flk-1(-/-) embryonic stem cells and embryos. *Proc Natl Acad Sci U S A* 1999;96:2159–2164.
52. Fong G, Zhang L, Bryce D, et al. Increased hemangioblast commitment, not vascular disorganization, is the primary defect in *flt-1* knock-out mice. *Development* 1999;126:3015–3025.
53. Hiratsuka S, Minowa O, Kuno J, et al. Flt-1 lacking the tyrosine kinase domain is sufficient for normal development and angiogenesis in mice. *Proc Natl Acad Sci U S A* 1998;95:9349–9354.
54. Drake C, Little C. Exogenous vascular endothelial growth factor induces malformed and hyperfused vessels during embryonic neovascularization. *Proc Natl Acad Sci U S A* 1995;92:7657–7661.
55. Springer M, Chen E, Kraft P, et al. VEGF gene delivery to muscle: potential role for vasculogenesis in adults. *Mol Cell* 1998;2:549–558.
56. Storkebaum E, Lambrechts D, Carmeliet P. VEGF: once regarded as a specific angiogenic factor, now implicated in neuroprotection. *Bioessays* 2004;26:943–954.

57. Oosthuyse B, Moons L, Storkebaum E, et al. Deletion of the hypoxia-response element in the vascular endothelial growth factor promoter causes motor neuron degeneration. *Nat Genet* 2001;28:131–138.

58. Dal Canto M, Gurney M. Neuropathological changes in two lines of mice carrying a transgene for mutant human Cu,Zn SOD, and in mice overexpressing wild type human SOD: a model of familial amyotrophic lateral sclerosis (FALS). *Brain Res* 1995;676:25–40.

59. Lambrechts D, Storkebaum E, Morimoto M, et al. VEGF is a modifier of amyotrophic lateral sclerosis in mice and humans and protects motoneurons against ischemic death. *Nat Genet* 2003;34:383–394.

60. LeCouter J, Kowalski J, Foster J, et al. Identification of an angiogenic mitogen selective for endocrine gland endothelium. *Nature* 2001;412:877–884.

61. Jussila L, Alitalo K. Vascular growth factors and lymphangiogenesis. *Physiol Rev* 2002;82:673–700.

62. Harvey N, Oliver G. Choose your fate: artery, vein or lymphatic vessel? *Curr Opin Genet Dev* 2004;14:499–505.

63. Oliver G. Lymphatic vasculature development. *Nat Rev Immunol* 2004;4:35–45.

64. Dumont D, Jussila L, Taipale J, et al. Cardiovascular failure in mouse embryos deficient in VEGF receptor-3. *Science* 1998;282:946–949.

65. Jeltsch M, Kaipainen A, Joukov V, et al. Hyperplasia of lymphatic vessels in VEGF-C transgenic mice. *Science* 1997;276:1423–1425.

66. Abtahian F, Guerriero A, Sebzda E, et al. Regulation of blood and lymphatic vascular separation by signaling proteins SLP-76 and Syk. *Science* 2003;299:247–251.

67. Hong Y, Foreman K, Shin J, et al. Lymphatic reprogramming of blood vascular endothelium by Kaposi sarcoma-associated herpesvirus. *Nat Genet* 2004;36:683–685.

68. Dumont D, Gradwohl G, Fong G, et al. Dominant-negative and targeted null mutations in the endothelial receptor tyrosine kinase, tek, reveal a critical role in vasculogenesis of the embryo. *Genes Dev* 1994;8:1897–1909.

69. Mustonen T, Alitalo K. Endothelial receptor tyrosine kinases involved in angiogenesis. *J Cell Biol* 1995;129:895–898.

70. Sato T, Qin Y, Kozak C, et al. Tie-1 and tie-2 define another class of putative receptor tyrosine kinase genes expressed in early embryonic vascular system. *Proc Natl Acad Sci U S A* 1993;90:9355–9358.

71. Davis S, Aldrich T, Jones P, et al. Isolation of angiopoietin-1, a ligand for the tie2 receptor, by secretion-trap expression cloning. *Cell* 1996;87:1161–1169.

72. Sato T, Tozawa Y, Deutsch U, et al. Distinct roles of receptor tyrosine kinases tie-1 and tie-2 in blood vessel formation. *Nature* 1995;376:70–74.

73. Gale N, Yancopoulos G. Growth factors acting via enotethelial cell-specific receptor tyrosine kinases: VEGFs, angiopoietins, and ephrins in vascular development. *Genes Dev* 1999;13:1055–1066.

74. Asahara T, Chen D, Takahashi T, et al. Tie2 receptor ligands, angiopoietin-1 and angiopoietin-2, modulate VEGF-induced postnatal neovascularization. *Circ Res* 1998;83:233–240.

75. Peters K. Vascular endothelial growth factor and the angiopoietins: working together to build a better blood vessel. *Circ Res* 1998;83:342–343.

76. Suri C, Jones P, Patan S, et al. Requisite role of angiopoietin-1, a ligand for the tie2 receptor, during embryonic angiogenesis. *Cell* 1996;87:1171–1180.

77. Meyer D, Birchmeyer C. Multiple essential functions of neuregulin in development. *Nature* 1995;378:386–390.

78. Koblizek T, Weiss C, Yancopoulos G, et al. Angiopoietin-1 induces sprouting angiogenesis *in vitro*. *Curr Biol* 1998;8:529–532.

79. Pereira F, Qiu Y, Zhou G, et al. The nuclear orphan receptor COUP-TFII is required for angiogenesis and heart development. *Genes Dev* 1999;13:1037–1049.

80. Bi W, Drake C, Schwarz J. The transcription factor MEF2C-null mouse exhibits complex vascular malformations and reduced cardiac expression of angiopoietin 1 and VEGF. *Dev Biol* 1999;211:255–267.

81. Lin Q, Lu J, Yanagisawa H, et al. Requirement of the MADS-box transcription factor MEF2C for vascular development. *Development* 1998;125:4565–4574.

82. Kullander K, Klein R. Mechanisms and functions of Eph and ephrin signalling. *Nat Rev Mol Cell Biol* 2002;3:475–486.

83. Wang H, Anderson D. Eph family transmembrane ligands can mediate repulsive guidance of trunk neural crest migration and motor axon outgrowth. *Neuron* 1997;18:383–396.

84. Durbin L, Brennan C, Shiomi K, et al. Eph signaling is required for segmentation and differentiation of the somites. *Genes Dev* 1998;12:3096–3109.

85. Wang H, Chen Z, Anderson D. Molecular distinction and angiogenic interaction between embryonic arteries and veins revealed by ephrin-B2 and its receptor Eph-B4. *Cell* 1998;93:741–753.

86. Torres-Vazquez J, Kamei M, Weinstein B. Molecular distinction between arteries and veins. *Cell Tissue Res* 2003;314:43–59.

87. Stein E, Lane A, Cerretti D, et al. Eph receptors discriminate specific ligand oligomers to determine alternative signaling complexes, attachment, and assembly responses. *Genes Dev* 1998;12:667–678.

88. Gale N, Baluk P, Pan L, et al. Ephrin-B2 selectively marks arterial vessels and neovascularization sites in the adult, with expression in both endothelial and smooth-muscle cells. *Dev Biol* 2001;230:151–160.

89. Shina D, Garcia-Cardenac G, Hayashid S, et al. Expression of ephrinB2 identifies a stable genetic difference between arterial and venous vascular smooth muscle as well as endothelial cells, and marks subsets of microvessels at sites of adult neovascularization. *Dev Biol* 2001;230:139–150.

90. Pandy A, Shao H, Marks R, et al. Role of B61, the ligand for the Eck receptor tyrosine kinase, in TNF-$\alpha$-induced angiogenesis. *Science* 1995;268:567–569.

91. Adams R, Wilkinson G, Weiss C, et al. Roles of ephrinB ligands and EphB receptors in cardiovascular development: demarcation of arterial/venous domains, vascular morphogenesis and sprouting angiogenesis. *Genes Dev* 1999;13:295–306.

92. Lawson N, Scheer N, Pham V, et al. Notch signaling is required for arterial-venous differentiation during embryonic vascular development. *Development* 2001;128:3675–3683.

93. Lawson N, Vogel A, Weinstein B. *sonic hedgehog* and *vascular endothelial growth factor* act upstream of the notch pathway during arterial endothelial differentiation. *Dev Cell* 2002;3:127–136.

94. Krebs L, Xue Y, Norton C, et al. Notch signaling is essential for vascular morphogenesis in mice. *Genes Dev* 2000;14:1343–1352.

95. Domenga V, Fardoux P, Lacombe P, et al. Notch3 is required for arterial identity and maturation of vascular smooth muscle cells. *Genes Dev* 2004;18:2730–2735.

96. Pepinsky R, Zeng C, Wen D, et al. Identification of a palmitic acid-modified form of human sonic hedgehog. *J Biol Chem* 1998;273:14037–14045.

97. van den Heuvel M. Hedgehog signaling: off the shelf modulation. *Curr Biol* 2003;13:R686–R688.

98. Zhang X, Ramalho-Santos M, McMahon A. Smoothened mutants reveal redundant roles for Shh and Ihh signaling including regulation of L/R asymmetry by the mouse node. *Cell* 2001;105:781–792.

99. Jia J, Tong C, Jiang J. Smoothened transduces hedgehog signal by physically interacting with Costal2/Fused complex through its C-terminal tail. *Genes Dev* 2003;17:2709–2720.

100. Lum L, Beachy P. The hedgehog response network: sensors, switches, and routers. *Science* 2004;304:1755–1759.

101. St-Jacques B, Hammerschmidt M, McMahon A. Indian hedgehog signaling regulates proliferation and differentiation of chondrocytes and is essential for bone formation. *Genes Dev* 1999;13:2072–2086.

102. Maye P, Becker S, Kasameyer E, et al. Indian hedgehog signaling in extraembryonic endoderm and ectoderm differentiation in ES embryoid bodies. *Mech Dev* 2000;94:117–132.

103. Dyer M, Farrington S, Mohn D, et al. Indian hedgehog activates hematopoiesis and vasculogenesis and can respecify prospecive neuroectodermal cell fate in the mouse embryo. *Development* 2001;128:1717–1730.

104. Byrd N, Becker S, Maye P, et al. Hedgehog is required for murine yolk sac angiogenesis. *Development* 2002;129:361–372.

105. Pola R, Ling L, Silver M, et al. The morphogen sonic hedgehog is an indirect angiogenic agent upregulating two families of angiogenic growth factors. *Nat Med* 2001;7:706–711.

106. Pola R, Ling L, Aprahamian T, et al. Postnatal recapitulation of embryonic hedgehog pathway in response to skeletal muscle ischemia. *Circulation* 2003;108:479–485.

107. Goshima Y, Ito T, Sasaki Y, et al. Semaphorins as signals for cell repulsion and invasion. *J Clin Invest* 2002;109:993–998.

108. Tamagnone L, Artigiani S, Chen H, et al. Plexins are a large family of receptors for transmembrane, secreted, and GPI-anchored semaphorins in vertebrates. *Cell* 1999;99:71–80.

109. Torres-Vazquez J, Gitler A, Fraser S, et al. Semaphorin-plexin signaling guides patterning of the developing vasculature. *Dev Cell* 2004;7:117–123.

110. Gitler A, Lu M, Epstein J. PlexinD1 and semaphorin signaling are required in endothelial cells for cardiovascular development. *Dev Cell* 2004;7:107–116.

111. Dickson M, Martin J, Cousins F, et al. Defective haematopoiesis and vasculogenesis in transforming growth factor-$\beta$1 knock out mice. *Development* 1995;121:1845–1854.

112. Shull M, Ormsby I, Kier A, et al. Targeted disruption of the mouse transforming growth factor-beta 1 gene results in multifocal inflammatory disease. *Nature* 1992;359:693–699.

113. Sanford L, Ormsby I, Gittenberger-de Groot A, et al. TGF$\beta$2 knockout mice have multiple developmental defects that are non-overlapping with other TGF$\beta$ knockout phenotypes. *Development* 1997;124:2659–2670.

114. LeLievre C, Le Douarin N. Mesenchymal derivatives of the neural crest: analysis of chimeric quail and chick embryos. *J Embryol Exp Morphol* 1975;34:125–154.

115. Topouzis S, Majesky M. Smooth muscle lineage diversity in the chick embryo: two types of aortic SMC differ in growth and receptor-mediated signaling responses to transforming growth factor-beta. *Dev Biol* 1996;178:430–445.

116. Proetzel G, Pawlowski S, Wiles M, et al. Transforming growth factor-$\beta$3 is required for secondary palate fusion. *Nat Genet* 1995;11:409–414.

117. Bottinger E, Factor V, Tsang M, et al. The recombinant proregion of transforming growth factor beta1 (latency-associated peptide) inhibits active transforming growth factor beta1 in transgenic mice. *Proc Natl Acad Sci U S A* 1996;93:5877–5882.

118. Dubois C, Laprise M, Blanchette F, et al. Processing of transforming growth factor beta 1 precursor by human furin convertase. *J Biol Chem* 1995;270:10618–10624.

119. Roebroek A, Umans L, Pauli I, et al. Failure of ventral closure and axial rotation in embryos lacking the proprotein convertase Furin. *Development* 1998;125:4863–4876.

120. Oshima M, Oshima H, Taketo M. TGF-β receptor type II deficiency results in defects of yolk sac hematopoiesis and vasculogenesis. *Dev Biol* 1996; 179:297–302.

121. Brown C, Boyer A, Runyan R, et al. Requirement of type III TGF-β receptor for endocardial cell transformation in the heart. *Science* 1999;283: 2080–2082.

122. Heldin C, Miyazono K, ten Dijke P. TGF-β signalling from cell membrane to nucleus through SMAD proteins. *Nature* 1997;390:465–471.

123. Massague J. TGF-β signal transduction. *Annu Rev Biochem* 1998;67: 753–791.

124. Wong C, Rougier-Chapman E, Frederick J, et al. Smad3-Smad4 and AP-1 complexes synergize in transcriptional activation of the c-jun promoter by transforming growth factor β. *Mol Cell Biol* 1999;19:1821–1830.

125. Chen X, Weisberg E, Fridmacher V, et al. Smad4 and FAST-1 in the assembly of activin-responsive factor. *Nature* 1997;389:85–89.

126. Topper J, Cai J, Qiu Y, et al. Vascular MADs: two novel MAD-related genes selectively inducible by flow in human vascular endothelium. *Proc Natl Acad Sci U S A* 1997;94:9314–9319.

127. Imamura T, Takase M, Nishihara A, et al. Smad6 inhibits signalling by the TGF-β superfamily. *Nature* 1997;389:622–626.

128. Nakao A, Afrakhte M, Moren A, et al. Identification of Smad7, a TGFβ-inducible antagonist of TGF-β signalling. *Nature* 1997;389:631–635.

129. Whitman M. Feedback from inhibitory SMADs. *Nature* 1997;389: 549–550.

130. Nomura M, Li E. Smad2 role in mesoderm formation, left-right patterning and craniofacial development. *Nature* 1998;393:786–790.

131. Datto M, Frederick J, Pan L, et al. Targeted disruption of Smad3 reveals an essential role in transforming growth factor β-mediated signal transduction. *Mol Cell Biol* 1999;19:2495–2504.

132. Zhu Y, Richardson J, Parada L, et al. Smad3 mutant mice develop metastatic colorectal cancer. *Cell* 1998;94:703–714.

133. Chang H, Huylebroeck D, Verschueren K, et al. Smad5 knockout mice die at mid-gestation due to multiple embryonic and extraembryonic defects. *Development* 1999;126:1631–1642.

134. Yang L, Qiu C, Ludlow A, et al. Active transforming growth factor-β in wound repair: determination using a new assay. *Am J Pathol* 1999;154: 105–111.

135. Lampugnani M, Resnati M, Raiteri M, et al. A novel endothelial-specific membrane protein is a marker of cell-cell contacts. *J Cell Biol* 1992;118: 1511–1522.

136. Carmeliet P, Lampugnani M-G, Moons L, et al. Targeted deficiency or cytosolic truncation of the VE-cadherin gene in mice impairs VEGF-mediated endothelial survival and angiogenesis. *Cell* 1999;98:147–157.

137. Gory-Faure S, Prandini M, Pointu H, et al. Role of vascular endothelial-cadherin in vascular morphogenesis. *Development* 1999;126:2093–2102.

138. Hoschuetsky H, Aberle H, Kemler R. β-catenin mediates the interaction of the cadherin-catenin complex with epidermal growth factor receptor. *J Cell Biol* 1994;127:1375–1380.

139. Yang J, Rayburn H, Hynes R. Cell adhesion events mediated by α4 integrins are essential in placental and cardiac development. *Development* 1995;121:549–560.

140. Kwee L, Baldwin H, Shen H, et al. Defective development of the embryonic and extraembryonic circulatory systems in vascular cell adhesion molecule (VCAM-1) deficient mice. *Development* 1995;121:489–503.

141. Goh K, Yang J, Hynes R. Mesodermal defects and cranial neural crest apoptosis in alpha5 integrin-null embryos. *Development* 1997;124:4309–4319.

142. Drake C, Cheresh D, Little C. An antagonist of alpha v beta 3 prevents maturation of blood vessels during embryonic neovascularization. *J Cell Sci* 1995;108:2655–2661.

143. Friedlander M, Brooks P, Shaffer R, et al. Definition of two angiogenic pathways by distinct av integrins. *Science* 1995;270:1500–1502.

144. Brooks P, Stromblad S, Klemke R, et al. Anti-integrin alpha v beta 3 blocks human breast cancer growth and angiogenesis in human skin. *J Clin Invest* 1995;96:1815–1822.

145. Diaz-Gonzalez F, Forsyth J, Steiner B, et al. Transdominant inhibition of integrin function. *Mol Biol Cell* 1996;7:1939–1951.

146. Hungerford J, Little C. Developmental biology of the vascular smooth muscle cell: building a multilayered vessel wall. *J Vasc Res* 1999;36:2–27.

147. Owens G, Kumar M, Wamhoff B. Molecular regulation of vascular smooth muscle cell differentiation in development and disease. *Physiol Rev* 2004;84: 767–801.

148. Hellstrom M, Kalen M, Lindahl P, et al. Role of PDGF-B and PDGFR-β in recruitment of vascular smooth muscle cells and pericytes during embryonic blood vessel formation in the mouse. *Development* 1999;126: 3047–3055.

149. Skalak T, Price R, Zeller P. Where do new arterioles come from? Mechanical forces and microvessel adaptation. *Microcirculation* 1998;5:91–94.

150. Yamashita J, Itoh H, Hirashima M, et al. Flk1-positive cells derived from embryonic stem cells serve as vascular progenitors. *Nature* 2000;408:92–96.

151. Choi K, Kennedy M, Kazarov A, et al. A common precursor for hematopoietic and endothelial cells. *Development* 1998;125:725–732.

152. Minasi M, Riminucci M, De Angelis L, et al. The meso-angioblast: a multipotent, self-renewing cell that originates from the dorsal aorta and differentiates into most mesodermal tissues. *Development* 2002;129:2773–2783.

153. Cossu G, Bianco P. Mesoangioblasts – vascular progenitors for extravascular mesodermal tissues. *Curr Opin Genet Dev* 2003;13:537–542.

154. DeRuiter M, Poelmann R, VanMunsteren J, et al. Embryonic endothelial cells transdifferentiate into mesenchymal cells expressing smooth muscle actins *in vivo* and *in vitro* [see comments]. *Circ Res* 1997;80:444–451.

155. Majesky M, Schwartz S. An origin for smooth muscle from endothelium? *Circ Res* 1997;80:601–603.

156. Folkman J, D'Amore P. Blood vessel formation: what is its molecular basis? *Cell* 1996;87:1153–1155.

157. Gittenberger-de Groot A, DeRuiter M, Bergwerff M, et al. Smooth muscle cell origin and its relation to heterogeneity in development and disease. *Arterioscler Thromb Vasc Biol* 1999;19:1589–1594.

158. Majesky M. Vascular smooth muscle diversity: insights from developmental biology. *Curr Atheroscler Rep* 2003;5:208–213.

159. Waldo K, Kirby M. Cardiac neural crest contribution to the pulmonary artery and sixth aortic arch artery complex in chick embryos aged 6 to 18 days. *Anat Rec* 1993;237:385–399.

160. Dettman R, Denetclaw W, Ordahl C, et al. Common epicardial origin of coronary vascular smooth muscle, perivascular fibroblasts, and intermyocardial fibroblasts in the avian heart. *Dev Biol* 1998;193:169–181.

161. Gittenberger-de Groot A, Vrancken Peeters M, Mentink M, et al. Epicardium-derived cells contribute a novel population to the myocardial wall and the atrioventricular cushions. *Circ Res* 1998;82:1043–1052.

162. Majesky M. Development of coronary vessels. *Curr Top Dev Biol* 2004;62: 225–259.

163. Mikawa T, Gourdie R. Pericardial mesoderm generates a population of coronary smooth muscle cells migrating into the heart along with ingrowth of the epicardial organ. *Dev Biol* 1996;174:221–232.

164. Gourdie R, Mima T, Thompson R, et al. Terminal diversification of the myocyte lineage generates Purkinje fibers of the cardiac conduction system. *Development* 1995;121:1423–1431.

165. Gourdie R, Wei Y, Kim D, et al. Endothelin-induced conversion of embryonic heart muscle cells into impulse-conducting Purkinje fibers. *Proc Natl Acad Sci U S A* 1998;95:6815–6818.

166. Hyer J, Johansen M, Prasad A, et al. Induction of Purkinje fiber differentiation by coronary arterialization. *Proc Natl Acad Sci U S A* 1999;96: 13214–13218.

167. Scott N, Cipolla G, Ross C, et al. Identification of a potential role for the adventitia in vascular lesion formation after balloon overstretch injury of porcine coronary arteries. *Circulation* 1996;93:2178–2187.

168. Shi Y, O'Brien J, Fard A, et al. Adventitial myofibroblasts contribute to neointimal formation in injured porcine arteries. *Circulation* 1996;94: 1655–1664.

169. Hirschi K, D'Amore P. Pericytes in the microvasculature. *Cardiovasc Res* 1996;32:687–698.

170. Gerhardt H, Betsholtz C. Endothelial-pericyte interactions in angiogenesis. *Cell Tissue Res* 2003;314:15–23.

171. Davies P. Flow-mediated endothelial mechanotransduction. *Physiol Rev* 1995;75:519–560.

172. Little T, Beyer E, Duling B. Connexin 43 and connexin 40 gap junctional proteins are present in arteriolar smooth muscle and endothelium *in vivo*. *Am J Physiol* 1995;268:H729–H739.

173. Price R, Owens G, Skalak T. Immunohistochemical identification of arteriolar development using markers of smooth muscle differentiation: evidence that capillary arterialization proceeds from terminal arterioles. *Circ Res* 1994;75:520–527.

174. Clark E. R, Clark E. L, Microscopic observations on the extraendothelial cells of living mammalian blood vessels. *Am J Anat* 1940;66:1–49.

175. Lindahl P, Johansson B, Leveen P, et al. *Pericyte loss and microaneurysm formation in PDGF-B-deficient mice. Science* 1997;277:242–245.

176. Lindahl P, Bostrom H, Karlsson L, et al. Role of platelet-derived growth factors in angiogenesis and alveogenesis. *Curr Top Pathol* 1999;93:27–33.

177. Crosby J, Seifert R, Soriano P, et al. Chimaeric analysis reveals role of Pdgf receptors in all muscle lineages. *Nat Genet* 1998;18:385–388.

178. Vikkula M, Boon L, Carraway K, et al. Vascular dysmorphogenesis caused by an activating mutation in the receptor tyrosine kinase TIE2. *Cell* 1996; 87:1181–1190.

179. Benjamin L, Hemo I, Keshet E. A plasticity window for blood vessel remodeling is defined by pericyte coverage of the preformed endothelial network and is regulated by PDGF-B and VEGF. *Development* 1998;125: 1591–1598.

180. Benjamin L, Golijanin D, Itin A, et al. Selective ablation of immature blood vessels in established human tumors follows vascular endothelial growth factor withdrawal [see comments]. *J Clin Invest* 1999;103:159–165.

181. Abramovitch R, Neeman M, Reich R, et al. Intercellular communication between vascular smooth muscle and endothelial cells mediated by heparin-binding epidermal growth factor–like growth factor and vascular endothelial growth factor. *FEBS Lett* 1998;425:441–447.

182. Altschul R. Histologic analysis of arateriosclerosis. *Arch Pathol* 1944;38: 305–312.

183. Arciniegas E, Sutton A, Allen T, et al. Transforming growth factor beta-1 promotes the differentiation of endothelial cells into smooth muscle–like cells *in vitro*. *J Cell Sci* 1992;103:521–529.

184. Sarkisov D, Kolokolchikova E, Kaem R, et al. Vascular changes in maturing granulation tissue. *Bull Exp Biol Med* 1988;105:604–605.

185. Tuder R, Groves B, Badesch D, et al. Exuberant endothelial growth and elements of inflammation are present in plexiform lesions of pulmonary hypertension. *Am J Pathol* 1994;144:275–285.

186. Markwald R, Mjaatvedt C, Krug E, et al. Inductive interactions in heart development. Role of cardiac adherons in cushion tissue formation. *Ann N Y Acad Sci* 1990;588:13–25.

187. Eisenberg L, Markwald R. Molecular regulation of atrioventricular valvuloseptal morphogenesis. *Circ Res* 1995;77:1–6.

188. De Angelis L, Berghella L, Coletta M, et al. Skeletal myogenic progenitors originating from embryonic dorsal aorta coexpress endothelial and myogenic markers and contribute to postnatal muscle growth and regeneration. *J Cell Biol* 1999;147:869–877.

189. Ordahl C. Myogenic shape-shifters. *J Cell Biol* 1999;147:695–697.

190. Pardanaud L, Luton D, Prigent M, et al. Two distinct endothelial lineages in ontogeny, one of them related to hemopoiesis. *Development* 1996;122:1363–1371.

191. Kuo C, Veselits M, Barton K, et al. The LKLF transcription factor is required for normal tunica media formation and blood vessel stabalization during murine embryogenesis. *Genes Dev* 1997;11:2996–3006.

192. Li D, Sorensen L, Brooke B, et al. Defective angiogenesis in mice lacking endoglin. *Science* 1999;284:1534–1537.

193. Solway J, Forsythe S, Halayko A, et al. Transcriptional regulation of smooth muscle contractile apparatus expression. *Am J Respir Crit Care Med* 1998;158:S100–S108.

194. Miano J. Serum response factor: toggling between disparate programs of gene expression. *J Mol Cell Cardiol* 2003;35:577–593.

195. Wang D, Olson E. Control of smooth muscle development by the myocardin family of transcriptional coactivators. *Curr Opin Genet Dev* 2004;14:558–566.

196. Li D, Brooke B, Davis E, et al. Elastin is an essential determinant of arterial morphogenesis. *Nature* 1998;393:276–280.

197. Cook C, Weiser M, Schwartz P, et al. Developmentally timed expression of an embryonic growth phenotype in vascular smooth muscle cells. *Circ Res* 1994;74:189–196.

198. Li D, Faury G, Taylor D, et al. Novel arterial pathology in mice and humans hemizygous for elastin. *J Clin Invest* 1998;102:1783–1787.

199. Koyama H, Raines E, Bornfeldt K, et al. Fibrillar collagen inhibits arterial smooth muscle proliferation through regulation of Cdk2 inhibitors. *Cell* 1996;87:1069–1078.

200. Stenmark K, Mecham R. Cellular and molecular mechanisms of pulmonary vascular remodeling. *Annu Rev Physiol* 1997;59:89–144.

201. Adams J, Watt F. Regulation of development and differentiation by the extracellular matrix. *Development* 1993;117:1183–1198.

202. Carey D. Control of growth and differentiation of vascular cells by extracellular matrix proteins. *Annu Rev Physiol* 1991;53:161–177.

203. Vernon R, Sage E. Between molecules and morphology: extracellular matrix and creation of vascular form. *Am J Pathol* 1995;147:873–882.

204. Holzenberger M, Lievre C, Robert L. Tropoelastin gene expression in the developing vascular system of the chicken: an in situ hybridization study. *Anat Embryol (Berl)* 1993;188:481–492.

205. Rosenquist T, McCoy J, Waldo K, et al. Origin and propagation of elastogenesis in the developing cardiovascular system. *Anat Rec* 1988;221:860–871.

206. Selmin O, Volpin D, Bressen G. Changes of cellular expression of mRNA for tropoelastin in the intraembryonic arterial vessels of developing chick by in situ hybridization. *Matrix* 1991;11:347–358.

207. Mecham R, Stenmark K, Parks W. Connective tissue production by vascular smooth muscle in development and disease. *Chest* 1991;99:43S–47S.

208. Rosenquist T, Beall A. Elastogenic cells in the developing cardiovascular system: smooth muscle, nonmuscle and cardiac neural crest. *Ann N Y Acad Sci* 1990;588:106–119.

209. Hungerford J, Owens G, Aargraves W, et al. Development of the aortic vessel wall as defined by vascular smooth muscle and extracellular markers. *Dev Biol* 1996;178:375–392.

210. Rongish B, Drake C, Argraves W, et al. Identification of the developmental marker, JB3-antigen, as fibrillin-2 and its de novo organization into embryonic microfibrous arrays. *Dev Dyn* 1998;212:461–471.

211. Zhang H, Timpl R, Sasaki T, et al. Fibulin-1 and fibulin-2 expression during organogenesis in the developing mouse embryo. *Dev Dyn* 1996;205:348–364.

212. Dietz H, Cutting G, Pyeritz R, et al. Marfan syndrome caused by a recurrent de novo missense mutation in the fibrillin gene. *Nature* 1991;352:337–339.

213. Park E, Putnam E, Chitayat D, et al. Clustering of FBN2 mutations in patients with congenital contractural arachnodactyly indicates an important role of the domains encoded by exons 24 through 34 during human development. *Am J Med Genet* 1998;78:350–355.

214. Ramirez F, Pereira L. The fibrillins. *Int J Biochem Cell Biol* 1999;31:255–259.

215. Gallagher B, Sakai L, Little C. Fibrillin delineates the primary axis of the early avian embryo. *Dev Dyn* 1993;196:70–78.

216. Bressen G, Daga-Gordini D, Colombatti A, et al. Emilin, a component of elastic fibers preferentially located at the elastin-microfibrils interface. *J Cell Biol* 1993;121:201–212.

217. Parmacek M. Transcriptional programs regulating vascular smooth muscle cell development and differentiation. *Curr Top Dev Biol* 2001;51:69–89.

218. Duband J, Gimona M, Scatena M, et al. Calponin and SM 22 as differentiation markers of smooth muscle: spatiotemporal distribution during avian embryonic development. *Differentiation* 1993;55:1–11.

219. Miano J, Cserjesi P, Ligon K, et al. Smooth muscle myosin heavy chain exclusively marks the smooth muscle lineage during mouse embryogenesis. *Circ Res* 1994;75:803–812.

220. Gromak N, Smith C. A splicing silencer that regulates smooth muscle specific alternative splicing is active in multiple cell types. *Nucleic Acids Res* 2002;30:3548–3557.

221. Shimizu R, Blank R, Jervis R, et al. The smooth muscle alpha-actin gene promoter is differentially regulated in smooth muscle versus non-smooth muscle cells. *J Biol Chem* 1995;270:7631–7643.

222. Solway J, Seltzer J, Samaha F, et al. Structure and expression of a smooth muscle cell-specific gene, SM22 alpha. *J Biol Chem* 1995;270:13460–13469.

223. Li L, Miano J, Mercer B, et al. Expression of the SM22α promoter in transgenic mice provides evidence for distinct transcriptional regulatory programs in vascular and visceral smooth muscle cells. *J Cell Biol* 1996;132:849–859.

224. Browning C, Culberson D, Aragon I, et al. The developmentally regulated expression of serum response factor plays a key role in the control of smooth muscle-specific genes. *Dev Biol* 1998;194:18–37.

225. Qian J, Kumar A, Szucsik J, et al. Tissue and developmental specific expression of murine smooth muscle gamma-actin fusion genes in transgenic mice. *Dev Dyn* 1996;207:135–144.

226. Herring B, Smith A. Telokin expression is mediated by a smooth muscle cell-specific promoter. *Am J Physiol* 1996;270:C1656–C1665.

227. Katoh Y, Loukianov E, Kopras E, et al. Identification of functional promoter elements in the rabbit smooth muscle myosin heavy chain gene. *J Biol Chem* 1994;269:30538–30545.

228. Johansen F, Prywes R. Serum response factor: transcriptional regulation of genes induced by growth factors and differentiation. *Biochim Biophys Acta* 1995;1242:1–10.

229. Croissant J, Kim J, Eichele G, et al. Avian serum response factor expression restricted primarily to muscle cell lineages is required for alpha-actin gene transcription. *Dev Biol* 1996;177:250–264.

230. Arsenian S, Weinhold B, Oelgeschlager M, et al. Serum response factor is essential for mesoderm formation during mouse embryogenesis. *EMBO J* 1998;17:6289–6299.

231. Shore P, Sharrocks A. The transcription factors Elk-1 and serum response factor interact by direct protein-protein contacts mediated by a short region of Elk-1. *Mol Cell Biol* 1994;14:3283–3291.

232. Triesman R. Ternary complex factors: growth factor regulated transcriptional activators. *Curr Opin Genet Dev* 1994;4:96–101.

233. Lilly B, Zhao B, Ranganayakulu G, et al. Requirement of MADS domain transcription factor D-MEF2 for muscle formation in Drosophila. *Science* 1995;267:688–693.

234. Blank R, McQuinn T, Yin K, et al. Elements of the smooth muscle alpha-actin promoter required in cis for transcriptional activation in smooth muscle. Evidence for cell type-specific regulation. *J Biol Chem* 1992;267:984–989.

235. Szucsik J, Lessard J. Cloning and sequence analysis of the mouse smooth muscle gamma-enteric actin gene. *Genomics* 1995;28:154–162.

236. Li L, Liu Z, Mercer B, et al. Evidence for serum response factor-mediated regulatory networks governing SM22alpha transcription in smooth, skeletal and cardiac muscle cells. *Dev Biol* 1997;187:311–321.

237. Zilberman A, Dave V, Miano J, et al. Evolutionarily conserved promoter region containing CArG*-like elements is crucial for smooth muscle myosin heavy chain gene expression. *Circ Res* 1998;82:566–575.

238. Yano H, Hayashi K, Momiyama T, et al. Transcriptional regulation of the chicken caldesmon gene: activation of gizzard-type caldesmon promoter requires a CArG box–like motif. *J Biol Chem* 1995;270:23661–23666.

239. Obata H, Hayashi K, Nishida W, et al. Smooth muscle cell phenotype-dependent transcriptional regulation of the α1-integrin gene. *J Biol Chem* 1997;272:26643–26651.

240. Kim S, Ip H, Lu M, et al. A serum response factor-dependent transcriptional regulatory program identifies distinct smooth muscle cell sublineages. *Mol Cell Biol* 1997;17:2266–2278.

241. Landerholm T, Dong X-R, Lu J, et al. A role for serum response factor in coronary smooth muscle differentiation from proepicardial cells. *Development* 1999;126:2053–2062.

242. Miano J, Ramanan N, Georger M, et al. Restricted inactivation of serum response factor to the cardiovascular system. *Proc Natl Acad Sci U S A* 2004;101:17132–17137.

243. Moessler H, Mericskay M, Li Z, et al. The SM-22 promoter directs tissue-specific expression in arterial but not in venous or visceral smooth muscle cells in transgenic mice. *Development* 1996;122:2415–2425.

244. Sotiropoulos A, Gineitis D, Copeland J, et al. Signal-regulated activation of serum response factor is mediated by changes in actin dynamics. *Cell* 1999;98:159–169.

245. Wang D, Chang P, Wang Z, et al. Activation of cardiac gene expression by myocardin, a transcriptional cofactor for serum response factor. *Cell* 2001;105:851–862.

246. Wang D, Li S, Hockemeyer D, et al. Potentiation of serum response factor activity by a family of myocardin-related transcription factors. *Proc Natl Acad Sci U S A* 2002;99:14855–14860.

247. Du K, Ip H, Li J, et al. Myocardin is a critical serum response factor cofactor in the transcriptional program regulating smooth muscle cell differentiation. *Mol Cell Biol* 2003;23:2425–2437.

248. Yoshida T, Sinha S, Dandre F, et al. Myocardin is a key regulator of CArG-dependent transcription of multiple smooth muscle markers. *Circ Res* 2003;92:856–864.

249. Li S, Wang D, Wang Z, et al. The serum response factor coactivator myocardin is required for vascular smooth muscle development. *Proc Natl Acad Sci U S A* 2003;100:9366–9370.

250. Miralles F, Posern G, Zaromytidou A, et al. Actin dynamics control SRF activity by regulation of its coactivator MAL. *Cell* 2003;113:329–342.

251. Selvaraj A, Prywes R. Megakaryoblastic leukemia-1/2, a transcriptional co-activator of SRF, is required for skeletal myogenic differentiation. *J Biol Chem* 2003;278:41977–41987.

252. Cen B, Selvaraj A, Prywes R. Myocardin/MKL family of SRF coactivators: key regulators of immediate early and muscle specific gene expression. *J Cell Biochem* 2004;93:74–82.

253. Chang DF, Belaguli NS, Iyer D, et al. Cysteine-rich LIM-only proteins CRP1 and CRP2 are potent smooth muscle differentiation cofactors. *Dev Cell* 2003;4:107–118.

# CHAPTER 42 ■ THE VASCULAR BIOLOGY OF NITRIC OXIDE AND NITRIC OXIDE SYNTHASES

DAVID M. DUDZINSKI AND THOMAS MICHEL

## NITRIC OXIDE CHEMISTRY

### Introduction

Nitric oxide (NO) is a ubiquitous and biologically versatile molecule that plays a central role in the biology of the vascular wall. The special chemical properties of NO render the molecule an ideal intercellular messenger in the vascular system, and are reflected in its key role as an endothelium-derived relaxing factor (EDRF) (1,2). The distinctive chemistry of NO is exploited in the modulation of diverse intercellular and intracellular reactions with pleiotropic effects on vascular function. As a small (30-Da) lipophilic gaseous molecule, NO easily traverses cell membranes and vascular layers (3–5). NO is also a labile free radical that may react with oxygen, proteins, thiols, metal centers, or other free radicals such as superoxide. Consequently, the short half-life (5 to 10 seconds) (6) of NO ensures both rapid and localized signaling effect (7,8), useful for exquisite temporal juxtacrine control of nearby cells. The constitutive synthesis of NO by the endothelial isoform of nitric oxide synthase (eNOS) serves to maintain vascular homeostasis, but this key enzyme itself is subject to close modulation by extracellular signals that modify eNOS and regulate endothelial function.

### Targets of Nitric Oxide

The chemistry of NO suggests many possibilities for its reactions with proteins via metallic centers and sulfhydryl groups, as well as reactions between NO and other radicals or with low-molecular-weight thiol compounds. The reactivity of NO with hemoproteins has been extensively characterized, yet additional targets of NO continue to be elucidated. NO produced by eNOS in the vascular endothelium rapidly diffuses both into the underlying layers of vascular smooth muscle and also into the vascular lumen where NO interacts with blood platelets. In both vascular smooth muscle cells and in platelets, NO binds to the heme prosthetic group of soluble guanylate cyclase, a signaling protein found ubiquitously in mammalian cells. Binding of NO to the heme group disrupts a nitrogen–iron interaction, freeing an axial histidine residue to participate in catalysis. Nanomolar concentrations of NO can lead to a 100-fold activation of the ability of guanylate cyclase to convert guanosine triphosphate (GTP) into cyclic guanosine monophosphate (cGMP). The primary intracellular target of cGMP in the vascular wall is the cGMP-dependent protein kinase, also known as protein kinase G (PKG). However, additional molecular targets for endothelium-derived NO have been more recently identified.

The relatively short half-life of NO has generated speculation about possible storage forms of NO that may help establish basal levels of NO and may permit actions of NO to occur at targets distant from its sites of synthesis (9). The redox reactivity of nitrogen oxides with sulfhydryl groups are well characterized, and various nitrosothiols, including proteins covalently modified by a NO adduct, appear to represent likely candidates for possible storage forms of NO *in vivo* (10). Both protein and nonprotein nitrosothiols have been found in cells and biological fluids *in vivo*. Compared with a free plasma NO concentration of approximately 3 nM, the concentration of plasma nitrosothiol is approximately 1 $\mu$M, of which 85% is nitrosoalbumin (11–13). *S*-nitrosothiols are endogenously formed in both the cardiovascular and pulmonary systems (14,15), and micromolar concentrations of *S*-nitrosoglutathione have been isolated from the lung (16). Plasma levels of *S*-nitrosothiols may be the subject of intricate regulation by supplementary metabolic pathways, for example, formaldehyde dehydrogenase (17).

Hemoglobin has been proposed to be a nitrosoprotein with potential biological relevance. Although it has been clearly established that hemoglobin has the capacity to bind NO at its heme moieties, it has been suggested that hemoglobin may also undergo nitrosation at Cys93 in the $\beta$ globin protein to form a protein nitrosothiol. The binding of NO by hemoglobin at heme and cysteinyl sites may allow nitrosated hemoglobin to serve as an endogenous NO-donating molecule by delivering NO to distant locales in the vascular system (18). However, the *in vivo* roles of nitrosothiols in the delivery of NO and regulation of vasomotor tone remain incompletely understood, and are under active investigation (19,20).

Nitrosothiols share a qualitatively similar pharmacodynamic profile with NO, such as stimulating soluble guanylate cyclase (21), inducing vascular relaxation and hypotension, and exerting antithrombogenic effects by the inhibition of platelet aggregation (22). However, the pathways whereby endogenous nitrosothiols exert their biological effects remain incompletely understood. Nitrosothiols may undergo spontaneous nonenzymatic decomposition to release NO, can cause transnitrosation of other proteins, or may directly exert nitrergic effects (23), although some evidence suggests that nitrosohemoglobin may release NO (24).

In addition to functioning as a storage reservoir of NO, NO-protein adducts may serve as important posttranslational modifications with signaling functions (25). For example, both prostaglandin H synthase and ribonucleotide reductase have been identified as 3-nitrotyrosine-modified proteins in which binding of NO may play an inhibitory role by binding to a tyrosyl radical in the active site (26). Recent studies demonstrate that eNOS undergoes dynamic S-nitrosation and denitrosation (27). It is the chemistry of NO that uniquely suits it to these putative roles because its small lipophilic nature allows it to penetrate the protein structure while exhibiting reactivity with a broad range of biomolecules.

Nitrosation pathways may also regulate proteins associated with hemostasis. *S*-nitrosoglutathione may interact with fibrinogen and impair fibrin cross-linking without chemically reacting with fibrinogen but possibly by inducing a conformational change in fibrinogen (28). Nitrosation of factor XIII may be an antihemostatic mechanism that could attenuate fibrin cross-linking and render a nascent clot more susceptible to fibrinolysis (29). Whereas nitrosation of tissue-type plasminogen activator (S-NO-tPA) has no effect on its interaction with fibrin or the catalytic activation of plasmin, S-NO-tPA may act as a nitrosothiol carrier of NO to inhibit platelets and cause vasodilatation at sites of thrombus where the local endothelium may be dysfunctional and produce insufficient quantities of NO (30).

Formation of NO adducts may be affected by cellular redox state, and in turn may influence the nature of redox-active species present in the vascular wall. The most prominent example of this phenomenon is the formation of peroxynitrite through the reaction of NO and superoxide. This process may be a mechanism of detoxifying superoxide, although peroxynitrite itself is a chemically reactive species that may modify cellular proteins.

# SOURCES OF NITRIC OXIDE

## Endogenous Sources: Nitric Oxide Synthases

NO is synthesized in mammalian tissues by a family of three nitric oxide synthase (NOS) isoforms, each being the product of a distinct gene. The mammalian NO synthases are homodimeric enzymes containing an *N*-terminal heme-binding domain and a *C*-terminal reductase domain, separated by a calmodulin-binding domain. The *N*-terminal domain, also known as the oxygenase domain, contains binding sites for heme (protoporphyrin IX), tetrahydrobiopterin, and the substrate L-arginine (31). The *C*-terminal flavoprotein oxidoreductase domain is structurally homologous to cytochrome P-450 reductase and binds flavin adenine dinucleotide (FAD), flavin mononucleotide (FMN), and reduced nicotinamide adenine dinucleotide phosphate (NADPH) (32). Because these mixed redox functions are often the products of separate polypeptides, the combination of the oxygenase and reductase functions of NOS suggests that the protein evolved by gene fusion. The calmodulin-binding domain may be important in "gating" the

flow of electrons from the reductase to the oxygenase domains (33). The fact that NOS binds five redox-active cofactors—more than any other enzyme known—suggests an intricate catalytic mechanism. NOS catalyzes the 5-electron oxidation of the guanidine nitrogen of L-arginine, although most reactions of NADPH and flavoproteins involve an even number of electrons. NOS catalysis proceeds in two distinct monooxygenation steps, each involving electron transfer to molecular oxygen. In the first step, 1 mol of NADPH transfers, via FAD and FMN (34), 2 mol of electrons to a heme-bound oxygen, which reacts with L-arginine to form 1 mol each of $\omega$-*N*-hydroxy-L-arginine and water (35). In the second step, 0.5 mol of NADPH transfers electrons to a second heme-bound oxygen, which reacts with $\omega$-*N*-hydroxy-L-arginine to release 1 mol each of NO and L-citrulline. The role of tetrahydrobiopterin as an enzymatic cofactor remains cryptic: Some experiments suggest that it is not used stoichiometrically but catalytically, whereas conflicting data indicate participation of this cofactor in each catalytic cycle as an electron donor (36). There is evidence, however, that the various NOS isozymes become uncoupled and produce superoxide instead of NO when tetrahydrobiopterin is deficient or oxidized (37).

Of the three distinct NOS isoforms that have been identified, two isoforms are constitutively expressed in their archetypal cells of origin: endothelial NOS (eNOS) in vascular endothelial cells and neuronal NOS (nNOS) in neurons. iNOS, or inducible iNOS, is an isoform found in immunoactivated cells, the levels of which can be upregulated by various stimuli (see Table 42-1). Such terminology is somewhat misleading because NOSs are expressed in diverse additional locations besides endothelium, neurons, and immunoactivated cells. The various *NOS* genes are expressed in multiple tissues, including discrete cell types within the vessel wall and in circulating blood cells, and are subject to a hierarchy of tissue-specific transcriptional and posttranslational controls that dictate the functional role of these enzymes. Furthermore, the designation of constitutive and inducible NOS expression patterns is not strictly maintained because nNOS and *eNOS* genes can undergo tissue-specific transcriptional regulation. The overall catalytic scheme of the three mammalian NOS isoforms is conserved, and the members of this gene family share similar gene structure and exhibit 50% to 60% mammalian amino acid sequence homology (38–40), as well as nearly identical locations of cofactor binding sites. The only notable heterogeneity among the isoforms is recognized at the *N*-termini where nNOS

## TABLE 42-1

### CELLULAR AND TISSUE LOCALIZATION OF NITRIC OXIDE SYNTHASE EXPRESSION

| eNOS (NOS 3) | iNOS (NOS 2) | nNOS (NOS 1) |
|---|---|---|
| Vascular endothelial cells, including arteries and veins | Immunoactivated cells, including: | "Nitrergic" nerves innervating large vessels in diverse vascular beds |
| Blood platelets | Macrophages | |
| Cardiomyocytes | Neutrophils | Central nervous system |
| Brain (hippocampus) | Vascular smooth muscle | Skeletal muscle |
| | Cardiomyocytes | Gastrointestinal system |
| | Small vessel endothelial cells | Genitourinary system |

NOS, nitric oxide synthase; eNOS, endothelial NOS; iNOS, inducible NOS; nNOS, neuronal NOS.

contains an additional sequence of approximately 290 amino acids not found in either eNOS or iNOS (41). The N-terminus of eNOS is distinguished from nNOS and iNOS by the presence of consensus sites for acylation that are thought to determine eNOS subcellular localization.

All three NOS isoforms catalyze the same chemical reaction and have similar redox cofactor requirements. A major difference lies in the isoforms' differential affinity for calmodulin: Although all three NOS isoforms are dependent on calmodulin binding for activity, there are important differences in the calcium dependence for calmodulin binding. Whereas eNOS and nNOS require elevated intracellular calcium levels in order to bind calmodulin and thereby become activated, the affinity of iNOS for calmodulin is comparatively so much greater that iNOS fully binds calmodulin and is activated even at resting intracellular calcium concentrations (42).

## Exogenous Sources: Nitrovasodilator Drugs and Nitric Oxide–Donating Molecules

Nitrovasodilator drugs encompass a chemically heterogenous group of molecules that have the ability to generate NO *in vivo*. As such, NO has been termed the *endogenous nitrovasodilator* and nitrovasodilator drugs have been dubbed *endothelial cell replacement therapy* (43). However, it is important to note that exogenous and endogenous sources of NO can differ significantly in their kinetics and reactivity. Of the various organic nitrovasodilators in clinical use, the NO-donating group is either a nitrate group, as in nitroglycerin, isosorbide dinitrate, and isosorbide mononitrate, or a nitrite group, as in amyl nitrite. The pathways whereby organic nitrovasodilators release NO are incompletely understood, but several mechanisms for the enzymatic transformation to NO have been proposed (44). Sodium nitroprusside is an organometallic compound that directly releases its NO ligand apparently in a nonenzymatic process. The nitrovasodilators also differ importantly in their bioavailability, route of administration, doses, elimination half-life, and side effects, but share common characteristics in their releasing NO as the principal bioactive product (45).

# VASCULAR FUNCTIONS OF ENDOTHELIAL NITRIC OXIDE SYNTHASE–DERIVED NITRIC OXIDE

## Endothelial Nitric Oxide Synthase, Nitric Oxide, and the Vessel Wall

NO is an essential endogenous vasodilator, platelet inhibitor, and antithrombogenic agent. Numerous experiments in both animal models and humans indicate that the physiologic role of eNOS is to produce NO in response to diverse extracellular stimuli and thereby both maintain a baseline level of systemic vasodilatation and establish vasomotor tone. Endothelium-derived NO also sustains the anticoagulant, antiadhesive, and antiproliferative properties of vascular endothelium. A wide range of pathophysiologic states appear to derange eNOS signaling, resulting in a tendency toward vasoconstriction, hypertension, and a prothrombotic state.

Analyses of mice in which the *eNOS* gene has been inactivated show elevated blood pressure, suggesting that tonic synthesis of NO by eNOS is a key determinant of vascular tone. Both knockout and overexpression experiments suggest a role of eNOS and NO in maintaining basal vascular homeostasis. eNOS[null] mice are hypertensive, and the characteristic vasodilatory response to acetylcholine is lost (46). These eNOS[null] mice also develop pulmonary hypertension, hypoxia, and right ventricular hypertrophy (47). Conversely, transgenic mice that overexpress eNOS show increased basal levels of NO and cGMP, associated with decreased blood pressure (48).

Injection of NOS inhibitors into brachial arteries in humans causes local vasoconstriction and decreased blood flow, suggesting a role for NO in controlling arterial and arteriolar blood flow (49–51). Endothelial dysfunction is implicated in many vascular diseases including atherosclerosis, hypertension, and diabetes. Endothelial dysfunction probably involves eNOS dysregulation and/or deficiencies in NO bioavailability, and a concomitant loss of NO's vasoprotective and antiatherogenic effects (52). In a murine model, eNOS expression was correlated with protecting aortic allografts against arteriosclerosis (53). Experiments with transgenic rabbits confirmed an antiatherogenic function of eNOS in a model of severe atherosclerosis, where it was found that eNOS improved vessel relaxation, stimulated cGMP production, and lowered levels of superoxide radicals (54).

Tetrahydrobiopterin may itself serve as a central regulator of eNOS by controlling the ability of the enzyme to produce either superoxide or NO as a function of the cellular oxidative state. Oxidative damage in the endothelium is correlated with endothelial dysfunction and hypertension (55). A role of tetrahydrobiopterin in connecting oxidative stress to endothelial dysfunction is based on the observation that tetrahydrobiopterin can operate as a redox sensor: In the presence of fully reduced tetrahydrobiopterin, eNOS synthesizes more NO than superoxide, but partially oxidized tetrahydrobiopterin appears to favor the synthesis of superoxide by eNOS (56). Therefore, the oxidation of tetrahydrobiopterin by a number of chemicals, including superoxide itself, may be an important factor in the phenomenon of endothelial dysfunction and may reduce NO levels in diverse vascular disease states by controlling the ratio of superoxide to NO (57,58).

A number of human studies have reported increased prevalence of eNOS polymorphisms in hypertensive cohorts (59). For example, the Glu298Asp polymorphism has been associated with decreased NOS activity in the renal artery (60), reduced basal production of NO (61), coronary vasospasm (62), essential hypertension (63,64), hypertension in pregnancy (65,66), elevated risk of atherosclerosis (67), and possible myocardial infarction (68,69). However, the relevance of changes in eNOS function to this genetic polymorphism remains to be determined.

## Pharmacodynamics of Nitric Oxide in Vascular Smooth Muscle Relaxation

NO produced in the endothelium stimulates production of cGMP by the soluble isoform of guanylate cyclase in smooth muscle, leading to activation of the cGMP-dependent protein kinase PKG. In vascular smooth muscle, a key target for PKG is myosin light chain phosphatase (MLCP). Phosphorylation of MLCP increases its activity, thereby converting myosin light chain into the dephosphorylated form (70,71). Dephosphorylated myosin light chains are unable to maintain tonic contraction via interactions with actin, leading to vascular smooth muscle relaxation and vessel dilation. Activation of MLCP also desensitizes the response of the smooth muscle contractile apparatus to calcium, providing an additional mechanism of smooth muscle relaxation and vessel dilation (72).

PKG also affects several targets in vascular smooth muscle that regulate intracellular calcium levels, including voltage-gated calcium channels, sodium/calcium exchangers, calcium-ATPase, phospholamban, the IP$_3$ receptor, and G proteins (73). cGMP may independently regulate monovalent cation channels and can influence the activity of other key regulatory proteins, including cyclic nucleotide phosphodiesterases. Alterations in cellular calcium levels may further influence the phosphorylation state of the myosin light chain under the control of the calcium/calmodulin–dependent enzyme, myosin light chain kinase.

NO may also induce important biologic effects through cGMP-independent pathways, including the activation of calcium-dependent potassium channels that serve to hyperpolarize vascular smooth muscle (74). NO can also rapidly and reversibly inhibit cytochrome $c$ oxidase (complex IV); additional evidence suggests that prolonged exposure to NO may persistently inhibit other heme or iron–sulfur cluster enzymes of the respiratory chain including aconitase, NADH–ubiquinone oxidoreductase (complex I), and succinate–ubiquinone oxidoreductase (complex II) (75). The rapid, reversible inhibition of cytochrome $c$ oxidase is believed to provide a mechanism whereby NO may limit cell respiration and available cellular ATP, thereby attenuating smooth muscle contraction and causing passive vasodilatation (76,77). Longer-term inhibition of other enzymes in the respiratory chain may lead to the suppression of key metabolic pathways and to pathologic changes in vascular smooth muscle cells (78).

## Endothelium-Derived Nitric Oxide as an Inhibitor of Vascular Smooth Muscle Proliferation

NO inhibits the migration and proliferation of vascular smooth muscle cells (79). Pharmacologic NO donors have been found to exhibit antiproliferative effects in *in vitro* systems (80) and the underlying mechanisms have been explored in a variety of studies. Vascular smooth muscle motility can be attenuated by a cGMP-dependent protein tyrosine phosphatase termed PTP-PEST (81). Elevated levels of cGMP can activate cAMP-dependent protein kinases, a pathway that may, at least in part, mediate the antiproliferative effect of NO (82).

Antiproliferative characteristics of NO-donating drugs may have an antiatherogenic effect in healthy endothelium by preventing formation of neointima and the other characteristic phenotypic changes in vascular smooth muscle. However, endogenous NO signaling pathways also have the ability to stimulate migration (83) and proliferation (84) of vascular smooth muscle. For example, VEGF-NO pathways can induce initial events in angiogenesis. Whether NO can exhibit proatherogenic roles is less clear, but the differentiation between antiatherogenic and proatherogenic potential of NO may depend upon the pathophysiologic state of the cellular environment, as well as on the chemical factors influenced by local NO concentration, kinetics, and subcellular localization.

## Nitric Oxide and Vascular Apoptosis

NO is one of the prominent mediators of apoptosis in various cell types, including endothelial cells and smooth muscle cells (85). The effects of NO on apoptotic processes appear to be concentration dependent in that low levels of NO exert protective antiapoptotic effects, whereas high NO levels result in apoptosis and cytotoxicity (86). Because of the concentration dependence of this NO effect, it is possible that eNOS mediates the protective antiapoptotic responses, whereas production of NO by iNOS promotes apoptosis. Moreover, because of its distinctive regulatory characteristics, eNOS in the endothelium appears to predominantly play an antiapoptotic role, whereas iNOS induced in either smooth muscle cells or macrophages in the vascular media has the capacity to generate proapoptotic effects, possibly pertinent to atherosclerosis.

The mechanisms whereby NO inhibits apoptosis in the endothelium appear to be independent of cGMP and may involve the increased expression of heat shock proteins (87), inhibition of apoptotic kinase cascades, and inhibition of a family of proapoptotic cysteine proteases (termed caspases) probably by cysteine sulfhydryl nitrosation and/or tyrosine nitrosation (88–90). Shear stress over the endothelial layer, which is an important determinant of basal NO synthesis by eNOS, may be an important antiapoptotic factor that serves to protect the endothelium against apoptosis in the initial stages of atherogenesis (91).

The ability of iNOS-derived NO to exert proapoptotic and antiproliferative effects on vascular smooth muscle may contribute to the putative role of iNOS in vascular wall remodeling (92). NO-induced apoptosis of vascular smooth muscle cells may also be important in atherogenesis and plaque instability (93,94). The proapoptotic functions of iNOS-derived NO also appear to be cGMP independent, and may relate to NO-induced oxidative damage of cytosine residues, which results in DNA fragmentation (95). Other mechanisms that have been proposed include increased formation of peroxynitrite, activation of caspases, activation of poly [adenosine 5'-diphosphate (ADP) ribose] polymerase, and increased mitochondrial permeability. Some evidence indicates an upregulation of p53 protein in apoptotic cells, and experiments demonstrate vascular smooth muscle from p53$^{null}$ mice are specifically more susceptible to NO-induced apoptosis than wild-type (96).

Endothelial expression of iNOS may also induce apoptosis in endothelium in diabetic vasculopathy, where circulating glycosylated albumin derivatives have been reported to upregulate iNOS activity in small vessels (97). Additionally, expression of iNOS has been suggested as a mechanism of neuronal apoptosis that contributes to cardiovascular autonomic depression in septic shock (98).

## Endothelial Nitric Oxide Synthase and Leukocyte–Endothelium Interactions

eNOS-derived NO exerts broad antiinflammatory and antithrombogenic effects that arise in large part by the inhibition by NO of leukocyte-endothelial interactions. NO downregulates expression of P selectin on endothelial cells (99). Normally, endothelial P selectin facilitates leukocyte rolling followed by cell adhesion, but NO-mediated inhibition of P selectin expression prevents the entire process of leukocyte recruitment. NO may also limit the expression of leukocyte adhesion molecules such as L selectin or CD11/CD18 (100). Because superoxide in the endothelium and leukocytes can promote oxidant-dependent adhesion, the inhibitory effects of NO on cell adhesion may be mediated in part by detoxification of superoxide (101). Inhibition of eNOS enzyme activity results in enhanced adherence of leukocytes to the vascular endothelium (102). Because monocyte adhesion may be one of the initial events in atherogenesis, eNOS may function as an antiatherogenic agent in part by inhibiting recruitment of leukocytes to endothelium. eNOS enzyme inhibition by arginine analogs also leads to increases in vascular permeability, extravasation of plasma proteins, and microvascular edema, involving both cGMP-dependent (103) and cGMP-independent pathways of vascular permeability (104). These increased vascular permeability responses may be mediated in part by the increased adherence of leukocytes to endothelium in the absence of NO (105).

## Endothelial Nitric Oxide Synthase Expression in Blood Platelets

The same eNOS isoform originally described in vascular endothelium is also expressed in blood platelets (106,107). Although the same eNOS isoform is expressed in both cell types, the vascular endothelium is quantitatively much more significant as a source of NO. Endothelial cell–derived NO is important to the regulation of platelet function, and is a key determinant of the balance between physiologically appropriate hemostasis and pathologic thrombosis. Nevertheless, platelet-derived NO from endogenous platelet eNOS may also play an important role in inhibiting platelet adhesion (108–110), aggregation (111), and activation. NO may affect platelets through several interrelated signaling pathways that variously involve cGMP, calcium, eicosanoids, and phosphoinositides as key effectors of the NO response.

Platelet adhesion to the endothelium depends on a number of adhesion molecules expressed on both cells, including ICAM-1 and $\alpha_V\beta_3$ integrin on the endothelium, and $\beta1$ integrin, P selectin, glycoprotein (GP) Ib, and glycoprotein IIb/IIIa on platelets (112). NO released by nitrovasodilator drugs inhibits expression of P selectin on platelets (113). In addition to antagonizing platelet–endothelial interactions, the downregulation of P selectin also inhibits platelet–leukocyte interactions. A PKG-modulated pathway also disrupts activation of GP IIb/IIIa, one of the more crucial mechanisms of platelet adhesion to the endothelium. In this pathway, cGMP-activated PKG phosphorylates both phospholipase C and vasodilator-simulated phosphoprotein (VASP) (114), which results in a decline in intraplatelet calcium level. cGMP can also lower intraplatelet calcium level by inhibiting release of intracellular calcium stores and by shuttling more calcium out of the cell while limiting extracellular calcium reabsorption (115). Low calcium level hinders protein kinase C signaling, impairing the activation of GP IIb/IIIa (116). The GP IIb/IIIa receptor is also necessary for aggregation of platelets in nascent thrombi by cross-linking platelets and fibrin. The potent platelet aggregating effects of thrombin are inhibited by NO (117) from eNOS, which may also be activated by insulin (118). In platelets, insulin stimulates the Akt-mediated phosphorylation of eNOS Ser1177 via phosphatidylinositol 3-kinase (PI 3-K) and AMP-activated protein kinase pathways (119). In addition to insulin's direct effects on eNOS in endothelial cells, it may also induce vasodilatation by activating platelet eNOS and PKG (120), resulting in release of vesicles containing the vasoactive substances ATP, adenosine, and serotonin, which may in turn activate endothelial eNOS (121). The lipid mediator sphingosine-1-phosphate (S1P) is involved in signaling between platelets and the endothelium: Activated platelets secrete S1P, which stimulates activation of endothelial eNOS, thereby releasing NO into the vascular lumen, which serves to attenuate platelet activity.

NO inhibits a number of arachidonic acid pathways that normally function to activate platelets. NO inhibits platelet release of ADP (122) as well as 12-lipoxygenase, thereby preventing formation of leukotrienes and hydroxyeicosatetraenoic acids. NO attenuates the activity of phospholipase A2, the rate-determining enzyme in the arachidonate pathway by which platelets ultimately produce thromboxane. PKG in platelets also impairs thromboxane-mediated signaling by directly phosphorylating the G protein–coupled $TxA_2$ receptors, further inhibiting thromboxane-mediated platelet activation via the downstream phospholipase C cascade (123). These mechanisms of thromboxane antagonism coordinately attenuate a potent stimulus of platelet activation and recruitment.

NO also positively affects the *in vivo* synthesis of prostacyclin, the physiologic antagonist of thromboxane (124). Synergy in the antiplatelet effects of prostacyclin and NO may result from cGMP-mediated inhibition of cAMP-specific phosphodiesterase III, which elevates intraplatelet cAMP and frustrates platelet activation. NO-mediated inhibition of platelet function may also occur by cGMP-independent mechanisms, as suggested for the NO-dependent suppression of thromboxane synthesis (125,126).

Platelets derived from eNOS[null] mice show several abnormalities in agonist-induced platelet aggregation (127), confirming the role of platelet eNOS-derived NO in normal hemostatic mechanisms. The loss of NO-cGMP signaling in these eNOS[null] mice shifts the balance of platelet function toward platelet adhesion and aggregation. In mice with normal endothelial eNOS but with eNOS-deficient platelets, bleeding time also decreased because NO-mediated inhibition of platelet-endothelial adhesion was lost (128). In humans, NO-mediated inhibition of platelet function results in decreased bleeding time (129), and it has been suggested that nitrovasodilator-mediated inhibition of platelet aggregation may affect the progression of coronary thrombosis in patients with unstable angina pectoris.

## Regulation of Endothelial Nitric Oxide Synthase in Endothelial Cells

Whereas endothelial cells constitute the predominant source of eNOS, other cells including platelets (130), mast cells, and neutrophils (131) express eNOS and release some NO on the luminal side of the vascular wall. The tissue-specific expression of eNOS has led to analyses of the eNOS promoter. The promoter for the *eNOS* gene lacks a prototypical TATA promoter and instead contains promoter sites for the binding of Sp-1 and GATA transcription factors, two mechanisms that are utilized by other constitutively expressed genes (132,133). Despite constitutive expression, the precise levels of eNOS protein are further controlled by specific transcriptional stimuli and by posttranscriptional modulation of eNOS messenger ribonucleic acid (mRNA) stability (134).

A key determinant of basal eNOS transcription is shear stress, the mechanical effect of blood flow over the surfaces of endothelial cells. The *eNOS* gene contains nine consensus shear stress response elements (135). The transcription factor KLF2 is specifically upregulated by shear stress in the endothelium (136), and KLF2 itself serves as an important regulator of basal eNOS transcription in response to laminar shear stress (137). Shear stress also activates induced eNOS transcription in a c-Src/NFκB–dependent pathway (138,139). The *eNOS* gene is also characterized by a stimulatory hypoxia-responsive element 5.3 kb upstream of the transcription start site (140). The role of hypoxia in regulating eNOS is not entirely clear because some evidence suggests that hypoxia could downregulate eNOS expression by the Rho kinase pathway (141). Cytokines, including TNF-α, downregulate eNOS transcription in part by inhibition of Sp-1 (142). High levels of oxidized low density lipoproteins (LDL) have been shown to impair eNOS mRNA stability (143). Statins, which may exert an indirect effect on eNOS mRNA via LDL-lowering properties, may also have an independent effect in increasing the level of eNOS mRNA (144,145), which may be mediated by limiting the cytokine-mediated downregulation of eNOS transcription (146) or by statin-mediated inhibition of Rho GTPases (147). Many other mediators exert effects at the level of eNOS transcription, including thrombin and Rho kinase, both of which attenuate the half-life of eNOS mRNA (148,149).

In endothelial cells, the eNOS enzyme is subject to an intricate scheme of modifications and controls that result in a dynamic pattern of stimulation and inhibition in response to a number of physiologic stimuli. Five themes have emerged from a wide variety of experiments that elucidate some of the biochemical systems controlling eNOS in vascular endothelial cells: (a) eNOS is targeted to plasmalemmal caveolae; (b) in the caveolae, eNOS is tonically inhibited by its interaction with the scaffolding-regulatory protein caveolin; (c) certain extracellular signals, including shear stress and specific agonists, establish a basal level of eNOS activity for NO signaling in the endothelium; (d) a diverse family of eNOS agonists—generally involving calcium- or phosphorylation-mediated pathways—dynamically regulates eNOS activity by promoting a relatively rapid, reversible eNOS activation *and* a relatively slower return of eNOS activity to basal levels; and (e) part of this inhibitory mechanism and return to baseline may involve subcellular translocation of eNOS from caveolae in a reversible agonist-mediated process.

Most eNOS in a resting endothelial cell is targeted to specialized plasmalemmal domains called *caveolae*. Caveolae are small invaginations of the plasma membrane that are relatively enriched with cholesterol and sphingolipids, and are further distinguished by the presence of the transmembrane scaffolding protein caveolin-1. The unique biochemical composition of caveolae generates an "ordered liquid phase," which may facilitate various protein–protein and protein–lipid interactions (150). Caveolae are now recognized as important domains for the sequestration of diverse receptors and signaling molecules, including G protein–coupled receptors and growth factor receptors, and their downstream activators, as well as calcium regulatory proteins, and sphingolipids. The targeting of eNOS to caveolae depends on dual acylations of the protein by myristoylation and palmitoylation. Myristoylation of eNOS is irreversible and cotranslational and occurs on the amino group of glycine-2 after removal of the *N*-terminal methionine; this modification is absolutely essential to caveolar targeting (151). Palmitoylation of eNOS is posttranslational and occurs at two cysteine residues, Cys15 and Cys26, near the *N*-terminus. The thiopalmitoyl bond is relatively labile, and palmitoylation is reversible in the presence of the enzyme acyl protein thioesterase-1 (APT-1) (152).

When anchored in caveolae, eNOS is tightly associated with caveolin-1 via protein–protein interaction; eNOS can be coimmunoprecipitated with anti–caveolin-1 antibodies. It is the association with caveolin that maintains eNOS in an inactive state in resting endothelial cells. Dynamic regulation of eNOS activity is achieved through various calcium- and phosphorylation/dephosphorylation-mediated pathways that appear to operate in tandem with cycles of enzyme acylation/deacylation. Regulation of intracellular calcium levels appears to provide the most rapid increase in eNOS activity through the binding of calcium/calmodulin to the enzyme. eNOS agonists, including acetylcholine (acting via M2 muscarinic receptors), bradykinin, and estradiol (153), are known to initiate receptor-specific intracellular signaling pathways in endothelial cells. For example, bradykinin and acetylcholine activate a Gq pathway that increases phospholipase C activity, leading to generation of inositol triphosphate and the release of calcium from intracellular stores (154). These agonist-induced transient increases in intracellular calcium level lead to the activation of the ubiquitous calcium regulatory protein calmoldulin. Binding by eNOS of the calcium–calmodulin complex disrupts the caveolin-eNOS inhibitory protein–protein interaction and increases the catalytic activity of eNOS, apparently by facilitating the transfer of electrons from the NADPH/FAD/FMN cofactors in the reductase domain to the oxygenase domain in eNOS. Displacement of caveolin from eNOS occurs in concert with the binding of calcium-calmodulin to the enzyme (155). In turn, calcium-calmoldulin binding to eNOS facilitates the depalmitoylation of eNOS catalyzed by the enzyme APT-1 (156). In the cytosol, eNOS activity is downregulated further, possibly by reversible phosphorylation at Ser116 (157). Recent evidence indicates that calmodulin itself is under control

of kinase CK2; phosphorylated calmodulin is less efficiently bound, and, therefore, the response of eNOS to intracellular calcium is abbreviated and eNOS activity attenuated. Because calmodulin levels in the cell are low relative to total capacity of calmodulin-binding proteins, this CK2 phosphorylation mechanism may serve to selectively displace calmodulin from eNOS without decreasing total cellular calmodulin levels or disturbing other signaling pathways (158).

In addition to these mechanisms involving acylation and calcium, the complete picture of eNOS regulation includes extensive pathways of phosphorylation and dephosphorylation at multiple sites on the enzyme (see Fig. 42-1). Phosphorylation at Ser1179 in bovine eNOS (Ser1177 in human eNOS) leads to enzyme activation, whereas phosphorylation at Thr497 and Ser116 leads to attenuation of eNOS activity. Recent studies suggest that Ser635 is a stimulatory phosphorylation site, possibly responsive to shear stress (159), whereas phosphorylation of Ser617 may sensitize eNOS to calmodulin binding (160).

Phosphorylation of eNOS Ser1179 is mediated directly by kinase Akt (also known as protein kinase B) (161), although numerous protein kinases have been implicated in phosphorylation of this site. Kinase Akt is itself activated by phosphorylation pathways downstream of PI 3-K. Although kinase Akt is predominantly found in the cytosol, membrane targeting of both eNOS and kinase Akt is necessary for eNOS to undergo phosphorylation at Ser1179 (162). Upon activation, Akt is known to translocate to the membrane because its upstream activators are membrane-associated. Several molecules superimpose another level of control on eNOS by interacting with kinase Akt in the vascular endothelium. Thrombin, acting by the Rho/Rho kinase pathway, inhibits Akt-mediated phosphorylation and activation of eNOS (163). The heat shock protein hsp90 appears to bind to eNOS and/or kinase Akt to promote eNOS activation (164). Adipocyte-released hormones appear to cause vasodilatation: Leptin may activate endothelial Akt in a tyrosine kinase–dependent mechanism (165), whereas adiponectin, an insulinomimetic, activates insulin receptor tyrosine kinases, leading to eNOS activation via a PI 3-K/AMPK pathway (166).

Part of the overall endothelial response to shear stress is mediated by phosphorylation of eNOS Ser1179. Shear stress is likely a key determinant of the tonic stimulation of NO production and the maintenance of basal vascular tone (167).

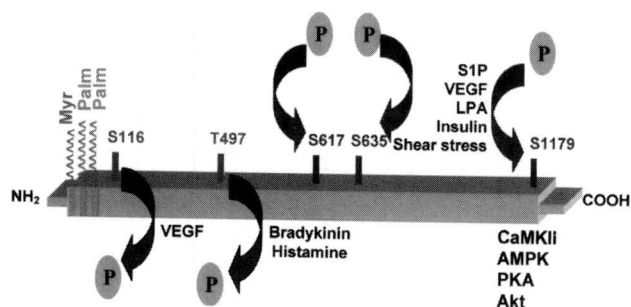

**FIGURE 42-1.** Endothelial nitric oxide synthase (eNOS) activity is regulated by agonist-mediated phosphorylation and dephosphorylation at a number of eNOS serine and threonine sites (amino acid sequence numbers refer to bovine eNOS). Phosphorylation at Ser1179 and Ser635 are believed to stimulate eNOS activity, whereas phosphorylation at Ser617 may promote calmodulin binding and therefore increase eNOS activity. Many eNOS agonists, including shear stress, vascular endothelial growth factor (VEGF), S1P, estrogen, and leptin, lead to phosphorylation at Ser1179. Phosphorylation at Ser116 or Thr497 attenuates eNOS catalytic activity. VEGF-induced dephosphorylation at Ser116 may increase eNOS activity; similarly, protein phosphatase 2A may dephosphorylate Thr497 and Ser1179 (see Color Fig. 42-1). LPA, lysophosphatidic acid; AMPK, AMP-activated protein kinase.

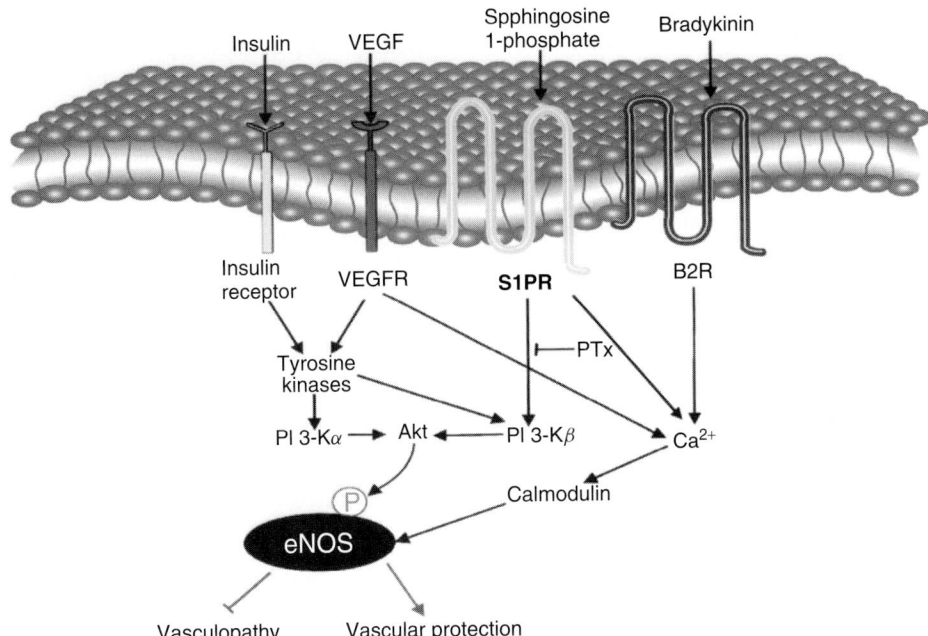

**FIGURE 42-2.** Diverse agonists affect various endothelial cell receptors and signaling pathways that activate endothelial nitric oxide synthase (eNOS) via calcium and/or phosphorylation. Agonists that activate eNOS by increasing intracellular calcium level include bradykinin, sphingosine 1-phosphate (S1P), and vascular endothelial growth factor (VEGF). VEGF, S1P, and insulin activate phosphoinositide-3-kinase (PI 3-K) isoforms, which then activate kinase Akt. Cross talk between the various agonist-mediated signaling pathways represents another key point of regulation. For example, VEGF induces both calcium- and phosphorylation-dependent pathways; VEGF also induces synthesis of S1P receptors (see Color Fig. 42-2). (From Igarashi J, Michel T. More sweetness than light: A search for the causes of diabetic vasculopathy. *J Clin Invest* 2001;108: 1425–1427, with permission.)

Shear stress is transduced via a mechanochemical coupling circuit that increases both calcium and potassium currents and leads to activation of the PI 3-K/Akt kinase pathway.

Vascular endothelial growth factor (VEGF), one of the more potent stimuli of eNOS activity, functions via kinase Akt-mediated phosphorylation at eNOS Ser 1179 (168). Activation of the VEGF receptor Kdr-1 results in PI 3-K α– and PI 3-K β–activation, and, ultimately, in increased activity of kinase Akt. In addition to its effects at Ser1179, VEGF induces dephosphorylation at eNOS Ser116 in a pathway that involves the activation of the phosphatase calcineurin. Because phosphorylation of eNOS at Ser116 appears to inhibit enzyme activity, the involvement of calcineurin in eNOS dephosphorylation may provide a clue to the hypertensive effects of the calcineurin inhibitor cyclosporin (169).

eNOS PI 3-K/Akt-phosphorylation cascades are also mediated by estrogen (170,171), VEGF, and a class of platelet-derived lipid mediators that includes S1P and lysophosphatidic acid (LPA) (172). In addition to S1P being released from activated platelets, PDGF induces its release from platelets into the extracellular space, where it activates endothelial cells through its interaction with G-protein–coupled S1P receptors (formerly known as EDG, or endothelial differentiation gene receptors). S1P, for example, has many functions in endothelial cells, including angiogenesis, vasorelaxation, and proliferation. S1P induces translocation of S1P receptors to caveolae (173). This translocation may facilitate coupling of the S1P receptor to downstream effectors that lead to eNOS Ser1179 phosphorylation via a PI 3-K β/Akt pathway (174).

LPA is released by platelets activated by agonists, including thrombin. Although LPA exerts actions similar to S1P, including phosphorylation of kinase Akt and eNOS, it acts independently of S1P receptors (175) and appears to bind the related family of LPA receptors (176). S1P and LPA signaling provides a paradigmatic example of cross talk between platelets and endothelial cells in the regulation of eNOS.

VEGF is a crucial regulator of eNOS in that it directly exerts effects via PI 3-K/Akt but also sensitizes the endothelium to the effects of lipid mediators (177). VEGF induces S1P receptor mRNA and receptor levels, and thereby augments eNOS

activity and endothelial responses to S1P. S1P and VEGF may synergize and coordinately promote angiogenesis by stimulating the migration of endothelial cells in angiogenesis.

PI 3-K/Akt pathways are but one of a number of phosphorylation cascades that modulate the activity of eNOS. VEGF, S1P, and bradykinin all stimulate various mediators in the MAP kinase pathway, especially ERK1 and ERK2 (178–181). The pleiotropic effects of various agonists evince a possible developing paradigm of complex temporal regulation of eNOS. A wide variety of protein kinases have been implicated in phosphorylation of eNOS. In addition to the role clearly established for kinase Akt, other reports have implicated PKA, PKC, PKG, MAP kinases, and the AMP-activated protein kinase (AMPK) in eNOS phosphorylation. The relative roles of different kinase pathways represent an active area of investigation, and it is safe to say that the pattern of eNOS regulation by protein kinases and phosphoprotein phosphatases is complex (see Fig. 42-2). The phosphorylation of eNOS at different sites has profound effects in stimulating and inhibiting eNOS activity, and it is clear that various phosphatases, as well as kinases, contribute to these processes. Part of the eNOS-activating effect of bradykinin may derive from calcineurin-mediated dephosphorylation of Thr497 (182). In addition to the phosphatase calcineurin, protein phosphatase 2A appears to be a key regulator with an overall inhibitory effect on eNOS activity that dephosphorylates eNOS on Thr497 and Ser1179 (183). Reciprocal control of phosphorylation at Thr497 may contribute to the balance of production of NO and superoxide, respectively, by eNOS (184).

Postranslational control of eNOS is now known to involve receptor-mediated dynamic S-nitrosation. When at basal levels, eNOS activity is tonically inhibited by S-nitrosation of cysteines in a zinc-tetrathiolate cluster. In response to agonists like VEGF and insulin, eNOS is rapidly denitrosated on a time course paralleling the increase in enzyme activity. Like the other activation pathways of eNOS, this period is transient and is followed by rapid renitrosation and a return to basal enzyme activity levels. Interestingly, membrane targeting of eNOS is required for the renitrosation, suggesting that this process may occur temporally after the other measures of eNOS deactivation and return to caveolae (27).

# INDUCIBLE NITRIC OXIDE SYNTHASE–DERIVED NITRIC OXIDE AND VASCULAR PHYSIOLOGY

iNOS has been isolated from macrophages, endothelial cells, hepatocytes, neutrophils, airway epithelium, fibroblasts, bone, microglia, retina, and mast cells; its prototypical function is as a component of the innate immune response to pathogens and tumor cells (185,186). iNOS is generally absent in quiescent cells, but in a wide range of cell types, cellular iNOS mRNA rises rapidly within hours after exposure to proinflammatory stimuli, including bacterial lipopolysaccharide, lipoteichoic acid, and some exotoxins like TSST-1; heat stress and hypoxia may induce similar transcriptional responses. Bacterial products induce proinflammatory cytokines including IFNγ, TNF-α, TNF-β, IL-1, IL-12, and PAF (187), which promote iNOS transcription through the action of NFκB at various cis-acting sites (188,189). Induction of iNOS leads to persistent NO production because the tight binding of calmodulin to iNOS at low levels of intracellular calcium leads to "constitutive activation" of this inducible enzyme once it is synthesized in response to proinflammatory stimuli. The relatively high concentrations of iNOS-derived NO destroy cellular structures and inhibit iron-containing enzymes. iNOS[null] mice are unable to destroy intracellular pathogens or combat proliferation of lymphoma tumor proliferation. Communication between the cyclooxygenase and NOS pathways has been described in several studies, and NO is known to stimulate prostaglandin production; this interconnection may promote inflammation.

In addition to its roles in inflammation and infection, iNOS has important roles in vascular biology, and iNOS-derived NO has been associated with several vascular disease states. In iNOS-deficient mice, cholesterol levels and the incidence of atherosclerotic plaques were found to be significantly increased (190). Several studies have reported that iNOS is induced in vascular smooth muscle within human atherosclerotic lesions, and the expression of iNOS in macrophages colocalizes with peroxidized lipids and necrotic cores in advanced atheromas (191,192). Recent studies have suggested that inhibition of iNOS in atherosclerotic plaques is associated with increased expression of matrix metalloproteinase-9 that may destabilize the lesion (193). However, the precise roles of iNOS in atherogenesis are still being defined, and it is yet unclear whether iNOS reflects a pathologic or protective response, or both. For example, iNOS-derived NO may possibly function as an antioxidant in atherosclerotic plaques (194). Additionally, by combating certain pathogens, iNOS may prevent the initiation or exacerbation of the inflammatory and immunologic reactions of atherosclerotic responses in the vascular wall (195). Statins have been demonstrated to upregulate iNOS mRNA levels in vascular smooth muscle, which may contribute to the atheroprotective effect of this class of therapeutics (196). Although these studies of iNOS in atherosclerosis suggest an atheroprotective role, iNOS expression has been correlated with decreased extracellular collagen content and plaque instability, possibly via a proapoptotic mechanism (197).

iNOS induction is linked with endotoxemia, sepsis, and circulatory shock, associated with the widespread induction of iNOS in macrophages, vascular smooth muscle, hepatocytes, and cardiomyocytes. It has been suggested that in sepsis there is a specific temporal course of early eNOS activation followed by delayed activation of iNOS via transcriptional induction. In any case, supraphysiologic induction of iNOS in macrophages and vascular smooth muscle significantly raises NO production in the vasculature, such that blood levels of NO and its metabolites can reach micromolar levels (198) that contribute to the systemic hypotension in septic shock. Septic shock is also characterized by a particular inability to respond to vasoconstrictors and by the formation of pathologic shunts, both of which may be consequences of the elevated intravascular levels of NO. iNOS[null] mice provide limited insight into the pathogenesis of sepsis. Induction of iNOS in sepsis models in mice appears to suppress eNOS and may lead to endothelial dysfunction; in iNOS[null] mice, this sepsis-induced endothelial dysfunction is less pronounced (199). Some experiments suggest that iNOS induction may impair the ability of blood vessels to undergo catecholamine-induced vasoconstriction; indeed, the iNOS[null] mice displayed improved early survival in a sepsis model (200). Another analysis of sepsis pathways in iNOS[null] mice proposed that iNOS was actually functioning in a protective role in sepsis by inducing thymocyte apoptosis (201). In addition to its vascular roles in shock, iNOS induction in the heart directly creates negative inotropic effects, thereby exacerbating hypotension, whereas NO may contribute to the end-organ injury in shock by mitochondrial inhibition or direct cytotoxicity.

iNOS may also play a role in the pathogenesis of hypertensive states including preeclampsia and essential hypertension. Inhibition of NO synthesis in pregnant rats causes symptoms similar to those in pregnancy-induced hypertension including proteinuria and thrombocytopenia (202). eNOS may play a role in placental vasoregulation (203), but it is likely that iNOS actually serves as a significant source of placental vascular NO, crucial in maternal–fetal vasoregulation and facilitating placental blood flow (204). This observation is consistent with observations that NO production in vessels and endothelial cells increases during pregnancy. In preeclampsia, NO production is significantly reduced, and trophoblasts from preeclamptic mothers show lowered levels of iNOS as compared with normotensive mothers. Inhibition of iNOS has been suggested to be a result of elevated endothelin-1 concentration (205). Other reports have suggested that preeclampsia is a result of reduced concentrations of the key NOS substrate (206). One study has suggested that a hypertension susceptibility locus on chromosome 17 is related to an iNOS promoter polymorphism (207), but the broader implications remain to be determined.

# NEURONAL NITRIC OXIDE AND VASOREGULATION

## Neuronal Nitric Oxide Synthase and Vasodilatation in Skeletal Muscle Vasculature

nNOS is found in relatively high concentrations in specific regions of the mammalian central nervous system (208). However, nNOS is also expressed in skeletal muscle and in parasympathetic nervous systems of the gastrointestinal tract, bladder, ureter, prostate, and the walls of corpus cavernosa large blood vessels (209). nNOS transcription is complexly regulated in pathways involving the p38 kinase (210) and OCT2 (211) transcription factors, whereas differential splicing of nNOS results in at least three tissue-specific variants (212,213). In neurons, nNOS localizes to both the rough endoplasmic reticulum and electron-dense postsynaptic areas. nNOS is expressed at high levels in mammalian skeletal muscle and is localized to the sarcolemma of fast-twitch (type I) muscle fibers (214,215). This interaction is facilitated by the N-terminal domain of nNOS, which is homologous to the syntrophin family of proteins that bind dystrophin via a conserved GLGF motif (216). Genetic deficiency of dystrophin causes Duchenne muscular dystrophy, a disease-specific degeneration of fast-twitch fibers. These patients also exhibit a selective loss of nNOS, which normally may serve to regulate blood flow in skeletal muscle by antagonizing alpha-adrenergic–mediated vasoconstriction (217). It is also possible that NO produced by nNOS may function to limit muscle contractile force.

## Neurogenic Vasodilatation Mediated by Nitric Oxide

Experiments demonstrating a vasodilatory response mediated by nonadrenergic, noncholinergic nerves that was not mediated by other well-known neurotransmitters was independent of denuded endothelium, and yet was susceptible to NOS inhibitors, led to the hypothesis that nitrergic (also termed *nitroxidergic*) nerves modulate local NO release to mediate vasodilatation (218). This phenomenon of nitrergic innervation has been revealed in the cerebral, mesenteric, temporal, and ophthalmic arteries and arterioles of dogs, cows, and monkeys, as well as the human uterine artery (219). Some evidence from experiments in humans suggests that NO functions in vasoneuronal coupling of cerebral blood flow to neuronal activity, which may be relevant to the maintenance of cerebral blood flow and to the pathophysiology of migraine (220). Nitrergic nerves may mediate hypercapnia-induced vasodilatation, although there is conflicting evidence on the role of the endothelium and cGMP in this response (221).

Nitrergic nerves, similar to noradrenergic nerves, directly innervate vascular smooth muscle. nNOS is localized to postsynaptic terminals of perivascular nerves (222), and there is immunohistochemical evidence for nNOS in the adventitia and outer media of nitrergic innervated vessels (223). Nitrergic nerves have been found to track along with other postsynaptic parasympathetic neurons using acetylcholine and vasoactive intestinal peptide transmitters, and some originate from the pterygopalatine ganglia (224). An electric potential from the nitrergic neuron triggers calcium influx into the nitrergic terminal, thereby activating NOS to synthesize NO. Dual innervation of vascular smooth muscle cells by noradrenergic and nitrergic nerves provides a mechanism for reciprocal neurogenic control of vasoconstriction and vasodilatation (225).

# IMPACT OF PHARMACOLOGIC SOURCES OF NITRIC OXIDE ON VASCULAR SIGNALING

The ability of nitrovasodilators to deliver NO and thereby dilate venous and coronary vessels is exploited in the treatment of hypertension, angina, and heart failure. Prolonged nitrate therapy generally leads to tolerance, characterized by a decreased sensitivity of vascular cells to the nitrovasodilator. Numerous theories have been advanced to account for the observation of tolerance, including vascular tolerance by feedback inhibition, sulfhydryl depletion, increased endothelial production of free radicals including superoxide, neurohumoral reflexes, and alteration in local vascular production of vasoactive compounds (226). The sulfhydryl hypothesis posits that tolerance is related to depletion of reactive sulfhydryl groups necessary for the enzymatic release of NO from nitrovasodilators (227). Tolerance could be related to inhibition of NO-cGMP signaling in response to elevated vascular NO levels (228). At least with respect to nitroglycerin, tolerance has been linked to downregulation of an enzyme reported to be involved in the metabolism of nitroglycerin to release NO, mitochondrial aldehyde dehydrogenase (229). Nitroglycerin also induces production of reactive oxygen species, which in

part blunt the response to vasodilatory agonists while sensitizing the vascular response to endogenous vasoconstricting agents (230).

Inhibitors of angiotensin converting enzymes (ACE) exert vasodilatory effects by blunting the renin-angiotensin-aldosterone pathway as well as by blocking the breakdown of the key eNOS agonist bradykinin. By inhibiting the catabolism of bradykinin by ACE, ACE inhibitors result in increased endothelial formation of NO in a bradykinin-dependent manner (231).

Beyond the effects of statins on HMG-CoA reductase and plaque stabilization, part of the antiatherogenic effect of statins may derive from the upregulation of eNOS mRNA and protein levels, which could ameliorate endothelial dysfunction in atherosclerotic lesions.

## CONCLUSION

NO, whether endogenously produced or derived from nitrovasodilator drugs, plays a vital role in vascular physiology and pathology. The vascular effects of NO predominantly result from the action of eNOS, with endothelial eNOS affecting signaling pathways in the endothelium and underlying vascular smooth muscle and with platelet eNOS primarily affecting platelets. eNOS itself is known to be regulated by a complex, interlinked network of agonists, calcium transients, phosphorylation and dephosphorylation cascades, and acylation. Healthy endothelium is characterized by robust eNOS activity, which is central to maintaining vascular tone as well as limiting the adhesion of platelets and leukocytes to the endothelium. The phenomenon of endothelial dysfunction is associated with a wide range of disease states and is linked with dysregulation of eNOS and NO-dependent vascular responses, thereby tipping the vascular balance toward vasoconstriction and thrombosis.

iNOS and nNOS also have central roles in vascular biology. iNOS appears to be involved in the maturation of atherosclerotic lesions and is intimately linked to vascular responses in sepsis and preeclampsia. nNOS assists in vasoneuronal coupling and the regulation of cerebral blood flow, as well as in modulating the tone of peripheral vessels by nitrergic neurons.

A more detailed understanding of molecular dynamics of NO and NO synthases is emerging from studies in a broad range of experimental systems. Nitrosothiol compounds may prolong the half-life of NO, deliver NO to locations distal to the site of its production, and may alter the biological consequences of NO synthesis. NO and its metabolites play a fundamental role in the modulation of vascular homeostasis and derangements in NO-dependent pathways have been implicated in a wide range of disease states. Advances in our understanding of NOS molecular regulation and NO chemistry may lead to the identification of new points for therapeutic intervention in vascular disease.

## *References*

1. Furchgott RF, Zawadzki JV. The obligatory role of endothelial cells in the relaxation of arterial smooth muscle by acetylcholine. *Nature* 1980;288: 373–376.
2. Ignarro LJ, Byrns RE, Buga GM, et al. Endothelium-derived relaxing factor from pulmonary artery and vein possesses pharmacologic and chemical properties identical to those of nitric oxide radical. *Circ Res* 1987;61: 866–879.
3. Kerwin JF, Lancaster JR, Feldman PR. Nitric oxide: a new paradigm for second messengers. *J Med Chem* 1995;38:4343–4362.
4. Lancaster JR. Simulation of the diffusion and reaction of endogenously produced nitric oxide. *Proc Natl Acad Sci U S A* 1994;91:8137–8141.
5. Galla H. Nitric oxide, NO, an intercellular messenger. *Angew Chem Int Ed Engl* 1993;32:378–382.
6. Moncada S, Palmer RMJ, Higgs EA. Nitric oxide: physiology, pathophysiology, and pharmacology. *Pharmacol Rev* 1991;43:109–142.

7. Lancaster JR. Simulation of the diffusion and reaction of endogenously produced nitric oxide. *Proc Natl Acad Sci U S A.* 1994;91:8137–8141.

8. Wood J, Garthwaite J. Models of the diffusional spread of nitric oxide: implications for neural nitric oxide signalling and its pharmacological properties. *Neuropharmacology* 1994;33:1235–1244.

9. Giustarini D, Milzani A, Colombo R, et al. Nitric oxide and S-nitrosothiols in human blood. *Clin Chim Acta* 2003;330:85–98.

10. Wink DA, Nims RW, Darbyshire JF, et al. Reaction kinetics for nitrosation of cysteine and glutathione in aerobic nitric oxide solutions at neutral pH. Insights into the fate and physiological effects of intermediates generated in the NO/O2 reaction. *Chem Res Toxicol* 1994;7:519–525.

11. Stamler JS, Jaraki O, Osborne J, et al. Nitric oxide circulates in mammalian plasma primarily as an S-nitroso adduct of serum albumin. *Proc Natl Acad Sci U S A* 1992;89:7674–7677.

12. Gaston B, Reilly J, Drazen JM, et al. Endogenous nitrogen oxides and bronchodilator S-nitrosothiols in human airways. *Proc Natl Acad Sci U S A* 1993;90:10957–10961.

13. Ishibashi T, Yoshida J, Nishio M. New methods to evaluate endothelial function: A search for a marker of nitric oxide (NO) *in vivo*: re-evaluation of NOx in plasma and red blood cells and a trial to detect nitrosothiols. *J Pharmacol Sci* 2003;93:409–416.

14. Stamler JS, Jaraki O, Osborne J, et al. Nitric oxide circulates in mammalian plasma primarily as an S-nitroso adduct of serum albumin. *Proc Natl Acad Sci U S A* 1992;89:7674–7677.

15. Gaston B, Reilly J, Drazen JM, et al. Endogenous nitrogen oxides and bronchodilator S-nitrosothiols in human airways. *Proc Natl Acad Sci U S A* 1993;90:10957–10961.

16. Gaston B, Reilly J, Drazen JM, et al. Endogenous nitrogen oxides and bronchodilator S-nitrosothiols in human airways. *Proc Natl Acad Sci U S A* 1993;90:10957–10961.

17. Haqqani AS, Do SK, Birnboim HC. The role of a formaldehyde dehydrogenase-glutathione pathway in protein S-nitrosation in mammalian cells. *Nitric Oxide* 2003;9:172–181.

18. Schechter AN, Gladwin MT. Hemoglobin and the paracrine and endocrine functions of nitric oxide. *N Engl J Med* 2003;348:1483–1485.

19. Gladwin MT, Shelhamer JH, Schechter AN, et al. Role of circulating nitrite and S-nitrosohemoglobin in the regulation of regional blood flow in humans. *Proc Natl Acad Sci U S A* 2000;97:11482–11487.

20. Muller B, Kleschyov AL, Alencar JL, et al. Nitric oxide transport and storage in the cardiovascular system. *Ann N Y Acad Sci* 2002;962:131–139.

21. Giustarini D, Milzani A, Colombo R, et al. Nitric oxide and S-nitrosothiols in human blood. *Clin Chim Acta* 2003;330:85–98.

22. Radomski MW, Rees DD, Dutra A, et al. S-nitroso-glutathione inhibits platelet activation *in vitro* and *in vivo*. *Br J Pharmacol* 1992;107:745–749.

23. Hothersall JS, Noronha-Dutra AA. Nitrosothiol processing by platelets. *Methods Enzymol* 2002;359:238–244.

24. Wolzt M, MacAllister RJ, Davis D, et al. Biochemical characterization of S-nitrosohemoglobin. Mechanisms underlying synthesis, NO release, and biological activity. *J Biol Chem* 1999;274:28983–28990.

25. Broillet MC. S-Nitrosylation of proteins. *Cell Mol Life Sci* 1999;55:1036–1042.

26. Guittet O, Roy B, Lepoivre M. Nitric oxide: A radical molecule in quest of free radicals in proteins. *Cell Mol Life Sci* 1999;55:1054–1067.

27. Erwin PA, Lin AJ, Golan DE, et al. Receptor-regulated dynamic S-nitrosylation of endothelial nitric oxide synthase in vascular endothelial cells. *J Biol Chem* 2005;280:19888–19894.

28. Akhter S, Vignini A, Wen Z, et al. Evidence for S-nitrosothiol-dependent changes in fibrinogen that do not involve transnitrosation or thiolation. *Proc Natl Acad Sci U S A* 2002;99:9172–9177.

29. Catani MV, Bernassola F, Rossi A, et al. Inhibition of clotting factor XIII activity by nitric oxide. *Biochem Biophys Res Commun* 1998;249:275–278.

30. Stamler JS, Simon DI, Jaraki O, et al. S-nitrosylation of tissue-type plasminogen activator confers vasodilatory and antiplatelet properties on the enzyme. *Proc Natl Acad Sci U S A* 1992;89:8087–8091.

31. Raman CS, Li H, Martasek P, et al. Crystal structure of constitutive endothelial nitric oxide synthase: a paradigm for pterin function involving a novel metal center. *Cell* 1998;95:939–950.

32. Porter TD, Beck TW, Kasper CB. NADPH-cytochrome P-450 oxidoreductase gene organization correlates with structural domains of the protein. *Biochemistry* 1990;29:9814–9818.

33. Abu-Soud HM, Feldman PL, Clark P, et al. Electron transfer in nitric-oxide synthases. Characterization of L-arginine analogs that block heme iron reduction. *J Biol Chem* 1994;269:32318–32326.

34. Vermilion JL, Ballou DP, Massey V, et al. Separate roles for FMN and FAD in catalysis by liver microsomal NADPH-cytochrome P-450 reductase. *J Biol Chem* 1981;256:266–277.

35. Steuhr DJ, Griffith OW. Mammalian nitric oxide synthases. *Adv Enzymol Relat Areas Mol Biol* 1992;65:287–346.

36. Witteveen CF, Giovanelli J, Kaufman S. Reactivity of tetrahydrobiopterin bound to nitric-oxide synthase. *J Biol Chem* 1999;274:29755–29762.

37. Alp NJ, Channon KM. Regulation of endothelial nitric oxide synthase by tetrahydrobiopterin in vascular disease. *Arterioscler Thromb Vasc Biol* 2004;24:445–450.

38. Lowenstein CJ, Glatt CS, Bredt DS, et al. Cloned and expressed macrophage nitric oxide synthase contrasts with the brain enzyme. *Proc Natl Acad Sci U S A* 1992;89:6711–6715.

39. Janssens SP, Simouchi A, Quertermous T, et al. Cloning and expression of a cDNA encoding human endothelium-derived relaxing factor/nitric oxide synthase. *J Biol Chem* 1992;267:14519–14522.

40. Michel T, Lamas S. Molecular cloning of constitutive endothelial nitric oxide synthase: evidence for a family of related genes. *J Cardiovasc Pharmacol* 1992;20(Suppl. 12):S45–S49.

41. Ponting CP, Phillips C. DHR domains in syntrophins, neuronal NO synthases and other intracellular proteins. *Trends Biochem Sci* 1995;20:102–103.

42. Cho HJ, Xie QW, Calaycay J, et al. Calmodulin is a subunit of nitric oxide synthase from macrophages. *J Exp Med* 1992;176:599–604.

43. Cohen RA. The role of nitric oxide and other endothelium-derived vasoactive substances in vascular disease. *Prog Cardiovasc Dis* 1995;38:105–128.

44. Parker JD. Nitrate tolerance, oxidative stress, and mitochondrial function: another worrisome chapter on the effects of organic nitrates. *J Clin Invest* 2004;113:352–354.

45. Parker JD, Parker JO. Nitrate therapy for stable angina pectoris. *N Engl J Med* 1998;338:520–531.

46. Huang PL, Huang Z, Mashimo H, et al. Hypertension in mice lacking the gene for endothelial nitric oxide synthase. *Nature* 1995;377:239–242.

47. Steudel W, Scherrer-Crosbie M, Bloch KD, et al. Sustained pulmonary hypertension and right ventricular hypertrophy after chronic hypoxia in mice with congenital deficiency of nitric oxide synthase 3. *J Clin Invest* 1998;101:2468–2477.

48. Ohashi Y, Kawashima S, Hirata K, et al. Hypotension and reduced nitric oxide-elicited vasorelaxation in transgenic mice overexpressing endothelial nitric oxide synthase. *J Clin Invest* 1998;102:2061–2071.

49. Vallance P, Collier J, Moncada S. Effects of endothelium-derived nitric oxide on peripheral arteriolar tone in man. *Lancet* 1989;2:997–1000.

50. Loscalzo J, Welch G. Nitric oxide and its role in the cardiovascular system. *Prog Cardiovasc Dis* 1995;38:87–104.

51. Cohen RA. The role of nitric oxide and other endothelium-derived vasoactive substances in vascular disease. *Prog Cardiovasc Dis* 1995;38:105–128.

52. Pieper GM, Peltier BA. Amelioration by L-arginine of a dysfunctional arginine/nitric oxide pathway in diabetic endothelium. *J Cardiovasc Pharmacol* 1995;25:397–403.

53. Lee PC, Wang ZL, Qian S, et al. Endothelial nitric oxide synthase protects aortic allografts from the development of transplant arteriosclerosis. *Transplantation* 2000;27:1186–1192.

54. Hayashi T, Sumi D, Juliet PA, et al. Gene transfer of endothelial NO synthase, but not eNOS plus inducible NOS, regressed atherosclerosis in rabbits. *Cardiovasc Res* 2004;61:339–351.

55. Kerr S, Brosnan MJ, McIntyre M, et al. Superoxide anion production is increased in a model of genetic hypertension: role of the endothelium. *Hypertension* 1999;33:1353–1358.

56. Vasquez-Vivar J, Martasek P, Whitsett J, et al. The ratio between tetrahydrobiopterin and oxidized tetrahydrobiopterin analogues controls superoxide release from endothelial nitric oxide synthase: an EPR spin trapping study. *Biochem J* 2003;362:733–739.

57. Landmesser U, Dikalov S, Price SR, et al. Oxidation of tetrahydrobiopterin leads to uncoupling of endothelial cell nitric oxide synthase in hypertension. *J Clin Invest* 2003;111:1201–1209.

58. Alp NJ, Mussa S, Khoo J, et al. Tetrahydrobiopterin-dependent preservation of nitric oxide-mediated endothelial function in diabetes by targeted transgenic GTP-cyclohydrolase I overexpression. *J Clin Invest* 2003;112:725–735.

59. Nakayama T, Soma M, Takahashi Y, et al. Association analysis of CA-repeat polymorphism of the endothelial nitric oxide synthase gene with essential hypertension in Japanese. *Clin Genet* 1997;51:26–30.

60. Persu A, Stoenoiu MS, Messiaen T, et al. Modifier effect of ENOS in autosomal dominant polycystic kidney disease. *Hum Mol Genet* 2002;11:229–241.

61. Veldman BA, Spiering W, Doevendans PA, et al. The Glu298Asp polymorphism of the NOS 3 gene as a determinant of the baseline production of nitric oxide. *J Hypertens* 2002;20:2023–2027.

62. Chang K, Baek SH, Seung KB, et al. The Glu298Asp polymorphism in the endothelial nitric oxide synthase gene is strongly associated with coronary spasm. *Coron Artery Dis* 2003;14:293–299.

63. Jachymova M, Horky K, Bultas J, et al. Association of the Glu298Asp polymorphism in the endothelial nitric oxide synthase gene with essential hypertension resistant to conventional therapy. *Biochem Biophys Res Commun* 2001;284:426–430.

64. Miyamoto Y, Saito Y, Kajiyama N, et al. Endothelial nitric oxide synthase gene is positively associated with essential hypertension. *Hypertension* 1998;32:3–8.

65. Kobashi G, Yamada H, Ohta K, et al. Endothelial nitric oxide synthase gene (NOS3) variant and hypertension in pregancy. *Am J Med Genet* 2001;103:241–244.

66. Savvidou MD, Vallance PJ, Nicolaides KH, et al. Endothelial nitric oxide synthase gene polymorphism and maternal vascular adaptation to pregnancy. *Hypertension* 2001;38:1289–1293.

67. Lembo G, De Luca N, Battagli C, et al. A common variant of endothelial nitric oxide synthase (Glu298Asp) is an independent risk factor for carotid atherosclerosis. *Stroke* 2001;32:735–740.

68. Hingorani AD, Liang CF, Fatibene J, et al. A common variant of endothelial nitric oxide synthase (Glu298Asp) is a major risk factor for coronary artery disease in the UK. *Circulation* 1999;100:1515–1520.

69. Shimasaki Y, Yasue H, Yoshimura M, et al. Association of the missense Glu298Asp variant of the endothelial nitric oxide synthase gene with myocardial infarction. *J Am Coll Cardiol* 1998;31:1506–1510.

70. Surks HK, Mochizuki N, Kasai Y, et al. Regulation of myosin phosphatase by a specific interaction with cGMP- dependent protein kinase Iα. *Science* 1999;286:1583–1587.

71. Etter EF, Eto M, Wardle RL, et al. Activation of myosin light chain phosphatase in intact arterial smooth muscle during nitric oxide-induced relaxation. *J Biol Chem* 2001;276:34681–34685.

72. Bolz S-S, Vogel L, Sollinger D, et al. Nitric oxide-induced decrease in calcium sensitivity of resistance arteries is attributable to activation of the myosin light chain phosphatase and antagonized by the rhoA/rho kinase pathway. *Circulation* 2003;107:3081–3087.

73. Loscalzo J, Welch G. Nitric oxide and its role in the cardiovascular system. *Prog Cardiovasc Dis* 1995;38:87–104.

74. Bolotina VM, Najibi S, Palacino JJ, et al. Nitric oxide directly activates calcium-dependent potassium channels in vascular smooth muscle. *Nature* 1994;368:850–853.

75. Henry Y, Guissani A. Interactions of nitric oxide with hemoproteins: roles of nitric oxide in mitochondria. *Cell Mol Life Sci* 1999;55:1013–1014.

76. Henry Y, Guissani A. Interactions of nitric oxide with hemoproteins: roles of nitric oxide in mitochondria. *Cell Mol Life Sci* 1999;55:1013–1014.

77. Brown GC. Nitric oxide regulates mitochondrial respiration and cell functions by inhibiting cytochrome oxidase. *FEBS Lett* 1995;369:136–139.

78. Henry Y, Guissani A. Interactions of nitric oxide with hemoproteins: roles of nitric oxide in mitochondria. *Cell Mol Life Sci* 1999;55:1013–1014.

79. Moncada S, Higgs A. The L-arginine-nitric oxide pathway. *N Engl J Med* 1993;329:2002–2012.

80. Mooradian DL, Hutsell TC, Keefer LK. Nitric oxide (NO) donor molecules: effect of NO release rate on vascular smooth muscle cell proliferation *in vitro*. *J Cardiovasc Pharmacol* 1995;25:674–678.

81. Lin Y, Ceacareanu AC, Hassid A. Nitric oxide-induced inhibition of aortic smooth muscle cell motility: role of PTP-PEST and adaptor proteins p130cas and Crk. *Am J Physiol Heart Circ Physiol* 2003;285:H710–H721.

82. Cornwell TL, Arnold E, Boerth NJ, et al. Inhibition of smooth muscle cell growth by nitric oxide and activation of cAMP-dependent protein kinase by cGMP. *Am J Physiol* 1994;267:C1405–C1413.

83. Chang Y, Ceacareanu B, Dixit M, et al. Nitric oxide-induced motility in aortic smooth muscle cells: role of protein tyrosine phosphatase SHP-2 and GTP-binding protein Rho. *Circ Res* 2002;91:390–397.

84. Wolfsgruber W, Feil S, Brummer S, et al. A proatherogenic role for cGMP-dependent protein kinase in vascular smooth muscle cells. *Proc Natl Acad Sci U S A* 2003;100:13519–13524.

85. Nishio E, Fukushima K, Shiozaki M, et al. Nitric oxide donor SNAP induces apoptosis in smooth muscle cells through cGMP-independent mechanism. *Biochem Biophys Res Commun* 1996;221:163–168.

86. Kim PK, Zamora R, Petrosko P, et al. The regulatory role of nitric oxide in apoptosis. *Int Immunopharmacol* 2001;1:1421–1441.

87. Kim YM, de Vera ME, Watkins SC, et al. Nitric oxide protects cultured rat hepatocytes from tumor necrosis factor-α-induced apoptosis by inducing heat shock protein 70 expression. *J Biol Chem* 1997;272:1402–1411.

88. Zech B, Kohl R, von Knethen A, et al. Nitric oxide donors inhibit formation of the Apaf-1/caspase-9 apoptosome and activation of caspases. *Biochem J* 2003;371:1055–1064.

89. Rossig L, Fichtlscherer B, Breitschopf K, et al. Nitric oxide inhibits caspase-3 by S-nitrosation *in vivo*. *J Biol Chem* 1999;274:6823–6826.

90. Kim JE, Tannenbaum SR. S-Nitrosation regulates the activation of endogenous procaspase-9 in HT-29 human colon carcinoma cells. *J Biol Chem* 2004;279:9758–9764.

91. Dimmeler S, Haendeler J, Nehls M, et al. Suppression of apoptosis by nitric oxide via inhibition of interleukin-1β-converting enzyme (ICE)-like and cysteine protease protein (CPP)-32-like proteases. *J Exp Med* 1997;185:601–607.

92. Iwashina M, Shichiri M, Marumo F, et al. Transfection of inducible nitric oxide synthase gene causes apoptosis in vascular smooth muscle cells. *Circulation* 1998;98:1212–1218.

93. Cai W, Devaux B, Schaper W, et al. The role of FAS/APO-1 and apoptosis in the development of human atherosclerotic lesions. *Atherosclerosis* 1997;131:177–186.

94. Kockx MM, De Meyer GR, Muhring J, et al. Apoptosis and related proteins in different stages of human atherosclerotic plaques. *Circulation* 1998;97:2307–2315.

95. Nguyen T, Brunson D, Crespi CL, et al. DNA damage and mutation in human cells exposed to nitric oxide *in vitro*. *Proc Natl Acad Sci U S A* 1992;89:3030–3034.

96. Kibbe MR, Li J, Nie S, et al. Potentiation of nitric oxide-induced apoptosis in p53-/- vascular smooth muscle cells. *Am J Physiol Cell Physiol* 2002;282:C625–C634.

97. Amore A, Cirina P, Conti G, et al. Amadori-configurated albumin induces nitric oxide-dependent apoptosis of endothelial cells: a possible mechanism of diabetic vasculopathy. *Nephrol Dial Transplant* 2004;19:53–60.

98. Sharshar T, Gray F, Lorin de la Grandmaison G, et al. Apoptosis of neurons in cardiovascular autonomic centres triggered by inducible nitric oxide synthase after death from septic shock. *Lancet* 2003;362:1799–1805.

99. Kubes P, Suzuki M, Granger DN. Nitric oxide: an endogenous modulator of leukocyte adhesion. *Proc Natl Acad Sci U S A* 1991;88:4651–4655.

100. Ahluwalia A, Foster P, Scotland RS, et al. Antiinflammatory activity of soluble guanylate cyclase: cGMP-dependent down-regulation of P-selectin expression and leukocyte recruitment. *Proc Natl Acad Sci U S A* 2004; 101:1386–1391.

101. Kubes P, Kanwar S, Niu XF, et al. Nitric oxide synthesis inhibition induces leukocyte adhesion via superoxide and mast cells. *FASEB J* 1993;7: 1293–1299.

102. Kubes P, Kanwar S, Niu XF, et al. Nitric oxide synthesis inhibition induces leukocyte adhesion via superoxide and mast cells. *FASEB J* 1993;7: 1293–1299.

103. Kubes P. Nitric oxide-induced microvascular permeability alterations: a regulatory role for cGMP. *Am J Physiol* 1993;265:H1909–H1915.

104. Johnston B, Gaboury JP, Suematsu M, et al. Nitric oxide inhibits microvascular protein leakage induced by leukocyte adhesion-independent and adhesion-dependent inflammatory mediators. *Microcirculation* 1999; 6:153–162.

105. Kubes P, Granger DN. Nitric oxide modulates microvascular permeability. *Am J Physiol* 1992;262:H611–H615.

106. Sase K, Michel T. Expression of constitutive endothelial nitric oxide synthase in human blood platelets. *Life Sci* 1993;57:2049–2055.

107. Chen LY, Mehta JL. Further evidence of the presence of constitutive and inducible nitric oxide synthase isoforms in human platelets. *J Cardiovasc Pharmacol* 1996;27:154–158.

108. Moncada S, Higgs A. The L-arginine-nitric oxide pathway. *N Engl J Med* 1993;329:2002–2012.

109. Radomski MW, Palmer RM, Moncada S. The role of nitric oxide and cGMP in platelet adhesion to vascular endothelium. *Biochem Biophys Res Commun* 1987;148:1482–1489.

110. Freedman JE, Sauter R, Battinelli EM, et al. Deficient platelet-derived nitric oxide and enhanced hemostasis in mice lacking the NOSIII gene. *Circ Res* 1999;84:1416–1421.

111. Moncada S, Higgs A. The L-arginine-nitric oxide pathway. *N Engl J Med* 1993;329:2002–2012.

112. Bombeli T, Schwartz BR, Harlan JM. Adhesion of activated platelets to endothelial cells: evidence for a GPIIbIIIa-dependent bridging mechanism and novel roles for endothelial intercellular adhesion molecule 1 (ICAM-1), $\alpha_v\beta_3$ integrin, and GPIbα. *J Exp Med* 1998;187:329–339.

113. Michelson AD, Benoit SE, Furman MI, et al. Effects of nitric oxide/EDRF on platelet surface glycoproteins. *Am J Physiol* 1996;270:H1640–H1648.

114. Becker EM, Schmidt P, Schramm M, et al. The vasodilator-stimulated phosphoprotein (VASP): target of YC-1 and nitric oxide effects in human and rat platelets. *J Cardiovasc Pharmacol* 2000;35:390–397.

115. Radomski MW, Rees DD, Dutra A, et al. S-nitroso-glutathione inhibits platelet activation *in vitro* and *in vivo*. *Br J Pharmacol* 1992;107:745–749.

116. Michelson AD, Benoit SE, Furman MI, et al. Effects of nitric oxide/EDRF on platelet surface glycoproteins. *Am J Physiol* 1996;270:H1640–H1648.

117. Pigazzi A, Heydrick S, Folli F, et al. Nitric oxide inhibits thrombin receptor-activating peptide-induced phosphoinositide 3-kinase activity in human platelets. *J Biol Chem* 1999;274:14368–14375.

118. Fleming I, Schulz C, Fichtlscherer B, et al. AMP-activated protein kinase (AMPK) regulates the insulin-induced activation of the nitric oxide synthase in human platelets. *Thromb Haemost* 2003;90:863–871.

119. Fleming I, Schulz C, Fichtlscherer B, et al. AMP-activated protein kinase (AMPK) regulates the insulin-induced activation of the nitric oxide synthase in human platelets. *Thromb Haemost* 2003;90:863–871.

120. Randriamboavonjy V, Schrader J, Busse R, et al. Insulin induces the release of vasodilator compounds from platelets by a nitric oxide-G kinase-VAMP-3-dependent pathway. *J Exp Med* 2004;199:347–356.

121. McDuffie JE, Coaxum SD, Maleque MA. 5-Hydroxytryptamine evokes endothelial nitric oxide synthase activation in bovine aortic endothelial cell cultures. *Proc Soc Exp Biol Med* 1999;221:386–390.

122. Radomski MW, Rees DD, Dutra A, et al. S-nitroso-glutathione inhibits platelet activation *in vitro* and *in vivo*. *Br J Pharmacol* 1992;107:745–749.

123. Wang GR, Zhu Y, Halushka PV, et al. Mechanism of platelet inhibition by nitric oxide: *in vivo* phosphorylation of thromboxane receptor by cyclic GMP-dependent protein kinase. *Proc Natl Acad Sci U S A* 1998;95: 4888–4893.

124. Davidge ST, Baker PN, Roberts JM. NOS expression is increased in endothelial cells exposed to plasma from women with preeclampsia. *Circ Res* 1995;77:274–283.

125. Tsikas D, Ikic M, Tewes KS, et al. Inhibition of platelet aggregation by S-nitroso-cysteine via cGMP-independent mechanisms: evidence of inhibition of thromboxane A2 synthesis in human blood platelets. *FEBS Lett* 1999;15:162–166.

126. Sogo N, Magid KS, Shaw CA, et al. Inhibition of human platelet aggregation by nitric oxide donor drugs: relative contribution of cGMP-independent mechanisms. *Biochem Biophys Res Commun* 2000;279:412–419.

127. Freedman JE, Sauter R, Battinelli EM, et al. Deficient platelet-derived nitric oxide and enhanced hemostasis in mice lacking the NOS3 gene. *Circ Res* 1999;84:1416–1421.

128. Freedman JE, Sauter R, Battinelli EM, et al. Deficient platelet-derived nitric oxide and enhanced hemostasis in mice lacking the NOSIII gene. *Circ Res* 1999;84:1416–1421.

129. Simon DI, Stamler JS. Effect of NOS inhibition on bleeding time in humans. *J Cardiovasc Pharmacol* 1995;26:339–342.

130. Sase K, Michel T. Expression of constitutive endothelial nitric oxide synthase in human blood platelets. *Life Sci* 1995;57:2049–2055.

131. de Frutos T, Sanchez de Miguel L, Farre J, et al. Expression of an endothelial-type nitric oxide synthase isoform in human neutrophils: modification by tumor necrosis factor-alpha and during myocardial infarction. *J Am Coll Cardiol* 2001;37:800–807.

132. Zhang R, Min W, Sessa WC. Functional analysis of the human endothelial nitric oxide synthase promoter. Sp1 and GATA factors are necessary for basal transcription in endothelial cells. *J Biol Chem* 1995;270:15320–15326.

133. Marsden PA, Heng HH, Scherer SW, et al. Control of cardiac muscle cell function by an endogenous nitric oxide signaling system. *Proc Natl Acad Sci U S A* 1993;90:347–351.

134. Tai SC, Robb GB, Marsden PA. Endothelial nitric oxide synthase: a new paradigm for gene regulation in the injured blood vessel. *Arterioscler Thromb Vasc Biol* 2004;24:405–412.

135. Loscalzo J, Welch G. Nitric oxide and its role in the cardiovascular system. *Prog Cardiovasc Dis* 1995;38:87–104.

136. Dekker RJ, van Soest S, Fontijn RD, et al. Prolonged fluid shear stress induces a distinct set of endothelial cell genes, most specifically lung Kruppel-like factor (KLF2). *Blood* 2002;100:1689–1698.

137. SenBanerjee S, Lin Z, Atkins GB, et al. Identification of KLF2 as a novel transcriptional regulator of endothelial proinflammatory activation. *J Exp Med* 2004;199:1305–1315.

138. Davis ME, Cai H, Drummond GR, et al. Shear stress regulates endothelial nitric oxide synthase expression through c-Src by divergent signaling pathways. *Circ Res* 2001;89(11):1073–1080.

139. Davis ME, Grumbach IM, Fukai T, et al. Shear stress regulates endothelial nitric-oxide synthase promoter activity through nuclear factor κB binding. *J Biol Chem* 2004;279:163–168.

140. Coulet F, Nadaud S, Agrapart M, et al. Identification of hypoxia-response element in the human endothelial nitric-oxide synthase gene promoter. *J Biol Chem* 2003;278:46230–46240.

141. Takemoto M, Sun J, Hiroki J, et al. Rho-kinase mediates hypoxia-induced downregulation of endothelial nitric oxide synthase. *Circulation* 2002; 106:57–62.

142. Anderson HD, Rahmutula D, Gardner DG. Tumor necrosis factor-alpha inhibits endothelial nitric-oxide synthase gene promoter activity in bovine aortic endothelial cells. *J Biol Chem* 2004;279:963–969.

143. Hernandez-Perera O, Perez-Sala D, Navarro-Antolin J, et al. Effects of the 3-hydroxy-3-methylglutaryl-CoA reductase inhibitors, atorvastatin and simvastatin, on the expression of endothelin-1 and endothelial nitric oxide synthase in vascular endothelial cells. *J Clin Invest* 1998;101:2711–2719.

144. Sumi D, Hayashi T, Thakur NK, et al. A HMG-CoA reductase inhibitor possesses a potent anti-atherosclerotic effect other than serum lipid lowering effects—the relevance of endothelial nitric oxide synthase and superoxide anion scavenging action. *Atherosclerosis* 2001;155:347–357.

145. Hernandez-Perera O, Perez-Sala D, Navarro-Antolin J, et al. Effects of the 3-hydroxy-3-methylglutaryl-CoA reductase inhibitors, atorvastatin and simvastatin, on the expression of endothelin-1 and endothelial nitric oxide synthase in vascular endothelial cells. *J Clin Invest* 1998;101:2711–2719.

146. Wagner AH, Schwabe O, Hecker M. Atorvastatin inhibition of cytokine-inducible nitric oxide synthase expression in native endothelial cells in situ. *Br J Pharmacol* 2002;136:143–149.

147. Laufs U, Liao JK. Post-transcriptional regulation of endothelial nitric oxide synthase mRNA stability by Rho GTPase. *J Biol Chem* 1998;273: 24266–24271.

148. Eto M, Barandier C, Rathgeb L, et al. Thrombin suppresses endothelial nitric oxide synthase and upregulates endothelin-converting enzyme-1 expression by distinct pathways: role of Rho/ROCK and mitogen-activated protein kinase. *Circ Res* 2001;89:583–590.

149. Ming XF, Viswambharan H, Barandier C, et al. Rho GTPase/Rho kinase negatively regulates endothelial nitric oxide synthase phosphorylation through the inhibition of protein kinase B/Akt in human endothelial cells. *Mol Cell Biol* 2002;22:8467–8477.

150. Brown DA, London E. Structure of detergent-resistant membrane domains: does phase separation occur in biological membranes? *Biochem Biophys Res Commun* 1997;240:1–7.

151. Gonzalez E, Kou R, Lin AJ, et al. Subcellular targeting and agonist-induced site-specific phosphorylation of endothelial nitric-oxide synthase. *J Biol Chem* 2002;277:39554–39560.

152. Yeh DC, Duncan JA, Yamashita S, et al. Depalmitoylation of endothelial nitric-oxide synthase by acyl-protein thioesterase 1 is potentiated by Ca$^{+2}$-calmodulin. *J Biol Chem* 1999;274:33148–33154.

153. Goetz RM, Thatte HS, Prabhakar P, et al. Estradiol induces the calcium-dependent translocation of endothelial nitric oxide synthase. *Proc Natl Acad Sci U S A* 1999;96:2788–2793.

154. Loscalzo J, Welch G. Nitric oxide and its role in the cardiovascular system. *Prog Cardiovasc Dis* 1995;38:87–104.

155. Michel JB, Feron O, Sase K, et al. Caveolin *versus* calmodulin. *J Biol Chem* 1997;272:25907–25912.

156. Yeh DC, Duncan JA, Yamashita S, et al. Depalmitoylation of endothelial nitric-oxide synthase by acyl-protein thioesterase 1 is potentiated by Ca$^{+2}$-calmodulin. *J Biol Chem* 1999;274:33148–33154.

157. Kou R, Greif D, Michel T. Dephosphorylation of endothelial nitric-oxide synthase by vascular endothelial growth factor. Implications for the vascular responses to cyclosporin A. *J Biol Chem* 2002;277:29669–29673.

158. Greif DM, Sacks DB, Michel T. Calmodulin phosphorylation and modulation of endothelial nitric oxide synthase catalysis. *Proc Natl Acad Sci U S A* 2004;101:1165–1170.

159. Boo YC, Hwang J, Sykes M, et al. Shear stress stimulates phosphorylation of eNOS at Ser(635) by a protein kinase A-dependent mechanism. *Am J Physiol Heart Circ Physiol* 2002;283:H1819–H1828.

160. Michell BJ, Harris MB, Chen ZP, et al. Identification of regulatory sites of phosphorylation of the bovine endothelial nitric-oxide synthase at serine 617 and serine 635. *J Biol Chem* 2002;277:42344–42351.

161. Fulton D, Gratton JP, McCabe TJ, et al. Regulation of endothelium-derived nitric oxide production by the protein kinase Akt. *Nature* 1999;399: 597–601.

162. Gonzalez E, Kou R, Lin AJ, et al. Subcellular targeting and agonist-induced site-specific phosphorylation of endothelial nitric-oxide synthase. *J Biol Chem* 2002;277:39554–39560.

163. Eto M, Barandier C, Rathgeb L, et al. Thrombin suppresses endothelial nitric oxide synthase and upregulates endothelin-converting enzyme-1 expression by distinct pathways: role of Rho/ROCK and mitogen-activated protein kinase. *Circ Res* 2001;89:583–590.

164. Garcia-Cardena G, Fan R, Shah V, et al. Dynamic activation of endothelial nitric oxide synthase by Hsp90. *Nature* 1998;392:821–824.

165. Vecchione E, Maffei A, Colella S, et al. Leptin effect on endothelial nitric oxide is mediated through Akt-endothelial nitric oxide synthase phosphorylation pathway. *Diabetes* 2002;51:168–173.

166. Chen H, Montagnani M, Funahashi T, et al. Adiponectin stimulates production of nitric oxide in vascular endothelial cells. *J Biol Chem* 2003; 278:450212–450216.

167. Dimmeler S, Fleming I, Fisslthaler B, et al. Activation of nitric oxide synthase in endothelial cells by Akt-dependent phosphorylation. *Nature* 1999; 399:601–605.

168. Kou R, Greif D, Michel T. Dephosphorylation of endothelial nitric-oxide synthase by vascular endothelial growth factor. Implications for the vascular responses to cyclosporin A. *J Biol Chem* 2002;277:29669–29673.

169. Kou R, Greif D, Michel T. Dephosphorylation of endothelial nitric-oxide synthase by vascular endothelial growth factor. Implications for the vascular responses to cyclosporin A. *J Biol Chem* 2002;277:29669–29673.

170. Simoncini T, Hafezi-Moghadam A, Brazil DP, et al. Interaction of oestrogen receptor with the regulatory subunit of phosphatidylinositol-3-OH-kinase. *Nature* 2000;407:538–541.

171. Kakui K, Itoh H, Sagawa N, et al. Augmented endothelial nitric oxide synthase (eNOS) protein expression in human pregnant myometrium: possible involvement of eNOS promoter activation by estrogen via both estrogen receptor (ER)α and ERβ. *Mol Hum Reprod* 2004;10:115–122.

172. Li H, Junk P, Huwiler A, et al. Dual effect of ceramide on human endothelial cells: induction of oxidative stress and transcriptional upregulation of endothelial nitric oxide synthase. *Circulation* 2002;106:2250–2266.

173. Igarashi J, Michel T. Agonist-modulated targeting of the EDG-1 receptor to plasmalemmal caveolae. *J Biol Chem* 2000;275:32363–32370.

174. Igarashi J, Michel T. Sphingosine-1-phosphate and isoform-specific activation of phosphoinositide 3-Kinase Beta. *J Biol Chem* 2000;276: 36281–36288.

175. Kou R, Igarashi J, Michel T. Lysophosphatidic acid and receptor-mediated activation of endothelial nitric-oxide synthase. *Biochemistry* 2002;41: 4982–4988.

176. Goetzl EJ, An S. Diversity of cellular receptors and functions for the lysophospholipid growth factors lysophosphatidic acid and sphingosine 1-phosphate. *FASEB J* 1998;12:1589–1598.

177. Igarashi J, Erwin PA, Dantas APV, et al. VEGF Induces S1P receptors in endothelial cells: implications for cross-talk between sphingolipid and growth factor receptors. *Proc Natl Acad Sci U S A* 2003;100:10664–10669.

178. Kou R, Greif D, Michel T. Dephosphorylation of endothelial nitric-oxide synthase by vascular endothelial growth factor. Implications for the vascular responses to cyclosporin A. *J Biol Chem* 2002;277:29669–29673.

179. Igarashi J, Thatte HS, Prabhakar P, et al. Calcium-independent activation of endothelial nitric-oxide synthase by ceramide. *Proc Natl Acad Sci U S A* 1999;96:12583–12588.

180. Igarashi J, Bernier SG, Michel T. Sphingosine-1-phosphate and activation of endothelial nitric-oxide synthase. *J Biol Chem* 2001;276:12420–12426.

181. Bernier SG, Haldar S, Michel T. Bradykinin-regulated interactions of the mitogen-activates protein kinase pathway with the endothelial nitric-oxide synthase. *J Biol Chem* 2000;276:30707–30715.

182. Harris MB, Ju H, Venema VJ, et al. Reciprocal phosphorylation and regulation of endothelial nitric-oxide synthase in response to bradykinin stimulation. *J Biol Chem* 2001;276:16587–16591.

183. Lin MI, Fulton D, Babbitt R, et al. Phosphorylation of threonine 497 in endothelial nitric-oxide synthase coordinates the coupling of L-arginine metabolism to efficient nitric oxide production. *J Biol Chem* 2003;278: 44719–44726.

184. Greif DM, Kou R, Michel T. Site-specific dephosphorylation of endothelial nitric oxide synthase by protein phosphatase 2A: evidence for crosstalk between phosphorylation sites. *Biochemistry* 2002;41:15845–15853.

185. Diefenbach A, Schindler H, Rollinghoff M, et al. Requirement for type 2 NO synthase for IL-12 signaling in innate immunity. *Science* 1999;284:951–955.

186. Nicholson S, Bonecini-Almeida Mda G, Lapa e Silva JR, et al. Inducible nitric oxide synthase in pulmonary alveolar macrophages from patients with tuberculosis. *J Exp Med* 1996;183:2293–2302.

187. Brightbill HD, Libraty DH, Krutzik SR, et al. Host defense mechanisms triggered by microbial lipoproteins through toll-like receptors. *Science* 1999;285:732–736.

188. Taylor BS, de Vera ME, Ganster RW, et al. Multiple NF-κB enhancer elements regulate cytokine induction of the human inducible nitric oxide synthase gene. *J Biol Chem* 1998;273:15148–15156.

189. Ganster RW, Taylor BS, Shao L, et al. Complex regulation of human inducible nitric oxide synthase gene transcription by Stat 1 and NF-κB. *Proc Natl Acad Sci U S A* 2001;98:8638–8643.

190. Ihrig M, Dangler CA, Fox JG. Mice lacking inducible nitric oxide synthase develop spontaneous hypercholesterolaemia and aortic atheromas. *Atherosclerosis* 2001;156:103–107.

191. Depre C, Havaux X, Renkin J, et al. Expression of inducible nitric oxide synthase in human coronary atherosclerotic plaque. *Cardiovasc Res* 1999;41:465–472.

192. Cromheeke KM, Kockx MM, De Meyer GR, et al. Inducible nitric oxide synthase colocalizes with signs of lipid oxidation/peroxidation in human atherosclerotic plaques. *Cardiovasc Res* 1999;15:744–754.

193. Knipp BS, Ailawadi G, Ford JW, et al. Increased MMP-9 expression and activity by aortic smooth muscle cells after nitric oxide synthase inhibition is associated with increased nuclear factor-κB and activator protein-1 activity. *J Surg Res* 2004;116:70–80.

194. Niu XL, Xia Y, Hoshiai K, et al. Inducible nitric oxide synthase knockout mouse macrophages disclose prooxidant effect of interferon-γ on low-density lipoprotein oxidation. *Nitric Oxide* 2000;4:363–371.

195. Chesebro BB, Blessing E, Kuo CC, et al. Nitric oxide synthase plays a role in Chlamydia pneumoniae-induced atherosclerosis. *Cardiovasc Res* 2003;60:170–174.

196. Kolyada AY, Fedtsov A, Madias NE. 3-Hydroxy-3-methylglutaryl coenzyme a reductase inhibitors upregulate inducible NO synthase expression and activity in vascular smooth muscle cells. *Hypertension* 2001;38:1024–1029.

197. Niu XL, Yang X, Hoshiai K, et al. Inducible nitric oxide synthase deficiency does not affect susceptibility of mice to atherosclerosis but increases collagen content in lesions. *Circulation* 2001;103:1115–1120.

198. Nathan CF. Nitric oxide as a secretory product of mammalian cells. *FASEB J* 1992;6:3051–3064.

199. Chauhan SD, Seggara G, Vo PA, et al. Protection against lipopolysaccharide-induced endothelial dysfunction in resistance and conduit vasculature of iNOS knockout mice. *FASEB J* 2003;17:773–775.

200. Hollenberg SM, Broussard M, Osman J, et al. Increased microvascular reactivity and improved mortality in septic mice lacking inducible nitric oxide synthase. *Circ Res* 2000;86:774–778.

201. Cobb JP, Hotchkiss RS, Swanson PE, et al. Inducible nitric oxide synthase (iNOS) gene deficiency increases the mortality of sepsis in mice. *Surgery* 1999;126:438–442.

202. Yallampalli C, Garfield RE. Inhibition of nitric oxide synthesis in rats during pregnancy produces signs similar to those of preeclampsia. *Am J Obstet Gynecol* 1993;169:1316–1320.

203. Buttery LD, McCarthy A, Springall DR, et al. Endothelial nitric oxide synthase in the human placenta: regional distribution and proposed regulatory role at the feto-maternal interface. *Placenta* 1994;15:257–265.

204. Napolitano M, Miceli F, Calce A, et al. Expression and relationship between endothelin-1 messenger ribonucleic acid (mRNA) and inducible/endothelial nitric oxide synthase mRNA isoforms from normal and preeclamptic placentas. *J Clin Endocrinol Metab* 2000;85:2318–2323.

205. Napolitano M, Miceli F, Calce A, et al. Expression and relationship between endothelin-1 messenger ribonucleic acid (mRNA) and inducible/endothelial nitric oxide synthase mRNA isoforms from normal and preeclamptic placentas. *J Clin Endocrinol Metab* 2000;85:2318–2323.

206. Noris M, Todeschini M, Cassis P, et al. L-arginine depletion in preeclampsia orients nitric oxide synthase toward oxidant species. *Hypertension* 2004;43:614–622.

207. Rutherford S, Johnson MP, Curtain RP, et al. Chromosome 17 and the inducible nitric oxide synthase gene in human essential hypertension. *Hum Genet* 2001;109:408–415.

208. Kharazia VN, Schmidt HH, Weinberg RJ. Type I nitric oxide synthase fully accounts for NADPH-diaphorase in rat striatum, but not cortex. *Neuroscience* 1994;62:983–987.

209. Burnett AL, Lowenstein CJ, Bredt DS, et al. Nitric oxide: a physiologic mediator of penile erection. *Science* 1992;257:401–403.

210. Raoul C, Estevez AG, Nishimune H, et al. Motoneuron death triggered by a specific pathway downstream of Fas. Potentiation by ALS-linked SOD1 mutations. *Neuron* 2002;35:1067–1083.

211. Deans Z, Dawson SJ, Xie J, et al. Differential regulation of the two neuronal nitric-oxide synthase gene promoters by the Oct-2 transcription factor. *J Biol Chem* 1996;271:32153–32158.

212. Lee MA, Cai L, Hubner N, et al. Tissue- and development-specific expression of multiple alternatively spliced transcripts of rat neuronal nitric oxide synthase. *J Clin Invest* 1997;100:1507–1512.

213. Xie J, Roddy P, Rife TK, et al. Two closely linked but separable promoters for human neuronal nitric oxide synthase gene transcription. *Proc Natl Acad Sci U S A* 1995;92:1242–1246.

214. Brenman JE, Chao DS, Xia H, et al. Nitric oxide synthase complexed with dystrophin and absent from skeletal muscle sarcolemma in Duchenne muscular dystrophy. *Cell* 1995;82:743–752.

215. Kobzik L, Reid MB, Bredt DS, et al. Nitric oxide in skeletal muscle. *Nature* 1994;372:546–548.

216. Ponting CP, Phillips C, Davies KE, et al. PDZ domains: targeting signalling molecules to sub-membranous sites. *Bioessays* 1997;19:469–479.

217. Sander M, Chavoshan B, Harris SA. Functional muscle ischemia in neuronal nitric oxide synthase-deficient skeletal muscle of children with Duchenne muscular dystrophy. *Proc Natl Acad Sci U S A* 2000;97:13818–13823.

218. Toda N, Okamura T. The pharmacology of nitric oxide in the peripheral nervous system of blood vessels. *Pharmacol Rev* 2003;55:271–324.

219. Toda N, Kimura T, Yoshida K, et al. Human uterine arterial relaxation induced by nitroxidergic nerve stimulation. *Am J Physiol* 1994;266:H1446–H1450.

220. White RP, Hindley C, Bloomfield PM, et al. The effect of the nitric oxide synthase inhibitor L-NMMA on basal CBF and vasoneuronal coupling in man: a PET study. *J Cereb Blood Flow Metab* 1999;19:673–678.

221. Toda N, Okamura T. Nitroxidergic nerve: regulation of vascular tone and blood flow in the brain. *J Hypertens* 1996;14:423–434.

222. Toda N, Okamura T. Nitroxidergic nerve: regulation of vascular tone and blood flow in the brain. *J Hypertens* 1996;14:423–434.

223. Toda N, Kimura T, Yoshida K, et al. Human uterine arterial relaxation induced by nitroxidergic nerve stimulation. *Am J Physiol* 1994;266:H1446–H1450.

224. Toda N, Okamura T. Nitroxidergic nerve: regulation of vascular tone and blood flow in the brain. *J Hypertens* 1966;14:423–434.

225. Toda N, Okamura T. The pharmacology of nitric oxide in the peripheral nervous system of blood vessels. *Pharmacol Rev* 2003;55:271–324.

226. Parker JD, Parker JO. Nitrate therapy for stable angina pectoris. *N Engl J Med* 1998;338:520–531.

227. Parker JD, Parker JO. Nitrate therapy for stable angina pectoris. *N Engl J Med* 1998;338:520–531.

228. Ohashi Y, Kawashima S, Hirata K, et al. Hypotension and reduced nitric oxide-elicited vasorelaxation in transgenic mice overexpressing endothelial nitric oxide synthase. *J Clin Invest* 1998;102:2061–2071.

229. Sydow K, Daiber A, Oelze M, et al. Central role of mitochondrial aldehyde dehydrogenase and reactive oxygen species in nitroglycerin tolerance and cross-tolerance. *J Clin Invest* 2004;113:482–489.

230. Sydow K, Daiber A, Oelze M, et al. Central role of mitochondrial aldehyde dehydrogenase and reactive oxygen species in nitroglycerin tolerance and cross-tolerance. *J Clin Invest* 2004;113:482–489.

231. Kaplan NM. Systemic hypertension: mechanisms and diagnosis. In: Braunwald E, ed. *Heart disease: a textbook of cardiovascular medicine*, 6th ed. St. Louis, MO: WB Saunders, 2001:988.

# CHAPTER 43 ■ VASCULAR ADAPTATIONS TO ALTERED BLOOD FLOW

MARC CHRETIEN, SABRENA F. NORIA, MOIRA JACKSON, AND B. LOWELL LANGILLE

The vascular system continuously remodels throughout development, first as primitive vessels form and reorganize, then as the circulation accommodates changing tissue perfusion requirements. This capacity of the blood vessels to restructure persists throughout life; it is expressed when the adult circulation adapts to many chronic changes in cardiovascular function, including those associated with exercise training, reproductive cycles, and pregnancy, and it is critical to the development of vascular pathologies, including hypertension, atherosclerosis, and restenosis.

The mechanical forces that are imposed on arterial tissue are important stimuli for vascular remodeling. Chronic changes in blood flow rates cause corresponding changes in arterial diameters, alterations in blood pressure affect wall thickness, and growth/hypertrophy of contiguous tissues stimulate longitudinal growth in the arterial tree. By these means, vascular structure continually adapts to changes in cardiovascular function. This remodeling is regulated by direct sensitivity of vascular tissues to fluid shear stress, in the case of flow; circumferential tensile stress, in the case of pressure; and lengthwise tensile stress when contiguous tissues grow. Tensile stress–related remodeling may be important sequelae to occlusive or partially occlusive thrombotic events; however, the primary effects of arterial occlusion relate to altered flow and shear stress. Therefore, this chapter focuses on arterial adaptations to perturbations in perfusion and the shear stresses that result from these perturbations. These adaptations are usually driven by the endothelium, which transduces the shear stress generated by blood flow; however, both endothelium and the underlying media exhibit remodeling in response to this mechanotransduction. How endothelial cells transduce shear stress, how these cells adapt to shear stress, and how the underlying media is restructured in response to shear are all important aspects of blood flow–induced arterial remodeling, and all are potential targets of future therapeutic interventions.

In recent years, many of the processes by which arteries remodel in response to altered blood flow rate have been defined. In addition, substantial success has been achieved in defining the multiple mechanisms by which vascular cells sense shear stress and in defining the effector pathways that are activated by shear, including gene transcription. Important areas in which current knowledge is weak include linking specific mechanotransducer mechanisms to the manifestations of arterial remodeling they elicit and defining the ways in which these outcomes are integrated to produce a coordinated reorganization of arterial wall constituents.

## TRANSDUCTION OF SHEAR STRESS BY ENDOTHELIUM

Shear stresses produced by flowing blood are imposed on the apical surface of endothelial cells; however, resulting cell deformation ensures that mechanical forces are transmitted to cell–cell junctions and, through the cytoskeleton, to intracellular sites, as well as to the basal cell membrane. Sensing of these forces may result from mechanical deformation of sensor molecules or structures, from mechanical disruption or induction of intermolecular (e.g., protein–protein) interactions, or from diffusion-limited interaction of endothelial releasates with their receptors on the cell surface. Shear stress can also cause substantial flow within the two-dimensional lipid bilayer of cell membranes (1), which could be important in bringing together or separating reactants at the cell surface. Current evidence indicates, not surprisingly, that shear stress is sensed through multiple mechanisms that drive multiple signal transduction pathways (see Fig. 43-1). We consider in the following text shear transduction pathways for which there is most evidence.

### Shear Sensors

#### Ion Channels

Two types of shear-sensitive endothelial ion currents have been described: a hyperpolarizing current that is principally carried by inward-rectifying $K^+$ channels (2,3) and a depolarizing current that is at least partly due to activation of outward-rectifying $Cl^-$ channels (4). Ion channels are important in the control of vasomotor tone, which is the first step in initiating flow-dependent arterial remodeling (5), and they likely regulate other aspects of endothelial cell biology. Blocking $K^+$ channels abrogates shear stress–induced expression of transforming growth factor (TGF)-$\beta_1$, an important regulator of cell proliferation, matrix synthesis, and tissue remodeling (6). Shear-sensitive channels also respond differentially to different shear regimens (7), a finding that may implicate them in localized vascular pathologies that localize to sites of unusual hemodynamics, notably atherosclerosis.

#### Caveolae

Caveolae are invaginations of the endothelial cell plasma membrane that constitute microdomains in which signaling molecules may be clustered to allow their interaction and subsequent signaling activity. Rizzo et al. report that endothelial cell nitric

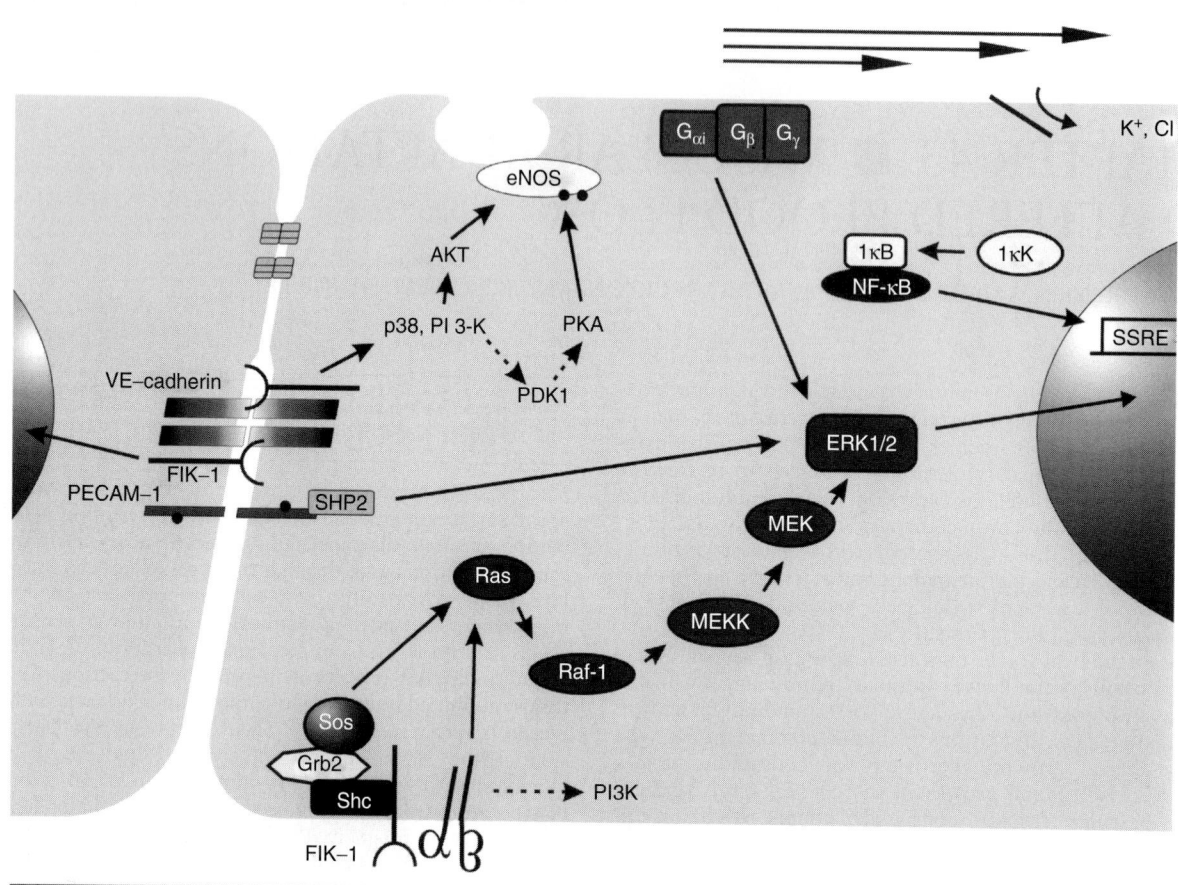

**FIGURE 43-1.** Multiple signaling pathways drive endothelial cell responses to shear stress. The sensitivity of the artery wall to changes in blood flow results from the collaboration of multiple signal transduction cascades that are initiated at cell membrane–associated structures, for example caveolae or G proteins, cell–cell junctional complexes such as platelet endothelial cell adhesion molecule-1 (PECAM-1) and vascular endothelial (VE)-cadherin, and integrin-mediated cell–matrix interactions. Also, signaling by growth factor receptors, for example VEGFR2 (Flk-1), is elicited by both VE-cadherin and integrins during responses to shear stress. See text for details.

oxide synthase (eNOS) is sequestered and inactivated in caveolae, by association with caveolin and that this association is disrupted by signaling related to shear stress (8). This is an important observation because nitric oxide (NO) production is largely responsible for flow-induced vasodilation in most arteries; furthermore, null mutation of the eNOS gene disrupts flow-induced arterial remodeling in adult mice (9).

There also is evidence that shear stress induces the rapid translocation of signaling molecules, such as c-Src and the adapter protein 14-3-3, to caveolae at the luminal surface of endothelial cells (10), and shear effects on caveolae ultimately may activate the mitogen activated protein (MAP) kinase pathway. Filipin, which induces disassembly of caveolae, abrogates ERK activation in response to flow (8). Several other signaling molecules that are involved in shear signaling are concentrated in caveolae, including protein kinase C (PKC) and G proteins. More recent evidence indicates that shear stress induces formation of caveolae and that conditioning to prolonged shear stress thereby modulates sensitivity of the mechanosensory responses (11,12).

## G Proteins

Activation of G protein–coupled receptors induces their interaction with heterotrimeric G proteins and the conversion of an inactive GDP-bound to an active GTP-bound $\alpha$ subunit and subsequent dissociation of the heterotrimer into a GTP-$\alpha$ subunit and a $\beta/\gamma$ dimer. These subunits activate second messengers and may modulate ion channels and focal adhesion/integrin-mediated signaling pathways. Roles in the flow-mediated regulation of endothelin 1, phospholipase C, and the phosphoinositol pathway have also been proposed (13). Shear-induced activation of ERK 1/2 and JNK can be abrogated by inhibitors of $G_{i2}$ and $G_{\beta/\gamma}$ subunits respectively (14). These findings implicate G proteins in shear-related signaling. However, a specific G protein–coupled receptor has not been implicated. Reports of shear-sensitive activity of G proteins that have been reconstituted in liposomes suggest receptor-independent activation (15).

## Integrin-Related Signaling

Focal adhesion plaques are areas of integrin clustering and linkage to the actin cytoskeleton. Multiple signaling molecules also associate with the cytoplasmic domains of integrins, and these respond to matrix–integrin interaction. As major mediators of mechanical attachment between cells and matrix, integrins and associated proteins are also strong candidates for sites of force transduction. In particular, shear forces imposed on the apical endothelial cell membrane may be concentrated at sites of integrin-mediated adhesion on the basal surface.

Matrix/integrin-mediated signal transduction involves recruitment of focal adhesion kinase (FAK), which can bind to the cytoplasmic domains of $\beta$ integrins. Autophosphorylation of FAK, and further subsequent phosphorylation by c-Src, allows FAK to interact, through Grb2, with the GDP/GTP exchange protein mSos and activate Ras and the MAP kinase cascade (see next section). Li et al. (16) reported shear-induced interaction of Fak/Grb2/Sos, and they found that dominant negative FAK and dominant negative Sos blocked shear-induced activation of the MAP kinases, ERK1/ERK2. These data implicate integrin signaling in an important shear transduction pathway. FAK signaling may converge with G protein signaling at the MAP kinase pathway because inhibitors of G protein signaling also greatly suppress shear-induced ERK1/ERK2 activity.

Members of the Rho family of small GTPases participate in shear stress–induced signaling. These molecular switches cycle between an active state (GTP-bound) and an inactive state (GDP-bound), and control cellular processes. Tzima et al. (17) have shown that $\alpha_v\beta3$ integrin changes from a low- to high-affinity state in the presence of shear stress, and this leads to new integrin-ECM connections, which are essential for Rho GTPase-induced signaling and for endothelial cell directional migration and alignment with shear stress. This group exploited a fluorescence resonance energy transfer–based probe to localize shear-activated Rac1 at the downstream poles of endothelium (18). Cortactin, a regulator of actin assembly, also localizes to this site (19), a finding that may reflect the role of Rac in shear-induced cytoskeletal (actin) remodeling (18). In total, a collaboration of Rac, Rho, and cdc42 activities induce massive actin reorganization in endothelial cells and polarization of the microtubule system (17,18,20,21). It appears that shear-dependent integrin signaling also links to activation of VEGFR2, a finding that is all the more intriguing because VEGFR2 is downstream of shear transduction at cell–cell junctions (see next section).

### Cell–Cell Junctions

Endothelial cell–cell adhesion sites also are important sites of mechanotransduction. Vascular endothelial (VE)-cadherin is an adhesive protein found at cell–cell junctions in endothelial cells. Shay-Salit et al. (22) have shown that VEGFR2 translocation to the nucleus, in response to shear stress or vascular endothelial growth factor (VEGF)-A, is VE-cadherin–dependent. Whereas nuclear translocation of VEGFR2 occurs hours after introduction of VEGF-A, it occurs within minutes in response to shear stress. Shear stress may promote collateral vessel development (arteriogenesis, see subsequent text) through this mechanism, but more acute physiologic roles are evident. Shear-induced p38 activation is abrogated in the absence of VE-cadherin, as is activation of the important downstream target of phosphatidylinositol 3-kinase (PI 3-K) signaling, AKT (protein kinase B). The collaboration of VEGFR2 and VE-cadherin in regulating AKT may impact directly on vasomotor control because others have shown that ligand-independent activation of VEGFR2 leads to phosphorylation/activation of eNOS and acute NO production, by AKT (23).

Platelet endothelial cell adhesion molecule-1 (PECAM-1) is also involved in transduction of shear stress. This transmembrane glycoprotein, with six extracellular Ig-like domains, is expressed by endothelial cells and localizes to cell–cell junctions, where it establishes homophilic binding with PECAM of neighboring cells. Shear stress–initiated recruitment of signaling proteins (SHP-2, and Gab1) to cell junctions in endothelial cells is PECAM-1–dependent (24). This study also established that direct application of force to PECAM-1 on the endothelial surface is required for the activation of the ERK signaling pathway. This finding underscores the importance of interactions between different shear-induced signaling pathways, including PECAM, G protein, and integrin signaling.

## Signal Transduction Pathways

### The Mitogen-Activated Protein Kinase Pathway

Mitogen-activated protein kinases (MAP kinases) are ubiquitously expressed serine/threonine kinases that are downstream activators of many signaling pathways, including pathways activated by shear stress. MAP kinases are important regulators of cell proliferation and differentiation, and they influence other important aspects of cell biology. Four principle cascades result in the dual phosphorylation and activation of extracellular signal related kinases 1 and 2 (ERK 1/2), jun-kinase (JNK), p38, and big MAP kinase 1 (BMK-1 or ERK-5). These activated proteins can act on cytoplasmic targets or translocate to the nucleus to activate transcription factors. Activation of ERK1/2 by shear stress is a rapid, transient response that reaches a maximum within 10 minutes of initiation of physiologic levels of shear and returns to basal levels by 15 minutes (16,25). Preconditioning endothelial cells to 12 dynes per cm$^2$ of shear for 24 hours followed by offloading shear also results in a transient ERK 1/2 activation 15 minutes after cessation of shear (our unpublished data). Therefore, MAP kinase signaling may not discriminate between increased and decreased shear stress.

As indicated previously, multiple pathways, including integrin, PECAM, and G protein signaling, can activate ERK. Inhibitor studies implicate PKC in driving MAP kinase activation, and antisense experiments point to a primary role for the isoform, PKC-$\varepsilon$, possibly through serine/threonine phosphorylation of Raf-1 (26).

Ras, upstream of Raf-1, is converted to its active GTP-bound state by interaction with the Grb2/mSos complex, and the shear-induced integrin signaling described earlier may drive this pathway. Ras also can be activated by G proteins, and it is also possible that Grb/Sos signaling originates from growth factor receptors that are activated by shear-induced ligand production or by ligand-independent shear sensitivity.

Activation of JNK in endothelial cells exposed to shear stress is slower than activation of ERK1/ERK2, with maximal activation occurring between 30 minutes and 4 hours (14). Interestingly, JNK is activated by very low shear stresses, but the level of activation does not depend on shear stress over a physiologic range. These findings suggest that JNK signaling is sensitive to stasis rather than to physiologic levels of shear; therefore, this signaling molecule may be particularly important in responses to thrombotic events.

BMK-1 has a similar activation motif to ERK 1/2 but is activated by MEK5 (27). In the presence of shear stress, BMK-1 has a delayed (onset at 10 minutes) yet sustained activation profile that peaks at 60 minutes (27). BMK-1 is part of a signal transduction pathway that is distinct from ERK. Unlike shear stress–induced activation of BMK-1, ERK 1/2 activation is c-Src–dependent. Furthermore, BMK-1 activation depends on increases in intracellular Ca$^{2+}$ concentrations, whereas ERK 1/2 activation does not. Shear-induced activation of different MAP kinases is likely to be important for control of gene expression (described subsequently).

### Phosphatidylinositol 3-Kinase

Signaling by PI 3-K regulates diverse cell activities. It is particularly important in endothelium in promoting cell survival. Because this pathway is activated by shear stress (28), low shear or stasis may be proapoptotic for endothelium. *In vivo*, low blood flow rates induce endothelial cell (and smooth muscle cell) apoptosis (29), but it is not clear whether this is a direct effect of shear or is secondary to shear-induced remodeling that produces a reduced vessel diameter.

PI 3-K phosphorylates membrane phospholipids to induce their association with protein kinase B (AKT), which is then activated by the serine and threonine phosphorylation by the kinases PDK-1 and PDK-2. AKT then may inhibit apoptosis by phosphorylating the proapoptotic protein Bad (30) or other substrates, for example, eNOS (see preceding text) or GSK-3$\beta$. PDK-1 is a constitutively active kinase; therefore, AKT regulation is thought to involve PDK-2. Autophosphorylation may occur after the PDK-1 site is phosphorylated (31); in addition, both integrin-linked kinase (ILK) (32) and a distinct membrane raft–associated kinase display PDK-2 activity (33). There are no published data concerning shear sensitivity of the activity of these kinases.

PI 3-K also appears to be important in other cell signaling pathways. Inhibition of PI 3-K–dependent signaling abrogates both ERK (our unpublished data) and JNK (34) activation in response to shear stress.

### Transcriptional Regulation

The nuclear factor activator protein 1 (AP-1) and the Rel-related nuclear factor kappa B (NF-$\kappa$B) are activated in cultured endothelial cells in response to shear stress. AP-1 factors comprise c-jun/c-jun homodimers or c-jun/c-fos heterodimers. Exposure of endothelial cells to arterial levels of shear stress results in a biphasic induction of AP-1 with DNA binding peaking after 10 to 20 minutes and 2 hours (35). Both c-fos and c-jun mRNA levels increase in human endothelial cells subjected to shear stress. AP-1 mediates shear-induced downregulation of endothelin and vascular cell adhesion module (VCAM)-1 transcription by shear stress (36), so this factor may promote vasoconstriction and leukocyte adhesion under low-flow conditions.

NF-$\kappa$B is particularly interesting given its prominent role in mediating (proatherogenic) inflammatory responses, whereas steady laminar shear is thought to be antiatherogenic. Cytoplasmic NF-$\kappa$B is kept inactive by association with I$\kappa$B, whereas steady laminar shear stress activates the kinases IKKa and IKKb, which then phosphorylate I$\kappa$B and target it for degradation. NF-$\kappa$B is then free to translocate to the nucleus and regulate gene transcription (37). NF-$\kappa$B regulates shear-dependent transcription of genes that are important for vessel remodeling [for example, platelet-derived growth factor (PDGF)-B chain, eNOS, and possibly TGF-$\beta$] and leukocyte-endothelial interaction [intercellular adhesion module (ICAM)-1, MCP-1] by binding a six base pair sequence (GAGACC) termed the shear stress responsive element (SSRE) (38–40). eNOS transcription is important because the antiinflammatory properties of nitric oxide may partly offset proinflammatory arms of the NF-$\kappa$B signaling pathway. In contrast to PDGF-B, PDGF-A transcription is regulated by shear stress by competition of egr1 with SP1 for overlapping sequences in its promoter region (41).

The role of NF-$\kappa$B in shear-dependent responses *in vivo* is further complicated by its differential sensitivity to temporal patterns of shear stress. Therefore, recent evidence associates NF-$\kappa$B expression with sites of atherosclerotic lesion formation, which occur near arterial bends and branches where shears are normally low but complex (42). The inference is that cells here are "primed" to respond to proatherosclerotic inflammatory stimuli even before the onset of disease.

# ENDOTHELIAL ADAPTATIONS TO SHEAR STRESS

Endothelial cells exhibit profound changes in gross cell morphology and in cytoskeletal organization in response to shear stress. These changes include adaptations that minimize variations in shear stress imposed on the cells or that enhance the capacity of endothelium to maintain integrity of the monolayer despite large mechanical loads. They also may change the sensitivity of the cells to mechanical signals. Finally, reorganization of cell structure/ultrastructure may affect the physiology of the cells either transiently, while cell morphologic changes are underway, or permanently.

## Endothelial Cell Shape

Many *in vivo* and *in vitro* studies have demonstrated that changes in shear stress cause endothelial cells to change their shape and orientation. Under low shear stress *in vivo*, or in static tissue culture, endothelial cells assume a cuboidal shape within a contact-inhibited monolayer, whereas cells elongate and their major axes align in the direction of flow under moderate to high shear conditions. Studies using atomic force microscopy (43) have also revealed major changes in the surface topography of endothelial cells exposed to shear stress. Undulations of the cell surface are reduced substantially in shear-aligned cells *in vitro*, when compared to static cultures. Endothelial cells therefore present a flatter, more streamlined surface to flow, and shear gradients on the cell surface are reduced by greater than 50%.

## Endothelial Cytoskeleton

The cell cytoskeleton consists of microfilaments, microtubules, and intermediate filaments. Collectively, the endothelial cell cytoskeleton functions in maintaining cell-shape, cell-adhesion, cell-migration, and in controlling permeability across the monolayer. There is evidence that all three components of the cytoskeleton are sensitive to shear stress.

### Actin Microfilaments

When endothelial cells form a confluent, contact-inhibited monolayer in static cultures, or when they line areas of low-to-moderate shear stress *in vivo* (44), F-actin is distributed predominantly around the periphery of the cells, in a circumferential dense peripheral band (DPB), as well as in short central microfilament bundles (see Fig. 43-2) (45,46). This morphology is thought to be important in cell–cell adhesion and in maintenance of the permeability barrier (47). Cell–cell adhesion is promoted primarily through actin association with proteins of the adherens junctions. At these junctions, homophilic binding occurs between transmembrane proteins, the cadherins (primarily VE-cadherin/cadherin-5 in endothelium), and the cytoplasmic domains of cadherins are linked to the cytoskeleton by additional proteins, termed catenins.

Permeability is controlled largely by tight junctions, which follow a similar, but less well-characterized pattern. Occludin is a transmembrane protein that undergoes homophilic binding at tight junctions, although a second transmembrane group of proteins, the claudins, may be more critical to permeability control, and claudin-5 has been implicated in the formation of endothelial tight junctions (48). Actin probably participates in

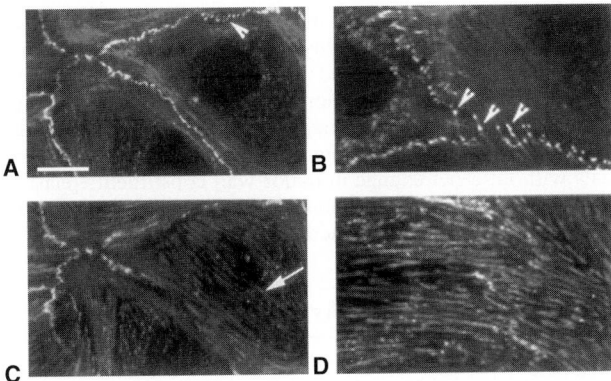

**FIGURE 43-2.** Endothelial microfilaments and adherens junctions reorganize during responses to shear stress. The adherens junctions (*arrowheads*) convert from continuous (**A**) to highly punctate (**B**) junctions during adaptation to shear stress (**B**). This junctional reorganization may underlie the elevation in endothelial monolayer permeability that occurs during responses to shear stress. At steady state, i.e., after 96 hours, junctions return to a linear morphology (not shown). Actin microfilaments concentrate at cell–cell junctions in static cultures (**A,C**) but much of this junctional localization is lost during responses to shear stress (**B**); instead, basal stress fibers become more prominent (**D** vs. **C**). Recent work has shown that assembly and reorientation of stress fibers drives endothelial cell elongation in the direction of shear stress (52). (Reprinted with permission from Noria S, Cowan DB, Gotlieb AI, Langille BL. Transient and steady state effects of shear stress on endothelial cell adherens junctions. *Circ Res* 1999;85:504–514.)

permeability control by influencing tight junction assembly, but there is also a direct role for actin/myosin-mediated contraction in control of the permeability barrier (49).

Tight junctions and adherens junctions do not function independently because assembly of adherens junctions appears to be a prerequisite for assembly of tight junctions, and disruption of the former compromises permeability control (50). Adherens junctions are partially disassembled as cells undergo shear-induced shape change (Fig. 43-2) (51,52). Consequently, thrombotic occlusive events that suppress or eliminate shear stress may have substantial effects on endothelial permeability control or other aspects of their physiology that are influenced by adherens junctions and the associated actin cytoskeleton.

In areas of spontaneously high shear stress, F-actin is not localized to cell junctional complexes; instead, it forms long, thick stress fibers that are aligned in the direction of flow (Fig. 43-2) (53). This pattern is seen at sights of spontaneously high shear stress *in vivo*; however, it can also be induced if shear stress is elevated by surgical manipulations, for example, coarctation (46,54). The large stress fibers that form when shear is high are important in cell-substratum adhesion and in migration during wound repair (47). Since stress fibers insert into focal adhesion plaques, it is also likely that F-actin redistribution influences shear-related signaling from these structures.

Shear-induced formation, growth, and realignment of stress fibers has another important function. It drives elongation of endothelial cells in the direction of shear stress (52). It is well established that actin assembly initiates many other modes of cell-shape change, but usually this is through formation of filopodia and lamellipodia (55). Shear responses of endothelium are the only known case where formation of stress fibers drives shape change.

## Microtubules

Microtubules are dynamic networks of tubulin filaments that emanate from perinuclear structures, the microtubule organizing center (MTOC), by polymerization of tubulin from a fast growing end (plus end), which is directed away from the MTOC, and a slow-growing (minus) end. In endothelial cells, as in many cell types, the MTOC and associated microtubules orient toward the direction of cell migration, for example, during repair of wounds to the endothelial monolayer (56). This polarity positions the microtubule system to deliver cargoes, for example, cell membrane, signaling molecules, and activators of signaling pathways, by microtubule-based motors to the leading edge of the cell, or to simply position microtubule-bound proteins at these sites. Cultured endothelial cells that are exposed to shear stress polarize with the centrosome downstream of the nucleus, a process that is controlled by the Rho GTPase, cdc42 (20). These findings cannot be directly extrapolated to *in vivo* conditions, for which the MTOC of both arterial and venous endothelium orient toward the heart-lung unit (57). Clearly, some *in situ* influence overrides the effects of shear stress. One hypothesis is that endothelial cells *in vivo* are engaged in continuous centripetal migration toward the heart (58), perhaps in response to trauma and cell turnover associated with contractile activity.

*In vivo*, endothelial cells that are undergoing migratory repair align at an angle that is intermediate between the direction of blood flow and the direction of repair. Thereby, influences of shear stress on cell morphology affect repair processes. In addition, when blood flow rate is suppressed, endothelial cells lose their well-defined orientation and appear to migrate into the wound as individual cells rather than as a monolayer (59). The reasons for the latter behavior are not understood.

## Intermediate Filaments

Intermediate filaments form a network that is distributed throughout the cytoplasm by microtubule-based motors and can ultimately link to adherens junctions through plakoglobin or the p120 catenin, p0071 [for review see (60)]. The intermediate filament system is deformed by shear stress (61), and it may provide structural stability for the endothelium to withstand these mechanical forces. Notably, *in vivo* studies demonstrated that there is a two- to threefold higher amount of vimentin in endothelial cells of arteries than in veins (62). This finding suggests that fluid shear stress may be involved in vimentin expression, and larger shear forces induce more vimentin expression (62).

Intermediate filaments also appear to be involved in shear-induced responses of endothelium. Accordingly, null mutation of the vimentin gene causes significant attenuation of flow-induced arterial dilation in resistance arteries (63). Flow-induced arterial dilation is mediated primarily by production of nitric oxide; therefore, the vimentin network must be involved in eliciting NO production in response to shear stress. Since chronically remodeling in response to altered shear stress is disrupted in mice with an eNOS null mutation, it will be of interest to see if the same is true in the vimentin knockout animals.

# Medial Remodeling

Increases and decreases in arterial blood flow rates (64,65) result in increases or decreases of vessel diameters, respectively, and thereby return shear stress toward normal levels (see Fig. 43-3). Chronic flow-induced remodeling, like acute vasomotor responses to altered flow, are endothelium-dependent

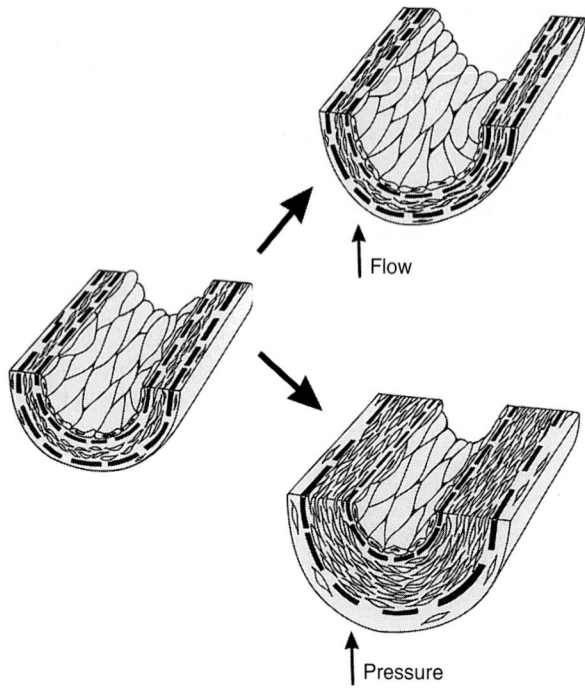

**Flow**

**Pressure**

**FIGURE 43-3.** Schematic illustration of arterial remodeling induced by chronic changes in mechanical loads. Chronically elevated arterial blood flow rate results in remodeling that increases arterial diameter, whereas elevated arterial pressure induces arterial wall thickening. Recent findings indicate that arteries also remodel in response to altered longitudinal forces, for example when contiguous tissue hypertrophy (see text). Therefore, arterial cells sense and respond independently to at least three forces imposed on them.

(65) and involve vasoregulation (66–68) followed by medial remodeling that alters the resting diameter of the artery (64,69). In most large arteries, the acute vasomotor responses that accompany altered flow are mediated by endothelium-derived NO production. As stated earlier, current evidence indicates that this early, NO-dependent vasoregulation is also critical for the long-term remodeling in response to altered flow. Rudic et al. (9) found that the capacity of arteries to remodel to a smaller diameter in response to reduced blood flow rate was lost in mice with null mutation of the eNOS gene; instead, these mice displayed a paradoxical wall thickening. It is unlikely, however, that all flow-induced remodeling depends on eNOS because this remodeling much influences normal arterial growth and development (70) and eNOS$^{-/-}$ mice do not show a striking developmental phenotype. Perhaps other mediators are important prior to maturity.

Vasomotor responses to altered flow rates are initiated very quickly and are amplified over a period of days or weeks (69,70). The mechanism for this amplification is unknown. If shear stress is sensed at focal adhesion sites, then formation of new, larger stress fibers and associated focal adhesions could enhance shear sensitivity when shear elevation is sustained. Alternatively, increased gap junction formation can enhance vasomotor responses (71). We have observed that shear stress upregulates connexin 43 expression, a major gap junctional protein in endothelial cells (72).

Arterial narrowing in response to decreased flow goes to completion rapidly, within 2 weeks in rabbit carotid arteries (69), whereas it may take months for diameters to stabilize after flow increases (64). The slower response to increased flow probably occurs because early vasodilator responses to increased flow are limited by the modest tone exhibited by most large arteries. Therefore, structural remodeling is required to

permit substantial diameter increases. In contrast, vasoconstriction in response to decreased blood flow rate usually reduces luminal diameter, and then structural modifications simply entrench these reductions and reset the working range of arterial diameter. Accordingly, remodeling responses to decreased blood flow rates can go to completion in mature animals without a net change in major wall constituents [elastin, total collagen, or DNA (cell number)], whereas responses to increased blood flow involve increased wall mass (73,74).

## Blood Flow and Arterial Development

In addition to simple growth, developing blood vessels undergo massive remodeling. After *de novo* formation of blood vessels (vasculogenesis) and budding of new vessels from preexisting vessels (angiogenesis), early restructuring includes radical reorganization. After the arterial system has taken on its final geometry, remodeling that shapes arterial growth involves a complex interplay of cell proliferation, cell death, cell migration, matrix synthesis, and matrix degradation. Many of these remodeling processes are reinitiated in vascular disease in adults.

Thoma (75) first proposed that changes in blood flow control the earliest development of the circulation after observing that those channels that carry the greatest flows within the developing area vasculosa of the chicken embryo enlarge to become conduit vessels, whereas those that carry modest flows frequently regress. Clark (76) speculated that the "blood flow over the endothelium" may be the stimulus for growth modulation. Much later experiments demonstrated that selective persistence or regression of embryonic arches could be modified by experimental interventions that alter central blood flow distribution through these vessels (77,78), although other factors contribute to selective survival among these vessels (44).

Sensitivity of arterial development to blood flow is not restricted to embryonic life; it is observed at all stages of development. The perinatal period is particularly instructive in this regard, because very large and abrupt developmental changes in blood flow rates occur at parturition (79). For example, there is a more than 90% decrease in blood flow in the subrenal abdominal aorta, subsequent to loss of placental perfusion, that is accompanied by a marked reduction in diameter of the vessel and a near arrest of wall tissue accumulation that lasts for weeks (80). Other arteries also display growth modulation that correlates with blood flow in this period. In particular, elastin accumulation in early postpartum life correlates with blood flow changes at birth (81). The sensitivity of elastin to changes in blood flow rate is not surprising. Elastin bears much of the tensile load at resting blood pressures. It is a primary determinant of normal vessel dimensions and, consequently, considerable remodeling of elastin is necessary to change vessel geometry.

During postnatal growth and development, experimental changes in blood flow modulate growth of vessel diameter. Unlike the remodeling of adult arteries, both increases and decreases in blood flow influence wall tissue contents. In particular, both smooth muscle and elastin accumulation are affected when flows are manipulated in the subnormal range. When 70% reductions in common carotid blood flows were induced in weanling rabbits by ligating the external carotid, DNA and elastin contents were substantially below those of control vessels 1 month later (69). However, smooth muscle content becomes relatively insensitive to flows that are above normal levels, whereas elastin accumulation continues to be affected. Twofold increases in carotid blood flows caused by contralateral common carotid ligation, again in young rabbits, resulted in a 50% elevation in elastin accumulation, whereas changes in cell number were insignificant (82).

## Pathologic Arterial Remodeling

The clinical consequences of arterial disease are most often due to compromised blood flow. Subsequent flow-induced diameter adjustments of arteries may significantly affect the progression of these diseases, as well as the efficacy of therapeutic interventions. The nature of these adaptations in a pathologic setting remain uncertain. Atherogenesis is affected by flow-induced vascular remodeling, and these effects may occur at several levels (see Fig. 43-4). Initially, atherosclerotic lesions narrow the vessel lumen, and the resulting acceleration of blood flow through the lesion site elevates shear stress. Glagov et al. (83) demonstrated "compensatory enlargement" in which the media subsequently expands to restore lumen diameter, presumably as a response to the increased shear associated with these accelerated flows. Therefore, flow-induced adaptations appear to limit encroachment on the vessel lumen early in lesion development. Nevertheless, growth of the lesion ultimately compromises blood flow, and adjacent, healthy segments of the vessel wall experience reduced shear. If these segments respond

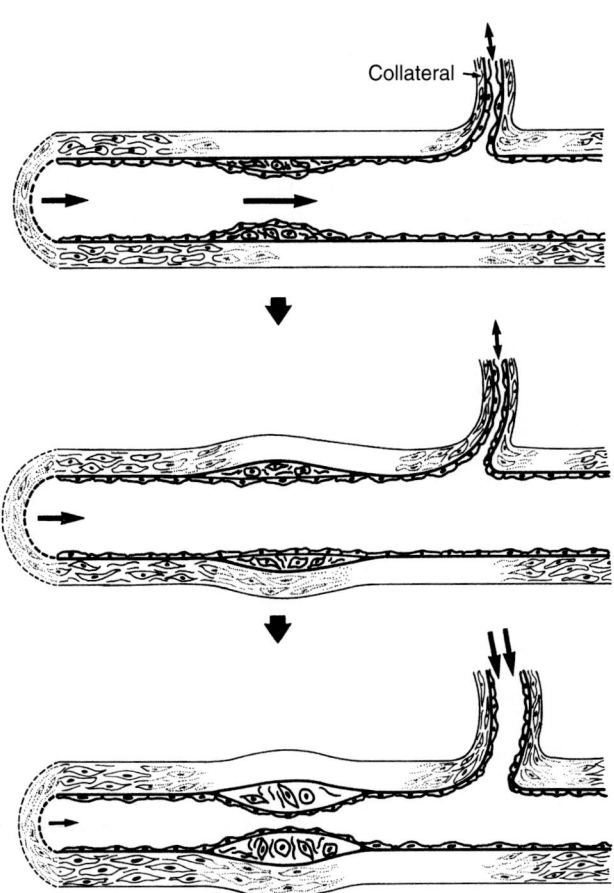

**FIGURE 43-4.** Early development of an atherosclerotic lesion (**Top**) leads to "compensatory enlargement" of vessel diameter (**Middle**), probably due to the acceleration of flow through the lesion site. Late in lesion development, compensation fails, the lumen is narrowed at the lesion site, and flow is compromised. Healthy artery upstream and downstream of the lesion then narrows in response to reduced flow (**Bottom**). Narrowing also establishes a pressure gradient across the lesion site, and reduced pressure downstream can enhance flow through collateral vessels (*double arrow*). Resulting increases in shear stress in these vessels can contribute to their enlargement. (Reprinted with permission from Langille BL, Gotlieb AI, Kim DW, et al. eds. *Vascular dynamics.* New York: Plenum Publishing, 1989:229–235.)

normally, then they remodel to a smaller diameter, a response that would exacerbate hypoperfusion. Consequently, "adaptive" remodeling may be advantageous during early atherogenesis but disadvantageous in later stages.

Normal, flow-induced remodeling can also affect the development of collateral supply in obstructive arterial disease. In the absence of arterial disease, collateral vessels carry little flow because there is little pressure gradient between the arteries they link; however, obstruction of one of these arteries upstream of the collateral vessel will depressurize that end of the collateral and initiate or enhance flow through it, thereby stimulating collateral growth (84,85). It is also noteworthy, but little studied, that bypass graft implantation should compromise flow through collaterals and through any residual lumen in the bypassed vessel segment by delivering central arterial pressure downstream of the obstruction. If collaterals and the obstructed vessel segment narrow in response to this flow reduction, then tissues perfused by the vessel may become more vulnerable if occlusion of the graft occurs.

These considerations implicitly assume that arteries will respond normally to changes in shear stress in the setting of vascular disease; however, quite novel responses can sometimes occur. Some well-controlled experiments have demonstrated the influence of changes in shear stress on intimal proliferative responses. Intimal proliferation after balloon injury of rat carotid arteries is greater under low-flow conditions than when flow rates are high (86). In addition, high blood flow rates inhibit intimal proliferation in endothelialized PTFE grafts in baboons (87,88). PDGF may contribute to these responses because both PDGF (B chain) and its receptor (β type) are upregulated by injury (89), and Kraiss et al. (90) have reported upregulated expression of PDGF when flow through prosthetic grafts is reduced in a baboon model. PDGF-A expression under low flow in the latter study was localized to endothelium (and subjacent smooth muscle) of the baboon grafts, a surprising finding given that PDGF-A expression is upregulated by *increased* shear stress in cultured endothelium (91). The role of PDGF in intimal proliferation is not completely understood, but it appears to be an important stimulus of migration of smooth muscle from the media to the intima (92). Furthermore, recent data indicates that blockade of both receptor subtypes causes atrophy of neointima; therefore, PDGF-mediated regulation of proliferation and survival may be an important therapeutic target (93).

## Mechanisms of Arterial Remodeling

The studies described in the preceding sections characterize arterial remodeling that adapts resting arterial diameters to changes in blood flow rates. This remodeling proceeds independently of other structural responses of large arteries, for example, the wall thickening that adapts these vessels to increased arterial pressure. The capacity to change vessel dimensions in a stimulus-specific manner raises intriguing questions concerning how the smooth muscle cells that populate the media achieve these changes. How do these cells selectively deposit new tissues (e.g., elastin, collagen, daughter cells after cell division) in the circumferential direction to increase diameter when flow increases, whereas these same cells deposit new tissues in the radial direction to thicken the media when pressure increases? If tissue is elaborated in the longitudinal direction, how is lengthening of the vessel prevented? In recent years, substantial progress has been made in defining the processes involved in remodeling in response to particular hemodynamic stimuli. It now appears that cell proliferation, cell death, matrix synthesis, and matrix degradation all contribute to this remodeling, and these processes are overviewed in the following section. Much of the discussion focuses on developing arteries because remodeling processes are most in evidence in these vessels, which are rapidly synthesizing new tissues; however, remodeling of mature vessels and developing arteries also are considered.

## Longitudinal Tension and Arterial Remodeling

One of the intriguing questions, raised in the preceding text, concerns how adaptive growth of arterial diameter or wall thickness can proceed without lengthening the vessel. It is counterintuitive that smooth muscle cells stimulated to produce new tissues, whether matrix or daughter cells, could do so without elaborating at least some of these tissues in the longitudinal direction. One possible resolution relates to the substantial longitudinal stretch that is imposed on most arteries (94). A consequence of lengthwise stretch is that longitudinal growth at one point along the vessel does not imply a longer vessel; it simply allows some retraction of stretched tissues at other longitudinal positions. Furthermore, this lengthwise retraction will result in thickening and/or increased circumference of the vessel; therefore, longitudinal elaboration of tissues is automatically translated into radial or circumferential growth. These effects of longitudinal stretch on remodeling are described in more detail elsewhere (44).

Recent evidence indicates arterial remodeling provides negative feedback regulation of lengthwise tension, just as shear and circumferential tension are regulated. Accordingly, surgical elevation of lengthwise tension was normalized within days through potent growth and remodeling responses (95). Therefore, cells in arteries sense and independently control three mechanical loads that are imposed on them.

## Flow-Related Remodeling of Extracellular Matrix

Collagen synthesis and accumulation contributes greatly to developmental remodeling of arteries in prenatal and postnatal life; however, it is surprisingly insensitive to changes in blood flow rate, at least after birth. We found that 70% reductions in blood flow rate had no effect on total collagen accumulation in immature rabbit carotid arteries even after 1 month, when substantial net effects on wall structure were detected. Similarly, doubling of flow rates in these arteries for even 12 weeks (3 to 15 weeks of age) had no considerable affect on total collagen contents. It remains possible that flow modulation has a large affect on the relative amounts of different types of collagen found in arteries without affecting total collagen content.

In contrast to collagen, elastin accumulation in developing arteries is highly sensitive to increases or decreases in blood flow rate. Sensitivity of elastin synthesis in large arteries to hemodynamic stresses is not surprising. Remodeling in response to these stresses changes the basic geometry of the vessel wall, and this geometry is sensitive to elastin content and organization because elastin bears much of resting wall tension. Consequently, remodeling of elastin probably is a prerequisite for producing large changes in resting arterial dimensions. Conversely, remodeling of elastin will impose dimensional changes on the other constituents of the vessel wall. However, the local mechanisms that translate mechanical forces into the regulation of elastin production are poorly understood. The elastin gene has been well characterized; it is a single copy gene of about 45 kb containing 35 (human) or 36 (bovine and rat) exons that are subject to alternative splicing. The promoter region contains multiple SP-1 and AP2 binding sites as well as putative glucocorticoid, cyclic adenosine monophosphate (cAMP), and TPA responsive elements. Expression is modulated by cortisol (96), insulinlike growth factor-1(IGF-1) (97,98) and transforming growth factor-$\beta$ (TGF-$\beta$) (99,100). Of these, TGF-$\beta$ is potentially important in flow-induced remodeling because its expression by endothelium is known to be shear-sensitive (6).

Precisely how elastin is reorganized during remodeling of large arteries is intriguing because this protein is laid down essentially in complete cylindrical shells within the vessel wall. Work by Davis (101) indicates that newly synthesized elastin accretes onto the inner and outer surfaces of lamellae, with preferential deposition occurring near the fenestrae that frequently perforate the lamellae. Such accretion could account for lamellar thickening during normal development or when blood pressure becomes chronically elevated, but does not explain how selective changes in lamellar circumference, as when flow is chronically altered, is achieved. However, important insights have been gained through recent application of laser scanning confocal microscopy to examine whole-mount arterial preparations that were perfusion-fixed at physiologic distension to preserve *in situ* morphology. The autofluorescence of elastin allowed direct examination of lamellar structure at various stages in the remodeling process. The first applications of this approach demonstrated that alterations to the fenestrae that perforate lamellae (102) are important in the remodeling of these structures. Lamellae increase several-fold both in size and number during postnatal growth, such that the space occupied by the fenestrae increases almost 20-fold between 3 weeks of age and adulthood (103). Enlargement of fenestrae occurs despite rapid accumulation of new elastin and despite evidence that newly synthesized elastin is deposited preferentially at fenestrae (101). Most notably, experimental increases and decreases in blood flow rate substantially influence the size of fenestrae in lamellae of developing arteries (see Fig. 43-5).

It is clear from these findings that changes to fenestrae contribute substantially to remodeling of elastic lamellae. The picture that emerges is of lamellar thickening proceeding through deposition of new elastin onto the inner and outer surfaces of lamellae and lamellar circumference (and length), increasing through formation of fenestrae. But how is the size of fenestrae altered? Elastolytic enzymes are obvious candidates. Expression of matrix metalloproteinase-2 (MMP-2) and MMP-9 are sensitive to mechanical forces and the latter has elastolytic activity.

There is no evidence pertaining to flow-induced changes in other matrix constituents, notably proteoglycans or glycoproteins, some of which may be particularly important in regulating smooth muscle and endothelial cell functions as remodeling proceeds (105).

## Cell Proliferation and Cell Death in Arterial Remodeling

Physiologic and developmental remodeling of tissues generally is achieved by resident cell types; therefore, control of intrinsic cell populations is vital to appropriate remodeling responses. Recent data indicate that alterations in blood flow rate modulate both cell proliferation and cell death (apoptosis), at least in developing arteries (29), and this is true for both endothelial and smooth muscle cells. Control over both processes is significant. A 70% decrease in blood flow rate suppresses cell proliferation and enhances apoptosis to the point where the cell populations are transiently decreased.

The role of smooth muscle cell death, and specifically apoptosis, in flow-induced remodeling of mature arteries is less well established given that DNA contents are not altered after flow reduction. However, a stronger case can be made for endothelial cell apoptosis. Endothelial cell apoptosis occurs after maturation in vessels of the regressing corpus luteum (106). Furthermore, endothelial cells are deleted from the walls of mature arteries adapting to flow reduction (69). Through this mechanism, substantial reductions in vessel diameter and luminal surface area are achieved without a net change in endothelial cell density.

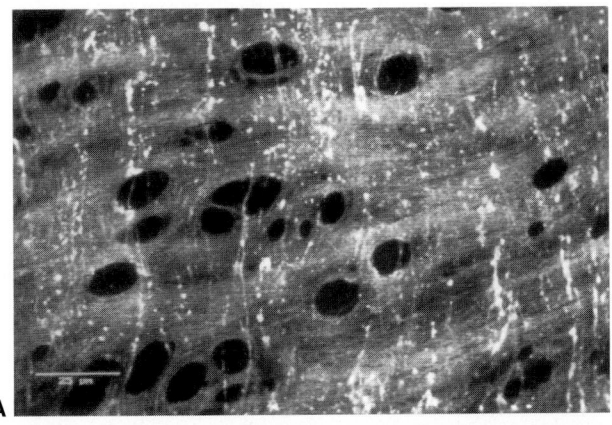
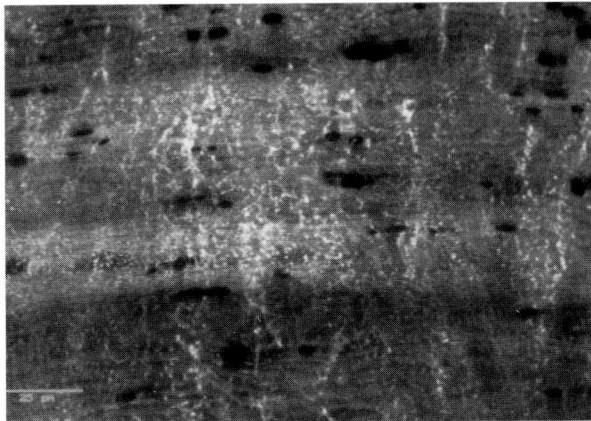
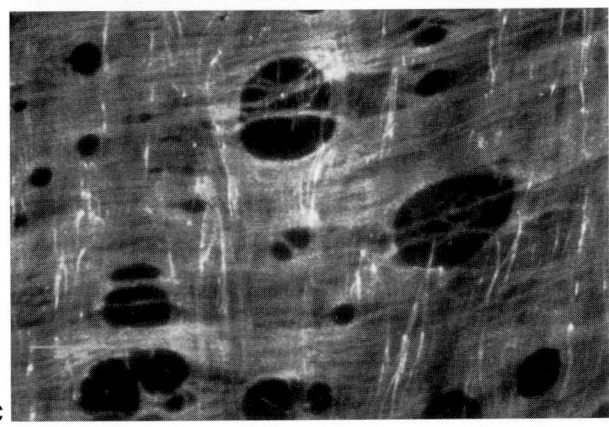

FIGURE 43-5. Internal elastic laminae of the carotid arteries of 15-week-old rabbits, viewed in whole-mount preparations by laser scanning confocal microscopy. Arteries are from (**A**) control animals and (**B**) animals in which flow was decreased by 70%, or (**C**) doubled for the preceding 5 weeks. Markers are 25 mm.

## Growth of Collateral Vessels (Arteriogenesis)

Fluid shear stress plays an integral part in the growth of collateral vessels after arterial occlusion, a process that has been renamed arteriogenesis and that causes arterioles to remodel into conductance vessels. The concept that the process is driven by shear stress is not new (Fig. 43-4) (84,85), and shear-induced remodeling has been studied extensively in large and small vessels. Furthermore, examination of collateral growth per se indicates that high shear stress increases the number and size of collateral vessels (107,108). However, intriguing recent data indicate that a variety of cell types participate in collateral vessel growth. Shear stress–activated endothelium upregulates monocyte chemoattractant MCP-1 expression and other adhesion molecules that contribute to adhesion and recruitment of monocytes (107). Most importantly, shear stress upregulates ICAM-1 expression *in vivo* (see Fig. 43-6) (109) and *in vitro* (110), and recent evidence indicates that this endothelial adhesion molecule is critical in recruiting monocytes to collateral vessels (111). Additionally, the effects of some growth factors (VEGF-A and placental growth factor) on collateral growth appear to be mediated through their effects on monocytes (107). Mast cells and T-lymphocytes aggregate in growing collateral vessels and may participate in arteriogenesis (112).

## Relation to Pressure-Induced Remodeling

The enlargement or reduction of vessel diameter when blood flow rates are chronically altered contrasts with the relative wall thickening that accompanies persistent increases in blood pressure. The adaptive significance of these two modes of remodeling is obvious, but it remains unclear how medial smooth muscle cells selectively deliver new tissue (daughter cells and matrix) in different directions under different mechanical stimuli. Part of the answer is likely related to early vasoregulatory changes that precede changes in structure. Increased/decreased flow rates induce early vasodilation/vasoconstriction, respectively; therefore, structural remodeling may simply entrench these changes, at least when flow alterations are modest. In contrast, increased luminal pressure tends to produce no vasomotor response in large arteries and myogenic constriction in resistance vessels. The latter response increases wall thickness to lumen ratio, thereby normalizing tensile loads; structural changes, therefore, may again only entrench this alteration to achieve the eutrophic (constant tissue volume) inward remodeling often seen in small arteries in hypertension. Recent investigations have elucidated two novel mechanisms that may underlie "entrenchment." Accordingly, Martinez-Lemus et al. showed that smooth muscle cells in resistance arteries with elevated tone can undergo elongation to restore cell length, whereas vessel diameter remains unchanged (113). Alternatively, early regulation of tissue transglutaminases appear to participate in entrenching vasoconstriction (114). Tissue transglutaminase probably functions in this context, at least partly, by cross-linking matrix elements; however, the enzyme is multifunctional, and other mechanisms may contribute (115).

When changes in pressure and flow are large, additional mechanisms take adjustments of vessel dimensions beyond those achievable by vasoregulation. We discussed earlier a mechanism by which selective accumulation/remodeling of elastin can contribute to pressure- versus flow-specific remodeling, and similar mechanisms may contribute to reorganization of other matrix elements. Much less is known about selective reorganization of cellular constituents, for example,

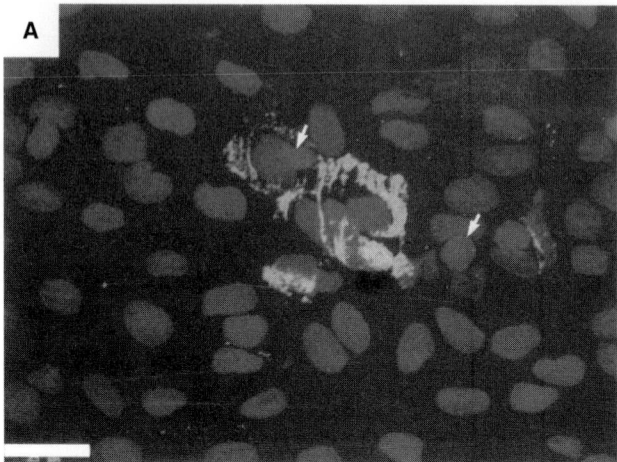

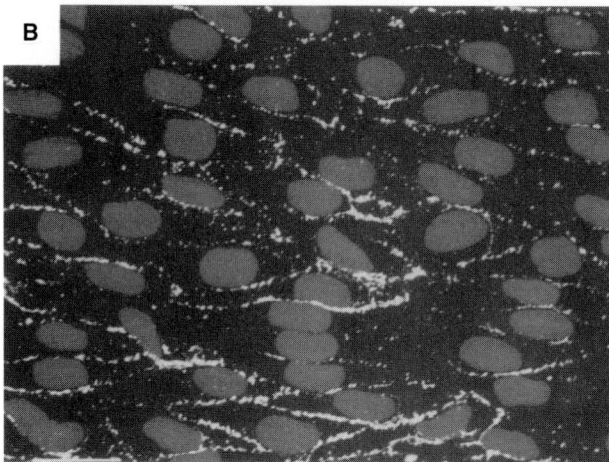

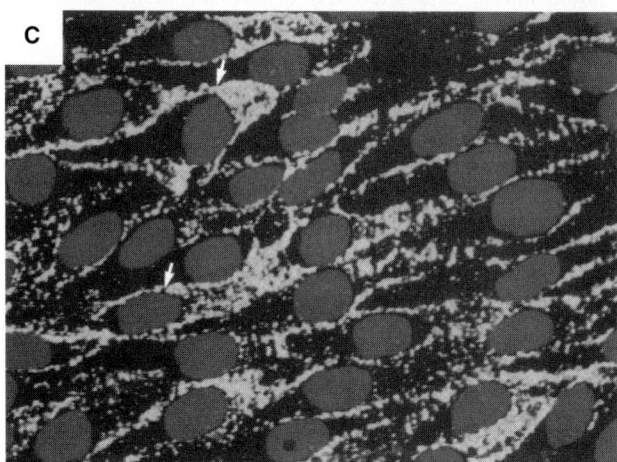

**FIGURE 43-6.** Intercellular adhesion module (ICAM-1) expression by endothelium is flow-sensitive in arteries. Rare, isolated cells display diffuse immuno-staining for ICAM-1 under low-flow (30% control) conditions in rabbit carotid arteries (**A**). Under normal-flow conditions, constitutively expressed ICAM-1 localizes to cell–cell junctions (**B**). Under high-flow conditions (200% of normal), cell junctional and overall expression of ICAM is substantially elevated (**C**). Nuclei are counterstained with propidium iodide. (Reprinted by permission from Walpola PL, Gotlieb AI, Cybulsky MI, Langille BL. Expression of ICAM-1 and VCAM-1 and monocyte adherence in arteries exposed to altered shear stress. *Arterioscler Thromb Vasc Biol* 1995;15:2–10.)

whether smooth muscle cells specifically target the direction of mitosis to deliver daughter cells in a force-specific direction or undergo hypertrophy such that changes in cell length or width are specific to the loads imposed on the cells.

## SUMMARY

Changes in blood flow rate through arteries, and the shear stress that blood flow exerts on the endothelial lining of the vessel wall, elicit endothelium-dependent remodeling that ultimately adjusts vessel diameter in accord with flow alterations. This remodeling is adaptive under normal physiologic conditions, but it can exacerbate pathologic conditions that compromise blood flow, such as thrombosis and atherosclerosis. Remodeling under the influence of blood flow and shear stress involves coordinated control of cell proliferation, cell death, matrix synthesis, and matrix degradation. Endothelial shear sensing and signal transduction mechanisms are now being defined, and the mediators of remodeling that they control are being elucidated; however, much more work is needed before the means by which shear-related signaling is integrated to produce a coherent remodeling response are understood.

## *References*

1. Schmid-Schonbein H, Wells R. Fluid drop–like transition of erythrocytes under shear. *Science* 1969;165:288–291.
2. Olesen S-P, Clapham DE, Davies PF. Haemodynamic shear stress activates a K+ current in vascular endothelial cells. *Nature Lond* 1988;221:168–170.
3. Hoger JH, Ilyin VI, Forsyth S, et al. Shear stress regulates the endothelial Kir2.1 ion channel. *Proc Natl Acad Sci U S A* 2002;99:7780–7785.
4. Qui WP, Hu Q, Paolocci N, et al. Differential effects of pulsatile versus steady flow on coronary endothelial membrane potential. *Am J Physiol Heart Circ Physiol* 2003;285:H341–H346.
5. Miura H, Wachtel RE, Liu Y, et al. Flow-induced dilation of human coronary arterioles: important role of Ca(2+)-activated K(+) channels. *Circulation* 2001;103:1992–1998.
6. Ohno M, Cooke JP, Dzau VJ, et al. Fluid shear stress induces endothelial transforming growth factor beta-1 transcription and production. Modulation by potassium channel blockade. *J Clin Invest* 1995;95:1363–1369.
7. Lieu DK, Pappone PA, Barakat AI. Differential membrane potential and ion current responses to different types of shear stress in vascular endothelial cells. *Am J Physiol Cell Physiol* 2004;286:C1367–C1375.
8. Rizzo V, McIntosh DP, Schnitzer JE, et al. In situ flow activates endothelial nitric oxide synthase in luminal caveolae of endothelium with rapid caveolin dissociation and calmodulin association. *J Biol Chem* 1998;273: 34724–34729.
9. Rudic RD, Shesely EG, Maeda N, et al. Direct evidence for the importance of endothelium-derived nitric oxide in vascular remodeling. *J Clin Invest* 1998;101:731–736.
10. Rizzo V, Sung A, Oh P, et al. Rapid mechanotransduction in situ at the luminal cell surface of vascular endothelium and its caveolae. *J Biol Chem* 1998;273:26323–26329.
11. Boyd NL, Park H, Hong Y, et al. Chronic shear induces caveolae formation and alters ERK and Akt responses in endothelial cells. *Am J Physiol Heart Circ Physiol* 2004;285:H1113–H1122.
12. Rizzo V, Morton C, DePaola N, et al. Recruitment of endothelial caveolae into mechanotransduction pathways by flow conditioning in vitro. *Am J Physiol Heart Circ Physiol* 2003;285:H1720–H1729.
13. Ishida T, Takahashi M, Corson MA, et al. Fluid shear stress-mediated signal transduction: how do endothelial cells transduce mechanical force into biological responses?. *Ann N Y Acad Sci* 1997;811:12–24.
14. Jo H, Sipos K, Go Y-M, et al. Differential effect of shear stress on extracellular signal-regulated kinase and N-terminal Jun kinase in endothelial cells Gi2- and G[beta]/[gamma]-dependent signaling pathways. *J Biol Chem* 1997;272(2):1395–1401.
15. Gudi S, Nolan JP, Frangos JA. Modulation of GTPase activity of G proteins by fluid dhear stress and phospholipid composition. *Proc Natl Acad Sci U S A* 1998;95(3):2515–2519.
16. Li S, Kim M, Hu Y-L, et al. Fluid shear stress activation of focal adhesion kinase—Linking to mitogen-activated protein kinases. *J Biol Chem* 1997; 272:30455–30462.
17. Tzima E, del Pozo A, Shattil SJ, et al. Activation of integrins in endothelial cells by fluid shear stress mediates Rho-dependent cytoskeletal alignment. *EMBO J* 2001;20:4639–4647.

18. Tzima E, Del Pozo MA, Kiosses WB, et al. Activation of Rac1 by shear stress in endothelial cells mediates both cytoskeletal reorganization and effects on gene expression. *EMBO J* 2002;21:6791–6800.

19. Birukov KG, Birukova AA, Dudek SM, et al. Shear stress-mediated cytoskeletal remodeling and cortactin translocation in pulmonary endothelial cells. *Am J Respir Cell Mol Biol* 2002;26:453–464.

20. Tzima E, Kiosses WB, Del Pozo MA, et al. Localized cdc42 activation, detected using a novel assay, mediates microtubule organizing center positioning in endothelial cells in response to fluid shear stress. *J Biol Chem* 2003;278(33):31020–31023.

21. Wojciak-Stothard B, Ridley AJ. Shear stress-induced endothelial cell polarization is mediated by Rho and Rac but not Cdc42 or PI 3-kinases. *J Cell Biol* 2003;161:429–439.

22. Shay-Salit A, Shushy M, Wolfovitz E, et al. VEGF receptor 2 and the adherens junction as a mechanical transducer in vascular endothelial cells. *Proc Natl Acad Sci U S A* 2002;99:9462–9467.

23. Jin ZG, Ueba H, Tanimoto T, et al. Ligand-independent activation of vascular endothelial growth factor receptor 2 by fluid shear stress regulates activation of endothelial nitric oxide synthase. *Circ Res* 2003;93(4):354–363.

24. Osawa M, Masuda M, Kusano K-I, et al. Evidence for a role of platelet endothelial cell adhesion molecule-1 in endothelial cell mechanosignal transduction: is it a mechanoresponsive molecule? *J Cell Biol* 2002;158:773–785.

25. Tseng H, Peterson TE, Berk BC. Fluid shear stress stimulates mitogen-activated protein kinase in endothelial cells. *Circ Res* 1995;77:869–878.

26. Traub O, Monia BP, Dean NM, et al. PKC-ε is required for mechanosensitive activation of ERK1/2 in endothelial cells. *J Biol Chem* 1997;272:31251–31257.

27. Yan C, Takahashi M, Okuda M, et al. Fluid shear stress stimulates big mitogen-activated protein kinase 1 (BMK1) activity in endothelial cells – dependence on tyrosine kinases and intracellular calcium. *J Biol Chem* 1999;274:143–150.

28. Dimmeler S, Assmus B, Hermann C, et al. Fluid shear stress stimulates phosphorylation of Akt in human endothelial cells—involvement in suppression of apoptosis. *Circ Res* 1998;83:334–341.

29. Cho A, Mitchell L, Koopmans D, et al. Effects of changes in blood flow rate on cell death and cell proliferation in carotid arteries of immature rabbits. *Circ Res* 1997;81:328–337.

30. Datta SR, Dudek H, Tao X, et al. Akt phosphorylation of BAD couples survival signals to the cell-intrinsic death machinery. *Cell* 1999;91(2):231–241.

31. Toker A, Newton AC. Akt/protein kinase B is regulated by autophosphorylation at the hypothetical PDK-2 site. *J Biol Chem* 2000;275:8271–8274.

32. Persad S, Attwell S, Gray V, et al. Regulation of protein kinase B/Akt-serine 473 phosphorylation by integrin-linked kinase. *J Biol Chem* 2001;276:27462–27469.

33. Hill MM, Feng J, Hemmings BA. Identification of a plasma membrane raft-associated PKB Ser473 kinase activity that is distinct from ILK and PDK1. *Curr Biol* 2002;12:1251–1255.

34. Go Y-M, Park H, Maland MC, et al. Phosphatidylinositol 3-kinase γ mediates shear stress-dependent activation of JNK in endothelial cells. *Am J Physiol Heart Circ Physiol* 1998;275:H1898–H1904.

35. Lan Q, Mercurius KO, Davies PF. Stimulation of transcription factors NF kappa B and AP1 in endothelial cells subjected to shear stress. *Biochem Biophys Res Commun* 1994;201(2):950–956.

36. Braddock M, Schwachtgen J-L, Houston P, et al. Fluid shear stress modulation of gene expression in endothelial cells. *News Physiol Sci* 1998;13:241–246.

37. Bhullar IS, Li YS, Miao H, et al. Fluid shear stress activation of IkappaB kinase is integrin-dependent. *J Biol Chem* 1998;273:30544–30549.

38. Davis ME, Grumbach IM, Fukai T, et al. Shear stress regulates endothelial nitric-oxide synthase promoter activity through nuclear factor kappa B binding. *J Biol Chem* 2004;279(1):163–168.

39. Resnick N, Collins T, Atkinson W, et al. Platelet-derived growth factor B chain promoter contains a cis-acting fluid shear-stress-responsive element. *Proc Natl Acad Sci U S A* 1993;90:4591–4595.

40. Khachigian LM, Resnick N, Gimbrone MA Jr, et al. Nuclear factor-kappaB interacts functionally with the platelet-derived growth factor B-chain shear-stress response element in vascular endothelial cells exposed to fluid shear stress. *J Clin Invest* 1995;96:1169–1175.

41. Khachigian LM, Anderson KR, Halnon NJ Jr, et al. Egr-1 is activated in endothelial cells exposed to fluid shear stress and interacts with a novel shear-stress-response element in the PDGF A-chain promoter. *Arterioscler Thromb Vasc Biol* 1997;17:2280–2286.

42. Hajra L, Evans AI, Chen M, et al. The NF-κB signal transduction pathway in aortic endothelial cells is primed for activation in regions predisposed to atherosclerotic lesion formation. *Proc Natl Acad Sci U S A* 2000;97:9052–9057.

43. Barbee KA, Mundel T, Lal R, et al. Subcellular distribution of shear stress at the surface of flow-aligned and nonaligned endothelial monolayers. *Am J Physiol Heart Circ Physiol* 1995;268:H1765–H1772.

44. Langille BL. Blood flow-induced remodeling of the artery wall. In: Bevan JA, Kaley G, Rubanyi G, eds. *Flow-dependent regulation of vascular function*, New York: Oxford University Press, 1995:277–299.

45. Kim DW, Langille BL, Wong MKK, et al. Patterns of endothelial microfilament distribution in the rabbit aorta in situ. *Circ Res* 1989;64:21–31.

46. Kim DW, Gotlieb AI, Langille BL. *In vivo* modulation of endothelial F-actin microfilaments by experimental alterations in shear stress. *Arteriosclerosis* 1989;9:439–445.

47. YU JCM, Gotlieb AI. Disruption of endothelial actin microfilaments by protein kinase C inhibitors. *Microvasc Res* 1992;43:100–111.

48. Morita K, Sasaki H, Furuse M, et al. Endothelial claudin: claudin-5/TMVCF constitutes tight junction strands in endothelial cells. *J Cell Biol* 1999;147:185–194.

49. Schnittler H-J, Wilke A, Gress T, et al. Role of actin and myosin in the control of paracellular permeability in pig, rat and human vascular endothelium. *J Physiol* 1991;431:379–401.

50. Dejana E. Endothelial adherens junctions: implications in the control of vascular permeability and angiogenesis. *J Clin Invest* 1996;98:1949–1953.

51. Noria S, Cowan DB, Gotlieb AI, et al. Transient and steady-state effects of shear stress on endothelial cell adherens junctions. *Circ Res* 1999;85:504–514.

52. Noria S, Xu F, McCue S, et al. Assembly and reorientation of stress fibers drives morphologic changes to endothelial cells exposed to shear stress. *Am J Pathol* 2004;164:1211–1223.

53. Grosso LE, Parks WC, Wu L, et al. Fibroblast adhesion to recombinant tropoelastin expressed as a protein A-fusion protein. *Biochem J* 1991;273:517–522.

54. Langille BL, Graham JJK, Kim D, et al. Dynamics of shear-induced redistribution of F-actin in endothelial cells *in vivo*. *Arterioscler Thromb* 1991;11:1814–1820.

55. Pollard TD, Borisy GG. Cellular motility driven by assembly and disassembly of actin filaments. *Cell* 2003;112:453–465.

56. Gotlieb AI, McBurnie-May L, Subrahmanyan L, et al. Distribution of microtubule organizing centers in migrating sheets of endothelial cells. *J Cell Biol* 1981;91:589–594.

57. Rogers KA, McKee NH, Kalnins VI. Preferential orientation of centrioles towards the heart in endothelial cells of major blood vessels is reestablished after reversal of a segment. *Proc Natl Acad Sci U S A* 1985;82:3272–3276.

58. Kiosses WB, McKee NH, Kalnins VI. Evidence for the migration of rat aortic endothelial cells toward the heart. *Arterioscler Thromb Vasc Biol* 1997;17:2891–2896.

59. Vyalov S, Langille BL, Gotlieb AI. Decreased blood flow rate disrupts endothelial repair *in vivo*. *Am J Pathol* 1996;149:2107–2118.

60. McCue S, Noria S, Langille BL. Shear-induced reorganization of endothelial cell cytoskeleton and adhesion complexes. *Trends Cardiovasc Med* 2004;14:143–151.

61. Helmke BP, Thakker DB, Goldman RD, et al. Spatiotemporal analysis of flow-induced intermediate filament displacement in living endothelial cells. *Biophys J* 2001;80:184–194.

62. Schnittler H-J, Schmandra T, Drenckhahn D. Correlation of endothelial vimentin content with hemodynamic parameters. *Histochem Cell Biol* 1998;110:161–167.

63. Henrion D, Terzi F, Matrougui K, et al. Impaired flow-induced dilation in mesenteric resistance arteries from mice lacking vimentin. *J Clin Invest* 1997;100:2909–2914.

64. Kamiya A, Togawa T. Adaptive regulation of wall shear stress to flow change in the canine carotid artery. *Am J Physiol* 1980;239:H14–H21.

65. Langille BL, O'Donnell F. Reductions in arterial diameter produced by chronic decreases in blood flow are endothelium-dependent. *Science* 1986;231:405–407.

66. Schretzenmayr A. Uber kreislaufregulatorische vorgange an den grossen arterien bei der muskelarbeit. *Pflugers Archiv Ges Physiol* 1933;232:743–748.

67. Smiesko V, Kozik J, Delezel S. Role of endothelium in the control of arterial diameter by blood flow. *Blood Vessels* 1985;22:247–251.

68. Pohl U, Holtz J, Busse R, et al. Crucial role of endothelium in the vasodilator response to increased flow *in vivo*. *Hypertension* 1986;8:38–44.

69. Langille BL, Bendeck MP, Keeley FW. Adaptations of carotid arteries of young and mature rabbits to reduced carotid blood flow. *Am J Physiol* 1989;256:H931–H939.

70. Langille BL. Remodelling of developing and mature arteries: endothelium, smooth muscle and matrix. *J Cardiovasc Pharmacol* 1993;21:S11–S17.

71. Christ GJ, Spray DC, El-Sabban M, et al. Gap junctions in vascular tissues: evaluating the role of intercellular communication in the modulation of vasomotor tone. *Circ Res* 1996;79:631–646.

72. Cowan DB, Langille BL. Cellular and molecular biology of vascular remodeling. *Curr Opin Lipidol* 1996;7:94–100.

73. Zarins CK, Zatina MA, Giddens DP, et al. Shear stress regulation of artery lumen diameter in experimental atherogenesis. *J Vasc Surg* 1987;5:413–420.

74. Lehman RM, Owens GK, Kassell NF, et al. Mechanism of enlargement of major cerebral collateral arteries in rabbits. *Stroke* 1991;22:499–504.

75. Thoma R. *Untersuchagen uberdie histogenese und histomechanik des gefassystems*. Stuttgart: Enke, 1893.

76. Clark ER. Studies on the growth of blood-vessels in the tail of the frog larva—by observation and experiment on the living animal. *Am J Anat* 1918;23:37–88.

77. Rychter Z. Experimental morphology of the aortic arches and heart loop in chick embryos. *Adv Morphog* 1962;2:333–371.

78. Stephan F. Les suppleances obtenues experimentalement dans le systeme des arcs aortiques de l'embryon d'oiseau. *Comptes Rendu* 1949;36:647–651.

79. Bendeck MP, Langille BL. Changes in blood flow distribution in the perinatal period in fetal sheep and lambs. *Can J Physiol Pharmacol* 1992;70:1576–1582.

80. Langille BL, Brownlee RD, Adamson SL. Perinatal aortic growth in lambs: relation to blood flow changes at birth. *Am J Physiol* 1990;259: H1247–H1253.

81. Bendeck MP, Keeley FW, Langille BL. Perinatal accumulation of arterial wall constituents: relation to hemodynamic changes at birth. *Am J Physiol* 1994;267:H2268–H2279.

82. Di Stefano I, Koopmans DR, Langille BL. Modulation of arterial growth of the rabbit carotid artery associated with experimental elevation of blood flow. *J Vasc Res* 1998;35:1–7.

83. Glagov S, Weisenberg E, Zarins CK, et al. Compensatory enlargement of human atherosclerotic coronary arteries. *N Engl J Med* 1987;316: 1371–1375.

84. Mulvihill DA, Harvey SC. The mechanism of the development of collateral circulation. *N Engl J Med* 1931;204:1031–1032.

85. Langille BL, Gotlieb AI, Kim DW. Vascular tissue response to experimentally altered local blood flow conditions. In: Westerhof N, Gross DR, eds. *Vascular dynamics*, New York: Plenum Publishing, 1989:229–235.

86. Kohler TR, Jawien A. Flow affects development of intimal hyperplasia after arterial injury in rats. *Circ Res* 1992;12:963–971.

87. Kohler TR, Kirkman TR, Kraiss LW, et al. Increased blood flow inhibits neointimal hyperplasia in endothelialized vascular grafts. *Circ Res* 1991;69:1557–1565.

88. Geary RL, Kohler TR, Vergel S, et al. Time course of flow-induced smooth muscle cell proliferation and intimal thickening in endothelialized baboon vascular grafts. *Circ Res* 1994;74:14–23.

89. Majesky MW, Reidy MA, Bowen-Pope DF, et al. PDGF ligand and receptor expression during repair of arterial injury. *J Cell Biol* 1990;111:2149–2158.

90. Kraiss LW, Geary RL, Mattsson EJR, et al. Acute reductions in blood flow and shear stress induce platelet-derived growth factor-a expression in baboon prosthetic grafts. *Circ Res* 1996;79:45–53.

91. Hsieh H-J, Li N-Q, Frangos JA. Shear-induced platelet-derived growth factor gene expression in human endothelial cells is mediated by protein kinase C. *J Cell Physiol* 1992;150:552–558.

92. Jackson CL, Raines EW, Ross R, et al. Role of endogenous platelet-derived growth factor in arterial smooth muscle cell migration after balloon catheter injury. *Arterioscler Thromb* 1993;13:1218–1226.

93. Englesbe MJ, Hawkins SM, Hsieh PC, et al. Concomitant blockade of platelet-derived growth factor receptors alpha and beta induces intimal atrophy in baboon PTFE grafts. *J Vasc Surg* 2004;39:440–446.

94. Learoyd BM, Taylor MG. Alterations with age in the viscoelastic properties of human arterial walls. *Circ Res* 1966;18:278–292.

95. Jackson ZS, Gotlieb AI, Langille BL. Wall tissue remodeling regulates longitudinal tension in arteries. *Circ Res* 2002;90:918–925.

96. Keeley FW, Johnson DJ. Age differences in the effect of hydrocortisone on the synthesis of insoluble elastin in aortic tissue of growing chicks. *Connect Tissue Res* 1987;16:259–268.

97. Rich CB, Ewton DZ, Martin BM, et al. IGF-I regulation of elastogenesis: comparison of aortic and lung cells. *Am J Physiol Lung Cell Mol Physiol* 1992;263:L276–L282.

98. Jensen DE, Rich CB, Terpstra AJ, et al. Transcriptional regulation of the elastin gene by insulin-like growth factor-I involves disruption of Sp1 binding. Evidence for the role of Rb in mediating Sp1 binding in aortic smooth muscle cells. *J Biol Chem* 1995;270:6555–6563.

99. Kahari V-M, Olsen DR, Rhudy RW, et al. Transforming growth factor-beta up-regulates elastin gene expression in human skin fibroblasts. *Lab Invest* 1992;66:580–588.

100. Marigo V, Volpin D, Vitale G, et al. Identification of a TGF-b responsive element in the human elastin promoter. *Biochem Biophys Res Commun* 1994;199:1049–1056.

101. Davis EC. Elastic lamina growth in the developing mouse aorta. *J Histochem Cytochem* 1995;43:1115–1123.

102. Campbell GJ, Roach MR. Fenestrations in the internal elastic lamina at bifurcations of human cerebral arteries. *Stroke* 1981;12:489–496.

103. Wong LCY, Langille BL. Developmental remodeling of the internal elastic lamina of rabbit arteries. Effect of blood flow. *Circ Res* 1996;78:799–805.

104. Zhu L, Wigle D, Hinek A, et al. The endogenous vascular elastase that governs development and progression of monocrotaline-induced pulmonary hypertension in rats is a novel enzyme related to the serine proteinase adipsin. *J Clin Invest* 1994;94:1163–1171.

105. Wight TN. The vascular extracellular matrix. In: Fuster V, Ross R, Topol EJ, eds. *Atherosclerosis and coronary artery disease*, Philadelphia, PA: Lippincott–Raven Publishers, 1996:421–440.

106. Azmi TI, O'Shea JD. Mechanism of deletion of endothelial cells during regression of the corpus luteum. *Lab Invest* 1984;51:206–217.

107. Schaper W, Scholz D. Factors regulating arteriogenesis. *Arterioscler Thromb Vasc Biol* 2003;23:1143–1151.

108. Helisch A, Schaper W. Arteriogenesis the development and growth of collateral arteries. *Microcirculation* 2003;10:83–97.

109. Walpola PL, Gotlieb AI, Cybulsky MI, et al. Expression of ICAM-1 and VCAM-1 and monocyte adherence in arteries exposed to altered shear stress. *Arterioscler Thromb Vasc Biol* 1995;15:2–10.

110. Nagel T, Resnick N, Atkinson WJ, et al. Shear stress selectively upregulates intercellular adhesion molecule-1 expression in cultured human vascular endothelial cells. *J Clin Invest* 1994;94:885–891.

111. Kevil CG, Orr AW, Langston W, et al. ICAM-1 regulates endothelial cell motility through an NO dependent pathway. *JBC* 2004;279:19230–19238.

112. Wolf C, Cai W-J, Vosschulte R, et al. Vascular remodeling and altered protein expression during growth of coronary collateral arteries. *J Mol Cell Cardiol* 1998;30:2291–2305.

113. Martinez-Lemus LA, Hill MA, Bolz SS, et al. Acute mechanoadaptation of vascular smooth muscle cells in response to continuous arteriolar vasoconstriction: implications for functional remodeling. *FASEB J* 2004;18: 708–710. Epub ahead of print.

114. Bakker ENTP, Buus CL, Spaan JAE, et al. Small artery remodeling depends on tissue-type transglutaminase. *Circ Res* 2005;96:119–126.

115. Langille BL, Dajnowiec D. Cross-linking vasomotor tone and vascular remodeling—A novel function for tissue transglutaminase? *Circ Res* 2005; 96(1):9–11.

# CHAPTER 44 ■ ANGIOGENESIS, LYMPHANGIOGENESIS, AND VASCULAR MORPHOGENESIS

JILLIAN A. HARRISON, RAPHAËLE BUSER, AND MICHAEL S. PEPPER

Angiogenesis and lymphangiogenesis refer to the growth of new capillary blood vessels from the preexisting blood and lymphatic vasculature, respectively. Until recently, lymphangiogenesis was overshadowed by the greater emphasis placed on the blood vascular system (angiogenesis), partly because of the lack of identification of lymphangiogenic factors, as well as suitable markers that allow the distinction of lymphatic from blood vascular endothelium. This situation has changed dramatically in the last few years and lymphangiogenesis has become more accessible from a molecular and experimental point of view.

Immature endothelial-lined tubes that arise during angiogenesis and lymphangiogenesis differentiate into capillaries or into larger vessels such as arteries, veins, collecting lymphatics, and the thoracic duct. The early phase of sprouting includes endothelial cell migration, proliferation, and extracellular proteolysis, and is mediated in part by the vascular endothelial growth factor (VEGF) family and its receptors. Reciprocal interactions then occur between pluripotent mesenchyme and endothelium, resulting in the differentiation of pericytes and smooth muscle cells. In the case of the blood vascular system, these interactions are mediated by the transforming growth factor-$\beta$ (TGF-$\beta$), platelet-derived growth factor (PDGF), and angiopoietin families and their respective receptor-tyrosine kinases (RTKs). A role in angiogenesis as well as a specification of arterial and venous vascular segments has been attributed to certain members of the ephrin family and their RTKs. In the case of lymphangiogenesis, a role for the VEGF and angiopoietin families has been defined.

## ANGIOGENESIS AND LYMPHANGIOGENESIS

The formation of new blood vessels can be ascribed to two interrelated but separable processes: vasculogenesis and angiogenesis. Vasculogenesis is a series of differentiation and morphogenetic events that occur during development and that result in the formation of a primary capillary plexus (1). Angiogenesis is the formation of new capillary blood vessels by a process of sprouting from preexisting vessels in a variety of developmental, physiologic, and pathologic settings (2). Although, by definition, vasculogenesis must precede angiogenesis, the two processes continue in parallel during early development. However, unlike vasculogenesis, which appears to be restricted to early development, angiogenesis is required for the maintenance of functional and structural integrity of the organism in postnatal life. A form of nonsprouting angiogenesis called *intussusceptive microvascular growth* (IMG) has been described. During this process, slender transcapillary tissue pillars are inserted into newly formed tubes, which subsequently grow into normal-sized capillary meshes.

IMG seems to be a ubiquitous process occurring in all species and in all organ systems investigated so far (3). The sequential stages of blood vessel formation that occur during development and in postnatal life are outlined in Table 44-1. No distinction has been made between angiogenesis and vasculogenesis.

In addition to its role during development, angiogenesis occurs during wound healing, in inflammation, in ischemia (i.e., heart, extremities, and central nervous system), and in female reproductive organs (i.e., in the ovary before ovulation and during corpus luteum formation; in the placenta and mammary gland during pregnancy) (see Table 44-2). Angiogenesis in these situations is tightly regulated and is limited by the metabolic demands of the tissues concerned. Angiogenesis also occurs in pathologic situations such as proliferative retinopathy, rheumatoid arthritis, psoriasis, and juvenile hemangioma (Table 44-2) (4,5).

Much of the interest in angiogenesis comes from the notion that for tumors to grow beyond a critical size, they must recruit endothelial cells from the surrounding stroma to form their own endogenous microcirculation (6). Therefore, during tumor progression, two phases can be recognized: a prevascular phase and a vascular phase. The transition from the prevascular to the vascular phase is referred to as the "angiogenic switch." The prevascular phase is characterized by an initial increase in tumor growth, followed by a plateau in which the rate of tumor cell proliferation is balanced by the rate of cell death (apoptosis). This phase may persist for many years and can be recognized clinically as carcinoma *in situ*, which is characterized by few or no metastases. During the vascular phase, which is characterized by exponential growth, tissue invasion, and the hematogenous spread of tumor cells, the rapid increase in tumor growth is largely due to a decrease in the rate of tumor cell apoptosis (7,8). An inverse relationship therefore exists between tumor cell apoptosis and tumor angiogenesis. In a sense, tumor angiogenesis might almost be considered as being "appropriate," in that newly formed vessels serve to meet the metabolic demands of the rapidly growing tumor. Although this may be beneficial to the tumor itself, it is clearly detrimental to the organism because it is permissive for tumor growth, for the dissemination of tumor cells, and for the formation of metastases.

A process analogous to angiogenesis occurs in the lymphatic system and is referred to as lymphangiogenesis. In response to molecular mediators, lymphatic endothelial cells proliferate and migrate through the extracellular matrix, followed by association of the endothelial cells into tubelike structures (9).

Production and realignment of the extracellular matrix and controlled apoptosis at appropriate sites are required for blood and lymphatic vessel formation. Blood and lymphatic vessels are closely associated *in vivo*. Blood vascular plexuses are often accompanied by lymphatic vessels (10), although the

**TABLE 44-1**

STAGES OF BLOOD VESSEL FORMATION

**DEVELOPMENT**
Angioblast/hemangioblast differentiation
Endothelial cell differentiation (primary capillary plexus)
Sprouting, intussusception, and regression
Smooth muscle cell and pericyte differentiation
Vessel wall assembly and maintenance
Organ-specific endothelial differentiation:
    Blood–brain barrier
    Fenestrated endothelium
    High endothelial venules
    Sinusoidal endothelium

**POSTNATAL LIFE**
Vessel wall disassembly
Endothelial cell activation (i.e., increased permeability,
    proteolysis, migration, and mitosis)
Capillarylike tube formation
Smooth muscle and pericyte differentiation
Vessel wall assembly and maintenance

**TABLE 44-2**

ANGIOGENESIS IN HEALTH AND DISEASE

**DEVELOPMENT**
Cardiovascular system
Organ vascularization

**PHYSIOLOGY**
Female hormonal cycle: ovary and uterus
Pregnancy: placenta and mammary gland
Wound healing and fracture repair
Inflammation
Ischemia-induced collateral formation
    (heart, extremities, brain)

**ANGIOGENESIS-ASSOCIATED DISEASES**
Tumor growth and metastasis
Ocular neovascularization
Hemangioma
Psoriasis
Inflammatory (rheumatoid) arthritis

ratio of lymphatic vessels to blood vessels varies, depending on tissue type and function (11). Direct lymphaticovenous connections do not occur outside the lymphoid system.

The lymphatic system consists of blind-ending initial thin-walled, low-pressure vessels, which drain into lymphatic collectors and the thoracic duct. Circulating lymphocytes and aggregations of lymphoid tissue, such as lymph nodes, spleen, tonsils, Peyer patches, and thymus, further constitute the lymphoid system (12–14). This extensive network of capillaries, collecting vessels, and ducts that permeate most organs is an open-ended, one-way transit system, unlike the blood vasculature that forms a continuous loop (15). Vessels collect extravasated fluid, macromolecules, and cells of the immune system within tissues and return them to the blood circulation (see Fig. 44-1). Larger lymphatic vessels are surrounded by a muscular layer that contracts automatically when the vessel becomes stretched with fluid. In addition, external factors such as skeletal muscle contractions or arterial pulsation compress the initial lymphatic vessels and increase the efficiency of fluid transport. When lymphatic circulation is compromised, lymphedema ensues. The lymphatic system is intimately associated with the immune system by continuously transporting lymphocytes and antigen-presenting cells between lymphoid organs.

Traditionally, lymphatic vessels have been identified by lymphangiography/lymphoscintigraphy, which is based on the ability of lymphatic capillaries to take up dyes and high-molecular-weight molecules from the interstitium. Most commonly used are vital dyes such as Evans, trypan, and patent blue; fluorescently labeled tracers; and radioactive colloids. The absence of a complete basement membrane (i.e., laminin, collagen IV, and collagen XVIII), the lack of Pathologische Anatomie Leiden-Endothelium (PAL-E) staining of CD31-positive endothelial cells, as well as 5′-nucleotidase activity, have been considered as lymphatic endothelial-specific criteria (16). In the last few years, several positive markers specific for lymphatic endothelium have been discovered. These markers include VEGFR-3, which is expressed in lymphatic endothelium early in development, although it is also expressed in a subset of blood vessels and can be reactivated in angiogenic vessels in certain pathologic conditions (17,18). Other transmembrane proteins such as podoplanin (19) and LYVE-1 (20) as well as the transcription factor Prox-1 (21) have been shown to be reliable in distinguishing lymphatic endothelium from

blood endothelium, although none is strictly endothelium specific (16). Recently, a β-chemokine receptor D6 was shown to be present in a subset of lymphatic vessels in the skin, intestine, and lymphoid tissues (22). The macrophage mannose receptor is also expressed by the lymphatic endothelium, in addition to macrophages and other nonendothelial cells (23).

# REGULATION OF ANGIOGENESIS AND LYMPHANGIOGENESIS

Endothelial cell turnover in the healthy adult organism is low. The maintenance of endothelial quiescence is due to the presence of endogenous negative regulators because positive regulators are frequently detected in adult tissues in which there is apparently no angiogenesis. The converse also is true—positive and negative regulators often coexist in tissues in which endothelial cell turnover is increased; this has led to the notion of the "angiogenic switch," where endothelial activation status is determined by a balance between positive and negative regulators: In activated (angiogenic) endothelium, positive regulators predominate, whereas endothelial quiescence is achieved and maintained by the dominance of negative regulators (24, 25). Used initially in the context of tumor progression to describe the passage from the prevascular to the vascular phase, the notion of the "switch" can also be applied to developmental, physiologic, and pathologic angiogenesis. The current working hypothesis is that the "switch" involves either the induction of a positive regulator or the loss of a negative regulator, or both. Although widely applied to angiogenesis, the notion of a "switch" is at present not applied to lymphangiogenesis.

Among the factors affecting endothelial cell activation status, either positively or negatively, are growth factors and cytokines (referred to collectively as cytokines), which are produced by normal and tumor cells. On the basis of the observation that a given tissue can profoundly influence the way in which its cellular components respond to a given cytokine, it has been suggested that cytokines should be seen as "specialized symbols in a language of intercellular communication, whose meaning is controlled by context" (26). Context is determined by (at least) four parameters: first, by the presence and concentration of other cytokines in the pericellular environment of the responding cell; second, by interactions between cells, cytokines, and the extracellular matrix; third,

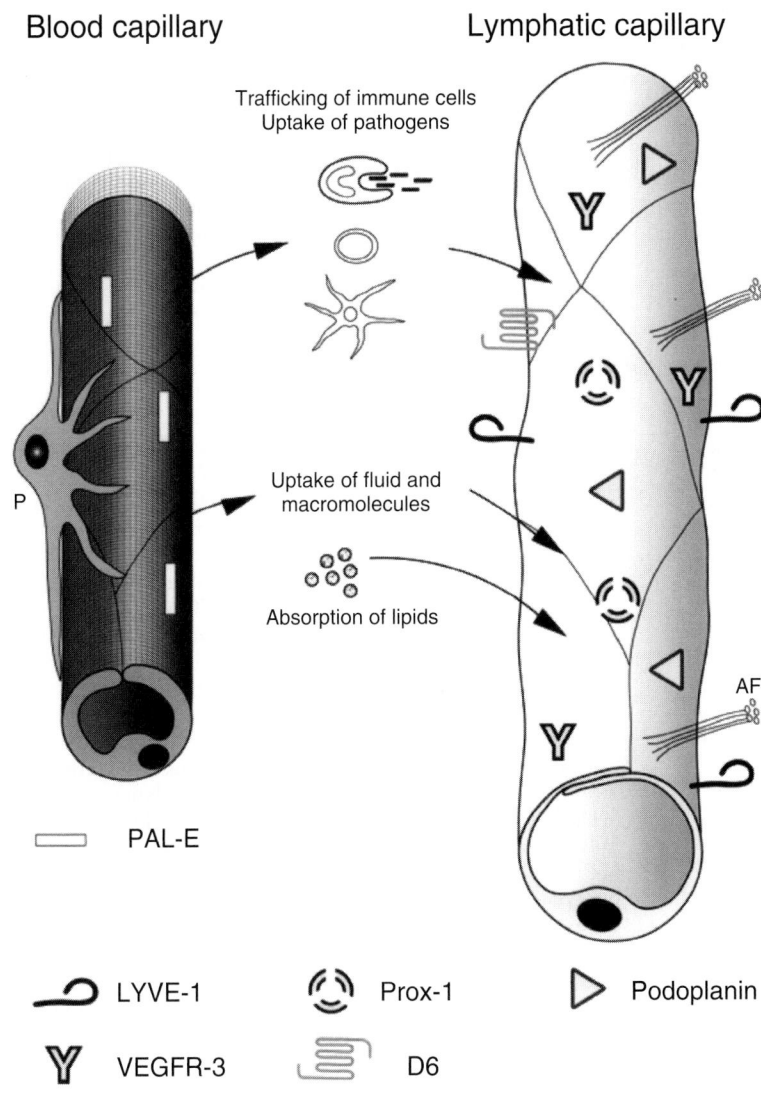

**Blood capillary**

**Lymphatic capillary**

Trafficking of immune cells
Uptake of pathogens

P

Uptake of fluid and
macromolecules

Absorption of lipids

AF

⬭ PAL-E

↻ LYVE-1      ⟲ Prox-1      ▷ Podoplanin

Υ VEGFR-3      ⟿ D6

**FIGURE 44-1.** Structure and function of blood and lymphatic capillaries. Lymphatic capillaries are uniquely adapted for the uptake of fluid, lipids, macromolecules, and cells from the interstitium. In contrast to blood capillaries, lymphatic capillaries have a poorly developed basal lamina and are devoid of pericytes. Lymphatic endothelium is highly attenuated. The cells are connected to each other by overlapping junctions, and directly to interstitial collagen by bundles of elastic fibers called *anchoring filaments*. A number of markers have been identified to distinguish lymphatic endothelium from blood vascular endothelium. Members of the vascular endothelial growth factor (VEGF) and fibroblast growth factor (FGF) families induce angiogenesis and lymphangiogenesis, although with regard to VEGF, angiogenesis is induced by vascular endothelial growth factor receptors (VEGFRs) -1 and -2, whereas lymphangiogenesis is induced by VEGFRs -2 and -3. (From Pepper MS, Skobe M. Lymphatic endothelium: morphological, molecular, and functional properties. *J Cell Biol* 2003;163:209–213, with permission.)

by the geometric configuration of the cells (and thereby their cytoskeleton); and fourth, by biomechanical forces imposed by circulating blood, particularly in the case of endothelial cells (see Table 44-3).

The most extensively studied cytokines involved in the positive regulation of angiogenesis belong to the VEGF and FGF families. However, although a regulatory role for VEGF in developmental, physiologic, and pathologic angiogenesis has been clearly defined (27–29), the relevance of FGF families to the endogenous control of angiogenesis is still ill defined. A large body of evidence, gained principally from gene deletion studies, negates the role of FGF families during development, although a role during inflammatory and tumor angiogenesis

cannot be excluded (30,31). Three additional families of cytokines have been implicated in new blood vessel formation, and their function appears to be particularly important for vessel wall assembly and the maintenance of vascular integrity. These families include PDGF and, in particular, PDGF-BB (32); TGF-$\beta$ (33); and the angiopoietins (34). A fourth family—the ephrins—has been identified, members of which are involved in angiogenesis and in the specification of the arterial and venous vascular beds (35) (see Table 44-4).

Two lymphangiogenic factors, which are members of the VEGF family, have been identified to date: VEGF-C and VEGF-D. VEGF-C and -D have the dual capacity to induce

**TABLE 44-3**

ANGIOGENESIS-REGULATING CYTOKINES: FACTORS THAT DETERMINE CONTEXT

Cytokines
Extracellular matrix
Geometry (i.e., cytoskeletal organization)
Biomechanical forces
Presence of other (i.e., nonendothelial) cell types

**TABLE 44-4**

CYTOKINE FAMILIES INVOLVED IN BLOOD VESSEL FORMATION

Vascular endothelial growth factors
Angiopoietins
Transforming growth factor-$\beta$s
Platelet-derived growth factors
Ephrins
Fibroblast growth factors?

lymphangiogenesis and angiogenesis, as demonstrated in a number of experimental systems including the chick chorioallantoic membrane (CAM), (36) the rabbit cornea assay (37), and transgenic mice (38). Other molecules that play an important role in the development of the lymphatic system include angiopoietin-2 (39), neuropilin-2 (40), and Prox-1 (21). FGF-2 has been shown to induce lymphangiogenesis as well as angiogenesis in several experimental systems (37), and to correlate positively with increased tumor lymphatic vessel density (41).

Once formed, immature endothelial-lined tubes in the blood vascular system subsequently differentiate into capillaries (after association with pericytes) or into larger vessels such as arteries and veins (after forming a media and adventitia). The absence of pericyte coverage renders newly formed vessels particularly susceptible to stimulatory or inhibitory factors. Once pericytes are in place, endothelial cells become refractory to these stimuli. These observations have given rise to the notion of the "window of endothelial plasticity" (42,43), during which growth and remodeling of the vascular tree is maximal. During this period, vessel density adapts to the needs of the tissue, principally through oxygen tension–mediated regulation of VEGF production. It is also during this period that newly formed capillary sprouts are likely to be most sensitive to pharmacologic manipulation, either positive or negative (see section, "Perspectives"). In the lymphatic system, initial capillaries are devoid of pericytes. However, collecting lymphatics and the thoracic duct are invested with one or several layers of smooth muscle cells. The precise mechanisms of vessel wall assembly in the lymphatic system remains to be elucidated.

# VASCULAR ENDOTHELIAL GROWTH FACTOR

VEGF was initially described as a tumor-secreted protein that increases the permeability of microvessels—hence, its alternate name, vascular permeability factor. VEGF is also a potent positive regulator of angiogenesis because it induces endothelial cell migration and proliferation and alters endothelial cell gene expression (including the production of matrix-degrading proteolytic enzymes) (27–29,44,45). Alterations in endothelial cell function induced by members of the VEGF family are mediated by transmembrane tyrosine kinase receptors (VEGFRs).

The importance of VEGF in experimental models of proliferative retinopathy and primary and metastatic tumor growth has been clearly demonstrated using a variety of approaches. In addition, the critical requirement for VEGF-induced angiogenesis for postnatal growth, survival, organ development, and corpus luteum formation has been reported (46,47). However, the most dramatic demonstration of the requirement for VEGF in the development of the vascular tree comes from genetic studies involving targeted gene disruption in mice. In a manner that is unprecedented for a gene that does not undergo imprinting, heterozygosity for VEGF inactivation was embryonically lethal (48,49). The observation that the phenotype of VEGF$^{-/-}$ mice was more severe than that of VEGF$^{+/-}$ mice demonstrates the existence of a dose-dependent requirement for VEGF during embryogenesis and implies that minimal amounts of VEGF are required in a tightly regulated manner for normal vascular development. Essentially, although endothelial cell development was delayed in VEGF-deficient mice, resulting in the formation of abnormal vascular structures and massive tissue necrosis, it was not entirely aborted.

Four proteins with structural homology to VEGF have been described. The first is VEGF-B (50) or, alternatively, VEGF-related factor (51). VEGF-B has two alternatively-spliced isoforms that differ in their C-termini, VEGF-B$_{167}$ and VEGF-B$_{186}$, with VEGF-B$_{167}$ being predominantly expressed. The overall genomic organization of VEGF-B is conserved between other members of the VEGF gene family [i.e., VEGF, placenta growth factor (PlGF), and PDGF]. VEGF-B$_{167}$ is secreted but remains cell associated, whereas VEGF-B$_{186}$ is freely secreted, lacking the heparin sulphate, proteoglycan, and neurophilin-1 (NRP-1) binding properties of VEGF$_{167}$ (52). VEGF-B is most highly expressed in heart and skeletal muscles, with relatively stable expression levels that are not altered by growth factors, hormones, hypoxia, or oncogenes. VEGF-B binds to VEGFR-1 (53); VEGFR-1 phosphorylation on binding VEGF-B$_{167}$ has only been demonstrated using rhVEGF-B in a matrigel plug model *in vivo* (54). The precise role of VEGF-B during development and postnatal life remains to be elucidated; however, on the basis of its tissue distribution pattern in the embryo, VEGF-B may be important for cardiac development. VEGF-B may also regulate the bioavailability of VEGF-A in a similar manner to PlGF by competing for VEGF-R1 and NRP-1 or by forming stable heterodimers with VEGF-A, thereby changing the relative availability of VEGF-A. VEGF-B$_{186}$ has been shown to be expressed at lower basal levels but to be upregulated in tumor cell lines, primary tumors (55), and in rheumatoid arthritis (56).

The second protein is VEGF-C (57) or, alternatively, VEGF-related protein (58), Flt-4 ligand (59), or VEGF-2 (60). VEGF-C displays a high degree of similarity to VEGF, including conservation of the eight cysteine residues involved in intra- and intermolecular disulfide bonding. The cysteine-rich C-terminal half increases the length of the VEGF-C polypeptide relative to other members of this family. VEGF-C messenger ribonucleic acid (mRNA) is first translated into a precursor from which the mature ligand is derived by cell-associated proteolytic processing (61). Partially processed VEGF-C binds to VEGFR-3, whereas fully processed VEGF-C binds to both VEGFRs -2 and -3; in both cases, binding is accompanied by receptor tyrosine phosphorylation (57,61). Patterns of VEGF-C expression during development suggest that this cytokine plays an important role in lymphangiogenesis [see (62), and the preceding section], and targeted overexpression of VEGF-C in the skin results in selective hypertrophy of lymphatic vessels (38). However, application of exogenous VEGF-C to the chick CAM induced either angiogenesis (i.e., growth of new blood capillaries) or lymphangiogenesis (36,63). Furthermore, when applied to the mouse cornea, recombinant VEGF-C induced angiogenesis (63), and when administered by a gene therapy approach in a model of rabbit hindlimb ischemia, VEGF-C was shown to induce formation of new blood vessels and improvement in functional parameters (64). Finally, an immunohistochemical study of VEGF-C and VEGFR-3 in breast cancer suggests that ligand and receptor may be associated with both angiogenesis and lymphangiogenesis in this setting (18). There is currently no explanation for the selective effects of VEGF-C on lymphangiogenesis versus angiogenesis, but it is possible that this depends on the repertoire of VEGFRs expressed at the time VEGF-C is present in the endothelial pericellular environment (including heterodimers between the different VEGFRs). Alternatively, selectivity may be mediated by interactions with other cytokines that induce synergistic interactions with VEGF-C, such as FGF-2 or VEGF (65).

The third protein with structural homology to VEGF is the c-fos-induced growth factor (66), or VEGF-D (67,68). VEGF-D contains the eight conserved cysteine residues characteristic of the VEGF family and has a cysteine-rich C-terminal extension similar to VEGF-C. Like VEGF-C, VEGF-D binds to and activates VEGFRs -2 and -3 with affinities that depend on post-translational proteolytic processing (68). VEGF-D expression has been shown to increase in certain tumors and correlates with cancer metastasis, its expression often localized to the leading edge of a tumor (69).

The fourth and most recent addition to the VEGF family is VEGF-E (70,71), or ORFV2-VEGF (72). VEGF-E was identified in the genome of the Orf virus, a parapoxvirus that affects sheep, goats, and, occasionally, humans, causing highly vascular lesions. VEGF-E has 25% similarity to mammalian VEGF and contains the conserved eight cysteine residues characteristic of the VEGF family. VEGF-E binds to and activates VEGFR-2 but not VEGFR-1 or NRP-1. *In vitro*, VEGF-E is an endothelial cell mitogen and induces endothelial cell chemotaxis and sprouting. *In vivo*, VEGF-E induces angiogenesis and increases vascular permeability.

VEGFRs are expressed at low levels in many adult tissues and are upregulated in endothelial cells during development and in certain angiogenesis-associated or -dependent pathologic situations, including tumor growth. VEGFR-1–, -2–, and -3–deficient mice die *in utero* during midgestation. With respect to VEGFR-1, which binds VEGF, VEGF-B, and PlGF, homozygous, deficient mice form endothelial cells, but their assembly into vessels is severely perturbed, resulting in the formation of disorganized vascular channels (73). Surprisingly, this formation has been attributed to an increase in hemangioblast commitment and hence to the number of endothelial progenitors (74). Even more surprising, mutant mice containing a tyrosine kinase–deficient VEGFR-1 undergo normal vascular development (75), indicating that tyrosine phosphorylation is dispensable. These findings have led to the suggestion that VEGFR-1 may serve as a reservoir for VEGF, thereby regulating VEGF bioavailability. Whether this is the sole function of VEGFR-1 remains to be determined. In contrast, VEGFR-2–deficient mice die because of abortive development of endothelial cell and hematopoietic precursors (76). VEGFR-2 binds VEGF, VEGF-C, VEGF-D, and VEGF-E. VEGFR-3–deficient mice die from abnormal vascular remodeling and pericardial defects; vasculogenesis and angiogenesis appear to occur normally in these mice (77). Although the interaction of VEGFR-3 with VEGF-C has been implicated in lymphangiogenesis, VEGFR-3–null embryos die before the development of the lymphatic system, suggesting that VEGFR-3 signaling is also required for the remodeling and maturation of primary vascular networks into larger blood vessels. VEGFR-3 also binds VEGF-D. Finally, in addition to the three VEGFRs described earlier, VEGF, PlGF-2, and VEGF-E also have been shown to bind to NRP-1 (72,78,79), a receptor of the collapsin/semaphorin family that mediates neuronal guidance. NRP-1–deficient mice display central nervous system defects but die *in utero* from cardiac defects (80), whereas overexpression of NRP-1 in chimeric mice induces anomalies in the nervous and cardiovascular systems, including an increase in the number and size (dilatation) of blood vessels, as well as malformed hearts (81).

# TRANSFORMING GROWTH FACTOR-$\beta$

Three isoforms of TGF-$\beta$ have been described in mammals. TGF-$\beta$s achieve their biological effects through binding to cell surface receptors (T$\beta$Rs), designated types I, II, and III. The role of TGF-$\beta$s and their receptors in the maintenance of vascular integrity has been clearly established by genetic studies in humans and mice. This ligand–receptor pair appears to be required for capillary sprout maturation and for the maintenance of vessel wall integrity by promoting the recruitment and differentiation of pericytes and smooth muscle cells. Targeted disruption of the TGF-$\beta_1$ (82), T$\beta$RII (83), and endoglin/CD105 (84) genes results in defective pericyte and smooth muscle cell recruitment, resulting, in turn, in the formation of vessels with increased wall fragility. The phenotype of vessel wall fragility is similar to the vascular lesions that occur in patients with hereditary hemorrhagic telangiectasia (HHT), an autosomal dominant single gene disorder characterized by multisystemic vascular dysplasia and recurrent hemorrhage. The earliest detectable change in the telangiectatic

lesions is dilatation of postcapillary venules in the upper dermis; the endothelial cells themselves, including intercellular junctions, appear to be normal (85). The genes for HHT have been identified, leading to the definition of two HHT subtypes. The gene for HHT type I is endoglin (86), which displays regions of structural homology to betaglycan, the type III T$\beta$R. The gene for HHT type 2 is ALK-1 (87), a T$\beta$RI expressed at high levels in endothelial cells (88,89). In the TGF-$\beta$ receptor complex there are two classes of receptors T$\beta$RI and T$\beta$RII. T$\beta$RII receptors transphosphorylate type I receptors when the receptors have heterotetramerized into a complex of two T$\beta$RII and two T$\beta$RI molecules. There is only one type II receptor in mammals, whereas there are two type I receptors, ALK-1 and ALK-5, that are believed to influence the proangiogenic or antiangiogenic balance. ALK-5 favors resolution of angiogenesis, whereas ALK-1 activates angiogenesis (90). Therefore, TGF-$\beta$ may have a pro- or antiangiogenic response depending on its concentration and the responsiveness of its target tissues.

TGF-$\beta$ superfamily intracellular signals are transduced to the nucleus in part by the Smad family of proteins (91,92) that consists of three subfamilies; receptor-regulated or R-Smads, common-partner or Co-Smads, and inhibitory Smads or I-Smads. The phenotype of mice deficient in Smad5, an R-Smad, has been described (93,94). These mice die in midgestation and display a marked reduction in yolk sac vasculature. In addition, intraembryonic blood vessels are dilated and surrounded by decreased numbers of vascular smooth muscle cells. Smad5 has been primarily implicated in the transduction of signals of the bone morphogenetic protein pathway. However, the similarity between the phenotypes of TGF-$\beta_1$–, T$\beta$RII-, and Smad5-deficient mice suggests that Smad5 may also relay TGF-$\beta$– signals during vascular morphogenesis.

The pathogenesis of the vascular lesions seen in TGF-$\beta$– and T$\beta$R-deficient mice as well as in individuals with HHT is not known. Nonetheless, because TGF-$\beta$ induces the synthesis and assembly of the endothelial cell extracellular matrix (33), one of the consequences of defective T$\beta$R signaling may be the formation of structurally-incompetent basement membranes. It is striking that with respect to the vasculature, the phenotype of mice lacking either fibronectin or the $\alpha_5$ integrin subunit (95,96) closely mimics the phenotype of TGF-$\beta$– and T$\beta$R-deficient mice, particularly because TGF-$\beta_1$ has been shown to increase expression of fibronectin and its specific integrin, $\alpha_5\beta_1$ (33). It is also noteworthy that vascular lesions in HHT are well localized and that vascular integrity is maintained outside of the lesions; these factors suggest that some local event, possibly trauma, initiates vascular repair, which, in the case of patients with HHT, is defective. An additional and intriguing possibility comes from the observation that a similar phenotype of vessel dilatation and increased vessel wall fragility occurs in mice deficient in PDGF-B or platelet-derived growth factor receptor (PDGFR)-$\beta$, or in angiopoietin-1 (Ang-1) or Tie2 (see section, "Angiopoietins"). It is therefore possible that the absence of TGF-$\beta$ signaling in endothelial cells may result in or from defective signaling by other cytokine–receptor pair interactions.

# PLATELET-DERIVED GROWTH FACTOR

PDGFs are homodimers or heterodimers of A and B chains or homodimers of the more recently described C and D chains that exert their functions by interacting with two related RTKs, PDGFR-$\alpha$ and PDGFR-$\beta$ (97–100). During development, the *PDGF-B* gene is expressed in endothelial cells of arteries and unperfused capillary sprouts (101). In contrast, the *PDGFR-$\beta$* gene is expressed in the mesenchyme of presumptive smooth muscle cells and pericytes (102). The importance of the

to be necessary for formation of new patent blood vessels (111). The extracellular matrix also plays an active role in angiogenesis, on one hand, being a store for growth factors and, on the other, being degraded and remodeled by matrix metalloproteinases (MMPs) and other proteases, which also activate and release growth factors (143). To balance endogenous activators of angiogenesis, there are endogenous inhibitors of angiogenesis such as thrombospondin-1. The precise role of environmental factors in the regulation of lymphangiogenesis remains to be assessed. However, there are substantial differences between the two processes. The lack of expression of the angiogenic repertoire of MMPs during lymphangiogenesis, the lack of expression of ets-1 transcription factor (144), and the lack of inhibition of lymphangiogenesis by thrombospondin (145) are recently described examples.

Like most other biological processes, angiogenesis (and probably lymphaniogenesis) is the result of subtle and often complex interactions between molecules that have regulatory (e.g., cytokines and their receptors) and effector (e.g., extracellular matrix, integrins, and proteases) functions. Under conditions of normal homeostasis, endothelial cell turnover in the healthy adult organism is low, owing in part to the activation of TGF-$\beta$ after endothelial cell–perivascular cell contact. Perivascular cell adhesion and the maintenance of the differentiated phenotype is mediated by Ang-1. At the onset of angiogenesis, the local induction of Ang-2 expression in endothelial cells by signals such as hypoxia and VEGF inactivates the stabilizing effect of Ang-1, thereby promoting the loosening of endothelial–perivascular cell contacts (vessel wall disassembly) and allowing endothelial cells to respond to incoming angiogenic signals such as VEGF. The result is endothelial cell activation, proliferation, and migration, which lead subsequently to the formation of capillary sprouts. Important interactions occur with the extracellular matrix, and these are mediated by integral membrane proteins including integrins, which provide a link between the extracellular matrix and the cytoskeleton, as well as by extracellular proteases and their inhibitors, which mediate focal degradation of the extracellular matrix during cellular invasion. In the resolution phase of angiogenesis, a local decrease in Ang-2 expression, possibly mediated by increased TGF-$\beta$ activity, reestablishes the Ang-1 signal. Ang-1, in contrast to Ang-2, is constitutively expressed in many organs and promotes the recruitment of perivascular cells and the maturation of newly formed vessels (vessel wall assembly). Perivascular cell recruitment is also likely to be mediated by endothelial cell–derived cytokines such as TGF-$\beta$ and PDGF-BB. Although the precise role of the ephrins and their receptors in vascular morphogenesis and pattern formation remains to be established, initial observations (see the section, "Ephrins") have set the stage for an exciting period of research in this area that is likely to lead to major discoveries in the physiology and pathology of the normal and diseased vascular tree. The precise sequence of events during lymphangiogenesis remains to be established, and it is likely that although there may be similarities, there will also be important differences.

Although an enormous amount of progress has been made in identifying the factors that regulate blood vessel formation either positively or negatively, many important fundamental questions remain. A number of issues that merit further investigation are discussed below.

First, it is currently assumed that vasculogenesis, which includes the differentiation of angioblasts from the presumptive (but still elusive) hemangioblast, is limited to early development. However, the observation that circulating endothelial cell precursors/angioblasts contribute to new blood vessel formation in postnatal life (146–148) suggests that at least this phase of vasculogenesis persists in the adult. From a mechanistic point of view, these findings suggest that our current definition of angiogenesis will have to be extended to account

for the inclusion of circulating angioblasts into newly forming vessels. From a therapeutic point of view, the existence of circulating precursors may have important implications both for stimulation and inhibition of angiogenesis (149).

Second, it is possible that endothelial cells are "sensors" of hypoxia in the intact organism. However, are endothelial cells, which are in constant contact with circulating blood, ever exposed to conditions of hypoxia? At least two pieces of evidence support the hypothesis that endothelial cells can, in fact, sense hypoxia *in vivo*. First, mice exposed to systemic hypoxia upregulate VEGFR-1 in endothelial cells in the lung, heart, brain, kidney, and liver (150), and hypoxia-responsive elements are known to be present in the VEGFR-1 promoter. Second, high levels of hypoxia-inducible factor (HIF)-1$\alpha$ protein have been detected in endothelial cells in hypoxic ferret lung; HIF-1$\alpha$ was undetectable in normoxic lungs (151). HIF-1$\alpha$ is a transcription factor expressed in response to hypoxia; regulation appears to be at the level of protein stabilization rather than transcription.

Third, we are entering an era in which a genetic approach to understanding the pathogenesis of vascular disorders (152) requires identification of mutations in endothelial cell RTKs (e.g., VEGFRs, TGF-$\beta$Rs, PDGFRs, Ties, and EphA receptors) and other molecules involved in new blood vessel formation. Mutations in these receptors are expected to be important in the pathogenesis of vascular malformations and may play a role in the development of chronic vasoproliferative disorders such as cancer, arthritis, and retinopathy, which are likely to be multigenic in origin. It is also possible that increased susceptibility or predisposition to some of these chronic disorders is linked to a genetically based proangiogenic state that results from increased activity of positive regulators (i.e., angiogenic factors and receptors) or decreased activity of inhibitors. With respect to the pathogenesis of vascular malformations, a clear relation has been established between mutations in the following molecules and the associated clinical condition: Tie2 and venous malformations, TGF-$\beta$ and HHT, and VEGFR-3 and lymphedema.

Finally, increased understanding of the mechanisms of angiogenesis, lymphangiogenesis, and vessel wall formation has opened up novel and exciting therapeutic opportunities, and considerable benefit can be envisaged in the clinical setting in the future from manipulating angiogenesis, either positively or negatively (see Table 44-5). Extensive clinical evaluation of novel therapeutic strategies will require testing in multicenter

---

## TABLE 44-5

MANIPULATION OF ANGIOGENESIS IN THE CLINIC

### STIMULATION OF ANGIOGENESIS
Induction of collateral vessel formation:

  Myocardial ischemia (i.e., coronary artery disease)
  Peripheral ischemia (i.e., peripheral arterial occlusive disease)
  Cerebral ischemia (i.e., cerebral vascular disease)

Wound healing and fracture repair
Reconstructive surgery: skin flaps
Organ transplantation (e.g., islets of Langerhans)

### INHIBITION OF ANGIOGENESIS
Tumor growth and metastasis
Ocular neovascularization
Hemangioma
Rheumatoid arthritis
Psoriasis
Atherosclerotic plaque neovascularization
Birth control?

trials. It also will be important to develop animal models that are relevant to angiogenesis-associated diseases that could be exploited in the search for novel therapeutic strategies. The current explosion in the field of angiogenesis, lymphangiogenesis, and vascular morphogenesis will undoubtedly ensure that we move rapidly to attain these objectives.

# References

1. Flamme I, Frolich T, Risau W. Molecular mechanisms of vasculogenesis and embryonic angiogenesis. *J Cell Physiol* 1997;173:206–210.
2. Risau W. Mechanisms of angiogenesis. *Nature* 1997;386:671–674.
3. Burri PH. Intussusceptive microvascular growth, a new mechanism of capillary network formation. *EXS* 1992;61:32–39.
4. Folkman J. Clinical applications of research on angiogenesis. *N Engl J Med* 1995;333:1757–1763.
5. Pepper MS. Manipulating angiogenesis: from basic science to the bedside. *Arterioscler Thromb Vasc Biol* 1997;17:605–619.
6. Folkman J. Tumor angiogenesis. *Adv Cancer Res* 1974;19:331–358.
7. Holmgren L, O'Reilly MS, Folkman J. Dormancy of micrometastases: balanced proliferation and apoptosis in the presence of angiogenesis suppression. *Nat Med* 1995;1:149–153.
8. O'Reilly MS, Holmgren L, Chen C, et al. Angiostatin induces and sustains dormancy of human primary tumors in mice. *Nat Med* 1996;2:689–692.
9. Witte MH, Way DL, Witte CL, et al. Lymphangiogenesis: mechanisms, significance and clinical implications. *EXS* 1997;79:65–112.
10. Witte MH, Bernas MJ, Martin CP, et al. Lymphangiogenesis and lymphangiodysplasia: from molecular to clinical lymphology. *Microsc Res Tech* 2001;55:122–145.
11. Skobe M, Detmar M. Structure, function, and molecular control of the skin lymphatic system. *J Investig Dermatol Symp Proc* 2000;5:14–19.
12. Casley-Smith JR, Florey HW. The structure of normal small lymphatics. *Q J Exp Physiol Cogn Med Sci* 1961;46:101–106.
13. Leak LV. Electron microscopic observations on lymphatic capillaries and the structural components of the connective tissue-lymph interface. *Microvasc Res* 1970;2:361–391.
14. Leak LV, Burke JF. Fine structure of the lymphatic capillary and the adjoining connective tissue area. *Am J Anat* 1966;118:785–809.
15. Ryan TJ, Mortimer PS, Jones RL. Lymphatics of the skin. Neglected but important. *Int J Dermatol* 1986;25:411–419.
16. Sleeman JP, Krishnan J, Kirkin V, et al. Markers for the lymphatic endothelium: in search of the holy grail? *Microsc Res Tech* 2001;55:61–69.
17. Partanen TA, Alitalo K, Miettinen M. Lack of lymphatic vascular specificity of vascular endothelial growth factor receptor 3 in 185 vascular tumors. *Cancer* 1999;86:2406–2412.
18. Valtola R, Salven P, Heikkila P, et al. VEGFR-3 and its ligand VEGF-C are associated with angiogenesis in breast cancer. *Am J Pathol* 1999;154:1381–1390.
19. Breiteneder-Geleff S, Soleiman A, Kowalski H, et al. Angiosarcomas express mixed endothelial phenotypes of blood and lymphatic capillaries: podoplanin as a specific marker for lymphatic endothelium. *Am J Pathol* 1999;154:385–394.
20. Banerji S, Ni J, Wang SX, et al. LYVE-1, a new homologue of the CD44 glycoprotein, is a lymph-specific receptor for hyaluronan. *J Cell Biol* 1999;144:789–801.
21. Wigle JT, Oliver G. Prox1 function is required for the development of the murine lymphatic system. *Cell* 1999;98:769–778.
22. Nibbs RJ, Kriehuber E, Ponath PD, et al. The beta-chemokine receptor D6 is expressed by lymphatic endothelium and a subset of vascular tumors. *Am J Pathol* 2001;158:867–877.
23. Linehan SA, Martinez-Pomares L, da Silva RP, et al. Endogenous ligands of carbohydrate recognition domains of the mannose receptor in murine macrophages, endothelial cells and secretory cells; potential relevance to inflammation and immunity. *Eur J Immunol* 2001;31:1857–1866.
24. Bouck N. Tumor angiogenesis: the role of oncogenes and tumor suppressor genes. *Cancer Cells* 1990;2:179–185.
25. Hanahan D, Folkman J. Patterns and emerging mechanisms of the angiogenic switch during tumorigenesis. *Cell* 1996;86:353–364.
26. Nathan C, Sporn M. Cytokines in context. *J Cell Biol* 1991;113:981–986.
27. Dvorak HF, Nagy JA, Feng D, et al. Vascular permeability factor/vascular endothelial growth factor and the significance of microvascular hyperpermeability in angiogenesis. *Curr Top Microbiol Immunol* 1999;237:97–132.
28. Ferrara N. Vascular endothelial growth factor: molecular and biological aspects. *Curr Top Microbiol Immunol* 1999;237:1–30.
29. Veikkola T, Alitalo K. VEGFs, receptors and angiogenesis. *Semin Cancer Biol* 1999;9:211–220.
30. Pepper MS, Mandriota SJ, Vassalli JD, et al. Angiogenesis regulating cytokines: activities and interactions. Attempts to understand metastasis formation. *Curr Top Microbiol Immunol* 1996;213:31–67.
31. Christofori G. The role of fibroblast growth factors in tumour progression and angiogenesis. In: Bicknell R, Lewis CE, Ferrara N, eds. *Tumour angiogenesis*, New York: Oxford University Press, 1997:201–237.
32. Lindahl P, Hellström M, Kalén M, et al. Endothelial-perivascular cell signalling in vascular development: lessons from knockout mice. *Curr Opin Lipidol* 1998;9:407–411.
33. Pepper MS. Transforming growth factor-beta: vasculogenesis, angiogenesis and vessel wall integrity. *Cytokine Growth Factor Res* 1997;8:21–43.
34. Davis S, Yancopoulos GD. The angiopoietins: yin and yang in angiogenesis. *Curr Top Microbiol Immunol* 1999;237:173–185.
35. Gale NW, Yancopoulos GD. Growth factors acting via endothelial cell-specific receptor tyrosine kinases: VEGFs, angiopoietins, and ephrins in vascular development. *Genes Dev* 1999;13:1055–1066.
36. Oh SJ, Jeltsch MM, Birkenhager R, et al. VEGF and VEGF-C: specific induction of angiogenesis and lymphangiogenesis in the differentiated avian chorioallantoic membrane. *Dev Biol* 1997;188:96–109.
37. Kubo H, Cao R, Brakenhielm E, et al. Blockade of vascular endothelial growth factor receptor-3 signaling inhibits fibroblast growth factor-2-induced lymphangiogenesis in mouse cornea. *Proc Natl Acad Sci U S A* 2002;99:8868–8873.
38. Jeltsch M, Kaipainen A, Joukov V, et al. Hyperplasia of lymphatic vessels in VEGF-C transgenic mice. *Science* 1997;276:1423–1425.
39. Gale NW, Thurston G, Hackett SF, et al. Angiopoietin-2 is required for postnatal angiogenesis and lymphatic patterning, and only the latter role is rescued by Angiopoietin-1. *Dev Cell* 2002;3:411–423.
40. Yuan L, Moyon D, Pardanaud L, et al. Abnormal lymphatic vessel development in neuropilin 2 mutant mice. *Development* 2002;129:4797–4806.
41. Straume O, Jackson DG, Akslen LA. Independent prognostic impact of lymphatic vessel density and presence of low-grade lymphangiogenesis in cutaneous melanoma. *Clin Cancer Res* 2003;9:250–256.
42. Benjamin LE, Hemo I, Keshet E. A plasticity window for blood vessel remodelling is defined by pericyte coverage of the preformed endothelial network and is regulated by PDGF-B and VEGF. *Development* 1998;125:1591–1598.
43. Benjamin LE, Golijanin D, Itin A, et al. Selective ablation of immature blood vessels in established human tumors follows vascular endothelial growth factor withdrawal. *J Clin Invest* 1999;103:159–165.
44. Breier G, Risau W. The role of vascular endothelial growth factor in blood vessel formation. *Trends Cell Biol* 1996;6:454–456.
45. Thomas KA. Vascular endothelial growth factor, a potent and selective angiogenic agent. *J Biol Chem* 1996;271:603–606.
46. Ferrara N, Chen H, Davis-Smyth T, et al. Vascular endothelial growth factor is essential for corpus luteum angiogenesis. *Nat Med* 1998;4:336–340.
47. Gerber HP, Hillan KJ, Ryan AM, et al. VEGF is required for growth and survival in neonatal mice. *Development* 1999;126:1149–1159.
48. Carmeliet P, Ferreira V, Breier G, et al. Abnormal blood vessel development and lethality in embryos lacking a single VEGF allele. *Nature* 1996;380:435–439.
49. Ferrara N, Carver-Moore K, Chen H, et al. Heterozygous embryonic lethality induced by targeted inactivation of the VEGF gene. *Nature* 1996;380:439–442.
50. Olofsson B, Pajusola K, Kaipainen A, et al. Vascular endothelial growth factor B, a novel growth factor for endothelial cells. *Proc Natl Acad Sci U S A* 1996;93:2576–2581.
51. Grimmond S, Lagercrantz J, Drinkwater C, et al. Cloning and characterization of a novel human gene related to vascular endo-thelial growth factor. *Genome Res* 1996;6:124–131.
52. Makinen T, Olofsson B, Karpanen T, et al. Differential binding of vascular endothelial growth factor B splice and proteolytic isoforms to neuropilin-1. *J Biol Chem* 1999;274:21217–21222.
53. Olofsson B, Korpelainen E, Pepper MS, et al. Vascular endothelial growth factor B (VEGF-B) binds to VEGF receptor-1 and regulates plasminogen activator activity in endothelial cells. *Proc Natl Acad Sci U S A* 1998;95:11709–11714.
54. Silvestre JS, Tamarat R, Ebrahimian TG, et al. Vascular endothelial growth factor-B promotes *in vivo* angiogenesis. *Circ Res* 2003;93:114–123.
55. Li X, Aase K, Li H, et al. Isoform-specific expression of VEGF-B in normal tissues and tumors. *Growth Factors* 2001;19:49–59.
56. Mould AW, Tonks ID, Cahill MM, et al. Vegfb gene knockout mice display reduced pathology and synovial angiogenesis in both antigen-induced and collagen-induced models of arthritis. *Arthritis Rheum* 2003;48:2660–2669.
57. Joukov V, Pajusola K, Kaipainen A, et al. A novel vascular endothelial growth factor, VEGF-C, is a ligand for the Flt4 (VEGFR-3) and KDR (VEGFR-2) receptor tyrosine kinases [Erratum appears in *EMBO J* 1996;15:1751]. *EMBO J* 1996;15:290–298.
58. Lee J, Gray A, Yuan J, et al. Vascular endothelial growth factor–related protein: a ligand and specific activator of the tyrosine kinase receptor FLT4. *Proc Natl Acad Sci U S A* 1996;93:1988–1992.
59. Fitz LJ, Morris JC, Towler P, et al. Characterization of murine Flt4 ligand/VEGF-C. *Oncogene* 1997;15:613–618.
60. Hu JS, Hastings GA, Cherry S, et al. A novel regulatory function of proteolytically cleaved VEGF-2 for vascular endothelial and smooth muscle cells. *FASEB J* 1997;11:498–504.
61. Joukov V, Sorsa T, Kumar V, et al. Proteolytic processing regulates receptor specificity and activity of VEGF-C. *EMBO J* 1997;16:3898–3911.
62. Kukk E, Lymboussaki A, Taira S, et al. VEGF-C receptor binding and pattern of expression with VEGFR-3 suggests a role in lymphatic vascular development. *Development* 1996;122:3829–3837.

63. Cao Y, Linden P, Farnebo J, et al. Vascular endothelial growth factor C induces angiogenesis *in vivo*. *Proc Natl Acad Sci U S A* 1998;95: 14389–14394.

64. Witzenbichler B, Asahara T, Murohara T, et al. Vascular endothelial growth factor-C (VEGF-C/VEGF-2) promotes angiogenesis in the setting of tissue ischemia. *Am J Pathol* 1998;153:381–394.

65. Pepper MS, Mandriota SJ, Jeltsch M, et al. Vascular endothelial growth factor (VEGF)-C synergises with basic fibroblast growth factor and VEGF in the induction of angiogenesis *in vitro*, and alters endothelial cell proteolytic properties. *J Cell Physiol* 1998;177:439–452.

66. Orlandini M, Marconcini L, Ferruzzi R, et al. Identification of a c-*fos*-induced gene that is related to the platelet-derived growth factor/vascular endothelial growth factor family. *Proc Natl Acad Sci U S A* 1996;93: 11675–11680.

67. Yamada Y, Nezu J, Shimane M, et al. Molecular cloning of a novel vascular endothelial growth factor, VEGF-D. *Genomics* 1997;42:483–488.

68. Achen MG, Jeltsch M, Kukk E, et al. Vascular endothelial growth factor D (VEGF-D) is a ligand for the tyrosine kinases VEGF receptor 2 (Flk1) and VEGF receptor 3 (Flt4). *Proc Natl Acad Sci U S A* 1998;95: 548–553.

69. Onogawa S, Kitadai Y, Tanaka S, et al. Expression of VEGF-C and VEGF-D at the invasive edge correlates with lymph node metastasis and prognosis of patients with colorectal carcinoma. *Cancer Sci* 2004;95:32–39.

70. Ogawa S, Oku A, Sawano A, et al. A novel type of vascular endothelial growth factor, VEGF-E (NZ-7 VEGF), preferentially utilizes KDR/Flk-1 receptor and carries a potent mitotic activity without heparin-binding domain. *J Biol Chem* 1998;273:31273–31282.

71. Meyer M, Clauss M, Lepple-Wienhues A, et al. A novel vascular endothelial growth factor encoded by Orf virus, VEGF-E, mediates angiogenesis via signalling through VEGFR-2 (KDR) but not VEGFR-1 (Flt-1) receptor tyrosine kinases. *EMBO J* 1999;18:363–374.

72. Wise LM, Veikkola T, Mercer AA, et al. Vascular endothelial growth factor (VEGF)–like protein from Orf virus NZ2 binds to VEGFR2 and neuropilin-1. *Proc Natl Acad Sci U S A* 1999;96:3071–3076.

73. Fong GH, Rossant J, Gertsenstein M, et al. Role of the Flt-1 receptor tyrosine kinase in regulating the assembly of vascular endothelium. *Nature* 1995;376:66–70.

74. Fong GH, Zhang L, Bryce DM, et al. Increased hemangioblast commitment, not vascular disorganization, is the primary defect in Flt-1 knockout mice. *Development* 1999;126:3015–3025.

75. Hiratsuka S, Minowa O, Kuno J, et al. Flt-1 lacking the tyrosine kinase domain is sufficient for normal development and angiogenesis in mice. *Proc Natl Acad Sci U S A* 1998;95:9349–9354.

76. Shalaby F, Rossant J, Yamaguchi TP, et al. Failure of blood-island formation and vasculogenesis in Flk-1-deficient mice. *Nature* 1995;376:62–66.

77. Dumont DJ, Jussila L, Taipale J, et al. Cardiovascular failure in mouse embryos deficient in VEGF receptor-3. *Science* 1998;282:946–949.

78. Soker S, Takashima S, Miao HQ, et al. Neuropilin-1 is expressed by endothelial and tumor cells as an isoform-specific receptor for vascular endothelial growth factor. *Cell* 1998;92:735–745.

79. Migdal M, Huppertz B, Tessler S, et al. Neuropilin-1 is a placenta growth factor-2 receptor. *J Biol Chem* 1998;273:22272–22278.

80. Kitsukawa T, Shimizu M, Sanbo M, et al. Neuropilin-semaphorin III/D–mediated chemorepulsive signals play a crucial role in peripheral nerve projection in mice. *Neuron* 1997;19:995–1005.

81. Kitsukawa T, Shimono A, Kawakami A, et al. Overexpression of a membrane protein, neuropilin, in chimeric mice causes anomalies in the cardiovascular system, nervous system and limbs. *Development* 1995;121: 4309–4318.

82. Dickson MC, Martin JS, Cousins FM, et al. Defective haematopoiesis and vasculogenesis in transforming growth factor-1 knock out mice. *Development* 1995;121:1845–1854.

83. Oshima M, Oshima H, Taketo MM. TGF-β receptor type II deficiency results in defects of yolk sac hematopoiesis and vasculogenesis. *Dev Biol* 1996;179:297–302.

84. Li DY, Sorensen LK, Brooke BS, et al. Defective angiogenesis in mice lacking endoglin. *Science* 1999;284:1534–1537.

85. Guttmacher AE, Marchuk DA, White RI. Hereditary hemorrhagic telangiectasia. *N Engl J Med* 1995;333:918–924.

86. McAllister KA, Grogg KM, Johnson DW, et al. Endoglin, a TGF-binding protein of endothelial cells, is the gene for hereditary haemorrhagic telangiectasia type 1. *Nat Genet* 1994;8:345–351.

87. Johnson DW, Berg JN, Baldwin MA, et al. Mutations in the activin receptor-like kinase 1 gene in hereditary haemorrhagic telangiectasia type 2. *Nat Genet* 1996;13:189–195.

88. Attisano L, Carcamo J, Ventura F, et al. Identification of human activin and TGF β type I receptors that form heteromeric kinase complexes with type II receptors. *Cell* 1993;75:671–680.

89. Roelen BA, van Rooijen MA, Mummery CL. Expression of ALK-1, a type 1 serine/threonine kinase receptor, coincides with sites of vasculogenesis and angiogenesis in early mouse development. *Dev Dyn* 1997;209:418–430.

90. Goumans MJ, Lebrin F, Valdimarsdottir G. Controlling the angiogenic switch: a balance between two distinct TGF-b receptor signaling pathways. *Trends Cardiovasc Med* 2003;13:301–307.

91. Christian JL, Nakayama T. Can't get no SMADisfaction: smad proteins as positive and negative regulators of TGF-β family signals. *BioEssays* 1999; 21:382–390.

92. Kawabata M, Miyazono K. Signal transduction of the TGF-beta superfamily by Smad proteins. *J Biol Chem* 1999;125:9–16.

93. Chang H, Huylebroeck D, Verschueren K, et al. Smad5 knockout mice die at mid-gestation due to multiple embryonic and extraembryonic defects. *Development* 1999;126:1631–1642.

94. Yang X, Castilla LH, Xu X, et al. Angiogenesis defects and mesenchymal apoptosis in mice lacking SMAD5. *Development* 1999;126:1571–1580.

95. Yang JT, Rayburn H, Hynes RO. Embryonic mesodermal defects in alpha 5 integrin–deficient mice. *Development* 1993;119:1093–1105.

96. George EL, Georges-Labouesse EN, Patel-King RS, et al. Defects in mesoderm, neural tube and vascular development in mouse embryos lacking fibronectin. *Development* 1993;119:1079–1091.

97. Rosenkranz S, Kazlauskas A. Evidence for distinct signalling properties and biological responses induced by the PDGF receptor alpha and beta subtypes. *Growth Factors* 1999;16:201–216.

98. Gilbertson DG, Duff ME, West JW, et al. Platelet-derived growth factor C (PDGF-C), a novel growth factor that binds to PDGF alpha and beta receptor. *J Biol Chem* 2001;276:27406–27414.

99. LaRochelle WJ, Jeffers M, McDonald WF, et al. PDGF-D, a new protease-activated growth factor. *Nat Cell Biol* 2001;3:517–521.

100. Li X, Eriksson U. Novel PDGF family members: PDGF-C and PDGF-D. *Cytokine Growth Factor Rev* 2003;14:91–98.

101. Lindahl P, Johansson BR, Levéen P, et al. Pericyte loss and microaneurysm formation in PDGF-B-deficient mice. *Science* 1997;277:242–245.

102. Crosby JR, Seifert RA, Soriano P, et al. Chimaeric analysis reveals role of PDGF receptors in all muscle lineages. *Nat Genet* 1998;18:385–388.

103. Levéen P, Pekny M, Gebre-Medhin S, et al. Mice deficient for PDGF B show renal, cardiovascular, and hematological abnormalities. *Genes Dev* 1994;8:1875–1887.

104. Soriano P. Abnormal kidney development and hematological disorders in PDGF β-receptor mutant mice. *Genes Dev* 1994;8:1888–1896.

105. Hellström M, Kalén M, Lindahl P, et al. Role of PDGF-B and PDGFR-beta in recruitment of vascular smooth muscle cells and pericytes during embryonic blood vessel formation in the mouse. *Development* 1999;126: 3047–3055.

106. Daniel TO, Gibbs VC, Milfay DF, et al. Agents that increase cAMP accumulation block endothelial c-*sis* induction by thrombin and transforming growth factor-β. *J Biol Chem* 1987;262:11893–11896.

107. Starksen NF, Harsh GR, Gibbs VC, et al. Regulated expression of the platelet-derived growth factor A chain gene in microvascular endothelial cells. *J Biol Chem* 1987;262:14381–14384.

108. Kavanaugh WM, Harsh GR, Starksen NF, et al. Transcriptional regulation of the A and B chains of platelet-derived growth factor in microvascular endothelial cells. *J Biol Chem* 1988;263:8470–8472.

109. Gronwald RGK, Seifert RA, Bowen-Pope DF. Differential regulation of expression of two platelet-derived growth factor receptor subunits by transforming growth factor-β. *J Biol Chem* 1989;264:8120–8125.

110. Battegay EJ, Raines EW, Seifert RA, et al. TGF-β induces bimodal proliferation of connective tissue cells via complex control of an autocrine PDGF loop. *Cell* 1990;63:515–524.

111. Cao R, Brakenhielm E, Pawliuk R, et al. Angiogenic synergism, vascular stability and improvement of hind-limb ischemia by a combination of PDGF-BB and FGF-2. *Nat Med* 2003;9:604–613.

112. Davis S, Aldrich TH, Jones PF, et al. Isolation of angiopoietin-1, a ligand for the TIE2 receptor, by secretion-trap expression cloning. *Cell* 1996;87: 1161–1169.

113. Suri C, Jones PF, Patan S, et al. Requisite role of angiopoietin-1, a ligand for the TIE2 receptor, during embryonic angiogenesis. *Cell* 1996;87:1171–1180.

114. Koblizek TI, Weiss C, Yancopoulos GD, et al. Angiopoietin-1 induces sprouting angiogenesis *in vitro*. *Curr Biol* 1998;8:529–532.

115. Maisonpierre PC, Suri C, Jones PF, et al. Angiopoietin-2, a natural antagonist for Tie2 that disrupts *in vivo* angiogenesis. *Science* 1997;277:55–60.

116. Stratmann A, Risau W, Plate KH. Cell type-specific expression of angiopoietin-1 and angiopoietin-2 suggests a role in glioblastoma angiogenesis. *Am J Pathol* 1998;153:1459–1466.

117. Mandriota SJ, Pepper MS. Regulation of angiopoietin-2 mRNA levels in bovine microvascular endothelial cells by cytokines and hypoxia. *Circ Res* 1998;83:852–859.

118. Oh H, Takagi H, Suzuma K, et al. Hypoxia and vascular endothelial growth factor selectively up-regulate angiopoietin-2 in bovine microvascular endothelial cells. *J Biol Chem* 1999;274:15732–15739.

119. Asahara T, Chen D, Takahashi T, et al. Tie2 receptor ligands, angiopoietin-1 and angiopoietin-2, modulate VEGF-induced postnatal neovascularization. *Circ Res* 1998;83:233–240.

120. Hanahan D. Signaling vascular morphogenesis and maintenance. *Science* 1997;277:48–50.

121. Puri MC, Rossant J, Alitalo K, et al. The receptor tyrosine kinase TIE is required for integrity and survival of vascular endothelial cells. *EMBO J* 1995;14:5884–5891.

122. Sato TN, Tozawa Y, Deutsch U, et al. Distinct roles of the receptor tyrosine kinases Tie-1 and Tie-2 in blood vessel formation. *Nature* 1995;367: 70–74.

123. Dumont DJ, Gradwohl G, Fong GH, et al. Dominant-negative and targeted null mutations in the endothelial receptor tyrosine kinase, tek, reveal a critical role in vasculogenesis of the embryo. *Genes Dev* 1994;8:1897–1909.

124. Vikkula M, Boon LM, Carraway KL, et al. Vascular dysmorphogenesis caused by an activating mutation in the receptor tyrosine kinase TIE2. *Cell* 1996;87:1181–1190.

125. Folkman J, D'Amore PA. Blood vessel formation: what is its molecular basis? *Cell* 1996;87:1153–1155.

126. Hirschi KK, Rohovsky SA, D'Amore PA. PDGF, TGF-beta, and heterotypic cell-cell interactions mediate endothelial cell-induced recruitment of 10T1/2 cells and their differentiation to a smooth muscle fate [published erratum in *J Cell Biol* 1998;141:1287]. *J Cell Biol* 1998;141:805–814.

127. Hirschi KK, Rohovsky SA, Beck LH, et al. Endothelial cells modulate the proliferation of mural cell precursors via platelet-derived growth factor-BB and heterotypic cell contact. *Circ Res* 1999;84:298–305.

128. Abramovitch R, Neeman M, Reich R, et al. Intercellular communication between vascular smooth muscle and endothelial cells mediated by heparin-binding epidermal growth factor-like growth factor and vascular endothelial growth factor. *FEBS Lett* 1998;425:441–447.

129. Holder N, Klein R. Eph receptors and ephrins: effectors of morphogenesis. *Development* 1999;126:2033–2044.

130. Holzman LB, Marks RM, Dixit VM. A novel immediate-early response gene of endothelium is induced by cytokines and encodes a secreted protein. *Mol Cell Biol* 1990;10:5830–5838.

131. Pandey A, Shao H, Marks RM, et al. Role of B61, the ligand for the Eck receptor tyrosine kinase, in TNF-alpha–induced angiogenesis. *Science* 1995;268:567–569.

132. Daniel TO, Stein E, Cerretti DP, et al. ELK and LERK-2 in developing kidney and microvascular endothelial assembly. *Kidney Int* 1996;(Suppl. 57):73–81.

133. Flenniken AM, Gale NW, Yancopoulos GD, et al. Distinct and overlapping expression patterns of ligands for Eph-related receptor tyrosine kinases during mouse embryogenesis. *Dev Biol* 1996;179:382–401.

134. McBride JL, Ruiz JC. Ephrin-A1 is expressed at sites of vascular development in the mouse. *Mech Dev* 1998;77:201–204.

135. Cheng N, Brantley DM, Liu H, et al. Blockade of EphA receptor tyrosine kinase activation inhibits vascular endothelial cell growth factor-induced angiogenesis. *Mol Cancer Res* 2002;1:2–11.

136. Wang HU, Chen ZF, Anderson DJ. Molecular distinction and angiogenic interaction between embryonic arteries and veins revealed by ephrin-B2 and its receptor EphB4. *Cell* 1998;93:741–753.

137. Adams RH, Wilkinson GA, Weiss C, et al. Roles of ephrinB ligands and EphB receptors in cardiovascular development: demarcation of arterial/venous domains, vascular morphogenesis, and sprouting angiogenesis. *Genes Dev* 1999;13:295–306.

138. Stein E, Lane AA, Cerretti DP, et al. Eph receptors discriminate specific ligand oligomers to determine alternative signaling complexes, attachment, and assembly responses. *Genes Dev* 1998;12:667–678.

139. Huynh-Do U, Stein E, Lane AA, et al. Surface densities of ephrin-B1 determine EphB1-coupled activation of cell attachment through alphavbeta3 and alpha5beta1 integrins. *EMBO J* 1999;18:2165–2173.

140. Arras M, Ito WD, Scholz D, et al. Monocyte activation in angiogenesis and collateral growth in the rabbit hindlimb. *J Clin Invest* 1998;101:40–50.

141. Wolf C, Cai WJ, Vosschulte R, et al. Vascular remodeling and altered protein expression during growth of coronary collateral arteries. *J Mol Cell Cardiol* 1998;30:2291–2305.

142. Ferrara N. Vascular endothelial growth factor: basic science and clinical progress. *Endocr Rev* 2004;25:581–611.

143. Pepper MS. Role of the matrix metalloproteinase and plasminogen activator-plasmin systems in angiogenesis. *Arterioscler Thromb Vasc Biol* 2001;21:1104–1117.

144. Wernert N, Okuducu AF, Pepper MS. Ets 1 is expressed in capillary blood vessels but not in lymphatics. *J Pathol* 2003;200:561–567.

145. Hawighorst T, Oura H, Streit M, et al. Thrombospondin-1 selectively inhibits early-stage carcinogenesis and angiogenesis but not tumor lymphangiogenesis and lymphatic metastasis in transgenic mice. *Oncogene* 2002;21:7945–7956.

146. Asahara T, Murohara T, Sullivan A, et al. Isolation of putative progenitor endothelial cells for angiogenesis. *Science* 1997;275:964–967.

147. Shi Q, Rafii S, Wu MH, et al. Evidence for circulating bone marrow–derived endothelial cells. *Blood* 1998;92:362–367.

148. Takahashi T, Kalka C, Masuda H, et al. Ischemia- and cytokine-induced mobilization of bone marrow–derived endothelial progenitor cells for neovascularization. *Nat Med* 1999;5:434–438.

149. Isner JM, Asahara T. Angiogenesis and vasculogenesis as therapeutic strategies for postnatal neovascularization. *J Clin Invest* 1999;103:1231–1236.

150. Marti HH, Risau W. Systemic hypoxia changes the organ-specific distribution of vascular endothelial growth factor and its receptors. *Proc Natl Acad Sci U S A* 1998;95:15809–15814.

151. Yu AY, Frid MG, Shimoda LA, et al. Temporal, spatial, and oxygen-regulated expression of hypoxia-inducible factor-1 in the lung. *Am J Physiol* 1998;275:L818–L826.

152. Shovlin CL, Scott J. Inherited diseases of the vasculature. *Annu Rev Physiol* 1996;58:483–507.

# CHAPTER 45 ■ MONOCYTE–PLATELET–ENDOTHELIAL INTERACTIONS

**KLAUS LEY**

Interactions between monocytes, platelets, and endothelial cells are intimately involved with and of key importance for the regulation of hemostasis, thrombosis, inflammation, and atherosclerosis. Although other cells such as neutrophils and T lymphocytes participate, the monocyte–platelet–endothelial cell axis has emerged as a predominant factor in vascular disease and thrombosis. This chapter introduces the molecular basis of the adhesive interactions among the three cell types; explores the cross talk between hemostasis, thrombosis, and inflammation; and discusses the pathophysiologic significance of these cell–cell interactions with an emphasis on vascular disease.

## CELLULAR AND MOLECULAR BASIS

### Monocytes

Monocytes are myeloid cells produced in the bone marrow. Although originally thought to be a homogeneous population, it has become clear that in human and mouse blood, at least two and probably more subpopulations of monocytes exist (1,2). One type is characterized by a more inflammatory phenotype, whereas the other type may be a precursor for tissue-resident macrophages and dendritic cells, which are the most important antigen-presenting cells of the immune system. It is not known whether only "inflammatory" monocytes or "resident-type" monocytes, or both interact with platelets and endothelial cells, but both types express molecules that would support such interactions (see Table 45-1).

Monocytes communicate with endothelial cells and platelets through the engagement of adhesion molecules, chemokine receptors, and cytokine receptors. Most adhesion molecules are integral transmembrane cell surface molecules that can bind the same (homotypic) or other cell surface molecules (heterotypic) or molecules in the extracellular matrix. Most adhesion molecules provide mechanical strength to the interaction between cells by mechanically linking the extracellular environment to the intracellular cytoskeleton through reversible interactions. Many, if not all, cell adhesion molecules also transduce signals into the cells upon engagement by extracellular ligand.

### Monocyte Adhesion Molecules

**Integrins.** Integrins are transmembrane $\alpha\beta$ heterodimers that bind many extracellular matrix proteins and certain immunoglobulinlike adhesion molecules on other cells (3,4). Most integrins require conformational activation to support binding. The mechanisms of integrin activation have been studied in detail for $\alpha_V\beta_3$ (5), an integrin also expressed on monocytes, and lymphocyte function-associated antigen (LFA)-1 (6), an integrin highly expressed on monocytes and other leukocytes. Integrin

activation is probably initiated by placing the head domain of the intracellular cytoskeletal adaptor molecule talin between the integrin $\alpha$ and $\beta$ chains (7), which causes a switchbladelike opening of the extracellular domain that exposes the ligand binding site (see Fig. 45-1A). This process is called inside-out signaling, because the change in the extracellular domain of the integrin is brought about by intracellular processes. The mechanism of activation-induced conformational change is thought to apply fairly generally to many, if not all, integrins (4). In addition, integrins can also rearrange in the plasma membrane to cluster and form patches, which results in enhanced binding (Fig. 45-1B). This rearrangement and clustering results in increased ligand binding and is called avidity change. It does not result in increased affinity for monovalent ligand (8). Under *in vivo* conditions, cell activation probably results in a combination of integrin affinity and avidity increase. Although this can be tested by looking at monovalent versus polyvalent ligand binding, the role of avidity and affinity regulation remains controversial (4,8,9). A third possibility suggests that integrins may undergo some conformational change through inside-out signaling, followed by ligand binding, which then causes outside-in signaling that leads to full activation and strong binding (9,10) (Fig. 45-1C).

Of the 24 known integrins, mature blood monocytes express only a few. The most abundant monocyte integrin is $\alpha_4\beta_1$ integrin, or VLA-4 (CD49d/CD29). It is composed of a 150-kDa $\alpha_4$ chain that can undergo proteolytic cleavage and a noncovalently associated 130-kDa $\beta_1$ chain. $\alpha_4\beta_1$ integrin is preferentially expressed on cell surface projections that are often called microvilli but resemble ridges rather than true villous processes (11). This position is believed to facilitate the interaction of $\alpha_4\beta_1$ integrin with its ligands under conditions of flow. The most important ligands for $\alpha_4\beta_1$ integrin include vascular cell adhesion molecule-1 (VCAM-1) on endothelial and other cells (see Table 45-2) and the heparin-binding region of alternatively spliced fibronectin expressed in the extracellular matrix and on the luminal surface of inflamed endothelial cells (12). Like other integrins, $\alpha_4\beta_1$ integrin can probably undergo conformational activation (13). This process of affinity regulation can be triggered by monocyte activation, for example, through chemokines. Gene-targeted mice lacking either $\alpha_4$ (14) or $\beta_1$ (15) are not viable. Blocking $\alpha_4\beta_1$ with a monoclonal antibody or a peptide based on the fibronectin sequence ILDV reduces atherosclerosis in mice (16), suggesting that $\alpha_4\beta_1$ is important in monocyte recruitment to atherosclerotic lesions.

The integrin $\alpha_M\beta_2$ (CD11b/CD18) is also known as Macrophage-1 or Mac-1. Mac-1 antibodies were some of the earliest monocyte-macrophage–specific antibodies described. Although Mac-1 is also expressed on neutrophils, most of its function seems to be related to monocyte-macrophages. First, Mac-1 participates in monocyte adhesion to various substrates, including endothelial cells. Second, Mac-1 is an important receptor for complement and is also known as complement

**TABLE 45-1**

CELL SURFACE MOLECULES ON MONOCYTES RELEVANT TO CELL–CELL INTERACTION

| Molecule | Inflammatory monocytes | | Resident monocytes | | Main function | Secondary function |
|---|---|---|---|---|---|---|
| | Mouse | Human | Mouse | Human | | |
| CD11a/CD18 ($\alpha_L \beta_2$, LFA-1) | + | + | + | + | Inducible adhesion to ICAM-1,2 | Reduces rolling velocity (neutrophils) |
| CD11b/CD18 ($\alpha_M \beta_2$, Mac-1) | + | + | + | + | Inducible adhesion to, C3bi, ICAM-1,2 fibrinogen | Phagocytosis |
| CD11c ($\alpha_x \beta_2$) | − | + | − | + | Complement binding | |
| CD14 | − | + | − | low | LPS coreceptor | |
| CD16 (Fc$\gamma$RIII) | + | − | + | + | Fc receptor for IgG | |
| CX3CR1 (fractalkine r.) | low | + | high | high | Binds fractalkine, activates monocyte | May mediate adhesion |
| CCR1 | n.d. | + | n.d. | − | Binds chemokines CCL3,5,7,14,15,16, 23; causes activation | Chemokine binding causes arrest of rolling cells |
| CCR2 | + | + | − | − | Binds chemokines CCL2,7,12,13; causes activation, chemotaxis | Soluble CCL2 can cause monocyte arrest |
| CCR4 | n.d. | + | n.d. | − | Binds chemokines CCL17,22 | |
| CCR7 | n.d. | + | n.d. | − | Binds chemokines CCL19,21 | Promotes macrophage migration to lymphatic organs |
| CXCR1 (IL-8 receptor) | − | low | − | − | Binds chemokines, mainly CXCL8 | |
| CXCR2 | n.d. | + | n.d. | − | Binds chemokines CXCL1,2,3,5,6,7,8 | Chemokine binding causes arrest |
| CXCR3 | n.d. | − | n.d. | − | Binds chemokines CXCL9,10,11 | Promotes type 1 inflammation |
| CXCR4 | n.d. | low | n.d. | + | Binds CXCL12, induces arrest | Release of cells from bone marrow |
| Gr1 (Ly6G/C) | + | − | low | − | No known function | |
| CD49b ($\alpha_2 \beta_1$, VLA2) | + | n.d. | − | n.d. | Inducible binding to collagen | |
| CD49d ($\alpha_4 \beta_1$, VLA4) | + | n.d. | + | n.d. | Inducible binding to VCAM-1, fibronectin | Monocyte arrest on atherosclerotic lesions |
| CD62L (L selectin) | + | n.d. | − | n.d. | Binds PSGL-1, secondary tethering | Binds PNAd, monocyte rolling in lymph nodes |
| CD162 (PSGL-1) | + | + | + | + | Binds P selectin on platelets, endothelial cells, microparticles | Binds L selectin for secondary tethering, binds E selectin |
| Tissue factor | Inducible, but unknown in which subsets | | | | Initiator of coagulation | Signaling into monocyte |
| PECAM-1 (CD31) | Most or all | | | | Transendothelial migration | Monocyte activation |

LFA, lymphocyte function–associated antigen; ICAM, intercellular adhesion module; CCR, corresponding chemokine receptors; LPS, lipopolysaccharide; VCAM, vascular cell adhesion molecule; PSGL, P selectin glycoprotein ligand; PECAM-1, Platelet/endothelial cell adhesion molecule-1; n.d., not determined.

receptor 3 (CR3). Mac-1 binds complement C3bi and is critically involved in phagocytosis of complement-coated bacteria and particles. Mac-1 engagement promotes a proinflammatory response, including a respiratory burst with vigorous oxygen radical production, actin polymerization, induction of nitric oxide synthase (iNOS), and shape change. Interestingly, under flow conditions such as those achieved in flow chambers *in vitro*, or isolated perfused vessels *ex vivo*, Mac-1 does not appear to contribute to monocyte adhesion to endothelial cells (17). Mac-1 has been shown to lower the rolling velocity of neutrophils (18), but the role of Mac-1 in monocyte rolling has not been studied. Mice lacking Mac-1, prepared by targeting

the gene for $\alpha_M$, are viable, fertile, and healthy under vivarium conditions (19). There is no evidence that these mice are protected from atherosclerosis, but their response to vascular injury is blunted (20). Like all $\beta_2$ integrins, Mac-1 has an I-domain with homology to the von Willebrand factor (VWF) A-domain inserted in its $\alpha$ subunit, which contains the ligand binding site. Mac-1 binds many other ligands, including fibrinogen and coagulation factor X (Table 45-2). Mac-1 is thought to be involved in assembling prothrombinase on the monocyte surface and may be able to support platelet binding to monocyte through a fibrinogen bridge between $\alpha_{IIb}\beta_3$ on platelets and Mac-1 on monocytes (21). Although Mac-1–deficient mice

Integrin activation

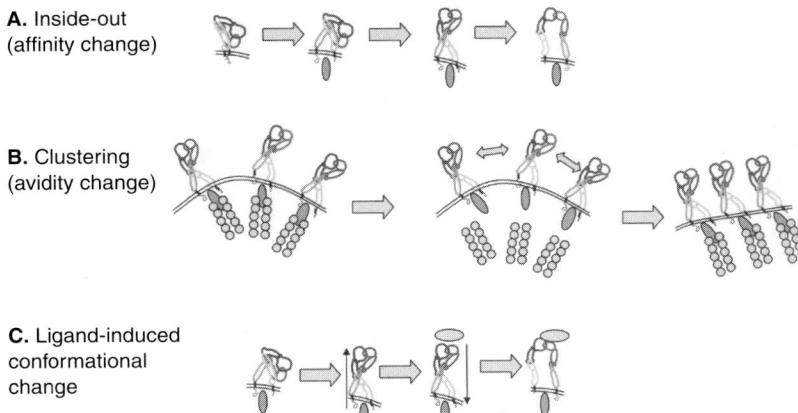

**A.** Inside-out
(affinity change)

**B.** Clustering
(avidity change)

**C.** Ligand-induced
conformational
change

**FIGURE 45-1.** Regulation of integrin ligand binding activity. **A:** Integrin affinity regulation by conformational changes in the $\alpha$ and $\beta$ chains (*red* and *blue*), resulting in increased affinity for monovalent ligands. Note that cytoplasmic tails move apart during affinity regulation, probably through interaction with talin (*green ellipse*). **B:** Integrin avidity regulation by lateral mobility/clustering. Transient release of integrins from cytoskeletal anchorage (actin filaments, represented as *strings of circles*) allows integrin rearrangement and clustering in the plane of the cell membrane, resulting in increased avidity for multivalent ligands. It is not known whether the release occurs at the level of talin–actin binding. Integrins bind actin through talin and various other linker proteins (not shown). **C:** Ligand-induced activation and outside-in signaling. After activation as in **A**, inside-out signaling, *arrow up*, ligand (*blue ellipse*) binding induces outside-in signaling (*arrow down*) and bond maturation (see Color Fig. 45-1).

have no obvious defect in hemostasis, Mac-1 could participate in monocyte activation and the delivery of tissue factor to sites of thrombosis (22). Human monocytes, but not mouse monocytes, also express a closely related integrin, $\alpha_x\beta_2$, which is also a complement receptor and alternatively known as CR4. Abundant $\alpha_x$ expression is found on dendritic cells. Like Mac-1, $\alpha_x\beta_2$ binds C3bi and denatured proteins (23).

The lymphocyte function–associated antigen LFA-1, or $\alpha_L\beta_2$ integrin (CD11a/CD18), is expressed on all leukocytes, including monocytes. Although LFA-1 is responsible for lymphocyte arrest and the sudden stopping of rolling cells upon activation (24), and it participates in neutrophil arrest under flow, little is known about its function in monocytes. LFA-1 binds to cell surface immunoglobulins, including intercellular

**TABLE 45-2**

LIGANDS FOR MONOCYTE AND PLATELET INTEGRINS

| Integrin | Ligands | Function |
|---|---|---|
| $\alpha_4\beta_1$ | VCAM-1 | Adhesion to endothelial cells |
| | Fibronectin | Adhesion to extracellular matrix |
| Mac-1 | Complement C3bi | Phagocytosis of opsonized particles |
| | Coagulation factor Xa | Assembly of prothrombinase complex |
| | Fibrinogen | Bridging between monocytes and platelets |
| | Intercellular adhesion molecule-1 (ICAM-1) | Adhesion to endothelial and other cells |
| | Intercellular adhesion molecule-2 (ICAM-2) | Adhesion to endothelial cells and platelets |
| | Denatured collagen | Migration, phagocytosis? |
| | Denatured albumin | Migration, phagocytosis? |
| | *Leishmania* GP63 | Uptake of *Leishmania* |
| | Bordetella FHA | Uptake of Bordetella |
| | Fibronectin | Adhesion to extracellular matrix |
| $\alpha_x\beta_2$ | Complement C3bi | Phagocytosis of opsonized particles |
| LFA-1 | Intercellular adhesion molecule-1 (ICAM-1) | Adhesion to endothelial and other cells |
| | Intercellular adhesion molecule-2 (ICAM-2) | Adhesion to endothelial cells and platelets |
| $\alpha_V\beta_3$ | Vitronectin | Bone remodeling? |
| | Entactin | Unknown |
| | L1 | Unknown |
| $\alpha_{IIb}\beta_3$ | Fibrinogen | Binds immobilized Fg without activation |
| | Fibronectin | |
| VWF | | Induced by GP Ib binding to VWF |
| | Vitronectin | |
| CD40L | | Promotes CD40L shedding |
| $\alpha_2\beta_1$ | Collagens | On platelets, requires activation by GP VI |

VCAM, vascular cell adhesion molecule; ICAM, intercellular adhesion module; LFA, lymphocyte function–associated antigen; GP, glycoprotein; VWF, von Willebrand factor.

adhesion molecules ICAM-1 and-2, and has no known extracellular matrix ligands. Mice lacking LFA-1 were prepared by targeting the gene for $\alpha_L$ (25) and are viable, healthy, and fertile under vivarium conditions. There are no reports of these mice having altered thrombosis, hemostasis, or atherosclerosis. Like the other $\beta_2$ integrins, LFA-1 has an I-domain and undergoes extensive conformational changes of the extracellular domain upon activation (6).

The integrin $\alpha_V\beta_3$ is expressed on blood monocytes at a low copy number. Its expression increases upon differentiation to osteoclastlike cells. This integrin was initially called leukocyte response integrin (26) because it participates in inducing the respiratory burst associated with nicotinamide adenine dinucleotide phosphate (NADPH) oxidase activation and oxygen free radical production in neutrophils. Ligands for $\alpha_V\beta_3$ integrin include vitronectin, entactin, and possibly the immunoglobulinlike adhesion molecule L1. Gene-targeted mice lacking $\alpha_V$ are not viable, whereas mice lacking $\beta_3$ have a defect in both $\alpha_V\beta_3$ on monocytes, neutrophils, and proliferating endothelial cells and $\alpha_{IIb}\beta_3$ on platelets, which share the common $\beta_3$ subunit. The phenotype of these mice is dominated by the platelet defect (Glanzmann thrombasthenialike), and these mice also have osteosclerosis, suggesting defective osteoclast function (27). Blood monocytes express low levels of $\alpha_V\beta_5$ integrin, which is also a vitronectin receptor. Monocytes express $\alpha_2\beta_1$ integrin, a collagen receptor, at the mRNA and protein levels. $\alpha_5\beta_1$, a fibronectin receptor, $\alpha_{10}\beta_1$, a collagen receptor, and $\alpha_E\beta_7$, a receptor for E-cadherin, are found at the message level, but functional data have not been published.

**Immunoglobulins.** Blood monocytes express many immunoglobulinlike molecules. Of importance for this chapter is ICAM-1, because it supports homotypic aggregation of monocytes by LFA-1 and Mac-1 and because it can bind fibrinogen (28). Mice with hypomorphic mutations in the ICAM-1 gene or

lacking ICAM-1 entirely have no overt defect in hemostasis or thrombosis, but are somewhat protected from atherosclerosis in the C57BL/6 and apolipoprotein E knockout models (29). However, these mice also lack ICAM-1 on endothelial cells, smooth muscle cells, lymphocytes, and many other cells. ICAM-2 and ICAM-3 are found in monocytes at the message level but they have no known function in monocytes.

PECAM-1 (CD31) is a homotypic adhesion molecule expressed on blood monocytes and has an important role in transendothelial migration and in monocyte activation (30, 31). Monocyte PECAM-1 interacts with PECAM-1 on endothelial cells during transmigration. PECAM-1-deficient C57BL/6 mice have no apparent defect in leukocyte and monocyte transmigration, demonstrating that PECAM-1–independent pathways of transmigration exist (32). However, PECAM-1–deficient mice show reduced monocyte recombinant when crossed into other backgrounds (33).

Other immunoglobulins expressed on monocytes include major histocompatibility complex (MHC) class II, which is important in antigen presentation but is not fully induced until monocytes differentiate to macrophages. CD8 and CD83 are also expressed but have no known function in monocytes.

**Selectins and Their Ligands.** L selectin (CD62L) is expressed on "inflammatory" blood monocytes and most other leukocytes. Its most important function is in lymphocyte homing to secondary lymphatic organs (34), but it also has an accessory function in inflammation (35). Like the other selectins, L selectin can mediate leukocyte rolling, a passive motion of leukocytes down a vessel wall driven by the blood flow and the forces exerted on the loosely attached cell. During rolling, molecular bonds form at the leading edge and continually break at the trailing edge of the cell, allowing the leukocyte to stay in contact with the endothelium without actually stopping (36) (see Fig. 45-2). Rolling is thought to

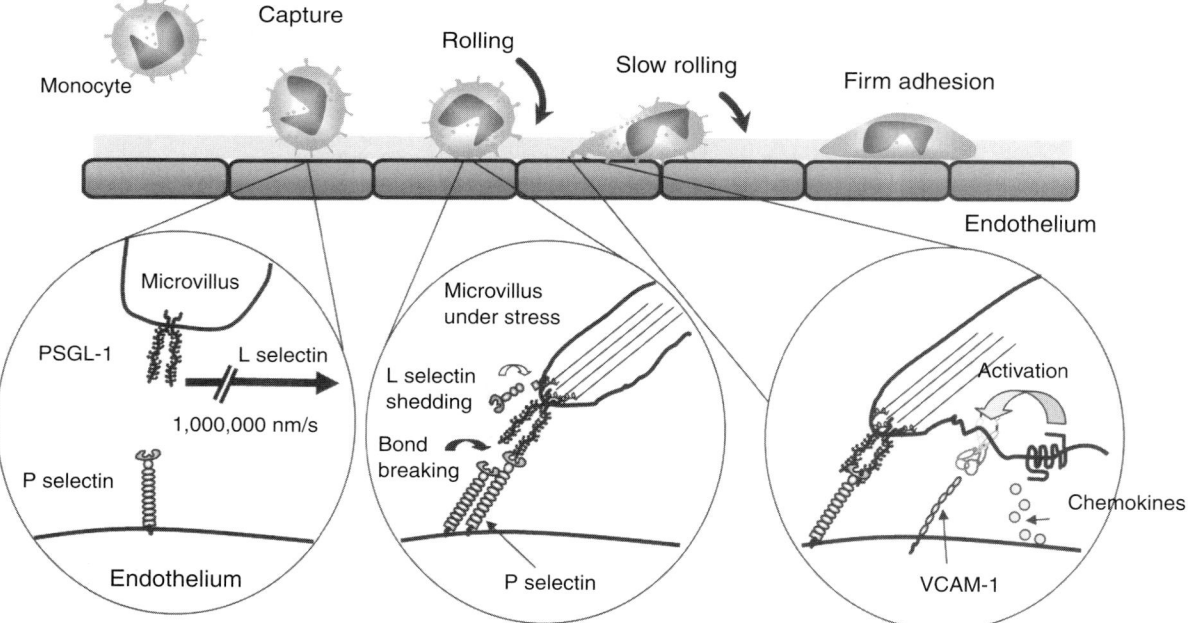

**FIGURE 45-2.** Sequence of monocyte capture, rolling, slow rolling, and adhesion on endothelial cells. Flow from left to right, endothelial surface layer shown in *light grey*. Primary capture or tethering is initiated by monocyte P selectin glycoprotein ligand (PSGL)-1 binding to endothelial P selectin (**left insert**). Note high velocity of monocyte (1 mm per second). The **middle insert** shows a P selectin/PSGL-1 bond at the trailing edge of a rolling monocyte. Applied stress induces faster bond breakage and may also activate cleavage of L selectin. The **right insert** shows VLA-4/vascular cell adhesion molecule (VCAM)-1–dependent bond required for slow rolling. Monocyte activation by surface-immobilized chemokine binding to chemokine receptor results in integrin affinity upregulation and firm binding to endothelial ligands such as VCAM-1 (shown here) (see Color Fig. 45-2). (Modified from Mammalian Carbohydrate Recognition Systems: Functions of Selectins, Kinsley, Figure 1, Page 180, © Springer Verlag Berlin, Heidelberg 2001.)

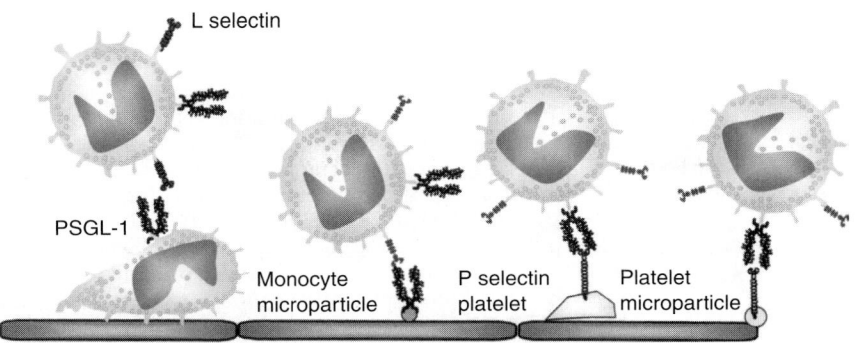

**FIGURE 45-3.** Secondary capture or secondary tethering. Monocytes can be captured by binding to other, already adherent monocytes or other leukocytes (**left**), or to monocyte-derived microparticles (**middle**). Both require L selectin on the circulating monocytes and P selectin glycoprotein ligand (PSGL)-1 on the adherent monocyte or microparticle. Monocytes can also adhere to platelets or platelet-derived microparticles (**right**), which requires monocyte PSGL-1 and platelet P selectin.

serve to "scan for" inflammatory stimuli, and rolling cells can stop (arrest) in response to appropriate stimuli (9,24,37). On neutrophils, L selectin is expressed on the tips of microvilli (38) and can be rapidly shed upon cell activation by a protease-dependent mechanism involving TACE (ADAM-17) (39). Although L selectin has been shown to support monocyte rolling on L selectin ligands in flow chambers, it is not known whether L selectin mediated monocyte rolling on endothelial cells serves a physiologic function. It is tempting to speculate that monocyte L selectin may enhance monocyte recruitment to atherosclerotic lesions by nucleating monocyte–monocyte interactions through binding to P selectin glycoprotein ligand-1 (PSGL-1, CD162, see subsequent text) in a process called secondary capture (40) (see Fig. 45-3). Secondary capture is initiated when a vessel wall–adherent monocyte or monocyte-derived microparticle exposes PSGL-1 to other monocytes that pass by in the free stream. These cells can transiently bind to the adherent monocyte through L selectin and then attach to the endothelium downstream from the nucleation site. Although this process is certainly plausible and has been observed to occur in mouse aortas (41), no direct evidence has been provided to support its importance in atherosclerosis, thrombosis, or hemostasis.

The most important selectin ligand on monocytes is PSGL-1, CD162. PSGL-1 is somewhat of a misnomer, because PSGL-1 also binds L and E selectins with affinity similar to P selectin (42). All monocytes, like most leukocytes, express

PSGL-1 protein on the cell surface, but not all cell surface–expressed PSGL-1 can bind selectins. PSGL-1 binding to selectins is regulated by a series of glycosyltransferases and sulfotransferases required to make it a functional selectin ligand (see Table 45-3). Blood monocytes express fucosyltransferase VII, core 2N-acetylglucosaminy-transferase-I, and at least one sialyltransferase. Therefore, PSGL-1 on monocytes is constitutively active and can bind all three selectins. PSGL-1 is a covalent homodimer and, like VLA-4 and L selectin, is expressed on microvilli (43).

Recently, PSGL-1 has been shown to be of key importance for the delivery of tissue factor to sites of thrombosis (45,46). PSGL-1–expressing microparticles, presumably derived from monocytes, deliver tissue factor to sites of thrombosis in a PSGL-1– and P selectin–dependent process. Apparently, the generation of these microparticles can be induced by soluble P selectin (47) in a process that requires PSGL-1 expression. Taken together, PSGL-1 is one of the most important molecules connecting inflammation with hemostasis and thrombosis. PSGL-1–deficient mice show reduced inflammatory responses in many models and have a remarkable defect in tissue factor recruitment to sites of vascular injury and thrombosis (45,46).

Recently, P selectin was also found to be expressed on peritoneal macrophages (48) and in foam cells found in the neointima formed after vascular injury in atherosclerotic mice (Sarembock, unpublished). There is no evidence for P selectin expression on blood monocytes.

**TABLE 45-3**

GLYCOSYLTRANSFERASES AND SULFOTRANSFERASES RELEVANT TO SELECTIN BINDING

| Enzyme | Abbreviation | Involved in ligands for | Expression |
|---|---|---|---|
| Fucosyltransferase-VII | FucT-VII | L, E, P | Myeloid, act. T cells, HEV |
| Fucosyltransferase-IV | FucT-IV | L, E, P[a] | Myeloid, some HEV |
| Core2 $\beta$1, 6 glucosaminyl transferase | C2GlcNAcT-I | L, P | Myeloid, act. T cells, B cells |
| Sialyl 3-galactosyltransferase | ST3Gal | L, E, P | Ubiquitous |
| $\beta$1, 4-galactosyl transferase | $\beta$1, 4GalT-I | P[b] | Ubiquitous |
| Tyrosine protein sulfotransferases 1,2 | TPST-1,2 | L, P | Ubiquitous |
| HEC-glucosaminyl sulfotransferase | HEC-GlcNAc6ST | L | HEV, chronically inflamed Ecs |

HEV, high endothelial venules; EC, endothelial cell.
[a]Only in myeloid cells, not T cells.
[b]Not yet tested for E, L; probably involved for L.
From Ley K, Kansas GS. Selectins in T-cell recruitment to non-lymphoid tissues and sites of inflammation. *Nat Rev Immunol* 2004;4:325–335, with permission.

**Integrin-Associated Molecules.** The urokinase plasminogen activator receptor (UPAR) is expressed on blood monocytes and sharply upregulated by activation. UPAR associates with $\alpha_L\beta_2$, $\alpha_M\beta_2$, and various other integrins. UPAR coexpression increases the affinity of integrins and can change ligand specificity (49). Tetraspanins have also been reported to associate with integrins and change their activation status (50). A third integrin-associated molecule is CD47, which is associated with leukocyte activation and transendothelial migration (51). These integrin-associated cell surface glycoproteins can change integrin affinity for ligand, can change ligand specificity, and can serve signaling functions (52,53).

## Monocyte Chemokines

Chemokines are small peptides that bind to G-protein–coupled receptors (GPCRs) on monocytes, lymphocytes, neutrophils, platelets, and many other cells (54). Most chemokines are classified according to the location of two conserved pairs of cysteins that either do (CXC) or do not (CC) have an intervening amino acid. Chemokines are named for their ability to induce a chemotactic response, that is, initiate migration of a receptor-bearing cell from areas of lower to areas of higher concentration of chemokines. However, chemokines have many other important functions. Some, but not all, can induce rapid integrin activation by inducing conformational changes and/or clustering of integrins (see preceding text). When chemokines act on rolling leukocytes, such integrin activation often results in arrest, converting the rolling motion to firm adhesion (37,55).

Inflammatory chemokines such as interleukin-8 (CXCL8) also induce degranulation of secondary and tertiary granules in neutrophils and monocytes, and induce a respiratory burst resulting in production of oxygen-derived free radicals. Stromal cell–derived factor-1$\alpha$ (SDF-1$\alpha$, CXCL12) has homeostatic functions in the bone marrow where it supports progenitor cells and hematopoiesis. Other chemokines participate in the organogenesis of lymphatic organs.

In the context of this chapter, we discuss chemokines elaborated by monocytes, platelets, and endothelial cells. These chemokines can have autocrine, paracrine, and remote effects. Monocytes express low levels of CCL2, 3, 4, and 20 and

CXCL8, which are heavily and immediately upregulated upon activation. CCL7 and 8 as well as CXCL9 and 10 show only modest upregulation. By contrast, CCL5 is downregulated in activated monocytes. CCL22 [macrophage-derived chemokine (MDC)] is an inflammatory chemokine that shows low expression on monocytes but is induced by macrophage differentiation. CCL2 [monocyte chemoattractant protein (MCP)-1], CCL3 [macrophage inflammatory protein (MIP)-1$\alpha$], CCL4 (MIP-1$\beta$), CCL7 (MCP-3), CCL8 (MCP-3), and CXCL8 (interleukin-8) are considered proinflammatory chemokines because they can activate neutrophils and monocytes. Injection of these chemokines into experimental animals results in a rapid and considerable accumulation of monocytes and/or neutrophils. CCL20 (LARC, MIP-3$\alpha$) is considered a constitutive chemokine that was first described to be expressed in the intestine and skin. Its function in monocytes is not known. CXCL9 (Mig) and CXCL10 (IP-10) are considered classical T-helper 1 chemokines that are proinflammatory and can attract effector T lymphocytes by binding to their CXCR3 receptor. Although CCL5 is considered an inflammatory chemokine, it is constitutively expressed in many organs, including the lung, and in some blood cells, predominantly platelets (56). Overall, it is clear that monocytes produce proinflammatory chemokines that can sustain and increase inflammation, and attract more monocytes, neutrophils, and inflammatory T cells. In the context of this chapter, it is interesting to note that monocytes can synthesize several chemokines, including MIP-1$\alpha$, regulated on activation, normal T cell expressed and secreted (RANTES), and MDC, that can help activate platelets and promote platelet aggregation in the presence of suboptimal concentrations of agonist. Platelets express the corresponding chemokine receptors (CCR) 1, 3, and 4 (see Table 45-4).

## Monocyte Chemokine Receptors

Chemokine receptors are GPCRs that transduce signals by phospholipase C (PLC) and phosphatidylinositol-3-kinase (PI 3-K). CCR2 is the main receptor for CCL2 (MCP-1) and is considered the most important monocyte chemokine receptor. MCP-1 was the first monocyte-specific chemoattractant to be discovered. Atherosclerosis-prone mice lacking MCP-1 (57) or CCR2 (58)

---

**TABLE 45-4**

**CELL SURFACE MOLECULES ON PLATELETS RELEVANT TO CELL–CELL INTERACTION**

| Molecule | Main function | Secondary function |
|----------|---------------|--------------------|
| GP Ib$\alpha$ | Binds VWF, mediates adhesion under high shear | Binds P selectin |
| GP IIb/IIIa | Promotes platelet aggregation by binding fibrinogen | Binds monocyte Mac-1 |
| GP VI | Main platelet receptor for collagen | |
| CD16 | Obligatory coreceptor for GP VI | Binds Fc |
| P selectin | Binds PSGL-1 on monocytes, microparticles, neutrophils | Anchors VWF |
| VWF | Binds GP Ib$\alpha$ on other platelets, binds P selectin | |
| ICAM-2 | Binds LFA-1 on monocytes, neutrophils, lymphocytes | |
| CCR1 | Receptor for MIP1$\alpha$, RANTES | Augments responses to low-dose ADP |
| CCR3 | Receptor for RANTES, eotaxin | |
| CCR4 | Receptor for MDC | |
| CXCR4 | Receptor for SDF-1$\alpha$ | |
| CD40L | Binds CD40 on monocytes and endothelial cells | GP IIb/IIIa on platelets |
| Fc$\gamma$RIIa | Binds Fc portion of IgG | Activates platelets |

GP, glycoprotein; VWF, von Willebrand factor; PSGL, P selectin glycoprotein ligand; ICAM, intercellular adhesion module; MIP, macrophage inflammatory protein; LFA, lymphocyte function–associated antigen; CCR, corresponding chemokine receptors; RANTES, regulated on activation, normal T cell expressed and secreted; ADP, adenosine 5'-diphosphate; MDC, macrophage-derived chemokine; SDF, stromal cell–derived factor.

are approximately 50% protected from atherosclerosis in all models tested. Beyond CCR2, monocytes express many other chemokine receptors, including CCR1 and 5 and CXCR1, 2, and 4. CXCR1 and 2 are of special interest, because they elicit no chemotactic response in monocytes but can very effectively activate monocyte integrins to promote arrest (17). In fact, CXCR2 on monocytes is the first example of a "pure" arrest chemokine receptor, because it induces arrest only of rolling monocytes, not of other responses like chemotaxis. CCR1 is up-regulated in activated monocytes and stays expressed in macrophages, which suggests possible autocrine effects of CCR1 chemokines such as MIP-1$\alpha$ and RANTES, which are also produced by monocytes. CCR1 is the receptor responsible for RANTES-induced monocyte arrest (59). CCR5 is also expressed on monocytes, another receptor for the chemokines RANTES, MIP-1$\alpha$, and MIP-1$\beta$. RANTES has been shown to induce platelet–monocyte and monocyte–endothelial interactions (56, 60). CCR7 is not highly expressed in monocytes, but induced upon macrophage differentiation. CCR7 binds and responds to the secondary lymphoid tissue–expressed chemokines CCL19 and CCL21, attracting macrophages (and dendritic cells) to lymph nodes and Peyer patches. CXCR4 is very highly expressed on resting monocytes and is downregulated upon activation. It stays low in macrophages. CXCR4 is believed to be involved in retaining monocytes in the bone marrow, but is also a very effective arrest chemokine (61) (Table 45-1).

## Endothelial Cells

Endothelial cells line all blood and lymph vessels. Endothelial cells are specialized by organ and even by vessel size (large artery, arteriole) or position in the circulatory system (arteriole, capillary, venule). The endothelial cell properties and molecules mentioned in subsequent text apply to endothelial cells in a general sense. Most data are derived from experimental systems using cultured human umbilical vein endothelial cells.

### Endothelial Cell Adhesion Molecules

Endothelial cells express a host of constitutive and inducible adhesion molecules, some chemokines and some chemokine receptors (see Table 45-5).

**P selectin.** In the context of this chapter, P selectin is probably the most important endothelial adhesion molecule. As a member of the selectin class of adhesion molecules, it mediates leukocyte rolling (Fig. 45-2). P selectin is prepackaged in Weibel-Palade bodies of endothelial cells, where it is intimately associated with VWF (46). From Weibel-Palade bodies, P selectin can be transported to the luminal surface by exocytosis induced by mild inflammatory stimuli. Endothelial P selectin, once surface-expressed, can also support platelet interactions with the endothelium (62). Once platelets are activated, it is platelet, not endothelial P selectin, that is responsible for platelet–endothelial interactions (56,60). Mice lacking P selectin are approximately 50% protected from atherosclerosis (63) and show almost no neointima formation in response to vascular injury (64). Experiments in bone marrow chimeric mice show that in both spontaneous atherosclerosis (65) and injury-accelerated neointima formation (66), it is mainly the platelet, not the endothelial P selectin, that is responsible for inflammatory cell recruitment and neointimal growth. In addition to cell surface expression, both endothelial and platelet P selectin can also be released into the plasma by alternative splicing and by a poorly understood proteolytic mechanism (67).

Most of the knowledge about endothelial P selectin function was derived from mouse experiments. However, the regulation of endothelial P selectin expression is different in mice and primates, where P selectin shows less sustained expression during inflammation (68). It is possible that the function of human P selectin is not quite as important as that of mouse P selectin. There is some evidence that E selectin is important for atherosclerosis in humans (69), but less so in mice (29). Human monocytes roll on human endothelial cells through P selectin under shear. Human PSGL-1, like its mouse counterpart, can transmit proinflammatory and prothrombotic signals into monocytes (70,71).

**E selectin.** Activated endothelial cells express E selectin, which binds PSGL-1 (72,73), but more importantly, another unidentified ligand (74). Like PSGL-1, this other ligand is heavily dependent on glycosylation by fucosyl transferase-VII and at least one sialyltransferase (75), but unlike PSGL-1 binding to P selectin, does not appear to require core 2GlcNAcT-I (76) or sulfyltransferases. Like the other selectins, E selectin supports leukocyte and monocyte rolling on inflamed endothelial

---

**TABLE 45-5**

CELL SURFACE MOLECULES ON ENDOTHELIAL CELLS RELEVANT TO CELL–CELL INTERACTION

| Molecule | Main function | Secondary function |
|---|---|---|
| P selectin | Leukocyte/monocyte rolling, binds PSGL-1 | Platelet rolling |
| E selectin | Leukocyte/monocyte slow rolling, binds PSGL-1 and unknown ligand | Leukocyte activation |
| PNAd | Lymphocyte rolling in HEV, binds L selectin | |
| ICAM-1 | Leukocyte/monocyte adhesion, binds LFA-1, Mac-1 | Binding Fg |
| ICAM-2 | Leukocyte/monocyte adhesion, binds LFA-1 | |
| VCAM-1 | Monocyte adhesion, binds $\alpha_4\beta_1$ | Slow rolling |
| Fibronectin | Monocyte adhesion, binds $\alpha_5\beta_1$, $\alpha_V\beta_3$ and $\alpha_4\beta_1$ | |
| VWF | Interaction with GP Ib/V/IX on platelets | |
| GP Ib$\alpha$ | Interaction with VWF | Binds Fg, Fn |
| CCL5 (RANTES) | Monocyte arrest through CCR1 | Chemotaxis |
| CXCL1 (GRO-$\alpha$) | Monocyte arrest through CXCR2 | |
| CXCR4 | Monocyte arrest through CXCR4 | Chemotaxis |

PSGL, P selectin glycoprotein ligand; HEV, high endothelial venules; ICAM, intercellular adhesion module; LFA, lymphocyte function–associated antigen; VCAM, vascular cell adhesion molecule; VWF, von Willebrand factor; RANTES, regulated on activation, normal T cell expressed and secreted; CCR, corresponding chemokine receptors.

cells *in vitro* and *in vivo*. E selectin–dependent rolling is typically slower than P or L selectin–dependent rolling, suggesting that cells rolling through E selectin can more closely scan the endothelial surface for activating signals. Endothelial E selectin does not support platelet interactions, but very efficiently binds neutrophils and monocytes. E selectin is required for an additional activating signal (77) that can arrest rolling neutrophils (78) and possibly monocytes. This signal is independent of G$\alpha$i-coupled receptors such as chemokine receptors and probably not directly transduced through the E selectin ligand molecule, because coimmobilization of E selectin with ICAM-1 does not support neutrophil arrest. E selectin–deficient mice have no spontaneous defect in inflammation, platelet aggregation, or thrombus formation, suggesting that E selectin function in mice overlaps with other rolling and activation molecules. Indeed, mice lacking both P and E selectin have a severe defect in neutrophil recruitment to sites of inflammation and show spontaneous pathology and altered hematopoiesis (79,80). In humans, a "hyperadhesive" polymorphism in the E selectin gene correlates with an increased incidence of myocardial infarctions (69), suggesting that E selectin may be involved in atherosclerosis in primates.

**ICAM-1.** Endothelial cells constitutively express ICAM-1 (see preceding text). Endothelial ICAM-1 expression is increased by inflammatory cytokines such as IL-1-$\beta$ and tumor necrosis factor (TNF)-$\alpha$ and further enhanced in the presence of IFN-$\gamma$. Endothelial ICAM-1 is thought to be the major ligand supporting the binding of the $\beta_2$ integrins LFA-1 and Mac-1, but other ligands exist (18). One of these other ligands is ICAM-2, a molecule with two extracellular immunoglobulin domains, that is constitutively expressed on the endothelial surface and platelets, and is not upregulated by inflammatory mediators.

**VCAM-1.** Most endothelial cells express vascular cell adhesion molecule-1 (VCAM-1) upon cytokine stimulation. VCAM-1 is an immunoglobulinlike cell adhesion molecule with six to seven immunoglobulin domains. VCAM-1 is the most important endothelial ligand for VLA-4 ($\alpha_4\beta_1$ integrin) and is intimately involved with monocyte recruitment to sites of inflammation and atherosclerosis. Mice deficient in VCAM-1 are not viable, but endothelial cell–specific knockouts and mice expressing a low level of a mutated VCAM-1 that lacks one of the VLA-4 binding sites have been prepared. These VCAM-1 hypomorphic mice are dramatically protected from atherosclerosis in all models tested (81,82).

**PECAM-1.** Endothelial cells constitutively express CD31 (PECAM-1) and CD99, both of which have been implicated in monocyte transmigration (83). C57BL/6 mice lacking CD31 have no transmigration defect, but on other genetic backgrounds, the migration defect is evident (33). Other endothelial-expressed adhesion molecules include JAM-1, JAM-2, and JAM-3 (84). They may function in monocyte and leukocyte transmigration.

**Other Adhesion Molecules.** Some specialized endothelial cells express adhesion molecules in an organ-specific manner. This includes MAdCAM-1 expressed by high endothelial venules (HEV) of the mesenteric lymph node and Peyer patches (85), E selectin expressed in resting skin endothelial cells (86), and PNAd expressed in HEV of peripheral lymph nodes (87). These region- and organ-specific adhesion molecules are not discussed further, because they have not been reported to be involved in platelet–monocyte–endothelial interactions.

The endothelial adhesion molecules mediating interactions with platelets are not well defined. Endothelial-expressed P selectin can support platelet rolling (88), but interaction of activated platelets with endothelial cells is dependent on platelet P selectin (60). The endothelial adhesion receptors responsible for binding P selectin are unknown. Activated endothelial cells secrete VWF as a very large multimer (ultralarge VWF), which can form long adhesive strings that can capture platelets by binding to platelet GP Ib$\alpha$ (89). The fluid drag force on the attached platelets stretches out VWF multimers, exposing a cleavage site that allows a plasma protease, ADAMTS-13, to cleave the multimers into shorter oligomers of VWF that are released into the plasma (90). This seems to be an important source of plasma VWF.

## Endothelial Cell Chemokines and Chemokine Receptors

Endothelial cells can express a number of proinflammatory chemokines, most notably of the IL-8 family (91). The endothelial isoform of IL-8 is slightly different from the monocyte-expressed isoform (92), but there are no known functional differences. IL-8 is immobilized on the endothelial cell surface, where it is in a strategic position to activate and arrest monocytes and neutrophils that may be rolling by. Although endothelial cells synthesize little MCP-1 or RANTES, RANTES can be delivered by rolling platelets and be immobilized on the endothelial surface (56,60). Immobilized RANTES triggers monocyte arrest, whereas MCP-1 immobilization is less efficient and triggers monocyte arrest in some (93), but not all, vascular beds (60). The ability of endothelial cells to produce other chemokines has not been tested systematically. Endothelial cells express the nonsignaling chemokine receptor Duffy antigen/receptor for chemokines (DARC), which probably augments chemokine immobilization and thereby helps transmigration. Endothelial cells may also express CCR2, the main receptor for MCP-1 (94).

## Platelets

Platelets are nonnucleated disks ($2 \times 0.5$ $\mu$m) derived from megakaryocytes. They are abundant in blood (approximately 300,000 per $\mu$L) and primarily responsible for hemostasis.

### Platelet Adhesion Molecules

**P Selectin.** Platelets express large amounts of P selectin, which is stored in $\alpha$ secretory granules (Table 45-4). Upon activation, platelet P selectin is translocated to the cell surface by exocytosis. In fact, platelet surface P selectin is a hallmark of platelet activation. P selectin–expressing platelets are found in patients with stable and unstable angina pectoris, myocardial infarction, and other cardiovascular diseases (95). P selectin is also found on the surface of a subset of blood platelets in apolipoprotein E–deficient mice (60), a standard model of atherosclerosis. Platelet P selectin is not only a marker of, but also an active participant in, vascular disease. Injecting activated platelets into apolipoprotein E–deficient mice exacerbates the size of atherosclerotic lesions (60). Similarly, preventing platelets from interacting with the vascular endothelium reduces atherosclerotic lesion size (96). In one report (97), platelets were found to also express PSGL-1, but this may have been caused by contamination of the platelet preparations used with monocyte-derived microparticles (98). There is no evidence for L or E selectin expression in platelets.

**Platelet Integrins.** Platelets express several integrin adhesion molecules. The most abundant, best known, and possibly most important of them is integrin $\alpha_{IIb}\beta_3$ (GP IIb/IIIa). Even in the resting state, GP IIb/IIIa can bind immobilized fibrinogen and fibrin. This integrin rapidly acquires ligand binding activity upon platelet activation (99). $\alpha_{IIb}\beta_3$ is well documented to change its conformation and express neoepitopes related to the ligand binding site (10,100). Platelets from patients or mice that do not express GP IIb/IIIa (Glanzmann thrombasthenia) show defects in platelet aggregation and clot retraction (27,101). VWF, vitronectin, and fibronectin bind GP IIb/IIIa through RGD sequences, fibrinogen binds through AGDV, and soluble CD40 ligand (sCD40L) uses a KGD sequence. In the context of this chapter, GP IIb/IIIa binding of fibrinogen is of particular interest, because it may provide a means to promote platelet–monocyte interactions through Mac-1, which can also bind fibrinogen (102). Blocking GP IIb/IIIa by antibodies or small molecules is a successful clinical treatment of coronary artery disease (103). In addition to inhibiting platelet adhesion and aggregation, the various GP IIb/IIIa antagonists also reduce formation of the proinflammatory sCD40L from platelets. Interestingly, deficiency in GP IIb/IIIa does not confer protection from atherosclerosis (104).

Other platelet integrins include $\alpha_5\beta_1$, which binds fibronectin, and the collagen receptor $\alpha_2\beta_1$ (GP Ia/IIa). Knockout mice have been prepared for both of these integrins but show no detectable platelet defect. Humans lacking $\alpha_2\beta_1$ have a mild bleeding tendency and decreased platelet adhesion to the subendothelium (105). $\alpha_2\beta_1$ appears to be activated by inside-out signaling secondary to GP VI binding (see subsequent text).

**Collagen Receptors.** The main platelet collagen receptor is GP VI, a 339–amino acid immunoglobulinlike collagen receptor with similarity to the natural killer receptors (106). GP VI ligation causes platelet activation and thereby initiates hemostasis. It associates through its transmembrane domain with the FcRγ chain, which has an ITAM domain (107) for signaling. There is some evidence that GP VI resides preferentially in so-called lipid rafts, domains of the platelet membrane that are rich in sphingolipids and cholesterol (108). Lipid rafts can merge and possibly give rise to platelet-derived microparticles (see subsequent text). A congenital defect in GP VI causes a mild bleeding tendency (109). There is no evidence that GP VI is involved in platelet interactions with other cells.

GP Ib, the main platelet receptor for VWF, is associated with GP V and IX in a GP Ibα/Ibβ/V/IX complex (110), also known as CD42bα/CD42bβ/CD42d/CD42a. All four glycoproteins belong to the leucine-rich repeat family. GP Ib/V/IX mediates platelet adhesion to VWF under high shear. GP Ibα also has binding sites for P selectin, Mac-1, thrombin, and coagulation factors XI and XIIa. Deficiency of GP Ib/V/IX in humans causes Bernard-Soulier syndrome, a relatively severe bleeding disorder. GP Ib/V/IX binding to VWF triggers intracellular signals that lead to activation of GP IIb/IIIa. Injecting apoE$^{-/-}$ mice with an antibody to GP Ibα reduces the size of atherosclerotic lesions (96), suggesting that the GP Ibα interaction with endothelial VWF may have proinflammatory consequences.

**Fc Receptors.** Platelets express one Fc-gamma receptor, FcγRIIa. Upon cross-linking by intact IgG, FcγRIIa relocates to lipid rafts and activates platelets through src-family kinases and adapter proteins. FcγRIIa associates with GP Ib (108).

**Von Willebrand Factor.** Platelet α-granules contain VWF, which is rapidly secreted upon activation and forms long strings that may be anchored to platelets by P selectin. Platelet VWF is very large and very thrombogenic. Deficiency in VWF protects from atherosclerosis in mice (111).

## Platelet Chemokines and G-Protein–Coupled Receptors

**Platelet Chemokines.** Platelets constitutively and abundantly express the chemokines CXCL4 (platelet factor 4, PF4) and RANTES (CCL5). Both are important in mediating monocyte–platelet–endothelial cell interactions. RANTES is deposited by transiently interacting platelets on inflamed endothelium *in vitro* (56) and on atherosclerotic endothelium and monocytes *in vivo* (60), where it promotes monocyte arrest and activation, most likely through CCR1 (59). PF4 is of importance in macrophage differentiation. It binds to and activates a splice variant of CXCR3 (112).

**Platelet Chemokine Receptors.** Platelets express the chemokine receptors CCR1, 3, and 4, and CXCR4 (Table 45-4). These receptors bind proinflammatory cytokines and SDF-1α, respectively. Chemokine receptor ligation can augment platelet responses to low doses of agonists (113). These chemokine receptors are modifiers rather than initiators of responses but are nevertheless important in the cross talk between inflammation, platelet aggregation, hemostasis, and thrombosis (see subsequent text).

**Other G-Protein–Coupled Receptors.** The most important activating GPCRs on platelets belong to the protease-activated receptor (PAR) and adenosine 5′-diphosphate (ADP)–receptor (P2Y) families. Of the four known PAR receptors, platelets express PAR-1 and -4 in humans, and PAR-3 and -4 in mice. These receptors are responsible for thrombin-induced platelet activation, a prominent event initiating platelet aggregation. The PAR receptors bear a tethered ligand, which becomes available to bind to and activate the receptor after cleavage by a specific protease such as thrombin (114). Details of PAR receptors on platelets are covered in Chapter 33. Platelets also express GPCRs for ADP, most prominently, P2Y$_1$ coupled to Gαq, and P2Y$_{12}$ coupled to Gαi. P2Y$_{12}$ is the molecular target of platelet aggregation inhibitors of the clopidogrel type. In the context of atherothrombosis and vascular disease, ADP may be released from red and other blood cells, triggering platelet aggregation. *Per se*, ADP is not a very strong stimulus for platelet activation, but it may synergize with other stimuli such as low-dose thrombin or chemokines. Blocking P2Y$_{12}$ also reduces formation of CD40L. Other platelet GPCRs include receptors for epinephrine and thromboxane A$_2$, a cyclooxygenase product that amplifies platelet aggregation. Some GPCRs, including PAR-1, are preferentially found in lipid rafts (108).

## Platelet Cytokines

The most important cytokine produced by platelets is the TNF-like CD40 ligand (CD40L), which has both prothrombotic and proinflammatory effects (99). CD40L is a type II transmembrane protein that binds CD40 on antigen-presenting cells and GP IIb/IIIa on platelets. GP IIb/IIIa binding promotes cleavage ("shedding") of CD40L by an unknown metalloproteinase in response to activation by collagen or thrombin. sCD40L also has proinflammatory and prothrombotic effects. Almost all CD40L in blood is on platelets, although some lymphocytes also express CD40L. Mice lacking CD40L have a thrombosis defect and are protected from atherosclerosis. sCD40L accumulates in stored platelet concentrates, and elevated levels of serum sCD40L are associated with thrombotic diseases, acute coronary syndrome, rheumatoid arthritis, lupus, and other inflammatory diseases. Platelets also contain platelet-derived growth factor (PDGF), a cytokinelike growth factor for smooth muscle and other cells.

## Small Molecules Secreted by Platelets

Thromboxane A$_2$ (TxA$_2$) and serotonine are powerful vasoconstrictors released by activated platelets. Both bind to receptors on smooth muscle and endothelial cells. TxA$_2$ also promotes platelet aggregation. TxA$_2$ is a cyclooxygenase-1 product, an enzyme that is inhibited by aspirin. Small molecules secreted by platelets are covered in more detail in Chapters 36 to 38.

## Microparticles

Blood contains a host of microparticles with diameters between 50 nm and 1 $\mu$m that can support platelet–monocyte–endothelial interactions (115). Most (approximately 90%) microparticles in normal human plasma are derived from platelets (116), but others come from monocytes, endothelial cells, smooth muscle cells, and other cells. Platelet-derived microparticles are very prothrombotic by providing a phosphatodylserine-rich surface on which coagulation factors can assemble (117). Monocyte-derived microparticles are a major source of tissue factor, which initiates intravascular coagulation during thrombus formation (115). The adhesion molecules used by microparticles to interact with endothelial cells, monocytes, and platelets are most likely derived from the cells from which the microparticles were generated. Indeed, the delivery of tissue factor to platelet aggregates has been shown to require PSGL-1 on monocyte-derived microparticles and to require P selectin on activated platelets (45,46).

## Plasma and Extracellular Matrix Proteins Relevant to Cell–Cell Interactions

Although platelet–monocyte–endothelial cell interaction is often studied in tissue culture media, these adhesive interactions occur naturally in blood, which is itself a rich source of other adhesive proteins. Plasma fibrinogen can bind to many cell adhesion receptors, including Mac-1, $\alpha_V\beta_3$ integrin, and ICAM-1 on monocytes, activated GP IIb/IIIa on platelets, and ICAM-1 on endothelial cells. Fibrinogen has multiple binding sites per molecule that can bridge between platelets, endothelial cells, and monocytes. Fibrinogen-deficient mice have a surprisingly mild bleeding defect (118) and demonstrate that fibrinogen is not strictly necessary for hemostasis.

Plasma contains VWF, most of which exists as dimers and oligomers. VWF is required for platelet adhesion under high shear stress. VWF deficient mice (119), and humans have a significant bleeding disorder (von Willebrand disease). By binding to platelet GP Ib/V/IX, VWF promotes platelet–endothelial interactions. Plasma also contains fibronectin, an adhesive protein that can bind to integrins $\alpha_5\beta_1$ and $\alpha_V\beta_3$ on endothelial cells and supports endothelial cell interaction with monocytes (through binding of $\alpha_4\beta_1$) and platelets (through binding to $\alpha_{IIb}\beta_3$). Mice lacking fibronectin are not viable (120). Upon coagulation, fibrin is formed from fibrinogen, forming a tight meshwork that can entrap all classes of blood cells, including poorly adhesive red blood cells. Fibrin shares some of its adhesive properties with fibrinogen, and immobilized fibrin can bind GP IIb/IIIa even in its nonactivated state.

When in the course of vascular injury the subendothelial matrix is exposed, various collagens, laminin, fibronectin, VWF, and other adhesive molecules become exposed. Collagen and VWF are very important for platelet binding. These interactions are treated in Chapters 46 and 47.

# CELL–CELL INTERACTIONS

## Shear Rate and Shear Stress

To understand the mutual interactions among platelets, monocytes, and endothelial cells, their attachment must be studied under shear flow conditions, because such conditions exist in almost all situations where these interactions occur in the flowing blood. Shear flow in the circulatory system is usually a pressure-driven flow through a series of distensible tubes. Owing to the physical principle of the no-slip condition at the fluid–solid interface, the fluid particles very near the vessel wall (and near each blood cell) do not move relative to that surface. In tube flow, there is a gradient of flow velocities such that the highest velocity is reached in the center of the vessel. The rate of change of flow velocity between adjacent fluid layers is called the shear rate and has units of meters per second (velocity) divided by meters (distance between layers), or per second. The change in velocity between adjacent layers of fluid is associated with a drag force (Newtons) that is calculated per unit surface area (square meters), which is defined as the shear stress (in N per m² or Pascals). The cgs unit, dyne per cm², is also used for shear stress, and 10 dynes per cm² is equal to 1 Pa. The ratio between shear

stress and shear rate is the viscosity, which is measured in Pa·S. An older unit, centipoise, is often used, where 1 centipoise is equal to 0.001 Pa·S. In blood, the viscosity is not constant across the cross section of a blood vessel, but changes as a function of hematocrit (121). The shear stress and shear rate along the vessel wall—the wall shear rate and wall shear stress—are most relevant for cell interactions with the vessel wall. When only one shear stress or shear rate is reported without a qualifier, this usually refers to the wall shear stress or wall shear rate.

## Endothelial Surface Layer

Under normal conditions, the luminal aspect of most endothelial cells is covered by a thick layer of extracellular matrix material called the glycocalyx. The thickness and composition of this layer probably varies between vascular beds, vessel sizes, and physiologic conditions, but most reports place its thickness between 0.3 and 0.6 $\mu$m (122). This layer contains proteoglycans, glycosaminoglycans, and hyaluronic acid. The mechanical properties of this layer are such that there is almost no fluid flow through this layer along the vessel surface (123). This means that the wall shear stress and wall shear rate on the surface of the endothelium of healthy blood vessels is nearly equal to zero (124). All known endothelial adhesion molecules are buried deep within this layer and hardly accessible to adhesion molecules on monocytes, platelets, and other cells in the flowing blood. However, as monocytes and other white blood cells pass through and exit from small capillaries, they can compress the endothelial surface layer sufficiently to initiate adhesive interactions and start rolling (125). In large vessels such as the aorta, carotid artery, or coronary arteries, where cells do not exit from capillaries, it is probably necessary that the endothelial surface layer is degraded before productive leukocyte–endothelial cell interactions can occur (126). It is not known whether cultured endothelial cells maintain a surface layer of similar size and composition as that found in vivo, although there is indirect evidence that they express some hydrodynamically relevant layer on their luminal surface. Recent evidence suggests that the glycocalyx layer is thinner in areas of disturbed flow, endothelial dysfunction, or under inflammatory conditions (127).

## Cell–Cell Interactions Under Shear

To study cell–cell interactions under shear, several in vitro and in vivo methods have been developed. A defined shear stress and shear rate can be applied to cells in suspension using a plate-and-cone apparatus, which produces a uniform shear throughout the fluid (128). A modification of this apparatus is the rheoscope, constructed of two counterrotating transparent cones, which allows the direct visualization of cell–cell interactions at a defined shear rate and shear stress (129). A very popular device is the parallel plate flow chamber (130), which combines excellent visibility because of its optical properties with versatile use of adhesion molecules, cultured endothelial cells, and other substrates. Leukocyte–endothelial and platelet–endothelial interactions have also been studied using capillary tubes (131), which mimic the radial symmetry of the flow profile in most blood vessels in vivo but have limited visibility due to optical diffraction. A specialized form of this method is the traveling capillary apparatus, in which the microscope stage is moved at a speed equal and opposite to that of the cell suspension flow such that the interacting cells appear to remain stationary (132). Other adhesion assays include the radial flow chamber (133) and the graded shear stress flow chamber (134). Recently, autoperfused flow chambers have been developed that allow the study of leukocyte and platelet interactions with adhesion molecules in their natural blood environment (135,136). In so-called static adhesion assays, adhesion occurs in the absence of shear stress, but non-adherent cells, are washed off with an undefined shear stress. Such assays are not suitable for studying blood cell interactions with each other or with endothelial cells. In some tissues and species, monocyte interaction can be studied by intravital microscopy. Relevant to this chapter, monocyte and platelet interactions have been studied with the mouse aorta (137), carotid artery (138), and femoral artery (Huo and Ley, 2004, unpublished) *in vivo*.

## Monocyte–Endothelial Interactions

Monocytes may encounter the endothelium in two fundamentally different situations. In the microcirculation, the initiation of monocyte interactions with the endothelium has not been studied systematically, but the process is probably similar to that described for neutrophils (139). In postcapillary venules, most leukocyte–endothelial interactions are initiated at the point where leukocytes enter the venules from capillaries. Because capillary diameters are smaller than leukocyte diameters in most organs, leukocytes must deform to pass, and in the process probably squeeze down the endothelial surface layer, which brings them in close contact with the endothelial adhesion molecules. Once engaged, these adhesion molecules (see Table 45-6) support stable rolling, during which the endothelial surface layer is probably continuously flattened. The layer appears to recover after the leukocyte has passed. In large vessels such as arteries, this mechanism is not operative because the vessel is much wider than the monocyte. In these cases, most monocyte–endothelial interaction is initiated by secondary capture (41).

### Monocyte Capture

In large vessels such as arteries, it is likely that the endothelial surface layer is damaged or reduced in thickness during the initiation of atherosclerosis or other forms of vascular inflammation. Monocyte interaction is largely P selectin– and PSGL-1–dependent (138). In these larger vessels, secondary capture is very important (41). Secondary capture or secondary tethering describes the transient interaction between a free-flowing blood cell and an already adherent blood cell that can greatly facilitate the initiation of monocyte interactions with the endothelial wall. Although this process was originally described as an interaction between like cells (131), monocyte capture onto the endothelial surface of inflamed arteries can also be initiated by platelets that transiently or stably interact with the vessel wall (60) (Fig. 45-3). In this case, the interaction requires platelet P selectin and monocyte PSGL-1. When a monocyte is captured through interaction with another monocyte, secondary capture probably requires PSGL-1 on the adherent monocyte and L selectin on the incoming monocyte. Secondary capture does not allow any predictions about whether or how rolling along the endothelium will ensue.

### Monocyte Rolling

In mouse models, monocyte rolling is almost entirely dependent on P selectin expressed by the inflamed, or atherosclerotic, endothelium and PSGL-1 on the monocytes. Monocyte rolling is slowed by transient $\alpha_4\beta_1$–VCAM-1 interactions (140). In human atherosclerotic lesions, E selectin expression has been described (141). Monocytes express E selectin ligands, which remain to be identified at the molecular level. With the exception of HEV in secondary lymphatic organs (93), monocyte rolling in small microvessels has not been studied systematically.

### Monocyte Arrest

Rolling *per se* is not sufficient to allow monocyte recruitment. Monocyte arrest is commonly triggered by specific arrest chemokines, chemokines that are deposited on the endothelial surface and can signal integrin activation by binding to GPCRs while the cell is rolling by. Identified arrest chemokines for monocytes include CXCL1, 2, and 3, all of which bind to CXCR2, and CCL5, which mediates arrest by binding to CCR1. In the human system, IL-8 (CXCL8), which binds to CXCR1 and CXCR2, can also act as an arrest chemokine (142). CXCL1, 2, 3, and 8 are synthesized by inflamed endothelial cells, whereas CCL5 is deposited by platelets that transiently interact with the vessel wall (56,60). Soluble CCL2 (MCP-1) can also trigger monocyte arrest, but the relevance for monocyte arrest of endothelial-bound CCR2 has not been demonstrated outside lymph node venules (17,93). The arrest function of many chemokines for monocytes has not been investigated, but it is likely that other chemokines may be able to trigger arrest. Of note, the arrest and chemoattractant functions of chemokines do not necessarily correlate with each other (143). Monocyte arrest does not require a change in intracellular free calcium ("calcium flux") or activation of mitogen-activated protein (MAP) kinase (143).

When a rolling monocyte is exposed to an arrest chemokine, its surface integrins are activated by inside-out signaling. In adhesion assays conducted in atherosclerotic vessels under shear flow conditions, monocyte arrest is triggered by $\alpha_4\beta_1$ integrin binding to VCAM-1 (17), but an arrest component through $\beta_2$ integrins has been described in a flow chamber system using cultured endothelial cells (142). Although it is clear that monocyte arrest is integrin-dependent, the detailed molecular mechanisms can currently only be inferred from studies in other cells (see preceding text). In addition to affinity regulation, integrins also cluster in the plane of the monocyte membrane, giving rise to patches of integrins with increased apparent affinity for multivalent ligands (avidity regulation, Fig. 45-1). The lateral movement of integrins requires their temporary release from cytoskeletal constraints and subsequent reattachment to cytoskeletal elements, an event that is unlikely to occur within milliseconds. A third possibility is that monocyte integrins undergo some limited conformational change, followed by ligand binding and outside-in signaling that leads to rapid bond maturation (9). The exact contribution of affinity and avidity regulation during monocyte arrest is controversial and awaits further experimentation.

### Outside-In Signaling

Once $\alpha_4$ and $\beta_2$ integrins are activated and engage their respective ligands, they transmit signals into the adherent

---

### TABLE 45-6

#### ENDOTHELIAL–MONOCYTE INTERACTIONS

| Endothelial cell | | Monocyte | Remarks |
|---|---|---|---|
| P selectin | $\longleftrightarrow$ | PSGL-1 | Rolling, monocyte activation? |
| VCAM-1 | $\longleftrightarrow$ | $\alpha_4\beta_1$ | Slow rolling, adhesion |
| Fibronectin CS-1 | $\longleftrightarrow$ | $\alpha_4\beta_1$ | Adhesion |
| ICAM-1 | $\longleftrightarrow$ | LFA-1, Mac-1 | Adhesion strengthening? |
| ICAM-2 | $\longleftrightarrow$ | LFA-1 | |
| E selectin | $\longleftrightarrow$ | Unknown ligand | Slow rolling? |
| GRO, IL-8 | $\longleftrightarrow$ | CXCR1, 2 | Monocyte activation |

PSGL, P selectin glycoprotein ligand; VCAM, vascular cell adhesion molecule; ICAM, intercellular adhesion module; LFA, lymphocyte function–associated antigen.

monocyte. These signals probably help the adhesive contact to mature, initiate cell crawling on the endothelial surface, and initiate transmigration into the subendothelial space. In neutrophils (139), but not monocytes (143), a gradual increase in intracellular free calcium has been shown during rolling, with a massive increase in intracellular free calcium upon arrest.

Cytoskeletal interactions of integrins are likely to be important not only for outside-in signaling but also for lending mechanical strength to the bonds between the adherent cells and the vascular endothelium. Many of the relevant monocyte–endothelial cell interactions in the arterial circulation occur in the presence of very high shear forces. $\alpha_4$ integrins attach to VCAM-1 and fibronectin. $\beta_2$ integrins attach to endothelial ICAM-1, ICAM-2, and other ligands. Although arrest of monocytes under moderate wall shear stress of 3 dynes per cm$^2$ was attributed to $\alpha_4$ integrins and did not require $\beta_2$ integrins (17), it is likely that $\beta_2$ integrins contribute to bond strengthening, migration, and transendothelial migration.

## Platelet–Monocyte Interactions Under Shear

Platelet–monocyte interactions are most commonly studied in plate-and-cone devices, which produce a uniform shear rate and shear stress throughout the cell suspension (144). It is clear that most, if not all, monocyte–platelet adhesion is mediated by P selectin on the activated platelet surface and PSGL-1 on the monocyte. That this interaction occurs *in vivo* is demonstrated by the presence of platelet–monocyte aggregates in patients with coronary heart disease (145). The abundance of these aggregates correlates with the incidence of unstable angina, myocardial infarction, and stroke (95). Platelet–monocyte aggregates are also found in the blood of apoE-deficient mice on a proatherogenic diet, but not in control mice (60,146).

Monocyte interactions have also been studied in flow chambers coated with platelet monolayers. This model is most relevant to the adhesion of monocytes at sites of vascular injury, where a platelet monolayer forms almost immediately. Monocyte interaction with platelet monolayers is strictly P selectin– and PSGL-1–dependent and shares many similarities with monocyte–endothelial cell interactions, with the exception that P selectin expression on monolayers of activated platelets is probably higher than on endothelial cells, and the rolling velocity is consequently lower. Monocytes can adhere to platelets by an interaction of monocyte Mac-1 with plasma fibrinogen and platelet GP IIb/IIIa (147). Platelets express ICAM-2, a known ligand for LFA-1, which is expressed on monocytes (see Fig. 45-4). The relative importance of these other pathways *in vivo* is not known. P selectin–PSGL-1 interactions seem to dominate platelet–monocyte interactions (see Table 45-7).

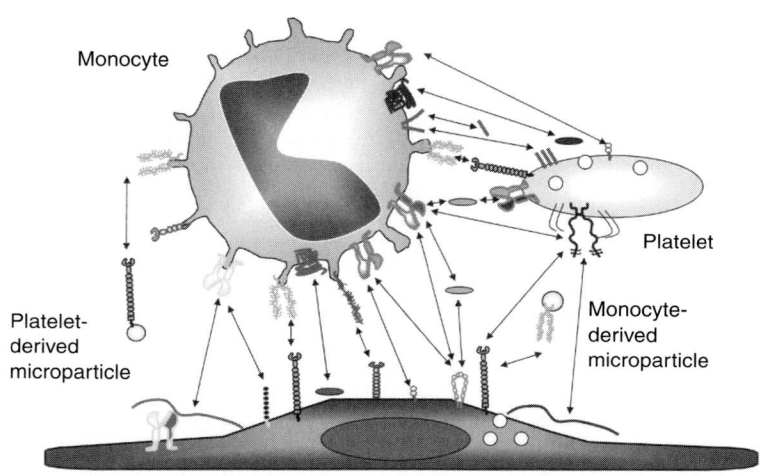

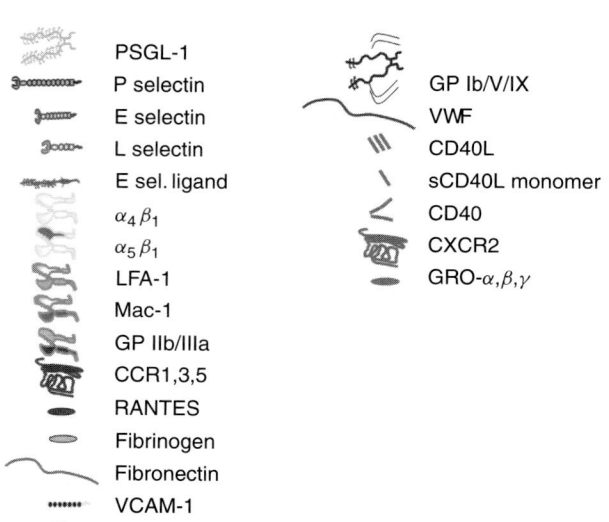

**FIGURE 45-4.** Monocyte–platelet–endothelial interactions. Each *arrow* shows a molecular interaction, legend for molecules indicated in figure. Monocyte- and platelet-derived microparticles are also shown. See text for details (see Color Fig. 45-4). PSGL, P selectin glycoprotein ligand; LFA, lymphocyte function–associated antigen; GP, glycoprotein; CCR, corresponding chemokine receptors; RANTES, regulated on activation, normal T cell expressed and secreted; VCAM, vascular cell adhesion molecule; ICAM, intercellular adhesion module; VWF, von Willebrand factor.

**TABLE 45-7**

PLATELET INTERACTIONS WITH ENDOTHELIAL CELLS AND MONOCYTES

| Endothelial cell | | Platelet | | Monocyte | | Remarks |
|---|---|---|---|---|---|---|
| Fibronectin | ⟷ | GP IIb/IIIa | ⟷ | Mac-1 | | IIb/IIIa with Mac-1 through Fg |
| CD40 | ⟷ | CD40L | ⟷ | CD40 | | Activates EC and monocytes |
| P selectin | ⟷ | GP Ib/V/IX | ⟷ | Mac-1 | ↕ | Also binds VWF |
| | | | | ICAM-1 | | Homotypic aggregation |
| | | ICAM-2 | ⟷ | LFA-1 | ↕ | Function not demonstrated |
| Unknown, maybe GP Ibα? | ⟷ | P selectin | ⟷ | PSGL-1 | ↕ | GP Ibα on EC controversial |
| | | | | L selectin | | Secondary capture |
| Proteoglycans | ⟷ | RANTES | ⟷ | CCR1,3,5 | | Activates monocytes |
| Proteoglycans | ⟷ | PF4 | ⟷ | CXCR3 variant | | Activates monocytes |
| VEGF-R | ⟷ | VEGF | ⟷ | | | Activates EC |

EC, endothelial cell; VWF, von Willebrand factor; ICAM, intercellular adhesion module; LFA, lymphocyte function-associated antigen; PSGL, P selectin glycoprotein ligand; GP, glycoprotein; RANTES, regulated on activation, normal T cell expressed and secreted; CCR, corresponding chemokine receptors; PF4, Platelet factor 4; VEGF, vascular endothelial growth factor.

## Platelet–Endothelial Interactions Under Shear

Platelets can roll on and adhere to endothelial cells through at least two mechanisms. One requires P selectin expression on inflamed endothelial cells and results in platelet rolling in microvessels (88). In this interaction, endothelial P selectin binds to a ligand on platelets, most likely GP Ibα (148). Another

**TABLE 45-8**

PROINFLAMMATORY AND PROTHROMBOTIC MOLECULES ON PLATELETS, MONOCYTES, AND ENDOTHELIAL CELLS

**PLATELETS**
Prothrombotic
VWF, IIb/IIIa, fibrinogen
CD40L, sCD40L: induces MCP-1, IL-6, IL-8 in monocytes, E selectin, VCAM-1, ICAM-1 in endothelial cells
Serotonin, thromboxane A$_2$
Proinflammatory
RANTES (CCL5), platelet factor 4 (CXCL4), P selectin
sCD40L, CD40L
VEGF

**MONOCYTES**
Prothrombotic
Tissue factor, Mac-1
Proinflammatory
Chemokine receptors CCR2, CXCR2, CCR1, CCR5, Mac-1, LFA-1, ICAM-1, chemokines
CD40

**ENDOTHELIAL CELLS**
Prothrombotic
VWF
Proinflammatory
P selectin, E selectin, VCAM-1, ICAM-1, ICAM-2

VWF, von Willebrand factor; MCP, monocyte chemoattractant protein; IL, interleukin; VCAM, vascular cell adhesion molecule; ICAM, intercellular adhesion module; RANTES, regulated on activation, normal T cell expressed and secreted; VEGF, vascular endothelial growth factor; LFA, lymphocyte function–associated antigen.

mechanism for platelet–endothelial cell interactions is found in large arteries and appears to be relevant for the process of atherosclerosis (60). It requires P selectin expression on platelets, which interact with an unknown ligand on endothelial cells (Table 45-7). A third candidate mechanism for platelet attachment to endothelial cells is dependent on platelet GP Ibα interacting with VWF, which is stored in Weibel-Palade bodies of endothelial cells and can be released as an ultralarge VWF upon activation (89).

## Enhanced Monocyte Adhesion by Platelets and Microparticles

Given these extensive interactions, the monocyte–platelet–endothelial cell system can be viewed as a synergistic proinflammatory and prothrombotic triad. Platelets enhance monocyte binding to inflamed endothelium, which is critically important in atherosclerosis (60,96). Conversely, monocytes rolling on endothelial cells can deliver platelets that are attached to them (145). Because each of these cell types brings critical components of the hemostasis, coagulation, and inflammation system, it is easy to see how the mutual interaction of these cells greatly enhances both inflammation and thrombosis (see Table 45-8). The intimate interaction between platelets, endothelial cells, and monocytes results in enhanced monocyte recruitment (see Fig. 45-5) and accelerated atherosclerosis (60).

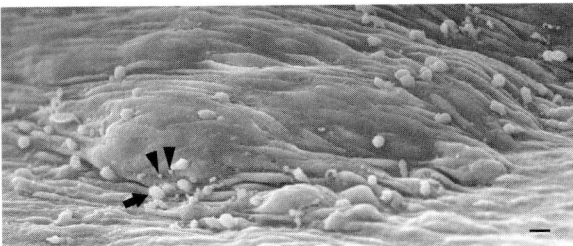

**FIGURE 45-5.** Monocyte and platelet adhesion in an atherosclerotic apoE$^{-/-}$ mouse carotid artery. Monocytes (*arrow*) and platelets (*arrowheads*) preferentially adhere in the shoulder region of this atherosclerotic plaque. Sample taken 30 min after intravenous infusion of activated mouse platelets. Scale bar indicates 10 μm. Scanning electron micrograph prepared by Jan Redick and Yuqing Huo, University of Virginia.

## Tissue Factor and Monocyte-Derived Microparticles

Tissue factor initiates coagulation (see Chapter 5). Although tissue factor is expressed in many extravascular cells, its expression is highest on activated monocytes. Monocytes continuously shed microparticles ranging in size from 0.05 to 1 $\mu$m. Monocyte-derived microparticles lack metabolic functions but are enriched in tissue factor and many other monocyte components (45,115). Microparticles of both platelet (149) and monocyte origin are abundant in human and mouse plasma, and their number can increase during disease states.

Some (150), if not most, of the "plasma" tissue factor is, in fact, contained in monocyte-derived microparticles (45,115). This source of tissue factor is available for incorporation into platelet aggregates, where it initiates coagulation. Monocyte-derived microparticles express PSGL-1, and activated platelets express P selectin. Because the P selectin–PSGL-1 interaction is critical for microparticle recruitment to sites of thrombosis, P selectin–deficient mice (151) and PSGL-1–deficient mice (152) both have a reduced propensity for intravascular thrombus formation with little evidence of an overt bleeding disorder. The formation of monocyte-derived particles can be induced by soluble P selectin (152), which has been proposed to be a useful mechanism for delivering procoagulant activity to patients with hemophilia.

# CROSS TALK BETWEEN INFLAMMATION AND HEMOSTASIS

## Monocyte Activation by Interaction with Platelets

Activated platelets can bind to monocytes and deposit chemokines such as RANTES, which cause an increase in $\alpha_4\beta_1$ integrin avidity (lateral clustering) and affinity (conformational change) (56,60). Platelet-induced chemokine deposition can also induce monocyte differentiation into macrophages, at least *in vitro* (153). Platelet CD40L, either surface-expressed or secreted, interacts with monocyte CD40, and causes monocyte activation (99). Chemokine-induced L selectin shedding on monocytes could potentially limit the inflammatory response. Chemokines can also induce a secretory response in monocytes, including release of specific, secretory and tertiary granules. Monocyte degranulation releases a wide variety of proinflammatory mediators and enzymes.

## Proinflammatory Effects of Coagulation Products

Not only does the inflammatory response enhance the coagulation response (discussed earlier), but the converse is also true. Many coagulation products are proinflammatory, including fibrin degradation products. Thrombin has strong proinflammatory effects, as has the binding of coagulation factor X to monocyte Mac-1 (154). This so-called cross talk between the inflammatory and coagulation systems is described in more detail in Chapter 53.

## References

1. Passlick B, Flieger D, Ziegler-Heitbrock HW. Identification and characterization of a novel monocyte subpopulation in human peripheral blood. *Blood* 1989;74:2527–2534.
2. Geissmann F, Jung S, Littman DR. Blood monocytes consist of two principal subsets with distinct migratory properties. *Immunity* 2003;19:71–82.
3. Hynes RO. Integrins: versatility, modulation, and signaling in cell adhesion. *Cell* 1992;69:11–25.
4. Hynes RO. Integrins: bidirectional, allosteric signaling machines. *Cell* 2002; 110:673–687.
5. Xiong JP, Stehle T, Diefenbach B, et al. Crystal structure of the extracellular segment of integrin $\alpha_V\beta_3$. *Science* 2001;294:339–345.
6. Lu C, Takagi J, Springer TA. Association of the membrane proximal regions of the $\alpha$ and $\beta$ subunit cytoplasmic domains constrains an integrin in the inactive state. *J Biol Chem* 2001;276:14642–14648.
7. Tadokoro S, Shattil SJ, Eto K, et al. Talin binding to integrin beta tails: a final common step in integrin activation. *Science* 2003;302:103–106.
8. Bazzoni G, Hemler ME. Are changes in integrin affinity and conformation overemphasized? *Trends Biochem Sci* 1998;23:30–34.
9. Alon R, Grabovsky V, Feigelson S. Chemokine induction of integrin avidity on rolling and arrested leukocytes: local signaling events or global stepwise activation? *Microcirculation* 2003;10:297–311.
10. Du X, Plow EF, Frelinger AL III, et al. Ligands "activate" integrin $\alpha_{IIb}\beta_3$ (platelet GPIIb-IIIa). *Cell* 1991;65:409–416.
11. Berlin C, Bargatze RF, Campbell JJ, et al. $\alpha_4$ integrins mediate lymphocyte attachment and rolling under physiologic flow. *Cell* 1995;80:413–422.
12. Elices MJ, Osborn L, Takada Y, et al. VCAM-1 on activated endothelium interacts with the leukocyte integrin VLA-4 at a site distinct from the VLA-4/fibronectin binding site. *Cell* 1990;60:577–584.
13. Chigaev A, Zwartz G, Graves SW, et al. $\alpha_4\beta_1$ integrin affinity changes govern cell adhesion. *J Biol Chem* 2003;278:38174–38182.
14. Yang YT, Rayburn H, Hynes RO. Cell adhesion events mediated by $\alpha_4$ integrins are essential in placental and cardiac development. *Development* 1995; 121:549–560.
15. Fassler R, Meyer M. Consequences of lack of beta 1 integrin gene expression in mice. *Genes Dev* 1995;9:1896–1908.
16. Shih PT, Brennan ML, Vora DK, et al. Blocking very late antigen-4 integrin decreases leukocyte entry and fatty streak formation in mice fed an atherogenic diet. *Circ Res* 1999;84:345–351.
17. Huo Y, Weber C, Forlow SB, et al. The chemokine KC, but not monocyte chemoattractant protein-1, triggers monocyte arrest on early atherosclerotic endothelium. *J Clin Invest* 2001;108:1307–1314.
18. Dunne JL, Ballantyne CM, Beaudet AL, et al. Control of leukocyte rolling velocity in TNF-$\alpha$ induced inflammation by LFA-1 and Mac-1. *Blood* 2002; 99:336–341.
19. Coxon A, Rieu P, Barkalow FJ, et al. A novel role for the beta-2 integrin CD11b/CD18 in neutrophil apoptosis - a homeostatic mechanism in inflammation. *Immunity* 1996;5:653–666.
20. Simon DI, Dhen Z, Seifert P, et al. Decreased neointimal formation in Mac-1(−/−) mice reveals a role for inflammation in vascular repair after angioplasty. *J Clin Invest* 2000;105:293–300.
21. Altieri DC, Mannucci PM, Capitanio AM. Binding of fibrinogen to human monocytes. *J Clin Invest* 1986;78:968–976.
22. Fan S-T, Edgington TS. Integrin regulation of leukocyte inflammatory functions: CD11b/CD18 enhancement of the tumor necrosis factor-$\alpha$ responses of monocytes. *J Immunol* 1993;150:2972–2980.
23. Davis GE. The Mac-1 and p150,95 $\beta_2$ integrins bind denatured proteins to mediate leukocyte cell substrate adhesion. *Exp Cell Res* 1992;200: 242–252.
24. Campbell JJ, Hedrick J, Zlotnik A, et al. Chemokines and the arrest of lymphocytes rolling under flow conditions. *Science* 1998;279:381–384.
25. Schmits R, Kündig TM, Baker DM, et al. LFA-1 deficient mice show normal CTL responses to virus but fail to reject immunogenic tumor. *J Exp Med* 1996;183:1415–1426.
26. Zhou M, Brown EJ. Leukocyte response integrin and integrin-associated protein act as a signal transduction unit in generation of a phagocyte respiratory burst. *J Exp Med* 1993;178:1165–1174.
27. Hodivala-Dilke KM, McHugh KP, Tsakiris DA, et al. Beta 3-integrin-deficient mice are a model for Glanzmann thrombasthenia showing placental defects and reduced survival. *J Clin Invest* 1999;103:229–238.
28. Duperray A, Languino LR, Plescia J, et al. Molecular identification of a novel fibrinogen binding site on the first domain of ICAM-1 regulating leukocyte-endothelium bridging. *J Biol Chem* 1997;272:435–441.
29. Collins RG, Velji R, Guevara NV, et al. P-selectin or ICAM-1 deficiency substantially protects against atherosclerosis in apo E deficient mice. *J Exp Med* 2000;191:189–194.
30. Muller WA, Weigl SA, Deng X, et al. PECAM-1 is required for transendothelial migration of leukocytes. *J Exp Med* 1993;178:449–460.
31. Elias CG, Spellberg JP, Karantamir B, et al. Ligation of CD31/PECAM-1 modulates the function of lymphocytes, monocytes and neutrophils. *Eur J Immunol* 1998;28:1948–1958.
32. Duncan GS, Andrew DP, Takimoto H, et al. Genetic evidence for functional redundancy of platelet/endothelial cell adhesion molecule-1 (PECAM-1): CD31- deficient mice reveal PECAM-1-dependent and PECAM-1-independent functions. *J Immunol* 1999;162:3022–3030.
33. Schenkel AR, Chew TW, Muller WA. Platelet endothelial cell adhesion molecule deficiency or blockade significantly reduces leukocyte emigration in a majoity of mouse strains. *J Immunol* 2004;173:6403–6408.
34. Arbones ML, Ord DC, Ley K, et al. Lymphocyte homing and leukocyte rolling and migration are impaired in L-selectin-deficient mice. *Immunity* 1994;1:247–260.

35. Lewinsohn DM, Bargatze RF, Butcher EC. Leukocyte-endothelial cell recognition: evidence of a common molecular mechanism shared by neutrophils, lymphocytes, and other leukocytes. *J Immunol* 1987;138: 4313–4321.

36. Tözeren A, Ley K. How do selectins mediate leukocyte rolling in venules? *Biophys J* 1992;63:700–709.

37. Ley K. Arrest chemokines. *Microcirculation* 2003;10:289–295.

38. von Andrian UH, Hasslen SR, Nelson RD, et al. A central role for microvillous receptor presentation in leukocyte adhesion under flow. *Cell* 1995;82: 989–999.

39. Peschon JJ, Slack JL, Reddy P, et al. An essential role for ectodomain shedding in mammalian development. *Science* 1998;282:1281–1284.

40. Lim YC, Snapp K, Kansas GS, et al. Important contributions of P-selectin glycoprotein ligand-1- mediated secondary capture to human monocyte adhesion to P- selectin, E-selectin, and TNF-alpha-activated endothelium under flow *in vitro*. *J Immunol* 1998;161:2501–2508.

41. Eriksson EE, Xie X, Werr J, et al. Importance of primary capture and L-selectin-dependent secondary capture in leukocyte accumulation in inflammation and atherosclerosis *in vivo*. *J Exp Med* 2001;194:205–218.

42. Yang J, Furie BC, Furie B. The biology of P-selectin glycoprotein ligand-1: its role as a selectin counterreceptor in leukocyte-endothelial and leukocyte- platelet interaction. *Thromb Haemost* 1999;81:1–7.

43. Moore KL, Patel KD, Breuhl RE, et al. P-selectin glycoprotein ligand-1 mediates rolling of human neutrophils on P-selectin. *J Cell Biol* 1995;128: 661–671.

44. Ley K, Kansas GS. Selectins in T-cell recruitment to non-lymphoid tissues and sites of inflammation. *Nat Rev Immunol* 2004;4:325–335.

45. Furie B, Furie BC. Role of platelet P-selectin and microparticle PSGL-1 in thrombus formation. *Trends Mol Med* 2004;10:171–178.

46. Cambien B, Wagner DD. A new role in hemostasis for the adhesion receptor P-selectin. *Trends Mol Med* 2004;10:179–186.

47. Andre P, Hartwell D, Hrachovinova I, et al. Pro-coagulant state resulting from high levels of soluble P-selectin in blood. *Proc Natl Acad Sci U S A* 2000;97:13835–13840.

48. Tchernychev B, Furie B, Furie BC. Peritoneal macrophages express both P-selectin and PSGL-1. *J Cell Biol* 2003;163:1145–1155.

49. Ossowski L, Aguirre-Ghiso JA. Urokinase receptor and integrin partnership: coordination of signaling for cell adhesion, migration and growth. *Curr Opin Cell Biol* 2000;12(5):613–620.

50. Hemler ME. Tetraspanin proteins mediate cellular penetration, invasion, and fusion events and define a novel type of membrane microdomain. *Annu Rev Cell Dev Biol* 2003;19:397–422.

51. Cooper D, Lindberg FP, Gamble JR, et al. Transendothelial migration of neutrophils involves integrin- associated protein (CD47). *Proc Natl Acad Sci U S A* 1995;92:3978–3982.

52. Porter JC, Hogg N. Integrins take partners: cross-talk between integrins and other membrane receptors. *Trends Cell Biol* 1998;8:390–396.

53. Sendo F, Araki Y. Regulation of leukocyte adherence and migration by glycosylphosphatidyl-inositol-anchored proteins. *J Leukoc Biol* 1999;66: 369–374.

54. Olson TS, Ley K. Chemokines and chemokine receptors in leukocyte trafficking. *Am J Physiol Regul Integr Comp Physiol* 2002;283:R7–R28.

55. Springer TA. Traffic signals for lymphocyte recirculation and leukocyte emigration: the multistep paradigm. *Cell* 1994;76:301–314.

56. Schober A, Manka D, von Hundelshausen P, et al. Deposition of platelet RANTES triggering monocyte recruitment requires P-selectin and is involved in neointima formation after arterial injury. *Circulation* 2002;106: 1523–1529.

57. Gu L, Okada Y, Clinton SK, et al. Absence of monocyte chemoattractant protein-1 reduces atherosclerosis in low density lipoprotein receptor-deficient mice. *Mol Cell* 1998;2:275–281.

58. Boring L, Gosling J, Cleary M, et al. Decreased lesion formation in CCR2$^{-/-}$ mice reveals a role for chemokines in the initiation of atherosclerosis. *Nature* 1998;394:894–897.

59. Weber C, Weber KS, Klier C, et al. Specialized roles of the chemokine receptors CCR1 and CCR5 in the recruitment of monocytes and T(H)1-like/CD45RO(+) T cells. *Blood* 2001;97:1144–1146.

60. Huo Y, Schober A, Forlow SB, et al. Circulating activated platelets exacerbate atherosclerosis in mice deficient in apolipoprotein E. *Nat Med* 2003;9: 61–67.

61. Peled A, Grabovsky V, Habler L, et al. The chemokine SDF-1 stimulates integrin-mediated arrest of CD34$^{+}$ cells on vascular endothelium under shear flow. *J Clin Invest* 1999;104:1199–1211.

62. Frenette PS, Moyna C, Hartwell DW, et al. Platelet-endothelial interactions in inflamed mesenteric venules. *Blood* 1998;91:1318–1324.

63. Johnson RC, Chapman SM, Dong ZM, et al. Absence of P-selectin delays fatty streak formation in mice. *J Clin Invest* 1997;99:1037–1043.

64. Manka DR, Collins RG, Ley K, et al. Absence of P-selectin, but not intercellular adhesion molecule-1, attenuates neointimal growth after arterial injury in apolipoprotein E-deficient mice. *Circulation* 2001;103: 1000–1005.

65. Burger PC, Wagner DD. Platelet P-selectin facilitates atherosclerotic lesion development. *Blood* 2003;101:2661–2666.

66. Manka DR, Forlow SB, Sanders JM, et al. Critical role of platelet P-selectin in the response to arterial injury in apolipoprotein-E–deficient mice. *Arterioscler Thromb Vasc Biol* 2004;24:1124–1129.

67. Berger G, Hartwell DW, Wagner DD. P-selectin and platelet clearance. *Blood* 1998;92:4446–4452.

68. Pan JL, Xia LJ, McEver RP. Comparison of promoters for the murine and human P-selectin genes suggests species-specific and conserved mechanisms for transcriptional regulation in endothelial cells. *J Biol Chem* 1998;273:10058–10067.

69. Wenzel K, Felix S, Kleber FX, et al. E-selectin polymorphism and atherosclerosis: an association study. *Hum Mol Genet* 1994;3:1935–1937.

70. Urzainqui A, Serrador JM, Viedma F, et al. ITAM-based interaction of ERM proteins with Syk mediates signaling by the leukocyte adhesion receptor PSGL-1. *Immunity* 2002;17:401–412.

71. Weyrich AS, Elstad MR, McEver RP, et al. Activated platelets signal chemokine synthesis by human monocytes. *J Clin Invest* 1996;97:1525–1534.

72. Xia L, Sperandio M, Yago T, et al. P-selectin glycoprotein ligand-1 deficient mice have impaired leukocyte tethering to E-selectin under flow. *J Clin Invest* 2002;109:939–950.

73. Zanardo RC, Bonder CS, Hwang JM, et al. A down regulatable E-selectin ligand is functionally important for PSGL-1-independent leukocyte-endothelial cell interactions. *Blood* 2004;104:3766–3773.

74. Ley K. Integration of inflammatory signals by rolling neutrophils. *Immunol Rev* 2002;186:8–18.

75. Wagers AJ, Lowe JB, Kansas GS. An important role for the alpha-1,3 fucosyltransferase, FucT-VII, in leukocyte adhesion to E-selectin. *Blood* 1996;88:2125–2132.

76. Snapp KR, Heitzig CE, Ellies LG, et al. Differential requirements for the O-linked branching enzyme core 2 2 β1-6-N-glucosaminyltransferase in biosynthesis of ligands for E-selectin and P-selectin. *Blood* 2001;97:3806–3811.

77. Simon SI, Hu Y, Vestweber D, et al. Neutrophil tethering on E-selectin activates beta 2 integrin binding to ICAM-1 through a mitogen-activated protein kinase signal transduction pathway. *J Immunol* 2000;164:4348–4358.

78. Smith ML, Olson TS, Ley K. CXCR2- and E-selectin-induced neutrophil arrest during inflammation *in vivo*. *J Exp Med* 2004;200:935–939.

79. Bullard DC, Kunkel EJ, Kubo H, et al. Infectious susceptibility and severe deficiency of leukocyte rolling and recruitment in E-selectin and P-selectin double mutant mice. *J Exp Med* 1996;183:2329–2336.

80. Frenette PS, Mayadas TN, Rayburn H, et al. Susceptibility to infection and altered hematopoiesis in mice deficient in both P- and E-selectins. *Cell* 1996; 84:563–574.

81. Huo Y, Ley K. Adhesion molecules and atherogenesis. *Acta Physiol Scand* 2001;173:35–43.

82. Dansky HM, Barlow CB, Lominska C, et al. Adhesion of monocytes to arterial endothelium and initiation of atherosclerosis are critically dependent on vascular cell adhesion molecule-1 gene dosage. *Arterioscler Thromb Vasc Biol* 2001;21:1662–1667.

83. Muller WA. The role of PECAM-1 (CD31) in leukocyte emigration: studies *in vitro* and *in vivo*. *J Leukoc Biol* 1995;57:523–528.

84. Chavakis T, Preissner KT, Santoso S. Leukocyte trans-endothelial migration: JAMs add new pieces to the puzzle. *Thromb Haemost* 2003;89:13–17.

85. Berlin C, Berg EL, Briskin MJ, et al. α$_4$β$_7$ integrin mediates lymphocyte binding to the mucosal vascular addressin MAdCAM-1. *Cell* 1993; 74:185–195.

86. Norris P, Poston RN, Thomas DS, et al. The expression of endothelial leukocyte adhesion molecule-1 (ELAM-1), intercellular adhesion molecule-1 (ICAM-1), and vascular cell adhesion molecule-1 (VCAM-1) in experimental cutaneous inflammation: a comparison of ultraviolet-B erythema and delayed hypersensitivity. *J Invest Dermatol* 1991;96:763–770.

87. Hemmerich S, Butcher EC, Rosen SD. Sulfation-dependent recognition of high endothelial venules (HEV)-ligands by L-selectin and MECA 79, an adhesion-blocking monoclonal antibody. *J Exp Med* 1994;180:2219–2226.

88. Frenette PS, Johnson RC, Hynes MR, et al. Platelets roll on stimulated endothelium *in vivo*: an interaction mediated by endothelial P-selectin. *Proc Natl Acad Sci U S A* 1995;92:7450–7454.

89. Padilla A, Moake JL, Bernardo A, et al. P-selectin anchors newly released ultralarge von Willebrand factor multimers to the endothelial cell surface. *Blood* 2004;103:2150–2156.

90. Lopez JA, Dong JF. Cleavage of von Willebrand factor by ADAMTS-13 on endothelial cells. *Semin Hematol* 2004;41:15–23.

91. Goebeler M, Yoshimura T, Toksoy A, et al. The chemokine repertoire of human dermal microvascular endothelial cells and its regulation by inflammatory cytokines. *J Invest Dermatol* 1997;108:445–451.

92. Hebert CA, Luscinskas FW, Kiely J-M, et al. Endothelial and leukocyte forms of IL-8: conversion by thrombin and interactions with neutrophils. *J Immunol* 1990;145:3033–3040.

93. Palframan RT, Jung S, Cheng G, et al. Inflammatory chemokine transport and presentation in HEV: a remote control mechanism for monocyte recruitment to lymph nodes in inflamed tissues. *J Exp Med* 2001;194:1361–1373.

94. Weber KSC, Nelson PJ, Grone HJ, et al. Expression of CCR2 by endothelial cells—implications for MCP-1 mediated wound injury repair and *in vivo* inflammatory activation of endothelium. *Arterioscler Thromb Vasc Biol* 1999; 19:2085–2093.

95. Michelson AD, Barnard MR, Krueger LA, et al. Circulating monocyte-platelet aggregates are a more sensitive marker of *in vivo* platelet activation than platelet surface P- selectin: studies in baboons, human coronary intervention, and human acute myocardial infarction. *Circulation* 2001;104: 1533–1537.

96. Massberg S, Brand K, Gruner S, et al. A critical role of platelet adhesion in the initiation of atherosclerotic lesion formation. *J Exp Med* 2002;196:887–896.

97. Frenette PS, Denis CV, Weiss L, et al. P-Selectin glycoprotein ligand 1 (PSGL-1) is expressed on platelets and can mediate platelet-endothelial interactions *in vivo*. *J Exp Med* 2000;191:1413–1422.

98. Sperandio M, Smith ML, Forlow SB, et al. P-selectin glycoprotein ligand-1 mediates L-selectin-dependent leukocyte rolling in venules. *J Exp Med* 2003;197:1355–1363.

99. Prasad KS, Andre P, Yan Y, et al. The platelet CD40L/GP IIb-IIIa axis in atherothrombotic disease. *Curr Opin Hematol* 2003;10:356–361.

100. Hato T, Pampori N, Shattil SJ. Complementary roles for receptor clustering and conformational change in the adhesive and signaling functions of integrin $\alpha_{IIb}\beta_3$. *J Cell Biol* 1998;141:1685–1695.

101. Tronik-Le Roux D, Roullot V, Poujol C, et al. Thrombasthenic mice generated by replacement of the integrin alpha(IIb) gene: demonstration that transcriptional activation of this megakaryocytic locus precedes lineage commitment. *Blood* 2000;96:1399–1408.

102. Altieri DC, Plescia J, Plow EF. The structural motif glycine-190-valine-202 of the fibrinogen-gamma chain interacts with CD11b/CD18 integrin ($\alpha_M\beta_2$, Mac-1) and promotes leukocyte adhesion. *J Biol Chem* 1993;268:1847–1853.

103. Caron A, Theoret JF, Mousa SA, et al. Anti-platelet effects of GPIIb/IIIa and P-selectin antagonism, platelet activation, and binding to neutrophils. *J Cardiovasc Pharmacol* 2002;40:296–306.

104. Shpilberg O, Rabi I, Schiller K, et al. Patients with Glanzmann thrombasthenia lacking platelet glycoprotein $\alpha_{IIb}\beta_3$ (GPIIb/IIIa) and $\alpha_V\beta_3$ receptors are not protected from atherosclerosis. *Circulation* 2002;105:1044–1048.

105. Nieuwenhuis HK, Akkerman JW, Houdijk WP, et al. Human blood platelets showing no response to collagen fail to express surface glycoprotein Ia. *Nature* 1985;318:470–472.

106. Nieswandt B, Watson SP. Platelet-collagen interaction: is GPVI the central receptor? *Blood* 2003;102:449–461.

107. Gibbins J, Asselin J, Farndale R, et al. Tyrosine phosphorylation of the Fc receptor gamma-chain in collagen-stimulated platelets. *J Biol Chem* 1996;271:18095–18099.

108. Bodin S, Tronchere H, Payrastre B. Lipid rafts are critical membrane domains in blood platelet activation processes. *Biochim Biophys Acta* 2003;1610:247–257.

109. Moroi M, Jung SM, Okuma M, et al. A patient with platelets deficient in glycoprotein VI that lack both collagen-induced aggregation and adhesion. *J Clin Invest* 1989;83:1440–1445.

110. Andrews RK, Gardiner EE, Shen Y, et al. Glycoprotein Ib-IX-V. *Int J Biochem Cell Biol* 2003;35:1170–1174.

111. Methia N, Andre P, Denis CV, et al. Localized reduction of atherosclerosis in von Willebrand factor- deficient mice. *Blood* 2001;98(5):1424–1428.

112. Lasagni L, Francalanci M, Annunziato F, et al. An alternatively spliced variant of CXCR3 mediates the inhibition of endothelial cell growth induced by IP-10, Mig, and I-TAC, and acts as functional receptor for platelet factor 4. *J Exp Med* 2003;197:1537–1549.

113. Gear AR, Camerini D. Platelet chemokines and chemokine receptors: Linking hemostasis, inflammation and host defense. *Microcirculation* 2003;10:335–350.

114. Kahn ML, Zheng YW, Huang W, et al. A dual thrombin receptor system for platelet activation. *Nature* 1998;394:690–694.

115. Falati S, Liu Q, Gross P, et al. Accumulation of tissue factor into developing thrombi in vivo is dependent upon microparticle P-selectin glycoprotein ligand 1 and platelet P-selectin. *J Exp Med* 2003;197:1585–1598.

116. Matsumoto N, Nomura S, Kamihata H, et al. Association of platelet-derived microparticles with C-C chemokines on vascular complication in patients with acute myocardial infarction. *Clin Appl Thromb Hemost* 2002;8:279–286.

117. Omoto S, Nomura S, Shouzu A, et al. Detection of monocyte-derived microparticles in patients with type II diabetes mellitus. *Diabetologia* 2002;45:550–555.

118. Xiao Q, Danton MJ, Witte DP, et al. Fibrinogen deficiency is compatible with the development of atherosclerosis in mice. *J Clin Invest* 1998;101:1184–1194.

119. Denis C, Methia N, Frenette PS, et al. A mouse model of severe von-Willebrand-disease—defects in hemostasis and thrombosis. *Proc Natl Acad Sci U S A* 1998;95:9524–9529.

120. Hynes RO. Targeted mutations in cell adhesion genes—what have we learned from them. *Dev Biol* 1996;180:402–412.

121. Long DS, Smith ML, Pries AR, et al. Microviscometry reveals reduced blood viscosity and altered shear rate and shear stress profiles in microvessels after hemodilution. *Proc Natl Acad Sci U S A* 2004;101:10060–10065.

122. Vink H, Duling BR. Identification of distinct luminal domains for macromolecules, erythrocytes, and leukocytes within mammalian capillaries. *Circ Res* 1996;79:581–589.

123. Damiano ER, Duling BR, Ley K, et al. Axisymmetric pressure-driven flow of rigid pellets through a cylindrical tube lined with a deformable porous wall layer. *J Fluid Mech* 1996;314:163–189.

124. Smith ML, Long Ds, Damiano ER, et al. Near-wall micro-PIV reveals a hydrodynamically relevant endothelial surface layer *in vivo*. *Biophys J* 2003;85:637–645.

125. Ley K, Adhesion molecules and the recruitment of leukocytes in postcapillary venules. In: Shepro D, ed. *Microvascular research: biology and pathology*, Burlington, MA: Elsevier Academic Press, 2005:317–322.

126. Vink H, Constantinescu AA, Spaan JA. Oxidized lipoproteins degrade the endothelial surface layer: implications for platelet-endothelial cell adhesion. *Circulation* 2000;101:1500–1502.

127. Henry CB, Duling BR. TNF-alpha increases entry of macromolecules into luminal endothelial cell glycocalyx. *Am J Physiol Heart Circ Physiol* 2000;279:H2815–H2823.

128. Ley K, Lundgren E, Berger EM, et al. Shear-dependent inhibition of granulocyte adhesion to cultured endothelium by dextran sulfate. *Blood* 1989;73:1324–1330.

129. Schmid-Schonbein H, von Gosen J, Heinich L, et al. A counter-rotating "rheoscope chamber" for the study of the microrheology of blood cell aggregation by microscopic observation and microphotometry. *Microvasc Res* 1973;6:366–376.

130. Lawrence MB, McIntire LV, Eskin SG. Effect of flow on polymorphonuclear leukocyte/endothelial cell adhesion. *Blood* 1987;70:1284–1290.

131. Bargatze RF, Kurk S, Butcher EC, et al. Neutrophils roll on adherent neutrophils bound to cytokine- induced endothelial cells via L-selectin on the rolling cells. *J Exp Med* 1994;180:1785–1792.

132. Goldsmith HL. Red cell motions and wall interactions in tube flow. *Fed Proc* 1971;30:1578–1588.

133. Cozens-Roberts C, Quinn JA, Lauffenburger DA. Receptor-mediated cell attachment and detachment kinetics. II. Experimental model studies with the radial-flow detachment assay. *Biophys J* 1990;58:857–872.

134. Usami S, Chen HH, Zhao Y, et al. Design and construction of a linear shear stress flow chamber. *Ann Biomed Eng* 1993;21:77–83.

135. Smith ML, Sperandio M, Galkina EV, et al. Autoperfused mouse flow chamber reveals synergistic neutrophil accumulation through P-selectin and E-selectin. *J Leukoc Biol* 2004;76:985–993.

136. Hafezi-Moghadam A, Thomas KL, Cornelssen C. A novel mouse-driven *ex vivo* flow chamber for the study of leukocyte and platelet function. *Am J Physiol Cell Physiol* 2004;286:C876–C892.

137. Eriksson EE, Werr J, Guo Y, et al. Direct observations *in vivo* on the role of endothelial selectins and $\alpha_4$ integrin in cytokine-induced leukocyte-endothelium interactions in the mouse aorta. *Circ Res* 2000;86:526–533.

138. Ramos CL, Huo Y, Jung U, et al. Direct demonstration of P-selectin and VCAM-1-dependent mononuclear cell rolling in early atherosclerotic lesions of apolipoprotein E-deficient mice. *Circ Res* 1999;84:1237–1244.

139. Kunkel EJ, Dunne JL, Ley K. Leukocyte arrest during cytokine-dependent inflammation *in vivo*. *J Immunol* 2000;164:3301–3308.

140. Huo Y, Hafezi-Moghadam A, Ley K. Role of vascular adhesion molecule-1 (VCAM-1) and fibronectin connecting segment-1 (CS-1) in monocyte adherence on early atherosclerotic lesions. *Circ Res* 2000;87:153–159.

141. Davies MJ, Gordon JL, Gearing AJH, et al. The expression of the adhesion molecules ICAM-1, VCAM-1, PECAM, and E-selectin in human atherosclerosis. *J Pathol* 1993;171:223–229.

142. Gerszten RE, Garcia-Zepeda EA, Lim YC, et al. MCP-1 and IL-8 trigger firm adhesion of monocytes to vascular endothelium under flow conditions. *Nature* 1999;398:718–723.

143. Smith DF, Galkina E, Ley K, et al. GRO family chemokines are specialized for monocyte arrest from flow. *Am J Physiol—Heart Circ Physiol*, 2005.

144. McIntire LV, Kukreti S, Konstantopoulos K. Biomechanics of cell interactions in shear fields. *Adv Drug Delivery Rev* 1998;33:1–2.

145. Gutensohn K, Geidel K, Brockmann M, et al. Binding of activated platelets to WBCs *in vivo* after transfusion. *Transfusion* 2002;42:1373–1380.

146. Huo Y, Ley KF. Role of platelets in the development of atherosclerosis. *Trends Cardiovasc Med* 2004;14:18–22.

147. Weber C, Springer TA. Neutrophil accumulation on activated, surface-adherent platelets in flow is mediated by interaction of Mac-1 with fibrinogen bound to $\alpha_{IIb}\beta_3$ and stimulated by platelet-activating factor. *J Clin Invest* 1997;100:2085–2093.

148. Romo GM, Dong JF, Schade AJ, et al. The glycoprotein Ib-IX-V complex is a platelet counterreceptor for P-selectin. *J Exp Med* 1999;190:803–813.

149. Forlow SB, McEver RP, Nollert MU. Leukocyte-leukocyte interactions mediated by platelet microparticles under flow. *Blood* 2000;95:1317–1323.

150. Bogdanov VY, Balasubramanian V, Hathcock J, et al. Alternatively spliced human tissue factor: a circulating, soluble, thrombogenic protein. *Nat Med* 2003;9:458–462.

151. Subramaniam M, Frenette PS, Saffaripour S, et al. Defects in hemostasis in P-selectin-deficient mice. *Blood* 1996;87:1238–1242.

152. Hrachovinova I, Cambien B, Hafezi-Moghadam A, et al. Interaction of P-selectin and PSGL-1 generates microparticles that correct hemostasis in a mouse model of hemophilia A. *Nat Med* 2003;9:1020–1025.

153. Weber C, Aepfelbacher M, Haag H, et al. Tumor necrosis factor induces enhanced responses to platelet- activating factor and differentiation in human monocytic Mono Mac 6 cells. *Eur J Immunol* 1993;23:852–859.

154. Altieri DC, Edgington TS. The saturable high affinity association of factor X to ADP-stimulated monocytes defines a novel function of the Mac-1 receptor. *J Biol Chem* 1988;263:7007–7015.

# CHAPTER 46 ■ STRUCTURE AND FUNCTION OF VON WILLEBRAND FACTOR

SANDRA L. HABERICHTER AND ROBERT R. MONTGOMERY

The most common hereditary bleeding disorder, with a prevalence estimated by some to be 1% or greater, is von Willebrand disease (VWD) (1,2). Its clinical manifestations are brought about by a reduction of two of the established functions of von Willebrand factor (VWF): First, its role in supporting the adhesion of platelets to damaged blood vessels and, second, postsynthetic association of VWF with factor VIII (FVIII) that protects FVIII from proteolysis. The clinical features of VWD are discussed in greater detail in Chapter 60.

## HISTORICAL PERSPECTIVE

In 1924, a 5-year-old girl from the Åland Islands off the coast of Finland was brought to the Deaconess Hospital in Helsinki, where she was evaluated by Dr. Erik von Willebrand for a severe bleeding disorder (3–5). After assessing the patient and 65 members of her family, von Willebrand concluded that she had a previously undescribed bleeding disorder that differed from hemophilia in three cardinal manifestations: Primarily, the affected individual had mucocutaneous hemorrhage rather than hemarthroses or deep muscle hemorrhage; the inheritance was consistent with autosomal dominant rather than X-linked recessive transmission; and in contrast to the normal bleeding times found in patients with hemophilia, these patients had prolonged bleeding times (3,6,7). Von Willebrand knew that thrombocytopenia could cause prolonged bleeding times, so he determined the patient's platelet counts and found them to be normal. *(Patients with certain von Willebrand variants, platelet-type pseudo-VWD, or type 2B VWD are now known to have mild thrombocytopenia.)* He, therefore, concluded that the patients had a qualitative disorder of platelet function, in particular, thrombus formation. What he could not determine was whether the abnormality in platelet function was intrinsic or extrinsic to the platelet. Subsequently, assays of platelet adhesiveness were developed and demonstrated a defect in platelet adhesiveness in patients with VWD (8,9).

Over the next several decades, numerous infusion studies were performed on patients with VWD, and these suggested that the major abnormality responsible for the failure of hemostasis resided in the plasma of these patients, and not in their platelets (10–14). In 1953, three separate groups reported a reduction in factor VIII (antihemophilic factor) in patients with VWD (15–17). Although this was the beginning of an era when hemophilia A and VWD were difficult to distinguish conceptually, studies demonstrating that hemophilic plasma transiently corrected the hemostatic defect in patients with VWD clearly established these as separate clinical entities. When plasma fractionation became available, both cryoprecipitate and Cohn fraction I-O corrected the factor VIII deficiency in hemophilia and VWD and corrected the bleeding time defect in VWD (18,19). The effect of subsequent modifications of plasma purification procedures on the products used

to treat these two disorders will be discussed in more detail subsequently in this chapter and in chapter 60.

Despite von Willebrand's initial demonstration of abnormal thrombus formation by platelets in VWD, most early attempts to define an *in vitro* abnormality in platelet physiology or function were unsuccessful. It was not until the subsequent discovery that the antibiotic ristocetin-induced platelet aggregation (RIPA) and platelet agglutination in the presence of normal concentrations of VWF that the role of VWF was understood more clearly (20–23).

### Terminology

It was not clearly understood until the 1970s that VWF and factor VIII were different proteins produced by different cells under different genetic control (21,24–26). Because the two proteins associate with one another in plasma, they may co-purify during cryoprecipitate fractionation and column chromatography. Therefore, the early terminology (1970s) referred to VWF as factor VIII–related antigen (27). This terminology led to the confusion that unfortunately persists today in some textbooks. VWF and factor VIII are distinct entities. Table 46-1 lists the terminology currently used to describe these proteins.

In 1977, a second antigen was found to be absent from the plasma, platelets, and endothelial cells of patients with severe VWD and was termed von Willebrand antigen II but now is termed as the VWF propeptide (VWFpp) (28). A complex of VWFpp and VWF was identified in endothelial cells that was subsequently demonstrated to be pro-VWF (29). Following the cloning of the *VWF* gene, the N-terminal sequence of VWFpp was found to be identical to that predicted for the gene encoding pro-VWF (30). Therefore, VWFpp is the large 741–amino acid propolypeptide cleaved from VWF that is released from platelets and endothelial cells at the same time that VWF is released. VWFpp is discussed later in this chapter.

## GENETICS

From the first description by Erik von Willebrand of the patients on the Åland Islands, this disorder was recognized as usually being inherited as an autosomal trait; therefore, both men and women seem to have a similar prevalence. Older descriptions of VWD describe only severe and moderately severe VWD, and therefore underestimate the frequency. Current estimates suggest a prevalence of 1% to 2% of the general population (1,2,31,32). The prevalence of severe type 3 VWD (homozygous) has been estimated to be 0.5 to 5.3 per million population (33); the expected calculated prevalence of heterozygotes, assuming random mating, would be 1.4 to 5.0 per 1,000. The effect of ABO blood type on VWF concentration (34), the

## TABLE 46-1

### TERMINOLOGY

| | |
|---|---|
| VWD | The autosomally inherited bleeding disorder with a reduced amount or function of VWF |
| VWF | The glycoprotein that is abnormal or present in reduced amounts in patients with VWD |
| VWF:Ag | VWF antigen, the detection and quantitation of VWF by immunoassay |
| VWF:Rco | Ristocetin cofactor, the detection or quantitation of VWF using the antibiotic ristocetin, which induces VWF binding to platelets |
| VWF multimers | The multiple molecular forms of VWF comprised of C-terminal–linked dimers assembled through subsequent N-terminal multimerization to produce high-molecular-weight VWF multimers |
| VWFpp | The large propeptide of VWF normally cleaved from pro-VWF during intracellular processing to produce a free VWFpp molecule (also previously called VW AgII) and mature VWF |
| FVIII | Factor VIII, the protein that is abnormal or reduced in patients with hemophilia A; VWF serves as an FVIII carrier protein in plasma, and, therefore, if VWF is reduced or its binding to FVII is abnormal, patients with VWD have reduced FVIII levels |
| FVIIIC:Ag | Factor VIII coagulant antigen, factor VIII antigen is measured by immunoassay |

VWD, von Willebrand disease; VWF, von Willebrand factor.
Used by permission, RR Montgomery.

calculation of normal ranges based on two standard deviations, and the variable precision of laboratory testing for VWF proteins contribute to the difficulty with establishing prevalence of VWD. When the gene for VWF was identified, it was hoped that more precise diagnosis would be possible. This prediction has been true for VWD variants, but most patients with type 1 VWD cannot be easily identified by genetic testing.

Numerous studies have demonstrated the autosomal inheritance pattern for VWD. Figure 46-1 demonstrates the expected inheritance pattern when one parent is affected and when both parents are affected. Swedish studies have estimated the penetrance to be between 73% and 90%, but clinical expression varies widely (35,36). In heterozygous type 1 VWD, the

expression may be affected by other variables such as blood type and other "gene modifiers" (34,37–39). If a patient has significant clinical symptoms, repeat testing may be required to identify the laboratory phenotype.

Several variants, including type IIC (old classification system), type 2N VWD (abnormal FVIII binding), and some cases of 2A or 2B, appear to be inherited as recessive traits (40–43). These patients should be studied by DNA analysis of allele-specific VWF gene repeats, termed variable number of tandem repeats (VNTR) (44–46). Such analysis identifies paternal and maternal alleles and their effect on phenotypic expression. It would be useful to repeat some early studies on variability in laboratory diagnosis with these newer genetic markers to determine the true variability of laboratory testing and subclassification (47–49).

# MOLECULAR AND STRUCTURAL BIOLOGY

Over the last 20 years, investigators have gained much insight into the structure and function of VWF through the delineation of its molecular and cellular biology. Such studies have helped us understand the clinical manifestations of VWF and develop assays for laboratory diagnosis, the classification of VWD and its variants, and the rationale for therapy.

## Molecular Biology

In 1985, the coding sequence for human VWF was identified in a cDNA library derived from endothelial mRNA by several independent groups (50–53). This cDNA sequencing demonstrated an 8.7-kb mRNA with an open reading frame that encodes a 2,813–amino acid protein, including a signal peptide of 22 amino acids, a large propolypeptide of 741 amino acids, and a mature VWF molecule containing 2,050 amino acids. Figure 46-2 demonstrates the relation of this cDNA to the VWF protein. Using the current numbering system, the initiating methionine codon is defined at nucleotide number one, and this

Inheritance of von Willebrand disease

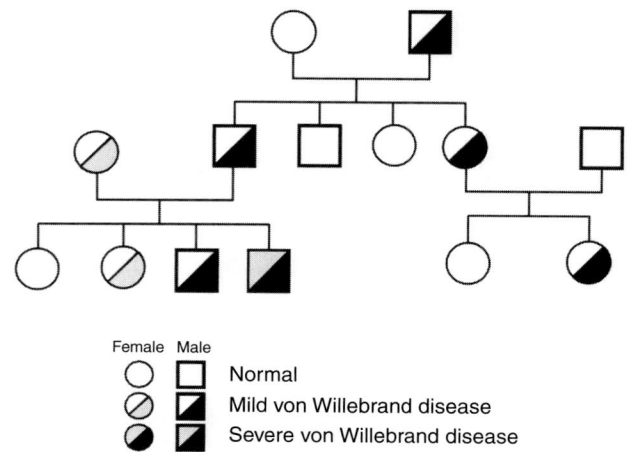

FIGURE 46-1. The autosomal inheritance of von Willebrand disease (VWD) is illustrated in this figure. Because low von Willebrand factor (VWF) has a frequency of 1% to 2%, some of these individuals are asymptomatic. Those with symptoms are said to have mild type 1 VWD. Patients with type 3 VWD are homozygous and inherit null alleles from each parent. (Used by permission, RR Montgomery.)

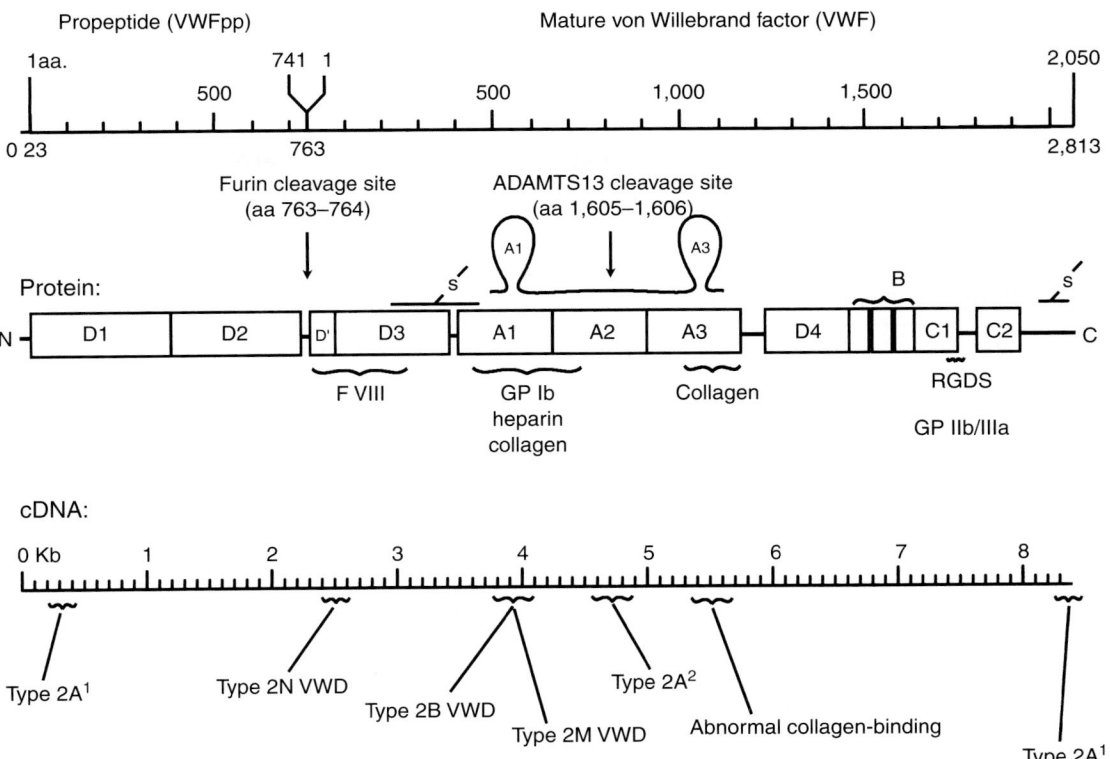

**FIGURE 46-2.** The von Willebrand factor (VWF) protein is initially synthesized as a 2,813–amino acid pro-VWF molecule whose synthesis is directed by an 8.5-kb RNA. The pre-pro-VWF is composed of a 22–amino acid signal peptide, a 741–amino acid propeptide (VWFpp), and a 2,050–amino acid mature VWF monomer. The pro-VWF is composed of A, B, C, and D repeats. Various functional domains have been identified and contain the sites of interaction with factor VIII, platelet glycoprotein GP Ib, GP IIb/IIIa, collagen, and heparin. On the basis of these functional domains, various genetic mutations have been mapped to discrete regions of the cDNA as illustrated. Two protease domains are illustrated: furin cleavage site (cleaves the VWFpp from VWF) and ADAMTS13 cleavage site that cleaves the A2 domain. This ADAMTS13 cleavage is increased by some VWF mutations that cause type 2A VWD caused by increased VWF proteolysis. Cleavage by ADAMTS13 is absent in patients with thrombotic thrombocytopenic purpura (TTP) either because of a deficiency of the enzyme (hereditary TTP) or an autoantibody that blocks its cleavage of VWF (acquired or sporadic TTP). Type 2 mutations are generally located in specific regions along the VWF protein. Types 2A, 2B, and 2M are primarily located within exon 28 that encodes for the A1 and A2 regions of VWF. The two different types of 2A are those that have increased proteolysis 2A[2] and those with abnormal multimer synthesis 2A[1]. Mutations with abnormal collagen binding are clustered in the region encoding the A3 domain. (Used by permission, RR Montgomery.)

methionine is also identified as amino acid number one. Analysis of the protein structure suggested areas of internal homology that have been termed A-, B-, C-, and D-domains (54,55). The A repeats have sequence similarity to complement factor B, type VI collagen, chicken cartilage matrix protein, and the "I-domain"-containing integrin α-subunit [Mac-1, VLA2, leukocyte function-associated antigen (LFA), p 150, 95] (56,57). Areas of the C repeat are similar to segments of procollagen and thrombospondin (58). Several functions of VWF have been mapped to specific domains. The D′- and D3 domains are important in FVIII binding and the D3 domain is also essential for multimerization. The A1 domain contains the site for glycoprotein (GP) Ibα binding. VWF binding to collagen occurs through interaction with the A1 and A3 domains. The C1 domain contains an Arg-Gly-Asp-Ser (RGDS) sequence that allows VWF to bind GP IIb/IIIa.

After the coding sequence for VWF was identified, the entire human *VWF* gene has been cloned and much of its structure defined. The gene is approximately 178 kb long and contains 51 introns (59). The localization and sequence of the intron–exon boundaries of these 51 introns has been determined. The gene

for VWF has been localized to the short arm of chromosome 12, although a pseudogene, representing approximately the middle third of the *VWF* gene, has been identified and mapped to chromosome 22 (60,61). The presence of this pseudogene can cause problems in determining the genetic structure of some of the VWD variants, but various strategies have been developed to avoid this problem (62). This pseudogene has approximately 98% homology to its corresponding portion of the authentic *VWF* gene on chromosome 12 (60).

Various genetic alterations of the *VWF* gene have been reported and include deletions, insertions, point mutations, alternative splice junctions, and premature transcription termination sites. Many of the molecular mutations reported are included in exon 28 (63). This exon encodes the region of VWF that interacts with platelet GP Ib and encodes the portion of the VWF protein containing the important N-terminal multimerization site(s) (54) and an important site where a metalloprotease cleaves VWF between Y1605 and M1606 (64). Most of the type 2A and 2B mutations have been localized within exon 28 (63). Type 2N mutations are clustered within the D′- and D3 domains of VWF (65–69).

Within intron 40, there are repetitive elements of variable length that have been termed VNTR or short tandem repeats (STR) (44,70). These repetitive elements can be amplified to define the allelic inheritance for unusual genetic phenotypes. These STRs may also be helpful for intrauterine diagnosis using amniocytes or chorionic villi cells with subsequent gene amplification of segments of the *VWF* gene using the polymerase chain reaction. Caution in amplifying this region must be exercised because of instability of this locus (71).

## von Willebrand Factor Promoter

Major progress has been made in defining the upstream regulatory elements that control VWF expression. Several consensus sequences for *cis*-acting elements have been identified in the immediate upstream promoter region and first exon, including two GATA-binding consensus sequences (72). The endothelial cell–specific expression appears to be regulated by a repressor-derepression mechanism and includes both an NF1-binding site and an Oct-1–binding site (72–76). A more complex mode of transcriptional regulation through vascular bed–specific signaling pathways has been recently defined. A 2200-bp 5′ flanking sequence together with the first intron and exon direct expression to microvascular endothelial cells of skeletal muscle and heart (77). Recently, cell type–specific regulation of VWF expression by the E4BP4 transcriptional repressor has been identified (78). Within the heart, a cardiomyocyte-dependent signaling pathway through platelet-derived growth factor (PDGF) has been defined (79). A single nucleotide polymorphism at nucleotide –1793 has been associated with plasma VWF:Ag levels (80). Therefore, *VWF* gene is regulated by both cell-specific elements as well as the environment in which these cells are growing (73,81).

## Molecular Diagnosis of von Willebrand Disease

Following the identification of the *VWF* gene, molecular biologic assays were undertaken to increase the sensitivity and specificity of the laboratory diagnosis of VWD. Unfortunately, the von Willebrand gene is very complex, and most molecular defects have not yet been identified. The most clearly defined molecular abnormalities are those involving types 2A, 2B, 2M, 2N VWD (82,83). These are discussed in more detail in Chapter 60.

### Analysis by Southern Blotting

After the gene for VWF was isolated, several laboratories undertook Southern blot analysis for gross abnormalities of the *VWF* gene (63,84–86). The most rewarding results came from the analysis of patients with inhibitors to VWF, many of whom were demonstrated to possess partial or complete gene deletions (61,63,87,88). Some have deletions encompassing the entire *VWF* gene, whereas others have deletions as small as 2.5 kb (exon 42) (63,88,89). This group of patients represents less than 1% of those with VWD; therefore, the diagnostic sensitivity of this form of testing is very low.

### Deoxyribonucleic Acid Sequencing of Specific Exons or Complementary Deoxyribonucleic Acid Regions

For some variants such as types 2A, 2B, 2M, and 2N VWD, there are defined regions of the *VWF* gene in which there are clusters of mutations; these regions can be amplified by the polymerase chain reaction and either directly sequenced or subjected to restriction enzyme digestion to define these mutations (63,82,90). A Web site was developed at the University of Michigan and now transferred to the University of Sheffield to catalog these mutations (*http://www.shef.ac.uk/vwf/vwd.html*). The clustering of variant mutations is graphically illustrated in Figure 46-2.

### Variable Number of Tandem Repeats Analysis

Repeats of a highly polymorphic tetranucleotide (TCTA) are present in intron 40 of the *VWF* gene (44,63,70,82,82,91). Within intron 40 there are three VNTR segments, each of which has multiple possible lengths in an individual allele. A recent study has demonstrated at least 94 different alleles in this region, with an observed heterozygosity rate of 98% (92). These regions have multiple repeats, and, therefore, caution must be exercised in interpretation because allele slippage can occur (71,93).

# CELL BIOLOGY

Although VWF is synthesized both in the megakaryocyte and the endothelial cell, most of our understanding of cellular biosynthesis is derived from the endothelial cell because of the ease of *in vitro* endothelial cell culture (94,95). Figure 46-3 illustrates the endothelial cell processing of VWF. Studies on megakaryocytes are limited (96). A few continuous or transformed cell lines and inference from the study of platelets suggest that platelet VWF production is similar to that in endothelial cells. One difference has been seen in dogs whose platelets have been shown by several laboratories to lack VWF (97), although one report identified VWF in canine platelets (98).

## Cellular Processing

Endothelial cells and platelets store VWF in secretory granules that are termed Weibel-Palade bodies (endothelial cells) and α-granules (megakaryocytes and platelets) (95,99,100). These secretory granules can be induced to release their contents by a variety of agonists such as calcium ionophore A23187, thrombin, adenosine diphosphate (ADP)/epinephrine (platelets), and histamine (endothelial cells) (101–103). *In vivo*, the vasopressin derivative desmopressin acetate (DDAVP) can induce the release of VWF into plasma (104). The cell from which it is released is presumably the endothelial cell, as evidenced by a lack of reduction in platelet VWF after DDAVP therapy and a loss of Weibel-Palade body VWF on immunostained tissue sections obtained after DDAVP administration (105). Much of our understanding of these endothelial cell events comes from the expression studies in model cell lines and is summarized in the following paragraphs (106–109).

VWF is synthesized as a 2,813–amino acid pre-pro-VWF molecule and contains a 22–amino acid signal peptide, 741–amino acid propeptide, and 2,050–amino acid mature VWF protein. VWF is subjected to extensive intracellular modifications. In the endoplasmic reticulum (ER), the signal peptide is removed, disulfide bonds are formed, and protein folding occurs. VWF is a cysteine-rich protein containing 234 cysteine residues, all of which appear to be paired in disulfide bonds. The pro-VWF forms C-terminal dimers in the ER. This results in a pro-VWF C-terminal–linked dimer, the protomeric species that later forms larger VWF multimers. On transport through the Golgi compartments, VWF undergoes carbohydrate modification. The mature VWF subunit is heavily glycosylated with 10 O-linked and 12 N-linked oligosaccharides (110–112). This glycosylation accounts for approximately 18% to 19% of the total protein mass. Sulfation of the VWF molecule has also been demonstrated (113). In the Golgi, the C-terminal–linked pro-VWF dimers form N-terminal linked multimers that may exceed 20 million Da in size. The VWF propeptide, a protein initially described in plasma as VW AgII, is also proteolytically

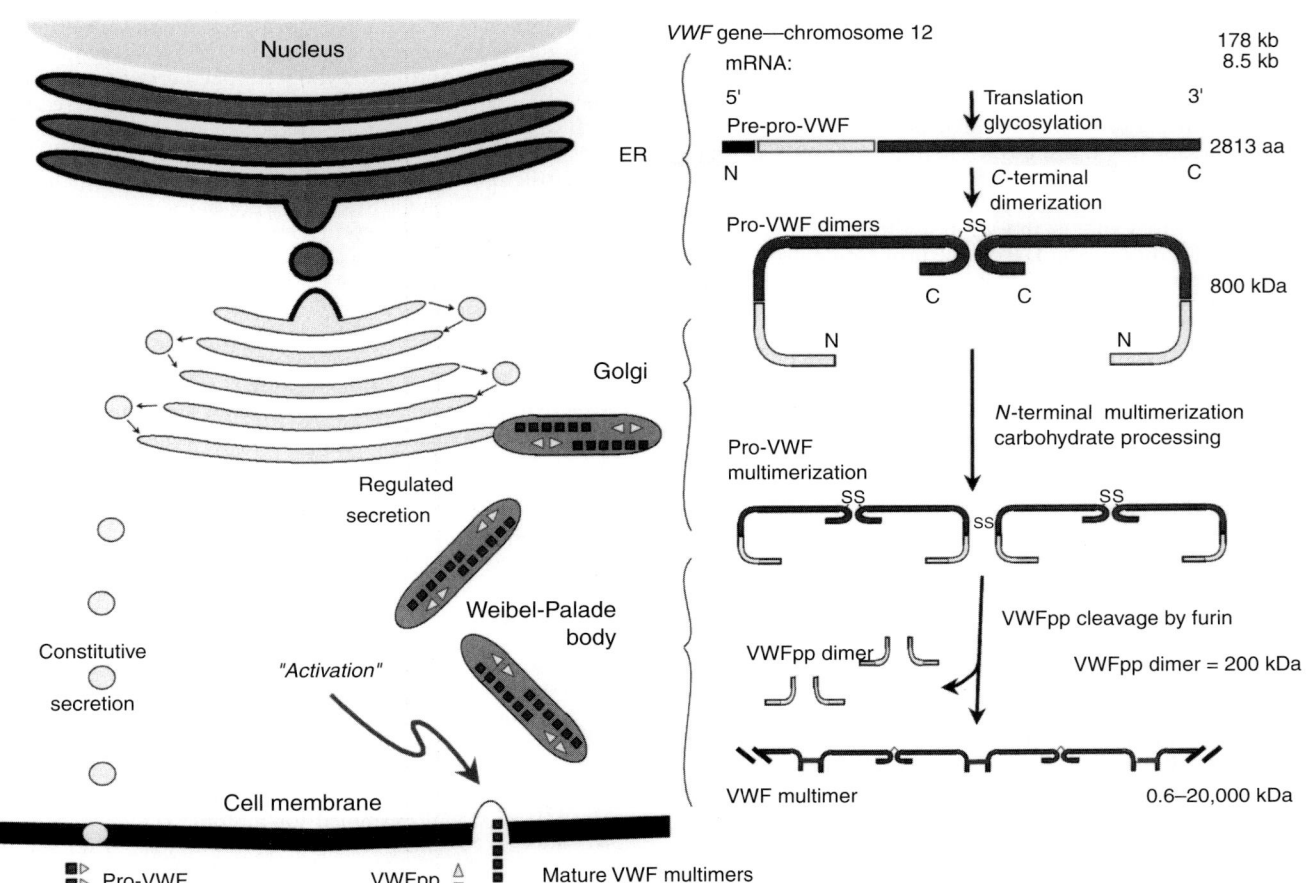

**FIGURE 46-3.** The sites of cellular biosynthesis are represented schematically in this illustration of endothelial cell biosynthesis. The von Willebrand factor (VWF)-protomer is synthesized as a pre-pro-VWF dimer that is a C-terminal disulfide-bonded dimer within the endoplasmic reticulum (ER). The 22–amino acid signal peptide is then cleaved. The carbohydrate is then processed into complex sugars within the Golgi compartment. N-linked multimerization by virtue of the self-association of the VWF propeptide (VWFpp) occurs in the acidic compartment of the late-Golgi and the VWFpp is cleaved from the mature VWF by furin. A pH-dependent association between VWFpp and VWF enables the packaging of both proteins into storage granules termed Weibel-Palade bodies. After activation of the endothelial cell, the regulated secretion of these proteins occurs, but at the neutral pH in plasma, there is no longer an association of VWFpp with VWF. A similar pathway is assumed to occur in megakaryocytes, but the α-granule contains more different types of proteins. In the absence of VWF, the Weibel-Palade body is not formed, but the α-granule is still present. (Used by permission, RR Montgomery.)

cleaved in the *trans*-Golgi. Processing of pro-VWF into VWFpp and the mature VWF is carried out by a paired amino acid–cleaving enzyme (PACE), or furin, that cleaves the propeptide from the mature VWF (114,115). The site of propeptide cleavage is targeted by the sequence motif Arg-Xxx-Arg/Lys-Arg at the C-terminal end of the propeptide (115). Because patients with hereditary persistence of pro-VWF have normal multimers, cleavage of the propeptide does not appear to be a prerequisite for multimerization or secretion (116). The cleavage of propeptide appears to be essentially completed in the Golgi, before regulated storage (117–119). Both portions of the molecule, the high-molecular-weight multimerized VWF and the cleaved propeptide, are stored in the Weibel-Palade body secretory granule.

VWF is subjected to extensive posttranslational modifications and mutations in the *VWF* gene can affect its intracellular processing. In the ER, protein misfolding (perhaps a result of aberrant disulfide bonding) can lead to intracellular retention and degradation resulting in reduced VWF secretion and low plasma VWF levels. Defective VWF multimerization results in reduced platelet binding as seen in type 2A VWD. Aberrant processing of carbohydrates may affect VWF function or its clearance from plasma. Defects in any of the many VWF intracellular processing steps may result in VWF intracellular retention, lack or secretion, defective regulated storage and secretion, or a functionally defective protein.

## von Willebrand Factor Multimerization and Regulated Storage

The assembly of VWF into *N*-linked multimers is a complex process involving interchain disulfide bonds. The first interchain disulfide bonds are formed during dimerization and involve cysteine residues located in the C-terminus region. Multimerization of C-terminal dimers involves cysteine residues located in the N-terminus region (D'- and D3 domains) (107,120). These studies have also shown that C-terminal dimerization is independent of multimerization. Initial glycosylation of the VWF protein and a low pH in the trans-Golgi network have been shown to be important for normal multimerization of VWF (108). The acidic pH in the trans-Golgi network appears to be of particular importance. The assembly of functional VWF multimers from purified VWF subunits can be triggered *in vitro* under low pH conditions, similar to the pH in the Golgi (121). The large propeptide plays an essential role in the VWF multimerization process. Deletion of either of the D1 or D2 propeptide domains, or the entire propeptide, results in a complete loss of normal VWF multimerization (122,123). When the propeptide and the "mature" VWF molecule (propeptide-deleted) were expressed as two separate gene constructs, normal multimerization was observed indicating the propeptide can function *in trans* to facilitate multimerization (123). The propeptide may facilitate VWF multimerization through areas of the propeptide that contain vicinal cysteine motifs similar to disulfide isomerase (124). Most recently, the propeptide was shown to act as an oxidoreductase, thereby promoting the multimerization of VWF in the Golgi apparatus (125).

The large VWF propeptide also plays a critical role in the regulated storage of VWF. VWF expression studies utilizing the AtT-20 cell line have examined the regulated storage of VWF (118,122,126). The AtT-20 cell line has an intact regulated storage pathway and correctly processes VWF. After the propeptide is furin-cleaved in the Golgi, the propeptide and VWF remain noncovalently associated and are trafficked to regulated storage in a propeptide-dependent process. Expression studies have shown that deletion of either of the D-domains abolishes the sorting of VWF to storage granules (122). When the entire propeptide is deleted (Δpro), regulated storage of the "mature" VWF protein is also abolished (see Fig. 46-4). In contrast, the propeptide sorts to endogenous

storage granules when it is expressed alone in AtT-20 cells. When the VWF propeptide and mature VWF (propeptide-deleted VWF or Δpro) are expressed together as two separate gene constructs, normal granular storage of VWF is reestablished (118,127). The propeptide contains the necessary sequence or conformation for sorting to storage granules and secondarily cotrafficks mature VWF multimers through noncovalent association (118). The nature of the noncovalent association between propeptide and mature VWF has been further defined. Two amino acids, Arg416 within the propeptide and Thr869 in the mature VWF protein, are essential for noncovalent association and regulated storage of VWF (128). The putative sorting signal for the propeptide may be located in the D2 domain. By using a series of propeptide truncation cDNA constructs (see Fig. 46-5), the sorting signal has be localized within amino acids 387 to 545 of the propeptide. The sorting signal within the VWF propeptide has been used to traffick an unrelated, nonsecretory granule protein (C3α) to the regulated storage pathway in AtT-20 cells and endothelial cells (119).

Although the propeptide plays a critical role in both the multimerization and storage of VWF, the two events are clearly independent. Expression of VWF with disrupted vicinal cysteine motifs demonstrated a lack of VWF multimerization but maintenance of VWF regulated storage (124). This was further demonstrated by expression studies utilizing human and canine VWF cDNA constructs. The canine propeptide was able to facilitate multimerization of human propeptide-deleted VWF (Δpro) but could not traffick the human VWF to regulated storage (118). In a study utilizing the cross-species storage difference, a large number of human/canine chimeric constructs were expressed and examined for multimerization and regulated storage. No correlation was found between VWF multimerization and granular trafficking (128). In many cases

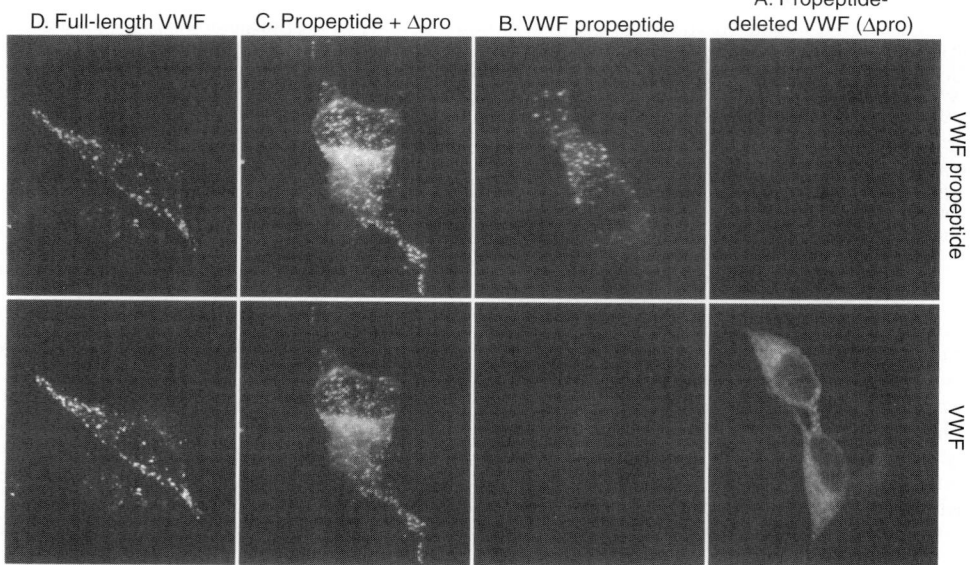

**FIGURE 46-4.** AtT-20 cells were transiently transfected with von Willebrand factor (VWF) expression plasmids, immunofluorescently stained, and examined by confocal microscopy. The panels on the top are immunostained for VWF propeptide and the panels on the bottom are stained for VWF. **A:** Cells expressing "mature," propeptide-deleted VWF (Δpro) demonstrate a diffuse staining pattern and no VWF containing granules are detected. **B:** Cells expressing only VWF propeptide demonstrate a granular staining pattern, indicating the propeptide trafficks independently to granules. **C:** When the "mature" VWF is coexpressed with VWF propeptide (two separate gene constructs), both VWF and propeptide traffick to granules, similar to the granular staining observed when full-length VWF is expressed (**D**). The propeptide contains the necessary signal for trafficking to storage granules and cotrafficks mature VWF through a noncovalent interaction. (Used by permission, RR Montgomery and SL Haberichter.)

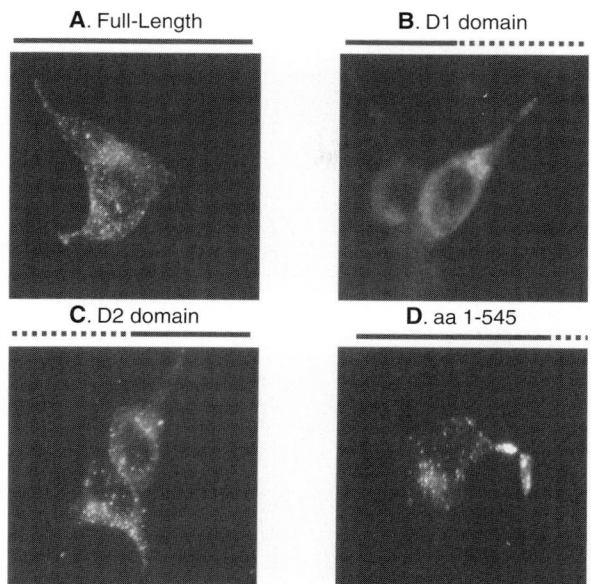

**A.** Full-Length    **B.** D1 domain

**C.** D2 domain    **D.** aa 1-545

**FIGURE 46-5.** AtT-20 cells were transiently transfected with von Willebrand factor (VWF) propeptide truncation expression plasmids, immunofluorescently stained, and examined by confocal microscopy. **A:** Cells expressing full-length propeptide demonstrate a granular staining pattern. **B:** Cells expressing only the D1 domain (amino acids 1 to 386) of the propeptide demonstrate a diffuse staining pattern with no granules detected. **C:** Cells expressing only the D2 domain (amino acids 386 to 763) of the propeptide demonstrate a granular staining pattern similar to full-length propeptide. **D:** Granular staining of a propeptide consisting of amino acids 1 to 545. The putative VWF propeptide sorting signal lies in the D2 domain within the region of amino acids 387 to 545. (Used by permission, RR Montgomery and SL Haberichter.)

normally multimerized VWF was not stored in granules and conversely, several VWF species that did not form multimers were trafficked to storage granules. A number of VWF mutations have been identified in patients with VWD, that disrupt VWF multimerization but did not affect the regulated storage of VWF (129,130). There have been no reported patient mutations that maintain normal VWF multimerization but eliminate regulated storage and secretion.

The regulated storage of VWF in Weibel-Palade bodies in endothelial cells is important physiologically. Patients with type 1 VWD are often treated with the vasopressin analog DDAVP (1-desamino-8-D-arginine vassopressin). Administration of DDAVP results in a rapid increase in plasma VWF levels resulting from release of VWF from Weibel-Palade bodies (131,132). VWF plays an essential role in the formation of Weibel-Palade bodies in endothelial cells. In the VWF-deficient mouse (e.g., Type 3 VWD), no Weibel-Palade bodies can be detected in endothelial cells and the membrane protein P selectin is routed to lysosomes (133). Similarly, cultured endothelial cells harvested from dogs with type 3 VWD demonstrated a lack of Weibel-Palade bodies (134). Expression studies using the endothelium from dogs with type 3 VWD have demonstrated that expression of VWF protein is necessary for the formation of Weibel-Palade bodies that contain the membrane protein, P selectin (see Fig. 46-6) (134). The full-length VWF protein is necessary for formation of Weibel-Palade bodies: Neither the propeptide nor mature VWF ($\Delta$pro) were sufficient for granule formation. These studies indicate that VWF may serve an active role in the recruitment of the leukocyte receptor, P selectin, to the Weibel-Palade body membrane. Although VWF is believed to be the most abundant protein in the Weibel-Palade body, additional components include

P selectin, the tetraspanin CD63, IL-8, and tPA (135–138). Although the site of synthesis of FVIII is unclear, FVIII can be stored together in a Weibel-Palade body when expressed with VWF (139). Therefore, VWF-dependent Weibel-Palade body biogenesis has significant biologic implications.

On appropriate agonist stimulation, endothelial cells and platelets release both VWF and the propeptide from Weibel-Palade bodies and $\alpha$-granules, respectively. The cleaved propeptide remains associated with VWF under acidic conditions similar to those observed in the late trans-Golgi network and Weibel-Palade bodies, but dissociates from VWF in when exposed to the higher pH found in plasma. The propeptide self-associates as a noncovalent dimer in plasma (140). VWF can be secreted both luminally into plasma and abluminally into the subendothelial cell matrix (106). Although the propeptide is also secreted, its extracellular function has not been delineated.

## Proteolysis of von Willebrand Factor

Once secreted, VWF multimers circulate in plasma at a concentration of approximately 10 $\mu$g per mL with a half-life of approximately 12 hours. The free propeptide circulates in normal human plasma at a concentration of approximately 1 $\mu$g per mL with a half-life of 2 to 3 hours. Little is known about the mechanisms underlying the normal clearance of VWF from circulation (141). Increased clearance from the circulation has been identified as a mechanism causing type 1 VWD (142,143). In these patients, VWF has a substantially decreased half-life. Two mutations have been reported that are linked with increased clearance, Arg1205His (142) and Ser2179Phe (Montgomery and Haberichter, unpublished data). The Ser2179Phe mutation was identified in several generations of affected members of two unrelated families with moderately severe type 1 VWD. These affected members have a significantly decreased VWF half-life (2 to 3 hrs). In these patients clearance was not dependent on multimer size because all multimers, small and large, disappeared quickly. An experimental model has been developed to examine clearance of human VWF from mouse circulation (144). These studies supported the role of the D'- and D3 domains in regulation of clearance. The relevance of this mechanism to the normal clearance of VWF is not known.

Degradation of VWF is also accomplished by the VWF-cleaving protease, ADAMTS13, a member of the "a disintigrinlike and metalloprotease with thrombospondin repeats" (145–148). VWF is proteolytically processed by ADAMTS13 by cleavage of the Tyr1605–Met1606 bond located within the A2 domain (149,150). VWF is resistant to ADAMTS13 cleavage under static conditions but is rapidly cleaved when subjected to high shear stress. The high shear conditions most likely expose the cleavage site. VWF released from endothelial cell Weibel-Palade bodies consists of ultralarge VWF multimers. If the ultralarge VWF multimers are released directly into plasma, platelets can spontaneously aggregate, resulting in thrombosis (151,152). The ultralarge multimers form long stringlike structures that remain tethered to the endothelial cell surface by interaction of the VWF with the membrane protein, P selectin (153). ADAMTS13 cleaves the tethered ultralarge VWF multimers rapidly under flow conditions (154,155). Recently, the binding of platelet GP Ib$\alpha$ to the VWF A1 domain was shown to stimulate the cleavage of the adjacent A2 domain by ADAMTS13 (156). A number of mutations in ADAMTS13 have been identified that affect its synthesis or function and cause a congenital form of thrombotic thrombocytopenic purpura TTP (148,157). In contrast, a number of mutations have been identified in VWF that increase the susceptibility of VWF to proteolysis by ADAMTS13, resulting in a loss of high-molecular-weight multimers in patient plasma and defective platelet binding (type 2A VWD)

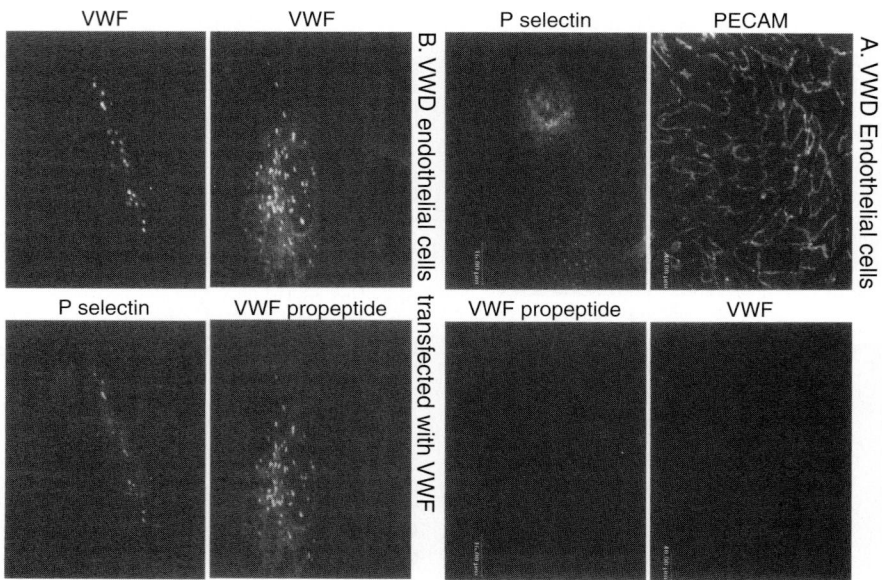

**FIGURE 46-6. A:** Endothelial cells were harvested from the aortas of dogs with type 3 von Willebrand disease (VWD), cultured, immunofluorescently stained, and examined by confocal microscopy. The cells were platelet/endothelial cell adhesion molecule (PECAM) (CD31)-positive, indicating that a homogenous population of endothelial cells had been cultured as shown. The cells were also found to be von Willebrand factor (VWF)-negative as shown. Staining for P selectin was faint and diffuse with many small granules, most likely lysosomes. The VWF propeptide could not be detected in these cells. Therefore, no apparent Weibel-Palade bodies were detected in the canine VWD aortic endothelial cells. **B:** The canine VWD aortic endothelial cells were transiently transfected with a VWF expression plasmid. Immunostaining of cells expressing VWF demonstrated a granular distribution of VWF and VWF propeptide as shown. Dual staining for VWF and P selectin revealed that the VWF was colocalized with P selectin in granules. Therefore, in the absence of VWF, no Weibel-Palade bodies are formed in endothelial cells. However, VWF expression induces the formation of Weibel-Palade bodies and the Weibel-Palade body distribution of endogenous P selectin is reestablished. (Used by permission, RR Montgomery and SL Haberichter.)

(64,158). The role of ADAMTS13 in normal degradation of VWF multimers is not well defined.

## Interaction with Platelets

VWF is known to bind to subendothelium, perhaps in part due to its interaction with collagen (159–161). Therefore, in the normal hemostatic system, an intact endothelium precludes the interaction between matrix-bound VWF and platelets. After vessel injury, however, this bound VWF can be induced to interact with the GP Ib receptor on platelets (162). *In vitro*, this interaction with platelets can be mimicked in platelet-rich plasma by the addition of the antibiotic ristocetin, by the venom protein botrocetin, or by subjecting the platelets to high shear stress, all of which promote the binding of VWF to GP Ib platelet (163–165). This interaction of VWF with GP Ib results both in the adhesion of platelets and the subsequent activation of platelets.

VWF can bind to a second receptor on platelets, the GP IIb/IIIa (or integrin $\alpha_{IIb}\beta_3$) complex (166–168). The GP IIb/IIIa receptor normally is the physiologic binding site for fibrinogen during *in vitro* aggregation, but in the absence of fibrinogen or after the local concentration of VWF is increased (platelet or endothelial cell secretion), VWF also may promote this platelet aggregation process (164). Monoclonal antibodies to these two separate platelet receptors demonstrate the differential binding brought about by selected agonists (163,164,166). The antibiotic ristocetin or the snake venom botrocetin induce VWF binding to GP Ib, which can be blocked by monoclonal antibodies to the GP Ib binding site for VWF (163,164,169). ADP/epinephrine or thrombin induces VWF binding to the GP IIb/IIIa receptor, and this interaction can be blocked by monoclonal antibodies directed against the GP IIb/IIIa complex (163,164,166–168,170,171). Therefore, immobilized VWF can bind to GP Ib and promote platelet aggregation through the GP IIb/IIIa receptor using either fibrinogen or VWF as its ligand.

Although the physiologic stimuli for the interaction of VWF with platelets are not fully defined, VWF may undergo a conformational change caused either by interaction with subendothelial matrix or by shear stress (162,172,173). As described in more detail in the subsequent text, shear-induced platelet aggregation or adhesion can be inhibited by monoclonal antibodies directed against both GP Ib and GP IIb/IIIa, suggesting that both receptors are physiologically relevant (172,174–181).

## Biochemistry

Numerous laboratories have purified normal human VWF, and there is general agreement concerning its structure and function relation (90,107,108,182–185). It is composed of a series of high-molecular-weight multimers that range between approximately 600,000 (VWF dimer) and 20 million Da. Using low-concentration agarose gels (0.65% to 1%), these multimers can be resolved, with the lowest band representing the dimer. Using high-concentration agarose gels (2% to 3%), each of these individual multimers can be resolved into several additional bands that are thought to result from subunits that have undergone partial proteolytic cleavage.

When the disulfide bonds are reduced, a single predominant band is seen on polyacrylamide gel electrophoresis with an apparent molecular weight estimated to be approximately 220,000 Da, plus some smaller bands caused by proteolytic degradation (186). The complete protein sequence has been determined and is identical to the protein sequence derived from the cDNA sequence with a molecular weight of 225,663 Da for just the amino acid sequence of the mature VWF (50–52,110). The carbohydrate component is estimated to add approximately 10% to 15% to the molecular mass; therefore, the true molecular weight of the monomer is approximately 255,000 Da, and its migration in polyacrylamide gel underestimates its true molecular weight.

The VWF multimers are extraordinarily large; the biggest are considerably larger than some virus particles. Electron microscopy of the VWF molecule after rotary shadowing reveals a flexible filamentous structure with irregularly spaced nodules that have been reported from several groups (187–189). These filaments are approximately 20 to 30 Å wide and as long as 11,500 Å, with an average length of 4,780 Å; for comparison, fibrinogen is 475 Å long. Under native conditions, these long filamentous strands are presumed to be wound together in a compact molecule. During activation, shear stress, or other *in vivo* modifications, portions of the VWF may be unwound, allowing exposure of multiple interactive sites that may participate in platelet adhesion. Decreasing the size of the multimers by partial reduction of disulfide bonds results in a dramatic decrease in the platelet agglutinating activity (187,190,191).

This molecular-weight–dependent heterogeneity of VWF is important when one compares the results of assays based on immunologic and platelet agglutinating activities. Although immunoassays recognize large and small multimers, estimates of VWF activity using the ristocetin cofactor (VWF R:Co) assay predominantly measure the function of high-molecular-weight multimers (191–194). In contrast, estimates of VWF activity using botrocetin-induced platelet binding correlate better with the immunoassays but may not represent functional activity *in vivo* (195). Individuals with hereditary conditions such as type 2A VWD, in which there is a reduction in multimeric size, often have more severe bleeding symptoms than individuals with a similar reduction in protein concentration but normal multimeric size (type 1 VWD); therefore, *in vivo*, multimeric size may correlate with function (192).

## Interaction with Factor VIII

Antihemophilic factor, factor VIII, circulates in plasma associated with VWF; this led investigators to conclude that VWF and factor VIII were the same molecules (25,196–200). Other investigators established that these were two independent molecules that circulated together in plasma as an associated complex (196–200). Although the initial name for VWF was factor VIII–related antigen, this is now an outdated and incorrect term (Table 46-1).

Early studies on patients with VWD demonstrated a reduced level of FVIII (6,7,201). When cryoprecipitate was infused into patients with VWD, there was a modest initial increase in FVIII that increased to even higher levels over several hours and then slowly declined. This contrasts sharply with the pattern seen in patients with hemophilia infused with the same product, who have a rapid increase in FVIII with a normal 12-hour half-life (201,202). Furthermore, early studies demonstrated that after cryoprecipitate or plasma prepared from patients with hemophilia containing no FVIII was infused into patients with VWD, it resulted in a paradoxic increase in plasma FVIII in the patient's plasma (7,201,203). Our current understanding is that these two proteins associate through a noncovalent interaction between the light chain of FVIII and the *N*-terminus of the VWF subunit (204,205). The

plasma concentration of VWF is approximately 10 μg per mL, and that for FVIII is only approximately 200 ng per mL. The paradoxical increase in FVIII in patients with VWD is caused by at least two mechanisms. The infused VWF associates with the endogenously produced FVIII to protect this FVIII from rapid degradation and removal, normalizing the short half-life of the endogenously produced FVIII (206,207). Also, VWF in plasma (or in culture media) facilitates the more efficient secretion of FVIII from the endoplasmic reticulum (207–211).

It is generally assumed that VWF is synthesized in endothelial cells and megakaryocytes (54,90,182,212) and that FVIII is synthesized in hepatocytes (213–215). When the drug DDAVP is administered, VWF is released from endothelial cells, and FVIII is found to increase in parallel with the VWF, although the source of this released FVIII remains controversial. It has been demonstrated that if FVIII is produced in a cell that also synthesizes and stores VWF (AtT-20 cells or endothelial cells), FVIII follows VWF into storage granules (216). In addition, patients with severe hemophilia A who are administered recombinant FVIII for prolonged periods have no increase in their FVIII after administration of DDAVP (217). Furthermore, the patient with severe VWD who is given only VWF, which results in normalization of FVIII, has been found to have no change in plasma FVIII after the administration of DDAVP. Therefore, FVIII and VWF must both be endogenously synthesized for FVIII to be released from storage sites. A study by Lollar et al. demonstrates that sinusoidal endothelial cells synthesize and store FVIII together with VWF in *ex vivo* cultured cells (215). Understanding the mechanism of VWF and FVIII association may be important for the most appropriate transfection strategy in the gene therapy for hemophilia A. The functional reason for the association of FVIII with VWF is not entirely clear, but one could theorize that VWF binding and delivery of FVIII to the phospholipid surface of platelets might be coordinated *in vivo*. Recent studies have demonstrated the potential for targeting FVIII expression to megakaryocytes and platelets for efficient delivery of FVIII to the site of platelet plug formation (218,219).

## Effects of Ristocetin on Binding of von Willebrand Factor to Platelets

The interaction of VWF with platelets is the biologic event that reflects a major interaction of VWF with the hemostatic system. Much of our knowledge about the normal interaction of VWF with platelets is derived from several assays that identify a functional abnormality in blood from patients with VWD: ristocetin-induced (or botrocetin-induced) platelet aggregation and agglutination, *ex vivo* interaction of platelets with blood vessel segments from which the endothelium has been denuded, and shear-induced platelet adhesion or aggregation.

Ristocetin, an antibiotic similar in structure and antimicrobial mechanism of action to vancomycin, was introduced as an antibiotic into clinical practice in the late 1950s. Shortly thereafter, it was noted to produce thrombocytopenia in recipients and was therefore withdrawn from clinical use. Approximately 10 years later, ristocetin was shown to aggregate normal platelets *in vitro* but to cause little or no aggregation of platelets from patients with VWD (220,221). This defect could be corrected with normal or hemophilic plasma and could be blocked by specific monoclonal antibodies directed against VWF. Furthermore, even after fixation, platelets still agglutinated in response to ristocetin in the presence of VWF, demonstrating that this event did not require metabolically active platelets (220,222). This observation permitted the development of a quantitative assay, the ristocetin cofactor assay (223). If fixed platelets, which lack metabolic activity, are used, the response to ristocetin is termed *ristocetin-induced platelet agglutination* (21). When ristocetin is used with metabolically active platelets in platelet-rich plasma, however, the overall response is termed *RIPA*. Once VWF binds to its receptor, it induces GP IIb/IIIa receptor–dependent aggregation (RIPA) that uses fibrinogen (or VWF) as a ligand (224–227).

## Interaction with Platelet Glycoprotein Ib

The platelet receptor for VWF during this agglutination process is platelet GP Ib, a GP receptor absent from the platelets of patients with the hereditary disorder Bernard-Soulier syndrome (228–230). Platelets from these patients do not aggregate with ristocetin, although their plasma has normal levels of VWF. Monoclonal antibodies to GP Ib block VWF binding and ristocetin-induced agglutination (140,163).

The GP Ib complex on the platelet surface is composed of at least four proteins. GP Ib$\alpha$ is disulfide-linked to GP Ib$\beta$. It appears that GP Ib$\beta$ is then noncovalently associated with GP IX. Two of these GP Ib$\alpha$/Ib$\beta$/IX complexes are then associated with one GP V molecule (231–235). Ristocetin induces the binding of VWF to the GP Ib complex by an alteration of electrostatic forces between GP Ib$\alpha$ and VWF (236–238). Ristocetin binds both to VWF and to platelet GP Ib$\alpha$, in which it induces a change in surface charge or structure that either is directly associated with the bridge between the ligand and the receptor or, perhaps more likely, modifies the structure of the ligand or receptor to facilitate spontaneous interaction. In support of this latter argument, molecular abnormalities of VWF (type 2B VWD) and GP Ib (platelet-type pseudo-VWD) can render the respective molecules capable of spontaneously forming a complex between ligand and receptor without the need for ristocetin.

The antibiotic ristocetin can also precipitate proteins such as fibrinogen and VWF (239). The concentration of ristocetin necessary to induce VWF binding to platelets and the concentration necessary to cause ristocetin-induced precipitation of plasma proteins are identical to the concentration required for ristocetin to spontaneously dimerize itself (240). When the concentration of ristocetin reaches approximately 1 mg per mL, ristocetin may dimerize with a second ristocetin molecule. This causes a conformational change in VWF that facilitates its binding to GP Ib. A variety of structurally unrelated polycations can substitute for ristocetin and demonstrate the importance of the positive charge on ristocetin (241,242).

## von Willebrand Factor Interactions Under High Shear Stress

To simulate more closely the conditions *in vivo* and to permit the differentiation between initial platelet adhesion to a surface in the subsequent platelet–platelet aggregation, a number of research models have been developed to study the effects of shear stress. Early studies on shear stress used the wall of an inverted rabid aorta that demonstrated the adherence of isolated platelets and subsequent platelet aggregate formation under the control of VWF and fibrinogen (243,244). The participation of VWF in this process was highly dependent on high shear forces (1,300 to 5,200 per second) (245,246). A number of laboratories have developed techniques to define the interaction between VWF and GP Ib$\alpha$, the necessary initial step that tethers platelets to damaged vascular surfaces (247,248). The immobilization of plasma VWF onto exposed subendothelial surfaces is thought to be the predominant mechanism that initiates platelet reponse in areas of vascular injury exposed to elevated shear forces.

Shear forces in the circulation may uncoil globular VWF proteins while they are bound transiently to vascular surfaces (249). The binding of GP Ib$\alpha$ to the A1 domain of VWF is the main interaction that can tether platelets to a surface, even under conditions of high flow velocity (250–252). Furthermore, the stable attachment of platelets requires the synergistic binding of integrins $\alpha_2\beta_1$ and $\alpha_{IIb}\beta_3$ to their respective substrates. Under abnormally elevated shear conditions (>5,000 per second), VWF is thought to participate in the binding to $\alpha_{IIb}\beta_3$ in addition to GP Ib$\alpha$ (165,253,254). Subsequent studies have demonstrated a role for VWF, fibrinogen, and possibly fibronectin, and CD40 ligand in the support of thrombus development (133,247,248,255–257). Under physiologic arterial shear rates, VWF is responsible for the immobilization of platelets on the surface. Irreversible attachment of these platelets to the surface requires both VWF and fibrinogen and involves both receptors GP Ib$\alpha$ and $\alpha_{IIb}\beta_3$.

## Interaction with Platelet Glycoprotein IIb/IIIa (Integrin $\alpha_{IIb}\beta_3$)

*In vitro*, if one uses washed platelets and purified VWF, platelet agonists such as ADP and thrombin can induce the binding of VWF to GP IIb/IIIa (167,168). This binding is blocked by monoclonal antibodies to GP IIb/IIIa but not by antibodies to GP Ib (140,164). In the presence of normal concentrations of fibrinogen, however, fibrinogen, not VWF, binds to this receptor (164). This may be in part a result of the fibrinogen concentration being much greater than the concentration of VWF (3 mg per mL vs. 10 $\mu$g per mL). In clinical conditions in which fibrinogen is reduced in concentration, VWF can be demonstrated to bind to this receptor and may partially support platelet aggregation in patients congenitally deficient in fibrinogen (afibrinogenemia) (171). *In vivo*, at local sites at which platelets and endothelial cells may participate in hemostasis, secretion of VWF from $\alpha$-granules and Weibel-Palade bodies may increase substantially the local concentration of VWF and facilitate VWF interaction with GP IIb/IIIa. In studies on shear-induced platelet aggregation both in a cone viscometer, as well as in flow chambers, VWF appears to participate with both the GP Ib receptor and the GP IIb/IIIa receptor (258,259).

Identification of the specific sites of interaction between VWF and platelets has been greatly facilitated by both the delineation of VWF genetic structure and by using specific VWF fragments, synthetic peptides, and recombinant proteins. A crucial interaction site for GP IIb/IIIa is the Arg-Gly-Asp (RGD) sequence at amino acid positions 2,507 to 2,509 on the C-terminal end of the VWF subunit (260,261). Initial studies indicated that the GP Ib binding site for VWF was localized to a disulfide-bonded loop at amino acids 1,226 to 1,684 of VWF, which is encoded by exon 28 of the *VWF* gene (262,263). More recently, the crystal structure of GP Ib$\alpha$ complexed with the A1 domain of VWF has been reported allowing a detailed analysis of the interaction site (251). Several type 2 molecular variants of VWF have been caused by mutations in this region of the molecule that either upregulate (type 2B VWD) or down-regulate (type 2M VWD) the interaction with GP Ib (264,265). Synthetic peptides whose sequences were derived from this region of VWF have been developed and used for inhibition (266).

## Asialo von Willebrand Factor

VWF binding to platelets induced either by ristocetin (GP Ib) or thrombin (GP IIb/IIIa) is agonist-dependent. Modified VWF molecules such as type 2B VWF, or normal VWF in which the negatively charged sialic acid residues are removed (asialo VWF), can bind directly to platelets even without any agonist activation. Studies on the mechanism of aggregation indicate that the initial binding of asialo VWF is to GP Ib, and that this binding results in the exposure of the GP IIb/IIIa receptor, the binding of fibrinogen, and the subsequent aggregation of platelets (224,227,267).

## Subendothelial Binding

The mechanism of VWF interaction with components of the blood vessel wall has been extensively studied. Endothelial cells not only secrete VWF but also deposit VWF on the abluminal surface in close association with the internal elastic lamina (268,269). Although there is *in vitro* evidence that VWF interacts specifically with collagen, it is unclear what role this plays *in vivo*, as treatment of subendothelium with collagenase does not decrease the VWF detection by immunofluorescence (270–273). Type VI collagen, which is resistant to collagenase, does bind to VWF, so it is a candidate for the collagen-resistant VWF binding site in the subendothelial matrix (274,275). Another subendothelial component that may function as a binding site for VWF is the elastin-associated microfibril; extracts of this material cause platelets to aggregate in the presence of VWF, which requires the presence of platelet GP Ib receptor (276,277). Further studies are necessary to fully delineate the various interactions of VWF required for normal hemostatic function.

## Effect of Blood Type on von Willebrand Factor Levels

There is a marked effect of ABO blood type on the VWF antigen (VWF:Ag) levels seen in healthy individuals (34,278). A study of more than 1,300 healthy blood donors revealed that patients with group A, B, and AB have a much greater mean VWF:Ag plasma concentration than blood group O individuals. The A, B, and H antigen (the unmodified H antigen is present in individuals with blood group O) has also been identified in VWF. The primary effect of this posttranslational carbohydrate modification appears to result in altered VWF survival *in vivo*. Symptoms of VWD appear to correlate with the absolute level of VWF. Table 46-2 lists the normal ranges for the different blood types reported in one study (34). In a retrospective analysis of samples from patients diagnosed with VWD, approximately 70% to 80% of individuals diagnosed as having VWD were blood group O (34). Because this bias might be caused by a difference in normal ranges, a prospective analysis of patients using blood type–specific normal ranges established that more than 65% of patients with VWD were blood group O; the reduced VWF in individuals with blood group O may cause them to have increased symptoms and result in a greater frequency of diagnostic evaluation and a greater likelihood of being diagnosed with VWD. The effect of ABO blood type on VWF is now recognized as a disease-modifying gene for VWD.

## Animal Models of von Willebrand Disease

Several animal species have been found to have VWD similar to the human disorder (canine and porcine). Recently, a "knockout" mouse model of VWD has also been developed (133). Porcine VWD has been identified for more than 20 years (279). This model was recently used to study both liver and bone marrow transplantation as a means of correcting endothelial (liver) or platelet VWF (bone marrow). Bone marrow corrected the platelet VWF but resulted in only a minimal increase in plasma VWF. Bleeding symptoms decreased and there was partial correction of the bleeding time. Liver transplantation caused a near normalization of plasma VWF levels and a normalization of the bleeding time. Such studies suggest that plasma VWF is primarily derived from endothelial cell VWF synthesis, but that platelet VWF also provides some benefit even if it is not accompanied by an increase in plasma VWF (280). Canine models of VWD are also available as either type 2 and type 1 VWD (98,281,282). Such models will be useful in studying gene therapy for VWD. The canine type 2 models are important for studying the variant forms, which are not present in the porcine model.

Studies on the porcine and murine model of VWD suggested a potential role for VWF in the development of atherosclerosis and endocarditis (283,284). Studies on human VWD have not yet identified a similar protection from atherosclerosis (285).

### TABLE 46-2

INFLUENCE OF ABO BLOOD GROUP ON VON WILLEBRAND FACTOR: VALUES IN VOLUNTEER BLOOD DONORS

| ABO type | N | Geometric values | Geometric mean ±2 SD |
|---|---|---|---|
| O | 456 | 74.8 | (35.6157.0) |
| A | 340 | 105.9 | (48.0233.9) |
| B | 196 | 116.9 | (56.8241.0) |
| AB | 109 | 123.3 | (63.8238.2) |

The groups were statistically significantly different from each other as follows: O versus A, B, AB, $P$ <0.01; A versus AB, $P$ <0.01; B versus A, $P$ <0.05.
Used by permission, RR Montgomery.

## References

1. Rodeghiero F, Castaman G, Dini E. Epidemiological investigation of the prevalence of von Willebrand's disease. *Blood* 1987;69:454–459.
2. Werner EJ, Broxson EH, Tucker EL, et al. Prevalence of von Willebrand disease in children: a multiethnic study. *J Pediatr* 1993;123:893–898.
3. Von Willebrand EA. Hereditary pseudohaemophilia. *Haemophilia* 1999;5: 223–231.
4. Jurgens R, Forsius H. On Willebrand-Jurgens constitutional thrombopathy in the Aland islands. *Schweiz Med Wochenschr* 1951;81:1248–1253.
5. Jorpes EJ. von Willebrand och von Willebrands sjukdom. *Nord Med* 1962; 67:729.
6. Nilsson IM, Blomback M, Jorpes EJ, et al. VWD and its correction with human plasma fraction I-O. *Acta Med Scand* 1957;159:179.
7. Biggs R, Matthews JM. The treatment of hemorrhage in VWD and the blood level of factor VIII (AHG). *Br J Haematol* 1963;9:203.
8. Salzman EW. Measurement of platelet adhesiveness: progress report. *Thromb Diath Haemorrh* 1967;26:303–307.
9. Meyer D, Larrieu MJ. Von Willebrand factor and platelet adhesiveness. *J Clin Pathol* 1970;23:228–231.
10. Cornu P. Willebrand's disease. *Pathol Biol* 1965;13:546–553.
11. Stefanini M, Dameshek W. *The hemorrhagic disorders.* New York: Grune & Stratton, 1955:56.
12. Schulman I, Smith CH, Erlandson M, et al. Vascular hemophilia. *Pediatrics* 1956;18:347.
13. Weiss HJ. The use of plasma and plasma fractions in the treatment of a patient with vWd. *Vox Sang* 1962;7:267.
14. Perkins HA. Correction of the hemostatic defects in vWd. *Blood* 1967;30: 375.
15. Alexander B, Goldstein R. Dual hemostatic defect in pseudo-hemophilia. *J Clin Invest* 1953;32:551.
16. Larrieu MJ, Soulier JP. Deficit en facteur antihemophilique a chez une fille, associe a un trouble du saignement. *Rev Hematol* 1953;8:361.
17. Quick AJ, Hussey CV. Hemophilic condition in the female. *J Lab Clin Med* 1953;42:929.
18. Borchgrevink CF, Egeberg O, Godal HC, et al. The effect of plasma and Cohn's fraction I on the Duke and Ivy bleeding times in vWd. *Acta Med Scand* 1963;173:235.

19. Bennett E, Dormandy K. Pool's cryoprecipitate and exhausted plasma in the treatment of vWd and factor XI deficiency. *Lancet* 1966;2:731.
20. Howard MA, Firkin BG. Ristocetin—a new tool in the investigation of platelet aggregation. *Thromb Diath Haemorrh* 1971;26:362–369.
21. Howard MA, Sawers RJ, Firkin BG. Ristocetin: a means of differentiating von Willebrand's disease into two groups. *Blood* 1973;41:687–690.
22. Tschopp TB, Weiss HG, Baumgartner HR. Decreased adhesion of platelets to subendothelium in vWd. *J Lab Clin Med* 1974;83:296.
23. Weiss HJ, Hoyer LW, Rickles FR, et al. Quantitative assay of a plasma factor deficient in von Willebrand's disease that is necessary for platelet aggregation. Relationship to factor VIII procoagulant activity and antigen content. *J Clin Invest* 1973;52:2708–2716.
24. Bouma BN, Mourik Jv, Wiegerinck Y, et al. Immunological characterization of anti-haemophilic factor A related antigen in haemophilia A. *Scand J Haematol* 1973;11:184–187.
25. Zimmerman TS, Edgington TS. Factor VIII coagulant activity and factor VIII-like antigen: independent molecular entities. *J Exp Med* 1973;138:1015–1020.
26. Bennett B, Forman WB, Ratnoff OD. Studies in the nature of antihemophilic factor (Factor VIII): further evidence relating the AHF-like antigens in normal and hemophilic plasmas. *J Clin Invest* 1973;52:2191.
27. Zimmerman TS, Ratnoff OD, Powell AE. Immunologic differentiation of classic hemophilia (Factor VIII deficiency) and vWd with observations on combined deficiencies of antihemophilic factor and proaccelerin (Factor V) and on an acquired circulating anticoagulant against antihemophilic factor. *J Clin Invest* 1971;50:244.
28. Montgomery RR, Zimmerman TS. vWd antigen II: a new plasma and platelet antigen deficient in severe vWd. *J Clin Invest* 1978;61:1498.
29. McCarroll DR, Levin EG, Montgomery RR. Endothelial cell synthesis of von Willebrand antigen II, vWf, and vWf/von Willebrand antigen II complex. *J Clin Invest* 1985;75:1089.
30. Fay PJ, Kawai Y, Wagner DD, et al. Propolypeptide of von Willebrand factor circulates in blood and is identical to von Willebrand antigen II. *Science* 1986;232:995–998.
31. Berliner SA, Seligsohn U, Zivelin A, et al. A relatively high frequency of severe (type III) von Willebrand's disease in Israel. *Br J Haematol* 1986;62:535–543.
32. Lenk H, Nilsson IM, Holmberg L, et al. Frequency of different types of von Willebrand's disease in the GDR. *Acta Med Scand* 1988;224:275–280.
33. Fischer RR, Lerner C, Bandinelli E, et al. Inheritance and prevalence of von Willebrand's disease severe form in a Brazilian population. *J Inherit Metab Dis* 1989;12:293–301.
34. Gill JC, Endres-Brooks J, Bauer PJ, et al. The effect of ABO blood group on the diagnosis of von Willebrand disease. *Blood* 1987;69:1691–1695.
35. Nilsson IM. *Haemorrhagic and thrombotic disease.* London: John Wiley and Sons, 1971.
36. Wahlberg T, Blomback M, Hall P, et al. Application of indicators, predictors and diagnostic indices in coagulation disorders. I. Evaluation of a self-administered questionnaire with binary questions. *Methods Inf Med* 1980;19:194–200.
37. Mohlke KL, Purkayastha AA, Westrick RJ, et al. Mvwf, a dominant modifier of murine von Willebrand factor, results from altered lineage-specific expression of a glycosyltransferase. *Cell* 1999;96:111–120.
38. Mohlke KL, Purkayastha AA, Westrick RJ, et al. Comparative mapping of distal murine chromosome 11 and human 17q21.3 in a region containing a modifying locus for murine plasma von Willebrand factor level. *Genomics* 1998;54:19–30.
39. Nichols WC, Cooney KA, Mohlke KL, et al. von Willebrand disease in the RIIIS/J mouse is caused by a defect outside of the von Willebrand factor gene [published erratum appears in Blood 1995 Sep 15;86(6):2461]. *Blood* 1994;83:3225–3231.
40. Batlle J, Lopez Fernandez MF, Lasierra J, et al. von Willebrand disease type IIC with different abnormalities of von Willebrand factor in the same sibship. *Am J Hematol* 1986;21:177–188.
41. Lopez-Fernandez MF, Blanco-Lopez MJ, Castineira MP, et al. Further evidence for recessive inheritance of von Willebrand disease with abnormal binding of von Willebrand factor to factor VIII [see comments]. *Am J Hematol* 1992;40:20–27.
42. Asakura A, Harrison J, Gomperts E, et al. Type IIA von Willebrand disease with apparent autosomal recessive inheritance. *Blood* 1987;69:1419–1420.
43. Donner M, Holmberg L, Nilsson IM. Type IIB von Willebrand's disease with probable autosomal recessive inheritance and presenting as thrombocytopenia in infancy. *Br J Haematol* 1987;66:349–354.
44. Standen GR, Bignell P, Bowen DJ, et al. Family studies in von Willebrand's disease by analysis of restriction fragment length polymorphisms and an intragenic variable number tandem repeat (VNTR) sequence. *Br J Haematol* 1990;76:242–249.
45. Eikenboom JC, Reitsma PH, Peerlinck KM, et al. Recessive inheritance of von Willebrand's disease type I [see comments]. *Lancet* 1993;341:982–986.
46. Eikenboom JC, Ploos van, Amstel HK, et al. Mutations in severe, type III von Willebrand's disease in the Dutch population: candidate missense and nonsense mutations associated with reduced levels of von Willebrand factor messenger RNA. *Thromb Haemost* 1992;68:448–454.
47. Miller CH, Graham JB, Goldin LR, et al. Genetics of classic vWd. I. Phenotypic variation within families. *Blood* 1979;54:117.
48. Miller CH, Graham JB, Goldin LR, et al. Genetics of classic von Willebrand's disease. II. Optimal assignment of the heterozygous genotype (diagnosis) by discriminant analysis. *Blood* 1979;54:137–145.
49. Abildgaard CF, Suzuki Z, Harrison J, et al. Serial studies in von Willebrand's disease: variability versus "variants". *Blood* 1980;56:712–716.
50. Lynch DC, Zimmerman TS, Collins CJ, et al. Molecular cloning of cDNA for human von Willebrand factor: authentication by a new method. *Cell* 1985;41:49–56.
51. Ginsburg D, Handin RI, Bonthron DT, et al. Human von Willebrand factor (vWF): isolation of complementary DNA (cDNA) clones and chromosomal localization. *Science* 1985;228:1401–1406.
52. Sadler JE, Shelton-Inloes BB, Sorace JM, et al. Cloning and characterization of two cDNAs coding for human von Willebrand factor. *Proc Natl Acad Sci U S A* 1985;82:6394–6398.
53. Verweij CL, Hofker M, Quadt R, et al. RFLP for a human von Willebrand factor (vWF) cDNA clone, pvWF1100 [published erratum appears in Nucleic Acid Res 1986 Feb 25;14(4):1930]. *Nucleic Acids Res* 1985;13:8289.
54. Ruggeri ZM, Ware J. The structure and function of von Willebrand factor. *Thromb Haemost* 1992;67:594–599.
55. Shelton-Inloes BB, Broze GJ Jr, Miletich JP, et al. Evolution of human von Willebrand factor: cDNA sequence polymorphisms, repeated domains, and relationship to von Willebrand antigen II. *Biochem Biophys Res Commun* 1987;144:657–665.
56. Koller E, Winterhalter KH, Trueb B. The globular domains of type VI collagen are related to the collagen-binding domains of cartilage matrix protein and von Willebrand factor. *EMBO J* 1989;8:1073–1077.
57. Sadler JE, Mancuso DJ, Randi AM, et al. Molecular biology of von Willebrand factor. *Ann N Y Acad Sci* 1991;614:114–124.
58. Hunt LT, Barker WC. von Willebrand factor shares a distinctive cysteine-rich domain with thrombospondin and procollagen. *Biochem Biophys Res Commun* 1987;144:876–882.
59. Mancuso DJ, Tuley EA, Westfield LA, et al. Structure of the gene for human von Willebrand factor. *J Biol Chem* 1989;264:19514–19527.
60. Mancuso DJ, Tuley EA, Westfield LA, et al. Human von Willebrand factor gene and pseudogene: structural analysis and differentiation by polymerase chain reaction. *Biochemistry* 1991;30:253–269.
61. Shelton-Inloes BB, Chehab FF, Mannucci PM, et al. Gene deletions correlate with the development of alloantibodies in von Willebrand disease. *J Clin Invest* 1987;79:1459–1465.
62. Ginsburg D, Konkle BA, Gill JC, et al. Molecular basis of human von Willebrand disease: analysis of platelet von Willebrand factor mRNA. *Proc Natl Acad Sci U S A* 1989;86:3723–3727.
63. Ginsburg D, Sadler JE. von Willebrand disease: a database of point mutations, insertions, and deletions. For the Consortium on von Willebrand Factor Mutations and Polymorphisms, and the Subcommittee on von Willebrand Factor of the Scientific and Standardization Committee of the International Society on Thrombosis and Haemostasis. *Thromb Haemost* 1993;69:177–184.
64. Tsai HM, Sussman II, Ginsburg D, et al. Proteolytic cleavage of recombinant type 2A von Willebrand factor mutants R834W and R834Q: inhibition by doxycycline and by monoclonal antibody VP-1. *Blood* 1997;89:1954–1962.
65. Kroner PA, Friedman KD, Fahs SA, et al. Abnormal binding of factor VIII is linked with the substitution of glutamine for arginine 91 in von Willebrand factor in a variant form of von Willebrand disease. *J Biol Chem* 1991;266:19146–19149.
66. Perez-Casal M, Daly M, Peake I, et al. A case of recessive type 2N von Willebrand's disease due to Arg 53 Trp substitution. *Am J Hematol* 1995;48:140.
67. Bowen DJ, Standen GR, Mazurier C, et al. Type 2N von Willebrand disease: rapid genetic diagnosis of G2811A (R854Q), C2696T (R816W), T2701A (H817Q) and G2823T (C858F)—detection of a novel candidate type 2N mutation: C2810T (R854W). *Thromb Haemost* 1998;80:32–36.
68. Gu J, Jorieux S, Lavergne JM, et al. A patient with type 2N von Willebrand disease is heterozygous for a new mutation: Gly22Glu. Demonstration of a defective expression of the second allele by the use of monoclonal antibodies. *Blood* 1997;89:3263–3269.
69. Hilbert L, Jorieux S, Fontenay-Roupie M, et al. Expression of two type 2N von Willebrand disease mutations identified in exon 18 of von Willebrand factor gene. *Br J Haematol* 2004;127:184–189.
70. Peake IR, Bowen D, Bignell P, et al. Family studies and prenatal diagnosis in severe von Willebrand disease by polymerase chain reaction amplification of a variable number tandem repeat region of the von Willebrand factor gene. *Blood* 1990;76:555–561.
71. Eikenboom JC, Reitsma PH, Peerlinck KM, et al. Recessive inheritance of von Willebrand's disease type I. *Lancet* 1993;341:982–986.
72. Guan J, Guillot PV, Aird WC. Characterization of the mouse von Willebrand factor promoter. *Blood* 1999;94:3405–3412.
73. Jahroudi N, Lynch DC. Endothelial-cell-specific regulation of von Willebrand factor gene expression. *Mol Cell Biol* 1994;14:999–1008.
74. Schwachtgen JL, Remacle JE, Janel N, et al. Oct-1 is involved in the transcriptional repression of the von willebrand factor gene promoter. *Blood* 1998;92:1247–1258.
75. Schwachtgen JL, Janel N, Barek L, et al. Ets transcription factors bind and transactivate the core promoter of the von Willebrand factor gene. *Oncogene* 1997;15:3091–3102.

76. Ardekani AM, Greenberger JS, Jahroudi N. Two repressor elements inhibit expression of the von Willebrand factor gene promoter *in vitro*. *Thromb Haemost* 1998;80:488–494.

77. Aird WC, Edelberg JM, Weiler-Guettler H, et al. Vascular bed-specific expression of an endothelial cell gene is programmed by the tissue microenvironment. *J Cell Biol* 1997;138:1117–1124.

78. Hough C, Cuthbert CD, Notley C, et al. Cell type-specific regulation of von Willebrand Factor expression by the E4BP4 transcriptional repressor. *Blood* 2005;105:1531–1539.

79. Edelberg JM, Aird WC, Wu W, et al. PDGF mediates cardiac microvascular communication. *J Clin Invest* 1998;102:837–843.

80. Harvey PJ, Keightley AM, Lam YM, et al. A single nucleotide polymorphism at nucleotide -1793 in the von Willebrand factor (VWF) regulatory region is associated with plasma VWF:Ag levels. *Br J Haematol* 2000;109: 349–353.

81. Collins CJ, Underdahl JP, Levene RB, et al. Molecular cloning of the human gene for von Willebrand factor and identification of the transcription initiation site. *Proc Natl Acad Sci U S A* 1987;84:4393–4397.

82. Sadler JE, Ginsburg D. A database of polymorphisms in the von Willebrand factor gene and pseudogene. For the Consortium on von Willebrand Factor Mutations and Polymorphisms and the Subcommittee on von Willebrand Factor of the Scientific and Standardization Committee of the International Society on Thrombosis and Haemostasis. *Thromb Haemost* 1993;69:185–191.

83. Sadler JE. A revised classification of von Willebrand disease. For the Subcommittee on von Willebrand Factor of the Scientific and Standardization Committee of the International Society on Thrombosis and Haemostasis. *Thromb Haemost* 1994;71:520–525.

84. Ngo KY, Glotz VT, Koziol JA, et al. Homozygous and heterozygous deletions of the von Willebrand factor gene in patients and carriers of severe von Willebrand disease. *Proc Natl Acad Sci U S A* 1988;85:2753–2757.

85. Inbal A, Kornbrot N, Zivelin A, et al. The inheritance of type I and type III von Willebrand's disease in Israel: linkage analysis, carrier detection and prenatal diagnosis using three intragenic restriction fragment length polymorphisms. *Blood Coagul Fibrinolysis* 1992;3:167–177.

86. Sadler JE, Gralnick HR. Commentary: a new classification for von Willebrand disease. *Blood* 1994;84:676–679.

87. Bernardi F, Marchetti G, Guerra S, et al. A de novo and heterozygous gene deletion causing a variant of von Willebrand disease. *Blood* 1990;75: 677–683.

88. Mancuso DJ, Tuley EA, Castillo R, et al. Characterization of partial gene deletions in type III von Willebrand disease with alloantibody inhibitors. *Thromb Haemost* 1994;72:180–185.

89. Peake IR, Liddell MB, Moodie P, et al. Severe type III von Willebrand's disease caused by deletion of exon 42 of the von Willebrand factor gene: family studies that identify carriers of the condition and a compound heterozygous individual. *Blood* 1990;75:654–661.

90. Sadler JE. Biochemistry and genetics of von Willebrand factor. *Annu Rev Biochem* 1998;67:395–424.

91. Gaiger A, Mannhalter C, Hinterberger W, et al. Detection of engraftment and mixed chimerism following bone marrow transplantation using PCR amplification of a highly variable region- variable number of tandem repeats (VNTR) in the von Willebrand factor gene. *Ann Hematol* 1991;63: 227–228.

92. Mercier B, Gaucher C, Mazurier C. Characterisation of 98 alleles in 105 unrelated individuals in the F8VWF gene. *Nucleic Acids Res* 1991;19: 4800.

93. Eikenboom JC, Reitsma PH, van der, et al. Instability of repeats of the von Willebrand factor gene variable number tandem repeat sequence in intron 40. *Br J Haematol* 1993;84:533–535.

94. Jaffe EA, Hoyer LW, Nachman RL. Synthesis of von Willebrand factor by cultured human endothelial cells. *Proc Natl Acad Sci U S A* 1974;71: 1906–1909.

95. Wagner DD, Olmsted JB, Marder VJ. Immunolocalization of von Willebrand protein in Weibel-Palade bodies of human endothelial cells. *J Cell Biol* 1982;95:355–360.

96. Sporn LA, Chavin SI, Marder VJ, et al. Biosynthesis of von Willebrand protein by human megakaryocytes. *J Clin Invest* 1985;76:1102–1106.

97. Nichols TC, Bellinger DA, Reddick RL, et al. The roles of von Willebrand factor and factor VIII in arterial thrombosis: studies in canine von Willebrand disease and hemophilia A. *Blood* 1993;81:2644–2651.

98. McCarroll DR, Waters DC, Steidley KR, et al. Canine platelet von Willebrand factor: quantification and multimeric analysis. *Exp Hematol* 1988; 16:929–937.

99. Slot JW, Bouma BN, Montgomery R, et al. Platelet factor VIII-related antigen: immunofluorescent localization. *Thromb Res* 1978;13:871–881.

100. Coller BS, Hirschman RJ, Gralnick HR. Studies on the factor VIII/von Willebrand factor antigen on human platelets. *Thromb Res* 1975;6:469–480.

101. Koutts J, Walsh PN, Plow EF, et al. Active release of human platelet factor VIII-related antigen by adenosine diphosphate, collagen, and thrombin. *J Clin Invest* 1978;62:1255–1263.

102. Scott JP, Montgomery RR. Platelet von Willebrand's antigen II: active release by aggregating agents and a marker of platelet release reaction *in vivo*. *Blood* 1981;58:1075–1080.

103. Hamilton KK, Sims PJ. Changes in cytosolic Ca2+ associated with von Willebrand factor release in human endothelial cells exposed to histamine.

104. Menon C, Berry EW, Ockelford P. Beneficial effect of DDAVP on bleeding-time in von Willebrand's disease. *Lancet* 1978;2:743–744.

105. Takeuchi M, Nagura H, Kaneda T. DDAVP and epinephrine-induced changes in the localization of von Willebrand factor antigen in endothelial cells of human oral mucosa. *Blood* 1988;72:850–854.

106. Wagner DD, Fay PJ, Sporn LA, et al. Divergent fates of von Willebrand factor and its propolypeptide (von Willebrand antigen II) after secretion from endothelial cells. *Proc Natl Acad Sci U S A* 1987;84:1955–1959.

107. Wagner DD, Lawrence SO, Ohlsson-Wilhelm BM, et al. Topology and order of formation of interchain disulfide bonds in von Willebrand factor. *Blood* 1987;69:27–32.

108. Wagner DD, Mayadas T, Marder VJ. Initial glycosylation and acidic pH in the Golgi apparatus are required for multimerization of von Willebrand factor. *J Cell Biol* 1986;102:1320–1324.

109. Wagner DD, Marder VJ. Biosynthesis of von Willebrand protein by human endothelial cells. Identification of a large precursor polypeptide chain. *J Biol Chem* 1983;258:2065–2067.

110. Titani K, Kumar S, Takio K, et al. Amino acid sequence of human von Willebrand factor. *Biochemistry* 1986;25:3171–3184.

111. Matsui T, Kihara C, Fujimura Y, et al. Carbohydrate analysis of human von Willebrand factor with horseradish peroxidase-conjugated lectins. *Biochem Biophys Res Commun* 1991;178:1253–1259.

112. Matsui T, Titani K, Mizuochi T. Structures of the asparagine-linked oligosaccharide chains of human von Willebrand factor. Occurrence of blood group A, B, and H(O) structures. *J Biol Chem* 1992;267:8723–8731.

113. Carew JA, Browning PJ, Lynch DC. Sulfation of von Willebrand factor. *Blood* 1990;76:2530–2539.

114. Wise RJ, Barr PJ, Wong PA, et al. Expression of a human proprotein processing enzyme: correct cleavage of the von Willebrand factor precursor at a paired basic amino acid site. *Proc Natl Acad Sci U S A* 1990;87: 9378–9382.

115. Hosaka M, Nagahama M, Kim WS, et al. Arg-X-Lys/Arg-Arg motif as a signal for precursor cleavage catalyzed by furin within the constitutive secretory pathway. *J Biol Chem* 1991;266:12127–12130.

116. Montgomery RR, Dent J, Schmidt W, et al. Hereditary persistence of circulating pro-vWf. *Circulation* 1986;74(Suppl. II):406.

117. Vischer UM, Wagner DD. von Willebrand factor proteolytic processing and multimerization precede the formation of Weibel-Palade bodies. *Blood* 1994;83:3536–3544.

118. Haberichter SL, Fahs SA, Montgomery RR. von Willebrand factor storage and multimerization: 2 independent intracellular processes. *Blood* 2000; 96:1808–1815.

119. Haberichter SL, Jozwiak MA, Rosenberg JB, et al. The von Willebrand factor propeptide (VWFpp) traffics an unrelated protein to storage. *Arterioscler Thromb Vasc Biol* 2002;22:921–926.

120. Voorberg J, Fontijn R, van Mourik JA, et al. Domains involved in multimer assembly of von willebrand factor (vWF): multimerization is independent of dimerization. *EMBO J* 1990;9:797–803.

121. Mayadas TN, Wagner DD. *In vitro* multimerization of von Willebrand factor is triggered by low pH. Importance of the propolypeptide and free sulfhydryls. *J Biol Chem* 1989;264:13497–13503.

122. Journet AM, Saffaripour S, Wagner DD. Requirement for both D domains of the propolypeptide in von Willebrand factor multimerization and storage. *Thromb Haemost* 1993;70:1053–1057.

123. Wise RJ, Pittman DD, Handin RI, et al. The propeptide of von Willebrand factor independently mediates the assembly of von Willebrand multimers. *Cell* 1988;52:229–236.

124. Mayadas TN, Wagner DD. Vicinal cysteines in the prosequence play a role in von Willebrand factor multimer assembly. *Proc Natl Acad Sci U S A* 1992;89:3531–3535.

125. Purvis AR, Sadler JE. A covalent oxidoreductase intermediate in propeptide-dependent von Willebrand factor multimerization. *J Biol Chem* 2004;279: 49982–49988.

126. Blagoveshchenskaya AD, Hannah MJ, Allen S, et al. Selective and signal-dependent recruitment of membrane proteins to secretory granules formed by heterologously expressed von Willebrand factor. *Mol Biol Cell* 2002;13:1582–1593.

127. Voorberg J, Fontijn R, Calafat J, et al. Biogenesis of von Willebrand factor-containing organelles in heterologous transfected CV-1 cells. *EMBO J* 1993;12:749–758.

128. Haberichter SL, Jacobi P, Montgomery RR. Critical independent regions in the VWF propeptide and mature VWF that enable normal VWF storage. *Blood* 2003;101:1384–1391.

129. Rosenberg JB, Haberichter SL, Jozwiak MA, et al. The role of the D1 domain of the von Willebrand factor propeptide in multimerization of VWF. *Blood* 2002;100:1699–1706.

130. Michaux G, Hewlett LJ, Messenger SL, et al. Analysis of intracellular storage and regulated secretion of three von Willebrands disease-causing variants of von Willebrand factor. *Blood* 2003;102:2452–2458.

131. Mannucci PM. Desmopressin (DDAVP) in the treatment of bleeding disorders: the first 20 years. *Blood* 1997;90:2515–2521.

132. Kaufmann JE, Oksche A, Wollheim CB, et al. Vasopressin-induced von Willebrand factor secretion from endothelial cells involves V2 receptors and cAMP. *J Clin Invest* 2000;106:107–116.

133. Denis C, Methia N, Frenette PS, et al. A mouse model of severe von Willebrand disease: defects in hemostasis and thrombosis. *Proc Natl Acad Sci U S A* 1998;95:9524–9529.

134. Haberichter SL, Merricks EP, Fahs SA, et al. Re-establishment of VWF-dependent Weibel-Palade bodies in VWD endothelial cells. *Blood* 2005;105: 145–152.

135. Huber D, Cramer EM, Kaufmann JE, et al. Tissue-type plasminogen activator (t-PA) is stored in Weibel-Palade bodies in human endothelial cells both *in vitro* and *in vivo*. *Blood* 2002;99:3637–3645.

136. Romani dW, de Leeuw HP, Rondaij MG, et al. Von Willebrand factor targets IL-8 to Weibel-Palade bodies in an endothelial cell line. *Exp Cell Res* 2003;286:67–74.

137. Wolff B, Burns AR, Middleton J, et al. Endothelial cell "memory" of inflammatory stimulation: human venular endothelial cells store interleukin 8 in Weibel-Palade bodies. *J Exp Med* 1998;188:1757–1762.

138. Vischer UM, Wagner DD. CD63 is a component of Weibel-Palade bodies of human endothelial cells. *Blood* 1993;82:1184–1191.

139. Rosenberg JB, Greengard JS, Montgomery RR. Genetic induction of a releasable pool of factor VIII in human endothelial cells. *Arterioscler Thromb Vasc Biol* 2000;20:2689–2695.

140. Kawai Y, Montgomery RR. Endothelial cell processing of von Willebrand proteins. *Ann N Y Acad Sci* 1987;509:60–70.

141. van Mourik JA, Boertjes R, Huisveld IA, et al. von Willebrand factor propeptide in vascular disorders: a tool to distinguish between acute and chronic endothelial cell perturbation. *Blood* 1999;94:179–185.

142. Casonato A, Pontara E, Sartorello F, et al. Reduced von Willebrand factor survival in type Vicenza von Willebrand disease. *Blood* 2002;99:180–184.

143. Brown SA, Eldridge A, Collins PW, et al. Increased clearance of von Willebrand factor antigen post-DDAVP in Type I von Willebrand disease: is it a potential pathogenic process? *J Thromb Haemost* 2003;1:1714–1717.

144. Lenting PJ, Westein E, Terraube V, et al. An experimental model to study the *in vivo* survival of Von Willebrand factor: basic aspects and application to the Arg1205His mutation. *J Biol Chem* 2003.

145. Gerritsen HE, Robles R, Lammle B, et al. Partial amino acid sequence of purified von Willebrand factor-cleaving protease. *Blood* 2001;98:1654–1661.

146. Fujikawa K, Suzuki H, McMullen B, et al. Purification of human von Willebrand factor-cleaving protease and its identification as a new member of the metalloproteinase family. *Blood* 2001;98:1662–1666.

147. Zheng X, Chung D, Takayama TK, et al. Structure of von Willebrand factor-cleaving protease (ADAMTS13), a metalloprotease involved in thrombotic thrombocytopenic purpura. *J Biol Chem* 2001;276:41059–41063.

148. Levy GG, Nichols WC, Lian EC, et al. Mutations in a member of the ADAMTS gene family cause thrombotic thrombocytopenic purpura. *Nature* 2001;413:488–494.

149. Tsai HM. Physiologic cleavage of von Willebrand factor by a plasma protease is dependent on its conformation and requires calcium ion. *Blood* 1996;87:4235–4244.

150. Furlan M, Robles R, Galbusera M, et al. von Willebrand factor-cleaving protease in thrombotic thrombocytopenic purpura and the hemolytic-uremic syndrome. *N Engl J Med* 1998;339:1578–1584.

151. Moake JL. Thrombotic microangiopathies. *N Engl J Med* 2002;347: 589–600.

152. Allford SL, Machin SJ. Current understanding of the pathophysiology of thrombotic thrombocytopenic purpura. *J Clin Pathol* 2000;53:497–501.

153. Padilla A, Moake JL, Bernardo A, et al. P-selectin anchors newly released ultra-large von Willebrand factor multimers to the endothelial cell surface. *Blood* 2004;103:2150–2156.

154. Dong JF, Moake JL, Nolasco L et al. ADAMTS-13 rapidly cleaves newly secreted ultra-large von Willebrand factor multimers on the endothelial surface under flowing conditions. *Blood* 2002;100:4033–4039.

155. Dong JF, Moake JL, Bernardo A et al. Adamts-13 metalloprotease interacts with the endothelial cell-derivd ultra-large von Willebrand factor. *J Biol Chem* 2003;278:29633–29639.

156. Nishio K, Fujimura Y, Nishida S, et al. Antiplatelet glycoprotein Ib monoclonal antibody (OP-F1) totally abolishes ristocetin-induced von Willebrand factor binding, but has minimal effect on the botrocetin-induced binding. *Haemostasis* 1991;21:353–359.

157. Furlan M, Robles R, Solenthaler M, et al. Deficient activity of von Willebrand factor-cleaving protease in chronic relapsing thrombotic thrombocytopenic purpura. *Blood* 1997;89:3097–3103.

158. Sutherland JJ, O'Brien LA, Lillicrap D, et al. Molecular modeling of the von Willebrand factor A2 domain and the effects of associated type 2A von Willebrand disease mutations. *J Mol Model (Online)* 2004;10:259–270.

159. Bockenstedt P, Greenberg JM, Handin RI. Structural basis of von Willebrand factor binding to platelet glycoprotein Ib and collagen. Effects of disulfide reduction and limited proteolysis of polymeric von Willebrand factor. *J Clin Invest* 1986;77:743–749.

160. Girma JP, Kalafatis M, Pietu G, et al. Mapping of distinct von Willebrand factor domains interacting with platelet GPIb and GPIIb/IIIa and with collagen using monoclonal antibodies. *Blood* 1986;67:1356–1366.

161. Pareti FI, Fujimura Y, Dent JA, et al. Isolation and characterization of a collagen binding domain in human von Willebrand factor. *J Biol Chem* 1986;261:15310–15315.

162. Inbal A, Loscalzo J. Glycocalicin binding to von Willebrand factor adsorbed onto collagen-coated or polystyrene surfaces. *Thromb Res* 1989; 56:347–357.

163. Ruggeri ZM, De Marco L, Gatti L, et al. Platelets have more than one binding site for von Willebrand factor. *J Clin Invest* 1983;72:1–12.

164. Schullek J, Jordan J, Montgomery RR. Interaction of von Willebrand factor with human platelets in the plasma milieu. *J Clin Invest* 1984;73:421–428.

165. Goto S, Salomon DR, Ikeda Y, et al. Characterization of the unique mechanism mediating the shear-dependent binding of soluble von Willebrand factor to platelets. *J Biol Chem* 1995;270:23352–23361.

166. Ruggeri ZM, Bader R, De Marco L. Glanzmann thrombasthenia: deficient binding of von Willebrand factor to thrombin-stimulated platelets. *Proc Natl Acad Sci U S A* 1982;79:6038–6041.

167. Fujimoto T, Ohara S, Hawiger J. Thrombin-induced exposure and prostacyclin inhibition of the receptor for factor VIII/von Willebrand factor on human platelets. *J Clin Invest* 1982;69:1212–1222.

168. Fujimoto T, Hawiger J. Adenosine diphosphate induces binding of von Willebrand factor to human platelets. *Nature* 1982;297:154–156.

169. Coller BS, Peerschke EI, Scudder LE, et al. Studies with a murine monoclonal antibody that abolishes ristocetin-induced binding of von Willebrand factor to platelets: additional evidence in support of GPIb as a platelet receptor for von Willebrand factor. *Blood* 1983;61:99–110.

170. Chen CS, Hawiger J. Reactivity of synthetic peptide analogs of adhesive proteins in regard to the interaction of human endothelial cells with extracellular matrix. *Blood* 1991;77:2200–2206.

171. Timmons S, Hawiger J. von Willebrand factor can substitute for plasma fibrinogen in ADP-induced platelet aggregation. *Trans Assoc Am Physicians* 1986;99:226–235.

172. Fressinaud E, Baruch D, Girma JP, et al. von Willebrand factor-mediated platelet adhesion to collagen involves platelet membrane glycoprotein IIb-IIIa as well as glycoprotein Ib. *J Lab Clin Med* 1988;112:58–67.

173. Goto S, Sakai H, Goto M, et al. Enhanced shear-induced platelet aggregation in acute myocardial infarction. *Circulation* 1999;99:608–613.

174. Baumgartner HR, Muggli R, Tschopp TB, et al. Platelet adhesion, release and aggregation in flowing blood: effects of surface properties and platelet function. *Thromb Haemost* 1976;35:124–138.

175. Tschopp TB, Weiss HJ, Baumgartner HR. Decreased adhesion of platelets to subendothelium in von Willebrand's disease. *J Lab Clin Med* 1974;83: 296–300.

176. Sugimoto M, Tsuji S, Kuwahara M, et al. Shear-dependent functions of the interaction between soluble von Willebrand factor and platelet glycoprotein Ib in mural thrombus formation on a collagen surface. *Int J Hematol* 1999;69:48–53.

177. Fredrickson BJ, Dong JF, McIntire LV, et al. Shear-dependent rolling on von Willebrand factor of mammalian cells expressing the platelet glycoprotein Ib-IX-V complex. *Blood* 1998;92:3684–3693.

178. Iijima K, Murata M, Nakamura K, et al. High shear stress attenuates agonist-induced, glycoprotein IIb/IIIa-mediated platelet aggregation when von Willebrand factor binding to glycoprotein Ib/IX is blocked. *Biochem Biophys Res Commun* 1997;233:796–800.

179. Gralnick HR, Kramer WS, McKeown LP, et al. Platelet adhesion at high shear rates: the roles of von Willebrand factor/GPIb and the beta 1 integrin alpha 2 beta 1. *Thromb Res* 1996;81:113–119.

180. Weiss HJ, Hoffmann T, Yoshioka A, et al. Evidence that the arg1744 gly1745 asp1746 sequence in the GPIIb-IIIa-binding domain of von Willebrand factor is involved in platelet adhesion and thrombus formation on subendothelium. *J Lab Clin Med* 1993;122:324–332.

181. Alevriadou BR, Moake JL, Turner NA, et al. Real-time analysis of shear-dependent thrombus formation and its blockade by inhibitors of von Willebrand factor binding to platelets. *Blood* 1993;81:1263–1276.

182. Ruggeri ZM. Structure and function of von Willebrand factor. *Thromb Haemost* 1999;82:576–584.

183. Ruggeri ZM. von Willebrand factor. *J Clin Invest* 1997;99:559–564.

184. Sadler JE. Von Willebrand factor. *J Biol Chem* 1991;266:22777–22780.

185. Wagner DD, Mayadas T, Urban-Pickering M, et al. Inhibition of disulfide bonding of von Willebrand protein by monensin results in small, functionally defective multimers. *J Cell Biol* 1985;101:112–120.

186. Zimmerman TS, Dent JA, Ruggeri ZM, et al. Subunit composition of plasma von Willebrand factor. Cleavage is present in normal individuals, increased in IIA and IIB von Willebrand disease, but minimal in variants with aberrant structure of individual oligomers (types IIC, IID, and IIE). *J Clin Invest* 1986;77:947–951.

187. Ohmori K, Fretto LJ, Harrison RL, et al. Electron microscopy of human factor VIII/Von Willebrand glycoprotein: effect of reducing reagents on structure and function. *J Cell Biol* 1982;95:632–640.

188. Fowler WE, Fretto LJ, Hamilton KK, et al. Substructure of human von Willebrand factor. *J Clin Invest* 1985;76:1491–1500.

189. Slayter H, Loscalzo J, Bockenstedt P, et al. Native conformation of human von Willebrand protein. Analysis by electron microscopy and quasi-elastic light scattering. *J Biol Chem* 1985;260:8559–8563.

190. Counts RB, Paskell SL, Elgee SK. Disulfide bonds and the quaternary structure of factor VIII/von Willebrand factor. *J Clin Invest* 1978;62: 702–709.

191. Gralnick HR, Williams SB, Morisato DK. Effect of multimeric structure of the factor VIII/von Willebrand factor protein on binding to platelets. *Blood* 1981;58:387–397.

192. Zimmerman TS, Roberts J, Edgington TS. Factor-VIII-related antigen: multiple molecular forms in human plasma. *Proc Natl Acad Sci U S A* 1975;72:5121–5125.

193. Nilsson IM, Peake IR, Bloom AL, et al. Report of the Working Party on Factor VIII Related Antigens. Addendum: the relationship between ristocetin co-factor activity (VIIIR:Cof) and Factor VIII related antigen (VIIIR:Ag). *Thromb Haemost* 1980;43:167–168.

194. Nilsson IM. Report of the working party on factor VIII-related antigens. *Thromb Haemost* 1978;39:511–520.

195. Hillery CA, Mancuso DJ, Evan SJ, et al. Type 2M von Willebrand disease: F606I and I662F mutations in the glycoprotein Ib binding domain selectively impair ristocetin- but not botrocetin-mediated binding of von Willebrand factor to platelets. *Blood* 1998;91:1572–1581.

196. Weiss HJ, Hoyer IW. Von Willebrand factor: dissociation from antihemophilic factor procoagulant activity. *Science* 1973;182:1149–1151.

197. Cooper HA, Wagner RH. The defect in hemophilic and von Willebrand's disease plasmas studied by a recombination technique. *J Clin Invest* 1974;54:1093–1099.

198. McKee PA, Andersen JC, Switzer ME. Molecular structural studies of human factor VIII. *Ann N Y Acad Sci* 1975;240:8–33.

199. Shapiro GA, Andersen JC, Pizzo SV, et al. The subunit structure of normal and hemophilic factor VIII. *J Clin Invest* 1973;52:2198–2210.

200. Switzer ME, McKee PA. Studies on human antihemophilic factor. Evidence for a covalently linked subunit structure. *J Clin Invest* 1976;57:925–937.

201. Cornu P, Larrieu MJ, Caen J, et al. Transfusion studies in vWd: effect on bleeding time and Factor VIII. *Br J Haematol* 1963;9:189.

202. Weiss HJ, Sussman II, Hoyer LW. Stabilization of factor VIII in plasma by the von Willebrand factor. Studies on posttransfusion and dissociated factor VIII and in patients with von Willebrand's disease. *J Clin Invest* 1977;60:390–404.

203. Bennett E, Dormandy K. Pool's cryoprecipitate and exhausted plasma in the treatment of von Willebrand's disease and factor-XI deficiency. *Lancet* 1966;2:731–732.

204. Kaufman RJ, Pipe SW. Regulation of factor VIII expression and activity by von Willebrand factor. *Thromb Haemost* 1999;82:201–208.

205. Pipe SW, Kaufman RJ. Factor VIII C2 domain missense mutations exhibit defective trafficking of biologically functional proteins. *J Biol Chem* 1996;271:25671–25676.

206. Koppelman SJ, van Hoeij M, Vink T, et al. Requirements of von Willebrand factor to protect factor VIII from inactivation by activated protein C. *Blood* 1996;87:2292–2300.

207. Fay PJ. Factor VIII structure and function. *Thromb Haemost* 1993;70:63–67.

208. Kaufman RJ, Pipe SW, Tagliavacca L, et al. Biosynthesis, assembly and secretion of coagulation factor VIII. *Blood Coagul Fibrinolysis* 1997;8(Suppl. 2):S3–14.

209. Kaufman RJ, Wasley LC, Davies MV, et al. Effect of von Willebrand factor coexpression on the synthesis and secretion of factor VIII in Chinese hamster ovary cells. *Mol Cell Biol* 1989;9:1233–1242.

210. Pittman DD, Tomkinson KN, Kaufman RJ. Post-translational requirements for functional factor V and factor VIII secretion in mammalian cells. *J Biol Chem* 1994;269:17329–17337.

211. Kaufman RJ. Biological regulation of factor VIII activity. *Annu Rev Med* 1992;43:325–339.

212. Zimmerman TS, Ruggeri ZM. von Willebrand's Disease. *Clin Haematol* 1983;12:175–200.

213. Gibson-D'Ambrosio RE, Crowe DL, Shuler CE, et al. The establishment and continuous subculturing of normal human adult hepatocytes: expression of differentiated liver functions. *Cell Biol Toxicol* 1993;9:385–403.

214. Ingerslev J, Christiansen BS, Heickendorff L, et al. Synthesis of factor VIII in human hepatocytes in culture. *Thromb Haemost* 1988;60:387–391.

215. Do H, Healey JF, Waller EK, et al. Expression of factor VIII by murine liver sinusoidal endothelial cells. *J Biol Chem* 1999;274:19587–19592.

216. Rosenberg JB, Foster PA, Kaufman RJ, et al. Intracellular trafficking of factor VIII to von Willebrand factor storage granules. *J Clin Invest* 1998;101:613–624.

217. Montgomery RR, Gill JC. Interactions between von Willebrand factor and factor VIII: where did they first meet. *J Pediatr Hematol Oncol* 2000;22:269–275.

218. Shi Q, Wilcox DA, Fahs SA, et al. Expression of human factor VIII under control of the platelet-specific alphaIIb promoter in megakaryocytic cell line as well as storage together with VWF. *Mol Genet Metab* 2003;79:25–33.

219. Wilcox DA, Shi Q, Nurden P, et al. Induction of megakaryocytes to synthesize and store a releasable pool of human factor VIII. *J Thromb Haemost* 2003;1:2477–2489.

220. Moake JL, Olson JD, Troll JH Jr, et al. Interaction of platelets, von Willebrand factor, and ristocetin during platelet agglutination. *J Lab Clin Med* 1980;96:168–184.

221. Weiss HJ, Rogers J, Brand H. Defective ristocetin-induced platelet aggregation in von Willebrand's disease and its correction by factor VIII. *J Clin Invest* 1973;52:2697–2707.

222. Jenkins CS, Clemetson KJ, Luscher EF. Studies on the mechanism of ristocetin-induced platelet agglutination: binding of ristocetin to platelets. *J Lab Clin Med* 1979;93:220–231.

223. Allain JP, Cooper HA, Wagner RH, et al. Platelets fixed with paraformaldehyde: a new reagent for assay of von Willebrand factor and platelet aggregating factor. *J Lab Clin Med* 1975;85:318–328.

224. De Marco L, Girolami A, Russell S, et al. Interaction of asialo von Willebrand factor with glycoprotein Ib induces fibrinogen binding to the glycoprotein IIb/IIIa complex and mediates platelet aggregation. *J Clin Invest* 1985;75:1198–1203.

225. Grainick HR, Williams SB, Coller BS. Asialo von Willebrand factor interactions with platelets. Interdependence of glycoproteins Ib and IIb/IIIa for binding and aggregation. *J Clin Invest* 1985;75:19–25.

226. Bastida E, Monteagudo J, Ordinas A, et al. Asialo von Willebrand factor enhances platelet adhesion to vessel subendothelium. *Thromb Haemost* 1988;60:30–34.

227. De Marco L, Shapiro SS. Properties of human asialo-factor VIII. A ristocetin-independent platelet-aggregating agent. *J Clin Invest* 1981;68:321–328.

228. Phillips DR. An evaluation of membrane glycoproteins in platelet adhesion and aggregation. *Prog Hemost Thromb* 1980;5:81–109.

229. George JN, Nurden AT, Phillips DR. Molecular defects in interactions of platelets with the vessel wall. *N Engl J Med* 1984;311:1084–1098.

230. Montgomery RR, Kunicki TJ, Taves C, et al. Diagnosis of Bernard-Soulier syndrome and Glanzmann's thrombasthenia with a monoclonal assay on whole blood. *J Clin Invest* 1983;71:385–389.

231. Calverley DC, Yagi M, Stray SM, et al. Human platelet glycoprotein V: its role in enhancing expression of the glycoprotein Ib receptor. *Blood* 1995;86:1361–1367.

232. Noda M, Fujimura K, Takafuta T, et al. Heterogeneous expression of glycoproteins Ib, IX and V in platelets from two patients with Bernard-Soulier syndrome caused by different genetic abnormalities. *Thromb Haemost* 1995;74:1411–1415.

233. Clemetson KJ, Clemetson JM. Platelet GPIb-V-IX complex. Structure, function, physiology, and pathology. *Semin Thromb Hemost* 1995;21:130–136.

234. Modderman PW, Admiraal LG, Sonnenberg A, et al. Glycoproteins V and Ib-IX form a noncovalent complex in the platelet membrane. *J Biol Chem* 1992;267:364–369.

235. Berndt MC, Gregory C, Chong BH, et al. Additional glycoprotein defects in Bernard-Soulier's syndrome: confirmation of genetic basis by parental analysis. *Blood* 1983;62:800–807.

236. Coller BS, Gralnick HR. Studies on the mechanism of ristocetin-induced platelet agglutination. Effects of structural modification of ristocetin and vancomycin. *J Clin Invest* 1977;60:302–312.

237. Coller BS. The effects of ristocetin and von Willebrand factor on platelet electrophoretic mobility. *J Clin Invest* 1978;61:1168–1175.

238. Coller BS. Biochemical and electrostatic considerations in primary platelet aggregation. *Ann N Y Acad Sci* 1983;416:693–708.

239. Scott JP, Montgomery RR, Retzinger GS. Dimeric ristocetin flocculates proteins, binds to platelets, and mediates von Willebrand factor-dependent agglutination of platelets. *J Biol Chem* 1991;266:8149–8155.

240. Cho YR, Maguire AJ, Try AC, et al. Cooperativity and anti-cooperativity between ligand binding and the dimerization of ristocetin A: asymmetry of a homodimer complex and implications for signal transduction. *Chem Biol* 1996;3:207–215.

241. Coller BS, Lundberg WB, Gralnick HR. Effects of vancomycin on platelets, plasma proteins and hepatitis B surface antigen. *Thromb Diath Haemorrh* 1975;34:83–93.

242. Coller BS. Polybrene-induced platelet agglutination and reduction in electrophoretic mobility: enhancement by von Willebrand factor and inhibition by vancomycin. *Blood* 1980;55:276–281.

243. Turitto VT, Weiss HJ, Baumgartner HR. Decreased platelet adhesion on vessel segments in von Willebrand's disease: a defect in initial platelet attachment. *J Lab Clin Med* 1983;102:551–564.

244. Turitto VT, Weiss HJ, Baumgartner HR. Platelet interaction with rabbit subendothelium in von Willebrand's disease: altered thrombus formation distinct from defective platelet adhesion. *J Clin Invest* 1984;74:1730–1741.

245. Turitto VT, Weiss HJ, Zimmerman TS, et al. Factor VIII/von Willebrand factor in subendothelium mediates platelet adhesion. *Blood* 1985;65:823–831.

246. Stel HV, Sakariassen KS, de Groot PG, et al. Von Willebrand factor in the vessel wall mediates platelet adherence. *Blood* 1985;65:85–90.

247. Sakariassen KS, Bolhuis PA, Sixma JJ. Platelet adherence to subendothelium of human arteries in pulsatile and steady flow. *Thromb Res* 1980;19:547–559.

248. Sixma JJ, de Groot PG. von Willebrand factor and the blood vessel wall. *Mayo Clin Proc* 1991;66:628–633.

249. Siedlecki CA, Lestini BJ, Kottke-Marchant KK, et al. Shear-dependent changes in the three-dimensional structure of human von Willebrand factor. *Blood* 1996;88:2939–2950.

250. Celikel R, Varughese KI, Madhusudan, et al. Crystal structure of the von Willebrand factor A1 domain in complex with the function blocking NMC-4 Fab. *Nat Struct Biol* 1998;5:189–194.

251. Huizinga EG, Tsuji S, Romijn RA, et al. Structures of glycoprotein Ibalpha and its complex with von Willebrand factor A1 domain. *Science* 2002;297:1176–1179.

252. Celikel R, Ruggeri ZM, Varughese KI. von Willebrand factor conformation and adhesive function is modulated by an internalized water molecule. *Nat Struct Biol* 2000;7:881–884.

253. Ruggeri ZM, Dent JA, Saldivar E. Contribution of distinct adhesive interactions to platelet aggregation in flowing blood. *Blood* 1999;94:172–178.

254. Goto S, Ikeda Y, Saldivar E, et al. Distinct mechanisms of platelet aggregation as a consequence of different shearing flow conditions. *J Clin Invest* 1998;101:479–486.

255. Ni H, Denis CV, Subbarao S, et al. Persistence of platelet thrombus formation in arterioles of mice lacking both von Willebrand factor and fibrinogen. *J Clin Invest* 2000;106:385–392.

256. Andre P, Prasad KS, Denis CV, et al. CD40L stabilizes arterial thrombi by a beta3 integrin—dependent mechanism. *Nat Med* 2002;8:247–252.

257. Moake JL, Turner NA, Stathopoulos NA, et al. Shear-induced platelet aggregation can be mediated by vWF released from platelets, as well as by exogenous large or unusually large vWF multimers, requires adenosine diphosphate, and is resistant to aspirin. *Blood* 1988;71:1366–1374.

258. Ikeda Y, Handa M, Kawano K, et al. The role of von Willebrand factor and fibrinogen in platelet aggregation under varying shear stress. *J Clin Invest* 1991;87:1234–1240.

259. O'Brien JR, Salmon GP. Shear stress activation of platelet glycoprotein IIb/IIIa plus von Willebrand factor causes aggregation: filter blockage and the long bleeding time in von Willebrand's disease. *Blood* 1987;70:1354–1361.

260. Beacham DA, Wise RJ, Turci SM, et al. Selective inactivation of the Arg-Gly-Asp-Ser (RGDS) binding site in von Willebrand factor by site-directed mutagenesis. *J Biol Chem* 1992;267:3409–3415.

261. Berliner S, Niiya K, Roberts JR, et al. Generation and characterization of peptide-specific antibodies that inhibit von Willebrand factor binding to glycoprotein IIb-IIIa without interacting with other adhesive molecules. Selectivity is conferred by Pro1743 and other amino acid residues adjacent to the sequence Arg1744-Gly1745-Asp1746. *J Biol Chem* 1988;263:7500–7505.

262. Azuma H, Dent JA, Sugimoto M, et al. Independent assembly and secretion of a dimeric adhesive domain of von Willebrand factor containing the glycoprotein Ib-binding site. *J Biol Chem* 1991;266:12342–12347.

263. Sugimoto M, Ricca G, Hrinda ME, et al. Functional modulation of the isolated glycoprotein Ib binding domain of von Willebrand factor expressed in Escherichia coli. *Biochemistry* 1991;30:5202–5209.

264. Kroner PA, Kluessendorf ML, Scott JP, et al. Expressed full-length von Willebrand factor containing missense mutations linked to type IIB von Willebrand disease shows enhanced binding to platelets. *Blood* 1992;79:2048–2055.

265. Mancuso DJ, Kroner PA, Christopherson PA, et al. Type 2M:Milwaukee-1 von Willebrand disease: an in-frame deletion in the Cys509-Cys695 loop of the von Willebrand factor A1 domain causes deficient binding of von Willebrand factor to platelets. *Blood* 1996;88:2559–2568.

266. Mohri H, Fujimura Y, Shima M, et al. Structure of the von Willebrand factor domain interacting with glycoprotein Ib. *J Biol Chem* 1988;263:17901–17904.

267. Lawrence JB, Gralnick HR. Asialo-von Willebrand factor inhibits platelet adherence to human arterial subendothelium: discrepancy between ristocetin cofactor activity and primary hemostatic function. *Blood* 1987;70:1084–1089.

268. Rand JH, Gordon RE, Sussman II, et al. Electron microscopic localization of factor-VIII–related antigen in adult human blood vessels. *Blood* 1982;60:627–634.

269. Sussman II, Rand JH. Subendothelial deposition of von Willebrand's factor requires the presence of endothelial cells. *J Lab Clin Med* 1982;100:526–532.

270. Rand JH, Sussman II, Gordon RE, et al. Localization of factor-VIII-related antigen in human vascular subendothelium. *Blood* 1980;55:752–756.

271. Tschopp TB, Baumgartner HR, Meyer D. Antibody to human factor VIII/von Willebrand factor inhibits collagen-induced platelet aggregation and release. *Thromb Res* 1980;17:255–259.

272. Baumgartner HR, Tschopp TB, Meyer D. Shear rate dependent inhibition of platelet adhesion and aggregation on collagenous surfaces by antibodies to human factor VIII/von Willebrand factor. *Br J Haematol* 1980;44:127–139.

273. Santoro SA. Adsorption of von Willebrand factor/factor VIII by the genetically distinct interstitial collagens. *Thromb Res* 1981;21:689–691.

274. Rand JH, Patel ND, Schwartz E, et al. 150-kD von Willebrand factor binding protein extracted from human vascular subendothelium is type VI collagen. *J Clin Invest* 1991;88:253–259.

275. Rand JH, Badimon L, Gordon RE, et al. Distribution of von Willebrand factor in porcine intima varies with blood vessel type and location. *Arteriosclerosis* 1987;7:287–291.

276. Legrand YJ, Fauvel F, Gutman N, et al. Microfibrils (MF) platelet interaction: requirement of von Willebrand factor. *Thromb Res* 1980;19:737–739.

277. Fauvel F, Grant ME, Legrand YJ, et al. Interaction of blood platelets with a microfibrillar extract from adult bovine aorta: requirement for von Willebrand factor. *Proc Natl Acad Sci U S A* 1983;80:551–554.

278. Percy ME, Rusk AC, Garvey MB, et al. Carrier detection in hemophilia A: ABO blood group, multiple measurements, and application of logistic discrimination. *Am J Med Genet* 1988;31:871–879.

279. Webster WP, Mandel SR, Strike LE, et al. Factor VIII synthesis: hepatic and renal allografts in swine with von Willebrand's disease. *Am J Physiol* 1976;230:1342–1348.

280. Brinkhous KM, Reddick RL, Read MS, et al. von Willebrand factor and animal models: contributions to gene therapy, thrombotic thrombocytopenic purpura, and coronary artery thrombosis. *Mayo Clin Proc* 1991;66:733–742.

281. Dodds WJ. Further studies of canine von Willebrand's disease. *Blood* 1975;45:221–230.

282. Johnson GS, Turrentine MA, Kraus KH. Canine von Willebrand's disease. A heterogeneous group of bleeding disorders. *Vet Clin North Am Small Anim Pract* 1988;18:195–229.

283. Bowie EJ, Fuster V, Fass DN, et al. The role of Willebrand factor in platelet/blood vessel interaction, including a discussion of resistance to atherosclerosis in pigs with von Willebrand disease. *Philos Trans R Soc Lond B Biol Sci* 1981;294:267–279.

284. Methia N, Andre P, Denis CV, et al. Localized reduction of atherosclerosis in von Willebrand factor-deficient mice. *Blood* 2001;98:1424–1428.

285. Mannucci PM, Bloom AL, Larrieu MJ, et al. Atherosclerosis and von Willebrand factor. I. Prevalence of severe von Willebrand's disease in western Europe and Israel. *Br J Haematol* 1984;57:163–169.

# CHAPTER 47 ■ PLATELET–VESSEL WALL INTERACTIONS IN FLOWING BLOOD

ZAVERIO M. RUGGERI AND BRIAN SAVAGE

Platelets respond to vascular injury by forming thrombi that, during hemostasis, seal severed vessels and limit blood loss after tissue trauma, and may also cause the acute occlusion of atherosclerotic arteries, resulting in life-threatening diseases such as myocardial infarction and stroke (1). Platelets interact with the vessel wall in the fluid dynamic environment of circulating blood, and forces generated by flow influence all aspects of their function, including initial contacts with reactive substrates, activation, and aggregation. A didactical distinction between "adhesion" and "aggregation" separates the process of bond formation between platelets and immobilized substrates from the cohesion of platelets with one another. In this regard the two events are distinct, although they share underlying mechanisms and are similarly influenced by hemodynamic forces. Most concepts on aggregation derive from *in vitro* experiments in which platelets are studied in suspension and are induced to interact with one another by appropriate stimuli in the absence of a reactive surface. *In vivo*, however, thrombi develop by the progressive accrual of circulating platelets onto those already attached to a vascular lesion and activated, therefore, as a result of continued adhesion to a dynamic substrate rather than cohesion of multiple platelets in suspension. Understanding these mechanisms requires a clarification of how adhesive surfaces are recognized and stable bonds are established, opposing the tendency of flow to keep platelets moving with blood.

## VASCULAR STRUCTURES THAT INTERACT WITH PLATELETS AT SITES OF INJURY

Platelets normally circulate in close contact with the inner surface of vessels without adhesion, but this equilibrium is altered when endothelial cells become reactive or when subendothelial structures are exposed. The response of platelets to traumatic injury is triggered primarily by thrombogenic subendothelial components (see Fig. 47-1). However, in diseased vessels the nonthrombogenic properties of the endothelium may cease to be fully effective, resulting in platelet adhesion to damaged endothelial cells even without exposure of subendothelial components.

## NORMAL ENDOTHELIAL CELLS ARE NONREACTIVE TOWARD PLATELETS

The endothelial cells lining the lumen of normal vessels do not support stable adhesion of circulating platelets, a key property that depends on several active functions (2). Important in this respect are physical characteristics, such as repulsive forces between negatively charged cell membranes, and biochemical attributes, such as synthesis and release of inhibitors of platelet activation. The latter include prostacyclin ($PGI_2$) and nitric oxide (NO), which are expressed constitutively and may act locally on platelets that are flowing in the vicinity of the vessel wall. In addition, substances expressed on the surface of endothelial cells may reduce the possibility of focal platelet activation through the removal of potential agonists. For example, ADPases degrade adenosine 5'-diphosphate (ADP) (3), heparan sulfate (a heparinlike glycosaminoglycan) participates in the inactivation of thrombin, and thrombomodulin induces a change in the substrate specificity of thrombin, rendering it incapable of stimulating platelets (4). The contribution of endothelial cells to the regulation of platelet activation is illustrated by the occurrence of cerebrovascular thrombotic episodes documented in two brothers whose platelets exhibited enhanced response to stimuli owing to decreased levels of NO (5).

## PLATELET INTERACTION WITH ALTERED ENDOTHELIAL CELLS

In the course of vascular disease, platelets may participate in pathologic processes involving endothelial cells that have lost the ability to inhibit thrombogenic responses but may do so without exposure of extracellular matrix components. A relevant example of such a situation occurs in the early stages of atherosclerotic lesions (1). Platelets adhere to dysfunctional endothelium as well as to exposed subendothelial structures and other vascular cells present in the developing plaque, such as monocytes, and form mural thrombi. Adherent platelets become activated and release cytokines and growth factors that contribute to the proliferation of smooth muscle cells and recruit more monocytes into the lesion (6). In such a manner, formation and organization of mural platelet thrombi becomes part of the process responsible for the progression from fatty plaques to unstable and thrombogenic lesions. Different stimuli have been found to alter the reactivity of endothelial cells toward platelets in experimental conditions, and many of them may act concurrently, although to variable extents, during the course of distinct disease processes. Viral transformation is a relevant example of endothelial perturbation resulting in enhanced interactions with platelets, caused at least in part by decreased $PGI_2$ production (7), accelerated rate of thrombin generation (8), and enhanced secretion of von Willebrand factor (VWF) (9). Viral as well as bacterial infections with subsequent immune and inflammatory reactions may play a considerable role in the etiology of vascular lesions (6,10).

The generation of α-thrombin on the surface of endothelial cells may have a considerable thrombogenic potential at sites of vascular injury. The outcome of this event may depend on the action of receptors such as thrombomodulin (4) that can change the

723

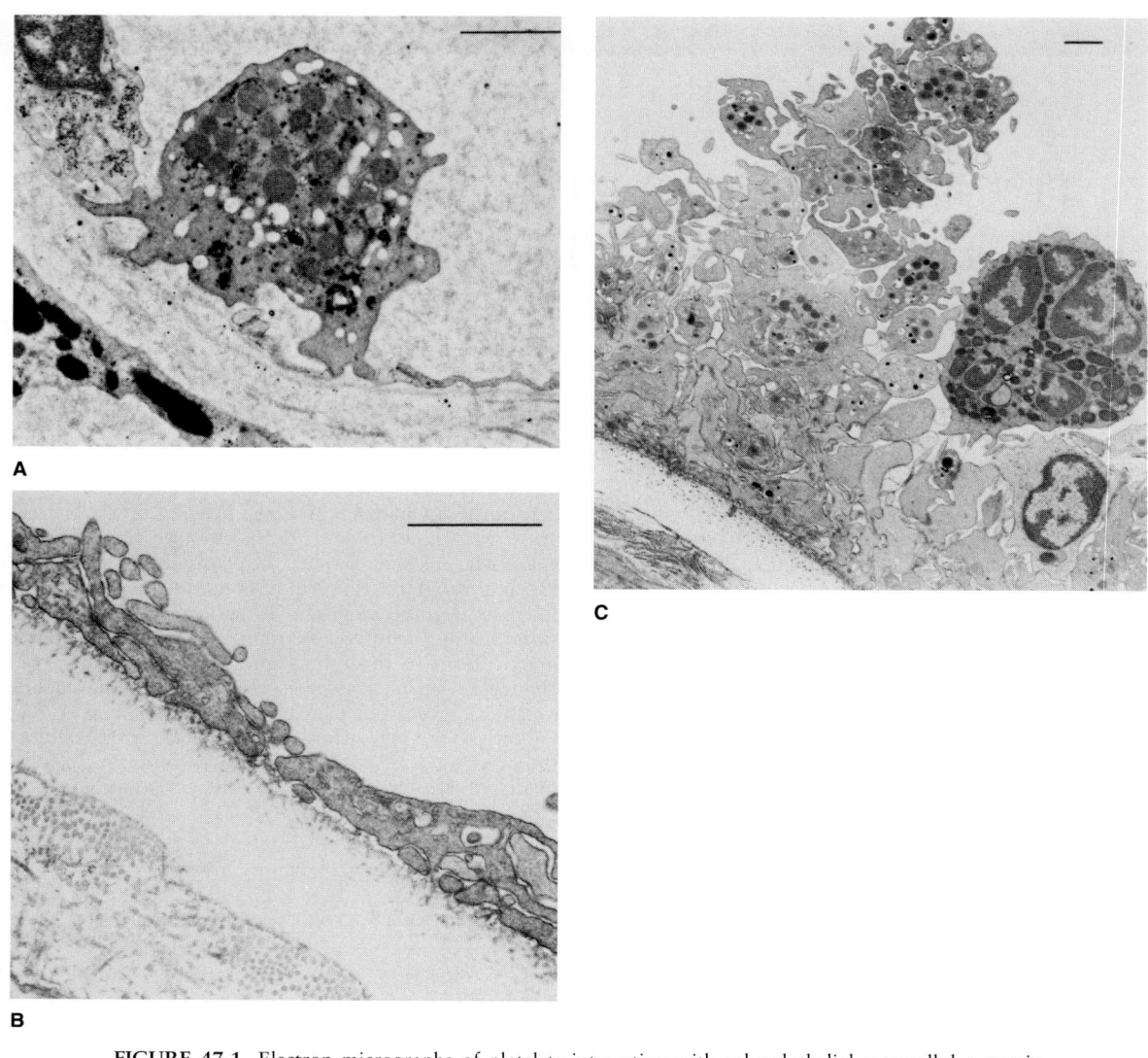

**FIGURE 47-1.** Electron micrographs of platelets interacting with subendothelial extracellular matrix components. **A:** A platelet fills the gap between two endothelial cells. **B:** Spread and interdigitated platelets adhere to the subendothelium. **C:** Platelet thrombus attaches to the subendothelium. The platelets near the surface are degranulated. Two leukocytes (seen in the lower right corner) are attached to the platelet mass. This specimen is fixed 10 minutes after removing the endothelium from rabbit aorta. The bars in each panel indicate a distance of 1 $\mu$m.

specificity of the enzyme, as well as on the interplay of distinct possible responses of both platelets and endothelial cells to the agonist. For example, activated platelets can influence the function of endothelial cells by releasing several vasoactive mediators, and these effects may precede direct intercellular interactions. Endothelial cells stimulated by $\alpha$-thrombin may be either prothrombotic, exposing adhesive substrates or receptors that can interact with platelets, or antithrombotic, inducing the release of a potent inhibitor of platelet activation, such as PGI$_2$. Experimental manipulation may highlight one or the other possibility, as demonstrated by the evidence that stimulation of endothelial cells with $\alpha$-thrombin *in vitro* may induce the attachment of aggregated platelets, particularly after inhibition of PGI$_2$ synthesis with aspirin (11). Similarly, a thrombogenic response was observed *in vivo* with otherwise ineffective doses of $\alpha$-thrombin if cell surface proteoglycans were simultaneously blocked with protamine or after administration of high doses of aspirin (12). After the first exposure to $\alpha$-thrombin, endothelial cells may become transiently refractory to further stimulation and secrete lower levels of PGI$_2$ than when under baseline conditions; accordingly,

during this time frame, activated platelets may adhere more promptly. Aspirin administered at lower doses displays a predominant effect on cyclooxygenase-dependent platelet activation rather than on endothelial cell PGI$_2$ synthesis, resulting in inhibition of platelet deposition onto the endothelium. These combined observations suggest that alterations in the antithrombotic potential of endothelial cells may be an early determinant of platelet deposition onto the vessel wall, particularly if powerful agonists of platelet activation are generated locally.

## ADHESIVE MOLECULES THAT SUPPORT THE INTERACTION OF PLATELETS WITH ALTERED ENDOTHELIAL CELLS

Endothelial cell membranes contain members of several major classes of adhesion receptors, such as integrins, cadherins, cell adhesion molecules (CAMs) of the immunoglobulin superfamily, and selectins. With the exception of the cadherins, these receptors are also present on platelet membranes (13–15). The levels of expression of these receptors may vary with cell activation or stimulation. Appropriate ligands are present on the membranes of vascular cells and on subendothelial structures, or may localize onto matrix components because of specific binding events. The precise roles played by different types of adhesion molecules in mediating platelet–endothelial cell interactions remain to be elucidated. Following thrombin stimulation, a number of mechanisms potentially involved in the process are evoked, but none has been proven unequivocally to be relevant *in vivo*. For example, soluble fibrinogen could serve as a bridge between activated $\alpha_{IIb}\beta_3$ on platelets and endothelial ICAM-1, whose level of expression is regulated by endothelial cell agonists. An equivalent pathway has been demonstrated to support adhesion of leukocytes to the endothelium by fibrinogen binding to leukocyte integrin $\alpha_M\beta_2$ (16). Endothelial cells themselves have a receptor for fibrinogen/fibrin, $\alpha_V\beta_3$, that could contribute to the initial localization of this adhesive substrate at injury sites, thereby mediating platelet attachment through $\alpha_{IIb}\beta_3$ (17). The expression of P selectin on activated endothelial cells appears to support a transient interaction (rolling) of platelets (18) in a manner reminiscent of that typically described for leukocytes. Platelets, like leukocytes, express known P selectin ligands, and this pathway may be important to localize platelets at sites of endothelial damage, with subsequent establishment of permanent adhesion if appropriate conditions develop. A similar mechanism can also be supported by VWF expressed on the surface of stimulated endothelial cells, as shown in the veins of mice by intravital microscopy (19).

# EXTRACELLULAR SUBENDOTHELIAL MOLECULES THAT INTERACT WITH PLATELETS

The main trigger of platelet thrombus formation after traumatic vascular injury is the exposure of extracellular matrix components of the vessel wall and surrounding tissues to flowing blood; these components are normally not in contact with the flowing blood. Moreover, circulating plasma proteins may become immobilized at sites of injury by interacting with subendothelial components, thereby adding to the diversity of thrombogenic substrates that are recognized by specific platelet receptors. The major basement membrane constituents in contact with the abluminal surface of endothelial cells, which are likely to be exposed to blood upon minimal disruption of vascular integrity, are proteoglycans (20), collagen type IV (21), nidogen (entactin) (22), laminin (23), and fibulin (24). Proteoglycans are generally considered as not being directly relevant in mediating adhesion, although they may be important in modulating platelet reactivity as well as coagulation reactions. Collagen type IV, like most other types (25), can initiate platelet interactions but may be less thrombogenic than the collagens found in deeper layers of the vessel wall. Laminins (23), a family of related glycoproteins (GPs) that includes merosin, are the major components of the subendothelial matrix. The GPs are associated with collagen type IV in a tight supramolecular assembly through the action of nidogen (entactin) and play a key role in controlling cell attachment and motility in all tissues. Platelets may adhere to laminin both under static conditions and under flow (26,27), but it is unclear whether the interaction is of pathophysiologic significance with regard to hemostasis and thrombosis. Fibulins (24,28) have attracted attention owing to their ability to assemble with fibronectin (29) and fibrinogen (30,31), possibly modulating the thrombogenic activity of these substrates. Certain forms of fibulin also circulate in

blood and may become localized at sites of vascular injury, potentially influencing platelet–platelet interactions in which fibrinogen is implicated.

Numerous other matrix components may become exposed to platelets when deeper injuries of the vessel wall occur, the most notable for thrombogenic potential being fibronectins, thrombospondins, fibrillar collagens type I and III, collagen type VI, and VWF. In contrast, elastin (32), a major component of the vessel wall, is nonreactive to platelets. Fibrinogen/fibrin and vitronectin are not directly synthesized by endothelial cells or other cells in the vascular wall. Both components, however, must be considered as potentially relevant substrates for the initiation of thrombogenesis because they become rapidly immobilized at sites of injury through specific interactions with the extracellular matrix. Vitronectin has been implicated in platelet function because of its ability to bind to $\beta_3$ integrins, in particular, to $\alpha_{IIb}\beta_3$ on platelets, and to support aggregation in experimental settings (33). There is no definitive evidence, however, that this molecule has a role in promoting platelet adhesion in the presence of all other plasma proteins. Indeed, exposure of whole blood to surfaces coated with vitronectin (or fibronectin) failed to result in platelet adhesion under conditions that prompted rapid attachment to immobilized fibrinogen (34). It should also be noted that obliteration of the vitronectin gene function in mice has no apparent consequences on hemostasis (35). A possible role for vitronectin in vascular disease processes involving platelet adhesion and aggregation is still being investigated.

Fibronectins (36) are modular macromolecules found in the vessel wall and in circulating blood. Evidence indicates that different splice variants have distinct functions (37). Studies performed under both static and flow conditions have demonstrated that platelets attach to and spread onto fibronectin, presumably through the $\alpha_5\beta_1$ receptor as well as through $\alpha_{IIb}\beta_3$ (38), although other experiments with whole blood have yielded conflicting results (34). Fibronectin contains distinct adhesive domains; the domain relevant for platelet interactions is the RGD sequence in the tenth type III repeat. Plasma fibronectin differs in several respects from the forms found in extracellular matrices and in cells, including platelet $\alpha$-granules (39), but all the forms contain the RGD sequence. Nonetheless, fibronectin fibrils in the matrix and fibronectin in the plasma may differ in their ability to interact with platelets. Optimal platelet adhesion to fibronectin may involve VWF and its GP Ib$\alpha$ receptor (40), a possible example of synergistic interaction between different adhesive substrates in the initiation of thrombus formation.

Thrombospondins are a group of related GPs present in extracellular matrices and involved in cell migration and attachment (41,42). Of the five known members of this family, thrombospondin-1 (TSP-1) and thrombospondin-2 (TSP-2) are homologous, disulfide-linked homotrimeric molecules composed of chains of approximately 145 kD with modular structure. In contrast, thrombospondin-3, thrombospondin-4, and thrombospondin-5 are homopentamers of smaller chains that lack many of the domains present in TSP-1 and TSP-2 subunits. The latter two subunits have been defined as *matricellular proteins* (42) to indicate their intimate relation with constitutive extracellular matrix components as well as their important association with the cell surface. Although matricellular proteins are not considered to be necessary structural elements in the extracellular matrix, deficiency of TSP-2 in mice has been found to result in disordered collagen fibrillogenesis (43). TSP-1 was initially described as a platelet $\alpha$-granule protein released upon activation, whereas TSP-2 is not present in platelets (44). TSP-1 is present in microfibrillar structures and is found in the subendothelial matrix where it interacts with several other constituents such as collagen; TSP-1 also binds proteins from blood, including VWF. TSP-1 has been implicated with the regulation of the size of the VWF multimer (45) and has been shown to mediate platelet adhesion at high shear rates (46). TSP-2, on the other hand, appears to be relevant for platelet and megakaryocyte function because mice with a targeted disruption of the corresponding gene exhibit a prolonged bleeding time from tail wounds and abnormal platelet formation in the bone marrow (43,47).

The role played by collagens in platelet adhesion and activation has been recognized for many years (48,49). Collagen types I, III, and VI have been extensively studied in experimental conditions because they are known to be present in different layers of the vessel wall—type III and VI being closer to the lumen, that is, more superficial than type I—and their thrombogenic potential has been established. Nevertheless, most, if not all, collagen types in native conditions may be capable of interacting with platelets (25).

The role of VWF in mediating platelet adhesive functions is well established, and all the domains responsible for known biologic activities have been identified (50). This large, polymeric molecule occupies an interesting position among adhesive substrates, being, at the same time, an insoluble subendothelial matrix component, a circulating plasma protein, and a platelet $\alpha$-granule protein that is released after activation. The structure of VWF in different compartments of the body differs with regard to the degree of polymerization, and multimers in the subendothelium (51) and in platelets (52) are larger than those in blood. The largest molecules are found "unusually" in the circulation, essentially only after acute release from endothelial cells (53) or in pathologic conditions (54). The presence of large molecules is likely to reflect an active mechanism that normally controls the size of VWF molecules in the circulation through regulated proteolysis (55,56). The metalloproteinase that cleaves VWF at the $Tyr^{842}$–$Met^{843}$ bond (57) has been identified as ADAMTS13 [A Disintegrinlike And Metalloprotease domain (reprolysin-type) with ThromboSpondin-type I motifs] (58,59), and the structure of the corresponding gene has been fully characterized (60,61). Because the prothrombotic activity of multimers is likely to be directly related to the degree of polymerization, the regulation of VWF size may serve to prevent interactions with platelets. There is evidence that VWF of a different anatomic origin participates in hemostatic processes; however, the circulating pool is probably the most important in initiating platelet adhesion. The reason for the importance of the circulating pool is that the distribution of subendothelial VWF is not homogeneous, with apparent lack of the protein in many vessels where platelet function is important for hemostasis (62). Moreover, platelet VWF is not released until after activation and may not be immediately available at the site of injury to promote adhesion, although its contribution to later phases of thrombus formation has been convincingly demonstrated (63). Plasma VWF is well suited to mediate early adhesion because it binds rapidly and tightly to collagen—and possibly to other matrix structures such as proteoglycans—whenever blood is exposed to the injured tissues. Differential reconstitution of VWF in body compartments of pigs with severe von Willebrand disease provides good support for these concepts (63). The distinctive mechanisms through which VWF mediates platelet adhesion and aggregation in flowing blood will be discussed in detail in subsequent text.

# PLATELET THROMBUS FORMATION IN FLOWING BLOOD

The complex events that determine the occurrence of a normal hemostatic response—including interactions that involve cells, the vessel wall, and molecules in solution—are influenced by

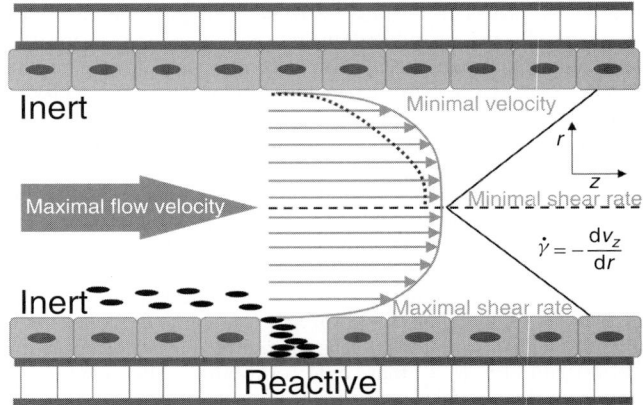

## Platelets respond to alterations in the vascular wall

$$\dot\gamma = -\frac{dv_z}{dr}$$

FIGURE 47-2. Normal endothelial cells are nonreactive to platelets, but exposed subendothelial structures induce rapid platelet adhesion. Subsequent thrombus growth is dependent on platelet–platelet interactions (aggregation). In either case, platelets are recruited from flowing blood and immobilized at a surface, first represented by matrix components and then by ligands bound to activated, adherent platelets. Blood flow in a cylindrical vessel can be visualized as a series of fluid layers (laminae) moving at different velocities. The laminae near the center of the vessel have greater velocity than those near the wall (depicted schematically by arrows of different lengths). The corresponding velocity profile (solid line) is more blunted than the parabolic profile expected with a homogeneous suspension (dotted line) because of cell depletion in the boundary layer near the wall. The shear rate is the rate of change of velocity with respect to the distance measured perpendicularly to the direction of flow. The negative sign indicates that the gradient is defined from the center (where velocity is maximal) to the wall (where velocity is minimal). (From Ruggeri ZM, Saldivar E. Platelets, hemostasis and thrombosis. In: Ruggeri ZM, ed. Von Willebrand factor and the mechanisms of platelet function. Berlin: Springer, 1998:1–32, with permission.)

the flow of blood. The velocity of blood near the wall is less than that at the center of the vessel, and this difference creates a shearing effect between adjacent layers of fluid (see Fig. 47-2). Therefore, "shear" is the consequence of the relative parallel motion between adjacent fluid "laminae" and is greatest at the luminal surface, decreasing progressively toward the center of the vessel. The shear rate, a difference in flow velocity as a function of distance from the wall, is expressed in cm/second per cm or the equivalent inverse seconds ($s^{-1}$). Fluid shear stress is force per unit area and is expressed in Pascal (Pa), equivalent to one Newton per $m^2$ (N per $m^2$), or in dynes per $cm^2$ (1 Pa = 10 dynes per $cm^2$). The shear rate is directly proportional to the shear stress and is inversely proportional to the fluid viscosity. In blood, therefore, where viscosity is approximately 0.004 Pa · second (or 0.04 dynes per $cm^2$ · second), a shear stress of 1 dyne per $cm^2$ corresponds to a shear rate of 25 $s^{-1}$. The force opposing stable adhesion and aggregation of platelets is greater with increasing shear rate. Consequently, it can be concluded that shear-dependent phenomena are of particular relevance in those regions of the vasculature where shear forces are greater, that is, in arteries, where the shear forces are more than those in veins, and, particularly, in arterioles. The highest wall shear rate in the normal circulation occurs in small arterioles of diameter 10 to 50 $\mu$m (see Fig. 47-3), where levels have been estimated to vary between 500 and 5,000 $s^{-1}$ (64). In vessels of this caliber, blood is assumed to behave as a Newtonian fluid with an essentially steady laminar flow that is not influenced by the cardiac cycle. Wall shear rates of 3,000 to 10,000 $s^{-1}$ have been measured at the top of

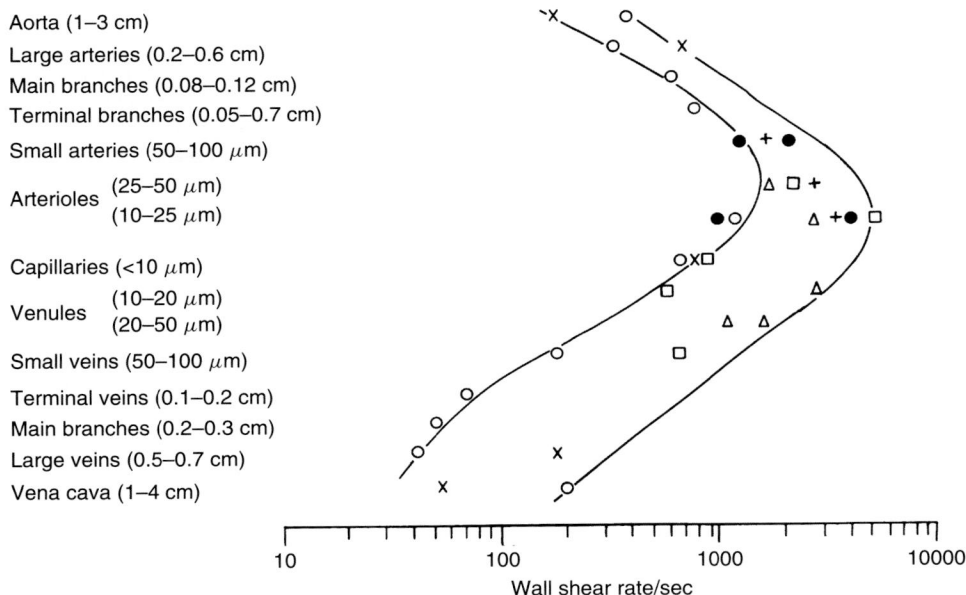

Aorta (1–3 cm)
Large arteries (0.2–0.6 cm)
Main branches (0.08–0.12 cm)
Terminal branches (0.05–0.7 cm)
Small arteries (50–100 µm)
Arterioles (25–50 µm)
(10–25 µm)
Capillaries (<10 µm)
Venules (10–20 µm)
(20–50 µm)
Small veins (50–100 µm)
Terminal veins (0.1–0.2 cm)
Main branches (0.2–0.3 cm)
Large veins (0.5–0.7 cm)
Vena cava (1–4 cm)

Wall shear rate/sec

**FIGURE 47-3.** Wall shear rates (γ) in different parts of the vasculature. Rates were calculated from values of average blood velocity and vessel diameter, assuming that fully established Newtonian flow existed in the vessels. The results are from different studies in humans (X) and dogs (O) (69); cats (+) and other species (●) (70); rabbit (△) (71) ; and cat (□) (72). [From Whitmore RL. *Rheology of the circulation*, 1st ed. Oxford: Pergamon Press Ltd, 1968; Fronek K, Zweifach W. Microvascular blood flow in cat tenuissimus muscle. *Microvasc Res* 1977;14:181–189; Schmid-Schoenbein GW, Zweifach BW. RBC velocity profiles in arterioles and venules of the rabbit omentum. *Microvasc Res* 1975;10(153):164; Lipowsky HH, Zweifach BW. Methods for the simultaneous measurement of pressure differentials and flow in single unbranched vessels of the microcirculation for rheological studies. *Microvasc Res* 1977;14:345–361, with permission.]

plaques causing 50% occlusion of coronary arteries (65), a degree of stenosis of moderate clinical significance (66,67). Higher shear rates develop with more severe occlusion; therefore, shear stress is of greater pathogenic relevance in conditions predisposing to acute arterial occlusion than it is in the course of normal hemostasis.

# INITIAL PLATELET ATTACHMENT TO THROMBOGENIC SURFACES

Stable platelet attachment to a reactive surface is essential to establish thrombus formation. Distinct ligand–receptor interactions are required to initiate thrombogenesis at sites of vascular injury, depending on the velocity of flowing blood; beyond a limiting shear rate—approximately 1,000 s$^{-1}$ such a function is absolutely dependent on VWF and its GP Ibα receptor. The structural features that support the unique adhesive properties of VWF have been elucidated, with the resolution of the atomic structures of the isolated A1 domain, both with native sequence (73,74) and with a gain of function mutation (75), and of the complex between VWF-A1 and the amino-terminal domain of GP Ibα (76,77). The interaction between these two molecules is characterized by a fast rate of bond formation and allows tethering of platelets to thrombogenic surfaces that present immobilized VWF even when the velocity of flowing blood relative to the vessel wall is elevated. However, the VWF–GP Ibα interaction is also characterized by a fast dissociation rate and cannot support irreversible adhesion (78), so that platelets tethered in such a manner to the vessel wall move constantly in the direction of flow (see Fig. 47-4). The translocation velocity, nonetheless, is

1/30th second (1 frame)    10 seconds (30 frames superimposed)

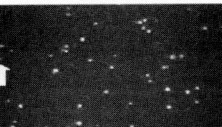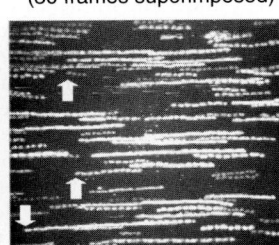

**FIGURE 47-4.** Time-lapse analysis of platelet movement on immobilized von Willebrand factor (VWF). Blood containing the thrombin inhibitor D-phenylalanyl-L-prolyl-L-arginine chloromethyl ketone dihydrochloride (PPACK; 40 µM final concentration) as anticoagulant as well as prostaglandin E$_1$ that inhibit platelet activation was perfused through a parallel plate flow chamber at 37°C. The bottom surface of the chamber exposed to blood was coated with purified VWF, and the wall shear rate during perfusion was 1,500 s$^{-1}$. Platelets were also treated with 100 µg per mL of the monoclonal antibody LJ-CP8 F(ab')$_2$ to block α$_{IIb}$β$_3$ receptor function. Platelets were visualized by epifluorescence videomicroscopy during perfusion using mepacrine, and images were recorded in real time (30 frames per second). The figure on the left is a single frame from the videotape recording, showing a snapshot of individual platelets interacting with the VWF-coated surface. The figure on the right shows the superimposition of 30 consecutive frames captured from the real-time recording at a sampling rate of 3 frames per second. The occurrence of platelet translocation on VWF is rendered by the streaking effect produced by moving platelets. (From Savage B, Saldivar E, Ruggeri ZM. Initiation of platelet adhesion by arrest onto fibrinogen or translocation on von Willebrand factor. *Cell* 1996;84:289–297, with permission.)

typically less than 2% of the free flow velocity of noninteracting platelets at the same distance from the luminal surface, and this slow motion allows additional bond formation and activation that eventually lead to the arrest of individual platelets and thrombus formation.

The transition from initial rolling to stable adhesion requires the intervention of other receptors and depends on the nature of the substrates onto which immobilized VWF is exposed to blood. The simplest condition is observed with purified VWF. In this case, platelet activation changes the recognition specificity of $\alpha_{IIb}\beta_3$ such that the latter acquires the ability to interact with the Arg-Gly-Asp (RGD) sequence at residues 1,744 to 1,747 in the C1 domain of the mature VWF subunit (79,80). Before activation, instead, $\alpha_{IIb}\beta_3$ can only interact with immobilized fibrinogen or fibrin (81). The characteristics of the initial platelet attachment to fibrinogen/fibrin highlight the biomechanical properties of the bonds mediated by $\alpha_{IIb}\beta_3$. Platelet adhesion to immobilized fibrinogen occurs promptly at relatively low but not high wall shear rates (78). Maximal surface coverage by single adherent platelets is typically observed between 50 and 500 s$^{-1}$, with progressive decrease observed at increasing shear rates and loss of considerable adhesion observed between 1,500 and 2,000 s$^{-1}$. The interaction of flowing platelets with immobilized fibrinogen, unlike that with immobilized VWF, is instantaneously irreversible (78). This interaction implies coupling between initial adhesion and signaling pathways that is necessary to induce and control the morphologic and biochemical responses that lead to spreading—the hallmark of firmly adherent platelets. The limiting factor responsible for the inability of fibrinogen/fibrin to support platelet adhesion at higher shear rates is likely to be a relatively slow rate of bond formation, preventing initiation of adhesion when the platelet–surface contact time is reduced as a consequence of high flow velocity.

The paradigm of platelet interaction with immobilized VWF and fibrinogen shows how distinct receptor–ligand pairs possess unique biomechanical properties that complement each other and are functionally integrated during thrombus growth under the influence of shear forces. One relevant example of this concept is provided by collagen type I fibrils that are by themselves capable of mediating platelet adhesion (25) and inducing activation and aggregation (82–84). At the wall shear rate of 1,500 s$^{-1}$, representative of flow conditions in vessels such as arterioles where platelets are essential for hemostasis (64), attachment to collagen fibrils occurs only if VWF and GP Ib$\alpha$ are functionally active (85) (see Fig. 47-5). The underlying mechanism depends on a specific interaction mediated by the A3 domain that leads to immobilization of plasma VWF onto the collagen fibrils. The atomic structure of VWF-A3 has been solved (86,87), and the specific site for collagen binding has been modeled on the basis of the structure of homologous receptors (88). The tethering of platelets to collagen-bound VWF occurs through an interaction of GP Ib$\alpha$, with the A1 domain exhibiting characteristics essentially identical to those observed with the purified protein (78,85). In contrast, at the lower shear rate of 500 s$^{-1}$, the binding of VWF is not required for inducing thrombogenesis (Fig. 47-5), an indication that platelet attachment to the surface can be mediated by the direct interaction with collagen of specific receptors, namely, $\alpha_2\beta_1$ and GP VI (49,89,90).

The nature of the substrate onto which the initial tethering mediated by VWF occurs at high shear rates influences the process that leads to irreversible adhesion by providing the possibility of different bonds capable of supporting stable attachment. Regardless of whether VWF is immobilized onto glass or adsorbed onto collagen, platelets exhibit rolling motion at low velocities but do not exhibit irreversible attachment when integrin function is blocked (see Fig. 47-6A). With normal platelets, in contrast, collagen type I fibrils exposed to blood flowing at 1,500 s$^{-1}$ become rapidly covered with firmly adherent platelets, and it is apparent that both $\alpha_{IIb}\beta_3$ and $\alpha_2\beta_1$ are involved in the transition from initial tethering to irreversible platelet adhesion. In fact, when $\alpha_{IIb}\beta_3$ function is blocked selectively, approximately 60% of first contact events still result in prolonged adhesion, with no translocation from the initial point of tethering. However, when $\alpha_{IIb}\beta_3$ and $\alpha_2\beta_1$ are blocked concurrently, approximately 90% of the platelets becoming tethered to the surface move within 4 seconds to a position different from the point of first contact. Interestingly, in this case, the velocity of rolling, approximately 5.5 $\mu$m per second (see Fig. 47-6B), is similar to that of platelets interacting with VWF immobilized onto glass (78). This observation indicates that the affinity of VWF for GP Ib$\alpha$ is regulated by intrinsic properties of the immobilized A1 domain and not by conformational changes specifically induced upon binding to collagen. On substrates that contain multiple potential sites of adhesion, such as the extracellular matrix secreted by endothelial cells, global inhibition of integrin function results in platelet tethering and rolling, mediated by VWF and GP Ib$\alpha$ but not in any stable attachment at high shear rates (85). In such a situation, $\alpha_{IIb}\beta_3$ and $\alpha_2\beta_1$ still provide a major contribution to firm adhesion following initial tethering, but additional anchorage to the surface can be provided by other integrin receptors, for example, $\alpha_5\beta_1$ interacting presumably with fibronectin (85). It is apparent, therefore, that the general mechanism responsible for initiating platelet thrombus formation in rapidly flowing blood always involves VWF and GP Ib$\alpha$ as the first tethering interaction, with the subsequent contribution of multiple stabilizing bonds mediated by diverse receptors.

An additional mechanism to explain the contribution of soluble plasma VWF to the process of platelet adhesion has been unveiled more recently (91). A process of self-association occurs at the interface between soluble and surface-bound VWF, such that the first layer of VWF multimers bound to matrix collagen supports the transient adsorption of additional multimers from plasma to which platelets can readily attach. This mechanism was demonstrated by binding a mutant VWF devoid of domain A1 to collagen, the mutant VWF thereby being unable to promote platelet adhesion and showing that GP Ib$\alpha$–mediated tethering was restored by the presence of soluble VWF in plasma (see Fig. 47-7). The adsorption of soluble VWF to immobilized VWF is a reversible process because the number of platelets–surface contacts on immobilized $\Delta$A1-VWF is rapidly reduced when the perfusing blood is replaced with a plasma-free blood suspension (91). Plasma VWF, therefore, has a dual role in mediating platelet adhesion under flow. One role involves the A3 domain through which tight binding to collagen is established, and the other role is a reversible self-association with immobilized VWF that can modulate and reinforce the adhesive properties of the latter. These findings demonstrate that a direct linkage between VWF and a surface such as collagen is not an absolute requisite for the expression of GP Ib$\alpha$ binding function.

# VON WILLEBRAND FACTOR–MEDIATED SIGNALING THROUGH GLYCOPROTEIN Ib$\alpha$ AND PLATELET ACTIVATION

The binding of the VWF A1 domain to GP Ib$\alpha$ elicits signals—including elevation of levels of cytosolic $Ca^{2+}$, activation of protein kinase C and tyrosine kinases—that contribute to platelet activation. These signals can be detected under static conditions (92–95), but may be particularly relevant for the activation of platelets exposed to high shear stress (96,97).

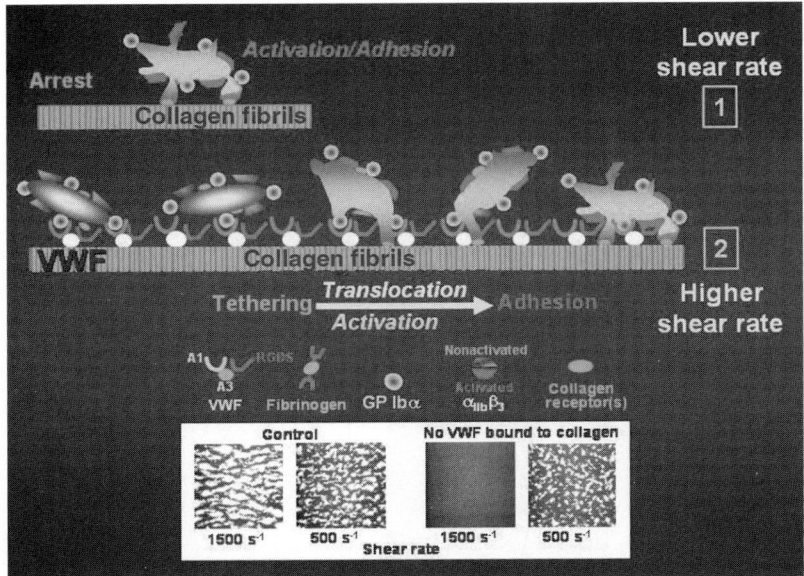

**A**

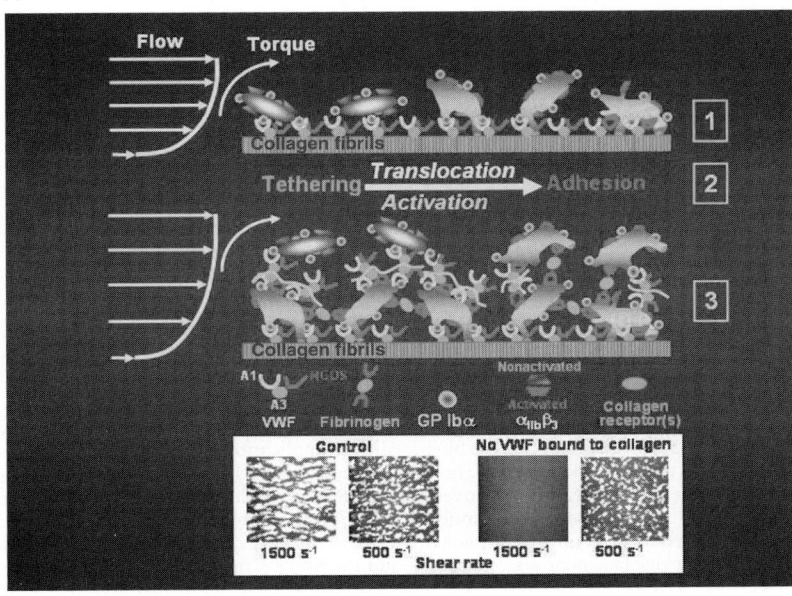

**B**

**FIGURE 47-5.** Schematic representation of the distinct biomechanical properties of bonds supporting platelet adhesion to collagen type I fibrils. *1*, lower shear rate. Initial attachment and subsequent irreversible adhesion are rapidly mediated by collagen receptors. The binding of von Willebrand factor (VWF) to collagen is not required to support thrombus formation, as shown in the **bottom panel** (VWF binding to collagen blocked by an antibody directed against VWF domain A3). *2*, higher shear rate. The first contact between platelets and the substrate is mediated by VWF bound to collagen. The VWFA1–GP Ibα bond forms rapidly and has high resistance to tensile stress (78) but a limited half-life; in the absence of other bonds, platelets detach at the tailing edge where tension is greatest and move forward with a rotational movement (rolling) because of the torque imposed by the flowing fluid. New VWFA1–GP Ibα bonds form as different regions of the membrane of rolling platelets come close to the surface; therefore platelets remain in contact with the substrate for extended periods of time while translocating at low velocity. In normal conditions, however, the initial tethering to VWF is rapidly followed by binding to collagen through specific receptors (namely, GP VI and $\alpha_2\beta_1$), and by firm adhesion, activation, and additional stable bonds being mediated by $\alpha_{IIb}\beta_3$. Note that thrombus formation on collagen exposed to a high shear rate is blocked if the interaction with VWF cannot take place (see **bottom panel**), demonstrating the role of the initial rapid tethering in permitting subsequent bonds (see Color Fig. 47-5).

Two distinct elevations of intracytoplasmic levels of $Ca^{2+}$ have been documented in association with platelet GP Ibα–mediated adhesion to immobilized VWF (97). A first rise in $[Ca^{2+}]_i$, designated an $\alpha/\beta$ peak, occurs during the initial contacts that are still potentially reversible and always precedes stable platelet attachment. Type $\alpha/\beta$ peaks involve $Ca^{2+}$ release from intracellular stores. A second $Ca^{2+}$ signal, designated a $\gamma$ peak, occurs in platelets that have established firm adhesion through the integrin $\alpha_{IIb}\beta_3$ and appears to be required for subsequent aggregation. Type $\gamma$ peaks involve a transmembrane $Ca^{2+}$ flux. Therefore, the initial GP Ibα interaction with the VWF A1 domain leads to a first level of $\alpha_{IIb}\beta_3$ activation sufficient for stable platelet adhesion to immobilized VWF but not for binding soluble VWF or fibrinogen (required for aggregation). Progression to thrombus formation requires further $\alpha_{IIb}\beta_3$ activation that is contingent on signal amplification associated with type $\gamma$ $[Ca^{2+}]_i$ peaks (see Fig. 47-8). Inhibition of PI 3-K activity or removal of ADP with apyrase blocks $\gamma$ peaks and prevents platelet aggregation (97–99).

Although apyrase has no effect on the frequency or amplitude of $\alpha/\beta$ peaks (97), the use of specific inhibitors highlights an important role of the $P2Y_1$ ADP receptor in reinforcing the initial signal induced by GP Ibα binding to VWF A1. Therefore, the latter interaction causes ADP release that acts rapidly through $P2Y_1$ in enhancing $Ca^{2+}$ release from intracellular stores, such that enzymatic degradation of ADP by apyrase is not sufficiently rapid to block this activity (100). In contrast, a subsequent effect of ADP required for platelet aggregation and mediated by a different receptor, $P2Y_{12}$, can also be blocked efficiently by apyrase (100).

Signaling dependent on the VWF A1 domain is thought to involve the cross-linking (receptor clustering) of GP Ibα subunits by multivalent VWF (94). A monomeric proteolytic fragment of VWF containing a single A1 domain binds to GP Ibα and inhibits binding of native VWF but does not induce cytoskeletal rearrangement and activation of $\alpha_{IIb}\beta_3$ (101–103). The observation that a subpopulation of platelet GP Ib/IX/V is associated with FcRγ chain, which contains an ITAM

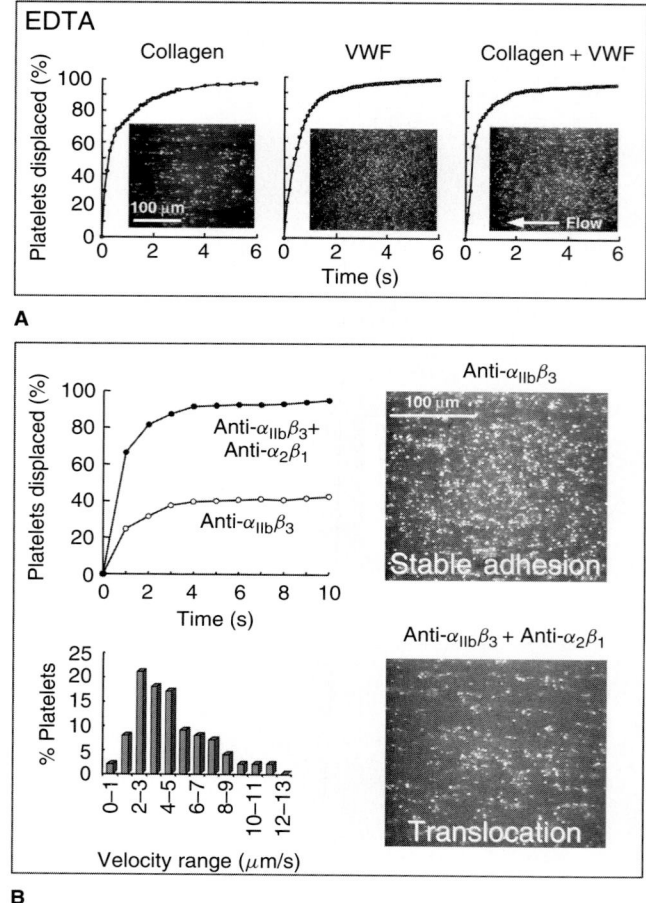

**FIGURE 47-6.** Integrins $\alpha_2\beta_1$ and $\alpha_{IIb}\beta_3$ contribute to stabilize the adhesion of platelets initially tethered to collagen-bound von Willebrand factor (VWF). **A:** Blood containing 5 mM ethylenediamine tetraacetic acid (EDTA) in order to inhibit integrin function was perfused at the wall shear rate of 1,500 s$^{-1}$ over a surface coated with fibrillar type I collagen (**left panel**), purified VWF (**middle panel**), or collagen preincubated with purified VWF before the onset of blood flow (**right panel**). After 2 minutes of perfusion, consecutive images were captured from videotapes and analyzed for platelet motion. A single-frame image, corresponding to an area of 65,536 $\mu$m$^2$, is shown for each condition tested. To estimate motion, the series of images was digitized at a sampling rate of 6 frames per second. The images were binarized after application of a threshold to distinguish platelets from the background. Time was calculated by referring to the frame number. The first two consecutive frames in a series were superimposed using the logical AND function, so that the resulting image represented only the overlapping areas of single platelets at two different times. The new image was then superimposed to the next frame, and the process was continued until the overlapping area was equal to zero. When this occurred, a platelet had moved by a distance greater than its diameter; if this did not occur, a platelet was considered firmly attached during the period of observation. The time for each individual platelet displacement was computed and the process repeated until either all the platelets in the microscopic field had moved, or for a preselected time interval, whichever occurred first. The percentage of platelets displaced from their initial position was calculated as a function of time relative to the total number of platelets attached to the surface in the first image analyzed. Note that greater than 90% of all platelets moved on the surface within 3 seconds of observation, indicative of predominantly transient attachment with surface translocation. In spite of the movement, most of the platelets remained persistently tethered to the surface. **B:** Perfusion over collagen-coated surfaces of blood containing 80 $\mu$M PPACK as anticoagulant and the function-blocking monoclonal antibodies of indicated specificity. The stability of platelet adhesion was evaluated after 2 minutes of perfusion. Note that approximately 90% of all platelets (indicated as platelets displaced) moved on the surface within 3 seconds of observation when $\alpha_{IIb}\beta_3$ and $\alpha_2\beta_1$ were inhibited concurrently, as opposed to greater than 60% of the platelets remaining stationary (40% displaced) after selective inhibition of $\alpha_{IIb}\beta_3$. The frequency distribution of the average velocity of individual platelets with blocked $\alpha_{IIb}\beta_3$ and $\alpha_2\beta_1$ moving on the surface is also shown. The two single-frame images on the right, each representing an area of 65,536 $\mu$m$^2$, depict surface coverage after perfusing for 2 minutes platelets with selective inhibition of $\alpha_{IIb}\beta_3$ (**top**) or combined inhibition of $\alpha_{IIb}\beta_3$ and $\alpha_2\beta_1$. (From Savage B, Almus-Jacobs F, Ruggeri ZM. Specific synergy of multiple substrate-receptor interactions in platelet thrombus formation under flow. *Cell* 1998;94:657–666, with permission.)

(immuno-receptor tyrosine-based activation motif) module (104–106), lends support to the cross-linking mechanism of signaling. FcR$\gamma$ chain and GP Ib$\alpha$ are proximal to within 10 nm of each other in the platelet membrane (107). Nevertheless, there is also evidence that VWF A1 domain–induced signaling through GP Ib$\alpha$ can activate $\alpha_{IIb}\beta_3$ in a manner that is independent of other receptors (95). In particular, mouse platelets expressing human GP Ib$\alpha$ but lacking the FcR$\gamma$ chain adhere to a dimeric VWF A1 domain and undergo Ca$^{2+}$ oscillations in a manner that is qualitatively similar, although slightly

impaired, to that seen with mouse platelets expressing both receptors. Therefore, the FcR$\gamma$ chain contributes to maximal elevations in Ca$^{2+}$ levels but is not absolutely required for the initiation of Ca$^{2+}$ responses.

The cytoplasmic region of GP Ib$\alpha$ is associated with actin-binding protein and 14-3-3$\zeta$ (108–110), which provide potential links to several signaling molecules including phosphatidylinositol 3-kinase (PI 3-K), focal adhesion kinase, Src-related tyrosine kinases (i.e., *Syk*, *Src*, *Fyn Lyn*, and *Yes*), GTPase-activating protein, and tyrosine phosphatases (i.e., PTP-1B and SHPTP10)

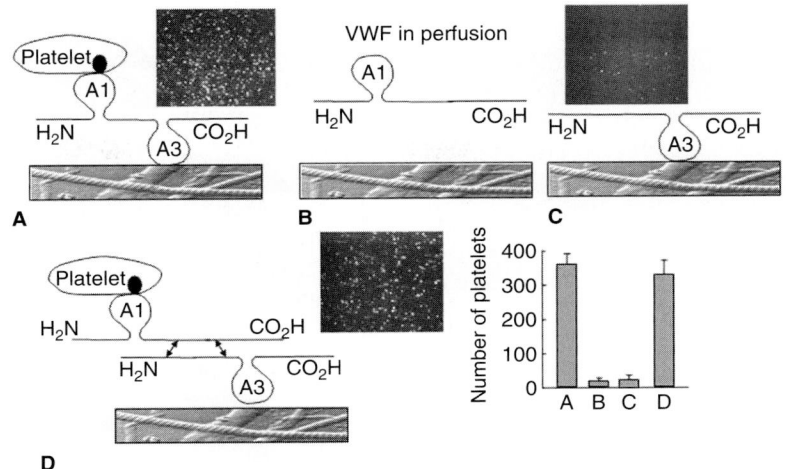

**FIGURE 47-7.** Role of soluble von Willebrand factor (VWF) A1 domain in mediating platelet interaction with surface-bound VWF. A washed blood cells suspension devoid of plasma proteins and containing ethylenediamine tetraacetic acid (EDTA) (to block integrin function in adhesion and aggregation) and prostaglandin $E_1$ (to block platelet activation) was perfused over immobilized collagen type I fibrils at the wall shear rate of 1,500 s$^{-1}$. **A:** Control experiment with normal multimeric VWF added to the cell suspension. The A3 domain mediates VWF binding to collagen, and the A1 domain interacts with platelet glycoprotein (GP) Ibα; tethered platelets are seen rolling on the surface, which is represented by an electron micrograph of collagen fibrils. **B:** Experiments performed after adding to the cell suspension recombinant VWF devoid of the A3 domain (ΔA3-VWF), which cannot bind to collagen; or (**C**) recombinant VWF devoid of the A1 domain (ΔA1-VWF), which binds to collagen but cannot interact with platelet GP Ibα. In either case, no platelets are seen tethered to the surface. **D:** The collagen fibrils were precoated with ΔA1-VWF multimers, which cannot initiate platelet tethering, and then exposed to the blood cell suspension containing ΔA3-VWF. Although the latter cannot bind directly to collagen (see **B**), it could compensate for the lack of A1 domain in the surface-bound VWF and restore platelet tethering. The association of VWF multimers with one another can explain this result; the two-sided arrows between multimers indicate that the association is reversible. The schemes presented with the images depict the soluble and immobilized VWF used in the experiments with respect to A1 and A3 domain presence and function. The images are single frames from a real-time recording representing an area of 65,536 μm$^2$. The bar graph shows the number of platelets tethered to the surface under the different experimental conditions described in preceding text (mean ± SEM of two separate experiments). (From Savage B, Sixma JJ, Ruggeri ZM. Functional self-association of von Willebrand factor during platelet adhesion under flow. *Proc Natl Acad Sci U S A* 2002;99:425–430, with permission.)

(111). Several studies indicate that 14-3-3ζ plays a crucial role in regulating signaling through GP Ib/IX/V, leading to the activation of $\alpha_{IIb}\beta_3$ (112–114). Chinese hamster ovary (CHO) cells coexpresssing GP Ib/IX and $\alpha_{IIb}\beta_3$ spread on a VWF-coated surface and bind fibrinogen in an $\alpha_{IIb}\beta_3$ activation-dependent manner (112). Both PI 3-K and protein kinase C play important roles in this process because their inhibition blocks cell spreading (112). Moreover, deletion of the 18 amino acids in the C-terminal of GP Ibα, containing the binding site for 14-3-3ζ, prevents cell spreading and fibrinogen binding to $\alpha_{IIb}\beta_3$. PI 3-K forms a constitutive complex with both GP Ib/IX/V and 14-3-3ζ in resting platelets (113) and may therefore play a key role in 14-3-3ζ signaling. Although dissociation of 14-3-3ζ from the GP Ib/IX/V complex is seen following platelet activation (113,114), it is unclear whether this is a direct effect of platelet activation, or a process that precedes activation.

# PLATELET ACTIVATION AND THROMBUS PROPAGATION UNDER FLOW

The response of platelets to vascular injury involves a series of coordinated reactions initiated by tethering to appropriate substrates linked to activation processes that promote the binding of soluble adhesive proteins and the recruitment of additional platelets. The time course of this sequence of events is influenced by the composition of the reactive surface exposed to flowing blood. For example, in experimental conditions where only purified VWF is the substrate and exogenous agonists are either not present or inhibited, demonstrable consequences of activation (i.e., thrombus formation) are typically seen only

after several minutes and only at high shear rates (78). In the setting of vascular lesions, however, subendothelial components, such as collagen, and soluble platelet agonists, such as ADP, epinephrine, and α-thrombin, may greatly enhance the efficiency of the hemostatic response by contributing synergistically to $\alpha_{IIb}\beta_3$ activation. It is apparent that soluble agonists may influence thrombus formation at sites of injury, but, in the early stages of the process, a relevant role is likely to be played by activation signals originating from engagement of adhesion receptors. Indeed, irreversible platelet adhesion to matrices containing collagen type I is essentially instantaneous even at the highest levels of shear stress, and thrombus formation ensues within seconds (85). Collagens, particularly type I, III, and VI, function in synergism with VWF to support platelet adhesion and aggregation in areas of the circulation with high velocity flow, but collagens alone are sufficient for efficient thrombus formation at lower shear rates (85). Domain A3 of VWF has a key role in mediating binding to collagen (115), but domain A1 may also be involved in the interaction (116–118), as shown particularly for binding to collagen type VI under flow conditions (119).

After platelet adhesion and activation onto a vascular lesion have taken place, thrombus growth proceeds through local accumulation of additional platelets in a process of homotypic aggregation. During this phase, activated adherent platelets bind soluble adhesive proteins, mainly fibrinogen, and VWF, that upon immobilization onto the cellular membrane become substrates for the adhesion of circulating platelets in successive layers (85). Activation of the newly recruited platelets continues the process until the thrombus mass grows sufficiently to arrest blood loss from an injured vessel or, in pathologic conditions, until regulatory mechanisms interrupt the cycle or until the vascular lumen is occluded. Therefore,

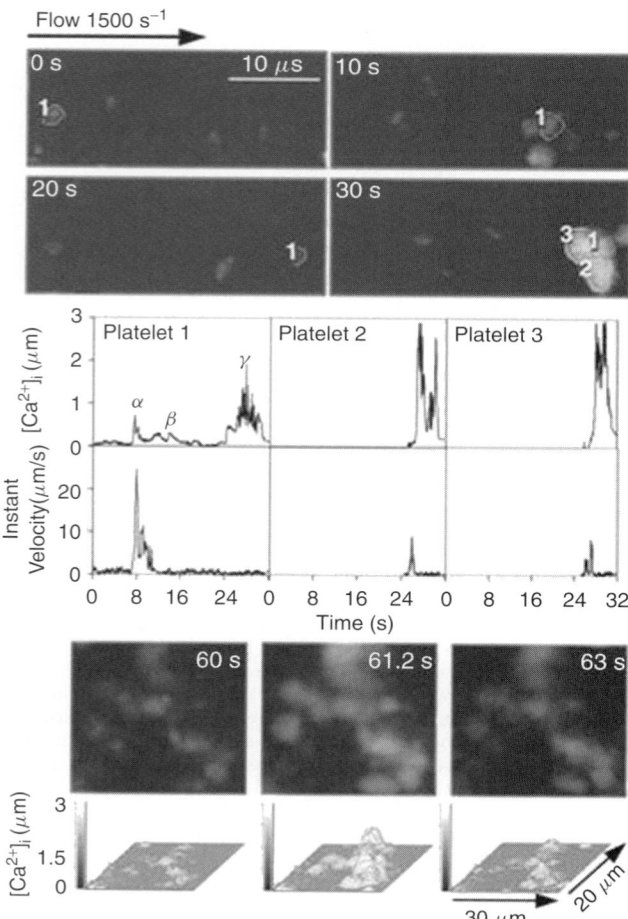

**FIGURE 47-8.** Real-time analysis of $[Ca^{2+}]_i$ during platelet translocation and aggregate formation on immobilized von Willebrand factor (VWF). Platelets loaded with fluo-3 AM ($2 \times 10^7$ per mL) were suspended with washed erythrocytes in homologous plasma and perfused over immobilized VWF for 3 minutes at the shear rate of 1,500 s$^{-1}$. The sequence of images at the top shows an example of aggregate formation. At 0 second, platelet 1 appears in the optical field; at 10 seconds, it has moved in the direction of flow by approximately 20 $\mu$m; at 20 seconds, it has moved by an additional few $\mu$m; at 30 seconds, it is in the same position, and two new platelets (2 and 3) are attached in close proximity, forming a small aggregate. The diagrams in the middle show $[Ca^{2+}]_i$ and instant velocity of platelets 1, 2, and 3. The translocation of platelet 1 occurs mostly during a few seconds of relatively rapid movement, coincident with the appearance of transient $[Ca^{2+}]_i$ peaks ($\alpha/\beta$); a higher and longer-lasting increase in $[Ca^{2+}]_i$ ($\gamma$) develops while the platelet is stationary. Cytosolic $Ca^{2+}$ oscillations appear also when platelets 2 and 3 arrest on the surface, without a clear sequence from $\alpha/\beta$ to $\gamma$. The images at the bottom, captured between 60 and 63 seconds after the appearance of platelet 1 in the field, show the long-lasting synchronous increase of $[Ca^{2+}]_i$ in platelets forming a large aggregate. The 3-D diagrams under each image show the measurement of $[Ca^{2+}]_i$ in all the platelets in the field. (From Mazzucato M, Pradella P, Cozzi MR, et al. Sequential cytoplasmic calcium signals in a two-stage platelet activation process induced by the glycoprotein Ib$\alpha$ mechanoreceptor. *Blood* 2002;100:2793–2800, with permission.)

notwithstanding the importance of initiating events, a thrombus is constituted essentially of platelets linked to one another but not directly to subendothelial components, and its development is strictly dependent on the formation of interplatelet bonds.

Fibrinogen bound to activated $\alpha_{IIb}\beta_3$ is generally considered the predominant adhesive bridge between aggregating

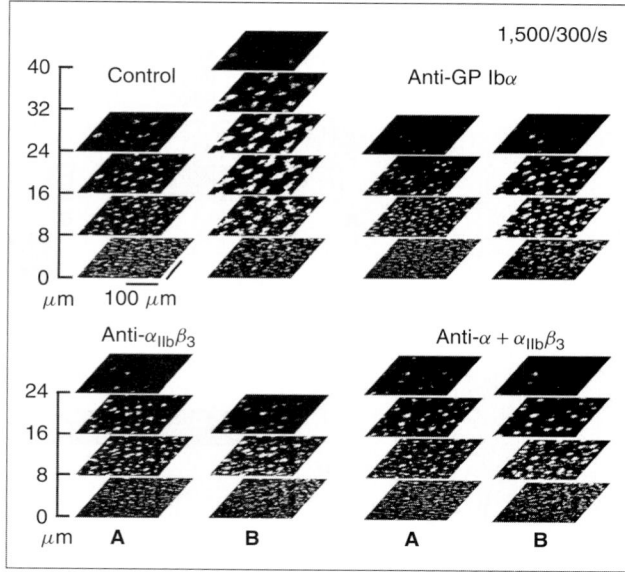

**FIGURE 47-9.** Progression of thrombus growth demonstrated in a two-stage experiment, first with perfusion of untreated blood over collagen type I fibrils at 1,500 s$^{-1}$ for 100 seconds, then continuing without interruption at 300 s$^{-1}$ with blood containing either buffer (control) or specific monoclonal antibodies, as indicated. Antibodies were incubated in blood for 10 minutes before initiating perfusion. Stacks of z sections labeled *A* show thrombi formed after 100 seconds of perfusion with blood containing no antibody at a wall shear rate of 1,500 s$^{-1}$. Stacks labeled *B* show the growth of thrombi after additional 740 seconds of perfusion at 300 s$^{-1}$ with blood containing either buffer or the indicated antibodies (total perfusion time of 840 seconds).

platelets (120). At elevated shear rates, typically in excess of 5,000 s$^{-1}$, VWF can also bind to platelets in a process that involves GP Ib$\alpha$ and $\alpha_{IIb}\beta_3$ sequentially (121) and is thought to mediate aggregation as an alternative to fibrinogen (122,123). Such concepts, however, have been suggested by the results of experiments with platelets in suspension not interacting with a reactive substrate. Studies on the bonds that link platelets to one another during thrombus development on collagen type I fibrils indicate a synergistic role for fibrinogen and VWF in supporting platelet aggregation. In the absence of fibrinogen, VWF-mediated thrombi grow rapidly at high shear rates, but are unstable; in the presence of VWF and fibrinogen, thrombi grow more slowly, but are stable (124). Unstable thrombi in the absence of fibrinogen have also been seen in the mouse circulation (125). These results provide a plausible explanation for the altered hemostatic properties of platelets from patients with isolated congenital deficiency of either fibrinogen (126) or VWF (127). Because neither protein by itself can sustain the full development of stable thrombi within the range of pathophysiologically relevant flow conditions, hemostasis cannot be normal unless both are present and are functional. Studies in genetically modified mice have indicated that thrombus formation may persist even in the absence of both fibrinogen and VWF (128), and evidence has been obtained that fibronectin, another ligand for activated $\alpha_{IIb}\beta_3$, may contribute to platelet aggregation within a thrombus (129). In this regard, therefore, it appears that several $\alpha_{IIb}\beta_3$ ligands support thrombus stability, including CD40 ligand (130).

The role of different adhesion receptors in mediating interplatelet contact has been analyzed with two-step perfusion experiments (see Fig. 47-9). These studies have shown that the height of a thrombus is limited by the inhibition of GP Ib$\alpha$ even when blood is initially perfused at shear rates permissive of adhesion to collagen without participation of the GP Ibα–VWF interaction. This limitation to the height is because the shear rate increases at the tip of a growing thrombus where the flow channel narrows, such that the threshold may be reached at which only a rapidly forming bond can capture flowing platelets. Therefore, the synergy between fibrinogen and VWF in supporting platelet aggregation depends on the recognized ability of each of these molecules to establish bonds with distinct adhesive properties. The initial function of VWF may depend primarily on its rapid rate of association with GP Ibα (78,85), which is particularly important in hemodynamic conditions characterized by high flow rates that increase the velocity differential between adjacent platelets. The subsequent interaction of multimeric VWF with both GP Ibα and activated $\alpha_{IIb}\beta_3$ (121,131) may temporarily stabilize interplatelet contacts and allow permanent bridging mediated by fibrinogen binding across activated platelet membranes (121). Therefore, adhesive interactions between platelets and a thrombogenic surface or between two platelets may depend essentially on the same mechanisms to oppose fluid dynamic forces generated by blood flow.

# CONCLUSIONS

New knowledge on the mechanisms of platelet adhesion and aggregation in flowing blood continues to accumulate, particularly with the use of specific models in genetically modified mice. Perhaps the most relevant directions for future research are the study of how differences in the composition of extracellular matrices influence the rate of thrombus formation and of how signaling networks link initial platelet adhesion to aggregation. Progress in these areas will enhance our ability to recognize the predisposition to thrombotic diseases and treat affected patients.

## *References*

1. Ruggeri ZM. Platelets in atherothrombosis. *Nat Med* 2002;8:1227–1234.
2. Ware JA, Heistad DD. Platelet-endothelium interactions. *N Engl J Med* 1993;328:628–635.
3. Marcus AJ, Broekman MJ, Drosopoulos JHF, et al. The endothelial cell ecto-ADPase responsible for inhibition of platelet function is CD39. *J Clin Invest* 1997;99(6):1351–1360.
4. Esmon NL, Carroll RC, Esmon CT. Thrombomodulin blocks the ability of thrombin to activate platelets. *J Biol Chem* 1983;258:12238–12242.
5. Freedman JE, Loscalzo J, Benoit SE, et al. Decreased platelet inhibition by nitric oxide in two brothers with a history of arterial thrombosis. *J Clin Invest* 1996;97(4):979–987.
6. Ross R. Atherosclerosis—an inflammatory disease. *N Engl J Med* 1999; 340:115–126.
7. Curwen KD, Gimbrone MA, Handin RI Jr. *In vitro* studies of thromboresistance. The role of prostacyclin (PGI₂) in platelet adhesion to cultured normal and virally transformed human vascular endothelial cells. *Lab Invest* 1980;42(3):366–374.
8. Visser MR, Tracy PB, Vercellotti GM, et al. Enhanced thrombin generation and platelet binding on herpes simplex virus-infected endothelium. *Proc Natl Acad Sci U S A* 1988;85:8227–8230.
9. Etingin OR, Silverstein RL, Hajjar DP. von Willebrand factor mediates platelet adhesion to virally infected endothelial cells. *Proc Natl Acad Sci U S A* 1993;90:5153–5156.
10. Ross R. The pathogenesis of atherosclerosis: a perspective for the 1990s. *Nature* 1993;362:801–809.
11. Czervionke RL, Hoak JC, Fry GL. Effect of aspirin on thrombin-induced adherence of platelets to cultured cells from the blood vessel wall. *J Clin Invest* 1978;62:847–856.
12. Shanberge JN, Kajiwara Y, Quattrociocchi-Longe T. Effect of aspirin and iloprost on adhesion of platelets to intact endothelium *in vivo. J Lab Clin Med* 1995;125(1):96–101.
13. Frenette PS, Wagner DD. Adhesion molecules—Part I. *N Engl J Med* 1996;334:1526–1529.
14. Frenette PS, Wagner DD. Adhesion molecules—Part II: blood vessels and blood cells. *N Engl J Med* 1996;335:43–45.
15. Carlos TM, Harlan JM. Leukocyte-endothelial adhesion molecules. [Review]. *Blood* 1994;84(7):2068–2101.

16. Languino LR, Plescia J, Duperray A, et al. Fibrinogen mediates leukocyte adhesion to vascular endothelium through an ICAM-1–dependent pathway. *Cell* 1993;73:1423–1434.
17. Cheresh DA, Berliner AS, Vicente V, et al. Recognition of distinct adhesive sites on fibrinogen by related integrins on platelets and endothelial cells. *Cell* 1989;58:945–953.
18. Frenette PS, Johnson RC, Hynes RO, et al. Platelets roll on stimulated endothelium *in vivo*: an interaction mediated by endothelial P-selectin. *Proc Natl Acad Sci U S A* 1995;92:7450–7454.
19. André P, Denis CV, Ware J, et al. Platelets adhere to and translocate on von Willebrand factor presented by endothelium in stimulated veins. *Blood* 2000;96:3322–3328.
20. Iozzo RV, Murdoch AD. Proteoglycans of the extracellular environment: clues from the gene and protein side offer novel perspectives in molecular diversity and function. *FASEB J* 1996;10:598–614.
21. Olsen BR. Basement membrane collagens (type IV). In: Kreis T, Vale R, eds. *Guidebook to the extracellular matrix and adhesion proteins.* Oxford: Oxford University Press, 1993:35–37.
22. Timpl R. Nidogen/entactin. In: Kreis T, Vale R, eds. *Guidebook to the extracellular matrix and adhesion proteins.* Oxford: Oxford University Press, 1993:75–76.
23. Timpl R, Brown JC. The laminins. *Matrix Biol* 1994;14:275–281.
24. Argraves WS, Tran H, Burgess WH, et al. Fibulin is an extracellular matrix and plasma glycoprotein with repeated domain structure. *J Cell Biol* 1990;111:3155–3164.
25. Saelman EUM, Nieuwenhuis HK, Hese KM, et al. Platelet adhesion to collagen types I through VIII under conditions of stasis and flow is mediated by GPIa/IIa ($\alpha_2\beta_1$-Integrin). *Blood* 1994;83(5):1244–1250.
26. Tandon NN, Holland EA, Kralisz U, et al. Interaction of human platelets with laminin and identification of the 67 kDa laminin receptor on platelets. *Biochem J* 1991;274:535–542.
27. Hindriks G, Ijsseldijk MJW, Sonnenberg A, et al. Platelet adhesion to laminin: role of Ca²⁺ and Mg²⁺ ions, shear rate, and platelet membrane glycoproteins. *Blood* 1992;79:928–935.
28. Pan TC, Sasaki T, Zhang RZ, et al. Structure and expression of fibulin-2, a novel extracellular matrix protein with multiple EGF-like repeats and consensus motifs for calcium-binding. *J Cell Biol* 1993;123:1269–1277.
29. Balbona K, Tran H, Godyna S, et al. Fibulin binds to itself and to the carboxy-terminal heparin-binding region of fibronectin. *J Biol Chem* 1992; 267:20120–20125.
30. Tran H, Tanaka A, Litvinovich SV, et al. The interaction of fibulin-1 with fibrinogen: a potential role in hemostasis and thrombosis. *J Biol Chem* 1995; 270:19458–19464.
31. Godyna S, Diaz-Ricart M, Argraves WS. Fibulin-1 mediates platelet adhesion via a bridge of fibrinogen. *Blood* 1996;88(7):2569–2577.
32. Mecham RP. Elastin. In: Kreis T, Vale R, eds. *Guidebook to the extracellular matrix and adhesion proteins.* Oxford: Oxford University Press, 1993:50–52.
33. Asch E, Podack E. Vitronectin binds to activated human platelets and plays a role in platelet aggregation. *J Clin Invest* 1990;85:1372–1378.
34. Zaidi TN, McIntire LV, Farrell DH, et al. Adhesion of platelets to surface-bound fibrinogen under flow. *Blood* 1996;88(8):2967–2972.
35. Zheng X, Saunders TL, Camper SA, et al. Vitronectin is not essential for normal mammalian development and fertility. *Proc Natl Acad Sci U S A* 1995;92(26):12426–12430.
36. Hynes RO. *Fibronectins*, 1st ed.. New York: Springer-Verlag, 1989.
37. Corbett SA, Schwarzbauer JE. Modulation of protein tyrosine phosphorylation by the extracellular matrix. *J Surg Res* 1997;69:220–225.
38. Beumer S, IJsseldijk MJ, de Groot PG, et al. Platelet adhesion to fibronectin in flow: dependence on surface concentration and shear rate, role of platelet membrane glycoproteins GP IIb/IIIa and VLA-5, and inhibition by heparin. *Blood* 1994;84(11):3724–3733.
39. Hynes RO. The complexity of platelet adhesion to extracellular matrices. *Thromb Haemost* 1991;66:40–43.
40. Beumer S, Heijnen HF, IJsseldijk MJ, et al. Platelet adhesion to fibronectin in flow: the importance of von Willebrand factor and glycoprotein Ib. *Blood* 1995;86(9):3452–3460.
41. Adams J, Lawler J. The thrombospondin family. *Curr Biol* 1993;3:188–190.
42. Bornstein P. Diversity of function is inherent in matricellular proteins: an appraisal of thrombospondin 1. *J Cell Biol* 1995;103:503–506.
43. Kyriakides TR, Zhu Y, Smith LT, et al. Mice that lack thrombospondin 2 display connective tissue abnormalities that are associated with disordered collagen fibrillogenesis, an increased vascular density, and a bleeding diathesis. *J Cell Biol* 1998;140(2):419–430.
44. Kyriakides TR, Zhu Y, Yang Z, et al. The distribution of the matricellular protein thrombospondin 2 in tissues of embryonic and adult mice. *J Histochem Cytochem* 1998;46(9):1007–1015.
45. Pimanda JE, Ganderton T, Maekawa A, et al. Role of thrombospondin-1 in control of von Willebrand factor multimer size in mice. *J Biol Chem* 2004;279:21439–21448.
46. Jurk K, Clemetson KJ, de Groot PG, et al. Thrombospondin-1 mediates platelet adhesion at high shear via glycoprotein IB (GPIb): an alternative/backup mechanism to von Willebrand factor. *FASEB J* 2003;17: 1490–1492.
47. Kyriakides TR, Rojnuckarin P, Reidy MA, et al. Megakaryocytes require thrombospondin-2 for normal platelet formation and function. *Blood* 2003;101:3915–3923.

48. Clemetson KJ, Clemetson JM. Platelet collagen receptors. *Thromb Haemost* 2001;86:189–197.

49. Nieswandt B, Watson SP. Platelet-collagen interaction: is GPVI the central receptor? *Blood* 2003;102:449–461.

50. Ruggeri ZM. Von Willebrand factor. *Curr Opin Hematol* 2003;10:142–149.

51. Sporn LA, Marder VJ, Wagner DD. Inducible secretion of large, biologically potent von Willebrand factor multimers. *Cell* 1986;46:185–190.

52. Lopez-Fernandez MF, Ginsberg MH, Ruggeri ZM, et al. Multimeric structure of platelet factor VIII/von Willebrand factor. The presence of larger multimers and their reassociation with thrombin-stimulated platelets. *Blood* 1982;60:1132–1138.

53. Ruggeri ZM, Mannucci PM, Federici AB, et al. Multimeric composition of factor VIII/von Willebrand factor following administration of DDAVP: implications for pathophysiology and therapy of von Willebrand's disease subtypes. *Blood* 1982;59:1272–1278.

54. Moake JL, Rudy CK, Troll JH, et al. Unusually large plasma factor VIII:von Willebrand factor multimers in chronic relapsing thrombotic thrombocytopenic purpura. *N Engl J Med* 1982;307:1432–1435.

55. Furlan M, Robles R, Lammle B. Partial purification and characterization of a protease from human plasma cleaving von Willebrand factor to fragments produced by *in vivo* proteolysis. *Blood* 1996;87(10):4223–4234.

56. Tsai HM. Physiologic cleavage of von Willebrand factor by a plasma protease is dependent on its conformation and requires calcium ion. *Blood* 1996;87(10):4235–4244.

57. Dent JA, Berkowitz SD, Ware J, et al. Identification of a cleavage site directing the immunochemical detection of molecular abnormalities in type IIA von Willebrand factor. *Proc Natl Acad Sci U S A* 1990;87:6306–6310.

58. Gerritsen HE, Robles R, Lämmle B, et al. Partial amino acid sequence of purified von willebrnad factor-cleaving protease. *Blood* 2001;98:1654–1661.

59. Fujikawa K, Suzuki H, McMullen B, et al. Purification of human von Willebrand factor-cleaving protease and its identification as a new member of the metalloproteinase family. *Blood* 2001;98:1662–1666.

60. Levy GG, Nichols WC, Lian EC, et al. Mutations in a member of the *ADAMTS* gene family cause thrombotic thrombocytopenic purpura. *Nature* 2001;413:488–494.

61. Zheng X, Chung D, Takayama TK, et al. Structure of von Willebrand factor-cleaving protease (ADAMTS13), a metalloprotease involved in thrombotic thrombocytopenic purpura. *J Biol Chem* 2001;276:41059–41063.

62. Bahnak BR, Wu Q-Y, Coulombel L, et al. Expression of von Willebrand factor in porcine vessels: heterogeneity at the level of von Willebrand factor mRNA. *J Cell Physiol* 1989;138:305–310.

63. Nichols TC, Samama CM, Bellinger DA, et al. Function of von Willebrand factor after crossed bone marrow transplantation between normal and von Willebrand disease pigs: effect on arterial thrombosis in chimeras. *Proc Natl Acad Sci U S A* 1995;92:2455–2459.

64. Tangelder GJ, Slaaf DW, Arts T, et al. Wall shear rate in arterioles *in vivo*: least estimates from platelet velocity profiles. *Am J Physiol* 1988;254: H1059–H1064.

65. Back CH, Radbill JR, Crawford DW. Analysis of pulsatile viscous blood flow through diseased coronary arteries of man. *J Biomech* 1977;10: 339–353.

66. Fuster V, Badimon L, Badimon JJ, et al. The pathogenesis of coronary artery disease and the acute coronary syndromes (1). *N Engl J Med* 1992; 326:242–250.

67. Fuster V, Badimon L, Badimon JJ, et al. The pathogenesis of coronary artery disease and the acute coronary syndromes (2). *N Engl J Med* 1992; 326:310–318.

68. Ruggeri ZM, Saldivar E. Platelets, hemostasis and thrombosis. In: Ruggeri ZM, ed. *Von Willebrand factor and the mechanisms of platelet function.* Berlin: Springer, 1998:1–32.

69. Whitmore RL. *Rheology of the circulation*, 1st ed..Oxford: Pergamon Press Ltd, 1968.

70. Fronek K, Zweifach W. Microvascular blood flow in cat tenuissimus muscle. *Microvasc Res* 1977;14:181–189.

71. Schmid-Schoenbein GW, Zweifach BW. RBC velocity profiles in arterioles and venules of the rabbit omentum. *Microvasc Res* 1975;10(153):164.

72. Lipowsky HH, Zweifach BW. Methods for the simultaneous measurement of pressure differentials and flow in single unbranched vessels of the microcirculation for rheological studies. *Microvasc Res* 1977;14: 345–361.

73. Celikel R, Varughese KI, Madhusudan YA, et al. Crystal structure of von Willebrand factor A1 domain in complex with the function blocking NMC-4 fab. *Nat Struct Biol* 1998;5:189–194.

74. Emsley J, Cruz M, Handin R, et al. Crystal structure of the von Willebrand factor A1 domain and implications for the binding of platelet glycoprotein Ib. *J Biol Chem* 1998;273:10396–10401.

75. Celikel R, Ruggeri ZM, Varughese KI. Von Willebrand factor conformation and adhesive function is modulated by an internalized water molecule. *Nat Struct Biol* 2000;7:881–884.

76. Huizinga EG, Tsuji S, Romijn RAP, et al. Structures of glycoprotein Ibα and its complex with von Willebrand factor A1 domain. *Science* 2002; 297:1176–1129.

77. Dumas JJ, Kumar R, McDonagh T, et al. Crystal structure of the wild-type von Willebrand factor A1-glycoprotein Ibα complex reveals conformation differences with a complex bearing von Willebrand disease mutations. *J Biol Chem* 2004;279:23327–22334.

78. Savage B, Saldivar E, Ruggeri ZM. Initiation of platelet adhesion by arrest onto fibrinogen or translocation on von Willebrand factor. *Cell* 1996;84: 289–297.

79. Ruggeri ZM, Bader R, De Marco L. Glanzmann thrombasthenia: deficient binding of von Willebrand factor to thrombin-stimulated platelets. *Proc Natl Acad Sci U S A* 1982;79:6038–6041.

80. Ruggeri ZM, De Marco L, Gatti L, et al. Platelets have more than one binding site for von Willebrand factor. *J Clin Invest* 1983;72:1–12.

81. Savage B, Ruggeri ZM. Selective recognition of adhesive sites in surface-bound fibrinogen by GP IIb-IIIa on nonactivated platelets. *J Biol Chem* 1991;266:11227–11233.

82. Polanowska-Grabowska R, Geanacopoulos M, Gear ARL. Platelet adhesion to collagen via the $\alpha_2\beta_1$ integrin under flow conditions causes rapid tyrosine phosphorylation of pp125$^{FAK}$. *Biochem J* 1993;296:543–547.

83. Keely PJ, Parise LV. The $\alpha_2\beta_1$ integrin is a necessary co-receptor for collagen-induced activation of syk and subsequent phosphorylation of phospholipase Cy2 in platelets. *J Biol Chem* 1996;271(43):26668–26676.

84. Ichinohe T, Takayama H, Ezumi Y, et al. Collagen-stimulated activation of syk but not c-src is severely compromised in human platelets lacking membrane glycoprotein VI. *J Biol Chem* 1997;272:63–68.

85. Savage B, Almus-Jacobs F, Ruggeri ZM. Specific synergy of multiple substrate-receptor interactions in platelet thrombus formation under flow. *Cell* 1998;94:657–666.

86. Bienkowska J, Cruz MA, Handin RI, et al. The von Willebrand factor A3 domain does not contain a metal ion-dependent adhesion site motif. *J Biol Chem* 1997;272:25162–25167.

87. Huizinga EG, van der Plas RM, Kroon J, et al. Crystal structure of the A3 domain of human von Willebrand factor: implications for collagen binding. *Structure* 1997;5:1147–1156.

88. Romijn RA, Westein E, Bouma B, et al. Mapping the collagen-binding site in the von Willebrand factor-A3 domain. *J Biol Chem* 2003;278:15035–15039.

89. Jarvis GE, Atkinson BT, Snell DC, et al. Distinct roles of GPVI and integrin $\alpha_2\beta_1$ in platelet shape change and aggregation induced by different collagens. *Br J Pharmacol* 2002;137:107–117.

90. Kato K, Kanaji T, Russell S, et al. The contribution of glycoprotein VI to stable platelet adhesion and thrombus formation illustrated by targeted gene deletion. *Blood* 2003;102:1701–1707.

91. Savage B, Sixma JJ, Ruggeri ZM. Functional self-association of von Willebrand factor during platelet adhesion under flow. *Proc Natl Acad Sci U S A* 2002;99:425–430.

92. Kroll MH, Harris TS, Moake JL, et al. Von Willebrand factor binding to platelet GPIb initiates signals for platelet activation. *J Clin Invest* 1991; 88:1568–1573.

93. Savage B, Shattil SJ, Ruggeri ZM. Modulation of platelet function through adhesion receptors: a dual role for glycoprotein IIb-IIIa (integrin $\alpha_{IIb}\beta_3$) mediated by fibrinogen and glycoprotein Ib-von Willebrand factor. *J Biol Chem* 1992;267:11300–11306.

94. Kasirer-Friede A, Ware J, Leng L, et al. Lateral clustering of platelet GP Ib-IX complexes leads to up-regulation of the adhesive function of integrin $\alpha_{IIb}\beta_3$. *J Biol Chem* 2002;277:11949–11956.

95. Kasirer-Friede A, Cozzi MR, Mazzucato M, et al. Signaling through GP Ib-IX-V activates $\alpha$IIb$\beta$3 independently of other receptors. *Blood* 2004; 103:3403–3411.

96. Kroll MH, Hellums JD, McIntire LV, et al. Platelets and shear stress. *Blood* 1996;88(5):1525–1541.

97. Mazzucato M, Pradella P, Cozzi MR, et al. Sequential cytoplasmic calcium signals in a two-stage platelet activation process induced by the glycoprotein Ibα mechanoreceptor. *Blood* 2002;100:2793–2800.

98. Yap CL, Anderson KE, Hughan SC, et al. Essential role for phosphoinositide 3-kinase in shear-dependent signaling between platelet glycoprotein Ib/V/IX and integrin $\alpha_{IIb}\beta_3$. *Blood* 2002;99:151–158.

99. Goto S, Tamura N, Eto K, et al. Functional significance of adenosine 5'-diphosphate receptor (P2Y$_{12}$) in platelet activation inititated by binding of von Willebrand factor to platelet Gp Ibα induced by conditions of high shear rate. *Circulation* 2002;105:2531–2536.

100. Mazzucato M, Cozzi MR, Pradella P, et al. Distinct roles of two ADP receptors in von Willebrand factor-mediated platelet signaling and activation under flow. *Blood* 2004;104:3221–3227. Epub.

101. Andrews RK, Berndt MC. Adhesion-dependent signalling and the initiation of haemostasis and thrombosis. *Histol Histopathol* 1998;13:837–844.

102. Satoh K, Asazuma N, Yatomi Y, et al. Activation of protein-tyrosine kinase pathways in human platelets stimulated with the A1 domain of von Willebrand factor. *Platelets* 2000;11:171–176.

103. Yanabu M, Ozaki Y, Nomura S, et al. Tyrosine phosphorylation and p72$^{syk}$ activation by an anti-glycoprotein Ib monoclonal antibody. *Blood* 1997; 89(5):1590–1598.

104. Falati S, Edmead CE, Poole AW. Glycoprotein Ib-V-IX, a receptor for von Willebrand factor, couples physically and functionally to the fc receptor gamma-chain, fyn, and lyn to activate human platelets. *Blood* 1999;94: 1648–1656.

105. Torti M, Bertoni A, Canobbio I, et al. Rap 1B and rap2B translocation to the cytoskeleton by von Willebrand factor involves fcgammaII receptor-mediated protein tyrosine physphorylation. *J Biol Chem* 1999;274: 13690–13697.

106. Wu Y, Suzuki-Inoue K, Satoh K, et al. Role of fc receptor gamma-chain in platelet glycoprotein Ib-mediated signaling. *Blood* 2001;97:3836–3845.

107. Sullam PM, Hyun W, Szollosi J, et al. Physical proximity and functional interplay of the glycoprotein Ib-IX-V complex and the fc receptor FcψRIIa on the platelet plasma membrane. *J Biol Chem* 1998;273(9):5331–5336.

108. Cunningham JG, Meyer SC, Fox JEB. The cytoplasmic domain of the α-subunit of glycoprotein (GP) Ib mediates attachment of the entire GP Ib-IX complex to the cytoskeleton and regulates von Willebrand factor-induced changes in cell morphology. *J Biol Chem* 1996;271(19):11581–11587.

109. Andrews RK, Fox JEB. Identification of a region in the cytoplasmic domain of the platelet membrane glycoprotein Ib-IX complex that binds to purified actin-binding protein. *J Biol Chem* 1992;267:18605–18611.

110. Du X, Harris SJ, Tetaz TJ, et al. Association of a phospholipase A₂ (14-3-3 protein) with the platelet glycoprotein Ib-IX complex. *J Biol Chem* 1994;269:18287–18290.

111. Andrews RK, Shen Y, Gardiner EE, et al. The glycoprotein Ib-IX-V complex in platelet adhesion and signaling. *Thromb Haemost* 1999;82:357–364.

112. Gu M, Xi X, Englund GD, et al. Analysis of the roles of 14-3-3 in the platelet glycoprotein Ib-IX-mediated activation of integrin alpha (IIB)beta(3) using a reconstituted mammalian cell expression model. *J Cell Biol* 1999;147:1085–1096.

113. Munday AD, Berndt MC, Mitchell CA. Phosphoinositide 3-kinase forms a complex with platelet membrane glycoprotein Ib-IX-V complex and 14-3-3zeta. *Blood* 2000;96:577–584.

114. Feng S, Christodoulides N, Resendiz JC, et al. Cytoplasmic domains of GpIbalpha and GpIbbeta regulate 14-3-3zeta binding to GpIb/IX/V. *Blood* 2000;95:551–557.

115. Cruz MA, Yuan H, Lee JR, et al. Interaction of the von Willebrand factor (VWF) with collagen. *J Biol Chem* 1995;270(18):10822–10827.

116. Roth GJ, Titani K, Hoyer LW, et al. Localization of binding sites within human von Willebrand factor for monomeric type III collagen. *Biochemistry* 1986;25:8357–8361.

117. Pareti FI, Fujimura Y, Dent JA, et al. Isolation and characterization of a collagen binding domain in human von Willebrand factor. *J Biol Chem* 1986;261:15310–15315.

118. Pareti FI, Niiya K, McPherson JM, et al. Isolation and characterization of two domains of human von Willebrand factor that interact with fibrillar collagen types I and III. *J Biol Chem* 1987;262:13835–13841.

119. Mazzucato M, Spessotto P, Masotti A, et al. Identification of domains responsible for von Willebrand factor type VI collagen interaction mediating platelet adhesion under high flow. *J Biol Chem* 1999;274:3033–3041.

120. Lefkovits J, Plow EF, Topol EJ. Platelet glycoprotein IIb/IIIa receptors in cardiovascular medicine. *N Engl J Med* 1995;332:1553–1559.

121. Goto S, Ikeda Y, Saldivar E, et al. Distinct mechanisms of platelet aggregation as a consequence of different shearing flow conditions. *J Clin Invest* 1998;101:479–486.

122. Peterson DM, Stathopoulos NA, Giorgio TD, et al. Shear-induced platelet aggregation requires von Willebrand factor and platelet membrane glycoproteins Ib and IIb-IIIa. *Blood* 1987;69:625–628.

123. Ikeda Y, Handa M, Kawano K, et al. The role of von Willebrand factor and fibrinogen in platelet aggregation under varying shear stress. *J Clin Invest* 1991;87:1234–1240.

124. Ruggeri ZM, Dent JA, Saldivar E. Contribution of distinct adhesive interactions to platelet aggregation in flowing blood. *Blood* 1999;94:172–178.

125. Ni H, Subbarao S, Denis C, et al. Distinct roles of von Willebrand factor and fibrinogen in thrombus growth in arterioles. *Thromb Haemost Suppl* 1999;82:411.

126. Weiss HJ, Rogers J. Fibrinogen and platelets in the primary arrest of bleeding-studies in two patients with congenital afibrinogenemia. *N Engl J Med* 1971;285:369–374.

127. Nichols WC, Cooney KA, Ginsburg D, et al. Von Willebrand disease. In: Loscalzo J, Schafer AI, eds. *Thrombosis and hemorrhage*. Philadelphia, PA: Lippincott Williams & Wilkins, 2003:539–559.

128. Ni H, Denis CV, Subbarao S, et al. Persistence of platelet thrombus formation in arterioles of mice lacking both von Willebrand factor and fibrinogen. *J Clin Invest* 2000;106:385–392.

129. Ni H, Yuen PS, Papalia JM, et al. Plasma fibronectin promotes thrombus growth and stability in injured arterioles. *Proc Natl Acad Sci U S A* 2003;100:2415–2419.

130. Andre P, Prasad KS, Denis CV, et al. CD40L stabilizes arterial thrombi by a β₃ integrin-dependent mechanism. *Nat Med* 2002;8:247–252.

131. Goto S, Salomon DR, Ikeda Y, et al. Characterization of the unique mechanism mediating the shear-dependent binding of soluble von Willebrand factor to platelets. *J Biol Chem* 1995;270:23352–23361.

# CHAPTER 48 ■ RHEOLOGY OF THROMBOSIS

SUZANNE G. ESKIN AND LARRY V. McINTIRE

Blood flow–induced shear stresses and pulsatile pressure–induced vessel wall strain can considerably modulate blood and vascular cell function. The kinetics of thrombus formation depends on the flow conditions present locally, with different cell receptors and ligands supporting cell–cell and cell–protein adhesion under arterial, venous, and pathologic shear conditions. Additionally, mass transport of cells and proteins to and from reactive surfaces, such as a damaged vessel wall, varies in different flow regimes. Studies (1–3) have demonstrated that local mechanical forces can directly alter the metabolism and gene expression of vascular cells. Understanding hemodynamics requires the application of the fundamentals of rheology, the science of deformation and flow of materials to the vascular system. Theoretical models of the vascular system have been developed by applying the governing principles of fluid flow and mass transport. On the basis of these relatively simple models, dynamic experimental systems have been designed that simulate vascular shear conditions. These systems are valuable tools for investigating the molecular mechanisms supporting vascular processes important to thrombosis under flow, as seen *in vivo*.

## BLOOD FLUID DYNAMICS

Blood flow conditions have long been considered as important to vascular function as the blood vessel and the circulating components. A simple, but relevant, model of the vascular system may be developed by considering the steady, pressure-driven laminar flow of an incompressible, Newtonian fluid through a long cylindrical tube with a constant cross-sectional area (4–7). Under these conditions, only an axial velocity field exists, and it depends on the radial position ($r$), the mean fluid velocity ($v$), and the vessel radius ($R$):

$$v_z = 2(v)\left[1 - \left(\frac{r}{R}\right)^2\right] \qquad (48\text{-}1)$$

As suggested by equation 48-1, the axial velocity, $v_z$, reaches a maximum at the center of the tube where $r$ is equal to zero (see Fig. 48-1). Moving away from this center position, velocity decreases as the wall of the tube is approached. The fluid is assumed not to slip along the wall; that is, the fluid velocity at the wall is assumed to be zero (5). *Shear* refers to the relative motion of the different fluid planes in the velocity profile. The shear rate ($\gamma$) is a measure of the velocity gradient and indicates the rate at which fluid layers are sliding past one another.

$$\gamma = \frac{dv_z}{dr} = \frac{4(v)r}{R^2} \qquad (48\text{-}2)$$

The units of the shear rate are inverse time, commonly reported as inverse seconds. Although the fluid velocity is greatest at the center of the tube, the velocity gradient, and therefore the shear rate, is zero there. Conversely, at the wall of the tube, the velocity gradient and therefore the shear rate reach a maximum (Fig. 48-1), but the actual velocity is zero. Important to the rheology of the vascular system is the shear rate at the wall of the tube ($r = R$), which corresponds to the shear rate at the vessel surface ($\gamma_w$):

$$\gamma_w = \frac{4(v)}{R} \qquad (48\text{-}3)$$

The mean fluid velocity, ($v_z$), may be expressed in terms of physical quantities as in equation 48-4:

$$(v) = \frac{Q}{\pi R^2} \qquad (48\text{-}4)$$

where $Q$ is the volumetric flow rate. Substituting equation 48-4 into the wall shear rate equation (equation 48-3) leads to a more practical expression of $\gamma_w$:

$$\gamma_w = \frac{4Q}{\pi R^3} \qquad (48\text{-}5)$$

As predicted from the range of vessel sizes and volumetric blood flow rates, the wall shear rates corresponding to the different regions of the vascular system can vary greatly (see Table 48-1).

In addition to shear rate, the fluid shear stress is commonly used to describe rheologic conditions in the vascular system. Shear stress is a measure of the force per unit area the flowing blood exerts as different fluid layers slide past one another. The shear stress is typically expressed in dynes per square centimeter (dyn per cm$^2$). For Newtonian fluids, the shear stress ($\tau_z$) is directly proportional to both the viscosity of the fluid ($\mu$) and the shear rate (6):

$$\tau_z = -\mu\frac{dv_z}{dr} = \mu\left(\frac{4(v)r}{R^2}\right) \qquad (48\text{-}6)$$

At the vessel wall, $r = R$, and equation 48-6 becomes the equation for the wall shear stress ($\tau_w$):

$$\tau_w = \mu\gamma_w = \mu\left(\frac{4Q}{\pi R^3}\right) \qquad (48\text{-}7)$$

Fluids resist shear, and so pressure gradients along the tube length are necessary to produce the work required to overcome the frictional resistance to flow. In fully developed laminar flow, a balance exists between the force generated by the pressure gradient (acting across the luminal surface) and the force of shear resistance generated by viscous drag (acting on the vessel wall) (4):

$$\frac{\Delta P}{\Delta z}\pi R^2 = 2\pi R\tau(R) \qquad (48\text{-}8)$$

where $\Delta P$ is the pressure difference across a given tube length in the axial direction, $\Delta z$. Substituting for $\tau(R)$, which equals $\tau_w$

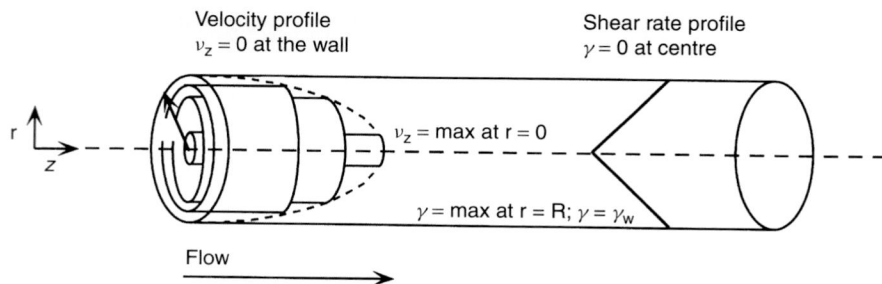

**FIGURE 48-1.** Velocity ($v_z$) and shear rate ($\gamma$) profiles produced by steady, laminar flow of an incompressible, Newtonian fluid through a long cylindrical tube with a constant cross-sectional area. Shear refers to the relative motion of the different fluid planes in the velocity profile. The shear rate indicates how fast the fluid layers are sliding past one another. The fluid velocity is greatest at the center of the tube while the shear rate is zero. Conversely, at the wall of the tube, the shear rate ($\gamma_w$) reaches a maximum and the fluid velocity is zero. $r$, radial position; $R$, vessel radius. (Modified from Alevriadou BR, McIntire LV. Rheology. In: Loscalzo J, Schafer AI, eds. *Thrombosis and hemorrhage.* Boston: Blackwell, 1994:369–381; Goldsmith HL, Turitto VT. Rheological aspects of thrombosis and haemostasis: basic principles and applications. ICTH9 Report—Subcommittee on Rheology of the International Committee on Thrombosis and Haemostasis. *Thromb Haemost* 1986;55:415–435.)

in equation 48-7, yields the Hagen-Poiseuille equation that relates the pressure drop along a vessel to the volumetric flow rate (6):

$$\frac{\Delta P}{\Delta z} = \frac{8\,\mu Q}{\pi R^4} \qquad (48\text{-}9)$$

This model of the vascular system describes flow regimes where viscous forces rather than inertial forces dominate. This type of flow is known as *Poiseuille flow* (4–6). The Reynolds number ($N_{Re}$) is a dimensionless parameter that describes the relative importance of the inertial and viscous forces present under flow (5):

$$N_{Re} = \frac{\text{inertial force}}{\text{viscous force}} = \frac{\rho(v)^2}{\left(\mu \dfrac{(v)}{2R}\right)} = \frac{2R(v)\rho}{\mu} \qquad (48\text{-}10)$$

where $\rho$ is the fluid density. When the viscous forces are dominant relative to the inertial forces, specifically when $N_{Re}$ is less than approximately 2,100, the fluid flow is laminar and equations 48-1 through 48-9 are valid descriptions of the velocity and shear profiles (4,6). This is nearly always the case in the straight portions of blood vessels, with the possible exception of the largest vessels with high blood flow rates, such as the ascending aorta, and in severly stenotic atherosclerotic vessels.

When $N_{Re}$ is greater than 2,100 the steady, Poiseuille flow becomes unstable and is replaced by complex, turbulent flow regimes (4–6). Under these conditions, the inertial forces required to accelerate and decelerate the fluid along its flow path dominate.

## TABLE 48-1

### SHEAR RATES IN THE VASCULAR SYSTEM

| Vessel | Shear rate (per second) |
|---|---|
| Large arteries | 300–800 |
| Veins | 20–200 |
| Arterioles | 500–1,600 |
| Stenotic vessels | 800–10,000 |

Modified from Alevriadou BR, McIntire LV. Rheology. In: Loscalzo J, Schafer AI, eds. *Thrombosis and hemorrhage.* Boston: Blackwell, 1994:369–381.

The pulsatile motion of blood flow contributes to the inertial forces present and a specific modified Reynolds number has been developed to determine when inertial forces resulting from the pulsations in the cardiac cycle must be considered. This dimensionless parameter is called the *Womersley alpha parameter* (4):

$$\alpha = R\left(\frac{\omega \rho}{\mu}\right)^{1/2} \qquad (48\text{-}11)$$

where $\omega$ is the frequency of the oscillation in radians per second. Pulsation effects predominately impact the flow regimes in major arteries that have large diameters and are located proximal to the heart where oscillations have not been significantly dampened by vascular compliance (4).

Adding to the complexity of flow in the vascular system is the elasticity of the blood vessels. As indicated by equations 48-5 and 48-9, the shear profiles and the pressure gradients required to produce flow are highly sensitive to changes in the vessel radius. Although most vessels do not substantially dilate under the oscillatory conditions of normal blood flow, very large vessels (e.g., the aortic and the pulmonic arteries) experience radial changes during the different phases of the cardiac cycle (4). Additionally, the velocity and shear profiles in a broad distribution of vessels are affected by events, such as vasoconstriction and vessel stenosis, that also lead to changes in vessel radius.

The model of the blood vessel as a long cylindrical tube is applicable to much of the vascular system, and in the straight portions of vessels, turbulence due to a Reynolds number higher than 2,100 is rarely observed. Even in the presence of physiologic shear rates, however, complex vessel geometries may change the flow from simple Poiseuille to a more complex laminar form. This complexity can induce a separation of streamlines, stagnant regions, transient flow reversal, and eddy formation (6,7). In the vascular system, recirculating flow conditions increase the residence time between the vessel wall and circulating cells and proteins, leading to a potential increase in the local deposition of the components necessary for plaque and thrombi formation. Common sites of vascular flow complexity include bifurcations, t-junctions, highly curved vessels, regions near valves, and vessels with abruptly changing diameters (see Fig. 48-2) (4,8–11). These sites correspond with areas of increased thrombi and plaque formation (12–18).

In addition to geometric and flow-rate influences, blood flow regimes vary because the viscosity of blood depends on the shear rate applied; that is, blood is not strictly a Newtonian fluid (19).

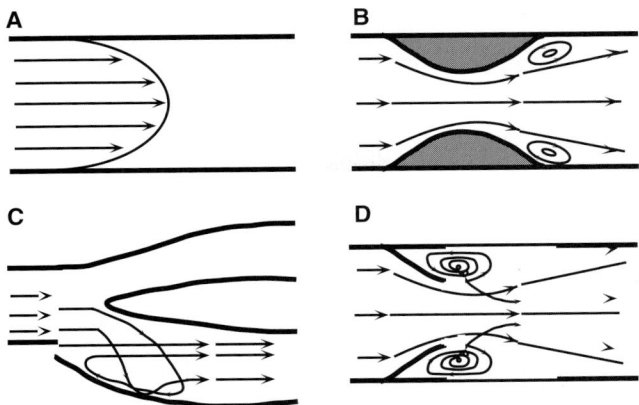

**FIGURE 48-2.** Streamlines in normal Poiseuille flow (**A**) and flow at sites of complex laminar flows, including vessels with abruptly changing diameters (**B**), bifurcations (**C**), and regions near valves (**D**). (Modified from Karino T, Goldsmith HL, Motomiya M, et al. Flow patterns in vessels of simple and complex geometries. *Ann N Y Acad Sci* 1987; 516:422–441.)

At very low shear rates, blood does not flow in response to the subthreshold levels of shear stress applied (19–21). This property of having a yield stress is characteristic of elastic materials rather than Newtonian fluids. After the yield stress is applied, blood flows and, as the shear rate is increased further, the viscosity of blood decreases (see Fig. 48-3) (19,22–24). In contrast to blood, plasma is a Newtonian fluid (20). Therefore, the non-Newtonian properties of blood can be attributed to the presence of cells and cell aggregation. All cells in the bloodstream experience shear from the flowing blood. If the cells were simply hard spheres, the shear would cause simple rotation and translation (25,26). Owing to the viscoelastic nature of cells, however, shear can twist, stretch, or compress the cells causing deformations (25,27). Red blood cells, constituting 99% of the blood cellular volume, contribute significantly to the non-Newtonian nature of blood. At low shear rates (<50 per second), fibrinogen mediates red cell aggregation into chains called *rouleaux* (4,19,28). As the

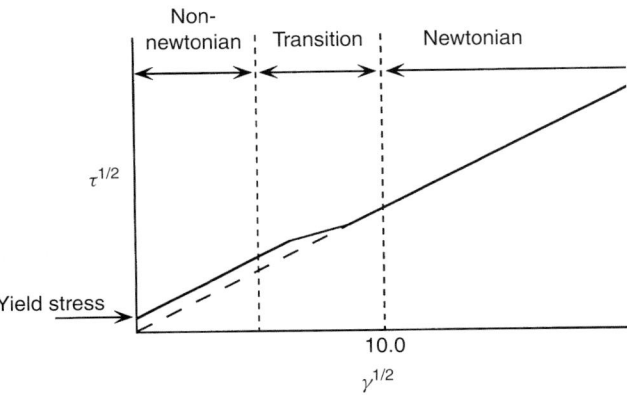

**FIGURE 48-3.** The non-Newtonian nature of blood. At very low shear rates ($\gamma$), blood will not flow in response to the subthreshold levels of shear stress ($\tau$) applied. After the yield stress is reached, blood will flow, and as the shear rate is increased further, the viscosity of blood will decrease, as indicated by the decrease in slope with increasing shear rate. For Newtonian fluids, the shear stress is directly proportional to the shear rate over the entire range of shear rates and no yield stress is present. Blood behaves as a Newtonian fluid at shear rates greater than 100 to 200 per second. (Modified from Merrill EW. Rheology of blood. *Physiol Rev* 1969;49:863–888.)

shear rate is increased, the rouleaux break down and the blood viscosity decreases (24,29,30). At shear rates greater than 20 per second, red cells deform and align in the direction of flow (31,32). Deformations on single cells in dilute suspensions lead to cell migration toward the center of the flow stream (31,32). In concentrated suspensions, crowding restricts the rotation and translational movements of the red cells and increases the number of red blood cell collisions. These crowding effects drive the cells toward the wall and offset the migration of deformable particles to the vessel center (31). In vessels with diameters larger than 100 $\mu$m, the flow of a suspension with a physiologic concentration of red cells will result in a cell-free layer of approximately 4 $\mu$m at the wall (4,31). Red cell crowding and collisions also complicate the flow paths of circulating white blood cells, platelets, and large plasma proteins (31,32). Additionally, under physiologic red cell concentrations, the velocity profile is no longer parabolic as in Poiseuille flow, but becomes blunted at the leading edge (4,31). Despite all these limitations, blood can normally be considered a homogeneous, Newtonian fluid for shear rates greater than 100 to 200 per second (4,19). At these shear rates, the viscosity of blood remains relatively constant and is determined primarily by the hematocrit, temperature, and the concentration of fibrinogen and other proteins (19).

The shear of flowing blood also influences the interactions between the vascular wall and adherent cells. The shear force and torque a cell experiences when it is tethered to a surface depend on the cell size, the fluid viscosity, and the shear rate (33–35). At higher shear forces, stronger cell–surface bonds are required to support firm cell adhesion. If the energy from shear in the bloodstream is high enough to deform the cell membrane and overcome the adhesive bond strength, cells will not adhere firmly to the wall (35). Under these conditions, rapid cell–surface bond formation may support transient adhesion, or rolling, on the vascular surface (see Fig. 48-4A). Cells that constitute the vascular wall itself, such as endothelial cells and smooth muscle cells, also experience tangential shear stress when exposed to flowing blood. Additionally, these cells may experience circumferential stress resulting from deformations caused by expansion and contraction of the blood vessel as well as compressive stress resulting from hydrodynamic pressure (Fig. 48-4B) (2,3).

## BLOOD TRANSPORT PROCESSES

The primary function of blood is to transport materials to and from the organs, thereby sustaining life. Although vital, this transport may also augment pathologic states such as thrombosis and atherosclerosis. The transport of materials occurs by two processes: diffusion and convection. *Diffusion* is the movement of material relative to the average fluid motion, irrespective of whether the fluid is flowing or stationary. Diffusion is random and results from Brownian motion of the particles. *Convection* is the movement of materials with the fluid and results from flow. Diffusion of materials is a very slow process in liquids, whereas convection can be very rapid. If flow is present, convection forces will dominate the mass transfer in blood, and diffusion effects will be negligible in the directions of flow. The *Peclet number* ($N_{Pe}$) is a dimensionless parameter that describes the relative importance of convection and diffusion in a given fluid stream (6,36):

$$N_{Pe} = \frac{\text{convection effects}}{\text{diffusion effects}} = \frac{(\nu)2R}{D} \qquad (48\text{-}12)$$

where $D$ is the molecular diffusion coefficient. Large Peclet numbers correspond to fluid flow where convection dominates, whereas for small Peclet numbers, diffusion is the dominant method of mass transport.

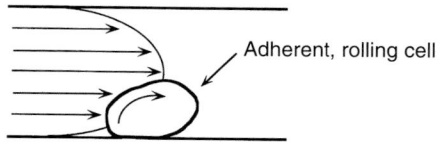

**A**

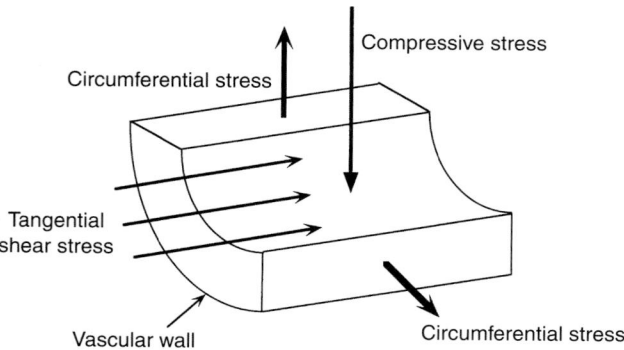

**B**

**FIGURE 48-4. A:** Shear forces acting on an adherent, rolling cell in a flow stream. **B:** Stresses acting on cells that constitute the vascular wall, such as endothelial cells and smooth muscle cells. Tangential shear stress results from the flow of blood over the vascular wall. Circumferential stress results from deformations caused by the expansion and contraction of the blood vessel, whereas compressive stress results from hydrodynamic pressure. (Modified from Papadaki M, Eskin SG. Effects of fluid shear stress on gene regulation of vascular cells. *Biotechnol Prog* 1997;13:209–221.)

Considering again the model of the vascular system using Poiseuille flow of a Newtonian fluid through a cylindrical tube of constant cross-sectional area, convection moves fluid along streamlines parallel to the wall and, therefore, the effects of diffusion are negligible in the axial direction. In the radial direction, convection does not occur and mass transfer is due solely to diffusion. The rate of mass transfer is proportional to the product of the molecular diffusivity and the local concentration gradient. Under these conditions, radial diffusion is required to transport material to the wall, and the steady state mass balance at any point in the tube for a single species reduces to (neglecting homogeneous reactions):

$$v_z \frac{\partial C}{\partial z} = \frac{1}{r}\frac{\partial}{\partial r}\left(rD\frac{\partial C}{\partial r}\right) \qquad (48\text{-}13)$$

where $C$ is the concentration of the species in the bulk fluid and $D$ is the effective diffusion coefficient (7,37). When turbulence, which generates an effective radial convection that directly pushes cells and soluble proteins to the wall (Fig. 48-2), is present, equation 48-13 does not apply. Turbulence and complex laminar flows in the vascular system most commonly result from complex vessel geometries or high-flow rates, although blood pulsations and vessel elasticity may also contribute to the development of secondary flows. Independent of its origin, any radial convection present greatly enhances the transfer of material from the bloodstream to the wall of the vessel.

Mass transfer processes are also significantly affected by the presence of red blood cells, even in steady, laminar flow regimes where blood can be considered Newtonian. Because red cells deform in response to shear, the cells align in the direction of flow and migrate to the center of the flow stream. This effect is less pronounced in blood with a normal hematocrit flowing at high shear rates, but even under these physiologic conditions, a thin red cell–free layer exists at the wall. Radial mixing of circulating platelets, white blood cells, and large protein components occurs as these components are pushed to the vessel surface by red cells crowding in the vessel center. Increasing hematocrit increases the frequency of platelet, white cell, and protein collisions with the vessel wall (4). Relative to Brownian motion alone, movements by red cells can increase the diffusivity of platelets by 2 to 3 orders of magnitude (38). The diffusion of platelets in response to red cells has been quantified and is a function of the shear rate (36–38):

$$D = \alpha\gamma^n \qquad (48\text{-}14)$$

where $\alpha$ is a proportionality constant and $n$ is a power law constant.

On a reactive surface, such as a damaged vessel wall, both fluid dynamics and reaction kinetics influence mass transport. To solve the mass transfer equations, the mass and the momentum boundary layers must first be evaluated (4,6). These boundary layers indicate the distance from the wall at which the concentration profile (mass boundary layer) or the velocity profile (momentum boundary layer) reaches maximum values. When the Peclet numbers are large, indicating convection forces are dominant, the height of the mass boundary layer is much smaller than the height of the momentum boundary layer. Under these conditions, it can be assumed that within the mass boundary layer the diffusion coefficient is essentially the diffusion coefficient at the wall and the velocity profile is a linear function of the distance from the wall. Applying these two assumptions, equation 48-13, developed for steady state, laminar, Poiseuille flow through a cylindrical tube with constant cross-sectional area, can be solved using the following boundary conditions (4,6):

$$C = C_\infty \text{ at } r \le \delta \qquad (48\text{-}15)$$

$$-D\frac{\partial C}{\partial r} = kC \text{ at } r = R \qquad (48\text{-}16)$$

where $\delta$ is the thickness of the boundary layer, $C_\infty$ is the concentration of the homogeneous reactant outside the boundary layer, and $k$ is the reaction rate constant. The boundary conditions also assume the reaction is first order and the surface does not become saturated or exhibit decreasing reactivity. Evaluation and substitution of these boundary conditions leads to the general solution for the steady state flux ($j$) of platelets at any point on the surface (3,36):

$$j = \left[-D\frac{\partial C}{\partial r}\right]_{r=R} = \frac{C_\infty}{\underbrace{\frac{1}{k}}_{\substack{\text{reaction}\\\text{control}}} + \frac{1.48}{\left(\dfrac{D^2\gamma_w}{2z}\right)^{1/3}}} = \frac{C_\infty}{\dfrac{1}{k} + \dfrac{1.48}{\left(\dfrac{D^2}{2z}\left(\dfrac{4(\nu)}{R}\right)\right)^{1/3}}}$$
$$(48\text{-}17)$$

As shown in equation 48-17, the flux of platelets at any point on the vessel surface is determined by the wall shear rate of the fluid ($\gamma_w$), the axial position ($z$), the reactant concentration in the homogeneous phase outside the boundary layer ($C_\infty$), the reaction rate constant ($k$), and the effective diffusion coefficient ($D$).

To investigate the thrombotic process, it is useful to determine the parameters controlling platelet transport to the surface under three different vascular conditions. The first condition occurs when platelets flow across an intact monolayer of endothelial cells. In this case, the surface is nonthrombogenic and $k \ll D$. Therefore, the flux of platelets at the vessel wall is limited by the reaction kinetics and no longer depends on the axial position or the shear rate:

$$j_z = kC_\infty \qquad (48\text{-}18)$$

The second condition occurs when platelets flow across a mildly reactive surface, $k \simeq D$, and equation 48-17 cannot be simplified. In this circumstance, in order to determine the flux of platelets at the wall, the equations of motion must be solved first. For simple cases, such as steady Poiseuille flow, these solutions can be found analytically. However, when more complex flow regimes are present, the equations of mass transfer must be determined simultaneously with the equations of motion, and an analytical solution is difficult (5,7).

The third condition occurs when platelets flow across a very reactive surface (e.g., exposed subendothelium), $D \ll k$, and the flux is limited by the diffusion of platelets to the surface (6,37):

$$j_z = 0.67C_\infty\left(\frac{D^2\gamma_w}{2z}\right)^{1/3} = 0.67C_\infty\left(\frac{D^2}{2z}\left(\frac{4(\nu)}{R}\right)\right)^{1/3} \quad (48\text{-}19)$$

In this case, flux depends on the shear rate, the axial position, and the effective diffusion coefficient. As shown in equation 48-14, the effective diffusion coefficient of platelets in flowing blood is a function of the shear rate. This indicates that for a given increase in shear rate, platelet flux at the vessel wall will increase by more than $\gamma_w^{1/3}$. The inverse relation between the axial position and the platelet flux is compounded by the depletion of platelets in the mass boundary layer as a result of upstream thrombi growth (39). In addition to platelets, circulating proteins and other soluble compounds that support platelet adhesion and growth of thrombi may become depleted in the mass boundary layer. Platelets partially offset the decrease in the delivery of soluble blood components by secreting activating factors and other necessary compounds that then accumulate downstream of the growing thrombi (40). Despite the presence of these secreted components, the rate of thrombus growth on the thrombogenic components of the subendothelial matrix is decreased in the axial direction (39).

## MODELS OF THROMBOSIS UNDER FLOW

Thrombosis in the vascular system may occur in the bulk fluid phase leading to circulating platelet aggregates or on the vessel wall leading to mural thrombus growth. To identify the molecular mechanisms supporting each type of thrombosis, the dynamic nature of the vascular system must be incorporated into experimental models. This requires the application of engineering principles to develop systems that are physiologically relevant to a number of conditions present in the vascular system.

The platelet aggregometer was one of the first experimental systems developed to study thrombosis occurring in the bulk fluid phase (41). In this system, aggregation in platelet-rich plasma can be monitored over time by measuring light scattering or particle counts. The observed platelet aggregation depends on the addition of chemical agonists to the platelet-rich plasma that induce platelet binding to fibrinogen or von Willebrand factor (VWF) (42–45). Agonists include substances present in the blood, such as adenosine diphosphate (ADP) (41), but nonphysiologic modulators, such as the antibiotic ristocetin (46) or the snake venom botrocetin (43), also induce aggregation, and have been used extensively to study thrombosis. Agitation is required for aggregation to occur, and, therefore, the system can be described as shear-dependent. However, the shear produced by the aggregometer is low and cannot be quantified with certainty owing to the variable flow patterns produced in response to agitation.

In contrast to the aggregometer, rotational viscometers can produce constant and uniform shear stress on all cells and proteins in liquid suspensions, independent of the individual particle location (5). The shear profiles in viscometer systems

are well characterized and can be varied widely to match a number of physiologic and pathologic vascular conditions. Shear stresses high enough to directly induce platelet aggregation can be developed in viscometer systems, so that the addition of chemical agonists is not necessary (47–51). In concentric, or Couette, viscometers, the sample to be investigated is placed between a stationary bob and a rotating outer cylindrical shell (see Fig. 48-5A). In cone-and-plate viscometers, the sample of interest is placed between a rotating cone and a stationary platen (Fig. 48-5B). To study arterial thrombosis, the rotating cone and stationary platen are separated by approximately 25 $\mu$m and the cone angle ranges from 0.3 degree to 1.0 degree. Over the range of shear stresses used to investigate arterial

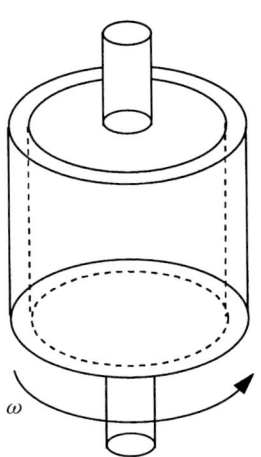

**A**

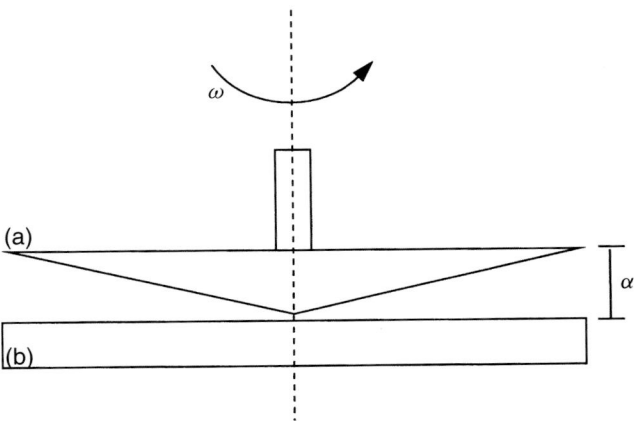

**B**

**FIGURE 48-5.** Schematic of a concentric, or Couette, viscometer (**A**) and cone-and-plate viscometer (**B**). These rotational viscometers can produce a constant and uniform shear stress on cells and proteins in liquid suspensions, independent of the individual particle location. In a Couette viscometer, samples are placed between a stationary bob and a rotating outer cylindrical shell. In a cone-and-plate viscometer, samples are placed between a rotating cone (*a*) and a stationary plate (*b*). The cone angle ($\alpha$) typically ranges from 0.3 to 1.0 degree. The shear stress that particles experience in a cone-and-plate viscometer depends on the cone angle, the rotation rate ($\omega$), and the fluid viscosity (equation 48-20). (Modified from Alevriadou BR, McIntire LV. Rheology. In: Loscalzo J, Schafer AI, eds. *Thrombosis and hemorrhage*. Boston: Blackwell, 1994:369–381; Wang LN, Keller KH. Augmented transport of extracellular solutes in concentrated erythrocyte suspensions in Couette flow. *J Colloid Interface Sci* 1985;103:210–225.)

thrombosis, blood viscosity is constant and the shear stress is varied by changing the shear rate. The shear rate in a cone-and-plate viscometer depends on the cone angle ($\alpha$) and the rotation rate of the cone ($\omega$):

$$\tau = \mu\gamma = \frac{\mu\omega}{\alpha} \qquad (48\text{-}20)$$

The extent of shear-induced platelet aggregation can be determined by directly comparing the number of single platelets in samples before and after exposure to shear (51–53). Additionally, the size of the platelet aggregates formed in response to shear can be quantified (54,55).

Platelet aggregation in the bulk fluid phase can be investigated in viscometer systems using whole blood, platelet-rich plasma, or washed platelet suspensions. The presence of other cellular and protein components will affect platelet function and, therefore, whole blood is particularly useful for studying samples from patients receiving therapeutics (56), recovering from a thrombotic event (57), or both. However, the use of washed platelets is extremely valuable to isolate and investigate distinct molecular mechanisms supporting the thrombotic process. For example, by using washed platelet suspensions in physiologic concentrations, it has been shown that shear stress induces the binding of VWF to the platelet glycoprotein (GP) Ib and GP IIb/IIIa receptors (58). More recently, using dilute suspensions of washed platelets, it has been determined that VWF binding to platelet GP Ib precedes binding to platelet GP IIb/IIIa (59). The cone-and-plate viscometer system can also be used to study cell–surface interactions by immobilizing cells or proteins on the stationary plate. This method has been used to study the response of smooth muscle cells and endothelial cells to shear by quantifying the released compounds and changes in gene expression (60–66).

Cell–surface interactions have also been investigated through the use of flow chambers. In these systems, whole blood or a cell suspension is perfused through the chamber across a surface of immobilized cells or proteins. Parallel plate (67–70), annular (71–75), and tubular (76–78) flow chamber geometries have been developed. The parallel plate flow chamber, consisting of a polycarbonate slab, a silicon gasket, and a glass coverslip, can be used to illustrate the fundamental principles of these systems (see Fig. 48-6). The glass coverslip forms the bottom side of the parallel plate flow chamber and cells or proteins may be immobilized on this surface. The thickness of the silicon gasket determines the height of the gap between the coverslip and the polycarbonate slab. Fluid is pumped across this gap through the chamber. The wall shear stress in the system depends on the height of the gap ($G$), the width of the chamber ($W$), the fluid viscosity ($\mu$), and the volumetric flow rate through the chamber ($Q$) (5,79):

$$\tau_{\omega} = \frac{6Q\mu}{G^2W} \qquad (48\text{-}21)$$

In the range of shear stresses applied to investigate arterial thrombosis, plane Poiseuille flow is developed and the velocity and shear profiles are similar to those shown in Figure 48-1. The use of washed platelets or platelet-rich plasma in flow chambers is limited because the absence of red blood cells considerably changes the mass transfer of platelets to the surface. Therefore, to study platelet-mediated events in arterial thrombosis, whole blood is generally perfused through the chambers across glass coverslips coated with thrombogenic components of the subendothelial matrix, such as collagen or VWF. Significant insight into the molecular mechanisms supporting mural thrombosis, including the roles of fibrinogen and VWF and the platelet receptors GP Ib and GP IIb/IIIa, has been gained through the use of whole blood in flow chambers (73–75,80–85). Distinct pathways in the thrombotic process are commonly investigated by the addition of blocking antibodies or by the use

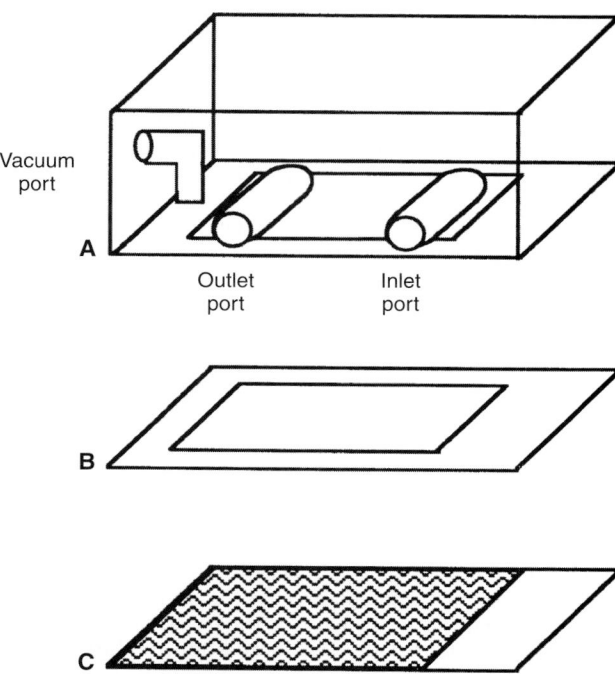

**FIGURE 48-6.** Schematic of a parallel plate flow chamber. The chamber consists of a polycarbonate slab (**A**), a silicon gasket (**B**), and a glass coverslip (**C**) held together by vacuum. The thickness of the silicon gasket determines the height of the gap between the coverslip and the polycarbonate slab. A syringe pump connected to the outlet port draws fluid across this gap through the chamber. The wall shear stress depends on the height of the gap, the width of the chamber, the fluid viscosity, and the flow rate through the chamber (equation 48-21).

of patient blood that is deficient in an individual component. Specific interactions may also be studied by using mammalian cells transfected with only the receptor or ligand of interest (86–88). The transfected cells may be in the fluid suspension, immobilized on the surface, or both. In addition to basic mechanism studies, flow chambers have been used to evaluate the effects of potential or current therapeutic compounds on mural thrombosis from patient samples under arterial shear conditions (89,90).

Both arterial and venous shear conditions can be produced using flow chambers of the same geometry with the only modification required being a change in the volumetric flow rate (equation 48-21). A wide range of laminar shear conditions has been used to study the interactions of platelets and leukocytes with immobilized proteins, endothelial cells, or transfected mammalian cells. Turbulent or complex laminar flow regimes, such as those in regions of stenoses or valves, may be produced by changing the geometry of the chamber or tube to resemble the complex geometry of interest. Under these conditions, the equations of Poiseuille flow (equations 48-1 through 48-10, 48-21) no longer apply.

Endpoint measurements of platelet deposition after perfusion of whole blood through a flow chamber may be measured either by fixing and staining the mural thrombi formed (80,91–94) or by using radiolabeled platelets reconstituted in blood (14,91,93,95,96). Using these methods, the total number of platelets deposited may be evaluated by observing thrombi morphology with light microscopy or by radioactive measurements and imaging. Although these methods provide a snapshot of thrombi growth at a specific point, direct visualization of platelet deposition over time may be determined by combining epifluorescent videomicroscopy and digital image processing (67,70,85,97–99). In this method, platelets are fluorescently labeled before perfusion through the flow chamber. Platelets can be labeled by adding the fluorescent dye mepacrine (100) or fluorescent platelet monoclonal antibodies (101) directly to whole blood. During experiments, the flow chamber is mounted on an inverted-stage microscope equipped with an epifluorescent illumination attachment and a silicon-intensified target video camera connected to a videocassette recorder. Whole blood is pumped through the chamber, and real-time growth of thrombi is recorded on videotape. The video data can be analyzed offline using digital image processing to obtain quantitative values for the number of platelets deposited and the total surface coverage over time (67,97). The use of videomicroscopy and digital image processing can be extended to evaluate the surface interactions with larger cells such as leukocytes and transfected mammalian cells. These larger cells are phase-bright, and fluorescent illumination is not necessary. Leukocytes and transfected mammalian cells in suspensions can be clearly distinguished by phase-contrast microscopy even if the suspensions are perfused over a cell monolayer immobilized on the surface. The mean velocity of rolling platelets or larger cells may be calculated by overlapping sequential digital images obtained from the video data and determining the distance the cells rolled during the period of the image acquisition (102).

# FLOW EFFECTS ON COAGULATION

The coagulation cascade is a complex series of linked enzymatic reactions that support the formation of mural thrombi by producing thrombin and fibrin at sites of vascular injury (103,104). The reactions are catalyzed by complexes composed of circulating proteases and surface-associated protein cofactors. The key regulating enzyme complexes and a number of the reaction products form on phospholipid surfaces (103–105). This surface requirement localizes reactions to certain elements in the subendothelial matrix, as well as membranes of endothelial cells (intact or damaged) and peripheral blood components such as platelets (105,106). The formation of enzyme complexes depends on the delivery of the required circulating protease to the vessel wall where the protein cofactor is immobilized. Under laminar flow conditions, the protease may only reach the wall by radial diffusion. Increasing velocity, and therefore increasing shear, enhances the mass transfer of the protease to the surface (78,105,107). Thrombin production measured in a phospholipid/cofactor-coated capillary tube clearly demonstrates the effects of mass transfer on the formation of surface-bound enzyme complexes in the coagulation cascade (107). The production of thrombin is accelerated by the phospholipid-bound enzyme complex, prothrombinase, formed by circulating factor Xa associating with surface-bound factor Va. In the capillary tube system, the steady state production level of thrombin can be limited by a low concentration of factor Va bound to the phospholipid surface. When factor Va is limiting, increasing the concentration of circulating factor Xa or increasing the shear does not change the final, steady state thrombin production values. However, under these conditions, the time to reach the steady state production values is reduced by increasing the concentration of circulating factor Xa or by increasing the shear rate. These results indicate that shear increases the formation of the prothrombinase complex by increasing the delivery of factor Xa to the surface. When the concentration of the circulating component rather than the surface component is limiting, increasing shear will lead to an increase in steady state production values. In addition to increasing the supply of circulating components to the vessel surface, increasing shear will increase the

removal of species produced at the wall but not bound to the vessel. This may explain the decrease in fibrin deposition on exposed subendothelium observed in response to increasing shear (108). Alternatively, the decrease in fibrin deposition may be attributed to shear-induced secretion of tissue-type plasminogen activator (tPA) by endothelial cells upstream of the wound (109).

# MOLECULAR MECHANISMS OF CELL–SURFACE AND CELL–CELL ADHESION UNDER FLOW

Endothelial cells lining the blood vessels constitute a non-thrombogenic surface over which platelets flow during normal homeostasis. When the endothelium is compromised after angioplasty, atherosclerotic plaque rupture, or other vascular injury, mural thrombi form on the thrombogenic components of the exposed subendothelial matrix. Platelets are transported to the injury site by convection. If platelet transport were the only determinant of thrombi growth, increasing shear would always increase the deposition of platelets. The growth of thrombi on some surface components isolated from the subendothelium is decreased by increasing shear, however, suggesting that the bonds between platelets and these components either are not strong enough to withstand the increasing drag force on the platelet or do not have a fast enough on rate to fully form during the decreased contact time between the cell and the surface. Increasing shear also decreases the local concentration of activating factors produced at the vascular wall, potentially decreasing the total number of platelets deposited. A final explanation for observed inverse relation between shear and growth of thrombi on these surfaces is that shear may change the affinity of platelet–surface interactions by directly affecting the structure of the ligand or the platelet receptor. Dynamic experimental models have been used successfully to determine the molecular mechanisms supporting thrombus formation under the different shear conditions present in the vascular system.

Under arterial shear conditions, VWF is the principal mediator of both initial platelet adhesion to exposed subendothelium and subsequent platelet aggregation on the vessel wall, although fibrinogen and other proteins may also participate (73–75,80,85,92,110–113). VWF is well suited to support platelet adhesion because a single platelet may form multiple bonds to the repeating subunits within the VWF molecule (114). Multiple bonds increase the strength of interaction, potentially allowing the platelet to remain attached to the vessel surface in the presence of high shear forces. Soluble VWF, released into the blood from the $\alpha$-granules of platelets and from the Weibel-Palade bodies of endothelial cells, is rapidly insolubilized on exposed subendothelial matrix (115). Endothelial cells may also secrete VWF directly into the subendothelium (115). Unusually large forms of VWF, not found in plasma but present in platelets and endothelial cells, are most effective in promoting thrombus formation (51). Further research is necessary to fully determine the primary components supporting the binding of soluble VWF to exposed subendothelial matrix, but it has been shown that collagen type I does play a role in the process (116).

The platelet GP Ib/IX/V complex binds immobilized VWF under high shear conditions mediating the initial step of platelet adhesion to the subendothelium of a damaged vessel (see Fig. 48-7) (85,92,110). This result has been demonstrated in flow chambers using patient blood deficient in GP Ib/IX/V (Bernard-Soulier syndrome) (92,110) and normal blood with added monoclonal GP Ib/IX/V antibodies (85). Aggregation to the initial and subsequent layers of platelets on a damaged

Background: thrombosis

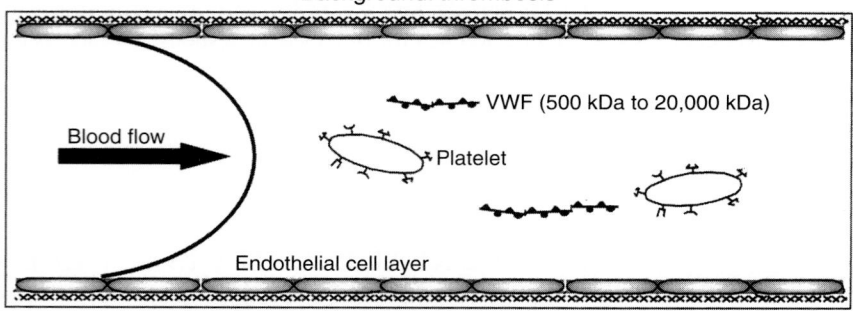

**FIGURE 48-7.** Schematic of platelet adhesion and aggregation on a denuded artery. After platelet activation by shear or chemical stimuli, the platelet receptor glycoprotein (GP) Ib binds von Willebrand factor (VWF) immobilized on collagen present in the subendothelial matrix. GP Ia/IIa (collagen receptor, integrin $\alpha_2\beta_1$) may also be required in the process. Aggregation to the initial and subsequent layers of platelets is mediated primarily by soluble VWF forming bridges between GP IIb/IIIa receptors on adjacent platelets, although other proteins, such as fibrinogen, may also be involved.

arterial wall is mediated by soluble VWF and possibly other proteins such as fibrinogen binding to GP IIb/IIIa complexes on adjacent platelets. This has been demonstrated in flow chambers using patient blood deficient in GP IIb/IIIa (Glanzmann thrombasthenia) (92,110) and normal blood with added monoclonal GP IIb/IIIa antibodies (Fig. 48-7) (85,89,90). Adhesion of platelets to the subendothelial matrix under high shear conditions may also involve platelet GP IIb/IIIa (92,117).

In contrast to thrombosis occurring in high shear conditions, mural thrombus formation under low shear conditions is supported mainly by fibrinogen-platelet rather than by VWF–platelet interactions (118,119). Collagen VI (120) and fibrillin (121) have also been shown to support mural thrombosis under low shear conditions only. Adhesion on these surfaces is supported by the platelet GP IIb/IIIa complex, although other platelet receptors may play a role (122). As with high shear conditions, the platelet GP IIb/IIIa complex is required for subsequent platelet aggregation.

Circulating platelet aggregates form in the presence of elevated shear conditions, such as are found in stenotic vessels, as a direct result of shear-induced platelet activation (47–51). This high shear–induced platelet aggregation depends on VWF binding to GP Ib and GP IIb/IIIa receptors (51,52,85,123). It has been established that calcium influx, platelet activation, and platelet GP Ib–VWF binding precede GP IIb/IIIa–VWF binding (58,59,124,125). Platelet–VWF binding is minimal in the absence of shear. Currently it is unknown whether a change in VWF itself or a change in the platelet complexes enhances VWF–platelet binding under high shear conditions, although evidence suggests the change occurs on the platelet receptors (51). Under low shear conditions ($<12$ dyn per cm$^2$), platelet–VWF binding becomes less important and platelet–fibrinogen binding predominantly supports the observed shear-induced platelet aggregation (126).

Leukocytes, which have been observed to accumulate in atherosclerotic plaques (127,128) and thrombotic clots (129,130) *in vivo*, may amplify the thrombotic process through the release of secretory products that activate platelets, promote vasoconstriction, aggravate endothelial damage, and increase local generation of thrombin and fibrin (131–134). Additionally, the physical presence of leukocytes on mural thrombi may augment the coagulation cascade by providing an assembly site for the prothrombinase complex (135,136). Monocytes may contribute further to the coagulation cascade because these cells express tissue factor after certain types of stimulation (137). The effect of shear on leukocyte adhesion to the vascular surface has been characterized using parallel plate flow chambers (102,138–146). Leukocyte rolling on stimulated, intact endothelium is mediated primarily by selectins, and rolling is optimal at wall shear stresses of 1 to 2 dyn per cm$^2$ (102,141). Under these conditions, firm adhesion (no rolling) of leukocytes to the stimulated endothelial cells requires the formation of integrin bonds (140, 141). At higher shear stresses, the number of rolling leukocytes decreases

rapidly and at 10 dyn per cm$^2$ is nearly zero (102,141). In contrast, P selectin expressed on activated platelet monolayers supports leukocyte rolling at higher levels of shear characteristic of the arterial system (145). Circulating leukocyte-platelet aggregates may also contribute to the vascular response to injury and have been observed to increase in number after percutaneous transluminal coronary angioplasty (133) or cardiopulmonary bypass (147,148). Shear enhances the formation of these circulating aggregates by activating platelets to express P selectin.

It is of interest that unactivated platelets appear to be able to bind to activated endothelium, perhaps through an interaction of GP Ib and endothelial cell P selectin (87). In addition, GP Ib can utilize the I-domain of the leukocyte Mac-1 integrin as a ligand, providing a mechanism for platelet accumulation at the site of activated leukocyte adhesion [see (149) and Fig. 48-8].

# BLOOD FLOW EFFECTS ON VASCULAR WALL FUNCTION

The role of endothelial cells in the vascular system extends beyond providing a simple cover for the thrombogenic components of the subendothelial matrix. Instead, endothelial cells, responding to both chemical and mechanical stimuli, express

Interaction of GP Ibα with Mac-1 and P selectin

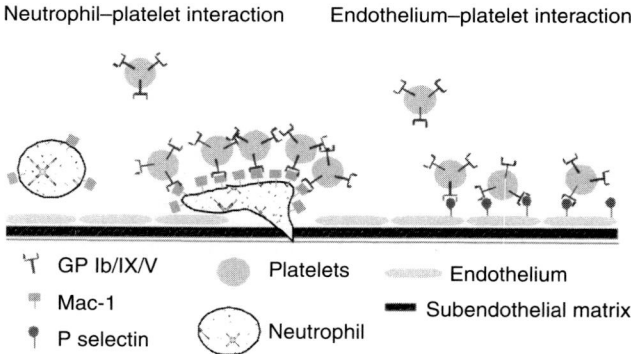

**FIGURE 48-8.** Additional ligands for platelet receptor GP Ib. Unactivated platelets can interact with activated endothelial cells through GP Ib/P selectin interactions or with activated leukocytes at sites of inflammation via GP Ib/Mac-1 binding through the I-domain of the α chain (CD 11b) of Mac-1. This provides another possible direct strong connection between thrombosis and inflammation.

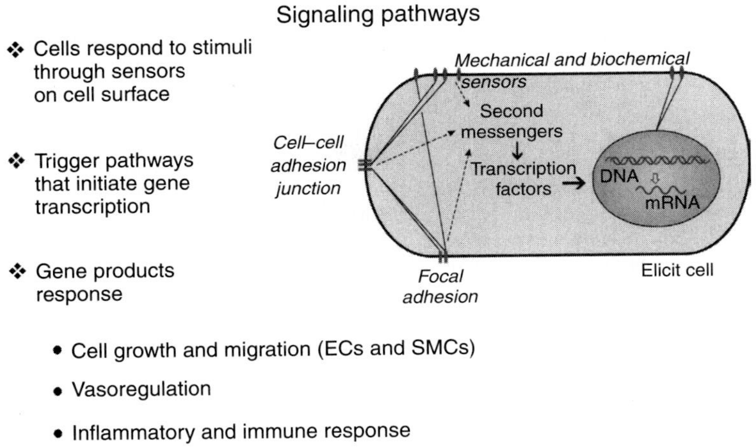

## Signaling pathways

- ❖ Cells respond to stimuli through sensors on cell surface
- ❖ Trigger pathways that initiate gene transcription
- ❖ Gene products response
  - Cell growth and migration (ECs and SMCs)
  - Vasoregulation
  - Inflammatory and immune response

FIGURE 48-9. Some of the possible mechanotransduction pathways in vascular cells. Putative mechanoreceptors on the luminal cell membrane may alter their conformation in response to mechanical stimuli, activating a signal transduction cascade involving diffusible second messengers. The cascade of chemical reactions leads to activation of gene transcription in the nucleus. Alternatively, mechanotransduction may be direct via elements of the cytoskeleton. Forces may be transmitted through these networks from the luminal cell membrane to focal adhesion sites, intracellular junctions, or directly to the nucleus. Translation of the mechanical force to a chemical signal at these sites would then lead to alterations of cell function and gene expression. ECs, endothelial cells; SMCs, smooth muscle cells.

and secrete a wide variety of molecules that regulate thrombosis, fibrinolysis, coagulation reactions, vasoconstriction, and leukocyte adhesion, and recruitment. The mechanical stimuli acting on endothelial cells include tangential, circumferential, and compressive stresses (Fig. 48-4B) (5,6). Circumferential stress is generated primarily by cyclic strain in compliant arterial vessels. Mechanoreceptors on endothelial cells respond to these stresses either by activating signal transducers or by altering the cytoskeletal structure. Mechanical stimuli, propagated through several cascade systems, may ultimately lead to increased gene expression and elevated secretion of molecules (see Fig. 48-9). Parallel plate flow chambers, cone-and-plate viscometers, and other dynamic models have been used to determine the molecular mechanisms that translate mechanical stresses into cellular responses. Both venous and arterial levels of shear stress and strain have been investigated.

Ion channels, G protein–linked receptors, tyrosine kinase receptors, and integrins have been identified as mechanoreceptors although it has not yet been determined if all of these receptors initiate the primary response, or whether some act downstream of additional mechanoreceptors (2). Mechanoresponsive ion channels include a nonselective stretch-responsive ion channel that depolarizes the cell on activation (150). Additionally, at least three shear-responsive ion channels have been identified. Two of the shear-responsive ion channels, an $HCO_3^-/Cl^-$ exchanger and an $Na^+/H^+$ exchanger, acidify the intracellular cytosol within minutes of endothelial cell exposure to shear (151). The third shear-responsive ion channel, a potassium channel, becomes activated within 10 seconds of exposing endothelial cells to shear (152,153). Activation of this potassium channel leads to hyperpolarization of the cell in contrast to the cell depolarization observed in response to cyclic strain. There is some evidence that this potassium channel is linked to a G protein that elevates intracellular guanosine 3',5'-cyclic monophosphate (cGMP) levels in response to shear (154). The presence of other mechanoresponsive G protein–linked receptors is suggested by the shear-induced elevation of the levels of other signal transducers, such as inositol 1,4,5-trisphosphate ($IP_3$) (155,156) and cyclic adenosine 3',5'-monophosphate (cAMP) (157), that are generated by the activation of G proteins. Cyclic strain also elevates the level of the G protein activation–dependent signal transducers, $IP_3$, and diacylglycerol (158,159). Direct shear-induced G protein activation has been observed within 1 second of endothelial cell exposure to shear (160). This fast activation process requires no mechanoreceptor and may be due to shear effects on membrane fluidity (161). The presence of tyrosine kinase mechanoreceptors is suggested by the shear-induced elevation of multiple protein kinases. The major protein kinases activated

by shear stress are extracellular signal-regulated kinase (ERK) 1/2, c-Jun NH$_2$-terminal kinase (JNK), and p38 mitogen-activated protein kinase MAPK/RK (2). Protein kinase C is also responsive to both cyclic strain (159,162) and shear stress (163,164). Integrins, transmembrane glycoproteins that link the cytoskeleton and extracellular adhesion proteins, may also serve as mechanoreceptors and transmit decentralized signals to the cell through the cytoskeleton (2,165). Shear has been shown to enhance the integrin-mediated activation of the MAPK, ERK 1/2 (164,166). Shear also enhances the integrin-mediated phosphorylation of the focal adhesion kinase, which may alter the cytoskeleton and lead to rearrangements of focal adhesion sites, eventually producing changes in the cell shape (166–168). Cytoskeletal changes also regulate the gene expression of a number of proteins, including the urokinase-type plasminogen activator (uPA) that modulates the generation of plasmin and, therefore, affects blood clot dissolution (169).

Changes in cellular pH, production of G protein activation-dependent signal transducers, and stimulation of protein kinases may impact cellular responses by regulating transcription factors that activate or inhibit gene expression by binding to promoter regions within DNA. Two transcription factor families have been shown to be shear-responsive: nuclear factor activator protein-1 (AP-1) and *Rel*-related nuclear factor κB (NFκB). AP-1 can bind cAMP response element (CRE) and tumor-promoting agent response element (TRE) promoter regions of DNA (2). In response to shear, AP-1 binding activity increases fourfold in the first 20 minutes, then falls back to basal levels (170). The shear-induced response of AP-1 is biphasic, however, and after 2 hours of shear exposure, the binding activity of AP-1 is increased substantially relative to both the basal level and the initial burst of activity (170). AP-1 has binding sites on the promoters of many proteins important to thrombosis and vascular wall function, including tPA, plasminogen activator inhibitor 1 (PAI-1), endothelin-1 (ET-1), monocyte chemotactic protein-1 (MCP-1), collagenase, intercellular adhesion molecule-1 (ICAM-1), transforming growth factor-$\beta_1$ (TGF-$\beta_1$), platelet-derived growth factor (PDGF)-A, and PDGF-B (61,171,172). However, only MCP-1 has been shown to depend on shear-induced AP-1/DNA binding (172). Binding of NFκB to DNA increases within 30 minutes of cell exposure to shear and reaches maximum levels of activity in 1 hour (170). Binding sites of NFκB have been identified on vascular cell adhesion molecule-1 (VCAM-1), E selectin, interleukin (IL)-1, IL-6, IL-8, *c*-myc, and tissue factor (173). NFκB has also been shown to interact with a shear stress responsive element (SSRE) in the promoter region in PDGF-B (174). This SSRE is distinct from other DNA binding sites of NFκB and is required for shear-induced elevation of PDGF-B messenger RNA levels in endothelial cells. Promoter regions with identical sequence homology to this SSRE are present on tPA, ICAM-1, and TGF-$\beta_1$, all of which are increased in response to shear (61,174).

Of particular importance to thrombus formation is the increase in tPA messenger RNA level in response to arterial levels of shear (109). Endothelial secretion of tPA also increases by a factor of three after 4 to 6 hours of exposure to arterial, but not venous, levels of shear (109). In contrast, neither arterial nor venous shear levels increase the secretion of the prothrombotic compound, PAI-1 (109). Further illustrating the selective response of endothelial cells to mechanical stimuli are the mechanisms that may support shear-induced vasodilation. Only minutes of arterial shear exposure are required to increase the production of prostacyclin (PGI$_2$), a potent platelet aggregation inhibitor and vasodilator (66,175,176). Within 4 hours, the production of the vasoconstrictor and smooth muscle mitogen, ET-1, decreases (177). Shear-induced vasodilation may also depend on nitric oxide production that increases with increasing shear (64,178–181). The synthesis of several other biomolecules is regulated by shear, including prostaglandin F$_2\alpha$ (182) and fibronectin (183). The response of endothelial cells to cyclic strain differs from their response to shear. Physiologic levels of cyclic strain increase the secretion of PAI-1, whereas the secretion of tPA is unchanged (184,185). Cyclic strain has also been shown to increase the secretion of both ET-1 and PGI$_2$ from endothelial cells (184–186).

Vascular smooth muscle cells also produce and secrete biomolecules in response to mechanical stimuli. Like endothelial cells, vascular smooth muscle cells are continually exposed to circumferential and compressive stresses. Direct smooth muscle cell exposure to tangential shear stress results from deep vessel injuries produced by angioplasty or atherosclerotic plaque rupture. Even in the presence of an intact endothelium, transmural pressure gradients lead to interstitial fluid flow that continuously produces a shear stress on smooth muscle cells under normal physiologic conditions (187). It has been found that either with (188) or without (189,190) an intact endothelium, increasing tangential shear stress reduces the proliferation of smooth muscle cells. Increasing shear also increases smooth muscle cell secretion of tPA, nitric oxide, prostaglandin E$_2$, PGI$_2$, PDGF, and basic fibroblast growth factor (3,189,191–193). The shear-induced release of mitogens may partially inhibit the observed shear-induced decrease in smooth muscle cell growth. Under dynamic conditions, however, it is more likely that mitogens released in high-shear regions will accumulate in low-shear regions downstream and potentiate the higher smooth muscle cell proliferation rates observed in regions of low shear. In addition to the secreted products discussed previously, in response to either shear or cyclic strain, smooth muscle cells release a factor, potentially carbon monoxide, that inhibits the ADP-induced aggregation of platelets (63). Activated smooth muscle cells may also express VCAM-1 and ICAM-1 that support leukocyte–smooth muscle cell binding (194–197). After angioplasty or atherosclerotic plaque rupture, expression of these surface molecules may recruit leukocytes to sites of vascular injury (198). The shear-induced mechanisms that lead to smooth muscle cell expression and secretion of biomolecules remain largely undetermined, but cellular pH may play a role. It has been shown that shear induces alkalinization of smooth muscle cells mediated by an Na$^+$/H$^+$ exchanger (199).

## SUMMARY

The process of thrombosis depends on complex interactions between fluid dynamics, convective mass transfer, reaction kinetics, and cell adhesion. Dynamic experimental models that mimic the local environment *in vivo* have been used successfully to determine the molecular mechanisms supporting thrombus formation under different shear conditions present in the vascular system. Under arterial shear conditions, it has been shown that mural thrombosis requires the binding of VWF to platelet GP Ib and GP IIb/IIIa receptors. Inhibiting these interactions during the onset of thrombosis not only decreases the formation of thrombi but also helps to prevent long-term restenosis of the vessel (200–202). The use of these dynamic models has been extended to investigate how shear modulates endothelial and smooth muscle cell metabolism, smooth muscle cell proliferation, the coagulation cascade, the inflammatory process, and tumor cell metastasis. All of these studies lead to the conclusion that the local rheologic environment can have a profound effect on the molecular mechanisms of thrombosis. Understanding the different molecular mechanisms supporting thrombosis and other vascular processes under different flow conditions will accelerate the development of novel, more potent therapeutic agents.

## ACKNOWLEDGMENTS

This work was supported by the National Institutes of Health Grants No. HL-18672 and HL-70537, and the Robert A. Welch Foundation Grant No. C-938.

## *References*

1. McCormick SM, Eskin SG, McIntire LV, et al. DNA microarray reveals changes in gene expression of shear stressed human umbilical vein endothelial cells. *Proc Natl Acad Sci U S A* 2001;98:8955–8960.
2. Frye SR, Yee A, Eskin SG, et al. cDNA microarray analysis of endothelial cells subjected to cyclic mechanical strain: importance of motion control. *Physiol Genomics* 2005;21:124–130.
3. Feng Y, Yang JH, Huang H, et al. Transcriptional profile of mechanically induced genes in human vascular smooth muscle cells. *Circ Res* 1999;85:1118–1123.
4. Goldsmith HL, Turitto VT. Rheological aspects of thrombosis and haemostasis: basic principles and applications. ICTH-Report—Subcommittee on Rheology of the International Committee on Thrombosis and Haemostasis. *Thromb Haemost* 1986;55:415–435.
5. McIntire LV, Yee A, Eskin SG. Mechanical forces on cells. In: Ratner BD, Hoffman AS, Schoen FS, eds. *Biomaterials science*. Amsterdam: Elsevier Academic Press, 2004:282–291.
6. Kao SH, McIntire LV. Rheology. In: Loscalzo J, Schafer AI, eds. *Thrombosis and hemorrhage*. Boston, MA: Lippincott Williams & Wilkins, 2002:294–314.
7. Levich VG. *Physicochemical hydrodynamics*. Englewood Cliffs, NJ: Prentice-Hall, 1962.
8. Back LH, Liem TK, Kwack EY, et al. Flow measurements in a highly curved atherosclerotic coronary artery cast of man. *J Biomech Eng* 1992;114:232–240.
9. Motomiya M, Karino T. Flow patterns in the human carotid artery bifurcation. *Stroke* 1984;15:50–56.
10. Karino T, Motomiya M. Flow visualization in isolated transparent natural blood vessels. *Biorheology* 1983;20:119–127.
11. Karino T, Goldsmith HL, Motomiya M, et al. Flow patterns in vessels of simple and complex geometries. *Ann N Y Acad Sci* 1987;516:422–441.
12. Glagov S, Zarins C, Giddens DP, et al. Hemodynamics and atherosclerosis. Insights and perspectives gained from studies of human arteries. *Arch Pathol Lab Med* 1988;112:1018–1031.
13. Ku DN, Giddens DP, Zarins CK, et al. Pulsatile flow and atherosclerosis in the human carotid bifurcation. Positive correlation between plaque location and low oscillating shear stress. *Arteriosclerosis* 1985;5:293–302.
14. Badimon L, Badimon JJ. Mechanisms of arterial thrombosis in nonparallel streamlines: platelet thrombi grow on the apex of stenotic severely injured vessel wall. Experimental study in the pig model. *J Clin Invest* 1989;84:1134–1144.
15. Zarins CK, Giddens DP, Bharadvaj BK, et al. Carotid bifurcation atherosclerosis. Quantitative correlation of plaque localization with flow velocity profiles and wall shear stress. *Circ Res* 1983;53:502–514.
16. Karino T, Goldsmith HL. Adhesion of human platelets to collagen on the walls distal to a tubular expansion. *Microvasc Res* 1979;17:238–262.
17. Karino T, Goldsmith HL. Role of blood cell-wall interactions in thrombogenesis and atherogenesis: a microrheological study. *Biorheology* 1984;21:587–601.

18. Packham MA, Rowsell HC, Jorgensen L, et al. Localized protein accumulation in the wall of the aorta. *Exp Mol Pathol* 1967;7:214–232.
19. Merrill EW. Rheology of blood. *Physiol Rev* 1969;49:863–888.
20. Merrill EW, Benis AM, Gilliland ER, et al. Pressure-flow relations of human blood in hollow fibers at low flow rates. *J Appl Physiol* 1965;20:954–967.
21. Cokelet GR, Merrill EW, Gilliland ER, et al. The rheology of human blood-measurement near and at zero shear rate. *Trans Soc Rheol* 1963;7:303–317.
22. Copley AL, Huang CR, King RG. Rheogoniometric studies of whole human blood at shear rates from 1000 to 0.0009 sec–1. I. Experimental findings. *Biorheology* 1973;10:17–22.
23. Copley AL, Huang CR, King RG. Rheogoniometric studies of whole human blood at shear rates down to 0.0009 sec–1. II. Mathematical interpretation. *Biorheology* 1973;10:23–28.
24. Schmid-Schonbein H, Gaehtgens P, Hirsch H. On the shear rate dependence of red cell aggregation *in vitro*. *J Clin Invest* 1968;47:1447–1454.
25. Brenner H, Bungay PM. Rigid-particle and liquid-droplet models of red cell motion in capillary tubes. *Fed Proc* 1971;30:1565–1577.
26. Brenner H. Pressure drop due to motion of neutrally buoyant particles in duct flows. *J Fluid Mech* 1970;43:641–660.
27. Brunn PO. The deformation of a viscous particle surrounded by an elastic shell in a general time-dependent linear flow field. *J Fluid Mech* 1983;126:533–544.
28. Fahraeus R. The suspension stability of the blood. *Physiol Rev* 1929; IX:241–274.
29. Usami S, King RG, Chien S, et al. Microcinephotographic studies on red cell aggregation in steady and oscillatory shear—a note. *Biorheology* 1975;12:323–325.
30. Copley AL, King RG, Chien S, et al. Microscopic observations of viscoelasticity of human blood in steady and oscillatory shear. *Biorheology* 1975;12:257–263.
31. Goldsmith HL. Red cell motions and wall interactions in tube flow. *Fed Proc* 1971;30:1578–1590.
32. Goldsmith HL. Microscopic flow properties of red cells. *Fed Proc* 1967;26:1813–1820.
33. Goldman AJ, Cox RG, Brenner H. Slow viscous motion of a sphere parallel to a plane wall—II. Couette flow. *Chem Eng Sci* 1967;22:653–660.
34. Tözeren A, Skalak R. Stress in a suspension near rigid boundaries. *J Fluid Mech* 1977;82:289–307.
35. Schmid-Schonbein GW, Skalak R, Simon SI, et al. The interaction between leukocytes and endothelium *in vivo*. *Ann N Y Acad Sci* 1987;516:348–361.
36. Grabowski EF, Friedman LI, Leonard EF. Effects of shear rate on the diffusion and adhesion of blood platelets to a foreign surface. *Ind Eng Chem Fundam* 1972;11:224–232.
37. Turitto VT, Baumgartner HR. Platelet deposition on subendothelium exposed to flowing blood: mathematical analysis of physical parameters. *Trans Am Soc Artif Intern Organs* 1975;21:593–601.
38. Wang LN, Keller KH. Augmented transport of extracellular solutes in concentrated erythrocyte suspensions in Couette flow. *J Colloid Interface Sci* 1985;103:210–225.
39. Sakariassen KS, Weiss HJ, Baumgartner HR. Upstream thrombus growth impairs downstream thrombogenesis in non-anticoagulated blood: effect of procoagulant artery subendothelium and non-procoagulant collagen. *Thromb Haemost* 1991;65:596–600.
40. Hubbell JA, McIntire LV. Platelet active concentration profiles near growing thrombi. A mathematical consideration. *Biophys J* 1986;50:937–945.
41. Born GV. Aggregation of blood platelets by adenosine diphosphate and its reversal. *Nature* 1962;194:927.
42. Fujimoto T, Hawiger J. Adenosine diphosphate induces binding of von Willebrand factor to human platelets. *Nature* 1982;297:154–156.
43. Read MS, Shermer RW, Brinkhous KM. Venom coagglutinin: an activator of platelet aggregation dependent on von Willebrand factor. *Proc Natl Acad Sci U S A* 1978;75:4514–4518.
44. Kao KJ, Pizzo SV, McKee PA. Demonstration and characterization of specific binding sites for factor VIII/von Willebrand factor on human platelets. *J Clin Invest* 1979;63:656–664.
45. Moake JL, Olson JD, Troll JH, et al. Binding of radioiodinated human von Willebrand factor to Bernard-Soulier, thrombasthenic and von Willebrand's disease platelets. *Thromb Res* 1980;19:21–27.
46. Howard MA, Firkin BG. Ristocetin—a new tool in the investigation of platelet aggregation. *Thromb Diath Haemorrh* 1971;26:362–369.
47. Brown CH, Leverett LB, Lewis CW, et al. Morphological, biochemical, and functional changes in human platelets subjected to shear stress. *J Lab Clin Med* 1975;86:462–471.
48. Belval T, Hellums JD, Solis RT. The kinetics of platelet aggregation induced by fluid-shearing stress. *Microvasc Res* 1984;28:279.
49. Fukuyama M, Sakai K, Itagaki I, et al. Continuous measurement of shear-induced platelet aggregation. *Thromb Res* 1989;54:253–260.
50. Giorgio TD, Hellums JD. A cone and plate viscometer for the continuous measurement of blood platelet activation. *Biorheology* 1988;25:605–624.
51. Moake JL, Turner NA, Stathopoulos NA, et al. Involvement of large plasma von Willebrand factor (VWF) multimers and unusually large VWF forms derived from endothelial cells in shear stress-induced platelet aggregation. *J Clin Invest* 1986;78:1456–1461.
52. Moake JL, Turner NA, Stathopoulos NA, et al. Shear-induced platelet aggregation can be mediated by VWF released from platelets, as well as by exogenous large or unusually large VWF multimers, requires adenosine diphosphate, and is resistant to aspirin. *Blood* 1988;71:1366–1374.
53. Konstantopoulos K, Wu KK, Udden MM, et al. Flow cytometric studies of platelet responses to shear stress in whole blood. *Biorheology* 1995;32:73–93.
54. Dewitz TS, Martin RR, Solis RT, et al. Microaggregate formation in whole blood exposed to shear stress. *Microvasc Res* 1978;16:263–271.
55. Jen CJ, McIntire LV. Characteristics of shear-induced aggregation in whole blood. *J Lab Clin Med* 1984;103:115–124.
56. Konstantopoulos K, Kamat SG, Schafer AI, et al. Shear-induced platelet aggregation is inhibited by *in vivo* infusion of an anti-glycoprotein IIb/IIIa antibody fragment, c7E3 Fab, in patients undergoing coronary angioplasty. *Circulation* 1995;91:1427–1431.
57. Konstantopoulos K, Grotta JC, Sills C, et al. Shear-induced platelet aggregation in normal subjects and stroke patients. *Thromb Haemost* 1995;74:1329–1334.
58. McCrary JK, Nolasco LH, Hellums JD, et al. Direct demonstration of radio-labeled von Willebrand factor binding to platelet glycoprotein Ib and IIb-IIIa in the presence of shear stress. *Ann Biomed Eng* 1995;23:787–793.
59. Konstantopoulos K, Chow TW, Turner NA, et al. Shear stress-induced binding of von Willebrand factor to platelets. *Biorheology* 1997;34:57–71.
60. Panaro NJ, McIntire LV. Flow and shear stress effects on endothelial cell function. In: Sumpio BE, ed. *Hemodynamic forces and vascular cell biology*. Georgetown, TX: R.G. Landes Company, 1993:47–65.
61. Malek AM, Izumo S. Control of endothelial cell gene expression by flow. *J Biomech* 1995;28:1515–1528.
62. Resnick N, Gimbrone MA Jr. Hemodynamic forces are complex regulators of endothelial gene expression. *FASEB J* 1995;9:874–882.
63. Wagner CT, Durante W, Christodoulides N, et al. Hemodynamic forces induce the expression of heme oxygenase in cultured vascular smooth muscle cells. *J Clin Invest* 1997;100:589–596.
64. Malek AM, Izumo S, Alper SL. Modulation by pathophysiological stimuli of the shear stress-induced up-regulation of endothelial nitric oxide synthase expression in endothelial cells. *Neurosurgery* 1998;45:334–344.
65. Matsumoto Y, Kawai Y, Watanabe K, et al. Fluid shear stress attenuates tumor necrosis factor-alpha-induced tissue factor expression in cultured human endothelial cells. *Blood* 1998;91:4164–4172.
66. Okahara K, Sun B, Kambayashi J. Upregulation of prostacyclin synthesis-related gene expression by shear stress in vascular endothelial cells. *Arterioscler Thromb Vasc Biol* 1998;18:1922–1926.
67. Hubbell JA, McIntire LV. Technique for visualization and analysis of mural thrombogenesis. *Rev Sci Instrum* 1986;57:892.
68. Muggli R, Baumgartner HR, Tschopp TB, et al. Automated microdensitometry and protein assays as a measure for platelet adhesion and aggregation on collagen-coated slides under controlled flow conditions. *J Lab Clin Med* 1980;95:195–207.
69. Sakariassen KS, Aarts PA, de Groot PG, et al. A perfusion chamber developed to investigate platelet interaction in flowing blood with human vessel wall cells, their extracellular matrix, and purified components. *J Lab Clin Med* 1983;102:522–535.
70. Folie BJ, McIntire LV, Lasslo A. Effects of a novel antiplatelet agent in mural thrombogenesis on collagen-coated glass. *Blood* 1988;72:1393–1400.
71. Baumgartner HR, Haudenschild C. Adhesion of platelets to subendothelium. *Ann N Y Acad Sci* 1972;27:22–36.
72. Anderson GH, Hellums JD, Moake J, et al. Platelet response to shear stress: changes in serotonin uptake, serotonin release, and ADP induced aggregation. *Thromb Res* 1978;13:1039–1047.
73. Weiss HJ, Turitto VT, Baumgartner HR. Effect of shear rate on platelet interaction with subendothelium in citrated and native blood. I. Shear rate-dependent decrease of adhesion in von Willebrand's disease and the Bernard-Soulier syndrome. *J Lab Clin Med* 1978;92:750–764.
74. Weiss HJ, Baumgartner HR, Tschopp TB, et al. Correction by factor VIII of the impaired platelet adhesion to subendothelium in von Willebrand disease. *Blood* 1978;51:267–279.
75. Tschopp TB, Weiss HJ, Baumgartner HR. Decreased adhesion of platelets to subendothelium in von Willebrand's disease. *J Lab Clin Med* 1974;83:296–300.
76. Badimon L, Turitto V, Rosemark JA, et al. Characterization of a tubular flow chamber for studying platelet interaction with biologic and prosthetic materials: deposition of indium 111-labeled platelets on collagen, subendothelium, and expanded polytetrafluoroethylene. *J Lab Clin Med* 1987;110:706–718.
77. Bell DN, Spain S, Goldsmith HL. Adenosine diphosphate-induced aggregation of human platelets in flow through tubes. I. Measurement of concentration and size of single platelets and aggregates. *Biophys J* 1989;56:817–828.
78. Gemmell CH, Turitto VT, Nemerson Y. Flow as a regulator of the activation of factor X by tissue factor. *Blood* 1988;72:1404–1406.
79. Slack SM, Turitto VT. Flow chambers and their standardization for use in studies of thrombosis. On behalf of the Subcommittee on Rheology of the Scientific and Standardization Committee of the ISTH. *Thromb Haemost* 1994;72:777–781.
80. Baumgartner HR, Tschopp TB, Meyer D. Shear rate–dependent inhibition of platelet adhesion and aggregation on collagenous surfaces by antibodies to human factor VIII/von Willebrand factor. *Br J Haematol* 1980;44:127–139.

81. Sixma JJ, Sakariassen KS, Beeser-Visser NH, et al. Adhesion of platelets to human artery subendothelium: effect of factor VIII-von Willebrand factor of various multimeric composition. *Blood* 1984;63:128–139.

82. Li F, Moake JL, McIntire LV. Characterization of von Willebrand interaction with collagens using surface plasmon resonance. *Ann Biomed Eng* 2002;30:1107–1116.

83. Turitto VT, Weiss HJ, Baumgartner HR. Platelet interaction with rabbit subendothelium in von Willebrand's disease: altered thrombus formation distinct from defective platelet adhesion. *J Clin Invest* 1984;74:1730–1741.

84. Turitto VT, Weiss HJ, Zimmerman TS, et al. Factor VIII/ von Willebrand factor in subendothelium mediates platelet adhesion. *Blood* 1985;65:823–831.

85. Alevriadou BR, Moake JL, Turner NA, et al. Real-time analysis of shear-dependent thrombus formation and its blockade by inhibitors of von Willebrand factor binding to platelets. *Blood* 1993;81:1263–1276.

86. Fredrickson BJ, Dong JF, McIntire LV, et al. Shear-dependent rolling on von Willebrand factor of mammalian cells expressing the platelet glycoprotein Ib-IX-V complex. *Blood* 1998;15:3684–3693.

87. Romo GM, Dong JF, Schade AJ, et al. The glycoprotein Ib-IX-V complex is a platelet counter receptor for P-selectin. *J Exp Med* 1999;190:803–814.

88. Kumar RA, Dong JF, Thaggard JA, et al. Kinetics of GP Ib-vWF-A1 tether bond formation under flow: effect of GP Ib mutations on the association and dissociation rates. *Biophys J* 2003;85:4099–4109.

89. Turner NA, Moake JL, Kamat SG, et al. Comparative real-time effects on platelet adhesion and aggregation under flowing conditions of *in vivo* aspirin, heparin, and monoclonal antibody fragment against glycoprotein IIb-IIIa. *Circulation* 1995;91:1354–1362.

90. Fredrickson BJ, Turner NA, Kleinman NS, et al. Effects of Abciximab, Ticlopidine and combined therapy on platelet and leukocyte function in patients undergoing coronary angioplasty. *Circulation* 2000;101:1122–1129.

91. Sixma JJ, Nievelstein PF, Houdijk WP, et al. Adhesion of blood platelets to isolated components of the vessel wall. *Ann N Y Acad Sci* 1987;509:103–117.

92. Weiss HJ, Turitto VT, Baumgartner HR. Platelet adhesion and thrombus formation on subendothelium in platelets deficient in glycoproteins IIb-IIIa, Ib, and storage granules. *Blood* 1986;67:322–330.

93. Sakariassen KS, Fressinaud E, Girma JP, et al. Mediation of platelet adhesion to fibrillar collagen in flowing blood by a proteolytic fragment of human von Willebrand factor. *Blood* 1986;67:1515–1518.

94. Sakariassen KS, Fressinaud E, Girma JP, et al. Role of platelet membrane glycoproteins and von Willebrand factor in adhesion of platelets to subendothelium and collagen. *Ann N Y Acad Sci* 1987;516:52–65.

95. Hanson SR, Kotze HF, Savage B, et al. Platelet interactions with Dacron vascular grafts. A model of acute thrombosis in baboons. *Arteriosclerosis* 1985;5:595–603.

96. Fressinaud E, Baruch D, Girma JP, et al. von Willebrand factor-mediated platelet adhesion to collagen involves platelet membrane glycoprotein IIb-IIIa as well as glycoprotein Ib. *J Lab Clin Med* 1988;112:58–67.

97. Hubbell JA, McIntire LV. Visualization and analysis of mural thrombogenesis on collagen, polyurethane and nylon. *Biomaterials* 1986;7:354–363.

98. Folie BJ, McIntire LV. Mathematical analysis of mural thrombogenesis. Concentration profiles of platelet-activating agents and effects of viscous shear flow. *Biophys J* 1989;56:1121–1141.

99. Owens CK, McIntire LV, Lasslo A. Inhibition of mural thrombus formation by novel nipecotoylpiperazine antiplatelet agents. *Biochim Biophys Acta* 1990;1052:351–359.

100. Dise CA, Burch JW, Goodman DB. Direct interaction of mepacrine with erythrocyte and platelet membrane phospholipid. *J Biol Chem* 1982;257:4701–4704.

101. Grabowski EF. Platelet aggregation in flowing blood at a site of injury to an endothelial cell monolayer: quantitation and real-time imaging with the TAB monoclonal antibody. *Blood* 1990;75:390–398.

102. Jones DA, Abbassi O, McIntire LV, et al. P-selectin mediates neutrophil rolling on histamine-stimulated endothelial cells. *Biophys J* 1993;65:1560–1569.

103. Jackson CM, Nemerson Y. Blood coagulation. *Annu Rev Biochem* 1980;49:765–811.

104. Mann KG, Jenny RJ, Krishnaswamy S. Cofactor proteins in the assembly and expression of blood clotting enzyme complexes. *Annu Rev Biochem* 1988;57:915–956.

105. Nemerson Y, Turitto VT. The effect of flow on hemostasis and thrombosis. *Thromb Haemost* 1991;66:272–276.

106. Mann KG, Nesheim ME, Church WR, et al. Surface-dependent reactions of the vitamin K-dependent enzyme complexes. *Blood* 1990;76:1–16.

107. Schoen P, Lindhout T, Willems G, et al. Continuous flow and the prothrombinase-catalyzed activation of prothrombin. *Thromb Haemost* 1990;64:542–547.

108. Weiss HJ, Turitto VT, Baumgartner HR. Role of shear rate and platelets in promoting fibrin formation on rabbit subendothelium. Studies utilizing patients with quantitative and qualitative platelet defects. *J Clin Invest* 1986;78:1072–1082.

109. Diamond SL, Eskin SG, McIntire LV. Fluid flow stimulates tissue plasminogen activator secretion by cultured human endothelial cells. *Science* 1989;243:1483–1485.

110. Sakariassen KS, Nievelstein PF, Coller BS, et al. The role of platelet membrane glycoproteins Ib and IIb-IIIa in platelet adherence to human artery subendothelium. *Br J Haematol* 1986;63:681–691.

111. Sakariassen KS, Bolhuis PA, Sixma JJ. Human blood platelet adhesion to artery subendothelium is mediated by factor VIII-von Willebrand factor bound to the subendothelium. *Nature* 1979;279:636–638.

112. Bolhuis PA, Sakariassen KS, Sander HJ, et al. Binding of factor VIII-von Willebrand factor to human arterial subendothelium precedes increased platelet adhesion and enhances platelet spreading. *J Lab Clin Med* 1981;97:568–576.

113. Polanowska-Grabowska R, Simon CG Jr, Gear AR. Platelet adhesion to collagen type I, collagen type IV, von Willebrand factor, fibronectin, laminin and fibrinogen: rapid kinetics under shear. *Thromb Haemost* 1999;81:118–123.

114. Ruggeri ZM, Ware J. The structure and function of von Willebrand factor. *Thromb Haemost* 1992;67:594–599.

115. Ruggeri ZM. von Willebrand factor. *J Clin Invest* 1997;99:559–564.

116. van Zanten GH, de Graaf S, Slootweg PJ, et al. Increased platelet deposition on atherosclerotic coronary arteries. *J Clin Invest* 1994;93:615–632.

117. Savage B, Almus-Jacobs F, Ruggeri ZM. Specific synergy of multiple substrate-receptor interactions in platelet thrombus formation under flow. *Cell* 1998;94:657–666.

118. Zaidi TN, McIntire LV, Farrell DH, et al. Adhesion of platelets to surface-bound fibrinogen under flow. *Blood* 1996;88:2967–2972.

119. Savage B, Saldivar E, Ruggeri ZM. Initiation of platelet adhesion by arrest onto fibrinogen or translocation on von Willebrand factor. *Cell* 1996;84:289–297.

120. Ross JM, McIntire LV, Moake JL, et al. Platelet adhesion and aggregation on human type VI collagen surfaces under physiological flow conditions. *Blood* 1995;85:1826–1835.

121. Ross JM, McIntire LV, Moake JL, et al. Fibrillin containing elastic microfibrils support platelet adhesion under dynamic shear conditions. *Thromb Haemost* 1998;91:155–161.

122. Ross JM, McIntire LV. Molecular mechanisms of mural thrombosis under dynamic flow conditions. *News Physiol Sci* 1995;10:117–122.

123. Peterson DM, Stathopoulos NA, Giorgio TD, et al. Shear-induced platelet aggregation requires von Willebrand factor and platelet membrane glycoproteins Ib and IIb-IIIa. *Blood* 1987;69:625–628.

124. Chow TW, Hellums JD, Moake JL, et al. Shear stress-induced von Willebrand factor binding to platelet glycoprotein Ib initiates calcium influx associated with aggregation. *Blood* 1992;80:113–120.

125. Ikeda Y, Handa M, Kamata T, et al. Transmembrane calcium influx associated with von Willebrand factor binding to GP Ib in the initiation of shear-induced platelet aggregation. *Thromb Haemost* 1993;69:496–502.

126. Ikeda Y, Handa M, Kawano K, et al. The role of von Willebrand factor and fibrinogen in platelet aggregation under varying shear stress. *J Clin Invest* 1991;87:1234–1240.

127. Jonasson L, Holm J, Skalli O, et al. Regional accumulations of T cells, macrophages, and smooth muscle cells in the human atherosclerotic plaque. *Arteriosclerosis* 1986;6:131–138.

128. Tsukada T, Rosenfeld M, Ross R, et al. Immunocytochemical analysis of cellular components in atherosclerotic lesions. Use of monoclonal antibodies with the Watanabe and fat-fed rabbit. *Arteriosclerosis* 1986;6:601–613.

129. Palabrica T, Lobb R, Furie BC, et al. Leukocyte accumulation promoting fibrin deposition is mediated *in vivo* by P-selectin on adherent platelets. *Nature* 1992;359:848–851.

130. Baumgartner HR. The role of blood flow in platelet adhesion, fibrin deposition, and formation of mural thrombi. *Microvasc Res* 1973;5:167–179.

131. Ikeda H, Nakayama H, Oda T, et al. Neutrophil activation after percutaneous transluminal coronary angioplasty. *Am Heart J* 1994;128:1091–1098.

132. De Servi S, Mazzone A, Ricevuti G, et al. Granulocyte activation after coronary angioplasty in humans. *Circulation* 1990;82:140–146.

133. Mickelson JK, Lakkis NM, Villarreal-Levy G, et al. Leukocyte activation with platelet adhesion after coronary angioplasty: a mechanism for recurrent disease? *J Am Coll Cardiol* 1996;28:345–353.

134. Ricevuti G, Mazzone A, Pasotti D, et al. Role of granulocytes in endothelial injury in coronary heart disease in humans. *Atherosclerosis* 1991;91:1–14.

135. Tracy PB, Eide LL, Mann KG. Human prothrombinase complex assembly and function on isolated peripheral blood cell populations. *J Biol Chem* 1985;260:2119–2124.

136. Tracy PB, Rohrbach MS, Mann KG. Functional prothrombinase complex assembly on isolated monocytes and lymphocytes. *J Biol Chem* 1983;258:7264–7267.

137. Prydz H, Allison AC. Tissue thromboplastin activity of isolated human monocytes. *Thromb Haemost* 1978;39:582–591.

138. Jones DA, Smith CW, McIntire LV. Leucocyte adhesion under flow conditions: principles important in tissue engineering. *Biomaterials* 1996;17:337–347.

139. Jones DA, McIntire LV, Smith CW, et al. A two-step adhesion cascade for T cell/endothelial cell interactions under flow conditions. *J Clin Invest* 1994;94:2443–2450.

140. Jones DA, Smith CW, McIntire LV. Flow effects on leukocyte adhesion to vascular endothelium. In: Richardson PD, Steiner M, eds. *Principles of cell adhesion*. Boca Raton, FL: CRC Press Inc, 1995:143–160.

141. Lawrence MB, Springer TA. Leukocytes roll on a selectin at physiologic flow rates: distinction from and prerequisite for adhesion through integrins. *Cell* 1991;65:859–873.

142. Kukreti S, Konstantopoulos K, Smith CW, et al. Molecular mechanisms of monocyte adhesion to interleukin-1 beta-stimulated endothelial cells under physiologic flow conditions. *Blood* 1997;89:4104–4111.

143. Moore KL, Patel KD, Bruehl RE, et al. P-selectin glycoprotein ligand-1 mediates rolling of human neutrophils on P-selectin. *J Cell Biol* 1995;128:661–671.

144. Kirchhofer D, Riederer MA, Baumgartner HR. Specific accumulation of circulating monocytes and polymorphonuclear leukocytes on platelet thrombi in a vascular injury model. *Blood* 1997;89:1270–1278.

145. Kuijper PH, Gallardo Torres HI, van der Linden JA, et al. Platelet-dependent primary hemostasis promotes selectin-and integrin-mediated neutrophil adhesion to damaged endothelium under flow conditions. *Blood* 1996;87:3271–3281.

146. Lalor P, Nash GB. Adhesion of flowing leucocytes to immobilized platelets. *Br J Haematol* 1995;89:725–732.

147. Rinder CS, Gaal D, Student LA, et al. Platelet-leukocyte activation and modulation of adhesion receptors in pediatric patients with congenital heart disease undergoing cardiopulmonary bypass. *J Thorac Cardiovasc Surg* 1994;107:280–288.

148. Rinder CS, Bonan JL, Rinder HM, et al. Cardiopulmonary bypass induces leukocyte-platelet adhesion. *Blood* 1992;79:1201–1205.

149. Simon DI, Chen Z, Li CQ, et al. Platelet glycoprotein Iba is a counter receptor for the leukocyte integrin Mac-1 (CD11b/CD18). *J Exp Med* 2000;192:193–204.

150. Lansman JB, Hallam TJ, Rink TJ. Single stretch-activated ion channels in vascular endothelial cells as mechanotransducers? *Nature* 1987;325:811–813.

151. Ziegelstein RC, Cheng L, Capogrossi MC. Flow-dependent cytosolic acidification of vascular endothelial cells. *Science* 1992;258:656–659.

152. Olesen SP, Clapham DE, Davies PF. Haemodynamic shear stress activates a K+ current in vascular endothelial cells. *Nature* 1988;331:168–170.

153. Alevriadou BR, Eskin SG, McIntire LV, et al. Effect of shear stress on 86Rb+ efflux from calf pulmonary artery endothelial cells. *Ann Biomed Eng* 1993;21:1–7.

154. Ohno M, Gibbons GH, Dzau VJ, et al. Shear stress elevates endothelial cGMP. Role of a potassium channel and G protein coupling. *Circulation* 1993;88:193–197.

155. Nollert MU, Eskin SG, McIntire LV. Shear stress increases inositol trisphosphate levels in human endothelial cells. *Biochem Biophys Res Commun* 1990;170:281–287.

156. Nollert MU, Diamond SL, McIntire LV. Hydrodynamic shear stress and mass transport modulation of endothelial cell metabolism. *Biotechnol Bioeng* 1991;38:588–602.

157. Reich KM, Gay CV, Frangos JA. Fluid shear stress as a mediator of osteoblast cyclic adenosine monophosphate production. *J Cell Physiol* 1990;143:100–104.

158. Rosales OR, Sumpio BE. Changes in cyclic strain increase inositol trisphosphate and diacylglycerol in endothelial cells. *Am J Physiol* 1992;262:C956–C962.

159. Isales C, Rosales O, Sumpio BE. Mediators and mechanisms of cyclic strain and shear stress-induced vascular responses. In: Sumpio BE, ed. *Hemodynamic forces and vascular cell biology*. Georgetown, TX: R.G. Landes Company, 1993:90–115.

160. Gudi SR, Clark CB, Frangos JA. Fluid flow rapidly activates G proteins in human endothelial cells. Involvement of G proteins in mechanochemical signal transduction. *Circ Res* 1996;79:834–839.

161. Berthiaume F, Frangos JA. Fluid flow increases membrane permeability to merocyanine 540 in human endothelial cells. *Biochim Biophys Acta* 1994;1191:209–218.

162. Rosales OR, Sumpio BE. Protein kinase C is a mediator of the adaptation of vascular endothelial cells to cyclic strain *in vitro*. *Surgery* 1992;112:459–466.

163. Hsieh HJ, Li NQ, Frangos JA. Shear-induced platelet-derived growth factor gene expression in human endothelial cells is mediated by protein kinase C. *J Cell Physiol* 1992;150:552–558.

164. Takahashi M, Berk BC. Mitogen-activated protein kinase (ERK1/ 2) activation by shear stress and adhesion in endothelial cells. *J Clin Invest* 1996;98:2623–2631.

165. Davies PF. Flow-mediated endothelial mechanotransduction. *Physiol Rev* 1995;75:519–560.

166. Ishida T, Peterson TE, Kovach NL, et al. MAP kinase activation by flow in endothelial cells. Role of beta 1 integrins and tyrosine kinases. *Circ Res* 1996;79:310–316.

167. Berk BC, Corson MA, Peterson TE, et al. Protein kinases as mediators of fluid shear stress stimulated signal transduction in endothelial cells: a hypothesis for calcium-dependent and calcium-independent events activated by flow. *J Biomech* 1995;28:1439–1450.

168. Malek AM, Izumo S. Mechanism of endothelial cell shape change and cytoskeletal remodeling in response to fluid shear stress. *J Cell Sci* 1996;109:713–726.

169. Botteri FM, Ballmer-Hofer K, Rajput B, et al. Disruption of cytoskeletal structures results in the induction of the urokinase-type plasminogen activator gene expression. *J Biol Chem* 1990;265:13327–13334.

170. Lan Q, Mercurius KO, Davies PF. Stimulation of transcription factors NF kappa B and AP1 in endothelial cells subjected to shear stress. *Biochem Biophys Res Commun* 1994;201:950–956.

171. Shyy YJ, Hsieh HJ, Usami S, et al. Fluid shear stress induces a biphasic response of human monocyte chemotactic protein 1 gene expression in vascular endothelium. *Proc Natl Acad Sci U S A* 1994;91:4678–4682.

172. Shyy JY, Lin MC, Han J, et al. The cis-acting phorbol ester "12-O-tetradecanoylphorbol 13-acetate"–responsive element is involved in shear stress-induced monocyte chemotactic protein 1 gene expression. *Proc Natl Acad Sci U S A* 1995;92:8069–8073.

173. Read MA, Whitley MZ, Williams AJ, et al. NF-kappa B and I kappa B alpha: an inducible regulatory system in endothelial activation. *J Exp Med* 1994;179:503–512.

174. Resnick N, Collins T, Atkinson W, et al. Platelet-derived growth factor B chain promoter contains a cis-acting fluid shear-stress-responsive element. *Proc Natl Acad Sci U S A* 1993;90:7908.

175. Frangos JA, Eskin SG, McIntire LV, et al. Flow effects on prostacyclin production by cultured human endothelial cells. *Science* 1985;227:1477– 1479.

176. Grabowski EF, Jaffe EA, Weksler BB. Prostacyclin production by cultured endothelial cell monolayers exposed to step increases in shear stress. *J Lab Clin Med* 1985;105:36–43.

177. Sharefkin JB, Diamond SL, Eskin SG, et al. Fluid flow decreases preproendothelin mRNA levels and suppresses endothelin-1 peptide release in cultured human endothelial cells. *J Vasc Surg* 1991;14:1–9.

178. Kuchan MJ, Frangos JA. Role of calcium and calmodulin in flow-induced nitric oxide production in endothelial cells. *Am J Physiol* 1994;266:C628–C636.

179. Cooke JP, Stamler J, Andon N, et al. Flow stimulates endothelial cells to release a nitrovasodilator that is potentiated by reduced thiol. *Am J Physiol* 1990;259:H804–H812.

180. Rubanyi GM, Romero JC, Vanhoutte PM. Flow-induced release of endothelium-derived relaxing factor. *Am J Physiol* 1986;250:H1145–H1149.

181. Papadaki M, Tilton RG, Eskin SG, et al. Nitric oxide production by cultured human aortic smooth muscle cells: stimulation by fluid flow. *Am J Physiol* 1998;274:H616–H626.

182. Nollert MU, Hall ER, Eskin SG, et al. The effect of shear stress on the uptake and metabolism of arachidonic acid by human endothelial cells. *Biochim Biophys Acta* 1989;1005:72–78.

183. Gupte A, Frangos JA. Effects of flow on the synthesis and release of fibronectin by endothelial cells. *In Vitro Cell Dev Biol* 1990;26:57–60.

184. Carosi JA, Eskin SG, McIntire LV. Cyclical strain effects on production of vasoactive materials in cultured endothelial cells. *J Cell Physiol* 1992;151:29–36.

185. Carosi JA, McIntire LV. Modulation of secretion of vasoactive materials from human and bovine endothelial cells by cyclic strain. *Biotechnol Bioeng* 1994;43:615–621.

186. Wang DL, Tang CC, Wung BS, et al. Cyclical strain increases endothelin-1 secretion and gene expression in human endothelial cells. *Biochem Biophys Res Commun* 1993;195:1050–1056.

187. Wang D, Tarbell J. Modeling interstitial flow in an artery wall allows estimation of wall shear stress on smooth muscle cells. *J Biomech Eng* 1995;117:358–363.

188. Kohler TR, Kirkman TR, Kraiss LW, et al. Increased blood flow inhibits neointimal hyperplasia in endothelialized vascular grafts. *Circ Res* 1991;69:1557–1565.

189. Sterpetti AV, Cucina A, D'Angelo LS, et al. Shear stress modulates the proliferation rate, protein synthesis, and mitogenic activity of arterial smooth muscle cells. *Surgery* 1993;113:691–699.

190. Papadaki M, McIntire LV, Eskin SG. Effects of shear stress on the growth kinetics of human aortic smooth muscle cells *in vitro*. *Biotechnol Bioeng* 1996;50:555–561.

191. Sterpetti AV, Cucina A, Fragale A, et al. Shear stress influences the release of platelet derived growth factor and basic fibroblast growth factor by arterial smooth muscle cells. *Eur J Vasc Surg* 1994;8:138–142.

192. Alshihabi SN, Chang YS, Frangos JA, et al. Shear stress-induced release of PGE2 and PGI2 by vascular smooth muscle cells. *Biochem Biophys Res Commun* 1996;224:808–814.

193. Rhodes DN, Eskin SG, McIntire LV. Fluid flow releases fibroblast growth factor-2 from human aortic smooth muscle cells. *Atherioscler Thromb Vasc Biol* 2000;20:416–421.

194. Wang X, Feuerstein GZ, Clark RK, et al. Enhanced leucocyte adhesion to interleukin-1 beta stimulated vascular smooth muscle cells is mainly through intercellular adhesion molecule-1. *Cardiovasc Res* 1994;28:1808–1814.

195. Wang X, Feuerstein GZ, Gu JL, et al. Interleukin-1 beta induces expression of adhesion molecules in human vascular smooth muscle cells and enhances adhesion of leukocytes to smooth muscle cells. *Atherosclerosis* 1995;115:89–98.

196. Barks JL, McQuillan JJ, Iademarco MF. TNF-alpha and IL-4 synergistically increase vascular cell adhesion molecule-1 expression in cultured vascular smooth muscle cells. *J Immunol* 1997;159:4532–4538.

197. Braun M, Pietsch P, Schror K, et al. Cellular adhesion molecules on vascular smooth muscle cells. *Cardiovasc Res* 1999;41:395–401.

198. Landry DB, Couper LL, Bryant SR, et al. Activation of the NF-kappa B and I kappa B system in smooth muscle cells after rat arterial injury. Induction of vascular cell adhesion molecule-1 and monocyte chemoattractant protein-1. *Am J Pathol* 1997;151:1085–1095.

199. Stamatas GN, Patrick CW Jr, McIntire LV. Intracellular pH changes of human aortic smooth muscle cells in response to fluid shear stress. *Tissue Eng* 1997;3:391–403.

200. Matsuno H, Kozawa O, Niwa M, et al. Inhibition of von Willebrand factor binding to platelet GP Ib by a fractionated aurintricarboxylic acid prevents restenosis after vascular injury in hamster carotid artery. *Circulation* 1997;96:1299–1304.

201. The EPIC Investigation. The EPIC investigators. Use of a monoclonal antibody directed against the platelet glycoprotein IIb/IIIa receptor in high-risk coronary angioplasty. *N Engl J Med* 1994;330:956–961.

202. Topol EJ, Califf RM, Weisman HF, et al. Randomised trial of coronary intervention with antibody against platelet IIb/IIIa integrin for reduction of clinical restenosis: results at six months. The EPIC Investigators. *Lancet* 1994;343:881–886.

# CHAPTER 49 ■ BIOMATERIAL-ASSOCIATED THROMBOSIS

MAUD B. GORBET AND MICHAEL V. SEFTON

Cardiovascular device manufacturers rely on elegant device designs and systemic pharmacologic agents to work wonders with existing materials despite their thrombogenicity. Adverse effects are minimized and existing devices are, if not risk free, providing sufficient benefit to outweigh the risks. The focus of research in biomaterials is to make better materials that pose fewer risks and offer greater benefits. Many strategies for lowering thrombogenicity have been identified, and all these strategies show a beneficial effect in at least one assay of thrombogenicity. However, the perfect material is yet to be identified.

Clinical manifestations of the bioincompatibility of cardiovascular devices are numerous (1,2): Sudden and complete occlusion of stents (3); acute and subacute thrombotic occlusion in medium sized grafts (4 to 6 mm) (2); embolic complications with artificial hearts (4), catheters (5), and prosthetic valves (6,7); and thrombotic complications during cardiopulmonary bypass (2) and angioplasty (8). Large-diameter vascular grafts remain thrombogenic for many years, but fewer thrombotic complications are observed because high flows disperse the clotting factors. Even if the risk of thrombotic complication appears to be low (varying between 2% and 10% depending on the device), the complications may have fatal outcomes, and the cost associated with the follow-up intervention is not negligible. Furthermore, these thrombotic complications with cardiovascular devices occur despite the use of antiplatelet and anticoagulant therapies. In the absence of nonthrombogenic materials, current devices rely on avoiding irregular flow geometries (i.e., sudden contractions, recirculation zones, and poor device streamlining) so that thrombi do not accumulate within the device (9,10). Coupled with this is the routine use of anticoagulants and antithrombotics [see Spinler et al. for guidelines (11) and Gorbet et al. for review (12)].

This chapter focuses on biomaterials and their interactions with blood. We consider how each component, including leukocytes and complement, is thought to interact with biomaterials to induce thrombosis.

# INTRODUCTION TO BIOMATERIAL-ASSOCIATED THROMBOSIS

## Overview

Cardiovascular devices (except endothelial cell–seeded vascular grafts) expose a foreign surface lacking the properties of the endothelium to the circulation. This exposure triggers a complex series of events, including protein adsorption, platelet and leukocyte activation/adhesion, and the activation of complement and coagulation; the events are highly interlinked in this simplified picture (see Fig. 49-1).

## Criteria for Nonthrombogenicity

Much of the effort in biomaterials research over the last 30 years has been directed toward the development of inert materials that do not react with platelets and coagulation factors. A number of approaches, often conflicting, have been developed. For example, there is still no consensus as to whether a surface should be hydrophilic or hydrophobic.

Thrombogenicity is defined (13) as the ability of a material to induce or promote the formation of thromboemboli. In the past, we have thought of a nonthrombogenic surface as one that prevented platelets adherence and did not shorten blood clotting time. These criteria are easily met by heparinized materials (4), but further studies have shown that some hydrogels, even with heparin, can activate platelets leading to high platelet consumption (5). The latter materials promote the formation of microthrombi, although the thrombi do not attach to the materials. A clotting time measurement is a reasonable way of assessing the effect of a material on coagulation. However, the importance of this assay for predicting thrombosis *in vivo* under normal and pathologic conditions is uncertain.

The criteria that we use as hallmarks of nonthrombogenicity are given in Table 49-1. Rather than a clotting time, a specific thrombin production rate constant, $k_p$, enables the extrapolation to indicate realistic situations. Experimental results suggest that $k_p$ is of the order of $10^{-3}$ per second for simple materials such as polyethylene (the same scale as mass transfer coefficients in flowing blood) but less than $10^{-4}$ per second for heparinized materials (14). According to a simple flow model (see Fig. 49-2), only the latter low $k_p$ materials can be expected to minimize fibrin production. This is one of the reasons heparinization and other active methods of inhibiting thrombin formation are so popular as strategies for imparting low thrombogenicity. There are, however, other criteria that must also be met. It is also a requirement that platelet interactions with the surface should not lead to thrombosis. Platelet activation and consumption may therefore be better indicators of platelet incompatibility than just deposition. Furthermore, some deposition may even be desirable since these deposits appear to passivate the surface to further activation. Although a nonthrombogenic surface should not support platelet adhesion, some *ex vivo* studies (15,16) have demonstrated that even in the absence of adhesion, platelets can be "consumed." That is, the platelets can be activated by the material and prematurely removed from the circulation (e.g., shorter platelet lifespan, decrease in systemic platelet count). This suggests that low platelet adhesion is not a sufficient criterion of *in vivo* platelet compatibility. Rather low thrombogenicity is characterized by both low platelet adhesion and low platelet activation. Leukocyte activation (and complement activation) may also be key components in thrombogenicity (see subsequent text); with further research, these factors too may

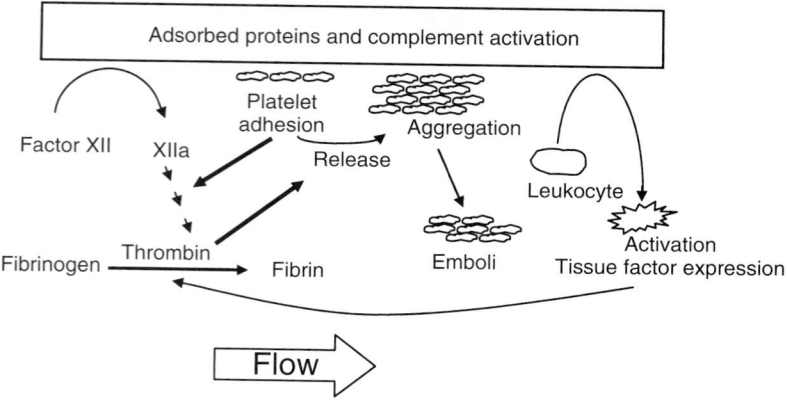

**FIGURE 49-1.** On or in the adsorbed protein layer, coagulation factors change their conformation or are converted into active enzymes and result in the generation of thrombin and fibrin. In parallel, platelets adhere to the surface (or adsorbed protein), become activated, change their shape, and form platelet aggregates. Both processes are linked most notably through thrombin generated on the activated platelet surface. Complement is activated on many biomaterials within the protein adsorbate and leukocytes are activated to express tissue factor (TF) and other procoagulant activities. Flow (shear rate) is a crucial factor affecting both transport coefficients (from bulk to the surface and reverse) and the activation of leukocytes and platelets.

become crucial parameters that define the thrombogenicity of the surface.

## Evaluation Methods

Microscopy and scanning electron microscopy (SEM) are often used as a means of assessing platelet and thrombus deposition on test materials. Lactate dehydrogenase (LDH) release is a more recent indicator for platelet adhesion (17). To assess platelet response in the bulk, standard clinical tests such as platelet aggregability and release of platelet factor 4 and $\beta$-thromboglobulin are used, whereas the generation of thrombin–antithrombin complexes (TAT) and prothrombin fragments (F1.2) are good indicators of coagulation. Flow cytometry is used to measure bulk (or circulating) activated platelets, platelet microaggregates, platelet microparticles, and activated leukocytes following blood–material contact (18,19); cytometry can also be used to assess the number and activation state of cells attached to small beads (20,21). The development of *in vitro* assays that predict *in vivo* thrombotic potential continues to be an elusive goal. Good surface characterization and careful attention being paid to preventing

endotoxin contamination are the hallmarks of current studies that augur well for future advances.

## Surface Modification Strategies

Many different materials are found in cardiovascular devices. Polymers such as silicone rubber, polytetrafluoroethylene, polyvinylchloride, polyethylene, or polyurethanes are used in catheters, vascular implants, ventricular assist devices, and oxygenator membranes. Stainless steel and nickel-titanium are found in heart valves, vena cava filters, and stents. Pyrolytic carbon coatings have been used on prosthetic heart valves to improve biocompatibility, whereas chemically treated natural tissues such as pig or cadaver heart valves are also implanted. To improve the blood compatibility of cardiovascular devices, various surface modifications, such as attachment of antithrombotic agents or the immobilization of polyethylene oxide (PEO), have been considered but their success has been limited. For example, radiofrequency glow discharge treatment of materials to silanize a surface, to deposit a fluorocarbon polymer on the surface, or to introduce functional groups for the subsequent attachment of biomolecules (e.g., antithrombotic agents) have been tried (22). PEO treatment to reduce protein adsorption and to prevent platelet adhesion has not reduced thrombogenicity (23). Heparin-releasing polymers (e.g., heparin ionically bound or dispersed in surfaces), polymers with immobilized heparin (covalently bound), and heparin–PEO polymer coatings have been developed (24). Heparinized surfaces have actually been used in cardiopulmonary bypass tubing

### TABLE 49-1

#### HALLMARKS OF NONTHROMBOGENICITY

| Conventional wisdom | Updated criteria |
|---|---|
| Prolonged clotting times | Thrombin production rate constant $k_p < 10^{-4}$ |
| Few adherent platelets or thrombi | Low platelet consumption; low degree of platelet activation (e.g., microparticle formation) |
| Spread platelets are a marker of blood incompatibility—it is better to have rounded, nonactivated platelets | Some platelet spreading (?) |
| Complement and leukocyte activation are not relevant to studies of thrombogenicity | Low complement and leukocyte activation (?) |

(?), the validity of these criteria is subject to further verification.

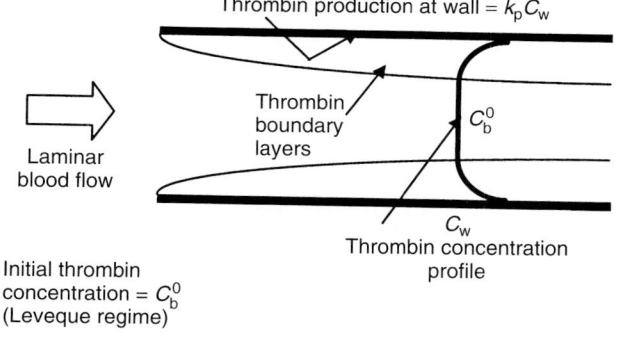

**FIGURE 49-2.** Model illustrating thrombin production at the surface of a tube as a balance between autoaccelerative production and mass transfer away from the wall. [From Rollasson G, Sefton MV. Measurement of the rate of thrombin production in human plasma in contact with different materials. *J Biomed Mater Res* 1992;26(5):675–693, with permission.]

(25) and in coronary stents. However, reports on the improvement of *in vivo* biocompatibility have been mixed (26–31). Heparinized cardiopulmonary bypass circuits appear to partially reduce the inflammatory response associated with cardiopulmonary bypass (31). But to date, heparin coatings have not been shown to significantly reduce the number of postoperative complications, improve patient outcome, or reduce hospital stay (26,27,32).

Seeding endothelial cells on biomaterials to enhance antithrombogenicity before implantation has been under investigation for over 30 years but remains at the research stage [for a complete review, see Pawlowski et al. (33)], although there has been clinical success in the hands of some investigators (34). To promote adhesion and to prevent detachment upon implantation, adsorption of adhesive proteins, such as fibronectin, (35) or specific peptide sequences, such as RGD (36) or YIGSR (37), have been explored. On the other hand, seeded endothelial cells on some materials express increased levels of E selectin and intercellular adhesion molecule-1 (ICAM-1) (38), perhaps leading to leukocyte infiltration, whereas some *in vitro* conditions lead to TF expression (39).

# MECHANISTIC DETAILS

The failure to create nonthrombogenic biomaterials is directly attributable to our limited understanding of the complexity of biomaterial-associated thrombosis. The variety of mechanisms that are involved are summarized here.

## Coagulation

In the past, the discussion of coagulation at the biomaterial–blood interface has focused on the intrinsic coagulation system and the effects of the adsorbed protein layer. Protein adsorption is certainly the first event in blood–material interactions, and adsorption of the contact-phase proteins may result in activation of the intrinsic cascade. Recent studies, however, demonstrate that TF and the extrinsic coagulation system are also involved.

Early studies that were focused on protein adsorption on glass or biomaterial surfaces showed how fibrinogen is replaced over time by high-molecular-weight kininogen (the Vroman effect), suggesting a possible role of the intrinsic pathway in material thrombosis (40). On the other hand, factor XII (FXII) adsorption has been observed in moderate amounts on materials used in vascular grafts (41) and hemodialysers (42) but has not been found in its activated form (43). In some instances, *in vitro* activation of FXII and kallikrein has been reported with biomaterials (44–46); whether this activation results in any significant coagulation is not known. Other studies have actually shown that only minute amounts of thrombin or thrombin–antithrombin III complex (TAT) are generated when biomaterials are incubated with undiluted plasma alone (47–49). Furthermore, the levels of adsorbed kallikrein and FXII on biomaterials do not correlate with TAT formation (47), suggesting that the contact-phase proteins, by themselves, play little role in the activation of coagulation. In fact, a study by Hong et al. (48) suggested that the presence of leukocytes is required for activation of the coagulation cascade. TAT formation on PVC was found to be negligible in both plasma and platelet-rich plasma, whereas significant levels of TAT were observed in whole blood. *In vivo*, a small increase of FXIIa is observed during cardiopulmonary bypass (50,51), but it appears to be in response to the surgical intervention. The establishment of extracorporeal circulation (i.e., exposure to the biomaterials of the circuit) does not further increase FXIIa levels (51). Furthermore, no significant

correlation has been observed between FXIIa and thrombin generation (51). *In vivo* results with hemodialysis also failed to show any significant increase of FXIIa (52). That a patient with a severe FXII deficiency showed levels of thrombin generation during cardiopulmonary bypass similar to normal patients (53) casts further doubt on the role of FXII in the initiation of coagulation with biomaterials. Taken together, these studies do not support the view that activation of the contact-phase proteins is important in the activation of coagulation by biomaterials. Rather a TF-dependent pathway of initiation for coagulation may be more important, and this is discussed in the context of leukocyte activation in subsequent text.

## Platelets

Platelet activation and adhesion is known to occur during cardiopulmonary bypass and hemodialysis, as well as in vascular grafts, stents, and catheters (1,9). The thrombotic complications associated with cardiovascular devices are clearly linked to their ability to activate platelets. Adherent platelets (54) and circulating platelet microparticles generated by material contact (55,56) have been shown to be procoagulant in nature. Association between platelets and leukocytes through P selectin occurs in the presence of cardiovascular devices (8), and such associations may directly or indirectly contribute to thrombin generation (by monocyte TF) or may participate in the removal of platelets from the circulation because several platelets can be bound to each neutrophil or monocyte.

Following contact with the layer of adsorbed proteins on the artificial surface, platelets will either adhere or "bounce off" (57), most likely depending on their state of activation and the ligands present at the interface (58). Many investigators have studied the influence of surface characteristics of biomaterials (i.e., hydrophilicity/hydrophobicity, surface free energy, chemistry, charge, and roughness) on platelet adhesion *in vitro*, but the results have been contradictory and adsorbed proteins remain the crucial factor in platelet adhesion. Few platelets are found on biomaterials that preferentially adsorb albumin. Preadsorbed fibrinogen, fibronectin, vitronectin, and von Willebrand factor (VWF) support platelet adhesion *in vitro* on biomaterials. However, initial platelet adhesion on surfaces *in vitro* is mediated mainly by fibrinogen and glycoprotein (GP) IIb/IIIa (59–61). No initial platelet activation is required, and binding of GP IIb/IIIa occurs through the amino-terminal of the $\gamma$ chain in fibrinogen (62). A very small amount of fibrinogen appears to be necessary to support platelet adhesion ($<30$ ng per cm$^2$) (59), suggesting that a biomaterial has to be extremely resistant to protein adsorption to prevent adhesion. Interaction with VWF (by GP Ib/IX/V) and fibronectin (by GP IIb/IIIa) is believed to improve platelet adhesion once adherent platelets have been activated (63–66). Adherent platelets on biomaterials become activated and undergo morphologic changes; the extent of platelet spreading or flattening is directly related to the increase in activation (67). The state of activation of adherent platelets is also dependent on the biomaterial (68,69). Activation of adherent platelets may result in degranulation, with the release of activation products such as $\beta$-thromboglobulin, thromboxane B$_2$, adenosine 5′-diphosphate (ADP) or serotonin (which can activate bulk platelets), and NAP-2 (which can activate leukocytes). In addition, adherent platelets express P selectin (translocated to the surface during release from the $\alpha$-granule), which promotes the binding of monocytes and neutrophils. The activated adherent platelet surface supports thrombin generation (i.e., prothrombinase and tenase formation) and can also shed procoagulant microparticles (MPs) from their plasma membrane.

The absence of significant platelet adhesion does not preclude platelet activation in the bulk as shown by the generation of platelet MPs with polyvinyl alcohol (PVA) hydrogel both *in vitro* (18) and *ex vivo* in a canine shunt model (70). In a baboon AV shunt model, the rate of platelet consumption was directly linked to the water content of hydrogels (15), despite the absence of significant adhesion. All materials that were tested, (71), not just hydrogels, were observed to activate platelets, resulting in their premature removal from the circulation.

It is not clear whether inhibition of platelet adhesion will reduce platelet consumption or inhibit the generation of platelet MPs. It appears that the effects of antiplatelet agents vary depending on the surface characteristics as shown by Spijker et al. (72). For example, abciximab is less effective in reducing platelet adhesion on hydrophilic surfaces than on hydrophobic surfaces. The strategies available to minimize platelet adhesion (e.g., polyethylene glycol immobilization) have not been sufficient to prevent platelet consumption (73). The mechanism of material-induced platelet activation is often presumed to be through the generation of thrombin due to activation of the intrinsic coagulation cascade or the release of ADP from damaged red blood cells or platelets. Even in the presence of heparin, small amounts of thrombin are generated and may activate platelets. However, the inability of thrombin and kallikrein inhibitors to reduce platelet activation suggests that platelet activation is at least mediated in part by other agonists (74). Unpublished studies in our lab have pointed to the beneficial effect of classical pathway complement inhibitors. Pentamidine (12 mg per kg, daily, i.m.) but neither Reopro nor low-molecular-weight heparin reduces PVA-induced platelet consumption in the canine AV shunt. A correlation between complement activation and thrombocytopenia has also been noted during dialysis (75,76).

Complement activation can lead to platelet activation in many ways. Platelets possess a receptor for C1q that induces GP IIb/IIIa activation, P selectin expression, and procoagulant activity (77). It is currently not known how classical complement activation leads to activated platelets, but *in vitro* results support a role for C1 (78). Insertion of C5b-9 in platelets has also been associated with increased platelet procoagulant activity (79). A role for complement in platelet activation mediated by biomaterials offers new strategies to improve the thombogenicity of surfaces.

## Leukocytes

Contact with biomaterials *in vivo* activates both neutrophils and monocytes. Indicators of leukocyte activation such as L-selectin shedding and CD11b upregulation on leukocytes have been widely observed following angioplasty (80,81), hemodialysis (82,83), and cardiopulmonary bypass (84–86) [for review, see Asimakopoulos and Taylor (87)]. Degranulation with the release of elastase and lactoferrin (88–90) and the presence of cytokines (86,91,92), such as IL-1 and TNF-α, have been associated with extracorporeal circulation and further demonstrate leukocyte activation. Activation of the respiratory burst is also a common response to hemodialysis (82,93).

Many clinical materials can activate isolated leukocytes suspended in plasma. Fibrinogen adsorption enhances this activation (94). Monocytes express TF after coming into contact with a biomaterial (21,95,96). Material-induced monocyte TF expression *in vitro* depends on complement activation and platelets (97). On the other hand, the removal of platelets or the blocking of GP IIb/IIIa by monoclonal antibody (7E3) has no effect on CD11b upregulation. Contact with materials such as PVA hydrogel (98) or pellethane (99) leads to a two-fold upregulation of CD11b, typical of the degree of leukocyte activation induced by phorbol esters. Both *in vitro* (21) and *in vivo* (100) studies have found that material-induced leukocyte activation is dependent on the exposed surface area.

Material-induced leukocyte activation results in increased adhesion to artificial surfaces. Because the biomaterial is larger than a microorganism and cannot therefore be engulfed by leukocytes, adherent neutrophils and monocytes respond with a frustrated attempt at phagocytosis, whereby these cells release their array of potent oxygen metabolites, growth factors, cytokines, and proteolytic enzymes (101). The state of adherent leukocyte activation depends on the type of surface, the protein ligands present at the interface (94,102,103), and the presence of adherent platelets (97,104). Hydrophobic surfaces tend to promote leukocyte adhesion and activation, whereas less activation is observed in leukocytes adherent to hydrophilic surfaces (105). *In vivo* studies have demonstrated activated leukocytes adhering to stents (106,107), oxygenators (108), and hemodialysis membranes (109,110).

Leukocytes adhere *in vitro* to fibrinogen, fibronectin, and IgG adsorbed to surfaces by means of the integrin receptors CD11b/CD18 (Mac-1), CD49e/CD29 (VLA-5), and Fc receptors. Fibrinogen appears to be an important ligand in leukocyte adhesion to artificial surfaces. Monocyte adhesion correlates positively with the amount of fibrinogen adsorbed to the surface (111). Fibrinogen is important for leukocyte adhesion *in vivo*. Fewer leukocytes are found on polymers implanted in hypofibrinogenemic mice (112). Leukocyte binding to fibrinogen occurs by a protein kinase C (PKC)-dependent pathway important for both initial and sustained adhesion. Adsorbed IgG does not seem to support macrophage adhesion directly on polymers but may play a role as a trigger for complement activation, which would then bind to the surface and provide ligand for leukocyte adhesion (113). On the other hand, on metals such as titanium, leukocytes adhere initially through the FcγIII receptor (CD16), making IgG the ligand of preference (114). Complement proteins (101,115) are also involved. C3a can mediate leukocyte adhesion on surfaces *in vitro* by the direct complexation with C3a receptors, whereas C5a appears to have a lesser role (116). The iC3b is a ligand for CD11b/CD18 and is present even on low complement-activating surfaces (117). The iC3b has been shown to play an important role in leukocyte adhesion to hemodialysis membranes (118).

Platelets on the surface have also been reported to mediate leukocyte adhesion by the interaction between P selectin and PSGL-1 and/or GP IIb/IIIa and CD11b (119,120). Before adhesion to the biomaterials, leukocyte may roll by shedding of the L selectin (similar to what happens on endothelial cells), but the mechanisms by which leukocytes sample a biomaterial before adhering to it have been less well characterized than with endothelial cells. The mechanisms of material-induced leukocyte activation as distinct from adhesion also remain unknown. Whether these leukocytes are directly activated by contact with a foreign surface, by complement activation, by kallikrein, or by platelet activation has not been fully determined. *In vitro* and *in vivo* investigations with protease inhibitors (74,121,122), complement inhibitors (98,123–126), and antiplatelet agents (127) suggest that they all play a role, but no inhibitor has consistently reduced material-induced leukocyte activation. Material-induced leukocyte activation may be mediated by several factors, and inhibition of just one pathway of activation may not be sufficient to result in a significant impact on leukocyte activation. For example, complement inhibition using sCR1 was only partially effective in reducing leukocyte activation (98). On the other hand, a combination of sCR1 and anti–GP IIb/IIIa (which blocks platelet activation) reduced material-induced leukocyte activation to almost background levels.

In addition to thrombotic consequences (e.g., through TF expression, see subsequent text), material-induced leukocyte activation contributes to the degradation of biomaterials and to the resistance of biomaterial-associated infection to antibiotics. Some materials, such as polyurethanes or polylactic-glycolic acid copolymers, are susceptible to *in vivo* hydrolysis and/or oxidation (128). In addition to enhancing hydrolysis by local lowering of pH, neutrophils and macrophages have a potent redox metabolism, which can be activated upon contact with a biomaterial and lead to the generation of superoxide anion and hypochlorous acid. Stress cracking is a consequence of oxidative degradation that affects biomaterial performance (128) of, for example, polyether urethanes used in pacing leads. Removal of the implant is sometimes the only effective solution to the antibiotic-resistant infections associated with medical devices. *Staphylococcus epidermis* strains, most common strain on infected devices (129), are weak activators of neutrophils when compared to strains of *Staphylococcus aureus*, which may explain the indolent and chronic course biomaterial infections caused by *S. epidermis* (60). Some studies have shown that bacteria are able to adhere to biomaterials even at high shear, whereas fewer leukocytes are found in such areas (130). High shear rates also appear to trigger apoptosis in adherent neutrophils, further compromising their capacity to kill bacteria (131). Another reason for the chronic infections may be that adherent leukocytes have already been activated by the biomaterial and have been depleted of their oxygen free radicals and granule products. The presence of defensins (small cationic antibacterial peptides contained in granules) has also been reported to impair the microbicidal function of both leukocytes adherent to biomaterials and freshly added leukocytes (61).

### Complement

Complement activation is generally treated as if it is part of the inflammatory response induced by biomaterials. For example, complement activation is known to occur during cardiopulmonary bypass and hemodialysis (132–134), and with catheters and prosthetic vascular grafts (135,136). It is recognized that, both in the short and long term, complement activation plays a role in the leukocyte-related clinical sequelae, such as leukopenia, hypotension, and pulmonary injury, which are associated with the use of cardiovascular devices (137,138). The presence of a biomaterial is believed to activate complement by the alternative pathway. On a nonactivating surface (139), negatively charged groups such as carboxyl and sulfate, sialic acid, and bound heparin appear to promote high-affinity association between bound C3b and factor H. On the other hand, an activating surface is usually characterized by the presence of nucleophiles such as hydroxyl and amino groups: These groups will allow covalent binding of C3b and promote formation of the C3 and C5 convertase (3,140). However, even in the absence of these activating groups on the surface, some biomaterials, such as polyacrylonitrile, are able to activate complement, suggesting that the mechanisms of material-induced complement activation due to nucleophilic groups is not the whole story. An alternative hypothesis places emphasis on interaction of factor H with the surface; an activating material is then defined by its capacity to bind factor B rather than factor H (140). Binding of factor H would lead to C3b inactivation by factor I and would therefore terminate the propagation of the complement cascade.

Some activating materials generate high levels of both C3b and C5b-9, whereas other materials will generate high levels of C3b but little C5b-9. The reason why the efficiency of C5 convertase formation relative to that of C3 formation differs from one activating surface to another is not well understood. However, even low amounts of C5b-9 are able to activate leukocytes (139) and, therefore, a low terminal complement-activating material may still induce a significant inflammatory response. The question remains as to what are the appropriate levels of complement activation that the host can accept without deleterious effect.

The hypothesis that material-induced complement activation occurs exclusively by the alternative pathway has been challenged. Reports of complement activation by the classical pathway during cardiopulmonary bypass (141,142) and a delay in complement activation observed with patients deficient in C4 who are undergoing hemodialysis (143) suggest that classical activation plays a role in material-induced activation. The presence of immune complexes may allow for a rapid onset of complement activation, and then subsequently the alternative pathway may also become activated. *In vitro* studies have also demonstrated activation of the classical pathway by some biomaterials (144–146). C1 inhibitors such as pentamidine and benzamidine are effective in lowering platelet adhesion and activation by polystyrene beads and polyethylene tubes, whereas sCR1, an inhibitor of both pathways at the level of C3, has no effect (20,78). Pentamidine is also effective in a canine chronic shunt by eliminating the thrombocytopenia seen with a platelet activating material (a PVA hydrogel) (Gemmell CH, 2000, unpublished data).

Although some of the consequences of complement activation are well understood, more work is needed to fully understand how a material activates complement. Controlling the differential adsorption of C3b, factor D, and factor H may be more important than preparing so-called nonfouling, low-adsorption surfaces. The latter may lower the adsorption of all proteins but it may be more important to alter the composition of the protein adsorbate.

### Leukocyte Activation and Coagulation

Circulating monocytes and neutrophils normally roll on the endothelium and adhere to damaged or stimulated endothelial cells or adherent platelets and further contribute to localized thrombogenesis through one or more mechanisms (147), some of which apply to biomaterials (21,97). Leukocytes have membrane-associated procoagulant activity, which is manifested by TF expression on the cell membrane (TF-dependent coagulation pathway), by TF-independent mechanisms through factor X binding to CD11b receptors leading to factor Xa generation or fibrinogen binding to CD11b, or by binding of the prothrombinase complex on the membrane. In addition, degranulation and oxidative products have the capacity to neutralize various anticoagulant proteins and activate platelets, whereas the association between platelets and neutrophils or monocytes may lead to mutual activation and to a microenvironment protected from inhibitors.

Many investigators think that the extrinsic pathway is not activated during blood–material interactions (1,9,148,149). However, blood contact with a material represents a stimulus to induce TF expression by monocytes (21,97), resulting potentially in blood coagulation through the extrinsic system. Material-induced TF expression on monocytes *in vitro* results in significantly shorter clotting times when compared to control (21). The TF expression appears to be strongly dependent on the presence of platelets and increases with material surface area (97). Following blood contact with cardiopulmonary bypass circuits or ventricular assist devices, TF expression on monocytes has been observed *in vitro* (150–152) and *in vivo* (95,96,151). It has also been shown that CD11b, upregulated on monocytes by cardiopulmonary bypass, is able to directly activate factor X (153) and platelet–leukocyte aggregates have been observed (154–156), as noted in the preceding passage. The number of studies that have tried to minimize thrombus formation by the administration of drugs specifically targeted at leukocytes underscores the potential role of leukocytes in thrombogenesis. Antibodies to block leukocyte adhesion may prove to be a reasonable therapeutic approach in the prevention of thrombus formation as demonstrated in *in vivo* baboon models (157,158). Complement inhibition may also become a successful approach to controlling thrombosis on biomaterials. Classical pathway complement inhibitors such as pentamidine and pyridoxal-5-phosphate inhibit platelet adhesion to polystyrene surfaces (20) and prevent platelet loss and MP formation in polyethylene tubing.

The initiation of the coagulation cascade by contact-phase activation and TF expression occur at different times after exposure of blood to a biomaterial. Because it is part of the protein adsorption "reaction," contact-phase activation occurs during the first few seconds after blood contact with a material. On the other hand, the induction of TF expression and thrombin generating activity in monocytes requires a minimum of 60 minutes (in a healthy patient). Thrombin generation by FXIIa on materials depends on flow (159), because of the effects of flow on mass transfer as well as direct effects of flow on platelet/leukocyte phenotype. Therefore, the relative roles of the intrinsic and extrinsic pathways in thrombin generation probably depend on both time and blood flow. More research is needed to clarify the potential contribution of leukocyte procoagulant activities to thrombogenesis and thrombotic complications associated with the use of biomaterials and cardiovascular devices.

## Fluid Dynamics

Fluid dynamics affect the growth of thrombi and the deposition of fibrin. The difference between arterial and venous thrombi is one example of this effect, although the underlying mechanisms are still not well understood. Thorough reviews are available (5,159–162) and we merely highlight a few key points for the purpose of completeness. Flow determines the rates of transport of cells and proteins to the surface; it can also change the level of receptor expression on platelets and leukocytes. Because platelets are an important part of the thrombus, the effect of shear on platelets has been studied extensively. Higher shear results in higher platelet and lower fibrin deposition, whereas at lower shear the inverse occurs (160). High shear in diseased, stenotic arteries is also able to induce platelet aggregation even in the absence of any other exogenous factors (163,164). Conflicting results have been obtained on the effect of flow on leukocyte adhesion, whereas little is known of its effect on leukocyte activation. High shear has been shown to reduce, increase, or leave unchanged leukocyte adhesion on different substrates (165–172). These conflicting results may be explained by differences in experimental conditions, including the presence of red blood cells (166), platelets (167,170,173) and plasma proteins (167), the surface studied (170), and the state of leukocyte activation (171).

As for the effects of flow on the coagulation cascade, it has been a subject of very little study. Current knowledge about biomaterials is limited to factor Xa generation initiated by the extrinsic pathway and thrombin generation initiated by the intrinsic pathway. Factor Xa generation by the complex TF:VIIa increases with shear rate (and shear stress) (174,175). For thrombin generation by the intrinsic pathway, modeling has identified three types of reactions (159): At low flow, a significant amount of thrombin is produced after a long time lag (more than 10 hours); at moderate flow, significant thrombin generation is produced in a short time (within minutes); at high flow, low levels of thrombin are produced within seconds.

Turbulent flow can be present at anastomoses, joints, and bifurcations of cardiovascular devices, and such turbulence also contributes to the observed thrombosis. It is believed to play an important role in the failure of mechanical heart valves, for example. Turbulent flow (in contrast to recirculation and stagnation zones, which may or may not have the characteristics of turbulence) results in hemolysis and/or cell

activation, but the mechanisms leading to thrombus formation are still poorly understood. Platelet deposition remains the focus of most studies (176), but the literature on turbulent flow and thrombus formation is more limited. Nonetheless, much effort has been devoted to the design of devices so that recirculation or stagnation zones are avoided because these are known loci for thrombus growth.

## CONCLUSIONS

Given the complexity of normal hemostatic events, it is not surprising that blood contact with artificial surfaces initiates a complex response, and the mechanism of biomaterial-associated thrombosis is not completely clear. The role of FXII is unclear, whereas that of TF has only barely been studied. The mechanisms of leukocyte and platelet activation by materials remain to be further elucidated. The timing of the events contributing to thrombin formation is also a complex issue. Both FXII activation and platelet activation are able to generate thrombin formation within minutes, whereas thrombin generation by leukocyte TF requires hours. The question of what happens over hours to days as leukocytes synthesize TF and thrombotic deposits become remodeled is almost beyond current experimental capacity. Whether thrombosis leads to passivation or embolization or some other long-term consequence is still largely unknown.

Thrombosis is viewed now more as a multicellular event rather than just a platelet event (177). The mechanism of material-induced platelet activation is often presumed to be by the generation of thrombin due to activation of the intrinsic coagulation cascade or the release of ADP from damaged red blood cells or platelets. A role for complement in activating platelets and the potential for complement to be activated by the fibrinolytic and kinin system have rarely been considered. If complement also plays a role in activating monocytes to express TF or directly generate fibrin (157) then this will certainly refocus strategies in order to reduce material thrombogenicity.

## *References*

1. Ratner BD. The blood compatibility catastrophe. *J Biomed Mater Res* 1993;27:283–287.
2. Clagett GP, Eberhart RC. Artificial devices in clinical practice. In: Colman RW, Hirsh J, Marder VJ et al., eds. *Hemostasis and thrombosis: basic principles and clinical practice*. Philadelphia, PA: JB Lippincott Co, 1994: 1486–1505.
3. Bittl JA. Coronary stent occlusion: thrombus horribilis. *J Am Coll Cardiol* 1996;28(2):368–370.
4. Bick RL. Hemostasis defects with cardiac surgery, general surgery and prosthetic devices. In: Bick RL, ed. *Disorders of hemostasis and thrombosis*. Chicago, IL: American Society of Clinical Pathologist Press, 1992:195–222.
5. Eberhart RC, Clagett CP. Catheter coatings, blood flow, and biocompatibility. *Semin Hematol* 1991;28(4 Suppl. 7):42–48.
6. Edmunds LHJ. Is prosthetic valve thrombogenicity related to design or material? *Tex Heart Inst J* 1996;23(1):24–27.
7. Geiser T, Sturzenegger M, Genewein U, et al. Mechanisms of cerebrovascular events as assessed by procoagulant activity, cerebral emboli and platelet microparticles in patients with prosthetic heart valves. *Stroke* 1998;29:1770–1777.
8. Mickelson JK, Lakkis NM, Villarreal-Levy G, et al. Leukocyte activation with platelet adhesion after coronary angioplasty: a mechanism for recurrent disease? *J Am Coll Cardiol* 1996;28(2):345–353.
9. Hanson SR. Device thrombosis and thromboembolism. *Cardiovasc Pathol* 1993;2(Suppl. 3):157S–165S.
10. Slack SM, Turitto VT. Fluid dynamic and hemorheologic considerations. *Cardiovasc Pathol* 1993;2(3):11S–21S.
11. Spinler SA, Hilleman DE, Cheng JWM, et al. New recommendations from the 1999 American College of Cardiology/American Heart Association acute myocardial infarction guidelines. *Ann Pharmacother* 2002;35:589–617.
12. Gorbet MB, Sefton MV. Biomaterial-associated thrombosis: roles of coagulation factors, complement, platelets and leukocytes. *Biomaterials* 2004; 25(26):5681–5703.
13. Williams DF. *The williams dictionary of biomaterials*. Liverpool: Liverpool University Press, 1999.

14. Rollasson G, Sefton MV. Measurement of the rate of thrombin production in human plasma in contact with different materials. *J Biomed Mater Res* 1992;26(5):675–693.

15. Hanson SR, Harker LA, Ratner BD, et al. *In vivo* evaluation of artificial surfaces with a nonhuman primate model of arterial thrombosis. *J Lab Clin Med* 1980;95(2):289–304.

16. Cholakis CH, Zingg W, Sefton MV. Effect of heparin-PVA hydrogel on platelets in a chronic canine AV shunt. *J Biomed Mater Res* 1989;23:417–441.

17. Tsai W-B, Grunkemeier JM, Horbett TA. Human plasma fibrinogen adsorption and platelet adhesion to polystyrene. *J Biomed Mater Res* 1999;44(2):130–139.

18. Gemmell CH, Ramirez SM, Yeo EL, et al. Platelet activation in whole blood by artificial surfaces: identification of platelet-derived microparticles and activated platelet binding to leukocytes as material-induced activation events. *J Lab Clin Med* 1995;125(2):276–287.

19. Baker LC, Davis WC, Autieri J, et al. Flow cytometric assays to detect platelet activation and aggregation in device-implanted calves. *J Biomed Mater Res* 1998;41(2):312–321.

20. Gemmell CH. Platelet adhesion onto artificial surfaces: inhibition by benzamidine, pentamidine, and pyridoxal-5-phosphate as demonstrated by flow cytometric quantification of platelet adhesion to microspheres. *J Lab Clin Med* 1998;131(1):84–92.

21. Gorbet MB, Sefton MV. Leukocyte activation and leukocyte procoagulant activities following blood contact with polystyrene and PEG-immobilized polystyrene beads. *J Lab Clin Med* 2001;137:345–355.

22. Ratner BD, Hoffman AS. Thin films, grafts, and coatings. In: Ratner BD, Hoffman AS, Schoen FJ et al., eds. *Biomaterials science: an introduction to materials in medicine.* San Diego, CA: Academic Press, 1996:105–118.

23. Park K, Shim HS, Dewanjee MK, et al. *In vitro* and *in vivo* studies of PEO-grafted blood contacting cardiovascular prostheses. *J Biomater Sci Polym Ed* 2000;11(11):1121–1134.

24. Kim SW. Nonthrombogenic treatments and strategies. In: Ratner BD, Hoffman AS, Schoen FJ et al., eds. *Biomaterials science: an introduction to materials in medicine.* San Diego, CA: Academic Press, 1996:297–308.

25. Wendel HP, Ziemer G. Coating techniques to improve the hemocompatibility of artificial devices used for extracorporeal circulation. *Eur J Cardiothorac Surg* 1999;16:342–350.

26. Sudkamp M, Melhorn U, Reza Raji M, et al. Cardiopulmonary bypass copolymer surface modification reduces neither blood loss nor transfusions in coronary artery surgery. *Thorac Cardiovasc Surg* 2002;50(1):5–10.

27. Isgro F, Kiessling AH, Mittelstaedt H, et al. Surface modification of extracorporeal circuits: is there really an impact on cerebral performance after cardiopulmonary bypass. *Thorac Cardiovasc Surg* 2001;49(2):65–69.

28. Moen O, Hogasen K, Fosse E, et al. Attenuation of changes in leukocyte surface markers and complement activation with heparin-coated cardiopulmonary bypass. *Ann Thorac Surg* 1997;63(1):105–111.

29. Muehrcke DD, McCarthy PM, Kottke-Marchant K, et al. Biocompatibility of heparin-coated extracorporeal bypass circuits: a randomized, masked clinical trial. *J Thorac Cardiovasc Surg* 1996;112(2):472–483.

30. Levy M, Hartman AR. Heparin-coated bypass circuits in cardiopulmonary bypass: improved biocompatibility or not. *Int J Cardiol* 1996;53(Suppl. 1):S81–S87.

31. Fosse E, Thelin S, Svennevig JL, et al. Duraflo II coating of cardiopulmonary bypass circuits reduces complement activation, but does not affect the release of granulocyte enzymes: a european multicentre study. *Eur J Cardiothorac Surg* 1997;11(2):320–327.

32. Videm V, Mollnes TE, Fosse E, et al. Heparin-coated cardiopulmonary bypass equipment. I. biocompatibility markers and development of complications in high risk population. *J Thorac Cardiovasc Surg* 1999;117(4):794–802.

33. Pawlowski KJ, Rittgers SE, Schmidt SP, et al. Endothelial cell seeding of polymeric vascular grafts. *Front Biosci* 2004;9:1412–1421.

34. Meinhart JG, Deutsch M, Fischlein T, et al. Clinical autologous *in vitro* endothelialization of 153 infrainguinal ePTFE grafts. *Ann Thorac Surg* 2001;71(Suppl. 5):S327–S331.

35. Bhat VD, Truskey GA, Reichert WM. Fibronectin and avidin-biotin as a heterogeneous ligand system for enhanced endothelial cell adhesion. *J Biomed Mater Res* 1998;41(3):377–385.

36. Fussell GW, Cooper SL. Endothelial cell adhesion on RGD-containing methacrylate polymers. *J Biomed Mater Res* 2004;70A(2):265–273.

37. Jun HW, West J. Development of a YIGSR-peptide modified polyurethaneurea to enhance endothelialization. *J Biomater Sci Polym Ed* 2004;15(1):73–94.

38. Imbert E, Poot AA, Figdor CG, et al. Expression of leukocyte adhesion molecules by endothelial cells seeded on various polymer surfaces. *J Biomed Mater Res* 2001;56(3):376–381.

39. Murugesan G, Rani MR, Ransohoff RM, et al. Endothelial cell expression of monocyte chemotactic protein-1, tissue factor and thrombomodulin on hydrophilic plasma polymers. *J Biomed Mater Res* 2000;49(3):396–408.

40. Horbett TA. Principles underlying the role of adsorbed plasma proteins in blood interactions with foreign materials. *Cardiovasc Pathol* 1993;2(3 Suppl.):137S–148S.

41. Ziats N, Pankowsky DA, Tierney BP, et al. Adsorption of hageman factor (factor XII) and other human plasma proteins to biomedical polymers. *J Lab Clin Med* 1990;116:687–696.

42. Mulzer SR, Brash JL. Identification of plasma proteins adsorbed to hemodialyzers during clinical use. *J Biomed Mater Res* 1989;23:1483–1504.

43. Cornelius RM, Brash JL. Identification of proteins adsorbed to hemodialyser membranes from heparinized plasma. *J Biomater Sci Polym Ed* 1993;4(3):291–304.

44. Matata BM, Courtney JM, Sundaram S, et al. Determination of contact phase activation by the measurement of the activity of supernatant and membrane surface-adsorbed factor XII: its relevance as a useful parameter for the *in vitro* assessment of haemodialysis membranes. *J Biomed Mater Res* 1993;31(1):63–70.

45. Elam J-H, Nygren H. Adsorption of coagulation proteins from whole blood on to polymer materials: relation to platelet activation. *Biomaterials* 1992;13(1):3–8.

46. Van der Kamp KWHJ, van Oweren W. Factor XII fragment and kallikrein generation in plasma during incubation with biomaterials. *J Biomed Mater Res* 1994;28:349–352.

47. Van der Kamp KWHJ, Kauch KD, Feijen J, et al. Contact activation during incubation of five different polyurethanes or glass in plasma. *J Biomed Mater Res* 1995;29(10):1303–1306.

48. Hong J, Nilsson Ekdahl K, Reynolds H, et al. A new *in vitro* model to study interaction between whole blood and biomaterials. Studies of platelet and coagulation activaton and the effect of aspirin. *Biomaterials* 1999;20:603–611.

49. Blezer R, Willems GM, Cahalan PT, et al. Initiation and propagation of blood coagulation at artificial surfaces studied in a capillary flow reactor. *Thromb Haemost* 1998;79:296–301.

50. Irvine L, Sundaram S, Courtney JM, et al. Monitoring of factor XII activity and granulocyte elastase release during cardiopulmonary bypass. *ASAIO Trans* 1991;XXXVII:569–571.

51. Boisclair MD, Lane DA, Philippou H. Mechanisms of thrombin generation during surgery and cardiopulmonary bypass. *Blood* 1993;82(11):3350–3357.

52. Boisclair MD, Philippou H, Lane DA. Thrombogenic mechanisms in the human: fresh insights obtained by immunodiagnostic studies of coagulation markers. *Blood Coagul Fibrinolysis* 1993;4:1007–1021.

53. Burman JF, Chung HI, Lane DA, et al. Role of factor XII in thrombin generation and fibrinolysis during cardiopulmonary bypass. *Lancet* 1994;344:1192–1193.

54. Grunkemeier JM, Tsai WB, Horbett TA. Hemocompatibility of treated polystyrene substrates: contact activation, platelet adhesion, and procoagulant activity of adherent platelets. *J Biomed Mater Res* 1998;41(4):657–670.

55. Nieuwland R, Bercmans RJ, Rotteveel-Eijkman RC, et al. Cell-derived microparticles generated in patients during cardiopulmonary bypass are highly procoagulant. *Circulation* 1997;96:3534–3541.

56. Gemmell CH. Assessment of material-induced procoagulant activity by a modified russell viper venom coagulation time test. *J Biomed Mater Res* 1998;42(4):611–616.

57. Godo MN, Sefton MV. Characterization of transient platelet contacts on a polyvinyl alcohol hydrogel by video microscopy. *Biomaterials* 1999;20(12):1117–1126.

58. Sheppard JI, McClung WG, Feuerstein IA. Adherent platelet morphology on adsorbed fibrinogen: effects of protein incubation time and albumin addition. *J Biomed Mater Res* 1994;28(10):1175–1186.

59. Tsai W-B, Grunkemeier JM, McFarland CD, et al. Platelet adhesion to polystyrene-based surfaces preadsorbed with plasmas selectively depleted in fibrinogen, fibronectin, vitronectin or von Willebrand's factor. *J Biomed Mater Res* 2002;60:348–359.

60. Nilsdotter-Augustinsson A, Wilsson A, Larsson J, et al. Staphylococcus aureus, but not stapylococcus epidermidis, modulates the oxidative response and induces apoptosis in human neutrophils. *APMIS* 2004;112(2):109–118.

61. Kaplan SS, Heine RP, Simmons RL. Defensins impair phagocytic killing by neutrophils in biomaterila-related infection. *Infect Immun* 1999;67(4):1640–1648.

62. Broberg M, Eriksson C, Nygren H. GPIIb/IIIa is the main receptor for initial platelet adhesion to glass and titanium surfaces in contact with whole blood. *J Lab Clin Med* 2004;139:163–172.

63. Chinn JA, Ratner BD, Horbett TA. Adsorption of baboon fibrinogen and the adhesion of platelets to a thin film polymer deposited by radio-frequency glow discharge of allylamine. *Biomaterials* 1992;13(5):322–332.

64. Hanson SR, Harker LA. Blood coagulation and blood-materials interactions. In: Ratner BD, Hoffman AS, Schoen FJ et al., eds. *Biomaterials science.* San Diego, CA: Academic Press, 1996:193–199.

65. Tsai WB, Grunkemeier JM, Horbett TA. Human plasma fibrinogen adsorption and platelet adhesion to polystyrene. *J Biomed Mater Res* 1999;44(2):130–139.

66. Bailly AL, Laurent A, Lu H, et al. Fibrinogen binding and platelet retention: relationship with the thrombogenicity of catheters. *J Biomed Mater Res* 1996;30:101–108.

67. Goodman SL, Grasel TG, Cooper SL, et al. Platelet shape change and cytoskeletal reorganization on polyurethanes. *J Biomed Mater Res* 1989;23(1):105–123.

68. Goodman SL, Lelah MD, Lambrecht LK, et al. *In vitro* vs. *ex vivo* platelet deposition on polymer surfaces. *Scan Electron Microsc* 1984;Pt 1:279–290.

69. Spijker HT, Bos R, Busscher HJ, et al. Platelet adhesion and activation on a shielded plasma gradient prepared on polyethylene. *Biomaterials* 2002;23:757–766.

70. Gemmell CH, Yeo EL, Sefton MV. Flow cytometric analysis of material-induced platelet activation in a canine model: elevated microparticle levels and reduced platelet life span. *J Biomed Mater Res* 1997;37(2):176–181.

71. Ip WF, Sefton MV. Platelet consumption by NHLBI reference materials and silastic. *J Biomed Mater Res* 1991;25:1321–1324.

72. Spijker HT, Busscher HJ, van Oeveren W. Influence of abciximab on the adhesion of platelets on a shielded plasma gradient prepared on polyethylene. *Thromb Res* 2002;108(1):57–62.

73. Llanos GR, Sefton MV. Immobilization of poly(ethylene glycol) onto poly(vinyl alcohol) hydrogel: 2. Evaluaton of thrombogenicity. *J Biomed Mater Res* 1993;27:1383–1391.

74. Wachtfogel YT, Bischoff R, Bauer R, et al. Alpha 1-antitrypsin Pittsburgh (Met358—>Arg) inhibits the contact pathway of intrinsic coagulation and alters the release of human neutrophil elastase during simulated extracorporeal circulation. *Thromb Haemost* 1994;72(6):843–847.

75. Simon P, Ang KS, Cam G. Enhanced platelet aggregation and membrane biocompatibility: possible influence on thrombosis and embolism in haemodialysis patients. *Nephron* 1987;45:172–173.

76. Hakim RM, Schafer AI. Hemodialysis-associated platelet activation and thrombocytopenia. *Am J Med* 1985;78:575–580.

77. Peerschke EIB, Ghebrehiwet B. Platelet receptors for the complement component C1q: implication for hemostasis and thrombosis. *Immunobiology* 1998;199(2):239–249.

78. Gemmell CH. Platelet-derived micropartcle formation: enhancement by early classical complement components abd inhibition by C1-INH. *Thromb Res* 2000 (submitted).

79. Sims PJ, Wiedmer T. Induction of cellular procoagulant activity by the membrane attack complex of complement. *Semin Cell Biol* 1995;6:275–282.

80. Takala AJ, Jousela IT, Takkumen OS, et al. Time course of $\beta_2$ integrin CD11b/CD18 upregulation on neutrophils and monocytes after coronary artery bypass grafting. *Scand J Thorac Cardiovasc Surg* 1996;30:141–148.

81. Inque T, Sakai Y, Morooka S, et al. Expression of polymorphonuclear adhesion molecules and its clinical significance in patients treated with percutaneous transluminal coronary angioplasty. *J Am Coll Cardiol* 1996;28(5):1127–1133.

82. Cristol JP, Canaud B, Rabesandratana H, et al. Enhancement of reactive oxygen species production and cell surface markers expression due to hemodialysis. *Nephrol Dial Transplant* 1994;9:389–394.

83. Von Appen K, Goolsby C, Mehl P, et al. Leukocyte adhesion molecule as biocompatibility markers for hemodialysis membranes. *ASAIO J* 1994;40:M609–M615.

84. El Habbal MH, Carter H, Smith L, et al. Neutrophil activation in paediatric extracorporeal circuits: effect of circulation and temperature variation. *Cardiovasc Res* 1995;29:102–107.

85. Gillinov AM, Bator JM, Zehr KJ, et al. Neutrophil adhesion molecule expression during cardiopulmonary bypass with bubble and membrane oxygenators. *Ann Thorac Surg* 1993;56:847–853.

86. Cameron DE. Initiation of white cell activation during cardiopulmonary bypass: cytokines and receptors. *J Cardiovasc Pharmacol* 1996;27(Suppl. 1):S1–S5.

87. Asimakopoulos G, Taylor KM. Effects of cardiopulmonary bypass on leukocyte and endothelial adhesion molecules. *Ann Thorac Surg* 1998;66:2135–2144.

88. Grooteman MP, van TA, van HA, et al. Hemodialysis-induced degranulation of polymorphonuclear cells: no correlation between membrane markers and degranulation products. *Nephron* 2000;85(3):267–274.

89. Haag-Weber M, Schollmeyer P, Horl WH. Beta-2-microglobulin and main granulocyte components in hemodialysis patients. *Artif Organs* 1989;13(2):92–96.

90. Stegmayr BG, Esbensen K, Gutierrez A, et al. Granulocyte elastase, $\beta$ thromboglobulin, and C3d during acetate or bicarbonate hemodialysis with hemophan compared to a cellulose acetate membrane. *Int J Artif Organs* 1992;15(1):10–18.

91. Peek GJ, Firmin RK. The inflammatory and coagulative response to prolonged extracorporeal membrane oxygenation. *ASAIO J* 1999;45:250–263.

92. Frering B, Philip I, Dehoux M, et al. Circulating cytokines in patients undergoing normothermic cardiopulmonary bypass. *J Thorac Cardiovasc Surg* 1994;108:636–641.

93. Himmelfarb J, Lazarus JM, Hakim R. Reactive oxygen species production by monocytes and polymorphonuclear leukocytes during dialysis. *Am J Kidney Dis* 1991;XVII(3):271–276.

94. Gorbet MB, Yeo EL, Sefton MV. Flow cytometric study of *in vitro* neutrophil activation by biomaterials. *J Biomed Mater Res* 1999;44(3):289–297.

95. Chung JH, Gikakis N, Rao K, et al. Pericardial blood activates the extrinsic coagulation pathway during clinical cardiopulmonary bypass. *Circulation* 1996;93:2014–2018.

96. Wilhelm CR, Ristich J, Kormos RL, et al. Monocyte tissue factor expression and ongoing complement generation in ventricular assist devices patients. *Ann Thorac Surg* 1998;65:1071–1076.

97. Gorbet MB, Sefton MV. Material-induced tissue factor expression but not CD11b depends on the presence of platelets. *J Biomed Mater Res* 2003;67A(3):792–800.

98. Gemmell CH, Black JP, Yeo EL, et al. Material-induced up-regulation of leukocyte CD11b during whole blood contact: material differences and a role for complement. *J Biomed Mater Res* 1996;32(1):29–35.

99. Sefton MV, Sawyer A, Gorbet MB, et al. Does surface chemistry affect thrombogenicity of surface modfied polymers. *J Biomed Mater Res.* 2001;55(4):447–459.

100. Gourlay T, Stefanou DC, Asimakopoulos G, et al. The effect of circuit surface area on CD11b (Mac-1) expression in a rat recirculation model. *Artif Organs* 2001;25(6):475–479.

101. Anderson JM. Mechanisms of inflammation and infection with implanted devices. *Cardiovasc Pathol* 1993;2(Suppl. 1):33S–41S.

102. Kaplan SS, Basford RE. Mechanisms of biomaterial induced superoxide release by neutrophils. *J Biomed Mater Res* 2000;28:377–386.

103. Kuwahara T, Markert M, Wauters JP. Proteins adsorbed on hemodialysis membranes modulate neutrophil activation. *Artif Organs* 1989;13(5):427–431.

104. Nimeri G, Ohman L, Elwing H, et al. The influence of plasma proteins and platelets on oxygen radical production and F-actin distribution in neutrophils adhering to polymer surfaces. *Biomaterials* 2002;23:1785–1795.

105. Brodbeck WG, Voskerician G, Ziats NP, et al. *In vivo* leukocyte cytokine mRNA responses to biomaterials are dependent on surface chemistry. *J Biomed Mater Res* 2003;64A(2):320–329.

106. Serruys PW, Strauss BH, van Beusekom HM, et al. Stenting of coronary arteries: has a modern Pandora's box been opened? *J Am Coll Cardiol* 1991;17(6):143B–154B.

107. van Beusekom HMM, van der Giessen WJ, Van Suylen RJ, et al. Histology after stenting of human saphenous vein bypass grafts: observations from surgically excised grafts 3 to 320 days after stent implantation. *J Am Coll Cardiol* 1993;21(1):45–54.

108. Jobes DR. Safety issues in heparin and protamine admistration for extracorporeal circulation. *J Cardiothorac Vasc Anesth* 1998;12(2 Suppl. 1):17–20.

109. Grooteman MPC, Bos JC, Van Houte AJ, et al. Mechanisms of intra-dialyser granulocyte activation: a sequential dialyser elution study. *Nephrol Dial Transplant* 1997;12:492–499.

110. Castiglione A, Pagliaro P, Romagnoni M, et al. Flow cytometric analysis of leukocytes eluted from haemodialysers. *Nephrol Dial Transplant* 1991;2(Suppl. 6):31–35.

111. Shen M, Horbett TA. The effects of surface chemistry and adsorbed proeitns on monocyte/macrophage adhesion to chemically modified polystyrene surfaces. *J Biomed Mater Res* 2001;57:336–345.

112. Tang L, Eaton JW. Fibrinogen mediates acute inflammatory responses to biomaterials. *J Exp Med* 1993;178:2147–2156.

113. Jenney CR, Anderson JM. Adsorbed IgG: a potent adhesive substrate for human macrophages. *J Biomed Mater Res* 2000;50(3):281–290.

114. Eriksson C, Nygren H. Adhesion receptors of polymorphonuclear granulocytes on titanium in contact with whole blood. *J Lab Clin Med* 2001;137:56–63.

115. Remes A, Williams DF. Immune response in biocompatibility. *Biomaterials* 1992;13(11):731–743.

116. Kao WJ. Evaluation of leukocyte adhesion on polyurethanes: the effect of shear stress and blood proteins. *Biomaterials* 2000;21:2295–2303.

117. Gorbet MB, Sefton MV. Complement inhibition reduces material-induced leukocyte activation with PEG modified polystyrene beads (Tentagel) but not polystyrene beads. *J Biomed Mater Res* 2005 (In press).

118. Cheung AK, Hohnholt M, Gilson J. Adherence of neutrophils to haemodialysis membranes: roles of complement receptors. *Kidney Int* 1991;40:1123–1133.

119. Eriksson O, Nygren H. Polymorphonuclear leukocytes in coagulating whole blood recognize hydrophilic and hydrophobic titanium surfaces by different adhesion receptors and show different patterns of receptor expression. *J Lab Clin Med* 2001;137:296–302.

120. Gorbet MB, Sefton MV. Role of complement and platelets in leukocyte activation induced by polystyrene and PEG-immobilized polystyrene beads in whole blood. Manuscript in preparation, 2005.

121. Wachtfogel YT, Kettner C, Hack CE, et al. Thrombin and human plasma kallikrein inhibition during simulated extracorporeal circulation block platelet and neutrophil activation. *Thromb Haemost* 1998;80(4):686–691.

122. Himmelfarb J, Holbrook D, McMonagle E. Effects of aprotinin on complement and granulocyte activation during *ex vivo* hemodialysis. *Am J Kidney Dis* 1994;24(6):901–906.

123. Fitch JC, Rollins S, Matis L, et al. Pharmacology and biological efficacy of a recombinant, humanized, single-chain antibody C5 complement inhibitor in patients undergoing coronary artery bypass graft surgery with cardiopulmonary bypass. *Circulation* 1999;100(25):2499–2506.

124. Himmelfarb J, McMonagle E, Holbrook D, et al. Soluble complement receptor 1 inhibits both complement and granulocyte activation during *ex vivo* hemodialysis. *J Lab Clin Med* 1995;126(4):392–400.

125. Gillinov AM, Redmond JM, Winkelstein JA, et al. Complement and neutrophil activation during cardiopulmonary bypass: a study in the complement-deficient dog. *Ann Thorac Surg* 1994;57(2):345–352.

126. Finn A, Morgan BP, Rebuck N, et al. Effects of inhibition of complement activation using recombinant soluble complement receptor 1 on neutrophil CD11b/CD18 and L-selectin expression and release of interleukin-8 and elastase in simulated cardiopulmonary bypass. *J Thorac Cardiovasc Surg* 1996;111:451–459.

127. Mickelson JK, Ali MN, Kleiman NS, et al. Chimeric 7E3 fab (reopro) decreases detectable CD11b on neutrophils from patients undergoing coronory angioplasty. *J Am Coll Cardiol* 1999;33:97–106.

128. Coury AJ. Chemical and biochemical degradation of polymers. In: Ratner BD, Hoffman AS, Schoen FJ et al., eds. *Biomaterials science: an introduction to materials in medicine.* San Diego, CA: Academic Press, 1996:243–260.

129. Gristina AG, Naylor PT. Implant-associated infection. In: Ratner BD, Hoffman AS, Schoen FJ et al., eds. *Biomaterials science: an introduction to materials in medicine.* San Diego, CA: Academic Press, 1996:205–214.

130. Shive MS, Hasan SM, Anderson JM. Shear stress effects on bacterial adhesion, leukocyte adhesion and leukocyte oxidative capacity on a polyetherurethane. *J Biomed Mater Res* 1999;46(4):511–519.

131. Shive MS, Salloum LM, Anderson JM. Shear stress induced apoptosis of adherent neutrophils: a mechanism for persistence of cardiovascular device infections. *Proc Natl Acad Sci U S A* 2000;97(12):6710–6715.

132. Chenoweth DE. Complement activation during hemodialysis: clinical observations, proposed mechanisms, and theoretical implications. *Artif Organs* 1984;8(3):281–290.

133. Johnson RJ. Complement activation during extracorporeal therapy: biochemistry, cell biology and clinical relevance. *Nephrol Dial Transplant* 1994;9(Suppl. 2):36–45.

134. Videm V, Fosse E, Mollnes TE, et al. Time for new concepts about measurement of complement activation by cardiopulmonary bypass? *Ann Thorac Surg* 1992;54:725–731.

135. Kottke-Marchant K, Anderson JM, Miller KM, et al. Vascular graft-associated complement activation and leukocyte adhesion in an artificial circulation. *J Biomed Mater Res* 1987;21:379–397.

136. Shepard AD, Gelfand JA, Callow AD, et al. Complement activation by synthetic vascular grafts. *J Vasc Surg* 1984;1:829–838.

137. Johnson RJ. Immunology and the complement system. In: Ratner BD, Hoffman AS, Schoen FJ et al., eds. *Biomaterials science.* San Diego, CA: Academic Press, 1996:173–188.

138. Craddock PR, Fehr J, Dalmasso AP, et al. Hemodialysis leukopenia. Pulmonary vascular leukostasis resulting from complement activation by dialyzer cellophane membranes. *J Clin Invest* 1977;59(5):879–888.

139. Kazatchkine MD, Carreno M-P. Activation of the complement system at the interface between blood and artificial surfaces. *Biomaterials* 1988;9:30–35.

140. Hakim RM. Complement activation by biomaterials. *Cardiovasc Pathol* 1993;2(Suppl. 3):187S–197S.

141. Tulunay M, Demiralp S, Tatsan S, et al. Complement (C3, C4) and C-reactive protein responses to cardiopulmonary bypass and protamine administration. *Anaesth Intensive Care* 1993;21:50–55.

142. Videm V, Mollnes TE, Bergh K, et al. Heparin-coated cardiopulmonary bypass equipment. II. Mechanisms for reduced complement activation *in vivo. J Thorac Cardiovasc Surg* 1999;117(4):803–809.

143. Lhotta K, Wurzner R, Kronenberg F, et al. Rapid activation of the complement system by cuprophane depends on complement component C4. *Kidney Int* 1998;53(4):1044–1051.

144. Thylen P, Fernvik E, Lundhal J, et al. Modulation of CD11b/CD18 on monocytes and neutrophils following hemodialysis membrane interaction *in vitro. Int J Artif Organs* 1996;19(3):156–163.

145. Nilsson UR, Larm O, Nilsson B, et al. Modification of the complement binding properties of polystyrene; effects of end-point heparin attachment. *Scand J Immunol* 1993;37(3):349–354.

146. Sefton MV, Gemmell CH, Gorbet MB. What really is blood compatibility. *J Biomater Sci Polym Ed* 2000;11(11):1165–1182.

147. Gorbet MB, Sefton MV. Leukocyte activation and procoagulant activities. In preparation, 2005.

148. Colman RW. Mechanisms of thrombus formation. *Cardiovasc Pathol* 1993;2(Suppl. 3):23S–31S.

149. Edmunds LH Jr. Is prosthetic valve thrombogenicity related to design or material? *Tex Heart Inst J* 1996;23(1):24–27.

150. Kappelmayer J, Bernabei A, Edmunds LH Jr, et al. Tissue factor is expressed on monocytes during simulated extracorporeal circulation. *Circ Res* 1993;72(5):1075–1081.

151. Barstad RM, Hamers MJAG, Moller A-S, et al. Monocyte procoagulant activity induced by adherence to an artificial surface is reduced by end-point immobilized heparin coating of the surface. *Thromb Haemost* 1998;79:302–305.

152. Stahl RF, Fisher CA, Kucich U, et al. Effects of simulated extracorporeal circulation on human leukocyte elastase release, superoxide generation and procoagulant activity. *J Thorac Cardiovasc Surg* 1991;101:230–239.

153. Parratt R, Hunt BJ. Direct activation of factor X by monocytes occurs during cardiopulmonary bypass. *Br J Haematol* 1998;101:40–46.

154. Rinder CS, Bonan JL, Rinder HM, et al. Cardiopulmonary bypass induces leukocyte-platelet adhesion. *Blood* 1992;79(5):1201–1205.

155. Gawaz M, Bogner C. Changes in platelet membrane glycoproteins and platelet leukocyte interactions during hemodialysis. *J Clin Invest* 1994;72:424–429.

156. May AE, Neumann F-J, Gavaz M, et al. Reduction of monocyte-platelet interaction and monocyte activation in patients receiving antiplatelet therapy after coronary stent implantation. *Eur Heart J* 1997;18:1913–1920.

157. Palabrica T, Lobb R, Furie BC, et al. Leukocyte accumulation promoting fibrin deposition is mediated *in vivo* by P-selectin on adherent platelets. *Nature* 1992;359:848–851.

158. Toombs CF, De Graaf GL, Martin JP, et al. Pretreatment with a blocking antibody to P-sel accelerates pharmacological thrombolysis in a primate model of arterial thrombosis. *J Pharmacol Exp Ther* 1995;275(2):941.

159. Basmadjian D, Sefton MV, Baldwin SA. Coagulation on biomaterials in flowing blood: some theoretical considerations. *Biomaterials* 1997;18:1511–1522.

160. Turitto VT, Weiss HJ, Baumgartner HR. The effect of shear rate on platelet interaction with subendothelium exposed to citrated human blood. *Microvasc Res* 1980;19:352–365.

161. Turitto VT, Hall CL. Mechanical factors affecting hemostasis and thrombosis. *Thromb Res* 1998;92:S25–S31.

162. Hanson SR, Sakariassen KS. Blood flow and antithrombotic drug effects. *Am Heart J* 1998;135:S132–S145.

163. O'Brien JR. Shear induced platelet aggregation. *Lancet* 1990;335:711–713.

164. Oda A, Yokoyama K, Murata M, et al. Protein tyrosine phosphorylation in human platelets during shear-stress induced aggregation (SIPA) is regulated by GPIb/IX as well as GPIIb/IIIa and requires intact cytskeleton and endogenous ADP. *Thromb Haemost* 1995;74:736–742.

165. Kujiper PHM, Gallardo Torres HI, van der Linden JAM, et al. Platelet-dependent primary hemostasis promotes selectin- and integrin-mediated neutrophil adhesion to damaged endothelium under flow conditions. *Blood* 1996;87(8):3271–3281.

166. Yeo EL, Sheppard J-OI, Feuerstein IA. Role of P-selectin and leukocyte activation in polymorphonuclear cell adhesion to surface adherent activated platelets under physiological shear conditions (an injury vessel wall model). *Blood* 1994;83(9):2498–2507.

167. Morley DJ, Feuerstein IA. Adhesion of polymorphonuclear leukocytes to protein-coated and platelet adherent surfaces. *Thromb Haemost* 1989;62(3):1023–1028.

168. Weber C, Springer TA. Neutrophil accumulation on activated, surface-adherent platelets in flow is mediated by interaction of MAc-1 with fibrinogen bound to αIIbβ3 and stimulated by platelet activating factor. *J Clin Invest* 1997;100:2085–2093.

169. Kujiper PHM, Gallardo Torres HI, Lammers J-WJ, et al. Platelet and fibrin deposition at the damaged vessel wall: cooperative substrates for neutrophil adhesion under flow conditions. *Blood* 1997;89(1):166–175.

170. Bruil A, Sheppard JI, Feijen J, et al. *In vitro* leukocyte adhesion to modified polyurethane surfaces: III effects of flow, fluid medium and platelets on PMN adhesion. In: Cooper SL, Bamford CH, Tsuruta T, eds. *Polymer biomaterials in solution, as interfaces and as solid,* Leiden, The Netherlands, VSP 1995:357–371.

171. Kujiper PHM, Gallardo Torres HI, van der Linden JAM, et al. Neutrophil adhesion to fibrinogen and fibrin under flow conditions is diminished by activation and L-selectin shedding. *Blood* 1997;89(6):2131–2138.

172. Hernandez MR, Escolar G, Bozzo J, et al. Inhibition of fibrin deposition on the subendothelium by a monoclonal antibody to polymorphonuclear leukocyte integrin CD11b. Studies in a flow system. *Haematologica* 1997;82:566–571.

173. Bahra P, Nash GB. Sparsely adherent platelets support capture and immobilization of flowing neutrophils. *J Lab Clin Med* 1998;132:223–228.

174. Gemmell CH, Nemerson Y, Turitto VT. The effects of shear rate on the enzymatic activity of the tissue factor–factor VIIa complex. *Microvasc Res* 1990;40:327–340.

175. Nemerson Y, Contino PB. Tissue factor, flow and the initiation of coagulation. In: Seghatchian MJ, Samana MM, Hecker SP, eds. *Hypercoagulable states*: CRC Press, Boca Raton, Florida 1996:21–28.

176. Bluestein D, Rambod E, Gharib M. Vortex shedding as a mechanism for free emboli formation in mechanical heart valves. *J Biomech Eng* 2000;122:125–134.

177. Marcus AJ. Thrombosis and inflammation as multicellular processes: significance of cell–cell interactions. *Semin Hematol* 2000;31(4):261–269.

# CHAPTER 50 ■ THE VASCULAR RESPONSE TO INJURY

## ALEXANDER W. CLOWES

When an artery is damaged, the injury is repaired by cells derived from the adjacent normal tissue. The reparative response often includes the development of a thickened intima. The intimal thickening induced by injury resembles the fibrous lesions found in atherosclerotic arteries and was first studied as a model of the human disease (1,2). The current rationale for studying the injury response is that all forms of vascular reconstruction inevitably damage vessels, and the healing that follows often narrows the reconstructed vessel. The information gained from these studies has provided insights into the regulation of vascular cell growth and function during normal development and in pathologic states. The ultimate goal of this research is to develop pharmacologic strategies to modify vascular scarring so that zones of injury are repaired without luminal narrowing. The ways to damage a blood vessel are innumerable and are bound only by the inventiveness of the investigator, but the ways in which the wall can respond are limited and depend mostly on the extent of the initial injury and whether the injury recurs.

## CLINICAL SIGNIFICANCE

The importance of vascular wound healing in vascular reconstructions became evident when vascular surgeons developed techniques for direct repair (e.g., patch angioplasty and endarterectomy) or bypass grafting (e.g., vein and synthetic). More recently, cardiologists and interventional radiologists have developed a similar appreciation for the injury response because they use less intrusive but, in the final analysis, more injurious intraluminal approaches to rebuilding blood vessels (i.e., balloon angioplasty, atherectomy and stent angioplasty). Each of these interventions can fail early because of technical misadventures, and later (i.e., 1 to 12 months), because of injury-induced scarring (3,4). Late (i.e., >12 months) failures occur because the underlying atherosclerotic process progresses during the period—a problem of great clinical importance. The morbidity and expense of further treatment are considerable because no adjuvant therapies exist to prevent luminal narrowing.

## BIOLOGIC ASPECTS OF REPAIR

A simple conclusion drawn from 40 years of investigation is that the response of the artery is in proportion to the magnitude and not to the type of injury (5). Cannulation of an artery for a short time strips some of the endothelium but has little impact on the structure and the function of the vessel, whereas stent angioplasty disrupts medial elastic layers and induces a scarring that makes the vessel thick and immobile. In the following sections, we explore the biologic and biochemical bases for these graded responses to injury.

### Mild Injury

The introduction of a nylon filament or moderate hydrostatic distension of the rat carotid artery causes focal loss of endothelium (6–8). Platelets adhere, spread, and degranulate at the site of injury and are rapidly replaced by regenerating endothelium, a process that involves both migration and proliferation. Although the media is not disrupted, a small fraction of the smooth muscle cells (SMCs) undergo one round of proliferation. If the endothelial layer is completely stripped, the reparative process is protracted, and endothelial regeneration may cease before the monolayer is fully reestablished. If endothelial repair is not complete by 1 week after injury, SMCs migrate from the media to the intima and form a small intimal thickening.

### Moderate Injury

The passage of a balloon embolectomy catheter in a rat carotid artery strips away the endothelium and stretches and damages the underlying media (see Fig. 50-1) (9–11). Approximately one fourth of the medial SMCs are destroyed by this maneuver. The pattern of response of the balloon- and filament-injured vessels is similar, except that the first wave of proliferation and subsequent intimal thickening are greater in the balloon-injured vessel. SMC proliferation, as detected by tritiated thymidine or bromodeoxyuridine labeling, begins between 24 and 48 hours after injury and is localized primarily to the inner layers of the media. By 4 days, SMCs start migrating from the media into the intima. These cells continue to divide for several more rounds before resuming the resting state. At the luminal surface, in regions not covered by endothelium, the SMCs can form a nonthrombogenic pseudoendothelium, although the intercellular junctions are leaky to macromolecules (12,13). These luminal SMCs proliferate. Because the proliferation is matched by cell death, no net accumulation of cells occurs, and the intima does not expand (1,14,15). The intimal cells synthesize and secrete extracellular matrix. In its final form, the intima is largely composed of matrix (approximately 80%) and is relatively acellular (10). Endothelial cells derived from the ends of the zone of injury regenerate a luminal surface by migration and proliferation. If the injured segment is long and if the remaining sources of endothelium are far apart (>4 cm), endothelial repair is not completed and stops at approximately 1.5 cm (11,16).

### Severe Injury

The procedures used to restore luminal patency in atherosclerotic arteries (balloon angioplasty, atherectomy, stent angioplasty) produce severe damage and induce a response that

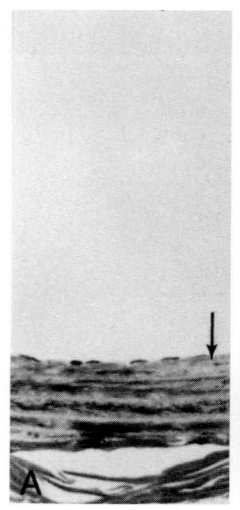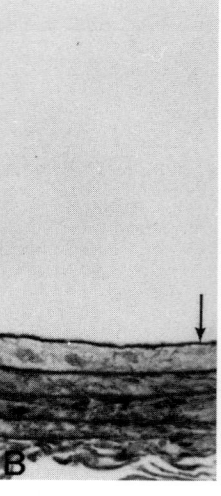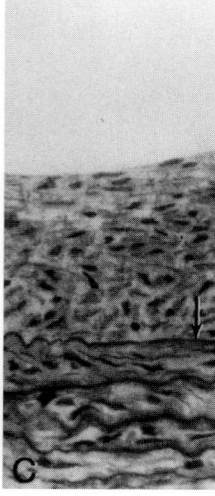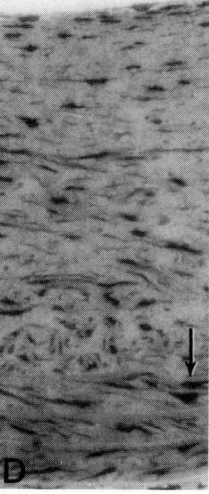

**FIGURE 50-1.** Histologic cross sections of rat carotid artery (**A**) before injury, (**B**) immediately after endothelial denudation with a balloon catheter, (**C**) 2 weeks after injury, and (**D**) 12 weeks after injury. Note the marked intimal thickening at 2 and 12 weeks. *Arrows* indicate internal elastic lamina. Lumen is at top. (From Clowes AW, Reidy MA, Clowes MM. Kinetics of cellular proliferation after arterial injury. I. Smooth muscle growth in the absence of endothelium. *Lab Invest* 1983; 49:327, with permission.)

differs considerably from what has been observed in arteries subjected to simple denuding injuries (17,18). Balloon angioplasty disrupts the elastin layers of the media and, in atherosclerotic vessels, creates tears in the intima. Thrombus forms rapidly in these rents and can cause vascular occlusion. The reparative phase involves an initial influx of macrophages and is followed by the accumulation of mesenchymal cells, which expresses SMC proteins at later stages. Although the neointimal cells might come from the media and diseased intima, they are also derived from adventitial cells that appear to be able to traverse the entire wall (19,20).

How the endothelial layer is reestablished has not been determined completely. Repair by ingrowth from adjacent artery is likely to proceed as it does in milder forms of injury. In addition, transected microvessels (vasa vasorum) and circulating stem cell precursors can serve as sources of endothelium and SMCs (21,22). Blood-borne progenitors have the potential to differentiate into endothelium and SMCs and to contribute to the formation of microvessels, the lesions of transplant atherosclerosis, and the neointima of arteries treated by angioplasty (23–25).

In the more severe forms of injury, luminal narrowing is a feature of the reparative process (see Figs. 50-2 and 50-3). Although originally thought to be a reflection of encroachment of the thickened intima, luminal narrowing is largely caused by vasoconstriction (often called *pathologic* or *geometric remodeling*) except in cases in which the vessel is stented open and vasomotor activity is abolished (26–29). The underlying mechanism has not been defined; it may be related to the formation and contraction of granulation tissue in the adventitia (30).

## Intimal Thickening in Chronically Injured Arteries and Vascular Grafts

A number of pathologic states are associated with chronic injury to the artery, including advanced atherosclerosis with or without stent angioplasty, aneurysmal degeneration, and transplant arteriosclerosis. These diseases are all characterized by inflammation and loss of tissue architecture in association with endothelial damage. The long-term outcome depends on the location and severity of the inflammation. The inflammation and pathologic narrowing are an intimal process in atherosclerosis, whereas in aneurysmal disease, the inflammation is transmural (31,32).

In stented atherosclerotic arteries, the inflammatory response following the intraluminal intervention persists, whereas after simple balloon angioplasty the response is transient (33). In some circumstances (e.g., following intraluminal irradiation), endothelial regeneration in the stented vessel is incomplete and renders the stented artery susceptible to late thrombosis, often with catastrophic consequences (34).

Neointimal thickening develops in synthetic vascular grafts, particularly at anastomoses. In the baboon, polytetrafluoroethylene (PTFE) grafts form a neointima composed of SMCs and lined by endothelium derived from adjacent arteries and microvessels arising from the surrounding granulation tissue that penetrate the graft matrix (4). The intima that is established under the high flow generated by a femoral arteriovenous fistula is thin and can be induced to thicken by ligating the fistula to return the flow to normal. Like the intima of the injured artery, this increase in neointimal thickening is associated with SMC proliferation and matrix deposition. Unlike the injured artery, it develops in the absence of endothelial denudation and platelet activation (4).

# MOLECULAR MECHANISMS

A detailed understanding of the molecular basis for the injury response has grown out of three primary observations: (a) medial SMC proliferation is in proportion to the severity of the injury—more injury causes more proliferation; (b) nearly all forms of injury cause endothelial denudation and accumulation of platelets on the subendothelium; and (c) serum derived from clotted blood contains factors that stimulate SMC growth and migration *in vitro*.

The magnitude of the first wave of SMC proliferation is linked to the damage inflicted on the arterial wall (35). In the rat carotid artery, the passage of an inflated embolectomy catheter strips away the endothelium and ruptures a significant proportion of the medial SMCs, thereby releasing growth-promoting factors, including basic fibroblast growth factor (bFGF). SMC proliferation can be suppressed either by displacing the bFGF with a bolus of heparin or by blocking it with an antibody (36–38). Administration of pharmacologic quantities of bFGF stimulates SMC proliferation. The induction of SMC growth might also be regulated by thrombin generated at the site of injury because inhibitors of tissue factor and thrombin are also able to inhibit DNA synthesis (39–42).

SMC migration is controlled by factors from platelets. Intimal thickening in case of animals rendered thrombocytopenic is largely blocked although the first wave of DNA synthesis is

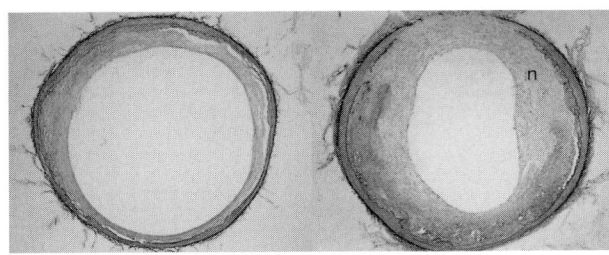

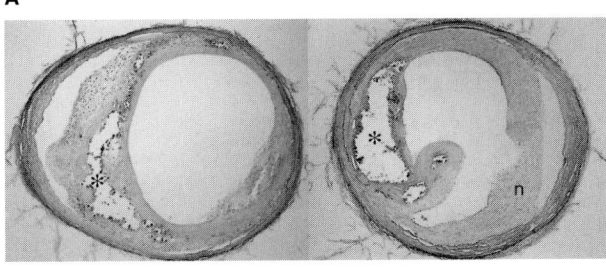

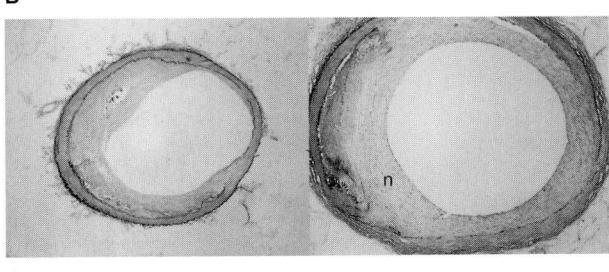

**FIGURE 50-2.** Photomicrographs of control (**left**) and of angioplastied (**right**) iliac arteries from three monkeys 28 days after unilateral iliac angioplasty. The lesions depicted are representative of the variation in primary iliac atherosclerosis (**left**) and of the injury response 28 days after angioplasty (**right**) in this model. **A:** Despite fracture of the plaque and media, artery size is similar to the control artery and significant neointimal hyperplasia (*n*) has decreased the lumen caliber. **B:** Large eccentric plaques with regions of necrosis and calcification (*asterisk*) are present in both arteries. Angioplasty has fractured and dissected the plaque, resulting in a complex lumen channel, which has been partly filled in with neointima (*n*). Lumen area is similar. **C:** Fracture of the plaque and media has led to the formation of a very large neointima (*n*). Although the external elastic lamina appears intact, artery size and lumen caliber have both increased (magnification ×40). (From Geary RI, Williams JK, Golden D, et al. Time course of cellular proliferation, intimal hyperplasia, and remodeling following angioplasty in monkeys with established atherosclerosis. A nonhuman primate model of restenosis. *Arterioscl Thromb Vasc Biol* 1996;16:34, with permission.)

unaffected (43,44). Furthermore, in injured animal arteries, SMC migration, and not SMC proliferation, is stimulated by platelet-derived growth factor (PDGF-BB) and is blocked by the administration of antibodies that recognize PDGF or inhibitors of the β form of the platelet-derived growth factor receptor (PDGFR-β) (45–49). Medial SMC proliferation is not affected by these manipulations. PDGF is not only liberated from platelets during degranulation but also synthesized and secreted by vascular wall cells (50). Viewed together, these observations support the conclusion that platelets and platelet factors control the recruitment and movement of SMC into the zone of injury, whereas factors from dead cells and, perhaps, the initial coagulation events initiate growth.

Other factors, including angiotensin II, transforming growth factor-β (TGF-β), norepinephrine, and endothelin, might play a role in stimulating intimal thickening (51–56). Some of these factors might act indirectly through costimulatory pathways involving the local release and paracrine action of heparin-binding growth factors (57). Blockade with angiotensin-converting enzyme (ACE) or angiotensin receptor antagonists retards intimal thickening by inhibiting SMC migration from the media to the intima. ACE inhibitors may act not only by blocking the formation of angiotensin II but also by preventing the degradation of bradykinin. Although the ACE inhibitors do not affect SMC proliferation, angiotensin II infused in pharmacologic amounts increases blood pressure and stimulates SMC–DNA replication in the media and the intima (58,59). Intimal thickening can be blocked by the administration of antibodies to TGF-β. Although TGF-β is a pleiotropic stimulant for SMCs in culture, it is not known as to what part of the intimal thickening process is affected by TGF-β *in vivo*. Factors secreted by macrophages might also play a role in intimal thickening (60–62).

The factors regulating intimal SMC growth and death as well as matrix deposition have not been determined for the injured rat carotid artery. For example, intimal SMC proliferation does not appear to be regulated by PDGF or bFGF although receptors for these growth factors are present. In baboon arterial bypass grafts, however, intimal thickening stimulated by a switch from high to normal blood flow can be inhibited by a chimeric blocking antibody against human PDGFR-β and can even be induced to atrophy if antibodies to both forms of the receptor are administered simultaneously (63,64).

PDGFR-β binds only PDGF-B or -D chain, whereas the other isoform of the receptor (PDGFR-α) binds PDGF-A, -B, or -C chain (65). The receptor forms a dimer and is activated in the presence of the appropriate dimeric ligand. PDGF-BB binds to PDGFR-ββ, -αβ, or -αα; PDGF-AB binds to PDGFR-αβ or -αα; and PDGF-AA binds only to PDGFR-αα. PDGF-CC binds to PDGFR-αα and -αβ, wheras PDGF-DD binds to PDGFR-ββ and -αβ. PDGFR-β is expressed by intimal SMCs. Therefore, the inhibition by an antibody to PDGFR-β demonstrates conclusively that PDGF-B or -D chain contributes to intimal thickening. The PDGFs are not only released from platelets but are also synthesized by endothelium, SMCs, and macrophages *in vitro*; in arterial and graft intima, PDGF-A predominates, although PDGF-B has been detected in endothelial cells under conditions of reduced flow (50,66–68).

It is important to link the mechanism of healing in adult animals to the development of vessels in the embryonic period. The disruption of the genes for PDGF-A, PDGF-B, PDGFR-α, or PDGFR-β leads to death in the embryonic period (50). In the PDGFR-β knockout mouse, endothelial tubes form but lack a complete pericyte/SMC coat. Therefore, PDGFR-β expression by the mesodermal cells destined to become SMCs is required for SMC recruitment by the nascent endothelial cells. This pattern of SMC activation is recapitulated in the adult in response to injury.

The program of gene induction in the embryo is described in detail in Chapter 41. Many of these genes are turned off in the neonatal period, only to be reinduced in the injured vessel (1). For example, elastin is expressed in the aorta beginning at fetal day 19 and is turned off at 4 weeks after birth in the rat. After balloon injury of the carotid artery, elastin is expressed by SMCs after they migrate into the intima (69,70). The elastin gene is also induced by acute hypertension (71).

A number of genes are expressed and are required for entry into the cell cycle (0 to 24 hours) and for migration into the intima (after 3 days). For example, in the rat, c-*myc* and c-*myb* blockade with antisense oligonucleotides inhibits DNA replication and intimal hyperplasia (72). The plasminogen activators, urokinase-type plasminogen activator (uPA) and tissue-type plasminogen activator, are expressed during the first 2 weeks; inhibition with tranexamic acid or local overexpression of the

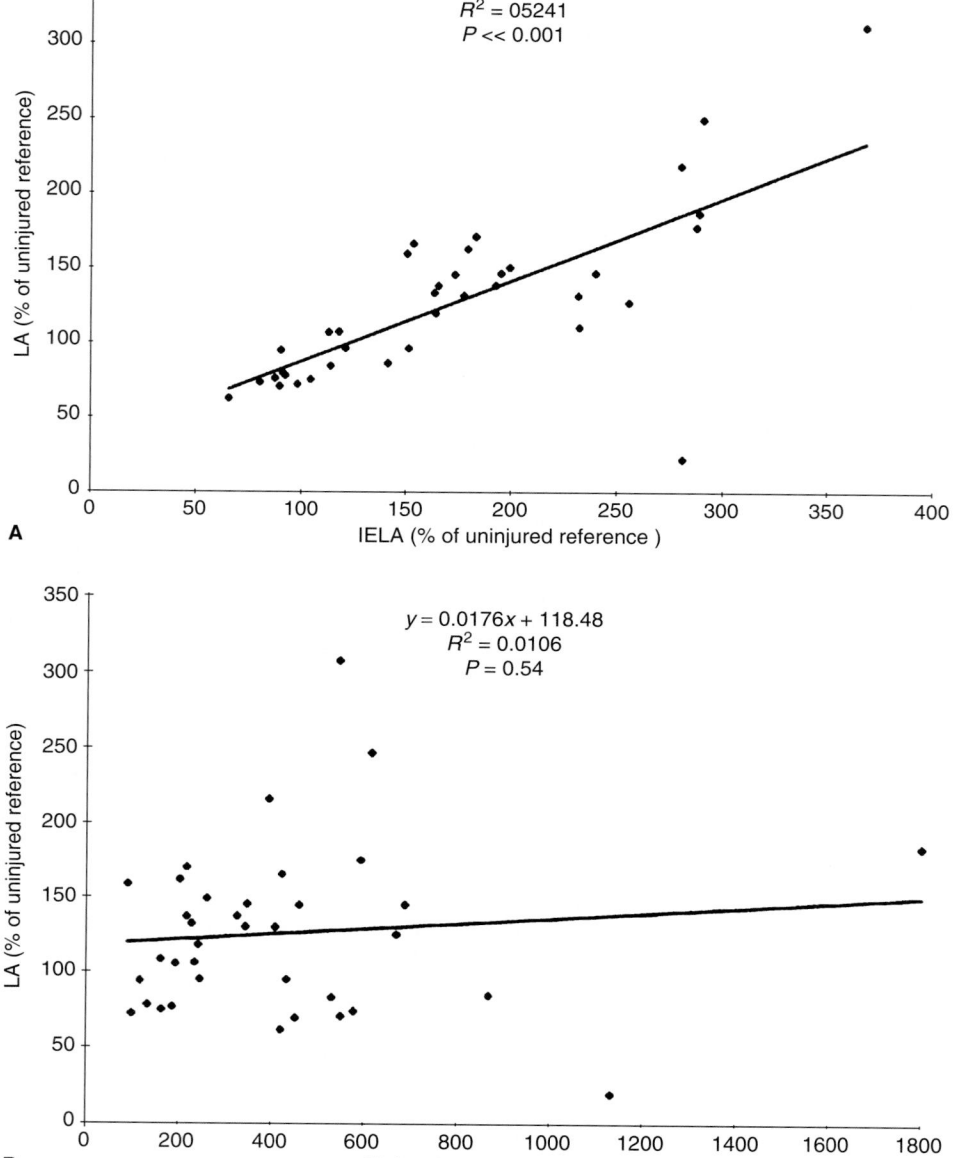

**FIGURE 50-3.** Scatter plots with regression lines for normalized luminal area (LA) compared with normalized internal elastic lamina area (IELA) **(A)** and compared with normalized intimal area (IA) **(B)** of injured iliac arteries from 37 atherosclerotic cynomolgus monkeys. Lumen caliber and artery size are closely related ($r = 0.72$), whereas a poor correlation exists between lumen caliber and intimal mass ($r = 0.10$). (From Mondy JS, Williams JK, Adams MR, et al. Structural determinants of lumen narrowing after angioplasty in atherosclerotic nonhuman primates. *J Vasc Surg* 1997;26:875, with permission.)

plasminogen activator inhibitor, PAI-1, suppresses SMC migration without affecting proliferation (73–75). Intimal thickening in response to injury is reduced in uPA and uPA receptor$^{-/-}$ mice, is increased in PAI-1$^{-/-}$ mice, and is not altered in tissue-type plasminogen activator$^{-/-}$ mice (76). Matrix metalloproteinases (MMPs) are also expressed and are required primarily for cell movement. Although gelatinase A (MMP-2) is expressed constitutively, gelatinase B (MMP-9) and stromelysin-1 (MMP-3) are induced early after injury (77–80). The administration of active site inhibitors or local overexpression of the tissue inhibitor of MMP-1 suppresses intimal thickening by inhibiting SMC migration. The cells also express and respond to provisional matrix proteins (i.e., vitronectin, fibronectin, osteopontin, and hyaluronan) (70,81–90). The proteins surround the cells and provide a necessary substrate for movement. Certain integrin receptors on SMCs (e.g., $\alpha_v\beta_3$) are similar to the receptors on platelets that mediate aggregation [e.g., glycoprotein (GP)

IIb/IIIa]. It is an intriguing possibility that pharmacologic antagonists of platelet aggregation (e.g., monoclonal antibody 7E3) may also have a significant and independent inhibiting effect on other injury responses, such as SMC migration (91).

## NEGATIVE GROWTH CONTROL

SMCs in healthy adult arteries have a very low rate of proliferation (<0.01% per day) and, therefore, turn over once every 30 years! Nevertheless, they can be induced to enter the growth cycle within 24 hours of injury. This observation is of great importance because it suggests that SMCs are relatively refractory to transient mitogenic stimuli, except under very well controlled circumstances. Indeed, a bolus of bFGF administered intravenously or locally has no stimulatory effect unless the wall has been disrupted (92,93).

What keeps SMC growth in check? Is it simply the lack of stimulatory factors, or is it because the growth inhibitors are present? The observation that injury sets the stage for SMC proliferation driven by bFGF provides support for the hypothesis that endothelial cells, or possibly SMCs, are a potential source of growth-controlling substances (94,95). In the embryonic period, the endothelial cells express PDGF, and the knockout experiments tell us that PDGF is essential for the recruitment of SMCs. Could endothelial cells also express inhibitors of SMC growth? In the rat, endothelial regeneration is associated with the cessation of SMC replication (7). On the other hand, in the baboon graft subjected to a decrease in blood flow, SMCs proliferate just underneath the endothelium and nowhere else in the neointima (96,97). These disparate findings can be reconciled if we propose that nitric oxide (NO) generated by the catalytic action of endothelial cell nitric oxide synthase (eNOS) on L-arginine is responsible for maintaining medial SMCs in the quiescent state (see Chapter 42). In the first situation (rat carotid injury), ballooning simply deletes the endothelial cells and the source of eNOS, whereas in the second situation (baboon graft), eNOS gene expression, and, therefore, NO production, is turned off by a switch in blood flow from high to normal (98). The eNOS gene is one of several endothelial genes induced by high shear stress. Other genes expressing inhibitors of SMC growth are also induced in endothelium by increased shear stress (e.g., cyclooxygenase-2) (99). Prostaglandins $I_2$ and $E_2$ are synthesized from arachidonic acid by cyclooxygenase-2. These molecules might also play a role in suppressing SMC growth under high flow conditions. Cyclooxygenase-2 and the inducible form of nitric oxide synthase (NOS) are expressed in injured arteries and might therefore help to limit intimal hyperplasia by blunting the activity of growth factors such as bFGF and PDGF (100–103). Interferon-γ is another potential negative regulator of SMC function. It is secreted by a small number of T cells in the intima, induces the expression of major histocompatibility complex class II antigens, and suppresses SMC replication (104,105).

Matrix molecules surrounding the medial SMCs might also regulate responsiveness to growth factors. For example, heparinlike heparan sulfates possess growth inhibitory activity (95,106,107). In mice expressing a mutant perlecan lacking heparan sulfates, the response to injury is markedly increased (108). Heparin suppresses SMC proliferation and migration *in vitro* and *in vivo*, possibly, by blocking autocrine heparin-binding growth factors (e.g., bFGF and heparin-binding epidermal growth factor–like growth factor) and by inhibiting the activation of mitogen-activated protein kinases as well as critical cell cycle genes (e.g., c-*myb*) and proteases required for matrix degradation (109–112). Polymerized interstitial collagen suppresses SMC growth by inducing endogenous cyclin inhibitors, whereas monomeric collagen has no effect (113). Perhaps, one of the functions of the proteases induced in SMCs as a part of the response to injury is to degrade the polymerized collagen in the neighborhood of the cells and to thereby potentiate the proliferative response. The matrix secreted in the intima as the SMCs stop growing might help maintain the quiescent state.

We think of intimal thickening as a process determined by the migration and proliferation of SMCs—cellular events controlled by the balance of positive and negative stimulants. Intimal thickening is probably also affected by cell death (apoptosis). Apoptosis is an important event in vasculogenesis and vascular remodeling (see Chapters 41 and 43) and may contribute to the termination of intimal thickening after injury (15,114–117). Although SMCs continue to replicate at the surface of vessels lacking endothelium, no net increase in SMC number occurs. Furthermore, an increase in apoptotic cells is readily detected in this region. Apoptosis can be induced in SMCs in vessels subjected to a permanent change in blood flow (98,118). For example, in synthetic PTFE grafts in baboons, a switch from normal to high flow causes the neointima to shrink, a process reflecting a net loss of cells and matrix (98). The intracellular mechanisms of apoptosis are being defined and appear to involve the activation of a sequence of proteases called *caspases* (119). The initiating events in whole vessels are not known and could include an increase in negative growth control factors (e.g., NO) and a decrease in growth or survival factors (e.g., PDGF and angiotensin II) (120).

# REGULATION OF THE RESPONSE TO INJURY IN HUMANS

At the beginning of the chapter, it was suggested that injury and the injury response were part of all forms of vascular reconstruction. In 30% to 50% of the reconstructions, the lumen of the vessel narrows (or renarrows) within 3 to 12 months after surgery. In some instances, the narrowing is attributable to intimal hyperplasia (e.g., arteries subjected to stent angioplasty, synthetic, or vein bypass grafts), whereas, in others, it is largely caused by vascular shrinkage (pathologic remodeling after angioplasty) (4,28,121). Pharmacologic approaches to prevent narrowing have focused on antithrombotic/anticoagulant agents (122,123). These drugs either have no effect or improve patency by inhibiting thrombosis immediately after surgery. If the administration of the drugs is delayed until several days after the intervention, they are of no benefit. However, a study comparing the effects of ticlopidine to placebo started between 3 and 14 days after peripheral vein bypass grafting reported a statistically significant improvement in patency (i.e., 82% vs. 63% at 24 months) (124). These results are surprising because thrombotic activity in vascular reconstructions declines rapidly after the first 24 hours (125,126). Therefore, either ticlopidine has some activity apart from inhibiting platelet aggregation or thrombotic activity persists in peripheral vein bypass grafts for a long time.

The most successful strategies for controlling luminal narrowing are mechanical. Stents improve patency simply because they brace the angioplastied vessel open and create an abnormally large lumen. Stenoses in vein bypass grafts are best treated by additional surgery (i.e., patch angioplasty or further bypass grafting) (127). All these re-reconstructions are subject to the injury response and luminal narrowing. Local irradiation has been proposed as a means of controlling intimal hyperplasia and restenosis in stented coronary arteries (128,129). Although radiation can suppress intimal thickening, it can also prevent endothelial repair and cause SMC proliferation at the boundary of the radiation field (129). It is still too early to know whether radiation will be of general use for controlling the injury response.

The problem of intimal hyperplasia and luminal narrowing in stented arteries has been controlled by drugs (e.g., rapamycin and paclitaxel) released from a gel coating on the stents. Systemic toxicity is avoided by using this local delivery approach. The drugs used are general cell cycle inhibitors and are not particularly targeted at SMCs. The results have been astonishing, and the recurrence rates extremely low (130–134). However, systemically administered therapies to control luminal narrowing in stented arteries or other kinds of vascular reconstruction are not yet available. Unfortunately, the systemic administration of a PDGFR-β antagonist failed to inhibit restenosis in stented human coronary arteries (135).

Adjuvant therapy to prevent luminal narrowing will make a more thorough use of what is known about positive and negative regulators of SMC growth. For example, we need to know whether vascular shrinkage (i.e., pathologic remodeling) is the vascular form of wound contraction and whether it will therefore respond to agents that prevent SMC or myofibroblast contraction. In addition, it is important to know what factors keep vessel growth in check and whether, like NO, these factors possess activities that affect both the growth and vasocontractile state of the vessel. Many of these factors are secreted by the endothelium but can still function in the absence of endothelium if supplied systemically or locally. The goal is to suppress excessive scarring and contracture while permitting normal wound healing and restoration of vascular integrity.

In summary, these observations provide support for the conclusion that SMC growth and death are regulated by positive and negative effectors. Under normal physiologic circumstances, the negative factors predominate and render the wall resistant to stimulants of growth. These conclusions should come as no surprise, given that many other physiologic activities (e.g., vasomotor activity and coagulation) are similarly regulated. Many of the inhibitors of vascular contraction and coagulation are also inhibitors of the injury response (e.g., NO, tissue factor inhibitors and heparin).

## References

1. Schwartz SM, DeBlois D, O'Brien ERM. The intima – soil for atherosclerosis and restenosis. *Circ Res* 1995;77:445–465.
2. Moore S. Injury mechanisms in atherogenesis. In: Moore S, ed. *Vascular injury and atherosclerosis.* New York: Marcel Dekker Inc, 1981:131–148.
3. Allaire E, Clowes AW. The intimal hyperplastic response. *Ann Thorac Surg* 1997;64(4):S38–S46.
4. Clowes AW. Intimal hyperplasia and graft failure. *Cardiovasc Pathol* 1993;2:179S–186S.
5. Reidy MA, Fingerle J, Lindner V. Factors controlling the development of arterial lesions after injury. *Circulation* 1992;86(Suppl. III):43–46.
6. Lindner V, Reidy MA, Fingerle J. Regrowth of arterial endothelium. Denudation with minimal trauma leads to complete endothelial cell regrowth. *Lab Invest* 1989;61:556–563.
7. Fingerle J, Au YPT, Clowes AW, et al. Intimal lesion formation in rat carotid arteries after endothelial denudation in absence of medial injury. *Arteriosclerosis* 1990;10:1082–1087.
8. Clowes AW, Clowes MM, Fingerle J, et al. Kinetics of cellular proliferation after arterial injury. V. Role of acute distension in the induction of smooth muscle proliferation. *Lab Invest* 1989;60:360–364.
9. Clowes AW, Reidy MA, Clowes MM. Kinetics of cellular proliferation after arterial injury. I. Smooth muscle growth in the absence of endothelium. *Lab Invest* 1983;49:327–333.
10. Clowes AW, Reidy MA, Clowes MM. Mechanisms of stenosis after arterial injury. *Lab Invest* 1983;49:208–215.
11. Reidy MA, Clowes AW, Schwartz SM. Endothelial regeneration. V. Inhibition of endothelial regrowth in arteries of rat and rabbit. *Lab Invest* 1983;49:569–575.
12. Clowes AW, Collazzo RE, Karnovsky MJ. A morphologic and permeability study of luminal smooth muscle cells after arterial injury in the rat. *Lab Invest* 1978;39:141–150.
13. Clowes AW, Clowes MM, Reidy MA. Kinetics of cellular proliferation after arterial injury. III. Endothelial and smooth muscle growth in chronically denuded vessels. *Lab Invest* 1986;54:295–303.
14. Han DKM, Haudenschild CC, Hong MK, et al. Evidence for apoptosis in human atherogenesis and in a rat vascular injury model. *Am J Pathol* 1995;147:267–277.
15. Bochaton-Piallat M-L, Gabbiani F, Redard M, et al. Apoptosis participates in cellularity regulation during rat aortic intimal thickening. *Am J Pathol* 1995;146:1059–1064.
16. Reidy MA. A reassessment of endothelial injury and arterial lesion formation. *Lab Invest* 1985;53:513–520.
17. Farb A, Weber DK, Kolodgie FD, et al. Morphological predictors of restenosis after coronary stenting in humans. *Circulation* 2002;105(25):2974–2980.
18. Geary RL, Williams JK, Golden D, et al. Time course of cellular proliferation, intimal hyperplasia, and remodeling following angioplasty in monkeys with established atherosclerosis – a nonhuman primate model of restenosis. *Arterioscler Thromb Vasc Biol* 1996;16:34–43.
19. Shi Y, O'Brien JE Jr, Fard A, et al. Adventitial myofibroblasts contribute to neointimal formation in injured porcine coronary arteries. *Circulation* 1996;94(7):1655–1664.
20. Wilcox JN, Waksman R, King SB, et al. The role of the adventitia in the arterial response to angioplasty: the effect of intravascular radiation. *Int J Radiat Oncol Biol Phys* 1996;36(4):789–796.
21. Wu MHD, Shi Q, Wechezak AR, et al. Definitive proof of endothelialization of a Dacron arterial prosthesis in a human being. *J Vasc Surg* 1995;21:862–867.
22. Shi Q, Wu H-D, Sauvage LR, et al. Reendothelialization of isolated segments of the canine carotid artery with reference to the possible role of the adventitial vasa vasorum. *J Vasc Surg* 1990;12:476–487.
23. Asahara T, Murohara T, Sullivan A, et al. Isolation of putative progenitor endothelial cells for angiogenesis. *Science* 1997;275(5302):964–967.
24. Hillebrands JL, Klatter FA, Rozing J. Origin of vascular smooth muscle cells and the role of circulating stem cells in transplant arteriosclerosis. *Arterioscler Thromb Vasc Biol* 2003;23(3):380–387.
25. Sata M. Circulating vascular progenitor cells contribute to vascular repair, remodeling, and lesion formation. *Trends Cardiovasc Med* 2003;13(6):249–253.
26. Bauters C, Van Belle E, Meurice T, et al. Prevention of restenosis – future directions. *Trends Cardiovasc Med* 1997;7(3):90–94.
27. Libby P. Lesion versus lumen. *Nat Med* 1995;1:17–18.
28. Hoffmann R, Mintz GS, Dussaillant GR, et al. Patterns and mechanisms of in-stent restenosis – a serial intravascular ultrasound study. *Circulation* 1996;94(6):1247–1254.
29. Mintz GS, Popma JJ, Pichard AD, et al. Arterial remodeling after coronary angioplasty – a serial intravascular ultrasound study. *Circulation* 1996;94:35–43.
30. Mondy JS, Williams JK, Adams MR, et al. Structural determinants of lumen narrowing after angioplasty in atherosclerotic nonhuman primates. *J Vasc Surg* 1997;26(5):875–883.
31. Libby P, Geng YJ, Sukhova GK, et al. Molecular determinants of atherosclerotic plaque vulnerability. *Ann N Y Acad Sci* 1997;811:134–145.
32. Shah PK. Inflammation, metalloproteinases, and increased proteolysis– an emerging pathophysiological paradigm in aortic aneurysm. *Circulation* 1997;96(7):2115–2117.
33. Welt FGP, Rogers C. Inflammation and restenosis in the stent era. *Arterioscler Thromb Vasc Biol* 2002;22(11):1769–1776.
34. Cheneau E, John MC, Fournadjiev J, et al. Time course of stent endothelialization after intravascular radiation therapy in rabbit iliac arteries. *Circulation* 2003;107(16):2153–2158.
35. Clowes AW, Clowes MM, Fingerle J, et al. Regulation of smooth muscle cell growth in injured artery. *J Cardiovasc Pharmacol* 1989;14(Suppl. 6):S12–S15.
36. Lindner V, Majack RA, Reidy MA. Basic fibroblast growth factor stimulates endothelial regrowth and proliferation in denuded arteries. *J Clin Invest* 1990;85:2004–2008.
37. Lindner V, Reidy MA. Proliferation of smooth muscle cells after vascular injury is inhibited by an antibody against basic fibroblast growth factor. *Proc Natl Acad Sci U S A* 1991;88:3739–3743.
38. Lindner V, Olson NE, Clowes AW, et al. Inhibition of smooth muscle cell proliferation in injured rat arteries. Interaction of heparin with basic fibroblast growth factor. *J Clin Invest* 1992;90:2044–2049.
39. Sarembock IJ, Gertz SD, Thome LM, et al. Effectiveness of hirulog in reducing restenosis after balloon angioplasty of atherosclerotic femoral arteries in rabbits. *J Vasc Res* 1996;33:308–314.
40. Walters TK, Gorog DA, Wood RFM. Thrombin generation following arterial injury is a critical initiating event in the pathogenesis of the proliferative stages of the atherosclerotic process. *J Vasc Res* 1994;31:173–177.
41. Harker LA, Hanson SR, Runge MS. Thrombin hypothesis of thrombus generation and vascular lesion formation. *Am J Cardiol* 1995;75:12B–17B.
42. Jang YS, Guzman LA, Lincoff AM, et al. Influence of blockade at specific levels of the coagulation cascade on restenosis in a rabbit atherosclerotic femoral artery injury model. *Circulation* 1995;92:3041–3050.
43. Fingerle J, Johnson R, Clowes AW, et al. Role of platelets in smooth muscle cell proliferation and migration after vascular injury in rat carotid artery. *Proc Natl Acad Sci U S A* 1989;86:8412–8416.
44. Sirois MG, Simons M, Kuter DJ, et al. Rat arterial wall retains myointimal hyperplastic potential long after arterial injury. *Circulation* 1997;96(4):1291–1298.
45. Jawien A, Bowen-Pope DF, Lindner V, et al. Platelet-derived growth factor promotes smooth muscle migration and intimal thickening in a rat model of balloon angioplasty. *J Clin Invest* 1992;89:507–511.
46. Rutherford C, Martin W, Salame M, et al. Substantial inhibition of neo-intimal response to balloon injury in the rat carotid artery using a combination of antibodies to platelet-derived growth factor-BB and basic fibroblast growth factor. *Atherosclerosis* 1997;130(1–2):45–51.
47. Ferns GAA, Raines EW, Sprugel KH, et al. Inhibition of neointimal smooth muscle accumulation after angioplasty by an antibody to PDGF. *Science* 1991;253:1129–1132.
48. Jackson CL, Raines EW, Ross R, et al. Role of endogenous platelet-derived growth factor in arterial smooth muscle cell migration after balloon catheter injury. *Arterioscler Thromb* 1993;13:1218–1226.
49. Sirois MG, Simons M, Edelman ER. Antisense oligonucleotide inhibition of PDGFR-β receptor subunit expression directs suppression of intimal thickening. *Circulation* 1997;95(3):669–676.
50. Betsholtz C, Karlsson L, Lindahl P. Developmental roles of platelet-derived growth factors. *Bioessays* 2001;23(6):494–507.
51. Pratt RE, Dzau VJ. Pharmacological strategies to prevent restenosis: lessons learned from blockade of the renin-angiotensin system. *Circulation* 1996;93:848–852.
52. Farhy RD, Carretero OA, Ho K-L, et al. Role of kinins and nitric oxide in the effects of angiotensin converting enzyme inhibitors on neointima formation. *Circ Res* 1993;72:1202–1210.

53. Wolf YG, Rasmussen LM, Ruoslahti E. Antibodies against transforming growth factor-β1 suppress intimal hyperplasia in a rat model. *J Clin Invest* 1994;93:1172–1178.

54. Smith JD, Bryant SR, Couper LL, et al. Soluble transforming growth factor-β type II receptor inhibits negative remodeling, fibroblast transdifferentiation, and intimal lesion formation but not endothelial growth. *Circ Res* 1999;84(10):1212–1222.

55. McKenna CJ, Burke SE, Opgenorth TJ, et al. Selective ET(A) receptor antagonism reduces neointimal hyperplasia in a porcine coronary stent model. *Circulation* 1998;97(25):2551–2556.

56. Teeters JC, Erami C, Zhang H, et al. Systemic α1A-adrenoceptor antagonist inhibits neointimal growth after balloon injury of rat carotid artery. *Am J Physiol Heart Circ Physiol* 2003;284(1):H385–H392.

57. Chan AK, Kalmes A, Hawkins S, et al. Blockade of the epidermal growth factor receptor decreases intimal hyperplasia in balloon-injured rat carotid artery. *J Vasc Surg* 2003;37(3):644–649.

58. Daemen MJAP, Lombardi DM, Bosman FT, et al. Angiotensin II induces smooth muscle cell proliferation in the normal and injured rat arterial wall. *Circ Res* 1991;68:450–456.

59. Van Kleef EM, Smits JFM, De Mey JGR, et al. α1-Adrenoreceptor blockade reduces the angiotensin II-induced vascular smooth muscle cell DNA synthesis in the rat thoracic aorta and carotid artery. *Circ Res* 1992;70:1122–1127.

60. Furukawa Y, Matsumori A, Ohashi N, et al. Anti-monocyte chemoattractant protein-1 monocyte chemotactic and activating factor antibody inhibits neointimal hyperplasia in injured rat carotid arteries. *Circ Res* 1999;84(3):306–314.

61. Schober A, Manka D, Von Hundelshausen P, et al. Deposition of platelet RANTES triggering monocyte recruitment requires P-selectin and is involved in neointima formation after arterial injury. *Circulation* 2002;106(12):1523–1529.

62. Phillips JW, Barringhaus KG, Sanders JM, et al. Single injection of P-selectin or P-selectin glycoprotein ligand-1 monoclonal antibody blocks neointima formation after arterial injury in apolipoprotein E-deficient mice. *Circulation* 2003;107(17):2244–2249.

63. Davies MG, Owens EL, Mason DP, et al. Effect of platelet-derived growth factor receptor-α and -β blockade on flow-induced neointimal formation in endothelialized baboon vascular grafts. *Circ Res* 2000;86(7):779–786.

64. Englesbe MJ, Hawkins SM, Hsieh PC, et al. Concomitant blockade of platelet-derived growth factor receptors α and β induces intimal atrophy in baboon PTFE grafts. *J Vasc Surg* 2004;39(2):440–446.

65. Hoch RV, Soriano P. Roles of PDGF in animal development. *Development* 2003;130(20):4769–4784.

66. Kraiss LW, Raines EW, Wilcox JN, et al. Regional expression of the platelet-derived growth factor and its receptors in a primate graft model of vessel wall assembly. *J Clin Invest* 1993;92:338–348.

67. Kraiss LW, Geary RL, Mattsson EJR, et al. Acute reductions in blood flow and shear stress induce platelet-derived growth factor-A expression in baboon prosthetic grafts. *Circ Res* 1996;79:45–53.

68. Mondy JS, Lindner V, Miyashiro JK, et al. Platelet-derived growth factor ligand and receptor expression in response to altered blood flow *in vivo*. *Circ Res* 1997;81(3):320–327.

69. Belknap JK, Grieshaber NA, Schwartz PE, et al. Tropoelastin gene expression in individual vascular smooth muscle cells – relationship to DNA synthesis during vascular development and after arterial injury. *Circ Res* 1996;78:388–394.

70. Nikkari ST, Järveläinen HT, Wight TN, et al. Smooth muscle cell expression of extracellular matrix genes after arterial injury. *Am J Pathol* 1994;144:1348–1356.

71. Keeley FW, Johnson DJ. The effect of developing hypertension on the synthesis and accumulation of elastin in the aorta of the rat. *Biochem Cell Biol* 1986;64:38–43.

72. Baek S, March KL. Gene therapy for restenosis–getting nearer the heart of the matter. *Circ Res* 1998;82(3):295–305.

73. Clowes AW, Clowes MM, Au YPT, et al. Smooth muscle cells express urokinase during mitogenesis and tissue-type plasminogen activator during migration in injured rat carotid artery. *Circ Res* 1990;67:61–67.

74. Jackson CL, Reidy MA. The role of plasminogen activation in smooth muscle cell migration after arterial injury. *Ann N Y Acad Sci* 1992;667:141–150.

75. Hasenstab D, Lea H, Clowes AW. Local plasminogen activator inhibitor type 1 overexpression in rat carotid artery enhances thrombosis and endothelial regeneration while inhibiting intimal thickening. *Arterioscler Thromb Vasc Biol* 2000;20(3):853–859.

76. Carmeliet P. Insights from gene-inactivation studies of the coagulation and plasminogen. *Fibrinolysis* 1997;11:181–191.

77. Hasenstab D, Forough R, Clowes AW. Plasminogen activator inhibitor type 1 and tissue inhibitor of metalloproteinases-2 increase after arterial injury in rats. *Circ Res* 1997;80(4):490–496.

78. Webb KE, Henney AM, Anglin S, et al. Expression of matrix metalloproteinases and their inhibitor TIMP-1 in the rat carotid artery after balloon injury. *Arterioscler Thromb Vasc Biol* 1997;17(9):1837–1844.

79. Bendeck MP, Irvin C, Reidy MA. Inhibition of matrix metalloproteinase activity inhibits smooth muscle cell migration but not neointimal thickening after arterial injury. *Circ Res* 1996;78:38–43.

80. Forough R, Koyama N, Hasenstab D, et al. Overexpression of tissue inhibitor of matrix metalloproteinase-1 inhibits vascular smooth muscle cell functions *in vitro* and *in vivo*. *Circ Res* 1996;79(4):812–820.

81. Geary RL, Wong JM, Rossini A, et al. Expression profiling identifies 147 genes contributing to a unique primate neointimal smooth muscle cell phenotype. *Arterioscler Thromb Vasc Biol* 2002;22(12):2010–2016.

82. Koyama H, Reidy MA. Expression of extracellular matrix proteins accompanies lesion growth in a model of intimal reinjury. *Circ Res* 1998;82(9):988–995.

83. Strauss BH, Robinson R, Batchelor WB, et al. *In vivo* collagen turnover following experimental balloon angioplasty injury and the role of matrix metalloproteinases. *Circ Res* 1996;79(3):541–550.

84. Srivatsa SS, Fitzpatrick LA, Tsao PW, et al. Selective αvβ3 integrin blockade potently limits neointimal hyperplasia and lumen stenosis following deep coronary arterial stent injury: evidence for the functional importance of integrin αvβ3 and osteopontin expression during neointima formation. *Cardiovasc Res* 1997;36(3):408–428.

85. Choi ET, Engel L, Callow AD, et al. Inhibition of neointimal hyperplasia by blocking αvβ3 integrin with a small peptide antagonist *GpenGRGDSPCA*. *J Vasc Surg* 1994;19:125–134.

86. Thyberg J, Blomgren K, Roy J, et al. Phenotypic modulation of smooth muscle cells after arterial injury is associated with changes in the distribution of laminin and fibronectin. *J Histochem Cytochem* 1997;45(6):837–846.

87. Ishiwata T, Aida T, Yokoyama M, et al. Fibronectin biosynthesis in endothelial regeneration after intimal injury. *Exp Mol Pathol* 1994;60:1–11.

88. Bauters C, Marotte F, Hamon M, et al. Accumulation of fetal fibronectin mRNAs after balloon denudation of rabbit arteries. *Circulation* 1995;92:904–911.

89. Liaw L, Lombardi DM, Almeida MM, et al. Neutralizing antibodies directed against osteopontin inhibit rat carotid neointimal thickening after endothelial denudation. *Arterioscler Thromb Vasc Biol* 1997;17(1):188–193.

90. Riessen R, Wight TN, Pastore C, et al. Distribution of hyaluronan during extracellular matrix remodeling in human restenotic arteries and balloon-injured rat carotid arteries. *Circulation* 1996;93:1141–1147.

91. Stouffer GA, Hu ZY, Sajid M, et al. β3 integrins are upregulated after vascular injury and modulate thrombospondin- and thrombin-induced proliferation of cultured smooth muscle cells. *Circulation* 1998;97(9):907–915.

92. Reidy MA. Neointimal proliferation: the role of basic FGF on vascular smooth muscle cell proliferation. *Thromb Haemost* 1993;70:172–176.

93. Cuevas P, Gonzalez AM, Carceller F, et al. Vascular response to basic fibroblast growth factor when infused onto the normal adventitia or into the injured media of the rat carotid artery. *Circ Res* 1991;69:360–369.

94. Nathan A, Nugent MA, Edelman ER. Tissue engineered perivascular endothelial cell implants regulate vascular injury. *Proc Natl Acad Sci U S A* 1995;92:8130–8134.

95. Bingley JA, Hayward IP, Campbell JH, et al. Arterial heparan sulfate proteoglycans inhibit vascular smooth muscle cell proliferation and phenotype change *in vitro* and neointimal formation *in vivo*. *J Vasc Surg* 1998;28(2):308–318.

96. Kraiss LW, Kirkman TR, Kohler TR, et al. Shear stress regulates smooth muscle proliferation and neointimal thickening in porous polytetrafluoroethylene grafts. *Arterioscler Thromb* 1991;11:1844–1852.

97. Geary RL, Kohler TR, Vergel S, et al. Time course of flow-induced smooth muscle cell proliferation and intimal thickening in endothelialized baboon vascular grafts. *Circ Res* 1994;74:14–23.

98. Mattsson EJR, Kohler TR, Vergel SM, et al. Increased blood flow induces regression of intimal hyperplasia. *Arterioscler Thromb Vasc Biol* 1997;17(10):2245–2249.

99. Topper JN, Cai JX, Falb D, et al. Identification of vascular endothelial genes differentially responsive to fluid mechanical stimuli: Cyclooxygenase-2, manganese superoxide dismutase, and endothelial cell nitric oxide synthase are selectively up-regulated by steady laminar shear stress. *Proc Natl Acad Sci U S A* 1996;93(19):10417–10422.

100. Chen L, Daum G, Fischer JW, et al. Loss of expression of the beta subunit of soluble guanylyl cyclase prevents nitric oxide-mediated inhibition of DNA synthesis in smooth muscle cells of old rats. *Circ Res* 2000;86(5):520–525.

101. Hansson GK, Geng Y, Holm J, et al. Arterial smooth muscle cells express nitric oxide synthase in response to endothelial injury. *J Exp Med* 1994;180:733–738.

102. Rimarachin JA, Jacobson JA, Szabo P, et al. Regulation of cyclooxygenase-2 expression in aortic smooth muscle cells. *Arterioscler Thromb* 1994;14:1021–1031.

103. Pritchard KA Jr, O'Banion MK, Miano JM, et al. Induction of cyclooxygenase-2 in rat vascular smooth muscle cells *in vitro* and *in vivo*. *J Biol Chem* 1994;269:8504–8509.

104. Hansson GK, Holm J. Interferon-gamma inhibits arterial stenosis after injury. *Circulation* 1991;84:1266–1272.

105. Wessely R, Hengst L, Jaschke B, et al. A central role of interferon regulatory factor-1 for the limitation of neointimal hyperplasia. *Hum Mol Genet* 2003;12(2):177–187.

106. Fritze LMS, Reilly CF, Rosenberg RD. An antiproliferative heparan sulfate species produced by postconfluent smooth muscle cells. *J Cell Biol* 1985;100:1041–1049.

107. Castellot JJ Jr, Favreau LV, Karnovsky MJ, et al. Inhibition of vascular smooth muscle cell growth by endothelial cell-derived heparin. Possible role of a platelet endoglycosidase. *J Biol Chem* 1982;257:11256–11260.

108. Tran PK, Tran-Lundmark K, Soininen R, et al. Increased intimal hyperplasia and smooth muscle cell proliferation in transgenic mice with heparan sulfate-deficient perlecan. *Circ Res* 2004;94(4):550–558.

109. Kalmes A, Daum G, Clowes AW. EGFR transactivation in the regulation of SMC function. *Ann N Y Acad Sci* 2001;947:42–54.

110. Kalmes A, Vesti BR, Daum G, et al. Heparin blockade of thrombin-induced smooth muscle cell migration involves inhibition of epidermal growth factor (EGF) receptor transactivation by heparin-binding EGF-like growth factor. *Circ Res* 2000;87(2):92–98.

111. Rauch BH, Millette E, Kenagy RD, et al. Thrombin- and factor Xa-induced DNA synthesis is mediated by transactivation of fibroblast growth factor receptor-1 in human vascular smooth muscle cells. *Circ Res* 2004;94(3):340–345.

112. Au YPT, Kenagy RD, Clowes MM, et al. Mechanisms of inhibition by heparin of vascular smooth muscle cell proliferation and migration. *Haemostasis* 1993;23(Suppl. 1):177–182.

113. Koyama H, Raines EW, Bornfeldt KE, et al. Fibrillar collagen inhibits arterial smooth muscle cell proliferation through regulation of Cdk2 inhibitors. *Cell* 1996;87(6):1069–1078.

114. Perlman H, Maillard L, Krasinski K, et al. Evidence for the rapid onset of apoptosis in medial smooth muscle cells after balloon injury. *Circulation* 1997;95(4):981–987.

115. Slomp J, Gittenberger-de Groot AC, Glukhova MA, et al. Differentiation, dedifferentiation, and apoptosis of smooth muscle cells during the development of the human ductus arteriosus. *Arterioscler Thromb Vasc Biol* 1997;17(5):1003–1009.

116. McCarthy NJ, Bennett MR. The regulation of vascular smooth muscle cell apoptosis. *Cardiovasc Res* 2000;45(3):747–755.

117. Berk BC. Vascular smooth muscle growth: autocrine growth mechanisms. *Physiol Rev* 2001;81(3):999–1030.

118. Langille BL. Blood flow-induced remodeling of the artery wall. In: Bevan JA, Kaley G, Rubanyi GM, eds. *Flow-dependent regulation of vascular function.* New York: Oxford University Press, 1995:277–299.

119. Schwartz SM. Cell death and the caspase cascade. *Circulation* 1998;97(3):227–229.

120. Pollman MJ, Yamada T, Horiuchi M, et al. Vasoactive substances regulate vascular smooth muscle cell apoptosis – countervailing influences of nitric oxide and angiotensin II. *Circ Res* 1996;79(4):748–756.

121. Mintz GS, Popma JJ, Hong MK, et al. Intravascular ultrasound to discern device-specific effects and mechanisms of restenosis. *Am J Cardiol* 1996;78:18–22.

122. Herrman J-PR, Hermans WRM, Vos J, et al. Pharmacological approaches to the prevention of restenosis following angioplasty: the search for the Holy Grail? (Part I). *Drugs* 1993;46:18–52.

123. Herrman J-PR, Hermans WRM, Vos J, et al. Pharmacological approaches to the prevention of restenosis following angioplasty: the search for the Holy Grail? (Part II). *Drugs* 1993;46:249–262.

124. Becquemin JP. Effect of ticlopidine on the long-term patency of saphenous-vein bypass grafts in the legs. *N Engl J Med* 1997;337(24):1726–1731.

125. Groves HM, Kinlough-Rathbone RL, Mustard JF. Development of nonthrombogenicity of injured rabbit aortas despite inhibition of platelet adherence. *Arteriosclerosis* 1986;6:189–195.

126. Ghigliotti G, Waissbluth AR, Speidel C, et al. Prolonged activation of prothrombin on the vascuplar wall after arterial injury. *Arterioscler Thromb Vasc Biol* 1998;18(2):250–257.

127. Bandyk DF, Schmitt DD, Seabrook GR, et al. Monitoring functional patency of in situ saphenous vein bypasses: the impact of a surveillance protocol and elective revision. *J Vasc Surg* 1989;9:286–296.

128. Sheppard R, Eisenberg MJ, Donath D, et al. Intracoronary brachytherapy for the prevention of restenosis after percutaneous coronary revascularization. *Am Heart J* 2003;146(5):775–786.

129. Kaluza GL, Ali NM, Raizner AE. Intracoronary radiotherapy for prevention of restenosis after percutaneous coronary interventions. *Ann Med* 2000;32(9):622–631.

130. Sousa JE, Serruys PW, Costa MA. New frontiers in cardiology – drug-eluting stents: Part II. *Circulation* 2003;107(18):2383–2389.

131. Sousa JE, Costa MA, Abizaid AC, et al. Sustained suppression of neointimal proliferation by sirolimus-eluting stents – one-year angiographic and intravascular ultrasound follow-up. *Circulation* 2001;104(17):2007–2011.

132. Park SJ, Shim WH, Ho DS, et al. A paclitaxel-eluting stent for the prevention of coronary restenosis. *N Engl J Med* 2003;348(16):1537–1545.

133. Moses JW, Leon MB, Popma JJ, et al. Sirolimus-eluting stents versus standard stents in patients with stenosis in a native coronary artery. *N Engl J Med* 2003;349(14):1315–1323.

134. Stone GW, Ellis SG, Cox DA, et al. A polymer-based, paclitaxel-eluting stent in patients with coronary artery disease. *N Engl J Med* 2004;350(3):221–231.

135. Serruys PW, Heyndrickx GR, Patel J, et al. Effect of an anti-PDGF-beta-receptor-blocking antibody on restenosis in patients undergoing elective stent placement. *Int J Cardiovasc Intervent* 2003;5(4):214–222.

# CHAPTER 51 ■ VESSEL WALL LIPIDS

JUDITH A. BERLINER

A number of human studies have demonstrated a role for vessel wall lipids in atherosclerosis and thrombosis. The sources of extracellular lipids that accumulate in the vessel wall are lipoproteins, vesicles shed from cells, and the cellular membranes of dying cells. Membranes of activated platelets are also a source of bioactive lipids. The early accumulation of lipoproteins in the vessel wall of experimental animals has been demonstrated using antibodies to the apoproteins of these animals. Studies on human specimens have determined that apoB [the low density lipoprotein (LDL) apoprotein], and apoA [the high density lipoprotein (HDL) apoprotein], lipoprotein (a) [Lp(a)] (an LDL-associated protein containing lipoproteins), and apoE [the major very low density lipoprotein (VLDL) apoprotein] accumulate in areas of the vessel wall susceptible to atherosclerosis. However, there are differences in accumulation of the different lipoproteins. Membrane vesicles from apoptotic cells and necrotic cells and from degranulated platelets accumulate in atherosclerotic lesions.

Lipids derived from lipoproteins have proatherogenic and prothrombotic effects, as summarized in Figure 51-1. Within the vessel wall, LDL is oxidized and aggregated. Specific lipids in the oxidized LDL activate endothelial cells to bind monocytes, and these monocytes then enter the vessel wall. Monocytes entering the vessel wall bind platelets, a process that may facilitate their entry (as discussed in Chapter 45). Once inside the vessel wall, macrophages produce cytokines that accelerate the process of smooth muscle cell proliferation. The macrophages also produce proteases that weaken the vessel wall. The macrophages and, to a smaller extent, smooth muscle cells, take up lipoproteins and become foam cells; tissue factor is highly induced in these cells, which subsequently die releasing their thrombotic contents. Breaks in the vessel wall expose the blood to the thrombotic contents of the vessel, resulting in a thrombus. Endothelial cells exposed to bioactive lipids are less able to support thrombolysis. It is increasingly recognized that lipoproteins and lipids derived from lipoproteins can have antiinflammatory effects that impact atherosclerosis and thrombosis. This chapter will focus on (a) the mechanism of accumulation of lipoproteins in the vessel wall, (b) identification of vessel wall lipids mediating inflammation, (c) identification of vessel wall lipids mediating thrombosis, and (d) formation and metabolism of bioactive lipids. Although this chapter will focus on atherosclerosis, it should be emphasized that the bioactive lipids found in atherosclerotic lesions are also present at other sites of chronic inflammation such as rheumatoid arthritis, lupus, and Alzheimer disease; these lipids may also play an important role in inflammation and thrombosis in these disorders.

# ACCUMULATION OF LIPOPROTEIN PARTICLES IN THE VESSEL WALL

Both transport and retention of lipoproteins in the vessel wall are important determinants of lipoprotein accumulation (1).

Lipoproteins are particles approximately 30 nm in diameter that contain a core of cholesterol ester and triglyceride surrounded by a phospholipid monolayer in which specific apoproteins and enzymes are embedded. Each type of lipoprotein has a characteristic lipid and protein distribution. Surprisingly, there is still considerable controversy as to how lipoproteins move from the blood into the vessel wall (2). The transport of LDL has received the most study because LDL accumulates to the greatest extent. LDL can be taken up by binding to the LDL receptor localized to coated vesicles that join with lysosomes, leading to metabolism of the lipoprotein within the endothelial cells. However, LDL can be taken up and transcytosed intact across the endothelium in uncoated vesicles. Within 2 hours of a bolus of LDL, these particles are seen under the endothelium within the matrix of the intima (see Fig. 51-2A) (3). Within a few hours, the lipoproteins become aggregated, and this aggregation continues in the arterial intima (see Fig. 51-2B). The LDL receptor is not the only receptor mediating LDL uptake into the vessel wall because LDL receptor–null mice demonstrate LDL accumulation in the vessel wall. In addition to transcytosis through vesicles, some studies suggest that lipoproteins may move through channels made up of temporarily fused vesicles or may move through temporarily opened tight junctions, although there is some evidence against this route in the aorta.

## Mechanisms of Lipoprotein Retention in the Artery Wall

A prominent feature of human atherosclerotic lesions is the accumulation of *extracellular* lipoproteins. The concentration of apoB in a vessel wall is equal to that in plasma and approximately one tenth of that found in other connective tissue (4). Several studies have addressed the mechanism of LDL accumulation in the vessel wall, initially focusing on components of the extracellular matrix that bind LDL. Lipoproteins accumulate in specific areas of the vessel wall where shear stress is low or disturbed. In these areas, the extracellular matrix differs from that in the nonsusceptible areas (5).

Earlier theories of atherosclerosis assumed that accumulation of lipoproteins in the arterial intima was the result of endothelial injury (6), which damaged the endothelial barrier and resulted in an increased ease of entry of lipoproteins into the intima. However, important studies by Schwenke and Carew demonstrated, using radiolabeled lipoproteins, that lipoprotein entry into the artery wall from plasma is similar in both atherosclerosis-resistant and atherosclerosis-prone regions (7,8). In contrast, atherosclerosis-prone regions have a lower rate of lipoprotein exit. Therefore, lipoprotein retention might be a result of the presence of cells or extracellular molecules unique to atherosclerosis-prone, as compared with atherosclerosis-resistant, sites.

Pathologic studies suggested that a specific class of extracellular matrix molecules—proteoglycans—might be responsible

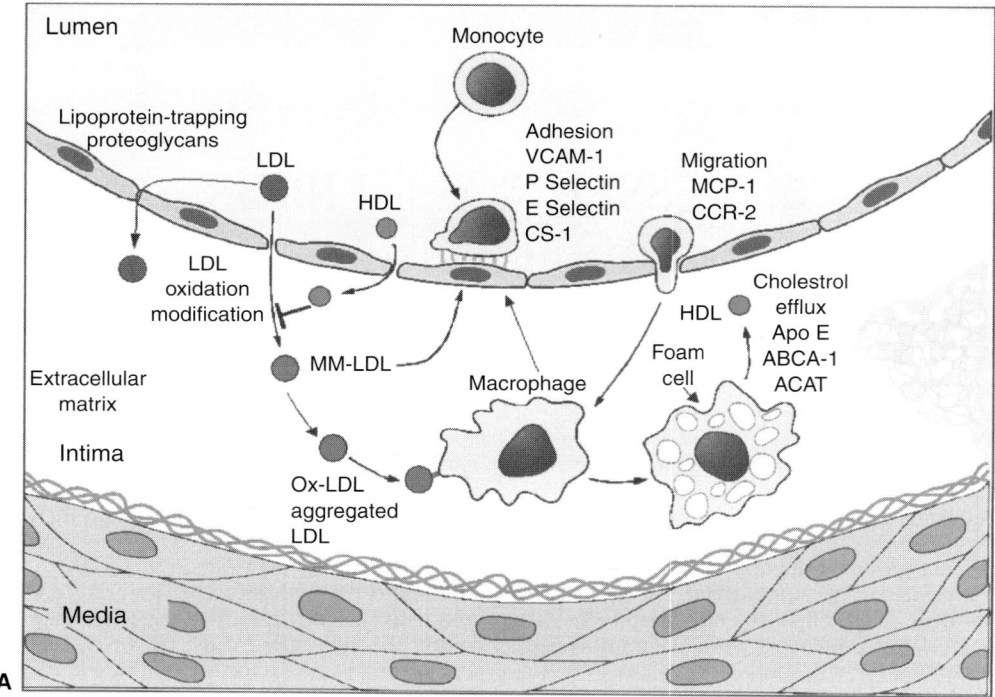

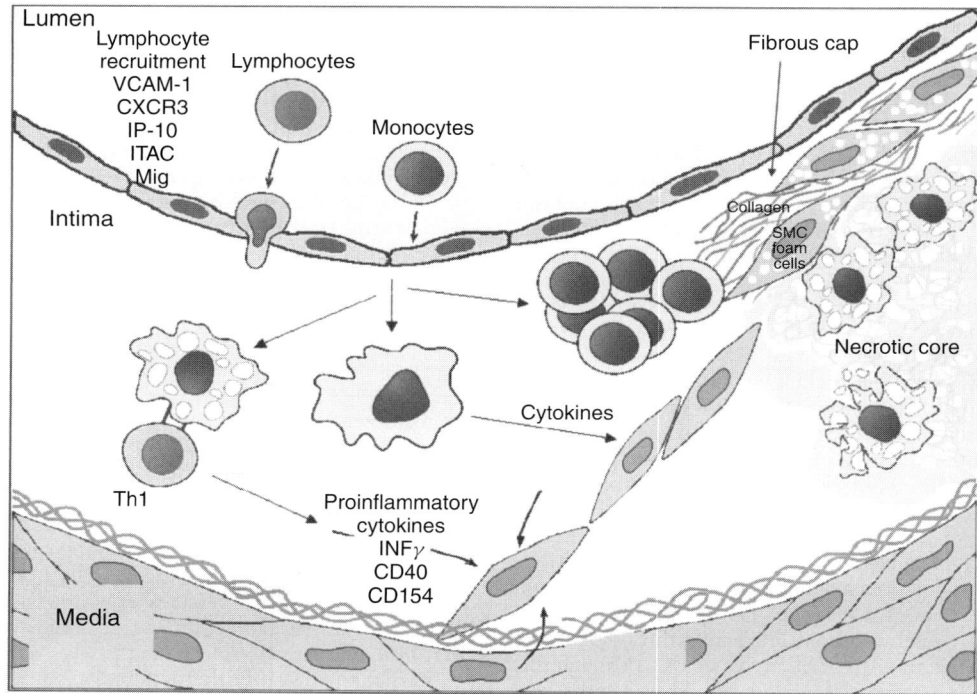

**FIGURE 51-1.** Stages in the development of the atherosclerotic lesion. **A:** Formation of the fatty streak. Lipoproteins enter the vessel wall and become oxidized. This oxidation can be inhibited by high density lipoproteins (HDL). Oxidized lipids increase monocyte endothelial interactions. Monocytes form foam cells by taking up highly oxidized low density lipoproteins (LDL). **B:** Development of the fibrous plaque. Monocytes and lymphocytes enter the vessel wall at the shoulder region. Smooth muscle cells (SMC) migrate from the media to the intima and proliferate in response to cytokines. They form the fibrous cap that covers dying foam cells. **C:** Plaque rupture. Monocytes that enter the lesion produce metalloproteinases that weaken the vessel wall. A break in the endothelium occurs, leading to thrombus formation by exposure to the high levels of tissue factor released from dying foam cells. These thrombi are stable because of the low levels of tissue-type plasminogen activator (tPA) and the high levels of plasminogen activator inhibitor (PAI) in the lesions (see Color Fig. 51-1). VCAM-1, vascular cell adhesion molecule-1; IP-10, Human interferon-inducible protein 10; INFγ, Interferon γ; MCP-1, monocyte chemoattractant protein-1; ACAT, acyl coenzyme A-cholesterol acyltransferase; MMPs, matrix metalloproteinases.

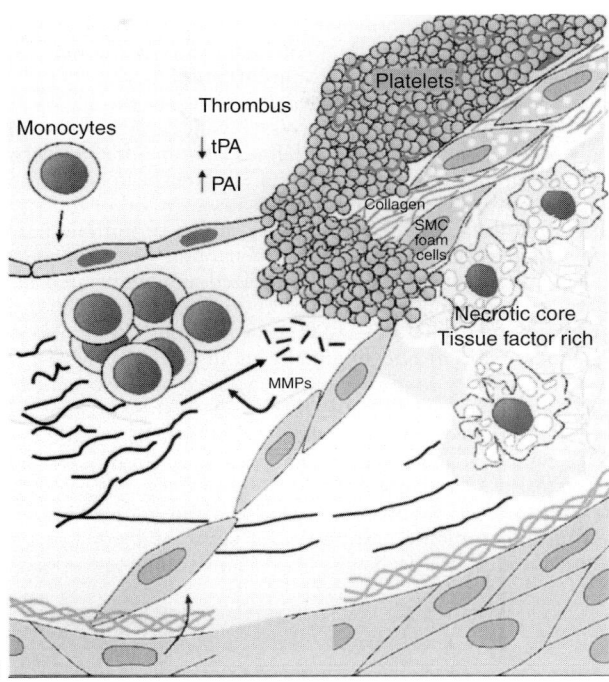

for the excess retention of lipoproteins (9). There are three major families of proteoglycans: (a) Chondroitin sulfate proteoglycans, such as versican, primarily synthesized by smooth muscle cells; (b) dermatan sulfate proteoglycans, such as biglycan and decorin, which may, among other things, participate in collagen fibrillogenesis; and (c) heparan sulfate proteoglycans, such as perlecan (a prominent component of basement membranes) and syndecan [a cell surface–associated heparan sulfate proteoglycan (10)]. Proteoglycans are a minor constituent of a healthy human arterial intima, but their content is increased in atherosclerosis-prone regions (9). The relative content of proteoglycans, in particular of the chondroitin sulfate– and dermatan sulfate–containing classes, is increased to an even greater extent in atherosclerotic lesions (5).

Several *in vitro* lines of evidence have demonstrated that proteoglycans can interact with lipoproteins. Chondroitin sulfate proteoglycans bind apolipoproteins, apoB in particular, through ionic interactions of the proteoglycans' negatively charged GAG side chains with positively charged amino acids of apoB (10). Lipoproteins containing apoB or apoE also can bind to dermatan sulfate proteoglycans, whereas apoA-I does not bind directly to these proteoglycan classes (11). Immunocytochemistry demonstrates that apolipoproteins colocalize primarily with the dermatan sulfate proteoglycan, biglycan, but not with the chondroitin sulfate proteoglycan, versican (11). Finally, elegant transgenic mouse studies have confirmed the central role of lipoprotein/proteoglycan interactions in atherogenesis. Mice made atherosclerosis

**FIGURE 51-1.** Continued.

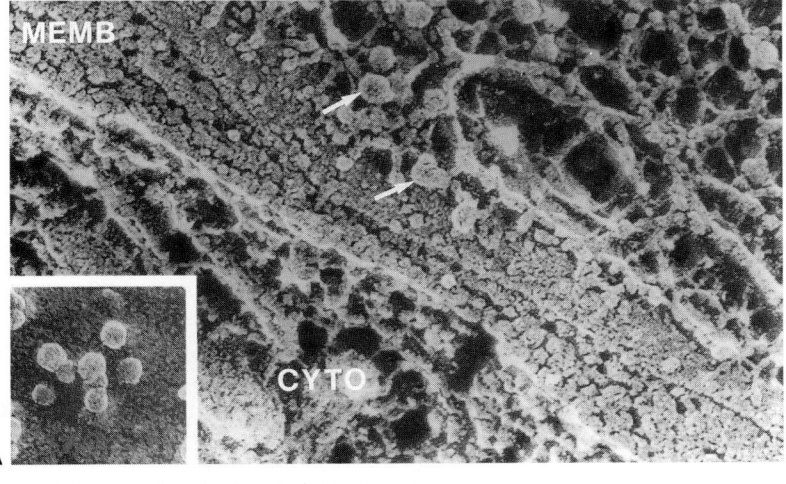

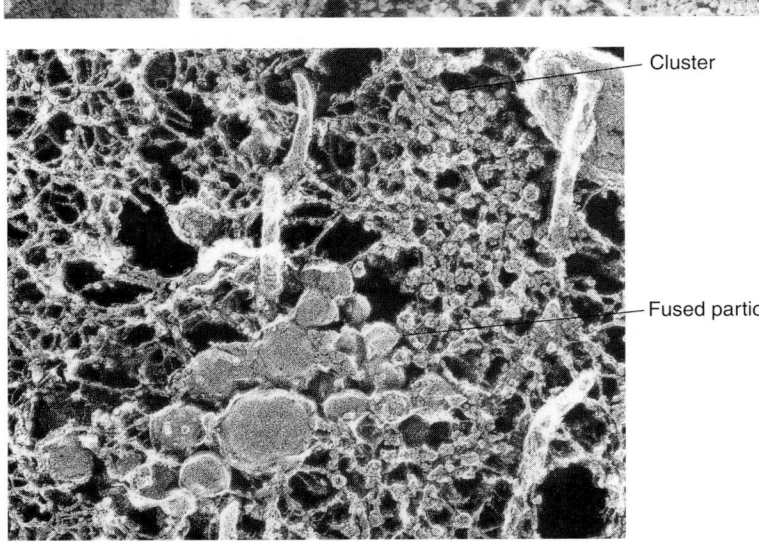

**FIGURE 51-2. A:** This freeze-etch electron micrograph shows the cytoplasm and fractured cell membrane of an endothelial cell as well as the subendothelial space (intima) from an isolated atrioventricular valve from an untreated rabbit. The valve was incubated with human low density lipoprotein (LDL) (**inset**) for 2 hours. *Arrows* point to 23-nm LDL particles just under the endothelial cell membrane. LDL particles are associated with matrix filaments. **Inset** shows an aliquot from human LDL (300 mg per mL) in the incubating medium that was ultrarapidly frozen and freeze etched. Note that the freeze-etch structure of the LDL aliquot and the LDL transported into the subendothelial space of the valve are the same (magnification ×220,000). **B:** This freeze-etch electron micrograph illustrates a portion of the intima within the atrioventricular valve of a rabbit exposed to a high-fat diet for 2 weeks. Clusters of LDL particles are observed. These fuse to form large lipid particle aggregates anchored in the matrix filaments of the intima (magnification ×65,000).

prone through overexpression of the human *apoB* gene have markedly diminished atherosclerotic lesion development if the proteoglycan-binding site of the apoB molecule (12) is altered by site-directed mutagenesis. It has also been observed that binding of lipoproteins can be facilitated by apoC-III, phospholipid transfer protein, and lipoprotein lipase (LPL), which may act as a bridge to the proteoglycans. Alternatively, the enzymes LPL and sphingomyelinase promote lipoprotein aggregation in the vessel wall that has been shown to promote retention.

# INFLAMMATORY EFFECTS OF VESSEL WALL LIPIDS

The importance of lipoprotein-derived lipids in the regulation of inflammation has been increasingly recognized (13,14). Lipoproteins contain cholesterol, cholesterol ester, triglycerides, and phospholipids. In addition, the levels of other lipids released from cells, such as lysophosphatidic acid (LPA), are increased in lipoproteins. Unmodified lipids have minimal inflammatory effects; however, modified lipids derived from all of the classes present in lipoproteins have been demonstrated to have proinflammatory and antiinflammatory effects. HDL particles, and the HDL apoprotein apoA-I in the blood and, perhaps to some extent, in the vessel wall, can protect against some of these effects of modified lipids (14). In addition, certain modified lipids present in oxidized LDL have been demonstrated to inhibit inflammatory effects caused by other lipids, cytokines, and bacterial products (15). Other antiinflammatory lipids form in cells in response to their uptake of lipoproteins.

The inflammatory effects of oxidized and aggregated LDL, as well as individual lipid oxidation products, have been determined. Oxidized LDL (Ox-LDL) (in which both lipids and proteins are oxidized) and minimally modified LDL (MM-LDL) (in which mainly lipids are oxidized) have been examined. In general, the effects of MM-LDL have been shown to be more proinflammatory than the effects of Ox-LDL. Small dense LDL, which is increased in diabetics, has proinflammatory characteristics similar to MM-LDL (16). The structures of several important bioactive lipids are shown in Figure 51-3; pro- and antiinflammatory properties of some of these lipids are summarized in Table 51-1. The proinflammatory effects of

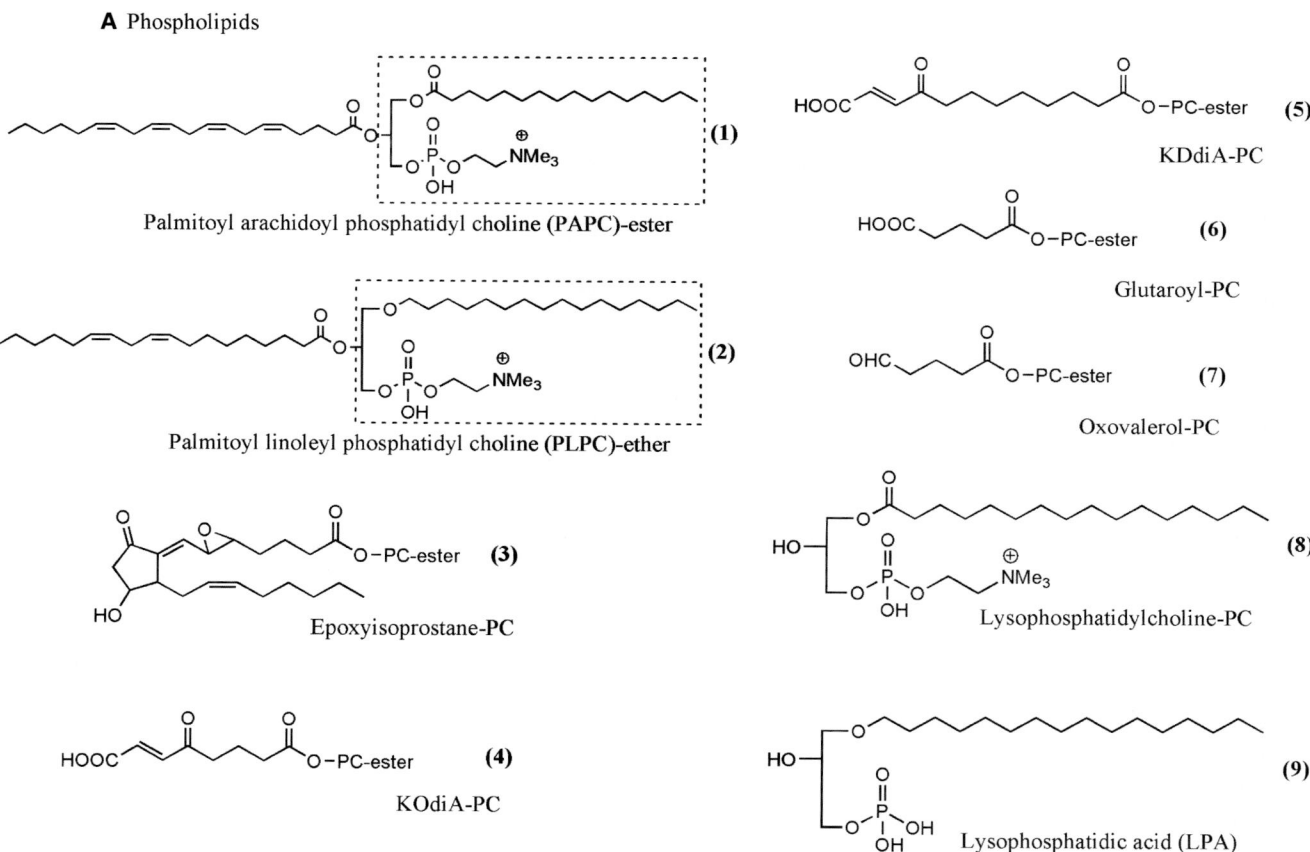

**A** Phospholipids

Palmitoyl arachidoyl phosphatidyl choline (PAPC)-ester **(1)**

Palmitoyl linoleyl phosphatidyl choline (PLPC)-ether **(2)**

Epoxyisoprostane-PC **(3)**

KOdiA-PC **(4)**

KDdiA-PC **(5)**

Glutaroyl-PC **(6)**

Oxovalerol-PC **(7)**

Lysophosphatidylcholine-PC **(8)**

Lysophosphatidic acid (LPA) **(9)**

**FIGURE 51-3.** Bioactive vessel wall lipids: Selected examples of bioactive vessel wall lipids derived from phospholipids, fatty acids, and cholesterol. **A:** Phospholipids. Bioactive lipids can be derived from ester- or ether-containing phospholipids (examples of these structures are demonstrated in *1* and *2*). (*1*) Palmitoyl arachidoyl phosphatidyl choline (PAPC): The lipid shown is a phosphatidylcholine (PC) ester with palmitate at the sn-1 and arachidonate at the sn-2. (*2*) Palmitoyl linoleyl phosphatidyl choline (PLPC): The lipid shown is an ether PC with palmitate at the sn-1 and linoleate at the sn-2. The *dotted line* shows the part of the molecule labeled "PC" in the bioactive phospholipids *3* to *9*. The bioactive lipids shown in this figure contain palmitate as the saturated fatty acid at the sn-1 and products of the unsaturated fatty acids arachidonate or linoleate at the sn-2. **B:** Bioactive fatty acid derivatives of arachidonic acid shown in *1*. Bioactive fatty acid derivatives are shown in *3* to *7*. **C:** Bioactive derivatives of cholesterol (*1*) are shown in *2* and *3*. Several of the bioactive lipids can be formed both nonenzymatically and enzymatically.

**B** Fatty acid derivatives

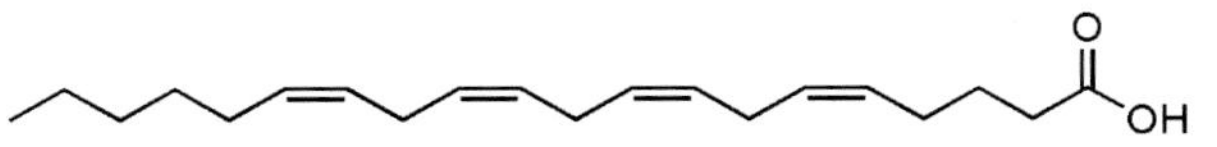

**C** Cholesterol derivatives

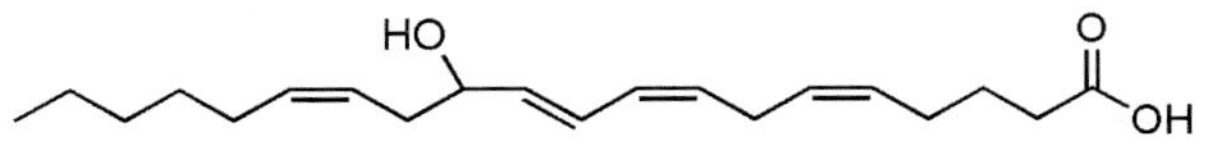

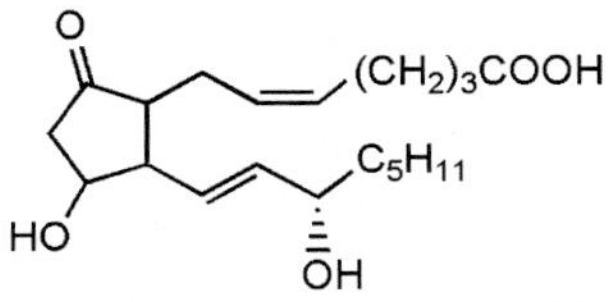

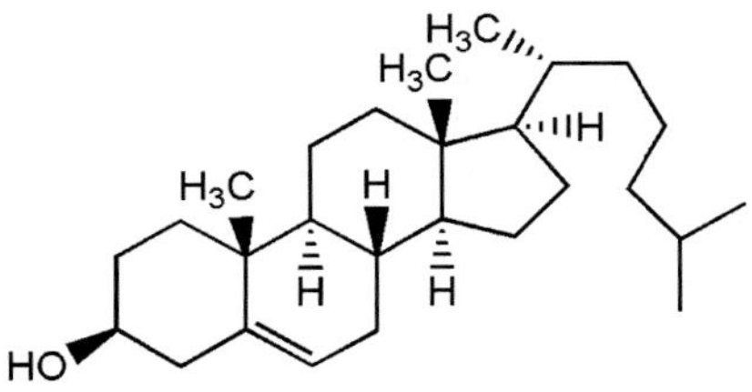

Arachidonic acid (1)

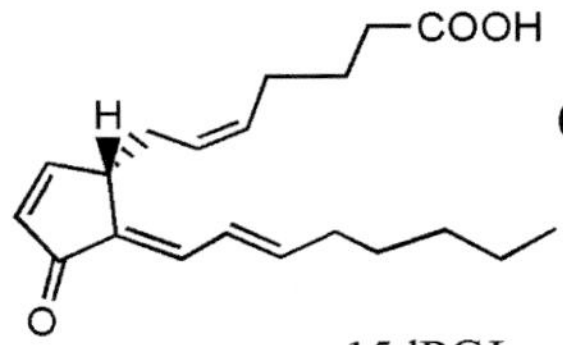

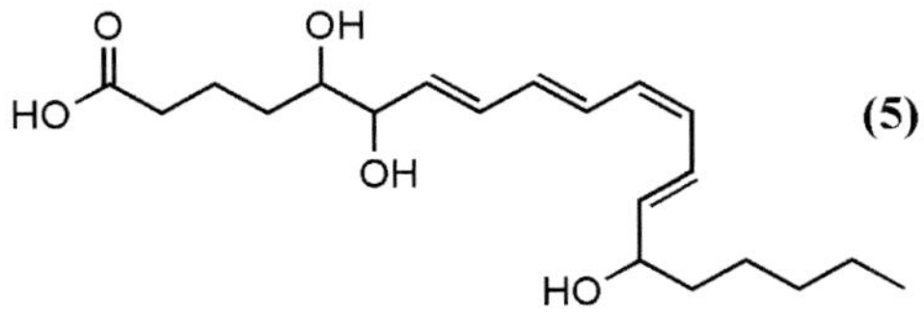

12-HETE (2)

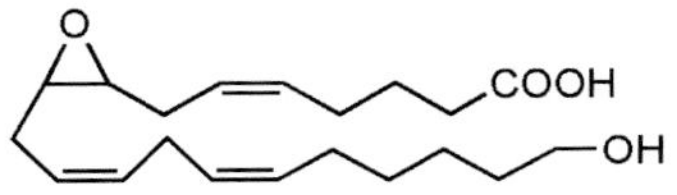

PGE$_2$ (3)

15dPGJ$_2$ (4)

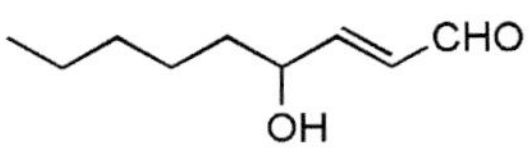

Lipoxin A4 (5)

20,8,9-HEET (6)

HNE (7)

Cholesterol (1)

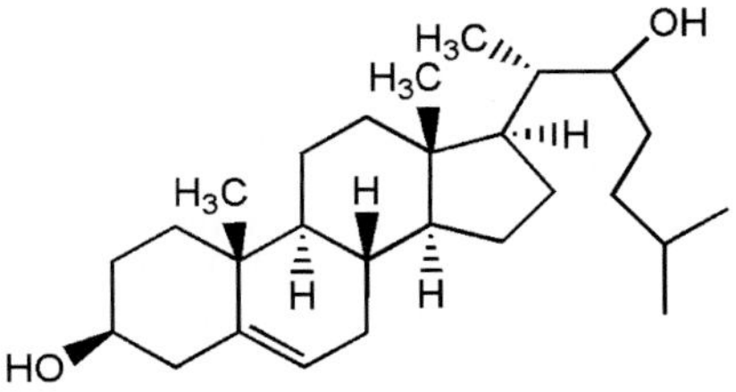

22-Hydroxycholesterol (2)

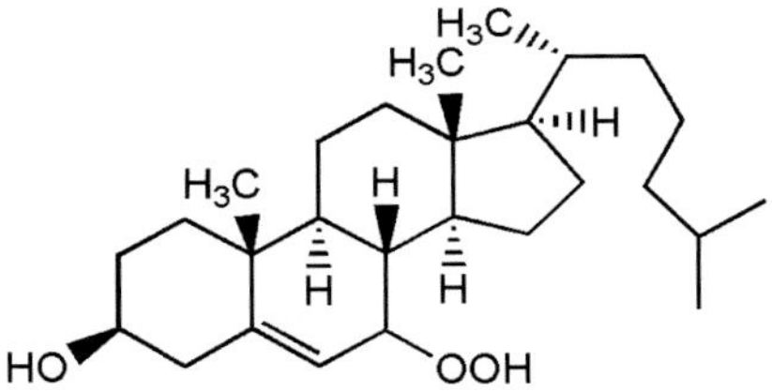

7-hydroperoxycholesterol (3)

FIGURE 51-3. Continued.

### TABLE 51-1

#### INFLAMMATORY EFFECTS OF VESSEL WALL LIPIDS

| Lipid | Pro | Anti |
|---|---|---|
| Ox-LDL | Cytokine synthesis by EC | Inhibits SMC proliferation |
| MM-LDL POVPC | Activates EC to bind monocytes | Inhibits LPS action |
| 12-HETE | Activates EC to bind monocytes | Inhibits TNF action on EC |
| Lipoxin 4 | Monocyte chemoattractant | Inhibits neutrophil binding |
| LPA | Prolongs macrophage life | Inhibits TNF action |
|  | Activates lymphocytes |  |

Ox-LDL, oxidized low density lipoprotein; MM-LDL, minimally modified low density lipoprotein; POVPC, palmitoyl-2-oxovaleroyl-*sn*-glycero-3-phosphoryl choline; LPA, lysophosphatidic acid; EC, endothelial cell; SMC, smooth muscle cell; LPS, lipopolysaccharide; TNF, tumor necrosis factor; HETE, hydroxytetraeicosenoic acid.

lipids include activation of endothelial cells to display leukocyte-binding molecules and synthesis of leukocyte chemotactic factors and monocyte maturation factors. Many of these inflammatory effects are also seen with MM-LDL. Oxidized palmitoyl arachidoyl phosphatidyl choline (PAPC) and its component phospholipid PEIPC (l-palmitoyl 2-epoxy isoprostane-*sn*-glycero-3-phosphoryl choline) (active at 100 nM) and POVPC (l-palmitoyl 2-oxovaleroyl-*sn*-glycero-3-phosphoryl choline) (active at 5 $\mu$M) increase endothelial cell expression of CS-1 fibronectin, a receptor for monocyte VLA4, and synthesis of monocyte chemotactic factors by endothelial cells and smooth muscle cells. There is no increase in neutrophil endothelial interactions (13). Comparable ethanolamine phospholipids have similar activity. Prostaglandins are bioactive fatty acids that are formed by cellular enzymes; they accumulate in both cells and lipoproteins. Several prostaglandins including PGE2 have been shown to have inflammatory effects *in vivo*. Isoprostaglandins including iso-PGE2 can be formed nonenzymatically and are also proinflammatory (17). LPA (10 $\mu$) (18) and lysophosphatidylcholine (LPC) (50 $\mu$) (19,20) increased VCAM-1 and E selectin expression on endothelial cells. At similar concentrations, LPA alters endothelial cell shape and increases monolayer permeability. Ox-LDL and PAF-like lipids present in Ox-LDL increase the proliferation of smooth muscle cells (21). Ox-LDL at higher concentrations is toxic to smooth muscle cells; the responsible lipid has been identified as 7-keto cholesterol (22). Lipids stimulate smooth muscle cells to produce leukocyte chemotactic factors (23). Furthermore, 12-HETE (12-hydroxytetraeicosenoic acid) increases hypertrophy and fibronectin transcription in smooth muscle cells (24). Bioactive lipids also activate leukocytes. Platelet-activating factor–like (PAF-like) phospholipids present in oxidized LDL and vesicles from activated endothelial cells bind to the PAF receptor on monocytes and neutrophils (25,26); activate integrins, leading to leukoctye binding and transmigration into the vessel wall; and stimulate the leukocyte synthesis of cytokines. POVPC can act as an antigen to stimulate B and T cell responses that play an important role in atherosclerosis (27,28). Antibodies reacting with this phospholipid and other phospholipid oxidation products have been detected in the plasma of individuals with atherosclerosis and a number of other chronic inflammatory diseases including diabetes, eclampsia, and rheumatoid arthritis (29).

Recently, a number of antiinflammatory effects of vessel wall lipids have been described. Some of these lipids are found in lipoproteins and vesicles, whereas others are formed in response to vessel wall lipids (15,30,31). A major antiinflammatory mechanism is the activation of peroxisome proliferator–activated receptors (PPARs); PPAR agonists have been shown to decrease inflammation *in vivo* and to decrease the responsiveness of endothelial cells to cytokine activators such as tumor necrosis factor (TNF) (32,33). Both PEIPC and particular PAF-like lipids are strong PPAR activators [reviewed in (15)]. Unidentified PPAR activators are formed by hydrolysis of VLDL by the enzyme LPL (34). Hydroxy-11,12-epoxyeicosatrienoic acids (HEETs) are formed in endothelial cells in response to treatment of the cells with high levels of LDL and minimally oxidized LDL and accumulate in lipoproteins, especially LDL (30). Although EETs are extensively studied as regulators of vascular tone, it is now recognized that the HEETs may also serve as PPAR agonists (35). Cyclopentanone prostaglandins, such as 15dPGJ2 and lipoxins, act by PPAR-independent pathways as inhibitors of neutrophil and monoctye accumulation, respectively [reviewed in (31,36)]. There is evidence that cyclopentanone prostaglandins, such as 15dpGJ2, act by selectively regulating the proteins of the NF$\kappa$B complex. LXR agonists, including 22-hydroxycholesterol, act by non-PPAR pathways to inhibit the action of both lipopolysaccharide (LPS) and TNF action (37). A number of phospholipid oxidation products specifically inhibit the action of both TLR4 agonists (such as LPS) and TLR2 agonists (such

as mycobacteria) [reviewed in (15)]. These products include POVPC, 5 keto-6-octendioic acid ester of 2 lyso PC (KOdiA PC), and 5-hydroxy-8-oxo-6-octenedioic acid ester of 2 lyso PC (HOOA PC) (38,39). One mechanism by which these lipids inhibit LPS action involves competitive binding to CD14, a component of the TLR4-receptor complex. Another mechanism of action may be an alteration in membrane trafficking, a necessary component of Toll receptor signaling. Therefore, vessel wall lipids act in a variety of ways to inhibit inflammatory responses, especially acute inflammation.

# EFFECT OF VESSEL WALL LIPIDS ON THROMBOSIS AND FIBRINOLYTIC ACTIVITY

Vessel wall lipids contribute to thrombotic potential of atherosclerotic lesions by several different mechanisms: (a) Contributing to the formation of foam cells; (b) contributing to the death of smooth muscle cells and macrophage foam cells, leading to the formation of the highly thrombogenic necrotic core; (c) activating the synthesis of matrix metalloproteinase (MMP) in macrophages and smooth muscle cells—these MMPs break down the vessel wall matrix, leading to plaque rupture; (d) stimulating endothelial cell synthesis of tissue factor and decreasing plasminogen activity; (e) increasing activation of platelets. Table 51-2 lists specific vessel wall lipids regulating some of these functions.

## Formation of Foam Cells

As noted previously, nearly all cells express LDL receptors. Therefore, in the normal circumstance, uptake of LDL by the LDL receptor is the major route by which peripheral cells take up exogenous cholesterol. However, increases in cell cholesterol content lead to downregulation of LDL-receptor expression at the cell surface, thereby protecting against accumulation of excess lipid derived from LDL. By contrast,

**TABLE 51-2**

THROMBOTIC ACTIVITIES OF VESSEL WALL LIPIDS

| Activity | Lipid |
|---|---|
| Foam cell formation; increase in scavenger receptors | KOdiA PC, 12-HETE |
| Foam cell formation; lipid alterations to increase uptake | Ox-LDL, sphingomyelinase treated LDL |
| Increase synthesis of MMPs | Ox-LDL |
| Increase tissue factor synthesis | MM-LDL, PGPC, LPA |
| Increase PAI expression and decreas PA and/or thrombomodulin | MM-LDL, Ox-LDL |
| Increase platelet activation | LPA (ether) |

MMP, matrix metalloproteinase; PC, phosphatidylcholine; Ox-LDL, oxidized low density lipoprotein; MM-LDL, minimally modified low density lipoprotein; LDL, low density lipoprotein; PGPC, l, palmotyl-2-glutaroyl-*sn*-glycero-3-phosphatidylcholine; LPA, lysophosphatidic acid; PAI, plasminogen activator inhibitor; KOdiA PC, 5 keto-6-octendioic acid ester of 2 lyso PC; 12-HETE, 12-hydroxytetraeicosenoic acid.

scavenger receptors on macrophages and smooth muscle cells take up modified LDL in an unregulated fashion. The principal scavenger receptors are SRA-1, CD 36, SRB-1, and LOX-1. These receptors recognize oxidized phospholipids on lipoproteins including POVPC (40), KOdiA, and KDdiA PC (41). Several additional mechanisms for cell cholesterol accumulation have been described. These include: (a) Aggregation of LDL, which may form through several mechanisms, including binding to fibronectin, collagen, or proteoglycans, as well as aggregation induced by the action of neutral sphingomyelinase (42); aggregated LDL can be taken up phagocytically by macrophages; (b) immune complexes, which could be composed of oxidized or glycosylated LDL and antibodies to epitopes present on these modified forms of lipoproteins, could bind to and be internalized by Fcγ R receptors on the surface of plaque macrophages (43); (c) C-reactive protein has also been demonstrated to bind oxidized phospholipids to load macrophages by the Fcγ RIIa receptor; and (d) the expression in plaques of "bridging" molecules that have the capacity to bind to both lipoproteins and cell surface proteoglycans. LPL represents one example of a potential bridging molecule (44). Therefore, both macrophages and smooth muscle cells become lipid loaded by multiple receptors. Vessel wall lipids such as hydroxynonenal may also affect foam cell formation by covalently binding and inactivating lysosomal enzymes that degrade lipids (45). HDL and apoA-1 from HDL can reduce lipid loading, probably by serving as a cholesterol acceptor. Therefore, the extent of foam cell formation is probably a balance between uptake of lipoproteins and removal of cholesterol.

## Death of Macrophages and Smooth Muscle Cells

An important determinant of plaque rupture is the thickness of the fibrous cap and the size of the necrotic core that represents cells that have died by apoptosis or necrosis. The necrotic core contains foam cells that have undergone apoptosis. Levels of active tissue factor are exceptionally high in this area. The thickness of the fibrous cap that overlies the necrotic core has been demonstrated to be a good predictor of resistance of the vessel to rupture. The size of the fibrous cap differs between lesions and probably represents a balance between smooth muscle cell proliferation and smooth muscle cell apoptosis. One factor contributing to macrophage and smooth muscle cell death is the uptake of lipids. Excessive loading of cells with free cholesterol has been demonstrated to be apoptotic to macrophages (46). Normally, cells metabolize excess cholesterol to the less toxic ester form. However, prolonged cholesterol uptake coupled with disturbances in vesicular processing may lead to excess accumulation of free cholesterol. 7-β hydroperoxy cholesterol, which accumulates in LDL, has been shown to be toxic to macrophages and smooth muscle cells in cell culture (47). Other bioactive lipids, such as the cyclopentenone prostaglandins, accelerate macrophage apoptosis by separate mechanisms (31).

## Increased Synthesis of Matrix Metalloproteinases by Macrophages and Smooth Muscle Cells

There is a strong accumulation of MMP-1 and MMP-3 in atherosclerotic lesions where they colocalize with Ox-LDL epitopes (48); these molecules have been demonstrated to degrade vessel wall matrix molecules. Synthesis of both MMP-1 and MMP-3 is increased by incubation of smooth muscle cells and macrophages with Ox-LDL (49,50). The specific lipid responsible for these effects has not been identified.

## Increasing Endothelial, Smooth Muscle Cell, and Macrophage Synthesis of Tissue Factor and Altering Thrombolytic Activity of Endothelial Cells

Atherosclerotic plaque lipids are intensely thrombogenic. One study, using an extracorporeal perfusion system, demonstrated that atherosclerotic plaque lipids were up to sixfold more potent in inducing platelet-rich thrombus formation than other plaque components (51). The most compelling data about plaque lipids and atherogenicity focus on the role of plaque lipids in the expression of tissue factor. Tissue factor, the predominant physiologic initiator of coagulation, is present in large amounts in human atherosclerotic plaques (52–54). It is expressed in plaques primarily by macrophage and smooth muscle foam cells and localizes predominantly to lipid-rich cores where Ox-LDL is also at high levels (52,54,55). Increased expression in endothelial cells is also seen by immunostaining.

MM-LDL, specifically the component lipid PGPC, has been shown to upregulate tissue factor expression in endothelial cells by increasing transcription (56). In smooth muscle cells, tissue factor expression is upregulated by both LDL and Ox-LDL and a component phospholipid LPA (57). In addition, the activity of tissue factor is increased by Ox-LDL even in the absence of increased tissue factor levels. As already discussed, hydroperoxy cholesterols also promote release of active tissue factor by induction of apoptosis in cells rich in tissue factor. In addition, tissue factor–rich microparticles derived from the membranes of apoptotic macrophages and lymphocytes are present in atherosclerotic plaques (55). Therefore, both normal and oxidized lipoproteins increase tissue factor expression and activity.

Modified lipids also contribute to deceased thrombolysis in atherosclerotic lesions. Both Ox-LDL and MM-LDL have been demonstrated to increase PAI expression and decrease the expression of thrombomodulin in endothelial cells and, for PAI, in smooth muscle cells (58,59). Furthermore, hypertriglyceridemia also has been positively correlated with raised fibrinopeptide A levels in a case–control study of patients with angina (60) and with raised levels of PAI-1. Triglyceride-rich lipoproteins isolated from patients with hypertriglyceridemia have been shown to impair in vitro fibrinolysis by decreasing plasminogen binding to endothelial cells (61) and by upregulating expression of PAI-1 (62,63). Lipoprotein lipase (LPL) has been implicated as a mediator of the prothrombotic actions of triglyceride-rich lipoproteins. It has been proposed that these fatty acids present at the surface of triglyceride-rich lipoproteins can provide the negative charge necessary for activation of the extrinsic pathway of coagulation (64). Interestingly, both triglyceride-rich lipoproteins (65,66) and LPL (67,68) are present in human atherosclerotic plaques. These observations raise the possibility that triglyceride-rich lipoproteins may act synergistically to enhance coagulation not only in the plasma but also within the atherosclerotic plaque.

## Lipoprotein (a)

Lp(a) is a class of lipoprotein particle similar in composition to LDL but containing an additional protein component, apoA. apoA is attached to the outer surface of the Lp(a) particle by a single disulfide linkage with apoB. Increased plasma concentrations of Lp(a) have been associated with an increased risk of atherosclerosis, particularly in the presence of elevated levels of LDL [reviewed in (69)]. Lp(a) has been detected in human atherosclerotic lesions (70), where it colocalizes with fibrin (71). The exact mechanisms responsible for Lp(a)'s atherogenicity are not known but may relate to the marked sequence similarity of apoA to plasminogen. Plasminogen contains a signal sequence, five kringles (triple-disulfide loop structures), and a serine protease domain. apoA contains a signal sequence, multiple copies of kringle 4, and a single kringle 5; but its protease domain is inactive (72,73). As a result, it has been proposed that Lp(a) might contribute to atherogenesis by interfering with the binding of plasminogen to endothelial cells and fibrin (73). This hypothesis is supported by the *in vitro* observation that Lp(a) and apoA inhibit plasminogen binding to, and tPA-dependent plasmin generation on, endothelial cells (74). Furthermore, apoA-overexpressing mice are resistant to the clot-lysing effect of tPA *in vivo* (75).

## Activation of Platelets by Lipid Oxidation Products

The increased activation of platelets in plasma from patients with hyperlipidemia is well recognized. It has recently been demonstrated that an ether-derived LPA and, to a lesser extent, ester-derived LPA can stimulate platelet activation and can increase platelet monocyte interaction (76). These activities may have significance at the surface of the vessel to promote platelet accumulation in the thrombus.

## Formation and Destruction of Bioactive Oxidation Products

Controlling the levels of bioactive oxidation products would seem to have a therapeutic potential in atherosclerosis and thrombosis; an understanding of the mechanism of formation and destruction of these lipids will be the key to development of such therapies. Many of the bioactive lipids are formed by oxidation, and several strategies to limit oxidation have been proposed. Eleven trials of antioxidants have been conducted mainly as secondary preventions. In all of the larger trials, with at least 400 IU of vitamin E, whether primary or secondary prevention, there were no demonstrated effects of vitamin E on lesion progression or coronary events [reviewed in (77)]. The ineffectiveness of vitamin E does not mean that other more powerful antioxidants will not be effective in limiting disease. Nonetheless, these studies suggest that additional strategies to limit oxidation will be necessary. Alternate strategies to limit oxidation may involve inhibiting enzymes that form oxidized lipids. Activated macrophages and neutrophils are rich sources of radicals that can oxidize polyunsaturated fatty acids present in LDL lipids and are present in cell membranes. Both myeloperoxidase (78) and nicotinamide adenine dinucleotide phosphate (NADPH) oxidase (79,80) enzymes, concentrated in activated inflammatory cells, have been demonstrated to produce a variety of lipid oxidation products. These enzymes are not inhibited by vitamin E. In addition, 12/15LO, a more widely distributed intracellular enzyme, has been demonstrated to attach to the cell membrane following prenylation and to cause oxidation of lipoproteins (81). Ingestion of a high fat meal has been demonstrated to induce the peroxidation of lipids (82); the oxidative increase probably relates to an elevated rate of mitochondrial metabolism of these lipids. Several studies have demonstrated that nitric oxide synthase can also become a radical generator in conditions similar to those found in atherosclerotic lesions (83). Polymorphisms of myeloperoxidase (MPO) (84) have been associated with human atherosclerosis. Furthermore, knockout of an NADPH oxidase (85) subunit and 12,15LO have been associated with decreased atherosclerosis in mice (81).

Low levels of oxidized lipoproteins are seen in plasma, and there is increasing evidence that oxidation of LDL may be initiated in protected compartments where antioxidants may be exhausted and not easily replenished. These compartments may be phagocytic vesicles of activated macrophages where products of myeloperoxidase (86) and NADPH oxidase are released (82). It may occur on lipoproteins bound to the extracellular matrix because specific matrix molecules have been demonstrated to interact with LDL (87). It may occur in other phagocytic compartments formed by a recently identified process termed *potocytosis* (88). The most important enzymes mediating formation of oxidized lipids and the compartments where they are formed need to be identified as part of devising therapeutic strategies.

Another important regulator of vessel wall lipid oxidation products is the destruction and removal of these lipids. A variety of enzymes, concentrated in HDL, destroy lipid oxidation products. PON-1 (peroxynitrite), PAF-AH [reviewed in (12)] and L-CAT (L-carnitine acetyltransferase) decrease the activity of many of the bioactive phospholipid oxidation products (89). Polymorphisms of these enzymes are associated with increased risk of atherosclerosis. Molecules such as SAA (serum amyloid A protein), which are increased in infection, displace protective enzymes from HDL. There are also several mechanisms to transport oxidized phospholipids out of cells. apoA-I associated with pre-β HDL has been demonstrated to deplete cells and LDL of lipid oxidation products (90). Cells exposed to oxidative stress have an alternate mechanism for removal of oxidized lipids involving formation of blebs that contain concentrated oxidized phospholipids (91). The destruction of cholesterol oxidation products has been less well studied. A balance between enzymes that synthesize and enzymes that destroy bioactive lipids appears to be an important key in determining levels of these bioactive molecules.

# SUMMARY

Vessel wall lipids play an important role in the homeostasis of the vessel wall. They are important mediators of inflammation and thrombosis. The bioactive lipids of the vessel wall are derived from lipoproteins, and membranes are derived from cells under oxidative stress. Cellular enzymes are involved in the formation of bioactive lipids, some of which may form in phagocytic vesicles into which the enzymes are secreted. Some lipids such as prostaglandins are carried by lipoproteins. Extracellular enzymes such as sphingomyelinases can also accelerate the formation of bioactive lipids. Some vessel wall lipids stimulate inflammation and thrombosis, whereas others are antiinflammatory. The balance between the proinflammatory and antiinflammatory lipids may shift during disease progression, suggesting that therapeutic strategies directed at one lipid may only be effective in particular settings. Targeting enzymes involved in their formation and destruction will likely represent an important therapeutic strategy.

## References

1. Williams KJ, Tabas I. The response-to-retention hypothesis of atherogenesis reinforced. *Curr Opin Lipidol* 1998;9:471–474.
2. Rippe B, Rosengren BI, Carlsson O, et al. Transendothelial transport: the vesicle controversy. *J Vasc Res* 2002;39:375–390.
3. Nievelstein PF, Fogelman AM, Mottino G, et al. Lipid accumulation in rabbit aortic intima 2 hours after bolus infusion of low density lipoprotein. A deep-etch and immunolocalization study of ultrarapidly frozen tissue. *Arterioscler Thromb* 1991;11:1795–1805.
4. Guyton JR, Klemp KF. Development of the atherosclerotic core region. Chemical and ultrastructural analysis of microdissected atherosclerotic lesions from human aorta. *Arterioscler Thromb* 1994;14:1305–1314.
5. Chait A, Wight TN. Interaction of native and modified low-density lipoproteins with extracellular matrix. *Curr Opin Lipidol* 2000;11:457–463.
6. Ross R. The pathogenesis of atherosclerosis: a perspective for the 1990s. *Nature* 1993;362:801–809.

7. Schwenke DC, Carew TE. Initiation of atherosclerotic lesions in choles-terol-fed rabbits. II. Selective retention of LDL vs. selective increases in LDL permeability in susceptible sites of arteries. *Arterioscler* 1989;9: 908–918.

8. Schwenke DC, Carew TE. Initiation of atherosclerotic lesions in choles-terol-fed rabbits. I. Focal increases in arterial LDL concentration precede development of fatty streak lesions. *Arterioscler* 1989;9:895–907.

9. Cardoso LE, Mourao PA. Glycosaminoglycan fractions from human arteries presenting diverse susceptibilities to atherosclerosis have different binding affinities to plasma LDL. *Arterioscler Thromb* 1994;14:115–124.

10. Wight TN. Cell biology of arterial proteoglycans. *Arterioscler* 1989;9: 1–20.

11. Olsson U, Camejo G, Hurt-Camejo E, et al. Possible functional interactions of apolipoprotein B-100 segments that associate with cell proteoglycans and the ApoB/E receptor. *Arterioscler Thromb Vasc Biol* 1997;17: 149–155.

12. Boren J, Olin K, Lee I, et al. Identification of the principal proteoglycan-binding site in LDL. A single-point mutation in apo-B100 severely affects proteoglycan interaction without affecting LDL receptor binding. *J Clin Invest* 1998;101:2658–2664.

13. Berliner J. Introduction. Lipid oxidation products and atherosclerosis. *Vascul Pharmacol* 2002;38:187–191.

14. Navab M, Hama SY, Reddy ST, et al. Oxidized lipids as mediators of coronary heart disease. *Curr Opin Lipidol* 2002;13:363–372.

15. Bochkov VN, Leitinger N. Anti-inflammatory properties of lipid oxidation products. *J Mol Med* 2003;81:613–626.

16. De Castellarnau C, Sanchez-Quesada JL, Benitez S, et al. Electronegative LDL from normolipemic subjects induces IL-8 and monocyte chemotactic protein secretion by human endothelial cells. *Arterioscler Thromb Vasc Biol* 2000;20:2281–2287.

17. Harris SG, Padilla J, Koumas L, et al. Prostaglandins as modulators of immunity. *Trends Immunol* 2002;23:144–150.

18. Rizza C, Leitinger N, Yue J, et al. Lysophosphatidic acid as a regulator of endothelial/leukocyte interaction. *Lab Invest* 1999;79:1227–1235.

19. Kohno M, Yokokawa K, Yasunari K, et al. Induction by lysophosphatidyl-choline, a major phospholipid component of atherogenic lipoproteins, of human coronary artery smooth muscle cell migration. *Circulation* 1998; 98:353–359.

20. Kume N, Cybulsky MI, Gimbrone MA Jr. Lysophosphatidylcholine, a component of atherogenic lipoproteins, induces mononuclear leukocyte adhesion molecules in cultured human and rabbit arterial endothelial cells. *J Clin Invest* 1992;90:1138–1144.

21. Heery JM, Kozak M, Stafforini DM, et al. Oxidatively modified LDL contains phospholipids with platelet-activating factor-like activity and stimulates the growth of smooth muscle cells. *J Clin Invest* 1995;96:2322–2330.

22. Agrawal S, Agarwal ML, Chatterjee-Kishore M, et al. Stat1-dependent, p53-independent expression of p21(waf1) modulates oxysterol-induced apoptosis. *Mol Cell Biol* 2002;22:1981–1992.

23. Klouche M, Rose-John S, Schmiedt W, et al. Enzymatically degraded, nonox-idized LDL induces human vascular smooth muscle cell activation, foam cell transformation, and proliferation. *Circulation* 2000;101:1799–1805.

24. Reddy MA, Thimmalapura PR, Lanting L, et al. The oxidized lipid and lipoxygenase product 12(S)-hydroxyeicosatetraenoic acid induces hypertrophy and fibronectin transcription in vascular smooth muscle cells via p38 MAPK and cAMP response element-binding protein activation. Mediation of angiotensin II effects. *J Biol Chem* 2002;277:9920–9928.

25. Marathe GK, Zimmerman GA, Prescott SM, et al. Activation of vascular cells by PAF-like lipids in oxidized LDL. *Vascul Pharmacol* 2002;38: 193–200.

26. Marathe GK, Prescott SM, Zimmerman GA, et al. Oxidized LDL contains inflammatory PAF-like phospholipids. *Trends Cardiovasc Med* 2001;11: 139–142.

27. Horkko S, Bird DA, Miller E, et al. Monoclonal autoantibodies specific for oxidized phospholipids or oxidized phospholipid-protein adducts inhibit macrophage uptake of oxidized low-density lipoproteins. *J Clin Invest* 1999;103:117–128.

28. Fei GZ, Huang YH, Swedenborg J, et al. Oxidised LDL modulates immune-activation by an IL-12 dependent mechanism. *Atherosclerosis* 2003;169:77–85.

29. Horkko S, Binder CJ, Shaw PX, et al. Immunological responses to oxidized LDL. *Free Radic Biol Med* 2000;28:1771–1779.

30. Pritchard KA Jr, Wong PY, Stemerman MB. Atherogenic concentrations of low-density lipoprotein enhance endothelial cell generation of epoxye-icosatrienoic acid products. *Am J Pathol* 1990;136:1383–1391.

31. Levy BD, Clish CB, Schmidt B, et al. Lipid mediator class switching during acute inflammation: signals in resolution. *Nat Immunol* 2001;2: 612–619.

32. Duval C, Chinetti G, Trottein F, et al. The role of PPARs in atherosclerosis. *Trends Mol Med* 2002;8:422–430.

33. Plutzky J. The potential role of peroxisome proliferator-activated receptors on inflammation in type 2 diabetes mellitus and atherosclerosis. *Am J Cardiol* 2003;92:34J–41J.

34. Ziouzenkova O, Asatryan L, Sahady D, et al. Dual roles for lipolysis and oxidation in peroxisome proliferation-activator receptor responses to electronegative low density lipoprotein. *J Biol Chem* 2003;278: 39874–39881.

35. Muller DN, Theuer J, Shagdarsuren E, et al. A peroxisome proliferator-activated receptor-alpha activator induces renal CYP2C23 activity and protects from angiotensin II–induced renal injury. *Am J Pathol* 2004;164: 521–532.

36. Lawrence T, Willoughby DA, Gilroy DW. Anti-inflammatory lipid mediators and insights into the resolution of inflammation. *Nature Rev Immunol* 2002;2:787–795.

37. Joseph SB, Castrillo A, Laffitte BA, et al. Reciprocal regulation of inflammation and lipid metabolism by liver X receptors. *Nat Med* 2003;9:213–219.

38. Subbanagounder G, Deng Y, Borromeo C, et al. Hydroxy alkenal phospholipids regulate inflammatory functions of endothelial cells. *Vascul Pharmacol* 2002;38:201–209.

39. Walton KA, Hsieh X, Gharavi N, et al. Receptors involved in the oxidized 1-palmitoyl-2-arachidonoyl-sn-glycero-3-phosphorylcholine-mediated synthesis of interleukin-8. A role for Toll-like receptor 4 and a glycosylphos-phatidylinositol-anchored protein. *J Biol Chem* 2003;278:29661–29666.

40. Boullier A, Gillotte KL, Horkko S, et al. The binding of oxidized low density lipoprotein to mouse CD36 is mediated in part by oxidized phospholipids that are associated with both the lipid and protein moieties of the lipoprotein. *J Biol Chem* 2000;275:9163–9169.

41. Podrez EA, Poliakov E, Shen Z, et al. A novel family of atherogenic oxidized phospholipids promotes macrophage foam cell formation via the scavenger receptor CD36 and is enriched in atherosclerotic lesions. *J Biol Chem* 2002;277:38517–38523.

42. Schissel SL, Tweedie-Hardman J, Rapp JH, et al. Rabbit aorta and human atherosclerotic lesions hydrolyze the sphingomyelin of retained low-density lipoprotein. Proposed role for arterial-wall sphingomyelinase in subendothelial retention and aggregation of atherogenic lipoproteins. *J Clin Invest* 1996;98:1455–1464.

43. Klimov AN, Denisenko AD, Popov AV, et al. Lipoprotein-antibody immune complexes. Their catabolism and role in foam cell formation. *Atherosclerosis* 1985;58:1–15.

44. Saxena U, Klein MG, Vanni TM, et al. Lipoprotein lipase increases low density lipoprotein retention by subendothelial cell matrix. *J Clin Invest* 1992;89:373–380.

45. Hoff HF, O'Neil J, Wu Z, et al. Phospholipid hydroxyalkenals: biological and chemical properties of specific oxidized lipids present in atherosclerotic lesions. *Arterioscler Thromb Vasc Biol* 2003;23:275–282.

46. Feng B, Yao PM, Li Y, et al. The endoplasmic reticulum is the site of cholesterol-induced cytotoxicity in macrophages. *Nat Cell Biol* 2003;5:781–792.

47. Chisolm GM, Ma G, Irwin KC, et al. 7 beta-hydroperoxycholest-5-en-3 beta-ol, a component of human atherosclerotic lesions, is the primary cytotoxin of oxidized human low density lipoprotein. *Proc Natl Acad Sci U S A* 1994;91:11452–11456.

48. Uzui H, Harpf A, Liu M, et al. Increased expression of membrane type 3-matrix metalloproteinase in human atherosclerotic plaque: role of activated macrophages and inflammatory cytokines. *Circulation* 2002;106: 3024–3030.

49. Huang Y, Mironova M, Lopes-Virella MF. Oxidized LDL stimulates matrix metalloproteinase-1 expression in human vascular endothelial cells. *Arterioscler Thromb Vasc Biol* 1999;19:2640–2647.

50. Rajavashisth TB, Xu XP, Jovinge S, et al. Membrane type 1 matrix metalloproteinase expression in human atherosclerotic plaques: evidence for activation by proinflammatory mediators. *Circulation* 1999;99:3103–3109.

51. Fernandez-Ortiz A, Badimon JJ, Falk E, et al. Characterization of the relative thrombogenicity of atherosclerotic plaque components: implications for consequences of plaque rupture. *J Am Coll Cardiol* 1994;23:1562–1569.

52. Wilcox JN, Smith KM, Schwartz SM, et al. Localization of tissue factor in the normal vessel wall and in the atherosclerotic plaque. *Proc Natl Acad Sci U S A* 1989;86:2839–2843.

53. Ardissino D, Merlini PA, Ariens R, et al. Tissue-factor antigen and activity in human coronary atherosclerotic plaques. *Lancet* 1997;349:769–771.

54. Toschi V, Gallo R, Lettino M, et al. Tissue factor modulates the thrombogenicity of human atherosclerotic plaques. *Circulation* 1997;95:594–599.

55. Mallat Z, Hugel B, Ohan J, et al. Shed membrane microparticles with procoagulant potential in human atherosclerotic plaques: a role for apoptosis in plaque thrombogenicity. *Circulation* 1999;99:348–353.

56. Bochkov VN, Mechtcheriakova D, Lucerna M, et al. Oxidized phospholipids stimulate tissue factor expression in human endothelial cells via activation of ERK/EGR-1 and Ca(++)/NFAT. *Blood* 2002;99:199–206.

57. Cui MZ, Zhao G, Winokur AL, et al. Lysophosphatidic acid induction of tissue factor expression in aortic smooth muscle cells. *Arterioscler Thromb Vasc Biol* 2003;23:224–230.

58. Kim JA, Tran ND, Berliner JA, et al. Minimally oxidized low-density lipoprotein regulates hemostasis factors of brain capillary endothelial cells. *J Neurol Sci* 2004;217:135–141.

59. Dichtl W, Stiko A, Eriksson P, et al. Oxidized LDL and lysophosphatidyl-choline stimulate plasminogen activator inhibitor-1 expression in vascular smooth muscle cells. *Arterioscler Thromb Vasc Biol* 1999;19:3025–3032.

60. Lowe GD. Haemostatic changes and the hypercoagulable state. *Lancet* 1991;338:1526.

61. Li XN, Koons JC, Benza RL, et al. Hypertriglyceridemic VLDL decreases plasminogen binding to endothelial cells and surface-localized fibrinolysis. *Biochemistry* 1996;35:6080–6088.

62. Li XN, Grenett HE, Benza RL, et al. Genotype-specific transcriptional regulation of PAI-1 expression by hypertriglyceridemic VLDL and Lp(a)

in cultured human endothelial cells. *Arterioscler Thromb Vasc Biol* 1997; 17:3215–3223.

63. Allison BA, Nilsson L, Karpe F, et al. Effects of native, triglyceride-enriched, and oxidatively modified LDL on plasminogen activator inhibitor-1 expression in human endothelial cells. *Arterioscler Thromb Vasc Biol* 1999;19:1354–1360.

64. Mitropoulos KA. Lipoprotein metabolism and thrombosis. *Curr Opin Lipidol* 1994;5:227–235.

65. Rapp JH, Lespine A, Hamilton RL, et al. Triglyceride-rich lipoproteins isolated by selected-affinity anti-apolipoprotein B immunosorption from human atherosclerotic plaque. *Arterioscler Thromb* 1994;14:1767–1774.

66. Chung BH, Tallis G, Yalamoori V, et al. Liposome-like particles isolated from human atherosclerotic plaques are structurally and compositionally similar to surface remnants of triglyceride-rich lipoproteins. *Arterioscler Thromb* 1994;14:622–635.

67. Yla-Herttuala S, Lipton BA, Rosenfeld ME, et al. Macrophages and smooth muscle cells express lipoprotein lipase in human and rabbit atherosclerotic lesions. *Proc Natl Acad Sci U S A* 1991;88:10143–10147.

68. O'Brien KD, Gordon D, Deeb S, et al. Lipoprotein lipase is synthesized by macrophage-derived foam cells in human coronary atherosclerotic plaques. *J Clin Invest* 1992;89:1544–1550.

69. Maher VM, Brown BG. Lipoprotein (a) and coronary heart disease. *Curr Opin Lipidol* 1995;6:229–235.

70. Rath M, Niendorf A, Reblin T, et al. Detection and quantification of lipoprotein(a) in the arterial wall of 107 coronary bypass patients. *Arterioscler* 1989;9:579–592.

71. Beisiegel U, Niendorf A, Wolf K, et al. Lipoprotein(a) in the arterial wall. *Eur Heart J* 1990;11(Suppl. E):174–183.

72. Lawn RM, Wade DP, Hammer RE, et al. Atherogenesis in transgenic mice expressing human apolipoprotein(a). *Nature* 1992;360:670–672.

73. Scanu AM, Lawn RM, Berg K. Lipoprotein(a) and atherosclerosis. *Ann Intern Med* 1991;115:209–218.

74. Hajjar KA, Gavish D, Breslow JL, et al. Lipoprotein(a) modulation of endothelial cell surface fibrinolysis and its potential role in atherosclerosis. *Nature* 1989;339:303–305.

75. Palabrica TM, Liu AC, Aronovitz MJ, et al. Antifibrinolytic activity of apolipoprotein(a) *in vivo*: human apolipoprotein(a) transgenic mice are resistant to tissue plasminogen activator-mediated thrombolysis. *Nat Med* 1995;1:256–259.

76. Haseruck N, Erl W, Pandey D, et al. The plaque lipid lysophosphatidic acid stimulates platelet activation and platelet-monocyte aggregate formation in whole blood: involvement of P2Y1 and P2Y12 receptors. *Blood* 2004;103:2585–2592.

77. Vivekananthan DP, Penn MS, Sapp SK, et al. Use of antioxidant vitamins for the prevention of cardiovascular disease: meta-analysis of randomised trials. *Lancet* 2003;361:2017–2023.

78. Brennan ML, Hazen SL. Emerging role of myeloperoxidase and oxidant stress markers in cardiovascular risk assessment. *Curr Opin Lipidol* 2003; 14:353–359.

79. Cai H, Griendling KK, Harrison DG. The vascular NAD(P)H oxidases as therapeutic targets in cardiovascular diseases. *Trends Pharmacol Sci* 2003;24:471–478.

80. Cathcart MK. Regulation of superoxide anion production by NADPH oxidase in monocytes/macrophages: contributions to atherosclerosis. *Arterioscler Thromb Vasc Biol* 2004;24:23–28.

81. Cyrus T, Witztum JL, Rader DJ, et al. Disruption of the 12/15-lipoxygenase gene diminishes atherosclerosis in apo E-deficient mice. *J Clin Invest* 1999;103:1597–1604.

82. Maxeiner H, Husemann J, Thomas CA, et al. Complementary roles for scavenger receptor A and CD36 of human monocyte-derived macrophages in adhesion to surfaces coated with oxidized low-density lipoproteins and in secretion of H2O2. *J Exp Med* 1998;188:2257–2265.

83. Vasquez-Vivar J, Hogg N, Martasek P, et al. Effect of redox-active drugs on superoxide generation from nitric oxide synthases: biological and toxicological implications. *Free Radic Res* 1999;31:607–617.

84. Nikpoor B, Turecki G, Fournier C, et al. A functional myeloperoxidase polymorphic variant is associated with coronary artery disease in French-Canadians. *Am Heart J* 2001;142:336–339.

85. Hayaishi-Okano R, Yamasaki Y, Kajimoto Y, et al. Association of NAD(P)H oxidase p22 phox gene variation with advanced carotid atherosclerosis in Japanese type 2 diabetes. *Diabetes Care* 2003;26:458–463.

86. Chisolm GM III, Hazen SL, Fox PL, et al. The oxidation of lipoproteins by monocytes-macrophages. Biochemical and biological mechanisms. *J Biol Chem* 1999;274:25959–25962.

87. Hurt-Camejo E, Olsson U, Wiklund O, et al. Cellular consequences of the association of apoB lipoproteins with proteoglycans. Potential contribution to atherogenesis. *Arterioscler Thromb Vasc Biol* 1997;17:1011–1017.

88. Kruth HS. Sequestration of aggregated low-density lipoproteins by macrophages. *Curr Opin Lipidol* 2002;13:483–488.

89. Forte TM, Subbanagounder G, Berliner JA, et al. Altered activities of anti-atherogenic enzymes LCAT, paraoxonase, and platelet-activating factor acetylhydrolase in atherosclerosis-susceptible mice. *J Lipid Res* 2002;43:477–485.

90. Navab M, Ananthramaiah GM, Reddy ST, et al. Thematic review series: the pathogenesis of atherosclerosis: the oxidation hypothesis of atherogenesis: the role of oxidized phospholipids and HDL. *J Lipid Res* 2004;45:993–1007.

91. Huber J, Vales A, Mitulovic G, et al. Oxidized membrane vesicles and blebs from apoptotic cells contain biologically active oxidized phospholipids that induce monocyte-endothelial interactions. *Arterioscler Thromb Vasc Biol* 2002;22:101–107.

# CHAPTER 52 ■ THROMBOPHILIA GENETICS

MARTINE AIACH AND JOSEPH EMMERICH

Each year, approximately 1 in 1,000 individuals in industrialized countries develops deep vein thrombosis (DVT) of the lower extremities (1,2). Between 1% and 2% of these patients die from pulmonary embolism, and as many as 25% suffer the chronic effects of the postthrombotic syndrome. It is therefore important to identify high-risk patients with a genetic predisposition to thrombosis, particularly among those individuals who have recurrent DVT. The terms "hypercoagulability" and "thrombophilia" refer to situations in which constitutional or acquired risk factors for thrombotic events are present (3).

Hereditary thrombophilia is associated with a higher risk of thrombosis (mainly venous thrombosis) and is the counterpart of hemophilia, a disease associated with a high risk of spontaneous hemorrhage. Female carriers of hemophilia have clotting factor levels approximately 50% of normal and are protected against thrombosis (4). In contrast, thrombophilia is an autosomal dominant trait mainly linked to heterozygous loss-of-function mutations affecting inhibitors of coagulation, or gain-of-function mutations affecting clotting factors. Interestingly, half-normal clotting factor levels are not associated with a bleeding tendency, whereas half-normal levels of coagulation inhibitors are associated with an increased risk of thrombosis.

As far back as 1856, Virchow postulated that thrombosis could be due to "changes in the composition of blood," yet it was only in 1965 that Egeberg published the first case of inherited antithrombin deficiency (5), and this was followed by similar reports of protein C (PC) and protein S (PS) deficiency (6–8). Hereditary thrombophilia was initially considered as a rare monogenic disorder, but this view was challenged in the mid 1980s (9,10). With the discovery of activated protein C resistance (APCR), a frequent factor V (FV) mutation known as FV$_{Leiden}$ became a paradigm of genetic risk factors for thrombophilia and paved the way for studies of gene–gene and gene–environment interactions (11,12). The main risk factors for venous thromboembolism (VTE) can be divided into acquired factors, genetic factors, and other factors that may vary due to genetic variations yet to be identified (13,14) (see Table 52-1). This chapter focuses on genetic risk factors, the main features of which are summarized in Table 52-2.

## COAGULATION INHIBITOR DEFICIENCY

### Antithrombin Deficiency

#### Biochemistry

Antithrombin (AT) is a 58-kDa plasma protein that regulates coagulation by inhibiting procoagulant serine proteases such as thrombin, activated (a) factor X, and factor IXa. AT belongs to the serpin family, members of which share structural features that allow them to form a stable stoichiometric complex with their target serine protease. The reaction between AT and thrombin involves the reactive center loop and the protease active site serine, and is increased approximately 1,000-fold by heparin and other glycosaminoglycans (e.g., heparan sulfate) that are present on the endothelial surface. Heparin binding to AT involves amino-terminal amino acids 1–47, the A helix, and the D helix (15). AT is synthesized by the liver and circulates at a concentration of approximately 2.5 $\mu$M; levels are decreased by estrogen and heparin therapy.

### Clinical Manifestations

AT deficiency is transmitted as an autosomal dominant trait (0.02% prevalence in the general population) and is associated with a high risk of VTE (approximately 1% per year) (16–18) and 2% of first VTE events (19) in asymptomatic members of thrombophilic families, a higher risk than in patients with other thrombophilic factors (20). Homozygous AT deficiency may cause death *in utero* or severe, life-threatening thrombotic problems in the perinatal period.

### Laboratory Diagnosis

There are two types of hereditary AT deficiency. Type I is the most frequent and is characterized by decreased activity in a heparin cofactor assay and a decreased protein concentration by immunoassay. Type II deficiencies are caused by functional defects, protein concentrations being normal or near normal in immunoassays. The dysfunction may affect the reactive site (II$_{RS}$) or the heparin-binding site (II$_{HBS}$) or both (II$_{PE}$) (pleiotropic effect) (21). Homozygosity is mostly present in patients with type II$_{HBS}$, with the exception of one patient with type II$_{PE}$ deficiency. Venous and arterial thrombosis may occur during infancy in such patients (22,23).

The ability of plasma to inhibit bovine thrombin and human FXa in the presence of heparin is the foundation for chromogenic heparin cofactor assays. Concentrations less than 80% (without heparin or estrogen treatment) call for further investigation, although only patients with severe deficiencies (<60%) are at high risk of thrombosis. Chromogenic assays distinguish type II deficiencies, in that type II$_{HBS}$ has normal activity whereas type II$_{RS}$ has low activity; the risk of VTE is very low in type II$_{HBS}$ deficiency (24).

### Molecular Basis

The human *AT* gene is located on chromosome arm 1q23-25 and it comprises 7 exons spanning 1.3 kb and containing 10 Alu repeats (25). A leader sequence of 32 amino acids is encoded by exon I and by the 5' end of exon II. The mature secreted polypeptide (432 amino acids) is encoded by exons II to VI. The reactive site, an Arg393–Ser394 bond, is located in the carboxy terminus of the protein and is encoded by exon VI. The heparin-binding

**TABLE 52-1**

## MAIN RISK FACTORS FOR VENOUS THROMBOSIS

| Acquired risk factors | Genetic risk factors | Other risk factors[a] |
|---|---|---|
| Age | Antithrombin deficiency | Hyperhomocysteinemia |
| History of venous thrombosis | Protein C deficiency | High levels of factor VIII |
| Surgery | Protein S deficiency | High levels of factor XI |
| Cancer | Factor V$_{Leiden}$ | High levels of factor IX |
| Hormonal treatment | Factor II G20210A | High levels of factor VII |
| Antiphospholipid syndrome | | |
| Myeloproliferative disorders | | |

[a]Possible genetic regulation.
From Chandler WL, Rodgers GM, Sprouse JT, et al. Elevated hemostatic factor levels as potential risk factors for thrombosis. *Arch Pathol Lab Med* 2002;126(11):1405–1414; Bertina RM. Genetic approach to thrombophilia. *Thromb Haemost* 2001;86(1):92–103, with permission.

site of AT is located in the amino-terminal domain and consists of two regions encoded by exon II and exon IIIa.

One of the two alleles is not expressed in type I deficiency, leading to a 50% reduction in the circulating protein. The database lists 80 different point mutations, including microinsertions and deletions, and partial or entire deletions have been found in 12 patients (21).

The type II$_{RS}$ mutations result from amino acid substitutions in the reactive site loop, comprising amino acids 378(P15) to 398(P5′), protruding from the surface of the protein. Mutations located in the hinge domain, affecting Ala382 or Ala384 (P10-P12), transform AT into a substrate for thrombin (24). The Ala384 Ser mutation is particularly frequent in the British population (25,26). Mutations affecting Gly392, Arg393, and Ser394 (P2, P1, P1′) prevent AT recognition by its target protease (25).

Most published mutations modifying AT affinity for heparin (type II$_{HBS}$) are located in the amino-terminal domain encoded by exon II or exon IIIa. Several patients have been found to be homozygous for the Arg47Cys mutation or the Leu99Phe mutation (21,22,27).

A cluster of mutations located on the carboxy-terminal side of the reactive loop, affecting residues 402, 404, 407, and 429, have a pleiotropic effect (type II$_{PE}$). The identification of an Asn187Asp mutation in a patient with recurrent thrombosis and apparently normal circulating AT is puzzling (27). Indeed, this AT variant has a normal function in its native form, but tends to adopt an inactive conformation during storage *in vitro*, leading the authors to suspect that the thrombotic episodes were provoked by fever.

We recently identified a Phe229Leu mutation in a 13-month-old child with cerebral thrombosis. This mutation appears to generate an unstable variant that spontaneously polymerises in the circulation (23). This observation confirms that conformationally altered AT variants with reduced thermostability can be associated with severe thrombosis (28).

## Protein C and Protein S Deficiencies

### Biochemistry

PC is a vitamin K–dependent zymogen that is activated at the endothelial surface when thrombin binds to thrombomodulin. This reaction transforms thrombin from a procoagulant enzyme

**TABLE 52-2**

## MAIN FEATURES OF HEREDITARY THROMBOPHILIA

| Protein affected | Antithrombin | Protein C | Protein S | Factor V | Factor II |
|---|---|---|---|---|---|
| Gene location | 1q23-25 | 2q13-14 | 3p11 | 1q21-22 | 11p11-q12 |
| Type of mutation(s) | Loss-of-function | | | Gain-of-function | |
| | Private mutations | | | Arg506Gln | G20210A |
| Frequency in the general population % | 0.02[a] | 0.2–0.4[a] | 0.7–2.3[a] | 2–10 | 2–4 |
| Type of assay | Heparin cofactor activity against FXa | Clotting assay or amidolytic assay | Clotting assay or immunoassay for free PS | APCR (second generation aPTT-based assay) or FV genotyping | FII genotyping |
| Functional effect | Thrombin and FXa inhibitor | Reduce thrombin generation by inactivating FVa and FVIIIa | | FV variant resistant to APC inactivation | Increase the circulating FII concentration |
| Risk of VTE | ×10 | ×4–5 | ×4–5 | ×4–5 | ×3–4 |

PS, protein S; APCR, activated protein C resistance; aPTT, activated partial thromboplastin time; APC, activated protein C; VTE, venous thromboembolism.
[a]From Seligsohn U, Lubetsky A. Genetic susceptibility to venous thrombosis. *N Engl J Med* 2001;344(16):1222–1231, with permission.

into an inhibitor, by activating PC to activated protein C (APC). PC binding to the endothelial protein C receptor (EPCR) augments its PC activation by the thrombin–thrombomodulin complex (29). In the presence of its cofactor PS, APC degrades activated FV (FVa) and FVIIIa, thereby impeding further thrombin generation (30). FV inactivation occurs in a biphasic reaction, with rapid cleavage at Arg506, followed by slower cleavage at Arg306. The first cleavage only partially affects FVa activity, whereas full inactivation occurs after the second cleavage at Arg306. PS markedly stimulates the second phase of the inactivation process, by a 20-fold enhancement of Arg306 hydrolysis (31). The anticoagulant activity of PS has also been attributed to interaction with the prothrombinase complex, independent of APC (32,33), but the physiologic relevance of this interaction remains to be demonstrated. The mechanism of FVIIIa inhibition by APC is also biphasic, with cleavage at Arg562 and then at Arg336. FVIIIa inactivation by APC is increased by PS and FV, which act synergistically as cofactors for the reaction (34).

PC is synthesized by hepatocytes and circulates at a concentration of approximately 70 nM, with a half-life of approximately 8 hours. APC forms inactive complexes with serine protease inhibitors, mainly protein C inhibitor (PCI), but also protease nexin 3, $\alpha_1$ antitrypsin, and $\alpha_2$ macroglobulin (35).

Although PS is mainly produced by hepatocytes, it is also detected in endothelial cells and platelets. In the circulation, PS forms inactive complexes with C4b-binding protein (C4b-BP). Free PS represents approximately 40% of the total circulating level, and only this fraction has APC cofactor activity. C4b-BP is a multimeric protein composed of 6 or 7 $\alpha$ chains, plus or minus a $\beta$ chain. Only isoforms with a $\beta$ chain (C4b-BP $\beta$+), which normally represent 80% of circulating C4b-BP, can bind PS. The interaction between PS and C4b-BP is reversible, but, in the presence of $Ca^{2+}$, the dissociation constant is less than $10^{-9}$ mol per L. All circulating C4b-BP $\beta$+ molecules carry one molecule of PS, so free plasma PS results from a molar excess of PS over that of C4b-BP $\beta$+ (36). PS plasma levels are lower in women younger than 45 years and in those who are pregnant or are using oral contraceptives (37). During acute-phase reactions, plasma C4b-BP concentrations increase after stimulation of the C4b-BP $\alpha$, C4b-BP $\beta$, and PROS1 genes by inflammatory cytokines.

## Clinical Manifestations of Protein C and Protein S Deficiencies

PC and PS deficiencies are transmitted as autosomal dominant traits with incomplete penetrance, and heterozygous subjects belonging to families with the disorder are at risk of recurrent VTE during adulthood. Hereditary PC deficiency was first identified in subjects who had about half the normal PC concentration and a family history of thrombosis. At 45 years of age, 65% of affected members of the family described by Bovill et al. (38) and 50% of affected members of the 24 families described by Allaart et al. (39) were still free of thrombotic events. In prospectively studied asymptomatic members of thrombophilic families, the incidence of VTE was approximately 0.5% per patient-year in patients with PC deficiency and between 0.5% and 1.65% in patients with PS deficiency (14–18).

The thrombotic risk associated with PC levels less than 67% was confirmed in a case–control study of unselected patients who developed DVT before 70 years of age, with a relative risk (RR) of approximately 3 (40). Homozygous patients with undetectable PC have a very severe clinical phenotype, including life-threatening thrombotic complications at birth, mainly neonatal purpura fulminans with large bruises that become necrotic and gangrenous. The parents and family members of these homozygous infants have about half the normal PC concentration and are asymptomatic (41,42). This form of genetically determined PC deficiency was believed to be recessively transmitted.

Heterozygous subjects belonging to families with PS deficiencies are at risk of recurrent thromboembolic disease in adulthood. In heterozygous subjects, the probability of being free of thrombotic events at 45 years of age is approximately 50% (43). We found that free PS and/or PS anticoagulant activity less than the 90th percentile of control values was indeed associated with a risk of developing VTE (44). Homozygous PS deficiency, such as homozygous PC deficiency, is a rare disease associated with severe thrombosis, including neonatal skin necrosis and purpura fulminans (45,46).

### Laboratory Diagnosis

Most clinical laboratories now use the snake venom protease Protac-based assay, allowing PC to be specifically and directly activated in plasma (47). Such one-step assays evaluate the APC generated after activation by Protac with synthetic substrates (amidolytic assays) or measure the prolongation of the activated partial thromboplastin time (aPTT) (anticoagulant assays). An immunoenzymatic assay measuring the protein concentration in plasma and functional assays measuring enzymatic or anticoagulant activity are used to distinguish several types of PC deficiency. In type I (quantitative) deficiency, which is caused by reduced synthesis of a normal protein, the plasma concentration is low in the three assays; this is the case in most PC deficiencies. Type II (qualitative) deficiency is characterized by normal synthesis of a nonfunctional protein that affects the amidolytic and coagulation assays when the mutation disturbs the catalytic site but is done so only by coagulation assays when the mutation disturbs the interaction of PC with calcium, phospholipids, or macromolecular substrates (FV and FVIII). Therefore, it is recommended to use coagulation assays to screen patients for PC deficiency. It is difficult to establish normal ranges, as PC levels in subjects with *PC* gene abnormalities overlap with levels in healthy subjects (47), and vary with age. According to Miletich (47), the increase in the PC concentration is approximately 4% per decade. Therefore, patients with PC concentrations less than 70% may have a hereditary deficiency, although values between 55% and 70% must be considered as borderline.

The diagnosis of PS deficiency is complicated by the presence in plasma of two molecular forms, that is, free PS and C4b-BP/PS complexes. Therefore, to measure the total circulating PS, immunoenzymatic assays have to be performed in conditions in which C4b-BP/PS complexes are dissociated, such as with highly diluted plasma in anti-PS–coated plates (48). PS deficiency characterized by a low free PS concentration but a normal total PS concentration was identified by Comp (48). A monoclonal antibody (MoAb)-based immunoenzymatic assay is now available to measure free PS specifically (49). APC cofactor activity can be evaluated in an aPTT assay after adding diluted plasma to PS-depleted plasma in the presence of purified APC and purified FVa.

According to the International Society on Thrombosis and Hemostasis (ISTH) standardization subcommittee, three types of PS deficiency have been defined on the basis of total PS levels, free PS levels, and APC cofactor activity. Type I deficiency is characterized by low total PS and free PS antigen levels; type II deficiency by normal free PS and low APC cofactor activity; and type III PS deficiency is characterized by low free PS levels and normal or near normal total PS levels. Type I and type III deficiencies in fact appear to be two phenotypic expressions of the same genetic disease (43), and free PS is used to diagnose PS deficiency in these cases. The lower normal limit of total and free PS levels is 65% of the level observed in a pool of normal plasmas. However, the reference range in women younger than 45 years is approximately 55% under the same conditions. Therefore, it is recommended to use both the clotting assay and the monoclonal-based immunoassay specific for free PS to screen patients for PS deficiency.

## Molecular Bases of Protein C and Protein S Deficiencies

The human *PC* gene maps to chromosome arm 2q13-q14, spans over 11 kb, and comprises a coding region (exons II to IX) and a 5′ untranslated region encompassing exon I (50). The protein domains encoded by exons II to IX show considerable homology with other vitamin K–dependent coagulation proteins such as factors VII, IX, and X. Exon II codes for a signal peptide, whereas exon III codes for a propeptide and a 38–amino acid sequence containing 9 Glu residues. Exons IV, V, and VI encode a short connecting sequence and two epidermal growth factor (EGF)-like domains, respectively. Exon VII encodes both a domain encompassing a 12–amino acid activation peptide that is released after activation of PC by thrombin, and dipeptide 156–157, which, when cleaved, yields the mature two-chain form of the protein. Exons VIII and IX encode the serine protease domain, with His211, Asp257 and Ser360, forming the catalytic triad.

The database published on behalf of the ISTH coagulation inhibitor subcommittee (51) lists 160 different mutations. The proportion of missense mutations is very high and the spectrum very wide, making the molecular basis of PC deficiencies similar to that of FIX deficiency (hemophilia B). The large spectrum of mutations responsible for PC deficiency is probably caused by a high rate of *de novo* mutations (52). Among 90 patients with point mutations, selected on the basis of PC levels less than 65% and with at least one episode of thrombosis, 76 bore a missense mutation. Interestingly, 4.4% of the patients with the missense mutation were homozygous or compound heterozygotes, of whom only one had purpura fulminans at birth (53). Homozygosity and compound heterozygosity may account for concentrations ranging from less than 1% to 25%. Only patients with concentrations less than 5% are at risk of purpura fulminans (53,54).

The amount of PC produced by the mutant allele (null or plus), as well as genetic status (heterozygous, homozygous, or compound heterozygous), partly accounts for the variable clinical expression. However, these factors do not explain why, in many families carrying a single *PC* gene mutation, more than 50% of the affected members remain asymptomatic. Other putative genetic factors may therefore favor thrombosis or protect against disease expression.

Two kinds of type II deficiency can be distinguished on the basis of plasma assays after PC activation by Protac. The substitution of different residues in the propeptide or the gamma carboxyglutamic acid (GLA) domain always resulted in low PC anticoagulant activity, whereas amidolytic activity was normal. It is not surprising that mutations giving rise to this biologic phenotype affect exon III because both the propeptide and the N-terminal region play a major role in the formation of the GLA domain, required for the anticoagulant activity of PC.

A few mutations in exon IX, which encodes the serine protease domain, also affected the coagulation assay but not the amidolytic assay, suggesting that, in addition to the catalytic pocket, this domain encompasses a region or regions required for PC anticoagulant activity. The other mutations in exon IX led to abnormal results in both the coagulation assay and the amidolytic assay (55–57). The possible structural impact of natural substitutions has been examined by Greengard et al. (57) using three-dimensional molecular modeling.

Two homologous genes for PS map to chromosome 3p11 (50) The active gene, *PROS1*, spans over 80 kb and comprises 15 exons. Because PROS2 has no open reading frame and shows multiple base changes, stop codons, and frameshifts, it is probably a pseudogene. The 5′ part of the *PROS1* gene shows strong homology with the other vitamin K–dependent proteins, particularly PC. Exon I encodes the signal peptide; exon II encodes the

propeptide and the GLA domain; exon III encodes a domain with a high aromatic amino acid content; exon IV encodes a thrombin-sensitive loop; and exons V to VIII encode four EGF-like domains. The 3′ part of the *PROS1* gene differs from that of all other known coagulation proteins: The last seven exons (IX to XV) encode a sex-hormone-binding-globulin (SHBG)-homologous domain (54). On screening consecutive patients with unexplained thrombosis and low PS levels, we found mutations in 70% of cases (58). Simmonds et al. (59) found a mutation in 41% of 34 patients with type I deficiency, selected using criteria similar to ours. The mutations observed in type I deficiency are distributed throughout the coding sequence. More than 131 different mutations are listed in the database (46,60). Other mechanisms may explain why one allele is not expressed in patients with type I deficiency who have no detectable mutation. Because the screening strategy is based on selective amplification of the *PROS1* gene, recombination events between the *PROS2* and *PROS1* genes are not detected by PCR-based techniques. However, only three *PS* gene abnormalities involving large deletions have been shown to be responsible for PS deficiencies (61). No mutations in the promoter domain have been identified (unpublished data).

A single mutation transforming Ser460 to Pro, first described by Bertina et al. as a polymorphism (62), was found in 28 of our 118 patients referred with unexplained thrombosis and PS type III deficiency; however, approximately 50% of the patients also carried the FV Arg506Gln mutation or a *PC* gene defect, suggesting a cooperative effect on clinical expression (58). The fact that the affected members of seven families carrying the Ser460Pro mutation were all asymptomatic (63) further suggests that this mutation is not itself a major cause of thrombosis. The type I and type III phenotypes were found to be associated with a similar thrombotic risk, and the two phenotypes coexisted in 14 families, leading the investigators to postulate that type I and type III are phenotypic variants of the same genotype (43). Taken together, these results show that type III phenotypes have a heterogeneous molecular basis and a wide range of clinical consequences.

PS type II deficiency is fairly infrequent, and only a few mutations have been identified in patients with normal PS concentrations and low APC cofactor activity. Most mutations giving rise to a type II phenotype are located in the amino-terminal part of PS, which is homologous to that of other vitamin K–dependent proteins and encodes the domains interacting with APC (60).

# FACTOR V$_{LEIDEN}$

## Biochemistry of Activated Protein C Resistance

In 1993, Dahlbäck described three families in whom APC did not yield the expected prolongation of the clotting time in an aPTT assay (64,65); this defined a new phenotype, called APCR. APCR was found in more than 15% of patients with DVT and in 2% to 10% of control subjects (66,67). The study by Bertina et al. showed that APCR cosegregated with the *FV* gene and with a single mutation (FV$_{Leiden}$, Arg506 Gln) affecting one of the APC cleavage sites (68). Most, but not all, cases of APCR are caused by FV$_{Leiden}$. In the Leiden Thrombophilia Study (LETS), after exclusion of patients with FV$_{Leiden}$, a relation was observed between APC sensitivity and the risk of thrombosis: The lower the normalized APC sensitivity ratio, the higher the associated risk. The adjusted (i.e., age, sex, and FVIII) odds ratio (OR) for the lowest quartile was 2.5 [95% confidence intervals (CI), 1.5 to 4.2] compared with the highest quartile (69). In another study, phenotypic resistance to APC was associated with VTE, independently of FV$_{Leiden}$ status; the age- and sex-adjusted OR for VTE was 1.7 (95% CI, 1.0 to 2.7) in participants who had a normalized APC sensitivity ratio of 0.50 to 0.84 compared with those who had a ratio of 0.85 to 1.3 (70). Clinical states with low APC sensitivity that are not caused by FV$_{Leiden}$ may also be acquired, as is the case during pregnancy, with the use of oral contraceptives, or in patients with lupus anticoagulant or high levels of FVIII.

## Molecular Basis of Activated Protein C Resistance

FV is a 330-kDa multidomain single-chain glycoprotein, with a plasma concentration of 20 nmol per L (0.007 g per L) (71). The FV gene (gene locus on chromosome arm 1q23) spans more than 80 kb and contains 25 exons. The complimentary DNA (cDNA) has a length of 6,672 bp and encodes a preprotein of 224 amino acids. Similar to FVIII, FV is organized into six domains (i.e., A1, A2, B, A3, C1, and C2). FV and FVIII share approximately 40% sequence identity in their A- and C-domains. Thrombin and FXa activate FV by a cleavage at peptide bonds at positions 709, 1,018 and 1,545, thereby releasing the B-domain, which connects the heavy chain (domains A1-A2) to the light chain (domains A3-C1-C2). Upon activation, FVa is formed by the heavy and light chains that are noncovalently associated by a Ca$^{2+}$ ion. FVa is an essential FXa cofactor; its presence in the prothrombinase complex enhances the rate of prothrombin activation 10$^3$- to 10$^5$-fold. Downregulation of the procoagulant activity of FVa is accomplished through its inactivation by APC at positions Arg306, Arg506 and Arg679. Cleavage at Arg506 is essential for optimal exposure of cleavage sites Arg306 and Arg679 but results in partial inactivation of FVa (approximately 40% of procoagulant activity remains). The slower Arg306 cleavage is required for complete inactivation of the protein, whereas the third cleavage site (Arg679) is less important. Therefore, any defect on one or more of these three cleavage sites (i.e., Arg506, Arg306, and Arg679) may potentially affect APC inactivation. In addition to its major role in the procoagulant process when activated, native FV also has an anticoagulant role as an APC cofactor (such as PS), downregulating FVIIIa activity. This latter molecular mechanism is poorly understood but seems to involve the B-domain and also APC-mediated cleavage of intact FV at position 506 (72). Therefore, this dual pathway involving both inactivation of procoagulant FVa by APC and partial proteolysis of intact FV generating an anticoagulant protein, is a complex and subtle regulatory system.

The genetic explanation for the APCR phenotype was obtained initially by Bertina in 1994, and almost concomitantly by three other groups (68,73–75). A single base mutation, guanine to adenine at position 1,691 of the FV gene, is responsible for the Arg506 Gln mutation known as FV$_{Leiden}$. This mutation results in a substantially reduced anticoagulant response to APC, because FV$_{Leiden}$ is inactivated about 10 times more slowly than normal FV. This impairment of FVa inactivation increases thrombin generation and explains more than 90% of clinical APCR phenotypes. However, other mechanisms may contribute to the hypercoagulable state, as suggested by similar inactivation of FVa and FVa$_{Leiden}$ by APC in the presence of PS, FXa, and high concentrations of FVa (65). The fact that FV$_{Leiden}$ is a much less active cofactor of APC than wild-type FV for FVIIIa inactivation may also explain the thrombophilic state. Impaired FVa inactivation and loss of APC cofactor activity contribute equally to the APCR phenotype in subjects with FV$_{Leiden}$ (76). Interestingly, two other mutations in FV affect the Arg306 cleavage site. Arg306 is replaced by Gly in FV$_{Hong Kong}$, and Arg306 is replaced by Thr in FV$_{Cambridge}$ (77,78). FV$_{Hong Kong}$ is prevalent (approximately 5%) among the Chinese in Hong Kong, but neither of these latter mutations is associated with an increased risk of developing venous thrombosis (79). The two FV mutations involving Arg306 yield identical mild APCR patterns. This observation is explained by stimulation of FVa cleavage after Arg679 in the presence of PS. It strongly argues for the importance of the loss of the APC cofactor activity of FV when Arg506 is mutated; it is also strengthened by the recent demonstration that a recombinant FVa, in which the three known APC cleavage sites have been mutated, is still inactivated by APC, although much more slowly than the wild-type protein (80).

## Epidemiology

The prevalence of FV$_{Leiden}$ is high in populations of white descent, but low in native populations of Asia, Africa, and Australia (81). All FV$_{Leiden}$ alleles are carried by the same haplotype, leading to the inference that the mutation occurred only once and spread by a founder effect. The estimated time of the mutation is approximately 30,000 years, implying that it took place after the out-of-Africa divergence that occurred approximately 100,000 years ago (82). Its spread among Whites and its high prevalence suggest that FV$_{Leiden}$ is associated with a survival advantage, such as a decrease in severe bleeding after delivery (83,84).

The frequency of FV$_{Leiden}$ in white populations is between 2 and 15% (66,67,85–92) (see Table 52-3). FV$_{Leiden}$ is very rare in China, Korea, Taiwan, and Japan (93–95). In the United

### TABLE 52-3

ODDS RATIO FOR VENOUS THROMBOEMBOLISM IN HETEROZYGOUS CARRIERS OF FACTOR V$_{Leiden}$

| Author (reference) | Number of cases | Number of cases with FV$_{Leiden}$ (%) | Number of controls | Number of controls with FV$_{Leiden}$ (%) | OR (95% CI) |
|---|---|---|---|---|---|
| Koster et al. (66) | 301 | 64 (21) | 301 | 14 (5) | 6.6 (3.6–12.0) |
| Svensson and Dahlback (67) | 104 | 34 (33) | 130 | 9 (7) | 6.5 (2.8–16.3) |
| Ridker et al. (85) | 121 | 14 (11.6) | 704 | 42 (6) | 2.7 (1.3–5.6) |
| Trossaert et al. (86) | 175 | 29 (17) | 50 | 2 (4) | 4.8 (1.2–42.5) |
| Hainaut et al. (87) | 126 | 27 (22) | 91 | 3 (3.3) | 8.0 (2.4–42.2) |
| Leroyer et al. (88) | 165 | 24 (14.5) | 200 | 7 (3.5) | 4.1 (1.8–9.4) |
| Lambropoulos et al. (89) | 172 | 48 (28.1) | 104 | 5 (4.8) | 7.6 (2.9–25.4) |
| Lindmarker et al. (90) | 467 | 118 (25.3) | 207 | 17 (8.2) | 4.4 (2.6–7.8) |
| Emmerich et al. (91)[a] | 2,310 | 428 (18.6) | 3,204 | 144 (4.5) | 4.9 (4.1–5.9) |
| Folsom et al. (92) | 229 | 39 (17) | 494 | 26 (5.3) | 3.7 (2.2–6.2) |

FV$_{Leiden}$, Factor V$_{Leiden}$; OR, odds ratio; CI, confidence interval.
[a]Pooled analysis of individual data from eight case–control studies.

States, $FV_{Leiden}$ is found in 2.21% of Hispanic Americans, in 1.23% of African Americans, in 0.45% of Asian Americans, and in 1.25% of American Indians (96). $FV_{Leiden}$ affects 15% to 25% of patients with DVT, and the risk of DVT in heterozygous carriers is approximately fivefold higher than in a control population. The association with pulmonary embolism is much weaker, with a prevalence of $FV_{Leiden}$ less than 10% (97), perhaps caused by the formation of a thrombus that is more stable and adherent, and less prone to embolism (98,99). Whatever be the reasons, this imbalance between the risk of DVT and pulmonary embolism is not caused by a bias in selection and is specific for $FV_{Leiden}$, as it has not been observed in carriers of the prothrombin G20210A mutation (99).

Familial and case–control studies show that $FV_{Leiden}$ is clearly a milder thrombophilic state than heterozygous AT, PC, or PS deficiency (16–18). The absolute risks of VTE events in subjects with AT, PC, and PS deficiency are between 0.5% and 1.5% per year, compared to only 0.1% to 0.3% per year in heterozygous carriers of $FV_{Leiden}$. On the basis of these data, it is estimated that the lifetime probability of developing thrombosis in heterozygous $FV_{Leiden}$ carriers is between 5% and 10% (70,100). A census-based screening study of 15,109 persons between 18 and 65 years of age suggested that the FV mutation could explain approximately 7% of all cases of venous thrombosis and could be responsible for at least 50 cases of VTE annually per million community-living adults (70).

The prevalence of $FV_{Leiden}$ homozygosity in the general population is approximately 1 in 2,500. The thrombotic complications are far less severe than in homozygous PC and PS deficiencies (101,102). $FV_{Leiden}$ homozygosity was found in 4.1% of 1,200 consecutive patients with juvenile VTE (103). In a pooled analysis of eight case–control studies on behalf of the ISTH coagulation inhibitor subcommittee, we found $FV_{Leiden}$ homozygosity in 1.3% of 2,310 cases and 0.13% of 3,204 controls (91). In homozygotes, the risk of venous thrombosis is increased 30- to 140-fold, yet an additional environmental or genetic risk factor is often present at the first thrombotic event (91,103). The risk of death among $FV_{Leiden}$ carriers is identical to that among noncarriers (104,105).

## Factor $V_{Leiden}$ and Recurrent Venous Thrombosis

Three studies showed an increased risk of recurrence in heterozygous carriers of $FV_{Leiden}$ (106–108), but nine other studies did not (see Table 52-4) (90,109–116). It seems unlikely that $FV_{Leiden}$ is associated with a significantly increased risk of recurrence compared to patients without other known permanent thrombophilic risk factors. For this reason, long-term anticoagulant therapy is not mandatory after a first thrombotic event in heterozygous carriers of $FV_{Leiden}$. The risk of recurrence in $FV_{Leiden}$ homozygotes appears to be increased, mainly from retrospective studies (22,90,102,103).

## Factor $V_{Leiden}$ and Arterial Thrombosis

The possible link between $FV_{Leiden}$ and arterial thrombosis is elusive (117–121). Most studies have shown no association between $FV_{Leiden}$ and myocardial infarction. Nevertheless, metaanalysis of 19 studies (17,500 individuals) suggests that $FV_{Leiden}$ may be associated with a 20% increase in the risk of myocardial infarction (117). In a case–control study of young women (18 to 44 years), the OR for myocardial infarction was 2.4 (95% CI, 1.0 to 5.9), the increased risk being largely confined to current smokers (122). A metaanalysis of five studies on premature myocardial infarction determined an OR of 1.54 (95% CI, 1.07 to 2.22) (117). Another metaanalysis of six studies determined an OR of 1.34 (95% CI, 0.94 to 1.91) associated with the $FV_{Leiden}$ and myocardial infarction before the age of 55 years (121). Two studies suggest that the prevalence of $FV_{Leiden}$ is higher in patients with myocardial infarction associated with nonsignificant stenosis or obstruction, as shown by coronary arteriography (123,124). Any association between myocardial infarction and $FV_{Leiden}$ would be weak and would not justify screening for the mutation in patients with coronary artery disease.

The prevalence of APCR or the $FV_{Leiden}$ mutation in patients who have had stroke has been examined in more than 30 studies, few of which showed a link with ischemic stroke (125,126).

## TABLE 52-4

### RISK OF RECURRENT VENOUS THROMBOEMBOLISM IN HETEROZYGOUS CARRIERS OF THE FACTOR $V_{LEIDEN}$ MUTATION

| Author (reference) | Number of patients studied/ number of recurrences | Follow-up (mo) | Prospective/ retrospective study | RR of recurrence in $FV_{Leiden}$ carriers (95% CI) |
|---|---|---|---|---|
| Ridker et al. (106) | 77/11 | 68 | Prospective | 4.7 ($P = 0.047$) |
| Simioni et al. (107) | 251/49 | 47 | Prospective | 2.4 (1.3–4.5) |
| Eichinger et al. (109) | 380/36 | 19 | Prospective | NS |
| Lindmarker et al. (90) | 534/92 | 48 | Prospective | NS |
| Kearon et al. (110) | 162/18 | 10 | Prospective | NS |
| De Stefano et al. (111) | 412/131 | – | Retrospective | NS |
| Margaglione et al. (112) | 542/82 | – | Retrospective | NS |
| Kyrle et al. (113) | 360/38 | 30 | Prospective | NS |
| Simioni et al. (108) | 251/68 | 99 | Prospective | 2.4 (1.4–4.1) |
| Eichinger et al. (114) | 287/61 | 72 | Prospective | NS |
| Baglin et al. (115) | 570/62 | 24 | Prospective | NS |
| Eichinger et al. (116) | 436/54 | 30 | Prospective | NS |

RR, relative risk; $FV_{Leiden}$, Factor $V_{Leiden}$; CI, confidence interval; NS, not significant.

In 100 patients younger than 45 years who survived an ischemic stroke without a cardiac embolic source, $FV_{Leiden}$ was not over-represented (126). $FV_{Leiden}$ is associated with cerebral vein thrombosis, with an OR of 3 to 4 (127–131).

## Laboratory Diagnosis

Two types of tests can be used for diagnosing APCR: the functional APCR assay and the genetic $FV_{Leiden}$ identification test. The functional test is based on aPTT prolongation after the addition of purified APC and is expressed as an APC sensitivity ratio: APTT($+$APC)/APTT($-$APC). A low APC sensitivity ratio defines APCR. Second-generation APCR tests, which use dilution of test plasma into FV-deficient plasma, have very good specificity and can even be used to test patients taking warfarin (119,132). It is mandatory to confirm a positive APCR test by direct detection of $FV_{Leiden}$. The most commonly used genetic test for $FV_{Leiden}$ is based on polymerase chain reaction (PCR) amplification of the FV gene exon 10. The presence or absence of the mutation can be determined with allele-specific probes or restriction enzymes. The advantage of genetic testing is that it avoids ambiguous results and determines heterozygous/homozygous status in patients with a low APC sensitivity ratio. Consensus recommendations by the College of American Pathologists on $FV_{Leiden}$ testing have been edicted in 2002.

# THE FII (PROTHROMBIN) G20210A MUTATION

## Biochemistry

Prothrombin has procoagulant, anticoagulant, and antifibrinolytic activities after its activation into thrombin by the prothrombinase complex. Thrombin acts by activating factors XIII, XI and VIII, V, PC, and the thrombin-activatable fibrinolysis inhibitor (TAFI) and by cleaving fibrinogen to fibrin. Prothrombin is a 72-kDa multidomain single-chain vitamin K–dependent glycoprotein. Prothrombin activation is mediated by FXa, which cleaves prothrombin at Arg271–Thr272 and Arg320–Ile321 to release the catalytic domain from the carboxy-terminal domain. Prothrombin activation is accelerated approximately 300,000-fold in the presence of FVa, phospholipids, and $Ca^{2+}$. Human thrombin contains an A chain of 36 amino acids and a B chain of 259 amino acids. The prothrombin gene is 21 kb in length and is encoded by chromosome 11 (position 11p11-q12) (134). The gene comprises 14 exons separated by 13 introns, with the 5′ and 3′ untranslated regions that may play regulatory roles in gene expression.

## Molecular Characteristics

By extensively screening the prothrombin genes of 28 families with unexplained venous thrombosis (133), Poort et al. found one heterozygous nucleotide transition (G to A) at position 20210 in the 3′ untranslated region in 5 probands (18%). In 474 unselected patients with a first episode of venous thrombosis and 474 controls of the LETS, the frequency of the mutation was 6.2% and 2.3%, respectively. In this study, the OR for thrombosis associated with the FII 20210A allele was 2.8 (95% CI, 1.4 to 5.6). Interestingly, the FII 20210A allele was associated with significantly higher prothrombin levels in heterozygotes than in noncarriers (1.32 U per mL and 1.05 U per mL, respectively). The plasma prothrombin level was an independent risk factor for thrombosis. Together, these risk factors

suggested that FII 20210A acts by increasing prothrombin levels, leading to increased thrombin generation (135,136). Another possible explanation for the role of the FII level in thrombosis is that elevated prothrombin levels can inhibit APC-mediated inactivation of FVa (137).

The mechanism by which the G20210A mutation influences prothrombin levels is controversial (138–142). The increase in protein synthesis could result from more efficient 3′-end formation, increased messenger ribonucleic acid (mRNA) stability, increased translation efficiency, or a combination of these mechanisms. Mutations of the poly(A) signal sequence commonly cause loss of gene function. FII G20210A is the only example of mutation in the cleavage site required for mRNA polyadenylation that increases 3′ end processing. Another rare FII mutation (FII C20221T) was found in a child with arterial thrombosis after allogenic kidney transplantation and in a 28-year-old man with Budd-Chiari syndrome (142–144). This paradoxical gain-of-function from mutations in the 3′ end of the FII gene was explained by unusual 3′ noncanonical sequence elements: The FII cleavage site for polyadenylation and uridine-rich elements in the 3′ flanking sequence seems less efficient than in other genes, thereby favoring gain-of-function mutations (142). The same authors demonstrated that, compared to the wild-type FII (FII 20210G), the 20210C and 20210T mutations led to a 40% to 50% increase in mRNA expression, and the 20210A mutation led to a 215% increase.

It was recently reported that an intronic FII gene polymorphism, A19911G, influences splicing efficiency and modulates the effects of the FII G20210A mutation on mRNA and protein expression (145). The 19911G allele is in linkage disequilibrium with the 20210A allele, and heterozygous carriers of the FII G20210A mutation who also have the 19911G mutation on the other allele (19911G homozygotes) have a higher risk of venous thrombosis.

## Epidemiology

The prevalence of the FII mutation is high in populations of white descent but low or nil in Asians, American Indians, and African Americans (146–148). As in the case of $FV_{Leiden}$, a founder effect explains the high prevalence of the factor II G20210A mutation in whites (148). Haplotyping suggests that the mutation arose 20,000 to 30,000 years ago, after the divergence of nonAfricans from Africans and Caucasoids from Mongoloid subpopulations. A survival advantage based on a protective prenatal effect of the FII G20210A genotype, such as improved embryonic implantation, has been suggested (149).

The estimated frequency of FII G20210A in white populations is between 1% and 6% (91,133,150–156) (see Table 52-5). This mutation is more common in southern than in northern Europe, a gradient opposite to that of $FV_{Leiden}$ (146). The risk of DVT is increased by threefold to fourfold in heterozygous carriers of FII G20210A compared to noncarriers. In two prospective studies, and in a large Italian cross-sectional survey, the risk of thrombosis was lower than in case–control studies (150,151, 155). In the rare FII G20210A homozygotes, the risk of thrombosis is only moderately increased (136,157–159), often associated with other genetic or acquired risk factors (159).

## FII G20210A and Recurrent Venous Thrombosis

Two studies showed an increased risk of DVT recurrence among heterozygous carriers of FII G20210A (108,160), but eight other studies did not (90,110,112,113,115,116,161,162) (see Table 52-6). Overall, it seems unlikely that FII G20210A is associated with a significantly increased risk of recurrence

TABLE 52-5

**TABLE 52-5**

ODDS RATIO FOR VENOUS THROMBOEMBOLISM IN HETEROZYGOUS CARRIERS OF THE FII G20210A MUTATION

| Author (reference) | Number of cases | Number of cases with FII G20210A (%) | Number of controls | Number of controls with FII G20210A (%) | OR (95% CI) |
|---|---|---|---|---|---|
| Poort et al. (133) | 474 | 29 (6.2) | 474 | 11 (2.3) | 2.8 (1.4–5.6) |
| Brown et al. (152) | 504 | 26 (5.2) | 508 | 13 (2.6) | 2.0 (1.0–4.0) |
| Leroyer et al. (153) | 366 | 17 (4.6) | 400 | 4 (1) | 3.7 (1.1–13.6) |
| Souto et al. (154) | 116 | 20 (17.2) | 201 | 13 (6.5) | 3.1 (1.4–6.6) |
| Ridker et al. (151)[a] | 218 | 14 (6.4) | 1,774 | 69 (3.9) | 1.7 (0.9–3.1) |
| Tosetto et al. (155) | 116 | 5 (4.3) | 232 | 8 (3.4) | 1.26 (0.4–3.9) |
| Adamczuk et al. (156) | 110 | 8 (7.2) | 200 | 4 (2) | 3.7 (1.0–13.7) |
| Emmerich et al. (91)[b] | 2,310 | 216 (9.4) | 3,204 | 93 (2.9) | 3.8 (3.0–4.9) |
| Folsom et al. (150)[a] | 231 | 12 (5.2) | 489 | 14 (2.9) | 1.9 (0.85–4.1) |

OR, odds ratio; CI, confidence interval.
[a]Prospective studies.
[b]Pooled analysis of individual data from eight case–control studies.

relative to patients with no other known permanent thrombophilic risk factors; long-term anticoagulant therapy is therefore not mandatory after a first thrombotic event. The risk of recurrence in FII G20210A homozygotes is probably increased, as in double heterozygotes carrying both $FV_{Leiden}$ and FII G20210A, in whom the risk of a primary VTE event is increased 20-fold (91,111,112,160).

## FII G20210A and Arterial Thrombosis

Similar to FV, any association of FII G20210A with arterial thrombosis would be very weak (118–121,163). Most studies have shown no association between FII G20210A and myocardial infarction or stroke. Nevertheless, in populations at low risk of arterial thrombotic events, such as young women, the OR for myocardial infarction is increased fourfold in FII 20210A carriers (122,164). A metaanalysis of three studies in patients with myocardial infarction before the age of 55 years found an OR associated with the FII G20210A mutation of 1.86 (95% CI, 0.99 to 3.51) (121).

More than a dozen studies have analyzed the association between the FII G20210A mutation and stroke and none has shown a link with ischemic events (125). One study, of 72 patients with ischemic stroke before the age of 50 years and no other risk factors, found a fourfold to fivefold increase in the risk of stroke in carriers of the FII G20210A mutation (165). This increased risk of stroke in young patients was not found in another study (126). The risk of cerebral venous thrombosis is also increased in carriers of the FII G20210A mutation (131).

## Laboratory Diagnosis

Although FII G20210A heterozygotes have 30% higher prothrombin levels than noncarriers on an average, this phenotype cannot be used to identify carriers of the mutation because of a large overlap of prothrombin levels. The only way to reliably detect the mutation is genetic screening after PCR amplification of the 3′ untranslated region of the *FII* gene. Several techniques

**TABLE 52-6**

RISK OF RECURRENT VENOUS THROMBOEMBOLISM IN HETEROZYGOUS CARRIERS OF THE FII G20210A MUTATION

| Author (reference) | Number of patients studied/ number of recurrences | Follow-up (mo) | Prospective/ retrospective study | RR of recurrence in FII G20210A carriers (95% CI) |
|---|---|---|---|---|
| Margaglione et al. (112) | 542/82 | – | Retrospective | NS |
| Eichinger et al. (161) | 492/55 | 24 | Prospective | NS |
| Lindmarker et al. (90) | 534/92 | 48 | Prospective | NS |
| Kearon et al. (110) | 162/18 | 10 | Prospective | NS |
| Simioni et al. (108) | 251/68 | 99 | Prospective | 2.4 (1.3–4.7) |
| Miles et al. (160) | 218/29 | 88 | Prospective | 4.93 (1.9–12.9) |
| De Stefano et al. (162) | 335/52 | – | Retrospective | NS |
| Kyrle et al. (113) | 360/38 | 30 | Prospective | NS |
| Baglin et al. (115) | 570/62 | 24 | Prospective | NS |
| Eichinger et al. (116) | 436/54 | 30 | Prospective | NS |

RR, relative risk; CI, confidence interval; NS, not significant.

are based on detection using specific restriction endonucleases, gel electrophoresis, or fluorescent probing (163). Multiplex PCR-based assay is valuable for concomitant detection of $FV_{Leiden}$ and FII G20210A (166).

# OTHER GENETIC RISK FACTORS

## The Protein C Gene Promoter Polymorphism

The 5′ untranslated region of the *PC* gene, which encompasses exon I, has polymorphic sites at positions −1654 (C/T), −1641 (A/G), and −1476 (A/T). Three haplotypes are commonly observed (CGT, TAA, and CAA). In the LETS, individuals homozygous for CGT had a higher risk of venous thrombosis than individuals with the TAA genotype (167). In the Paris Thrombosis Study (PATHROS), we found that both homozygotes and heterozygotes for the CG haplotype had lower PC concentrations than noncarriers. The CG allelic frequency was considerably higher in patients with VTE than in controls (168).

## The FXIII α Chain Gene Polymorphism

The replacement of Val34 by Leu in the α chain of FXIII modifies the activation process and results in faster activation by thrombin (169). Unexpectedly, this polymorphism had a protective effect on myocardial infarction (170,171). In venous thrombosis, several case–control studies failed to show any effect of the FXIII polymorphism; however, in a metaanalysis of four of these studies, we found a weak protective effect, with ORs of 0.86 (95% CI, 0.74 to 0.99) and 0.58 (95% CI, 0.41 to 0.82) in heterozygotes and homozygotes, respectively (172).

## Future Directions

FVIII and other coagulation factors such as FXI, FIX, and FVII were found to be independent risk factors for thrombosis (14); this was also observed for APCR in noncarriers of $FV_{Leiden}$ (69). The genetic studies have not yet identified the molecular basis for high levels of the coagulation factor (except in patients with FII A20210) and for APCR (except in patients with $FV_{Leiden}$). However, ongoing studies confirm that genetic mechanisms account for these observations (173–178). Genetic analysis of idiopathic thrombophilia (GAIT) is a modern family-based genetic study involving 398 individuals belonging to 21 pedigrees. The results published to date offer three main insights: (a) The heritability of many quantitative hemostatic variables is high and significant (173), (b) the heritability of susceptibility to thrombosis is confirmed whatever the underlying mechanism (174), and (c) quantitative hemostasis variables correlate with the risk of thrombosis (174). In the GAIT study, the heritability of APCR was high, pointing to genetic control independent of $FV_{Leiden}$. The GAIT study group recently identified a new locus on chromosome 18 linked to both APCR and FVIII activity, as well as to thrombotic susceptibility (175). We used a very simple approach to detect several functional genetic polymorphisms that influence either platelet function or coagulation regulation (179,180). We thereby identified a new polymorphism in the gene encoding the EPCR, which was strongly associated with circulating levels of soluble EPCR (sEPCR). This variable was evaluated in 100 healthy men aged 20 to 35 years from whom blood samples were taken twice, one week apart. One of the three haplotypes identified (A3) was always present in subjects with sEPCR levels greater than 200 ng per L; A3 carriers were also found to have a higher risk of DVT in the PATHROS study (181).

# ASSOCIATION OF GENETIC AND ACQUIRED RISK FACTORS

## Oral Contraception

The level of thrombotic risk using progestin–ethinylestradiol contraceptive combinations is low, approximately 2 to 4 cases per 10,000 woman-years and depends on the dose of estradiol, the type of progestin, and individual factors (182–184). The first oral contraceptive contained more than 50 μg of ethinyl estradiol (EE). Most of the currently available oral contraceptives contain 30 μg of EE, yet the most recent studies suggest that this dose still increases the risk of VTE threefold to sixfold. Epidemiologic studies show that the risk is increased twofold to threefold in women using pills with third-generation progestins compared with those using pills with other progestins. Desogestrel, gestoden, and norgestimate belong to the third generation, norgestrel and levogestrel to the second generation, and lynestrenol and norethynodrel to the first generation. Another type of progestin, cyproterone, with antiandrogenic properties (used to treat acne and hirsutism), increases the risk of VTE threefold to fourfold when compared to levonorgestrel in a case–control study including oral contraception users with VTE (185).

The interaction between oral contraceptives and thrombophilia was first established in the LETS study, by selecting 155 cases aged between 15 and 49 years with a first episode of VTE and 169 matched controls. In this study, the use of oral contraceptives by women carrying $FV_{Leiden}$ led to a 30-fold increase in the risk of VTE, which strongly suggested a synergistic effect (186). In a metaanalysis of several case–control studies (91), the risks of using oral contraceptives in $FV_{Leiden}$ carriers were estimated in 517 women aged 15 years through 49 years and in 518 controls. The OR (10.28) clearly indicates a supraadditive effect of the association $FV_{Leiden}$ and oral contraception. The risk of using oral contraceptives associated with FII G20210 was also evaluated in this metaanalysis (OR, 7.14). As already observed (187), the latter mutation was found to interact synergistically with oral contraception.

The risk of thrombosis is also high in women with AT, PC, and PS deficiencies or homozygous for $FV_{Leiden}$ who use oral contraceptives, particularly in case of AT deficiency, with an annual incidence of 3.4% per person (vs. 0.75% in nonusers) (188,189). Analysis of the LETS dataset led to the conclusion that women with inherited thrombophilia ($FV_{Leiden}$, FII G20210, and AT, PC and PS deficiencies) develop VTE not only more often but also earlier than other women (190). FVIII, FV, and FXI levels more than the 90th percentile and FXII levels less than the 10th percentile in patients whose first VTE episode occurred when they were taking oral contraceptives were associated with ORs of 10 to 12. However, the joint effect of these risk factors did not exceed the sum of separate effects (additive but not synergistic) (191).

These observations raise the question of whether asymptomatic young women should be tested for thrombophilic factors before the first use of oral contraceptives. Most authors agree that such tests in young women is not desirable because the absolute risk is very low in this population (to prevent one death by pulmonary embolism would require tests on approximately 500,000), although it might be justified in some cases (192).

## Hormone Replacement Therapy

Several observational studies have shown that women taking conjugated or natural estrogen therapy have an increased risk of VTE (183,193). Few studies have been designed to evaluate the risk of such replacement therapies in thrombophilic postmenopausal women. In the Estrogen in Venous Thromboembolism Trial (EVTET) study (194), 144 women younger than 70 years were randomly allocated to receive a dosage of 2 mg per day of 17-β-oestradiol, norethisterone, or placebo in a double-blind study. Eight of the women receiving hormone replacement therapy (HRT) had recurrent VTE, compared to only one woman in the placebo group. In this study, which was interrupted for safety reasons, $FV_{Leiden}$ carriers did not experience more frequent VTE than noncarriers, suggesting that this thrombophilic risk factor was not predictive of recurrence during HRT. In another study, 77 postmenopausal women who had had VTE were compared to 163 controls. The ORs (95% CI) were 3.9 (1.3 to 11.2), 3.2 (1.7 to 6.0), and 15.5 (3.1 to 76.7) in $FV_{Leiden}$ carriers, HRT users, and in $FV_{Leiden}$ carriers taking HRT, respectively, suggesting a synergistic effect (195).

There is no strong evidence that genetic thrombophilic factors can be used to identify a subpopulation at high risk of VTE. The risk of VTE is very high in HRT users with prior VTE, whatever be the underlying mechanism.

## Pregnancy

Pregnancy is an acquired risk factor for VTE, multiplying the risk fivefold. In families with inherited thrombophilia, asymptomatic carriers have an increased probability of VTE onset during pregnancy relative to noncarriers. Women carrying two risk alleles, such as homozygotes for $FV_{Leiden}$ and double heterozygotes for $FV_{Leiden}$ and FII G20210A, have a particularly high risk (196).

In another approach, women with a history of VTE during pregnancy were compared with age-matched women with a prior pregnancy free of VTE. The results confirm that the probability of pregnancy-related thrombosis is high in women with homozygous $FV_{Leiden}$ or with double $FV_{Leiden}$ and FII G20210A mutations (197,198). Unequivocal PC deficiency (<50%) and AT deficiency (<60%) were also associated with an increased risk of VTE during pregnancy.

# COMBINATIONS OF GENETIC RISK FACTORS

## Combined Defects

There is an increased risk of VTE in patients carrying more than one genetic defect. Indeed, in two studies, 19% and 9.5% of symptomatic probands carrying a *PC* gene mutation also carried the $FV_{Leiden}$ mutation (199,200). Similar frequencies of combined defects were found in the probands of thrombophilic families carrying a *PS* gene mutation (58,59). In family members with AT deficiency, coinheritance of $FV_{Leiden}$ increased the risk of DVT (201). A metaanalysis confirmed that the RR of thrombosis was much higher in carriers of both $FV_{Leiden}$ and FII G20210A (91). Patients heterozygous for a single genetic risk factor, with the possible exception of AT deficiency, have the lowest risk (RR 3 to 5). These patients may have DVT during adulthood, the risk increasing with age and, often, with acquired risk factors such as prolonged immobilization, surgery, pregnancy, and estrogen therapy. Combined genetic defects are associated with a stronger risk (RR 10 to 20) and may lead to thrombosis in early adulthood; this includes patients carrying two risk alleles, such as homozygotes for $FV_{Leiden}$ and heterozygotes for $FV_{Leiden}$ plus any of the other four genetic risk factors. Finally, homozygosity for PC, PS, or some types of AT deficiency is often associated with very severe early onset thrombotic disease. Patients carrying two risk alleles have a much

higher risk of severe and early thrombosis and are likely to benefit from continuous or discontinuous preventive antithrombotic therapy. Because 10% to 30% of thrombophilic family probands have combined defects, the thrombotic phenotype may not be transmitted as a dominant trait.

## Other Genes Possibly Influencing the Thrombophilic Phenotype

Noncarrier members of $FV_{Leiden}$ families have a higher frequency of DVT than the general population do (73,202), and the Vermont family study showed that PC deficiency penetrance was controlled by other (unknown) gene(s) (203). The role of *FV* gene polymorphisms also illustrates the complexity of the mechanisms that may increase the penetrance of genetic thrombophilic factors, and available data show an influence of the HR2 haplotype on the penetrance of $FV_{Leiden}$. The A4070G polymorphism in exon 13 of the *FV* gene, which replaces His by Arg at position 1,299 of the B-domain, influences circulating FV levels and contributes to the APCR phenotype. This polymorphism is in high-linkage disequilibrium with several other polymorphisms of the *FV* gene, defining two haplotypes designated HR1 and HR2 (204). The Arg506Gln mutation is always carried by the R1 allele, whereas the R2 allele influences APCR in the absence of the FV Arg506Gln mutation (205). Carriers of both FV Arg506Gln and the R2 allele have a pseudohomozygous plasma phenotype (205). The HR2 haplotype includes an amino acid change in the FV C2 domain, which influences the ratio of two FV glycoforms (206); this may explain the association of R2 with mild APC resistance (205,207–210). Faioni et al. (209) reported that coinheritance of the R2 allele with $FV_{Leiden}$ increased the risk of DVT in thrombophilic families, but we failed to confirm this finding in another series of thrombophilic families (202).

# THROMBOPHILIA SCREENING AND MANAGEMENT

There is no consensus on the subsets of subjects who qualify for thrombophilia screening, the types of laboratory test to use, or the clinical treatment of patients with thrombophilia. The most salient recommendations are summarized here (19,20,211–213). Most guidelines are not very useful in clinical practice because they consider each genetic risk factor on its own and do not consider thrombophilia as a single clinical entity (214–216).

Thrombophilia is mainly associated with venous thrombosis rather than arterial thrombosis. Venous thrombosis most commonly occurs as DVT and/or pulmonary embolism, and a given case of thrombosis is not associated with a peculiar genetic thrombophilic state. Less common clinical forms such as superficial, upper limb, cerebral, and visceral vein thrombosis (i.e., portal, mesenteric, hepatic, and renal) should be screened because these forms are often associated with thrombophilia (217,218).

The predictive value of a family history for identifying patients with a thrombophilic state is unreliable, and the absence of a family history does not preclude the need to screen for $FV_{Leiden}$, FII G20210A, and coagulation inhibitor deficiencies (192,219–221). The multifactorial nature of venous thrombosis explains why thrombotic events in carriers of thrombophilic factors are triggered in half of the cases by acquired risk factors (12,19). Therefore, venous thrombosis associated with an acquired risk factor does not preclude the need for screening. It makes sense to restrict screening after a first thrombotic event in young patients and in patients experiencing recurrences after withdrawal of oral anticoagulants (222,223). Finally, testing for

**TABLE 52-7**

RECOMMENDATIONS CONCERNING SCREENING FOR THROMBOPHILIA

1. Thrombophilia screening is recommended in patients with:
   - A history of recurrent VTE
   - A first VTE at younger than 50 yr of age
   - A first unprovoked VTE at any age
   - A first VTE at an unusual anatomic site, such as the upper limb, cerebral, mesenteric, portal, or hepatic
   - A first VTE related to pregnancy, the puerperium, contraceptive, or hormone replacement therapy
   - Women with two or more unexplained pregnancy losses
2. Testing for thrombophilia is controversial in:
   - Young women smokers (age <50 yr) with a myocardial infarction
   - Elderly patients (age >50 yr) with a first provoked VTE event in the absence of cancer or an intravascular device
   - A first VTE related to SERMs or tamoxifen
   - Selected cases of women with unexplained severe preeclampsia, placenta abruptio, or intrauterine growth retardation
3. Testing for thrombophilia may be indicated in:
   - Asymptomatic adult family members of probands with known coagulation inhibitor deficiency and maybe in $FV_{Leiden}$ families (especially those with a strong family history of thrombosis at a young age)
   - Asymptomatic female family members who are pregnant or are considering oral contraceptives or pregnancy
4. Thrombophilia testing is not recommended:
   - As a general population screen
   - As a routine initial test prior to or during oral contraceptive use, hormone replacement therapy or SERMs therapy
   - As a prenatal test, newborn initial test, or as a routine test in asymptomatic prepubescent children
   - As a routine initial test in patients with arterial thrombotic events; however, testing can be considered in certain unusual situations, such as in patients with unexplained arterial thrombosis without atherosclerosis or in young patients

VTE, venous thromboembolism; SERMs, selective estrogen receptor modulators; $FV_{Leiden}$, Factor $V_{Leiden}$.

thrombophilia would be useful if we were able to identify patients who are particularly prone to recurrence, but the risk of recurrence is not increased for $FV_{Leiden}$ or FII G20210A. Recommendations for testing are shown in Table 52-7.

## Management of Thrombophilia

### Management of a First Acute Thrombotic Episode

The initial management of DVT or pulmonary embolism in patients with heritable thrombophilia is not different from the management of venous thrombosis in any other patient according to the British Society of Haematology (216).

### Duration of Anticoagulant Therapy

Identification of the most prevalent forms of heritable thrombophilia, heterozygosity for $FV_{Leiden}$ or FII G20210A, should not influence decisions about the duration of anticoagulant therapy (usually 3 to 6 months after a first event).

Longer duration or long-term anticoagulation may be recommended in antithrombin deficiency, homozygotes for $FV_{Leiden}$, and double heterozygotes.

### Management of Recurrent Venous Thrombosis

In general, patients who have had two or more apparently spontaneous venous thrombotic events and genetic thrombophilia need to be considered for indefinite anticoagulant thromboprophylaxis.

### Management of Acute Venous Thromboembolism during Pregnancy

The management of VTE occurring during pregnancy in a woman with thrombophilia is no different from the management of VTE in a pregnant woman.

### Thrombosis Prevention

Patients with history of VTE and a thrombophilic defect need short-term thromboprophylaxis to cover periods of increased thrombotic risk, for example, surgery, trauma, plaster casts, or immobilization.

Affected asymptomatic relatives of patients with thrombophilia merit consideration for short-term thromboprophylaxis to cover similar periods of increased thrombotic risk.

### Contraceptive Advice

The use of a combined oral contraceptive pill is not recommended in women who have a personal history of venous thrombosis. Women who have a family history of at least one first-degree relative with a history of proven venous thrombosis should consider using a contraceptive method other than the combined pill as the first choice.

### Management during Pregnancy

All women should be encouraged to wear graduated compression stockings throughout their pregnancy and for 6 weeks after delivery.

Women at high risk of pregnancy-associated VTE are those who are on long-term anticoagulant thromboprophylaxis or who have type I AT deficiency or a type II reactive site AT defect. Treatment is with adjusted doses of low-molecular-weight heparin (LMWH) or unfractionated heparin.

Women at moderately increased risk of pregnancy-associated VTE are those with a previous history of VTE and a thrombophilic defect, or asymptomatic women with a familial history of venous thrombosis who are heterozygous for PC or PS deficiency, or homozygous for $FV_{Leiden}$ or the FII G20210A mutation, or a combination of defects. Treatment is a fixed prophylactic dose of LMWH or unfractionated heparin.

Patients at a slightly increased risk of pregnancy-associated VTE are those who are asymptomatic with a familial history of venous thrombosis and are heterozygous for FV$_{Leiden}$ or FII G20210A. These patients do not require anticoagulant thromboprophylaxis antenatally, but anticoagulant prophylaxis following delivery should be considered.

# References

1. Rosendaal FR. Thrombosis in the young: epidemiology and risk factors. A focus on venous thrombosis. *Thromb Haemost* 1997;78(1):1–6.
2. Oger E. Incidence of venous thromboembolism: a community-based study in Western France. EPI-GETBP Study Group. Groupe d'Etude de la thrombose de bretagne occidentale. *Thromb Haemost* 2000;83(5):657–660.
3. Bertina RM. Introduction: hypercoagulable states. *Semin Hematol* 1997; 34(3):167–170.
4. Sramek A, Kriek M, Rosendaal FR. Decreased mortality of ischaemic heart disease among carriers of haemophilia. *Lancet* 2003;362(9381):351–354.
5. Egeberg O. Inherited antithrombin deficiency causing thrombophilia. *Thromb Diath Haemorrh* 1965;13:516–530.
6. Comp PC, Nixon RR, Cooper MR, et al. Familial protein S deficiency is associated with recurrent thrombosis. *J Clin Invest* 1984;74(6):2082–2088.
7. Griffin JH, Evatt B, Zimmerman TS, et al. Deficiency of protein C in congenital thrombotic disease. *J Clin Invest* 1981;68(5):1370–1373.
8. Schwarz HP, Fischer M, Hopmeier P, et al. Plasma protein S deficiency in familial thrombotic disease. *Blood* 1984;64(6):1297–1300.
9. Miletich J, Sherman L, Broze G Jr. Absence of thrombosis in subjects with heterozygous protein C deficiency. *N Engl J Med* 1987; 317(16):991–996.
10. Miletich JP, Prescott SM, White R, et al. Inherited predisposition to thrombosis. *Cell* 1993;72(4):477–480.
11. Rosendaal FR. Risk factors for venous thrombosis: prevalence, risk, and interaction. *Semin Hematol* 1997;34(3):171–187.
12. Rosendaal FR. Venous thrombosis: a multicausal disease. *Lancet* 1999; 353(9159):1167–1173.
13. Chandler WL, Rodgers GM, Sprouse JT, et al. Elevated hemostatic factor levels as potential risk factors for thrombosis. *Arch Pathol Lab Med* 2002; 126(11):1405–1414.
14. Bertina RM. Genetic approach to thrombophilia. *Thromb Haemost* 2001; 86(1):92–103.
15. Carrell RW, Stein PE, Fermi G, et al. Biological implications of a 3 A structure of dimeric antithrombin. *Structure* 1994;2(4):257–270.
16. Bucciarelli P, Rosendaal FR, Tripodi A, et al. Risk of venous thromboembolism and clinical manifestations in carriers of antithrombin, protein C, protein S deficiency, or activated protein C resistance: a multicenter collaborative family study. *Arterioscler Thromb Vasc Biol* 1999;19(4):1026–1033.
17. Martinelli I, Mannucci PM, De Stefano V, et al. Different risks of thrombosis in four coagulation defects associated with inherited thrombophilia: a study of 150 families. *Blood* 1998;92(7):2353–2358.
18. Simioni P, Sanson BJ, Prandoni P, et al. Incidence of venous thromboembolism in families with inherited thrombophilia. *Thromb Haemost* 1999; 81(2):198–202.
19. Seligsohn U, Lubetsky A. Genetic susceptibility to venous thrombosis. *N Engl J Med* 2001;344(16):1222–1231.
20. Crowther MA, Kelton JG. Congenital thrombophilic states associated with venous thrombosis: a qualitative overview and proposed classification system. *Ann Intern Med* 2003;138(2):128–134.
21. Lane DA, Bayston T, Olds RJ, et al. Antithrombin mutation database: 2nd (1997) update. For the Plasma Coagulation Inhibitors Subcommittee of the Scientific and Standardization Committee of the International Society on Thrombosis and Haemostasis. *Thromb Haemost* 1997;77(1):197–211.
22. Kuhle S, Lane DA, Jochmanns K, et al. Homozygous antithrombin deficiency type II (99 Leu to Phe mutation) and childhood thromboembolism. *Thromb Haemost* 2001;86(4):1007–1011.
23. Picard V, Dautzenberg MD, Villoutreix BO, et al. Antithrombin Phe229Leu: a new homozygous variant leading to spontaneous antithrombin polymerization *in vivo* associated with severe childhood thrombosis. *Blood* 2003;102(3): 919–925.
24. Molho-Sabatier P, Aiach M, Gaillard I, et al. Molecular characterization of antithrombin III (ATIII) variants using polymerase chain reaction. Identification of the ATIII Charleville as an Ala 384 Pro mutation. *J Clin Invest* 1989;84(4):1236–1242.
25. van Boven HH, Lane DA. Antithrombin and its inherited deficiency states. *Semin Hematol* 1997;34(3):188–204.
26. Perry DJ, Daly ME, Tait RC, et al. Antithrombin Cambridge II (Ala384Ser): clinical, functional and haplotype analysis of 18 families. *Thromb Haemost* 1998;79(2):249–253.
27. Bruce D, Perry DJ, Borg JY, et al. Thromboembolic disease due to thermolabile conformational changes of antithrombin Rouen-VI (187 Asn → Asp). *J Clin Invest* 1994;94(6):2265–2274.
28. Carrell RW, Huntington JA, Mushunje A, et al. The conformational basis of thrombosis. *Thromb Haemost* 2001;86(1):14–22.
29. Esmon CT. The protein C anticoagulant pathway. *Arterioscler Thromb* 1992;12(2):135–145.
30. Esmon CT. The endothelial cell protein C receptor. *Thromb Haemost* 2000; 83(5):639–643.
31. Rosing J, Hoekema L, Nicolaes GA, et al. Effects of protein S and factor Xa on peptide bond cleavages during inactivation of factor Va and factor VaR506Q by activated protein C. *J Biol Chem* 1995;270(46):27852–27858.
32. Heeb MJ, Mesters RM, Tans G, et al. Binding of protein S to factor Va associated with inhibition of prothrombinase that is independent of activated protein C. *J Biol Chem* 1993;268(4):2872–2877.
33. Heeb MJ, Rosing J, Bakker HM, et al. Protein S binds to and inhibits factor Xa. *Proc Natl Acad Sci U S A* 1994;91(7):2728–2732.
34. Shen L, Dahlback B. Factor V and protein S as synergistic cofactors to activated protein C in degradation of factor VIIIa. *J Biol Chem* 1994;269(29): 18735–18738.
35. Heeb MJ, Espana F, Griffin JH. Inhibition and complexation of activated protein C by two major inhibitors in plasma. *Blood* 1989;73(2):446–454.
36. Griffin JH, Gruber A, Fernandez JA. Reevaluation of total, free, and bound protein S and C4b-binding protein levels in plasma anticoagulated with citrate or hirudin. *Blood* 1992;79(12):3203–3211.
37. Boerger LM, Morris PC, Thurnau GR, et al. Oral contraceptives and gender affect protein S status. *Blood* 1987;69(2):692–694.
38. Bovill EG, Bauer KA, Dickerman JD, et al. The clinical spectrum of heterozygous protein C deficiency in a large New England kindred. *Blood* 1989;73(3):712–717.
39. Allaart CF, Poort SR, Rosendaal FR, et al. Increased risk of venous thrombosis in carriers of hereditary protein C deficiency defect. *Lancet* 1993; 341(8838):134–138.
40. Koster T, Rosendaal FR, Briet E, et al. Protein C deficiency in a controlled series of unselected outpatients: an infrequent but clear risk factor for venous thrombosis (Leiden Thrombophilia Study). *Blood* 1995;85(10):2756–2761.
41. Marciniak E, Wilson HD, Marlar RA. Neonatal purpura fulminans: a genetic disorder related to the absence of protein C in blood. *Blood* 1985; 65(1):15–20.
42. Dreyfus M, Magny JF, Bridey F, et al. Treatment of homozygous protein C deficiency and neonatal purpura fulminans with a purified protein C concentrate. *N Engl J Med* 1991;325(22):1565–1568.
43. Zoller B, Garcia de Frutos P, Dahlback B. Evaluation of the relationship between protein S and C4b-binding protein isoforms in hereditary protein S deficiency demonstrating type I and type III deficiencies to be phenotypic variants of the same genetic disease. *Blood* 1995;85(12):3524–3531.
44. Borgel D, Reny JL, Fischelis D, et al. Cleaved protein S (PS), total PS, free PS, and activated protein C cofactor activity as risk factors for venous thromboembolism. *Clin Chem* 2003;49(4):575–580.
45. Gomez E, Ledford MR, Pegelow CH, et al. Homozygous protein S deficiency due to a one base pair deletion that leads to a stop codon in exon III of the protein S gene. *Thromb Haemost* 1994;71(6):723–726.
46. Gandrille S, Borgel D, Ireland H, et al. Protein S deficiency: a database of mutations. For the Plasma Coagulation Inhibitors Subcommittee of the Scientific and Standardization Committee of the International Society on Thrombosis and Haemostasis. *Thromb Haemost* 1997;77(6):1201–1214.
47. Miletich JP. Laboratory diagnosis of protein C deficiency. *Semin Thromb Hemost* 1990;16(2):169–176.
48. Comp PC. Laboratory evaluation of protein S status. *Semin Thromb Hemost* 1990;16(2):177–181.
49. Amiral J, Grosley B, Boyer-Neumann C, et al. New direct assay of free protein S antigen using two distinct monoclonal antibodies specific for the free form. *Blood Coagul Fibrinolysis* 1994;5(2):179–186.
50. Aiach M, Borgel D, Gaussem P, et al. Protein C and protein S deficiencies. *Semin Hematol* 1997;34(3):205–216.
51. Reitsma PH, Bernardi F, Doig RG, et al. Protein C deficiency: a database of mutations, 1995 update. On behalf of the Subcommittee on Plasma Coagulation Inhibitors of the Scientific and Standardization Committee of the International Society on Thrombosis and Haemostasis. *Thromb Haemost* 1995;73(5):876–889.
52. Gandrille S, Jude B, Alhenc-Gelas M, et al. First *de novo* mutations in the protein C gene of two patients with type I deficiency: a missense mutation and a splice site deletion. *Blood* 1994;84(8):2566–2570.
53. Gandrille S, Aiach M, The French INSERM Network on Molecular Abnormalities Responsible for Protein C and Protein S Deficiencies. Identification of mutations in 90 of 121 consecutive symptomatic French patients with a type I protein C deficiency. *Blood* 1995;86(7):2598–2605.
54. Aiach M, Gandrille S, Emmerich J. A review of mutations causing deficiencies of antithrombin, protein C and protein S. *Thromb Haemost* 1995; 74(1):81–89.
55. Gandrille S, Alhenc-Gelas M, Gaussem P, et al. Five novel mutations located in exons III and IX of the protein C gene in patients presenting with defective protein C anticoagulant activity. *Blood* 1993;82(1):159–168.
56. Alhenc-Gelas M, Gandrille S, Aubry ML et al., French INSERM Network on Molecular Abnormalities Responsible for Protein C and Protein S. Thirty-three new mutations in the protein C gene. *Thromb Haemost* 2000;83(1):86–92.
57. Greengard JS, Fisher CL, Villoutreix B, et al. Structural basis for type I and type II deficiencies of antithrombotic plasma protein C: patterns revealed by three-dimensional molecular modelling of mutations of the protease domain. *Proteins* 1994;18(4):367–380.
58. Borgel D, Duchemin J, Alhenc-Gelas M et al. The French Network on Molecular Abnormalities Responsible for Protein C and Protein S Deficiencies. Molecular basis for protein S hereditary deficiency: genetic defects observed in 118 patients with type I and type IIa deficiencies. *J Lab Clin Med* 1996;128(2):218–227.

59. Simmonds RE, Ireland H, Kunz G et al., Protein S Study Group. Identification of 19 protein S gene mutations in patients with phenotypic protein S deficiency and thrombosis. *Blood* 1996;88(11):4195–4204.

60. Gandrille S, Borgel D, Sala N, et al. Protein S deficiency: a database of mutations—summary of the first update. *Thromb Haemost* 2000;84(5): 918.

61. Borgel D, Gandrille S, Aiach M. Protein S deficiency. *Thromb Haemost* 1997;78(1):351–356.

62. Bertina RM, Ploos van Amstel HK, van Wijngaarden A, et al. Heerlen polymorphism of protein S, an immunologic polymorphism due to dimorphism of residue 460. *Blood* 1990;76(3):538–548.

63. Duchemin J, Gandrille S, Borgel D, et al. The Ser 460 to Pro substitution of the protein S alpha (*PROS1*) gene is a frequent mutation associated with free protein S (type IIa) deficiency. *Blood* 1995;86(9):3436–3443.

64. Dahlback B, Carlsson M, Svensson PJ. Familial thrombophilia due to a previously unrecognized mechanism characterized by poor anticoagulant response to activated protein C: prediction of a cofactor to activated protein C. *Proc Natl Acad Sci U S A* 1993;90(3):1004–1008.

65. Dahlback B. The discovery of activated protein C resistance. *J Thromb Haemost* 2003;1(1):3–9.

66. Koster T, Rosendaal FR, de Ronde H, et al. Venous thrombosis due to poor anticoagulant response to activated protein C: Leiden Thrombophilia Study. *Lancet* 1993;342(8886-8887):1503–1506.

67. Svensson PJ, Dahlback B. Resistance to activated protein C as a basis for venous thrombosis. *N Engl J Med* 1994;330(8):517–522.

68. Bertina RM, Koeleman BP, Koster T, et al. Mutation in blood coagulation factor V associated with resistance to activated protein C. *Nature* 1994; 369(6475):64–67.

69. de Visser MC, Rosendaal FR, Bertina RM. A reduced sensitivity for activated protein C in the absence of factor V Leiden increases the risk of venous thrombosis. *Blood* 1999;93(4):1271–1276.

70. Rodeghiero F, Tosetto A. Activated protein C resistance and factor V Leiden mutation are independent risk factors for venous thromboembolism. *Ann Intern Med* 1999;130(8):643–650.

71. Nicolaes GA, Dahlback B. Factor V and thrombotic disease: description of a janus-faced protein. *Arterioscler Thromb Vasc Biol* 2002;22(4):530–538.

72. Thorelli E, Kaufman RJ, Dahlback B. Cleavage of factor V at Arg 506 by activated protein C and the expression of anticoagulant activity of factor V. *Blood* 1999;93(8):2552–2558.

73. Zoller B, Dahlback B. Linkage between inherited resistance to activated protein C and factor V gene mutation in venous thrombosis. *Lancet* 1994;343(8912):1536–1538.

74. Voorberg J, Roelse J, Koopman R, et al. Association of idiopathic venous thromboembolism with single point-mutation at Arg506 of factor V. *Lancet* 1994;343(8912):1535–1536.

75. Greengard JS, Sun X, Xu X, et al. Activated protein C resistance caused by Arg506Gln mutation in factor Va. *Lancet* 1994;343(8909):1361–1362.

76. Castoldi E, Brugge JM, Nicolaes GA, et al. Impaired APC-cofactor activity of factor V plays a major role in the APC resistance associated with the factor V Leiden (R506Q) and R2 (H1299R) mutations. *Blood* 2004;103: 4173–4179.

77. Chan WP, Lee CK, Kwong YL, et al. A novel mutation of Arg306 of factor V gene in Hong Kong Chinese. *Blood* 1998;91(4):1135–1139.

78. Williamson D, Brown K, Luddington R, et al. Factor V Cambridge: a new mutation (Arg306 → Thr) associated with resistance to activated protein C. *Blood* 1998;91(4):1140–1144.

79. Norstrom E, Thorelli E, Dahlback B. Functional characterization of recombinant FV Hong Kong and FV Cambridge. *Blood* 2002;100(2): 524–530.

80. van der Neut Kolfschoten M, Dirven RJ, Vos HL, et al. Factor Va is inactivated by activated protein C in the absence of cleavage sites at Arg-306, Arg-506, and Arg-679. *J Biol Chem* 2004;279(8):6567–6575.

81. Rees DC, Cox M, Clegg JB. World distribution of factor V Leiden. *Lancet* 1995;346(8983):1133–1134.

82. Zivelin A, Griffin JH, Xu X, et al. A single genetic origin for a common Caucasian risk factor for venous thrombosis. *Blood* 1997;89(2):397–402.

83. Lindqvist PG, Svensson PJ, Dahlback B, et al. Factor V Q506 mutation (activated protein C resistance) associated with reduced intrapartum blood loss—a possible evolutionary selection mechanism. *Thromb Haemost* 1998;79(1):69–73.

84. Lindqvist PG, Zoller B, Dahlback B. Improved hemoglobin status and reduced menstrual blood loss among female carriers of factor V Leiden—an evolutionary advantage? *Thromb Haemost* 2001;86(4):1122–1123.

85. Ridker PM, Hennekens CH, Lindpaintner K, et al. Mutation in the gene coding for coagulation factor V and the risk of myocardial infarction, stroke, and venous thrombosis in apparently healthy men. *N Engl J Med* 1995;332(14):912–917.

86. Trossaert M, Conard J, Horellou MH, et al. Resistance to activated protein C in venous thromboembolic complications. Incidence and clinical manifestations. *Presse Med* 1995;24(4):209–212.

87. Hainaut P, Azerad MA, Lehmann E, et al. Prevalence of activated protein C resistance and analysis of clinical profile in thromboembolic patients. A Belgian prospective study. *J Intern Med* 1997;241(5):427–433.

88. Leroyer C, Mercier B, Escoffre M, et al. Factor V Leiden prevalence in venous thromboembolism patients. *Chest* 1997;111(6):1603–1606.

89. Lambropoulos AF, Foka Z, Makris M, et al. Factor V Leiden in Greek thrombophilic patients: relationship with activated protein C resistance

test and levels of thrombin-antithrombin complex and prothrombin fragment 1 + 2. *Blood Coagul Fibrinolysis* 1997;8(8):485–489.

90. Lindmarker P, Schulman S, Sten-Linder M et al., DURAC Trial Study Group. Duration of Anticoagulation. The risk of recurrent venous thromboembolism in carriers and non-carriers of the G1691A allele in the coagulation factor V gene and the G20210A allele in the prothrombin gene. *Thromb Haemost* 1999;81(5):684–689.

91. Emmerich J, Rosendaal FR, Cattaneo M, et al. Study Group for Pooled-Analysis in Venous Thromboembolism. Combined effect of factor V Leiden and prothrombin 20210A on the risk of venous thromboembolism—pooled analysis of 8 case-control studies including 2310 cases and 3204 controls. *Thromb Haemost* 2001;86(3):809–816.

92. Folsom AR, Cushman M, Tsai MY, et al. A prospective study of venous thromboembolism in relation to factor V Leiden and related factors. *Blood* 2002;99(8):2720–2725.

93. Herrmann FH, Koesling M, Schroder W, et al. Prevalence of factor V Leiden mutation in various populations. *Genet Epidemiol* 1997;14(4):403–411.

94. Ko YL, Hsu TS, Wu SM, et al. The G1691A mutation of the coagulation factor V gene (factor V Leiden) is rare in Chinese: an analysis of 618 individuals. *Hum Genet* 1996;98(2):176–177.

95. Kodaira H, Ishida F, Shimodaira S, et al. Resistance to activated protein C and Arg 506 Gln factor V mutation are uncommon in eastern Asian populations. *Acta Haematol* 1997;98(1):22–25.

96. Ridker PM, Miletich JP, Hennekens CH, et al. Ethnic distribution of factor V Leiden in 4047 men and women. Implications for venous thromboembolism screening. *JAMA* 1997;277(16):1305–1307.

97. Bounameaux H. Factor V Leiden paradox: risk of deep-vein thrombosis but not of pulmonary embolism. *Lancet* 2000;356(9225):182–183.

98. Bajzar L, Kalafatis M, Simioni P, et al. An antifibrinolytic mechanism describing the prothrombotic effect associated with factor V Leiden. *J Biol Chem* 1996;271(38):22949–22952.

99. Meyer G, Emmerich J, Helley D, et al. Factors V leiden and II 20210A in patients with symptomatic pulmonary embolism and deep vein thrombosis. *Am J Med* 2001;110(1):12–15.

100. Press RD, Bauer KA, Kujovich JL, et al. Clinical utility of factor V leiden (R506Q) testing for the diagnosis and management of thromboembolic disorders. *Arch Pathol Lab Med* 2002;126(11):1304–1318.

101. Rosendaal FR, Koster T, Vandenbroucke JP, et al. High risk of thrombosis in patients homozygous for factor V Leiden (activated protein C resistance). *Blood* 1995;85(6):1504–1508.

102. Emmerich J, Alhenc-Gelas M, Aillaud MF, et al. Clinical features in 36 patients homozygous for the ARG 506 → GLN factor V mutation. *Thromb Haemost* 1997;77(4):620–623.

103. Ehrenforth S, Nemes L, Mannhalter C, et al. Impact of environmental and hereditary risk factors on the clinical manifestation of thrombophilia in homozygous carriers of factor V:G1691A. *J Thromb Haemost* 2004;2(3): 430–436.

104. Heijmans BT, Westendorp RG, Knook DL, et al. The risk of mortality and the factor V Leiden mutation in a population-based cohort. *Thromb Haemost* 1998;80(4):607–609.

105. Hille ET, Westendorp RG, Vandenbroucke JP, et al. Mortality and causes of death in families with the factor V Leiden mutation (resistance to activated protein C). *Blood* 1997;89(6):1963–1967.

106. Ridker PM, Miletich JP, Stampfer MJ, et al. Factor V Leiden and risks of recurrent idiopathic venous thromboembolism. *Circulation* 1995;92(10): 2800–2802.

107. Simioni P, Prandoni P, Lensing AW, et al. The risk of recurrent venous thromboembolism in patients with an Arg506 → Gln mutation in the gene for factor V (factor V Leiden). *N Engl J Med* 1997;336(6):399–403.

108. Simioni P, Prandoni P, Lensing AW, et al. Risk for subsequent venous thromboembolic complications in carriers of the prothrombin or the factor V gene mutation with a first episode of deep-vein thrombosis. *Blood* 2000;96(10):3329–3333.

109. Eichinger S, Pabinger I, Stumpflen A, et al. The risk of recurrent venous thromboembolism in patients with and without factor V Leiden. *Thromb Haemost* 1997;77(4):624–628.

110. Kearon C, Gent M, Hirsh J, et al. A comparison of three months of anticoagulation with extended anticoagulation for a first episode of idiopathic venous thromboembolism. *N Engl J Med* 1999;340(12):901–907.

111. De Stefano V, Martinelli I, Mannucci PM, et al. The risk of recurrent deep venous thrombosis among heterozygous carriers of both factor V Leiden and the G20210A prothrombin mutation. *N Engl J Med* 1999;341(11): 801–806.

112. Margaglione M, D'Andrea G, Colaizzo D, et al. Coexistence of factor V Leiden and factor II A20210 mutations and recurrent venous thromboembolism. *Thromb Haemost* 1999;82(6):1583–1587.

113. Kyrle PA, Minar E, Hirschl M, et al. High plasma levels of factor VIII and the risk of recurrent venous thromboembolism. *N Engl J Med* 2000; 343(7):457–462.

114. Eichinger S, Weltermann A, Mannhalter C, et al. The risk of recurrent venous thromboembolism in heterozygous carriers of factor V Leiden and a first spontaneous venous thromboembolism. *Arch Intern Med* 2002; 162(20):2357–2360.

115. Baglin T, Luddington R, Brown K, et al. Incidence of recurrent venous thromboembolism in relation to clinical and thrombophilic risk factors: prospective cohort study. *Lancet* 2003;362(9383):523–526.

116. Eichinger S, Weltermann A, Minar E, et al. Symptomatic pulmonary embolism and the risk of recurrent venous thromboembolism. *Arch Intern Med* 2004;164(1):92–96.

117. Juul K, Tybjaerg-Hansen A, Steffensen R, et al. Factor V Leiden: the Copenhagen city heart study and 2 meta-analyses. *Blood* 2002;100(1):3–10.

118. Sykes TC, Fegan C, Mosquera D. Thrombophilia, polymorphisms, and vascular disease. *Mol Pathol* 2000;53(6):300–306.

119. Lee R. Factor V Leiden: a clinical review. *Am J Med Sci* 2001;322(2):88–102.

120. Lane DA, Grant PJ. Role of hemostatic gene polymorphisms in venous and arterial thrombotic disease. *Blood* 2000;95(5):1517–1532.

121. Boekholdt SM, Bijsterveld NR, Moons AH, et al. Genetic variation in coagulation and fibrinolytic proteins and their relation with acute myocardial infarction: a systematic review. *Circulation* 2001;104(25):3063–3068.

122. Rosendaal FR, Siscovick DS, Schwartz SM, et al. Factor V Leiden (resistance to activated protein C) increases the risk of myocardial infarction in young women. *Blood* 1997;89(8):2817–2821.

123. Mansourati J, Da Costa A, Munier S, et al. Prevalence of factor V Leiden in patients with myocardial infarction and normal coronary angiography. *Thromb Haemost* 2000;83(6):822–825.

124. Van de Water NS, French JK, Lund M, et al. Prevalence of factor V Leiden and prothrombin variant G20210A in patients age <50 years with no significant stenoses at angiography three to four weeks after myocardial infarction. *J Am Coll Cardiol* 2000;36(3):717–722.

125. Bushnell CD, Goldstein LB. Diagnostic testing for coagulopathies in patients with ischemic stroke. *Stroke* 2000;31(12):3067–3078.

126. Lopaciuk S, Bykowska K, Kwiecinski H, et al. Factor V Leiden, prothrombin gene G20210A variant, and methylenetetrahydrofolate reductase C677T genotype in young adults with ischemic stroke. *Clin Appl Thromb Hemost* 2001;7(4):346–350.

127. Zuber M, Toulon P, Marnet L, et al. Factor V Leiden mutation in cerebral venous thrombosis. *Stroke* 1996;27(10):1721–1723.

128. Deschiens MA, Conard J, Horellou MH, et al. Coagulation studies, factor V Leiden, and anticardiolipin antibodies in 40 cases of cerebral venous thrombosis. *Stroke* 1996;27(10):1724–1730.

129. Ludemann P, Nabavi DG, Junker R, et al. Factor V Leiden mutation is a risk factor for cerebral venous thrombosis: a case-control study of 55 patients. *Stroke* 1998;29(12):2507–2510.

130. de Bruijn SF, Stam J, Koopman MM et al., The Cerebral Venous Sinus Thrombosis Study Group. Case-control study of risk of cerebral sinus thrombosis in oral contraceptive users and in [correction of who are] carriers of hereditary prothrombotic conditions. *BMJ* 1998;316(7131):589–592.

131. Martinelli I, Sacchi E, Landi G, et al. High risk of cerebral-vein thrombosis in carriers of a prothrombin-gene mutation and in users of oral contraceptives. *N Engl J Med* 1998;338(25):1793–1797.

132. Trossaert M, Conard J, Horellou MH, et al. Modified APC resistance assay for patients on oral anticoagulants. *Lancet* 1994;344(8938):1709.

133. Poort SR, Rosendaal FR, Reitsma PH, et al. A common genetic variation in the 3′-untranslated region of the prothrombin gene is associated with elevated plasma prothrombin levels and an increase in venous thrombosis. *Blood* 1996;88(10):3698–3703.

134. Degen SJ, Davie EW. Nucleotide sequence of the gene for human prothrombin. *Biochemistry* 1987;26(19):6165–6177.

135. Butenas S, van't Veer C, Mann KG. "Normal" thrombin generation. *Blood* 1999;94(7):2169–2178.

136. Kyrle PA, Mannhalter C, Beguin S, et al. Clinical studies and thrombin generation in patients homozygous or heterozygous for the G20210A mutation in the prothrombin gene. *Arterioscler Thromb Vasc Biol* 1998;18(8):1287–1291.

137. Smirnov MD, Safa O, Esmon NL, et al. Inhibition of activated protein C anticoagulant activity by prothrombin. *Blood* 1999;94(11):3839–3846.

138. Gehring NH, Frede U, Neu-Yilik G, et al. Increased efficiency of mRNA 3′ end formation: a new genetic mechanism contributing to hereditary thrombophilia. *Nat Genet* 2001;28(4):389–392.

139. Carter AM, Sachchithananthan M, Stasinopoulos S, et al. Prothrombin G20210A is a bifunctional gene polymorphism. *Thromb Haemost* 2002;87(5):846–853.

140. Pollak ES, Lam HS, Russell JE. The G20210A mutation does not affect the stability of prothrombin mRNA *in vivo*. *Blood* 2002;100(1):359–362.

141. Ceelie H, Spaargaren-Van Riel CC, De Jong M, et al. Functional characterization of transcription factor binding sites for HNF1-alpha, HNF3-beta (FOXA2), HNF4-alpha, Sp1 and Sp3 in the human prothrombin gene enhancer. *J Thromb Haemost* 2003;1(8):1688–1698.

142. Danckwardt S, Gehring NH, Neu-Yilik G, et al. The prothrombin 3′ end formation signal reveals a unique architecture that is sensitive to thrombophilic gain-of-function mutations. *Blood* 2004;104(2):428–435.

143. Wylenzek M, Geisen C, Stapenhorst L, et al. A novel point mutation in the 3′ region of the prothrombin gene at position 20221 in a Lebanese/Syrian family. *Thromb Haemost* 2001;85(5):943–944.

144. Balim Z, Kosova B, Falzon K, et al. Budd-Chiari syndrome in a patient heterozygous for the point mutation C20221T of the prothrombin gene. *J Thromb Haemost* 2003;1(4):852–853.

145. von Ahsen N, Oellerich M. The intronic prothrombin 19911A > G polymorphism influences splicing efficiency and modulates effects of the 20210G > A polymorphism on mRNA amount and expression in a stable reporter gene assay system. *Blood* 2004;103(2):586–593.

146. Rosendaal FR, Doggen CJ, Zivelin A, et al. Geographic distribution of the 20210 G to A prothrombin variant. *Thromb Haemost* 1998;79(4):706–708.

147. Hessner MJ, Luhm RA, Pearson SL, et al. Prevalence of prothrombin G20210A, factor V G1691A (Leiden), and methylenetetrahydrofolate reductase (MTHFR) C677T in seven different populations determined by multiplex allele-specific PCR. *Thromb Haemost* 1999;81(5):733–738.

148. Zivelin A, Rosenberg N, Faier S, et al. A single genetic origin for the common prothrombotic G20210A polymorphism in the prothrombin gene. *Blood* 1998;92(4):1119–1124.

149. Hundsdoerfer P, Vetter B, Stover B, et al. Homozygous and double heterozygous Factor V Leiden and Factor II G20210A genotypes predispose infants to thromboembolism but are not associated with an increase of foetal loss. *Thromb Haemost* 2003;90(4):628–635.

150. Folsom AR, Cushman M, Tsai MY, et al. Prospective study of the G20210A polymorphism in the prothrombin gene, plasma prothrombin concentration, and incidence of venous thromboembolism. *Am J Hematol* 2002;71(4):285–290.

151. Ridker PM, Hennekens CH, Miletich JP. G20210A mutation in prothrombin gene and risk of myocardial infarction, stroke, and venous thrombosis in a large cohort of US men. *Circulation* 1999;99(8):999–1004.

152. Brown K, Luddington R, Williamson D, et al. Risk of venous thromboembolism associated with a G to A transition at position 20210 in the 3′-untranslated region of the prothrombin gene. *Br J Haematol* 1997;98(4):907–909.

153. Leroyer C, Mercier B, Oger E, et al. Prevalence of 20210 A allele of the prothrombin gene in venous thromboembolism patients. *Thromb Haemost* 1998;80(1):49–51.

154. Souto JC, Coll I, Llobet D, et al. The prothrombin 20210A allele is the most prevalent genetic risk factor for venous thromboembolism in the Spanish population. *Thromb Haemost* 1998;80(3):366–369.

155. Tosetto A, Missiaglia E, Frezzato M, et al. The VITA project: prothrombin G20210A mutation and venous thromboembolism in the general population. *Thromb Haemost* 1999;82(5):1395–1398.

156. Adamczuk Y, Iglesias Varela ML, Forastiero R, et al. Factor V Leiden and prothrombin G20210A variant are risk factors for venous thromboembolism in the Argentinean population. *Thromb Haemost* 2000;83(3):509–510.

157. Zawadzki C, Gaveriaux V, Trillot N, et al. Homozygous G20210A transition in the prothrombin gene associated with severe venous thrombotic disease: two cases in a French family. *Thromb Haemost* 1998;80(6):1027–1028.

158. Alatri A, Franchi F, Moia M. Homozygous G20210A prothrombin gene mutation without thromboembolic events: a case report. *Thromb Haemost* 1998;80(6):1028–1029.

159. Kosch A, Junker R, Wermes C, et al. Recurrent pulmonary embolism in a 13-year-old male homozygous for the prothrombin G20210A mutation combined with protein S deficiency and increased lipoprotein (a). *Thromb Res* 2002;105(1):49–53.

160. Miles JS, Miletich JP, Goldhaber SZ, et al. G20210A mutation in the prothrombin gene and the risk of recurrent venous thromboembolism. *J Am Coll Cardiol* 2001;37(1):215–218.

161. Eichinger S, Minar E, Hirschl M, et al. The risk of early recurrent venous thromboembolism after oral anticoagulant therapy in patients with the G20210A transition in the prothrombin gene. *Thromb Haemost* 1999;81(1):14–17.

162. De Stefano V, Martinelli I, Mannucci PM, et al. The risk of recurrent venous thromboembolism among heterozygous carriers of the G20210A prothrombin gene mutation. *Br J Haematol* 2001;113(3):630–635.

163. McGlennen RC, Key NS. Clinical and laboratory management of the prothrombin G20210A mutation. *Arch Pathol Lab Med* 2002;126(11):1319–1325.

164. Rosendaal FR, Siscovick DS, Schwartz SM, et al. A common prothrombin variant (20210 G to A) increases the risk of myocardial infarction in young women. *Blood* 1997;90(5):1747–1750.

165. De Stefano V, Chiusolo P, Paciaroni K, et al. Prothrombin G20210A mutant genotype is a risk factor for cerebrovascular ischemic disease in young patients. *Blood* 1998;91(10):3562–3565.

166. Endler G, Kyrle PA, Eichinger S, et al. Multiplexed mutagenically separated PCR: simultaneous single-tube detection of the factor V R506Q (G1691A), the prothrombin G20210A, and the methylenetetrahydrofolate reductase A223V (C677T) variants. *Clin Chem* 2001;47(2):333–335.

167. Spek CA, Koster T, Rosendaal FR, et al. Genotypic variation in the promoter region of the protein C gene is associated with plasma protein C levels and thrombotic risk. *Arterioscler Thromb Vasc Biol* 1995;15(2):214–218.

168. Aiach M, Nicaud V, Alhenc-Gelas M, et al. Complex association of protein C gene promoter polymorphism with circulating protein C levels and thrombotic risk. *Arterioscler Thromb Vasc Biol* 1999;19(6):1573–1576.

169. Balogh I, Szoke G, Karpati L, et al. Val34Leu polymorphism of plasma factor XIII: biochemistry and epidemiology in familial thrombophilia. *Blood* 2000;96(7):2479–2486.

170. Kohler HP, Grant PJ. Clustering of haemostatic risk factors with FXIIIVal34Leu in patients with myocardial infarction. *Thromb Haemost* 1998;80(5):862.

171. Elbaz A, Poirier O, Canaple S, et al. The association between the Val34Leu polymorphism in the factor XIII gene and brain infarction. *Blood* 2000;95(2):586–591.

172. Alhenc-Gelas M, Reny JL, Aubry ML, et al. The FXIII Val 34 Leu mutation and the risk of venous thrombosis. *Thromb Haemost* 2000;84(6): 1117–1118.

173. Souto JC, Almasy L, Borrell M, et al. Genetic determinants of hemostasis phenotypes in Spanish families. *Circulation* 2000;101(13):1546–1551.

174. Souto JC, Almasy L, Borrell M, et al. Genetic susceptibility to thrombosis and its relationship to physiological risk factors: the GAIT study. Genetic Analysis of Idiopathic Thrombophilia. *Am J Hum Genet* 2000;67(6):1452–1459.

175. Soria JM, Almasy L, Souto JC, et al. A new locus on chromosome 18 that influences normal variation in activated protein C resistance phenotype and factor VIII activity and its relation to thrombosis susceptibility. *Blood* 2003;101(1):163–167.

176. Vossen CY, Hasstedt SJ, Rosendaal FR, et al. Heritability of plasma concentrations of clotting factors and measures of a prethrombotic state in a protein C-deficient family. *J Thromb Haemost* 2004;2(2):242–247.

177. de Lange M, Snieder H, Ariens RA, et al. The genetics of haemostasis: a twin study. *Lancet* 2001;357(9250):101–105.

178. Ariens RA, de Lange M, Snieder H, et al. Activation markers of coagulation and fibrinolysis in twins: heritability of the prethrombotic state. *Lancet* 2002;359(9307):667–671.

179. Dupont A, Fontana P, Bachelot-Loza C, et al. An intronic polymorphism in the PAR-1 gene is associated with platelet receptor density and the response to SFLLRN. *Blood* 2003;101(5):1833–1840.

180. Fontana P, Dupont A, Gandrille S, et al. Adenosine diphosphate-induced platelet aggregation is associated with P2Y12 gene sequence variations in healthy subjects. *Circulation* 2003;108(8):989–995.

181. Saposnik B, Reny JL, Gaussem P, et al. A haplotype of the EPCR gene is associated with increased plasma levels of sEPCR and is a candidate risk factor for thrombosis. *Blood* 2004;103(4):1311–1318.

182. Vandenbroucke JP, Rosing J, Bloemenkamp KW, et al. Oral contraceptives and the risk of venous thrombosis. *N Engl J Med* 2001;344(20):1527–1535.

183. Rosendaal FR, Van Hylckama Vlieg A, Tanis BC, et al. Estrogens, progestogens and thrombosis. *J Thromb Haemost* 2003;1(7):1371–1380.

184. Martinelli I, Battaglioli T, Mannucci PM. Pharmacogenetic aspects of the use of oral contraceptives and the risk of thrombosis. *Pharmacogenetics* 2003;13(10):589–594.

185. Vasilakis-Scaramozza C, Jick H. Risk of venous thromboembolism with cyproterone or levonorgestrel contraceptives. *Lancet* 2001;358(9291): 1427–1429.

186. Vandenbroucke JP, Koster T, Briet E, et al. Increased risk of venous thrombosis in oral-contraceptive users who are carriers of factor V Leiden mutation. *Lancet* 1994;344(8935):1453–1457.

187. Martinelli I, Taioli E, Bucciarelli P, et al. Interaction between the G20210A mutation of the prothrombin gene and oral contraceptive use in deep vein thrombosis. *Arterioscler Thromb Vasc Biol* 1999;19(3):700–703.

188. Pabinger I, Schneider B, The GTH Study Group on Natural Inhibitors. Thrombotic risk of women with hereditary antithrombin III-, protein C- and protein S-deficiency taking oral contraceptive medication. *Thromb Haemost* 1994;71(5):548–552.

189. Rintelen C, Mannhalter C, Ireland H, et al. Oral contraceptives enhance the risk of clinical manifestation of venous thrombosis at a young age in females homozygous for factor V Leiden. *Br J Haematol* 1996;93(2):487–490.

190. Bloemenkamp KW, Rosendaal FR, Helmerhorst FM, et al. Higher risk of venous thrombosis during early use of oral contraceptives in women with inherited clotting defects. *Arch Intern Med* 2000;160(1):49–52.

191. van Hylckama Vlieg A, Rosendaal FR. Interaction between oral contraceptive use and coagulation factor levels in deep venous thrombosis. *J Thromb Haemost* 2003;1(10):2186–2190.

192. Cosmi B, Legnani C, Bernardi F, et al. Role of family history in identifying women with thrombophilia and higher risk of venous thromboembolism during oral contraception. *Arch Intern Med* 2003;163(9):1105–1109.

193. Rosendaal FR, Helmerhorst FM, Vandenbroucke JP. Female hormones and thrombosis. *Arterioscler Thromb Vasc Biol* 2002;22(2):201–210.

194. Hoibraaten E, Qvigstad E, Andersen TO, et al. The effects of hormone replacement therapy (HRT) on hemostatic variables in women with previous venous thromboembolism—results from a randomized, double-blind, clinical trial. *Thromb Haemost* 2001;85(5):775–781.

195. Rosendaal FR, Vessey M, Rumley A, et al. Hormonal replacement therapy, prothrombotic mutations and the risk of venous thrombosis. *Br J Haematol* 2002;116(4):851–854.

196. Martinelli I, Legnani C, Bucciarelli P, et al. Risk of pregnancy-related venous thrombosis in carriers of severe inherited thrombophilia. *Thromb Haemost* 2001;86(3):800–803.

197. Gerhardt A, Scharf RE, Beckmann MW, et al. Prothrombin and factor V mutations in women with a history of thrombosis during pregnancy and the puerperium. *N Engl J Med* 2000;342(6):374–380.

198. Gerhardt A, Scharf RE, Zotz RB. Effect of hemostatic risk factors on the individual probability of thrombosis during pregnancy and the puerperium. *Thromb Haemost* 2003;90(1):77–85.

199. Koeleman BP, Reitsma PH, Allaart CF, et al. Activated protein C resistance as an additional risk factor for thrombosis in protein C-deficient families. *Blood* 1994;84(4):1031–1035.

200. Gandrille S, Greengard JS, Alhenc-Gelas M et al., The French Network on the behalf of INSERM. Incidence of activated protein C resistance caused by the ARG 506 GLN mutation in factor V in 113 unrelated symptomatic protein C-deficient patients. *Blood* 1995;86(1):219–224.

201. van Boven HH, Vandenbroucke JP, Briet E, et al. Gene-gene and gene-environment interactions determine risk of thrombosis in families with inherited antithrombin deficiency. *Blood* 1999;94(8):2590–2594.

202. Le Cam-Duchez V, Gandrille S, Tregouet D, et al. Influence of three potential genetic risk factors for thrombosis in 43 families carrying the factor V Arg 506 to Gln mutation. *Br J Haematol* 1999;106(4):889–897.

203. Hasstedt SJ, Bovill EG, Callas PW, et al. An unknown genetic defect increases venous thrombosis risk, through interaction with protein C deficiency. *Am J Hum Genet* 1998;63(2):569–576.

204. Lunghi B, Iacoviello L, Gemmati D, et al. Detection of new polymorphic markers in the factor V gene: association with factor V levels in plasma. *Thromb Haemost* 1996;75(1):45–48.

205. Bernardi F, Faioni EM, Castoldi E, et al. A factor V genetic component differing from factor V R506Q contributes to the activated protein C resistance phenotype. *Blood* 1997;90(4):1552–1557.

206. Castoldi E, Rosing J, Girelli D, et al. Mutations in the R2 FV gene affect the ratio between the two FV isoforms in plasma. *Thromb Haemost* 2000; 83(3):362–365.

207. Alhenc-Gelas M, Nicaud V, Gandrille S, et al. The factor V gene A4070G mutation and the risk of venous thrombosis. *Thromb Haemost* 1999; 81(2):193–197.

208. de Visser MC, Guasch JF, Kamphuisen PW, et al. The HR2 haplotype of factor V: effects on factor V levels, normalized activated protein C sensitivity ratios and the risk of venous thrombosis. *Thromb Haemost* 2000; 83(4):577–582.

209. Faioni EM, Franchi F, Bucciarelli P, et al. Coinheritance of the HR2 haplotype in the factor V gene confers an increased risk of venous thromboembolism to carriers of factor V R506Q (factor V Leiden). *Blood* 1999; 94(9):3062–3066.

210. Mingozzi F, Legnani C, Lunghi B, et al. A FV multiallelic marker detects genetic components of APC resistance contributing to venous thromboembolism in FV Leiden carriers. *Thromb Haemost* 2003;89(6):983–989.

211. De Stefano V, Rossi E, Paciaroni K, et al. Screening for inherited thrombophilia: indications and therapeutic implications. *Haematologica* 2002; 87(10):1095–1108.

212. Kearon C, Crowther M, Hirsh J. Management of patients with hereditary hypercoagulable disorders. *Annu Rev Med* 2000;51:169–185.

213. Anderson FA Jr. Spencer FA: risk factors for venous thromboembolism. *Circulation* 2003; 107(23 Suppl.1): I9–16.

214. Van Cott EM, Laposata M, Prins MH. Laboratory evaluation of hypercoagulability with venous or arterial thrombosis. *Arch Pathol Lab Med* 2002;126(11):1281–1295.

215. Carraro P. Guidelines for the laboratory investigation of inherited thrombophilias. Recommendations for the first level clinical laboratories. *Clin Chem Lab Med* 2003;41(3):382–391.

216. British Society for Haematology Investigation and Management of Heritable Thrombophilia. *Br J Haematol* 2001; 114(3):512–528.

217. Bombeli T, Basic A, Fehr J. Prevalence of hereditary thrombophilia in patients with thrombosis in different venous systems. *Am J Hematol* 2002; 70(2):126–132.

218. Heron E, Lozinguez O, Alhenc-Gelas M, et al. Hypercoagulable states in primary upper-extremity deep vein thrombosis. *Arch Intern Med* 2000; 160(3):382–386.

219. Schambeck CM, Schwender S, Haubitz I, et al. Selective screening for the factor V Leiden mutation: is it advisable prior to the prescription of oral contraceptives? *Thromb Haemost* 1997;78(6):1480–1483.

220. Heijboer H, Brandjes DP, Buller HR, et al. Deficiencies of coagulation-inhibiting and fibrinolytic proteins in outpatients with deep-vein thrombosis. *N Engl J Med* 1990;323(22):1512–1516.

221. Briet E, van der Meer FJ, Rosendaal FR, et al. The family history and inherited thrombophilia. *Br J Haematol* 1994;87(2):348–352.

222. Lensen RP, Rosendaal FR, Koster T, et al. Apparent different thrombotic tendency in patients with factor V Leiden and protein C deficiency due to selection of patients. *Blood* 1996;88(11):4205–4208.

223. Bauer KA. The thrombophilias: well-defined risk factors with uncertain therapeutic implications. *Ann Intern Med* 2001;135(5):367–373.

# CHAPTER 53 ■ INFLAMMATION AND ATHEROTHROMBOSIS

PETER LIBBY, DANIEL I. SIMON, AND PAUL M. RIDKER

Accumulating evidence supports a key role for inflammation in the pathogenesis of atherosclerosis and its thrombotic complications. This chapter reviews the emerging links between these three processes, classically considered separately. Indeed, the tendency to view atherosclerosis and thrombosis as distinct has deep historical roots. During the mid-19th century, Karl von Rokitansky postulated that incorporation of thrombi into the artery wall caused atherosclerosis (1); the celebrated cellular pathologist Rudolph Virchow ridiculed this view (2). Virchow considered atherosclerosis a disease predicated on proliferation and death of vascular wall cells. Virchow's eminence deterred acceptance of the relation between thrombosis and atherogenesis.

The role of thrombosis in atherogenesis has resurfaced periodically since the time of these pioneers. Duguid, in the middle of the 20th century, revived von Rokitanksy's view that accorded a key role to the incorporation of thrombi in the formation of atheromatous lesions (3). Hand and Chandler found that induction of thrombi could induce lesions resembling atheroma in experimental animals (4). Various investigators who used increasingly sophisticated biochemical methods, including Smith and Bini, localized products of thrombosis such as fibrin in human atheromatous plaques (5,6).

We now recognize that this polarized debate scarcely pertains to atherogenesis and that both views of atherosclerosis apply to the human disease. Thrombosis and the behavior of artery wall cells intimately and inextricably intertwine. Although the very earliest lesions of atherosclerosis may not involve thrombosis, which nonetheless contributes to all subsequent stages of atherosclerosis. Indeed, recent experimental evidence suggests a role for platelets even in early murine aterosclerosis (7). Moreover, compelling laboratory and clinical evidence now provides growing support for the role of inflammation in both atherogenesis and the pathophysiology of its thrombotic complications. This discussion highlights the interactions between inflammation, thrombosis, and atherosclerosis during various stages of atherogenesis.

Several themes recur while considering the interfaces between inflammation, thrombosis, and atherosclerosis. First, the pathogenic effects of thrombosis in the context of atherogenesis reflect an inappropriate expression of fundamental biological mechanisms important in normal homeostasis. The products of coagulation can alter the functions of vascular wall cells in a manner that promotes fibrosis and healing. Substances released from activated platelets, such as platelet-derived growth factor (PDGF) and transforming growth factor $\beta$ (TGF-$\beta$), can augment synthesis of collagen by smooth muscle cells (SMC) (8). PDGF is a potent chemoattractant that stimulates the migration of SMC (9–12). Thrombin, generated during the clotting cascade is both a potent smooth muscle mitogen and an agonist that regulates the expression of many other genes

that may influence lesion healing as well as a proinflammatory mediator (13–16). All of these processes may prove essential during wound healing and tissue repair. However, these usually salutary functions can become pathogenic in the context of the artery wall. Therefore, considering the interface of atherosclerosis with thrombosis invokes the same conundrum that applies to the inflammatory aspects of atherosclerosis. Normal homeostatic mechanisms expressed inappropriately or in excess actually contribute to the pathogenesis of atheroma.

Another recurring theme concerns the balance between stimulatory and inhibitory limbs of regulatory pathways. This concept, which is used when considering proteases versus antiproteases and thrombosis versus fibrinolysis, is quite familiar to students of thrombosis. We see subsequently how altered balances between such pathways contribute to atherogenesis.

A third recurring theme has emerged more recently. We increasingly recognize that inflammation can heighten thrombosis and that mediators of thrombosis can play roles not only in clot formation but also in augmenting inflammation. For example, thrombin can elicit inflammatory mediators, notably CD40 ligand (CD154), that can induce tissue factor expression on vascular cells and macrophages (M$\Phi$), the principal source of this potent procoagulant in the atheroma (17,18). In turn, platelets, when activated, can release CD40 ligand; regulated on activation, normal T cell expressed and secreted (RANTES); and other proinflammatory mediators (19). Therefore, reciprocal reinforcement of inflammation by thrombosis, and vice versa, can amplify these pathologic processes (see Fig. 53-1).

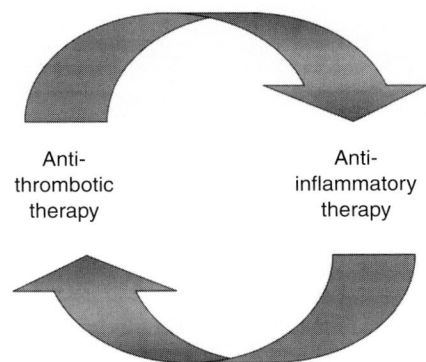

**FIGURE 53-1.** Accumulating data linking inflammation and thrombosis support the hypothesis illustrated here that antiinflammatory therapies may limit thrombosis and that antithrombotic therapies may reduce vascular inflammation. (From Libby P, Simon DI. Inflammation and thrombosis: the clot thickens. *Circulation* 2001;103:1718–1720, with permission.)

# INITIATION OF ATHEROSCLEROTIC LESIONS

As noted earlier, the very first steps in the evolution of atheroma may be the only aspects of this disease that do not involve thrombosis. Atherosclerosis usually develops in the context of elevated risk factors. An altered pattern of plasma lipoproteins is a well-established risk factor for lesion initiation. We have learned much about the earlier stages of atherogenesis by studying experimental animals, which develop atheromatous lesions when they consume diets enriched with cholesterol and saturated fat. Such animal experiments likely represent a caricature of human atherosclerosis because the levels of lipoproteins achieved exceed by far those found in most human patients with atherosclerosis. Despite the convenience of hypercholesterolemic models of atherogenesis, many other risk factors contribute to this disease. Nonetheless, these well-studied experimental preparations have afforded considerable insight into one pathway for lesion initiation.

Extracellular lipid tends to accumulate in the intima when high levels of plasma lipoproteins bearing cholesterol circulate in plasma (see Fig. 53-2) (20). Part of this accumulation may result from increased permeability of the endothelial layer to lipoproteins at sites of lesion predilection (21,22), undoubtedly related to hydrodynamic changes at these locations, which are typically branch or flow dividers in the arterial tree. In addition to increased penetration into the artery wall, increased retention of lipoprotein particles can contribute to accumulation of lipid

(23). Whatever the mechanism that causes them to accumulate in the intima, lipoproteins provoke biological reactions that seem to initiate atherogenesis (24). Lipoprotein particles undergo modification in the arterial intima (25). In particular, binding of lipoproteins to proteoglycan in the intima may both retard the egress of these particles and render them more susceptible to modification by oxidation (26,27). Glycation in the presence of hyperglycemia represents another form of modification of low density lipoprotein (LDL) particles in the intima (28).

Modified lipoproteins can elicit inflammatory mediators, such as proinflammatory cytokines, from the resident cell types in the normal artery: endothelial cells (EC) and SMC (29–31). Such cytokines, protein mediators of inflammation, can elicit the expression of leukocyte adhesion molecules on the surface of EC. Leukocytes attached to such "activated" EC at sites of lesion predilection can enter the intima by diapedesis between EC junctions (32,33). Chemotactic cytokines, such as macrophage chemoattractant protein-1 (MCP-1) and other chemokines, probably cause such directed migration of the leukocytes. Atheromata overexpress these mediators, probably in some measure in response to modified lipoprotein particles. Once resident in the intima, mononuclear phagocytes can imbibe the modified lipoproteins that have accumulated extracellularly. The phagocytic cells bind and internalize these modified lipoprotein particles by a number of "scavenger receptors" (34). The lipid-laden MΦ so produced constitutes the foam cell, the hallmark of the initial lesion of atherosclerosis, the fatty streak (Fig. 53-2).

We owe much of our knowledge about the initiation of atherosclerosis to studies in well-defined animal preparations,

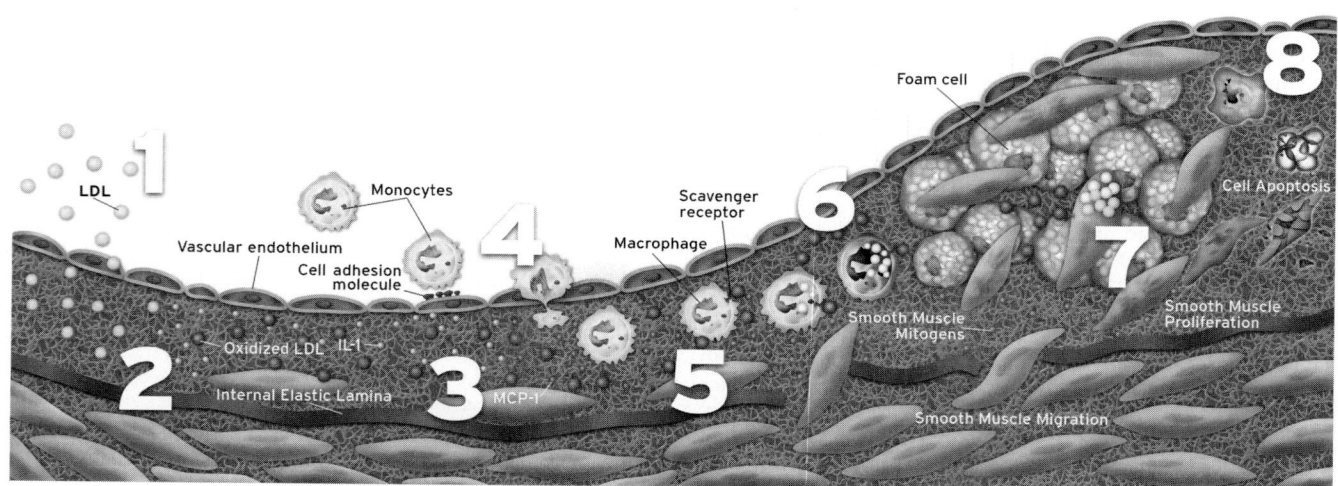

**FIGURE 53-2.** Schematic of the evolution of the atherosclerotic plaque.
1. Accumulation of lipoprotein particles in the intima. The modification of these lipoproteins is depicted by the *darker color*. Modifications include oxidation and glycation.
2. Oxidative stress, including products found in modified lipoproteins, can induce local cytokine elaboration.
3. The cytokines thereby induced increase expression of adhesion molecules for leukocytes that cause their attachment and chemoattractant molecules that direct their migration into the intima.
4. Blood monocytes, upon entering the artery wall in response to chemoattractant cytokines such as monocyte chemoattractant protein 1 (MCP-1) encounter stimuli such as macrophage-colony–stimulating factor (M-CSF) that can augment their expression of scavenger receptors.
5. Scavenger receptors mediate the uptake of modified lipoprotein particles and promote the development of foam cells. Macrophage foam cells are a source of mediators such as further cytokines and effector molecules such as hypochlorous acid, superoxide anion ($O_2^-$), and matrix metalloproteinases.
6. Smooth muscle cells in the intima divide. Other smooth muscle cells migrate into the intima from the media.
7. Smooth muscle cells can then divide and elaborate extracellular matrix, promoting extracellular matrix accumulation in the growing atherosclerotic plaque. In this manner, the fatty streak can evolve into a fibro-fatty lesion.
8. In later stages, calcification can occur (not depicted), and fibrosis continues, sometimes accompanied by smooth muscle cell death (including programmed cell death, or apoptosis) yielding a relatively acellular fibrous capsule surrounding a lipid-rich core that may also contain dying or dead cells and their detritus. (From Libby P. The vascular biology of atherosclerosis. In: Zipes DP, Libby P, Bonow RO, et al. eds. *Braunwald's heart disease: a textbook of cardiovascular medicine*, 7th ed. Philadelphia: Elsevier Saunders, 2005:921–937, with permission.)

as noted earlier. However, none of the available animal models perfectly mimic human atherosclerosis, not even the powerful mouse models discussed later. Hence, the concurrent study of human lesions has proven an important complement to the animal work. With regard to the initiation of lesions, a number of human studies have furnished insight. Autopsy studies on young Americans, including those killed in armed conflicts in the 1950s and 1960s, showed a high prevalence of fatty streaks and even raised lesions in coronary arteries (35,36). Systematic study of arteries collected from Americans younger than 35 years and dying of noncardiac causes has affirmed the high prevalence of nascent atheroma in humans in the third and fourth decades of life (37,38). The general pattern of disease morphology agrees with the inferences made by extrapolation from atherosclerotic animals.

# COMPLICATION OF THE ATHEROSCLEROTIC LESION

During formation of the fatty streak, the endothelium generally remains intact, albeit activated, as gauged by the expression of markers such as the leukocyte adhesion molecules (39–42). As MΦ continue to accumulate in the intima and inflammation persists, small areas of endothelial desquamation occur. Careful examination of the arteries of cholesterol-fed monkeys by scanning electron microscope shows microthrombi occurring at such sites of very focal and limited EC loss (43). Typically, these microthrombi consist of clusters of platelets adherent to MΦ foam cells that have been uncovered by the desquamated EC. Scanning electron microscopic studies of human hearts with severe but stable atherosclerosis, removed at the time of cardiac transplantation for ischemic cardiomyopathy and perfusion-fixed immediately, also disclose frequent microthrombi resembling those seen in the cholesterol-fed nonhuman primate (44–47). The platelets at these sites of microthrombosis, upon degranulation, release mediators that promote SMC migration (e.g., PDGF), collagen synthesis (e.g., TGF-β), and inhibit fibrinolysis [e.g., plasminogen activator inhibitor-1 (PAI-1)]. Such altered behavior of SMC probably initiates the evolution of the fatty streak toward a more fibrous lesion consisting of an admixture of SMC, with mononuclear leukocytes, and increasing accumulation of interstitial forms of collagen, one of the major extracellular proteins of the advanced atherosclerotic plaque. Local inhibition of fibrinolysis caused by deposition of PAI-1 may also promote fibrosis of plaques (48). Observations on advanced human atheroma have documented the presence of each of these platelet-derived mediators in atheroma, although cells within the lesion can also elaborate PDGF, TGF-β, and PAI-1 (49,50).

Initially, the SMC that migrate and secrete collagen may derive from SMC resident in the human arterial intima early in life. Other SMC may migrate into the intima from the tunica media in response to chemoattractant factors such as PDGF, released from platelets (9,12). EC, among other cell types in the artery wall, can also produce PDGF in response to such stimuli as thrombin, which is generated during thrombosis and likely present at the sites of early mural microthrombosis (51).

Curiously, during much of the early life history of a given atheromatous plaque, growth of the atheroma proceeds in an abluminal direction. This compensatory enlargement, or "positive remodeling," permits the growth of the atheroma without impinging on the lumen (52,53). In this manner, the lesion can grow without causing clinical symptoms related to reduced blood flow. This finding may account for the prolonged and usually clinically silent period of asymptomatic

progression of atherosclerosis. It may also explain why atherosclerosis not infrequently presents as an acute thrombotic complication without prior warning because of luminal narrowing. Lesions very likely grow in size and eventually encroach upon the lumen because of bouts of local microhemorrhage with healing and fibrosis.

The growth of new microvessels within the evolving atheroma may contribute to lesion complication. Neovascularization of the atheroma likely occurs in response to angiogenic growth factors such as acidic fibroblast and vascular endothelial growth factor (54–56). These microvessels seem to arise by extension of vasa vasorum in the adventitia and outer third of the tunica media of many arteries. These neovessels may be friable and easily disrupted, as those in the diabetic retina. Therefore, the plaque's microvessels may provide a nidus for hemorrhage *in situ* within the plaque. Such breeches in microvascular integrity might well entrain local microthrombosis within the atherosclerotic intima, producing local lesion growth by the fibrogenic mechanisms familiar from the earlier discussion, including PDGF, TGF-β release, and the consequences of thrombin generation.

As the atherosclerotic lesion evolves, the constituents of the extracellular matrix tend to accumulate. In addition to interstitial collagen previously alluded to, such matrix constituents include proteoglycans, elastin, and microfibrillar proteins (57). The extracellular matrix of the atheroma may actually constitute most of the volume of certain atherosclerotic plaques, particularly at later or more advanced stages. These matrix constituents interact with the thrombotic and hemostatic mechanisms in several ways. Collagen is a classical platelet activator and hence may promote thrombosis when exposed to the blood. On the other hand, endogenous heparin sulfate molecules may bind and activate antithrombin III, acting as an anticoagulant.

Complex atherosclerotic lesions often contain calcium. The mechanisms of calcification are currently under intense scrutiny (58,59). Interestingly, binding of calcium to proteins with carboxyl glutamate residues may contribute to lesion calcification. This chemistry resembles that which operates in proteins of the coagulation system.

# PLAQUE DISRUPTION AND THROMBOSIS

As lesions evolve, larger patches of endothelial denudation may occur, giving rise to larger mural thrombi. Even such superficial erosions of coronary arteries can lead to occlusive thrombosis and sudden death (60). The degree to which these desquamative lesions arise at bland or inflamed areas remains controversial (60,61). In a highly selected population of individuals who have died suddenly and then been referred for consultation to a cardiac pathology group by medical examiners, such superficial erosions with occlusive thrombi account for up to one third of sudden death cases caused by acute myocardial infarction (MI). Careful study of the clinical variables in these cases suggests that such superficial erosions occur more frequently in women than in men (62). Other associations with superficial erosions as the nidus for thrombosis include hypertriglyceridemia, a low high density lipoprotein (HDL), and diabetes mellitus (63).

A fracture of the plaque's fibrous cap causes most acute MI (see Fig. 53-3) (64–66). Sites of fibrous cap fracture invariably bear signs of inflammation (61,67). The type of atheroma that typically causes thrombosis on the substrate of a fissured fibrous cap includes the presence of numerous mononuclear phagocytes and large lipid pools. The MΦ in the lipid-rich core of such atheroma contains high levels of tissue factor

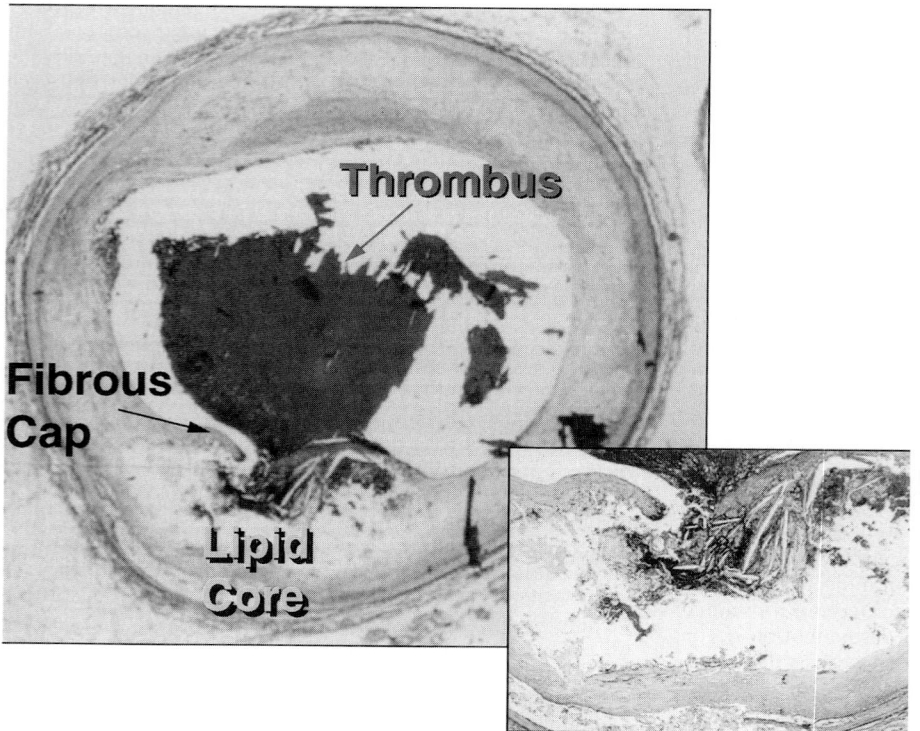

**FIGURE 53-3.** Plaque rupture: a common cause of coronary thrombosis. The fibrous cap overlying the lipid core of this plaque has ruptured, allowing the blood to contact the plaque's thrombogenic lipid core. Note that the lumen of this plaque is not critically narrowed. The **inset** shows a detail of the site of rupture, illustrating the fracture of the collagenous fibrous cap that caused the thrombus. This is how approximately two thirds of fatal coronary thrombi form. (Courtesy of Dr. Maria de Lourdes Higuchi, Department of Pathology, University of São Paulo, Brazil.)

(68,69). Because it can bind labeled factors VIIa and Xa *in situ*, tissue factor in atheroma retains biologic activity.

When the plaque's protective fibrous cap ruptures, coagulation factors in blood gain access to tissue factor that can trigger thrombus formation. Moreover, as noted earlier, the collagen within the atheroma can activate platelets, further aggravating thrombus formation. Such fibrous cap fractures cause approximately two thirds of acute MI as determined in autopsy studies. However, as noted earlier, plaque disruption appears commonplace in patients with atherosclerosis, and most plaque disruptions do not cause sustained occlusive thrombi such as those that produce acute MI in the coronary circulation (70,71).

The balance between procoagulant and anticoagulant factors and fibrinolytic and antifibrinolytic factors likely determines the consequence of any given plaque disruption. In the presence of a robust fibrinolytic system, a mural thrombus might undergo rapid lysis, limiting its clinical consequences. In the presence of prothrombotic factors such as a high fibrinogen, or when levels of the fibrinolytic inhibitor PAI-1 pertain, growth of a thrombus to occlusion may occur more frequently. The fate of the nonocclusive mural thrombus, whether produced by superficial erosion or fracture of the fibrous cap, may indeed be incorporation into the plaque as hypothesized by von Rokitansky in the 19th century (1). Indeed, human atheromata contain considerable fibrin (5,6). By means of the fibrogenic mechanisms detailed earlier, mural thrombi may promote smooth muscle migration, proliferation, and matrix secretion. This mechanism could ultimately lead to the evolution of a lipid-rich lesion into one of much more fibrotic character. Such episodes of thrombosis-induced plaque growth may lead to the formation of stenotic lesions capable of producing limitation of blood flow and thereby producing clinical symptoms.

The dichotomy of so-called vulnerable versus stable plaques is useful conceptually, but it substantially oversimplifies reality (see Fig. 53-4). Indeed, lesions of both morphologies often coexist in a given arterial tree and can even occur serially within a given artery, in close proximity or side-by-side at branch points (72). Therefore, the arterial tree of a patient with atherosclerosis probably includes lesions of diverse morphologies: uncomplicated fatty streaks, raised lesions not complicated by thrombosis, lesions that have disrupted causing acute mural thrombosis, and lesions that have evolved to a more fibrous character, perhaps by healing due to a previous mural thrombosis.

## PATHOPHYSIOLOGY OF PLAQUE DISRUPTION

In view of the importance of plaque disruption as a substrate for thrombosis, consideration of some current notions regarding the pathophysiology of this process seems worthwhile. As noted earlier, two major mechanisms of plaque disruption account for most coronary thromboses: superficial erosion and rupture of the fibrous cap.

A local denudation of EC characterizes superficial erosion of the arterial intima. Indeed, denuding injury of endothelium was considered primary in the pathogenesis of atherosclerosis for many years (73). Although we now recognize that the endothelium remains largely intact over atheroma, patchy areas of denudation do occur and represent an important substrate for thrombosis. Initially, mechanical injury was considered most important as a cause of denuding endothelial injury. Mechanical denudation certainly applies to atherogenic endothelial injury such as those produced by interventions such as balloon angioplasty or stenting. Endothelial desquamation due to hemodynamic stresses was also considered a cause for endothelial denudation. However, sites where plaques actually form are generally considered areas of low shear stress. Although circumferential or "hoop" stresses may be increased in hypertension, the effect of hypertension on endothelial desquamation focally remains uncertain.

Biological rather than mechanical mechanisms, very likely apoptosis or death of EC at areas of lesion predilection, might

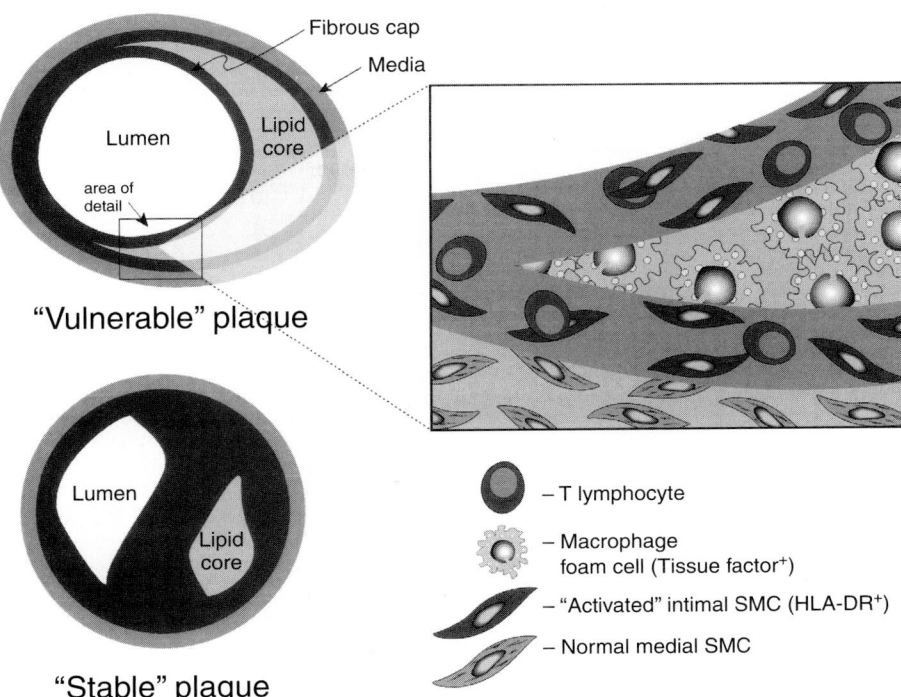

- – T lymphocyte
- – Macrophage foam cell (Tissue factor⁺)
- – "Activated" intimal SMC (HLA-DR⁺)
- – Normal medial SMC

"Vulnerable" plaque

"Stable" plaque

**FIGURE 53-4.** The characteristics of "vulnerable" plaques and "stable" plaques. Vulnerable plaques often have a well-preserved lumen, because plaques grow outward initially (compensatory enlargement or "positive remodeling"). The vulnerable plaque usually has a large lipid core and a thin fibrous cap separating the tissue factor in macrophages and other cells from circulating coagulation factors. Sites of lesion disruption often contain activated smooth muscle cells, detected by their expression of the histocompatibility antigen HLA-DR. In contrast, stable plaques tend to have a relatively thick fibrous cap protecting the lipid core from contact with the blood. (From Libby P. The molecular vases of the acute coronary syndromes. *Circulation* 1995;91:2844–2850, with permission.)

furnish one such pathway to focal endothelial denudation. Although apoptosis is generally considered a noninflammatory process, during atherogenesis inflammation, it may actually prove common as a mechanism for precipitating apoptosis (74). Proteolysis could also sever the proteins involved in adhesive interactions of EC with their substrate. EC can overexpress matrix-degrading proteinases, including the matrix metalloproteinases (MMPs) inducibly in response to inflammatory mediators or oxidized lipids known to localize in atheroma (75–77). In addition, enzymes generally considered important in fibrinolysis, such as urokinase-type plasminogen activator and tissue-type plasminogen activators (uPA, tPA), may influence matrix degradation in two ways. Plasmin generated by these PAs can directly degrade components of the arterial extracellular matrix (78,79). Moreover, plasmin can process the inactive zymogen forms of MMPs into their enzymatically active forms. Thrombin can activate latent MMP-2, a matrix-degrading enzyme constitutively produced by vascular cells (80). The typical basement membrane constituent Type IV collagen is a classical substrate for active MMP-2. Therefore, both thrombin and fibrinolytic enzymes may participate in the regulation of proteolysis that could render EC prone to desquamation.

Proteolysis may also play an important role in fracture of the fibrous cap, the other major mechanism of plaque disruption (see Figs. 53-5 and 53-6). The inflammatory cells that appear quite numerous in rupture-prone atherosclerotic plaques can also produce enzymes capable of degrading structurally important constituents of the extracellular matrix of the plaque's protective fibrous cap (81). For example, MΦ in human atheroma overexpress interstitial collagenases (including MMP-1 and MMP-13) (82–84). These cells can also produce the elastolytic enzymes, cathepsins S and K (85). Additionally, MΦ in atheromatous lesions overexpress gelatinases, including MMP-2 and MMP-9 (82). Further contributions to elastolysis in atheroma can derive from overexpression of MMP-12, matrix metalloelastase (86).

The interstitial forms of collagen that lend strength to the plaque's fibrous cap can also diminish in vulnerable plaques because of decreased *de novo* synthesis by SMC. T lymphocytes comprise an important component of the leukocytic infiltrate in human atheroma. T cells, when activated, can secrete interferon γ (IFN-γ), an inhibitor of smooth muscle cell collagen synthesis (8). Considerable evidence supports the activation of T cells in human atheroma and the presence of IFN-γ (87). Therefore, impaired ability of the SMC to synthesize new collagen to reinforce and maintain the extracellular matrix of the fibrous cap can also lead to thinning and weakening of the structure, characteristics of the plaques that tend to rupture and cause thrombosis (88).

Indeed, SMC may serve an important function as protectors of the plaque's fibrous cap due to their ability to synthesize collagen and other structurally important components of the arterial extracellular matrix (Figs. 53-5 and 53-6). In this regard, death of SMC within atheroma may promote plaque disruption (89). As noted earlier, inflammatory pathways in

**Factors increasing stress**
- Thin fibrous cap
- Large lipid pool
- Less stenotic lesions
- ↑ (ester/free) cholesterol

**Factors weakening the cap**
- ↓ collagen synthesis
- ↑ collagen degradation
- ↑ macrophages, T cells
- ↓ smooth muscle cells

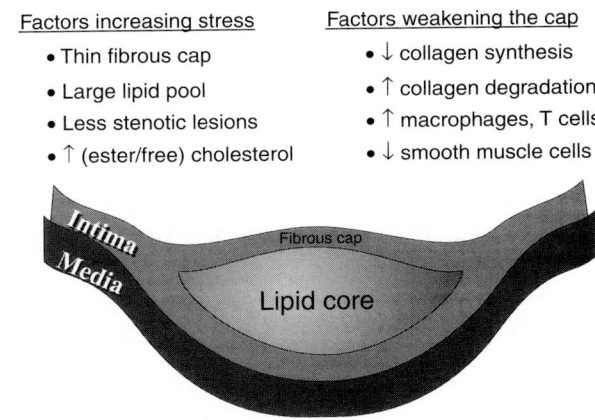

**FIGURE 53-5.** Biomechanical and biochemical features contribute to disruption of atheromatous plaques and their thrombotic complications. See text for explanation. (From Lee R, Libby P. The unstable atheroma. *Arterioscler Thromb Vasc Biol* 1997;17:1859–1867, with permission.)

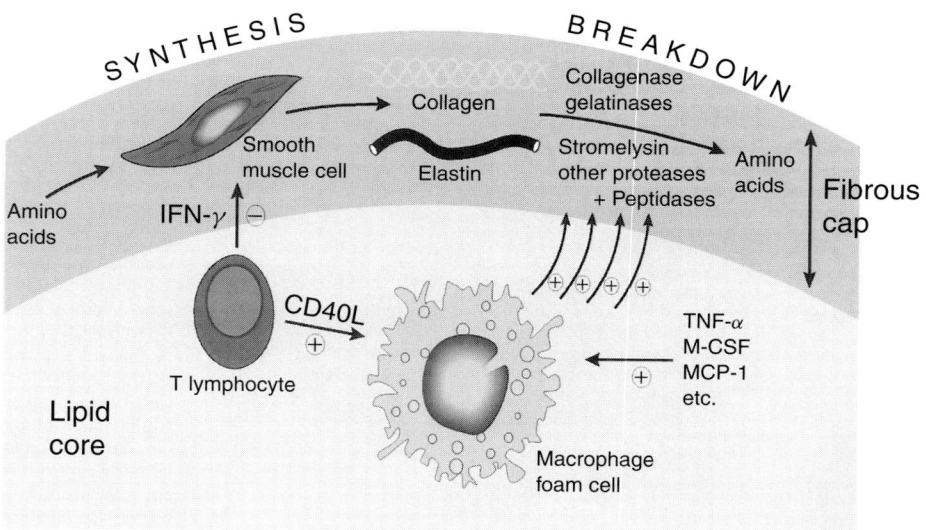

**FIGURE 53-6.** Molecular mechanisms regulating the stability of atheroma. The vascular smooth muscle cell synthesizes the collagen and elastin in the atheroma's fibrous cap. When inflammation is present, as characteristic of plaques that cause fatal thromboses, interferon γ (IFN-γ) secreted by activated T cells may inhibit collagen synthesis, impeding the repair and maintenance of the collagenous framework of the plaque's fibrous cap. The activated macrophage secretes proteinases that can degrade both collagen and elastin. The breakdown of these structural molecules of the extracellular matrix can weaken the fibrous cap, rendering it particularly susceptible to rupture and precipitation of the thrombotic complications of atheroma. The macrophage, in turn, undergoes activation by IFN-γ derived from the T lymphocytes and by CD40 ligand (CD154) expressed on the surface of these cells. Platelets also can express active CD40 ligand. Plaques contain other activators of macrophages not derived from T cells, including tumor necrosis factor-α (TNF-α), macrophage-colony–stimulating factor (M-CSF), and macrophage chemoattractant protein-1 (MCP-1), among others. (From Libby P. The molecular bases of the acute coronary syndromes. *Circulation* 1995;91:2844–2850, with permission.)

atheroma likely promote apoptosis. In particular, combinations of inflammatory cytokines can trigger cell death by apoptosis in human SMC *in vitro* (90). Moreover, the activated T cells within lesions, by expression of Fas ligand, can engage Fas on the surface of SMC and, in conjunction with inflammatory cytokines including IFN-γ, trigger death of these cells (74). Therefore, just as in the case of superficial erosion where the target is EC, fibrous cap rupture may depend on both proteolysis and cell death. Inflammatory pathways appear to participate importantly in the destabilization of the plaque that triggers thrombosis in both superficial erosion and fibrous cap rupture.

# INSIGHTS INTO PATHOPHYSIOLOGY OF ATHEROSCLEROSIS AFFORDED BY STUDY OF GENETICALLY ALTERED MICE

Studies of rabbits and other animals have provided invaluable insight into elements of the pathogenesis of atherosclerosis, as illustrated earlier. The current availability of useful mouse models of atherosclerosis has afforded an opportunity to test hypotheses about the causal nature of various mediators suggested by observational work in animals and humans. Recent studies in genetically altered mice have furnished evidence supporting causative roles of specific inflammatory mediators and other molecules in elements of the pathogenesis of atheromatous lesions.

Mice with mutations introduced by homologous recombination in genes encoding apolipoprotein E or the LDL receptor (LDLr) develop arterial lesions that recapitulate many features thought to pertain to human atherogenesis (91–93). The study of compound mutant mice bearing one or more of these atherosclerosis-susceptibility conferring mutations and also lacking function of a particular gene implicated in atherogenesis permits evaluation of the role of the candidate gene product in this process. For example, such an approach has shown that MCP-1 indeed regulates mononuclear cell recruitment (94) and that macrophage-colony–stimulating factor (M-CSF) promotes lesion formation (95–97). Other such studies have demonstrated a role for γ interferon in plaque fibrosis and evolution (98), and of MΦ scavenger receptors in foam cell accumulation in experimentally produced atheroma in mice (99). Mice with bone-marrow chimerism can explore the roles of mediators derived from cells of hematogenous lineages in atherogenesis. This approach has particular value in cases where global lack of a particular mediator yields a lethal phenotype. For example, such studies have demonstrated that lack of PDGF B chain does not alter lesion size but markedly alters the character of lesions, yielding less fibrotic but not smaller plaques (100,101).

The availability of genetically altered mice with susceptibility to develop atherosclerosis has provided a model for investigating mechanisms of complications of atheroma as well. For example, physiologic stressors such as hypoxia or fright can cause myocardial ischemia and perhaps thrombotic occlusion of coronary arteries (102). Older ApoE deficient mice can develop plaque disruption with thrombosis particularly in the brachiocephalic branches of the proximal aorta (103,104). However, the consistency and reproducibility of such plaque disruptions remains a matter of debate.

# THERAPEUTIC CONSIDERATIONS WITH EMPHASIS ON THE ACUTE CORONARY SYNDROMES

The current approach to treatment of patients with acute MI and unstable angina focuses on thrombus formation following plaque rupture, the fundamental event in the acute clinical manifestation of coronary artery disease (105,106). This section provides a broad overview of treatment strategies for acute ischemic syndromes that include thrombolytic, antiplatelet, and antithrombotic agents. Other chapters review extensive pharmacologic and preclinical data as well as clinical trial experience with these effective cardiovascular therapeutics, development of which is based on a thorough understanding of basic mechanisms of endogenous fibrinolysis, platelet function, and coagulation.

Prolonged thrombotic occlusion of the infarct-related artery results in myocardial necrosis. The rationale of reperfusion therapy rests on the concept that the longer coronary occlusion persists, the more irreversible ischemic injury will occur in cardiac myocytes. Therefore, ischemic but viable myocardium is available for pharmacologic or direct mechanical [i.e., percutaneous coronary intervention (PCI)] salvage. This "wavefront phenomenon" of ischemic cell death was advanced by the early observations of Reimer et al. demonstrating that irreversible injury develops at variable times with a wave of cell death that begins in the subendocardium and progresses toward the subepicardium (107,108). In various experimental studies, reperfusion preserved viable myocytes and resulted in smaller average transmural infarcts if reperfusion occurred up to approximately 6 hours (109). These preclinical studies form the experimental basis for current reperfusion therapy (thrombolysis or primary revascularization with PCI) in MI.

DeWood's landmark angiographic trial ushered in the thrombolytic era by unequivocally demonstrating that thrombotic occlusion of the infarct-related artery causes acute MI and by reestablishing the safety of cardiac catheterization and angiography in the setting of MI (105). Prospective, randomized trials have shown that thrombolytic agents such as streptokinase (SK) tPA, which promote clot lysis by generating the fibrinolytic enzyme plasmin, reduce 30-day mortality in ST-segment elevation MI by 18% on average [95% confidence interval (CI), 13% to 23%; 2P <0.00001]. Substantial benefits are observed with treatment from 0 to 12 hours after the onset of symptoms (see Fig. 53-7) (110).

Although they provide an important survival benefit, contemporary thrombolytic strategies still have substantial limitations. Angiographic studies evaluating coronary artery patency within 90 minutes of intravenous thrombolytic administration have shown infarct-related artery patency [defined as Thrombolysis in Myocardial Infarction (TIMI) grade ≥2] flow in approximately 80% of cases. The studies also show that normal flow (TIMI grade 3 flow), which predicts the most favorable outcome from a survival standpoint, follows in only 30% to 50% of cases, and that reocclusion of the coronary artery following successful thrombolysis occurs in at least 10% of cases (111). While allowing for convenient bolus administration, the development and clinical testing of new "third-generation" thrombolytic agents, such as TNK-tPA and rPA, have not resulted in enhanced coronary artery patency or improvement in clinical endpoints (112). Furthermore, thrombolytic therapy has not had a beneficial effect on the treatment of patients with unstable angina or acute MI unaccompanied by ST segment elevation (i.e., non–Q-wave), as illustrated by the results of the TIMI IIIb trial, which showed a trend toward increased mortality and (re)infarction rates in patients who received tPA (113). Possible explanations for the deficiencies of current thrombolytic regimens include (a) plasminogen activator resistance due to high levels of the naturally occurring inhibitor, PAI-1, in platelet-rich thrombi; (b) concomitant thrombin generation induced by plasmin; and (c) inadequate adjunctive antiplatelet and antithrombotic agents to permit efficient and rapid fibrinolysis by inhibiting further thrombus formation.

Attempts to improve reperfusion strategies have explored two widely disparate approaches: (a) Direct mechanical reperfusion with primary PCI and (b) adjunctive therapy with more potent antiplatelet and antithrombin agents, in addition to thrombolysis. Primary PCI is associated with high procedural success rates, achieving TIMI 3 flow in greater than 90% of patients, and low in-hospital mortality (<7%) rates in randomized trials (114). More than 20 head-to-head randomized trials have randomly assigned approximately 8,000 thrombolytic-eligible patients with ST segment elevation myocardial infarction (STEMI) to primary PCI (balloon angioplasty or stenting) or thrombolytic therapy (115). Recent metaanalysis of these trials showed that primary PCI was better than thrombolytic therapy at reducing short-term death (7% vs. 9%, P = 0.0002), nonfatal reinfarction (3% vs. 7%, P <0.0001), stroke (1% vs. 2%, P = 0.0004), and the combined endpoint of death, nonfatal reinfarction, and stroke (8% vs. 14%, P <0.0001) (115). The results yielded by primary PCI remained better than those with thrombolytic therapy during long-term follow-up and did not depend on the type of thrombolytic agent used or whether or not the patient was transferred for primary PCI. This metaanalysis suggests that for every 1,000 patients treated with primary angioplasty rather than thrombolytic therapy, an additional 20 lives are saved, 43 reinfarctions are prevented, 10 fewer strokes occur, and 13 intracranial hemorrhages are prevented. Myocardial salvage is greater with PCI, and primary PCI gives better results than thrombolytic therapy even in community hospitals without on-site surgical backup (116). Most importantly, primary PCI reduces death, recurrent MI, or stroke compared with front-loaded tPA (14.2% vs. 8.5%, P <0.002) even if patients must be transferred by ambulance for up to 150 minutes to reach an intervention center.

Unfortunately, the current average door-to-balloon times in the United States exceed the 90-minute goal, and transfer patients average more than 3 hours (118). Efforts to improve clinical outcome when timely angioplasty is unavailable have focused on "facilitated angioplasty," which denotes the combination of pharmacologic reperfusion with mechanical revascularization (119). However, four randomized trials have found that facilitated angioplasties are either inferior to or no better than primary PCI alone (120).

To enhance further infarct artery-related patency and to reduce the risk of embolization of thrombotic and atherosclerotic debris, interventional cardiologists have also turned to a variety of newer device strategies, including rheolytic thrombectomy (121) as well as distal embolic protection balloons (122) and filters (123).

Efforts to improve reperfusion strategies have also focused on adjunctive therapy with new antiplatelet (glycoprotein (GP) IIb/IIIa inhibitors) and antithrombotic [direct thrombin inhibitors and low-molecular-weight heparins (LMWHs)] agents in combination with thrombolysis or PCI. The pivotal role of platelet activation and aggregation in the formation of coronary thrombus was confirmed in the Second International Study of Infarct Survival (ISIS-2), which showed that the administration of aspirin up to 24 hours after the onset of symptoms of suspected acute MI reduced 5-week mortality by 23% when compared with the placebo control group. Nonfatal MI was reduced by 49% and nonfatal stroke by 46% (111). Importantly, the effect of aspirin was equal to that of SK alone and additive when used in combination.

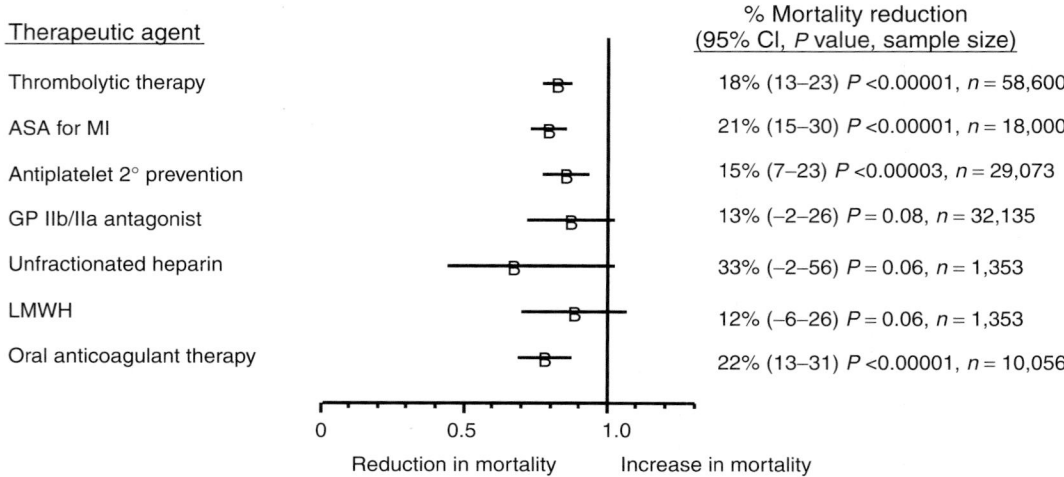

**FIGURE 53-7.** Antithrombotic and thrombolytic therapies improve clinical outcomes in the acute coronary syndromes. This graph illustrates the effects of therapeutic agents on mortality in acute ischemic syndromes. Odds ratios or relative risk and their 95% confidence intervals, derived from metaanalyses cited subsequently, are plotted. In the case of unfractionated heparin, the odds ratio for the combined cardiovascular endpoint of death and myocardial infraction (MI) is plotted. The odds ratio for low-molecular-weight heparin (LMWH) represents a comparison of LMWH to unfractionated heparin for death at 30 days in the thrombolysis in myocardial infarction (TIMI) 11b and Efficacy and Safety of Subcutaneous Enoxaparin in Non–Q-wave Coronary Events (ESSENCE) trials. (Elliott Antman, MD, Brigham and Women's Hospital, *personal communication.*)

However, aspirin is not a strong antiplatelet agent, interfering principally with thromboxane $A_2$–dependent platelet activation. Other agonist-induced pathways remain relatively unaffected. A new class of potent antiplatelet agents, the GP IIb/IIIa inhibitors, has revolutionized the treatment of patients with acute ischemic syndromes. These agents (e.g., abciximab, eptifibatide, and tirofiban) block platelet fibrinogen and von Willebrand factor (VWF) binding, the final common molecular pathway of platelet aggregation, and considerably reduce death and MI in the treatment of a variety of clinical syndromes, including unstable angina and acute MI with and without concomitant PCI (124). GP IIb/IIIa inhibitors have been shown to reduce major adverse cardiac events (death, MI, and urgent revascularization) by 35% to 50% in patients undergoing PCI (125). Although no single study demonstrated a significant reduction in mortality alone with GP IIb/IIIa inhibitors, metaanalysis suggests that these agents as a class reduce death by 20% to 30% (125). The mechanism by which GP IIb/IIIa inhibitors reduce long-term mortality is unclear and cannot be explained solely by its ability to reduce periprocedural death or MI other than in conventional balloon angioplasty. Investigators have postulated that this therapy may also be associated with significant antiinflammatory properties that may favorably influence the course of atherothrombotic disease (126,127), a contention that remains unproven.

Results from pilot trials that examined the use of GP IIb/IIIa inhibitors in conjunction with reduced doses of thrombolytic agents suggest that they may significantly enhance coronary artery patency (128) and augment perfusion of the microvasculature (129). However, improvement of hard clinical endpoints using this combination with (130) and without (131) mandated PCI remains undetermined.

Thrombin occupies a pivotal position in the coagulation cascade and also potently activates platelets. Heparin, which inactivates thrombin activity through binding to antithrombin III, has been a staple in pharmacologic management of acute coronary syndromes (ACS). However, the inability of unfractionated heparin to inactivate clot-bound thrombin limits its efficacy (132), as does an unpredictable, highly variable anticoagulant response due to heparin binding to plasma proteins (133). Direct thrombin inhibitors (e.g., hirudin, bivalirudin, argatroban), which may allow for complete inhibition of thrombin activity by inhibiting both fluid-phase and clot-bound thrombin, have also been developed and evaluated in patients with ACS. Results with these direct thrombin inhibitors have been largely disappointing in the non-PCI setting (134,135), but recent clinical trial experience with bivalirudin in PCI showing noninferiority to the combination of unfractionated heparin and GP IIb/IIIa inhibitors (136) has prompted a reevaluation of this class of agents in ACS.

LMWHs offer potential advantages over unfractionated heparin because they have excellent bioavailability and a more predictable anticoagulant response that allows for subcutaneous administration and obviates the need for anticoagulant blood monitoring. In addition, LMWHs possess a higher anti-Xa:anti-IIa activity ratio compared with unfractionated heparin, thereby possibly providing enhanced inhibition of coagulation by inhibiting thrombin generation and activity (137). Although the LMWH enoxaparin plus aspirin was more effective than unfractionated heparin plus aspirin in reducing the 30-day composite endpoint of death, MI, or recurrent angina/urgent revascularization in two older medical treatment trials of unstable angina (138,139), there appears to be no advantage of LMWH over unfractionated heparin in patients treated with an invasive strategy mandating angiography and revascularization with PCI or coronary artery bypass surgery in most patients (140).

Antiplatelet therapy is also a cornerstone of primary and secondary prevention of acute ischemic syndromes. Aspirin reduces the risk of first MI (primary prevention) by 44% (141) and, in the post-MI setting (secondary prevention), aspirin reduced the risk of vascular death by 13%, nonfatal reinfarction by 31%, and nonfatal stroke by 42% (142). However, despite state-of-the-art secondary prevention regimens with aspirin, β-blockers, aggressive cholesterol-lowering agents, and angiotensin converting enzyme inhibitors (143), recurrent fatal and nonfatal MI and stroke continue to occur at rates approaching 5% per year in patients who have had prior MI (144). Intensifying antiplatelet therapy may further reduce clinical events. The Clopidogrel in Unstable Angina to Prevent Recurrent Ischemic Events (CURE) trial found that treatment with the thienopyridine derivative clopidogrel, an inhibitor of platelet aggregation induced by adenosine diphosphate, in combination with aspirin was superior to aspirin alone, reducing overall cardiovascular events by 20% (145).

The early experience with coronary stenting was notable for unacceptably high rates of subacute stent thrombosis, occurring in 3% to 5% of patients and associated with MI, need for urgent coronary artery bypass grafting, and/or death. Aggressive anticoagulation regimens [including intravenous heparin and dextran, warfarin, acetylsalicylic acid (ASA), and dipyridamole] to minimize the risk of stent thrombosis led to frequent bleeding complications and prolonged hospitalizations. Several studies have demonstrated a dramatic, approximately fivefold reduction in acute and subacute stent thrombosis when ASA in combination with a thienopyridine was used post-PCI compared with ASA alone or in combination with warfarin (146,147).

Chronic oral GP IIb/IIIa antagonism did not offer more effective antiplatelet therapy for primary and secondary prevention of cardiovascular disease. Combining chronic oral (warfarin) or subcutaneous (LMWH) anticoagulation with antiplatelet therapy may also be effective in further reducing the rate of recurrent ischemic events in patients with acute ischemic syndromes (138,148). Despite effective therapy with newer antiplatelet and antithrombotic agents, adverse cardiovascular event rates remain high in the active treatment groups, approaching 20% at 6 months in modern ACS trials (149). While vascular biologists aggressively pursue therapy that focuses on preventing plaque rupture, clinical investigators are moving ahead with adjunctive agents that attack other key mediators of thrombosis, including GP Ib/IX (platelet adhesion), tissue factor (a potent procoagulant overexpressed in atherosclerotic plaques) (150), and more selective inhibitors of factor Xa (e.g., fondaparinux) (151).

# THE CLINICAL APPLICATION OF INFLAMMATORY BIOMARKERS AND THE ATHEROTHROMBOTIC PROCESS

As described earlier, inflammation plays an important role in plaque initiation, progression, and rupture. In particular, increased expression of cell adhesion molecules, including sICAM-1, sVCAM-1, and P selectin, are triggered by inflammatory cytokines such as interleukin-1 and tumor necrosis factor-α (TNF-α), leading to early leukocyte adhesion on the endothelium and enhancing fatty streak formation. Mononuclear cells within this infiltrate subsequently express growth factors that lead to proliferation of SMC, whereas other proinflammatory cytokines such as CD40 ligand can induce tissue factor and promote thrombosis. In the aggregate, interactions of multiple inflammatory pathways contribute importantly to plaque growth and instability.

Current approaches to disease detection exploit this role of inflammation in atherothrombosis, and measurement of inflammatory biomarkers has become increasingly common in clinical practice. To date, several inflammatory biomarkers, including tumor necrosis factor (TNF) (152), sICAM-1 (153,154), P selectin (155), macrophage inhibitory cytokine (MIC-1) (156), lipoprotein-associated phospholipase (LP-PL) A2 (157,158), interleukins-1, -6, and -8 (159–161), myeloperoxidase (162,163), pregnancy-associated plasma protein A (PAPP-A) (164), and CD40 ligand (165,166), have all shown promise either in the setting of primary disease detection or in acute coronary ischemia. However, because of both its ease of measurement and long-term stability, the simple downstream acute-phase reactant C-reactive protein (CRP) has emerged as the most important of these inflammatory biomarkers and is the only marker endorsed by the Centers for Disease Control for clinical use (167,168).

Circulating CRP consists of five 23-kDa subunits and belongs to the pentraxin family of molecules that play major roles in human innate immunity. Although largely derived from hepatocytes in response to interleukin-6 stimulation, human coronary arteries can also produce CRP, and accumulating evidence indicates that CRP plays a direct role in atherothrombosis through complement activation, induction of local adhesion molecule expression, increased thrombogenicity, and reduced endothelial nitric oxide availability. Recent work in transgenic mice further suggests that CRP may directly enhance intravascular thrombosis and promote atherogenesis (169). Although hepatic induction by IL-6 has long been considered the only source of CRP production during the acute-phase response, more recent data indicates that CRP can be produced locally by cellular components of the vascular endothelium and SMC within the vessel wall, both under basal conditions and after stimulation by inflammatory cytokines. Translational studies have also reported local generation of CRP, serum amyloid A (SAA), and IL-6 in arterial segments undergoing angioplasty that have been isolated from the systemic vasculature. Whether or not this local production is important and its relative contribution to the systemic inflammatory response during acute ischemia are areas of ongoing research.

## C-Reactive Protein in Primary Prevention

To date, more than 20 prospective epidemiologic studies have evaluated CRP with "high sensitivity" assays. In each of these, CRP levels were increased at baseline among apparently healthy individuals at high risk for future MI, stroke, peripheral arterial disease, and sudden cardiac death. Several large primary prevention studies have also shown that CRP adds important prognostic information at all levels of LDL cholesterol and across the full spectrum of Framingham Risk Scores (see Fig. 53-8) (158,170–176).

Importantly, CRP levels do not correlate with total or LDL cholesterol, and therefore, the addition of CRP evaluation to cholesterol screening has emerged as a powerful new method for vascular risk detection. Individuals with elevated levels of CRP but low levels of LDL cholesterol have higher absolute and relative risks of developing future vascular disease than those with elevated levels of LDL cholesterol but low levels of CRP (see Fig. 53-9), an observation important to global risk prediction algorithms (171). CRP levels do track with obesity, hypofibrinolysis, and insulin resistance, and thereby increase with prevalence of metabolic syndrome (177). In this regard, several

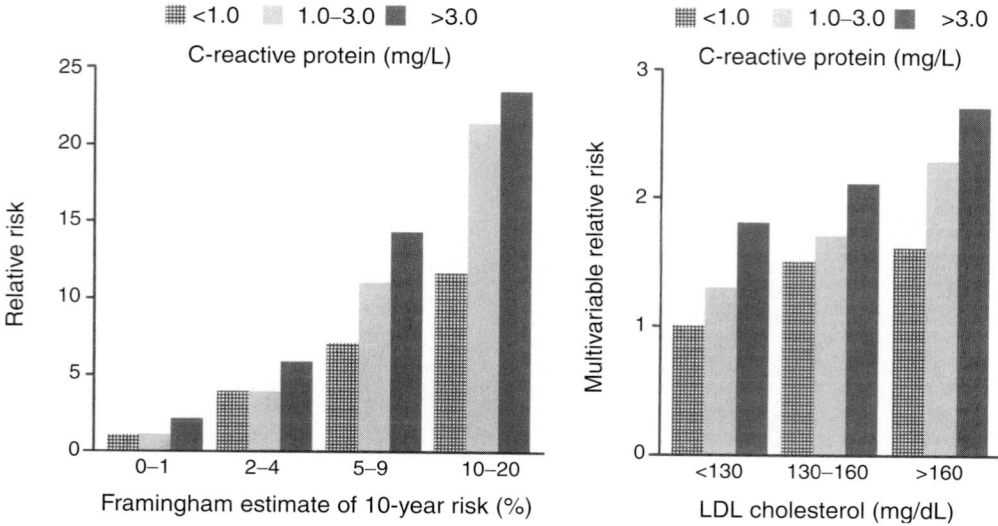

**FIGURE 53-8.** C-reactive protein levels add prognostic information on risk of future cardiovascular events at all levels of low density lipoprotein (LDL) cholesterol (*right*) and at all levels of calculated Framingham risk (*left*). (From Ridker PM, Rifai N, Rose L, et al. Comparison of C-reactive protein and low density lipoprotein cholesterol levels in the prediction of first cardiovascular events. *N Engl J Med* 2002;347:1557–1565, with permission.)

major studies have also shown that CRP levels add prognostic information on risk at all levels of metabolic syndrome (see Fig. 53-10) (177,178). Moreover, CRP levels in healthy individuals predict future development of hypertension (179) and of type 2 diabetes (180–183). On this basis, the formal definition of metabolic syndrome may change to include CRP.

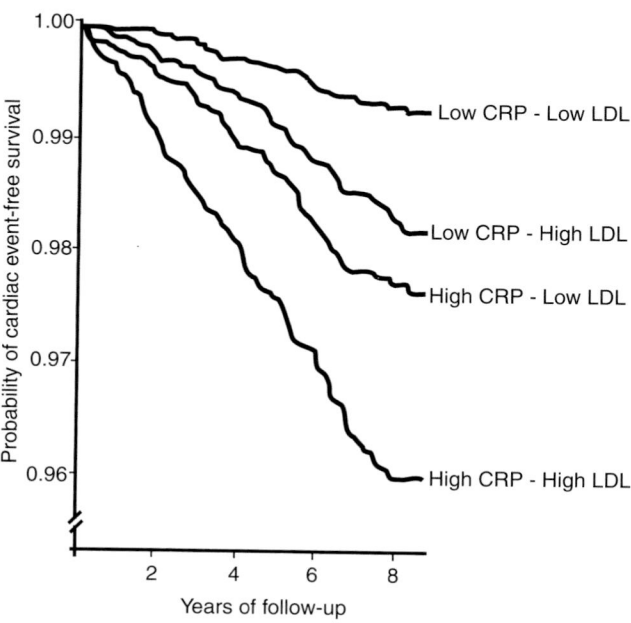

**FIGURE 53-9.** Cardiovascular event–free survival among healthy individuals, according to baseline levels of low density lipoprotein cholesterol and C-reactive protein. (From Ridker PM, Rifai N, Rose L, et al. Comparison of C-reactive protein and low density lipoprotein cholesterol levels in the prediction of first cardiovascular events. *N Engl J Med* 2002;347:1557–1565, with permission.)

Recognizing the importance of these data, the Centers for Disease Control and the American Heart Association issued the first clinical guidelines for use of high-sensitivity CRP (hsCRP) and suggested that this biomarker be used among those identified as "intermediate risk" according to usual measures of global vascular risk (168). Following analyses from both the Physicians Health Study (PHS) (170) and the Women's Health Study (WHS) (152,161), those initial guidelines indicated that hsCRP levels of less than 1 mg per L, 1 to 3 mg per L, and greater than 3 mg per L represented lower, moderate, and higher vascular risks, respectively. These values have proven highly consistent across major cohorts. Categorization of hsCRP values provides incremental information on vascular risk in all major studies to date, even after full adjustment for all components of the Framingham risk score (see Fig. 53-11). More recent data indicates that those with marked elevations of CRP (values chronically in excess of 10 mg per L) are at even higher absolute risk and therefore false-positive elevations of CRP are rare (184).

## C-Reactive Protein in Acute Coronary Ischemia, Chronic Stable Angina, and Secondary Prevention

In addition to a predictive role in primary prevention, CRP levels have utility as an adjunct to troponin in the setting of acute coronary ischemia. Multiple studies have shown that those who present with acute ischemia and elevated levels of CRP are at increased short- and long-term risk of vascular death, even when troponin levels are normal. Early data from Liuzzo et al. demonstrate that patients with unstable angina with CRP levels in excess of 3 mg per L have significantly higher rates of coronary death, recurrent MI, and need for revascularization as compared to those with lower levels (185). Since then, investigators in the TIMI, c7E3 Antiplatelet Therapy in Unstable Angina (CAPTURE), and Fast Revascularization During Instability in Coronary Artery Disease (FRISC) trials have all found that CRP independently predicts recurrent event rates in ACS and that this effect is additive to and independent of troponin (186–188).

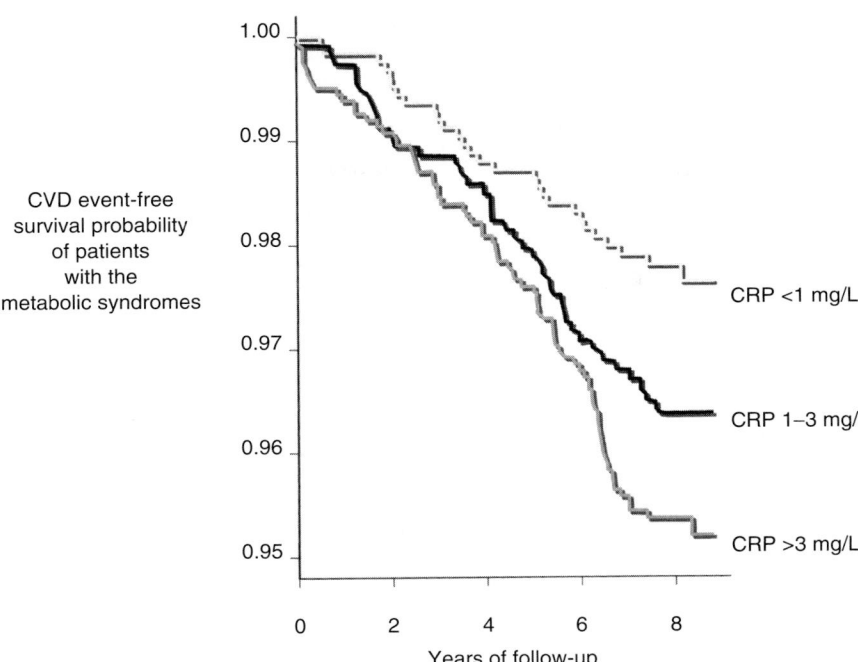

FIGURE 53-10. Cardiovascular event–free survival among individuals with metabolic syndrome by adenosine triphosphate III criteria, according to plasma C-reactive protein (CRP) levels. CVD, cardiovascular disease. (From Ridker PM, Buring JE, Cook NR, et al. C-reactive protein, the metabolic syndrome, and risk of incident cardiovascular events: an 8-year follow-up of 14,719 initially healthy American women. *Circulation* 2003;107: 391–397, with permission.)

Moreover, the level of inflammation in the setting of unstable angina predicts the need for aggressive revascularization therapies, particularly primary angioplasty (189). These observations have led many centers to use a multimarker approach to the detection of vascular risk in the ACS setting that includes troponin (as a marker of myocyte necrosis), brain natriuretic peptide (as a marker for heart failure), and CRP (as a marker of inflammation) (184).

Patients with chronic stable angina (190), prior MI (191, 192), or prior stent procedures (193–195) who express elevated levels of CRP also have increased risk for recurrent coronary events and cardiovascular death. These data are particularly important, because CRP relates only weakly to measures of atherosclerotic burden such as carotid intima medial thickness, ankle-brachial indices, or coronary calcification. Further, autopsy reports indicate higher CRP levels among those who died with frankly ruptured plaques compared to those with eroded plaques (196). Therefore, CRP appears more closely related to plaque vulnerability and the propensity to undergo acute occlusive events than to the extent of underlying disease. CRP determination can also identify those who might benefit more or less from specific therapeutic interventions including aspirin, thiazolidinediones, GP IIb/IIIa inhibitors, and most importantly from a clinical perspective, HMG CoA reductase inhibitors (statins).

## C-Reactive Protein Levels and Statin Therapy

In addition to its role in the detection of cardiovascular risk, data has emerged suggesting that CRP levels can be used to improve the targeting of statin therapy. The observation that

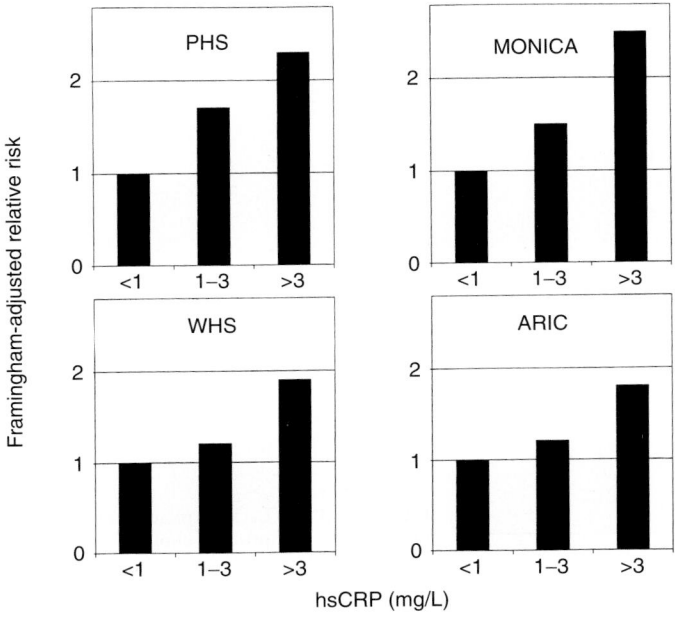

FIGURE 53-11. Framingham-adjusted relative risks of future coronary events according to baseline levels of hsCRP less than 1, 1 to 3, and greater than 3 mg/L in four major cohort studies. (From Ridker PM, Wilson WF, Grundy SM. Should C-reactive protein be added to metabolic syndrome and to assessment of global cardiovascular risk? *Circulation* 2004;109:2818–2825, with permission.)

statins lower CRP levels first emerged from analysis of the Cholesterol and Recurrent Events (CARE) trial in which the long-term use of pravastatin reduced CRP levels in a largely LDL-independent manner (197). Further, this effect had clinical relevance for event reduction in that the benefit of pravastatin in secondary prevention was greatest among those with the highest CRP levels (191). Subsequent studies have shown this to be a class effect with all statins lowering CRP levels (198,199).

Whether or not to use CRP levels to target statin therapy in primary prevention remains highly controversial and is the topic of an ongoing multinational clinical trial (200). *Post hoc* analyses of the Air Force Coronary Atherosclerosis Prevention Study/Texas Coronary Atherosclerosis Prevention Study (AF-CAPS/TexCAPS) clinical trial demonstrate that those with elevated levels of CRP but low levels of LDL cholesterol are not only at high risk for first vascular events but also appear to benefit from statin therapy (201). This observation suggests that statin therapy reduces vascular risk even among those without hyperlipidemia. It is important to recognize, however, that there was no evidence of benefit from statin therapy among those within the AFCAPS/TexCAPS trial who had neither increased lipids nor increased CRP, a group representing approximately 25% of the general population.

Until very recently, no clinical data demonstrated that CRP reduction achieved with statin therapy had prognostic importance independent of LDL reduction also achieved with these agents. However, analyses performed within the Pravastatin or Atorvastatin Evaluation and Infection Therapy (PROVE IT-TIMI-22) clinical trial comparing atorvastatin 80 mg to pravastatin 40 mg, among 3,745 patients with ACS, has recently provided this information (149). In this analysis, "achieved" levels of both LDL cholesterol and CRP were defined as those levels attained after 30 days of therapy, a period adequate for the effects of statin therapy to be seen for both LDL and CRP and for alterations due to the acute event to resolve.

Several important observations regarding LDL, CRP, and statin therapy emerge from this recent analysis of the PROVE IT trial (149). First, levels of achieved LDL as well as achieved CRP were highly associated with recurrent event rates: specifically, among those who achieved LDL levels above and below the approximate median value of 70 mg per dL, rates of recurrent MI or cardiovascular death were 4.0 and 2.7 events per 100 person-years, respectively (P <0.01). However, almost identical recurrent event rates were observed among those with achieved CRP levels above or below the approximate study median of 2 mg per L (3.9 vs. 2.8 events per 100 person-years, P <0.01). This latter effect is important because there was minimal relation between achieved LDL and achieved CRP, data consistent with prior work indicating that the change in CRP associated with statin therapy lacks a relation to changes in LDL cholesterol (see Fig. 53-12). Therefore, patients who had reduced CRP levels as a result of statin therapy had better clinical outcomes than those with higher CRP levels, an effect observed at all levels of achieved LDL.

This new evidence bears directly on the inflammatory hypothesis of atherothrombosis because it provides the first demonstration that CRP reduction per se may in fact result in improved clinical outcomes. Moreover, within the PROVE IT trial, the best cardiovascular event–free survival was observed among those who not only lowered LDL levels below 70 mg per dL, but who also lowered CRP levels below 2 mg per L (see Fig. 53-13). These observations have given rise to the hypothesis that the best use of statin therapy will be a "dual goal" strategy that monitors both LDL and CRP.

CRP analyses from PROVE IT not only demonstrate that CRP reduction lowers vascular risk but also provides insight into the mechanisms by which statin therapy lowers vascular risk. Within the PROVE IT trial as a whole, random allocation to atorvastatin 80 mg significantly lowered vascular event rates compared to pravastatin 40 mg (202). However, while atorvastatin 80 mg was more likely than pravastatin 40 mg to achieve the dual goals of LDL less than 70 mg per dL and CRP less than 2 mg per L, there was no evidence that one statin had a relative advantage over the other once target levels of LDL and CRP were met. Therefore, reducing LDL cholesterol and reducing CRP were of greater clinical importance for individual patients than was the specific choice of statin therapy.

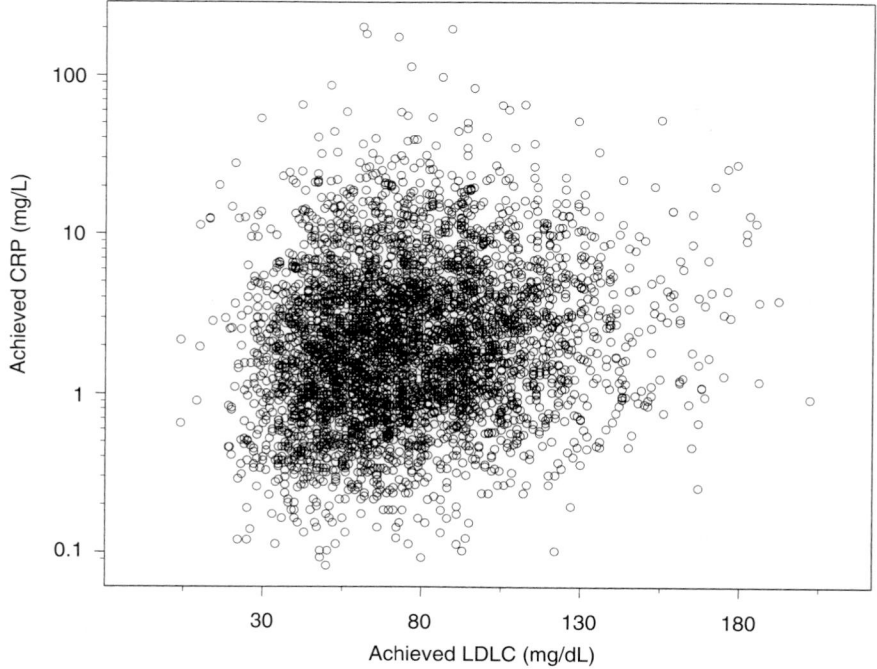

**FIGURE 53-12.** Lack of relation of achieved low density lipoprotein cholesterol (LDLC) levels and achieved C-reactive protein (CRP) levels after 30 days of statin therapy. (From Ridker et al. *N Engl J Med* 2005;325:20–28.)

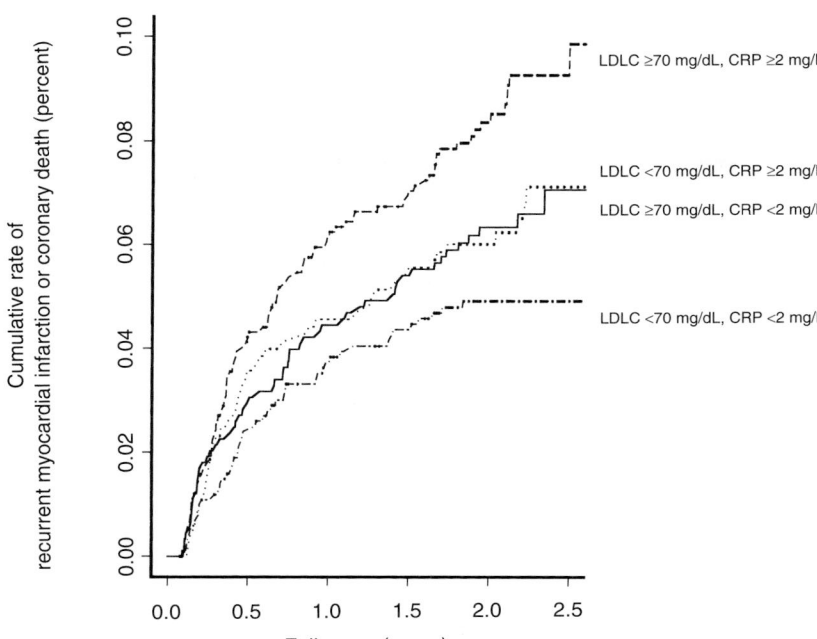

FIGURE 53-13. Incidence rates of recurrent cardiovascular events among patients with acute coronary syndrome, treated with statin therapy according to achieved low density lipoprotein cholesterol (LDLC) and achieved C-reactive protein (CRP) levels. (From Ridker et al. *N Engl J Med* 2005;325: 20–28.)

## SUMMARY

The interrelationships between inflammation, thrombosis, and atherosclerosis have recently come into sharper focus. Current thinking accords a crucial role for thrombosis in the evolution, complication, and acute manifestations of atherosclerosis. In turn, inflammatory signaling pathways appears central in regulating both the formation and thrombotic complications of atherosclerotic lesions. Advances in therapeutics targeting the hemostatic pathways described earlier have already permitted reductions in morbidity and mortality in patients with acute MI. The refinements currently under evaluation should provide further inroads in reducing the ravages of late-stage atheroma. In the long run, the use of antiplatelet therapy (e.g., aspirin) in "primary prevention" might even slow down lesion evolution and progression by limiting asymptomatic mural thrombosis that may stimulate arterial fibrosis and plaque growth. Because platelets can elaborate inflammatory mediators and thrombin can stimulate inflammatory functions of cells involved in atherosclerosis, antiplatelet and anticoagulant therapy might even quell aspects of the inflammatory processes that operate during atherogenesis and plaque complication. Loss of myocardium caused by coronary ischemia is a major cause of heart failure. By mitigating the consequences of plaque thrombosis, and perhaps also by slowing lesion progression, antithrombotic therapy can be viewed as a preventive measure against heart failure, the leading cause for hospitalization in the elderly. The past, studded with controversy about the role of thrombosis in atherosclerosis, has given way to an era in which the intimate links between these processes are not only widely acknowledged but have also given rise to major therapeutic advances. The links between inflammation and atherothrombosis are yielding practical applications that help hone risk stratification and also guide and monitor therapy in the clinic. Few areas of medical investigation have witnessed such rapid translation to practice, and the pace of progress in this area promises continued acceleration in the coming years.

## References

1. Rokitansky K. The organs of circulation. In: Swaine W, Moore C, Sleveking E, et al., eds. *A manual of pathological anatomy*, Philadelphia, PA: Blanchard & Lea, 1855:201–208.
2. Virchow R. *Cellular pathology*. London: John Churchill, 1858.
3. Duguid J. Thrombosis as a factor in the pathogenesis of coronary atherosclerosis. *J Pathol* 1946;58:208–212.
4. Hand R, Chandler A. Atherosclerotic metamorphosis of autologous pulmonary thromboemboli in the rabbit. *Am J Pathol* 1962;40:469–486.
5. Smith EB. Fibrin deposition and fibrin degradation products in atherosclerotic plaques. *Thromb Res* 1994;75:329–335.
6. Bini A, Kudryk BJ. Fibrinogen and fibrin in the arterial wall. *Thromb Res* 1994;75:337–341.
7. Massberg S, Brand K, Gruner S, et al. A critical role of platelet adhesion in the initiation of atherosclerotic lesion formation. *J Exp Med* 2002;196: 887–896.
8. Amento EP, Ehsani N, Palmer H, et al. Cytokines and growth factors positively and negatively regulate interstitial collagen gene expression in human vascular smooth muscle cells. *Arterioscler Thromb Vasc Biol* 1991;11:1223–1230.
9. Fingerle J, Johnson R, Clowes AW, et al. Role of platelets in smooth muscle cell proliferation and migration after vascular injury in rat carotid artery. *Proc Natl Acad Sci U S A* 1989;86:8412–8416.
10. Koyama N, Hart CE, Clowes AW. Different functions of the platelet-derived growth factor-alpha and -beta receptors for the migration and proliferation of cultured baboon smooth muscle cells. *Circ Res* 1994; 75:682–691.
11. Bornfeldt KE, Raines EW, Nakano T, et al. Insulin-like growth factor-I and platelet-derived growth factor-BB induce directed migration of human arterial smooth muscle cells via signaling pathways that are distinct from those of proliferation. *J Clin Invest* 1994;93:1266–1274.
12. Jawien A, Bowen PDF, Lindner V, et al. Platelet-derived growth factor promotes smooth muscle migration and intimal thickening in a rat model of balloon angioplasty. *J Clin Invest* 1992;89:507–511.
13. McNamara CA, Sarembock IJ, Gimple LW, et al. Thrombin stimulates proliferation of cultured rat aortic smooth muscle cells by a proteolytically activated receptor. *J Clin Invest* 1993;91:94–98.
14. Kranzhöfer R, Clinton SK, Ishii K, et al. Thrombin potently induces cytokine production by human vascular smooth muscle cells but not in mononuclear phagocytes. *Circ Res* 1996;79:286–294.
15. Coughlin SR. Sol Sherry lecture in thrombosis: how thrombin 'talks' to cells: molecular mechanisms and roles *in vivo*. *Arterioscler Thromb Vasc Biol* 1998;18:514–518.
16. Coughlin SR. How the protease thrombin talks to cells. *Proc Natl Acad Sci U S A* 1999;96:11023–11027.
17. Mach F, Schoenbeck U, Bonnefoy J-Y, et al. Activation of monocyte/macrophage functions related to acute atheroma complication by ligation

of CD40. Induction of collagenase, stromelysin, and tissue factor. *Circulation* 1997;96:396–399.

18. Schonbeck U, Mach F, Sukhova GK, et al. CD40 ligation induces tissue factor expression in human vascular smooth muscle cells. *Am J Pathol* 2000;156:7–14.

19. Libby P, Simon DI. Inflammation and thrombosis: the clot thickens. *Circulation* 2001;103:1718–1720.

20. Kruth HS. The fate of lipoprotein cholesterol entering the arterial wall. *Curr Opin Lipidol* 1997;8:246–252.

21. Schwenke DC, Carew TE. Initiation of atherosclerotic lesions in cholesterol-fed rabbits. I. Focal increases in arterial LDL concentration precede development of fatty streak lesions. *Arteriosclerosis* 1989;9:895–907.

22. Schwenke DC, Carew TE. Initiation of atherosclerotic lesions in cholesterol-fed rabbits. II. Selective retention of LDL vs. selective increases in LDL permeability in susceptible sites of arteries. *Arteriosclerosis* 1989;9:908–918.

23. Herrmann RA, Malinauskas RA, Truskey GA. Characterization of sites with elevated LDL permeability at intercostal, celiac, and iliac branches of the normal rabbit aorta. *Arterioscler Thromb* 1994;14:313–323.

24. Williams KJ, Tabas I. The response-to-retention hypothesis of atherogenesis reinforced. *Curr Opin Lipidol* 1998;9:471–474.

25. Tabas I. Nonoxidative modifications of lipoproteins in atherogenesis. *Annu Rev Nutr* 1999;19:123–139.

26. Nievelstein PF, Fogelman AM, Mottino G, et al. Lipid accumulation in rabbit aortic intima 2 hours after bolus infusion of low density lipoprotein. A deep-etch and immunolocalization study of ultrarapidly frozen tissue. *Arterioscler Thromb* 1991;11:1795–1805.

27. Camejo G, Hurt-Camejo E, Wiklund O, et al. Association of apo B lipoproteins with arterial proteoglycans: pathological significance and molecular basis. *Atherosclerosis* 1998;139:205–222.

28. Witztum JL, Steinbrecher UP, Fisher M, et al. Nonenzymatic glucosylation of homologous low density lipoprotein and albumin renders them immunogenic in the guinea pig. *Proc Natl Acad Sci U S A* 1983;80: 2757–2761.

29. Rajavashisth TB, Andalibi A, Territo MC, et al. Induction of endothelial cell expression of granulocyte and macrophage colony-stimulating factors by modified low-density lipoproteins. *Nature* 1990;344:254–257.

30. Clinton S, Underwood R, Sherman M, et al. Macrophage-colony stimulating factor gene expression in vascular cells and in experimental and human atherosclerosis. *Am J Pathol* 1992;140:301–316.

31. Berliner J, Leitinger N, Watson A, et al. Oxidized lipids in atherogenesis: formation, destruction and action. *Thromb Haemost* 1997;78:195–199.

32. Poole JCF, Florey HW. Changes in the endothelium of the aorta and the behavior of macrophages in experimental atheroma of rabbits. *J Path Bacteriol* 1958;75:245–253.

33. Faggiotto A, Ross R, Harker L. Studies of hypercholesterolemia in the nonhuman primate. I. Changes that lead to fatty streak formation. *Arteriosclerosis* 1984;4:323–340.

34. Hajjar DP, Haberland ME. Lipoprotein trafficking in vascular cells. Molecular Trojan horses and cellular saboteurs. *J Biol Chem* 1997;272: 22975–22978.

35. Virmani R, Robinowitz M, Geer JC, et al. Coronary artery atherosclerosis revisited in Korean war combat casualties. *Arch Pathol Lab Med* 1987; 111:972–976.

36. Joseph A, Ackerman D, Talley JD, et al. Manifestations of coronary atherosclerosis in young trauma victims—an autopsy study. *J Am Coll Cardiol* 1993;22:459–467.

37. Strong JP, Malcom GT, Oalmann MC, et al. The PDAY Study: natural history, risk factors, and pathobiology. Pathobiological determinants of atherosclerosis in youth. *Ann N Y Acad Sci* 1997;811:226–235.

38. Komatsu A, Sakurai I, The Pathobiological Determinants of Atherosclerosis in Youth (PDAY) Research Group. A study of the development of atherosclerosis in childhood and young adults: risk factors and the prevention of progression in Japan and the USA. *Pathol Int* 1996;46: 541–547.

39. Cybulsky MI, Gimbrone MA Jr. Endothelial expression of a mononuclear leukocyte adhesion molecule during atherogenesis. *Science* 1991;251: 788–791.

40. Davies MJ, Gordon JL, Gearing AJ, et al. The expression of the adhesion molecules ICAM-1, VCAM-1, PECAM, and E-selectin in human atherosclerosis. *J Pathol* 1993;171:223–229.

41. Li H, Cybulsky MI, Gimbrone MA Jr, et al. An atherogenic diet rapidly induces VCAM-1, a cytokine regulatable mononuclear leukocyte adhesion molecule, in rabbit endothelium. *Arterioscler Thromb* 1993;13: 197–204.

42. Nakashima Y, Raines EW, Plump AS, et al. Upregulation of VCAM-1 and ICAM-1 at atherosclerosis-prone sites on the endothelium in the apoE-deficient mouse. *Arterioscler Thromb Vasc Biol* 1998;18:842–851.

43. Faggiotto A, Ross R. Studies of hypercholesterolemia in the nonhuman primate. II. Fatty streak conversion to fibrous plaque. *Arteriosclerosis* 1984;4:341–356.

44. Davies MJ, Woolf N, Rowles PM, et al. Morphology of the endothelium over atherosclerotic plaques in human coronary arteries. *Br Heart J* 1988;60:459–464.

45. Davies MJ. A macro and micro view of coronary vascular insult in ischemic heart disease. *Circulation* 1990;82:II38–II46.

46. Davies MJ. Anatomic features in victims of sudden coronary death. Coronary artery pathology. *Circulation* 1992;85:I19–I24.

47. Davies MJ. The investigation of sudden cardiac death. *Histopathology* 1999;34:93–98.

48. Robbie LA, Booth NA, Brown AJ, et al. Inhibitors of fibrinolysis are elevated in atherosclerotic plaque. *Arterioscler Thromb Vasc Biol* 1996;16: 539–545.

49. Wilcox JN, Smith KM, Williams LT, et al. Platelet-derived growth factor mRNA detection in human atherosclerotic plaques by in situ hybridization. *J Clin Invest* 1988;82:1134–1143.

50. Loskutoff DJ, Van Mourik JA, Erickson LA, et al. Detection of an unusually stable fibrinolytic inhibitor produced by bovine endothelial cells. *Cell Biol* 1983;80:2956–2960.

51. Harlan JM, Thompson PJ, Ross RR, et al. Alpha-thrombin induces release of platelet-derived growth factor-like molecule(s) by cultured human endothelial cells. *J Cell Biol* 1986;103:1129–1133.

52. Glagov S, Weisenberg E, Zarins C, et al. Compensatory enlargement of human atherosclerotic coronary arteries. *N Engl J Med* 1987;316: 371–375.

53. Clarkson TB, Prichard RW, Morgan TM, et al. Remodeling of coronary arteries in human and nonhuman primates. *JAMA* 1994;271:289–294.

54. Brogi E, Winkles J, Underwood R, et al. Distinct patterns of expression of fibroblast growth factors and their receptors in human atheroma and nonatherosclerotic arteries: association of acidic FGF with plaque microvessels and macrophages. *J Clin Invest* 1993;92:2408–2418.

55. Inoue M, Itoh H, Ueda M, et al. Vascular endothelial growth factor (VEGF) expression in human coronary atherosclerotic lesions: possible pathophysiological significance of VEGF in progression of atherosclerosis. *Circulation* 1998;98:2108–2116.

56. Ramos MA, Kuzuya M, Esaki T, et al. Induction of macrophage VEGF in response to oxidized LDL and VEGF accumulation in human atherosclerotic lesions. *Arterioscler Thromb Vasc Biol* 1998;18:1188–1196.

57. Wight TN. The extracellular matrix and atherosclerosis. *Curr Opin Lipidol* 1995;6:326–334.

58. Demer LL. A skeleton in the atherosclerosis closet. *Circulation* 1995; 92:2029–2032.

59. Giachelli CM. Vascular calcification mechanisms. *J Am Soc Nephrol* 2004; 15:2959–2964.

60. Farb A, Burke A, Tang A, et al. Coronary plaque erosion without rupture into a lipid core. A frequent cause of coronary thrombosis in sudden coronary death. *Circulation* 1996;93:1354–1363.

61. van der Wal AC, Becker AE, van der Loos CM, et al. Site of intimal rupture or erosion of thrombosed coronary atherosclerotic plaques is characterized by an inflammatory process irrespective of the dominant plaque morphology. *Circulation* 1994;89:36–44.

62. Burke AP, Farb A, Malcom GT, et al. Effect of risk factors on the mechanism of acute thrombosis and sudden coronary death in women. *Circulation* 1998;97:2110–2116.

63. Virmani R, Farb A, Burke AP. Risk factors in the pathogenesis of coronary artery disease. *Compr Ther* 1998;24:519–529.

64. Constantinides P. Plaque hemorrhages, their genesis and their role in supraplaque thrombosis and atherogenesis. In: Glagov S, Newman WP, Schaffer SA, eds. *Pathobiology of the Human Atherosclerotic Plaque*. New York: Springer-Verlag, 1989:393–412.

65. Falk E. Plaque rupture with severe pre-existing stenosis precipitating coronary thrombosis characteristics of coronary atherosclerotic plaques underlying fatal occlusive thrombi. *Br Heart J* 1983;50:127–134.

66. Davies MJ, Thomas T. The pathological basis and microanatomy of occlusive thrombus formation in human coronary arteries. *Philos Trans R Soc Lond B Biol Sci* 1981;294:225–229.

67. Davies M. The composition of coronary-artery plaques. *N Engl J Med* 1997;336:1312–1314.

68. Wilcox JN, Smith KM, Schwartz SM, et al. Localization of tissue factor in the normal vessel wall and in the atherosclerotic plaque. *Proc Natl Acad Sci U S A* 1989;86:2839–2843.

69. Drake TA, Morrissey JH, Edgington TS. Selective cellular expression of tissue factor in human tissues. Implications for disorders of hemostasis and thrombosis. *Am J Pathol* 1989;134:1087–1097.

70. Davies MJ. Stability and instability: the two faces of coronary atherosclerosis. The Paul Dudley White Lecture, 1995. *Circulation* 1996;94: 2013–2020.

71. Libby P, Theroux P. Pathophysiology of coronary artery disease. *Circulation* 2005;111:3481–3488.

72. Falk E, Shah P, Fuster V. Coronary plaque disruption. *Circulation* 1995; 92:657–671.

73. Ross R. Atherosclerosis: the role of endothelial injury, smooth muscle proliferation and platelet factors. *Triangle* 1976;15:45–51.

74. Geng Y-J, Henderson L, Levesque E, et al. Fas is expressed in human atherosclerotic intima and promotes apoptosis of cytokine-primed humann vascular smooth muscle cells. *Arterioscler Thromb Vasc Biol* 1997;17: 2200–2208.

75. Hanemaaijer R, Koolwijk P, le Clercq L, et al. Regulation of matrix metalloproteinase expression in human vein and microvascular endothelial cells. Effects of tumour necrosis factor alpha, interleukin 1 and phorbol ester. *Biochem J* 1993;296:803–809.

76. Mach F, Schonbeck U, Fabunni RP, et al. T lymphocytes induce endothelial cell matrix metalloproteinase expression by a CD40L-dependent mechanism: implications for tubule formation. *Am J Pathol* 1999;154: 229–238.

77. Rajavashisth TB, Liao JK, Galis ZS, et al. Inflammatory cytokines and oxidized low density lipoproteins increase endothelial cell expression of

membrane type 1-matrix metalloproteinase. *J Biol Chem* 1999;274: 11924–11929.

78. Sperti G, van Leeuwen RT, Quax PH, et al. Cultured rat aortic vascular smooth muscle cells digest naturally produced extracellular matrix. Involvement of plasminogen-dependent and plasminogen-independent pathways. *Circ Res* 1992;71:385–392.

79. Carmeliet P, Moons L, Lijnen R, et al. Urokinase-generated plasmin activates matrix metalloproteinases during aneurysm formation. *Nat Genet* 1997;17:439–444.

80. Galis Z, Kranzhoefer R, Fenton JI, et al. Thrombin promotes activation of matrix metalloproteinase-2 produced by cultured vascular smooth muscle cells. *Arterioscler Thromb Vasc Biol* 1997;17:483–489.

81. Henney AM, Wakeley PR, Davies MJ, et al. Localization of stromelysin gene expression in atherosclerotic plaques by in situ hybridization. *Proc Natl Acad Sci U S A* 1991;88:8154–8158.

82. Galis Z, Sukhova G, Lark M, et al. Increased expression of matrix metalloproteinases and matrix degrading activity in vulnerable regions of human atherosclerotic plaques. *J Clin Invest* 1994;94:2493–2503.

83. Nikkari ST, O'Brien KD, Ferguson M, et al. Interstitial collagenase (MMP-1) expression in human carotid atherosclerosis. *Circulation* 1995; 92:1393–1398.

84. Sukhova GK, Schonbeck U, Rabkin E, et al. Evidence for increased collagenolysis by interstitial collagenases-1 and -3 in vulnerable human atheromatous plaques. *Circulation* 1999;99:2503–2509.

85. Sukhova GK, Shi GP, Simon DI, et al. Expression of the elastolytic cathepsins S and K in human atheroma and regulation of their production in smooth muscle cells. *J Clin Invest* 1998;102:576–583.

86. Curci JA, Liao S, Huffman MD, et al. Expression and localization of macrophage elastase (matrix metalloproteinase-12) in abdominal aortic aneurysms. *J Clin Invest* 1998;102:1900–1910.

87. Hansson GK, Libby P, Schonbeck U, et al. Innate and adaptive immunity in the pathogenesis of atherosclerosis. *Circ Res* 2002;91:281–291.

88. Libby P. The molecular bases of the acute coronary syndromes. *Circulation* 1995;91:2844–2850.

89. Geng Y-J, Libby P. Evidence for apoptosis in advanced human atheroma. Co-localization with interleukin-1 b-converting enzyme. *Am J Pathol* 1995;147:251–266.

90. Geng Y-J, Wu Q, Muszynski M, et al. Apoptosis of vascular smooth muscle cells induced by *in vitro* stimulation with interferon-gamma, tumor necrosis factor-alpha, and interleukin-1-beta. *Arterioscler Thromb Vasc Biol* 1996;16:19–27.

91. Plump AS, Smith JD, Hayek T, et al. Severe hypercholesterolemia and atherosclerosis in apolipoprotein E-deficient mice created by homologous recombination in ES cells. *Cell* 1992;71:343–353.

92. Zhang SH, Reddick RL, Piedrahita JA, et al. Spontaneous hypercholesterolemia and arterial lesions in mice lacking apolipoprotein E. *Science* 1992;258:468–471.

93. Ishibashi S, Brown MS, Goldstein JL, et al. Hypercholesterolemia in low density lipoprotein receptor knockout mice and its reversal by adenovirus-mediated gene delivery. *J Clin Invest* 1993;92:883–893.

94. Gu L, Okada Y, Clinton S, et al. Absence of monocyte chemoattractant protein-1 reduces atherosclerosis in low-density lipoprotein-deficient mice. *Mol Cell* 1998;2:275–281.

95. Smith JD, Trogan E, Ginsberg M, et al. Decreased atherosclerosis in mice deficient in both macrophage colony-stimulating factor (op) and apolipoprotein E. *Proc Natl Acad Sci U S A* 1995;92:8264–8268.

96. Qiao JH, Tripathi J, Mishra NK, et al. Role of macrophage colony-stimulating factor in atherosclerosis: studies of osteopetrotic mice. *Am J Pathol* 1997;150:1687–1699.

97. Rajavashisth T, Qiao JH, Tripathi S, et al. Heterozygous osteopetrotic (op) mutation reduces atherosclerosis in LDL receptor-deficient mice. *J Clin Invest* 1998;101:2702–2710.

98. Gupta S, Pablo AM, Jiang X, et al. IFN-gamma potentiates atherosclerosis in ApoE knock-out mice. *J Clin Invest* 1997;99:2752–2761.

99. Suzuki H, Kurihara Y, Takeya M, et al. A role for macrophage scavenger receptors in atherosclerosis and susceptibility to infection. *Nature* 1997; 386:292–296.

100. Kozaki K, Kaminski WE, Tang J, et al. Blockade of platelet-derived growth factor or its receptors transiently delays but does not prevent fibrous cap formation in ApoE null mice. *Am J Pathol* 2002;161: 1395–1407.

101. Raines EW, Ross R. Platelet-derived growth factor. I. High yield purification and evidence for multiple forms. *J Biol Chem* 1982;257:5154–5160.

102. Caligiuri G, Levy B, Pernow J, et al. Myocardial infarction mediated by endothelin receptor signaling in hypercholesterolemic mice. *Proc Natl Acad Sci U S A* 1999;96:6920–6924.

103. Rosenfeld ME, Polinsky P, Virmani R, et al. Advanced atherosclerotic lesions in the innominate artery of the ApoE knockout mouse. *Arterioscler Thromb Vasc Biol* 2000;20:2587–2592.

104. Williams H, Johnson JL, Carson KG, et al. Characteristics of intact and ruptured atherosclerotic plaques in brachiocephalic arteries of apolipoprotein E knockout mice. *Arterioscler Thromb Vasc Biol* 2002;22: 788–792.

105. DeWood MA, Spores J, Notske R, et al. Prevalence of total coronary occlusion during the early hours of transmural myocardial infarction. *N Engl J Med* 1980;303:897–902.

106. Sherman CT, Litvack F, Grundfest W, et al. Coronary angioscopy in patients with unstable angina pectoris. *N Engl J Med* 1986;315:913–919.

107. Reimer KA, Lowe JE, Rasmussen MM, et al. The wavefront phenomenon of ischemic cell death. I. Myocardial infarct size vs duration of coronary occlusion in dogs. *Circulation* 1977;56:786–794.

108. Reimer KA, Jennings RB. The "wavefront phenomenon" of myocardial ischemic cell death: II. Transmural progression of necrosis within the framework of ischemic bed size (myocardium at risk) and collateral flow. *Lab Invest* 1979;40:633–644.

109. Maroko P, Libby P, Ginks W, et al. Coronary artery reperfusion: I. Early effects on local myocardial function and the extent of myocardial necrosis. *J Clin Invest* 1972;51:2710–2717.

110. Fibrinolytic Therapy Trialists' (FTT) Collaborative Group. Indications for fibrinolytic therapy in suspected acute myocardial infarction: collaborative overview of early mortality and major morbidity results from all randomised trials of more than 1000 patients. *Lancet* 1994;343:311–322.

111. ISIS-2, Collaborative, Group. Randomized trial of IV streptokinase, oral aspirin, both, or neither among 17,187 cases of suspected acute myocardial infarction. *Lancet* 1988;2:349–360.

112. Thrombolytic AotSaEoaN, Investigators. Single-bolus tenecteplase compared with front-loaded alteplase in acute myocardial infarction: the AS-SENT-2 double-blind randomized trial. *Lancet* 1999;354:716–722.

113. Antiplatelet Trialists' Collaboration. Secondary prevention of vascular disease by prolonged antiplatelet treatment. *Br Med J (Clin Res Ed)* 1988; 296:320–331.

114. Grines CL, Cox DA, Stone GW et al, Stent Primary Angioplasty in Myocardial Infarction Study Group. Coronary angioplasty with or without stent implantation for acute myocardial infarction. *N Engl J Med* 1999;341:1949–1956.

115. Keeley EC, Boura JA, Grines CL. Primary angioplasty versus intravenous thrombolytic therapy for acute myocardial infarction: a quantitative review of 23 randomized trials. *Lancet* 2003;361:13–20.

116. Aversano T, Aversano LT, Passamani E, et al. Thrombolytic therapy vs primary percutaneous coronary intervention for myocardial infarction in patients presenting to hospitals without on-site cardiac surgery: a randomized controlled trial. *JAMA* 2002;287:1943–1951.

117. Andersen HR, Nielsen TT, Rasmussen K, et al. A comparison of coronary angioplasty with fibrinolytic therapy in acute myocardial infarction. *N Engl J Med* 2003;349:733–742.

118. Antman EM, Anbe DT, Armstrong PW, et al. ACC/AHA guidelines for the management of patients with ST-elevation myocardial infarction—executive summary: a report of the American College of Cardiology/American Heart Association Task Force on Practice Guidelines (Writing Committee to Revise the 1999 Guidelines for the Management of Patients With Acute Myocardial Infarction). *Circulation* 2004;110:588–636.

119. Herrmann HC. Triple therapy for acute myocardial infarction: combining fibrinolysis, platelet IIb/IIIa inhibition, and percutaneous coronary intervention. *Am J Cardiol* 2000;85:10C–16C.

120. Stone GW. Primary angioplasty versus "earlier" thrombolysis—time for a wake-up call. *Lancet* 2002;360:814–816.

121. Stone GW, Cox DA, Babb J, et al. Prospective, randomized evaluation of thrombectomy prior to percutaneous intervention in diseased saphenous vein grafts and thrombus-containing coronary arteries. *J Am Coll Cardiol* 2003;42:2007–2013.

122. Baim D, Wahr D, George B, et al. Randomized trial of a distal embolic protection device during percutaneous intervention of saphenous vein aorto-coronary bypass grafts. *Circulation* 2002;105:1285–1290.

123. Stone G, Rogers C, Ramee S, et al. Distal filter protection during saphenous vein graft stenting: technical and clinical correlates of efficacy. *J Am Coll Cardiol* 2002;40:1882–1888.

124. Topol EJ, Byzova TV, Plow EF. Platelet GPIIb-IIIa blockers. *Lancet* 1999;353:227–231.

125. Karvouni E, Katritsis DG, Ioannidis JP. Intravenous glycoprotein IIb/IIIa receptor antagonists reduce mortality after percutaneous coronary interventions. *J Am Coll Cardiol* 2003;41:26–32.

126. Lincoff AM, Kereiakes DJ, Mascelli MA, et al. Abciximab suppresses the rise in levels of circulating inflammatory markers after percutaneous coronary revascularization. *Circulation* 2001;104:163–167.

127. Welt FG, Rogers SD, Zhang X, et al. GP IIb/IIIa inhibition with eptifibatide lowers levels of soluble CD40L and RANTES after percutaneous coronary intervention. *Catheter Cardiovasc Interv* 2004;61:185–189.

128. Antman EM, Giugliano RP, Gibson CM, et al. Abciximab facilitates the rate and extent of thrombolysis: results of the thrombolysis in myocardial infarction (TIMI) 14 trial. *Circulation* 1999;99:2720–2732.

129. Gibson CM, Cannon CP, Murphy SA, et al. Relationship of TIMI myocardial perfusion grade to mortality after administration of thrombolytic drugs. *Circulation* 2000;101:125–130.

130. Kastrati A, Mehilli J, Schlotterbeck K, et al. Early administration of reteplase plus abciximab vs abciximab alone in patients with acute myocardial infarction referred for percutaneous coronary intervention: a randomized controlled trial. *JAMA* 2004;291:947–954.

131. Lincoff AM, Califf RM, Van de Werf F, et al. Mortality at 1 year with combination platelet glycoprotein IIb/IIIa inhibition and reduced-dose fibrinolytic therapy vs conventional fibrinolytic therapy for acute myocardial infarction: GUSTO V randomized trial. *JAMA* 2002;288: 2130–2135.

132. Weitz JI, Hudoba M, Massel D, et al. Clot-bound thrombin is protected from inhibition by heparin-antithrombin III but is susceptible to inactivation by antithrombin III-independent inhibitors. *J Clin Invest* 1990; 86: 385–391.

133. Hirsh J, Dalen JE, Deykin D, et al. Heparin: mechanism of action, pharmacokinetics, dosing considerations, monitoring, efficacy, and safety. *Chest* 1992;102:337S–351S.
134. Antman EM. Hirudin in acute myocardial infarction. Thrombolysis and thrombin inhibition in myocardial infarction (TIMI) 9B trial. *Circulation* 1996;94:911–921.
135. Investigators. TGUoStOOAGI. A comparison of recombinant hirudin with heparin for the treatment of acute coronary syndromes. *N Engl J Med* 1996;335:775–782.
136. Lincoff AM, Bittl JA, Harrington RA, et al. Bivalirudin and provisional glycoprotein IIb/IIIa blockade compared with heparin and planned glycoprotein IIb/IIIa blockade during percutaneous coronary intervention: REPLACE-2 randomized trial. *JAMA* 2003;289:853–863.
137. Hirsh J, Levine MN. Low molecular weight heparin. *Blood* 1992; 79: 1–17.
138. Cohen M, Demers C, Gurfinkel EP, et al. A comparison of low-molecular-weight heparin with unfractionated heparin for unstable coronary artery disease. *N Engl J Med* 1997;337:447–452.
139. Antman EM, McCabe CH, Gurfinkel EP, et al. Enoxaparin prevents death and cardiac ischemic events in unstable angina/non-Q-wave myocardial infarction results of the Thrombolysis in Myocardial Infarction (TIMI) 11B Trial. *Circulation* 1999;100:1593–1601.
140. Ferguson JJ, Califf RM, Antman EM, et al. Enoxaparin vs unfractionated heparin in high-risk patients with non-ST-segment elevation acute coronary syndromes managed with an intended early invasive strategy: primary results of the SYNERGY randomized trial. *JAMA* 2004;292:45–54.
141. Physicians', Health, Study, Research, Group. Final report on the aspirin component of the ongoing Physicians' Health Study. Steering Committee of the Physicians' Health Study Research Group. *N Engl J Med* 1989;321: 129–135.
142. Antiplatelet, Trialists', Collaboration. Collaborative overview of randomized trials of antiplatelet therapy—1. Prevention of death, myocardial infarction, and stroke by prolonged antiplatelet therapy in various categories of patients. *Br Med J* 1994;308:81–106.
143. Yusuf S, Sleight P, Pogue J et al. The Heart Outcomes Prevention Evaluation Study Investigators. Effects of an angiotensin-converting-enzyme inhibitor, ramipril, on cardiovascular events in high-risk patients. *N Engl J Med* 2000;342:145–153.
144. Sacks FM, Pfeffer MA, Moye LA, et al. The effect of pravastatin on coronary events after myocardial infarction in patients with average cholesterol levels. Cholesterol and Recurrent Events Trial Investigators. *N Engl J Med* 1996;335:1001–1009.
145. Yusuf S, Zhao F, Mehta SR, et al. Effects of clopidogrel in addition to aspirin in patients with acute coronary syndromes without ST-segment elevation. *N Engl J Med* 2001;345:494–502.
146. Schomig A, Neumann FJ, Kastrati A, et al. A randomized comparison of antiplatelet and anticoagulant therapy after the placement of coronary-artery stents. *N Engl J Med* 1996;334:1084–1089.
147. Leon MB, Baim DS, Popma JJ et al. Stent Anticoagulation Restenosis Study Investigators. A clinical trial comparing three antithrombotic-drug regimens after coronary-artery stenting. *N Engl J Med* 1998;339:1665–1671.
148. Anand SS, Yusuf S, Pogue J, et al. Long-term oral anticoagulant therapy in patients with unstable angina or suspected non-Q-wave myocardial infarction: organization to assess strategies for ischemic syndromes (OASIS) pilot study results. *Circulation* 1998;98:1064–1070.
149. Ridker PM, Cannon CP, Morrow D, et al. C-reactive protein levels and outcomes after statin therapy. *N Engl J Med* 2005;352:20–28.
150. Moons AH, Peters RJ, Bijsterveld NR, et al. Recombinant nematode anticoagulant protein c2, an inhibitor of the tissue factor/factor VIIa complex, in patients undergoing elective coronary angioplasty. *J Am Coll Cardiol* 2003;41:2147–2153.
151. Wong NN. Fondaparinux: a synthetic selective factor-Xa inhibitor. *Heart Dis* 2003;5:295–302.
152. Ridker PM, Rifai N, Pfeffer M, et al. Elevation of tumor necrosis factor-alpha and increased risk of recurrent coronary events after myocardial infarction. *Circulation* 2000;101:2149–2153.
153. Ridker PM, Hennekens CH, Roitman-Johnson B, et al. Plasma concentration of soluble intercellular adhesion molecule 1 and risks of future myocardial infarction in apparently healthy men. *Lancet* 1998;351:88–92.
154. Pradhan AD, Rifai N, Ridker PM. Soluble intercellular adhesion molecule-1, soluble vascular adhesion molecule-1, and the development of symptomatic peripheral arterial disease in men. *Circulation* 2002;106:820–825.
155. Ridker PM, Buring JE, Rifai N. Soluble P-selectin and the risk of future cardiovascular events. *Circulation* 2001;103:491–495.
156. Brown DA, Breit SN, Buring J, et al. Concentration in plasma of macrophage inhibitory cytokine-1 and risk of cardiovascular events in women: a nested case-control study. *Lancet* 2002;359:2159–2163.
157. Packard CJ, O'Reilly DS, Caslake MJ et al, West of Scotland Coronary Prevention Study Group. Lipoprotein-associated phospholipase A2 as an independent predictor of coronary heart disease. *N Engl J Med* 2000; 343:1148–1155.
158. Ballantyne CM, Hoogeveen RC, Bang H, et al. Lipoprotein-associated phospholipase A2, high-sensitivity C-reactive protein, and risk for incident coronary heart disease in middle-aged men and women in the Atherosclerosis Risk in Communities (ARIC) Study. *Circulation* 2004;109: 837–842.
159. Biasucci LM, Liuzzo G, Fantuzzi G, et al. Increasing levels of interleukin (IL)-1Ra and IL-6 during the first 2 days of hospitalization in unstable angina are associated with increased risk of in-hospital coronary events. *Circulation* 1999;99:2079–2084.
160. Ridker PM, Rifai N, Stampfer MJ, et al. Plasma concentration of interleukin-6 and the risk of future myocardial infarction among apparently healthy men. *Circulation* 2000;101:1767–1772.
161. Boekholdt SM, Peters RJ, Hack CE, et al. IL-8 plasma concentrations and the risk of future coronary artery disease in apparently healthy men and women: the EPIC-Norfolk prospective population study. *Arterioscler Thromb Vasc Biol* 2004;24:1503–1508.
162. Zhang R, Brennan ML, Fu X, et al. Association between myeloperoxidase levels and risk of coronary artery disease. *JAMA* 2001;286:2136–2142.
163. Brennan ML, Penn MS, Van Lente F, et al. Prognostic value of myeloperoxidase in patients with chest pain. *N Engl J Med* 2003;349:1595–1604.
164. Bayes-Genis A, Conover CA, Overgaard MT, et al. Pregnancy-associated plasma protein A as a marker of acute coronary syndromes. *N Engl J Med* 2001;345:1022–1029.
165. Schonbeck U, Varo N, Libby P, et al. Soluble CD40L and cardiovascular risk in women. *Circulation* 2001;104:2266–2268.
166. Varo N, Vicent D, Libby P, et al. Elevated plasma levels of the atherogenic mediator soluble CD40 ligand in diabetic patients: a novel target of thiazolidinediones. *Circulation* 2003;107:2664–2669.
167. Ridker PM. Clinical application of C-reactive protein for cardiovascular disease detection and prevention. *Circulation* 2003;107:363–369.
168. Pearson TA, Mensah GA, Alexander RW, et al. Markers of inflammation and cardiovascular disease: application to clinical and public health practice: a statement for healthcare professionals from the Centers for Disease Control and Prevention and the American Heart Association. *Circulation* 2003;107:499–511.
169. Danenberg HD, Szalai AJ, Swaminathan RV, et al. Increased thrombosis after arterial injury in human C-reactive protein-transgenic mice. *Circulation* 2003;108:512–515.
170. Ridker PM, Cushman M, Stampfer MJ, et al. Inflammation, aspirin, and the risk of cardiovascular disease in apparently healthy men. *N Engl J Med* 1997;336:973–979.
171. Ridker PM, Rifai N, Rose L, et al. Comparison of C-reactive protein and low-density lipoprotein cholesterol levels in the prediction of first cardiovascular events. *N Engl J Med* 2002;347:1557–1565.
172. Ridker PM, Hennekens CH, Buring JE, et al. C-reactive protein and other markers of inflammation in the prediction of cardiovascular disease in women. *N Engl J Med* 2000;342:836–843.
173. Ridker PM, Stampfer MJ, Rifai N. Novel risk factors for systemic atherosclerosis: a comparison of C-reactive protein, fibrinogen, homocysteine, lipoprotein(a), and standard cholesterol screening as predictors of peripheral arterial disease. *JAMA* 2001;285:2481–2485.
174. Koenig W, Lowel H, Baumert J, et al. C-reactive protein modulates risk prediction based on the Framingham Score: implications for future risk assessment: results from a large cohort study in southern Germany. *Circulation* 2004;109:1349–1353.
175. Albert MA, Glynn RJ, Ridker PM. Plasma concentration of C-reactive protein and the calculated Framingham Coronary Heart Disease Risk Score. *Circulation* 2003;108:161–165.
176. Danesh J, Wheeler JG, Hirschfield GM, et al. C-reactive protein and other circulating markers of inflammation in the prediction of coronary heart disease. *N Engl J Med* 2004;350:1387–1397.
177. Ridker PM, Buring JE, Cook NR, et al. C-reactive protein, the metabolic syndrome, and risk of incident cardiovascular events: an 8-year follow-up of 14,719 initially healthy American women. *Circulation* 2003;107:391–397.
178. Sattar N, Gaw A, Scherbakova O, et al. Metabolic syndrome with and without C-reactive protein as a predictor of coronary heart disease and diabetes in the West of Scotland Coronary Prevention Study. *Circulation* 2003;108:414–419.
179. Sesso HD, Buring JE, Rifai N, et al. C-reactive protein and the risk of developing hypertension. *JAMA* 2003;290:2945–2951.
180. Pradhan AD, Cook NR, Buring JE, et al. C-reactive protein is independently associated with fasting insulin in nondiabetic women. *Arterioscler Thromb Vasc Biol* 2003;23:650–655.
181. Freeman DJ, Norrie J, Caslake MJ, et al. C-reactive protein is an independent predictor of risk for the development of diabetes in the West of Scotland Coronary Prevention Study. *Diabetes* 2002;51:1596–1600.
182. Pradhan AD, Manson JE, Rifai N, et al. C-reactive protein, interleukin 6, and risk of developing type 2 diabetes mellitus. *JAMA* 2001;286: 327–334.
183. Festa A, D'Agostino R Jr, Tracy RP, et al. Elevated levels of acute-phase proteins and plasminogen activator inhibitor-1 predict the development of type 2 diabetes: the insulin resistance atherosclerosis study. *Diabetes* 2002; 51:1131–1137.
184. Sabatine MS, Morrow DA, de Lemos JA, et al. Multimarker approach to risk stratification in non-ST elevation acute coronary syndromes: simultaneous assessment of troponin I, C-reactive protein, and B-type natriuretic peptide. *Circulation* 2002;105:1760–1763.
185. Liuzzo G, Biasucci LM, Gallimore JR, et al. The prognostic value of C-reactive protein and serum amyloid A protein in severe unstable angina. *N Eng J Med* 1994;331:417–424.
186. Morrow DA, Rifai N, Antman EM, et al. C-reactive protein is a potent predictor of mortality independently of and in combination with troponin T in acute coronary syndromes: a TIMI 11A substudy. Thrombolysis in Myocardial Infarction. *J Am Coll Cardiol* 1998;31:1460–1465.

187. Lindahl B, Toss H, Siegbahn A et al. FRISC Study Group. Fragmin during Instability in Coronary Artery Disease. Markers of myocardial damage and inflammation in relation to long-term mortality in unstable coronary artery disease. *N Engl J Med* 2000;343:1139–1147.

188. Heeschen C, Hamm CW, Bruemmer J, et al. Predictive value of C-reactive protein and troponin T in patients with unstable angina: a comparative analysis. CAPTURE Investigators. Chimeric c7E3 AntiPlatelet Therapy in Unstable angina REfractory to standard treatment trial. *J Am Coll Cardiol* 2000;35:1535–1542.

189. Lindmark E, Diderholm E, Wallentin L, et al. Relationship between interleukin 6 and mortality in patients with unstable coronary artery disease: effects of an early invasive or noninvasive strategy. *JAMA* 2001;286: 2107–2113.

190. Haverkate F, Thompson SG, Pyke SD et al. European Concerted Action on Thrombosis and Disabilities Angina Pectoris Study Group. Production of C-reactive protein and risk of coronary events in stable and unstable angina. *Lancet* 1997;349:462–466.

191. Ridker PM, Rifai N, Pfeffer MA et al. Cholesterol and Recurrent Events (CARE) Investigators. Inflammation, pravastatin, and the risk of coronary events after myocardial infarction in patients with average cholesterol levels. . *Circulation* 1998;98:839–844.

192. Retterstol L, Eikvar L, Bohn M, et al. C-reactive protein predicts death in patients with previous premature myocardial infarction—a 10 year follow-up study. *Atherosclerosis* 2002;160:433–440.

193. Chew DP, Bhatt DL, Robbins MA, et al. Incremental prognostic value of elevated baseline C-reactive protein among established markers of risk in percutaneous coronary intervention. *Circulation* 2001;104:992–997.

194. de Winter RJ, Koch KT, van Straalen JP, et al. C-reactive protein and coronary events following percutaneous coronary angioplasty. *Am J Med* 2003;115:85–90.

195. Dibra A, Mehilli J, Braun S, et al. Association between C-reactive protein levels and subsequent cardiac events among patients with stable angina treated with coronary artery stenting. *Am J Med* 2003;114:715–722.

196. Burke AP, Tracy RP, Kolodgie F, et al. Elevated C-reactive protein values and atherosclerosis in sudden coronary death: association with different pathologies. *Circulation* 2002;105:2019–2023.

197. Ridker PM, Rifai N, Pfeffer MA et al. The Cholesterol and Recurrent Events (CARE) Investigators. Long-term effects of pravastatin on plasma concentration of C-reactive protein. *Circulation* 1999;100:230–235.

198. Ridker PM, Rifai N, Lowenthal SP. Rapid reduction in C-reactive protein with cerivastatin among 785 patients with primary hypercholesterolemia. *Circulation* 2001;103:1191–1193.

199. Kinlay S, Timms T, Clark M, et al. Comparison of effect of intensive lipid lowering with atorvastatin to less intensive lowering with lovastatin on C-reactive protein in patients with stable angina pectoris and inducible myocardial ischemia. *Am J Cardiol* 2002;89:1205–1207.

200. Ridker PM. Rosuvastatin in the primary prevention of cardiovascular disease among patients with low levels of low-density lipoprotein cholesterol and elevated high-sensitivity C-reactive protein: rationale and design of the JUPITER trial. *Circulation* 2003;108:2292–2297.

201. Ridker PM, Rifai N, Clearfield M, et al. Measurement of C-reactive protein for the targeting of statin therapy in the primary prevention of acute coronary events. *N Engl J Med* 2001;344:1959–1965.

202. Cannon CP, Braunwald E, McCabe CH, et al. Intensive versus moderate lipid lowering with statins after acute coronary syndromes. *N Engl J Med* 2004;350:1495–1504.

# CHAPTER 54 ■ HISTOPATHOLOGY OF ATHEROSCLEROSIS

RENU VIRMANI, ALLEN P. BURKE, AND FRANK D. KOLODGIE

In this manner *destruction, demolition, ulceration* is produced, and ultimately the *atheromatous ulcer*—It is a product of the atheromatous deposit, but it no longer contains any formed elementary parts.

Cellular Pathology by *Rudolph Virchow* 1858 (1)

The descriptive studies of atherosclerosis detailed by the 19th century pathologists still hold true today. The use of elaborate discriminating immunohistochemical stains coupled with the ability to peer through powerful microscopes has confirmed the works of Virchow, Rokitansky, and Aschoff. In this chapter, the authors review the plaque morphology underlying various causes of thrombosis in symptomatic and asymptomatic coronary artery disease.

Until the American Heart Association (AHA) classification of atherosclerosis proposed by Stary et al. in 1994, atherosclerotic lesions were primarily classified as fatty streak or atheromatous plaque, also referred to as fibrous, fibrofatty, lipid, or fibrolipid plaque (2,3). The word atheroma—the Greek word for gruel—means yellow grumous fluid, which is considered the hallmark of the fibroatheroma even today. The fully mature fibroatheroma may develop complications of calcification, ulceration, thrombosis, hemorrhage, and aneurysms. Atherosclerotic material is composed of cellular and acellular elements. The cellular elements consistently present during lesion formation and progression constitute smooth muscle cells, macrophages, lymphocytes, and luminal endothelial cells. Those elements that are variably present include endothelial cells as part of neoangiogenesis, neutrophils, mast cells, platelets, and erythrocytes. Tissue matrix (acellular) components include collagen, fibrin, elastic fibers, and proteoglycans; it also includes calcium (generally in the form of calcium apatite), lipid (including cholesterol crystals), and iron (typically in the form of hemosiderin). Together, the assembly of these essential components produces a wide array of plaque morphologies, which have been classified by the authors and by others into various lesion types (see Table 54-1).

In the classification scheme by Stary et al., atherosclerotic plaques are grouped into six lesion types: type I, intimal lesion; type II, fatty streak; type III, intermediate (transitional or preatheroma); type IV, atheroma; type V, fibroatheroma; and type VI, complicated plaques with surface defects, and/or hematoma–hemorrhage, and/or thrombosis (2,3). In the authors' morphologic studies of coronary lesions from sudden deaths, this classification was inadequate because it was derived solely from the assumption that luminal thrombi occurred exclusively from plaque rupture. Moreover, there is the perception that lesion growth occurs through sequential stages involving specific lesion morphologies.

The modified classification scheme developed by the authors for atherosclerotic lesions is based on the works of Stary et al. (4). Rather than referring to the lesions as lesion types I to IV, the roman numerals have been substituted with descriptive terminology. In this classification, lesion types I and II are referred to as intimal thickening and intimal xanthoma, respectively. The latter lesion is considered nonprogressive and is common to all populations. Intimal xanthomas tend to regress in most locations. On the other hand, transitional lesions, referred to as pathologic intimal thickening, will, with time, become fibroatheromas. The term fibrous-cap (FC) atheroma pertains to the definition of atheroma by Stary et al. and the term thin-cap fibroatheroma (TCFA) applies to the precursor lesion of plaque rupture. Notably, coronary thrombosis occurs in the presence of three different morphologies: *plaque rupture, erosion*, and *calcified nodule* (4). Plaque rupture is defined by an area of FC disruption or break where the overlying thrombus is in continuity with the underlying necrotic core (NC) (5). Plaque erosion is identified when serial sectioning of a thrombosed artery fails to show any contact with the NC when present; the endothelium is absent and the intima is rich in smooth muscle cells in a proteoglycan matrix (6). The least frequent morphology is the calcified nodule in which the luminal thrombus is in contact with eruptive, dense, calcified bodies (4). Descriptive terms for lesions that show specific morphologies with implications for disease progression or stabilization have also been introduced. For example, plaque hemorrhage is recognized as a distinct lesion because it signifies plaque progression. In direct contrast, fibrocalcific plaques correspond to lesions with greater than 75% cross-sectional luminal narrowing and represent end-stage (burned out) stable disease because of healed ruptures. Further, the term fibrous plaque implies a progression to luminal narrowing in response to an organizing propagated thrombus, possibly arising from a rupture at a proximal site.

## VARIOUS CORONARY PLAQUE MORPHOLOGIES

The various coronary plaque morphologies include adaptive intimal thickening, intimal xanthomas, pathologic intimal thickening, fibroatheroma, and TCFA (see Fig. 54-1).

### Adaptive Intimal Thickening

The appearance of *adaptive intimal thickening* is the first change that occurs in the vessel wall of a human coronary artery (7). This condition, usually localized to branch points, is caused by the accumulation of smooth muscle cells and proteoglycans. Although these lesions are not grossly visible, microscopically, they may contain lipid droplets. Adaptive intimal thickening occurs

The opinions or assertions contained herein are the private views of the authors and are not to be construed as official or as reflecting the views of the Department of the Army, the Department of the Air Force, or the Department of Defense.

TABLE 54-1

ATHEROSCLEROTIC PLAQUE CLASSIFICATIONS

| Plaque morphologies | Traditional classification | Stary et al. | Virmani et al. | |
|---|---|---|---|---|
| | | | Initial | Progression |
| Early plaques | | Type I: Microscopic detection of lipid droplets in intima and small groups of macrophage foam cells | Intimal thickening | None |
| | Fatty streak | Type II: Fatty streaks visible on gross inspection, layers of foam cells, occasional lymphocytes, and mast cells | Intimal xanthoma | None |
| | | Type III (intermediate): Extracellular lipid pools present among layers of smooth muscle cells | Pathologic intimal thickening | Thrombus (erosion) |
| Intermediate plaque Late lesions | Atheroma | Type IV: Well-defined lipid core; may develop surface disruption (fissure) | Fibrous-cap atheroma | Thrombus (erosion)[a] |
| | | | Thin fibrous-cap atheroma | Thrombus (rupture) hemorrhage/fibrin[b] |
| | | Type Va: New fibrous tissue overlying lipid core (multilayered fibroatheroma)[c] | Healed plaque rupture, erosion | Repeated rupture or erosion with or without total occlusion |
| | | Type Vb: Calcification[d] | Fibrocalcific plaque (with or without necrotic core) | |
| | Fibrous plaque | Type Vc: Fibrotic lesion with minimal lipid (could be result of organized thrombi) | | |
| Miscellaneous/complicated features | Complicated/advanced plaques | Type VIa: Surface disruption | | |
| | | Type VIb: Intraplaque hemorrhage Type VIc: Thrombosis | | |
| | | | Calcified nodule | Thrombus (usually nonocclusive) |

[a]May further progress with healing (healed erosion).
[b]May further progress with healing (healed rupture).
[c]May overlap with healed plaque ruptures.
[d]Occasionally referred to as type VII lesion.
From Burke AP, Virmani R, Galis Z, et al. 34th Bethesda Conference: Task Force #2—what is the pathologic basis for new atherosclerosis imaging techniques? *J Am Coll Cardiol* 2003;41:1874–1886, with permission.

in 30% of neonates, and the distribution and development of intimal masses correlates with the existence of atherosclerotic plaques later in life (8). Cell replication is relatively low at these sites and the plaques that develop later in life may be clonal in origin (8). Tabas et al. have proposed that the extracellular matrix in early lesions contains enzymes capable of retaining lipids, a step toward early NC formation (9). However, there are few published studies on the early evolution of intimal masses in humans, and these studies do not clarify the precise pathologic mechanism(s) that occurs during development.

## Intimal Xanthomas

*Intimal xanthomas* ("fatty streaks" in the AHA classification) correspond to a lesion with lipid-laden macrophages (2). Unlike adaptive intimal thickening, these lesions are visible as yellow-colored streaks, dots, or patches, flush with the intimal surface

of the artery and they stain positive for neutral lipids with Sudan III or IV. Microscopically, these lesions contain foamy macrophages with occasional lymphocytes and mast cells. Smooth muscle cells are also present and may contain neutral lipids; however, most of the lipid is present in the macrophages (2). In humans, these lesions are common in the thoracic aorta of young individuals (<35 years) whereas advanced lesions are usually absent in the thoracic aorta of the adult (>40 years) (10). Therefore, fatty streaks do not represent "true" atherosclerotic process because most lesions regress with age (11).

## Pathologic Intimal Thickening

*Pathologic intimal thickening* or AHA type III lesions are thought to constitute the morphologic and chemical basis for progression from the intimal mass lesion (2). These plaques are characterized by smooth muscle cells often located near

## Development of human coronary atherosclerosis

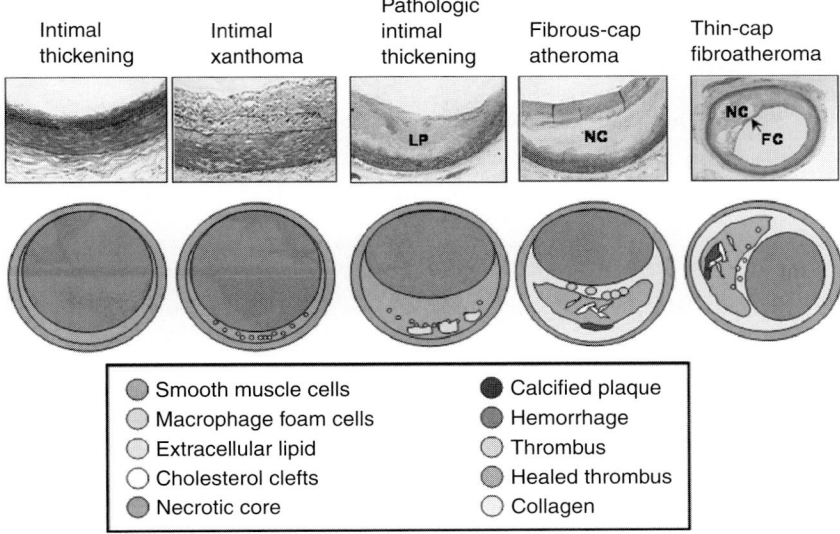

| Intimal thickening | Intimal xanthoma | Pathologic intimal thickening | Fibrous-cap atheroma | Thin-cap fibroatheroma |

Smooth muscle cells
Macrophage foam cells
Extracellular lipid
Cholesterol clefts
Necrotic core

Calcified plaque
Hemorrhage
Thrombus
Healed thrombus
Collagen

**Figure 54-1.** Intimal thickening and intimal xanthoma: preatherosclerotic coronary lesions. Lesions are uniformly present in all populations, although intimal xanthomas (fatty streaks) are more prevalent with exposure to a standard American diet. Both lesions occur soon after birth; the intimal xanthoma (fatty streak) is known to regress. Intimal thickening consists mainly of smooth muscle cells (SMCs) in a proteoglycan matrix, whereas intimal xanthomas primarily contain macrophage-derived foam cell, T lymphocytes, and varying degrees of SMCs. Pathologic intimal thickening versus atheroma: Pathological intimal thickening (PIT) is a poorly defined entity, referred to in the literature as "intermediate" lesion. True necrosis is not apparent, and there is no evidence of cellular debris; lipid pools (*LP*) are seen deep in the lesion. The tissue over the lipid pools is rich in SMCs and proteoglycans—some scattered macrophages and lymphocytes may also be present. The more definitive lesions, the fibrous-cap (*FC*) atheroma, classically shows a necrotic core (*NC*) containing cholesterol esters, free cholesterol, phospholipids, and triglycerides. The FC consists of SMCs in a proteoglycan–collagen matrix, with a variable number of macrophages and lymphocytes. The TCFA (vulnerable plaque): TCFAs are lesions with large NCs containing numerous cholesterol clefts. The overlying FC is thin ($<65 \mu$m) and heavily infiltrated by macrophages; SMCs are rare and microvessels are generally present in the adventitia and intima (see Color Fig. 54-1). (From Virmani R, Kolodgie FD, Burke AP, et al. Lessons from sudden coronary death: a comprehensive morphological classification scheme for atherosclerotic lesions. *Arterioscler Thromb Vasc Biol* 2000;20:1262–1275, with permission.)

the medial layer surrounded by pools of extracellular lipid and proteoglycan matrix (4). Few viable smooth muscle cells are found within lipid pools (LP); empty shells, identified by periodic acid-Schiff (PAS) staining, represent the basement membranes of earlier cells (12). On electron microscopy, sites of attenuated smooth muscle cells show plasma membrane remnants, apoptotic bodies, and free or membrane bound lipid droplets. LP may also contain free cholesterol appearing as fine cholesterol clefts in a paraffin section (13). Special calcium stains reveal speckled granular calcification, often underappreciated by hematoxylin and eosin. Proteoglycans including dermatan sulfate (i.e., decorin and biglycan) accumulate in the intima during this phase (14). Other negatively charged proteoglycans containing chondroitin sulfate participate in the binding and retention of apo B-100 (15). Scattered intact lipid-laden macrophages, in addition to T lymphocytes, are often found above the lipid pool (16). In contrast, B lymphocytes are restricted mostly to the adventitia; only a few are found within the developing plaque. Similarly, mast cells may also be present, but these cells are far fewer than other cell types (17). Notably, no necrosis is present although these lesions do contain free cholesterol, fatty acid, sphingomyelin, lysolecithin, and triglycerides (18).

## Fibroatheroma

Unlike the aforementioned lesions, *fibroatheroma* has a distinct layer of superficial fibrous tissue confining an area of defined necrosis. The FC consists of smooth muscle cells and

proteoglycan–collagen matrix, with varying degrees of inflammatory cells, mostly macrophages and lymphocytes. The thickness of FC primarily distinguishes the fibroatheroma from the thin FC atheroma (classic "vulnerable" plaque) (4). Moreover, the authors have recently subtyped fibroatheromas with "early" and "late" necrosis (Fig. 54-1) (19). The "early fibroatheroma" contains a lipid-rich matrix composed of proteoglycans, versican, hyaluronan, and type III collagen interspersed with intact foamy macrophages. On the other hand, cores with late necrosis show numerous cholesterol clefts, cellular debris, and an absence of extracellular matrix (especially, versican and hyaluronan and type III collagen) (19). Within the center and perimeter of the necrotic area, ghosts of CD68-positive macrophages with ill-defined cell membranes are found, and the picrosirius red staining for collagen is negative.

## Thin-Cap Fibroatheroma

The *thin-cap fibroatheroma* is specifically characterized as a separate lesion morphology because this entity was unrecognized by the AHA classification. These lesions contain FC, which measures less than 65 $\mu$m in thickness, that are heavily infiltrated by macrophages, lymphocytes, and rare smooth muscle cells (see Table 54-2; Fig. 54-2) (5,20). A separate classification for this lesion is paramount because its early recognition as a precursor to rupture may help reduce the incidence of sudden coronary death and cardiac morbidity. In the sudden death population, the authors found that TCFAs were most frequently found in patients with acute myocardial infarction and were

**TABLE 54-2**

MORPHOLOGIC CHARACTERISTICS OF PLAQUE RUPTURE AND THIN-CAP FIBROATHEROMA

| Plaque type | Necrotic core (%) | Fibrous cap thickness (μm) | Mφs (%) | SMCs (%) | T lymph | Calcification score |
|---|---|---|---|---|---|---|
| Rupture | 34 ± 17 | 23 ± 19 | 26 ± 20 | 0.002 ± 0.004 | 4.9 ± 4.3 | 1.53 ± 1.03 |
| TCFA | 23 ± 17 | <65 | 14 ± 10 | 6.6 ± 10.4 | 6.6 ± 10.4 | 0.97 ± 1.1 |
| P value | NS | | 0.005 | | NS | 0.014 |

Mφs, macrophages; SMCs, smooth muscle cells; T lymph, T lymphocytes; TCFA, thin-cap fibroatheroma; NS, not significant.
Mean values represent ± standard deviation.
From Kolodgie FD, Burke AP, Farb A, et al. The thin-cap fibroatheroma: a type of vulnerable plaque: the major precursor lesion to acute coronary syndromes. *Curr Opin Cardiol* 2001;16:285–292, with permission.

uncommon in those with erosion or in those who died from noncardiac causes. In the same patients the distribution of plaque rupture was similar to that of thin-cap atheromas, with approximately 60% occurring in proximal segments, 30% in midarterial segments, and 10% in distal segments (20,21).

# NECROTIC CORE AND ITS ENLARGEMENT ARE CRITICAL FOR PLAQUE RUPTURE: ROLE OF PLAQUE HEMORRHAGE

Macrophage infiltration is the first step toward the eventual formation of an atherosclerotic plaque and NC (3,4,22,23). *In vitro* studies have shown that oxidation facilitates the uptake of low density lipoprotein (LDL) by the macrophage (24,25). This two-step process begins with mild oxidation of lipid followed by oxidation by apolipoprotein B, a modification required for the recognition of the lipid by the scavenger receptor that is unaffected by the cholesterol content of the cell (26). Foam cells contain cholesterol esters and free cholesterol and

are no different from a nonfoamy macrophage (17). However, as plaques progress, the free cholesterol content of the lesion increases and the cholesteryl ester content decreases (18). Felton et al., in a study of atherosclerotic plaques in human aorta, found that the progression of the plaques from a nondisrupted to a disrupted lesion was associated with an increase in free cholesterol, cholesterol esters, and ratio of free-to-esterified cholesterol but with no change in triglyceride content (18). Further, the percentage of cholesterol clefts was greater in lesions that have ruptured than in fibrocalcific plaques (see Table 54-3) (4,20).

Although in the first half of the 20th century several leading pathologists believed intraplaque hemorrhage to be a major contributor to the progression of coronary atherosclerosis, the precise nature of this relation was not well understood (27–29). In an effort to further understand the importance of hemorrhage in plaque progression, several human coronary plaque morphologies were examined at autopsy for evidence of erythrocyte membranes (19). It was of interest to the authors that the areas of extravasated erythrocytes outside the vasculature, such as those found in atrial hemangioma, hemorrhagic pericarditis, and pulmonary hemorrhage, showed atherogenic changes including the accumulation of free cholesterol, foamy macrophages, and iron with fibrosis (30–32). Because the cholesterol content of the erythrocyte membrane exceeds that of all other cells in the body, with lipid constituting 40% of the weight, the red blood cell itself may contribute to the accumulation of free cholesterol within a plaque (33,34).

In a recent study from the authors' laboratory, glycophorin A (Gp A), a protein specific to erythrocyte membranes, was used to stain coronary arteries for the determination of previous hemorrhagic events. The frequency of previous hemorrhages was greater in coronary atherosclerotic lesions with late necrosis and in those lesions prone to rupture than those lesions with early necrosis or pathologic intimal thickening (19). The amount of Gp A and the level of iron deposits in the plaque corresponded to the size of the NC, and changes in these variables paralleled an increase in lesional macrophages, suggesting that the hemorrhage itself serves as an inflammatory stimulus (see Table 54-4; Fig. 54-3) (19). Intraplaque hemorrhage is believed to occur from the disruption of thin-walled microvessels (*vasa vasorum*) that are lined by a discontinuous endothelium without supporting smooth muscle cells (35). Many investigators including some from the authors' laboratory have suggested that intraplaque hemorrhage and plaque rupture are associated with an increased density of microvessels (36–38). Although the precise mechanism of how red blood cells leak into the NC is poorly understood, the authors and others have described diffuse perivascular staining of the

A nonhemodynamically limiting
thin-cap fibroatheroma

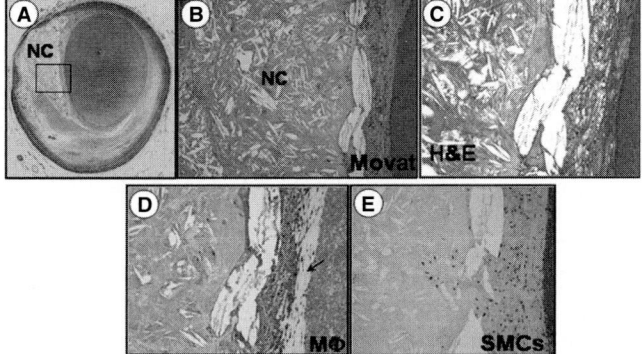

**FIGURE 54-2.** A nonhemodynamically limiting thin-cap fibroatheroma (TCFA). **A:** A TCFA having a necrotic core (*NC*) and an overlying thin fibrous cap (<65 μm). **B:** The high power view of the **boxed area** in A; note that an advanced NC with a large number of cholesterol clefts with surrounding loss of matrix and no cellular infiltration is seen. The fibrous cap is infiltrated by macrophages, better seen in (**C**) when stained by hematoxylin and eosin (*H&E*). (**D**) and (**E**) show macrophage (*Mφ*) infiltration (CD68-positive) and rare staining of smooth muscle cells (*SMCs*) (α-actin positive) in the fibrous cap (see Color Fig. 54-2).

**TABLE 54-3**

COMPARISON OF NECROTIC CORE SIZE, NUMBER OF CHOLESTEROL CLEFTS, MACROPHAGE INFILTRATION, NUMBER OF VASA VASORUM, AND HEMOSIDERIN-LADEN MACROPHAGES IN CULPRIT PLAQUES

| Plaque type | Necrotic core (%) | No. of cholesterol clefts (%) | Macrophage infiltration of fibrous cap (%) | Mean no. of vasa vasorum | Mean no. of hemosiderin-laden macrophages |
|---|---|---|---|---|---|
| Rupture | $34 \pm 17^{\Omega, \ni}$ | $12 \pm 12^{*, \wedge}$ | $26 \pm 20^{\psi, \tau, \varpi}$ | $44 \pm 22^{\varphi, \perp, \partial}$ | $18.9 \pm 11\delta, \lambda, \notin$ |
| TCFA | $24 \pm 17$ | $8 \pm 9$ | $14 \pm 10^{\psi}$ | $26 \pm 23^{\varphi}$ | $4.4 \pm 3.6\delta$ |
| Erosion | $14 \pm 14^{\Omega}$ | $2 \pm 5^{*}$ | $10 \pm 12^{\tau}$ | $28 \pm 18^{\perp}$ | $4.3 \pm 4.7\lambda$ |
| Stable | $12 \pm 25^{\ni}$ | $4 \pm 6^{\wedge}$ | $3 \pm 0.7^{\varpi}$ | $13 \pm 9^{\partial}$ | $5.0 \pm 9.3 \notin$ |
| $P$ value | $\Omega$ 0.003, $\ni$ 0.01 | *0.002, $\wedge$0.04 | $\psi$ 0.005, $\tau < 0.0001$, $\varpi$ 0.0001 | $\varphi$ 0.07, $\perp$ 0.02, $\partial$ 0.01 | $\delta$ 0.001, $\lambda < 0.0001$, $\notin$ 0.03 |

TCFA, thin-cap fibroatheroma.
Greek symbols are used to show significant differences between groups.
From Virmani R, Kolodgie FD, Burke AP, et al. Lessons from sudden coronary death: a comprehensive morphological classification scheme for atherosclerotic lesions. *Arterioscler Thromb Vasc Biol* 2000;20:1262–1275, with permission.

**TABLE 54-4**

MORPHOMETRIC ANALYSIS OF 365 PLAQUES IN CORONARY ARTERIES FROM PATIENTS WHO DIED SUDDENLY OF CORONARY CAUSES[a]

| Type of plaque | No. of plaques | Glycophorin A score[b] | Iron score[b] | Size of necrotic core (mm²) | Extent of macrophage infiltration |
|---|---|---|---|---|---|
| Plaque with pathologic intimal thickening | 129 | $0.09 \pm 0.04$ | $0.07 \pm 0.05$ | — | $0.002 \pm 0.001$ |
| Fibroatheroma | | | | | |
| Core in early stage of necrosis | 79 | $0.23 \pm 0.11$ | $0.17 \pm 0.08$ | $0.06 \pm 0.02$ | $0.018 \pm 0.004$ |
| Core in late stage of necrosis | 105 | $0.94 \pm 0.11^{c}$ | $0.14 \pm 0.09^{c}$ | $0.84 \pm 0.08^{c}$ | $0.059 \pm 0.007^{c}$ |
| Thin-cap fibroatheroma | 52 | $1.60 \pm 0.20^{c}$ | $1.24 \pm 0.24^{c}$ | $1.95 \pm 0.30^{c}$ | $0.142 \pm 0.016^{c}$ |

[a]Plus-minus values are mean ± SE.
[b]Scores can range form 0 to 4, with higher scores indicating greater proportion of the analyte.
[c]$P < 0.01$ for comparison with fibroatheromas whose scores were in an early stage of necrosis.
From Kolodgie FD, Gold HK, Burke AP, et al. Intraplaque hemorrhage and progression of coronary atheroma. *New Engl J Med* 2003;349:2314–2323, with permission.

Fibrous-cap atheroma (late necrosis)

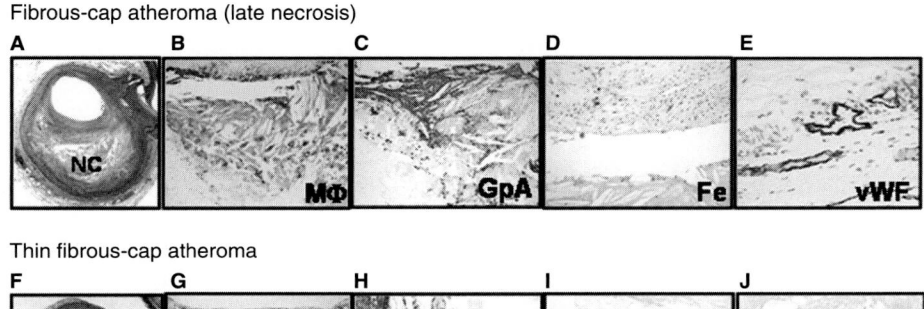

Thin fibrous-cap atheroma

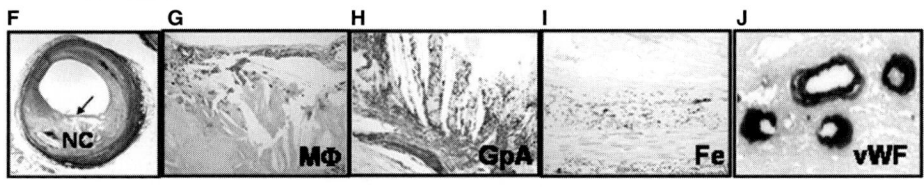

**Figure 54-3.** Late core (A–E) and thin fibrous-cap atheroma (TCFA) (F–J) showing intraplaque hemorrhage. A: Shows a low-power view of a fibrous-cap (FC) atheroma with a late necrotic core (NC) (Movat Pentachrome ×20). B: Intense staining of CD68-positive macrophages is seen within the NC. C: Shows extensive glycophorin A (*Gp A*)–positive erythrocyte membranes colocalized with numerous cholesterol clefts within the necrotic core (×200). D: Iron deposits (*blue*) are seen within macrophage foam cells (×200). E: Microvessels bordering the NC show perivascular von Willebrand factor (*VWF*) deposition (×400). F: Shows a low-power view of a fibroatheroma with a thin FC (*arrow*) overlying a relatively large NC (Movat Pentachrome, ×20). G: The FC is devoid of smooth muscle cells (not shown) and is heavily infiltrated by CD68-positive macrophages (*Mφ*, × 200). H: Intense Gp A staining of erythrocyte membranes within the NC colocalized with cholesterol clefts (×100). I: Adjacent coronary segment with accumulated iron (*blue pigment*) in a macrophage-rich region deep within the plaque (×200). J: Perivascular diffuse deposits of VWF in microvessels, indicates leaky vessels bordering the NC (×400) (see Color Fig. 54-3). (From Kolodgie FD, Gold HK, Burke AP, et al. Intraplaque hemorrhage and progression of coronary atheroma. *N Engl J Med* 2003;349:2316–2325, with permission.)

von Willebrand factor (VWF) of intraplaque vasa vasorum, suggestive of microvascular disruption or leakiness (19). Plaque fissures could also account for the accumulation of erythrocytes; however, fissures are often accompanied by luminal thrombi, which were absent in the authors' studies (39).

## LESIONS WITH THROMBI

Lesions of the thrombi include plaque rupture, erosions, and calcified nodule (see Fig. 54-4).

### Plaque Rupture

Plaque rupture is caused by fibrous cap disruption, allowing blood to come in contact with the thrombogenic NC, resulting in thrombus formation. Although the thrombus develops at the site of rupture and consists predominantly of platelets, it may propagate proximally or distally to the nearest branch (see Figs. 54-5 and 54-6). In areas of propagation, the thrombus mostly consists of layers of fibrin separated by layers of erythrocytes (Fig. 54-6). Ruptured lesions typically show larger NCs, with disrupted FCs heavily infiltrated by macrophages (Fig. 54-5). Plaque ruptures are found in 60% of individuals dying suddenly, are associated with luminal thrombi, and are probably the most frequent cause of death in young men (<50 years) and older women (>50 years). The trigger for plaque rupture is likely related to conditions that result in FC thinning along with local hemodynamics and emotional status that cause surges in sympathetic activity (40). Angiographic findings of luminal surface irregularities in coronary arteries correlate with plaque rupture. The extent of luminal narrowing is often minimal (<50% diameter stenosis) at the site of thrombosis (41,42). Macrophage density at rupture sites is typically very high; although in atypical cases, macrophages may be relatively sparse. In the authors' experience and in the experience of Becker et al., occasional neutrophils are also

seen in plaque rupture. Myeloperoxidase (MPO)-positive cells are more frequent in ruptured plaques than in fibroatheroma (43). As shown in the laboratory, significantly greater MPO-positive cells in the thrombus are associated with occlusive rather than nonocclusive thrombi (44). In the authors' laboratory, T lymphocytes were present in 75% of ruptures (6). Although macrophage density is maximal in plaque rupture, the number of T lymphocytes varies among culprit lesions and is significantly higher in patients with diabetes, especially those with type I diabetes (45).

### Erosion

Plaque disruption and thrombosis in the absence of fibrous cap thinning characterizes plaque erosion. Angiographically, there is less narrowing and irregularity of the luminal surface in erosion (see Fig. 54-7). The morphologic characteristics include an abundance of smooth muscle cells and proteoglycan matrix, especially versican and hyaluronan, and disruption of the surface endothelium (6,46). In erosion, a necrotic core is often absent, and, if present, it is a negligible part of the plaque. Compared to TCFAs, plaque erosion contains relatively few or no macrophages and T cells compared with ruptures (46). Erosions account for approximately 40% of cases of thrombotic sudden coronary death and are especially common in young women (45 ± 8 years) and men (53 ± 10 years). Eroded lesions are usually eccentric and normally show less severe luminal narrowing than plaque ruptures; calcification is rare (see Table 54-5). Currently, the authors have little understanding of the mechanisms of erosion. In addition to the thrombus, the most striking aspects are the absence of endothelium and "activated" appearance of the underlying smooth muscle cells. Smooth muscle cells at the plaque–thrombus interface are bizarre in shape and contain hyperchromatic nuclei with prominent nucleoli. The matrix is strongly positive for hyaluronan and proteoglycan versican, with little reactivity to biglycan and decorin (46). Hyaluronan may interfere with

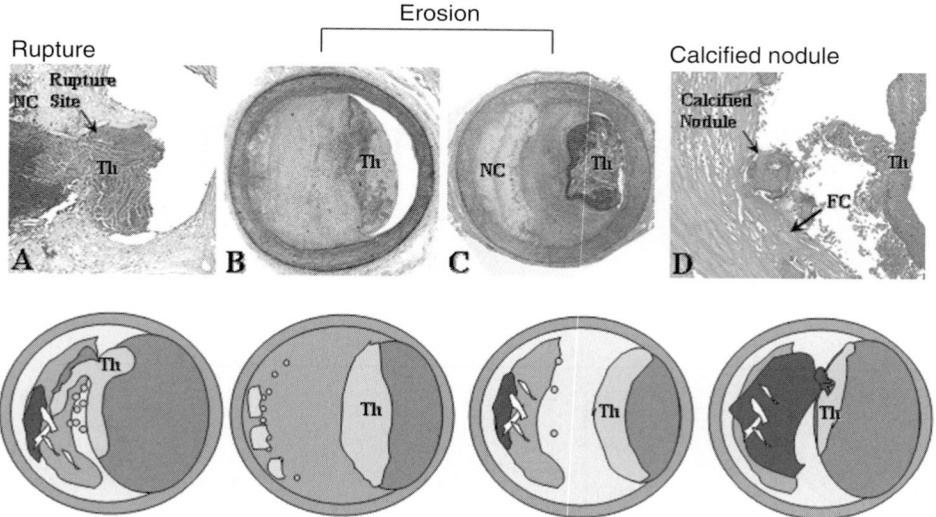

**FIGURE 54-4.** Atherosclerotic lesions with luminal thrombi. **A:** Ruptured plaques are thin fibrous-cap atheromas with luminal thrombi (*Th*). These lesions usually have an extensive necrotic core (*NC*) containing large numbers of cholesterol crystals and a thin fibrous-cap (*FC*) (<65 μm) infiltrated by foamy macrophages and T lymphocytes. The FC is thinnest at the site of rupture and consists of a few collagen bundles and rare smooth muscle cells. The luminal thrombus is in communication with the lipid-rich necrotic core. **B and C:** Erosions occur over lesions rich in smooth muscle cells and proteoglycans. Luminal Th overlie areas lacking surface endothelium. The deep intima of the eroded plaque often shows extracellular lipid pools, but NCs are uncommon; when present, the NC does not communicate with the luminal thrombus. Inflammatory infiltrate is usually absent, but, if present, it is sparse and consists of macrophages and lymphocytes. **D:** Calcified nodules are plaques with luminal Th showing calcified nodule protruding into the lumen through a disrupted thin FC. An endothelium is absent at the site of the thrombus, and inflammatory cells (macrophages, T lymphocytes) are absent (see Color Fig. 54-4).

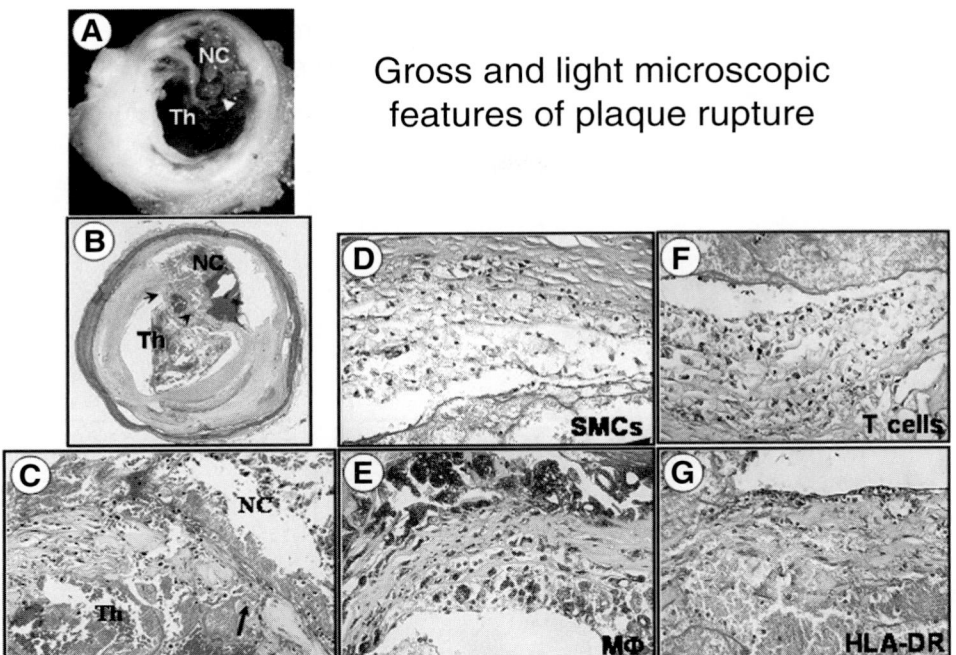

## Gross and light microscopic features of plaque rupture

**FIGURE 54-5.** Gross photograph and histologic composition of plaque rupture. **A:** Gross photograph of a coronary artery cut in cross section showing the site of plaque rupture (*arrow*) with an underlying necrotic core (*NC*) and luminal thrombus (*Th*). **B:** Histologic section of the artery in (**A**) showing rupture site, necrotic core, and luminal thrombus. (Movat ×20) **C:** High-power view of the area of the fibrous cap disruption (*arrow*), and there is communication of the thrombus (*Th*) with the underlying NC (×200). **D:** High-power view of the thin fibrous cap (FC) showing a paucity of smooth muscle cells (α-actin, ×200). **E and F:** The FC is heavily infiltrated by macrophages and T lymphocytes (CD68 and CD45Ro, respectively, ×200). **G:** Shows the strong expression of HLA-DR antigens, particularly in macrophages and T cells of the FC (see Color Fig. 54-5). (From Farb A, Burke AP, Tang AL, et al. Coronary plaque erosion without rupture into a lipid core. A frequent cause of coronary thrombosis in sudden coronary death. *Circulation* 1996;93:1354–1363, with permission.)

## Thrombus propagation in plaque rupture

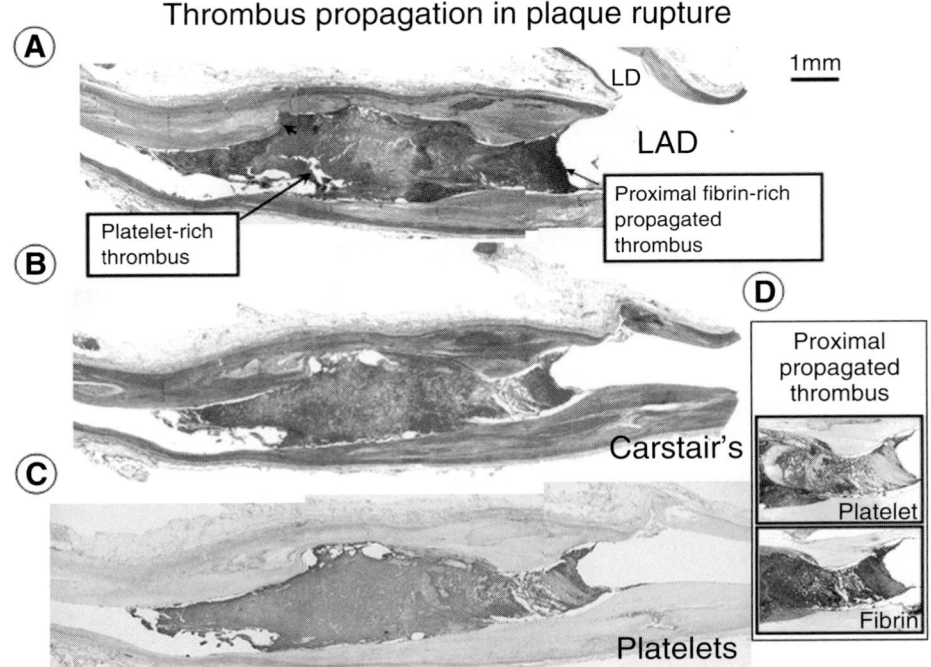

**FIGURE 54-6.** Thrombus propagation in plaque rupture. **A:** Composite of a longitudinal section of aleft anterior descending (*LAD*) coronary artery with plaque rupture; the rupture site is marked by the arrowhead (Movat pentachrome, original magnification ×20). **B:** Shows the same longitudinal section as in **A** stained with Carstair method for the detection of fibrin (*dark red*) and platelets (*blue-grey*). The proximal thrombus consists predominantly of fibrin whereas the more distal portion at the rupture site is platelet-rich. **C:** The presence of platelets was further confirmed using an antibody directed against glycoprotein IIIa. **D:** Proximal propagated portion of the thrombus showing mostly fibrin; mild layered reactivity is seen for platelets (see Color Fig. 54-6).

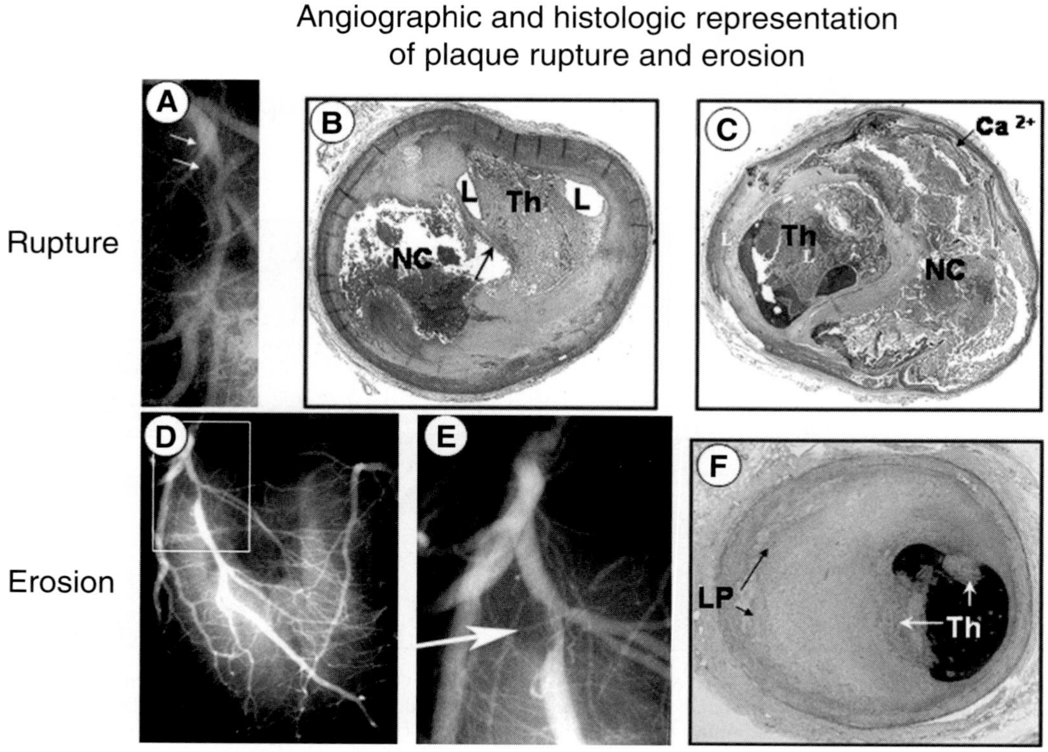

## Angiographic and histologic representation of plaque rupture and erosion

FIGURE 54-7. Angiographic and histologic representation of plaque rupture and erosion. A 43-year-old white man with no known history of risk factors was found unresponsive in the bathroom. **A:** Postmortem angiogram shows the left anterior descending (LAD) coronary artery at the origin of the left diagonal with near total occlusion. Sections taken from these sites show a plaque rupture [*arrow*, and (**B**)] with an underlying necrotic core (*NC*). The occluded artery shows an organizing thrombus with small lumens (*L*). In (**C**), the fibrous cap is intact with a large underlying NC with peripheral calcification (*Ca²⁺*), and the lumen shows organizing thrombus (*Th*) with small lumens (*L*). At autopsy, there was a healing transmural myocardial infarction present in the distribution of the LAD. Postmortem angiogram (**D** and **E**) and corresponding photomicrograph (**F**) of a 38-year-old man, who died of sudden coronary thrombosis. A focal stenosis is present in the left anterior coronary artery (**boxed area**), which is highlighted in (**A**) and an arrow points to the area of narrowing at the take off of the left diagonal. In (**F**), acute nonocclusive luminal thrombus (*Th*) is present on the surface of an erosive plaque rich in proteoglycans, and the underlying plaque shows pathologic intimal thickening with lipid pools (*LP*) (see Color Fig. 54-7). (From Farb A, Tang AL, Burke AP, et al. Sudden coronary death. Frequency of active coronary lesions, inactive coronary lesions, and myocardial infarction. *Circulation* 1995;92:1701–1709, with permission.)

### TABLE 54-5

CORONARY THROMBOSIS WITH RUPTURE INTO A LIPID CORE COMPARED WITH THROMBOSIS ASSOCIATED WITH PLAQUE EROSION

|  | Plaque rupture (*n* = 28) | Plaque erosion (*n* = 22) | *P* value |
|---|---|---|---|
| Male:female | 23:5 | 11:11 | 0.03 |
| Age (years) | 53 ± 10 | 44 ± 7 | <0.02 |
| % Stenosis | 78 ± 12 | 70 ± 11 | <0.03 |
| Calcified plaque | 19 (69%) | 5 (23%) | 0.002 |
| Occlusive: Nonocclusive thrombus | 12:16 (43%:57%) | 4:18 (18%:82%) | 0.08 |
| Concentric: Eccentric | 13:15 (46%:54%) | 4:18 (18%:82%) | 0.07 |
| Macrophages | 28 (100%) | 11 (50%) | <0.0001 |
| T cells | 21 (75%) | 7 (32%) | <0.004 |
| Smooth muscle cells | 11 (33%) | 21 (95%) | <0.0001 |
| HLA-DR–positive | 25 (89%) | 8 (36%) | 0.0002 |

Macrophages, T cells, smooth muscle cells, and HLA-DR–positive refer to cellular collections at plaque rupture of erosion site.
From Farb A, Burke AP, Tang AL, et al. Coronary plaque erosion without rupture into a lipid core. A frequent cause of coronary thrombosis in sudden coronary death. *Circulation* 1996;93:1354–1363.

adherence, growth, and survival of endothelial cells. CD44 is localized along the plaque–thrombus interface, staining smooth muscle cells, inflammatory cells, and platelets. The ligation of hyaluronan to CD44 may be critical for smooth muscle cell migration to the wounded edge. It has been postulated that erosions result from vasospasm, and they are often found in cigarette smokers (5,47).

## Calcified Nodule

Calcified nodules are fibrous lesions that contain multiple dense calcific bodies that can erupt into the lumen and cause thrombosis (4). The plaque underneath the calcified nodule usually contains calcified plates, and the NC, when present, is generally small. These lesions typically show healed plaque ruptures and are present where torsion stress is maximal, especially in the mid right coronary artery and in older individuals. The fragmentation of calcified matrix may contribute to the formation of calcified nodules.

# THROMBUS ORGANIZATION AND HEALING

Pathologists use the term "healing" to describe two types of scar tissue in atherosclerotic plaques. The first of these types, representing a newly formed scar, is characteristically rich in proteoglycan, with highly arborized smooth muscle cells with cytoplasm-rich perikaryons containing prominent endoplasmic reticulum. Regions suggestive of nascent scar tissue and a recent response to injury are often found in atherectomy specimens obtained within days to weeks after a percutaneous intervention (48,49). The second type of tissue representing a healed old scar contains smooth muscle cells with less abundant processes and cytoplasm with dense collagen as a substitute for the proteoglycan matrix (50). This type of tissue is often found in layers separated by areas of old hemorrhage or thrombotic debris, implying previous thrombotic events followed by healing.

Healed ruptures are characterized as lesions with a disrupted fibrous cap (rich in type I collagen) filled in by smooth muscle cells, proteoglycans, and type III collagen (see Fig. 54-8) (51,52). The matrix within the healed fibrous cap defect may, with time, be replaced by type I collagen as part of the late phase of healing. Healed ruptures commonly exhibit multiple layers of NC with overlying smooth muscle cells and extracellular matrix, suggestive of previous episodes of thrombosis (52). Other healed lesions lack evidence of preexisting fibrous cap rupture, and, instead of an NC, there are distinct layers of dense collagen interspersed with smooth muscle cells and proteoglycans along with fibrin and/or platelets; these lesions may correspond to healed erosions. Similarly, a healed propagated thrombus in areas of minimal or no atherosclerosis will histologically appear as fibrous lesions, which in some instances may produce severe luminal narrowing. These lesions can form proximal and distal to the site of a nonocclusive thrombus.

The role of cellular proliferation in healing atherosclerotic lesions is uncertain. Although pathologists often refer to the smooth muscle cell response as characteristic of healing, analysis of cell kinetics in plaques and restenotic areas have consistently shown minimal or no replication (49,53–55). This finding conforms to the very limited replicative life span seen with plaque smooth muscle cells *in vitro* and *in vivo* (56–58). Nonetheless, it is difficult to explain healing unless some smooth muscle cell replication occurs. The authors have shown greater smooth muscle cell replication at healed repair sites; although the proliferative response is generally less

### Healed plaque rupture

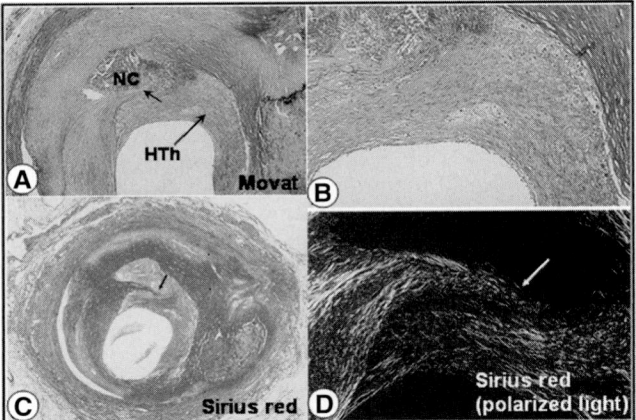

**FIGURE 54-8.** Healed plaque rupture. **A:** Areas of intraintimal lipid-rich core with hemorrhage and cholesterol clefts; an old area of necrosis (*NC*) is seen underlying a healed thrombus (*HTh*). **B:** Higher magnification showing extensive smooth muscle cells (SMCs) within a collagenous proteoglycan-rich neointima (healed thrombus) with clear demarcation from the fibrous region of old plaque to right. **C** and **D:** Layers of collagen by Sirius red staining. **C:** Note area of dense, dark collagen surrounding lipid hemorrhagic cores seen in corresponding view in **A. D:** Image taken with polarized light. Dense collagen (type I) that forms the fibrous cap is disrupted (*arrow*), with newer greenish type III collagen on the right and above the rupture site; (**A**) and (**B**), Movat pentachrome (see Color Fig. 54-8). (From Burke AP, Kolodgie FD, Farb A, et al. Healed plaque ruptures and sudden coronary death: evidence that subclinical rupture has a role in plaque progression. *Circulation* 2001;103:934–940, with permission.)

than 1%, this reaction usually exceeds beyond other areas of the plaque (52).

## Fresh Occlusion

Fresh occlusion is caused by an acute luminal thrombus containing platelet aggregates interspersed with inflammatory cells and a paucity of red cells. The thrombus, however, often propagates from its original site and becomes fibrin-rich with interspersed red blood cells and leukocytes. Little is known of the mechanism(s) involved in thrombus propagation. In a fresh thrombus, there is no evidence of invasion by endothelial cells and/or smooth muscle cells. With time, the thrombus becomes invaded by endothelial and smooth muscle cells and begins to heal. It is very common to see some degree of thrombus healing in erosions (80%), whereas healing is infrequent in acute plaque rupture.

## Old Total Occlusion

In healed total occlusions, the lumen is obstructed by dense collagen and/or proteoglycans interspersed with capillaries, arterioles, smooth muscle cells, and inflammatory cells. These lesions may also demonstrate earlier phases of organizing thrombi containing fibrin, red blood cells, and granulation tissue, especially in the mid portion of a long, occluded arterial segment. Healing is more rapid in small total occlusions, but in long total occlusions it is maximal at the two ends, and the mid portion may show persistence of fibrin thrombus and minimal invasion by macrophages and smooth muscle and endothelial cells. Lesions of total occlusion often show less calcification but almost always demonstrate negative remodeling (arterial shrinkage).

## Fibrocalcific Plaques

Fibrocalcific plaques often have a thick fibrous cap and extensive accumulation of calcium that result in severe luminal narrowing (>75% cross-sectional area luminal narrowing). The NC, when present, is often an insignificant part of the lesion. These plaques are frequently found in patients with stable angina and in 20% of cases of sudden coronary deaths without acute or healed ruptures and 10% of individuals dying a noncoronary death (4). Fibrocalcific lesion may represent an end stage process of atheromatous plaque rupture and/or erosion with healing and calcification. Angiographically, these lesions demonstrate severe stenosis of the diameter and a smooth luminal surface.

## Atherothrombotic Emboli

Patients dying with luminal thrombi may show distal emboli. Distal emboli in intramyocardial coronary arteries have been described in patients dying with plaque rupture (59,60). Davies et al. found intramural thrombi in 54% of patients with a history of unstable angina compared to 20% of patients with no record of angina. In the sudden death population, platelet-rich emboli were found in 60% of patients dying suddenly with epicardial coronary thrombi (59). This incidence was highest in vessels exhibiting plaque erosion (74%) rather than with those exhibiting plaque rupture (40%, $P < 0.03$) Atheroemboli were uncommon in the authors' series of sudden coronary deaths. Approximately 89% of intramyocardiac emboli occur in arteries less than or equal to 120 $\mu$m in diameter, 7% in vessels 120 to 200 $\mu$m, and 4% in those greater than 200 $\mu$m (60). Focal myocardial necrosis is seen in 57% of hearts with emboli, and 83% of these cases are associated with multiple emboli.

# RISK FACTORS AND PLAQUE MORPHOLOGY

Traditional risk factors such as hyperlipidemia, smoking, diabetes mellitus, and hypertension are associated with accelerated atherosclerosis; their relation to thrombi with different plaque etiologies has only recently been investigated (5,47,61). In an autopsy study from their laboratory, the authors assessed risk factors in 113 men with sudden coronary death (5). Serum analysis of total cholesterol (TC), high density lipoprotein cholesterol (HDL-C), TC/high density lipoprotein (HDL) ratio, and thiocyanate (surrogate marker for smoking) were measured along with red blood cell glycosylated hemoglobin to determine diabetic status. Together, the risk factors were evident in 96.5% of sudden coronary deaths, and smoking was a consistent predictor of acute thrombosis regardless of plaque etiology. The incidence of plaque rupture correlated with high total cholesterol, low HDL-cholesterol, and high TC/HDL-cholesterol ratio (5). Increased serum TC also correlated with the extent of macrophage infiltration, NC size, and a greater frequency of TCFAs. In contrast, however, greater macrophage infiltration and NC size in patients with type I and II diabetes was independent of hyperlipidemia. T lymphocytes were also more prominent in coronary lesions from patients with diabetes, in particular those with type I diabetes (45). Increased inflammatory cells in type I and II diabetic lesions were associated with greater HLA-DR expression, suggestive of an ongoing inflammatory process (45).

In women, plaque erosion is highly associated with smoking and occurs with a greater frequency in individuals younger than 50 years. In contrast, plaque rupture is more frequent in women older than 50 years and is associated with elevated total cholesterol (47). TCFAs are more frequently seen in women older than 50 years. Stable plaque with healed myocardial infarction is more frequently observed in women with greater than 10% glycohemoglobin (47).

The link between risk factors and morphologic diversity of lesions with coronary thrombosis suggests an underlying pathogenic basis for atherosclerotic disease. The finding that plaque erosion is independent of elevated cholesterol levels may explain why some individuals with normal lipid profiles still suffer from severe coronary disease. Although the precise risk factors related to erosion still remain elusive, unpublished data suggest that thrombotic factors, in addition to vasospasm, may be important to its etiology. Cigarette smoking appears to increase the likelihood of fatal thrombosis, regardless of the underlying plaque. Recently described inflammatory markers such as high sensitivity C-reactive protein (hs-CRP) correlate with the incidence of sudden coronary death (62). Finally, high serum homocysteine correlates with the incidence of sudden coronary death. Homocysteine levels were highest in patients with healed myocardial infarcts or those with healed plaque ruptures (63).

# SUMMARY

Plaque rupture involves lesions with NCs and thin disrupted fibrous caps heavily infiltrated by macrophages, lymphocytes, and occasional smooth muscle cells. The fibrous cap is focally discontinuous, and the luminal thrombus is in communication with the NC. Ruptured plaques are associated with positive remodeling, and approximately 50% of sudden coronary deaths attributed to plaque rupture occur in lesions with less than 50% diameter stenosis. Healed plaque ruptures, which may or may not be clinically silent, are likely to be responsible for plaque progression. NC expansion may occur from intraplaque hemorrhage through the accumulation of free cholesterol derived from erythrocyte membranes and the recruitment of macrophages. Although the trigger for plaque rupture is poorly understood, the destruction of extracellular matrix by metalloproteinases together with local rheological forces and vasospasm is likely to be involved. Risk factors closely associated with rupture are hypercholesterolemia, smoking, age, and high serum levels of hs-CRP.

In contrast, plaque erosion is seen in 40% of patients who die suddenly and is most frequent in women who are younger than 50 years and who smoke. The least frequent cause of thrombosis is a calcified nodule, which is often seen in the right coronary artery and in older individuals with heavily calcified arteries. The precursor lesion to plaque rupture is a thin-cap fibroatheroma, which is identified by an NC with an overlying thin-fibrous cap less than 65 $\mu$m in thickness and is heavily infiltrated by macrophages. The lesion most associated with severe narrowing is the fibrocalcific plaque that usually has a thick fibrous cap and is heavily calcified.

## *References*

1. Virchow R. Cellular pathology. In: Virchow R, ed. *Cellular pathology as based upon physiological and pathological histology*, Birmingham, AL: The Classics of Medicine Library, 1858:362.
2. Stary HC, Chandler AB, Glagov S, et al. A definition of initial, fatty streak, and intermediate lesions of atherosclerosis. A report from the Committee on Vascular Lesions of the Council on Arteriosclerosis, American Heart Association. *Circulation* 1994;89:2462–2478.
3. Stary HC, Chandler AB, Dinsmore RE, et al. A definition of advanced types of atherosclerotic lesions and a histological classification of atherosclerosis. A report from the Committee on Vascular Lesions of the Council on Arteriosclerosis, American Heart Association. *Circulation* 1995;92:1355–1374.

4. Virmani R, Kolodgie FD, Burke AP, et al. Lessons from sudden coronary death: a comprehensive morphological classification scheme for atherosclerotic lesions. *Arterioscler Thromb Vasc Biol* 2000;20:1262–1275.

5. Burke AP, Farb A, Malcom GT, et al. Coronary risk factors and plaque morphology in men with coronary disease who died suddenly. *N Engl J Med* 1997;336:1276–1282.

6. Farb A, Burke AP, Tang AL, et al. Coronary plaque erosion without rupture into a lipid core. A frequent cause of coronary thrombosis in sudden coronary death. *Circulation* 1996;93:1354–1363.

7. Velican D, Velican C. Study of fibrous plaques occurring in the coronary arteries of children. *Atherosclerosis* 1979;33:201–205.

8. Schwartz SM, deBlois D, O'Brien ER. The intima: soil for atherosclerosis and restenosis. *Circ Res* 1995;77:445–465.

9. Tabas I, Marathe S, Keesler GA, et al. Evidence that the initial up-regulation of phosphatidylcholine biosynthesis in free cholesterol-loaded macrophages is an adaptive response that prevents cholesterol-induced cellular necrosis. Proposed role of an eventual failure of this response in foam cell necrosis in advanced atherosclerosis. *J Biol Chem* 1996;271:22773–22781.

10. McGill HC Jr, McMahan CA, Herderick EE, et al. Origin of atherosclerosis in childhood and adolescence. *Am J Clin Nutr* 2000;72:1307S–1315S.

11. Velican D, Velican C. Atherosclerotic involvement of the coronary arteries of adolescents and young adults. *Atherosclerosis* 1980;36:449–460.

12. Kockx MM, De Meyer GR, Bortier H, et al. Luminal foam cell accumulation is associated with smooth muscle cell death in the intimal thickening of human saphenous vein grafts. *Circulation* 1994;94:1255–1262.

13. Tanimura A, McGregor DH, Anderson HC. Calcification in atherosclerosis. I. Human studies. *J Exp Pathol* 1986;2:261–273.

14. Hoff HF, Heideman CL, Gaubatz JW, et al. Correlation of apolipoprotein B retention with the structure of atherosclerotic plaques from human aortas. *Lab Invest* 1978;38:560–567.

15. Radhakrishnamurthy B, Tracy RE, Dalferes ER, et al. Proteoglycans in human coronary arteriosclerotic lesions. *Exp Mol Pathol* 1998;65:1–8.

16. Hansson GK. Immune mechanisms in atherosclerosis. *Arterioscler Thromb Vasc Biol* 2001;21:1876–1890.

17. Libby P, Hansson GK, Schonbeck U, et al. Inflammation in atherosclerosis. *Nature* 2002;420:868–874.

18. Felton CV, Crook D, Davies MJ, et al. Relation of plaque lipid composition and morphology to the stability of human aortic plaques. *Arterioscler Thromb Vasc Biol* 1997;17:1337–1345.

19. Kolodgie FD, Gold HK, Burke AP, et al. Intraplaque hemorrhage and progression of coronary atheroma. *N Engl J Med* 2003;349:2316–2325.

20. Kolodgie FD, Burke AP, Farb A, et al. The thin-cap fibroatheroma: a type of vulnerable plaque: the major precursor lesion to acute coronary syndromes. *Curr Opin Cardiol* 2001;16:285–292.

21. Burke AP, Virmani R, Galis Z, et al. 34th Bethesda Conference: Task Force #2—what is the pathologic basis for new atherosclerosis imaging techniques? *J Am Coll Cardiol* 2003;41:1874–1886.

22. Kruth HS. Localization of unesterified cholesterol in human atherosclerotic lesions. Demonstration of filipin-positive, oil-red-O-negative particles. *Am J Pathol* 1984;114:201–208.

23. Guyton JR, Klemp KF. Transitional features in human atherosclerosis. Intimal thickening, cholesterol clefts, and cell loss in human aortic fatty streaks. *Am J Pathol* 1993;143:1444–1457.

24. Yuan XM, Brunk UT, Olsson AG. Effects of iron- and hemoglobin-loaded human monocyte-derived macrophages on oxidation and uptake of LDL. *Arterioscler Thromb Vasc Biol* 1995;15:1345–1351.

25. Coffey MD, Cole RA, Colles SM, et al. *In vitro* cell injury by oxidized low density lipoprotein involves lipid hydroperoxide-induced formation of alkoxyl, lipid, and peroxyl radicals. *J Clin Invest* 1995;96:1866–1873.

26. Steinberg D. Atherogenesis in perspective: hypercholesterolemia and inflammation as partners in crime. *Nat Med* 2002;8:1211–1217.

27. Wartman WB. Occlusion of the coronary arteries by hemorrhage into their walls. *Am Heart J* 1938;15:459–470.

28. Winternitz MC, Thomas RM, Le Compte PM. Thrombosis. In: Thomas CC, ed. *The biology of atherosclerosis*. Springfield, IL: Charles C Thomas, 1938:94–103.

29. Patterson JC. The reaction of the arterial wall to intramural hemorrhage. *Symposium of atherosclerosis*. Washington, DC: National Academy of Sciences, 1954:65–73.

30. Virmani R, Roberts WC. Pulmonary arteries in congenital heart disease: a structure-function analysis. In: Roberts WC, ed. *Adult congenital heart disease*. Philadelphia, PA: F.A. Davis Co, 1987:77–130.

31. Virmani R, Burke AP, Farb A. Non-neoplastic diseases of the pericardium. *Atlas of cardiovascular pathology*. Philadelphia, PA: WB Saunders, 1996:103–110.

32. Arbustini E, Morbini P, D'Armini AM, et al. Plaque composition in plexogenic and thromboembolic pulmonary hypertension: the critical role of thrombotic material in pultaceous core formation. *Heart* 2002;88:177–182.

33. Bloch K. Cholesterol: evolution of structure and function. In: Vance DE, Vance JE, eds. *Biochemistry of lipids, lipoproteins and membranes*. Amsterdam: Elsevier Science, 1991:363–381.

34. Yeagle PL. Cholesterol and the cell membrane. *Biochim Biophys Acta* 1985;822:267–287.

35. Virmani R, Narula J, Farb A. When neoangiogenesis ricochets. *Am Heart J* 1998;136:937–939.

36. Burke AP, Farb A, Malcom GT, et al. Plaque rupture and sudden death related to exertion in men with coronary artery disease. *JAMA* 1999;281:921–926.

37. McCarthy MJ, Loftus IM, Thompson MM, et al. Angiogenesis and the atherosclerotic carotid plaque: an association between symptomatology and plaque morphology. *J Vasc Surg* 1999;30:261–268.

38. Mofidi R, Crotty TB, McCarthy P, et al. Association between plaque instability, angiogenesis and symptomatic carotid occlusive disease. *Br J Surg* 2001;88:945–950.

39. Davies MJ, Woolf N, Rowles P, et al. Lipid and cellular constituents of unstable human aortic plaques. *Basic Res Cardiol* 1994;89:33–39.

40. Muller JE, Tofler GH, Stone PH. Circadian variation and triggers of onset of acute cardiovascular disease. *Circulation* 1989;79:733–743.

41. Falk E, Shah PK, Fuster V. Coronary plaque disruption. *Circulation* 1995;92:657–671.

42. Farb A, Tang AL, Burke AP, et al. Sudden coronary death. Frequency of active coronary lesions, inactive coronary lesions, and myocardial infarction. *Circulation* 1995;92:1701–1709.

43. Sugiyama S, Okada Y, Sukhova GK, et al. Macrophage myeloperoxidase regulation by granulocyte macrophage colony-stimulating factor in human atherosclerosis and implications in acute coronary syndromes. *Am J Pathol* 2001;158:879–891.

44. Burke AP, Kolodgie FD, Farb A, et al. Role of circulating myeloperoxidase positive monocytes and neutrophils in occlusive coronary thrombi. *J Am Coll Cardiol* 2002;39:256A.

45. Burke AP, Kolodgie FD, Zieske A, et al. Morphologic findings of coronary atherosclerotic plaques in diabetics: a post-mortem study. *Arterioscler Thromb Vasc Biol* 2004;24:1266–1271.

46. Kolodgie FD, Burke AP, Farb A, et al. Differential accumulation of proteoglycans and hyaluronan in culprit lesions: insights into plaque erosion. *Arterioscler Thromb Vasc Biol* 2002;22:1642–1648.

47. Burke AP, Farb A, Malcom GT, et al. Effect of risk factors on the mechanism of acute thrombosis and sudden coronary death in women. *Circulation* 1998;97:2110–2116.

48. Haft JI, Mariano DL, Goldstein J. Comparison of the histopathology of culprit lesions in chronic stable angina, unstable angina, and myocardial infarction. *Clin Cardiol* 1997;20:651–655.

49. Chung IM, Gold HK, Schwartz SM, et al. Enhanced extracellular matrix accumulation in restenosis of coronary arteries after stent deployment. *J Am Coll Cardiol* 2002;40:2072–2081.

50. Zaman AG, Helft G, Worthley SG, et al. The role of plaque rupture and thrombosis in coronary artery disease. *Atherosclerosis* 2000;149:251–266.

51. Mann J, Davies MJ. Mechanisms of progression in native coronary artery disease: role of healed plaque disruption. *Heart* 1999;82:265–268.

52. Burke AP, Kolodgie FD, Farb A, et al. Healed plaque ruptures and sudden coronary death: evidence that subclinical rupture has a role in plaque progression. *Circulation* 2001;103:934–940.

53. O'Brien ER, Urieli-Shoval S, Garvin MR, et al. Replication in restenotic atherectomy tissue. *Atherosclerosis* 2000;152:117–126.

54. Glover C, Ma X, Chen YX, et al. Human in-stent restenosis tissue obtained by means of coronary atherectomy consists of an abundant proteoglycan matrix with a paucity of cell proliferation. *Am Heart J* 2002;144:702–709.

55. Braun-Dullaeus RC, Ziegler A, Bohle RM, et al. Quantification of the cell-cycle inhibitors p27(Kip1) and p21(Cip1) in human atherectomy specimens: primary stenosis versus restenosis. *J Lab Clin Med* 2003;141:179–189.

56. Scott S, O'Sullivan M, Hafizi S, et al. Human vascular smooth muscle cells from restenosis or in-stent stenosis sites demonstrate enhanced responses to p53: implications for brachytherapy and drug treatment for restenosis. *Circ Res* 2002;90:398–404.

57. Boyle JJ, Bowyer DE, Weissberg PL, et al. Human blood-derived macrophages induce apoptosis in human plaque-derived vascular smooth muscle cells by Fas-ligand/Fas interactions. *Arterioscler Thromb Vasc Biol* 2001;21:1402–1407.

58. Bennett MR, Littlewood TD, Schwartz SM, et al. Increased sensitivity of human vascular smooth muscle cells from atherosclerotic plaques to p53-mediated apoptosis. *Circ Res* 1997;81:591–599.

59. Davies MJ, Thomas AC, Knapman PA, et al. Intramyocardial platelet aggregation in patients with unstable angina suffering sudden ischemic cardiac death. *Circulation* 1986;73:418–427.

60. Farb A, Burke AP, Kolodgie FD, et al. Platelet-rich intramyocardial thromboemboli are frequent in acute coronary thrombosis, especially plaque erosions. *Circulation* 2000;102:II-774.

61. Burke AP, Farb A, Pestaner J, et al. Traditional risk factors and the incidence of sudden coronary death with and without coronary thrombosis in blacks. *Circulation* 2002;105:419–424.

62. Burke AP, Tracy RP, Kolodgie F, et al. Elevated C-reactive protein values and atherosclerosis in sudden coronary death: association with different pathologies. *Circulation* 2002;105:2019–2023.

63. Burke AP, Fonseca V, Kolodgie F, et al. Increased serum homocysteine and sudden death resulting from coronary atherosclerosis with fibrous plaques. *Arterioscler Thromb Vasc Biol* 2002;22:1936–1941.

# CHAPTER 55 ■ LABORATORY MARKERS OF PLATELET ACTIVATION

ALAN D. MICHELSON

Platelet activation results in a complex series of changes including a physical redistribution of receptors, changes in the molecular conformation of receptors, secretion of granule contents, development of a procoagulant surface, generation of platelet-derived microparticles, and formation of leukocyte–platelet aggregates. Each of these changes can potentially be used as a marker of platelet activation. Whole blood flow cytometry (1) is the method of choice for the measurement of all these changes, except for the secretion of soluble molecules, which are usually measured by enzyme-linked immunosorbent assay (ELISA). Whole blood flow cytometry has many advantages—only minuscule volumes (approximately 5 $\mu$L) of blood are required; platelets are directly analyzed in their physiologic milieu of whole blood; the minimal manipulation of samples prevents artifactual *in vitro* activation and potential loss of platelet subpopulations; both the activation state of circulating platelets and the reactivity of circulating platelets can be determined; and a spectrum of different activation-dependent changes can be determined.

## PRINCIPLES OF FLOW CYTOMETRY

Flow cytometry rapidly measures the specific characteristics of a large number of individual cells (2). Before flow cytometric analysis, cells in suspension are labeled, typically with a fluorescent conjugated monoclonal antibody. In the flow cytometer, the suspended cells pass through a flow chamber, and, at a rate of 1,000 to 10,000 cells per minute, through the focused beam of a laser. After the laser light activates the fluorophore at the excitation wavelength, detectors process the emitted fluorescence and light-scattering properties of each cell (2). The intensity of the emitted light is directly proportional to the antigen density or the characteristics of the cell being measured.

Clinical studies that utilize flow cytometric assays of washed platelets or platelet-rich plasma are, like other assays of platelet function, potentially susceptible to artifactual *in vitro* platelet activation because of the obligatory separation procedures. The introduction of whole blood flow cytometry by Shattil et al. (3) was therefore a major step toward the application of flow cytometry to clinical settings.

A typical schema of sample preparation for whole blood flow cytometry is shown in Figure 55-1. The anticoagulant is usually buffered sodium citrate. The purpose of the dilution is to minimize the formation of platelet aggregates (see subsequent text). A minimum of two monoclonal antibodies is used, each conjugated with a different fluorophore. A wide variety of fluorophores is available for antibody conjugation [e.g., phycoerythrin, fluorescein, peridinin chlorophyll protein (PerCP), phycoerythrin-Cy5, phycoerythrin-Texas Red (Red-670), and allophycocyanin (APC)]. The "test" monoclonal antibody (which recognizes the antigen to be measured) is added

at a saturating concentration. The "platelet identifier" monoclonal antibody [e.g., glycoprotein (GP) Ib-, integrin $\alpha_{IIb}$-, or integrin $\beta_3$-specific] is added at a near saturating concentration. Physiologic agonists can be used in the assay, including thrombin, thrombin receptor–activating peptide (TRAP), adenosine diphosphate (ADP), collagen, the complement fraction C5b-9, and thromboxane $A_2$ analogs. Nonphysiologic agonists include phorbol myristate acetate and the calcium ionophore A23187. Samples are stabilized by fixation, typically with a final concentration of 1% paraformaldehyde. Antibodies can be added after fixation, provided fixation does not interfere with antibody binding (4) (see subsequent text). Samples are then analyzed in a flow cytometer. After identification of platelets both by their characteristic light scatter and by phycoerythrin positivity, binding of the fluorescein isothiocyanate (FITC)–conjugated test monoclonal antibody is determined by analyzing 5,000 to 10,000 individual platelets.

For specific methodologic protocols of whole blood flow cytometric assays of platelet function, the reader is referred to (5) and (6).

## MEASUREMENT OF PLATELET ACTIVATION

In the absence of an added exogenous platelet agonist, whole blood flow cytometry can determine the activation state of circulating platelets, as judged by the binding of an activation-dependent monoclonal antibody. In addition to this assessment of platelet function *in vivo*, the inclusion of an exogenous agonist in the assay enables analysis of the reactivity of circulating platelets *in vitro*. In the latter application, whole blood flow cytometry is a physiologic assay of platelet function, in that an agonist results in a specific functional response by the platelets: a change in the surface expression of a physiologic receptor (or other antigen or bound ligand), as determined by a change in the binding of a monoclonal antibody. In addition, as discussed below, whole blood flow cytometric enumeration of monocyte–platelet aggregates and procoagulant platelet-derived microparticles are also sensitive markers of *in vivo* platelet activation.

## MARKERS OF PLATELET ACTIVATION

### Activation-Dependent Monoclonal Antibodies

Laboratory markers of platelet activation include activation-dependent conformational changes in integrin $\alpha_{IIb}\beta_3$ (the GP IIb/IIIa complex, CD41/CD61), exposure of granule membrane proteins, platelet surface binding of secreted platelet

Blood
↓
Anticoagulant
↓
Dilution
↓
Test monoclonal antibody (labeled with fluorophore)
+ platelet identifier monoclonal antibody (labeled with different fluorophore)
+ agonist or buffer
↓
Fixation and dilution
↓
Analysis

**FIGURE 55-1.** A typical schema of sample preparation for analysis of platelets by whole blood flow cytometry.

proteins, and development of a procoagulant surface (see Table 55-1). The two most widely studied types of activation-dependent monoclonal antibodies are those directed against conformational changes in $\alpha_{IIb}\beta_3$, and those directed against granule membrane proteins.

Integrin $\alpha_{IIb}\beta_3$ is a receptor for fibrinogen and von Willebrand factor that is essential for platelet aggregation (31). Whereas most monoclonal antibodies directed against $\alpha_{IIb}\beta_3$ bind to resting platelets, monoclonal antibody PAC1 is directed against the fibrinogen-binding site exposed by a conformational change in $\alpha_{IIb}\beta_3$ of activated platelets (see Fig. 55-2 and Table 55-1) (7). Therefore, PAC1 only binds to activated platelets amd not to resting platelets. Other $\alpha_{IIb}\beta_3$-specific activation-dependent monoclonal antibodies are directed against either ligand-induced conformational changes in $\alpha_{IIb}\beta_3$ (ligand-induced binding sites; LIBS) (8) or receptor-induced conformational changes in the bound ligand (fibrinogen) (receptor-induced binding sites; RIBS) (11) (Table 55-1). Rather

than integrin $\alpha_{IIb}\beta_3$-specific monoclonal antibodies, fluorescein-conjugated fibrinogen can also be used in flow cytometric assays to detect the activated form of platelet surface $\alpha_{IIb}\beta_3$ (32,33), but the concentration of unlabeled plasma fibrinogen and unlabeled fibrinogen released from platelet $\alpha$-granules must also be considered in these assays.

The most widely studied type of activation-dependent monoclonal antibodies directed against granule membrane proteins are P selectin (CD62P)–specific. P selectin is a component of the $\alpha$-granule membrane of resting platelets that is only expressed on the platelet surface membrane after $\alpha$-granule secretion. Therefore, a P selectin–specific monoclonal antibody only binds to degranulated platelets, not to resting platelets. The activation-dependent increase in platelet surface P selectin is not reversible over time *in vitro* (34,35). However, *in vivo* circulating degranulated platelets rapidly lose their surface P selectin but continue to circulate and function (36,37). Platelet surface P selectin is therefore not an ideal marker for the detection of circulating degranulated platelets, unless (a) the blood sample is drawn immediately distal to the site of platelet activation, (b) the blood sample is drawn within 5 minutes of the activating stimulus, or (c) there is continuous activation of platelets. The length of time that other activation-dependent surface markers remain expressed on the platelet surface *in vivo* has not yet been definitively determined.

## Leukocyte–Platelet Aggregates

P selectin mediates the initial adhesion of activated platelets to monocytes and neutrophils by the P selectin glycoprotein ligand-1 (PSGL-1) counter-receptor on the leukocyte surface (38). Monocyte–platelet and neutrophil–platelet aggregates are readily identified by whole blood flow cytometry (6,39).

## TABLE 55-1

ACTIVATION-DEPENDENT MONOCLONAL ANTIBODIES—THAT IS, ANTIBODIES THAT BIND TO ACTIVATED BUT NOT RESTING PLATELETS

| Activation-dependent surface change | Prototypic antibodies | References |
|---|---|---|
| **CONFORMATIONAL CHANGES IN INTEGRIN $\alpha_{IIb}\beta_3$** | | |
| Activation-induced conformational change in integrin $\alpha_{IIb}\beta_3$ resulting in exposure of the fibrinogen-binding site | PAC1 | 7 |
| LIBS on integrin $\alpha_{IIb}\beta_3$ | PM 1.1.; LIBS1; LIBS6 | 8–10 |
| RIBS on bound fibrinogen | 2G5; 9F9; F26 | 11–13 |
| **EXPOSURE OF GRANULE MEMBRANE PROTEINS** | | |
| P selectin ($\alpha$-granules) | S12; AC1.2 | 14,15 |
| GMP-33 ($\alpha$-granules) | RUU-SP 1.77 | 16,17 |
| CD63 (lysosomes) | CLB-gran/12 | 18 |
| LAMP-1 (lysosomes) | H5G11 | 19 |
| LAMP-2 (lysosomes) | H4B4 | 20 |
| CD40L | TRAP1 | 21 |
| LOX-1 | JTX68 | 22 |
| **PLATELET SURFACE BINDING OF SECRETED PLATELET PROTEINS** | | |
| Thrombospondin | P8; TSP-1 | 23,24 |
| Multimerin | JS-1 | 25,26 |
| **DEVELOPMENT OF A PROCOAGULANT SURFACE**[a] | | |
| Factor V/Va binding | V237 | 27 |
| Factor X/Xa binding | 5224 | 28 |
| Factor VIII binding | 1B3 | 29 |

LIBS, ligand-induced binding sites; RIBS, receptor-induced binding sites; LOX-1, lectinlike oxidized low density lipoprotein receptor.
[a]Development of a procoagulant platelet surface can also be detected by the binding of annexin V to phosphatidylserine (30).

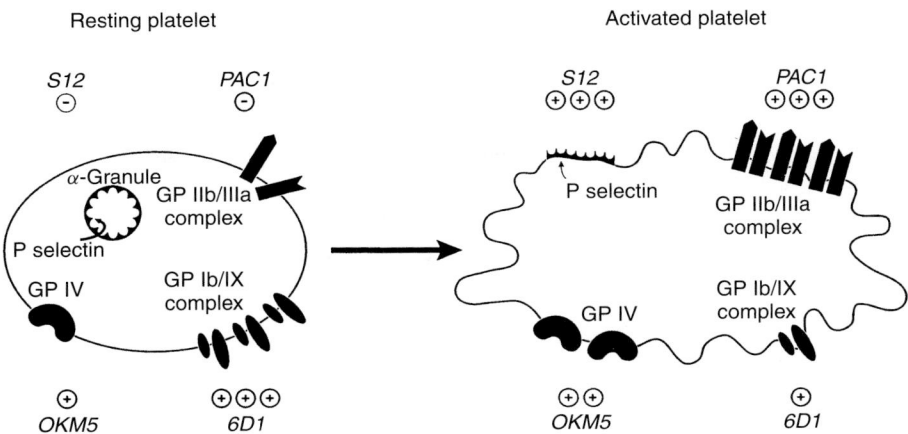

**FIGURE 55-2.** Effect of platelet activation on monoclonal antibody binding. The cartoon depicts the binding of monoclonal antibodies (*in italics*) to resting platelets and the relative change in the binding of these antibodies after thrombin activation. S12 is directed at the α-granule membrane protein P selectin (CD62P). P selectin is not detectable on the surface of resting platelets. After thrombin activation, P selectin is translocated to the platelet plasma membrane. Therefore, S12 only binds to the surface of activated platelets. PAC1 is directed at the fibrinogen-binding site on the GP IIb/IIIa complex (integrin $\alpha_{IIb}\beta_3$). This fibrinogen-binding site is not exposed on resting platelets. Thrombin stimulation results in a conformational change in the GP IIb/IIIa complex that exposes the fibrinogen-binding site. Therefore, PAC1 only binds to the surface of activated platelets. OKM5 is directed at the thrombospondin-binding site on GP IV. OKM5 binds to resting platelets, but binding is increased following thrombin stimulation. 6D1 is directed at the von Willebrand factor–binding site on GP Ib. In contrast to the other monoclonal antibodies, the binding of 6D1 is markedly reduced following thrombin stimulation (40). (From Kestin AS, Ellis PA, Barnard MR, et al. The effect of strenuous exercise on platelet activation state and reactivity. *Circulation* 1993;88:1502–1511, with permission.)

Tracking of autologous infused biotinylated platelets in baboons by three color whole blood flow cytometry enabled us (39) to directly demonstrate *in vivo* that (a) platelets degranulated by thrombin very rapidly (within 1 minute) form circulating aggregates with monocytes and neutrophils (see Fig. 55-3, upper panel), (b) the percentage of monocytes with adherent infused platelets is greater than the percentage of neutrophils with adherent infused platelets (Fig. 55-3, upper panel), and (c) the *in vivo* half-life of detectable circulating monocyte–platelet aggregates (approximately 30 minutes) is longer than both the *in vivo* half-life of neutrophil–platelet aggregates (approximately 5 minutes) and the previously reported (36) rapid loss of surface P selectin from nonaggregated infused platelets (Fig. 55-3, upper panel).

All these findings suggested that measurement of circulating monocyte–platelet aggregates may be a more sensitive indicator of *in vivo* platelet activation than either circulating neutrophil–platelet aggregates or circulating P selectin–positive nonaggregated platelets. We therefore performed two clinical studies in patients with acute coronary syndromes (39). In the first study, after percutaneous coronary intervention (PCI), there was more circulating monocyte–platelet (and, to a lesser extent, neutrophil–platelet) aggregates, but not P selectin–positive platelets, in peripheral blood. In the second study, of patients presenting to an Emergency Department with chest pain, patients with acute myocardial infarction had more circulating monocyte–platelet aggregates than patients without acute myocardial infarction and healthy controls. However, circulating P selectin–positive platelets were not increased in chest pain patients with or without acute myocardial infarction (39).

In summary, we have demonstrated by five independent means [*in vivo* tracking of activated platelets in baboons (Fig. 55-3, upper panel) (39), human PCI (39), human acute myocardial infarction (39), human stable coronary artery disease (41) (discussed in subsequent text), and human chronic venous insufficiency (42) (discussed in subsequent text)] that circulating monocyte–platelet aggregates are more sensitive markers of *in vivo* platelet activation than platelet surface P selectin.

## Platelet-Derived Microparticles

As determined by flow cytometry, *in vitro* activation of platelets by some agonists (e.g., C5b-9, collagen/thrombin, and the calcium ionophore A23187) in the presence of extracellular calcium ions results in platelet-derived microparticles (defined by low forward-angle light scatter and binding of a platelet-specific monoclonal antibody) that are procoagulant (determined by binding of monoclonal antibodies to activated factors V or VIII or by annexin V) (27,29,30). These findings suggest that procoagulant platelet-derived microparticles may have an important role in the assembly of the "tenase" and "prothrombinase" components of the coagulation system *in vivo*. A flow cytometric method for the direct detection of procoagulant platelet-derived microparticles in whole blood has been developed (43).

## Platelet-Derived Plasma Markers

Platelet-derived plasma markers are usually measured by ELISA. Platelet secretion results in the release of numerous soluble molecules from intracellular granules into plasma. Of these molecules, the most commonly measured as markers of platelet activation are the α-granule constituents: soluble P selectin (44), β-thromboglobulin (β-TG) (45,46), and platelet factor 4 (PF4) (45,46). However, because of the obligatory plasma separation procedures, these assays are particularly vulnerable to artifactual *in vitro* platelet activation (45,46). Furthermore, soluble P selectin in plasma may be of endothelial cell origin (44). Lumiaggregometry can be used to measure the *ex vivo* release of adenosine triphosphate (ATP) from dense granules in response to an exogenous agonist (47).

Proteolysis of platelet surface molecules results in the generation of plasma markers of platelet activation. Platelet surface GP V is proteolyzed by thrombin (48–50), releasing a soluble form of GP V (sGP V) into plasma (51). Release of soluble CD40 ligand (sCD40L) by the activation-induced proteolysis of platelet surface CD40L (52,53) is the predominant source of plasma sCD40L (52). sCD40L shows prothrombotic action by stabilization of arterial thrombi by a $\beta_3$ integrin–dependent

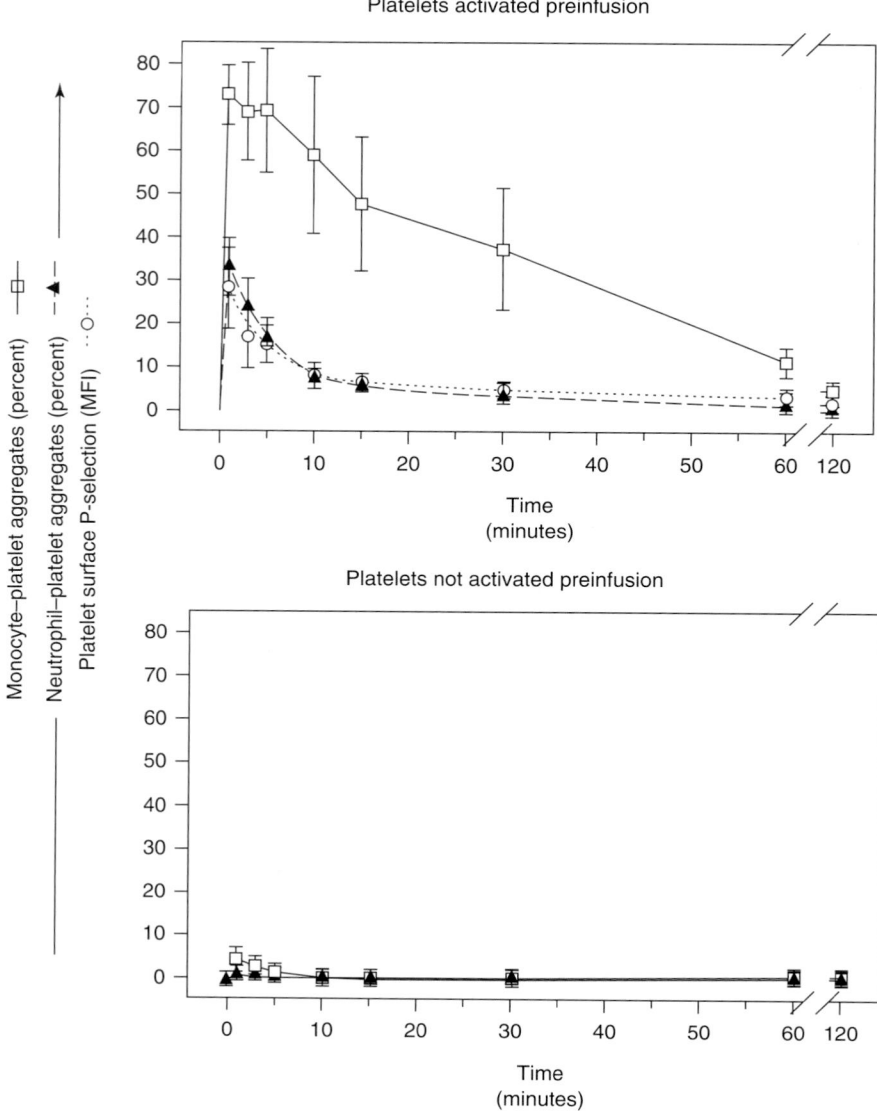

FIGURE 55-3. *In vivo* tracking of platelets. Baboons were infused with autologous, biotinylated platelets that were (**upper panel**) or were not (**lower panel**) thrombin-activated preinfusion. Surface P selectin on the infused platelets and participation of the infused platelets in circulating monocyte–platelet and neutrophil–platelet aggregates was determined by three-color whole blood flow cytometric analysis of peripheral blood samples drawn at the indicated time points. The "0" time point refers to blood samples taken immediately preinfusion. Platelet surface P selectin is expressed as mean fluorescence intensity (MFI), as a percentage of the fluorescence of a preinfusion maximally activated (10 U per mL) thrombin control sample. Monocyte–platelet and neutrophil–platelet aggregates are expressed as the percent of all monocytes and neutrophils with adherent infused platelets. Data are mean ± S.E.M. (From Michelson AD, Barnard MR, Krueger LA, et al. Circulating monocyte–platelet aggregates are a more sensitive marker of *in vivo* platelet activation than platelet surface P selectin: studies in baboons, human coronary intervention, and human acute myocardial infarction. *Circulation* 2001;104:1533–1537, with permission.)

mechanism (54) and proinflammatory action by induction of leukocyte chemokine production (55) and endothelial cell adhesive proteins (56) [although not all studies agree on this latter point (52)]. An important practical point is that many published studies on sCD40L levels of patients performed the assay in serum. However, blood clotting in a serum tube results in platelet activation and the *ex vivo* release of large amounts of sCD40L into the serum. Therefore, accurate measurement of *in vivo* circulating sCD40L requires assay in plasma rather than serum (57).

Plasma and urine assays for thromboxane $A_2$ metabolites also have utility in the measurement of platelet activation (58–60).

## Platelet Activation in Clinical Disorders

### Acute Coronary Syndromes

Platelets play an important role in the pathogenesis of coronary artery disease including unstable angina and acute myocardial infarction (61,62). Angiography (63) and angioscopy

(64) during acute coronary ischemic syndromes frequently reveal intracoronary arterial thrombi, which pathologic studies have found to be rich in platelets (65). In large clinical trials, antiplatelet agents have been shown to reduce the incidence of cardiovascular ischemic events, supporting the concept of an association between platelet activation and cardiovascular ischemia (66). Furthermore, some investigators have found biochemical markers of platelet activation to be elevated during episodes of acute cardiac ischemia (58,67), which may identify patients who could benefit from additional antiplatelet therapy (67).

Whole blood flow cytometric studies have demonstrated circulating activated platelets, as determined by activation-dependent monoclonal antibodies, in patients with stable angina, unstable angina, and acute myocardial infarction (41,68–71). In addition, as determined by activation-dependent monoclonal antibodies, PCI results in platelet activation in coronary sinus blood (72,73).

Flow cytometric analysis of platelet activation–dependent markers can be used to determine optimal antiplatelet therapy in clinical settings, for example, in acute coronary syndromes (74,75) and after coronary stenting (76,77). Flow cytometric analysis of platelet activation markers before PCI can predict an increased risk of acute and subacute ischemic events after PCI (78–81). Flow cytometrically detected exposure of LIBS is strongly associated with the development and progression of heart transplant vasculopathy (82).

The Pl[A2] polymorphism of GP IIIa has been reported to be associated with ischemic coronary syndromes (83). Flow cytometry has been used to demonstrate that (a) Pl[A2]-positive platelets display a lower threshold for activation, and (b) platelets heterozygous for Pl[A] alleles show increased sensitivity to antiplatelet drugs (84).

Circulating leukocyte–platelet aggregates are increased in stable coronary artery disease (41), unstable angina (68), acute myocardial infarction (85,86), and cardiopulmonary bypass (87). Circulating leukocyte–platelet aggregates also increase after PCI, with a greater magnitude in patients experiencing late clinical events (88). As discussed in the previous text, circulating monocyte–platelet aggregates (but not neutrophil–platelet aggregates) are a more sensitive marker of *in vivo* platelet activation than platelet surface P selectin in the clinical settings of stable coronary artery disease (41), PCI (39), and acute myocardial infarction (39). Furthermore, circulating monocyte–platelet aggregates are an early marker of acute myocardial infarction (89).

Platelet-derived microparticles are increased in acute coronary syndromes (90) and in cardiopulmonary bypass (12,91).

Elevated plasma levels of sCD40L have been demonstrated in unstable angina (92), PCI (92), and cardiopulmonary bypass (93). GP IIb/IIIa antagonists inhibit the release of sCD40L from platelets both in *vitro* (53,94) and in *vivo* (95). Measurement of sCD40L in the first 12 hours after the onset of ischemic symptoms in patients with unstable angina identifies a subgroup of patients who experience a much greater clinical benefit from abciximab treatment (96). High plasma concentrations of sCD40L may be associated with increased cardiovascular risk in apparently healthy women (97).

Elevated plasma levels of sGP V have also been demonstrated in patients with coronary artery disease (51).

## Cerebrovascular Ischemia

Increased circulation of P selectin–positive, CD63-positive, activated $\alpha_{IIb}\beta_3$-positive platelets, and platelet-derived microparticles have been reported in acute cerebrovascular ischemia (98–102). This platelet activation is evident 3 months after the acute event, suggesting the possibility of an underlying prothrombotic state (100,102,103). Furthermore, increased expression of surface P selectin on platelets is a risk factor for silent cerebral infarction in patients with atrial fibrillation (104).

Platelet-derived microparticles are increased after transient ischemic attacks (12,105). Increased platelet-derived microparticles and procoagulant activity occur in symptomatic patients with prosthetic heart valves and provide a potential pathophysiologic explanation of cerebrovascular events in this patient group (106).

## Peripheral Vascular Disease

Circulating activated platelets and platelet hyperreactivity (as determined by P selectin expression, platelet aggregates, and platelet-derived microparticle formation) are increased in patients with peripheral arterial occlusive disease compared with healthy volunteers (107,108). In addition, plasma levels of sCD40L (109) and sGP V (51) are elevated in peripheral arterial occlusive disease.

With regard to peripheral venous disease, Peyton et al. demonstrated more circulating monocyte–platelet aggregates in patients with chronic venous stasis ulceration than in control individuals without venous disease. Interestingly, these changes were present not only in blood drawn from the lower extremity veins of affected individuals but also in blood drawn from their arm veins, suggesting that the changes are systemic rather than localized to the lower extremities (42). Powell et al. (110) further characterized these findings as being related to the presence of chronic venous disease rather than the presence of venous ulceration because increased numbers of monocyte–platelet aggregates were noted in patients with all classes of venous disease and not just in patients with deep venous valvular insufficiency. Furthermore, increased levels of monocyte–platelet aggregates were noted even in patients with only superficial venous stasis disease manifested by the presence of varicose veins. Even more intriguing is the fact that the number of monocyte–platelet aggregates remains elevated 6 weeks after total correction of the venous insufficiency by stripping of the abnormal veins, leaving normal venous physiology as documented by postoperative duplex scanning (111). This finding suggests an underlying predisposition to the development of chronic venous disease in these patients, perhaps mediated by monocyte–platelet interactions.

## Other Clinical Disorders Associated with Platelet Hyperreactivity and/or Circulating Activated Platelets

Other conditions in which whole blood flow cytometric measurement of platelet hyperreactivity, circulating activated platelets, and/or circulating leukocyte–platelet aggregates may prove to have a clinical role include diabetes mellitus (112), preeclampsia (113,114), placental insufficiency (115), nephrotic syndrome (116), hemodialysis (117), sickle cell disease (118), systemic inflammatory response syndrome (119), septic multiple organ dysfunction syndrome (120,121), antiphospholipid syndrome (122), systemic lupus erythematosus (122), rheumatoid arthritis (122), myeloproliferative disorders (123,124), and Alzheimer disease (125). High levels of circulating monocyte–platelet aggregates can predict rejection episodes after orthotopic liver transplantation (126). Uremic patients with thrombotic events have higher numbers of circulating platelet-derived microparticles than those without thrombotic events (127).

## Quality Control of Stored Platelet Concentrates in the Blood Bank

As determined by P selectin, CD63, and integrin $\alpha_{IIb}\beta_3$, flow cytometric studies of platelets stored in the blood bank before transfusion have provided direct evidence of a time-dependent platelet activation (128–130). These changes correlated with modifications in platelet morphology (decrease in swirling), leakage of lactate dehydrogenase, and release of $\beta$-thromboglobulin (128). It has been suggested that platelet surface P selectin may be useful as a quality control measurement, on the basis of correlations between the platelet surface expression of P selectin in stored blood bank platelets and (a) posttransfusion platelet counts (131), (b) platelet survival determined by In (129),(132) and (c) clearance of P selectin–positive platelets from the recipient (129).

## Platelet Hyporeactivity

Although there are currently few published studies in this area, whole blood flow cytometry may be useful in the clinical assessment of platelet hyporeactivity. For example, compared to adults, the platelets of very low birth weight preterm neonates are markedly hyporeactive to thrombin, ADP/epinephrine, and thromboxane $A_2$, as determined by flow cytometric detection of (a) the exposure of the fibrinogen-binding site on integrin $\alpha_{IIb}\beta_3$, (b) fibrinogen binding, (c) the increase in platelet surface P selectin, and (d) the decrease in platelet surface GP Ib (133). This platelet hyporeactivity may contribute to the risk of intraventricular hemorrhage in neonates with very low birth weight (134).

# SPECIFIC METHODOLOGIC ISSUES OF WHOLE BLOOD FLOW CYTOMETRY

## Blood Drawing

After discarding the first 2 mL of blood, collection of blood into a 3.2% sodium citrate Vacutainer (Becton Dickinson) does not result in significant platelet activation (135). However, each laboratory should determine whether their method of collection, including the drawing of samples through PCI and other catheters, results in artifactual *in vitro* platelet activation, as determined by the binding of activation-dependent monoclonal antibodies.

Although sodium citrate (a weak calcium chelator) is the most commonly used anticoagulant, other anticoagulants have been successfully used, for example, corn trypsin inhibitor (an inhibitor of activated factor XII) (136). Ethylenediaminetetraacetic acid (EDTA) (a strong calcium chelator) should be avoided because it uncomplexes $\alpha_{IIb}\beta_3$. Nonchelating anticoagulants [e.g., D-Phe-Pro-Arg-chloromethylketone (PPACK) (a direct thrombin inhibitor)] may be preferable for the monitoring of GP IIb/IIIa antagonist therapy (137).

## Minimizing Platelet Aggregates

Platelet aggregates can be minimized in the preparation of platelets for whole blood flow cytometry by a combination of the following methods: (a) preparing reagents in advance and avoiding delays in procedure; (b) using a light tourniquet and a needle not narrower than 21 gauge to collect blood; (c) smooth, easy flow from the blood draw; (d) discarding the first 2 mL of blood; (e) using polypropylene (or siliconized glass) tubes or syringes; (f) immediate mixing with the anticoagulant; (g) no washing, centrifugation, gel filtration, vortexing, or stirring steps; (h) reducing the platelet count by dilution of the samples; (i) if thrombin is the agonist, including the synthetic tetrapeptide Gly-Pro-Arg-Pro (GPRP) in the assay (see subsequent text); (j) mixing gently after addition of agonist, then incubating undisturbed; and (k) fixing (see subsequent text). RGD-containing peptides have also been used to minimize platelet aggregates (138) but these peptides may interfere with the binding of detecting antibodies (e.g., PAC1) and result in exposure of LIBS (8,9).

Each sample should be monitored for evidence of platelet aggregation ["smearing" of the platelets into the upper right quadrant of the log-side (orthogonal) light scatter vs. log-forward light scatter histogram].

## Use of Thrombin in Whole Blood Assays

Platelet activation by thrombin, one of the most physiologically important platelet activators (139–141), can be directly measured in whole blood through the use of the synthetic peptide GPRP (142). In the absence of GPRP, addition of thrombin to whole blood results in a fibrin clot, thereby precluding the use of thrombin as an agonist in the whole blood assay. Furthermore, thrombin is a potent inducer of platelet-to-platelet aggregation, which precludes analysis by flow cytometry of activation-dependent changes in individual platelets. However, addition to whole blood of GPRP together with thrombin inhibits both fibrin polymerization and, to a lesser extent, platelet-to-platelet aggregation, without affecting thrombin-induced platelet activation (40,142,143). An alternative to the use of thrombin and GPRP in a whole blood flow cytometric assay is the use of TRAP. TRAP is a peptide fragment of the protease-activated receptor 1 (PAR1) "tethered ligand" receptor for thrombin (144). Without the need for GPRP, TRAP directly activates platelets in whole blood without resulting in a fibrin clot (145). However, TRAP may not reflect all aspects of thrombin-induced platelet activation, because PAR1 is not the only platelet receptor for thrombin (146).

## Detection of the Activation-Dependent Decrease in the Platelet Surface Expression of the GP Ib/IX/V Complex

Whole blood flow cytometric assays frequently employ a GP Ib– or GP IX–specific monoclonal antibody to identify platelets. Because GP Ib and GP IX are not present on any circulating blood cell except platelets (147,148), the activation-induced decrease in the platelet surface expression of GP Ib/IX (143,143,149,150) generally does not result in fluorescence lesser than the threshold used to distinguish platelets from other cells and debris (3,40). Therefore, no subpopulations of platelets are excluded. A method of avoiding the activation-induced decrease in binding of a GP Ib–specific monoclonal antibody is to add a direct conjugate of the GP Ib–specific antibody before addition of the agonist [(151); see subsequent text].

To specifically analyze the activation-induced decrease in the platelet surface expression of the GP Ib/IX complex in whole blood, an $\alpha_{IIb}$- or $\beta_3$-specific monoclonal antibody can be employed as the platelet-identifying reagent (135).

There is an important methodologic point that needs to be emphasized in the flow cytometric detection of the activation-induced decrease in the platelet surface expression of the GP Ib/IX complex (151). If a FITC-conjugated GP Ib/IX–specific test monoclonal antibody is added before the platelet agonist (as in the typical schema shown in Fig. 55-1), the activation-induced redistribution of GP Ib/IX to the surface-connected canalicular system (152) will not result in a significant decrease in platelet fluorescence because a flow cytometer can detect FITC fluorescence irrespective of whether the conjugated antibody is on the surface or the interior of the platelet. Therefore, in flow cytometric assays examining platelet surface GP Ib/IX modulation, GP Ib/IX–specific antibodies that are directly conjugated (e.g., with FITC) must be added to the assay *after* the addition of the agonist.

## Fixation

Sample fixation is very advantageous in a clinical setting where there may not be immediate access to a flow cytometer. Fixation prevents subsequent artifactual *in vitro* platelet activation. For most antibodies, the "antibody labeling before fixation" method described in previous text, and shown in Figure 55-1, results in no significant differences in fluorescence intensity between samples analyzed immediately and samples analyzed within 24 hours of fixation (143). A "fixation before antibody labeling" method also results in no significant differences in fluorescence intensity between samples analyzed immediately and samples analyzed within 24 hours of antibody labeling (135). However, fixation is an important variable to be controlled for, especially in a "fixation before antibody labeling" method because the binding of activation-dependent monoclonal antibodies to fixed platelets is often decreased compared to unfixed platelets (4). Furthermore, the binding of some antibodies further decreases after fixation in a time-dependent manner. The optimal fixation method for each new monoclonal antibody must therefore be defined by each laboratory.

A compelling argument in favor of immediate sample fixation is that activation-dependent changes are often time-dependent, at least *in vitro*. For example, the platelet surface expression of the GP Ib/IX/V complex decreases within 30 seconds of platelet activation, reaching a nadir at approximately 5 minutes, but, approximately in the next 45 minutes, the platelet surface expression of the GP Ib/IX/V complex returns to normal (34). The activation-dependent increase in the platelet surface expression of integrin $\alpha_{IIb}\beta_3$ and CD40 ligand (CD40L and CD154) are also reversible with time (21,35). In contrast, although circulating degranulated platelets rapidly lose their surface P selectin *in vivo* (36), the activation-dependent increase in platelet surface P selectin is not reversible over time *in vitro* (34,35).

## Choice of Antibodies

Because the exposure of different antigens reflect different aspects of platelet activation, it may be preferable to use a panel of monoclonal antibodies. Monoclonal antibodies are preferable to polyclonal antibodies in whole blood flow cytometry because these (a) can more reliably saturate all specific epitopes and (b) result in less nonspecific binding. Platelet-specific monoclonal antibodies are now available from a wide variety of commercial sources and can often be purchased already conjugated to fluorescein, biotin, phycoerythrin, PerCP, APC, or a tandem conjugate (e.g., phycoerythrin-Cy5 or RED-670). Alternatively, unlabeled antibodies can be FITC-conjugated by the method of Rinderknecht (153) or (easier and more rapidly) by a kit method (commercially available from, e.g., Boehringer Mannheim, Molecular Probes, and Sigma-Aldrich). Antibodies can be biotinylated as described by Shattil et al. (3) or by following the biotin manufacturer's directions. The use of antibodies that are directly conjugated with fluorescein, phycoerythrin, PerCP, APC, or tandem conjugates eliminates the requirement for the addition of secondary antibodies, thereby avoiding time-consuming additional incubations and washing procedures, which, in unfixed samples, may result in artifactual *in vitro* activation of platelets. Furthermore, the use of secondary antibodies is likely to result in increased background fluorescence, and decreased sensitivity of the assay. Finally, the use of directly conjugated antibodies allows multiple-color analysis with, for example, a number of differently conjugated murine antibodies.

$F_{ab}$ fragments of monoclonal antibodies can be used to avoid $F_c$-mediated binding and the $F_c$-induced platelet activation that has been reported with some monoclonal antibodies (154). However, the use of $F_{ab}$ fragments is usually unnecessary, provided: (a) The absence of antibody-induced binding of other activation-dependent monoclonal antibodies is demonstrated in control samples or the problem is avoided by fixation before test antibody binding, (b) the $F_c$-mediated and nonspecific binding obtained from parallel samples with isotypic species–specific immunoglobulin is subtracted from the binding of the test antibody, or (c) the Fc$\gamma$RIIa receptor–specific monoclonal antibody IV.3, immunoglobulins, or $F_c$ fragments are used as blocking reagents.

The saturating concentration of each antibody for platelet binding must be specifically determined by each laboratory. This concentration is typically between 0.25 and 20 $\mu$g per mL. In addition, when more than one monoclonal antibody is used in the same assay (as is standard in whole blood flow cytometry), it

is necessary to determine that these antibodies do not interfere each other's binding to the platelet surface.

Platelets can be detected in whole blood by light scatter only. However, some of the particles falling within the light scatter gate for platelets may not bind any platelet-specific monoclonal antibody. It is therefore recommended that a minimum two-color/two-antibody technique be used for whole blood flow cytometry: One monoclonal antibody (e.g., GP Ib–, GP IX–, $\alpha_{IIb}$-, or $\beta_3$-specific, typically phycoerythrin-conjugated) is used to identify a particle as a platelet; another monoclonal antibody (typically FITC-conjugated) is used to quantify the expression of the GP of interest.

## Expression of Antibody Binding

Antibody binding can be expressed as MFI (mean fluorescence intensity) or as the percentage of platelets staining positive for a particular antibody [on the basis of a positive analysis region placed just to the right of the negative (isotype) control fluorescence histogram]. Depending on the experimental circumstances and the physiologic nature of the antigen being measured, either MFI or percent-positive platelets may have more relevance than the other. Unlike the MFI method, the "percent-positive platelets" method is independent of variations in signal amplification [e.g., because of changes in photomultiplier tube (PMT) voltage or gain] because the negative control signal increases in proportion with the test sample. The "percent-positive platelets" method may detect subpopulations of platelets arising from a local *in vivo* insult. However, it is important to realize that "antibody-positive" platelets may have very little antigen expressed on their surface. For example, in a given clinical setting, the data may be reported as 20% circulating activated platelets, on the basis of P selectin positivity. However, if each P selectin–positive platelet expresses only 10% of maximal platelet surface P selectin, then the overall average increase in platelet surface P selectin is only 2%. If the goal is to determine the total amount of platelet surface antigen, MFI is the preferred method of data presentation. For activation-dependent antibodies, inclusion of a control sample maximally activated by thrombin, TRAP, or phorbol myristate acetate assists in the quantification of the amount of surface antigen per platelet. The activation-dependent decrease in platelet surface GP Ib/IX/V (143) should be quantified by MFI rather than by the "percent-positive platelets" method because the decrease in platelet surface GP Ib/IX/V on each platelet is usually insufficient to result in a "negative" platelet.

Although standard flow cytometry does not result in a measure of the absolute number of binding sites, Shattil et al. (3) and Johnston et al. (155) used monoclonal antibodies double-labeled with $^{125}$I and biotin to demonstrate a linear relation between the number of antibody binding sites per platelet, as determined by $^{125}$I-labeled and (after incubation with phycoerythrin-streptavidin) fluorescent-labeled antibody. Once this relation is known for a given monoclonal antibody, it is possible to use subsequent batches of the biotinylated or FITC-conjugated antibody for binding site quantitation, provided that the molar ratio of fluorescein to antibody is known.

Commercial kits (e.g., Quantum and Sigma-Aldrich) containing a set of calibrated fluorescent standards and software can be used to determine molecules of equivalent soluble fluorochrome (MESF). Use of these standards allows: (a) quantitation of the fluorescence intensity of samples in MESF, (b) determination of the fluorescence threshold of the instrument, (c) determination of the linearity and stability of the instrument, and, most important, (d) data comparison over time and between different instruments and laboratories (156). Furthermore, flow cytometric methods are now available for the absolute quantitation of the number of antibodies bound per cell (e.g., Quantum Simply Cellular Microbeads Kit, Sigma-Aldrich, and BioCytex). The lower limit of detection of antibody binding by flow cytometry is approximately 500 antibody molecules per platelet.

# References

1. Michelson AD, Barnard MR, Krueger LA, et al. Flow cytometry. In: Michelson AD, ed. *Platelets*. New York: Academic Press/Elsevier Science, 2002.
2. Givan AL. *Flow cytometry. First principles*. New York: Wiley-Liss, 1992.
3. Shattil SJ, Cunningham M, Hoxie JA. Detection of activated platelets in whole blood using activation-dependent monoclonal antibodies and flow cytometry. *Blood* 1987;70:307–315.
4. Michelson AD, Barnard MR, Benoit SE, et al. Characterization of platelet binding of blind panel mAb. In: Schlossman SF, Boumsell L, Gilks W et al., eds. *Leucocyte typing V*. Oxford: Oxford University Press, 1995.
5. Krueger LA, Barnard MR, Frelinger AL III, et al. Immunophenotypic analysis of platelets. In: Robinson JP, Darzynkiewicz Z, Dean PN, et al., eds. *Current protocols in cytometry*. New York: John Wiley and Sons, 2002.
6. Barnard MR, Krueger LA, Frelinger AL III, et al. Whole blood analysis of leukocyte-platelet aggregates. In: Robinson JP, Darzynkiewicz Z, Dean PN, et al., eds. *Current protocols in cytometry*. New York: John Wiley and Sons, 2003.
7. Shattil SJ, Hoxie JA, Cunningham M, et al. Changes in the platelet membrane glycoprotein IIb-IIIa complex during platelet activation. *J Biol Chem* 1985;260:11107–11114.
8. Frelinger AL, Lam SC, Plow EF, et al. Occupancy of an adhesive glycoprotein receptor modulates expression of an antigenic site involved in cell adhesion. *J Biol Chem* 1988;263:12397–12402.
9. Frelinger AL, Cohen I, Plow EF, et al. Selective inhibition of integrin function by antibodies specific for ligand-occupied receptor conformers. *J Biol Chem* 1990;265:6346–6352.
10. Ginsberg MH, Frelinger AL, Lam SC, et al. Analysis of platelet aggregation disorders based on flow cytometric analysis of membrane glycoprotein IIb-IIIa with conformation-specific monoclonal antibodies. *Blood* 1990;76:2017–2023.
11. Zamarron C, Ginsberg MH, Plow EF. Monoclonal antibodies specific for a conformationally altered state of fibrinogen. *Thromb Haemost* 1990;64:41–46.
12. Abrams CS, Ellison N, Budzynski AZ, et al. Direct detection of activated platelets and platelet-derived microparticles in humans. *Blood* 1990;75:128–138.
13. Gralnick HR, Williams SB, McKeown L, et al. Endogenous platelet fibrinogen: its modulation after surface expression is related to size-selective access to and conformational changes in the bound fibrinogen. *Br J Haematol* 1992;80:347–357.
14. Stenberg PE, McEver RP, Shuman MA, et al. A platelet alpha-granule membrane protein (GMP-140) is expressed on the plasma membrane after activation. *J Cell Biol* 1985;101:880–886.
15. Larsen E, Celi A, Gilbert GE, et al. PADGEM protein: a receptor that mediates the interaction of activated platelets with neutrophils and monocytes. *Cell* 1989;59:305–312.
16. Metzelaar MJ, Heijnen HF, Sixma JJ, et al. Identification of a 33-kD protein associated with the alpha-granule membrane (GMP-33) that is expressed on the surface of activated platelets. *Blood* 1992;79:372–379.
17. Damas C, Vink T, Nieuwenhuis HK, et al. The 33-kDa platelet alpha-granule membrane protein (GMP-33) is an N-terminal proteolytic fragment of thrombospondin. *Thromb Haemost* 2001;86:887–893.
18. Nieuwenhuis HK, van Oosterhout JJ, Rozemuller E, et al. Studies with a monoclonal antibody against activated platelets: evidence that a secreted 53,000-molecular weight lysosome-like granule protein is exposed on the surface of activated platelets in the circulation. *Blood* 1987;70:838–845.
19. Febbraio M, Silverstein RL. Identification and characterization of LAMP-1 as an activation-dependent platelet surface glycoprotein. *J Biol Chem* 1990;265:18531–18537.
20. Silverstein RL, Febbraio M. Identification of lysosome-associated membrane protein-2 as an activation-dependent platelet surface glycoprotein. *Blood* 1992;80:1470–1475.
21. Henn V, Slupsky JR, Grafe M, et al. CD40 ligand on activated platelets triggers an inflammatory reaction of endothelial cells. *Nature* 1998;391:591–594.
22. Chen M, Kakutani M, Naruko T, et al. Activation-dependent surface expression of LOX-1 in human platelets. *Biochem Biophys Res Commun* 2001;282:153–158.
23. Boukerche H, McGregor JL. Characterization of an anti-thrombospondin monoclonal antibody (P8) that inhibits human blood platelet functions. Normal binding of P8 to thrombin-activated Glanzmann thrombasthenic platelets. *Eur J Biochem* 1988;171:383–392.
24. Aiken ML, Ginsberg MH, Plow EF. Mechanisms for expression of thrombospondin on the platelet cell surface. *Semin Thromb Hemost* 1987;13:307–316.
25. Hayward CP, Smith JW, Horsewood P, et al. p-155, a multimeric platelet protein that is expressed on activated platelets. *J Biol Chem* 1991;266:7114–7120.
26. Hayward CP, Bainton DF, Smith JW, et al. Multimerin is found in the alpha-granules of resting platelets and is synthesized by a megakaryocytic cell line. *J Clin Invest* 1993;91:2630–2639.
27. Sims PJ, Faioni EM, Wiedmer T, et al. Complement proteins C5b-9 cause release of membrane vesicles from the platelet surface that are enriched in the membrane receptor for coagulation factor Va and express prothrombinase activity. *J Biol Chem* 1988;263:18205–18212.
28. Holme PA, Brosstad F, Solum NO. Platelet-derived microvesicles and activated platelets express factor Xa activity. *Blood Coagul Fibrinolysis* 1995;6:302–310.
29. Gilbert GE, Sims PJ, Wiedmer T, et al. Platelet-derived microparticles express high affinity receptors for factor VIII. *J Biol Chem* 1991;266:17261–17268.
30. Furman MI, Krueger LA, Frelinger AL III, et al. GPIIb-IIIa antagonist-induced reduction in platelet surface factor V/Va binding and phosphatidylserine expression in whole blood. *Thromb Haemost* 2000;84:492–498.
31. Hato T, Ginsberg MH, Shattil SJ. Integrin alphaIIb-beta3. In: Michelson AD, ed. *Platelets*. New York: Academic Press/Elsevier Science, 2002.
32. Faraday N, Goldschmidt-Clermont P, Dise K, et al. Quantitation of soluble fibrinogen binding to platelets by fluorescence-activated flow cytometry. *J Lab Clin Med* 1994;123:728–740.
33. Heilmann E, Hynes LA, Burstein SA, et al. Fluorescein derivatization of fibrinogen for flow cytometric analysis of fibrinogen binding to platelets. *Cytometry* 1994;17:287–293.
34. Michelson AD, Benoit SE, Kroll MH, et al. The activation-induced decrease in the platelet surface expression of the glycoprotein Ib-IX complex is reversible. *Blood* 1994;83:3562–3573.
35. Ruf A, Patscheke H. Flow cytometric detection of activated platelets: comparison of determining shape change, fibrinogen binding, and P-selectin expression. *Semin Thromb Hemost* 1995;21:146–151.
36. Michelson AD, Barnard MR, Hechtman HB, et al. *In vivo* tracking of platelets: circulating degranulated platelets rapidly lose surface P-selectin but continue to circulate and function. *Proc Natl Acad Sci U S A* 1996;93:11877–11882.
37. Berger G, Hartwell DW, Wagner DD. P-selectin and platelet clearance. *Blood* 1998;92:4446–4452.
38. McEver RP. P-selectin/PSGL-1 and other interactions between platelets, leukocytes, and endothelium. In: Michelson AD, ed. *Platelets*. New York: Academic Press/Elsevier Science, 2002.
39. Michelson AD, Barnard MR, Krueger LA, et al. Circulating monocyte-platelet aggregates are a more sensitive marker of *in vivo* platelet activation than platelet surface P-selectin: studies in baboons, human coronary intervention, and human acute myocardial infarction. *Circulation* 2001;104:1533–1537.
40. Kestin AS, Ellis PA, Barnard MR, et al. The effect of strenuous exercise on platelet activation state and reactivity. *Circulation* 1993;88:1502–1511.
41. Furman MI, Benoit SE, Barnard MR, et al. Increased platelet reactivity and circulating monocyte-platelet aggregates in patients with stable coronary artery disease. *J Am Coll Cardiol* 1998;31:352–358.
42. Peyton BD, Rohrer MJ, Furman MI, et al. Patients with venous stasis ulceration have increased monocyte-platelet aggregation. *J Vasc Surg* 1998;27:1109–1115.
43. Michelson AD, Rajasekhar D, Bednarek FJ, et al. Platelet and platelet-derived microparticle surface factor V/Va binding in whole blood: differences between neonates and adults. *Thromb Haemost* 2000;84:689–694.
44. Chong BH, Murray B, Berndt MC, et al. Plasma P-selectin is increased in thrombotic consumptive platelet disorders. *Blood* 1994;83:1535–1541.
45. Kaplan KL, Owen J. Radioimmunoassays of platelet alpha-granule proteins. In: Harker LA, Zimmerman TS, eds. *Measurements of platelet function*. Edinburgh: Churchill Livingstone, 1983.
46. Levine SP. Secreted platelet proteins as markers for pathological disorders. In: Phillips DR, Shuman MA, eds. *Biochemistry of platelets*. Orlando, FL: Academic Press, 1986.
47. Feinman RD, Lubowsky J, Charo I, et al. The lumi-aggregometer: a new instrument for simultaneous measurement of secretion and aggregation by platelets. *J Lab Clin Med* 1977;90:125–129.
48. Berndt MC, Phillips DR. Purification and preliminary physicochemical characterization of human platelet membrane glycoprotein V. *J Biol Chem* 1981;256:59–65.
49. Modderman PW, Admiraal LG, Sonnenberg A, et al. Glycoproteins V and Ib-IX form a noncovalent complex in the platelet membrane. *J Biol Chem* 1992;267:364–369.
50. Phillips DR, Agin PP. Platelet plasma membrane glycoproteins. Identification of a proteolytic substrate for thrombin. *Biochem Biophys Res Commun* 1977;75:940–947.
51. Blann AD, Lanza F, Galajda P, et al. Increased platelet glycoprotein V levels in patients with coronary and peripheral atherosclerosis—the influence of aspirin and cigarette smoking. *Thromb Haemost* 2001;86:777–783.
52. Henn V, Steinbach S, Buchner K, et al. The inflammatory action of CD40 ligand (CD154) expressed on activated human platelets is temporally limited by coexpressed CD40. *Blood* 2001;98:1047–1054.
53. Furman MI, Krueger LA, Barnard MR, et al. Release of soluble CD40L from platelets is regulated by GPIIb-IIIa and actin polymerization. *J Am Coll Cardiol* 2004;43:2319–2345.

54. Andre P, Prasad KS, Denis CV, et al. CD40L stabilizes arterial thrombi by a beta3 integrin-dependent mechanism. *Nat Med* 2002;8:247–252.

55. Kiener PA, Moran-Davis P, Rankin BM, et al. Stimulation of CD40 with purified soluble gp39 induces proinflammatory responses in human monocytes. *J Immunol* 1995;155:4917–4925.

56. Hollenbaugh D, Mischel-Petty N, Edwards CP, et al. Expression of functional CD40 by vascular endothelial cells. *J Exp Med* 1995;182:33–40.

57. Conde ID, Kleiman NS. Soluble CD40 ligand in acute coronary syndromes. *N Engl J Med* 2003;348:2575–2577.

58. Fitzgerald DJ, Roy L, Catella F, et al. Platelet activation in unstable coronary disease. *N Engl J Med* 1986;315:983–989.

59. Oates JA, FitzGerald GA, Branch RA, et al. Clinical implications of prostaglandin and thromboxane A2 formation. *N Engl J Med* 1988;319:689–698.

60. Eikelboom JW, Hirsh J, Weitz JI, et al. Aspirin-resistant thromboxane biosynthesis and the risk of myocardial infarction, stroke, or cardiovascular death in patients at high risk for cardiovascular events. [See comment]. *Circulation* 2002;105:1650–1655.

61. Fuster V, Badimon L, Badimon JJ, et al. The pathogenesis of coronary artery disease and the acute coronary syndromes. *N Engl J Med* 1992;326:242–250.

62. Flores NA, Sheridan DJ. The pathophysiological role of platelets during myocardial ischaemia. *Cardiovasc Res* 1994;28:295–302.

63. Williams AE, Freeman MR, Chisholm RJ, et al. Angiographic morphology in unstable angina pectoris. *Am J Cardiol* 1988;62:1024–1027.

64. Sherman CT, Litvack F, Grundfest W, et al. Coronary angioscopy in patients with unstable angina pectoris. *N Engl J Med* 1986;315:913–919.

65. DeWood MA, Spores J, Notske R, et al. Prevalence of total coronary occlusion during the early hours of transmural myocardial infarction. *N Engl J Med* 1980;303:897–902.

66. Antiplatelet Trialists' Collaboration. Secondary prevention of vascular disease by prolonged antiplatelet treatment. *Br Med J* 1988;296:320–331.

67. Hamm CW, Lorenz RL, Bleifeld W, et al. Biochemical evidence of platelet activation in patients with persistent unstable angina. *J Am Coll Cardiol* 1987;10:998–1006.

68. Ott I, Neumann FJ, Gawaz M, et al. Increased neutrophil-platelet adhesion in patients with unstable angina. *Circulation* 1996;94:1239–1246.

69. Becker RC, Tracy RP, Bovill EG et al, TIMI-III Thrombosis and Anticoagulation Group. The clinical use of flow cytometry for assessing platelet activation in acute coronary syndromes. *Coron Artery Dis* 1994;5:339–345.

70. Coulter SA, Cannon CP, Ault KA, et al. High levels of platelet inhibition with abciximab despite heightened platelet activation and aggregation during thrombolysis for acute myocardial infarction: results from TIMI (thrombolysis in myocardial infarction) 14. *Circulation* 2000;101:2690–2695.

71. Schultheiss HP, Tschoepe D, Esser J, et al. Large platelets continue to circulate in an activated state after myocardial infarction. *Eur J Clin Invest* 1994;24:243–247.

72. Scharf RE, Tomer A, Marzec UM, et al. Activation of platelets in blood perfusing angioplasty-damaged coronary arteries. Flow cytometric detection. *Arterioscler Thromb* 1992;12:1475–1487.

73. Langford EJ, Brown AS, Wainwright RJ, et al. Inhibition of platelet activity by S-nitrosoglutathione during coronary angioplasty. *Lancet* 1994;344:1458–1460.

74. Langford EJ, Wainwright RJ, Martin JF. Platelet activation in acute myocardial infarction and unstable angina is inhibited by nitric oxide donors. *Arterioscler Thromb Vasc Biol* 1996;16:51–55.

75. Ault KA, Cannon CP, Mitchell J, et al. Platelet activation in patients after an acute coronary syndrome: results from the TIMI-12 trial. Thrombolysis in myocardial infarction. *J Am Coll Cardiol* 1999;33:634–639.

76. Gawaz M, Neumann FJ, Ott I, et al. Platelet activation and coronary stent implantation. Effect of antithrombotic therapy. *Circulation* 1996;94:279–285.

77. Neumann FJ, Gawaz M, Dickfeld T, et al. Antiplatelet effect of ticlopidine after coronary stenting. *J Am Coll Cardiol* 1997;29:1515–1519.

78. Tschoepe D, Schultheiss HP, Kolarov P, et al. Platelet membrane activation markers are predictive for increased risk of acute ischemic events after PTCA. *Circulation* 1993;88:37–42.

79. Gawaz M, Neumann FJ, Ott I, et al. Role of activation-dependent platelet membrane glycoproteins in development of subacute occlusive coronary stent thrombosis. *Coron Artery Dis* 1997;8:121–128.

80. Kabbani SS, Watkins MW, Ashikaga T, et al. Platelet reactivity characterized prospectively: a determinant of outcome 90 days after percutaneous coronary intervention. *Circulation* 2001;104:181–186.

81. Kabbani SS, Watkins MW, Ashikaga T, et al. Usefulness of platelet reactivity before percutaneous coronary intervention in determining cardiac risk one year later. *Am J Cardiol* 2003;91:876–878.

82. Fateh-Moghadam S, Bocksch W, Ruf A, et al. Changes in surface expression of platelet membrane glycoproteins and progression of heart transplant vasculopathy. *Circulation* 2000;102:890–897.

83. Afshar-Kharghan V, Bray PF. Platelet polymorphisms. In: Michelson AD, ed. *Platelets*. New York: Academic Press/Elsevier Science, 2002.

84. Michelson AD, Furman MI, Goldschmidt-Clermont P, et al. Platelet GP IIIa Pl(A) polymorphisms display different sensitivities to agonists. *Circulation* 2000;101:1013–1018.

85. Gawaz M, Reininger A, Neumann FJ. Platelet function and platelet-leukocyte adhesion in symptomatic coronary heart disease. Effects of intravenous magnesium. *Thromb Res* 1996;83:341–349.

86. Neumann FJ, Marx N, Gawaz M, et al. Induction of cytokine expression in leukocytes by binding of thrombin-stimulated platelets. *Circulation* 1997;95:2387–2394.

87. Rinder CS, Bonan JL, Rinder HM, et al. Cardiopulmonary bypass induces leukocyte-platelet adhesion. *Blood* 1992;79:1201–1205.

88. Mickelson JK, Lakkis NM, Villarreal-Levy G, et al. Leukocyte activation with platelet adhesion after coronary angioplasty: a mechanism for recurrent disease? *J Am Coll Cardiol* 1996;28:345–353.

89. Furman MI, Barnard MR, Krueger LA, et al. Circulating monocyte-platelet aggregates are an early marker of acute myocardial infarction. *J Am Coll Cardiol* 2001;38:1002–1006.

90. Katopodis JN, Kolodny L, Jy W, et al. Platelet microparticles and calcium homeostasis in acute coronary ischemias. *Am J Hematol* 1997;54:95–101.

91. George JN, Pickett EB, Saucerman S, et al. Platelet surface glycoproteins. Studies on resting and activated platelets and platelet membrane microparticles in normal subjects, and observations in patients during adult respiratory distress syndrome and cardiac surgery. *J Clin Invest* 1986;78:340–348.

92. Aukrust P, Muller F, Ueland T, et al. Enhanced levels of soluble and membrane-bound CD40 ligand in patients with unstable angina. Possible reflection of T lymphocyte and platelet involvement in the pathogenesis of acute coronary syndromes. *Circulation* 1999;100:614–620.

93. Nannizzi-Alaimo L, Rubenstein MH, Alves VL, et al. Cardiopulmonary bypass induces release of soluble CD40 ligand. *Circulation* 2002;105:2849–2854.

94. Nannizzi-Alaimo L, Alves VL, Phillips DR. Inhibitory effects of glycoprotein IIb/IIIa antagonists and aspirin on the release of soluble CD40 ligand during platelet stimulation. *Circulation* 2003;107:1123–1128.

95. Michelson AD, Krueger LA, Barnard MR, et al. GPIIb-IIIa antagonists reduce thromboinflammatory processes in patients with acute coronary syndromes undergoing percutaneous coronary intervention. *J Thromb Haemost* 2003;1(Suppl. 1):1767.

96. Heeschen C, Dimmeler S, Hamm CW, et al. Soluble CD40 ligand in acute coronary syndromes. *N Engl J Med* 2003;348:1104–1111.

97. Schonbeck U, Varo N, Libby P, et al. Soluble CD40L and cardiovascular risk in women. *Circulation* 2001;104:2266–2268.

98. Grau AJ, Ruf A, Vogt A, et al. Increased fraction of circulating activated platelets in acute and previous cerebrovascular ischemia. *Thromb Haemost* 1998;80:298–301.

99. Zeller JA, Tschoepe D, Kessler C. Circulating platelets show increased activation in patients with acute cerebral ischemia. *Thromb Haemost* 1999;81:373–377.

100. Meiklejohn DJ, Vickers MA, Morrison ER, et al. *In vivo* platelet activation in atherothrombotic stroke is not determined by polymorphisms of human platelet glycoprotein IIIa or Ib. *Br J Haematol* 2001;112:621–631.

101. Yamazaki M, Uchiyama S, Iwata M. Measurement of platelet fibrinogen binding and p-selectin expression by flow cytometry in patients with cerebral ischemia. *Thromb Res* 2001;104:197–205.

102. Cherian P, Hankey GJ, Eikelboom JW, et al. Endothelial and platelet activation in acute ischemic stroke and its etiological subtypes. *Stroke* 2003;34:2132–2137.

103. Marquardt L, Ruf A, Mansmann U, et al. Course of platelet activation markers after ischemic stroke. [See comment]. *Stroke* 2002;33:2570–2574.

104. Minamino T, Kitakaze M, Sanada S, et al. Increased expression of P-selectin on platelets is a risk factor for silent cerebral infarction in patients with atrial fibrillation: role of nitric oxide. *Circulation* 1998;98:1721–1727.

105. Lee YJ, Jy W, Horstman LL, et al. Elevated platelet microparticles in transient ischemic attacks, lacunar infarcts, and multiinfarct dementias. *Thromb Res* 1994;72:295–304.

106. Geiser T, Sturzenegger M, Genewein U, et al. Mechanisms of cerebrovascular events as assessed by procoagulant activity, cerebral microemboli, and platelet microparticles in patients with prosthetic heart valves. *Stroke* 1998;29:1770–1777.

107. Zeiger F, Stephan S, Hoheisel G, et al. P-selectin expression, platelet aggregates, and platelet-derived microparticle formation are increased in peripheral arterial disease. *Blood Coagul Fibrinolysis* 2000;11:723–728.

108. Cassar K, Bachoo P, Ford I, et al. Platelet activation is increased in peripheral arterial disease. *J Vasc Surg* 2003;38:99–103.

109. Tsakiris DA, Tschopl M, Wolf F, et al. Platelets and cytokines in concert with endothelial activation in patients with peripheral arterial occlusive disease. *Blood Coagul Fibrinolysis* 2000;11:165–173.

110. Powell CC, Rohrer MJ, Barnard MR, et al. Chronic venous insufficiency is associated with increased platelet and monocyte activation and aggregation. *J Vasc Surg* 1999;30:844–851.

111. Rohrer MJ, Claytor RB, Garnette CSC, et al. Platelet-monocyte aggregates in patients with chronic venous insufficiency remain elevated following correction of reflux. *Cardiovasc Surg* 2002;10:464–469.

112. Tschoepe D, Roesen P, Esser J, et al. Large platelets circulate in an activated state in diabetes mellitus. *Semin Thromb Hemost* 1991;17:433–438.

113. Janes SL, Goodall AH. Flow cytometric detection of circulating activated platelets and platelet hyper-responsiveness in pre-eclampsia and pregnancy. *Clin Sci* 1994;86:731–739.

114. Konijnenberg A, van der Post JA, Mol BW, et al. Can flow cytometric detection of platelet activation early in pregnancy predict the occurrence of

preeclampsia? A prospective study. *Am J Obstet Gynecol* 1997;177: 434–442.

115. Trudinger B, Song JZ, Wu ZH, et al. Placental insufficiency is characterized by platelet activation in the fetus. *Obstet Gynecol* 2003;101:975–981.

116. Sirolli V, Ballone E, Garofalo D, et al. Platelet activation markers in patients with nephrotic syndrome. A comparative study of different platelet function tests. *Nephron* 2002;91:424–430.

117. Gawaz MP, Mujais SK, Schmidt B, et al. Platelet-leukocyte aggregates during hemodialysis: effect of membrane type. *Artif Organs* 1999;23:29–36.

118. Wun T, Cordoba M, Rangaswami A, et al. Activated monocytes and platelet-monocyte aggregates in patients with sickle cell disease. *Clin Lab Haematol* 2002;24:81–88.

119. Ogura H, Kawasaki T, Tanaka H, et al. Activated platelets enhance microparticle formation and platelet-leukocyte interaction in severe trauma and sepsis. *J Trauma* 2001;50:801–809.

120. Gawaz M, Dickfeld T, Bogner C, et al. Platelet function in septic multiple organ dysfunction syndrome. *Intensive Care Med* 1997;23:379–385.

121. Russwurm S, Vickers J, Meier-Hellmann A, et al. Platelet and leukocyte activation correlate with the severity of septic organ dysfunction. *Shock* 2002;17:263–268.

122. Joseph JE, Harrison P, Mackie IJ, et al. Increased circulating platelet-leucocyte complexes and platelet activation in patients with antiphospholipid syndrome, systemic lupus erythematosus and rheumatoid arthritis. *Br J Haematol* 2001;115:451–459.

123. Jensen MK, de Nully BP, Lund BV, et al. Increased circulating platelet-leukocyte aggregates in myeloproliferative disorders is correlated to previous thrombosis, platelet activation and platelet count. *Eur J Haematol* 2001;66:143–151.

124. Villmow T, Kemkes-Matthes B, Matzdorff AC. Markers of platelet activation and platelet-leukocyte interaction in patients with myeloproliferative syndromes. *Thromb Res* 2002;108:139–145.

125. Sevush S, Jy W, Horstman LL, et al. Platelet activation in Alzheimer disease. *Arch Neurol* 1998;55:530–536.

126. Vanacore R, Guida C, Urciuoli P, et al. High levels of circulating monocyte-platelet aggregates can predict rejection episodes after orthotopic liver transplantation. *Transplant Proc* 2003;35:1019.

127. Ando M, Iwata A, Ozeki Y, et al. Circulating platelet-derived microparticles with procoagulant activity may be a potential cause of thrombosis in uremic patients. *Kidney Int* 2002;62:1757–1763.

128. Fijnheer R, Modderman PW, Veldman H, et al. Detection of platelet activation with monoclonal antibodies and flow cytometry. Changes during platelet storage. *Transfusion* 1990;30:20–25.

129. Rinder HM, Murphy M, Mitchell JG, et al. Progressive platelet activation with storage: evidence for shortened survival of activated platelets after transfusion. *Transfusion* 1991;31:409–414.

130. Divers SG, Kannan K, Stewart RM, et al. Quantitation of CD62, soluble CD62, and lysosome-associated membrane proteins 1 and 2 for evaluation of the quality of stored platelet concentrates. *Transfusion* 1995;35:292–297.

131. Triulzi DJ, Kickler TS, Braine HG. Detection and significance of alpha granule membrane protein 140 expression on platelets collected by apheresis. *Transfusion* 1992;32:529–533.

132. Ault KA, Mitchell J, Hillman RS. Appearance of P-selectin (CD62) during labeling is responsible for the majority of the variability in recovery of In111 labeled platelets. *Blood* 1992;80:496a.

133. Rajasekhar D, Barnard MR, Bednarek FJ, et al. Platelet hyporeactivity in very low birth weight neonates. *Thromb Haemost* 1997;77:1002–1007.

134. Setzer ES, Webb IB, Wassenaar JW, et al. Platelet dysfunction and coagulopathy in intraventricular hemorrhage in the premature infant. *J Pediatr* 1982;100:599–605.

135. Kestin AS, Valeri CR, Khuri SF, et al. The platelet function defect of cardiopulmonary bypass. *Blood* 1993;82:107–117.

136. Schneider DJ, Tracy PB, Mann KG, et al. Differential effects of anticoagulants on the activation of platelets *ex vivo*. *Circulation* 1997;96:2877–2883.

137. Phillips DR, Teng W, Arfsten A, et al. Effect of Ca2+ on GP IIb-IIIa interactions with integrilin: enhanced GP IIb-IIIa binding and inhibition of platelet aggregation by reductions in the concentration of ionized calcium in plasma anticoagulated with citrate. *Circulation* 1997;96:1488–1494.

138. Evangelista V, Manarini S, Rotondo S, et al. Platelet/polymorphonuclear leukocyte interaction in dynamic conditions: evidence of adhesion cascade and cross talk between P-selectin and the beta 2 integrin CD11b/CD18. *Blood* 1996;88:4183–4194.

139. Hanson SR, Harker LA. Interruption of acute platelet-dependent thrombosis by the synthetic antithrombin PPACK. *Proc Natl Acad Sci U S A* 1988;85:3184–3188.

140. Eidt JF, Allison P, Nobel S, et al. Thrombin is an important mediator of platelet aggregation in stenosed canine coronary arteries with endothelial injury. *J Clin Invest* 1989;84:18–27.

141. Kelly AB, Marzec UM, Krupski W, et al. Hirudin interruption of heparin-resistant arterial thrombus formation in baboons. *Blood* 1991;77:1006–1012.

142. Michelson AD. Platelet activation by thrombin can be directly measured in whole blood through the use of the peptide GPRP and flow cytometry: methods and clinical studies. *Blood Coagul Fibrinolysis* 1994;5: 121–131.

143. Michelson AD, Ellis PA, Barnard MR, et al. Downregulation of the platelet surface glycoprotein Ib-IX complex in whole blood stimulated by thrombin, ADP or an *in vivo* wound. *Blood* 1991;77:770–779.

144. Vu T-KH, Hung DT, Wheaton VI, et al. Molecular cloning of a functional thrombin receptor reveals a novel proteolytic mechanism of receptor activation. *Cell* 1991;64:1057–1068.

145. Michelson AD, Benoit SE, Furman MI, et al. The platelet surface expression of glycoprotein V is regulated by two independent mechanisms: proteolysis and a reversible cytoskeletal-mediated redistribution to the surface-connected canalicular system. *Blood* 1996;87:1396–1408.

146. Kahn ML, Zheng YW, Huang W, et al. A dual thrombin receptor system for platelet activation. *Nature* 1998;394:690–694.

147. Coller BS, Peerschke EI, Scudder LE, et al. Studies with a murine monoclonal antibody that abolishes ristocetin-induced binding of von Willebrand factor to platelets: additional evidence in support of GPIb as a platelet receptor for von Willebrand factor. *Blood* 1983;61:99–110.

148. Montgomery RR, Kunicki TJ, Taves C, et al. Diagnosis of Bernard-Soulier syndrome and Glanzmann's thrombasthenia with a monoclonal assay on whole blood. *J Clin Invest* 1983;71:385–389.

149. Michelson AD, Barnard MR. Thrombin-induced changes in platelet membrane glycoproteins Ib, IX, and IIb-IIIa complex. *Blood* 1987;70: 1673–1678.

150. Michelson AD. Thrombin-induced down-regulation of the platelet membrane glycoprotein Ib-IX complex. *Semin Thromb Hemost* 1992;18:18–27.

151. Michelson AD, Barnard MR. Flow cytometric detection of the redistribution of the glycoprotein Ib-IX complex on thrombin-stimulated platelets is dependent on the type of antibody conjugate used. *Blood* 1993;81: 1408–1409.

152. Hourdille P, Heilmann E, Combrie R, et al. Thrombin induces a rapid redistribution of glycoprotein Ib-IX complexes within the membrane systems of activated human platelets. *Blood* 1990;76:1503–1513.

153. Rinderknecht H. Ultra-rapid fluorescent labelling of proteins. *Nature* 1962; 193:167–168.

154. Horsewood P, Hayward CP, Warkentin TE, et al. Investigation of the mechanisms of monoclonal antibody-induced platelet activation. *Blood* 1991;78:1019–1026.

155. Johnston GI, Pickett EB, McEver RP, et al. Heterogeneity of platelet secretion in response to thrombin demonstrated by fluorescence flow cytometry. *Blood* 1987;69:1401–1403.

156. Poon RYM, Johnson R, Stanton T, et al. Calibration of fluorescent intensity microbead standards and assignment of effective fluorescein/protein ratios to the fluorescein isothiocyanate (FITC)-conjugated secondary antibodies used in the fifth workshop. In: Schlossman SF, Boumsell L, Gilks, W, et al., eds. *Leucocyte typing V*. Oxford: Oxford University Press, 1995.

# CHAPTER 56 ■ LABORATORY MARKERS OF COAGULATION AND FIBRINOLYSIS

KENNETH A. BAUER

Clinicians have long sought blood tests to predict thrombotic events in high-risk patients or to confirm or exclude the presence of thrombosis. Advances in our knowledge of the biochemistry of coagulation and fibrinolysis have facilitated the development of sensitive and specific assays that are able to detect platelet activation, the generation of coagulation enzymes, and products of intravascular fibrin formation or dissolution in the human circulation. This chapter focuses on the latter two groups of laboratory markers.

Many of the protein components of the hemostatic mechanism are zymogens that are converted to serine proteases. For coagulation system enzymes to be generated at any significant rate, a zymogen, a cofactor, and a converting enzyme must form a multimolecular complex on a natural surface. These transformations are suppressed if the converting enzyme is inhibited, the protein cofactor is destroyed, or the surface receptors that are essential for the assembly of the macromolecular complex are sequestered. It has not been possible so far to measure directly the levels of most hemostatic enzymes *in vivo*. Many of the enzymes are not available for quantification in blood because they are neutralized rapidly by naturally occurring protease inhibitors or bound to cellular receptors in the locale in which they are generated. Faced with these obstacles, immunochemical assays have been developed for peptides that are liberated with the activation of coagulation enzymes or enzyme-inhibitor complexes. The assays that have been developed along with the reported *in vivo* half-lives for some of the species are listed in Table 56-1 and described in detail in a later section (see sections, "Assays for Coagulation Activation" and "Assays for Fibrinopeptides"). Most of these assays were initially developed in research laboratories, but some are now available commercially in kit form using either polyclonal or monoclonal antibodies.

The assay formats for these markers are generally of two types. The first is a competitive radioimmunoassay procedure. This requires an antibody population that recognizes antigenic determinants on the activation fragment or enzyme-inhibitor complex that are hidden in the parent zymogen or inhibitor. The need for highly specific antibodies to the marker of interest can sometimes be obviated by devising sample processing procedures that efficiently remove the cross-reacting species in plasma before assay. The second approach is the enzyme-linked immunosorbent assay (ELISA). In most instances, immunoglobulin G (IgG) or F(ab′)2 fragments directed toward epitopes on one region of the marker are bound to wells of plastic microtiter plates to "capture" the antigen from the plasma specimens. After washing away unbound species, a second IgG or F(ab′)2 population recognizing epitopes in a different domain of the molecule is added to the wells. These antibodies are coupled to an enzyme capable of cleaving a suitable colorimetric substrate, allowing the development of a titration curve.

Two coagulation enzymes, activated protein C and factor VIIa, have relatively slow *in vivo* inactivation mechanisms. It has therefore been possible to develop techniques to measure these species directly in plasma. The test for activated protein C uses an immunoenzymatic procedure (23–25), whereas the procedure for factor VIIa uses a clotting assay using recombinant tissue factor that has undergone a C-terminal truncation (51,52). This tissue factor mutant maintains cofactor activity toward factor VIIa but does not support factor VII activation.

The execution of clinical investigations seeking to establish a relation between markers of coagulation, fibrinolysis and thromboembolic disease is difficult. First, one must ensure that the selected assays are specific for the products of interest and possess sufficient sensitivity. Second, the tests must be properly standardized so that the assays perform in a reproducible manner. Third, care must be taken to ensure that technical factors do not introduce *in vitro* artifacts that can significantly alter the immunoassay results (e.g., drawing of blood samples through indwelling intravenous catheters). These include the venipuncture quality, choice of anticoagulant, sample processing procedure (if required), and plasma storage conditions. Fourth, objective endpoints must be used to establish a diagnosis of thrombosis, bias in patient selection should be avoided, and an appropriate control group of patients must be chosen for comparison.

## ASSAYS FOR COAGULATION ACTIVATION

Although the blood coagulation mechanism was initially described as functionally independent extrinsic and intrinsic pathways that separately activate factor X and generate thrombin, the contact factors responsible for initiating the intrinsic cascade are not physiologically important in triggering downstream reactions of the cascade (53). The contact factors rather play a role in inflammation and fibrinolysis, and may actually be antithrombotic (see Chapter 6). It is now appreciated that the factor VII–tissue factor mechanism is important in initiating coagulation by virtue of its ability to activate factor IX, as well as factor X. Factor XI can be activated by thrombin, thereby providing a physiologic mechanism for its conversion to an active enzyme, which is involved in sustaining thrombin generation (54). The components of the intrinsic system include factor XI, as well as factors IX and VIII. The factor Xa that is generated by either the factor VII–tissue factor or factor IXa–factor VIIIa–cell surface complex then is able to convert prothrombin to thrombin by binding to factor Va on activated platelets.

Contact system activation can be monitored by immunoassays for factor XIIa, factor XIIa–C1 inhibitor complex, kallikrein–C1 inhibitor, and kallikrein–$\alpha_2$-macroglobulin. Factor XIa activation can be measured as factor XIa and factor XIa–factor XIa inhibitor ($\alpha_1$-antitrypsin, antithrombin, C1 inhibitor, and $\alpha_2$-antiplasmin) complexes (1–3,6,7). The activation of factor IX can

835

## TABLE 56-1

### IMMUNOCHEMICAL MARKERS OF COAGULATION AND FIBRINOLYSIS

| Biochemical step | Marker (reference) | T1/2 (reference) |
|---|---|---|
| **COAGULATION** | | |
| Factor XII–factor XIIa | Factor XIIa (1) | |
| | Factor XIIa–C1 inhibitor complex (2,3) | |
| Prekallikrein-kallikrein | Kallikrein–C1 inhibitor complex (3,4) | |
| | Kallikrein–$\alpha_2$-macroglobulin complex (5) | |
| Factor XI–factor XIa | Factor XIa–XIa inhibitor complexes (6,7) | |
| Factor IX–factor IXa | Factor IX activation peptide (8) | 15 min |
| | Factor IX–antithrombin complex (9) | 30 min |
| Factor X–factor Xa | Factor X activation peptide (10) | 30 min |
| | Factor X–antithrombin complex (11) | |
| Prothrombin-thrombin | Prothrombin activation fragment F1+2 (12–15) | 90 min (16) |
| | Thrombin–antithrombin complex (17–19) | 15 min (20,21) |
| Protein C–activated protein C | Protein C activation peptide (22) | 5 min (22) |
| | Activated protein C (23–26) | |
| | Inhibitor complex (27) | 40 min (28) |
| | Activated protein C–$\alpha_1$-antitrypsin complex (29) | 140 min (28) |
| | Activated protein C–$\alpha_2$-macroglobulin complex (30) | |
| Fibrinogen-fibrin | Fibrinopeptide A (31–33) | 3–5 min (32) |
| | Fibrinopeptide B (34,35) | |
| **FIBRINOLYSIS** | | |
| Plasminogen-plasmin | Plasmin–$\alpha_2$-antiplasmin complex (36–42) | |
| | Plasmin–$\alpha_2$-macroglobulin complexes (38) | |
| Plasmin action on fibrin I | B$\beta$1–42 fragment (43,44) | |
| Plasmin action on fibrin II | B$\beta$15–42 fragment (45) | |
| Plasmin action on fibrinogen/fibrin | Fibrinogen (fibrin) degradation products (46,47) | |
| Plasmin action on cross-linked fibrin | D-dimer (48,49) | 8 h (50) |

be monitored by measuring the levels of the factor IX activation peptide (8,55) or factor IXa–antithrombin complexes (9). These assays reflect the action of factor XIa or the factor VII–tissue factor complex, or both, on factor IX (Fig. 56-1). Factor X activation mediated by the extrinsic or intrinsic pathways can be monitored by measuring the factor X activation peptide (10).

Thrombin generation takes place at an appreciable rate under physiologic conditions only in the presence of factor Xa, factor Va, calcium ions, and activated platelets. During this process, the amino-terminus of the prothrombin molecule is released as the F1+2 fragment (see Figs. 56-1 and 56-2). Once evolved, this serine protease converts fibrinogen into fibrin, releasing fibrinopeptides A and B, or it can be inhibited by the endogenous heparan sulfate–antithrombin mechanism to form thrombin–antithrombin TAT complex, a stable enzyme-inhibitor complex (Fig. 56-2). Immunoassays have been developed for the F1+2 fragment (12–15,56) and the TAT complex (17,18,57) that can be used as indices of thrombin generation *in vivo*.

Alternatively, thrombin can also rapidly activate protein C by binding to thrombomodulin on vascular endothelial cells, and assays have been developed to monitor this transformation (Fig. 56-2). These immunoassays include measurements of the protein C activation peptide (22) and activated protein C inhibitor complexes (27,29,30). The plasma inhibitors of activated protein C include protein C inhibitor, $\alpha_1$-proteinase inhibitor, and $\alpha_2$-macroglobulin.

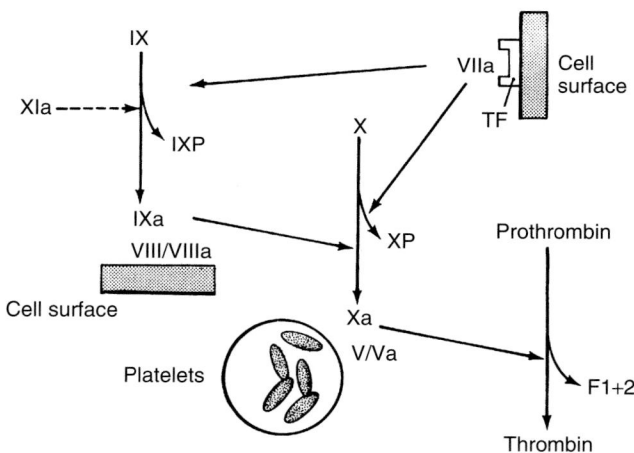

**FIGURE 56-1.** Pathways of coagulation activation. The activation of factor IX by factor XIa or the factor VII–tissue factor (TF) mechanism liberates the factor IX activation peptide (IXP). The conversion of factor X to factor Xa by the factor IXa–factor VIII/VIIIa–cell surface complex releases the factor X activation peptide (XP). The generation of thrombin from prothrombin is mediated by factor Xa in the presence of factor Va, and activated platelets. During this process, the F1+2 fragment is released.

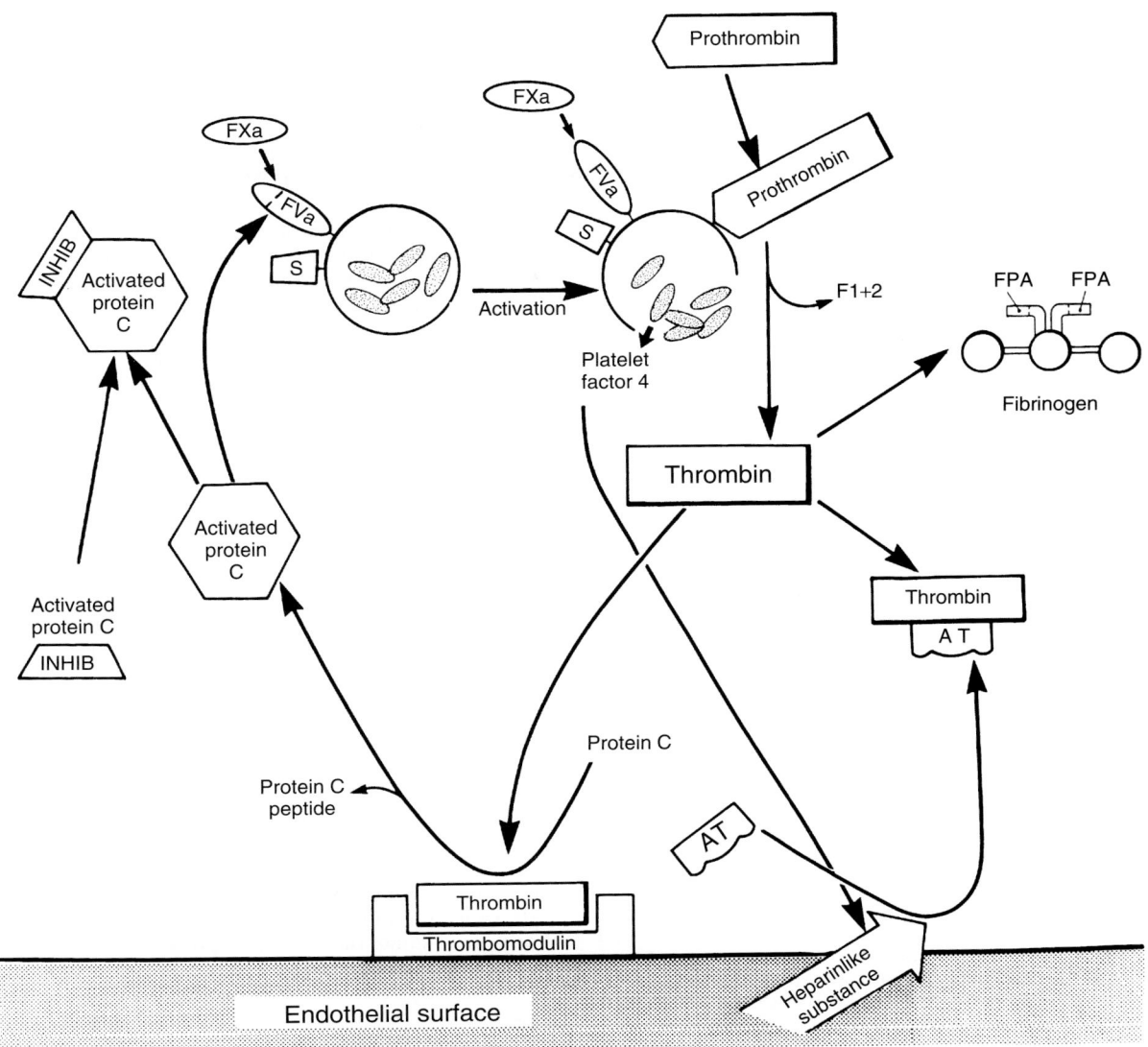

**FIGURE 56-2.** Regulation of thrombin generation by the natural anticoagulant mechanisms of the endothelium. Factor Xa, factor Va, protein S, prothrombin activation fragment F1+2, fibrinopeptide A, antithrombin, and activated protein C inhibitor(s) are designated as FXa, FVa, S, F1+2, FPA, AT, and activated protein C inhibitor, respectively. Thrombin may be inactivated by forming 1:1 stoichiometric complexes with its major physiologic inhibitor, antithrombin, thereby resulting in the formation of thrombin–antithrombin (TAT) complexes. Activated protein C can be neutralized by inhibitors of activated protein C (e.g., protein C inhibitor, $\alpha_1$-proteinase inhibitor, and $\alpha_2$-macroglobulin), which results in the generation of activated protein C inhibitor complexes.

## ASSAYS FOR FIBRINOPEPTIDES

Thrombin cleaves fibrinopeptides A and B from the amino-terminal regions of the A$\alpha$ and B$\beta$ chains of fibrinogen, respectively (58), thereby converting fibrinogen to fibrin (see Fig. 56-3A). The rate of fibrinopeptide A release from fibrinogen is considerably faster than that of fibrinopeptide B (34,58,59). Cleavage of fibrinopeptide A from fibrinogen generates an intermediate known as *fibrin I* that can polymerize but cross-links poorly (60,61). Further proteolysis of fibrin I can occur through the action of either thrombin or plasmin. If thrombin action predominates, fibrinopeptide B is released, and fibrin II is formed. Alternatively, plasmin action on fibrin I releases B$\beta$1–42 from the amino-terminus of the B$\beta$ chain and cleaves the carboxyl terminus of the A$\alpha$ chains, thereby generating fragment X (62) (Fig. 56-3B). In contrast, plasmin

proteolysis of fibrin II results in the release of B$\beta$15–42 rather than B$\beta$1–42 because fibrinopeptide B has already been removed by the action of thrombin.

Assays for fibrinopeptide A (31–33,63–66) and fibrinopeptide B (34,35) provide an index of thrombin action on fibrinogen. Plasma levels of B$\beta$1–42 (43,44) and B$\beta$15–42 (45), peptides released by the proteolytic action of plasmin on fibrinogen and fibrin, respectively, have been used as indices of *in vivo* plasmin activity. The antisera used in these assays show significant, but not absolute, specificity for the various fibrinopeptides relative to fibrinogen. Consequently, fibrinogen must be removed from plasma samples before analysis using techniques that do not alter the levels of the peptides (32,64).

The initial assay for B$\beta$1–42 was indirect and involved measurement of fibrinopeptide B immunoreactivity before and after thrombin addition to fibrinogen-depleted plasma. The resultant

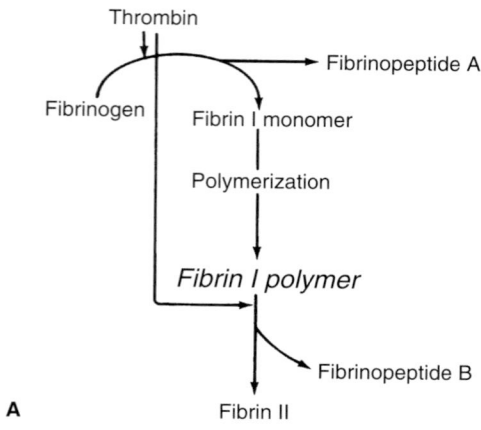

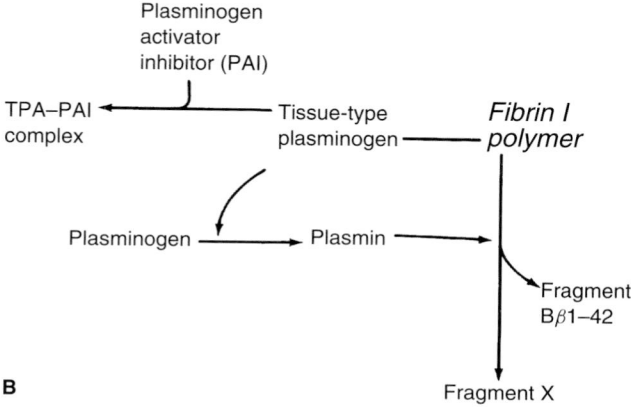

**FIGURE 56-3.** The actions of thrombin (**A**) and plasmin (**B**) on fibrin I polymer. **A:** The conversion of fibrinogen to fibrin II polymer by thrombin. **B:** The action of plasmin on fibrin I polymer. The fibrinolytic capacity of human plasma is determined primarily by the activity of tissue-type plasminogen activator (tPA) and its inhibitor [plasminogen activator inhibitor 1 (PAI)], which are released from vascular endothelial cells. tPA is able to bind to fibrin I polymer, which allows plasminogen to be activated to plasmin at an increased rate.

increase in immunoreactivity, termed thrombin-increasable fibrinopeptide B, reflects the presence of Bβ1–42, a fibrinopeptide B-containing fragment (67). Assays were subsequently developed that directly measured the levels of Bβ1–42 with either a polyclonal (44) or a monoclonal antibody (43). These antisera are specific for Bβ1–42 and do not cross-react with fibrinopeptide B or Bβ15–42. An alternative approach is to use an antiserum raised against Bβ15–42 that cross-reacts completely with Bβ1–42 because it recognizes the carboxyl-terminal region of these peptides (68). However, the Bβ1–42/Bβ15–42 assay may underestimate the circulating levels of Bβ1–42 because release of the carboxyl-terminal arginine residue by circulating carboxypeptidases decreases the immunoreactivity of the peptide when measured with a carboxyl-terminal–directed antisera (44).

Using a monoclonal antibody, a specific assay for Bβ15–42 has been developed (45) that provides a marker of plasmin action on fibrin II. However, two factors may limit the clinical utility of this test. First, because the antibody exhibits some cross-reactivity with Bβ1–42, the assay may not be a specific marker of fibrin proteolysis in patients with marked fibrinogenolysis (69). Second, only low levels of Bβ15–42 are generated during thrombolysis (70,71), probably because the Bβ42–43 bond of fibrin II is not cleaved as readily by plasmin as is the same bond of fibrinogen or fibrin I. Exploiting this phenomenon, the fibrin

specificity of thrombolytic agents has been increased by linking them to monoclonal antibodies against the Bβ15–42 domain of fibrin, thereby targeting them to fibrin (72,73).

# ASSAYS FOR DERIVATIVES OF FIBRINOGEN AND FIBRIN

The levels of fibrinogen or fibrin degradation products (FDPs) can be measured using a variety of immunologic techniques (46,47) or by use of the staphylococcal clumping reaction (74). Most of the antisera used in these assays cross-react with fibrinogen, and the tests therefore must be performed on serum samples. These assays, like those for fragment E (75,76), a degradation product found in most high-molecular-weight derivatives produced by plasmin proteolysis of fibrinogen or fibrin, do not differentiate between fibrin and fibrinogen degradation products. Furthermore, serum FDP measurements can be problematic (77) because incomplete removal of fibrinogen falsely elevates FDP levels, whereas adsorption of degradation products to the clot results in a spurious reduction in FDP values (78). These limitations have prompted the development of antibodies against neoantigenic determinants on plasmin-derived fibrinogen or fibrin fragments that do not cross-react with fibrinogen. Both polyclonal and monoclonal antibodies against neoantigens on fragments D and E (79–82) have been developed for this purpose. Although some clinical testing has been done with these assays (83,84), they have been replaced largely by assays for D-dimer.

Plasmin-induced lysis of cross-linked fibrin results in the formation of a variety of degradation products, the smallest of which is D-dimer. This fibrin derivative is comprised of two fragment D moieties covalently linked by their γ chains (85,86). D-dimer levels in whole blood can be measured by red cell agglutination, whereas levels in plasma can be quantified using an enzyme immunoassay (EIA) or latex bead agglutination. All assays use monoclonal antibodies that recognize neoepitopes on D-dimer that are not expressed on the D-domains of non–cross-linked fibrinogen or fibrin (48,49). Although agglutination assays can be done more rapidly than the EIA, latex agglutination assays are less sensitive and provide only semiquantitative results.

The performance of each D-dimer assay differs, depending on the specificity of the monoclonal antibodies used in the test, variability in the cutoff value selected to identify positive results, and heterogeneity of the patient populations in which the test was evaluated (87–89). Commercial D-dimer assays use different units for D-dimer measurement. Although most use authentic D-dimer as the reference standard, others use fibrinogen. When a fibrinogen standard is used, results are reported as fibrinogen equivalent units, with two of these units approximately equivalent to a single D-dimer. The use of different standards makes it difficult to compare study results because the units for D-dimer measurement are rarely specified.

The concept that D-dimer is derived only from the breakdown of cross-linked fibrin in thrombi has been challenged, because it has been observed that the levels of D-dimer in patients undergoing coronary thrombolysis are higher than those that would be predicted given the volume of the coronary thrombus (90). In addition, D-dimer levels can be elevated in the absence of concomitant evidence of angiographic reperfusion (90). There are two potential explanations for these findings. The first is that a flaw in the design of D-dimer assays can limit its specificity and lead to higher than expected plasma levels (69,91). Although a monoclonal antibody is used to "capture" the D-dimer in plasma, a panspecific antibody is sometimes used to identify the bound antigen. Cross-reactivity of this "tag" antibody with fibrinogen degradation products would lead to an overestimate of D-dimer levels in the setting of thrombolytic therapy. A second possibility is that soluble cross-linked fibrin may provide an alternative source of D-dimer (69). Rather than reflecting clot lysis, the elevated D-dimer levels after thrombolytic therapy may reflect proteolysis of large amounts of circulating cross-linked fibrin, thereby explaining the increased D-dimer levels that occur in the absence of angiographic evidence of reperfusion (90).

As an alternative to D-dimer, plasma levels of soluble fibrin monomer, a complex of fibrin monomer with fibrinogen, can be measured as an index of thrombin action on fibrinogen. Early assays used protamine sulfate to precipitate soluble fibrin monomers (92), but newer tests use monoclonal antibodies against fibrin-specific epitopes on the $\alpha$ or $\gamma$ chains, or examine the cofactor activity of fibrin monomer in a tissue-type plasminogen activator (tPA)–induced plasminogen activation assay (93). The two types of assays yield different results, highlighting the need for standardization. Theoretically, assays for soluble fibrin monomer may be superior to D-dimer assays if patients with thrombosis have reduced fibrinolytic activity, as has been suggested by some investigators (94).

## ASSAYS FOR PLASMIN–$\alpha_2$-ANTIPLASMIN COMPLEXES

$\alpha_2$-Antiplasmin, the major plasma inhibitor of plasmin, forms a 1:1 stoichiometric complex with the enzyme (95–99). The reaction between plasmin and $\alpha_2$-antiplasmin is extremely rapid and the enzyme-inhibitor complex is stable and devoid of enzyme activity (36,100,101). Assays that measure the plasma levels of plasmin–$\alpha_2$-antiplasmin complexes have been developed and can be used as an index of *in vivo* plasmin generation (36–42). Increased levels of complex have been detected in patients with intravascular coagulation (102), consistent with the activation of fibrinolysis that occurs in this disorder.

## APPLICATIONS

### Influence of Physiologic Factors and Organ Dysfunction

A number of variables can result in overlap of assay results between individuals with a pathologic condition or altered physiologic status and healthy individuals. Although values further from the mean of the normal distribution are more likely to be abnormal, appropriate interpretation requires an appreciation of the factors that can influence measurements.

The normal aging process alters coagulation activation in a predictable fashion (103–105). With advancing age from 45 to 70 years, an increasing number of patients who are otherwise healthy exhibit elevated levels of prothrombin activation fragment F1+2. Elevated F1+2 levels reflect increased thrombin generation rather than decreased clearance of the fragment because clearance of radiolabeled F1+2 is unchanged (103). The levels of the factor IX and X activation peptides also increase with advancing age (8). Significant, but somewhat less striking, positive correlations have been observed between increasing age and the levels of fibrinopeptide A and protein C activation peptide (103).

It has been reported that strenuous exercise in the form of long-distance running leads to increased TAT complex levels without elevations in the levels of fibrinopeptide A (106). Cigarette smoking has been associated with elevations in activation markers of blood coagulation (107).

Certain medications that are not known to have a direct effect on blood coagulation can alter these assays. Caine et al. (108)

showed that administration of conjugated equine estrogen daily to menopausal women for 3 months increased the levels of prothrombin activation fragment F1+2 in a dose-dependent manner. The activity of fibrinopeptide A also increased, and levels of protein S and antithrombin were decreased as compared to placebo treatment. In women who had undergone oophorectomy, Kroon et al. (109) confirmed that 0.625 mg of conjugated equine estrogen, as well as 0.05 transdermal 17$\beta$-estradiol daily for 6 weeks increased levels of F1+2. Scarabin et al. (110) found that 2 mg of estrogen valerate daily with cyclic progesterone increased F1+2 levels and decreased antithrombin III activity levels, whereas transdermal estrogen (2.5 mg 17$\beta$-estradiol daily with cyclic progesterone) did not. The treatment of patients with coronary heart disease with gemfibrozil, a drug used to lower serum cholesterol and triglyceride concentrations, reduces F1+2 levels by approximately 25% (111).

In healthy volunteers, postprandial elevations in the levels of factors VIIa and IX activation peptide have been demonstrated, but no changes were observed in the levels of factor XIIa or indices of thrombin generation (112–114). The roles of factors XII, XI, and IX in factor VII activation were evaluated by investigating patients with isolated deficiencies of these factors after a fatty meal (112,114). Factor VIIa levels increased postprandially in patients with factor XII deficiency but did not change in those with factor IX deficiency. In patients with factor XI deficiency, Miller et al. (112) found that factor VIIa levels rose postprandially, whereas Silveira et al. (114) did not observe significant alterations. From these studies, it can be concluded that factor IX plays a critical role in the events linking postprandial lipemia to factor VII activation, but factor XII does not. This implies that factor XII is not involved in the activation of factor VII by lipolysis of triglyceride-rich lipoproteins.

Dysfunction in normal physiologic clearance mechanisms can also result in substantial elevations in the levels of activation peptides. For F1+2, this has been demonstrated in patients with chronic renal failure on dialysis (56,115). Therefore, one must be cautious in interpreting an elevated level of a marker as evidence of heightened coagulation or fibrinolytic activity in disorders associated with renal (e.g., thrombotic thrombocytopenic purpura, systemic lupus erythematosus, nephrotic syndrome, renal transplant rejection) or hepatic dysfunction.

### Disseminated Intravascular Coagulation

A number of factors can trigger disseminated intravascular coagulation (DIC), and increased coagulation system activation and secondary fibrinolysis are cardinal features of the disorder. The aforementioned assays should therefore be sensitive markers of acute or chronic DIC syndromes, and elevations in levels of factor X activation peptide (10), protein C activation markers (22,29,30), F1+2 (13,116), TAT complex (13,117–119), fibrinopeptide A (32,33,63,66,116,120), fibrinopeptide B (34, 35,67), and B$\beta$1–42 (67) have been observed in such patients. However, the sensitivity and specificity of these assays for the diagnosis of DIC have yet to be determined, and the diagnosis of DIC can usually be made with more routine laboratory tests.

Nossel et al. used radioimmunoassays for fibrinopeptide A B, and B$\beta$1–42 (measured as thrombin-increasable fibrinopeptide B) to investigate the pathophysiology of DIC in patients receiving hypertonic saline to terminate pregnancy (67). Immediately after intrauterine infusion, there was a marked increase in fibrinopeptide A levels, an index of thrombin action on fibrinogen. This was followed by a rise in the concentration of B$\beta$1–42, a measure of plasmin action on non–cross-linked fibrin I polymer. On the basis of these observations, it was hypothesized that the relative rates of proteolysis of the B$\beta$ chain of fibrinogen by thrombin and plasmin were determinants for venous thrombosis (62). Supporting this concept, a study of patients undergoing neurosurgery and craniotomy found that individuals who developed venous thrombosis exhibited fibrinopeptide A levels that were considerably greater than those of B$\beta$1–42 during the 4 days preceding the onset of this disorder (121). These observations suggest that thrombosis occurs at a time when thrombin action predominates over that of plasmin. Studies also have been carried out to determine whether elevated levels of plasmin–$\alpha_2$-antiplasmin complexes before surgery are predictive of postoperative venous thrombosis (122,123).

## Deep Vein Thrombosis

Levels of F1+2 (14,124,125), TAT complex (117,119,124,125), fibrinopeptide A (32,63,126,127) and B (34,35), and protein C activation peptide (22) are frequently elevated in symptomatic patients with venous thrombosis, pulmonary embolism, or both. Although these parameters are sensitive indices of hemostatic enzyme generation, the tests are not specific for intravascular thrombosis. Elevated values have been reported in nonpathologic, as well as in pathologic conditions, including localized and generalized infections, cancer, and connective tissue disease (see Table 56-2).

Fibrinopeptide A was the first coagulation activation marker to be developed and evaluated for its diagnostic utility in patients with venous thromboembolism. A study by Yudelman et al. (126) found that 89% of symptomatic patients presenting with positive venographic or lung scan findings, or both, had elevated fibrinopeptide A levels (>1.3 nM). The levels were generally highest in patients presenting with symptoms for 24 hours or less. However, 15% of patients without documented thrombosis had fibrinopeptide A levels in the normal range, highlighting the limitations of this assay as a diagnostic test for venous thromboembolism.

Studies using F1+2 and TAT complex assays for the diagnosis of venous thrombosis indicate that these tests also have limitations (117,124,143). F1+2 assays are less sensitive than EIAs for D-dimer (124,144,145). Although levels of TAT complex are increased in patients with venous thromboembolism (18,117,146), there is considerable overlap between patients and healthy controls (18,124,147). Furthermore, the relation between levels of TAT complexes and extent of thrombosis or duration of symptoms is inconsistent (117,124, 147–149). Therefore, TAT complex assays have inadequate sensitivity and specificity for venous thromboembolism to be useful clinically.

The D-dimer tests with the highest sensitivity are those that use the EIA format. Although initial EIA technology was cumbersome, time consuming, and only amenable for batch assays, subsequent tests can be done rapidly and samples can be assayed individually (150–152). The accuracy of rapid EIA is similar to that of the original, more cumbersome assays, and these tests are considered to be the gold standard for measuring D-dimer levels.

A whole blood, red cell agglutination assay also has high negative predictive value, rendering it useful to exclude venous thromboembolism (153–157). In contrast, plasma-based latex agglutination assays have insufficient sensitivity and specificity to be useful screening tests in patients with suspected venous thromboembolism (88,89).

Serial noninvasive testing with impedance plethysmography or compression ultrasonography is a safe alternative to venography for the diagnosis of deep vein thrombosis (DVT). However, this approach is inefficient because most patients with negative noninvasive tests at presentation do not have thrombosis and are unnecessarily subjected to serial noninvasive studies. D-dimer testing is emerging as a cost-effective strategy

## TABLE 56-2

CONDITIONS ASSOCIATED WITH ELEVATED LEVELS OF MARKERS OF COAGULATION ACTIVATION (EXCLUDING THROMBOSIS OR DISSEMINATED INTRAVASCULAR COAGULATION)

| Condition | Marker (reference) |
|---|---|
| **PHYSIOLOGIC** | |
| Normal aging | F1+2 (103–105), FPA (103), PCP (103), factor IX activation peptide (8) |
| Strenuous exercise | TAT (106) |
| Alimentary lipemia | Factor VIIa (112–114), factor IX activation peptide (114) |
| Normal pregnancy | F1+2 (128) |
| **PATHOLOGIC** | |
| Cigarette smoking | Activation peptides of factor IX and X, F1+2 (107) |
| Postmenopausal estrogen use | F1+2, FPA (108) |
| Systemic lupus erythematosus | FPA (33,129) |
| Malignancy | F1+2, FPA (130–132) |
| Acute myelogenous leukemia | F1+2, FPA (116,133,134) |
| Sickle cell disease | F1+2, FPA, D-dimer (135–138) |
| Prothrombin complex concentrate administration in hemophilia B | Factor X activation peptide, F1+2, TAT, FPA (139–141) |
| Hemolytic uremic syndrome in children | F1+2, TAT (142) |

FPA, fibrinopeptide A; PCP, protein C activation peptide; TAT, thrombin–antithrombin complex.

because it helps exclude the diagnosis of acute venous thromboembolism, thereby obviating the need for serial testing.

Clinical management studies have confirmed the utility of at least three D-dimer assays. In a prospective multicenter cohort study, a whole blood, red cell agglutination D-dimer assay (SimpliRED assay) was tested as an adjunct to impedance plethysmography for the diagnosis of DVT (158). A total of 401 patients with suspected venous thrombosis underwent a priori pretest probability assessment, D-dimer testing, and impedance plethysmography at presentation. Patients with negative D-dimer and impedance plethysmography results were not treated and underwent no further testing. Those with other combinations of results underwent additional investigations with compression ultrasonography, venography, or both. The negative predictive value for a normal D-dimer test alone was 97.1%. With a normal D-dimer and impedance plethysmography result, the negative predictive value was 98.5%, whereas it was 99.4% for a low pretest probability and normal D-dimer. These findings confirm the results of accuracy studies and suggest that a negative SimpliRED D-dimer together with a low clinical suspicion, or a normal result in combination with a negative noninvasive test, reliably excludes acute DVT, obviating the need for serial testing.

Similar results have been obtained using a rapid D-dimer EIA as an adjunct to compression ultrasonography in 946 patients with suspected DVT (159). D-dimer was measured in 686 patients who had a normal ultrasound at presentation, and repeat ultrasonography was performed only in those with a positive test. Documented venous thromboembolism occurred in only one of 598 patients with a normal ultrasound and D-dimer at presentation. In a randomized prospective study of more than 1,000 patients, it was demonstrated that DVT can be ruled out with a negative D-dimer test in patients who are judged clinically unlikely to have this diagnosis; furthermore, ultrasound testing for DVT could be safely omitted in such patients (160). These results provide further support for the concept that a normal D-dimer in conjunction with a negative noninvasive test reliably excludes DVT (26,161).

Although assays for fibrin monomer have accuracies similar to those for D-dimer (147,162,163), they have yet to be tested in clinical management studies. It is important to point out that each assay is different, and results obtained with one assay cannot be extrapolated to another (87,164). Consequently, each individual assay must be evaluated in prospective management studies before it can be adopted into clinical practice.

## Pulmonary Embolism

Numerous studies have examined the accuracy of various D-dimer assays in patients with clinically suspected pulmonary embolism. Although some investigators used pulmonary angiography as the reference standard (165,166), most of them used decision-making algorithms that combined clinical assessment with ventilation/perfusion lung scans, noninvasive studies of the legs (using impedance plethysmography or compression ultrasonography), and clinical follow-up. A summary of these studies indicates that the performance characteristics of EIAs for D-dimer in patients with suspected pulmonary embolism are similar to those in patients with DVT (88). These results prompted two prospective management trials to determine the clinical utility of D-dimer testing in patients with suspected pulmonary embolism.

Perrier et al. (167) evaluated consecutive patients presenting to the emergency department with clinically suspected pulmonary embolism. Patients were managed using a sequential algorithm that involved clinical assessment, lung scanning, D-dimer testing, and bilateral compression ultrasonography. Pulmonary angiography was done only in those with nondiagnostic results. Of 308 patients, 109 (35%) were diagnosed with pulmonary embolism at presentation, whereas two of the remaining 199 subjects had documented venous thromboembolism during the 6-month follow-up period. No patient with a normal D-dimer level had a thromboembolic event during follow-up. With this strategy, a definitive diagnosis was possible in 62% of patients with a nondiagnostic lung scan, and 53% of patients were spared the need for pulmonary angiography.

A rapid D-dimer EIA test has been evaluated in 918 consecutive outpatients who presented with suspected venous thromboembolism (168). All patients underwent clinical assessment, D-dimer testing, lower limb compression ultrasonography, and lung scanning. A normal D-dimer level ruled out venous thromboembolism in 286 subjects (35%). By combining D-dimer testing with other noninvasive tests, a diagnosis was possible in 94% of the study cohort, thereby obviating the need for more invasive studies.

Although likely to be useful in outpatients with suspected pulmonary embolism, D-dimer testing is unlikely to be as helpful in hospitalized medical or surgical patients, for whom it has lower sensitivity (146,169,170). Further studies are needed to evaluate the utility of D-dimer testing in patients who are hospitalized with suspected pulmonary embolism.

## Sepsis

Septicemia frequently results in disturbances of the hemostatic mechanism. In septic shock, DIC can lead to the deposition of fibrin in the microvasculature and the failure of multiple organs. Endotoxin, a lipopolysaccharide present in the outer membrane of Gram-negative bacteria, plays an important role in the development of the clinical and laboratory manifestations of septicemia. The intravenous administration of *Escherichia coli* endotoxin to healthy volunteers under controlled conditions increases thrombin generation, as monitored by the $F1+2$ and TAT complex assays, that is maximal 3 to 4 hours after infusion without evidence of contact system activation (171). Evidence exists that this activation is driven by the tissue factor pathway (see subsequent text). Factor XI, interposed between the contact system and factor IX, is activated after endotoxin infusion (6). The fibrinolytic system also is triggered by endotoxin, as evidenced by increased levels of tPA and plasmin–$\alpha_2$-antiplasmin complex at 2 to 3 hours (171,172). This rise in fibrinolytic activity subsequently is offset by the release of plasminogen activator inhibitor-1 (PAI-1).

Many of endotoxin's biologic effects appear to be mediated by cytokines synthesized and released by macrophages and monocytes. High levels of cytokines, tumor necrosis factor (TNF), and interleukin-6 (IL-6) have been observed within the first 2 hours of administering endotoxin to healthy subjects (171,173,174). Bauer et al. (130) showed that TNF has a potent procoagulant effect *in vivo* by studying the changes in the levels of $F1+2$, protein C activation peptide, and fibrinopeptide A after the administration of the recombinant cytokine to patients with cancer. In healthy volunteer studies, the early dynamics and route of coagulation activation in response to TNF administration were investigated (175). This resulted in the early activation of factor X, probably by the factor VII–tissue factor pathway. Infusion of recombinant IL-6 into patients with renal cell carcinoma results in elevated plasma concentrations of $F1+2$ and TAT complexes; fibrinolysis is not affected (174).

Because the immunoreactivities of coagulation system zymogens and their respective activation peptides are virtually identical in humans and chimpanzees, it has been possible to reproduce a coagulopathic response to intravenous endotoxin in this animal that is similar to that in humans (176). To investigate the molecular pathways elicited by endotoxin, pentoxifylline, a xanthine oxidase inhibitor that interrupts "immediate early" gene activation by monocytes, or a potent monoclonal antibody that rapidly neutralizes tissue factor–mediated initiation of coagulation, were administered to chimpanzees just before infusing endotoxin. Pentoxifylline markedly inhibited the endotoxin-elicited increases in serum levels of TNF and IL-6, as well as the effects on coagulation (as measured by assays for $F1+2$, TAT complex, and fibrinopeptide A) and fibrinolysis (as monitored by assays for plasminogen activator activity and plasmin–$\alpha_2$-antiplasmin complexes). In contrast, the monoclonal antibody to tissue factor completely abrogated the augmentation in thrombin generation but had no effect on cytokine levels or the fibrinolytic response. These data indicate that the fibrinolytic response triggered by endotoxin is not dependent on the generation of thrombin and that cytokines may be important in mediating the activation of both the coagulation and the fibrinolytic mechanisms *in vivo*. In addition, treatment with an antibody to IL-6 prevents coagulation activation after administration of a low dose of endotoxin to chimpanzees and does not affect activation of the fibrinolytic system (174). IL-6 probably augments coagulation by an indirect mechanism, because this cytokine has not been reported to influence the hemostatic properties of vascular endothelium or monocytes *in vitro*. Studies of administration of live *E. coli* to primates (baboons) indicate that, although an antibody to factor XII can inhibit activation of the contact system, it has no effect on the manifestations of DIC (see Chapter 6).

# Hereditary Deficiencies of Coagulation Factors

The investigation of patients with hereditary coagulation factor deficiencies using the activation peptide assays has generated information about the pathways responsible for coagulation activation *in vivo* under basal conditions (i.e., the absence of thrombosis or provocative stimuli). Patients with factor VII deficiency, but not factor XI deficiency, have reduced levels of factor IX activation (8,9), whereas patients with deficiencies of factor VIII or factor IX have normal levels of factor X and prothrombin activation (10). The administration of relatively small doses of recombinant factor VIIa (10 to 20 $\mu$g per kg of body weight) to patients with factor VII deficiency results in substantial elevations in the plasma concentrations of the factor IX activation peptide, factor X activation peptide, and prothrombin fragment F1+2 (177). Therefore, these data demonstrate that the factor VII–tissue factor pathway is largely responsible for the activation of factor IX, as well as factor X in the basal state (8,10,177). Using a clotting assay for factor VIIa, patients with severe factor IX deficiency were found to have circulating levels of enzyme less than 10% of those in healthy individuals (51,178). This suggests that factor IXa is the principal activator of factor VII *in vivo* under basal conditions.

To provide direct proof that basal level activation of the hemostatic mechanism occurs via factor VIIa–dependent activation of factor X, a monoclonal antibody directed against human tissue factor was administered to normal chimpanzees before infusing relatively high concentrations of recombinant factor VIIa (approximately 50 $\mu$g per kg body weight) (179). The monoclonal antibody used in this study is a potent inhibitor of factor VIIa–tissue factor complex function *in vitro* (180). The administration of antibody before factor VIIa abolished the significant increases in the plasma levels of factor IX activation peptide, factor X activation peptide, and F1+2 mediated by the infused recombinant protein alone, and also suppressed basal level activation of factor IX and factor X.

Infusions of a monoclonal antibody–purified factor IX concentrate to individuals with hemophilia B increase plasma factor IX activation peptide levels that are initially greatly decreased but do not change factor X activation peptide or F1+2 measurements (177). Administration of highly purified factor VIII concentrates to patients with hemophilia A results in no significant change in concentrations of factor X activation peptide and F1+2 (177). These observations therefore indicate that the factor IXa–factor VIIIa–cell surface complex is unable to activate factor X under basal conditions. In response to vascular injury or thrombotic stimuli, it is surmised that increased formation of free thrombin or factor Xa via the action of the factor VII–tissue factor pathway generates factor VIIIa or a natural surface (e.g., activated platelets) on which assembly of the factor IXa–factor VIIIa complex takes place. This hypothesis is consistent with the severe bleeding tendency of most patients with factor VIII or factor IX deficiency and with the insensitivity of the factor X activation peptide and F1+2 assays to significant deficiencies of these two proteins.

The earlier mechanistic findings derived from studies of patients with coagulation factor deficiencies have significant potential implications about the utility of basal coagulation system markers in diagnosing patients with prethrombotic disorders (177). It follows that the conversion of a prethrombotic state to a thrombotic event occurs due to small increases in the generation rates of hemostatic enzymes that exceed the inhibitory threshold of an individual's endogenous anticoagulant mechanisms. It remains to be determined whether persons with elevated basal levels of coagulation system markers are more likely to respond in a hypersensitive fashion to environmental stimuli. Because the activity of the blood coagulation mechanism in such individuals is closer to the threshold of normal inhibitory processes, they may generate slightly more thrombin by the extrinsic pathway. This thrombin could then be used to ignite the dormant intrinsic cascade, which could ultimately result in the generation of large amounts of free thrombin and the development of arterial or venous thrombosis.

# Hereditary Thrombotic Disorders

Hereditary deficiencies of proteins C, S, antithrombin, and activated protein C resistance caused by the factor V–Arg506Gln mutation have all been associated with hypercoagulable states, and coagulation activation has been investigated in patients with each of these disorders. In asymptomatic individuals with heterozygous deficiencies of protein C or protein S, the mean F1+2 level is significantly increased as compared to age-matched controls (181–184). Approximately one third of patients have levels greater than the upper limit of normal controls (defined as the mean + 2 standard deviations) (181,182). The elevated F1+2 concentrations are not caused by diminished clearance of the polypeptide (181). Fibrinopeptide A levels are elevated in approximately 20% of subjects (181,182).

Protein C activation as measured by its peptide or an immunoenzymatic assay for activated protein C is reduced to approximately 50% of normal in asymptomatic persons with heterozygous protein C deficiency (22,23). In two adult patients with homozygous protein C deficiency, it was shown that the levels of protein C activation peptide as well as F1+2 can be normalized by administration of a monoclonal antibody–purified protein C concentrate (185). Therefore, augmented activity of the protein C anticoagulant pathway can inhibit prothrombin activation *in vivo*, and protein C activation by the thrombin–thrombomodulin complex is a tonically active mechanism in the regulation of coagulation system activation.

Markers of thrombin generation have been measured in patients with nonanticoagulated venous thrombosis and their relatives with the factor V–Arg506Gln mutation. Martinelli et al. (183) reported that the median levels of F1+2 and TAT complex were significantly elevated in 69 heterozygotes from 23 families as compared to age- and sex-matched controls (for F1+2 and TAT complexes, 1.24 nM and 3.3 ng per L vs. 1.08 nM and 2.4 ng per mL, $P < 0.005$, respectively). Similar results were obtained by Zoller et al. (184) for F1+2 in 38 nonanticoagulated patients (1.7 nM vs. 1.3 nM, $P < 0.001$). In the Second Northwick Park Heart Study, a prospective cardiovascular survey of healthy men between ages 50 and 61, with no antecedent history of thrombosis, the mean levels of F1+2 were found to be significantly increased among heterozygous carriers of either the factor V–Arg506Gln mutation or the prothrombin G20210A mutation (186). The factor V–Arg506Gln mutation causes factor Va to be relatively resistant to inactivation by activated protein C, thereby facilitating an increased rate of prothrombin to thrombin conversion by the factor Xa–factor Va–activated platelet complex; heterozygosity for the prothrombin G20210A mutation results in an increase in the plasma prothrombin concentration of approximately 30% as compared to healthy subjects.

In asymptomatic patients with hereditary antithrombin deficiency, it was initially reported that F1+2 levels are frequently increased as compared to age-matched unaffected siblings (16). Fibrinopeptide A measurements were similar in both groups. The plasma antithrombin concentrations were reduced to approximately 50% of normal. Subsequently, it was shown that the high concentrations of the fragment resulted from an *in vitro* effect due to the presence of low amounts of heparin (final concentration of 4 U per mL) in the anticoagulant cocktail used for sample collection in the presence of reduced blood levels of antithrombin (187). Other studies of antithrombin-deficient subjects did not demonstrate significant elevations in plasma F1+2 or fibrinopeptide A levels (182,188). An investigation of asymptomatic persons from a single large family with functional antithrombin deficiency (antithrombin Hamilton, a type II mutation having diminished serine protease reactivity) found significantly higher results in affected family members (189). However, the mean F1+2 value was within the normal range, and the majority had normal levels. The mean levels of TAT complex and fibrinopeptide A were not significantly different between the antithrombin–deficient individuals and their unaffected family members (189). The reason for this apparent paradox in patients with heterozygous antithrombin deficiency, which is generally considered as the most prothrombotic disorder among the hereditary thrombophilias, is unknown.

## LUPUS ANTICOAGULANTS

Ginsberg et al. (190) found that the presence of anticardiolipin antibodies in patients with systemic lupus erythematosus is associated with a prothrombotic state as measured by the F1+2 and fibrinopeptide A assays. This relation was maintained even after excluding from analysis those individuals with prior thrombotic histories. Another study by Tripodi et al. (191) of patients with systemic lupus erythematosus and lupus anticoagulants found significant elevations in fibrinopeptide A but not F1+2.

## ACUTE CORONARY SYNDROMES

This section reviews data about coagulation activation markers in patients with cardiac ischemic syndromes and describes how this information has helped to clarify the pathophysiology of coronary artery thrombosis. Most patients with acute myocardial infarction and unstable angina have high plasma levels of fibrinopeptide A (192,193). The levels of fibrinopeptide A in spot urine samples and 24-hour urine collections from these patients also have been found to be elevated (194,195). These findings are consistent with the results of angiographic, angioscopic, and pathologic studies that have clearly shown that intracoronary thrombosis plays a pivotal role in the pathogenesis of these coronary syndromes (196). Abnormally high plasma F1+2 or fibrinopeptide A levels are found in approximately 50% of patients during the acute phase of the disease, the prevalence being higher in those with unstable angina (197) or angiographic evidence of intracoronary thrombosis. No difference in the levels of these peptides has been observed between patients with unstable angina and those with acute myocardial infarction (197). This may indicate that plasma F1+2 and fibrinopeptide A levels are not dependent on the characteristics of the thrombus (which is subocclusive and platelet-rich in unstable angina, but occlusive and fibrin-rich in myocardial infarction) (198), but rather reflect a systemic condition of hypercoagulability.

The degree of coagulation activation seems to be related to prognosis. Ardissino et al. (199) measured both plasma and urinary fibrinopeptide A levels in patients with unstable angina on hospital admission and found that elevated plasma levels were associated with a higher risk of developing primary (death or myocardial infarction) or secondary (refractory angina requiring emergency coronary revascularization) clinical endpoints during hospitalization. Granger et al. (200) found that higher baseline levels of F1+2 were associated with an increased likelihood of death or myocardial reinfarction during a 30-day follow-up period in patients with myocardial infarction receiving thrombolytic therapy.

The serial measurement of coagulation activation peptides over time has provided interesting information concerning the pathophysiology of acute coronary syndromes. Merlini et al. (197) measured F1+2 and fibrinopeptide A plasma levels in patients with unstable angina or acute myocardial infarction during the acute phase and 6 months after their initial acute presentation. Levels of F1+2 and fibrinopeptide A both were elevated during the acute ischemic episode, thereby reflecting the presence of an intracoronary thrombosis. However, in patients with an uneventful clinical course at 6 months, fibrinopeptide A levels had returned to the normal range, whereas F1+2 levels remained high. This observation of a decrease in plasma levels of fibrinopeptide A without substantial change in F1+2 indicates that increased thrombin generation persists after initial coronary ischemic episodes but is not sufficient to initiate fibrin formation and deposition. It is not known whether the presence of such biochemical hypercoagulability state is a risk factor for the occurrence (or recurrence) of coronary events, but studies to address this question in both healthy populations without prior cardiac events, as well as patients with recent prior coronary events are ongoing.

Coronary angioplasty mechanically causes plaque disruption that may evoke a thrombotic response, and abrupt coronary artery occlusion still represents one of the major complications of the procedure. Tearing of the atherosclerotic plaque might induce cap rupture that exposes the procoagulant matrix of the plaque itself to blood flow, giving rise to thrombosis. Marmur et al. (201) measured arterial blood F1+2 and fibrinopeptide A during uncomplicated coronary angioplasty. Although no changes occurred in most patients, seven of 32 showed an increase in F1+2, which was associated with an increase in fibrinopeptide A in four. These data show that most patients do not experience heightened coagulation system activation during uncomplicated coronary angioplasty under antithrombotic treatment with heparin; however, a few do, and this could be due to the biochemical characteristics of the plaque itself (202) or to deeper trauma of the vessel wall induced by the angioplasty procedure. In another series of patients undergoing mechanical revascularization, Oltrona et al. (203) showed that a failure to normalize fibrinopeptide A levels during the procedure (heparin resistance) was associated with a higher risk of complications.

## ATRIAL FIBRILLATION

Chronic atrial fibrillation predisposes to thromboembolism, and cardioversion itself also is associated with cerebral, systemic, and pulmonary embolic events. The mechanism underlying the occurrence of embolic episodes after the restoration of sinus rhythm in these patients is poorly understood. The reduction in the incidence of cardioversion-related embolic events induced by the administration of warfarin has led to the widespread recommendation that anticoagulation should be prescribed for several weeks before and after cardioversion in patients with chronic atrial fibrillation. The use of anticoagulants, however, is not recommended in patients with acute atrial fibrillation lasting fewer than 48 hours who undergo cardioversion, although definitive data about the risk of postcardioversion embolism in these patients are scanty. The finding of atrial thrombosis in 14% of patients with recent-onset atrial fibrillation suggests that these individuals also are at risk for developing embolic events (204). Oltrona et al. (205) measured the plasma concentrations of TAT complex and fibrinopeptide A in a series of patients with acute nonvalvular atrial fibrillation and found a significant increase in the plasma concentrations of both markers early after pharmacologic cardioversion as compared to hospital admission; the levels decreased toward baseline values 1 month after restoration of sinus rhythm. This finding of a hypercoagulable state early after cardioversion in patients with recent-onset atrial fibrillation thereby raises the important question as to whether prophylactic antithrombotic treatment also should be adopted for these cases.

# ANTITHROMBOTIC THERAPY

Intravenous heparin, a mainstay in the treatment of patients with acute coronary syndromes, acts by inhibiting thrombin and activated factors X and IX, and less potently activated factors XI and XII. The anticoagulant action of heparin is due primarily to its ability to bind antithrombin, thereby accelerating the rate of inhibition of the major coagulation enzymes, particularly thrombin. Biochemical studies of patients with acute coronary syndromes have demonstrated clearly that intravenous heparin rapidly inhibits the action of thrombin on fibrinogen and lowers plasma fibrinopeptide A levels to within the normal range (206–208). Merlini et al. (209) showed that intravenous heparin at doses giving an activated partial thromboplastin time of more than double its baseline value reduced plasma fibrinopeptide A levels, but did not lower plasma prothrombin fragment F1+2 levels in most patients. Studies have shown that hirudin, a high-affinity direct thrombin inhibitor, does not decrease thrombin generation in patients with stable angina or acute coronary syndromes (210). Because thrombin plays a critical role in the amplification of the coagulation cascade by activating factor V and factor VIII, persistent thrombin generation may contribute partly to the persistent thrombotic risk that exists despite anticoagulation. Plasma levels of both fibrinopeptide A and F1+2 have been found to be higher in patients developing infarction, reinfarction, or refractory ischemia, suggesting that the presence of a persistent hypercoagulable state in patients with acute coronary syndromes, notwithstanding heparin therapy at the usual dose, still may be associated with an unfavorable outcome (200,209).

The measurement of coagulation peptides after the discontinuation of heparin or hirudin has revealed the presence of a so-called rebound phenomenon. Gallino et al. (207) have shown that, although a decrease in plasma fibrinopeptide A levels occurs during heparin infusions, a sharp increase occurs once the infusion is over, which suggests a reactivation of coagulation system activity. This finding has been confirmed by Granger et al. (211), who found the same phenomenon for F1+2 and activated protein C levels (which also reflect, in part, increased thrombin generation). A similar effect has been observed after the discontinuation of argatroban, another direct thrombin inhibitor (212). It is tempting to speculate that the increase in clinical events observed after the cessation of heparin or argatroban therapy is linked to this rebound in coagulation (212,213), most likely due to the persistence of the original procoagulant activity that necessitated anticoagulation in the first place.

The failure to achieve reperfusion and the occurrence of subsequent reocclusion after successful thrombolysis are major limitations of thrombolytic therapy in acute myocardial infarction. The measurement of coagulation activation markers during thrombolytic therapy has demonstrated the prothrombotic effect of thrombolytic therapy (214). In patients receiving streptokinase or recombinant tissue plasminogen activator, there is an increase in the plasma levels of fibrinopeptide A, TAT complex, and F1+2 (215). Although the concomitant administration of heparin prevents fibrinopeptide A levels from increasing (216), F1+2 levels increase in most patients despite the associated anticoagulant therapy (217). These findings raise the question of the role of hypercoagulability in the pathogenesis of the failure of reperfusion or postthrombolytic reocclusion. The possibility exists that this may be contributed to by the ability of plasmin's ability to activate platelets. In patients receiving thrombolytic therapy, the behavior of coagulation activation markers after treatment seems to be predictive of outcome. Gulba et al. (218)

have shown that patients in whom plasma TAT complex levels increase 90 minutes after the start of thrombolytic therapy are those with no reperfusion or in whom reocclusion occurs. Granger et al. (200) have assessed the relation of fibrinopeptide A and F1+2 levels with subsequent reinfarction and death in patients who received either recombinant tissue plasminogen activator or streptokinase; lower levels of fibrinopeptide A or F1+2 after 12 hours were associated with a trend toward a lower likelihood of subsequent reinfarction.

Merlini et al. (219) found that there was an increase in F1+2 levels in patients with unstable angina who received thrombolytic therapy in addition to heparin. In the patients who developed refractory angina or infarction, higher fibrinopeptide A levels also were measured, thereby suggesting that the hypercoagulable state induced by thrombolytic therapy may be detrimental in the setting of the subocclusive thrombosis typical of unstable angina. This perhaps explains the unfavorable results of this therapy in such patients.

In most patients with venous thromboembolism, treatment with adequate doses of heparin rapidly inhibits thrombin action on fibrinogen and lowers elevated fibrinopeptide A levels into the normal range (32,220). Thrombin generation, as measured by the F1+2 and TAT complex assays, declines gradually over the first several days of heparin treatment but often can remain elevated compared with levels in healthy controls even after a week of treatment (125). This observation may reflect that factor Xa in the prothrombinase complex is relatively protected from inhibition by heparin bound to plasma (221).

Therapy with oral anticoagulants such as warfarin suppresses prothrombin activation *in vivo* as measured by the F1+2 (222–224). In patients with prior thrombotic histories and high F1+2 levels, Conway et al. (220) demonstrated that stable anticoagulation at moderate intensity as reflected by international normalized ratios (INRs) of 2.5 to 3.5, produces five- to 10-fold reductions in the extent of prothrombin activation. It also has been shown that the mean values of F1+2 decrease in parallel with the intensity of warfarin therapy. A study has demonstrated that a target INR range as low as 1.3 to 1.6 results, on average, in a 50% reduction in prothrombin activation from baseline levels (224). It is important to note that the findings of these studies cannot be translated into clinical practice because the F1+2 level that confers antithrombotic protection has yet to be determined.

Although F1+2 levels often are suppressed below normal in stably anticoagulated patients on oral agents, this has not been observed for TAT complexes and fibrinopeptide A. However, it has been observed that plasma fibrinopeptide A concentrations increase above the normal range in patients with a history of myocardial infarction several weeks after the cessation of the drug (225).

On the basis of these data, clinical studies have been carried out in situations in which the monitoring of coagulation system function by standard methods has been unsatisfactory (e.g., the prophylaxis of subacute thrombosis after stent implantation). The main problem of intracoronary stenting is subacute thrombosis, which often occurs unpredictably even in conditions of optimal anticoagulation according to classic standard coagulation tests. It has been shown that an increase in F1+2 levels, despite optimal anticoagulation, is a sensitive indicator of subacute thrombosis (226). In a case–control study (227), a study population on oral anticoagulants was investigated using F1+2 measurements, as well as classic coagulation tests and compared to a control population in which only the classical tests were used to monitor the level of anticoagulation. It was found that the incidence of subtotal occlusion was 3.5% in the study group, but 17% in the control group. For elective and nonelective stenting, the monitoring of F1+2 levels therefore may be associated with a reduced rate of subacute thrombosis (227).

## Extracorporeal Circulation

Using activation markers of coagulation, Boisclair et al. (55, 56,188) have examined whether extracorporeal circulation in patients undergoing hemodialysis for chronic renal failure or cardiopulmonary bypass for coronary artery bypass grafting activates the contact system. They did not find that exposure of blood to foreign surfaces triggers coagulation activation and rather postulated it to be a consequence of defective neutralization of downstream coagulation proteases (e.g., factor Xa, thrombin) caused by the absence of normal vascular endothelium. In patients undergoing cardiopulmonary bypass, it was suggested that the surgery itself was primarily responsible for increased factor VII–tissue factor mechanism function and the subsequent generation of factor Xa and thrombin (55). These findings, however, must be reconciled with the observations of increased kallikrein- and factor XIIa–C1 inhibitor complexes during bypass (see Chapter 6).

## Thrombolytic Therapy

The availability of biochemical markers that reflect the activation of the coagulation and fibrinolytic systems has led to a number of important observations in patients receiving thrombolytic therapy. For example, there is increasing evidence that plasminogen activators induce a procoagulant state characterized by increased levels of fibrinopeptide A (214,215,228,229). The procoagulant state is likely to be multifactorial in origin. One trigger may be thrombin bound to fibrin, which is enzymatically active and protected from fluid-phase inhibitors (230, 231). As the clot undergoes progressive lysis, increasingly more of the clot-bound thrombin is exposed, thereby increasing the procoagulant stimulus (232). In addition, thrombin bound to soluble FDPs generated in the vicinity of the lysing thrombus also is protected from inactivation by circulating inhibitors (233). Plasmin-mediated activation of the coagulation mechanism also may contribute to the procoagulant state. It has been shown that plasmin is able to activate contact factors (234), factor V (235), and possibly prothrombin (236), thereby promoting thrombin generation. Further investigation is needed to determine the contribution of the procoagulant state to reocclusion that can occur after successful thrombolysis, and it has been suggested that persistent elevation of levels of TAT or fibrinopeptide A may be predictive of this complication (228).

The validity of using plasma fibrinopeptide A and B levels as specific markers of thrombin activity in the setting of thrombolytic therapy has been questioned on the basis of observations that tPA and urokinase have direct catalytic activity against fibrinogen. Under plasminogen-free conditions, tPA releases fibrinopeptides A and B from fibrinogen, but unlike thrombin action on fibrinogen, the rate of tPA–induced fibrinopeptide B release is faster than that of fibrinopeptide A, and release of both fibrinopeptides is unaffected by heparin (237). Urokinase also has catalytic activity against fibrinogen but only releases fibrinopeptide B (238). Although pharmacologic concentrations of tPA may directly cleave fibrinopeptide A from fibrinogen, the observation that therapy with either streptokinase or tPA leads to increased levels of fibrinopeptide A (214,215,228,229) that are rapidly lowered with high doses of heparin (229) suggests that thrombin is the major mediator of the elevated fibrinopeptide A levels in this setting.

Using concomitant measurements of B$\beta$1–42 and B$\beta$15–42 in patients receiving tPA therapy, Eisenberg et al. (70) demonstrated that the fibrinolytic effect of tPA therapy persists for some time after fibrinogenolysis ceases. This finding is consistent with the results of studies in experimental animals showing that tPA–induced clot lysis continues after the drug is cleared from the circulation (239), likely reflecting enzymatically active tPA bound to the thrombus. In accord with these findings, it is of interest to note that the rapid administration of tPA in an animal model produces an enhanced thrombolytic effect with reduced bleeding, as compared to more prolonged infusions (240). Despite the affinity of tPA for fibrin, its administration to patients with acute myocardial infarction or venous thromboembolic disease causes significant fibrinogenolysis. Using plasma levels of B$\beta$1–42 as an index of fibrinogenolysis, Owen et al. (241) demonstrated that streptokinase, a plasminogen activator without fibrin specificity, as well as tPA produced significant fibrinogen proteolysis. Although it was predicted that high doses of tPA would produce systemic fibrinogen breakdown, studies have provided a mechanism by which even physiologic concentrations of tPA can induce fibrinogenolysis. It has been shown that soluble FDPs, particularly (DD)E, potentiate tPA–induced plasminogen activation by binding both plasminogen and tPA (242,243). These findings are not surprising given the potentiating activity of cyanogen bromide fragments of fibrin or fibrinogen (244–248) that are frequently used as stimulators in commercial tPA activity assays. Studies indicate that tPA binds to (DD)E with an affinity similar to fibrin. Likewise, plasminogen also binds to (DD)E with high affinity, suggesting that, like fibrin, (DD)E serves as a template to which both tPA and plasminogen bind (249).

The interaction of tPA with (DD)E is mediated by its second kringle domain (249). In contrast, tPA binds to fibrin mainly by its finger domain (249,250). These findings rationalize the greater fibrin-selectivity of vampire bat plasminogen activator (b-PA) relative to tPA. Although structurally similar to tPA, b-PA lacks a second kringle domain (251). Consequently, unlike tPA, b-PA does not bind to (DD)E (249).

## Other Conditions Associated with Elevated Levels of Markers of Coagulation Activation

Elevated levels of markers of coagulation activation have been reported in settings in which thrombosis or DIC is not evident clinically. A list of some of these disorders is shown in Table 56-2.

## *References*

1. Ford RP, Esnouf MP, Burgess AI, et al. An enzyme-linked immunosorbent assay (ELISA) for the measurement of activated factor XII (Hageman factor) in human plasma. *J Immunoassay* 1996;172:119–131.
2. Kaplan AP, Gruber B, Harpel PC. Assessment of Hageman factor activation in human plasma: quantification of activated Hageman factor–C1 inactivator complexes by an enzyme-linked differential antibody immunosorbent assay. *Blood* 1985;66:636–641.
3. Nuijens JH, Huijbregts CC, Eerenberg-Belmer AJ, et al. Quantification of plasma factor XIIa–Cl(-)-inhibitor and kallikrein–Cl(-)-inhibitor complexes in sepsis. *Blood* 1988;72:1841–1848.
4. Lewin MF, Kaplan AP, Harpel PC. Studies of C1 inactivator-plasma kallikrein complexes in purified systems and in plasma. *J Biol Chem* 1983;258:6415–6421.
5. Kaufman N, Page JD, Pixley RA, et al. Alpha2–macroglobulin–kallikrein complexes detect contact system activation in hereditary angioedema and human sepsis. *Blood* 1991;77:2660–2667.
6. Minnema MC, Pajkrt D, Wuillemin WA, et al. Activation of clotting factor XI without detectable contact activation in experimental human endotoxemia. *Blood* 1998;92:3294–3301.
7. Wuillemin WA, Minnema M, Meijers JC, et al. Inactivation of factor XIa in human plasma assessed by measuring factor XIa–protease inhibitor complexes: major role for C1-inhibitor. *Blood* 1995;85:1517–1526.
8. Bauer KA, Kass BL, ten Cate H, et al. Factor IX is activated *in vivo* by the tissue factor mechanism. *Blood* 1990;764:731–736.
9. Takahashi I, Kato K, Sugiura I, et al. Activated factor IX-antithrombin III complexes in human blood: quantification by an enzyme-linked differential antibody immunoassay and determination of the *in vivo* half-life. *J Lab Clin Med* 1991;118:317–325.
10. Bauer KA, Kass BL, ten Cate H, et al. Detection of factor X activation in humans. *Blood* 1989;746:2007–2015.

11. Jesty J, Morrison SA, Harpel PC. Measurement of human activated factor X–antithrombin complex by an enzyme-linked differential antibody immunosorbent assay. *Anal Biochem* 1984;139:158–167.
12. Lau HK, Rosenberg JS, Beeler DL, et al. The isolation and characterization of a specific antibody population directed against the prothrombin activation fragments $F_2$ and $F_{1+2}$. *J Biol Chem* 1979;254:8751–8761.
13. Teitel JM, Bauer KA, Lau HK, et al. Studies of the prothrombin activation pathway utilizing radioimmunoassays for the $F_2/F_{1+2}$ fragment and thrombin-antithrombin complex. *Blood* 1982;59:1086–1097.
14. Pelzer H, Schwart A, Stuber W. Determination of human prothrombin activation fragment 1+2 in plasma in plasma with an antibody against a synthetic peptide. *Thromb Haemost* 1991;65:153–159.
15. Hursting MJ, Butman BT, Steiner JP, et al. Monoclonal antibodies specific for prothrombin fragment 1.2 and their use in a quantitative enzyme-linked immunosorbent assay. *Clin Chem* 1993;39:583–591.
16. Bauer KA, Goodman TL, Kass BL, et al. Elevated factor Xa activity in the blood of asymptomatic patients with congenital antithrombin deficiency. *J Clin Invest* 1985;76:826–836.
17. Lau HK, Rosenberg RD. The isolation and characterization of a specific antibody population directed against the thrombin–antithrombin complex. *J Biol Chem* 1980;255:5885–5893.
18. Pelzer H, Schwarz A, Heimburger N. Determination of human thrombin-antithrombin III complex in plasma with an enzyme-linked immunosorbent assay. *Thromb Haemost* 1988;59:101–106.
19. Collen D, De Cock F, Verstraete M. Quantitation of thrombin–antithrombin III complexes in human blood. *Eur J Clin Invest* 1977;7:407–411.
20. Shifman MA, Pizzo SV. The *in vivo* metabolism of antithrombin III and antithrombin III complexes. *J Biol Chem* 1982;257:3243–3248.
21. Leonard B, Bies R, Carlson T, et al. Further studies of the turnover of dog antithrombin III. Study of 131I-labeled antithrombin protease complexes. *Thromb Res* 1983;30:165–177.
22. Bauer KA, Kass BL, Beeler DL, et al. Detection of protein C activation in humans. *J Clin Invest* 1984;74:2033–2041.
23. Gruber A, Griffin JH. Direct detection of activated protein C in blood from human subjects. *Blood* 1992;799:2340–2348.
24. Orthner CL, Kolen B, Drohan WN. A sensitive and facile assay for the measurement of activated protein C activity levels *in vivo*. *Thromb Haemost* 1993;695:441–447.
25. Liaw PC, Ferrell G, Esmon CT. A monoclonal antibody against activated protein C allows rapid detection of activated protein C in plasma and reveals a calcium ion dependent epitope involved in factor Va inactivation. *J Thromb Haemost* 2003;1:662–670.
26. Stein PD, Hull RD, Patel KC, et al. D-dimer for the exclusion of acute venous thrombosis and pulmonary embolism. A systematic review. *Ann Intern Med* 2004;140:589–602.
27. Espana F, Griffin JH. Determination of functional and antigenic protein C inhibitor and its complexes with activated protein C in plasma by ELISA's. *Thromb Res* 1989;556:671–682.
28. Espana F, Gruber A, Heeb MJ, et al. *In vivo* and *in vitro* complexes of activated protein C with two inhibitors in baboons. *Blood* 1991;778:1754–1760.
29. Espana F, Vicente V, Tabernero D, et al. Determination of plasma protein C inhibitor and of two activated protein C–inhibitor complexes in normals and in patients with intravascular coagulation and thrombotic disease. *Thromb Res* 1990;593:593–608.
30. Scully MF, Toh CH, Hoogendoorn H, et al. Activation of protein C and its distribution between its inhibitors, protein C–inhibitor, alpha 1-antitrypsin and alpha 2-macroglobulin, in patients with disseminated intravascular coagulation. *Thromb Haemost* 1993;69:448–453.
31. Nossel HL, Younger LR, Wilner GD, et al. Radioimmunoassay of human fibrinopeptide A. *Proc Natl Acad Sci U S A* 1971;68:2350–2353.
32. Nossel HL, Yudelman I, Canfield RE, et al. Measurement of fibrinopeptide A in human blood. *J Clin Invest* 1974;54:43–53.
33. Cronlund M, Hardin J, Burton J, et al. Fibrinopeptide A in plasma of normal subjects and patients with disseminated intravascular coagulation and systemic lupus erythematosus. *J Clin Invest* 1976;58:142–151.
34. Bilezikian SB, Nossel HL, Butler VP Jr, et al. Radioimmunoassay of human fibrinopeptide B and kinetics of cleavage by different enzymes. *J Clin Invest* 1975;56:438–445.
35. Eckhardt T, Nossel HL, Hurlet-Jensen A, et al. Measurement of desarginine fibrinopeptide B in human blood. *J Clin Invest* 1981;67:809–816.
36. Collen D, De Cock F. A tanned red cell hemagglutination inhibition immunoassay (TRCHII) for the quantitative estimation of thrombin-antithrombin III and plasmin–alpha2-antiplasmin complexes in human plasma. *Thromb Res* 1975;7:235–238.
37. Collen D, de Cock F, Cambiaso CL, et al. A latex agglutination test for rapid quantitative estimation of the plasmin–antiplasmin complex in human plasma. *Eur J Clin Invest* 1977;7:21–26.
38. Harpel PC. $\alpha_2$-Plasmin inhibitor and $\alpha_2$-macroglobulin–plasmin complexes in plasma: quantification by an enzyme-linked differential antibody immunosorbent assay. *J Clin Invest* 1981;68:46–55.
39. Wiman B, Jacobsson L, Anderson M, et al. Determination of plasmin–alpha2-antiplasmin complex in plasma samples by means of a radioimmunoassay. *Scand J Lab Clin Invest* 1983;43:27–33.
40. Mimuro J, Koike Y, Sumi Y, et al. Monoclonal antibodies to discrete regions in a2-plasmin inhibitor. *Blood* 1987;69:446–453.
41. Holvoet P, de Boer A, Verstreken M, et al. An enzyme linked immunosorbent assay (ELISA) for the measurement of PAP complexes in human plasma: application to the detection of *in vivo* activation of the fibrinolytic system. *Thromb Haemost* 1986;56:124–127.
42. Levi M, de Boer JP, Roem D, et al. Plasminogen activation *in vivo* upon intravenous infusion of DDAVP. Quantitative assessment of plasmin–alpha2-antiplasmin complex with a novel monoclonal antibody based radioimmunoassay. *Thromb Haemost* 1992;67:111–116.
43. Kudryk B, Rohoza A, Ahadi M, et al. A monoclonal antibody with ability to distinguish between NH2-terminal fragments derived from fibrinogen and fibrin. *Mol Immunol* 1983;20:1191–1200.
44. Weitz JI, Koehn JA, Canfield RW, et al. Development of a radioimmunoassay for the fibrinogen-derived peptide Bβ1-42. *Blood* 1986;67:1014–1022.
45. Kudryk B, Rohoza A, Ahadi M, et al. Specificity of a monoclonal antibody for the NH2-terminal region of fibrin. *Mol Immunol* 1984;21:89–94.
46. Merskey C, Kleiner GJ, Johnson AJ. Quantitative estimation of split products of fibrinogen in human serum, relation to diagnosis and treatment. *Blood* 1966;28:1–18.
47. Marder VJ, Matchett MO, Sherry S. Detection of serum fibrinogen and fibrin degradation products. Comparison of six technics using purified products and application in clinical studies. *Am J Med* 1971;51:71–82.
48. Rylatt DB, Blake AS, Cottis LE, et al. An immunoassay for human D dimer using monoclonal antibodies. *Thromb Res* 1983;31:767–778.
49. Whitaker AN, Elms MJ, Masci PP, et al. Measurement of crosslinked fibrin derivatives in plasma: an immunoassay using monoclonal antibodies. *J Clin Pathol* 1984;37:882–887.
50. Franks JJ, Kirsch RE, Kao B. Fibrinogen and fibrinogen related peptides in cancer. In: Mariani G, ed. *Pathophysiology of plasma protein metabolism*, London: McMillan, 1984:265–269.
51. Wildgoose P, Nemerson Y, Hansen LL, et al. Measurement of basal levels of factor VIIa in hemophilia A and B patients. *Blood* 1992;801:25–28.
52. Morrissey JH, Macik BG, Neuenschwander PF, et al. Quantitation of activated factor VII levels in plasma using a tissue factor mutant selectively deficient in promoting factor VII activation. *Blood* 1993;813:734–744.
53. Davie EW, Fujikawa K, Kisiel W. The coagulation cascade: initiation, maintenance, and regulation. *Biochemistry* 1991;30:10363–10370.
54. Gailani D, Broze GJ Jr. Factor XI activation in a revised model of blood coagulation. *Science* 1991;253:909–912.
55. Boisclair MD, Lane DA, Philippou H, et al. Mechanisms of thrombin generation during surgery and cardiopulmonary bypass. *Blood* 1993;82:3 350–3357.
56. Boisclair MD, Lane DA, Philippou H, et al. Thrombin production, inactivation and expression during open heart surgery measured by assays for activation fragments including a new ELISA for prothrombin fragment F1+2. *Thromb Haemost* 1993;70:253–258.
57. Boisclair MD, Lane DA. A microtitre plate ELISA to measure thrombin-antithrombin complex using pan-specific antibodies. *Blood Coagul Fibrinolysis* 1992;3:795–802.
58. Blomback B, Hessel B, Hogg D, et al. A two-step fibrinogen-fibrin transition in blood coagulation. *Nature* 1978;275:501–505.
59. Hurlet-Jensen A, Cummins HZ, Nossel HL, et al. Fibrin polymerization and release of fibrinopeptide B by thrombin. *Thromb Res* 1982;27:419–427.
60. Kanaide H, Shainoff JR. Crosslinking of fibrinogen and fibrin by fibrin-stabilizing factor (factor XIIIa). *J Lab Clin Med* 1975;85:574–597.
61. Brosstad F. Lower susceptibility of human des-AA versus des-AABB fibrin towards fibrin stabilizing factor. *Thromb Res* 1978;13:799–803.
62. Nossel HL. Relative proteolysis of the fibrinogen B beta chain by thrombin and plasmin as a determinant of thrombosis. *Nature* 1981;291:165–167.
63. Nossel HL, Ti M, Kaplan KL, et al. The generation of fibrinopeptide A in clinical blood samples: Evidence for thrombin activity. *J Clin Invest* 1976;58:1136–1144.
64. Kockum C, Frebelius S. Rapid radioimmunoassay of human fibrinopeptide A—removal of cross-reacting fibrinogen with bentonite. *Thromb Res* 1980;19:589–598.
65. Soria J, Soria C, Ryckewaert JJ. A solid phase immuno enzymological assay for the measurement of human fibrinopeptide A. *Thromb Res* 1980;20:425–435.
66. Woodhams BJ, Kernoff PBA. Rapid radioimmunoassay for fibrinopeptide A in plasma. *Thromb Res* 1981;22:407–416.
67. Nossel HL, Wasser J, Kaplan KL, et al. Sequence of fibrinogen protolysis and platelet release after intrauterine infusion of hypertonic saline. *J Clin Invest* 1979;64:1371–1378.
68. Kudryk B, Robinson D, Netre C, et al. Measurement in human blood of fibrinogen/fibrin fragments containing the B beta 15-42 sequence. *Thromb Res* 1982;25:277–291.
69. Lawler CM, Bovill EG, Stump DC, et al. Fibrin fragment D-dimer and fibrinogen B beta peptides in plasma as markers of clot lysis during thrombolytic therapy in acute myocardial infarction. *Blood* 1990;76:1341–1348.
70. Eisenberg PR, Sherman LA, Tiefenbrunn AJ, et al. Sustained fibrinolysis after administration of t-PA despite its short half-life in the circulation. *Thromb Haemost* 1987;57:35–40.
71. Ring ME, Butman SM, Bruck DC, et al. Fibrin metabolism in patients with acute myocardial infarction during and after treatment with tissue-type plasminogen activator. *Thromb Haemost* 1987;60:428–433.
72. Bode C, Matsueda GR, Hui KY, et al. Antibody-directed urokinase: a specific fibrinolytic agent. *Science* 1985;229:765–767.

73. Runge MS, Bode C, Matsueda GR, et al. Conjugation to an antifibrin monoclonal antibody enhances the fibrinolytic potency of tissue plasminogen activator *in vitro. Biochemistry* 1988;27:1153–1157.

74. Hawiger J, Niewiarowski S, Gurewich V, et al. Measurement of fibrinogen and fibrin degradation products in serum by staphylococcal clumping test. *J Lab Clin Med* 1970;75:93–108.

75. Gordon YB, Martin MJ, McNeile AT, et al. Specific and sensitive determination of fibrinogen degradation products by radioimmunoassay. *Lancet* 1973;2:1168–1170.

76. Gordon YB, Martin MJ, McNeile AT, et al. The development of radioimmunoassays for fibrinogen degradation products: fragments D and E. *Br J Haematol* 1975;29:109–119.

77. Gaffney PJ, Perry MJ. Unreliability of current serum fibrin degradation product (FDP) assays. *Thromb Haemost* 1985;53:301–302.

78. Koopman J, Haverkate F, Koppert P, et al. New enzyme immunoassays of fibrin-fibrinogen degradation products in plasma using a monoclonal antibody. *J Lab Clin Med* 1987;109:75–84.

79. Plow E, Edgington TS. Immunobiology of fibrinogen. Emergence of neoantigenic expression during physiologic cleavage *in vitro* and *in vivo. J Clin Invest* 1973;52:273–282.

80. Plow EF, Hougie C, Edgington TS. Neoantigenic expressions engendered by plasmin cleavage of fibrinogen. *J Immunol* 1971;107:1496–1500.

81. Plow EF, Edgington TS. Localization and characterization of the cleavage-associated neoantigen locus in the E domain of fibrinogen. *J Biol Chem* 1979;254:672–678.

82. Chen JP, Shurley HM. A simple efficient production of neoantigenic antisera against fibrinolytic degradation products: radioimmunoassay of fragment E. *Thromb Res* 1975;7:425–434.

83. Chen JP, Hanna WT, Williams TK, et al. Radioimmunoassay of fragment E-related neoantigen: validation studies and clinical application. *Br J Haematol* 1984;57:133–144.

84. Zielinsky A, Hirsh J, Stranmanis G. The diagnostic value of the fibrinogen/fibrin fragment E antigen assay in clinically suspected deep vein thrombosis. *Blood* 1982;59:346–350.

85. Gaffney PJ, Brasher M. Subunit structure of the plasmin-induced degradation products of cross-linked fibrin. *Biochim Biophys Acta* 1973;295:308–313.

86. Pizzo SV, Taylor LM Jr, Schwartz ML, et al. Subunit structure of fragment D from fibrinogen and cross-linked fibrin. *J Biol Chem* 1973;248:4584–4590.

87. van Beek EJ, van den Ende B, Berckmans RJ, et al. A comparative analysis of D-dimer assays in patients with clinically suspected pulmonary embolism. *Thromb Haemost* 1993;70:408–413.

88. Bounameaux H, de Moerloose P, Perrier A, et al. Plasma measurements of D-dimer as diagnostic aid in suspected venous thromboembolism: an overview. *Thromb Haemost* 1994;71:1–6.

89. Becker DM, Philbrick JT, Bachhuber TL, et al. D-dimer testing and acute venous thromboembolism: a shortcut to accurate diagnosis? *Arch Intern Med* 1996;156:939–946.

90. Francis CW, Connaghan DG, Marder VJ. Assessment of fibrin degradation products during fibrinolytic therapy for acute myocardial infarction. *Circulation* 1986;74:1027–1036.

91. Eisenberg PR, Jaffe AS, Stump DC, et al. Validity of enzyme-linked immunosorbent assays of cross-linked fibrin degradation products as a measure of clot lysis. *Circulation* 1990;82:1159–1168.

92. Gurewich V, Hume M, Patrick M. The laboratory diagnosis of venous thromboembolic disease by measurement of fibrinogen/fibrin degradation products and fibrin monomer. *Chest* 1973;64:585–590.

93. Dempfle CE, Pfitzner SA, Dollman M, et al. Comparison of immunological and functional assays for measurement of soluble fibrin. *Thromb Haemost* 1995;74:673–679.

94. Prins MH, Hirsh J. A critical review of the evidence supporting a relationship between impaired fibrinolytic activity and venous thromboembolism. *Arch Intern Med* 1991;151:1721–1731.

95. Moroi M, Aoki N. Isolation and characterization of alpha2-antiplasmin inhibitor from human plasma. A novel proteinase inhibitor which inhibits activator-induced clot lysis. *J Biol Chem* 1976;251:5956–5965.

96. Collen D. Identification and some properties of a new fast-reacting plasmin inhibitor in human plasma. *Eur J Biochem* 1976;69:209–216.

97. Mullertz S, Clemmensen I. The primary inhibitor of plasmin in human plasma. *Biochem J* 1976;159:545–553.

98. Wiman B, Collen D. Purification and characterization of human antiplasmin, the fast-acting plasmin inhibitor in plasma. *Eur J Biochem* 1977;78:19–26.

99. Aoki N, Harpel PC. Inhibitors of the fibrinolytic enzyme system. *Semin Thromb Hemost* 1984;10:24–41.

100. Wiman B, Collen D. On the mechanism of the reaction between human alpha2-antiplasmin and plasmin. *J Biol Chem* 1979;254:9291–9297.

101. Christensen U, Clemmensen I. Kinetic properties of the primary inhibitor of plasmin from human plasma. *Biochem J* 1977;163:389–391.

102. Brower MS, Harpel PC. Alpha1-antitrypsin-human leukocyte elastase complexes in blood: quantification by an enzyme-linked differential antibody immunosorbent assay and comparison with alpha2-plasmin inhibitor–plasmin complexes. *Blood* 1983;61:842–849.

103. Bauer KA, Weiss LM, Sparrow D, et al. Aging-associated changes in indices of thrombin generation and protein C activation in humans. Normative aging study. *J Clin Invest* 1987;80:1527–1534.

104. Hursting MJ, Stead AG, Crout FV, et al. Effects of age, race, sex and smoking on plasma prothrombin fragment 1.2 levels in a healthy population. *Clin Chem* 1993;39:683–686.

105. Mari D, Mannucci PM, Coppola R, et al. Hypercoagulability in centenarians: the paradox of successful aging. *Blood* 1995;85:3144–3149.

106. Bartsch P, Haeberli A, Straub PW. Blood coagulation after long distance running: antithrombin III prevents fibrin formation. *Thromb Haemost* 1990;63:430–434.

107. Miller GJ, Bauer KA, Cooper JA, et al. Activation of the coagulant pathway in cigarette smokers. *Thromb Haemost* 1998;79:549–553.

108. Caine YG, Bauer KA, Barzegar S, et al. Coagulation activation following estrogen administration to postmenopausal women. *Thromb Haemost* 1992;68:392–395.

109. Kroon U-B, Silfverstolpe G, Tengborn L. The effects of transdermal estradiol and oral conjugated estrogens on haemostasis variables. *Thromb Haemost* 1994;71:420–423.

110. Scarabin PY, Alhenc-Gelas M, Plu-Bureau G, et al. Effects of oral and transdermal estrogen/progesterone regimens on blood coagulation and fibrinolysis in post-menopausal women. A randomized controlled trial. *Arterioscler Thromb Vasc Biol* 1997;17:3071–3078.

111. Wilkes HC, Meade TW, Barzegar S, et al. Gemfibrozil reduces plasma prothrombin fragment F1+2 concentration, a marker of coagulability, in patients with coronary heart disease. *Thromb Haemost* 1992;67:503–506.

112. Miller GJ, Martin JC, Mitropoulos KA, et al. Activation of factor VII during alimentary lipemia occurs in healthy adults and patients with congenital factor XII or factor XI deficiency, but not in patients with factor IX deficiency. *Blood* 1996;87:4187–4196.

113. Kapur R, Hoffman CJ, Bhushan V, et al. Postprandial elevation of elevated factor VII in young adults. *Arterioscler Thromb Vasc Biol* 1996;16:1327–1332.

114. Silveira A, Karpe F, Johnsson H, et al. *In vivo* demonstration in humans that large postprandial triglyceride-rich lipoproteins activate coagulation factor VII through the intrinsic coagulation pathway. *Arterioscler Thromb Vasc Biol* 1996;16:1333–1339.

115. Weinstein MJ, Chute LE, Schmitt GW, et al. Abnormal factor VIII coagulant antigen in patients with renal dysfunction and in those with disseminated intravascular coagulation. *J Clin Invest* 1985;76:1406–1411.

116. Bauer KA, Rosenberg RD. Thrombin generation in acute promyelocytic leukemia. *Blood* 1984;64:791–796.

117. Hoek JA, Sturk A, ten Cate JW, et al. Laboratory and clinical evaluation of an assay of thrombin–antithrombin III complexes in plasma. *Clin Chem* 1988;34:2058–2062.

118. Asakura H, Saito M, Ito K, et al. Levels of thrombin–antithrombin III complex in plasma in cases of acute promyelocytic leukemia. *Thromb Res* 1988;50:895–899.

119. Boisclair MD, Lane DA, Wilde JT, et al. A comparative evaluation of assays for markers of activated coagulation and/or fibrinolysis: thrombin-antithrombin complex, D-dimer and fibrinogen/fibrin fragment E antigen. *Br J Haematol* 1990;74:471–479.

120. Neame PB, Kelton JG, Walker IR, et al. Thrombocytopenia in septicemia: the role of disseminated intravascular coagulation. *Blood* 1980;56:88–92.

121. Owen J, Kvam D, Nossel HL, et al. Thrombin and plasmin activity and platelet activation in the development of venous thrombosis. *Blood* 1983;61:476–482.

122. Mellbring G, Dahlgren S, Reiz S, et al. Fibrinolytic activity in plasma and deep vein thrombosis after major abdominal surgery. *Thromb Res* 1983;32:575–584.

123. Mellbring G, Dahlgren S, Wiman B. Prediction of deep vein thrombosis after extensive abdominal operations by the quotient between plasmin–alpha2-antiplasmin complex and fibrinogen concentration in plasma. *Surg Gynecol Obstet* 1985;161:339–342.

124. Boneu B, Bes G, Pelzer H, et al. D-dimers, thrombin antithrombin III complexes and prothrombin fragments 1+2: diagnostic value in clinically suspected deep vein thrombosis. *Thromb Haemost* 1991;65:28–31.

125. Estivals M, Pelzer H, Sie P, et al. Prothrombin fragment 1+2, thrombin-antithrombin III complexes and D-dimers in acute deep vein thrombosis: effects of heparin treatment. *Br J Haematol* 1991;78:421–424.

126. Yudelman IM, Nossel HL, Kaplan KL, et al. Plasma fibrinopeptide A levels in symptomatic venous thromboembolism. *Blood* 1978;51:1189–1195.

127. Yudelman I, Greenberg J. Factors affecting fibrinopeptide-A levels in patients with venous thromboembolism during anticoagulant therapy. *Blood* 1982;59:787–792.

128. Bauer KA, Rosenberg RD. Assays for thrombin generation in humans with prethrombotic states. *Thromb Haemost* 1983;50:159.

129. Hardin JA, Cronlund M, Haber E, et al. Activation of blood clotting in patients with systemic lupus erythematosus. Relationship to disease activity. *Am J Med* 1978;65:430–436.

130. Bauer KA, ten Cate H, Barzegar S, et al. Tumor necrosis factor infusions have a procoagulant effect on the hemostatic mechanism of humans. *Blood* 1989;741:165–172.

131. Peuscher FW, Cleton FJ, Armstrong L, et al. Significance of plasma fibrinopeptide A (FpA) in patients with malignancy. *J Lab Clin Med* 1980;96:5–14.

132. Goldenberg N, Kahn SR, Solymoss S. Markers of coagulation activation and angiogenesis in cancer-associated venous thromboembolism. *J Clin Oncol* 2003;21:4194–4199.

133. Myers TJ, Rickles FR, Barb C, et al. Fibrinopeptide A in acute leukemia: relationship of activation of blood coagulation to disease activity. *Blood* 1981; 57:518–525.

134. Gugliotta L, Vigano S, D'Angelo A, et al. High fibrinopeptide A (FPA) levels in acute non-lymphocytic leukemia are reduced by heparin administration. *Thromb Haemost* 1984;52:301–304.

135. Leichtman D, Brewer G. Elevated plasma levels of fibrinopeptide A during sickle cell anemia pain crisis—evidence for intravascular coagulation. *Am J Hematol* 1978;5:183–190.

136. Green D, Scott JP. Is sickle cell crisis a thrombotic event? *Am J Hematol* 1986;23:317–321.

137. Devine DV, Kinney TR, Thomas PF, et al. Fragment D-dimer levels: an objective marker of vaso-occlusive crisis and other complications of sickle cell disease. *Blood* 1986;68:317–319.

138. Tomer A, Harker LA, Kasey S, et al. Thrombogenesis in sickle cell disease. *J Lab Clin Med* 2001;137:398–407.

139. Mannucci PM, Bauer KA, Gringeri A, et al. Thrombin generation is not increased in the blood of hemophilia B patients after the infusion of a purified factor IX concentrate. *Blood* 1990;76:2540–2545.

140. Mannucci PM, Bauer KA, Gringeri A, et al. No activation of the common pathway of the coagulation cascade after a highly purified factor IX concentrate. *Br J Haematol* 1991;79:606–611.

141. Philippou H, Adami A, Lane DA, et al. High purity factor IX and prothrombin complex concentrate (PCC): pharmacokinetics and evidence that factor IXa is the thrombogenic trigger in PCC. *Thromb Haemost* 1996;76:23–28.

142. Nevard CHF, Jurd KM, Lane DA, et al. Activation of coagulation and fibrinolysis in childhood diarrhoea-associated haemolytic uraemic syndrome. *Thromb Haemost* 1997;78:1450–1453.

143. Hoek JA, Nurmohamed MT, ten Cate JW, et al. Thrombin–antithrombin III complexes in the prediction of deep vein thrombosis following total hip replacement. *Thromb Haemost* 1989;62:1050–1052.

144. The DVTENOX Study Group. Markers of hemostatic activation in acute deep venous thrombosis. Evolution during the first days of treatment. *Thromb Haemost* 1993;70:909–914.

145. Bouman CS, Ypma ST, Sybesma JP. Comparison of the efficacy of D-dimer, fibrin degradation products and prothrombin fragment 1+2 in clinically suspected deep venous thrombosis. *Thromb Res* 1995;77:225–234.

146. Demers C, Ginsberg JS, Johnston M, et al. D-dimer and thrombin–antithrombin III complexes in patients with clinically suspected pulmonary embolism. *Thromb Haemost* 1992;67:408–412.

147. Hansson PO, Eriksson H, Eriksson E, et al. Can laboratory testing improve screening strategies for deep venous thrombosis at an emergency unit? *J Intern Med* 1994;235:143–151.

148. Speiser W, Mallek R, Koppensteiner R, et al. D-dimer and TAT measurement in patients with deep venous thrombosis: utility in diagnosis and judgment of anticoagulant treatment. *Thromb Haemost* 1990;64:196–201.

149. Tengborn L, Palmblad S, Wojciechowski J, et al. D-dimer and thrombin/antithrombin III complex—diagnostic tools in deep venous thrombosis? *Haemostasis* 1994;24:344–350.

150. Gogstad GO, Dale S, Brosstad F, et al. Assay of D-dimer based on immunofiltration and staining with gold colloids. *Clin Chem* 1993;39: 2070–2076.

151. Vissac A, Grimaux M, Chartier S, et al. A new sensitive membrane based ELISA technique for instantaneous D-dimer evaluation in emergency. *Thromb Res* 1995;78:341–352.

152. Pittet JL, De Moerloose P, Reber G, et al. VIDAS D-dimer: fast quantitative ELISA for measuring D-dimer in plasma. *Clin Chem* 1996;42:410–415.

153. Brenner B, Pery M, Lanir N, et al. Application of a bedside whole blood D-dimer assay in the diagnosis of deep venous thrombosis. *Blood Coagul Fibrinolysis* 1995;6:219–222.

154. Ginsberg JS, Wells PS, Brill-Edwards P, et al. Application of a novel and rapid whole blood assay for D-dimer in patients with clinically suspected pulmonary embolism. *Thromb Haemost* 1995;73:35–38.

155. Wells PS, Brill-Edwards P, Stevens P, et al. A novel and rapid whole-blood assay for D-dimer in patients with clinically suspected deep vein thrombosis. *Circulation* 1995;91:2184–2187.

156. Turkstra F, van Beek EJR, ten Cate JW, et al. Reliable rapid blood test for the exclusion of venous thromboembolism in symptomatic outpatients. *Thromb Haemost* 1996;76:9–11.

157. Mayer W, Hirschwehr R, Hippman G, et al. Whole blood immunoassay (SimpliRED) versus plasma immunoassay (NycoCard) for the diagnosis of clinically suspected deep vein thrombosis. *Vasa* 1997;26:97–101.

158. Ginsberg JS, Kearon C, Douketis J, et al. The use of D-dimer testing and impedance plethysmographic examination in patients with clinical indications of deep vein thrombosis. *Arch Intern Med* 1997;157:1077–1081.

159. Bernardi E, Prandoni P, Lensing AW, et al. D-dimer testing as an adjunct to ultrasonography in patients with clinically suspected deep vein thrombosis: prospective cohort study. The Multicentre Italian D-dimer Ultrasound Study Investigators Group. *Br Med J* 1998;317:1037–1040.

160. Wells PS, Anderson DR, Rodger M, et al. Evaluation of D-dimer in the diagnosis of suspected deep-vein thrombosis. *N Eng J Med* 2003;349: 1227– 1235.

161. Tick LW, Ton E, van Voorthuizen T, et al. Practical diagnostic management of patients with clinically suspected deep vein thrombosis by clinical probability test, compression ultrasonography, and d-dimer test. *Am J Med* 2002;113:630–635.

162. Ginsberg JS, Siragusa S, Douketis J, et al. Evaluation of a soluble fibrin assay in patients with suspected pulmonary embolism. *Thromb Haemost* 1996;75: 551–554.

163. Ginsberg JS, Siragusa S, Douketis J, et al. Evaluation of a soluble fibrin assay in patients with suspected deep vein thrombosis. *Thromb Haemost* 1995;74:833–836.

164. Charles LA, Edwards T, Macik BG. Evaluation of sensitivity and specificity of six D-dimer latex assays. *Arch Pathol Lab Med* 1994;118:1102–1105.

165. Bounameaux H, Schneider PA, Slosman D, et al. Plasma D-dimer in suspected pulmonary embolism: a comparison with pulmonary angiography and perfusion-ventilation scintigraphy. *Blood Coagul Fibrinolysis* 1990;1: 577–579.

166. Goldhaber SZ, Simons GR, Elliott CG, et al. Quantitative plasma D-dimer levels among patients undergoing pulmonary angiography for suspected pulmonary embolism. *JAMA* 1993;270:2819–2822.

167. Perrier A, Bounameaux H, Morabia A, et al. Diagnosis of pulmonary embolism by a decision analysis-based strategy including clinical probability, D-dimer levels, and ultrasonography: a management study. *Arch Intern Med* 1996;156:531–536.

168. Perrier A, Desmarais S, Miron MJ, et al. Non-invasive diagnosis of venous thromboembolism in outpatients. *Lancet* 1999;353:190–195.

169. Rowbotham BJ, Carroll P, Whitaker AN, et al. Measurement of crosslinked fibrin derivatives: use in the diagnosis of venous thrombosis. *Thromb Haemost* 1987;57:59–61.

170. Ginsberg JS, Brill-Edwards PA, Demers C, et al. D-dimer in patients with clinically suspected pulmonary embolism. *Chest* 1993;104:1679–1684.

171. van Deventer SJH, Buller HR, ten Cate JW, et al. Experimental endotoxemia in humans: analysis of cytokine release and coagulation, fibrinolytic, and complement pathways. *Blood* 1990;76:2520–2526.

172. Suffredini AF, Harpel PC, Parrillo JE. Promotion and subsequent inhibition of plasminogen activation after administration of intravenous endotoxin to normal subjects. *N Engl J Med* 1989;320:1165–1172.

173. Michie HR, Manogue KR, Spriggs DR, et al. Detection of circulating tumor necrosis factor after endotoxin administration. *N Engl J Med* 1988; 318:1481–1486.

174. ten Cate JW, van der Poll T, Levi M, et al. Cytokines: triggers of clinical thrombotic disease. *Thromb Haemost* 1997;78:415–419.

175. van der Poll T, Buller HR, ten Cate H, et al. Coagulation activation following tumor necrosis factor administration to normal subjects. *N Engl J Med* 1990;322:1622–1627.

176. Levi M, ten Cate H, Bauer KA, van der Poll T, Edgington TS, Büller HR, et al. Inhibition of endotoxin-induced activation of coagulation and fibrinolysis in chimpanzees by pentoxyfylline or by a nonclonal anti-tissue factor antibody in chimpanzees. *J Clin Invest* 1994;93:114–120.

177. Bauer K, Mannucci P, Gringeri A, et al. Factor IXa–factor VIIIa–cell surface complex does not contribute to the basal activation of the coagulation mechanism *in vivo*. *Blood* 1992;798:2039–2047.

178. Eichinger S, Mannucci PM, Tradati F, et al. Determinants of plasma factor VIIa levels in humans. *Blood* 1995;86:3021–3025.

179. ten Cate H, Bauer KA, Levi M, et al. The activation of factor X and prothrombin by recombinant factor VIIa *in vivo* is mediated by tissue factor. *J Clin Invest* 1993;92:1207–1212.

180. Ruf W, Edgington TS. An anti-tissue factor monoclonal antibody which inhibits TF-VIIa complex is a potent anticoagulant in plasma. *Thromb Haemost* 1991;66:529–533.

181. Bauer KA, Broekmans AW, Bertina RM, et al. Hemostatic enzyme generation in the blood of patients with hereditary protein C deficiency. *Blood* 1988;71:1418–1426.

182. Mannucci PM, Tripodi A, Bottasso B, et al. Markers of procoagulant imbalance in patients with inherited thrombophilic syndromes. *Thromb Haemost* 1992;67:200–202.

183. Martinelli I, Bottasso B, Duca F, et al. Heightened thrombin generation in individuals with resistance to activated protein C. *Thromb Haemost* 1996;755: 703–705.

184. Zöller B, Holm J, Svensson P, et al. Elevated levels of prothrombin activation fragment 1+2 in plasma from patients with heterozygous Arg[506] to Gln mutation in the factor V gene (APC-resistance) and/or inherited protein S deficiency. *Thromb Haemost* 1996;752:270–274.

185. Conard J, Bauer KA, Gruber A, et al. Normalization of markers of coagulation activation with a purified protein C concentrate in adults with homozygous protein C deficiency. *Blood* 1993;824:1159–1164.

186. Bauer KA, Humphries S, Smillie B, et al. Prothrombin activation is increased among asymptomatic carriers of the prothrombin G20210A and factor V Arg506Gln mutations. *Thromb Haemost* 2000;84:396–400.

187. Bauer KA, Barzegar S, Rosenberg RD. Influence of anticoagulants used for blood collection on plasma prothrombin fragment $F_{1+2}$ measurements. *Thromb Res* 1991;63:617–628.

188. Boisclair MD, Philippou H, Lane DA. Thrombogenic mechanisms in the human: fresh insights obtained by immunodiagnostic studies of coagulation markers. *Blood Coagul Fibrinolysis* 1993;4:1007–1021.

189. Demers C, Ginsberg JS, Hirsh J, et al. Thrombosis in antithrombin-III-deficient persons. Report of a large kindred and literature review. *Ann Intern Med* 1992;1169:754–761.

190. Ginsberg JS, Demers C, Brill-Edwards P, et al. Increased thrombin generation and activity in patients with systemic lupus erythematosus and

anticardiolipin antibodies: evidence for a prothrombotic state. *Blood* 1993;8111: 2958–2963.

191. Tripodi A, Mannucci PM, Chantarangkul V, et al. Markers of procoagulant imbalance in patients with localized melanomas and autoimmune disorders. *Br J Haematol* 1993;84:670–674.

192. van Hulsteijn H, Kolff J, Briet E, et al. Fibrinopeptide A and beta thromboglobulin in patients with angina pectoris and acute myocardial infarction. *Am Heart J* 1984;107:39–45.

193. Theroux P, Latour JG, Leger-Gautier C, et al. Fibrinopeptide A plasma levels and platelet factor 4 levels in unstable angina pectoris. *Circulation* 1987;75: 156–162.

194. Wilensky RL, Bourdillon PD, Vix VA, et al. Intracoronary artery thrombus formation in unstable angina: a clinical, biochemical and angiographic correlation. *J Am Coll Cardiol* 1993;21:692–699.

195. Ardissino D, Gamba MG, Merlini PA, et al. Fibrinopeptide A excretion in urine: a marker of cumulative thrombin activity in stable versus unstable angina patients. *Am J Cardiol* 1991;68:58B–63B.

196. Fuster V, Badimon L, Badimon JJ, et al. The pathogenesis of coronary artery disease and the acute coronary syndromes. *N Eng J Med* 1992;326: 242–250, 310–318.

197. Merlini PA, Bauer KA, Oltrona L, et al. Persistent activation of the coagulation mechanism in unstable angina and myocardial infarction. *Circulation* 1994;90:61–68.

198. Mizuno K, Satomura K, Miyamoto A, et al. Angioscopic evaluation of coronary artery thrombi in acute coronary syndromes. *N Eng J Med* 1992;326: 287–291.

199. Ardissino D, Merlini PA, Gamba G, et al. Thrombin activity and early outcome in unstable angina patients. *Circulation* 1996;93:1634–1639.

200. Granger CB, Becker R, Tracy RP, et al. Thrombin generation, inhibition, and clinical outcomes in patients with acute myocardial infarction treated with thrombolytic therapy and heparin: results from the GUSTO-1 trial. GUSTO-1 Hemostasis Substudy Group. Global Utilization of Streptokinase a TPA for Occluded Coronary Arteries. *J Am Coll Cardiol* 1998;31:497–505.

201. Marmur JD, Merlini PA, Sharma SK, et al. Thrombin generation in human coronary arteries after percutaneous transluminal balloon angioplasty. *J Am Coll Cardiol* 1994;24:1484–1491.

202. Ardissino D, Merlini PA, Ariens R, et al. Tissue factor antigen and activity of human coronary atherosclerotic plaques. *Lancet* 1997;349:769–771.

203. Oltrona L, Eisenberg PR, Lasala JM, et al. Association of heparin-resistant thrombin activity with acute ischemic complications of coronary interventions. *Circulation* 1996;94:2064–2071.

204. Stoddard MF, Dawkins PR, Prince CR, et al. Left atrial appendage thrombus is not uncommon in patients with acute atrial fibrillation and a recent embolic event: a transesophageal echocardiographic study. *J Am Coll Cardiol* 1995;25:452–459.

205. Oltrona L, Broccolino M, Merlini PA, et al. Activation of the hemostatic mechanism following pharmacological cardioversion of acute nonvalvular atrial fibrillation. *Circulation* 1996;95:2003–2006.

206. Mombelli G, Im Hof V, Haeberli A, et al. Effect of heparin on plasma fibrinopeptide A in patients with acute myocardial infarction. *Circulation* 1984;69:684–689.

207. Gallino A, Haeberli A, Hess T, et al. Fibrin formation and platelet aggregation in patients with acute myocardial infarction: effect of intravenous and subcutaneous low-dose heparin. *Am Heart J* 1986;112:285–290.

208. Neri Serneri GG, Gensini G, Poggesi L, et al. Effect of heparin, aspirin, or alteplase in reduction of myocardial ischemia in refractory unstable angina. *Lancet* 1990;335:615–618.

209. Merlini PA, Ardissino D, Bauer KA, et al. Persistent thrombin generation during heparin therapy in acute coronary syndromes. *Arterioscler Thromb Vasc Biol* 1997;17:1325–1330.

210. Zoldhelyi P, Bichler J, Owen WG, et al. Persistent thrombin generation in humans during specific thrombin inhibition with hirudin. *Circulation* 1994; 90:2671–2678.

211. Granger CB, Miller JM, Bovill EG, et al. Rebound increase in thrombin generation and activity after cessation of intravenous heparin in patients with acute coronary syndromes. *Circulation* 1995;91:1929–1935.

212. Gold HK, Torres FW, Garabedian HD, et al. Evidence for a rebound coagulation phenomenon after cessation of a 4-hour infusion of a specific thrombin inhibitor in patients with unstable angina pectoris. *J Am Coll Cardiol* 1993;21:1039–1047.

213. Theroux P, Waters D, Lam J, et al. Reactivation of unstable angina after discontinuation of heparin. *N Eng J Med* 1992;327:141–145.

214. Eisenberg PR, Sherman LA, Jaffe AS. Paradoxic elevation of fibrinopeptide A: evidence for continued thrombosis despite intensive fibrinolysis. *J Am Coll Cardiol* 1987;10:527–529.

215. Owen J, Friedman KD, Grossman BA, et al. Thrombolytic therapy with tissue-type plasminogen activator or streptokinase induces transient thrombin activity. *Blood* 1988;72:616–620.

216. Rapold HJ, de Bono D, Arnold AE et al, The European Cooperative Group. Plasma fibrinopeptide A levels in patients with acute myocardial infarction treated with alteplase. Correlation with concomitant heparin, coronary artery patency, and recurrent ischemia. *Circulation* 1992;85:928–934.

217. Merlini PA, Bauer KA, Oltrona L, et al. Thrombin generation and activity during thrombolysis and concomitant heparin therapy in patients with acute myocardial infarction. *J Am Coll Cardiol* 1995;25:203–209.

218. Gulba DC, Barthels M, Westhoff-Bleck M, et al. Increased thrombin levels during thrombolytic therapy in acute myocardial infarction. Relevance of the success of therapy. *Circulation* 1991;83:937–944.

219. Merlini PA, Ardissino D, Bauer KA, et al. Activation of the hemostatic mechanism during thrombolysis in patients with unstable angina pectoris. *Blood* 1995;86:3327–3332.

220. Peuscher FW, van Aken WG, Flier OTN, et al. Effect of anticoagulant treatment measured by fibrinopeptide A (fpA) in patients with venous thrombo-embolism. *Thromb Res* 1980;18:33–43.

221. Teitel JM, Rosenberg RD. The protection of factor Xa from neutralization by the heparin–antithrombin complex. *J Clin Invest* 1983;71:1383–1391.

222. Conway EM, Bauer KA, Barzegar S, et al. Suppression of hemostatic system activation by oral anticoagulants in the blood of patients with thrombotic diatheses. *J Clin Invest* 1987;80:1535–1544.

223. Elias A, Bonfils S, Daoud-Elias M, et al. Influence of long term oral anticoagulants upon prothrombin fragment 1 + 2, thrombin–antithrombin III complex and D-dimer levels in patients affected by proximal deep vein thrombosis. *Thromb Haemost* 1993;69:302–305.

224. Millenson MM, Bauer KA, Kistler JP, et al. Monitoring 'mini-intensity' anticoagulation with warfarin: Comparison of the prothrombin time using a sensitive thromboplastin with prothrombin fragment F1 + 2 levels. *Blood* 1992;79:2034–2038.

225. Harenberg J, Haas R, Zimmermann R. Plasma hypercoagulability after termination of oral anticoagulants. *Thromb Res* 1983;29:627–633.

226. Hafner G, Swars H, Erbel R, et al. Monitoring prothrombin fragment 1 + 2 during initiation of oral anticoagulant therapy after intracoronary stenting. *Ann Hematol* 1992;65:83–87.

227. Haude M, Hafner G, Jablonka A, et al. Guidance of anticoagulation after intracoronary implantation of Palmaz-Schatz stents by monitoring prothrombin and prothrombin fragment 1 + 2. *Am Heart J* 1995;130:228–238.

228. Eisenberg PR, Sherman LA, Rich M, et al. Importance of continued activation of thrombin reflected by fibrinopeptide A to the efficacy of thrombolysis. *J Am Coll Cardiol* 1986;7:1255–1262.

229. Rapold HJ, Grimaudo V, Declerck PJ, et al. Plasma levels of plasminogen activator inhibitor type 1, beta-thromboglobulin, and fibrinopeptide A before, during, and after treatment of acute myocardial infarction with alteplase. *Blood* 1991;78:1490–1495.

230. Hogg PJ, Jackson CM. Fibrin monomer protects thrombin from inactivation by heparin-antithrombin III: implications for heparin efficacy. *Proc Natl Acad Sci U S A* 1989;86:3619–3623.

231. Weitz JI, Hudoba M, Massel D, et al. Clot-bound thrombin is protected from inhibition by heparin–antithrombin III but is susceptible to inactivation by antithrombin III–independent inhibitors. *J Clin Invest* 1990;86:385–391.

232. Mirshahi M, Soria J, Soria C, et al. Evaluation of the inhibition by heparin and hirudin of coagulation activation during rt-PA–induced thrombolysis. *Blood* 1989;74:1025–1030.

233. Weitz JI, Leslie B, Hudoba M. Thrombin binds to soluble fibrin degradation products where it is protected from inhibition by heparin–antithrombin but susceptible to inactivation by antithrombin-dependent inhibitors. *Circulation* 1998;97:544–552.

234. Ewald GA, Eisenberg PR. Plasmin-mediated activation of contact system in response to pharmacological thrombolysis. *Circulation* 1995;91:28–36.

235. Lee CD, Mann KG. Activation/inactivation of human factor V by plasmin. *Blood* 1989;73:185–190.

236. Eisenberg PR, Miletich JP, Sobel BE, et al. Differential effects of activation of prothrombin by streptokinase compared with urokinase and tissue-type plasminogen activator (t-PA). *Thromb Res* 1988;50:707–717.

237. Weitz JI, Cruickshank MK, Thong B, et al. Human tissue-type plasminogen activator releases fibrinopeptides A and B from fibrinogen. *J Clin Invest* 1988;82:1700–1707.

238. Weitz JI, Leslie B. Urokinase has direct catalytic activity against fibrinogen and renders it less clottable by thrombin. *J Clin Invest* 1990;86:203–212.

239. Agnelli G, Buchanan MR, Fernandez F, et al. Sustained thrombolysis with DNA-recombinant tissue-type plasminogen activator in rabbits. *Blood* 1985;66:399–401.

240. Agnelli G, Buchanan MR, Fernandez F, et al. The thrombolytic and hemorrhagic effects of tissue-type plasminogen activator: influence of dosage regimens in rabbits. *Thromb Res* 1985;40:769–777.

241. Owen J, Friedman KD, Grossman BA, et al. Quantitation of fragment X formation during thrombolytic therapy with streptokinase or tissue plasminogen activator. *J Clin Invest* 1987;79:1642–1647.

242. Weitz JI, Leslie B, Ginsberg J. Soluble fibrin degradation products potentiate tissue plasminogen activator-induced fibrinogen proteolysis. *J Clin Invest* 1991; 87:1082–1090.

243. Weitz JI, Leslie B, Hirsh J, et al. Alpha 2-antiplasmin supplementation inhibits tissue plasminogen activator-induced fibrinogenolysis and bleeding with little effect on fibrinolysis. *J Clin Invest* 1993;91:1343–1350.

244. Nieuwenhuizen W, Vermond A, Voskuilen M, et al. Identification of a site in fibrin(ogen) which is involved in the acceleration of plasminogen activation by tissue-type plasminogen activator. *Biochim Biophys Acta* 1983; 748:86–92.

245. Verheijen J, Nieuwenhuizen W, Traas DW, et al. Differences in effects of fibrin(ogen) fragments on the activation of 1-glu-plasminogen and 442-val-plasminogen by tissue-type plasminogen activator. *Thromb Res* 1983; 32:87–92.

246. Verheijen JH, Nieuwenhuizen W, Wijngaards G. Activation of plasminogen by tissue activator is increased specifically in the presence of certain soluble fibrin(ogen) fragments. *Thromb Res* 1982;27:377–385.

247. Nieuwenhuizen W, Verheijen JH, Vermond A, et al. Plasminogen activation by tissue activator is accelerated in the presence of fibrin(ogen) cyanogen bromide fragments FCB-2. *Biochim Biophys Acta* 1983;755:531–533.

248. Voskuilen M, Vermond A, Veeneman GH, et al. Fibrinogen lysine residue Aa157 plays a crucial role in the fibrin-induced acceleration of plasminogen activation catalyzed by tissue-type plasminogen activator. *J Biol Chem* 1987;262:5944–5946.

249. Stewart RJ, Fredenburgh JC, Weitz JI. Characterization of the interactions of plasminogen and tissue and vampire bat plasminogen activators with fibrinogen, fibrin, and the complex of D-dimer noncovalently linked to fragment E. *J Biol Chem* 1998;273:18292–18299.

250. Nesheim M, Fredenburgh JC, Larsen GR. The dissociation constants and stoichiometries of the interactions of Lys-plasminogen and chloromethyl ketone derivatives of tissue plasminogen activator and the variant FEIX with intact fibrin. *J Biol Chem* 1990;265:21541–21548.

251. Gardell SJ, Duong LT, Diehl RE, et al. Isolation, characterization, and cDNA cloning of a vampire bat salivary plasminogen activator. *J Biol Chem* 1989;264:17947–17952.

# CHAPTER 57 ■ MALIGNANCY AND HEMOSTASIS

HAROLD F. DVORAK AND FREDERICK R. RICKLES

The important association between malignant disease and hemostasis has been recognized for almost 150 years (1). In 1865, Trousseau observed that unexplained episodes of migratory thrombophlebitis in patients with gastrointestinal symptoms tipped the diagnostic balance in favor of malignancy (2). Unlike thrombosis from other causes, which generally affects deep veins of the lower extremities and tends to be solitary, venous thrombosis associated with cancer can be migratory, may involve superficial as well as deep veins, may affect unusual sites such as the arms and chest, and may be relatively unresponsive to standard anticoagulant therapy. As Trousseau sadly observed in his own case, venous thrombosis may also be the first indication of malignancy in an otherwise healthy individual, antedating the clinical detection of tumor by months or even years. Trousseau wrote to his student, Peter, "I am lost; the phlebitis that has just appeared tonight leaves me no doubt about the nature of my illness." Six months after the development of idiopathic deep vein thrombosis (DVT) in his left arm, Trousseau died of gastric cancer (3). Indeed, the diagnosis of idiopathic venous thromboembolism (VTE), including both DVT and pulmonary embolism, even in the absence of the migratory component, carries with it a significantly increased risk of occult malignancy, often manifest within months of the initial thrombotic episode (4). This classic observation of Trousseau has been validated in several retrospective, population-based studies and in well-designed prospective studies (5). It is now agreed that the clotting system is activated systemically in most of the patients with cancer and that such activation contributes importantly to morbidity and mortality. Thromboembolism may be the earliest manifestation of cancer and is one of its most frequent complications. However, thromboembolism is not the only form of abnormal hemostasis found in patients with cancer. Also of importance is the bleeding diathesis that results from consumption of platelets and clotting factors as occurs in disseminated intravascular coagulation (DIC). Finally, a new relation has been found between clotting and cancer in recent years: Cross-linked fibrin (XLF) and fibrinogen-related proteins (FRP) are deposited extravascularly within tumor stroma and there exert important roles in the pathogenesis of tumor growth and spread.

This chapter reviews the current understanding of the mechanisms by which clotting is initiated in cancer and the significance of abnormal hemostasis for tumor angiogenesis, stroma generation, and metastasis. More clinical aspects concerning the prevention and treatment of thromboembolism in cancer, as well as strategies for the use of anticoagulation as an approach to cancer therapy, are discussed elsewhere in this textbook (see Chapter 85).

## EPIDEMIOLOGY

### Systemic Abnormalities of Hemostasis in Cancer

Many types of hemostatic disorders occur with increased frequency in patients with cancer (6). In general, the distribution of specific cancers associated with such disorders follows the frequency of cancer in the general population. However, it is increasingly recognized that cancer is not a single disease but rather a group of related diseases that manifest themselves in many different ways depending on the organ and cell of origin. More than 300 different types of cancer have been identified, each with its own distinct properties, and it therefore should not be surprising that some cancers cause greater aberrations in hemostasis than others. Patients at greatest risk for VTE include those with mucin-secreting tumors (e.g., adenocarcinomas arising in the pancreas and gastrointestinal tract); cancers of the lung, kidney, brain, prostate, and ovary; acute promyelocytic leukemia; myeloproliferative disorders; and lymphomas (2,6,7). Malignancies with the lowest incidence of thrombosis include cancers of the head and neck, bladder, breast, esophagus, uterus, and cervix (8).

The most common hemostatic disorder in patients with cancer is VTE, which may be migratory or, much more commonly, confined to deep veins. DVT is of course a common source of pulmonary emboli. VTE has been found at autopsy in as many as half of patients dying of cancer, although it is recognized clinically in a much smaller fraction, for example, as low as 0.1% of the patients with stage I breast cancer and as high as 18% in patients with stage III/IV disease treated with hormones and chemotherapy and hormones (6,9,10). The best data indicate that 10% to 20% of patients presenting with a new diagnosis of idiopathic (as opposed to secondary) VTE have previously diagnosed cancer (4,6). Overall, VTE is estimated to be the second-most common cause of death in patients with cancer, with more than half of thromboembolic deaths occurring at an otherwise favorable time in the history of cancer (11). Arterial thrombosis is relatively less common although more frequent in patients with myeloproliferative disorders (6). The newly formed blood vessels that arise in tumor angiogenesis are particularly susceptible to thrombosis (see subsequent text).

Another common manifestation of abnormal hemostasis in patients with cancer is DIC. The incidence of DIC in patients with cancer sufficiently severe to require intervention has been estimated at 9% to 15% but is much more frequent in its subclinical compensated form, detectable only by abnormal blood tests (12). Severe DIC is primarily associated with acute leukemias and results in hemorrhage caused by excessive consumption of clotting factors and platelets (12). DIC is commonly exacerbated by cancer therapy.

## Abnormal Laboratory Values in Patients with Cancer

Clinically overt thromboembolism and hemorrhage are only the tip of the iceberg of systemic clotting abnormalities in patients with cancer. Much more common are hemostatic abnormalities recognized only as the result of laboratory testing. These fall into several categories: markers of a hypercoagulable state, DIC, and abnormalities in the number and/or state of platelets (see Chapters 55 and 56).

## Hypercoagulable State and Disseminated Intravascular Coagulation

The underlying principle in patients with cancer is that the clotting system is activated systemically, clotting factors are consumed, and fibrinolysis is activated. Approximately half of all patients with cancer, and as many as 90% of those with metastases, exhibit abnormalities in one or more routine coagulation parameters (13–16) (see Table 57-1). The most common abnormalities are thrombocytosis (present in 30% to 60% of patients with cancer) and increased levels of plasma fibrinogen and fibrinopeptide A (FPA), a pattern that is consistent with what has been termed *overcompensated* DIC.

In some patients with cancer, clotting abnormalities are detected only with more sophisticated tests. Therefore, the reported incidence of hemostatic abnormalities is not only a function of the type of tumor, the extent of tumor burden,

### TABLE 57-1

#### ABNORMALITIES OF BLOOD CLOTTING TESTS IN CANCER

Shortening or prolongation of the prothrombin time and activated partial thromboplastin time with either elevation or depression of plasma fibrinogen and clotting factors V, VIII, IX, XI, and XII (2,15,17–22)
Increased fibrinogen–fibrin cleavage products, including fibrinopeptide A, D-dimer, Bβ 15–42, and fibrin monomers (2,15,17,20,23–30)
Abnormally rapid fibrinogen turnover (31–33)
Increased plasma levels of prothrombin F1 + 2 or thrombin–antithrombin complexes (27,29,34–38)
Decreased levels of circulating antithrombin (20,39–42), protein C (14,40,42,43), and free protein S (43)
Activated protein C resistance (± factor V$_{Leiden}$) (37,44)
Increased plasminogen activator inhibitor activity with impaired fibrinolysis (28,45–48)
Increased plasma prekallikrein and high-molecular-weight kininogen (49)
Increased plasma levels of markers of endothelial cell activation: von Willebrand factor, thrombomodulin, tPA, PAI-1 (26,47,50,51)
Increased plasma levels of tissue factor, VIIa, or tissue factor pathway inhibitor (52,53)
Elevated plasma β-thromboglobulin levels (54)

tPA, tissue-type plasminogen activator; PAI-1, plasminogen activator inhibitor.

and treatment; it may also be highly dependent on the sensitivity and specificity of the laboratory tests used. Among the newer tests are sensitive assays of the delicate balance between procoagulant and anticoagulant pathways, including circulating prothrombin activation fragment (F1+2), thrombin–antithrombin complexes, FPA, protein C and its activation peptide, tissue factor pathway inhibitor (TFPI), and β-thromboglobulin (2,15,17,18,23–29,34–37,52,53). FPA, with a normal circulation time in plasma of less than 4 minutes, is not unexpectedly a sensitive prognostic indicator of changing clinical status. Several studies have revealed elevated levels of plasma FPA in virtually all patients with acute leukemia or with extensive solid tumor burden (15,31,34,55) and in a smaller fraction of patients with more limited disease (56). Many other clotting abnormalities have been reported in patients with cancer, as summarized in Table 57-1 and described in greater detail elsewhere (12,16,19,57).

These seemingly variable and even contradictory laboratory findings are to be anticipated in a disease in which excessive, but generally low-grade, coagulation, fibrinolysis, and compensatory homeostatic mechanisms are proceeding at different and changing rates. Individual patients with cancer may lie at any point along a spectrum that extends from a "prethrombotic" or "hypercoagulable" state to DIC of varying degrees of severity and compensation. Patients with cancer exhibit widely varying levels of DIC, from milder, more chronic forms without bleeding sequelae to severe forms with catastrophic bleeding. However, prospective studies indicate that overt DIC is unusual, even during treatment (15). Nonetheless, hypercoagulability increases as patients are followed up prospectively over time, consistent with a semiquantitative relation between tumor burden and activation of clotting (55,56,58).

None of the clotting tests currently available is specific for cancer. For instance, plasma fibrinogen may be elevated as part of an acute-phase response, and thrombocytosis may occur as the result of hemorrhage or iron deficiency. However, abnormal clotting values may offer a sensitive measure of tumor burden. Serial determinations indicating a trend are generally far more useful than a single measurement in evaluating tumor remission or progression. For example, FPA levels typically fall after successful treatment, only to rise again before clinical evidence of tumor relapse. There is disagreement in the literature as to whether hemostatic abnormalities, which often appear early in the course of the disease, have predictive value for the later development of thrombotic or hemorrhagic complications (14,28,29). Similar conflicting results have been generated in studies attempting to determine if patients with cancer who develop thrombosis have an underlying predisposition because of hereditary defects of one or more of the anticoagulation pathway proteins [see (59) for review].

## Thrombocytopenia and Thrombocytopathy

*Quantitative* platelet abnormalities occur frequently in patients with cancer, especially in those with solid tumors such as carcinomas of the lung and liver, both Hodgkin and non-Hodgkin lymphomas, and chronic myelocytic leukemia (16,20,45). As already mentioned, modestly increased platelet counts are a common finding, but thrombocytopenia occurs in a smaller fraction of patients with cancer (estimated 4% to 11%) and is a principal cause of bleeding (60). Thrombocytopenia may reflect impaired generation, increased use, or accelerated destruction of platelets or their sequestration within an enlarged spleen (45). Impaired generation follows replacement of bone marrow by tumor cells, sepsis, vitamin B$_{12}$ or folate deficiency, or ineffective thrombopoiesis, and may result from the elaboration by tumor cells of mediators that inhibit platelet production (16,20,45,61). DIC is the most common cause of increased platelet consumption, and platelet counts, whether elevated or depressed, reflect the overall degree to which DIC is compensated. As the result of activation, circulating platelets often exhibit increased expression of markers such as P selectin, CD63, and von Willebrand factor (50).

A symptom complex resembling idiopathic thrombocytopenic purpura with accelerated, apparently immune destruction of platelets has been reported repeatedly in patients with a variety of tumors, including Hodgkin disease, acute and chronic lymphocytic leukemia, and carcinomas of many types; in these patients, thrombocytopenia may precede clinical evidence of neoplasia (16,45,62–64). Thrombocytopenia may also occur as the result of thrombotic microangiopathy, especially in patients with gastric and less commonly other types of adenocarcinoma (16,65,66).

The platelets of patients with cancer may also exhibit *qualitative* abnormalities, including reduced adhesion; impaired, increased, or spontaneous aggregation; and poor clot retraction (67). Qualitative platelet abnormalities are particularly common in dysproteinemias, in which clinical hemorrhage is more commonly attributable to tumor-secreted paraproteins that coat platelets and interfere with their function than to either thrombocytopenia or clotting factor deficiencies (20). As many as 15% of patients with immunoglobulin G (IgG) myeloma, more than 38% of patients with IgA myeloma, and more than 60% of patients with Waldenström macroglobulinemia exhibit such abnormalities. Several studies have indicated that platelets from patients with cancer show enhanced adenosine diphosphate (ADP)–induced platelet aggregation and reduced sensitivity to prostacyclin [reviewed in (50)]. Other authors have measured an acquired storage-pool defect and other selective biochemical defects in the platelets of patients with cancer (68,69).

# MECHANISMS RESPONSIBLE FOR SYSTEMIC ACTIVATION OF CLOTTING IN CANCER

The pathogenesis of the hypercoagulability that is observed in patients with cancer is incompletely understood but is often multifactorial and may result from one or more defects in the normal host defense against thrombosis. Clotting defects have been usefully classified under the rubric known as the *Virchow triad* (70). This triad can be restated and summarized as follows: (i) Defects in blood flow resulting in *stasis*; (ii) defects in the normal balance between procoagulant and anticoagulant proteins in the blood with resultant *activation of clotting proteins*; and (iii) defects (alterations) in the blood vessel lining that result in a shift from an anticoagulant to a *procoagulant endothelium*. All three of these defects may occur in patients with cancer and together form a helpful framework for understanding the hypercoagulability observed in such patients (57,71).

Systemic activation of clotting may result from both *tumor-related* and *tumor-unrelated* mechanisms (discussed in the subsequent text) as well as from *therapy* (see Chapter 85). Examples of tumor-unrelated factors that render patients with cancer susceptible to clotting include age greater than 40 (the incidence of many cancers increases exponentially with age), immobility caused by ill health or hospitalization, comorbidities (e.g., obesity), and acute-phase response from complications such as infection (with resulting increased levels of plasma fibrinogen and other clotting factors). Tumors themselves activate clotting by two mechanisms, *indirectly* by secreting cytokines that activate host cells and *directly* by expressing procoagulant activities.

## Tumor Cell Interactions with Host Endothelial Cells, Platelets, and Leukocytes

Tumor cells commonly activate host endothelial cells, platelets, and leukocytes that are present within the vasculature or within tumor stroma by direct contact or by secreting cytokines and other factors.

### Tumor–Platelet Interactions

The elevated platelet counts commonly found in patients with cancer likely result from tumor-secreted factors such as interleukin (IL)-6, IL-11, stem cell factor, and thrombopoietin (72–75). Tumor cells can also activate blood platelets and induce their aggregation directly by adhesion, by releasing soluble factors such as ADP or a cathepsinlike cysteine protease, or, most important, by activating clotting and generating thrombin (76,77). Activated platelets serve as a surface template for prothrombinase generation, a late step in the clotting cascade. They also adhere to other vascular elements (endothelial cells, leukocytes), favoring local thrombosis, and to blood-borne tumor cells, thereby facilitating metastasis (see subsequent text) (78,79).

### Tumor–Endothelial Cell Interactions

The quiescent endothelial cells lining normal blood vessels exert an important anticoagulant function. However, in patients with cancer, the vascular endothelium is often activated and rendered procoagulant (80–83). This is evidenced by elevated plasma levels of such endothelial cell-specific markers as von Willebrand factor, E selectin, tissue-type plasminogen activator (tPA), and plasminogen activator inhibitor (PAI-1) (80,84). This activation is thought to be mediated by tumor cell–secreted products, particularly tumor necrosis factor (TNF-$\alpha$) and interleukin-$\beta$ (IL-1-$\beta$), which induce endothelial cells to express tissue factor (TF) and PAI-1 while downregulating the expression of thrombomodulin (TM), the high-affinity endothelial cell surface receptor for thrombin that leads to activation of the anticoagulant protein C system (50,80). In addition, tumor cell–secreted vascular endothelial growth factor-A (VEGF-A) induces endothelial cell TF expression (85–87). These findings can be replicated experimentally. IL-1 given to rabbits causes endothelium to develop thrombogenic properties, for example, a 10-fold increase in TF generation and a 72% decrease in thrombin-mediated protein C activation (88).

### Tumor–Leukocyte Interactions

Tumor-secreted cytokines attract and activate monocytes and macrophages, variable numbers of which are regular components of tumor stroma. TNF-$\alpha$ and IL-1-$\beta$ upregulate TF in tumor-associated macrophages, just as they do in endothelial cells (85,89–91). Indeed, TF antigen and procoagulant activity (PCA) are expressed by macrophages in tumor stroma, and TF expression correlates with deposition of XLF (58,92–94). Peripheral blood monocytes isolated from patients with cancer also express TF (95). In addition, VEGF-A and other members of the vascular permeability factor/vascular endothelial growth factor (VPF/VEGF) family of tumor-secreted cytokines are chemotactic for monocytes and macrophages and induce these cells to express TF; TF, in turn, may increase macrophage VEGF-A transcription just as in endothelial cells.

Neutrophils may also be present in the stroma of solid tumors and can promote tumor growth and metastasis (50,96,97). Tumor cell–derived factors can activate neutrophils by upregulating the expression of adhesion molecules

(CD11b/CD18), promoting binding to tumor cells, and facilitating tumor cell migration through endothelium (98). Neutrophils may also release reactive oxygen species and proteases that may activate both endothelial cells and platelets (99).

## Tumor Cell Procoagulants

Tumor cells, like many normal cells, express procoagulant activities and, because tumors commonly exhibit zones of necrosis even in the absence of therapy, local activation of clotting would not be unexpected. Of greater importance, however, are procoagulant activities expressed by viable tumor cells. These have been described in an extensive literature dating back to the 1950s (100–106), and their properties have been compiled in detailed registries maintained by the International Society for Thrombosis and Haemostasis (107,108). A brief, updated summary of human PCAs appears in Table 57-2. The two principal and best-characterized tumor cell procoagulants are *TF* (see Chapter 5) and *cancer procoagulant* (CP). TF is a transmembrane, nonproteolytic cofactor and cell surface receptor for clotting factor VII (and VIIa); CP is a soluble, cysteine protease that cleaves factor X directly in the absence of factor VII (or VIIa). Isolated reports of thrombinlike and factor XIII–like activities await further confirmation, although data are consistent with the presence of thrombin-activated factor XIII, or at least a tissue transglutaminase, in human tumor cells (109,110). In addition, tumor cells, like platelets, can provide a phospholipid-rich surface for prothrombinase assembly, a critical step in the clotting cascade (111).

### Tumor-Associated Tissue Factor Activity

Many types of tumor cells express TF constitutively (Table 57-2). Other tumors induce TF expression in host macrophages and endothelial cells (113,119). As a result, the TF PCA found in solid tumors can come from either or both tumor and host cells, and the relative contribution of each is difficult to ascertain in any given case. Nonetheless, abundant TF PCA is present in most malignant tumor cells and has been identified in sonicates, extracts, whole cell populations, and shed vesicles obtained from human and animal tumors and derived cell lines (104,107,108,120). Human tumors reported to express TF include carcinomas of the breast, adenocarcinomas of the colon and pancreas, large cell carcinomas of the lung, prostate cancer, transitional carcinomas of the bladder, squamous carcinomas of the head and neck, and malignant gliomas (87). Also, the PCA expressed by purified tumor cell populations is, on the basis of mass, thought to be predominantly TF (121). Moreover, increasing TF expression in tumors often correlates with the multidrug resistance phenotype, increased angiogenesis, advanced stage of disease, and poor patient survival. Guan et al. (122) recently correlated TF expression levels in human gliomas by quantitative reverse transcription-polymerase chain reaction methodology and found that TF was strongly positive in 90%, 58%, 43%, and 20% of grade IV, grade III, grade II, and grade I cases, respectively. Increased vascular density in these specimens was also directly correlated with tumor grade. Similar results have been reported in colorectal cancer (123). Studies of non–small-cell lung carcinoma also demonstrated a correlation between TF expression, microvascular density, and VEGF-A expression. In a comparison between seven malignant and 10 benign breast tumors, TF as detected by *in situ* hybridization was found in the vascular endothelial cells (VECs) and tumor cells only in the malignant tumors (86).

An interesting property of many tumor cells is that they shed vesicles composed of portions of their plasma membranes when grown in tissue culture or in ascites form (104,120); these vesicles commonly express TF activity (104,120,124). As a result, it is not surprising that PCA with the properties of

TF can be found in the cell-free fraction of plasma drawn from patients with cancer (125,126). On the other hand, platelets may also shed vesicles (microparticles) into plasma in patients with cancer (127), and these could account for some of the circulating PCA observed.

### Tumor-Associated Factor X Activators

Falanga et al. identified the factor X activator CP in extracts of the rabbit V2 carcinoma (128) and subsequently in tumor cells isolated from patients with acute leukemia (129,130) and a variety of other solid tumors, including breast and colon cancer (124) and melanoma (131) (Table 57-2). CP is a 68-kDa cysteine protease that cleaves the heavy chain of factor X independent of factor VIIa and at a site distinct from that of other factor X activators. CP may contribute to local tumor fibrin deposition (92), and CP antigen has been found in the circulation of patients with cancer (50). However, when CP and TF are identified in crude extracts of both human and experimental animal tumors, the bulk of the PCA can be attributed to TF (e.g., factor VII–dependent and phospholipase-sensitive), even in those tumors from which CP has been purified (121). Therefore, although CP can surely be isolated from tumor extracts, its pathophysiologic significance *in vivo*, including in patients with acute leukemia, remains to be defined.

### Tumor Cell–Mediated Assembly of the Prothrombinase Complex

Prothrombinase activity, occurring late in the clotting cascade, is essential for thrombin and therefore for fibrin generation. Prothrombin is activated by the formation of the prothrombinase complex, a complex of clotting factors Xa, Va, and prothrombin on an appropriate phospholipid membrane template in the presence of calcium ions. Assembly of the prothrombinase complex results in a marked increase in the rate of prothrombin activation over that produced by factor Xa alone. Platelet membrane phospholipid is generally accepted to be the template for prothrombinase complex assembly in normal intravascular hemostasis (132). However, other cells—including leukocytes, endothelial cells, and tumor cells—have been shown to be capable of binding factors Va and Xa, with subsequent assembly of the prothrombinase complex (111,118,133–137). Van DeWater et al. first described the binding of factors Va and Xa to guinea pig hepatocarcinoma cell lines with resultant cell-mediated assembly of the prothrombinase complex (111). Sakai and Kisiel demonstrated that human factor Xa can bind to receptors on human bladder cancer cells topographically close to but independent of cell surface factor Va (134). The nature of this high-affinity factor Xa receptor has not been clarified, although it is likely to prove to be *effector cell protease receptor-1* (EPR-1), which has also been described on monocytes, endothelial cells, and smooth muscle cells (118,133). The presence of EPR-1 on the surface of other human tumor cells is less certain (118,134), although Zhou et al. (138) have reported prothrombin binding to human melanoma cells, and Leach et al. (135) have characterized a unique prothrombinase activator on a hepatoma-derived cell line. In any event, tumor cells appear capable of independent binding of both factors Va and Xa and can thereby enhance the rate of local blood coagulation. We predict that other receptors for clotting proteins and additional proteases capable of cleaving clotting proteins, such as the prothrombinase activator described in a human hepatoma-derived cell line, will be found in tumor cells (135).

### Procoagulant Activities in Leukemia

If leukemic cells behaved as many solid tumor cells, massive DIC would be expected as the rule because circulating leukemic cells are continually in contact with plasma. However, although

**TABLE 57-2**

HUMAN TUMOR PROCOAGULANTS[a]

| Tumor type | Tissue factor | Procoagulant type/cancer procoagulant | Other[b] |
|---|---|---|---|
| **EPITHELIAL TUMORS** | | | |
| Lung[c] | | | |
| Squamous cell | Yes | Yes | ? |
| Adenocarcinoma | Yes | ? | Yes |
| Large cell | Yes | Yes | ? |
| Small cell | Yes[d] | ? | ? |
| Breast (adenocarcinoma) | Yes[e] | Yes | ? |
| Cervical/Vaginal (squamous) | Yes | ? | ? |
| Endometrial (adenocarcinoma) | Yes | ? | ? |
| Ovarian adenocarcinoma | Yes | ? | ? |
| Dysgerminoma | Yes | ? | ? |
| Testis embryonal cell | Yes | ? | ? |
| Seminoma | Yes | ? | ? |
| Renal adenocarcinoma | Yes[f] | Yes | ? |
| Wilms tumor | No | ? | ? |
| Neuroblastoma | ? | Yes | ? |
| Bladder (transitional) | Yes | ? | Yes |
| Prostate (adenocarcinoma) | No | ? | ? |
| Head and neck (squamous) | Yes | ? | ? |
| Thyroid (papillary) | Yes | ? | ? |
| Colon (adenocarcinoma) | Yes | Yes | ? |
| Hepatoma | Yes | Yes | Yes |
| Pancreatic (adenocarcinoma) | Yes | ? | ? |
| Gastric (adenocarcinoma) | Yes | ? | ? |
| Melanoma | Yes[g] | Yes | Yes |
| **MESENCHYMAL TUMORS** | | | |
| Sarcoma | Yes[h] | Yes[h] | ? |
| **TUMORS OF MIXED ORIGIN** | | | |
| Teratoma/Teratocarcinoma | Yes[i] | ? | ? |
| **BRAIN TUMORS** | | | |
| Glioblastoma | Yes[j] | ? | ? |
| **HEMATOPOIETIC TUMORS** | | | |
| ANLL | Yes | Yes | ? |
| ALL | Yes[k] | Yes | ? |
| Lymphoma | Yes[l] | ? | Yes[l] |

ALL, acute lymphocytic leukemia; ANLL, acute nonlymphocytic leukemia; ?, not known.
[a]Determined by measuring procoagulant activity in cell extracts or by immunohistochemical localization *in situ.*
[b]Factor Xa–like activity, Xa-binding activity, prothrombinase, and so on.
[c]Lung tumors classified according to reference (112).
[d]Small cell carcinoma of the lung positive for tissue in two studies (113,114); negative in one (92).
[e]Breast cancer positive for tissue factor in several studies (86,113,115); negative in one study (113).
[f]Renal cell cancer positive for tissue factor in one study (113); negative in one study (114).
[g]Melanoma positive for tissue factor in two studies (113,116); negative in one study (114).
[h]Only one sixth of tumors examined was positive for tissue factor (114); subtypes examined for CP included osteosarcoma, chondrosarcoma, and liposarcoma (117).
[i]It should be noted that in two studies, with the exception of a single teratoma, all benign tumors (of the limited number studied) were negative for tissue factor by immunohistochemical techniques (86,114).
[j]Glioblastoma cell lines positive for tissue factor by functional assays (108), but two tumors negative for tissue factor by immunohistochemical analysis (114).
[k]Lymphocytic leukemic cell lines express only small amounts of tissue factor in comparison to cell lines derived from patients with either monocytic leukemia or promyelocytic leukemia, which may be related to lineage infidelity of these cells in tissue culture (117,118).
[l]A few lymphoma cell lines in tissue culture express tissue factor, but immunohistochemical analysis failed to confirm tissue factor in the malignant cell in Hodgkin disease or non-Hodgkin lymphoma (94,114).
Modified and adapted from (68,74,90,94,393,395).

hemostatic abnormalities commonly accompany leukemias, fulminant DIC is only rarely observed in untreated patients (34,139). The reasons for this discrepancy between solid and liquid tumors have not been fully investigated, although data suggest that the "relative differentiation" of leukemic cells may play a role (71,140). Leukemias are derived from the precursors of normal circulating leukocytes, which for obvious reasons do not normally express PCAs on their surfaces. Although macrophages can express TF, the circulating monocytes from which they differentiate do not in the absence of specific stimulation (141). Similarly, although the *TF* gene is commonly expressed by leukemic cells, gene expression may not translate into surface expression of TF PCA (140,142).

Nonetheless, it has been known since 1954 that some human leukemia cells do express PCA (143). It was not until 1973, however, that Gralnick and Abrell identified TF-like activity in the buffy coat of patients with progranulocytic leukemia (144). Subsequently, others demonstrated that the PCA of peripheral blood cells from some patients with acute progranulocytic leukemia (APL) was neutralized by a polyclonal antibody raised against brain TF (145). Bauer et al. described TF gene expression in some, but not all, leukemic myeloblasts (142). The relatively high incidence of bleeding and thrombotic abnormalities in patients with APL in the era before the introduction of therapy with all-*trans* retinoic acid (146) has been attributed to activation of systemic blood coagulation by *TF* expressed by APL cells with resultant DIC (147). Indeed, one of the likely reasons for the efficacy of all-*trans* retinoic acid in ameliorating the coagulopathy of APL is its ability to downregulate expression of the *TF* gene in the malignant cells (71,139,140,146). Some studies, however, have suggested alternatives to tumor cell–mediated TF generation as the primary mechanism for the coagulopathy, at least in some patients with APL, for example, CP (130) or IL-1 (148). Like solid tumors, leukemia cells may also shed plasma membrane vesicles into the circulation, but at least in an initial study, these supported prothrombinase assembly but failed to express TF PCA (149).

# FIBRINOGEN-RELATED PROTEINS AND CROSS-LINKED FIBRIN AS COMPONENTS OF TUMOR STROMA

The preceding sections have been largely concerned with systemic activation of the clotting system in cancer. We now turn to the activation of clotting that commonly occurs locally in and around solid tumors. Such clotting may be of two types: Those that occur within tumor blood vessels (thrombosis) and those that occur extravascularly in tumor stroma.

## Selective Thrombosis of Tumor Blood Vessels

It has been known since the time of Billroth in the latter part of the 19th century that tumor vessels are particularly susceptible to thrombosis (150). There are a number of reasons for this. First, solid tumors form masses that may compress tumor microvessels externally, resulting in stasis of flow and thrombosis. Second, tumor cells may invade the vasculature and directly expose the plasma to tumor procoagulants. Third, the cytokines secreted by tumor cells that activate platelets, endothelial cells, and monocytes are obviously in high concentration in the microvessels immediately surrounding tumors. Last, the new vessels that tumors induce are abnormal with respect to structure and function. They are characteristically

hyperpermeable (see Fig. 57-1), leading to extravasation of plasma proteins and, consequently, increased hematocrit and blood viscosity, stasis of flow, and proclivity to thrombosis (151). In addition, as discussed in subsequent text, tumor blood vessels may have an irregular surface lining that promotes turbulent flow and therefore a tendency to thrombosis (151,152).

The potential importance of VEC TF in the generation of XLF in the tumor microenvironment was investigated by Zhang et al. and Huang et al. (153,154). Both groups developed novel strategies for targeting the tumor vasculature, taking advantage of the apparently selective expression of TF in the neoangiogenic vessels of experimental murine tumors, as has also been shown for human breast cancer (86). Zhang et al. demonstrated that even in those tumors in which the cancer cells themselves expressed little or no TF, the VECs expressed TF on induction with tumor necrosis factor, resulting in tumor vessel thrombosis (153). Tumor blood flow could be restored with somatic gene transfer of antisense TF constructs. Huang et al. treated neuroblastomas in mice by intravenous administration of a bifunctional immunoconjugate of a truncated, soluble form of TF (which retained only limited PCA) targeted with a monoclonal antibody to an expressed antigen specific for murine tumor endothelium (154). This conjugate resulted in thrombosis of tumor vessels and complete tumor regression in 38% of the treated mice (154). A similar strategy was used successfully by Hu et al., who regressed human melanoma in immunodeficient mice using an inactivated factor VIIa conjugate that targeted TF in the endothelium of the angiogenic vessels (155). These studies illustrate the possible significance of tumor VEC TF both in the pathogenesis of tumor-associated XLF formation and as a possible target of cancer therapy.

## Extravascular Accumulation of Fibrinogen-Related Proteins and Cross-Linked Fibrin

In the late 1950s, the Irish pathologist O'Meara proposed that FRP were deposited within the substance of solid tumors (156). Better evidence for intratumor FRP came later from studies demonstrating that systemically administered fibrinogen and antifibrinogen antibodies were selectively concentrated in both animal and human tumors (157–159). Several groups demonstrated FRPs in rat and human neoplasms by immunofluorescence (160,161). For a time, there was reluctance to accept these findings. Valid questions were raised as to the specificity of the antibodies used, the generality of the observations, and the possibility that the entire phenomenon was an artifact resulting from accumulation of FRPs either during postmortem or as tissues were being removed surgically. More recent work has laid these doubts to rest. Immunohistochemical, electron microscopic, and biochemical studies have shown that the FRPs deposited in several autochthonous and transplantable human and animal tumors represent XLF (i.e., fibrin similar or identical to that which forms when fibrinogen is clotted with thrombin in the presence of clotting factor XIII) (86,162–173) (see Figs. 57-1B, C, and 57-2).

Before defining the intratumor localization of FRP and XLF, a bit of background about tumor structure will be helpful. Normal tissues are composed of two interdependent compartments: parenchyma (generally epithelium) and stroma. Stroma is the vascular connective tissue on which epithelial cells depend for structure, support, nutrient supply, gas exchange, and clearance of waste metabolic products (172–174). Components include blood vessels, fibroblasts, and other mesenchymal cells, inflammatory cells, matrix proteins, proteoglycans, hyaluronan, and so on. Parenchyma and stroma appear as distinct compartments early in the developing embryo and engage in continuous cross-talk throughout life to maintain homeostasis at the level of the tissue, the organ, and the organism. Like

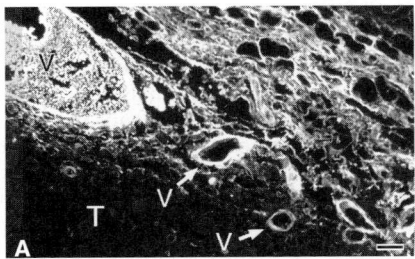 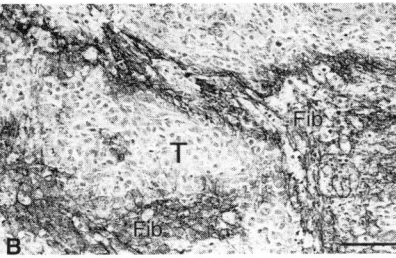 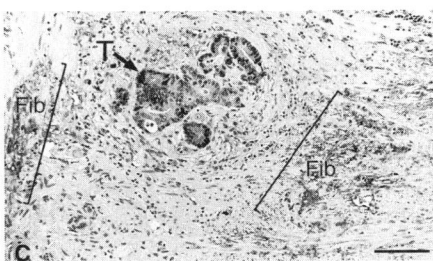

**FIGURE 57-1.** Hyperpermeability of tumor blood vessels resulting in plasma fibrinogen extravasation and extravascular clotting. **A:** Fluorescence image illustrating extravasation of circulating macromolecular fluorescein isothiocyanate-labeled dextran from tumor blood vessels (*V*). **B, C:** Immunoperoxidase staining demonstrates abundant fibrin (*Fib*) in stroma of guinea pig line 10 hepatocarcinoma and human colorectal adenocarcinoma. *T*, tumor. Scale bar: 50 μm. (Reprinted in revised form from Dvorak HF, How tumors make bad blood vessels and stroma, *Am J Pathol* 2003;162:1747, with permission.)

normal tissues, tumors are composed of these same two compartments. In tumors, neoplastic cells comprise the parenchyma, and the new vascular connective tissue that tumors induce serves as stroma. Whether transplanted experimentally or arising autochthonously, tumors require stroma for survival and must generate new stroma to grow beyond minimal size. Like tumor cells themselves, tumor blood vessels and other components of tumor stroma are highly abnormal and more closely resemble the composition of healing wounds than that of normal adult tissues (151,166,172,174).

The anatomic distribution of FRPs varies somewhat depending on the tumor type. In carcinomas, FRPs are deposited in tumor stroma and may be particularly abundant at the tumor periphery (i.e., at the tumor–host interface) (162,163,166,170–174). FRPs are generally less prominent in older, more central zones of tumor stroma characterized by sclerotic collagenous connective tissue. In lymphomas, FRP deposits may be observed between individual malignant tumor cells, as well as among reactive benign lymphoid elements (Fig. 57-2) and in zones of tumor sclerosis, as in the nodular sclerosis form of Hodgkin disease (165). Certain other generalizations deserve

mention. First, no evident relation exists between the amount of FRP deposited in tumors and the degree of tumor malignancy. However, fibrin deposits appear to correlate with and likely determine sites of subsequent collagen deposition (165). On the basis of studies of a small number of animal tumors, it appears likely that the extent of net fibrin accumulation is a predictor of the extent of mature tumor stroma formation and desmoplasia. Transplantable tumors have revealed another important principle: The pattern and extent of fibrin deposition are characteristic for a given tumor and remain constant over multiple transplant generations (166–171). Therefore, fibrin provides a characteristic and reproducible signature for tumors in much the same way that certain other histologic features do (tumor cell morphology, stromal pattern, and so forth) (166,171–174).

The nature of the FRP deposited in solid tumors has been the subject of several investigations. The heteroantibodies originally used for immunohistochemical identification of FRP recognize fibrinogen and a variety of related proteins, including non–cross-linked and factor XIIIa–crossl-inked XLF, as well as various fibrinogen and fibrin degradation products. Therefore, by themselves, these reagents cannot distinguish among the various types of tumor-associated FRPs. However, biochemical characterization of the fibrin extracted from tumors has revealed fibrin γ–γ dimers and polymerized fibrin α chains (167–169), conclusive evidence of XLF. This conclusion is also supported by immunohistochemical staining with monoclonal antibodies specific for fibrin, that is, antibodies that recognize fibrin but not fibrinogen (86,92,113,166,175) (Fig. 57-1C). Although some controversy exists regarding which human tumors contain stromal XLF (and, therefore, by inference, active extravascular clotting) and which do not (86,92,113), considerable heterogeneity probably exists, and the balance between tumor procoagulant and fibrinolytic activities likely determines the amounts of fibrin that are present.

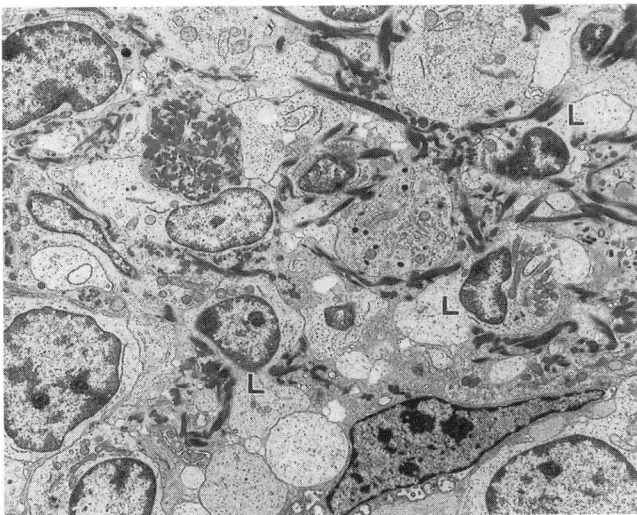

**FIGURE 57-2.** Electron micrograph illustrating fibrin deposition in a lymph node with Hodgkin disease. A prominent intercellular meshwork of fibrin (dark fibrillar material) separates benign small and medium lymphocytes. Some lymphocytes (*L*) appear to be compressed or indented at points of contact with fibrin (magnification ×7,000). (From Harris NL, Dvorak AM, Smith J, et al. Fibrin deposits in Hodgkin disease. *Am J Pathol* 1982;108:119, with permission.)

## PATHOGENESIS OF INTRATUMOR FIBRINOGEN-RELATED PROTEINS AND FIBRIN DEPOSITION

A few tumors have been found to synthesize fibrinogen *in vitro* (176,177), but aside from well-differentiated hepatocellular carcinomas, such expression has not been demonstrated in cancer *in vivo*. Therefore, it follows that plasma fibrinogen is nearly always the source of the FRP and fibrin that are found in most solid tumors. In normal tissues, very little fibrinogen escapes from plasma. Therefore, for fibrinogen and its derivatives to enter tumors, the local blood vessels must be rendered hyperpermeable (see Fig. 57-3). Also, for fibrin to be

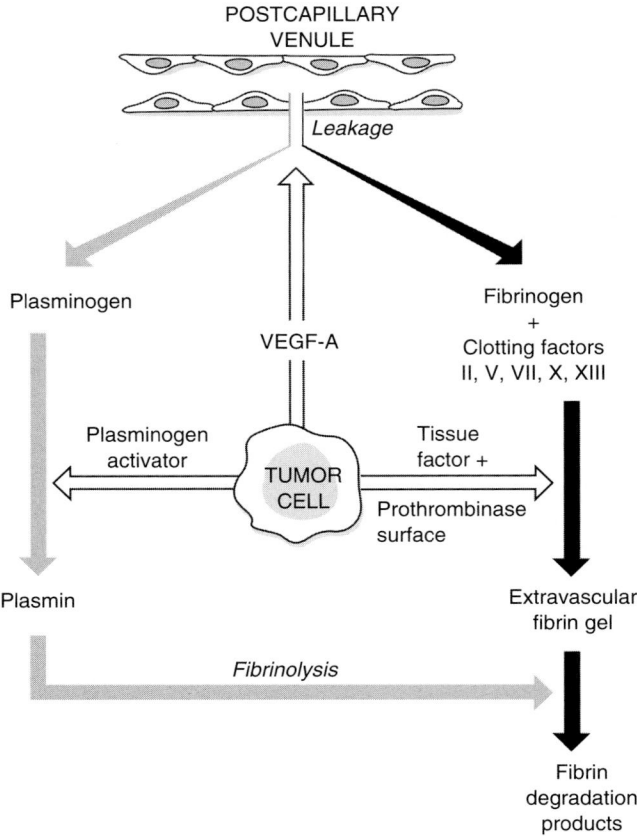

**FIGURE 57-3.** Schematic diagram illustrating the relations among tumor cell–secreted VEGF-A, vascular hyperpermeability, and extravascular fibrin deposition and degradation.

deposited in tumors, still another event must take place: activation of the clotting system in the extravascular space. The latter is mediated by the cells and mechanisms that have already been described, that is, procoagulant activities associated with tumor cells themselves and with tumor-associated host mesenchymal cells, macrophages, and endothelial cells.

## Increased Vascular Permeability

It has been known for some time that the microvasculature supplying tumors exhibits substantially increased permeability to plasma proteins but not, unless injured, to formed elements (162,163,166,167,178,179). This fact has been documented by tracer studies in a variety of experimental tumors. Various mechanisms have been proposed to account for this hyperpermeability, including release of histamine from tissue mast cells, kinins, and the activities of fibrin and fibrin degradation products (180–184). Mast cells are irregular components of tumors, and their presence does not correlate with increased vessel permeability. Unusual kinins have been reported in tumors, but these may have resulted from unphysiologic manipulations (181), although more recent work suggests that the contact system and bradykinin generation may play a role in tumor angiogenesis (185). Fibrin and specific fibrin degradation products do cause increased vascular permeability, generally at high concentrations and by provoking either histamine release from mast cells or perhaps by inducing IL-8 release from endothelial cells; however, such breakdown products would be expected to be present only after vessels had already become leaky and extravascular fibrin was deposited (184).

One possible exception, discussed more fully elsewhere (183), may be the induction of endothelial cell damage by fibrin at concentrations readily achieved in tumor microvessels.

Although any or all of these mechanisms may play a role in some tumors, it is now clear that the predominant mechanism by which the tumor microvasculature is rendered hyperpermeable is through the expression and secretion of members of the VPF/VEGF family of cytokines, and particularly one of its members, VEGF-A (151,162,163,166,186–188). However, before discussing VEGF-A and the VPF/VEGF protein family, it will be useful to document the significance of increased microvascular permeability and its relation to extravascular clotting.

## Consequences of Increased Microvascular Hyperpermeability

Whether in normal tissues or tumors, increased microvascular permeability has a number of consequences. One of these, the proclivity to intravascular clotting that results from increased hematocrit and blood viscosity, has already been mentioned. There are additional consequences. First among these is accumulation of plasma protein–rich edema fluid in the extravascular compartment, a characteristic feature of tumors, healing wounds, and other pathologies in which VEGF-A is overexpressed (151,166,174). This fluid includes a representative sample of plasma proteins, including all of those necessary for clot formation, that is, clotting factors V, VII, X, and prothrombin (factor II) as well as fibrinogen. In the case of solid tumors, extravascular fluid accumulation is generally limited by increasing interstitial tissue pressure (189). However, when tumor cells grow in body cavities such as the peritoneum, the restraints imposed by tissue pressure are minimal, and very large amounts of fluid can accumulate (190,191).

Another and related consequence of increased vascular permeability and plasma extravasation is that the clotting system is activated extravascularly, leading to deposition of an extravascular fibrin gel (192). This gel retards clearance of edema fluid and thereby contributes to increased interstitial tissue pressure. When vascular permeability is increased in normal tissues, extravascular clotting is initiated by TF that is expressed primarily on stromal fibroblasts (192). This pathway is also triggered in tumors as tumor cells, as well as stromal macrophages and VECs, come to express TF. As was already discussed, tumor cells may also express other procoagulants such as CP. The relative contribution of tumor and host cells to initiation of clotting likely varies among different tumors and their stage of growth. Immunohistochemical studies of human tumors have demonstrated an association between TF expressed by macrophages and deposition of XLF (86). However, studies of tumors at early intervals after transplantation, before infiltration of macrophages, associate XLF with TF-expressing tumor cells (163,170). As was already mentioned, tumor and/or stromal cells have a second role in extravascular clotting, that of providing a surface for prothrombinase assembly, a function normally played by platelets in intravascular clotting.

## Fibrin as Provisional Matrix for Tumor Angiogenesis and Stroma Generation

The XLF deposited in solid tumors has at least three important functions that favor the establishment of tumors and their growth, invasion, and metastasis (166,171–174): (i) Imposition of initial structure; (ii) provision of a three-dimensional matrix that supports the migration of tumor and host cells; and (iii) induction of angiogenesis and mature stroma. By providing a provisional matrix, the first of these functions, fibrin organizes tumors into discrete clumps of malignant cells that are separated from each other by a serum-rich gel that provides structural support as well as nutrients (151).

Fibrin's second function is that of providing a favorable temporary or provisional matrix for tumor and host cell migration (151). Mammalian cells do not "swim"—they "walk" on solid surfaces, and fibrin offers particular advantages in this regard because it possesses binding sites for many different cell types, including leukocytes (193), endothelial cells (194), tumor cells (195), and fibroblasts (196). To a large extent, cells bind to fibrin via integrins. Integrin binding sites are located at A$\alpha$95-98 (RGDF) and A$\alpha$572-575 (RGDS) of human fibrinogen (197). However, other proteins, such as fibronectin, are commonly integrated into fibrin gels, expanding the repertoire of available cell-binding sites. On the one hand, tumor cells make use of these sites to invade host tissues and eventually to enter lymphatics and the circulating blood. On the other hand, host mesenchymal cells (e.g., endothelial cells, pericytes, and fibroblasts) and leukocytes (monocytes, neutrophils, lymphocytes) use these same binding sites to enter developing tumors, to generate vascularized stroma, and in some cases, to provide a defense against tumor growth.

Fibrin also has nonintegrin binding sites that facilitate cell migration. One is the N-terminal $\beta$15-42 sequence exposed after thrombin cleavage of fibrinopeptide B (FPB) (198); this site binds VE-cadherin expressed on the surface of endothelial cells and is thought to have roles in endothelial cell spreading (199), proliferation (200), and capillary tube formation (201). Other sites are the ICAM-1 binding site at $\gamma$117-133 (202) and the heparin-binding domains on the N-terminal $\beta$ chain (203).

Platelets also bind to fibrin by the integrin $\alpha_{IIb}\beta_3$ and also by another site at $\gamma$400-411 (204,205). Such binding is important for platelet spreading and clot formation. Although platelets uncommonly escape from blood vessels (206), growth factors and other products released by activated platelets may diffuse from the vasculature to modulate stroma formation.

Fibrin also favors angiogenesis and mature stroma formation in other, subtler ways that have not as yet been fully elucidated. When fibrin gels prepared from highly purified fibrinogen are formed *in vitro* and implanted in animals without tumor cells, new blood vessels and fibroblasts grow in, digest the fibrin, and replace it over time with vascular fibrous connective tissue (207). This response resembles wound healing, but in this setting formation of fibrin gel occurs without the platelets and related growth factors such as platelet derived growth factor (PDGF), VEGF-A, and others that are associated with the latter. This implies that fibrin gels in some way impart information to cells, an unexpected conclusion because most chemotactic and chemokinetic activities described to date have been soluble molecules. Even in the early 1990s, this last idea appeared radical. However, increasing evidence now suggests that the extracellular matrix can indeed regulate the function of cells that impinge on it (208–210).

How might insoluble fibrin mediate such functions? Several possibilities exist. First, fibrin binds and sequesters a number of growth factors including bFGF and the larger isoforms of VEGF-A; this protects them from degradation and makes their activity available for release as fibrin is gradually degraded and replaced by mature stroma (211–213). Fibrin can also sequester IGF-1 by its association with IGF-binding protein 3, which binds directly to fibrin (87). At least *in vitro*, fibrin has been shown to induce the synthesis and secretion of proangiogenic factors such as IL-8 in some tumor cells (214) and endothelial cells (119). Fibrin structure and spatial organization may also be important (215). For example, fibrinogen$_{Nieuwegein}$ forms a more dense fibrin gel that is less susceptible than normal fibrin to proteolytic cleavage and less permeable to infiltrating microvascular endothelial cells (216). Last, physiologic levels of fibrin have been shown to potently induce TF expression in human vascular endothelial cells (HUVECs). This response required

direct contact between insoluble fibrin and endothelial cells because separation of cells from fibrin in transwell chambers was not stimulatory (217).

In summary, the fibrin deposited in tumors is not an inert matrix, but one that provides important feedback signaling functions. It contributes to additional activation of clotting in the tumor milieu and to tumor growth and angiogenesis. Nonetheless, studies with fibrinogen-null mice have demonstrated that fibrinogen is not always required because two transplantable tumors were found to grow comparably with equivalent angiogenesis in both null and control mice (217, 218). Interestingly, however, tumor metastasis was greatly reduced in the fibrinogen-null animals. These findings indicate that tumor growth, invasion, and metastasis are extremely complex events subject to regulation at many different levels.

## Fibrinolysis and Replacement of Fibrin by Mature Stroma

It has been known for more than a century that tumor cells digest fibrin clots, and in more recent times, this activity has been shown to be mediated by tumor-secreted plasminogen activators (119,219,220). Tumor stromal macrophages, fibroblasts, and endothelial cells also express plasminogen activators. Increased urokinase-type plasminogen activator (uPA) and tissue-type plasminogen activator (tPA) activity have been demonstrated in a number of tumors and have been linked to unfavorable prognosis [reviewed in (119)]. Angiogenic factors, including bFGF and VEGF-A, upregulate the expression of plasminogen activators along with the plasminogen activator receptor (u-PAR) and inhibitor (PAI-1) (219,221–223). Paradoxically, overexpression of PAI-1 in cancer also correlates with poor prognosis, suggesting that an optimal balance of proteolysis regulates tumor growth (119). Both uPA and tPA cleave plasminogen to generate plasmin, a potent protease that degrades fibrin and other proteins. Plasminogen, of course, is a plasma protein that, like plasma clotting factors, extravasates from leaky tumor blood vessels into the tissues, where it can serve as a substrate for plasminogen activators (Fig. 57-3). Tumor and stromal cells also express other proteases, notably matrix metalloproteases (MMPs), that also contribute to the degradation of fibrin and other matrix proteins (224).

Fibrinolysis in tumors is important for several reasons. First, localized fibrinolysis is thought to be necessary for cell migration in fibrin matrix, and uPA has been localized to the leading front of migrating monocytes and invading tumor cells (225). More generally, fibrin is only a provisional matrix and is degraded as it is being replaced by mature connective tissue stroma. Therefore, the fibrin present in tumors is in a dynamic state, undergoing simultaneous deposition and dissolution (167,174,226). The amount of fibrin matrix present in tumors at any point of time reflects a balance between clotting and fibrinolysis. Each tumor has a characteristic amount of fibrin matrix that is thought to be predictive of the amount of mature stroma that will eventually replace it. Parenthetically, the mature stroma that tumors generate is highly abnormal and includes elements such as fetal fibronectins, tenascin, abnormal proteoglycans, and degradative enzymes that are not normally found in normal adult connective tissues (172–174,227,228); however, many of these elements are also found in the equally abnormal stroma found in healing wounds, supporting the concept that "tumors are wounds that do not heal" (166).

Fibrinolysis is also important because it generates fragments with biologic activities. *Fibrin* fragment E, resulting from plasmin degradation of fibrin, stimulates angiogenesis *in vitro* (229) and in the chorioallantoic membrane (CAM) assay *in vivo* (230). That this fragment may have biologic significance was demonstrated by the finding that treatment with an antifragment E antibody in an animal model resulted in tumor regression and long-term survival (231). Conversely, *fibrinogen* fragment E, resulting from plasmin degradation of fibrinogen, inhibits endothelial cell proliferation and tubule formation (229) and does so with a potency equivalent to that of the well-known angiogenesis inhibitor endostatin.

Plasminogen activators and plasmin can influence tumors in ways that are independent of fibrinolysis. For example, uPA can activate the proform of hepatocyte growth factor (HGF) (232), a regulator of VEGF-A expression and an angiogenesis factor in its own right (233). Plasmin can activate latent TGF-$\beta$ (234), and liberate the cell-membrane-bound VEGF-A [(212),(235), also see subsequent text].

One additional point must be made. Proteolysis of plasminogen by MMPs and other proteases generates a family of antiangiogenic agents, the best known of which is angiostatin (236,237).

# ROLES OF VASCULAR PERMEABILITY FACTOR/VASCULAR ENDOTHELIAL GROWTH FACTOR FAMILY CYTOKINES IN TUMOR ANGIOGENESIS

VEGF-A was discovered in the late 1970s as the result of a targeted search for a tumor-secreted factor that increased microvascular permeability (162,163,186). It is the founding member of the VPF/VEGF family of proteins, a family that also includes VEGFs B, C, and D, as well as placenta growth factor (PLGF) and a related viral protein, VEGF-E (151,238–241). Of these, VEGF-A has so far been studied most intensively. It is a highly conserved, disulfide-bonded glycoprotein of $M_r$ approximately 45 kDa, composed of two chains that are joined together by disulfide bonds and arranged in antiparallel fashion with receptor binding sites at either end (242–244). VEGF-A is essential for the development and organization of the vascular system (vasculogenesis) and for both physiologic and pathologic angiogenesis. Mice lacking even one copy of the *VEGF-A* gene are embryonic lethals (245,246).

The human *VEGF-A* gene is located on the short arm of chromosome 6 and is differentially spliced to yield predominant isoforms encoding polypeptides of 189, 165, and 121 amino acids in human cells (corresponding murine proteins are one amino acid shorter) (242,243,247,248). These different isoforms have distinct physical properties. VEGF-A[121] (144) is acidic, freely soluble, and does not bind heparin. By contrast, the 165 and 189 isoforms of VEGF-A have increasing basic charge and bind heparin with increasing affinity; in fact, VEGF-A[188] was originally purified on the basis of its affinity for heparin (186–188). The different VEGF-A isoforms have largely identical biological activities *in vitro*, and all can potently increase vascular permeability. However, there is increasing evidence for distinctive functions for each isoform *in vivo*. Tumors expressing one or another VEGF-A isoform induce significantly different vascular patterns (249,250), and mice engineered to express only the 120 or 188 isoforms develop severe vascular anomalies (241,251,252).

VEGF-A is expressed constitutively at low levels in many normal adult tissues and is highly expressed by most human and animal carcinomas, where it is thought to be the prime mover of tumor angiogenesis (151,238,242). Most VEGF-A in solid tumors is expressed by the malignant cells, but VEGF-A can also be expressed by tumor stromal cells, including fibroblasts and macrophages (151,238,253–255). Different tumors express the several VEGF-A isoforms in different proportions,

but VEGF-A[165] is generally predominant. VEGF-A is also overexpressed in some important premalignant lesions (e.g., precursor lesions of breast, cervix, and colon cancers), and expression levels increase in parallel with malignant progression (238,256,257). Some benign tumors also express VEGF-A, but this has been less well studied (238).

VEGF-A expression in tumors and normal tissues is regulated by a number of different mechanisms, including local hypoxia; low pH; oncogenes (src, ras); tumor suppressor genes [p53, p73, von Hippel-Lindau (vHL)]; hormones (estrogen, insulin); and by numerous growth factors, cytokines, and lipid mediators (e.g., EGF, TGF-$\alpha$, bFGF, TGF-$\beta$, PDGF, keratinocyte growth factor, TNF-$\alpha$, IL-1 and -6, insulinlike growth factor 1, HGF, and prostaglandins E1 and E2) (242,258–261).

## Biological Activities of VEGF-A

VEGF-A was originally discovered because of its ability to permeabilize microvessels, primarily postcapillary venules and small veins, to circulating macromolecules (162,163,186). Permeability becomes evident within a minute following a single intradermal injection of VEGF-A protein and persists for approximately 20 minutes. The ability to enhance microvascular permeability is VEGF-A's most distinctive property, and the nearly universal hyperpermeability of tumor blood vessels to plasma proteins is largely attributable to tumor cell expression of VEGF-A. VEGF-A is among the most potent vascular permeabilizing agents known, acting at concentrations below 1 nM and with a potency approximately 50,000 times that of histamine on a molar basis (162,186,258). Other members of the VPF/VEGF family, notably VEGF-C and PlGF, also exert vascular permeability-enhancing activity but are less potent and less widely expressed than VEGF-A (262,263).

VEGF-A's vascular permeabilizing activity occurs within a matter of minutes, but VEGF-A is a multifunctional cytokine whose many other effects on vascular endothelium take place over the course of hours to days. Therefore, VEGF-A alters cell morphology, stimulates endothelial cell proliferation and migration, is an endothelial cell survival factor (antiapoptotic effect), and delays endothelial cell senescence (238,243,264,265). Many of these activities are mediated through reprogramming endothelial cell gene expression. For example, VEGF-A upregulates the expression of MMPs, the GLUT-1 glucose transporter, nitric oxide synthase, numerous mitogens, and a number of antiapoptotic factors. Of particular relevance to this chapter, VEGF-A increases the expression of a number of proteins associated with clotting and fibrinolysis, including TF, uPA, tPA, PAI-1, and the urokinase receptor urokinase plasminogen activator receptor (uPAR) [reviewed in (238)]. Also, TF feeds back to upregulate VEGF-A expression, generating a vicious cycle (see subsequent text).

## Anatomic Basis of Vascular Endothelial Growth Factor-A's Permeability-Enhancing Activity

VECs are the primary barrier to extravasation of plasma proteins from the circulation, and VEGF-A induces its permeability effects by a direct action on these cells. However, although nearly all endothelial cells express VEGF-A receptors, VEGF-A induces permeability selectively on postcapillary venules and on tumor blood vessels derived from venules. There is disagreement in the literature as to the pathway that circulating macromolecules follow in traversing endothelium [reviewed in (238,258)]. Some investigators hold that vasoactive agents cause venular endothelial cells to pull apart from one another, creating an interendothelial cell gap through which macromolecules extravasate (266). Although consistent with tissue culture data, evidence for an intercellular extravasation pathway *in vivo* is less convincing. More recent studies have shown that macromolecules cross tumor and normal venular endothelium by means of a transendothelial cell pathway that involves a newly recognized structure unique to venular endothelium, the vesiculo-vacuolar organelle (VVO) (267–271) (see Fig. 57-4). VVOs comprise interconnecting cytoplasmic vesicles and vacuoles that extend from the endothelial cell lumen to the ablumen and that open to form continuous transendothelial cell channels in response to VEGF-A and other vascular permeabilizing agents such as histamine. These vesicles and vacuoles are joined to each other and to the luminal and albuminal plasma membranes by stomata that are normally closed by thin diaphragms, the composition of which is only now coming to be understood (272). VVOs are typically parajunctional, and this location may account for the confusion as to whether the openings generated by VEGF-A and other permeabilizing agents are trans- or intercellular. VEGF-A also induces endothelial fenestrations that provide an additional transcellular pathway for solute and protein extravasation (271,273).

## VEGF-A Receptors and VEGF-A Signaling

VEGF-A mediates its effects primarily by interacting with two high-affinity transmembrane tyrosine kinase receptors, VEGFR-1 (Flt-1) and VEGFR-2 (KDR, Flk-1), that are selectively expressed on normal endothelial cells (242,258,274). VEGFR-1 is also expressed on monocytes and at least on some tumor cells, raising the possibility that VEGF-A exerts autocrine effects that enhance tumor cell motility and survival (275–278). A truncated soluble form of VEGFR-1 (sFLT) that results from alternative splicing is found in serum and retains VEGF-A binding activity [reviewed in (279)]. Both VEGFR-1 and VEGFR-2 are commonly upregulated in endothelial cells in the course of angiogenesis (242,258,280); hypoxia, which also upregulates VEGF-A expression, may play a role. VEGFs A and B and both isoforms of PLGF bind to VEGFR-1,whereas VEGFs A, C, D, and E bind to VEGFR-2 [reviewed in (238)].

A third, nonkinase VEGF-A receptor, neuropilin (NRP), has recently been found (281). NRP is also a receptor for the semaphorin/collapsin family of neuronal guidance mediators and is expressed widely on nonendothelial cells, including some tumor cells (282). NRP potentiates VEGF-A[188] binding to VEGFR-2 but recently has been shown to have independent signaling functions (283). VEGF-A[188], B, E, and PLGF bind to NRP, but VEGF-A (144) does not. Mice null for any of the three VEGF-A receptors are embryonic lethals, with death being attributable to failures of vascular development [reviewed in (238,282)].

Most of the biologic activities mediated by VEGF-A on endothelial cells (e.g., proliferation, migration, vascular permeability, antiapoptosis) are mediated through VEGFR-2, an important exception being induction of TF expression (see subsequent text). VEGFR-2 also has an important role in the development of endothelial cell precursors present in the bone

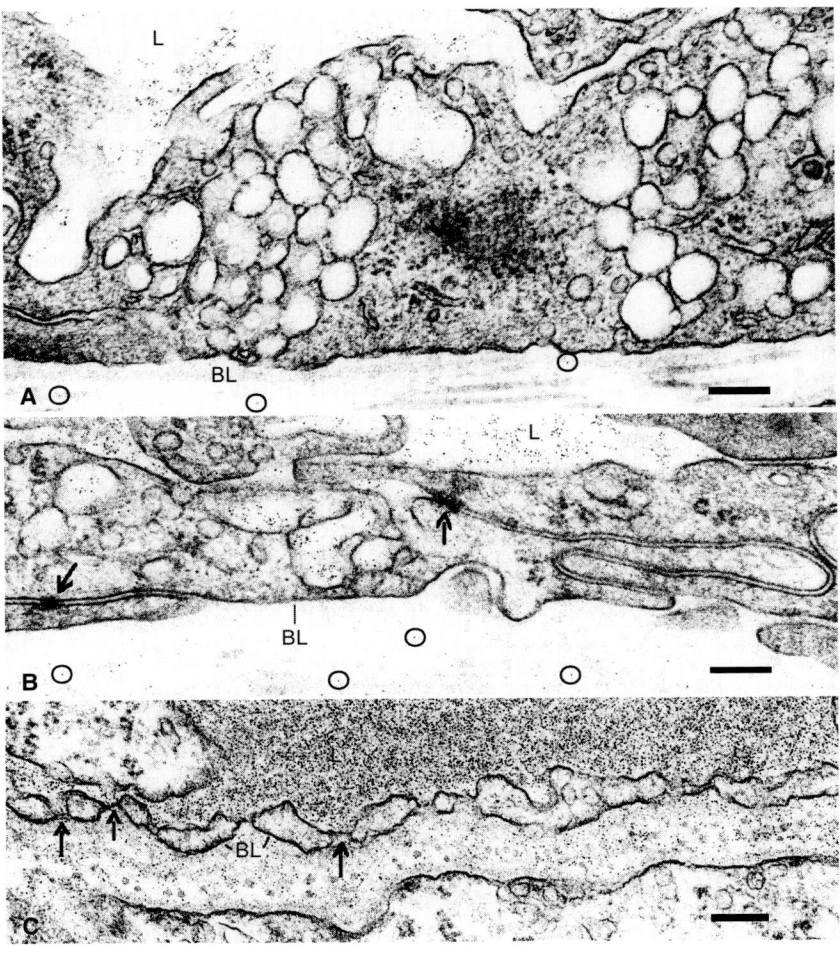

**FIGURE 57-4.** Electron micrographs illustrating vesiculo-vacuolar vesicles (VVOs) in normal postcapillary venule endothelial cell (**A**), thinned mother vessel endothelial cell with reduced VVO vesicles (**B**), and fenestrae (**C**). L, lumen; BL, basal lamina. (Reprinted from Pettersson A, Nagy JA, Brown LF et al, Heterogeneity of the angiogenic response induced in different normal adult tissues by vascular permeability factor/vascular endothelial growth factor. *Lab Invest* 2000;80:99, with permission.)

marrow and circulating in blood (284). Upon binding to VEGFR-2, VEGF-A initiates a cascade of events that begins with receptor dimerization and autophosphorylation, followed by phosphorylation of numerous downstream proteins, an increase in intracellular calcium, and IP$_3$ accumulation (279). Very recently, G proteins have been implicated in VEGF-A signaling (285).

Although binding to VEGF-A with very high affinity, VEGFR-1 induces only minimal stimulation of kinase activity in vascular endothelium (279); as a result, downstream signaling pathways have had to be worked out in endothelial cells that were engineered to overexpress this receptor (286,287). These studies have revealed that activation of the VEGFR-1 pathway exerts inhibitory effects on the VEGFR-2 signaling pathway and does not stimulate endothelial cell proliferation or chemotaxis. However, VEGFR-1 signaling is responsible for inducing chemotactic activity in monocytes (which also express this receptor) and for inducing expression of TF in both monocytes and endothelial cells (85,288). TF expression has been shown to be regulated by activation of the transcription factor *early growth response-1 (egr-1)* gene, apparently by a pathway that involves decreased PI 3-K activity concurrent with increased p38 and Erk-1/2 MAP kinase activity (87,289,290). In agreement with these results, angiopoietin-1, an activator of PI 3-K/Akt signaling, inhibits VEGF-A and TNF-α–induced expression of TF in endothelial cells (291).

## Tumor Angiogenesis and Lymphangiogenesis

The multiple activities exerted by VEGF-A and other members of the VPF/VEGF family result in the generation of new blood vessels and lymphatics. However, the new blood vessels and lymphatics that form are highly abnormal (151,174,292). Unlike normal blood vessels, those induced by VEGF-A in tumors are nonuniformly distributed, branch irregularly, form A-V shunts, are structurally and functionally heterogeneous, and do not conform to a clear hierarchical pattern. In addition, and as already discussed, they are hyperpermeable to plasma proteins and display an activated, procoagulant phenotype as the result of exposure to tumor cell and macrophage secreted cytokines such as TNF-α, IL-1, and VEGF-A.

Recent studies have defined the properties of these vessels in more detail, making use of adenoviral vectors to express VEGF-A and other cytokines in order to induce tumor surrogate blood vessels, that is, vessels with all of the properties of tumor vessels but in the absence of tumor cells (151,152, 293,294). These studies have shown that the vessels formed are quite heterogeneous but develop in a highly reproducible and carefully scripted fashion. The first new vessels to form are called *mother vessels* (see Fig. 57-5). These are greatly enlarged, thin-walled, serpentine, pericyte-poor, hyperpermeable, and strongly VEGFR-2–positive sinusoids. Vessels of this description are commonly found in animal and human tumors and are also transiently present in healing wounds (151,295, 296). Mother vessels arise from the extensive enlargement of preexisting venules (approximately a fourfold increase in cross-sectional area) by a process that involves degradation of vascular basement membrane, extensive endothelial cell thinning, and a substantial increase in surface area that is made possible by transfer of VVO membranes to the plasma membrane (Fig. 57-4). Like their counterparts in tumors, mother vessels induced by adenoviruses expressing VEGF-A commonly thrombose, a not surprising finding given their high hematocrit and irregular surface endothelium that predisposes to sluggish and turbulent blood flow.

Mother vessels are transient structures that evolve over time into several different types of daughter blood vessels (151). Among these are glomeruloid vascular proliferations,

arterio-venous malformations, and relatively normal capillaries. Both mother vessels and glomeruloid vascular proliferations are hyperpermeable to plasma, although their content of VVOs is reduced in both number and size; the explanation seems to be that the extensive endothelial cell thinning involved in their formation greatly reduces the transendothelial cell pathway length that solutes must traverse in crossing from the vascular lumen to the extravascular space. Both types of vessels also exhibit fenestrations over a small portion of their surface, providing another route for transvascular passage of solute.

VEGF-C and VEGF-D have been known to induce the formation of new lymphatics (239), and recently, VEGF-A has also been found to induce lymphangiogenesis (297). The lymphatics induced by VEGF-A have been carefully studied and, like VEGF-A–induced mother vessels, are highly abnormal in structure and function (297). Most relevant to this chapter is the finding that they commonly thrombose. The extensive microvascular permeability induced by VEGF-A leads to extravasation of fibrinogen and other soluble plasma clotting factors in sufficient concentration to reach not only the extravascular space but also to enter lymphatics. The mechanisms by which clotting is initiated within lymphatics have not been investigated. It is possible that VEGF-A activates TF expression in lymphatic endothelium just as it does in VECs. In any event, lymphatic endothelial cells invade the luminal fibrin matrix, dividing it into smaller channels; a similar process is thought to occur when mother vessels evolve to generate daughter blood capillaries (151).

# ROLES OF TISSUE FACTOR, THROMBIN, AND OTHER CLOTTING PROTEINS IN TUMOR ANGIOGENESIS: CLOTTING-DEPENDENT AND CLOTTING-INDEPENDENT MECHANISMS

Although VPF/VEGF family members, and particularly VEGF-A, are thought to be the most important inducers of tumor angiogenesis, recent evidence suggests that two clotting proteins, TF and thrombin, also have important roles and act by both clotting-dependent as well as clotting-independent means.

## Tissue Factor

TF is a 47-kDa immediate early response gene whose capacity to activate factor VIIa is the initial step in triggering both the intravascular and extravascular clotting that accompany cancer (see Chapter 5). Clotting leads to thrombin generation, platelet activation, and fibrin formation, all of which support tumor angiogenesis and stroma generation, as previously discussed (86,92,116,262,298–300). In fact, a close correlation has been demonstrated between microvascular density and expression of both TF and VEGF-A in a variety of human tumors, including carcinomas of the breast, colon, rectum, and lung (92,123,301,302). TF has also been shown to increase VEGF-A expression in various cell types by a *coagulation-dependent* mechanism that required binding of TF to factor VIIa and generation of both factor Xa and thrombin (300,303–306).

TF can also upregulate the expression of VEGF-A (and possibly other growth factors) by *coagulation-independent* mechanisms. This was first shown by Zhang et al. (299), who found that TF increased VEGF-A transcription in murine tumor cells while downregulating transcription of thrombospondin-2, generally regarded as an angiogenesis inhibitor. Subsequently,

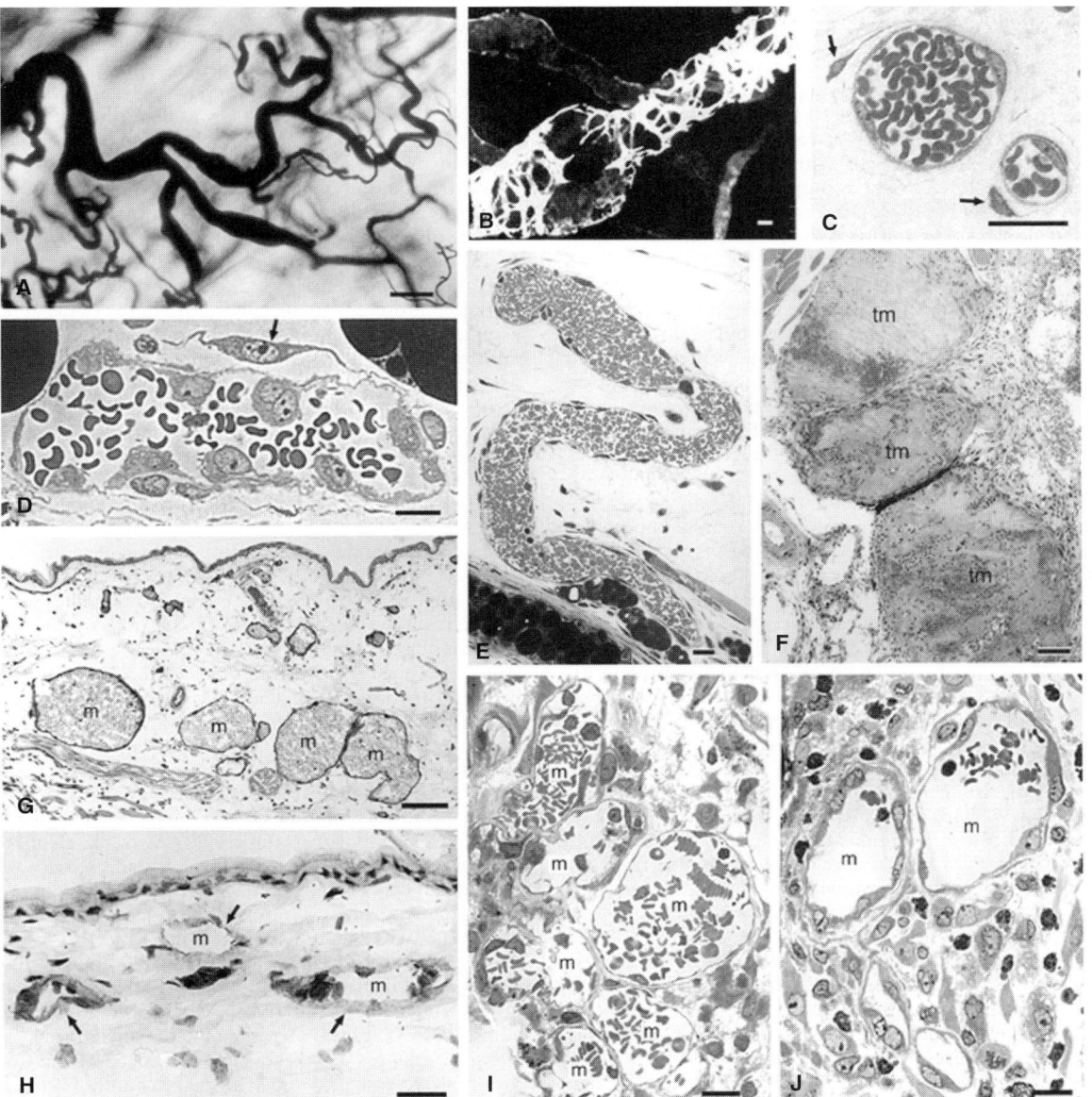

**FIGURE 57-5.** Typical "mother" vessels induced by Ad-VEGF-A (187) (**A–H**) or by mouse tumor cells secreting VEGF-A (187). **A:** Whole mount of colloidal carbon-perfused vascular bed. Mother vessels appear as enlarged segments of much smaller, normal venules. **B:** Confocal microscopic image of mother vessel stained for pericytes with an antibody to α smooth muscle actin. Note incomplete pericyte covering, especially over segments of greatest vessel enlargement. **C:** Developing mother vessels illustrating pericyte detachment (*arrows*). **D:** Mother vessel with detached pericyte (*arrow*) and activated endothelial cells whose large nuclei bulge into the vascular lumen, creating a highly irregular surface. **E:** Serpentine mother vessels with irregular luminal surface. **F:** Thrombosed mother vessels (*tm*). **G:** Mother vessels (*m*) embedded in fibrin gel provisional stroma. **H:** Loss of laminin staining (*arrows*) in developing mother vessels (*m*). **I** and **J:** Mother vessels (*m*) in mouse MOT ovarian and TA3/St mammary carcinomas. Note transluminal endothelial bridging in I. Scale bars, **A, F:** 100 $\mu$m; all others 20 $\mu$m. [**A, B** Reprinted from Nagy JA, Vasile E, Feng D et al., VEGF-A induces angiogenesis, arteriogenesis, lymphangiogenesis, and vascular malformations. *Cold Spring Harbor Symposia on Quantitative Biology* 2002;67:227–237, with permission. **C, E, F, H** Reprinted from Pettersson A, Nagy JA, Brown LF et al., Heterogeneity of the angiogenic response induced in different normal adult tissues by vascular permeability factor/vascular endothelial growth factor. *Lab Invest* 2000;80(1):99–115, with permission. **I, J** Reprinted from Feng D, Nagy JA, Dvorak AM and Dvorak HF, Microvasc Res 2000;59:24, with permission.]

Abe et al. showed that human melanoma cell lines expressing high levels of TF and VEGF-A formed highly vascular tumors in mice, whereas lines expressing low levels of these factors formed relatively avascular tumors (116). However, transfection of full-length TF cDNA into cell lines expressing low levels of TF and VEGF-A caused these cells to express high levels of both; transfection of the cells with a cytoplasmic domain deleted mutant TF cDNA failed to support the expression of either TF or VEGF-A (116). Mutation of two lysine sites in the extracellular domain of TF, critical for TF-mediated activation of factor X, did not affect the ability of the transfected cells to support expression of both TF and VEGF-A. Bromberg et al. (307) also reported that VEGF-A expression in some, but not all, melanoma lines was regulated by the cytoplasmic tail of TF, not the ligand-binding extracellular domain. Whether induced by clotting-dependent or -independent means, the upregulation of VEGF-A induced by TF has the potential to set up a self-perpetuating feedback loop because VEGF-A expression also upregulates that of TF in a number of cell types (85,87).

That TF is capable of upregulating VEGF-A expression through signaling mechanisms should not be surprising because TF is a true cell surface receptor that shares homologies with members of the cytokine receptor superfamily (308). In addition to its 219–amino acid extracellular factor VII–binding domain, TF has a 29–amino acid hydrophobic transmembrane domain and a 21–amino acid intracellular tail containing three putative serine phosphorylation sites (309). There is good evidence that the cytoplasmic domain of TF activates protein kinase C–dependent signaling, which then upregulates VEGF-A synthesis in response to different stimuli (119,310).

Another important line of evidence that TF has important, clotting-independent vascular functions comes from genetic experiments. Mice rendered null for TF are embryonic lethals by day 10.5 (311–313). Although the mechanisms are not fully understood, TF-null animals die from impaired vascular integrity and defects in blood vessel development in the yolk sac long before the clotting system has become functional. Therefore, TF has important roles in vasculogenesis as well as in pathologic angiogenesis.

Finally, mention should be made of another TF-related protein that has an impact on angiogenesis, the *TFPI*. TFPI is a Kunitz-type serine proteinase inhibitor that forms a quaternary complex on cell membranes with TF, factor VIIa, and factor Xa (314), resulting in internalization and inactivation of factor Xa clotting activity (315). Recombinant TFPI has been shown to inhibit bFGF-induced angiogenesis in the CAM assay and to greatly reduce melanoma and colon and lung carcinoma–induced angiogenesis [reviewed in (119)]. Also, patients bearing solid tumors (but apparently not leukemias) have increased levels of both free and total forms of TFPI (316,317). An antiangiogenic role has also been proposed for a second TF inhibitor, TFPI-2 (119).

## Thrombin

Many tumors activate the clotting cascade and generate thrombin (see Chapter 10). Also, thrombin is reported to be expressed by a variety of tumor cells, including melanoma and carcinomas of the lung, kidney, ovary, larynx, pancreas, and stomach [reviewed in (119,318)]. Like TF, thrombin has been found to affect tumor angiogenesis in many ways. For example, fibrin that results from clotting has been found to stabilize $\alpha_V\beta_3$ mRNA in endothelial cells, thereby favoring their migration and protecting them from apoptosis (319). Some of these functions of thrombin, therefore, involve its role in clotting and fibrin generation. However, increasing evidence indicates that in addition to actions that involve clotting, thrombin modulates angiogenesis by cleaving and thereby activating *protease activated receptors* (PARs). PARs are a family of seven transmembrane spanning G protein–coupled receptors that are expressed on the surfaces of many different cells, including platelets, tumor cells, endothelial cells, vascular smooth muscle cells, and macrophages in the tumor environment (320–324). At least four PARs have been identified, of which PAR-1 (expressed on endothelial cells, platelets, leukocytes, and some mesenchymal cells and tumor cells) is most important for the present discussion.

Accumulating evidence relates thrombin activation of PAR receptors to angiogenesis (325). Tsopanoglou et al. reported that thrombin promotes angiogenesis both in the CAM and Matrigel assays. The angiogenesis induced was thrombin-dose–dependent and required that the catalytic site of thrombin be functional. Moreover, the angiogenic effect was blocked by heparin and hirudin and could be mimicked by the *thrombin receptor activating peptide* (TRAP), which activates the PAR-1 receptor by a nonproteolytic mechanism (325). Further, $\gamma$ thrombin, a thrombin analog that is catalytically active but cannot generate fibrin, also promoted angiogenesis. Together, these experiments indicate that the proangiogenic action of thrombin is receptor-mediated and presumably independent of fibrin generation.

How does thrombin achieve these proangiogenic effects? There appears to be no single answer to this question. Thrombin exerts a diverse set of actions on platelets, endothelial cells, and tumor cells that individually and collectively promote angiogenesis; the relative importance of these actions has not yet been fully worked out. The actions of thrombin on platelets have already been mentioned briefly and involve promotion of intercellular adhesion and release of granule contents. As discussed further in the section on metastasis, tumor cells form heteroaggregates with platelets, and tumor-activated platelets release products that favor tumor cell–endothelial cell adhesion both locally and at metastatic sites. Also, platelets are important reservoirs and transporters of a wide variety of growth factors and other tumor-secreted products, including those that are proangiogenic and antiangiogenic: VEGF-A, VEGF-C, bFGF, PD-ECGF, PDGF, IGF-1, IGF-2, EGF, TGF-$\beta$1, Ang-1, PAI-1, thrombospondin, platelet factor 4, endostatin, and domains of HGF [reviewed in (119)]. Patients with cancer frequently have increased numbers of circulating platelets; in addition, the platelets of patients with cancer often contain increased amounts of these factors and, upon activation by thrombin, release them from storage granules (326–329).

Thrombin acts on vascular cells through PAR receptors to induce the expression of many genes that regulate angiogenesis, including VEGF-A, VEGFR-1, VEGFR-2, TF, bFGF, and MMP-2 (325). Upregulation of TF, of course, promotes thrombin generation and also contributes to nonhemostatic TF activities (119). One early effect, evident within 5 minutes of addition of thrombin in tissue culture, is inhibition of endothelial cell attachment to basement membrane proteins such as collagen IV and laminin (325); it is thought that endothelial cells must undergo similar detachment from basement membrane in the early stages of sprouting angiogenesis *in vivo*. Thrombin also activates MMP-2, an enzyme that degrades collagen IV (330) and releases tPA and PAI-1 (225). These effects are likely to be important because angiogenesis requires breakdown of the vascular basement membrane (152). Also, proteolytic digestion of extracellular matrix is likely to liberate bound growth factors such as bFGF that stimulate angiogenesis (331).

Thrombin exerts yet other effect on endothelial cells. It increases vascular permeability by mechanisms that apparently involve Rac, myosin light chain kinase, VE-cadherin, and protein tyrosine kinases (332–334). Thrombin also inhibits fibrinolysis by activating tissue-type PAI-1 (335,336). It upregulates the expression of VEGFR-1 as well as VEGFR-2, the VEGF receptor thought to be most important for mediating angiogenesis, and also leads to an increase in functional VEGR-2 protein (325); increased expression of VEGFR-2 is commonly observed in pathologic angiogenesis (280) and likely potentiates the activities of VEGF-A and other VEGF family members that bind to it (325). In addition, thrombin increases the availability of VEGF-A by upregulating its expression by tumor cells (337). Thrombin also releases bFGF from endothelial cells (338) and stimulates them to synthesize Ang-2 (339). In addition, thrombin induces endothelial cell division by both catalytic (thrombin receptor–dependent) and nonproteolytic signaling pathways (338,340–342). Thrombin can also upregulate VEGF-A transcription by mechanisms that seem to involve oxygen reactive species and hypoxia inducible factor-1 (333).

Another way in which thrombin may alter endothelial cell function is through modulating integrin expression. The $\alpha_V\beta_3$ integrin is commonly expressed by the endothelium lining tumor blood vessels. Thrombin increases the expression of the $\beta_3$ integrin subunit at both the mRNA and protein levels and does so in a time- and concentration-dependent manner (325). $\alpha_V\beta_3$ is a "promiscuous" integrin that interacts with a variety of substrates, including fibrin, fibronectin, vitronectin, thrombospondin, and osteopontin (343). Ligand binding to $\alpha_V\beta_3$ induces intracellular signals that favor cell attachment, migration, and proliferation and that prevent apoptosis (344). Recently, thrombin has been proposed as an additional $\alpha_V\beta_3$ ligand because endothelial cells cultured on thrombin-coated plates are protected from apoptosis (325). However, binding of $\alpha_V\beta_3$ to thrombin, although saturable and specific, apparently does not involve thrombin's catalytic site because DIP-thrombin is equally effective in binding $\alpha_V\beta_3$. Endothelial cells have been shown to migrate toward immobilized thrombin, an effect that is likely $\alpha_V\beta_3$-dependent because it can be blocked by the RGD peptide. This interaction could be important in the recanalization of thrombosed blood vessels because thrombin bound to and immobilized by fibrin is protected from degradation and therefore may serve as a haptotactic stimulus to endothelial cell migration.

Most of the effects of thrombin summarized so far have been proangiogenic. However, thrombin has also been reported to have antiangiogenic properties. For example, thrombin can cleave antithrombin (AT) to generate a potent inhibitor of VEGF-A– and bFGF-induced endothelial cell proliferation *in vitro* and angiogenesis *in vivo* (345,346). Some recent reports suggest that native AT itself can block thrombin-induced mitogenicity (347), inhibit endothelial cell expression of TF (348), and block VEGF-A–induced endothelial cell proliferation (349). Thrombin's proenzyme, prothrombin, also has antiangiogenic properties. The prothrombin kringle 2 domain is reported to inhibit angiogenesis in the CAM assay (350), and prothrombin fragment F1+2, formed as a byproduct during thrombin generation, inhibits bFGF-induced endothelial cell proliferation and angiogenesis in the CAM assay (351). Thrombin itself has been reported to inhibit endothelial cell tube formation (although at rather high concentrations) (352). Also, peptide activators of PAR-1 inhibit endothelial cell tube formation *in vitro* and bFGF-induced angiogenesis *in vivo* (352). Finally, when bound to TM, thrombin loses its ability to cleave fibrinogen and instead activates protein C, which inactivates factors VIIIa and Va, downregulating clotting and thereby further tipping the balance against angiogenesis. VEGF-A increases TM synthesis in EC and attenuates downregulation of TM induced by IL-1 and TGF-$\beta$; in turn, this may lead to a decrease in thrombin clotting activity. Overall, the effects of thrombin on tumor growth and angiogenesis are exceedingly complex and subject to local environmental factors.

## Other Fibrinolytic and Clotting-Related Proteins

The role of the fibrinolytic system in angiogenesis has not as yet been well investigated. However, recent studies indicate that urokinase and plasminogen (but not uPAR) knockout mice have impaired angiogenesis in response to growth factors such as bFGF and VEGF-A (353). In addition, at least five proteins that participate in the hemostatic system contain cryptic antiangiogenic fragments: angiostatin (plasminogen fragment), antiangiogenic AT, domain 5 of the high-molecular-weight kininogen, and prothrombin fragments 1 and 2 (354).

# PLATELETS, CLOTTING, AND TUMOR METASTASIS

Tumor metastasis has been likened to a decathlon in the sense that, to metastasize, individual tumor cells must satisfactorily complete in succession a number of very different and difficult tasks; failure at any one step precludes successful metastasis (355). Critical steps in the metastatic process include at least the following: intravasation of tumor cells into lymphatics or directly into the blood vasculature; survival in the circulation; extravasation from the vasculature; and growth and stroma generation to form new tumors at distant sites. Platelets and clotting are likely to have important roles at each of these steps.

As already noted, fibrin provides a favorable substrate for tumor cell migration and therefore allows tumor cells to migrate toward and to enter lymphatics and blood vessels. On entering the vasculature, tumor cells commonly initiate clotting by mechanisms that were discussed earlier. In some instances, as in the case of renal cell carcinoma, intravascular clotting may be extensive, with tumor cells becoming enmeshed in thrombi that fill the renal vein; these may extend to thrombose the inferior vena cava. In other instances, tumor cells entering the blood stream detach and circulate individually or in small clumps. However, passage through the circulation provides a challenge for many types of cancer cells, especially those of epithelial origin whose well-organized cytoskeleton is not designed for the compression and distortion encountered in passing through capillary beds. Most circulating cancer cells are cleared and destroyed in the first capillary bed they encounter, for example, in the lungs for cancer cells that enter the general venous circulation. It is not surprising, therefore, that metastasis is a highly inefficient process. Circulating tumor cells clearly need help if they are going to survive in the circulation, and they receive such help from platelets and activation of clotting.

## Role of Platelets in Metastasis

It has been known for many years that platelets have an important role in experimental tumor metastasis [reviewed in (16)]. Gasic et al. demonstrated in the late 1960s that thrombocytopenic mice developed fewer lung metastases following bolus intravenous injection of tumor cells. These experiments can be criticized because they do not closely mimic spontaneous tumor metastasis in which small numbers of tumor cells enter the circulation repeatedly over a long period of time. Nonetheless, a great deal of subsequent evidence has supported an association between platelets and tumor metastasis (356–358) and this relation may be very important given that patients with cancer commonly have increased numbers of activated platelets. Several classes of drugs that inhibit platelets, such as pyrimido–pyrimidine compounds (359) and prostacyclin (PGI$_2$), have been found to prevent tumor metastases (360).

The prometastatic effects of platelets relate in part to the fact that tumor cells activate platelets and form heteroaggregates with them by a variety of mechanisms, including platelet integrin glycoprotein (GP) IIb/IIIa ($\alpha_2\beta_3$), fibronectin, and von Willebrand factor (16,361); also, antibodies against von Willebrand factor or GP IIb/IIIa strikingly reduce hematogenous metastases in mice (356,361). P selectin, which mediates leukocyte adhesion to vascular endothelium and platelets under flow conditions, is also involved in the initial phase of adhesion of tumor cells to platelets (16,362), and P selectin–deficient mice exhibit decreased tumor growth and metastasis (363). Also, heparin, which among other activities inhibits tumor cell–platelet associations, also inhibits tumor metastasis (364). Thrombin may render tumor cells more adhesive to platelets and to endothelium not only by activating clotting, but also through activation of the PAR-1 receptor, which is present on some tumor cells (321,365–369).

Tumor cell–platelet heteroaggregates are thought to favor metastasis by at least four different mechanisms (361,362, 367,370): (a) They prolong the otherwise extremely short survival of tumor cells in the circulation, perhaps by shielding the tumor cells from host defense mechanisms (e.g., from NK cells) but also possibly by protecting tumor cells from physical forces as they pass through constricting capillary beds. (b) Activated platelets provide an adhesive surface that facilitates attachment to vascular endothelium, thereby facilitating downstream tumor cell extravasation. (c) Heteroaggregates form microemboli that damage downstream endothelial cells, again facilitating tumor cell extravasation by facilitating attachment to the subendothelial cell matrix. (d) Activated, tumor cell–associated platelets provide a source of cytokines that, along with tumor cell products, can permeabilize the vessel wall, promote the growth of arrested tumor cells, and stimulate the angiogenesis needed for tumor cell colonization.

## Roles of Clotting and Fibrinolysis in Metastasis

It is difficult to separate the roles of clotting from those of platelets in metastasis because platelets play such a central role in intravascular clotting. Nonetheless, there is a substantial literature documenting beneficial effects of anticoagulants in the prevention of metastases in experimental animals and also some evidence of benefit in the treatment of patients with cancer (371–375) (see Chapter 85). However, these studies are complicated by the fact that all of the agents tested have multiple activities, not all related to clotting.

Warfarin has been much used to reduce spontaneous tumor metastasis in animals (376). It is unlikely that the beneficial response observed can be attributed to an effect on primary tumor growth, but it is also uncertain if warfarin's effect can be attributed solely to its anticoagulant action (377). Warfarin interferes with the vitamin K–dependent, posttranslational carboxylation of glutamic acid residues. Many proteins in addition to the plasma procoagulant clotting factors VII, IX, X, and prothrombin require this modification for biologic function (378). For example, both of the natural anticoagulant proteins—protein C and protein S, which inactivate factors V and VIII and promote fibrinolysis—require vitamin K (379). Therefore, warfarin, long regarded as an anticoagulant, may also act in some circumstances to interfere with endogenous anticoagulant and fibrinolytic function and has many other biologic effects as well (372). Which, if any, of these actions accounts for its antimetastatic effects is unknown (113,372,380).

Heparin has been less consistently effective than warfarin in preventing tumor metastasis in animal models (376,381,

382). In some systems, heparin has been beneficial; in others, it has actually led to increased metastasis and even to the more rapid growth of primary tumors. However, the heparins are a diverse family of negatively charged proteoglycans, and not all heparins possess anticoagulant activity (383). Like warfarin, heparin has other biologic effects that may not relate to clotting. These include electrostatic binding to a wide variety of proteins; interference with lymphocyte recirculation; regulation of smooth muscle growth; effects on tumor cell proliferation; adhesion to vascular endothelium; migration and invasion; and angiogenesis [reviewed in (384)]. Therefore, some of the variability of the effects of heparin in these tumor models might be explained by the relative concentrations of different molecular species of heparins in the preparations used. Studies with low-molecular-weight heparin have been encouraging [see (385), Chapter 85 for review].

More recent studies have found that blocking the coagulation cascade at the levels of TF, factor Xa, or thrombin by more specific agents can also inhibit hematogenous metastasis (307,317,386–392). These studies made use of reagents such as antibodies to TF, the specific thrombin inhibitor hirudin, and the TFPI. They also demonstrated that the effects of TF on metastasis can be mediated both by activation of clotting (TF extracellular domain) and by cell signaling (cytoplasmic domain) (307,369,387,391,392).

Finally, a small number of studies have been performed with fibrinolytic and antifibrinolytic agents. One report demonstrated a reduction in pulmonary metastases if streptokinase or recombinant tPA was administered within 30 minutes after inoculating rats with mammary carcinoma cells (393). Also, synthetic peptides based on the uPA-inhibited spontaneous metastases arising from the highly malignant mouse Lewis lung carcinoma but were ineffective in other cancers (394). Of interest, agents that inhibit fibrinolysis have also been found to be of benefit in at least some instances; therefore, tumor growth and metastasis can be blocked by antibodies against uPA, suggesting that metastatic success or failure is determined by an optimal balance of fibrinolytic activity (395).

## SUMMARY

This chapter has reviewed the evidence that abnormal hemostasis is a fundamental property of malignant disease, not merely an epiphenomenon attributable to therapy or to chronic illness. Data supporting this view have developed rapidly in recent years and are now quite convincing. Tumor cells commonly express procoagulants such as TF and act again late in the coagulation pathway to provide a surface for prothrombinase generation. In addition, tumor cells activate platelets and secrete mediators that stimulate expression of procoagulants in host stromal macrophages and endothelial cells. Together, these activities create a systemic hypercoagulable state that frequently manifests itself in the form of abnormal laboratory tests and clinical thromboembolic disease (the second-most common cause of death in patients with cancer). Also, tumor cells and the stromal cells they activate secrete VEGF-A and other members of the VPF/VEGF family. These factors permeabilize the blood vessels supplying tumors, allowing fibrinogen and other plasma clotting proteins to leak into the extravascular space where tumor and host cell procoagulants initiate clotting. The resulting fibrin gel provides a surface for tumor and host cell migration and serves as a provisional matrix that is replaced over time by mature stroma. VEGF-A is also the prime mover of tumor angiogenesis. However, its activities are supplemented by those of other growth factors and by clotting proteins, particularly TF and thrombin, that act by both clotting-dependent and clotting-independent mechanisms.

Tumor cells entering the blood also activate the clotting system and form heteroaggregates with platelets that favor their ability to survive and colonize at distant sites. Taken together, it is clear that the clotting system plays a central role in the biology of tumor growth, invasion, and metastasis. Much more needs to be learned, but it is already clear that exciting times lie ahead for investigators working at the interface between tumor biology and hemostasis.

# ACKNOWLEDGMENTS

Preparation of this chapter was supported by U.S. Public Health Service grants CA-50453, HL-59316, and P01CA-92644 and by a contract from the National Foundation for Cancer Research (Dr. Dvorak) and by U.S. Public Health Service grants CA22202, CA60429, and the Centers for Disease Control and Prevention (Dr. Rickles).

## *References*

1. Trousseau A. *Plegmasia alba dolens*, Vol 3. Paris: JB Balliere et Fils, 1865.
2. Sack GH Jr, Levin J, Bell WR. Trousseau's syndrome and other manifestations of chronic disseminated coagulopathy in patients with neoplasms: clinical, pathophysiologic, and therapeutic features. *Medicine (Baltimore)* 1977;56(1):1–37.
3. Stolinsky DC. Trousseau's phenomenon. *Blood* 1983;62(6):1304.
4. Prins M, Otten H-M. Thrombosis and cancer: a short history of Trousseau's syndrome. In: Lugassy G, Fanlanga A, Kakkar A, et al., eds. *Thrombosis and cancer*. London: Taylor & Francis, 2004:1–10.
5. Rickles FR, Levine MN. Venous thromboembolism in malignancy and malignancy in venous thromboembolism. *Haemostasis* 1998;28(Suppl. 3):43–49.
6. Lugassy G, Yoffe B. Thrombotic complications of overt cancer. In: Lugassy G, Fanlanga A, Kakkar A, et al., eds. *Thrombosis and cancer*, London: Taylor & Francis, 2004:109–115.
7. Levine M, Gent M, Hirsh J, et al. A comparison of low-molecular-weight heparin administered primarily at home with unfractionated heparin administered in the hospital for proximal deep-vein thrombosis. *N Engl J Med* 1996;334(11):677–681.
8. Levitan N, Dowlati A, Remick SC, et al. Rates of initial and recurrent thromboembolic disease among patients with malignancy versus those without malignancy. Risk analysis using Medicare claims data. *Medicine (Baltimore)* 1999;78(5):285–291.
9. Levine MN, Gent M, Hirsh J, et al. The thrombogenic effect of anticancer drug therapy in women with stage II breast cancer. *N Engl J Med* 1988;318(7):404–407.
10. Rickles FR, Patierno S, Fernandez PM. Tissue factor, thrombin, and cancer. *Chest* 2003;124(Suppl. 3):58S–68S.
11. Kakkar A, Petralia G. Thromboprophylaxis in cancer surgery. In: Lugassy G, Fanlanga A, Kakkar A, et al., eds. *Thrombosis and cancer*. London: Taylor & Francis, 2004:163–178.
12. Levi M. Systemic microangiopathies in the cancer patient. In: Lugassy G, Fanlanga A, Kakkar A, et al., eds. *Thrombosis and cancer*. London: Taylor & Francis, 2004:117–127.
13. Luzzatto G, Schafer AI. The prethrombotic state in cancer. *Semin Oncol* 1990;17(2):147–159.
14. Nand S, Fisher SG, Salgia R, et al. Hemostatic abnormalities in untreated cancer: incidence and correlation with thrombotic and hemorrhagic complications. *J Clin Oncol* 1987;5(12):1998–2003.
15. Edwards RL, Rickles FR, Moritz TE, et al. Abnormalities of blood coagulation tests in patients with cancer. *Am J Clin Pathol* 1987;88(5):596–602.
16. Klepfish A, Schattner A, Lugassy G. Platlets and cancer. In: Lugassy G, Fanlanga A, Kakkar A, et al., eds. *Thrombosis and cancer*. London: Taylor & Francis, 2004:31–46.
17. Rickles FR, Levine M, Edwards RL. Hemostatic alterations in cancer patients. *Cancer Metastasis Rev* 1992;11(3-4):237–248.
18. Green D, Maliekel K, Sushko E, et al. Activated-protein-C resistance in cancer patients. *Haemostasis* 1997;27(3):112–118.
19. Goad KE, Gralnick HR. Coagulation disorders in cancer. *Hematol Oncol Clin North Am* 1996;10(2):457–484.
20. Steingart RH. Coagulation disorders associated with neoplastic disease. *Recent Results Cancer Res* 1988;108:37–43.
21. Rivkin SE, Green S, Metch B, et al. Adjuvant CMFVP versus tamoxifen versus concurrent CMFVP and tamoxifen for postmenopausal, node-positive, and estrogen receptor-positive breast cancer patients: a Southwest Oncology Group study. *J Clin Oncol* 1994;12(10):2078–2085.
22. Miller SP, Sanchez-Avalos J, Stefanski T, et al. Coagulation disorders in cancer. I. Clinical and laboratory studies. *Cancer* 1967;20(9):1452–1465.
23. Hunt FA, Rylatt DB, Hart RA, et al. Serum crosslinked fibrin (XDP) and fibrinogen/fibrin degradation products (FDP) in disorders associated with activation of the coagulation or fibrinolytic systems. *Br J Haematol* 1985;60(4):715–722.
24. Wilde JT, Kitchen S, Kinsey S, et al. Plasma D-dimer levels and their relationship to serum fibrinogen/fibrin degradation products in hypercoagulable states. *Br J Haematol* 1989;71(1):65–70.
25. McCulloch P, Douglas J, Lowe GD, et al. *In vivo* measurements of fibrin formation and fibrinolysis in operable breast cancer. *Thromb Haemost* 1989;61(2):318–321.
26. Gadducci A, Baicchi U, Marrai R, et al. Pretreatment plasma levels of fibrinopeptide-A (FPA), D-dimer (DD), and von Willebrand factor (vWF) in patients with ovarian carcinoma. *Gynecol Oncol* 1994;53(3):352–356.
27. Falanga A, Ofosu FA, Delaini F, et al. The hypercoagulable state in cancer patients: evidence for impaired thrombin inhibitions. *Blood Coagul Fibrinolysis* 1994;5(Suppl. 1):S19–S23; discussion 59–64.
28. von Tempelhoff GF, Dietrich M, Hommel G, et al. Blood coagulation during adjuvant epirubicin/cyclophosphamide chemotherapy in patients with primary operable breast cancer. *J Clin Oncol* 1996;14(9):2560–2568.
29. Falanga A, Levine MN, Consonni R, et al. The effect of very-low-dose warfarin on markers of hypercoagulation in metastatic breast cancer: results from a randomized trial. *Thromb Haemost* 1998;79(1):23–27.
30. Carr JM, McKinney M, McDonagh J. Diagnosis of disseminated intravascular coagulation. Role of D-dimer. *Am J Clin Pathol* 1989;91(3):280–287.
31. Mombelli G, Roux A, Haeberli A, et al. Comparison of 125I-fibrinogen kinetics and fibrinopeptide A in patients with disseminated neoplasias. *Blood* 1982;60(2):381–388.
32. Robson EB, Murawski GF, Bettigole RE. Use of 125I-fibrinogen kinetic data to detect disseminated intravascular coagulation and deposition of fibrin in patients with metastatic cancer. *Thromb Haemost* 1977;37(3):484–508.
33. Yoda Y, Abe T. Fibrinopeptide A (FPA) level and fibrinogen kinetics in patients with malignant disease. *Thromb Haemost* 1981;46(4):706–709.
34. Bauer KA, Rosenberg RD. Thrombin generation in acute promyelocytic leukemia. *Blood* 1984;64(4):791–796.
35. Costantini V, De Monte P, Cazzato AO, et al. Systemic thrombin generation in cancer patients is correlated with extrinsic pathway activation. *Blood Coagul Fibrinolysis* 1998;9(1):79–84.
36. Iversen LH, Okholm M, Thorlacius-Ussing O. Pre- and postoperative state of coagulation and fibrinolysis in plasma of patients with benign and malignant colorectal disease—a preliminary study. *Thromb Haemost* 1996;76(4):523–528.
37. Tricerri A, Vangeli M, Errani AR, et al. Plasma thrombin-antithrombin complexes, latent coagulation disorders and metastatic spread in lung cancer: a longitudinal study. *Oncology* 1996;53(6):455–460.
38. Okamoto K, Takaki A, Takeda S, et al. Coagulopathy in disseminated intravascular coagulation due to abdominal sepsis: determination of prothrombin fragment 1 + 2 and other markers. *Haemostasis* 1992;22(1):17–24.
39. Honegger H, Anderson N, Hewitt LA, et al. Antithrombin III profiles in malignancy, relationship primary tumors and metastatic sites. *Thromb Haemost* 1981;46(2):500–503.
40. Rodeghiero F, Mannucci PM, Vigano S, et al. Liver dysfunction rather than intravascular coagulation as the main cause of low protein C and antithrombin III in acute leukemia. *Blood* 1984;63(4):965–969.
41. Rubin RN, Kies MS, Posch JJ Jr. Measurements of antithrombin III in solid tumor patients with and without hepatic metastases. *Thromb Res* 1980;18(3-4):353–360.
42. Wajima T. Fibrinolytic profiles in patients with small cell carcinoma of the lung. *Semin Thromb Hemost* 1991;17(3):280–285.
43. Troy K, Essex D, Rand J, et al. Protein C and S levels in acute leukemia. *Am J Hematol* 1991;37(3):159–162.
44. Feffer SE, Carmosino LS, Fox RL. Acquired protein C deficiency in patients with breast cancer receiving cyclophosphamide, methotrexate, and 5-fluorouracil. *Cancer* 1989;63(7):1303–1307.
45. Ratnoff OD. Hemostatic emergencies in malignancy. *Semin Oncol* 1989;16(6):561–571.
46. Rocha E, Paramo JA, Fernandez FJ, et al. Clotting activation and impairment of fibrinolysis in malignancy. *Thromb Res* 1989;54(6):699–707.
47. Khoo SK, Rylatt DB, Parsons P, et al. Serial D-dimer levels in the assessment of tumor mass and clinical outcome in ovarian cancer. *Gynecol Oncol* 1988;29(2):188–198.
48. Uchiyama T, Matsumoto M, Kobayashi N. Studies on the pathogenesis of coagulopathy in patients with arterial thromboembolism and malignancy. *Thromb Res* 1990;59(6):955–965.
49. Simonneau G, Charbonnier B, Decousus H, et al. Subcutaneous low-molecular-weight heparin compared with continuous intravenous unfractionated heparin in the treatment of proximal deep vein thrombosis. *Arch Intern Med* 1993;153(13):1541–1546.
50. Falanga A, Marchetti M, Vignoli A. Pathogenesis of thrombosis in cancer. In: Lugassy G, Fanlanga A, Kakkar A, et al., eds. *Thrombosis and cancer*. London: Taylor & Francis, 2004:11–29.
51. Sweeney JD, Killion KM, Pruet CF, et al. von Willebrand factor in head and neck cancer. *Cancer* 1990;66(11):2387–2389.

52. Lindahl AK, Jacobsen PB, Sandset PM, et al. Tissue factor pathway inhibitor with high anticoagulant activity is increased in post-heparin plasma and in plasma from cancer patients. *Blood Coagul Fibrinolysis* 1991;2(6):713–721.

53. Kakkar AK, DeRuvo N, Chinswangwatanakul V, et al. Extrinsic-pathway activation in cancer with high factor VIIa and tissue factor. *Lancet* 1995; 346(8981):1004–1005.

54. Schernthaner G, Ludwig H, Silberbauer K. Elevated plasma beta-thromboglobulin levels in multiple myeloma and in polycythaemia vera. *Acta Haematol* 1979;62(4):219–222.

55. Myers TJ, Rickles FR, Barb C, et al. Fibrinopeptide A in acute leukemia: relationship of activation of blood coagulation to disease activity. *Blood* 1981;57(3):518–525.

56. Peuscher FW, Cleton FJ, Armstrong L, et al. Significance of plasma fibrinopeptide A (fpA) in patients with malignancy. *J Lab Clin Med* 1980; 96(1):5–14.

57. Green K, Silverstein R. Hypercoagulability and cancer. *Hematol Oncol Clin North Am* 1996;10:499–530.

58. Edwards RL, Rickles FR, Cronlund M. Abnormalities of blood coagulation in patients with cancer. Mononuclear cell tissue factor generation. *J Lab Clin Med* 1981;98(6):917–928.

59. Hoffman R, Brenner B. Thrombophilia and the risk of venous thromboembolism in cancer. In: Lugassy G, Fanlanga A, Kakkar A, et al., eds. *Thrombosis and cancer*. London: Taylor & Francis, 2004:129–136.

60. Goldsmith G. Hemostatic disorders associated with neoplasia. In: Ratnoff O, Forbes C, eds. *Disorders of hemostasis*. Philadelphia, PA: Grunde and Stratton, 1991:352–368.

61. Kies MS, Posch JJ Jr, Giolma JP, et al. Hemostatic function in cancer patients. *Cancer* 1980;46(4):831–837.

62. Rutherford CJ, Frenkel EP. Thrombocytopenia. Issues in diagnosis and therapy. *Med Clin North Am* 1994;78(3):555–575.

63. Porrata LF, Alberts S, Hook C, et al. Idiopathic thrombocytopenic purpura associated with breast cancer: a case report and review of the current literature. *Am J Clin Oncol* 1999;22(4):411–413.

64. Bachmeyer C, Audouin J, Bouillot JL, et al. Immune thrombocytopenic purpura as the presenting feature of gastric MALT lymphoma. *Am J Gastroenterol* 2000;95(6):1599–1600.

65. Lesesne JB, Rothschild N, Erickson B, et al. Cancer-associated hemolytic-uremic syndrome: analysis of 85 cases from a national registry. *J Clin Oncol* 1989;7(6):781–789.

66. Kwaan HC, Gordon LI. Thrombotic microangiopathy in the cancer patient. *Acta Haematol* 2001;106(1-2):52–56.

67. Francis JL. Haemostasis and cancer. *Med Lab Sci* 1989;46(4):331–346.

68. Boneu B, Bugat R, Boneu A, et al. Exhausted platelets in patients with malignant solid tumors without evidence of active consumption coagulopathy. *Eur J Cancer Clin Oncol* 1984;20(7):899–903.

69. Sloand EM, Kenney DM, Chao FC, et al. Platelet antithrombin defect in malignancy: platelet protein alterations. *Blood* 1987;69(2):479–485.

70. Virchow R. *Cellular pathology*. London: Churchill Livingstone, 1866.

71. Falanga A, Rickles FR. Pathophysiology of the thrombophilic state in the cancer patient. *Semin Thromb Hemost* 1999;25(2):173–182.

72. Hollen CW, Henthorn J, Koziol JA, et al. Elevated serum interleukin-6 levels in patients with reactive thrombocytosis. *Br J Haematol* 1991;79(2):286–290.

73. Kaser A, Brandacher G, Steurer W, et al. Interleukin-6 stimulates thrombopoiesis through thrombopoietin: role in inflammatory thrombocytosis. *Blood* 2001;98(9):2720–2725.

74. Komura E, Matsumura T, Kato T, et al. Thrombopoietin in patients with hepatoblastoma. *Stem Cells* 1998;16(5):329–333.

75. Hsu HC, Tsai WH, Jiang ML, et al. Circulating levels of thrombopoietic and inflammatory cytokines in patients with clonal and reactive thrombocytosis. *J Lab Clin Med* 1999;134(4):392–397.

76. Grignani G, Jamieson GA. Platelets in tumor metastasis: generation of adenosine diphosphate by tumor cells is specific but unrelated to metastatic potential. *Blood* 1988;71(4):844–849.

77. Varon D, Brill A. Platelets cross-talk with tumor cells. *Haemostasis* 2001; 31(Suppl. 1):64–66.

78. Felding-Habermann B. Tumor cell-platelet interaction in metastatic disease. *Haemostasis* 2001;31(Suppl. 1):55–58.

79. Poggi A, Rossi C, Beviglia L, et al. Platelet-tumor cell interactions. In: Joseph M, ed. *The handbook of immunopharmacology*. London: Academic Press, 1995:151–165.

80. Bevilacqua MP, Pober JS, Majeau GR, et al. Recombinant tumor necrosis factor induces procoagulant activity in cultured human vascular endothelium: characterization and comparison with the actions of interleukin 1. *Proc Natl Acad Sci U S A* 1986;83(12):4533–4537.

81. Moore KL, Esmon CT, Esmon NL. Tumor necrosis factor leads to the internalization and degradation of thrombomodulin from the surface of bovine aortic endothelial cells in culture. *Blood* 1989;73(1):159–165.

82. Falanga A, Marchetti M, Giovanelli S, et al. All-trans-retinoic acid counteracts endothelial cell procoagulant activity induced by a human promyelocytic leukemia-derived cell line (NB4). *Blood* 1996;87(2):613–617.

83. Maiolo A, Tua A, Grignani G. Hemostasis and cancer: tumor cells induce the expression of tissue factor-like procoagulant activity on endothelial cells. *Haematologica* 2002;87(6):624–628.

84. van Hinsbergh VW, Bauer KA, Kooistra T, et al. Progress of fibrinolysis during tumor necrosis factor infusions in humans. Concomitant increase in tissue-type plasminogen activator, plasminogen activator inhibitor type-1, and fibrin(ogen) degradation products. *Blood* 1990;76(11):2284–2289.

85. Clauss M, Gerlach M, Gerlach H, et al. Vascular permeability factor: a tumor-derived polypeptide that induces endothelial cell and monocyte procoagulant activity, and promotes monocyte migration. *J Exp Med* 1990;172(6):1535–1545.

86. Contrino J, Hair G, Kreutzer DL, et al. In situ detection of tissue factor in vascular endothelial cells: correlation with the malignant phenotype of human breast disease. *Nat Med* 1996;2(2):209–215.

87. Fernandez PM, Patierno SR, Rickles FR. Tissue factor and fibrin in tumor angiogenesis. *Semin Thromb Hemost* 2004;30(1):31–44.

88. Clauss M, Murray JC, Vianna M, et al. A polypeptide factor produced by fibrosarcoma cells that induces endothelial tissue factor and enhances the procoagulant response to tumor necrosis factor/cachectin. *J Biol Chem* 1990;265(12):7078–7083.

89. Nawroth PP, Handley DA, Esmon CT, et al. Interleukin 1 induces endothelial cell procoagulant while suppressing cell-surface anticoagulant activity. *Proc Natl Acad Sci U S A* 1986;83(10):3460–3464.

90. Miyauchi S, Moroyama T, Kyoizumi S, et al. Malignant tumor cell lines produce interleukin-1-like factor. *In Vitro Cell Dev Biol* 1988;24(8):753–758.

91. Nawroth P, Handley D, Matsueda G, et al. Tumor necrosis factor/cachectin-induced intravascular fibrin formation in meth A fibrosarcomas. *J Exp Med* 1988;168(2):637–647.

92. Shoji M, Hancock WW, Abe K, et al. Activation of coagulation and angiogenesis in cancer: immunohistochemical localization in situ of clotting proteins and vascular endothelial growth factor in human cancer. *Am J Pathol* 1998;152(2):399–411.

93. Morgan D, Edwards RL, Rickles FR. Monocyte procoagulant activity as a peripheral marker of clotting activation in cancer patients. *Haemostasis* 1988;18(1):55–65.

94. Costantini V, Zacharski LR, Memoli VA, et al. Fibrinogen deposition and macrophage-associated fibrin formation in malignant and nonmalignant lymphoid tissue. *J Lab Clin Med* 1992;119(2):124–131.

95. Semeraro N, Colucci M. Tissue factor in health and disease. *Thromb Haemost* 1997;78(1):759–764.

96. Aeed PA, Nakajima M, Welch DR. The role of polymorphonuclear leukocytes (PMN) on the growth and metastatic potential of 13762NF mammary adenocarcinoma cells. *Int J Cancer* 1988;42(5):748–759.

97. Welch DR, Schissel DJ, Howrey RP, et al. Tumor-elicited polymorphonuclear cells, in contrast to "normal" circulating polymorphonuclear cells, stimulate invasive and metastatic potentials of rat mammary adenocarcinoma cells. *Proc Natl Acad Sci U S A* 1989;86(15):5859–5863.

98. Wu QD, Wang JH, Condron C, et al. Human neutrophils facilitate tumor cell transendothelial migration. *Am J Physiol Cell Physiol* 2001;280(4):C814–C822.

99. Falanga A, Marchetti M, Evangelista V, et al. Neutrophil activation and hemostatic changes in healthy donors receiving granulocyte colony-stimulating factor. *Blood* 1999;93(8):2506–2514.

100. Boggust WA, O'Meara RA, Fullerton WW. Diffusible thromboplastins of human cancer and chorion tissue. *Eur J Cancer* 1968;3(6):467–473.

101. Gordon SG, Lewis BJ. Comparison of procoagulant activity in tissue culture medium from normal and transformed fibroblasts. *Cancer Res* 1978;38(8):2467–2472.

102. Curatolo L, Colucci M, Cambini AL, et al. Evidence that cells from experimental tumours can activate coagulation factor X. *Br J Cancer* 1979;40(2):228–233.

103. Gordon SG, Cross BA. A factor X-activating cysteine protease from malignant tissue. *J Clin Invest* 1981;67(6):1665–1671.

104. Dvorak HF, Van DeWater L, Bitzer AM, et al. Procoagulant activity associated with plasma membrane vesicles shed by cultured tumor cells. *Cancer Res* 1983;43(9):4434–4442.

105. Semeraro N, Donati M. Pathways of blood clotting initiation by cancer cells. In: Donati M, Davidson J, Garattini S, eds. *Malignancy and the hemostatic system*. New York: Raven Press, 1981:1–32.

106. Gordon S. Evidence for a tumor proteinase in blood coagulation. In: Honn K, Sloane B, eds. *Hemostatic mechanisms and metastasis*. Boston, MA: Martinus Nijhoff, 1984:72–83.

107. Edwards RL, Morgan DL, Rickles FR. Animal tumor procoagulants: registry of the Subcommittee on Haemostasis and Malignancy of the Scientific and Standardization Committee, International Society of Thrombosis and Haemostasis. *Thromb Haemost* 1990;63(1):133–138.

108. Edwards RL, Silver J, Rickles FR. Human tumor procoagulants: registry of the Subcommittee on Haemostasis and Malignancy of the Scientific and Standardization Committee, International Society on Thrombosis and Haemostasis. *Thromb Haemost* 1993;69(2):205–213.

109. Laki K, Tyler HM, Yancey ST. Clot forming and clot stabilizing enzymes from the mouse tumor YPC-1. *Biochem Biophys Res Commun* 1966;22(5):776–781.

110. Hettasch JM, Bandarenko N, Burchette JL, et al. Tissue transglutaminase expression in human breast cancer. *Lab Invest* 1996;75(5):637–645.

111. Van De Water L, Tracy PB, Aronson D, et al. Tumor cell generation of thrombin via functional prothrombinase assembly. *Cancer Res* 1985;45(11 Pt 1):5521–5525.

112. Kreyberg L. Histologic typing of lung tumors. In: Kreyberg L, ed. *International histologic classification of tumors*, No. 1. Geneva: World Health Organization, 1967:19–36.

113. Zacharski LR, Wojtukiewicz MZ, Costantini V, et al. Pathways of coagulation/fibrinolysis activation in malignancy. *Semin Thromb Hemost* 1992;18(1):104–116.

114. Callander NS, Varki N, Rao LV. Immunohistochemical identification of tissue factor in solid tumors. *Cancer* 1992;70(5):1194–1201.

115. Luther T, Flossel C, Mackman N, et al. Tissue factor expression during human and mouse development. *Am J Pathol* 1996;149(1):101–113.

116. Abe K, Shoji M, Chen J, et al. Regulation of vascular endothelial growth factor production and angiogenesis by the cytoplasmic tail of tissue factor. *Proc Natl Acad Sci U S A* 1999;96(15):8663–8668.

117. Gordon SG, Chelladurai M. Non-tissue factor procoagulants in cancer cells. *Cancer Metastasis Rev* 1992;11(3-4):267–282.

118. Adida C, Ambrosini G, Plescia J, et al. Protease receptors in Hodgkin's disease: expression of the factor Xa receptor, effector cell protease receptor-1, in Reed-Sternberg cells. *Blood* 1996;88(4):1457–1464.

119. Wojtukiewicz MZ, Sierko E, Rak J. Contribution of the hemostatic system to angiogenesis in cancer. *Semin Thromb Hemost* 2004;30(1):5–20.

120. Dvorak HF, Quay SC, Orenstein NS, et al. Tumor shedding and coagulation. *Science* 1981;212(4497):923–924.

121. Edwards R, Brande W. Tissue factor procoagulant activity is expressed by fibroblast- and monocyte-free preparations of the VX2 carcinoma grown in nude mice. *Clin Res* 1989;47:406a; (Abstract).

122. Guan M, Su B, Lu Y. Quantitative reverse transcription-PCR measurement of tissue factor mRNA in glioma. *Mol Biotechnol* 2002;20(2):123–129.

123. Nakasaki T, Wada H, Shigemori C, et al. Expression of tissue factor and vascular endothelial growth factor is associated with angiogenesis in colorectal cancer. *Am J Hematol* 2002;69(4):247–254.

124. Grignani G, Jamieson GA. Tissue factor-dependent activation of platelets by cells and microvesicles of SK-OS-10 human osteogenic sarcoma cell line. *Invasion Metastasis* 1987;7(3):172–182.

125. Maruyama M, Yagawa K, Hayashi S, et al. Presence of thrombosis-inducing activity in plasma from patients with lung cancer. *Am Rev Respir Dis* 1989;140(3):778–781.

126. Ogino H, Hayashi S, Kawasaki M, et al. Association of thrombosis-inducing activity (TIA) with fatal hypercoagulable complications in patients with lung cancer. *Chest* 1994;105(6):1683–1686.

127. Kim HK, Song KS, Park YS, et al. Elevated levels of circulating platelet microparticles, VEGF, IL-6 and RANTES in patients with gastric cancer: possible role of a metastasis predictor. *Eur J Cancer* 2003;39(2):184–191.

128. Falanga A, Gordon SG. Isolation and characterization of cancer procoagulant: a cysteine proteinase from malignant tissue. *Biochemistry* 1985;24(20):5558–5567.

129. Alessio MG, Falanga A, Consonni R, et al. Cancer procoagulant in acute lymphoblastic leukemia. *Eur J Haematol* 1990;45(2):78–81.

130. Falanga A, Alessio MG, Donati MB, et al. A new procoagulant in acute leukemia. *Blood* 1988;71(4):870–875.

131. Donati MB, Gambacorti-Passerini C, Casali B, et al. Cancer procoagulant in human tumor cells: evidence from melanoma patients. *Cancer Res* 1986;46(12 Pt 1):6471–6474.

132. Tracy PB, Nesheim ME, Mann KG. Coordinate binding of factor Va and factor Xa to the unstimulated platelet. *J Biol Chem* 1981;256(2):743–751.

133. Nicholson AC, Nachman RL, Altieri DC, et al. Effector cell protease receptor-1 is a vascular receptor for coagulation factor Xa. *J Biol Chem* 1996;271(45):28407–28413.

134. Sakai T, Kisiel W. Binding of human factors X and Xa to HepG2 and J82 human tumor cell lines. Evidence that factor Xa binds to tumor cells independent of factor Va. *J Biol Chem* 1990;265(16):9105–9113.

135. Leach ME, Bolton P, Sethi M, et al. Characterisation of a prothrombinase activator on the hepatoma derived cell-line, PLC/PRF/5. *Biochem Soc Trans* 1998;26(1):S14.

136. Tracy PB, Eide LL, Mann KG. Human prothrombinase complex assembly and function on isolated peripheral blood cell populations. *J Biol Chem* 1985;260(4):2119–2124.

137. Stern D, Nawroth P, Handley D, et al. An endothelial cell-dependent pathway of coagulation. *Proc Natl Acad Sci U S A* 1985;82(8):2523–2527.

138. Zhou H, Gabazza EC, Takeya H, et al. Prothrombin and its derivatives stimulate motility of melanoma cells. *Thromb Haemost* 1998;80(3):407–412.

139. Tallman MS, Hakimian D, Kwaan HC, et al. New insights into the pathogenesis of coagulation dysfunction in acute promyelocytic leukemia. *Leuk Lymphoma* 1993;11(1-2):27–36.

140. Hair GA, Padula S, Zeff R, et al. Tissue factor expression in human leukemic cells. *Leuk Res* 1996;20(1):1–11.

141. Drake TA, Ruf W, Morrissey JH, et al. Functional tissue factor is entirely cell surface expressed on lipopolysaccharide-stimulated human blood monocytes and a constitutively tissue factor-producing neoplastic cell line. *J Cell Biol* 1989;109(1):389–395.

142. Bauer KA, Conway EM, Bach R, et al. Tissue factor gene expression in acute myeloblastic leukemia. *Thromb Res* 1989;56(3):425–430.

143. Eiseman G, Stefanini M. Thromboplastic activity of leukemic white cells. *Proc Soc Exp Biol Med* 1954;86(4):763–765.

144. Gralnick HR, Abrell E. Studies of the procoagulant and fibrinolytic activity of promyelocytes in acute promyelocytic leukaemia. *Br J Haematol* 1973;24(1):89–99.

145. Gouault Heilmann M, Chardon E, Sultan C, et al. The procoagulant factor of leukaemic promyelocytes: demonstration of immunologic cross reactivity with human brain tissue factor. *Br J Haematol* 1975;30(2):151–158.

146. Barbui T, Finazzi G, Falanga A. The impact of all-trans-retinoic acid on the coagulopathy of acute promyelocytic leukemia. *Blood* 1998;91(9):3093–3102.

147. Stone RM, Mayer RJ. The unique aspects of acute promyelocytic leukemia. *J Clin Oncol* 1990; 8(11):1913–1921.

148. Cozzolino F, Torcia M, Miliani A, et al. Potential role of interleukin-1 as the trigger for diffuse intravascular coagulation in acute nonlymphoblastic leukemia. *Am J Med* 1988;84(2):240–250.

149. Carr JM, Dvorak AM, Dvorak HF. Circulating membrane vesicles in leukemic blood. *Cancer Res* 1985;45(11 Pt 2):5944–5951.

150. Billroth T. *Lectures on surgical pathology and therapeutics (translated from the 8th edition).* London: The New Sydenham Society, 1878.

151. Dvorak HF. Rous-Whipple Award Lecture. How tumors make bad blood vessels and stroma. *Am J Pathol* 2003;162(6):1747–1757.

152. Pettersson A, Nagy JA, Brown LF, et al. Heterogeneity of the angiogenic response induced in different normal adult tissues by vascular permeability factor/vascular endothelial growth factor. *Lab Invest* 2000;80(1):99–115.

153. Zhang Y, Deng Y, Wendt T, et al. Intravenous somatic gene transfer with antisense tissue factor restores blood flow by reducing tumor necrosis factor-induced tissue factor expression and fibrin deposition in mouse meth-A sarcoma. *J Clin Invest* 1996;97(10):2213–2224.

154. Huang X, Molema G, King S, et al. Tumor infarction in mice by antibody-directed targeting of tissue factor to tumor vasculature. *Science* 1997; 275(5299):47–550.

155. Hu Z, Sun Y, Garen A. Targeting tumor vasculature endothelial cells and tumor cells for immunotherapy of human melanoma in a mouse xenograft model. *Proc Natl Acad Sci U S A* 1999;96(14):8161–8166.

156. O'Meara RA. Coagulative properties of cancers. *Ir J Med Sci* 1958;394:474–479.

157. Spar IL, Bale WF, Marrack D, et al. 131-I-labeled antibodies to human fibrinogen. Diagnostic studies and therapeutic trials. *Cancer* 1967;20(5):865–870.

158. Day ED, Planinsek JA, Pressman D. Localization *in vivo* of radio-iodinated anti-rat-fibrin antibodies and radio-iodinated rat fibrinogen in the Murphy rat lymphosarcoma and in other transplantable rat tumors. *J Natl Cancer Inst* 1959;22(2):413–426.

159. Marrack D, Kubala M, Corry P, et al. Localization of intracranial tumors. Comparative study with 131-I-labeled antibody to human fibrinogen and neohydrin-203Hg. *Cancer* 1967;20(5):751–755.

160. Hiramoto R, Bernecky J, Jurandowski J, et al. Fibrin in human tumors. *Cancer Res* 1960;20:592–593.

161. Kodama Y, Tanaka K. Effect of urokinase on growth and metastases of rabbit V2 carcinoma. *Gann* 1978;69(1):9–18.

162. Dvorak HF, Orenstein NS, Carvalho AC, et al. Induction of a fibrin-gel investment: an early event in line 10 hepatocarcinoma growth mediated by tumor-secreted products. *J Immunol* 1979;122(1):166–174.

163. Dvorak HF, Dvorak AM, Manseau EJ, et al. Fibrin gel investment associated with line 1 and line 10 solid tumor growth, angiogenesis, and fibroplasia in guinea pigs. Role of cellular immunity, myofibroblasts, microvascular damage, and infarction in line 1 tumor regression. *J Natl Cancer Inst* 1979; 62(6):1459–1472.

164. Dvorak HF, Dickersin GR, Dvorak AM, et al. Human breast carcinoma: fibrin deposits and desmoplasia. Inflammatory cell type and distribution. Microvasculature and infarction. *J Natl Cancer Inst* 1981;67(2):335–345.

165. Harris NL, Dvorak AM, Smith J, et al. Fibrin deposits in Hodgkin's disease. *Am J Pathol* 1982;108(1):119–129.

166. Dvorak HF. Tumors: wounds that do not heal. Similarities between tumor stroma generation and wound healing. *N Engl J Med* 1986;315(26):1650–1659.

167. Dvorak HF, Harvey VS, McDonagh J. Quantitation of fibrinogen influx and fibrin deposition and turnover in line 1 and line 10 guinea pig carcinomas. *Cancer Res* 1984;44(8):3348–3354.

168. Brown LF, Van de Water L, Harvey VS, et al. Fibrinogen influx and accumulation of cross-linked fibrin in healing wounds and in tumor stroma. *Am J Pathol* 1988;130(3):455–465.

169. Brown LF, Asch B, Harvey VS, et al. Fibrinogen influx and accumulation of cross-linked fibrin in mouse carcinomas. *Cancer Res* 1988;48(7):1920–1925.

170. Nagy JA, Meyers MS, Masse EM, et al. Pathogenesis of ascites tumor growth: fibrinogen influx and fibrin accumulation in tissues lining the peritoneal cavity. *Cancer Res* 1995;55(2):369–375.

171. Nagy JA, Brown LF, Senger DR, et al. Pathogenesis of tumor stroma generation: a critical role for leaky blood vessels and fibrin deposition. *Biochim Biophys Acta* 1989;948(3):305–326.

172. Dvorak HF, Nagy JA, Dvorak AM. Structure of solid tumors and their vasculature: implications for therapy with monoclonal antibodies. *Cancer Cells* 1991;3(3):77–85.

173. Dvorak HF, Senger DR, Dvorak AM. Fibrin as a component of the tumor stroma: origins and biological significance. *Cancer Metastasis Rev* 1983; 2(1):41–73.

174. Dvorak H, Nagy J, Feng D. Tumor architecture and targeted delivery. In: Abrams P, Fritzberg A, eds. *Radioimmunotherapy of cancer.* New York: Marcel Dekker Inc, 2000:107–135.

175. Hui KY, Haber E, Matsueda GR. Monoclonal antibodies to a synthetic fibrin-like peptide bind to human fibrin but not fibrinogen. *Science* 1983;222(4628):1129–1132.

176. Simpson-Haidaris PJ, Rybarczyk B. Tumors and fibrinogen. The role of fibrinogen as an extracellular matrix protein. *Ann N Y Acad Sci* 2001; 936:406–425.

177. Lee SY, Lee KP, Lim JW. Identification and biosynthesis of fibrinogen in human uterine cervix carcinoma cells. *Thromb Haemost* 1996;75(3): 466–470.

178. Dvorak HF, Nagy JA, Dvorak JT, et al. Identification and characterization of the blood vessels of solid tumors that are leaky to circulating macromolecules. *Am J Pathol* 1988;133(1):95–109.

179. Underwood JC, Carr I. The ultrastructure and permeability characteristics of the blood vessels of a transplantable rat sarcoma. *J Pathol* 1972;107(3): 157–166.

180. Tanooka H, Kitamura Y, Sado T, et al. Evidence for involvement of mast cells in tumor suppression in mice. *J Natl Cancer Inst* 1982;69(6): 1305–1309.

181. Greenbaum LM. Pepstatin, an inhibitor of acid kininogenases and ascites retardant in neoplastic disease. *Fed Proc* 1979;38(13):2788–2791.

182. Matsumura Y, Kimura M, Yamamoto T, et al. Involvement of the kinin-generating cascade in enhanced vascular permeability in tumor tissue. *Jpn J Cancer Res* 1988;79(12):1327–1334.

183. Contrino J, Goralnick S, Qi J, et al. Fibrin induction of tissue factor expression in human vascular endothelial cells. *Circulation* 1997;96(2):605–613.

184. Gerdin B, Saldeen T. Effect of fibrin degradation products on microvascular permeability. *Thromb Res* 1978;13(6):995–1006.

185. Colman RW. The contact system and angiogenesis: potential for therapeutic control of malignancy. *Semin Thromb Hemost* 2004;30(1):45–61.

186. Senger DR, Galli SJ, Dvorak AM, et al. Tumor cells secrete a vascular permeability factor that promotes accumulation of ascites fluid. *Science* 1983; 219(4587):983–985.

187. Senger DR, Perruzzi CA, Feder J, et al. A highly conserved vascular permeability factor secreted by a variety of human and rodent tumor cell lines. *Cancer Res* 1986;46(11):5629–5632.

188. Senger DR, Connolly DT, Van de Water L, et al. Purification and NH2-terminal amino acid sequence of guinea pig tumor-secreted vascular permeability factor. *Cancer Res* 1990;50(6):1774–1778.

189. Boucher Y, Leunig M, Jain RK. Tumor angiogenesis and interstitial hypertension. *Cancer Res* 1996;56(18):4264–4266.

190. Nagy JA, Herzberg KT, Dvorak JM, et al. Pathogenesis of malignant ascites formation: initiating events that lead to fluid accumulation. *Cancer Res* 1993;53(11):2631–2643.

191. Nagy JA, Masse EM, Herzberg KT, et al. Pathogenesis of ascites tumor growth: vascular permeability factor, vascular hyperpermeability, and ascites fluid accumulation. *Cancer Res* 1995;55(2):360–368.

192. Dvorak HF, Senger DR, Dvorak AM, et al. Regulation of extravascular coagulation by microvascular permeability. *Science* 1985;227(4690): 1059–1061.

193. Altieri DC, Mannucci PM, Capitanio AM. Binding of fibrinogen to human monocytes. *J Clin Invest* 1986;78(4):968–976.

194. Dejana E, Languino LR, Polentarutti N, et al. Interaction between fibrinogen and cultured endothelial cells. Induction of migration and specific binding. *J Clin Invest* 1985;75(1):11–18.

195. Felding-Habermann B, Ruggeri AM, Cheresh DA. Distinct biological consequences of integrin alpha v beta 3-mediated melanoma cell adhesion to fibrinogen and its plasmic fragments. *J Biol Chem* 1992;267(8):5070–5077.

196. Brown LF, Lanir N, McDonagh J, et al. Fibroblast migration in fibrin gel matrices. *Am J Pathol* 1993;142(1):273–283.

197. Henschen A, Lottspeich F, Kehl M, et al. Covalent structure of fibrinogen. *Ann N Y Acad Sci* 1983;408:28–43.

198. Gorlatov S, Medved L. Interaction of fibrin(ogen) with the endothelial cell receptor VE-cadherin: mapping of the receptor-binding site in the NH2-terminal portions of the fibrin beta chains. *Biochemistry* 2002;41(12): 4107–4116.

199. Bunce LA, Sporn LA, Francis CW. Endothelial cell spreading on fibrin requires fibrinopeptide B cleavage and amino acid residues 15-42 of the beta chain. *J Clin Invest* 1992;89(3):842–850.

200. Sporn LA, Bunce LA, Francis CW. Cell proliferation on fibrin: modulation by fibrinopeptide cleavage. *Blood* 1995;86(5):1802–1810.

201. Martinez J, Ferber A, Bach TL, et al. Interaction of fibrin with VE-cadherin. *Ann N Y Acad Sci* 2001;936:386–405.

202. Altieri DC, Duperray A, Plescia J, et al. Structural recognition of a novel fibrinogen gamma chain sequence (117-133) by intercellular adhesion molecule-1 mediates leukocyte-endothelium interaction. *J Biol Chem* 1995;270(2):696–699.

203. Odrljin TM, Francis CW, Sporn LA, et al. Heparin-binding domain of fibrin mediates its binding to endothelial cells. *Arterioscler Thromb Vasc Biol* 1996;16(12):1544–1551.

204. Phillips DR, Charo IF, Parise LV, et al. The platelet membrane glycoprotein IIb-IIIa complex. *Blood* 1988;71(4):831–843.

205. Shattil SJ, Kashiwagi H, Pampori N. Integrin signaling: the platelet paradigm. *Blood* 1998;91(8):2645–2657.

206. Feng D, Nagy JA, Pyne K, et al. Platelets exit venules by a transcellular pathway at sites of F-met peptide-induced acute inflammation in guinea pigs. *Int Arch Allergy Immunol* 1998;116(3):188–195.

207. Dvorak HF, Harvey VS, Estrella P, et al. Fibrin containing gels induce angiogenesis. Implications for tumor stroma generation and wound healing. *Lab Invest* 1987;57(6):673–686.

208. van den Hooff A. Stromal involvement in malignant growth. *Adv Cancer Res* 1988;50:159–196.

209. Bissell MJ, Hall HG, Parry G. How does the extracellular matrix direct gene expression? *J Theor Biol* 1982;99(1):31–68.

210. Ruoslahti E. The Walter Herbert Lecture. Control of cell motility and tumour invasion by extracellular matrix interactions. *Br J Cancer* 1992;66(2): 239–242.

211. Fernandez P, Patierno S, Rickles F. Tumor angiogenesis and blood coagulation. In: Lugassy G, Fanlanga A, Kakkar A, et al., eds. *Thrombosis and cancer*. London: Taylor & Francis, 2004:69–98.

212. Sahni A, Francis CW. Vascular endothelial growth factor binds to fibrinogen and fibrin and stimulates endothelial cell proliferation. *Blood* 2000;96(12): 3772–3778.

213. Sahni A, Baker CA, Sporn LA, et al. Fibrinogen and fibrin protect fibroblast growth factor-2 from proteolytic degradation. *Thromb Haemost* 2000; 83(5):736–741.

214. Lalla RV, Goralnick SJ, Tanzer ML, et al. Fibrin induces IL-8 expression from human oral squamous cell carcinoma cells. *Oral Oncol* 2001;37(3): 234–242.

215. van Hinsbergh VW, Collen A, Koolwijk P. Role of fibrin matrix in angiogenesis. *Ann N Y Acad Sci* 2001;936:426–437.

216. Collen A, Maas A, Kooistra T, et al. Aberrant fibrin formation and cross-linking of fibrinogen Nieuwegein, a variant with a shortened Aalpha-chain, alters endothelial capillary tube formation. *Blood* 2001;97(4):973–980.

217. Palumbo JS, Kombrinck KW, Drew AF, et al. Fibrinogen is an important determinant of the metastatic potential of circulating tumor cells. *Blood* 2000;96(10):3302–3309.

218. Palumbo JS, Degen JL. Fibrinogen and tumor cell metastasis. *Haemostasis* 2001;31(Suppl. 1):11–15.

219. Mandriota SJ, Seghezzi G, Vassalli JD, et al. Vascular endothelial growth factor increases urokinase receptor expression in vascular endothelial cells. *J Biol Chem* 1995;270(17):9709–9716.

220. Goldberg GI, Frisch SM, He C, et al. Secreted proteases. Regulation of their activity and their possible role in metastasis. *Ann N Y Acad Sci* 1990;580:375–384.

221. Gualandris A, Presta M. Transcriptional and posttranscriptional regulation of urokinase-type plasminogen activator expression in endothelial cells by basic fibroblast growth factor. *J Cell Physiol* 1995;162(3):400–409.

222. Mignatti P, Mazzieri R, Rifkin DB. Expression of the urokinase receptor in vascular endothelial cells is stimulated by basic fibroblast growth factor. *J Cell Biol* 1991;113(5):1193–1201.

223. Bikfalvi A, Klein S, Pintucci G, et al. Biological roles of fibroblast growth factor-2. *Endocr Rev* 1997;18(1):26–45.

224. Dano K, Romer J, Nielsen BS, et al. Cancer invasion and tissue remodeling—cooperation of protease systems and cell types. *APMIS* 1999; 107(1):120–127.

225. Levin EG, Stern DM, Nawroth PP, et al. Specificity of the thrombin-induced release of tissue plasminogen activator from cultured human endothelial cells. *Thromb Haemost* 1986;56(2):115–119.

226. Dvorak HF, Form DM, Manseau EJ, et al. Pathogenesis of desmoplasia. I. Immunofluorescence identification and localization of some structural proteins of line 1 and line 10 guinea pig tumors and of healing wounds. *J Natl Cancer Inst* 1984;73(5):1195–1205.

227. Yeo TK, Brown L, Dvorak HF. Alterations in proteoglycan synthesis common to healing wounds and tumors. *Am J Pathol* 1991;138(6):1437–1450.

228. Vlodavsky I, Goldshmidt O, Zcharia E, et al. Mammalian heparanase: involvement in cancer metastasis, angiogenesis and normal development. *Semin Cancer Biol* 2002;12(2):121–129.

229. Bootle-Wilbraham CA, Tazzyman S, Marshall JM, et al. Fibrinogen E-fragment inhibits the migration and tubule formation of human dermal microvascular endothelial cells *in vitro*. *Cancer Res* 2000;60(17):4719–4724.

230. Thompson WD, Smith EB, Stirk CM, et al. Angiogenic activity of fibrin degradation products is located in fibrin fragment E. *J Pathol* 1992;168(1): 47–53.

231. Schlager SI, Dray S. Complete local tumor regression with antibody to fibrin Fragment E. *J Immunol* 1975;115(4):976–981.

232. Naldini L, Tamagnone L, Vigna E, et al. Extracellular proteolytic cleavage by urokinase is required for activation of hepatocyte growth factor/scatter factor. *EMBO J* 1992;11(13):4825–4833.

233. Gille J, Khalik M, Konig V, et al. Hepatocyte growth factor/scatter factor (HGF/SF) induces vascular permeability factor (VPF/VEGF) expression by cultured keratinocytes. *J Invest Dermatol* 1998;111(6):1160–1165.

234. Sato Y, Tsuboi R, Lyons R, et al. Characterization of the activation of latent TGF-beta by co-cultures of endothelial cells and pericytes or smooth muscle cells: a self-regulating system. *J Cell Biol* 1990;111(2):757–763.

235. Ferrara N. Vascular endothelial growth factor: molecular and biological aspects. *Curr Top Microbiol Immunol* 1999;237:1–30.

236. O'Reilly MS, Holmgren L, Chen C, et al. Angiostatin induces and sustains dormancy of human primary tumors in mice. *Nat Med* 1996;2(6):689–692.

237. Cao Y. Therapeutic potentials of angiostatin in the treatment of cancer. *Haematologica* 1999;84(7):643–650.

238. Dvorak HF. Vascular permeability factor/vascular endothelial growth factor: a critical cytokine in tumor angiogenesis and a potential target for diagnosis and therapy. *J Clin Oncol* 2002;20(21):4368–4380.

239. Jussila L, Alitalo K. Vascular growth factors and lymphangiogenesis. *Physiol Rev* 2002;82(3):673–700.

240. Carmeliet P, Moons L, Luttun A, et al. Synergism between vascular endothelial growth factor and placental growth factor contributes to angiogenesis and plasma extravasation in pathological conditions. *Nat Med* 2001;7(5):575–583.

241. Carmeliet P, Collen D. Role of vascular endothelial growth factor and vascular endothelial growth factor receptors in vascular development. *Curr Top Microbiol Immunol* 1999;237:133–158.

242. Brown LF, Detmar M, Claffey K, et al. Vascular permeability factor/vascular endothelial growth factor: a multifunctional angiogenic cytokine. *EXS* 1997;79:233–269.

243. Ferrara N. Molecular and biological properties of vascular endothelial growth factor. *J Mol Med* 1999;77(7):527–543.

244. Muller YA, Li B, Christinger HW, et al. Vascular endothelial growth factor: crystal structure and functional mapping of the kinase domain receptor binding site. *Proc Natl Acad Sci U S A* 1997;94(14):7192–7197.

245. Ferrara N, Carver-Moore K, Chen H, et al. Heterozygous embryonic lethality induced by targeted inactivation of the VEGF gene. *Nature* 1996;380(6573):439–442.

246. Carmeliet P, Ferreira V, Breier G, et al. Abnormal blood vessel development and lethality in embryos lacking a single VEGF allele. *Nature* 1996;380(6573):435–439.

247. Claffey KP, Senger DR, Spiegelman BM. Structural requirements for dimerization, glycosylation, secretion, and biological function of VPF/VEGF. *Biochim Biophys Acta* 1995;1246:1–9.

248. Tischer E, Mitchell R, Hartman T, et al. The human gene for vascular endothelial growth factor. Multiple protein forms are encoded through alternative exon splicing. *J Biol Chem* 1991;266:11947–11954.

249. Grunstein J, Masbad JJ, Hickey R, et al. Isoforms of vascular endothelial growth factor act in a coordinate fashion to recruit and expand tumor vasculature. *Mol Cell Biol* 2000;20(19):7282–7291.

250. Yu JL, Rak JW, Klement G, et al. Vascular endothelial growth factor isoform expression as a determinant of blood vessel patterning in human melanoma xenografts. *Cancer Res* 2002;62(6):1838–1846.

251. Ruhrberg C, Gerhardt H, Golding M, et al. Spatially restricted patterning cues provided by heparin-binding VEGF-A control blood vessel branching morphogenesis. *Genes Dev* 2002;16(20):2684–2698.

252. Maes C, Carmeliet P, Moermans K, et al. Impaired angiogenesis and endochondral bone formation in mice lacking the vascular endothelial growth factor isoforms VEGF164 and VEGF188. *Mech Dev* 2002;111(1-2):61–73.

253. Hlatky L, Tsionou C, Hahnfeldt P, et al. Mammary fibroblasts may influence breast tumor angiogenesis via hypoxia-induced vascular endothelial growth factor up-regulation and protein expression. *Cancer Res* 1994;54:6083–6086.

254. Detmar M, Brown LF, Berse B, et al. Hypoxia regulates the expression of vascular permeability factor/vascular endothelial growth factor (VPF/VEGF) and its receptors in human skin. *J Invest Dermatol* 1997;108(3):263–268.

255. Fukumura D, Xavier R, Sugiura T, et al. Tumor induction of VEGF promoter activity in stromal cells. *Cell* 1998;94(6):715–725.

256. Guidi AJ, Schnitt SJ, Fischer L, et al. Vascular permeability factor (vascular endothelial growth factor) expression and angiogenesis in patients with ductal carcinoma in situ of the breast. *Cancer* 1997;80(10):1945–1953.

257. Guidi AJ, Abu-Jawdeh G, Berse B, et al. Vascular permeability factor (vascular endothelial growth factor) expression and angiogenesis in cervical neoplasia. *J Natl Cancer Inst* 1995;87(16):1237–1245.

258. Dvorak HF, Nagy JA, Feng D, et al. Vascular permeability factor/vascular endothelial growth factor and the significance of microvascular hyperpermeability in angiogenesis. *Curr Top Microbiol Immunol* 1999;237:97–132.

259. Mukhopadhyay D, Tsiokas L, Zhou XM, et al. Hypoxic induction of human vascular endothelial growth factor expression through c-Src activation. *Nature* 1995;375(6532):577–581.

260. Rak J, Filmus J, Finkenzeller G, et al. Oncogenes as inducers of tumor angiogenesis. *Cancer Metastasis Rev* 1995;14(4):263–277.

261. Fukumura D, Xu L, Chen Y, et al. Hypoxia and acidosis independently up-regulate vascular endothelial growth factor transcription in brain tumors *in vivo*. *Cancer Res* 2001;61(16):6020–6024.

262. Kadambi A, Carreira CM, Yun CO, et al. Vascular endothelial growth factor (VEGF)-C differentially affects tumor vascular function and leukocyte recruitment: role of VEGF-receptor 2 and host VEGF-A. *Cancer Res* 2001;61(6):2404–2408.

263. Odorisio T, Schietroma C, Zaccaria ML, et al. Mice overexpressing placenta growth factor exhibit increased vascularization and vessel permeability. *J Cell Sci* 2002;115(Pt 12):2559–2567.

264. Benjamin LE, Golijanin D, Itin A, et al. Selective ablation of immature blood vessels in established human tumors follows vascular endothelial growth factor withdrawal [see comments]. *J Clin Invest* 1999;103(2):159–165.

265. Watanabe Y, Lee SW, Detmar M, et al. Vascular permeability factor/vascular endothelial growth factor (VPF/VEGF) delays and induces escape from senescence in human dermal microvascular endothelial cells. *Oncogene* 1997;14(17):2025–2032.

266. McDonald DM, Thurston G, Baluk P. Endothelial gaps as sites for plasma leakage in inflammation. *Microcirculation* 1999;6(1):7–22.

267. Kohn S, Nagy JA, Dvorak HF, et al. Pathways of macromolecular tracer transport across venules and small veins. Structural basis for the hyperpermeability of tumor blood vessels. *Lab Invest* 1992;67(5):596–607.

268. Dvorak AM, Kohn S, Morgan ES, et al. The vesiculo-vacuolar organelle (VVO): a distinct endothelial cell structure that provides a transcellular pathway for macromolecular extravasation. *J Leukoc Biol* 1996;59(1):100–115.

269. Feng D, Nagy JA, Hipp J, et al. Vesiculo-vacuolar organelles and the regulation of venule permeability to macromolecules by vascular permeability factor, histamine, and serotonin. *J Exp Med* 1996;183(5):1981–1986.

270. Feng D, Nagy JA, Hipp J, et al. Reinterpretation of endothelial cell gaps induced by vasoactive mediators in guinea-pig, mouse and rat: many are transcellular pores. *J Physiol* 1997;504(Pt 3):747–761.

271. Feng D, Nagy JA, Dvorak AM, et al. Different pathways of macromolecule extravasation from hyperpermeable tumor vessels. *Microvasc Res* 2000;59(1):24–37.

272. Stan RV, Tkachenko E, Niesman IR. PV1 is a key structural component for the formation of the stomatal and fenestral diaphragms. *Mol Biol Cell* 2004;15(8):3615–3630.

273. Roberts WG, Palade GE. Increased microvascular permeability and endothelial fenestration induced by vascular endothelial growth factor. *J Cell Sci* 1995;108(Pt 6):2369–2379.

274. Mustonen T, Alitalo K. Endothelial receptor tyrosine kinases involved in angiogenesis. *J Cell Biol* 1995;129:895–898.

275. Clauss M, Weich H, Breier G, et al. The vascular endothelial growth factor receptor Flt-1 mediates biological activities. Implications for a functional role of placenta growth factor in monocyte activation and chemotaxis. *J Biol Chem* 1996;271(30):17629–17634.

276. Mercurio AM, Bachelder RE, Bates RC, et al. Autocrine signaling in carcinoma: VEGF and the alpha6beta4 integrin. *Semin Cancer Biol* 2004;14(2):115–122.

277. Bates RC, Goldsmith JD, Bachelder RE, et al. Flt-1-dependent survival characterizes the epithelial-mesenchymal transition of colonic organoids. *Curr Biol* 2003;13(19):1721–1727.

278. Bachelder RE, Lipscomb EA, Lin X, et al. Competing autocrine pathways involving alternative neuropilin-1 ligands regulate chemotaxis of carcinoma cells. *Cancer Res* 2003;63(17):5230–5233.

279. Cross MJ, Dixelius J, Matsumoto T, et al. VEGF-receptor signal transduction. *Trends Biochem Sci* 2003;28(9):488–494.

280. Feng D, Nagy JA, Brekken RA, et al. Ultrastructural localization of the vascular permeability factor/vascular endothelial growth factor (VPF/VEGF) receptor-2 (FLK-1, KDR) in normal mouse kidney and in the hyperpermeable vessels induced by VPF/VEGF-expressing tumors and adenoviral vectors. *J Histochem Cytochem* 2000;48(4):545–556.

281. Soker S, Takashima S, Miao HQ, et al. Neuropilin-1 is expressed by endothelial and tumor cells as an isoform-specific receptor for vascular endothelial growth factor. *Cell* 1998;92(6):735–745.

282. Klagsbrun M, Takashima S, Mamluk R. The role of neuropilin in vascular and tumor biology. *Adv Exp Med Biol* 2002;515:33–48.

283. Wang L, Zeng H, Wang P, et al. Neuropilin-1-mediated vascular permeability factor/vascular endothelial growth factor-dependent endothelial cell migration. *J Biol Chem* 2003;278(49):48848–48860.

284. Rafii S, Lyden D, Benezra R, et al. Vascular and haematopoietic stem cells: novel targets for anti-angiogenesis therapy? *Nat Rev Cancer* 2002;2(11):826–835.

285. Mukhopadhyay D, Zeng H. Involvement of G proteins in vascular permeability factor/vascular endothelial growth factor signaling. *Cold Spring Harb Symp Quant Biol* 2002;67:275–283.

286. Rahimi N, Dayanir V, Lashkari K. Receptor chimeras indicate that the vascular endothelial growth factor receptor-1 (VEGFR-1) modulates mitogenic activity of VEGFR-2 in endothelial cells. *J Biol Chem* 2000;275(22):16986–16992.

287. Zeng H, Zhao D, Mukhopadhyay D. Flt-1-mediated down-regulation of endothelial cell proliferation through pertussis toxin-sensitive G proteins, beta gamma subunits, small GTPase CDC42, and partly by Rac-1. *J Biol Chem* 2002;277(6):4003–4009.

288. Clauss M, Grell M, Fangmann C, et al. Synergistic induction of endothelial tissue factor by tumor necrosis factor and vascular endothelial growth factor: functional analysis of the tumor necrosis factor receptors. *FEBS Lett* 1996;390(3):334–338.

289. Mechtcheriakova D, Wlachos A, Holzmuller H, et al. Vascular endothelial cell growth factor-induced tissue factor expression in endothelial cells is mediated by EGR-1. *Blood* 1999;93(11):3811–3823.

290. Blum S, Issbruker K, Willuweit A, et al. An inhibitory role of the phosphatidylinositol 3-kinase-signaling pathway in vascular endothelial growth factor-induced tissue factor expression. *J Biol Chem* 2001;276(36):33428–33434.

291. Kim I, Oh JL, Ryu YS, et al. Angiopoietin-1 negatively regulates expression and activity of tissue factor in endothelial cells. *FASEB J* 2002;16(1):126–128.

292. Warren BA. The vascular morphology of tumors. In: Peterson H-I, ed. *Tumor blood circulation: angiogenesis, vascular morphology and blood flow of experimental and human tumors.* Boca Raton, FL: CRC Press, 1979:1–47.

293. Sundberg C, Nagy JA, Brown LF, et al. Glomeruloid microvascular proliferation follows adenoviral vascular permeability factor/vascular endothelial growth factor-164 gene delivery. *Am J Pathol* 2001;158(3):1145–1160.

294. Nagy JA, Vasile E, Feng D, et al. VEGF-A induces angiogenesis, arteriogenesis, lymphangiogenesis, and vascular malformations. *Cold Spring Harb Symp Quant Biol* 2002;67:227–237.

295. Brown LF, Yeo KT, Berse B, et al. Expression of vascular permeability factor (vascular endothelial growth factor) by epidermal keratinocytes during wound healing. *J Exp Med* 1992;176(5):1375–1379.

296. Ren G, Michael LH, Entman ML, et al. Morphological characteristics of the microvasculature in healing myocardial infarcts. *J Histochem Cytochem* 2002;50(1):71–79.

297. Nagy JA, Vasile E, Feng D, et al. Vascular permeability factor/vascular endothelial growth factor induces lymphangiogenesis as well as angiogenesis. *J Exp Med* 2002;196(11):1497–1506.

298. Abdulkadir SA, Carvalhal GF, Kaleem Z, et al. Tissue factor expression and angiogenesis in human prostate carcinoma. *Hum Pathol* 2000;31(4):443–447.

299. Zhang Y, Deng Y, Luther T, et al. Tissue factor controls the balance of angiogenic and antiangiogenic properties of tumor cells in mice. *J Clin Invest* 1994;94(3):1320–1327.

300. Ollivier V, Bentolila S, Chabbat J, et al. Tissue factor-dependent vascular endothelial growth factor production by human fibroblasts in response to activated factor VII. *Blood* 1998;91(8):2698–2703.

301. Guan M, Jin J, Su B, et al. Tissue factor expression and angiogenesis in human glioma. *Clin Biochem* 2002;35(4):321–325.

302. Koomagi R, Volm M. Tissue-factor expression in human non-small-cell lung carcinoma measured by immunohistochemistry: correlation between tissue factor and angiogenesis. *Int J Cancer* 1998;79(1):19–22.

303. Camerer E, Rottingen JA, Iversen JG, et al. Coagulation factors VII and X induce Ca2+ oscillations in Madin-Darby canine kidney cells only when proteolytically active. *J Biol Chem* 1996;271(46):29034–29042.

304. Camerer E, Huang W, Coughlin SR. Tissue factor- and factor X-dependent activation of protease-activated receptor 2 by factor VIIa. *Proc Natl Acad Sci U S A* 2000;97(10):5255–5260.

305. Prydz H, Camerer E, Rottingen JA, et al. Cellular consequences of the initiation of blood coagulation. *Thromb Haemost* 1999;82(2):183–192.

306. Ollivier V, Chabbat J, Herbert JM, et al. Vascular endothelial growth factor production by fibroblasts in response to factor VIIa binding to tissue factor involves thrombin and factor Xa. *Arterioscler Thromb Vasc Biol* 2000;20(5):1374–1381.

307. Bromberg ME, Sundaram R, Homer RJ, et al. Role of tissue factor in metastasis: functions of the cytoplasmic and extracellular domains of the molecule. *Thromb Haemost* 1999;82(1):88–92.

308. Edgington TS, Mackman N, Brand K, et al. The structural biology of expression and function of tissue factor. *Thromb Haemost* 1991;66(1):67–79.

309. Bazan JF. Structural design and molecular evolution of a cytokine receptor superfamily. *Proc Natl Acad Sci U S A* 1990;87(18):6934–6938.

310. Zioncheck TF, Roy S, Vehar GA. The cytoplasmic domain of tissue factor is phosphorylated by a protein kinase C-dependent mechanism. *J Biol Chem* 1992;267(6):3561–3564.

311. Carmeliet P, Mackman N, Moons L, et al. Role of tissue factor in embryonic blood vessel development. *Nature* 1996;383(6595):73–75.

312. Bugge TH, Xiao Q, Kombrinck KW, et al. Fatal embryonic bleeding events in mice lacking tissue factor, the cell-associated initiator of blood coagulation. *Proc Natl Acad Sci U S A* 1996;93(13):6258–6263.

313. Toomey JR, Kratzer KE, Lasky NM, et al. Targeted disruption of the murine tissue factor gene results in embryonic lethality. *Blood* 1996;88(5):1583–1587.

314. Bajaj MS, Birktoft JJ, Steer SA, et al. Structure and biology of tissue factor pathway inhibitor. *Thromb Haemost* 2001;86(4):959–972.

315. Sevinsky JR, Rao LV, Ruf W. Ligand-induced protease receptor translocation into caveolae: a mechanism for regulating cell surface proteolysis of the tissue factor-dependent coagulation pathway. *J Cell Biol* 1996;133(2):293–304.

316. Iversen N, Lindahl AK, Abildgaard U. Elevated plasma levels of the factor Xa-TFPI complex in cancer patients. *Thromb Res* 2002;105(1):33–36.

317. Lorenzet R, Donati MB. Blood clotting activation, angiogenesis and tumor metastasis: any role for TFPI? *Thromb Haemost* 2002;87(6):928–929.

318. Zacharski LR, Memoli VA, Morain WD, et al. Cellular localization of enzymatically active thrombin in intact human tissues by hirudin binding. *Thromb Haemost* 1995;73(5):793–797.

319. Feng X, Clark RA, Galanakis D, et al. Fibrin and collagen differentially regulate human dermal microvascular endothelial cell integrins: stabilization of alphav/beta3 mRNA by fibrin1. *J Invest Dermatol* 1999;113(6):913–919.

320. Wojtukiewicz MZ, Tang DG, Ben-Josef E, et al. Solid tumor cells express functional "tethered ligand" thrombin receptor. *Cancer Res* 1995;55(3):698–704.

321. Even-Ram S, Uziely B, Cohen P, et al. Thrombin receptor overexpression in malignant and physiological invasion processes. *Nat Med* 1998;4(8):909–914.

322. Macfarlane SR, Seatter MJ, Kanke T, et al. Proteinase-activated receptors. *Pharmacol Rev* 2001;53(2):245–282.

323. Coughlin SR. Thrombin signalling and protease-activated receptors. *Nature* 2000;407(6801):258–264.

324. D'Andrea MR, Derian CK, Santulli RJ, et al. Differential expression of protease-activated receptors-1 and -2 in stromal fibroblasts of normal, benign, and malignant human tissues. *Am J Pathol* 2001;158(6):2031–2041.

325. Tsopanoglou NE, Maragoudakis ME. Role of thrombin in angiogenesis and tumor progression. *Semin Thromb Hemost* 2004;30(1):63–69.

326. Mohle R, Green D, Moore MA, et al. Constitutive production and thrombin-induced release of vascular endothelial growth factor by human megakaryocytes and platelets. *Proc Natl Acad Sci U S A* 1997;94(2):663–668.

327. Pinedo HM, Verheul HM, D'Amato RJ, et al. Involvement of platelets in tumour angiogenesis? *Lancet* 1998;352(9142):1775–1777.

328. Adams J, Carder PJ, Downey S, et al. Vascular endothelial growth factor (VEGF) in breast cancer: comparison of plasma, serum, and tissue VEGF and microvessel density and effects of tamoxifen. *Cancer Res* 2000;60(11):2898–2905.

329. George ML, Eccles SA, Tutton MG, et al. Correlation of plasma and serum vascular endothelial growth factor levels with platelet count in colorectal cancer: clinical evidence of platelet scavenging? *Clin Cancer Res* 2000;6(8):3147–3152.

330. Maragoudakis ME, Kraniti N, Giannopoulou E, et al. Modulation of angiogenesis and progelatinase a by thrombin receptor mimetics and antagonists. *Endothelium* 2001;8(3):195–205.

331. Benezra M, Vlodavsky I, Ishai-Michaeli R, et al. Thrombin-induced release of active basic fibroblast growth factor-heparan sulfate complexes from subendothelial extracellular matrix. *Blood* 1993;81(12):3324–3331.

332. Ukropec JA, Hollinger MK, Salva SM, et al. SHP2 association with VE-cadherin complexes in human endothelial cells is regulated by thrombin. *J Biol Chem* 2000;275(8):5983–5986.

333. Richard DE, Vouret-Craviari V, Pouyssegur J. Angiogenesis and G-protein-coupled receptors: signals that bridge the gap. *Oncogene* 2001;20(13):1556–1562.

334. Bogatcheva NV, Garcia JG, Verin AD. Molecular mechanisms of thrombin-induced endothelial cell permeability. *Biochemistry (Mosc)* 2002;67(1):75–84.

335. Zacharski LR, Costantini V, Wojtukiewicz MZ, et al. Anticoagulants as cancer therapy. *Semin Oncol* 1990;17(2):217–227.

336. Gaffney PJ, Edgell TA, Whitton CM. The haemostatic balance — Astrup revisited. *Haemostasis* 1999;29(1):58–71.

337. Yamahata H, Takeshima H, Kuratsu J, et al. The role of thrombin in the neo-vascularization of malignant gliomas: an intrinsic modulator for the up-regulation of vascular endothelial growth factor. *Int J Oncol* 2002;20(5):921–928.

338. Herbert JM, Dupuy E, Laplace MC, et al. Thrombin induces endothelial cell growth via both a proteolytic and a non-proteolytic pathway. *Biochem J* 1994;303(Pt 1):227–231.

339. Huang YQ, Li JJ, Hu L, et al. Thrombin induces increased expression and secretion of angiopoietin-2 from human umbilical vein endothelial cells. *Blood* 2002;99(5):1646–1650.

340. Belloni PN, Carney DH, Nicolson GL. Organ-derived microvessel endothelial cells exhibit differential responsiveness to thrombin and other growth factors. *Microvasc Res* 1992;43(1):20–45.

341. Naldini A, Carney DH, Pucci A, et al. Thrombin regulates the expression of proangiogenic cytokines via proteolytic activation of protease-activated receptor-1. *Gen Pharmacol* 2000;35(5):255–259.

342. Wojtukiewicz MZ, Sierko E, Zacharski LR. Interfering with hemostatic system components: possible new approaches to antiangiogenic therapy. *Semin Thromb Hemost* 2004;30(1):145–156.

343. Ruoslahti E. RGD and other recognition sequences for integrins. *Annu Rev Cell Dev Biol* 1996;12:697–715.

344. Giancotti FG, Ruoslahti E. Integrin signaling. *Science* 1999;285(5430):1028–1032.

345. O'Reilly MS, Pirie-Shepherd S, Lane WS, et al. Antiangiogenic activity of the cleaved conformation of the serpin antithrombin. *Science* 1999;28(5435):1926–1928.

346. Prox D, Becker C, Pirie-Shepherd SR, et al. Treatment of human pancreatic cancer in mice with angiogenic inhibitors. *World J Surg* 2003;27(4):405–411.

347. Pahl MV, Vaziri ND, Oveisi F, et al. Antithrombin III inhibits mesangial cell proliferation. *J Am Soc Nephrol* 1996;7(10):2249–2253.

348. Souter PJ, Thomas S, Hubbard AR, et al. Antithrombin inhibits lipopolysaccharide-induced tissue factor and interleukin-6 production by mononuclear cells, human umbilical vein endothelial cells, and whole blood. *Crit Care Med* 2001;29(1):134–139.

349. Bombeli T, Mueller M, Haeberli A. Anticoagulant properties of the vascular endothelium. *Thromb Haemost* 1997;77(3):408–423.

350. Lee TH, Rhim T, Kim SS. Prothrombin kringle-2 domain has a growth inhibitory activity against basic fibroblast growth factor-stimulated capillary endothelial cells. *J Biol Chem* 1998;273(44):28805–28812.

351. Rhim TY, Park CS, Kim E, et al. Human prothrombin fragment 1 and 2 inhibit bFGF-induced BCE cell growth. *Biochem Biophys Res Commun* 1998;252(2):513–516.

352. Chan B, Merchan JR, Kale S, et al. Antiangiogenic property of human thrombin. *Microvasc Res* 2003;66(1):1–14.

353. Oh CW, Hoover-Plow J, Plow EF. The role of plasminogen in angiogenesis in vivo. *J Thromb Haemost* 2003;1(8):1683–1687.

354. Browder T, Folkman J, Pirie-Shepherd S. The hemostatic system as a regulator of angiogenesis. *J Biol Chem* 2000;275(3):1521–1524.

355. Fidler IJ. The pathogenesis of cancer metastasis: the 'seed and soil' hypothesis revisited. *Nat Rev Cancer* 2003;3(6):453–458.

356. Gasic GJ, Gasic TB, Stewart CC. Antimetastatic effects associated with platelet reduction. *Proc Natl Acad Sci U S A* 1968;61(1):46–52.

357. Gasic GJ, Gasic TB, Galanti N, et al. Platelet-tumor-cell interactions in mice. The role of platelets in the spread of malignant disease. *Int J Cancer* 1973;11(3):704–718.

358. Pearlstein E, Salk PL, Yogeeswaran G, et al. Correlation between spontaneous metastatic potential, platelet-aggregating activity of cell surface extracts, and cell surface sialylation in 10 metastatic-variant derivatives of a rat renal sarcoma cell line. *Proc Natl Acad Sci U S A* 1980;77(7): 4336–4339.

359. Gastpar H. Platelet-cancer cell interaction in metastasis formation: a possible therapeutic approcach to metastasis prophylaxis. *J Med* 1977;8(2): 103–114.

360. Honn K, Onoda J, Menter D. Prostacyclin/thromboxanes and tumor cell metastasis. In: Honn K, Sloane B, eds. *Hemostatic mechanisms and metastasis.* Boston, MA: Martinus Nijhoff, 1984:207–231.

361. Nierodfish ML, Klepfish A, Karpatkin S. Role of platelets, thrombin, integrin IIb-IIIa, fibronectin and von Willebrand factor on tumor adhesion *in vitro* and metastasis *in vivo. Thromb Haemost* 1995;74(1):282–290.

362. Dardik R, Savion N, Kaufmann Y, et al. Thrombin promotes platelet-mediated melanoma cell adhesion to endothelial cells under flow conditions: role of platelet glycoproteins P-selectin and GPIIb-IIIA. *Br J Cancer* 1998;77(12):2069–2075.

363. Kim YJ, Borsig L, Varki NM, et al. P-selectin deficiency attenuates tumor growth and metastasis. *Proc Natl Acad Sci U S A* 1998;95(16):9325–9330.

364. Varki NM, Varki A. Heparin inhibition of selectin-mediated interactions during the hematogenous phase of carcinoma metastasis: rationale for clinical studies in humans. *Semin Thromb Hemost* 2002;28(1):53–66.

365. Nierodzik ML, Bain RM, Liu LX, et al. Presence of the seven transmembrane thrombin receptor on human tumour cells: effect of activation on tumour adhesion to platelets and tumor tyrosine phosphorylation. *Br J Haematol* 1996;92(2):452–457.

366. Nierodzik ML, Chen K, Takeshita K, et al. Protease-activated receptor 1 (PAR-1) is required and rate-limiting for thrombin-enhanced experimental pulmonary metastasis. *Blood* 1998;92(10):3694–3700.

367. Klepfish A, Greco MA, Karpatkin S. Thrombin stimulates melanoma tumor-cell binding to endothelial cells and subendothelial matrix. *Int J Cancer* 1993;53(6):978–982.

368. Bromberg ME, Bailly MA, Konigsberg WH. Role of protease-activated receptor 1 in tumor metastasis promoted by tissue factor. *Thromb Haemost* 2001;86(5):1210–1214.

369. Ruf W, Mueller BM. Tissue factor signaling. *Thromb Haemost* 1999;82(2): 175–182.

370. Wojtukiewicz MZ, Tang DG, Ciarelli JJ, et al. Thrombin increases the metastatic potential of tumor cells. *Int J Cancer* 1993;54(5):793–806.

371. Bastida E. The metastatic cascade: potential approaches for the inhibition of metastasis. *Semin Thromb Hemost* 1988;14(1):66–72.

372. Zacharski LR, Henderson WG, Rickles FR, et al. Effect of warfarin on survival in small cell carcinoma of the lung. Veterans Administration Study No. 75. *JAMA* 1981;245(8):831–835.

373. Chahinian AP, Propert KJ, Ware JH, et al. A randomized trial of anticoagulation with warfarin and of alternating chemotherapy in extensive small-cell lung cancer by the Cancer and Leukemia Group B. *J Clin Oncol* 1989;7(8):993–1002.

374. Torngren S, Rieger A. The influence of heparin and curable resection on the survival of colorectal cancer. *Acta Chir Scand* 1983;149(4): 427–429.

375. Kramer B. Historical overview of clinical experience with anticoagulant therapy. In: Honn K, Sloane B, eds. *Hemostatic mechanisms and metastasis.* Boston, MA: Martinus Nijhoff, 1984:355–368.

376. Hilgard P. Evidence for the antimetastatic effects of coumarin derivatives. In: Honn K, Sloane B, eds. *Hemostatic mechanisms and metastasis.* Boston, MA: Martinus Nijhoff, 1984:259–265.

377. McCulloch P, George WD. Warfarin inhibits metastasis of Mtln3 rat mammary carcinoma without affecting primary tumour growth. *Br J Cancer* 1989;59(2):179–183.

378. Gallop PM, Lian JB, Hauschka PV. Carboxylated calcium-binding proteins and vitamin K. *N Engl J Med* 1980;302(26):1460–1466.

379. Comp PC, Jacocks RM, Ferrell GL, et al. Activation of protein C *in vivo. J Clin Invest* 1982;70(1):127–134.

380. McNiel NO, Morgan LR Jr. Effects of sodium warfarin and sodium heparin plus anticancer agents on growth of rat C6 glioma cells. *J Natl Cancer Inst* 1984;73(1):169–176.

381. Temple W, Ketcham A. Current clinical trials with anticoagulant therapy in the management of cancer patients. In: Honn K, Sloane B, eds. *Hemostatic mechanisms and metastasis.* Boston, MA: Martinus Nijhoff, 1984:381–408.

382. Chan SY, Pollard M. Metastasis-enhancing effect of heparin and its relationship to a lipoprotein factor. *J Natl Cancer Inst* 1980;64(5):1121–1125.

383. Weitz JI. Low-molecular-weight heparins. *N Engl J Med* 1997;337(10): 688–698.

384. Smorenburg SM, Van Noorden CJ. The complex effects of heparins on cancer progression and metastasis in experimental studies. *Pharmacol Rev* 2001;53(1):93–105.

385. Breddin H, Bauersachs R. Prevention and treatment of thrombosis in cancer patients. In: Lugassy G, Fanlanga A, Kakkar A, et al., eds. *Thrombosis and cancer.* London: Taylor & Francis, 2004:187–206.

386. Mueller BM, Reisfeld RA, Edgington TS, et al. Expression of tissue factor by melanoma cells promotes efficient hematogenous metastasis. *Proc Natl Acad Sci U S A* 1992;89(24):11832–11836.

387. Mueller BM, Ruf W. Requirement for binding of catalytically active factor VIIa in tissue factor-dependent experimental metastasis. *J Clin Invest* 1998;101(7):1372–1378.

388. Esumi N, Fan D, Fidler IJ. Inhibition of murine melanoma experimental metastasis by recombinant desulfatohirudin, a highly specific thrombin inhibitor. *Cancer Res* 1991;51(17):4549–4556.

389. Bromberg ME, Konigsberg WH, Madison JF, et al. Tissue factor promotes melanoma metastasis by a pathway independent of blood coagulation. *Proc Natl Acad Sci U S A* 1995;92(18):8205–8209.

390. Walz DA, Fenton JW. The role of thrombin in tumor cell metastasis. *Invasion Metastasis* 1994;14(1-6):303–308.

391. Ott I, Fischer EG, Miyagi Y, et al. A role for tissue factor in cell adhesion and migration mediated by interaction with actin-binding protein 280. *J Cell Biol* 1998;140(5):1241–1253.

392. Francis JL, Amirkhosravi A. Effect of antihemostatic agents on experimental tumor dissemination. *Semin Thromb Hemost* 2002;28(1):29–38.

393. Brown DC, Purushotham AD, George WD. Inhibition of pulmonary tumor seeding by antiplatelet and fibrinolytic therapy in an animal experimental model. *J Surg Oncol* 1994;55(3):154–159.

394. Kobayashi H, Gotoh J, Fujie M, et al. Inhibition of metastasis of Lewis lung carcinoma by a synthetic peptide within growth factor-like domain of urokinase in the experimental and spontaneous metastasis model. *Int J Cancer* 1994;57(5):727–733.

395. Dunbar SD, Ornstein DL, Zacharski LR. Cancer treatment with inhibitors of urokinase-type plasminogen activator and plasmin. *Expert Opin Investig Drugs* 2000;9(9):2085–2092.

# PART II ■ CLINICAL APPLICATIONS

# CHAPTER 58 ■ OVERVIEW OF INHERITED HEMORRHAGIC DISORDERS

HAROLD R. ROBERTS AND ALICE D. MA

## HEREDITARY COMPONENTS OF THE CLOTTING SYSTEM

Normal hemostasis requires adequate levels of soluble clotting factors, quantitatively and qualitatively normal platelets, and normal vessel wall components including the endothelium, connective tissues, and other constituents. Hereditary abnormalities in any of these components may result in abnormal bleeding. The purpose of this overview is to describe briefly the inherited hemorrhagic disorders and how they can be distinguished and treated.

## DISORDERS OF SOLUBLE CLOTTING FACTORS

Table 58-1 depicts the disorders of soluble clotting factors and some of their characteristics. All of these disorders occur in mild, moderate, and severe forms. The hemorrhagic manifestations include easy bruising and bleeding from mucous membranes, but the most characteristic feature is the formation of hematomas that involve subcutaneous or deeper muscle and connective tissues. In patients who are severely affected, hematomas have a tendency to dissect and involve adjacent tissues.

Although classic hemophilia (factor VIII deficiency) and hemophilia B (factor IX deficiency) are the best known examples of soluble clotting factor deficiencies, the following overview discusses each deficiency in the numerical order ascribed by the Roman numeral classification system.

### Fibrinogen (Factor I) Abnormalities

Fibrinogen abnormalities are inherited in an autosomal pattern and occur in two main forms: afibrinogenemia and dysfibrinogenemia (1). afibrinogenemia is a very rare disorder that occurs when any one of the three genes coding for the $\alpha$, $\beta$, or $\gamma$ chains that make up the fibrinogen dimer is mutated. If the mutation is sufficient to disrupt formation or secretion of any of the three chains, afibrinogenemia results (2). Patients who are afibrinogenemic have a severe bleeding disorder manifested by bleeding after trauma into subcutaneous and deeper tissues that may result in dissection. Bleeding from the umbilical stump is very frequent. Oddly enough, although hemarthroses occur in these patients, they do not occur as frequently as they do in severe forms of hemophilia A and B. Diagnosis is usually apparent with lack of clot formation in screening clotting tests such as the prothrombin time (PT), partial thromboplastin time (PTT), or the thrombin clotting time (TCT). The bleeding time (BT) is also prolonged because of the absence of fibrinogen in the platelet $\alpha$ granule. Treatment consists of transfusing cryoprecipitate to raise the fibrinogen level to the range of approximately 100 mg per dL. Each bag of cryoprecipitate contains approximately 100 mg of fibrinogen, but the amount of fibrinogen in each bag may be quite variable. There are a few reports of antifibrinogen antibodies occurring in patients with afibrinogenemia who have been exposed repeatedly to fibrinogen replacement.

Dysfibrinogenemia is also rare, but it is more common than afibrinogenemia, with most patients being heterozygous for the disorder (3). The dysfibrinogens are the result of missense, nonsense, or splice junction mutations. Several hundred different mutations have been recorded, many of which do not result in a hemorrhagic or thrombotic state. Other dysfibrinogens, however, are associated with bleeding episodes, whereas a few may be associated with venous or arterial thrombosis. Diagnosis is usually suspected by the observation of abnormal appearing clots in the PT, PTT, and TCT, with the clotting time in all three tests being prolonged. In those dysfibrinogens associated with thrombosis, the TCT may be shortened. It is best to also perform a reptilase time on plasmas of patients suspected of having an abnormal fibrinogen because this test may be more sensitive than the TCT. Specific diagnosis requires DNA sequencing of the fibrinogen gene. Patients who are bleeding should be treated with infusions of cryoprecipitate. In patients predisposed to thrombosis, anticoagulation with warfarin or heparin may be required.

### Prothrombin (Factor II) Deficiency

Inherited prothrombin deficiency is rare, with fewer than 50 distinct mutations being reported (4). It is an autosomal recessive disorder, and heterozygotes have no bleeding symptoms. Symptomatic patients may be homozygous or double heterozygotes. Bleeding in patients who are affected varies from mild to severe, depending on the prothrombin level. The complete absence of prothrombin probably leads to embryonic lethality. Diagnosis depends on a high index of suspicion in patients with a prolonged PT and PTT who do not have other known clotting factor defects. Specific diagnosis requires an assay for prothrombin.

### Factor V Deficiency

Factor V deficiency is an autosomal recessive disorder caused by defects in the factor V gene (4). Heterozygotes are asymptomatic, whereas homozygotes or combined heterozygotes may have mild to moderately severe bleeding symptoms. Although approximately 40 mutations in the factor V gene have been reported, they seem to occur less frequently than in genes for other clotting factors (4–6). Even when factor V levels are

**TABLE 58-1**

DISORDERS OF SOLUBLE CLOTTING FACTORS

| Defect | Inheritance pattern | Bleeding manifestations | Diagnostic testing | | | | Treatment |
|---|---|---|---|---|---|---|---|
| | | | PT | PTT | TCT | BT | |
| Fibrinogen abnormalities — Afibrinogenemia | Autosomal | Severe, but less so than severe Hemophilia A and B | Infinite | Infinite | Infinite | Prolonged | Cryoprecipitate |
| Dysfibrinogenemia | Autosomal | Variable bleeding and/or clotting | Prolonged | Prolonged | Prolonged or shortened | Normal | Cryoprecipitate |
| Prothrombin deficiency | Autosomal | Varies with prothrombin levels | Prolonged | Prolonged | Normal | Normal | PCCs |
| Factor V deficiency | Autosomal | Mild-moderate | Prolonged | Prolonged | Normal | Prolonged | FFP, potential need for exchange transfusion |
| Factor VII deficiency | Autosomal | Moderate-severe | Prolonged | Normal | Normal | Normal | Recombinant activated factor VII |
| Hemophilia A | X-linked recessive | Variable, depending on factor VIII level | Normal | Prolonged | Normal | Normal | Factor VIII concentrates, DDAVP in mild cases |
| Hemophilia B | X-linked recessive | Variable, depending on factor IX level | Normal | Prolonged | Normal | Normal | Factor IX concentrates |
| Factor X deficiency | Autosomal | Variable, depending on factor X level | Prolonged | Prolonged | Normal | Normal | Plasma or PCCs |
| Factor XI deficiency | Autosomal | Variable, but *not* dependent on Factor XI levels | Normal | Prolonged | Normal | Normal | Plasma or recombinant activated factor VII |
| Deficiency of factor XII, prekallikrein, or high-molecular-weight kininogen | Autosomal | None | Normal | Prolonged | Normal | Normal | None needed |
| Factor XIII deficiency | Autosomal | Severe | Normal | Normal | Normal | Normal | Cryoprecipitate |
| Deficiency of $\alpha_2$ plasmin inhibitor or plasminogen activator inhibitor-1 | Autosomal | Severe | Normal | Normal | Normal | Normal | Antifibrinolytic agents (epsilon aminocaproic acid or tranexamic acid) |

PT, prothrombin time; PTT, partial thromboplastin time; TCT, thrombin clotting time; BT, bleeding time; PCCs, prothrombin complex concentrates; DDAVP, 1-deamino-8-D-arginine vasopressin.

less than 1% of normal, bleeding does not seem to be as severe as that seen in severe classic hemophilia, perhaps because no patients who have factor V deficiency have been reported with complete deletions of the gene. This is supported by murine studies showing that complete knockout of the factor V gene is lethal in mice, but introduction of a "mini-gene" of factor V DNA expressing less than 1% factor V will rescue the "knockout" mice from lethality (7).

Factor V deficiency is another disorder that results in a long BT, presumably because of the lack of platelet factor V. It has been reported that 20% of the circulating factor V mass resides in the platelet $\alpha$-granule. Bleeding manifestations are similar to those seen in classic hemophilia, except that they tend to be milder, and hemarthroses are less common, although they do occur. The PT, PTT, and BT are prolonged in this disease, but the TCT is normal. Treatment consists of replacing factor V with fresh frozen plasma. It is difficult to raise the factor V level higher than 15% to 20% of normal, using plasma transfusions alone because of danger of volume overload. Exchange transfusion using fresh frozen plasma may therefore be needed when factor V levels above 15% or 20% of normal are required. Inhibitor antibodies against factor V in congenital deficiency are rare.

## Factor VII Deficiency

Factor VII deficiency is an autosomal recessive bleeding disorder that occurs in mild, moderate, and severe forms (8,9). Factor VII with its cofactor, tissue factor, is the main initiator of the clotting mechanism. More than 100 mutations in the gene for factor VII have been reported (9). Bleeding manifestations vary, but in patients who are severely affected bleeding can be as severe as that seen in severe classic hemophilia including the occurrence of crippling hemarthroses (8). Factor VII levels of 10% of normal may be sufficient to control most bleeding episodes, but, in some cases, higher levels may be required for hemostasis. There are a few patients with almost no measurable factor VII who express very few hemorrhagic manifestations. The reason for this is not clear.

In patients with factor VII deficiency, the PT is prolonged, whereas the PTT, TCT, and BT are normal. This is the only soluble clotting factor deficiency in which only the PT is prolonged. It is best to use human tissue factor in the PT assay, because tissue factor from other species may give spurious results. The best replacement therapy is factor VII concentrates. Many physicians now prefer to use recombinant activated factor VII that has been shown to provide hemostasis in patients who are bleeding when given in doses of 15 to 20 $\mu$g per kg of body weight. [Note: This indication has not been approved by the U.S. Food and Drug Administration (FDA).] Inhibitor antibodies against factor VII occur, usually in those patients whose genetic mutation results in virtual absence of factor VII protein.

## Hemophilia A and Hemophilia B (Classic Hemophilia and Christmas Disease)

Hemophilia A and B result from abnormalities in factors VIII and IX, respectively. Factors VIII and IX are necessary for the normal rapid conversion of prothrombin to thrombin. Hemophilia A and B are the only two soluble clotting factor deficiencies that are inherited as X-linked recessive disorders. Several hundred distinct mutations in each gene have been reported (4,5,10). These mutations result in mild, moderate, and severe forms of hemophilia, and the clinical manifestations of hemophilia A and B are, for all practical purposes, indistinguishable. In the severe form, both disorders are characterized by recurrent hemarthroses that result in chronic crippling hemarthropathy unless treated by replacing the deficient factor on a prophylactic basis. Hematomas are also common and may affect almost any organ or tissue in the body, except for the myocardium and penis, where hemorrhage is unusual. Bleeding episodes may be "spontaneous," but, on close questioning, bleeding usually can be related to trauma. Central nervous system hemorrhage is especially hazardous and remains one of the leading causes of death. Any trauma to the head in a patient with either severe or moderate hemophilia A or B should be treated with appropriate replacement therapy as soon as possible before beginning diagnostic procedures. Even if a patient with hemophilia is asymptomatic for a few hours after head trauma, it is prudent to treat the patient prophylactically by raising the factor VIII or IX level to normal, because hemorrhage may be delayed in these patients.

The diagnosis of hemophilia A or B should be suspected in any male patient with hemarthroses, severe bleeding, or excessive bleeding after trauma or surgery. The PTT is prolonged, and the PT, TCT, and BT are normal. Specific diagnosis requires assays for factors VIII and IX.

Safe and effective replacement therapy is available for both hemophilia A and B in the form of highly purified factor VIII or IX concentrates, prepared either from large pools of human plasma or by recombinant DNA technology. Most physicians prefer to use recombinant products, although others prefer highly purified plasma–derived products that have been treated to inactivate potential transmissible infectious agents such as hepatitis and human immune deficiency viruses. Nonplasma products such as desmopressin (1-desamino 8-D-arginine vasopressin; DDAVP) may be used for mild or moderate hemophilia, but some physicians still prefer specific replacement therapy, even in patients who are mildly affected. Prophylactic therapy to prevent bleeding complications is now the treatment of choice for both types of hemophilia. For hemophilia A, 25 to 40 U of factor VIII per kg body weight, three times weekly is recommended; for hemophilia B, 40 U of factor IX per kg body weight, twice weekly is recommended.

The main complication of therapy at the present time is the development of inhibitors to factor VIII, which occurs with a frequency between 10% and 30% of patients who have undergone treatment. Factor IX antibody inhibitors occur in approximately 3% of patients who are severely affected, usually in those patients whose mutation results in undetectable factor IX antigen. Some patients with factor IX inhibitors develop anaphylaxis and/or the nephrotic syndrome when exposed to factor IX. Patients with hemophilia A and B who develop inhibitors can be treated with inhibitor-bypassing agents including recombinant activated factor VII (NovoNordisk) or FEIBA (Baxter Bioscience). However, patients with factor IX deficiency who develop anaphylaxis when exposed to factor IX–containing materials should not receive FEIBA, as this material contains factor IX among its other constituents. Patients who are hemophilic with inhibitors to factor VIII or IX are resistant to treatment; hence, they are subject to more complications and have subsequent increased morbidity and mortality.

## Factor X Deficiency

Factor X deficiency was initially confused with factor VII deficiency until it was found that the PTT was prolonged in the initial patient with factor X deficiency. Like factor VII deficiency, the disorder is inherited in an autosomal recessive fashion and can be mild, moderate, or severe. Numerous mutations have been recorded (4). Patients who are severely affected have symptoms similar to severe classic hemophilia, including hemarthroses and chronic crippling hemarthropathy unless treated prophylactically with factor X–containing concentrates.

The PT and the PTT are both prolonged, and the BT and the TCT are normal. Treatment consists of replacement therapy using either plasma or prothrombin complex concentrates (PCCs) that contain all the vitamin K–dependent factors. The biologic half-life of the factor is approximately 40 hours, so plasma therapy is reasonable, although overload of the circulation can be a problem. We prefer to use PCCs containing factor X, being careful not to raise the factor X level to more than 50% of normal, so as to avoid possible thromboembolic events. Inhibitor antibodies to factor X occur, but are not common.

## Factor XI deficiency

Factor XI deficiency is an autosomal recessive disorder that commonly occurs in patients of Ashkenazi Jewish descent. The deficiency generally produces a mild bleeding tendency. The lack of clinical severity may be explained by the fact that patients with factor XI deficiency have normal levels of factors VIII and IX to form the tenase complex and normal levels of factors V and X to form the prothrombinase complex (11). This is not to say that patients with factor XI deficiency never experience severe bleeding. For example, some patients with factor XI deficiency may bleed extensively after surgery, but, as a general rule, during everyday activity, these patients have very few bleeding symptoms and rarely experience hemarthroses. It appears that some patients with factor XI deficiency do not bleed as much as others, and some patients with severe deficiency may have no history of bleeding. There are reports of a few patients with 1% or so of measurable factor XI clotting activity that have been placed on coumarin for arterial thrombosis. Whether or not patients with factor XI deficiency bleed may depend on differences in their ability to generate thrombin, the ability to activate the thrombin activatable fibrinolytic inhibitor (TAFI), or the activity of the fibrinolytic system. In this disorder, the PT and TCT are normal, whereas the PTT is prolonged. Specific diagnosis depends on an assay for factor XI.

The deficiency can be treated with either plasma replacement or recombinant activated factor VII, the latter being preferred by some physicians (12). Inhibitor antibodies to factor XI have developed in patients with deficiency rendering treatment with plasma ineffective. In these patients, treatment with recombinant activated factor VII is usually effective. (Note: This indication has not been approved by the FDA.)

## Deficiencies of Factor XII, Prekallikrein and High-Molecular-Weight Kininogen

Deficiencies of factors XII, prekallikrein (PK), and high-molecular-weight kininogen (HK) (the so-called contact factors) cause a marked prolongation of the PTT, but other screening tests of coagulation are normal. These defects are inherited in an autosomal recessive fashion. They are not associated with bleeding even after trauma or surgery, even though the prolonged PTT may cause a great deal of consternation amongst those not familiar with these defects. A good history revealing the absence of bleeding in these patients and their family members despite a long PTT is the best indication that one is dealing with one of these defects. A specific assay for each is needed for the exact diagnosis. Factor replacement therapy is not needed. The precise role of these factors in hemostasis, if any, is not clear. Furthermore, these patients do not appear to have any other disease associated with defects in these factors.

## Factor XIII Deficiency

Factor XIII deficiency is caused by a defect in plasma transglutaminase that is necessary for the covalent cross-linking of fibrin α and γ chains to form an impermeable fibrin clot. Although a clot may form in the absence of factor XIII and be held together by hydrogen bonds, this clot is permeable to blood and is easily lysed by the fibrinolytic system. The clot formed in the absence of factor XIII does not form a normal framework for wound healing, and abnormal scar formation may occur. Factor XIII consists of two A chains and two B chains. The complete molecule is an $A_2B_2$ tetramer with the A chains containing the active site and the B chains acting as a carrier for the A subunits. Platelet α-granules contain A chains, but no B chains. Factor XIII deficiency may result from mutations in the genes coding for either the A or B chains, with A chain mutations being more common (13). Autosomal genes govern hepatic synthesis of the factor, and the disease is expressed as a recessive disorder.

Bleeding manifestations are generally severe, and hemorrhage can occur into any tissue. Umbilical stump bleeding is common in factor XIII deficiency. All the screening tests of clotting function are normal in this disorder, so the diagnosis requires a high index of suspicion, especially in patients with a striking lifelong history of excessive bleeding and in whom the PT, PTT, and TCT are normal. Screening for the diagnosis is done by taking the clot from one of the tests mentioned earlier, placing it in a 5 M urea solution or a dilute solution of trichloroacetic acid and measuring the time required for its dissolution. If the clot dissolves within minutes to an hour or so, then factor XIII deficiency is almost certainly present. However, these screening tests are not very sensitive, and specific diagnosis rests on an assay for plasma transglutaminase such as measuring incorporation of putrescine into casein.

The plasma half-life of factor XIII is several days, and so weekly prophylactic treatment with cryoprecipitate is practical. Cryoprecipitate is the replacement therapy of choice in the United States, although factor XIII concentrates are available in Europe.

## Multiple Clotting Factor Deficiencies

The two most common multiple clotting factor deficiencies are a combined deficiency of factors V and VIII and a combined deficiency of the vitamin K–dependent factors (prothrombin and factors VII, IX, X, and protein C and S) (14,15).

A combined deficiency of factors V and VIII is inherited in an autosomal recessive fashion and can be distinguished from a combined inheritance of mild classic hemophilia and mild factor V deficiency by family studies or by genetic analysis. The disorder is caused by defects in one of two genes: the *LMAN1* gene and a newly discovered gene called the "multiple clotting factor deficiency 2 (*MCFD2*)" gene (15). There are multiple mutations in both genes, but the most common ones occur in the *LMAN1* gene. The products of both genes play an important role in the transport of factors V and VIII from the endoplasmic reticulum to the Golgi apparatus and are necessary for normal secretion of these factors. The disorder results in a mild to moderate bleeding tendency with factors V and VIII levels ranging from 5% to 30% of normal. When both the PT and PTT are prolonged, and either factor V or VIII is found to be decreased, the combined deficiency should be suspected. Factor VIII is easily replaced using factor VIII concentrates, but the only readily available factor V replacement is fresh frozen plasma, which is limited in its ability to normalize the factor V level. In some cases, plasma exchange is necessary to raise the factor V to hemostatic levels.

Combined deficiencies of the vitamin K–dependent factors can be caused by defects in either the gene for vitamin K–dependent carboxylase or the gene for vitamin K epoxide reductase (9). This is an autosomal recessive disorder that may be associated with severe deficiency of prothrombin, factors VII, IX, and X, as well as protein CS and S (15). In this syndrome, both the PT and PTT are prolonged, and assays for the individual factors that influence these tests are necessary. The diagnosis must be distinguished from surreptitious ingestion of coumarin drugs, which is an acquired disorder with bleeding manifestations of recent onset. Large doses of vitamin K may partially correct the hereditary defect in some, but not in all cases. Some bleeding episodes will require replacement with PCCs.

## von Willebrand Disease

The most common hereditary clotting factor deficiency arises from abnormalities in von Willebrand factor (VWF). VWF occurs in plasma as multimers of a 240,000 D subunit, with molecular weights ranging from approximately 1 million to 20 million D. The main functions of VWF are to act as a carrier for clotting factor VIII and to mediate platelet adhesion to the injured vessel wall. VWF binds to glycoprotein (GP) Ib on the platelet surface and also to collagen in the vessel wall. VWF also cross-links platelets together by binding to GP IIb/IIIa.

There are three main types of von Willebrand disease (VWD): type 1, 2, and 3 (16). Type 1 is autosomal dominant and represents a quantitative deficiency of VWF. Type 3 is autosomal recessive, with patients having a near absence of VWF. Type 2 VWD usually occurs as an autosomal dominant disorder with abnormalities in VWF function. Type 2 occurs in four major forms, 2A, 2B, 2N, and 2M. Types 2A and 2B are characterized by absence of the higher-molecular-weight multimers of VWF. Type 2B is also associated with thrombocytopenia as a result of a gain of function mutation resulting in a VWF molecule with higher affinity for the GP Ib receptor, thereby enhancing platelet agglutination. Patients with type 2M show reduced binding of their VWF to GP Ib.

Type 2N VWD is a rare autosomal recessive disorder arising from a mutation in the factor VIII–binding site on the VWF molecule. Without the protection provided by VWF binding, factor VIII levels fall because of a markedly decreased half-life. VWF multimers and antigen and activity levels may be normal, whereas the factor VIII levels are low enough so that this type of VWD may be confused with classic hemophilia. Specific diagnosis either requires demonstrating the lack of binding of VWF to factor VIII or genetic analysis.

Although VWD is a defect in a soluble clotting factor, bleeding in patients with this disorder is more similar to that produced by a defect in platelets. The bleeding manifestations tend to be more of the "oozing and bruising" variety, with hematoma formation being rare. Bleeding in types 1 and 2 VWD is usually mild to moderate, although severe bleeding may occur with trauma and surgery. Some patients with type 1 VWD may be relatively asymptomatic. Table 58-2 lists the diagnostic features of the various types of VWD.

One of the most troublesome complications of VWD is the tendency of patients to develop arteriovenous malformations (AVMs) in the gastrointestinal tract, leading to chronic blood loss and iron deficiency. This complication is difficult to treat. Although bleeding may be temporarily controlled by infusion of VWF-rich concentrates (e.g., Humate-P), gastrointestinal bleeding tends to be recurrent. These AVMs are more common in types 2 and 3 VWD, but they can also occur in type 1.

## TABLE 58-2

### VON WILLEBRAND DISEASE SUBTYPES

| | | Inheritance pattern | Bleeding manifestations | Diagnostic testing | | | | Treatment |
|---|---|---|---|---|---|---|---|---|
| | | | | VWF antigen | VWF activity | Factor VIII activity | VWF multimers | |
| Type 1 | | Autosomal dominant | Generally mild | Low | Low | Low | All multimers present but at decreased concentration | DDAVP, factor VIII concentrates rich in VWF |
| Type 2 | 2A | Autosomal dominant | Mild-moderate | Low | Lower than antigen | Variable | Absent high-molecular-weight forms | Factor VIII concentrates rich in VWF |
| | 2B[a] | Autosomal dominant | Mild-moderate | Low | Lower than antigen | Variable | Absent high-molecular-weight forms | Factor VIII concentrates rich in VWF |
| | 2N[b] | Autosomal recessive | Mild | Normal | Normal | Low | Normal | Factor VIII concentrates rich in VWF |
| | 2M | Autosomal dominant | Mild-moderate | Normal | Lower than antigen | Normal | Normal | DDAVP, factor VIII concentrates rich in VWF |
| Type 3 | | Autosomal recessive | Severe | Near absent | Near absent | Near absent | Absent | Factor VIII concentrates rich in VWF |

VWF, von Willebrand factor; DDAVP, 1-deamino-8-D-arginine vasopressin.
[a]Type 2B is associated with thrombocytopenia.
[b]Type 2N may be confused with mild hemophilia A.

The diagnosis of VWD should be suspected in any patient with abnormal bruising, bleeding from mucosal surfaces, menorrhagia, or excessive bleeding after surgery, dental work, or trauma. The PT and TCT should be normal. The PTT is variably prolonged, depending on the degree to which the factor VIII level is reduced. The BT is prolonged, except in patients with type 2N VWD. A new diagnostic test, the PFA-100, is another test of primary hemostasis and is said to be more sensitive and specific for diagnosis of VWD. The presence of a low factor VIII level as the sole laboratory abnormality in a woman with no family history of hemophilia A should lead one to suspect the presence of type 2N VWD.

Treatment of type 1 and type 2A VWD usually consists of administration of desmopressin (DDAVP), either parenterally or by intranasal administration. It can be used for 3 to 5 days, but in time the drug loses its efficacy by depleting endothelial stores of VWF, a process termed "tachyphylaxis." DDAVP is theoretically contraindicated in type 2B VWD because thrombocytopenia can be worsened as release of type 2B VWF with enhanced affinity for platelet membrane GP 1b results in further *in vivo* platelet agglutination. In type 2b and type 3 VWD, factor VIII concentrates rich in VWF should be used for treatment.

VWF is synthesized in endothelial cells and it is secreted as a very large molecular weight protein that normally does not circulate. The secreted VWF is cleaved by ADAMTS 13, (a disintegrin and metalloproteinase with thrombospondin repeats), which is a member of a family of proteases that cleave proteins under high shear rates. When this protease is lacking or inhibited, larger than normal VWF multimers appear in the circulation and result in platelet aggregation *in vivo*, a situation that results in thrombotic thrombocytopenic purpura (TTP). Familial deficiency of ADAMTS 13 occurs and leads to hereditary TTP (17).

## Inherited Deficiency of Inhibitors of the Fibrinolytic System

There are two main inhibitors of the fibrinolytic system: the $\alpha_2$ plasmin inhibitor ($\alpha_2$-antiplasmin) and the plasminogen activator inhibitor 1 (PAI-1). The genes for both have been identified and sequenced, and mutations within each have been described (18,19). Deficiency of either inhibitor results in excessive fibrinolysis and hence to severe bleeding, including hemarthroses and hematoma formation that often occurs following trauma or surgery. Both disorders are inherited in an autosomal pattern and, in most cases, bleeding occurs in homozygotes. The diagnosis is suspected when a patient gives a lifelong history of bleeding, often after trauma, and when the usual screening tests of coagulation are normal. In such cases, a euglobulin lysis test should be performed, and if the clot lyses within a few hours (normal lysis times are >24 hours), specific assays for $\alpha_2$-plasmin inhibitor and PAI-1 should be considered. Bleeding episodes respond to administration of antifibrinolytic agents, either epsilon aminocaproic or tranexamic acid (20).

Table 58-3 gives a salient summary and clinical pearls regarding defects in soluble clotting factors.

## TABLE 58-3

### DEFECTS IN SOLUBLE CLOTTING FACTORS—CLINICAL PEARLS

- The most common hereditary bleeding disorder is VWD with type 1 VWD the most common subtype
  - VWD is inherited as an autosomal dominant trait and is expressed in the heterozygous state
  - Bleeding in this disorder resembles the type of bleeding seen with thrombocytopenia, with bruising and hemorrhage from mucous membranes
  - Menorrhagia is common, and women with this common complaint should be screened for VWD
- The only two soluble clotting factors deficiencies that are inherited as sex-linked recessive characteristics are hemophilia A and B, resulting from defects in factors VIII and IX, respectively
  - The occurrence of severe bleeding in men, especially associated with hemarthropathy, is strongly suggestive of one of these disorders
  - Hemophilia A and B can be clinically indistinguishable, but classic hemophilia is much more common than hemophilia B
  - Inhibitor antibodies occur more frequently in hemophilia A, and patients with such inhibitors are resistant to treatment and have increased morbidity and mortality
- The other deficiencies of soluble clotting factors are inherited in an autosomal recessive fashion, and bleeding occurs when the patient is homozygous or a combined heterozygote
- Deficiencies of factors XII, PK, and HK are not associated with bleeding, even after trauma or surgery
- A prolonged PT with a normal PTT and TCT suggests factor VII deficiency, whereas a prolonged PTT with a normal PT and TCT in a patient who is bleeding suggests a factor VIII or IX deficiency if the bleeding is confined to men or factor XI deficiency if the bleeding is mild and occurs in both sexes
- If all screening tests of coagulation are normal, deficiency of factor XIII, $\alpha_2$-plasmin inhibitor or PAI-1 should be suspected, although these are very rare disorders
- When both the PT and PTT are prolonged, one should suspect deficiency of either factor V or factor X; bleeding from prothrombin deficiency and combined factor deficiencies can also present with these laboratory values, but these cases are more rare and can be easily diagnosed with assays for individual factors
- When the TCT as well as the PT and PTT are prolonged, dysfibrinogenemia should be suspected; when no clot is detected, afibrinogenemia is likely
- Acquired bleeding disorders can be confused with hereditary defects but are usually not lifelong and can be distinguished by a careful medical history

VWD, von Willebrand disease; PK, prekallikrein; HK, high-molecular-weight kininogen; PT, prothrombin time; PTT, partial thromboplastin time; TCT, thrombin clotting time; PAI-1, plasminogen activator inhibitor 1.

# INHERITED PLATELET DISORDERS

Hereditary disorders of platelets as causes of bleeding are more rare than diseases related to defects in the soluble clotting factors. These disorders are often complex, and some are not completely understood. The hereditary platelet diseases can be characterized in several ways. One convenient classification is to divide them into hereditary thrombocytopenias, hereditary nonthrombocytopenic diseases, and hereditary abnormalities of platelet secretion or signaling, which may or may not be associated with thrombocytopenia. These abnormalities may be the result of defects in growth factors controlling platelet production, platelet membrane abnormalities, or abnormalities in subcellular structures or intracellular proteins.

The hallmark of bleeding from a disorder of platelets is mucocutaneous bleeding. Bruising, epistaxis, oral bleeding, gastrointestinal bleeding, and menorrhagia are seen. Unlike hemophilia and similar conditions, hematoma formation is very rare in platelet disorders.

## Hereditary Thrombocytopenias

These are a complicated group of diseases of variable severity arising from a number of genetic defects (21). Only the most common disorders is described in this overview.

### Giant Platelet Syndromes

The best characterized syndrome associated with mild to moderate thrombocytopenia with macrothrombocytes is the Bernard-Soulier syndrome. This disorder is autosomal recessive and arises from defects in any of three genes encoding components of the platelet GP Ib/IX/V complex (GP Ibα, GP Ibβ, or GP IX). Clinical manifestations are usually mild to moderate and consist of bruising and bleeding from mucous membranes. The platelets of these patients show a normal pattern of aggregation to all agonists, but agglutination in response to ristocetin is absent. Patients can be treated by transfusion of normal platelets, but one should first try DDAVP or recombinant activated factor VII because of the risk of inducing platelet alloantibodies. There will be times when transfusions of normal platelets may be needed, so it is better to avoid alloimmunization for as long as possible. Recombinant activated factor VII is not always efficacious, but recent reports suggest that it is worth trying. (Note: This indication has not been approved by the FDA.)

There are several macrothrombocytopenias secondary to defects in the MYH9 gene resulting in the May-Hegglin anomaly and the Fechtner, Epstein, and Sebastian syndromes. The May-Hegglin anomaly is the most common of these disorders. Patients have mild thrombocytopenia, with platelet counts ranging from 20 to $100 \times 10^3$ per mm$^3$, and their peripheral blood smears show Döhle-like inclusion bodies in the neutrophils, eosinophils, and monocytes. The finding of mild thrombocytopenia of long duration should prompt examination of the peripheral smear, looking for these bluish inclusion bodies. The May-Hegglin anomaly may otherwise be confused with immune thrombocytopenia, and patients with May-Hegglin have been erroneously treated with steroids and splenectomy. Platelets are giant, sometimes exceeding the size of the red cells, and the total platelet mass may be normal. Bleeding symptoms are typically mild. The Fechtner, Epstein, and Sebastian syndromes are rare and can be suspected if there is associated hearing loss, cataracts, or nephritis. Patients who are bleeding respond to platelet transfusions.

### Other Hereditary Thrombocytopenias without Giant Platelets

Perhaps the most common hereditary thrombocytopenia with small platelets is the Wiskott-Aldrich syndrome, a disorder associated with the triad of immune deficiency, eczema, and thrombocytopenia. This syndrome is X-linked and results from mutations in the gene for Wiskott-Aldrich syndrome protein (WASP). Platelets, as well as T lymphocytes show defective function, and clinical manifestations vary widely. Definitive treatment requires allogeneic stem cell transplantation.

Other rare syndromes include: the familial thrombocytopenia that may lead to acute myelogenous leukemia caused by mutations in the AML1 gene; the Paris-Trousseau syndrome associated with motor retardation and skeletal abnormalities caused by a haplodeficiency of chromosome 11; the thrombocytopenia and absent radius syndrome (TAR syndrome); the thrombocytopenia with radio-ulnar synostosis secondary to mutations in the HOXA11 gene; GATA-1 related thrombocytopenia with dyserythropoiesis; and congenital amegakaryocytic thrombocytopenia caused by defects in the thrombopoietin receptor (c-Mpl), which may eventually result in marrow failure.

## Hereditary Nonthrombocytopenic Disorders

Glanzmann thrombasthenia is the hallmark of the nonthrombocytopenic purpuras (22). This disorder is caused by one of multiple defects in the platelet membrane GP complex IIb/IIIa, also known as the integrin $\alpha_{2b} \beta_3$. The disease is autosomal recessive and may arise from abnormalities in the genes for either GP IIb or IIIa. There are multiple mutations in either gene that can give rise to a similar phenotype and, as such, the disorder is a prime example of genetic heterogeneity. The molecular defects lead to absent platelet aggregation when patient's platelets are exposed to platelet agonists such as adenosine 5'-diphosphate (ADP), collagen, thrombin, and epinephrine. Platelet adhesion, as reflected by agglutination of platelets in the presence of ristocetin is normal, indicating that GP Ib is unaffected. Bleeding symptoms are usually severe and include purpura, bleeding from mucous membranes, and menorrhagia. Hemarthroses and hematoma formation are rare. Bleeding from major surgery can be quite severe, and patients should be pretreated with normal platelets unless previous use of platelets has resulted in alloimmunization. Although patients may respond to transfusions of normal platelets early in the course of the disease, one can expect patients to become refractory when antibodies develop against that part of the GP IIb/IIIa complex that is absent. In such patients, antifibrinolytic therapy or therapy with recombinant activated factor VII may be of benefit. (Note: This indication has not been approved by the FDA.)

## Hereditary Platelet Disorders with Abnormal Platelet Secretion and/or Signaling (Qualitative Platelet Defects)

Many of the syndromes associated with abnormal secretion or signaling defects are incompletely understood. Only those syndromes that are more common will be discussed in this section. Most of these disorders are caused by defects in signaling and are characterized by abnormal platelet aggregation to one or more platelet agonists including thrombin, collagen, epinephrine, ADP, and several others. The mechanisms are heterogeneous and are discussed in detail in Chapter 64. These disorders must be distinguished from the effects of drugs such as aspirin, whose ingestion can produce similar effects on platelet function.

## Storage Pool Deficiency

There are two main types of subcellular organelles in the platelet that have been linked to disease, the $\delta$-, or dense, granules [containing mainly nonmetabolic ADP, adenosine triphosphate (ATP), calcium, and serotonin] and $\alpha$-granules. $\alpha$-Granules contain fibrinogen, factor V, thrombospondin, platelet-derived growth factor, multimerin, fibronectin, factor XIII A chains, HK, and VWF among other proteins.

Failure to secrete the contents of $\delta$-granules on platelet activation results in $\delta$ storage pool disease, which can be diagnosed by failure to detect these dense bodies on electron microscopy. The absence of a second wave of aggregation in response to epinephrine or exogenous ADP suggests the defect. Patients with $\delta$ storage pool deficiency have a mild bleeding tendency.

The Hermansky-Pudlak syndrome is the association of $\delta$ storage pool deficiency with oculocutaneous albinism and increased ceroid in the reticuloendothelial system. There are several subtypes of the Hermansky-Pudlack syndrome resulting from at least seven different mutations. The syndrome is inherited in an autosomal recessive pattern.

The Chediak-Higashi syndrome is also associated with storage pool deficiency and is characterized by oculocutaneous albinism, neurologic abnormalities, immune deficiency with a tendency to infections, and giant inclusions in the cytoplasm of platelets and leukocytes. The disorder is rare, and bleeding manifestations are relatively mild. The syndrome is caused by mutations in the *LYST* (lysosomal trafficking regulator) gene. Patients who are affected are homozygous, whereas heterozygotes are clinically normal.

The gray platelet syndrome is caused by a lack of $\alpha$-granules and can usually be recognized by examination of a Wright-Giemsa stained peripheral blood smear showing platelets that appear gray without the usual red-staining granules. Electron microscopy is a better way to diagnose the syndrome and shows a depletion of $\alpha$-granules. The syndrome is therefore classified with the other platelet secretion defects, but the disorder may also be classified with the macrothrombocytopenias. In this disorder, platelets may be slightly larger than usual, but they are not as large as those seen in the giant platelet disorders described earlier. Furthermore, the platelet count is only moderately depressed and bleeding symptoms are mild. Patients with this disorder may develop early onset myelofibrosis in addition to their defect in platelet function.

## Other Rare Platelet Disorders

Several other platelet disorders deserve mention. The Quebec platelet disorder is associated with a normal to slightly low platelet count with a mild bleeding disorder caused by abnormal proteolysis of $\alpha$-granule proteins. It was first recognized as a deficiency of platelet factor V, with normal concentrations of plasma factor V. The platelets appear normal on peripheral blood smears under the light microscope and diagnosis depends on showing decreased $\alpha$-granule proteins.

The Scott syndrome also deserves mention. In this disorder, platelets, when activated, cannot translocate phosphatidylserine from the inner to the outer platelet membrane when the "flip-flop" of the membrane leaflet occurs, presumably because of defects in the "scramblase" enzyme activity. The Scott syndrome is characterized by a mild bruising and bleeding tendency.

Several platelet receptor defects resulting in a mild bleeding disorder have been described and include defects in platelet receptors for collagen, ADP, epinephrine, and thromboxane $A_2$, as well as intracellular signaling molecules. The platelet count in these disorders is normal and diagnosis is difficult, but it should be suspected in patients whose history of bleeding suggests a platelet-type disorder and in whom measurements of VWF antigen and activity are normal. Platelet aggregation tests are abnormal, and their pattern of abnormality may give clues to the diagnosis.

Table 58-4 gives a salient summary and clinical pearls regarding defects in platelet number or function.

## TABLE 58-4

### DEFECTS IN PLATELET NUMBER AND/OR FUNCTION—CLINICAL PEARLS

- Bleeding caused by defects in platelet number or function is characterized by bruising and bleeding from mucous membranes, including epistaxis, menorrhagia, gastrointestinal bleeding; hematomas and hemarthroses are rare; the bleeding time is prolonged, but other screening tests, such as the PT and PTT, are normal
- Storage pool deficiency can affect either the $\alpha$- or the $\delta$-granules in platelets and produces a mild bleeding disorder
  - $\delta$ storage pool disorders can be found in association with oculocutaneous albinism and other systemic abnormalities in the Hermansky-Pudlak syndrome and the Chediak-Higashi syndrome
  - Signaling defects may be the most common inherited disorders of platelet function and occur much more commonly than either Glanzmann thrombaesthenia or Bernard-Soulier syndrome
  - Patients with qualitative platelet abnormalities may respond to desmopressin (DDAVP)
  - The effect of ingestion of aspirin or other nonsteroidal antiinflammatory agents should be carefully excluded
- The May-Hegglin anomaly produces mild thrombocytopenia with macrothrombocytes, along with Döhle-like inclusion bodies in granulocytes and monocytes; the peripheral smear should be examined in all patients with thrombocytopenia, in order to differentiate this diagnosis from immune thrombocytopenia
- Bernard-Soulier syndrome is a rare autosomal recessive syndrome produced by defects in the GP Ib/IX/V complex causing impaired or absent binding to VWF; macrothrombocytopenia is present; platelet transfusions may be ineffective in patients who have developed alloantibodies, which are directed against the GP Ib/IX/V complex
- Glanzmann thrombasthenia is an autosomal recessive disorder arising from defects in the GP IIb/IIIa complex, producing a defect in platelet aggregation in response to all platelet agonists except for ristocetin; it is not associated with thrombocytopenia; platelet transfusions may be ineffective in patients who have developed alloantibodies, which are directed against the GP IIb/IIIa complex
- The Wiskott-Aldrich syndrome is an X-linked disorder associated with the triad of immune deficiency, eczema, and thrombocytopenia

PT, prothrombin time; PTT, partial thromboplastin time; GP, glycoprotein.

## TABLE 58-5

### DEFECTS IN THE VESSEL WALL—CLINICAL PEARLS

Defects in the vessel wall should be suspected when unusual bleeding is not explained by defects in soluble clotting factors or platelets

Hereditary hemorrhagic telangiectasia should be suspected when bleeding is due to epistaxis and gastrointestinal bleeding; or when telangiectasia are visible on cutaneous tissues or mucous membranes

If laboratory tests of hemostasis are normal and rupture of vessels occurs, type IV Ehlers-Danlos syndrome should be suspected

# INHERITED VASCULAR DISORDERS

There are several inherited bleeding disorders that are not caused by clotting factor defects or by platelet disorders but, rather, are caused by the abnormalities in the blood vessels themselves. These include hereditary hemorrhagic telangiectasia (HHT) and Ehlers-Danlos syndrome (EDS). Marfan syndrome and pseudoxanthoma elasticum may occasionally be associated with bleeding, but these are not primary hemorrhagic disorders and will not be discussed here.

## Hereditary Hemorrhagic Telangiectasia ( Osler-Weber-Rendu Syndrome)

HHT is an autosomal dominant disorder that is associated with AVMs of the small vessels of the skin, oropharynx, lungs, gastrointestinal tract, and other tissues. The syndrome is often suspected by the presence of epistaxis, gastrointestinal bleeding, telangiectasias on the lips and fingertips, and iron deficiency anemia. It is caused by one of several mutations involving either the endoglin gene (chromosome 9, HHT-1) or the Alk1 gene (chromosome 12, HHT-2). These genes code for proteins that influence intracellular signaling by transforming growth factor-$\beta$ and probably exert their effect by vascular remodeling (23). Defects in or absence of these protein products lead to AVMs in which endothelial cells form thin-walled vessels connecting the arterial and venous beds. Such malformed vessels are easily injured, producing a tendency to easy bleeding. Although bleeding does not occur at birth, it may begin in childhood, and by age 16 most patients will experience hemorrhagic symptoms. Treatment is difficult, but some patients respond to antifibrinolytic agents, local pressure (when possible) or to recombinant activated factor VII, although the last has not been tried extensively. (Note: This indication has not been approved by the FDA.)

## Ehlers-Danlos Syndrome

This disorder is characterized by easy bruising and hemorrhage from ruptured blood vessels and is caused by one of several genetic defects (24). The classic Ehlers-Danlos syndrome (EDS) causing joint hypermotility and hyperextensibility of the skin

may be associated with bruising, but it is not likely to result in massive bleeding. The vascular type IV EDS is the most likely to result in considerable bruising and is caused by a defect in type III collagen resulting from defects in the *COL3A1* gene. In this type of EDS, bruising can be very extensive and vascular rupture can result in death. The skin may be thin and wrinkled, but hyperextensibility of the skin is not common. The bruising is sufficient to make one suspect a platelet disorder, but tests of platelet and coagulant function are normal. Diagnosis is dependent on demonstration of the genetic abnormality or the demonstration of abnormal type III collagen.

Table 58-5 gives a salient summary and clinical pearls regarding defects in the vessel wall.

## References

1. Roberts HR, Stinchcombe TE, Gabriel DA. The dysfibrinogenaemias. *Br J Haematol* 2001;114(2):249–257.
2. Anwar M, Iqbal H, Gul M, et al. Congenital afibrinogenemia: report of three cases. *J Thromb Haemost* 2005;3(2):407–409.
3. Cunningham MT, Brandt JT, Laposata M, et al. Laboratory diagnosis of dysfibrinogenemia. *Arch Pathol Lab Med* 2002;126(4):499–505.
4. Stenson PD, Ball EV, Mort M, et al. Human Gene Mutation Database (HGMD): 2003 update. *Hum Mutat* 2003;21(6):577–581.
5. Kemball-Cook G. The Haemophilia A Mutation, Structure, Test and Resource Site. In: http://europium.csc.mrc.ac.uk; 2003.
6. Kemball-Cook G. FVII Mutation Database. In. Website ed. http://europium.csc.mrc.ac.uk; 2004.
7. Yang TL, Cui J, Taylor JM, et al. Rescue of fatal neonatal hemorrhage in factor V deficient mice by low level transgene expression. *Thromb Haemost* 2000;83(1):70–77.
8. Mariani G, Herrmann FH, Dolce A, et al. Clinical phenotypes and factor VII genotype in congenital factor VII deficiency. *Thromb Haemost* 2005; 93(3):481–487.
9. Li T, Chang CY, Jin DY, et al. Identification of the gene for vitamin K epoxide reductase. *Nature* 2004;427(6974):541–544.
10. Oldenburg J, Ananyeva NM, Saenko EL. Molecular basis of haemophilia A. *Haemophilia* 2004;10(Suppl. 4):133–139.
11. Oliver JA, Monroe DM, Roberts HR, et al. Thrombin activates factor XI on activated platelets in the absence of factor XII. *Arterioscler Thromb Vasc Biol* 1999;19(1):170–177.
12. Roberts HR, Monroe DM, White GC. The use of recombinant factor VIIa in the treatment of bleeding disorders. *Blood* 2004;104(13):3858–3864.
13. Ariens RA, Lai TS, Weisel JW, et al. Role of factor XIII in fibrin clot formation and effects of genetic polymorphisms. *Blood* 2002;100(3):743–754.
14. McMillan C, Roberts H. Congenital combined deficiency of coagulation factors II, VII, IX and X. *N Engl J Med* 1966;274:1313–1315.
15. Zhang B, Ginsburg D. Familial multiple coagulation factor deficiencies: new biologic insight from rare genetic bleeding disorders. *J Thromb Haemost* 2004;2(9):1564–1572.
16. Sadler JE. New concepts in von Willebrand disease. *Annu Rev Med* 2005; 56:173–191.
17. Tsai HM. Deficiency of ADAMTS-13 in thrombotic and thrombocytopenic purpura. *J Thromb Haemost* 2003;1(9):2038–2040; discussion 2040–2045.
18. Fay WP, Shapiro AD, Shih JL, et al. Brief report: complete deficiency of plasminogen-activator inhibitor type 1 due to a frame-shift mutation. *N Engl J Med* 1992;327(24):1729–1733.
19. Favier R, Aoki N, de Moerloose P. Congenital alpha(2)-plasmin inhibitor deficiencies: a review. *Br J Haematol* 2001;114(1):4–10.
20. Morimoto Y, Yoshioka A, Imai Y, et al. Haemostatic management of intraoral bleeding in patients with congenital deficiency of alpha2-plasmin inhibitor or plasminogen activator inhibitor-1. *Haemophilia* 2004;10(5): 669–674.
21. Drachman JG. Inherited thrombocytopenia: when a low platelet count does not mean ITP. *Blood* 2004;103(2):390–398.
22. Nurden AT, Nurden P. Inherited defects of platelet function. *Rev Clin Exp Hematol* 2001;5(4):314–334; quiz following 431.
23. Brusgaard K, Kjeldsen AD, Poulsen L, et al. Mutations in endoglin and in activin receptor-like kinase 1 among danish patients with hereditary haemorrhagic telangiectasia. *Clin Genet* 2004;66(6):556–561.
24. De Paepe A, Malfait F. Bleeding and bruising in patients with Ehlers-Danlos syndrome and other collagen vascular disorders. *Br J Haematol* 2004; 127(5):491–500.

# CHAPTER 59 ■ CLINICAL MANIFESTATIONS AND THERAPY OF THE HEMOPHILIAS

CRAIG M. KESSLER AND GUGLIELMO MARIANI

## HEMOPHILIAS

The hemophilias comprise a category of hereditary bleeding disorders resulting from congenital deficiencies in proteins involved in blood coagulation. The most frequently encountered deficiencies involve factor VIII (antihemophilic factor), associated with hemophilia A, and factor IX (Christmas factor), associated with hemophilia B; both X-linked recessive diseases are characteristically recognized almost exclusively in male hemizygotes. Factor XI (plasma thromboplastin antecedent) deficiency, associated with hemophilia C, is transmitted as an autosomal recessive abnormality and is most commonly observed in Jewish individuals of Eastern European ancestry. Hemophilia A, accounting for 80% to 85% of the cases (one per 5,000 male births), is four to six times more prevalent than hemophilia B (one per 30,000 male births) and is 100 times more common than factor XI deficiency in the general population (one per million births, but one per 500 Ashkenazi Jewish births).

## Carrier Detection and Prenatal Diagnosis

Carrier detection is useful for all obligate women regardless of whether they are of child-bearing potential. Their factor VIII or IX activities may be low enough to place them at greatly increased risk for severe hemorrhagic complications during surgical procedures or after major trauma. Carriers also may experience easy bruisability, menorrhagia, or both. Phenotypic analysis (FVIII:C/VWF: Ag ratio, FIX:C) for the hemophilia carrier state is very sensitive and is specific for obligate carriers of hemophilia A but is much less so for hemophilia B carriers (approximately 20%). Ratios less than 0.5 can identify 91% to 99% of hemophilia A carriers (1). Genotype assessment by DNA polymorphism analysis is superior to phenotypic analysis because it usually provides a definitive diagnosis (when informative) and identifies the pathogenic mutation in the factor VIII or IX gene. Physiologically meaningless mutations in the factor VIII gene and the presence of mosaicism (a mixture of healthy and mutation-carrying cells) in some families may confound the confirmation of carrier status. If the gene mutation is uninformative for diagnostic purposes, the use of linked polymorphic markers [restriction fragment length polymorphisms (RFLP)] to trace the inheritance of the abnormal hemophilia gene within a pedigree may be helpful. Linkage analysis is limited because of uninformative patterns of polymorphic markers, ethnic variation, linkage disequilibrium, and the need for participation of family members. It is not helpful in families with spontaneous mutations of the factor VIII gene, which constitute approximately 30% of the hemophilia families.

Direct gene mutation analysis for the intron 22 inversion is recommended as first-line testing for carrier detection in families with severe hemophilia A and may be helpful when affected family members are not available (2). Intrachromosomal recombinations, involving F8A in intron 22 of the factor VIII gene and one of two homologous regions 500 kb in length on the 5′ region of the factor VIII gene, may result in large inversions of DNA at the tip of the X chromosome. The factor VIII gene becomes dysfunctional, causing severe hemophilia A. Two inversions are possible, distal and proximal, depending on which homologous region is involved in the recombination event. In a group of 85 patients with severe hemophilia A, 47% of the patients had an inversion, of which 80% was of the distal type. If the intron 22 inversion is not detected in the family or the obligate carrier, intragenic and extragenic linkage analysis of DNA polymorphisms (3) can be achieved after digestion with specific enzymes (RFLP). Polymerase chain reaction amplification of DNA and screening for the specific mutation within the coding sequence of the factor VIII gene is theoretically possible but is extremely cumbersome. These gene-tracking techniques provide up to 99.9% precision, but only when an affected male patient and intervening family members are available for analysis (4).

Because the factor IX gene is approximately one third the size of the factor VIII complementary DNA, factor IX genetic mutations are more easily identifiable in carriers or affected men. More than 300 unique mutations have been reported, predominantly single base-pair substitutions (5). Ninety-five percent of families with moderate to severe disease and 40% of those with mild disease have independent mutations (6). RFLP and direct gene mutation analysis have been successful in hemophilia B–carrier detection (7). Only 60% to 70% of hemophilia B carriers can be detected by the measurement of reduced plasma factor IX activity (8). As in the case of hemophilia A, up to one third of cases of hemophilia B are associated with spontaneous mutations with no affected family members.

Because detection of hemophilia A and B is possible using linkage studies or direct gene mutation analysis, prenatal diagnosis can be performed at most high-risk obstetric centers either by chorionic villous sampling at 12 weeks gestation or, less preferably, by amniocentesis after the sixteenth week (9). These procedures can determine the sex of the fetus and whether a male infant is affected with hemophilia. The presence of maternal factor IX (but not factor VIII) in the amniotic fluid may confound neonatal diagnosis of hemophilia B. If DNA markers are not available, fetal blood sampling by fetoscopy can be performed at 20 weeks, gestation for direct measurement of fetal factor VIII activity. Because of the physiologically low levels of factor IX in newborns, this technique is less applicable for the diagnosis of hemophilia B. Maternal–fetal combined complication rates for amniocentesis and chorionic villous sampling are 0.5% to 1% and 1% to 2%, respectively. Fetoscopy is associated with risk of fetal death ranging from 1% to 6% (10). These techniques should be discussed in routine prenatal genetic counseling performed through comprehensive hemophilia treatment centers (11). Furthermore, the severity of the coagulation deficiency in the mother should be considered. Because most of the significant hemorrhages occur in carriers with prepregnancy factor levels below 50%, replacement therapy immediately before and following delivery may be necessary. Prenatal diagnosis may increase the safety of delivery because the use of vacuum extraction, forceps delivery, and prolonged labor are associated with increased intracranial bleeding and hemolysis and severe cephalhematoma formation in affected infants and therefore should be avoided. The risk of intracranial hemorrhage with normal vaginal delivery is small and has proven to be as safe as cesarean delivery. One recent report documented the successful use of intrauterine infusion of recombinant factor VIII concentrate to reduce the risk of intracranial peripartum hemorrhage in a fetus with documented hemophilia A. Interestingly, an alloantibody inhibitor was detected against factor VIII shortly after birth, emphasizing a potential deleterious outcome of exposing an immature immune system to a non–self antigen (1).

## Postnatal Diagnosis

Hemophilia A and B are clinically heterogeneous disorders; however, symptoms, family history, or the results of global coagulation assays, such as the activated partial thromboplastin time (aPTT), cannot distinguish hemophilia A from hemophilia B. The postnatal diagnosis depends on direct assays of plasma levels of factor VIII or IX activity. Factor VIII activity can be measured specifically by clot-based or chromogenic substrate methodologies. von Willebrand factor (VWF) assays should be performed to distinguish hemophilia A from von Willebrand disease (VWD) and its variants. Factor IX activity is measured using clot detection assays. Factors VIII and IX activity levels are expressed in international units per milliliter of plasma (IU per mL) or as a percentage of the activity determined in normal pooled plasma with 1 IU per mL corresponding to 100% of the coagulation factor activity found in 1 mL of pooled normal plasma. Normal plasma activity levels range from 0.5 IU per mL to 1.5 IU per mL (50% to 150%). The levels of factor activity define the degree of severity that characterizes the clinical spectrum of hemophilic bleeding. Severe hemophilia is defined by factor VIII or IX activity levels of less than 1% (<0.01 IU per mL) and occurs in approximately 50% of affected patients. Moderate-severity hemophilia occurs in approximately 10% of patients, with factor activity levels between 2% and 5% (0.02 to 0.05 IU per mL). Mild hemophilia comprises 30% to 40% of patients, with factor activity levels greater than 5% (>0.05 IU per mL).

Severe hemophilia is characterized by recurrent hemorrhages, occurring spontaneously or after surgery and minimal trauma. In the absence of a family history, infants often present with postcircumcision bleeding. There also is a 2% to 8% risk of intracranial and extracranial (subgaleal and cephalhematoma) bleeds at the time of labor and delivery (12). Most of these events occur with vaginal delivery (87%) and are independent of the mode of delivery (e.g., spontaneous vs. forceps or vacuum extraction). Only intracranial hemorrhages result in neurologic deficits (15%) and late neurologic sequelae (38%).

Otherwise, infants with severe hemophilia begin to develop palpable subcutaneous ecchymoses at 3 or 4 months of age, with more significant bleeding complications becoming evident by toddling and walking age. Large hematomas also may follow deep intramuscular injections of routine vaccinations;

these children should either receive subcutaneous vaccinations or be pretreated with replacement clotting factor concentrate. Oral bleeding predominantly from lip and tongue biting becomes apparent by the age of 2 years and continues into childhood, with loss of deciduous teeth. At 3 to 4 years of age, intraarticular and intramuscular bleeding becomes problematic. Major hemorrhage can occur in severely affected individuals at any anatomic site after mild or unknown trauma. As the use of primary prophylaxis protocols becomes more widespread, the clinical spectrum of bleeding in children with hemophilia will likely be altered.

Moderately severe hemophilia is not associated with spontaneous hemorrhage, but bleeding usually is precipitated by surgery or minor trauma. The first symptoms become apparent between 1 and 2 years of age. Mild disease may present with significant bleeding after major trauma or surgery, but, more often, these patients are identified immediately before elective surgery when routine screening coagulation assays reveal an incidentally prolonged aPTT.

# CLINICAL PRESENTATIONS IN HEMOPHILIA

## Intraarticular Bleeding: Hemarthroses and Hemophilic Arthropathy

Ninety percent of all bleeding episodes in individuals with hemophilia A and B occur into the joints and muscles. In order of involvement, the joints most commonly affected include the knees (>50% of all events), followed by the elbows, ankles, shoulders, and wrists (13). Knees and elbows are particularly vulnerable to bleeding because, as relatively unstable hinge articulations, they must withstand rotatory and angulatory stresses (14). After an acute intraarticular bleed, autolysis of erythrocytes results in the deposition of cytoplasmic iron in the synovium and chondrocytes of the articular cartilage (15). Within 4 days, the inflammatory and proliferative effects induced by the bleed become apparent as focal areas of villous formation develop on the synovial surface. Recurrent hemarthroses stimulate more synovial hyperplasia, which is friable and more likely to rebleed with minimal stress (e.g., weight bearing or trauma). A vicious cycle of rebleeding may become established, creating a *target joint*. The progressive pathobiology of hemophilic arthropathy is likely propagated by molecular changes induced by iron, mediated by the overexpression of mdm2 (a p53-binding protein) and c-myc oncogenes and by the elaboration of various cytokines (16). Eventually, these processes lead to chronic synovitis, articular fibrosis, progressive joint stiffness and compromised range of motion, and constant pain (13). Obesity in patients with hemophilia exacerbates arthropathy and mitigates the benefits of prophylactic or treatment strategies. The fear of precipitating bleeds with exercise and the resulting sedentary lifestyle to "protect" the joints contribute to this phenomenon; however, this is counterintuitive to the observed benefits of primary prophylaxis regimens and regular exercise, which are associated with less frequent bleeding events and improved joint mobility.

The hallmark of an acute intraarticular bleed is pain, which is immediately followed by swelling. Individuals with hemophilia frequently describe a premonitory prickly sensation and warmth within the joint shortly before the onset of overt pain or swelling (17). The joint becomes fixed in a flexed position until swelling and pain subside enough to allow movement. It is therefore crucial that the acute bleed be treated rapidly with factor VIII or IX concentrates to prevent accumulation of large amounts of blood in the closed joint space and to minimize articular pain and damage. Occasionally, repeat infusions of clotting factor concentrate are required for pain control or to treat target joints. This is more likely to occur for weight-bearing joints (e.g., ankle, knee, and hips) rather than non–weight-bearing joints. A short course of corticosteroids sometimes is attempted to reduce the pain and swelling in children with limited joint disease but is used infrequently in adults. Joint aspirations for routine hemarthroses should not be performed unless there is severe, intractable pain despite adequate replacement therapy (18) or unless the patient appears toxic with a fever (body temperature >39°C) and septic arthritis is suspected (19). Adequate replacement therapy should be administered before aspiration is attempted (20); aspiration should be avoided in patients with an inhibitor (21). For some target joints, a regimen of secondary prophylaxis consisting of twice- or thrice-weekly administration of factor VIII or IX concentrates for at least 3 months is necessary to break the bleeding cycle. If this does not improve the situation, synovectomy can be considered, but this procedure is more effective before there is significant hemarthropathy (see subsequent text). The initiation of primary prophylaxis regimens immediately after the first or second articular bleed may, in the least, impede development of joint destruction and, at the most, prevent it altogether (see subsequent text).

In individuals with chronic synovitis as a component of early progressive hemophilic arthropathy, surgical or radionuclide synovectomy (RSV) may be considered as effective means to reduce recurrent joint bleeds and to relieve joint pain. Surgical synovectomy is very effective in the short-term reduction of pain, reduction in clotting factor consumption, and preservation of joint mobility; however, progression of the hemophilic arthropathy is not halted. In contrast to surgical synovectomy, RSV requires no anesthesia, requires minimal clotting factor replacement therapy, and is considerably less expensive. Furthermore, protracted physical therapy is not needed after RSV to preserve the range of motion of the affected joint, and the patient remains ambulatory. The non-surgical RSV approach is most likely to benefit hemophilic arthropathy refractory to aggressive replacement therapy with factor concentrate or in those who have previously failed arthroscopic synovectomy. Clinical trials indicate that RSV is ideal to provide sustained relief from joint pain and that it reduces bleeding frequency by at least 80% in those with alloantibody inhibitors and increased propensity to hemorrhagic complications despite replacement therapy and in those with human immunodeficiency virus (HIV), in whom joint surgery is associated with significantly increased postoperative infections. If three consecutive synoviortheses (repeated every 3 months) fail to relieve or prevent synovitis symptoms, a surgical synovectomy (open or by arthroscopy) should be pursued. RSV should not be used in those with end-stage hemophilic arthropathy (advanced beyond Arnold-Hilgartner stage 4 or 5) because the pain, bleeding frequency, and impaired mobility of the joint will not be sufficiently ameliorated. Although numerous radiocolloids have been employed [e.g., rhenium 186 ($^{186}$Re), gold 189 ($^{189}$Au), and yttrium 90 ($^{90}$Y)], phosphorus 32 ($^{32}$P) is the only radionuclide used for RSV in the United States because of its larger particle size, pure $\beta$-emission profile, and longer half-life. Two cases of acute lymphoblastic leukemia (precursor B cell and T cell) have been reported to occur in young men within a year of their synoviortheses. The intraarticular instillation of radionuclides has not been associated with leakage or with excessive chromosomal damage to the synovium; however, theoretical leukemic potential must be considered when deciding to proceed with RSV. Chemical synovectomy using osmic acid and rifampicin has also been attempted in a few subjects with hemophilic synovitis. The results appear inferior to RSV, and the delayed effects of chemical synovectomy remain to be established.

Surgical replacement of the affected joint with a prosthesis is recommended when joint destruction has progressed to the point that the patient with hemophilia experiences constant pain and disability due to compromised range of motion despite aggressive clotting factor replacement to assure that the pain is not due to an acute bleeding event. When performed in a comprehensive hemophilia treatment center, the surgical results are good or excellent in over 95% of patients. Joint pain is reduced in all recipients, and significantly increased physical activity and capacity are achieved, particularly if rigorous postoperative physical therapy rehabilitation regimens have been adhered to. Recurrent hemarthroses in the replaced joint are infrequent. In a very small percentage of severe hemophiliacs and a larger percentage of mild cases, the surgical procedure may precipitate the development of an alloantibody inhibitor directed against the patient's deficient clotting factor protein. This certainly complicates the postoperative care and may be the result of immune stimulation by inflammation or, perhaps, by the intensive exposure to large quantity of clotting factor protein administered intraoperatively and during the convalescent period. Typically, all quality-of-life measures improve following surgical joint replacement in the hemophiliac. The decreased consumption of clotting factor is often not immediately appreciated because of the large cumulative requirement for factor replacement to protect the joint during the prolonged and rigorous physical therapy recovery period. Over the long term, joint replacements are cost effective; however, the ultimate goal is to prevent the development of severe hemophilic arthropathy, perhaps achievable by initiating primary prophylaxis of clotting factor early in the life of the patient with hemophilia.

The most experience in patients with hemophilia has been gained with total knee and hip prostheses, which have a 10-year overall survival rate of over 80%. Increasing experience is emerging in patients with hemophilia who present with prosthetic shoulders, elbows, and ankles. The complex range of motion of these latter joints has hindered their widespread use. For elbows, the more successful approach for severe pain and joint destruction is synovectomy combined with resection of the radial head. The most common complication of surgical joint replacements is late infection, with an approximate incidence of 15%. Several series have reported considerably higher rates of infection in patients with hemophilia who are also HIV infected, but careful patient selection and maintenance of highly active antiretroviral therapy (HAART) minimize this risk. In contrast to other populations undergoing total knee or hip replacements, patients with hemophilia do not appear to develop the venous thromboembolic (VTE) complications of orthopedic procedures in the absence of anticoagulation prophylaxis. The use of VTE prophylaxis regimens in patients with hemophilia in this scenario remains controversial from the risk-to-benefit perspective but currently is rarely used.

Aggressive clotting factor replacement therapy and postoperative physical therapy are critical to the successful recovery of range of motion and long-term survival of the prosthetic joint. It also adds substantially to the expense of surgery and convalescence. The administration of clotting factor concentrates by continuous infusion rather than bolus injection following orthopedic procedures in the patient with hemophilia may reduce the cumulative requirement for overall factor needs, and therefore the cost of care, without sacrificing safety or benefit. Larger randomized studies are underway to confirm this hypothesis. Concurrent joint replacements in the same surgical session (e.g., contralateral joints, ipsilateral hip, and knee) are becoming more commonplace and are cost effective as far as overall clotting factor consumption, complication rates, and rehabilitation time are concerned. Furthermore, this approach avoids the delay inherent to staged procedures in achieving a totally functional limb. If the joint or adjacent bone is destroyed beyond the ability of the surgeon to implant a prosthesis, an arthrodesis (fusion) procedure provides an alternative method to relieve pain and/or to support weight bearing.

## Intramuscular Hemorrhage

Intramuscular hemorrhages are the second most prevalent type of bleeding event in severe hemophilia, accounting for approximately 30% of bleeding episodes (22). Hemorrhages into large muscles generally resolve without complication but may be quite extensive because they diffuse along fascial planes. In contrast, a much smaller amount of bleeding in a closed fascial compartment may cause significant compression of vital structures with attendant distal ischemia, possible gangrene, flexion contractures, and neuropathy (compartment syndrome) (23). Intramuscular hematomas typically present with localized tenderness and pain, either on movement or at rest (24), and may also be associated with low-grade fevers, elevations in serum lactate dehydrogenase levels, and large ecchymoses. They are the most common hemorrhagic complication in the hands and forearms, as compared to hemarthroses in other parts of the musculoskeleton (25). Hematomas of the psoas muscle and the retroperitoneal space are particularly problematic and produce sudden onset of severe inguinal pain and compromised range of motion of the ipsilateral hip, which assumes a markedly flexed position, usually with lateral rotation (26). Bleeding may be spontaneous or posttraumatic and can become life threatening because of the large volume of blood that can be lost in the soft tissues of the retroperitoneal space. Unless bleeding is contained by aggressively raising and maintaining factor VIII or IX levels to 80% to 100% of normal levels for 48 to 72 hours (14), hypotension and femoral nerve entrapment and compression will occur. Paresthesias or anesthesia proximal to the patella or along the medial aspect of the thigh, loss of the patellar reflex, quadriceps weakness, and hip flexion contractures are characteristic complications (26). Pelvic ultrasonography and computed tomography scan can confirm the diagnosis.

## Hematuria and Renal Disease

Spontaneous gross hematuria occurs frequently in individuals with severe hemophilia and generally is a benign and painless condition unless accompanied by intraureteral clots (27). Trauma, exertion, and ingestion of nonsteroidal antiinflammatory drugs (NSAIDs) may provoke bleeding. Approximately 36% to 58% of patients with acute hematuria have abnormal intravenous pyelograms showing pelvic clots, obstructive hydronephrosis, small collecting systems, or retroperitoneal fibrosis (28). The exact mechanism for spontaneous hemophilic hematuria is unknown but is thought to reflect direct tubular damage by circulating immune complexes. HIV infection and hemophilia-related factors, including alloantibody inhibitors to factor VIII or IX and kidney bleeds, are strongly associated with development of hypertension and acute and/or chronic renal disease (29).

Nephrotic syndrome may develop in a subset of hemophilia B patients with alloantibody inhibitors to factor IX. These individuals may experience life-threatening anaphylactic reactions during the administration of factor IX replacement concentrates. These complications also are mediated by circulating immune complexes. Patients with large gene deletions appear to be most vulnerable. All infectious, neoplastic, and lithogenic etiologies of hematuria should be considered before attributing nephrotic syndrome to severe hemophilia. Currently, hematuria due to nephrolithiasis most commonly affects patients with hemophilia who are also HIV-infected and are taking the HIV protease inhibitor indinavir (Crixivan), which produces crystalluria and calculi consisting of the intact drug. In developing countries, patients with severe and moderately severe hemophilia may be at a higher risk of urolithiasis because of prolonged recumbency, which is necessitated by recurrent joint bleeds and inadequate replacement therapy (30).

The treatment of hematuria depends on the etiology; however, hydration and factor replacement are basic elements. There are conflicting data on the benefits of short courses of high-dose steroids (31,32); however, the only randomized, double-blinded study revealed no appreciable benefit in the steroid-treated group (32). Hematuria persisting over several days despite aggressive hydration should be treated with replacement therapy to raise the factor VIII or IX level to 50%. Antifibrinolytic agents, such as ε-aminocaproic acid (EACA) or tranexamic acid, should be administered judiciously (27) because intraureteral clots may form and cause obstruction with renal colic, anuria, or both. Sporadic, transient hemospermia is not rare in patients with hemophilia and, as with noncoagulopathic individuals, is a benign condition, with mostly idiopathic or inflammatory causes. Factor VIII or IX replacement therapy is occasionally required to treat the bleeding.

## Intracranial Hemorrhage

Central nervous system (CNS) bleeding was the leading cause of death in the hemophilia population (33,34) until the beginning of the acquired immunodeficiency syndrome (AIDS) epidemic in the early 1980s. The incidence of spontaneous CNS bleeds varies between 2.6% and 13.8% (33,35–37). Intracranial hemorrhage almost always is preceded by head trauma in children, whereas in adults more than 50% of intracranial hemorrhages occur without prior head injury (33,38). The risk of spontaneous CNS bleeding is increased significantly in adults with AIDS taking HIV–protease inhibitor drugs. Approximately 30% of CNS events result in death; more than 50% of the survivors develop long-term neurologic sequelae (33,39). The most frequent presenting symptom of intracranial bleeding is headache, often with vomiting and seizure (33). CNS bleeding can be subdural, subarachnoid, intraspinal, or intracerebral, and all should be treated aggressively and rapidly with administration of factor VIII or IX concentrates to achieve 100% of normal activity. This must precede diagnostic testing in any patient with hemophilia who has a suspected head-bleed, even in the absence of head trauma or symptoms (33). Treatment should not be reserved solely for trauma that produces lacerations, hematomas, or neurologic deficits (21); less than 5% of acute head injuries produce early computed tomographic scan abnormalities, and when they are present, they are usually accompanied with signs and symptoms of increased intracranial pressure. Patients with mild hemophilia generally need treatment only for significant trauma (33). If a diagnostic lumbar puncture is necessary, factor VIII or IX levels should be raised to 100% with a dose of clotting factor concentrate given 30 minutes earlier. The risks of postpartum or intrapartum intracranial hemorrhage in a fetus with known hemophilia can be minimized by the administration of factor VIII or factor IX concentrate immediately after delivery. Alternatively, the successful use of an intrauterine infusion of factor VIII has been reported in a fetus with documented hemophilia A (40). The neonatal or intrauterine use of clotting factor replacement for prophylaxis or treatment of acute bleeds in patients with severe hemophilia remains controversial because exposure to exogenous factor VIII or IX concentrate so early in life may stimulate the production of alloantibody inhibitors (40).

## Oropharyngeal and Gastrointestinal Bleeding

Excessive bleeding from mucous membranes is common in severe hemophilia, but if it occurs in mildly affected individuals, the diagnosis of VWD should be excluded. Traumatic hemorrhage in the oropharynx may lead to life-threatening upper airway obstruction; retropharyngeal bleeds are particularly dangerous and require 80% to 100% replacement factor levels (41). Epistaxis and bleeding from tooth extractions can be treated with fibrin sealants, microfibrillar collagen, or topical or systemic antifibrinolytic agents (42). For extensive dental procedures, particularly those requiring nerve block, factor levels should be raised to approximately 25% of normal, and antifibrinolytic agents can be given for prophylaxis.

Gastrointestinal (GI) bleeding occurs in approximately 15% to 20% of adults with severe hemophilia. The rate of *Helicobacter pylori* infection and dyspepsia in patients with hemophilia is similar to the prevalence in the healthy population, but symptomatic bleeding from gastric ulcers (20% vs. 5%) and duodenal ulcers (7% vs. 5%) is more common in patients who have coagulopathy (43). GI bleeding has also increased because of the frequent use of NSAIDs for chronic arthritis and because of the rising incidence of esophageal varices resulting from portal hypertension due to chronic hepatitis and cirrhosis. Concurrent use of proton-pump inhibitors and the switch to COX-2 inhibitors (not withstanding their potential arterial hypercoagulable risks) have mitigated GI bleeding precipitated by NSAIDs while allowing for marked pain relief from hemophilic arthropathy and for significant sparing of clotting factor replacement requirements. For severe bleeds and for diagnostic endoscopic procedures, factor VIII and IX activity levels should be raised to more than 50% of normal (44).

# TREATMENT

## Replacement Therapy with Coagulation Factor Concentrates

The mainstay of successful hemophilia therapy either for treatment or prevention of acute hemorrhage is prompt and sufficient intravenous replacement of factor VIII or IX to hemostatically adequate plasma levels. Early treatment, at the first onset of symptoms, limits both the amount of the bleeding and the extent of the ensuing tissue damage.

Replacement products are derived either from normal pooled plasma or mammalian cell lines genetically engineered to synthesize recombinant human proteins (see Tables 59-1 and 59-2). All replacement products appear to have equivalent clinical efficacy but are classified according to their final purity, defined as specific activity (international units of specific clotting factor activity per milligram relative to the amount of total protein in the preparation); by the source of origin of the purified clotting factor (from source or recovered pooled normal donor plasma vs. those synthesized by genetically engineered mammalian cell lines); by the method of viral attenuation; and by the presence or absence of extraneous mammalian proteins in the nutrient milieu of the genetically engineered cells and in the final formulation of purified clotting protein. Intermediate purity products have relatively low specific clotting factor activity (<50 IU per mg) because they are contaminated with extraneous plasma proteins, such as fibrinogen, VWF protein, and other noncoagulant proteins (45). High-purity (>50 IU per mg) and ultra–high-purity (>3,000 IU per mg for factor VIII concentrates; >160 IU per mg for factor IX concentrates) products contain little or virtually no contaminating plasma proteins

other than albumin that are added as a stabilizer. Viral inactivation methods include single-step or combination dry heating, pasteurization, or solvent detergent extraction (45–48), and are enhanced by immunoaffinity chromatography (49) (monoclonal antibody purification), nanofiltration, and gel filtration chromatography (50) added in tandem to manufacturing techniques used to isolate the desired therapeutic clotting factor protein.

Viral-attenuated plasma-derived products are considered virtually free of lipid-enveloped pathogenic viruses, such as HIV; hepatitis B (HBV), hepatitis C virus (HCV), and G (GB virus C) viruses; and West Nile virus. No transmission of these viruses has been documented in the United States since 1985 for factor VIII concentrates and since 1990 for factor IX concentrates. Unfortunately, non–lipid-coated viruses, such as parvovirus B19, transfusion transmitted virus (TTV), hepatitis A virus (HAV), and prions, are not susceptible to these processes. The seroprevalence of patient with hemophilia treated with plasma-derived products approaches 80% for B19; data from a multicenter hemophilia cohort indicate that the risk of B19 seroconversion was ninefold greater in children who received plasma-derived factor only versus recombinant clotting factor. Children who were anti-B19 seropositive also demonstrated less overall range of motion in their joints affected by hemophilia-related bleeds (51). TTV, another hepatotropic DNA virus associated with the transfusion of plasma proteins, infected approximately 70% of recipients of plasma-derived factor VIII concentrates, regardless of whether the concentrate was viral attenuated. Factor VIII recombinant concentrates stabilized by human albumen probably do not— and second- and third-generation (human protein–free) factor VIII concentrates and plasma-derived, viral attenuated, and recombinant factor IX concentrates certainly do not—transmit TTV (52,53). Fortunately, TTV does not appear to be pathogenic and does not cause or exacerbate chronic hepatitis.

Sporadic cases of HAV have been reported with a plasma-derived high-purity factor IX concentrate; however, nanofiltration has since been added to the purification process of plasma-derived factor IX concentrates and has proven to be very effective in removing HAV and parvovirus B19.

Nanofiltration is not effective in removing small viruses from high-molecular-weight protein preparations like plasma-derived factor VIII concentrates because the size of the protein is similar to that of viruses. The introduction of viral nucleic acid amplification testing (NAT) of plasma pools for potential viral contamination has reinforced the viral safety of plasma-derived concentrates.

Transfusion transmitted hepatitis A and B should be problems of the past for patients with hemophilia if vaccinations for these two viruses are administered routinely in infancy. Recombinant clotting factor concentrates are considered virus free, although there has been concern that the first-generation products, which are stabilized in human albumen, along with plasma-derived factor concentrates, theoretically possess the potential to transmit the prion-related new-variant Creutzfeldt-Jakob disease (vCJD). To date, no cases of vCJD are known to have been transmitted by any plasma product and no person with hemophilia has been diagnosed with vCJD. As an extra measure of safety, plasma-derived concentrates no longer employ source plasma from the United Kingdom, where most of the cases of vCJD have been diagnosed, and fractionation processes have been shown to partition substantial amounts of vCJD from plasma in spiking experiments. Longitudinal epidemiologic surveillance and autopsy studies analyzing brain tissue from patients with hemophilia who died with neurologic symptoms mostly associated with HIV seropositivity, reassuringly have not yielded any evidence for transmission of vCJD despite their repeated exposures to blood components or factor replacement products. No evidence of spongiform

**TABLE 59-1**

FACTOR VIII CONCENTRATES AVAILABLE IN THE UNITED STATES

| Product name (manufacturer) | Viral inactivation procedure(s) | Purity/Specific activity (IU factor VIII activity/mg total protein) before addition of stabilizer |
|---|---|---|
| **HUMAN PLASMA–DERIVED CONCENTRATES** | | |
| Humate-P (ZLB Behring, Inc.) (contains von Willebrand factor protein) | Pasteurization (heating in solution, 60°C, 10 h) | Intermediate (1-10 IU/mg) |
| Alphanate SD (Grifols, Inc.) (contains von Willebrand factor protein) | Solvent detergent (TNBP/ Polysorbate 80) Affinity chromatography Dry heat (80°C, 72 h) | High (50–100 IU/mg) (>400 IU/mg after correcting for VWF content) |
| Koate-DVI (Bayer, Inc.) (contains von Willebrand factor protein) | Solvent detergent (TNBP/ Polysorbate 80) Dry heat (80°C, 72 h) | High (50–100 IU/mg) |
| **MONOCLONAL ANTIBODY, PURIFIED (IMMUNOAFFINITY PURIFIED FROM HUMAN PLASMA, NO INTACT VON WILLEBRAND FACTOR PROTEIN)** | | |
| Monarc M (Baxter/Immuno, Inc., using recovered plasma from the American Red Cross) | Solvent detergent (TNBP/ Octoxynol 9) Immunoaffinity chromatography | Ultra high (>3,000 IU/mg) |
| Hemofil M (Baxter/Immuno, Inc.) | Solvent detergent (TNBP/ Octoxynol 9) Immunoaffinity chromatography | Ultra high (>3,000 IU/mg) |
| Monoclate-P (ZLB Behring, Inc.) | Pasteurization (heated in solution, 60°C, 10 h) Immunoaffinity chromatography | Ultra high (>3,000 IU/mg) |
| **RECOMBINANT (GENETIC ENGINEERED)/FIRST GENERATION** | | |
| Recombinate (Baxter/Immuno, Inc.) (human albumin as a stabilizer) | Immunoaffinity, ion exchange chromatography Bovine serum albumin used in culture medium for Chinese hamster ovary cells | Ultra high (>4,000 IU/mg) |
| **RECOMBINANT/SECOND GENERATION (HUMAN ALBUMIN–FREE FINAL FORMULATIONS)** | | |
| Kogenate FS (Bayer, Inc.) Helixate FS (Bayer for ZLB Behring, Inc.) (sucrose as a stabilizer) | Immunoaffinity chromatography Ion exchange Solvent detergent (TNBP/ polysorbate 80) Ultrafiltration | Ultra high (>4,000 IU/mg) |
| Refacto (Wyeth, Inc.) B-domain deleted (sucrose as a stabilizer) | Immunoaffinity chromatography Ion exchange Solvent detergent (TNBP/Triton X-100) nanofiltration | Ultra high (>11,200–15,500 IU/mg), measured by chromogenic assay technique |
| **RECOMBINANT/THIRD GENERATION (NO HUMAN OR ANIMAL PROTEIN USED IN THE CULTURE MEDIUM OR MANUFACTURING PROCESS)** | | |
| Advate (Baxter/Immuno, Inc.) (trehalose as a stabilizer) | Immunoaffinity chromatography Ion exchange Solvent detergent (TNBP/ polysorbate 80) | Ultra high (>4,000–10,000 IU/mg) |

TNBP, tri-N-butyl phosphate; VWF, von Willebrand factor.

encephalopathy was found, and the immunocytochemistry was negative for PrP in all brains (54,55).

The choice of which factor VIII concentrate any individual should use primarily is made on the basis of the perception of the degree of viral safety and cost of product. For example, second-generation (albumen-free final formulations) and third-generation (free of mammalian protein throughout manufacturing and no albumen stabilization of the final product) recombinant factor VIII concentrates are considered by many physicians and patients to be more viral-safe than

**TABLE 59-2**

COAGULATION FACTOR IX REPLACEMENT PRODUCTS AVAILABLE IN THE UNITED STATES

| Product name (manufacturer) | Viral inactivation procedure(s) | Purity/Specific activity (IU FIX activity/mg protein) |
|---|---|---|
| **PLASMA-DERIVED PROTHROMBIN COMPLEX CONCENTRATES/FACTOR IX COMPLEX CONCENTRATES (NONACTIVATED)** | | |
| Bebulin VH (Baxter/Immuno) | Vapor heat (60°C, 10 h at 190 mbar pressure plus 1 h at 80°C, 375 mbar) | Intermediate (<50 IU/mg) |
| Profilnine SD (Grifols) | Solvent detergent (TNBP/polysorbate 80) | Intermediate (<50 IU/mg) |
| Proplex-T (Baxter/Immuno) | Dry heat (60°C, 144 h) | Intermediate (<50 IU/mg) |
| **PLASMA-DERIVED PROTHROMBIN COMPLEX CONCENTRATES/FACTOR IX COMPLEX CONCENTRATES (ACTIVATED)** | | |
| FEIBA (Baxter/Immuno) | Vapor heating (60°C, 10 h, 1,160 mbar) | Intermediate (<50 IU/mg) |
| **PLASMA-DERIVED COAGULATION FACTOR IX (HUMAN) CONCENTRATES** | | |
| AlphaNine SD (Grifols) | Dual affinity chromatography Solvent detergent (TNBP/polysorbate 80) nanofiltration (viral filter) | High (>200 IU/mg) |
| Mononine (ZLB Behring) | Monoclonal antibody immunoaffinity chromatography Sodium thiocyanate Ultrafiltration | High (>160 IU/mg) |
| BeneFIX (Wyeth) (no animal- or human-derived protein in cell line; no albumin added to final product) | Affinity chromatography Ultrafiltration | Ultra high (>200 IU/mg) |

TNBP, tri-N-butyl phosphate.

first-generation recombinant factor VIII products (synthesized in the presence of mammalian proteins and stabilized in human albumen) and viral attenuated plasma-derived concentrates. Cost of the products is directly proportional to specific activity and the sophistication of the production and viral attenuation technology used. HIV and HCV status, the age of the patient, and the possible association of alloantibody inhibitor development with use of ultra–high-purity and recombinant factor VIII or IX products in previously untreated patients (PUPs) (see subsequent text) are additional considerations. The perception that these concentrates may be more antigenic has not been confirmed in adequately powered, randomized studies (56). Most physicians believe this increased incidence is related to more frequent laboratory surveillance using more sensitive assays for the detection of inhibitors rather than to increased clotting factor protein antigenicity (56).

The general order of priority for the exclusive use of recombinant factor concentrates is: (i) PUPs; (ii) HIV- and HCV-negative patients; (iii) HIV-negative, HCV-positive patients; (iv) HIV-positive patients. These guidelines for recombinant concentrate use have been adopted by most economically accomplished countries; recombinant factor VIII and IX concentrates are used by over 90% of all patients with hemophilia in the United States. However, it must be appreciated that 80% to 90% of the world's hemophilia population do not receive adequate or any replacement therapy for their acute bleeds. The currently available plasma-derived concentrates are virtually viral-safe, except for the limitations discussed earlier; are considerably less expensive than the recombinant alternatives; and are equally efficacious in promoting adequate hemostasis. Their favorable pricing and cost-to-benefit profile should facilitate their use in countries with limited health care resources to reduce the morbidity and mortality associated with hemophilia.

The choice of factor IX replacement products has been influenced by the fact that intermediate purity factor IX complex concentrates [previously designated *prothrombin complex concentrates* (PCCs)] contain significant amounts of activated vitamin K–dependent factors VII, X, and prothrombin. When administered at frequent intervals or over a prolonged period, they may produce hypercoagulable complications, such as disseminated intravascular coagulation, VTE, stroke, or myocardial infarction (57). Because of their high specific activities and absence of extraneous activated clotting factors, recombinant factor IX and plasma-derived ultra–high-purity factor IX concentrates have little or no thrombogenic potential (58) and are the products of choice for surgery, prophylactic regimens, immune tolerance induction (ITI), and for those who have experienced prior thrombotic complications.

Factor replacement therapy in hemophilia is based on plasma volume and distribution of the clotting protein between intravascular or extravascular compartments, the circulating retention time (half-life or survival) in plasma, and the optimal level of clotting factor required to terminate or prevent hemorrhage. Dosing can be calculated simply by assuming that 1 U per kg body weight of factor VIII replacement raises the plasma activity by approximately 0.02 U per mL (2%). Its circulating half-life is biphasic, averaging approximately 12 hours. One U per kg of factor IX, which has a larger volume distribution, increases plasma levels by 0.01 U per mL (1%). Approximately one third of patients receiving recombinant factor IX require dosing at least 20% higher than calculated because of its low recovery (i.e., lower-than-expected increment of factor IX activity 15 to 30 minutes after factor IX infusion). Factor IX has a plasma half-life up to 24 hours (59).

Optimal hemostatic plasma levels for factors VIII and IX and various clinical scenarios are presented in Table 59-3. In general, 30% to 50% of normal factor levels are required for most bleeding episodes of less severity. Usually one, and occasionally

**TABLE 59-3**

GUIDELINES FOR FACTOR REPLACEMENT THERAPY

| Type of bleeding | Factor VIII dose (U/kg) | Factor IX dose (U/kg) | Hemostatic factor level |
|---|---|---|---|
| Acute hemarthrosis | 10–20 qd as needed | 15 q.o.d. as needed | 30%–50% |
| Intramuscular | 20–30, q12h | 40–60, q.o.d. as needed | 40%–50% |
| Central nervous system | 50 q12h, or continuous infusion | 100, then 50 q12h | 100% initially; 50%–100% 10–14 d |
| Trauma or surgery | 50 q12h, or continuous infusion | 100, then q24h | 100%, then 50% until wound healing begins, then 30% until wound healing complete |
| Retropharyngeal | 50 q12h, 4 d | 40, 4 d | 50%–70% |
| Gastrointestinal | 50, 3 d, or until bleeding subsides | 40, 3 d, or until bleeding subsides | 50%–100% |
| Hematuria | 40, 3–5 d | 40, 3 d | 50% |
| Mouth | 40 once, then Amicar 100 mg/kg for 6 d | 20 once, then Amicar 100 mg/kg for 6 d | 30%–40% |
| Tooth extraction, dental procedures | 40 once, then Amicar 100 mg/kg for 7–10 d | 30 once, then Amicar 100 mg/kg for 6 d | 50% |
| Retroperitoneal | 50, q12h for 6 d | 40, 12 h for 6 d | 100% initially, then 50% until complete resolution of hematoma |

Adapted from Schramm W. Experience with prophylaxis in Germany. *Semin Hematol* 1993;30(Suppl 2):12–15.

two, doses of factor VIII or IX are sufficient to control bleeding, prevent secondary hemorrhage, and initiate tissue healing. Between 50% and 100% of activity levels are necessary to treat or prevent life-threatening or limb-threatening hemorrhage or surgical bleeding. Factor replacement can be delivered either by bolus or continuous infusion as part of demand, primary or secondary prophylaxis, or ITI regimens. Continuous infusion maintains a constant therapeutic factor level not subject to the peaks and troughs observed with bolus injections and may decrease total dosing by as much as 30% (60). Widespread use of continuous infusion regimens has become feasible with the advent of ultra–high-purity plasma-derived and recombinant concentrates (61).

## Cryoprecipitate

Cryoprecipitate, prepared from fresh frozen plasma after slowly thawing at 4°C, is rich in factor VIII, VWF, and fibrinogen. Viral attenuation techniques have not been applied to cryoprecipitate. Photochemical inactivation of DNA and RNA viruses by methylene blue or psoralen derivatives appears very effective except against prions, but are associated with substantial losses of factor VIII (approximately 25%) and VWF (approximately 15%) activities. Therefore, administration of cryoprecipitate should be limited to urgent replacement in hemophilia A or VWD when other more viral-safe products are not available or responses to 1-deamino 8-D-arginine vasopressin (DDAVP) are not adequate. Cryoprecipitate lacks factor IX and is not useful in treating hemophilia B.

## Ancillary Therapies

### Desmopressin Acetate

DDAVP stimulates a transient fourfold increase in plasma factor VIII and VWF protein levels (62) by causing an almost immediate release of factor VIII/VWF from storage sites (63–65). This synthetic drug also raises factor XI levels and enhances platelet

adhesion and spreading at injury sites (63,64). Providing an effective alternative non–plasma-based therapy for most patients with mild hemophilia, DDAVP (Stimate) can be administered intravenously, at a dose of 0.3 μg per kg of body weight in 50 mL of normal saline over 15 to 20 minutes, or as a concentrated intranasal spray administered in one puff (150 μg per nostril) with efficacy similar to the intravenous preparation. The peak effect of the intravenous preparation occurs 30 to 60 minutes after infusion, whereas the intranasal product peaks later at 60 to 90 minutes after administration (66,67). DDAVP can be given every 12 to 24 hours to treat or prevent bleeding, although many individuals may develop tachyphylaxis (62). DDAVP should not be used in patients with severe hemophilia because they do not have any storage pools of factor VIII. The most common side effects of DDAVP are inconsequential facial flushing and fluctuations of blood pressure (65). Severe hyponatremia may precipitate seizures, particularly in infants and children receiving large amounts of free water. Therefore, oral and intravenous fluids should be limited and serum sodium levels monitored. Angina pectoris, coronary artery thrombosis, and stroke have been reported in elderly patients after receiving DDAVP (68); cause-and-effect relationships remain unclear (69).

### Antifibrinolytic Agents

Antifibrinolytic agents are useful ancillary therapies that stabilize clot formation by inhibiting the clot's lysis by plasmin. They are especially helpful for the prevention or treatment of hemorrhage emanating from mucous membranes (i.e., oropharynx, nose, genitourinary tract, among others) because their secretions contain fibrinolytic enzymes. Two drugs—EACA (Amicar) and tranexamic acid (Cyklokapron)—are available for intravenous or oral administration (17) and often are used in conjunction with DDAVP to reverse the thrombolytic effects generated by the release of tissue plasminogen activator.

Topical agents, such as fibrin sealants, have successfully reduced blood loss and requirements for replacement therapy with factor concentrates in individuals with severe hemophilia A or B undergoing minor and major surgical procedures. Very few controlled clinical trials have been published, which has limited their widespread use in these clinical scenarios.

## Prophylactic Factor Replacement

The prevention of recurrent hemarthrosis, subsequent irreversible joint damage, and long-term disability and pain should be the goals of therapy for patients with hemophilia. Because individuals with moderately severe hemophilia develop few spontaneous bleeding episodes, it was hypothesized that maintaining factor VIII or IX levels between 1% and 5% of normal may alter the clinical phenotype of patients with severe hemophilia and provide for adequate hemostasis (70). Swedish investigators have been testing this theory since the 1950s by initiating primary prophylaxis regimens in patients with severe hemophilia aged 1 to 3 years or after the first spontaneous bleed, whichever occurs first (71). Individuals who maintained factor VIII or IX trough levels greater than 1% to 2% (25 to 40 IU per kg concentrate administered three times weekly for hemophilia A and twice weekly for hemophilia B) experienced fewer than one spontaneous joint bleed per year and demonstrated normal joint structure and function on standardized orthopedic and radiologic evaluations over a 10-year observation period. This resulted in significantly enhanced performance status but was accomplished with more than a fourfold increased consumption of clotting factor concentrate over the average on-demand usage for individuals with severe hemophilia. In contrast, when prophylaxis was started after the development of arthropathy, the overall number of bleeds decreased, but the development of arthropathy was not halted. In one center, the mean number of major bleeds was reduced dramatically from 15.5 per year on on-demand replacement therapy to 1.9 per year on primary prophylaxis, with a significant decrease in target joints, emergency department visits, and hospitalizations (72). Despite these apparent benefits, primary prophylaxis has been adopted as standard treatment for hemophilia in only few countries because of concerns about the complications associated with central venous access devices (thrombosis and infections) to achieve compliance with primary prophylaxis protocols and concerns about the substantial increased cost of clotting factor replacement. Although the results from prospective, randomized cost-benefit outcomes studies are being collected, efforts to fine-tune primary prophylaxis regimens are being pursued. One strategy individualizes the regimen by initiating primary prophylaxis with once-weekly infusions through peripheral veins with rapid escalation to full-dose prophylaxis or dose escalation based on frequency of bleeding (73,74). This regimen is based on observations that some patients do not bleed in spite of a trough level of less than 1% and others did bleed in spite of trough levels greater than 3%.

Secondary prophylaxis regimens, instituted at a later age to break the cycle of target joint bleeding or to minimize progression of early arthropathy, dramatically improves quality of life but does not prevent future episodes of joint hemorrhage or eliminate progression of joint damage (74,75).

# TREATMENT COMPLICATIONS

## Acquired Alloantibody Inhibitors in Individuals with Hemophilia A or B

### Epidemiology

The sudden occurrence of refractoriness to treatment with clotting factor replacement products is usually associated with the appearance of an alloantibody inhibitor, which directly targets the FVIII:C or factor IX protein and neutralizes its coagulant activity (76). The standardized Bethesda unit assay is utilized to quantitate the potency of FVIII:C and FIX inhibitors (77), and the more sensitive Nemejgen modification of the Bethesda assay detects low-level FVIII:C alloantibody inhibitor titers (78). The Nemejgen assay is reserved predominantly for clinical research situations rather than for therapeutic decision making.

Although a systematic retrospective review revealed the overall prevalence of FVIII:C alloantibody inhibitors to range between 5% and 7% in an unselected hemophilic population (79), the prevalence is higher, approximately 13%, when only severe cases (<1% FVIII:C activity) are considered (80,81). Longitudinal, prospective studies of well-defined cohorts indicate an incidence of allo-FVIII:C antibody inhibitor development in approximately 28% of previously treated patients (PTPs) and up to 39% of PUPs (82). Subsequent analyses have revealed that individuals with large factor VIII:C gene deletions, affecting more than one domain of the FVIII:C molecule, have a threefold higher risk of developing an allo-FVIII:C antibody inhibitor compared with single-domain deletions (88% vs. 24%) (83). In persons with hemophilia B, alloantibodies occur in only 1% to 3% of severely affected individuals (84).

**Genetic Factors.** Allo-FVIII:C antibodies occur twice as commonly in African Americans and in Hispanics than in whites, whereas Scandinavians are at higher risk than other populations to develop allo-factor IX antibodies (83,85). Furthermore, sibling pairs with hemophilia are significantly more likely than distant relatives to develop alloantibody inhibitors. That alloinhibitor formation may be discordant in sibling pairs or even in identical monozygotic twins, despite similar gene defects, suggests that other factors must be contributory, perhaps those involving immune system responses. Major histocompatibility gene (MHC) classes, which may influence how peptides of FVIII:C or FIX are presented to the antigen processing lymphocyte, have been proposed as potential mediators, but studies have been inconclusive. FVIII:C and FIX gene polymorphisms definitely are critical to the development of alloantibody inhibitors. Severe FVIII:C and FIX gene lesions (intron 22 inversion of the FVIII:C gene and large deletions, and nonsense mutations in both FVIII:C and FIX genes), which are unlikely to produce detectable circulating clotting protein in the plasma, are associated with a higher risk of developing alloantibody inhibitors (21% to 88% prevalence in hemophilia A vs. 6% to 60% in hemophilia B) in comparison to missense mutations, splice-site mutations, and small deletions (83), which are associated with the synthesis of small amounts of endogenous, nonfunctional coagulation factor antigen. Intron 22 inversion, the most prevalent gene mutation responsible for severe hemophilia A, accounting for up to 60% of severely affected individuals, is associated with 21% allo-FVIII:C antibody inhibitor prevalence (83). A current compilation of all of the hemophilic gene mutations is contained in the Hemophilia A Mutation, Structure, Test and Resource Site (HAM-SteRS) mutation registry, which is accessible at http://europium.csc.mrc.ac.uk. Similarly, null mutations and large deletions in the factor IX gene (presumably, circulating plasma clotting protein negative) are associated with an allo-factor IX antibody inhibitor prevalence of up to 60% versus approximately 6% in nonsense mutations and small deletions in the factor IX gene (detectable plasma factor IX clotting protein) (83). The marked difference between the high versus low prevalence for alloantibody inhibitor development in hemophilia A and B, respectively, may be related to the homology of factor IX with other vitamin K–dependent clotting factors (83).

**Clinical Severity of the Coagulopathy.** The phenotypic expression of clinical disease severity is a definite risk factor for alloantibody inhibitor development in hemophilia A and B; however, this may be linked directly to their associated genetic polymorphisms. The incidence of allo-FVIII:C antibody inhibitors is significantly greater in patients with severe hemophilia (23%), compared to patients with moderately severe hemophilia (8%) (79,86,87). Anecdotal cases of allo-FVIII:C antibody inhibitors in individuals with mild hemophilia have been described and are related to missense mutations. The discrepant incidences of acquired allo-FVIII:C antibody inhibitors in severe and moderate severity hemophilia A also could reflect the significantly greater cumulative exposures to antigenic protein (clotting factor replacement therapies) required by patients severely affected with hemophilia.

**Properties of the Clotting Factor Replacement Product.** Observed differences in the cumulative risks of acquiring allo-FVIII:C antibody inhibitors have been attributed by some investigators to the type (plasma-derived vs. recombinant full-length FVIII:C vs. B-domain deleted FVIII:C) and purity (presence vs. absence of VWF protein) of factor VIII concentrates administered to the patients. Only 0% to 7% of PUPs treated exclusively with cryoprecipitate or intermediate purity FVIII:C products (containing intact and functional VWF protein) developed allo-FVIII:C antibodies (86,88–90). Preliminary results from an ongoing prospective, multicenter PUP-study in Europe have revealed slightly higher inhibitor development ($P = 0.08$) in patients severely affected by hemophilia A treated with recombinant FVIII:C concentrates compared to intermediate purity FVIII:C products (91). Both these studies involve very few patients and/or limited monitoring for acquired allo-FVIII:C antibody inhibitors (see subsequent text); statistically reliable statements therefore cannot be made from these data. Most of the physicians treating hemophilia believe that no differences exist in the immunogenic potentials among the various FVIII:C replacement products (92). In considerably larger PUP studies, predominant use of plasma-derived, high-purity FVIII:C products (lacking intact or functional VWF protein) was associated with an overall allo-FVIII:C antibody inhibitor incidence ranging from 20% to 33% (87,93–97), comparable to the exclusive use of recombinant products (also lacking intact or functional VWF protein) (25% to 39%) (82,98,99). Furthermore, no significant difference in inhibitor incidence has been found in PUP studies conducted with full-length FVIII:C or B-domain deleted recombinant products.

The true immunogenic potential of a clotting factor replacement product is determined by the development of alloantibody inhibitor formation in PTPs with hemophilia A or B. In a well-conducted trial, the switch to a recombinant FVIII:C concentrate in hemophilic PTPs previously treated with plasma-derived products was not associated with an increased incidence of allo-FVIII:C antibody inhibitors (2% to 3% over 2 years for both products) (100). On the other hand, untoward immunogenicity was induced in PTPs, who experienced a five-fold increase in allo-FVIII:C antibody inhibitor development after receiving a new type of plasma-derived FVIII:C product, which had undergone pasteurization during its manufacture (101,102). Whether the heat treatment produced a neoantigenic FVIII:C molecule was never established; however, the allo-FVIII:C antibodies disappeared spontaneously and did not recur when the affected PTPs were rechallenged with other plasma-derived FVIII:C concentrates.

**Inhibitor Testing Schedules: Frequency and Duration of Laboratory Assessment.** Comparison of published studies indicates that the more frequently alloantibodies are tested for, the more commonly they will be detected because transient and low-titer inhibitors occur not infrequently and would have been missed or underreported with less frequent monitoring (82,87,98,99). Laboratory testing for alloantibody inhibitors should occur over an extended fixed time period or for a predetermined number of exposure days when evaluating the potential immunogenicity of any replacement therapy in a clinical trial. In nonstudy situations, laboratory monitoring for alloantibody development should be accomplished intermittently over the patient's lifespan and is certainly indicated whenever multiple spontaneous bleeding events occur in association with a previously effective therapeutic regimen. Recent, well-designed, prospective PUP trials with recombinant FVIII:C concentrates reveal that approximately 25% of patients with severe hemophilia A will develop allo-FVIII:C antibody inhibitors over a median of 9 to 15 exposure days and 5 years of observation (103). New inhibitors rarely develop after 100 to 150 exposure days (2% to 3% incidence) (100).

**Miscellaneous Variables.** Miscellaneous variables, which have been associated epidemiologically with development of alloantibody inhibitors, include the age at first exposure to clotting factor replacement therapy; the administration of the clotting factor concentrate in a continuous infusion mode; and activation of the immune system by surgery, vaccination, bacterial or viral illnesses, or chronic inflammatory states. Allo-FVIII:C antibody inhibitors were detected with a 41% cumulative incidence within 3 years from first factor VIII exposure before the age of 6 months compared to 29% inhibitor incidence when replacement therapy was initiated between 6 and 12 months of age, and 12% in those starting therapy beyond 1 year of age ($P = 0.03$). This observation, if confirmed, suggests that the liberal, early use of FVIII:C or FIX concentrates (e.g., primary prophylaxis regimens) may be imprudent. Breast feeding does not appear to reduce the development of alloantibody inhibitors in hemophilic infants, and there is no evidence that breast milk induces oral immune tolerance to factor VIII:C (104).

## Pathophysiology of Allo-FVIII:C/FIX Antibody Inhibitors: Mechanisms of Neutralization

Allo- and auto-FVIII:C and FIX antibody inhibitors neutralize the procoagulant activities of FVIII:C and FIX in a similar fashion, interfering with the participation of those coagulant proteins in the formation of the tenase complex. Allo- (and auto-) FVIII:C antibody inhibitors interact with the FVIII:C molecule (see Fig. 71-1) with remarkable consistency and fidelity to predominant epitopes on the A2 and C2 domains and a minor epitope on A3. This results in disruption of conformational relationships and physical binding of FVIII:C to phospholipid, VWF protein (VWF), factor X (and Xa), and factor IX (and IXa).

Inhibitory antibodies, which are directed against the A3 and C2 domains, impede VWF protein binding to FVIII:C, leading to the permissive proteolysis and subsequent inactivation of FVIII:C by Factor IXa, activated protein C, and factor Xa. In addition, FVIII:C circulating unchaperoned by VWF in plasma is susceptible to proteolysis by plasmin. If the specificity of the alloantibody (or autoantibody) targets the thrombin- or factor Xa–binding site on the C2 domain, activation of FVIII:C is inhibited. Other inhibitory antibodies interact with epitopes on the C2 domain and block FVIII:C interactions with the phospholipid component of the tenase complex. Antibodies against A1 epitopes are thought to interfere with FVIIIa–FX interactions in the tenase complex. Inhibitory antibodies against certain areas of the A2 and A3 domains interfere with FVIII:C binding to multiple regions on FIXa.

In contrast to auto-FVIII:C inhibitory antibodies, which usually are directed against single epitopes on either the C2 or A2 domains (62%), allo-FVIII:C inhibitors typically target multiple epitopes (85%) (105). Another class of allo-FVIII:C antibodies possesses proteolytic properties, which degrade FVIII:C and impede it from expressing its procoagulant activity (106). Proteolytic antibodies, which are detected in more than 50% of plasmas from patients with severe hemophilia and with allo-FVIII:C antibody inhibitors, have not been noted in individuals with acquired auto-FVIII:C antibody inhibitors.

The inhibitory mechanisms of allo-factor IX antibody inhibitors have not been studied as intensively; however, they are probably similar to the FVIII:C alloantibody situation.

## Clinical Bleeding Manifestations of Allo-FVIII:C/FIX Antibody Inhibitors

The hemorrhagic manifestations associated with acquired allo-factors VIII and IX antibody inhibitors are indistinguishable clinically from those that occur in individuals with severe hemophilia A or B, uncomplicated by inhibitors. Spontaneous onset of mucocutaneous bleeds, hemarthroses (knees and elbows > ankles > shoulders > hips), and intramuscular bleeds (flexors > extensors) predominate. This is in contrast to the bleeding complications associated with the autoimmune hemophilias (auto-FVIII:C or FIX antibody inhibitors), which typically present in individuals with previously normal coagulation as large ecchymoses and intramuscular bleeds rather than hemarthroses. Profuse bleeding can be iatrogenically precipitated at sites of invasive diagnostic or therapeutic procedures in the presence of either alloantibody or autoantibody inhibitors. Allo-FVIII:C and FIX antibody inhibitors should be suspected clinically when the patient with previously well-controlled hemophilia demonstrates poor control of bleeding events after receiving heretofore adequate doses of clotting factor replacement therapy. Pain and bleeding may persist despite administration of multiple treatments. Pharmacokinetic studies reveal suboptimal recovery (lower than expected FVIII:C or FIX incremental rises after intravenous infusion of the respective clotting factor replacement product) and reduced circulating survival (half-life) of the achieved FVIII:C or FIX activities. In addition, an allo-factor IX antibody inhibitor should be suspected when an individual with hemophilia B experiences anaphylaxis or a severe allergic reaction early into the infusion of any type of factor IX–containing product. This phenomenon usually develops after relatively few exposures to factor IX and is observed in approximately half of those who develop allo-factor IX antibody inhibitors. This is unique to acquired allo-factor IX antibody inhibitors, which fix complement. Once suspected, the specific clotting factor target of the alloantibody inhibitor should be identified, and the potency of the inhibitor should be determined. The isolated prolongation of the aPTT assay, characteristic for clotting factor deficiencies (factors XII, XI, IX, or VIII) in the intrinsic pathway of coagulation, will not normalize when alloantibody-containing patient plasma is mixed with normal plasma for 1 to 2 hours at 37°C. Specific assays for FVIII:C or FIX activity will usually reveal total neutralization (<1% normal clotting activity) of FVIII:C or FIX function (auto-FVIII:C antibody inhibitor plasma usually has residual FVIII:C activity detectable); serial dilutions of patient plasma eventually decrease the concentration of the alloantibody so that FVIII:C or FIX activity can be expressed. This forms the basis of the Bethesda assay, which is used to quantitate the potency of antibody (alloimmune or autoimmune) neutralization of clotting factor activity (1,5). By definition, one Bethesda unit (BU) is the amount of antibody that will neutralize 50% of normal plasma FVIII:C or FIX clotting activity in mixing studies performed as described previously. If the maximum titer of alloantibody (or autoantibody) inhibitor never exceeds 5 BU (low-titer inhibitor), the patient is classified as a "low responder." Reexposure to FVIII:C or FIX replacement products is not associated with an anamnestic response (e.g., the titer of alloantibody or autoantibody inhibitor does not increase); these products therefore can be used successfully to treat or prevent clinical bleeding complications, albeit at higher than conventional doses. Alloantibody (or autoantibody) inhibitor titers, which are consistently above 5 BU (high-titer inhibitor), occur in high responders, and reexposure to the specific clotting

factor antigen will result in an anamnestic rise in the inhibitor titer, peaking within 2 to 4 weeks after exposure to clotting factor product. The use of FVIII:C or FIX concentrates, even in extraordinarily increased doses, typically cannot "overwhelm" high-titer inhibitor–mediated neutralization of clotting factor activity. Therefore, the treatment or prevention of hemorrhage in high-titer high responders is predicated on the administration of "bypassing" agents, which promote thrombin generation independent of the contribution of FVIII:C or FIX. When monitoring patients longitudinally for the presence and titer of alloantibody (or autoantibody) inhibitors, the time elapsed between the last challenge with FVIII:C or FIX must be considered because the inhibitor in unchallenged individuals decreases over time according to the circulating half-life of the IgG4 antibody (approximately 20 days). An apparent low-titer inhibitor patient may actually possess a quiescent high-titer inhibitor, which is unmasked after reexposure to FVIII:C or FIX.

A special category of alloantibody (or autoantibody) inhibitor is the transient inhibitor, which is usually low-titer and disappears over a few months, notwithstanding continuation of clotting factor replacement. Very low-titer alloantibody and autoantibody inhibitors may not be detected by the traditional Bethesda assay. The more sensitive Nijmegen modification of the Bethesda assay is used in this situation, and, arbitrarily, 0.6 BU or higher is considered positive and clinically significant. Pharmacokinetic studies will reveal recoveries of less than 60% of calculated incremental rise in the specific clotting factor activity after infusion of replacement products.

## Control of Bleeding in the Allo-FVIII:C/FIX Antibody Inhibitor Patient

The pattern and character of clinical hemorrhage in individuals with alloantibody inhibitors against FVIII:C (hemophilia A) or FIX (hemophilia B) is indistinguishable from classical severe hemophilia. The frequency of bleeding is not significantly higher and is not influenced by the titer of the alloantibody inhibitor. In contrast, the titer of inhibitor does determine how acute bleeding episodes should be treated. The following treatment strategies (see Table 59-4) should be considered for the acute hemorrhagic complications associated with development of alloantibody inhibitors against FVIII:C or FIX: (a) administration of high doses of FVIII:C or FIX concentrates; (b) administration of factor IX complex concentrates (unactivated and activated), which are designated as "bypassing agents"; (c) administration of activated recombinant factor VII (rFVIIa) concentrate; (d) implementation of immunoadsorption and/or plasmapheresis techniques to physically remove the neutralizing alloantibody inhibitor from the patient's circulating plasma; and (e) induction of immune tolerance to eradicate the alloantibody inhibitor as a long-term objective.

**Administration of High Doses of FVIII:C or FIX Concentrates.** FVIII:C or FIX concentrates are useful to treat or prevent acute bleeding problems only in patients with hemophilia with low-responding/low-titer (≤5 BU) alloantibody inhibitors. The goal of these products is twofold: to overwhelm the circulating neutralizing alloantibody inhibitor and to recover sufficiently high concentrations of VIII:C or FIX activity in the circulation to achieve adequate hemostasis. It is difficult to predict the dose required to stop or to prevent bleeding in any individual patient with low-titer alloinhibitors because response to dosing is not influenced by the titer of antibody across the defined range of low-titer inhibitors. Typically, dosing for low-titer/low-responding alloantibody inhibitors is initiated at 200 IU per kg and is titrated according to clinical response and to the level of FVIII:C or FIX incremental rises postadministration. No matter what the incremental improvement, the circulating survival of FVIII:C or FIX is considerably shorter than that found in patients without alloantibody

**TABLE 59-4**

**FACTOR VIII (AND/OR FACTOR IX) CONCENTRATES USEFUL IN TREATMENT OF ALLOANTIBODY INHIBITOR-RELATED BLEEDING**

| Product name (manufacturer) | Viral inactivation method | Dosage |
|---|---|---|
| Recombinant factor VIIa (genetically engineered) | Affinity chromatography | 90 $\mu$g/kg intravenous bolus every 2–3 h until bleeding ceases (larger dosing regimens are experimental but may be useful in refractory bleeding); this product is the treatment of choice for individuals with allo-factor IX antibody inhibitors and anaphylaxis and/or renal disease associated with the use of factor IX–containing concentrates |
| NovoSeven (Novo Nordisk, Inc.) (Stabilized in mannitol; bovine calf serum used in culture medium) | Solvent/detergent (TNBP/polysorbate 80) | |
| FEIBA-VH (Baxter Immuno, Inc.) (human plasma–derived) | Vapor heated (10 h, 60°C, 190 mbar plus 1 h, 80°C, 375 mbar) | 50–100 IU/kg not to exceed 200 IU/kg/24 h (for factor VIII and IX inhibitors) |
| Porcine plasma–derived factor VIII concentrate (Hyate C) (Ibsen Biomeasure, Inc.) | No longer available | >50 IU/mg (for factor VIII inhibitors only) |

TNBP, tri-N-butyl phosphate.

inhibitors. Recombinant and plasma-derived FVIII:C and FIX concentrates appear to be equally effective in the treatment of low-titer alloantibody inhibitors. A potential treatment complication in individuals with low-titer alloantibody inhibitors may occur in surgery scenarios when the administration of high doses of FVIII:C or FIX concentrates unmasks the presence of a high-titer/high-responding alloantibody inhibitor with a rapid anamnestic rise in antibody formation and subsequent loss of hemostatic effect with these concentrates. Therefore, in low-titer alloantibody inhibitor patients undergoing surgery, inhibitor titers should be determined frequently and the incremental response to concentrate administration monitored carefully to detect the emergence of brisk anamnesis and rising antibody titers.

FVIII:C concentrates derived from pooled porcine plasma (PFVIII:C) had been used successfully for decades to treat or prevent acute bleeding problems in allo-FVIII:C antibody inhibitor patients. This strategy was based on the observation that PFVIII:C has reduced crossreactivity (less neutralizing potential) with allohuman (or autohuman) FVIII:C antibodies compared to interactions between administered human FVIII:C and circulating allohuman or autohuman FVIII:C antibody inhibitors. Specific anti-PFVIII:C antibodies did occasionally develop in these patients (15% to 40%) within 7 to 14 days, but the PFVIII:C concentrate provided adequate hemostasis as long as the anti-PFVIII inhibitor titer remained less than 15 BU. (For more details, read Chapter 71.) Currently, PFVIII:C concentrates are not available because of the difficulties inherent with the screening and inactivation of porcine-derived viruses.

Intranasal (150 $\mu$g per nostril in adults) or intravenous desmopressin (0.3 $\mu$g per kg) may raise FVIII:C activity to adequate hemostatic levels in selected individuals with low-titer allo-FVIII:C antibody inhibitors.

**Administration of Factor IX Complex Concentrates.** Bypassing products, including unactivated PCCs (Bebulin and Profilnine) and activated prothrombin complex concentrates (APCCs) [Autoplex (no longer available commercially) and FEIBA], have been available to treat patients with allo- and auto-FVIII:C or

FIX antibody inhibitor since the early 1980s. Their hemostatic efficacy in the presence of inhibitors remains somewhat obscure; however, their content of activated vitamin K–dependent factors II (prothrombin), X(a), and trace amounts of VII(a) and IX(a), probably promote thrombin generation in vivo and can "bypass" the inhibitor effect. There may also be a component of platelet activation by these products, which contributes to their hemostatic effects. The titer of alloantibody or autoantibody inhibitor does not influence the likelihood of achieving adequate hemostasis in vivo.

Both PCCs and APCCs are produced from pooled human-derived plasma and therefore contain trace amounts of FVIII:C, which may elicit anamnesis. This will not necessarily alter the hemostatic effectiveness of future infusions of PCCs or APCCs. Individuals with severe hemophilia B complicated with allo-factor IX antibody inhibitors may experience anaphylaxis or severe allergic reactions on infusion of any type of factor IX–containing product. Nephrotic syndrome may also develop. The treatment of choice for acute bleeding episodes in these patients is rFVIIa concentrate. For patients with hemophilia B with allo-factor IX antibody inhibitors not complicated by allergic reactions to factor IX, bleeding episodes can be treated with PCCs, APCCs, or rFVIIa.

Randomized clinical trials (107,108) have demonstrated variable efficacy of the PCCs to control or prevent bleeding in patients with allo-FVIII:C or FIX antibody inhibitor (range of effectiveness 29% to 63%), mostly with hemarthroses. There are limited and inconclusive data examining the use of PCCs in general and oral surgery scenarios. The hemostatic efficacy of the APCCs appears slightly higher than PCCs in randomized, controlled studies [Autoplex efficacy was 52% (109); FEIBA efficacy was 64% (110)] and markedly higher in uncontrolled studies [Autoplex efficacy was 87% (111); FEIBA efficacy was 81% (112)]. The major adverse effect of the PCCs is their propensity to precipitate thrombotic complications (acute myocardial infarction, deep vein thrombosis, pulmonary embolism, disseminated intravascular coagulopathy), particularly after repeated and frequent dosing (113–115).

Anamnesis with rises in factor VIII or IX antibody titers can also occur with these products. Theoretically, the PCCs and APCCs, as human plasma–derived products, can transmit pathogenic blood-borne viruses and prions; however, there have been no cases reported.

Currently, APCCs predominate for the treatment of inhibitors, usually with initial bolus intravenous injections of 50 to 100 IU per kg, followed by repeat dosing every 8 to 12 hours, depending on clinical response. When frequent and repeated dosing is provided, the patient should be carefully monitored for the development of thrombogenic complications.

Currently, there are no laboratory techniques available to monitor or predict the hemostatic effectiveness of the APCCs; there are also no coagulation assays, which predict the onset of thromboembolic complications potentially associated with their use.

**Administration of Activated Recombinant factor VII Concentrate.** Recombinant human factor VIIa (rFVIIa, NovoSeven) is a genetically engineered concentrate consisting of activated factor VII, essentially indistinguishable from the native form, which circulates in human plasma in very low concentrations (5 to 10 ng per mL). The high concentration of rFVIIa in the commercial product renders it stable, with a long shelf-life and suitable for pharmaceutical use. rFVIIa is considered another "bypass" agent for the treatment or prevention of bleeding complications associated with alloantibody or autoantibody inhibitors against FVIII:C or FIX. Its administration in large intravenous bolus doses produces supraphysiological levels of factor VIIa in blood and promotes thrombin generation indirectly through tissue factor cell–based and platelet activation–mediated mechanisms (116). In the absence of FVIII:C or FIX, such as in individuals with alloantibody (or autoantibody) inhibitors against these coagulation factor proteins, rFVIIa binds to activated platelets and subsequently activates factor X to factor Xa, which, in turn, incorporates into a prothrombinase complex to generate a thrombin "burst." As with PCCs and APCCs, the hemostatic efficacy of rFVIIa concentrate is achieved in a manner that is not influenced by the titer of the alloantibody (or autoantibody) FVIII:C or FIX inhibitor. In multiple randomized, prospective trials in patients with hemophilia and with allo-FVIII:C antibody inhibitors, rFVIIa administered at bolus intravenous doses of 90 $\mu$g per kg every 2 to 3 hours effectively stopped active bleeds 79% to 93% of the time in a self-administered homecare protocol. Efficacy correlates directly with timeliness of treatment and the number of doses utilized (117,118). Life- and limb-threatening bleeds in inhibitor patients responded successfully to rFVIIa in 69% to 88% of episodes (119,120). Similarly, rFVIIa administered prophylactically at 90 $\mu$g per kg prior to major surgery and then every 2 to 3 hours achieved good hemostasis in over 83% of the patients with alloantibody inhibitors (121). Therapy with rFVIIa for patients with hemophilia and with inhibitors remains logistically challenging because multiple infusions of rFVIIa every 2 to 3 hours are necessary to achieve and sustain hemostatic activity over an extended time period, and there is no way to predict in advance whether rFVIIa will effectively reverse or prevent bleeding complications. The safety and efficacy of combining rFVIIa with APCCs have been mixed in those with bleeding refractory to rFVIIa or APCCs alone. This option may be effective but should be reserved for desperate situations because the risks of life-threatening thrombogenicity, such as disseminated intravascular coagulopathy, VTE, or stroke, appear significantly increased.

Continuous infusion of rFVIIa (initial bolus of 90 $\mu$g per kg followed by fixed rate of 50 $\mu$g/kg/hour) reduces the number of micrograms and the cost of replacement therapy by 25% to 30% (122). However, it is not an approved delivery method; its bioequivalence, safety, and superiority in comparison to multiple-bolus administration remain to be documented; and the approach appears counterintuitive to the "thrombin burst" theory of hemostasis. Continuous infusion rFVIIa regimens may not be optimal for acute or surgical oral cavity bleeds (123), perhaps related to insufficient inhibition of local fibrinolytic enzymes.

Recently, single, high-dose rFVIIa regimens ("megadose," i.e., >200 to 300 $\mu$g per kg) have been proposed to exaggerate the thrombin "burst" and thereby achieve quicker resolution of bleeding episodes, reduced frequency of rFVIIa dosing, and decreased cumulative drug consumption. Preliminary data, to date, have revealed response rates (83% to 87%) very similar to standard dose regimens (124,125).

As with the PCCs and APCCs, there is no laboratory assay that can predict adequacy of rFVIIa dosing. This has led to incomplete information on optimal dosing of rFVIIa. In addition, no assays can predict whether patients will develop thrombotic complications after receiving rFVIIa. Known factors predisposing to thrombosis were present in 20 of the 25 (80%) patients with hemophilia who were reported spontaneously or who developed a thrombosis during a clinical trial (126).

Although it is difficult to make a comparison with the PCCs and the APCCs, the incidence of thrombotic complications appears to be lower with rFVIIa and certainly not different from that observed in the general population (1 to 2 events per 1,000 individuals per year) (126). At any rate, caution is advised when administering rFVIIa, PCCs, or APCCs in a repetitive, sequential (to achieve synergistic effects of both classes of products), or prolonged manner. This is particularly critical in elderly patients with alloantibody (or autoantibody) inhibitors because their underlying coagulopathy does not appear to protect them from the potential thrombogenicity associated with prolonged and frequent treatment with these hemostatic agents (127).

**Immunoadsorption/Plasmapheresis.** The most efficient and rapid method to reduce high titers of alloantibody (or autoantibody) inhibitors directed against FVIII:C or FIX, consists of plasmapheresis combined with extracorporeal adsorption of the IgG inhibitory antibody to staphylococcal protein A coupled to a Sepharose matrix (128). This technique can reduce the inhibitor titer by 96%, although transiently. Immunoadsorption requires specialized personnel and good venous access and should be reserved for urgent clinical situations in which control or prevention of intractable bleeding requires the rapid reduction of the inhibitor titer followed by short-term, high-dose FVIII:C or FIX (i.e., to perform surgery or to reverse bleeding). Immunoadsorption has also been utilized to minimize the initial titer of alloantibody inhibitor in anticipation of implementing an ITI protocol.

**Immune Tolerance Induction.** Early attempts to achieve tolerance to exogenous sources of FVIII:C in patients with hemophilia with alloantibody inhibitors and to suppress anamnesis to the FVIII:C involved the use of immunosuppressive medication (e.g., corticosteroids, cyclophosphamide, or azathioprine) and resulted in frequent failures or, at best, unpredictable outcomes. Subsequently, a standardized approach to treat allo-FVIII:C or FIX antibody inhibitors with very high doses of FVIII:C or FIX concentrate (up to 200 IU per kg twice daily) produced remarkable reductions in inhibitor titer so that hemorrhage could be controlled (Bonn protocol) (56). When anamnesis occurred, acute bleeding events were treated with APCCs. The suppression of inhibitor titers has also been observed with lower FVIII:C doses administered three times weekly (van Creveld protocol), but with less predictability (129). In the absence of prospective clinical trials, data collected from registries have revealed a 50% to 100% success rate for ITI. Maximum historical titer of alloantibody inhibitor, inhibitor titer immediately before initiating ITI, and age were inversely related to attainment of tolerance. Controversy and contradictory results exist as to the optimal dosing regimen for FVIII:C or FIX concentrate for ITI; however, the overall impression is that high FVIII:C doses generally are associated with higher success rates (129,130). Treatment duration for ITI over 1 year appears to be crucial to success in most of the published reports.

Remaining to be determined is the role of VWF protein in ITI. Patients with allo-FVIII:C antibody inhibitor and with failing ITI responses to treatment with FVIII:C concentrates containing very little or no VWF increased their success rate up to 90% when they were changed over to concentrates containing high amounts of VWF (56). This requires verification.

Elimination of alloantibody inhibitors to FVIII:C and FIX from plasma by immunoadsorption followed by aggressive multimodality immune suppression (Malmo protocol) has also been achieved with approximately 60% success rate (131).

Long-term eradication of acquired alloimmune FVIII:C and FIX antibody inhibitors has been attempted by eliminating the offending clone(s) of lymphocytes responsible for antibody generation. Cytotoxic agents, such as cyclophosphamide, used alone or in combination with corticosteroids, certainly induce lymphopenia but have not been demonstrated conclusively to be either necessary or synergistic to the success of ITI for alloantibody inhibitors. Furthermore, there is concern that the immunosuppressive and leukemogenic potential of these medications should be avoided, particularly because most allo-FVIII:C or FIX antibody inhibitors occur in very young patients with hemophilia. On the basis of its potential for elimination of autoreactive B-cell clones and its success in the auto-FVIII:C antibody scenario for acquired hemophilia, rituximab, a chimeric anti-CD20 monoclonal antibody, was administered to two hemophilic children with alloantibodies to FVIII:C or FIX, which failed to respond to conventional ITI therapy. Anecdotally, rituxan successfully eradicated the allo-FVIII:C antibody inhibitor but had no effect on the allo-factor IX antibody (132). More experience will be necessary to determine if rituximab has a role for this clinical problem.

## Human Immunodeficiency Virus

The first three cases of AIDS in the hemophilia population were noted in 1981 and 1982, and reported in 1983 (133,134). By 1984, almost 90% of patients with severe hemophilia A and 50% of patients with hemophilia B, were HIV-seropositive by virtue of being obligate recipients of plasma-derived replacement products. The eradication of HIV from the pooled plasma-derived clotting factor concentrates was achieved when various high-heat and pasteurization techniques, nanofiltration, and solvent detergent treatment were applied to eradicate this lipid-enveloped virus. This, the examination of plasma pools by NAT testing, and the availability of genetically engineered recombinant clotting factor concentrates have resulted in no new documented HIV-seroconversions in patients with hemophilia A since 1986 and patients with hemophilia B since 1989. HIV infection in patients with hemophilias differs little from HIV infection in other populations. Kaposi sarcoma is an extremely rare, malignant complication in patients with hemophilia and AIDS, but similar to other high-risk HIV groups, there has been an increased incidence of lymphoproliferative malignancies. Asymptomatic autoimmune thrombocytopenia occurs in 25% to 45% of patients with hemophilia who are HIV-seropositive and frequently precedes the development of AIDS (94,95). Although thrombocytopenia may exacerbate hemophilia-related bleeding, particularly when HIV protease inhibitors are being used, it does not necessarily portend a poor prognosis and may respond to steroids and splenectomy without increased morbidity or mortality. Ritonavir has been associated with the highest incidence of serious bleeding, including

intracerebral hemorrhagic catastrophes, followed by indinavir and combination therapy with lopinavir–ritonavir (135).

Approximately 50% of individuals with hemophilia who were infected with HIV have died; however, the administration of HAART with protease inhibitors has changed the profile of the disease. Most of the patients with hemophilia who were HIV-infected and who remain alive are chronically infected with HCV, which has implications for their prognosis and choice of HAART. HAART has stabilized the progression of HIV, and most patients have fared well, with low HIV viral titers, CD4 counts greater than $200 \times 10^6$ per L, few opportunistic infections, and an excellent performance status over many years. In fact, because a substantial number of patients with hemophilia are coinfected with both HIV and HCV, HIV has been shown to accelerate the course of HCV chronic liver disease, and there is evidence that HCV infection may worsen the prognosis of HIV (136). From 1977 to 1984, the overall annual mortality rate in patients with severe hemophilias was 0.9%. For HIV-seropositive patients with hemophilia, the annual mortality peaked to over 10% from 1993 to 1996, before falling to 5% in 1997 to 1999 when HAART became available. Currently, the predominant cause of death in HIV-seropositive patients with hemophilia is end-stage liver disease related (137).

HIV-positive patients with hemophilia, demonstrate an unusually high vaccination failure rate to hepatitis A and B and *Pneumococcus pneumoniae* immunizations. Up to 50% of vaccinated patients do not develop protective antibody titers. HIV-seropositve patients with hemophilia also may lose their preexisting alloantibody inhibitors, only for them to reemerge once their immune systems reconstitute with HAART.

## Hepatitis and Parvovirus B19

Before the introduction of the hepatitis B vaccine, 70% to 90% of patients with hemophilia were found to have antibody to hepatitis B surface antigen, and between 5% and 15% became chronic carriers of the hepatitis B surface antigen. The prevalence of HCV seropositivity exceeds 90% of patients with hemophilia treated before 1985 (138). In a cohort study of 138 HCV-seropositive patients with hemophilia followed-up for 22 years after HIV exposure infection, 19% developed cirrhosis, and 9% developed liver failure (139).

HIV coinfection with HCV accelerates the rate of progression of liver disease and the incidence of hepatic failure. HCV ribonucleic acid levels are substantially increased in coinfected individuals compared with those who are HCV-seropositive only. Similarly, concurrent HCV exacerbates the clinical course of HIV. Initiating HAART is crucial in these coinfected individuals to prevent opportunistic infections, to preserve absolute CD4 lymphocyte counts over $200 \times 10^6$ per L, and to allow for the initiation of pegylated interferon-$\alpha$ (IFN-$\alpha$) and ribavarin combination therapy for chronic HCV. Hemophiliacs exposed to clotting factor concentrates derived from North American sources or recovered plasma were infected primarily by HCV genotypes 1 and 4, which are relatively more difficult to eradicate with IFN-$\alpha$. Clinical trials are in progress to determine the degree of superiority of pegylated IFN-$\alpha$ versus conventional IFN-$\alpha$ in coinfected patients with hemophilia.

There is a 30-fold increased incidence of hepatocellular carcinoma (HCC) in the HCV-seropositive hemophilia population (140). The overall incidence rate of HCC is 239 per 100,000 per year, with HCC risk increased 12.9-fold with alcohol intake more than 80 g per day and 15.2-fold with $\alpha$-fetoprotein (AFP) levels higher than 11 ng per mL (141). Successful repeat chemoembolization followed by orthotopic liver transplantation has been reported for HCC. HCV-seropositive patients with hemophilia, particularly when coninfected with HIV, should undergo periodic abdominal ultrasounds to screen for HCC.

Chronic liver disease has emerged as a major cause of morbidity and mortality in patients who are HIV-seronegative and HIV-positive and can be exacerbated by concurrent use of ethanol, acetaminophen (in large quantities), and numerous hepatotoxic antiretroviral medications.

Although the transmission of HCV from men with hemophilia to their sexual partners occurs at a low rate (<3%), the incidence of hepatitis C transmission was increased fivefold in women who are HIV-seropositive, suggesting that HIV may be cofactor in the acquisition of HCV (142).

Human parvovirus B19 is a non–lipid-enveloped DNA virus that is invulnerable to all available viral attenuation techniques used for plasma-derived factor VIII and IX concentrates. Therefore, the seroprevalence of parvovirus B19 in patients with hemophilia using these products approaches 80% (51), and approximately 30% of those with progressive hemarthropathy have evidence of parvovirus B19 DNA in their synovial tissue by nested (polymerase chain reaction) PCR (143). Infection with parvovirus B19 usually is asymptomatic in adults; however, its potential transmission from plasma-derived products is representative of the risks posed to patients with hemophilia by any other pathogenic non–lipid-coated viruses that may contaminate the blood supply. Furthermore, parvovirus B19 can be transmitted vertically to the unborn fetus of pregnant hemophilic carriers, with resulting spontaneous miscarriage, hydrops fetalis, and pure red cell aplasia. These potential complications provide compelling arguments in favor of the exclusive use of recombinant factor concentrates in the hemophilia population.

# OTHER HEREDITARY COAGULATION DEFICIENCIES

## Factor XI Deficiency (Hemophilia C)

Factor XI deficiency should be considered in the differential diagnosis for a patient with mild to moderate bleeding with a prolonged aPTT or for a previously asymptomatic individual with an incidental prolongation of the aPTT. The frequency and severity of bleeding manifestations often do not correlate with the clotting factor XI level. That is, some homozygotes with factor XI activity levels less than 20% may not bleed even after surgery, whereas some heterozygotes with factor XI levels between 50% to 70% may bleed. The previous hemorrhagic histories of the patient and that of his or her family may be useful predictors of clinical symptomatology. Replacement therapy can certainly be justified for major surgical procedures regardless of prior history. Bleeding events often are mucosal in origin, including epistaxis, menorrhagia, or hematuria, or are related to trauma and surgery, occasionally first presenting at circumcision (144). Coexisting coagulopathies, particularly VWD, have been described in association with factor XI deficiency and may be the more critical precipitant of bleeding complications in factor XI heterozygotes.

Treatment of symptomatic bleeding due to factor XI deficiency and surgical prophylaxis usually can be achieved satisfactorily by raising the factor XI level to 30% to 45% of normal. Infusions of fresh frozen plasma are the mainstay of management but expose the recipients to potentially pathogenic blood-borne viruses. The volume of plasma required to raise factor XI levels to an adequate range may produce symptomatic intravascular volume overload and requires substantial infusion time. The circulating half-life of transfused factor XI is estimated to be between 50 and 80 hours. Plasma-derived high-purity factor XI concentrates, available for use in the United Kingdom and France, can be administered rapidly and effectively and appear to be safe at low doses (145). However, life-threatening thrombotic complications, including disseminated intravascular coagulation and arterial thrombi, have been observed to occur in approximately 10% of treated patients, particularly in older patients (with preexisting coronary or peripheral arterial disease) receiving doses more than 40 U per kg (146). Often, the use of antifibrinolytic agents alone or as an adjuvant treatment is indicated to prevent bleeding episodes, particularly mucosal-based surgery in the oropharynx and prostate. Desmopressin administration is also a reasonable treatment modality for selected symptomatic, heterozygous factor XI patients to raise levels to the low–normal range (147).

# THE PROMISE AND REALITY OF GENE THERAPY FOR HEMOPHILIA A AND B

The hemophilias were recognized early on as good candidates for cure by gene therapy strategies. The single defective genes responsible for disease manifestations are well characterized, and 1% to 2% incremental rises in factor VIII or IX levels in plasma dramatically improve the phenotype of the diseases. Six Phase I/II clinical gene transfer trials have been initiated since 1999 for both hemophilia A and B, and all have been terminated prematurely. They have yielded promising results, but their limited benefits, their complications (actual and theoretical), and the technical difficulties involved with the development of an efficient, safe vector to induce sustained and high expression of factor VIII or IX have forced the trials to close. The proof of principle has been established despite the slow clinical progress. Most of the success to date has been associated with clinical trials utilizing an adeno-associated viral (AAV) vector for gene transfer of factor IX in hemophilia B. The factor IX cDNA is considerably smaller than factor VIII cDNA and is therefore more amenable for incorporation into the vector.

The first gene therapy trial for severe hemophilia B consisted of a dose-escalation study, employing intramuscular injections of a human factor IX construct integrated into AAV (148). Only transient rises of factor IX activity in the 1% to 5% range, well below therapeutic needs, were detected in one of eight participants. The benign nature of this approach was encouraging, but the necessity of administering such large doses of vector to skeletal muscle to affect hemostasis was impractical, and the study was abandoned in favor of delivering the AAV-factor IX construct directly to the liver by bolus infusion into the hepatic artery (149). The considerably larger doses of vector resulted in transient but modest rises in factor IX activity (1% to 3%) in two of six patients in the study. The trial was discontinued after vector genome was detectable in the semen of all patients for up to 3 months after administration. Hypertransaminasemia also was noted, bringing into question the safety of the AAV vector. A unique approach to factor IX gene therapy has been developed in China, where autologous fibroblasts, genetically modified ex vivo to secrete human factor IX, were implanted subcutaneously in two patients with moderate severity hemophilia B (2% factor IX) and produced a sustained (>420 days) rise in factor IX levels (150). Repeat treatment also was successful.

Three small hemophilia A gene therapy trials have been conducted, and all are closed to further enrollment. Retroviral vectors have been used in two of the studies, one of which delivered full-length factor VIII constructs by peripheral venipuncture (151), and the other one, a B-domain–deleted factor VIII construct (152). There is concern that these retroviral vectors could be leukemogenic in their own right. Both trials resulted in unsustained slight rises in factor VIII activity (1% to 3%), and the "gutless" AAV containing full-length factor VIII produced a transient inflammatory response, which was associated with elevated liver enzymes in one patient. These trials were not pursued any further in anticipation that a less immunogenic and oncogenic vector would soon become available. A third approach avoided the use of a viral vector, employing electroporation of autologous fibroblasts *ex vivo* with factor VIII gene with subsequent implantation into the omentum of six individuals with severe hemophilia A (153). This produced transient increases in factor VIII activity up to 8% of normal in four of six subjects with duration of effect noted up to 10 months. In summary, some slow progress has been made in the development of treatment strategies for the gene therapy for hemophilia A and particularly for hemophilia B. Incremental rises of clotting factor activity are transient, and the viral vectors used to achieve those increments are problematic. Nevertheless, the challenges of gene therapy for the patients with hemophilia are becoming better defined and the proof of principle has been firmly fulfilled so that the likelihood of eventual success is evident.

## *References*

1. Gilchrist GS, Wilke JL, Muehlenbein LR, et al. Intrauterine correction of factor VIII (FVIII) deficiency. Intrauterine correction of factor VIII (FVIII) deficiency. *Haemophilia* 2001;7:497–499.
2. Jenkins PV, Collins PW, Goldman E, et al. Analysis of intron 22 inversions of the factor VIII gene in severe hemophilia A: implications for genetic counseling. *Blood* 1994;84:2197–2201.
3. Lillicrap DP, White BN, Holden JJ, et al. Carrier detection in the hemophilias. *Am J Hematol* 1987;26(3):285–296.
4. Pecorara M, Casarino L, Mori PG, et al. A carrier detection and prenatal diagnosis by DNA analysis. *Blood* 1987;70:531–535.
5. Giannelli F, Green PM, Sommer SS, et al. Hemophilia B: database of point mutations and short additions and deletions—fifth edition. *Nucleic Acids Res* 1994;22:3534–3546.
6. Sommer SS. Assessing the underlying pattern of human germline mutations: lessons from the factor IX gene. *FASEB J* 1992;6:2767–2774.
7. Wang NS, Zhang M, Thompson AR. A new mutation in the calcium binding domain of factor IX resulting in severe hemophilia B. *Thromb Haemost* 1990;63:24–26.
8. Graham JB. Genotype assignment (carrier detection) in the hemophilias. *Clin Haematol* 1978;8:11545.
9. Gitschier J, Lawn RM, Rotblat F, et al. Antenatal diagnosis and carrier detection of hemophilia A using factor VIII gene probe. *Lancet* 1985;1(8437):1093–1094.
10. Hoyer LW, Carta CA, Golbus MS, et al. Prenatal diagnosis of classic hemophilia (hemophilia A) by immunoradiometric assays. *Blood* 1985;65:1312–1317.
11. Dalton ME, DeCherny AH. Prenatal diagnosis. *N Engl J Med* 1993;328:114–120.
12. Kulkarni R, Lusher JM. Intracranial and extracranial hemorrhages in newborns with hemophilia: a review of the literature. *J Pediatr Hematol Oncol* 1999;21:289–295.
13. Handelsman JE. The knee joint in hemophilia. *Orthop Clin North Am* 1979;10:13973.
14. Hoskinson J, Duthie RB. Management of musculoskeletal problems in the hemophilias. *Orthop Clin North Am* 1978;9(2):455–480.
15. Stein H, Duthie RB. The pathogenesis of chronic haemophilic arthropathy. *J Bone Joint Surg* 1981;63B:601–609.
16. Hakobyan N, Kazarian T, Jabbar AA, et al. Pathobiology of hemophilic synovitis I: overexpression of mdm2 oncogene. *Blood* 2004;104:2060–2064.
17. Furie B, Limentani SA, Rosenfield CG. A practical guide to the evaluation and treatment of hemophilia. *Blood* 1994;84(1):3–9.
18. Gilbert MS, Aledort LM, Seremetis S, et al. Long term evaluation of septic arthritis in hemophilic patients. *Clin Ortop* 1996;328:54–59.
19. Goldsmith JC, Silberstein PT, Fromm RE Jr, et al. Hemophilic arthropathy complicated by polyarticular septic arthritis. *Acta Haemol* 1983;71:121–123.
20. Lurie A, Bailey BP. The management of acute hemophilic hemarthrosis and muscle hematoma. *S Afr Med J* 1972;46:656–659.
21. Gill FM. Congenital bleeding disorders: hemophilia and von Willebrand's disease. *Med Clin North Am* 1984;68:601–615.
22. Handelsman JE, Glasser RA. Pathogenesis and treatment of hemophilic arthropathy and deep muscle hemorrhages. *Prog Clin Biol Res* 1990;324:199–206.
23. Gilbert MS. Musculoskelatal manifestations of hemophilia. *Mt Sinai J Med (NY)* 1977;44:339–358.
24. Railton GT, Aronstam A. Early bleeding into upper limb muscles in severe hemophilia. *J Bone Joint Surg Br* 1987;69:100–102.
25. Lancourt JE, Gilbert MS, Posner ME. Management of bleeding and associated complications of hemophilia in the hand and forearm. *J Bone Joint Surg Am* 1977;59:451–460.
26. Goodfellow J, Fearn CB, Matthew JM, et al. Iliacus haematoma: a common complication of hemophilia. *J Bone Joint Surg* 1967;49:748–756.
27. Prentice GRM, Lindsay RM, Barr RD, et al. Renal complications in hemophilia and Christmas disease. *Q J Med* 1971;40:47–61.
28. Small M, Rose PE, McMillan N, et al. Haemophilia and the kidney: assessment after 11 year follow-up. *Br Med J* 1982;285:1609–1611.
29. Kulkarni R, Soucie JM, Evatt B. Renal disease among males with haemophilia. *Haemophilia* 2003;9:703–710.
30. Ghosh K, Jijina F, Mohanty D. Haematuria and urolithiasis in patients with haemophilia. *Eur J Haematol* 2003;70:410–412.
31. Abildgaard CF, Simone JV, Schulman I. Steroid treatment of hemophilic hematuria. *J Pediatr* 1965;66:117–119.
32. Rizza CR, Kernoff PBA, Matthews JM, et al. A comparison of coagulation factor replacement with and without prednisolone in the treatment of haematuria in haemophilia and Christmas disease. *Thromb Haemost* 1977;37:86–90.
33. Eyster ME, Gillo FM, Blott PM, et al. Central nervous system bleeding in hemophiliacs. *Blood* 1978;51:1179–1188.
34. Pierce GF, Lusher JM, Brownstein AP, et al. The use of purified clotting factor concentrates in hemophilia. Influence of viral safety, cost, and supply on therapy. *JAMA* 1989;261:3434–3438.
35. Anders WA, Wulff K, Smith WB. Head trauma in hemophilia: a prospective study. *Arch Intern Med* 1984;144:1981–1983.
36. Blattner RJ. Recent developments in the management of hemophilia with particular reference to intracranial bleeding. *J Pediatr* 1967;70:449–452.
37. de Tezanos Pinto M, Fernandez J, Perez Bianco PR. Update of 156 episodes of central nervous system bleeding in hemophiliacs. *Haemostasis* 1992;22:259–267.
38. Bray GL, Luban NLC. Hemophilia presenting with intracranial hemorrhage: an approach to the infant with intracranial bleeding and coagulopathy. *Am J Dis Child* 1987;141:1215–1217.
39. Frederici A, Mannucci PM, Minetti D, et al. Intracranial bleeding in hemophilia. A study of 11 cases. *J Neurosurg Sci* 1983;27:31–35.
40. Gilchrist GS, Wilke JL, Muehlenbein LR, et al. Intrauterine correction of factor VIII (FVIII) deficiency. *Haemophilia* 2001;7:497–499.
41. Bray G, Nugent D. Hemorrhage involving the upper airway in hemophilia. *Clin Pediatr* 1986;25:436–439.
42. Logan LJ. Management of von Willebrand's disease. *Prog Clin Biol Res* 1990;324:279–290.
43. Braden B, Wenke A, Karich HJ, et al. Risk of gastrointestinal bleeding associated with Helicobacter pylori infection in patients with hemophilia or von Willebrand's syndrome. *Helicobacter* 1998;3:184–187.
44. Roberts HR, Jones MR. Hemophilia and related conditions—congenital deficiencies of prothrombin (factor II), factor V and factors VII to XII. In: Williams AWJ, Beutler E, Erslev AJ et al., eds. *Hematology*, 4th ed. New York: McGraw-Hill, 1990:1453–1473.
45. Bray GL. Recent advances in the preparation of plasma-derived and recombinant coagulation factor VIII. *J Pediatr* 1990;117(3):503–507.
46. Gomperts ED. Procedures for the inactivation of viruses in clotting factor concentrates. *Am J Hematol* 1986;23:295–305.
47. Schimpf K, Mannucci PM, Kreutz W, et al. Absence of hepatitis after treatment with pasteurized factor VIII concentrate in patients with hemophilia and no previous transfusion. *N Engl J Med* 1987;316:918–922.
48. Zimmerman TS. Purification of VIII by monoclonal antibody affinity chromatography. *Semin Hematol* 1988;25(Suppl. 1):25–26.
49. Epstein JS, Fricke WA. Current safety of clotting factor concentrates. *Arch Pathol Lab Med* 1990;114:335–340.
50. Mannucci PM. Modern treatment of hemophilia: from the shadows towards the light. *Thromb Haemost* 1993;70:17–23.
51. Soucie JM, Siwak EB, Hooper WC, et al. Human parvovirus B19 in young male patients with hemophilia A: associations with treatment product exposure and joint range of motion limitation. *Transfusion* 2004;44: 1179–1185.
52. Azzi A, De Santis R, Morfini M, et al. TT virus contaminates first-generation recombinant factor VIII concentrates. *Blood* 2001;98:2571–2573.
53. Kreil TR, Zimmermann K, Pable S, et al. TT virus does not contaminate first-generation recombinant factor VIII concentrate. *Blood* 2002;100: 2271–2272.
54. Lee CA, Ironside JW, Bell JE, et al. Retrospective neuropathological review of prion disease in UK haemophilic patients. *Thromb Haemost* 1998;80:909–911.
55. Evatt B, Austin H, Barnhart E, et al. Surveillance for Creutzfeldt-Jakob disease among persons with hemophilia. *Transfusion* 1998;38:817–820.
56. Kreuz W, Ettingshausen CE, Auerswald G et al. GTH PUP Study Group. Epidemiology of inhibitors and current treatment strategies. *Haematologica* 2003;88:EREP04.

57. Lusher JM. Prediction and management of adverse events associated with the use of factor IX complex concentrates. *Semin Hematol* 1993;30 (Suppl. 1):36–40.

58. Kim HC, McMillan CW, White GC, et al. Purified factor IX using monoclonal immunoaffinity technique: clinical trials in hemophilia B and comparison with prothrombin complex concentrates. *Blood* 1992;79: 568–575.

59. Pfaff JA, Geninatti M. Hemophilia. *Emerg Med Clin North Am* 1993; 11:337–363.

60. Hathaway WE, Christian MJ, Clarke SL, et al. Comparison of continuous and intermittent factor VIII concentrate therapy in hemophilia A. *Am J Hematol* 1984;17:85–88.

61. Kim HC, Smith C, Matts L, et al. Continuous infusion of factor IX in a patient undergoing surgical procedure. *Blood* 1993;82(Suppl. 1):154A.

62. Mannucci PM, Ruggeri ZM, Pareti FI, et al. 1-Deamino-8-D-arginine vasopressin: a new pharmacological approach to the management of hemophilia and von Willebrand's disease. *Lancet* 1977;1:869–872.

63. Barnhart MI, Chen S, Lusher JM. DDAVP—does the drug have a direct effect on the vessel wall? *Thromb Res* 1983;31:239–253.

64. Mannucci PM. Desmopressin (DDAVP) for treatment of disorders of hemostasis. *Prog Hemost Thromb* 1986;8:19–45.

65. Lethagen S. Desmopressin (DDAVP) and hemostasis. *Ann Hematol* 1994; 69:173–180.

66. Lethagen S, Harris AS, Nilsson IM. Intranasal desmopressin (DDAVP) by spray in mild hemophilia A and von Willebrand's disease type 1. *Blut* 1990;60:187–191.

67. Rose EH, Aledort LM. Nasal spray desmopressin (DDAVP) for mild hemophilia A and von Willebrand disease. *Ann Intern Med* 1991;114: 563–568.

68. Chavin SI, Siegel DM, Rocco TA, et al. Acute myocardial infarction during treatment with an activated prothrombin complex concentrate in a patient with factor VIII deficiency and factor VIII inhibitor. *Am J Med* 1988; 85:245–249.

69. Mannucci PM, Carlsson S, Harris AS. Desmopressin, surgery and thrombosis. *Thromb Haemost* 1994;71:154–155.

70. Ahlberg Å. Haemophilia in Sweden. VII. Incidence, treatment, and prophylaxis of arthropathy and other musculoskeletal manifestations of hemophilia A and B. *Acta Orthop Scand* 1965;77(Suppl.):3–132.

71. Berntorp E, Astermark J, Bjorkman S, et al. Consensus perspectives on prophylactic therapy for haemophilia: summary statement. *Haemophilia* 2003;9(Suppl. 1):1–4.

72. Panicker J, Warrier I, Thomas R, et al. The overall effectiveness of prophylaxis in severe haemophilia. *Haemophilia* 2003;9:272–278.

73. Blanchette VS, Manco-Johnson M, Santagostino E, et al. Optimizing factor prophylaxis for the haemophilia population: where do we stand? *Haemophilia* 2004;10(Suppl. 4):97–104.

74. van den Berg HM, Fischer K. Prophylaxis for severe haemophilia: experience from Europe and the United States. *Semin Thromb Hemost* 2003;29: 49–54.

75. Valento LA. Secondary prophylaxis therapy: what are the benefits, limitations and unknowns? *Haemophilia* 2004;10:147–157.

76. Hall M. Haemophilia complicated by an acquired circulating anticoagulant: a report of three cases. *Br J Haematol* 1961;7:340–348.

77. Kasper CK, Aledort L, Aronson D, et al. A more uniform measurement of FVIII inhibitors. *Thromb Diath Haemorrh* 1975;34:612.

78. Verbuggen B, Novakova I, Wessel H, et al. The Neimegen modification of the Bethesda assay for factor VIII:C inhibitors: improved specificity and reliability. *Thromb Haemost* 1995;73:247–251.

79. Wight J, Paisley S. The epidemiology of inhibitors in hemophilia A: a systematic review. *Haemophilia* 2003;4:418–435.

80. Rizza CR, Spooner R, Giangrande PLF. Treatment of hemophilia in the United Kingdom 1981–1006. *Haemophilia* 2001;7:349–359.

81. Sutan Y, French Haemophilia Study Group. Prevalence of inhibitors in a population of 3455 haemophilia patients in France. *Thromb Haemost* 1992;67:600–602.

82. Rothschild C, Laurian Y, Satre EP, et al. French previously untreated patients with severe hemophilia A after exposure with recombinant factor VIII: Incidence of inhibitors and evaluation of immune tolerance. *Thromb Haemost* 1998;80:769–783.

83. Oldenburg J, Schroeder J, Brackmann HH, et al. Environmental and genetic factors influencing inhibitor development. *Semin Hematol* 2004;41: 82–88.

84. Briet E, Reisner HM, Roberts HR. Inhibitors in Christmas disease. *Prog Clin Biol Res* 1984;150:123–139.

85. Aledort LM, DiMichele DM. Inhibitors occur more frequently in Afro-American and Latino hemophiliacs. *Haemophilia* 1998;4:68.

86. Perlinck K, Rosendaal FR, Vermylen J. Incidence of inhibitor development in a group of young hemophilia A patients treated exclusively with lyophilized cryoprecipitate. *Blood* 1993;81:3332–3335.

87. Ehrenforth S, Kreuz W, Scharrer I, et al. Incidence of development of FVIII and FIX inhibitors in hemophiliacs. *Lancet* 1992;339:594–598.

88. Guerois C, Laurian Y, Rothschild C, et al. Incidence of factor VIII inhibitor development in severe hemophilia A patients treated only with one brand of highly purified plasma-derived concentrates. *Thromb Haemost* 1995;73:215–218.

89. Yee TT, Williams MD, Hill FG, et al. Absence of inhibitors in previously untreated patients with severe hemophilia A after exposure to a single, intermediate purity factor VIII product. *Thromb Haemost* 1997;78: 1027–1029.

90. Schimpf K, Schwartz P, Kunschack M. Zero incidence of inhibitors in previously untreated patients who received intermediate purity factor VIII concentrate or factor IX complex. *Thromb Haemost* 1995;73:553–555.

91. Kreuz W, Ettingshausen CE, Auerswald G, et al. Epidemiology of inhibitors and current treatment strategies. *Haematologica* 2003;88: EREP04.

92. Lusher JM. Is the incidence and prevalence of inhibitors greater with recombinant products? No. *J Thromb Haemost* 2004;2:863–865.

93. de Biasi R, Rocino A, Papa ML, et al. Incidence of factor VIII inhibitor development in hemophilia A patients treated with less pure plasma derived concentrates. *Thromb Haemost* 1994;71:544–547.

94. Schwarzinger I, Pabinger I, Korninger C, et al. Incidence of inhibitors in patients with severe and moderate hemophilia A treated with factor VIII concentrates. *Am J Hematol* 1987;24:241–245.

95. Rasi V, Ikkala E. Hemophiliacs with factor VIII inhibitors in Finland: prevalence, incidence and outcome. *Br J Haematol* 1990;76:369–371.

96. Lorenzo JI, Garcia R, Molina R. Factor VIII and FIX inhibitors in hemophiliacs. *Lancet* 1992;339:1550–1551.

97. Addiego JE, Kasper C, Abilgaard C, et al. Frequency of inhibitor development in hemophiliacs treated with low-purity factor VIII. *Lancet* 1993; 342:462–464.

98. Lusher JM, Arkin S, Abilgaard CF et al. Kogenate Previously Untreated Patient Study Group. Recombinant factor VIII for the treatment of previously untreated patients with hemophilia A. Safety, efficacy, and development of inhibitors. *N Engl J Med* 1993;328:453–459.

99. Bray GL, Gomperts ED, Courter SG. A multicenter study of recombinant factor VIII (Recombinate): safety, efficacy and inhibitor risk in previously untreated patients. *Blood* 1997;83:2428–2435.

100. Giles AR, Rivard GE, Teitel J, et al. Surveillance for factor VIII inhibitor development in the Canadian Hemophilia A population following the widespread introduction of recombinant factor VIII replacement therapy. *Transfus Sci* 1998;19:139–148.

101. Rosendaal FR, Nieuwenhuis HK, van den Berg HM et al. Dutch Hemophilia Study Group. A sudden increase in FVIII inhibitor in multi-transfused hemophilia A patients in the Netherlands. *Blood* 1993;81:2180–2186.

102. Perlinck K, Arnout J, Gilles JG, et al. A higher than expected incidence of factor VIII inhibitors in multi-transfused hemophilia A patients treated with an intermediate purity pasteurized factor VIII concentrate. *Thromb Haemost* 1993;69:115–118.

103. Lusher J, Abildgaard C, Arkin S, et al. Human recombinant DNA-derived antihemophilic factor in the treatment of previously untreated patients with hemophilia A: final report on a hallmark clinical investigation. *J Thromb Haemost* 2004;2:574–583.

104. Knobe KE, Tengborn LI, Petrini P, et al. Breastfeeding does not influence the development of inhibitors in haemophilia. *Haemophilia* 2002;8:657–659.

105. Prescott R, Nakai H, Saenko EL, et al. The inhibitor antibody response is more complex in hemophilia A patients than in most nonhemophiliacs with Factor VIII autoantibodies. *Blood* 1997;89:3663–3671.

106. Lacroix-Desmazes S, Bayry J, Misra N, et al. The prevalence of proteolytic antibodies against Factor VIII in hemophilia A. *N Engl J Med* 2002; 346:662–667.

107. Gomperts ED, Fannon RB, Lee ML, et al. Proplex vs. Proplex SX: a controlled double blind study of the effectiveness in treating acute hemarthroses in hemophilia A patients with inhibitors to FVIII. *Thromb Res* 1986;42: 789–796.

108. Lusher JM, Shapiro SS, Palascak JE, et al. Effect of prothrombin-complex concentrates in hemophiliacs with antibodies to factor VIII: a multicenter therapeutic trial. *N Engl J Med* 1980;303:421–425.

109. Lusher JM, Blatt PM, Penner J, et al. Autoplex versus Proplex: a controlled, double-blind study of effectiveness in acute hemarthroses in hemophiliacs with inhibitors to factor VIII. *Blood* 1983;62:1135–1138.

110. Sjamsoedin LJ, Heijnen L, Mauser-Bunschoten EP, et al. The effect of activated prothrombin-complex concentrate (FEIBA) on joint and muscle bleeding in patients with hemophilia A and antibodies to FVIII. A double-blind clinical trial. *N Engl J Med* 1981;305:717–721.

111. Kantrowitz JL, Lee ML, McClure DA, et al. Early experience with the use of anti-inhibitor coagulant complex to treat bleeding in hemophiliacs with inhibitors to factor VIII. *Clin Ther* 1987;9:405–419.

112. Negrier C, Goudemand J, Sultan Y, et al. Multicenter retrospective study on the utilization of FEIBA in France in patients with factor VIII and factor IX inhibitors. *Thromb Haemost* 1997;77:1113.

113. Kohler M. Thrombogenicity of prothrombin complex concentrates. *Thromb Res* 1999;95:13–17.

114. Philippou H, Adami A, Lane DA, et al. High purity factor IX and prothrombin complex concentrate (PCC): pharmacokinetics and evidence that factor IXa is the thrombogenic trigger in PCC. *Thromb Haemost* 1996;76:23–28.

115. Ehrlich HJ, Henzl MJ, Gomperts ED. Safety of factor VIII inhibitor bypass activity (FEIBA):10-year compilation of thrombotic adverse events. *Haemophilia* 2002;8:83–90.

116. Hoffmann M, Monroe DM. The action of high-dose factor VIIa in a cell-based model of hemostasis. *Semin Hemost* 2001;38(4 Suppl. 12):6–9.

117. Key NS, Aledort LM, Beardsley D, et al. Home treatment of mild to moderate bleeding episodes using recombinant factor VIIa (Novoseven) in hemophiliacs with inhibitors. *Thromb Haemost* 1998;80:912–918.
118. Santagostino E, Gringeri A, Mannucci PM. Home treatment with recombinant activated factor VII in patients with factor VIII inhibitors: the advantage of early intervention. *Br J Haematol* 1999;104:22–26.
119. Lusher J. Recombinant factor VIIa (Novoseven) in the treatment of internal bleeding in patients with factor VII and IX inhibitors. *Haemostasis* 1996;26:S124–S130.
120. Liebman HA, Chediak J, Fink KI, et al. Activated, recombinant human coagulation factor VII (rFVIIa) therapy for abdominal bleeding in patients with inhibitor antibodies to factor VIII. *Am J Hematol* 2000;63:109–113.
121. Shapiro AD, Gilchrist GS, Hoots WK, et al. Prospective, randomized trial of two doses of rFVIIa (Novoseven) in hemophilia patients with inhibitors undergoing surgery. *Thromb Haemost* 1998;80:773–778.
122. Ludlam CA, Smith MP, Morfini M, et al. A prospective study of recombinant activated factor VII administered by continuous infusion to inhibitor patients undergoing elective major orthopaedic surgery: a pharmacokinetic and efficacy evaluation. *Br J Haematol* 2003;120:808–813.
123. Mauser-Bunschoten EP, Koopman MM, Goede-Bolder AD, et al. Efficacy of recombinant factor VIIa administered by continuous infusion to haemophilia patients with inhibitors. *Haemophiliia* 2002;8:649–656.
124. Parameswaran R, Shapiro AD, Gill JC, et al. Dose effect and efficacy of rFVIIa in the treatment of haemophilia patients with inhibitors: analysis from the Hemophilia and Thrombosis Research Society Registry. *Haemophilia* 2005;11:100–106.
125. Kenet G, Lubetski A, Luboshitz J, et al. A new approach to treatment of bleeding episodes in young hemophilia patients: a single bolus megadose of recombinant activated factor VII (Novoseven). *J Thromb Haemost* 2003;1:450–455.
126. Abshire T, Kenet G. Recombinant factor VIIa: review of efficacy, dosing regimens and safety in patients with congenital and acquired factor VIII or IX inhibitors. *J Thromb Haemost* 2004;2:899–909.
127. Mariani G, Herrmann FH, Schulman S et al. International Factor VII Deficiency Study Group. Thrombosis in inherited factor VII deficiency. *J Thromb Haemost* 2003;1:2153–2158.
128. Freedman J, Garvey MB. Immunoadsorption of factor VIII inhibitors. *Curr Opin Hematol* 2004;11:327–333.
129. Mariani G, Siragusa S, Kroner BL. Immunetolerance induction in hemophilia A: a review. *Semin Thromb Hemost* 2003;29:69–76.
130. Wight J, Paisley S, Knight C. Immunetolerance induction in patients with haemophilia A with inhibitors: a systematic review. *Haemophilia* 2003;9: 436–463.
131. Carlborg E, Astermark J, Lethagen S, et al. The Malmo model for immune tolerance induction: impact of previous treatment on outcome. *Haemophilia* 2000;6:639–642.
132. Mathias M, Khair K, Hann I, et al. Rituximab in the treatment of alloimmune factor VIII and IX antibodies in two children with severe haemophilia. *Br J Haematol* 2004;125:366–368.
133. Davis KC, Horsburgh CR Jr, Hasiba U, et al. AIDS in a patient with hemophilia. *Ann Intern Med* 1983;98:284–286.
134. Elliott JL, Hoppes WL, Platt MS, et al. AIDS and MAI bacteremia in a patient with hemophilia. *Ann Intern Med* 1983;98:290–293.
135. Yazdanpanah Y, Viget N, Cheret A, et al. Increased bleeding in HIV-positive haemophiliac patients treated with lopinavir–ritonavir. *AIDS* 17; 2003:2397–2399.
136. Wilde JT. HIV and HCV coinfection in haemophilia. *Haemophilia* 2004; 10:1–8.
137. Darby SC, Kan SW, Spooner RJ, et al. The impact of HIV on mortality rates in the complete UK haemophilia population. *AIDS* 2004;18:525–533.
138. Zakrzewska K, Azzi A, De Biasi E, et al. Persistence of parvovirus B19 DNA in synovium of patients with haemophilic arthritis. *J Med Virol* 2001; 65:402–407.
139. Troisi CL, Hollinger FB, Hoots WK, et al. A multicenter study of viral hepatitis in a United States hemophilic population. *Blood* 1993;81: 412–418.
140. Makris M, Preston FE, Rosendaal FR, et al. The natural history of chronic hepatitis C in haemophiliacs. *Br J Haematol* 1996;94:746–752.
141. Colombo M, Mannucci PM, Brettler DB, et al. Hepatocellular carcinoma in hemophilia. *Am J Hematol* 1991;37:243–246.
142. Santagostino E, Colombo M, Rivi M, et al. A 6-month versus a 12-month surveillance for hepatocellular carcinoma in 559 hemophiliacs infected with the hepatitis C virus. *Blood* 2003;102:78–82.
143. Eyster ME, Alter HJ, Aledort LM, et al. Heterosexual co-transmission of hepatitis C and HIV. *Ann Intern Med* 1991;115:764–768.
144. Seligsohn U. Factor XI deficiency. *Thromb Haemost* 1993;70:68–71.
145. Lusher JM. Transfusion therapy in congenital coagulopathies. *Hematol Oncol Clin North Am* 1994;8:1167–1180.
146. Richards EM, Makris MM, Cooper P, et al. *In vivo* coagulation activation following infusion of highly purified factor XI concentrate. *Br J Haematol* 1997;96:293–297.
147. Castaman G, Ruggeri M, Rodeghiero F. Clinical usefulness of desmopressin for prevention of surgical bleeeding in patients with symptomatic heterozygous factor XI deficiency. *Br J Haematol* 1996;94:168–170.
148. Manno CS, Chew AJ, Hutchison S, et al. AAV-mediated factor IX gene transfer to skeletal muscle in patients with severe hemophilia B. *Blood* 2003;101:2963–2972.
149. High K, Manno CS, Sabatino DE, et al. Immune response to AAV and to factor IX in a Phase 1 study of AAV-mediated liver directed gene transfer for hemophilia B. *Mol Ther* 2004;9:S383–S384 (abstract).
150. Qiu X, Lu D, Zhou J, et al. Implantation of autologous skin fibroblast genetically modified to secrete clotting factor IX partially corrects the hemorrhagic tendencies in two hemophilia B patients. *Chin Med J (Engl)* 1996;109:832–839.
151. Nathwani AC, Nienhuis AW, Davidoff AM. Current status of gene therapy for hemophilia. *Curr Hematol Rep* 2003;2:319–327.
152. Powell JS, Ragni MV, White GC, et al. Phase 1 trial of FVIII gene transfer for severe hemophilia A using a retroviral construct administered by peripheral intravenous infusion. *Blood* 2003;102:2038–2045.
153. Roth DA, Nicholas ET, O'Brien JM, et al. Nonviral transfer of the gene encoding the coagulation factor VIII in patients with severe hemophilia A. *N Engl J Med* 2001;344:1735–1742.

# CHAPTER 60 ■ VON WILLEBRAND DISEASE: DIAGNOSIS, CLASSIFICATION, AND TREATMENT

J. EVAN SADLER AND MOREY BLINDER

Von Willebrand disease (VWD) was discovered by Erik von Willebrand, a Finnish internist who investigated a family living in Föglö, one of the Åland Islands in the Gulf of Bothnia, separating Sweden and Finland (1,2). The proband was a 5-year-old girl with a severe bleeding tendency. Four of her affected sisters died of hemorrhage before the age of 4 years, and the proband herself died at the age of 13 years with her fourth menstrual period (3). The parents and several other relatives of both sexes had mild bleeding symptoms, suggesting autosomal inheritance. The severity of bleeding was variable throughout this large pedigree, and some obligate heterozygous individuals were asymptomatic. The most common sites of bleeding were skin, uterus and mucous membranes rather than deep tissues. Patients had a prolonged bleeding time, but had normal coagulation time, clot retraction, and platelet count. Von Willebrand distinguished this condition from hemophilia and Glanzmann thrombasthenia but was unable to determine whether the defect lay in the blood, the vasculature, or the platelets.

Considerable progress has been made in understanding the pathophysiology of VWD. In the 1950s, patients with VWD were reported to have low levels of blood clotting factor VIII (FVIII), and transfusions with plasma fractions from healthy individuals or patients with hemophilia were shown to correct the bleeding tendency in VWD (4–8). These observations suggested that VWD was caused by abnormalities in a plasma protein, now known as von Willebrand factor (VWF). In 1972, VWF was purified (9), and genetic variants of VWD were identified and correlated with structural differences in VWF (10). The development of multimer gel electrophoresis (11–13) uncovered additional heterogeneity in VWD. In 1985, the structure of VWF was determined by protein sequencing and cDNA cloning (14–17). This was followed almost immediately by the characterization of mutations that cause severe VWD (18,19). Today hundreds of mutations in many subtypes of VWD have been described (20,21). An on-line database of VWD mutations is maintained by Dr. Ian Peake et al. at the University of Sheffield and is accessible at http://www.shef.ac.uk/vwf/index.html.

We now understand many aspects of VWF biosynthesis, structure, and function, as discussed in Chapter 46. VWF is a multimeric blood protein that performs two major roles in hemostasis; it mediates the adhesion of platelets to sites of vascular injury, and it is a carrier protein for FVIII. These activities require the assembly of VWF into large multimers and interactions with several ligands. Inherited defects in VWF may interfere with biosynthetic processing, or disrupt specific ligand-binding sites, thereby causing bleeding by impairing either platelet adhesion or blood clotting. Depending on the disease mechanism, VWF mutations may cause autosomal dominant or recessive VWD. This knowledge provides a framework to understand the pathogenesis and classify the many variants of VWD.

## DIAGNOSIS AND CLASSIFICATION OF VON WILLEBRAND DISEASE

Three major categories of VWD are distinguished: partial quantitative deficiency (type 1), qualitative deficiency (type 2), and total deficiency (type 3) (see Table 60-1) (22). Qualitative type 2 VWD is divided further into four variants (2A, 2B, 2M, and 2N) on the basis of details of the clinical phenotype. These six categories correspond to distinct pathophysiologic mechanisms and they correlate with distinct clinical features and therapeutic requirements, as discussed in a subsequent section. The laboratory features of VWD subtypes are summarized in Table 60-2.

### von Willebrand Disease Type 1

VWD type 1 includes partial quantitative deficiency of VWF and is commonly inherited as an autosomal dominant trait. VWD type 1 appears to account for more than 70% of all VWD, although the prevalence of VWD type 1 is not known precisely. Symptomatic VWD that leads to medical treatment appears to affect approximately 35 to 100 per million individuals, which is comparable to the prevalence of hemophilia A (23). Screening programs often identify many more individuals with low VWF and mild symptoms, and suggest that VWD could have a prevalence of approximately 1% (24), but very few patients identified by population screening subsequently have significant bleeding (25). VWD type 1 includes variants previously designated as type IA (26); type I-1, I-2, and I-3 (27); type I-platelet normal and type I-platelet low (28); and VWD Vicenza. Whether VWD Vicenza should be classified as VWD type 1 or type 2M is somewhat controversial, although the consensus appears to favor classifying it as VWD type 1. Most studies indicate that VWF Vicenza has a normal VWF:RCo/VWF:Ag ratio (29,30), but some suggest the protein is dysfunctional (31).

Many factors can make VWD type 1 difficult to diagnose with confidence. Mild bleeding symptoms are sufficiently common that coincidental association with low VWF levels also is common, even when patients have a positive family history of bleeding (32). Furthermore, bleeding symptoms are not specific for VWD, and apparent transmitters of low VWF or a bleeding phenotype may themselves be phenotypically normal. Therefore, the criteria used for diagnosis are important determinants of the apparent prevalence of VWD type 1.

## TABLE 60-1

### CLASSIFICATION OF VON WILLEBRAND DISEASE

1. Type 1 VWD refers to partial quantitative deficiency of VWF
   Type 2 VWD refers to qualitative deficiency of VWF
   Type 3 VWD refers to virtually complete deficiency of VWF
2. Type 2A VWD refers to qualitative variants with decreased platelet-dependent function that is associated with the absence of high molecular weight VWF multimers
3. Type 2B VWD refers to qualitative variants with increased affinity for platelet GP Ib
4. Type 2M VWD refers to qualitative variants with decreased platelet-dependent function that is not caused by the absence of high molecular weight VWF multimers
5. Type 2N VWD refers to qualitative variants with markedly decreased affinity for FVIII
6. When recognized, a mixed phenotype caused by compound heterozygosity is indicated by separate classification of each allele separated by a slash (/)

VWD, von Willebrand disease; VWF, von Willebrand factor; GP, glycoprotein.
Adapted from Sadler JE. A revised classification of von Willebrand disease. *Thromb Haemost* 1994;71:520–525.

To address these issues, an epidemiologic approach to VWF level and bleeding risk has been proposed (32), in which "VWD type 1" is reserved for dominant, symptomatic, and relatively severe VWF deficiency. A VWF level that is only slightly decreased can instead be treated as a biomarker for a modestly increased risk of bleeding, thereby avoiding the false-positive diagnosis of an inherited bleeding disease in relatively healthy individuals.

### Bleeding Symptoms

Few large studies of symptoms in VWD have been published, and they rarely distinguish among subtypes of VWD. For example, the extensive compilations of Silwer (33) and of Buchanan and Leavell (34) include patients with all variants of VWD. Because other variants are relatively uncommon, these surveys remain useful guides to the clinical features of VWD type 1. The most common symptoms (see Table 60-3) are epistaxis, skin bruises, and hematomas, prolonged bleeding from trivial wounds, oral cavity bleeding, and excessive menstrual bleeding.

Gastrointestinal bleeding appears to be relatively rare, but may be serious when it occurs.

Epistaxis may be severe and prolonged. Easy bruising is common in VWD but is not specific. Prolonged bleeding after minor trauma to skin or mucous membranes is characteristic of VWD. Severe hemorrhage after major surgery may occur up to several weeks after surgery. Prolonged oral bleeding is common from gums, or with biting of the tongue or lips. Heavy bleeding also is common after tooth extraction or other oral surgery such as tonsillectomy and adenoidectomy. Menorrhagia a very common presenting symptom in women with VWD, but also is common in otherwise healthy women (33).

Coexistent conditions or drug interactions can strongly influence the severity of symptoms in VWD. Bleeding may be exacerbated by the use of aspirin or corticosteroids, and decreased by the use of oral contraceptives. Treatment with sodium valproate for epilepsy can lower the level of VWF and induce bleeding (35). The risk of hemorrhage may be increased by liver disease, uremia, defects in connective tissue such as Ehlers-Danlos syndrome (36), hypothyroidism (37),

## TABLE 60-2

### SELECTED LABORATORY FEATURES OF VON WILLEBRAND DISEASE SUBTYPES

| VWD | FVIII | VWF:Ag | VWF:RCo or VWF:CB | RIPA | Multimer structure |
|-----|-------|--------|-------------------|------|--------------------|
| Type 1 | Decreased | Decreased | Decreased | Decreased | Normal in plasma and platelets |
| Type 2A | Decreased or normal | Decreased or normal | Decreased relative to VWF:Ag | Decreased relative to VWF:Ag | Large and intermediate multimers absent from plasma; variable in platelets |
| Type 2B | Decreased or normal | Decreased or normal | Decreased or normal | Increased at low ristocetin concentration | Large and intermediate multimers absent from plasma; normal in platelets |
| Type 2M | Decreased or normal | Decreased or normal | Decreased relative to VWF:Ag | Decreased relative to VWF:Ag | Large and intermediate multimers present in plasma and platelets |
| Type 2N | Moderately decreased (<20 IU/dL) | Normal | Normal | Normal | Normal in plasma and platelets |
| Type 3 | Moderately decreased (<20 IU/dL) | Absent or trace | Absent | Absent | None or trace in plasma or platelets |

VWD, von Willebrand disease; VWF, von Willebrand factor; RIPA, ristocetin-induced platelet aggregation.

## TABLE 60-3

### FREQUENCY (%) OF BLEEDING SYMPTOMS IN VON WILLEBRAND DISEASE

| Symptoms | Swedish series[b] (264 cases) | Buchanan and Leavell[a] | | |
| --- | --- | --- | --- | --- |
| | | Men (95 cases) | Women (104 cases) | Normal[b] (500 cases) |
| Nose bleeding | 62.5 | 73 | 64.5 | 4.6 |
| Menorrhagia | 60[c] | — | 51 | 25.3[c] |
| Bleeding after tooth extraction | 51.5 | 28.5 | 38 | 4.8 |
| Ecchymoses and hematomas | 49.2 | — | — | 11.8 |
| Ecchymoses | — | 55.7 | 67 | — |
| Hematomas | — | 8.5 | 7.5 | — |
| Bleeding from minor cuts or abrasions | 36 | 37 | 33.5 | 0.2 |
| Gingival bleeding | 34.8 | 33 | 36 | 7.4 |
| Postoperative bleeding | 28 | 19 | 20 | 1.4 |
| Bleeding at delivery | 23.3[c] | — | 10.5 | 19.5[c] |
| Gastrointestinal bleeding | 14 | 24.5 | 9 | 0.6 |
| Traumatic oral and lip bleeding | 11.7 | — | — | 0.6 |
| Petechiae | 11.5 | 16 | 18.5 | 1.2 |
| Joint bleeding | 8.3 | 12.5 | 5 | 0 |
| Hematuria | 6.8 | 7.5 | 2 | 0.6 |
| Ovarian bleeding | 6.8[c] | — | — | — |
| Bleeding after tonsillectomy | 6.1 | — | — | — |
| Bleeding during shedding of teeth | 4.9 | — | — | — |
| Bleeding at abortion | 3.8[c] | — | — | — |
| Intramuscular, deep subcutaneous, or submucosal bleeding | 2.7 | — | — | — |

[a]Data of Buchanan JC, Leavell BS. Pseudohemophilia: report of 13 new cases and statistical review of previously reported cases. *Ann Intern Med* 1956;44:241–256.
[b]Data of Silwer J. von Willebrand's disease in Sweden. *Acta Paediatr Scand Suppl* 1973;238:1–159.
[c]For women older than 15 years.

and focal lesions such as gastric or duodenal ulcers, or gastrointestinal angiodysplasia (38).

## Laboratory Testing

The goal of laboratory testing in VWD type 1 is to exclude other causes of bleeding, document VWF deficiency, and exclude qualitative VWF defects. As a complete laboratory evaluation for VWD is quite elaborate, the efficiency of testing can be increased by using initial screening tests for VWD. VWF levels vary with physiologic stress, and where possible, tests should not be performed in proximity to hemorrhagic events, pregnancy, acute infection, or strenuous exercise. Optimal testing strategies have not yet been validated experimentally, and the approach described here is an attempt to synthesize various expert opinions.

Initial tests for any hemostatic disorder include a complete blood count with platelet count, prothrombin time (PT), and activated partial thromboplastin time (aPTT). Additional tests specific for VWD include ristocetin cofactor activity (VWF:RCo), collagen binding activity (VWF:CB), VWF antigen (VWF:Ag), and FVIII level. Blood counts and clotting tests may identify other causes of bleeding and indicate the severity of anemia, if present.

VWF:RCo is a useful initial assay for VWF concentration and platelet binding function (24), but the test is difficult to standardize and is not very precise. Therefore, VWF:Ag may be used to confirm any low values obtained for VWF:RCo. Like the VWF:RCo test, VWF:CB also depends on VWF concentration but measures the interaction of VWF with immobilized collagen.

VWF:CB tests are not as widely available as VWF:RCo, but are useful for a comprehensive evaluation of VWF functional defects (39,40). Discrepancies between VWF:RCo and VWF:Ag, or between VWF:CB and VWF:Ag, suggest a qualitative VWF defect that should be investigated along with other tests, as discussed in the section, "von Willebrand Disease type 2."

VWF levels may be normal intermittently in VWD, and abnormal results should be confirmed (41). For example, the PT, aPTT, FVIII, and VWF tests may be repeated after an interval of 2 weeks. If the results are inconsistent, they may be performed again. Unfortunately, such repeated testing is impractical or not feasible for many patients. With the limitations discussed in the subsequent text, VWD is excluded by arriving at repeated normal values of FVIII, concordant VWF:RCo, VWF:CB, and VWF:Ag on serial testing. If these initial tests are abnormal, other tests are indicated.

An abnormal aPTT is evaluated in concert with the FVIII level. A FVIII that is disproportionately lower than the VWF:Ag would suggest either hemophilia A, a defect that impairs VWF ability to bind FVIII (VWF:FVIIIB) as occurs in VWD type 2N, or another cause of FVIII deficiency such as an anti–FVIII antibody. If the FVIII is normal, then other causes of a prolonged aPTT should be considered.

Low values for VWF by any test can be hard to evaluate because the range of normal values for plasma VWF concentration is very broad. VWF levels also depend on ABO blood type (see Table 60-4), and the mean VWF:Ag level is approximately 25% lower for individuals of blood type O compared to other blood types (42). Some additional variation has been attributed to the Secretor locus that specifies some oligosaccharide

**TABLE 60-4**

INFLUENCE OF ABO BLOOD GROUPS ON VWF:AG
IN VOLUNTEER BLOOD DONORS

| ABO type | n | VWF:Ag (percentage of pooled normal plasma standard) | |
|---|---|---|---|
| | | Geometric Mean | Geometric Mean ± 2 SD |
| O | 456 | 74.8 | 35.6–157.0 |
| A | 340 | 105.9 | 48.0–233.9 |
| B | 196 | 116.9 | 56.8–241.0 |
| AB | 109 | 123.3 | 63.8–238.2 |

VWF, von Willebrand factor.
The groups were statistically different from each other as follows:
O versus A, B, and AB, $P < 0.01$; A versus AB, $P < 0.01$; B versus A,
$P < 0.05$.
From Gill JC, Endres-Brooks J, Bauer PJ, et al. The effect of ABO
blood group on the diagnosis of von Willebrand disease. *Blood* 1987;
69:1691–1695.

antigens of the Lewis blood group system (43,44). However, most of the variation in VWF levels is due to unknown factors other than either VWD or blood type. The problem is illustrated in Figure 60-1, using data for blood type O. For this population of normal type O blood donors, the mean level of VWF:Ag was 0.75 IU per mL, with a range (±2 SD) of 0.36 to 1.57 IU per mL (42). Therefore, blood type O alone can cause VWF levels low enough to suggest the diagnosis of VWD. By halving the values for this normal population, the distribution for individuals of blood type O and only one functional VWF allele can be estimated to have a mean VWF:Ag of 0.37 IU per mL (see Fig. 60-1), but there is considerable overlap with the normal distribution. Because individuals heterozygous for VWD mutations constitute much less than 1% of the population (23), moderately low VWF levels cannot reliably identify patients with VWD. Whether blood type adjusted means should be used routinely remains controversial, and additional studies on this point would be helpful. Furthermore, comparison of functional assays with the level of VWF:Ag must not suggest a qualitative abnormality

of VWF, as discussed in the section on VWD type 2. If available, ristocetin-induced platelet aggregation (RIPA) should not indicate abnormal sensitivity to ristocetin, and the plasma VWF multimer distribution should have a normal complement of large multimers.

The template bleeding time has been used to diagnose VWD, but its value for this purpose is difficult to demonstrate. A prolonged bleeding time is not specific for VWD, and does not predict bleeding at surgery (45–47). The bleeding time is subject to even greater normal variation than VWF levels, has poor reproducibility, and often is normal in VWD (41). The test can distinguish populations that are defined independently, but generally is not useful when applied to individuals. The bleeding time may be helpful for assessing the efficacy of therapeutic interventions in selected patients with VWD, but it does not appear to have sufficient sensitivity or reproducibility to contribute strongly to the diagnosis or exclusion of VWD.

A platelet function analyzer (PFA)-100 has been developed to test platelet plug formation *in vitro* by forcing a sample of citrated whole blood through a porous membrane coated with collagen plus adenosine 5'-diphosphate (ADP) or collagen plus epinephrine. Normal platelets become activated upon contact with the membrane and form occlusive aggregates. The time required for blood flow to stop is termed the closure time, which is prolonged by defects in VWF or platelet function. The PFA-100 has been proposed as a sensitive and reproducible alternative to the bleeding time, but lack of specificity remains a concern and the clinical utility of PFA-100 testing remains uncertain (48,49). As previously reported for the bleeding time (45–47), a prolonged PFA-100 closure time was not found to predict increased surgical bleeding (50).

Other VWF tests may be performed in specialized diagnostic or research laboratories. Approximately 15% of VWF in the blood is located within the α-granules of platelets and is secreted upon platelet activation (51). Platelet VWF can be assayed by methods similar to those used for plasma VWF, and the results can help identify some variants of VWD type 1 (28). Botrocetin is a snake venom protein that binds VWF (52,53). Like ristocetin, botrocetin induces high-affinity binding to platelet glycoprotein (GP) Ibα. Tests of botrocetin-induced platelet aggregation or "botrocetin cofactor activity" have been developed that are analogous to VWF assays employing ristocetin, although botrocetin and ristocetin affect VWF function by distinct mechanisms (54). A variant of the VWF:RCo assay has been described that replaces platelets with recombinant GP Ibα immobilized on microtiter plates. This enzyme-linked immunosorbent assay (ELISA) style test is very precise and sensitive compared to conventional VWF:RCo assays (55), but is not available commercially.

## Criteria for Diagnosis of von Willebrand Disease Type 1

No matter what criteria are used, the extreme range of normal VWF levels complicates the diagnosis of VWD type 1, and a satisfactory general answer to this dilemma has not yet been devised. Because of this diagnostic uncertainty, the risk and benefit of specifically diagnosing VWD type 1 should be balanced for each patient.

The diagnosis of VWD type 1 is easy to make, when the patient has significant mucocutaneous bleeding, the VWF level is very low (e.g., <20 IU per dL), and the family history is strongly positive with high penetrance. Such families usually show clear coinheritance of low VWF with bleeding symptoms, and usually, mutations in the VWF gene can be found (28,56–58). For these patients, a diagnosis of VWD type 1 seems appropriate because they often can benefit from changes in lifestyle, or from specific treatment to prevent or control bleeding. Also, genetic counseling is straightforward when the inheritance of the disorder can be predicted with confidence. Unfortunately, this combination of features is relatively rare.

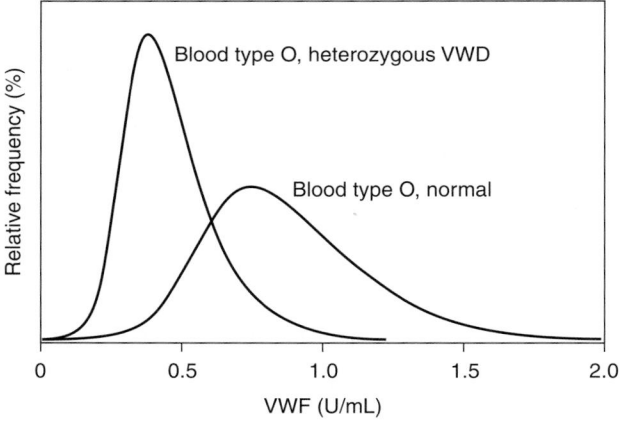

**FIGURE 60-1.** Distribution of VWF:Ag levels in normal blood donors of blood type O, and hypothetical distribution of VWF:Ag levels in individuals of blood type O who are heterozygous for VWF null alleles. The reference normal value of 1 IU per mL is based on the World Health Organization standard pooled plasma (42). (Adapted from tabulated data of Gill JC, Endres-Brooks J, Bauer PJ, et al. The effect of ABO blood group on the diagnosis of von Willebrand disease. *Blood* 1987; 69:1691–1695.)

More commonly, patients have a medical history of only menorrhagia or other infrequent mild bleeding, their VWF levels are borderline low (e.g., 25 to 50 IU per dL), and their family members do not consistently have either low VWF or bleeding symptoms. In such cases, low VWF level and bleeding are likely to associate coincidentally rather than causally (32). Family studies usually show that bleeding symptoms and low VWF levels are not coinherited, and linkage to the *VWF* gene mutations cannot be demonstrated (25,59,60). VWF levels that are slightly more than 2 SD below the population mean confer a relatively small relative risk of menorrhagia or other bleeding (32), and do not correlate with increased bleeding at surgery (61). To label these patients as VWD type 1 has little clinical utility. It may, in fact, harm them by affecting their relationship with employers and insurance providers, by causing unnecessary change in lifestyle, and by inducing unjustified fear of transmitting a genetic disease. A modestly low VWF level may be treated instead, as a biomarker for modestly increased bleeding risk. Patients with "low VWF" may be told they fall at one end of the normal range of VWF levels and may have a slightly higher than average tendency for bleeding. Empiric therapy to raise VWF may be considered for these patients with low VWF if they should bleed.

## Molecular Defects in von Willebrand Disease Type 1

VWD type 1 can sometimes be caused by frameshifts, nonsense mutations, or deletions that are similar or identical to mutations found in patients with VWD type 3 (62–64). As first shown by von Willebrand, some heterozygous members of such families may not have bleeding symptoms, so that possession of a single such mutant allele does not consistently cause bleeding symptoms. In some families, the variation in symptoms has been attributed to chance coinheritance of a second mutated VWF allele. For example, in two families in the Netherlands, compound heterozygosity for VWD type 1 and VWD type 2N was found in patients with substantial bleeding, whereas relatives with either single mutant allele were asymptomatic (65).

VWD type 1 occasionally appears to be inherited as an autosomal dominant trait with very high penetrance, and the molecular basis for this strongly dominant phenotype appears to be distinct from that of the more common form of VWD type 1 with low and variable penetrance. In one family a Cys1149Arg missense mutation was identified that caused the retention of mutant subunits in the endoplasmic reticulum and inhibited the secretion of normal VWF subunits, possibly by causing the intracellular retention of heterodimers between mutant and normal subunits (57,66). Another missense mutation at a cysteine residue, Cys1130Arg, was found in two other families with a similar dominant phenotype, although the effect on VWF biosynthesis was not reported (57). This mechanism provides a plausible biochemical explanation for the dominant transmission of exceptionally low VWF levels and bleeding symptoms with high penetrance.

Quantitative VWF deficiency also can be caused by mutations that lead to the increased clearance of VWF from the blood, provided that the clearance mechanism does not exhibit a strong preference for large multimers (67). For example, the mutation R1205H causes VWD Vicenza, which is characterized by VWF:Ag less than 15 IU per dL and plasma VWF multimers that are even larger than those found in normal plasma, and VWF Vicenza appears to be cleared from the blood approximately fivefold more rapidly than normal VWF (30).

---

## von Willebrand Disease Type 2

For VWF to perform its hemostatic functions, it must be assembled into large multimers and functional binding sites must be constructed for FVIII, for platelet receptors, and for ligands in connective tissue. Mutations in VWD type 2 can disrupt any of these properties, and VWD type 2 accounts for between 7% and 30% of all VWD in various reports. Such qualitative abnormalities of VWF often are associated with discrepancies between the level of VWF:Ag and functional assays such as VWF:RCo, VWF:CB, or VWF:FVIIIB. Four subtypes are currently recognized (Tables 60-1, 60-2). The prevalence of the subtypes appears to be increasing as awareness of them increases, although the distribution of subtypes differs considerably among treatment centers. A recent survey in France found that patients with VWD type 2 were divided as 30% type 2A, 28% type 2B, 8% type 2M (or unclassified), and 34% type 2N (68). A similar study in Germany found 74% type 2A, 10% type 2B, 13% type 2M, and 3.5% type 2N (69).

Discrimination between qualitatively normal VWF and abnormal VWF can be difficult by laboratory testing, especially because VWF:RCo assays become somewhat unreliable when the VWF:Ag level is less than 20 IU per dL. A common strategy is to compare values obtained in functional assays (VWF:RCo, VWF:CB, VWF:FVIIIB) with VWF:Ag; a ratio less than 0.6 (70) or less than 0.7 (71,72) the VWF value is inferred to be abnormal, and a ratio larger than the selected value is interpreted as normal. This approach seems reasonable, although the sensitivity and specificity of a particular ratio would depend on the performance characteristics of the individual assays.

### von Willebrand Disease Type 2A

A disproportionately low VWF:RCo or VWF:CB, relative to VWF:Ag, may reflect decreased affinity of VWF for platelets or collagen, respectively. The most common cause of this defect is the absence of large VWF multimers (see Fig. 60-2), which is characteristic of VWD type 2A. This subtype can be diagnosed by the combination of markedly reduced VWF:RCo or VWF:CB and compatible multimer gel analysis (Fig. 60-2). VWD type 2A appears to account for most of VWD type 2 (73). VWD type 2A includes variants previously designated as type IIA (12); type IIA-1, IIA-2, and IIA-3 (27); type I-platelet discordant (28); type IB (26); type IIC (74); type IID (75); type IIE (76); type IIF (77); type IIG (78); type IIH (79); and type II-I (80).

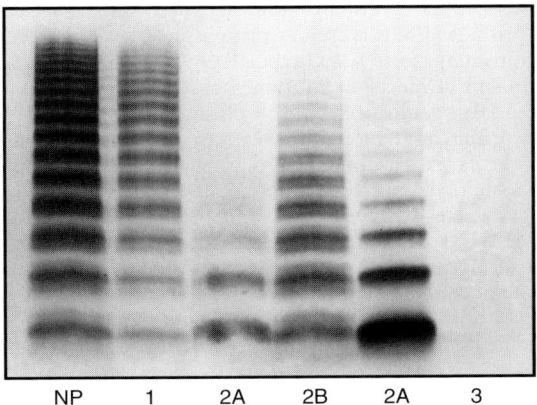

FIGURE 60-2. Multimer patterns in von Willebrand disease (VWD). Samples of plasma from a normal individual (*N*) and from patients with VWD types 1, 2A (two unrelated patients), 2B, and 3 were electrophoresed through a 1.3% agarose/SDS gel and von Willebrand factor (VWF) was detected by Western blotting. (Reprinted with permission from Sadler JE. von Willebrand disease. In: Bloom AL, Forbes CD, Thomas DP, et al., eds. *Haemostasis and thrombosis*, 3rd ed. Edinburgh: Churchill-Livingstone; 1994: 843–857.)

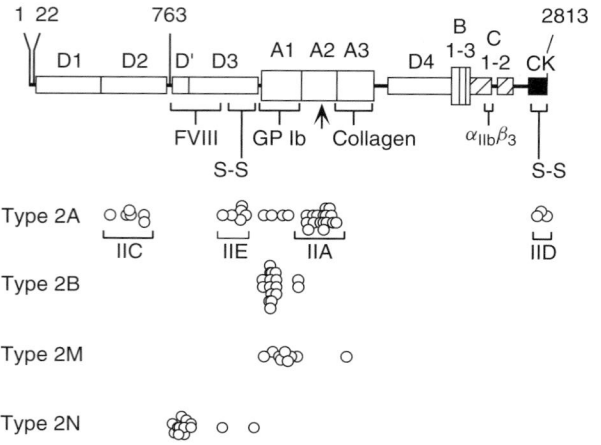

**FIGURE 60-3.** Mutations in von Willebrand disease (VWD) type 2. Amino acid residues are numbered by codon number 1 to 2813 for preproVWF. The signal peptide contains residues 1–22, the propeptide contains residues 23–763, and the mature subunit contains residues 764–2813. The locations of conserved structural domains (A, B, C, D, and CK) are indicated. Intersubunit disulfide bonds (not shown) connect CK to CK domains, and D3 domains to D3 domains. The locations of binding sites are indicated for FVIII, platelet glycoprotein (GP) Ib, collagen, and platelet $\alpha_{IIb}\beta_3$. The metalloprotease ADAMTS13 cleaves a Tyr–Met bond in domain A2 (*arrow*). *Circles* mark the positions of mutations that cause the VWD phenotypes noted at the left. For VWD type 2A, the *labeled brackets* show the location of mutations that correspond to variants with characteristic multimer patterns discussed in the text. These include variants with increased sensitivity to proteolysis (*IIA*) or by defective multimer assembly due to mutations in the propeptide (*IIC*), the D3 domain (*IIE*), or the CK domain (*IID*). References to the individual mutations can be found in the database of VWD mutations (20) maintained by Ian Peake et al. (University of Sheffield) and accessible at http://www.shef.ac.uk/vwf/index.html. (Reproduced with permission from White GC, II, Sadler JE. Von Willebrand disease: Clinical aspects and therapy. In: Hoffman R, Benz EJ, Shattil SJ, eds. *Hematology: Basic principles and practice.* 4th ed. Philadelphia: Elsevier Churchill Livingstone; 2005:2121–2136.)

VWD type 2A usually is a dominant disorder and often is caused by single amino acid substitutions in or near domain A2 (residues 1480-1672) of the mature VWF subunit (20) (see Fig. 60-3). These mutations lead to the absence of large VWF multimers either by impairing intracellular multimer assembly or by promoting intravascular proteolysis of VWF (81). Some mutations may cause VWD type 2A by a combination of these mechanisms. Defects in multimer assembly produce an absence of large multimers in both plasma and platelet VWF. In contrast, increased susceptibility to proteolysis selectively depletes the large multimers of plasma VWF because platelet VWF is relatively protected from proteolysis. The plasma metalloprotease, a disintegrin and metalloprotease with thrombospondin type 1 motif 13 (ADAMTS13), cleaves the Tyr1605–Met1606 bond within domain A2 of VWF (82,83), and this cleavage accounts for the major proteolytic fragments of the VWF subunit that are found in plasma VWF (84). Mutations that increase the susceptibility of VWF to ADAMTS13 cause the loss of large, hemostatically effective multimers from plasma and leads to bleeding. Conversely, deficiency of ADAMTS13 causes thrombotic thrombocytopenic purpura associated with unusually large VWF multimers, as discussed in Chapter 111.

A similar dominant phenotype is caused by mutations within the cystine knot motif at the carboxyl terminus of the VWF subunit. These mutations disrupt the initial dimerization of proVWF subunits in the endoplasmic reticulum. The mutant subunits remain capable of forming disulfide bonds in the

Golgi apparatus, and the VWF found in the blood consists of small multimers comprised mainly of an even number of subunits, with prominent abnormal intermediate bands composed of an odd number of subunits (85–88). VWD type 2A caused by mutations in the cystine knot domain corresponds to the variant originally named "type IID" (Fig. 60-3) (75,89).

VWD type 2A also may result from defective multimerization within the Golgi. Mutations in the D3 region can cause a dominant phenotype characterized by small multimers that are indistinct or "smeary," suggesting heterogeneity of the disulfide bond arrangements that probably is caused by disruption of normal intersubunit disulfide bond formation (69,86,88). These mutations correspond to the variant, originally named "type IIE" (Fig. 60-3) (76). A recessive form of VWD type 2A is caused by mutations within the VWF propeptide that impair the assembly of disulfide bond-linked multimers (Fig. 60-3) (88,90–93). The small plasma VWF multimers in these patients are characterized by an exceptionally clean appearance, lacking the usual intermediate or "satellite" bands that are associated with proteolysis *in vivo*; these mutations correspond to the variant originally named "type IIC" (74,76).

These studies indicate that VWD type 2A can be caused by several distinct defects in VWF biosynthesis or proteolytic susceptibility, and some can be distinguished by multimer gel electrophoresis. These various defects are united, however, by a common mechanism of impaired hemostasis resulting from the absence of large VWF multimers, and currently, they cannot be distinguished clinically by differences in severity of bleeding or response to therapy.

### von Willebrand Disease Type 2B

The mutant VWF in VWD type 2B has increased affinity for platelets (13). This causes spontaneous binding of large VWF multimers to platelets *in vivo*, followed by removal of the large VWF multimers and a variable decrease in the platelet count. The remaining small multimers are not hemostatically effective, and patients with VWD type 2B have a bleeding diathesis that may seem disproportionately severe for their VWF level. Thrombocytopenia in VWD type 2B can be intermittent, and is frequently exacerbated by stress factors, such as infection or pregnancy (94–99). VWD type 2B has been misdiagnosed and treated as autoimmune thrombocytopenia (95–97,99–102). VWD type 2B includes variants previously designated as VWD type IIB (13), type I New York (103), and Malmö (104).

The results of initial laboratory tests may be difficult to interpret in VWD type 2B. VWF levels occasionally are in the normal range, but VWF:Ag usually is decreased (13). VWF:RCo may be decreased more than VWF:Ag and suggest a diagnosis of VWD type 2A. Less commonly, VWF:Ag and VWF:RCo are decreased proportionately, which suggests a diagnosis of VWD type 1. In most cases of VWD type 2B the plasma VWF lacks the largest multimers, and multimer gels may not reliably distinguish VWD type 2B from VWD type 2A (Fig. 60-2).

The diagnosis of VWD type 2B depends on the results of RIPA. In platelet-rich plasma (PRP) from normal controls, RIPA requires VWF and exhibits a characteristic dose response to ristocetin (see Fig. 60-4). In VWD type 2B, brisk platelet aggregation occurs at low concentrations of ristocetin that has little or no effect on PRP from normal controls (13). Positive results in this test are found in one other rare disease, platelet-type or pseudo-VWD, in which mutations in platelet GP Ibα cause a phenotype very similar to VWD type 2B. Increased RIPA at low ristocetin concentrations is sensitive and fairly specific for VWD type 2B. The RIPA test is not sensitive to moderate decreases in VWF concentration (105), and therefore is not an effective screening assay for other subtypes of VWD.

In the absence of RIPA data, the only sign pointing to VWD type 2B may be thrombocytopenia. For patients misdiagnosed

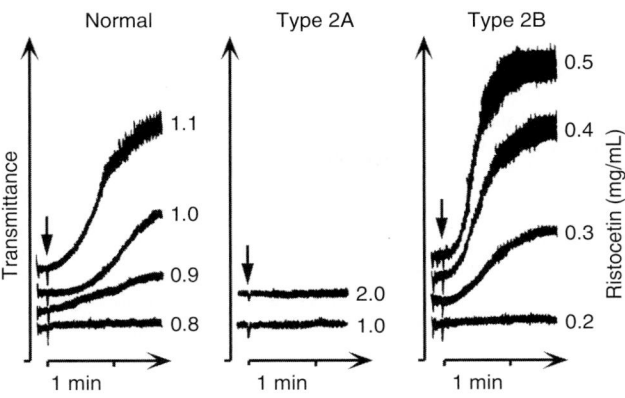

**FIGURE 60-4.** Ristocetin-induced platelet aggregation (RIPA) in a healthy control and patients with von Willebrand disease (VWD) type 2A and 2B. Stirred samples of platelet-rich plasma were supplemented at the time marked with the *arrow* (↓) with the indicated concentrations of ristocetin and light transmission was recorded as a function of time. Normal samples always required more ristocetin than did VWD type 2B samples to achieve comparable rates of platelet agglutination. (Adapted from Ruggeri ZM, Pareti FI, Mannucci PM, et al. Heightened interaction between platelets and factor VIII/von Willebrand factor in a new subtype of von Willebrand disease. *N Engl J Med* 1980;302: 1047–1051.)

as VWD type 1, the correct diagnosis of VWD type 2B may be discovered accidentally by finding that thrombocytopenia develops or is markedly worsened by desmopressin (1-deamino-8-D-arginine vasopressin, DDAVP) (94). For this reason, the platelet count should be followed in all patients who receive their first diagnostic or therapeutic trial of desmopressin.

The binding site on VWF for platelet GP Ib is within VWF domain A1, between amino acid residues 1226-1479. At least 14 mutations are known to cause VWD type 2B and all of them are within domain A1 (Fig. 60-3). The crystal structure of a complex between VWF domain A1 and a fragment of GP Ibα suggests that large conformational changes occur in both proteins when they bind (106). The locations of VWD type 2B mutations indicate that they are likely to stabilize the bound conformation of domain A1, which could allow binding to platelet GP Ib in the absence of vascular injury and thereby cause the observed dominant, "gain-of-function" phenotype (106).

### von Willebrand Disease Type 2M

VWD type 2M ("M" for "multimer") includes variants in which platelet adhesion is impaired but the VWF multimer distribution is normal. This phenotype may be produced by mutations that inactivate specific binding sites for ligands on platelets or in connective tissue (22). For example, several VWD type 2M mutations that impair binding to platelet GP Ib have been reported within VWF domain A1 (Fig. 60-3) (68,88,107–109). Only one mutation that impairs binding to collagen has been reported in VWF domain A3 (110), although the apparent low prevalence of domain A3 mutations might reflect the relatively limited use of VWF:CB assays compared to VWF:RCo assays. Screening laboratory results generally are similar to those in VWD type 2A (Table 60-2), but multimer gel analysis shows that large multimers are present. VWD type 2M includes variants previously designated as type B (111), type IC (112), and type ID (113).

### von Willebrand Disease Type 2N

The FVIII binding site on VWF is near the amino-terminus of the mature subunit. Missense mutations that selectively inactivate this binding site (Fig. 60-3) produce an interesting autosomal recessive VWD phenotype in which the platelet-dependent functions of VWF are preserved and the multimer pattern appears normal, but FVIII levels are low, often less than 10 IU per dL (114, 115). This autosomal mimic of hemophilia A is named VWD "type 2N" after "Normandy," the birth province of one index case. The correct diagnosis is made by demonstrating that the patient's VWF has markedly decreased binding affinity for FVIII in VWF:FVIIIB assays.

The prevalence of VWD type 2N is not known, but it might be higher than currently appreciated. For example, 31 affected families were identified between 1990 and 1995 in France, where only two centers perform VWF:FVIIIB assays (116). Some of these patients with VWD type 2N had been misdiagnosed with hemophilia A or as carriers of hemophilia A. Screening of patients with hemophilia A has shown that a small percentage of those with apparent mild hemophilia A may instead have VWD type 2N (117).

Although VWD type 2N superficially resembles mild hemophilia A, or a hemophilia carrier state with low FVIII levels due to extreme lyonization, the therapeutic requirements in VWD type 2N are quite distinct. In particular, highly purified or recombinant FVIII preparations give poor FVIII recovery and survival *in vivo* because the patient's endogenous VWF cannot stabilize it normally (118,119). For the same reason, treatment with desmopressin often does not effectively increase plasma FVIII levels (119). This behavior may incorrectly suggest the presence of a FVIII inhibitor. Furthermore, genetic counseling for an autosomal recessive disease is very different from that for an X chromosome–linked disease. Because of these important points, the differential diagnosis of VWD type 2N versus hemophilia A should be considered in any patient with low FVIII levels in whom the evidence for X-linked inheritance is incomplete, or in whom initial therapy with desmopressin or pure FVIII gives unexpectedly poor results.

### von Willebrand Disease Type 3

VWD type 3 is a recessive disorder in which VWF protein is essentially absent. Total deficiency of VWF causes a secondary deficiency of FVIII, and such patients have a severe combined defect in platelet adhesion and blood clotting. Laboratory testing show undetectable VWF:RCo and VWF:Ag, as well as a prolonged aPTT that is explained by a low FVIII level. If the condition is congenital, other testing is not usually necessary to make the diagnosis.

Heterozygous relatives of patients with VWD type 3 usually are phenotypically normal, but may have mild bleeding symptoms and meet criteria for VWD type 1 (120–123). Review of published data for 117 obligate heterozygotes indicated that they had a mean plasma VWF level of 45 IU per dL with a range of 5 IU per dL to 130 IU per dL; some had mild bruising, epistaxis, menorrhagia, or bleeding after tooth extraction (32). Such variability was evident in the first report by von Willebrand—the proband was one of five siblings with VWD type 3 and both parents had mild symptoms, but several relatives who could transmit the disease appeared to be unaffected (1). Similar variability in symptoms is evident in many other families in whom mutations have been characterized. VWD type 3 appears to be caused mainly by deletion, frameshift, and nonsense mutations (20,62–64,123). The mutation in the original Åland Islands families studied by von Willebrand was shown to be a single nucleotide deletion in exon 18, causing a frameshift and premature termination within the propeptide (124).

Questions regarding the "expressivity" or "penetrance" of VWD in the relatives of type 3 patients are related to questions concerning the pathophysiology of VWD type 1. For example, the prevalence of VWD type 3 is reported to be 2.5 to 3 per million in Scandinavian countries and is 0.1 to 1.6 per million in many counties of Europe and the Middle East (125). An intermediate prevalence of approximately 1.5 per million was reported for the United States and Canada (126). These figures provide approximate values for $q^2$, where q is the gene frequency for type 3 alleles; therefore, the prevalence of heterozygous individuals (2pq) is 660 to 3,400 per million. The prevalence of heterozygotes could be even higher because of the shortened life expectancy in VWD type 3. However, the prevalence of symptomatic VWD type 1 appears to be less than 10% of these values. Therefore, a single nonfunctional VWF allele may sometimes be associated with VWD type 1, but rarely is sufficient to cause disease.

## DIFFERENTIAL DIAGNOSIS OF VON WILLEBRAND DISEASE

VWD types 2 and 3 are relatively easy to diagnose and appear at present to be genetic diseases of a single locus, the VWF gene. The most common variant, VWD type 1, often is difficult to diagnose and appears to involve factors other than mutations in the VWF gene. Some of these modifying factors are known. For example, the ABO locus affects the level of plasma VWF, and the combination of a VWF mutation and blood type O may be associated with bleeding symptoms. Other genetic and possibly nongenetic factors remain uncharacterized.

Mucocutaneous bleeding symptoms and low VWF levels are both common, and a major diagnostic problem is to determine for a given patient, whether low VWF levels merit a diagnosis of VWD type 1 or should instead be managed as a biomarker for mildly increased bleeding risk. In addition, VWD must be distinguished from other inherited or acquired disorders of platelet function or FVIII deficiency. A few conditions are characterized by laboratory features that are remarkably like certain VWD subtypes, and therefore pose special diagnostic challenges.

### Acquired von Willebrand Syndrome

Acquired von Willebrand syndrome (AVWS) refers to VWF deficiency that is not inherited but is secondary to another cause. AVWS is usually a chronic condition in which patients may have mucocutaneous bleeding symptoms and laboratory parameters consistent with the diagnosis of VWD. Although the incidence of AVWS is unclear, a survey of 260 patients with myeloproliferative or lymphoproliferative disorders identified 25 patients with a ristocetin cofactor activity of less than 40 IU per dL, eight of whom had evidence of a VWF inhibitor (127). In many cases, a multimer pattern consistent with type 2A VWD was identified, suggesting an increased effect on high-molecular-weight multimers. AVWS typically is caused by one of three mechanisms: autoimmune clearance, proteolysis induced by increased fluid shear stress, or binding to cell surfaces (128,129).

Autoimmune clearance probably accounts for the common association of AVWS with monoclonal gammopathy of unknown significance (MGUS). Other conditions thought to induce immune clearance of VWF include lymphoproliferative diseases such as non-Hodgkin lymphoma and multiple myeloma, and autoimmune diseases such as systemic lupus erythematosus and autoimmune thyroiditis. Antibodies to VWF have been demonstrated in a few patients tested, suggesting the assays are insensitive or the mechanism of disease may not always involve circulating antibodies (128,129).

Cardiovascular conditions with pathologically increased fluid shear stress will promote the cleavage of circulating large VWF multimers by ADAMTS13, thereby causing AVWS. A classic presentation of AVWS is associated with aortic stenosis and bleeding from intestinal angiodysplasia. The AVWS and bleeding resolve upon surgical replacement of the stenotic valve (130). AVWS also has been described in patients with mitral valve prolapse, pulmonary hypertension, ventricular septal defect, and patent ductus arteriosus (128,129,131–133).

AVWS caused by increased VWF binding to platelets has been described in reactive thrombocytosis and in thrombocytosis associated with myeloproliferative diseases including essential thrombocythemia, polycythemia vera, and chronic myelogenous leukemia. The platelet count correlates inversely with the level of large VWF multimers, and reducing the platelet count can restore a normal VWF multimer distribution (134,135). VWF binding to malignant lymphocytes and other cancer cells has also been described, sometimes associated with the expression of platelet GP Ib or other VWF binding proteins on the tumor cell surface (128,129).

Hypothyroidism may sometimes cause decreased VWF levels attributed to decreased VWF synthesis, and the levels return to normal with thyroid replacement therapy (37). Certain drugs including sodium valproate (35) and ciprofloxacin (136) are reported to be associated with AVWS.

### Platelet-Type Pseudo–von Willebrand Disease

VWD type 2B is characterized by exaggerated affinity of plasma VWF for platelets, and this defect is demonstrated in the RIPA assay as increased platelet aggregation at low concentrations of ristocetin. The VWD type 2B phenotype is mimicked closely by an analogous but relatively rare gain-of-function defect in platelet GP Ib that is referred to as "platelet-type" or "pseudo" VWD (137–139). Both VWD type 2B and platelet-type pseudo-VWD are associated with decreased plasma VWF and FVIII, increased sensitivity to ristocetin in the RIPA assay, the absence of the largest VWF multimers from plasma, and the presence of all sizes of multimers within platelets. Furthermore, administration of desmopressin to patients with either disorder can cause transient thrombocytopenia and spontaneous platelet aggregation (94,140). Platelet-type pseudo-VWD can be distinguished from VWD type 2B by suitable mixing experiments: Addition of normal VWF (e.g., in normal plasma) to patient platelets causes platelet aggregation in platelet-type pseudo-VWD, but not in VWD type 2B (138,140,141). Three mutations in the platelet GP Ibα subunit have been described in patients with platelet-type pseudo-VWD: Gly233Val (142), Gly233Ser (143), and Met239Val (144). The affected residues are located in a small region that changes structure and adopts a β-sheet conformation upon binding to VWF domain A1. The mutations that cause platelet-type pseudo-VWD appear to enhance the affinity of binding, by stabilizing this β-sheet conformation (106).

### Hemophilia A

As discussed in the preceding text, VWD type 2N may be misdiagnosed as hemophilia A, particularly if the family history does not provide clear evidence for X chromosome–linked inheritance of FVIII deficiency. Conversely, patients with hemophilia A who also have platelet dysfunction, commonly caused by aspirin use, can have mucocutaneous bleeding similar to that of patients with VWD (145).

### Other Disorders

Because patients with VWD type 2B may present with thrombocytopenia, this subtype of VWD has been misdiagnosed as autoimmune thrombocytopenia in adults and infants (95–97,99–102).

# TREATMENT OF VON WILLEBRAND DISEASE AND ACQUIRED VON WILLEBRAND SYNDROME

## Agents Used in the Treatment of von Willebrand Disease

### Desmopressin

Desmopressin (DDAVP) is a synthetic analog of vasopressin that has less than 1% of the pressor effect of the natural hormone. Originally used as replacement therapy for central diabetes insipidus, this agent was shown to successfully treat bleeding in hemophilia A and VWD (146–148). Administration of desmopressin results in a rapid increase in plasma levels of FVIII and VWF in normal individuals and those with type 1 VWD. The rapid rise suggests an effect on preformed VWF that is released from the Weibel-Palade bodies of the endothelium, but the mechanism of this effect is uncertain.

Desmopressin may be administered intravenously, subcutaneously, or as an intranasal spray. When given intravenously the usual dose is 0.3 $\mu$g per kg diluted in 50 mL of 0.9% sodium chloride and infused over 30 minutes. The maximal response in the VWF levels occurs in 30 to 60 minutes and generally persists for at least 6 hours. When indicated, repeat doses are usually given every 12 to 24 hours (147,149,150). The response is consistent in any one individual and usually results in a twofold to fourfold increase in VWF. This response often is associated with an improvement in the bleeding time. Several early reports suggested that patients developed tachyphylaxis (decreased response) to repeated doses of desmopressin and this is thought to be caused by depletion of VWF from its storage sites. On an average, the increment in VWF is approximately 30% less with a second dose given 24 hours subsequent to the initial dose, but the response was not reduced further after one or two additional doses (151). Repeated dosing at intervals of less than 24 hours is also more likely to cause tachyphylaxis. Three to four days after desmopressin is stopped, a full response can again be anticipated with readministration of the drug. If suitably concentrated preparations of injectable desmopressin are available, a subcutaneous dose is approximately as effective as the same intravenous dose, providing a feasible route of administration for home therapy (152).

In some countries a highly concentrated form of desmopressin containing 1.5 mg per mL (Stimate, ZLB Behring) is available as an intranasal spray. The recommended adult dose is 300 $\mu$g given in divided doses, 150 $\mu$g in each nostril. In children and adults weighing less than 50 kg, the recommended dose is 150 $\mu$g. Preparations of intranasal desmopressin used for diabetes insipidus or enuresis are too dilute as intranasal therapy for bleeding in VWD. The therapeutic levels achieved with this approach are thought to be similar to a dose of approximately 0.2 $\mu$g per kg intravenous desmopressin (147). For patients with type 1 VWD, peak responses in VWF activity occur in 1 to 2 hours and the plasma concentrations of VWF generally are not as high as with intravenous desmopressin. The responses are also less predictable than with intravenous therapy (153). Nevertheless, this approach is useful for patients who are in remote settings or who require treatment of minor recurrent bleeding (e.g., menorrhagia). The medication should be stored under refrigeration but appears stable for up to 3 weeks when stored at room temperature for use during travel.

Because the response to desmopressin varies among individuals, a trial dose should be evaluated before any therapeutic or prophylactic use of desmopressin. Blood samples are obtained for baseline measurement of VWF:Ag, VWF:RCo (or VWF:CB) and FVIII. Then a single dose of desmopressin, 0.3 $\mu$g per kg in 50 mL of normal saline, is given intravenously over 30 minutes. The subject should be monitored for vital signs, flushing, and headache. Additional samples for measurement of VWF:Ag, VWF:RCo and FVIII should be obtained at 1 hour and 4 hours after the start of the infusion. Values at 1 hour represent the maximum response. Values at 4 hours allow calculation of the circulatory half-life of the released factors. Some authors recommend monitoring the bleeding time, but bleeding time changes may not correlate with clinical efficacy.

Target plasma levels of VWF and FVIII depend on the hemostatic challenge. Minor bleeding and minor surgical procedures may be covered satisfactorily with increases of VWF and FVIII to at least 30 IU per dL at 1 hour after desmopressin, provided the half-life is normal. Major bleeding and major surgery may require levels greater than 100 IU per dL that remain greater than 50 IU per dL before the next dose.

Useful responses to desmopressin are common in VWD type 1 and rare in VWD type 2 variants (148). The percentage of patients with VWD type 1 that responds to intravenous desmopressin varies from 90% (149) to approximately 30% (31). Some of this variation reflects different definitions of response.

It is generally recommended that a test dose of intranasal desmopressin also be evaluated before the clinical use of this form of the drug, even in patients who have previously responded to intravenous desmopressin.

The most common adverse reaction to intravenous desmopressin, occurring in up to 10% of patients, is vasodilatation with facial flushing and, less commonly, headache and mild hypotension. Extending the period of infusion from 30 to 60 minutes generally lessens these side effects. Intranasal desmopressin is associated with similar reactions and may also be associated with local reactions including nasal congestion, rhinitis, and upper respiratory symptoms. Hyponatremia, the result of the antidiuretic effect of desmopressin, tends to occur in children younger than 2 years, and in elderly patients who have received several doses. Hyponatremia has been described with either intravenous or intranasal desmopressin and, when severe, may cause seizures (150,154). Monitoring of the serum sodium level and fluid restriction should be instituted for patients receiving more than two to three doses. Hyponatremia resolves rapidly after desmopressin is discontinued. There have been several isolated reports of stroke and myocardial infarction among patients receiving desmopressin. However, a retrospective review of patients receiving desmopressin for major surgery found no difference in thrombotic events between patients who did and did not receive the drug (155). Most cases of thrombosis have been described in older men who have other thrombotic risk factors so that a concern remains in these patients requiring therapy.

Unlike vasopressin, desmopressin does not appear to cause uterine contractions. Nevertheless, because of the concern over a possible oxytocinlike effect, desmopressin is rarely used in pregnancy. Safety in nursing mothers has not been defined.

### Plasma-Derived von Willebrand Factor

Cryoprecipitate is prepared from plasma and is enriched in FVIII, VWF, and fibrinogen. Blood collected for the preparation of cryoprecipitate is screened for a number of infectious agents including human immunodeficiency virus (HIV), hepatitis B and hepatitis C, but at present is not virucidally treated. Therefore, a small risk of viral contamination remains, similar to that of red cell transfusions. One unit of blood yields approximately 8 to 10 mL of cryoprecipitate containing 100 to 150 IU of VWF. When prepared from single donors and processed individually, cryoprecipitate contains VWF multimeric structure similar to that found in plasma (156). Cryoprecipitate is given as an intravenous infusion and a typical dose is 1 to 2 "bags" per 10 kg of body weight. Matching for ABO type is not necessary and the product does not need to be given through a leukocyte-depleting filter. Cryoprecipitate was once the preferred plasma-derived product for the treatment of bleeding in VWD. However, concern over viral transmission has led to the abandonment of cryoprecipitate in favor of virucidally treated FVIII concentrates in most circumstances.

FVIII-containing products are either derived from plasma or prepared as a recombinant product from cultured cells. Plasma-derived products are virucidally treated and available data suggest that the risks of transmitting HIV, hepatitis B, and hepatitis C have been essentially eliminated. Highly purified or "monoclonal" plasma FVIII concentrates and recombinant FVIII products lack sufficient VWF to be useful in the treatment of any form of VWD. In contrast, plasma-derived FVIII concentrates that contain 15 to 200 IU FVIII per mg protein (commonly described as "intermediate purity") also contain substantial amounts of VWF. Because these products are virucidally treated, they have become the preferred products for the treatment of VWD.

When examined by gel electrophoresis, the VWF present in plasma-derived FVIII concentrates generally shows some evidence of limited degradation compared to fresh plasma VWF. Nevertheless, these products can correct the hemostatic defect in patients with VWD (157,158). Humate-P (ZLB Behring) has recently been licensed in the United States for use in VWD. The drug appears effective for the prevention of bleeding perioperatively and for the treatment of other bleeding episodes. Each vial of Humate-P is labeled with both FVIII units and VWF units (ristocetin cofactor units) so that particular attention is paid to this information to ensure correct dosing. Examples of treatment guidelines are shown in Table 60-5. Monitoring of VWF activity may be helpful to reduce the

hemostatic risk of underdosing and the extra cost of overdosing (159). Humate-P is generally well tolerated with few adverse events (159). Continuous infusion of Humate-P may be considered because this appears effective and consumes approximately one half of the total dose required when given by intermittent bolus injection (160).

Data with Alphanate (Alpha Therapeutics) and other plasma-derived FVIII concentrates suggest that these products are also effective in correcting the VWF activity level and therefore may be considered for use in VWD (157,158). Because the concentration of VWF in these products is not yet standardized in the United States, dosing is determined in units of FVIII activity. Initial treatment with 40 FVIII IU per kg intravenously every 12 hours is usually sufficient to maintain the VWF activity level greater than 50 IU per dL. However, dosing based on FVIII content is likely to be less reliable than dosing based upon assayed VWF content.

Concentrates that contain both VWF and FVIII have the potential to cause disproportionately high plasma FVIII levels when administered to patients with VWD. Both the transfused FVIII and endogenously synthesized FVIII are stabilized by binding to the transfused VWF, and after several days of therapy the VWF level may be normal but the FVIII level may exceed 400 IU per dL (148). These levels of FVIII may be associated with venous thrombosis and pulmonary embolism in patients with VWD (148,161,162), and standard measures for thromboprophylaxis should be considered.

A virucidally treated, highly purified VWF concentrate that contains little FVIII has been used successfully to increase the levels of VWF in patients with VWD (157,158, 163,164). This product is not yet available in the United States. Because the FVIII content is so low, the normalization of FVIII levels depends on endogenous FVIII production and may require 12 hours in patients with severe VWD. Therefore, prophylactic treatment with purified VWF should be given 12 to 24 hours before any elective procedure, and acute correction

---

## TABLE 60-5

### USAGE OF PLASMA-DERIVED FVIII CONCENTRATES IN THE TREATMENT OF VON WILLEBRAND DISEASE

| Hemostatic challenge | Therapy |
|---|---|
| Major surgery or bleeding | 50 IU FVIII or VWF:RCo/kg body weight, followed by 25 to 40 IU/kg every 12 or 24 h, adjusted to keep the nadir level of FVIII or VWF:RCo >50 IU/dL until healing is progressing, typically for 5 to 10 d |
| Minor surgery | 40 IU FVIII or VWF:RCo/kg body weight every 24 or 48 h, adjusted to keep the nadir level of FVIII or VWF:RCo >30 IU/dL until healing is progressing, typically for 2 to 4 d |
| Dental extraction | 30 IU FVIII or VWF:RCo/kg body weight as a single dose, to maintain the level of FVIII or VWF:RCo >50 IU/dL for 12 h |
| Spontaneous minor bleeding | 25 IU FVIII or VWF:RCo/kg body weight every 24 h to keep the nadir level of FVIII or VWF:RCo >30 IU/dL until bleeding stops, usually for 2 to 4 d |
| Labor and delivery | 40 IU FVIII or VWF:RCo/kg body weight daily, adjusted to maintain the FVIII or VWF:RCo >50 IU/dL h on the day of delivery and for 3 to 4 d postpartum |

FVIII, factor VIII; VWF, von Willebrand factor.
Doses may be increased 20% for subjects younger than 18 years, to compensate for their increased plasma volume.
Adapted from Mannucci PM, Chediak J, Hanna W, et al. Treatment of von Willebrand disease with a high-purity factor VIII/von Willebrand factor concentrate: a prospective, multicenter study. *Blood* 2002;99:450–456.

of both FVIII and VWF levels requires concomitant treatment with a source of FVIII.

Recombinant human VWF has been evaluated in dog models of VWD, and it appears to be safe and effective (165). This product currently is not available for use in humans.

### Antifibrinolytic Agents

Tranexamic acid and ε-aminocaproic acid (Amicar) inhibit fibrinolysis and may be used alone or in combination with other hemostatic agents. These agents are most useful in oropharyngeal bleeding and menorrhagia. They are generally contraindicated in urinary tract hemorrhage because of the risk of a fibrin clot obstructing the urinary outflow tract. Tranexamic acid (10 to 15 mg per kg every 8 to 12 hours) or ε-aminocaproic acid (50 to 60 mg per kg every 4 to 6 hours) may be given orally or by intravenous infusion (166). These agents may also be used as a mouthwash for oral bleeds or dental procedures. Tranexamic acid mouthwash, 10 mL of a 4.8% solution given as a "swish and spit" may be better tolerated than ε-aminocaproic acid in some patients (150,167).

### Other Therapy

Short courses of conjugated estrogens have been used in surgical prophylaxis and for treatment of bleeding associated with angiodysplasia (168). Platelet transfusions and recombinant factor VIIa have been used in specific circumstances to treat VWD type 3, as discussed in the subsequent section, "von Willebrand Disease Type 3."

## Therapy for von Willebrand Disease Subtypes

Although the bleeding in VWD is usually mild, particular care to achieve adequate hemostasis should always be taken in patients undergoing invasive procedures and in those with trauma. In addition to the severity of bleeding (or potential surgical bleeding), treatment is guided by the VWD subtype, so that whenever possible the correct subtype should be established prior to therapy. Because the bleeding time is a poor reflection of bleeding risk and other laboratory testing such as the VWF:Ag and VWF:RCo levels may be difficult to obtain in a timely fashion, intervention may be guided by clinical criteria. In general, with appropriate therapy, adequate hemostasis should be obtained so that surgical procedures may be safely undertaken in all forms of VWD.

### von Willebrand Disease Type 1

Surgical prophylaxis and treatment of minor bleeding can usually be accomplished with desmopressin. Treatment should be administered approximately 1 hour before a planned procedure or as soon as possible after bleeding is identified. In some patients a repeat dose 12 to 24 hours after a procedure, such as a tooth extraction, is necessary. Home therapy with intranasal desmopressin should be considered for patients who respond to the intranasal preparation, and this is particularly useful for patients with menorrhagia or intermittent epistaxis. Although a useful adjunct for patients with mild hemophilia A, antifibrinolytic therapy with ε-aminocaproic acid or tranexamic acid usually is not required for oral surgery or other mucosal bleeding in VWD patients treated with desmopressin. For patients who do not tolerate or respond adequately to desmopressin, treatment with plasma-derived VWF such as Humate-P may be necessary.

For patients undergoing surgical procedures or those with more severe bleeding, postoperative treatment should be considered for 5 to 10 days or until wound healing has progressed. Under these circumstances, initial treatment with plasma-derived VWF, rather than desmopressin, should be considered.

One approach to limit the expense and exposure to blood products in these patients is to switch to desmopressin after hemostasis has been established and the patient has been stable for several days.

Women with type 1 VWD rarely require therapy during pregnancy because the plasma levels increase in most individuals, particularly in the third trimester. However, factor levels decline rapidly in the postpartum period and patients are at risk of hemorrhage in the first week after delivery (169,170). When hemostatic treatment is needed, plasma-derived VWF is generally recommended for therapy during pregnancy and desmopressin is generally recommended postpartum.

### von Willebrand Disease Type 2A

A few patients with VWD type 2A have a useful response to desmopressin and these patients may be identified by their response to a test dose. In responsive patients, desmopressin can be sufficient to achieve adequate hemostasis for minor bleeding or surgical procedures (171,172). In the absence of test data or in a patient undergoing major surgery or trauma, treatment with plasma-derived VWF is recommended (Table 60-5). Limited data are available on the treatment of type 2A VWD during pregnancy, but an approach similar to that for patients with type 1 VWD is reasonable.

### von Willebrand Disease Type 2B

When given to patients with VWD type 2B, desmopressin increases the levels of VWF and FVIII, but also causes or exacerbates thrombocytopenia. For this reason, plasma-derived VWF products are generally recommended for use in VWD type 2B (Table 60-5). Nevertheless, a few patients have received desmopressin for surgical prophylaxis and bleeding episodes, with good hemostatic responses and no unexpected bleeding or thrombosis (173,174). Therefore, if plasma product therapy must be avoided, desmopressin could be considered after evaluation of the response to a test infusion. Platelet transfusions are not likely to be helpful in the treatment of thrombocytopenia associated with type 2B VWD (175).

During pregnancy, the VWF concentration increases during the third trimester, possibly in response to endogenous estrogens. Consequently, progressive pregnancy-associated thrombocytopenia is common and may be the presenting manifestation of VWD type 2B (97). Increased bleeding has not been reported to accompany pregnancy-associated thrombocytopenia in VWD type 2B.

### von Willebrand Disease Type 2M

Little published experience exists to guide the treatment of patients with VWD type 2M. On the basis of these case reports, an approach similar to that for patients with VWD type 2A appears reasonable.

### von Willebrand Disease Type 2N

Administration of desmopressin to patients with VWD type 2N is associated with the expected two to threefold increase in VWF:Ag and VWF:RCo. Patients with very severe FVIII binding defects have baseline FVIII levels of $8.4 \pm 5.2$ IU per dL (116); their FVIII response to desmopressin usually is small and transient with a half-life of only 2 to 3 hours. Therefore, desmopressin cannot be generally recommended for this subtype (176,177). Patients with the mutation R854Q are fairly common and have a less severe FVIII binding defect. Their baseline FVIII levels are much higher, $21.8 \pm 9.8$ IU per dL (116) and they may have a therapeutically useful FVIII response to desmopressin (31,176).

If the distinction between mild hemophilia A or type 2N VWD is uncertain, Humate-P or another plasma-derived concentrate containing VWF would be appropriate for either diagnosis, and is recommended for surgical prophylaxis or bleeding (Table 60-5). Highly purified or recombinant FVIII products are inappropriate in VWD type 2N because they will circulate with a short half-life. Bleeding in pregnancy or in the postpartum period should be treated with a product that contains VWF, such as an intermediate purity FVIII concentrate (177).

### von Willebrand Disease Type 3

Treatment of VWD type 3 usually requires a plasma-derived concentrate containing VWF for both minor and major bleeding episodes. Most of the published clinical experience is with Humate-P but other plasma-derived products containing VWF should also be effective, including high purity VWF concentrate. In emergencies, high purity VWF concentrate should not be considered as the sole therapy because a satisfactory increase in FVIII activity may require 12 to 24 hours. Almost all patients with type 3 VWD are insensitive to desmopressin and do not have a therapeutically useful response.

The therapeutic role of platelet transfusions is not well defined but data suggest a rapid improvement in the bleeding time after platelet transfusion despite an incomplete response to a prior infusion of plasma-derived VWF (178). Both platelet and plasma VWF contribute to hemostasis (179), and platelet transfusion (e.g., a plateletpheresis collection of 4 to $5 \times 10^{11}$ platelets) may be considered as adjunctive therapy for bleeding that is refractory to treatment with FVIII concentrate (180).

Alloantibody inhibitors of VWF are rare complications of transfusion therapy in VWD type 3, reportedly occurring in 3% to 10% of patients (181,182). Large VWF gene deletions appear to correlate with the risk of developing inhibitors (182). With one possible exception, the few inhibitors that have been characterized were polyclonal Ig (immunoglobulin) G antibodies (182). Patients with VWF inhibitors often have severe allergic reactions to transfused VWF that can include back pain, abdominal pain, hypotension, and anaphylaxis (181,183). These patients have been treated with purified plasma or recombinant FVIII that contains no VWF. The infused FVIII is cleared rapidly, but therapeutic levels (40 to 60 IU per mL) can be maintained by administering FVIII at a total dose of 700 to 900 IU/kg/day intravenously by continuous infusion or bolus infusions every 4 hours (184,185). Recombinant factor VIIa (NovoSeven) also has been used to treat surgical or postpartum bleeding by continuous infusion (approximately 20 $\mu$g/kg/hour) or bolus infusion (approximately 90 $\mu$g per kg every 4 hours) (185,186).

## Therapy for Problems Specific to Women with von Willebrand Disease

The incidence of VWD in women is disproportionate as compared to that in men, representing approximately two thirds of all patients (33,59), although autosomal inheritance requires an equal frequency of mutant gene transmission to both sexes. The increased impact of VWD on women of childbearing age is a consequence of the repeated hemostatic challenges of ovulation, menstruation, pregnancy, and delivery. Bleeding into the corpus luteum may occur after ovulation, and midcycle pain may be severe enough to prompt surgical exploration (33,187). The prevalence of menorrhagia in VWD is not known precisely because few studies have used quantitative measures of blood loss and bias in patient selection is possible. With these limitations in mind, approximately 65% of women with VWD appear to have menorrhagia (>80 mL blood loss per menstrual cycle), compared to 9% to 14% of controls, and

menorrhagia for women with VWD often begins at menarche (33,188,189).

Conversely, in one study approximately 13% of 150 women with menorrhagia were found to have VWF levels more than 2 SD below the mean (188). Independent of whether subjects meet criteria for diagnosing VWD, a low VWF level appears to be a modest risk factor for menorrhagia, with a relative risk of approximately 3.9 for VWF levels below approximately 50 IU per dL (32).

Excluding patients with VWD type 3, intranasal desmopressin every 12 to 24 hours for up to 3 days may be effective for menorrhagia in VWD, if the side effects can be tolerated (190). Two randomized placebo-controlled trials in a total of 44 women, approximately half with VWD, reported a trend in favor of desmopressin for menstrual bleeding, but the differences between the two arms were not statistically significant (191,192). A larger open-label study in 90 women, many with VWD, reported shortened or decreased bleeding in 88% of treated menstrual cycles (193).

Menorrhagia in all types of VWD may be treated successfully with hormonal therapy (danazol, progesterone, or oral contraceptive pills) (189,194). In appropriate patients, desmopressin and hormonal therapy can be combined.

Antifibrinolytic agents can be effective for menorrhagia (195) and, although experience is limited in VWD, case reports suggest these agents could be useful alone or as adjuncts to other treatments (196). Tranexamic acid has been used at 1 g every 6 hours for 5 days (195), or 4 g in a single daily dose for 3 to 5 days (196). ε-Aminocaproic acid has been used at dosages of 5 g three times daily for 5 days (197), or 3 g every 6 hours for 3 to 5 days (198). Occasional side effects include nausea, diarrhea, and orthostatic hypotension. ε-Aminocaproic acid is thought to reduce fertility by inhibiting embryo implantation although the data are scanty. For this reason, antifibrinolytics generally are not recommended during the first trimester of pregnancy or for patients considering pregnancy.

Pregnancy usually is tolerated well by patients with VWD. In most patients, except for those with VWD type 3, VWF levels increase during the third trimester and protect against hemorrhage late in pregnancy. However, miscarriage or therapeutic abortion early in pregnancy, while VWF and FVIII levels are low, carries an increased risk of maternal hemorrhage (199,200). Provided the levels of both VWF and FVIII are greater than 50 IU per dL, the risk of hemorrhage during labor and delivery does not appear to be increased. Exceptions to this generalization may occur for patients with VWD type 2. Retrospective series that include both VWD type 1 and type 2 suggest that primary postpartum hemorrhage (>500 mL blood loss in the first 24 hours) occurs in approximately 16% (201) to approximately 18.5% (200) of patients. After delivery, the levels of FVIII and VWF fall rapidly over several days and secondary postpartum bleeding (bleeding after 24 hours in excess of "normal" lochial loss) may occur with an incidence of 20% (200) to 25% (201). Therefore, patients should be monitored for at least 1 week postpartum, and they should be advised that bleeding may occur up to 3 weeks after delivery.

Maternal hemorrhagic complications can be minimized by prophylactic therapy to raise factor levels to greater than 50 IU per dL at delivery and to maintain them at that level for 3 to 4 days postpartum (170,181,200). Factor levels greater than 50 IU per dL appear to be sufficient to administer epidural anesthesia safely (200,202). In general, FVIII-VWF concentrates are used prior to delivery, switching to desmopressin if appropriate after delivery. FVIII concentrate may reverse the thrombocytopenia and correct the bleeding tendency of VWD type 2B for delivery (99). In all patients, complete uterine evacuation and contraction after delivery are important to prevent bleeding (170).

# Treatment of Acquired von Willebrand Syndrome

Treatment of AVWS involves consideration of both the underlying disease and the bleeding disorder. Because the mechanism of AVWS is variable, identifying effective therapy can be difficult (128).

The optimal treatment of AVWS associated with autoimmune disease is yet to be defined. Immunosuppressive therapy with oral prednisone, 1 mg/kg/day, or intravenous cyclophosphamide, 700 mg per M² monthly has been used successfully (203,204). For patients with malignant lymphoproliferative disorders such as non-Hodgkin lymphoma or multiple myeloma, successful treatment of the underlying disease with cytotoxic chemotherapy or surgical removal of the tumor typically results in resolution of the AVWS. In a few cases, the return of AVWS heralded a relapse (205–208). For patients with MGUS, treatment of the associated clonal lymphoid disorder with cytotoxic or immunosuppressive chemotherapy usually does not alter the course so that prevention and treatment of bleeding represents the mainstay of therapy.

Intravenous immunoglobulin (IVIG) was first proposed in 1976 for the treatment of AVWS (209), and many reports describe the success of this approach for patients with AVWS caused by immune-mediated clearance of VWF (128,205, 210–214). Active bleeding may be treated with IVIG 1 g/kg/day for 1 to 2 days with resolution of the hemorrhage within several days of the infusion. Repeated prophylactic infusions of IVIG 1 g per kg every 3 to 4 weeks have been used successfully in the prevention of bleeding (213,214). IVIG appears to be more effective for patients with IgG, than IgM MGUS (213). Patients in whom no underlying disease is identified may respond to IVIG, suggesting that an underlying immune-mediated disorder may be responsible.

Desmopressin or FVIII concentrate is effective in up to one third of patients with AVWS associated with MGUS or malignant lymphoproliferative diseases, although the primary mechanism of disease is increased clearance. A test dose of desmopressin can be helpful to identify responsive patients (128).

For patients with myeloproliferative disease or other solid malignancies, treatment of the underlying disease with surgery or chemoradiation therapy appears to be effective. Control of the platelet count in myeloproliferative disease seems to be effective in increasing the plasma concentration of large VWF multimers (215,216). An unusual association of AVWS with Wilms tumor has been described and the bleeding disorder resolved with the successful treatment of the malignancy (217). Cases of AVWS associated with medications resolve when the drug has been discontinued, and those associated with hypothyroidism resolve with thyroid hormone replacement therapy (37).

Patients with AVWS caused by increased fluid shear stress generally do not respond to desmopressin, FVIII concentrates, or IVIG, but require correction of the underlying cardiovascular abnormality to normalize VWF function (128). For example, AVWS associated with aortic stenosis typically resolves upon successful repair of the defective valve (130).

## References

1. von Willebrand EA. Hereditär pseudohemofili. *Fin Laekaresaellsk Hand* 1926;68:87–112.
2. von Willebrand EA. Über hereditäre pseudohæmophilie. *Acta Med Scand* 1931;76:521–549.
3. von Willebrand EA. Über eine neue Bluterkrankheit, die konstitutionelle Thrombopathie. *Klin Wochenschr* 1933;12:414.
4. Alexander B, Goldstein B. Dual hemostatic defect in pseudohemophilia. *J Clin Invest* 1953;32:551.
5. Larrieu MJ, Soulier JP. Déficit en facteur antihémophilique A chez une fille associé à un trouble saignement. *Rev Hematol* 1953;8:361–370.
6. Quick AJ, Hussey CV. Hemophilic condition in the female. *J Lab Clin Med* 1953;42:929–930.
7. Nilsson IM, Blombäck M, von Francken I. On an inherited autosomal hemorrhagic diathesis with antihemophilic globulin (AHG) deficiency and prolonged bleeding time. *Acta Med Scand* 1957;159:35–57.
8. Cornu P, Larrieu MJ, Caen J, et al. Transfusion studies in von Willebrand's disease: effect on bleeding time and factor VIII. *Br J Haematol* 1963;9:189–202.
9. Bouma BN, Wiegerinck Y, Sixma JJ, et al. Immunological characterization of purified anti-haemophilic factor A (factor VIII) which corrects abnormal platelet retention in von Willebrand's disease. *Nat New Biol* 1972;236:104–106.
10. Holmberg L, Nilsson IM. Genetic variants of von Willebrand's disease. *Br Med J* 1972;3:317–320.
11. Hoyer LW, Shainoff JR. Factor VIII-related protein circulates in normal human plasma as high molecular weight multimers. *Blood* 1980;55:1056–1059.
12. Ruggeri ZM, Zimmerman TS. Variant von Willebrand's disease. Characterization of two subtypes by analysis of multimeric composition of factor VIII/von Willebrand factor in plasma and platelets. *J Clin Invest* 1980;65:1318–1325.
13. Ruggeri ZM, Pareti FI, Mannucci PM, et al. Heightened interaction between platelets and factor VIII/von Willebrand factor in a new subtype of von Willebrand's disease. *N Engl J Med* 1980;302:1047–1051.
14. Sadler JE, Shelton-Inloes BB, Sorace JM, et al. Cloning and characterization of two cDNAs coding for human von Willebrand factor. *Proc Natl Acad Sci U S A* 1985;82:6394–6398.
15. Lynch DC, Zimmerman TS, Collins CJ, et al. Molecular cloning of cDNA for human von Willebrand factor: authentication by a new method. *Cell* 1985;41:49–56.
16. Ginsburg D, Handin RI, Bonthron DT, et al. Human von Willebrand factor (vWF): isolation of complementary DNA (cDNA) clones and chromosomal localization. *Science* 1985;228:1401–1406.
17. Verweij CL, de Vries CJ, Distel B, et al. Construction of cDNA coding for human von Willebrand factor using antibody probes for colony-screening and mapping of the chromosomal gene. *Nucleic Acids Res* 1985;13:4699–4717.
18. Shelton-Inloes BB, Chehab FF, Mannucci PM, et al. Gene deletions correlate with the development of alloantibodies in von Willebrand disease. *J Clin Invest* 1987;79:1459–1465.
19. Ngo K-Y, Glotz VT, Koziol JA, et al. Homozygous and heterozygous deletions of the von Willebrand factor gene in patients and carriers of severe von Willebrand's disease. *Proc Natl Acad Sci U S A* 1988;85:2753–2757.
20. Ginsburg D, Sadler JE. von Willebrand disease: a database of point mutations, insertions, and deletions. *Thromb Haemost* 1993;69:177–184.
21. Sadler JE, Ginsburg D. A database of polymorphisms in the von Willebrand factor gene and pseudogene. *Thromb Haemost* 1993;69:185–191.
22. Sadler JE. A revised classification of von Willebrand disease. *Thromb Haemost* 1994;71:520–525.
23. Sadler JE, Mannucci PM, Berntorp E, et al. Impact, diagnosis and treatment of von Willebrand disease. *Thromb Haemost* 2000;84:160–174.
24. Rodeghiero F, Castaman G, Dini E. Epidemiological investigation of the prevalence of von Willebrand's disease. *Blood* 1987;69:454–459.
25. Castaman G, Eikenboom JCJ, Bertina RM, et al. Inconsistency of association between type 1 von Willebrand disease phenotype and genotype in families identified in an epidemiological investigation. *Thromb Haemost* 1999;82:1065–1070.
26. Hoyer LW, Rizza CR, Tuddenham EG, et al. Von Willebrand factor multimer patterns in von Willebrand's disease. *Br J Haematol* 1983;55:493–507.
27. Weiss HJ, Piétu G, Rabinowitz R, et al. Heterogeneous abnormalities in the multimeric structure, antigenic properties, and plasma-platelet content of factor VIII/von Willebrand factor in subtypes of classic (type I) and variant (type IIA) von Willebrand's disease. *J Lab Clin Med* 1983;101:411–425.
28. Mannucci PM, Lombardi R, Bader R, et al. Heterogeneity of type I von Willebrand disease: evidence for a subgroup with an abnormal von Willebrand factor. *Blood* 1985;66:796–802.
29. Mannucci PM, Lombardi R, Castaman G, et al. von Willebrand disease "Vicenza" with larger-than-normal (supranormal) von Willebrand factor multimers. *Blood* 1988;71:65–70.
30. Casonato A, Pontara E, Sartorello F, et al. Reduced von Willebrand factor survival in type Vicenza von Willebrand disease. *Blood* 2002;99:180–184.
31. Federici AB, Mazurier C, Berntorp E, et al. Biologic response to desmopressin in patients with severe type 1 and type 2 von Willebrand disease: results of a multicenter European study. *Blood* 2004;103:2032–2038.
32. Sadler JE. Von Willebrand disease type 1: a diagnosis in search of a disease. *Blood* 2003;101:2089–2093.
33. Silwer J. von Willebrand's disease in Sweden. *Acta Paediatr Scand Suppl* 1973;238:1–159.
34. Buchanan JC, Leavell BS. Pseudohemophilia: report of 13 new cases and statistical review of previously reported cases. *Ann Intern Med* 1956;44:241–256.
35. Kreuz W, Linde R, Funk M, et al. Valproate therapy induces von Willebrand disease type I. *Epilepsia* 1992;33:178–184.

36. Clough V, MacFarlane IA, O'Connor J, et al. Acquired von Willebrand's syndrome and Ehlers-Danlos syndrome presenting with gastro-intestinal bleeding. *Scand J Haematol* 1979;22:305–310.

37. Dalton RG, Dewar MS, Savidge GF, et al. Hypothyroidism as a cause of acquired von Willebrand's disease. *Lancet* 1987;1:1007–1009.

38. Fressinaud E, Meyer D. International survey of patients with von Willebrand disease and angiodysplasia. *Thromb Haemost* 1993;70:546.

39. Favaloro EJ, Grispo L, Exner T, et al. Development of a simple collagen based ELISA assay aids in the diagnosis of, and permits sensitive discrimination between type I and type II, von Willebrand's disease. *Blood Coagul Fibrinolysis* 1991;2:285–291.

40. Favaloro EJ. Collagen binding assay for von Willebrand factor (VWF:CBA): detection of von Willebrand disease (VWD), and discrimination of VWD subtypes, depends on collagen source. *Thromb Haemost* 2000;83:127–135.

41. Abildgaard CF, Suzuki Z, Harrison J, et al. Serial studies in von Willebrand's disease: variability versus "variants". *Blood* 1980;56:712–716.

42. Gill JC, Endres-Brooks J, Bauer PJ, et al. The effect of ABO blood group on the diagnosis of von Willebrand disease. *Blood* 1987;69:1691–1695.

43. Ørstavik KH, Kornstad L, Reisner H, et al. Possible effect of secretor locus on plasma concentration of factor VIII and von Willebrand factor. *Blood* 1989;73:990–993.

44. O'Donnell J, Boulton FE, Manning RA, et al. Genotype at the secretor blood group locus is a determinant of plasma von Willebrand factor level. *Br J Haematol* 2002;116:350–356.

45. Rodgers RPC, Levin J. A critical reappraisal of the bleeding time. *Semin Thromb Hemost* 1990;16:1–20.

46. Lind SE. The bleeding time does not predict surgical bleeding. *Blood* 1991; 77:2547–2552.

47. De Caterina R, Lanza M, Manca G, et al. Bleeding time and bleeding: an analysis of the relationship of the bleeding time test with parameters of surgical bleeding. *Blood* 1994;84:3363–3370.

48. Fressinaud E, Veyradier A, Truchaud F, et al. Screening for von Willebrand disease with a new analyzer using high shear stress: a study of 60 cases. *Blood* 1998;91:1325–1331.

49. Nitu-Whalley IC, Lee CA, Brown SA, et al. The role of the platelet function analyser (PFA-100) in the characterization of patients with von Willebrand's disease and its relationships with von Willebrand factor and the ABO blood group. *Haemophilia* 2003;9:298–302.

50. Lasne D, Fiemeyer A, Chatellier G, et al. A study of platelet functions with a new analyzer using high shear stress (PFA 100) in patients undergoing coronary artery bypass graft. *Thromb Haemost* 2000;84:794–799.

51. Nachman RL, Jaffe EA. Subcellular platelet factor VIII antigen and von Willebrand factor. *J Exp Med* 1975;141:1101–1113.

52. Read MS, Shermer RW, Brinkhous KM. Venom coagglutinin: an activator of platelet aggregation dependent on von Willebrand factor. *Proc Natl Acad Sci U S A* 1978;75:4514–4518.

53. Fukuda K, Doggett TA, Bankston LA, et al. Structural basis of von Willebrand factor activation by the snake toxin botrocetin. *Structure (Camb)* 2002;10:943–950.

54. Sugimoto M, Mohri H, McClintock RA, et al. Identification of discontinuous von Willebrand factor sequences involved in complex formation with botrocetin. *J Biol Chem* 1991;266:18172–18178.

55. Vanhoorelbeke K, Cauwenberghs N, Vauterin S, et al. A reliable and reproducible ELISA method to measure ristocetin cofactor activity of von Willebrand factor. *Thromb Haemost* 2000;83:107–113.

56. Castaman G, Eikenboom JC, Missiaglia E, et al. Autosomal dominant type 1 von Willebrand disease due to G3639T mutation (C1130F) in exon 26 of von Willebrand factor gene: description of five Italian families and evidence for a founder effect. *Br J Haematol* 2000;108:876–879.

57. Eikenboom JCJ, Matsushita T, Reitsma PH, et al. Dominant type 1 von Willebrand disease caused by mutated cysteine residues in the D3 domain of von Willebrand factor. *Blood* 1996;88:2433–2441.

58. Bodó I, Katsumi A, Tuley EA, et al. Mutations causing dominant type 1 von Willebrand disease with high penetrance. *Blood* 1999;94 (Suppl.1): 373a.

59. Miller CH, Graham JB, Goldin LR, et al. Genetics of classic von Willebrand's disease. I. Phenotypic variation within families. *Blood* 1979;54: 117–136.

60. Casaña P, Martínez F, Haya S, et al. Significant linkage and non-linkage of type 1 von Willebrand disease to the von Willebrand factor gene. *Br J Haematol* 2001;115:692–700.

61. Biron C, Mahieu B, Rochette A, et al. Preoperative screening for von Willebrand disease type 1: low yield and limited ability to predict bleeding. *J Lab Clin Med* 1999;134:605–609.

62. Zhang ZP, Lindstedt M, Falk G, et al. Nonsense mutations of the von Willebrand factor gene in patients with von Willebrand disease type III and type I. *Am J Hum Genet* 1992;51:850–858.

63. Zhang ZP, Blombäck M, Egberg N, et al. Characterization of the von Willebrand factor gene (VWF) in von Willebrand disease type III patients from 24 families of Swedish and Finnish origin. *Genomics* 1994;21:188–193.

64. Schneppenheim R, Krey S, Bergmann F, et al. Genetic heterogeneity of severe von Willebrand disease type III in the German population. *Hum Genet* 1994;94:640–652.

65. Eikenboom JC, Reitsma PH, Peerlinck KMJ, et al. Recessive inheritance of von Willebrand's disease type I. *Lancet* 1993;341:982–986.

66. Bodó I, Katsumi A, Tuley EA, et al. Type 1 von Willebrand disease mutation Cys1149Arg causes intracellular retention and degradation of heterodimers:

67. a possible general mechanism for dominant mutations of oligomeric proteins. *Blood* 2001;98:2973–2979.

68. Brown SA, Eldridge A, Collins PW, et al. Increased clearance of von Willebrand factor antigen post-DDAVP in Type 1 von Willebrand disease: is it a potential pathogenic process? *J Thromb Haemost* 2003;1: 1714–1717.

68. Meyer D, Fressinaud E, Gaucher C, et al. Gene defects in 150 unrelated French cases with type 2 von Willebrand disease: from the patient to the gene. INSERM network on molecular abnormalities in von Willebrand disease. *Thromb Haemost* 1997;78:451–456.

69. Budde U, Drewke E, Mainusch K, et al. Laboratory diagnosis of congenital von Willebrand disease. *Semin Thromb Hemost* 2002;28:173–190.

70. Caron C, Mazurier C, Goudemand J. Large experience with a factor VIII binding assay of plasma von Willebrand factor using commercial reagents. *Br J Haematol* 2002;117:716–718.

71. Nitu-Whalley IC, Riddell A, Lee CA, et al. Identification of type 2 von Willebrand disease in previously diagnosed type 1 patients: a reappraisal using phenotypes, genotypes and molecular modelling. *Thromb Haemost* 2000;84:998–1004.

72. Riddell AF, Jenkins PV, Nitu-Whalley IC, et al. Use of the collagen-binding assay for von Willebrand factor in the analysis of type 2M von Willebrand disease: a comparison with the ristocetin cofactor assay. *Br J Haematol* 2002;116:187–192.

73. Holmberg L, Nilsson IM. von Willebrand's disease. *Eur J Haematol* 1992; 48:127–141.

74. Ruggeri ZM, Nilsson IM, Lombardi R, et al. Aberrant multimeric structure of von Willebrand factor in a new variant of von Willebrand's disease (type IIC). *J Clin Invest* 1982;70:1124–1127.

75. Kinoshita S, Harrison J, Lazerson J, et al. A new variant of dominant type II von Willebrand's disease with aberrant multimeric pattern of factor VIII-related antigen (type IID). *Blood* 1984;63:1369–1371.

76. Zimmerman TS, Dent JA, Ruggeri ZM, et al. Subunit composition of plasma von Willebrand factor. Cleavage is present in normal individuals, increased in IIA and IIB von Willebrand disease, but minimal in variants with aberrant structure of individual oligomers (types IIC, IID, and IIE). *J Clin Invest* 1986;77:947–951.

77. Mannucci PM, Lombardi R, Federici AB, et al. A new variant of type II von Willebrand disease with aberrant multimeric structure of plasma but not platelet von Willebrand factor (type IIF). *Blood* 1986;68:269–274.

78. Gralnick HR, Williams SB, McKeown LP, et al. A variant of type II von Willebrand disease with an abnormal triplet structure and discordant effects of protease inhibitors on plasma and platelet von Willebrand factor structure. *Am J Hematol* 1987;24:259–266.

79. Federici AB, Mannucci PM, Lombardi R, et al. Type II H von Willebrand disease: new structural abnormality of plasma and platelet von Willebrand factor in a patient with prolonged bleeding time and borderline levels of ristocetin cofactor activity. *Am J Hematol* 1989;32:287–293.

80. Castaman G, Rodeghiero F, Lattuada A, et al. A new variant of von Willebrand disease (type II I) with a normal degree of proteolytic cleavage of von Willebrand factor. *Thromb Res* 1992;65:343–351.

81. Lyons SE, Bruck ME, Bowie EJW, et al. Impaired intracellular transport produced by a subset of type IIA von Willebrand disease mutations. *J Biol Chem* 1992;267:4424–4430.

82. Furlan M, Robles R, Lämmle B. Partial purification and characterization of a protease from human plasma cleaving von Willebrand factor to fragments produced by *in vivo* proteolysis. *Blood* 1996;87:4223–4234.

83. Tsai H-M. Physiologic cleavage of von Willebrand factor by a plasma protease is dependent on its conformation and requires calcium ion. *Blood* 1996;87:4235–4244.

84. Dent JA, Berkowitz SD, Ware J, et al. Identification of a cleavage site directing the immunochemical detection of molecular abnormalities in type IIA von Willebrand factor. *Proc Natl Acad Sci U S A* 1990;87:6306–6310.

85. Schneppenheim R, Brassard J, Krey S, et al. Defective dimerization of von Willebrand factor subunits due to a Cys ∅ Arg mutation in type IID von Willebrand disease. *Proc Natl Acad Sci U S A* 1996;93:3581–3586.

86. Schneppenheim R, Budde U, Obser T, et al. Expression and characterization of von Willebrand factor dimerization defects in different types of von Willebrand disease. *Blood* 2001;97:2059–2066.

87. Enayat MS, Guilliatt AM, Surdhar GK, et al. Aberrant dimerization of von Willebrand factor as the result of mutations in the carboxy-terminal region: identification of 3 mutations in members of 3 different families with type 2A (phenotype IID) von Willebrand disease. *Blood* 2001;98:674–680.

88. Meyer D, Fressinaud E, Hilbert L, et al. Type 2 von Willebrand disease causing defective von Willebrand factor-dependent platelet function. *Best Pract Res Clin Haematol* 2001;14:349–364.

89. Hill FG, Enayat MS, George AJ. Investigation of a kindred with a new autosomal dominantly inherited variant type von Willebrand's disease (possible type II). *J Clin Pathol* 1985;38:665–670.

90. Gaucher C, Diéval J, Mazurier C. Characterization of von Willebrand factor gene defects in two unrelated patients with type IIC von Willebrand disease. *Blood* 1994;84:1024–1030.

91. Schneppenheim R , Thomas KB, Krey S, et al. Identification of a candidate missense mutation in a family with von Willebrand disease type IIC. *Hum Genet* 1995;95:681–686.

92. Gaucher C, Uno H, Yamazaki T, et al. A new candidate mutation (N528S) within the von Willebrand factor propeptide identified in a Japanese patient

with phenotype IIC of von Willebrand disease. *Eur J Haematol* 1998;61:145–148.

93. Holmberg L, Karpman D, Isaksson C, et al. Ins405AsnPro mutation in the von Willebrand factor propeptide in recessive type 2A (IIC) von Willebrand's disease. *Thromb Haemost* 1998;79:718–722.

94. Holmberg L, Nilsson IM, Borge L, et al. Platelet aggregation induced by 1-desamino-8-D-arginine vasopressin (DDAVP) in Type IIB von Willebrand's disease. *N Engl J Med* 1983;309:816–821.

95. Saba HI, Saba SR, Dent J, et al. Type IIB Tampa: a variant of von Willebrand disease with chronic thrombocytopenia, circulating platelet aggregates, and spontaneous platelet aggregation. *Blood* 1985;66:282–286.

96. Rick ME, Williams SB, Sacher RA, et al. Thrombocytopenia associated with pregnancy in a patient with type IIB von Willebrand's disease. *Blood* 1987;69:786–789.

97. Giles AR, Hoogendoorn H, Benford K. Type IIB von Willebrand's disease presenting as thrombocytopenia during pregnancy. *Br J Haematol* 1987;67:349–353.

98. Hultin MB, Sussman II. Postoperative thrombocytopenia in type IIB von Willebrand disease. *Am J Hematol* 1990;33:64–68.

99. Ieko M, Sakurama S, Sagawa A, et al. Effect of a factor VIII concentrate on type IIB von Willebrand's disease-associated thrombocytopenia presenting during pregnancy in identical twin mothers. *Am J Hematol* 1990;35:26–31.

100. Sakariassen KS, Nieuwenhuis HK, Sixma JJ. Differentiation of patients with subtype IIb-like von Willebrand's disease by means of perfusion experiments with reconstituted blood. *Br J Haematol* 1985;59:459–470.

101. Donnér M, Holmberg L, Nilsson IM. Type IIB von Willebrand's disease with probable autosomal recessive inheritance and presenting as thrombocytopenia in infancy. *Br J Haematol* 1987;66:349–354.

102. Valster FAA, Feijen HL, Hutten JW. Severe thrombocytopenia in a pregnant patient with platelet-associated IgM, and known von Willebrand's disease; a case report. *Eur J Obstet Gynecol Reprod Biol* 1990;36:197–201.

103. Weiss HJ, Sussman II. A new von Willebrand variant (type I, New York): increased ristocetin-induced platelet aggregation and plasma von Willebrand factor containing the full range of multimers. *Blood* 1986;68:149–156.

104. Holmberg L, Berntorp E, Donnér M, et al. von Willebrand's disease characterized by increased ristocetin sensitivity and the presence of all von Willebrand factor multimers in plasma. *Blood* 1986;68:668–772.

105. Weiss HJ. Abnormalities of factor VIII and platelet aggregation—use of ristocetin in diagnosing the von Willebrand syndrome. *Blood* 1975;45:403–412.

106. Huizinga EG, Tsuji S, Romijn RAP, et al. Structures of glycoprotein Ibα and its complex with von Willebrand factor A1 domain. *Science* 2002;297:1176–1179.

107. Rabinowitz I, Tuley EA, Mancuso DJ, et al. von Willebrand disease type B: a missense mutation selectively abolishes ristocetin-induced von Willebrand factor binding to platelet glycoprotein Ib. *Proc Natl Acad Sci U S A* 1992;89:9846–9849.

108. Mancuso DJ, Kroner PA, Christopherson PA, et al. Type 2M:Milwaukee-1 von Willebrand disease: an in-frame deletion in the Cys509-Cys695 loop of the von Willebrand factor A1 domain causes deficient binding of von Willebrand factor to platelets. *Blood* 1996;88:2559–2568.

109. Hillery CA, Mancuso DJ, Sadler JE, et al. Type 2M von Willebrand disease: F606I and I662F mutations in the glycoprotein Ib binding domain selectively impair ristocetin- but not botrocetin-mediated binding of von Willebrand factor to platelets. *Blood* 1998;91:1572–1581.

110. Ribba AS, Loisel I, Lavergne JM, et al. Ser968Thr mutation within the A3 domain of von Willebrand factor (VWF) in two related patients leads to a defective binding of VWF to collagen. *Thromb Haemost* 2001;86:848–854.

111. Howard MA, Salem HH, Thomas KB, et al. Variant von Willebrand's disease type B–revisited. *Blood* 1982;60:1420–1428.

112. Ciavarella G, Ciavarella N, Antoncecchi S, et al. High-resolution analysis of von Willebrand factor multimeric composition defines a new variant of type I von Willebrand disease with aberrant structure but presence of all size multimers (type IC). *Blood* 1986;66:1423–1429.

113. Lopez-Fernandez MF, Gonzalez-Boullosa R, Blanco-Lopez MJ, et al. Abnormal proteolytic degradation of von Willebrand factor after desmopressin infusion in a new subtype of von Willebrand disease (ID). *Am J Hematol* 1991;36:163–170.

114. Nishino M, Girma J-P, Rothschild C, et al. New variant of von Willebrand disease with defective binding to factor VIII. *Blood* 1989;74:1591–1599.

115. Mazurier C, Dieval J, Jorieux S, et al. A new von Willebrand factor (vWF) defect in a patient with factor VIII (FVIII) deficiency but with normal levels and multimeric patterns of both plasma and platelet vWF. Characterization of abnormal vWF/FVIII interaction. *Blood* 1990;75:20–26.

116. Mazurier C, Meyer D. Factor VIII binding assay of von Willebrand factor and the diagnosis of type 2N von Willebrand disease. Results of an international survey. *Thromb Haemost* 1996;76:270–274.

117. Schneppenheim R, Budde U, Krey S, et al. Results of a screening for von Willebrand disease type 2N in patients with suspected haemophilia A or von Willebrand disease type 1. *Thromb Haemost* 1996;76:598–602.

118. Mazurier C, Gaucher C, Jorieux S, et al. Evidence for a von Willebrand factor defect in factor VIII binding in three members of a family previously misdiagnosed mild haemophilia A and haemophilia A carriers: consequences for therapy and genetic counselling. *Br J Haematol* 1990;76:372–379.

119. Lopez-Fernandez MF, Blanco-Lopez MJ, Castiñeira MP, et al. Further evidence for recessive inheritance of von Willebrand disease with abnormal

binding of von Willebrand factor to factor VIII. *Am J Hematol* 1992;40:20–27.

120. Mannucci PM, Lattuada A, Castaman G, et al. Heterogeneous phenotypes of platelet and plasma von Willebrand factor in obligatory heterozygotes for severe von Willebrand disease. *Blood* 1989;74:2433–2436.

121. Inbal A, Kornbrot N, Zivelin A, et al. The inheritance of type I and type III von Willebrand's disease in Israel: linkage analysis, carrier detection and prenatal diagnosis using three intragenic restriction fragment length polymorphisms. *Blood Coagul Fibrinolysis* 1992;3:167–177.

122. Zhang Z, Lindstedt M, Blomback M, et al. Effects of the mutant von Willebrand factor gene in von Willebrand disease. *Hum Genet* 1995;96:388–394.

123. Eikenboom JC, Castaman G, Vos HL, et al. Characterization of the genetic defects in recessive type 1 and type 3 von Willebrand disease patients of Italian origin. *Thromb Haemost* 1998;79:709–717.

124. Zhang ZP, Blömbäck M, Nyman D, et al. Mutations of von Willebrand factor gene in families with von Willebrand disease in the Åland Islands. *Proc Natl Acad Sci U S A* 1993;90:7937–7940.

125. Mannucci PM, Bloom AL, Larrieu MJ, et al. Atherosclerosis and von Willebrand factor. I. Prevalence of severe von Willebrand's disease in western Europe and Israel. *Br J Haematol* 1984;57:163–169.

126. Weiss HJ, Ball AP, Mannucci PM. Incidence of severe von Willebrand's disease. *N Engl J Med* 1982;307:127.

127. Mohri H, Motomura S, Kanamori H, et al. Clinical significance of inhibitors in acquired von Willebrand syndrome. *Blood* 1998;91:3623–3629.

128. Federici AB, Rand JH, Bucciarelli P, et al. Acquired von Willebrand syndrome: data from an international registry. *Thromb Haemost* 2000;84:345–349.

129. Veyradier A, Jenkins CS, Fressinaud E, et al. Acquired von Willebrand syndrome: from pathophysiology to management. *Thromb Haemost* 2000;84:175–182.

130. Vincentelli A, Susen S, Le Tourneau T, et al. Acquired von Willebrand syndrome in aortic stenosis. *N Engl J Med* 2003;349:343–349.

131. Veyradier A, Nishikubo T, Humbert M, et al. Improvement of von Willebrand factor proteolysis after prostacyclin infusion in severe pulmonary arterial hypertension. *Circulation* 2000;102:2460–2462.

132. Rauch R, Budde U, Koch A, et al. Acquired von Willebrand syndrome in children with patent ductus arteriosus. *Heart* 2002;88:87–88.

133. Gill JC, Wilson AD, Endres-Brooks J, et al. Loss of the largest von Willebrand factor multimers from the plasma of patients with congenital cardiac defects. *Blood* 1986;67:758–761.

134. Budde U, Scharf RE, Franke P, et al. Elevated platelet count as a cause of abnormal von Willebrand factor multimer distribution in plasma. *Blood* 1993;82:1749–1757.

135. van Genderen PJ, Budde U, Michiels JJ, et al. The reduction of large von Willebrand factor multimers in plasma in essential thrombocythaemia is related to the platelet count. *Br J Haematol* 1996;93:962–965.

136. Castaman G, Lattuada A, Mannucci PM, et al. Characterization of two cases of acquired transitory von Willebrand syndrome with ciprofloxacin: evidence for heightened proteolysis of von Willebrand factor. *Am J Hematol* 1995;49:83–86.

137. Takahashi H. Studies on the pathophysiology and treatment of von Willebrand's disease. IV. Mechanism of increased ristocetin-induced platelet aggregation in von Willebrand's disease. *Thromb Res* 1980;19:857–867.

138. Miller JL, Castella A. Platelet-type von Willebrand's disease: Characterization of a new bleeding disorder. *Blood* 1982;60:790–794.

139. Weiss HJ, Meyer D, Rabinowitz R, et al. Pseudo-von Willebrand's disease. An intrinsic platelet defect with aggregation by unmodified human factor VIII/von Willebrand factor and enhanced adsorption of its high-molecular-weight multimers. *N Engl J Med* 1982;306:326–333.

140. Takahashi H, Handa M, Watanabe K, et al. Further characterization of platelet-type von Willebrand's disease in Japan. *Blood* 1984;64:1254–1262.

141. Miller JL, Kupinski JM, Castella A, et al. von Willebrand factor binds to platelets and induces aggregation in platelet-type but not type IIB von Willebrand disease. *J Clin Invest* 1983;72:1532–1542.

142. Miller JL, Cunningham D, Lyle VA, et al. Mutation in the gene encoding the α chain of platelet glycoprotein Ib in platelet-type von Willebrand disease. *Proc Natl Acad Sci U S A* 1991;88:4761–4765.

143. Matsubara Y, Murata M, Sugita K, et al. Identification of a novel point mutation in platelet glycoprotein Ibalpha, Gly to Ser at residue 233, in a Japanese family with platelet-type von Willebrand disease. *J Thromb Haemost* 2003;1:2198–2205.

144. Russell SD, Roth GJ. Pseudo-von Willebrand disease: a mutation in the platelet glycoprotein Ib alpha gene associated with a hyperactive surface receptor. *Blood* 1993;81:1787–1791.

145. Kaneshiro MM, Mielke CH Jr, Kasper CK, et al. Bleeding time after aspirin in disorders of intrinsic clotting. *N Engl J Med* 1969;281:1039–1042.

146. Mannucci PM, Ruggeri ZM, Pareti FI, et al. 1-Deamino-8-D-arginine vasopressin: a new pharmacological approach to the management of haemophilia and von Willebrands' diseases. *Lancet* 1977;1:869–872.

147. Mannucci PM. Desmopressin (DDAVP) in the treatment of bleeding disorders: the first 20 years. *Blood* 1997;90:2515–2521.

148. Mannucci PM. Treatment of von Willebrand's disease. *N Engl J Med* 2004;351:683–694.

149. de la Fuente B, Kasper CK, Rickles FR, et al. Response of patients with mild and moderate hemophilia A and von Willebrand's disease to treatment with desmopressin. *Ann Int Med* 1985;103:6–14.

150. Phillips MD, Santhouse A. von Willebrand disease: recent advances in pathophysiology and treatment. *Am J Med Sci* 1998;316:77–86.

151. Mannucci PM, Bettega D, Cattaneo M. Patterns of development of tachyphylaxis in patients with haemophilia and von Willebrand disease after repeated doses of desmopressin (DDAVP). *Br J Haematol* 1992;82:87–93.

152. Rodeghiero F, Castaman G, Mannucci PM. Prospective multicenter study on subcutaneous concentrated desmopressin for home treatment of patients with von Willebrand disease and mild or moderate hemophilia A. *Thromb Haemost* 1996;76:692–696.

153. Rose EH, Aledort LM. Nasal spray desmopressin (DDAVP) for mild hemophilia A and von Willebrand disease. *Ann Intern Med* 1991;114:563–568.

154. Sutor AH. Desmopressin (DDAVP) in bleeding disorders of childhood. *Semin Thromb Hemost* 1998;24:555–566.

155. Mannucci PM, Lusher JM. Desmopressin and thrombosis. *Lancet* 1989;2:675–676.

156. Mannucci PM, Lattuada A, Ruggeri ZM. Proteolysis of von Willebrand factor in therapeutic plasma concentrates. *Blood* 1994;83:3018–3027.

157. Mannucci PM, Tenconi PM, Castaman G, et al. Comparison of four virus-inactivated plasma concentrates for treatment of severe von Willebrand disease: a cross-over randomized trial. *Blood* 1992;79:3130–3137.

158. Lethagen S, Berntorp E, Nilsson IM. Pharmacokinetics and hemostatic effect of different factor VIII/von Willebrand factor concentrates in von Willebrand's disease type III. *Ann Hematol* 1992;65:253–259.

159. Dobrkovska A, Krzensk U, Chediak JR. Pharmacokinetics, efficacy and safety of Humate-P in von Willebrand disease. *Haemophilia* 1998;4 (Suppl. 3):33–39.

160. Lubetsky A, Schulman S, Varon D, et al. Safety and efficacy of continuous infusion of a combined factor VIII-von Willebrand factor (vWF) concentrate (Haemate-P) in patients with von Willebrand disease. *Thromb Haemost* 1999;81:229–233.

161. Mannucci PM. Venous thromboembolism in von Willebrand disease. *Thromb Haemost* 2002;88:378–379.

162. Makris M, Colvin B, Gupta V, et al. Venous thrombosis following the use of intermediate purity FVIII concentrate to treat patients with von Willebrand's disease. *Thromb Haemost* 2002;88:387–388.

163. Goudemand J, Mazurier C, Marey A, et al. Clinical and biological evaluation in von Willebrand's disease of a von Willebrand factor concentrate with low factor VIII activity. *Br J Haematol* 1992;80:214–221.

164. Goudemand J, Negrier C, Ounnoughene N, et al. Clinical management of patients with von Willebrand's disease with a VHP vWF concentrate: the French experience. *Haemophilia* 1998;4 (Suppl. 3):48–52.

165. Turecek PL, Gritsch H, Pichler L, et al. *In vivo* characterization of recombinant von Willebrand factor in dogs with von Willebrand disease. *Blood* 1997;90:3555–3567.

166. Mannucci PM. Hemostatic drugs. *N Engl J Med* 1998;339:245–253.

167. Derkay CS, Werner E, Plotnick E. Management of children with von Willebrand disease undergoing adenotonsillectomy. *Am J Otolaryngol* 1996;17:172–177.

168. Alperin JB. Estrogens and surgery in women with von Willebrand's disease. *Am J Med* 1982;73:367–371.

169. Walker ID, Walker JJ, Colvin BT, et al. Investigation and management of haemorrhagic disorders in pregnancy. Haemostasis and Thrombosis Task Force. *J Clin Pathol* 1994;47:100–108.

170. Conti M, Mari D, Conti E, et al. Pregnancy in women with different types of von Willebrand disease. *Obstet Gynecol* 1986;68:282–285.

171. Gralnick HR, Williams SB, McKeown LP, et al. DDAVP in type IIA von Willebrand's disease. *Blood* 1986;67:465–468.

172. Rodeghiero F, Castaman G, Mannucci PM. Clinical indications for desmopressin (DDAVP) in congenital and acquired von Willebrand disease. *Blood Rev* 1991;5:155–161.

173. Casonato A, Pontara E, Dannhaeuser D, et al. Re-evaluation of the therapeutic efficacy of DDAVP in type IIB von Willebrand's disease. *Blood Coagul Fibrinolysis* 1994;5:959–964.

174. Fowler WE, Berkowitz LR, Roberts HR. DDAVP for type IIB von Willebrand disease. *Blood* 1989;74:1859–1860.

175. Mauz-Korholz C, Budde U, Kruck H, et al. Management of severe chronic thrombocytopenia in von Willebrand's disease type 2B. *Arch Dis Child* 1998;78:257–260.

176. Mazurier C, Gaucher C, Jorieux S, et al. Biological effect of desmopressin in eight patients with type 2N ('Normandy') von Willebrand disease. *Br J Haematol* 1994;88:849–854.

177. Nishino M, Nishino S, Sugimoto M, et al. Changes in factor VIII binding capacity of von Willebrand factor and factor VIII coagulant activity in two patients with type 2N von Willebrand disease after hemostatic treatment and during pregnancy. *Int J Hematol* 1996;64:127–134.

178. Castillo R, Monteagudo J, Escolar G, et al. Hemostatic effect of normal platelet transfusion in severe von Willebrand disease patients. *Blood* 1991;77:1901–1905.

179. Mannucci PM. Platelet von Willebrand factor in inherited and acquired bleeding disorders. *Proc Natl Acad Sci U S A* 1995;92:2428–2432.

180. Castillo R, Escolar G, Monteagudo J, et al. Hemostasis in patients with severe von Willebrand disease improves after normal platelet transfusion and normalizes with further correction of the plasma defect. *Transfusion* 1997;37:785–790.

181. Lak M, Peyvandi F, Mannucci PM. Clinical manifestations and complications of childbirth and replacement therapy in 385 Iranian patients with type 3 von Willebrand disease. *Br J Haematol* 2000;111:1236–1239.

182. Mannucci PM, Federici AB. Antibodies to von Willebrand factor in von Willebrand disease. *Adv Exp Med Biol* 1995;386:87–92.

183. Mannucci PM, Ruggeri ZM, Ciavarella N, et al. Precipitating antibodies to factor VIII/von Willebrand factor in von Willebrand's disease: effects on replacement therapy. *Blood* 1981;57:25–31.

184. Bergamaschini L, Mannucci PM, Federici AB, et al. Posttransfusion anaphylactic reactions in a patient with severe von Willebrand disease: role of complement and alloantibodies to von Willebrand factor. *J Lab Clin Med* 1995;125:348–355.

185. Boyer-Neumann C, Dreyfus M, Wolf M, et al. Multi-therapeutic approach to manage delivery in an alloimmunized patient with type 3 von Willebrand disease. *J Thromb Haemost* 2003;1:190–192.

186. Ciavarella N, Schiavoni M, Valenzano E, et al. Use of recombinant factor VIIa (NovoSeven) in the treatment of two patients with type III von Willebrand's disease and an inhibitor against von Willebrand factor. *Haemostasis* 1996;26 (Suppl. 1):150–154.

187. Greer IA, Lowe GD, Walker JJ, et al. Haemorrhagic problems in obstetrics and gynaecology in patients with congenital coagulopathies. *Br J Obstet Gynaecol* 1991;98:909–918.

188. Kadir RA, Economides DL, Sabin CA, et al. Frequency of inherited bleeding disorders in women with menorrhagia. *Lancet* 1998;351:485–489.

189. Kouides PA. Females with von Willebrand disease: 72 years as the silent majority. *Haemophilia* 1998;4:665–676.

190. Lethagen S, Ragnarson Tennvall G. Self-treatment with desmopressin intranasal spray in patients with bleeding disorders: effect on bleeding symptoms and socioeconomic factors. *Ann Hematol* 1993;66:257–260.

191. Kadir RA, Lee CA, Sabin CA, et al. DDAVP nasal spray for treatment of menorrhagia in women with inherited bleeding disorders: a randomized placebo-controlled crossover study. *Haemophilia* 2002;8:787–793.

192. Edlund M, Blomback M, Fried G. Desmopressin in the treatment of menorrhagia in women with no common coagulation factor deficiency but with prolonged bleeding time. *Blood Coagul Fibrinolysis* 2002;13:225–231.

193. Leissinger C, Becton D, Cornell C Jr, et al. High-dose DDAVP intranasal spray (Stimate) for the prevention and treatment of bleeding in patients with mild haemophilia A, mild or moderate type 1 von Willebrand disease and symptomatic carriers of haemophilia A. *Haemophilia* 2001;7:258–266.

194. Foster PA. The reproductive health of women with von Willebrand Disease unresponsive to DDAVP: results of an international survey. *Thromb Haemost* 1995;74:784–790.

195. Bonnar J, Sheppard BL. Treatment of menorrhagia during menstruation: randomised controlled trial of ethamsylate, mefenamic acid, and tranexamic acid. *Br Med J* 1996;313:579–582.

196. Ong YL, Hull DR, Mayne EE. Menorrhagia in von Willebrand disease successfully treated with single daily dose tranexamic acid. *Haemophilia* 1998;4:63–65.

197. Nilsson L, Rybo G. Treatment of menorrhagia with epsilon aminocaproic acid. A double blind investigation. *Acta Obstet Gynecol Scand* 1965;44:467–473.

198. Kasonde JM, Bonnar J. Aminocaproic acid and menstrual loss in women using intrauterine devices. *Br Med J* 1975;4:17–19.

199. Punnonen R, Nyman D, Grönroos M, et al. Von Willebrand's disease and pregnancy. *Acta Obstet Gynecol Scand* 1981;60:507–509.

200. Kadir RA, Lee CA, Sabin CA, et al. Pregnancy in women with von Willebrand's disease or factor XI deficiency. *Br J Obstet Gynaecol* 1998;105:314–321.

201. Ramsahoye BH, Davies SV, Dasani H, et al. Obstetric management in von Willebrand's disease: a report of 24 pregnancies and a review of the literature. *Haemophilia* 1995;1:140–144.

202. Cohen S, Daitch JS, Amar D, et al. Epidural analgesia for labor and delivery in a patient with von Willebrand's disease. *Reg Anesth* 1989;14:95–97.

203. Viallard JF, Pellegrin JL, Vergnes C, et al. Three cases of acquired von Willebrand disease associated with systemic lupus erythematosus. *Br J Haematol* 1999;105:532–537.

204. Igarashi N, Miura M, Kato E, et al. Acquired von Willebrand's syndrome with lupus-like serology. *Am J Pediatr Hematol Oncol* 1989;11:32–33.

205. Tefferi A, Hanson CA, Kurtin PJ, et al. Acquired von Willebrand's disease due to aberrant expression of platelet glycoprotein Ib by marginal zone lymphoma cells. *Br J Haematol* 1997;96:850–853.

206. Mohri H, Noguchi T, Kodama F, et al. Acquired von Willebrand disease due to inhibitor of human myeloma protein specific for von Willebrand factor. *Am J Clin Pathol* 1987;87:663–668.

207. Rao KP, Kizer J, Jones TJ, et al. Acquired von Willebrand's syndrome associated with an extranodal pulmonary lymphoma. *Arch Pathol Lab Med* 1988;112:47–50.

208. Richard C, Cuadrado MA, Prieto M, et al. Acquired von Willebrand disease in multiple myeloma secondary to absorption of von Willebrand factor by plasma cells. *Am J Hematol* 1990;35:114–117.

209. Handin RI, Martin V, Moloney WC. Antibody-induced von Willebrand's disease: a newly defined inhibitor syndrome. *Blood* 1976;48:393–405.

210. Macik BG, Gabriel DA, White GC II, et al. The use of high-dose intravenous gamma-globulin in acquired von Willebrand syndrome. *Arch Pathol Lab Med* 1988;112:143–146.

211. Hanley D, Arkel YS, Lynch J, et al. Acquired von Willebrand's syndrome in association with a lupus-like anticoagulant corrected by intravenous immunoglobulin. *Am J Hematol* 1994;46:141–146.

212. van Genderen PJ, Terpstra W, Michiels JJ, et al. High-dose intravenous immunoglobulin delays clearance of von Willebrand factor in acquired von Willebrand disease. *Thromb Haemost* 1995;73:891–892.

213. Federici AB, Stabile F, Castaman G, et al. Treatment of acquired von Willebrand syndrome in patients with monoclonal gammopathy of uncertain significance: comparison of three different therapeutic approaches. *Blood* 1998;92:2707–2711.

214. Castaman G, Tosetto A, Rodeghiero F. Effectiveness of high-dose intravenous immunoglobulin in a case of acquired von Willebrand syndrome with chronic melena not responsive to desmopressin and factor VIII concentrate. *Am J Hematol* 1992;41:132–136.

215. van Genderen PJ, Michiels JJ, van der Poel-van de Luytgaarde SC, et al. Acquired von Willebrand disease as a cause of recurrent mucocutaneous bleeding in primary thrombocythemia: relationship with platelet count. *Ann Hematol* 1994;69:81–84.

216. Budde U, van Genderen PJ. Acquired von Willebrand disease in patients with high platelet counts. *Semin Thromb Hemost* 1997;23:425–431.

217. Scott JP, Montgomery RR, Tubergen DG, et al. Acquired von Willebrand's disease in association with Wilm's tumor: regression following treatment. *Blood* 1981;58:665–669.

# CHAPTER 61 ■ INHERITED DISORDERS OF PROTHROMBIN CONVERSION

HAROLD R. ROBERTS AND MIGUEL A. ESCOBAR

The procoagulants and their cofactors are necessary for the normal rate of conversion of prothrombin to thrombin. When these factors are deficient or defective, thrombin generation is retarded and contributes to the hemorrhagic manifestations observed in patients. The purpose of this chapter is to review the clinical aspects of inherited disorders of prothrombin conversion caused by deficiencies of prothrombin and of factors V, VII, and X. All these are synthesized in the liver, and, except for factor V, all depend on vitamin K for complete synthesis. The biochemistry of these factors and their interactions with the other clotting factors that are necessary for the normal rate of prothrombin conversion are reviewed elsewhere (see Chapters 7–10).

## PROTHROMBIN

### History

The historical account of prothrombin as a precursor of thrombin was reviewed by Morawitz in 1905; an English translation by Hartmann and Guenther was published in 1958 (1). An earlier name for prothrombin was *thrombogen*, postulated to be the precursor of "fibrin ferment," later known as *thrombin*. Pure preparations of prothrombin were first obtained by Seegers et al. (2). Subsequently, the prothrombin gene has been shown to be on chromosome 11, and the complete amino acid sequence has been determined (3–6).

After the discovery of prothrombin and the development of methods for its assay, reports of patients with hypoprothrombinemia appeared (6–14). Initially, it was not known whether the hypoprothrombinemia was due to a true deficiency of prothrombin or to the presence of abnormal molecules with decreased functional activity. In 1967, a case of hereditary hypoprothrombinemia due to a true deficiency of prothrombin was reported (15). Later, the existence of dysprothrombinemia, an inherited defect of prothrombin manifested by the presence of abnormal prothrombin molecules lacking functional activity but retaining antigenic activity, was described (16).

Therefore, inherited disorders of prothrombin, like other inherited procoagulant deficiencies, are genetically heterogeneous. Several families have been described that apparently are heterozygous for both dysprothrombinemia and hypoprothrombinemia (combined heterozygotes) (6,17–21). Some of the reported hereditary hypoprothrombinemias, as measured by clotting assays, have not been characterized in terms of the specific genetic defect. In any case, the incidence of congenital prothrombin deficiency of any sort is rare (1 in 2 million). Fewer than 40 kindreds have been reported (6). In homogeneous population, the frequency of a mutation may be higher, as is the case with the recently described Puerto Rico I defect (one in 700) (22).

### Genetics and Biology

The mode of inheritance of hypoprothrombinemia and dysprothrombinemia is autosomal recessive, with no known predilection for ethnic background (23). Individuals who are combined heterozygotes or who are homozygous for the condition may be symptomatic and may have functional levels of prothrombin ranging from 1% to 25% of normal. The reason for the variation in levels of functional prothrombin is unclear, but like other hereditary clotting factor defects, it probably represents a compilation of defects at the molecular level (24–26). The decrease in prothrombin antigen is due to decreased synthesis or increased clearance of a poorly functional protein. Functional and immunologic assays for prothrombin correlate well in true hypoprothrombinemia. Individuals heterozygous for hypoprothrombinemia have prothrombin activity levels of 50% or more and antigen levels that are normal or nearly normal. Complete absence of prothrombin seems to be incompatible with life, as demonstrated in knockout mice (27,28).

Selected abnormal prothrombins are listed in Table 61-1 (29–55). Although the biochemistry and molecular biology of prothrombin are discussed in detail elsewhere in this text (see Chapter 10), a brief synopsis may help with the understanding of the dysprothrombinemias. Prothrombin is divided into five functional domains: the propeptide, the $\gamma$-carboxyglutamic acid (Gla), two kringle, and the catalytic. The propeptide domain is thought to function in the processing, targeting, carboxylation, and secretion of the nascent polypeptide. The Gla domain is a product of the action of the vitamin K–dependent carboxylase enzyme system and functions to bind calcium and mediate phospholipid binding. Kringle domains are folded structures with multiple disulfide bonds thought to be involved in protein–protein interactions. The catalytic domain contains the active site, composed of serine, histidine, and aspartic acid (56–58). The dysprothrombinemias most likely exhibit defective function related to one or more of these domains. For example, prothrombin Shanghai has a defect affecting the function of the Gla region. This prothrombin shows abnormalities in calcium binding (49), whereas others show either defective activation by factor Xa or defects ascribed to the catalytic region. Prothrombin Corpus Christi is characterized by the substitution of a cysteine for an arginine at position 382. This mutation results in a thrombin molecule with markedly reduced fibrinogen clotting activity and normal amidolytic activity, suggesting a functional defect within the fibrinogen-binding exosite. The preserved ability to activate platelets may explain the absence of a significant bleeding tendency relative to its noticeably reduced fibrinogen clotting activity (54).

Prothrombins Quick I and II were described in a single patient heterozygous for each of the two types (43–46). The

## TABLE 61-1

### VARIANTS OF PROTHROMBIN

| Prothrombin variant | Coagulation assay (% *normal*) | Immunologic assay (% *normal*) | Genotype | Hemorrhagic symptoms | Functional or molecular defect |
|---|---|---|---|---|---|
| Barcelona/ Madrid/Obihiro | 10 | 100 | Homozygous | Yes | Arg271 → Cys |
| Brussels | 46 | 88 | Heterozygous | Yes | Unknown |
| Cardeza | 50 | 100 | Heterozygous | No | Impaired factor Xa proteolysis |
| Clamart | 50 | 100 | Heterozygous | No | Impaired factor Xa proteolysis |
| Corpus Christi | 2 | 25 | Compound heterozygous[a] | No | Arg382 → Cys |
| Denver | 5 | 21 | Compound heterozygous[a] | Yes | Glu300 → Lys Glu309 → Lys |
| Greenville | 51 | 102 | Heterozygous | No | Arg517 → Gly |
| Habana | <10 | 50 | Compound heterozygous[a] | Yes | Unknown |
| Himi | 10 | 100 | Compound heterozygous[a] | No | Met337 → Thr Arg388 → His |
| Magdeburg | 45 | 105 | Heterozygous | Yes | Unknown |
| Metz | 10 | 50 | Compound heterozygous[a] | Yes | Defective thrombin active site |
| Mexico City | <10 | <10 | Compound heterozygous[a] | No | (?) Abnormal activation by factor Xa |
| Molise | 10 | 50 | Compound heterozygous[a] | Yes | Arg418 → Trp |
| Padua | 50 | 100 | Heterozygous | Yes | Arg271 → His |
| Perija | 2 | 70 | Homozygous | Yes | Gly548 → Ala |
| Poissy | 2 | 50 | Homozygous | Yes | (?)Abnormal activation by factor Xa |
| Puerto Rico I | 17 | 35 | Homozygous | Yes | Arg457 → Gln |
| Puerto Rico II | 9 | 35 | Compound heterozygote[a] | Yes | Arg457 → Gln Gla16 → Gln |
| Quick I and II | <2 | 34 | Compound heterozygous for two abnormal alleles | Yes | Arg382 → Cys Gly558 → Val |
| Salatka/Frankfurt | 15 | 100 | Homozygous | No/Yes | Glu466 → Ala |
| Segovia | 7 | 100 | Homozygous | Yes | Gly319 → Arg |
| Shanghai | 7 | 32 | Homozygous | Yes | Gla29 → Gly |
| Tokushima | 12 | 42 | Homozygous | Yes | Arg418 → Tyr |
| Unnamed | 20 | 26 | Compound heterozygote[a] | Yes | Arg271 → His His562 → Arg -GT 20062-20063 |
| Unnamed | — | — | Heterozygous or homozygous | Patients predisposed to venous thrombosis | G to A transition at nucleotides 20210 in 3′ untranslated region |

[a]Patients affected by both dysprothrombinemia and hypoprothrombinemia.

mutation in Quick I is a cysteine substituted for an arginine at position 382 (45). After it is activated, prothrombin Quick I possesses decreased or abnormal activity in cleaving fibrinogen, with a marked decrease in the release of fibrinopeptide A. In addition, thrombin Quick I exhibits decreased ability to aggregate platelets and decreased ability to stimulate the production of prostaglandin I$_2$ by cultured endothelial cells (44). The arginine at position 382, therefore, is not only an important residue in determining the specificity of thrombin for fibrinogen but also appears critical in some of the cell receptor–mediated functions of thrombin. Prothrombin Quick II is a substitution of a valine for a glycine at position 558 (46). After it is activated, prothrombin Quick II shows no functional activity toward fibrinogen. The mutation in prothrombin Quick II is thought to affect the primary substrate binding pocket of the catalytic domain. Clinically, the patient with the mutation has less than 2% clotting activity with 34% antigen. Patients with elevated prothrombin levels due to a genetic variation (G to A at base 20210) in the 3′ untranslated region of the prothrombin gene also have been described (59). These patients have an increased predisposition to venous thrombosis (60). A detailed database of the mutations can be found on the Web site (61).

## Clinical Manifestations

The signs and symptoms of both hypoprothrombinemia and dysprothrombinemia vary roughly with the level of functional prothrombin. Heterozygous patients with approximately 50% functional activity usually have no bleeding symptoms, although there have been occasional reports of epistaxis and bleeding after dental extraction. Patients with lower prothrombin levels exhibit easy bruising, epistaxis, menorrhagia, postpartum hemorrhage, and hemorrhage after surgery or trauma. Intracranial hemorrhage has been reported in patients with the lowest prothrombin levels. Hemarthroses are not usually observed but have been reported. Bleeding may be exacerbated by ingestion of aspirin. Some members of the family with prothrombin Cardeza have coexistent Ehlers-Danlos syndrome, but the occurrence of these two disorders in the same family may be coincidental. In the family affected with prothrombin Mexico City, the dysprothrombinemia is either linked or associated coincidentally with a gene for multiple exostoses (21).

## Diagnosis

The diagnosis of inherited hypoprothrombinemia or dysprothrombinemia is suggested by an appropriate family history of excessive bleeding in the presence of variable prolongation of the prothrombin time (PT) and activated partial thromboplastin time (aPTT) and a normal thrombin time. These screening tests are not specific because a deficiency of factors V and X would result in the same abnormalities. Definitive diagnosis depends on specific assays for functional or immunologic prothrombin, or both. In true hypoprothrombinemia, both the functional assay and the immunologic assay show decreased prothrombin levels. The normal functional level of prothrombin is approximately 250 to 350 NIH U per mL plasma (one unit equals the amount of thrombin that clots a standard fibrinogen solution in 15 seconds), and affected patients generally have 2% to 25% of this level. In dysprothrombinemia, the coagulation assay measuring functional prothrombin activity is decreased, but the immunologic assay may reveal near-normal levels of prothrombin antigen. Compound heterozygotes have immunologic prothrombin assays that approach 50% of normal. Assays of other clotting factors are usually normal, although mild decreases in factor VII levels have been reported.

## Differential Diagnosis

Hypoprothrombinemia or dysprothrombinemia must be distinguished from vitamin K deficiency, as in hemorrhagic disease of the newborn, malabsorption, or therapeutic or surreptitious warfarin intoxication with either coumadin or one of the newer "super" warfarin rodenticides such as brodifacoum (62). Low levels of prothrombin also have been associated with many antimicrobials. Cephalosporins containing the N-methyl-thiotetrazole (NMTT) side chain impair the vitamin K–dependent γ-carboxylation of glutamic acid residues required for production of normal prothrombin and other vitamin K–dependent proteins (62,63). Hereditary defects in prothrombin also must be distinguished from the hypoprothrombinemia of liver disease or antibodies against prothrombin (64,65). In vitamin K deficiency or warfarin ingestion, functional prothrombin is variably decreased, whereas immunologic levels of prothrombin are approximately 50% of normal, presumably because of a shorter half-life of the descarboxy form of prothrombin. Immunologic levels of prothrombin also may be decreased in liver disease. In acquired prothrombin deficiency, there should be no family history of a bleeding diathesis, and laboratory evaluation of coagulation

in family members should be normal. Also, in all of the preceding cases except specific antibodies to prothrombin, levels of other vitamin K–dependent factors would be decreased.

Isolated acquired deficiencies of prothrombin are rare. Acquired antibodies against prothrombin have been described in association with infection, medications, and cancer (66–69). In the last the IgG antibody disappeared after treatment of the lymphoma. Mild to severe hypoprothrombinemia has been reported primarily in systemic lupus erythematosus and is due to antiprothrombin antibodies, some of which appear to be directed toward certain domains of the prothrombin molecule (70–73). Although these antibodies bind to prothrombin, they may not actually neutralize the coagulant activity of prothrombin in vitro; rather, antigen/antibody complexes formed in vivo are rapidly cleared from the circulation, resulting in hypoprothrombinemia. A similar type of antibody to prothrombin also has been reported in a patient without evidence of systemic lupus erythematosus (72). Treatment with corticosteroids resulted in an increase in prothrombin activity and a decrease in bleeding symptoms.

Treatment of an acquired prothrombin inhibitor in a patient with systemic lupus erythematosus using danazol has been reported to increase prothrombin antigen and activity (74).

A peculiar congenital defect of prothrombin consumption also has been described in five families (75–77). The rate of conversion of prothrombin to thrombin was slow and appeared as an isolated defect, with the results of all conventional coagulation assays, including platelet function tests, being normal. In one patient, both plasma and platelet transfusions were required to correct the defect. The nature of the abnormality is unclear. Transfusion with fresh frozen plasma corrected the abnormal prothrombin consumption of one patient. In addition, crossed immunoelectrofocusing of the patient's prothrombin showed an abnormal isoelectric point, suggesting the presence of an abnormal prothrombin molecule (76).

## Treatment

The treatment of hypoprothrombinemia or dysprothrombinemia depends on the severity of the disorder and the type of bleeding. Bruises or mild superficial bleeding need not be treated with replacement therapy because such bleeding usually responds to conservative therapy. Replacement therapy may be used for major bleeding episodes. Fresh frozen plasma in loading doses of 10 to 20 mL per kg body weight, followed by 3 mL per kg body weight every 24 hours, is probably sufficient for the average adult. Because the biologic half-life of prothrombin is approximately 3 days, the need for replacement therapy is infrequent and should be monitored by specific assays and clinical response. The risk of transmission of viral diseases via blood transfusion must always be considered and is reviewed in Chapter 50 (78,79). When using large volumes of plasma for replacement therapy, the patient's cardiovascular status should be carefully monitored to avoid circulatory overload and subsequent congestive heart failure.

Prothrombin complex concentrates (PCCs) have been available commercially for several years. They have been prepared by a variety of fractionation procedures, but most preparations contain significant amounts of prothrombin as well as factors VII, IX, and X. The content of these factors in several PCCs is shown in Table 61-2. Advantages of such concentrates include a prolonged shelf life, ease of administration, and the ability to achieve high levels of clotting factors without attendant fluid overload. All currently available PCCs have been treated by various methods to inactivate the human immunodeficiency and hepatitis B and C viruses but not parvovirus or hepatitis A virus. Prions also are not inactivated by current procedures, but there is no known transmission of

TABLE 61-2

**PROTHROMBIN COMPLEX CONCENTRATES**

| Product | Prothrombin | Factor VII | Factor IX | Factor X |
|---|---|---|---|---|
| Konyne 80 | 100 | 20 | 100 | 140 |
| Profilnine SD | 148 | 11 | 100 | 64 |
| Proplex T | 50 | 400 | 100 | 50 |
| Bebulin VH | 120 | 13 | 100 | 140 |

All factor levels are expressed relative to 100 U of factor IX. Other prothrombin complex concentrates available in Europe.

prion diseases by blood or blood products. Some of these products have been associated with thromboembolic phenomena, so care must be taken to use the smallest effective dose (80,81).

# FACTOR V (LABILE FACTOR, PROACCELERIN, ACCELERAT, OR GLOBULIN)

## History

The presence of a "convertibility" factor in plasma (which may have been factor V), different from prothrombin and other known clotting factors, was suspected as early as 1939. It was then shown that there was a substance in plasma, not adsorbable to magnesium hydroxide or barium salts, that was necessary for the conversion of prothrombin to thrombin. Later, it was determined that the one-stage PT of aged plasma was prolonged and that this prolongation could be corrected by fresh plasma obtained from animals receiving coumarin drugs and presumably deficient in prothrombin and other vitamin K–dependent factors (82).

Although these data suggested the presence of a hitherto unrecognized clotting factor, it remained for Owren to clearly characterize factor V, which was deficient in a 21-year-old woman with a lifelong bleeding history (83–85). The patient was discovered during the Nazi occupation of Norway, and it was not until after World War II that the importance of Owren's discovery was appreciated and reported. He showed that the clotting factor missing in his patient was found in the normal plasma from which vitamin K–dependent factors were adsorbed and that such plasma shortened the prolonged PT of the patient's plasma.

A factor similar to that described by Owren was also reported by others (86–88). Since then, human factor V has been isolated, and the structure and amino acid sequence of the molecule have been described (89–93). The biochemistry and physiology of factor V are reviewed in Chapter 9.

## Genetics and Biology

Factor V deficiency is inherited as an autosomal recessive trait (94–98). Heterozygotes are not always detectable by clotting assays. In some patients with factor V deficiency, other congenital disorders have been described (95,96,99). The estimated prevalence is one in 1 million (100).

Patients with hereditary factor V deficiency fall roughly into three groups: those in which both factor V antigen and clotting activity are undetectable; those with variably reduced, but not

absent, factor V antigen and activity; and those in which the factor V antigen is within normal limits, whereas factor V functional activity is reduced (101–106). The specific genetic defect in most of these patients has not been identified. One abnormal factor V has been labeled factor V$_{New Brunswick}$, characterized by an Ala221 to Val substitution as the result of a C to T transition in codon 51. The patient exhibited this transition on one allele, whereas the second allele was silent (107).

It has been suggested the factor V level in platelets may better predict the likelihood of bleeding in any particular patient (104,108). Factor V$_{Quebec}$ has been described in a family that exhibits an autosomal dominant disorder with severe bleeding after trauma (108). This disorder is characterized by mild thrombocytopenia, plasma factor V activity levels of 40% to 60%, plasma factor antigen levels of 65% to 75%, normal amounts of platelet factor V antigen, but low (2% to 4%) platelet factor V activity levels. Platelet ultrastructural studies in two of the patients with factor V$_{Quebec}$ were completely normal. It is now known that the platelet α-granule contents in these patients exhibits low concentrations of factor V, as well as fibrinogen, von Willebrand factor (VWF), and osteopontin. These proteins also are significantly degraded, suggesting that the low factor V level is associated with an unknown defect that causes proteolytic degradation of the proteins in platelet α-granules (109).

Complete deficiency of factor V in knockout mice results in neonatal death. This defect can be corrected by insertion of a minigene expressing factor V levels below the detectable threshold of standard clotting assays (<0.1%) (110).

A combined deficiency of factors V and VIII has been reported in a number of families and is often referred to as *familial multiple clotting factor deficiency type I* (111) (see subsequent text).

Several polymorphisms have been reported in the factor V gene, one leading to reduced factor activity (112). Factor V$_{Leiden}$ (Arg506Gln) has now been reported in numerous patients, but it is associated with a tendency to venous thrombosis while clotting activity is normal (113,114). In some patients, the factor V$_{Leiden}$ defect has been associated with a simultaneous deficiency of both factor V activity and antigen, type I factor V deficiency. These patients theoretically may be at greater risk for thrombotic events in that they resemble homozygotes in clotting tests designed to detect resistance to activated protein C (115).

## Clinical Manifestations

Patients having congenital factor V deficiency with levels ranging from undetectable to approximately 10% of normal usually have hemorrhagic manifestations but may be asymptomatic for long periods of time. The hemorrhagic manifestations associated with factor V deficiency include ecchymoses, epistaxis, menorrhagia, and bleeding from the gingiva, gastrointestinal tract, umbilicus, and central nervous system. Hemarthroses are uncommon but do occur. The severity of bleeding in patients with factor V deficiency may be related more to platelet-associated factor V than to the level of plasma factor V, but as yet this observation has not been fully explained (104).

As in some of the other factor deficiencies, thromboembolic phenomena have been reported in several patients and include myocardial infarction, thrombophlebitis, and pulmonary embolism (116,117). Factor V activity in these patients ranged from 10% to 14%, with normal levels of protein C, protein S, and plasminogen. Some patients with factor V deficiency have associated congenital abnormalities that may be coincidental (118).

## Diagnosis

A history of lifelong bleeding tendency is common, and occasionally there may be a family history of bleeding in siblings. Both the PT and PTT are prolonged, whereas the thrombin clotting time is normal. The diagnosis of factor V deficiency can be suspected if the patient's PT is corrected by normal plasma adsorbed with aluminum hydroxide or barium salts, but definitive diagnosis depends on a specific factor V assay.

Approximately one third of patients with hereditary factor V deficiency have a long bleeding time. This is an interesting observation, because it is known that factor V is stored in the $\alpha$-granules of platelets. Approximately 18% to 25% of the body pool of factor V is found in platelets (105,119,120). Platelet factor V is not synthesized by megakaryocytes but is acquired from plasma (121). Activated factor V on the platelet surface serves as part of the factor Xa receptor, but the precise relation between this and the long bleeding time is unknown (104). Platelet aggregation with the usual agonists is normal in patients with factor V deficiency. Typical laboratory observations are shown in Table 61-3.

Some patients with a congenital factor V deficiency develop specific antibodies to the factor (122). These can be detected by showing a prolongation both of the PT and PTT performed on a mixture of the patient's inhibitor plasma and normal plasma. In the presence of an inhibitor, these tests are not corrected by the addition of normal plasma. Inhibitors of factor V are time dependent; in this respect they resemble inhibitors of factor VIII (123). The inhibitor is usually an IgG antibody. Acquired inhibitors in patients without a congenital deficiency have been either IgG or a mixture of IgG and IgM (122). One case has been described with a monoclonal antibody (IgG$_4$, $\lambda$) against factor V (124). In another patient, the inhibitor was found to be active against plasma and platelet factor V, with a marked increase in platelet-associated IgG (125). In one individual with an acquired neutralizing antibody to factor V, circulating immune complexes containing the antibody and the factor V antigen were documented. The antibody was directed to the heavy chain of factor Va (126). Neutralizing factor V antibodies directed against the light chain have also been described (127,128).

## Differential Diagnosis

Acquired factor V deficiency usually is due to the appearance of specific antibodies that may be idiopathic or associated with a variety of underlying diseases, including pancreatitis, carcinoma, bone fracture, cholecystitis, autoimmune disorders, pulmonary tuberculosis, and other causes (129–131). Aminoglycoside antibiotics (e.g., streptomycin, gentamicin, or kanamycin) have been implicated in several patients with acquired factor V inhibitor antibodies. Bleeding in an acquired deficiency may vary from mild to severe but is usually transient because the inhibitor tends to disappear with time. Evidence exists that platelet factor V is inaccessible to the inhibitor even in the face of almost complete inhibition of plasma factor V (132). The relative inaccessibility of platelet factor V to an inhibitor may account for the lack of bleeding symptoms in some patients.

Antibodies to both factor V and thrombin have been described in patients undergoing surgery who have been exposed to topical bovine thrombin. Bovine factor V is a contaminant in this preparation. Some of these patients bleed because of actual inhibition of human factor V and thrombin due to the cross-reaction of antibovine antibodies with the human proteins. Bovine thrombin is a potent antigen that can induce antibodies to multiple human coagulation factors in up to 80% of exposed patients. Usually, these antibodies are transient and respond to intravenous $\gamma$-globulin (133,134).

Acquired factor V deficiency may also be seen in severe liver disease and, when present, suggests severe hepatocellular deficiency. It also is frequently decreased in patients experiencing disseminated intravascular coagulation. In these cases, other clotting factors also are decreased, and the clinical picture itself is usually sufficient to exclude a congenital deficiency.

## Treatment

Bleeding episodes in factor V deficiency should be treated with fresh frozen plasma. Major surgery, including cholecystectomy, osteotomy, resection of pseudotumors, and other procedures, have been performed on patients with factor V deficiency under cover of plasma replacement therapy (134,135). Generally, the factor V level is raised to 25% to 30% just before surgery, using a loading dose of plasma of up to 20 mL of plasma per kg body weight. Maintenance infusions of plasma (approximately 3 to 6 mL per kg body weight every 12 hours) are usually given for 5 to 10 days or until healing is well underway. As with all blood products, there is

## TABLE 61-3

TYPICAL LABORATORY TESTS IN PATIENTS WITH FACTOR V DEFICIENCY

| Test | Patient | Healthy subject |
|---|---|---|
| Prothrombin time (sec) | 40–50 | 10.5–13 |
| Activated partial thromboplastin time (sec) | 50–60 | 27–36 |
| Prothrombin time mix (sec) (mixture of one part patient plasma + one part normal plasma) | 13 | 12 |
| Thrombin clotting time (sec) | 12–15 | 12–15 |
| Template bleeding time (min) | 5–20 | <10 |
| Factor V activity (%) (severe) | <1 | 100 |
| Other procoagulants | Normal | Normal |

risk of the transmission of viral diseases even after the plasma is screened for viral contamination. When adequate factor V levels cannot be attained with plasma infusions alone, plasma exchange may be used (136). After the exchange, transfusion factor V levels can be maintained with plasma infusions.

The biologic half-life of transfused factor V is apparently variable, because there are reports of a half-life from 4.5 to 36 hours; most authors accept the longer half-life (137). In some individuals, platelet transfusions have been reported to decrease bleeding (138,139). However, platelet transfusions are usually not indicated for treatment because of the possible development of platelet isoantibodies. Aspirin should be avoided in all patients with factor V deficiency. Cryoprecipitate does not contain sufficient factor V to be used in therapy, but the supernatant plasma remaining after cryoprecipitate removal contains sufficient factor V to be used for treatment. Treatment of acquired inhibitors may not be necessary in patients with mild bleeding because, in most cases, the inhibitor disappears spontaneously in 4 to 6 weeks. If bleeding is severe, treatment with immunosuppressive drugs has been useful. Intravenous immunoglobulin and steroids may also be of benefit in patients with antibodies against the factor (134).

# COMBINED FACTOR V AND FACTOR VIII DEFICIENCY

A combined factor V and factor VIII deficiency is the most commonly reported compound hereditary deficiency of clotting factors, sometimes referred to as *familial multiple clotting factor deficiency type I*. Fewer than 100 families have been reported (140–152). Levels of factors V and VIII as low as 8% and 4%, respectively, have been observed in patients, but levels of approximately 15% for both factors seem to be more common. Patients with ostensibly mild factor V or factor VIII deficiency should be studied for the combined defect because some of these patients may be misdiagnosed as having either mild classic hemophilia or mild factor V deficiency.

The inheritance pattern of the combined deficiency is autosomal recessive. Usually factor V and factor VIII clotting and antigenic activity are concordant. The genetic defect leading to the combined deficiency has been localized to a small region of chromosome 18(q21) (153,154). A gene for LMAN1 (lectin mannose 1), also called ERGIC (ERGIC-53), a component of the endoplasmic reticulum (ER)-Golgi intermediate compartment, appears to function as a chaperone protein for factors V and VIII as they are transported through the ER-Golgi compartment (155,156). Mutations in LMAN1 can be found in approximately two thirds of affected individuals (157). Mutations in the MCFD2 gene (multiple coagulation factor deficiency 2) can also cause combined deficiency of factor V and factor VIII, phenotipically undistinguishable from that caused by LMAN1 (158). It appears that the LMAN1–MCFD2 complex plays a key role in ER to Golgi transport of certain proteins. Several different mutations leading to the combined deficiency have now been identified in both genes (158,159). Patients with the combined disorder usually have a mild bleeding tendency that occurs with surgery or trauma. Prolonged bleeding after dental extractions or after tonsillectomy may be the first manifestation of the disorder. Spontaneous bleeding is unusual (160).

Diagnosis of the combined defect can be suspected in patients who exhibit a mild, moderately prolonged PT and PTT and who have a lifelong history of mild bleeding tendency.

Three families with combined factor V, factor VIII, and VWF deficiency have been described (161–163). In one family, not all individuals deficient in factors V and VIII are also deficient in VWF. One family has a VWF multimer pattern consistent with

type I von Willebrand disease. Another individual had concomitant hypothyroidism.

Treatment of combined factor V and VIII deficiency involves the use of plasma as a source of factor V and cryoprecipitate as a source of factor VIII. DDAVP (1-deamino-8-D-arginine vasopressin) infusions in one family with the combined deficiency resulted in a threefold increase in factor VIII but only a variable rise in factor V (164). An 8-year-old boy underwent succesful circumcision with the use of DDAVP (165). One group has shown little difference in factor VIII response between mild hemophiliacs and factor V/VIII–deficient patients after DDAVP is given intranasally (166). Therefore, DDAVP, in combination with plasma infusion, may provide adequate treatment (167). In some cases in which severe bleeding is expected, however, exchange transfusion is necessary to raise factor V levels, and factor VIII concentrates have also been valuable (136).

# FACTOR VII (SERUM PROTHROMBIN CONVERSION ACCELERATOR, STABLE FACTOR, PROCONVERTIN, AUTO-PROTHROMBIN I)

## History

Although the fact that tissue substances accelerate the coagulation of whole blood was known before Morawitz's work in the early twentieth century, a better understanding of the role of tissue factor awaited the elucidation of the various accelerators of prothrombin conversion to thrombin. A new factor necessary for normal generation of thrombin was first reported in 1951 and was called "serum prothrombin conversion accelerator," now known as factor VII (168). Factor VII was subsequently shown to interact with tissue factor in the so-called extrinsic system of coagulation. After the initial patient was transfused with normal plasma, factor VII was noted to have a half-life of approximately 3.0 to 3.5 hours. The cardinal findings in the initial case were a prolonged PT with a normal prothrombin consumption test. These findings suggested a defect in an "early phase" of prothrombin conversion to thrombin.

Subsequently, reports of congenital syndromes (other than hypoprothrombinemia and factor V deficiency) with prolonged PT appeared (169). Initially, all these cases were considered to represent deficiencies of factor VII. Later, it was determined that some patients previously diagnosed as being deficient in factor VII were, in fact, deficient in factor X (Stuart factor) (170). In factor VII deficiency, the PTT is normal, whereas this test is prolonged in factor X deficiency.

## Genetics and Biology

The entire primary sequence of factor VII has been determined from complementary DNA (cDNA) clones (171). The factor VII gene also has been localized to chromosome 13, close to the gene for factor X. It is composed of eight exons and seven intervening sequences and is similar in organization to other vitamin K–dependent clotting factors (171–174).

Factor VII combines with tissue factor in a 1:1 stoichiometry. For activity, factor VII must be activated, perhaps by factor Xa, although it can be activated by other serine proteases such as factor IXa, factor XIIa, and thrombin (174). The importance of the tissue factor–factor VII pathway in coagulation and hemostasis has been emphasized by several authors (175–180). It is now generally accepted that the tissue factor–factor VII complex initiates coagulation by autoactivation and plays a role in both the so-called intrinsic and extrinsic pathways by activating both factor IX and factor X. The factor Xa and factor IXa resulting from tissue factor–factor VIIa activity play specific and distinct roles in clotting reactions leading to platelet activation and thrombin generation (181).

An inhibitor to the extrinsic pathway has been described and purified (182,183). This inhibitor, now termed *tissue factor pathway inhibitor*, binds first to factor Xa and then to the factor VIIa–tissue factor–Xa complex, resulting in inactivation of both factors Xa and VIIa. Under this circumstance, the predominant pathway for factor X activation is by factor IXa/VIIIa complex.

The inheritance of factor VII deficiency has been shown to be autosomal recessive (184,185). At the level of molecular genetics, factor VII deficiency is a heterogeneous disorder. The frequency has been estimated to be one per 500,000 persons (185).

Numerous genetic variants leading to functional factor VII deficiency have been described and are listed on the Internet (186,187). Illustrative variants are shown in Table 61-4 (186, 188,189). Some variants result in a severe hemorrhagic disorder, whereas others result in moderate to mild bleeding. Patients with less than 1% functional activity rarely are asymptomatic. It is important to emphasize, however, that the clotting activity may vary depending on the source of the tissue factor (i.e., whether it is human, bovine, or rabbit). Mutant factor VII molecules exhibit a variety of functional abnormalities, ranging from decreased secretion from the hepatocyte to point mutations in the molecule, that result in defective activation or defective interaction with substrates, or both.

The association between hereditary factor VII deficiency and Dubin-Johnson syndrome has been reported (190,191). One of three patients with the Rotor syndrome was deficient in factor VII. An association also is possible between Gilbert syndrome and factor VII deficiency (192). Combined deficiency of factors VII and X have been reported with familial carotid body tumors.

Several chromosomal abnormalities are associated with factor VII deficiency and, occasionally, concurrent factor X deficiency. Two patients were found to have a translocation and loss of the distal tip of the long arm of chromosome 13 (172). Both patients were deficient in factors VII and X and had multiple congenital abnormalities. Some patients with trisomy 8 mosaicism have factor VII deficiency (173). The mechanism for this is not clear, but it is postulated that some sort of regulatory gene for factor VII resides on chromosome 8.

Associated factor VII and IX deficiency has been reported (193,194). In an extensive study of the genetic variants of hemophilia B, significantly reduced levels of factor VII and other vitamin K–dependent clotting factors were found in some patients (195,196).

Combined deficiencies of factor VII and VIII (familial multiple factor deficiency type IV) have been reported but are rare (111). Several reports are consistent with the coincident occurrence of hemophilia A and factor VII deficiency, but in two families the disease appears to be an autosomal disorder, like combined factor V/VIII deficiency. In some patients, factor VII coagulant activity was much less than antigenic activity, implying an abnormal factor VII molecule, but the true nature of combined factor VII/VIII deficiency has not been defined. A single Japanese family has been found to have concurrent factor VII and protein C deficiencies. The nature of the genetic abnormality is unclear (197).

## Clinical Manifestations

Wide variation exists in the reported hemorrhagic manifestations of factor VII deficiency. For example, there are reports that some patients with low factor VII clotting activity have little or no bleeding, whereas other patients with the same activity may have severe bleeding. It should be emphasized, however, that assays of factor VII activity may vary according to the source of tissue factor used in the clotting assay. Therefore, factor VII levels determined using human tissue factor may not be the same as those determined using rabbit tissue factor. Despite reported clinical heterogeneity, however, several generalizations can be made about patients with factor VII deficiency. Those with less than 1% clotting activity may have severe hemorrhagic manifestations equivalent to those seen in severe hemophilia A and B. There are exceptions to this generalization; for example, as shown in Table 61-4, some patients with less than 1% activity have been asymptomatic. Patients with factor VII levels of greater than 5% generally have moderate or mild hemorrhagic episodes. Most patients who bleed usually have hemorrhagic episodes before adulthood. Some exhibit bleeding in the first few days of life (i.e., bleeding from the umbilical stump and cephalohematoma). Hemorrhage commonly occurs from the nose and gums. Easy bruising is a common observation. Hemarthroses sometimes occur, usually in patients with factor VII activity less than 1% of normal. A clinical radiologic study of the joints of some patients severely affected with factor VII deficiency indicated the presence of severe arthropathy equal to that seen in hemophilia A and B. Hematuria, gastrointestinal bleeding, splenic hematomas, pulmonary hemorrhage, bloody tears, intracranial hemorrhage, and subarachnoid hemorrhage also have been reported. A review of the literature revealed 12 cases of central nervous system hemorrhage in 75 cases of factor VII deficiency (198).

Interestingly, some severely affected patients seem to tolerate surgical procedures strikingly well. In a retrospective study of 17 individuals with inherited factor VII deficiency (FVII: C ≤0.1 IU per mL), a previous history of hemorrhage (hemarthroses, large

## TABLE 61-4

ILLUSTRATIVE GENETIC VARIANTS OF FACTOR VII

| Variant | Functional activity | Antigen | Severity | Molecular defect | Functional defect |
|---------|--------------------|---------|----------|------------------|-------------------|
| Charlotte | <1% | 100% | Severe | Arg79 → Gln | Decreased binding to tissue factor |
|  |  |  |  | Arg152 → Gln | Abolition of cleavage site |
| Central | <1% | 38% | Severe | Phe328 → Ser | Impaired activation |
| Toyama | <1.6% | 2% | Severe | Thr359 → Met | Coagulant activity |
| Unnamed | <1% | 2% | Severe | Asn57 → Ile | Epidermal growth factor 1 |
| Unnamed | <2% | 4% | Moderate | Ala294 → Val | Defect in catalytic domain |
| Unnamed | 6 | 85% | Mild | Met298 → Ile | Defect in catalytic domain |
| Unnamed | <5 | 25% | Asymptomatic | Ala191 → Thr | Defect in catalytic domain |
| Mie | 28% | 26% | Asymptomatic | Arg247 → His | Impaired secretion |

hematomas, severe epistaxis) was the most important predictive risk of surgical bleeding. No clinical correlation was seen with the factor VII level nor the factor VII genotype (199).

The issue of thrombotic complications in patients with factor VII deficiency has been reported (116,200,201). In a review of thrombotic events, nine such patients with thrombotic complications were identified (200). These episodes include superficial and deep-vein thrombosis, pulmonary embolism, central nervous sytem infarct, and overt disseminated intravascular coagulation. Thrombophilia markers were found in two cases. Interestingly, the allele frequency Ala294Val was more common in individuals with thrombotic events. A patient with factor VII deficiency and coronary artery disease has been studied, and *in vitro* assays demonstrated a brisk monocyte procoagulant response (202).

In contrast to low factor VII levels, data from the Northwick Park Heart Study suggest that the elevation of factor VII coagulant activity in middle-aged men is associated with increased risk of ischemic heart disease (203). Unaffected first-degree relatives of these individuals are found to have elevated levels of factor VII (204). However, the relation of elevated factor VII levels to coronary heart disease remains controversial because other studies have shown no relation to factor VII levels and cardiovascular disease (205).

## Diagnosis

The diagnosis of congenital factor VII deficiency is suggested by the presence of a prolonged PT and normal PTT and thrombin clotting times. Factor VII deficiency is the only inherited clotting factor defect in which only the PT is prolonged. The thromboplastin generation test and Stypven (Russell viper venom) time are normal. The prolonged PT is corrected by aged normal serum but not by plasma or serum from patients known to be deficient in factor VII. Definitive diagnosis rests upon a specific assay. Laboratory data on a typical patient with factor VII deficiency are shown in Table 61-5.

## Differential Diagnosis

Causes of acquired factor VII deficiency include liver disease and vitamin K antagonism by coumarin drugs or vitamin K deficiency. In these situations, multiple factor deficiencies occur, and the underlying disease is usually evident. Acquired factor VII deficiency secondary to antibodies is rare, but several cases have been reported in the literature (206–210). In one case, a patient with aplastic anemia had an isolated factor VII deficiency due to a nonneutralizing antibody (211). This patient had complete resolution of the deficiency with immunosuppressive therapy and allogeneic marrow transplantation.

Although factor X deficiency is the most common clotting factor decreased in systemic amyloidosis, a patient with combined factor VII and factor X deficiency with amyloidosis due to multiple myeloma has been reported (212). Intensive chemotherapy for the multiple myeloma resulted in a gradual rise in both factors VII and X. Acquired factor VII deficiency has been described in homocystinuria, with factor VII levels ranging from 20% to 44% (213). In most patients, a strict low-methionine diet and concurrent pyridoxine and folate administration resulted in an increase in the factor VII level.

## Treatment

Replacement therapy in patients with factor VII deficiency depends on the severity of hemorrhage. Bleeding is common after dental extraction in severely affected patients; such patients should receive appropriate prophylactic therapy with ε-aminocaproic acid and, if necessary, factor replacement. Other surgical procedures in severely affected patients, although not always associated with hemorrhage, usually require prophylactic replacement of factor VII.

The biologic half-life of factor VII, studied by a variety of methods, has been shown to be between 3.0 and 3.5 hours (214). Generally, an appropriate factor VII level between 10% and 20% is adequate for most bleeding episodes (215).

The therapeutic materials available for replacement therapy include recombinant factor VIIa (NovoSeven), plasma, and PCCs that contain factor VII (Table 61-2). Recombinant factor VIIa (NovoSeven) has been recently approved in European countries for the treatment of inherited factor VII deficiency. In the United States, its only approved use is for patients with hemophilia and inhibitors. This product has been used successfully to treat patients with factor VII deficiency and has been found to be both safe and effective (216,217). Doses that range between 15 and 30 $\mu$g per kg of body weight administered every 4 to 8 hours appear to be sufficient to maintain hemostasis during bleeding or surgical procedures. Antibodies following treatment with recombinant factor VII have been described but are quite rare (218).

# FACTOR X (STUART-PROWER FACTOR)

## History

In 1905, Morawitz postulated a central role for a factor ("thromboplastin") that interacted with thrombogen (prothrombin) and calcium to yield thrombin (1). In the 1940s and

## TABLE 61-5

### LABORATORY DATA IN TYPICAL PATIENTS WITH FACTOR VII DEFICIENCY

| Test | Patient | Healthy subject |
|---|---|---|
| Prothrombin time (sec) | 40 | 10.5–13 |
| Activated partial thromboplastin time (sec) | 30 | 27–36 |
| Prothrombin time mix (sec) (mixture one part patient plasma + one part normal plasma) | 13 | 12 |
| Thrombin clotting time (sec) | 12–15 | 12–15 |
| Stypven (Russell viper venom) time (sec) | 15 | 15 |
| Factor VII activity (%) (severe) | <1% | 100% |
| Other procoagulant assays | Normal | Normal |

1950s, a substance known as *thrombokinase* was shown to convert prothrombin to thrombin (219). It is possible that this substance actually represented activated factor X. In 1955, other investigators demonstrated that coumarin anticoagulants diminished a serum factor that was distinct from factors VII and IX (220). This factor was called *factor X* before the official Roman numeral nomenclature was established, but probably corresponds to the clearly delineated factor X that was given its official numerical assignment in 1959.

Inherited deficiency of factor X was first reported independently by two groups studying patients with a hemorrhagic disease resembling factor VII deficiency. A patient (Prower) with a hemorrhagic disease clinically resembling factor VII deficiency, but with an abnormal thromboplastin generation test, was reported (221). More definitive studies on factor X were provided independently by Hougie et al. who noted the heterogeneity of the patient populations reported as having factor VII deficiency (170). They reported a patient surnamed Stuart who was previously thought to have factor VII deficiency, but whose plasma corrected the clotting defect of the original patient with factor VII deficiency. The characteristics of plasma deficiency in Stuart factor were impaired prothrombin use, prolonged PT and PTT, a serum abnormality in the thromboplastin generation test, and a prolonged (Russell viper venom) Stypven time.

## Genetics and Biology

Factor X has been purified to homogeneity and biochemically characterized. The gene coding for factor X is found adjacent to that coding for factor VII on chromosome 13 (222). The factor X gene structure has been characterized and is highly homologous to that of other vitamin K–dependent coagulation factors (223). The amino acid sequence of the protein was deduced both from the cDNA sequence and amino acid analysis (224).

Congenital factor X deficiency is inherited as an autosomal recessive characteristic (185,225).

Numerous kindreds have been identified with factor X deficiency. The exact frequency of the defect has not been established, although a homozygous incidence of 1:1,000,000 has been described (226).

With the availability of the factor X gene sequence, many mutants have been characterized at the molecular level (227,228) (see Table 61-6). The original Stuart factor has a substitution of methionine for valine at position 104 in the heavy chain. Interestingly, factor X antigen cannot be detected in Stuart plasma. On the other hand, the original patient Prower reportedly had circulating factor X antigen, suggesting that the first two described cases of factor X deficiency were in fact genetically different (229,230).

Factor $X_{Vorarlberg}$ has two single-point mutations resulting in single amino acid substitutions (231). One mutation results in a substitution of a lysine for a glutamic acid at position 14 of the protein. This glutamic acid residue normally undergoes carboxylation of the $\gamma$ carbon after posttranslational modification by vitamin K–dependent carboxylase. The other mutation results in a lysine replacing glutamic acid at position 102. When this family was studied, the severity of the phenotypic coagulation defect correlated with the substitution at position 14. Therefore, the replacement of a $\gamma$-carboxyglutamic acid with a lysine accounts for the factor X clotting defect; the other mutation most likely is a benign polymorphism and has no clinical effect. The family history of patients with factor $X_{Vorarlberg}$ is remarkable for mild bruising. Tooth extraction, an appendectomy, and a hysterectomy have been performed on members of the Vorarlberg kindred without serious bleeding complications. The factor X antigen level in a homozygote is 20% of normal, whereas the clotting activity is 5% of normal. The reason for the decreased antigen is unclear but may be due to decreased synthesis of an aberrant protein, increased

## TABLE 61-6

VARIANTS OF FACTOR X DEFICIENCY

| Variant | Amino acid substitution | Genotype | Factor X:C[a] (percentage of normal) | Factor X:Ag[b] | Bleeding |
|---|---|---|---|---|---|
| Friuli | Pro343 → Ser | Homozygous | 4–9 | 100 | Moderate |
| Ketchikan | Gla14 → Gly | Homozygous | 5–10 | 20 | Mild |
| Leicester | Ile411 → Phe | Homozygous | <1 | 8 | Severe |
| Marseille | Ser334 → Pro | Homozygous | 21–26 | 100 | Asymptomatic |
| Kurayoshi | Arg139 → Ser | Homozygous | 77–90 | 72 | Asymptomatic |
| Roma | Thr318 → Met | Homozygous | 3 | 80 | Moderate |
| Tokyo | Gla32 → Gln | Homozygous | 3 | 61 | Moderate |
| San Antonio | Stop codon 272 Arg366 → Cys | Double heterozygote | 14 | 36 | Severe |
| Santo Domingo | Gly20 → Arg | Homozygous | <1 | <5 | Severe |
| Stuart | Val289 → Met | Homozygous | <1 | <1 | Severe |
| Nagoya 1 | Arg306 → Cys | Homozygous | 3 | <10 | Mild |
| Nagoya 2 | Gly366 → Ser | Heterozygous | 34 | 80 | Mild |
| Vienna | Gly201 → Glu | Homozygous | 1 | 5 | Severe |
| Vorarlberg | Gla14 → Lys | Homozygous | 5 | 20 | Mild |
| Wenatchee I | Arg139 → Cys Asn57 → Thr | Double heterozygote | 10–20 | 30–35 | Mild |
| Wenatchee II | Asn57 → Thr | Heterozygous | 40–72 | 120 | None |
| Unnamed | Glu102 → Lys Gla14 → Lys | Double homozygous | <1 | 20 | None |

[a]Coagulant activity.
[b]Antigen level.

**TABLE 61-7**

TYPICAL LABORATORY DATA IN A PATIENT WITH FACTOR X DEFICIENCY

| Test | Patient | Healthy subject |
|---|---|---|
| Prothrombin time (sec) | 35 | 10.5–13 |
| Activated partial thromboplastin time (sec) | 65 | 27–36 |
| Stypven (Russell viper venom) time (sec) | 50 | 15 |
| Thrombin clotting time (sec) | 12 | 12 |
| Factor X (%) (severe) | <1 | 100 |
| Other clotting assays | Normal | Normal |

intracellular destruction, or decreased secretion. Functional studies in a purified system have shown that factor $X_{Vorarlberg}$ has a defect in calcium binding.

The patient affected with factor $X_{San Antonio}$ appeared to have two distinct mutations at the DNA level, with only one protein species found in the patient's plasma (232). The protein in the patient's plasma corresponded in size to normal factor X. The allele encoding this protein had a DNA base change of C to T, resulting in the production of a factor X variant with an arginine replacing a cysteine at position 326. This substitution in the heavy chain probably results in conformational changes in the catalytic domain, resulting in decreased factor X activity. The second mutation involving a deletion of a cytidine results in a frameshift at amino acid 272 that in turn results in a termination signal. This mutation, presumed to be present on the second allele, was predicted to encode a shortened factor X molecule. It is likely that this protein is either degraded rapidly or not synthesized, because none of this shortened moiety could be detected in the patient's plasma. The affected patient had factor X activity of 14%.

Factor $X_{Santo Domingo}$ is characterized by a mutation in the signal peptide resulting in a severe hemorrhagic disorder (233). The affected patient was homozygous for the mutation and had factor X activity of less than 1%. The mutation, an arginine substituting for a glycine at position 20, was thought to interfere with signal peptide cleavage and function. That function, as in other proteins, is to target the nascent polypeptide to the ER or Golgi apparatus, or both, for further processing and secretion.

Factor $X_{Friuli}$ is a variant with Pro344-Ser transition that results in moderate hemorrhagic symptoms in homozygous patients, with factor X levels that range from 6% to 9% of normal (234–236).

Other factor X variants are listed in Table 61-6 (227,229, 237). Combined factor X and factor VII deficiencies also have been reported, sometimes but not always associated with carotid body tumors (238). A notable association between familial carotid body tumors and factor X deficiency has been reported in four generations of one affected family, with 60 of 242 patients showing mild to moderate factor X deficiency. The relation of this syndrome to inherited factor X deficiency is unknown. Excision of tumors in familial cases of carotid body tumors with factor X deficiency did not result in an increase in factor X activity.

## Clinical Manifestations

Clinical manifestations of factor X deficiency may occur at virtually any age, with more severely affected patients exhibiting more severe hemorrhagic symptoms early in life. Less severely affected patients and "symptomatic" heterozygotes may bleed only after more severe challenge to the hemostatic system, as in a trauma or during surgery. Some cases are discovered incidentally in routine screening or family studies. Bleeding sites vary according to the severity of the deficiency (239). Umbilical stump bleeding may be an early manifestation of factor X deficiency. Soft tissue hemorrhages, including menorrhagia in women, are common in affected patients. Hemarthrosis, exsanguinating postoperative hemorrhage, pseudotumors, and central nervous system hemorrhage have been reported in severely affected patients. Mildly affected patients experience easy bruising and excessive bleeding after trauma or surgery.

## Diagnosis

In general, the diagnosis of congenital factor X deficiency is suggested by an appropriate family history in a situation in which PT and activated PTT are prolonged and acquired causes have been excluded. The Russell viper venom time also is prolonged. However, specific diagnosis rests on a specific assay for factor X. The bleeding time is generally normal, but there are isolated reports of its prolongation in otherwise typical cases. Typical laboratory results are shown in Table 61-7.

The most widely used factor X assay uses human factor X–deficient substrate, to which are added dilutions of normal or test plasmas, and the corrective effect is compared in assays based on either the PT or activated PTT (240).

## Differential Diagnosis

The differentiation of inherited factor X deficiency from acquired deficiency should include consideration of liver disease and vitamin K deficiency (malabsorption, warfarin ingestion, propylthiouracil administration), although these clinical situations generally do not involve isolated factor X deficiency but also deficiency of other vitamin K–dependent clotting factors. One well-documented case of acquired, reversible factor X deficiency occurred in a patient exposed to methylbromide (241). Other causes or associations with isolated factor X deficiency have included upper respiratory infections, viral pneumonias, spindle-cell thymoma, fungicide exposure, renal and adrenal adenocarcinoma, and idiopathic and relapsed acute myeloid leukemia (242–244). Two cases have been described in patients with leprosy in association with an acquired inhibitor (245). Acquired inhibitor antibodies against factor X are uncommon, but several other cases have been reported (246).

The inhibitors are antibodies that neutralize factor X clotting activity. They are detected by demonstrating that patients' plasma prolongs the PT and PTT of normal plasma and by demonstrating a low factor X level by a specific assay (246).

An association of amyloidosis with acquired deficiency of factor X was first reported in 1962, and scattered similar case reports have subsequently appeared, documenting the association and confirming a rapid *in vivo* loss of exogenously administered factor X (247–254). The enhanced disappearance of factor X from the plasma of a patient with amyloidosis has been investigated (248). In this case, immobilization of radio-labeled human and bovine factor X was noted within the vasculature. It also has been pointed out that factor X deficiency is generally associated with amyloidosis of the primary type and that the specific amino acid side chain overlying the pleated sheet conformation could be responsible for distinguishing amyloid fibrils that bind factor X from those that do not (249). Factor X binds directly to amyloid fibrils (250). It is hypothesized that the development of factor X deficiency depends on the affinity of the particular amyloid protein for factor X and the quantity of amyloid directly exposed to the circulating blood.

## Treatment

The need for factor X replacement should naturally be guided by the severity of the hemorrhagic episode. The intravascular half-life of transfused factor X is in the range of 24 to 40 hours (255,256).

Treatment consists of fresh frozen plasma or PCCs. Generally, a factor level of 10% to 40% has been considered adequate for hemostasis. Because of the long biologic half-life of factor X, the level of the factor can be built up in the circulation by infusions of plasma every 12 hours. PCCs containing factor X can be used in patients before surgery or to treat serious bleeding (Table 61-2). These concentrates are treated so as to inactivate transmissible viruses. Because of the risk of thromboembolic phenomena, it is suggested that factor X levels should not exceed 50% of normal.

Treatment of the underlying cause of the amyloidosis has limited usefulness but may result in improvement of the factor X deficiency (253). Splenectomy has been reported to be of some benefit in correcting the factor X deficiency, presumably because the spleen usually acts as a large repository of amyloid material (251). Therapy with plasma products may not be effective in the treatment of acquired factor X deficiency of amyloidosis because the half-life of factor X infused in these patients is extremely short (248). PCCs rich in factor X and recombinant factor VIIa have been helpful in achieving hemostasis during splenectomy.

# CONGENITAL DEFICIENCY OF FACTORS II, VII, IX, AND X

Several reports have described combined congenital deficiencies of factors II, VII, IX, and X, as well as diminished protein C- and S-levels (257–264). The first case was described in a baby girl who had markedly prolonged PT and PTT (100 seconds and 200 seconds, respectively). Initial assays revealed low to undetectable levels of factors II, VII, IX, and X, although there was no evidence of liver disease, malabsorption, or ingestion of coumarin drugs. The patient partially responded to high doses of parenteral vitamin K, but her vitamin K–dependent factors never completely returned to normal. The patient has been followed for many years, during which time her PT has remained in the range of 20 seconds (control of 12 seconds) while taking large doses of oral vitamin K. Withdrawal of vitamin K results in bleeding and marked reduction in circulating levels of the vitamin K–dependent factors. It has been demonstrated that even while the patient is on vitamin K therapy, functional prothrombin activity is 7% of normal, whereas antigenic activity is approximately 50% of normal. At least part of her prothrombin lacks detectable $\gamma$-carboxyglutamic acid residues. The defect in this patient is unclear, but it is now known that the vitamin K–dependent carboxylase enzyme is normal (265). Therefore, it is possible

that the patient has a defective vitamin K reductase enzyme. In the other patients affected with this disorder, bleeding has ranged from mild to severe. A defect in the vitamin K–dependent carboxylase has been reported in one patient with Leu394Arg substitution (265). As yet, no defect in the vitamin K reductase gene has been noted.

Treatment of this deficiency has included large doses of oral vitamin K, which have produced a variable increase in factor levels and decreased bleeding episodes in two patients. In a third patient, vitamin K had no effect, suggesting that this syndrome is heterogeneous (259). Transfusions with normal plasma in one patient produced peak activities and duration in peak levels several times greater than the predicted values (261).

The deficiency of all vitamin K–dependent factors must be differentiated from such conditions as liver disease, malabsorption, and surreptitious ingestion of warfarin or warfarin derivatives. The diagnosis of liver disease and malabsorption is usually suspected on clinical and laboratory grounds. Surreptitious ingestion of warfarin may be much more difficult to detect. Several reports in the literature have appeared describing surreptitious ingestion of "super" warfarins now in use in rat poisons (266). These compounds, brodifacoum and difenacoum, have extremely long half-lives (several days), with clinical effects lasting up to several months. Large doses of vitamin K are needed to reverse their effect. "Super" warfarins are undetectable in routine laboratory assays for warfarin (266).

## References

1. Morawitz P. *The chemistry of blood coagulation*, Translators Hartmann RA, Guenther PF. Springfield, IL: Charles C Thomas Publisher, 1958.
2. Seegers WH, Brinkhous KM, Smith HP, et al. The purification of thrombin. *J Biol Chem* 1938;126:91.
3. Degen SJF, MacGillivray RTA, Davie EW. Characterization of the complementary deoxyribonucleic acid and gene coding for human prothrombin. *Biochemistry* 1983;22:2087.
4. Royale NJ, Irwin DM, Koschinsky ML, et al. Human genes encoding prothrombin and ceruloplasmin map to 11p11q–12 and 3q21–24, respectively. *Somat Cell Mol Genet* 1987;13:285.
5. Degen SJF, Davie EW. Nucleotide sequence of the gene for human prothrombin. *Biochemistry* 1987;26:6165.
6. Degen SJF. Prothrombin. In: High KA, Roberts HR, eds. *Molecular basis of thrombosis and hemostasis*. New York: Marcel Dekker Inc, 1995:75–99.
7. Landwehr G, Lang H, Alexander B. Congenital hypoprothrombinemia: a case study with particular reference to the role of non-prothrombin factors in the conversion of prothrombin. *Am J Med* 1950;8:255.
8. Van Creveld S. Congenital idiopathic hypoprothrombinemia. *Acta Pediat Scan* 1954;100(Suppl. 43):245.
9. Biggs R, Douglas AS. The measurement of prothrombin in plasma: a case of prothrombin deficiency. *J Clin Pathol* 1953;6:15.
10. Quick AJ, Pisciotta AV, Hussey CV. Congenital hypoprothrombinemic states. *Arch Intern Med* 1955;95:2.
11. Borchgrevink CF, Egeberg O, Pool JG, et al. A study of a case of congenital hypoprothrombinemia. *Br J Haematol* 1959;5:294.
12. Pool JG, Desai R, Kropatkin M. Severe congenital hypoprothrombinemia in a Negro boy. *Thromb Diath Haemorrh* 1962;8:235.
13. De Bastos O, Reno RS, Correa OT. A study of three cases of familial congenital hypoprothrombinemia (factor II deficiency). *Thromb Diath Haemorrh* 1964;11:497.
14. Josso F, Prou-Wartelle O, Soulier JP. Itude d'un cas d'hypoprothrombinemie congenitale. *Nouv Rev Fr Hematol* 1962;2:647.
15. Josso F, Lavergne JM, Weilland C, et al. Etude immunologique de la prothrombine et de la thrombine humaines. *Thromb Diath Haemorrh* 1967;18:311.
16. Shapiro SS, Martinez J, Holburn RR. Congenital dysprothrombinemia: an inherited structural disorder of human prothrombin. *J Clin Invest* 1969;48:2251.
17. Lefkowitz JB, Haver T, Clarke S, et al. The prothrombin Denver patient has two different prothrombin point mutations resulting in Glu-300 → Lys and Glu-309 → Lys substitutions. *Br J Haematol* 2000;108:182–187.
18. Josso F, Rio Y, Beguin S. A new variant of human prothrombin: prothrombin Metz demonstration in a family showing double heterozygosity for congenital hypoprothrombinemia and dysprothrombinemia. *Haemostasis* 1982;12:309.
19. Girolami A, Cocheri S, Palareti G, et al. Prothrombin Molise: a "new" congenital dysprothrombinemia, double heterozygosis with an abnormal prothrombin and true prothrombin deficiency. *Blood* 1978;52:115.

20. Rubio R, Almagro D, Cruz A, et al. Prothrombin Habana: a new dysfunctional molecule of human prothrombin associated with a true prothrombin deficiency. *Br J Haematol* 1983;54:553.

21. Valls de Ruiz M, Ruiz-Arguelles A, Ruiz-Arguelles GJ, et al. Prothrombin Mexico City, an asymptomatic autosomal dominant prothrombin variant. *Am J Hematol* 1987;24:229.

22. Lefkowitz JB, Weller A, Nuss R, et al. A common mutation, Arg457 → Gln, links prothrombin deficiencies in the Puerto Rican population. *J Thromb Haemost* 2003;1:2381–2388.

23. Girolami A, Scarano L, Saggiorato G, et al. Congenital deficiencies and abnormalities of prothrombin. *Blood Coagul Fibrinolysis* 1998;9:557–569.

24. Girolami A. The hereditary transmission of congenital "true" hypoprothrombinemia. *Br J Haematol* 1971;21:695.

25. White GC, Shoemaker CB. Factor VIII gene and hemophilia a. *Blood* 1989;73:1.

26. Thompson AR. Structure, function, and molecular defects of factor IX. *Blood* 1986;67:565.

27. Xue J, Wu Q, Westfield LA, et al. Incomplete embryonic lethality and fatal neonatal hemorrhage caused by prothrombin deficiency in mice. *Proc Natl Acad Sci U S A* 1998;95:7603–7607.

28. Sun WY, Witte DP, Degen JL, et al. Prothrombin deficiency results in embryonic and neonatal lethality in mice. *Proc Natl Acad Sci U S A* 1998;95: 7597–7602.

29. Guillin MC, Bezeaud A, Rabiet MJ, et al. Congenitally abnormal prothrombin and thrombin. *Ann N Y Acad Sci* 1986;485:56.

30. Huisse MG, Dreyfus M, Guillin MC. Prothrombin Clamart. Prothrombin variant with defective Arg322-Ile cleavage by factor Xa. *Thromb Haemost* 1985;54:46.

31. Josso F, Monasterio de Sanchez J, Lavergne JM, et al. Congenital abnormality of the prothrombin molecule (factor II) in four siblings: prothrombin Barcelona. *Blood* 1971;38:9.

32. Rabiet MJ, Furie BC, Furie B. Molecular defect of prothrombin Barcelona, substitution of cysteine for arginine at residue 273. *J Biol Chem* 1986;261: 15045.

33. Akhavan S, Mannucci PM, Lak M, et al. Identification and three-dimensional structural analysis of nine novel mutations in patients with prothrombin deficiency. *Thromb Haemost* 2000;84:989–997.

34. Guillin MC, Bezeaud A. Characterization of a variant of human prothrombin: prothrombin Madrid. *Ann N Y Acad Sci* 1981;370:414.

35. Diuguid DL, Rabiet MJ, Furie BC, et al. Molecular defects of factor IX Chicago 2 (Arg145His) and prothrombin Madrid (Arg271 Cys). Arginine mutations that preclude zymogen activation. *Blood* 1989;74:193.

36. Kahn MJP, Gouaerts A. Prothrombin Brussels. A new congenital defective protein. *Thromb Res* 1974;5:141.

37. Miyata T, Morita T, Inomoto T, et al. Prothrombin Tokushima, a replacement of arginine 418 by tryptophan that impairs the fibrinogen clotting activity of derived thrombin Tokushima. *Biochemistry* 1987;26:1118.

38. Akhavan S, Luciani M, Lavoretano S, et al. Phenotypic and genetic analysis of a compound heterozygote for dys- and hypoprothrombinaemia. *Br J Haematol* 2003;120:142–144.

39. Morishita E, Saito M, Kumabashiri I, et al. Prothrombin Himi: a compound heterozygote for two dysfunctional prothrombin molecules (Met-337 → Thr and Arg-388 → His). *Blood* 1992;80:2275–2280.

40. Girolami A, Bareggi G, Brunetti A, et al. Prothrombin Padua: a "new" congenital dysprothrombinemia. *J Lab Clin Med* 1974;84:654.

41. Dumont MD, Tapon-Bretaudiere J, Fischer A-M, et al. Prothrombin Poissy: a new variant of human prothrombin. *Br J Haematol* 1987;66:239.

42. Sekine O, Sugo T, Ebisawa K, et al. Substitution of Gly-548 to Ala in the substrate binding pocket of prothrombin Perija leads to the loss of thrombin proteolytic activity. *Thromb Haemost* 2002;87:282–287.

43. Henriksen RA, Owen WG, Nesheim ME, et al. Identification of a congenital dysthrombin, thrombin quick. *J Clin Invest* 1980;66:934.

44. Henriksen RA, Brotherton AFA. Evidence that activation of platelets and endothelium by thrombin involves distinct sites of interaction: studies with the dysthrombin, thrombin quick I. *J Biol Chem* 1983;258:13717.

45. Henriksen RA, Mann KG. Identification of the primary defect in the dysthrombin quick I: substitution of cysteine for arginine 382. *Biochemistry* 1988;27:9160.

46. Henriksen RA, Mann KG. Substitution of valine for glycine 558 in the congenital dysthrombin thrombin quick II alters primary substrate specificity. *Biochemistry* 1989;28:2078.

47. Miyata T, Aruga R, Umeyama H, et al. Prothrombin Salakta: substitution of glutamic acid-466 by alanine reduces the fibrinogen clotting activity and the esterase activity. *Biochemistry* 1992;31:7457–7462.

48. Akhavan S, Rocha E, Zeinali S, et al. Gly319 → arg substitution in the dysfunctional prothrombin Segovia. *Br J Haematol* 1999;105:667–669.

49. Wang W, Fu Q, Zhou R, et al. Prothrombin Shanghai: hypoprothrombinaemia caused by substitution of Gla29 by Gly. *Haemophilia* 2004;10: 94–97.

50. Rocha E, Paramo JA, Bascones C, et al. Prothrombin Segovia: a new congenital abnormality of prothrombin. *Scand J Haematol* 1986;36:444.

51. Lutze G, Frick U, Topfer G, et al. Hereditaire dysprothrombinie mit geringer blutungsneigung prothrombin magdeburg. *Dtsch Med Wochenschr* 1989; 114:288.

52. Henricksen RA, Durham CK, Miller LD, et al. Prothrombin Greenville, Arg 517 Gln, identified in an individual heterozygous for dysprothrombinemia. *Blood* 1997;91:337.

53. Tamarg H, Sucreg S, Augustin J, et al. Molecular analysis of a compound heterozygote for hypoprothrombinemia and dysprothrombinemia (-G7248-7249) and Arg 340 Trp. *Blood Coagul Fibrinolysis* 1997;8:337.

54. O'Marcaigh AS, Nichols WC, Hassinger NL, et al. Genetic analysis and functional characterization of prothrombin Corpus Christi, Arg 382 Cys, Dhahran Arg271(His) and hypoprothrombinemia. *Blood* 1996;88:2611.

55. Poort SR, Landolfi R, Bertina R. Compound heterozygosity for two novel missense mutations in the prothrombin gene in a patient with a severe bleeding tendency. *Thromb Haemost* 1997;77:610.

56. Leung LLK, Biggs CS. Modulation of thrombin's procoagulant and anticoagulant properties. *Thromb Hemost* 1997;78:577.

57. Fenton JW, Witting JI. Thrombin active-site regions. *Semin Thromb Hemost* 1986;12:200.

58. Krishnaswamy S, Mann KG, Nesheim ME. The prothrombinase-catalyzed activation of prothrombin proceeds through the intermediate meizothrombin in an ordered, sequential reaction. *J Biol Chem* 1986;261:8977.

59. Poort SR, Rosendaal EH, Reitsma PH, et al. A common genetic variation of the 3' untranslated region of the prothrombin gene is associated with elevated plasma prothrombin levels and an increase in venous thrombosis. *Blood* 1996;88:3698.

60. Kyrle PA, Mannhalter C, Beguin S, et al. Clinical studies and thrombin generation in patients homozygous or heterozygous for the G20210A mutation in the prothrombin gene. *Arterioscler Thromb Vasc Biol* 1998;18: 1287–1291.

61. http://archive.uwcm.ac.uk/uwcm/mg/hgmd0.html

62. Roberts HR, Liles D. Deficiencies of the vitamin K-dependent clotting factors. In: Brain MC, Carbone PP, eds. *Current therapy in hematology-oncology*, 5th ed. St Louis, MO: Mosby, 1995:171–176.

63. Bechtold H, Andrassy K, Jahnchen E, et al. Evidence for impaired hepatic vitamin K1 metabolism in patients treated with N-methyl-thiotetrazole cephalosporins. *Thromb Haemost* 1984;51:358–361.

64. Roberts HR, Cederbaum AI. The liver and blood coagulation: physiology and pathology. *Gastroenterology* 1972;63:297–320.

65. Scully MF, Ellis V, Kakkar W, et al. An acquired inhibitor to factor II. *Br J Haematol* 1982;50:655.

66. Lewis RM, Zeitler KD, Blatt PM, et al. Immunology of inhibitors to blood-clotting proteins. In: Rose NR, Friedman H, eds. *Manual of clinical immunology*, 2nd ed. Washington, DC: American Society of Microbiology, 1980.

67. Harrison RL, Alperin JB, Kumar D. Concurrent lupus anticoagulants and prothrombin deficiency due to phenytoin use. *Arch Pathol Lab Med* 1987;111:719.

68. Collazos J, Egurbide MV, Atucha K, et al. Transient acquired factor II deficiency with mycoplasma pneumoniae infection. *J Infect Dis* 1991;164: 434–435.

69. Lee ES, Hibsman BK, Liebman HA. Acquired bleeding disorder in a patient with malignant lymphoma: antibody-mediated prothrombin deficiency. *Cancer* 2001;91:636–641.

70. Erkan D, Bateman H, Lockshin MD. Lupus anticoagulant-hypoprothrombinemia syndrome associated with systemic lupus erythematosus: report of 2 cases and review of literature. *Lupus* 1999;8(7):560–564.

71. Bajaj SP, Rapaport SI, Fierer DS, et al. A mechanism for the hypoprothrombinemia of the acquired hypoprothrombinemia-lupus anticoagulant syndrome. *Blood* 1983;61:684.

72. Bajaj SP, Rapaport SI, Barclay S, et al. Acquired hypoprothrombinemia due to non-neutralizing antibodies to prothrombin. Mechanism and management. *Blood* 1985;65:1538.

73. Amural J, Aronis S, Adamtziki E, et al. Association of lupus anticoagulant with transient antibodies to prothrombin. *Thromb Res* 1997;86:73.

74. Williams S, Linardic C, Wilson O, et al. Acquired hypoprothrombinemia: effects of danazol treatment. *Am J Hematol* 1996;53:272–276.

75. Parry DH, Giddings JC, Bloom AL. Familial haemostatic defect associated with reduced prothrombin consumption. *Br J Haematol* 1980;44: 323.

76. Rocha E, Paramo JA, Cuesta B, et al. Inherited haemorrhagic disease with abnormal prothrombin consumption. *Br J Haematol* 1985;61:177.

77. Robinson AJ, Aggeler PM, McNicol GP, et al. An atypical genetic haemorrhagic disease with increased concentration of a natural inhibitor of prothrombin consumption. *Br J Haematol* 1967;13:510.

78. Vrielink H, Reesink HW. Transfusion-transmissible infections. *Curr Opin Hematol* 1998;5:396–405.

79. Glynn SA, Kleinman SH, Schreiber GB, et al. Retrovirus Epidemiology Donor Study (REDS). Trends in incidence and prevalence of major transfusion-transmissible viral infections in US blood donors, 1991 to 1996. *JAMA* 2000;284:229–235.

80. Blatt PM, Lunblad RL, Kingdon HS, et al. Thrombogenic materials in prothrombin complex concentrates. *Ann Intern Med* 1974;81:766.

81. Kohler M. Thrombogenicity of prothrombin complex concentrates. *Thromb Res* 1999;95(Suppl. 1):S13–S17.

82. Quick AJ. On the constitution of prothrombin. *Am J Physiol* 1943;140: 212.

83. Owren PA. The coagulation of blood. Investigations on a new clotting factor. *Acta Med Scand* 1947;194(Suppl.):1.

84. Owren PA, Cooper T. Parahemophilia. *Arch Intern Med* 1955;95:194.

85. Owren PA. Parahemophilia: hemorrhagic diathesis due to absence of a previously unknown factor. *Lancet* 1947;1:446.

86. Quick AJ, Stefanini M. The concentration of component A in blood, its assay and relation to the labile factor. *J Lab Clin Med* 1949;34:973.

87. Ware AG, Murphy RAC, Seegers WH. The function of AC-globulin in blood clotting. *Science* 1947;106:618.
88. Fantl P, Nance M. Acceleration of thrombin formation by a plasma component. *Nature* 1946;158:708.
89. Dahlback B. Human coagulation factor V purification and thrombin-catalyzed activation. *J Clin Invest* 1980;66:583.
90. Kane WH, Ichinose A, Hagen FS, et al. Cloning of cDNAs coding for the heavy chain region and connecting region of human factor V, a blood coagulation factor with four types of internal repeats. *Biochemistry* 1987;26:6508.
91. Jenny RJ, Pittman DD, Toole JJ, et al. Complete cDNA and derived amino acid sequence of human factor V. *Proc Natl Acad Sci U S A* 1987;84:4846.
92. Rosing J, Tans G. Coagulant factor V: an old star shines again. *Thromb Haemost* 1997;78:427.
93. Ortel TL, Keller FG, Kane WH. Factor V. In: High KA, Roberts HR, eds. *Molecular biology of thrombosis and hemostasis.* New York: Marcel Dekker Inc, 1995:119–146.
94. Colman RW. Factor V. *Prog Hemost Thromb* 1976;3:109.
95. Terheggen HG. Faktor V–mangel bei einem 8 monate alten mdchen. *Monatsschr Kinderheilkd* 1971;119:627.
96. Seeler RA. Parahemophilia. Factor V deficiency. *Med Clin North Am* 1972;56:119.
97. Mammen EF. Factor V deficiency. *Semin Thromb Hemost* 1983;9:17.
98. Fischer RR, Pereira WV, Pereira DV, et al. Inherited factor V deficiency: study of a Brazilian family. *Hum Hered* 1984;34:226.
99. De Vries A, Matoth Y, Shamir Z. Familial congenital labile factor deficiency with syndactylism. *Acta Haematol* 1951;5:129.
100. Peyvandi F, Duga S, Akhavan S, et al. Rare coagulation deficiencies. *Haemophilia* 2002;8:308–321.
101. Feinstein DI, Rapaport SI, McGehee WG, et al. Factor V anticoagulants. Clinical, biochemical and immunological observations. *J Clin Invest* 1970;49:1578.
102. Fratantoni JC, Hilgartner M, Nachman RL. Nature of the defect in congenital factor V deficiency: study in a patient with an acquired circulating anticoagulant. *Blood* 1972;39:751.
103. Giddings JC, Shearn SAM, Bloom AL. The immunological localization of factor V in human tissue. *Br J Haematol* 1975;29:57.
104. Miletich JP, Majerus DW, Majerus PW. Patients with congenital factor V deficiency have decreased factor Xa binding sites on their platelets. *J Clin Invest* 1978;62:824.
105. Tracy PB, Eide LL, Bowie EJW, et al. Radioimmunoassay of factor V in human plasma and platelets. *Blood* 1982;60:59.
106. Chiu HC, Whitaker E, Colman RW. Heterogeneity of human factor V deficiency: evidence for the existence of antigen-positive variants. *J Clin Invest* 1983;72:493.
107. Murray JM, Rand MP, Egen JO, et al. New Brunswick: Ala 221 Val substitution results in reduced cofactor activity. *Blood* 1995;86:1820.
108. Tracy PB, Giles AR, Mann KG, et al. Factor V (Quebec). A bleeding diathesis associated with a qualitative platelet factor V deficiency. *J Clin Invest* 1984;74:1221.
109. Janeway CM, Rwand GE, Tracy PB, et al. Factor V Quebec revisited. *Blood* 1996;87:3571.
110. Yang TL, Cui J, Taylor JM, et al. Rescue of fatal neonatal hemorrhage in factor V deficient mice by low level transgene expression. *Thromb Haemost* 2000;83:70–77.
111. Soff GA, Levin J. Familial multiple coagulation factor deficiencies. I. Review of the literature: differentiation of single hereditary disorders associated with multiple factor deficiencies from coincidental concurrence of single factor deficiency states. *Semin Thromb Hemost* 1981;7:112.
112. Lunghi B, Iacoviello L, Gemmati D, et al. Detection of new polymorphic markers in the factor V gene. Association with factor V levels in plasma. *Thromb Haemost* 1996;75:45.
113. Bertina RM, Koeleman BPC, Koster T, et al. Mutation in blood coagulation factor V associated with activated protein C. *Nature* 1994;369:64.
114. Greengard JS, Sun X, Xu X, et al. Activated protein C resistance caused by a Arg506 Gln mutation in factor Va. *Lancet* 1994;343:1361.
115. Guasch JF, Leusen RP, Bertina RM. Molecular characterization of a type I quantitative factor V deficiency in a thrombosis patient that is "pseudo-homozygous" for activated protein C resistance. *Thromb Haemost* 1997;77:232.
116. Goodnough LT, Saito H, Ratnoff OD. Thrombosis or myocardial infarction in congenital clotting factor abnormalities and chronic thrombocytopenias: a report of 21 patients and a review of 50 previously reported cases. *Medicine* 1983;62:248.
117. Manotti C, Quintavalla R, Pini M, et al. Thromboembolic manifestations and congenital factor V deficiency: a family study. *Haemostasis* 1989;19:331.
118. Tsuda H, Mizuno Y, Hara T, et al. A case of congenital factor V deficiency combined with multiple congenital anomalies: successful management of palatoplasty. *Acta Haematol* 1990;83:49.
119. Chiu HC, Schick P, Colman RW. Biosynthesis of coagulation factor V by megakaryocytes. *J Clin Invest* 1985;75:339.
120. Bode AP, Sandberg H, Dombrose FA, et al. Association of factor V activity with membranous vesicles released from human platelets: requirement for platelet stimulation. *Thromb Res* 1985;39:49.
121. Camire RM, Pollak ES, Kaushansky K, et al. Secretable human platelets-derived factor V originates from the plasma pool. *Blood* 1998;92:3035.
122. Feinstein DI. Acquired inhibitors of factor V. *Thromb Haemost* 1978;39:663.
123. Shapiro SS, Hultin M. Acquired inhibitors to the blood coagulation factors. *Semin Thromb Hemost* 1975;1:366.
124. Hurtubise PE, Coots MC, Jacob DJ, et al. A monoclonal IgG$_4$ (lambda) antibody with factor V inhibitory activity. *J Immunol* 1979;122:2119.
125. Grigg AP, Dauer R, Thurlow PJ. Bleeding due to an acquired inhibitor of platelet associated factor V. *Aust N Z J Med* 1989;19:310.
126. Annamalai A, Rao AK, Chiu HC, et al. Epitope mapping of functional domains of human factor Va with human and murine monoclonal antibodies; evidence for the interaction of the heavy chain with factor Xa and calcium. *Blood* 1987;70:139.
127. Coots MC, Muhleman AF, Glueck HI. Hemorrhagic death associated with a high-titer factor V inhibitor. *Am J Hematol* 1978;4:193.
128. Roberts HR, Sallah S. Immunology of inhibitors to clotting factors with emphasis on factor VIII. In: Silberstein LE, ed. *Autoimmune disorders of blood.* Bethesda, MD: American Association of Blood Banks, 1997:1551.
129. Shanahan F, Aburajab A, Goodacre R, et al. Factor V deficiency and its reversal with gluten restriction in a patient with celiac disease. *Arch Intern Med* 1983;143:2009.
130. Cornett PA, Wold HG, Mansour RP, et al. Acquired factor V deficiency associated with agnogenic myeloid metaplasia: spontaneous increase in factor V activity following splenectomy. *Blood* 1985;66:320a.
131. Gomez P, Phillips W, Cornett P, et al. Factor V deficiency associated with extramedullary hematopoiesis: spontaneous normalization of factor V level following splenectomy. *Blood* 1988;72:297a.
132. Nesheim ME, Nichols WC, Cote TC. Isolation and study of an acquired inhibitor to factor V. *J Clin Invest* 1986;77:405.
133. Ortel TL, Charles LA, Keller FG, et al. Topical thrombin and acquired coagulation factor deficiencies. Clinical spectrum and laboratory diagnosis. *Am J Hematol* 1994;45:128.
134. Streiff MB, Ness PM. Acquired FV inhibitors: a needless iatrogenic complication of bovine thrombin exposure. *Transfusion* 2002;42:18–26.
135. Rush B, Ellis H. The treatment of patients with factor V deficiency. *Thromb Diath Haemorrh* 1965;14:74.
136. Sallah AS, Anchaisuksiri P, Roberts HR. Use of plasma exchange in hereditary deficiency of factor V and factor VIII. *Am J Hematol* 1996;52:229.
137. Webster WP, Roberts HR, Penick GD. Hemostasis in factor V deficiency. *Am J Med Sci* 1964;248:194.
138. Chediak J, Ashenhurst JB, Garlick I, et al. Successful management of bleeding in a patient with factor V inhibitor by platelet transfusions. *Blood* 1980;56:835.
139. Raman B, Batchev C, Shurafa M. Acquired factor V inhibitors showing positive platelet neutralization test and responding to platelet transfusions: report of four cases. *Thromb Haemost* 1995;73:1426.
140. Rotoli B, D'Avino R, Chiurazzi F. Combined factor V and factor VIII deficiency. *Acta Haematol* 1983;69:117.
141. Seligsohn U, Zivelin A, Zwang E. Combined factor V and factor VIII deficiency among non-Ashkenazi Jews. *N Engl J Med* 1982;307:1191.
142. Giddings JC, Seligsohn U, Bloom AL. Immunological studies in combined factor V and factor VIII deficiency. *Br J Haematol* 1977;37:257.
143. Mazzone D, Fichera A, Pratico G, et al. Combined congenital deficiency of factor V and factor VIII. *Acta Haematol* 1982;68:337.
144. Girolami A, Gastaldi G, Patrassi G, et al. Combined congenital deficiency of factor V and factor VIII: a report of a further case with some considerations on the hereditary transmission of this disorder. *Acta Haematol (Basel)* 1976;55:234.
145. Jones JM, Rizza CR, Hardisty RM, et al. Combined deficiency of factor V and factor VIII (antihemophilic globulin): a report of three cases. *Br J Haematol* 1962;8:120.
146. Gobbi F, Ascari E, Barbieri U. Congenital combined deficiency of factor VIII (antihaemophilic globulin) and factor V (proaccelerin) in two siblings. *Thromb Diath Haemorrh* 1967;17:194.
147. Saito H, Shihoa H, Koie K, et al. Congenital combined deficiency of factor V and factor VIII. A case report and the effect of transfusion of normal plasma and hemophilic blood. *Thromb Diath Haemorrh* 1969;22:316.
148. Seligsohn U, Ramot B. Combined factor V and factor VIII deficiency: report of four cases. *Br J Haematol* 1969;16:475.
149. Smit Sibinga CTH, Gokemeyer JDM, ten Kate LP, et al. Combined deficiency of factor V and factor VIII: report of a family and genetic analysis. *Br J Haematol* 1972;23:467.
150. Faioni EM, Fontana G, Carpani G, et al. Review of clinical, biochemical and genetic aspects of combined factor V and factor VIII deficiency, and report of a new affected family. *Thromb Res* 2003;112:269–271.
151. Dansako H, Ishimaru F, Takai Y, et al. Molecular characterization of the ERGIC-53 gene in two Japanese patients with combined factor V-factor VIII deficiency. *Ann Hematol* 2001;80:292–294.
152. Shetty S, Madkaikar M, Nair S, et al. Combined factor V and VIII deficiency in Indian population. *Haemophilia* 2000;6:504–507.
153. Nichols WC, Seligsohn U, Zivelin A, et al. Linkage of combined factors V and VIII deficiency to chromosome 18q by homozygosity mapping. *J Clin Invest* 1997;99:596.
154. Neerman-Arbez M, Antonarakis SE, Blouin JL, et al. The locus for combined factor V-factor VIII deficiency (F5F8D) maps to 18q21, between D18S849 and D18S1103. *Am J Hum Genet* 1997;61:143–150.

155. Cunningham MA, Pipe SW, Zhang B, et al. LMAN1 is a molecular chaperone for the secretion of coagulation factor VIII. *J Thromb Haemost* 2003;1:2360–2367.

156. Moussalli M, Pipe SW, Hauri HP, et al. Mannose-dependent endoplasmic reticulum (ER)-Golgi intermediate compartment-53-mediated ER to Golgi trafficking of coagulation factors V and VIII. *J Biol Chem* 1999; 274: 32539–32542.

157. Neerman-Arbez M, Johnson KM, Morris MA, et al. Molecular analysis of the ERGIC-53 gene in 35 families with combined factor V-factor VIII deficiency. *Blood* 1999;93:2253–2260.

158. Zhang B, Cunningham MA, Nichols WC, et al. Bleeding due to disruption of a cargo-specific ER-to-Golgi transport complex. *Nat Genet* 2003;34: 220–225.

159. Nichols WC, Terry VH, Wheatley MA, et al. ERGIC-53 gene structure and mutation analysis in 19 combined factors V and VIII deficiency families. *Blood* 1999;93:2261–2266.

160. Peyvandi F, Tuddenham EG, Akhtari AM, et al. Bleeding symptoms in 27 Iranian patients with the combined deficiency of factor V and factor VIII. *Br J Haematol* 1998;100:773–776.

161. Fischer RR, Giddings JC, Rosenberg I. Hereditary combined deficiency of clotting factors V and VIII with involvement of von Willebrand factor. *Clin Lab Haematol* 1988;10:53.

162. Akutsu Y, Mori K, Suzuki S, et al. A new disorder characterized by factor V deficiency and molecular abnormality of von Willebrand antigen. *Thromb Haemost* 1987;58:133.

163. Setian N, Tanaka CM, Damiani D, et al. Hypopituitarism, deficiency of factors V and VIII and von Willebrand factor: an uncommon association. *J Pediatr Endocrinol Metab* 2002;15:331–333.

164. Hill FGH, Giddings JC, Williams CE, et al. Combined deficiency of factor V and VIII: study of a family and response to cryoprecipitate and DDAVP infusions including protein C inhibitor measurements. *Thromb Haemost* 1982;50:210.

165. Devecioglu O, Eryilmaz E, Celik D, et al. Circumcision in a combined factor V and factor VIII deficiency using desmopressin (DDAVP). *Turk J Pediatr* 2002;44:146–147.

166. Garcia VV, Silva IA, Borrasca AL. Response of factor VIII/von Willebrand factor to intranasal DDAVP in healthy subjects and mild haemophiliacs (with observations in patients with combined deficiency of factors V and VIII). *Thromb Haemost* 1982;48:91.

167. Chuansumrit A, Mahaphan W, Pintadit P, et al. Combined factor V and factor VIII deficiency with congenital heart disease: response to plasma and DDAVP infusion. *Southeast Asian J Trop Med Public Health* 1994; 25:217–220.

168. Alexander B, Goldstein R, Landwehr G, et al. Congenital SPCA deficiency: a hitherto unrecognized coagulation defect with hemorrhage rectified by serum and serum fractions. *J Clin Invest* 1951;30:596.

169. Miller SP. Congenital deficiency of proconvertin: a clinical and laboratory report. *Blood* 1959;14:1322.

170. Hougie C, Barrow EM, Graham JB. Stuart clotting defect. I. Segregation of an hereditary hemorrhagic state from the heterogeneous group heretofore called "stable factor" (SPCA, proconvertin, factor VII) deficiency. *J Clin Invest* 1957;36:485.

171. Hagen FS, Gray CL, O'Hara P, et al. Characterization of a cDNA coding for human factor VII. *Proc Natl Acad Sci U S A* 1986;83:2412.

172. Pfeiffer RA, Ott R, Gilgenkrantz S, et al. Deficiency of coagulation factors VII and X associated with deletion of a chromosome 13(q34): evidence from two cases with 46,XY,t(13;Y)(q11;q34). *Hum Genet* 1982;58:358.

173. de Grouchy J, Dautzenberg M-D, Turleau C, et al. Regional mapping of clotting factors VII and X to 13q34: expression of factor VII through chromosome 8. *Hum Genet* 1984;66:230.

174. Petersen LC, Wildgoose P, Hedner U. Factor VII. In: High KA, Roberts HR, eds. *Molecular basis of thrombosis and hemostasis*. New York: Marcel Dekker Inc, 1995:147–165.

175. Mackman N. Role of tissue factor in hemostasis, thrombosis, and vascular development. *Arterioscler Thromb Vasc Biol* 2004;24:1015–1022.

176. Østerud B. Factor VII and hemostasis. *Blood Coagul Fibrinolysis* 1990; 1:175.

177. Davie EW, Fujikawa K, Kisiel W. The coagulation cascade, initiation, maintenance, and regulation. *Biochemistry* 1990;36:10363.

178. Broze GJ. Tissue factor pathway inhibitor and a revised hypothesis of blood coagulation. *Trends Cardiovasc Med* 1992;2:72.

179. Rapaport SI, Rao LVM. Initiation and regulation of tissue factor dependent coagulation. *Arterioscler Thromb* 1992;12:111.

180. Giesen PL, Nemerson Y. Tissue factor on the loose. *Semin Thromb Hemost* 2000;26:379–384.

181. Hoffman M, Monroe DM, Oliver JA, et al. Factor IXa and Xa play distinct roles in tissue factor dependent initiation of coagulation. *Blood* 1995;86:1794.

182. Novotny WF, Girard TJ, Miletich JP, et al. Purification and characterization of the lipoprotein-associated coagulation inhibitor from human plasma. *J Biol Chem* 1989;264:18832.

183. Rapaport SI. Inhibition of factor VIIa/tissue factor-induced blood coagulation, with particular emphasis upon a factor Xa-dependent inhibitory mechanism. *Blood* 1989;73:359.

184. Perry DJ. Factor VII deficiency. *Br J Haematol* 2002;118:689–700.

185. Mannucci PM, Duga S, Peyvandi F. Recessively inherited coagulation disorders. *Blood* 2004;104(5):1243–1252.

186. McVey JH, Boswell E, Mumford AD, et al. Factor VII deficiency and the FVII mutation database. *Hum Mutat* 2001;17:3–17.

187. http://europium.csc.mrc.ac.uk, Accessed June 6, 2004.

188. Herrmann FH, Wulff K, Auberger K, et al. Molecular biology and clinical manifestation of hereditary factor VII deficiency. *Semin Thromb Hemost* 2000;26:393–400.

189. Wulff K, Herrmann FH. Twenty two novel mutations of the factor VII gene in factor VII deficiency. *Hum Mutat* 2000;15:489–496.

190. Seligsohn U, Shani M, Ramot B, et al. Hereditary deficiency of blood clotting factor VII and Dubin-Johnson syndrome in an Israeli family. *Isr J Med Sci* 1959;5:1060.

191. Levanon M, Rimon S, Shani M, et al. Active and inactive factor VII in Dubin-Johnson syndrome with factor VII deficiency, hereditary factor VII deficiency, and coumadin administration. *Br J Haematol* 1972;23:669.

192. Seligsohn U, Shani M, Ramot B. Gilbert syndrome and factor VII deficiency. *Lancet* 1970;1:1398.

193. Bell WH, Alton HG. Christmas disease associated with factor VII deficiency. Case report with family survey. *Br Med J* 1955;1:330.

194. Girolami A, Sticchi A, Burul A, et al. An immunological investigation of hemophilia B with a tentative classification of the disease into five variants. *Vox Sang* 1977;32:230.

195. Verstraete M, Vermylen J, Vandenbroucke J. Hemophilia B associated with a decreased factor VII activity. *Am J Med Sci* 1962;243:20.

196. Kasper C, Østerud B, Minami J, et al. Hemophilia B: characterization of genetic variants and detection of carriers. *Blood* 1977;50:351.

197. Takeuchi Y, Saito Y, Ikenouchi H, et al. Combined factor VII and protein C deficiency found in a patient with peripheral pulmonary artery stenosis accompanied by progressive pulmonary hypertension and hemoptysis. *Thromb Res* 1988;51:117.

198. Ragni MV, Lewis JH, Spero JA, et al. Factor VII deficiency. *Am J Hematol* 1981;10:79.

199. Giansily-Blaizot M, Biron-Andreani C, Aguilar-Martinez P, et al. Inherited factor VII deficiency and surgery: clinical data are the best criteria to predict the risk of bleeding. *Br J Haematol* 2002;117:172–175.

200. Mariani G, Herrmann FH, Schulman S, et al. International Factor VII Deficiency Study Group. Thrombosis in inherited factor VII deficiency. *J Thromb Haemost* 2003;1:2153–2158.

201. Escobar M, Ulmasov B, Kuppuswamy MN, et al. Congenital factor VII deficiency and thrombosis. Description of a novel mutation. *J Thromb-Haemost* 2003;(Suppl. 1), P1178.

202. Zacharski LR, Delprete SA, Kisiel W, et al. Atherosclerosis and coronary bypass surgery in hereditary factor VII deficiency. *Am J Med* 1988; 84:955.

203. Meade TW, Brozovic M, Chakrabarti RR, et al. Haemostatic function and ischaemic heart disease. Principal results of the Northwick Park Heart Study. *Lancet* 1986;II:533.

204. Hoffman CJ, Miller RH, Lawson WE, et al. Elevation of factor VII activity and mass in young adults at risk of ischemic heart disease. *J Am Coll Cardiol* 1989;14:941.

205. Doggen CJ, Manger Cats V, Bertina RM, et al. A genetic propensity to high factor VII is not associated with the risk of myocardial infarction in men. *Thromb Haemost* 1998;80:281–285.

206. Delmer A, Horellou MH, Andreau G, et al. Life-threatening intracranial bleeding associated with the presence of an antifactor VII autoantibody. *Blood* 1989;74:229.

207. Campbell E, Sanal S, Mattson J, et al. Factor VII inhibitor. *Am J Med* 1980;68:962.

208. Brunod M, Chatot-Henry C, Mehdaoui H, et al. Acquired anti-factor VII (proconvertin) inhibitor: hemorrhage and thrombosis. *Thromb Haemost* 1998;79:1065–1066.

209. Okajima K, Ishii M. Life-threatening bleeding in a case of autoantibody-induced factor VII deficiency. *Int J Hematol* 1999;69:129–132.

210. Aguilar C, Lucia JF, Hernandez P. A case of an inhibitor autoantibody to coagulation factor VII. *Haemophilia* 2003;9:119–120.

211. Weisdorf D, Hasegawa D, Fair DS. Acquired factor VII deficiency associated with aplastic anaemia: correction with bone marrow transplantation. *Br J Haematol* 1989;71:409.

212. Elezovic I, Djukanovic R, Rolovic Z. Successful treatment of hemorrhagic syndrome due to an acquired, combined deficiency of factors VII and X in a patient with multiple myeloma and amyloidosis. *Eur J Haematol* 1989; 42:105.

213. Palareti G, Coccheri S. Lowered antithrombin III activity and other clotting changes in homocystinuria: effects of a pyridoxine- folate regimen. *Haemostasis* 1989;19(Suppl. 1):24.

214. Wildgoose P, Nemerson Y, Hansen LL, et al. Measurement of basal levels of factor VIIa in hemophilia A and B patients. *Blood* 1992;80:25–28.

215. Greene WB, McMillan CW. Surgery for scoliosis in congenital factor VII deficiency. *Am J Dis Child* 1982;136:411.

216. Mariani G, Testa MG, Di Paolantonio T, et al. Use of recombinant, activated factor VII in the treatment of congenital factor VII deficiencies. *Vox Sang* 1999;77:131–136.

217. Hunault M, Bauer KA. Recombinant factor VIIa for the treatment of congenital factor VII deficiency. *Semin Thromb Hemost* 2000;26:401–405.

218. Nicolaisen EM. Antigenicity of activated recombinant factor VII followed through nine years of clinical experience. *Blood Coagul Fibrinolysis* 1998; 9(Suppl. 1):S119–S123.

219. Milstone JH. Thrombokinase as a prime activator of prothrombin: historical perspectives and present status. *Fed Proc* 1964;23:742.

220. Duckert F, Flükiger P, Matter M, et al. Clotting factor X. Physiologic and physiochemical properties. *Proc Soc Exp Biol Med* 1955;90:17.

221. Telfer TP, Denson KW, Wright DR. A "new" coagulation defect. *Br J Haematol* 1956;2:308.

222. Scambler PJ, Williamson R. The structural gene for human coagulation factor X is located on chromosome 13q34. *Cytogenet Cell Genet* 1985; 39:231.

223. Leytus SP, Foster DC, Kurachi K, et al. Gene for human factor X. A blood coagulation factor whose gene organization is essentially identical with that of factor IX and protein C. *Biochemistry* 1986;25:5098.

224. Leytus S, Chung DW, Kisiel W, et al. Characterization of a cDNA coding for human factor X. *Proc Natl Acad Sci U S A* 1984;81:3699.

225. Lechler E, Webster WP, Roberts HR, et al. The inheritance of Stuart disease: investigation of a family with factor X deficiency. *Am J Med Sci* 1965;249:191.

226. Uprichard J, Perry DJ. Factor X deficiency. *Blood Rev* 2002;16:97–110.

227. Peyvandi F, Menegatti M, Santagostino E, et al. Gene mutations and three-dimensional structural analysis in 13 families with severe factor X deficiency. *Br J Haematol* 2002;117:685–692.

228. Perry DJ. Factor X and its deficiency states. *Haemophilia* 1997; 3:159–172.

229. Cooper DN, Millar DS, Wacey A, et al. Inherited factor X deficiency: molecular genetics and pathophysiology. *Thromb Haemost* 1997;78:161.

230. Girolami A. Tentative and updated classification of factor X variants. *Acta Haematol* 1986;75:58.

231. Watzke HH, Lechner K, Roberts HR, et al. Molecular defect (Gla14 to Lys) and its functional consequences in a hereditary factor X deficiency (factor X "Vorarlberg"). *J Biol Chem* 1990;265:11980.

232. Reddy S, Zhou ZQ, Rao KJ, et al. Molecular characterization of human factor X San Antonio. *Blood* 1989;74:1486.

233. Watzke HH, Wallmark A, Hamaguchi N, et al. Factor X Santo Domingo: evidence that the severe clinical phenotype arises from a mutation blocking secretion. *J Clin Invest* 1991;88:1685.

234. Girolami A, Brunetti A, Bareggi G, et al. Abnormal factor X (factor X Friuli) coagulation disorder, the heterozygote population: a study of 57 subjects. *Acta Haematol* 1974;51:40.

235. Girolami A, Molaro G, Lazzarini M, et al. A "new" congenital haemorrhagic condition due to the presence of an abnormal factor X (factor X Friuli). Study of a large kindred. *Br J Haematol* 1970;19:179.

236. Fair DS, Revak DJ, Hubbard JG, et al. Isolation and characterization of the factor X Friuli variant. *Blood* 1989;73:2108.

237. Watzke HH, High KA, Factor X. In: High KA, Roberts HR, eds. *Molecular basis of thrombosis and hemostasis*. New York: Marcel Dekker Inc, 1995:239–255.

238. Kroll AJ, Alexander B, Cochizo F, et al. Hereditary deficiencies of clotting factors VII and X associated with carotid body tumors. *N Engl J Med* 1964;270:6.

239. Peyvandi F, Mannucci PM, Lak M, et al. Congenital factor X deficiency: spectrum of bleeding symptoms in 32 Iranian patients. *Br J Haematol* 1998;102:626–628.

240. Fair DS, Edgington TS. Heterogeneity of hereditary and acquired factor X deficiency by combined immunochemical and functional analyses. *Br J Haematol* 1985;59:235.

241. Graham JB, Barrow EM, Wynne TR. Stuart clotting defect III: an acquired case with complete recovery. In: Brinkhous KM, ed. *Hemophilia and other hemorrhagic states*. Chapel Hill, NC: University of North Carolina Press, 1958.

242. Nora RE, Bell WR, Noe DA, et al. Novel factor X deficiency. Normal partial thromboplastin time and associated spindle cell thymoma. *Am J Med* 1985;79:122.

243. Henson K, Files JC, Morrison FS. Transient acquired factor X deficiency. Report of the use of activated clotting concentrate to control a life-threatening hemorrhage. *Am J Med* 1989;87:583.

244. Carter C, Winfield DA. Factor X deficiency during treatment of relapsed acute myeloid leukaemia with amsacrine. *Clin Lab Haematol* 1988; 10:225.

245. Ness PM, Hymes PG, Gesme D, et al. An unusual factor X inhibitor in leprosy. *Am J Hematol* 1980;8:397.

246. Smith SV, Liles DK, White GC II, et al. Successful treatment of transient acquired factor X deficiency by plasmapheresis with concomitant intravenous immunoglobulin and steroid therapy. *Am J Hematol* 1998;57:245.

247. Korsan-Bengtsen L, Hjort PF, Ygge J. Acquired factor X deficiency in a patient with amyloidosis. *Thromb Diath Haemorrh* 1962;7:558.

248. Furie B, Greene E, Furie BC. Syndrome of acquired factor X deficiency and systemic amyloidosis: *in vivo* studies of the metabolic fate of factor X. *N Engl J Med* 1977;297:81.

249. Glenner G. Factor X deficiency and systemic amyloidosis. *N Engl J Med* 1977;297:108.

250. Furie B, Voo L, McAdam K, et al. Mechanism of factor X deficiency in systemic amyloidosis. *N Engl J Med* 1981;304:827.

251. Roberts HR, Lechler E, Webster WP, et al. Survival of transfused factor X in patients with Stuart disease. *Thromb Diath Haemorrh* 1965;18:305.

252. Mumford AD, O'Donnell J, Gillmore JD, et al. Bleeding symptoms and co-agulation abnormalities in 337 patients with AL-amyloidosis. *Br J Haematol* 2000;110:454–460.

253. Choufani EB, Sanchorawala V, Ernst T, et al. Acquired factor X deficiency in patients with amyloid light-chain amyloidosis: incidence, bleeding manifestations, and response to high-dose chemotherapy. *Blood* 2001;97: 1885–1887.

254. Glaspy JA. Hemostatic abnormalities in multiple myeloma and related disorders. *Hematol Oncol Clin North Am* 1992;6:1301–1314.

255. Bohrer H, Waldherr R, Martin E, et al. Splenectomy in an arsenic patient with acquired factor X deficiency due to AL-amyloidosis. *Nephrol Dial Transplant* 1998;13:190.

256. Biggs R, Denson KWE. The fate of prothrombin and factors VII, IX, and X transfused to patients deficient in these factors. *Br J Haematol* 1963; 9:532.

257. McMillan CW, Roberts HR. Congenital combined deficiency of coagulation factors II, VII, IX, and X. *N Engl J Med* 1966;274:1313.

258. Chung KS, Bezeaud A, Goldsmith JC, et al. Congenital deficiency of blood clotting factors II, VII, IX, and X. *Blood* 1979;53:776.

259. Johnson CA, Chung KS, McGrath KM, et al. Characterization of a variant prothrombin in a patient congenitally deficient in factors II, VII, IX, and X. *Br J Haematol* 1980;44:461.

260. Samama M, Bertina RM, Conard J, et al. Combined congenital deficiency in protein C and in factors II, VII, IX, and X. *Thromb Haemost* 1983;50:359.

261. Goldsmith GH, Pence RE, Ratnoff OD, et al. Studies on a family with combined deficiencies of vitamin K–dependent coagulation factors. *J Clin Invest* 1982;69:1253.

262. Soff GA, Levin J. Familial multiple coagulation deficiencies. Combined factor II, VII, IX, and X deficiency. *Semin Thromb Hemost* 1981;7:133.

263. Vincente V, Maia R, Alberca I, et al. Congenital deficiency of vitamin K–dependent coagulation factors and protein C. *Thromb Haemost* 1984; 51:343.

264. Bergmann F, Losoya G, Chediak J. Acquired prothrombin complex deficiency requiring high doses of vitamin K. *Blood* 1988;72: 290a.

265. Wu SM, Stanley TB, Mutucumarana P, et al. Characterization of gamma-glutamyl carboxylase. *Thromb Haemost* 1997;78:599.

266. Felice LJ, Murphy MJ. The determination of the anticoagulant rodenticide brodifacoum in blood serum by liquid chromatography with fluorescence detection. *J Anal Toxicol* 1989;13:229.

# CHAPTER 62 ■ AFIBRINOGENEMIAS AND DYSFIBRINOGENEMIAS

JENNIFER L. MOEN AND SUSAN T. LORD

Fibrinogen is a central participant in hemostasis; consequently, the absence of fibrinogen or alterations in the fibrinogen molecule can lead to aberrant coagulation. Both inherited and acquired disorders of fibrinogen have been described; this chapter reviews the molecular alterations found in the inherited defects. The inherited disorders fall into two categories: afibrinogenemias and dysfibrinogenemias. Individuals with afibrinogenemias have no fibrinogen in the circulation. These individuals are commonly identified at or shortly after birth, when significant bleeding events are manifest. The diagnoses are based on coagulation tests that show indefinitely prolonged bleeding times and undetectable fibrinogen antigen, usually less than 10 $\mu$g per mL. Individuals with dysfibrinogenemias have normal levels of fibrinogen (i.e., 1.5 to 4.0 mg per mL), with abnormal fibrinogen molecules in the circulation. Individuals with dysfibrinogenemias show a heterogeneous clinical presentation: Approximately half of them are asymptomatic, one fourth are associated with thrombotic events, and one fourth are associated with bleeding events. Most diagnoses are based on prolonged clotting times or abnormal fibrinogen levels, which are measured by a functional assay, and normal fibrinogen antigen levels. Individuals with reduced antigen levels and variant fibrinogen molecules in the circulation have a subcategory of dysfibrinogenemias, called *hypodysfibrinogenemias*. These individuals have clinical presentations similar to those for dysfibrinogens, with diagnoses based on prolonged clotting times and reduced levels of fibrinogen antigen. Individuals with reduced antigen levels and only normal fibrinogen molecules in the circulation have a subcategory of afibrinogenemias, called *hypofibrinogenemias*. These individuals are often asymptomatic, although several patients have been identified with hepatic fibrinogen storage and liver disease (1).

Inherited fibrinogen disorders were first identified by analysis of the plasma protein. The first afibrinogenemia to be identified was described by Rabe and Salomon in 1920 (2), although the molecular etiology of this disease was unknown. The first defect to be identified as a cause of dysfibrinogenemia was determined by Mammen et al. in 1969 (3); they identified the homozygous substitution of A$\alpha$ Arg19 with Ser by protein sequence analysis. More recently, genetic techniques have been used to identify these disorders, the first of which was dysfibrinogen Vlissingen, described by Koopman et al. in 1991 (4). With the advances in mass spectrometry, it is now relatively straightforward to corroborate expression of the variant fibrinogen identified by genetic techniques. Most recently, genetic techniques have enabled identification of the precise defects responsible for afibrinogenemias. The first case, described by Neerman-Arbez et al. in 1999, identified an 11-kb deletion in the FGA gene that eliminated synthesis of the A$\alpha$ chain (5). Subsequent studies have identified more than 30 novel mutations associated with afibrinogenemia and more than 300 novel mutations associated with dysfibrinogenemia. These genetic defects and their associated phenotypic effects are summarized here.

Fibrinogen is encoded by three genes found in a 50-kb cluster on chromosome 4 (q28). The genes, FGA, FGB, and FGG, encode three polypeptide chains, A$\alpha$, B$\beta$, and $\gamma$, respectively. Transcription of the genes is coordinately regulated and occurs predominantly in hepatocytes, where fibrinogen messages represent approximately 3% of the total mRNA. Translation occurs in the rough endoplasmic reticulum, where the three polypeptides are assembled into a dimer of six chains linked by 17 intrachain disulfide bonds. Two alternatively spliced messages lead to the synthesis of minor amounts of alternate polypeptides, $\gamma'$ and $\alpha_E$, which make up 10% and 2% of the population of each chain, respectively. Mutations have been identified in all three genes. The synthesis of fibrinogen and its structure and functions are described in detail in Chapter 16.

## AFIBRINOGENEMIAS

Inherited afibrinogenemia is a rare autosomal recessive disorder, with an estimated prevalence of 1:1,000,000 (6). Because individuals must have two affected alleles, either homozygous or compound heterozygous, to manifest this defect; the allelic frequency of causative mutations is approximately 1:1,000. This allelic frequency is approximately tenfold higher than the allelic frequency of causative mutations in the X-linked F8C gene that leads to the well-known bleeding disorder hemophilia A. From this data, we deduce that in men the prevalence of hemophilia A (approximately 1:10,000) is much greater than that of afibrinogenemia, while in women the prevalence of afibrinogenemia likely exceeds that of hemophilia A. Therefore, afibrinogenemia is rare because it is autosomal recessive, rather than because the mutations are unusually rare. As with other recessive diseases, afibrinogenemia often arises from consanguineous marriages. In the 5 years since the first report in 1999, more than 30 novel mutations have been identified as causative for afibrinogenemia.

Causative mutations have been identified in all three genes, with changes in FGA being the most frequent. Many of these are described in a recent review (6). Afibrinogenemias have not been associated with defects in the promoter regions of the three genes, or in the regulatory molecules that control expression of these three genes, or in the proteins that are necessary for the proper assembly and secretion of fibrinogen. The nature of the causative mutations is diverse, including two large deletions (i.e., 11 and 1.2 kb), seven small deletions (1 or 2 bp), two single base insertions, eleven nonsense substitutions, four missense substitutions, and eight mutations that could cause aberrant splicing. Because liver biopsies of patients are rarely performed, alternative splicing associated with mutations in splice-sites has not been directly confirmed. In several cases, however, expression of mutant genes has been compared to expression of the normal gene in transfected cultured cells and aberrant splicing was detected (6,7). Transfection studies have also shown that the outcome of

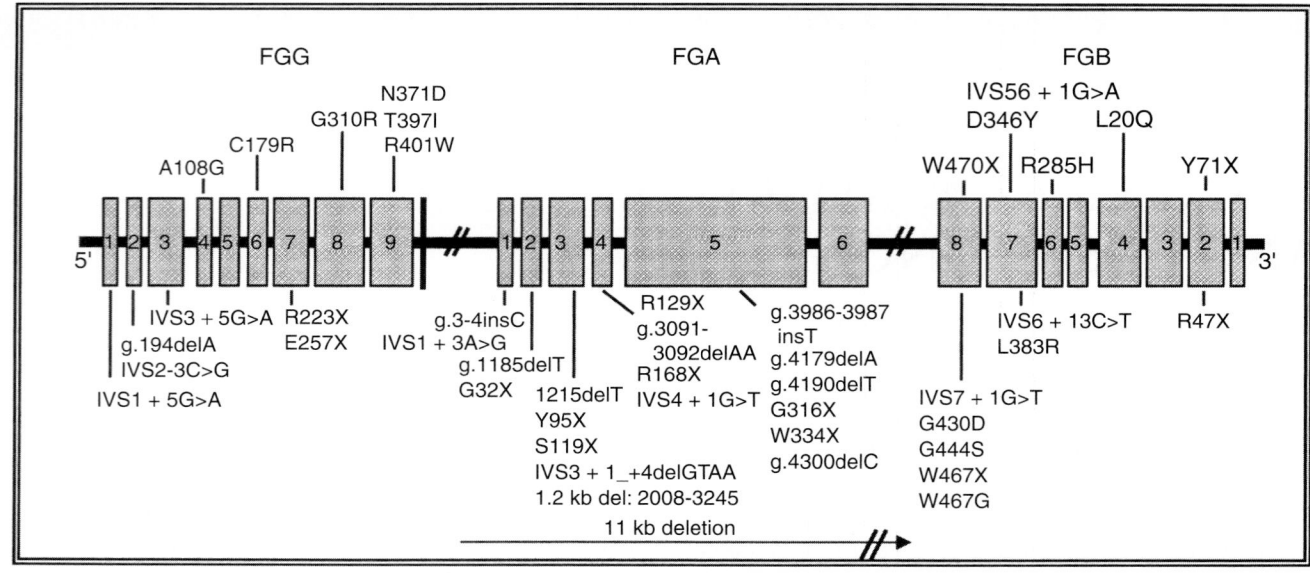

**FIGURE 62-1.** Schematic of genes encoding for the fibrinogen chains, Aα (FGA), Bβ (FGB), and γ (FGG). Mutations resulting in afibrinogenemia are listed below the gene, whereas hypofibrinogens are listed above the gene. Exons are in *gray* and are approximately to scale, and introns are represented by the *black line* and are not to scale.[1]

splice-site mutations varies with the order of splicing events and that in FGA intron 3 was spliced first, followed by intron 2, intron 4, and intron 1 (8). Except for the four missense substitutions, all these mutations lead to premature termination and, therefore, encode shorter polypeptide chains, which, by definition, are not found in circulation. The schematic shown in Figure 62-1 indicates the locations of these mutations; the specific mutations are listed in Table 62-1.

## Deletions

The first reported causative genetic defect was a homozygous 11-kb deletion from a breakpoint within FGA intron 1 to a breakpoint within the FGA-FGB intragenic region (Fig. 62-1) (5). This deletion eliminates most of the FGA gene, with the loss of the Aα polypeptide and the absence of fibrinogen in the circulation. It is remarkable that the first causative mutation discovered in humans is analogous to the earlier targeted disruption of the mouse FGA gene (9). The targeted gene was transmitted with a normal Mendelian pattern, and the mice had no circulating fibrinogen. Therefore, when the FGA deletion was discovered in humans, it was not surprising that this defect would cause afibrinogenemia. This deletion has been found in multiple unrelated individuals on multiple haplotypes, as expected for a relatively common recurrent mutation (6).

Subsequently, several deletions have been identified in the FGA gene. Another large 1238-bp deletion begins at a breakpoint in intron 3 and ends at a breakpoint in intron 4 (2008-3245del[1]) (10). This deletion was found in a 14-day-old Japanese infant with umbilical bleeding. Although the parents

were not related, both were heterozygous for the same deletion. Nevertheless, plasma fibrinogen levels in the parents were normal (1.9 to 2.0 mg per mL), whereas the level in the patient was less than 0.1 mg per mL. Synthesis of a normal mRNA from this deleted gene was not examined. Assuming exon 3 would be joined to exon 5, the resulting frameshift would produce a truncated 13.4-kDa Aα chain; such a truncated protein was not detected by immunoblot analysis of the patient's or his parents' plasmas.

A 2-bp deletion in FGA has been found in three patients, two that are compound heterozygotes and one that likely is a homozygote because his parents are related. This deletion in exon 4, g.3091-3092delAA, causes a frameshift, with a stop codon that is 15 codons downstream in the same exon. Single-base deletions have been found in exon 2 (g.1185delT), exon 3 (1215delT), and exon 5 (g.4179delA, g.4190delT, and g.4300delC) in FGA and exon 2 (g.194delA) in FGG. All these result in a frameshift, with stop codons encoded within the same exon (6,7). Interestingly, the FGA deletions g.4179delA and g.4190delT lead to the same frameshift, encoding long polypeptide additions of 108 and 104 amino acids, with the last 102 being the same (6,11).

## Insertions

Two single-base insertions have been identified, in exons 1 and 5 of FGA. The insertion in exon 1, g.3-4insC, results in an in-frame stop codon in exon 2. This mutation occurred in a compound heterozygous individual, in conjunction with the 2-bp deletion, g.3091- 3092delAA, in FGA (6). The insertion in exon 5, g.3986-3987insT, changed the Phe codon AAG to the stop codon TAA (12).

## Nonsense Mutations

Nonsense mutations have been identified in all three genes, 7 in FGA, 2 in FGB, and 2 in FGG. Mutations in FGA exon 3 (Y95X

---

[1]Mutations denoted by g.XXX are numbered with the A in ATG as nt #1; mutations without the g. are numbered according to GenBank #M64982 for FGA, #M64983 for FGB, and #M10014 for FGG. Nonsense and missense mutations are numbered by the amino acid, and include the signal sequences of 19 for Aα, 30 for Bβ, and 26 for γ.

TABLE 62-1

## REPORTED MUTATIONS RESULTING IN AFIBRINOGENEMIA OR HYPOFIBRINOGENEMIA

| Mutation Gene | Protein | | Genotype | | | | Clinical presentation | | | Hypo | Reference |
|---|---|---|---|---|---|---|---|---|---|---|---|
| | Native | Mature | Type | Ho | Ht | As | Th | Bl | Afb | | |
| **A. MUTATIONS IN FGA** | | | | | | | | | | | |
| 34insC (g.3-4insC) | | | INS | | X | | | X | X | | 13 |
| 11-kb deletion | | | DEL | X | X | | | X | X | | 14 |
| IVS1+3A → G | | | SS | | X | | | X | X | | 6 |
| g.1185delT | | | DEL | | X | | | X | X | | 6 |
| 1193G → T | G32X | G13X | NS | | X | | | X | X | | 7 |
| 1215delT | | | DEL | | X | | | X | X | | 7 |
| nr | Y95X | Y76X | NS | X | | | | X | X | | 15 |
| 1914C → G | S119X | S100X | NS | X | | | | X | X | | 7 |
| 2008-3245del (1.2-kb deletion) | | | DEL | X | | | | X | X | | 10 |
| IVS3+1_+4delGTAA | | | SS | X | | | | X | X | | 6 |
| 3075C → T | R129X | R110X | NS | X | | X | | X | X | | 7 |
| g.3091-3092delAA (3121delAA) | | K125X | DEL | X | X | | | X | X | | 9,16 |
| 3192C → T | R168X | R149X | NS | X | | | | X | X | | 6,7,17 |
| IVS4+1G → T | | | SS | X | X | | | X | X | | 9 |
| g.3986-3987insT | | | INS | X | | | | X | X | | 12 |
| g.4179delA; 4209delA | | | DEL | | X | | | X | X | | 11,15 |
| g.4190delT; 4220delT | | | DEL | X | | | | X | X | | 11,15 |
| nr | G316X | G297X | NS | | X | | | X | X | | 13 |
| nr | W334X | W315X | NS | | X | | | X | X | | 13 |
| g.4300delC (4329delC) | | | DEL | | X | | | X | X | | 13 |
| **B. MUTATIONS IN FGB** | | | | | | | | | | | |
| 3282C → T | R47X | R17X | NS | X | | | | X | X | | 11 |
| 3356T → G | Y71X | Y41X | NS | | X | X | | | | X | 18 |
| 5157T → A | L202Q | L172Q w/R17X | MS/NS | | X | | | X | | X | 19 |
| 6654G → A | R285H | R255H w/K148N | MS/MS | | X | | | X | | X | 20 |
| IVS6+13C → T | | | SS | X | | | | X | X | | 21 |
| IVS6+1G → A | | | SS | | X | X | | | | X | 22 |
| nr | D346Y | D316Y | MS | | X | | | X | | X | 23 |
| 7156T → G | L383R | L353R | MS | X | | | | X | X | | 24 |
| IVS7+1G → T | | | SS | X | | | | | X | | 21 |
| 7915G → A | G430D | G400D | MS | X | | | | X | X | | 24 |
| nr | G444S | G414S | MS | | X | | X | X | X | | 25 |
| nr | W467X | W437X | NS | | X | | | X | X | | 26 |
| 8025T → G | W467G | W437G | MS | X | | | | X | X | | 27 |
| 8035G → A | W470X | W440X | NS | | X | X | | | | X | 28 |
| **C. MUTATIONS IN FGG** | | | | | | | | | | | |
| g.194delA | | | DEL | X | | | | X | X | | 6 |
| IVS1+5G → A | | | SS | X | | | | X | X | | 29 |
| IVS2-3C → G | | | SS | X | | | | X | X | | 15 |
| IVS3+5G → A | | | SS | X | | | | X | X | | 30 |
| 2525C → G | A108G | A82G | MS | | X | | | X | | X | 31,32 |
| 2900T → C | C179R | C153R | MS | | X | X | | X | | X | 33 |
| nr | R223X | R197X | NS | X | | | | X | X | | 15 |
| 5860G → T | R257X | R231X | NS | X | | | | X | X | | 34 |
| nr | G310R | G284R | MS | | X | * | | | | X | 35 |
| 7685A → G | N371D | N345D | MS | | X | X | | | | X | 36 |
| 9502C → T | T397I | T371I | MS | | X | | | X | | X | 37 |
| nr | R401W | R375W | MS | | X | * | | | | X | 38 |

Mutations are ordered from 5' to 3' and those denoted by g.XXX are numbered with the A in ATG as nt #1; mutations without the g., are numbered according to GenBank #M64982 for FGA, #M64983 for FGB, and #M10014 for FGG; nr, not reported. Nonsense and missense mutations are numbered by the amino acid, and native numbers include the signal sequences of 19 for Aα, 30 for Bβ and 26 for γ; the numbers for the mature protein correspond to locations in the circulating molecule, if they were synthesized and secreted. The types of mutations are DEL, deletion; INS, insertion; MS, missense; NS, nonsense; and SS, splice-site. Genotypes are represented by homozygous (Ho) or heterozygous (Ht). Clinical presentations are asymptomatic (As), thrombotic (Th), or bleeding (Bl), and these mutations result in afibrinogenemia (Afb) or hypofibrinogenemia (Hypo). Boxes marked with X indicate the genotype and clinical presentation that correspond to each mutation. AAs encoded by each exon include (Aα) E1: −19 to (−2); E2: −1 to 41; E3:42 to 102; E4:103 to 151; E5:152 to 625; E6:612 to 847(αE). Bβ CHAIN: E1: −16 to 8; E2:9 to 72; E3:73 to 133; E4:134 to 209; E5:210 to 247; E6:248 to 289; E7:290 to 385; E8:386 to 461; γ CHAIN: E1: −26 to (−1); E2:1 to 15; E3:16 to 76; E4:77 to 108; E5:109 to 151; E6:152 to 196; E7:197 to 258; E8:259 to 350; E9:351 to 427(γ'); E10:408 to 411(γ). *variant fibrinogen inappropriately stored in endoplasmic reticulum of hepatocytes.

and S119X) and exon 4 (R168X) were homozygous, mostly in known consanguineous patients; interestingly, the exon 4 mutation has been identified in five separate families (6,7). Another FGA mutation, R129X in exon 4, was also found in two homozygous, but clearly unrelated families (7). Mutations in FGA exon 5 (G316X and W334X) were identified as compound heterozygotes: G316X with the common splice-site mutation (IVS4 + 1G > T) in FGA, and W334X with the two residue deletions in FGA (g.3091-3092delAA) (6). A mutation in exon 2 of FGA, G32X, was identified as a heterozygous mutation; the assumed second mutation was not identified, although Southern blot analysis showed no large deletions (7). Although premature termination codons can alter mRNA stability, analysis of four of these nonsense mutants by transient transfection showed no change in message stability (7).

The nonsense mutations in FGB are R47X, identified in an Iranian patient (18), and W467X, identified in a Palestinian patient (25), both from consanguineous unions. In the second case, the encoded polypeptide is only 24 residues shorter than the full-length Bβ chain; therefore, the loss of fibrinogen in the plasma was surprising. Expression of the altered Bβ chain along with normal Aα and γ chains in COS-7 cells demonstrated that the truncated chain is synthesized and assembled intracellularly but is not secreted into the media (25). Interestingly, a nearby nonsense mutation, W470X, was identified in a hypofibrinogenemic individual who was heterozygous for the mutation (27). Because the encoded shorter Bβ chain was not detected in this patient's plasma, it is reasonable to assume that this mutation would also cause afibrinogenemia in homozygous or compound heterozygous individuals.

Two nonsense mutations have been identified in FGG: R223X (11) and E257X (33). Although both were homozygous, only the R223X patient was known to come from a consanguineous pedigree. Because in vitro studies that examined fibrinogen expression in CHO cells have shown that the C-terminus of the γ chain is essential for assembly and secretion of fibrinogen, it is not surprising that these shortened γ chains caused afibrinogenemia (39).

## Missense Mutations

Interestingly, missense mutations have only been identified in FGB. These mutations encode the Bβ-chain substitutions L383R, G430D, G444S, and W467G. The first two substitutions were identified in two patients, each of whose parents were first cousins (23). To assess whether these substitutions could cause afibrinogenemia, transient expression of the mutant fibrinogens was examined in COS-1 cells. These experiments demonstrated that the mutant Bβ chains were synthesized and that the fibrinogen molecules were assembled in the cells, but in contrast to expression of normal fibrinogen, these two variant molecules were not detected in the culture media. Pulse-chase experiments confirmed this conclusion because both radiolabeled variant fibrinogens remained intracellular, whereas radiolabeled normal fibrinogen was chased into the culture medium. Similar experiments on W467G showed normal assembly and a marked reduction in the secretion of the variant (26). The G444S substitution was identified in a compound heterozygous patient, where the second mutation was the Bβ-chain nonsense mutation, R47X (24). Transient expression in COS-7 cells demonstrated that fibrinogen molecules containing the mutant Bβ chain did assemble in the cell but were not secreted into the culture medium. These four cases, along with the nonsense mutation W467X, suggest that the β-domain in the distal D nodule of fibrinogen has a critical role in secretion.

## Splice-Site Mutations

Splice-site mutations have been identified in all three genes, with FGA mutations in both homozygous and heterozygous patients and FGB and FGG mutations only in homozygous patients. The most common afibrinogenemia mutation, first identified by Neerman-Arbez et al., is a donor splice mutation in intron 4 (IVS4 + 1G > T) (9). Haplotype analyses demonstrate that this mutation is likely recurrent, because it occurs on multiple discrete haplotypes (6). Two other donor splice mutations have been identified in intron 1 (IVS1 + 3G > A) and intron 3 (IVS3 + 1 + 4delGTAA) of FGA (6). In vitro expression of these mutant genes has shown that multiple aberrant mRNA molecules may be associated with each mutation and that the different outcomes reflect the order of intron removal in processing the FGA encoded mRNA (6,8). Two splice-site mutations have been identified in FGB, in intron 6 (IVS6 + 13C > T) and intron 7 (IVS7 + 1G > T), by Spena et al. (20). In vitro expression of Bβ-chain minigenes in transfected HeLa cells showed the intron 6 mutation activated a new donor splice-site 11 nucleotides downstream from the physiologic one whereas the intron 7 mutation resulted in multiple aberrant splicings. Three splice-site mutations have also been found in FGG: in intron 1 (IVS1 + 5G > A), intron 2 (IVS2 − 3C > G), and intron 3 (IVS3 + 5G > A) (11,28,29). Asselta et al. showed the intron 1 mutation led to the retention of intron 1 in the mRNA (28). Margaglione et al. showed exon 3 was missing from the mRNA transcribed from the mutated gene (29). In all cases, the alternatively spliced messages encode novel amino acids, with or without a frameshift, before a stop codon, such that expressed polypeptides would be shorter than normal.

# HYPOFIBRINOGENEMIAS

When found in heterozygous individuals, mutations that prevent the assembly and/or secretion of variant fibrinogen molecules cause low circulating levels of fibrinogen. The parents of most, but not all, patients with afibrinogenemia show hypofibrinogenemia, with fibrinogen levels reported as approximately 50% of normal. In addition, hypofibrinogenemia has been independently identified in individuals with mutations in the FGB or FGG genes.

Within the FGB gene missense, nonsense, and splice-site mutations have been found. Two missense mutations, R285H (19) and D346Y (22), and one nonsense mutation, W470X (27), lead to changes in the β-domain of the distal D nodule of fibrinogen, suggesting impaired secretion of assembled molecules, as observed in several afibrinogenemia cases with missense and nonsense mutations in this domain. A second nonsense mutation, Y71X (17), likely leads to impaired assembly because the encoded protein completely lacks the β-domain of the distal D nodule. A single splice-site mutation at the 5′ site of intron 6 (IVS6 + 1G > A) results in a frameshift after Pro319 adding 18 novel residues prior to a stop codon (21). As with other mutations in this region, the variant fibrinogen is probably assembled but not secreted into the circulation. A third missense mutation, L202Q, was found in a compound heterozygous individual with the Bβ nonsense mutation R47X (18). This missense mutation caused hypofibrinogenemia by a novel mechanism. When the L202Q mutation was introduced into a cDNA vector, expression of the variant protein was normal. In contrast, expression from a genomic vector demonstrated that the mutation activates a cryptic splice site, resulting in a truncated Bβ chain and impaired expression.

Within the FGG gene, only missense mutations have been identified in individuals with hypofibrinogenemia. C179R resulted in hypofibrinogenemia with none of the variant chains present in circulation (32). *In vitro* expression in CHO cells showed that mutation of Cys to either Arg or Ala eliminated secretion of the variant fibrinogen. The substitution G310R was found in a patient with liver cirrhosis and hypofibrinogenemia (34). Upon examination, the variant chains were not found in circulation, but rather in inclusion bodies in the liver, suggesting the variant chains were not secreted, but rather were stored inappropriately. Defective polymerization of plasma fibrinogen from this patient was attributed to hypersialylation of normal fibrinogen, which is characteristic of the acquired dysfibrinogenemia associated with liver disease (40). Another substitution, N371D (35), was found in an individual with low fibrinogen levels, but with normal purified fibrin polymerization, suggesting that this mutation caused the hypofibrinogenemia. Further analysis is needed to confirm that the variant protein is not present in circulation. Two mutations in the C-terminal region of the γ chain, T397I (36) and R401W (37), also cause hypofibrinogenemia with variant chains undetectable in circulation. The R401W fibrinogen is not secreted, but rather accumulated in the endoplasmic reticulum. One mutation, A108G, has been seen in two unrelated propositi with hypofibrinogenemia and bleeding (30,31). In both cases, the direct correlation between this mutation and phenotype was complicated because another mutation was present: either the substitution BβP265L or a FGG splice-site mutation (IVS2 + 1G > A). When considered together, the data suggest that variant γ chains with single residue substitutions would likely be synthesized but not assembled into fibrinogen, supporting a role for the γ chain in early assembly of γβ and γα dimers (41).

# DYSFIBRINOGENEMIAS

Inherited dysfibrinogenemia is a relatively rare disorder that most commonly occurs in a heterozygous state. Historically, dysfibrinogens have been named after the town where they were discovered; the dysfibrinogens described here are named after the amino acid changes in the circulating polypeptides, usually with reference to the earlier local name. Although some dysfibrinogenemias were identified in individuals with thrombosis (approximately 25%) or bleeding (approximately 25%), most cases are discovered by chance during routine coagulation assays. Because fibrinogen has a central role in hemostasis, it is somewhat surprising that a causative mutation has been clearly identified in only a few cases. Indeed, several mutations, including AαR16H, AαR16C, γR275H, and γN308K, are associated with multiple clinical phenotypes: thrombosis, bleeding, and asymptomatic. The correlation between clinical presentation and specific mutations, including AαS532C, AαQ328X (with AαIVS4 + 1G > T), BβA68T, and γD364V, has been made in multiple individuals within a single family. Although this correlation is suggestive of dysfibrinogenemias, the clinical presentation may be dependent on other traits within the specific families. In only one case has a specific genotype been associated with a single clinical phenotype in multiple families: AαR554C found in Dusart, Chapel Hill III, and, most recently, Nashville, which strengthens the relation between this mutation and thrombosis (42–48). Recently, one group has screened 217 individuals with a history of thrombosis but with normal hemostasis parameters and fibrinogen levels; they identified two novel variants, Aα272ins39residues (Champagne au Mont d'Or) and BβY236X (Lozanne) (49). Similar screening will likely reveal many dysfibrinogens, providing useful information to further our understanding of their structure and function *in vivo*.

Mutations have been identified in all three genes, although none within the exons arising from alternative splicing (αE and γ'). Missense, deletion, and insertion mutations have all been found. The schematic shown in Figure 62-2 indicates the locations of these mutations; the specific mutations are listed in Table 62-2. Most dysfibrinogenemias were discovered in clinical assays that demonstrated delayed fibrin clot formation; these mutations impair either (a) the conversion of fibrinogen to fibrin monomer or (b) the conversion of fibrin monomers to polymers. In several cases, the level of the variant fibrinogen chain is substantially lower than the level of the comparable normal chain; these cases are called hypodysfibrinogenemias. Although the level of variant protein is not routinely quantitated, in some cases, investigators have reported these levels. Dysfibrinogens with low expression of the variant chains (hypodysfibrinogens) include the following: γC326S, γC326Y, γA327T, γM336I, γY354C, and several with truncations in the Aα chain. A few dysfibrinogenemias were discovered in renal amyloidosis; these will be described at the end of this section. And, one fibrinogen, BβK148N (Merivale II), was discovered coincidentally in a heterozygous patient with hypofibrinogenemia; the K148N substitution had no effect on fibrin polymerization (19).

## Cases That Impair the Conversion of Fibrinogen to Fibrin

These variants are located within the central E nodule and affect either thrombin binding or fibrinopeptide cleavage. Substitutions at both thrombin cleavage sites, AαArg16 and BβArg14, have been identified in multiple cases. Substitutions in Aα16 are the most common, with over 65 cases of AαR16H or AαR16C reported to date (56). Diagnostically, the R16H cases show markedly delayed FpA release, whereas the R16C cases show decreased FpA release, with half the normal levels of FpA being released in heterozygous cases. Both substitutions have been found in homozygous cases: Geissen I (151) and Bicetre I (152) for R16H and Metz (153) for R16C; Geissen I and Metz were associated with hemorrhagic symptoms and Bicetre I was asymptomatic. In heterozygous individuals the clinical presentations range from asymptomatic to bleeding or thrombosis. Substitutions at the thrombin cleavage site of FpB are less common, and only Cys substitutions have been identified. These dysfibrinogens are thrombotic (84,85) or asymptomatic (86). In these cases, the release of FpA is normal and release of FpB is half-normal, because all individuals are heterozygous. Studies on Fb Seattle have shown that polymerization with reptilase was also impaired, suggesting that it was not the lack of FpB release, but rather the mutation itself that impaired polymerization (86). Further studies on Fb Ijmuiden identified multiple species in the BβR14C population, with 40% of the variant chains being disulfide-linked to albumin, 36% in free sulfhydryl form and 30% in high-molecular-weight protein complexes, suggesting Fb–Fb dimers (85). Taken together, these results suggest that the Bβ chain is important for polymerization, but it is not evident whether the bound albumin or the mutation itself leads to the altered polymerization.

Studies with substitutions in FpA, AαD7N, AαL9P, AαE11G, and AαG12V, illustrate the importance of the structure of this region on efficient thrombin cleavage, because each dysfibrinogen has delayed FpA release. Indeed, both nuclear magnetic resonance (NMR) solution studies and x-ray crystallography studies have shown a specific structure for this region bound to thrombin (154). The AαD7N substitution (Lille) disrupts a critical electrostatic interaction (50). The AαL9P substitution (Magdeburg I) introduces a Pro into the

**TABLE 62-2**

REPORTED MUTATIONS RESULTING IN DYSFIBRINOGENEMIA OR HYPODYSFIBRINOGENEMIA

| Mutation | Name | Genotype | | Clinical presentation | | | Impaired features | | | Reference |
|---|---|---|---|---|---|---|---|---|---|---|
| | | Ho | Ht | As | Th | Bl | Fp | Polym | Other | |
| **A. DYSFIBRINOGENS WITH MUTATIONS IN THE Aα CHAIN** | | | | | | | | | | |
| AαAsp7Asn | Lille | | X | X | | | X | X | | 50,51 |
| AαLeu9Pro | Magdeburg | | X | X | | | X | | | 52 |
| AαGlu11Gly | Mitaka II | | X | | | X | X | X | 1 | 53 |
| AαGly12Val | Rouen | X | | | | X | X | | | 54 |
| | Saint-Germain | | X | X | | | X | | | 55 |
| AαArg16His | Many | X | X | X | X | X | X | X | 1,5 | 56 |
| AαArg16Cys | Many | X | X | X | X | X | X | X | 2,5 | 56 |
| AαGly17Val | Bremen | | X | | X | X | X | X | | 57 |
| AαPro18Leu | Kanazawa | | X | X | | | | X | | 58 |
| | Kyoto II | | X | | X | | | X | | 59 |
| AαArg19Gly | Aarhus | X | | X | | | X | X | | 60 |
| | Mannheim I | | X | | X | | X | | 4 | 61 |
| | Matsumoto V | | X | X | | | X | X | | 62 |
| | Milano XIII | | X | | X | | | X | | 63 |
| | Oslo IV | | X | X* | | | | X | 8 | 64,65 |
| AαArg19Asn | Munich I | | | | X | | X | X | | 66 |
| AαArg19Ser | Detroit | X | | | X | | X | X | | 3 |
| AαVal20Asp | Canterbury | | X | | X | | X | X | | 67 |
| Aα Arg141Ser | Lima | X | | | X | | | X | 6 | 68,69 |
| AαArg268QEPstop | Otago | X | | | X | | | X | | 70 |
| Aα272 insert 39 amino acids | Champagne au Mont d'Or | | X | | X | | | | | 49 |
| AαGln328stop (with Aα IVS4+1 G > T) | Keokuk | | X | | X | X | | | | 71 |
| AαSer434Asn | Caracas II | | X | X | | | X | X | 5,6 | 72,73 |
| Aα Ile451 Wstop | Milano III | X | | | X | | | X | 2,5 | 74,75 |
| AαAsp454stop | Nieuwegein | X | | X | | | | X | 2,5 | 76 |
| AαLys461stop | Marburg | X | | | | X | | X | 2,7 | 77 |
| AαAla475 HCLA stop | Lincoln | | X | | X | | | X | | 78 |
| Aα494 frameshift + 23 residues, trunc. at 517 | Perth | | X | | X | | | X | 2 | 79 |
| AαAla499; frameshift stop at 518 | San Giovanni Rotondo | | X | X | | | | X | 2 | 80 |
| AαSer532Cys | Caracas V | | X | | X | | | X | 2,4,5 | 81,82 |
| AαArg554Cys | Nashville | | X | | X | | | X | | 42 |
| | Chapel Hill III | | X | | X | | | X | 2,4 | 45,46 |
| | Paris V (Dusart) | | X | | X | | | X | 2,4,5 | 42–45,47,48 |
| **B. DYSFIBRINOGENS WITH MUTATIONS IN THE Bβ CHAIN** | | | | | | | | | | |
| Bβ9-72 deleted | New York I | | X | | X | | X | X | 1,3 | 83 |
| BβArg14Cys | Christchurch II | | X | | X | | X | X | | 84 |
| | Christchurch III | | X | | X | | X | X | | 84 |
| | Ijmuiden | | X | | X | X | X | X | 2 | 85 |
| | Seattle I | | X | X | | | X | X | | 86,87 |
| BβGly15Cys | Fukuoka II | | X | X | | | X | X | 2 | 88 |
| | Ise | | X | X | | | X | X | | 89 |
| | Kosai | | X | X | | | X | X | 2,5 | 90 |
| | Ogasa | | X | X | | | X | X | 2,5 | 90 |
| BβArg44Cys | Nijmegen | | X | | X | | | X | 2,3,4 | 85,91 |
| BβAla68Thr | Naples | X | | | X | | X | X | 1 | 92–94 |
| BβLys148Asn (with BβArg255His) | Merivale II | | X | ** | | | | | | 19 |
| BβAsn160Ser | Niigata | | X | X | | | | X | 5,6 | 95 |
| BβArg166Cys | Longmont | | X | | X | | | X | | 96–98 |
| BβTyr236stop | Lozanne | | X | | X | | | | | 49 |
| BβAla335Thr | Pontoise | | X | X | | | | X | 6 | 99 |
| Bβstop462 → 12 residue extension stop SPMRRFLLFCM | Osaka VI | | X | | X | | | X | 5 | 100 |

(continued)

## TABLE 62-2

CONTINUED

| Mutation | Name | Genotype | | Clinical presentation | | | Impaired features | | | Reference |
|---|---|---|---|---|---|---|---|---|---|---|
| | | Ho | Ht | As | Th | Bl | Fp | Polym | Other | |
| **C. DYSFIBRINOGENS WITH MUTATIONS IN THE γ CHAIN** | | | | | | | | | | |
| γGly165Arg (with AαArg16Cys) | Milano XII | | X | X | | | X | X | 2 | 101 |
| γGly268Glu | Kurashiki | X | | X | | | | X | 4 | 102 |
| γArg275Cys | Many | | X | X | X | | X | X | 2,4,5,8 | 56 |
| γArg275His | Many | | X | X | X | X | X | X | 4 | 56 |
| γArg275Ser | Kamogawa | | X | X | | | | X | 4 | 103 |
| γAla279Asp | Auckland | | X | | X | | | X | | 104 |
| γTyr280Cys | Banks Peninsula | | X | | X | | | X | | 105 |
| γGly292Val | Baltimore I | | X | | X | X | | X | 8 | 106–109 |
| | St. Gallen | | X | | X | | | X | 4,9 | 110 |
| γAsn308Ile | Baltimore III | | X | X | | | | X | | 111,112 |
| γAsn308Lys | Bicetre II | | X | | X | | | X | | 113 |
| | Kyoto I | | X | | X | | | X | | 114,115 |
| | Matsumoto II | | X | | | X | | X | | 116 |
| | Matsumoto VI | | X | X | | | | | | 117 |
| γGly309Asp | Hillsborough | | X | X | | | | X | | 118 |
| γMet310Thr | Asahi | | X | | X | | | X | 6,8 | 115,119–121 |
| γAsp318Tyr | Bastia | | X | X | | | | X | 9 | 122 |
| γAsp318Gly | Giessen IV (Kassel) | | X | | X | X | | | | 123 |
| ΔγAsn319, Asp320 | Vlissingen/ Frankfurt IV | | X | | X | | | X | 9,10 | 4,123,124 |
| | Otsu I | | X | X | | | | X | | 125 |
| γCys326Ser | Cordoba | | X | | X | | | X | | 126,127 |
| γCys326Tyr | Suhl | | X | | X | | | X | 2,5,9 | 35 |
| γAla327Thr | Tokyo V | | X | | X | | | X | 4,5,6,9 | 128 |
| γGln329Arg | Nagoya | | X | X | | | | X | | 129,130 |
| γAsp330Val | Ales | X | | | X | | | X | | 131 |
| | Milano I | | X | X | | | | X | | 132 |
| γAsp330Tyr | Kyoto III | | X | X | | | | X | | 115,133 |
| γMet336Ile | Hannover VI | | X | | X | | | X | 9 | 35 |
| γAsn337Lys | Bern I | | X | X | | | | X | 9 | 134,135 |
| γ350/G351S insert 15 aa's MCGEALPM LKDPCY | Paris I | | X | | | X | | X | 8 | 136–141 |
| γTyr354Cys | Homburg VII | | X | | X | | | X | 2,5,9 | 35 |
| γSer358Cys | Jena | | X | | | | X | X | | 142 |
| | Milano VII | | X | X | | | | X | 2 | 143 |
| γAsn361Lys | Poissy II | | X | | | X | X | X | 8 | 144 |
| γAsp364His | Matsumoto I | | X | X | | | | X | | 124,145 |
| γAsp364Val | Melun | | X | | X | | X | | | 146 |
| γArg375Gly | Osaka V | | X | X | | | | X | 4,8,9,10 | 147,148 |
| γLys380Asn | Kaiserslautern I | X | | | X | | | X | 5,6 | 149,150 |

The genotypes are represented by homozygous (Ho) or heterozygous (Ht). Clinical presentations are asymptomatic (As), thrombotic (Th), or bleeding (Bl). Impaired features are fibrinopeptide release (Fp), fibrin polymerization (Polym), and others: (1) decreased thrombin binding; (2) binds albumin; (3) impaired tPA binding; (4) impaired fibrinolysis; (5) abnormal fibrin clot structure; (6) extra glycosylation; (7) abolished endothelial cell binding; (8) impaired factor XIII cross-linking; (9) impaired protective effect of calcium on plasminolysis; or (10) decreased calcium binding. Each of the preceding items is noted in the Impaired features column. Boxes marked with X indicate the genotype and clinical presentation and features that are impaired in the propositus with each dysfibrinogen.

*, obscure pulmonary ailment may be related; **, present in compound heterozygote with mutation R285H, which is not secreted, thus resulting in hypofibrinogenemia.

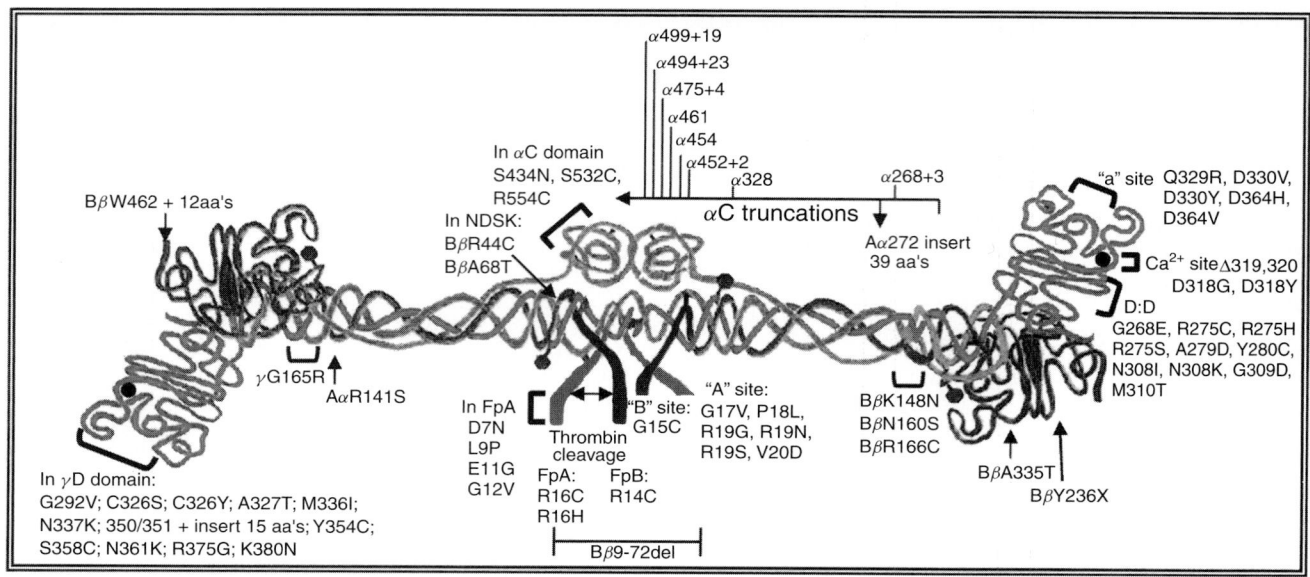

**FIGURE 62-2.** Schematic representation of the fibrinogen molecule with dysfibrinogens denoted. The γ, Aα, and Bβ chains are featured in *red*, *blue*, and *green*, respectively. Locations of dysfibrinogens are approximate based on known crystal structures of the D fragment. The N-termini of the Aα and Bβ chains are depicted with (left pair) and without (right pair) fibrinopeptides, to show the mutations within the Fp's and the exposed "A" and "B" knobs, respectively. Truncations of the αC domains are listed as the residue where the mutation occurs, followed by the number of residues added because of frameshift, before termination. *Purple* hexagons represent carbohydrate additions and *black* circles represent calcium (see Color Fig. 62-2). (From Cote HC, Lord ST, Pratt KP. γ chain dysfibrinogenemias: molecular structure–function relationships of naturally occurring mutations in the γ chain of human, fibrinogen. *Blood* 1998;92(7):2195–2212, with permission.)

α-helical stretch between residues Aα7 and 10 likely causing conformational changes that inhibit interaction with thrombin (52). Similarly, the AαG12V substitution (Rouen) disrupts the β turn involving Glu11 and Gly12 and slightly displaces Gly13 and Gly14 (54). In contrast, the AαE11G substitution (Mitaka II) not only destabilizes this β turn but also directly alters the fibrinogen-thrombin interaction by disrupting the salt bridge between AαE11 and R173 of thrombin (155). Interestingly, whereas Fbs Lille and Magdeburg are asymptomatic, Fbs Mitaka II and Rouen show a bleeding tendency. Another AαG12V dysfibrinogen, Saint-Germain, was found in an asymptomatic boy. Unlike Rouen, this variant showed delayed FpB release and an abnormal reptilase time (55).

Two other dysfibrinogens, both in the N-terminal region of the Bβ chain, show delayed fibrinopeptide release linked to impaired thrombin binding. The well-characterized homozygous substitution BβA68T (Naples) shows impaired thrombin binding (<10%) to fibrin and greatly delayed FpA and FpB release (92). Recent crystallographic data show that this substitution likely impairs interactions between fibrinogen and exosite I on thrombin (156). Other recent studies indicate that binding of thrombin to low-affinity sites is abolished with this mutation and high-affinity binding to the γ' chain is impaired (93). The second dysfibrinogen is a large deletion of residues Bβ9 to 72, which are encoded by exon 2 in FGB. This dysfibrinogen (New York I) was identified in heterozygous individuals (83). Biochemical analyses of purified fibrinogen showed delayed FpA release, and delayed and reduced release of FpB, indicating that thrombin binding was impaired. Both the homozygous BβA68T substitution and the heterozygous Bβ9 to 72 deletion were found in association with a thrombotic phenotype, indicating that the loss of thrombin binding may lead to thrombosis.

## Cases That Impair the Spontaneous Conversion of Fibrin Monomers to Polymers

This conversion has traditionally been described as a two-step process: the formation of half-staggered, double-stranded protofibrils and the lateral association of protofibrils into fibers. More recently, the specific interactions that mediate fiber formation have been elucidated in x-ray crystallographic structures of fibrinogen fragments D and FXIIIa–cross-linked fragment D–D in the presence of the peptides GPRPam and GHRPam, which mimic the N-terminal regions of the α and β chains of fibrin (157–160). Because many of the substitutions identified in dysfibrinogenemias are found within these crystal structures, it is now possible to correlate the clinical and biochemical data for these variants with the three-dimensional structure of fibrinogen. These cases are described first, within the context of interactions revealed by the new structural data. The remaining dysfibrinogenemias that impair polymerization—large insertions or deletions, changes in carbohydrate addition, changes within the C-terminal region of the Aα chain and changes related to novel Cys residues—will be described thereafter.

### "A:a" Interactions

Upon cleavage of FpA, the N-terminus of the α chain, called the "A" polymerization site, is exposed. This site binds noncovalently to a complementary polymerization site, called the "a" site, in the C-terminal region in the γ chain of another fibrin(ogen) molecule. This interaction, which leads to the formation of half-staggered, double-stranded protofibrils, is modeled in the crystal structures obtained in the presence of GPRPam. Substitutions at each of the "A" site residues have been identified in dysfibrinogenemias: G17V (Bremen), P18L (Kanazawa and Kyoto II), R19S (Detroit), R19G (Oslo IV, Aarhus, Mannheim I, Matsumoto V, and Milano XIII), R19N (Munich I) and V20D (Canterbury). The structure data indicate that the free amino group of the "A" mimic (GPRPam) interacts directly with the side chain of residue γD364 in the "a" site, suggesting that the nature of the side chain is less critical (158). Indeed, substitution of a Val residue for Gly17 likely impairs both thrombin-catalyzed FpA release and polymerization because the peptide Val-Pro-Arg-Val only partially inhibits normal polymerization (57). The structure data show that the positively charged side chain of Arg19 interacts directly with residues in the "a" site, particularly, γD330. Therefore, substitutions with Gly, Ser, or Asn will obliterate these interactions. The substitution of Leu for Pro18 likely alters the overall structure of the "A" site and thereby compromises the strength of the "A:a" interaction. The AαV20D substitution (67) presented an unanticipated abnormality because the extent of FpA release from this heterozygous variant was approximately 50% of normal. Further examination revealed that this Asp substitution created a novel furin cleavage site, such that cleavage of Aα1 to 20 by furin removed the "A" site and thereby impaired polymerization. Although this dysfibrinogen does not show a role for Val20 in "A:a" interactions, it does emphasize the many mechanisms by which altered fibrinogen can disrupt hemostasis.

Several dysfibrinogens have been found in γ-chain residues that make up the "a" site. The crystallographic studies showed that Q329 shifts on GPRPam binding; the substitution of γQ329R (Nagoya) may disrupt this shift, thereby impairing polymerization (129). Substitutions for γD330, D330V [Ales (131) and Milano I (132)], and D330Y [Kyoto III (133)] disrupt the ionic interactions with AαArg19. Biochemical analyses of these variants demonstrate that this residue is critical for polymerization (131,133). Similarly, substitutions at γD364, to His and Val [Matsumoto I (145) and Melun (146), respectively] disrupt ionic interactions with the free amino group of the "A" mimic. Biochemical analyses of both patient and recombinant variants at this site (145,161) demonstrate impaired polymerization.

### "B:b" Interactions

Upon cleavage of FpB, the N-terminus of the β chain, called the "B" polymerization site, is exposed. This site binds noncovalently to a complementary polymerization site, called the "b" site, in the C-terminal region in the β chain of another fibrin(ogen) molecule. This interaction is modeled in the crystal structures obtained in the presence of GHRPam. There are no reports of fibrinogen variants in the "b" site, and only one substitution has been found in the "B" site: BβG15C (Ise, Fukuoka II, Kosai, and Ogasa). Biochemical analyses of these dysfibrinogenemias showed normal FpA release, approximately 50% of FpB release, impaired thrombin- and reptilase-catalyzed polymerization, and impaired desA- and desAB-fibrin monomer repolymerization (88,90). Therefore, this "B" site mutation impaired both thrombin-catalyzed release of FpB and polymerization. These dysfibrinogens varied in the chemistries of the new sulfhydryl group, with some present in complexes with albumin, some in intramolecular fibrinogen dimers, some in intermolecular fibrinogen dimers, and some as free sulfhydryls. Although this variant showed significantly impaired polymerization, these dysfibrinogenemias were all found in asymptomatic individuals, indicating that the "B:b" interaction may be functionally insignificant at least in heterozygous individuals.

### Calcium Binding Sites

Calcium binding is known to enhance fibrin polymerization, (162) and multiple calcium binding sites have been identified in the crystal structures (157–160,163). One high-affinity site is found in fragment D, where the side chains of γD318 and γD320 provide ligands for the $Ca^{2+}$. This site is disrupted by two substitutions, γD318Y (Bastia) and γD318G (Giessen IV), and by a two-residue deletion, γΔ319,320 (Vlissingen/Frankfurt IV and Otsu). These dysfibrinogens show impaired polymerization, decreased calcium binding, and decreased protective effect of $Ca^{2+}$ on plasmic degradation (4,122). These results indicate that these $Ca^{2+}$ binding site residues are important for maintaining the proper structural conformation of the polymerization site "a."

### The D:D Interface

End-to-end alignment of fibrin monomers occurs through the D:D interface, which was seen first in the crystal structure of D:D (157). Several dysfibrinogens have been reported with mutations in this area: γG268E (Kurashiki), γR275C (Tokyo II and many others), γR275H (many), γR275S (Kamogawa), γA279D (Auckland), γY280C (Banks Peninsula), γN308I (Baltimore III), γN308K (several), γG309D (Hillsborough), and γM310T (Asahi). Biochemical analyses of fibrinogen Tokyo II showed normal D:E interactions and normal FXIII cross-linking, whereas electron microscopic images of factor XIII–cross-linked Tokyo II showed clearly that the clot structure was altered by this mutation (164,165). These findings, along with many other studies of γArg275 mutants, reiterate the importance of residue 275 in the D:D interface and the importance of the D:D interaction in fibrin polymerization. Recent studies of two neighboring dysfibrinogens, γA279D and γY280C, were also characterized by impaired polymerization, most likely because of the alteration of the D:D interactions. Indeed, the structure data show a direct interaction between γ280 and γ275 (157). The crystal structure also shows residues 308 to 310 lying on the surface of the γD domain, juxtaposed to residue 275. Therefore, it is not surprising that these variants have similar biochemical properties. Nevertheless, the clinical manifestations of the dysfibrinogens in this region are quite different: Baltimore III, Matsumoto VI, Kurashiki, Kamogawa, and Hillsborough were asymptomatic; Bicetre II and Kyoto I were thrombotic; and Matsumoto II, Auckland, Banks Peninsula, and Asahi were hemorrhagic. These differences emphasize that many factors combine to manifest clinically in different ways.

### Other Substitutions within the γ Chain in Fragment D

Several additional substitutions have been identified within the γ chain in fragment D: γG165R, γG292V, γC326S, γC326Y, γM336I, γN337K, γN361K, and γR375G. The γG165R substitution was found in an individual (Milano XII) with a second mutation, AαR16C, that likely led to the analysis of this individual, and the Aα-chain substitution may be fully responsible for abnormal polymerization of this dysfibrinogen (101). Nevertheless, analysis of the novel γ-chain mutation by circular dichroism showed that this substitution altered folding of the C-terminal part of the γ chain, likely because the mutation falls between the disulfide-bound residues γ153 and γ182. The γG292V substitution has been found in two cases, Baltimore I and St Gallen I (106,110). Molecular modeling of the latter variant suggested that the Val substitution altered the structure such that the loop containing the plasmin cleavage site γ302 to 303 is spread, and the site is more accessible to plasmin cleavage (110). Modeling also suggested that the impaired polymerization is caused by disruption of hydrogen bonds between γ297 and γ375, which destabilizes the A:a interactions (110). Both γ326 mutations [γC326S (126) and γC326Y (35)] have impaired polymerization, and γC326Y is found bound to albumin, because of its unpaired cysteine. Both γM336I (35) (Hannover VI) and γN337K (134) (Bern I) are located near the high-affinity $Ca^{2+}$

binding site and the "a" polymerization site; therefore, these substitutions likely alter the structure, disrupting one or both of these interactions to impair polymerization. Impaired polymerization but normal cross-linking of γN361K (144) (Poissy II) suggests that residue 361 contributes to the "A:a" interaction. Complete correction of impaired polymerization at increased $Ca^{2+}$ concentrations suggests that this mutation also affects $Ca^{2+}$ binding. The γR375G (Osaka V) dysfibrinogen was similar to γN361K (147,148), with impaired polymerization that can be corrected with $Ca^{2+}$ addition, an impaired protective effect of $Ca^{2+}$ on plasmin degradation, and reduced high-affinity $Ca^{2+}$ binding, indicating a role for γ375 in $Ca^{2+}$ binding and the polymerization "a" site (147).

## Large Insertions

Two large insertions have been identified in dysfibrinogens associated with impaired polymerization: an insertion of 12 residues at the C-terminus of the Bβ chain when the normal stop codon was changed to encode Trp462 (Osaka VI) and an insertion of 15 residues between γ350Q and γ351G, with a concomitant change of Gly351 to Ser (Paris I). Both inserts add novel Cys residues. In the Bβ insert, the single cysteine forms disulfide bonds between variant molecules forming homodimers of the variant Bβ chains (100). Clots of this variant had thinner fibers in a lacy meshwork with large pores. Compaction and permeation studies showed that these clots were more fragile and compressible. The γ-chain insertion was first noted in the protein and subsequently defined by genetic analyses (136,137). It has two cysteine residues that likely form a disulfide bond, which would alter the conformation of the region around residues γ350 and γ351 (136). Deficiencies in polymerization (138), factor XIII cross-linking, and platelet binding (141) have all been reported for this dysfibrinogenemia.

## Novel Carbohydrate Addition

In several cases, single residue substitutions have generated a consensus sequence for carbohydrate addition and, therefore, these dysfibrinogens contain novel carbohydrate additions: AαR141S (Lima), AαS434N (Caracas II), BβN160S (Niigata), BβA335T (Pontoise), γM310T (Asahi), γA327T (Tokyo V), and γK380N (Kaiserslautern I). The γM310T substitution was discussed in the preceding text because this residue is part of the D:D interface. Electron microscopic analysis of clots formed with this dysfibrinogen showed that the markedly abnormal clot structure could essentially be normalized by enzymatic removal of carbohydrate from this variant (121). Even so, the thrombin clotting time remained delayed. Both AαR141S (68,69) and BβN160S (95) lie in the coiled-coil region of the fibrinogen molecule, such that the novel carbohydrate could impair polymerization by blocking proper alignment of the monomers into protofibrils or the protofibrils into fibers. Polymerization of BβN160S remained impaired after deglycosylation at residue 158, indicating that the Ser substitution and/or the deglycosylation itself was associated with the impairment. In contrast, in Fb Lima, deglycosylation of AαAsn139 corrected the polymerization defect, suggesting that the novel glycosylation was responsible for the impaired polymerization (68). The impaired polymerization of the AαS434N dysfibrinogen suggests a role for the αC domain in the polymerization process; this suggestion is corroborated by studies with other dysfibrinogens located in this domain as described in the following text (72,73). Impaired polymerization of Fb Kaiserslautern (γLys380Asn), with a new glycosylation site at Asn380, was corrected by the removal of the sialic acids with neuraminidase, suggesting that the extra sialylation was responsible for the impaired polymerization (149). Studies with Fb Pontoise (BβA335T) showed impaired fibrin polymerization but normal factor XIII cross-linking and fibrinopeptide release (99).

## Changes within the C-Terminal Region of the Aα Chain

The C-terminal region of the Aα chain, commonly called the αC domain, extends from the distal D nodules of fibrinogen and folds back toward the center of the fibrinogen molecule, with the most C-terminal portions forming a globular domain that associates with the central E nodule (166). Upon release of FpA, the αC domains are released from the E nodule and likely facilitate interactions with other fibrinogen molecules and, therefore, the lateral aggregation of protofibrils (166,167). Because dysfibrinogens within the αC domains are associated with defective polymerization, it is logical to conclude these domains have a significant role in this process. One single residue substitution in the αC domain, AαS434N, was described in the preceding text because this variant has a novel carbohydrate addition. Two single residue substitutions, AαS532C (Caracas V) and AαR554C (Dusart, Chapel Hill III, and Nashville), introduce a novel Cys residue. In both cases, albumin has been found to be disulfide-linked to the novel Cys. Electron microscopy of Fb Caracas V and Dusart show abnormal fibrin clot structures (81,43). These data are of particular interest because the Dusart mutation is the only one that has been associated with a clinical phenotype, thrombosis, in multiple families. It has been speculated that the thrombotic symptoms are associated with the altered clot structure, leading to impaired fibrinolysis.

There are seven reported truncations in the αC domains, ranging from a 56% truncation [terminating at residue 271, Otago (70)] to a 15% truncation [terminating at residue 518, San Giovanni Rotondo (80)]. The Otago mutation, a frame shift mutation encoding AαR268QEP, is homozygous with the shortened chain at a concentration of only 0.1 mg per mL in the circulation, indicating a severe hypodysfibrinogenemia and suggesting a role for the αC domains in fibrinogen assembly and secretion. Similarly, low expression levels of hypodysfibrinogens Keokuk (10%, AαQ328X in the simple heterozygote) (71), Marburg (10% to 20%, homozygous AαK461X) (77), Lincoln (20%, a heterozygous frameshift mutation, AαA475HCLA) (78), and Perth (15%, a heterozygous frameshift with 23 novel residues after Aα494) (79) suggest that the αC domains are important for fibrinogen synthesis. In contrast, two homozygous truncations at Aα454 (Milano III and Nieuwegein) circulate at normal levels of 2.6 mg per mL and 1.7 mg per mL, respectively. These two fibrinogens differ from one another in their terminating residues because the Milano III (74,75) is a frameshift change in which two novel residues, Trp453 and Ser454, follow AαGly452 mutation before a novel stop codon, whereas the Nieuwegein (76) results from a nucleotide insertion at Pro453, resulting in a premature stop codon at 454. Turbidity studies indicate that each of these truncations displays decreased lateral aggregation. This finding supports the proposal that the αC domains contribute to lateral aggregation (166,167), but the binding of albumin to these dysfibrinogens by the free cysteine residue at Aα442 complicates interpretation of these data. Studies with Fb Lincoln showed that despite the new Cys residue, the variant chain is not found in albumin-bound complexes (78). Interestingly, the AαQ328X truncation (Keokuk) occurs in a compound heterozygote with an FGA (IVS1 + 4A > G) splice-site mutation, which causes hypofibrinogenemia. Therefore, only the variant α chain is found in the circulation. Studies of this compound heterozygote (effectively homozygous) show a drastic decrease in lateral aggregation by turbidity. The combined results of these studies indicate that the lack of the αC domains, and not just the presence of albumin, leads to a polymerization abnormality. The clinical presentation of the αC truncations varies from asymptomatic to bleeding and/or thrombosis. Bleeding occurred in most cases of αC truncations, but Milano III was found in a patient with thrombosis, whereas San Giovanni Rotondo and Nieuwegein were asymptomatic.

### Changes Related to Novel Cysteines

As mentioned in several cases in the preceding text, the addition of a novel Cys residue can lead to changes in the normal disulfide pairs or to additions of abnormal molecules by disulfide linkages, thereby generating remarkably abnormal molecules. Novel Cys residues have been found in five cases, in addition to those described previously. In one case, disulfide-linked fibrinogen dimers [BβArg166Cys (Longmont)] were found in the circulation (96). Studies of the variant fibrinogen showed that impaired polymerization remained even after the dimeric molecules were removed from the analyses. In the remaining four cases—BβR44C (85) (Nijmegen), γC326Y (35) (Suhl), γY354C (35) (Homburg VII), and γS358C (143) (Milano VII)—the novel Cys has been found complexed with other molecules including albumin, glutathione, and cysteine. It appears logical that these mixtures of molecules would lead to impaired polymerization, and, indeed, scanning electron micrographs of fibrinogens Suhl and Homburg VII show abnormal clot structures (35).

# HEREDITARY RENAL AMYLOIDOSIS

Hereditary renal amyloidosis, which is characterized by extracellular deposits of amyloid protein and is clinically presented as nephropathy during varied stages of life, is known to occur as a result of several mutations in the αC domains of fibrinogen. These mutations include AαR554L (168), AαE526V (169), and two frameshift mutations that encode truncations: a mutation at codon 524, resulting in termination at 548 (170), and a mutation at codon 522, resulting in termination at 548 (171). Currently, the mechanism of amyloid deposition is not well understood. Recent retrospective DNA and tissue analysis of 350 cases of systemic amyloidosis have shown that in 18 cases amyloid deposition was due to the AαE526V mutation. The presence of fibrinogen within the amyloid deposits was confirmed in these 18 cases (172). These results indicate that amyloidosis due to fibrinogen mutations is more prevalent than anticipated. Therefore, screening for fibrinogen mutations should be routine in the characterization of hereditary renal amyloidosis.

# CONCLUSION

Mutations in the fibrinogen genes clearly cause disease: bleeding in afibrinogenemia, but perhaps also in dysfibrinogenemias in some individuals; thrombosis in multiple families with the AαR554C substitution; and renal amyloidosis in some individuals with specific mutations encoding the αC domain. As genetic analyses become even more efficient, we anticipate a dramatic rise in the number of mutations identified within these three genes. This additional information should allow for an enhanced understanding of the fibrinogen structures that are critical for hemostasis. Moreover, these data will facilitate future diagnoses of hereditary afibrinogenemias and dysfibrinogenemias and enable prenatal diagnosis for parents who so desire. Although the incidence of these mutations is rare, the proper diagnosis of clinically relevant defects may enable novel treatments for specific mutations.

## References

1. Medicina D, Fabbretti G, Brennan SO, et al. Genetic and immunological characterization of fibrinogen inclusion bodies in patients with hepatic fibrinogen storage and liver disease. *Ann N Y Acad Sci* 2001;936: 522–525.
2. Rabe F, Saloman E. Ueber-faserstoffmangel im blute bei einem falle von hamophilie. *Arch Int Med* 1920;95:2–14.
3. Mammen EF, Prasad AS, Barnhart MI, et al. Congenital dysfibrinogenemia: fibrinogen Detroit. *J Clin Invest* 1969;48:235–249.
4. Koopman J, Haverkate F, Briet E, et al. A congenitally abnormal fibrinogen (Vlissingen) with a 6-base deletion in the gamma-chain gene, causing defective calcium binding and impaired fibrin polymerization. *J Biol Chem* 1991;266:13456–13461.
5. Neerman-Arbez M, Honsberger A, Antonarakis SE, et al. Deletion of the fibrinogen alpha-chain gene (FGA) causes congenital afibrogenemia. *J Clin Invest* 1999;103:215–218.
6. Neerman-Arbez M. The molecular basis of inherited afibrinogenaemia. *Thromb Haemost* 2001;86:154–163.
7. Asselta R, Duga S, Spena S, et al. Congenital afibrinogenemia: mutations leading to premature termination codons in fibrinogen a alpha-chain gene are not associated with the decay of the mutant mRNAs. *Blood* 2001;98: 3685–3692.
8. Attanasio C, David A, Neerman-Arbez M. Outcome of donor splice site mutations accounting for congenital afibrinogenemia reflects order of intron removal in the fibrinogen alpha gene (FGA). *Blood* 2003;101: 1851–1856.
9. Suh TT, Holmback K, Jensen NJ, et al. Resolution of spontaneous bleeding events but failure of pregnancy in fibrinogen-deficient mice. *Genes Dev* 1995;9:2020–2033.
10. Watanabe K, Shibuya A, Ishii E, et al. Identification of simultaneous mutation of fibrinogen alpha chain and protein C genes in a Japanese kindred. *Br J Haematol* 2003;120:101–108.
11. Asselta R, Spena S, Duga S, et al. Analysis of Iranian patients allowed the identification of the first truncating mutation in the fibrinogen Bbeta-chain gene causing afibrinogenemia. *Haematologica* 2002;87:855–859.
12. Vlietman JJ, Verhage J, Vos HL, et al. Congenital afibrinogenaemia in a newborn infant due to a novel mutation in the fibrinogen Aalpha gene. *Br J Haematol* 2002;119:282–283.
13. Neerman-Arbez M, de Moerloose P, Bridel C, et al. Mutations in the fibrinogen Aalpha gene account for the majority of cases of congenital afibrinogenemia. *Blood* 2000;96:149–152.
14. Neerman-Arbez M, Antonarakis SE, Honsberger A, et al. The 11 kb FGA deletion responsible for congenital afibrinogenaemia is mediated by a short direct repeat in the fibrinogen gene cluster. *Eur J Hum Genet* 1999;7: 897–902.
15. Neerman-Arbez M, de Moerloose P, Honsberger A, et al. Molecular analysis of the fibrinogen gene cluster in 16 patients with congenital afibrinogenemia: novel truncating mutations in the FGA and FGG genes. *Hum Genet* 2001;108:237–240.
16. Remijn JA, van Wijk R, Nieuwenhuis HK, et al. Molecular basis of congenital afibrinogenaemia in a Dutch family. *Blood Coagul Fibrinolysis* 2003;14:299–302.
17. Fellowes AP, Brennan SO, Holme R, et al. Homozygous truncation of the fibrinogen a alpha chain within the coiled coil congenital afibrinogenemia. *Blood* 2000;96:773–775.
18. Mimuro J, Hamano A, Tanaka T, et al. Hypofibrinogenemia caused by a nonsense mutation in the fibrinogen B beta chain gene. *J Thromb Haemost* 2003; 1:2356–2359.
19. Asselta R, Duga S, Spena S, et al. Missense or splicing mutation? The case of a fibrinogen B{beta}-chain mutation causing severe hypofibrinogenemia. *Blood* 2004;103:3051–3054.
20. Maghzal GJ, Brennan SO, Fellowes AP, et al. Familial hypofibrinogenaemia associated with heterozygous substitution of a conserved arginine residue; Bbeta255 Arg → His (Fibrinogen Merivale). *Biochim Biophys Acta* 2003; 1645:146–151.
21. Spena S, Duga S, Asselta R, et al. Congenital afibrinogenemia: first identification of splicing mutations in the fibrinogen B beta-chain gene causing activation of cryptic splice sites. *Blood* 2002;100:4478–4484.
22. Homer VM, Brennan SO, George PM. Novel fibrinogen B beta gene mutation causing hypofibrinogenaemia. *Thromb Haemost* 2002;88: 1066–1067.
23. Brennan SO, Wyatt JM, May S, et al. Hypofibrinogenemia due to novel 316 Asp → Tyr substitution in the fibrinogen B beta chain. *Thromb Haemost* 2001;85:450–453.
24. Duga S, Asselta R, Santagostino E, et al. Missense mutations in the human beta fibrinogen gene cause congenital afibrinogenemia by impairing fibrinogen secretion. *Blood* 2000;95:1336–1341.
25. Vu D, Bolton-Maggs PH, Parr JR, et al. Congenital afibrinogenemia: identification and expression of a missense mutation in FGB impairing fibrinogen secretion. *Blood* 2003;102:4413–4415.
26. Neerman-Arbez M, Vu D, Abu-Libdeh B, et al. Prenatal diagnosis for congenital afibrinogenemia caused by a novel nonsense mutation in the FGB gene in a Palestinian family. *Blood* 2003;101:3492–3494.
27. Spena S, Asselta R, Duga S, et al. Congenital afibrinogenemia: intracellular retention of fibrinogen due to a novel W437G mutation in the fibrinogen Bbeta-chain gene. *Biochim Biophys Acta* 2003;1639:87–94.
28. Homer VM, Brennan SO, Ockelford P, et al. Novel fibrinogen truncation with deletion of Bbeta chain residues 440-461 causes hypofibrinogenaemia. *Thromb Haemost* 2002;88:427–431.
29. Asselta R, Duga S, Simonic T, et al. Afibrinogenemia: first identification of a splicing mutation in the fibrinogen gamma chain gene leading to a major gamma chain truncation. *Blood* 2000;96:2496–2500.

30. Margaglione M, Santacroce R, Colaizzo D, et al. A G-to-A mutation in IVS-3 of the human gamma fibrinogen gene causing afibrinogenemia due to abnormal RNA splicing. *Blood* 2000;96:2501–2505.

31. Wyatt J, Brennan SO, May S, et al. Hypofibrinogenaemia with compound heterozygosity for two gamma chain mutations-gamma 82 Ala → Gly and an intron two GT → AT splice site mutation. *Thromb Haemost* 2000; 84:449–452.

32. Brennan SO, Fellowes AP, Faed JM, et al. Hypofibrinogenemia in an individual with 2 coding (gamma82 A → G and Bbeta235 P → L) and 2 non-coding mutations. *Blood* 2000;95:1709–1713.

33. Terasawa F, Okumura N, Kitano K, et al. Hypofibrinogenemia associated with a heterozygous missense mutation gamma153Cys to Arg (Matsumoto IV): *in vitro* expression demonstrates defective secretion of the variant fibrinogen. *Blood* 1999;94:4122–4131.

34. Iida H, Ishii E, Nakahara M, et al. A case of congenital afibrinogenemia: fibrinogen Hakata, a novel nonsense mutation of the fibrinogen gamma-chain gene. *Thromb Haemost* 2000;84:49–53.

35. Brennan SO, Wyatt J, Medicina D, et al. Fibrinogen Brescia: hepatic endoplasmic reticulum storage and hypofibrinogenemia because of a gamma284 Gly → Arg mutation. *Am J Pathol* 2000;157:189–196.

36. Meyer M, Franke K, Richter W, et al. New molecular defects in the gamma subdomain of fibrinogen D-domain in four cases of (hypo)dysfibrinogenemia: fibrinogen variants Hannover VI, Homburg VII, Stuttgart and Suhl. *Thromb Haemost* 2003;89:637–646.

37. Brennan SO, Wyatt JM, Fellowes AP, et al. Gamma371 Thr → Ile substitution in the fibrinogen gammaD domain causes hypofibrinogenaemia. *Biochim Biophys Acta* 2001;1550:183–188.

38. Brennan SO, Maghzal G, Shneider BL, et al. Novel fibrinogen gamma375 Arg → Trp mutation (fibrinogen Aguadilla) causes hepatic endoplasmic reticulum storage and hypofibrinogenemia. *Hepatology* 2002;36:652–658.

39. Okumura N, Terasawa F, Tanaka H, et al. Analysis of fibrinogen gamma-chain truncations shows the C-terminus, particularly gammaIle387, is essential for assembly and secretion of this multichain protein. *Blood* 2002; 99:3654–3660.

40. Martinez J, MacDonald KA, Palascak JE. The role of sialic acid in the dysfibrinogenemia associated with liver disease: distribution of sialic acid on the constituent chains. *Blood* 1983;61:1196–1202.

41. Redman CM, Xia H. Fibrinogen biosynthesis. Assembly, intracellular degradation, and association with lipid synthesis and secretion. *Ann N Y Acad Sci* 2001;936:480–495.

42. Tarumi T, Martincic D, Thomas A, et al. Familial thrombophilia associated with fibrinogen Paris V: Dusart syndrome. *Blood* 2000;96:1191–1193.

43. Collet JP, Woodhead JL, Soria J, et al. Fibrinogen Dusart: electron microscopy of molecules, fibers and clots, and viscoelastic properties of clots. *Biophys J* 1996;70:500–510.

44. Koopman J, Haverkate F, Grimbergen J, et al. Molecular basis for fibrinogen Dusart (A alpha 554 Arg → Cys) and its association with abnormal fibrin polymerization and thrombophilia. *J Clin Invest* 1993;91:1637–1643.

45. Wada Y, Lord ST. A correlation between thrombotic disease and a specific fibrinogen abnormality (a alpha 554 Arg → Cys) in two unrelated kindred, Dusart and Chapel Hill III. *Blood* 1994;84:3709–3714.

46. Carrell N, Gabriel DA, Blatt PM, et al. Hereditary dysfibrinogenemia in a patient with thrombotic disease. *Blood* 1983;62:439–447.

47. Collet JP, Soria J, Mirshahi M, et al. Dusart syndrome: a new concept of the relationship between fibrin clot architecture and fibrin clot degradability: hypofibrinolysis related to an abnormal clot structure. *Blood* 1993;82: 2462–2469.

48. Siebenlist KR, Mosesson MW, DiOrio JP, et al. The polymerization of fibrinogen Dusart (a alpha 554 Arg → Cys) after removal of carboxy terminal regions of the a alpha-chains. *Blood Coagul Fibrinolysis* 1993;4: 61–65.

49. Hanss MM, Ffrench PO, Mornex JF, et al. Two novel fibrinogen variants found in patients with pulmonary embolism and their families. *J Thromb Haemost* 2003;1:1251–1257.

50. Zheng Z, Ashton RW, Ni F, et al. Thrombin hydrolysis of an N-terminal peptide from fibrinogen Lille: kinetic and NMR studies. *Biochemistry* 1992; 31:4426–4431.

51. Denninger MH, Finlayson JS, Reamer LA, et al. Congenital dysfibrinogenemia: fibrinogen Lille. *Thromb Res* 1978;13:453–466.

52. Meyer M, Kutscher G, Sturzebecher J, et al. Fibrinogen Magdeburg I: a novel variant of human fibrinogen with an amino acid exchange in the fibrinopeptide a (Aalpha 9, Leu → Pro). *Thromb Res* 2003;109: 145–151.

53. Niwa K, Yaginuma A, Nakanishi M, et al. Fibrinogen Mitaka II: a hereditary dysfibrinogen with defective thrombin binding caused by an a alpha Glu-11 to Gly substitution. *Blood* 1993;82:3658–3663.

54. Ni F, Konishi Y, Bullock LD, et al. High-resolution NMR studies of fibrinogen-like peptides in solution: structural basis for the bleeding disorder caused by a single mutation of Gly(12) to Val(12) in the A alpha chain of human fibrinogen Rouen. *Biochemistry* 1989;28:3106–3119.

55. Mathonnet F, Peltier JY, Detruit H, et al. Fibrinogen Saint-Germain I: a case of the heterozygous Aalpha GLY 12 → VAL fibrinogen variant. *Blood Coagul Fibrinolysis* 2002;13:149–153.

56. Hanss M, Biot F. A database for human fibrinogen variants. *Ann N Y Acad Sci* 2001;936:89–90.

57. Wada Y, Niwa K, Maekawa H, et al. A new type of congenital dysfibrinogen, fibrinogen Bremen, with an A alpha gly-17 to Val substitution associated

58. Uotani C, Miyata T, Kumabashiri I, et al. Fibrinogen Kanazawa: a congenital dysfibrinogenaemia with delayed polymerization having a replacement of proline-18 by leucine in the a alpha-chain. *Blood Coagul Fibrinolysis* 1991;2:413–417.

59. Yoshida N, O kuma M, Hirata H, et al. Fibrinogen Kyoto II, a new congenitally abnormal molecule, characterized by the replacement of a alpha proline-18 by leucine. *Blood* 1991;78:149–153.

60. Hessel B, Stenbjerg S, Dyr J, et al. Fibrinogen aarhus—a new case of dysfibrinogenemia. *Thromb Haemost* 1986;42:21–37.

61. Dempfle C-E, Henschen A Fibrinogen Mannheim I—identification of an Aa19Arg → Gly substitution in dysfibrinogenemia associated with bleeding tendency. In: Matsuda M, Iwanaga S, Takada A et al., eds. *Fibrinogen 4. Current basic and clinical aspects.* Amsterdam: Elsevier Science, 1990:159.

62. Tanaka H, Terasawa F, Ito T, et al. Fibrinogen Matsumoto V: a variant with Aalpha19 Arg → Gly (AGG → GGG). Comparison between fibrin polymerization stimulated by thrombin or reptilase and fibrin monomer polymerization. *Thromb Haemost* 2001;85:108–113.

63. Bolliger-Stucki B, Buccierelli P, Lammle B, et al. Fibrinogen Milano XIII (Aalpha 19 Arg → Gly): a dysfunctional variant with an amino acid substitution in the N-terminal polymerization site. *Thromb Res* 1999;96:399–405.

64. Brennan SO, Ridgway H, Stormorken H, et al. Characterisation of fibrinogen Oslo IV by electrospray mass spectrometry. *Thromb Haemost* 1997;77:1040–1041.

65. Stormorken H, Brosstad F, Seim H. A new dysfibrinogenemia: fibrinogen Oslo IV. *Thromb Haemost* 1983;49:120–122.

66. Marx R, Schramm W. On dysfibrinogenemia. In: Henschen A, Graeff H, Lottspeich F, eds. *Fibrinogen—recent biochemical and medical aspects.* Berlin: de Gruyter, 1982:123.

67. Brennan SO, Hammonds B, George PM. Aberrant hepatic processing causes removal of activation peptide and primary polymerisation site from fibrinogen Canterbury (A alpha 20 Val → Asp). *J Clin Invest* 1995;96:2854–2858.

68. Maekawa H, Yamazumi K, Muramatsu S, et al. Fibrinogen Lima: a homozygous dysfibrinogen with an A alpha-arginine-141 to serine substitution associated with extra N-glycosylation at A alpha-asparagine-139. Impaired fibrin gel formation but normal fibrin-facilitated plasminogen activation catalyzed by tissue-type plasminogen activator. *J Clin Invest.* 1992;90:67–76.

69. Arocha-Pinango CL, Rodriguez S, Nagy H, et al. Fibrinogen Lima. A new dysfibrinogenaemia with a high-molecular-weight alpha-chain and effective polymerization. *Blood Coagul Fibrinolysis* 1990;1:561–565.

70. Ridgway HJ, Brennan SO, Faed JM, et al. Fibrinogen Otago: a major alpha chain truncation associated with severe hypofibrinogenaemia and recurrent miscarriage. *Br J Haematol* 1997;98:632–639.

71. Lefebvre P, Velasco PT, Dear A, et al. Severe hypodysfibrinogenemia in compound heterozygotes of the fibrinogen A{alpha}IVS4+1 G > T mutation and an A{alpha}Gln328 truncation (fibrinogen Keokuk). *Blood* 2004;130:2571–2576.

72. Maekawa H, Yamazumi K, Muramatsu S, et al. An a alpha Ser-434 to N-glycosylated Asn substitution in a dysfibrinogen, fibrinogen Caracas II, characterized by impaired fibrin gel formation. *J Biol Chem* 1991;266: 11575–11581.

73. Woodhead JL, Nagaswami C, Matsuda M, et al. The ultrastructure of fibrinogen Caracas II molecules, fibers, and clots. *J Biol Chem* 1996;271: 4946–4953.

74. Furlan M, Steinmann C, Jungo M, et al. A frameshift mutation in Exon V of the a alpha-chain gene leading to truncated a alpha-chains in the homozygous dysfibrinogen Milano III. *J Biol Chem* 1994;269:33129–33134.

75. Furlan M, Steinmann C, Jungo M, et al. Binding of calcium ions and their effect on clotting of fibrinogen Milano III, a variant with truncated a alpha-chains. *Blood Coagul Fibrinolysis* 1996;7:331–335.

76. Collen A, Maas A, Kooistra T, et al. Aberrant fibrin formation and cross-linking of fibrinogen Nieuwegein, a variant with a shortened Aalpha-chain, alters endothelial capillary tube formation. *Blood* 2001;97:973–980.

77. Koopman J, Haverkate F, Grimbergen J, et al. Fibrinogen Marburg: a homozygous case of dysfibrinogenemia, lacking amino acids a alpha 461-610 (Lys 461 AAA → stop TAA). *Blood* 1992;80:1972–1979.

78. Ridgway HJ, Brennan SO, Gibbons S, et al. Fibrinogen Lincoln: a new truncated alpha chain variant with delayed clotting. *Br J Haematol* 1996; 93:177–184.

79. Homer VM, Mullin JL, Brennan SO, et al. Novel Aalpha chain truncation (fibrinogen Perth) resulting in low expression and impaired fibrinogen polymerization. *J Thromb Haemost* 2003;1:1245–1250.

80. Margaglione M, Vecchione G, Santacroce R, et al. A frameshift mutation in the human fibrinogen Aalpha-chain gene (Aalpha(499)Ala frameshift stop) leading to dysfibrinogen San Giovanni Rotondo. *Thromb Haemost* 2001;86:1483–1488.

81. Marchi R, Mirshahi SS, Soria C, et al. Thrombotic dysfibrinogenemia. Fibrinogen "Caracas V" relation between very tight fibrin network and defective clot degradability. *Thromb Res* 2000;99:187–193.

82. Marchi R, Lundberg U, Grimbergen J, et al. Fibrinogen Caracas V, an abnormal fibrinogen with an Aalpha 532 Ser → Cys substitution associated with thrombosis. *Thromb Haemost* 2000;84:263–270.

83. Liu CY, Koehn JA, Morgan FJ Characterization of fibrinogen New York 1. A dysfunctional fibrinogen with a deletion of b beta(9-72) corresponding exactly to exon 2 of the gene. *J Biol Chem.* 1985;260:4390–4396.

84. Brennan SO, Hammonds B, Spearing R, et al. Electrospray ionisation mass spectrometry facilitates detection of fibrinogen (Bbeta 14 Arg → Cys) mutation in a family with thrombosis. *Thromb Haemost* 1997;78:1484–1487.

85. Koopman J, Haverkate F, Grimbergen J, et al. Abnormal fibrinogens Ijmuiden (B beta Arg14—Cys) and Nijmegen (B beta Arg44—Cys) form disulfide-linked fibrinogen-albumin complexes. *Proc Natl Acad Sci U S A* 1992;89:3478–3482.

86. Branson HE, Schmer G, Dillard DH. Fibrinogen Seattle: a qualitatively abnormal fibrinogen in a patient with tetralogy of Fallot. *Am J Clin Pathol* 1977;67:236–240.

87. Branson HE, Schmer G, Theodor I, et al. Fibrinogen Seattle releases half the normal amount of fibrinopeptide B. *Acta Haematol* 1983;70:257–263.

88. Kamura T, Tsuda H, Yae Y, et al. An abnormal fibrinogen Fukuoka II (Gly-B beta 15 → Cys) characterized by defective fibrin lateral association and mixed disulfide formation. *J Biol Chem* 1995;270:29392–29399.

89. Yoshida N, Wada H, Morita K, et al. A new congenital abnormal fibrinogen Ise characterized by the replacement of b beta glycine-15 by cysteine. *Blood* 1991;77:1958–1963.

90. Hirota-Kawadobora M, Terasawa F, Yonekawa O, et al. Fibrinogens Kosai and Ogasa: Bbeta 15Gly → Cys (GGT → TGT) substitution associated with impairment of fibrinopeptide B release and lateral aggregation. *J Thromb Haemost* 2003;1:275–283.

91. Engesser L, Koopman J, de Munk G, et al. Fibrinogen Nijmegen: congenital dysfibrinogenemia associated with impaired t-PA mediated plasminogen activation and decreased binding of t-PA. *Thromb Haemost* 1988;60:113–120.

92. Koopman J, Haverkate F, Lord ST, et al. Molecular basis of fibrinogen Naples associated with defective thrombin binding and thrombophilia. Homozygous substitution of B beta 68 Ala—Thr. *J Clin Invest* 1992;90:238–244.

93. Meh DA, Mosesson MW, Siebenlist KR, et al. Fibrinogen Naples I (B beta A68T) nonsubstrate thrombin-binding capacities. *Thromb Res* 2001;103:63–73.

94. Haverkate F, Koopman J, Kluft C, et al. Fibrinogens "Milano II"-and "Naples". *Thromb Haemost* 1987;57:375.

95. Sugo T, Nakamikawa C, Takano H, et al. Fibrinogen Niigata with impaired fibrin assembly: an inherited dysfibrinogen with a Bbeta Asn-160 to Ser substitution associated with extra glycosylation at Bbeta Asn-158. *Blood* 1999;94:3806–3813.

96. Lounes KC, Lefkowitz JB, Henschen-Edman AH, et al. The impaired polymerization of fibrinogen Longmont (Bbeta 166Arg → Cys) is not improved by removal of disulfide-linked dimers from a mixture of dimers and cysteine-linked monomers. *Blood* 2001;98:661–666.

97. Lefkowitz JB, DeBoom T, Weller A, et al. Fibrinogen Longmont: a dysfibrinogenemia that causes prolonged clot-based test results only when using an optical detection method. *Am J Hematol* 2000;63:149–155.

98. Lounes KC, Lefkowitz JB, Coates AI, et al. Fibrinogen Longmont. A heterozygous abnormal fibrinogen with b beta Arg-166 to Cys substitution associated with defective fibrin polymerization. *Ann N Y Acad Sci* 2001;936:129–132.

99. Kaudewitz H, Henschen A, Soria J, et al. Fibrinogen Pontoise-A genetically abnormal fibrinogen with defective fibrin polymerization and normal fibrinopeptide release. In: Lane DA, Henschen A, Jasani MK, eds. *Fibrinogen-fibrin formation and fibrinolysis*, Vol 4. Berlin: Walter de Gruyter, 1986:91.

100. Sugo T, Nakamikawa C, Yoshida N, et al. End-linked homodimers in fibrinogen Osaka VI with a B beta-chain extension lead to fragile clot structure. *Blood* 2000;96:3779–3785.

101. Bolliger-Stucki B, Lord ST, Furlan M. Fibrinogen Milano XII: a dysfunctional variant containing 2 amino acid substitutions, Aalpha R16C and gamma G165R. *Blood* 2001;98:351–357.

102. Niwa K, Takebe M, Sugo T, et al. A gamma Gly-268 to Glu substitution is responsible for impaired fibrin assembly in a homozygous dysfibrinogen Kurashiki I. *Blood* 1996;87:4686–4694.

103. Mimuro J, Kawata Y, Niwa K, et al. A new type of Ser substitution for gamma Arg-275 in fibrinogen Kamogawa I characterized by impaired fibrin assembly. *Thromb Haemost* 1999;81:940–944.

104. Brennan SO, Wyatt JM, Ockelford P, et al. Defective fibrinogen polymerization associated with a novel gamma 279Ala → Asp mutation. *Br J Haematol* 2000;108:236–240.

105. Fellowes AP, Brennan SO, Ridgway HJ, et al. Electrospray ionization mass spectrometry identification of fibrinogen Banks Peninsula (gamma 280Tyr → Cys): a new variant with defective polymerization. *Br J Haematol* 1998;101:24–31.

106. Bantia S, Mane SM, Bell WR, et al. Fibrinogen Baltimore I: polymerization defect associated with a gamma 292Gly--Val (GGC--GTC) mutation. *Blood* 1990;76:2279–2283.

107. Brown CH, Crowe MF. Defective alpha-polymerization in the conversion of fibrinogen Baltimore to fibrin. *J Clin Invest* 1975;55:1190–1194.

108. Beck EA, Charache P, Jackson DP. A new inherited coagulation disorder caused by an abnormal fibrinogen ('fibrinogen Baltimore'). *Nature* 1965;208:143–145.

109. Mosesson MW, Beck EA. Chromatographic, ultracentrifugal, and related studies of fibrinogen "Baltimore". *J Clin Invest* 1969;48:1656–1662.

110. Stucki B, Schmutz P, Schmid L, et al. Fibrinogen St. Gallen I (gamma 292 Gly → Val): evidence for structural alterations causing defective polymerization and fibrinogenolysis. *Thromb Haemost* 1999;81:268–274.

111. Ebert RF, Bell WR. Fibrinogen Baltimore III: congenital dysfibrinogenemia with a shortened gamma-subunit. *Thromb Res* 1988;51:251–258.

112. Bantia S, Bell WR, Dang CV. Polymerization defect of fibrinogen Baltimore III due to a gamma Asn308--Ile mutation. *Blood* 1990;75:1659–1663.

113. Grailhe P, Boyer-Neumann C, Haverkate F, et al. The mutation in fibrinogen Bicetre II (gamma Asn 308 → Lys) does not affect the binding of t-PA and plasminogen to fibrin. *Blood Coagul Fibrinolysis* 1993;4:679–687.

114. Yoshida N, Terukina S, Okuma M, et al. Characterization of an apparently lower molecular weight gamma-chain variant in fibrinogen Kyoto I. The replacement of gamma-asparagine 308 by lysine which causes accelerated cleavage of fragment D1 by plasmin and the generation of a new plasmin cleavage site. *J Biol Chem* 1988;263:13848–13856.

115. Mimuro J, Muramatsu S, Maekawa H, et al. Gene analyses of abnormal fibrinogens with a mutation in the gamma chain. *Int J Hematol* 1992;56:129–134.

116. Okumura N, Furihata K, Terasawa F, et al. Fibrinogen Matsumoto II: gamma 308 Asn → Lys (AAT → AAG) mutation associated with bleeding tendency. *Br J Haematol* 1996;94:526–528.

117. Terasawa F, Fujita K, Tozuka M, et al. Identification of a dysfibrinogen, the substitution of gamma308Asn(AAT) to Lys(AAG), using coagulation tests, immunoblot analysis, and allele-specific polymerase chain reaction. *Clin Chim Acta* 2000;295:77–85.

118. Mullin JL, Brennan SO, Ganly PS, et al. Fibrinogen hillsborough: a novel gammaGly309Asp dysfibrinogen with impaired clotting. *Blood* 2002;99:3597–3601.

119. Yamazumi K, Shimura K, Terukina S, et al. A gamma methionine-310 to threonine substitution and consequent N-glycosylation at gamma asparagine-308 identified in a congenital dysfibrinogenemia associated with posttraumatic bleeding, fibrinogen Asahi. *J Clin Invest* 1989;83:1590–1597.

120. Yamazumi K, Shimura K, Maekawa H, et al. Delayed intermolecular gamma-chain cross-linking by factor XIIIa in fibrinogen Asahi characterized by a gamma-Met-310 to Thr substitution with an N-glycosylated gamma-Asn-308. *Blood Coagul Fibrinolysis* 1990;1:557–559.

121. Sugo T, Sekine O, Nakamikawa C, et al. Mode of perturbation of Asahi fibrin assembly by the extra oligosaccharides. *Ann N Y Acad Sci* 2001;936:223–225.

122. Lounes KC, Soria C, Valognes A, et al. Fibrinogen Bastia (gamma 318 Asp → Tyr) a novel abnormal fibrinogen characterized by defective fibrin polymerization. *Thromb Haemost* 1999;82:1639–1643.

123. Haverkate F, Samama M. Familial dysfibrinogenemia and thrombophilia. Report on a study of the SSC subcommittee on fibrinogen. *Thromb Haemost* 1995;73:151–161.

124. Hogan KA, Lord ST, Okumura N, et al. A functional assay suggests that heterodimers exist in two C-terminal gamma-chain dysfibrinogens: Matsumoto I and Vlissingen/Frankfurt IV. *Thromb Haemost* 2000;83:592–597.

125. Terasawa F, Hogan KA, Kani S, et al. Fibrinogen Otsu I:a gammaAsn319, Asp320 deletion dysfibrinogen identified in an asymptomatic pregnant woman. *Thromb Haemost* 2003;90:757–758.

126. Guglielmone HA, Sanchez MC, Abate Daga D, et al. A new heterozygous mutation in gamma fibrinogen gene leading to 326 Cys → Ser substitution in fibrinogen Cordoba is associated with defective polymerization and familial hypofibrinogenemia. *J Thromb Haemost* 2004;2:352–354.

127. Guglielmone HA, Sanchez MC, Quinonez M, et al. Fibrinogen Cordoba: biochemical characterization of a new congenital hypodysfibrinogenemia. *Clin Chim Acta* 2002;317:239–240.

128. Hamano A, Mimuro J, Aoshima M, et al. Thrombophilic dysfibrinogen Tokyo V with the amino acid substitution of {gamma} Ala-327 to Thr: formation of fragile but fibrinolysis-resistant fibrin clots and its relevance to arterial thromboembolism. *Blood.* 2004;103:3045–3050.

129. Miyata T, Furukawa K, Iwanaga S, et al. Fibrinogen Nagoya, a replacement of glutamine-329 by arginine in the gamma-chain that impairs the polymerization of fibrin monomer. *J Biochem (Tokyo)* 1989;105:10–14.

130. Mizuochi T, Taniguchi T, Asami Y, et al. Comparative studies on the structures of the carbohydrate moieties of human fibrinogen and abnormal fibrinogen Nagoya. *J Biochem (Tokyo)* 1982;92:283–293.

131. Lounes KC, Soria C, Mirshahi SS, et al. Fibrinogen ales: a homozygous case of dysfibrinogenemia (gamma-Asp(330) → Val) characterized by a defective fibrin polymerization site "a". *Blood* 2000;96:3473–3479.

132. Reber P, Furlan M, Rupp C, et al. Characterization of fibrinogen Milano I: amino acid exchange gamma 330 Asp—Val impairs fibrin polymerization. *Blood* 1986;67:1751–1756.

133. Terukina S, Yamazumi K, Okamoto K, et al. Fibrinogen Kyoto III: a congenital dysfibrinogen with a gamma aspartic acid-330 to tyrosine substitution manifesting impaired fibrin monomer polymerization. *Blood* 1989;74:2681–2687.

134. Steinmann C, Reber P, Jungo M, et al. Fibrinogen Bern I: substitution gamma 337 Asn → Lys is responsible for defective fibrin monomer polymerization. *Blood* 1993;82:2104–2108.

135. Rupp C, Kuyas C, Haeberli A, et al. [Fibrinogen Bern I and fibrinogen Bern II: 2 hereditary fibrinogen variants with diverse biochemical properties]. *Schweiz Med Wochenschr* 1981;111:1543–1545.

136. Rosenberg JB, Newman PJ, Mosesson MW, et al. Paris I dysfibrinogenemia: a point mutation in intron 8 results in insertion of a 15 amino acid sequence in the fibrinogen gamma-chain. *Thromb Haemost* 1993;69:217–220.

137. Budzynski AZ, Marder VJ, Menache D, et al. Defect in the gamma polypeptide chain of a congenital abnormal fibrinogen (Paris I). *Nature* 1974;252:66–68.

138. Guillin MC, Menache D. Fetal fibrinogen and fibrinogen Paris I: comparative fibrin monomers aggregation studies. *Thromb Res* 1973;3:117–135.

139. Budzynski AZ, Marder VJ. Plasmic degradation of fibrinogen Paris I. *J Lab Clin Med* 1976;88:817–825.

140. Finlayson JS, Reamer LA, Mosesson MW, et al. Fibrinopeptide release from fibrinogen Paris I. *Thromb Res* 1980;17:577–579.

141. Denninger MH, Jandrot-Perrus M, Elion J, et al. ADP-induced platelet aggregation depends on the conformation or availability of the terminal gamma chain sequence of fibrinogen. Study of the reactivity of fibrinogen Paris 1. *Blood* 1987;70:558–563.

142. Maak B. Hereditary dysfibrinogenaemia (fibrinogen Jena)—report of a family study. *Folia Haematol Int Mag Klin Morphol Blutforsch* 1988; 115:519–522.

143. Steinmann C, Bogli C, Jungo M, et al. A new substitution, gamma 358 Ser → Cys, in fibrinogen Milano VII causes defective fibrin polymerization. *Blood* 1994;84:1874–1880.

144. Mathonnet F, Guillon L, Detruit H, et al. Fibrinogen Poissy II (gammaN361K): a novel dysfibrinogenemia associated with defective polymerization and peptide B release. *Blood Coagul Fibrinolysis* 2003;14:293–298.

145. Okumura N, Furihata K, Terasawa F, et al. Fibrinogen Matsumoto I: a gamma 364 Asp → His (GAT → CAT) substitution associated with defective fibrin polymerization. *Thromb Haemost* 1996;75:887–891.

146. Bentolila S, Samama MM, Conard J, et al. [Association of dysfibrinogenemia and thrombosis. Apropos of a family (fibrinogen Melun) and review of the literature]. *Ann Med Interne (Paris)* 1995;146:575–580.

147. Yoshida N, Hirata H, Morigami Y, et al. Characterization of an abnormal fibrinogen Osaka V with the replacement of gamma-arginine 375 by glycine. The lack of high affinity calcium binding to D-domains and the lack of protective effect of calcium on fibrinolysis. *J Biol Chem* 1992;267: 2753–2759.

148. Yoshida N, Hirata H, Imaoka S, et al. Effect of calcium on the mobility of gamma-chain from fibrinogen Osaka V on sodium dodecyl sulfate-polyacrylamide gel electrophoresis. *Thromb Res* 1994;73:79–82.

149. Ridgway HJ, Brennan SO, Loreth RM, et al. Fibrinogen Kaiserslautern (gamma 380 Lys to Asn): a new glycosylated fibrinogen variant with delayed polymerization. *Br J Haematol* 1997;99:562–569.

150. Brennan SO, Loreth RM, George PM. Oligosaccharide configuration of fibrinogen Kaiserslautern: electrospray ionisation analysis of intact gamma chains. *Thromb Haemost* 1998;80:263–265.

151. Alving BM, Henschen AH. Fibrinogen Giessen I: a congenital homozygously expressed dysfibrinogenemia with a alpha 16 Arg—His substitution. *Am J Hematol* 1987;25:479–482.

152. Henschen A, Kehl M, Southan C. Genetically abnormal fibrinogens-some current characterization strategies. In: Haverkate F HA, Nieuwenhuizen W, Straub PW, eds. *Fibrinogen: structure, functional aspects, metabolism.* Berlin: Walter de Gruyter, 1983:125.

153. Soria J, Soria C, Samama M, et al. Fibrinogen treys—fibrinogen Metz. Two new cases of congenital dysfibrinogenemia. *Thromb Diath Haemorrh* 1972;27:619–633.

154. Binnie CG, Lord ST. The fibrinogen sequences that interact with thrombin. *Blood* 1993;81:3186–3192.

155. Stubbs MT, Oschkinat H, Mayr I, et al. The interaction of thrombin with fibrinogen. A structural basis for its specificity. *Eur J Biochem* 1992;206: 187–195.

156. Pechik I, Madrazo J, Mosesson MW, et al. Crystal structure of the complex between thrombin and the central "E" region of fibrin. *Proc Natl Acad Sci U S A* 2004;101:2718–2723.

157. Spraggon G, Everse SJ, Doolittle RF. Crystal structures of fragment D from human fibrinogen and its crosslinked counterpart from fibrin. *Nature* 1997;389:455–462.

158. Everse SJ, Spraggon G, Veerapandian L, et al. Crystal structure of fragment double-D from human fibrin with two different bound ligands. *Biochemistry* 1998;37:8637–8642.

159. Everse SJ, Spraggon G, Veerapandian L, et al. Conformational changes in fragments D and double-D from human fibrin(ogen) upon binding the peptide ligand Gly-His-Arg-Pro-amide. *Biochemistry* 1999;38:2941–2946.

160. Kostelansky MS, Betts L, Gorkun OV, et al. 2.8 A crystal structures of recombinant fibrinogen fragment D with and without two peptide ligands: GHRP binding to the "b" site disrupts its nearby calcium-binding site. *Biochemistry.* 2002;41:12124–12132.

161. Okumura N, Gorkun OV, Lord ST. Severely impaired polymerization of recombinant fibrinogen gamma-364 Asp → His, the substitution discovered in a heterozygous individual. *J Biol Chem* 1997;272:29596–29601.

162. Furlan M, Rupp C, Beck EA, et al. Effect of calcium and synthetic peptides on fibrin polymerization. *Thromb Haemost* 1982;47:118–121.

163. Yee VC, Pratt KP, Cote HC, et al. Crystal structure of a 30 kDa C-terminal fragment from the gamma chain of human fibrinogen. *Structure* 1997;5: 125–138.

164. Mosesson MW, Siebenlist KR, DiOrio JP, et al. The role of fibrinogen D domain intermolecular association sites in the polymerization of fibrin and fibrinogen Tokyo II (gamma 275 Arg → Cys). *J Clin Invest* 1995;96: 1053–1058.

165. Matsuda M, Baba M, Morimoto K, et al. "Fibrinogen Tokyo II". An abnormal fibrinogen with an impaired polymerization site on the aligned DD domain of fibrin molecules. *J Clin Invest* 1983;72:1034–1041.

166. Veklich YI, Gorkun OV, Medved LV, et al. Carboxyl-terminal portions of the alpha chains of fibrinogen and fibrin. Localization by electron microscopy and the effects of isolated alpha C fragments on polymerization. *J Biol Chem* 1993;268:13577–13585.

167. Gorkun OV, Veklich YI, Medved LV, et al. Role of the alpha C domains of fibrin in clot formation. *Biochemistry* 1994;33:6986–6997.

168. Benson MD, Liepnieks J, Uemichi T, et al. Hereditary renal amyloidosis associated with a mutant fibrinogen alpha-chain. *Nat Genet* 1993;3:252–255.

169. Uemichi T, Liepnieks JJ, Benson MD. Hereditary renal amyloidosis with a novel variant fibrinogen. *J Clin Invest* 1994;93:731–736.

170. Uemichi T, Liepnieks JJ, Yamada T, et al. A frame shift mutation in the fibrinogen a alpha chain gene in a kindred with renal amyloidosis. *Blood* 1996;87:4197–4203.

171. Hamidi Asl L, Liepnieks JJ, Uemichi T, et al. Renal amyloidosis with a frame shift mutation in fibrinogen Aalpha-chain gene producing a novel amyloid protein. *Blood* 1997;90:4799–4805.

172. Lachmann HJ, Booth DR, Booth SE, et al. Misdiagnosis of hereditary amyloidosis as AL (primary) amyloidosis. *N Engl J Med* 2002;346: 1786–1791.

# CHAPTER 63 ■ FAMILIAL MULTIPLE COAGULATION FACTOR DEFICIENCIES

BIN ZHANG AND DAVID GINSBURG

The familial multiple coagulation factor deficiencies are a group of rare inherited disorders characterized by a simultaneous decrease in the levels of two or more coagulation factors. Earlier reports of deficiencies in various combinations of coagulation factors prompted Scoff and Levin (1) in 1981, to classify these disorders into six types [familial multiple factor deficiency (FMFD) I-VI]. Combined deficiency of FV and FVIII (F5F8D, or FMFD I) and combined deficiency of vitamin K–dependent clotting factors (VKCFD, or FMFD III) are the best known, and comprise most of the reported cases of familial multiple coagulation factor deficiencies. This chapter focuses on these two disorders. Little is known about other types of multiple coagulation factor deficiencies, because few new cases have been reported since 1981. As a consequence, this old classification is of limited relevance today and not generally used in practice.

## COMBINED DEFICIENCY OF FACTOR V AND FACTOR VIII

### History

Combined deficiency of factors V and VIII (F5F8D) was first described in a pair of Swiss siblings in 1954 (2). Since then, a number of additional families have been identified around the world. To our knowledge, at least 140 patients in 81 families have been diagnosed with F5F8D to date, with more than half the families from the Mediterranean region. However, it is likely that F5F8D is underdiagnosed, in part because of its often mild bleeding manifestations. Some patients with F5F8D may be misdiagnosed as having mild hemophilia A or parahemophilia (FV deficiency). F5F8D appears to be particularly prevalent among Middle Eastern Jews and non-Jewish Iranians, estimated at approximately 1:100,000 (3–5). This high frequency is probably caused, at least in part, by the high incidence of consanguineous marriages in these populations. Founder effect may also contribute to higher frequency in Middle Eastern Jews (6,7).

The molecular basis of F5F8D was a mystery until recently. Initial speculation centered on a defect in a precursor protein for both factors V and VIII (2), but no such precursor could be identified. A low level of protein C inhibitor activity in plasma of patients who were affected was reported in 1980 (8), suggesting that excessive degradation of factors V and VIII by the unopposed action of activated protein C (APC) as the cause of the disease. However, further studies by the original group and others found normal levels of protein C inhibitor activity and antigenicity, and demonstrated that the earlier findings were caused by an artifactual loss of protein C inhibitor in frozen samples (9–12). Recent genetic studies identified the cause of this disorder as deficiencies in a unique secretory pathway shared by FV and FVIII (6,13,14).

### Genetics and Biology

A comprehensive review of the biology of coagulation factors V and VIII can be found in Chapters 8 and 9. Here, we briefly discuss the similarities and differences between these two proteins. Factor V (FV) and factor VIII (FVIII) are two large plasma glycoproteins that function as essential cofactors for the proteolytic activation of prothrombin and factor X, respectively. FV is synthesized primarily in hepatocytes in humans (15,16), although also in megakaryocytes in rodents (17–19), and is found in the plasma and $\alpha$-granules of platelets as a 330-kDa single chain polypeptide (20). The primary tissue source for the biosynthesis of FVIII is less clear. Although earlier results suggested the hepatocyte (21–24), a recent study identified liver sinusoidal endothelial cell as a significant source of circulating FVIII (25). FVIII is processed upon secretion to a heterodimer consisting of an 80-kDa light chain in association with a 200-kDa heavy chain fragment (26). The light chain is bound through noncovalent interactions to a primary binding site at the amino-terminus of von Willebrand factor (VWF). Interaction with VWF is required to stabilize FVIII in plasma. FV and FVIII circulate as inactive precursors that are activated through limited proteolysis by thrombin. FV and FVIII share similar domain structure (A1-A2-B-A3-C1-C2), and undergo similar extensive posttranslational modifications, including signal peptide cleavage, formation of conserved disulfide bonds, addition of multiple oligosaccharide structures, and sulfation of specific tyrosine residues (27). Both protein cofactors are also inactivated through proteolysis by APC. Despite these similarities, the plasma concentration of FVIII is two orders of magnitude lower than that of FV.

Inheritance of F5F8D is autosomal, recessive, and distinct from the coinheritance of both FV deficiency and FVIII deficiency. Heterozygotes are asymptomatic and the plasma levels of FV and FVIII are indistinguishable from normal. Using homozygosity mapping and positional cloning approaches, the first gene for F5F8D was identified in 1998 (6) as *LMAN1* (also known as *ERGIC-53*) of previously unknown function (28,29). To date, 17 different *LMAN1* mutations have been identified (6,30–32). All but one are either nonsense or frameshift alleles whose truncated protein products would be predicted to lack normal *LMAN1* function (see Fig. 63-1A). The only missense mutation substitutes a threonine for the initiator methionine, also predicted to result in the absence of a protein product. The diverse nature of the mutations indicates multiple independent genetic origins. However, founder mutations may account for all or most F5F8D in some isolated populations. For example, one of the two original reported

953

mutations was found to be prevalent in Jews originating from the island of Djerba in Tunisia, whereas this mutation was not found among North African Jews (6,7).

Mutations in *LMAN1* account for approximately 70% of patients with F5F8D. No *LMAN1* mutations could be identified in approximately 30% of affected families (31,32). The second cause of F5F8D was identified in these families as mutations in a novel gene that was named *MCFD2* (multiple coagulation factor deficiency gene 2) (13). Seven different mutations have been identified to date in *MCFD2* (13), including splice-site mutation, frameshift deletions, as well as two missense mutations (Fig. 63-1B). Together, mutations in *LMAN1* and *MCFD2* account for nearly all cases of F5F8D.

LMAN1 is a 53-kDa homo-hexameric transmembrane protein that belongs to a recently defined class of animal lectins (33–36) with homology to leguminous mannose-binding lectins (34–36). MCFD2 is an EF-hand domain protein that colocalizes with LMAN1 in the ER-Golgi intermediate compartment (ERGIC). MCFD2 interacts with LMAN1 to form a stable complex in a calcium-dependent manner. This interaction also serves as a mechanism to retain MCFD2 in the *ERGIC*. Missense mutations within the second MCFD2 EF-hand domain disrupt this interaction and result in F5F8D (13).

One of the central problems in cell biology is how newly synthesized proteins are sorted for transport to their final destinations. An increasingly accepted model envisions that "cargo receptors," localized to the ER membrane, selectively package secreted proteins into "vesicles" for transport to the Golgi (37–39). The finding of *LMAN1* gene mutations as a cause of F5F8D provided the first direct evidence for a mammalian ER cargo receptor, suggesting that LMAN1 specifically mediates export of FV and FVIII from ER to Golgi (see Fig. 63-2). To date, the LMAN1-MCFD2 complex remains the only cargo receptor identified in higher eukaryotes, although two potential cargo receptors were recently described in yeast (40,41). LMAN1 and MCFD2 have been shown to directly bind to FV and FVIII (42). The heavily glycosylated

B-domains of FV and FVIII may be important in mediating secretion through the LMAN1-MCFD2 pathway (43). An interesting question is whether the ER to Golgi transport of other proteins is also altered in patients with F5F8D. This seems likely, given the ubiquitous expression patterns of both LMAN1 and MCFD2, as well as the presence of LMAN1 and MCFD2 orthologs in lower eukaryotes without a blood clotting system. Indeed, two other proteins have been identified to either interact with LMAN1 (44) or exhibit delayed secretion in cultured cells with a dysfunctional LMAN1 (45). However, transport deficiency in other proteins is likely to be at a level insufficient to produce a clinical phenotype, because no other abnormalities other than the deficiencies of FV and FVIII have been identified in patients with F5F8D.

## Clinical Manifestations

Seligsohn et al. (3) studied 14 patients in 7 families of Middle Eastern Jews. Peyvandi et al. (4) and Mansouritorgabeh et al. (5) studied a total of 46 patients from 23 families of non-Jewish Iranians. In addition to these relatively large studies, a number of case reports have also been published (46–66). Patients with this disorder exhibit plasma FV and FVIII activity level at approximately 10% of normal, with a range of 5% to 30%, although factor level as low as 2% have been reported (4). FV and FVIII clotting activity and antigenic level are both concordantly decreased (1,64,67). Bleeding symptoms appear to be comparable to those observed in patients with single deficiencies of FV or FVIII (3,4). No abnormalities outside of these hemostatic changes have been identified in F5F8D. Spontaneous bleeding symptoms are common, including easy bruising, epistaxis, and menorrhagia. Hemarthroses are less frequent, although they have been observed in up to one third of patients in some series (4,5,46). In contrast, gastrointestinal bleeding, hematuria, and intracranial bleeding are only rarely observed. Excessive bleeding is particularly common during or after trauma, tooth extraction, surgery, or labor. Postcircumcision bleeding was reported

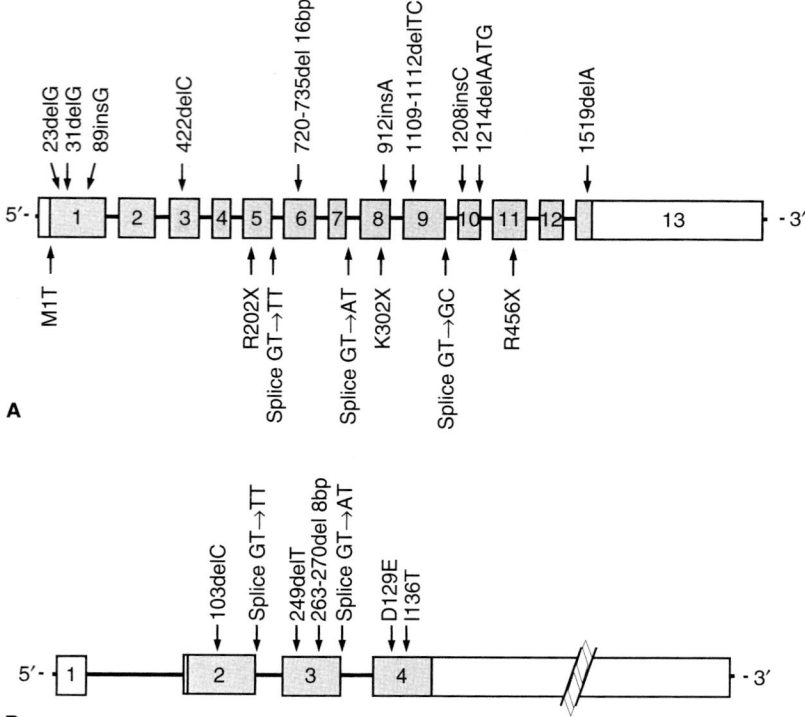

**FIGURE 63-1.** Structures of *LMAN1* and *MCFD2* genes and mutations identified in combined deficiency of factor V and factor VIII. **A:** All mutations in *LMAN1* identified to date are predicted to result in complete loss of protein function. Deletions and insertions are indicated above the gene, while nonsense mutations, splicing defects and the mutation that abolishes the initiation codon are indicated below the gene. **B:** Most mutations in *MCFD2* are predicted to result in frameshifts preceding the second EF-hand domain. Two missense mutations also occur in the second EF hand and were shown to abolish binding to *LMAN1 (13)*. Exons are numbered and drawn to scale. Shaded rectangles represent the coding regions of the genes, with the open portions of exons 1 and 13 in *LMAN1* and exons 1, 2, and 4 in *MCFD2* representing the 5' and 3' untranslated regions.

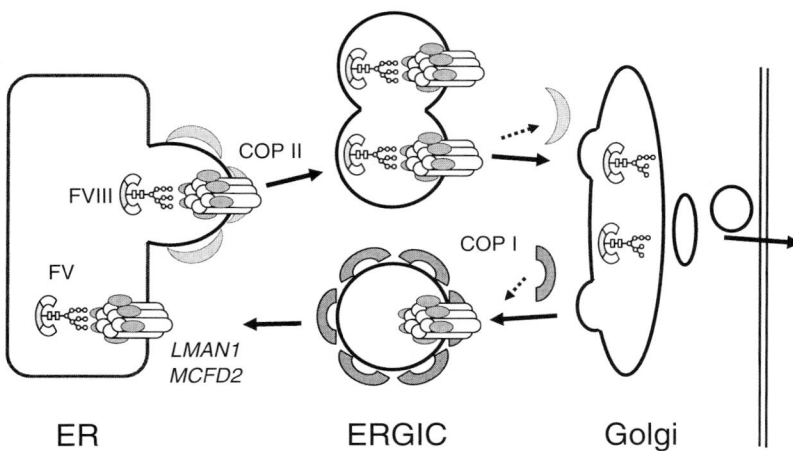

**FIGURE 63-2.** Model of receptor-mediate ER to Golgi transport of factor V (FV) and factor VIII (FVIII). Correctly folded FV/FVIII molecules are recruited to the COPII-coate d vesicles budding from the ER, by binding to the LMAN1–(MCFD2) complex. Upon budding, these vesicles uncoat and fuse with each other to form the ER-Golgi intermediate compartment (*ERGIC*). Release of FV/FVIII from LMAN1–MCFD2 occurs in the ERGIC. The LMAN1–MCFD2 complex is recycled back to the ER in COPI-coated retrograde vesicles as FV and FVIII are transported to the Golgi.

to be common among Iranian patients (4), but rare among Jewish patients (3), possibly because of the age at which circumcision is performed (at birth among Jews and usually at 5 to 7 years of age among Muslims). In contrast to hemophilia A, the levels of FV and FVIII correlate poorly with bleeding severity.

## Diagnosis and Differential Diagnosis

The diagnosis of F5F8D should be suspected in patients with a prolonged prothrombin time (PT) and partial thromboplastin time (PTT) and a history of mild to moderate bleeding beginning in childhood. Diagnosis is confirmed by the demonstration of FV and FVIII levels in the 5% to 30% range. A positive family history, if present, should be consistent with autosomal recessive inheritance. All other routine laboratory results would be expected to be normal. Differential diagnosis includes coinheritance of hemophilia and parahemophilia, although this is extremely rare. Coinheritance of FV deficiency and type 1 von Willebrand disease (VWD) may be more common (47,54), given the higher frequency of VWD (68). VWF levels could be determined to exclude this possibility.

## Treatment

Because of the small number of patients, only limited experience is available to guide therapy (51,52,55,61,63,66,69), although severe or life-threatening bleeding is fortunately rare. Fresh frozen plasma has been effective in F5F8D, and should be used for the treatment of life-threatening hemorrhage. DDAVP (1-deamino-8-D-arginine vasopressin) has been used for mild to moderate bleeding, and results in up to a threefold increase in FVIII, but does not alter the FV level. DDAVP has also been used in combination with plasma infusion. Overall, treatment must be individualized to the specific patient and the severity of clinical bleeding.

# COMBINED DEFICIENCY OF VITAMIN K–DEPENDENT CLOTTING FACTORS

## History

The first case of VKCFD was described in 1966 in an infant girl who exhibited significant bleeding from the first week of life (70). The proband was found to have low or undetectable

levels of factors II, VII, IX, and X, with no evidence of hepatic disease or malabsorption. High doses of vitamin K partially restored clotting factor levels with clinical improvement (71). At least 16 additional cases of VKCFD have been reported since than (72–87).

## Genetics and Biology

γ-glutamyl carboxylase (GGCX) catalyzes a posttranslational modification of glutamate (Glu) residues into γ-carboxyglutamate (Gla) residues (88,89) (90,91). This carboxylation is required for the activities of coagulation factors II, VII, IX, and X, as well as the anticoagulant factors protein C, protein S and protein Z (92,93). Carboxylation occurs at Glu residues located in a homologous, approximately 45–amino acid "Gla domain." The presence of Gla residues is thought to enable these proteins to adapt to a calcium-dependent conformation that allows binding to phospholipids. Other proteins known to undergo γ-carboxylation include osteocalcin (94), matrix Gla protein (94), Gas6 (95), nephrocalcin A-D (96), as well as several putative carboxylated proteins identified through nucleotide database screening (PRGP1, PRGP2, TMG3 and TMG4) (97,98). Vitamin K is an essential cofactor for γ-carboxylase (88,89). As carbon dioxide is added to Glu to form Gla, the reduced form of vitamin K (vitamin K hydroquinone) is oxygenated to form vitamin K 2,3 epoxide. Another enzyme, vitamin K epoxide reductase (VKOR), is required to regenerate the vitamin K hydroquinone, completing the so-called vitamin K cycle (see Fig. 63-3).

VKCFD is an autosomal recessive disorder characterized by deficiency of all vitamin K–dependent clotting factors. It is a heterogeneous disorder with two subtypes. VKCFD1 is defined by defective γ-carboxylase (GGCX) activity, first demonstrated in Devon Rex cats (100). Recently, five different mutations in the *GGCX* gene have been reported in human families. Two different homozygous point mutations were found in three consanguineous families (74,76,79). The first mutation results in the substitution of arginine for leucine at residue 394 (L394R) in four members of an Arab kindred. The second mutation that changes a tryptophan at residue 501 to serine (W501S) was reported in two Lebanese families. Two heterozygote mutations were identified in a German boy of nonconsanguineous parents (85). One is a splice-site mutation that results in early truncation of GGCX, and the other is a missense mutation that changes a conserved arginine at residue 485 to proline (R485P). In addition, another family was found to have an 8 nucleotide deletion in the first intron of *GGCX*, which may disrupt a *cis* transcriptional element (80). GGCX carrying the L394R mutation demonstrated a

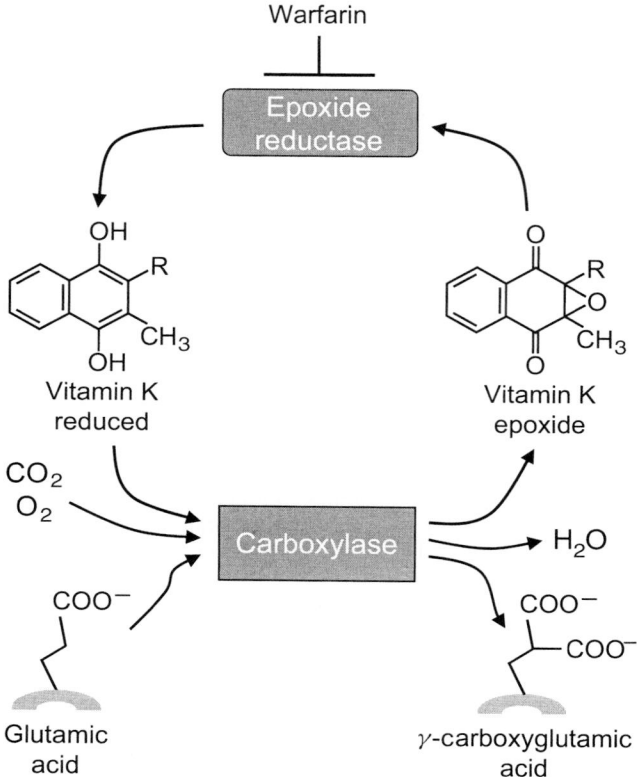

**FIGURE 63-3.** Vitamin K cycle. Vitamin K is an essential cofactor for γ-carboxylase (GGCX). GGCX adds a carbon dioxide to glutamic acid, to form γ-carboxyglutamic acid, at the same time that the reduced form of vitamin K (vitamin K hydroquinone) is oxygenated to form vitamin K 2,3 epoxide. Vitamin K epoxide reductase (VKOR) is required to regenerate the vitamin K hydroquinone, completing the vitamin K cycle. Warfarin inhibits VKOR to limit the carboxylation of vitamin K–dependent coagulation factors. (Modified by permission from Sadler JE. K is for koagulation. *Nature* 2004;427:493–494, copyright 2003, Macmillan Publishers Ltd.)

threefold reduced activity compared with the wild-type protein (74). L394 is in a 25–amino acid stretch of the enzyme that is highly conserved among all species with a known *GGCX* gene (89). The primary defect associated with L394R appears to be reduced glutamate-substrate binding (101,102). L394 may be directly involved in glutamate binding or may stabilize the binding site. The effects of the W501S and R485P mutations are still under investigation, although it has been suggested that they may affect propeptide binding (76) or vitamin K binding (85).

VKCFD2 results from functional deficiency of vitamin K 2,3-epoxide reductase (VKOR) (77,82), which is also the target of the oral anticoagulant warfarin (103). VKOR activity was identified 30 years ago (104). However, the gene for one of the subunits was only recently cloned (105–108) and named the VKOR complex subunit 1 (*VKORC1*). This gene was so named because of evidence suggesting that VKOR is a multisubunit complex (109,110). VKORC1 is a small protein of 163 amino acids (approximately 18-kDa) with up to three potential transmembrane domains. Like γ-carboxylase, it is localized to the ER by the *C*-terminal dilysine ER retention motif (107). Expression of VKORC1 alone in insect cells confers warfarin-sensitive VKOR activity, raising the possibility that VKOR activity may be encoded by a single gene (108). A homozygous point mutation that changes an arginine at residue 98 to tryptophan (R98W) was identified in two families of Lebanese and German origin and shown to decrease

VKOR activity. Multiple missense mutations were identified in warfarin-resistant rats, and were shown to result in VKOR resistance to warfarin. Administration of warfarin during pregnancy results in warfarin embryopathy, characterized by a spectrum of birth defects including abnormal midfacial development, stippling of the epiphyses, and mental retardation (77,111–113). Patients with VKORC1 mutations do not resemble those of warfarin embryopathy, except for bone deformation in some patients (77). These phenotypic differences may be explained by maternal complementation in patients with VKCFD2 of the fully γ-carboxylated form of the protein responsible for the teratogenic effect.

The rarity of VKCFD and the fact that only missense mutations in GGCX and VKORC1 have been identified suggest that complete deficiency in either of these enzymes has severe consequences. Indeed, deletion of the *GGCX* gene in mice results in partial embryonic lethality. Null mice surviving to term died uniformly at birth of massive intraabdominal hemorrhage (114). These results exclude the existence of a redundant carboxylase pathway and indicate a role for γ-carboxylated proteins in early mammalian development.

## Clinical Manifestations

Clinical symptoms of VKCFD vary widely, although they are roughly correlated with procoagulant protein levels (82). Large amounts of vitamin K can partially correct the bleeding symptoms in most, but not all patients. (81,87) Reported bleeding in VKCFD has included episodes of intracranial hemorrhage in the first weeks of life, sometimes leading to a fatal outcome. Hemarthroses and mucocutaneous bleeding may follow antibiotic therapy, because of decreased vitamin K production by gut bacteria. Skeletal defects have been reported in some probands, presumably resulting from undercarboxylation of bone Gla-proteins (72,77). Central nervous system abnormalities and mental retardation were also reported in some cases (84,115).

## Diagnosis and Differential Diagnosis

The hallmark of VKCFD2 is the simultaneous decrease of FII, FVII, FIX, and FX, although the levels range widely. Diagnosis of familial VKCFD2 requires differentiation from acquired forms of the disorder that can be caused by intestinal malabsorption of vitamin K or liver and renal dysfunction, or treatment with warfarin.

## Treatment

Large doses of vitamin K are the standard treatment. Suspected patients should be started on vitamin K therapy as soon as possible. Response to vitamin K varies from complete correction to no effect. The underlying mechanism for this variability is unknown. Treatment with fresh frozen plasma is the only alternative, if the response to vitamin K is inadequate.

# OTHER INHERITED DISEASES WITH MULTIPLE COAGULATION FACTOR DEFICIENCIES

Deficiencies of other combinations of coagulation factors have been reported (1,56,116–130), most probably caused by rare chance inheritance of two different disease genes. However, several other inherited diseases may exhibit a secondary coagulation abnormality. Most notable are the congenital disorders of glycosylation (CDG), a rare but rapidly growing family of inherited diseases affecting many of the steps involved in glycosylation of proteins in the ER and Golgi (131, 132). CDG types 1a and 1b are associated with abnormal coagulation levels, including a decreased activity of factor XI and of the coagulation inhibitors antithrombin III and protein C (133), probably caused by hypoglycosylation of these factors.

# References

1. Soff GA, Levin J. Familial multiple coagulation-factor deficiencies.1. Review of the literature–differentiation of single hereditary disorders associated with multiple factor deficiencies from coincidental concurrence of single factor deficiency states. *Semin Thromb Hemost* 1981;7:112–148.
2. Oeri J, Matter M, Isenschmid H, et al. Angeborener mangel an factor V (parahaemophilie) verbunden mit echter haemophilie A bein zwei brudern. *Med Probl Paediatr* 1954;1:575–588.
3. Seligsohn U, Zivelin A, Zwang E. Combined factor V and factor VIII deficiency among non-Ashkenazi Jews. *N Engl J Med* 1982;307:1191–1195.
4. Peyvandi F, Tuddenham EG, Akhtari AM, et al. Bleeding symptoms in 27 Iranian patients with the combined deficiency of factor V and factor VIII. *Br J Haematol* 1998;100:773–776.
5. Mansouritorgabeh H, Rezaieyazdi Z, Pourfathollah AA, et al. Haemorrhagic symptoms in patients with combined factors V and VIII deficiency in north-eastern Iran. *Haemophilia* 2004;10:271–275.
6. Nichols WC, Seligsohn U, Zivelin A, et al. Mutations in the ER-Golgi intermediate compartment protein ERGIC-53 cause combined deficiency of coagulation factors V and VIII. *Cell* 1998;93:61–70.
7. Segal A, Zivelin A, Rosenberg N, et al. A mutation in LMAN1 (ERGIC-53) causing combined factor V and factor VIII deficiency is prevalent in Jews originating from the island of Djerba in Tunisia. *Blood Coagul Fibrinolysis* 2004;15:99–102.
8. Marlar RA, Griffin JH. Deficiency of protein C inhibitor in combined factor V/VIII deficiency disease. *J Clin Invest* 1980;66:1186–1189.
9. Gardiner JE, Griffin JH. Studies on human protein C inhibitor in normal and factor V/VIII deficient plasmas. *Thromb Res* 1984;36:197–203.
10. Suzuki K, Nishioka J, Hashimoto S, et al. Normal titer of functional and immunoreactive protein-c inhibitor in plasma of patients with congenital combined deficiency of factor-V and factor-Viii. *Blood* 1983;62:1266–1270.
11. Canfield WM, Kisiel W. Evidence of normal functional levels of activated protein-C inhibitor in combined factor-V/VIII deficiency disease. *J Clin Invest* 1982;70:1260–1272.
12. Giddings JC, Sugrue A, Bloom AL. Quantitation of coagulant antigens and inhibition of activated protein-c in combined factor-V-VIII deficiency. *Br J Haematol* 1982;52:495–502.
13. Zhang B, Cunningham MA, Nichols WC, et al. Bleeding due to disruption of a cargo-specific ER-to-Golgi transport complex. *Nat Genet* 2003;34:220–225.
14. Zhang B, Ginsburg D. Familial multiple coagulation factor deficiencies: new biologic insight from rare genetic bleeding disorders. *J Thromb Haemost* 2004;2:1564–1572.
15. Wilson DB, Salem HH, Mruk JS, et al. Biosynthesis of coagulation-factor V by a human hepatocellular-carcinoma cell-line. *J Clin Invest* 1984;73:654–658.
16. Camire RM, Pollak ES, Kaushansky K, et al. Secretable human platelet-derived factor V originates from the plasma pool. *Blood* 1998;92:3035–3041.
17. Chiu HC, Schick PK, Colman RW. Biosynthesis of factor V in isolated guinea pig megakaryocytes. *J Clin Invest* 1985;75:339–346.
18. Sun H, Yang TL, Yang A, et al. The murine platelet and plasma factor V pools are biosynthetically distinct and sufficient for minimal hemostasis. *Blood* 2003;102:2856–2861.
19. Yang TL, Pipe SW, Yang A, et al. Biosynthetic origin and functional significance of murine platelet factor V. *Blood* 2003;102:2851–2855.
20. Tracy PB, Eide LL, Bowie EJW, et al. Radioimmunoassay of Factor V in human plasma and platelets. *Blood* 1982;60:59–63.
21. Bontempo FA, Lewis JH, Gorenc TJ, et al. Liver-transplantation in hemophilia-A. *Blood* 1987;69:1721–1724.
22. Kelly DA, Summerfield JA, Tuddenham EGD. Localization of factor-VIIIc-antigen in guinea-pig tissues and isolated liver-cell fractions. *Br J Haematol* 1984;56:535–543.
23. Wion KL, Kelly D, Summerfield JA, et al. Distribution of factor-VIII messenger-RNA and antigen in human-liver and other tissues. *Nature* 1985;317:726–729.
24. Zelechowska MG, Vanmourik JA, Brodniewiczproba T. Ultrastructural-localization of factor-VIII procoagulant antigen in human-liver hepatocytes. *Nature* 1985;317:729–730.
25. Do H, Healey JF, Waller EK, et al. Expression of factor VIII by murine liver sinusoidal endothelial cells. *J Biol Chem* 1999;274:19587–19592.
26. Kaufman RJ, Wasley LC, Dorner AJ. Synthesis, processing, and secretion of recombinant human factor VIII expressed in mammalian cells. *J Biol Chem* 1988;263:6352–6362.
27. Kaufman RJ. Post-translational modifications required for coagulation factor secretion and function. *Thromb Haemost* 1998;79:1068–1079.
28. Saraste J, Palade GE, Farquhar MG. Antibodies to rat pancreas Golgi subfractions: identification of a 58-kD cis-Golgi protein. *J Cell Biol* 1987;105:2021–2029.
29. Schweizer A, Fransen JAM, Bachi T, et al. Identification, by A Monoclonal-Antibody, of A 53-Kd protein associated with a tubulo-vesicular compartment at the Cis-side of the golgi-apparatus. *J Cell Biol* 1988;107:1643–1653.
30. Dansako H, Ishimaru F, Takai Y, et al. Molecular characterization of the ERGIC-53 gene in two Japanese patients with combined factor V-factor VIII deficiency. *Ann Hematol* 2001;80:292–294.
31. Neerman-Arbez M, Johnson KM, Morris MA, et al. Molecular analysis of the ERGIC-53 gene in 35 families with combined factor V factor VIII deficiency. *Blood* 1999;93:2253–2260.
32. Nichols WC, Terry VH, Wheatley MA, et al. ERGIC-53 gene structure and mutation analysis in 19 combined factors V and VIII deficiency families. *Blood* 1999;93:2261–2266.
33. Hauri H, Appenzeller C, Kuhn F, et al. Lectins and traffic in the secretory pathway. *FEBS Lett* 2000;476:32–37.
34. Fiedler K, Simons K. A putative novel class of animal lectins in the secretory pathway homologous to leguminous lectins. *Cell* 1994;77:625–626.
35. Arar C, Carpentier V, Le Caer JP, et al. ERGIC-53, a membrane protein of the endoplasmic reticulum-Golgi intermediate compartment, is identical to MR60, an intracellular mannose-specific lectin of myelomonocytic cells. *J Biol Chem* 1995;270:3551–3553.
36. Itin C, Roche AC, Monsigny M, et al. ERGIC-53 is a functional mannose-selective and calcium-dependent human homologue of leguminous lectins. *Mol Biol Cell* 1996;7:483–493.
37. Kuehn MJ, Herrmann JM, Schekman R. COPII-cargo interactions direct protein sorting into ER-derived transport vesicles. *Nature* 1998;391:187–190.
38. Muniz M, Morsomme P, Riezman H. Protein sorting upon exit from the endoplasmic reticulum. *Cell* 2001;104:313–320.
39. Nehls S, Snapp EL, Cole NB, et al. Dynamics and retention of misfolded proteins in native ER membranes. *Nat Cell Biol* 2000;2:288–295.
40. Belden WJ, Barlowe C. Role of Erv29p in collecting soluble secretory proteins into ER-derived transport vesicles. *Science* 2001;294:1528–1531.
41. Muniz M, Nuoffer C, Hauri HP, et al. The Emp24 complex recruits a specific cargo molecule into endoplasmic reticulum-derived vesicles. *J Cell Biol* 2000;148:925–930.
42. Cunningham MA, Pipe SW, Zhang B, et al. LMAN1 is a molecular chaperone for the secretion of coagulation factor VIII. *J Thromb Haemost* 2003;1:2360–2367.
43. Moussalli M, Pipe SW, Hauri HP, et al. Mannose-dependent endoplasmic reticulum (ER)-Golgi intermediate compartment-53-mediated ER to Golgi trafficking of coagulation factors V and VIII. *J Biol Chem* 1999;274:32539–32542.
44. Appenzeller C, Andersson H, Kappeler F, et al. The lectin ERGIC-53 is a cargo transport receptor for glycoproteins. *Nat Cell Biol* 1999;1:330–334.
45. Vollenweider F, Kappeler F, Itin C, et al. Mistargeting of the lectin ERGIC-53 to the endoplasmic reticulum of HeLa cells impairs the secretion of a lysosomal enzyme. *J Cell Biol* 1998;142:377–389.
46. Shetty S, Madkaikar M, Nair S, et al. Combined factor V and VIII deficiency in Indian population. *Haemophilia* 2000;6:504–507.
47. Akutsu Y, Mori K, Suzuki S, et al. A family of congenital combined deficiency of factor V and von Willebrand factor. *Rinsho Ketsueki* 1990;31:365–370.
48. Bartlett JA, Sweeney JD, Sadowsky D. Exodontia in combined factor V and factor VIII deficiency. *J Oral Maxillofac Surg* 1985;43:537–539.
49. Bauer F, Schapira M, Mannucci PM, et al. In vivo inactivation of factor V by a vitamin K-dependent factor. Study of an individual with combined factor V/VIII deficiency. *Thromb Res* 1983;29:453–457.
50. Brown JM, Selik NR, Voelpel MJ, et al. Combined factor V/VIII deficiency: a case report including levels of factor V and factor VIII coagulant and antigen as well as protein C inhibitor. *Am J Hematol* 1985;20:401–407.
51. Chuansumrit A, Mahaphan W, Pintadit P, et al. Combined factor V and factor VIII deficiency with congenital heart disease:response to plasma and DDAVP infusion. *Southeast Asian J Trop Med Public Health* 1994;25:217–220.
52. Devecioglu O, Eryilmaz E, Celik D, et al. Circumcision in a combined factor V and factor VIII deficiency using desmopressin (DDAVP). *Turk J Pediatr* 2002;44:146–147.
53. Faioni EM, Fontana G, Carpani G, et al. Review of clinical, biochemical and genetic aspects of combined factor V and factor VIII deficiency, and report of a new affected family. *Thromb Res* 2003;112:269–271.
54. Fischer RR, Giddings JC, Roisenberg I. Hereditary combined deficiency of clotting factors V and VIII with involvement of von Willebrand factor. *Clin Lab Haematol* 1988;10:53–62.
55. Garcia VV, Silva IA, Borrasca AL. Response of factor VIII/von Willebrand factor to intranasal DDAVP in healthy subjects and mild haemophiliacs (with observations in patients with combined deficiency of factors V and VIII). *Thromb Haemost* 1982;48:91–93.
56. Hellstern P, Mannhalter C, Kohler M, et al. Combined dys-form of homozygous factor XI deficiency and heterozygous factor XII deficiency. *Haemostasis* 1985;15:215–219.

57. Hultin MB, Eyster ME. Combined factor V-VIII deficiency: a case report with studies of factor V and VIII activation by thrombin. *Blood* 1981;58:983–985.

58. Mazzone D, Fichera A, Pratico G, et al. Combined congenital deficiency of factor V and factor VIII. *Acta Haematol* 1982;68:337–338.

59. Rahim Adam KA, Al Rahman F, el Seed A, et al. Combined factor V and factor VIII deficiency with normal protein C and protein C inhibitor. A family study. *Scand J Haematol* 1985;34:401–405.

60. Shukla J, Singhal R, Garbyal RS, et al. Hereditary combined coagulation factor V and factor VIII deficiency: report of two Indian families from Varanasi. *Indian J Pathol Microbiol* 2002;45:151–154.

61. Takai Y, Hayashi H, Ishimaru F, et al. DDAVP administration in a case of congenital combined factor V and factor VIII deficiency. *Rinsho Ketsueki* 1989;30:2035–2040.

62. Tsurumi H, Takahashi T, Moriwaki H, et al. Congenital combined deficiency of factor V and factor VIII with acquired ichthyosis, epidermodysplasia verruciformis, and immunological abnormalities. *Am J Hematol* 1992;40:320–321.

63. Ueno H, Asami M, Yoneda R, et al. Management of cesarean section under replacement therapy with factor VIII concentrates in a pregnant case with congenital combined deficiency of factor V and factor VIII. *Rinsho Ketsueki* 1991;32:981–985.

64. Bern MM, Suzuki K, Mann K, et al. Response of protein-C and protein-C inhibitor to warfarin therapy in patient with combined deficiency of factor-V and factor-VIII. *Thromb Res* 1984;36:485–495.

65. Karimi M, Yarmohammadi H, Ardeshiri R, et al. Inherited coagulation disorders in southern Iran. *Haemophilia* 2002;8:740–744.

66. Sallah AS, Angchaisuksiri P, Roberts HR. Use of plasma exchange in hereditary deficiency of factor V and factor VIII. *Am J Hematol* 1996;52:229–230.

67. Seligsohn U, Zivelin A, Zwang E. Decreased factor-VIII clotting antigen levels in the combined factor-V and factor-VIII deficiency. *Thromb Res* 1984;33:95–98.

68. Ginsburg D. Hemophilia and other disorders of hemostasis. In: Rimoin DL, Connor JM, Pyeritz RE, eds. *Emery and rimoin's principles and practice of medical genetics*, Vol. II. New York: Churchill Livingstone, 2002:1926–1958.

69. Hill FGH, Gidding JC, Williams CE, et al. Combined deficiency of factor-V and factor-VIII - study of a family and response to cryoprecipitate and DDAVP infusions including protein-C inhibitor measurement. *Thromb Haemost* 1983;50:210.

70. Mcmillan CW, Roberts HR. Congenital combined deficiency of coagulation factors II, VII, IX and X - report of a case. *N Engl J Med* 1966;274:1313.

71. Chung KS, Bezeaud A, Goldsmith JC, et al. Congenital deficiency of blood-clotting factor-II, factor-VII, factor-IX, and factor-X. *Blood* 1979;53:776–787.

72. Boneh A, BarZiv J. Hereditary deficiency of vitamin K-dependent coagulation factors with skeletal abnormalities. *Am J Med Genet* 1996;65:241–243.

73. Brenner B, Tavori S, Zivelin A, et al. Hereditary deficiency of all vitamin K-dependent procoagulants and anticoagulants. *Br J Haematol* 1990;75:537–542.

74. Brenner B, Sánchez-Vega B, Wu S-M, et al. A missense mutation in γ-glutamyl carboxylase gene causes combined deficiency of all vitamin K-dependent blood coagulation factors. *Blood* 1998;92:4554–4559.

75. Goldsmith GH Jr., Pence RE, Ratnoff OD, et al. Studies on a family with combined functional deficiencies of vitamin K-dependent coagulation factors. *J Clin Invest* 1982;69:1253–1260.

76. Mousallem M, Spronk HM, Sacy R, et al. Congenital combined deficiencies of all vitamin K-dependent coagulation factors. *Thromb Haemost* 2001;86:1334–1336.

77. Pauli RM, Lian JB, Mosher DF, et al. Association of congenital deficiency of multiple vitamin K-dependent coagulation factors and the phenotype of the warfarin embryopathy: clues to the mechanism of teratogenicity of coumarin derivatives. *Am J Hum Genet* 1987;41:566–583.

78. Pechlaner C, Vogel W, Erhart R, et al. A new case of combined deficiency of vitamin-K dependent coagulation-factors. *Thromb Haemost* 1992;68:617.

79. Spronk HM, Farah RA, Buchanan GR, et al. Novel mutation in the gamma-glutamyl carboxylase gene resulting in congenital combined deficiency of all vitamin K-dependent blood coagulation factors. *Blood* 2000;96:3650–3652.

80. Thomas A, Stirling D. Four factor deficiency. *Blood Coagul Fibrinolysis* 2003;14(Suppl. 1):S55–S57.

81. Vicente V, Maia R, Alberca I, et al. Congenital deficiency of vitamin K-dependent coagulation factors and protein C. *Thromb Haemost* 1984;51:343–346.

82. Oldenburg J, von Brederlow B, Fregin A, et al. Congenital deficiency of vitamin K dependent coagulation factors in two families presents as a genetic defect of the vitamin K-epoxide-reductase-complex. *Thromb Haemost* 2000;84:937–941.

83. Mickleson KN, Whyte G. Severe deficiency of vitamin K dependent coagulation factors in an infant. *N Z Med J* 1979;90:291–292.

84. Puetz J, Knutsen A, Bouhasin J. Congenital deficiency of vitamin K-dependent coagulation factors associated with central nervous system anomalies. *Thromb Haemost* 2004;91:819–821.

85. Rost S, Fregin A, Koch D, et al. Compound heterozygous mutations in the gamma-glutamyl carboxylase gene cause combined deficiency of all vitamin K-dependent blood coagulation factors. *Br J Haematol* 2004;126:546–549.

86. Ekelund H, Lindeberg L, Wranne L. Combined deficiency of coagulation factors II, VII, IX, and X: a case of probable congenital origin. *Pediatr Hematol Oncol* 1986;3:187–193.

87. Johnson CA, Chung KS, Mcgrath KM, et al. Characterization of a variant prothrombin in a patient congenitally deficient in factor-II, factor-VII, factor-IX and factor-X. *Br J Haematol* 1980;44:461–469.

88. Furie B, Bouchard BA, Furie BC. Vitamin K-dependent biosynthesis of γ-carboxyglutamic acid. *Blood* 1999;93:1798–1808.

89. Presnell SR, Stafford DW. The Vitamin K-dependent carboxylase. *Thromb Haemost* 2002;87:937–946.

90. Wu SM, Morris DP, Stafford DW. Identification and purification to near homogeneity of the vitamin K-dependent carboxylase. *Proc Natl Acad Sci U S A* 1991;88:2236–2240.

91. Wu S-M, Cheung W-F, Frazier D, et al. Cloning and expression of the cDNA for human gamma-glutamyl carboxylase. *Science* 1991;254:1634–1636.

92. Furie B, Furie BC. Molecular basis of vitamin K-dependent gamma-Carboxylation. *Blood* 1990;75:1753–1762.

93. Han X, Fiehler R, Broze GJ. Isolation of a protein Z-dependent plasma protease inhibitor. *Proc Natl Acad Sci U S A* 1998;95:9250–9255.

94. Hauschka PV, Lian JB, Cole DEC, et al. Osteocalcin and Matrix Gla Protein-Vitamin K-Dependent Proteins in Bone. *Physiol Rev* 1989;69:990–1047.

95. Stitt TN, Conn G, Gore M, et al. The anticoagulation factor protein S and its relative, Gas6, are ligands for the Tyro 3/Axl family of receptor tyrosine kinases. *Cell* 1995;80:661–670.

96. Mustafi D, Nakagawa Y. Characterization of calcium-binding sites in the kidney-stone inhibitor glycoprotein nephrocalcin with vanadyl ions - electron-paramagnetic-resonance and electron-nuclear double-resonance spectroscopy. *Proc Natl Acad Sci U S A* 1994;91:11323–11327.

97. Kulman JD, Harris JE, Haldeman BA, et al. Primary structure and tissue distribution of two novel proline-rich gamma-carboxyglutamic acid proteins. *Proc Natl Acad Sci U S A* 1997;94:9058–9062.

98. Kulman JD, Harris JE, Xie L, et al. Identification of two novel transmembrane gamma-carboxyglutamic acid proteins expressed broadly in fetal and adult tissues. *Proc Natl Acad Sci U S A* 2001;98:1370–1375.

99. Sadler JE. Medicine: K is for koagulation. *Nature* 2004;427:493–494.

100. Soute BAM, Ulrich MMW, Watson ADJ, et al. Congenital deficiency of all vitamin K-dependent blood coagulation factors due to a defective vitamin K-dependent carboxylase in Devon Rex cats. *Thromb Haemost* 1992;68:521–525.

101. Mutucumarana VP, Stafford DW, Stanley TB, et al. Expression and characterization of the naturally occurring mutation L394R in human gamma-glutamyl carboxylase. *J Biol Chem* 2000;275:32572–32577.

102. Mutucumarana VP, Acher F, Straight DL, et al. A conserved region of human vitamin K-dependent carboxylase between residues 393 and 404 is important for its interaction with the glutamate substrate. *J Biol Chem* 2003;278:46488–46493.

103. Wallin R, Martin LF. Vitamin-K-dependent carboxylation and vitamin-K metabolism in liver - effects of warfarin. *J Clin Invest* 1985;76:1879–1884.

104. Zimmerma A, Matschin JT. Biochemical basis of hereditary resistance to warfarin in rat. *Biochem Pharmacol* 1974;23:1033–1040.

105. Fregin A, Rost S, Wolz W, et al. Homozygosity mapping of a second gene locus for hereditary combined deficiency of vitamin K-dependent clotting factors to the centromeric region of chromosome 16. *Blood* 2002;100:3229–3232.

106. Kohn MH, Pelz HJ. A gene-anchored map position of the rat warfarin-resistance locus, Rw, and its orthologs in mice and humans. *Blood* 2000;96:1996–1998.

107. Rost S, Fregin A, Ivaskevicius V, et al. Mutations in VKORC1 cause warfarin resistance and multiple coagulation factor deficiency type 2. *Nature* 2004;427:537–541.

108. Li T, Chang CY, Jin DY, et al. Identification of the gene for vitamin K epoxide reductase. *Nature* 2004;427:541–544.

109. Begent LA, Hill AP, Steventon GB, et al. Characterization and purification of the vitamin K1 2,3 epoxide reductases system from rat liver. *J Pharm Pharmacol* 2001;53:481–486.

110. Cain D, Hutson SM, Wallin R. Assembly of the warfarin-sensitive vitamin K 2,3-epoxide reductase enzyme complex in the endoplasmic reticulum membrane. *J Biol Chem* 1997;272:29068–29075.

111. Hall JG, Pauli RM, Wilson KM. Maternal and fetal sequelae of anticoagulation during pregnancy. *Am J Med* 1980;68:122–140.

112. Howe AM, Lipson AH, deSilva M, et al. Severe cervical dysplasia and nasal cartilage calcification following prenatal warfarin exposure. *Am J Med Genet* 1997;71:391–396.

113. Menger H, Lin AE, Toriello HV, et al. Vitamin K deficiency embryopathy: a phenocopy of the warfarin embryopathy due to a disorder of embryonic vitamin K metabolism. *Am J Med Genet* 1997;72:129–134.

114. Zhu A, Raymond R, Zheng X, et al. Abnormalities of development and hemostasis in γ-carboxylase deficient mice. *Blood* 1998;92:152a (Abstract)

115. Ghosh K, Shetty S, Mohanty D. Inherited deficiency of multiple vitamin K-dependent coagulation factors and coagulation inhibitors presenting as hemorrhagic diathesis, mental retardation, and growth retardation. *Am J Hematol* 1996;52:67.

116. Machin SJ, Miller BR. Congenital combined factor VII and factor VIII deficiency. *Acta Haematol* 1980;63:167–169.
117. Soff GA, Levin J, Bell WR. Familial multiple coagulation-factor deficiencies .2. combined factor-VIII, factor-IX, and factor-XI deficiency and combined factor-IX and factor-XI deficiency—2 previously uncharacterized familial multiple factor deficiency syndromes. *Semin Thromb Hemost* 1981;7:149–169.
118. Sano M, Saito H, Shimamoto Y, et al. Combined hereditary factor XI (plasma thromboplastin antecedent) deficiency, von Willebrand's disease, and xeroderma pigmentosum in a Japanese family. *Am J Hematol* 1993;44:129–133.
119. Batra VV, Saxena R, Sharma LM, et al. Combined occurrence of von Willebrand's disease and factor XIII deficiency: a case report. *Indian J Pathol Microbiol* 2003;46:217–219.
120. Beard J, Dudley JM, Holland LJ, et al. Combined von Willebrand's disease and factor XII deficiency in a carrier of haemophilia B. *Clin Lab Haematol* 1989;11:139–141.
121. Berg LP, Varon D, Martinowitz U, et al. Combined factor VIII/factor XI deficiency may cause intra-familial clinical variability in haemophilia A among Ashkenazi Jews. *Blood Coagul Fibrinolysis* 1994;5:59–62.
122. Berube C, Ofosu FA, Kelton JG, et al. A novel congenital haemostatic defect: combined factor VII and factor XI deficiency. *Blood Coagul Fibrinolysis* 1992;3:357–360.
123. Bux-Gewehr I, Morgenschweis K, Zotz RB, et al. Combined von Willebrand factor deficiency and factor XII deficiency. *Thromb Haemost* 2000;83:514–516.
124. De Angelis V, Orazi BM, Santarossa L, et al. Combined factor VIII and factor XI congenital deficiency: a case report. *Haematologica* 1990;75:272–273.
125. Girolami A, Zanon E, Bertomoro A, et al. Combined factor V and factor VII deficiency due to an independent segregation of the two defects. *Clin Appl Thromb Hemost* 1999;5:136–138.
126. Matsushita T, Takamatsu J, Kagami K, et al. A female hemophilia A combined with hereditary coagulation factor XII deficiency: a case report. *Am J Hematol* 1992;39:137–141.
127. Menegatti M, Karimi M, Garagiola I, et al. A rare inherited coagulation disorder: combined homozygous factor VII and factor X deficiency. *Am J Hematol* 2004;77:90–91.
128. Rotoli B, D'Avino R, Chiurazzi F. Combined factor V and factor VII deficiency. Report of a case with a record on combined defects and considerations on the relevance of partial deficiency of coagulation factors. *Acta Haematol* 1983;69:117–122.
129. Shetty S, Ghosh K, Parekh S, et al. Combined factor VIII and IX deficiency in a family. *Clin Lab Haematol* 2001;23:201–204.
130. Tavori S, Brenner B, Tatarsky I. The effect of combined factor XI deficiency with von Willebrand factor abnormalities on haemorrhagic diathesis. *Thromb Haemost* 1990;63:36–38.
131. Marquardt T, Denecke J. Congenital disorders of glycosylation: review of their molecular bases, clinical presentations and specific therapies. *Eur J Pediatr* 2003;162:359–379.
132. Jaeken J, Carchon H. Congenital disorders of glycosylation: a booming chapter of pediatrics. *Curr Opin Pediatr* 2004;16:434–439.
133. Van Geet C, Jaeken J. A unique pattern of coagulation abnormalities in carbohydrate-deficient glycoprotein syndrome. *Pediatr Res* 1993;33:540–541.

# CHAPTER 64 ■ HEREDITARY DISORDERS OF PLATELET SECRETION AND SIGNAL TRANSDUCTION

A. KONETI RAO

Patients with inherited disorders of platelet function are characterized by longstanding mucocutaneous bleeding manifestations. Aberrations in the platelet mechanisms in hemostasis constitute the basis for the bleeding diathesis in these patients. Delineation of the abnormal platelet mechanisms in such patients has provided invaluable insights into the key aspects of platelet physiology and hemostasis. Following injury to the blood vessel, platelets adhere to exposed subendothelium by a process (adhesion) that involves the interaction of a plasma protein, von Willebrand factor (VWF), and a specific protein on the platelet surface, glycoprotein (GP) Ib (see Fig. 64-1). Adhesion is followed by recruitment of additional platelets, which form clumps, a process called aggregation (cohesion). This platelet–platelet interaction involves binding of fibrinogen to a specific platelet surface integrin—a complex composed of GP IIb/IIIa. In the resting state, platelets do not bind fibrinogen; platelet receptor activation induces "inside-out" signaling, resulting in a conformational change in the GP IIb/IIIa complex, fibrinogen binding, and aggregation. Activated platelets release contents of their granules (secretion or release reaction), such as adenosine diphosphate (ADP) and serotonin from the dense granules, which cause recruitment of additional platelets. In addition, activated platelets play a major role in coagulation mechanisms by providing the surface on which several of the key reactions occur. Platelets have an active machinery for production and use of adenosine triphosphate (ATP). The adenine nucleotides (i.e., ATP and ADP) in platelets exist in two compartments: the storage (secretable) pool within the dense granules and the metabolic (cytoplasmic) pool outside the granules (1). A number of physiologic agonists interact with specific receptors on platelet surface to induce responses, including shape change, aggregation, secretion, and thromboxane $A_2$ ($TxA_2$) formation.

## SIGNAL TRANSDUCTION MECHANISMS

Selected aspects of the complex sequence of events that occur on platelet activation are summarized here. They are presented in detail elsewhere in this book (see Chapter 39). Interaction of platelets with an agonist initiates the production or release of several intracellular messenger molecules, including $Ca^{2+}$ ions, products of phosphoinositide (PI) hydrolysis (diacylglycerol, DAG, and inositol 1,4,5-trisphosphate, $InsP_3$), $TxA_2$, and cyclic nucleotides [cyclic adenosine monophosphate (cAMP)] (Fig. 64-1). These induce or modulate the various platelet responses

of $Ca^{2+}$ mobilization, protein phosphorylation, aggregation, secretion, and liberation of arachidonic acid. The interaction between the agonist receptors and some of the intracellular effector enzymes [e.g., phospholipases $A_2$ and C, adenylyl cyclase (AC)] are mediated by a group of GTP-binding proteins that are modulated by GTP and serve as molecular on-and-off switches. Platelet activation results in a rise in cytoplasmic ionized calcium concentration; $InsP_3$ functions as a messenger to mobilize $Ca^{2+}$ from intracellular source. A $Ca^{2+}$-dependent process in platelets is the release of arachidonic acid from phospholipids by phospholipase $A_2$ ($PLA_2$). The free arachidonic acid is converted by cyclooxygenase (CO) to prostaglandins $G_2$ and $H_2$, and subsequently by thromboxane synthetase to $TxA_2$. DAG activates protein kinase C (PKC), which results in the phosphorylation of a host of proteins, including a 47-kDa protein pleckstrin. PKC activation is considered to play a major role in platelet secretion and in the activation of the platelet surface GP IIb/IIIa complexes. Numerous other mechanisms, such as phosphorylation of proteins by nonreceptor tyrosine kinases (TKs), also play a major role in signal transduction.

## CONGENITAL DISORDERS OF PLATELET FUNCTION

### Clinical Aspects and Classification

Disorders of platelet function are characterized by bleeding manifestations that are highly variable among individual patients and with different underlying defects. The manifestations are mucocutaneous in nature, and excessive hemorrhage may follow surgical procedures or trauma. Platelet counts and morphology are normal in most patients but may be decreased in a few. Most patients, but not all, have a prolonged bleeding time. Platelet aggregation and secretion studies provide evidence for the defect; however, these parameters are not generally predictive of the severity of clinical manifestations. In studies performed using platelet-rich plasma (PRP), as is the practice in most clinical laboratories, platelet aggregation in response to increasing concentrations of agonists such as ADP, epinephrine, and platelet-activating factor (PAF) consists of two phases—the initial wave of aggregation (primary aggregation) resulting from the interaction of the agonist with the platelet receptors and the secondary irreversible aggregation related to the release of dense granule contents and $TxA_2$ production (2). Therefore, patients with impaired release of dense

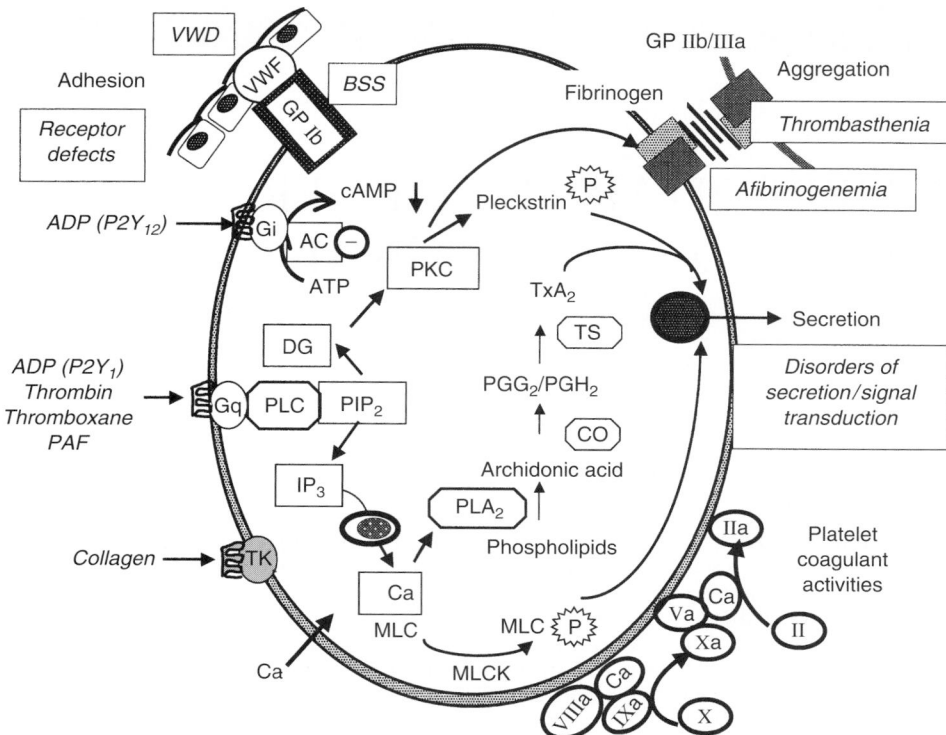

**FIGURE 64-1.** A schematic representation of selected platelet responses to activation and the congenital disorders of platelet function. cAMP, cyclic adenosine monophosphate; ADP, adenosine diphosphate; AC, adenylyl cyclase; BSS, Bernard-Soulier syndrome; CO, cyclooxygenase; DAG, diacylglycerol; G, GTP-binding protein; $IP_3$, inositoltris-phosphate; MLC, myosin light chain; MLCK, myosin light chain kinase; $PIP_2$, phosphatidylinositol bisphosphate; PKC, protein kinase C; PLC, phospholipase C; TK, tyrosine kinase; $PLA_2$, phospholipase $A_2$; TS, thromboxane synthase; VWF, von Willebrand factor; VWD, von Willebrand disease. The Roman numerals in the circles represent coagulation factors. (Rao AK. Congenital disorders of platelet function: disorders of signal transduction and secretion. *Am J Med Sci* 1998; 316:69–76.)

granule contents or $TxA_2$ production generally demonstrate a primary wave but not the second wave of aggregation in response to ADP.

Inherited platelet dysfunction may arise by diverse mechanisms (see Table 64-1). Despite tremendous advances in our knowledge of the normal platelet mechanisms, the specific molecular mechanisms underlying the altered function remain unknown in most patients with congenital disorders of platelet function. Table 64-1 provides a classification based on the platelet function or responses that are abnormal, and these responses are depicted in Figure 64-1. In patients with defects in platelet–vessel wall interaction, adhesion of platelets to subendothelium is abnormal. The two disorders in this group are the von Willebrand disease (VWD), due to a deficiency or abnormality in plasma VWF (see Chapter 60), and the Bernard-Soulier syndrome (see Chapter 66), in which platelets are deficient in GP Ib (and GP V and IX) and the binding of VWF to platelets is abnormal. Disorders of platelet–platelet interaction (aggregation) are characterized by severe deficiency of plasma fibrinogen (congenital afibrinogenemia) or by quantitative or qualitative abnormalities of the GP IIb/IIIa complex (Glanzmann thrombasthenia, see Chapter 66). Patients with defects in platelet secretion and signal transduction are a heterogeneous group lumped together for convenience of classification rather than on the basis of an understanding of the specific underlying abnormality (3). The major common characteristics in these patients, as currently perceived, are blunted aggregation responses and diminished release of granule contents upon activation of PRP with agonists ADP, epinephrine, collagen, and PAF. The second wave of aggregation is generally diminished or absent, whereas the primary wave is present, although it may also be impaired in some patients. Such patients are encountered far more frequently than the other groups represented in Table 64-1 with the exception of VWD. A small proportion of these patients have a deficiency of dense granule stores [storage pool deficiency (SPD)]. In some patients, the impaired secretion results from aberrations in the signal

transduction events that govern end responses such as secretion and aggregation (3). The final group are the patients who have abnormalities in interactions of platelets with proteins of the coagulation system, the best described being the Scott syndrome (4). In addition to these groups, there are patients who have abnormalities in platelet function associated with specific disorders such as Down syndrome and the May-Hegglin anomaly, in which the specific aberrant mechanisms in platelets still need to be delineated. This chapter focuses on patients with impaired secretion and signal transduction.

# DISORDERS OF PLATELET SECRETION, GRANULES, AND SIGNAL TRANSDUCTION

Patients in this remarkably heterogeneous group of platelet secretion defects generally manifest decreased aggregation and absence of the second wave of aggregation upon stimulation of PRP with ADP and epinephrine and impaired secretion of dense granule contents; responses to collagen, thromboxane analog (U46619), arachidonic acid, and PAF may also be impaired. Conceptually, platelet function is abnormal either when the granule or the granule contents are diminished (SPD) or when there are aberrations in the activation mechanisms governing aggregation and secretion.

During the late 1960s, several investigators (5–9) described patients with bleeding disorders associated with abnormalities in platelet aggregation induced by collagen, ADP, and epinephrine. In some of these patients, the abnormal platelet responses were attributed to a defect in the secretion of ADP (6–8). In 1969, Weiss et al. (9) reported a family with impaired platelet aggregation whose platelets had decreased amounts of ADP. Holmsen and Weiss (10,11) subsequently established that the defect in this family was a deficiency in the nonmetabolic pool of ADP stored in the dense granules, leading to the entity being called *storage*

**TABLE 64-1**

CLASSIFICATION OF INHERITED DISORDERS OF PLATELET FUNCTION

**DEFECTS IN PLATELET–VESSEL WALL INTERACTION (DISORDERS OF ADHESION)**
- von Willebrand disease (deficiency or defect in plasma VWF)
- Bernard-Soulier syndrome (deficiency or defect in GP Ib)

**DEFECTS IN PLATELET–PLATELET INTERACTION (DISORDERS OF AGGREGATION)**
- Congenital afibrinogenemia (deficiency of plasma fibrinogen)
- Glanzmann thrombasthenia (deficiency or defect in GP IIb/IIIa)

**DISORDERS OF PLATELET SECRETION AND ABNORMALITIES OF GRANULES**
- Storage pool deficiency
- Quebec platelet disorder

**DISORDERS OF PLATELET SECRETION AND SIGNAL TRANSDUCTION DEFECTS (PRIMARY SECRETION DEFECTS)**
- Defects in platelet–agonist interaction (receptor defects)
  - Receptor defects: thromboxane $A_2$, collagen, ADP, epinephrine
- Defects in G protein activation
  - $G\alpha q$ deficiency
  - $G\alpha s$ abnormalities
  - $G\alpha i1$ deficiency
- Defects in phosphatidylinositol metabolism
  - Phospholipase C-$\beta_2$ deficiency
  - Defects in calcium mobilization
  - Defects in protein phosphorylation (pleckstrin)
  - PKC-$\theta$ deficiency
- Abnormalities in arachidonic acid pathways and thromboxane $A_2$ synthesis
  - Impaired liberation of arachidonic acid
  - Cyclooxygenase deficiency
  - Thromboxane synthase deficiency

**DEFECTS IN CYTOSKELETAL REGULATION**
- Wiskott-Aldrich syndrome

**DISORDERS OF PLATELET COAGULANT–PROTEIN INTERACTION (MEMBRANE PHOSPHOLIPIDS DEFECTS)**
- Scott syndrome

**MISCELLANEOUS DISORDERS**

---

VWF, von Willebrand factor; GP, glycoprotein; ADP, adenosine diphosphate; PKC, protein kinase C isozyme.
Modified with permission from Rao AK. Congenital disorders of platelet function: disorders of signal transduction and secretion. *Am J Med Sci* 1998;316:69–76.

---

*pool deficiency* (SPD). In 1982, Rao et al. (12) reported five patients with a lifelong bleeding diathesis whose platelets had decreased aggregation and diminished dense granule and acid hydrolase secretion although their platelets had normal granule stores, thrombin-induced release of arachidonic acid, and thromboxane production. Such impairments in patients without SPD or defective TxA$_2$ production were subsequently referred to as *primary secretion defects* (2,13,14) and described in several reports (15–18). Patients with primary secretion defects are far more common than those with thrombasthenia, the Bernard-Soulier syndrome, SPD, or defects in TxA$_2$ production. In some of them, abnormalities have been documented in the specific signaling proteins or events that precede and regulate aggregation and secretion.

## Abnormalities of Granules

Studies in patients with SPD reveal a considerable heterogeneity (19). The term SPD now encompasses patients with deficiencies in the platelet contents of dense granules ($\delta$-SPD), alpha-granules ($\alpha$-SPD) (Gray platelet syndrome), or both types of granules ($\alpha\delta$-SPD). Another granule disorder is the Quebec platelet disorder (QPD), which is an autosomal dominant

disorder associated with abnormal proteolysis of several $\alpha$-granule proteins, deficiency of platelet $\alpha$-granule multimerin (a factor V binding protein), and markedly impaired aggregation with epinephrine alone (20).

### $\delta$-Storage Pool Deficiency

Patients with $\delta$-SPD have a mild to moderate bleeding diathesis associated with a prolonged bleeding time. In the platelet studies, the second wave of aggregation in response to ADP and epinephrine is absent or blunted, and the collagen response is markedly impaired. The response to the divalent ionophore A23187 is also abnormal (21). However, both impaired (22–24) and normal (25) aggregation responses to arachidonic acid have been noted. These conflicting observations may be related to the severity of platelet ADP deficiency (24). The responses to epinephrine may also be variable; a second wave of aggregation is noted in some patients (26,27). Interestingly, $\delta$-SPD has been documented (28,29) in a number of patients with prolonged bleeding times and normal aggregation responses. In one study (28), almost one fourth of the patients with SPD had normal aggregation responses to epinephrine, ADP, and collagen. Normal bleeding times have also been observed in $\delta$-SPD. Thrombin-induced secretion of acid hydrolases is impaired in SPD platelets (30); this is corrected by addition of exogenous ADP, suggesting that the primary defect in δ-SPD platelets is dense granule ADP deficiency (31).

Normal platelets possess three to eight dense granules (each 200 to 300 nm in diameter) (29). Under the electron microscope, dense granules are decreased in SPD platelets (29,32,33). Other methods to demonstrate a decrease in the dense granules include fluorescence microscopy after staining platelets with mepacrine (quinacrine), which localizes in the dense granules due to high affinity for ATP (34,35), and specific staining by uranyl ions (uranaffin reaction) of both the membrane and core of the dense granules (36,37). By direct biochemical measurements, the total platelet and granule ATP and ADP contents are decreased (1,10,11) along with other dense granule constituents, calcium, pyrophosphate, and serotonin (19,38). Two thirds of platelet ATP and ADP resides in the dense granules, with a smaller amount in the metabolic pool, and there is proportionally greater ADP than ATP in dense granules (1). Therefore, in δ-SPD platelets, the ratio of total ATP to ADP increases (>2.5) compared to normal platelets (1). An inverse correlation has been reported (39) between the granule-bound ATP and ADP and the bleeding time in patients with SPD.

Incubation of normal platelets with $^{14}$C-serotonin results in its incorporation into dense granules, and subsequent secretion upon activation. In SPD platelets, the initial rate of uptake of $^{14}$C serotonin is normal, but the saturation levels are decreased (7,40). In normal platelets, the incorporated $^{14}$C-serotonin remains in the platelet over a period of 4 to 6 hours of incubation, being protected from the mitochondrial monoamine oxidases because of its sequestration in the dense granules. In δ-SPD platelets, a significant proportion of the amine is metabolized by the monoamine oxidases to 5-hydroxyindoleacetic acid and 5-hydroxytryptophol, resulting in the loss of the radioactive label from the platelets (40,41). The inability to store the amine within the granules has been attributed to a lack of metal–nucleotide complexes that normally bind serotonin (42).

**Other Abnormalities in δ-SPD.** In some studies, synthesis of prostaglandins (43), TxA$_2$ (22), and malondialdehyde (24) was defective in δ-SPD platelets activated with collagen and epinephrine, but not arachidonate (27). Another study (44) reported an impaired liberation of arachidonic acid from membrane phospholipids in δ-SPD platelets with the Hermansky-Pudlak syndrome (HPS). Interestingly, enhanced ADP, but not thrombin-induced, rise in cytoplasmic Ca$^{2+}$ levels have been noted in SPD platelets (45). Platelet procoagulant activity (prothrombinase activity) induced upon activation has been reported to be impaired in association with an inability of these platelets to maintain elevated intracellular Ca$^{2+}$ levels (46). Both the Ca$^{2+}$ defect and the decreased prothrombinase activity are corrected by addition of exogenous ADP (46), indicating that dense granule constituents may play a role in the full development of prothrombinase activity.

δ-SPD has been reported in association with other inherited disorders such as the Hermansky-Pudlak syndrome (HPS) (oculocutaneous albinism and increased reticuloendothelial ceroid) (7,41,47–50), the Chediak-Higashi syndrome (CHS) (51–54), the Wiskott-Aldrich syndrome (WAS) (50,55), the thrombocytopenia-absent-radii (TAR) syndrome (56), and the Griscelli syndrome (50,57). The simultaneous occurrence of δ-SPD and defects in skin pigment granules, as in the HPS, point to the interrelatedness of the two kinds of granules with respect to genetic control. This concept has been further advanced by studies in animal models (50,58–60).

**Pathogenesis.** Using bone marrow transplantation in mouse models, Novak et al. (60) demonstrated that SPD involves a defect in the platelet precursor cells; normal mice demonstrated the SPD when transplanted with the mutant marrow. In line with this, megakaryocytes from cattle with the SPD and CHS have been shown to be deficient in dense granule precursors

(61). Studies in CHS cattle (61), mice (34,62,63), and patients with SPD (64–67) suggest that dense granule abnormalities may occur by different mechanisms. Dense granules are absent in megakaryocytes of CHS cattle that also have a pigmentary disorder (61), suggesting that a defective organelle development could be the basis for the SPD. However, in the mouse model (also having a pigment disorder), platelets have been found to have a substantial or normal number of mepacrine-positive granules (34,62,63), suggesting that there may be functional defect leading to impaired localization of the nucleotides rather than a lack of granule formation. In line with this dichotomy, ultrastructural studies have shown that patients with HPS and δ-SPD have a marked decrease in dense granules, suggesting an abnormality in granule development, whereas non-HPS patients have the presence of uranaffin and mepacrine-positive granules but with a lack of dense core (empty granules), suggesting a more qualitative granule defect (64). Other studies in patients with SPD have also demonstrated uranaffin-positive empty granules (65). Dense granule membranes possess the lysosomal proteins LAMP2 (lysosomal-associated membrane protein-2) and CD63 (granulophysin or LAMP3) (68,69), as well as P selectin and GP IIb/IIIa. Granulophysin is deficient in HPS platelets (66). Studies with antigranulophysin antibody demonstrated the presence of a normal number of granules in platelets of two nonalbino patients with SPD (67); these patients have the granules but with reduced contents.

A substantial amount of our information in SPD has been obtained from patients with the HPS, which is characterized by oculocutaneous albinism, platelet SPD, and lipofuscinosis (47,50). There is a large group of patients with HPS in northwest Puerto Rico, where HPS occurs in one of every 1,800 individuals (gene frequency one in 21) (70). There are at least seven known HPS-causing genes leading to seven subtypes of human HPS, with most of the patients being in HPS-1 and from Puerto Rico (50). There are at least 14 mouse models of HPS reported to date; seven of these constitute models for the human subtypes (50). Together, the human and mouse models have been an invaluable source of information on vesicle formation and trafficking. All of the human HPS subtypes are autosomal recessive, and the heterozygotes have no clinical findings. In addition to the albinism that is variable between the HPS subtypes, most patients have congenital nystagmus and decreased visual acuities. There are two additional manifestations in patients with HPS. Approximately 15% of the patients develop granulomatous colitis (49), which resembles Crohn disease in pathology and in response to treatment. The second manifestation is pulmonary fibrosis (49), which appears to be a crippling end result of an inflammatory process. An investigational antifibrotic agent, pirfenidone, appears to slow the progression of pulmonary fibrosis (71). Of the seven HPS subtypes, HPS-1 is the most severe and most prevalent form of HPS. It arises from mutations in *HPS-1* gene; the most frequent HPS-1 mutation is a 16-bp duplication in exon 15, although other mutations have been noted. In general, with one exception (HPS-2) caused by mutations in *AP3B1*, all of the HPS-causing genes encode novel proteins with no recognizable homology to other proteins. The gene defective in HPS-2, *AP3B1*, codes for the β3A subunit of AP3, a heterotetrameric complex responsible for vesicle formation from the trans-Golgi network (50). Details regarding the various *HPS* genes and the mouse models of HPS have been reviewed elsewhere (50).

CHS is a rare autosomal recessive disorder characterized by SPD, oculocutaneous albinism, immune deficiency, neurologic dysfunction, and the presence of giant cytoplasmic inclusions in different cells (58). Patients with CHS have defective cytotoxic T and NK cell function. CHS arises from mutations in the lysosomal trafficking regulator (*LYST*) gene on chromosome 1. The protein coded by this gene interacts with several proteins, including the SNARE complex protein

HRS and signaling proteins, and participates in intracellular membrane fusion reactions and vesicle trafficking (72).

## α-Granule Storage Pool Deficiency (The Gray Platelet Syndrome)

The rubric Gray platelet syndrome (GPS) has been derived from the initial observation by Raccuglia in 1971 (73) of a gray appearance of platelets with paucity of granules in peripheral blood smears from a patient with a lifelong bleeding disorder. The earliest cases of SPD involved dense granule abnormalities, but isolated deficiency of α-granule contents (GPS) may also lead to a bleeding diathesis (19,74,75). These patients have a lifelong bleeding diathesis of autosomal recessive inheritance, mild thrombocytopenia, and a prolonged bleeding time. Under the electron microscope, platelets and megakaryocytes reveal absent or markedly decreased α-granules (75). The platelets are severely and selectively deficient in α-granule proteins: platelet factor-4, β-thromboglobulin, VWF, thrombospondin, fibronectin, factor V, high-molecular-weight kininogen, and platelet-derived growth factor (PDGF) (74–76). Platelet aggregation responses have been variable. Responses to ADP and epinephrine were normal in most patients; in some patients, aggregation responses to thrombin, collagen, and ADP have been impaired (74,75,77). One patient has been reported (78) with a severe deficiency of GP VI, which provides a cogent explanation for the impaired collagen responses. Impaired thrombin-induced $Ca^{2+}$ mobilization (77), and an increase in $Ca^{2+}$ transport (79) has been reported in some patients.

The pathogenesis of the platelet granule abnormality remains to be elucidated. Plasma levels of PF-4 and βTG have been found to be raised (74,75) indicating that the defect is not in their synthesis by the megakaryocytes but in their packaging into granules. Small α-granules and α-granule membranes have been noted in the platelets and megakaryocytes (80–82) with this disorder and provide evidence that the fundamental defect may be in the targeting of endogenously synthesized secretory proteins to developing α-granules. Studies on megakaryocytes cultured from peripheral blood of three patients with GPS show that VWF is synthesized but is secreted into extracellular space instead of normal α-granule packaging (83). The neutrophils from these patients also had decreased granules. There is increased reticulin in the bone marrow from patients with GPS (75,82); this has been attributed to elevated plasma PDGF levels. Using cDNA microarrays, Hyman et al. (84) found upregulation of cytoskeletal proteins, including fibronectin 1, thrombospondins 1 and 2, and collagen VIα in fibroblasts from a patient with GPS. There was also a robust increase in fibronectin staining in the fibroblasts, suggesting a molecular basis for the myelofibrosis in GPS.

## Quebec Platelet Disorder

The QPD is an autosomal dominant disorder associated with delayed bleeding and abnormal proteolysis of α-granule proteins due to increased amounts of platelet urokinase type plasminogen activator (85–87). These patients are characterized by normal to reduced platelet counts, proteolytic degradation of soluble and membrane proteins of the α-granules, deficiency of α-granule factor V binding protein called multimerin, and defective aggregation selectively with epinephrine. Platelet factor V, but not plasma factor V, is degraded along with several other α-granule proteins, including fibrinogen, VWF, thrombospondin, osteonectin, fibronectin, and P selectin (85). The platelets contain increased fibrinolytic activity (86). In contrast to the GPS, platelets appear morphologically normal under the light microscope. Patients with QPD suffer from mucocutaneous bleeding, which is often delayed by 12 to 24 hours following injury and unresponsive to platelet transfusions (85) but responsive to fibrinolytic inhibitors (87).

# Defects in Platelet Signal Transduction (Primary Secretion Defects)

Signal transduction events encompass processes that are triggered by the interaction of agonists with specific platelet receptors and result in the activation of effectors, such as phospholipase C (PLC) and $PLA_2$, leading ultimately to aggregation and secretion. The link between the surface receptors and the effector enzymes is provided in many instances by G proteins. If the key components of platelet signal transduction mechanisms are the surface receptors, the G proteins, and the effectors, evidence now exists for specific platelet abnormalities at each of these levels.

## Defects in Platelet–Agonist Interaction: Receptor Defects

Impaired platelet responses because of an abnormality in platelet surface receptors have been documented for $TxA_2$, collagen, ADP, and epinephrine. One patient has been described with diminished responses to PAF alone (88). Because ADP and $TxA_2$ play a synergistic role in amplifying the platelet responses to several agonists, patients with specific defects at the ADP or $TxA_2$ receptor have impaired responses to other agonists, including collagen and thrombin.

**Thromboxane $A_2$ Receptor Defect.** In some patients with platelet dysfunction (89–91), the abnormal aggregation responses have been attributed to an impaired platelet responsiveness to $TxA_2$, although it is synthesized in normal amounts. The primary molecular defect in these patients has not been fully established. The existence of specific mutations in the platelet $TxA_2$ receptor has been established by Hirata et al. (92), who described an Arg60 to Leu mutation in the first cytoplasmic loop of the $TxA_2$ receptor in two unrelated patients. This Arg60 corresponds to a highly conserved basic residue among G protein–coupled receptors (92). These patients had a mild bleeding disorder with an autosomal dominant pattern of inheritance. Aggregation responses to several agonists were impaired with the exception of thrombin (93). The binding of $TxA_2$ analogs to platelets was normal (93,94). GTPase activity on activation with a $TxA_2$ analog, but not thrombin, was diminished (94,95), suggesting a defect in $TxA_2$ receptor–G protein coupling. $TxA_2$-induced activation of PLC (measured as $Ca^{2+}$ mobilization and inositol trisphosphate and phosphatidic acid formation) was impaired, whereas $PLA_2$ activation and $TxA_2$ production were normal. Less than half the number of $TxA_2$ receptors are sufficient for irreversible aggregation with $TxA_2$ agonist (96). The finding that the aggregation responses were impaired in the heterozygous family members (92) suggests a dominant negative effect of the mutation. Absent aggregation response to $TxA_2$ has also been observed in patients without evidence for a defect of $TxA_2$ receptor (97). In line with these observations, $TxA_2$ receptor knockout mice have a mild bleeding disorder and impaired aggregation with $TxA_2$ analogs, as well as collagen (98).

**Collagen Receptor Defects.** At least two platelet receptors are implicated in collagen-induced responses: $\alpha2\beta1$ (GP Ia/IIa) and GP VI (99). Platelets from the patient described by Nieuwenhuis et al. (100,101) had approximately 15% to 25% of normal platelet GP Ia and failed to aggregate with collagen or adhere and spread normally to subendothelial surfaces. In another patient (102), collagen-induced platelet aggregation was markedly reduced, and the platelets were deficient in GP Ia and thrombospondin. In both patients, the bleeding times were prolonged, and platelet aggregation responses to agonists other than collagen were preserved. Selective impairment in collagen responses and a mild bleeding disorder have also been related to a deficiency of platelet GP VI (103–105). In GP VI–deficient platelets collagen-stimulated activation of Syk but not c-Src is impaired. (106).

Another platelet glycoprotein, GP IV (CD 36), has also been implicated in platelet–collagen interactions, but not fully established. Platelets lacking GP IV have been reported to have reduced adhesion to collagen in flowing whole blood (107). However, individuals lacking platelet GP IV in the Japanese population (approximately 3% of the population) and the US population (approximately 0.3%) do not have a bleeding disorder (108) and have normal collagen-induced platelet aggregation (108), $Ca^{2+}$ mobilization, and tyrosine phosphorylation (109). In several subjects with GP IV deficiency, a Pro90 to Ser mutation has been reported in the GP IV gene (110), and GP IV mRNA has been detected in platelets (110,111).

**Defect in Platelet Adenosine Diphosphate Receptors ($P2Y_1$, $P2Y_{12}$, and $P2X_1$).** At least three receptors (i.e., $P2Y_1$, $P2Y_{12}$, and $P2X_1$) mediate ADP interaction with platelets (112). $P2Y_1$ receptors induce PLC activation, intracellular $Ca^{2+}$ mobilization, and shape change; $P2Y_{12}$ receptors mediate inhibition of cAMP formation by AC. ADP-induced aggregation requires coactivation of both $P2Y_1$ and $P2Y_{12}$ receptors. $P2X_1$ receptors function as cation channels. Cattaneo et al. (113,114) and Nurden et al. (115) have described patients with $P2Y_{12}$ receptor abnormality characterized by blunted platelet aggregation response to ADP and diminished ability of ADP to suppress $PGE_1$-induced elevation in cAMP; ADP-stimulated shape change was normal. ADP-stimulated $Ca^{2+}$ mobilization (113) and tyrosine phosphorylation in response to ADP and $TxA_2$ (116) were abnormal in the patient studied. The platelet binding of radiolabeled ADP (113) or the ADP analog 2-methylthio-ADP (114,115) was decreased in these patients. Decreased platelet 2-methylthio-ADP binding has also been reported (18) in additional patients with impaired aggregation and secretion in response to several agonists, including ADP.

The genetic defect has been unraveled in some of these patients. One of the previously mentioned patients (115) has a mutation in one allele in the $P2Y_{12}$ gene with deletion of two nucleotides in the coding region (at amino acid 240), resulting in a frameshift and a premature stop codon (117). Interestingly, although this patient has one $P2Y_{12}$ allele with normal coding region, the patient's platelets have an almost complete lack of $P2Y_{12}$ ADP receptors. The $P2Y_{12}$ transcripts in the platelet RNA are derived entirely from the mutant allele, suggesting a repression of the wild-type allele. In contrast, platelets from the patient's daughter have an intermediate number of ADP-binding sites (115), normal ADP responses, and one frame-shifted allele and one wild-type allele, suggesting that the mutant allele does not act in a dominant negative manner. Studies in a second patient (118) revealed a compound heterozygous state with one allele containing a G-to-A transition resulting in an Arg256-to-Gln codon substitution, and the other allele containing a C to T transition and Arg265-to-Trp codon substitution. Both mutations occurred in the third extracellular loop of the receptor. In patient platelets, the binding of $^{33}P$-2MeS ADP was normal. In expression studies in Chinese hamster ovary (CHO) cells, neither mutation affected the translocation of the $P2Y_{12}$ receptor to cell surface, but ADP-induced inhibition of AC was partially inhibited, indicating presence of a dysfunctional receptor. In three other patients (113,114), homozygous deletions of one to two base pairs have been demonstrated (119) in the $P2Y_{12}$ locus, resulting in premature termination and a lack of demonstrable protein in the platelet lysates. In line with these findings, $P2Y_{12}$ null mice have a prolonged bleeding time, and the platelets aggregate poorly and fail to inhibit adenybyl cyclase in response to ADP (120).

One patient has been briefly described (121) with a defect in the $P2Y_1$ platelet receptor, which is coupled to PLC and ADP-induced calcium mobilization. This patient also had impaired platelet aggregation in response to ADP and other agonists. $P2Y_1$-deficient mice have decreased platelet aggregation and a prolonged bleeding time (122).

Oury et al. (123) have reported a patient with a selective impairment of ADP-induced aggregation associated with a dominant negative mutation in $P2X_1$ receptor due to deletion of one leucine residue within a stretch of four leucine residues in the second transmembrane domain. The association of a bleeding disorder with alterations in this receptor (a ATP-gated ion channel) suggests hitherto unrecognized physiologic role of $P2X_1$ in hemostasis.

**Selective Impairment in Platelet Responsiveness to Epinephrine.** Epinephrine-induced aggregation, mediated by $\alpha_2$-adrenergic receptors ($\alpha_2AR$), may be variable or even impaired in some presumably normal individuals. The second wave of aggregation was noted to be absent in 10% to 15% of normal subjects in one study (27). Studies in twins suggest that platelet $\alpha_2AR$ is under genetic control (124). Rao et al. (125) have described a family in which several members had impaired aggregation and secretion in response to only epinephrine associated with a decreased number of platelet $\alpha_2AR$. Three family members had a history of easy bruising with minimally prolonged bleeding times. Despite the diminished aggregation response, epinephrine inhibition of adenylate cyclase was normal, indicating that the receptor requirements for these two platelet responses are different. Although other families with an epinephrine defect have been reported (126), the relation of the selective epinephrine defect to bleeding manifestations needs to be defined. The isolated impaired aggregation response to epinephrine in some patients may be related to the Quebec platelet syndrome (20) or a platelet $G\alpha z$ deficiency (127) (see subsequent text).

## Defects in GTP-Binding Proteins

GTP-binding proteins (consisting of $\alpha$, $\beta$, and $\gamma$ subunits) link surface receptors and intracellular enzymes. Because of their role as molecular switches, G proteins constitute a potential locus for aberrations leading to platelet dysfunction. Abnormalities involving $G\alpha q$, $G\alpha i_2$, and $G\alpha s$ have been described in human platelets. A human platelet deficiency of $G\alpha z$ has not been documented to date; $G\alpha z$-deficient mice have impaired epinephrine responses (127).

**$G\alpha q$ Deficiency.** Gabbeta et al. (128) have described, in a patient with a mild bleeding disorder, abnormal aggregation and secretion in response to a number of agonists, and diminished GTPase activity (a reflection of $\alpha$-subunit function) on activation. The binding of $^{35}S$-GTP$\gamma$S to platelet membranes was diminished, and there was a selective decrease in platelet membrane $G\alpha q$ with normal levels of $G\alpha_{i2}$, $G\alpha_{12}$, $G\alpha_{13}$, and $G\alpha_z$. This patient had abnormalities in other downstream events, including activation of the GP IIb/IIIa complex, $Ca^{2+}$ mobilization (129), and release of arachidonic acid from phospholipids on platelet activation (130). Responses to both protease-activated receptor PAR-1 (SFLLRN) and PAR-4 (GYPGKF) peptide agonists were impaired, demonstrating that $G\alpha q$ mediates the responses on PAR1 and PAR 4 activation. Genetic studies show that the $G\alpha q$ coding sequence in this patient is intact and the $G\alpha q$ mRNA levels are decreased in platelets but not in neutrophils, which have normal responses and $G\alpha q$ protein. (131). The findings in this patient with respect to platelet function have been corroborated by essentially identical abnormal responses in the $G\alpha q$-deficient mice (132).

**$G\alpha s$ Hyperfunction and Genetic Variation in Extra-Large $G\alpha s$.** Activation of $G\alpha s$ results in increased platelet cAMP levels and inhibition of platelet responses to activation. Freson et al. (133) have described two unrelated families with inducible hyperactivity of Gαs. The three patients reported to have had a bleeding diathesis, prolonged bleeding times, variable mental retardation, and mild skeletal malformations. Platelet aggregation responses to usual agonists were reportedly normal, but the platelets showed increased sensitivity to inhibition by agents that elevate cAMP levels. Exposure to $PGE_1$, $PGI_2$, or adenosine resulted in an enhanced increase in cAMP associated with an increased platelet Gαs protein. The Gαs gene (GNAS1) has three alternative promoters and exons in addition to the Gαs, and this includes the extra-large Gαs (XLαs). The XLαs is expressed only from the paternal allele. A heterozygous 36-bp insertion and two basepair substitutions were identified in the exon 1 of XLαs gene in these patients. Because XLαs is not activated by activation of the usual platelet Gαs–coupled receptors, the mechanisms leading to the increased cAMP levels and the enhanced expression of Gαs protein in the patients remain unclear. Interestingly, 2.2% of control subjects also revealed the mutations detected in the patients along with evidence of inducible Gαs-hyperfunction and increased platelet Gαs protein.

Interestingly, Freson et al. (134) have described Gαs deficiency in platelets from a patient with psuedohypoparathyroidism Ib (PHPIb) in association with disturbed imprinting and altered methylation in the GNAS1 gene cluster that encompasses the four GNAS1 splice variants, including the Gαs subunit. This patient showed a functional platelet Gαs defect with decreased cAMP formation upon Gαs-receptor activation and Gαs-protein deficiency; the Gαs-coding sequence was normal. The authors do not indicate whether the patient had a bleeding diathesis.

**Gαi1 Deficiency.** Patel et al. (135) have documented a patient with platelet Gαi1 deficiency who presented with a bleeding disorder, abnormal aggregation, and dense granule secretion on activation with multiple agonists, including ADP, U46619, collagen, and epinephrine. Additionally, ADP-induced GP IIb/IIIa activation was diminished, providing evidence for the role of Gαi1 in this response. A major platelet response mediated by Gαi is inhibition of AC and cAMP levels (Fig. 64-1). In the patient's platelets, no inhibition of forskolin-stimulated cAMP levels was observed on exposure to ADP, thrombin, or epinephrine. In contrast, Gαq-mediated responses (reflected by activation of PLC-β2, $Ca^{2+}$ mobilization, and pleckstrin phosphorylation) were normal following addition of ADP, thrombin, or collagen. By Western blotting, platelet expression of Gαi1 was decreased by 75%; other members of the Gαi family (Gαi2, Gαi3, Gαiz) or Gαq were normal. These studies suggest an important physiologic role in human platelet responses and hemostasis for Gαi1. Mouse platelets appear to lack Gαi1, indicating differences in the expression of the various Gαi members from human platelets.

## PLC-β2 Deficiency and Defects in Phospholipase C Activation, Calcium Mobilization, and Protein Phosphorylation

Several investigators have described patients with a relatively mild bleeding diathesis, impaired aggregation, and dense granule secretion, even though their platelets have normal granule stores and synthesize substantial amounts of $TxA_2$ (15–17, 136). An early event on platelet stimulation is activation of PLC, leading to the formation of other intracellular mediators, including $InsP_3$ and DAG (Fig. 64-1), and to mechanisms such as $Ca^{2+}$ mobilization and PKC-induced protein phosphorylation. Defects in some of these specific responses have been documented. Both PKC-induced pleckstrin phosphorylation and cytoplasmic $Ca^{2+}$ mobilization play a major role in secretion and aggregation on activation. Yang et al. (17) reported detailed studies in eight patients with abnormal aggregation and secretion in response to several different surface receptor-mediated agonists. Receptor-mediated $Ca^{2+}$ mobilization and/or

pleckstrin phosphorylation were abnormal in seven of the eight patients. It was postulated that platelet activation with a combination of a direct PKC activator $DIC_8$ (1,2, dioctonoyl-sn-glycerol) and ionophore A23187, which possibly bypass the surface receptors and the two major intracellular mediators ($InsP_3$, DAG), may induce normal dense granule secretion in these patients who have diminished secretion on activation with receptor-mediated agonists. In line with this, platelet activation with a combination of ADP with $DIC_8$ or A23187 improved secretion in four of eight patients. However, combination of $DIC_8$ and A23187 induced normal secretion in PRP in all patients. These studies suggest that the ultimate process of exocytosis or secretion per se is intact in these patients, and impaired secretion and aggregation result from upstream abnormalities in early signaling events. True to this supposition, specific defects at the level of PLC-β2 (137,138), Gαq (128), and PKC-θ (139) have been shown in these eight patients.

Lages and Weiss (15) have described eight patients who had decreased initial rates and extents of aggregation in response to weak agonists, ADP, epinephrine, and U44069; they postulated defects in early platelet activation events to explain the abnormal responses. They subsequently demonstrated a defect in phosphatidylinositol hydrolysis and phosphatidic acid formation (140), and in pleckstrin phosphorylation (141) in one patient.

Cytoplasmic $Ca^{2+}$ mobilization is an early response to platelet stimulation. Attention was therefore focused initially on this process to explain the impaired platelet function (17,129, 142). Studies in two related patients (142) with impaired aggregation and secretion responses revealed decreased peak $Ca^{2+}$ concentrations following activation with ADP, collagen, PAF, or thrombin, with abnormalities in intracellular release and in the influx of extracellular $Ca^{2+}$ (129). Formation of $InsP_3$, the key intracellular mediator of $Ca^{2+}$ release, as well as DAG formation and pleckstrin phosphorylation, were diminished upon platelet activation (137), indicating a defect in PLC activation (Fig. 64-1). Human platelets contain at least seven PLC isozymes in the quantitative order PLC-γ2 > PLC-β2 > PLC-β3 > PLC-β 1 > PLC-γ1 > PLC-δ1> PLC-β4 (138). Studies in one of these patients with impaired PLC activation revealed a selective decrease in only the PLC-β2 isozyme (138). The decreased platelet PLC-β2 protein levels were associated with a normal coding sequence but with diminished PLC-β2 mRNA levels in platelets, but not in neutrophils, suggesting a hematopoietic lineage-specific defect in PLC-β2 gene regulation (143). These studies provide direct validation in human platelets of the importance in hemostasis of PLC-β2. In line with these findings in platelets, agonist-induced $Ca^{2+}$ mobilization and inositol phosphate production in neutrophils is impaired in PLC-β2–deficient mice (144). These authors did not assess platelet responses. However, in mice deficient in both PLC-β2 and PLC-β3, the platelet responses are impaired (145).

Abnormalities in these signal transduction pathways have also been reported in other studies. Defects in phosphatidylinositol metabolism and protein phosphorylation have been described in such patients (94,140,141,146–148), although the primary protein abnormality remains unknown. Holmsen et al. (146) described a patient with abnormalities in platelet aggregation and dense granule secretion who had impaired PI hydrolysis and release of free arachidonic acid from phospholipids on thrombin activation; in addition, the platelets had reduced membrane GP IIb and GP IIIa. In another patient, the impaired platelet responses and diminished PI metabolism were attributed to abnormal membrane phospholipid composition (147). Fuse et al. (94) have reported a patient with a mild bleeding disorder whose platelets had impaired aggregation, secretion, $InsP_3$ formation, and $Ca^{2+}$ mobilization in response to a $TxA_2$ mimetic ($STA_2$) associated with a normal

TxA$_2$ formation. Interestingly, GTPase activity upon activation with STA$_2$ was also impaired, suggesting an abnormality in coupling between TxA$_2$ receptors and PLC. In the patient described by Mitsui (148), the abnormal platelet aggregation was associated with decreased TxA$_2$-induced InsP$_3$ formation but with normal GTPase activity and normal platelet TxA$_2$ receptors (including their cDNA sequence), suggesting that the abnormality in PLC activity was downstream of the surface receptor. Overall, these patients provide evidence for aberrations in the signal transduction pathways in patients with diminished platelet aggregation and secretion.

**Defects in Protein Phosphorylation: PKC-θ Deficiency.** PKC isozymes, a family of serine and threonine specific protein kinases, comprise at least 12 related isozymes that phosphorylate a wide array of proteins involved in signal transduction. Activation of PKC has been linked to several critical aspects of platelets, including GP IIb/IIIa activation and secretion, and megakaryocyte differentiation. Recently, a deficiency of a human platelet PKC isozyme (PKC-θ) has been described (139). This patient has been previously reported (149) to have lifelong mucocutaneous bleeding manifestations, mild thrombocytopenia, and markedly abnormal platelet aggregation (including primary wave) and dense granule secretion in response to multiple agonists. Phosphorylation of pleckstrin and myosin light chain (MLC) was diminished in the patient's platelets upon activation with PAF and thrombin. By flow cytometry, the patient's platelets had a full complement of GP IIb/IIIa complexes, but signal transduction–dependent activation of GP IIb/IIIa was impaired on stimulation with receptor-mediated agonists. More recently, Sun et al. (139) have demonstrated in this subject a heterozygous mutation in a transcription factor, core-binding factor A2 (CBFA2, also called RUNX1, AML1), suggesting that proteins regulated by this transcription factor play a role in the activation of GP IIb/IIIa. In addition, they showed that the platelets were deficient in one of the PKC isozymes, PKC-θ. This deficiency provides a cogent explanation for not only the impaired protein phosphorylation but also the thrombocytopenia (because of the role of PKC in megakaryopoiesis). Of note, the platelet albumin and IgG levels were decreased, suggesting a role for PKC in the uptake of α-granule proteins from plasma.

Protein phosphorylation by other kinases (TKs) is important in platelet signaling events. In thrombasthenia (150,151) and the Scott syndrome (152), tyrosine phosphorylation of several proteins is impaired on platelet activation. In these disorders, this defect is likely secondary to the primary abnormality in the GP IIb/IIIa complex and in phospholipids scrambling, respectively. Interestingly, in patients with the thrombocytopenia with absent radii (TAR) syndrome, thrombopoietin-induced tyrosine phosphorylation has been reported to be markedly abnormal (153).

## Signal Transduction Defects and Activation of GP IIb/IIIa

Activation of GP IIb/IIIa complex and fibrinogen-binding to platelets is a signal transduction–dependent process and has been linked to PKC activation (154). Therefore, it is likely that abnormalities in signaling mechanisms would impair activation of GP IIb/IIIa on platelets. Evidence for this is provided by the report (155) of a patient with markedly abnormal platelet aggregation and receptor-activated pleckstrin phosphorylation who had decreased activation of the platelet GP IIb/IIIa complexes despite the presence of normal numbers of these platelet receptors with intact ligand (fibrinogen) binding capacity. This patient has recently been shown to have deficiency in platelet PKC-θ (139). Abnormal activation of GP IIb/IIIa has also been observed in the patient with Gαq deficiency (128) and Gαi1 deficiency (135). Defective GP IIb/IIIa activation due

to abnormalities in upstream signaling events may be a more common mechanism for blunted aggregation than specific defects in the GP IIb/IIIa complex per se (156) and may explain the diminished initial aggregation responses noted in several patients by Lages and Weiss (15).

## Abnormalities in Platelet Arachidonic Acid Pathways and Thromboxane A$_2$ Production

Thromboxane A$_2$ production forms an important positive feedback, enhancing the overall activation process. In the absence of TxA$_2$ synthesis, dense granule secretion is decreased following stimulation of PRP with ADP, epinephrine, and low concentrations of collagen and thrombin. In general, most patients with defects in TxA$_2$ production have had mild to moderate bleeding manifestations.

**Defects in the Liberation of Arachidonic Acid from Phospholipids.** Patients have been described with abnormalities in mobilization of free arachidonic acid from membrane-bound phospholipids by PLA$_2$, the initial and rate-limiting step in TxA$_2$ synthesis. In four such patients (130), aggregation and secretion were abnormal, and TxA$_2$ production was diminished during stimulation with ADP and thrombin but was normal with free arachidonic acid. In $^3$H-arachidonic acid labeled platelets, thrombin-induced mobilization of free arachidonic acid from phospholipids was impaired in these patients. Subsequent studies in one of the patients showed that the platelet PLA$_2$ levels (both membrane and cytosolic) were normal but agonist-induced Ca$^{2+}$ mobilization (129) was impaired due to a platelet Gαq deficiency (128). Other reports have also documented patients with an impaired release of arachidonic acid (157).

**Deficiencies of Cyclooxygenase and Thromboxane Synthetase.** In 1975, Malmsten et al. (158) reported platelet CO deficiency in a patient with a mild bleeding disorder and impaired aggregation responses to ADP, epinephrine, collagen, and arachidonic acid but with normal response to PGG$_2$. Subsequently, several other patients have been described with a similar defect in TxA$_2$ synthesis (159–164). Because CO also mediates the endothelial production of prostacyclin (PGI$_2$), Pareti et al. (161) examined the PGI$_2$ production in a patient with CO deficiency and found it also to be impaired. Interestingly, this patient with defects in both platelet and vessel wall CO had predominantly bleeding symptoms and not thrombotic events. The patient reported by Rak and Boda (162) had progressive arteriosclerosis as evidenced by cerebrovascular and cardiac events. Using a radioimmunoassay, Roth and Machuga (163) found normal levels of CO in five of six patients suspected to have a deficiency, suggesting that these patients may have a functionally abnormal molecule. Three patients have been described (164) with impaired platelet responses and markedly decreased ability to convert arachidonic acid, but not PGH$_2$, to TxA$_2$. Using specific antibodies, the authors demonstrated decreased platelet cyclooxygenase-1 levels in two patients and normal levels in the third; levels of thromboxane synthase (TS) were normal in all three. Therefore, platelet CO deficiency is manifested either by undetectable enzyme protein levels (type 1) or as an antigenically detectable but functionally abnormal molecule (type 2) (164).

Two patients have been described with thromboxane synthetase deficiency (165,166). Another patient has been described (167) with bleeding manifestations, whose platelets had impaired aggregation, dense granule secretion, and TxA$_2$ production upon activation. Liberation of arachidonic acid from phospholipids was normal, and TxA$_2$ synthesis was markedly diminished during stimulation of PRP with thrombin, but substantial TxA$_2$ production was noted on activation of patient's platelets suspended in a buffer containing no albumin. These findings suggest that the platelets had diminished levels of enzyme activity, which could express itself adequately only in the absence of albumin; albumin binds free arachidonic acid avidly. Although the exact site of the enzyme defect was not elucidated, these studies reflect the modulating role of albumin on platelet arachidonate metabolism.

## Defects in Cytoskeletal Assembly

The Wiskott-Aldrich syndrome (WAS) is an X-linked inherited disorder affecting T lymphocytes and platelets and characterized by thrombocytopenia, small platelets with decreased survival, eczema, and immunodeficiency. The bleeding manifestations are variable. Several platelet abnormalities have been reported, including dense granule SPD; deficiencies of GP Ib, GP Ia, and GP IIb/IIIa; diminished activation of GP IIb/IIIa; impaired aggregation responses and expression of P selectin and abnormalities in platelet energy metabolism (168,169). In addition, resting cytoplasmic $Ca^{2+}$ levels have been reported to be elevated along with enhanced phosphotidylserine expression on platelet surface and microparticle formation in patients with WAS (170). WAS and the related X-linked thrombocytopenia (XLT) arise from mutations of the X-chromosome gene (location Xp11.22) called *WASP*, which encodes a novel intracellular proline-rich 53-kDa protein of 502 amino acids (168,171). This multifaceted WAS protein (WASp) appears to constitute a link between the cytoskeleton and signal transduction pathways and regulates actin polymerization. WASp has been shown to bind to a host of proteins, including F-actin, SH3-containing adapter proteins NCK and Grb2, TKs, PLC-$\gamma$1; the active GTP-complexed form of Cdc42, a member of the small GTP-hydrolyzing proteins (GTPases); and phosphatidylinositol bisphosphate (PIP-2) (168,172). WASp is a key regulator of actin polymerization and cytoskeletal assembly, leading to the unifying concept of WAS as a cytoskeletal disease (168,172). However, platelets from patients with WAS and from WASp-deficient mice change shape, elaborate filopodia, spread lamellae, and assemble actin identical to normal platelets, indicating a more specialized role of WASp (173). In terms of therapy, splenectomy usually improves the thrombocytopenia in WAS, and bone marrow transplantation has been curative (168,174).

## Platelet Function Abnormalities and Transcription Factor Deficiencies

Transcription factors regulate expression of proteins in megakaryocytes and platelets. Several reports have associated platelet function abnormalities with transcription factor CBFA2 (core-binding factor A2) haplodeficiency, including abnormalities in aggregation and secretion, dense granule deficiency, $\alpha$-granule deficiency, and, most recently, PKC-$\theta$ deficiency (139,175,176). These subjects have been initially recognized by an association between autosomal dominant thrombocytopenia and an increased predisposition to leukemia, which has been linked to a CBFA2 haplodeficiency (177). Patients with transcription factor GATA-1 mutations may have not only X-linked thrombocytopenia, but also large platelets and impaired responses to collagen and ristocetin (178) related to abnormalities in GP Ib$\beta$. Aggregation in response to ADP and thrombin were normal. Interestingly, one of the patients also had diminished levels of platelet G$\alpha$S protein and mRNA (178). In mouse models, NF-E2 deficiency is associated with thrombocytopenia, impaired activation of platelet GP IIb/IIIa in megakaryocytes, and a deficiency of thromboxane synthetase (179,180). Overall, these reports suggest that transcription factor abnormalities are associated with platelet dysfunction in addition to thrombocytopenia.

## Miscellaneous Disorders Associated with Platelet Function Defects

Platelet function abnormalities have been reported in inherited connective tissue disorders such as osteogenesis imperfecta, the Ehlers-Danlos syndrome, and the Marfan syndrome (181–184), which are associated with bleeding manifestations more likely due to the underlying connective tissue defect rather than the platelet dysfunction. Abnormal platelet responses have been reported in patients with hexokinase deficiency (185); glucose-6 phosphatase deficiency (glycogen storage disease, type I) (186,187); Epstein syndrome characterized by thrombocytopenia, hereditary nephritis, and nerve deafness (188,189); and Down syndrome (190). In glucose-6 phosphatase deficiency, the platelet abnormalities were reversed following total parenteral nutrition in these patients for 10 to 12 days (186,187), indicating that the platelets may be intrinsically normal. The May-Hegglin anomaly is characterized by giant platelets, thrombocytopenia, and basophilic granulocyte inclusions. Some patients with this anomaly have platelet function and ultrastructural abnormalities (191,192). Despite the large platelet size, the surface membrane glycoproteins appear to be normal (193). Markedly impaired platelet responses to multiple agonists have been reported with partial trisomy 18p associated with three copies of the PACAP (pituitary adenylate cyclase-activating polypeptide) gene and elevated plasma levels of PACAP, which induces increased platelet cAMP levels by the stimulation of G $\propto$s (194).

## Relative Frequency of Various Platelet Abnormalities

Thrombasthenia, the Bernard-Soulier syndrome, and afibrinogenemia are rare disorders. It is generally accepted that VWD is the most common congenital platelet function disorder, although the severe forms are rare. The heterogeneous category of defects in platelet secretion and signal transduction are probably the most frequently encountered inherited platelet function abnormalities, excluding VWD. Although frequently considered, dense granule SPD (10% to 15%) and defects in $TXA_2$ production (10% to 20%) occur in a small proportion of these patients. We have analyzed our findings in 62 patients with abnormal platelet function on an inherited basis studied in our laboratory (Rao AK, unpublished). All patients had impaired aggregation and $^{14}$C-serotonin secretion in studies using PRP; dense granule contents (ATP, ADP) and $TXA_2$ production on activation with thrombin and arachidonic acid were measured in all. Ten patients had a dense granule SPD (16%). Twenty-five patients (40%) had clear-cut abnormalities in the aggregation (generally, absent second wave) and secretion on activation but had normal dense granule stores and thromboxane production. These patients may have defects in the signaling mechanisms. In this highly heterogeneous group, there is a pressing need for detailed studies to delineate the mechanisms. In this series, thrombasthenia was detected in one patient.

# THERAPY FOR PATIENTS WITH CONGENITAL PLATELET FUNCTION DISORDERS

Patients with VWD and afibrinogenemia are managed during bleeding episodes and surgical procedures by methods aimed at elevating the deficient factor levels in plasma and are discussed in Chapters 60 and 62, respectively. Platelet transfusions and 1-desamino-8-D-arginine vasopressin (DDAVP) are the mainstays of therapy for patients with inherited platelet defects. Because of the wide disparity in bleeding manifestations, therapeutic approaches must be individualized. Platelet transfusions are effective in controlling the bleeding manifestations but come with potential risks associated with blood products, including alloimmunization. Patients with thrombasthenia may develop antibodies (195,196) against GP IIb/IIIa that compromise the efficacy of subsequent platelet transfusions. A viable alternative to platelet transfusions is intravenous administration of DDAVP, which shortens the bleeding time in a substantial number of patients with platelet function defects (197–200). This response appears to be dependent on the abnormalities leading to the platelet dysfunction (197,199,200). Most patients with thrombasthenia have not responded to DDAVP infusion with a shortening of the bleeding time (197,199–201), with exceptions (202). However, it is unknown whether DDAVP improves hemostasis in these patients despite a lack of shortening of the bleeding time. Responses in patients with SPD have been variable with a shortening of the bleeding time in some patients (200,203,204) but not others (197,199). In uncontrolled studies, it has been feasible to manage select patients with congenital platelet defects undergoing surgical procedures with DDAVP alone (197,199). However, this approach must be individualized based on the nature of the surgery and the intensity of bleeding symptoms, and platelet transfusions must be readily available for use in the event of excess hemorrhage. The mechanisms by which DDAVP enhances hemostasis in patients with platelet defects are unclear (198). Its administration induces a rise in plasma VWF, FVIII, and tissue plasminogen activator. The abnormal *in vitro* platelet aggregation or secretion responses in patients with platelet defects are not corrected by DDAVP (199).

Several investigators have reported the successful use of recombinant factor VIIa (rFVIIa) in the management of bleeding events in patients with inherited platelet defects, including thrombasthenia, the Bernard-Soulier syndrome (BSS), and SPD (205–208). Additional larger studies of rFVIIa are warranted in such patients.

The other approaches that have been utilized to improve hemostasis in patients with inherited platelet defects include a short 3- to 4-day course of prednisone (20 to 50 mg) (209) and the administration of antifibrinolytic agents epsilon-aminocaproic acid or tranexamic acid, which have been successfully used in patients with coagulation disorders (198, 210,211). Although allogeneic bone marrow transplantation has been successfully performed with complete correction in patients with thrombasthenia (212) and the Wiskott-Aldrich syndrome (168,174), such a therapy is rarely required in patients with congenital platelet function disorders.

## Future Directions

In the vast majority of patients with a familial bleeding diathesis and abnormalities in agonist-mediated platelet aggregation and secretion, the underlying molecular mechanisms leading to the platelet dysfunction are unknown. The generally thought-of entities such as thrombasthenia, the BSS, and storage pool deficiencies are uncommon in the overall group of patients with familial platelet dysfunction. Evidence is now available that some of the patients have specific abnormalities in the signaling events that regulate the end responses, such as aggregation and secretion. The larger group of poorly characterized patients who are currently lumped as "primary secretion defects or activation defects" represents an untapped reservoir of valuable new information into signaling mechanisms. There is a pressing need for concerted studies with state-of-the-art techniques to unravel the aberrant pathways in these patients.

# ACKNOWLEDGMENTS

This work was supported by grant R01 HL056724 from NIH-NHLBI. The excellent secretarial assistance of Ms. Denise Tierney is gratefully acknowledged.

## *References*

1. Holmsen H. Secretable storage pools in platelets. *Annu Rev Med* 1979;30: 119–134.
2. Day HJ, Rao AK. Platelet function testing. *Semin Hematol* 1986;23:89–101.
3. Rao AK. Inherited defects in platelet signaling mechanisms. *J Thromb Haemost* 2003;1:671–681.
4. Solum NO. Procoagulant expression in platelets and defects leading to clinical disorders. *Arterioscler Thromb Vasc Biol* 1999;19:2841–2846.
5. Caen JP, Sultan Y, Larrieu M. New familial platelet disease. *Lancet* 1968;1:203.
6. Hardisty RM, Hutton RA. Bleeding tendency associated with "new" abnormality of platelet behavior. *Lancet* 1967;1:983.
7. Hardisty RM, Mills DCB, Ketsa-Ard K. The platelet defect associated with albinism. *Br J Haematol* 1972;23:672.
8. Sahud MA, Aggeler PM. Platelet dysfunction—differentiation of a newly recognized primary type from that produced by aspirin. *N Engl J Med* 1969;280:453–459.
9. Weiss HJ, Chervenick PA, Zalusky R, et al. A familial defect in platelet function associated with impaired release of adenosine diphosphate. *N Engl J Med* 1969;281:1264–1270.
10. Holmsen H, Weiss HJ. Hereditary defect in the platelet release reaction caused by a deficiency in the storage poool of platelet adenine nucelotides. *Br J Haematol* 1970;19:643–649.
11. Holmsen H, Weiss HJ. Further evidence for a deficient storage pool of adenine nucleotides in platelets from some patients with thrombocytopathia-"storage pool disease." *Blood* 1972;39:197.
12. Rao AK, Willis J, Hassell B, et al. Congenital platelet secretion defects with normal storage pools and arachidonate metabolism. *Circulation* 1982;66:299.
13. Rao AK, Holmsen H. Congenital disorders of platelet function. *Semin Hematol* 1986;23:102–118.
14. Rao AK, Gabbeta J. Congenital disorders of platelet signal transduction. *Arterioscler Thromb Vasc Biol* 2000;20:285–289.
15. Lages B, Weiss HJ. Heterogeneous defects of platelet secretion and responses to weak agonists in patients with bleeding disorders. *Br J Haematol* 1988;68:53–62.
16. Koike K, Rao AK, Holmsen H, et al. Platelet secretion defect in patients with the attention deficit disorder and easy bruising. *Blood* 1984;63:427–433.
17. Yang X, Sun L, Gabbeta J, et al. Platelet activation with combination of ionophore A23187 and a direct protein kinase C activator induces normal secretion in patients with impaired receptor mediated secretion and abnormal signal transduction. *Thromb Res* 1997;88:317–328.
18. Cattaneo M, Lombardi R, Zighetti ML, et al. Deficiency of ($^{33}$)P-2MeS-ADP binding sites on platelets with secretion defect, normal granule stores and normal thromboxane A$_2$ production. *Thromb Haemost* 1997;77: 986–990.
19. Weiss HJ, Witte LD, Kaplan KL, et al. Heterogeneity in storage pool deficiency: studies on granule-bound substances in 18 patients including variants deficient in -granules, platelet factor-4, β-thromboglobulin and platelet-derived growth factor. *Blood* 1979;54:1296.
20. Hayward CPM. Inherited disorders of platelet α-granules. *Platelets* 1997;8:197–209.
21. Lages B, Holmsen H, Weiss HJ, et al. Thrombin and ionophore A23187-induced dense granule secretion in storage pool deficient patients: evidence for impaired nucleotide storage as the primary dense granule defect. *Blood* 1983;61:154.
22. Malmsten C, Kindahl H, Samuelsson B, et al. Thromboxane synthesis and the platelet release reaction in Bernard-Soulier syndrome, thrombasthenia Glanzmann and Hermansky-Pudlack syndrome. *Br J Haematol* 1977;35:511.
23. Weiss HJ, Willis AL, Kuhn D, et al. Prostaglandin E2 potentiation of platelet aggregation induced by LASS endoperoxide: absent in storage pool disease, normal after aspirin ingestion. *Br J Haematol* 1976;32:257–272.
24. Weiss HJ, Lages B. Platelet malondialdehyde production and aggregation responses induced by arachidonate, prostaglandin-G$_2$, collagen, and epinephrine in 12 patients with storage pool deficiency. *Blood* 1981;58:27–33.
25. Ingerman CM, Smith JB, Shapiro S, et al. Hereditary abnormality of platelet aggregation attributable to nucleotide storage pool deficiency. *Blood* 1978;52:332–344.
26. Lages B, Weiss HJ. Biphasic aggregation responses to ADP and epinephrine in some storage pool deficient platelets: relationship to the role of endogenous ADP in platelet aggregation and secretion. *Thromb Haemost* 1980;43:147.
27. Weiss HJ, Lages B. The response of platelets to epinephrine in storage pool deficiency—evidence pertaining to the role of adenosine diphosphate in mediating primary and secondary aggregation. *Blood* 1988;72:1717–1725.

28. Nieuwenhuis HK, Akkerman JWN, Sixma JJ. Patients with a prolonged bleeding time and normal aggregation tests may have storage pool deficiency: studies on one hundred six patients. *Blood* 1987;70:620–623.

29. Israels SJ, McNicol A, Robertson C, et al. Platelet storage pool deficiency: diagnosis in patients with prolonged bleeding times and normal platelet aggregation. *Br J Haematol* 1990;75:118–121.

30. Holmsen H, Setkowsky CA, Lages B, et al. Content and thrombin-induced release of acid hydrolases in gel-filtered platelets from patients with storage pool disease. *Blood* 1975;46:131–142.

31. Lages B, Dangelmaier CA, Holmsen H, et al. Specific correction of impaired acid hydrolase secretion in storage pool-deficient platelets by adenosine diphosphate. *J Clin Invest* 1988;81:1865–1872.

32. White JG, Edson JR, Desnick SJ, et al. Studies on platelets in a variant of the Hermansky-Pudlak syndrome. *Am J Pathol* 1971;63:319.

33. Weiss HJ, Ames RP. Ultrastructural findings in storage-pool disease and aspirin-like defects of platelets. *Am J Pathol* 1973;71:447.

34. Lorez HP, Da Prada M, Rendu F, et al. Mepacrine, a tool for investigating the 5-hydroxytryptamine organelles of blood platelets by fluorescence microscopy. *J Lab Clin Med* 1977;89:200–206.

35. Skaer RJ, Flemans RJ, McQuilkan S. Mepacrine stains the dense bodies of human platelets and not platelet lysosomes. *Br J Haematol* 1981;49:435–438.

36. Richards JG, Da Prada M. Uranaffin reaction: a new cytochemical technique for the localization of adenine nucleotides in organelles storing biogenic amines. *J Histochem Cytochem* 1977;25:1322–1326.

37. Payne CM. A quantitative ultrastructural evaluation of the cell organelle specificity of the uranaffin reaction in normal human platelets. *Am J Clin Pathol* 1984;81:62–70.

38. Lages B, Scrutton MC, Holmsen H, et al. Metal ion contents of gel-filtered platelets from patients with storage pool disease. *Blood* 1975;46:119–129.

39. Akkerman JWN, Nieuwenhuis HK, Mommersteeg-Leautaud ME, et al. ATP-ADP compartmentation in storage pool deficient platelets: correlation between granule-bound ADP and the bleeding time. *Br J Haematol* 1983;55:135–143.

40. Weiss HJ, Tschopp TB, Brand H, et al. Studies on platelet 5-hydroxytryptamine (serotonin) in patients with storage-pool disease and alibinism. *J Clin Invest* 1974;54:421.

41. Pareti FI, Day HJ, Mills DCB. Nucelotide and scrotonin metabolism in platelets with defective secondary aggregation. *Blood* 1974;44:789–800.

42. Ugurbil K, Fukami M, Holmsen H. Proton NMR studies of nucleotide and amine storage in the dense granules of pig platelets. *Biochemistry* 1984;23:416.

43. Willis AL, Weiss HJ. A congenital defect in platelet prostaglandin production associated with impaired hemostasis in storage pool disease. *Prostaglandins* 1973;4:783.

44. Rendu F, Breton-Gorius J, Trugnan G, et al. Studies on a new variant of the Hermansky-Pudlak syndrome: qualitative, ultrastructural, and functional abnormalities of the platelet-dense bodies associated with a phospholipase A defect. *Am J Hematol* 1978;4:387–399.

45. Lages B, Weiss HJ. Enhanced increases in cytosolic Ca2 + in ADP-stimulated platelets from patients with δ-storage pool deficiency—a possible indicator of interactions between granule-bound ADP and the membrane ADP receptor. *Thromb Haemost* 1997;77:376–382.

46. Weiss HJ, Lages B. Platelet prothrombinase activity and intracellular calcium responses in patients with storage pool deficiency, glycoprotein IIb-IIIa deficiency, or impaired platelet coagulant activity—a comparison with Scott syndrome. *Blood* 1997;89:1599–1611.

47. Hermansky F, Pudlak P. Albinism associated with hemorrhagic diathesis and unusual pigmented reticular cells in the bone marrow: report of two cases with histochemical studies. *Blood* 1959;14:162.

48. Logan LJ, Rapaport SI, Maher I. Albinism and abnormal platelet function. *N Engl J Med* 1971;284:1340–1345.

49. Gahl WA, Brantly M, Kaiser-Kupfer MI, et al. Genetic defects and clinical characteristics of patients with a form of oculocutaneous albinism (Hermansky-Pudlak syndrome). *N Engl J Med* 1998;338:1258–1264.

50. Gunay-Aygun M, Huizing M, Gahl W. Molecular defects that affect platelet dense granules. *Semin Thromb Hemost* 2004;30:537–548.

51. Apitz-Castro R, Cruz MR, Ledezma E, et al. The storage pool deficiency in platelets from humans with the Chediak-Higashi syndrome: study of six patients. *Br J Haematol* 1985;59:471–483.

52. Boxer GJ, Holmsen H, Robkin L, et al. Abnormal platelet function in Chediak-Higashi syndrome. *Br J Haematol* 1977;35:521.

53. Buchanan GR, Handin RI. Platelet function in the Chediak-Higashi syndrome. *Blood* 1976;47:941.

54. Costa JL, Fauci AS, Wolff SM. A platelet abnormality in the Chediak-Higashi syndrome of man. *Blood* 1976;48:517.

55. Grottum KA, Hovig T, Holmsen H, et al. Wiskott-Aldrich syndrome: qualitative platelet defects and short platelet survival. *Br J Haematol* 1969;17:373–388.

56. Day HJ, Holmsen H. Platelet adenine nucleotide "storage pool deficiency" in thrombocytopenia absent radii syndrome. *JAMA* 1972;221:1053.

57. Menasche G, Pastural E, Feldmann J, et al. Mutations in RAB27A cause Griscelli syndrome associated with haemophagocytic syndrome. *Nat Genet* 2000;25:173–176.

58. Huizing M, Anikster Y, Gahl WA. Hermansky-Pudlak syndrome and Chediak-Higashi syndrome: disorders of vesicle formation and trafficking. *Thromb Haemost* 2001;86:233–245.

59. Novak EK, Swank RT, Hui SW. Platelet storage pool deficiency in mouse pigment mutations associated with seven distinct genetic loci. *Blood* 1984;63:536–544.

60. Novak EK, McGarry MP, Swank RT. Correction of symptoms of platelet storage pool deficiency in animal models for Chediak-Higashi syndrome and Hermansky-Pudlak syndrome. *Blood* 1985;66:1196.

61. Menard M, Meyers KM. Storage pool deficiency in cattle with the Chediak-Higashi syndrome results from an absence of dense granule precursors in ther megakaryocytes. *Blood* 1988;72:1726–1734.

62. Reddington M, Novak EK, Hurley E, et al. Immature dense granules in platelets from mice with platelet storage pool disease. *Blood* 1987;69:1300–1306.

63. Novak EK, Sweet HO, Prochazka M, et al. Cocoa: a new mouse model for platelet storage pool deficiency. *Br J Haematol* 1988;69:371–378.

64. Weiss HJ, Lages B, Vicic W, et al. Heterogeneous abnormalities of platelet dense granule ultrastructure in 20 patients with congenital storage pool deficiency. *Br J Haematol* 1993;83:282–295.

65. Lorez HP, Richards JG, DaPrada M, et al. Storage pool disease: comparative flourescence microscopical, cytochemical and biochemical studies on amine-storing organelles of human blood platelets. *Br J Haematol* 1979;43:297–305.

66. Gerrard JM, Lint D, Sims PJ, et al. Identification of a platelet dense granule membrane protein that is deficient in a patient with the Hermansky-Pudlak syndrome. *Blood* 1991;77:101–112.

67. McNicol A, Israels SJ, Robertson C, et al. The empty sack syndrome: a platelet storage pool deficiency associated with empty dense granules. *Br J Haematol* 1994;86:574–582.

68. Israels SJ, McMillan EM, Robertson C, et al. The lysosomal granule membrane protein, LAMP-2, is also present in platelet dense granule membranes. *Thromb Haemost* 1996;75:623–629.

69. Nishibori M, Cham B, McNicol A, et al. The protein CD63 is in platelet dense granules, is deficient in a patient with Hermansky-Pudlak syndrome, and appears identical to granulophysin. *J Clin Invest* 1993;91:1775–1782.

70. Witkop CJ, Babcock MN, Rao GHR, et al. Albinism and Hermansky-Pudlak syndrome in Puerto Rico. *Bol Asoc P Rico-Agosto* 1990;82:333–339.

71. Gahl WA, Brantly M, Troendle J, et al. Effect of pirfenidone on the pulmonary fibrosis of Hermansky-Pudlak syndrome. *Mol Genet Metab* 2002;76:234–242.

72. Tchernev VT, Mansfield TA, Giot L, et al. The Chediak-Higashi protein interacts with SNARE complex and signal transduction proteins. *Mol Med* 2002;8:56–64.

73. Raccuglia G. Gray platelet syndrome: a variety of qualitative platelet disorder. *Am J Med* 1971;51:818.

74. Gerrard JM, Phillips DR, Rao GHR, et al. Biochemical studies of two patients with the gray platelet syndrome: selective deficiency of platelet α granules. *J Clin Invest* 1980;66:102.

75. Levy-Toledano S, Caen JP, Breton-Gorius J, et al. Gray platelet syndrome: α-granule deficiency: its influence on platelet function. *J Lab Clin Med* 1981;98:831.

76. Nurden AT, Kunicki TJ, Dupuis D, et al. Specific protein and glycoprotein deficiencies in platelets isolated from two patients with the gray platelet syndrome. *Blood* 1982;59:709.

77. Srivastava PC, Powling MJ, Nokes TJC, et al. Gray platelet syndrome: studies on α granules, lysosomes and defective response to thrombin. *Br J Haematol* 1987;65:441–446.

78. Nurden P, Jandrot-Perrus M, Combrie R, et al. Severe deficiency of glycoprotein VI in a patient with gray platelet syndrome. *Blood* 2004;104:107–114.

79. Enouf J, Lebret M, Bredoux R, et al. Abnormal calcium transport into microsomes of gray platelet syndrome. *Br J Haematol* 1987;65:437.

80. Rosa JP, George JN, Bainton DF, et al. Gray platelet syndrome. Demonstration of α granule membranes that can fuse with the cell surface. *J Clin Invest* 1987;80:1138–1146.

81. Cramer EM, Vainchenker W, Vincin G, et al. Gray platelet syndrome: immunoelectron microscopic localization of fibrinogen and von Willebrand factor in platelets and megakaryocytes. *Blood* 1985;66:1309–1316.

82. Breton-Gorius J, Vainchenker W, Nurden A, et al. Defective α-granule production in megakaryocytes from gray platelet syndrome: ultrastructural studies of bone marrow cells and megakaryocytes growing in culture from blood precursors. *Am J Pathol* 1981;102:10.

83. Drouin A, Favier R, Masse JM, et al. Newly recognized cellular abnormalities in the gray platelet syndrome. *Blood* 2001;98:1382–1391.

84. Hyman T, Huizing M, Blumberg PM, et al. Use of a cDNA microarray to determine molecular mechanisms involved in grey platelet syndrome. *Br J Haematol* 2003;122:142–149.

85. Hayward CPM, Rivard GE, Kane WH. An autosomal dominant, qualitative platelet disorder associated with multimerin deficiency, abnormalities in platelet factor V, thrombospondin, von Willebrand factor, and fibrinogen, and an epinephrine aggregation defect. *Blood* 1996;87:4967–4978.

86. Kahr WH, Zheng S, Sheth PM, et al. Platelets from patients with the Quebec platelet disorder contain and secrete abnormal amounts of urokinase-type plasminogen activator. *Blood* 2001;98:257–265.

87. McKay H, Derome F, Haq MA, et al. Bleeding risks associated with inheritance of the Quebec platelet disorder. *Blood* 2004;104:159–165.

88. Pelczar-Wissner CJ, McDonald EG, Sussman II. Absence of platelet activating factor (PAF) mediated platelet aggregation: a new platelet defect. *Am J Hematol* 1984;16:419–422.

89. Lages B, Malmsten C, Weiss HJ, et al. Impaired platelet response to thromboxane-A$_2$ and defective calcium mobilization in a patient with a bleeding disorder. *Blood* 1981;57:545–552.

90. Samama M, Lecrubier C, Conard J, et al. Constitutional thrombocytopathy with subnormal response to thromboxane A$_2$. *Br J Haematol* 1981;48:293–303.

91. Wu KK, Le Breton GC, Thai HH, et al. Abnormal platelet response to thromboxane A$_2$. *J Clin Invest* 1981;67:1801–1804.

92. Hirata T, Kakizuka A, Ushikubi F, et al. Arg60 to Leu mutation of the human thromboxane A2 receptor in a dominantly inherited bleeding disorder. *J Clin Invest* 1994;94:1662–1667.

93. Ushikubi F, Okuma M, Kanaji K, et al. Hemorrhagic thrombocytopathy with platelet thromboxane A2 receptor abnormality: defective signal transduction with normal binding activity. *Thromb Hemostas* 1987;57:158–164.

94. Fuse I, Mito M, Hattori A, et al. Defective signal transduction induced by thromboxane A2 in a patient with a mild bleeding disorder: impaired phospholipase C activation despite normal phospholipase A2 activation. *Blood* 1993;81:994–1000.

95. Ushikubi F, Ishibashi T, Narumiya S, et al. Analysis of the defective signal transduction mechanism through the platelet thromboxane A$_2$ receptor in a patient with polycythemia vera. *Thromb Hemostas* 1992;67:144–146.

96. Armstrong RA, Jones RL, Peesapati V, et al. Competitive antagonism at thromboxane receptors in human platelets. *Br J Pharmacol* 1985;84:595–607.

97. Fuse I, Hattori A, Mito M, et al. Pathogenetic analysis of five cases with a platelet disorder characterized by the absence of thromboxane A2 (TXA2)-induced platelet aggregation in spite of normal TXA2 binding activity. *Thromb Hemostas* 1996;76:1080–1085.

98. Thomas DW, Mannon RB, Mannon PJ, et al. Coagulation defects and altered hemodynamic responses in mice lacking receptors for thromboxane A2. *J Clin Invest* 1998;102:1994–2001.

99. Kahn M. Platelet-collagen responses: molecular basis and therapeutic promise. *Semin Thrombos Hemostas* 2004;30:419–426.

100. Nieuwenhuis HK, Akkerman JWN, Houdijk WPM, et al. Human blood platelets showing no response to collagen fail to express surface glycoprotein Ia. *Nature (London)* 1985;318:470–472.

101. Nieuwenhuis HK, Sakariassen KS, Houdijk WPM, et al. Deficiency of platelet membrane glycoprotein Ia associated with a decreased platelet adhesion to subendothelium: a defect in platelet spreading. *Blood* 1986;68:692–695.

102. Kehrel B, Balleisen L, Kokott R, et al. Deficiency of intact thrombospondin and membrane glycoprotein Ia in platelets with defective collagen-induced aggregation and spontaneous loss of disorder. *Blood* 1988;71:1074–1078.

103. Moroi M, Jung SM, Okuma M, et al. A patient with platelets deficient in glycoprotein VI that lack both collagen-induced aggregation and adhesion. *J Clin Invest* 1989;84:1440–1445.

104. Ryo R, Yoshida A, Sugano W, et al. Deficiency of P62, a putative collagen receptor, in platelet from a patient with defective collagen-induced platelet aggregation. *Am J Hematol* 1992;38:25–31.

105. Arai M, Yamamoto N, Moroi M, et al. Platelets with 10% of the normal amount of glycoprotein VI have an impaired response to collagen that results in a mild bleeding tendency. *Br J Haematol* 1995;89:124–130.

106. Ichinohe T, Takayama H, Ezumi Y, et al. Collagen-stimulated activation of Syk but not c-Src is severely compromised in human platelets lacking membrane glycoprotein VI. *J Biol Chem* 1997;272:63–68.

107. Diaz-Ricart M, Tandon NN, Carretero M, et al. Platelets lacking functional CD36 (glycoprotein IV) show reduced adhesion to collagen in flowing whole blood. *Blood* 1993;82:491–496.

108. Yamamoto N, Ikeda H, Tandon NN, et al. A platelet membrane glycoprotein (GP) deficiency in healthy blood donors: Nak$^{a-}$ platelets lack detectable GPIV (CD36). *Blood* 1990;76:1698–1703.

109. Daniel JL, Dangelmaier C, Strouse R, et al. Collagen induces normal signal transduction in platelets deficient in CD36 (platelet glycoprotein IV). *Thromb Hemostas* 1994;71:353–356.

110. Kashiwagi H, Honda S, Tomiyama Y, et al. A novel polymorphism in glycoprotein IV (replacement of proline-90 by serine) predominates in subjects with platelet GPIV deficiency. *Thromb Hemostas* 1993;69:481–484.

111. Lipsky R, Sobieski DA, Tandon NN, et al. Detection of GPIV (CD36) mRNA in Nak$^{a-}$ platelets. *Thromb Hemostas* 1991;65:456–457.

112. Dorsam RT, Kunapuli SP. Central role of the P2Y12 receptor in platelet activation. *J Clin Invest* 2004;113:340–345.

113. Cattaneo M, Lecchi A, Randi AM, et al. Identification of a new congenital defect of platelet function characterized by severe impairment of platelet responses to adenosine diphosphate. *Blood* 1992;80:2787–2796.

114. Cattaneo M, Lecchi A, Lombardi R, et al. Platelets from a patient heterozygous for the defect of P2(CYC) receptors for ADP have a secretion defect despite normal thromboxane A(2) production and normal granule stores : further evidence that some cases of platelet 'Primary Secretion Defect' are heterozygous for a defect of P2(CYC) receptors. *Arterioscler Thromb Vasc Biol* 2000;20:E101–E106.

115. Nurden P, Savi P, Heilmann E, et al. An inherited bleeding disorder linked to a defective interaction between ADP and its receptor on platelets. Its influence on glycoprotein IIb-IIIa complex function. *J Clin Invest* 1995;95:1612–1622.

116. Levy-Toledano S, Maclouf J, Rosa JP, et al. Abnormal tyrosine phosphorylation linked to a defective interaction between ADP and its receptor on platelets. *Thromb Haemost* 1998;80:463–468.

117. Hollopeter G, Jantzen HM, Vincent D, et al. Identification of the platelet ADP receptor targeted by antithrombotic drugs. *Nature* 2001;409:202–207.

118. Cattaneo M, Zighetti ML, Lombardi R, et al. Molecular bases of defective signal transduction in the platelet P2Y12 receptor of a patient with congenital bleeding. *Proc Natl Acad Sci U S A* 2003;100:1978–1983.

119. Conley PB, Jurek MM, Vincent D, et al. Unique mutations of the P2Y$_{12}$ locus of patients with previously described defects in ADP-dependent aggregation. *Blood* 2001;98:43b.

120. Foster CJ, Prosser DM, Agans JM, et al. Molecular identification and characterization of the platelet ADP receptor targeted by thienopyridine antithrombotic drugs. *J Clin Invest* 2001;107:1591–1598.

121. Oury C, Lenaerts T, Peerlinck K, et al. Congenital deficiency of the phospholipase C coupled platelet P2Y1 receptor leads to a mild bleeding disorder. *Thromb Haemost* 1999;82:20–21.

122. Leon C, Hechler B, Freund M, et al. Defective platelet aggregation and increased resistance to thrombosis in purinergic P2Y(1) receptor-null mice. *J Clin Invest* 1999;104:1731–1737.

123. Oury C, Toth-Zsamboki E, Van Geet C, et al. A natural dominant negative P2X1 receptor due to deletion of a single amino acid residue. *J Biol Chem* 2000;275:22611–22614.

124. Propping P, Friedl W. Genetic control of adrenergic receptors on human platelets. A twin study. *Hum Genet* 1983;64:105.

125. Rao AK, Willis J, Kowalska MA, et al. Differential requirements for epinephrine induced platelet aggregation and inhibition of adenylate cyclase. Studies in familial α$_2$-adrenergic receptor defect. *Blood* 1988;71:494–501.

126. Tamponi G, Pannocchia A, Arduino C, et al. Congenital deficiency of α-2-adrenoreceptors on human platelets: description of two cases. *Thromb Haemost* 1987;58:1012–1016.

127. Yang J, Wu J, Kowalska MA, et al. Loss of signaling through the G protein, Gz, results in abnormal platelet activation and altered responses to psychoactive drugs. *Proc Natl Acad Sci U S A* 2000;97:9984–9989.

128. Gabbeta J, Yang X, Kowalska MA, et al. Platelet signal transduction defect with Gα subunit dysfunction and diminished Gαq in a patient with abnormal platelet responses. *Proc Natl Acad Sci U S A* 1997;94:8750–8755.

129. Rao AK, Disa J, Yang X. Concomitant defect in internal release and influx of calcium in patients with congenital platelet dysfunction and impaired agonist-induced calcium mobilization: thromboxane production is not required for internal release of calcium. *J Lab Clin Med* 1993;121:52–63.

130. Rao AK, Koike K, Willis J, et al. Platelet secretion defect associated with impaired liberation of arachidonic acid and normal myosin light chain phosphorylation. *Blood* 1984;64:914–921.

131. Gabbeta J, Vaidyula VR, Dhanasekaran DN, et al. Human platelet Gαq deficiency is associated with decreased Gαq gene expression in platelets but not neutrophils. *Thromb Haemost* 2002;87:129–133.

132. Offermanns S, Toombs CF, Hu YH, et al. Defective platelet activation in Gαq-deficient mice. *Nature* 1997;389:183–186.

133. Freson K, Hoylaerts MF, Jaeken J, et al. Genetic variation of the extra-large stimulatory G protein alpha-subunit leads to Gs hyperfunction in platelets and is a risk factor for bleeding. *Thromb Haemost* 2001;86:733–738.

134. Freson K, Thys C, Wittevrongel C, et al. Pseudohypoparathyroidism type Ib with disturbed imprinting in the GNAS1 cluster and Gsalpha deficiency in platelets. *Hum Mol Genet* 2002;11:2741–2750.

135. Patel YM, Patel K, Rahman S, et al. Evidence for a role for Galphai1 in mediating weak agonist-induced platelet aggregation in human platelets: reduced Galphai1 expression and defective Gi signaling in the platelets of a patient with a chronic bleeding disorder. *Blood* 2003;101:4828–4835.

136. Cattaneo M. Inherited platelet-based bleeding disorders. *J Thromb Haemost* 2003;1:1628–1636.

137. Yang X, Sun L, Ghosh S, et al. Human platelet signaling defect characterized by impaired production of 1,4,5 inositoltrisphosphate and phosphatidic acid, and diminished pleckstrin phosphorylation. Evidence for defective phospholipase C activation. *Blood* 1996;88:1676–1683.

138. Lee SB, Rao AK, Lee K-H, et al. Decreased expression of phospholipase C-β2 isozyme in human platelets with impaired function. *Blood* 1996;88:1684–1691.

139. Sun L, Mao G, Rao AK. Association of CBFA2 mutation with decreased platelet PKC-{theta} and impaired receptor-mediated activation of GPIIb-IIIa and pleckstrin phosphorylation: proteins regulated by CBFA2 play a role in GPIIb-IIIa activation. *Blood* 2004;103:948–954.

140. Lages B, Weiss HJ. Impairment of phosphatidylinositol metabolism in a patient with a bleeding disorder associated with defects of initial platelet responses. *Thromb Haemost* 1988;59:175–179.

141. Speiser-Ellerton S, Weiss HJ. Studies on platelet protein phosphorylation in patients with impaired responses to platelet agonists. *J Lab Clin Med* 1990;115:104–111.

142. Rao AK, Kowalska MA, Disa J. Impaired cytoplasmic ionized calcium mobilization in inherited platelet secretion defects. *Blood* 1989;74:664–672.

143. Mao GF, Vaidyula VR, Kunapuli SP, et al. Lineage-specific defect in gene expression in human platelet phospholipase C-beta2 deficiency. *Blood* 2002;99:905–911.
144. Jiang H, Kuang Y, Wu Y, et al. Roles of phospholipase C β2 in chemoattractant-elicited responses. *Proc Natl Acad Sci U S A* 1997;94:7971–7975.
145. Lian L, Wang Y, Draznin J, et al. The relative role of PLCβ and PI3Kγ in platelet activation. *Blood* 2005;106:110–117.
146. Holmsen H, Walsh PN, Koike K, et al. Familial bleeding disorder associated with deficiencies in platelet signal processing and glycoproteins. *Br J Haematol* 1987;67:335–344.
147. Cartwright J, Hampton KK, Macneil S, et al. A haemorrhagic platelet disorder associated with altered stimulus-response coupling and abnormal membrane phospholipid composition. *Br J Haematol* 1994;88:129–136.
148. Mitsui T. Defective signal transduction through the thromboxane A₂ receptor in a patient with a mild bleeding disorder. Deficiency of the inositol 1,4,5-triphosphate formation despite normal G-protein activation. *Thromb Haemost* 1997;77:991–995.
149. Gabbeta J, Yang X, Sun L, et al. Abnormal inside-out signal transduction-dependent activation of glycoprotein IIb-IIIa in a patient with impaired pleckstrin phosphorylation. *Blood* 1996;87:1368–1376.
150. Ferrell JE, Martin GS. Tyrosine-specific protein phosphorylation is regulated by glycoprotein IIb-IIIa in platelets. *Proc Natl Acad Sci U S A* 1989;86:2234–2238.
151. Golden A, Brugge JS, Shattil SJ. Role of platelet membrane glycoprotein IIb-IIIa in agonist-induced tyrosine phosphorylation of platelet proteins. *J Cell Biol* 1990;111:3117–3127.
152. Dekkers DW, Comfurius P, Vuist WM, et al. Impaired Ca2+-induced tyrosine phosphorylation and defective lipid scrambling in erythrocytes from a patient with Scott syndrome: a study using an inhibitor for scramblase that mimics the defect in Scott syndrome. *Blood* 1998;91:2133–2138.
153. Ballmaier M, Schulze H, Cremer M, et al. Defective c-Mpl signaling in the syndrome of thrombocytopenia with absent radii. *Stem Cells* 1998;16:177–184.
154. Shattil SJ, Kashiwagi H, Pampori N. Integrin signaling: the platelet paradigm. *Blood* 1998;91:2645–2657.
155. Gabbeta J, Yang X, Sun L, et al. Abnormal inside-out signal transduction-dependent activation of GPIIb-IIIa in a patient with impaired pleckstrin phosphorylation. *Blood* 1996;87:1368–1376.
156. Gabbeta J, Rao AK. Impaired platelet aggregation and abnormal activation of GPIIb-IIIa. *Thromb Haemost* 1997;78:1302.
157. Rao AK. Congenital disorders of platelet secretion and signal transduction. In: Colman RW, Hirsh J, Marder VJ et al., eds. *Hemostasis and thrombosis: basic principles and clinical practice*, 4th ed. Philadelphia, PA: Lippincott Williams & Wilkins, 2001:890–904.
158. Malmsten C, Hamberg M, Svensson J. Physiological role of an endoperoxide in human platelets: hemostatic defect due to platelet cyclooxygenase deficiency. *Proc Natl Acad Sci U S A* 1975;72:1446–1450.
159. Horellou MH, Lecompte T, Lecrubier C, et al. Familial and constitutional bleeding disorder due to platelet cyclooxygenase deficiency. *Am J Hematol* 1983;14:1–9.
160. Lagarde M, Byron PA, Vargaftig BB, et al. Impairment of platelet thromboxane A₂ generation and of the platelet release reaction in two patients with congenital deficiency of platelet cyclooxygenase. *Br J Haematol* 1978;38:251–266.
161. Pareti FI, Mannucci PM, D'Angelo A, et al. Congenital deficiency of thromboxane and prostacyclin. *Lancet* 1980;1:898–901.
162. Rak K, Boda Z. Hemostatic balance in congenital deficiency of platelet cyclooxygenase. *Lancet* 1980;2:44.
163. Roth GJ, Machuga R. Radioimmune assay of human platelet prostaglandin synthetase. *J Lab Clin Med* 1982;99:187–196.
164. Matijevic-Aleksic N, McPhedran P, Wu KK. Bleeding disorder due to platelet prostaglandin H synthase-1 (PGHS-1) deficiency. *Br J Haematol* 1996;92:212–217.
165. Defryn G, Machin SJ, Carreras LD, et al. Familial bleeding tendency with partial platelet thromboxane synthetase deficiency: reorientation of cyclic endoperoxide metabolism. *Br J Haematol* 1981;49:29–41.
166. Mestel F, Oetliker O, Beck E, et al. Severe bleeding associated with defective thromboxane synthetase. *Lancet* 1980;1:157.
167. Rao AK, Koike K, Day HJ, et al. Bleeding disorder associated albumin-dependent partial deficiency in platelet thromboxane production. Effect of albumin on arachidonate metabolism in platelets. *Am J Clin Pathol* 1985;83:687–696.
168. Remold-ODonnell E, Rosen FS, Kenney DM. Defects in Wiskott-Aldrich syndrome blood cells. *Blood* 1996;87:2621–2631.
169. Semple JW, Siminovitch KA, Mody M, et al. Flow cytometric analysis of platelets from children with the Wiskott-Aldrich syndrome reveals defects in platelet development, activation and structure. *Br J Haematol* 1997;97:747–754.
170. Shcherbina A, Rosen FS, Remold-O'Donnell E. Pathological events in platelets of Wiskott-Aldrich syndrome patients. *Br J Haematol* 1999;106:875–883.
171. Zhu Q, Watanabe C, Liu T, et al. Wiskott-Aldrich syndrome/X-linked thrombocytopenia: WASP gene mutations, protein expression, and phenotype. *Blood* 1997;90:2680–2689.
172. Zigmond SH. How WASP regulates actin polymerization. *J Cell Biol* 2000;150:117–120.
173. Falet H, Hoffmeister KM, Neujahr R, et al. Normal Arp2/3 complex activation in platelets lacking WASp. *Blood* 2002;100:2113–2122.
174. Mullen CA, Anderson KD, Blaese RM. Splenectomy and/or bone marrow transplantation in the management of the Wiskott-Aldrich syndrome: long-term follow-up of 62 cases. *Blood* 1993;82:2961–2966.
175. Michaud J, Wu F, Osato M, et al. *In vitro* analyses of known and novel RUNX1/AML1 mutations in dominant familial platelet disorder with predisposition to acute myelogenous leukemia: implications for mechanisms of pathogenesis. *Blood* 2002;99:1364–1372.
176. Ho CY, Otterud B, Legare RD, et al. Linkage of a familial platelet disorder with a propensity to develop myeloid malignancies to human chromosome 21q22.1-22.2. *Blood* 1996;87:5218–5224.
177. Song WJ, Sullivan MG, Legare RD, et al. Haploinsufficiency of CBFA2 causes familial thrombocytopenia with propensity to develop acute myelogenous leukaemia. *Nat Genet* 1999;23:166–175.
178. Freson K, Devriendt K, Matthijs G, et al. Platelet characteristics in patients with X-linked macrothrombocytopenia because of a novel GATA1 mutation. *Blood* 2001;98:85–92.
179. Shivdasani RA. Molecular and transcriptional regulation of megakaryocyte differentiation. *Stem Cells* 2001;19:397–407.
180. Shiraga M, Ritchie A, Aidoudi S, et al. Primary megakaryocytes reveal a role for transcription factor NF-E2 in integrin αIIbβ3 signaling. *J Cell Biol* 1999;147:1419–1430.
181. Estes JW. Platelet abnormalities in heritable disorders of connective tissue. *Ann N Y Acad Sci* 1972;201:445–450.
182. Evensen SA, Myhre L, Stormorken H. Haemostatic studies in osteogenesis imperfecta. *Scand J Haematol* 1984;33:177–179.
183. Hathaway WE, Solomons CC, Ott JE. Platelet function and pyrophosphates in osteogenesis imperfecta. *Blood* 1972;39:500–509.
184. Onel D, Ulutin SB, Ulutin ON. Platelet defect in a case of Ehlers-Danlos syndrome. *Acta Haematol* 1973;50:238–244.
185. Akkerman JWN, Rijksen G, Gorter G, et al. Platelet functions and energy metabolism in a patient with hexokinase deficiency. *Blood* 1984;63:147–153.
186. Corby DG, Putnam CW, Greene HL. Impaired platelet function in glucose-6-phosphatase deficiency. *J Pediatr* 1974;85:71–76.
187. Czapek EE, Deykin D, Salzman EW. Platelet dysfunction in glycogen storage disease type I. *Blood* 1973;41:235–247.
188. Bernheim J, Dechavanne M, Byron PA, et al. Thrombocytopenia, macrothrombocytopathia, nephritis and deafness. *Am J Med* 1976;61:145–150.
189. Epstein CJ, Sahud MA, Piel CF, et al. Hereditary macrothrombocytopathia, nephritis and deafness. *Am J Med* 1972;52:299–310.
190. Boullin DJ, O'Brien RA. Abnormalities of 5-hydroxytryptamine uptake and binding by blood platelets from children with Down's syndrome. *J Physiol* 1971;212:287–297.
191. Hamilton RW, Shaikh BS, Ottie JN, et al. Platelet function, ultrastructure, and survival in the May-Heggelin anomaly. *Am J Clin Pathol* 1980;74:663–668.
192. Lusher JM, Schneider J, Mizukami I, et al. The May-Heggelin anomaly: platelet function, ultrastructure and chromosome studies. *Blood* 1968;32:950.
193. Coller BS, Zarrabi MH. Platelet membrane studies in the May-Heggelin anomaly. *Blood* 1981;58:279–284.
194. Freson K, Hashimoto H, Thys C, et al. The pituitary adenylate cyclase-activating polypeptide is a physiological inhibitor of platelet activation. *J Clin Invest* 2004;113:905–912.
195. Degos L, Dautigny A, Brouet JC, et al. A molecular defect in thrombasthenic platelets. *J Clin Invest* 1975;56:236–240.
196. George JN, Caen JP, Nurden AT. Glanzmann's thrombasthenia: the spectrum of clinical disease. *Blood* 1990;75:1383–1395.
197. Mannucci PM. Desmopressin (DDAVP) in the treatment of bleeding disorders; the first 20 years. *Blood* 1997;90:2515–2521.
198. Mannucci PM. Hemostatic drugs. *N Engl J Med* 1998;339:245–253.
199. Rao AK, Ghosh S, Sun L, et al. Effect of mechanism of platelet dysfunction on response to DDAVP in patients with congenital platelet function defects. A double-blind placebo-controlled trial. *Thromb Haemost* 1995;74:1071–1078.
200. Kobrinsky NL, Israels ED, Gerrard JM, et al. Shortening of bleeding time by 1-deamino-8-D-arginine vasopressin in various bleeding disorders. *Lancet* 1984;1:1145–1148.
201. Schulman S, Johnson H, Egberg N, et al. DDAVP-induced correction of prolonged bleeding time in patients with congenital platelet function defects. *Thromb Res* 1987;45:165–174.
202. DiMichele DM, Hathaway WE. Use of DDAVP in inherited and acquired platelet dysfunction. *Am J Hematol* 1990;33:39–45.
203. Mannucci PM. *Desmopression (DDAVP) for treatment of disorders of hemostasis. Progress in hemostasis and thrombosis.* Orlando, FL: Grune & Stratton, 1986:19–44.
204. Nieuwenhuis HK, Sixma JJ. 1-Desamino-8-d-arginine vasopressin (Desmopressin) shortens the bleeding time in storage pool deficiency. *Ann Intern Med* 1988;108:65–67.

205. Poon MC, d'Oiron R. Recombinant activated factor VII (NovoSeven) treatment of platelet-related bleeding disorders. International Registry on Recombinant Factor VIIa and Congenital Platelet Disorders Group. *Blood Coagul Fibrinolysis* 2000;11(Suppl. 1):S55–S68.

206. Poon MC, Demers C, Jobin F, et al. Recombinant factor VIIa is effective for bleeding and surgery in patients with Glanzmann thrombasthenia. *Blood* 1999;94:3951–3953.

207. del Pozo Pozo AI, Jimenez-Yuste V, Villar A, et al. Successful thyroidectomy in a patient with Hermansky-Pudlak syndrome treated with recombinant activated factor VII and platelet concentrates. *Blood Coagul Fibrinolysis* 2002;13:551–553.

208. Almeida AM, Khair K, Hann I, et al. The use of recombinant factor VIIa in children with inherited platelet function disorders. *Br J Haematol* 2003;121:477–481.

209. Mielke CH Jr, Levine PH, Zucker S. Preoperative prednisone therapy in platelet function disorders. *Thromb Res* 1981;21:655–662.

210. Berliner S, Horowitz I, Martinowitz U, et al. Dental surgery in patients with severe factor XI deficiency without plasma replacement. *Blood Coagul Fibrinolysis* 1992;3:465–468.

211. Sindet-Pedersen S, Ramstrom G, Bernvil S, et al. Hemostatic effect of tranexamic acid mouthwash in anticoagulant-treated patients undergoing oral surgery. *N Engl J Med* 1989;320:840–843.

212. Bellucci S, Devergie A, Gluckman E, et al. Complete correction of Glanzmann's thrombasthenia by allogeneic bone-marrow transplantation. *Br J Haematol* 1985;59:635–641.

# CHAPTER 65 ■ INHERITED THROMBOCYTOPENIAS

PAQUITA NURDEN, JAMES N. GEORGE, AND ALAN T. NURDEN

Bleeding syndromes that arise through an inherited defect of platelet production constitute a widely known but heterogeneous group of rare platelet disorders of growing importance (1–4). Some, such as Bernard-Soulier syndrome (BSS) and Wiskott-Aldrich syndrome (WAS), associate a low circulating platelet count with a deficiency in a known functional protein of platelets. In others, platelet dysfunction has not been shown, and the genetic cause lies in the inability of megakaryocytes to mature and to produce platelets in sufficient numbers. In one group, there is an increased tendency toward the development of leukemia; in others, the defects extend outside megakaryocytopoiesis and interfere with the development and/or functioning of major organs. A unique characteristic is that in most of these rare diseases, the low platelet count is accompanied by profound changes in platelet morphology. Recent advances are beginning to identify their genetic basis. They are also providing basic knowledge of how megakaryocytes develop from the pluripotent hematopoietic stem cell (HSC) under the influence of thrombopoietin (TPO). Our review deals with the biology, genetics, clinical management, and prognosis of inherited thrombocytopenias. The fundamental aspects of thrombocytopoiesis are dealt with in Chapter 25. Most important in this group of patients is the need to assure correct diagnosis and to avoid inappropriate therapy such as steroid treatment and splenectomy.

## PSEUDOTHROMBOCYTOPENIA

When a low platelet count is encountered unexpectedly in hematology, it is first necessary to exclude changes subsequent to blood sampling. So-called *pseudothrombocytopenia* occurs in both apparently healthy subjects and patients (1,2) and is not associated with any disorder or medication. As reviewed in Chapter 78 of the fourth edition of this book, a number of surveys have evaluated its incidence in routine blood testing as between 0.09% and 0.21%. Confirmation of the validity of a low platelet count is therefore necessary by microscopic examination of a blood smear. *In vitro* platelet clumping is most often encountered in blood collected into ethylenediaminetetraacetic acid (EDTA) anticoagulant. Platelets may also show EDTA-dependent attachment to leukocytes (termed *platelet rosetting* or *satellitism*). With electronic counters, falsely low platelet counts (and elevated leukocyte counts) can also occur in patients with giant platelet syndromes (see subsequent text). Examination of the blood film should therefore also include an examination of platelet size. Although normal platelet counts are often restored when using citrate anticoagulant, this is not always so. Platelet clumping is typically caused by a naturally occurring antibody (agglutinin) binding to an epitope exposed on the glycoprotein (GP) GP IIb/IIIa complex ($\alpha_{IIb}\beta_3$ integrin)

in the presence of EDTA (5,6). EDTA removes $Ca^{2+}$ from the integrin, and it may even dissociate the subunits at 37°C. In one series of 88 patients with EDTA-dependent thrombocytopenia, 56 also had anticardiolipin antibodies, and their removal by adsorption led to a loss in platelet clumping, suggesting additional epitopes for the agglutinating antibodies (7). For clumping to occur, bivalent antibodies have to react with epitopes on adjacent platelets; alternatively, bound antibodies may cross-link platelets by binding secondarily via the FcγRII receptor.

## CLASSIFICATION OF HEREDITARY THROMBOCYTOPENIA

The heterogeneity within this group of disorders is such that their classification is difficult. Drachman (1) classified the disorders on the basis of their mode of inheritance, whereas Geddis and Kaushansky (2) emphasized the phenotypic differences. We have attempted to combine both approaches (see Table 65-1). In the text, we deal with the disorders one by one and refrain from putting them into an artificial classification, although related disorders are grouped together wherever possible. Although the autosomal recessive BSS may be considered the first familial thrombocytopenia to have its molecular basis defined (2), the deficiency of the GP Ib/IX/V complex means that it is also a qualitative disorder of platelet adhesion and as such has been included in Chapter 66. Classic BSS is not discussed further here. We also only briefly discuss inherited diseases with general bone marrow failure such as Fanconi anemia.

## MEDITERRANEAN MACROTHROMBOCYTOPENIA

As recently as 1975, a large series of 145 subjects from Italy and the Balkan peninsula were reported to have what was termed Mediterranean macrothrombocytopenia (8). The diagnostic criteria included a moderately low platelet count (70,000 to 150,000 per μL) and increased mean platelet volume (MPV). Other European authors also reported series of patients with chronic isolated macrothrombocytopenia and reduced platelet production (8–10). In general, these patients have autosomal dominant inheritance with mild mucocutaneous to no bleeding, normal platelet function, and normal megakaryocyte numbers. A defective production of TPO was ruled out (11). A series of 12 unrelated Italian families were subsequently studied by linkage analysis and mutation screening (12). In six of the families, a heterozygous

**TABLE 65-1**

INHERITED THROMBOCYTOPENIAS CLASSIFIED BY GENETIC MUTATIONS AND ASSOCIATED PHENOTYPE

| Syndrome | Gene mutation | Chromosomal location inheritance | Associated phenotype |
|---|---|---|---|
| MYH9-related thrombo-cytopenia; May-Hegglin anomaly; Fechtner, Epstein, and Sebastian syndromes | MYH9 | 22q11<br>Autosomal dominant | Various combinations of neutrophil inclusions, sensorineural hearing loss, nephritis, cataracts (see text) Giant platelets |
| Mediterranean macrothrombocytopenia | GP Ibα, possibly others | 17per-p12<br>Autosomal dominant | Giant platelets |
| Bernard-Soulier syndrome | GP Ibα, GP Ibβ, GP IX | 17, 22, and 3<br>Autosomal recessive | Giant platelets, platelet dysfunction |
| DiGeorge/velocardiofacial syndrome (CATCH 22) | Hemizygous microdeletion including GP Ibβ | 22q11<br>Autosomal dominant (on occasion) | Cardiac, facial, parathyroid, and thymus anomalies, cognitive/learning impairment |
| Familial platelet disorder/acute myelogenous leukemia | RUNX (CBAF2, AML1) | 21q22.2<br>Autosomal dominant | Myelodysplasia, acute myeloid leukemia, platelet dysfunction |
| Chromosome 10/THC2 | FLJ14813 | 10p12-11.2<br>Autosomal dominant | Not reported |
| Paris-Trousseau and Jacobsen syndromes | Hemizygous deletion including FLI1 | 11q23<br>Autosomal dominant | Psychomotor retardation, facial anomalies (Jacobsen syndrome) Enlarged platelets with abnormal granules |
| Gray platelet syndrome | Unknown | Unknown<br>Autosomal dominant or recessive | Myelofibrosis, enlarged platelets, platelet dysfunction |
| Congenital amegakaryocytic thrombocytopenia | c-Mpl | 1p34<br>Autosomal recessive | Marrow failure during second decade |
| Thrombocytopenia and absent radii | Unknown, c-Mpl signaling affected | Unknown<br>Autosomal recessive | Shortened/absent radii bilaterally |
| Thrombocytopenia with radio-ulnar synostosis | HOXA11 | 7p15-p14.2<br>Autosomal dominant | Fused radius, incomplete range of motion |
| Wiskott-Aldrich syndrome | WAS | Xp11.23-p11.22<br>X-linked | Immunodeficiency, eczema, lymphoma, small platelets Defective platelet and lymphocyte function |
| X-linked thrombocytopenia | WAS | Xp11.23-p11.22<br>X-linked | Small platelets, no immune problems |
| GATA-1–related thrombocytopenia with dyserythropoiesis | GATA-1 | Xp11.23<br>X-linked | Dyserythropoiesis ± anemia, thalassemia in some patients (XLT) Platelet dysfunction, enlarged platelets |

GP, glycoprotein; XLT, X-linked thrombocytopenia.
Data adapted from Drachman JG. Inherited thrombocytopenia: when a low platelet count does not mean ITP. *Blood* 2004;103:390.

A156V missense substitution was identified in *GP Ibα*, whereas in eight of 10 patients, GP Ib/IX density on platelets was at levels reduced to those of BSS heterozygotes. Interestingly, the A156V missense mutation was first reported in homozygous form in an Italian patient with presumed variant form BSS (13) (see Chapter 66). In this patient, GP Ibα expression was much reduced, and the receptor was unable to bind to its ligand, von Willebrand factor (VWF). However, BSS is classically a disorder with autosomal recessive inheritance, and while both a low platelet count and an increased percentage of large platelets has been reported in obligate carriers, this is not an absolute rule (3) (see Chapter 66). Notwithstanding, the A136V mutation, suggesting that these patients may represent heterozygous BSS, may account for up to 30% of patients with congenital macrothrombocytopenia in Italy. There is no evidence, however, that this trait extends beyond the mediterranean region.

# DIGEORGE OR VELOCARDIOFACIAL SYNDROME

Some clues on the origin of macrothrombocytopenias may come from studies on the DiGeorge/velocardiofacial syndromes (14). These can have autosomal dominant inheritance but most often appear to arise spontaneously. They are seen in approximately 1:4,000 births. The phenotype arises from a chromosome 22q11.2 microdeletion on one of a pair of chromosomes. Phenotypic features can include conotruncal cardiac abnormalities, learning disabilities, velopharyngeal insufficiency, immunodeficiency, facial dysmorphology, and thymic hypoplasia. A haploinsufficiency of a single gene, *Tbx1* (encoding a T-box containing transcription factor), largely accounts for the phenotype (15). Surveys of patients with DiGeorge syndrome have confirmed that mild thrombocytopenia and platelets of increased size affect about 20% of the patients (14,16). Adjacent to *Tbx1* is the gene encoding *GP Ibβ*, and its deletion can give rise to BSS when accompanied by a pathologic *GP Ibβ* mutation on the second allele (see Chapter 71). One possibility is that only those patients that have a microdeletion extending to the *GP Ibβ* gene show macrothrombocytopenia. However, a study of the literature suggests that the microdeletion likely includes *GP Ibβ* loss in many patients and that other factors combine with hemizygous *GP Ibβ* loss to designate macrothrombocytopenia. Defining these factors would help clarify the origin of enlarged platelets in inherited thrombocytopenias. Bleeding is not a noted characteristic of DiGeorge syndrome, similar to the absence of bleeding in heterozygous BSS.

# *MYH9*-RELATED THROMBOCYTOPENIA SYNDROMES

May-Hegglin anomaly, Fechtner syndrome, Sebastian syndrome, and Epstein syndrome constitute a group of disorders with autosomal dominant inheritance and giant platelets sometimes even larger than red cells (Table 65-1) (1,2,4,17,18). May-Hegglin anomaly was historically the first to be described and is the most common of the macrothrombocytopenias. Large Döhle-like bodies in neutrophils and eosinophils, and in some monocytes, are a characteristic of this disease (see Fig. 65-1A) (18). Thrombocytopenia is often mild; bleeding is infrequent and rarely life-threatening. In fact, because of the very large size of the platelets, circulating platelet mass may be near normal. As the disorder is asymptomatic, diagnosis may await adulthood. Variations of this disease are defined on the basis of the presence or absence of Döhle-like bodies and the presence or absence of abnormalities similar to those in Alport syndrome (nephritis, sensorineural hearing loss, cataracts) (17–23). Sebastian syndrome is a very rare condition, associating macrothrombocytopenia with neutrophilic inclusions that differ in morphology from those in May-Hegglin anomaly (22). Fechtner syndrome adds hearing loss, nephritis, and cataracts, whereas in Epstein syndrome, neither neutrophilic inclusions nor cataracts are present (19,21,23). Thrombocytopenia can be very severe in these disorders and the platelets truly giant. As a result, platelets and mature megakaryocytes show distinct morphologic abnormalities with zones of internal membranes grouped in specific areas. Megakaryocytes fail to show the normal distribution of the demarcation membrane system (DMS) (24,25). The ultrastructure of the leukocyte inclusions can also aid the diagnosis; in May-Hegglin anomaly, they are composed of segments of rough endoplasmic reticulum, and parallel, 7- to 10-nm filaments can sometimes be seen to orientate along the long axis, whereas in Sebastian syndrome and Fechtner syndrome, they can be cross-striated and contain ribosomes (26).

Molecular genetics has confirmed a similar molecular defect in these four syndromes. First the affected gene was mapped to chromosome 22q12-13, then it was identified as *MYH9* encoding the nonmuscle myosin heavy-chain IIA (NMMHC-IIA) (27–29). NMMHC-IIA is classified as a class II conventional myosin. It is a hexameric enzyme composed of two heavy chains and two pairs of light chains. Dimerization of two heavy chains results in a polar structure with two distinct regions. The amino-terminus forms a globular head that binds to actin and adenosine triphosphate (ATP), has ATPase activity, and is required for motor activity. The *C*-terminal α-helical domain features a coiled-coil and a single rodlike tail that allows the molecules to polymerize into bipolar filaments. NMMHC-IIA is in platelets, monocytes, and granulocytes and is found in tissues including kidney, eye, and cochlea (30,31). A spectrum of *MYH9* gene mutations gives rise to amino acid

substitutions or other defects affecting the rod or the globular head [see (29)]. Some reported mutations were repeated within unrelated families, although haplotype analysis suggested that common ancestors may sometimes be the cause. Presumed *de novo* mutations were found in sporadic cases. Some mutations are repeated in different phenotypes. A good example is a D1424N substitution in the coiled-coil found first in May-Hegglin anomaly and then in Fechtner and Sebastian syndromes (29,32). Another is an E1841K substitution found in May-Hegglin anomaly and Fechtner syndrome (28,29). A third example is an exon 16 mutation (R702C), which has been located in Epstein syndrome and Fechtner syndrome as well as in a variant of Alport syndrome (29). N93K and R702C mutations found in May-Hegglin anomaly and Fechtner syndrome affect amino acids conserved in smooth and nonmuscle myosins of vertebrates and lie in the myosin head domain. Myosin molecules expressing these mutations were observed to have 4% and 25% of the maximal ATPase activity and failed to translocate actin filaments in an *in vitro* motility assay (33). An inability of the contractile system to assure normal development and organization of the membrane systems during megakaryocyte maturation and/or platelet production may be at the basis of the giant platelet syndromes.

The nature of the mutation may nevertheless play a role in governing phenotype. In two Epstein syndrome families (no Döhle-like bodies), an R702H substitution was found (34), whereas the above-mentioned R702C mutation had previously been shown to be present in a patient with Fechtner syndrome (with Döhle-like bodies). It was suggested that the additional cysteine (C) in the patient with Fechtner syndrome facilitated intermolecular bridges and myosin aggregate formation. But the question of phenotypic variability remains unclear. Do other genetic and/or environmental factors also intervene, as suggested, for example, by studies on a large family with Fechtner syndrome where five out of 10 affected members showed no signs of renal lesions at the time of study (23). In a survey of autosomal dominant macrothrombocytopenia in Asia, 14 patients possessed heterozygous *MYH9* mutations, but the data failed to show clear phenotype-genotype relationships within May-Hegglin anomaly, Sebastian syndrome, and Fechtner syndrome (32). Mutations (E1841K and D1424N) located in patients with Epstein syndrome had previously been found in May-Hegglin anomaly (31). Notwithstanding, sequence analysis of *MYH9* in a family with nonsyndromic hereditary deafness showed that a R705H substitution cosegregated with the hearing loss phenotype and yet giant platelets were not present (30).

*MHY9* mutations can affect myosin filament assembly or stability as well as function. Aggregates of the mutant protein resulting from impaired filament assembly may give rise to the characteristic leukocyte inclusions with their paracrystalline arrays. These diseases can be clearly distinguished from the Alport syndrome in which nephropathy occurs without giant platelets or thrombocytopenia and which arises from abnormalities within the *COL4A5* gene (for the predominant X-linked form) or other genes affecting type IV collagen expression (35,36). The question arises as to how can the MHY9 molecular abnormalities can account for the different phenotypes. Why does a given mutation in *MYH9* not affect all of the tissues in which the protein is present? One proposed explanation is that additional II-B and II-C NMMHC isoforms can compensate, at least in part, for the malfunction of defective NMMHC-IIA isoform when they are expressed in the same tissues (37). These alternative isoforms are not located in platelets or leukocytes, but at least one of them is found in kidneys, eyes, or ears, all of which may either show late abnormalities or no defects. The potential role of another gene, *fibulin-1*, encoding an extracellular matrix protein as a disease modifier, has recently been underlined (38). Eight unrelated families with autosomal dominant giant platelet syndromes

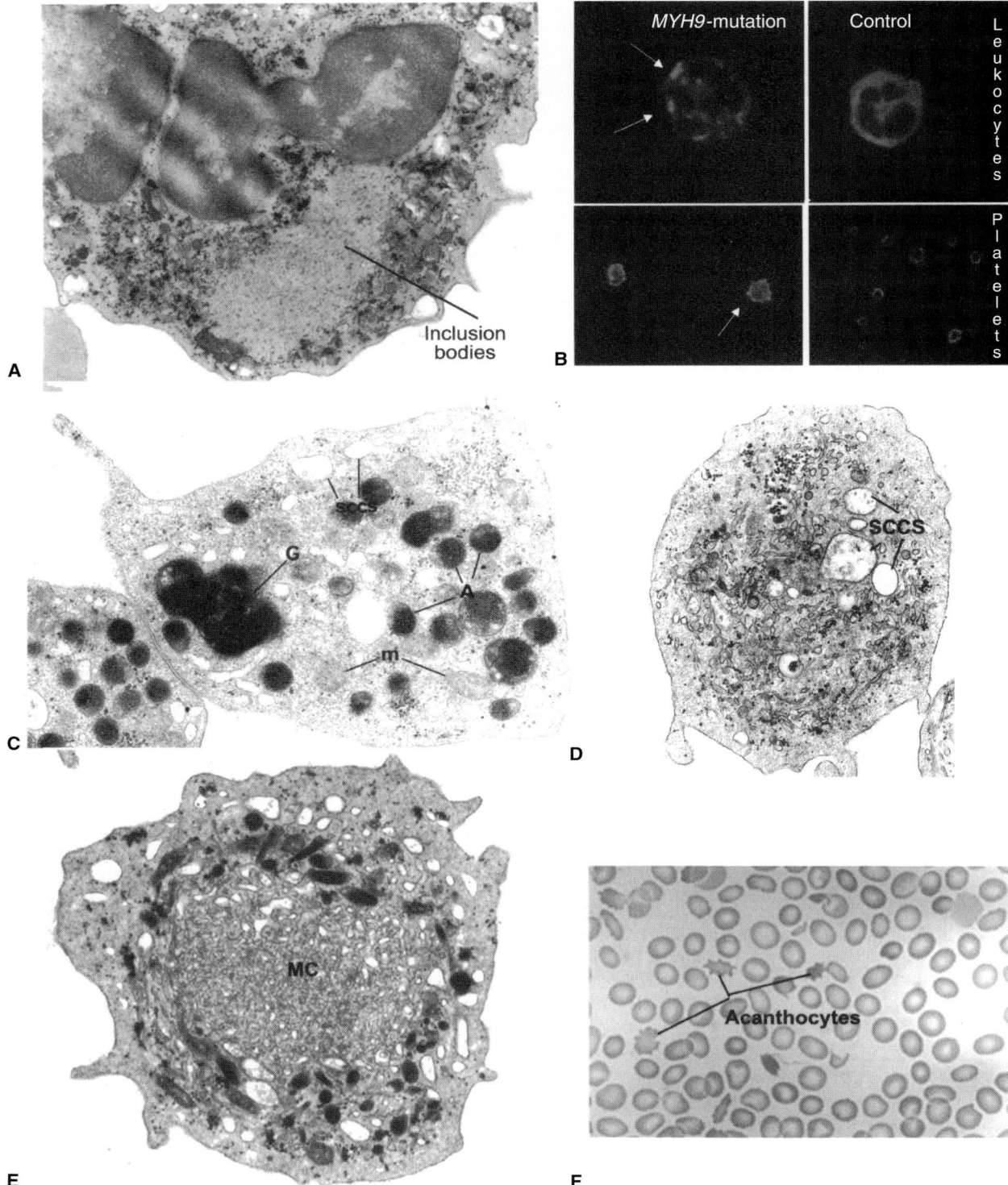

**FIGURE 65-1.** Composite illustration showing some of the striking ultrastructural characteristics of blood cells in selected inherited thrombocytopenias (see Color Fig. 65-1). (**A**) shows an electron micrograph of a Döhle-like body inclusion in a neutrophil from one of the first patients with May-Hegglin anomaly to be characterized (from Dr. A. Greinacher and courtesy of Dr. J.G. White, published from Greinacher A, Bux J, Kiefel V, et al. May-Hegglin anomaly: a rare cause of thrombocytopenia. *Eur J Pediatr* 1992;151:668, with permission). (**B**) shows the typical changes in NMMHC-IIA localization as detected using immunofluorescence in leukocytes and giant platelets from a patient with Sebastian syndrome (from Dr. A. Greinacher). (**C**) shows a typical giant α-granule in the enlarged platelets of a patient with Paris-Trousseau syndrome [from Dr. Elizabeth Cramer, published from Favier R, Jondeau K, Boutard P, et al. Paris-Trousseau syndrome: clinical, hematological, molecular data of 10 new cases. *Thromb Haemost* 2003;90:893, with permission (39)]. (**D**) presents a round and enlarged platelet from a Bordeaux patient with gray platelet syndrome. The absence of α-granules is to be noted. (**E**) shows an electron micrograph of a large round platelet with a cytoplasmic cluster of smooth endoplasmic reticulum membranes and membrane complexes, and (**F**) is a light microscopy slide of May-Grünweld-Giemsa stained blood cells showing dysmorphic red blood cells, both from a patient with X-linked macrothrombocytopenia due to a *GATA-1* mutation. G, giant granule; m, mitochondria; A, α-granule; SCCS, surface connected canalicular system; MC, membrane complexes. [From Kathleen Freson and Chris Van Geet, published with permission from Freson K, Devriendt K, Matthijs G, et al. Platelet characteristics in patients with X-linked macrothrombocytopenia because of a novel *GATA1* mutation. *Blood* 2001;98:85 (40).]

were studied for DNA sequence mutations and expression of the four *fibulin-1* splice variants (A-D). A mutation in the splice acceptor site of *fibulin-1* exon 19 was found in affected individuals of an Israeli Fechtner syndrome family, whereas no *MYH9* mutations were identified. Unexpectedly, *fibulin-1* variant D expression was absent in affected individuals from all eight families and coupled with expression of a putative antisense RNA (38). It is too early to know whether this finding is common or whether other cytoskeletal proteins may be similarly affected. It also remains to be seen whether the disorders result from a haploinsufficiency or a dominant negative effect of the mutated protein.

Diagnosis requires skilled reading of stained blood smears, and although electron microscopy is the procedure of choice, it is not readily available to all. It was a help when immunofluorescence procedures were developed for conventional air-dried peripheral blood smears to study the NMMHC-IIA localization in platelets and granulocytes of patients with *MYH9* disorders (41). A nonhomogeneous subcellular localization of myosin was observed in neutrophils from every individual with a *MYH9* mutation, whether May-Hegglin anomaly, Sebastian syndrome, or Fechtner syndrome. This procedure is illustrated in Figure 65-1B. For granulocytes, the localization is mostly in the form of spots, which represented the Döhle-like bodies. In platelets, the immunofluorescence is also not always homogeneous, and there is often a surface-oriented patch. Significantly, patients with Epstein syndrome and isolated macrothrombocytopenia with normal myosin localization did not have *MYH9* mutations (41). Immunofluorescence analysis of neutrophil NMMHC-IIA is useful as a novel screening test in the differential diagnosis of macrothrombocytopenia and aids the hematopathological classification of *MYH9* gene disorders.

Platelet transfusions remain the treatment as a precaution prior to surgery. Significantly, the presence of functionally normal giant platelets was speculated to compensate for the thrombocytopenia in reducing bleeding risk and also to account for the risk of myocardial infarction in patients with May-Hegglin anomaly (42) (P.N., personal observation). In Fechtner and Epstein syndromes, special care is required; hereditary nephritis leads to end-stage renal failure in middle age, necessitating dialysis and renal transplantation [reviewed in (18)]. High-frequency hearing loss and eye defects include juvenile glaucoma, and cataracts may also develop. Bleeding occurs but is variable in severity.

## MONTREAL PLATELET SYNDROME

In the Montreal platelet syndrome, severe macrothrombocytopenia (5 to $40 \times 10^9$ per L) is associated with spontaneous platelet aggregation in calcium-containing media and excessive bleeding (43). As far as it can be measured, platelets aggregate in response to agonists, although the response to thrombin may be reduced. Interestingly, a reduced platelet expression of a calcium-dependent protease, calpain, was reported, although the molecular basis for this and its relation to the phenotype remain unknown (44). Platelet membrane glycoproteins are basically normal.

## AUTOSOMAL DOMINANT THROMBOCYTOPENIA WITH PLATELETS OF NORMAL SIZE

An early report showed the presence of lifelong moderate to severe thrombocytopenia but with normal-sized platelets in large kindred with autosomal dominant inheritance (45). The inheritance pattern could be traced back over several generations. Studies of 30 members of a single American family linked the genetic defect to a 17-centimorgan region of the short arm of chromosome 10 (10p11-12) (46). Linkage to chromosome 10 was also established by a group in Italy working on an Italian family with an apparently identical phenotype (47). This chromosomal localization ruled out known candidate genes for inherited thrombocytopenias such as those encoding TPO, mpl, NF-E2, CBFA2, and GATA-1. Bone marrow and peripheral blood from the patients were enriched for megakaryocyte colony formation (CFU-MK). Megakaryocyte polyploidy failed to develop beyond 8N, and the cells were unable to achieve normal ultrastructural maturation after 11 days in liquid culture. TPO levels were moderately increased. A late block in terminal differentiation of megakaryocytes was indicated. Clinical manifestations were a propensity to easy bruising and increased bleeding at times of hemostatic stress. Myeloid or erythropoid cells were not affected, and there was no progression to aplastic anemia. A recent report has identified a novel putative kinase, *FLJ14813*, as a candidate gene mutated in this disorder (48). A missense mutation encoding an amino acid substitution (E167D) segregated perfectly with the thrombocytopenia in this family. Despite these studies, many families with uncharacterized autosomal dominant thrombocytopenia make this one of the more common inherited thrombocytopenia.

## FAMILIAL THROMBOCYTOPENIA WITH A PREDISPOSITION TO ACUTE MYELOGENOUS LEUKEMIA

Approximately 20 years ago, studies on a large kindred linked a bleeding tendency to an autosomal dominant disorder of platelet production and function and a propensity to develop myeloid leukemia (49). Thrombocytopenia was moderate and platelet size normal. Linkage to markers on chromosome 21q identified an 880-kb interval containing the disease gene. Further analysis of the disease gene and other families revealed nonsense mutations, missense mutations, or intragenic deletion of one allele of the hematopoietic transcription factor *RUNX1 (CBFA2, AML1)* gene, abnormalities that cosegregated with the disease in affected families (50,51). *RUNX1* is thought to have an important role in HSC differentiation. It may also act as a tumor suppressor. The haplodeficiency and missense or nonsense mutations interfering with DNA binding appear to lead to a decreased CFU-MK and insufficient production of platelets from birth. Mice with a targeted deletion of *RUNX1* showed primitive erythropoiesis but died at the embryonic stage because of a complete absence of hematopoiesis (52). Hemizygous deletion also affected erythroid and myeloid colonies. Mutated *RUNX1*, when present, may heterodimerize with normal protein and lead to loss of function. The propensity to develop leukemia requires that patients have a higher tendency to develop a second mutation either in *CBFA2* or another gene (51). This may be aided by the presence of an expanded population of undifferentiated HSCs. A recently described interaction between *RUNX1* protein and the GATA-1 and FLI1 transcription factors could be causally related to the thrombocytopenia (53). When platelets of these patients were examined, findings included decreased amounts of CBFA2, protein kinase C-θ, albumin, and IgG; impaired protein phosphorylation; and abnormal GP IIb/IIIa activation (54). HSC transplantation is an obvious therapeutic choice, although potential sibling donors must be screened for the family mutation.

# GRAY PLATELET SYNDROME

A mild bleeding disorder for which both autosomal recessive and autosomal dominant inheritance have been described, gray platelet syndrome is characterized by the platelet's inability to store α-granule proteins (17). Platelets are enlarged in this disorder but not giant (Fig. 65-1D). Thrombocytopenia is moderate, and the absence of α-granule contents gives the platelets a typical gray appearance on blood smears. One report has stated that patients with gray platelet syndrome also have gray neutrophils, but this finding has been challenged and said to be atypical (55,56). A feature of most patients is the early onset of myelofibrosis (which remains stable), a finding attributed to the inability of megakaryocytes to store newly synthesised platelet-derived growth factors, which, as a result, are released into the marrow (57). There is a tendency for secretion-dependent platelet aggregation to be abnormal. Collagen-induced platelet aggregation appears particularly affected in a cohort of patients with a low expression of the collagen receptor GP VI (58). This absence may be acquired and contribute to a more severe bleeding diathesis. Immunoelectron microscopy has shown that the α-granules in gray platelets and megakaryocytes are small and almost empty rather than absent, and many vacuoles are seen (Fig. 65-1D) (59). Residual α-granule proteins can be detected in the surface-connected canalicular system (SCCS), and the basic defect appears to involve packaging or storage of the α-granule contents (see also Chapter 64). Dense granules and their contents are normal. Emperipolesis (passage of other blood cells through megakaryocytes) has also been described in the gray platelet syndrome, perhaps linked to an abnormal surface expression of P selectin (60). The basic molecular defect(s) in this syndrome remains unknown, but probably it is a heterogenous disorder with more than one molecular cause. The importance of an altered $Ca^{2+}$ homeostasis and rap 1 protein phosphorylation (61) remains to be determined.

# WISKOTT-ALDRICH SYNDROME

WAS is an X-linked recessive disease characterized by moderate to severe thrombocytopenia with small platelets, a predisposition to infection, and eczema due to immune deficiency (1,2,17,62). Despite the thrombocytopenia, megakaryocyte numbers are normal. The small platelets (3.5 to 5.0 fL; normal 7 to 11 fL) may even result from modifications after release, for megakaryocyte maturation and proplatelet formation *in vitro* appear normal (63). A milder form without the immune problems is known as hereditary X-linked thrombocytopenia (XLT). WAS platelets show a decreased aggregation to adenosine 5′-diphosphate (ADP), epinephrine, and collagen, and their platelets have a reduced dense granule number. The disease is not exclusive to platelets, and T lymphocytes, among other blood cells, also show defective function. The gene responsible for WAS has been cloned and consists of 12 exons that encode a 502–amino acid protein (P) termed Wiskott-Aldrich syndrome protein (WASp) (64). WASp is selectively expressed in HSC lineages and is involved in cell signaling and regulation of the actin cytoskeleton. A secondary defect in WAS is abnormal expression of CD43 (sialophorin), a membrane glycoprotein of T-lymphoid cells. A wide range of genetic defects occur in WAS that localize throughout the gene and result either in the decreased expression of WASp or its absence (65,66). Mutations in exons 1, 2, and 3 were reported to more likely result in hereditary XLT. This finding may be because of a high prevalence of missense mutations in this region; a comprehensive phenotype-genotype study in Japan confirmed that the clinical phenotype depended on the presence or absence of WASp (67). WASp can be evaluated in platelets by flow cytometry and/or Western blotting; WASp-negative patients show a much higher susceptibility to infection and eczema and have a greater tendency for malignancies. The presence of residual levels of mutated or truncated WASp may be protective and translate into a more favorable outcome for patients. Total absence of WASp can give rise to a more severe phenotype. Recent evidence points to WASp having an early role in lymphocyte maturation (68).

WASp is a multifunctional protein involved in signal transduction, possessing tyrosine phosphorylation sites and adapter protein function. It binds through proline-rich motifs to SH3-containing proteins such as Fyn, Lck, PLC-γ, and Grb2 (62). WASp has a subtle role in cytoskeleton formation, and following activation by the Rho-family GTPase, Cdc42, and phosphatidylinositol 4,5-biphosphate it stimulates actin assembly by the Arp2/3 complex (69). Because of this, WAS has been termed a disorder of the cytoskeleton.

An autosomal dominant variant of WAS has been described (70). Although female heterozygotes for classic WAS have no clinical signs, because of preferential selection of the normal nonmutated X-chromosome in hematopoietic cells, X-linked WAS has been reported in young women presumably owing to coinheritance of a trait causing skewed X inactivation (71). Infections (often bacterial) and malignancies are major causes of death in WAS, and hemorrhage can also be a considerable problem. Overall, prognosis remains poor. However, clinical manifestations may vary greatly, even within the same family. Antibiotic prophylaxis, IVIgG infusions, or splenectomy can raise life expectancy, and splenectomy can increase platelet numbers. When possible, allogeneic HSC transplantation is the optimal treatment of the immunologic as well as the hematologic manifestations, with excellent outcomes using matched sibling donors and sometimes good results with closely matched donors (72,73). The development of a knockout mouse model for WAS has allowed the testing of retroviral gene transfer, and the successful transplantation of WASp-transduced HSCs improved T-cell signaling, offering long-term hope for gene therapy in WAS (74).

# PARIS-TROUSSEAU SYNDROME

The Paris-Trousseau syndrome is a rare disorder in which a low platelet production and a mild hemorragic tendency are associated with a haplodeficiency of chromosome 11 (deletion at 11q23.3-24) (39,75). Thrombocytopenia can be chronic (<50 × 10⁹ per L), and despite a normal platelet survival, the platelet aggregation response may be decreased. Paris-Trousseau syndrome is said to have autosomal dominant inheritance, although several isolated cases have been described in which *de novo* chromosome breakage cannot be excluded. Most reports concern children. Bone marrow dysmegakaryopoiesis is a constant feature; circulating platelets are often enlarged, and some have giant α-granules visible on Giemsa-stained blood smears (Fig. 65-1C). Two morphologically distinct populations of megakaryocytes are present: one composed of normal cells and the other of large numbers of small, immature cells with hypolobulated nucleus and arrested maturation. These cells appear susceptible to spontaneous lysis. Occasionally, platelet count may rapidly increase after birth and even normalize. The giant α-granules are a feature of platelets rather than megakaryocytes and may represent granule fusion after platelet release. Paris-Trousseau syndrome is a variant of the much more frequently encountered Jacobsen syndrome in which an 11q.23 deletion can give rise to congenital heart defects, trigonocephaly, mental retardation, respiratory infections, and malfunctions of multiple organs (76,77). Pancytopenia and/or thrombocytopenia are also seen in some, but not all, patients with Jacobsen syndrome. A feature of the deletion that occurs within 11q23-q24 is that it affects but one allele. Of variable length, the deletion includes two ETS transcription factor genes,

*ETS-1* and *FLI1*. FLI1 protein stimulates GATA-1/Friend of GATA (FOG-1)-dependent transcription of the *GP IIb* gene, and its interaction with GATA-1 also mediates synergistic expression of *GP IX* and *GP Ibα* (78,79). Studies on transgenic mouse models favor a role for FLI1 deficiency rather than ETS1 in the pathogenesis of Paris-Trousseau syndrome (80,81).

Recently, it has been shown that lentivirus-mediated overexpression of FLI1 in CD34$^+$ cells from a patient with Paris-Trousseau syndrome restores megakaryocytopoiesis *in vitro*, thereby proving that FLI1 hemizygous deletion contributes to the hematopoietic defects (82). Using RNA-FISH and single-cell RT-PCR, the authors elegantly showed that FLI1 expression is transiently monoallelic in CD41$^+$CD42$^-$ progenitors from normal donors, whereas it is predominantly biallelic in the other stages of megakaryocytopoiesis. In Paris-Trousseau syndrome cells, a half-reduction in *FLI1* gene dosage generated a subpopulation of CD41$^+$CD42$^-$ cells completely lacking *FLI1* transcription. The decreased FLI1 protein was suggested to prevent megakaryocyte differentiation and to explain the presence of a subpopulation of micromegakaryocytes that fail to reach the platelet production stage. The transient monoallelic expression of a gene essential for differentiation in the genesis of human haploinsufficiency-associated disease is a novel finding and requires a further molecular explanation, whereas short RNA interference of gene expression is something to exclude. The question now is whether this hypothesis can be expanded to other dominantly inherited disorders with haploinsufficiency.

## CONGENITAL AMEGAKARYOCYTIC THROMBOCYTOPENIA

In congenital amegakaryocytic thrombocytopenia (CAMT), severe thrombocytopenia at birth develops into a pancytopenia and severe aplastic anemia. With autosomal recessive inheritance, it is important to rule out immune-related thrombocytopenias during diagnosis. Over 50 families have been characterized (1,2). Affected patients have low numbers of megakaryocytes in their marrow from birth but show no physical abnormalities. Aplastic marrow evolves with age. The defects concern the incapacity of TPO to fulfill its normal thrombopoietic role as a result of abnormalities in the *c-Mpl* gene that encodes the TPO receptor. The first reported *c-Mpl* gene defect concerned a Japanese girl with compound heterozygosity associating a Q186X nonsense mutation in exon 4 and a delT in exon 10 (83). In a 2-year-old Italian boy, heterozygous R257C and P635L amino acid substitutions were speculated to give rise to a c-Mpl protein with qualitative defects of ligand binding and signaling (84). Ballmaier et al. (85) defined heterogeneity in CAMT, distinguishing patients with a severe form and early development into pancytopenia and a second group with mild thrombocytopenia in the first year of life but which then worsens over a 10-year period, with pancytopenia occuring in later life. Of eight point mutations detected in this study, frameshift or nonsense mutations predicted a complete loss of c-Mpl in five patients with severe disease. Missense mutations in three patients possessing residual c-Mpl were associated with a slower progression of the disease.

The fact that neither platelets nor haematopoietic progenitor cells show reactivity to TPO means that plasma TPO levels are highly elevated (>10-fold normal amounts), and this is a diagnostic feature of CAMT along with a lack of expression of c-Mpl on platelets (85,86). The absence of c-Mpl–bearing cells leads to a defective response to TPO in megakaryocyte colony formation. An early exhaustion of multipotential progenitors may account for the pancytopenia. Mice that are genetically null for c-Mpl are thrombocytopenic, and although they do not develop aplasia, marrow cell assays reveal a severe reduction in

precursors for all haematopoietic lineages (87). Allogeneic bone marrow transplantation is a recommended treatment for this disorder, although potential donors among relatives need to be screened for mutations that may limit megakaryocyte colony formation even in the heterozygous state (85).

Most interesting is the recent report of the presence of an activating mutation of the *c-Mpl* gene giving rise to familial essential thrombocythemia (88). This was a heterozygous S505N substitution inherited in an autosomal dominant manner and found in the transmembrane domain of c-Mpl protein. The mutation gave rise to upregulated and spontaneous intracellular signaling, activated megakaryocytopoiesis, and excessive platelet production. The long intracytoplasmic domain of Mpl is in fact organized into distinct functional elements.

The kinase JAK2 is critical for c-Mpl function, phosphorylating Mpl, and other signaling molecules, while leading to the activation of the Jak/signal transducer and activator of transcription (STAT) and Ras/Raf/Mek1/2-Mapk-Erk pathways. The JAK/STAT pathway is essential for TPO-stimulated proliferation, whereas the activation of Mapk promotes differentiation (89). A role for Src family kinases in Mpl signaling has also been shown, and these kinases, in particular Lyn kinase, negatively regulate TPO-induced proliferation and megakaryocytopoiesis by regulating the magnitude of Mapk (Mek1/2, Erk 1/2) activity (90). All of this raises the question of whether we are looking at the tip of the iceberg: Can defects in proteins of c-Mpl–stimulated signaling pathways lead to mild forms of inherited thrombocytopenias?

## AMEGAKARYOCYTIC THROMBOCYTOPENIA WITH RADIO-ULNAR SYNOSTOSIS

Three unrelated families were recently reported in which family members associated bone marrow failure and radioulnar synostosis (and other skeletal abnormalities) but with what appeared to be autosomal dominant inheritance (2,91,92). In some children, symptomatic thrombocytopenia with bleeding required correction by bone marrow or umbilical cord stem cell transplantation. Marrow studies had shown few or no megakaryocytes. Pancytopenia developed in some, but not all, individuals. Significantly, a heterozygous mutation was found in exon 2 of the homeobox gene, *HOXA11*. This mutation was found only in affected individuals and occurred in a domain critical for DNA binding. Studies on mice had previously shown that targeted disruption of the *HOXA10* and *HOXA11* genes affected forearm development in the embryo but did not extend to thrombocytopenia [reviewed in (2)]. However, it is so far unclear if both the skeletal and hematologic problems relate to *HOXA11* gene deficiency, although a predisposition to pancytopenia suggests an abnormality at the level of the HSC. It should be emphasized that radio-ulnar synostosis gives rise to mildly deformed forearms rather than their absence as in thrombocytopenia with absent radii (see subsequent text). The phenotype should also be distinguished from Fanconi anemia, in which skeletal abnormalities often affecting forearms, a predisposition to malignancies, and progressive pancytopenia are characteristic features (3).

## X-LINKED THROMBOCYTOPENIA WITH DYSERYTHROPOIESIS WITH OR WITHOUT ANEMIA

A special category of familial thrombocytopenia segregates XLT with dyserythropoiesis with or without anemia. Immunodeficiency and eczema are absent, and platelets are often large.

Thrombocytopenia ranges from moderate to severe (10,000 to 40,000 platelets per $\mu$L); splenomegaly, reticulocytosis, and unbalanced hemoglobin chain synthesis resembling $\beta$-thalassemia minor may be present. Bleeding times are prolonged and platelet function moderately affected. The gene responsible for this combination of defects was first mapped to the X-chromosome (Xp11-12) (93). The transcription factor GATA-1 together with its cofactor FOG-1 regulates erythropoiesis and megakaryocytopoiesis. GATA-1 is highly expressed in erythroid cells, megakaryocytes, mast cells, and eosinophilic cells (94). The GATA-1 gene is located at Xp11-12 and was found to be mutated in a series of families with XLT and dyserythropoiesis (40,95–98). GATA-1 contains two zinc fingers, the C-terminal which accounts for sequence-specific DNA binding and the N-terminal for both stabilization of DNA binding and for the interaction with FOG-1.

Nichols et al. (95) described a patient whose marrow showed numerous small dysplastic megakaryocytes and an abundance of large multinucleated erythroid precursors. Megakaryocytes displayed few $\alpha$-granules, an abnormal membrane development, and a paucity of demarcation membranes in mature cells. Circulating platelets were enlarged, had few $\alpha$-granules, and contained an abundance of membrane complexes. Erythrocytes were abnormal in size and shape (poikilocytosis and anisocytosis). The two affected male half-siblings were both severely anemic and thrombocytopenic at birth and thereafter. Their mother had mild chronic thrombocytopenia, but three female siblings were asymptomatic. A V205M substitution was found in GATA-1 that abrogated its interaction with FOG-1 and inhibited the ability of GATA-1 to rescue erythroid differentiation in a transfected erythroid cell line. The findings underscored the importance of FOG-1:GATA-1 associations in both megakaryocyte and erythroid development.

Freson et al. (40) studied a family with XLT without anemia (but with some dyserythropoietic features). A D218G substitution in GATA-1 affected its interaction with FOG1, although GATA-1 binding to DNA was normal. The bone marrow showed an increased number of large megakaryocytes. Structurally abnormal and enlarged platelets and dysmorphic red cells were present (Fig. 65-1E, F). Semiquantitative RNA analysis revealed a low transcription of the GATA-1 target genes, GP Ib$\beta$ and GP IX, and a reduced transcription of late megakaryocyte maturation markers. Flow cytometry revealed a subpopulation of very immature platelets with much reduced levels of membrane glycoproteins. Platelet function was affected with a poor response to ristocetin. GATA-1–regulated gene expression can result from GATA-1–DNA binding for some genes, whereas others require an intact GATA-1–FOG-1 complex. Interestingly, the same group later reported a family with a D218F mutation and a more severe phenotype showing that the nature of the substituted amino acid can be of crucial importance (96). A defect of GATA-1 self-association was observed as was a variable loss of expression of GATA-1–dependent genes. Skewed X inactivation in female carriers was also reported.

In the family studied by Mehaffey et al. (97), the effect of a G208S substitution on erythropoiesis was also less severe than was observed in the family with the V205M mutation. For three affected brothers, the degree of dyserythropoiesis was mild to moderate, but macrothrombocytopenia was again seen. This combination of thrombocytopenia with increased megakaryocytes in the bone marrow was considered as idiopathic thrombocytopenic purpura (ITP) for years. At the molecular level, this mutation causes disruption of binding primarily to FOG finger 9, whereas V205M results in reduced binding to fingers 1, 6, and 9. This report confirmed that normal platelet production may be more sensitive than that of erythrocytes to incomplete disruption of the GATA-1–FOG interaction.

Yu et al. (98) then reported a R216Q substitution in the N-terminal finger of GATA-1 in the family that originally led to the description of XLT and where red cell abnormalities were consistent with $\beta$-thalassemia (XLTT). Studies with recombinant GATA-1 showed that the mutation destabilized its binding to palindromic DNA sites but did not affect FOG-1 binding. This was the first report of $\beta$-thalassemia in humans caused by a mutation in an erythroid transcription factor. Platelet aggregation was normal, and platelet morphology showed enlarged platelets, but not for all affected individuals. The mutation allows programming of erythroid differentiation, although somewhat less efficiently than with wild-type protein. Balduini et al. (99) found the same R216Q substitution in an Italian family with XLTT. The propositus associated mild macrothrombocytopenia and defective maturation of megakaryocytes with mild dyserythropoiesis and red cell hemolysis. There was a bleeding tendency, and Hemoglobin studies were consistent with heterozygous $\beta$-thalassemia. Again, platelets contained few $\alpha$-granules and had an abundant and dilated SCCS. Immunofluorescence studies showed that TSP-1 and PF4 were not packed in the granules and that tubulin had an abnormal diffuse distribution. Platelet GP Ib/IX/V levels were higher than in controls, whereas GP IIb/IIIa was lower. These studies confirm that the mutation changes rather than abrogates the expression of GATA-1–dependent target genes. Studies on marrow showed that mature megakarocytes were often small and profoundly dysmorphic, whereas immature cells retained a capacity to proliferate. It is possible that the R216Q change caused GATA-1 to react with lower affinity only to palindromic and not to single GATA binding sites.

Overall, a defective interaction of GATA-1 with either DNA or FOG-1 can disrupt hematopoiesis and give rise to disorders sharing common themes but with diverging phenotypes. The role of GATA-1 was confirmed by transgenic mouse models with immature low ploidy megakaryocyte progenitors proliferating profusely in vitro as a result of a unique megakaryocyte differentiation arrest, a finding associated with dyserythropoietic anemia (100,101). Transgenic rescue of GATA-1 deficient mice with GATA-1 lacking a FOG-1 association site (GATA-1V205G) phenocopied patients with a V205 mutation (102). Studies on GATA-1 (and NF-E2) deficient mice showed increased bone mass due to megakaryocyte-stimulated osteoblast proliferation (103); it will therefore be interesting to examine bone mass in patients with GATA-1 defects. Transfusion therapy is given if bleeding is severe, or alternatively, HSC transplantation may be performed if an appropriate donor is available.

# THROMBOCYTOPENIA WITH ABSENT RADII

Thrombocytopenia and absent radii (TAR) syndrome is a rare congenital defect with severe hypomegakaryocytic thrombocytopenia and osteodysgenesis, namely shortened (or absent) forearms due to bilateral radial aplasia (1,2,104). Although other skeletal anomalies can be present, hands and fingers are unaffected. Inheritance appears to be autosomal recessive, for parents are not affected. Thrombocytopenia is very severe at birth (and most affected babies show purpura), but platelet numbers increase during childhood and platelet count can be near normal in adulthood. Intracranial hemorrhage is a particular risk in early life when mortality is at its greatest. Parents are normally healthy, although reports of a rare autosomal dominant variant of TAR can be found. TPO levels are elevated in the serum, and platelets of patients with TAR failed to respond to recombinant TPO as measured by testing TPO synergism to suboptimal concentrations of platelet activators (105). Studies on in vitro megakaryocyte differentiation and expression of the *c-Mpl* gene in six patients showed a profound defect in megakaryocyte progenitors (106). This was associated with a blockage in megakaryocyte differentiation with cells expressing GP Ib without GP IIb/IIIa. Megakaryocyte differentiation was poorly stimulated by TPO or other cytokines, and this was associated with a decrease in *c-Mpl* transcripts and Mpl protein. However, screening the *c-Mpl* gene has so far failed to show mutations, and a defect in the early events of Mpl signal transduction has been proposed to explain the disorder. Furthermore, sequencing of the *HOXA10*, *HOXA11*, and *HOXD11* nucleotide coding sequences of 10 patients with TAR syndrome revealed no mutations (107). The molecular defect underlying TAR syndrome therefore is currently unknown.

Bleeding risk is especially important in early life when the thrombocytopenia is most severe. Patients generally do not require platelet transfusions when adult, but bleeding risk during surgery led to an assessment of the use of erythropoietin (EPO) in a patient with TAR syndrome about to undergo hip replacement therapy (108). Moderate increases in platelet count (48–50 to 80–84 $\times$ 10$^9$ per L) suggested that EPO may reduce the need for platelet transfusions in such situations.

## OTHER DISORDERS

In some reports, insufficient evidence has been obtained to allow a complete classification of what may be a very rare defect. This is the case for the disorder associating giant platelets with abnormal surface glycoprotein and mitral valve insufficiency (109). In this apparently autosomal recessive disorder, a mild bleeding diathesis and moderate macrothrombocytopenia was associated with poorly defined defects in membrane glycoproteins. Even more unusual is a report of hereditary macrothombocytopenia with the atypical expression of glycophorin A on the surface of the giant platelets together with the usual platelet glycoproteins (110). Hearing loss developed in later life. No genetic defect has been described, although chromosomal crossover may be a possibility. Another example is the case reported by Willig et al. (111) in which a young boy died from complications associated with macrothrombocytopenia and mild neutropenia. Morphologic abnormalities of megakaryocytes included an abnormal fragmentation of megakaryocyte cytoplasm and the presence of giant membrane complexes. GP Ib appeared selectively decreased, but no sequencing abnormalities were found in the genes encoding GP Ib/IX. Significantly, there was a complete lack of sialyl-Lewis-X antigen on polymorphonuclear leukocytes from the patient, and the authors concluded that a posttranslational modification of membrane glycoproteins was at the origin of the defect (111). Recently, White (112) has described a woman and her son with lifelong macrothrombocytopenia and platelets with two types of large, opaque bodies originating from channels of the dense tubular system in megakaryocytes. These were additional aberrant structures distinct from dense and $\alpha$-granules. The molecular bases of this and the other disorders mentioned in the preceding text remain to be determined.

## DIFFERENTIAL DIAGNOSIS

Knowledge of the duration and severity of symptoms will help diagnosis. When thrombocytopenia is severe and/or is associated with platelet dysfunction, the condition is most often detected at birth or within the first year of life. Mild thrombocytopenia may yield sporadic symptoms, particularly at times of hemostatic stress. Sometimes there is no past history of bleeding, and moderate/mild thrombocytopenia is detected in routine testing (1–3). A detailed family history helps determine the inheritance pattern and gives clues to

bleeding risk. The coexpression of other phenotypic abnormalities can help define clinically recognized syndromes (see previous text), but sometimes the thrombocytopenia is isolated. The presence of macrothrombocytopenia will help diagnosis, as will morphologic studies of platelet granules and leukocyte inclusions. Plasma TPO levels should be measured. Balduini et al. (4), working on behalf of an Italian Study Group, have recently published a series of algorithms aimed at improving diagnosis of inherited thrombocytopenias, particularly those with giant platelets, and the reader is referred to this excellent publication for further details. It is necessary to eliminate inherited disorders of platelet dysfunction often with a normal platelet count but where an added acquired factor can cause or aggravate the thrombocytopenia. Analysis of the molecular defect is the final step, although mostly this requires the involvement of specialist centers.

First and foremost is the need to exclude an acquired cause. Among the many causes of acquired thrombocytopenia are autoimmune diseases, increased platelet consumption, splenomegaly, and marrow suppression or failure (Table 65-2). Neonatal alloimmune thrombocytopenia (NAIT) and ITP must be excluded to avoid incorrect treatment (corticosteroids or even splenectomy). It is necessary to know if the thrombocytopenia is persistent. Viral infection is a common cause of thrombocytopenia among children, whereas drug-induced thrombocytopenia is an increasingly recognized cause among adults. The list of drugs giving rise to drug-dependent antibodies is long (113); perhaps the most studied is heparin-induced thrombocytopenia (114). More recent is the description of thrombocytopenia induced following the administration of drugs inhibiting GP IIb/IIIa in cardiology. Here, the thrombocytopenia can occur in a matter of hours through the action of preexisting antibodies recognizing conformation-dependent epitopes on GP IIb/IIIa or can be delayed, requiring new antibody production (115, 116). The detection of plasma or serum alloantibodies and

---

**TABLE 65-2**

**CAUSES TO EXCLUDE OR TAKE INTO ACCOUNT WHEN DIAGNOSING INHERITED THROMBOCYTOPENIAS**

Immune thrombocytopenic purpura
    Childhood acute
    Adult chronic
Posttransfusion purpura
Drug-induced thrombocytopenia
    Heparin-induced thrombocytopenia
    Anti–GP IIb/IIIa drugs
    Other medicaments
Antiphospholipid syndrome
Gestational thrombocytopenia during pregnancy
    Preeclampsia and eclampsia
    HELLP syndrome
    TTP-HUS
Viral and bacterial infections
Increased platelet consumption
    Splenomegaly
    Disseminated intravascular coagulation and thrombosis
Myelodysplastic syndromes and myeloproliferative disease
Drug-induced marrow suppression and/or chemotherapy
Cancer and hematologic malignancy

GP, glycoprotein; HELLP, hemolysis, elevated liver, low platelet; TTP, thrombotic thrombocytopenic purpura; HUS, hemolytic-uremic syndrome.

autoantibodies requires immunologic testing readily available in specialized centers. But in ITP, the detection of an antibody does not guarantee that it is responsible for the thrombocytopenia, while the "nondetection" of an antibody does not rule out the presence of an antibody reacting with a minor component of platelets, so diagnosis may not be easy. Markedly elevated levels of circulating reticulated platelets may be an indicator of ITP in children (117).

Systemic lupus erythematosus (SLE) is an often encountered but complex disease in which the detection of antinuclear antibodies is a sensitive diagnostic feature (see Chapter 112). Thrombocytopenia can be severe and is a risk factor for mortality; other organs can be affected as well. To complicate matters, thrombocytopenia in SLE can also have a severe familial phenotype with genetic linkages at 1q22 and 11p13 (118). Whether this linkage involves genetic polymorphisms or mutations directly implicated in the pathogenesis of the disease is unknown. Similarly, familial acquired thrombotic purpura has been reported with ADAMTS inhibitory autoantibodies in identical twins (119). Antibodies associated with thrombocytopenia need not necessarily be directed against platelets. Neutralizing antibodies to granulocyte-macrophage colony stimulating factor (GM-CSF) or TPO have been detected in patients with amegakaryocytopenic purpura (AMTP) (120,121).

Although analysis of megakaryopoiesis *in vitro* requires specialized procedures, it is an essential part of a complete diagnosis for disorders such as Paris-Trousseau syndrome. For certain disorders, such as congenital amegakaryocytopoiesis, screening of the *c-Mpl* gene is now available. Care has to be taken not to misdiagnose disorders such as Type 2B von Willebrand disease. Although thrombocytopenia is an often described feature, giant platelets were reported for a patient by Moll et al. (122). Although this observation was thought to be a coincidence, platelets with a morphology typical of giant platelet syndromes were later described in three French patients with different mutations in exon 28 of the *VWF* gene (123). VWF was located on the platelet surface, but platelets did not show obvious signs of activation despite a tendency to agglutinate.

The surface expression of GP Ib/IX/V has been reported to be specifically decreased on giant platelets from patients with MHY9-related disorders, and this may cause confusion with BSS heterozygotes (124). One possible explanation is a retained intracellular localization of the complex due to the abnormal localization of the cytoskeleton with which it is attached. Interestingly, in the rare acquired Tn syndrome, a disorder characterized by the polyagglutination of blood cells, an incomplete glycosylation of GP Ibα results in thrombocytopenia, but changes in platelet morphology were not observed (125). Here, platelets abnormally expose α-N-acteyl-D-galactosamine residues through a defect in a galactosyltransferase.

## PROGNOSIS

Platelet transfusions remain the most commmon treatment of severe bleeding in inherited disorders of platelet production, although 1-deamino-8-D-arginine vasopressin (DDAVP) has been successfully used in a patient with Fechtner syndrome (126), and the use of recombinant human factor VIIa is a potentially new approach (127). The long-term treatment of CAMT is HSC transplanation with a matched donor. But the genetic basis of this disease suggests that it will be an excellent candidate for gene therapy, because even a small population of targeted stem cells may be able to proliferate in response to TPO and repopulate the marrow. Splenectomy may be an option in WAS, but its efficacy in other inherited thrombocytopenias has been questioned, although it may remain an option when HSC therapy is not possible (1,128).

## ACKNOWLEDGMENTS

We would like to thank Andreas Greinacher (Institute for Immunology and Transfusion Medicine, Ernst-Moritz-Arndt-University, Greifswald, Germany); Kathleen Freson and Christel van Geet (Center of Molecular and Vascular Biology and Department of Pediatrics, University Hospital Gasthuisberg, Leuven, Belgium); and Elizabeth Cramer (Laboratoire d'Hématologie, Hôpital Cochin, Paris, France) for generously providing electron micrographs or other material for use in Figure 65-1.

## *References*

1. Drachman JG. Inherited thrombocytopenia: when a low platelet count does not mean ITP. *Blood* 2004;103:390.
2. Geddis AE, Kaushansky K. Inherited thrombocytopenias: toward a molecular understanding of disorders of platelet production. *Curr Opin Pediatr* 2004;16:15.
3. Nurden AT. Qualitative disorders of platelets and megacaryocytes. *J Thromb Haemost* 2005 (*in press*).
4. Balduini C, Cattaneo M, Fabris F, et al. Inherited thrombocytopenias: a proposed diagnostic algorithm from the Italian Gruppoe di Studio delle Piastrine. *Haematologica* 2003;88:582.
5. Casonato A, Bertomoro A, Pontara E, et al. EDTA-dependent pseudothrombocytopenia caused by antibodies against the cytoadhesive receptor of platelet GPIIb-IIIa. *J Clin Pathol* 1994;47:625.
6. Fiorin F, Steffan A, Pradella P, et al. IgG platelet antibodies in EDTA-dependent pseudothrombocytopenia bind to platelet membrane glycoprotein IIb. *Am J Clin Pathol* 1998;110:178.
7. Bizzaro N, Brandalise M. EDTA-dependent pseudothrombocytopenia: association with antiplatelet and antiphospholipid antibodies. *Am J Clin Pathol* 1995;103:103.
8. Von Behrens WE. Mediterranean macrothrombocytopenia. *Blood* 1975; 46:199.
9. Najean Y, Lecompte T. Genetic thrombocytopenia with autosomal dominant transmission: a report of 54 cases. *Br J Haematol* 1990;74:203.
10. Fabris F, Cordiano I, Salvan F, et al. Chronic isolated macrothrombocytopenia with autosomal dominant transmission: a morphological and qualitative platelet disorder. *Eur J Haematol* 1997;58:40.
11. Fabris F, Cordianao I, Steffan A, et al. Indirect study of thrombopoiesis (TPO, reticulated platelets, glycocalicin) in patients with hereditary macrothrombocytopenia. *Eur J Haematol* 2000;64:151.
12. Savoia A, Balduini CL, Savino M, et al. Autosomal dominant macrothrombocytopenia in Italy is most frequently a type of heterozygous Bernard-Soulier syndrome. *Blood* 2001;97:1330.
13. Ware J, Russel SR, Marchese F, et al. Point mutation in a leucine-rich repeat of platelet glycoprotein Ibα resulting in the Bernard-Soulier syndrome. *J Clin Invest* 1993;92:1213.
14. Lawrence S, McDonald-McGinn DM, Zackai E, et al. Thrombocytopenia in patients with chromosome 22q11.2 deletion syndrome. *J Pediatr* 2003;143:277.
15. Kelly RG, Jerome-Majewska LA, Papaioannou VE. The del 22q11.2 gene Tbx1 regulates branchiomeric myogenesis. *Hum Mol Genet* 2004;13: 2829.
16. Kato T, Kosaka K, Kimura M, et al. Thrombocytopenia in patients with 22q11.2 deletion syndrome and its association with glycoprotein Ibb. *Genet Med* 2003;5:113.
17. Nurden AT, Nurden P. Inherited disorders of platelet function. In: Michelson AD, ed. *Platelets*. San Diego: Elsevier Science, 2002:681.
18. Mhawech P, Saleem A. Inherited giant platelet disorders. Classification and literature review. *Am J Clin Pathol* 2000;113:176.
19. Epstein CJ, Sahud MA, Piel CF, et al. Hereditary macrothrombocytopenia, thrombocytopenia and deafness. *Am J Med* 1972;52:299.
20. Greinacher A, Bux J, Kiefel V, et al. May-Hegglin anomaly: a rare cause of thrombocytopenia. *Eur J Pediatr* 1992;151:668.
21. Heynen JM, Blockmans D, Verwilghen LR, et al. Congenital macrothrombocytopenia, leukocyte inclusions, deafness and proteinuria: functional and electron microscopic observations on platelets and megakaryocytes. *Br J Haematol* 1998;70:441.
22. Greinacher A, Nieuwenhuis HK, White JG. Sebastian platelet syndrome: a new variant of herditary macrothrombocytopenia with leukocyte inclusions. *Blut* 1990;61:282.
23. Ghiggarei GM, Caridi G, Magrini U, et al. Genetics, clinical and pathological features of glomerulonephritis associated with mutations of nonmuscle myosin IIA (Fechtner syndrome). *Am J Kidney Dis* 2003;41:95.
24. Nurden P, Nurden A. Giant platelets, megakaryocytes and the expression of glycoprotein Ib-IX complexes. *CR Acad Sci Paris* 1996;319:717.
25. White JG. Use of the electron microscope for diagnosis of platelet disorders. *Semin Thromb Hemost* 1998;24:163.

26. Pujol-Moix N, Kelley MJ, Hernandez A, et al. Ultrastructural analysis of granulocyte inclusions in genetically confirmed MYH9-related disorders. *Haematologica* 2004;89:330.

27. Seri M, Cusano R, Gangarossa S, et al. The May-Hegglin/Fechtner Syndrome Consortium. Mutations in MYH9 result in the May-Hegglin anomaly, and Fechtner and Sebastian syndromes. *Nat Genet* 2000;26:103.

28. Kelley MJ, Jawien W, Ortel TL, et al. Mutation of MYH9, encoding non-muscle myosin heavy chain A, in May-Hegglin anomaly. *Nat Genet* 2000;26:106.

29. Heath KE, Campos-Barros A, Toren A, et al. Nonmuscle myosin heavy chain IIa mutations define a spectrum of autosomal dominant macrothrombocytopenias: May-Hegglin anomaly, and Fechtner, Sebastian, Epstein, and Alport-like syndromes. *Am J Hum Genet* 2001;69:1033.

30. Lalwani A, Goldstein JA, Kelley MJ, et al. Human nonsyndromic hereditary deafness DFNA17 is due to a mutation in nonmuscle myosin MYH9. *Am J Hum Genet* 2000;67:1121.

31. Arondel C, Vodovar N, Knebelmann B, et al. Expression of the nonmuscle myosin heavy chain IIA in the human kidney and screening for MYH9 mutations in Epstein and Fechtner syndromes. *J Am Soc Nephrol* 2001;13:65.

32. Kunishima S, Matsushita T, Kojima T, et al. Identification of six novel MYH9 mutations and genotype-phenotype relationships in autosomal dominant macrothrombocytopenia with leukocyte inclusions. *J Hum Genet* 2001;46:722.

33. Hu A, Wang F, Sellers JR. Mutations in human nonmuscle myosin IIA found in patients with May Hegglin anomaly and Fechtner syndrome result in impaired enzymatic function. *J Biol Chem* 2002;277:46512.

34. Seri M, Savino M, Bordo D, et al. Epstein syndrome: another renal disorder with mutations in the nonmuscle myosin heavy chain 9 gene. *Hum Genet* 2002;110:182.

35. Knebelmann B, Breillat C, Forestier L, et al. Spectrum of mutations in the COL4A5 collagen gene in X-linked Alport syndrome. *Am J Hum Genet* 1996;59:1221.

36. Boye E, Mollet G, Forestier L, et al. Determination of the genomic structure of the COL4A4 gene and of novel mutations causing autosomal recessive Alport syndrome. *Am J Hum Genet* 1998;63:1329.

37. Marigo V, Nigro A, Pecci A, et al. Correlation between the clinical phenotype of MYH9-related disease and tissue distribution of class II nonmuscle myosin heavy chains. *Genomics* 2004;83:1125.

38. Toren A, Rozenfeld-Granot G, Heath KE, et al. MYH9 spectrum of autosomal-dominant giant platelet syndromes: unexpected association with fibulin-1 variant-D inactivation. *Am J Hematol* 2003;74:254.

39. Favier R, Jondeau K, Boutard P, et al. Paris-Trousseau syndrome: clinical, hematological, molecular data of ten new cases. *Thromb Haemost* 2003;90:893.

40. Freson K, Devriendt K, Matthijs G, et al. Platelet characteristics in patients with X-linked macrothrombocytopenia because of a novel GATA1 mutation. *Blood* 2001;98:85.

41. Pecci A, Noris P, Invernizzi R, et al. Immunocytochemistry for the heavy chain of the non-muscle myosin IIA as a diagnostic tool for MYH9-related disorders. *Br J Haematol* 2002;117:164.

42. Goto S, Kasahara H, Saka H, et al. Functional compensation of the low platelet count by increased individual platelet size in a pateint with May-Hegglin anomaly presenting with acute myocardial infarction. *Int J Cardiol* 1998;64:171.

43. Milton JG, Frojmovic MM, Stang SS, et al. Spontaneous platelet aggregation in a hereditary giant platelet syndrome (MPS). *Am J Pathol* 1984;114:336.

44. Okita JR, Frojmovic MM, Kristopeit S, et al. Montreal platelet syndrome: a defect in calcium-activated neutral proteinase (calpain). *Blood* 1989;74:715.

45. Bithell TC, Didisheim P, Cartwright GE, et al. Thrombocytopenia inherited as an autosomal dominant trait. *Blood* 1965;25:231.

46. Drachman JG, Jarvik GP, Mehaffey MG. Autosomal dominant thrombocytopenia: incomplete megakaryocyte differentiation and linkage to human chromosome 10. *Blood* 2000;96:118.

47. Savoia A, Del Vecchio M, Totaro A, et al. An autosomal dominant thrombocytopenia gene maps to chromosomal region 10p. *Am J Hum Genet* 1999;65:1401.

48. Gandhi MJ, Cummings CL, Drachman JG, et al. FLJ14813 missense mutation; a candidate for autosomal dominant thrombocytopenia on human chromosome 10. *Hum Hered* 2003;55:68.

49. Ho CY, Otterud B, Lagare RD, et al. Linkage of a familial platelet disorder with a propensity to develop myeloid malignancies to human chromosome 21q22.1-22.2. *Hum Mol Genet* 1996;4:763–766.

50. Song W-J, Sullivan MG, Legare RD, et al. Haploinsufficiency of CBFA2 causes familial thrombocytopenia with propensity to develop acute myelogenous leukaemia. *Nat Genet* 1999;29:166.

51. Michaud J, Wu F, Osato M, et al. *In vitro* analyses of known and novel RUNX1/AML1 mutations in dominant familial platelet disorder with predisposition to acute myelogenous leukemia: implications for mechanisms of pathogenesis. *Blood* 2002;99:1364.

52. Yergeau DA, Hetherington CJ, Wang Q, et al. Embryonic lethality and impairment of hematopoiesis in mice heterozygous for an AMLI-ETO fusion gene. *Nat Genet* 1997;15:303.

53. Elagib KE, Racke FL, Mogass M, et al. RUNX1 and GATA-1 coexpression and cooperation in megakaryocytic differentiation. *Blood* 2003;101:4333.

54. Sun L, Mao G, Rao AL. Association of CBFA2 mutation with decreased platelet PKC-theta and impaired receptor-mediated activation of GPIIb-IIIa and plekstrin phosphorylation: proteins regulated by CBFA2 play a role in GPIIb-IIIa activation. *Blood* 2004;103:948.

55. Drouin A, Favier RM, Massé JM, et al. Newly recognized cellular abnormalities in the gray platelet syndrome. *Blood* 2001;98:1382.

56. White JG, Brunning RD. Neutrophils in the gray platelet syndrome. *Platelets* 2004;15:333.

57. Breton-Gorius J, Vainchenker W, Nurden A, et al. Defective α-granule production in megakaryocytes from gray platelet syndrome. Ultrastructural studies on bone-marrow cells and megakaryocytes growing in culture from blood precursors. *Am J Pathol* 1981;102:10.

58. Nurden P, Jandrot-Perrus M, Combrie R, et al. Severe deficiency of glycoprotein VI in a patient with gray platelet syndrome. *Blood* 2004;104:107.

59. Cramer EM, Vainchenker W, Vinci G, et al. Gray platelet syndrome: immunoelectron microscopic localization of fibrinogen and von Willebrand factor in platelets and megakaryocytes. *Blood* 1985;66:1309.

60. Falik-Zaccai T, Anikster Y, Rivera CE, et al. A new genetic isolate of gray platelet syndrome (GPS): clinical, cellular and hematologic characteristics. *Mol Genet Metab* 2001;74:303.

61. Enouf J, Corvazier E, Papp B, et al. Abnormal cAMP-induced phosphorylation of rap 1 protein in grey platelet syndrome platelets. *Br J Haematol* 1994;86:338.

62. Remold-O'Donnell E, Rosen FS, Kenney DM. Defects in Wiskott-Aldrich syndrome blood cells. *Blood* 1996;87:2671.

63. Haddad E, Cramer EM, Rivière C, et al. The thrombocytopenia of Wiskott-Aldrich syndrome is not related to a defect in proplatelet formation. *Blood* 1999;94:509.

64. Derry JMJ, Ochs HD, Francke U. Isolation of a novel gene mutated in Wiskott-Aldrich syndrome. *Cell* 1994;78:635.

65. Zhu QL, Zhang M, Blaese RM, et al. The Wiskott-Aldrich syndrome and X-linked thrombocytopenia are caused by mutations of the same gene. *Blood* 1995;86:3797.

66. Zhu QL, Watanabe C, Liu T, et al. Wiskott-Aldrich syndrome/X-linked thrombocytopenia: WASP gene mutations, protein expression and phenotype. *Blood* 1997;90:2680.

67. Imai K, Morio T, Jin Y, et al. Clinical course of patients with WASP gene mutations. *Blood* 2004;103:456.

68. Park JY, Kob M, Prodeus AP, et al. Early deficit of lymphocytes in Wiskott-Aldrich syndrome: possible role of WASP in human lymphocyte maturation. *Clin Exp Immunol* 2004;136:104.

69. Kim AS, Kakalis LT, Abdul-Manan N, et al. Autoinhibition and activation mechanisms of the Wiskott-Aldrich syndrome protein. *Nature* 2000;404:151.

70. Rocca B, Bellacosa A, De Cristofaro R, et al. Wiskott-Aldrich syndrome: report of an autosomal dominant variant. *Blood* 1996;87:4538.

71. Parolini O, Ressmann G, Haas OA, et al. X-linked Wiskott-Aldrich syndrome in a girl. *N Engl J Med* 1998;338:290.

72. Mullen CA, Anderson KD, Blaese RM, et al. Splenectomy and/or bone marrow transplantation in the management of the Wiskott-Aldrich syndrome: long-term follow-up of 62 cases. *Blood* 1993;82:2961.

73. Filipovich AH, Stone JV, Tomany SC, et al. Impact of donor type on outcome of bone marrow transplanation for Wiskott-Aldrich syndrome: collaborative study of the International Bone Marrow Transplant Registry and the National Marrow Donor Program. *Blood* 2001;97:1598.

74. Klein C, Nguyen D, Liu C-H, et al. Gene therapy for Wiskott-Aldrich syndrome: rescue of t-cell signaling and amelioration of colitis upon transplantation of retrovirally transduced hematopoietic stem cells in mice. *Blood* 2003;101:2159.

75. Breton-Gorius J, Favier R, Guichard J, et al. A new congenital dysmegakaryopoietic thrombocytopenia (Paris-Trousseau) associated with giant platelet alpha granules and chromosome 11 deletion at 11q23. *Blood* 1995;85:1805.

76. Krishnamurti L, Neglia JP, Nagarajan R, et al. Paris-Trousseau syndrome platelets in a child with Jacobsen's syndrome. *Am J Hematol* 2001;65:295.

77. Grossfeld PD, Mattina T, Lai Z, et al. The 11q terminal deletion disorder: a prospective study of 110 cases. *Am J Med Genet* 2004;129A:51.

78. Wang X, Crispino JD, Letting DL, et al. Control of megakaryocyte-specific gene expression by GATA-1 and FOG-1: role of Ets transcription factors. *EMBO J* 2002;21:5225.

79. Eisbacher M, Holmes ML, Newton A, et al. Protein-protein interaction between Fli-1 and GATA-1 mediates synergistic expression of megakaryocyte-specific genes through cooperative DNA binding. *Mol Cell Biol* 2003;23:3427.

80. Hart A, Melet F, Grossfeld P, et al. Fli-1 is required for murine vascular and megakaryocytic development and is hemizygously deleted in patients with thrombocytopenia. *Immunity* 2000;13:167.

81. Bartel FO, Higuchi T, Spyropoulos DD. Mouse models in the study of the Ets family of transcription factors. *Oncogene* 2000;19:6443.

82. Raslova H, Komura E, Le Couédic JP, et al. FLI1 monoallelic expression combined with its hemizygous loss underlies Paris-Trousseau/Jacobsen thrombopenia. *J Clin Invest* 2004;114:77.

83. Ihara K, Ishii E, Eguchi M, et al. Identification of mutations in the c-mpl gene in congenital amegakaryocytic thrombocytopenia. *Proc Natl Acad Sci U S A* 1999;96:3133.

84. Tonelli R, Scardovi AL, Pession A, et al. Compound heterozygosity for two different amino-acid substitution mutations in the thrombopoietin receptor (*c-mpl* gene) in congenital amegakaryocytic thrombocytopenia (CAMT). *Hum Genet* 2000;107:225.

85. Ballamaier M, Germeshausen M, Schulze H, et al. c-mpl mutations are the cause of congenital amegakaryocytic thrombocytopenia. *Blood* 2001;97:139.

86. van den Oudenrijn S, Bruin M, Folman CC, et al. Three parameters, plasma thrombopoietin levels, plasma glycocalicin levels and megakaryocyte culture, distinguish between different causes of congenital thrombocytopenia. *Br J Haematol* 2002;117:390.

87. Kimura S, Roberts AW, Metcalf D, et al. Hematopoietic stem cell deficiencies in mice lacking c-Mpl, the receptor for thrombopoietin. *Proc Natl Acad Sci U S A* 1998;95:1195.

88. Ding J, Komatsu H, Wakita A, et al. Familial essential thrombocythemia associated with a dominant-positive activating mutation of the *c-MPL* gene, which encodes for the receptor for thrombopoietin. *Blood* 2004;103:4198.

89. Rouyez MC, Boucheron C, Gisselbrecht S, et al. Control of thrombopoietin-induced magakaryocytic differentiation by the mitogen-activated protein kinase pathway. *Mol Cell Biol* 1997;17:4991.

90. Lannutti BJ, Drachman JG. Lyn tyrosine kinase regulates thrombopoietin-induced proliferation of hematopoietic cell lines and primary megakaryocytic progenitors. *Blood* 2004;103:3743.

91. Thompson AA, Nguyen LT. Amegakaryocytic thrombocytopenia and radio-ulnar synostosis are associated with *HOXA11* mutation. *Nat Genet* 2000;26:397.

92. Thompson AA, Woodruff K, Feig SA, et al. Congenital thrombocytopenia and radio-ulnar synostosis: a new familial syndrome. *Br J Haematol* 2001;113:866.

93. Raskind WH, Niakan KK, Wolff J, et al. Mapping of a syndrome of X-linked thrombocytopenia with thalassemia to band Xp11-12: further evidence of genetic heterogeneity of X-linked thrombocytopenia. *Blood* 2000;95:2262.

94. Weiss MJ, Orkin SH. GATA transcription factors: key regulators of hematopoiesis. *Exp Hematol* 1995;23:99.

95. Nichols KE, Crispino JD, Poncz M, et al. Familial dyserythropoietic anaemia and thrombocytopenia due to an inherited mutation in *GATA1*. *Nat Genet* 2000;24:266.

96. Freson K, Matthijs G, Thys C, et al. Different substitutions at residue D218 of the X-linked transcription factor GATA1 lead to altered clinical severity of macrothrombocytopenia and anemia and are associated with variable skewed X inactivation. *Hum Mol Genet* 2002;11:147.

97. Mehaffey MG, Newton AL, Gandhi MJ, et al. X-linked thrombocytopenia caused by a novel mutation of GATA-1. *Blood* 2001;98:2681.

98. Yu C, Niakan KK, Matsushita M, et al. X-linked thrombocytopenia with thalassemia from a mutation in the amino finger of GATA-1 affecting DNA binding rather than FOG-1 interaction. *Blood* 2002;100:2040.

99. Balduini CL, Pecci A, Loffredo G, et al. Effects of the R216Q mutation of GATA-1 on erythropoiesis and megakaryocytopoiesis. *Thromb Haemost* 2004;91:129.

100. Vyas P, Ault K, Jackson CW, et al. Consequences of GATA-1 deficiency in megakaryocytes and platelets. *Blood* 1999;93:2867.

101. Fujiwara Y, Browne CP, Cunniff K, et al. Arrested development of embryonic red cell precursors in mouse embryos lacking transcription factor GATA-1. *Proc Natl Acad Sci U S A* 1996;93:12355.

102. Shimiza R, Ohneda K, Engel JD, et al. Transgenic rescue of GATA-1-deficient mice with GATA-1 lacking a FOG-1 association site phenocopies patients with X-linked thrombocytopenia. *Blood* 2004;103:2560.

103. Kacena MA, Shivdasani RA, Wilson K, et al. Megakaryocyte-osteoblast interaction revealed in mice deficient in transcription factors GATA-1 and NF-E2. *J Bone Miner Res* 2004;19:652.

104. Hedberg VA, Lipton JM. Thrombocytopenia with absent radii. A review of 100 cases. *Am J Pediatr Hematol Oncol* 1988;10:50.

105. Ballmaier M, Schulze H, Cremer M, et al. Defective c-Mpl signaling in the syndrome of thrombocytopenia with absent radii. *Stem Cells* 1998;16:177.

106. Letestu R, Vitrat N, Massé A, et al. Existence of a differential blockage at the stage of amegakaryocyte precursor in the thrombocytopenia and absent radii (TAR) syndrome. *Blood* 2000;95:1633.

107. Fleischman RA, Letestu R, Mi X, et al. Absence of mutations in the *HoxA10*, *HoxA11* and *HoxD11* coding sequences in thrombocytopenia with absent radius syndrome. *Br J Haematol* 2002;116:367.

108. Decompte C-E, Burck C, Grützmacher T, et al. Increase in platelet count in response to rHuEpo in a patient with thrombocytopenia and absent radii syndrome. *Blood* 2001;97:2189.

109. Becker SP, Clavell AL, Beardsley DS. Giant platelets with abnormal surface glycoproteins: a new familial disorder associated with mitral valve insufficiency. *J Pediatr Hematol Oncol* 1998;20:69.

110. Gilman AL, Sloand E, White JG, et al. A novel hereditary thrombocytopenia. *J Pediatr Hematol Oncol* 1995;17:296.

111. Willig TN, Breton-Gorius J, Elbim C, et al. Macrothrombocytopenia with abnormal demarcation membranes in megakaryocytes and neutropenia with a complete lack of sialyl-Lewis-X antigen in leukocytes-a new syndrome. *Blood* 2001;97:826.

112. White JG. Giant electron-dense chains, clusters and granules in megakaryocytes and platelets with normal dense bodies: an inherited thrombocytopenic disorder. *Platelets* 2003;14:109.

113. George JN, Raskob GE, Shah SR, et al. Drug-induced thrombocytopenia: a systematic review of published case reports. *Ann Intern Med* 1998;129:886–890.

114. Warkentin TE. Heparin-induced thrombocytopenia: pathogenesis and management. *Br J Haematol* 2003;121:535.

115. Bougie DW, Wilker PR, Wuitschick ED, et al. Acute thrombocytopenia after treatment with tirofiban or eptifibatide is associated with antibodies specific for ligand-occupied GPIIb/IIIa. *Blood* 2002;100:2071.

116. Nurden P, Clofent-Sanchez G, Jais C, et al. Delayed immunologic thrombocytopenia induced by abciximab. *Thromb Haemost* 2004;92:820.

117. Rajentie J, Javela K, Joutsi-Korhonen L, et al. Chronic thrombocytopenia of childhood: use of nonivasive methods in clinical evaluation. *Eur J Haematol* 2004;72:268.

118. Scofield RH, Bruner GR, Kelly JA, et al. Thrombocytopenia identifies a severe familial phenotype of systemic lupus erythematosus and reveals genetic linkages at 1q22 and 11p13. *Blood* 2003;101:992.

119. Studt J-D, Hovinga JAK, Radonic R, et al. Familial acquired thrombotic thrombocytopenic purpura: ADAMTS13 inhibitory autoantibodies in identical twins. *Blood* 2004;103:4195.

120. Hoffman R, Briddell RA, van Besien K, et al. Acquired cyclic amegakaryocytic thrombocytopenia associated with an immunoglobulin blocking the action of granulocyte-macrophage colony-stimulating factor. *N Engl J Med* 1989;321:97.

121. Shiozaki H, Miyawaki S, Kuwaki T, et al. Autoantibodies neutralizing thrombopoietin in a patient with amegakaryocytic thrombocytopenic purpura. *Blood* 2000;95:2187.

122. Moll S, Lazarowski AR, White GC II. Giant platelet disorder in a patient with type 2B von Willebrand's disease. *Am J Hematol* 1998;57:62.

123. Nurden P, Chretien F, Poujol C, et al. Platelet ultrastructural abnormalities in three patients with type 2B von Willebrand disease. *Br J Haematol* 2000;110:704.

124. Di Pumpo M, Noris P, Pecci A, et al. Defective expression of GPIb/IX/V complex in platelets from patients with May-Hegglin anomaly and Sebastian syndrome. *Haematologica* 2002;87:943.

125. Nurden AT, Dupuis D, Pidard D, et al. Surface modifications in the platelets of a patient with a-N-acetyl-D-galactosamine residues, the Tn-syndrome. *J Clin Invest* 1982;70:1281.

126. Matzdorff AC, White JG, Malzahn K, et al. Perioperative management of a patient with Fechtner syndrome. *Ann Hematol* 2001;80:436.

127. Kjalke M, Johannessen M, Hedner U. Effect of recombinant factor VIIa (Novoseven) on thrombocytopenia-like conditions *in vitro*. *Semin Hematol* 2001;38:15.

128. Balduini CL. Role of splenectomy in inherited thrombocytopenias. *Blood* 2004;104:1227.

# CHAPTER 66 ■ INHERITED ABNORMALITIES OF THE PLATELET MEMBRANE: GLANZMANN THROMBASTHENIA, BERNARD-SOULIER SYNDROME, AND OTHER DISORDERS

ALAN T. NURDEN AND JAMES N. GEORGE

Glanzmann thrombasthenia (GT) and the Bernard-Soulier syndrome (BSS) are the best characterized inherited disorders of platelet membrane glycoproteins (GPs) (1-4). GT is a disease of the GP IIb/IIIa complex ($\alpha$IIb$\beta$3 integrin), resulting in absent platelet aggregation and, in most cases, defective clot retraction. BSS is caused by abnormalities of the GP Ib/IX/V complex, resulting in a much decreased platelet adherence to vessel wall subendothelium and a decreased platelet sensitivity to thrombin. Also highly significant are inherited defects of primary receptors such as $P2Y_{12}$ and TP$\alpha$, whose dysfunction leads to deficient platelet function with adenosine 5'-diphosphate (ADP) and thromboxane A2 ($TxA_2$), respectively (5). Clinical observations in these syndromes show that mucocutaneous bleeding is symptomatic. Historically, molecular studies on these diseases have been important because these studies have identified the function of platelet membrane GPs. In doing so, the studies have led not only to an improved understanding of the molecular pathways of primary hemostasis but also to the development of new strategies for antithrombotic therapy. This chapter describes the spectrum of clinical bleeding manifestations, the current diagnostic criteria, and the molecular and functional defects behind this highly significant group of rare inherited diseases (see Fig. 66-1). Other inherited disorders of platelets including those affecting platelet production (see Chapter 65), their ultrastructure (see Chapter 26), signaling pathways, and platelet secretion (see Chapter 64) are dealt with in other chapters of this book.

## GLANZMANN THROMBASTHENIA

This disease was described by Glanzmann in 1918 as "hereditary hemorrhagic thrombasthenia" (6). Although the patients in his report were heterogeneous, some certainly had what we now define as GT. As reviewed by the authors in previous editions of this book, a prolonged bleeding time, an isolated rather than clumped appearance of platelets on peripheral blood smears, platelets of normal morphology and number that failed to spread onto a surface or aggregate, and a lack of clot retraction were progressively described (7). The absence of platelet aggregation in thrombasthenia was confirmed in the classic report of the clinical and laboratory abnormalities of 15 patients by Caen et al. (8), who, for the first time, clearly established the diagnostic features of this disorder. Autosomal recessive inheritance was suggested by an equal incidence in both sexes, no excessive bleeding in the parents, and frequent consanguinity. Early reports also emphasized the clinical variability of GT: Some patients had only minimal bruising, whereas others had frequent, severe, and potentially fatal hemorrhages.

## Platelet Function Abnormality

### Platelet Aggregation

Absence of platelet aggregation in response to all physiologic agonists remains the hallmark of GT (8). GP Ib–dependent binding of von Willebrand factor (VWF) to thrombasthenic platelets is normal (9). Platelet agglutination induced by ristocetin and VWF is also initially normal, although it may be reversible and may occur in cycles (10). GT distinguishes an initial VWF binding to GP Ib from the subsequent responses mediated by GP IIb/IIIa.

### Platelet Adhesion, Secretion, and Procoagulant Activity

Thrombasthenic platelets bind to collagen and the initial attachment to exposed subendothelial tissue is also normal. However, platelet spreading on the vessel wall surface is defective, showing an early role for GP IIb/IIIa in the platelet–vessel wall interaction (11,12). Recently, the dynamics of GP IIb/IIIa–mediated thrombus formation on collagen were addressed by high-resolution time-lapsed video microscopy, although under static conditions (13). Results for normal donors showed the initial adhesion and spreading of "vanguard" platelets. The recruitment of "follower" platelets to and around the monolayer then led to thrombus formation. In GP IIb/IIIa deficiency, partially spread platelets were present as isolated forms in large numbers on the collagen, but "follower" platelet interactions were not seen. Notwithstanding, other authors have shown that in the presence of some residual (and presumably functional) GP IIb/IIIa, platelets can form small thrombi through a fibrin-dependent pathway (14). With strong agonists at high doses, dense granule and $\alpha$-granule secretion are normal. At low agonist concentrations, decreased granule secretion and thromboxane formation may result. A decreased phosphorylation of several proteins was observed when GT platelets were stimulated by thrombin (15). These phosphorylations are dependent on fibrinogen-binding and/or on aggregation in normal platelets and result from the participation of GP IIb/IIIa in "outside-in" signaling across the membrane.

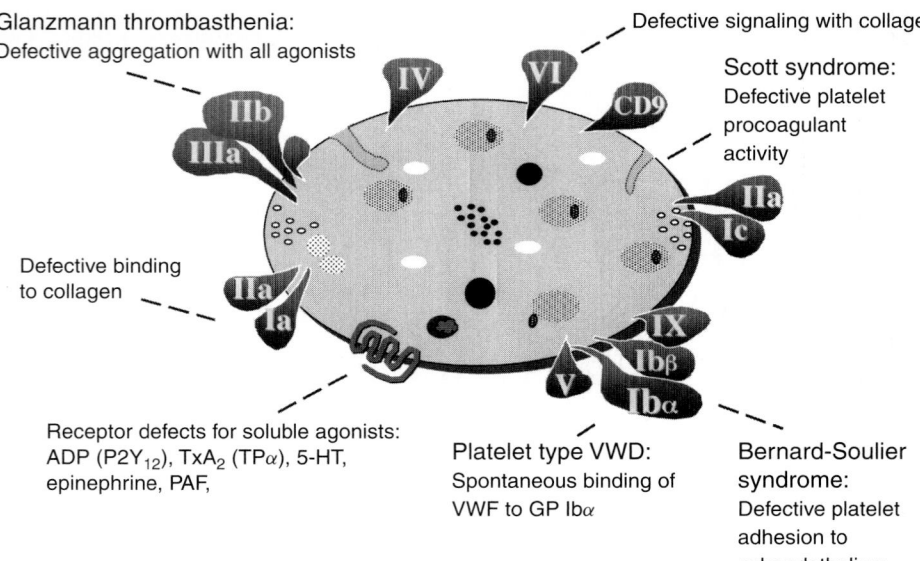

**FIGURE 66-1.** Cartoon identifying major membrane glycoproteins of human platelets and listing the principal inherited defects in the glycoproteins that lead to an altered platelet function and a hemorrhagic bleeding syndrome. ADP, adenosine 5'-diphosphate; TxA2, thromboxane A2; PAF, platelet activating factor; VWF, von Willebrand factor; GP, glycoprotein.

Platelet procoagulant activity was said to be deficient in early studies on GT, designated as platelet factor 3 [see (7)]. However, prothrombinase activity was normal in four patients, both for unstimulated platelets and for platelets stimulated with thrombin or with thrombin and collagen (16). Furthermore, fibrin formation was actually enhanced when thrombasthenic platelets adhered to subendothelium under flow (17). Published variations in prothrombinase activity of activated thrombasthenic platelets were linked to their ability to sustain increased cytoplasmic $Ca^{2+}$ levels under different experimental conditions, with shear being a key factor (18). Significantly, a defective ability of stimulated thrombasthenic platelets to produce procoagulant microvesicles was reported and could contribute to the hemostatic defect (19).

### Platelet Fibrinogen and α-Granule Proteins

Although early reports suggested fibrinogen synthesis by megakaryocytes (MK), subsequent data have demonstrated that MK contain little or no messenger RNA (mRNA) for this protein (20). Platelet fibrinogen is acquired by receptor-mediated endocytosis through GP IIb/IIIa and is stored in the α-granules (21). Platelets from many patients with GT lack fibrinogen, in spite of the usual plasma fibrinogen levels. For aggregation, platelet binding of exogenous fibrinogen requires the induction of fibrinogen receptor activity on GP IIb/IIIa by agonists such as ADP, epinephrine, and thrombin (see Chapter 30). There may be no activation requirement for uptake. Patient heterogeneity in GT (see Table 66-1) extends to both platelet GP IIb/IIIa and fibrinogen content. Therefore, in the subgroup with type I GT, patients have platelets that are totally unable to transport fibrinogen to the α-granules (1,2). Patients with type II thrombasthenia with platelets that express 5% to 15% of GP IIb/IIIa tend to have α-granule fibrinogen in readily detectable amounts, suggesting integrin recycling and active transport. Some variants have normal platelet fibrinogen, whereas in others it is completely lacking. Other α-granule proteins such as platelet factor 4, β-thromboglobulin, VWF, and thrombospondin are normally present in GT.

### Clot Retraction

This defect first appeared to correlate with the absence of α-granule fibrinogen. However, the cause is now known to be an insufficiency or nonfunctioning of GP IIb/IIIa in the platelets.

Patients with type II disease with residual GP IIb/IIIa can demonstrate partial clot retraction despite the lack of aggregation (2). This apparent paradox may be linked to the ability of fibrin fibers to cross-link a low density of GP IIb/IIIa receptors that serve as bridges linking the clot to the intracellular cytoskeleton.

## Platelet Membrane Glycoprotein Deficiencies

Nurden and Caen first demonstrated that platelets from patients with GT lacked specific membrane GPs (22,23). The deficiency was confirmed by Phillips and Poh Agin (24), and the affected GPs were identified as GP IIb and GP IIIa. Platelets are produced from MK, and because GT is an inherited disease, the GP deficiencies extend to these bone marrow cells. Early studies mostly used surface GP radiolabeling and gel electrophoresis to show the platelet deficiency of

**TABLE 66-1**

**CLASSIFICATION IN GLANZMANN THROMBASTHENIA**

| | |
|---|---|
| Type I disease: | Patients with no platelet aggregation, no α-granule storage pool of Fg, no clot retraction, and platelet GP IIb/IIIa levels <5% |
| Type II disease: | Patients with no platelet aggregation, readily detectable but often subnormal α-granule pools of Fg, residual clot retraction, and GP IIb/IIIa levels in the 5%–15% range |
| Variant disease: | Patients with no or very abnormal aggregation but, in most cases, with GP IIb or GP IIIa gene defects allowing GP IIb/IIIa expression but preventing ligand binding; Fg storage and clot retraction are variously affected |

Fg, fibrinogen; GP, glycoprotein.
From George JN, Caen J-P, Nurden AT. Glanzmann's thrombasthenia: the spectrum of clinical disease. *Blood* 1990;75:1383, with permission.

GP IIb and GP IIIa [reviewed in (1)]. A major advance occurred when the affected GPs were shown to be present as a heterodimeric complex, an observation initially shown by crossed immunoelectrophoresis. GT is now rapidly diagnosed using monoclonal antibodies (MoAbs) to GP IIb, GP IIIa, and the intact GP IIb/IIIa complex in flow cytometry (25). For normal donors, 40,000 to 100,000 copies of GP IIb/IIIa are accessible on circulating platelets. In GT, detecting and comparing the migration of residual GP IIb and/or GP IIIa in platelets using Western blotting (26) can help identify the affected gene (see subsequent text).

## Gene Expression and Transgenic Models

A key event was the recognition that GP IIb/IIIa is a member of the integrin family of cell surface receptors (see Chapter 30). Expression of the GP IIb gene (and therefore of GP IIb/IIIa complexes) is restricted to cells of the MK lineage in humans. GP IIIa is more widespread in distribution because it is also a component of the vitronectin receptor (VnR; $\alpha_V\beta_3$). VnR is present in many cell types, including endothelial cells (EC), osteoblasts, monocytes, and activated B lymphocytes. VnR is present in MK but decreases in abundance during maturation. In the normal platelet, VnR is a rare component, approximately 50 copies being found at the surface, although this number can double in patients with GT with GP IIb gene defects (27). VnR is concentrated in vesicular structures of unknown origin in platelets, whereas GP IIb/IIIa is densely distributed on the surface membrane as well as abundantly present in membranes of the surface-connected canalicular system and in membranes of storage organelles (28,29).

Transgenic mice lacking GP IIb or GP IIIa have confirmed the relation between the genotype and phenotype in GT because deletion of either gene results in a lack of platelet aggregation with all physiologic agonists and a bleeding syndrome (30,31). GP IIIa gene deletion and absent VnR function in mice is also associated with placental defects and reduced survival, the development of osteosclerosis with age, and enhanced tumor growth with increased vascularization (32,33). It is possible that in GT, particularly for women, $\beta3$ gene defects can give rise to added complications (discussed subsequently).

## Relation Between Thrombasthenia and the Functioning of GP IIb/IIIa

Following platelet activation, GP IIb/IIIa complexes acquire a high-affinity state for adhesive protein ligands including fibrinogen and VWF. Although fibrinogen is the predominant ligand in plasma, VWF binds under high shear, and animal models also support the participation of fibronectin and even CD40L in platelet aggregation (34,35). The importance of the quaternary structure of GP IIb/IIIa for its ligand-binding activity has been emphasized from computer models of the extracellular domains of VnR and GP IIb/IIIa, partially on the basis of the results of crystallography (36–38). The N-terminal region of the $\alpha$ subunits is composed of seven repeats of about 60 amino acids (AA) each and contain FG (phenylalanyl-glycyl) and GAP (glycyl-alanyl-prolyl) consensus sequences. Putative-$Ca^{2+}$– and ligand-binding sites have been assigned within these sequences, which form a $\beta$-propeller conformation. Ligands are predicted to bind to the upper face of the propeller, which is in intimate contact with a $\beta$ I-like domain of GP IIIa. $Ca^{2+}$ bind essentially to the lower face of the propeller. In classic GT, many mutations interfere with the processing and expression of the integrin. In variant GT (Table 66-1), rare patients retain the potential to process GP IIb/IIIa with varying degrees of efficacy. Here, mutations affect the structure of the integrin and interfere with its function.

Normal platelet aggregation and the absence of bleeding characterize obligate heterozygotes for type I and type II GT,

with approximately 50% of normal GP IIb/IIIa (1,2). One exception often observed is a decreased platelet aggregation to collagen in obligate carriers (39). In 1990, the analysis of the experience at the Hôpital Lariboisière in Paris (2) showed that 50 of 64 patients had type I disease, nine patients had type II, and five patients were classified as variant GT. Ion influx into normal platelets appears to occur through a channel associated with and regulating GP IIb/IIIa (40). Because GP IIb/IIIa binding of adhesive protein ligands leads to "outside-in" signaling, an altered ion exchange in thrombasthenia could contribute to platelet function deficiencies.

## The Genetic Defect

GT is an autosomal recessive disease. Consanguinity in affected families is frequent, and this in turn is reflected by an increased incidence in populations where marriage among close relatives is an accepted custom. Therefore, in our review of 177 patients in 1990 (2), 55 were from Israel and Jordan and 42 were from South India. In certain ethnic groups, such as South Indian Hindus, Iraqi Jews, French "Manouche" gypsies, and Jordanian nomads, thrombasthenia may actually be a common hereditary hemorrhagic disorder. The frequency of reported consanguinity among 84 patients from the literature surveyed in 1990 was 67%.

A database available on the Internet lists the mutations giving rise to GT (http://sinaicentral.mssm.edu/intranet/research/glanzmann). Many of these patients were reviewed by French (41), but only selected and newly reported defects will be discussed here. It should be noted that GP IIb is synthesized in MK as a single-chain precursor, termed pro-GP IIb, which forms a complex with GP IIIa in the ER (42). The pro-GP IIb/IIIa complex is transported to the Golgi apparatus where both subunits undergo glycosylation changes and pro-GP IIb is cleaved into heavy and light chains that remain linked by a disulfide. Pro-GP IIb alone is unstable and rapidly degraded. Noncomplexed GP IIb or GP IIIa is not processed in GT. The detection of residual GP IIIa (and not GP IIb) in platelets using Western blotting almost always is because of the presence of VnR. The defect in type II GT may imply residual but slow processing of GP IIb/IIIa in the ER and/or Golgi. The classification of types I and II has been a convenient way to group together patients with thrombasthenia, but they do not represent distinct categories of disease.

### Abnormalities in the GP IIb Gene

The GP IIb gene is composed of 30 exons, and its organization is shown in Figure 66-2, as is the location of a large series of missense mutations, insertions, inversions, and other defects giving rise to GT. Large deletions are rare, despite the fact that a 4.5-kb deletion resulting in alternative splicing of exon 1 and premature termination within intron 1 was one of the first reported abnormalities (43). Splice defects within the gene are fairly common. In a classic study, three Israeli Arab kindreds were shown to possess a 13-bp deletion encompassing the splice acceptor site of exon 4, which resulted in alternative splicing to a downstream nucleotide AG receptor, producing a six-AA deletion in the GP IIb protein (44). VnR was present in twice normal amounts (27). A 6-bp deletion and 31-bp insertion in exon 25 in an Iranian–Jewish family created an alternative splice site and an inframe deletion of 10 AA (45). Here, addition of eight new AA close to the proteolytic cleavage site in GP IIb affected complex formation and normal maturation of pro-GP IIb. A common type I haplotype within a gypsy population in France resulted from a G → A substitution at the splice donor site of intron 15 (46). A reading-frame shift and a premature stop codon led to the synthesis of a severely truncated GP IIb. Worthy of special mention is a novel homozygous splice junction mutation

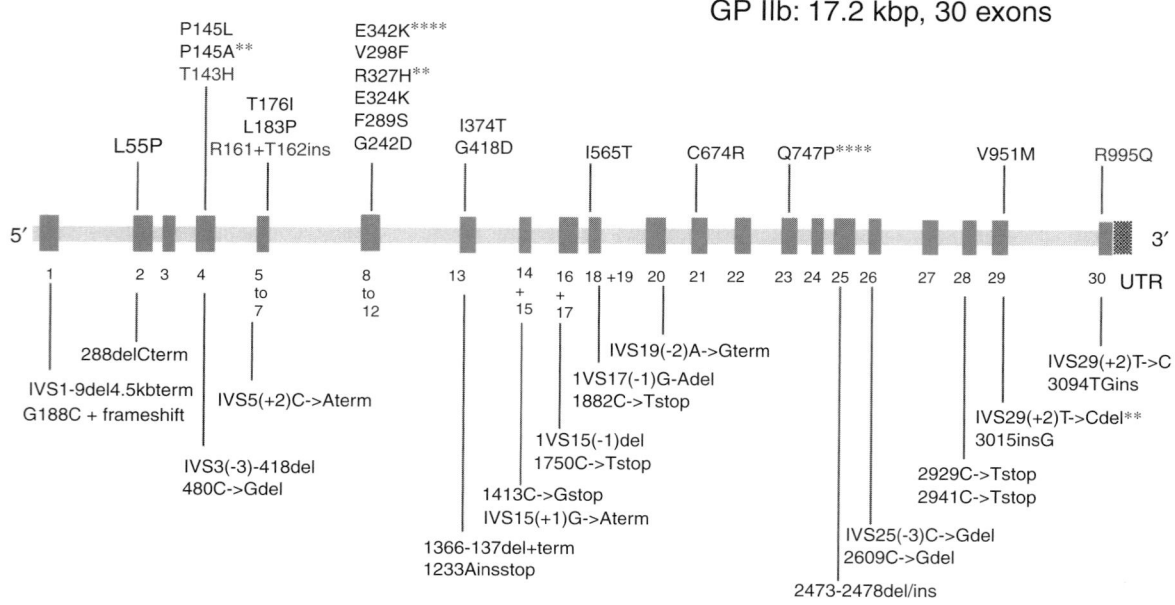

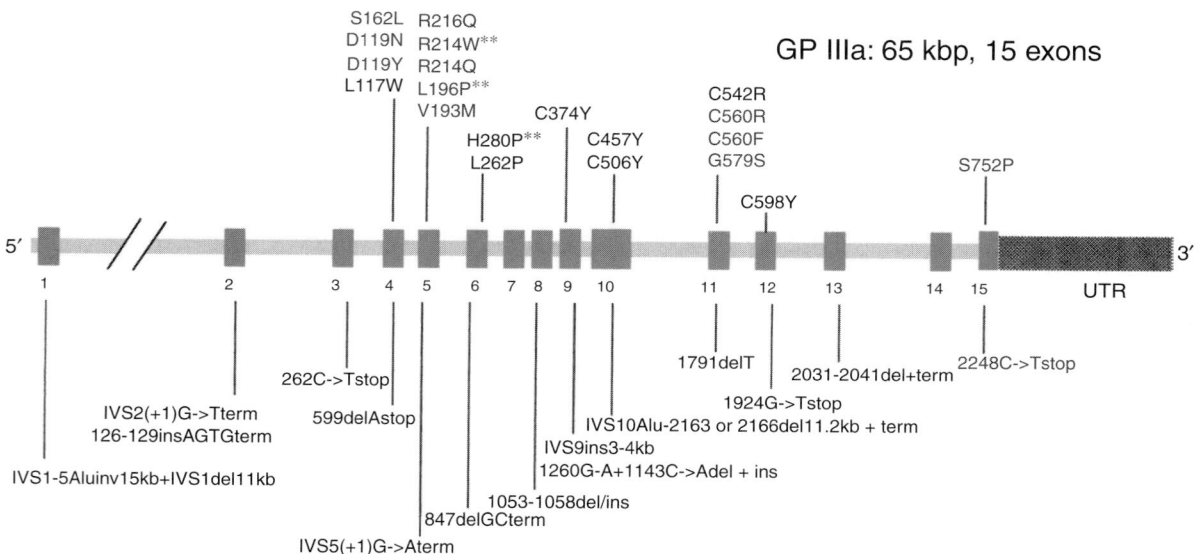

**FIGURE 66-2.** Schematic representation of the structure of the GP IIb and GP IIIa genes together with a representative spectrum of the types of genetic abnormalities that give rise to GT. The defects responsible for variant forms of the disease are represented by *brown* symbols; those that prevent GP IIb/IIIa complex expression are in *green*. *Asterisks* indicate the number of times that the same genetic defect has been described in apparently unrelated families. Mutations in *blue* refer to variant forms; those in *green* are characteristic of different ethnic groups. Note that abnormalities are distributed about equally in both genes and that no part of the gene appears to be exempt. In contrast, variant forms are more likely to have GP IIIa gene defects (see also Table 66-2). Only some of the illustrated mutations are discussed in the text (see Color Fig. 66-2). UTR, untranslated region; ins, insertion; inv, inversion; del, deletion; term, termination; stop, stop codon.

in GP IIb (G188A[1]) associated with alternative splicing, nonsense-mediated decay of GP IIb-mRNA, and type II GT (47). Inframe nonsense mutations giving rise to truncated GP IIb are common (Fig. 66-2). For example, a stop codon in exon

17 within codon 553 of the GP IIb gene of a Chinese patient resulted in a shortened protein seemingly unable to complex with GP IIIa (48). This mutation was subsequently reported in several unrelated families in the Far East.

Missense mutations within the N-terminal β-propeller domain of GP IIb are a frequent source of type I GT (49–52). Site-directed mutation of recombinant GP IIb/IIIa expressed in heterologous cell lines shows that these mutations do not prevent assembly of GP IIb/IIIa complexes but inhibit transport of the mutated complexes from the ER to the Golgi apparatus

---

[1]The mutation nomenclature used here for GP IIb and GP IIIa gene nucleotide sequences is without the leader sequences; in isolated cases this notation differs from that which the authors used in their original publications where leader sequences have been included.

and/or export to the cell surface [data reviewed in (53)]. In one patient, sufficient mutated GP IIb/IIIa was processed to produce a type II phenotype (51). A Glu324 → Lys mutation identified a mutation hot spot (54–56), that has now been found in unrelated patients over three continents. Milet-Marsal et al., in Bordeaux, substituted Glu324 with a series of AAs and examined the effect on the maturation and surface expression of recombinant GP IIb/IIIa in transiently transfected Cos-7 cells (55). Glu324 occupies a highly conserved *N*-terminal position in the third β strand of blade 5 of the GP IIb β propeller. Maturation efficiency depends on the electric charge as well as on the size of the side chain of the AA present. Therefore, the GT phenotype may depend not only on the AA substituted but also on its replacement. Mitchell et al. (57) showed how Val298 → Phe and Ile374 → Thr substitutions slowed down pro-GP IIb maturation and interfered with calcium binding. The structural integrity of the β-propeller domain of GP IIb is therefore essential for heterodimer stability.

Compound heterozygosity resulting from two defects within the GP IIb gene is a common cause of type I disease in the absence of consanguinity. For the case reported by Kato et al. (58), a C → T mutation in exon 17 of one allele resulted in trace amounts of mRNA; the second defect, a splicing mutation at the acceptor site of exon 26 (CAG → GAG), resulted in exon skipping, a single-chain polypeptide with a 42-AA deletion, and the absence of proteolytic cleavage into the heavy and light chains. In the example reported by Gonzalez-Manchon et al. (59), a splice-junction defect on one allele led to unstable mutant-mRNA, and this was associated with a Cys674 → Arg substitution that disrupted the 674–687 disulfide bridge of GP IIb. The net result was a type II phenotype. Recently, triple heterozygosity was reported in GP IIb in a young Canadian girl with type I disease (60). A maternally inherited G → A transition at a splice-site of exon 19 was associated with two paternal G → A transitions in exon 29; these led to Val951 → Met and Arg958 → Thr AA substitutions that cosegregated across three generations. Transient expression experiments showed that Val951 → Met alone gave a much reduced surface expression of GP IIb/IIIa and a block in the maturation of pro-GP IIb; this showed the importance of the membrane proximal calf-2 domain of GP IIb in integrin processing. Major mutations in calf-1 and calf-2 domains of GP IIb have also been shown by Rosenberg et al. to impair transport of GP IIb/IIIa from the ER to the Golgi apparatus (61).

### Abnormalities in the GP IIIa Gene

The organization of the GP IIIa gene is shown in Figure 66-2, as is a representative selection of the defects within this gene that give rise to GT. A GP IIIa abnormality was first described in six Iraqi Jews with type I disease; in each of these patients, an 11-base deletion within what was termed exon 12 (it is now exon 13) of the GP IIIa gene resulted in a DNA nucleotide frameshift leading to protein termination shortly before the transmembrane domain of GP IIIa (44). This defect prevented membrane insertion of the GP IIb/IIIa complex and also VnR expression in platelets and other cells. Splice-site mutations, DNA deletions and inversions, and nonsense mutations resulting in premature terminations are all found in the GP IIIa gene. Defects that affect GP IIIa transcript levels have been reported, such as the type I patient where mRNA for GP IIIa was undetectable because of a 3- to 4-kb deletion in intron 9 (62). In another patient, a compound heterozygote, one allele possessed a highly unusual 15-kb inversion immediately preceding a 1-kb deletion. This inversion resulted from homologous recombination among three intragene Alu sequences (63). A 6-bp deletion in exon 7 of a patient with type I disease led to the identification of Ile351Pro352Gly353 as a GP IIIa domain important for αβ subunit interaction (64).

Splice mutations working in cooperation resulted in a deletion of exon 9 and a 5-bp insertion that restored the reading-frame and led to a truncated GP IIIa unable to pair with GP IIb (65). Examination of DNA microsatellite dinucleotide polymorphisms suggested the presence of two identical or nearly identical copies of the maternal chromosome, suggesting disomy.

Preceding sections explained how missense mutations can affect GP IIb/IIIa biosynthesis and/or function. The key is the situation of the mutations in the three-dimensional structure of the integrin. Grimaldi et al. (66) showed how a Leu183 → Pro mutation in the W3 2-3 loop of GP IIb was associated with a surface expression of GP IIb/IIIa of about 12% of normal. An improved surface expression of about 60% of normal was seen in transfected Chinese hamster ovary (CHO) cells; nevertheless, the transfected cells failed to bind to fibrinogen. Closely situated in the integrin but within the MIDAS-like domain of GP IIIa is a Leu196 → Pro mutation located in two unrelated families (67,68). This mutation gave rise to a much lower expression of an abnormal integrin that failed to bind fibrinogen or PAC-1 when platelets were stimulated. A homozygous Leu117 → Trp mutation in the GP IIIa gene of a patient with type I disease led to a surface deficiency because of intracellular retention of malfolded GP IIb/IIIa complexes (69). Missense mutations in GP IIIa can have different impacts on the expression and function of GP IIb/IIIa compared to VnR; an example is a His280 → Pro GP IIIa mutation where platelets failed to express GP IIb/IIIa but contained 50% levels of VnR, a finding confirmed in expression studies (70). The hypothesis that disulfides maintain the conformation of GP IIIa is consistent with mutations affecting cysteines, causing abnormal GP IIIa structure and affecting its capacity to complex with GP IIb. A large deletion flanked by intron 10 and exon 14 created a frameshift and led to premature termination in the middle of the EGF-repeats and a type I phenotype affecting GP IIb/IIIa and VnR (71). Studies in Bordeaux revealed a type I phenotype with a homozygous Cys542 → Arg GP IIIa missense mutation (72). GP IIb/IIIa and VnR levels were affected. Site-directed mutagenesis and metabolic labeling confirmed that a novel Cys457 → Tyr mutation detected in another patient and the Cys542 → Arg mutation mentioned earlier, present in the GP IIIa EGF-1 and EGF-3 domains, respectively, strongly affected maturation of the pro-GP IIb/IIIa complex in the cell (73).

### Variant Thrombasthenia

Patients with variant GT are highly heterogeneous both in their molecular and clinical manifestations: Platelet fibrinogen levels and clot retraction range from absent to normal; bleeding symptoms range from severe to none (see Table 66-2). The first report described a family from Guam (designated Cam, case 1 in Table 66-2) [see (2)]. Three family members had normal levels of platelet GP IIb/IIIa but both platelet aggregation and clot retraction were absent. Their platelets were unable to bind fibrinogen, VWF, or fibronectin when stimulated. Stimulated Cam platelets also fail to bind either PAC-1 or anti–ligand-induced binding sites (LIBS) antibodies in the presence of fibrinogen (74,75). The IgM MoAb, PAC-1, identifies the activated conformation of GP IIb/IIIa and recognizes the fibrinogen-binding domain, whereas anti-LIBS antibodies bind to epitopes that are only accessible on GP IIb/IIIa after fibrinogen (or, in some cases, fibrinogen-derived peptides) has bound. An Asp119 → Tyr substitution within GP IIIa accounted for the phenotype and crucially permitted the identification of a site critical for the binding of the adhesive tripeptide, RGD, of fibrinogen, fibronectin, and VWF, to the integrin (74). This mutation falls within the "MIDAS-like" (see preceding text) or I-domain on GP IIIa (see Fig. 66-3).

Three patients from unrelated families (cases 2 to 4, Table 66-2), in whom the platelet GP IIb/IIIa content approaches normal, have GP IIb and GP IIIa subunits with facilitated dissociation in

**TABLE 66-2**

## MOLECULAR ABNORMALITIES AND PLATELET CHARACTERISTICS IN SELECTED PATIENTS WITH VARIANT GLANZMANN THROMBASTHENIA

| Case | Plt agg | CR | GP IIb/IIIa content | GP IIb/IIIa structure | Fg or PAC-1 binding | Platelet Fg | Mutation GP IIb | Mutation GP IIIa | Bleeding tendency | Reference |
|---|---|---|---|---|---|---|---|---|---|---|
| 1. | 0 | 0 | N | Abn | 0 | 0 | | Asp119 → Tyr | Severe | 74,75 |
| 2. | 0 | 0 | N | Unstable[b] | 0 | 0 | | Arg214 → Trp | Moderate | 76,79 |
| 3. | 0 | Sub | N | Unstable[b] | 0 | 0 | | Arg214 → Gln | Moderate | 77 |
| 4. | 0 | 0 | N | Unstable[b] | 0 | 0 | | Arg214 → Trp | Severe | 78,80 |
| 5. | Abn | Sub | 50%/18%[a] | N | Yes | Yes | Arg995 → Gln | | Mild | 81,82 |
| 6. | 0 | Sub | 60%[a] | Abn | 0 | Yes | | Ser752 → Pro | Mild | 85–88 |
| 7. | 0 | NR | 50%[a] | Abn | 0 | NR | | Arg724 stop | Severe | 92 |
| 8. | Abn | Sub | 50%/20%[a] | Abn | Yes | Yes | | Cys560 → Arg | Mild | 94 |
| 9. | 0 | Sub | 40%[a] | Abn | No | NR | Tyr143 → His | | Moderate | 96 |
| 10. | 0 | Sub | N | Abn | No | NR | Arg-Thr ins (161-162) | | Severe | 97 |
| 11. | 0 | N | 30% | Abn | No | NR | | Ser162 → Leu | Moderate | 99 |

Data are presented for selected patients described as variant Glanzmann thrombasthenia (GT) with GP IIb/IIIa complexes in amounts normally expected to allow aggregation. Platelet aggregation (Plt agg) was absent in all patients except in cases 5 and 8, in which it was significantly decreased. CR (clot retraction) was assessed as absent (0), subnormal (Sub) or normal (N). Platelet GP IIb/IIIa content was estimated by standard gel electrophoresis procedures and/or flow cytometry. Percentage values refer to the estimated content relative to normal platelets. When two values are given, the first is the total platelet content and the second the surface pool. GP IIb/IIIa complex structure was studied by CIE, using radiolabeled MoAbs or by flow cytometry. Abn means mutation-induced changes in conformation. Exogenous fibrinogen (Fg) binding was measured with radioiodinated exogenous fibrinogen or by using FITC-fibrinogen in flow cytometry. PAC-1 binding was determined on activated platelets by flow cytometry. Platelet Fg refers to the α-granule storage pool. Mutations are given and described according to the nomenclature in ref (41). Bleeding tendency was estimated from the data presented in the original publications. NR, not reported.

[a]is when the GP IIb/IIIa is from a single expressed allele.
[b]"Unstable" refers to abnormal dissociation of the subunits in the presence of ethylenediaminetetraacetic acid (EDTA).

## 'Variant-type' GT

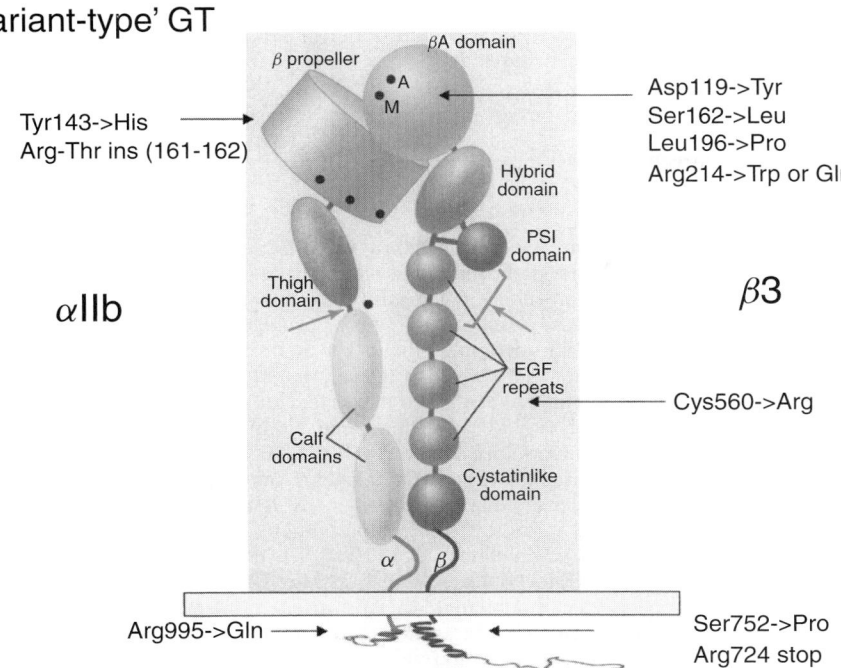

Tyr143->His
Arg-Thr ins (161-162)

Asp119->Tyr
Ser162->Leu
Leu196->Pro
Arg214->Trp or Gln

αIIb

β propeller

βA domain

A
M

Hybrid
domain

PSI
domain

Thigh
domain

EGF
repeats

Calf
domains

Cystatinlike
domain

α    β

β3

Cys560->Arg

Arg995->Gln

Ser752->Pro
Arg724 stop

**FIGURE 66-3.** Schematic representation of the GP IIb/IIIa complex (integrin αIIbβ3) showing the different structural domains of the integrin, as identified by computer modeling and crystallography of this and related integrins. Amino acid (AA) substitutions giving rise to variant GT are shown here. *Black dots* identify cation binding sites, *arrows* show regions of flexibility. M, metal ion–dependent adhesion site; A, an adjacent site; PSI, plexin-semaphorin-integrin domain; EFG, epidermal growth factor domains. [The structural model: from Humphries MJ, Mould AP. Structure. An anthropomorphic integrin. *Science* 2001;294:316, with permission; the figure was prepared with the help of Dr. David Wilcox (Medical College of Wisconsin, USA).]

the presence of calcium chelators (76–80). Studies on these patients have shown the codon for Arg214 of the GP IIIa gene to be a mutational hotspot. In two cases, Arg214 is substituted by a Trp, whereas, for the third patient, a Gln is in this position. The sequence containing Arg214 regulates the structure of the GP IIIa I-domain (Fig. 66-3) and thereby influences both the stability of the GP IIb/IIIa complex and its activation. Platelets from these patients do not bind fibrinogen when stimulated by ADP or other agonists and contain little or no platelet fibrinogen. They also do not bind PAC-1 or anti-LIBS antibodies when stimulated. Their platelets bind fibrinogen and aggregate after treatment with dithiothreitol, a disulfide-reducing agent that directly modifies integrin structure (see subsequent text) (80). Platelets from this type of variant possess GP IIb/IIIa complexes in an abnormal conformation, with the fibrinogen-binding domains failing to be expressed under physiologic stimulation.

Case 5 is unusual and has what should be termed a thrombasthenialike syndrome because clot retraction occurs, and aggregation is not absent but is delayed and is very much reduced in intensity (81). Total platelet GP IIb/IIIa is approximately 50% of normal, but the surface pool is decreased to approximately 18% of normal, yet binds fibrinogen when platelets are stimulated. Therefore, this patient has a surface pool at the threshold of that required to support normal platelet aggregation. The molecular explanation for this phenotype is complex. First, an unidentified defect in the GP IIb gene led to an unexpressed allele and an approximately 50% reduction in the total GP IIb/IIIa content of the patient's platelets. On the second allele, a Arg995 → Gln substitution in the GFFKR region of the cytoplasmic domain of GP IIb was identified (Fig. 66-3) (82). Interestingly, this domain is involved in regulating the activation state of the complex, although there is also evidence that the complex assembly might be impaired when the GFFKR region is mutated (83). In this patient, the mutated recombinant GP IIb formed complexes with a marginally greater capacity to bind PAC-1 (82). One intriguing possibility is that the conserved Arg995 → Gln substitution retains the salt bond between Asp723 of GP IIIa and Arg995 of GP IIb (84) but perturbs a recognition signal involved in integrin trafficking between membrane systems.

Case 6 is an Argentinian man whose platelets fail to bind fibrinogen when stimulated, despite a 50% GP IIb/IIIa content (85). The platelets do, however, support clot retraction and store fibrinogen in α-granules. During secretion, some fibrinogen is translocated to the exterior bound to intracellular GP IIb/IIIa, suggesting that integrin affinity is regulated differently between internal and external pools (86). The patient has an unexpressed allele for GP IIIa and a Ser752 → Pro mutation on the second allele, a substitution that also affects the cytoplasmic domain (Fig. 66-3). Transfection studies confirm that Pro752 interferes with GP IIb/IIIa–mediated cell spreading on immobilized fibrinogen or VWF (87,88). Yet, the purified complexes retain an ability to bind to immobilized RGD ligands, showing that RGD binding sites are still present. The presence of Pro752 has a marked effect on the conformation of the GP IIIa cytoplasmic domain, and "outside-in" and "inside-out" signaling are affected. Therefore, long-range signals are no longer transmitted and high-affinity extracellular ligand-binding sites are not induced. Talin binding to GP IIIa cytoplasmic tails is now known to be part of the activating process, leading to conformational rearrangements in the extracellular domains (89). Talin binding to the mutated β3 may be abnormal. Recently, β3Pro752 has been shown to prevent c-Src SH3 domain interaction with β3 and Src kinase activation following integrin clustering, thereby explaining the defective "outside-in" signaling (90). A normal clot retraction in this patient implies that fibrin interaction with his platelets involves sites other than the high-affinity recognition site for fibrinogen. Similarly, fibrin-dependent thrombus formation can occur for this patient (14). The Ser752 → Pro mutation also affects VnR, and studies on a mouse model show that it impairs osteoclast function (91). For case 7, a mutation in the maternal allele of the GP IIIa gene results in a stop codon at position 724 and in the biosynthesis of a truncated protein containing only the first eight of the 47 AAs normally present in the cytoplasmic domain (92). A second mutation in exon 10 is associated with an apparent lack of transcription of the paternal allele; therefore, as in cases 5 and 6, only the abnormal complex is present in the platelets. The truncated complex fails to bind fibrinogen when platelets are stimulated. CHO cells expressing the truncated integrin bind to immobilized fibrinogen, although downstream events such as cytoskeletal-mediated cell spreading and tyrosine phosphorylation of FAK fail to occur (92). A central role for the GP IIIa cytoplasmic domain in outside-in signaling is therefore confirmed.

Site-directed mutagenesis involving GP IIIa first showed that gain-of-function mutations might lead to constitutively activated integrins in pathology (93). In case 8, platelets spontaneously bind PAC-1 and fibrinogen (94). This patient has a homozygous Cys560 → Arg substitution in the EGF-repeats of GP IIIa (Fig. 66-3) and in the platelets that express about 20% of the normal level of surface GP IIb/IIIa. This situation recalls platelet-type von Willebrand disease (VWD) where VWF multimers spontaneously bind to a mutated GP Ibα subunit (see subsequent text). The question is why this patient presented with a bleeding rather than a thrombotic syndrome. One possible explanation is that plasma fibrinogen binds spontaneously to the surface-exposed GP IIb/IIIa so that unoccupied counterreceptors are no longer available to form platelet-to-platelet bridges. It is also interesting that the Cys560 → Arg substitution affects GP IIb/IIIa expression as well as upregulates its function. This is even more so for a patient with type II disease with a Cys598 → Tyr GP IIIa substitution, where activated integrin is only detected in transfected cells (95).

Case 9 is a newly reported Japanese variant (also known as Osaka-12), where a heterozygous Tyr143 → His substitution in the W3 4-1 loop of the β-propeller blade 4 domain of GP IIb is associated with 36% to 41% of normal platelet levels of GP IIb/IIIa (96). These platelets fail to bind soluble ligands or PAC-1 but retain the ability to mediate clot retraction and cell adhesion to fibrinogen. In contrast, both a two-AA Arg-Thr insertion between residues 160 and 161 in the same W3 4-1 loop of GP IIb (case 10) and an induced Asp163 → Ala mutation, although failing to affect GP IIb/IIIa expression, prevent binding of soluble ligands and adhesion interactions of transfected 293 cells (96,97). For case 11, a Ser162 → Leu substitution within GP IIIa results in an unstable GP IIb/IIIa complex that retains partial function (98). The platelets of this patient express 30% of the normal GP IIb/IIIa content and support clot retraction but do not aggregate. Transfection experiments show that the mutation induces a partial biosynthetic blockage in the maturation of the complex. Somewhat similar findings are reported for a Leu262 → Pro mutation giving a type II phenotype, where the mutated GP IIb/IIIa is able to bind fibrin but not fibrinogen (99). Patients such as these are at the interface between the type II and variant groups. Also to be taken into account are patients expressing nonfunctional GP IIb/IIIa and where mutations in the GP IIb and GP IIIa genes are not present (100). This leaves open the possibility that defects in other nonidentified genes can give rise to the GT phenotype.

### Association of Thrombasthenialike Disorders with Other Systemic Abnormalities

Patients in whom GT is associated with skeletal and other systemic abnormalities were reviewed by the authors previously (7). For example, cases have been described where platelet GP IIb/IIIa deficiency is associated with skeletal abnormalities and deafness or with Friedreich ataxia. Ruan et al. (72) have reported a homozygous GP IIIa defect and a type I phenotype in a young girl who is also symptomatic for tuberous sclerosis. Osteopetrosis, an autosomal recessive disease with defective bone resorption, and GT have been detected in a child in Turkey (101). It is unknown whether these are chance observations. An exciting recent development is the report of a novel form of integrin dysfunction involving β1, β2, and β3 integrins (102). The patient in question has a normal expression of the integrins, yet associates a GT-like syndrome with

leukocyte adhesion deficiency-1 and increased susceptibility to infection. A common defect linked to inside-out signaling is hypothesized.

## Clinical Manifestations

### Patient Sex and Age

Our review in 1990 of 177 patients with GT, for whom clinical data had been published, showed that 102 (58%) patients were women (2). The slightly greater proportion of female patients possibly reflects the serious problem with menorrhagia. The average age (at the time of the literature report) of the 113 patients for whom age was given was only 20 years. In fact, most patients are diagnosed in early childhood, many at birth or in early infancy. Because therapeutic inhibition of platelet GP IIb/IIIa function prevents thrombosis (103), it has been speculated that patients with thrombasthenia may be protected from atherosclerotic disease. However, GP IIIa deficiency actually promoted atherosclerosis and pulmonary inflammation in high-fat–fed, hyperlipidemic mice (104). When six Israeli patients with GT (45 to 66 years of age), lacking both GP IIb/IIIa and VnR, underwent bilateral carotid artery ultrasonography, five showed signs of early atherosclerosis (105). Therefore, while reports of myocardial infarction or stroke in patients with thrombasthenia are lacking, this may be influenced by the low average age of registered patients. Rare reports of venous thrombosis in GT include an episode of superficial thrombophlebitis in a young female patient with type I disease (2) and severe proximal deep vein thrombosis (DVT) in an adult male with variant-type disease (patient 6 in Table 66-2) (106). A patient with type I disease who developed recurrent proximal DVT was heterozygous for factor $V_{Leiden}$ (107), a finding that was not repeated for the other two patients mentioned in the preceding text (AT Nurden, unpublished finding).

### Hemorrhagic Symptoms

The types of bleeding in GT are clearly defined: Purpura, epistaxis, gingival hemorrhage, and menorrhagia are constant features; gastrointestinal bleeding and hematuria are less common; and hemarthroses and deep visceral hematomas occur rarely (see Table 66-3). Spontaneous petechiae are rare, and diffuse petechial hemorrhage has only been reported at birth (2,108). However, most newborn infants with GT show no signs of excessive bleeding (109). Epistaxis is a common cause of severe bleeding in thrombasthenia, and is typically more severe in childhood, perhaps an exaggeration of the often observed mild epistaxis among healthy children aged between 4 and 10 years. Severe epistaxis is unusual in adult patients, and bleeding in thrombasthenia most often decreases with age. Gingival bleeding, often reflecting poor dental hygiene, is rarely associated with major blood loss, but it is a common cause of iron deficiency. Menorrhagia can be a critical hemorrhagic problem. Bleeding at menarche represents a particular risk (110) and can require transfusions. This is consistent with the more prolonged bleeding that occurs with the first menstrual period in healthy adolescent women and is another physiologic explanation for the apparent greater risk of bleeding in younger patients.

Gastrointestinal hemorrhage and hematuria may occur in some patients. Intracranial hemorrhage is rare, but has been reported in two patients following trauma (2). Spontaneous deep visceral hematomas that are characteristic of disorders of coagulation have not been described. Therefore, unprovoked major bleeding may actually be uncommon in GT. In contrast, bleeding following trauma or surgical procedures can be severe. In one series, 10 of 12 infants undergoing circumcision

## TABLE 66-3

### BLEEDING IN PATIENTS WITH GLANZMANN THROMBASTHENIA

|  | Number of affected patients | Frequency (%) |
|---|---|---|
| **SYMPTOMS** | | |
| Menorrhagia | 54/55 | 98 |
| Easy bruising, purpura | 152/177 | 86 |
| Epistaxis | 129/177 | 73 |
| Gingival bleeding | 97/177 | 55 |
| Gastrointestinal hemorrhage | 22/177 | 12 |
| Hematuria | 10/177 | 6 |
| Hemarthrosis | 5/177 | 3 |
| Intracranial hemorrhage | 3/177 | 2 |
| Visceral hematoma | 1/177 | 1 |
| | | |
| **SEVERITY** | | |
| Requirement for red cell transfusions | 86/112 | 77 |

Data as published for 113 patients described in case reports in the literature, and in 64 patients studied in Paris (2). The frequency of each type of bleeding in the published reports was often noted only in concise comments or tables and may represent only the more prominent symptoms. The actual occurrence of purpura, epistaxis, and gingival bleeding may be nearly universal among these patients if careful observations are performed over a long time. It is not clear from the available data whether spontaneous hemarthroses, intracranial hemorrhages, or visceral hematomas occur. When these hemorrhages were fully described, a predisposing cause was apparent or suspected. Fifty-four of 64 patients from the Paris series required red cell transfusions; data on transfusions were available for only 48 of the 113 patients described in the literature, and these data may be incomplete.
From George JN, Caen J-P, Nurden AT. Glanzmann's thrombasthenia: the spectrum of clinical disease. *Blood* 1990;75:1383, with permission.

## TABLE 66-4

### PREGNANCY AND DELIVERY IN PATIENTS WITH GLANZMANN THROMBASTHENIA

| | |
|---|---|
| Patients | 16 |
| Pregnancies | 21 |
| Complications of pregnancy | 3 |
|   Vaginal hemorrhage | 1 |
|   Spontaneous abortion | 1 |
|   Cesarean delivery of dead fetus | 1 |
| Live births | 19 |
|   Cesarean section | 6 |
|     Hemorrhagic complications | 0 |
|   Vaginal delivery | 13 |
|     Postpartum hemorrhage | 6 |

Twelve patients are from the patients reported from the Paris study (2), four patients are from other reports [see (7)]. A patient in the Paris study, who had vaginal bleeding during her second trimester, is the only patient who required transfusion during pregnancy. Two other patients in the Paris study had pregnancy complications that were managed with platelet transfusions without excessive bleeding—a spontaneous abortion and the delivery of a dead fetus. Four cesarean deliveries were performed on three patients in the Paris study and on two other patients with both preoperative and postoperative platelet transfusions without excessive bleeding. Thirteen vaginal deliveries were performed on nine patients in the Paris study and on two other patients with platelet transfusions. Severe postpartum hemorrhage occurred in four patients in the Paris study, and in both deliveries in one patient from another study [see (7)].

without platelet transfusion had excessive bleeding (111). Tooth extractions without platelet transfusions are also commonly associated with excessive bleeding, which can be severe even with the spontaneous loss of deciduous teeth. Pregnancy may be a serious risk; but vaginal bleeding severe enough to require transfusions was reported only once in 21 reviewed pregnancies (see Table 66-4) (7). Nevertheless, our literature review in 1990 showed complications during delivery caused by severe hemorrhage in six of 19 occasions (2). Platelet transfusions are required before delivery and should be continued for at least a week because severe postpartum vaginal hemorrhage can also be delayed (2,111). None of the six patients who delivered by cesarean section, with platelet transfusions being continued until wound healing was complete, suffered from excessive bleeding.

### Clinical Severity

GT is certainly a severe hemorrhagic disease because most patients require blood transfusions (Table 66-3). Nevertheless, bleeding severity is unpredictable and occassional patients never have serious bleeding, and even more patients are healthy and free of bleeding complications once they reach adulthood. The unpredictability of severe hemorrhage is emphasized by the inconsistency between siblings, who presumably share the same genetic defect. One study examined whether polymorphisms normally associated with a thrombotic tendency such as factor $V_{Leiden}$ or a mutation in the 3'-UT region (20210G → A) of the prothrombin gene could provide a protective effect with increased survival or less bleeding in individual patients, but no evidence was obtained to support

this hypothesis (112). The observations that allele-dependent transcriptional regulation of the $\alpha2$ gene can markedly affect $\alpha_2\beta_1$ density on platelets (113), and that this in turn represents an increased risk factor for bleeding in VWD (114) indicate the regulation of bleeding tendency in congenital platelet disorders by the score of risk factors implicating multiple receptors on platelets and other vascular cells. Notwithstanding, an initial evaluation of the major polymorphisms affecting platelet membrane GPs in patients with GT failed to show changes in their distribution compared to a healthy population (115). Interestingly, in a result different from that published for the mouse model (32), upregulation of osteoclast $\alpha_2\beta_1$ integrin compensates for lack of VnR in these cells in Iraqi-Jewish patients with GT, suggesting that abnormalities of bone resorption, mediated by VnR, may not be seen in GT linked to GP IIIa gene defects (116).

### Isoantibody Formation

A frequent complication of transfusion therapy in GT is the development of an isoantibody against GP IIb/IIIa. The first such antibody to be characterized blocked platelet aggregation and reacted primarily with complex-dependent determinants on GP IIb/IIIa (1,117). Isoantibodies from other patients bound complex-dependent determinants on GP IIb/IIIa or specifically to GP IIIa (7,118). Interestingly, two antibodies recognized trace amounts of intracellular GP IIIa present in the patients' own platelets; therefore, in the strict sense of the term, they were autoantibodies (118). Another isoantibody (termed Ab1) recognized an epitope on GP IIb/IIIa involved in the binding of adhesive proteins (119). An antiidiotype antibody prepared against Ab1 recognized an isoantibody from an unrelated patient with GT but not the isoantibodies from two others, suggesting that such antibodies are heterogeneous. Jacobin et al. (120) studied the molecular nature of the humoral response to immunization in GT using combinatorial libraries of single-chain IgG fragments created from a patients' B cells.

Structural diversity in the variable-chain region confirmed that the patient had formed polyclonal antibodies by way of an antigen-driven immune response. These antibodies represent a major clinical problem because they cause the patients to become refractory to platelet transfusions, although the presence of such antibodies may not influence bleeding frequency *per se*. Because most patients will have received red cell or platelet transfusions, precautionary screening for these antibodies is highly recommended.

## Relation Between Genotype and Phenotype

The bleeding problems of patients with type II thrombasthenia demonstrate that more than 10% to 15% functional integrin is required for platelets to provide adequate primary hemostasis for severe challenges, such as obstetric delivery or after trauma. For obligate heterozygotes, a 50% content is normally sufficient. Nevertheless, it is still too early to say whether specific cohorts of patients with a defined bleeding risk can be identified or to even compare patients with GP IIb or GP IIIa gene defects. In type II GT, the phenotype may depend on whether the residual integrin is fully functional or not. Unfortunately, only a minority of patients have been genotyped so far. Setting up of national networks may accelerate this process and provide patient groups of sufficient size to evaluate if phenotype-genotype correlations exist. As a start, a recent report has described the genotyping of 30 patients in Italy (121).

## Current Diagnostic Criteria

The current diagnostic criteria for GT are as follows:

- an autosomal recessive trait, with no significant bleeding in heterozygous subjects
- bleeding symptoms that usually include purpura, epistaxis, gingival bleeding, and menorrhagia, without hemarthroses and deep visceral hematomas
- bleeding severity that ranges from mild bruising to severe, recurrent mucocutaneous bleeding beginning at birth
- normal platelet count and morphology
- long bleeding time or a grossly prolonged PFA-100 closure time
- absent or severely diminished platelet aggregation in response to ADP, collagen, thrombin, and epinephrine
- clot retraction, ranging from absent to subnormal in most patients
- normal but possibly reversible platelet agglutination by ristocetin and VWF.

The expected laboratory abnormalities are summarized in Table 66-5. These criteria can usually provide a firm diagnosis of GT with readily available clinical laboratory procedures and platelet function testing. Because thrombasthenia is a recessive trait, a family history of bleeding most likely only involves siblings, but consanguinity is a common feature, and this emphasizes a geographic bias in the occurrence of the disease (2). Flow cytometry (25) is the current method of choice for confirmation of the diagnosis; procedures exist both for quantitative assessment of the residual GP IIb/IIIa content of platelets and for testing the ability of variant GP IIb/IIIa to express activation-dependent epitopes (recognized by antibodies such as PAC-1 or FITC-fibrinogen) [previously illustrated by the authors in (7)]. Western blotting test will allow the detection of residual GP IIb and GP IIIa as well as reveal subunits with abnormal migration (26,73). As the authors have shown, the growing list of mutations reveals that the genetic origin of GT is highly variable (Fig. 66-2). Therefore, it is necessary to

### TABLE 66-5

**LABORATORY ASSESSMENT OF PLATELET FUNCTION IN PATIENTS WITH GLANZMANN THROMBASTHENIA AND BERNARD-SOULIER SYNDROME**

| Laboratory study | Glanzmann thrombasthenia | Bernard-Soulier syndrome |
|---|---|---|
| Platelet count | N | Low |
| Platelet size on blood smear | N | Large |
| Bleeding time | Abn | Abn |
| Platelet adhesion to subendothelium | N (but no spreading) | Abn |
| Platelet shape change to ADP | N | N |
| Platelet aggregation | | |
| ADP | Abs | N |
| Collagen | Abs | N |
| Epinephrine | Abs | N |
| Thrombin | Abs | Abn |
| Ristocetin–VWF | N[a] | Abs[a] |
| Platelet secretion by thrombin ($^{14}$C-5HT) | N[b] | N[b] |
| Clot retraction | Abn | N |

ADP, adenosine 5′-diphosphate; VWF, von Willebrand factor; N, normal; Abn, abnormal; Abs, absent.
Results are given for typical cases.
[a]Ristocetin-induced platelet agglutination may occur in cycles in thrombasthenia. In Bernard-Soulier syndrome, it is absent even in the presence of normal plasma.
[b]In thrombasthenia secretion may be reduced with low doses of agonists. In Bernard-Soulier syndrome, it is delayed with thrombin but not with other agonists.

determine the nature of the genetic lesion for each new case. The situation is complicated by the fact that new patients have a high chance of being compound heterozygotes, inheriting a distinct abnormal allele from each parent. Only in ethnic groups, where consanguinity is high, can procedures permitting the rapid screening of given mutations be used, as is the case of the Iraqi-Jewish and Arab groups in Israel and of a French gypsy population (see subsequent text). Here, rapid screening includes applying PCR-SSCP (single-strand conformation polymorphism) analysis of exons likely to carry preidentified mutations or performing allele-specific restriction enzyme analysis (ASRA) (41,122).

## Carrier Analysis and Prenatal Diagnosis

Initial studies attempted to diagnose carriers for GT by measuring the number of GP IIb/IIIa receptors on platelets or the GP IIb/IIIa content of platelet extracts. However, an occasional overlap between obligate heterozygotes and ostensibly healthy donors whose platelets had a low GP IIb/IIIa expression made interpretation of the results difficult. Prenatal diagnosis performed on platelets from cord blood has been attempted but is accompanied by a high risk of bleeding and of spontaneous abortion (123). Once the nature of the genetic lesion has been determined, carrier diagnosis can be determined with relative ease, particularly if sites are created (or lost) for restriction enzymes. Genetic counseling can be given with the following reservations: (i) when screening is followed for a single mutation, the presence of another Glanzmann defect would go undetected and (ii) individuals with the same genetic lesion may differ widely in the frequency and severity of bleeding (discussed in the preceding text). Peretz et al. (124) first used restriction digest analysis of polymerase chain reaction (PCR)–amplified fragments from DNA isolated from blood or urine to screen subjects for the Iraqi-Jewish and Arab mutations. These mutations could also be confirmed in prenatal diagnosis using DNA extracted from chorionic villi [see French (41)]. Ruan et al. (122) reported carrier detection within the French gypsy populations using ASRA methodology. Finally, prenatal diagnosis within GT has been achieved using the polymorphic markers BRCA1 and THRA1 on chromosome 17 (125).

## Differential Diagnosis

The differential diagnosis of GT includes disorders of platelet function associated with a normal platelet count and normal platelet morphology. Absent platelet aggregation in response to all physiologic stimuli is pathognomonic for thrombasthenia, and abnormal clot retraction is rarely observed in other disorders. Patients with dense granule deficiencies have abnormal secretion-dependent platelet aggregation, but their clot retraction is normal and the inheritance pattern is typically autosomal dominant (4,5). Similarly, patients belonging to the increasingly large family of disorders of platelet signaling mechanisms have platelets that respond well to different agonists (126). The bleeding time may be prolonged in congenital afibrinogenemia, but the results of coagulation tests are abnormal, and if the blood clots, the clot retracts (127). Here, platelet aggregation is also restored if exogenous fibrinogen is added. Because the bleeding symptoms of thrombasthenia are similar to those of VWD, and because VWD is much more common in most parts of the world, the latter disease is frequently the initial clinical impression. This is also the case if a prolonged closure time is seen in the PFA-100 system (128) or in assessing platelet adhesion to VWF under flow conditions, as in the so-called cone and plate(let) analyzer (129). However, VWD is easily ruled out by the abnormal platelet aggregation, while a platelet agglutination response to ristocetin and VWF is seen in GT.

### Acquired Thrombasthenia

A disorder identical to GT can be acquired, for example, through an autoantibody that inhibits the fibrinogen receptor function of platelet GP IIb/IIIa. Patients have been reported with autoantibodies to GP IIb/IIIa whose clinical manifestations resemble those described here for GT (130–132). One patient had multiple myeloma and a monoclonal paraprotein with antibody specificity for GP IIIa (130). Gastrointestinal bleeding was noted in at least two of these patients, although there is no firm evidence that the antibody was a primary cause. An antibody against GP IIb that blocked platelet aggregation was found in a patient with Evans syndrome; unusually, its production was increased after splenectomy (133). Acquired GT has been reported to be associated with lymphoproliferative disease, for example, in Hodgkin lymphoma where platelet-associated IgM antibody was the cause (134). A most unusual case was reported by Macchi et al. (135), in which an inhibitory autoantibody to GP IIb/IIIa was identified in a patient with thrombocytopenic whose platelets contained elevated amounts of GP Ib but a generalized decrease in the amounts of other GPs. Acquired GT is also observed during treatment of patients with anti–GP IIb/IIIa drugs such as abciximab, eptifibatide, and tirofiban, but this situation is beyond the scope of this review (see Chapter 120).

Platelet GP IIb/IIIa deficiency and abnormal platelet aggregation characteristic of GT have been reported in patients with acute promyelocytic leukemia (136). Here, the etiology of this acquired disorder is probably a chromosome 15–17 translocation, which is characteristic of this condition (137). Although the breakpoint region on chromosome 17 is heterogeneous in acute promyelocytic leukemia, in some patients it occurs at 17q21, the location of the genes for GP IIb and GP IIIa (138). Platelet GP IIb/IIIa deficiency can be severe in acute promyelocytic leukemia, although the chromosomal abnormality affects only one allele, probably because of selective expression of the leukemic clone of hematopoietic cells. Abnormal GP IIb has also been noted in a patient with a myelodysplastic syndrome, dysmegakaryocytopoiesis, and an abnormality of chromosome 3 (139).

## Management

Platelet transfusions before invasive procedures are indicated even in patients with minimal past hemorrhagic symptoms. Neither the clinical history nor biologic tests can adequately predict the bleeding risk; therefore, therapeutic management is largely supportive care and maintenance of sufficient hemostasis to arrest hemorrhage (or prevent it in case of surgery). The potential risk of platelet alloimmunization by human leukocyte antigen (HLA) antigens is as for any patient receiving transfusion; however, precautions need to be taken if isoantibodies against GP IIb/IIIa are present because they considerably worsen therapeutic management and prognosis (140). Plasma exchange and Protein A Sepharose immunoadsorption can restore the efficacy of platelet concentrates by temporally removing the antibody (141), but this is a cumbersome and specialized treatment that only a few centers can provide. Antifibrinolytic drugs, α-aminocaproic acid (EACA) and tranexamic acid, have been reported to be effective in controlling hemorrhage in patients with thrombocytopenia (7), but their efficacy in thrombasthenia remains anecdotal. Desmopressin (1-deamino-8-D-arginine vasopressin; DDAVP) has been tried in some patients with GT with variable success (142,143). DDAVP acts by inducing the release of VWF and tPA from endothelium, and plasma levels of FVIII increase too (143). The relevance of this mechanism of action on GT is unclear, although VWF–GP Ib interactions could be enhanced, as could platelet interaction with fibrin where VWF is also present. Infusion of recombinant FVIIa (NovoSeven, Novo Nordisk) is now often used to stop bleeding in GT and is particularly useful for patients with isoantibodies and/or patients undergoing invasive procedures, although thrombotic complications have been reported at high doses (144,145). It has been used in children with GT with variable success for stopping severe bleeding (in 12 of 22 acute episodes the response was judged as good or excellent), whereas in three out of three cases it prevented bleeding during surgery (145). Recombinant FVIIa enhances deposition of platelets to the vessel wall and even restores an aggregation response by stimulating tissue factor–independent thrombin generation and fibrin formation (146,147).

Local bleeding can almost always be treated by local measures. Epistaxis, gingival bleeding, or other superficial wounds are successfully controlled in most patients by nasal packing or by applying gelatin sponge or gauze soaked in topical thrombin. Patients with recurrent, severe nasal hemorrhage may require embolic occlusion of the internal maxillary artery. Regular dental care is essential to prevent gingival bleeding. For teeth extractions, or for hemorrhage accompanying the loss of deciduous teeth, hemostasis can be significantly improved by the application of individually prepared plastic splints that provide physical support for hemostasis. The use of autologous fibrin glue has been suggested (148). Systemic EACA administration is the conventional therapy for managing teeth extractions in patients with hemophilia, and it should be used as an adjunct to platelet transfusions in patients with thrombasthenia.

Life-threatening and intractable bleeding from gastrointestinal telangiectactic lesions continued in a patient with anti–GP IIb/IIIa antibodies despite tranexamic acid, oral iron, omeprazole, and platelet transfusions, although the situation was improved by using oral norethisterone (149). Gastrointestinal angiodysplasia and spontaneous duodenal hematoma have both been reported (150,151). Control of menstrual bleeding is a major problem. Severe menorrhagia, usually associated with an excessively proliferative endometrium caused by estrogen dominance, can be effectively treated with high doses of progesterone. Bleeding usually stops within 24 hours, the progesterone dose can then be decreased and continued at the decreased dose for several weeks. Menstrual bleeding will occur on withdrawal but it should not be severe. Maintenance treatment with birth control pills should then begin. More than one pill daily may be required to prevent breakthrough bleeding. Birth control pills control menorrhagia by causing progressively more atrophic endometrium during the initial cycles; in healthy women who take birth control pills, menstrual blood loss is typically reduced by half. Packing the uterine cavity for 48 hours halted the bleeding and avoided the necessity for a hysterectomy in a particularly severe case (110).

The frequent occurrence of iron deficiency anemia, which can develop insidiously with gingival oozing or minor menorrhagia, must be emphasized. During periods of rapid growth in infants and adolescents, when iron requirements are greater, iron deficiency is expected and oral iron supplements should be given. The rare coexistence of GT with other inherited diseases such as mild VWD in Saudi Arabian and Canadian families (60,152) can accentuate the clinical severity of bleeding.

Finally, drugs interfering with platelet function such as aspirin are contraindicated.

## Prognosis

Although thrombasthenia can be a severe hemorrhagic disease, the prognosis is excellent with careful supportive care. Most adult patients are healthy and their disease has minimal effect on their daily lives. Four of 64 patients followed up in Paris for over 30 years (2), have died. Causes were an apparently spontaneous intrahepatic hematoma in a 22-year-old woman, hemorrhage from an unknown site in a 9-year-old girl in 1963 (for whom records are not available), and hemorrhage in two patients caused by separate motor vehicle crashes many years ago. Only one other hemorrhagic death had occurred among the 113 patients, as reviewed in the literature up to 1990 (2). In contrast, it is not uncommon for newly diagnosed patients to report previous hemorrhagic deaths among siblings. Mostly, these deaths were reported among young children and involved gastrointestinal bleeding, epistaxis, tongue laceration, hemorrhage following traumatic surgery, and circumcision (7). Presumably, this mortality will decrease as early diagnosis becomes common. In rare patients, the condition was sufficiently grave, with repeated and life-threatening hemorrhage or severe alloimmunization in cases of allogenic bone marrow transplantation (153–156). The donors were HLA-identical siblings, and on each occasion, the transplantation was reported to be successful. The question for the future is whether GT is a suitable disease for gene therapy. Studies have shown that bone marrow stem cells can be given sufficient genetic information to induce abnormal MK from GT patients to synthesize transgene GP IIb and GP IIIa products [see (157)]. A lentivirus vector encoding GP IIIa has been prepared and shown to induce functional GP IIb/IIIa synthesis in abnormal MK lacking GP IIIa, so technology is advancing fast and studies on the correction of both canine and mouse models of GT are underway (157). A 20% GP IIb/IIIa expression may be sufficient, although it remains to be seen whether patient immune systems will tolerate newly expressed GP IIb/IIIa.

# BERNARD-SOULIER SYNDROME

BSS was first described in 1948 with the report of an infant who had severe mucocutaneous bleeding, a prolonged bleeding time with a normal platelet count, and abnormally large platelets (158). Additional patients were reported over the following years, and the initial diagnostic criteria of autosomal recessive inheritance, a prolonged bleeding time, thrombocytopenia in most patients, giant platelets, a defective ristocetin-induced platelet agglutination, and normal clot retraction were progressively established (3,159,160). The platelet counts in BSS range from 50,000 per $\mu$L to near normal; occasionally, patients may have platelet counts as low as 20,000 per $\mu$L (161). BSS is a rarer disease than GT, perhaps linked to the compactness of the genes and the lack of introns (3).

## Platelet Structure Abnormality

Large platelets are the most prominent morphologic feature of BSS. The platelets on the stained peripheral blood smear can be up to 20 $\mu$ in diameter. The large platelet size is also evident from its increased content of protein and dense granules (162). In one study of two families, the platelet size abnormalities of the two affected siblings in each family were similar to each other, with mean platelet diameters being about twice normal and with 30% to 80% giant platelets ($>3.5$ $\mu$, normal $= 2.1$ $\mu$) (161). In these two families, the platelets of some of the parents were also significantly larger than normal but not as large as those of their affected children. In addition to being giant, platelets in BSS are often spheroid rather than discoid (163,164) and more deformable (165). Increased deformability may be related to the deficiency of membrane GP Ib/IX complexes, causing less attachment of the surface membrane to the membrane cytoskeleton. Electron microscopic studies have demonstrated complexes in the platelets of most patients, in addition to the increased size, cytoplasmic vacuoles, and abnormal domains of membrane (166,167). Platelet survival has been described as being markedly decreased in this syndrome, although it is occasionally normal or only moderately shortened (7).

Studies on MK have been reported in only a few patients with BSS. In addition to the morphologic abnormalities described in platelets, the demarcation membrane system has an irregular appearance in most cells that often also show increased numbers of vacuoles (166–168). The significance of these observations is speculative, but the modifications may contribute to the thrombocytopenia and the formation of the abnormally large platelets (see discussion on transgenic models of BSS).

## Platelet Function Abnormality

It was first noted that although Bernard-Soulier platelets aggregated normally in response to ADP, epinephrine, and collagen, they failed to aggregate when stimulated with bovine fibrinogen. It is now known that bovine VWF, present in this preparation, causes a direct agglutination of normal human platelets. Subsequently, lack of aggregation in response to ristocetin (169,170) and lack of binding of radiolabeled human VWF in the presence of ristocetin were demonstrated (171). Botrocetin-induced VWF binding and the direct binding of asialo-von Willebrand factor to Bernard-Soulier platelets are also absent or are markedly decreased. These observations led to the discovery that platelet adhesion to subendothelium is markedly reduced, an abnormality similar to that observed in VWD (172,173). Studies of *in vitro* platelet adhesion to subendothelium consistently demonstrate that the attachment of Bernard-Soulier platelets is severely abnormal at all shear rates tested (25). Bernard-Soulier platelets specifically do not adhere to immobilized VWF, whose A1 domain expresses epitopes able to react with GP Ib and which are inaccessible on freely circulating VWF multimers [see (3)]. Ristocetin (or botrocetin) mimics the adhesion process by making these epitopes on VWF accessible. VWF binding stimulated by ADP or thrombin, which occurs on GP IIb/IIIa rather than GP Ib, is normal in Bernard-Soulier platelets (9), which is consistent with other evidence that GP IIb/IIIa receptor function is unmodified. Therefore, in the presence of ADP, collagen, and arachidonic acid, Bernard-Soulier platelets respond by binding fibrinogen, secreting their granule contents, and aggregating (174). Thrombin is a special case (see subsequent text). The platelet adhesion defect in BSS shows just how important the initial attachment by way of the GP Ib/VWF axis is. This step is an essential prerequisite for the adhesion process, which for normal primary hemostasis requires the stabilization of the interaction through the secondary involvement of GP IIb/IIIa and/or the collagen receptors $\alpha 2\beta 1$ and GP VI (175).

The response of Bernard-Soulier platelets to $\alpha$ thrombin is abnormal, as demonstrated by decreased thrombin binding and decreased aggregation following a prolonged lag phase (176,177). GP Ib$\alpha$ contains high-affinity thrombin binding sites located within the N-terminal domain and in particular to an anionic sulfated-tyrosine sequence (178). The diminished response of Bernard-Soulier platelets is related to the absence of these sites. Therefore, $\gamma$ thrombin, a proteolytic product of $\alpha$ thrombin that does not bind to GP Ib$\alpha$, induces a response in normal platelets that is similar to that in BSS (177). The residual response to thrombin of BSS platelets is presumably mediated through the moderate-affinity receptors of the protease activated receptor (PAR) family (PAR-1, PAR-4) (179). Although little is known of PAR-4 expression in the BSS, platelets from patients possessed PAR-1 and aggregated normally to thrombin-receptor activating peptide (TRAP) that is reactive with PAR-1 and gave a normal intracellular $Ca^{2+}$ response (180). Therefore, GP Ib$\alpha$ plays a role in accelerating the speed and the intensity of the response to low doses of thrombin. A reported postreceptor defect in phospholipase C activation may be related to a role for this pathway in GP Ib–mediated signaling (181,182).

An abnormal prothrombin consumption, diminished collagen-induced coagulant activity, and an inability to bind factor XI were featured in early studies of Bernard-Soulier platelets (7). In a cascade mechanism, fibrin polymerization appears to be crucial for optimal thrombin generation in platelet-rich plasma, as are thrombin binding to GP Ib and adhesive protein binding to GP IIb/IIIa (183). The fact that GP Ib on normal platelets mediates localization of factor XI to lipid rafts in the platelet membrane, thereby facilitating its cleavage by thrombin, may also help explain the decreased thrombin generation in BSS (184). High-molecular-weight kininogen has also been shown to react with platelets through GP Ib, so this interaction too is defective (185). Yet, other reports have suggested that Bernard-Soulier platelets have increased prothrombinase activity following stimulation, and this was suggested to be linked to their greater size and an increased expression of phosphatidylserine (PS) on their surface (16,186). Further studies are required to understand the apparent contradictions between published studies. It is as yet unclear how these abnormalities relate to the hemorrhagic tendency.

Bernard-Soulier platelets react poorly with quinine- and quinidine-dependent antibodies [reviewed in (187)]. This is because the epitopes for these drug-dependent antibodies are present on GP Ib/IX/V, although some of the antibodies may

also react with GP IIb/IIIa complexes. Bernard-Soulier platelets have normal Fc$\gamma$RII (IgG Fc receptor) expression, demonstrated by normal aggregation and secretion induced by IgG-coated latex particles (188).

## Platelet Membrane Glycoprotein Abnormality

In 1975, Nurden and Caen (23) demonstrated a specific decrease of platelet membrane GP Ib concentration, and this was confirmed by single and two-dimensional SDS-PAGE (Sodium **do**decyl sulfate–polyacrylamide gel electrophoresis) of $^{125}$I-labeled platelets (189), crossed immunoelectrophoresis, (1) and radiolabeled MoAbs in binding studies (190,191). The early observations on this syndrome were important in establishing that GP Ib was a platelet receptor for VWF [reviewed in (1,3)]. Further studies involving techniques to radiolabel platelet surface carbohydrate residues demonstrated that, in addition to GP Ib, Bernard-Soulier platelets were also deficient in GP IX and GP V (192,193). Because GP Ib is composed of two separate gene products linked by an extracellular disulfide, four distinct genes (i.e., Ib$\alpha$, Ib$\beta$, IX, and V) are necessary to produce the complex whose structure is illustrated in Figure 66-4. In fact, binding studies with subunit-specific MoAbs suggest that Ib$\alpha$, Ib$\beta$, IX, and V are present with a stoichiometry of 2:2:2:1, respectively [see (3)]. Patients were described whose platelets contained residual amounts of GP Ib when $^3$H-labeling of surface GPs was followed by SDS-PAGE and fluorography (192,193). This sensitive procedure detects the heavily glycosylated GP Ib$\alpha$ chain. The development of Western blot assay and enzyme-linked immunosorbent assay (ELISA) also permitted the detection of residual amounts of GP Ib$\alpha$ in the platelets of some patients with BSS, thereby confirming heterogeneity of the disease (194,195). In general, a quantitative deficiency of GP Ib$\alpha$ is accompanied by parallel decreases in GP Ib$\beta$, GP IX, and GP V, showing, as in GT, that complex formation is a prerequisite for efficient transport of each gene product to the cell surface. The development of MoAbs against each component of the GP Ib/IX/V complex allows their individual assessment on Bernard-Soulier platelets by flow cytometry (25). The advantage of simultaneously detecting epitopes on GP Ib$\alpha$, GP IX, and GP V is that determination of residual amounts of these subunits can indicate candidate genes for screening. In this regard, GP Ib$\beta$ has a limited accessibility to antibodies on platelets, but these antibodies can be used in Western blotting (196). As well as studying GP expression, flow cytometry allows an evaluation of platelet size, while double labeling allows the dual assessment of GP Ib/IX/V and GP IIb/IIIa levels (197).

Flow cytometry is most useful in characterizing the rare cases of variant BSS where qualitative defects lead to a nonfunctional GP Ib/IX/V complex. Therefore, De La Salle et al. (198) reported a patient (variant Nancy I) whose GP Ib$\alpha$ was recognized by two MoAbs (LJIb$\alpha$1 and Ib4) but which did not react with several others (e.g., AP1, SZ2, AN51), whereas antibodies to GP IX and GP V showed significant binding. The morphologically giant platelets of this patient aggregated normally with ADP but failed to agglutinate with ristocetin. Platelets of the "Bolzano" variant failed to react with the MoAbs LJ-1b1 and AP-1 in flow cytometry, yet the binding of LJ-1b10, was about 50% of normal (199). Immunoblotting confirmed the presence of GP Ib$\alpha$ and GP IX in the platelets of the patient, although a low molecular mass form of GP Ib$\alpha$ was also observed. Significantly, the binding of thrombin to the patient's platelets was normal, yet the ability to bind VWF had been lost. The platelets of this patient do not show the lag phase to thrombin, characteristic of the platelets of other patients.

The GP defects characteristic of Bernard-Soulier platelets also extend to the MK (168,197). Many MK have a highly vacuolar appearance with fragments resembling large platelets attached to the surface. According to one report, mature MK in BSS show an increased ploidy suggestive of stimulated thrombopoiesis caused by decreased platelet survival (197).

There are reports of GP Ib/IX/V expression in EC (200,201). A role for endothelial cell attachment to VWF has been proposed. However, others have failed to detect GP Ib (202), and there is no evidence to support an abnormal endothelial cell function in BSS. There are also no suggestions that other cell types are affected in this syndrome or express GP Ib/IX/V under normal conditions.

## The Genetic Defect of Bernard-Soulier Syndrome

In contrast to GT, in which the two involved subunits of GP IIb/IIIa are transcribed from closely linked genes on chromosome 17, the receptor affected in Bernard-Soulier platelets is composed of the products of four distinct genes located within different parts of the genome. The genes for the two disulfide-linked peptides GP Ibα and GP Ibβ are on chromosomes 17 and 22, respectively, whereas the gene for GP IX is on chromosome 3 as is the gene for GP V (203–207). Each of the coded proteins is a member of the leucine-rich motif superfamily, suggesting that they arose from a common ancestral gene. The genes share other structural features; only the gene encoding GP IX has more than one intron. GP Ibβ contains a single intron of 10 bases after the start of the coding sequence. This simplified gene structure limits the potential for splicing defects, which represent a significant proportion of the gene abnormalities giving rise to GT.

### Defects of the GP Ibα Gene

Abnormalities of the gene for GP Ibα are most frequent in BSS (see database: www.bernard-soulier.org). Truncation of GP Ibα with loss of the transmembrane domain is a common cause. For example, a homozygous deletion of T317 at codon 76 causes a frameshift, a premature stop codon after 19 altered AAs, and a severely truncated molecule (208). In another family, a homozygous C → A substitution resulted in a truncated GP Ibα, stopping at Ser444 and lacking the transmembrane and cytoplasmic domains (209). This shortened molecule was normally glycosylated and secreted into the plasma. Another patient had a nucleotide transition, changing the Trp-343 codon (TGG) to a nonsense codon (TGA) and resulting in GP Ibα lacking the transmembrane and cytoplasmic domains (210). However, both mutant and normal codons were found in this patient who was thought to be a compound heterozygote with a still unidentified defect in the other GP Ibα allele. A homozygous dinucleotide deletion within the TGTG repeat at cDNA number 972 to 975 in the GP Ibα gene caused a frameshift after Thr294 in a Swedish patient; a truncated protein was produced and detected in the plasma (211). Missense mutations also occur. Hourdillé et al. (168) first reported, in a Spanish patient, a homozygous single base pair mutation giving a Cys209 → Ser substitution, which was revealed by a nucleotide sequence analysis of the coding region of GP Ibα. It was suggested that absent disulfide bonding altered the folding of GP Ibα, thereby preventing the formation of the complex (and liaison with GP Ibβ) (212). Compound heterozygosity of the GP Ibα gene was reported for two related Spanish patients by Gonzalez-Manchon et al. (213). In this case, the maternal allele possessed a T insertion at position 1418, causing a translational frameshift and a premature polypeptide termination. The paternal allele had a T → A substitution changing Cys209 to Ser, as mentioned in the preceding text. Transfection experiments confirmed that both mutations were contributing to the BSS phenotype.

The mechanism of the noncovalent heterodimer association of GP Ib/IX is not yet completely defined, but transfection studies have demonstrated that cDNAs for GP Ibα, GP Ibβ, and GP IX are required for cell surface expression of the intact GP Ib/IX complex (214). GP V is the only one of the four polypeptides that can be expressed alone on the surface of transfected cells, although its expression is increased if the rest of the complex is present (215). Therefore, it would be expected that a defect in any of the three distinct genes for GP Ibα, GP Ibβ, and GP IX would produce the BSS phenotype. A deficiency of GP V may not do so, and abnormalities in the GP V gene have not been reported (see section on transgenic models of BSS).

### Defects of the GP Ibβ and GP IX Genes

Budarf et al. (216) were the first to demonstrate a defect in the GP Ibβ gene, and they did so in a patient who also had the DiGeorge/Velocardiofacial syndrome (see Chapter 65). The patient was a compound heterozygote—one abnormal allele resulted from a deletion in 22q11.2, the zone of localization of the GP Ibβ gene—and a region known to be affected in the DiGeorge syndrome (217). The other abnormality was a single point mutation (C → G) at −133, a site for the GATA-1 transcription factor (218). This was also the first report of BSS related to a promoter defect and severely reduced transcription. Since then, a homozygous 13-bp deletion in the signal peptide-coding region has been reported in the GP Ibβ gene of a Japanese patient (219). As well as GP Ibβ, GP IX was nearly absent from the giant platelets of this patient whereas GP Ibα and GP V were detectable. A unique feature in this patient was that some platelet α-granules were enlarged. Results for three novel hemizygous BSS mutations emphasized how the importance of the interaction of GP Ibβ with GP IX is essential for the functional expression of GP Ibα (196,220,221). In each patient, one allele had a 22q11.2 deletion symptomatic of DiGeorge syndrome, suggesting a link between this disease and BSS. In the first patient, Pro29 was substituted by a Leu (196). In the second case, the second GP Ibβ allele possessed a single nucleotide deletion at codon 80 (220). The result was a transitional frameshift that encodes for 86 altered AAs and a predicted stop codon. In the third patient, there was a novel Pro96 → Ser change in the leucine-rich repeat C-flanking region of GP Ibβ (221). The results for this patient led the authors to suggest that GP Ibβ actually participates in VWF binding. Transfection experiments showed that GP Ib/IX surface expression was severely reduced for each mutation. Homozygous missense mutations in the GP Ibβ gene giving rise to BSS include Asn64 → Thr, Pro74 → Arg, and Tyr88 → Cys; in each case the GP Ibβ defect led to a severe decrease in GP IX and, as a consequence, in GP Ib/IX (222–224). In the patient studied by Strrassel et al. (222), residual expression of an incompletely glycosylated form of GP Ibα was detected on his platelets. In a stable CHO cell line, wild-type GP Ibα and mutated GP Ibβ were largely confined to the ER and little GP IX was seen. Therefore, the mutation led to an early block on GP Ib/IX maturation and transport to the Golgi apparatus.

GP IX gene defects have also been described and they largely concern point mutations. Wright et al. (225), first described double heterozygosity in three siblings with a typical BSS phenotype. Missense mutations were observed in the coding region of the GP IX gene: (i) an A → G transition in codon 21, resulting in an Asp → Gly conversion and (ii) an A → G change in codon 45 that converts Asn → Ser. These mutations alter conserved residues in or flanking the single GP IX leucine-rich GP motif. Immunoblotting and flow cytometry failed to detect GP IX but showed small residual amounts of GP Ibα on the platelets. The Asn45 → Ser substitution is the object of several reports and is common among BSS patients in Finland and Germany; it may be an ancient mutation shared by patients of North European ancestry (226–228). A homozygous Phe55 → Ser substitution within the leucine-rich repeat was reported by Noris et al. (229). Again, it was speculated that conformational changes induced in GP IX prevented stable assembly of the GP Ib/IX complex. This was also the hypothesis for a homozygous Cys73 → Tyr detected in two unrelated Japanese families by Noda et al. (230). In another report by Noda et al. (231), a stop codon at Try126 led to a truncated protein without the transmembrane domain, preventing insertion of GP IX into the membrane. Therefore, the transmembrane and/or cytoplasmic domains of both GP Ibα and GP IX are necessary for GP Ib/IX/V complex formation. To prove the association between the Asp21 → Gly and Asn45 → Ser mutations and the Bernard-Soulier phenotype, Sae-Tung et al. (232), introduced each mutation into the cDNA for GP IX by site-directed mutagenesis and examined the associations of the mutants with wild-type GP Ibα and Ibβ subunits in transfected CHO cells. Evidence pointed to an important role of the leucine-rich motif of GP IX in the association with GP Ibβ, a defect that accounted for the lack of surface expression of the complex. Finally, a Leu7 → Pro mutation in the signal peptide of GP IX was shown to abolish surface expression of the GP Ib/IX/V complex by incorrect insertion of GP IX into the ER and/or defective signal peptide cleavage (233). It is now clear from BSS that both GP Ibβ and GP IX are necessary chaperones to ensure the correct transport of the GP Ibα subunit onto the cell surface.

### Variant-Type Bernard-Soulier Syndrome

Qualitative defects affecting GP Ib/IX/V function while allowing normal or subnormal expression are shown in Figure 66-4.

The first variant to be described occurred in a family with a unique autosomal dominant form of the disease caused by a heterozygous substitution of Leu57 → Phe within the first leucine tandem repeat (234). The patient had enlarged platelets but ristocetin-induced platelet agglutination was only slightly decreased, suggesting residual GP Ib function. Although GP Ibα was present in the patient's platelets, it was more susceptible to proteolysis. For the Bolzano variant (199,235), a point mutation gave rise to a homozygous Ala156 → Val substitution within a leucine-rich repeat of the extracellular N-terminal domain of GP Ibα. In fact, the VWF binding function of GP Ibα is now known to involve both a disulfide-bonded double loop region subterminal to the leucine repeats and the leucine-rich repeat domain itself [see (236) and Chapter 31]. This zone is held well away from the platelet surface by the highly glycosylated macroglycopeptide domain of GP Ibα. A causal effect of the Ala156 → Val substitution was confirmed by site-directed mutagenesis and functional studies on recombinant GP Ibα fragments (235). Each leucine-rich repeat is thought to form a short β strand parallel to an α helix. Conformational changes may also account for the loss of the epitopes for some, but not all, MoAbs reactive with GP Ibα. A somewhat similar situation was seen for the variant Nancy I where a three-base deletion resulted in the loss of Leu179 in a highly conserved region of the seventh leucine-rich repeat of GP Ibα (198,237). Similar results were also obtained by Li et al. (238) on two patients where platelets showed about 40% of residual VWF binding. In both cases, a point mutation in codon 129 of the GP Ibα gene resulted in a Leu → Pro substitution. This is within a leucine repeat sequence of GP Ibα. Transient transfection experiments in mouse L-cells transfected with wild-type GP Ibβ and GP IX genes proved that Pro129 in GP Ibα was responsible for the

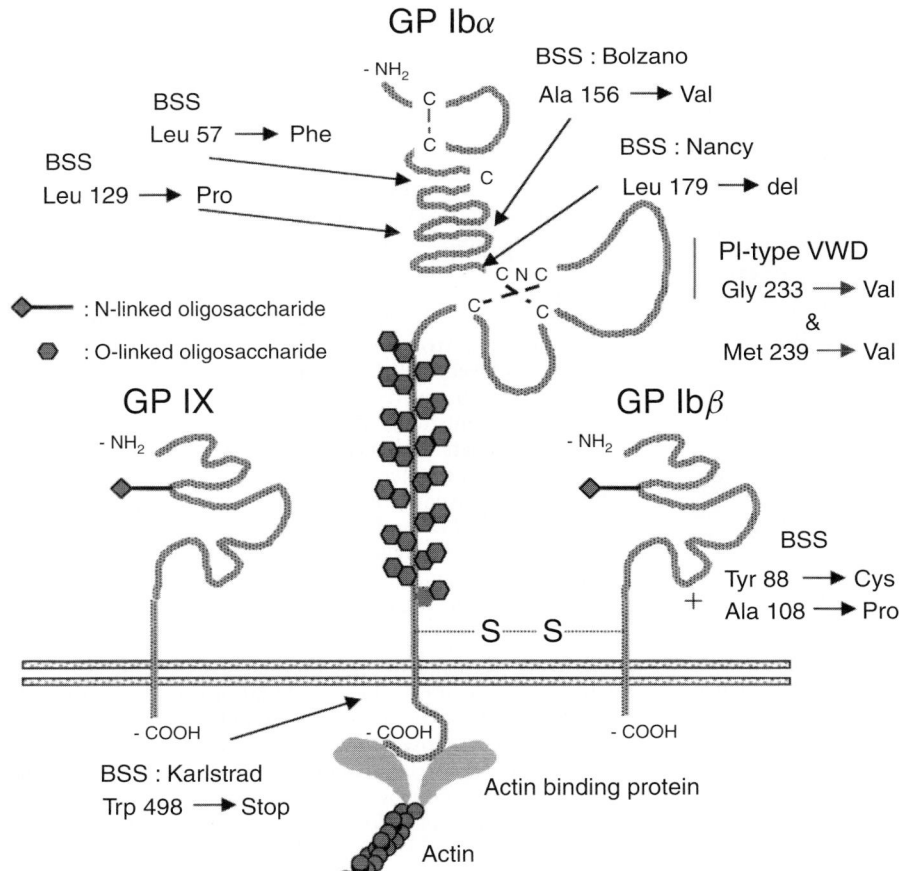

**FIGURE 66-4.** Schematic representation showing amino acid (AA) substitutions or other defects giving rise to downregulated function of glycoprotein (GP) Ib/IX [variant-type Bernard-Soulier syndrome (BSS)] or upregulated function [platelet-type von Willebrand disease (VWD), Pl-type VWD]. The cases are described in the text.

patients' phenotype. Mutations in the leucine-rich domain of GP Ibα appear as a likely cause of variant form of the disease.

Kunishima et al. (239) have reported a Japanese patient in whom most of the GP Ibα was not disulfide-linked to GP Ibβ. This unusual variant was because of two missense mutations in the GP Ibβ gene: (i) Tyr88 → Cys and (ii) Ala108 → Pro. Despite this, the biosynthesis of GP Ibβ was not greatly affected; only its capacity to form a disulfide with GP Ibα was altered. The presence of a noncovalent interaction between GP Ibα and GP IX was suggested, although noncovalent interactions with GP Ibβ were not excluded. Variants such as this provide novel data about the structure/function of the GP Ib/IX/V complex.

### Transgenic Models

Transgenic models have confirmed the genotype/phenotype relation as seen for patients in BSS. This was first shown by the generation of a murine knockout model for GP Ibα that recapitulated all the hallmarks of BSS (240). Moreover, using transgenic technology the murine Bernard-Soulier phenotype was rescued by expression of a human GP Ibα subunit on the surface of circulating mouse platelets. The availability of the GP Ibα knockout mouse enabled an examination of MK ultrastructure and maturation by electron microscope analysis of bone marrow samples (241). Abnormal membrane development was confirmed, and although the mature MK normally migrated to and crossed the endothelial barrier, their migration was accompanied by the production of unusually large MK fragments or proplatelets (Propl) in the vascular sinus (see Fig. 66-5). The impression given was that the proplatelets spontaneously broke up into giant platelets. Significantly, rescue with the human GP Ibα transgene corrected the morphologic

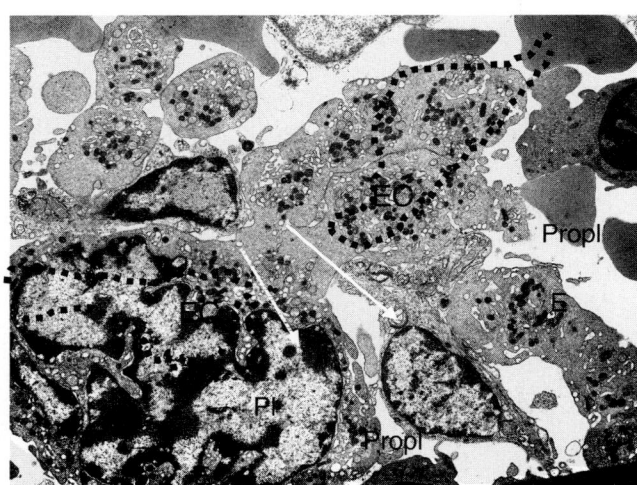

**FIGURE 66-5.** A megakaryocyte (MK) normally migrating into the vascular sinus in a transgenic glycoprotein (GP) Ibα–null mouse. Despite the absence of GP Ib/IX/V, the megakaryocyte has normally migrated to the endothelial cell barrier and extruded large processes or proplatelets (*Propl*) into the vascular sinus, which were still attached to the cell body (*direction of flow indicated by arrows*). Two endothelial cells (*EC*) have been highlighted. The Propl have an abnormal structure with a heterogeneous distribution of granules and regions containing packed membrane complexes. They may also be prone to fragmentation *in situ*, and giant platelets showing a typical BSS morphology can be seen in the bottom left-hand corner (bar = 2 μm). (From Poujol C, Ware J, Nieswandt B, et al. Absence of GP Ibα is responsible for aberrant membrane development during megakaryocyte maturation: ultrastructural study using a transgenic model. *Exp Hematol* 2002;30:352, with permission.)

abnormalities (241). None of the ultrastructural characteristics were seen in the GP V knockout mouse whose platelets did not show a BSS phenotype, confirming that GP V mutations are unlikely to be a source of this disease (242). Amelioration of the macrothrombocytopenia associated with the murine BSS was achieved using a mouse model in which platelets were engineered to express GP Ibα in which most of the extracellular domain was replaced by that of the human interleukin-4 receptor (243). The results were interpreted to show a role for the intracytoplasmic domain of GP Ibα in megakaryocyte maturation and platelet development, presumably through its ability to link to cytoskeletal elements. Very recently, the BSS phenotype was also seen in the GP Ibβ knockout mouse where an additional and unexpected feature was an increased α-granule size (244), a rare finding in human BSS (219).

## Clinical Manifestations

The data reported on 88 patients by Lopez et al. (3) show that both sexes are equally affected and that clinical observations are relatively consistent in this syndrome. The frequent presence of a homozygous trait and the rare gene frequency are reflections of the presence of consanguinity in many kindreds (5,160). The bleeding symptoms in BSS are the same as in GT. The severity of bleeding is unpredictable, as seen in GT; however, most patients have required transfusion at some time. Fatal hemorrhage is rare. Occasionally, patients have been reported to have very mild bleeding symptoms (239). As in GT, the explanation for the unpredictable severity of bleeding symptoms is unknown but appears to be independent of the residual content of functional GP Ibα and, therefore, probably depends on a range of vascular factors. The presence of severe thrombocytopenia, even as low as 20,000 per μL, does not appear to cause a greater risk of bleeding.

## Current Diagnostic Criteria

The diagnostic criteria for BSS are:

- an autosomal recessive trait, with no significant bleeding in most heterozygous subjects
- bleeding symptoms that usually include purpura, epistaxis, gingival bleeding, and menorrhagia, without hemarthroses and deep visceral hematomas
- bleeding severity that ranges from mild bruising, indistinguishable from normal, to severe, recurrent mucocutaneous bleeding from birth
- moderate to severe thrombocytopenia, although occasional patients have near normal platelet counts
- large platelets with a heterogeneous size distribution on the stained peripheral blood smear
- abnormal bleeding time, longer than that predicted for the degree of thrombocytopenia
- normal platelet aggregation in response to ADP, collagen, and epinephrine (but not thrombin)
- absent platelet agglutination by ristocetin and VWF that is not corrected by normal plasma.

These criteria can establish the diagnosis of BSS with reasonable certainty in routine clinical laboratory testing (Table 66-5). Additional observations are that clot retraction, plasma VWF, and bone marrow structure are all normal. Platelet aggregation can be difficult to assess because of thrombocytopenia and the problems of recovering the larger, more dense platelets in platelet-rich plasma. Flow cytometry is now the screening procedure of choice (25,197,222) because the analysis of whole blood samples allows even the largest platelets to be included in the analysis (197). It can be anticipated from the experience with GT that more patients with variant forms will be described in whom platelet GP Ib/IX and GP V are present in up to normal amounts but with abnormal VWF binding and defective platelet adhesion to vascular subendothelium because of qualitative defects.

Heterozygous subjects basically have low to normal platelet counts and normal platelet function, but occasionally platelets can be abnormally large (3,161). However, the situation has been complicated by the report that autosomal dominant macrothrombocytopenia in Italy is most frequently associated with the presence of heterozygous BSS linked to the Ala156 → Val (Bolzano variant mutation) (discussed further in Chapter 65) (245). Obligate heterozygotes for the classic form of BSS have intermediate concentrations of GP Ib/IX/V but usually have autosomal recessive inheritance.

## Differential Diagnosis

BSS must be differentiated from other congenital thrombocytopenias and diseases associated with giant platelets. The *May-Hegglin anomaly* is a rare autosomal dominant disorder characterized by large platelets, variable thrombocytopenia, and Döhle bodies seen in leukocytes on peripheral blood smears (246,247). Platelet function and platelet membrane GPs are normal, and most patients have no bleeding symptoms in spite of moderate thrombocytopenia. The autosomal dominant association of thrombocytopenia and large platelets with nephritis and deafness, termed *Epstein syndrome*, has been described in several reports (166,248). The bleeding time was prolonged and, in some patients, platelet aggregation in response to epinephrine and collagen was abnormal. *Fechtner syndrome* was described as macrothrombocytopenia, with normal platelet function, nephritis, deafness, cataracts, and leukocyte inclusions and said to be a variant of the *Alport syndrome* (249,250). When such features as nephritis, deafness, and cataracts are absent, but where giant platelets and morphologically distinct neutrophil inclusions are retained, the disorder is known as the *Sebastian platelet syndrome* (251). These syndromes are now considered as a spectrum of diseases defined by nonmuscle myosin heavy-chain IIA mutations (246,247). *Montreal platelet syndrome* is an autosomal dominant disorder characterized by moderate thrombocytopenia with giant platelets, a prolonged bleeding time and normal clot retraction (252,253). Spontaneous platelet microaggregates may form with stirring of platelet-rich plasma in patients with Montreal platelet syndrome. Platelet membrane GPs are normal, but deficient platelet calpain activity has been reported (253). The *gray platelet syndrome* is a rare disorder with mostly autosomal recessive inheritance, large platelets, mild thrombocytopenia, normal platelet membrane GPs, and a severe deficiency in α-granule contents, particularly of the endogenously synthesized proteins (254,255). Recent evidence points to a cohort of patients lacking the collagen receptor, GP VI (255).

Other than the above disorders, there are many isolated reports of *familial macrothrombocytopenia*. Some patients may represent unique syndromes, others may be as yet uncharacterized variant forms of BSS, perhaps with autosomal recessive inheritance. These and the familial thrombocytopenias linked to genetic defects of transcription factors are discussed in Chapter 65. Finally, the increasing number of patients with BSS associating hemizygous GP Ibβ defects with DiGeorge syndrome merits highlighting because, in DiGeorge syndrome alone, thrombocytopenia can be associated with increases in mean platelet volume and, interestingly, in some cases with an increased risk of schizophrenia (217).

### Acquired Bernard-Soulier Syndrome

Rarely, patients have been described in whom some of the clinical features of BSS were caused by acquired autoantibodies to GP Ib. Autoantibodies to GP Ib are quite common in ITP (256). One patient had a lymphoproliferative disorder and an autoantibody that inhibited ristocetin-induced platelet agglutination (257). Another patient developed an autoantibody during therapy with procainamide that inhibited ristocetin-induced platelet agglutination but not ADP-induced aggregation and that immunoprecipitated both GP Ib and GP V (258). Acquired BSS associated with antibodies to GP IX (259) has also been described. Acquired BSS can be associated with liver disease (260,261). In the latter report, anticardiolipin antibodies were also present. Korte et al. (262) presented a patient who had autoantibodies to GP Ib/IX/V, only residual amounts of GP Ib/IX/V in his platelets, and antiphospholipid antibodies suggesting coexistence of autoimmune thrombocytopenia and BSS. Interestingly, infusion of rat antibodies to murine GP Ib/IX (but not to GP V) into mice led to acute thrombocytopenia, with ultrastructural changes in both MK and platelets during the recovery phase, confirming that accurate diagnosis of BSS in isolated cases requires elimination of the presence of anti–GP Ib/IX antibodies (263).

BSS may also be acquired by somatic mutations within bone marrow stem cells. The first report was a 9-year-old girl who developed macrothrombocytopenia during the evolution of a myelodysplastic syndrome (264). Her disorder was associated with chromosomal abnormalities, monosomy 7 and trisomy 21. In fact, two populations of platelets were present in the blood, one of normal size with normal amounts of GP Ib/IX/V and the second population of platelets were large and lacked these GPs. In a second report, two children with a Bernard-Soulier–like functional defect were described in Turkey, one with a myelodysplastic syndrome and the second with acute myeloblastic leukemia (265).

## Management

Management of patients with BSS is much the same as described for GT. Treatment for bleeding episodes consists of local measures and the judicious use of platelet transfusions. Because bleeding complications are unpredictable and can be severe, platelet transfusions are indicated for invasive procedures. The appearance of isoantibodies with specificity for GP Ib (266) has been reported and, if present at a sufficient titer, these may render transfusion therapy inefficient. Because of the combination of thrombocytopenia and normal numbers of marrow MK, splenectomies have been performed in patients with probable BSS and in occasional patients with well-documented disease [see (3)]. A transient increase in the platelet count can follow splenectomy, but a sustained clinical benefit has not been reported and therefore, splenectomy should not be performed. Correct diagnosis of BSS is essential. Corticosteroid therapy and antifibrinolytic agents have been tried unsuccessfully (183). Other treatments include the use of DDAVP and r factor VIIa (145,267,268). Evidence was provided for a partial correction of platelet deposition on subendothelium after DDAVP infusion with increased fibrin formation (267). Arguments for the possible use of gene therapy for BSS are as for GT, and the evaluation of experimental models is already at an advanced stage (157). Although BSS patients may be thought to be protected against atherosclerosis through decreased platelet reactivity with the vessel wall, this has not been proven. Indeed, atherosclerosis and unstable angina in a patient with BSS has been reported, although this could be an isolated case (269).

## Platelet-Type von Willebrand Disease

Platelet-type or pseudo–von Willebrand disease is also associated with an abnormality of the platelet GP Ib/IX/V complex (3). However, in this disease, there is an unusual gain-of-function phenotype and spontaneous binding of plasma VWF to platelets. Initially, the mutations giving rise to this disorder were identified as Gly233 → Val and Met239 → Val (270,271). More recently, a novel Gly233 → Ser mutation has been described in a Japanese family (272). These AA substitutions occur within the disulfide-bonded double loop region of GP Ibα (Fig. 66-4). The mutant GP Ibα binds normal human VWF multimers spontaneously so that the latter are cleared from the plasma, and the result is a clinical condition that resembles VWD. Site-directed mutagenesis and expression of mutated GP Ibα in heterologous cells has confirmed that the mutations confirm a gain-of-function phenotype with facilitated binding of soluble VWF to GP Ibα and increased platelet adhesion to surface-bound VWF (236,273,274). This disorder is also discussed in Chapter 60.

# OTHER INHERITED DISORDERS OF THE PLATELET MEMBRANE

## Collagen-Receptor Deficiency

The collagen receptor α2β1 (previously known as GP Ia/IIa), a member of the β1 subfamily of the integrin family of adhesion receptors (see Chapter 34), is present on many cell types as well as platelets. A patient has been described with a mild, life-long bleeding disorder, selective absence of aggregation by collagen or adhesion to collagen, and a deficiency of GP Ia/IIa (275,276). Platelet responses to all other agonists were normal. A similar defect was subsequently reported in a woman with a lifelong history of severe mucocutaneous bleeding, but where a selective deficiency of platelet responses to collagen and absent platelet GP Ia and absent thrombospondin (277). This patient was remarkable in that a remission of both the bleeding symptoms and the platelet GP Ia and thrombospondin deficiencies were observed during the period of study. The current situation concerning the platelet–collagen interaction is of a two-step model, with a second receptor, termed GP VI, having a central role (278). GP VI is a member of the immunoglobulin class of receptors. Moroi et al. (279) described a patient deficient in GP VI and lacking the collagen-induced aggregation response. More recently, a patient with the Gray platelet syndrome has also been shown to be refractory to collagen and to lack GP VI (255). An abnormal platelet response to collagen is often seen in routine platelet function testing when it is almost always attributed to aspirin intake or to a storage pool defect. Until now, only rarely have patients been shown to have a congenital defect of a collagen receptor, suggesting that improved screening is required. Although targeted gene deletion in mice has confirmed the roles for α2β1 and GP VI in the platelet collagen response (280,281), the animals show little hemostatic disruption, and bleeding time was relatively normal. So, in the absence of trauma, patients may not bleed because one receptor may back up the other. Care must be taken, however, to also rule out an acquired condition caused by the presence of a blocking autoantibody to GP Ia or GP VI (282,283). This caution is particularly important for GP VI, where the presence of autoantibody can actually lead to loss of GP VI from the platelets (284). Care must also be taken to rule out changes in the platelet response to collagen, linked to changes in receptor density, because both genes are highly polymorphic (285,286).

## Adenosine Diphosphate and Other Primary Receptors

For many years, a single ADP receptor was postulated to account for the platelet response to this agonist and was often referred to as P2T. It is now known that the platelet has three receptors for purine nucleotides: P2X$_1$ for ATP, an ion channel linked to Ca$^{2+}$ influx; P2Y$_1$ thought to mediate ADP-induced Ca$^{2+}$ mobilization and shape change; and P2Y$_{12}$, responsible for ADP-induced macroscopic platelet aggregation and linked to adenylate cyclase (5,287). Two groups have reported patients with hereditary disease linked to a much decreased platelet aggregation to ADP despite a normal ADP-induced shape change and Ca$^{2+}$ mobilization (5,288,289). The much reduced binding of radiolabeled 2-MeS-ADP (a stable analog of ADP) together with the specific inability of ADP to lower the cyclic adenosine monophosphate (cAMP) content of PGE$_1$-stimulated platelets, suggested that the third receptor was affected, and this proved true. Studies on the French family in fact helped to the cloning and molecular characterization of the P2Y$_{12}$ receptor (290). The French patient was shown to have a silent allele for P2Y$_{12}$, whereas the second allele had a two-nucleotide deletion at position 240 followed by a frameshift and a stop codon, leading to a truncated protein. Since then, the molecular defects have been defined in four other families (5,291). Homozygous base pair deletions and stop codons were detected in three families, whereas in the fourth family heterozygous missense mutations (Arg256 → Gln and Arg265 → Trp) led to the normal expression of a mutated P2Y$_{12}$ with defective signaling (5,291). Although, the ADP response is specifically affected, the synergistic role of ADP in the platelet response to low doses of most stimuli means that the platelet abnormality may also be manifested by a decreased sensitivity to agonists such as collagen and TxA$_2$ (288,289,292). The net result is a much decreased thrombus formation on subendothelial components under flow (293). Studies on transgenic mice lacking P2Y$_{12}$ have confirmed the phenotype as defined for the patients and have shown that the animals are protected against arterial thrombosis (294). Interestingly, subjects who are heterozygous for a P2Y$_{12}$ defect, have been claimed to have an associated "primary secretion defect" (295), although the mechanism behind this is unknown. No human P2Y$_1$ deficiency has yet been described, and while a dominant negative P2X$_1$ receptor produced by the deletion of a single AA residue has been reported, the platelet aggregation response to ADP has not been defined (296).

A specifically defective response to TxA$_2$ has also been reported rarely patients, and an Arg60 → Leu mutation has been identified in the TxA$_2$ receptor (297,298). This receptor is present in two isoforms in platelets that differ only in their carboxyl-terminal tails and in their capacity to activate adenylate cyclase. Interestingly, patients with the mutated α form show an impaired TxA$_2$–induced phospholipase C activation and a reduced adenylate cyclase stimulation (297). Further studies showed that subjects who were homozygous for this mutation showed defective TxA$_2$–induced Ca$^{2+}$ mobilization, whereas heterozygotes did not (298). Congenital defects of the α$_2$-adrenergic receptor associated with a decreased platelet response to adrenaline (299,300) have also been described; the platelet also contains receptors for platelet activating factor (PAF) and serotonin, the pathophysiology of which is beyond the scope of this review. All of these receptors are GPs and belong to the seven transmembrane domain receptor family of which the classic examples in human platelets are the thrombin receptors PAR-1 and PAR-4, which have both been cloned [see (301)]. So far, pathologies of these receptors have not been described. It is to be expected that the number of patients shown with these disorders of primary receptors will increase as methods permitting their identification improve and become more widely applicable. However, for each case, the question will be whether the receptor itself is affected or whether the abnormality concerns a later step of a signal transduction mechanism into which the receptor is locked—a mutated G protein, impaired phosphorylation pathway or impaired phospholipase C activation—to quote but three examples of recently reported pathologies [reviewed in (126)].

# SCOTT SYNDROME

Scott syndrome is a rare inherited disorder of calcium-induced phospholipid scrambling and assembly of the prothombinase complex on blood cells including platelets (302–304). In brief, Scott platelets fail to transport PS from the inner to the outer phospholipid leaflet of the membrane bilayer, with the result that factors Va and Xa fail to bind, leading to the incapacity of the activated cell surface to transform prothrombin to thrombin. This lack of thrombin generation is probably related to the patients' mild bleeding diathesis. Stimuli that induce this translocation under physiologic conditions include a thrombin and collagen mixture and the complement proteins C5b-9. PS expression, which can be readily measured by flow cytometry using FITC-annexin V (305), is accompanied by microvesiculation and the diffusion of the procoagulant activity. An altered protein tyrosine phosphorylation showed that platelet activation was modified (305). Some evidence suggests that the defect in this disorder concerns the activation of the scramblase enzyme thought to be responsible for PS mobilization, while a defective store-mediated $Ca^{2+}$ entry was described for one family (306,307).

Nevertheless, despite intensive study, the molecular basis for the molecular defect remains elusive.

## References

1. George JN, Nurden AT, Phillips DR. Molecular defects in interactions of platelets with the vessel wall. *N Engl J Med* 1984;311:1084.
2. George JN, Caen J-P, Nurden AT. Glanzmann's thrombasthenia: the spectrum of clinical disease. *Blood* 1990;75:1383.
3. Lopez JA, Andrews RK, Afshar-Kharghan V, et al. Bernard-Soulier syndrome. *Blood* 1998;91:4397.
4. Nurden A, Nurden P. Inherited disorders of platelet function. In: Michaelson AD, ed. *Platelets*, San Diego, CA: Academic Press, 2003:681.
5. Cattaneo M. Inherited platelet-based bleeding disorders. *J Thromb Haemost* 2003;1:1628.
6. Glanzmann E. Hereditare hamorrhagische thrombasthenie: Ein Beitrag zur Pathologie der Blutplattchen. *J Kinderkranken* 1918;88:113.
7. Nurden AT, George JN. Inherited abnormalities of the platelet membrane: Glanzmann thrombasthenia, Bernard-Soulier syndrome, and other disorders. In: Colman RW, Hirsh J, Marder VJ, et al. eds. *Hemostasis and thrombosis. basic principles and clinical practice.* Philadelphia, PA: Lippincott Williams & Wilkins, 2001:921.
8. Caen JP, Castaldi PA, Leclerc JC, et al. Congenital bleeding disorders with long bleeding time and normal platelet count. I. Glanzmann's thrombasthenia. *Am J Med* 1966;41:4.
9. Ruggeri ZM, DeMarco L, Gatti L, et al. Platelets have more than one binding site for von willebrand factor. *J Clin Invest* 1983;72:1.
10. Cohen I, Glaser T, Seligsohn U. Effects of ADP and ATP on bovine fibrinogen- and ristocetin-induced platelet aggregation in Glanzmann's thrombasthenia. *Br J Haematol* 1975;31:343.
11. Baumgartner H, Tschopp TB, Weiss HJ. Platelet interaction with collagen fibrils in flowing blood. II. Impaired adhesion-aggregation in bleeding disorders: a comparison with subendothelium. *Thromb Haemost* 1977;37:17.
12. Weiss HJ, Hawiger J, Ruggeri ZM, et al. Fibrinogen-independent platelet adhesion and thrombus formation on subendothelium mediated by glycoprotein IIb-IIIa complex at high shear rates. *J Clin Invest* 1989;83:288.
13. Patel D, Vaananen H, Jirouskova M, et al. Dynamics of GP IIb/IIIa-mediated platelet-platelet interactions in platelet adhesion/thrombus formation on collagen *in vitro* as revealed by videomicroscopy. *Blood* 2003;101:929.
14. Hainud P, Brouland J-P, André P, et al. Dissociation between fibrinogen and fibrin interaction with platelets in patients with different subtypes of Glanzmann's thrombasthenia: studies in an *ex vivo* perfusion chamber model. *Br J Haematol* 2002;119:998.
15. Rosa J-P, Artçanuthurry V, Grelac F, et al. Reassessment of protein tyrosine phosphorylation in thrombasthenic platelets: evidence that phosphorylation of cortactin and a 64 kDa protein is dependent on thrombin activation and integrin αIIbβ3. *Thromb Haemost* 1997;89:4385.
16. Bevers EM, Comfurius P, Nieuwenhuis HK, et al. Platelet prothrombin converting activity in hereditary disorders of platelet function. *Br J Haematol* 1986;63:335.
17. Weiss HJ, Turitto VT, Baumgartner HR. The role of shear rate and platelets in promoting fibrin formation on rabbit subendothelium. Studies utilizing patients with quantitative and qualitative platelet defects. *J Clin Invest* 1986;78:1072.
18. Weiss HJ, Lages B. Platelet prothrombinase activity and intracellular calcium responses in patients with storage pool deficiency, glycoprotein IIb-IIIa deficiency, or impaired platelet coagulant activity-A comparison with Scott syndrome. *Blood* 1997;89:1599.
19. Gemmell CH, Sefton MV, Yeo EL. Platelet-derived microparticle formation involves glycoprotein IIb-IIIa. Inhibition by RGDS and a Glanzmann's thrombasthenia defect. *J Biol Chem* 1993;268:14586.
20. Handagama PJ, Rappoole DA, Werb Z, et al. Platelet α-granule fibrinogen, albumin and immunoglobulin G are not synthesized by rat and mouse megakaryocytes. *J Clin Invest* 1990;86:1364.
21. Harrison P, Wilbourn BR, Debili N, et al. Uptake of plasma fibrinogen into the alpha granules of human megakaryocytes and platelets. *J Clin Invest* 1989;84:1320.
22. Nurden AT, Caen JP. An abnormal platelet glycoprotein pattern in three cases of Glanzmann's thrombasthenia. *Br J Haematol* 1974;28:253.
23. Nurden AT, Caen JP. Specific roles for surface membrane glycoproteins in platelet function. *Nature* 1975;255:720.
24. Phillips DR, Poh Agin P. Platelet membrane defects in Glanzmann's thrombasthenia. Evidence for decreased amounts of two major glycoproteins. *J Clin Invest* 1977;60:535.
25. Michelson A. Flow cytometry: a clinical test of platelet function. *Blood* 1996;87:4925.
26. Nurden AT, Didry D, Kieffer N, et al. Residual amounts of glycoproteins IIb and IIIa may be present in the platelets of most patients with Glanzmann's thrombasthenia. *Blood* 1985;65:1021.
27. Coller BS, Cheresh DA, Asch E, et al. Platelet vitronectin receptor expression differentiates Iraqi-Jewish from Arab patients with Glanzmann thrombasthenia in Israel. *Blood* 1991;77:75.
28. Poujol C, Nurden AT, Nurden P. Ultrastructural analysis of the distribution of the vitronectin receptor (αvβ3) in human platelets and megakaryocytes reveals an intracellular pool and labelling of the α-granule membrane. *Br J Haematol* 1997;96:823.
29. Nurden P, Poujol C, Durrieu-Jais C, et al. Labeling of the internal pool of GPIIb-IIIa in platelets by c7E3 Fab fragments (abciximab): flow and endocytic mechanisms contribute to the transport. *Blood* 1999;93:1622.
30. Hodivala-Dilke KM, McHugh KP, Tsakiris DA, et al. β3-integrin-deficient mice are a model for Glanzmann thrombasthenia showing placental defects and reduced survival. *J Clin Invest* 1999;103:229.
31. Tronik-Le Roux D, Roullot V, Poujol C, et al. Thrombasthenic mice generated by replacement of the integrin αIIb gene: demonstration that transcriptional activation of this megakaryocytic locus precedes lineage commitment. *Blood* 2000;96:1399.
32. McHugh KP, Hodilvala-Dilke K, Zheng M-H, et al. Mice lacking β3 integrins are osteosclerotic because of dysfunctional osteoclasts. *J Clin Invest* 2000;105:433.
33. Reynolds LE, Wyder L, Lively JC, et al. Enhanced pathological angiogenesis in mice lacking β3 integrin or β3 and β5 integrins. *Nature Med* 2002;8:27.
34. Ni H, Denis CV, Subbarao S, et al. Persistence of platelet thrombus formation in arterioles of mice lacking both von Willebrand factor and fibrinogen. *J Clin Invest* 2000;106:385.
35. Ni H, Papalla JM, Degen JL, et al. Control of thrombus embolization and fibronectin internalization by integrin αIIbβ3 engagement of the fibrinogen γ chain. *Blood* 2003;102:3609.
36. Springer TA. Folding of the N-terminal, ligand-binding region of integrin α-subunits into a β-propeller domain. *Proc Natl Acad Sci U S A* 1997;94:65.
37. Xiong J-P, Stehle T, Diefenbach B, et al. Crystal structure of the extracellular segment of integrin αvβ3. *Science* 2001;2000:339.
38. Adair BD, Yeager M. Three-dimensional model of the human platelet integrin αIIbβ3 based on electron microscopy and x-ray crystallography. *Proc Natl Acad Sci U S A* 2002;90:14059.
39. Nurden A, Jacquelin B, Tuleja E, et al. Reduced collagen-induced platelet aggregation in obligate heterozygotes of a Glanzmann thrombasthenia variant with a β3 mutation. *Thromb Haemost* 2002;88:364.
40. Larkin D, Murphy D, Reilly DF, et al. Icln, a novel integrin αIIbβ3-associated protein, functionally regulates platelet activation. *J Biol Chem* 2004;279:27286.
41. French DL. The molecular genetics of Glanzmann's thrombasthenia. *Platelets* 1998;9:5.
42. Rosa J-P, McEver RP. Processing and assembly of the integrin, glycoprotein IIb-IIIa, in HEL cells. *J Biol Chem* 1989;264:12596.
43. Burk CD, Newman PJ, Lyman S, et al. A deletion in the gene for glycoprotein IIb associated with Glanzmann's thrombasthenia. *J Clin Invest* 1991;87:270.
44. Newman PJ, Seligsohn U, Lyman S, et al. The molecular genetic basis of Glanzmann thrombasthenia in the Iraqi-Jewish and Arab populations in Israel. *Proc Natl Acad Sci U S A* 1991;88:3160.
45. Peretz H, Rosenberg N, Usher S, et al. Glanzmann's thrombasthenia associated with deletion-insertion and alternative splicing in the glycoprotein IIb gene. *Blood* 1995;85:414.
46. Schlegel N, Gayet O, Morel-Kopp MC, et al. The molecular genetic basis of Glanzmann's thrombasthenia in a gypsy population in France: identification of a new mutation on the αIIb gene. *Blood* 1995;86:977.

47. Gonzalez-Manchon C, Arias-Salgado EG, Butta N, et al. A novel homzygous splice junction mutation in GP IIb associated with alternative splicing, nonsense-mediated decay of GPIIb mRNA, and type II Glanzmann's thrombasthenia. *J Thromb Haemost* 2003;1:1071.

48. Gu JM, Xu WF, Wang XD, et al. Identification of a nonsense mutation at amino acid 584-arginine of platelet glycoprotein IIb in patients with type I Glanzmann thrombasthenia. *Br J Haematol* 1993;83:442.

49. Poncz M, Rifat S, Coller BS, et al. Glanzmann thrombasthenia secondary to a Gly273Asp mutation adjacent to the first calcium-binding domain of platelet glycoprotein IIb. *J Clin Invest* 1994;93:172.

50. Wilcox DA, Wautier JL, Pidard D, et al. A single amino acid substitution flanking the fourth calcium binding domain of $\alpha_{IIb}$ prevents maturation of the integrin $\alpha$IIb$\beta$3 complex. *J Biol Chem* 1994;269:4450.

51. Wilcox DA, Paddock CM, Lyman S, et al. Glanzmann thrombasthenia resulting from a single amino acid substitution between the second and third calcium-binding domain of GP IIb. *J Clin Invest* 1995;95:1553.

52. Basani RB, Vilaire G, Shattil SJ, et al. Glanzmann thrombasthenia due to a two amino acid deletion in the fourth calcium-binding domain of $\alpha$IIb: demonstration of the importance of calcium-binding domains in the conformation of $\alpha$IIb$\beta$3. *Blood* 1996;88:167.

53. French DL, Seligsohn U. Platelet glycoprotein IIb/IIIa receptors and Glanzmann's thrombasthenia. *Arterioscler Thromb Vasc Biol* 2000;20:607.

54. Ruan J, Peyruchaud O, Alberio L, et al. Double heterozygosity of the GP IIb gene in a Swiss patient with Glanzmann's thrombasthenia. *Br J Haematol* 1998;102:918.

55. Milet-Marsal S, Breillat C, Peyruchaud O, et al. Analysis of the amino acid requirement for a normal $\alpha$IIb$\beta$3 maturation at $\alpha$IIbGlu324 commonly mutated in Glanzmann thrombasthenia. *Thromb Haemost* 2002;88:655.

56. Tao J, Arias-Salgado EG, Gonzalez-Manchon C, et al. A1063G → A mutation in exon 12 of glycoprotein (GP)IIb associated with a thrombasthenic phenotype: mutation analysis of (324E)GP IIb. *Br J Haematol* 2000;111:965.

57. Mitchell WB, Li JH, Michelson AD, et al. Two novel mutations in the $\alpha$IIb calcium-binding domains identify hydrophobic regions essential for $\alpha$IIb$\beta$3 biogenesis. *Blood* 2003;101:2268.

58. Kato A, Yamamoto K, Miyazaki S, et al. Molecular basis for Glanzmann's thrombasthenia (GT) in a compound heterozygote with glycoprotein IIb gene: a proposal for the classification of GT based on the biosynthetic pathway of glycoprotein IIb-IIIa complex. *Blood* 1992;79:3212.

59. Gonzalez-Manchon C, Fernandez-Pinel M, Arias-Salgada EG, et al. Molecular genetic analysis of a compound heterozygote for the glycoprotein (GP) IIb gene associated with Glanzmann's thrombasthenia: disruption of the 674-687 disulfide bridge in GP IIb prevents surface exposure of GP IIb-IIIa complexes. *Blood* 1999;93:866.

60. Nurden AT, Breillat C, Jacquelin B, et al. Triple heterozygosity in the integrin $\alpha$IIb subunit in a patient with Glanzmann thrombasthenia. *J Thromb Haemost* 2004;2:813.

61. Rosenberg N, Yatuf R, Sobolev V, et al. Major mutations in calf-1 and calf-2 domains of glycoprotein IIb in patients with Glanzmann thrombasthenia enable GP IIb/IIIa complex formation, but impair its transport from the endoplasmic reticulum to the Golgi apparatus. *Blood* 2003;101:4808.

62. Djaffar I, Caen JP, Rosa J-P. A large alteration in the human platelet glycoprotein IIIa (integrin $\beta$3) gene associated with Glanzmann's thrombasthenia. *Hum Mol Genet* 1993;2:183.

63. Li L, Bray P. Homologous recombination among three intragene Alu sequences causes an inversion-deletion resulting in the hereditary bleeding disorder Glanzmann thrombasthenia. *Am J Hum Genet* 1993;53:140.

64. Morel-Kopp M-C, Kaplan C, Proulle V, et al. A three amino acid deletion in glycoprotein IIIa is responsible for type I Glanzmann's thrombasthenia: importance of residues Ile$^{325}$Pro$^{326}$Gly$^{327}$ for $\beta$3 integrin subunit association. *Blood* 1997;90:669.

65. Jin Y, Dietz HC, Montgomery RA, et al. Glanzmann thrombasthenia. Cooperation between sequence variants in Cis during splice selection. *J Clin Invest* 1996;98:1745.

66. Grimaldi CM, Chen F, Wu C, et al. Glycoprotein IIb Leu214Pro mutation produces Glanzmann thrombasthenia with both quantitative and qualitative abnormalities in GP IIb/IIIa. *Blood* 1998;91:1562.

67. Morel-Kopp M-C, Melchior C, Chen P, et al. A naturally occurring point mutation in the $\beta$3 integrin MIDAS-like domain affects differently $\alpha$v$\beta$3 and $\alpha$IIb$\beta$3 receptor function. *Thromb Haemost* 2001;86:1425.

68. Nurden AT, Ruan J, Pasquet J-M, et al. A novel $^{196}$Leu to Pro substitution in the $\beta$3 subunit of the $\alpha$IIb$\beta$3 integrin in a patient with a variant form of Glanzmann thrombasthenia. *Platelets* 2002;13:101.

69. Basani RB, Brown DL, Vilaire G, et al. A Leu117 → Trp mutation within the RGD-peptide cross-linking region of $\beta$3 results in Glanzmann thrombasthenia by preventing $\alpha$IIb$\beta$3 export to the platelet surface. *Blood* 1997;90:3082.

70. Tadokoro S, Tomiyama Y, Honda S, et al. Missense mutations in the $\beta$3 subunit have a different impact on the expression and function between $\alpha$IIb$\beta$3 and $\alpha$v$\beta$3. *Blood* 2002;99:931.

71. Rosenberg N, Yatuv R, Orion Y, et al. Glanzmann thrombasthenia caused by a 11.2-kb deletion in the glycoprotein IIIa ($\beta$3) is a second mutation in Iraqi jews that stemmed from a distinct founder. *Blood* 1993;82:2281.

72. Ruan J, Schmugge M, Clemetson KJ, et al. Homozygous Cys$^{542}$ → Arg substitution in the GP IIIa gene in a Swiss patient with type I Glanzmann's thrombasthenia. *Br J Haematol* 1999;105:523.

73. Milet-Marsal S, Breillat C, Peyruchaud O, et al. Two different $\beta$3 cysteine substitutions alter $\alpha$IIb$\beta$3 maturation and result in Glanzmann thrombasthenia. *Thromb Haemost* 2002;88:104.

74. Loftus JC, O'Toole TE, Plow EF, et al. A $\beta$3 integrin mutation abolishes ligand binding and alters divalent cation-dependent conformation. *Science* 1990;249:925.

75. Ginsberg MH, Frelinger AL, Lam SC. Analysis of platelet aggregation disorders based on flow cytometric analysis of membrane glycoprotein IIb-IIIa with conformation-specific monoclonal antibodies. *Blood* 1990;76:2017.

76. Nurden AT, Rosa JP, Fournier D, et al. A variant of Glanzmann's thrombasthenia with abnormal GP IIb-IIIa complexes in the platelet membrane. *J Clin Invest* 1987;79:962.

77. Bajt ML, Ginsberg MH, Frelinger AL III, et al. A spontaneous mutation of integrin $\alpha$IIb$\beta$3 (platelet glycoprotein IIb-IIIa) helps define a ligand-binding site. *J Biol Chem* 1992;267:3789.

78. Lanza F, Stierlé A, Fournier D, et al. A new variant of Glanzmann's thrombasthenia (Strasbourg I). Platelets with functionally defective glycoprotein IIb-IIIa complexes and a glycoprotein IIIa 214Arg → Trp mutation. *J Clin Invest* 1992;89:1995.

79. Djaffar I, Rosa J-P. A second case of variant of Glanzmann's thrombasthenia due to substitution of platelet GP IIIa (integrin $\beta$3) 214Arg by Trp. *Hum Mol Genet* 1993;2:2179.

80. Kouns WC, Steiner B, Kunicki TJ, et al. Activation of the fibrinogen binding site on platelets isolated from a patient with the Strasbourg I variant of Glanzmann's thrombasthenia. *Blood* 1994;84:1108.

81. Hardisty R, Pidard D, Cox A, et al. A defect of platelet aggregation associated with an abnormal distribution of glycoprotein IIb-IIIa complexes within the platelet. *Blood* 1992;80:696.

82. Peyruchaud O, Nurden AT, Milet S, et al. R to Q aminoacid substitution in the GFFKR sequence of the cytoplasmic domain of the integrin $\alpha$IIb subunit in a patient with a Glanzmann's thrombasthenia-like syndrome. *Blood* 1998;92:4178.

83. Low E, Qi W, Vilaire G, et al. Effect of cytoplasmic domain mutations on the agonist-stimulated ligand-binding activity of the platelet integrin $\alpha$IIb$\beta$3. *J Biol Chem* 1996;271:30233.

84. Vinogradova O, Velyvis A, Velyvienne A, et al. A structural mechanism of integrin $\alpha$IIb$\beta$3 "inside-out" activation as regulated by its cytoplasmic face. *Cell* 2002;110:587.

85. Chen Y, Djaffar I, Pidard D, et al. Ser752 → Pro mutation in the cytoplasmic domain of integrin $\beta$3 subunit and defective activation of platelet integrin $\alpha$IIb$\beta$3 (glycoprotein IIb-IIIa) in a variant of Glanzmann's thrombasthenia. *Proc Natl Acad Sci U S A* 1992;89:10169.

86. Nurden P, Poujol C, Winckler J, et al. A Ser752 → Pro substitution in the cytoplasmic domain of $\beta$3 in a Glanzmann thrombasthenia variant fails to prevent interactions between the $\alpha$IIb$\beta$3 integrin and the platelet granule pool of fibrinogen. *Br J Haematol* 2002;118:1143.

87. Chen Y-P, O'Toole TE, Ylänne J, et al. A point mutation in the integrin $\beta$3 cytoplasmic domain (S752 → P) impairs bidirectional signaling through $\alpha$IIb$\beta$3 (platelet glycoprotein IIb-IIIa). *Blood* 1994;84:1857.

88. Perrault C, Mekrache M, Schoevaert D, et al. Ser752 mutation to Pro or Ala in the $\beta$3 integrin subunit differentially affects the kinetics of cell spreading to von Willebrand factor and fibrinogen. *Cell Adhes Commun* 1998;6:335.

89. Tadokoro S, Shattil SJ, Tai V, et al. Talin binding to integrin $\beta$ tails: a common step in integrin activation. *Science* 2003;302:103.

90. Arias-Salgado EG, Liziano S, Sarkar S, et al. Src kinase activation by direct interaction with the integrin $\beta$ cytoplasmic domain. *Proc Natl Acad Sci U S A* 2003;100:13298.

91. Feng X, Novack DV, Faccio R, et al. A Glanzmann's mutation in $\beta$3 integrin specifically impairs osteoclast function. *J Clin Invest* 2001;107:1137.

92. Wang R, Shattil SJ, Ambruso DR, et al. Truncation of the cytoplasmic domain of $\beta$3 in a variant form of Glanzmann thrombasthenia abrogates signaling through the $\alpha$IIb$\beta$3 complex. *J Clin Invest* 1977;100:2393.

93. Kashiwagi H, Tomiyama Y, Tadokoro S, et al. A mutation in the extracellular cysteine-rich repeat region of the $\beta$-subunit activates integrins $\alpha$IIb$\beta$3 and $\alpha$v$\beta$3. *Blood* 1999;93:2559.

94. Ruiz C, Liu C-Y, Sun Q-H, et al. A point mutation in the cysteine-rich domain of glycoprotein (GP) IIIa results in the expression of a GP IIb-IIIa ($\alpha$IIb$\beta$3) integrin receptor locked in a high affinity state and a Glanzmann thrombasthenia-like phenotype. *Blood* 2001;98:2432.

95. Chen P, Melchior C, Brons NH, et al. Probing conformational changes in the I-like domain and the cysteine-rich repeat of human $\beta$3 integrins following disulfide bond disruption by cysteine mutations: identification of cysteine 598 involved in $\alpha$IIb$\beta$3 activation. *J Biol Chem* 2001;276:38628.

96. Kiyoi T, Tomiyama Y, Honda S, et al. A naturally occurring Tyr143His $\alpha$IIb mutation abolishes $\alpha$IIb$\beta$3 function for soluble ligands but retains its ability for mediating cell adhesion and clot retraction: comparison with other mutations causing ligand-binding defects. *Blood* 2003;101:3485.

97. Honda S, Tomiyama Y, Shiraga M, et al. A two-amino acid insertion in the Cys146-Cys167 loop of the $\alpha$IIb subunit is associated with a variant of Glanzmann thrombasthenia. *J Clin Invest* 1998;102:1183.

98. Jackson DE, White MM, Jennings LK, et al. A Ser$_{162}$ → Leu mutation within glycoprotein (GP) IIIa (integrin $\beta$3) results in an unstable $\alpha$IIb$\beta$3 complex that retains partial function in a novel form of type II Glanzmann thrombasthenia. *Thromb Haemost* 1998;80:46.

99. Ward CM, Kestin AS, Newman PJ. A Leu262Pro mutation in the integrin β3 subunit results in an αIIbβ3 complex that binds fibrin but not fibrinogen. *Blood* 2000;96:161.
100. Tomiyama Y, Shiraga M, Kinoshita S, et al. A Glanzmann thrombasthenia-like phenotype caused by a defect in inside-out signaling through the integrin αIIbβ3. *Thromb Haemost* 1998;80:735.
101. Yarah N, Fisgin T, Duru F, et al. Osteopetrosis and Glanzmann's thrombasthenia in a child. *Ann Hematol* 2003;82:254.
102. McDowall A, Inwald D, Leitinger B, et al. A novel form of integrin dysfunction involving β1, β2, and β3 integrins. *J Clin Invest* 2003;111:51.
103. Coller BS. Platelet GP IIb/IIIa antagonists: the first anti-integrin receptor therapeutics. *J Clin Invest* 1997;100:S57.
104. Weng S, Zemany L, Standley KN, et al. β3 integrin deficiency promotes atherosclerosis and pulmonary inflammation in high-fat-fed, hyperlipidemic mice. *Proc Natl Acad Sci U S A* 2003;100:6730.
105. Shpilberg O, Rabi I, Schiller K, et al. Patients with Glanzmann thrombasthenia lacking platelet glycoprotein αIIbβ3 (GP IIb/IIIa) and αvβ3 receptors are not protected from atherosclerosis. *Circulation* 2002;105:1044.
106. Gruel Y, Pacouret G, Bellucci S, et al. Severe proximal deep vein thrombosis in a Glanzmann thrombasthenia variant successfully treated with a low molecular weight heparin. *Blood* 1997;90:888.
107. Ten Cate H, Brandies DPM, Smits PHM, et al. The role of platelets in venous thrombosis: a patient with Glanzmann's thrombasthenia and a factor V Leiden mutation suffering from deep vein thrombosis. *Thromb Haemost* 2003;1:394.
108. Reichert N, Seligsohn U, Ramot B. Clinical and genetic studies of Glanzmann's thrombasthenia in Israel. *Thromb Diath Haemorrh* 1975;34:806.
109. Awidi AS. Delivery of infants with a followup of 39 patients. *Am J Hematol* 1992;40:1.
110. Markovitch O, Ellis M, Holzinger M, et al. Severe juvenile vaginal bleeding due to Glanzmann's thrombasthenia: case report and review of the literature. *Am J Hematol* 1998;57:225.
111. Seligsohn U, Rososhansky S. A Glanzmann's thrombasthenia cluster among Iraqi jews in Israel. *Thromb Haemost* 1984;52:230.
112. Guyonnet Duperat V, Vergnes C, Nurden P, et al. Screening for Factor V Leiden and a prothrombin gene polymorphism in patients with Glanzmann's thrombasthenia. *Br J Haematol* 1998;101:592.
113. Jacquelin B, Tarantino MD, Kritzik M, et al. Allele-dependent transcriptional regulation of the human integrin α2 gene. *Blood* 2001;97:1721.
114. DiPaola J, Frederici AB, Mannucci PM, et al. Low platelet α2β1 levels in patients with von Willebrand disease type I represent an increased risk factor for bleeding. *Blood* 1999;93:3578.
115. Jacquelin B, Tuleja E, Kunicki TJ, et al. Analysis of platelet membrane glycoprotein polymorphisms in Glanzmann thrombasthenia showed the French gypsy mutation in the αIIb gene to be strongly linked to the HPA-1b polymorphism in β3. *J Thromb Haemost* 2003;1:573.
116. Horton MA, Massey HM, Rosenberg N, et al. Upregulation of osteoclast α2β1 integrin compensates for lack of αvβ3 vitronectin receptor in Iraqi-Jewish-type Glanzmann thrombasthenia. *Br J Haematol* 2003;122:950.
117. Rosa JP, Kieffer N, Didry D, et al. The human platelet membrane glycoprotein complex GP IIb-IIIa express antigenic sites not exposed on the dissociated glycoprotein. *Blood* 1984;64:1246.
118. Jallu V, Diaz-Ricart M, Ordinas A, et al. Two human antibodies reacting with different epitopes on integrin β3 of platelets and endothelial cells. *Eur J Biochem* 1994;222:743.
119. Gruel Y, Brojer E, Nugent DJ, et al. Further characterization of the thrombasthenia-related idiotype OG. Antiidiotype defines a novel epitope(s) shared by fibrinogen B beta chain, vitronectin, and von Willebrand factor and required for binding to β3. *J Exp Med* 1994;180:2259.
120. Jacobin MJ, Laroche-Traineau J, Little M, et al. Human IgG monoclonal anti-αIIbβ3-binding fragments derived from immunized donors using phage display. *J Immunol* 2002;168:2035.
121. D'Andrea G, Colaizzo D, Vecchione G, et al. Glanzmann's thrombasthenia: identification of 19 new mutations in 30 patients. *Thromb Haemost* 2002;87:1034–1042.
122. Ruan J, Peyruchaud O, Nurden P, et al. Family screening for a Glanzmann's thrombasthenia mutation using PCR-SSCP. *Platelets* 1998;9:129.
123. Seligsohn U, Milbashan RS, Rodeck CH, et al. Prenatal diagnosis in Glanzmann's thrombasthenia. *Lancet* 1985;2:1419.
124. Peretz H, Seligsohn U, Zwang E, et al. Detection of the Glanzmann's thrombasthenia mutations in Arab and Iraqi-Jewish patients by polymerase chain reaction and restriction analysis of blood and urine samples. *Thromb Haemost* 1991;616:500.
125. French D, Coller BS, Usher S, et al. Prenatal diagnosis of Glanzmann thrombasthenia using the polymorphic markers BRCA1 and THRAI on chromosome 17. *Br J Haematol* 1998;102:582.
126. Rao AK. Inherited defects in platelet signaling mechanisms. *J Thromb Haemost* 2003;1:671.
127. Weiss HJ, Rogers J. Fibrinogen and platelets in the primary arrest of bleeding: studies in two patients with congenital afibrinogenemia. *N Engl J Med* 1971;285:369.
128. Mammen EF, Comp PC, Gosselin R, et al. PFA-100 system: a new method for assessment of platelet dysfunction. *Semin Thromb Hemost* 1998;24:195.
129. Varon D, Lashevski I, Brenner B, et al. Cone and plate(let) analyzer: monitoring glycoprotein IIb/IIIa antagonists and von Willebrand disease replacement therapy by testing platelet deposition under flow conditions. *Am Heart J* 1998;135:S187.
130. DiMinno G, Coraggio F, Cerbone AM, et al. A myeloma paraprotein with specificity for platelet glycoprotein IIIa in a patient with a fatal bleeding disorder. *J Clin Invest* 1986;77:157.
131. Niessner H, Clemetson KJ, Panzer S, et al. Acquired thrombasthenia due to GP IIb-IIIa specific autoantibodies. *Blood* 1986;68:571.
132. Deckmyn H, Vanhoorelbeke K, Peerlink K. Inhibitory and activating human antiplatelet antibodies. *Baillières Clin Haematol* 1998;11:343.
133. Fuse I, Higuchi W, Narita M, et al. Overproduction of antiplatelet antibody against glycoprotein IIb after splenectomy in a patient with Evans syndrome resulting in acquired thrombasthenia. *Acta Haematol* 1998;99:83.
134. Malik U, Dutcher JP, Oleksowicz L. Acquired Glanzmann's thrombasthenia associated with Hodgkin's lymphoma: a case report and review of the literature. *Cancer* 1998;82:1764.
135. Macchi L, Nurden P, Marit G, et al. Autoimmune thrombocytopenic purpura (AITP) and acquired thrombasthenia due to autoantibodies to GP IIb-IIIa in a patient with an unusual platelet membrane glycoprotein composition. *Am J Hematol* 1998;57:164.
136. Chen Y, Wu QY, Wang Z, et al. Abnormalities of platelet membrane glycoproteins in acute nonlymphoblastic leukemia (abstract). *Thromb Haemost* 1989;62:176.
137. Garson OM, Hagemeijer A, Kondo K, et al. Chromosomes in acute promyelocytic leukemia. Fourth International Workshop on chromosomes in leukemia. *Cancer Genet Cytogenet* 1984;11:288.
138. Bray PF, Barsh G, Rosa JP, et al. Physical linkage of the genes for platelet membrane glycoproteins IIb and IIIa. *Proc Natl Acad Sci U S A* 1988;85:8683.
139. Yufu Y, Hashimoto M, Muta K, et al. Abnormality of platelet membrane glycoprotein GP IIb in a myelodysplastic syndrome with 3q inversion presenting with marked dysmegakaryopoiesis. *Acta Haematol* 1990;83:107.
140. Bellucci S, Caen J. Molecular basis of Glanzmann's thrombasthenia and current strategies in treatment. *Blood Rev* 2002;16:193.
141. Martin I, Kriaa F, Proulle V, et al. Protein A Sepharose immunoadsorption can restore the efficacy of platelet concentrates in patients with Glanzmann's thrombasthenia and anti-glycoprotein IIb-IIIa antibodies. *Br J Haematol* 2002;119:991.
142. Mannucci PM. Desmopressin: a nontransfusional form of treatment for congenital and acquired bleeding disorders. *Blood* 1988;72:1449.
143. Kaufmann JE, Vischer UM. Cellular mechanisms of the hemostatic effects of desmopressin (DDAVP). *J Thromb Haemost* 2003;1:682.
144. Poon MC, d'Oiron R, Von Depka M, et al. Prophylactic and therapeutic recombinant factor VIIa administration to patients with Glanzmann's thrombasthenia: results of an international survey. *J Thromb Haemost* 2004;38:21.
145. Almeida AM, Khair K, Hann I, et al. The use of recombinant factor VIIa in children with inherited platelet function disorders. *Br J Haematol* 2001;121:477.
146. Lisman T, Moschatsis S, Adelmeijer J, et al. Recombinant factor VIIa enhances deposition of platelets with congenital or acquired αIIbβ3 deficiency to endothelial cell matrix and collagen under conditions of flow via tissue factor-independent thrombin generation. *Blood* 2003;101:1864.
147. Lisman T, Adelmaier J, Heijnen HFG, et al. Recombinant factor VIIa restores aggregation of αIIbβ3-deficient platelets via tissue factor-independent fibrin generation. *Blood* 2004;103:1720.
148. Rakocz M, Lavie G, Martinowitz U. Glanzmann's thrombasthenia: the use of autologous fibrin glue in tooth extractions. *ASDC J Dent Child* 1995;62:129.
149. Leach M, Makris M, Hampton KK, et al. Norethisterone therapy for bleeding due to gastrointestinal telangiectases in Glanzmann's thrombasthenia. *Br J Haematol* 1998;100:594.
150. Okamura T, Kanaji T, Osaki K, et al. Gastrointestinal angiodysplasia in congenital platelet dysfunction. *Int J Hematol* 1996;65:79.
151. DeRose JJ, Diamond S, Bergman K. Spontaneous duodenal hematoma in a patient with Glanzmann's thrombasthenia. *J Pediatr Surg* 1997;32:1341.
152. Nounou R, Spence D. Glanzmann's thrombasthenia with mild von Willebrand's disease. *J Clin Pathol* 1993;46:1134.
153. Bellucci S, Devergie A, Gluckman E, et al. Complete correction of Glanzmann's thrombasthenia by allogeneic bone-marrow transplantation. *Br J Haematol* 1985;59:635.
154. Johnson A, Goodall AH, Downie CJ, et al. Bone marrow transplantation for Glanzmann's thrombasthenia. *Bone Marrow Transplant* 1994;14:147.
155. McColl MD, Gibson BES. Sibling allogeneic bone marrow transplantation in a patient with type I Glanzmann thrombasthenia. *Br J Haematol* 1997;99:58.
156. Bellucci S, Damaj G, Boval B, et al. Bone marrow transplantation in severe Glanzmann's thrombasthenia with antiplatelet alloimmunization. *Bone Marrow Transplant* 2000;25:327.
157. Wilcox DA, White GC, II Gene therapy for platelet disorders: studies with Glanzmann's thrombasthenia. *J Thromb Haemost* 2003;1:2300.
158. Bernard J, Soulier JP. Sur une nouvelle varieté de dystrophie thrombocytaire hémorragipare congénitale. *Sem Hôp Paris* 1948;24:2317.
159. Bithell TC, Parekh SJ, Strong RR. Platelet-function studies in the Bernard-Soulier syndrome. *Ann N Y Acad Sci* 1972;201:145.
160. Bellucci S, Tobelem G, Caen JP. Inherited platelet disorders. *Prog Hematol* 1983;131:223.

161. George JN, Reimann TA, Moake JL, et al. Bernard-Soulier disease. A study of four patients and their parents. *Br J Haematol* 1981;48:459.

162. Rendu F, Nurden AT, Lebret M, et al. Further investigations on Bernard-Soulier abnormalities. A study of 5-hydroxytryptamine uptake and mepacrine fluorescence. *J Lab Clin Med* 1981;97:689.

163. Bernard J, Caen J, Jeanneau C, et al. La dystrophie thrombocytaire hémorragipare. *Acta Haematol* 1974;8:3.

164. McGill M, Jamieson GA, Drouin J, et al. Morphometric analysis of platelets in Bernard-Soulier syndrome: size and configurations in patients and carriers. *Thromb Haemost* 1984;52:37.

165. White JG, Burris SM, Hasegawa D, et al. Micropipette aspiration of human platelets: a defect in Bernard-Soulier syndrome. *Blood* 1984;63:1249.

166. Nurden P, Nurden AT. Giant platelets, megakaryocytes and the expression of glycoprotein Ib-IX complexes. *CR Acad Sci Paris* 1996;319:717.

167. White JG. Use of the electron microscope for diagnosis of platelet disorders. *Semin Thromb Hemost* 1998;24:163.

168. Hourdillé P, Pico M, Jandrot-Perrus M, et al. Studies on the megakaryocytes of the Bernard-Soulier syndrome. *Br J Haematol* 1990;76:521.

169. Howard MA, Hutton RA, Hardisty RM. Hereditary giant platelet syndrome: a disorder of a new aspect of platelet function. *Br Med J* 1973;12:586.

170. Caen JP, Levy-Toledano S. Interaction between platelets and von Willebrand factor provides a new scheme for primary hemostasis. *Nature* 1973;244:159.

171. Moake J, Olson J, Trol JH, et al. Binding of radioiodinated human von Willebrand factor to Bernard-Soulier, thrombasthenic and von Willebrand's disease platelets. *Thromb Res* 1980;19:21.

172. Caen JP, Nurden AT, Jeanneau C, et al. Bernard-Soulier syndrome: a new platelet glycoprotein abnormality, its relationship with platelet adhesion to subendothelium and with the factor VIII von Willebrand protein. *J Lab Clin Med* 1976;87:586.

173. Weiss HJ, Turitto VT, Baumgartner HR. Effects of shear rate on platelet interaction with subendothelium in citrated and native blood. I. Shear-rate dependent decrease of adhesion in von Willebrand's disease and the Bernard-Soulier syndrome. *J Lab Clin Med* 1978;92:750.

174. Peerschke EI, Zucker MB, Grant RA, et al. Correlation between fibrinogen binding to human platelets and platelet aggregability. *Blood* 1980;55:841.

175. Savage B, Almus-Jacobs F, Ruggeri ZM. Specific synergy of multiple substrate-receptor interactions in platelet thrombus formation under flow. *Cell* 1998;94:657.

176. Jamieson GA, Okumura T. Reduced thrombin binding and aggregation in Bernard-Soulier platelets. *J Clin Invest* 1978;61:861.

177. Jandrot-Perrus M, Rendu F, Caen JP, et al. The common pathway for alpha- and gamma-thrombin-induced platelet activation is independent of GP Ib: a study of Bernard-Soulier platelets. *Br J Haematol* 1990;75:385.

178. De Marco L, Mazzucato M, Masotti A, et al. Localization and characterization of an α-thrombin-binding-site on platelet glycoprotein Ibα. *J Biol Chem* 1994;269:6478.

179. Kahn ML, Zheng Y-W, Huang W, et al. A dual thrombin receptor system for platelet activation. *Nature* 1998;394:690.

180. McNichol A, Sutherland M, Zou R, et al. Defective thrombin-induced calcium changes and aggregation of Bernard-Soulier platelets are not associated with deficient moderate-affinity receptors. *Arterioscler Thromb Vasc Biol* 1996;16:628.

181. McNicol A, Drouin J, Clemetson KJ, et al. Phospholipase C activity in platelets from Bernard-Soulier syndrome patients. *Arterioscler Thromb* 1993;13:1567.

182. Suzuki-Inoue K, Wilde JL, Andrews RK, et al. Glycoproteins VI and Ib-IX-V stimulate tyrosine phosphorylation of tyrosine kinase syk and phospholipaseCγ2 at distinct sites. *Biochem J* 2003;378:1023.

183. Beguin S, Keulars I, Al Dieri R, et al. Fibrin polymerization is crucial for thrombin generation in platelet-rich plasma in a VWF-GP Ib-dependent process, defective in Bernard-Soulier syndrome. *J Thromb Haemost* 2004;2:170.

184. Baglia FA, Shrimpton CN, Lopez JA, et al. The glycoprotein Ib-IX-V complex mediates localization of factor XI to lipid rafts on the platelet membrane. *J Biol Chem* 2003;278:21744.

185. Bradford HN, Dela Cadena RA, Kunapuli SP, et al. Human kininogens regulate thrombin binding to platelets through the glycoprotein Ib-IX-V complex. *Blood* 1997;90:1508.

186. Perret B, Levy-Toledano S, Plantavid M, et al. Abnormal phospholipid organization in Bernard-Soulier platelets. *Thromb Res* 1983;31:529.

187. Burgess JK, Lopez JA, Berndt MC, et al. Quinine-dependent antibodies bind a restricted set of epitopes on the glycoprotein Ib-IX complex: characterization of the epitopes. *J Biol Chem* 1998;273:2366.

188. Pfueller SL, Kerlero de Rosbo N, Bilston RA. Platelets deficient in glycoprotein I have normal Fc receptor expression. *Br J Haematol* 1984;56:607.

189. Nurden AT, Dupuis D, Kunicki TJ, et al. Analysis of the glycoprotein and protein composition of Bernard-Soulier platelets by single and two-dimensional sodium dodecyl sulfate-polyacrylamide gel electrophoresis. *J Clin Invest* 1981;67:1431.

190. Coller BS, Peerschke EI, Scudder LE, et al. Studies with a murine monoclonal antibody that abolishes ristocetin-induced binding of von Willebrand factor to platelets: additional evidence in support of GP Ib as a platelet receptor for von Willebrand factor. *Blood* 1983;61:99.

191. McMichael AJ, Rust NA, Pilch JR. Monoclonal antibody to human platelet glycoprotein I. I. Immunological studies. *Br J Haematol* 1981;49:501.

192. Clemetson KJ, McGregor JL, James E, et al. Characterization of the platelet membrane glycoprotein abnormalities in Bernard-Soulier syndrome and comparison with normal by surface-labeling techniques and high-resolution two-dimensional gel electrophoresis. *J Clin Invest* 1982;70:304.

193. Berndt M, Gregory C, Chong BH, et al. Additional glycoprotein defects in Bernard-Soulier syndrome: confirmation of genetic basis by parental analysis. *Blood* 1983;62:800.

194. Drouin J, McGregor JL, Parmentier S, et al. Residual amounts of glycoprotein Ib concomitant with near-absence of glycoprotein IX in platelets of Bernard-Soulier patients. *Blood* 1988;72:1086.

195. Poulson LO, Taaning E. Variation in surface platelet glycoprotein Ib expression in Bernard-Soulier syndrome. *Haemostasis* 1990;20:155.

196. Hillman A, Nurden A, Nurden P, et al. A novel hemizygous Bernard-Soulier syndrome (BSS) mutation in the amino terminal domain of glycoprotein (GP)Ibβ. Platelet characterization and transfection studies. *Thromb Haemost* 2002;88:1026.

197. Tomer A, Scharf RE, McMillan R, et al. Bernard-Soulier syndrome: quantitative characterization of megakaryocytes and platelets by flow cytometric and platelet kinetic measurements. *Eur J Haematol* 1994;52:193.

198. De La Salle C, Baas M-J, Lanza F, et al. A three-base deletion removing a leucine residue in a leucine-rich repeat of platelet glycoprotein Ibα associated with a variant of Bernard-Soulier syndrome (Nancy I). *Br J Haematol* 1995;89:386.

199. De Marco L, Mazzucato M, Fabris F, et al. Variant Bernard-Soulier syndrome type Bolzano. A congenital bleeding disorder due to a structural and functional abnormality of the platelet glycoprotein Ib-IX complex. *J Clin Invest* 1990;86:25.

200. Wu G, Essex DW, Meloni FJ, et al. Human endothelial cells in culture and in vivo express on their surface all four components of the glycoprotein Ib/IX/V complex. *Blood* 1997;90:2660.

201. Beacham DA, Cruz MA, Handin RI. Glycoprotein Ib can mediate endothelial cell attachment to a von Willebrand factor substratum. *Thromb Haemost* 1995;73:309.

202. Perrault C, Lankhof H, Pidard D, et al. Relative importance of the glycoprotein Ib-binding domain and the RGD sequence of von Willebrand factor for its interaction with endothelial cells. *Blood* 1997;90:2335.

203. Wenger RH, Kieffer N, Wicki AN, et al. Structure of the human blood platelet membrane glycoprotein Ibα gene. *Biochem Biophys Res Commun* 1988;156:389.

204. Hickey MJ, Roth GJ. Characterization of the gene encoding human platelet glycoprotein IX. *J Biol Chem* 1993;268:3438.

205. Yagi M, Edelhoff S, Disteche CM, et al. Structural characterization and chromosomal location of the gene encoding human platelet glycoprotein Ibβ. *J Biol Chem* 1994;269:17424.

206. Lanza F, Morales M, de la Salle C, et al. Cloning and characterization of the gene encoding the human platelet glycoprotein V. A member of the leucine-rich glycoprotein family cleaved during thrombin-induced platelet activation. *J Biol Chem* 1993;268:20801.

207. Yagi M, Edelhoff S, Disteche CM, et al. Structural characterization and chromosomal localization of the gene encoding human platelet glycoprotein Ibβ. *J Biol Chem* 1994;269:17424.

208. Simsek S, Admiraal LG, Modderman PW, et al. Kr: identification of a homozygous single base pair deletion in the gene coding for the human platelet glycoprotein Ibα causing Bernard-Soulier syndrome. *Thromb Haemost* 1994;72:444.

209. Kunishima S, Miura H, Fukutani H, et al. Bernard-Soulier syndrome Kagoshima: Ser444 → stop mutation of glycoprotein (GP) Ibα resulting in circulating truncated GPIbα and surface expression of GPIbβ and GP IX. *Blood* 1994;84:3356.

210. Ware J, Russell SR, Vicente V, et al. Nonsense mutation in the glycoprotein Ibα coding sequence associated with Bernard-Soulier syndrome. *Proc Natl Acad Sci U S A* 1990;87:2026.

211. Kanaji T, Okamura T, Kurolwa M, et al. Molecular and genetic analysis of two patients with Bernard-Soulier syndrome identification of new mutations in glycoprotein Ib alpha gene. *Thromb Haemost* 1977;77:1055.

212. Simsek S, Noris P, Lozano M, et al. Cys209Ser mutation in the platelet membrane glycoprotein Ibα gene is associated with Bernard-Soulier syndrome. *Br J Haematol* 1994;88:839.

213. Gonzalez-Manchon C, Larrucea S, Pastor AL, et al. Compound heterozygosity of the GPIbα gene associated with Bernard-Soulier syndrome. *Thromb Haemost* 2001;86:1385.

214. Lopez JA, Leung B, Reynolds CC, et al. Efficient plasma membrane expression of a functional platelet glycoprotein Ib-IX complex requires the presence of its three subunits. *J Biol Chem* 1992;267:12851.

215. Li CQ, Dong J-F, Lanza F, et al. Expression of platelet glycoprotein (GP) V in heterologous cells and evidence for its association with GP Ibα in forming a GP Ib-IX-V complex on the cell surface. *J Biol Chem* 1995;270:16302.

216. Budarf ML, Konkle BA, Ludlow LB, et al. Identification of a patient with a Bernard-Soulier syndrome and a deletion in the DiGeorge/Velo-cardio-facial chromosomal region in 22q11.2. *Hum Mol Genet* 1995;4:763.

217. Kato T, Kosaka K, Kimura M, et al. Thrombocytopenia in patients with 22q11.2 deletion syndrome and its association with glycoprotein Ibβ. *Genet Med* 2003;5:113.

218. Ludlow LB, Schick BP, Budarf ML, et al. Identification of a mutation in a GATA binding site of the platelet glycoprotein Ibβ promoter resulting in the Bernard-Soulier syndrome. *J Biol Chem* 1996;271:22076.

219. Watanabe R, Ishibashi T, Saitoh Y, et al. Bernard-Soulier syndrome with a homozygous 13 base pair deletion in the signal peptide-coding region of the platelet glycoprotein Ibβ gene. *Blood Coagul Fibrinolysis* 2003;14:387.

220. Kenny D, Morateck PA, Gill JC, et al. The critical interaction of glycoprotein (GP) Ibβ with GP IX—a genetic cause of Bernard-Soulier syndrome. *Blood* 1999;93:2968.

221. Tang J, Stern-Nezer S, Liu P-C, et al. Mutation in the leucine-rich repeat C-flanking region of platelet glycoprotein Ibβ impairs assembly of von Willebrand factor receptor. *Thromb Haemost* 2004;92:75.

222. Strassel C, Pasquet J-M, Alessi M-C, et al. A novel missense mutation shows that GPIbβ has a dual role in controlling the processing and stability of the platelet GP Ib-IX adhesion receptor. *Biochemistry* 2003;42:4452.

223. Kunishima S, Tomiyama Y, Honda S, et al. Homozygous Pro74 → Arg mutation in the platelet glycoprotein Ibβ gene associated with Bernard-Soulier syndrome. *Thromb Haemost* 2000;84:112.

224. Kurokawa Y, Ishida F, Kamijo T, et al. A missense mutation (Tyr88 to Cys) in the platelet membrane glycoprotein Ibβ gene affects GP Ib/IX complex expression. Bernard-Soulier syndrome in the homozygous form and giant platelets in the heterozygous form. *Thromb Haemost* 2001;86:1249.

225. Wright SD, Michaelides K, Johnson DJD, et al. Double heterozygosity for mutations in the platelet glycoprotein IX gene in three siblings with Bernard-Soulier syndrome. *Blood* 1993;81:2339.

226. Clemetson KJ, Kyrie PA, Brenner B, et al. Variant Bernard-Soulier syndrome associated with a homozygous mutation in the leucine-rich domain of glycoprotein IX. *Blood* 1994;84:1124.

227. Koskela S, Javela K, Jouppila J, et al. Variant Bernard-Soulier syndrome due to homozygous Asn45Ser mutation in the platelet glycoprotein (GP) IX in seven patients of five unrelated Finnish families. *Eur J Haematol* 1999;62:256.

228. Sachs UJH, Kroll H, Matzdorff AC, et al. Bernard-Soulier syndrome due to the homozygous Asn-45Ser mutation in GP IX: an unexpected finding in Germany. *Br J Haematol* 2003;123:127.

229. Noris P, Simsek S, Stibbe J, et al. A phenylalanine-55 to serine amino acid substitution in the human glycoprotein IX leucine-rich repeat is associated with Bernard-Soulier syndrome. *Br J Haematol* 1997;97:312.

230. Noda M, Fujimura K, Takafuta T, et al. A point mutation in glycoprotein IX coding sequence Cys73(TGT) to Tyr(TAT) causes impaired surface expression of GP Ib/IX/V complex in two families with Bernard-Soulier syndrome. *Thromb Haemost* 1996;76:874.

231. Noda M, Fujimura K, Takafuta T, et al. Heterogeneous expression of glycoprotein Ib, IX and V in platelets from two patients with Bernard-Soulier syndrome caused by different genetic abnormalities. *Thromb Haemost* 1995;74:1411.

232. Sae-Tung G, Dong JF, Lopez JA. Biosynthetic defect in platelet glycoprotein IX mutants associated with Bernard-Soulier syndrome. *Blood* 1996;87:1361.

233. Lanza F, De La Salle C, Baas M-J, et al. A Leu7Pro mutation in the signal peptide of platelet glycoprotein (GP)IX in a case of Bernard-Soulier syndrome abolishes surface expression of the GP Ib-V-IX complex. *Br J Haematol* 2002;118:260.

234. Miller JL, Lyle VA, Cunningham D. Mutation of leucine-57 to phenylalanine in a platelet glycoprotein Ibα leucine tandem repeat occurring in patients with an autosomal dominant variant of Bernard-Soulier disease. *Blood* 1992;79:439.

235. Ware J, Russell SR, Marchese P, et al. Point mutation in a leucine-rich repeat of platelet glycoprotein Ibα resulting in the Bernard-Soulier syndrome. *J Clin Invest* 1993;92:1213.

236. Huizinga EG, Tsuji S, Romijn RAP, et al. Structures of glycoprotein Ibα and its complex with von Willebrand factor A1 domain. *Science* 2002;297:1176.

237. Ulsemer P, Lanza F, Baas MJ, et al. Role of the leucine-rich domain of platelet GPIbα in correct post-translational processing—the Nancy I Bernard-Soulier mutation expressed on CHO cells. *Thromb Haemost* 2000;84:104.

238. Li C, Martin SE, Roth GJ. The genetic defect in two well-studied cases of Bernard-Soulier syndrome: a point mutation in the fifth leucine-rich repeat of platelet glycoprotein Ibα. *Blood* 1995;86:3805.

239. Kunishima S, Lopez JA, Kobayashi S, et al. Missense mutations of the glycoprotein (GP) Ibβ gene impairing the GP Ib α/β disulfide linkage in a family with giant platelet disorder. *Blood* 1997;89:2404.

240. Ware J, Russell S, Ruggeri ZM. Generation and rescue of a murine model of platelet dysfunction: the Bernard-Soulier syndrome. *Proc Natl Acad Sci U S A* 2000;97:2803.

241. Poujol C, Ware J, Nieswandt B, et al. Absence of GPIbα is responsible for aberrant membrane development during megakaryocyte maturation: ultrastructural study using a transgenic model. *Exp Hematol* 2002;30:352.

242. Poujol C, Ramakrishnan V, Deguzman F, et al. Ultrastructural analysis of megakaryocytes in GP V knockout mice. *Thromb Haemost* 2000;84:312.

243. Kanaji T, Russell S, Ware J. Amelioration of the macrothrombocytopenia with the murine Bernard-Soulier syndrome. *Blood* 2002;100:2102.

244. Kato K, Martinez C, Russell S, et al. Genetic deletion of mouse platelet glycoprotein Ibβ produces a Bernard-Soulier phenotype with increased α-granule size. *Blood* 2004;104:2339.

245. Savoia A, Balduini CL, Savino M, et al. Autosomal dominant macrothrombocytopenia in Italy is most frequently a type of heterozygous Bernard-Soulier syndrome. *Blood* 2001;97:1330.

246. Heath KE, Campos-Barros A, Toren A, et al. Nonmuscle myosin heavy chain IIA mutations define a spectrum of autosomal dominant macrothrombocytopenias: May Hegglin Anomaly and Fechtner, Sebastian, Epstein, and Alport-like Syndromes. *Am J Hum Genet* 2001;69:1033.

247. Balduini CL, Cattaneo M, Fabris M, et al. Inherited thrombocytopenias: a proposed diagnostic algorithm from the *Italian Gruppo di Studio delle Piastrine*. *Haematologica* 2003;88:582.

248. Epstein CJ, Sahud MA, Piel CF, et al. Hereditary macrothrombocytopathia, nephritis and deafness. *Am J Med* 1972;52:299.

249. Peterson LC, Rao KV, Crosson JT, et al. Fechtner syndrome—A variant of Alport's syndrome with leukocyte inclusions and macrothrombocytopenia. *Blood* 1985;65:397.

250. Heynen MJ, Blackmans D, Verwilghen RL, et al. Congenital macrothrombocytopenia, leukocyte inclusions deafness and proteinuria : functional and electron microscopic observations on platelets and megakaryocytes. *Br J Haematol* 1988;70:441.

251. Greinacher A, Nieuwenhuis HK, White JG. Sebastian platelet syndrome: a new variant of hereditary macrothrombocytopenia with leukocyte inclusions. *Blut* 1990;61:282.

252. Milton JG, Frojmovic MM, Tang SS, et al. Spontaneous platelet aggregation in a hereditary giant platelet syndrome (MPS). *Am J Pathol* 1984;114:336.

253. Okita JR, Frojmovic MM, Kristopeit S, et al. Montreal platelet syndrome: a defect in calcium-activated neutral protease (calpain). *Blood* 1989;74:715.

254. Nurden AT, Kunicki TJ, Dupuis D, et al. Specific protein and glycoprotein deficiencies in platelets isolated from two patients with the gray platelet syndrome. *Blood* 1982;59:709.

255. Nurden P, Jandrot-Perrus M, Combrié R, et al. Severe deficiency of glycoprotein VI in a patient with gray platelet syndrome. *Blood* 2004;104:107.

256. He R, Reid DM, Jones CE, et al. Extracellular epitopes of platelet glycoprotein Ibα reactive with serum antibodies from patients with chronic idiopathic thrombocytopenic purpura. *Blood* 1995;86:3789.

257. Stricker RB, Wong D, Saks SR, et al. Acquired Bernard-Soulier syndrome. *J Clin Invest* 1985;76:1274.

258. Devine DV, Currie MS, Rosse WF, et al. Pseudo-Bernard-Soulier syndrome: thrombocytopenia caused by autoantibody to platelet glycoprotein Ib. *Blood* 1987;70:428.

259. Varon D, Gitel SN, Varon N, et al. Immune Bernard-Soulier–like syndrome associated with anti-glycoprotein-IX antibody. *Am J Hematol* 1992;41:67.

260. Sanchez Roig MJ, Rivera J, Moraleda JM, et al. An acquired Bernard-Soulier–like platelet defect in a patient with liver cirrhosis. *Eur J Haematol* 1994;52:240.

261. Beales Il. An acquired-pseudo Bernard-Soulier syndrome occurring with autoimmune chronic active hepatitis and anti-cardiolipin antibody. *Postgrad Med J* 1994;70:305.

262. Korte W, Baumgartner C, Feldges A, et al. Coincidence of familial platelet glycoprotein Ib/IX deficiency (Bernard-Soulier syndrome), idiopathic autoantibody against platelet glycoprotein Ib/IX, familial appearance of antiphospholipid antibodies, and familial factor XII deficiency. *Ann Hematol* 1994;68:101.

263. Poujol C, Bergmeier W, Nurden P, et al. Effect of infusing rat monoclonal antibodies to the murine GP Ib-IX-V complex on platelet and megakaryocyte morphology in mice. *Platelets* 2003;14:35.

264. Berndt MC, Kabral A, Grimsley P, et al. An acquired Bernard-Soulier-like defect associated with juvenile myelodysplastic syndrome. *Br J Haematol* 1988;68:97.

265. Hicsonmez G, Gumruk F, Cetin M, et al. Bernard-Soulier-like functional platelet defect in myelodysplastic syndrome and in acute myeloblastic leukemia associated with trilineage myelodysplasia. *Turk J Pediatr* 1995;37:425.

266. Degos L, Tobelem G, Lethielleux P, et al. Molecular defects in platelets from patients with Bernard-Soulier syndrome. *Blood* 1977;50:899.

267. Lozano M, Escolar G, Bellucci S, et al. 1-Deamino (8-D-arginine) vasopressin infusion partially corrects platelet deposition in Bernard-Soulier syndrome: the role of factor VIII. *Platelets* 1999;10:141.

268. Peters M, Heijboer H. Treatment of a patient with Bernard-Soulier syndrome and recurrent nosebleeds with recombinant factor VIIa. *Thromb Haemost* 1998;80:352.

269. Humphries JE, Yirinec BA, Hess CE. Atherosclerosis and unstable angina in Bernard-Soulier syndrome. *Am J Clin Pathol* 1992;97:652.

270. Miller JL, Cunningham D, Lyle VA, et al. Mutation in the gene encoding the alpha chain of platelet glycoprotein Ib in platelet-type von Willebrand disease. *Proc Natl Acad Sci U S A* 1991;88:4761.

271. Russell SD, Roth GJ. Pseudo-von Willebrand disease: a mutation in the platelet glycoprotein Ib gene associated with a hyperactive surface receptor. *Blood* 1993;81:1787.

272. Matsubara Y, Murata M, Sugita K, et al. Identification of a novel point mutation in platelet glycoprotein Ibα, Gly to Ser at residue 233, in a Japanese family with platelet-type von Willebrand disease. *J Thromb Haemost* 2003;1:2198.

273. Dong J-F, Schader AJ, Romo GM, et al. Novel gain-of-function mutations of platelet glycoprotein Ibα by valine mutagenesis in the Cys209-Cys248 disulfide loop. Functional analysis under static and dynamic conditions. *J Biol Chem* 2000;275:27663.

274. Doggett TA, Girdhar G, Lawshe A, et al. Alterations in the intrinsic properties of the GPIbα-VWF tether bond define the kinetics of the platelet-type von Willebrand disease mutation, Gly233Val. *Blood* 2003;102:152.

275. Nieuwenhuis HK, Akkerman JWN, Houdijk WPM, et al. Human blood platelets showing no response to collagen fail to express surface glycoprotein Ia. *Nature* 1985;318:470.

276. Nieuwenhuis HK, Sakariassen KS, Houdijk WPM, et al. Deficiency of platelet membrane glycoprotein Ia associated with a decreased platelet adhesion to subendothelium: a defect in platelet spreading. *Blood* 1986;68:692.

277. Kehrel B, Balleisen L, Kokott R, et al. Deficiency of intact thrombospondin and membrane glycoprotein Ia in platelets with defective collagen-induced aggregation and spontaneous loss of disorder. *Blood* 1988; 71:1074.

278. Nieswandt B, Watson SP. Platelet-collagen interaction: is GP VI the central receptor. *Blood* 2003;102:449.

279. Moroi M, Jung SM, Okuma M, et al. A patient with platelets deficient in glycoprotein VI that lack both collagen-induced aggregation and adhesion. *J Clin Invest* 1989;84:1440.

280. Holtkotter O, Nieswandt B, Smyth N, et al. Integrin α2-deficient mice develop normally, are fertile, but display partially defective platelet interaction with collagen. *J Biol Chem* 2002;277:10789.

281. Kato K, Kanaji T, Russell S, et al. The contribution of glycoprotein VI to stable platelet adhesion and thrombus formation illustrated by targeted gene deletion. *Blood* 2003;102:1701.

282. Deckmyn H, Chew SL, Vermylen J. Lack of platelet response to collagen associated with an autoantibody against glycoprotein Ia: a novel cause of acquired qualitative platelet dysfunction. *Thromb Haemost* 1990;64:74.

283. Sugiyama T, Okuma M, Ushikubi F, et al. A novel platelet aggregating factor found in a patient with defective collagen-induced platelet aggregation and autoimmune thrombocytopenia. *Blood* 1987;69:1712.

284. Boylan B, Chen H, Rathore V, et al. Anti-GP VI-associated ITP: an acquired platelet disorder caused by autoantibody-mediated clearance of the GPVI/FcRγ-chain complex from the human platelet surface. *Blood* 2004; 104:1350.

285. Di Paula J, Federici AB, Mannucci PM, et al. Low platelet α2β1 levels in type I von Willebrand disease correlate with impaired platelet function in a high shear stress system. *Blood* 1999;93:3578.

286. Joutsi-Korhonen L, Smethurst PA, Rankin A, et al. The low-frequency allele of the platelet collagen signaling receptor glycoprotein VI is associated with reduced functional responses and expression. *Blood* 2003;101:4372.

287. Gachet C. ADP receptors of platelets and their inhibition. *Thromb Haemost* 2001;86:222.

288. Cattaneo M, Lecchi A, Randi AM, et al. Identification of a new congenital defect of platelet function characterized by severe impairment of platelet responses to adenosine diphosphate. *Blood* 1992;80:2787.

289. Nurden P, Savi P, Heilmann E, et al. An inherited bleeding disorder linked to a defective interaction between ADP and its receptor on platelets. *J Clin Invest* 1995;95:1612.

290. Hollopeter G, Jantzen H-M, Vincent D, et al. Identification of the platelet ADP receptor targeted by antithrombotic drugs. *Nature* 2001;409:202.

291. Cattaneo M, Zighetti ML, Lombardi R, et al. Molecular bases of defective signal transduction in the platelet P2Y12 receptor of a patient with congenital bleeding. *Proc Natl Acad Sci U S A* 2003;100:1978.

292. Levy-Toledano S, Maclouf J, Rosa JP, et al. Abnormal tyrosine phosphorylation linked to a defective interaction between ADP and its receptor on platelets. *Thromb Haemost* 1998;80:463.

293. Remijn JA, Wu Y-P, Jeninga EH, et al. Role of ADP receptor P2Y12 in platelet adhesion and thrombus formation in flowing blood. *Arterioscler Thromb Vasc Biol* 2002;22:68.

294. André P, Delaney SM, LaRocca T, et al. P2Y12 regulates platelet adhesion/activation, thrombus growth, and thrombus stability in injured arteries. *J Clin Invest* 2003;112:398.

295. Cattaneo M, Lecchi A, Lombardi R, et al. Platelets from a patient heterozygous for the defect of P2CYC receptors for ADP have a secretion defect despite normal thromboxane A2 production and normal granule stores: further evidence that some cases of platelet primary secretion defect are heterozygous for a defect of P2YCYC receptors. *Arterioscler Thromb Vasc Biol* 2000;20:101.

296. Oury C, Toth-Zsamboki E, Van Geet C, et al. A natural dominant negative P2X1 receptor due to deletion of a single amino acid residue. *J Biol Chem* 2000;275:23611.

297. Hirata T, Ushikubi F, Kakizuka A, et al. Two thromboxane A2 receptor isoforms in human platelets. Opposite coupling to adenylate cyclase with different sensitivity to Arg⁶⁰ to leu mutation. *J Clin Invest* 1996;97:949.

298. Higuchi W, Fuse I, Hattori A, et al. Mutations of the platelet thromboxane A2 (TXA2) receptor in patients characterized by the absence of TXA2-induced platelet aggregation despite normal TXA2 binding activity. *Thromb Haemost* 1999;82:1528.

299. Tamponi G, Pannocchia A, Arduino C, et al. Congenital deficiency of alpha-2-adrenoceptors on human platelets: description of two cases. *Thromb Haemost* 1987;58:1012.

300. Rao AK, Willis J, Kowalska MA, et al. Differential requirements for platelet aggregation and inhibition of adenylate cyclase by epinephrine. Studies of a familial platelet α2-adrenergic receptor defect. *Blood* 1988;71:494.

301. Coughlin SR. Protease-activated receptors in vascular biology. *Thromb Haemost* 2001;86:298.

302. Sims PJ, Wiedmer T, Esmon CT, et al. Assembly of the platelet prothrombinase complex is linked to vesiculation of the platelet plasma membrane. Studies in Scott syndrome: an isolated defect in platelet procoagulant activity. *J Biol Chem* 1989;264:17049.

303. Toti F, Satta N, Fressinaud E, et al. Scott syndrome characterized by impaired transmembrane migration of procoagulant phospholipids and hemorrhagic complications, is a genetic disorder. *Blood* 1996;87:1409.

304. Zwaal RF, Comfurius P, Bevers EM. Scott syndrome, a bleeding disorder caused by a defective scrambling of membrane phospholipids. *Biochim Biophys Acta* 2004;1636:119.

305. Dachary-Prigent J, Pasquet JM, Fressinaud E, et al. Aminophospholipid exposure, microvesiculation and abnormal protein tyrosine phosphorylation in the platelets of a patient with Scott syndrome: a study using physiologic agonists and local anaesthetics. *Br J Haematol* 1997;99:959.

306. Zhou Q, Sims PJ, Wiedmer T. Expression of proteins controlling transbilayer movement of plasma membrane phospholipids in the B lymphocytes from a patient with Scott syndrome. *Blood* 1998;92:1707.

307. Martinez MC, Martin S, Toti F, et al. Significance of capacitative Ca²⁺ entry in the regulation of phosphatidylserine expression at the surface of stimulated cells. *Biochemistry* 1999;38:10092.

308. Humphries MJ, Mould AP. Structure. An anthropomorphic integrin. *Science* 2001;294:316.

# CHAPTER 67 ■ PRIMARY VASCULAR DISORDERS

MARC ZUMBERG AND CRAIG S. KITCHENS

Confined to the vascular system, blood comes into contact only with endothelial cells, which line all macrovascular, microvascular, and sinusoidal systems. Disruption of this closed system leads to bleeding, either to gross bleeding (characteristic of macrovascular hemorrhage) or to extravasation into tissue (more typical of microvascular leakage). As outlined in Table 67-1, the nature, causes, consequences, therapeutic approaches, and even the physicians addressing these issues are distinct. Bleeding occurs chiefly by at least one of the three possible mechanisms: trauma, physical disruption, or hemostatic failure, none of which are necessarily exclusive. This chapter focuses on hemorrhagic processes that are caused by nontraumatic weakening of the vascular wall. The primary goal of the chapter is development of the differential diagnosis of purpura, and an approach to patients treated for purpura. Treatment of each disease is not feasible and the reader is referred to more in-depth reviews of each disease.

Sudden hemorrhage (which is characteristic of macrovascular disruption) leads to alterations in blood volume, with patients often presenting with shock and usually with pain. Purpura, ecchymoses, and especially petechiae are not characteristic. In microvascular disruption, leakage of red cells from extravasated blood displayed as petechiae and purpura is characteristic, whereas alterations in blood volume and blood pressure from blood loss are generally not characteristic. Less commonly, shock caused by infectious causes of purpura may occur. During histories and physical examinations, complaints of purpura are quite common, with up to 65% of healthy women and 25% of healthy men stating that they bruise easier than normal (1). Accordingly, this is a common complaint in general medical practice. Much of what is considered by patients as being excessive bleeding is actually mild traumatic purpura. Three defining characteristics of these benign "normal" lesions are that they are never true (i.e., palpable) hematomas, they number no more than four to six on the body at one time, and usually lesions are no larger than approximately 3 cm.

Petechiae are pinpoint lesions that are brilliant "cayenne pepper red" when they first appear. Petechiae are usually less than 2 mm in diameter. They soon fade to salmon color in a few days, and then finally become brownish because of the hemosiderin retained from extravasated blood, unless a new crop occurs.

Ecchymosis refers to larger extravasations, which occur either from coalescence of separate petechial lesions or, more commonly, from a bleed from a slightly larger vessel.

Purpura can be the obvious presentation of a variety of illnesses, which is further discussed in the section on microvascular disruption. Any leakage of blood may well have hematologic causes, and therefore the hematologist may be consulted. However, as often as not, there is not a true hemostatic defect, and therefore the hematologist must retain a broad base in medical knowledge and interest. Establishing the diagnosis from a broad differential perspective, as well as opening various therapeutic and prognostic windows is key and oftentimes the essence of treatment.

A modicum of hemostatic tests should be done at the initiation of the consultation. These tests, combined with the history and physical examination, usually differentiate the hematologic causes from the other causes (see Table 67-2). A thorough list of prescribed, nonprescribed, borrowed, and over-the-counter medications to include herbal and alternative medicines should be elicited. Systemic symptoms such as weight loss, chills, fevers, and night sweats, as well as malaise, are key indicators. Thorough examination, including auscultation of the heart, and examination for lymphadenopathy and splenomegaly, should be undertaken.

## MACROVASCULAR DISRUPTION

Macrovascular disruption most often occurs suddenly as a result of trauma or severe atherosclerotic processes, such as a ruptured abdominal aortic aneurysm. Whereas management of macrovascular hemorrhage is beyond the scope of this text, reference is made to disease processes for which the hematologist may be asked to consult and assist.

Macrovascular hemorrhage may occur primarily as a result of one of the six broad categories (see Table 67-3). The first two, trauma and atherosclerotic processes, are not discussed here. The four broad categories that may be termed as primary vascular disorders of the macrocirculation include disorders of connective tissue, infiltration of macrovascular vessels with amyloid, inflammatory processes involving the macrocirculation, and certain arteriovenous malformations. The assignment of disorders to either microvascular or macrovascular disorders is imperfect because some processes fit into either niche.

## TRUE DISORDERS OF CONNECTIVE TISSUE

### Ehlers-Danlos Syndrome

Ehlers-Danlos syndrome (EDS) encompasses the clinical manifestations of a true collagen-vascular disease (2). (In this section, we are not discussing rheumatic diseases such as lupus erythematosus, which previously was regarded as a collagen-vascular disease.) This clinically and genetically heterogeneous connective tissue disorder is characterized by abnormalities in the genetic coding of the various subtypes of collagen. Advances in the basic understanding of abnormalities of the various subtypes of EDS have been reviewed (3,4). In brief, there are nine

**TABLE 67-1**

CHARACTERISTICS OF MACROVASCULAR AND MICROVASCULAR VESSEL BLEEDING

|  | Large vessel | Small vessel |
|---|---|---|
| Vessel | Typically named | Typically unnamed |
| Nature of bleeding | Sudden gush | Slow ooze |
| Primary promoter | Vessel wall | Hemostatic system |
| Pathophysiology | Trauma, disruption | Hemostatic failure |
| Physician | Surgeon | Hematologist |
| Therapeutic approach | Ligature, cautery | Diagnose cause |
|  |  | Enhance hemostasis |

identifiable subtypes, each with specific genetic abnormalities, six of which are considered to be primary clinical variants and three to be primary biochemical variants (5).

Several groups have studied kindreds with EDS seeking disorders of the hemostatic system, yet have discovered no thematic defects (6,7). Anstey et al. studied a group of 51 patients, and found that although only 8% demonstrated any type of abnormal bleeding, 82% of the entire group showed normal results for plasma-based coagulation tests (7). The abnormalities in the results of hemostatic tests of the remaining 18% of these patients were thought not to be of clinical significance. Therefore, general consensus is that bleeding is caused by alterations in the structure of collagen allowing for weakened collagen and/or collagen that does not adequately enhance hemostasis. Most of the "bleeding" that these patients exhibit is the general tendency for their skin to be weak, thin, and to heal poorly, leading to tears with subcutaneous bruising. These abnormalities lead to the so-called cigarette paper skin characteristic of some EDS subtypes. Other problems reflecting the underlying connective tissue disorder are the spontaneous dislocation of joints and the tendency to be "double jointed."

Among the several subtypes of EDS, type IV appears to be one of the rarest, and yet it has the worst hemorrhagic potential in relation to arterial hemorrhage (8,9). Type IV EDS is the

disorder the hematologist is most likely to encounter. Median survival appears to be 48 years in this autosomal-dominant subtype. The specific abnormality in type IV EDS is the production of abnormal type III collagen. This abnormality accounts for the structural compromise of these vessels, which, in turn, accounts for their tendency to rupture.

The primary causes for death in EDS are rupture of large named intraabdominal arteries followed by colonic perforation. Freeman et al. (10) reviewed 90 surgical procedures encountered over a 20-year period of which 41 were for colonic perforations, 17 for arterial aneurysm repair, and 17 for spontaneous hemorrhages from ruptured arteries. Twenty-three percent of his patients died from a gastrointestinal (GI) problem and 30% died from vascular complications. Their review showed that treatment with fresh frozen plasma, cryoprecipitate, or any other hemostatic agent did not aid the patient's situation. They also noted that while attempting to repair these large muscular arteries, the use of vascular clamps was fraught with complications. Maltz et al. (11) concluded that hemorrhaging vessels should be ligated and none should be clamped. Other conservative methods were advocated, such as a great reluctance to operate, use of bedrest, and the generous and continued use of external compression.

**TABLE 67-2**

EVALUATION OF THE PATIENT WITH PETECHIAE, PURPURA, OR ECCHYMOSIS

After a complete history and physical examination, the following laboratory examinations should be considered.

| | |
|---|---|
| Always | Complete blood count and review of blood smear |
| | Partial thromboplastic time and prothrombin time |
| Additional tests to be considered if diagnosis not apparent | Thrombin time |
| | Fibrinogen level |
| | Analyses for fibrin degradation products and D-dimers |
| Additional tests to be considered in cases of cutaneous vasculitis | Skin biopsy |
| | Hepatitis B and C |
| | Antinuclear antibody (ANA) |
| | Antineutrophilic cytoplasmic antibody (ANCA) |
| | Rheumatoid factor (RF) |
| | Serum protein electrophoresis (SPEP) |
| | Complement |
| | HIV |
| Additional tests to be considered in obscure cases | Blood cultures |
| | Viral studies |
| | Bone marrow aspirate/biopsy |

## TABLE 67-3

MACROVASCULAR DISORDERS THAT MAY LEAD
TO HEMORRHAGE

1. Trauma
2. Atherosclerosis
3. Disorders of connective tissue
   a. Ehlers-Danlos syndrome
   b. Osteogenesis imperfecta
   c. Pseudoxanthoma elasticum
   d. Marfan syndrome and cystic medial degeneration
4. Infiltration with amyloid
5. Inflammatory vasculitis
   a. Syphilis
   b. Tuberculosis
   c. Mycotic aneurysms
   d. Rheumatic disorders (RA, SLE, PAN, etc.)
   e. Kawasaki disease
6. Arteriovenous malformations
   a. Hemangiomas
   b. Kaposiform hemangioendothelioma
   c. Hereditary hemorrhagic telangiectasia

RA, rheumatiod arthritis; SLE, systemic lupus erythematosus;
PAN, polyarteridis nodusa.

## Osteogenesis Imperfecta

Osteogenesis imperfecta (OI) is another true collagen-vascular disorder, as type I collagen is defective because of several described defects in the genes encoding for type I procollagen (12). Type I collagen is found primarily in bone, ligaments, tendons, skin, and sclerae, as well as dentin. Type I collagen is not a major component of blood vessels and therefore disorders of type I collagen are not typically hemorrhagic in their presentation. Although OI is occasionally mentioned as a collagen–vascular disease having hemorrhagic tendencies and presenting with purpuric lesions, the bruising is so minimal that it hardly serves any diagnostic purpose in the management of OI. Indeed, modern reviews of this disorder fail to mention clinical hemostatic defects, despite the several surgical needs presented by OI (12,13).

## Pseudoxanthoma Elasticum

Pseudoxanthoma elasticum (PXE) is another disease resulting from derangement of tensile strength in connective tissues that occasionally may be associated with subcutaneous evulsion of tissue resulting in minimal purpura. Purpura and bleeding, however, are not cardinal manifestations of this disease. PXE appears to be caused by homozygous (or double heterozygous) inheritance of mutations involving the *ABCC6* gene leading to degeneration of elastic fibers in the skin, retina, and cardiovascular system. The primary artery that ruptures is that of the gastric mucosa and therefore GI bleeding may occur. This disease has recently been reviewed (14,15).

## Marfan Syndrome and Cystic Medial Degeneration

Marfan syndrome results from mutations in genes encoding for production of fibrillin-1, a component of normal connective tissue (16). This autosomal-dominant syndrome has several defining features, such as a marked tendency toward dissection of the aorta with aneurysmal formation, the chief cause of death in this syndrome. Bleeding or bruising of the skin is rare and hemostatic defects are not encountered, despite the enormity of corrective cardiothoracic surgery in this disorder (17).

The histologic lesion that is uniformly seen in the aortic wall of Marfan syndrome is termed as cystic medial degeneration. There are many patients who have the identical histologic lesion, but they do not share any of the other features of Marfan syndrome. Most often these are patients who are older than those with Marfan syndrome and there appears to be no familial pattern of inheritance. The cause of their cystic medial degeneration of the aorta is unknown, but the effect on the aorta and resultant aneurysmal formation and its treatment are the same as for Marfan syndrome.

## LARGE VESSEL INFILTRATION

Amyloidosis and its hemorrhagic manifestations are generally microvascular in nature but may involve the great vessels of the brain and therefore are included here. Amyloidosis is not a single disorder but a series of disorders, all of which have in common the misfolding of any number of proteins giving rise to β-pleated sheets that reside beneath the basement membrane of multiple structures, to include blood vessels. All these proteins have in common a birefringent apple green color on staining effected tissue with Congo red in polarized light, as well as the typical pattern of microfibrils on electron microscopy (18). More than 20 types of amyloid have been described and each abnormality has subtle variations in its clinical manifestations (19). Vessel wall strength may be reduced and therefore simple mechanical stress or sheer force may result in bleeding which is seen in 28% of patients with amyloidosis (20). Purpura about the face seems especially common in amyloidosis and is discussed more in the section on microvascular purpura of this chapter. Of interest, spontaneous rupture of the spleen has been described in AL amyloidosis and in fact may be the presenting symptom (21).

A unique subset of amyloidosis that clearly has hemorrhagic macrovascular ramifications is cerebral amyloid angiopathy (CAA), which in the past has also been referred to as congophilic angiopathy. There are several subtypes of CAA, to include sporadic and familiar subtypes, all of which have as yet undetermined causes (22,23). In CAA, amyloid deposition of the cerebral arteries is characteristic. CAA is extremely common, and may be present in approximately half of all elderly individuals at autopsy. This is one of the leading causes of spontaneous cerebral hemorrhage, accounting for approximately 10% to 15% of all such bleeds (23). CAA has medical–legal implications, because many older patients are receiving chronic anticoagulation therapy, and this is often blamed for the occurrence of the hemorrhagic event, whereas the true underlying cause is more likely CAA (24). There also is a peculiar and uncertain relation between CAA and Alzheimer disease because cerebral vessels containing amyloid are seen in 80% of patients with Alzheimer disease (23).

## INFLAMMATORY PROCESSES

Any one of the several inflammatory processes may involve large vessels and subsequently lead to their rupture and hemorrhage.

Infectious causes have classically included syphilitic aortitis and although rarely seen now, in previous eras, it was the prevalent cause of aortic aneurysms. Tuberculous arteritis can conceivably affect any artery (25). Mycotic aneurysms (26) may accompany almost any infection, but are classically seen in subacute bacterial endocarditis (27), and unfortunately lead to hemorrhage, particularly in the central nervous system (CNS). HIV infection has been implicated as a cause of inflammatory vasculitis causing large vessel damage (28).

Any of the classic inflammatory rheumatic diseases, such as rheumatoid arthritis, periarteritis nodosa, relapsing polychondritis, Behçet syndrome (29), giant cell arteritis (30), and systemic lupus erythematosus (SLE) (31) occasionally involve large vessels with inflammation, weakening, and eventual rupture and sudden hemorrhage. Probably the best understood relation is with rheumatoid vasculitis (32), which, paradoxically, may occur in older patients with quiescent arthritic manifestations, yet may perforate large arteries. Kawasaki disease is an inflammatory process of the arteries that occurs in childhood and in a small number of patients; panvasculitis occurs with particular reference to coronary vessels, which may lead to aneurysmal dilation of these vessels (33).

# ARTERIOVENOUS MALFORMATIONS/ HEMANGIOMAS

Recent discoveries have changed our knowledge and understanding of the pathogenesis of this autonomic disorder. Whereas, in the past, most of the terms used to define these entities as separate diseases were based on epidemiology, clinical presentations, or even treatment, an explosion of the understanding of the basic science of vascular endothelial growth has already begun to change not only our understanding but even the classification of these disorders. Ultimately, there is no doubt that new treatments will be discovered as our knowledge increases. Accordingly, processes as diverse as Kaposi sarcoma, hereditary hemorrhagic telangiectasia, and diabetic retinopathy may have more in common than we would otherwise ever have imagined (34).

Many of these processes have at their core, abnormal and sustained proliferation of endothelial cells caused by either upregulation of growth-promoting factors and/or inhibition of growth-promoting apoptosis (35). Indeed, in hereditary hemorrhagic telangiectasia (HHT), circulating levels of vascular endothelial cell growth factor (VEGF) are consistently higher than normal and there is a tendency toward even higher levels among those patients with HHT who bleed more than other patients with HHT (36). It is hypothesized that most features of HHT are caused by the persistence of the activation phase of angiogenesis caused by perturbations in VEGF.

These understandings have realigned our thinking about hemangiomas, particularly those occurring in children (37). The International Society for the Study of Vascular Anomalies has produced a new classification scheme, based on whether the lesion is a tumor (caused by vascular proliferation), or a malformation (caused by structural abnormalities associated with slow endothelial cell turnover) (38). This group carefully dissected what was previously (and probably erroneously) considered to be two manifestations of the same process, namely localized disseminated intravascular coagulation (DIC) and "cavernous hemangioma" (previously known as the Kasabach-Merritt syndrome.) These students who are researching on this disease now argue that what we have to this point called Kasabach-Merritt syndrome is actually a localized form of coagulation activation producing thrombocytopenia and arguably DIC, but it is confined mostly to a unique vascular anomaly, namely, Kaposiform hemangioendothelioma (KHE) (39). Most vascular lesions, particularly the common hemangiomas of infancy, do not exhibit the Kasabach-Merritt phenomena, namely, localized DIC and DIC-like changes.

Mullikien et al. defined the differences between KHE and otherwise benign infantile hemangioma (40). Vascular lesions, whether KHE or not, that exhibit the Kasabach-Merritt phenomenon, have recently been reviewed by Hall (41). These lesions were initially described by Kasabach and Merritt in 1940 (42) and were thought to be seen only in approximately 1% of cases of hemangiomas. Neither the site nor the size of the vascular lesion predicts the syndrome. The Kasabach-Merritt phenomenon is very serious, with approximately a 40% mortality. Patients can "bleed into" these very vascular tumors. Understandably, not very many are biopsied, but most patients who have true Kasabach-Merritt phenomena actually have KHE, and not benign hemangiomas. Therapy includes arterial embolization and general support of the patient with FFP and/or platelet infusions. Many have advocated the use of glucocorticosteroids, 2 to 3 mg/kg/day. It is hoped that breakthroughs in antiangiogenic sciences may allow for antiangiogenic strategies to be therapeutically employed.

## Hereditary Hemorrhagic Telangiectasia

Whereas most of the hemangiomas that appear in infancy spontaneously involute over the years, the lesions of HHT [Osler-Weber-Rendu (OWR) syndrome] slowly progress over decades. As mentioned earlier, perturbations of VEGF are most certainly associated with the slow, continued hyperproliferation of microcirculatory endothelial cells giving rise to the characteristic telangiectasia (see Fig. 67-1). As blood remains intravascular in HHT, the lesions are easily blanched by external pressure, a key feature distinguishing telangiectasia from purpura.

HHT remains arguably the most understood and most common of this group of vascular proliferative lesions. Understanding of the molecular basis of this disease has resulted in division into two types of HHT, namely HHT-1 and HHT-2. The disorders of endoglin, located on chromosome 9q33-34, are those that determine that a kindred has HHT-1, whereas genes encoding for activin A receptor, which are encoded on chromosomes 12q13, comprise those kindred having HHT-2. Both these genes are heavily expressed in endothelial cells. Most lesions have in common loss-of-function mutations (43). Rapid growth in this field, as in other areas of human genetics, is documented by the cataloging of at least 57 genetic defects leading to HHT-1 and 50 defects leading to HHT-2 (44).

With extensive experience with HHT, the long-appreciated but poorly appreciated interrelations between the cutaneous

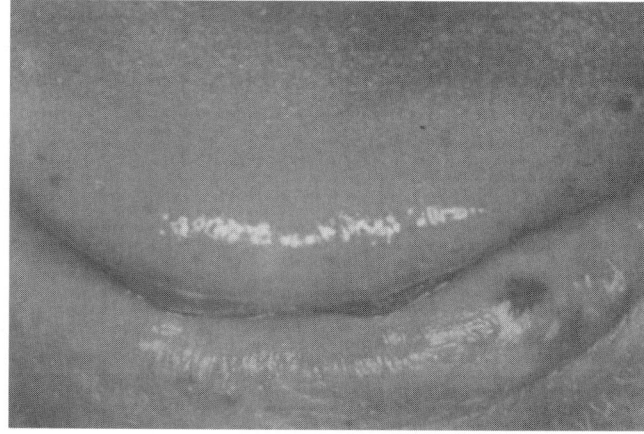

**FIGURE 67-1.** Telangiectases of the tongue and lower lip in a patient with hereditary hemorrhagic telangiectasia (see Color Fig. 67-1).

bothersome otolaryngologic (ENT) lesions of HHT and systemic arterial venous malformations (AVMs) has been solidified. Jacobson (45) estimated that 70% of all patients with pulmonary AVMs have as their root cause HHT, either type 1 or type 2, as do 10% of all patients with CNS AVMs.

Pulmonary AVMs in HHT can cause considerable morbidity and mortality ranging from high cardiac output heart failure to massive intrathoracic hemorrhage (46). These, as well as other AVMs may worsen with pregnancy especially given the increase in blood volume and cardiac output in pregnancy (47). Diagnosis and management of this situation in pregnancy has been addressed with the conclusion that embolotherapy is effective and safe in pregnancy (48).

The primary symptoms that lead to the diagnosis and treatment of HHT remain persistent ENT bleeding (see Table 67-4). In a study of recalcitrant epistaxis, Shah et al. (49) noticed among their 76 patients, that 66% of patients had mild epistaxis (correlating with one or two short episodes of epistaxis per week), 21% had moderate epistaxis (meaning one or two brief episodes per day), and 13% had severe (daily bleeds longer than 30 minutes) epistaxis. Their perceived requirement for red cell transfusion among their 76 patients with HHT, mirrored the degree of bleeding; among those patients labeled as having mild epistaxis, none required transfusions; those labeled as moderate, required one to 10 transfusions per year, and those labeled severe, required more than 10 U of blood per year.

The pathophysiology is explained by increased elaboration of VEGF leading to enhanced microcirculatory growth, which slowly increases over the decades, leading to AVMs that slowly grow into frank telangiectases characteristic of the disorder. The architecture of these AVMs is that of abnormally large capillaries, meaning that there is no smooth muscle investiture of these very large, even visible vessels that still have the architectural makeup of capillaries. Hence vasoconstriction to minimize bleeding is not possible.

Multiple methods to arrest bleeding have been advocated such as packing, electrocautery, cryosurgery, arterial embolization, arterial ligation, and hormonal manipulation. Others use various types of laser apparatus. Although each of these methods have been recommended, the fact that none of them have clearly been established as having precedence over the others is problematic. None of these treatments has been studied in any evidence-based format and one's local otolaryngologists' preferences and resources may well determine the approach taken until the best treatment for epistaxis of HHT is determined.

One group has developed a diagnostic criteria for HHT. Each finding is given a score of one. Findings include epistaxis, the presence of telangiectases, visceral AVMs, and a positive history of a first-degree relative with similar findings. A score of two leads to possible diagnosis of HHT, whereas a score of three or four is definitive (50).

Although the ENT manifestations of this disease are most problematic, it is now becoming clear that systemic AVMs are equally serious. Primary causes of death in HHT are hemorrhage caused by pulmonary AVMs and CNS AVMs. The CNS AVMs, in particular, may become sites of abscesses and therefore prophylactic administration of antibiotics in a manner similar to the prevention of endocarditis has been advocated by many for dental work and GI/genitourinary procedures (51).

The AVMs of HHT are cumulative and progressive. Abdulla et al. noted that 26% of a cohort having HHT-1 developed visceral lesions on screening, whereas 30% of those having HHT-2 had similar lesions (52). Lesions of the liver can be sought by ultrasound. One group (53) found that if the diameter of the hepatic artery is greater than 7 mm then there was a high probability of hepatic hypervascularity, whereas if the hepatic artery was less than 7 mm, such a phenomenon was not found. The average size among patients with hepatic AVMs caused by HHT was 11.3 mm, whereas the controls were 4.6 mm and only 4.8 mm in patients with cirrhosis. Larson (54) found 30% of patients having liver disease secondary to AVMs of HHT developed signs of high cardiac output congestive heart failure, portal hypertension, biliary ischemia, liver failure, and, some developed hepatic encephalopathy. There is debate as to whether embolization of large hepatic AVMs is less dangerous than liver transplantation in patients who are affected. Embolization of hepatic AVMs has complications in up to 40% of patients undergoing that procedure (54).

Elsewhere in the GI tract, telangiectases are common along the large and small intestine and a frequent cause of persistent GI hemorrhage and iron deficiency. Longacre et al. (55) found a correlation between the number of lesions seen in the GI tract on endoscopy and the number of transfusions per year. Those patients having fewer than seven lesions visible, required 9 U of blood per year; those with seven to 19 lesions required an average of 13 U of blood per year, and patients with more than 20 lesions used an average of 28 U of blood per year. Neither estrogen therapy, danazol, epsilon aminocaproic acid, nor any combination thereof yielded reproducible or dependable success; apparently 50% of patients responded to any therapeutic maneuver. Standard of care remains elusive. Video capsule endoscopy has been successful in finding the etiology (to include HHT) of obscure chronic GI hemorrhage (56).

CNS lesions occur less frequently, namely 5% to 10% of patients with HHT and these tend to occur later in life. Obviously, the seriousness of hemorrhage is high. It is estimated that the mortality of a CNS bleed from an AVM is between 53% and 81% (57). From their database, it appears that men have approximately a four times higher risk than women in developing a spontaneous CNS bleed with the entire group having a 1.8% chance per year of developing this complication.

These data have caused considerable debate in the literature about screening for CNS lesions. Students from the United Kingdom studying about this disorder (58), strongly suggest that the magnetic resonance imaging be used to screen even asymptomatic patients who have HHT. Maher et al. (59) in the United States, in their review of patients from the Mayo Clinic, found a low incidence (4%) of CNS AVMs in HHT patients having no symptoms of CNS AVMs. They argue that this figure is low and also that the outcome after a CNS bleed may not be as bleak as originally thought; therefore, they do not favor screening asymptomatic patients. However, among a cadre of patients with HHT known to have pulmonary AVMs, 30% had had symptoms from transient ischemic attacks and/or infarction of the brain, and so CNS screening of patients known to have pulmonary AVMs is quite rational.

## TABLE 67-4

### CHARACTERISTICS OF PATIENTS WITH HEREDITARY HEMORRHAGE TELANGIECTASIA

| | |
|---|---|
| Positive family history | 70%–95% |
| Epistaxis | 90%–95% |
| Cutaneous telangiectasia | 70%–75% |
| Visceral involvement | 20%–25% |
| Gastrointestinal | 12%–15% |
| Hepatic AVMs | 8%–30% |
| Pulmonary AVMs | 5%–20% |
| Central nervous system AVMs | 4%–10% |

AVMS, arterial venous malformations.
Republished with permission from Larson AM. Liver disease in hereditary hemorrhagic telangiectasia. *J Clin Gastroenterol* 2003;36: 149–158.

Despite several excellent reviews on the management of HHT (51,55,60) very little mention is made of aggressive replacement of iron in the form of intravenous iron. The anemia of HHT is caused by profound iron deficiency. Iron replacement in its least efficient form, namely transfusion of blood, however, is the prevalent method of treating severe anemia. Given that the rate of maximal absorption of iron from the GI tract through medicines and/or food is sufficient only to make 8 to 12 mL of blood a day even in the most compliant of patients, it is understandable that oral replenishment of iron is sufficient only in the mildest of cases of HHT. Appreciating that hemorrhagic loss from ENT and GI bleeding is lifelong and progressive, the routine administration of parenteral iron is rational. We at this institution follow our patients' serum ferritin levels, and as soon as they begin to drop, but before the development of microcytic anemia, we routinely infuse total replacement doses of iron in the form of 2 g of iron dextran, iron that is enough to generate the equivalent 8 U of blood. An average patient with HHT requires one to two such infusions per year, whereas some other patients require four to six infusions per year. Using periodic iron infusion, it is the exception that patients with HHT require transfusions (61). The rare patient who is intolerant to iron infusion may have to have oral iron replacement supplemented occasionally by transfusion. Given that the patient will need such treatment over his lifetime, once it can be established that a patient is tolerant to intravenous iron, outpatient maintenance therapy becomes much more rational and acceptable to all individuals involved. Additionally, the specter of blood-borne infections and multiple alloantibody formation are minimized.

# MICROVASCULAR HEMORRHAGE

Hemorrhage from the microcirculation is caused by rupture of the smallest vessels. Because the etiology may be hematologic in nature, the hematologist is frequently consulted. Processes associated with microvascular hemorrhage are listed in Table 67-5.

Purpura results from the extravasation of red cells from the confines of the endothelial-lined microcirculation. Purpura characteristically occurs from leaks in the microcirculation, that is, arterioles, capillaries, and venules. In the microcirculation, surface area-to-volume ratios are very high, thereby allowing fibrin formation, as well as platelet aggregation and adhesion to play major roles, whereas their roles in macrovascular hemorrhage are negligible.

Because of the acute and dramatic presentation of petechiae and purpura characteristic of immune thrombocytopenic purpura (ITP), ITP is the prototypic diagnosis in purpura. The primary cause of hematologic purpura is acute ITP, which is covered more thoroughly in Chapter 72.

In acute ITP, the platelet count suddenly drops to less than 10,000 mm$^3$ and through mechanisms that are not totally clear, blood extravasates from the microcirculation. Whereas one cause for extravasation is clearly the inability of platelets to participate in the repair of microvascular lesions, the concept of capillary fragility requires more explanation. Capillary fragility is the spontaneous bleeding without trauma, usually seen as epistaxis, oral petechiae, mucosal hemorrhagic blisters, and linear purpura, which can occur with the slightest of trauma, such as the pressure generated by a cuff during determination of blood pressure (see Fig. 67-2). Thrombocytopenia appears to alter the endothelial component of the microvascular circulation. By unclear mechanisms, the administration of glucocorticosteroids may ameliorate capillary fragility (62) and account for the frequently noted rapid clearance of active epistaxis and new petechial formation following initiation of glucocorticosteroid therapy even before any detectable improvement in the platelet count.

| TABLE 67-5 |
| --- |
| **MICROVASCULAR DISORDERS THAT MAY LEAD TO HEMORRHAGE** |

1. Hematologic causes
   a. Immune thrombocytopenic purpura (ITP)
   b. Disorders of platelet function
   c. Coagulation disorders
2. Nonhematologic causes
   a. Physical causes of purpura
   b. Factitious purpura
   c. Progressive pigmented purpuras
   d. Infectious processes
      i. Parvo B19 virus
      ii. Rickettsial agents
      iii. Febrile hemorrhagic disease
   e. Vasculitis/leukocytoclastic vasculitis
   f. Infiltration with amyloid
   g. Disorders of collagen metabolism
      i. Scurvy
      ii. Hypercortisolism
      iii. "Senile," "atrophic," or "actinic" purpura
   h. Microthrombi
      i. Disseminated intravascular coagulation (DIC)
      ii. Warfarin skin necrosis
      iii. Fat embolism
      iv. Thrombotic thrombocytopenic purpura (TTP)
      v. Heparin-induced thrombocytopenia (HIT)
      vi. Cholesterol emboli
   i. Endothelial malignancies
   j. Telangiectasia
      i. Hereditary hemorrhagic telangiectasia (HHT)
      ii. Others (CREST syndrome, postradiation, pregnancy)

CREST, calcinosis, Raynaud phenomenon, esophageal motility disorders, sclerodactyly, and telangiectasia.

Occasionally, petechial and purpuric lesions may be seen not only caused by abnormalities of platelet count but also by abnormalities of platelet function. Several diseases, especially Bernard-Soulier syndrome and Glanzmann thrombasthenia and other disorders of platelet function, may present with

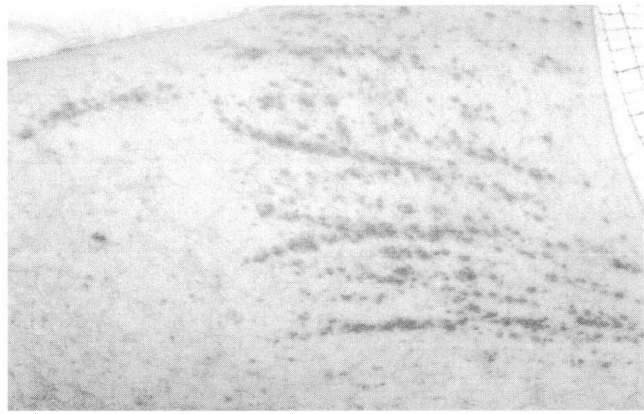

**FIGURE 67-2.** Scratch purpura demonstrating capillary fragility. This patient awoke and noted these linear petechiae on his thigh as the presenting sign of autoimmune thrombocytopenic purpura (see Color Fig. 67-2).

purpuric lesions. These disorders are covered more thoroughly in Chapter 66. Ecchymoses may also be seen with disorders of coagulation to include the classic hemophilias, and especially the development of acquired factor VIII inhibitors (see Chapters 59 and 71) (see Fig. 67-3). Excessive anticoagulation with either heparin or vitamin K antagonists may be detected by the development of purpura.

In the physiologic situation, the strength of the microvascular unit is comprised primarily of healthy endothelium, subendothelial membrane, collagen, and the few surrounding structural cells, chief of which are pericytes and, in the case of arterioles and venules, the strength of the microvascular unit is buttressed by a modicum of smooth muscle cells, which serve to regulate the flow in and out of adjacent capillary beds. By anatomical definition, capillaries do not have smooth muscle cells around them. The capillary microvascular unit must be thin and permeable enough to allow diffusion of nutrients, fluid, ions, and many proteins, but sufficient to withhold the cellular elements.

Physical stressors may overcome the limits of the perfectly normal microvascular unit. Approximately 200 mm Hg of suction can disrupt the normal microcirculation (63,64). Hanging upside down, for even as briefly as a minute, can result in petechiae around the eyelids and conjunctivae (65). Petechiae can be seen in victims of choking, asphyxiation, or can be seen following seizures (66–68).

The term "factitious purpura" is used for patients who, for their own reasons, use physical methods to induce trauma, usually to gain attention to themselves or for some other secondary gain. Blunt trauma can be employed with sticks, brushes, or various tools; other traumatic causes are limited only by the creativity of the patient. A peculiar subset of factitious purpura has been called "psychogenic purpura" (69,70). Because of the enormous complexity of the psychopathology in the bulk of these patients, this poorly understood purpura had been previously considered as a separate category of purpura. As most patients who have been followed-up for long periods of time, have not shown progression of disease, hemorrhage, associated illnesses, or death, it is now held more to be caused by a psychiatric illness, with factitious purpura as a chief and characteristic component. It is intricately intertwined with the psychiatric diagnosis of borderline personality and the only treatment that may work is psychiatric therapy (71). Such patients have normal coagulation studies and no evidence of underlying medical illness. Purpura may be severe for a while, only to undergo remission for long periods. The distribution of purpura is of diagnostic interest, appearing only in areas that the patient can reach.

There is a variety of dermatologic illnesses grouped under the heading progressive pigmented purpura (PPP), which is considered as a benign dermatologic condition but may cause considerable symptomatology in patients because of its cosmetic effects, and considerable concern on the part of physicians trying to find underlying causes. In this group of disorders, the purpura is petechial and pinpoint. The skin may show hyperpigmented areas caused by hemosiderin deposits remaining from prior extravasations. On biopsy one does find a capillaritis with a limited amount of round cell infiltration and extravasated red cells but essentially no signs of frank vasculitis or leukocytoclastic vasculitis (LCV). This process has been reviewed recently (72,73). By virtue of case series, PPP is still considered as both benign in etiology and absent of any long-term systemic effects. The etiology remains totally unknown, although in one series (73) the administration of vitamin C and rutin seemed to decrease the purpura in some patients. Because the process may last for decades, it is unlikely that this is a result of a transient infection. As the name implies, it is progressive.

Infections directly involving the microvascular structural unit may result in breakdown of the hemostatic barrier with subsequent extravasation of red cells and development of purpura. Infection with parvo B19 virus has been associated with a purpura occurring in a peculiar "socks-and-gloves" distribution. Biopsy of these lesions does not show vasculitis or LCV, but does show a mild lymphocyte infiltration, and therefore is slightly reminiscent of skin biopsies of PPP; however, the purpura is self-limited and it is not considered as a severe systemic infection.

Infection with rickettsial agents obviously can cause severe illnesses, such as Rocky Mountain spotted fever and typhus. In these illnesses, rickettsial organisms reside in the endothelial cells causing endothelial death with disruption of the vascular integrity of the microcirculation followed by red cell extravasation and subsequent purpura. These diseases may be associated with fever, organ dysfunction, and mild thrombocytopenia. In general, the thrombocytopenia is not held as being causal in the purpura, because platelet counts are not typically extremely low.

Other agents cause viral hemorrhagic fever with severe organ damage. These include Rift Valley fever, Lassa fever, Marburg agent, and the deadly Ebola viral fever. In these disorders, microvascular disease is systemic and is advanced to the point that organ dysfunction and even death occur.

## Cutaneous Vasculitis

If immune complexes are deposited between the endothelium and the basement membrane, the immune system may be activated, polymorphonucleocytes may infiltrate the area, and, by

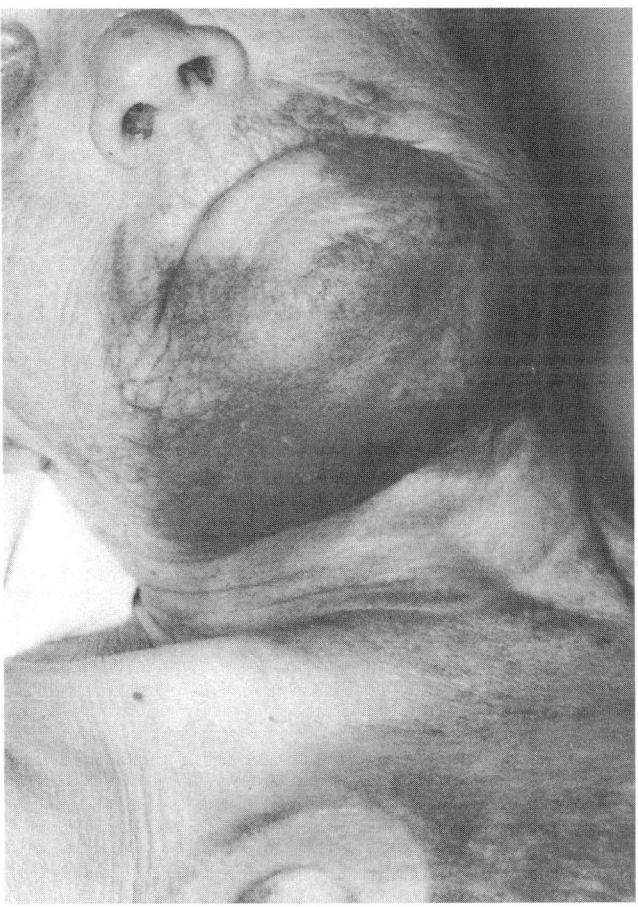

**FIGURE 67-3.** Ecchymosis in a patient with a spontaneous inhibitor to factor VIII. A small oral lesion bled into the floor of the mouth and with gravity dissected along the subcutaneous planes of the neck and chest (see Color Fig. 67-3).

way of their degradation enzymes, may result in the disintegration of the vasculature. When this happens in small vessels of the skin, it leads to a clinical condition commonly known as "palpable purpura," the histologic hallmark of which is LCV. Palpable purpura is now more often referred to as cutaneous vasculitis (CV), the term used in this chapter. Very commonly drug hypersensitivity reactions giving rise to immune complexes are the cause. The multiple systemic disorders that are associated with CV and LCV are generally considered to be autoimmune or rheumatic in nature, but the hematologist may be asked to see such patients initially because of the sudden onset of profound purpura (see Fig. 67-4). The purpura is maximal in areas of dependency, and so, in general, spares the face and arms. The lack of concomitant vascular fragility (expressed as scratch purpura, epistaxis, or purpura following minor trauma such as the skin beneath a blood pressure cuff), as well as normality of the coagulation system and platelet count turns the focus away from hemostatic failure.

As broad as the categories of diseases associated with CV, the prognosis and treatment are equally broad. Treatment will not be covered in these areas, and one should refer to treatises of rheumatic diseases for such treatment. Table 67-6 lists several of these classically regarded disorders in the differential diagnosis of the etiology of CV.

LCV has been thoroughly reviewed (74). When patients with CV are encountered, and the hematologist is consulted, tests that help in the discernment of the broad differential diagnosis include the complete blood count, erythrocyte sedimentation rate, cryoglobulins, antibodies against hepatitis B and C virus, serum protein electrophoresis (SPEP), rheumatoid factor (RF), antinuclear antibody (ANA) and related serologies, antineutrophilic cytoplasmic antibody (ANCA) and complement levels (Table 67-2). Blood cultures are strongly suggested to evaluate for infectious endocarditis despite absence of signs and symptoms usually suggestive of endocarditis. Tests that assist the practitioner in both the diagnosis and assessment for complications of immune complex deposition above and beyond the

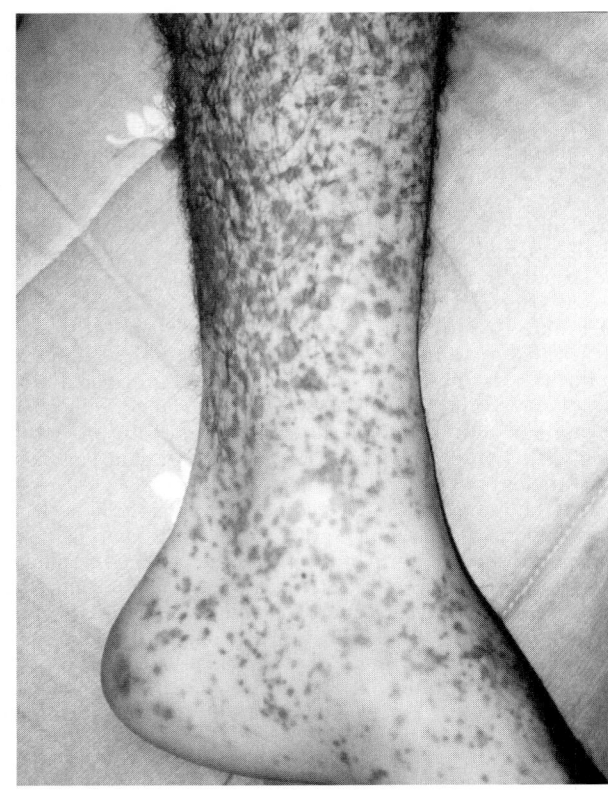

**FIGURE 67-4.** Cutaneous vasculitis in Henoch-Schönlein purpura (HSP). This 18-year-old boy had an upper respiratory tract infection 1 week prior. He awoke with this purpuric rash, knee pain, and vague abdominal pain. Protein and red cells were in his urine. All manifestations were cleared within 10 days without therapy (see Color Fig. 67-4).

**TABLE 67-6**

DISORDERS ASSOCIATED WITH CUTANEOUS VASCULITIS

| Primary | Secondary |
| --- | --- |
| Idiopathic | Systemic lupus erythematosus |
| Hypersensitivity reaction[a] | Chronic hepatitis B |
| Upper respiratory tract infection, viral or bacterial | Chronic hepatitis C |
| | Cryoglobulinemia |
| Drugs: | Sjögren syndrome |
| Penicillin | Polyarteritis nodosa |
| Iodine | Rheumatoid arthritis |
| Aspirin | Mixed connective tissue syndrome |
| Antibiotics | Subacute bacterial endocarditis |
| Analgesics | Wegener granulomatosis |
| NSAIDs | Churg-Strauss syndrome |
| Thiazides | Hypergammaglobulinemic purpura of Waldenstrom |
| Colchicine | Myelodysplastic syndromes |
| | Malignancies |

NSAIDs, nonsteroidal antiinflammatory drugs.
[a]Hypersensitivity reactions frequently are termed Henoch-Schönlein purpura (HSP) if the patient has colicky gastrointestinal (GI) symptoms, GI bleeding, hematuria or other evidence of nephritis, and large-joint arthralgias or swelling, and not on medication known to be associated with hypersensitivity vasculitis.

cutaneous manifestations include tests for renal function, hepatic function, chest x-ray, and urinalysis.

The morbidity and mortality of all the diseases of CV are determined by the underlying cause and the extent and chronicity of organ involvement; the purpura itself is harmless.

There has been considerable discussion in the body of literature on this subject about the importance of even distinguishing the variable etiologies from one another (74–76). Stone and Nousari (75) argue that the size and location of the vessel that is involved in LCV retains diagnostic and prognostic significance. Overlap and some degree of uncertainty still exists, because within any single diagnostic group one can have a wide variety of prognoses, some of which require little if any therapy, whereas others, seemingly with the same diagnosis, require aggressive therapy with immunosuppressives and cytotoxic agents.

One unusual and fairly rare cause of LCV is benign hypergammaglobulinemic purpura of Waldenstrom (77). This process is seen chiefly in women with episodic bursts of palpable purpura that are clearly dependent in distribution and exacerbated by prolonged standing or the wearing of tight clothes. As its name implies, the hallmark is a broad-based polyclonal increase in immunoglobulins that does not appear to be associated with any other known disease, and therefore, by definition, is negative for evidence of chronic viral hepatitis. The ANA and other serologic tests for lupus may be positive, as well as analysis for RF and ANCA. Treatment is rarely indicated and the process is not known to progress to any other disease.

One of the more common causes of CV is mixed cryoglobulinemic purpura, which is nearly exclusively associated with chronic hepatitic C, one of the autoimmune sequelae of that disorder. In the past, it was claimed that mixed cryoglobulinemic purpura was also associated with chronic hepatitis B, but with more modern serologic testing it appears to be much more commonly if not exclusively associated with chronic hepatitis C, which is found in 70% of all cases of mixed cryoglobulinemic purpura. Treatment and prognosis depend on the ability to address and control the underlying liver disease.

There has been similar confusion around what traditionally has been called Henoch-Schönlein purpura (HSP), the triad of purpura, large-joint arthralgias, and abdominal colic. Traditionally, this was regarded as a fairly benign disease in children and is still regarded as the most common CV in children (78). However, the process can be associated, even in the pediatric population, with nephritis, which can progress to end-stage renal disease (79). Others have noticed that by the diagnostic criterion of cutaneous microvascular deposition of IgA that the similarity with IgA nephropathy is noteworthy, and that the separation, if any, between IgA nephrology and HSP nephritis may be very blurred, if nonexistent (80–82). Kitoh et al. (83) described clinical situations that looked like HSP because of abdominal pain, nephritis, and CV, but because of asthmatic symptoms and increased levels in serum IgE, one had to consider Churg-Strauss syndrome. Treatment of these disorders most likely depends more on the degree and chronicity of organ involvement rather than on the precise moniker that is given to the individual clinical presentation.

Other diseases characterized by immune complexes may present with CV. These include subacute bacterial endocarditis, for which the hematologist may be consulted not only because of purpura but also because of hypergammaglobulinemia, anemia, and azotemia, a combination of findings that may initially mimic plasma cell dyscrasias.

## Infiltration with Amyloid

In addition to macrovascular infiltration, which was covered in previous paragraphs, amyloid infiltration weakens the tensile strength of the microvasculature. Purpura, especially of the face and upper body, are frequently seen in cases of amyloid and may serve as a diagnostic clue in difficult cases. So-called raccoon eyes results from bilateral periorbital purpura from coughing or similar maneuvers. It has also been observed after prolonged inverted positioning, which is characteristic of maneuvers such as sigmoidoscopy. Minimal trauma of the skin, such as by pinching, can result in the appearance of a new purpuric lesion within a few minutes. This phenomenon has been called "pinch purpura." The lack of dependence of the purpuric distribution in amyloidosis is noteworthy.

Coagulation defects are common in amyloidosis and can present with a variety of patterns of prolongation of the PT and/or partial thromboplastic time (PTT). Some plasma coagulation factors, notably factor X, may be depleted (20). Involved factors are thought to be adsorbed onto the amyloid fibrils; therefore, vitamin K administration is not usually effective. Therapeutic efforts must be aimed at the underlying amyloidosis.

## Disorders of Collagen Metabolism

### Scurvy

Scurvy is of historical interest, being the first purpuric disorder to be understood and successfully treated. The hemorrhagic manifestations of scurvy are due to vitamin C's role in converting proline into hydroxyproline in order to cross-link collagen molecules into its normal helical structure. The lack of cross-linking leads to the structural weakness, which is manifest by perifollicular hemorrhage (see Fig. 67-5). Large, flat platelike ecchymoses may occur on the legs or trunk. Typically, the gums are extremely spongy and bleed, with the teeth becoming loose. The disease is primarily seen in alcoholics with extremely poor nutritional intake, but it has been described in both pediatric populations (84) and in persons who may eat a very limited amount of carbohydrates, subsisting mostly on meat (85).

The diagnosis is made more by the clinical appearance of bleeding with the large platelike ecchymotic areas being essentially unique to that population. The history will normally disclose that foods containing vitamin C are, for some reason or another, not ingested. Whereas either plasma or cellular contents of vitamin C can be measured, the prompt response to administration of vitamin C followed by sound dietary measures not only confirms the clinical suspicion but also proves therapeutic.

### Hypercorticosolism

Exposure to glucocorticosteroids from either external (pharmacologic) or internal (paraneoplastic) sources leads to excessive breakdown of collagen. With the breakdown of collagen, microvascular tensile strength decreases and extravasation of blood may occur as a result of capillary fragility. Ecchymotic lesions are frequent, especially in the extensor surfaces of the forearms. Administration of vitamin C does not help.

### "Senile," "Atrophic," or "Actinic" Purpura

Solar exposure hastens breakdown of collagen. This explains the characteristic pattern of purpura on the forearms, particularly in those whose occupation or avocation results in sun exposure. With aging or chronic catabolic diseases, the turnover of collagen caused by normal breakdown may outstrip the production of new replacement collagen. In any of these processes, the skin appears very thin with the hemorrhage, often extensive, seemingly nearly on the surface of the skin. Should skin be biopsied, the rete pegs are flattened. Vitamin C administration is not efficacious. The process itself is benign.

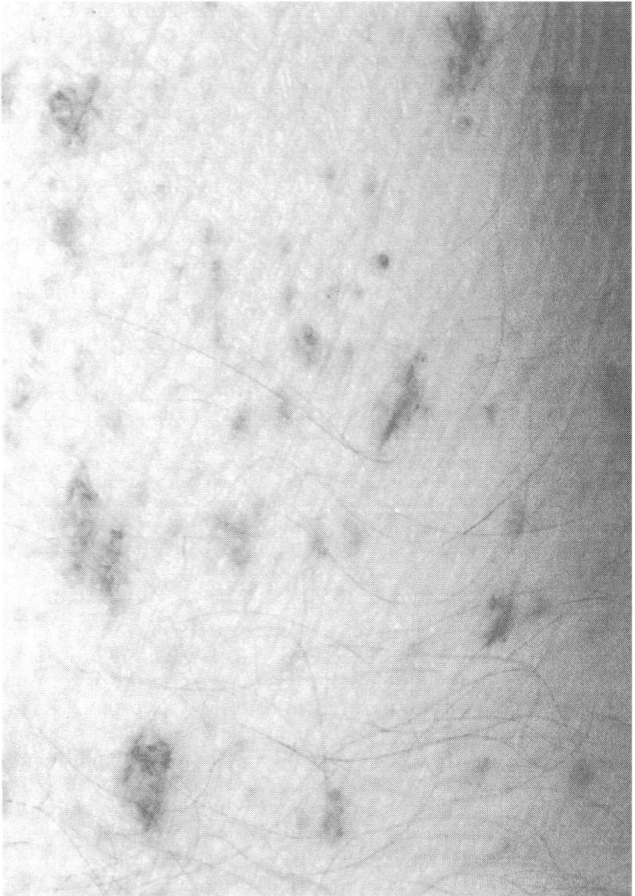

FIGURE 67-5. Perifollicular hemorrhages on the thigh in a patient with scurvy. He had subsisted on beer alone for 4 months (see Color Fig. 67-5).

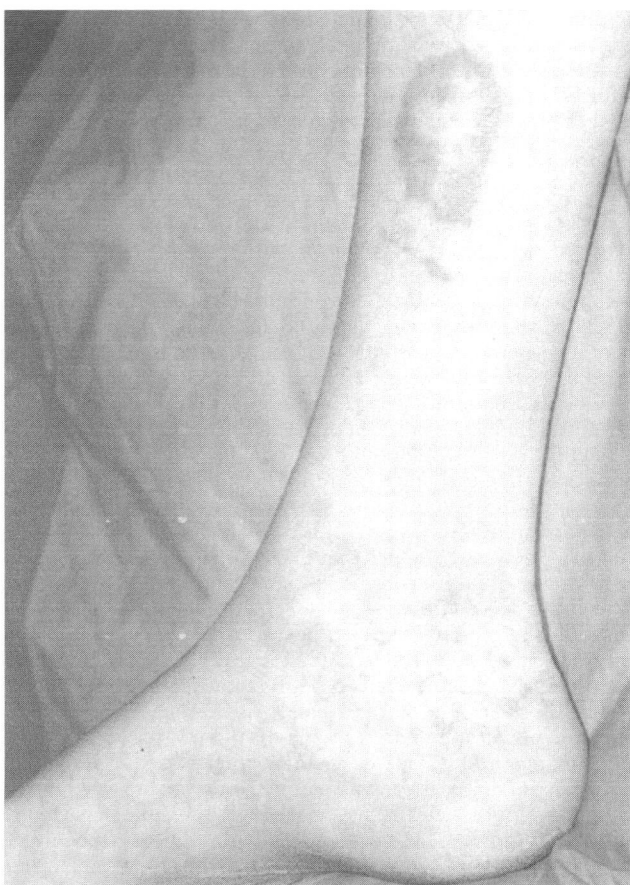

FIGURE 67-6. Expanding necrosing ("gunmetal gray") purpuric lesions of disseminated intravascular coagulation in a postsplenectomy patient with sepsis due to *Capnocytophaga*. Note the linear purpura lesion 2 cm distal to the necrotizing area; this was one of multiple scratches caused by a new pet dog and one of the presumed portals of entry for this bacterium (see Color Fig. 67-6).

## Purpura Associated with Microthrombi

If capillaries become obstructed with embolic material (either clot or other substances) the structural integrity of these thin-walled vessels can be overcome with extravasation of blood into the skin, which expresses itself as purpura. In extreme forms, this is called purpura fulminans (PF). Whereas this process is obviously clearly visible in the skin, it must be recalled that similar processes are occurring systemically and simultaneously in multiple vessels and the association of PF with multiorgan dysfunction syndrome is noteworthy.

### Disseminated Intravascular Coagulation

Disseminated intravascular coagulation (DIC) is associated with a host of causes and is thoroughly covered in Chapter 109. When the thromboconsumptive process involves the skin, purpura occurs. The most frequent cause of DIC resulting in PF is overwhelming infection. These infections may be caused by bacterial, rickettsial, viral, or even protozoan agents. In common with all causes of PF is the intense deposition of fibrin in the microcirculation giving rise to ischemia, disruption, extravasation, and local skin death, all of which are seen as PF. PF generally starts out with small petechial lesions and then rapidly spreads into coalescing necrotic lesions, often described as "gunmetal gray" in color. Prototypic examples of PF are disseminated meningococcemia and postsplenectomy overwhelming sepsis syndrome (see Fig. 67-6).

Overwhelming sepsis may follow either the asplenic or hyposplenic state, PF may occur in patients of all ages, with multiple diseases, and even many years or decades after the splenectomy (86). As many as 4% of patients with asplenia-hyposplenia may become septic, and of those, 25% (therefore 1% of all patients who are asplenic) may die per year. Concerning the cause of the asplenic state, it appears that PF and death caused by asplenia occurs most commonly in those who are asplenic as a result of thalassemia, portal hypertension following staging splenectomy for Hodgkin disease, and hereditary spherocytosis whereas it occurs less frequently in patients with sickle cell disease, splenectomy for ITP, or incidental splenectomies associated with general surgical procedures.

Esmon (87) has reviewed the key role of protein C in maintaining patency of the microcirculation, especially in the face of hypercoagulable challenges. Protein C, and particularly activated protein C, decrease the elaboration and secretion of tumor necrosis factor (TNF) in monocytes and also causes an antiinflammatory reaction by inhibiting selectin binding to neutrophils.

TNF seems to be particularly associated with decreases in components of the fibrinolytic system. Significant decreases in protein C (88), protein S (89), and factor VII activity have been documented (90). In a population of children with septic shock, 80% survived, but 19% developed PF, with many of those losing either their life or limb. Cremer et al. (90) found in their series that the most discriminate predictor of those who developed

PF was factor VII activity. Those patients who developed PF had no detectable plasma factor VII activity as a result of the enhanced secretion of tissue factor (TF) from the septic process, whereas the average factor VII activity in those patients who did not develop PF was 19%. Using fairly common and readily available laboratory tests, Gamper et al. (91) found that elevations of the thrombin time (TT) were the best predictors of those patients with sepsis-associated PF. The TT averaged 15 seconds in those patients who survived, and 75 seconds in those who died. Among those who died, platelet counts were lower, as were fibrinogen levels, whereas lactic acid levels were higher. They found that in such patients these tests predicted morbidity and mortality better than APACHE or Glasgow Coma Scores. Others have opined that those patients having higher degrees of morbidity and mortality caused by sepsis were patients who had higher than usual increase in the acute phase reactant plasminogen activator inhibitor 1 (PAI-1) (92). There is also the possibility that those patients faring poorly may have an additional burden of hypercoagulable disorders such as factor $V_{Leiden}$ or the prothrombin 20210 mutation.

## Warfarin Skin Necrosis

The skin necrosis that one sees with the initiation or alteration of warfarin therapy appears to be unique to the skin, as multiorgan dysfunction syndrome has not been described. Warfarin skin necrosis is thought to occur because of a precipitous drop in protein C levels following initiation of warfarin administration, as its half-life is much shorter than the aggregate of half-lives of the other vitamin K–dependent procoagulant factors II, VII, IX, and X, as well as protein S.

Clinically, this begins with a stinging and burning sensation in areas that are particularly characterized by generous adipose tissues, such as breast, buttocks, and thighs. The pain is thought to be the result of ischemia. If this condition is recognized, and especially if it occurs with the initiation or even reinitiation of warfarin therapy, warfarin should be stopped and the patient should be administered heparin and vitamin K as soon as possible. As prompt reductions of protein C are thought to be causal, theoretically, infusion of activated protein C products may be indicated. It occurs more frequently in patients who have an underlying acute thrombosis (therefore protein C levels may be low because of the thrombosis) and especially in patients who have congenital protein C deficiency as a cause of their hypercoagulability. Warfarin skin necrosis also can occur in patients who have been on chronic warfarin therapy that has been held and then restarted after an interruption for some procedure or oversight on the part of the patient.

In patients who have had warfarin skin necrosis, if it is deemed that warfarin is still indicated, warfarin can be readministered using heparin coverage for the first 4 to 6 days until warfarin therapy is stabilized (93,94).

## Fat Embolism Syndrome

Petechiae are characteristic of fat embolism syndrome. These petechiae have a fairly unusual distribution in that they are scattered mostly about the neck, shoulders, and especially the axillary folds in the upper chest area. They are occasionally seen on the conjunctivae. It is thought that this distribution may be because these are counterdependent areas of the body. Therefore, circulating fat particles may rise and embolize in this pattern. These petechiae rarely represent a problem in and of themselves, but their observation may serve to suggest or diagnose fat embolism syndrome (95–97).

Fat embolism is apparently much more common than fat embolism syndrome. If one looks for fat embolism particularly by using bronchioalveolar lavage (BAL) and stain pulmonary macrophages for neutral fat, fat may be seen in as many as 60% of patients who undergo instrumentation of long bone fractures.

Fat can also be seen traversing the cardiac circulation using transesophageal echocardiography at the time of long bone manipulation. Fat embolism can also be seen following liposuction.

Among trauma cases, fat embolism syndrome is diagnosed in approximately 0.5% of all trauma cases, if not actively sought; however, it is diagnosed in 10% to 20% of all trauma cases if evidence is prospectively sought, namely by examining patients with trauma and hypoxemia more closely. Fat embolism syndrome is seen in up to 60% of autopsies involving blunt trauma.

The fat embolism syndrome is characterized by petechiae in the characteristic distribution in 60% of patients, and shortness of breath and hypoxia in 50% of patients. Thirty percent of patients have confusion or coma. There may be retinal changes, and the platelet count may drop slightly in 50% of the cases. Fever is characteristic. The diagnosis hinges on recognizing the probability of this syndrome. Its peak incidence is between 24 and 72 hours following the traumatic event.

Treatment is thought to be nonspecific and supportive. Because of the apparent association (if not even a precipitating factor) with hypovolemic shock, low blood pressure should be aggressively treated. Hypoxemia needs to be addressed. Putative treatments include steroids, heparin, or aspirin. Although all of these may have some efficacy, there is no evidence-based study to prove their efficacy (98).

## Thrombotic Thrombocytopenic Purpura

Thrombotic thrombocytopenic purpura (TTP) is discussed thoroughly in Chapter 111. Despite its name, petechiae or purpura are not pronounced in TTP. If carefully looked for, petechiae and some infarcted lesions can be seen in the skin, but the process is more apparent in its manifestations of the internal organs that are extensively thrombosed, which is flagrantly apparent on autopsy in those who do not survive.

## Heparin-Induced Thrombocytopenia

Heparin-induced thrombocytopenia (HIT) and its diagnostic criteria are discussed in Chapter 114. Petechiae are not common and bleeding is peculiarly absent despite severe reduction in platelet count. Even patients who have recently undergone surgery typically do not bleed. Accordingly, many authorities dissuade the transfusion of platelets in HIT. Discoloration and pain of digits is extremely common demonstrating the underlying arteriolar thrombotic problem.

## Cholesterol Emboli Syndrome

Arterial depositions of cholesterol from atherosclerotic lesions may shower and embolize downstream, producing an inflammatory vasculitis of smaller arteries. Fever, anemia, eosinophilia, and an elevated erythrocyte sedimentation rate are characteristic. The skin lesions may appear petechial but more commonly appear to resemble advanced livedo reticularis. This process can go on to become infarctive with through-and-through necrosis of the toes and legs; therefore, it may be painful. Whereas it may occur spontaneously from any atherosclerotic area, it occurs more commonly following trauma or instrumentation of atheromatous vessels, such as following operation or arterial catheterization. In perplexing cases, skin biopsy can be performed revealing evidence of cholesterol crystal deposition in the microcirculation. Treatment is directed at the underlying disease, which is usually quite advanced by the time this syndrome is recognized. The role of heparin therapy is unclear (99).

# Endothelial Malignancies

Endothelial cells may cause various tumors ranging from growths that have been deemed nonmalignant, such as those discussed in earlier sections, namely hemangiomas and KHE. Frank malignancies of the microvascular to include the endothelium do exist (35). Primary tumors involving large vessels are rare, but they include sarcomas (100). Angiosarcomas (101) are rare but often occur in chronic lymphedematous areas, particularly in women who have been treated for breast cancer, and there appears to be an enhancement with concomitant radiotherapy (102).

However, the prototype of endothelial cell sarcomas is Kaposi sarcoma. This previously was a rare tumor, and then, at the beginning of the acquired immunodeficiency syndrome (AIDS) epidemic, was quite common, but now again less common, seen only in approximately 10% of patients with AIDS. In its first stage, when Kaposi sarcoma is seen as reddish vascular macules, it may be considered in the differential diagnosis of purpura. These purpuric lesions do not blanch on external pressure. As it matures into larger plaques and tumors, it is less likely to be considered a purpuric disorder.

Kaposi sarcoma is thought to be causally related to human herpesvirus 8 (HHV8), which is also known as Kaposi sarcoma-related herpesvirus (KSHV) (103). On biopsy, these tumors are extremely vascular with slitlike aborted vascular channels that extravasate red cells and cause the initial characteristic purpuric-appearing lesion. The disease appears to be quite well treated by highly active antiretroviral therapy (HAART), as well as interferon-$\alpha$ (104).

## Telangiectasia

Telangiectasia as a result of any cause first appears to be purpuric, but the distinguishing hallmark is that these lesions are totally blanchable. HHT has already been discussed in the macrovascular section of this chapter. Also known as OWR syndrome, HHT lesions are typically on the face, lips, hands, as well as the mucosa of the GI and genitourinary tracts. As discussed in the macrovascular section, HHT is also associated with larger AVMs, particularly in the pulmonary and CNS circulations.

Telangiectasia, however, may also be seen without the other features of HHT. They can appear individually. They can also be seen in skin that has previously undergone radiotherapy or solar damage. Telangiectasia is associated with scleroderma, particularly in the CREST syndrome of advanced scleroderma. A few telangiectases can be seen in normal pregnancy.

Spider angiomata are common in end-stage liver disease. These lesions are differentiated from either petechiae or telangiectases in that they have a large central feeding arteriole, which if pressed, quickly eliminates the "arms" of the spider, which reappears as soon as the pressure is taken off the central feeding arteriole.

## References

1. Lackner H, Karpatkin S. On the "easy bruising" syndrome with normal platelet count. *Ann Intern Med* 1975;83:190–196.
2. Myllyharju J, Kivirikko KI. Collagens and collagen-related diseases. *Ann Med* 2001;33:4–6.
3. Mao JR, Bristow J. The Ehlers-Danlos syndrome: on beyond collagens. *J Clin Invest* 2001;107:1063–1069.
4. de Paepe A. The Ehlers-Danlos syndrome: a heritable collagen disorder as cause of bleeding. *Thromb Haemost* 1996;75:379–386.
5. Solomon JA, Abrams L, Lichtenstein GR. GI manifestations of Ehlers-Danlos syndrome. *Am J Gastroenterol* 1996;91:2282–2288.
6. Nuss R, Manco-Johnson M. Hemostasis in Ehlers-Danlos syndrome. Patient report and literature review. *Clin Pediatr* 1995;34:552–555.
7. Anstey A, Mayne K, Winter M, et al. Platelet and coagulation studies in Ehlers-Danlos syndrome. *Br J Dermatol* 1991;125:155–163.
8. Germain DP. Clinical and genetic features of vascular Ehlers-Danlos syndrome. *Ann Vasc Surg* 2002;16:391–397.
9. Dowton SB, Pincott S, Demmer L. Respiratory complications of Ehlers-Danlos syndrome type IV. *Clin Genet* 1996;50:510–514.
10. Freeman RK, Swegle J, Sise MJ. The surgical complications of Ehlers-Danlos syndrome. *Am Surg* 1996;62:869–873.
11. Maltz SB, Fantus RJ, Mellett MM, et al. Surgical complications of Ehlers-Danlos syndrome type IV: case report and review of the literature. *J Trauma* 2001;51:387–390.
12. Byers PH. Osteogenesis imperfecta: Perspectives and opportunities. *Curr Opin Pediatr* 2000;12:603–609.
13. Cole WG. Advances in osteogenesis imperfecta. *Clin Orthop* 2002;401:6–16.
14. Ohtani T, Furukawa F. Pseudoxanthoma elasticum. *J Dermatol* 2002;29:615–620.
15. Ringpfeil F, Pulkkinen L, Uitto J. Molecular genetics of pseudoxanthoma elasticum. *Exp Dermatol* 2001;10:221–228.
16. Aburawi EH, O'Sullivan J, Hasan A. Marfan's syndrome: a review. *Hosp Med* 2001;62:153–157.
17. Hopkins RA. Aortic valve leaflet sparing and salvage surgery: evolution of techniques for aortic root reconstruction. *Eur J Cardiothorac Surg* 2003;24:886–897.
18. Skinner M, Falk RH. The systemic amyloidoses. An overview. *Adv Intern Med* 2000;45:107–137.
19. Merlini G, Bellotti V. Molecular mechanisms of amyloidosis. *N Engl J Med* 2003;349:583–596.
20. Mumford AD, O'Donnell J, Gillmore JD, et al. Bleeding symptoms and coagulation abnormalities in 337 patients with AL-amyloidosis. *Br J Haematol* 2000;110:454–460.
21. Oran B, Wright DG, Seldin DC, et al. Spontaneous rupture of the spleen in AL amyloidosis. *Am J Hematol* 2003;74:131–135.
22. Rensink AAM, deWaal RM, Kremer B, et al. Pathogenesis of cerebral amyloid angiopathy. *Brain Res Brain Res Rev* 2003;43:207–223.
23. Revesz T, Ghiso J, Lashley T, et al. Cerebral amyloid angiopathies: a pathologic, biochemical and genetic view. *J Neuropathol Exp Neurol* 2003;62:885–898.
24. Rosano J, Hyler EM, O'Donnell HC, et al. Warfarin-associated hemorrhage and cerebral amyloid angiopathy: a genetic and pathologic study. *Neurology* 2000;55:947–951.
25. Long R, Guzman G, Greenberg H, et al. Tuberculous mycotic aneurysm of the aorta: review of published medical and surgical experience. *Chest* 1999;115:522–531.
26. Cina CS, Arena GO, Fiture AO, et al. Ruptured mycotic thoracoabdominal aortic aneurysms: a report of three cases and a systematic review. *J Vasc Surg* 2001;33:861–867.
27. Chukwudelunzu F, Brown RD Jr, Wijdicks EF, et al. Subarachnoid haemorrhage associated with endocarditis: case report and literature review. *Eur J Neurol* 2002;9:423–427.
28. Chetty R, Batitang S, Nair R. Large artery vasculopathy in HIV-positive patients: another vasculitic enigma. *Hum Pathol* 2000;31:374–379.
29. Cakir O, Eren N, Ulku R, et al. Bilateral subclavian arterial aneurysm and ruptured aorta pseudoaneurysm in Behçet's disease. *Ann Vasc Surg* 2002;16:516–520.
30. Neunninghoff DM, Hunder GG, Christianson JH, et al. Incidence and predictors of large-artery complications (aortic aneurysm, aortic dissection, and/or large-artery stenosis) in patients with giant cell arteritis. A population-based study over 50 years. *Arthritis Rheum* 2003;48:3522–3531.
31. Ohara N, Miyata T, Kurata A, et al Ten years' experience of aortic aneurysm associated with systemic lupus erythematosus. *Eur J Vasc Endovasc Surg* 2000;19:288–293.
32. Turesson C, O'Fallon WM, Crowson CS, et al. Extra-articular disease manifestations in rheumatoid arthritis: Incidence, trends and risk factors over 46 years. *Ann Rheum Dis* 2003;62:722–727.
33. Burns JC, Kushner HI, Bastian JF, et al. Kawasaki disease. A brief history. *Pediatrics* 2000;106:E27.
34. Timar J, Dome B, Fazekas K, et al. Angiogenesis-dependent diseases and angiogenesis therapy. *Pathol Oncol Res* 2001;7:85–94.
35. Bell CD. Endothelial cell tumors. *Microsc Res Tech* 2003;60:165–170.
36. Cirulli A, Liso A, D'Ovidio F, et al. Vascular endothelial growth factor serum levels are elevated in patients with hereditary hemorrhagic telangiectasia. *Acta Haematol* 2003;110:29–32.
37. Drolet BA, Esterly NB, Frieden IJ. Hemangiomas in children. *N Engl J Med* 1999;341:173–181.
38. Enjolras O, Mulliken JB. Vascular tumors and vascular malformations (new issues). *Adv Dermatol* 1997;13:375–423.
39. Tsung WYW, Chan JKC. Kaposi-like infantile hemangioendothelioma: a distinctive vacular neoplasm of the retroperitoneum. *Am J Surg Pathol* 1991;15:982–989.
40. Mulliken JB, Anupindi S, Ezekowitz RAB, et al. Case records of the Massachusetts General Hospital. A newborn girl with a large cutaneous lesion, thrombocytopenia and anemia. *N Engl J Med* 2004;350:1764–1775.
41. Hall GW. Kasabach-Merritt syndrome: pathogenesis and management. *Br J Haematol* 2001;112:851–862.
42. Kasabach HH, Merritt KK. Capillary hemangioma with extensive purpura: report of a case. *Am J Dis Child* 1940;59:1063–1070.
43. Marchuk DA, Srinivasan S, Squire TL, et al. Vascular morphogenesis: tales of two syndromes. *Hum Mol Genet* 2003;12:R97–R112.
44. van den Driesche S, Mummery CL, Westermann CJ. Hereditary hemorrhagic telangiectasia: an update on transforming growth factor beta signaling in vasculogenesis and angiogenesis. *Cardiovasc Res* 2003;58:20–31.

45. Jacobson BS. Hereditary hemorrhagic telangiectasia. A model for blood vessel growth and enlargement. *Am J Pathol* 2000;156:737–742.

46. Gammon RB, Miksa AK, Keller FS. Osler-Weber-Rendu disease and pulmonary arteriovenous fistulas. *Chest* 1990;98:1522–1524.

47. Shovlin CL, Winstock AR, Peters AM, et al. Medical complications of pregnancy in hereditary hemorrhagic telangiectasia. *Q J Med* 1995;88:879–887.

48. Gershon AS, Faughnan ME, Chon KS, et al. Transcatheter embolotherapy of maternal pulmonary arteriovenous malformations during pregnancy. *Chest* 2001;119:470–477.

49. Shah RK, Dhingra JK, Shapshay SM. Hereditary hemorrhagic telangiectasia: a review of 76 cases. *Laryngoscope* 2002;112:767–773.

50. Shovlin CL, Guttmacher AE, Buscarini E, et al. Diagnostic criteria for hereditary hemorrhagic telangiectasia (Rendu-Osler-Weber syndrome). *Am J Med Genet* 2000;91:66–67.

51. Begbie ME, Wallace GM, Shovlin CL. Hereditary haemorrhagic telangiectasia (Osler-Weber-Rendu syndrome): a view from the 21st century. *Postgrad Med J* 2003;79:18–24.

52. Abdalla SA, Geisthoff UW, Bonneau D, et al. Visceral manifestations in hereditary haemorrhagic telangiectasia type 2. *J Med Genet* 2003;40:494–502.

53. Caselitz M, Bahr MJ, Bleck JS, et al. Sonographic criteria for the diagnosis of hepatic involvement in hereditary hemorrhagic telangiectasia (HHT). *Hepatology* 2003;37:1139–1146.

54. Larson AM. Liver disease in hereditary hemorrhagic telangiectasia. *J Clin Gastroenterol* 2003;36:149–158.

55. Longacre AV, Gross CP, Gallitelli M, et al. Diagnosis and management of gastrointestinal bleeding in patients with hereditary hemorrhagic telangiectasia. *Am J Gastroenterol* 2003;98:59–65.

56. Ali A, Santisi JM, Vargo J. Video capsule endoscopy: a voyage beyond the end of the scope. *Cleve Clin J Med* 2004;71:415–425.

57. Easey AJ, Wallace GM, Hughes JM, et al. Should asymptomatic patients with hereditary haemorrhagic telangiectasia (HHT) be screened for cerebral vascular malformations? Data from 22,061 years of HHT patient life. *J Neurol Neurosurg Psychiatry* 2003;74:743–748.

58. Mandzia J, Henderson K, Faughnan M, et al. Compelling reasons to screen brain in HHT. *Stroke* 2001;32:2957–2958.

59. Maher CO, Piepgras DG, Brown RD Jr, et al. Cerebrovascular manifestations in 321 cases of hereditary hemorrhagic telangiectasia. *Stroke* 2001;32:877–882.

60. Sabba C, Pasculli G, Cirulli A, et al. Rendu-Osler-Weber disease: experience with 56 patients. *Ann Ital Med Int* 2002;17:173–179.

61. Silverstein SB, Rodgers GM. Parental iron therapy options. *Am J Hematol* 2004;76:74–78.

62. Kitchens CS, Pendergast JF. Human thrombocytopenia is associated with structural abnormalities of the endothelium which are ameliorated by glucocorticosteroid administration. *Blood* 1986;67:203–206.

63. Elliott RHE. The suction test for capillary resistance in thrombocytopenic purpura. *JAMA* 1938;110:1177–1179.

64. Urkin I, Katz M. Suction purpura. *Isr Med Assoc J* 2000;2:711 (only).

65. Friberg TR, Weinreb RN. Ocular manifestations of gravity inversion. *JAMA* 1985;253:1755–1757.

66. Ely SF, Hirsch CS. Asphyxial deaths and petechiae: a review. *J Forensic Sci* 2000;45:1274–1277.

67. Maxeiner H. Congestion bleedings of the face and cardiopulmonary resuscitation—an attempt to evaluate their relationship. *Forensic Sci Int* 2001;117:191–198.

68. Grunfeld J, Klein C. Seizure-induced purpura: a rare but useful clue. *Isr Med Assoc J* 2001;3:779 (only).

69. Uthman IW, Moukarbel GV, Salman SM, et al. Autoerythrocyte sensitization (Gardner-Diamond) syndrome. *Eur J Haematol* 2000;65:144–147.

70. Yucel B, Kiziltan E, Aktan M. Dissociative identity disorder presenting with psychogenic purpura. *Psychosomatics* 2000;41:279–281.

71. Ratnoff OD. Psychogenic purpura (autoerythrocyte sensitization): an unsolved dilemma. *Am J Med* 1989;87(Suppl. 3N):16N–21N.

72. Tristani-Firouzi P, Meadows KP, Vanderhooft S. Pigmented purpuric eruptions of childhood: a series of cases and review of literature. *Pediatr Dermatol* 2001;18:299–304.

73. Reinhold U, Seiter S, Ugurel S, et al. Treatment of progressive pigmented purpura with oral bioflavonoids and ascorbic acid: an open pilot study in 3 patients. *J Am Acad Dermatol* 1999;41:207–208.

74. Koutkia P, Mylonakis E, Rounds S, et al. Leucocytoclastic vasculitis: an update for the clinician. *Scand J Rheumatol* 2001;30:315–322.

75. Stone JH, Nousari HC. "Essential" cutaneous vasculitis: what every rheumatologist should know about vasculitis of the skin. *Curr Opin Rheumatol* 2001;13:23–34.

76. Jennette JC, Falk RJ. Do vasculitis categorization systems really matter? *Curr Rheumatol Rep* 2000;2:430–438.

77. Malaviya AN, Kaushik P, Budhiraja S, et al. Hypergammaglobulinemic purpura of Waldenstrom: report of 3 cases with a short review. *Clin Exp Rheumatol* 2000;18:518–522.

78. Saulsbury FT. Henoch-Schönlein purpura. *Curr Opin Rheumatol* 2001;13:35–40.

79. Hattori M, Ito K, Konomoto T, et al. Plasmapheresis as the sole therapy for rapidly progressive Henoch-Schönlein purpura nephritis in children. *Am J Kidney Dis* 1999;33:427–433.

80. Rauta V, Tornroth T, Gronhage-Riska C. Henoch-Schönlein nephritis in adults-clinical features and outcomes in Finnish patients. *Clin Nephrol* 2002;58:1–8.

81. Pillebout E, Thervet E, Hill G, et al. Henoch-Schönlein purpura in adults: outcome and prognostic factors. *J Am Soc Nephrol* 2002;13:1271–1278.

82. Davin JC, Ten Berge IJ, Weening JJ. What is the difference between IgA nephropathy and Henoch-Schönlein purpura nephritis? *Kidney Int* 2001;59:823–834.

83. Kitoh A, Nobuhara S, Takahashi K, et al. Churg-Strauss syndrome with renal involvement: a case report. *J Dermatol* 2001;28:71–74.

84. Weinstein M, Babyn P, Zlotkin S. An orange a day keeps the doctor away: scurvy in the year 2000. *Pediatrics* 2001;108:E55.

85. Levin NA, Greer KE. Scurvy in an unrepentant carnivore. *Cutis* 2000;66:39–44.

86. Hansen K, Singer DB. Asplenic-hyposplenic overwhelming sepsis: postsplenectomy sepsis revisited. *Pediatr Dev Pathol* 2001;4:105–121.

87. Esmon CT. Protein C anticoagulant pathway and its role in controlling microvascular thrombosis and inflammation. *Crit Care Med* 2001;29(Suppl. 7):S48–S51.

88. Canpolat C, Bakir M. A case of purpura fulminans secondary to transient protein C deficiency as a complication of chickenpox infection. *Turk J Pediatr* 2002;44:148–151.

89. van Ommen CH, van Wijnen M, de Groot FG, et al. Postvaricella purpura fulminans caused by acquired protein S deficiency resulting from antiprotein S antibodies: search for the epitopes. *J Pediatr Hematol Oncol* 2002;24:413–416.

90. Cremer R, Leclerc F, Jude B, et al. Are there specific haemostatic abnormalities in children surviving septic shock with purpura and having skin necrosis or limb ischaemia that need skin grafts or limb amputations? *Eur J Pediatr* 1999;158:127–132.

91. Gamper G, Oschatz E, Herkner H, et al. Sepsis-associated purpura fulminans in adults. *Wien Klin Wochenschr* 2001;113:107–112.

92. Smith OP, White B. Infectious purpura fulminans: diagnosis and treatment. *Br J Haematol* 1999;104:202–207.

93. Ng T, Tillyer ML. Warfarin-induced skin necrosis associated with Factor V Leiden and protein S deficiency. *Clin Lab Haematol* 2001;23:261–264.

94. Jillella AP, Lutcher CL. Reinstating warfarin in patients who develop warfarin skin necrosis. *Am J Hematol* 1996;52:117–119.

95. Muller C, Rahn BA, Pfister U, et al. The incidence, pathogenesis, diagnosis and treatment of fat embolism. *Orthop Rev* 1994;23:107–117.

96. Pell ACH, Hughes D, Keating J, et al. Fulminating fat embolism syndrome caused by paradoxical embolism through a patent foramen ovale. *N Engl J Med* 1993;329:926–929.

97. Fabian TC. Unraveling the fat embolism syndrome. *N Engl J Med* 1993;329:961–963.

98. Mellor A, Soni N. Fat embolism. *Anaesthesia* 2001;56:145–154.

99. Sallah S, Thomas DP, Roberts HR. Warfarin and heparin-induced skin necrosis and the purple toe syndrome: infrequent complications of anticoagulant treatment. *Thromb Haemost* 1997;78:785–790.

100. Chiche L, Mongredien B, Brocheriou I, et al. Primary tumors of the thoracoabdominal aorta: surgical treatment of 5 patients and review of the literature. *Ann Vasc Surg* 2003;17:354–364.

101. Budd GT. Management of angiosarcoma. *Curr Oncol Rep* 2002;4:515–519.

102. Patel SR. Radiation-induced sarcoma. *Curr Treat Options Oncol* 2000;1:258–261.

103. Bubman D, Cesarman E. Pathogenesis of Kaposi's sarcoma. *Hematol Oncol Clin North Am* 2003;17:717–745.

104. Von Roenn JH. Clinical presentations and standard therapy of AIDS-related Kaposi's sarcoma. *Hematol Oncol Clin North Am* 2003;17:747–762.

# CHAPTER 68 ■ HEMOSTATIC ABNORMALITIES IN LIVER DISEASE

CHARLES S. EBY AND J. HEINRICH JOIST[1]

Abnormal bleeding manifested primarily by gastrointestinal bleeding, as well as epistaxis, ecchymoses, and gingival bleeding, is common in patients with acute, fulminant hepatic failure and advanced liver cirrhosis. These symptoms are consistent with the liver's central role in hemostasis. It is the sole or major site of synthesis of all of the recognized blood coagulation factors [except von Willebrand factor (VWF)], important regulatory proteins of the coagulation system (i.e., antithrombin, protein C, and protein S), and components of the fibrinolytic system (i.e., thrombin activatable fibrinolysis inhibitor, plasminogen, and $\alpha_2$-antiplasmin). In addition to decreased synthesis of hemostatic factors, severe liver disease can lead to synthesis of abnormal fibrinogen and functionally impaired vitamin K–dependent clotting factors, vitamin K deficiency due to intrahepatic cholestasis, thrombocytopenia, platelet dysfunction, and accelerated intravascular coagulation and fibrinolysis. The liver also functions as an important site for clearance from the circulation of activated coagulation factors, enzyme–inhibitor complexes, and fibrin degradation products. Owing to the substantial overlap in the hemostatic abnormalities observed in patients with acute infectious or toxic hepatitis, chronic hepatitis, and cirrhosis, the severity of hepatocellular dysfunction is typically more important than the etiology.

Hepatocellular injury and loss lead to alterations in the delicately controlled hemostatic system, affecting primary and secondary hemostasis, fibrinolysis, and natural anticoagulants (see Fig. 68-1). The clinical consequences of these changes depend upon the presence of additional acquired hemostatic disturbances and on the coexisting hemodynamic alterations in selected vascular beds and include an asymptomatic state, variceal bleeding, and portal vein thrombosis. Laboratory evaluation of hemostatic function to assess bleeding risk for invasive procedures in patients with liver disease is recommended but is inaccurate with the currently available tests. Prophylaxis and treatment of bleeding complications consists primarily of empiric infusions of plasma, platelets, and red cells. The appropriate indications and dosing of recombinant factor VIIa requires further clinical investigation.

## THROMBOCYTOPENIA

In patients with acute infectious, drug-induced, or toxic hepatitis, thrombocytopenia is uncommon unless complicated by acute liver failure (ALF) (1,2), when as many as 71% of patients have thrombocytopenia at some point during hospitalization (3). Typically, thrombocytopenia readily resolves with recovery of liver function. The pathogenesis is varied, including splenic sequestration, impaired platelet production, and thrombin-mediated platelet consumption (4). Rare case reports

of severe thrombocytopenia without ALF during or shortly after acute infections with hepatitis A (5), B (6), and C (7) support an immune-mediated mechanism of increased platelet destruction. Profound thrombocytopenia may occasionally develop, sometimes as a feature of aplastic anemia, several weeks or months after the onset of acute infectious hepatitis, presumably as a result of viral destruction of marrow stem cells (8,9).

Thrombocytopenia is uncommon in patients with chronic hepatitis, with the exception of patients infected with hepatitis C virus (HCV). In the Third National Health and Nutrition Examination Survey (NHANES III), 2.4% of adults were anti-HCV positive, 4% of this group had a platelet count less than $100 \times 10^9$ per L, and approximately 20% of adults with a platelet count less than $100 \times 10^9$ per L were anti-HCV positive (10), highlighting the necessity to screen all patients suspected of having immune thrombocytopenia for anti-HCV antibodies. Clinically significant HCV-asssociated thrombocytopenia is rare [seven out of 3,440 at one referral center (11)], and the interval between HCV exposure from blood transfusion to diagnosis of thrombocytopenia ranges from 10 to 40 years (11,12).

Possible mechanisms for HCV-induced thrombocytopenia include splenic sequestration due to portal hypertension in patients with advanced fibrosis or cirrhosis, decreased platelet production due to viral infection of megakaryocytes, and platelet destruction due to autoimmune mechanisms. Chronic HCV infection is associated with multiple autoimmune complications (11), and immune-mediated platelet destruction is supported by several case series reporting positive specific (11,13) or nonspecific (14,15) antiplatelet antibody assays in HCV patients with thrombocytopenia, and responses to immune suppression with steroids, IVIG, or cyclophosphamide (11,16). Alternatively, other investigators have reported on thrombocytopenic HCV patients with negative platelet-associated immunoglobin G (PAIgG) results who failed a trial of steroids (12). In general, Interferon alpha (INF-$\alpha$) therapy for chronic HCV is associated with approximately 30% decline in platelet count (17). However, a platelet count less than $50 \times 10^9$ per L occurred in 10% of patients in the original INF-$\alpha$ trials (18) and in approximately 1.5% of patients in both arms of a prospective trial comparing INF-$\alpha$ to pegylated INF (19). INF-$\alpha$–induced thrombocytopenia is typically due to a direct myelosuppressive affect (20), or, less likely, an autoimmune mechanism (21,22) There is limited experience with splenectomy to reverse thrombocytopenia in patients with HCV before or during INF-$\alpha$ treatment. In a series of 11 Child's class A patients with cirrhotic HCV, laparoscopic splenectomy was associated with no serious complications and platelet count improved from a mean of $55 \times 10^9$ per L to $439 \times 10^9$ per L (23).

Mild to moderate thrombocytopenia may be observed in one third or more of patients with liver cirrhosis (24–26), and approaches 90% in patients with end-stage liver disease (27). Splenic sequestration of platelets due to portal hypertension

---

[1]Deceased

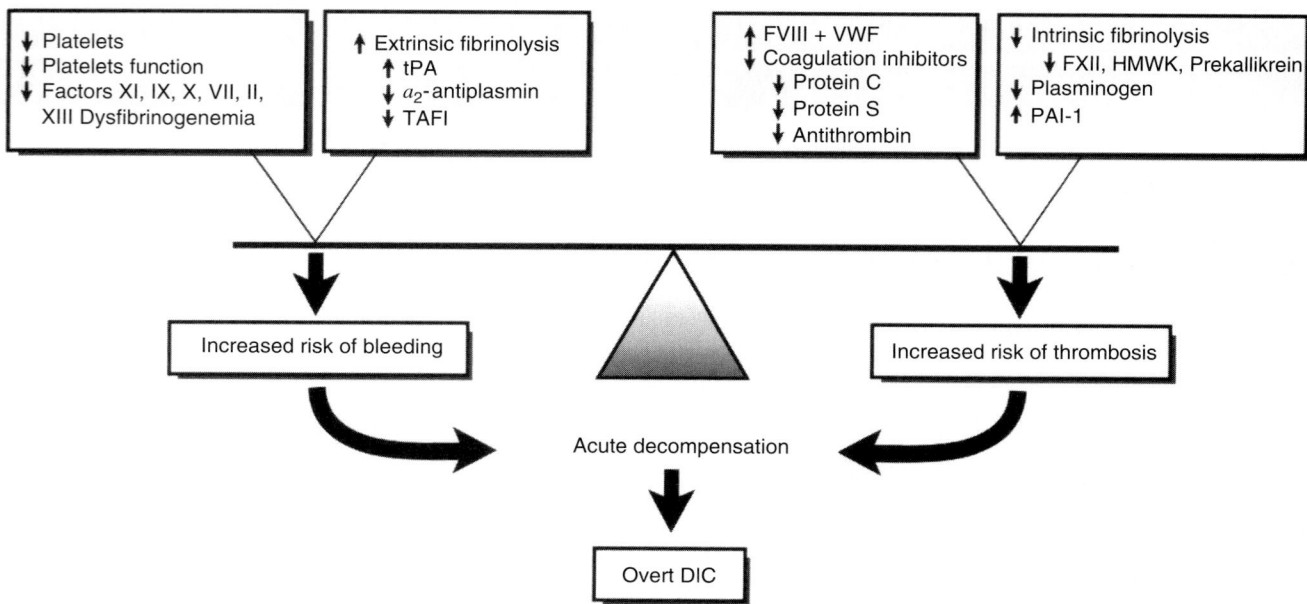

**FIGURE 68-1.** Hemostatic changes in liver disease may predispose for hemorrhagic or thrombotic complications when combined with acute, destabilizing events, tPA, tissue-type plasminogen activator; TAFI, thrombin-activatable fibrinolysis inhibitor; VWF, von Willebrand factor; HMWK, high-molecular-weight kininogen, PAI-1, plasminogen activator inhibitor-1; DIC, disseminated intravascular coagulopathy.

is typically proposed as the primary mechanism (28), although increased consumption and decreased production are also likely to contribute to varying degrees. In general, bone marrow megakaryocytes are adequate, estimates of platelet survival are shortened (29,30), and between 50% and 90% of total platelet mass may be sequestered in the spleen (29,30) secondary to portal and splenic vein hypertension (25,28,30). Reduction of splenic mass by partial splenic embolization (31) and laparoscopic splenectomy (32) improves platelet counts, whereas portal caval shunting (33) and transjugular intrahepatic portosystemic shunt (TIPS) (34,35) interventions reduce portal hypertension, but do not reliably improve platelet counts, suggesting that other mechanisms are involved in hypersplenism.

Total platelet IgG concentration is elevated in patients with cirrhosis and thrombocytopenia, and is positively correlated with serum IgG concentration (36), consistent with fluid-phase endocytosis of whole plasma by megakaryocytes and with incorporation of proteins into α-granules rather than evidence for immune-mediated platelet destruction (37). However, small increases in platelet surface–bound IgG that do not correlate with serum IgG concentration and are of unknown clinical significance have been reported in patients with cirrhosis (36). Increased PAIgG concentration has been described in patients with thrombocytopenia, chronic hepatitis, and cirrhosis due to a variety of underlying causes (15,38,39), and is inversely related to platelet count in some series (29,38). Nonspecific binding of IgG or immune complexes to platelets is the most likely mechanism, although antibodies to glycoprotein IIb/IIIa have been eluted from the platelets of patients with thrombocytopenic cirrhosis (13). However, the exact role of PAIgG in advanced liver disease–associated thrombocytopenia remains uncertain. This is, in part, due to the inadvertent measurement of total platelet IgG with some methods employed to measure platelet surface IgG (37). In the appropriate clinical setting, such as sepsis or peritoneal venous shunting of ascites, thrombin-mediated platelet consumption can also be an important factor.

Although some patients with compensated cirrhosis maintain normal platelet counts by increasing platelet production despite splenic sequestration or shortened survival (40), ineffective platelet production due to impaired hepatic synthesis of

thrombopoietin (TPO) may contribute to thrombocytopenia in more advanced cases of liver fibrosis (41). In patients with thrombocytopenia undergoing orthotopic liver transplantation, preoperative TPO concentrations are reduced or undetectable, begin to rise steadily 1 to 3 days posttransplantation, and are quickly followed by increasing platelet counts (42,43). Within 2 to 4 weeks posttransplantation, most patients are no longer thrombocytopenic and TPO levels have declined to within normal ranges (42,43). These findings are consistent with a major role for decreased production of platelets due to decreased hepatic synthesis of TPO in end-stage liver disease–associated thrombocytopenia rapidly reversed by normal TPO production from the transplanted liver.

However, TPO concentrations in stable patients with thrombocytopenic cirrhosis range from decreased (44), equivalent (38,45) or elevated (46) levels compared to control groups, with no clear relation between TPO levels and platelet counts. Some of the variability is due to the dynamic processes that affect TPO serum concentrations: rate of hepatic synthesis, binding to circulating and sequestered platelets, and platelet survival. The lack of any standardization of TPO enzyme–linked immunosorbent assay (ELISA) methods may also be a factor.

Other potential causes of thrombocytopenia in patients with alcoholic liver disease who continue to drink include folic acid deficiency, due to inadequate dietary intake, or direct toxic effects of ethanol on megakaryocyte proliferation (47,48).

## PLATELET DYSFUNCTION

Platelet abnormalities in patients with severe encephalopathy with fulminant hepatitis include bleeding time prolongation out of proportion to the extent of thrombocytopenia, impaired *in vitro* platelet aggregation to adenosine diphosphate (ADP) and collagen, and abnormal platelet ultrastructure (49,50). However, hospitalized patients with acute hepatitis who are not encephalopathic have both normal platelet counts and function (49,50).

Various platelet functional abnormalities have been described in patients with chronic liver disease, including reduced adhesion to subendothelium (51) and impaired platelet aggregation to ADP (52–54), epinephrine (55), thrombin (53), and ristocetin (56), with no clear relation to the severity of thrombocytopenia (52). Similarly, both prolonged and normal bleeding times in patients with cirrhosis have been reported with either no (52) or only a weak inverse (57) relation to platelet count. One study assessed whole blood primary hemostasis function in patients with cirrhosis (mean platelet count and hematocrit $126 \times 10^9$ per L and 27%, respectively) using the Platelet Function Analyzer (PFA-100, Dade-Berhing, Miami) (58). Mean closure times with collagen-ADP and collagen epinephrine cartridges were mildly prolonged compared to healthy controls, and normalized when autologous red cells were added to increase the hematocrit to an average of 32%, suggesting that correction of anemia in patients with cirrhosis could improve *in vivo* primary hemostasis.

The platelet function abnormalities in chronic liver disease have been attributed to the extrinsic inhibitory effect of elevated fibrin(ogen) degradation products (FDP) on platelet aggregation (52,53), abnormal high density lipoproteins (59), or ethanol (48). However, other data indicate that the platelet functional defect is intrinsic (60) and not inducible by short-term incubation of normal platelets in plasma from patients with cirrhosis (55). Other possible mechanisms are a decrease in arachadonic acid available for formation of thromboxane $A_2$ (60,61), a decrease in platelet adenine nucleotides (acquired storage pool deficiency) (54), increased cholesterol content of the platelet plasma membrane (55), and impairment of platelet transmembrane signaling mechanisms (60). Neither the nature of platelet dysfunction nor its clinical importance is clear (62). Uremia and medications that impair platelet function are also important contributors to acquired platelet dysfunction patients with liver disease.

# COAGULATION ABNORMALITIES

In acute liver disease, the extent of coagulation abnormalities, reflected most sensitively by the prothrombin time (PT), correlates well with the severity of hepatocellular damage, as well as with the occurrence of abnormal bleeding and the overall prognosis, irrespective of the etiology (1,2). In hospitalized patients with acute hepatitis, the PT and activated partial thromboplastin time (aPTT) were prolonged in 41% and 10% of patients without liver failure and in 100% of patients with liver failure, respectively (1). In some studies, the PT was found to be a better predictor of outcome than bilirubin, transaminase, or albumin concentration (63). In moderate and severe acute hepatitis, the plasma activities of vitamin K–dependent factors VII, X, and II are diminished due to decreased hepatic synthesis (64) and are more severely reduced than that of factor IX (1,65) and factor XI (65). Factor V activity is also reduced in acute hepatitis (65), and progressive decline in factor V activity is thought to be a clinically useful predictor of poor outcome and an indicator for liver transplantation (66). Factor VIII and VWF activity are stable or increased during fulminant hepatic failure in humans (67), yet in acetaminophen-induced murine hepatic failure, FVIII activity and VWF antigen concentration decline 90% and 62%, respectively (68). Although the human liver is the predominant, if not exclusive, site of FVIII production, the tissue location and regulation of FVIII synthesis remains obscure. Changes in VWF levels reflect release from vascular endothelium in response to hepatic injury, although the humoral signals and organ-specific vascular sites involved have not been defined. The plasma concentration of the contact activation system factors, factor XII, prekallikrein, and high-molecular-weight (HMW) kininogen, may be reduced in patients with acute liver disease, although

factor XII appears to be less affected (69). Plasma fibrinogen concentration is typically normal or increased in acute hepatitis, except for patients with liver failure (1,65). Hypofibrinogenemia most likely is a consequence of impaired hepatic synthesis, although some patients with ALF exhibit elevated levels of markers of thrombin generation and fibrinolysis consistent with a consumptive coagulopathy possibly initiated by cytokine-mediated release of tissue factor (65).

Progressive loss of liver parenchymal cells in chronic liver disease is associated with decreases of the procoagulant and anticoagulant components of the hemostatic system. In patients with stable chronic liver disease, the aPTT is typically normal and the PT is normal or slightly prolonged, reflecting a decrease in factor VII activity (70). Of the vitamin K–dependent clotting factors, factors VII, X, and II usually are decreased proportionately, and to a greater degree, than factor IX (4) and non-vitamin K–dependent factors (63), correlating with the severity of disease (71).

Hypogammacarboxylated forms of prothrombin (72,73) and protein C (74) have been demonstrated in some patients with liver cirrhosis, consistent with impaired utilization of vitamin K.

Factor V activity declines with progressive hepatic insufficiency, roughly paralleling changes in the vitamin K–dependent factors (65,75). Both VWF and factor VIII levels are elevated in patients with chronic liver disease (76). Increased VWF levels are positively correlated with severity of cirrhosis and nitric oxide production (77), as well as endotoxin concentrations (78). Although mild decreases in von Willebrand cleaving metalloproteins levels have been reported in patients with liver disease (79), unusually large VWF multimers are absent (80). The levels of the contact system coagulation factors, factors XII and XI, prekallikrein, and HMW kininogen, are mildly to moderately decreased in advanced chronic liver disease (81,82), probably as a result of decreased synthesis, as is the level of factor XIII (83), but the clinical importance of these abnormalities is also unknown.

Fibrinogen is normal or increased in most patients with stable disease, but hypofibrinogenemia may be seen with advanced cirrhosis (2,71) because of impaired synthesis, loss into extravascular spaces, increased fibrinogen catabolism, or massive hemorrhage. Acquired dysfibrinogenemia, characterized by abnormal fibrin polymerization and a prolonged thrombin time in the presence of a fibrinogen level greater than 100 mg per dL and normal or only slightly elevated FDP levels, is common in patients with chronic hepatitis, liver cirrhosis, and primary hepatomas (53,84,85) and is related to an excessive content of sialic acid (86,87). There is no definitive evidence that dysfibrinogenemia contributes to abnormal bleeding.

With the possible exception of tissue factor pathway inhibitor (88), diminished plasma levels of both vitamin K–dependent (proteins C, S, and Z) and –independent (antithrombin, heparin cofactor II, and $\alpha_2$ macroglobulin) coagulation-regulating proteins occur in patients with chronic liver disease (80). Global coagulation tests (PT and aPTT) and factor activity assays provide an incomplete assessment of *in vivo* thrombin generation potential in patients with liver disease because protein C activation and subsequent neutralization of factors Va and VIIIa is excluded. Tripodi et al. devised a more physiologic method for measuring thrombin generation by adding recombinant thrombomodulin to test plasma to simulate *in vivo* activation of protein C (89). Thrombin generation without thrombomodulin was impaired in cirrhotic plasma compared to controls, but in the presence of thrombomodulin, thrombin generation was equivalent in the two groups. These preliminary results suggest that the coagulopathy of advanced liver disease may be muted *in vivo* by a concurrent decrease in anticoagulant activity, and they deserve further investigation.

Prolonged biliary tract obstruction by neoplasms, by stones, or from primary biliary cirrhosis may lead to impairment of bile salt–dependent absorption of vitamin $K_1$ in the small intestine and deficiencies of factors VII, X, II, IX, protein C, and protein S. In patients with vitamin K deficiency or with primary biliary obstruction, levels of non-vitamin K–dependent coagulation factors remain normal, or may even be elevated, particularly factor VIII, factor V, and fibrinogen, until liver injury advances to cirrhosis (90,91). In addition, fibrinolysis may be impaired (92). Compared to patients with other causes of end-stage liver failure awaiting transplant, patients with primary biliary cirrhosis tend to have milder coagulopathies (93).

# DISSEMINATED INTRAVASCULAR COAGULATION AND HYPERFIBRINOLYSIS

In some patients with fulminant hepatitis, marked hypofibrinogenemia is observed in association with thrombocytopenia, increased levels of FDP, and shortened survival of radiolabeled fibrinogen (94,95). This has given rise to the concept that disseminated intravascular coagulopathy (DIC) contributes to these hemostatic abnormalities, as well as to the decreased levels of factors V and VIII and antithrombin (96). DIC in patients with acute, severe hepatocellular damage may be triggered by the release of procoagulant substances from necrotic hepatocytes (95,97) and expression of inflammatory mediators and tissue factor on blood mononuclear cells or endothelial cells induced by toxins (65) or viral infection (98). DIC may be facilitated by impaired clearance by the liver of activated coagulation factors (99) and decreased levels of major regulatory proteins of blood coagulation, such as antithrombin (100), protein C (101) protein S (102), and heparin cofactor II (103).

The concept that DIC is an important mechanism in the coagulopathy of acute liver disease has been questioned (104–106). Therefore, each of the hemostatic abnormalities generally thought to be characteristic of DIC may be explained by other mechanisms known to be operative in liver disease. For example, thrombocytopenia may be due to hypersplenism; hypofibrinogenemia may be due to impaired synthesis or loss into the extravascular space such as ascites; elevated serum FDP may reflect increased intravascular degradation of fibrinogen rather than fibrin; and low levels of antithrombin, protein C, protein S, and heparin cofactor II may be due to impaired synthesis by the liver rather than consumption. Furthermore, little, if any, morphologic evidence of organ microthrombi due to DIC has been found on liver biopsy or at autopsy in patients with acute hepatitis (104,107).

Low-grade DIC has been postulated to occur commonly in patients with chronic active hepatitis and cirrhosis (108,109). This concept is supported by findings such as shortened fibrinogen survival (24,97), which may be reversed following heparin (110) and antithrombin (111) infusions and elevated levels of sensitive markers of accelerated intravascular coagulation and fibrinolysis such as fibrinopeptide A (FPA), thrombin/antithrombin complexes, plasmin/antiplasmin complexes, and D-dimer (112,113), which may be lowered by heparin (114). However, others have found only infrequent and marginal abnormalities of DIC in patients with cirrhosis (115,116) and normal fibrinogen survival (117), leading some to question the existence of DIC in liver cirrhosis (105,115–117). Perhaps it is reasonable to conclude that advanced liver disease is accompanied by an asymptomatic acceleration of intravascular coagulation and fibrinolysis and that patients with additional prothrombotic risk factors, such as endotoxemia or trauma, may develop overt DIC or thrombosis (118,119). For instance, entry of clot-promoting, intestine-derived endotoxins in the congested portal system

(120) could be a possible triggering mechanism for portal vein thrombosis (119), which is consistent with the concept of regional hypercoagulability in the portal circulation (121). In addition, peritoneovenous shunt insertion in patients with intractable ascites is commonly associated with laboratory evidence of DIC and with occasionally immediate bleeding complications (122). Induction of DIC following shunt insertion has been attributed to cellular (123–125) and soluble (126) procoagulants and with platelet activators (125) in ascitic fluid.

Accelerated fibrinolysis has long been recognized in patients with cirrhosis of the liver (127–129). This hyperfibrinolytic state, indicated by a shortened whole blood or euglobulin clot lysis time and an increase in serum FDP, has been attributed mainly to increased concentrations of plasminogen activators (130–133) because of impaired hepatic clearance and lack of a compensatory increase in plasminogen activator inhibitors, especially plasminogen activator inhibitor-1 (PAI-1). Decreased levels of other naturally occurring fibrinolytic inhibitors, such as $\alpha_2$-antiplasmin (134) and histidine-rich glycoprotein, also occur (135). This combination of abnormalities could contribute to decreased plasminogen concentration (133,136), elevated FDP level (134), and the presence of plasmin/$\alpha_2$-antiplasmin complexes (137). Hyperfibrinolysis may be a predictor of mucosal/gastrointestinal bleeding (138,139) and poor outcome, particularly fatal hemorrhagic complication (140).

# HEMOSTASIS TESTING, PROGNOSIS, AND INVASIVE PROCEDURES

The PT is a component of short-term prognostic scoring systems for patients with acute hepatic failure (141) and cirrhosis (142). Abdominal surgery in patients with advanced liver disease and major hemostatic abnormalities is associated with a high incidence of bleeding and hemorrhagic death. In one series of patients with cirrhosis undergoing laparotomies, mortality rates were 7% versus 47% for patients with normal and prolonged PTs, respectively (143). The mortality rate for biliary tract surgery in cirrhotics can be 15% (144), although laparoscopic cholecystectomy may be associated with fewer complications (145).

Despite suggestions to the contrary (83,146), there is no conclusive evidence that bleeding or overall prognosis is better predicted by the results of specific coagulation factor assays than by the PT. The PT may be more valuable as a long-term (up to 2 years) predictor of hepatocellular failure in patients with cirrhosis than measurements of albumin, acetylcholinesterase, and cholesterol (147).

Percutaneous liver biopsy is an invasive procedure commonly carried out in patients with chronic liver disease and associated hemostatic defects. Because a liver biopsy carries a small risk of serious hemorrhage (148) and death (149), prophylactic transfusion strategies have been proposed based on empiric thresholds for hemostasis test results (150–152) despite minimal evidence of a strong correlation between abnormal results and risk of bleeding (153). Proposed tolerance limits include PT prolongation of no more than 3 to 7 seconds above the upper limit of the reference range, INR less than 1.5, and platelet counts no lower than 56 to 80 × $10^9$ per L (76). Variable sensitivities of commercial PT reagents to liver failure–related coagulopathies make it impractical to adopt institution-specific guidelines for general use. Unfortunately, conversion of the PT to an INR does not resolve this dilemma because interlaboratory INR precision in patients with liver disease is poor (154,155), possibly due to variable decreases in factor V (75). The utility of bleeding time to predict risk of hemorrhagic complications after liver biopsy is controversial (76). If liver biopsy is clearly indicated and hemostatic defects are judged to be significant, PT should be corrected by the administration of fresh frozen plasma (FFP) and thrombocytopenia corrected with platelet infusion. Although 1-desamino-8-D-arginine vasopressin (DDAVP) shortens the bleeding time in patients with cirrhosis who do not have bleeding, the efficacy of DDAVP for prevention of bleeding after liver biopsy is unproven (156, 157). Alternatively, a transvenous biopsy approach (158), percutaneous liver biopsy with plugging of the needle tract with an absorbable material (159), and laparoscopic liver biopsy (160) have also been used successfully.

The empiric approaches outlined here for percutaneous liver biopsy probably also apply to other invasive procedures where detection of severe bleeding may be delayed and where direct interventions are invasive, such as in thoracentesis, lumbar puncture, and placement of central venous catheters (161). The risk of severe bleeding is likely to be lower for paracentesis (162) and dental extraction, and bleeding may be easily controlled, so prophylactic administration of plasma or platelets is generally not indicated. Nevertheless, close monitoring of the patient after such procedures is essential.

## LIVER TRANSPLANTATION

Severe hemostatic alterations are commonly observed with orthotopic liver transplant, the most critical periods being the anhepatic phase and during the early hours after restoration of circulation to the graft (163). The acute coagulopathy is thought to be primarily due to the loss of coagulation factor synthesis (164) with release of thromboplastic substances (165) and decreased hepatic clearance of activated coagulation factors (166). Increased fibrinolytic activity due to increased plasma tissue-type plasminogen activator concentration and decreased PAI-1 concentration occurs with variable frequency and severity both during the anhepatic phase (167,168) and after graft reperfusion (169). Whereas some (168,170) have suggested that increased fibrinolysis is associated with increased bleeding and with increased use of blood products and therefore should be treated with antifibrinolytic agents, others (167) have concluded that this abnormality is rapidly reversible after graft reperfusion, making the use of antifibrinolytic agents unnecessary. Initial randomized trials to evaluate the efficacy of the serine protease and fibrinolytic inhibitor aprotinin were initially contradictory, but two recent studies confirmed a reduction in intraoperative red cell transfusions in patients who received aprotinin (171,172).

Platelet counts commonly fall during and early after liver transplant (163), and severe thrombocytopenia may contribute substantially to perioperative bleeding. Resolution of thrombocytopenia is frequently observed after transplantation, probably in part due to restoration of normal TPO production (42). The severity and duration of acute coagulopathy appear closely related to the primary quality and preservation of the transplanted liver (170). Release of endogenous, heparinlike substances during and early after liver transplantation may also contribute to the coagulopathy and abnormal bleeding (173). No information is available about the impact of plasma exchange on blood product utilization, graft, and patient survival when it is performed immediately before liver transplantation to temporarily improve the underlying coagulopathy in patients with end-stage liver failure. Plasma exchange, combined with hemofiltration (174) or charcoal perfusion (175), temporarily improves the coagulopathy and encephalopathy in some patients with fulminant hepatic failure awaiting liver transplantation.

The intraoperative use of blood components (176) has decreased considerably because of improvements in organ preservation and anesthetic and surgical techniques: 24% to 32% of recent liver transplant recipients received no intraoperative red cell transfusions at selected medical centers (177). There is no conclusive evidence that hemostatic laboratory monitoring to guide blood component substitution is effective in reducing perioperative blood loss or blood component usage (178). Similarly, it remains controversial whether and to what extent preoperative hemostatic evaluation predicts intraoperative blood loss, overall prognosis, and survival (179). Nevertheless, use of the thromboelastogram point of care instrument to monitor whole blood hemostasis parameters is felt by some clinicians to provide timely guidance for blood component replacement during liver transplant surgery (180)

Although coagulation factors and fibrinolytic activities generally return to normal within 1 to 3 days of transplantation, delayed recovery of the levels of the major regulatory proteins of coagulation, protein C, protein S, and antithrombin and elevated levels of thrombin/antithrombin complexes may be observed in adults during this later phase (181). During this period of apparent hemostatic imbalance, hepatic artery thrombosis, a catastrophic complication requiring emergency retransplantation, occurs in 2% to 12% of patients (182), and it has been suggested (181), but not confirmed, that prophylactic administration of low-dose heparin and plasma, or antithrombin and protein C concentrates, as well as maintenance of a low hematocrit (183) may be beneficial in preventing such thrombotic events.

## MANAGEMENT OF BLEEDING IN LIVER DISEASE

Many factors and mechanisms contribute to the hemorrhagic diathesis of acute and chronic liver disease, and in a particular patient it may be difficult to determine which of these contributes most to bleeding. The therapeutic approach should be tailored to the nature, site, and extent of bleeding. In addition, attempts at correction of the hemostatic disorder must be coordinated with other measures to correct the underlying vascular lesions, such as banding or sclerotherapy of esophageal varices, reduction of gastric acid secretion, and surgical, endovascular, or pharmacologic interventions to reduce portal pressure.

Multiple acquired coagulation factor deficiencies, reflected in a prolonged PT, and frequently accompanied by a prolonged aPTT, thrombin time, and hypofibrinogenemia, require prompt interventions. Vitamin K deficiency is uncommon in patients with hepatic failure, despite their frequently poor nutritional state. Nevertheless, it is prudent to administer 5 to 15 mg of vitamin $K_1$ by slow intravenous infusion to minimize hypotensive complications (184). Intramuscular and subcutaneous routes are not recommended because the former carries the risk of hematoma and the latter is associated with unpredictable absorption. Any improvement should be evident within 12 hours (184).

FFP contains all of the coagulation factors and inhibitors present in circulating blood and is theoretically the most suitable agent for correction of the multiple defects found in liver disease. In practice, however, effective replacement is difficult because the large amounts of plasma required to substantially correct a prolonged PT [840 to 1,400 mL for a 70-kg adult; based on a guideline of 12 to 20 mL per kg (184)] are frequently not well tolerated, due to intravascular volume expansion. Furthermore, because of the short biologic half-life of factor VII, additional infusions every 6 to 12 hours may be required to maintain partial correction of the PT. Fibrinogen can be efficiently restored with infusions of cryoprecipitate. A typical guideline is one U of cryoprecipitate (10 to 20 mL) per 10 kg body weight for a fibrinogen concentration less than 100 mg per dL (76).

Prothrombin-complex concentrates (PCCs) contain high concentrations of factor IX and variable concentrations of factors X, VII, and II and protein C, and, therefore, correct deficiencies of vitamin K–dependent factors but not of factor V or fibrinogen. Although the risk of transmitting hepatitis viruses and HIV has been largely eliminated with the introduction of highly purified, heat-treated and solvent/detergent-treated PCCs, these concentrates contain variable amounts of activated coagulation factors (IXa, Xa, VIIa, IIa) (185) that may not be adequately neutralized in patients with liver disease because of impaired hepatic clearance and reduced concentrations of antithrombin. The administration of PCCs has been associated with thromboembolic complications, including deep vein thrombosis, pulmonary embolism, and DIC (186–188). PCCs have been used to successfully treat or prevent bleeding complications in select patients with liver disease–induced coagulopathies without immediate thrombotic complications (189,190). However, some patients received concurrent infusions of antithrombin concentrate (190) or FFP (189) to mitigate the risk of thrombotic complications.

Recombinant factor VIIa (rFVIIa) would appear to be a reasonable treatment option to correct the coagulopathy in bleeding patients with liver disease, theoretically accelerating thrombin generation at the site of vascular injury without producing a systemic hypercoagulable state. Preliminary studies have reported temporary correction of prolonged PTs in nonbleeding patients with cirrhosis following infusions of 5, 20, or 80 $\mu$g per kg of rFVIIa (191), achievement of hemostasis within 10 minutes after the laparoscopic liver biopsy in 66 patients with cirrhosis following a single dose of rFVIIa (range 5 to 120 $\mu$g per kg) (192), and temporary control of variceal bleeding in 10 patients with cirrhosis after a single dose of 80 $\mu$g per kg (193). However, the only prospective, randomized study evaluating the safety and efficacy of rFVIIa in patients with cirrhosis who had active bleeding found that eight doses, each of 100 $\mu$g per kg, had no effect on control of bleeding within 24 hours or of rebleeding and mortality rates at 5 days (194); thromboembolic events were rare and were balanced between treatment groups. Additionally, preliminary results comparing a single preoperative dose of rFVIIa (20, 40, or 80 $\mu$g per kg) to placebo in patients undergoing orthotopic liver transplantation showed no difference in red cell transfusions or thromboembolic complications (195). Although studies of alternative rFVIIa dosing strategies are under way, it is still premature to recommend routine use of rFVIIa to prevent or treat bleeding complications in patients with liver disease.

Platelet transfusions may be helpful in patients with marked thrombocytopenia and serious bleeding. The platelet increment after transfusion may be markedly less than the expected increase of 8,000 to 10,000 per $\mu$L per U of random donor platelets transfused in an average adult because of sequestration of transfused platelets in the enlarged, congested spleen. Anecdotal reports of platelet count improvement in response to interleukin-11 stimulated megakaryopoiesis (196,197) and propanolol-induced changes in splenic hemodynamics (198) require further study. Novel TPO receptor agonists are under development, but have not been evaluated in patients with hepatic disease.

In a randomized, controlled trial of terlipressin with or without DDAVP in patients with cirrhosis and bleeding varices, there was no benefit to treatment with DDAVP (199). Synthetic fibrinolytic inhibitors such as $\varepsilon$-aminocaproic acid and tranexamic acid may be considered for some patients, particularly those with mucosal bleeding and laboratory abnormalities indicating a hyperfibrinolytic state.

## References

1. Gallus A, Lucas C, Hirsh J. Coagulation studies in patients with acute infectious hepatitis. *Br J Haematol* 1972;22:761.
2. Lechner K, Niessner H, Thaler E. Coagulation abnormalities in liver disease. *Semin Thromb Hemost* 1977;4:40.
3. Schiodt FV, Balko J, Schilsky M, et al. Thrombopoietin in acute liver failure. *Hepatology* 2003;37:558–561.
4. Deutsch E. Blood coagulation changes in liver disease. *Prog Liver Dis* 1965;2:69.
5. Avci Z, Turul T, Catal F, et al. Thrombocytopenia and emperiopolesis in a patient with hepatitis A infection. *Pediatr Hematol Oncol* 2002;19:67–70.
6. Ozaras R, Celik A, Kisacik B, et al. Acute hepatitis B and isolated thrombocytopenia. *J Clin Gastroenterol* 2003;37(letter):87–88.
7. Narita R, Asaumi H, Abe S, et al. Idiopathic thrombocytopenic purpura with acute hepatitis C viral infection. *J Gastroenterol Hepatol* 2003;18(letter):462–472.
8. Baranski B, Young N. Hematologic consequences of viral infection. *Hematol Oncol Clin North Am* 1987;1:167.
9. Zeldis J, Dienstag J, Gale R. Aplastic anemia and non-A, non-B hepatitis. *Am J Med* 1983;74:64.
10. Streiff M, Mehta S, Thomas D. Peripheral blood count abnormalities among patients with hepatitis C in the United States. *Hepatology* 2002;35:947–952.
11. Pockros P, Duchini A, McMillian R, et al. Immune thrombocytopenic purpura in patients with chronic hepatitis C virus infection. *Am J Gastroenterol* 2002;97:2040–2045.
12. Garcia-Suarez J, Burgaleta C, Hernanz N, et al. HCV-associated thrombocytopenia: clinical characteristics and platelet response after recombinant $\alpha$2b-interferon therapy. *Br J Haematol* 2000;110:98–103.
13. Kajihara M, Kato S, Okazaki Y, et al. A role of autoantibody-medicated platelet destruction in thrombocytopenia in patients with cirrhosis. *Hepatology* 2003;37:1267–1276.
14. Hernandez F, Blanquer A, Linares M, et al. Autoimmune thrombocytopenia associated with hepatitis C virus infection. *Acta Haematol* 1998;99:217–220.
15. Samuel H, Nardi M, Karpatkin M, et al. Differentiation of autoimmune thrombocytopenia from thrombocytopenia associated with immune complex disease: systemic lupus erythematosus, hepatitis-cirrhosis, and HIV-1 infection by platelet and serum immunological mesurements. *Br J Haematol* 1999;105:1086–1091.
16. Ramos-Casals M, Garcia-Carrasco M, Lopez-Medrano F, et al. Severe autoimmune cytopenias in treatment-naive hepatits C virus infection clinical description of 35 cases. *Medicine* 2003;82:87–96.
17. Peck-Radosavljevic M, Wichlas M, Pidlich J, et al. Blunted thrombopoietin response to interferon alfa-induced thrombocytopenia during treatment for hepatitis C. *Hepatology* 1998;28:1424–1329.
18. Poynard T, Bedossa P, Chevallier M, et al. A comparison of three interferon alfa-2b regimens for the long-term treatment of chronic non-A, non-B hepatitis. Multicenter Study Group. *N Engl J Med* 1995;332:1457–1462.
19. Zeuzem S, Feinman V, Rasenack J, et al. Peginterferon alfa-2a in patients with chronic hepatitis C. *N Engl J Med* 2000;343:1666–1672.
20. Hoofnagle J. Thrombocytopenia during interferon alfa therapy. *J Am Med Assoc* 1991;266:849–855.
21. Dourakis S, Deutsch M, Hadziyannis S. Immune thrombocytopenia and alpha-interferon therapy. *J Hepatol* 1996;25:972–975.
22. Sevastianos V, Deutsch M, Dourakis S, et al. Pegylated interferon-2b-associated autoimmune thrombocytopenia in a patient with chronic hepatitis C. *Am J Gastroenterol* 2003;98:706–707.
23. Kercher K, Carbonell A, Heniford B, et al. Laparoscopic splenectomy reverses thrombocytopenia in patients with hepatitis C cirrhosis and portal hypertension. *J Gastrointest Surg* 2004;8:120–126.
24. Stein S, Harker L. Kinetic and functional studies of platelets, fibrinogen, and plasminogen in patients with hepatic cirrhosis. *J Lab Clin Med* 1986;99:217.
25. Toghill P, Green S, Ferguson R. Platelet dynamics in chronic liver disease with special reference to the role of the spleen. *J Clin Pathol* 1977;30:367.
26. Bashour F, Teran J, Mullen K. Prevalence of peripheral blood cytopenias (hypersplenism) in patients with nonalcoholic liver disease. *Am J Gastroenterol* 2000;95:2936–2939.
27. Bontempo F, Lewis J, van Thiel D, et al. The relation of preoperative coagulation findings to the diagnosis, blood usage, and survival in adult liver transplantation. *Transplantation* 1985;39:532–536.
28. Aster R. Pooling of platelets in the spleen: role in the pathogenesis of "hypersplenic" thrombocytopenia. *J Clin Invest* 1966;45:645–657.
29. Aoki Y, Hidai K, Tanikawa K. Mechanisms of thrombocytopenia in liver cirrhosis; kinetics of indium-111 tropolone labelled platelets. *Eur J Nucl Med* 1993;20:123–129.
30. Schmidt K, Rasmussen J, Bekker C, et al. Kinetics and *in vitro* distribution of indium-III labeled autologous platelets in chronic hepatic disease: mechanisms of thrombocytopenia. *Scand J Gastroenterol* 1985;34:39.
31. Sangro B, Bilbao I, Herrero I, et al. Parital splenic embolization for the treatment of hypersplenism in cirrhosis. *Hepatology* 1993;18:309–314.
32. Hashizume M, Tomikawa M, Akahoshi T, et al. Laparoscopic splenectomy for portal hypertension. *Hepatogastroenterology* 2002;49:847–852.
33. Mutchnick M, Lerner E, Conn H. Effect of portacaval anastomosis on hypersplenism. *Dig Dis Sci* 1980;25:929–938.
34. Jabbour N, Zajko A, Orons P, et al. Does transjugular intrahepatic portosystemic shunt (TIPS) resolve thrombocytopenia associated with cirrhosis? *Dig Dis Sci* 1998;43:2459–2462.

35. Karasu Z, Guraker A, Kerwin B, et al. Effect of transjugular intrahepatic portosystemic shunt on thrombocytopenia associated with cirrhosis. *Dig Dis Sci* 2000;45:1971–1976.

36. George J, Saucerman S. Platelet IgG, IgA, IgM, and albumin: correlation of platelet and plasma concentrations in normal subjects and in patients with ITP or dysproteinemia. *Blood* 1988;72:362–365.

37. George J. Platelet immunoglobin G: its significance for the evaluation of thrombocytopenia and for understanding the origin of alpha granule proteins. *Blood* 1990;76:859–870.

38. Sanjo A, Saito H, Ohnishi A, et al. Role of elevated platelet-associated immunoglobin G and hypersplenism in thrombocytopenia of chronic liver disease. *J Gastroenterol Hepatol* 2003;18:638–644.

39. Bassendine M, Collins J, Stephenson J. Platelet associated immunoglobins in primary biliary cirrhosis: a cause of thrombocytopenia? *Gut* 1985;26:1074.

40. Panasiuk A, Prokopowicz D, Zak J, et al. Reticulated platelets as a marker of megakaryopoiesis in liver cirrhosis: relation to thrombopoietin and hepatocyte growth factor serum concentration. *Hepatogastroenterology* 2004; 51:1124–1128.

41. Adinolfi L, Giodano M, Andreana A, et al. Hepatic fibrosis plays a central role in the pathogenesis of thrombocytopenias in patients with chronic viral hepatitis. *Br J Haematol* 2001;113:590–595.

42. Martin T, Somberg K, Meng G, et al. Thrombopioetin levels in patients with cirrhosis before and after orthotopic liver thransplantation. *Ann Intern Med* 1997;127:285–288.

43. Peck-Radosavlijevic M, Wichlas M, Zacheri J, et al. Thrombopoietin induces rapid resolution of thrombocytopenia after orthotopic liver transplantation through increased platelet production. *Blood* 2000;95(3): 795–701.

44. Koruk M, Onuk M, Akcay F, et al. Serum thrombopoietin levels in patinets with chronic hepatitis and liver cirrhosis, and its relationship with circulating thrombocyte counts. *Hepatogastroenterology* 2002;49:1645–1648.

45. Espanol I, Gallego A, Enriquez J, et al. Thrombocytopenia associated with liver cirrhosis and hepatitis C infection: role of thrombopoietin. *Hepatogastroenterology* 2000;47:1404–1406.

46. Freni M, Spadaro A, Ajello A, et al. Serum thrombopoietin in chronic liver disease: relation to severity of the disease and spleen size. *Hepatogastroenterology* 2002;49:1382–1385.

47. Hillborn M, Neiman J. Platelet thromboxane formation capacity after ethanol withdrawal in chronic alcoholism. *Haemostasis* 1988;18:170.

48. Cowan D. Effects of alcoholism on hemostasis. *Semin Hematol* 1980; 17:119.

49. Weston M, Langley P, Rubin M. Platelet function in fulminant hepatic failure. *Gut* 1977;18:897.

50. Rubin M, Weston M, Bullock G. Abnormal platelet function and ultrastructure in fulminant hepatic failure. *Q J Med* 1977;46:339.

51. Ordinas A, Escolar G, Cirera I, et al. Existence of a platelet-adhesion defect in patients with cirrhosis independent of hematocrit: studies under flow conditions. *Hepatology* 1996;24:1137–1142.

52. Ballard H, Marcus A. Platelet aggregation in portal cirrhosis. *Arch Intern Med* 1976;136:316.

53. Thomas D, Ream V, Stuart R. Platelet aggregation in patients with Laennac's cirrhosis of the liver. *N Engl J Med* 1967;276:1342–1348.

54. Ingeberg S, Jacobsen P, Fischer E, et al. Platelet aggregation and release of ATP in patients with hepatic cirrhosis. *Scand J Gastroenterol* 1985;20: 285–288.

55. Owen J, Hutton R, Day R, et al. Platelet lipid composition and platelet aggregation in human liver disease. *J Lipid Res* 1981;22:423.

56. Castillo R, Maragall S, Rodes J, et al. Increased factor VIII complex and defective ristocetin-induced platelet aggregation in liver disease. *Thromb Res* 1977;11:899.

57. Blake J, Sprengers D, Grech P, et al. Bleeding time in patients with hepatic cirrhosis. *Br Med J* 1990;301:12–15.

58. Escolar G, Cases A, Vinas M, et al. Evaluation of acquired platelet dysfunctions in uremic and cirrhotic patients using the platelet function analyzer (PFA-100): influence of hematocrit elevation. *Haematologica* 1999; 84(7):614–619.

59. Desai K, Mistry P, Bagget C. Inhibition of platelet aggregation by abnormal high density lipoprotein particles in plasma from patients with hepatic cirrhosis. *Lancet* 1989;1:693.

60. Laffi G, Cominelli F, Ruggiero M. Altered platelet function in cirrhosis of the liver: impairment of inositol lipid and arachidonic acid metabolism in response to agonists. *Hepatology* 1988;8:1620.

61. Davi G, Migneco G, Vigneri S. Platelet thromboxane production in liver cirrhosis. *Prostaglandins Leukot Med* 1985;19:99.

62. Burroughs A, McCormick P, Sprengers D. Assessment of bleeding risk in chronic liver disease. *Fibrinolysis* 1988;2:56.

63. Koller F. Theory and experience behind the use of coagulation tests in diagnosis and prognosis of liver disease. *Scand J Gastroenterol* 1973;8 (Suppl. 19):51.

64. Pereira S, Langley P, Williams R. The management of abnormalities of hemostasis in acute liver failure. *Semin Liver Dis* 1996;16(4):403–414.

65. Kerr R, Newsome P, Germain L, et al. Effects of acute liver injury on blood coagulation. *J Thromb Haemost* 2003;1(4):754–759.

66. Williams R, Wendon J. Indications for orthotopic liver transplantation in fulminant liver failure. *Hepatology* 1994;20:5S–9S.

67. Langley P, Hughes R, Williams R. Increased factor VIII complex in fulminant hepaic failure. *Thromb Haemost* 1985;54:693.

68. Doering C, Nichols C, Lollar P. Decreased factor VIII levels during acetaminophen-induced murine fulminant hepatic failure. *Blood* 2003; 102:1743–1744.

69. Deutsch W, Dragosics B, Kopsa H. Prekallikrein, HMW-kininogen and factor XII in various disease states. *Thromb Res* 1983;31:351.

70. Green G, Potter L, Thomson J, et al. Factor VII as a marker of hepatocellular synthetic function in liver disease. *J Clin Pathol* 1976;29:971.

71. Spector I, Corn M. Laboratory tests of hemostasis: the relation to hemorrhage in liver disease. *Arch Intern Med* 1967;119:577.

72. Corrigan J, Jeter M, Earnest D. Prothrombin antigen and coagulant activity in patients with liver disease. *J Am Med Assoc* 1982;248:1736.

73. Blanchard R, Furie B, Jorgensen M, et al. Acquired vitamin K-dependent carboxylation deficiency in liver disease. *N Engl J Med* 1981; 305:242.

74. Yoshikawa Y, Sakata Y, Toda G, et al. The acquired vitamin K-dependent gamma-carboxylation deficiency in hepatocellular carcinoma invovles not only prothombin, but also protein C. *Hepatology* 1988;8: 524–530.

75. Deitcher S. Interpretation of the international normalised ratio in patients with liver disease. *Lancet* 2002;359:47–48.

76. Amitrano L, Guardascione M, Brancaccio V, et al. Coagulation disorders in liver disease. *Semin Liver Dis* 2002;22(1):83–96.

77. Albornoz L, Alvarez D, Otasa J, et al. von Willebrand factor could be an index of endothelial dysfunction in patients with cirrhosis; relationship to degree of liver failure and nitric oxide levels. *J Hepatol* 1999;30:451–455.

78. Ferro D, Quintarelli C, Lattuada A, et al. High plasma levels of von Willebrand factor as a marker of endothelial perturbation in cirrhosis: relationship to endotoxemia. *Hepatology* 1996;23:1377–1383.

79. Mannucci P, Canciani M, Forza I, et al. Changes in health and disease of the metalloprotease that cleaves von Willebrand factor. *Blood* 2001;98: 2730–2735.

80. Lisman T, Leebeek F. Haemostatic abnormalities in patients with liver disease. *J Hepatol* 2002;37(2):280–287.

81. Saito H, Goldsmith G, Waldman A. Fitzgerald factor (high molecular weight kininogen) clotting activity in human plasma in health and disease. *Blood* 1976;48:941.

82. Walker I, Milner R, Johnson M. Factors XI and XII are low in subjects with liver disease. *Dig Dis Sci* 1983;28:967.

83. Biland L, Duckert S, Prisender S, et al. Quantitative estimation of coagulation factors in liver disease. The diagnostic and prognostic value of factor XIII, factor V and plasminogen. *Thromb Haemost* 1978;39:646–656.

84. Gralnick H, Givelber H, Abrams E. Dysfibrinogenemia associated with hepatoma: increased carbohydrate content of the fibrinogen molecule. *N Engl J Med* 1978;299:221.

85. Lane D, Scully J, DP T. Acquired dysfibrinogenemia in acute and chronic liver disease. *Br J Haematol* 1977;35:301.

86. Francis J, Armstrong D. Fibrinogen-bound sialic acid levels in the dysfibrinogenemias of liver disease. *Haemostasis* 1982;11:215.

87. Martinez J, Palascak J, Kwasniak D. Abnormal sialic acid content of the dysfibrinogenemia associated with liver disease. *J Clin Invest* 1978; 61:535.

88. Bajaj M, Rana S, Wysolmerski R, et al. Inhibitor of the factor VII tissue factor complex is reduced in patients with disseminated intravascular coagulation but not in patients with severe hepatocellular disease. *J Clin Invest* 1987;79:1874–1878.

89. Tripodi A, Salerno F, Chantarangkul V, et al. Evidence of normal thrombin generation in cirrhosis despite abnormal conventional coagulation tests. *Hepatology* 2005;41:553–558.

90. Cederblad G, Korsan-Bengtsen K, Olson R. Observations of increased levels of blood coagulation factors and other plasma proteins in cholestatic liver disease. *Scand J Gastroenterol* 1976;11:391.

91. Rapaport S, Ames S, Mikkelsen S, et al. Plasma clotting factors in chronic hepatocellular disease. *N Engl J Med* 1960;263:278.

92. Colucci M, Altomare D, Chetta G. Impaired fibrinolysis in obstructive jaundice. Evidence from clinical and experimental studies. *Thromb Haemost* 1988;60:25.

93. Segal H, Cottam S, Potter D, et al. Coagulation and fibrinolysis in primary biliary cirrhosis compared with other liver disease and during orthotopic liver transplantation. *Hepatology* 1997;25(3):683–688.

94. Blomback B, Carlson L, Franzen S, et al. Turnover of I-labeled fibrinogen in man: studies in normal subjects, in congenital coagulation factor deficiency states, in liver disease, in polycythemia vera, and in epidermolysis bullosa. *Acta Med Scand* 1966;179:557.

95. Rake M, Flute P, Panell G, et al. Intravascular coagulation in acute hepatic necrosis. *Lancet* 1970;1:533.

96. Singh R, Singh M, Hazra D. A study of disseminated intravascular coagulation in hepatic coma complicating acute viral hepatitis. *Angiology* 1983;34:470.

97. Verstraete M, Vermylen J, Collen D. Intravascular coagulation in liver disease. *Annu Rev Med* 1974;25:447.

98. Levy G, Helin H, Edgington T. The pathobiology of viral hepatitis and immunologic activation of the coagulation protease network. *Semin Liver Dis* 1984;4:59.

99. Deykin D. The role of liver in serum induced hypercoagulability. *J Clin Invest* 1966;45:256.
100. Rodzynek J, Urbain D, Leautaud P, et al. Antithrombin III, plasminogen and alpha-2-antiplasmin in jaundice. Clinical usefulness and prognostic significance. *Gut* 1984;25:1050.
101. Langley P, Williams R. The effect of fulminant hepatic failure on protein C antigen and activity. *Thromb Haemost* 1988;59:316.
102. D'Angelo A, Vigano-D'Angelo S, Esmon C, et al. Acquired deficiencies of protein S. Protein S activity during oral anticoagulation in liver disease, and in disseminated intravascular coagulation. *J Clin Invest* 1988;81:1441.
103. Tollefsen D, Pestka C. Heparin cofactor II activity in patients with disseminated intravascular coagulation and hepatic failure. *Blood* 1985;66:769.
104. Hillenfrand P, Parbhoo S, Jedrychowski A, et al. Significance of intravascular coagulation in fibrinolysis in acute hepatic failure. *Gut* 1974;15:83.
105. Straub P. Diffuse intravascular coagulation in liver disease? *Semin Thromb Haemost* 1997;4:29–39.
106. Straub P. Intravascular coagulation in acute hepatic necrosis. *Lancet* 1970; 760:1339.
107. Oka K, Tanaka K. Intravascular coagulation in autopsy cases with liver disease. *Thromb Haemost* 1979;42:564.
108. Clark R, Gazzard B, Lewis M, et al. Fibrinogen metabolism in acute hepatitis and active chronic hepatitis. *Br J Haematol* 1975;30:95.
109. Tytgat G, Collen D, Verstraete M. Metabolism of fibrinogen in cirrhosis of the liver. *J Lab Clin Med* 1974;50:1690.
110. Coleman M, Finlayson N, Bettigole R. Fibrinogen survival in cirrhosis: improvement by low-dose heparin. *Ann Intern Med* 1975;83:79–81.
111. Schipper H, Ten Cate J. Antithrombin III transfusion in patients with hepatic cirrhosis. *Br J Haematol* 1982;52:25–33.
112. Bakker C, Knot E, Stibbe J. Disseminated intravascular coagulation in liver cirrhosis. *Hepatology* 1992;25:330–335.
113. Wilde J, Kitchen S, Kinsey S. Plasma D-dimer levels and their relationship to serum fibrinogen/fibrin degradation products in hypercoagulable states. *Br J Haematol* 1989;71:65.
114. Cordova C, Musca A, Viola F. Improvement of some blood coagulation factors in cirrhotic patients treated with low doses of heparin. *Scand J Haematol* 1982;29:235.
115. Ben-Ari Z, Osman E, Hutton R, et al. Disseminated intravascular coagulation in liver cirrhosis: fact or fiction? *Am J Gastroenterol* 1999;94(10): 2977–2982.
116. Mombelli G, Fiori G, Monotti R. Fibrinopeptide A in liver cirrhosis: evidence against a major contribution of disseminated intravascular coagulation to coagulopathy of chronic liver disease. *J Lab Clin Med* 1992;121: 83–90.
117. Ardaillou N, Yvart J, Le Bras P, et al. Catabolism of human fibrinogen fragment D in normal subjects and patients with liver cirrhosis. *Thromb Haemost* 1980;44:46.
118. Joist J. AICF and DIC in liver cirrhosis: expressions of a hypercoagulable state. *Am J Gastroenterol* 1999;94:2801–2803.
119. Belli L, Romani F, Sansalone C, et al. Portal thrombosis in cirrhotics. A retrospective analysis. *Ann Surg* 1986;203:286–291.
120. Violi F, Ferro D, Basili S. Association between low-grade disseminated intravascular coagulation and endotoxemia in patients with liver cirrhosis. *Gastroenterology* 1995;109:531–539.
121. Violi F, Ferro D, Basili S, et al. Ongoing prothrombotic state in the portal circulation of cirrhotic patients. *Thromb Haemost* 1997;77(1):44–47.
122. Lerner R, Nelson J, Corines P, et al. Disseminated intravascular coagulation: complications of peritoneovenous shunts. *JAMA* 1978;240:2064.
123. Holm A, Halpern N, Aldrete J. Peritoneovenous shunt for intractable ascites of hepatic, nephrogenic, and malignant causes. *Am J Surg* 1989;158:162.
124. Tempero M, Davis R, Reed E, et al. Thrombocytopenia and laboratory evidence of disseminated intravascular coagulation after shunts for ascites in malignant disease. *Cancer* 1985;55:2718.
125. Salem H, Koutts J, Handley C. The aggregation of human platelets by ascitic fluid: a possible mechanism for disseminated intravascular coagulation complicating LeVeen shunts. *Am J Hematol* 1981;11:153.
126. Baele G, Rasquin K, Barbier F. Coagulant, fibrinolytic and aggregating activity in ascitic fluid. *Am J Gastroenterol* 1986;81:440.
127. Fletcher A, Biederman O, Moore D. Abnormal plasminogen-plasmin system activity (fibrinolysis) in patients with hepatic cirrhosis: its cause and consequences. *J Clin Invest* 1964;43:681.
128. Ratnoff O. Studies on a proteolytic enzyme in human plasma. IV. The rate of lysis of plasma clots in normal and diseased individuals with particular reference to hepatic disease. *Bull Johns Hopkins Hosp* 1949;84:29.
129. Goodpasture E. Fibrinolysis in chronic hepatic insufficiency. *Bull Johns Hopkins Hosp* 1914;25:330.
130. Tran-Thang C, Fasel-Felly J, Pralong G. Plasminogen activators and plasminogen activator inhibitors in liver deficiencies caused by chronic alcoholism or infectious hepatitis. *Thromb Haemost* 1989;62:651.
131. Hersch S, Kunelis T, Francis R. The pathogenesis of accelerated fibrinolysis in liver cirrhosis: a critical role for tissue plasminogen activator inhibition. *Blood* 1987;69:1315.
132. Francis R, Seyfert U. Tissue plasminogen activator antigen and activity in disseminated intravascular coagulation: clinicopathologic correlation. *J Lab Clin Med* 1987;110:541.
133. Tytgat G, Collen D, DeVreker R, et al. Investigations on the fibrinolytic system in liver cirrhosis. *Acta Haematol (Basel)* 1968;40:265.
134. Marongiu F, Mamusa A, Mameli C. Alpha 2-antitrypsin and DIC in liver cirrhosis. *Thromb Res* 1985;37:287.
135. Saito H, Goodnough L, Boyle J, et al. Reduced histidine-rich glycoprotein levels in plasma of patients with advanced liver cirrhosis: possible implications of enhanced fibrinolysis. *Am J Med* 1982;73:179.
136. Collen D, Bouvier J, Chamone D, et al. Turnover of radiolabeled plasminogen and prothrombin cirrhosis of the liver. *Eur J Clin Invest* 1978; 8:185.
137. Takahashi H, Tatewaki W, Wada K. Thrombin and plasminogen in patients with liver disease. *Am J Hematol* 1989;36:30–35.
138. Violi F, Basili S, Ferro D. Association between high levels of D-dimer and tissue-plasminogen activator activity and first gastrointestinal bleeding in cirrhotic patients. CALC group. *Thromb Haemost* 1996;76:177–183.
139. Francis R, Feinstein D. Clinical significance of accelerated fibrinolysis in liver disease. *Haemostasis* 1984;14:460.
140. Ferro D, Saliola M, Quintarelli C, et al. 1 year survey of patients with advanced liver cirrhosis. Prognostic value of clinical and laboratory indexes identified by the cox regression model. *Scand J Gastroenterol* 1992;27: 852–856.
141. O'Grady J, Alexander G, Hayllat K. Early indicators of prognosis in fulminant hepatic failure. *Gastroenterology* 1989;97:439–445.
142. Pugh R, Murray-Lyon I, Dawson J. Transection of the oesophagus for bleeding oesophageal varices. *Br J Haematol* 1973;60:646–649.
143. Garrison R, Cryer H, Howard D. Classification of risk factors for abdominal operations in patients with hepatic cirrhosis. *Ann Surg* 1984;199:648.
144. Schwartz W. Biliary tract surgery and cirrhosis: a critical combination. *Surgery* 1981;90:577.
145. Yerdel M, Koksoy C, Aras N. Laproscopic versus open cholecystectomy in cirrhotic patients: a prospective study. *Surg Laparosc Endosc* 1997;7: 483–486.
146. Ragni M, Lewis J, Spero J. Bleeding and coagulation abnormalities in alcoholic cirrhotic liver disease. *Alcohol Clin Exp Res* 1982;6:267–274.
147. Christensen E, Schlichting P, Fauerholdt L, et al. Changes of laboratory variables with time in cirrhosis: prognostic and therapeutic significance. *Hepatology* 1985;5:843.
148. Hegarty J, Williams R. Liver biopsy: techniques, clinical applications and complications. *Br Med J* 1984;188:1254.
149. Piccinino F, Sagnelli E, Pasquale G. Complications following percutaneous liver biopsy. *J Hepatol* 1986;2:165–172.
150. Garcia-Tsao G, Boyer J. Outpatient liver biopsy: how safe is it? *Ann Intern Med* 1993;118:150–153.
151. Janes C, Lindon K. Outcome of patients hospitalized for complications after outpatient liver biopsy. *Ann Intern Med* 1993;118:96–98.
152. Westaby D, MacDougall B, Williams R. Liver biopsy as a day-case procedure: selection and complications in 200 consecutive patients. *Br Med J* 1980;281:1331–1332.
153. Ewe K. Bleeding after liver biopsy does not correlate with indices of peripheral coagulation. *Dig Dis Sci* 1981;26:388–393.
154. Kovacs M, Wong A, Mackinnon K, et al. Assessment of the validity of the INR system for patients with liver impairment. *Thromb Haemost* 1994; 71:727–730.
155. Robert A, Chazouilleres O. Prothombin time in liver failure: time, ratio, activity percentage, or international normalized ratio? *Hepatology* 1996; 24:1392–1394.
156. Mannucci P, Vicente V, Vianello L. Controlled trial of desmopressin in liver cirrhosis and other conditions associated with a prolonged bleeding time. *Blood* 1986;67:1148–1153.
157. Burroughs A, Matthews K, Qadiri M, et al. Desmopressin and bleeding time in patients with cirrhosis. *Br Med J* 1985;291:1377–1381.
158. Macelo G, Maia J, Gomez A. The role of transjugular liver biopsy in a liver transplant center. *J Clin Gastroenterol* 1999;29:155–157.
159. Tobin M, Gilmore I. Plugged liver biopsy in patients with impaired coagulation. *Dig Dis Sci* 1989;34:13.
160. Farrell R, Smiddy P, Pilkington R. Guided versus blind liver biopsy for chronic hepatitis C: clinical benefits and costs. *J Hepatol* 1999;30:580–587.
161. Friedman E, Sussman II. Safety of invasive procedures in patients with the coagulopathy of liver disease. *Clin Lab Haematol* 1989;11:199.
162. Grabau C, Crago S, Hoff L, et al. Performance standards for therapeutic abdominal paracentesis. *Hepatology* 2004;40:484–488.
163. Lewis J, Bontempo F, YG K. Liver transplantation: intraoperative changes in coagulation factors in 100 first transplants. *Hepatology* 1989;9:710.
164. Otto G, Wolf H, Uerlings I, et al. Preservation damage in liver transplantation. Influence of rapid cooling. *Transplantation* 1986;42:122.
165. Suzumura N, Monden M, Gotoh M. Mechanisms involved in coagulation disorders during orthotopic liver transplantation. *Transplant Proc* 1988; 20:622.
166. Porte R, Knot E, Bontempo F. Hemostasis in liver transplantation. *Gastroenterology* 1989;97:488–501.
167. Arnoux D, Boutiere B, Houvenaeghel M. Intraoperative evolution of coagulatin parameters and t-PA/PAI 1 balance in orthotopic liver transplantation. *Thromb Res* 1989;55:319.
168. Dzik W, Arkin C, Jenkins R, et al. Fibrinolysis during liver transplantation in humans. Role of tissue plasminogen activator. *Blood* 1988;71:1090.
169. Harper P, Luddington R, Jennings I. Coagulation changes following hepatic revascularization during liver transplantation. *Transplantation* 1989; 48:603.

170. Porte R, Bontempo F, Knot E. Systemic effects of tissue plasminogen activator-associated fibrinolysis and its relation to thrombin generation in orthotopic liver transplantation. *Transplantation* 1989;47:978.

171. Porte R, et al. Aprotinin and transfusion requirements in orthotopic liver transplantation: a multicenter randomised double-blind study. *Lancet* 2000; 355:1303–1309.

172. Findlay J, Rettke S, Ereth M, et al. Aprotinin reduces red blood cell transfusion in orthotopic liver transplantation: a prospective, randomized, double-blind study. *Liver Transpl* 2001;7:802–807.

173. Harding S, Mallett S, Peachey T, et al. Use of heparinase modified thromboelastography in liver transplantation. *Br J Anaesth* 1997;78:175–179.

174. Biancofiore L, DBindi L, Catalano A, et al. Combined twice-daily plasma exchange and continuous veno-venous hemodiafiltration for bridging severe acute liver failure. *Transplant Proc* 2003;35:3011–3014.

175. Wang Y, He Z, Niu R, et al. Assessment of the combined effect of plasma exchange and plasma perfusion on patients with severe hepatitis awaiting orthotopic liver transplantation. *Int J Artif Organs* 2004;27:40–44.

176. Motchman T, Taswell H, Brecher M, et al. Blood bank support of a liver transplantation program. *Mayo Clin Proc* 1989;64:103.

177. Massicotte L, Sassine M, Lenis S, et al. Transfusion predictors in liver transplant. *Anesth Analg* 2004;98:1245–1251.

178. Bontempo F. Monitoring of coagulation during liver transplantation. How much is enough? *Mayo Clin Proc* 1987;62:848.

179. Ritter D, Owen C, Bowie E. Evaluation of preoperative hematology-coagulation screening in liver transplantation. *Mayo Clin Proc* 1989;64:216.

180. Giles B. Thromboelastography and liver transplantation. *Semin Thromb Hemost* 1995;21(suppl. 4):45–49.

181. Stahl R, Duncan A, Hooks M. A hypercoagulable state follows orthotopic liver transplantation. *Hepatology* 1990;12:553.

182. Lemmons H, Neumann U, Bechstein W. Incidence and outcome of arterial complications after orthotopic liver transplantation. *Transpl Int* 1996; 9(suppl. 1):S178–S181.

183. Buckels J, Tisone G, Gunson B, et al. Low hematocrit reduces hepatic artery thrombosis after liver transplantation. *Transplant Proc* 1989;21:2460.

184. Fiore L, Brophy M, Deykin D. Hemostasis. In: Zakim D, Boyer T, eds. *Hepatology a textbook of liver disease*. Philadelphia, PA: Saunders, 2003: 549–580.

185. Hultin M. Activated clotting factors in factor IX concentrates. *Blood* 1979; 54:1028.

186. Lusher J. Thrombogenicity associated with factor IX complex concentrates. *Semin Hematol* 1991;28:3.

187. Marassi A, Manzullo V, DiCarlo V, et al. Thromboembolism following prothrombin complex concentrate and major surgery in severe liver disease. *Thromb Haemost* 1978;39:787.

188. Kohler M, Hellstern P, Lechner E. Thromboembolic complications associated with the use of prothrombin complex and factor IX concentrates. *Thromb Haemost* 1998;80:395–402.

189. Mannucci P, Franchi F, Dioguardi N. Correction of abnormal coagulation in chronic liver disease by combined use of fresh-frozen plasma and prothrombin complex concentrates. *Lancet* 1976;2:542.

190. Lorenz R, Kienast J, Otto U, et al. Efficacy and safety of a prothrombin complex concentratre with two virus-inactivation steps in patients with severe liver damage. *Eur J Gastroenterol Hepatol* 2003;15(1):15–20.

191. Bernstein D, Jeffers L, Erhardtsen E. Recombinant factor VIIa corrects prothrombin time in cirrhotic patients: a preliminary study. *Gastroenterology* 1997;113:1930–1937.

192. Jeffers L, Chalasani N, Balart L, et al. Safety and efficacy of recombinant factor VIIa in patients with liver disease undergoing labaroscopic liver biopsy. *Gastroenterology* 2002;123:118–126.

193. Ejlersen E, Melsen T, Ingerslev J, et al. Recombinant activated factor VII (rFVlla) acutely normalizes prothrombin time in patients with cirrhosis during bleeding from oesophageal varices. *Scand J Gastroenterol* 2001;36 (10):1081–1085.

194. Bosch J, Thabut D, Bendtsen F, et al. Recombinant factor VIIa for upper gastrointestinal bleeding in patients with cirrhosis: a randomized, double-blind trial. *Gastroenterology* 2004;127:1123–1130.

195. Plainsic R, Test G, Emre S, et al. Safety and efficacy of single bolus dose of recombinant factor VIIa in patients undergoing orthotopic liver transplantation: a randomized multi-center study. *Hepatology* 2002;36: 660A.

196. Ustun C, Deiner P, Faguet G. Interleukin-11 administration normalizes the platelet count in a hypersplenic cirrhotic patient. *Ann Hematol* 2002;81: 609–610.

197. Ghalib R, Levine C, Hassan M, et al. Recombinant human interleukin-11 improves thrombocytopenia in patients with cirrhosis. *Hepatology* 2003; 37:1165–1167.

198. Sakai K, Iwao G, Oho K, et al. Propranolol ameliorates thrombocytopenia in patients with cirrhosis. *J Gastroenterol* 2002;37:112–118.

199. de Franchis R, Arcidiancono P, Carpinelli P. Randomized controlled trial of desmopressin plus terlipressin and terlipressin alone for the treatment of acute variceal hemrrohage in cirrhotic patients: a multicenter, double blind study. *Hepatology* 1993;18:1102–1107.

# CHAPTER 69 ■ CLINICAL DISORDERS OF FIBRINOLYSIS

CHARLES W. FRANCIS AND VICTOR J. MARDER

Excessive inhibition of fibrinolysis interferes with the hemostatic balance and can lead to thrombosis by inhibiting clot dissolution while clot formation occurs unimpeded. The contribution of defective fibrinolysis to thrombotic disease has been difficult to evaluate because available plasma screening tests are generally less sensitive to decreased activity compared to increased activity, and because thrombosis is common in the population and typically involves a component of primary vascular pathology of complex pathogenesis. However, increasing evidence indicates that impaired fibrinolysis contributes to thrombosis in rare inherited deficiencies and also in more common acquired hypofibrinolytic states.

The inherited disorders are rare and typically caused by a single molecular defect. They have provided critical information about the role of specific molecules within the fibrinolytic system. More common are acquired bleeding disorders associated with heightened fibrinolysis as either the primary or contributing mechanism. These may be due to the increased secretion of plasminogen activator, to decreased inhibitory factors, or to a combination of both. Improved management of these more common bleeding disorders requires an appreciation of the potential of hyperfibrinolysis to cause bleeding, followed by the appropriate diagnostic tests and careful use of available therapies.

Intuitively, defective fibrinolysis would be expected to contribute to thrombotic disease, and thrombosis occurring in patients with single gene defects (as indicated in preceding text) and in knockout mouse models supports this concept. However, hypofibrinolysis may also contribute to thrombotic disease in more common conditions with complex, multifactor pathogenesis. Deciphering the specific contribution of hypofibrinolysis in these conditions is difficult because the regulation of fibrinolysis interacts with many metabolic and hormonal systems and is also influenced by genetic polymorphism.

## INHERITED DISORDERS

Inherited fibrinolytic disorders that cause bleeding are shown in Table 69-1.

### Inherited Bleeding Disorders

#### $\alpha_2$-Antiplasmin Deficiency

Inherited deficiency of $\alpha_2$-antiplasmin is a rare autosomal recessive condition resulting in a bleeding disorder (1–6). $\alpha_2$-Antiplasmin is the principal inhibitor of the fibrinolytic enzyme, plasmin, and patients with deficiency exhibit heightened fibrinolytic activity. A mouse knockout model has been developed,

which demonstrates enhanced endogenous fibrinolytic activity, but the mice, unlike humans, do not have an overt bleeding tendency, reflecting somewhat different regulatory mechanisms in different species (7). Congenital deficiency of $\alpha_2$-antiplasmin inhibitor is rare, but the true prevalence is unknown. Several different mutations causing congenital deficiency have been elucidated (8–12). Two types of deficiency are recognized: Type I represents a quantitative disorder, with similar decreases in functional and immunologic assays. Type II deficiency results from a structural change causing lower activity than reflected by the antigen concentration.

Homozygous deficiency was first reported in 1978 (1) in a patient with nearly undetectable plasma $\alpha_2$-antiplasmin inhibitor and a severe lifelong bleeding disorder with hemothorax, hemarthrosis, gingival bleeding, easy bruising, and prolonged bleeding after minor injury. Tests of *in vitro* clot lysis were accelerated, but plasma fibrinogen was normal. Fibrinogen degradation products were not elevated, indicating that bleeding was caused by premature lysis of hemostatic plugs and not the result of systemic plasminemia. The phenotype in the reported cases is variable, with most patients having severe bleeds in childhood and occasionally umbilical bleeding as the first manifestation. Other cases are less severe, presenting with only moderate bleeding disorders. A Dutch family with a bleeding disorder due to synthesis of a dysfunctional antiplasmin molecule with a mutation near the reactive site has been reported (13). Intramedullary hematoma in the diaphyses of long bones has occurred in several cases of $\alpha_2$-antiplasmin inhibitor, representing a perhaps unique site of bleeding (14,15).

Individuals with heterozygous $\alpha_2$-antiplasmin inhibitor deficiency may be either asymptomatic or exhibit a mild bleeding tendency that may worsen with advancing age (16–18). Diagnosis depends upon clinical suspicion and on performing the specific assay after ruling out more common disorders. Treatment with the antifibrinolytic agents tranexamic acid or epsilon aminocaproic acid has been successful in both preventing bleeding in patients undergoing invasive procedures and in treating bleeding complications. Fresh frozen plasma has also been used as an alternative to antifibrinolytic agents, and $\alpha_2$-antiplasmin exhibited an *in vivo* half-life of more than 20 hours following transfusion (19). The choice of the specific plasma preparation to use is important because solvent/detergent treatment may render $\alpha_2$-antiplasmin inactive (20).

#### Plasminogen Activator Inhibitor-1 Deficiency

Plasminogen activator inhibitor-1 (PAI-1) is the primary inhibitor of tissue plasminogen activator, and deficiency may result in increased fibrinolysis, premature lysis of hemostatic plugs, and a bleeding tendency. Several reports of congenital bleeding disorder related to PAI-1 deficiency describe multiple episodes of serious bleeding primarily after surgery or trauma

## TABLE 69-1

### INHERITED FIBRINOLYTIC DISORDERS CAUSING BLEEDING OR THROMBOSIS

| Bleeding | Characteristics |
|---|---|
| $\alpha_2$-Antiplasmin deficiency | Homozygous: severe bleeding |
| | Heterozygous: asymptomatic or mild bleeding |
| | Premature lysis of hemostatic plugs |
| | No systemic plasminemia |
| | Improves with antifibrinolytic agents |
| Plasminogen activator inhibitor-1 deficiency | Moderate to severe bleeding |
| | Short lysis times; reduced fibrinogen, plasminogen, and $\alpha_2$-antiplasmin |
| | Improves with antifibrinolytic therapy |
| Quebec platelet disorder | Moderate to severe delayed bleeding |
| | Increased intraplatelet uPA |
| | Degradation of $\alpha$-granule proteins |
| | Platelet dysfunction and premature lysis of hemostatic plugs |
| | Improves with antifibrinolytic therapy |
| **THROMBOSIS** | |
| Plasminogen deficiency | Low risk of thrombosis |
| | Ligneous conjunctivitis with severe deficiency |
| Dysfibrinogenemia | Structural changes result in defective interaction with fibrinolytic proteins |
| | Dusart and Chapel Hill III–A$\alpha$ R554C |
| | Caracas V–A$\alpha$ S532C |
| | New York I–del B$\beta$9-71 |
| | Tampere |
| | Belingham–$\gamma$R275C |

uPA, urokinase plasminogen activator.

(21–23). Screening tests, including the prothrombin time (PT), partial thromboplastin time (PTT), thrombin time, platelet count, and bleeding time, have all been normal. In two cases, PAI-1 antigen and activity were both low, whereas in the third the activity was low, but the antigen was within the normal range, suggesting synthesis of a dysfunctional protein. In all cases, the euglobulin clot lysis time was shortened, and fibrinogen, plasminogen, and $\alpha_2$-antiplasmin levels were reduced, albeit to variable degrees.

Deficiency of PAI-1 was due to a frameshift mutation in one case, in which a large family study showed that only homozygously affected individuals were symptomatic. A bleeding disorder due to dysfunctional PAI-1 molecule with reduced tissue plasminogen activator (tPA) inhibiting activity has been described in a patient with a lifelong history of bleeding (24). Clot lysis times were abnormally short, and plasminogen and $\alpha_2$-antiplasmin were low, although plasma tPA levels were normal. Use of antifibrinolytic agents has been effective in treating bleeding complications (25,26).

### Increased Tissue Plasminogen Activator

A congenital hemorrhagic disorder due to increasing circulating levels of plasminogen activator has been described in two cases, and fatal intracranial hemorrhage occurred in one (27, 28). The patients in both reports had shortened clot lysis times, low fibrinogen, and evidence of increased plasma tPA levels. In one case, treatment with epsilon aminocaproic acid or tranexamic acid resulted in improvement in laboratory markers of hyperfibrinolysis with normalization of clot lysis times and an increase in fibrinogen and $\alpha_2$-antiplasmin.

### Quebec Platelet Disorder

The Quebec platelet disorder is a rare autosomal dominant condition with the unusual clinical features of moderate to severe delayed bleeding, typically starting at 12 to 24 hours after surgery or trauma (29). Affected individuals may have large bruises, joint bleeds, and bleeding following dental extractions or trauma. The disorder was initially designated as *Factor V Quebec* because of abnormalities in platelet factor V (30). More recent investigation has identified other platelet abnormalities, including reduced to low-normal platelet counts, defective aggregation with epinephrine, and evidence of proteolytic degradation of $\alpha_2$-granule–contained and intrinsic membrane proteins (29,31–33). Characteristically, such patients have elevated levels of fibrinogen degradation products in the serum, derived from secretion of platelet fibrinogen degradation products, but the concentration of fibrinogen degradation products and D-dimer in plasma is normal. Platelets of affected individuals show excessive degradation of both plasma-derived and megakaryocyte-synthesized proteins stored in $\alpha$-granules, but external membrane, dense-granule, and cytoplasmic platelet proteins are not affected (29,31). This proteolytic degradation is the result of large amounts of urokinase-type plasminogen activator (uPA) present within a platelet secretory component. Although uPA is not increased in plasma, it is elevated more than 100-fold in platelets, in parallel with increased uPA mRNA, thereby causing generation of plasmin and proteolysis of $\alpha$-granule proteins (34,35). The bleeding disorder is likely to be caused by both defective platelet function and release of excess uPA, resulting in both poor clot formation and accelerated dissolution of hemostatic plugs, that can be improved by fibrinolytic inhibitors (36).

## Inherited Thrombotic Disorders

### Plasminogen Deficiency

Plasminogen is the zymogen of the active fibrinolytic enzyme plasmin, and inherited deficiency of plasminogen has been associated with thrombotic disease. The first case was described by Aoki et al. in a patient with recurrent venous thrombotic disease over a period of 15 years who had a normal plasma plasminogen antigen concentration, but approximately 50% functional activity (37). The defect was identified as an amino acid substitution occurring two residues from the active site histidine, resulting in an absence of proteolytic activity (38); the same defect has been found in additional cases (39). The occurrence of the variant plasminogen in several other family members suggested an autosomal dominant inheritance. Because no other family members, including one homozygous individual, experienced clinically significant disease, the contribution of the plasminogen variant to the pathogenesis of the recurrent thrombosis in the propositus remains unexplained. Several other abnormal plasminogen variants have been characterized by normal or slightly reduced antigen concentration with decreased functional activity (40–43). The index case usually presented with deep vein thrombosis (DVT) at an early age.

A study of the gene frequencies for abnormal plasminogens used electrofocusing to screen plasma samples and found a racial difference, with a relatively high frequency of 0.018 in the Japanese population, but no cases in a Caucasian-American population (44). The first appearance of DVT after trauma may indicate that the abnormal plasminogen does not by itself cause thrombotic disease, but rather predisposes to or exacerbates an existing thrombophilic state by interfering with thrombus resolution. A review of published studies suggests that the relative risk of thrombosis is low in individuals who are plasminogen deficient and may not be significantly higher than in unaffected persons (45).

A study in Scotland found familial plasminogen deficiency at a frequency of 2.9 per 1,000 (46). A common missense mutation, K19E in the plasminogen gene, was found in most of the propositi, but none of the individuals with plasminogen deficiency developed venous thrombosis, suggesting that the risk is low. Some studies suggest an association with cerebral vein thrombosis, particularly in children (47,48). In a large referral center, plasminogen deficiency was identified in 23 per 1,192 subjects, corresponding to an overall prevalence of venous thrombosis in 2.2% and arterial events in 1.4% (49). Of the 23 plasminogen-deficient individuals, eight had additional thrombophilic defects and four had relevant circumstantial risk factors. The evidence from this center suggests that plasminogen deficiency is a rare cause of thrombophilia and not as strong a thrombotic risk factor as a single defect. In a large database of 2,132 consecutive patients with venous thromboembolism, 16 (0.75%) had plasminogen deficiency (50).

Although the association with thrombotic disease is controversial, severe Type I plasminogen deficiency is associated with ligneous conjunctivitis, a rare disease characterized by woodlike pseudomembranes developing on the ocular and extraocular mucosa (51–53). Other findings are impaired wound healing, hyperviscous nasopharyngeal and bronchial secretions and hydrocephalus. All of theses manifestations have been attributed to defective fibrinolysis, and the conjunctival lesions contain fibrin without plasminogen, suggesting that deficient fibrinolysis in tears is the likely cause of the fibrinous pseudomembranes. A plasminogen knockout mouse model confirms this

association (54). Schott et al. demonstrated that the ligneous lesions in patients could be reversed by plasminogen infusion, with changes noted within 3 days and restored to normal after 2 weeks of treatment (55). Recurrence was prevented by daily injections of plasminogen sufficient to achieve plasma concentrations to approximately 40%. Treatment with topical plasminogen has also been successful and resulted in dramatic improvement and complete resolution of the membranes (56). In two young women patients with ligneous conjunctivitis and moderate hypoplasminogenemia, treatment with oral contraceptives resulted in a marked increase in plasminogen levels and some resolution of the pseudomembrane (57). Ligneous conjunctivitis has been related to homozygous type I plasminogen deficiency and also to compound heterozygous mutations, with the severity of clinical symptoms depending on the amount of residual functional plasminogen activity (53).

### Dysfibrinogenemia

Dysfibrinogenemia is usually asymptomatic but may be associated with bleeding, pregnancy loss, or, occasionally, a familial thrombotic disease (see Chapter 62). Some specific structural abnormalities in fibrinogen alter its interaction with fibrinolytic proteins and may represent the basis for clinical thrombotic disease. Fibrinogen Chapel Hill III was identified in a patient with recurrent venous thrombosis in a family with several other affected members (58). The fibrinogen exhibited defective polymerization and relative resistance to plasmic degradation and formed abnormally rigid fibrin gels. Defective thrombolysis may also account for the recurrent venous thrombosis and pulmonary embolism seen in patients with fibrinogen Dusart (59). This fibrinogen demonstrated abnormal fibrin monomer polymerization, decreased binding of plasminogen to fibrin, and reduction in the capacity of fibrin to enhance fibrinogen activation by tPA (60–62). The abnormality is due to a single-base change, Aα Arg554 Cys, the same as in fibrinogen Chapel Hill III, and resulting in cross-linking of albumin to the new residue at the C-terminus of the α chain (63). Electron microscopy showed that the αC domain was associated with albumin (61). Abnormal polymerization leading to tight fibrin gels with fibrinolytic resistance may also contribute to thrombosis in patients with fibrinogen Tampere (64). Fibrinogen New York I was identified in a family with a thrombotic tendency associated with abnormal fibrinolysis and defective potentiation of plasminogen activation by tPA (65). Characterization of the fibrinogen demonstrated a deletion of residues 9 to 69 of the β chain corresponding to exon 2 for the fibrinogen gene and providing evidence for the involvement of the sequence in interaction with tPA (66). Fibrinogen Caracas V occurred in a Venezuelan family with thrombophilia and exhibited prolonged thrombin and reptilase times (67). The accelerating capacity of the patient's fibrin on tPA-induced plasminogen activation was decreased, and the affinity of fibrinogen for plasmin was diminished (68). The mutation induced an Aα Ser532 Cys change, resulting in altered polymerization and generation of a tight fibrin network with decreased flow permeation leading to defective fibrinolysis. A dysfibrinogen with R 275 C alteration in the γ chain was identified in a propositus with recurrent venous thromboemboli and a positive family history of thrombosis (69). This dysfibrinogen revealed markedly abnormal thrombin-catalyzed polymerization and delayed fibrinolysis. These studies reveal the importance of fibrinogen as a mediator of fibrinolysis and provide insight into fibrinogen structures that interact with key fibrinolytic proteins.

### Defective Vascular Response

Familial thrombotic disease has been associated with a defective fibrinolytic response to stimulation from venous occlusion or 1-deamino-8-D-arginine vasopressin (DDAVP). In a large family studied by Johansson et al., DVT had occurred in 13 out of 17 members available for study, and 12 of these 13 had reduced plasma fibrinolytic activity after venous occlusion or DDAVP infusion (70). Vessel wall fibrinolytic activity as assayed histochemically was normal, suggesting that the defect was a decreased release of tPA or an increase of PAI-1 with autosomal dominant inheritance. A similar defect with a high incidence of venous thrombotic disease was described by Jorgensen et al. in three generations of a family; six members studied showed a subnormal increase in fibrinolytic activity after venous occlusion or exercise (71). A report by Stead et al. described a family with five members in two generations in whom venous thrombosis developed at an early age (72). Plasma fibrinolytic activity after venous occlusion was markedly deficient in all five subjects. Because it was associated with a subnormal increase in von Willebrand factor (VWF), a combined endothelial cell defect in processing or storage of VWF and tPA was suggested. These studies predated the availability of accurate assays for tPA, uPA, and PAI-1, so the contribution of decreased activator release or increased inhibitor to the reduced fibrinolytic activity still requires detailed investigation of additional cases.

# ACQUIRED DISORDERS

The acquired conditions that are associated with bleeding caused by hyperfibrinolysis are shown in Table 69-2.

## Acquired Bleeding Disorders

### Liver Disease

Severe liver disease frequently results in clinically significant bleeding and a coagulopathy with complex pathophysiology, including decreased synthesis of coagulation factors zymogens, inhibitors, and cofactors; synthesis of abnormal proteins; defective clearance of activated factors; and thrombocytopenia or thrombocytopathy. Accelerated fibrinolysis is common, and in some cases this may represent the primary coagulation

abnormality causing considerable bleeding. Patients with cirrhosis may have elevated levels of tPA with a decrease in $\alpha_2$-plasmin inhibitor and PAI-1 (73–77). Accelerated fibrinolysis identified by short clot lysis times has been correlated with increased plasma tPA activity and decreased $\alpha_2$-plasmin inhibitor (75). The limited capacity of plasma PAI-1 to inhibit increased tPA levels may be an important determinant in the development of excessive fibrinolysis in liver disease.

Heightened fibrinolysis as reflected by elevated tPA and D-dimer levels may be predictive of upper gastrointestinal bleeding in patients with cirrhosis. In a study of 112 cirrhotic patients with esophageal varices and without previous upper gastrointestinal bleeding who were followed-up for 3 years, multivariate analysis disclosed hyperfibrinolysis as the only marker predictive of bleeding (78). In a study of 86 consecutive patients referred to a tertiary center with cirrhosis, 31% showed hyperfibrinolysis as reflected by shortened euglobulin clot lysis times, and this correlated with evidence of more severe liver disease (79). Increased fibrinolysis was more frequently seen in patients with hepatic decompensation and mucocutaneous bleeding (79). Thrombin activatable fibrinolysis inhibitor (TAFI) is an important fibrinolytic regulator (see Chapter 20), and its level is reduced in cirrhosis (80,81). Low levels reflect defective TAFI$_a$ generation results from both reduced TAFI synthesis and impaired thrombin generation, and may contribute to bleeding associated with cirrhosis (82).

Laboratory findings reflecting the hyperfibrinolytic state include a shortened euglobulin lysis time and increase in plasma D-dimer and/or fibrinogen degradation products. tPA may be elevated because of decreased clearance, and the important inhibitors, PAI-1 and $\alpha_2$-plasmin, as well as plasminogen, are reduced, reflecting decreased synthesis and increased consumption. All of these findings are consistent with hyperfibrinolysis but can be difficult to distinguish from disseminated intravascular coagulation (DIC). However, macrovascular and microvascular thrombosis, typical of DIC, is rarely seen in cirrhosis. Treatment with fibrinolytic inhibitors such as epsilon aminocaproic acid, tranexamic acid, and aprotinin may be useful, particularly in patients with mucosal or gastrointestinal bleeding, but there are no prospective controlled studies demonstrating their effectiveness, and they should be used in conjunction with replacement therapy for optimum results.

**TABLE 69-2**

ACQUIRED CONDITIONS ASSOCIATED WITH BLEEDING DUE TO HYPERFIBRINOLYSIS

| | |
|---|---|
| Liver disease | Elevated activator, D-dimer and FDP, decreased antiplasmin and PAI-1 and TAFI |
| | Hyperfibrinolysis common in liver transplantation, especially in anhepatic phase |
| | Favorable response to antifibrinolytic therapy |
| Consumption coagulopathy | Fibrinolysis usually compensatory |
| | Antifibrinolytic therapy occasionally helpful when used with replacement and heparin |
| Acute promyelocytic leukemia | Elements of DIC, fibrinolysis, and elastase proteolysis may be present |
| | Marked improvement follows ATRA |
| Menorrhagia | Local endometrial hyperfibrinolysis is common |
| | Favorable response to antifibrinolytic therapy |
| Amyloidosis | Primary fibrinolysis occurs occasionally |
| | Favorable response to antifibrinolytic therapy |

FDP, fibrin degradation products; PAI-1, plasminogen activator inhibitor-1; TAFI, thrombin activatable fibrinolysis inhibitor; DIC, disseminated intravascular coagulation; ATRA, all trans-retinoic acid.

Pathologic hyperfibrinolysis may also contribute to severe hemorrhage seen in some cases of orthotopic liver transplantation, especially during the anhepatic phase of surgery (83,84). Accelerated fibrinolysis during transplantation has been associated with increased plasma tPA activity and antigen, depletion of fibrinogen and $\alpha_2$-plasmin, and elevated fibrin(ogen) degradation products (85). Both reduced hepatic clearance of activated tPA and systemic release of activator may contribute to the accelerated fibrinolysis, which improves after revascularization of the transplant. Treatment with fibrinolytic inhibitors can be useful. In a double-blind, randomized, placebo-controlled study of 45 patients, those who received tranexamic acid had less intraoperative blood loss and reduced intraoperative need for plasma, platelets, and cryoprecipitate (86). Porte et al. showed in a double-blind study of liver transplant recipients that treatment with aprotinin significantly reduced blood loss with no increase in thrombosis or change in mortality (87). Hyperfibrinolysis resolves after revascularization of the transplant liver, but continued antifibrinolytic therapy for up to 2 hours after reperfusion may be beneficial. The use of recombinant factor VIIa during transplantation results in localized thrombin generation without evidence of systemic coagulation activation (88). The coagulopathy during liver transplantation is complex, reflecting the severity of preexisting coagulopathy, thrombocytopenia and thrombocytopathy, hemostatic activation, and consumption related to surgery, and the pronounced synthetic defects during the anhepatic phase. Hyperfibrinolysis and the use of antifibrinolytic therapy should be considered in the overall context of blood and plasma component therapy.

## Secondary Fibrinolysis in Consumption Coagulopathy

The fibrinolytic activation typically seen in DIC is a secondary response to the marked hemostatic activation and microvascular thrombotic occlusion and serves an important compensatory function in maintaining vascular patency. Local release of tPA from endothelial cells may be stimulated by microvascular occlusion or systemic stress. The stimulation of plasminogen activation by tPA associated with fibrin degradation products (FDP) also contributes to systemic activation of fibrinolysis and to fibrinogen degradation (89). The abnormal hemostasis in DIC is therefore due to a combination of primary systemic activation of coagulation and secondary effects of accelerated fibrinolysis. Diagnostic evaluation requires assessment of both the hemostatic activation (DIC) and fibrinolysis. The pathogenesis of DIC relates primarily to enhanced tissue factor–mediated thrombin generation with concurrent dysfunction of inhibitory mechanisms resulting in excessive fibrin formation (90). The fibrinolytic system is activated as a compensatory mechanism but may be insufficient because the initial profibrinolytic response is accompanied by a sustained increase in plasma PAI-1 (89). Activation of TAFI by increased thrombin generation may further impair the fibrinolytic activation. Local fibrinolytic activation is reflected by increased plasma levels of fibrin(ogen) degradation and reduced plasminogen and $\alpha_2$-plasmin, reflecting their consumption. Plasmin–antiplasmin complexes increase, and global measures of fibrinolysis such as the euglobulin clot lyses time may be shortened. Secondary inhibitors such as $\alpha_2$-macroglobulin, $\alpha_1$-antitripsin, and C1-inhibitor may also be reduced with severe DIC, and plasma levels of PAI-1 are typically elevated, particularly in sepsis.

Hyperfibrinolysis may play a role in bleeding complications of DIC, and pharmacologic inhibition of fibrinolysis has been used successfully to treat bleeding. This, however, must be considered carefully because activation of fibrinolysis serves to maintain patency of the circulation under stress of thrombin generation and fibrin formation. Consequently, fibrinolytic inhibition may exacerbate thrombosis and worsen or precipitate ischemic symptoms. Use of a fibrinolytic inhibitor such as

tranexamic acid or epsilon aminocaproic acid may be useful in selected cases, such as in patients with severe bleeding who are unresponsive to the usual treatments, including replacement therapy (see Chapter 79). Antifibrinolytic therapy may be useful in such cases when given in conjunction with an anticoagulant such as heparin to prevent excessive coagulation.

The consumption coagulopathy and organ dysfunction seen with sepsis is associated with endotoxin released from Gram-negative bacteria. Administration of *Escherichia coli* endotoxin to normal volunteers results in rapid elevation of tPA and active fibrinolysis, reflected by elevated plasmin–antiplasmin complexes and by a subsequent rise in PAI-1, preventing further fibrinolysis (91,92). The overall response to endotoxin was biphasic, with initial activation and subsequent inhibition of fibrinolysis. Infection with *Rickettsia rickettsii* also results in a profibrinolytic response manifested by elevated tPA and decreased antiplasmin with increased fibrin(ogen) degradation products (92). Fibrinolysis may also play a central role in the pathogenesis of hemorrhage with African swine virus and dengue fever (93–95).

## Primary (Systemic) Hyperfibrinolysis

In some cases, the fibrinolytic activation seems out of proportion to the extent of coagulation activation, and in these cases, fibrinolysis may play an important role in consumption and bleeding. For example, the shock and bleeding symptoms of dengue infections are perhaps due to direct activation of plasminogen by the virus (93,95). Heat stroke is characterized by a markedly elevated core body temperature, central nervous dysfunction, an exaggerated acute-phase response, and multiorgan failure (96). A hemorrhagic diathesis with widespread microvascular thrombosis is commonly seen (97). However, manifestations of hyperfibrinolysis (increased tPA and D-dimer associated with decreases in plasminogen and increased plasmin–antiplasmin complexes) may reflect an exaggerated release of endothelial cell tPA causing a primary hemorrhagic disorder without the initial thrombotic events that characterize DIC syndromes (see Chapters 23 and 109). Activation of both coagulation and fibrinolysis occurs early and is improved by cooling. The hemorrhagic disorder may be transient, reflecting clearance of tPA, and in the absence of concomitant DIC, therapy may include an antifibrinolytic agent and replacement of consumed coagulation factors, especially fibrinogen. A similar transient clinical bleeding disorder may occur acutely after coronary artery bypass grafting surgery (98,99).

## Acute Promyelocytic Leukemia

Acute promyelocytic leukemia (APL) represents a malignant clonal expansion of immature myeloid cells exhibiting characteristic morphologic features and a balanced translocation t(15; 17), resulting in expression of a chimeric protein derived from the fusion of genes for the nuclear retinoic acid receptor on chromosome 17 and a transcription factor (PML) on chromosome 15 (100). Patients with APL exhibit characteristic clinical features including a hemorrhagic diathesis that frequently results in severe and often fatal bleeding early in its course. Before the introduction of modern therapy with all trans-retinoic acid (ATRA), hemorrhage was a major cause of morbidity and mortality. In a study of 268 consecutive patients, hemorrhagic deaths occurred in 14% of patients during induction therapy (101). This bleeding disorder exhibits complex features with important elements of thrombocytopenia, DIC, and fibrinolysis, each of which may contribute to bleeding (102,103).

However, the relative importance of primary fibrinolysis, DIC, and elastase proteolysis in the coagulopathy of APL is controversial, primarily because laboratory markers are nonspecific. Leukemic cells contain tPA, uPA, and elastase, and elevated levels have been found in patients with accelerated fibrinolysis and

APL (104–107). Leukemic blasts also produce inflammatory cytokines, including TNF-$\alpha$ and IL$-1\beta$ (108,109), which can downregulate endothelial anticoagulant properties and upregulate procoagulant tendencies. APL blasts also have abnormally high expression of the membrane receptor annexin II, which stimulates the generation of cell surface–oriented, tPA-dependent plasmin (110). Because plasmin formed on cell surfaces is protected from inhibition by $\alpha_2$-plasmin inhibitor (111), fibrinolytic overexpression on the cell surface related to annexin II may be particularly important in causing hemorrhage.

Before the introduction of ATRA, chemotherapy typically exacerbated bleeding (100,112). However, ATRA use leads to the decrease or normalization of hemostatic abnormalities in the first week of therapy, with improvement in all laboratory parameters, and a significant reduction in hemorrhagic events and death (102). Furthermore, with the use of ATRA, treatment with either heparin or antifibrinolytic agents is usually unnecessary. Although studies demonstrating the benefits of fibrinolytic inhibitors were published before the introduction of ATRA for induction therapy, contemporary treatment should focus on the optimal use of ATRA, and fibrinolytic inhibitors should be considered only in patients who are unresponsive, relapsed, or refractory to treatment, and who have prominent evidence of hyperfibrinolysis.

### Menorrhagia

Disorders of primary and secondary hemostasis, as well as of fibrinolysis may result in menorrhagia. Most women treated for menorrhagia have no anatomic pathology, and up to one third undergoing hysterectomies for heavy menstrual bleeding have anatomically normal uteri (113,114). An increase in plasminogen activator has been found in the endometrium and menstrual fluid in women with heavy menstrual bleeding compared to those with normal menstrual loss. Gleeson found that women with menorrhagia without a clear anatomic diagnosis had higher endometrial tPA levels in the menstrual flow compared to controls, and endometrial tPA levels were higher in both the late secretory and menstrual phases in essential menorrhagia than in women with normal menstrual flow. Edlund et al. found a significant correlation between the amount of menstrual blood loss and fibrinolytic activity in the menstrual fluid of six women with menorrhagia and in that of six healthy women (115). Increased fibrinolytic activity has been identified in the endometrium of women with an intrauterine device associated with menorrhagia, in comparison with controls or women who have normal menstrual flow with an intrauterine device (116). Treatment with antifibrinolytic agents has been effective in reducing menorrhagia associated with an intrauterine device.

A systematic review evaluated 15 randomized, controlled trials of women of reproductive age treated with antifibrinolytic agents versus placebo for regular, heavy menstrual bleeding (113). Seven of the trials were included in a metaanalysis, which found that treatment with an antifibrinolytic agent compared to placebo resulted in a considerable reduction in mean blood loss. Antifibrinolytic agents were compared to other nonsurgical therapies, including mefenamic acid, norethisterone, and ethamsylate, and there was a strong, although nonsignificant, trend in favor of antifibrinolytic agents in the participants' perception of improvement of menstrual blood loss. There was no significant difference in the frequency of the side effects with tranexamic acid. This review concluded that antifibrinolytic therapy causes a greater reduction and objective measurements of heavy menstrual bleeding when compared to placebo or other medical therapies without an increase in side effects.

### Amyloidosis

Occasionally, patients with systemic amyloidosis present with a bleeding disorder that can be due to direct filtration of blood vessels or to hemostatic abnormalities, including acquired factor X deficiency (117). Several reports also describe bleeding due to hyperfibrinolysis associated with increased levels of plasminogen activator (117,118,119), with findings of shortened euglobulin clot lysis time; decreased fibrinogen, plasminogen, and $\alpha_2$-plasmin inhibitor levels; and moderately increased fibrin(ogen) degradation products. Some reports relate hyperfibrinolysis primarily to deficiency of $\alpha_2$-plasmin inhibitor (118,120). Patients with amyloidosis and hyperfibrinolysis typically respond well to antifibrinolytic therapy (117–120). Hemostasis has also been characterized in the specific disorder, hereditary cerebral hemorrhage with amyloidosis-Dutch type, an autosomal dominant disorder caused by a point mutation in the $\beta$-amyloid gene and characterized by excessive deposition of amyloid in small cerebral vessels. However, there was no clear association of cerebral hemorrhage with decreased $\alpha_2$-antiplasmin, histidine-rich glycoprotein, plasminogen activator, PAI-1 fibrinogen, or fibrin(ogen) degradation products, indicating that a fibrinolytic disorder did not underlie the clinical manifestations of this type of amyloidosis (121).

## Acquired Thrombotic Disorders

Table 69-3 outlines disorders of hypofibrinolysis and thrombosis.

### Atherothrombtic Disease

In atherosclerotic disease, fibrin deposition occurs in the arterial wall, and thrombotic events resulting from plaque rupture lead to vessel obstruction. The fibrinolytic system is an important regulator of fibrin deposition, and hypofibrinolysis might be expected to increase fibrin deposition and promote thrombus formation. This hypothesis has formed the basis of studies that examine the regulation of fibrinolysis in coronary artery disease. Patients with coronary artery disease have elevated PAI-1 (122), and Hamsten et al. found that elevated PAI-1 is a risk factor for reinfarction in young survivors of myocardial infarction (MI) (123,124). Several reports have also linked elevated blood concentrations of PAI-1 with increased risk of acute MI or ischemic stroke. For example, Juhan-Vague et al. summarized results from the cooperative study of 3,043 patients with angina pectoris and found significant correlations of elevated PAI-1 with subsequent MI or sudden coronary death (125). Similarly, there was a strong correlation between low plasma fibrinolytic activity and coronary artery disease in the Northwick Park Heart Study (126), and in a Swedish case–control study, high plasma PAI-1 concentration predicted

### TABLE 69-3

#### HYPOFIBRINOLYSIS AND THROMBOTIC DISEASE

| | |
|---|---|
| Atherosclerosis | Elevated PAI-1 common |
| | Frequently part of metabolic syndrome |
| | Insulin, lipids, estrogens regulate PAI-1 synthesis |
| Surgery | Postoperative hypofibrinolysis contributes to thrombotic risk |
| | Pneumatic compression stimulates fibrinolysis |
| Pregnancy | Hypofibrinolysis caused by elevated PAI-1 and PAI-2 (produced by placenta) |

PAI, plasminogen activator inhibitor.

the occurrence of the first MI (127). High plasma PAI-1 concentrations are also associated with progressive coronary artery disease diagnosed angiographically in young men with the history of MI (128,129).

Elevated levels of tPA have also been associated with the development and progression of coronary artery disease, a finding apparently contradictory to the association with hypofibrinolysis. For example, Ridker et al. analyzed subjects from the Physicians Health Study in whom an MI occurred and found a significant risk associated with elevated tPA antigen concentration (130). However, most tPA in the circulation exists in a complex with PAI-1, and elevated levels primarily reflect an elevated concentration of this complex. Elevated antigenic tPA levels were associated with atherosclerosis risk in other studies, but these associations likely reflect elevated PAI-1 levels primarily (127,131–135).

The principal features of a syndrome of insulin resistance, termed the "metabolic syndrome," first described in 1983 by Reaven, include insulin resistance, hyperinsulinemia, impaired glucose metabolism, hypertiglyceridemia, low HDL-cholesterol concentrations, obesity, and hypertension (136). Since the original description, high plasma PAI-1 concentrations have also found a place in this cluster, likely due to mechanisms of PAI-1 regulation. Therefore, both glucose and insulin increase the synthesis of PAI-1 in endothelial cells (137,138); unsaturated fatty acids and very low density lipoprotein increase endothelial cell secretion of PAI-1 (139,140); and VLDL increase the production of PAI-1 by hepatocytes (141). These relations are the result of regulatory elements in PAI-1 gene responsive to insulin, lipids, and estrogens (142). The association is further complicated by PAI-1 gene polymorphisms that influence translational regulation, including a common single-base polymorphism resulting in the presence of either four or five guanine bases in the promoter region of the gene (4G/5G). Individuals homozygous for the 4G allele have higher plasma PAI-1 concentrations and are more sensitive to upregulation by hypertriglyceridemia (142–144). This relation may explain the higher prevalence of the 4G allele with cardiovascular disease in some studies. For example, in 2,565 subjects who underwent coronary angiography, the 4G PAI-1 genotype was related to the presence of atheroma (145). A metaanalysis suggests a small but significant effect of PAI-1 genotype on risk of MI (146). PAI-1 also has important effects in the vessel wall, where it functions to regulate proteolysis, and increased PAI-1 can be found in atherosclerotic lesions (147). Considerable evidence suggests an association of elevated PAI-1 levels with arterial vascular disease, possibly mediated through heightened systemic or local inhibition of fibrinolysis.

## Postoperative Thrombosis

Surgical trauma results in rapid activation of hemostasis followed by a postoperative reduction of fibrinolytic activity related in part to an increase in PAI-1 (148–150). This pattern has clear benefit in preventing excessive bleeding at the surgical site, but may also contribute to the increased risk of postoperative venous thromboembolism. The development of postoperative venous thrombosis has been related both to preoperative deficiencies of fibrinolysis and to excessive inhibition of fibrinolysis postoperatively, although the association is not strong enough to be of clinical predictive value (148–155). Pneumatic leg compression devices are effective in reducing the risk of postoperative venous thromboembolism, and stimulation of fibrinolytic activity may be one mechanism underlying this benefit (155–161).

## Pregnancy

Pregnancy results in significant changes in the hemostatic system with increases in procoagulants, decreases in protein S, and alterations in fibrinolysis, all of which prepare for the hemostatic challenges of delivery and allow for normal placental implantation and development (162–168). Although increases in plasma levels of plasminogen activators occur during pregnancy, these are overwhelmed by greater increases in PAI-1 and PAI-2, the latter of which is produced by the placenta (169–171). TAFI levels are also higher in pregnant than in nonpregnant women with a progressive increase in activity until approximately 20 weeks of gestation, maintenance of levels until delivery, after which there is a rapid decrease (172,173). PAI-1 also decreases rapidly after delivery, whereas PAI-2 remains elevated for several days postpartum. Compared to women with normal pregnancies, preeclampsia is associated with greater elevations of PAI-1 and lower PAI-2; PAI-1 elevations correlate with the severity of placental damage seen with preeclampsia (174–176).

## Administration of Fibrinolytic Inhibitors

Thrombosis due to hypofibrinolysis from excessive fibrinolytic inhibition may result from administration of antifibrinolytic agents such as epsilon aminocaproic acid to predisposed patients, including those with DIC or with the thrombophilia of malignancy. Intravascular coagulation normally leads to activation of compensatory fibrinolysis, presumably due in part to stimulation of plasminogen activator release from endothelial cells. This response contributes to the maintenance of vascular patency, and inhibition of fibrinolysis in patients with DIC or those developing thrombosis may disrupt the balance between thrombosis and fibrinolysis and exacerbate the thrombotic process with serious effects (177–179). Because epsilon aminocaproic acid is excreted in the urine and can inhibit normal urinary fibrinolysis, thrombosis may develop in the urinary collecting system in patients who have urinary tract bleeding and may result in ureteral obstruction; therefore, antifibrinolytic therapy must be used with great caution in patients with hematuria.

## References

1. Koie K, Kamiya T, Ogata K, et al. Alpha2-plasmin-inhibitor deficiency (Miyasato disease). *Lancet* 1978;2(8104-5):1334–1336.
2. Aoki N, Saito H, Kamiya T, et al. Congenital deficiency of alpha 2-plasmin inhibitor associated with severe hemorrhagic tendency. *J Clin Invest* 1979;63(5):877–884.
3. Kluft C, Vellenga E, Brommer EJ. Homozygous alpha 2-antiplasmin deficiency. *Lancet* 1979;2(8135):206.
4. Miles LA, Plow EF, Donnelly KJ, et al. A bleeding disorder due to deficiency of alpha 2-antiplasmin. *Blood* 1982;59(6):1246–1251.
5. Kettle P, Mayne EE. A bleeding disorder due to deficiency of alpha 2-antiplasmin. *J Clin Pathol* 1985;38(4):428–429.
6. Favier R, Aoki N, de Moerloose P. Congenital alpha(2)-plasmin inhibitor deficiencies: a review. *Br J Haematol* 2001;114(1):4–10.
7. Lijnen HR, Okada K, Matsuo O, et al. Alpha2-antiplasmin gene deficiency in mice is associated with enhanced fibrinolytic potential without overt bleeding. *Blood* 1999;93(7):2274–2281.
8. Holmes WE, Lijnen HR, Nelles L, et al. Alpha 2-antiplasmin Enschede: alanine insertion and abolition of plasmin inhibitory activity. *Science* 1987;238(4824):209–211.
9. Miura O, Sugahara Y, Aoki N. Hereditary alpha 2-plasmin inhibitor deficiency caused by a transport-deficient mutation (alpha 2-PI-Okinawa). Deletion of Glu137 by a trinucleotide deletion blocks intracellular transport. *J Biol Chem* 1989;264(30):18213–18219.
10. Miura O, Hirosawa S, Kato A, et al. Molecular basis for congenital deficiency of alpha 2-plasmin inhibitor. A frameshift mutation leading to elongation of the deduced amino acid sequence. *J Clin Invest* 1989;83(5):1598–1604.
11. Yoshinaga H, Hirosawa S, Chung DH, et al. A novel point mutation of the splicing donor site in the intron 2 of the plasmin inhibitor gene. *Thromb Haemost* 2000;84(2):307–311.
12. Lind B, Thorsen S. A novel missense mutation in the human plasmin inhibitor (alpha2-antiplasmin) gene associated with a bleeding tendency. *Br J Haematol* 1999;107(2):317–322.
13. Kluft C, Nieuwenhuis HK, Rijken DC, et al. Alpha 2-antiplasmin Enschede: dysfunctional alpha 2-antiplasmin molecule associated with an autosomal recessive hemorrhagic disorder. *J Clin Invest* 1987;80(5):1391–1400.
14. Takahashi Y, Tanaka T, Nakajima N, et al. Intramedullary multiple hematomas in siblings with congenital alpha-2-plasmin inhibitor deficiency: orthopedic surgery with protection by tranexamic acid. *Haemostasis* 1991; 21(5):321–327.

15. Devaussuzenet VM, Ducou-le-Pointe HA, Doco AM, et al. A case of intramedullary haematoma associated with congenital alpha2-plasmin inhibitor deficiency. *Pediatr Radiol* 1998;28(12):978–980.

16. Kordich L, Feldman L, Porterie P, et al. Severe hemorrhagic tendency in heterozygous alpha 2-antiplasmin deficiency. *Thromb Res* 1985;40(5):645–651.

17. Leebeek FW, Stibbe J, Knot EA, et al. Mild haemostatic problems associated with congenital heterozygous alpha 2-antiplasmin deficiency. *Thromb Haemost* 1988;59(1):96–100.

18. Ikematsu S, Fukutake K, Aoki N. Heterozygote for plasmin inhibitor deficiency developing hemorrhagic tendency with advancing age. *Thromb Res* 1996;82(2):129–136.

19. Yoshioka A, Kamitsuji H, Takase T, et al. Congenital deficiency of alpha 2-plasmin inhibitor in three sisters. *Haemostasis* 1982;11(3):176–184.

20. Mast AE, Stadanlick JE, Lockett JM, et al. Solvent/detergent-treated plasma has decreased antitrypsin activity and absent antiplasmin activity. *Blood* 1999;94(11):3922–3927.

21. Schleef RR, Higgins DL, Pillemer E, et al. Bleeding diathesis due to decreased functional activity of type 1 plasminogen activator inhibitor. *J Clin Invest* 1989;83(5):1747–1752.

22. Dieval J, Nguyen G, Gross S, et al. A lifelong bleeding disorder associated with a deficiency of plasminogen activator inhibitor type 1. *Blood* 1991;77(3):528–532.

23. Fay WP, Shapiro AD, Shih JL, et al. Brief report: complete deficiency of plasminogen-activator inhibitor type 1 due to a frame-shift mutation. *N Engl J Med* 1992;327(24):1729–1733.

24. Fay WP, Parker AC, Condrey LR, et al. Human plasminogen activator inhibitor-1 (PAI-1) deficiency: characterization of a large kindred with a null mutation in the PAI-1 gene. *Blood* 1997;90(1):204–208.

25. Matsui H, Takahashi Y, Matsunaga T, et al. Successful arthroscopic treatment of pigmented villonodular synovitis of the knee in a patient with congenital deficiency of plasminogen activator inhibitor-1 and recurrent haemarthrosis. *Haemostasis* 2001;31(2):106–112.

26. Minowa H, Takahashi Y, Tanaka T, et al. Four cases of bleeding diathesis in children due to congenital plasminogen activator inhibitor-1 deficiency. *Haemostasis* 1999;29(5):286–291.

27. Booth NA, Bennett B, Wijngaards G, et al. A new life-long hemorrhagic disorder due to excess plasminogen activator. *Blood* 1983;61(2):267–275.

28. Aznar J, Estelles A, Vila V, et al. Inherited fibrinolytic disorder due to an enhanced plasminogen activator level. *Thromb Haemost* 1984;52(2):196–200.

29. Hayward CP, Rivard GE, Kane WH, et al. An autosomal dominant, qualitative platelet disorder associated with multimerin deficiency, abnormalities in platelet factor V, thrombospondin, von Willebrand factor, and fibrinogen and an epinephrine aggregation defect. *Blood* 1996;87(12): 4967–4978.

30. Tracey P, Giles A, Mann K, et al. Factor V (Quebec): a bleeding diathesis associated with a qualitative platelet factor V deficiency. *J Clin Invest* 1984;74:1221–1228.

31. Hayward CP, Cramer EM, Kane WH, et al. Studies of a second family with the Quebec platelet disorder: evidence that the degradation of the alpha-granule membrane and its soluble contents are not secondary to a defect in targeting proteins to alpha-granules. *Blood* 1997;89(4):1243–1253.

32. Hayward CP, Welch B, Bouchard M, et al. Fibrinogen degradation products in patients with the Quebec platelet disorder. *Br J Haematol* 1997;97(2):497–503.

33. Weiss HJ, Lages B, Zheng S, et al. Platelet factor V New York: a defect in factor V distinct from that in factor V Quebec resulting in impaired prothrombinase generation. *Am J Hematol* 2001;66(2):130–139.

34. Kahr WH, Zheng S, Sheth PM, et al. Platelets from patients with the Quebec platelet disorder contain and secrete abnormal amounts of urokinase-type plasminogen activator. *Blood* 2001;98(2):257–265.

35. Sheth PM, Kahr WH, Haq MA, et al. Intracellular activation of the fibrinolytic cascade in the Quebec platelet disorder. *Thromb Haemost* 2003;90(2):293–298.

36. McKay H, Derome F, Haq MA, et al. Bleeding risks associated with inheritance of the Quebec platelet disorder. *Blood* 2004;104(1):159–165.

37. Aoki N, Moroi M, Sakata Y, et al. Abnormal plasminogen. A hereditary molecular abnormality found in a patient with recurrent thrombosis. *J Clin Invest* 1978;61(5):1186–1195.

38. Miyata T, Iwanaga S, Sakata Y, et al. Plasminogen Tochigi: inactive plasmin resulting from replacement of alanine-600 by threonine in the active site. *Proc Natl Acad Sci U S A* 1982;79(20):6132–6136.

39. Miyata T, Iwanaga S, Sakata Y, et al. Plasminogens Tochigi II and Nagoya: two additional molecular defects with Ala-600→Thr replacement found in plasmin light chain variants. *J Biochem (Tokyo)* 1984; 96(2):277–287.

40. Wohl RC, Summaria L, Robbins KC. Physiological activation of the human fibrinolytic system. Isolation and characterization of human plasminogen variants, Chicago I and Chicago II. *J Biol Chem* 1979;254(18):9063–9069.

41. Soria J, Soria C, Bertrand O, et al. Plasminogen Paris I: congenital abnormal plasminogen and its incidence in thrombosis. *Thromb Res* 1983;32 (2):229–238.

42. Scharrer IM, Wohl RC, Hach V, et al. Investigation of a congenital abnormal plasminogen, Frankfurt I, and its relationship to thrombosis. *Thromb Haemost* 1986;55(3):396–401.

43. Liu Y, Lyons RM, McDonagh J. Plasminogen San Antonio: an abnormal plasminogen with a more cathodic migration, decreased activation and associated thrombosis. *Thromb Haemost* 1988;59(1):49–53.

44. Aoki N. Genetic abnormalities of the fibrinolytic system. *Semin Thromb Hemost* 1984;10(1):42–50.

45. Prins MH, Hirsh J. A critical review of the evidence supporting a relationship between impaired fibrinolytic activity and venous thromboembolism. *Arch Intern Med* 1991;151(9):1721–1731.

46. Tefs K, Tait CR, Walker ID, et al. A K19E missense mutation in the plasminogen gene is a common cause of familial hypoplasminogenaemia. *Blood Coagul Fibrinolysis* 2003;14(4):411–416.

47. Stolz E, Kemkes-Matthes B, Potzsch B, et al. Screening for thrombophilic risk factors among 25 German patients with cerebral venous thrombosis. *Acta Neurol Scand* 2000;102(1):31–36.

48. Vielhaber H, Ehrenforth S, Koch HG, et al. Cerebral venous sinus thrombosis in infancy and childhood: role of genetic and acquired risk factors of thrombophilia. *Eur J Pediatr* 1998;157(7):555–560.

49. Demarmels Biasiutti F, Sulzer I, Stucki B, et al. Is plasminogen deficiency a thrombotic risk factor? A study on 23 thrombophilic patients and their family members. *Thromb Haemost* 1998;80(1):167–170.

50. Mateo J, Oliver A, Borrell M, et al. Laboratory evaluation and clinical characteristics of 2,132 consecutive unselected patients with venous thromboembolism—results of the Spanish multicentric study on thrombophilia (EMET-study). *Thromb Haemost* 1997;77(3):444–451.

51. Mingers AM, Heimburger N, Zeitler P, et al. Homozygous type I plasminogen deficiency. *Semin Thromb Hemost* 1997;23(3):259–269.

52. Schuster V, Mingers AM, Seidenspinner S, et al. Homozygous mutations in the plasminogen gene of two unrelated girls with ligneous conjunctivitis. *Blood* 1997;90(3):958–966.

53. Schuster V, Seidenspinner S, Zeitler P, et al. Compound-heterozygous mutations in the plasminogen gene predispose to the development of ligneous conjunctivitis. *Blood* 1999;93(10):3457–3466.

54. Drew AF, Kaufman AH, Kombrinck KW, et al. Ligneous conjunctivitis in plasminogen-deficient mice. *Blood* 1998;91(5):1616–1624.

55. Schott D, Dempfle CE, Beck P, et al. Therapy with a purified plasminogen concentrate in an infant with ligneous conjunctivitis and homozygous plasminogen deficiency. *N Engl J Med* 1998;339(23):1679–1686.

56. Heidemann DG, Williams GA, Hartzer M, et al. Treatment of ligneous conjunctivitis with topical plasmin and topical plasminogen. *Cornea* 2003;22(8):760–762.

57. Teresa Sartori M, Saggiorato G, Pellati D, et al. Contraceptive pills induce an improvement in congenital hypoplasminogenemia in two unrelated patients with ligneous conjunctivitis. *Thromb Haemost* 2003;90(1):86–91.

58. Carrell N, Gabriel DA, Blatt PM, et al. Hereditary dysfibrinogenemia in a patient with thrombotic disease. *Blood* 1983;62(2):439–447.

59. Soria J, Soria C, Caen JP. A new type of congenital dysfibrinogenaemia with defective fibrin lysis—Dusard syndrome: possible relation to thrombosis. *Br J Haematol* 1983;53(4):575–586.

60. Mosesson MW, Siebenlist KR, Hainfeld J, et al. The relationship between the fibrinogen D domain self-association/cross-linking site (gammaXL) and the fibrinogen Dusart abnormality (Aalpha R554C-albumin): clues to thrombophilia in the "Dusart syndrome." *J Clin Invest* 1996;97(10): 2342–2350.

61. Collet JP, Woodhead JL, Soria J, et al. Fibrinogen Dusart: electron microscopy of molecules, fibers and clots, and viscoelastic properties of clots. *Biophys J* 1996;70(1):500–510.

62. Lijnen HR, Soria J, Soria C, et al. Dysfibrinogenemia (fibrinogen Dusard) associated with impaired fibrin-enhanced plasminogen activation. *Thromb Haemost* 1984;51(1):108–109.

63. Wada Y, Lord ST. A correlation between thrombotic disease and a specific fibrinogen abnormality (A alpha 554 Arg → Cys) in two unrelated kindred, Dusart and Chapel Hill III. *Blood* 1994;84(11):3709–3714.

64. Hessel B, Silveira AM, Carlsson K, et al. Fibrinogenemia Tampere—a dysfibrinogenemia with defective gelation and thromboembolic disease. *Thromb Res* 1995;78(4):323–339.

65. Al-Mondhiry H, Bilezikian SB, Nossel HL. Fibrinogen "New York"—an abnormal fibrinogen associated with thromboembolism: functional evaluation. *Blood* 1975;45(5):607–619.

66. Liu CY, Koehn JA, Morgan FJ. Characterization of fibrinogen New York 1. A dysfunctional fibrinogen with a deletion of B beta(9-72) corresponding exactly to exon 2 of the gene. *J Biol Chem* 1985;260(7):4390–4396.

67. Marchi R, Lundberg U, Grimbergen J, et al. Fibrinogen Caracas V, an abnormal fibrinogen with an Aalpha 532 Ser → Cys substitution associated with thrombosis. *Thromb Haemost* 2000;84(2):263–270.

68. Marchi R, Mirshahi SS, Soria C, et al. Thrombotic dysfibrinogenemia. Fibrinogen "Caracas V" relation between very tight fibrin network and defective clot degradability. *Thromb Res* 2000;99(2):187–193.

69. Linenberger ML, Kindelan J, Bennett RL, et al. Fibrinogen bellingham: a gamma-chain R275C substitution and a beta-promoter polymorphism in a thrombotic member of an asymptomatic family. *Am J Hematol* 2000; 64(4):242–250.

70. Johansson L, Hedner U, Nilsson IM. A family with thromboembolic disease associated with deficient fibrinolytic activity in vessel wall. *Acta Med Scand* 1978;203(6):477–480.

71. Jorgensen M, Mortensen JZ, Madsen AG, et al. A family with reduced plasminogen activator activity in blood associated with recurrent venous thrombosis. *Scand J Haematol* 1982;29(3):217–223.

72. Stead NW, Bauer KA, Kinney TR, et al. Venous thrombosis in a family with defective release of vascular plasminogen activator and elevated plasma factor VIII/von Willebrand's factor. *Am J Med* 1983;74(1):33–39.

73. Comp PC, Jacocks RM, Rubenstein C, et al. A lysine-absorbable plasminogen activator is elevated in conditions associated with increased fibrinolytic activity. *J Lab Clin Med* 1981;97(5):637–645.

74. Booth NA, Anderson JA, Bennett B. Plasminogen activators in alcoholic cirrhosis: demonstration of increased tissue type and urokinase type activator. *J Clin Pathol* 1984;37(7):772–777.

75. Hersch SL, Kunelis T, Francis RB Jr. The pathogenesis of accelerated fibrinolysis in liver cirrhosis: a critical role for tissue plasminogen activator inhibitor. *Blood* 1987;69(5):1315–1319.

76. Tran-Thang C, Fasel-Felley J, Pralong G, et al. Plasminogen activators and plasminogen activator inhibitors in liver deficiencies caused by chronic alcoholism or infectious hepatitis. *Thromb Haemost* 1989;62(2):651–653.

77. Aoki N, Yamanaka T. The alpha2-plasmin inhibitor levels in liver diseases. *Clin Chim Acta* 1978;84(1-2):99–105.

78. Violi F, Basili S, Ferro D, et al. Association between high values of D-dimer and tissue-plasminogen activator activity and first gastrointestinal bleeding in cirrhotic patients. CALC Group. *Thromb Haemost* 1996;76(2):177–183.

79. Hu KQ, Yu AS, Tiyyagura L, et al. Hyperfibrinolytic activity in hospitalized cirrhotic patients in a referral liver unit. *Am J Gastroenterol* 2001;96(5):1581–1586.

80. Lisman T, Leebeek FW, Mosnier LO, et al. Thrombin-activatable fibrinolysis inhibitor deficiency in cirrhosis is not associated with increased plasma fibrinolysis. *Gastroenterology* 2001;121(1):131–139.

81. Van Thiel DH, George M, Fareed J. Low levels of thrombin activatable fibrinolysis inhibitor (TAFI) in patients with chronic liver disease. *Thromb Haemost* 2001;85(4):667–670.

82. Colucci M, Binetti BM, Branca MG, et al. Deficiency of thrombin activatable fibrinolysis inhibitor in cirrhosis is associated with increased plasma fibrinolysis. *Hepatology* 2003;38(1):230–237.

83. Kang Y. Coagulation and liver transplantation: current concepts. *Liver Transpl Surg* 1997;3(4):465–467.

84. Ozier Y, Steib A, Ickx B, et al. Haemostatic disorders during liver transplantation. *Eur J Anaesthesiol* 2001;18(4):208–218.

85. Dzik WH, Arkin CF, Jenkins RL, et al. Fibrinolysis during liver transplantation in humans: role of tissue-type plasminogen activator. *Blood* 1988;71(4):1090–1095.

86. Boylan JF, Klinck JR, Sandler AN, et al. Tranexamic acid reduces blood loss, transfusion requirements, and coagulation factor use in primary orthotopic liver transplantation. *Anesthesiology* 1996;85(5):1043–1048; discussion 30A–31A.

87. Porte RJ, Molenaar IQ, Begliomini B, et al. Aprotinin and transfusion requirements in orthotopic liver transplantation: a multicentre randomised double-blind study. EMSALT Study Group. *Lancet* 2000;355(9212):1303–1309.

88. Meijer K, Hendriks HG, De Wolf JT, et al. Recombinant factor VIIa in orthotopic liver transplantation: influence on parameters of coagulation and fibrinolysis. *Blood Coagul Fibrinolysis* 2003;14(2):169–174.

89. Taylor FB Jr. Response of anticoagulant pathways in disseminated intravascular coagulation. *Semin Thromb Hemost* 2001;27(6):619–631.

90. Levi M, de Jonge E, Meijers J. The diagnosis of disseminated intravascular coagulation. *Blood Rev* 2002;16(4):217–223.

91. Suffredini AF, Harpel PC, Parrillo JE. Promotion and subsequent inhibition of plasminogen activation after administration of intravenous endotoxin to normal subjects. *N Engl J Med* 1989;320(18):1165–1172.

92. Rao AK, Schapira M, Clements ML, et al. A prospective study of platelets and plasma proteolytic systems during the early stages of Rocky Mountain spotted fever. *N Engl J Med* 1988;318(16):1021–1028.

93. Monroy V, Ruiz BH. Participation of the Dengue virus in the fibrinolytic process. *Virus Genes* 2000;21(3):197–208.

94. Villeda CJ, Gomez-Villamandos JC, Williams SM, et al. The role of fibrinolysis in the pathogenesis of the haemorrhagic syndrome produced by virulent isolates of African swine fever virus. *Thromb Haemost* 1995;73(1):112–117.

95. Wills BA, Oragui EE, Stephens AC, et al. Coagulation abnormalities in Dengue hemorrhagic fever: serial investigations in 167 Vietnamese children with Dengue shock syndrome. *Clin Infect Dis* 2002;35(3):277–285.

96. Bouchama A, Bridey F, Hammami MM, et al. Activation of coagulation and fibrinolysis in heatstroke. *Thromb Haemost* 1996;76(6):909–915.

97. Bouchama A, Knochel JP. Heat stroke. *N Engl J Med* 2002;346(25):1978–1988.

98. Kucuk O, Kwaan HC, Frederickson J, et al. Increased fibrinolytic activity in patients undergoing cardiopulmonary bypass operation. *Am J Hematol* 1986;23(3):223–229.

99. Chandler WL, Velan T. Secretion of tissue plasminogen activator and plasminogen activator inhibitor 1 during cardiopulmonary bypass. *Thromb Res* 2003;112(3):185–192.

100. Warrell RP Jr, de The H, Wang ZY, et al. Acute promyelocytic leukemia. *N Engl J Med* 1993;329(3):177–189.

101. Rodeghiero F, Avvisati G, Castaman G, et al. Early deaths and anti-hemorrhagic treatments in acute promyelocytic leukemia. A GIMEMA retrospective study in 268 consecutive patients. *Blood* 1990;75(11):2112–2117.

102. Barbui T, Finazzi G, Falanga A. The impact of all-trans-retinoic acid on the coagulopathy of acute promyelocytic leukemia. *Blood* 1998;91(9):3093–3102.

103. Falanga A, Rickles FR. Pathogenesis and management of the bleeding diathesis in acute promyelocytic leukaemia. *Best Pract Res Clin Haematol* 2003;16(3):463–482.

104. Bennett B, Booth NA, Croll A, et al. The bleeding disorder in acute promyelocytic leukaemia: fibrinolysis due to u-PA rather than defibrination. *Br J Haematol* 1989;71(4):511–517.

105. Francis RB Jr, Seyfert U. Tissue plasminogen activator antigen and activity in disseminated intravascular coagulation: clinicopathologic correlations. *J Lab Clin Med* 1987;110(5):541–547.

106. Stephens R, Alitalo R, Tapiovaara H, et al. Production of an active urokinase by leukemia cells: a novel distinction from cell lines of solid tumors. *Leuk Res* 1988;12(5):419–422.

107. Oudijk EJ, Nieuwenhuis HK, Bos R, et al. Elastase mediated fibrinolysis in acute promyelocytic leukemia. *Thromb Haemost* 2000;83(6):906–908.

108. Griffin JD, Rambaldi A, Vellenga E, et al. Secretion of interleukin-1 by acute myeloblastic leukemia cells *in vitro* induces endothelial cells to secrete colony stimulating factors. *Blood* 1987;70(4):1218–1221.

109. Cozzolino F, Torcia M, Miliani A, et al. Potential role of interleukin-1 as the trigger for diffuse intravascular coagulation in acute nonlymphoblastic leukemia. *Am J Med* 1988;84(2):240–250.

110. Menell JS, Cesarman GM, Jacovina AT, et al. Annexin II and bleeding in acute promyelocytic leukemia. *N Engl J Med* 1999;340(13):994–1004.

111. Plow EF, Freaney DE, Plescia J, et al. The plasminogen system and cell surfaces: evidence for plasminogen and urokinase receptors on the same cell type. *J Cell Biol* 1986;103(6 Pt 1):2411–2420.

112. Fenaux P. Management of acute promyelocytic leukemia. *Eur J Haematol* 1993;50(2):65–73.

113. Lethaby A, Farquhar C, Cooke I. *Antifibrinolytics for heavy menstrual bleeding*. Cochrane Database Syst Rev 2000; CD000249.

114. Gleeson NC. Cyclic changes in endometrial tissue plasminogen activator and plasminogen activator inhibitor type 1 in women with normal menstruation and essential menorrhagia. *Am J Obstet Gynecol* 1994;171(1):178–183.

115. Edlund M, Blomback M, He S. On the correlation between local fibrinolytic activity in menstrual fluid and total blood loss during menstruation and effects of desmopressin. *Blood Coagul Fibrinolysis* 2003;14(6):593–598.

116. Khanna A, Biswas AK, Dubey B, et al. Fibrinolytic activity in bleeding associated with intrauterine contraceptive devices. *Indian J Med Res* 1992;96:147–149.

117. Sane DC, Pizzo SV, Greenberg CS. Elevated urokinase-type plasminogen activator level and bleeding in amyloidosis: case report and literature review. *Am J Hematol* 1989;31(1):53–57.

118. Liebman HA, Carfagno MK, Weitz IC, et al. Excessive fibrinolysis in amyloidosis associated with elevated plasma single-chain urokinase. *Am J Clin Pathol* 1992;98(5):534–541.

119. Takahashi H, Koike T, Yoshida N, et al. Excessive fibrinolysis in suspected amyloidosis: demonstration of plasmin-alpha 2-plasmin inhibitor complex and von Willebrand factor fragment in plasma. *Am J Hematol* 1986;23(2):153–166.

120. Meyer K, Williams EC. Fibrinolysis and acquired alpha-2 plasmin inhibitor deficiency in amyloidosis. *Am J Med* 1985;79(3):394–396.

121. Haan J, Kluft C, Leebeek FW, et al. Hereditary cerebral hemorrhage with amyloidosis-Dutch type: a study of fibrinolysis. *Thromb Haemost* 1992;67(1):16–18.

122. Kohler HP, Grant PJ. Plasminogen-activator inhibitor type 1 and coronary artery disease. *N Engl J Med* 2000;342(24):1792–1801.

123. Hamsten A, Wiman B, de Faire U, et al. Increased plasma levels of a rapid inhibitor of tissue plasminogen activator in young survivors of myocardial infarction. *N Engl J Med* 1985;313(25):1557–1563.

124. Hamsten A, de Faire U, Walldius G, et al. Plasminogen activator inhibitor in plasma: risk factor for recurrent myocardial infarction. *Lancet* 1987;2(8549):3–9.

125. Juhan-Vague I, Pyke SD, Alessi MC, et al. Fibrinolytic factors and the risk of myocardial infarction or sudden death in patients with angina pectoris. ECAT Study Group. European Concerted Action on Thrombosis and Disabilities. *Circulation* 1996;94(9):2057–2063.

126. Meade TW, Ruddock V, Stirling Y, et al. Fibrinolytic activity, clotting factors, and long-term incidence of ischaemic heart disease in the Northwick Park Heart Study. *Lancet* 1993;342(8879):1076–1079.

127. Thogersen AM, Jansson JH, Boman K, et al. High plasminogen activator inhibitor and tissue plasminogen activator levels in plasma precede a first acute myocardial infarction in both men and women: evidence for the fibrinolytic system as an independent primary risk factor. *Circulation* 1998;98(21):2241–2247.

128. Held C, Hjemdahl P, Rehnqvist N, et al. Fibrinolytic variables and cardiovascular prognosis in patients with stable angina pectoris treated with verapamil or metoprolol. Results from the angina prognosis study in Stockholm. *Circulation* 1997;95(10):2380–2386.

129. Bavenholm P, de Faire U, Landou C, et al. Progression of coronary artery disease in young male post-infarction patients is linked to disturbances of carbohydrate and lipoprotein metabolism and to impaired fibrinolytic function. *Eur Heart J* 1998;19(3):402–410.

130. Ridker PM, Vaughan DE, Stampfer MJ, et al. Endogenous tissue-type plasminogen activator and risk of myocardial infarction. *Lancet* 1993;341(8854):1165–1168.

131. Juhan-Vague I, Alessi MC. PAI-1, obesity, insulin resistance and risk of cardiovascular events. *Thromb Haemost* 1997;78(1):656–660.

132. Smith FB, Lee AJ, Fowkes FG, et al. Hemostatic factors as predictors of ischemic heart disease and stroke in the Edinburgh artery study. *Arterioscler Thromb Vasc Biol* 1997;17(11):3321–3325.

133. Carter AM, Catto AJ, Grant PJ. Determinants of tPA antigen and associations with coronary artery disease and acute cerebrovascular disease. *Thromb Haemost* 1998;80(4):632–636.

134. Macko RF, Kittner SJ, Epstein A, et al. Elevated tissue plasminogen activator antigen and stroke risk: the stroke prevention in young women study. *Stroke* 1999;30(1):7–11.

135. van der Bom JG, de Knijff P, Haverkate F, et al. Tissue plasminogen activator and risk of myocardial infarction. The Rotterdam Study. *Circulation* 1997;95(12):2623–2627.

136. Reaven G. Role of insulin resistance in human disease. *Diabetes* 1983;37:1595–1607.

137. Maiello M, Boeri D, Podesta F, et al. Increased expression of tissue plasminogen activator and its inhibitor and reduced fibrinolytic potential of human endothelial cells cultured in elevated glucose. *Diabetes* 1992;41(8):1009–1015.

138. Pandolfi A, Iacoviello L, Capani F, et al. Glucose and insulin independently reduce the fibrinolytic potential of human vascular smooth muscle cells in culture. *Diabetologia* 1996;39(12):1425–1431.

139. Nilsson L, Gafvels M, Musakka L, et al. VLDL activation of plasminogen activator inhibitor-1 (PAI-1) expression: involvement of the VLDL receptor. *J Lipid Res* 1999;40(5):913–919.

140. Nilsson L, Banfi C, Diczfalusy U, et al. Unsaturated fatty acids increase plasminogen activator inhibitor-1 expression in endothelial cells. *Arterioscler Thromb Vasc Biol* 1998;18(11):1679–1685.

141. Sironi L, Mussoni L, Prati L, et al. Plasminogen activator inhibitor type-1 synthesis and mRNA expression in HepG2 cells are regulated by VLDL. *Arterioscler Thromb Vasc Biol* 1996;16(1):89–96.

142. Eriksson P, Kallin B, van 't Hooft FM, et al. Allele-specific increase in basal transcription of the plasminogen-activator inhibitor 1 gene is associated with myocardial infarction. *Proc Natl Acad Sci U S A* 1995;92(6):1851–1855.

143. Mansfield MW, Stickland MH, Grant PJ. Environmental and genetic factors in relation to elevated circulating levels of plasminogen activator inhibitor-1 in Caucasian patients with non-insulin-dependent diabetes mellitus. *Thromb Haemost* 1995;74(3):842–847.

144. Eriksson P, Nilsson L, Karpe F, et al. Very-low-density lipoprotein response element in the promoter region of the human plasminogen activator inhibitor-1 gene implicated in the impaired fibrinolysis of hypertriglyceridemia. *Arterioscler Thromb Vasc Biol* 1998;18(1):20–26.

145. Gardemann A, Lohre J, Katz N, et al. The 4G4G genotype of the plasminogen activator inhibitor 4G/5G gene polymorphism is associated with coronary atherosclerosis in patients at high risk for this disease. *Thromb Haemost* 1999;82(3):1121–1126.

146. Iacoviello L, Burzotta F, Di Castelnuovo A, et al. The 4G/5G polymorphism of PAI-1 promoter gene and the risk of myocardial infarction: a meta-analysis. *Thromb Haemost* 1998;80(6):1029–1030.

147. Sobel BE, Taatjes DJ, Schneider DJ. Intramural plasminogen activator inhibitor type-1 and coronary atherosclerosis. *Arterioscler Thromb Vasc Biol* 2003;23(11):1979–1989.

148. Knight MT, Dawson R, Melrose DG. Fibrinolytic response to surgery. Labile and stable patterns and their relevance to post-operative deep venous thrombosis. *Lancet* 1977;2(8034):370–373.

149. Paramo JA, Alfaro MJ, Rocha E. Postoperative changes in the plasmatic levels of tissue-type plasminogen activator and its fast-acting inhibitor—relationship to deep vein thrombosis and influence of prophylaxis. *Thromb Haemost* 1985;54(3):713–716.

150. Eriksson BI, Eriksson E, Gyzander E, et al. Thrombosis after hip replacement. Relationship to the fibrinolytic system. *Acta Orthop Scand* 1989;60(2):159–163.

151. Clayton JK, Anderson JA, McNicol GP. Preoperative prediction of postoperative deep vein thrombosis. *Br Med J* 1976;2(6041):910–912.

152. Rakoczi I, Chamone D, Collen D, et al. Prediction of postoperative leg-vein thrombosis in gynaecological patients. *Lancet* 1978;1(8062):509–510.

153. Gordon-Smith IC, Hickman JA, Le Quesne LP. Postoperative fibrinolytic activity and deep vein thrombosis. *Br J Surg* 1974;61(3):213–218.

154. Comp PC, Jacocks RM, Taylor FB Jr. The dilute whole blood clot lysis assay: a screening method for identifying postoperative patients with a high incidence of deep venous thrombosis. *J Lab Clin Med* 1979;93(1):120–127.

155. Allenby F, Boardman L, Pflug JJ, et al. Effects of external pneumatic intermittent compression on fibrinolysis in man. *Lancet* 1973;2(7843):1412–1414.

156. Tarnay TJ, Rohr PR, Davidson AG, et al. Pneumatic calf compression, fibrinolysis, and the prevention of deep venous thrombosis. *Surgery* 1980;88(4):489–496.

157. Comerota AJ, Chouhan V, Harada RN, et al. The fibrinolytic effects of intermittent pneumatic compression: mechanism of enhanced fibrinolysis. *Ann Surg* 1997;226(3):306–313; discussion 13–14.

158. Christen Y, Wutschert R, Weimer D, et al. Effects of intermittent pneumatic compression on venous haemodynamics and fibrinolytic activity. *Blood Coagul Fibrinolysis* 1997;8(3):185–190.

159. Kessler CM, Hirsch DR, Jacobs H, et al. Intermittent pneumatic compression in chronic venous insufficiency favorably affects fibrinolytic potential and platelet activation. *Blood Coagul Fibrinolysis* 1996;7(4):437–446.

160. Killewich LA, Cahan MA, Hanna DJ, et al. The effect of external pneumatic compression on regional fibrinolysis in a prospective randomized trial. *J Vasc Surg* 2002;36(5):953–958.

161. Murakami M, Wiley LA, Cindrick-Pounds L, et al. External pneumatic compression does not increase urokinase plasminogen activator after abdominal surgery. *J Vasc Surg* 2002;36(5):917–921.

162. Bonnar J, McNicol GP, Douglas AS. Coagulation and fibrinolytic mechanisms during and after normal childbirth. *Br Med J* 1970;2(703):200–203.

163. Walker JE, Gow L, Campbell DM, et al. The inhibition by plasma of urokinase and tissue activator-induced fibrinolysis in pregnancy and the puerperium. *Thromb Haemost* 1983;49(1):21–23.

164. Clark P. Changes of hemostasis variables during pregnancy. *Semin Vasc Med* 2003;3(1):13–24.

165. Bremme KA. Haemostatic changes in pregnancy. *Best Pract Res Clin Haematol* 2003;16(2):153–168.

166. Sattar N, Greer IA, Rumley A, et al. A longitudinal study of the relationships between haemostatic, lipid, and oestradiol changes during normal human pregnancy. *Thromb Haemost* 1999;81(1):71–75.

167. Cerneca F, Ricci G, Simeone R, et al. Coagulation and fibrinolysis changes in normal pregnancy. Increased levels of procoagulants and reduced levels of inhibitors during pregnancy induce a hypercoagulable state, combined with a reactive fibrinolysis. *Eur J Obstet Gynecol Reprod Biol* 1997;73(1):31–36.

168. Nakashima A, Kobayashi T, Terao T. Fibrinolysis during normal pregnancy and severe preeclampsia relationships between plasma levels of plasminogen activators and inhibitors. *Gynecol Obstet Invest* 1996;42(2):95–101.

169. Kruithof EK, Tran-Thang C, Gudinchet A, et al. Fibrinolysis in pregnancy: a study of plasminogen activator inhibitors. *Blood* 1987;69(2):460–466.

170. Gore M, Eldon S, Trofatter KF, et al. Pregnancy-induced changes in the fibrinolytic balance: evidence for defective release of tissue plasminogen activator and increased levels of the fast-acting tissue plasminogen activator inhibitor. *Am J Obstet Gynecol* 1987;156(3):674–680.

171. Estelles A, Gilabert J, Aznar J, et al. Changes in the plasma levels of type 1 and type 2 plasminogen activator inhibitors in normal pregnancy and in patients with severe preeclampsia. *Blood* 1989;74(4):1332–1338.

172. Watanabe T, Minakami H, Sakata Y, et al. Changes in activity of plasma thrombin activatable fibrinolysis inhibitor in pregnancy. *Gynecol Obstet Invest* 2004;58(1):19–21.

173. Chabloz P, Reber G, Boehlen F, et al. TAFI antigen and D-dimer levels during normal pregnancy and at delivery. *Br J Haematol* 2001;115(1):150–152.

174. Bellart J, Gilabert R, Fontcuberta J, et al. Coagulation and fibrinolytic parameters in normal pregnancy and in pregnancy complicated by intrauterine growth retardation. *Am J Perinatol* 1998;15(2):81–85.

175. Schjetlein R, Haugen G, Wisloff F. Markers of intravascular coagulation and fibrinolysis in preeclampsia: association with intrauterine growth retardation. *Acta Obstet Gynecol Scand* 1997;76(6):541–546.

176. Kanfer A, Bruch JF, Nguyen G, et al. Increased placental antifibrinolytic potential and fibrin deposits in pregnancy-induced hypertension and preeclampsia. *Lab Invest* 1996;74(1):253–258.

177. Gralnick HR, Greipp P. Thrombosis with epsilon aminocaproic acid therapy. *Am J Clin Pathol* 1971;56(2):151–154.

178. Naeye RL. Thrombotic state after a hemorrhagic diathesis, a possible complication of therapy with epsilon-aminocapproic acid. *Blood* 1962;19:694–701.

179. Charytan C, Purtilo D. Glomerular capillary thrombosis and acute renal failure after epsilon-amino caproic acid therapy. *N Engl J Med* 1969;280(20):1102–1104.

# CHAPTER 70 ■ ACQUIRED QUALITATIVE PLATELET DEFECTS

A. KONETI RAO

Platelets play a major role in hemostasis, and defects in platelet function may lead to a bleeding diathesis. These defects may be inherited or, far more commonly, acquired. Alterations in platelet function occur in many acquired disorders of diverse etiologies. The specific biochemical and pathophysiologic aberrations leading to platelet dysfunction in hemostasis are poorly understood in most of these disorders. In several disorders, abnormalities have been described in multiple aspects of platelet function, including adhesion, aggregation, and secretion, and in the platelet contribution to the blood coagulation reactions. Although it would be preferable to consider the acquired platelet function disorders on the basis of the nature of the specific biochemical defect, the presence of multiple and poorly characterized platelet abnormalities even in a single disease state makes such a classification difficult. In this chapter, the acquired qualitative platelet disorders are described according to the disease states in which they are recognized (see Table 70-1). The platelet abnormalities in these diseases arise because of a variety of factors. In some, such as the myeloproliferative disorders (MPD), there is production of intrinsically abnormal platelets by the bone marrow. In others, the dysfunction results from interaction of platelets with exogenous factors such as pharmacologic agents, artificial surfaces [cardiopulmonary bypass (CPB)], compounds that accumulate in plasma because of impaired renal function, and antibodies. Some of the acquired causes of platelet dysfunction are described in detail elsewhere in this book: uremia and liver disease (see Chapter 68) and CPB (see Chapter 74).

In acquired disorders of platelet dysfunction, the bleeding is usually mucocutaneous in nature. There is a wide and often unpredictable spectrum with respect to the impact on hemostasis and of bleeding manifestations. The bleeding symptoms are generally mild to moderate, but the potential for severe life-threatening bleeding exists. The usual laboratory tests that lead to the identification of the platelet dysfunction are the bleeding time and in vitro platelet aggregation studies performed using platelet-rich plasma. The bleeding time can be variably prolonged and often normal even in individuals with impaired platelet aggregation responses. For example, aspirin ingestion impairs platelet aggregation and secretion responses to commonly used agonists (such as adenosine 5'-diphosphate (ADP), epinephrine, arachidonic acid, and low doses of collagen) in almost all individuals but prolongs the bleeding time in only about half of the subjects (1,2). Overall, the correlation between the abnormalities observed in platelet aggregation studies and clinical bleeding (or prolongation of the bleeding time) remains weak.

## MYELOPROLIFERATIVE DISEASES

Bleeding tendency, thromboembolic complications, and qualitative platelet defects are recognized in all MPD, which include essential thrombocythemia (ET), polycythemia vera (PV), agnogenic myeloid metaplasia (AMM), and chronic myelogenous leukemia (CML) (3–6). Although these stem cell disorders share common features, the observed platelet defects and clinical features may vary. The platelet abnormalities most likely result from their development from an abnormal clone of stem cells, but some of the alterations may be secondary to enhanced platelet activation in vivo. The clinical impact of the in vitro qualitative platelet defects is often unclear, with divergent findings in different studies. Platelet defects are demonstrable even in asymptomatic patients. Bleeding and thrombotic events may occur in the same patient, which creates further complexity in the interpretation of the laboratory findings. Overall, platelet abnormalities likely contribute to the excessive morbidity and mortality of these disorders, but the precise mechanisms are poorly understood.

## Clinical Features

Both hemorrhagic and thrombotic complications occur in patients with MPD, with a greater impact of the latter on the resulting morbidity (3,4). Bleeding and thrombosis are less frequent in CML compared to other MPD. Bleeding appears more prevalent in AMM, whereas patients with other MPD are more prone to thrombosis. Bleeding is chiefly mucocutaneous with particular involvement of the gastrointestinal (GI) and genitourinary tracts. Deep hematomas, hemarthrosis, and retroperitoneal hemorrhages are distinctly unusual. The risk of spontaneous hemorrhage may be increased with platelet counts in excess of 2 million per $\mu$L (7). Although the major mechanism for the hemorrhage is the disease-related alterations in platelets, aspirin ingestion is an important contributing factor (8).

Thrombotic events encompass both arterial and venous events and may occur at unusual sites, such as the splenic, hepatic, and mesenteric vessels and cerebral venous sinuses. Deep vein thrombosis, pulmonary embolism, and arterial events involving the peripheral, coronary, and cerebral vessels have been documented (3–6). In addition to the often underappreciated large vessel thrombosis (9), MPD are associated with microcirculatory arterial events resulting in

**TABLE 70-1**

CONDITIONS IN WHICH ACQUIRED DEFECTS
IN PLATELET FUNCTION ARE RECOGNIZED

Uremia
Myeloproliferative disorders
    Essential thrombocythemia
    Polycythemia vera
    Chronic myelogenous leukemia
    Agnogenic myeloid metaplasia
Acute leukemias and myelodysplastic syndromes
Dysproteinemias
Cardiopulmonary bypass
Acquired von Willebrand disease
Acquired storage pool deficiency
Antiplatelet antibodies
Liver disease
Drugs and other agents

erythromelalgia and neurologic symptoms. Erythromelalgia is characterized by intense burning or throbbing pain in the extremities, predominantly the feet, and is associated with warmth and mottled erythema (10). Erythromelalgia occurs predominantly in ET and may progress to digital ischemia and necrosis. The arterial pulses in the extremities are generally normal in these patients. Histologically, erythromelalgia is characterized by fibromuscular intimal proliferation, endothelial swelling, and thrombotic occlusions (10). Platelet survival is decreased in patients with ET and erythromelalgia compared to patients with asymptomatic ET and reactive thrombocytosis (10). Aspirin effectively relieves the symptoms of erythromelalgia (3,5,10) and reverses the shortened platelet survival (11), indicating the role of platelet aggregates in erythromelalgia. Neurologic symptoms are frequently noted in patients with MPD and span a wide spectrum of symptoms, from nonspecific headaches and dizziness to focal neurologic events, such as transient ischemic events, seizures, and monocular blindness (4,5,12). The transient neurologic events are also highly responsive to aspirin therapy (12).

Risk factors for thrombosis identified in patients with ET include increasing age, a prior thrombotic event, inadequate control of thrombocytosis, presence of risk factors for atherosclerotic heart disease, and *in vitro* occurrence of spontaneous megakaryocyte colony formation (5,6,8,13–18). Neither the degree of thrombocytosis (8,13,14,19) nor the abnormal *in vitro* platelet responses (7,13,14) correlate with risk of thrombosis in patients with MPD. However, the degree of erythrocytosis in PV correlates with an increased risk of thrombosis, which has been attributed to rheologic factors associated with the increase in red cells (20). In patients with thrombocytosis, there is a correlation between thrombosis and increased platelet turnover (21), as measured by circulating reticulated platelets.

Initial presentation of hepatic vein and/or portal vein thrombosis may be observed in patients with MPD, especially PV. MPD constitute a frequent underlying disease in patients presenting with the Budd-Chiari syndrome and portal vein thrombosis (3,22). This association is supported by the finding of a high frequency of endogenous erythropoietin-independent erythroid colony growth in patients presenting with thrombosis in these areas (22). Other abnormalities reported in MPD include an increased risk of recurrent spontaneous abortions, fetal growth retardation, premature deliveries, and *abruptio placentae* in patients with ET (5).

Despite the hemorrhagic and thrombotic events, life expectancy in patients with ET is normal (23). In a historical

cohort of 100 patients, the incidence of thrombosis in ET has been estimated at 6.6 episodes per 100 patient-years of observation (8). In different studies, 20% to 50% of the patients with ET have had thrombotic events (4). In CML, the prognosis is primarily determined by progression to blast crisis. The incidence of thrombotic and hemorrhagic complications is low in the chronic phase (4); bleeding increases in the accelerated phase, largely owing to thrombocytopenia. Survival in AMM is determined by the progression of the hematologic disease with increasing spleen size, decreasing hemoglobin, and marrow failure. Bleeding is common in the advanced thrombocytopenic stage. Patients with PV have a prolonged survival and, as in ET, morbidity and mortality are influenced by vascular events. In two large trials (24,25) in patients with PV, thrombotic events occurred in 34% and 41% of patients, respectively.

## Morphologic and Functional Abnormalities in Myeloproliferative Disorders

Several studies have examined platelet function and morphology in patients with MPD (3–6,26). Under the light microscope, there is a heterogeneity in platelet size and morphology. This heterogeneity is corroborated by alterations in mean platelet volume and in its distribution obtained from electronic platelet counters (27,28). Under the electron microscope, the findings include reduction in the number of dense and $\alpha$-granules, alterations in the open canalicular and dense tubular systems, and a reduction of mitochondria levels (29). An acquired storage-pool deficiency (SPD) in MPD platelets is also documented by direct demonstration of decreased dense-granule content of ADP, adenosine 5'-triphosphate (ATP), and serotonin (30–33). The decreased level of platelet buoyant density described in patients with MPD may reflect the dense-granule SPD (34).

The bleeding time is prolonged in approximately 17% of patients with MPD and appears to be more often prolonged in AMM than in other MPD (3,35). It does not correlate with an increased risk of bleeding symptoms (3,35,36). Platelet aggregation responses are also highly variable in patients with MPD and often vary in the same patient over time. Decreased platelet responses are more common (37), although some patients demonstrate enhanced responses to agonists or spontaneous aggregation even without addition of an agonist (38,39). In one analysis (3), responses to ADP, collagen, and epinephrine were decreased in 39%, 37%, and 57% of patients, respectively. The impairment in aggregation in response to epinephrine has been more commonly encountered than with other agonists; however, a diminished response to epinephrine is not pathognomonic of an MPD because it may be encountered in some otherwise healthy subjects and as a familial defect (see Chapter 64). The impaired responsiveness to epinephrine in MPD has been attributed to a decrease in the number of platelet $\alpha_2$-adrenergic receptors, which has been observed in some studies (40–42) but not others (30), and has depended on the ligand used: $^3$H-dihydroergocryptine (40,42) or $^3$H-yohimbine (30). In addition to aggregation, epinephrine induces several other responses, including the inhibition of adenylyl cyclase and cyclic adenosine monophosphate (cAMP) levels. Even in patients with impaired aggregation response, epinephrine-induced inhibition of adenylyl cyclase has been normal (43,44), reflecting the differential receptor requirements for the two responses. Diminished epinephrine-induced thromboxane $A_2$ (TxA_2) production, dense-granule secretion, and $Ca^{2+}$ mobilization have also been reported in patients with impaired epinephrine-induced aggregation response (30,44). The finding that dense-granule contents are also decreased in some of these patients suggests that the impaired functional responses may not necessarily be due to a decrease in the surface receptors alone.

GP IIb/IIIa complexes on platelets play an essential role in platelet aggregation. On the platelet surface, decreases in GP IIb/IIIa complexes and GP Ib have been documented (45–49) in patients with MPD. In some studies (46,50,51), there is decreased platelet fibrinogen binding, indicating a functional concomitant of the decrease in GP IIb/IIIa levels. Moreover, there is evidence for impaired signal transduction-dependent activation of GP IIb/IIIa (49) in addition to the decrease in the number of these receptors. One patient has been described (52) with deficiency of GP Ia/IIa and markedly abnormal response to collagen. The level of platelet GP IV (CD36), another membrane GP related to platelet-collagen and platelet–thrombospondin interactions, has been noted to be increased in ET (53–55); increased thrombospondin binding to MPD platelets has been noted in some (53) but not other studies (54,56). Interestingly, the number of platelet receptors for the Fc portion of IgG are increased in MPD platelets (57).

Platelet activation results in the release of free arachidonic acid, which is metabolized by two well-recognized pathways: the cyclooxygenase pathway leading to $TxA_2$ production and the 12-lipoxygenase pathway leading to formation of 12-hydroperoxy-eicosatetraenoic acid (12 HPETE) and 12-hydroxy-eicosatetraenoic acid (12-HETE). Reduced platelet formation of lipoxygenase products has been reported in patients with MPD (58–60), and this was associated with enhanced $TxA_2$ production (60). Another study demonstrated substantial production of 12-HETE following aspirin treatment of MPD platelets to block the cyclooxygenase pathway (61). Agonist-induced platelet $TxA_2$ production in MPD platelets has been normal in some studies (30,60,62); however, there is evidence for an enhanced $TxA_2$ production *in vivo* (61,63–65), suggesting an ongoing platelet activation. A lipoxygenase deficiency has also been described (66) in leukocytes from patients with MPD. Although a selective lipoxygenase deficiency with intact or enhanced cyclooxygenase may intuitively suggest enhanced platelet function, patients with the lipoxygenase deficiency have had bleeding rather than thrombotic symptoms (60). The biological functions of the lipoxygenase products 12 HETE and 12 HPETE are not fully understood; however, platelets produce other products (lipoxins) related to the action of the 12-lipoxygenase that have diverse biologic effects, including antagonistic effects on leukotrienes (67–69). MPD platelets deficient in 12-lipoxygenase have a defect not only in the conversion of arachidonic acid to 12-HPETE and 12-HETE but also in the production of lipoxins from leukotriene A4. In one study (70), the most striking deficiency in lipoxin synthesis was observed in the blast crisis of CML, and this improved during conversion to a second chronic phase.

Patients with MPD have been reported to have defects in platelets signaling mechanisms, including calcium mobilization and $Ca^{2+}$ fluxes across platelet membranes (71), signaling through the $TxA_2$ receptor (72), and protein phosphorylation due to deficiency of cGMP-dependent protein kinase (73). In normal platelets, prostaglandin (PG) $D_2$ induces an increase in cyclic AMP levels due to stimulation of adenylyl cyclase, which results in inhibition of platelet responses. Cooper et al. (74) reported a decrease in $PGD_2$-induced activation of adenylyl cyclase associated with a 50% reduction in the number of platelet $PGD_2$ receptors; responses to $PGE_2$ and $PGI_2$ were normal. This finding suggests an impairment in the platelet-inhibitory mechanisms in MPD. In another study (75), the cAMP response to these three inhibitory PGs was blunted. Platelets from patients with PV and idiopathic myelofibrosis, but not ET or CML, have been shown to have reduced expression of the thrombopoietin receptor (Mpl) and reduced thrombopoietin-induced tyrosine phosphorylation of proteins (76). Thrombin-induced tyrosine phosphorylation was preserved. Finally, CML platelets have enhanced constitutive tyrosine phosphorylation of the adapter protein, Crkl, which is normally phosphorylated on platelet activation (77).

Abnormalities in plasma von Willebrand factor (VWF) have been documented in patients with MPD (and likely contribute to the hemostatic defect in MPD). Plasma VWF, particularly the large VWF multimers, are decreased, inversely related to the platelet counts, and have improved following cytoreduction (78). These changes in plasma VWF occur in patients with reactive thrombocytosis as well.

## Therapy

Guidelines for the therapy for patients with MPD are still evolving and remain controversial. The two major pharmacologic approaches are cytoreduction and platelet inhibition. However, it is still somewhat unclear which patients with MPD require therapy—an uncertainty arising due to the lack of adequate data on efficacy and the recognition of potential side effects of the agents, including serious hemorrhage and leukemogenesis. Patients with PV clearly benefit by reduction in red cell mass. The prognosis in patients with AMM is dictated by the effects of increasing marrow fibrosis. Much of the discussion revolves around patients with ET who have a healthy life span, but thrombohemorrhagic events occur in a substantial number of patients. There is general consensus that treatment is indicated in patients with ET with a history of a thromboembolic event because these patients have an increased risk of recurrent thrombosis (7,8,14,15,79). Although previous studies have suggested that lowering of platelet counts prevents recurrence of events (7,8,15), strong evidence comes from the study of Cortelazzo et al. (79) who randomly assigned 114 patients with ET at a high risk of thrombosis (age >60 years or previous thrombotic events) to receive hydroxyurea (target platelet count <600,000 per $\mu$L) or no myelosuppression. Treatment with antiplatelet agents (aspirin and ticlopidine) was continued and comparable in both groups. Thrombotic events occurred in two patients (3.6%; one stroke, one myocardial infarction) treated with hydroxyurea and in 14 patients (24%; $P = 0.003$) in the control group (one stroke, five transient ischemic attacks, five peripheral arterial occlusions, one deep vein thrombosis, and two cases of superficial thrombophlebitis). Multivariate analysis did not reveal a significant effect of antiplatelet drugs on thrombotic events. In addition to patients with a previous thrombotic event, patients with cardiovascular risk factors are at high risk for thrombosis and are candidates for specific therapy (17). In asymptomatic patients without the risk factors mentioned in the preceding text, the role of cytoreduction remains to be established.

The various pharmacologic agents for cytoreduction in MPD include hydroxyurea, anagrelide, $\alpha$-interferon, alkylating agents (busulfan), and $^{32}$P. The leukemogenic risk conferred by use of hydroxyurea alone remains unclear, and perhaps low. However, it is an important consideration in its use in asymptomatic patients or young patients. The use of busulfan and $^{32}$P in ET has been largely abandoned because of the leukemogenic potential. A rapid reduction of extremely elevated platelet counts in ET with a life-threatening event can be achieved by platelet pheresis.

Anagrelide, a nonmutagenic, orally active quinazoline derivative, inhibits cyclic AMP phosphodiesterase (80). It inhibits maturation of megakaryocytes with a decrease in size of recognizable megakaryocytes in bone marrow biopsy specimens (81).

More than 90% of patients with ET respond to anagrelide with a decline in platelet counts (82). The side effects of anagrelide include palpitations, fluid retention, nausea, diarrhea, anemia, headache, dizziness, confusion and, in a small number of patients, congestive heart failure (82). The selective reduction in platelet counts without affecting the white cell count is an advantage of this agent over hydroxyurea, although the side effects may restrict its use in some older patients. In a retrospective series of 35 young patients with ET (aged 17 to 48 years) on anagrelide for a median of 10.8 years, 24% of patients developed a decrease in hemoglobin of greater than 3 g per dL; thrombotic and hemorrhagic events each occurred in 20% of patients, and these occurred at a platelet count greater than 400,000 per $\mu$L (83). Anagrelide is not recommended for use during pregnancy. In the only randomized trial (Medical Research Council PT1 Trial) (84) comparing hydroxyurea with anagrelide (809 patients with ET randomized; median follow-up 39 months), the long-term control of the platelet count and overall survival were not different, but anagrelide was associated with an excess rate of arterial thrombosis, major hemorrhage, and myelofibrotic transformation, with a decreased rate of venous thrombosis. Both groups received aspirin as well. These results suggest that hydroxyurea should remain the first-line therapy in patients with ET at high risk for vascular events.

Another agent shown to be effective in reducing platelet counts, as well as splenomegaly, in ET and other patients with MPD is interferon-alpha (IFN-$\alpha$), which has a potent antiproliferative effect on the hematopoietic stem cells. It is nonmutagenic and nonleukemogenic, but its widespread use has been limited because of the cost and side effects such as fever and flulike symptoms (85,86).

The role of aspirin in MPD is not well defined. Its use has been associated with serious bleeding, particularly at high doses (3,6,87). On the other hand, aspirin is effective in controlling microvascular complications, digital ischemia, erythromelalgia, and neurologic events (10,12). Aspirin is indicated in patients with arterial thrombotic events and microvascular events, but the potential for hemorrhage needs to be recognized. Its role in asymptomatic patients has been unclear. In a recently reported double-blind placebo-controlled randomized trial in 518 patients, low-dose aspirin (100 mg daily) prophylaxis reduced the risk of the combined endpoint of nonfatal myocardial infarction (MI), nonfatal stroke, pulmonary embolism, major venous thrombosis, or death from cardiovascular causes (relative risk, 0.40; $P = 0.03$); there was no increase in major bleeding episodes (88). In this primary prevention trial, the patients were heavily pretreated to normalize the platelet count, and in a quarter of the patients, the hematocrit was greater than 48%. These two features need to be taken into account in translating the findings to clinical practice. Nevertheless, this trial provides information that supports the use of prophylactic aspirin in at least some subsets of patients with PV. It is effective and safe in PV when platelet counts are normal. Aspirin has been considered to be relatively contraindicated in patients with previous bleeding episodes and those with platelet counts over 1.5 million per $\mu$L (5).

# ACUTE LEUKEMIAS AND MYELODYSPLASTIC SYNDROMES

The major cause of bleeding in leukemias and myelodysplastic syndromes (MDS) is thrombocytopenia. However, in patients with normal or elevated platelet counts, bleeding complications may be associated with platelet dysfunction (89–96). Acquired platelet defects associated with clinical bleeding are more common in acute myelogenous leukemia, but have been reported in acute lymphoblastic and myelomonoblastic leukemias, hairy cell leukemia, and MDS (93–99).

Reduced aggregation responses to ADP, epinephrine, and collagen have been reported (90,91,95,100). These abnormalities have been associated with diminished nucleotide secretion, serotonin uptake and release, $TxA_2$ production, and platelet PDGF

and $\beta$-thromboglobulin (59,91,94,97,98,100–102). Impaired platelet procoagulant activities have been described in both acute leukemias and MDS (89–91,94,95,97,99). Acquired forms of von Willebrand disease (VWD) and the Bernard-Soulier–like platelet defect have been described in hairy cell leukemia and juvenile MDS, respectively (103,104).

In acute leukemias and MDS, platelets may be large and morphologically abnormal, with a balloonlike appearance (105). Ultrastructural studies have shown decreased microtubules, reduced number and abnormal sizes of dense granules, and excessive membranous systems (91,94,95,99). In acute leukemias and MDS, megakaryocytes exhibit dysplasia (94,105), and the platelet abnormalities reflect this. Bleeding in the acute leukemias and MDS usually responds to transfusion of platelets.

# DYSPROTEINEMIAS

Excessive clinical bleeding may occur in patients with dysproteinemias and appears to be related to multiple mechanisms, including platelet dysfunction, specific coagulation abnormalities, hyperviscosity, and alterations in blood vessels due to amyloid deposition (106–111). Qualitative platelet defects occur in 33% of patients with IgA myeloma or Waldenstrom macroglobulinemia, 15% of patients with IgG multiple myeloma, and infrequently in monoclonal gammopathy of undetermined significance (107–112). Coagulation abnormalities reported in patients with dysproteinemias include factor X deficiency related to amyloidosis (113,114), a circulating heparinlike anticoagulant (115,116), and impaired fibrin polymerization (111). Abnormal clot retraction has been reported in IgG myeloma and appears to be due to altered fibrin structure rather than platelet dysfunction (117). An acquired form of VWD has been described in some patients (118–120).

## Platelet Defects and Pathogenesis

The platelet dysfunction is demonstrated by prolonged bleeding time, impaired platelet glass-bead retention and aggregation, and reduced platelet procoagulant activity (107–111,121). It has been proposed that binding of the paraprotein to the platelet membrane interferes with normal platelet membrane functions. In some cases, the paraprotein bound specifically to platelet GP IIIa (121) or interfered with VWF or its interaction with platelet GP Ib (118,120).

## Therapy

The impaired platelet function appears to correlate with the serum paraprotein levels (107,122). Acute bleeding episodes can be managed by lowering the paraprotein levels by plasmapheresis, and chronic bleeding may be controlled by chemotherapy aimed at reducing the concentration of the abnormal protein. Cryoprecipitate, 1-desamino-8-D-vasopressin (DDAVP, desmopressin acetate), or plasmapheresis may be transiently effective in patients with acquired von Willebrand disease (AVWD) (118–120). Intravenous immunoglobulin has also been used in patients with AVWD (see subsequent text).

# ACQUIRED VON WILLEBRAND DISEASE

Although most cases of VWD are inherited (see Chapter 60), there are several reports of patients with a mild to moderate bleeding disorder in whom this disease appears acquired. Most patients with AVWD have been older than 40 years without previous manifestations or a family history of a bleeding diathesis. The associated disorders in these patients have been diverse, including both benign and malignant hematologic disorders (123,124). About half of the patients have had an underlying lymphoproliferative disorder or plasma cell proliferative disorder (124). Dysproteinemias, including monoclonal gammopathy of unknown significance (MGUS), multiple myeloma, and Waldenstrom macroglobulinemia, constitute the most frequently observed association. AVWD has been reported in chronic lymphocytic leukemia, hairy cell leukemia, acute myeloid and lymphoblastic leukemias, and non-Hodgkin lymphoma. In patients with myeloproliferative diseases (CML, ET, PV) and in reactive thrombocytosis, there is an impressive correlation between the abnormalities in plasma VWF and the elevated platelet counts (78,125,126). AVWD has been reported in patients with autoimmune disorders including systemic lupus erythematosus (SLE), scleroderma and mixed connective tissue disease, hypothyroidism, and antiphospholipid antibody syndrome (123,124). Several therapeutic agents have been associated with AVWD: ciprofloxacin (127), valproic acid (128), griseofulvin (129), and a plasma expander hydroxyethyl starch (130,131). AVWD has been reported in patients with solid tumors, most notably Wilms tumor, but case reports have associated with others as well (adrenocortical carcinoma, lung carcinoma, gastric carcinoma) (123,132). Patients with aortic stenosis and congenital valvular heart disease may have excess bleeding (particularly GI), and several reports have documented AVWD in such patients (133,134). Vincentelli et al. (134) studied 50 consecutive patients with aortic stenosis and found skin or mucosal bleeding in 21% of patients with severe aortic stenosis; abnormal platelet function using the platelet function analyzer (PFA-100), decreased VWF collagen-binding activity, and the loss of the largest multimers, or a combination of these occurred in 67% to 92% of patients with severe aortic stenosis. The abnormalities were corrected on the first day after surgery, providing evidence of the causal role of the valvular defect in the pathogenesis of AVWD.

The AVWD arises by diverse mechanisms. Some patients (especially those with dysproteinemias, lymphoproliferative, and myeloproliferative diseases) have had antibodies directed against functional domains of VWF (123,135). In such patients, the patient's plasma inhibited the ristocetin cofactor activity in normal plasma. In some patients with AVWD, the enhanced clearance of VWF has been mediated by antibodies that are not targeted to a functional VWF region. Increased proteolysis of VWF, induced by exposure of VWF to high stress, is another mechanism leading to AVWD, as in patients with severe aortic stenosis (134,136) and congenital cardiac diseases (133), for example. In some patients, cellular adsorption and removal of VWF by malignant or other cells (platelets in myeloproliferative diseases) has been considered the main mechanism (123). Nonimmunologic binding and precipitation of VWF has been noted following administration of hydroxyethyl starch (130). Finally, decreased VWF synthesis has been invoked in patients with hypothyroidism (137) and those receiving valproate (128).

## Laboratory Findings and Pathogenesis

Laboratory findings in patients with AVWD have included various combinations of prolonged bleeding times and decreased plasma levels of VWF (VWF antigen and ristocetin cofactor activity) and FVIIIC. Several studies have documented a selective reduction in the large VWF multimers in plasma. Decreased levels of VWF antigen II have also been noted (138).

## Therapy

There are two goals of treatment in patients with AVWD. The first includes approaches to quickly raise plasma VWF levels to treat or prevent bleeding, and the second encompasses therapeutic modalities targeted to the underlying associated conditions. The first is achieved by administration of DDAVP (78,123,124,135) or FVIII concentrates that contain VWF. Cryoprecipitate is also effective but is associated with the risk of transfusion-transmitted diseases. Recombinant factor VIIa has also been used to control bleeding in a patient with AVWD (139). Several reports have found intravenous immunoglobulin (IVIG) to be effective, including in patients with MGUS (123,124,135,140,141). A major advantage of IVIG is the sustained increase in VWF, lasting several weeks, which contrasts with that of DDAVP, lasting only a few hours. Other modalities utilized in AVWD include measures to lower the pathogenetic antibody levels in plasma using plasma exchange (119) and extracorporeal immunoadsorption (142).

Treatment of the underlying disorder is an important aspect of management of patients with AVWD. In patients with MPD and elevated platelet counts, cytoreduction is effective in reversing the plasma VWF abnormalities (78,143,144) as well as the decreased half-life (78,145). In other patients with AVWD, remissions have occurred spontaneously and after therapy for the underlying disease, such as lymphoproliferative disease, Wilms tumor, multiple myeloma, hypothyroidism, CML, and the cardiac valve abnormalities (123,134).

# ACQUIRED STORAGE-POOL DISEASE

Congenital deficiency of the platelet dense-granule pool of ATP and ADP (SPD) is associated with impaired platelet function and a bleeding diathesis (see Chapter 64). Several patients have been reported in whom the dense-granule SPD appears to be acquired. In general, this defect probably reflects *in vivo* release of platelet dense-granule contents due to activation or a hematopoietic abnormality with abnormal platelets being produced by the marrow. Acquired SPD may therefore occur in diverse clinical states. Zahavi and Marder described a patient with a circulating antiplatelet antibody and SPD in whom the platelet defect was corrected by steroid therapy (146). Weiss et al. described five patients, including two with SLE and one with chronic idiopathic thrombocytopenic purpura (ITP), who had abnormal platelet aggregation responses, elevated platelet-associated antibodies, and deficiency in dense- and α-granule contents (147). SPD has also been reported in patients with disseminated intravascular coagulation (DIC), ITP, hemolytic-uremic syndrome, renal transplant rejection, multiple congenital cavernous hemangioma, MPD, CML, hairy cell leukemia, and acute nonlymphocytic leukemia (31,59,94,148–152). Depletion of platelet granule contents has also been reported in patients with severe valvular disease and with Dacron aortic grafts, in patients undergoing CPB, and in platelet concentrates stored for transfusion (153–156).

# ANTIPLATELET ANTIBODIES AND PLATELET FUNCTION

Binding of an antibody to platelets may induce several effects, including accelerated destruction, platelet activation, cell lysis, aggregation, secretion of granule contents, and expression of platelet factor-3 activity. Platelet–antibody interaction may lead to impaired function, both as a consequence of activation and due to antibody binding to specific platelet glycoproteins. Platelets can bind immune complexes, mediated by the platelet Fc receptors, and activation of the complement system (c5b-9) on cell surface can contribute to the platelet activation (157). The overall impact of the antibodies may be thrombocytopenia and/or impaired platelet function, as noted in a wide range of autoimmune disorders, including ITP, collagen vascular diseases, and AIDS.

Patients with ITP have decreased platelet survival, with increased platelet-associated antibodies present in most patients (158–161). Because of the increased rate of thrombopoiesis, it has been suggested that these patients have young platelets in circulation with an enhanced functional ability. Harker and Slichter reported the bleeding times to be disproportionately shortened in relation to the platelet counts in patients with ITP compared with those with regenerative thrombocytopenia (162). However, patients with ITP may have impaired platelet function and abnormally prolonged bleeding times even at adequate counts. Clancy et al. reported defective in vitro platelet aggregation in nine of 11 patients with chronic ITP (163). Serum globulin fractions isolated from some of the patients inhibited the aggregation responses of normal platelets to collagen and ADP. Impaired platelet aggregation responses to agonists (ADP, epinephrine, collagen) with and without prolonged bleeding times have been reported in ITP and in disorders such as SLE and Graves disease, which are associated with increased platelet-associated antibodies (146,147,164–170).

Antibodies can induce platelet dysfunction by multiple mechanisms. In many patients, the antibodies are directed against specific platelet surface membrane glycoproteins GP Ib (171, 172), GP IIb/IIIa (173,174), GP Ia/IIa (175,176), GP IV (177), GP VI (178,179), and glycosphingolipids (180,181). In some patients, the antibody specifically blocked platelet aggregation induced by collagen alone through interaction with GP VI (178), GP IV (177), or GP Ia/IIa (175,176). In one report, the anti-GP VI antibody induced a clearance of the GP VI/FcRr complex from the platelet surface (179). Antibodies against GP Ib/IX and GP IIb/IIIa have been detected in 5% to 29 % and 10% to 75% of patients with ITP, respectively (171,173,182). These antibodies in effect induced acquired forms of the Bernard-Soulier syndrome and thrombasthenia, respectively. One study noted that the severity of thrombocytopenia was not related to the glycoprotein specificity of the autoantibody (183). Most of the platelet antibodies in ITP have been IgG, with IgM and IgA occurring less frequently (184). Stuart et al. have reported impaired platelet arachidonate metabolism as reflected by increased lipoxygenase activity and decreased cyclooxygenase products (TxA$_2$ and hydroxyheptadecatrienoic acid) in patients with ITP (167). They noted an inverse correlation between the bleeding times and the TxA$_2$ production. Another defect is the antibody-induced deficiency of platelet granule contents in some patients with ITP and collagen vascular diseases (146,147,185). Overall, antiplatelet antibodies not only induce thrombocytopenia but may also impair platelet function.

# MISCELLANEOUS CONDITIONS WITH IMPAIRED PLATELET FUNCTION

Alterations in platelet function have been described in several other disease states, such as severe vitamin B$_{12}$ deficiency (186) and eosinophilia (187–189); in some patients with atopy (190) and patients with asthma and hay fever (190,191); and in

Bartter syndrome (192). The clinical importance and pathogenesis of the platelet defects in these disorders remain uncertain.

# DRUGS THAT INHIBIT PLATELET FUNCTION

Many drugs affect platelet function (see Table 70-2). For several drugs, the effects on platelets have been studied in vitro, and the relevance of such findings to the drug levels achieved in clinical practice is not well established. Even among those shown to alter platelet responses ex vivo, the impact on hemostasis remains unclear for many. Moreover, the impact of concomitant administration of multiple drugs, each with a mild effect on platelet function, is unknown, although this impact is clinically relevant.

## Aspirin and Nonsteroidal Antiinflammatory Agents

Because of its widespread use, aspirin is an important cause of platelet inhibition in clinical practice.

Its ingestion results in inhibition of platelet aggregation and secretion upon stimulation with ADP, epinephrine, and low concentrations of collagen. Aspirin irreversibly acetylates and inactivates the platelet cyclooxygenase, leading to the inhibition of synthesis of endoperoxides (PGG$_2$ and PGH$_2$) and TxA$_2$. Much of this effect of orally administered aspirin on platelet cyclooxygenase occurs in the presystemic (portal) circulation (193). As little as a single 80-mg tablet is adequate to block platelet TxA$_2$ production (194,195). The impressive efficacy of aspirin in the primary and secondary prevention of arterial vascular events is well established (196,197). The efficacy of aspirin as an antithrombotic agent and its effects in impairing primary hemostasis are both related to the inhibition of platelet TxA$_2$ production. Although aspirin inhibits platelet aggregation responses in all but a few individuals (198), the overall effect in otherwise normal individuals is a mild impairment of hemostasis. Aspirin prolongs the bleeding time in many normal individuals, and this is influenced by the direction of the incision on the forearm and the application of venostasis during the procedure (199). Ethanol ingestion potentiates the effect of aspirin on the bleeding time (200). Evidence for aspirin's adverse effect on hemostasis, particularly on the risk of major extracranial and intracranial bleeds, comes from the larger aspirin trials. In general, the overall risk of major bleeding is low (<1% per year) (197). Ingestion of aspirin during pregnancy has been reported to result in excessive maternal and neonatal bleeding at delivery (201–203). In the Physicians' Health Study, 22,071 healthy, male physicians were randomized to receive placebo or aspirin (325 mg every other day); over a 5-year follow-up, there was a significantly higher incidence of easy bruising, mucosal bleeding (including GI bleeding), and blood transfusion requirement (204). The rate of hemorrhagic stroke was higher with aspirin (0.04% per year) compared to placebo (0.02% per year, $P = 0.06$) (204), but this was not statistically significant. Preoperative ingestion of aspirin increases blood loss, transfusions, and repeated operations in patients undergoing cardiac surgery (205,206). However, a recent large study (207) on the early use of aspirin after coronary artery bypass grafting (CABG) showed that patients who received aspirin during the first 48 hours had a 60% lower mortality rate compared to those who did not, and the rates of other nonfatal ischemic events were also lower. Of particular interest, the frequency of bleeding complications and reoperations was significantly lower among aspirin-treated patients. If confirmed, this study may change the generally held reluctance to use aspirin in the immediate CABG postoperative period.

**TABLE 70-2**

DRUGS THAT AFFECT PLATELET FUNCTION

Drugs that inhibit thromboxane synthesis
Cyclooxygenase inhibitors
    Aspirin
    Nonsteroidal antiinflammatory agents
      Indomethacin, phenylbutazone, ibuprofen, sulfinpyrazone, sulindac, meclofenamic acid
ADP receptor antagonists
    Ticlopidine, clopidogrel
GP IIb/IIIa receptor antagonists
    c7E3 (Abciximab), tirofiban, eptifibatride
Drugs that increase platelet cyclic AMP or cyclic GMP
    Adenylate cyclase activators
      Prostaglandins $I_2$, $D_2$, $E_1$ and analogs
    Phosphodiesterase inhibitors
      Dipyridamole
      Cilostazol
      Anagrelide
      Milrinone
      Methyl xanthines
      Caffeine, theophylline, aminophylline
Nitric oxide and nitric oxide donors
Antimicrobials
    Penicillins
    Cephalosporins
    Nitrofurantoin
    Hydroxychloroquine
    Miconazole
Cardiovascular drugs
    $\beta$-adrenergic blockers (propranolol)
    Vasodilators (nitroprusside, nitroglycerin)
    Diuretics (furosemide)
    Calcium-channel blockers
    Quinidine
    Angiotensin-converting enzyme inhibitors
Anticoagulants
    Heparin
Thrombolytic agents
    Streptokinase, tissue plasminogen activator, urokinase
Psychotropics and anesthetics
    Tricyclic antidepressants
      Imipramine, amitryptyline, nortriptyline
    Phenothiazines
      Chlorpromazine, promethazine, trifluoperazine
    Local anesthetics
    General anesthesia (halothane)
Chemotherapeutic agents
    Mithramycin
    BCNU
    Daunorubicin
Miscellaneous agents
    Dextrans and hydroxyethyl starch
    Lipid-lowering agents (clofibrate, halofenate)
    $\varepsilon$-aminocaproic acid
    Antihistaminics
    Ethanol
    Vitamin E
    Radiographic contrast agents
    Food items ($\omega$-3 fatty acids, vitamin E, onions, garlic, ginger, cumin, tumeric, clove,
      black tree fungus, Ginko)

ADP, adenosine diphosphate; AMP, adenosine monophosphate; GMP, guanosine monophosphate; BCNU, 1,3-bis (2-chloroethyl)-1-nitrosurea.

GI bleeding is a major adverse effect of aspirin (197,204, 208–212). Aspirin-induced GI toxicity, but not its antithrombotic effect, is dose-related in the range 30 mg to 1,300 mg daily (197,208). However, even at low doses (30 to 50 mg daily), aspirin can cause serious GI bleeding (209,210). The overall relative risks of GI complications with the use of nonsteroidal antiinflammatory drugs (NSAIDs), including aspirin, have been estimated to be between threefold and fivefold as compared to nonusers (212).

Subjects who may develop considerable postoperative or even spontaneous bleeding during aspirin ingestion are those with underlying hemostatic defects such as VWD, hemophilia, mild platelet function defects, uremia, and those on oral anticoagulant therapy. In these patients, aspirin ingestion may lead to a striking prolongation of the bleeding time and increase in bleeding manifestations, and should be avoided. In otherwise healthy subjects who are on aspirin and require elective surgery, aspirin should be discontinued 7 to 10 days before the procedure. Given the widespread use of aspirin as an antithrombotic agent, this is often not feasible in patients with arterial diseases. In patients undergoing CABG, one set of guidelines recommend starting 325 mg of aspirin 6 hours after the surgery (213). On the basis of the recent report of beneficial effects of early administration of aspirin (207), there is a need to reevaluate the current practice regarding use of antiplatelet agents in the immediate post-CABG period (214). If excessive perioperative hemorrhage is encountered, it is generally responsive to platelet transfusions. Moreover, DDAVP infusion shortens the prolongation in bleeding time with aspirin (215).

Several other NSAIDs also impair platelet function by inhibiting the cyclooxygenase enzyme and may prolong the bleeding time. These include indomethacin, ibuprofen, sulfinpyrazone, meclofenamic acid, phenylbutazone, and sulindac (197,216–219). Compared with aspirin, the inhibition of cyclooxygenase by these agents is generally short-lived and reversible. For example, the effect of indomethacin is not detectable after 6 hours (217). In contrast, the effect of piroxicam may last for several days, related to its long half-life (220). Exposure to NSAIDs other than aspirin also increases the risk of upper GI bleeding and/or perforation. However, this effect is variable with different NSAIDs (211,212). One analysis (211) found the relative risk to be lowest for ibuprofen and diclofenac; intermediate for aspirin, indomethacin, naproxen, and sulindac; and higher for azapropazone, tolmetin, ketoprofen, and piroxicam. These findings may be relevant to the choice of the drug for use in patients with impaired hemostasis. Ibuprofen has been administered to patients with hemophilia without a major increase in bleeding (221,222). However, enhanced bleeding has been noted in HIV-positive hemophiliacs receiving a combination of ibuprofen and zidovudine (223). Most of these NSAIDs, such as aspirin, inhibit both forms of cyclooxygenase (cyclooxygenase-1 and -2). The concomitant administration of ibuprofen (but not acetaminophen, rofecoxib, or diclofenal) antagonizes the irreversible platelet inhibition by aspirin, which may affect the efficacy of aspirin in cardiovascular diseases (224). The three commercially available selective cyclooxygenase-2 inhibitors, celecoxib, rofecoxib, and valdecoxib, have no antiplatelet activity because mature platelets lack cyclooxygenase-2. The widely used analgesic acetaminophen does not impair platelet function at levels attained *in vivo*, although in some subjects, it may inhibit *in vitro* platelet responses as a weak, reversible cyclooxygenase inhibitor (225).

## Ticlopidine and Clopidogrel: Adenosine Diphosphate P2Y$_{12}$ Receptor Antagonists

Ticlopidine and its analog clopidogrel are orally administered thienopyridine derivatives that inhibit platelet function

by inhibiting the binding of ADP to the platelet P2Y$_{12}$ receptor (197,226,227). Platelet aggregation responses to several agonists, including ADP, collagen, epinephrine, and thrombin, are inhibited to various extents depending on agonist concentrations. The effects of both agents are mediated by active metabolites generated *in vivo* by hepatic transformation. With repeated twice-daily dosing of ticlopidine, plasma ticlopidine levels increase by about threefold over a period of 2 to 3 weeks because of drug accumulation. Likewise, the elimination half-life is up to 96 hours after 14 days of repeated dosing. Clopidogrel differs from ticlopidine in its pharmacokinetics. It is rapidly metabolized, and the main carboxylic derivative has a plasma elimination half-life of approximately 8 hours. On repeated daily dosing (50 to 100 mg) in healthy volunteers, ADP-induced platelet aggregation is inhibited from the second day of treatment and steady state is reached after 4 to 7 days (197). After a single dose of 400 mg clopidogrel, inhibition of platelet aggregation is noted at 2 hours and persists up to 48 hours. The platelet-inhibitory effect persists for 7 to 10 days after therapy with these agents is discontinued. Both ticlopidine and clopidogrel prolong the bleeding time by 1.5 to two times over control (227–229), but more striking prolongations have been noted. Because of their prolonged effect, these drugs need to be discontinued for 7 to 10 days before elective surgery. Both drugs have been associated with thrombotic thrombocytopenic purpura (230–232).

## Glycoprotein IIb/IIIa Receptor Antagonists

Platelet activation results in a conformational change in platelet GP IIb/IIIa complex, which then binds fibrinogen, a prerequisite for platelet aggregation. GP IIb/IIIa receptor antagonists are a class of compounds that inhibit fibrinogen binding and platelet aggregation (197,233). These include a monoclonal antibody against the GP IIb/IIIa receptor c7E3 [abciximab, (ReoPro)], a synthetic peptide containing the KGD sequence [eptifibatide (Integrilin)], and a peptidomimetics [tirofiban, (Aggrastat)]. These agents are used in acute coronary syndromes and in the context of percutaneous coronary interventions (197,233). They are potent inhibitors of aggregation (both primary and secondary) in response to all of the usual agonists; they all prolong the bleeding time (197) and are far more potent as platelet inhibitors than aspirin. Not unexpectedly, bleeding is a potential complication with these agents, and it is responsive to platelet transfusions. In addition to their platelet-inhibitory effect, immune thrombocytopenia (secondary to drug-dependent antibodies) is another potential complication of the GP IIb/III antagonists (197,234).

## Drugs That Increase Platelet Cyclic Adenosine Monophosphate or Cyclic Guanosine Monophosphate

Elevation of intracellular cAMP levels by agents that activate adenylate cyclase (PGE$_1$, PGI$_2$, PGD$_2$) or inhibit the cyclic nucleotide phosphodiesterases results in inhibition of platelet responses. Intravenous infusion of prostacyclin (PGI$_2$) or its stable analogs inhibits platelet aggregation responses and prolongs the bleeding time (235,236). Dipyridamole, a weak phosphodiesterase inhibitor, appears not to inhibit aggregation responses to collagen, epinephrine, and ADP at usual doses, but has a synergistic effect with aspirin in prolonging the shortened platelet survival in thromboembolic disorders (237). Cilostazol, a cyclic nucleotide phosphodiesterase 3 inhibitor, suppresses platelet aggregation and is currently being used for therapy for peripheral arterial disease (238,239). It does not prolong the bleeding time (229). Anagrelide (80) and milrinone (240) are also inhibitors of cAMP phosphodiesterase. Other weak phosphodiesterase inhibitors, such as caffeine, theophylline, and aminophylline, inhibit ADP-induced platelet aggregation *in vitro* but may not have clinical significance (241). Sildenafil, a selective inhibitor of cyclic nucleotide phosphodiesterase 5, was found not to have a direct effect on platelet function but potentiated the *in vitro* antiaggregatory effect of sodium nitroprusside (242).

Platelets produce nitric oxide (NO) and NO donors. NO and NO donors inhibit platelet activation and responses by elevating cyclic guanosine monophosphate (cGMP) levels (243–247). Administration of NO is associated with a prolonged bleeding time (243,245). NO donors are currently being developed as platelet-inhibitory agents for clinical use.

## Antimicrobial Agents

$\beta$-lactam antibiotics, including penicillins and cephalosporins, have been shown to inhibit platelet aggregation responses, and some induce a bleeding diathesis when given in high doses. These include carbenicillin, penicillin G, ticarcillin, ampicillin, nafcillin, cloxacillin, mezlocillin, oxacillin, and piperacillin (248–258). The platelet inhibition is dose-dependent, taking approximately 2 to 3 days to manifest and 3 to 10 days to abate after discontinuation of the drug (248,253,254,257,258). Penicillins lacking the $\alpha$-carboxy group (mezlocillin, piperacillin, apalcillin) appear to affect platelet function adversely less often than carboxypenicillins or moxalactam (257). Cephalosporins also impair platelet function (257,259,260). Moxalactam has been reported to induce platelet dysfunction associated with prolonged bleeding times and clinical hemorrhage (257,260). However, other third-generation cephalosporins appear to show little effect on normal platelet function (257). Several antibiotics (moxalactam, cefamandole, cefoperazone) induce hypoprothrombinemia, which contributes to hemorrhage (257,260).

Several generalizations can be made regarding the overall effects of $\beta$-lactam antibiotics. First, the effects on platelet function and hemostasis appear to be dose dependent and time dependent with effects becoming discernible over several days (248,253,254,257,258). Second, the patients at particular risk of bleeding appear to be those with concurrent illnesses, including sepsis, malnourishment, thrombocytopenia, and malignancy, as is often the case in the intensive care units. The platelet-inhibitory effect of $\beta$-lactam antibiotics is influenced by plasma albumin concentration. Both the platelet binding of the antibiotic and the impact on platelet responses are inversely related to albumin concentration (261). Third, the impairment in hemostasis noted with some of the $\beta$-lactam antibiotics (e.g., moxalactam, cefamandole, cefoperazone) is related to a concomitant inhibitory effect on synthesis of vitamin K–dependent coagulation factors (257,259,260).

A number of mechanisms have been invoked to explain the effects of $\beta$-lactam antibiotics on platelet function. These drugs inhibit platelet aggregation and secretion as well as platelet adherence to subendothelial structures and collagen-coated surfaces (252). Of note, many of the studies have evaluated the effects on platelets only *in vitro* at concentrations more than those attained *in vivo*. Short-term *in vitro* exposure of platelets to penicillin has been reported to result in impaired aggregation responses and decreased binding of agonists to specific platelet receptors (ADP, VWF, $\alpha_2$-adrenergic) (262,263). The latter effect of penicillins was found to be rapidly reversible (262,263). However, the platelet-inhibitory effect of $\beta$-lactam antibiotics persists for several days after discontinuation, indicating that other mechanisms may also be responsible. Other effects reported include inhibition of intracellular signaling events, calcium mobilization (264) and TxA$_2$ synthesis (263,264), and alterations in activation-induced changes in membrane glycoproteins

GP IIb/IIIa and GP Ib/IX (265). In general, because of the concomitant factors (thrombocytopenia, disseminated intravascular coagulation (DIC), vitamin K deficiency), it is often difficult to define the precise role of the antimicrobials in the observed bleeding. Discontinuation of a specifically indicated antibiotic is often not an option nor is it necessary. Supportive measures using blood products and other interventions (correcting metabolic abnormalities, vitamin K deficiency) are indicated in the overall management. In addition to the $\beta$-lactam antibiotics, other antimicrobials shown to inhibit platelet function include nitrofurantoin (266), hydroxychloroquine (267), and miconazole (268).

## Cardiovascular Drugs

Propranolol is a weak inhibitor of platelet function and does not influence the bleeding time. *In vitro*, it inhibits the aggregation responses of normal platelets to ADP and epinephrine only at relatively high concentrations (269). At lower concentrations, it inhibits secondary aggregation and secretion in patients whose platelets are responsive to a low-threshold concentration of agonists, but not uniformly in all patients taking the drug (269,270). At conventional doses, it inhibits and normalizes the increased sensitivity to agonists of platelets from patients with angina pectoris (271). The mechanism by which propranolol alters platelet behavior is probably unrelated to its $\beta$-blocking effects and may be due to an effect on platelet membranes (269,270). The drug inhibits the release of free amino acids from phospholipids and TxA$_2$ production during platelet activation (272,273). Other $\beta$-blockers (pindolol, atenolol, metoprolol) have also been reported to inhibit platelet responses when added *in vitro* (274). Other cardiovascular drugs known to inhibit platelet responses include furosemide (275), nitroprusside (276–278), nitroglycerin, and isosorbide dinitrate (277,279). Quinidine can prolong the bleeding time and has an effect on the platelet $\alpha_2$-adrenergic receptors (280,281). Although calcium-channel blockers (nifedipine, verapamil, diltiazem) inhibit platelet responses, this is seen *in vitro* at drug concentrations higher than those achieved during therapy (282–286). Inhibition of platelet $\alpha_2$-adrenergic receptors has been demonstrated with these agents (284,285).

Some angiotensin-converting enzyme (ACE) inhibitors, [captopril (287,288), perindopril (289), and fosinopril (290)], but not others [quinapril (289), enalapril (291) and lisinopril (292)], have been reported to inhibit platelet aggregation in human studies (293). Some ACE inhibitors [captopril, (288,291) and fosinopril (291)] decreased TxA$_2$ production. Interestingly, reduced circulating levels of plasma fibrinogen, factor XII, factor XI, tissue plasminogen activator, and plasminogen activator inhibitor-1 have been observed with the use of ACE inhibitors (293).

## Anticoagulants and Thrombolytic Agents

The interactions of heparin with platelets are complex and diverse, ranging from potentiation or impairment of *in vitro* platelet responses to severe thrombocytopenia. Heparin binds to platelets (294), and *in vitro* enhances aggregation responses to platelet agonists (295). However, bolus injection of heparin into healthy subjects prolongs the bleeding time (296) and inhibits VWF-dependent platelet responses *in vitro* and *in vivo* (297). The overall impact of these disparate effects on hemostatic mechanisms during heparin therapy remains unclear. The effects of heparin are described in further detail in Chapter 15. Protamine sulfate, widely used to neutralize heparin, also inhibits thrombin-induced platelet responses *in vitro* (298). The major complication following the administration of thrombolytic agents, streptokinase, urokinase, and recombinant tissue plasminogen activator (rt-PA), is hemorrhage, which arises from multiple mechanisms, including the effect of plasmin on the plasma coagulation system and platelets and the dissolution of blood clots, providing hemostasis at the site of vascular breach. The bleeding time in patients receiving rt-PA may be prolonged (299). *In vitro* plasmin induces several effects in platelets: initial platelet activation followed by inhibition, cleavage of membrane glycoproteins, inhibition of $TxA_2$ production, and disaggregation of platelet clumps (300–304). Urinary metabolites of $TxA_2$ are increased during thrombolytic therapy with rt-PA or streptokinase, indicating *in vivo* activation of platelets (305,306). Several other factors may contribute to platelet inhibition in patients receiving thrombolytic therapy, including radiographic contrast media, other medications (e.g., aspirin, nitrates, heparin), and the elevated levels of fibrin(ogen) degradation products.

## Psychotropic Drugs and Anesthetics

This heterogeneous group of drugs includes the tricyclic antidepressants, such as imipramine, amitriptyline, and nortriptyline, which have been reported to inhibit the aggregation and secretion responses to ADP, epinephrine, and collagen (307,308). Phenothiazines (chlorpromazine, promethazine, trifluoperazine) inhibit platelet responses to stimulation *in vitro* and perhaps *in vivo* (309–313). Trifluoperazine may impair platelet responses by inhibiting calmodulin-dependent platelet processes (312). Increased bleeding times during general anesthesia with halothane have been reported (314). Thiopental appears to inhibit platelet responses in patients who have undergone cardiac surgery (315).

## Miscellaneous Drugs

Dextrans are branched polysaccharides of 40,000 or 70,000 Da that have been used as antithrombotic agents. They induce prolongation of the bleeding time after infusion and inhibit platelet factor 3 (PF3) availability, glass-bead retention, aggregation, and secretion (316,317). The prolongation of bleeding time and inhibition of platelet function are most pronounced at 4 to 8 hours after transfusion (316). The mechanisms by which dextrans induce platelet dysfunction are unclear. They are also considered to adsorb to platelets as well as decrease levels of plasma factor VIII/VWF (317,318). However, it is not established that their use, even in the perioperative state, is associated with excessive hemorrhage (319). In one multicenter study in surgical patients, prophylaxis with dextran-70 was associated with less bleeding than with low-dose heparin (320). Another plasma expander, hydroxyethyl starch, can induce a hemostatic defect and prolonged bleeding time, and it also induces alterations in blood coagulation (321,322) and AVWD (130,131).

Other drugs that impair platelet function include lipid-lowering agents (clofibrate and halofenate) (323,324); chemotherapeutic agents such as daunomycin, mithramycin, and 1,3-bis (2-chloroethyl)-1-nitrosurea (BCNU) (325–328); and antihistaminics (329,330). Interestingly, the fibrinolytic inhibitor epsilon aminocarpoic acid [EACA (Amicar)], which has been used in patients with subarachnoid hemorrhage, can prolong the bleeding time at the generally administered doses (331).

Ethanol inhibits platelet responses *in vitro* (332–334). Although by itself it does not prolong bleeding time, acute ingestion of 50 g of ethanol potentiates aspirin-induced prolongation of bleeding time even in otherwise healthy subjects (200). Other agents reported to inhibit platelet function include radiographic contrast agents (335–337), although some contrast agents activate platelets (338); vitamin E (339–341); fish oil and $\omega$-3 fatty acids (342); and food items and their extracts,

such as onions (343–345), garlic (345,346), ginger (347), cumin (348), turmeric (348,349), clove (350), black tree fungus (351,352), and Chinese food. Inhibition of eicosanoid synthesis appears to be the mechanism of action for several of the spices, although they have other effects, such as lowering of plasma lipids. There is little evidence that these diverse agents induce a significant hemostatic defect. Herbal medicines, such as Gingko (*Gingko biloba*) and garlic (*Allium sativum*), inhibit platelet function and have been associated with increased bleeding, particularly when administered concomitantly with other medicines (warfarin and aspirin) (353). Given the increasing use of herbal medicines and food supplements, their role and interaction with pharmaceutical drugs needs to be considered in the evaluation of patients with unexplained bleeding.

# ACKNOWLEDGMENTS

Supported by Grant HL56724 from the National Heart Lung and Blood Institute. The excellent secretarial assistance of Ms. Mary Merrick and Ms. Denise Tierney is gratefully acknowledged.

## References

1. Mielke CH, Kaneshiro MM, Maher IA, et al. The standardized normal Ivy bleeding time and its prolongation by aspirin. *Blood* 1969;34:204–215.
2. Mielke CH. Influence of aspirin on platelets and the bleeding time. *Am J Med* 1983;74:72–78.
3. Schafer AI. Bleeding and thrombosis in myeloproliferative disorders. *Blood* 1984;64:1–12.
4. Wehmeier A, Sudhoff T, Meierkord F. Relation of platelet abnormalities to thrombosis and hemorrhage in chronic myeloproliferative disorders. *Semin Thromb Hemost* 1997;23:391–402.
5. Ravandi-Kashani F, Schafer AI. Microvascular disturbances, thrombosis, and bleeding in thrombocythemia: current concepts and perspectives. *Semin Thromb Hemost* 1997;23:479–488.
6. Landolfi R, Marchioli R, Patrono C. Mechanisms of bleeding and thrombosis in myeloproliferative disorders. *Thromb Haemost* 1997;78:617–621.
7. Fenaux P, Simon M, Caulier MT, et al. Clinical course of essential thrombocythemia in 147 cases. *Cancer* 1990;66:549–556.
8. Cortelazzo S, Viero P, Finazzi G, et al. Incidence and risk factors for thrombotic complications in a historical cohort of 100 patients with essential thrombocythemia. *J Clin Oncol* 1990;8:556–562.
9. Johnson M, Gernsheimer T, Johansen K. Essential thrombocytosis: underemphasized cause of large-vessel thrombosis. *J Vasc Surg* 1995;22:443–447; discussion 9–448.
10. van Genderen PJ, Michiels JJ. Erythromelalgia: a pathognomonic microvascular thrombotic complication in essential thrombocythemia and polycythemia vera. *Semin Thromb Hemost* 1997;23:357–363.
11. van Genderen PJ, Michiels JJ, van Strik R, et al. Platelet consumption in thrombocythemia complicated by erythromelalgia: reversal by aspirin. *Thromb Haemost* 1995;73:210–214.
12. Koudstaal PJ, Koudstaal A. Neurologic and visual symptoms in essential thrombocythemia: efficacy of low-dose aspirin. *Semin Thromb Hemost* 1997;23:365–370.
13. Tefferi A, Hoagland HC. Issues in the diagnosis and management of essential thrombocythemia. *Mayo Clin Proc* 1994;69:651–655.
14. Colombi M, Radaelli F, Zocchi L, et al. Thrombotic and hemorrhagic complications in essential thrombocythemia. A retrospective study of 103 patients. *Cancer* 1991;67:2926–2930.
15. Lahuerta-Palacios JJ, Bornstein R, Fernandez-Debora FJ, et al. Controlled and uncontrolled thrombocytosis. Its clinical role in essential thrombocythemia. *Cancer* 1988;61:1207–1212.
16. Juvonen E, Ikkala E, Oksanen K, et al. Megakaryocyte and erythroid colony formation in essential thrombocythaemia and reactive thrombocytosis: diagnostic value and correlation to complications. *Br J Haematol* 1993;83:192–197.
17. Watson KV, Key N. Vascular complications of essential thrombocythaemia: a link to cardiovascular risk factors. *Br J Haematol* 1993;83:198–203.
18. Besses C, Cervantes F, Pereira A, et al. Major vascular complications in essential thrombocythemia: a study of the predictive factors in a series of 148 patients. *Leukemia* 1999;13:150–154.
19. Wehmeier A, Daum I, Jamin H, et al. Incidence and clinical risk factors for bleeding and thrombotic complications in myeloproliferative disorders. A retrospective analysis of 260 patients. *Ann Hematol* 1991;63:101–106.

20. Pearson TC. Hemorheologic considerations in the pathogenesis of vascular occlusive events in polycythemia vera. *Semin Thromb Hemost* 1997; 23:433–439.
21. Rinder HM, Schuster JE, Rinder CS, et al. Correlation of thrombosis with increased platelet turnover in thrombocytosis. *Blood* 1998;91:1288–1294.
22. De Stefano V, Teofili L, Leone G, et al. Spontaneous erythroid colony formation as the clue to an underlying myeloproliferative disorder in patients with Budd-Chiari syndrome or portal vein thrombosis. *Semin Thromb Hemost* 1997;23:411–418.
23. Rozman C, Giralt M, Feliu E, et al. Life expectancy of patients with chronic nonleukemic myeloproliferative disorders. *Cancer* 1991;67:2658–2663.
24. Berk PD, Wasswerman LR, Fruchtman SM. Treatment of polycythemia vera: a summary of clinical trials conducted by the polycythemia vera study group. In: Wasserman LR, Berk PD, Berlin NI, eds. *Polycythemia vera and the myeloproliferative disorders*. Philadelphia, PA: WB Saunders, 1995:166–194.
25. Gruppo Italiano Studio Policitemia Polycythemia vera: the natural history of 1213 patients followed for 20 years. *Ann Intern Med* 1995; 123:656–654.
26. Rao AK, Carvalho A. Acquired qualitative platelet defects. In: Colman RW, Hirsh J, Marder VJ et al., eds. *Hemostasis and thrombosis: basic principles and clinical practice*, 3rd ed. Philadelphia, PA: JB Lippincott Co, 1994:685–704.
27. Small BM, Bettigole RE. Diagnosis of myeloproliferative disease by analysis of the platelet volume distribution. *Am J Clin Pathol* 1981;76:685–691.
28. Van der Lelie J, Von dem Borne AK. Platelet volume analysis for differential diagnosis of thrombocytosis. *J Clin Pathol* 1986;39:129–133.
29. Maldonado JE, Pintado T, Pierre RV. Dysplastic platelet and circulating megakaryocytes in chronic myeloproliferative diseases. I. The platelets: ultrastructure and peroxidase reaction. *Blood* 1974;43:797–809.
30. Swart SS, Pearson D, Wood JK, et al. Functional significance of the platelet $\alpha$ 2-adrenoceptor: studies in patients with myeloproliferative disorders. *Thromb Res* 1984;33:531–541.
31. Rendu F, Lebret M, Nurden A, et al. Detection of an acquired platelet storage pool disease in three patients with a myeloproliferative disorder. *Thromb Haemost* 1979;42:794–796.
32. Caranobe C, Sie P, Nouvel C, et al. Platelets in myeloproliferative disorders. II. Serotonin uptake and storage: correlation with mepacrine labelled dense bodies and with platelet density. *Scand J Haematol* 1980;25: 289–295.
33. Malpass TW, Savage B, Hanson SR, et al. Correlation between prolonged bleeding time and depletion of platelet dense granule ADP in patients with myelodysplastic and myeloproliferative disorders. *J Lab Clin Med* 1984; 103:894–904.
34. Holme S, Murphy S. Studies of the platelet density abnormality in myeloproliferative disease. *J Lab Clin Med* 1984;103:373–383.
35. Murphy S, Davis JL, Walsh PN, et al. Template bleeding time and clinical hemorrhage in myeloproliferative disease. *Arch Intern Med* 1978;138: 1251–1253.
36. Boneu B, Nouvel C, Sie P, et al. Platelets in myeloproliferative disorders. I. A comparative evaluation with certain platelet function tests. *Scand J Haematol* 1980;25:214–220.
37. Balduini CL, Bertolino G, Noris P, et al. Platelet aggregation in platelet-rich plasma and whole blood in 120 patients with myeloproliferative disorders. *Am J Clin Pathol* 1991;95:82–86.
38. Waddell CC, Brown JA, Repinecz YA. Abnormal platelet function in myeloproliferative disorders. *Arch Pathol Lab Med* 1981;105:432–435.
39. Wu KK. Platelet hyperaggregability and thrombosis in patients with thrombocythemia. *Ann Intern Med* 1978;88:7–11.
40. Kaywin P, McDonough M, Insel PA, et al. Platelet function in essential thrombocythemia: decreased ephinephrine responsiveness associated to $\alpha$ adrenergic receptors. *N Engl J Med* 1978;299:505–509.
41. Pfeifer MA, Ward K, Malpass T, et al. Variations in circulating catecholamines fail to alter human platelet $\alpha$-2-adrenergic receptor number or affinity for [3H]yohimbine or [3H]dihydroergocryptine. *J Clin Invest* 1984;74:1063–1072.
42. Swart SS, Wood JK, Barnett DB. Differential labeling of platelet $\alpha$ 2 adrenoceptors by 3H dihydroergocryptine and 3H yohimbine in patients with myeloproliferative disorders. *Thromb Res* 1985;40:623–629.
43. Swart SS, Maguire M, Wood JK, et al. $\alpha$ 2-adrenoceptor coupling to adenylate cyclase in adrenaline insensitive human platelets. *Eur J Pharmacol* 1985;116:113–119.
44. Ushikubi F, Okuma M, Ishibashi T, et al. Deficient elevation of the cytoplasmic calcium ion concentration by epinephrine in epinephrine-insensitive platelets of patients with myeloproliferative disorders. *Am J Hematol* 1990; 33:96–100.
45. Gugliotta L, Pickering C, Greaves M, et al. Abnormality of platelet membrane glycoproteins in essential thrombocythemia. *Thromb Haemost* 1983;50:216.
46. Mazzucato M, De Marco L, De Angelis V, et al. Platelet membrane abnormalities in myeloproliferative disorders: decrease in glycoproteins Ib and IIb/IIIa complex is associated with deficient receptor function. *Br J Haematol* 1989;73:369–374.
47. Eche N, Sie P, Caranobe C, et al. Platelets in myeloproliferative disorders. III: glycoprotein profile in relation to platelet function and platelet density. *Scand J Haematol* 1981;26:123–129.

48. Clezardin P, McGregor JL, Dechavanne M, et al. Platelet membrane glycoprotein abnormalities in patients with myeloproliferative disorders and secondary thrombocytosis. *Br J Haematol* 1985;60:331–344.
49. Kaplan R, Gabbeta J, Sun L, et al. Combined defect in membrane expression and activation of platelet GP IIb-IIIa complex without primary sequence abnormalities in myeloproliferative disease. *Br J Haematol* 2000; 111:954–964.
50. Landolfi R. Bleeding and thrombosis in myeloproliferative disorders. *Curr Opin Hematol* 1998;5:327–331.
51. Mistry R, Cahill M, Chapman C, et al. 125I-fibrinogen binding to platelets in myeloproliferative disease. *Thromb Haemost* 1991;66:329–333.
52. Handa M, Watanabe K, Kawai Y, et al. Platelet unresponsiveness to collagen: involvement of glycoprotein Ia-IIa ($\alpha$ 2b 1 integrin) deficiency associated with a myeloproliferative disorder. *Thromb Haemost* 1995;73:521–528.
53. Legrand C, Bellucci S, Disdier M, et al. Platelet thrombospondin and glycoprotein IV abnormalities in patients with essential thrombocythemia: effect of $\alpha$-interferon treatment. *Am J Hematol* 1991;38:307–313.
54. Thibert V, Bellucci S, Cristofari M, et al. Increased platelet CD36 constitutes a common marker in myeloproliferative disorders. *Br J Haematol* 1995;91:618–624.
55. Bolin RB, Okumura T, Jamieson GA. Changes in the distribution of platelet membrane glycoproteins in patients with myeloproliferative disorders. *Am J Hematol* 1977;3:63–71.
56. Wehmeier A, Tschope D, Esser J, et al. Circulating activated platelets in myeloproliferative disorders. *Thromb Res* 1991;61:271–278.
57. Moore A, Nachman RL. Platelet Fc receptor: increased expression in myeloproliferative disease. *J Clin Invest* 1981;67:1064–1071.
58. Okuma M, Uchino H. Altered arachidonate metabolism by platelets in patients with myeloproliferative disorders. *Blood* 1979;54:1258–1271.
59. Russel NH, Salmon J, Keenan JP, et al. Platelet adenine nucleotides and arachidonic acid metabolism in the myeloproliferative disorders. *Thromb Res* 1981;22:389–397.
60. Schafer AI. Deficiency of platelet lipoxygenase activity in myeloproliferative disorders. *N Engl J Med* 1982;306:381–386.
61. van Genderen PJ, Michiels JJ, Zijlstra FJ. Lipoxygenase deficiency in primary thrombocythemia is not a true deficiency. *Thromb Haemost* 1994; 71:803–804.
62. Smith IL, Martin TJ. Platelet thromboxane synthesis and release reactions in myeloproliferative disorders. *Haemostasis* 1982;11:119–127.
63. Zahavi J, Zahavi M, Firsteter E, et al. An abnormal pattern of multiple platelet function abnormalities and increased thromboxane generation in patients with primary thrombocytosis and thrombotic complications. *Eur J Haematol* 1991;47:326–332.
64. Rocca B, Ciabattoni G, Tartaglione R, et al. Increased thromboxane biosynthesis in essential thrombocythemia. *Thromb Haemost* 1995;74: 1225–1230.
65. Landolfi R, Ciabattoni G, Patrignani P, et al. Increased thromboxane biosynthesis in patients with polycythemia vera: evidence for aspirin-suppressible platelet activation in vivo [see comments]. *Blood* 1992;80:1965–1971.
66. Takayama H, Okuma M, Kanaji K, et al. Altered arachidonate metabolism by leukocytes and platelets in myeloproliferative disorders. *Prostaglandins Leukot Med* 1983;12:261–272.
67. Samuelsson B, Dahlen SE, Lindgren JA, et al. Leukotrienes and lipoxins: structures, biosynthesis, and biological effects. *Science* 1987;237: 1171–1176.
68. Badr KF, DeBoer DK, Schwartzberg M, et al. Lipoxin A4 antagonizes cellular and in vivo actions of leukotriene D4 in rat glomerular mesangial cells: evidence for competition at a common receptor. *Proc Natl Acad Sci U S A* 1989;86:3438–3442.
69. Brady HR, Persson U, Ballermann BJ, et al. Leukotrienes stimulate neutrophil adhesion to mesangial cells: modulation with lipoxins. *Am J Physiol* 1990;259:F809–F815.
70. Stenke L, Edenius C, Samuelsson J, et al. Deficient lipoxin synthesis: a novel platelet dysfunction in myeloproliferative disorders with special reference to blastic crisis of chronic myelogenous leukemia. *Blood* 1991;78: 2989–2995.
71. Fujimoto T, Fujimura K, Kuramoto A. Abnormal $Ca^{2+}$ homeostasis in platelets with myeloproliferative disorders: low levels of $Ca^{2+}$ influx and efflux across the plasma membrane and increased $Ca^{2+}$ accumulation into the dense tubular system. *Thromb Res* 1989;53:99–108.
72. Ushikubi F, Ishibashi T, Narumiya S, et al. Analysis of the defective signal transduction mechanism through the platelet thromboxane $A_2$ receptor in a patient with polycythemia vera. *Thromb Haemost* 1992;67:144–146.
73. Eigenthaler M, Ullrich H, Geiger J, et al. Defective nitrovasodilator-stimulated protein phosphorylation and calcium regulation in cGMP-dependent protein kinase-deficient human platelets of chronic myelocytic leukemia. *J Biol Chem* 1993;268:13526–13531.
74. Cooper B, Schafer AI, Puchalsky D, et al. Platelet resistance to prostaglandin D2 in patients with myeloproliferative disorders. *Blood* 1978; 52:618–626.
75. Cortelazzo S, Galli M, Castagna D, et al. Increased response to arachidonic acid and U-46619 and resistance to inhibitory prostaglandins in patients with chronic myeloproliferative disorders. *Thromb Haemost* 1988;59:73–76.
76. Moliterno AR, Siebel KE, Sun AY, et al. A novel thrombopoietin signaling defect in polycythemia vera platelets. *Stem Cells* 1998;16:185–192.

77. Best D, Pasquet S, Littlewood TJ, et al. Platelet activation via the collagen receptor GP VI is not altered in platelets from chronic myeloid leukaemia patients despite the presence of the constitutively phosphorylated adapter protein CrkL. *Br J Haematol* 2001;112:609–615.

78. Budde U, van Genderen PJ. Acquired von Willebrand disease in patients with high platelet counts. *Semin Thromb Hemost* 1997;23:425–431.

79. Cortelazzo S, Finazzi G, Ruggeri M, et al. Hydroxyurea for patients with essential thrombocythemia and a high risk of thrombosis. *N Engl J Med* 1995;332:1132–1136.

80. Tefferi A, Silverstein MN, Petitt RM, et al. Anagrelide as a new platelet-lowering agent in essential thrombocythemia: mechanism of action, efficacy, toxicity, current indications. *Semin Thromb Hemost* 1997;23:379–383.

81. Solberg LA Jr, Tefferi A, Oles KJ, et al. The effects of anagrelide on human megakaryocytopoiesis. *Br J Haematol* 1997;99:174–180.

82. Petitt RM, Silverstein MN, Petrone ME. Anagrelide for control of thrombocythemia in polycythemia and other myeloproliferative disorders. *Semin Hematol* 1997;34:51–54.

83. Storen EC, Tefferi A. Long-term use of anagrelide in young patients with essential thrombocythemia. *Blood* 2001;97:863–866.

84. Green A, Campbell P, Buck G, et al. The medical research council PT1 trial in essential thrombocythemia. *Blood* 2004;104:5a–6a.

85. Elliott MA, Tefferi A. Interferon-α therapy in polycythemia vera and essential thrombocythemia. *Semin Thromb Hemost* 1997;23:463–472.

86. Gisslinger H, Ludwig H, Linkesch W, et al. Long-term interferon therapy for thrombocytosis in myeloproliferative diseases. *Lancet* 1989;1:634–637.

87. Tartaglia AP, Goldberg JD, Berk PD, et al. Adverse effects of antiaggregating platelet therapy in the treatment of polycythemia vera. *Semin Hematol* 1986;23:172–176.

88. Landolfi R, Marchioli R, Kutti J, et al. Efficacy and safety of low-dose aspirin in polycythemia vera. *N Engl J Med* 2004;350:114–124.

89. Friedman IA, Schwarts SO, Leithold SL. Platelet function defects with bleeding early manifestations of acute leukemia. *Arch Intern Med* 1964;113:177.

90. Caen J, Rendu F, Sultan Y, et al. Platelet aggregation and populations in acute leukemias. *Haemostasis* 1972;1:61.

91. Cowan DH, Haut JJ. Platelet function in acute leukemia. *J Lab Clin Med* 1972;79:893–905.

92. Sultan Y, Caen JP. Platelet dysfunction in preleukemia states and in various types of leukemia. *Ann N Y Acad Sci* 1972;201:300–306.

93. Cowan DH, Graham RC Jr. Structural-functional relationships in platelets in acute leukemia and related disorders. *Ser Haematol* 1975;8:68–100.

94. Cowan DH, Graham RC Jr, Baunach D. The platelet defect in leukemia, platelet ultrastructure, adenine nucleotide metabolism and the release reaction. *J Clin Invest* 1975;56:188–200.

95. Stuart JJ, Lewis JC. Platelet aggregation and electron microscopic studies of platelets in preleukemia. *Arch Pathol Lab Med* 1982;106:458–461.

96. Levine PH, Katayama I. The platelet in leukemic reticuloendotheliosis. Functional and morphological evidence of a qualitative disorder. *Cancer* 1975;36:1353–1358.

97. Nouvel C, Caronobe C, Sie P, et al. Platelet volume, density and 5HT organelles (mepacrine test) in acute leukemia. *Scand J Haematol* 1978;21:421–426.

98. Russell NH, Keenan JP, Bellingham AJ. Platelet adenine nucleotides and arachidonic acid metabolism in myeloproliferative diseases. *Thromb Res* 1981;22:389–397.

99. Maldonado JE, Pierre RV. The platelets in preleukemia and myelomonocytic leukemia. Ultrastructural cytochemistry and cytogenetics. *Mayo Clin Proc* 1975;50:573–587.

100. Raman BK, VanSlyck EJ, Riddle J, et al. Platelet function and structure in myeloproliferative disease, myelodysplastic syndrome and secondary thrombocytosis. *Am J Clin Pathol* 1989;91:647–655.

101. Baker RI, Manoharan A. Platelet function in myeloproliferative disorders: and sequential studies show multiple platelet abnormalities and change with time. *Eur J Haematol* 1988;40:267–272.

102. Meschengieser S, Blanco A, Woods A, et al. Intraplatelet levels of vWF:Ag and fibrinogen in myeloproliferative disorders. *Thromb Res* 1987;48:311–319.

103. Roussi JH, Houbouyan LL, Alterscu R, et al. Acquired von Willebrand's Syndrome associated with hairy cell leukemia. *Br J Haematol* 1980;46:503–506.

104. Berndt MC, Kabral A, Grimsley P, et al. An acquired Bernard-Soulier–like platelet defect associated with juvenile myelodysplastic syndrome. *Br J Haematol* 1988;68:97–101.

105. Widell S, Hast R. Balloon platelets in myelodysplastic sydromes—a feature of dysmegakaryopoiesis. *Leuk Res* 1987;11:747–752.

106. Robert F, Mignucci M, McCurdy SA, et al. Hemostatic abnormalities associated with monoclonal gammopathies. *Am J Med Sci* 1993;306: 359–366.

107. Perkins HA, McKenzie MR, Fudenberg HH. Hemostatic defects in dysproteinemias. *Blood* 1970;35:695–707.

108. Saraya AK, Kasturi J, Kishan R. A study of hemostasis in macroglobulinemia. *Acta Haematol* 1972;47:33.

109. Rozenberg MD, Dintenfass L. Platelet aggregation in Waldenstrom's macroglobulinemia. *Thromb Diath Haemorrh* 1965;14:202.

110. Penny R, Castaldi PA, Whitsead HM. Inflammation and hemostasis in paraproteinemias. *Br J Haematol* 1971;20:35–44.

111. Lackner H. Hemostatic abnormalities associated with dysproteinemias. *Semin Hematol* 1973;10:125–133.

112. Kasturi J, Saraya AK. Platelet functions in dysproteinemia. *Acta Haematol* 1978;59:104–113.

113. Furie B, Greene E, Furie BC. Syndrome of acquired factor X deficiency and systemic amyloidosis in vivo studies of the metabolic fate of factor X. *N Engl J Med* 1977;297:81–85.

114. McPherson RA, Onstad JW, Ugoretz RJ, et al. Coagulopathy in amyloidosis: combined deficiency of factors IX and X. *Am J Hematol* 1977;3:225–235.

115. Palmer RN, Rick ME, Rick PD, et al. Circulating heparan sulfate anticoagulant in a patient with a fatal bleeding disorder. *N Engl J Med* 1984;310:1696–1699.

116. Chapman GS, George CB, Danley DL. Heparin-like anticoagulant associated with plasma cell myeloma. *Am J Clin Pathol* 1985;83:764–766.

117. Carr ME Jr, Zekert SL. Abnormal clot retraction, altered fibrin structure, and normal platelet function in multiple myeloma. *Am J Physiol* 1994;266:H1195–H1201.

118. Mohri H, Noguchi T, Kodoma F, et al. Acquired von Willebrand disease due to inhibitor of human myeloma protein specific for von Willebrand factor. *Am J Pathol* 1987;97:663–668.

119. Bovill EG, Ershler WB, Golden EA, et al. A human myeloma-produced monoclonal protein directed against the active subpopulation of von Willebrand factor. *Am J Clin Pathol* 1986;85:115–123.

120. Takahashi H, Nagayama R, Tanabe Y, et al. DDAVP in acquired von Willebrand syndrome associated with multiple myeloma. *Am J Hematol* 1986;22:421–429.

121. DiMinno G, Coraggio F, Cerbone AM, et al. A myeloma paraprotein with specificity for platelet glycoprotein IIIa in a patient with a fatal bleeding disorder. *J Clin Invest* 1986;77:157–164.

122. McGrath KM, Stuart JJ, Richards FD. Correlation between serum IgG, platelet membrane IgG, and platelet function in hypergammaglobulinaemic states. *Br J Haematol* 1979;42:585–591.

123. Kumar S, Pruthi RK, Nichols WL. Acquired von Willebrand disease. *Mayo Clin Proc* 2002;77:181–187.

124. Federici AB, Rand JH, Bucciarelli P, et al. Acquired von Willebrand syndrome: data from an international registry. *Thromb Haemost* 2000;84: 345–349.

125. Budde U, Scharf RE, Franke P, et al. Elevated platelet count as a cause of abnormal von Willebrand factor multimer distribution in plasma. *Blood* 1993;82:1749–1757.

126. van Genderen PJ, Budde U, Michiels JJ, et al. The reduction of large von Willebrand factor multimers in plasma in essential thrombocythaemia is related to the platelet count. *Br J Haematol* 1996;93:962–965.

127. Castaman G, Lattuada A, Mannucci PM, et al. Characterization of two cases of acquired transitory von Willebrand syndrome with ciprofloxacin: evidence for heightened proteolysis of von Willebrand factor. *Am J Hematol* 1995;49:83–86.

128. Kreuz W, Linde R, Funk M, et al. Induction of von Willebrand disease type I by valproic acid. *Lancet* 1990;335:1350–1351.

129. Conrad ME, Latour LF. Acquired von Willebrand's disease, IgE polyclonal gammopathy and griseofulvin therapy. *Am J Hematol* 1992;41:143.

130. Lazarchick J, Conroy JM. The effect of 6% hydroxyethyl starch and desmopressin infusion on von Willebrand factor: ristocetin cofactor activity. *Ann Clin Lab Sci* 1995;25:306–309.

131. Dalrymple-Hay M, Aitchison R, Collins P, et al. Hydroxyethyl starch induced acquired von Willebrand's disease. *Clin Lab Haematol* 1992;14: 209–211.

132. Jonge Poerink-Stockschlader AB, Dekker I, Risseeuw-Appel IM, et al. Acquired Von Willebrand disease in children with a Wilms' tumor. *Med Pediatr Oncol* 1996;26:238–243.

133. Gill JC, Wilson AD, Endres-Brooks J, et al. Loss of the largest von Willebrand factor multimers from plasma of patients with congenital cardiac defects. *Blood* 1986;67:758–761.

134. Vincentelli A, Susen S, Le Tourneau T, et al. Acquired von Willebrand syndrome in aortic stenosis. *N Engl J Med* 2003;349:343–349.

135. Mohri H, Motomura S, Kanamori H, et al. Clinical significance of inhibitors in acquired von Willebrand syndrome. *Blood* 1998;91:3623–3629.

136. Sadler JE. Aortic stenosis, von Willebrand factor, and bleeding. *N Engl J Med* 2003;349:323–325.

137. Levesque H, Borg JY, Cailleux N, et al. Acquired von Willebrand's syndrome associated with decrease of plasminogen activator and its inhibitor during hypothyroidism. *Eur J Med* 1993;2:287–288.

138. Scott JP, Montgomery RR, Tubergen DG, et al. Acquired von Willebrand's disease in association with Wilm's tumor: regression following treatment. *Blood* 1981;58:665–669.

139. Friederich PW, Wever PC, Briet E, et al. Successful treatment with recombinant factor VIIa of therapy-resistant severe bleeding in a patient with acquired von Willebrand disease. *Am J Hematol* 2001;66:292–294.

140. Federici AB, Stabile F, Castaman G, et al. Treatment of acquired von Willebrand syndrome in patients with monoclonal gammopathy of uncertain significance: comparison of three different therapeutic approaches. *Blood* 1998;92:2707–2711.

141. Agarwal N, Klix MM, Burns CP. Successful management with intravenous immunoglobulins of acquired von Willebrand disease associated with monoclonal gammopathy of undetermined significance. *Ann Intern Med* 2004;141:83–84.

142. Uehlinger J, Button GR, McCarthy J, et al. Immunoadsorption for coagulation factor inhibitors. *Transfusion* 1991;31:265–269.

143. Budde U, Schaefer G, Mueller N, et al. Acquired von Willebrand's disease in the myeloproliferative syndrome. *Blood* 1984;64:981–985.

144. Budde U, Dent JA, Berkowitz SD, et al. Subunit composition of plasma von Willebrand factor in patients with myeloproliferative syndrome. *Blood* 1986;68:1213–1217.

145. van Genderen PJ, Prins FJ, Lucas IS, et al. Decreased half-life time of plasma von Willebrand factor collagen binding activity in essential thrombocythaemia: normalization after cytoreduction of the increased platelet count. *Br J Haematol* 1997;99:832–836.

146. Zahavi J, Marder VJ. Acquired storage pool disease of platelets associated with circulating anti-platelet antibodies. *Am J Med* 1974;56:883–889.

147. Weiss HJ, Rosove MH, Lages BA, et al. Acquired storage pool deficiency with increased platelet-associated IgG. Report of five cases. *Am J Med* 1980;69:711–717.

148. Pareti FI, Gugliotta L, Mannucci L, et al. Biochemical and metabolic aspects of platelet dysfunction in myeloproliferative disorders. *Thromb Haemost* 1982;47:84–89.

149. Pareti FI, Capitanio A, Mannucci PM. Acquired storage pool disease in platelets during disseminated intravascular coagulation. *Blood* 1976;48:511–515.

150. Pareti FI, Capitanio A, Mannucci C, et al. Acquired dysfunction due to circulation of "exhausted" platelets. *Am J Med* 1980;69:235–240.

151. Khurana MS, Lian ECY, Harkness DR. Storage pool disease of platelets. Association with multiple congenital cavernous hemangiomas. *J Am Med Assoc* 1980;244:169–171.

152. Nenci GG, Gresele P, Agnetti F, et al. Intrinsically defective or exhausted platelets in hairy cell leukemia? *Thromb Haemost* 1981;46:572.

153. Harker LA, Malpass TW, Branson HE, et al. Mechanism of abnormal bleeding in patients undergoing cardiopulmonary bypass: acquired transient platelet dysfunction associated with selective α granule release. *Blood* 1980;55:824–834.

154. Beurling-Harbury C, Galvan CA. Acquired decreased in platelet secretory ADP associated with increased postoperative bleeding in postcardiopulmonary bypass patients and in patients with severe valvular heart disease. *Blood* 1978;52:13–23.

155. Savage B, Malpass TW, Stratton JR, et al. Platelet adenine nucleotide levels in patients with dacron vascular prostheses. *Thromb Res* 1983;32:365–372.

156. Rao AK, Niewiarowski S, Murphy S. Acquired granular pool defect in stored platelets. *Blood* 1981;57:203–208.

157. Wiedmer T, Ando B, Sims PJ. Complement C5b-9-stimulated platelet secretion is associated with a Ca²⁺-initiated activation of cellular protein kinases. *J Biol Chem* 1987;262:13674–13681.

158. Kelton JG, Gibbons S. Autoimmune platelet destruction: idiopathic thrombocytopenic purpura. *Semin Thromb Hemost* 1982;8:83–104.

159. Harker LA. Thrombokinetics in idiopathic thrombocytopenic purpura. *Br J Haematol* 1970;19:95–104.

160. Branehog I, Jutti J, Weinfeld A. Platelet survival and platelet production in idiopathic thrombocytopenic purpura (ITP). *Br J Haematol* 1974;27:127–143.

161. Kelton JG, Neame PB, Bishop J, et al. The direct assay for platelet-associated IgG (PAIgG): lack of association between antibody level and platelet size. *Blood* 1979;53:73–80.

162. Harker LA, Slichter SJ. The bleeding time as a screening test for evaluation of platelet function. *N Engl J Med* 1972;287:155–159.

163. Clancy R, Jenkins E, Firkin B. Qualitative platelet abnormalities in idiopathic thrombocytopenic purpura. *N Engl J Med* 1972;286:622–626.

164. Karpatkin S, Lackner HL. Association of antiplatelet antibody with functional platelet disorders: autoimmune thrombocytopenic purpura, systemic lupus erythematosus and thrombopathia. *Am J Med* 1975;59:599–604.

165. Lackner HL, Karpatkin S. On the "easy brusing" syndrome with normal platelet count. A study of 75 patients. *Ann Intern Med* 1975;83:190–196.

166. Heyns A, Fraser J, Retief FP. Platelet aggregation in chronic idiopathic thrombocytopenic purpura. *J Clin Pathol* 1978;31:1239–1243.

167. Stuart MJ, Kelton JG, Allen JB. Abnormal platelet function and arachidonate metabolism in chronic idiopathic thrombocytopenic purpura. *Blood* 1981;58:326–329.

168. Regan MG, Lackner HL, Karpatkin S. Platelet function and coagulation profile in lupus erythematosus. *Ann Intern Med* 1974;81:462–468.

169. Dorsch CA, Meyerhoff J. Mechanisms of abnormal platelet aggregation in systemic lupus erythematosus. *Arthritis Rheum* 1982;25:966–973.

170. Kurata Y, Nishioeda Y, Tsubakio T, et al. Thrombocytopenia in Grave's disease: effect of T3 on platelet kinetics. *Acta Haematol* 1980;63:185–190.

171. Woods VL Jr, Kurata Y, Montgomery RR, et al. Autoantibodies against platelet glycoprotein Ib in patients with chronic immune thrombocytopenic purpura. *Blood* 1984;64:156–160.

172. Szatkowski NS, Kunicki TJ, Aster RH. Identification of glycoprotein Ib as a target for autoantibody in idiopathic (autoimmune) thrombocytopenic purpura. *Blood* 1986;67:310–315.

173. Woods VL Jr, Oh EH, Mason D, et al. Autoantibodies against the platelet glycoprotein IIb/IIIa complex in patients with chronic ITP. *Blood* 1984;63:368–375.

174. Berchtold P, McMillan R, Tani P, et al. Autoantibodies against platelet membrane glycoproteins in children with acute and chronic immune thrombocytopenic purpura. *Blood* 1989;74:1600–1602.

175. Deckmyn H, Zhang J, Van Houtte E, et al. Production and nucleotide sequence of an inhibitory human IgM autoantibody directed against platelet glycoprotein Ia/IIa. *Blood* 1994;84:1968–1974.

176. Dromigny A, Triadou P, Lesavre P, et al. Lack of platelet response to collagen associated with autoantibodies against glycoprotein (GP) Ia/IIa and Ib/IX leading to the discovery of SLE. *Hematol Cell Ther* 1996;38:355–357.

177. Rao AK, Kowalska MA, Karczewski J, et al. Impaired platelet response to collagen and human antibody against an 88 kilo-dalton platelet membrane glycoprotein. *Thromb Haemost* 1989;62:506.

178. Sugiyama T, Okuma M, Ushikubi F, et al. A novel platelet aggregating factor found in a patient with defective collagen-induced platelet aggregation and autoimmune thrombocytopenia. *Blood* 1987;69:1712–1720.

179. Boylan B, Chen H, Rathore V, et al. Anti-GP VI-associated ITP: an acquired platelet disorder caused by autoantibody-mediated clearance of the GP VI/FcRgamma-chain complex from the human platelet surface. *Blood* 2004;104:1350–1355.

180. van Vliet HH, Kappers-Klunne MC, van der Hel JW, et al. Antibodies against glycosphingolipids in sera of patients with idiopathic thrombocytopenic purpura. *Br J Haematol* 1987;67:103–108.

181. Koerner TA, Weinfeld HM, Bullard LS, et al. Antibodies against platelet glycosphingolipids: detection in serum by quantitative HPTLC-autoradiography and association with autoimmune and alloimmune processes. *Blood* 1989;74:274–284.

182. McMillan R, Tani P, Millard F, et al. Platelet-associated and plasma antiglycoprotein autoantibodies in chronic ITP. *Blood* 1987;70:1040–1045.

183. Kiefel V, Santoso S, Kaufmann E, et al. Autoantibodies against platelet glycoprotein Ib/IX: a frequent finding in autoimmune thrombocytopenic purpura. *Br J Haematol* 1991;79:256–262.

184. Kiefel V, Freitag E, Kroll H, et al. Platelet autoantibodies (IgG, IgM, IgA) against glycoproteins IIb/IIIa and Ib/IX in patients with thrombocytopenia. *Ann Hematol* 1996;72:280–285.

185. Meyerhoff J, Dorsch CA. Decreased platelet serotonin levels in systemic lupus erythematosus. *Arthritis Rheum* 1981;24:1495–1500.

186. Ingeberg S, Stoffersen E. Platelet dysfunction in patients with vitamin B12 deficiency. *Acta Haematol* 1979;61:75–79.

187. Laosombat V, Wongchanchailert M, Sattayasevana B, et al. Acquired platelet dysfunction with eosinophilia in children in the south of Thailand. *Platelets* 2001;12:5–14.

188. Lim SH, Tan CE, Agasthian T, et al. Acquired platelet dysfunction with eosinophilia: review of seven adult cases. *J Clin Pathol* 1989;42:950–952.

189. Poon MC, Ng SC, Coppes MJ. Acquired platelet dysfunction with eosinophilia in white children. *J Pediatr* 1995;126:959–961.

190. Solinger A, Bernstein IL, Glueck HI. The effect of epinephrine on platelet aggregation in normal and atopic patients. *J Allergy Clin Immunol* 1973;51:29–34.

191. Szczeklik A, Milner PC, Birch J, et al. Prolonged bleeding time, reduced platelet aggregation, altered PAF-acether sensitivity and increased platelet mass are a trait of asthma and hay fever. *Thromb Haemost* 1986;56:283–287.

192. Stoff JS, Stomerman M, Steer M, et al. A defect in platelet aggregation in Bartter's syndrome. *Am J Med* 1980;68–80:171.

193. Pedersen AK, Fitzgerald GA. Dose-related kinetics of aspirin. Presystemic acetylation of platelet cyclooxygenase. *N Engl J Med* 1984;311:1206–1211.

194. Patrigrani P, Filabozzi P, Patrono C. Selective cumulative inhibition of platelet thromboxane production by low-dose aspirin in healthy subjects. *J Clin Invest* 1982;69:1366–1372.

195. Weksler BB, Pett SB, Alonso D, et al. Differential inhibition of aspirin in vascular prostaglandin synthesis in atherosclerotic patients. *N Engl J Med* 1983;308:800–805.

196. Antiplatelet Trialists' Collaboration. Collaborative meta-analysis of randomised trials of antiplatelet therapy for prevention of death, myocardial infarction, and stroke in high risk patients. *BMJ* 2002;324:71–86.

197. Patrono C, Coller B, Dalen JE, et al. Platelet-active drugs: the relationships among dose, effectiveness, and side effects. *Chest* 2001;119:39S–63S.

198. Patrono C. Aspirin resistance: definition, mechanisms and clinical readouts. *J Thromb Haemost* 2003;1:1710–1713.

199. Mielke CH. Aspirin prolongation of the template bleeding time: influence of venostasis and direction of incision. *Blood* 1982;60:1139–1142.

200. Deykin D, Janson P, McMahon L. Ethanol potentiation of aspirin-induced prolongation of the bleeding time. *N Engl J Med* 1982;306:852–854.

201. Rumack CM, Guggenheim MA, Rumack BH, et al. Neonatal intracranial hemorrhage and maternal use of aspirin. *Obstet Gynecol* 1981;58:52S–56S.

202. Bleyer WA, Breckenridge RT. Studies on the detection of adverse drug reactions in the newborn. II. The effects of prenatal aspirin on newborn hemostasis. *J Am Med Assoc* 1970;213:2049–2053.

203. Stuart MJ, Gross SJ, Elrad H, et al. Effects of acetylsalicylic-acid ingestion on maternal and neonatal hemostasis. *N Engl J Med* 1982;307:909–912.

204. Steering Committee of the Physicians' Health Study Research Group. Final report on the aspirin component of the ongoing Physicians' Health Study. *N Engl J Med* 1989;321:129–135.

205. Merritt JC, Bhatt DL. The efficacy and safety of perioperative antiplatelet therapy. *J Thromb Thrombolysis* 2002;13:97–103.

206. Sethi GK, Copeland JG, Goldman S, et al. Implications of preoperative administration of aspirin in patients undergoing coronary artery bypass

grafting. Department of Veterans Affairs Cooperative Study on Antiplatelet Therapy. *J Am Coll Cardiol* 1990;15:15–20.

207. Mangano DT. Aspirin and mortality from coronary bypass surgery. *N Engl J Med* 2002;347:1309–1317.

208. Roderick PJ, Wilkes HC, Meade TW. The gastrointestinal toxicity of aspirin: an overview of randomised controlled trials. *Br J Clin Pharmacol* 1993;35: 219–226.

209. Diener HC, Cunha L, Forbes C et al, European Stroke Prevention Study. 2. Dipyridamole and acetylsalicylic acid in the secondary prevention of stroke. *J Neurol Sci* 1996;143:1–13.

210. The Dutch TIA Trial Study Group. A comparison of two doses of aspirin (30mg vs 823 mg a day) in patients after a transient ischemic attack or minor ischemic stroke. *N Engl J Med* 1991;325:1261–1266.

211. Garcia Rodriguez LA, Cattaruzzi C, Troncon MG, et al. Risk of hospitalization for upper gastrointestinal tract bleeding associated with ketorolac, other nonsteroidal anti-inflammatory drugs, calcium antagonists, and other antihypertensive drugs. *Arch Intern Med* 1998;158:33–39.

212. Henry D, Lim LL, Garcia Rodriguez LA, et al. Variability in risk of gastrointestinal complications with individual non-steroidal anti-inflammatory drugs: results of a collaborative meta-analysis. *Br Med J* 1996;312: 1563–1566.

213. Stein PD, Dalen JE, Goldman S, et al. Antithrombotic therapy in patients with saphenous vein and internal mammary artery bypass grafts. *Chest* 2001;119:278S–282S.

214. Topol EJ. Aspirin with bypass surgery—from taboo to new standard of care. *N Engl J Med* 2002;347:1359–1360.

215. Mannucci PM. Desmopressin (DDAVP) in the treatment of bleeding disorders: the first 20 years. *Blood* 1997;90:2515–2521.

216. Simon LS, Mills JA. Drug therapy: nonsteroidal antiinflammatory drugs (first of two parts). *N Engl J Med* 1980;302:1179–1185.

217. OBrien JR, Finch W, Clark E. A comparison of an effect of different anti-inflammatory drugs on human platelets. *J Clin Pathol* 1970;23:522–525.

218. Nishizawa EE, Wynalda DJ. Inhibitory effect of ibuprofen (motrin) on platelet function. *Thromb Res* 1981;21:347–356.

219. Green D, Given KM, Ts'ao CH, et al. The effect of a new non-steroidal anti-inflammatory agent, sulindac, on platelet function. *Thromb Res* 1977;10: 283–289.

220. McQueen EG, Facoory B. Non-steroidal anti-inflammatory drugs and platelet function. *N Z Med J* 1986;99:358–360.

221. Thomas P, Hepburn B, Kim HC, et al. Nonsteroidal anti-inflammatory drugs in the treatment of hemophilic arthropathy. *Am J Hematol* 1982; 12:131–137.

222. McIntyre BA, Philp RB, Inwood MJ. Effect of ibuprofen on platelet function in normal subjects and hemophiliac patients. *Clin Pharmacol Ther* 1978;24:616–621.

223. Ragni MV, Miller BJ, Whalen R, et al. Bleeding tendency, platelet function, and pharmacokinetics of ibuprofen and zidovudine in HIV(+) hemophilic men. *Am J Hematol* 1992;40:176–182.

224. Catella-Lawson F, Reilly MP, Kapoor SC, et al. Cyclooxygenase inhibitors and the antiplatelet effects of aspirin. *N Engl J Med* 2001;345:1809–1817.

225. Lages B, Weiss HJ. Inhibition of human platelet function in vitro and ex vivo by acetaminophen. *Thromb Res* 1989;53:603–613.

226. Sharis PJ, Cannon CP, Loscalzo J. The antiplatelet effects of ticlopidine and clopidogrel. *Ann Intern Med* 1998;129:394–405.

227. Coukell AJ, Markham A. Clopidogrel. *Drugs* 1997;54:745–750.

228. Mills DC, Puri R, Hu CJ, et al. Clopidogrel inhibits the binding of ADP analogues to the receptor mediating inhibition of platelet adenylate cyclase. *Arterioscler Thromb* 1992;12:430–436.

229. Wilhite DB, Comerota AJ, Schmieder FA, et al. Managing PAD with multiple platelet inhibitors: the effect of combination therapy on bleeding time. *J Vasc Surg* 2003;38:710–713.

230. Bennett CL, Connors JM, Carwile JM, et al. Thrombotic thrombocytopenic purpura associated with clopidogrel. *N Engl J Med* 2000;342: 1773–1777.

231. Bennett CL, Weinberg PD, Rozenberg-Ben-Dror K, et al. Thrombotic thrombocytopenic purpura associated with ticlopidine. A review of 60 cases. *Ann Intern Med* 1998;128:541–544.

232. Bennett C, Kiss J, Weinberg P, et al. Thrombotic thrombocytopenic purpura after stenting and ticlopidine. *Lancet* 1998;352:1036–1037.

233. Coller BS. Anti-GP IIb/IIIa drugs: current strategies and future directions. *Thromb Haemost* 2001;86:427–443.

234. Aster R, Curtis BR, Boutie DW. Thrombocytopenia resulting from sensitivity to GP IIb/IIIa inhibitors. *Semin Thromb Hemost* 2004;30:569–577.

235. Szczeklik A, Gryglewski RJ, Nizankowski R, et al. Circulatory and antiplatelet effects of intravenous prostacyclin in healthy men. *Pharmacol Res Commun* 1978;10:545–556.

236. Fitzgerald GA, Friedman LA, Miyamori I, et al. A double blind placebo controlled crossover study of prostacylin in man. *Life Sci* 1979;25:665–672.

237. Fitzgerald GA. Dipyridamole. *N Engl J Med* 1987;316:1247–1257.

238. Kim JS, Lee KS, Kim YI, et al. A randomized crossover comparative study of aspirin, cilostazol and clopidogrel in normal controls: analysis with quantitative bleeding time and platelet aggregation test. *J Clin Neurosci* 2004;11:600–602.

239. Dawson DL, Cutler BS, Meissner MH, et al. Cilostazol has beneficial effects in treatment of intermittent claudication: results from a multicenter, randomized, prospective, double-blind trial. *Circulation* 1998;98:678–686.

240. Jeremy JY, Gill J, Mikhailidis D. Effect of milrinone on thromboxane A2 synthesis, cAMP phosphodiesterase and 45Ca$^{2+}$ uptake by human platelets. *Eur J Pharmacol* 1993;245:67–73.

241. Ardlie NG, Glew G, Schultz BG, et al. Inhibition and reversal of platelet aggregation by methylxanthines. *Thromb Diath Haemorrh* 1968;18:670.

242. Wallis RM, Corbin JD, Francis SH, et al. Tissue distribution of phosphodiesterase families and the effects of sildenafil on tissue cyclic nucleotides, platelet function, and the contractile responses of trabeculae carneae and aortic rings in vitro. *Am J Cardiol* 1999;83:3C–12C.

243. Cheung PY, Salas E, Schulz R, et al. Nitric oxide and platelet function: implications for neonatology. *Semin Perinatol* 1997;21:409–417.

244. Freedman JE, Loscalzo J, Barnard MR, et al. Nitric oxide released from activated platelets inhibits platelet recruitment. *J Clin Invest* 1997;100: 350–356.

245. Hogman M, Frostell C, Arnberg H, et al. Bleeding time prolongation and NO inhalation. *Lancet* 1993;341:1664–1665.

246. Samama CM, Diaby M, Fellahi JL, et al. Inhibition of platelet aggregation by inhaled nitric oxide in patients with acute respiratory distress syndrome. *Anesthesiology* 1995;83:56–65.

247. Gries A, Bode C, Peter K, et al. Inhaled nitric oxide inhibits human platelet aggregation, P-selectin expression, and fibrinogen binding in vitro and in vivo. *Circulation* 1998;97:1481–1487.

248. Brown CH III, Natelson EA, Bradshaw MW, et al. The hemostatic defect produced by carbenicillin. *N Engl J Med* 1974;291:265–270.

249. Haburchak DR, Head DR, Everett ED. Postoperative hemorrhage associated with carbenicillin administration—report of two cases and review of the literature. *Am J Surg* 1977;134:630–634.

250. Brown CH III, Bradshaw MW, Natelson EA, et al. Defective platelet function following the administration of penicillin compounds. *Blood* 1976; 47:949–956.

251. Andrassy K, Ritz E, Hasper B, et al. Penicillin-induced coagulation disorder. *Lancet* 1976;2:1039–1041.

252. Cazenave JP, Guccione MA, Packham MA, et al. Effects of cephalothin and penicillin G on platelet function in vitro. *Br J Haematol* 1977;35: 135–152.

253. Fass RJ, Copelan EA, Brandt JT, et al. Platelet mediated bleeding caused by broad spectrum penicillins. *J Infect Dis* 1987;155:1242–1248.

254. Brown CH III, Natelson EA, Bradshaw MW. A study of the effects of ticarcillin on blood coagulation and platelet function. *Antimicrob Agents Chemother* 1975;7:652–657.

255. Pillgram-Larsen J, Wisloff F, Jorgensen JJ, et al. Effect of high-dose ampicillin and cloxacillin on bleeding time and bleeding in open-heart surgery. *Scand J Thorac Cardiovasc Surg* 1985;19:45–48.

256. Alexander DP, Russo ME, Fohrman DE, et al. Nafcillin induced platelet dysfunction and bleeding. *Antimicrob Agents Chemother* 1983;23:59–62.

257. Sattler FR, Weitekamp MR, Ballard JO. Potential for bleeding with the new β-lactam antibiotics. *Ann Intern Med* 1986;105:924–931.

258. Johnson GJ. Platelets, penicillins, and purpura: what does it all mean. *J Lab Clin Med* 1993;121:531–533.

259. Natelson EA, Brown CH III, Bradshaw MW, et al. Influence of cephalosporin antibiotics on blood coagulation and platelet function. *Antimicrob Agents Chemother* 1976;9:91–93.

260. Weitekamp MR, Aber RC. Prolonged bleeding times and bleeding diathesis associated with moxalactam administration. *J Am Med Assoc* 1983;249:69–71.

261. Sloand EM, Klein HG, Pastakia KB, et al. Effect of albumin on the inhibition of platelet aggregation by β- lactam antibiotics. *Blood* 1992;79: 2022–2027.

262. Shattil SJ, Bennett JS, McDonaugh M, et al. Carbenicillin and penicillin G inhibit platelet function in vitro by impairing the interaction of agonists with the platelet surface. *J Clin Invest* 1980;65:329–337.

263. Burroughs SF, Johnson GJ. β-Lactam antibiotic-induced platelet dysfunction: evidence for irreversible inhibition of platelet activation *in vitro* and *in vivo* after prolonged exposure to penicillin. *Blood* 1990;75:1473–1480.

264. Burroughs SF, Johnson GJ. β-lactam antibiotics inhibit agonist-stimulated platelet calcium influx. *Thromb Haemost* 1993;69:503–508.

265. Pastakia KB, Terle D, Prodouz KN. Penicillin-induced dysfunction of platelet membrane glycoproteins. *J Lab Clin Med* 1993;121:546–554.

266. Rossi EC, Levin NW. Inhibition of primary ADP-induced platelet aggregation in normal subjects after administration of nitrofurtoin (furadantin). *J Clin Invest* 1973;52:2457–2467.

267. Cummins D, Faint R, Yardumian DA, et al. The in-vitro and ex-vivo effects of chloroquine sulphate on platelet function: implications for malaria prophylaxis in patients with impaired haemostasis. *J Trop Med Hyg* 1990;93:112–115.

268. Ishikawa S, Manabe S, Wada O. Miconazole inhibition of platelet aggregation by inhibiting cyclooxygenase. *Biochem Pharmacol* 1986;35: 1787–1792.

269. Weksler BB, Gillik M, Pink J. Effect of propranolol on platelet function. *Blood* 1977;49:185–196.

270. Leon R, Tiarks CY, Pechet L. Some observations on the in vivo effect of propranolol on platelet aggregation and release. *Am J Hematol* 1978;5: 117–121.

271. Frishman WH, Weksler B, Christodoulo JB, et al. Reversal of abnormal platelet aggregability and change in exercise tolerance in patients with angina pectoris. *Circulation* 1974;50:887–896.

272. Vanderhoek JY, Feinstein MB. Local anesthetics, chlorpromazine and propranolol inhibit stimulus-activation of phospholipase A$_2$ in human platelets. *Mol Pharm* 1979;16:171–180.

273. Mehta J, Mehta P. Effects of propranolol therapy on platelet release and prostaglandin generation in patients with coronary heart disease. *Circulation* 1982;66:1294–1299.

274. Srivastava KC. Influence of some β blockers (pindolol, atenolol, timolol and metoprolol) on aggregation and arachidonic acid metabolism in human platelets. *Prostaglandins Leukot Med* 1987;29:79–84.

275. Ingerman CM, Smith JB, Silver MJ. Inhibition of the platelet release reaction and platelet prostaglandin synthesis by furosemide. *Thromb Res* 1976;8:417–419.

276. Hines R, Barash PG. Infusion of sodium nitroprusside induces platelet dysfunction in vitro. *Anesthesiology* 1989;70:611–615.

277. Pfister B, Imhof P. Influence of vasodilators used in the therapy of heart failure on platelet aggregation. *Agents Actions* 1979;9:217–219.

278. Mehta J, Mehta P. Platelet function in heart disease. VI. Enhanced platelet aggregate formation activity in congestive heart failure. Inhibition by sodium nitroprusside. *Circulation* 1979;60:497–503.

279. Schafer AJ, Alexander RW, Handin RI. Inhibition of platelet function by organic nitrate vasodilators. *Blood* 1980;55:649–654.

280. Lawson D, Mehta J, Mehta P, et al. Cumulative effects of quinidine and aspirin on bleeding time and platelet α2-adrenoreceptors: potential mechanism of bleeding diathesis in patients receiving this combination. *J Lab Clin Med* 1986;108:581–586.

281. Motulsky HJ, Maisel AS, Snavely MD, et al. Quinidine is a competitive antagonist at α1- and α2- adrenergic receptors. *Circ Res* 1984;55:376–381.

282. Ring ME, Corrigan JJ Jr, Fenster PE. Effects of oral diltiazem on platelet function: alone and in combination with "low dose" aspirin. *Thromb Res* 1986;44:391–400.

283. Ware JA, Johnson PC, Smith M, et al. Inhibition of human platelet aggregation and cytoplasmic calcium response by calcium antagonists: studies with aequorin and quin2. *Circ Res* 1986;59:39–42.

284. Barnathan ES, Addonizio VP, Shattil SJ. Interaction of verapamil with human platelet α-adrenergic receptors. *Am J Physiol* 1982;242:H19–H23.

285. Johnson GJ, Leis LA, Francis GS. Disparate effects of the calcium-channel blockers, nifedipine and verapamil, on α2-adrenergic receptors and thromboxane A$_2$-induced aggregation of human platelets. *Circulation* 1986;73:847–854.

286. Glusa E, Bevan J, Heptinstall S. Verapamil is a potent inhibitor of 5-HT-induced platelet aggregation. *Thromb Res* 1989;55:239–245.

287. Ambrosioni E, Borghi C. Potential use of ACE inhibitors after acute myocardial infarction. *J Cardiovasc Pharmacol* 1989;14:S92–S94.

288. James IM, Dickenson EJ, Burgoyne W, et al. Treatment of hypertension with captopril: preservation of regional blood flow and reduced platelet aggregation. *J Hum Hypertens* 1988;2:21–25.

289. Okrucka A, Pechan J, Kratochvilova H. Effects of the angiotensin-converted enzyme inhibitor perindopril on endothelial and platelet function in essential hypertension. *Platelets* 1998;9:395–396.

290. Keidar S, Oiknine J, Leiba A, et al. Fosinopril reduces ADP-induced platelet aggregation in hypertensive patients. *J Cardiovasc Pharmacol* 1996;27:183–186.

291. Moser L, Callahan KS, Cheung AK, et al. ACE inhibitor effects on platelet function in stages I-II hypertension. *J Cardiovasc Pharmacol* 1997;30:461–467.

292. Zannad F, Bray-Desboscs L, el Ghawi R, et al. Effects of lisinopril and hydrochlorothiazide on platelet function and blood rheology in essential hypertension: a randomly allocated double-blind study. *J Hypertens* 1993;11:559–564.

293. Jagroop IA, Papadaksi JA, Mikhailidis DP. Effects of the angiotensin-converting enzyme inhibitor perindopril on endotheial and platelet function in essential hypertension. *Platelets* 1998;9:395–396.

294. Horne MK III, Chao ES. Heparin binding to resting and activated platelets. *Blood* 1989;74:238–243.

295. Salzman EW, Rosenberg RD, Smith MH, et al. Effect of heparin and heparin fractions on platelet aggregation. *J Clin Invest* 1980;65:64–73.

296. Heiden D, Mielke CH Jr, Rodvien R. Impairment by heparin of primary haemostasis and platelet [14C]5-hydroxytryptamine release. *Br J Haematol* 1977;36:427–436.

297. Sobel M, McNeill PM, Carlson PL, et al. Heparin inhibition of von Willebrand factor-dependent platelet function in vitro and in vivo. *J Clin Invest* 1991;87:1787–1793.

298. Lindblad B, Wakefield TW, Whitehouse WM, et al. The effect of protamine sulfate on platelet function. *Scand J Thorac Cardiovasc Surg* 1988;22:55–58.

299. Gimple LW, Gold HK, Leinbach RC, et al. Correlation between template bleeding times and spontaneous bleeding during treatment of acute myocardial infarction with recombinant tissue-type plasminogen activator. *Circulation* 1989;80:581–588.

300. Coller BS. Platelets and thrombolytic therapy. *N Engl J Med* 1990;322:33–42.

301. Schafer AI, Adelman B. Plasmin inhibition of platelet function and of arachidonic acid metabolism. *J Clin Invest* 1985;75:456–461.

302. Schafer AI, Maas AK, Ware JA, et al. Platelet protein phosphorylation, elevation of cytosolic calcium, and inositol phospholipid breakdown in platelet activation induced by plasmin. *J Clin Invest* 1986;78:73–79.

303. Penny WF, Ware JA. Platelet activation and subsequent inhibition by plasmin and recombinant tissue-type plasminogen activator. *Blood* 1992;79:91–98.

304. Loscalzo J, Vaughan DE. Tissue plasminogen activator promotes platelet disaggregation in plasma. *J Clin Invest* 1987;79:1749–1755.

305. Fitzgerald DJ, Catella F, Roy L, et al. Marked platelet activation in vivo after intravenous streptokinase in patients with acute myocardial infarction. *Circulation* 1988;77:142–150.

306. Kerins DM, Roy L, FitzGerald GA, et al. Platelet and vascular function during coronary thrombolysis with tissue-type plasminogen activator. *Circulation* 1989;80:1718–1725.

307. Mills DCB, Roberts GCK. Membrane active drugs and the aggregation of human blood platelets. *Nature* 1967;213:35.

308. Mills DCB, Robb IA, Roberts GCK. The release of nucleotides, 5-hydroxytryptamine and enzymes from human blood platelets during aggregation. *J Physiol* 1968;195:715–729.

309. Rysanek R, Svehla C, Spankova H, et al. The effect of tricyclic antidepresive drugs on adrenaline and adenosine diphosphate induced platelet aggregation. *J Pharmacol Exp Ther* 1966;18:616.

310. OBrien JR. The adhesiveness of native platelets and its prevention. *J Clin Pathol* 1961;14:140.

311. Jain MF, Eskow E, Kuchibhotla J, et al. Correlation of inhibition of platelet aggregation by phenothiazines and local anesthetics with their effects on a phospholipid bilayer. *Thromb Res* 1978;13:1067–1075.

312. White GC, Raynor ST. The effects of trifluoroperazine, an inhibitor of calmodulin on platelet function. *Thromb Res* 1980;18:279–284.

313. Warlow C, Ogston D, Douglas AS. Platelet function after administration of chloropromazine to human subjects. *Haemostasis* 1976;5:21–26.

314. Dalsgaard-Nielsen J, Risbo A, Simmelkjaer P, et al. Impaired platelet aggregation and increased bleeding time during general anesthesia with halothane. *Br J Anaesth* 1981;53:1039–1042.

315. Parolari A, Guarnieri D, Alamanni F, et al. Platelet function and anesthetics in cardiac surgery: an in vitro and ex vivo study. *Anesth Analg* 1999;89:26–31.

316. Weiss HJ. The effect of clinical dextran on platelet aggregation, adhesion and ADP release in man: in vivo and in vitro studies. *J Lab Clin Med* 1967;69:37–46.

317. Evans RJ, Gordon JD. Mechanisms of the antithrombotic action of dextran. *N Engl J Med* 1974;290:748.

318. Aberg M, Hedner U, Bergentz SE. Effect of dextran 70 on factor VIII and platelet function in von Willebrand's disease. *Thromb Res* 1978;12:629–634.

319. Kelton JG, Hirsch J. Bleeding associated with antithrombotic therapy. *Semin Hematol* 1980;17:259–291.

320. Gruber UF, Saldeen T, Brokop T, et al. Incidences of fatal postoperative pulmonary embolism after prophylaxis with dextran 70 and low-dose heparin: an international multicentre study. *Br Med J* 1980;280:69–72.

321. Cope JT, Banks D, Mauney MC, et al. Intraoperative hetastarch infusion impairs hemostasis after cardiac operations. *Ann Thorac Surg* 1997;63:78–82; discussion 82–83.

322. Ruttmann TG, James MF, Aronson I. In vivo investigation into the effects of haemodilution with hydroxyethyl starch (200/0.5) and normal saline on coagulation. *Br J Anaesth* 1998;80:612–616.

323. Favis GR, Colman RW. The action of halofenate on platelet shape change and prostaglandin synthesis. *J Lab Clin Med* 1978;92:45–52.

324. Colman RW, Bennett JS, Sheridan JS, et al. Halofenate: a potent inhibitor of normal and hypersensitive platelets. *J Lab Clin Med* 1976;88:282–291.

325. Pogliani EM, Fantasia R, Lambertenghi-Deliliers G, et al. Daunorubicin and platelet function. *Thromb Haemost* 1981;45:38–42.

326. Ahr DJ, Scialla SJ, Kimball DB Jr. Acquired platelet dysfunction following mithramycin therapy. *Cancer* 1974;41:448–454.

327. McKenna R, Ahmad T, Ts'ao CH, et al. Glutathione reductase deficiency and platelet dysfunction induced by 1,3-bis (2-chloroethyl)-1-nitrosourea. *J Lab Clin Med* 1983;102:102–115.

328. Karolak L, Chandra A, Khan W, et al. High-dose chemotherapy-induced platelet defect: inhibition of platelet signal transduction pathways. *Mol Pharmacol* 1993;43:37–44.

329. Thomson C, Forbes CD, Prentice CRM. A comparison of the effects of antihistamines on platelet function. *Thromb Diath Haemorrh* 1973;30:547–556.

330. Herrmann RG, Frank JD. Effect of adenosine derivatives and antihistamines on platelet aggregation. *Proc Soc Exp Biol Med* 1966;123:654–660.

331. Green D, Ts'ao CH, Cerullo L, et al. Clinical and laboratory investigation of the effects of E-aminocaproic acid on hemostasis. *J Lab Clin Med* 1985;105:321–327.

332. Rubin R, Rand ML. Alcohol and platelet function. *Alcohol Clin Exp Res* 1994;18:105–110.

333. Rand ML, Packham MA, Kinlough-Rathbone RL, et al. Effects of ethanol on pathways of platelet aggregation in vitro. *Thromb Haemost* 1988;59:383–387.

334. Mikhailidis DP, Barradas MA, Jeremy JY. The effect of ethanol on platelet function and vascular prostanoids. *Alcohol* 1990;7:171–180.

335. Rao AK, Rao VM, Willis J, et al. Inhibition of platelet function by contrast media. Iopamidol and hexabrix are less inhibitory then Conray-60. *Radiology* 1985;156:311–313.

336. Li X, Gabriel DA. Differences between contrast media in the inhibition of platelet activation by specific platelet agonists. *Acad Radiol* 1997;4:108–114.

337. Parvez Z, Moncada R, Fareed J, et al. Antiplatelet action of intravascular contrast media. Implications in diagnostic procedures. *Invest Radiol* 1984;19:208–211.

338. Grabowski EF, Jang IK, Gold H, et al. Variability of platelet degranulation by different contrast media. *Acad Radiol* 1996;3(Suppl. 3):S485–S487.

339. Srivastava KC. Vitamin E exerts antiaggregatory effects without inhibiting the enzymes of the arachidonic acid cascade in platelets. *Prostaglandins Leukot Med* 1986;21:177–185.

340. Violi F, Micheletta F, Iuliano L. Vitamin E, atherosclerosis and thrombosis. *Thromb Haemost* 2001;85:766–770.

341. Freedman JE, Farhat JH, Loscalzo J, et al. $\alpha$-tocopherol inhibits aggregation of human platelets by a protein kinase C-dependent mechanism. *Circulation* 1996;94:2434–2440.

342. Goodnight SH Jr. Effects of dietary fish oil and omega-3 fatty acids on platelets and blood vessels. *Semin Thromb Hemost* 1988;14:285–289.

343. Srivastava KC. Onion exerts antiaggregatory effects by altering arachidonic acid metabolism in platelets. *Prostaglandins Leukot Med* 1986;24:43–50.

344. Phillips C, Poyser NL. Inhibition of platelet aggregation by onion extracts. *Lancet* 1978;1:1051–1052.

345. Makheja AN, Vanderhock JY, Bailey JM. Inhibition of platelet aggregation and thromboxane synthesis by onion and garlic. *Lancet* 1979;1:781.

346. Bordia A, Verma SK, Srivastava KC. Effect of garlic (Allium sativum) on blood lipids, blood sugar, fibrinogen and fibrinolytic activity in patients with coronary artery disease. *Prostaglandins Leukot Essent Fatty Acids* 1998;58:257–263.

347. Bordia A, Verma SK, Srivastava KC. Effect of ginger (Zingiber officinale Rosc.) and fenugreek (Trigonella foenumgraecum L.) on blood lipids, blood sugar and platelet aggregation in patients with coronary artery disease. *Prostaglandins Leukot Essent Fatty Acids* 1997;56:379–384.

348. Srivastava KC. Extracts from two frequently consumed spices—cumin (cuminum cyminum) and turmeric (curcuma longa)—inhibit platelet aggregation and alter eicosanoid biosynthesis in human blood platelets. *Prostaglandins Leukot Essent Fatty Acids* 1989;37:57–64.

349. Srivastava KC, Bordia A, Verma SK. Curcumin, a major component of food spice turmeric (curcuma longa) inhibits aggregation and alters eicosanoid metabolism in human blood platelets. *Prostaglandins Leukot Essent Fatty Acids* 1995;52:223–227.

350. Srivastava KC. Antiplatelet principles from a food spice clove (syzygium aromaticum L). *Prostaglandins Leukot Essent Fatty Acids* 1993;48:363–372.

351. Dorso CR, Levin RI, Eldor A, et al. Chinese food and platelets. *N Engl J Med* 1980;303:756–757.

352. Hammerschmidt DE. Szechwan purpura. *N Engl J Med* 1980;302:1191–1193.

353. Fugh-Berman A. Herb-drug interactions. *Lancet* 2000;355:134–138.

# CHAPTER 71 ■ ACQUIRED DISORDERS OF COAGULATION: THE IMMUNE COAGULOPATHIES

CRAIG M. KESSLER, PETER ACS, AND GUGLIELMO MARIANI

The formation of a blood clot is the final result of a cascade of interactions among multiple plasma proteins that ultimately results in the conversion of fibrinogen to fibrin, and cross-linking of fibrin by activated factor XIII, which stabilizes the formed clot. Qualitative or quantitative deficiencies of any of the coagulation factors involved in these reactions may be associated with clinically significant bleeding disorders. Circulating immunoglobulins, usually, but not exclusively, composed of immunoglobulin (Ig) G, may develop in the plasma of individuals whose coagulation mechanism was previously normal and may function as a circulating anticoagulant when directed against a specific clotting factor protein. In this scenario, these immunoglobulins are designated as autoantibody inhibitors, in contrast to alloantibody inhibitors, which arise in individuals with congenital factor deficiencies as a consequence of replacement therapy (1,2).

Although autoantibody inhibitors have been described to neutralize each of the coagulation factor proteins, their incidence is very rare in the general population. Nevertheless, when they do occur, they frequently produce life- and/or limb-threatening bleeding episodes. Acquired hemophilia A (factor VIII:C deficiency) is the most common of the acquired autoantibodies against specific clotting factors but is much less prevalent than the lupuslike autoanticoagulant, which usually is directed against a protein-phospholipid complex. In fact, the acquired autoantibody, which characterizes the lupus anticoagulant (LAC), is an *in vitro* anticoagulant only, and is actually associated with clinical hypercoagulability *in vivo*.

Autoantibodies targeting specific coagulation factor proteins are often associated with more profound bleeding manifestations and often demonstrate different pharmacokinetics and binding affinities compared to alloantibodies directed against the same protein. Autoantibody inhibitors may arise in association with a number of benign diseases, such as autoimmune, chronic inflammatory and infectious states, and in pregnancy. The development of autoantibody inhibitors may also complicate lymphoproliferative and, to a lesser degree, solid tumor malignancies. Incidental associations have occurred in the context of certain antibiotics and bone marrow transplantation, but many patients have no obvious underlying pathology.

From a laboratory perspective, the diagnosis of autoantibody inhibitors, similar to alloantibodies, is based on the inability of plasma from normal individuals to correct prolonged clotting assays produced by patient plasma in mixing studies. The potency of the inhibitor and the target of the inhibitor determine the mode of treatment of acute bleeding episodes (see Table 71-1).

## ACQUIRED INHIBITORS TO FVIII:C

### Autoantibodies to FVIII: The Acquired Hemophilia Syndrome

In contrast to the development of alloantibody inhibitors, directed specifically against FVIII:C in individuals with congenital hemophilia and arising as a side effect of FVIII:C replacement therapy, autoantibody FVIII:C inhibitors appear spontaneously in subjects with previously normal hemostatic function. Designated as *acquired hemophilia*, this rare immune coagulopathy occurs with an approximate incidence of 0.2 to 1.0 case per 1 million individuals per year (3). This figure, however, may be a significant and historic underestimate because of the vagaries of diagnostic accuracy. Many low-titer (<5 BU) inhibitors, in fact, may remain undetected unless patients experience severe bruising or bleed after surgery or trauma. Acquired hemophilia is being diagnosed more frequently now that there is increased awareness that this syndrome complicates a wide variety of autoimmune and malignant diseases. Also, the availability of improved and specific treatment options for acquired hemophilia has increased the urgency of accurately diagnosing this potentially severe and morbid condition.

#### Epidemiology and Clinical Settings

The age distribution of autoantibodies to FVIII:C is biphasic with a small peak in young, fertile women between 20 and 30 years of age (associated with pregnancy and the postpartum state and collagen vascular disorders) and a major peak in older age groups, predominantly men older than 60 years, with lymphoproliferative and solid tumor malignancies (4–6). Overall, there does not seem to be a gender difference in prevalence, although the sex distribution reflects the age of dominating associated disease states. Inhibitors to FVIII have also been reported in nonhemophilic children (7).

In approximately 50% of individuals with autoantibodies to FVIII:C, there is no obvious underlying disease state ("idiopathic" inhibitors) (4–6). Among the remaining 50%, a distinct group (10% to 15% of total cases) comprises mostly primiparous women in whom acquired hemophilia typically occurs within 3 months postpartum (8,9). The remaining heterogeneous group (35% to 40% of total cases) comprises:

■ Autoimmune disorders/collagen vascular diseases, including systemic lupus erythematosus (SLE), rheumatoid arthritis, temporal arteritis, multiple sclerosis, Sjögren syndrome, myasthenia gravis, autoimmune hypothyroidism and hyperthyroidism, ulcerative colitis, graft versus host disease, and vaccinations (10–15).

- Solid tumor malignancies, including that of prostate, breast, lung, gastric, pancreas, colon, head and neck, and renal cell (16).
- Hematologic malignancies, including chronic lymphocytic leukemia (CLL), non-Hodgkin lymphoma, multiple myeloma, Waldenstrom macroglobulinemia, myelofibrosis, and myelodysplastic syndromes (17).
- Allergic diseases/drug reactions, including asthma; allergies to penicillin, sulfonamides, phenytoin, chloramphenicol, and methyldopa; treatment with fludarabine, interferon-α; and antipsychotic medications (18,19).
- Autoimmune dermatologic diseases, including pemphigus and psoriasis.

Spontaneous remissions of the autoimmune antibody inhibitor targeting FVIII:C are not rare events, occurring in approximately one third of cases, mostly in scenarios with low-titer inhibitors, and usually after months to years of involvement (5). The acquired hemophilia syndrome associated with pregnancy and the postpartum state is an exception to this observation because spontaneous disappearance of the inhibitor against factor VIII occurs in most cases (20). Despite this optimistic characterization of the natural history of acquired autoimmune FVIII:C antibody inhibitors, the published mortality rates associated with this condition have ranged between 7.9% to 22% of cases (5,6,21,22), with most deaths related to uncontrolled hemorrhage within the first few weeks after presentation. These deaths are often precipitated by intractable bleeding after invasive diagnostic and therapeutic procedures are performed (22); however, delayed diagnosis and inappropriate treatment also contribute significantly to the early high mortality rate. Infectious complications, secondary to immunosuppressive therapy, account for most of the late deaths. A review of more recent studies reveals a trend toward decreasing mortality, which may be related to the availability of improved management options (22–24).

## TABLE 71-1

**ACQUIRED INHIBITORS: CLINICAL AND LABORATORY FEATURES AND THERAPEUTIC APPROACHES TO BLEEDING EPISODES**

| Targeted factor | Associated conditions | Lab findings | Symptoms | Therapeutic options for acute bleeds |
|---|---|---|---|---|
| V | Autoimmune antibodies<br>  Postoperative state<br>  Fibrin-glue application<br>  Aminoglycosides<br>  β-lactam antibiotics<br>  Malignancy<br>  Collagen vascular disease<br>  Idiopathic<br>Alloimmune antibodies<br>  Transfusions of fresh frozen<br>    plasma and platelets | PT ↑↑↑<br>aPTT ↑↑↑<br>Mixing studies:<br>  no correction<br>TT normal<br>dRVVT ↑<br>Factor V antigen: ↓<br>Factor V activity: ↓ | Variable: ranging<br>  from minor to fatal<br>  bleeding<br>Titer of inhibitory<br>  antibody correlates<br>  with severity of<br>  bleeding episodes | Fresh frozen plasma<br>Platelet transfusions<br>Prothrombin<br>  complex concentrate<br>Plasmapheresis<br>Extracorporeal<br>  immunoadsorption<br>? IVIg<br>Recombinant FVIIa<br>  concentrate |
| II<br>Prothrombin | SLE | PT ↑<br>aPTT ↑<br>Mixing studies:<br>  no correction<br>Factor II antigen ↓<br>Factor II activity ↓ | Thrombophilia:<br>  predominant<br>Rare bleeding | If excessive clotting:<br>  anticoagulation<br><br>If excess bleeding:<br>  corticosteroids +<br>  high-dose IVIg<br>Androgens |
| IIa<br>Thrombin | Topical application of fibrin<br>  sealant preparations<br>  containing bovine thrombin<br>Collagen vascular disease<br>Drug-induced SLE<br>Hepatic cirrhosis<br>Monoclonal gammopathies | PT ↑<br>aPTT ↑<br>TT ↑↑↑<br>Mixing studies:<br>  no correction<br>Factor II antigen ↓<br>Factor II activity ↓ | Bleeding: variable<br>  frequency and severity<br>Thrombophilia:<br>  very rare | Fresh frozen plasma<br>Prothrombin<br>  complex concentrate<br>Intravenous<br>  γ globulin<br>? Methylene blue |
| IX | Autoimmune antibodies<br>  Collagen vascular disease<br>  Postpartum state<br>  Malignancy<br>Alloimmune antibodies<br>  Congenital hemophilia B | aPTT ↑↑<br>PT, TT normal<br>Mixing studies:<br>  no correction<br>Factor IX antigen ↓<br>Factor IX activity ↓ | Bleeding: variable<br>  frequency and<br>  severity; may be fatal<br>Severe bleeding into<br>  skin, muscles, GI, GU<br>  sites very common | Prothrombin<br>  complex concentrate<br>Recombinant FVIIa<br>Factor IX<br>  concentrates (<5 BU)<br>FEIBA<br>(Note: in alloantibody<br>  inhibitor patients,<br>  severe anaphylaxis<br>  or nephritic syndrome |

*(continued)*

**TABLE 71-1**

CONTINUED

| Targeted factor | Associated conditions | Lab findings | Symptoms | Therapeutic options for acute bleeds |
|---|---|---|---|---|
| | | | | may occur after exposure to factor IX–containing replacement therapies; rFVIIa is therapy of choice in this situation) Prednisone High dose Intravenous γ globulin |
| VWF protein | Autoimmune antibodies Monoclonal gammopathies (MGUS, MM, WM) Lymphoproliferative diseases Collagen vascular disease Hypothyroidism (↓ synthesis component also may be contributory to ↓ VWF activity) Malignancy Alloantibody antibodies Congenital type 3 (severe) Drug-induced Pesticides Valproate Ciprofloxacin Griseofulvin Tetracyclines Hydroxyethyl starch Mechanical or proteolytic) mechanisms (nonimmune) Thrombolytic agents Angiodysplasia Acquired and congenital heart disease Myeloproliferative disease (adsorption of VWF to ↑↑↑ platelets) | VWF:Ag ↓↓↓ Ristocetin cofactor activity ↓↓↓ Ristocetin-induced platelet aggregation (RIPA): inhibited FVIII activity ↓ aPTT ↑ Bleeding time ↑ SPEP and/or immunofixationel ectropheresis monoclonal spikes | Excessive bruising Bleeding may be life threatening | Based on etiology: Desmopressin (DDAVP) VWF/FVIII conc. High-dose IVIg Corticosteroids Treatment of underlying disease Remove offending medication Rituximab (experimental and anecdotal) |
| VII | Autoimmune antibodies Penicillins Cephalosporins Myeloma Malignancy Antithymocyte globulin Interleukin 2 Aplastic anemia Alloimmune antibodies Severe congenital FVII deficiency: postreplacement therapy with fresh frozen plasma, prothrombin complex concentrates, or recombinant FVIIa Acquired (nonimmune) Vitamin K deficiency Liver disease | PT ↑↑↑ aPTT, TT: normal Mixing studies: no correction except in vitamin K deficient states Factor VII antigen ↓ Factor VII activity ↓ | Bleeding is very variable Mucous membrane bleeding (similar to platelet dysfunction) CNS bleeding is common, often fatal | Recombinant FVIIa Prothrombin complex concentrate (caution in severe liver disease) Fresh frozen plasma Platelet transfusions Desmopressin (DDAVP): to reverse platelet dysfunction component of bleeding in liver disease Vitamin K replacement Treatment of underlying disease |

*(continued)*

**TABLE 71-1**

CONTINUED

| Targeted factor | Associated conditions | Lab findings | Symptoms | Therapeutic options for acute bleeds |
|---|---|---|---|---|
| | Sepsis | | | Removal of offending medication Intravenous γ globulin Immunosuppression with corticosteroids or cytotoxic agents |
| X | Autoimmune antibodies Lupus anticoagulant Respiratory infection Inflammatory GI diseases Malignancy Acquired (nonimmune mechanisms) Systemic amyloidosis (adsorption to amyloid fibrils) Extensive burns (consumption and proteolysis) | PT ↑↑↑ aPTT ↑↑↑ TT ↑ Reptilase time ↑ Mixing studies: no correction In presence of antibody inhibitor; Correction in acquired nonimmune-based deficiencies Factor X antigen ↓ Factor X activity ↓ | Bleeding severity and frequency are variable CNS bleeding is common and often fatal | In amyloidosis: Factor IX complex concentrate Prothrombin complex concentrate Recombinant FVIIa Splenectomy FX Autoimmune inhibitors: Fresh frozen plasma Prothrombin complex concentrate Recombinant factor VIIa Plasmapheresis Intravenous γ globulin Corticosteroids |
| XI | Autoimmune antibodies SLE Chronic lymphocytic leukemia Inflammatory GI diseases Chlorpromazine Phenothiazines Alloimmune antibodies Severe congenital hemophilia C with type II gene polymorphism: post replacement therapy with fresh frozen plasma or factor XI concentrate | aPTT ↑↑↑ PT, TT normal Mixing studies: No correction Factor XI antigen ↓ Factor XI activity ↓ | Spontaneous bleeding: uncommon Injury-related bleeding: typical Bleeding with surgery (particularly on mucosal surfaces): very common | Corticosteroids Factor XI concentrate (if low-titer inhibitor; unavailable in USA) Recombinant FVIIa concentrate Treat underlying disease state Remove offending medication |
| XII | Lupus anticoagulant Liver disease | aPTT ↑↑↑ PT, TT normal Mixing studies: No correction Factor XII antigen ↓ Factor XII activity ↓ | No bleeding ? thrombosis ? fetal loss | ? Anticoagulation |
| Fibrinogen fibrin | Autoimmune antibodies Idiopathic SLE Monoclonal gammopathies Pregnancy | aPTT ↑ PT ↑ TT ↑ Reptilase time ↑ Fibrinogen ↓↓↓ (in afibrinogenemia) | Bleeding frequency and severity: variable | Fresh frozen plasma Cryoprecipitate ? Recombinant factor VIIa Corticosteroids Treat underlying disease state |

*(continued)*

**TABLE 71-1**

CONTINUED

| Targeted factor | Associated conditions | Lab findings | Symptoms | Therapeutic options for acute bleeds |
|---|---|---|---|---|
| | Alloimmune antibodies Congenital afibrinogenemia: post replacement therapy with fresh frozen plasma or cryoprecipitate | | | |
| XIII | Autoimmune antibodies SLE Henoch-Schönlein purpura Colitis Gastritis Monoclonal gammopathies Acute leukemias Isoniazid Procainamide Practolol Alloimmune antibodies Congenital severe factor XIII deficiency: post replacement with fresh frozen plasma, cryoprecipitate, or factor XIII concentrate | Abnormal urea clot solubility test Abnormal dansylcadaverine incorporation assay PTT normal PT normal TT normal Fibrinogen normal Factor XIII antigen ↓ | Bleeding: recurrent, severe, spontaneous, and some times fatal, particularly intracerebral hemorrhage Easy bruising, soft tissue bleeding are common | Cryoprecipitate Factor XIII concentrate (if available) Plasmapheresis with exchange Removal of offending medication Treatment underlying disease state Corticosteroids Cyclophosphamide |

PT, prothrombin time; aPTT, activated-partial-thromboplastin time; TT, thrombin time; dRVVT, dilute Russells viper venom time; SLE, systemic lupus erythematosus; GI, gastrointestinal; GU, genitourinary; IVIg, intravenous immunoglobulin; VWF, von Willebrand factor; MGUS, monoclonal gammopathy of unknown significance; MM, multiple myeloma; WM, Waldenström macroglobulinemia; SPEP, serum protein electrophoresis; DDAVP, 1-deamino-8-D-arginine vasopressin; CNS, central nervous system.

## Clinical Manifestations and Salient Features of Acquired Autoimmune FVIII:C Inhibitors

The occurrence of an acquired inhibitor to FVIII:C typically is heralded by spontaneous, often life- and limb-threatening bleeding manifestations, in individuals without a previous coagulopathic history. In contrast to the predominant sites of intramuscular and joint hemorrhage observed in individuals with allo-FVIII:C antibody inhibitors, intramuscular (superficial or retroperitoneal) bleeds are infrequent and hemarthrosis is unusual in acquired autoimmune inhibitors to FVIII:C. The most common bleeding episodes in these patients involve soft tissues and the mucous membranes (skin and subcutaneous tissue, epistaxis, hematuria, melena, menorrhagia). Spontaneous bleeding into the central nervous system is also infrequent; however, even minor bleeds in the acquired hemophilia setting may become severe if not rapidly recognized clinically or properly treated.

The clinical features of acquired autoimmune FVIII:C inhibitors associated with pregnancy deviate from the usual pattern of this disease state. These autoimmune inhibitors appear most frequently (up to 80%) in primiparous women within 3 months after delivery (9) [median onset of 2 months postpartum (25)]; however, severe uterine bleeding during labor or delivery does occur and may require hysterectomy. These

acquired autoantibody inhibitors are very sensitive to treatment with corticosteroids alone and may remit spontaneously in most of the cases (up to 76%), compared to the very low rate of spontaneous remissions observed with autoimmune hemophilia associated with other etiologies or allo-FVIII:C antibody inhibitors. Another distinctive feature of acquired hemophilia in pregnancy is its very low mortality rate (<5%) (9,25) compared to other autoimmune hemophilia-associated disease states (13% to 22%). Recurrence of the autoantibody FVIII:C inhibitor with subsequent pregnancies is not unusual and possibly could cause life-threatening hemorrhages in the fetus because of the transplacental transfer of IgG autoantibody responsible for neutralizing FVIII:C (26).

In contrast to pregnancy-associated acquired hemophilia, individuals with autoimmune FVIII:C antibody inhibitors due to other etiologies usually have high-titer inhibitors (>5 BU) that rarely resolve spontaneously or with corticosteroids alone. Cytotoxic agents (azathioprine or cyclophosphamide) or more aggressive treatment protocols increase the chance of successful remission, with the prognosis clearly dependent on the response of the underlying disease state to the immunosuppressive regimen (25). Autoantibodies to FVIII:C have been acquired by patients with a wide array of solid tumor malignancies (16) and tend to be low-titer. The titer of autoantibody to FVIII:C does not correlate with tumor size, aggressiveness, or likelihood of response to chemotherapy or radiation. The development of an autoantibody inhibitor to FVIII:C in the presence of a malignancy forebodes a poor overall prognosis. Successful suppression of the autoantibody inhibitor occurs in only approximately 20% of cases and appears to require eradication of the underlying tumor (16). If the autoantibody FVIII:C inhibitor does remit, it may recur and is not a reliable marker of tumor recurrence. Acquired hemophilia occurs much more frequently in association with lymphoproliferative malignancies than with solid tumors, which testifies to the importance of lymphocyte and immune system dysfunction in the etiology of this autoimmune epiphenomenon. CLL, non-Hodgkin lymphoma, multiple myeloma, and Waldenstrom macroglobulinemia are the most frequent hematologic malignancies associated with the development of autoimmune FVIII:C inhibitors. Although autoantibody and alloantibody inhibitors to FVIII:C are usually of the IgG variety, IgA and IgM monoclonal antibodies have been described with multiple myeloma and CLL. Other hematologic diseases, including myelodysplastic syndromes, myelofibrosis, and erythroleukemia, also have been complicated by autoimmune inhibitors to FVIII:C, but the association is mainly anecdotal.

Allergic reactions to medications, particularly sulfonamides and rarely penicillin, have been implicated in the development of an autoimmune response to FVIII:C. The prognosis in these cases is favorable because the neutralizing inhibitory antibody usually disappears shortly after withdrawal of the offending drug. Of interest is the fact that acquired inhibitors to FVIII:C have also been observed after treatment with medications known to interfere with the immune system, such as interferon-α and fludarabine.

### Laboratory Diagnosis of Autoimmune FVIII:C Antibody Inhibitors

The laboratory assessment of autoantibody inhibitors to FVIII:C is similar to that of alloantibody inhibitors. The suspicion that a previously noncoagulopathic individual has acquired hemophilia is strengthened by detecting a prolonged activated-partial-thromboplastin time (aPTT) and reduced FVIII:C activity levels (which do not normalize in prolonged mixing studies at 37°C) in the presence of significant bruising or bleeding. The diagnosis is confirmed with a formal Bethesda assay, possibly modified following the Nijmegen recommendations for low-titer inhibitors. However, the Bethesda measurement of autoantibodies against FVIII:C is less reliable as compared to the assay for alloantibodies in hemophilia because of their different kinetics (type II), which, also in contrast to alloantibody inhibitors, often result in residual FVIII:C activity measuring up to 25% of normal levels in these patients' plasmas.

### Immunochemistry of Autoantibody Inhibitors to FVIII:C

At variance with alloantibodies detected in hemophilia, which are oligoclonal in nature and belong to IgG1 and IgG4 subclasses, autoantibody inhibitors to FVIII:C are usually polyclonal, belong to the IgG4 subclass, and more often than not are directed against one epitope on the FVIII:C molecule. Another distinctive feature is that the autoimmune autoantibody inhibitors rarely may be monoclonal IgA or IgM antibodies and shifting immunoglobulin profiles have been observed, for example, shifting from IgM to IgG.

Systematic epitope mapping has indicated that autoantibodies are usually directed against either the A2 or C2 domain of the FVIII:C molecule (62%) but rarely to both epitopes as observed with alloantibodies, which overwhelmingly interact with both

A2 and C2 domains (27). There appears to be preferential targeting of FVIII:C autoantibodies to the C2 domain (67%). The A3 epitope is targeted much less commonly. Both alloantibodies and autoantibodies bind to the same epitopes on the A2 and C2 domains. Autoantibodies may exert their inhibitory activity by interfering with thrombin cleavage sites on A2 or by impeding the interactions between FVIII:C and phospholipid or von Willebrand factor (VWF) protein on C2 (see Figs. 71-1 and 71-2). This may result in increased FVIII:C catabolism and increased susceptibility of FVIII:C to degradation by activated protein C and factors IX and X.

### Management and Prevention of Bleeding Complications

Figure 71-3 shows an algorithm for treatment of bleeding complications.

Management of patients with autoimmune inhibitors to FVIII:C depends in large part upon the natural history of the concurrent underlying associated disease state, if any, and upon the extent and severity of hemorrhagic complications. As with alloantibody FVIII:C inhibitors, the inhibitor titer is also a critical component in determining the therapeutic strategy. Cohorts of patients with postpartum or drug-induced inhibitors and mild bleeding/bruising may require only close observation because the autoimmune inhibitor tends to disappear spontaneously within a few months after delivery or drug discontinuation. Otherwise, treatment strategies should focus on the urgent control of bleeding complications and on the ultimate suppression of the inhibitor (4,25). Long-term success will parallel the treatment, control, and, if possible, the eradication of the underlying disease. Practical management issues include the avoidance of intramuscular injections and the use of aspirin, nonsteroidal antiinflammatory drugs (NSAIDS), anticoagulants, and so on. Any invasive diagnostic or therapeutic procedure should be carried out with caution and certainly under adequate hemostatic cover.

**Factor VIII:C Concentrates.** Whenever possible, optimal control of bleeding in acquired hemophilia should be achievable by normalizing FVIII:C activity levels in plasma. The effectiveness of FVIII:C replacement therapy depends on the inhibitor titer. Human FVIII:C concentrates should be used only if the maximum inhibitor titer, including peak anamnestic response (low responder), is consistently less than 5 BU so that the neutralizing capacity of the autoimmune inhibitor can be overwhelmed and sufficiently high levels of VIII:C can be attained in plasma. Human plasma-derived FVIII:C concentrates, which are characterized as being of intermediate purity by virtue of their substantial content of VWF protein, theoretically may be less susceptible to inactivation by the autoimmune FVIII:C inhibitor directed against the C2 domain (28); however, this premise has not been confirmed in clinical studies.

Another source of FVIII:C concentrate, which has proven extremely useful for the treatment of autoimmune FVIII:C neutralizing antibodies, is derived from pooled porcine-derived plasma. Porcine FVIII:C concentrate has been extensively used since the early eighties, but recently its availability has been hampered by the fact that it is not virally inactivated. Although porcine FVIII:C concentrate was never implicated in the transmission of pathogens dangerous to human recipients, it is no longer manufactured. The ongoing development of a recombinant porcine FVIII:C molecule promises to provide an important treatment strategy for this disease because it will be virtually devoid of any risk of blood-borne pathogens and will obviate the need for quarantined herds of pigs for source plasma. The clinical effectiveness of porcine FVIII:C provides insight into the mechanism(s) by which human FVIII:C is neutralized by its specific inhibitory antibody and how neutralization can be circumvented clinically.

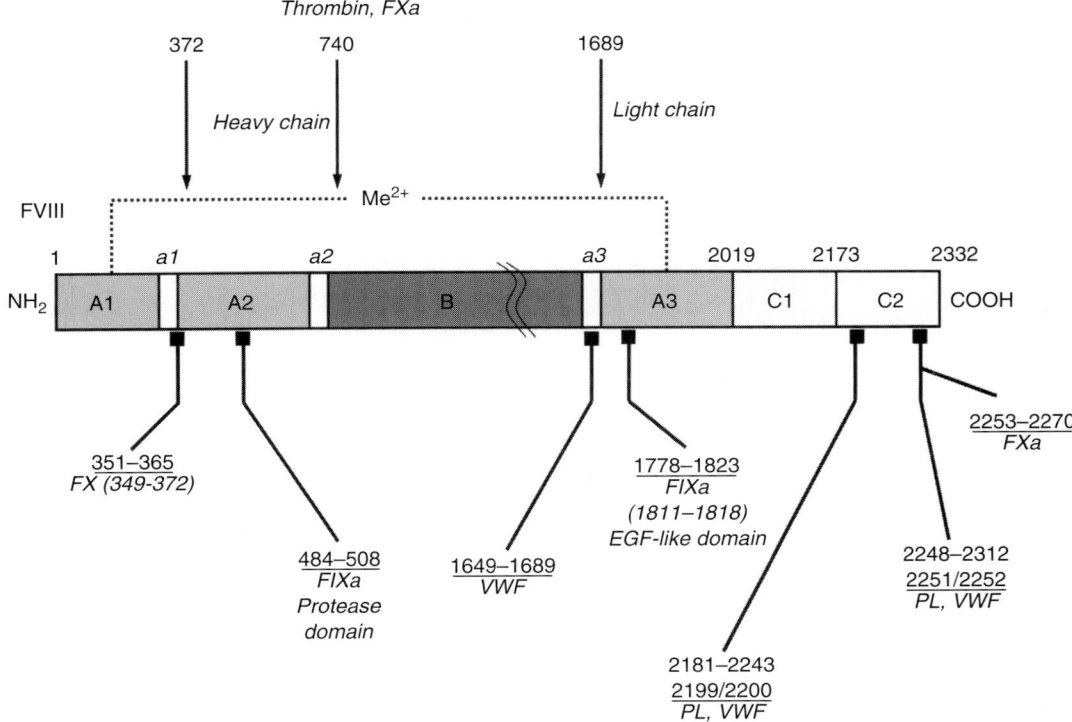

**FIGURE 71-1.** Factor VIII structure and epitopes for anti-FVIII:C antibody inhibitors. VWF, von Willebrand factor protein; PL, phospholipids; FIXa, activated factor IX; FX, factor X; FXa, activated factor X; EGF, epidermal growth factor. (From Ananyeva NM, Lacroix-Desmazes S, Hauser CA, et al. Inhibitors in hemophilia A: mechanisms of inhibition, management and perspectives. *Blood Coagul Fibrinolysis.* 2004;15:109–124, with permission.)

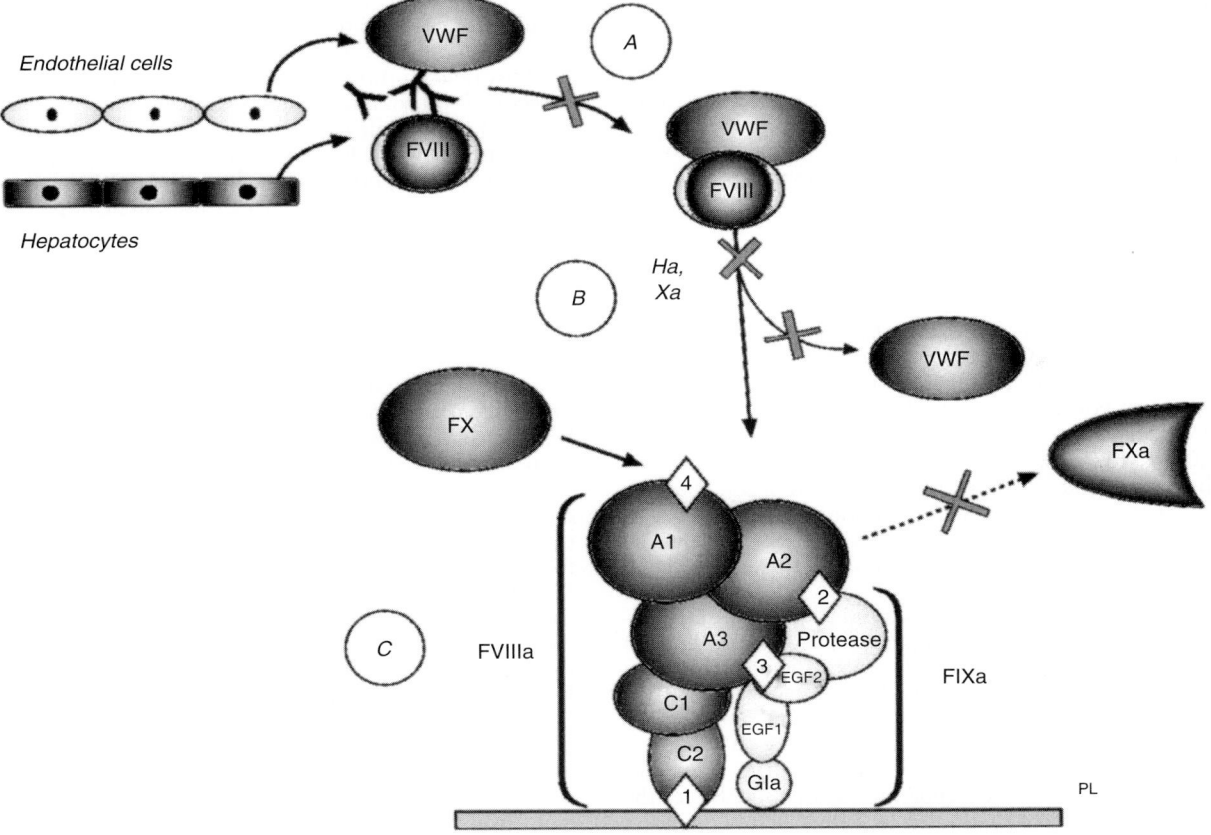

**FIGURE 71-2.** Hypothetical structure of FVIII:C and inhibitory mechanisms of anti-FVIII:C antibodies. VWF, von Willebrand factor; FVIII; FX, Factor X;FXa, activated factorX; EGF, epidermal growth factor; FVIIIa, activated factor VIII. (From Ananyeva NM, Lacroix-Desmazes S, Hauser CA, et al. Inhibitors in hemophilia A: mechanisms of inhibition, management and perspectives. *Blood Coagul Fibrinolysis.* 2004;15:109–124, with permission.)

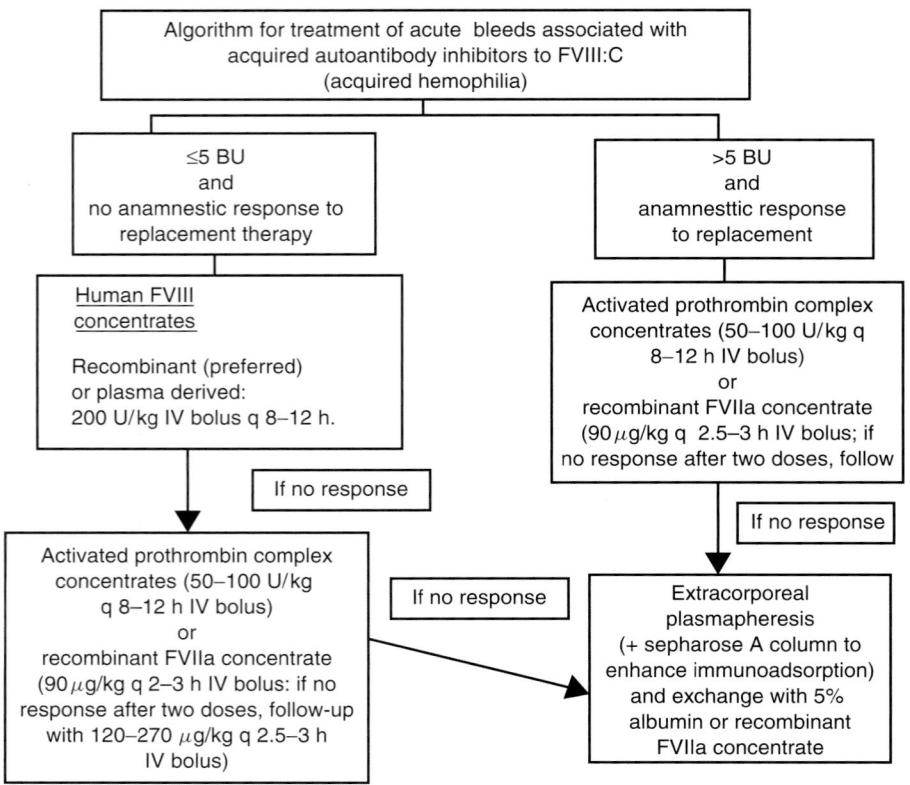

**FIGURE 71-3.** Algorithm for treatment of acute bleeds associated with acquired autoantibody inhibitors to FVIII:C. FIX, factor IX; BU, Bethesda units; rFVIIa, recombinant factor VIIa; PCC, prothrombin complex concentrate; DDAVP, 1-deamino-8-D-arginine vasopressin.

The practical benefits underlying the use of porcine FVIII:C include the fact that heterologous FVIII:C has significantly reduced cross-reactivity with antihuman FVIII:C antibody inhibitors (alloantibodies and autoantibodies) compared with human FVIII:C concentrates. Therefore, neutralization of the porcine FVIII:C activity will be reduced.

Clinical trials have consistently revealed evidence of hemostatic efficacy with porcine FVIII:C despite extremely high antihuman FVIII:C autoantibody inhibitor titers (22,28). Less impressive and reliable results have been observed in allo-FVIII:C antibodies arising in congenital hemophilia (29). The cross-reactivity of antihuman FVIII:C antibodies (allo or auto) with porcine FVIII:C may vary widely, necessitating *in vitro* cross-reactivity testing with the patient's plasma before administration. Porcine FVIII:C concentrate may not be hemostatically effective if the cross-reactive inhibitor titer is greater than 40 BU. An initial bolus of 75 to 100 IU porcine FVIII:C is recommended with subsequent dosing determined by the level of FVIII:C activity achieved and the durability of the response. FVIII:C levels of at least 30% to 50% are desirable. Porcine FVIII:C is the only one of the replacement options that will yield a measurable FVIII:C activity level in recipient plasma for clinical monitoring in the setting of high-titer inhibitors (22,23).

**Desmopressin (1-deamino-8-D-Arginine Vasopressin).** Administration of 1-deamino-8-D-arginine vasopressin (DDAVP) (desmopressin) either intravenously or subcutaneously at the dose of 0.3 $\mu$g per kg induces a rapid rise of VWF and FVIII:C activities in normal individuals and those with mild uncomplicated hemophilia A and von Willebrand disease (VWD) (30, 31). DDAVP may also induce a rapid rise of FVIII:C in individuals with low-titer inhibitors, rendering the drug suitable for the treatment of minor, non–life-threatening bleeds or for prevention of potential bleeding secondary to mild surgical procedures in the context of acquired hemophilia (32). Potential patients should receive a test dose of DDAVP in advance of their surgery to determine their responsiveness.

**Activated Prothrombin Complex Concentrates and Nonactivated Prothrombin Complex Concentrates.** Nonactivated prothrombin complex concentrates (PCCs) (Proplex, Konyne, Profilnine, Bebulin) have been used since the seventies with success rates of approximately 50% in the treatment of acute bleeding episodes, mainly hemarthroses, in hemophiliacs with allo-FVIII:C antibody inhibitors. The postulated mechanism of action is that of "bypassing" the obstruction to coagulation caused by the neutralizing inhibitor of FVIII:C. This is accomplished through their content of trace amounts of serine proteases (activated factors IX, X, VII, and thrombin). The "fully activated" PCCs [activated prothrombin complex concentrate (aPCC), that is, FEIBA, Autoplex (recently withdrawn from the market)] are perceived to be more active than PCCs in patients with alloantibody and this perception has been extrapolated to the autoantibody situation even though no prospective, controlled studies on the efficacy of these concentrates in acquired hemophilia are available. Retrospective analyses of patient cohorts with alloantibodies and autoantibodies have revealed efficacy rates of approximately 80% for both FEIBA (average dose of 70 IU per kg) (33) and Autoplex (average dose of >50 IU per kg) (34), but their dosages and schedules are arbitrary and there are no laboratory methods that predict or correlate with clinical efficacy. Furthermore, bolus doses higher than 200 IU per kg or frequent repeat dosing of aPCC significantly increases the risks of thrombotic adverse events (35). Another drawback of these products as plasma derivatives is their capacity to induce anamnesis of the FVIII:C inhibitor because of residual contamination with FVIII:C. No HIV or HCV seroconversions have occurred with their use.

**Recombinant FVIIa Concentrate.** Recombinant FVIIa (rFVIIa, Novoseven) is a genetically engineered replacement product composed of high concentrations of activated FVII protein, indistinguishable from the native form, which circulates in plasma in very low concentrations (5 to 10 ng per mL). rFVIIa concentrate is generally administered as an intravenous bolus, resulting in supraphysiologic levels of FVIIa activity in blood. In individuals with normal coagulation, it is hypothesized that thrombin is generated after FVIIa interacts with tissue factor on mononuclear cell surfaces (monocytes and macrophages) and subsequently activates FX to participate in the tenase and prothrombinase complexes. This small quantity of thrombin is adequate only to activate platelets and to cleave VWF protein from FVIII:C, but this results in a self-amplification process in which rFVIIa binds to the surface of the activated platelet, activates FX in the presence of FVIII and FIX, and produces an extraordinary "thrombin burst" to affect fibrin formation (36). Pertinent to the clinical situation with autoantibody FVIII:C or FIX inhibitors, large amounts of administered rFVIIa may bind nonspecifically to the platelet surface and activate FX in a TF-independent manner and in absence of FVIII:C and/or FIX.

The recommended dose of rFVIIa concentrate to reverse active bleeding or to prevent bleeding associated with either low-titer or high-titer autoantibody FVIII:C or FIX inhibitors consists of an intravenous bolus of 90 $\mu$g per kg, administered every 2 to 3 hours because of its short circulating half-life. Replacement therapy with rFVIIa should continue until durable hemostasis is achieved, which may require days. This dosing regimen is similar to that used for bleeding related to alloantibody FVIII:C or FIX inhibitors. In the largest clinical trial in acquired hemophilia, rFVIIa, employed as frontline replacement therapy, reversed symptomatic bleeding 100% of the time, whereas rFVIIa, used as salvage or rescue therapy, yielded a 75% response rate (24). If bleeding is not successfully reversed within the initial 24 hours of treatment with rFVIIa, the patient is likely to remain unresponsive to further rFVIIa and an alternative regimen should be considered.

Recent studies using rFVIIa at doses greater than 200 $\mu$g per kg in children with alloantibody inhibitors suggest that high-dose regimens may not only be more effective, but may also reduce the number of doses required or reverse bleeding that is refractory to standard doses of rFVIIa. This high dose of rFVIIa is believed to further accelerate clot formation by enhancing the thrombin burst on the surface of activated platelets. However, before supratherapeutic dosing schedules become more widely used, particularly in older adults with autoantibody inhibitors, the risks of potential hypercoagulability must be assessed. Continuous infusion regimens for rFVIIa replacement remain to be standardized.

Overall, very few side effects, including episodes of thrombosis, have been reported for rFVIIa concentrate use in autoimmune hemophilia. A finite risk does exist, however, and cases of myocardial infarction, disseminated intravascular coagulation, and venous thromboembolism (VTE) have been reported (37). No laboratory methods are available to monitor the hemostatic efficacy or safety of rFVIIa.

## Immunosuppression Regimens

The most important long-term goal for the treatment of autoimmune hemophilia is the ultimate eradication of the autoantibody inhibitor directed against FVIII:C or FIX. Often, for acquired hemophilia, this final cure of the syndrome will depend on the cure or control of the underlying associated disease state. Nevertheless, because autoantibody production represents lymphocyte response, various approaches to immune suppression have been pursued to affect disease progression and symptomatology.

These include administration of: (i) corticosteroids; (ii) corticosteroids plus cytotoxic agents (cyclophosphamide, azathioprine, CVP, 6-MP); (iii) immunosuppression/immune tolerance induction regimens; (iv) cyclosporin A; (v) high-dose intravenous immunoglobulin (IVIg); (vi) anti-CD20 monoclonal antibody (Rituximab); (vii) inhibition of CD40 ligand; (viii) plasmapheresis/immunoabsorption.

Because autoantibodies may disappear spontaneously, the true efficacy of any given immunosuppression regimen in acquired hemophilia is difficult to assess. In addition, the low incidence of acquired hemophilia has rendered any therapeutic strategy difficult to study. At any rate, corticosteroids, as single agent therapy, have produced an average complete remission rate of 60% (range 33% to 88%) (6,16,21,25,38–41). When corticosteroids have failed as a single agent, cytotoxic medications are often administered alone; in combination with corticosteroids; or as a cocktail of agents, similar to regimens used for the treatment of lymphoproliferative malignancies, such as cyclophosphamide, vincristine and prednisone or 2-chlorodeoxyadenosine. Complete remissions and eradication of the autoantibody FVIII:C or FIX inhibitors range between 74% to 89%, compared to corticosteroids alone; however, this marginal advantage of cytotoxic agents over single-agent corticosteroids is mitigated in terms of neutropenia and infection-induced morbidity and mortality. Therefore, these cytotoxic, myelosuppressive regimens are usually reserved for those autoantibody inhibitors associated with known underlying lymphoproliferative malignancies or for salvage therapy in the face of corticosteroid failure (6,16,17,25, 38,41,42).

The experience with cyclosporine A (CsA) to eradicate autoantibody FVIII:C and FIX inhibitors is anecdotal but provocative for its success in single case reports. CsA has usually been administered as second- or third-line treatment, most often in combination with steroids (43,44).

The mechanism of action of high-dose intravenous immunoglobulin (IVIg) preparations has been discussed earlier for alloantibody FVIII:C inhibitors. Similarly, IVIg has had a relatively low success rate (<20%) in eradicating autoantibody FVIII:C and FIX inhibitors and then has been beneficial only in individuals with low-titer autoimmune antibody inhibitors (45–47). IVIg combined with corticosteroids appears to provide no advantages over corticosteroids alone in treating autoimmune inhibitory antibodies (40,47).

Extracorporeal immunoadsorption of FVIII:C antibodies using Sepharose matrix columns coupled with staphylococcal protein A was reported over 2 decades ago. This technique for removing FVIII:C or FIX alloantibodies and autoantibodies of the IgG subtypes is definitely efficient, but is expensive, only temporizing in its benefits, labor intensive, and considered for those with very high-titer inhibitors refractory to classical immunosuppression. Excellent hemostatic successes have been reported in autoantibody FVIII:C or FIX inhibitor scenarios in which active bleeding was not responsive to upfront administration of bypass replacement therapies. Immunoadsorption temporarily reduces the titer of the autoantibody inhibitor, enabling replacement (high doses of human- or porcine-derived FVIII:C concentrates) or bypass (aPCCs, rFVIIa) therapy for several days. A few long-term remissions have been described after extracorporeal plasmapheresis and immunoadsorption alone although immunosuppressive and cytotoxic medications are usually started in conjunction with this procedure. This maneuver has also been applied as a preliminary measure immediately prior to initiating immune tolerance induction for acquired hemophilia (48–50).

There is limited experience with immune tolerance induction regimens to suppress autoimmune FVIII:C antibody inhibitors. The successful eradication of autoantibodies appears dependent on FVIII:C "priming" combined with immunosuppression, similar to the immune tolerance induction for alloantibody FVIII:C or FIX inhibitors (51,52). One very promising protocol, combining tapering doses of corticosteroids with limited exposure to cyclophosphamide and daily infusions of FVIII:C concentrate, obtained a remarkably high complete remission rate of 95% (19/20 patients) over a median time for inhibitor disappearance of 4.7 weeks (51). This regimen remains to be studied in a prospective, randomized manner, but provides a very provocative and cost-efficient approach to this difficult and expensive clinical disease. It is difficult to ascertain whether these protocols are successful because of immunosuppression, FVIII:C concentrate administration, or both, as similar results have been obtained without FVIII:C priming (53).

Acquired autoantibody inhibitors to FVIII:C, which are refractory to conventional immunosuppressive therapy, may respond favorably to purine analog monotherapy (54). 2-chlorodeoxyadenosine (2-CDA), administered at a dose of 0.1 mg per kg as a 24-hour continuous infusion for a total of 7 days, induced complete remissions of autoantibody production in six individuals with heretofore resistant acquired hemophilia (54). No major toxicity was observed.

Another successful method to eradicate autoantibody FVIII:C inhibitors has included the administration of rituximab, a chimeric monoclonal antibody, which targets the CD20 antigen on B lymphocytes and blocks their proliferation. The largest series with 10 patients describes an 80% complete response in autoantibody FVIII:C inhibitor eradication with normalization of FVIII:C activity levels in plasma. The remaining two (extremely high-titer inhibitors) responded after the addition of pulses of cyclophosphamide. In this series and in scattered case reports (total of 15 patients to date), complete disappearance of the autoantibody has occurred rapidly (4 to 12 weeks) and is durable. Relapses generally have responded successfully to repeat doses of rituximab (55). Rituximab administration appears to be safe and despite severe depletion of CD19$^+$ cells, no infectious sequelae have been reported in this patient population. Nevertheless, reactivation of hepatitis B remains a potential adverse event. It is unlikely that adequately powered, prospective, randomized trials can be accomplished in this rare disease state to determine whether rituximab will be useful as up-front therapy and which patients will be the optimal candidates for its use. However, there are reports that indicate that not all patients will respond favorably, perhaps because of extremely high-titer inhibitors (56).

A potential alternative strategy to inhibit the production of antifactor VIII:C autoantibody inhibitors consists of blocking T-cell/B-cell interactions that are required to generate humoral responses. This was attempted in the allo-FVIII:C antibody inhibitor scenario employing monthly injections of a humanized mouse monoclonal antibody to human CD40L (hu5c8*) (57). Although anamnestic responses to FVIII:C concentrate exposure was blocked in some allo-FVIII:C inhibitor patients, the study was terminated for safety reasons before it could be determined that tolerance had developed to FVIII:C concentrate in the absence of hu5c8 coadministration. Such approaches may be useful for the patients on autoantibody as well, if a safe antibody product can be made available. Therefore, immunosuppression and lymphocyte and antibody depletion are mainstays for the treatment of acquired hemophilia with autoantibody inhibitors against FVIII:C or FIX. Those with postpartum or drug-related inhibitors with mild bleeding may be kept under observation, because their autoantibodies may remit spontaneously. Immunosuppression and clinical eradication of the autoantibody in other situations clearly reduce the mortality rate in acquired hemophilia, but the overall survival and the disease-free survival are not improved because of the side effects related with the use of myelosuppressive and immunosuppressive agents (25). Figure 71-4 offers an algorithmic approach to the complex and challenging care of patients with acquired hemophilia.

# INHIBITORS OF PROTHROMBIN AND THROMBIN

Thrombin (factor IIa) is a serine protease that performs multiple functions in blood coagulation (58). Its most important action is converting fibrinogen into fibrin monomers, which then polymerize to form the fibrin clot. Thrombin also participates in the activation of factors V, VIII, and XIII, as well as of platelets (59). A crucial role of thrombin in the regulation of coagulation is to bind to thrombomodulin on vascular endothelial cells to form a complex that activates protein C, thereby limiting the extent of an emerging clot (60). Cleavage of the inactive zymogen precursor to thrombin, prothrombin (factor II), is required to generate functionally active thrombin. The essential final step of blood coagulation is the enzymatic conversion of prothrombin to an active enzyme, thrombin.

Patients with hereditary abnormalities of prothrombin generate decreased amounts of thrombin, which typically results in a lifelong bleeding disorder (61). On the other hand, acquired inhibitors of thrombin or prothrombin may have variable effects on the blood coagulation system. Antibodies to thrombin, in general, lead to bleeding diathesis and rarely clotting, whereas the presence of antibodies to prothrombin is a frequent cause of thrombophilia. In fact, nonneutralizing, antiprothrombin antibodies are the most common inhibitors that lead to a prothrombotic state that is associated with the LAC in patients with SLE and various other diseases (62). Antiphospholipid antibodies are a heterogeneous group of antibodies that can be detected as anti-$\beta$2-glycoprotein I antibodies, antiprothrombin antibodies, and LAC (63). A study of 96 patients with SLE by Nojima et al. found that the prevalence of antiprothrombin antibodies in these patients is as high as 51% (64). They have shown that the coexistence of IgG antiprothrombin antibodies and LAC activity is the most significant risk factor for the prevalence of activated protein C resistance and correlates best with a history of VTE in patients with SLE (64). In rare cases of SLE, severe bleeding may occur because of antibodies causing acquired hypoprothrombinemia-lupus anticoagulant syndrome (HLAS) (65). In this reported case, treatment with corticosteroids and high-dose immunoglobulin succeeded in reestablishing normal prothrombin time (PT) values. Another patient responded to danazol treatment with an increase in factor II activity and antigen to 50% in 10 days (66).

In general, inhibitors of blood coagulation include abnormal immunoglobulins that specifically bind to coagulation factors and either neutralize their procoagulant activity (67), accelerate their clearance from the circulation (68), or have proteolytic activity to degrade them into inactive polypeptides (69). A novel mechanism was observed in case of an autoantibody that was directed toward prothrombin and induced proteaselike activity to facilitate a stable stoichiometric complex formation with its physiologic inhibitor antithrombin III without thrombin conversion (70). This resulted in potent inhibition of coagulation that manifested in a bleeding diathesis that was associated with recurrent bleedings, including retroperitoneal and pulmonary hematoma, in the apparent absence of underlying disease.

In contrast to antiprothrombin antibodies, neutralizing autoantibodies against thrombin rarely occur. Most acquired inhibitors of thrombin appear in patients exposed to topical preparations of bovine thrombin or fibrin "glue" during major surgery; these antibodies react mainly with bovine coagulation proteins (71–74). Acquired inhibitors directed primarily against human thrombin are usually associated with predisposing conditions (73) and are extremely rare in patients

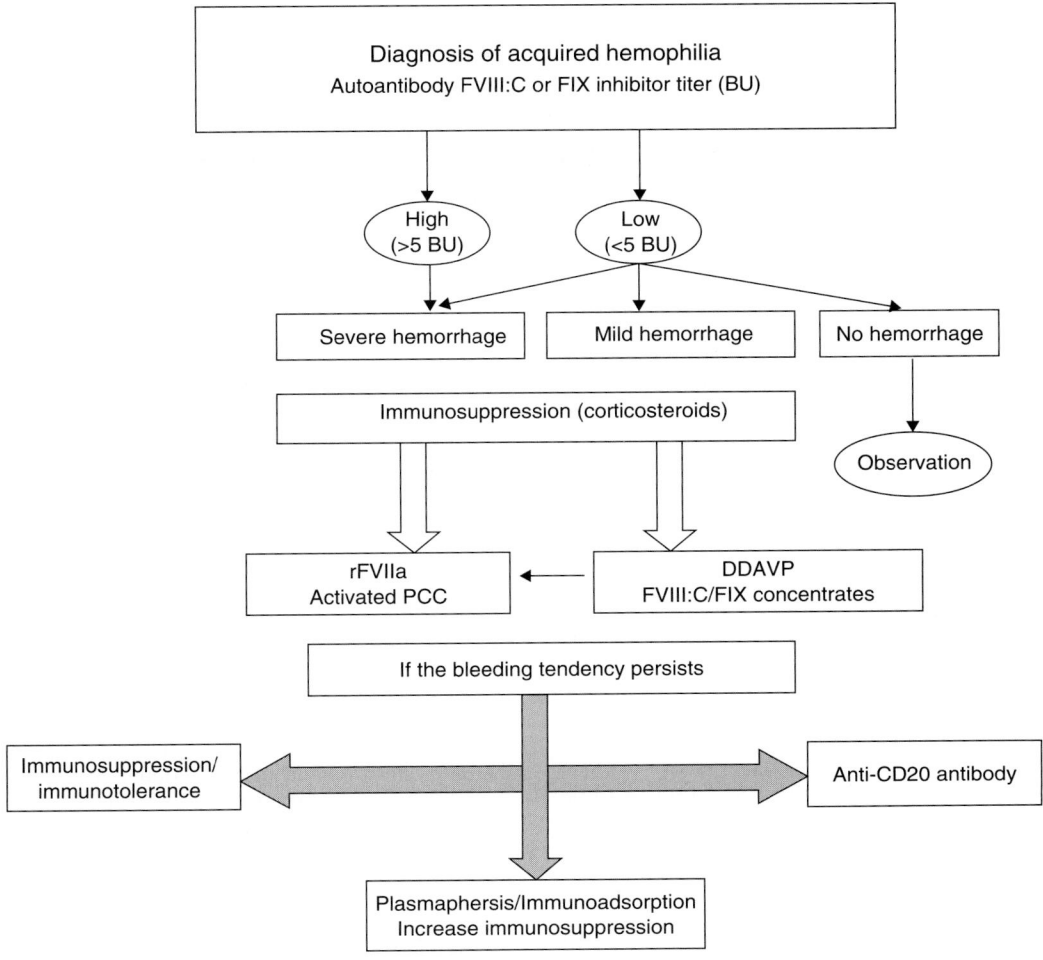

**FIGURE 71-4.** Algorithmic approach to the care of autoimmune FVIII:C/FIX antibody inhibitors. BU, Bethesda units.

without an underlying disease. The underlying condition is frequently of the autoimmune type (73). Indeed, the first characterized inhibitor of thrombin was found in a patient with rheumatoid arthritis in 1957 (75). In 1964, Hawiger et al. (76) isolated an inhibitor of thrombin from a patient with SLE. An acquired inhibitor of thrombin has also been described in a patient in whom a lupuslike syndrome developed during procainamide therapy (77). Other than collagen vascular diseases, isolated cases of antithrombin autoantibodies have been reported in patients with liver cirrhosis, or even without any apparent disease (78,79). Some patients with either monoclonal or polyclonal gammopathies occasionally have inhibitors of thrombin (80–83). In some instances, these inhibitors have been associated with a serious bleeding disorder (68,84–86). On the other hand, in certain cases, the acquired thrombin inhibitor binds to a site involved in the molecule's anticoagulant function and produces thrombotic disease (87).

Apart from these sporadic cases, most examples of acquired thrombin inhibitors occur in patients exposed to bovine topical thrombin or fibrin-glue preparations during major surgery (73). Prospective studies have shown that one third to one half of such patients become immunized to bovine thrombin and bovine factor Va and have abnormal clotting-based coagulation (74,88). Most of these patients are asymptomatic, but some with thrombin inhibitors that cross-react strongly with human thrombin have severe hemostatic complications and may even bleed to death (88).

The suspicion of the presence of antithrombin antibodies should arise if coagulation tests reveal a prolonged PT, a prolonged aPTT, and a markedly prolonged thrombin time (TT). In patients with acquired thrombin inhibitors as opposed to antiprothrombin antibodies, the TT is more prolonged than the PT and clinically a bleeding diathesis is more typical. Factor-activity levels are markedly decreased, and mixing studies suggest the presence of an inhibitor of thrombin. Given the possibility of an unfavorable outcome, in the presence of prolonged PT, aPTT, and TT, with normal platelet count and fibrinogen, a search for an inhibitor of thrombin should be pursued in patients with either bleeding or thrombosis. Timely diagnosis and the initiation of prompt aggressive treatment may result in reduced morbidity and mortality in these patients.

Acute bleeding episodes associated with autoantibody inhibitors against prothrombin or thrombin may be difficult to reverse and there is no consensus on the best approach to replacement therapy. The administration of "bypassing" agents, such as aPCC and rFVIIa concentrate, used alone or in combination with each other or with plasmapheresis and exchange transfusions with fresh frozen plasma (FFP), probably constitutes the best strategy (89,90). The concurrent use of antifibrinolytic agents, such as epsilon amino caproic acid, tranexamic acid, and so on, and human derived fibrin glues may enhance fibrin formation. Corticosteroid use has also been reported to be helpful for the long-term attempt to reverse the coagulopathy and to suppress autoantibody formation (89).

# INHIBITORS OF VON WILLEBRAND FACTOR PROTEIN

## Acquired von Willebrand Disease

When autoantibodies develop against VWF protein in individuals with previously absent personal and family histories of abnormal bleeding, a clinical disorder arises that resembles congenital VWD. Acquired von Willebrand disease or syndrome (AVWS) is an extremely rare disease condition with an estimated, although probably underdiagnosed, prevalence of 0.04% of the population (91). The mean age at diagnosis is usually more than 60 years and most individuals present with spontaneous or postoperative bleeding complications, predominantly involving the gastrointestinal tract and other mucous membranes, such as epistaxis (91). AVWS is often an epiphenomenon of other underlying diseases, most commonly lymphoproliferative (92–95) and lymphoplasmacytic malignancies (96,97); monoclonal gammopathies, including monoclonal gammopathy of unknown significance (MGUS) (98–104) and multiple myeloma (104–108); autoimmune diseases, such as hypothyroidism (109–112) and SLE (113–115); and myeloproliferative disorders (116–120). Less frequent etiologic associations with AVWS have included chronic graft versus host disease post bone marrow transplantation (121); postvaccination prodromes (15); solid tumor nonhematologic malignancies such as Wilms tumors (122–127) and peripheral neuroectodermal tumors (PNET) (128); angiodysplasia of the gastrointestinal tract (129–133); and acquired or congenital heart disease (134,135). Finally, AVWS has iatrogenic associations with the use of valproic acid (136,137), ciprofloxacin (138), griseofulvin (139), and hydroxyethyl starch (140,141).

The proposed pathogenic mechanisms underlying AVWS are variable and include the following:

1. Development of specific anti-VWF antibodies that neutralize VWF activities
2. Adsorption of VWF protein, particularly the high-molecular-weight multimeric forms, onto surfaces of tumor cells, platelets, or endothelial cells of abnormal blood vessels
3. Development of nonspecific immunoglobulin antibodies that form circulating complexes with VWF protein and induce accelerated clearance from the circulating plasma, mediated by Fc-bearing cells in the reticuloendothelial system and by the increased proteolytic degradation of VWF protein (108,112,114,142–144)
4. Decreased synthesis of the VWF protein (111,112)

AVWS is classified according to the multimeric composition of the VWF protein, a feature which usually correlates with the etiology of the syndrome and which has important implications for management.

Type 1 AVWS is associated with decreased levels of VWF activities but with normal VWF protein multimeric structure. The prototypic etiology of type 1 AVWS is untreated hypothyroidism, in which the synthesis of VWF is decreased but in which FVIII:C and VWF have normal circulating half-lives in plasma. These patients respond well to administration of desmopressin (110) and their VWF activities can be normalized by treatment with thyroxine (109,110,112,145).

Type II AVWS is characterized by normal factor VIII:C activity and VWF antigen levels accompanied by reduced VWF activity (ristocetin cofactor and/or collagen-binding activities) and loss of the highest and intermediate size VWF multimers on SDS polyacrylamide gel electropheresis. The loss of the VWF multimers is mediated by their physical adsorption to cell surfaces, by the proteolytic or mechanical degradation of the native

VWF protein, or by the accelerated physical removal of VWF high-molecular-weight multimers from the circulation after complexing to immunoglobulins. The adsorption phenomenon is illustrated clinically by the myeloproliferative disease essential thrombocythemia, in which there exists enhanced platelet-dependent adsorption of VWF multimers when platelet counts are extremely high. There may also be a component of platelet-mediated proteolysis of VWF in this clinical condition. The VWF multimeric composition and activities usually normalize and the VWF symptomatology disappears when the platelet count is reduced below 1 million per $\mu$L.

Specific neutralizing and nonneutralizing anti-VWF autoantibodies, usually IgG, may bind to the intermediate and high-molecular-weight VWF multimers and produce a type II multimeric pattern after the autoantibody–VWF antigen complexes are cleared from the circulation. Type II patterns have been observed in AVWS associated with SLE and in benign MGUS (146). These patients usually have prolonged bleeding time and aPTT and decreased or absent VWF and FVIII:C activity. Similarly, enzymatic degradation of VWF by neuraminidase released from Wilms tumor cells and the mechanical destruction of large VWF multimers, probably mediated by high shear rate activation of the fibrinolytic system in cardiac valve defects, will both result in type II VWF patterns.

Consistent with the mechanisms responsible for the decreased VWF activities in type II AVWS, treatment with desmopressin, cryoprecipitates, or VWF/FVII:C concentrates may yield lower than expected and unsustained VWF incremental increases and poor clinical responses. In contrast, administration of high-dose intravenous immunoglobulin may correct the FVIII:C and VWF activity parameters, albeit this response may be transient, lasting only for a few weeks (147,148). It is unclear whether this improvement is related to binding of the offending IgG by antiidiotype antibodies in the intravenous gammaglobulin, or whether improvement is due to blockade of the Fc receptors in the reticuloendothelial system with decelerated clearance of the VWF from the circulation. Low-dosage intravenous immunoglobulin regimens have also proven to be effective for planned surgery (103,149). As would be anticipated, high-dose intravenous gammaglobulin is not effective in patients with IgM-MGUS states (103). The use of antifibrinolytic agents, such as ε-aminocaproic acid or tranexamic acid, may reverse VWF proteolysis associated with activation of fibrinolysis induced by mechanical or damaged heart valves. Corticosteroids may effectively suppress the autoimmune and malignant lymphoproliferative etiologies of type II AVWS and expedite long-term normalization of VWF structure and function.

Type III AVWS is rare but has been observed in association with Wilms tumors and essential thrombocytosis. This type of AVWS occurs in the complete absence of inhibitors against VWF and is characterized by markedly deficient VWF activities and protein concentration, which, if detectable at all, has a normal multimeric structure. The etiologies for type III AVWS respond to chemotherapy and/or tumor resection (95, 122,124,144).

Although corticosteroids, thyroid replacement, chemotherapy, surgical removal of Wilms tumor or other solid tumors, and more recently, the administration of rituximab provide suitable long-range strategies to eliminate the underlying etiologies of AVWS, the immediate treatment goal involves reversal or prevention of bleeding complications. For this, the infusion of FFP, cryoprecipitate, or preferably, high doses of viral-attenuated FVIII:C/VWF concentrate is the treatment of choice for types I and III AVWS, even though they may not produce the sustained or anticipated increases in VWF activity or the expected secondary rise in factor VIII activity, characteristic of congenital VWD or its variants. Administration of DDAVP should be reserved for patients with type I AVWS or selected type II patients with residual VWF activities. A transient and blunted rise in VWF and factor VIII may result, such that effective hemostasis may be achieved.

The laboratory diagnosis of AVWS is not always as straightforward or as obvious as it is with hereditary VWD, although the two entities may be indistinguishable from a clinical perspective. In both cases, the hallmark findings are low levels of plasma VWF antigen and ristocetin cofactor with impaired ristocetin-induced platelet aggregation. In patients with AVWS, mixing studies coupled with these assays would be expected to detect interfering substances (antibodies). In fact, most of these patients test negative for an inhibitor of ristocetin cofactor activity (91). Occasionally, anti-VWF autoantibodies can be demonstrated by a competitive enzyme-linked immunoassay (150). With rare exceptions (151), autoantibody inhibitors directed against VWF protein do not inhibit FVIII:C, even though FVIII:C activity levels are typically depressed, by virtue of the fact that VWF serves as a carrier for FVIII:C and protects it from proteolytic degradation *in vivo* (152). Bleeding time is prolonged in most patients with AVWS, particularly if there are associated marked reductions in plasma VWF antigen and ristocetin cofactor activity levels. Subsequent analysis of plasma VWF multimer distribution is useful for further definition of the AVWS and for determination of appropriate treatment strategies. Type II AVWS, in contrast to type IIB variant of VWD, is not accompanied by thrombocytopenia or hyperreactivity of platelet-rich plasma to low doses of ristocetin in the platelet aggregation assay. Once AVWS is suspected, serum protein electrophoresis with immunofixation and radiologic imaging studies are helpful to detect an underlying etiology.

## Alloantibody Inhibitors to von Willebrand Factor Protein in Hereditary von Willebrand Disease

Analogous to severe hemophilia A, alloantibody inhibitors may develop against the congenitally absent or severely deficient VWF protein after repeated transfusions with plasma-derived replacement therapies containing VWF (153–155). These alloantibodies have been characterized as polyclonal IgG, have weak or no activity against FVIII:C, and strongly inhibit ristocetin cofactor activity. They most commonly arise in severe type III VWD, but in contrast to hemophiliacs with alloantibody inhibitors, the appearance of an alloantibody inhibitor in patients with VWD, does not always significantly complicate therapy. There may be a familial tendency to develop these alloantibody VWF inhibitors (156).

Replacement of VWF protein in the presence of alloantibody inhibitors to VWF follows the same strategies as for AVWS with VWF/FVIII:C concentrates available as the mainstay of treatment.

# ACQUIRED INHIBITORS TO FACTOR V

## Etiology and Natural History

Coagulation factor V is an essential component of the prothrombinase complex, which activates the zymogen prothrombin to thrombin. Alloantibody inhibitors directed against factor V rarely occur in individuals even after repeated replacement therapy for severe hereditary deficiencies of factor V (157). Development of autoantibodies, which specifically target and neutralize factor V, historically have been very unusual; however,

the increasing use of hemostatic products containing bovine thrombin has been associated with a resurgence in the clinical appearance of these rare autoantibodies. Acquired factor V inhibitors have occurred primarily in previously noncoagulopathic elderly individuals (158) who had received treatment with $\beta$ lactam or aminoglycoside antibiotics (streptomycin and gentamicin) or who had malignant diseases (159–161). More recently, approximately two thirds of factor V inhibitors have developed after a surgical procedure (159,160), during which topical bovine thrombin alone or fibrin glue prepared with bovine thrombin was applied. Both of these bovine-derived products are contaminated with small amounts of bovine factor V, stimulating the production of antibovine thrombin or factor V antibodies that cross-react with human thrombin and factor V (162). Hemorrhagic complications due to acquired neutralizing factor V antibodies usually have occurred after repeated exposures to bovine thrombin products, but one case of severe hemorrhage after only a single exposure to bovine thrombin products has been reported (89). A factor V inhibitor has also been reported after injection of human thrombin (Tissucol) into a bleeding peptic ulcer (163).

On the basis of 105 cases, Knöbl and Lechner have divided the pathogenesis of the factor V inhibitors into five groups: patients exposed to bovine thrombin, postoperative patients without exposure to bovine proteins, miscellaneous associated conditions, idiopathic inhibitors, and alloantibody inhibitors in congenital severe factor V deficiency (160). The overall clinical prognosis for factor V inhibitors is generally good; however, the best prognosis exists in patients exposed to bovine thrombin and the worst prognosis is associated with "idiopathic" inhibitors.

Most factor V inhibitors are polyclonal IgG, although mixed IgG associated with IgM (164) or IgA (165) have been reported. Autoimmune factor V antibody inhibitors usually disappear spontaneously within 8 to 10 weeks after their first appearance. Their mechanism(s) of inhibition are variable and in some respects resemble antibodies directed against FVIII:C, this not being surprising because considerable homology exists between the structures of both clotting factor proteins. The inhibitor may be directed to epitopes on the C2 domain of factor V, thereby interfering with the interaction of factor Va with phospholipids and disrupting formation of the prothrombinase complex (166). Alternatively, antifactor V IgG autoantibodies have been detected in both patient plasma and platelets and neutralized factor V procoagulant activity by reacting with an epitope contained on the factor V light chain (167). The autoimmune nature of the factor V autoantibody inhibitor is epitomized by its association in one patient with Hashimoto thyroiditis, primary biliary cirrhosis, and membranous nephropathy (168). Curiously, acquired antifactor V autoantibodies rarely may mediate the development of a paradoxical hypercoagulable state. Thrombotic rather than hemorrhagic manifestations were described in a woman in whom severe activated protein C resistance occurred by virtue of the blockade of crucial factor Va proteolytic cleavage sites by an acquired antifactor V antibody. The patient's factor V coagulation protein activity was unaffected; however, her purified antifactor V antibody produced a "factor $V_{Leiden}$-like" defect when incubated *in vitro* with normal plasma (169).

Acquired factor V deficiency, unassociated with the presence of an autoantibody inhibitor, has been described as a complication of primary systemic amyloidosis (170).

## Clinical Presentation

In general, the bleeding manifestations of autoantibody inhibitors to factor V are similar to those observed in congenital factor V deficiency. The severity of clinical bleeding varies considerably and typically correlates with the inhibitor titer. Counterintuitively, in some instances, little, if any bleeding is observed even in surgical settings, despite overtly abnormal *in vitro* laboratory findings (170). The propensity to clinical hemorrhage induced by antifactor V antibodies may be related to the content of factor V in the $\alpha$-granule of the platelet and the susceptibility of that factor V to neutralization by the circulating antibody (171,172). Platelet factor V may be relatively protected from interacting with neutralizing antifactor V antibodies in whole blood, even though plasma factor V is completely neutralized (171). The potential role of platelet factor V in maintaining hemostatic competency in the presence of a factor V inhibitor is supported by the efficacy of platelet concentrates in individuals with autoimmune factor V antibodies (173). In contrast, severe bleeding complications have been observed when antifactor V IgG was present in both the patient's plasma and platelets (167).

The clinical presentation of factor V deficiency due to autoantibody inhibitors ranges from mild epistaxis, or gingival bleeding, to life-threatening retroperitoneal hemorrhage (170). Other reported presentations include hematospermia, hematuria, and severe gastrointestinal bleeding (167).

## Diagnosis

An inhibitor to factor V should be suspected when mixing studies with patient and pooled normal plasma do not correct the abnormally prolonged aPTT and PT in patient plasma. Factor V activity should be absent in the patient plasma and the mixture with normal plasma but progressive dilutions of patient plasma with factor V–deficient plasma will eventually allow for the expression of factor V activity as the inhibitor is sufficiently diluted out. An additional confirmatory laboratory assay for autoimmune factor V antibody inhibitors includes a prolonged dilute Russell viper venom time (dRVVT), which, in contrast to the situation with LACs, does not shorten after incubation of patient plasma with an excess of phospholipids. Disseminated intravascular coagulation should be ruled out because high levels of circulating D-dimers also may prolong these coagulation assays and allow for misinterpretation of results.

## Treatment of Factor V Inhibitors

As with congenital factor V deficiency, patients with acquired factor V inhibitors can usually be managed adequately with transfusions of FFP or platelets (173,174). Platelet transfusions appear to be an especially effective means of "bypassing" the inhibitor because platelet factor V does not become accessible to the inhibitor until platelets are activated (173). A number of salvage therapies are available for those unusual bleeding scenarios, which are unresponsive to FFP or platelets. These include the administration of aPCC or rFVIIa concentrate (24) to bypass the inhibitor to factor V. Alternatively, the anecdotal use of high-dose IVIG has also been successful in the management of acquired FV autoimmune inhibitors, with normalization of factor V levels and disappearance of the inhibitor within a few days after infusion (175). For those particularly refractory autoimmune antifactor V inhibitory antibodies associated with persistent and life-threatening bleeding, physical removal of the antibody by plasmapheresis with extracorporeal immunoadsorption methods may be necessary to effect a rapid reduction of the inhibitor titer (176).

Because most autoimmune factor V antibody inhibitors disappear spontaneously over weeks to months, it is uncertain whether immunosuppressive regimens actually hasten the disappearance of the inhibitor. Combination treatment with plasmapheresis and corticosteroids (89); corticosteroids, azathioprine,

and plasmapheresis (168); or prednisone and cyclophosphamide have all been reported to reverse the coagulation defect over time, but the effect of these agents on the natural history of this disorder is not yet known.

# AUTOIMMUNE ANTIBODY INHIBITORS TO FACTOR XII

The contact phase coagulation factor protein, factor XII, is no longer believed to be responsible for the initiation of the intrinsic coagulation pathway, but may be an important component in the intrinsic fibrinolytic pathway. Most cases of autoantibodies directed against factor XII have been described in the presence of an LAC (177,178) or antiphospholipid syndrome (APS) (179). In one study, 21 of 42 patients with APS had either IgG or IgM autoantibodies targeting factor XII (179) as per enzyme-linked immunosorbent assays (ELISA) and four of the 21 individuals had decreased factor XII levels (179).

The clinical significance of these autoantibodies is not entirely clear. Severe factor XII deficiency does not cause clinical bleeding and, in fact, has been associated with thrombotic complications (180,181) although factor XII deficiency is not considered an independent risk factor for developing thrombosis (182,183). Similarly, autoantibody inhibitors to factor XII do not cause bleeding but have been implicated as a hypercoagulability cause of excessive fetal loss (184,185), independent of a concurrent LAC or $\beta_2$-glycoprotein antibodies. Acquired inhibitors directed against factor XII have also been described in association with various liver diseases: metastatic liver disease from gastric carcinoma, autoimmune hepatitis, and severe chronic hepatitis B (186). The coagulation abnormalities corrected after partial hepatectomy, corticosteroid treatment, and hydroxychloroquine therapy, respectively (186).

Therefore, there is no need to administer plasma products to replace the deficient factor XII coagulation protein because there is no associated bleeding diathesis. However, long-term anticoagulation with unfractionated heparin or low-molecular-weight heparin should be considered, particularly in the context of pregnancy following multiple miscarriages.

# ACQUIRED AUTOIMMUNE ANTIBODY INHIBITORS OF FACTOR XI

Inherited factor XI deficiency is a relatively unusual bleeding disorder except for its increased prevalence among the Ashkenazi [due to either a nonsense mutation Glu117 Stop (termed type II), a missense mutation Phe283Leu (termed type III), or a compound heterozygous state], and Iraqi Jews (associated with type II mutations only). The development of alloantibodies to factor XI occurs in individuals with inherited severe factor XI deficiency, following FFP infusions to replace the deficient clotting factor. Alloantibodies to factor XI are recognized in approximately 10% of all severely affected and previously treated individuals, but this incidence is very likely to be an underestimate because low-titer and transient alloantibody inhibitors probably do not come to clinical attention and do not affect replacement therapy (187). Interestingly, the incidence of recognized alloantibodies in homozygotes with the Glu117Stop gene mutation approaches 33% (187).

These alloantibodies are typically IgG, complexing with factor XI and interfering with its proteolytic activation of factor IX or its own activation by thrombin or factor XIIa (187). Most patients on alloantibodies do not bleed spontaneously; however, serious bleeding can occur during or after surgery. Because a relatively high proportion of severely deficient patients appear vulnerable to alloantibody development, poor or no response to bleeding after replacement therapy should alert the clinician to rule out the presence of an alloantibody. On the other hand, when assessing severely deficient patients prior to surgery, genotyping may provide useful predictive information and alternatives to plasma-based infusion therapy should be considered. For example, for minor procedures, antifibrinolytic agents and topical fibrin glue should be used instead of FFP (188). For major surgery, factor IX concentrate or FFP may be unavoidable. If an alloantibody inhibitor has developed, the administration of rFVIIa concentrate is an effective alternative replacement therapy (189). Theoretically, as with other acquired inhibitors, the use of plasmapheresis and exchange with a factor XI–containing replacement product could be helpful in desperate situations, though no literature support exists.

Factor XI concentrate (Bio Products Lab, UK), a viral attenuated, plasma-derived replacement product available in the United Kingdom and Canada, but not in the United States, provides another effective alternative for the treatment of major bleeding complications associated with acquired factor XI (190). Its repeated use, particularly in surgical settings in older patients, has been associated with thrombotic phenomena despite the fact that the concentrate contains a small amount of both heparin and antithrombin III. The risk of thromboembolism appears to be higher in those with a history of cardiovascular disease, hereditary thrombophilia, or underlying malignancy (191).

Autoimmune antibody inhibitors typically arise spontaneously in patients with no prior history of factor XI deficiency (192–198), most frequently in association with an underlying collagen vascular disease, such as SLE (193,194,196,198). Sporadic autoantibody inhibitors, directed against factor XI, have also complicated CLL (199) and chronic myelomonocytic leukemia (200), and autoimmune gastrointestinal diseases (201) and have arisen iatrogenically in association with phenothiazine antipsychotic therapy (195,202).

The autoimmune antibody inhibitor against factor XI usually results in decreased activities of all the plasma clotting factors in the intrinsic pathway and interferes with the contact phase of coagulation. These inhibitors rarely produce excessive bleeding and typically are detected only through routine coagulation testing for other reasons, such as prolonged aPTT. Autoantibody-induced factor XI deficiency improved after corticosteroid therapy in patients with SLE (196) and resolved after the patient with CLL received pulsed methylprednisolone and chlorambucil (199). The patient with chronic myelomonocytic leukemia required small doses of recombinant activated factor VIIa concentrate to achieve adequate hemostasis for an invasive procedure (200).

# ACQUIRED FACTOR X DEFICIENCY

Acquired factor X deficiency, a rare condition that is associated with a tendency to precipitate significant bleeding, in general, on the basis of etiology, can be divided into two categories: with and without evidence of circulating antibodies. Most of the individuals with acquired factor X deficiency fall into the latter category and are affected by systemic amyloidosis. Only a few cases of true autoantibody factor X inhibitors have been reported.

Factor X deficiency is the most common coagulopathy acquired in association with systemic amyloidosis (AL-Amyloidosis) (203–217). The apparent factor X deficiency is the result of factor X adsorption and rapid clearance from the circulation by interacting amyloid fibrils in the vasculature and

organs of the reticuloendothelial system (208,210,215). The severity of the factor X deficiency usually varies between 2% and 50% of normal activity; bleeding and bruising are unlikely until the factor X level falls to less than 25% (215). Typically, the factor X deficiency is an isolated abnormality, but occasional patients have combined deficiencies with other vitamin K–dependent clotting factors, including factor IX and X (209,211,213) or factor VII and X (212). Isolated acquired factor V deficiency in the absence of a specific circulating antibody inhibitor was associated with a fatal bleed in one case of systemic amyloidosis.

The bleeding tendency in patients with systemic amyloidosis cannot be attributed solely to acquired factor X deficiency or to combined clotting factor deficiencies. There is also probably a synergistic contribution to impaired hemostasis by the physical changes in the integrity of the microvasculature caused by the amyloid deposition (215,218).

There are approximately 10 published reports of transient factor X deficiency not associated with systemic amyloidosis (219–221). Evidence of specific factor X inhibition was demonstrated in the plasma of only one of these transient cases, a woman with pneumonia following the use of erythromycin (221). Otherwise, specific autoimmune antifactor X inhibitory antibodies are extremely rare (201,221–225) and have been detected in three elderly, previously healthy individuals who experienced sudden onset of bleeding diatheses (222, 223,225) without any underlying disease states; three cases of inflammatory bowel disease or gastrointestinal malignancy (201); a child with extensive burns (224); and the aforementioned woman whose pneumonia was being treated with erythromycin (221). In three cases, the antifactor X inhibitor was characterized as an IgG antibody (222,223,225). The best characterized IgG autoimmune factor X inhibitor antibody inhibited activation of factor X by VIIa/tissue factor (TF), by IXa/VIIIa/phospholipid complex, and by Russell viper venom (223). The IgG failed to inhibit the proteolytic activity of factor Xa toward a chromogenic substrate. However, under reaction conditions of limited factor Xa availability, the IgG could be shown to impair hemostatic functions of factor Xa that require the participation of its light chain: activation of prothrombin by prothrombinase; activation of factor VII bound to TF; and inhibition of VIIa/TF activity by factor Xa/tissue factor pathway inhibitor complexes (223).

Nonspecific nonneutralizing inhibitors of factor X activity, which were associated with transient factor X deficiency and major hemorrhagic complications, have been detected in two individuals in conjunction with a lupuslike anticoagulant (226). Because no specific neutralizing antibodies were isolated from their plasmas, it was surmised that the nonspecific, nonneutralizing antibodies formed factor X–IgG immune complexes and mediated the accelerated clearance of factor X from the circulation (226).

The laboratory diagnosis of acquired factor X deficiency, whether due to specific or nonspecific neutralizing autoantibody inhibitors or due to accelerated clearance from the circulation by amyloid fibril binding, is not always straightforward. In those with acquired factor X deficiency in the context of systemic, the most common abnormalities of global coagulation assays are prolongations of the TT, the PT, and the aPTT (227). The prolonged PT was most predictive of clinical bleeding but was independent of whole body amyloid load. Prolongations of the reptilase time accompany the prolonged TTs in most individuals, and the prolonged TTs appear to be associated with hepatic amyloid infiltration and the presence of the nephrotic syndrome (214,227). The prolonged PT and aPTT are explained by reduced factor X activity without evidence of an inhibitor; however, the corresponding factor X antigen levels are discordantly and consistently higher than the corresponding decreased factor X activity levels (median FX:Ag/FX:C = 2.5).

The etiology of this phenomenon has not been explained (227). Because multiple clotting factor deficiencies may occur in conjunction with decreased factor X activity in the context of systemic amyloidosis, for example, factors VII, IX, and V (227), other specific clotting factor assays may be called for. In those whose decreased factor X levels do not correct with mixing studies, serial dilutions for specific clotting factor assays will indicate if a specific neutralizing autoimmune antifactor X antibody inhibitor or a nonspecific lupuslike antibody exists.

Treatment strategies for patients with acquired factor X deficiency must be individualized and depends on the presumed etiology of the coagulopathy. For example, immediate reversal of clinical bleeding due to acquired factor X deficiency secondary to systemic amyloidosis is often challenging because of the extremely rapid clearance of the factor X protein contained in replacement products. The administration of PCCs (inactivated or activated) may be temporarily effective and may be useful if there are other vitamin K–dependent factor deficiencies present. Splenectomy may result in a significant rise in the plasma factor X level; however, surgery may not be possible unless adequate hemostasis can be guaranteed. There are anecdotal successes employing rFVIIa concentrate to control or to prevent bleeding and to facilitate splenectomy (228,229). These replacement products, which are viral attenuated, obviate the administration of less viral safe and effective FFP, unless deficiency of factor V or other clotting factor complicates the clinical picture. FFP is utilized in plasmapheresis and exchange protocols intended to expedite factor X replacement, or when the physical removal of autoimmune anti–factor X antibody inhibitors is deemed necessary to control bleeding (230).

Although spontaneous resolution of amyloid-associated factor X deficiency may occur rarely (231), the usual course of the coagulopathy is linked to the ability to eradicate the underlying plasma cell dyscrasia in systemic amyloidosis. Therefore, aggressive treatment with high-dose melphalan chemotherapy, with or without corticosteroids, has emerged as the treatment of choice for systemic amyloidosis and in those patients with good performance status, autologous stem cell transplantation should follow. This approach usually reverses or at least ameliorates the factor X deficiency (215,216,232).

Acquired circulating autoantibody inhibitors, which specifically neutralize factor Xa, are usually transient so that long-term eradication strategies are not usually necessary (222,223). Active bleeding is treated optimally with rFVIIa, PCCs (221), or daily therapeutic plasma exchange (plasmapheresis) with concomitant administration of intravenous immunoglobulin and steroids (225). Intravenous γ globulin alone may facilitate the disappearance of an autoimmune factor X antibody inhibitor (224). One patient with acquired autoimmune factor X antibody inhibitor successfully and gradually raised his factor X activity level over time with the administration of danazol, a nonvirilizing androgenic analog (233).

# ACQUIRED DEFICIENCIES AND INHIBITORS OF FACTOR IX

Similar to hemophilia A, inhibitors to factor IX develop in those with congenital deficiencies of factor IX due to alloimmunization after replacement therapy, albeit at a considerably lower incidence. The overall incidence of alloantibody inhibitors complicating hemophilia B is approximately 3% (234–236) with an incidence of 12% in those with severe hemophilia B (234). Individuals with major gene deletions or nonsense mutations, who do not have demonstrable plasma factor IX protein, are especially susceptible to production of factor IX alloantibody inhibitors (237,238). Factor IX alloantibody inhibitors are unusual in association with missense mutations (238).

In general, factor IX alloantibody inhibitors are polyclonal IgG4 immunoglobulins (234,239,240), although rarely a monoclonal gammopathy is detected (239–242).

## Laboratory Evaluation of Factor IX Alloantibody Inhibitors

The presence of a factor IX alloantibody inhibitor should be suspected in a patient with hemophilia B if there is less than expected incremental rise in factor IX activity after transfusion of a factor IX replacement product, if there is shortened circulating survival of factor IX activity, or both. In the laboratory an inhibitor, whether alloantibody- or autoantibody-derived, will present as a noncorrecting aPTT or factor IX activity assay in mixing studies with normal plasma. The in vitro kinetics of allo- and auto-factor IX inhibitors differ from FVIII:C inhibitors in that factor IX inhibitors produce an immediate loss of factor IX activity with no progressive loss of activity with prolonged incubation at 37°C (243–245). In addition, antifactor IX alloantibodies, in contrast to antifactor VIII:C alloantibodies, may form circulating immune complexes, which are capable of precipitating anaphylactic reactions when the patient is reexposed to factor IX containing replacement products. Specificity of the factor IX alloantibody or autoantibody inhibitor can be confirmed in factor IX coagulation assays, and the degree of inhibition can be quantified by a modified Bethesda assay (246,247).

## Clinical Presentation and Treatment of Acquired Alloantibody Inhibitors to Factor IX

The clinical course and symptomatology of alloantibody inhibitors directed against factor IX in patients with hemophilia B are identical to the hemophilia A alloantibody inhibitor situation. Patients with factor IX alloantibodies present most commonly with intraarticular bleeds and, counterintuitively, the frequency of bleeding events in the context of alloantibodies may be decreased from the basal, noninhibitor state. In contrast, hemorrhagic complications with autoimmune antifactor IX inhibitors rarely involve joints and mainly consist of severe and extensive ecchymoses and intramuscular bleeds, as well as gastrointestinal and genitourinary bleeds (248).

The mainstay of therapy for patients with hemophilia B and with high-titer factor IX inhibitory alloantibodies, is the administration of PCC, replacement concentrates (activated or inactivated), which possess "bypassing" activity. For low-titer inhibitors (<5 BU), purified plasma-derived or recombinant factor IX concentrates can be used to overwhelm the inhibitor. Recombinant FVIIa (249–254) is an excellent salvage therapy and has emerged as the treatment of choice for those at high risk (large factor IX gene deletions) to develop anaphylactic reactions, for those who have previously experienced anaphylaxis, or for those who have developed nephrotic syndrome after exposure to any source of factor IX protein. These treatment products are used in regimens similar to those for FVIII:C alloantibody inhibitors and are equally effective (248,249,253–256) with an 80% complete and partial response rate (257). Factor IX activity cannot be measured accurately in the plasma after their use. Treatment failures require alternative strategies, such as combining the PCCs with rFVIIa (258). Patients who are high responders with low-titer alloantibodies may experience an anamnestic response to any source of infused factor IX protein within 2 to 5 days. Occasionally, in high-titer inhibitor situations, plasmapheresis or extracorporeal immunoadsorption is necessary to transiently decrease inhibitor titers and facilitate control of acute bleeding

(248). For long-term control, regimens for induction of immune tolerance have been initiated for allo-FIX antibody inhibitors, as for allo-factor VIII:C antibody inhibitors, with and without the use of high doses of intravenous IgG and cyclophosphamide and sometimes preceded by extracorporeal immunoadsorption (259,260). Successful immune tolerance is achieved in approximately 30% of factor IX alloantibodies with normalization of factor IX pharmacokinetics after replacement therapy and complete disappearance of the inhibitor (261). Successful immune tolerance for autoantibodies to factor IX is anecdotal.

For those with life-threatening anaphylactic or anaphylactoid reactions upon exposure to factor IX protein (262,263), acute bleeding episodes have been managed successfully with rFVIIa concentrate. Immune tolerance induction regimens yield poor results in these patients on alloantibodies.

## Autoimmune Acquired Factor IX Inhibitors

Spontaneously acquired factor IX autoantibody inhibitors are extremely rare (239,240,244,264,265). The associated disease states are quite similar to those underlying acquired factor VIII inhibitors. Three cases of autoimmune factor IX antibodies have been described in the context of SLE and two others have occurred during the postpartum state. Adenocarcinoma of the colon was the presumed trigger in another case (266). Most autoimmune factor IX inhibitors resolve spontaneously within 1 to 7 months of onset, but whether immunosuppressive therapy alters the natural history is unclear. The use of corticosteroids with or without high-dose intravenous immunoglobulin (400 mg/kg/day for 5 consecutive days by intravenous infusion), has been successful anecdotally (267). Furthermore, the extirpation of a malignant tumor may allow for spontaneous resolution of an autoimmune factor IX antibody inhibitor (266). Recurrence of the autoantibody is unusual after successful treatment. As a general rule the strategies for treatment of acquired autoimmune hemophilia A can be applied for acquired autoimmune factor IX antibody inhibitors.

## Acquired Nonimmune Factor IX Deficiency

Acquired isolated factor IX deficiency due to nonimmune mechanisms are more common than autoantibody inhibitors causing factor IX deficiency. This coagulopathy has been associated with the proteinuria of nephrotic syndrome (268,269), primary amyloidosis (270), Gaucher disease (271), and pituitary insufficiency (272). Laboratory assessment confirms the absence of an inhibitor and bleeding manifestations are treated with factor IX replacement in the form of PCCs (activated or unactivated), ultra-high purity plasma-derived or recombinant factor IX concentrates, or rFVIIa for salvage therapy. The replaced factor IX protein usually has accelerated plasma clearance in these situations, except for pituitary insufficiency, which was treated successfully with administration of thyroxine.

# ACQUIRED FACTOR VII DEFICIENCY

Although congenital or inherited factor VII deficiency is a relatively rare coagulopathy, acquired deficiencies of factor VII associated with warfarin, antibiotics, hepatic disease, or malabsorption are commonplace events in patient care. Acquired factor VII deficiency due to the development of autoimmune antibody inhibitors is an anecdotal phenomenon and a clinical curiosity.

The pattern of bleeding complications in individuals with acquired autoimmune factor VII deficiency tends to be more severe and is more likely to be life-threatening compared to inherited factor VII deficiency (273–277). This may reflect selection bias in publishing the most dramatic cases of acquired autoimmune factor VII deficiency because intracerebral hemorrhage has been reported in 15% to 60% of patients with severe congenital factor VII deficiency and is frequently fatal (273–277). Hemarthroses are uncommon in either congenital or autoimmune factor VII deficiencies.

Isolated acquired autoimmune factor VII deficiency has developed in association with varied clinical scenarios, including aplastic anemia with the use of antithymocyte globulin (278); medication administration, including penicillins, cephalosporins, and interleukin 2 (IL-2) therapy (277,279); septicemia (280); pancreatitis (281); and malignancy, such as multiple myeloma (282). A specific factor VII autoimmune antibody has also been isolated from the plasma of an AIDS patient with a concurrent lupuslike anticoagulant (283).

These acquired factor VII autoantibody inhibitors are predominantly IgG and most are neutralizing antibodies (276,284). Rarely, factor VII deficiency has occurred because of IgG-factor VIII complex formation with accelerated clearance of the immune complex (278). Alloantibody formation has been reported in several individuals with severe hereditary factor VII deficiency after being treated with rFVIIa concentrate (285).

Acquired deficiencies of factor VII, not related to autoimmune antibody inhibitor formation, are most commonly due to vitamin K deficiency states associated with hepatic diseases (severe cirrhosis, ethanol or acetaminophen toxicity, Dubin-Johnson syndrome, Rotor syndrome, Gilbert disease, etc.) (286,287) or with medications classified as vitamin K antagonists (warfarin and coumarin derivatives). Factor VII deficiency has also accompanied amyloidosis (288,289), presumably caused by adsorption of the clotting factor to amyloid fibrils.

Laboratory analysis of plasma samples from individuals with specific autoimmune factor VII antibody inhibitors usually reveals isolated prolongations of the PT assays and factor VII activity assays, which do not correct with mixing studies performed with normal plasma. The aPTTs are typically normal. In contrast, for factor VII deficiency due to hepatic disease or warfarin effects, mixing studies with patient and normal plasmas should show immediate normalization of prolonged PTs and aPTTs (reflecting deficiencies in all vitamin K–dependent clotting factor proteins) and depressed factor VII activity assays.

Because of the rarity of autoimmune acquired factor VII deficiency due to circulating inhibitors, there is no consensus on the best treatment strategy for significant bleeding complications. Anecdotal reports indicate that eradication of the associated underlying disease state is clearly crucial over the long term, for example, normalization of autoimmune factor VII deficiency which occurred after an allogenic bone marrow transplant cured aplastic anemia (278) and after tumor regression by chemotherapy. Factor VII activities decreased again when the tumor relapsed (282). For significant active bleeding, administration of plasma-derived or genetically-engineered factor VII concentrates is probably the most efficient and consistently effective first-line treatment strategy to overcome the inhibitor (257). FFP has limited usefulness because of the large volumes required, the prolonged administration time, the possible transmission of blood-borne pathogens, and the low likelihood that the factor VII inhibitor can be overwhelmed. PCCs may be of value but also may induce hypercoagulability with repeated doses. When these strategies are unsuccessful in reversing bleeding or if achieved factor VII increments after replacement therapy are shortlived because of the inhibitory antibody, extracorporeal plasmapheresis with or without concomitant intravenous gammaglobulin may be lifesaving

(286,290). Antifibrinolytic agents and fibrin glues may be useful adjunctive therapies.

The prompt reversal of bleeding related to warfarin or to liver disease can be achieved with administration of PCCs (50 to 100 U per kg every 8 to 12 hours until bleeding ceases), with the same *caveat*s as mentioned in preceding text. Recombinant factor VIIa concentrate (20 to 30 $\mu$g per kg IV as a single bolus, with repeat dosing every 2 to 3 hours as necessary) has been used successfully in these situations as well, but has been reserved primarily as salvage therapy for patients who fail to respond to other treatment modalities (291,292). No controlled clinical studies have been conducted to compare the relative risks and benefits of these approaches. FFP can also be used and vitamin K repletion provides a longer-term adjunctive strategy for these other modalities.

# ACQUIRED AUTOIMMUNE INHIBITORS OF FIBRIN FORMATION, FIBRIN POLYMERIZATION, AND FACTOR XIII

The final stages of blood coagulation consist of fibrin formation, mediated by thrombin cleavage of fibrinopeptides A and B from fibrinogen, followed by polymerization of fibrin monomers, and ultimately concludes with the covalent cross-linking of the $\alpha$ and $\gamma$ chains of adjacent fibrin molecules by factor XIIIa (293). Spontaneously acquired neutralizing inhibitory antibodies, many with autoimmune origins, have been identified to target each of these reactions specifically and have been associated with the development of severe clinical bleeding complications.

Alloantibody inhibitors, which target fibrinogen, rarely may develop in individuals who have received transfusions of FFP or cryoprecipitate as replacement therapy for their hereditary afibrinogenemia (294). Considerably more common than alloantibody formation to fibrinogen is the occurrence of acquired autoimmune antibodies, which complex with fibrinogen and fibrin monomers and impede fibrin polymerization and thrombus stabilization. Acquired polyclonal IgG autoantibodies have been shown to inhibit both thrombin-mediated release of fibrinopeptide A from fibrinogen (295) and fibrin monomer formation (296) without interfering with subsequent fibrin polymerization or cross-linking. The affected individuals presented with a severe hemorrhagic syndrome reminiscent of congenital afibrinogenemia. Allo and autoantibodies targeting fibrinogen initially should be suspected when the aPTT, PT, TT, and reptilase time coagulation assays are all prolonged and chronometric assays for fibrinogen quantitation reveal substantially reduced concentrations. Subsequently, the TT, which measures clot formation *in vitro* following the addition of exogenous thrombin, will remain significantly prolonged when mixing studies are performed with patient plasma (or the isolated inhibitory monoclonal IgG antibody) added to normal plasma.

Impaired fibrin polymerization also has been reported in individuals with acquired monoclonal and polyclonal IgG autoantibody inhibitors. These antibodies were targeted specifically against nonfibrinopeptide epitopes on fibrinogen (297–300) and/or fibrin monomers (298–300). Clinical bleeding was consistent with dysfibrinogenemia, but their purified fibrinogens were functionally and structurally normal and their isolated inhibitors did not interfere with fibrinopeptide cleavage or fibrin cross-linking (298,299). These acquired autoimmune neutralizing autoantibody inhibitors were detected in individuals with *de novo* coagulation defects arising in association with chronic aggressive hepatitis, postnecrotic cirrhosis, and ulcerative colitis

(298), SLE (299), and benign and malignant monoclonal gammopathies (300–302). In one study, autoantibodies directed specifically against fibrinogen and fibrinogen fragments X, Y, and D were detected in pregnant and postpartum women, particularly in those who are Rh immunized, and their newborns (303). Laboratory abnormalities were observed, but the significance of these "physiologic" antibodies remains unclear because no hemorrhagic diathesis was apparent.

Acquired antibodies, which inhibit cross-linking of fibrin polymers, would be expected to target epitopes on the factor XIII molecule or cross-linking sites on fibrin. Acquired alloantibody inhibitors have been reported only anecdotally in individuals with congenital factor XIII deficiency and typically have occurred after replacement therapy for bleeding complications. In contrast, acquired factor XIII deficiency, caused by development of autoantibody inhibitors in previously noncoagulopathic individuals, has been described in association with varied disease states (304–309) and medications (310–313). Most of the underlying accompanying illnesses have been autoimmune in nature, including SLE, Henoch-Schonlein purpura, inflammatory bowel diseases, psoriatic arthritis, IgG monoclonal gammopathies, and acute leukemias (promyelocytic, lymphoblastic, and myeloid) (314,315). Long-term isoniazid administration is the most important drug therapy associated with the spontaneous development of a specific autoantibody inhibitor to factor XIII. The increasing use of isoniazid to combat a worldwide rise in the incidence of tuberculosis is anticipated to raise the recognized incidence of factor XIII inhibitors. Procainamide, penicillins, diphenylhydantoin, and practolol have also been implicated in the development of clinically relevant autoimmune antifactor XIII antibody inhibitors.

Autoimmune factor XIII deficiency can be produced by autoantibody inhibitors directed against factor XIII. These inhibitors, which are principally IgG immunoglobulins, neutralize factor XIII clotting activity through three predominant molecular mechanisms: inhibition of factor XIII activation by thrombin (type I inhibitor) (306,316), interference of factor XIIIa–mediated transamidase activity and fibrin polymer cross-linking (type II), and blockade of factor XIIIa binding sites on fibrin (type III) (317–320).

Acquired factor XIII deficiency can also develop by nonimmunologic mechanisms. The venom of caterpillars in the *Lonomia* species produces a severe hemorrhagic syndrome due to direct proteolysis of the factor XIII molecule (321,322). The crude salivary gland extract of the giant Amazon leech, *Haementeria ghilianii*, contains a unique peptide, named tridegin, which specifically inhibits the transglutaminase function of plasma factor XIIIa (323). This is the most potent, naturally occurring inhibitor of factor XIIIa yet described. Synthetic, low-molecular-weight inhibitors (nonspecific thiol reagents and specific azol derivatives and azolium salts) exert their factor XIII inhibitory effects at nanomolar concentrations (305).

Generally, the presence of acquired autoimmune antibodies and nonimmunologic inhibitors of factor XIIIa can be detected *in vitro* by the ability of the patient's plasma or purified IgG fraction to inhibit the cross-linking of $\alpha$ chains of fibrin in a mixture with normal plasma (306,324). There is also reduced fibrin clot stability in dissociating agents, such as 5 M urea (urea clot solubility test) (306,324). Global coagulation assays, such as aPTT, PT, TT, and fibrinogen levels, are usually normal although the thromboelastogram device may reveal a pattern consistent with factor XIII deficiency. Decreased factor XIII activity can be quantitated specifically by the dansyl-cadaverine incorporation assay.

From a clinical perspective, the severe, recurrent, and spontaneous hemorrhagic complications (307–318,325) caused by acquired potent inhibitors against factor XIII or fibrin stabilization are associated with a high mortality rate. Gastrointestinal, genitourinary, pulmonary, and intraperitoneal bleeding often occur in combination with dramatic soft tissue hematomas and ecchymoses. Intracranial hemorrhage also has been described (310) and emphasizes the need for prompt diagnosis and treatment. The bleeding events precipitated by acquired autoimmune factor XIII deficiency are considerably more severe than those typically occurring in the context of congenital factor XIII deficiency, such as hemarthroses, poor wound healing, recurrent miscarriage, and so on, although fatal intracranial bleeds occur in both.

The treatment of acute hemorrhagic events due to inhibitors targeting factor XIII or other areas of fibrin stabilization, whether alloantibody or autoantibody in nature, is based on the requirement to replenish factor XIII activity or fibrinogen substrate in plasma. Cryoprecipitate is more suited to accomplish this than FFP but neither may be adequate to overcome inhibitor effects. Intravenous bolus administration of large doses of plasma derived, viral-attenuated factor XIII concentrate appears to be the safest and most effective and efficient alternative method of controlling or preventing acute episodes of bleeding in patients with acquired FXIII deficiency (326,327). Two such factor XIII concentrates are currently in production. The first, Fibrogammin P, (ZLB Behring, King of Prussia, Pennsylvania, USA, and Marburg, Germany) is marketed in Europe, South America, South Africa, and Japan and is distributed in the United States only under a Food and Drug Administration Investigational New Drug Application. A second factor XIII concentrate (Bio Products Laboratory, Elstree, UK) is available for use only on a "named patient" compassionate basis in the United Kingdom. Occasionally, more aggressive measures, such as extracorporeal plasmapheresis to physically remove the inhibitor, followed by exchange transfusion with factor XIII concentrate, cryoprecipitate, or FFP, are necessary to reverse refractory bleeding. This is an inefficient and temporizing option because most of these antibodies are IgG. Longer-term care is directed at eradication of antibody production, which can be approached with immunosuppressive drug regimens employing corticosteroids and alkylating agents (309,319). A significant number of patients may experience the spontaneous remission of their antibody production, particularly after offending medications are discontinued.

One published case report describes the treatment of acquired autoimmune factor XIII deficiency with cryoprecipitate to arrest the acute hemorrhagic event, followed by administration of cyclophosphamide. The antibody titer was reduced enough so that the patient's clot became insoluble in urea and close to normal cross-linking of the $\gamma$–$\gamma$ and $\alpha(n)$-fibrin chains was restored. Nevertheless, the patient still had detectable anti-FXIII autoantibody titers and remained at risk for hemorrhage (315).

In another anecdotal report, infusions of cryoprecipitate successfully controlled the bleeding associated with a serious subcutaneous hematoma precipitated by an autoimmune factor XIII inhibitor; however, subsequent treatment with cyclophosphamide and prednisone, followed by extracorporeal immunoadsorption over a staphylococcal protein A column, did not reduce the inhibitor titer. Plasma exchange therapy reduced the inhibitor titer to undetectable levels but failed to restore factor XIII activity. Infusions of factor XIII concentrate repeatedly raised the factor XIII activity into the hemostatic range and did not provoke an anamnestic rise in the titer of the autoimmune inhibitory antibody (318).

## References

1. Green D, ed. *Anticoagulants-physiologic, pathologic, pharmacologic.* Boca Raton, FL: CRC Press, 1994:282.
2. Hay CR, Baglin TP, Collins PW, et al. The diagnosis and management of factor VIII and IX inhibitors: a guideline from the UK Haemophilia Centre Doctors' Organization (UKHCDO). *Br J Haematol* 2000;111:78.
3. Collins P, Macartney N, Davies R, et al. A population based, unselected, consecutive cohort of patients with acquired hemophilia A. *Br J Haematol* 2004;124:86.
4. Cohen AJ, Kessler CM. Acquired inhibitors. *Baillieres Clin Haematol* 1996;9:331.
5. Green D, Lechner K. A survey of 215 non-hemophilic patients with inhibitors to factor VIII. *Thromb Haemost* 1981;45:200.
6. Yee TT, Taher A, Pasi KJ, et al. A survey of patients with acquired hemophilia in a hemophilia centre over a 28-year period. *Clin Lab Haematol* 2000;22:275.
7. Brodeur GM, O'Neill PJ, Wiliams JA. Acquired inhibitors of coagulation in non-hemophilic children. *J Pediatr* 1980;96:439.
8. Solymoss S. Postpartum acquired factor VIII inhibitors: results of a survey. *Am J Hematol* 1998;59:1.
9. Hauser I, Schneider B, Lechner K. Post-partum factor VIII inhibitors: a review of the literature with special reference to the value of steroid and immunosuppressive treatment. *Thromb Haemost* 1995;73:1.
10. Soriano RM, Mathews JM, Guerado-Parra E. Acquired haemophilia and rheumatoid arthritis. *Br J Rheumatol* 1987;26:381.
11. Hoyle C, Ludlam C. Acquired factor VIII inhibitor associated with multiple sclerosis, successfully treated with porcine factor VIII. *Thromb Haemost* 1987;57:233.
12. Vignes S, Le Moing V, Meekel P, et al. Acquired hemophilia: a rare complication of Sjögren's syndrome. *Clin Exp Rheumatol* 1996;14:559.
13. Sievert R, Goldstein ML, Surks MI. Graves' disease and autoimmune factor VIII deficiency. *Thyroid* 1996;6:245.
14. Seidler CW, Mills LE, Flowers ME, et al. Spontaneous factor VIII inhibitor occurring in association with chronic graft-versus-host disease. *Am J Hematol* 1994;45:240.
15. Ferri GM, Vaccaro F, Caccavo D, et al. Development of factor VIII:C inhibitors following vaccination. *Acta Haematol* 1996;96:110.
16. Sallah S, Wan JY. Inhibitors against factor VIII in patients with cancer. *Cancer* 2001;91:1067.
17. Sallah S, Nguien NP, Abdallah JM, et al. Acquired hemophilia in patients with hematologic malignancies. *Arch Pathol Lab Med* 2004;124:730.
18. Sallah S, Wan JY. Inhibitors against factor VIII associated with the use of interferon-alpha and fludarabine. *Thromb Haemost* 2001;86:1119.
19. Stewart AJ, Manson LM, Dasani H, et al. Acquired haemophilia in recipients of depot thioxanthenes. *Haemophilia* 2000;6:709.
20. Michiels J. Acquired hemophilia A in women postpartum: clinical manifestations, diagnosis, and treatment. *Clin Appl Thromb Hemost* 2000;6:82.
21. Bossi P, Cabane J, Ninet J, et al. Acquired haemophilia due to factor VIII inhibitors in 34 patients. *Am J Med* 1998;105:400.
22. Morrison AE, Ludlam CA, Kessler C. Use of porcine factor VIII in the treatment of patients with acquired hemophilia. *Blood* 1993;81:1513.
23. Kessler CM, Nemes L. Acquired inhibitors to factor VIII. In: Rodriguez-Merchan EC, Lee CA, eds. *Inhibitors in patients with haemophilia.* Oxford: Blackwell Science, 2002:98.
24. Hay CRM, Negrier C, Ludlam CA. The treatment of bleeding in acquired hemophilia with recombinant factor VIIa: a multicenter study. *Thromb Haemost* 1997;78:1463.
25. Delgado J, Yimenez-Yuste V, Hernandez-Navarro F, et al. Acquired haemophilia: review and meta-analysis focused on therapy and prognostic factors. *Br J Haematol* 2003;121:21.
26. Baudo F, de Cataldo F. Acquired factor VIII inhibitors in pregnancy: data from the Italian Haemophilia Register relevant to clinical practice. *BJOG* 2003;110:311.
27. Prescott R, Nakai H, Saenko EL, et al. The inhibitor antibody response is more complex in hemophilia A patients than in most nonhemophiliacs with factor VIII autoantibodies. *Blood* 1997;89:3663.
28. Suzuki T, Arai M, Amano K, et al. Factor VIII inhibitor antibodies with C2 domain specificity are less inhibitory to FVIII complexed with von-Willebrand factor. *Thromb Haemost* 1996;76:749.
29. Brettler BD, Forsberg AD, Levine PH, et al. The use of porcine factor VIII concentrates (Hyate:C) in the treatment of patients with inhibitor antibodies to FVIII. A multicenter US experience. *Arch Intern Med* 1989;149:1381.
30. Mannucci PM. Desmopressin (DDAVP) in the treatment of bleeding disorders: the first 20 years. *Blood* 1997;90:2515.
31. De Sio L, Mariani G, Mazzucconi MG, et al. Comparison between subcutaneous and intravenous DDAVP in mild and moderate hemophilia A. *Thromb Haemost* 1985;54:387.
32. Mudad R, Kane WH. DDAVP in acquired hemophilia A: case report and review of the literature. *Am J Hematol* 1993;43:295.
33. Negrier C, Goudemand J, Sultan Y, et al. Multicenter retrospective study on the utilization of FEIBA in France in patients with factor VIII and factor IX inhibitors. *Thromb Haemost* 1997;77:1113.
34. Penner JA. Management of haemophilia in patients with high-titre inhibitors: focus on the evolution of activated prothrombin complex concentrate AUTOPLEX T. *Haemophilia* 1999;5:1.
35. Ehrlich HJ, Henzl MJ, Gomperts ED. Safety of factor VIII inhibitor bypass activity (FEIBA): 10-year compilation of thrombotic adverse events. *Haemophilia* 2002;8:83.
36. Hoffmann M, Monroe DM, Roberts HR. Activated factor VII activates FIX and X on the surface of activated platelets: thoughts on the mechanism of action of high-dose activated FVII. *Blood Coagul Fibrinolysis* 1998;9:861.

37. Abshire T, Kenet G. Recombinant factor VIIa: review of efficacy, dosing regimens and safety in patients with congenital and acquired factor VIII or IX inhibitors. *J Thromb Haemost* 2004;2:899.

38. Di Bona E, Schiavoni M, Castaman G. Acquired hemophilia: experience of two Italian centres with 17 new cases. *Haemophilia* 1997;3:183.

39. Spero JA, Lewis JH, Hasiba U. Corticosteroid therapy for acquired FVIII:C inhibitors. *Br J Haematol* 1981;48:635.

40. Mazzucconi MG, Bizzoni L, Giorgi A, et al. Postpartum inhibitor to FVIII: treatment with high dose immunoglobulin and dexamethasone. *Haemophilia* 2001;7:422.

41. Grunewald M, Beneke H, Guthner C, et al. Acquired haemophilia: experiences with a standardized approach. *Haemophilia* 2001;7:164.

42. Pruthi RK, Nichols WL. Autoimmune factor VIII inhibitors. *Curr Opin Hematol* 1999;6:314.

43. Zakarija A, Green D. Acquired hemophilia: diagnosis and management. *Curr Hematol Rep* 2002;1:27.

44. Petrovic M, Derom E, Baele G. Cyclosporine treatment of acquired hemophilia due to factor VIII antibodies. *Haematologica* 2000;85:895.

45. Sultan Y, Kazatchkine MD, Maissonneuve P, et al. Anti-idiotypic suppression of autoantibodies to factor VIII (antihaemophilic factor) to high-dose intravenous gammaglobulin. *Lancet* 1984;2:765.

46. Schwartz RS, Gabriel DA, Aledort LM, et al. A prospective study of treatment of acquired (autoimmune) factor VIII inhibitors with high-dose intravenous gammaglobulin. *Blood* 1995;86:797.

47. Dykes AC, Walker ID, Lowe GD, et al. Combined prednisolone and intravenous immunoglobulin treatment for acquired factor VIII inhibitors. *Haemophilia* 2001;7:160.

48. Rivard GE. Use of Protein-A column and porcine factor VIII. *Haemophilia* 2002;8(Suppl. 1):20.

49. Freedman J, Rand ML, Russell O, et al. Immunoadsorption may provide a cost-effective approach to management of patients with inhibitors to FVIII. *Transfusion* 2003;43:1508.

50. Jansen M, Schmaldienst S, Banyai S, et al. Treatment of coagulation inhibitors with extracorporeal immunoadsorption (Ig-Therasorb). *Br J Haematol* 2001;112:91.

51. Nemes L, Pitlik E. New protocol for immune-tolerance induction in acquired hemophilia. *Haematologica* 2000;85:64.

52. Lian EC, Larcada AF, Chiu AY. Combination immunosuppressive therapy after FVIII infusion for acquired FVIII inhibitors. *Ann Intern Med* 1989;110:774.

53. Lian EC, Villar MJ, Noy LI, et al. Acquired factor VIII inhibitor treated with cyclophosphamide, vincristine and prednisone. *Am J Hematol* 2002;69:294.

54. Sallah S, Wan JY. Efficacy of 2-chlorodeoxyadenosine in refractory factor VIII inhibitors in persons without hemophilia. *Blood* 2003;101:943.

55. Stasi R, Brunetti M, Stipa E, et al. Selective B-cell depletion with rituximab for the treatment of patients with acquired hemophilia. *Blood* 2004;103: 4424.

56. Fischer KG, Deschler B, Lubbert M. Acquired high-titer factor VIII inhibitor: fatal bleeding despite multimodal treatment including rituximab preceded by multiple plasmaphereses. *Blood* 2003;101:3753.

57. Ewenstein BM, Hoots WK, Lusher JM, et al. Inhibition of CD40 ligand (CD154) in the treatment of factor VIII inhibitors. *Haematologica* 2000;85 (Suppl. 10):35.

58. Colman RW, Marder VJ, Salzman EW. Overview of hemostasis. In: Colman RW, Hirsh J, Marder VJ, et al., eds. *Hemostasis and thrombosis: basic principles and clinical practice*, 3rd ed. Philadelphia, PA: JB Lippincott Co, 1994:3.

59. Mann KG. Prothrombin and thrombin. In: Colman RW, Hirsh J, Marder VJ, et al., eds. *Hemostasis and thrombosis: basic principles and clinical practice*, 3rd ed. Philadelphia: JB Lippincott Co, 1994:184.

60. Esmon CT, Owen WG. Identification of an endothelial cell cofactor for thrombin-catalyzed activation of protein C. *Proc Natl Acad Sci U S A* 1981; 78:2249.

61. Rabiet MJ, Furie BC, Furie B. Molecular defect of prothrombin Barcelona: substitution of cysteine for arginine at residue 273. *J Biol Chem* 1983;261: 15045.

62. Fleck RA, Rapaport SI, Rao VM. Anti-prothrombin antibodies and the lupus anticoagulant. *Blood* 1988;72:512.

63. Roubey RA. Autoantibodies to phospholipid-binding plasma proteins: a new view of lupus anticoagulants and other "anti-phospholipid" autoantibodies. *Blood* 1994;84:2854.

64. Nojima J, Kuratsune H, Suehisa E, et al. Acquired activated protein C resistance is associated with the co-existence of anti-prothrombin antibodies and lupus anticoagulant activity in patients with systemic lupus erythematosus. *Br J Haematol* 2002;118:577.

65. Vivaldi P, Rossetti G, Galli M, et al. Severe bleeding due to acquired hypoprothrombinemia-lupus anticoagulant syndrome. Case report and review of literature. *Haematologica* 1997;82:345.

66. Williams S, Linardic C, Wilson O, et al. Acquired hypoprothrombinemia: effects of danazol treatment. *Am J Hematol* 1996;53:272.

67. Margolius A, Jackosn DP, Rantoff OD. Circulating anticoagulants: a study of 40 cases and a review of the literature. *Medicine* 1960;40: 145.

68. Bajaj SP, Rapaport SI, Barclay S, et al. Acquired hypoprothrombinemia due to nonneutralizing antibodies to prothrombin: mechanism and management. *Blood* 1985;65:1538.

69. Lacroix-Desmazes S, Moreau A, Sooryanarayana, et al. Catalytic activity of antibodies against factor VIII in patients with hemophilia A. *Nat Med* 1999;5:1044.

70. Madoiwa S, Nakamura Y, Mimuro J, et al. Autoantibody against prothrombin aberrantly alters the proenzyme to facilitate formation of a complex with its physiological inhibitor antithrombin III without thrombin conversion. *Blood* 2001;97:3783.

71. Stricker RB, Lane PK, Leffert JD, et al. Development of antithrombin antibodies following surgery in patients with prosthetic cardiac valves. *Blood* 1988;72:1375.

72. Flaherty MJ, Henderson R, Wener MH. Iatrogenic immunization with bovine thrombin: a mechanism for prolonged thrombin times after surgery. *Ann Intern Med* 1989;111:631.

73. Lawson JH, Pennell BJ, Olson JD, et al. Isolation and characterization of an acquired antithrombin antibody. *Blood* 1990;76:2249.

74. Banninger H, Hardegger T, Tobler A, et al. Fibrin glue in surgery: frequent development of inhibitors of bovine thrombin and human factor V. *Br J Haematol* 1993;85:528.

75. Loeliger A, Hers JFP. Chronic antithrombinaemia (antithrombin V) with haemorrhagic diathesis in a case of rheumatoid arthritis with hypergammaglobulinaemia. *Thromb Diath Haemorrh* 1957;1:499.

76. Hawiger J, Hanicki Z, Struzik T. On the immunologic nature of antithrombin in the course of lupus erythematosus disseminatus. *Acta Med Pol* 1964;5:53.

77. Galanakis DK, Newman J, Summers D. Circulating thrombin time anticoagulant in a procainamide-induced syndrome. *JAMA* 1978;239:1873.

78. Struzik TZ, Hanicki J, Hawiger J, et al. Cryo-coagulopathy with presence of immunoantithrombin in the course of lupus erythematosus disseminatus. *Acta Med Pol* 1964;19:61.

79. Barthels M, Heimburger N. Acquired thrombin inhibitor in a patient with liver cirrhosis. *Haemostasis* 1985;15:395.

80. Gabriel DA, Carr ME, Cook L, et al. Spontaneous antithrombin in a patient with benign paraprotein. *Am J Hematol* 1987;25:85.

81. Craddock CG Jr, Adams WS, Figueroa WG. Interference with fibrin formation in multiple myeloma by an unusual protein found in blood and urine. *J Lab Clin Med* 1953;42:847.

82. Frick PG. Inhibition of conversion of fibrinogen to fibrin by abnormal proteins in multiple myeloma. *Am J Clin Pathol* 1955;25:1263.

83. Perkins HA, MacKenzie MR, Fudenberg HH. Hemostatic defects in dysproteinemias. *Blood* 1970;35:695.

84. Scully MF, Ellis V, Kakkar VV, et al. An acquired coagulation inhibitor to factor II. *Br J Haematol* 1982;50:655.

85. Sie P, Bezeaud A, Dupouy D, et al. An acquired antithrombin autoantibody directed toward the catalytic center of enzyme. *J Clin Invest* 1991; 88:290.

86. La Spada AR, Skalhegg BS, Henderson R, et al. Fatal hemorrhage in a patient with an acquired inhibitor of human thrombin. *N Engl J Med* 1995; 333:494.

87. Arnaud E, Lafay M, Gaussem P, et al. An autoantibody directed against human thrombin anion-binding exosite in a patient with arterial thrombosis: effects on platelets, endothelial cells, and protein C activation. *Blood* 1994; 84:1843.

88. Nichols WL, Daniels TM, Fisher PK, et al. Antibodies to bovine thrombin and coagulation factor V associated with surgical use of topical bovine thrombin or fibrin "glue:" a frequent finding. *Blood* 1993;82(Suppl. 1):59a.

89. Kajitani M, Ozdemir A, Aguinaga M, et al. Severe hemorrhagic complication due to acquired factor V inhibitor after single exposure to bovine thrombin product. *J Card Surg* 2000;15:378.

90. Giovannini L, Appert A, Monpoux F, et al. Successful use of recombinant factor VIIa for management of severe menorrhagia in an adolescent with an acquired inhibitor of human thrombin. *Acta Paediatr* 2004;93:841.

91. Kumar S, Pruthi RK, Nichols WL. Acquired von Willebrand's syndrome: a single institution experience. *Am J Hematol* 2003;72:243.

92. Mannucci PM, Lombardi R, Bader R, et al. Studies of the pathophysiology of acquired von Willebrand's disease in seven patients with lymphoproliferative disorders or benign monoclonal gammopathies. *Blood* 1984;64:614.

93. Tran-Thang C, Mannucci PM, Schneider P, et al. Profound alterations of the multimeric structure of von Willebrand factor in a patient with malignant lymphoma. *Br J Haematol* 1985;61:307.

94. Kao KP, Kizer J, Jones TJ, et al. Acquired von Willebrand's syndrome associated with an extranodal pulmonary lymphoma. *Arch Pathol Lab Med* 1988; 112:47.

95. Tefferi A, Hanson CA, Kurtin PJ, et al. Acquired von Willebrand's disease due to aberrant expression of platelet glycoprotein Ib by marginal zone lymphoma cells. *Br J Haematol* 1997;96:850.

96. Brody JL, Harder ME, Rossman RE. A hemorrhagic syndrome in Waldenström's macroglobulinemia secondary to immuno-adsorption of factor VIII. *N Engl J Med* 1979;300:408.

97. Mazurier C, Parquet-Gernez A, Descamps J, et al. Acquired von Willebrand's syndrome in the course of Waldenström's disease. *Thromb Haemost* 1980;44:315.

98. Mant MJ, Hirsh J, Gauldie J, et al. Von Willebrand's syndrome presenting as an acquired bleeding disorder in association with a monoclonal gammopathy. *Blood* 1973;42:429.

99. Castaman G, Rodeghiero F, Di Bona E, et al. Clinical effectiveness of desmopressin in a case of acquired von Willebrand's syndrome associated with benign monoclonal gammopathy. *Blut* 1989;58:211.

100. Scrobohaci ML, Daniel MT, Levy Y, et al. Expression of GpIb on plasma cells in a patient with monoclonal IgG and acquired von Willebrand disease. *Br J Haematol* 1993;84:471.

101. Michiels JJ, van Vliet HH. Acquired von Willebrand disease in monoclonal gammopathies: effectiveness of high-dose intravenous gamma globulin. *Clin Appl Thromb Hemost* 1999;5:152.

102. Federici AB, Rand JH, Bucciarelli P, et al. Acquired von Willebrand syndrome: data from an international registry. On behalf of the subcommittee on von Willebrand factor. *Thromb Haemost* 2000;84:345.

103. Hayashi T, Yagi H, Suzuki H, et al. Low-dosage intravenous immunoglobulin in the management of a patient with acquired von Willebrand syndrome associated with monoclonal gammopathy of undetermined significance. *Pathophysiol Haemost Thromb* 2002;32:33.

104. Lamboley V, Zabranecki L, Sie P, et al. Myeloma and monoclonal gammopathy of uncertain significance associated with acquired von Willebrand's syndrome. Seven new cases with a literature review. *Joint Bone Spine* 2002; 69:62.

105. Bovill EG, Ershler WB, Golden EA, et al. A human myeloma-produced monoclonal protein directed against the active subpopulation of von Willebrand factor. *Am J Clin Pathol* 1986;85:115.

106. Takahashi H, Nagayama R, Tanabe Y, et al. DDAVP in acquired von Willebrand syndrome associated with multiple myeloma. *Am J Hematol* 1986; 22:421.

107. Mohri H, Noguchi T, Kodama F, et al. Acquired von Willebrand disease due to inhibitor of human myeloma protein specific for von Willebrand factor. *Am J Clin Pathol* 1987;88:663.

108. Richard C, Cuadrado MA, Prieto M, et al. Acquired von Willebrand disease in multiple myeloma secondary to absorption of von Willebrand factor by plasma cells. *Am J Hematol* 1990;35:114.

109. Dalton RG, Dewar MS, Savidge GF, et al. Hypothyroidism as a cause of acquired von Willebrand's disease. *Lancet* 1987;1:1007.

110. Bruggers CS, McElligott K, Rallison ML. Acquired von Willebrand disease in twins with autoimmune hypothyroidism: response to desmopressin and L-thyroxine therapy. *J Pediatr* 1994;125:911.

111. Nitu-Whalley IC, Lee CA. Acquired von Willebrand syndrome—report of 10 cases and review of the literature. *Haemophilia* 1999;5:318.

112. Michiels JJ, Schroyens W, Berneman Z, et al. Acquired von Willebrand syndrome type 1 in hypothyroidism: reversal after treatment with thyroxine. *Clin Appl Thromb Hemost* 2001;7:113.

113. Niiya M, Niiya K, Takazawa Y, et al. Acquired type 3-like von Willebrand syndrome preceded full-blown systemic lupus erythematosus. *Blood Coagul Fibrinolysis* 2002;13:361.

114. Simone JV, Cornet JA, Abildgaard CF. Acquired von Willebrand's syndrome in systemic lupus erythematosus. *Blood* 1968;31:806.

115. Igarashi N, Miura M, Kato E, et al. Acquired von Willebrand's syndrome with lupus-like serology. *Am J Pediatr Hematol Oncol* 1989; 11:32.

116. Budde U, Schaefer G, Mueller N, et al. Acquired von Willebrand's disease in the myeloproliferative syndrome. *Blood* 1984;64:981.

117. Mohri H, Ohkubo T. Acquired von Willebrand's syndrome due to an inhibitor of IgG specific for von Willebrand's factor in polycythemia rubra vera. *Acta Haematol* 1987;78:258.

118. Murakawa M, Okamura T, Tsutsumi K, et al. Acquired von Willebrand's disease in association with essential thrombocythemia: regression following treatment. *Acta Haematol* 1992;87:83.

119. Carter C, Boughton BJ. Acquired von Willebrand's disease in myeloproliferative syndrome: spontaneous remission during pregnancy. *Thromb Haemost* 1992;67:387.

120. van Genderen PJ, Michiels JJ, van der Poel-van de Luytgaarde SC, et al. Acquired von Willebrand disease as a cause of recurrent mucocutaneous bleeding in primary thrombocythemia: relationship with platelet count. *Ann Hematol* 1994;69:81.

121. Seidler C. Spontaneous factor VIII inhibitor occurring in association with chronic graft-versus-host disease. *Am J Hematol* 1994;24:241.

122. Scott JP, Montgomery RR, Tubergen DG, et al. Acquired von Willebrand's disease in association with Wilms' tumor: regression following treatment. *Blood* 1981;58:665.

123. Coppes MJ, Zandvoort SW, Sparling CR, et al. Acquired von Willebrand disease in Wilms' tumor patients. *J Clin Oncol* 1992;10:422.

124. Barr RD, Winthrop A, deSa D, et al. Child with Wilms' tumor and von Willebrand disease at diagnosis and apparent complete response to chemotherapy after multiple relapses. *Med Pediatr Oncol* 1996;26:64.

125. Jonge Poerink-Stockschlader AB, Dekker I, Risseeuw-Appel IM, et al. Acquired von Willebrand disease in children with a Wilms' tumor. *Med Pediatr Oncol* 1996;26:238.

126. Delmer A, Horellou MH, Brechot JM, et al. Acquired von Willebrand disease: correction of hemostatic defect by high-dose intravenous immunoglobulins. *Am J Hematol* 1992;40:151.

127. Michiels J, Schroyens W, Berneman Z, et al. Atypical variant of acquired von Willebrand syndrome in Wilms tumor: is hyaluronic acid secreted by nephroblastoma cells the cause? *Clin Appl Thromb Hemost* 2001; 7:102.

128. Nowak-Gottl U, Kehrel B, Budde U, et al. Acquired von Willebrand disease in malignant peripheral neuroectodermal tumor (PNET). *Med Pediatr Oncol* 1995;25:117.

129. Wautier JL, Caen JP, Rymer R. Angiodysplasia in acquired von Willebrand disease. *Lancet* 1976;2:973.

130. McGrath KM, Johnson CA, Stuart JI. Acquired von Willebrand's disease associated with an inhibitor to factor VIII antigen and gastrointestinal telangiectasia. *Am J Med* 1979;67:693.

131. Inbal A. Acquired von Willebrand's disease, plasma cell dyscrasia, and angiodysplasia: more than a coincidence? *Isr J Med Sci* 1990;26:518.

132. Inbal A, Bank I, Zivelin A, et al. Acquired von Willebrand disease in a patient with angiodysplasia resulting from immune-mediated clearance of von Willebrand factor. *Br J Haematol* 1997;96:179.

133. Warkentin TE, Moore JC, Anand SS, et al. Gastrointestinal bleeding, angiodysplasia, cardiovascular disease, and acquired von Willebrand syndrome. *Transfus Med Rev* 2003;17:272.

134. Takahashi H, Tatewaki W, Nagayama R, et al. Acquired and congenital von Willebrand factor abnormalities in congenital cardiac defects. *Thromb Haemost* 1986;56:111.

135. Gill JC, Wilson AD, Endres-Brooks J, et al. Loss of the largest von Willebrand factor multimers from the plasma of patients with congenital cardiac defects. *Blood* 1986;67:758.

136. Kreuz W, Linde R, Funk M, et al. Valproate therapy induces von Willebrand disease type I. *Epilepsia* 1992;33:178.

137. Serdaroglu G, Tutuncuoglu S, Kavakli K, et al. Coagulation abnormalities and acquired von Willebrand's disease type 1 in children receiving valproic acid. *J Child Neurol* 2002;17:41.

138. Castaman G, Lattuada A, Mannucci PM, et al. Characterization of two cases of acquired transitory von Willebrand syndrome with ciprofloxacin: evidence for heightened proteolysis of von Willebrand factor. *Am J Hematol* 1995;49:83.

139. Conrad ME, Latour LF. Acquired von Willebrand's disease, IgE polyclonal gammopathy and griseofulvin therapy. *Am J Hematol* 1992; 41:143.

140. Dalrymple-Hay M, Aitchison R, Collins P, et al. Hydroxyethyl starch induced acquired von Willebrand's disease. *Clin Lab Haematol* 1992;14:209.

141. Jonville-Bera AP, Autret-Leca E, Gruel Y. Acquired type 1 von Willebrand's disease associated with highly substituted hydroxyethyl starch. *N Engl J Med* 2001;345:622.

142. Tefferi A, Nichols WL. Acquired von Willebrand disease: concise review of occurrence, diagnosis, pathogenesis, and treatment. *Am J Med* 1997; 103:536.

143. Handin RI, Martin V, Moloney WC. Antibody-induced von Willebrand's disease: a newly defined inhibitor syndrome. *Blood* 1976;48:393.

144. Facon T, Caron C, Courtin P, et al. Acquired type II von Willebrand's disease associated with adrenal cortical carcinoma. *Br J Haematol* 1992; 80:488.

145. Levesque H, Borg JY, Cailleux N, et al. Acquired von Willebrand's syndrome associated with decrease of plasminogen activator and its inhibitor during hypothyroidism. *Eur J Med* 1993;2:287.

146. Sitbon N, Horellou MH, Conard J, et al. Acquired Willebrand factor deficiency associated with monoclonal IgG kappa gammopathy: presence of an inhibitor of ristocetin cofactor (authors' trans). *Nouv Presse Med* 1981;10: 2171.

147. Castaman G, Tosetto A, Rodeghiero F. Effectiveness of high-dose intravenous immunoglobulin in a case of acquired von Willebrand syndrome with chronic melena not responsive to desmopressin and factor VIII concentrate. *Am J Hematol* 1992;41:132.

148. Federici AB, Stabile F, Castaman G, et al. Treatment of acquired von Willebrand syndrome in patients with monoclonal gammopathy of uncertain significance: comparison of three different therapeutic approaches. *Blood* 1998;92:2707.

149. Mohri H, Motomura S, Kanamori H, et al. Clinical significance of inhibitors in acquired von Willebrand syndrome. *Blood* 1998;91:3623.

150. Stewart MW, Etches WS, Shaw AR, et al. VWF inhibitor detection by competitive ELISA. *J Immunol Methods* 1997;200:113.

151. Stableforth P, Tamagnin GL, Dormandy KM. Acquired von Willebrand syndrome with inhibitors to factor VIII clotting activity and ristocetin-induced platelet aggregation. *Br J Haematol* 1976;33:365.

152. Ruggeri ZM, Ware J. von Willebrand factor. *FASEB J* 1993;7:308.

153. Egberg N, Blomback M. On the characterization of acquired inhibitors to ristocetin-induced platelet aggregation found in patients with von Willebrand's disease. *Thromb Res* 1976;9:927.

154. Maragall S, Castillo R, Ordinas FL, et al. Inhibition of von Willebrand factor in von Willebrand's disease. *Thromb Res* 1979;14:495.

155. Mannucci PM, Ruggeri ZM, Ciavarella N, et al. Precipitating antibodies to factor VIII/von Willebrand factor in von Willebrand's disease: effects on replacement therapy. *Blood* 1981;57:25.

156. Ruggeri ZM, Ciavarella N, Mannucci PM, et al. Familial incidence of precipitating antibodies in von Willebrand's disease: a study of four cases. *J Lab Clin Med* 1979;94:60.

157. Feinstein DI. Acquired inhibitors of factor V. *Thromb Haemost* 1978;39: 663.

158. Feinstein D, Rapaport SI, McGehee WG, et al. Factor V anticoagulants: clinical, biochemical, and immunological observations. *J Clin Invest* 1970;49:1578.

159. Knöbl P, Tribl K, Lechner K. Acquired factor V inhibitors: a review of the literature. *Thromb Haemost* 1997;78:594.

160. Knöbl P, Lechner K. Acquired factor V inhibitors. *Baillieres Clin Haematol* 1998;11:305.

161. Shastri KA, Ho C, Logue G. An acquired factor V inhibitor: clinical and laboratory features. *J Med* 1999;30:357.

162. Zehnder JL, Leung LL. Development of antibodies to thrombin and factor V with recurrent bleeding in a patient exposed to topical bovine thrombin. *Blood* 1990;76:2011.

163. Caers J, Reekmans A, Jochmans K, et al. Factor V inhibitor after injection of human thrombin (tissucol) into a bleeding peptic ulcer. *Endoscopy* 2003; 35:542.

164. Crowell EB Jr. Observations on a factor-V inhibitor. *Br J Haematol* 1975; 29:397.

165. Lane TA, Shapiro SS, Burke ER. Factor V antibody and disseminated intravascular coagulation. *Ann Intern Med* 1978;89:182.

166. Ortel TL, Quinn-Allen MA, Charles LA, et al. Characterization of an acquired inhibitor to coagulation factor V. Antibody binding to the second C-type domain of factor V inhibits the binding of factor V to phosphatidylserine and neutralizes procoagulant activity. *J Clin Invest* 1992; 90:2340.

167. Ajzner E, Balogh I, Haramura G, et al. Anti-factor V auto-antibody in the plasma and platelets of a patient with repeated gastrointestinal bleeding. *J Thromb Haemost* 2003;1:943.

168. Takahashi H, Fuse I, Abe T, et al. Acquired factor V inhibitor complicated by Hashimoto's thyroiditis, primary biliary cirrhosis and membranous nephropathy. *Blood Coagul Fibrinolysis* 2003;14:87.

169. Kalafatis M, Simioni P, Tormene D, et al. Isolation and characterization of an antifactor V antibody causing activated protein C resistance from a patient with severe thrombotic manifestations. *Blood* 2002;99:3985.

170. Emori Y, Sakugawa M, Niiya K, et al. Life-threatening bleeding and acquired factor V deficiency associated with primary systemic amyloidosis. *Blood Coagul Fibrinolysis* 2002;13:555.

171. Nesheim ME, Nichols WL, Cole TK, et al. Isolation and study of an acquired inhibitor of human coagulation factor V. *J Clin Invest* 1986; 77:405.

172. Miletich JP, Majerus DW, Majerus PW. Patients with congenital factor V deficiency have decreased factor Xa binding sites on their platelets. *J Clin Invest* 1978;62:824.

173. Chediak J, Ashenhurst JB, Garlick I, et al. Successful management of bleeding in a patient with factor V inhibitor by platelet transfusion. *Blood* 1980; 56:835.

174. Onoura CA, Lindenbaum J, Nossel HJ. Massive hemorrhage associated with circulating antibodies to factor V. *Am J Med Sci* 1973;265:407.

175. de Roucourt E, Barbier C, Sinda P, et al. High-dose intravenous immunoglobulin treatment in two patients with acquired factor V inhibitors. *Am J Hematol* 2003;74:187.

176. Tribl B, Knöbl P, Derfler K, et al. Rapid elimination of a high-titer spontaneous factor V antibody by extracorporeal antibody-based immunoadsorption and immunosuppression. *Ann Hematol* 1995;71:199.

177. Gallimore MJ, Jones DW, Winter M. Factor XII determinations in the presence and absence of phospholipid antibodies. *Thromb Haemost* 1998;79:87.

178. Jones DW, Gallimore MJ, Harris SL, et al. Antibodies to factor XII associated with lupus anticoagulant. *Thromb Haemost* 1999;81:387.

179. Jones DW, Gallimore MJ, MacKie IJ, et al. Reduced factor XII levels in patients with the antiphospholipid syndrome are associated with antibodies to factor XII. *Br J Haematol* 2000;110:721.

180. Goodnough LT, Saito H, Ratnoff OD. Thrombosis or myocardial infarction in congenital clotting factor abnormalities and chronic thrombocytopenias: a report of 21 patients and a review of 50 previously reported cases. *Medicine (Baltimore)* 1983;62:248.

181. Winter M, Gallimore M, Jones DW. Should factor XII assays be included in thrombophilia screening? *Lancet* 1995;346:52.

182. Koster T, Rosendaal FR, Briet E, et al. John Hageman's factor and deep-vein thrombosis: Leiden thrombophilia Study. *Br J Haematol* 1994;87:422.

183. Zeerleder S, Schloesser M, Redondo M, et al. Reevaluation of the incidence of thromboembolic complications in congenital factor XII deficiency—a study on 73 subjects from 14 Swiss families. *Thromb Haemost* 1999;82:1240.

184. Jones DW, MacKie IJ, Gallimore MJ, et al. Antibodies to factor XII and recurrent fetal loss in patients with the anti-phospholipid syndrome. *Br J Haematol* 2001;113:550.

185. Jones DW, Gallimore MJ, Winter M. Antibodies to factor XII: a possible predictive marker for recurrent foetal loss. *Immunobiology* 2003;207:43.

186. Chalkiadakis G, Kyriakou D, Oekonomaki E, et al. Acquired inhibitors to the coagulation factor XII associated with liver disease. *Am J Gastroenterol* 1999;94:2551.

187. Salomon O, Zivelin A, Livnat T, et al. Prevalence, causes, and characterization of factor XI inhibitors in patients with inherited factor XI deficiency. *Blood* 2003;101:4783.

188. Berliner S, Horowitz I, Martinowitz U, et al. Dental surgery in patients with severe factor XI deficiency without plasma replacement. *Blood Coagul Fibrinolysis* 1992;3:465.

189. Lawler P, White B, Pye S, et al. Successful use of recombinant factor VIIa in a patient with inhibitor secondary to severe factor XI deficiency. *Haemophilia* 2002;8:145.

190. Bolton-Maggs PH, Wensley RT, Kernoff PB, et al. Production and therapeutic use of a factor XI concentrate from plasma. *Thromb Haemost* 1992; 67: 314.

191. Bolton-Maggs PHB, Colvin BT, Satchi G, et al. Thrombogenic potential of factor XI concentrate. *Lancet* 1994;344:748.

192. Goldsmith GH, Silverman P Jr. Inhibitors of plasma thromboplastin antecedent (factor XI): studies on mechanism of inhibition. *J Lab Clin Med* 1985;106:279.

193. Castro O, Farber LW, Clyne LP. Circulating anticoagulants against factors IX and XI in systemic lupus erythematosus. *Ann Intern Med* 1972;77:543.

194. Krieger H, Leddy JP, Breckenridge RT. Studies on a circulating anticoagulant in systemic lupus erythematosus: evidence for inhibition of the function of activated plasma thromboplastin antecedent (factor XIa). *Blood* 1975; 46:189.

195. Zucker S, Zarrabi MH, Romano GS, et al. IgM inhibitors of the contact activation phase of coagulation in chlorpromazine-related patients. *Br J Haematol* 1978;40:447.

196. Vercellotti GM, Mosher DF. Acquired factor XI deficiency in systemic lupus erythematosus. *Thromb Haemost* 1982;48:250.

197. Reece EA, Clyne LP, Romero R, et al. Spontaneous factor XI inhibitors: seven additional cases and a review of the literature. *Arch Intern Med* 1984; 144:525.

198. Poon MC, Saito H, Koopman WJ. A unique precipitating autoantibody against plasma thromboplastin antecedent associated with multiple apparent plasma clotting factor deficiencies in a patient with systemic lupus erythematosus. *Blood* 1984;63:1309.

199. Goodrick MJ, Prentice AG, Copplestone JA, et al. Acquired factor XI inhibitor in chronic lymphocytic leukaemia. *J Clin Pathol* 1992;45:352.

200. Billon S, Le Niger C, Escoffre-Barbe M, et al. The use of recombinant factor VIIa (NovoSeven) in a patient with a factor XI deficiency and a circulating anticoagulant. *Blood Coagul Fibrinolysis* 2001;12:551.

201. Kyriakou DS, Alexandrakis MG, Passam FH, et al. Acquired inhibitors to coagulation factors in patients with gastrointestinal diseases. *Eur J Gastroenterol Hepatol* 2002;14:1383.

202. Canoso RT, Hutton RA, Deykin D. A chlorpromazine-induced inhibitor of blood coagulation. *Am J Hematol* 1977;2:183.

203. Korsan-Bengtsen K, Hjort P, Ygge J. Acquired factor X deficiency in a patient with amyloidosis. *Thromb Diath Haemorrh* 1962;7:558.

204. Howell M. Acquired factor X deficiency associated with systemized amyloidosis – a report of a case. *Blood* 1963;21:739.

205. Pechet L, Kastrul JJ. Amyloidosis associated with factor X (Stuart) deficiency. *Ann Intern Med* 1964;61:315.

206. Galbraith PA, Sharma N, Parker WL, et al. Acquired factor X deficiency: altered plasma antithrombin activity and association with amyloidosis. *JAMA* 1974;230:1658.

207. Spero JA, Lewis JH, Hasiba U, et al. Treatment of amyloidosis associated with factor X deficiency. *Thromb Haemost* 1976;35:377.

208. Furie B, Greene E, Furie BC. Syndrome of acquired factor X deficiency and systemic amyloidosis. *N Engl J Med* 1977;297:81.

209. McPherson RA, Onstad JW, Ugoretz RJ, et al. Coagulopathy in amyloidosis: combined deficiency of factors IX and X. *Am J Hematol* 1977; 3:225.

210. Cohen D, Pras M, Franklin EC, et al. Characterization of amyloid deposits and P component from a patient with factor X deficiency reveals proteins derived from a lambda VI light chain. *Am J Med* 1983;74:513.

211. Greipp PR, Kyle RA, Bowie EJW. Factor X deficiency in primary amyloidosis. *N Engl J Med* 1979;301:1050.

212. Furie B, Voo L, McAdam K, et al. Mechanism of factor X deficiency in systemic amyloidosis. *N Engl J Med* 1981;304:827.

213. Rosenstein ED, Itzkowitz SH, Penziner AS, et al. Resolution of factor X deficiency in primary amyloidosis following splenectomy. *Arch Intern Med* 1983;143:597.

214. Butler WM, Baldwin PE. Prolongation of thrombin and reptilase times in patients with amyloidosis and acquired factor X deficiency. *South Med J* 1984; 77:648.

215. Choufani EB, Sanchorawala V, Ernst T, et al. Acquired factor X deficiency in patients with amyloid light-chain amyloidosis: incidence, bleeding manifestations, and response to high-dose chemotherapy. *Blood* 2001; 97:1885.

216. Sanchorawala V, Wright DG, Seldin DC, et al. An overview of the use of high-dose melphalan with autologous stem cell transplantation for the treatment of AL amyloidosis. *Bone Marrow Transplant* 2001;28:637.

217. Uprichard J, Perry DJ. Factor X deficiency. *Blood Rev* 2002;16:97.

218. Bohler A, Lammle B. Decreased Quick percentage, acquired factor X deficiency, hemarthrosis and ecchymosis: amyloidosis. *Ther Umsch* 1999; 56:523.

219. Peuscher FW, van Aken WG, van Mourik JA, et al. Acquired, transient factor X (Stuart) deficiency in patient with mycoplasma pneumonia infection. *Scand J Haematol* 1979;23:257.

220. Currie MS, Stein AM, Rustagi PK, et al. Transient acquired factor X deficiency associated with pneumonia. *N Y State J Med* 1984;84:572.

221. Mulhare PE, Tracy PB, Golden EA, et al. A case of acquired factor X deficiency with *in vivo* and *in vitro* evidence of inhibitor activity directed against factor X. *Am J Clin Pathol* 1991;96:196.

222. Lankiewicz MW, Bell WR. A unique circulating inhibitor with specificity for coagulation factor X. *Am J Med* 1992;93:343.

223. Rao LV, Zivelin A, Iturbe I, et al. Antibody-induced acute factor X deficiency: clinical manifestations and properties of the antibody. *Thromb Haemost* 1994;72:363.

224. Matsunaga AT, Shafer FE. An acquired inhibitor to factor X in a pediatric patient with extensive burns. *J Pediatr Hematol Oncol* 1996;18:223.

225. Smith SV, Liles DK, White GC II, et al. Successful treatment of transient acquired factor X deficiency by plasmapheresis with concomitant intravenous immunoglobulin and steroid therapy. *Am J Hematol* 1998;57:245.

226. Ashrani AA, Aysola A, Al-Khatib H, et al. Lupus anticoagulant associated with transient severe factor X deficiency: a report of two patients presenting with major bleeding complications. *Br J Haematol* 2003;121:639.

227. Mumford AD, O'Donnell J, Gillmore JD, et al. Bleeding symptoms and coagulation abnormalities in 337 patients with AL-amyloidosis. *Br J Haematol* 2000;110:454.

228. Boggio L, Green D. Recombinant human factor VIIa in the management of amyloid-associated factor X deficiency. *Br J Haematol* 2001;112:1074.

229. Takabe K, Holman PR, Herbst KD, et al. Successful perioperative management of factor X deficiency associated with primary amyloidosis. *J Gastrointest Surg* 2004;8:358.

230. Beardell FV, Varma M, Martinez J. Normalization of plasma factor X levels in amyloidosis after plasma exchange. *Am J Hematol* 1997;54:68.

231. le Quellec A, Sotto A, Ciurana AJ. Spontaneous resolution of acquired factor X deficiency in amyloidosis. *J Intern Med* 1993;234:329.

232. Breems DA, Sonneveld P, de Man RA, et al. Successful treatment of systemic amyloidosis with hepatic involvement and factor X deficiency by high dose melphalan chemotherapy and autologous stem cell reinfusion. *Eur J Haematol* 2004;72:181.

233. Ghosh K, Shetty S, Pawar A, et al. Danazol therapy in factor X deficiency: more questions than answers. *Haemophilia* 2002;8:61.

234. Shapiro SS, Hultin M. Acquired inhibitors to the blood coagulation factors. *Semin Thromb Hemost* 1975;1:336.

235. Biggs R. Jaundice and antibodies directed against factor VIII and IX in patients treated for haemophilia or Christmas disease in the United Kingdom. *Br J Haematol* 1974;26:313.

236. Briet E, Reisner HM, Roberts HR. Inhibitors in Christmas disease. In: Hoyer LW, ed. *Factor VIII inhibitors.* New York: Alan R. Liss, 1984:123.

237. Gianelli F, Choo KH, Rees DJG, et al. Gene deletions in patients with hemophilia B and anti-factor IX antibodies. *Nature* 1983;303:181.

238. Ljung RC. Gene mutations and inhibitor formation in patients with hemophilia B. *Acta Haematol* 1995;94:49.

239. Reisner MM, Roberts HR, Krumhold S, et al. Immunochemical characterization of a polyclonal human antibody to factor IX. *Blood* 1977;50:11.

240. Pike IM, Yount WJ, Puritz EM, et al. Immunochemical characterization of a monoclonal gamma G4-lambda human antibody to factor IX. *Blood* 1972;40:1.

241. Giddings JC, Bloom AL, Kelly MA, et al. Human factor IX inhibitors: immunochemical characteristics and treatment with activated concentrate. *Clin Lab Haematol* 1983;5:165.

242. Orstavik KH. Alloantibodies to factor IX in hemophilia B characterized by crossed immunoelectrophoresis and enzyme-conjugated antisera to human immunoglobulins. *Br J Haematol* 1981;48:15.

243. Lusher JM, Arkin S, Abilgaard CF, et al. Recombinant factor VIII for the treatment of previously untreated patients with hemophilia A. Safety, efficacy and development of inhibitors. Kogenate Previously untreated patient Study Group. *N Engl J Med* 1993;328:453.

244. Lechner K. Factor IX inhibitors: report of two cases and a study of the biological, chemical, and immunological properties of the inhibitors. *Thromb Diath Haemorrh* 1971;25:447.

245. Roberts HR. Hemophiliacs with inhibitors, therapeutic options. *N Engl J Med* 1981;305:757.

246. Kasper CK, Aledort L, Aronson D, et al. A more uniform measurement of FVIII inhibitors. *Thromb Diath Haemorrh* 1975;34:612.

247. Kasper CK. Blood—its derivatives and its problems: factor IX. *Ann NY Acad Sci* 1975;240:172.

248. Boggio LN, Green D. Acquired hemophilia. *Rev Clin Exp Hematol* 2001;5:389.

249. Hedner U, Kisiel W. Use of human factor VIIa in the treatment of two hemophilia A patients with high-titer inhibitors. *J Clin Invest* 1983;71:1836.

250. Hedner U. Recombinant activated factor VII as a universal haemostatic agent. *Blood Coagul Fibrinolysis* 1998;9(Suppl. 1):S147.

251. Hedner U. Recombinant factor VIIa (Novoseven) as a hemostatic agent. *Semin Hematol* 2001;38(4 Suppl. 12):43.

252. Tomokiyo K, Teshima K, Nakatomi Y, et al. Induction of acquired factor IX inhibitors in cynomolgus monkey (Macaca fascicularis): a new primate model of hemophilia B. *Thromb Res* 2001;102:363.

253. Hedner U. Recombinant factor VIIa (NovoSeven) as a hemostatic agent. *Dis Mon* 2003;49:39.

254. Lusher JM, Roberts HR, Davignon G, et al. A randomized, double-blind comparison of two dosage levels of recombinant factor VIIa in the treatment of joint, muscle and mucocutaneous haemorrhages in persons with haemophilia A and B, with and without inhibitors. rFVIIa Study Group. *Haemophilia* 1998;4:790.

255. Lusher J. Recombinant factor VIIa (Novoseven) in the treatment of internal bleeding in patients with factor VII and IX inhibitors. *Haemostasis* 1996;26:S124.

256. Shapiro AD. American experience with home use of NovoSeven: recombinant factor VIIa in hemophiliacs with inhibitors. *Haemostasis* 1996;26(Suppl. 1):143.

257. Scharrer I. Recombinant factor VIIa for patients with inhibitors to factor VIII or IX or FVII deficiency. *Haemophilia* 1999;5:253.

258. Tomokiyo K, Nakatomi Y, Araki T, et al. A novel therapeutic approach combining human plasma-derived factors VIIa and X for haemophiliacs with inhibitors: evidence of a higher thrombin generation rate *in vitro* and more sustained haemostatic activity *in vivo* than obtained with factor VIIa alone. *Vox Sang* 2003;85:290.

259. Nilsson IM. Immune tolerance. *Semin Hematol* 1994;11:44.

260. Nilsson IM, Berntorp E, Zitterval O. Induction of split tolerance and clinical cure in high responding hemophiliacs with factor IX antibodies. *Proc Natl Acad Sci U S A* 1986;83:9169.

261. DiMichele DM, Kroner BL. The North American Immune Tolerance Registry: practices, outcomes, outcome predictors. *Thromb Haemost* 2002;87:52.

262. Sawamoto Y, Shima M, Yamamoto M, et al. Measurement of antifactor IX IgG subclasses in haemophilia B patients who developed inhibitors with episodes of allergic reactions to factor IX concentrates. *Thromb Res* 1996;83:279.

263. Warrier I, Ewenstein BM, Koerper MA, et al. Factor IX inhibitors and anaphylaxis in hemophilia B. *J Pediatr Hematol Oncol* 1997;19:23.

264. Largo R, Sigg P, Von Felten A, et al. Acquired factor-IX inhibitor in a non-hemophiliac patient with autoimmune disease. *Br J Haematol* 1974;26:129.

265. Miller K, Neeley JE, Krivit W, et al. Spontaneously acquired factor IX inhibitor in a nonhemophiliac child. *J Pediatr* 1978;93:232.

266. Collins HW, Gonzalez MF. Acquired factor IX inhibitor in a patient with adenocarcinoma of the colon. *Acta Haematol* 1984;71:49.

267. Mazzucconi MG, Peraino M, Bizzoni L, et al. Acquired inhibitor against factor IX in a child: successful treatment with high-dose immunoglobulin and dexamethasone. *Haemophilia* 1999;5:132.

268. Hinojosa-Lezama M, Bello-Gonzalez A, Munoz-Arizpe R, et al. Acquired coagulation factor IX deficiency in a patient with idiopathic nephrotic syndrome. *Bol Med Hosp Infant Mex* 1987;44:492.

269. Rahman F, Zanger B, Natelson EA. Factor IX deficiency in the nephrotic syndrome: studies with prothrombin complex concentrate. *J Urol* 1975;113:853.

270. Hanley JP, MacLean FR, Evans JL, et al. Hemorrhagic lymphadenopathy as a presenting feature of primary amyloidosis. *Pathology* 2000;32:21.

271. Billett HH, Rizvi S, Sawitsky A. Coagulation abnormalities in patients with Gaucher's disease: effect of therapy. *Am J Hematol* 1996;51:234.

272. Woodcock BE, Preston FE. Haemorrhage and factor IX deficiency in pituitary insufficiency. *Acta Haematol* 1983;70:205.

273. Peyvandi F, Mannucci PM, Asti D, et al. Clinical manifestations in 28 Italian and Iranian patients with severe Factor VII deficiency. *Haemophilia* 1997;3: 242.

274. Mariani G, Lo Coco L, Bernardi F, et al. Molecular and clinical aspects of factor VII deficiency. *Blood Coagul Fibrinolysis* 1998;9(Suppl. 1):S83.

275. Bernardi F, Liney DL, Patracchini P, et al. Molecular defects in CRM+ factor VII deficiencies: modelling of missense mutations in the catalytic domain of FVII. *Br J Haematol* 1994;86:610.

276. Kamikubo Y, Miyamoto S, Iwasa A, et al. Purification and characterization of factor VII inhibitor found in a patient with life threatening bleeding. *Thromb Haemost* 2000;83:60.

277. Mehta J, Singhal S, Mehta BC. Factor VII inhibitor. *J Assoc Physicians India* 1992;40:44.

278. Weisdorf D, Hasegawa D, Fair DS. Acquired factor VII deficiency associated with aplastic anaemia: correction with bone marrow transplantation. *Br J Haematol* 1989;71:409.

279. Birchfield GR, Rodgers GM, Girodias KW, et al. Hypoprothrombinemia associated with interleukin-2 therapy: correction with vitamin K. *J Immunother* 1992;11:71.

280. Biron C, Bengler C, Gris JC, et al. Acquired isolated factor VII deficiency during sepsis. *Haemostasis* 1997;27:51.

281. Martinez C, Mateo J, Perez M, et al. Severe bleeding in a patient with spontaneous factor VIII inhibitor and acute exacerbation of chronic pancreatitis. *Intensive Care Med* 1996;22:1278.

282. de Raucourt E, Dumont MD, Tourani JM, et al. Acquired factor VII deficiency associated with pleural liposarcoma. *Blood Coagul Fibrinolysis* 1994;5:833.

283. Ndimbie OK, Raman BK, Saeed SM. Lupus anticoagulant associated with specific inhibition of factor VII in a patient with AIDS. *Am J Clin Pathol* 1989;91:491.

284. Delmer A, Andreu G, Horellou MH, et al. Acquired factor VII inhibitor: treatment using high-dose immunoglobulins, corticotherapy and plasma exchange. *Ann Med Interne* 1988;139(Suppl. 1):48.

285. Nicolaisen EM, Hansen LL, Poulsen F, et al. Immunological aspects of recombinant factor VIIa (rFVIIa) in clinical use. *Thromb Haemost* 1996;76:200.

286. Mammen EF. Coagulation defects in liver disease. *Med Clin North Am* 1994;78:545.

287. Bernstein D. Effectiveness of the recombinant factor VIIa in patients with the coagulopathy of advanced Child's B & C cirrhosis. *Semin Thromb Hemost* 2000;26:437.

288. Uematsu M, Tsukaguchi M, Kinman K, et al. Case of factor VII deficiency with systemic amyloidosis having a unique clinical course such as splenic rupture. *Nippon Naika Gakkai Zasshi* 1997;86:314.

289. Elezovic I, Djukanovic R, Rolovic Z. Successful treatment of hemorrhagic syndrome due to an acquired, combined deficiency of factors VII and X in a patient with multiple myeloma and amyloidosis. *Eur J Haematol* 1989;42:105.

290. Delmer A, Horellou MH, Andreu G, et al. Life-threatening intracranial bleeding associated with the presence of an antifactor VII autoantibody. *Blood* 1989;74:229.

291. Deveras RA, Kessler CM. Reversal of warfarin-induced excessive anticoagulation with recombinant human factor VIIa concentrate. *Ann Intern Med* 2002;137:884.

292. Freeman WD, Brott TG, Barrett KM, et al. Recombinant factor VIIa for rapid reversal of warfarin anticoagulation in acute intracranial hemorrhage. *Mayo Clin Proc* 2004;79:1495.

293. McDonagh J, Duckert F. The influence of fibrin crosslinking on the kinetics of urokinase-induced clot lysis. *Br J Haematol* 1971;21:323.

294. DeVries A, Rosenberg T, Kochwa S, et al. Precipitating antifibrinogen antibody appearing after fibrinogen infusions in a patient with congenital afibrinogenemia. *Am J Med* 1961;30:486.

295. Marciniak E, Greenwood MF. Acquired coagulation inhibitor delaying fibrinopeptide release. *Blood* 1979;53:81.

296. Gris JC, Schved JF, Branger B, et al. Autoantibody to plasma fibrinopeptide A in a patient with a severe acquired haemorrhagic syndrome. *Blood Coagul Fibrinolysis* 1992;3:519.

297. Hoots WK, Carrell NA, Wagner RH, et al. A naturally occurring antibody that inhibits fibrin polymerization. *N Engl J Med* 1981;304:857.

298. Galanakis DK, Ginzler EM, Fikrig SM. Monoclonal IgG anticoagulants delaying fibrin aggregation in two patients with systemic lupus erythematosus (SLE). *Blood* 1978;52:1037.

299. Ghosh S, McEvoy P, McVerry BA. Idiopathic autoantibody that inhibits fibrin monomer polymerization. *Br J Haematol* 1983;53:65.

300. Lackner H. Hemostatic abnormalities associated with dysproteinemias. *Semin Hematol* 1973;10:125.

301. Cohen I, Amir J, Ben-Shaul Y, et al. Plasma cell myeloma associated with an unusual myeloma protein causing impairment of fibrin aggregation and platelet function in a patient with multiple malignancies. *Am J Med* 1970;48:766.

302. Coleman M, Vigliano EM, Weksler ME, et al. Inhibition of fibrin monomer polymerization by lambda myeloma globulins. *Blood* 1972;39:210.

303. Kondera-Anasz Z. Antibodies against fibrinogen in pregnant women, in post delivery women and in the newborns. *Thromb Haemost* 1998;79:963.

304. Board PG, Losowsky MS, Miloszewski KJ. Factor XIII: inherited and acquired deficiency. *Blood Rev* 1993;7:229.

305. Prasa D, Sturzebecher J. Inhibitors of factor XIIIa. *Hamostaseologie* 2002;22:43.

306. Lorand L, Jacobsen A, Bruner-Lorand J. A pathological inhibitor of fibrin cross-linking. *J Clin Invest* 1968;47:268.

307. Rosenberg RD, Colman RW, Lorand L. A new haemorrhagic disorder with defective fibrin stabilization and cryofibrinogenaemia. *Br J Haematol* 1974;26:269.

308. Ahmad F, Solymoss S, Poon MC, et al. Characterization of an acquired IgG inhibitor of coagulation factor XIII in a patient with systemic lupus erythematosus. *Br J Haematol* 1996;93:700.

309. Lorand L, Velasco PT, Hill JM, et al. Intracranial hemorrhage in systemic lupus erythematosus associated with an autoantibody against actor XIII. *Thromb Haemost* 2002;88:919.

310. Otis PT, Feinstein DI, Rapaport SI, et al. An acquired inhibitor of fibrin stabilization associated with isoniazid therapy: clinical and biochemical observations. *Blood* 1974;44:771.

311. Krumdieck R, Shaw DR, Huang ST, et al. Hemorrhagic disorder due to an isoniazid-associated acquired factor XIII inhibitor in a patient with Waldenstrom's macroglobulinemia. *Am J Med* 1991;90:639.

312. Lorand L, Campbell LK, Robertson BJ. Enzymatic coupling of isoniazid to proteins. *Biochemistry* 1972;11:434.

313. Milner GR, Holt PJ, Bottomley J, et al. Practolol therapy associated with a systemic lupus erythematosus-like syndrome and an inhibitor to factor XIII. *J Clin Pathol* 1977;30:770.

314. Dombret H, Scrobohaci ML, Ghorra P, et al. Coagulation disorders associated with acute promyelocytic leukemia: corrective effect of all-trans retinoic acid treatment. *Leukemia* 1993;7:2.

315. Rodeghiero F, Barbui T, Dal Belin-Peruffo A, et al. Defective fibrin crosslinking in acute leukemia. *Thromb Haemost* 1984;52:343.

316. Godal HC, Ly B. An inhibitor of activated factor XIII, inhibiting fibrin cross-linking but not incorporation of amine into casein. *Scand J Haematol* 1977;19:443.

317. Taubenfeld SM, Song Y, Sheng D, et al. A monoclonal antibody against a peptide sequence of fibrinogen gamma chain acts as an inhibitor of factor XIII-mediated crosslinking of human fibrin. *Thromb Haemost* 1995;74:923.

318. Lorand L, Maldonado N, Fradera J, et al. Haemorrhagic syndrome of autoimmune origin with a specific inhibitor against fibrin stabilizing factor (factor XIII). *Br J Haematol* 1972;23:17.

319. Tosetto A, Rodeghiero F, Gatto E, et al. An acquired hemorrhagic disorder of fibrin crosslinking due to IgG antibodies to FXIII, successfully treated with FXIII replacement and cyclophosphamide. *Am J Hematol* 1995;48:34.

320. Lorand L, Velasco PT, Rinne JR, et al. Autoimmune antibody (IgG Kansas) against the fibrin stabilizing factor (factor XIII) system. *Proc Natl Acad Sci U S A* 1988;85:232.

321. Arocha-Pinango CL, Guerrero B. Hemorrhagic syndrome induced by caterpillars. Clinical and experimental studies. *Invest Clin* 2003;44:155.

322. Arocha-Pinango CL, Guerrero B. Lonomia genus caterpillar envenomation: clinical and biological aspects. *Haemostasis* 2001;31:288.

323. Finney S, Seale L, Sawyer RT, et al. Tridegin, a new peptidic inhibitor of factor XIIIa, from the blood-sucking leech Haementeria ghilianii. *Biochem J* 1997;324:797.

324. Lorand L, Velasco PT, Murthy SN, et al. Autoimmune antibody in a hemorrhagic patient interacts with thrombin-activated factor XIII in a unique manner. *Blood* 1999;93:909.

325. Nakamura S, Kato A, Sakata Y, et al. Bleeding tendency caused by IgG inhibitor to factor XIII, treated successfully by cyclophosphamide. *Br J Haematol* 1988;68:313.

326. Green D. Spontaneous inhibitors to coagulation factors. *Clin Lab Haematol* 2000;22(Suppl. 1):21.

327. Gootenberg JE. Factor concentrates for the treatment of factor XIII deficiency. *Curr Opin Hematol* 1998;5:372.

# CHAPTER 72 ■ IMMUNE THROMBOCYTOPENIC PURPURA

JAMES N. GEORGE AND KIARASH KOJOURI

Immune thrombocytopenic purpura (ITP) is an acquired disease of children and adults, defined as isolated thrombocytopenia with no clinically apparent associated conditions or other causes of thrombocytopenia (1–3). No specific criteria establish the diagnosis of ITP; the diagnosis relies on the exclusion of other causes of thrombocytopenia (1). The clinical features of ITP in children and adults are distinct: childhood ITP typically has an acute onset and spontaneously resolves in most children within 6 months; ITP in adults typically has an insidious onset and spontaneous resolution is uncommon (1–3). Both sexes are equally affected in children (4,5). In adults, a female predominance is often described, but among older adults the incidence may be equal in women and men (6,7). Race is not mentioned in standard texts or reviews of ITP; a recent observation suggests that in the United States, ITP may be less common among blacks (8).

With the practice of routine platelet counts during the last 25 years, the apparent incidence of ITP has increased (6,7). Currently 30% to 40% of adult patients with ITP are asymptomatic, diagnosed only by the incidental observation of a low platelet count (6,7,9,10). The incidence of ITP in adults is estimated to be approximately 16 to 38 new cases per million population per year (6,7); in children the incidence is estimated to be approximately 53 new cases per million population per year (11). This discussion focuses on ITP in adults; ITP in children is discussed in Chapter 76.

## PATHOGENESIS

### Platelet Production and Destruction

Accelerated platelet destruction in ITP was first demonstrated by the legendary experiments of Harrington et al. in 1951 (12,13). When these investigators infused whole blood or plasma from patients with ITP into healthy volunteers, severe thrombocytopenia occurred. Subsequent studies by Shulman et al. (14,15) demonstrated that increasing doses of plasma caused more severe thrombocytopenia in healthy volunteers (see Fig. 72-1). In further experiments, these investigators were able to show that the ability to induce thrombocytopenia in healthy volunteers was greater with plasma from patients with more severe ITP, refractory to prednisone and splenectomy; in these experiments, they were able to establish a "titer" of ITP autoantibody (14). Higher doses of ITP plasma were required to cause thrombocytopenia in volunteers who had splenectomy than were required in healthy subjects, suggesting that the spleen is the major site of platelet destruction (Fig. 72-1) (15). Administration of prednisone to healthy subjects also diminished the thrombocytopenia caused by ITP plasma, but was not as protective as splenectomy (Fig. 72-1) (15). The protective effect of prednisone was different when different ITP plasmas were used, perhaps related to the autoantibody titer (15). Infusion of

ITP plasma into recipients with hereditary spherocytosis resulted in less thrombocytopenia despite their larger spleens, suggesting that platelet removal is reduced when reticuloendothelial clearance is saturated by accelerated red cell destruction, anticipating the therapeutic mechanism of intravenous γ globulin (IVIg) and anti-Rh(D) globulin (14). Shulman et al. also identified the plasma factor causing thrombocytopenia as a γ globulin, supporting its characterization as an antibody (15). These studies (14,15), from a different era of human investigation, established ITP as an immunologic disorder and provided the basis for understanding many of the clinical features of ITP and its treatment that were described during the subsequent 40 years.

Platelet kinetic studies using radiolabeled autologous platelets have demonstrated shortened intravascular survival consistent with platelet destruction as the primary mechanism of thrombocytopenia. Body surface imaging with $^{111}$In-oxine-labeled platelets has demonstrated splenic sequestration as the major site of platelet clearance in ITP (16–18). Platelet kinetic studies have also demonstrated that most patients have either normal or diminished platelet production rather than the anticipated compensatory increased platelet production (16,17,19,20). Diminished platelet production has been demonstrated in spite of the presence of normal or increased numbers of megakaryocytes with increased cell cycle activity (16). These data from platelet kinetic studies using autologous platelets may be more accurate than earlier studies using homologous platelets, which have a shorter survival in patients with ITP and therefore had suggested greater platelet turnover and production (16). However, autologous platelets may have a longer survival, and therefore underestimate platelet production, because they are a select population of younger platelets that have survived immunologic damage.

Serum thrombopoietin levels are normal in patients with ITP, not increased as in patients with amegakaryocytic thrombocytopenia or aplastic anemia, because of thrombopoietin binding to the normal or increased numbers of marrow megakaryocytes (21,22). Ineffective platelet production has been suggested morphologically by the demonstration of paraapoptosis in megakaryocytes from patients with ITP (23) and may be caused by the effect of antiplatelet antibodies on megakaryocytes and their progenitors (24–26). These observations may explain the apparent diminished platelet production response to the thrombocytopenia documented by platelet kinetic studies (16) and are the basis for current investigation of exogenous thrombopoietin as treatment of ITP (27,28).

### Antiplatelet Antibodies

Most platelet IgG is not antiplatelet antibody. Normal platelets contain two distinct pools of IgG: approximately 100 molecules of IgG on their surface and approximately 20,000 IgG molecules contained within α-granules (29). The α-granule contents of

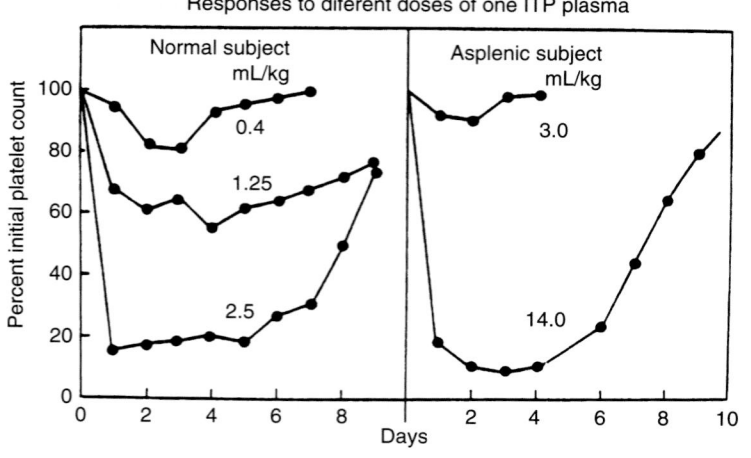

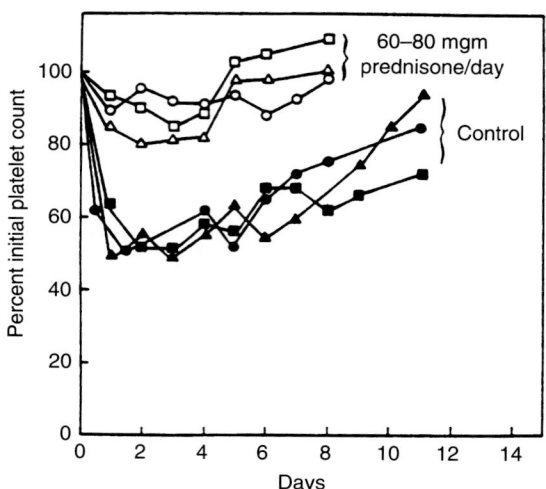

**FIGURE 72-1.** Response to infusions of plasma from patients with immune thrombocytopenic purpura (ITP) into healthy subjects. The **two left panels** illustrate the occurrence of thrombocytopenia in a healthy subject following different doses of plasma from a patient with ITP, and the results of infusion of the same ITP plasma into a splenectomized subject. Note that the ITP plasma dose that did not produce thrombocytopenia in the splenectomized subject was greater than the dose that produced marked thrombocytopenia in the healthy subject. The **right panel** illustrates the effect of prednisone on the response to ITP plasma. Plasma from one patient with ITP was infused into three healthy subjects without and with treatment with prednisone, 60 to 80 mg per day. Prednisone was begun 3 hours, 1 day, or 3 days before the plasma infusion and continued for a minimum of 7 days. The control infusions were given 1 and 2 months before, and 3 weeks after, the infusion with prednisone. (Adapted from Shulman NR, Weinrach RS, Libre EP, et al. The role of the reticuloendothelial system in the pathogenesis of idiopathic thrombocytopenic purpura. *Trans Assoc Am Physicians* 1965;78:374–390, with permission.)

IgG, IgA, IgM, and albumin are acquired by pinocytosis, and their concentrations mirror the plasma concentrations of these proteins (30). Patients with ITP have increased platelet concentrations of IgG as well as IgA, IgM, and albumin (30), probably due to increased platelet volume (31,32); many patients with apparently nonimmune etiologies for their thrombocytopenia also have high platelet concentrations of IgG (29,33).

Measures of antibody binding to specific platelet membrane glycoproteins detect antibodies in most patients with ITP, primarily with specificity for glycoprotein (GP) IIb/IIIa and/or GP Ib/IX (34–36). Viral infections, which commonly precede the onset of acute ITP in children (2), may exacerbate antiplatelet antibody–mediated thrombocytopenia through macrophage activation by γ-interferon production (37). Production of antiplatelet antibodies in ITP may be enhanced by the endogenous CD154 on the surface of activated platelets, which can drive CD40-dependent proliferation of B lymphocytes (38).

Assays for antiplatelet antibodies in ITP remain investigational and are not important for either diagnosis or management (1,2). In two studies that addressed the correlation between antiplatelet antibody tests results and clinical diagnosis, ITP could not be distinguished from gestational thrombocytopenia (39) or thrombocytopenias with a demonstrable alternative etiology (40). Another study reported that six of 18 patients with thrombocytopenia of apparent nonimmune etiology had serum antibodies to platelet GP IIb/IIIa (41), perhaps because neoepitopes are exposed on membrane proteins during accelerated platelet destruction by any mechanism, consistent with the observation that some antibodies to GP IIb/IIIa in patients with ITP react with normally concealed cytoplasmic epitopes (42).

### Platelet Function

Platelet function is typically normal or enhanced in patients with ITP (43). However, some patients appear to have impaired platelet function, perhaps related to antibody binding to epitopes close to the fibrinogen-binding site of GP IIb/IIIa (36).

Autoantibodies to GP IIb/IIIa and GP Ib/IX can cause functional platelet disorders indistinguishable from Glanzmann thrombasthenia (44) and Bernard-Soulier syndrome (45), respectively, but these disorders are rare. These observations suggest that platelet function may vary depending on the epitope specificity of the antiplatelet antibodies, and this may be partially responsible for the variable bleeding severity among patients with ITP with similar platelet counts.

## DIAGNOSIS

Isolated thrombocytopenia is the essential abnormality of ITP. The diagnosis is established by excluding pseudothrombocytopenia and other causes of true thrombocytopenia (1–3). The diagnosis of ITP is based principally on the history, physical examination, complete blood count, and examination of the peripheral blood smear. Further diagnostic studies are generally not indicated in the routine evaluation of patients with suspected ITP, assuming that the history, physical examination, and blood counts are compatible with the diagnosis of ITP and do not include atypical findings that are uncommon in ITP or suggest other etiologies (1). Marrow morphology in ITP is normal, with normal or increased numbers of megakaryocytes as well as normal erythropoiesis and myelopoiesis. Bone marrow examination is not necessary in most patients (46); however it may be appropriate for patients aged above 60 years because of concern for myelodysplasia (1), which may rarely present with isolated thrombocytopenia (47–49).

### Differential Diagnosis of Isolated Thrombocytopenia

#### Pseudothrombocytopenia

Multiple studies have reported a consistent incidence of pseudothrombocytopenia, 0.09% to 0.21%, in all subjects, healthy or ill, who have platelet counts (50–55). The falsely low platelet count is caused by *in vitro* clumping, detected by examination of the blood film made from the routine clinical laboratory EDTA-anticoagulated sample. Platelet clumps often appear in the leukocyte histogram and may cause a false elevation of the white blood cell count (55). The giant platelets of hereditary syndromes (see Chapters 65 and 66) may also cause falsely low platelet counts with corresponding falsely elevated white blood cell counts.

Platelet clumping is typically caused by a "naturally occurring" antibody to an epitope exposed on platelets by EDTA (56–58). The platelet epitope has been identified on GP IIb/IIIa by immunochemical techniques (59) and by the absence of clumping with platelets from patients with Glanzmann thrombasthenia (60,61). These platelet agglutinins appear to have no clinical importance; no abnormalities of hemostasis or thrombosis have been reported (57).

### Drug-Induced Thrombocytopenia

Drug-induced thrombocytopenia (see Chapter 73) may account for some of the acute thrombocytopenias that are diagnosed as ITP and appear to resolve spontaneously (7,62,63).

### Hereditary Thrombocytopenias

Hereditary thrombocytopenias (see Chapters 65 and 66) are usually recognized in infancy, but occasionally they may not be discovered until a later age, even adulthood, often after a mistaken diagnosis of ITP (64).

### Gestational Thrombocytopenia

The frequency of gestational thrombocytopenia in women admitted for labor and delivery is approximately 5% (65). Platelet counts are typically more than 70,000 per $\mu$L, with two thirds being between 130,000 and 150,000 per $\mu$L (65). When initially evaluating a woman with thrombocytopenia during pregnancy, the distinction between gestational thrombocytopenia and ITP is not possible because the diagnosis of both disorders requires the exclusion of other etiologies (1). In some women, gestational thrombocytopenia may not resolve for several months following delivery, further confusing the distinction from ITP (66–68). When

thrombocytopenia is initially encountered during pregnancy, ITP is the more likely diagnosis if thrombocytopenia occurs early during pregnancy or if the platelet count is less than 50,000 per $\mu$L during the third trimester or at term (1). For women whose platelet count recovers, thrombocytopenia may recur with a subsequent pregnancy (66). Because ITP, like other autoimmune disorders (69), can exacerbate during pregnancy, perhaps because of higher estrogen levels (70), it is possible that some women with gestational thrombocytopenia actually have mild and unrecognized ITP.

### Other Etiologies of Isolated Thrombocytopenia

Other conditions that may mimic ITP are chronic liver disease with hypersplenism, myelodysplastic syndromes (47–49), disseminated intravascular coagulation (71), and indolent infections such as tuberculosis (72).

## CLINICAL COURSE

The clinical features of ITP in adults can be estimated from large case series with long follow-up (see Table 72-1) (7,73). Although patients at any age who have an acute onset of thrombocytopenia may have a spontaneous remission, approximately one third of adults with ITP fail to achieve a complete remission following treatment with steroids and splenectomy (74,75). Data on mortality are imprecise. Although some experience suggests that ITP, even with severe thrombocytopenia, is a benign condition that very rarely causes hemorrhagic death (76), other estimates suggest a 5-year mortality rate of 2% among young adults and a much higher mortality among older adults (77). More recent case series (7,73) report lower mortality than earlier case series (77), probably because of better supportive care and the diagnosis of more patients with less severe ITP (Table 72-1). Bleeding symptoms are rare unless the thrombocytopenia is severe, less than 10,000 per $\mu$L, and even at this level most patients do not experience major bleeding episodes (78). At equivalent platelet counts, major hemorrhagic complications may be more common in patients aged above 60 years (9,79), but other observations suggest that older age does not increase the risk for bleeding (76). In patients who

### TABLE 72-1

#### THE CLINICAL COURSE OF IMMUNE THROMBOCYTOPENIC PURPURA

| Case series | Portielje et al. (73) | Neylon et al. (7) |
|---|---|---|
| Total patients | 134 | 245 |
| Patient accrual | 1974–1994 | 1993–1999 |
| Patients splenectomized | 78 (58%) | 30 (12%) |
| Patients with incomplete response to splenectomy | 27 (35%) | 7 (23%) |
| Patients who required additional treatment after splenectomy | NA | 0 |
| Deaths | 6 (4%) deaths related to ITP<br>2 (1%) caused by bleeding (1, early in course of ITP; 1, intracranial hemorrhage in a patient refractory to additional treatment following splenectomy)<br>4 (3%) caused by infection (1, pneumococcal sepsis after splenectomy; 3, related to immunosuppressive treatment) | 4 (2%) deaths related to ITP<br>3 (1%), gastrointestinal hemorrhage (1 at initial admission; 1 with lymphoma; 1 on warfarin) 1, postsplenectomy sepsis |

NA, data not reported.
The reports by Portielje et al. (73) and Neylon et al. (7) are inception cohorts of consecutive patients in their regions who had an initial diagnosis of immune thrombocytopenic purpura (ITP).

have persistent, severe, and symptomatic thrombocytopenia in spite of treatment, including splenectomy, mortality may be high (80,81). The treatment of ITP may actually be a more common cause of death than bleeding, as a result of immunosuppression and opportunistic infections (Table 72-1) (73,82).

# MANAGEMENT

## Initial Management

### Observation

Most patients who are incidentally discovered to have mild or moderate thrombocytopenia with no or negligible bleeding symptoms can be safely followed up with no treatment. The risk that more severe thrombocytopenia will subsequently develop is estimated by one case series to be 15%; in this series another 15% of patients with asymptomatic, incidentally discovered ITP recovered spontaneously; the remaining patients had persistent asymptomatic thrombocytopenia (10). Patients with platelet counts more than 30,000 per $\mu$L may be observed without treatment and without risk for significant hemorrhage (7,9,73). Patients with platelet counts more than 50,000 per $\mu$L do not have clinically important bleeding (78) and may safely undergo invasive procedures (83).

### Glucocorticoids

Glucocorticoids, typically given as oral prednisone, 1 mg/kg/day as a single dose, are appropriate for patients with symptomatic thrombocytopenia and for most adult patients who are initially diagnosed with platelet counts below 30,000 per $\mu$L (1). Most patients will increase their platelet count, reflecting increased production (84), as well as diminished platelet destruction (Fig. 72-1) (14). An alternative initial glucocorticoid regimen is dexamethasone, 40 mg per day for 4 days (85). In this study (85), 106 (85%) of 125 patients whose initial platelet counts were less than 20,000 per $\mu$L responded to platelet counts more than 50,000 per $\mu$L; 53 (50%) of the responding patients

maintained this safe platelet count with no further treatment. Long-term glucocorticoid treatment is not appropriate because of the high risk of osteoporosis, often within 3 months and even with a prednisone dose of only 5 mg per day (86).

### Intravenous Immunoglobulin (IVIg) and Anti-Rh(D)

Initial treatment with IVIg or anti-D has no advantage over prednisone for inducing a durable remission or preventing the need for splenectomy (87,88). These agents are appropriate therapy for attaining a prompt, transient increase of the platelet count to manage severe bleeding or to prepare a patient for an invasive procedure.

### Splenectomy

Splenectomy was an effective treatment of ITP for many years before the introduction of glucocorticoids in 1950 (89), resulting in durable complete responses, defined by a normal platelet count with no requirement for further treatment, in two thirds of patients (75). Common practice is to consider splenectomy in patients with persistent severe thrombocytopenia despite 4 to 6 weeks of glucocorticoid therapy (1). Splenectomy was performed much less frequently in the case series by Neylon et al. (7) (12% of all patients) than in the case series by Portielje et al. (73) (50% of all patients) (Table 72-1). This may reflect more recent patient accrual, 1993–1999 (7) compared to 1974–1994 (73) and recognition of more asymptomatic or minimally symptomatic patients. The major effects of splenectomy are (a) removal of the major site of destruction of antibody-sensitized platelets (Fig. 72-1) (14), explaining the prompt recovery of thrombocytopenia, and (b) removal of a major site of antibody synthesis. No preoperative features can accurately predict the response to splenectomy (75). Surgical complications are uncommon, especially with current laparoscopic techniques (see Table 72-2) (75).

Splenectomy is associated with surgical complications in approximately 10% of patients and surgery-related death in 0.2% to 0.75% of patients (Table 72-2). Surgery-related deaths are often attributed to bleeding complications in patients with severe ITP refractory to treatment; the higher mortality with laparotomy, compared to laparoscopy, may be because laparotomy is performed on patients with more severe ITP (75). Splenectomy

---

**TABLE 72-2**

RESULTS OF SPLENECTOMY FOR IMMUNE THROMBOCYTOPENIC PURPURA

**COMPLETE REMISSION FOLLOWING SPLENECTOMY:**
3,506 of 5,086 patients (69%) in 85 case series; complete remission was defined as a normal platelet count on no treatment for the total duration of observation following splenectomy

**DURABILITY OF COMPLETE REMISSIONS FOLLOWING SPLENECTOMY:**
Durability was documented by the observation that there was no correlation between complete response rates and duration of follow-up, 1–153 mo

**COMPLICATIONS OF SPLENECTOMY:**
Laparotomy: 12.9%
Laparoscopy: 9.6%

**DEATHS ATTRIBUTED TO SPLENECTOMY:**
Laparotomy:
  48 deaths among 4,955 patients (1%) in 81 case series; to compare laparotomy with laparoscopy during the same period, there was one death among 134 patients (0.75%) in five case series that accrued patients after 1991, the year of the earliest reported laparoscopic splenectomy
Laparoscopy:
  3 deaths among 1,301 patients (0.2%) in 29 case series

Data adapted from Kojouri K, Vesely SK, Terrell DR, et al. Splenectomy for adult patients with idiopathic thrombocytopenic purpura: a systematic literature review to assess long-term platelet count responses, prediction of response, and surgical complications. *Blood* 2004;104:2623–2634.

is associated with a small but significantly increased risk for severe infectious complications throughout the remainder of the patient's life (90). Therefore, it is recommended that all patients be immunized with polyvalent pneumococcal vaccine, *Haemophilus influenzae* b vaccine, and quadrivalent meningococcal polysaccharide vaccine at least 2 weeks before splenectomy (91). Splenectomy may also increase risk for thrombotic disorders, such as stroke, myocardial infarction, and pulmonary hypertension, many decades later (92–94).

## Management of Chronic Refractory Immune Thrombocytopenic Purpura

The proper management of adult patients who have not responded to glucocorticoids and splenectomy remains a dilemma (74). Many different treatment therapies have been reported, all with a suggestion of success (80,81). However the efficacy of all therapies is uncertain because the number of reported patients with severe thrombocytopenia is small, and many of these additional treatments have significant risks (74). Table 72-3 documents the results of a comprehensive search of all published reports on the treatment of patients with chronic refractory ITP, from 1966 through September 2003 (74). Articles were searched to identify patients who had ITP for more than 3 months, who had had splenectomy, and whose platelet count was less than 10,000 per μL. These are the patients who are at greatest risk for bleeding, who are most in need of treatment, but who are also most refractory to treatment. For all therapies, very few patients could be identified using these criteria (74). Table 72-3 reports the results of this literature analysis for 10 commonly considered therapies. The surprising result is how few patients with severe refractory ITP have been reported (74). This absence of information explains why management of these patients remains difficult and empirical.

### Observation

Because the goal of treatment of ITP is a safe platelet count, not a normal platelet count, it is appropriate to withhold further treatment in patients who have no or minimal bleeding symptoms and whose platelet counts are more than 10,000 to 20,000 per μL (1,7,73,78,105–107). Treatment decisions must include assessment of lifestyle, as well as other medical conditions that may influence the risks of bleeding and risks of immunosuppressive treatment.

### Immunosuppressive Regimens

In recent case series and reviews describing treatment of patients who were refractory to splenectomy (80,81,105,108), many different regimens were reported. If therapy is restricted to patients with severe and symptomatic thrombocytopenia, then therapy should be based on intensive immunosuppression. Less intensive therapies, such as *Helicobacter pylori* eradication, danazol, dapsone, colchicine, and many others, are most often reported in patients who may be satisfactorily managed with observation alone (80,81,105). An example of an intensive immunosuppressive regimen is the combination of cyclophosphamide (750 to 1,000 mg per m$^2$ by intravenous bolus on day 1) (109), vincristine (2 mg by intravenous bolus on day 1), and methylprednisolone (1,000 mg by intravenous bolus on days 1–3) (110), a regimen commonly used for low-grade lymphoma. High-dose cyclophosphamide (50 mg/kg/day for 4 days) with autologous peripheral blood stem cell support has been successful to achieve long-term responses for patients with refractory ITP and life-threatening bleeding complications (111).

### Rituximab

A more selective immunosuppressive agent is the anti-CD20 monoclonal antibody, rituximab, that was developed for patients

---

**TABLE 72-3**

RESPONSE TO TREATMENT OF PATIENTS WITH CHRONIC REFRACTORY IMMUNE THROMBOCYTOPENIC PURPURA

| Treatment | Patients | Response | | |
|---|---|---|---|---|
| | | CR | PR | NR |
| Rituximab | 21 | 6 | 7 | 8 |
| Cyclophosphamide | 20 | 8 | 7 | 9 |
| Azathrioprine | 16 | 4 | 12 | 0 |
| Danazol | 15 | 0 | 14 | 1 |
| Dexamethasone | 11 | 3 | 7 | 1 |
| Vinca alkaloids | 8 | 0 | 5 | 3 |
| High-dose cyclophosphamide with stem cell support | 5 | 2 | 2 | 1 |
| Interferon | 3 | 1 | 1 | 1 |
| Accessory splenectomy | 2 | 2 | 0 | 0 |
| Cyclosporine | 1 | 0 | 1 | 0 |

Chronic refractory immune thrombocytopenic purpura (ITP) was defined as thrombocytopenia with a platelet count less than 50,000 per μL following splenectomy and duration of at least 3 months since diagnosis of ITP (74). Complete response (CR) was defined as achievement and maintenance of a normal platelet count (>150,000 per μL, or as defined in the original report) on no treatment for at least 3 months and for the duration of observation. Partial response (PR) was defined as achievement of a platelet count more than 50,000 per μL for any duration, with or without additional treatment, excluding patients who qualified for CR. No response (NR) was defined as failure to increase the platelet count to more than 50,000 per μL.
Data are adapted from Vesely SK, Perdue JJ, Rizvi MA, et al. Management of adult patients with idiopathic thrombocytopenic purpura after failure of splenectomy. A systematic review. *Ann Intern Med* 2004;140:112–120. Data for rituximab have been updated by review of additional case series published through October 2005 and described in detail in Table 72-4.

with low-grade B-cell lymphoma and has been used for a variety of autoimmune disorders. The advantage of rituximab is the targeted elimination of B cells, avoiding the risk of marrow suppression that may occur with nonspecific immunosuppressive agents that may also cause diminished platelet production. Although severe adverse reactions caused by rituximab have been reported, including allergic reactions, immunosuppression (112), interstitial pneumonitis (113), and severe neutropenia (114), these are rare. Rituximab has also been reported to cause thrombocytopenia (115). Table 72-4 presents a summary of case series of patients with ITP treated with rituximab, describing results of treatment for patients who had platelet counts less than 30,000 per $\mu$L and less than 10,000 per $\mu$L. More than half of patients in these case series had platelet counts above 30,000 per $\mu$L and some therefore may have been safely managed by observation alone. These data suggest that rituximab results in complete remissions in approximately 30% of patients, equivalent to the best reported results using other immunosuppressive agents (Table 72-3) (74). Therefore, rituximab may be appropriate initial therapy for patients who have persistent, severe, and symptomatic thrombocytopenia after splenectomy.

## Investigational Therapy

A novel approach to the management of patients with ITP is to increase platelet production by administration of a thrombopoietic agent. The value of this approach is avoidance of the risk for immune suppression and suppression of platelet production. The basis for this approach is the observations that most patients with ITP do not have maximum platelet production (16,17,19,20) and their serum thrombopoietin levels are not increased (21,22). The initial report of efficacy in four patients with ITP used pegylated recombinant human megakaryocyte growth and development factor (27). A potential risk of this agent is the development of antibodies that can neutralize native thrombopoietin, causing prolonged thrombocytopenia or pancytopenia (116). To avoid this risk, a thrombopoietic protein has been developed that has no sequence homology to native thrombopoietin but still stimulates megakaryocytopoiesis by binding to the thrombopoietin receptor, Mpl (117). Experience with this compound has demonstrated platelet count responses in both healthy subjects and patients with ITP (28).

## TABLE 72-4

RESULTS OF RITUXIMAB TREATMENT FOR PATIENTS WITH CHRONIC REFRACTORY IMMUNE THROMBOCYTOPENIC PURPURA

| Case series | Patients (no.) | Follow-up (mo) | CR | PR | NR |
|---|---|---|---|---|---|
| Perotta (96) | 10 | 1–14 | | | |
| Platelet counts <30,000 | 6 | | 2 | 3 | 1 |
| Platelet counts <10,000 | 4 | | 2 | 1 | 1 |
| Grossi (97) | 5 | 6 | | | |
| Platelet counts <30,000 | 3 | | 1 | 0 | 2 |
| Platelet counts <10,000 | 3 | | 1 | 0 | 2 |
| Saleh (98) | 12 | 3 | | | |
| Platelet counts <30,000 | 3 | | 0 | 1 | 4 |
| Platelet counts <10,000 | 3 | | 0 | 0 | 1 |
| Stasi (99) | 25 | 3 | | | |
| Platelet counts <30,000 | 8 | | 1 | 5 | 2 |
| Platelet counts <10,000 | 2 | | 0 | 2 | 0 |
| Giagounidis (100) | 12 | 10 | | | |
| Platelet counts <10,000 | 11 | | 4 | 4 | 3 |
| Stasi (101) | 7 | 4 | | | |
| Platelet counts <30,000 | 3 | | 1 | 2 | 0 |
| Platelet counts <10,000 | 2 | | 1 | 1 | 0 |
| Zaja (102) | 20 | 6 | | | |
| Platelet counts <30,000 | 2 | | 1 | 1 | 0 |
| Platelet counts <10,000 | 0 | | – | – | – |
| Shanafelt (103) | 12 | 1–10 | | | |
| Platelet counts <30,000 | 9 | | 2 | 3 | 4 |
| Platelet counts <10,000 | 9 | | 2 | 3 | 4 |
| All case series: | 103 | | | | |
| Platelet counts <30,000 | 47 | | 12 (26%) | 19 (40%) | 16 (34%) |
| Platelet counts <10,000 | 21 | | 6 (29%) | 7 (33%) | 8 (33%) |

Chronic refractory immune thrombocytopenic purpura (ITP) was defined as thrombocytopenia with a platelet count less than 30,000 per $\mu$L following splenectomy and duration of at least 3 months since diagnosis of ITP (74). Patients with these clinical features were selected from the case series for presentation in this table. Additional analyses were done on patients with platelet counts greater than 10,000 per $\mu$L. Complete response (CR) was defined as achievement and maintenance of a normal platelet count (>150,000 per $\mu$L, or as defined in the original report) on no treatment for at least 3 months and for the duration of observation. Partial response (PR) was defined as achievement of a platelet count more than 30,000 per $\mu$L for any duration, with or without additional treatment, excluding patients who qualified for CR. No response (NR) was defined as failure to increase the platelet count to more than 30,000 per $\mu$L (74). Only case series with five or more patients treated with rituximab were included in this analysis. Duration of ITP before treatment with rituximab was not mentioned in case series reported by Perotta (96), Grossi (97), Saleh (98), and Giagounidis (100). An additional case series describing 57 patients with ITP treated with rituximab was not included in Table 72-3 because it combined 32 previously reported patients (99,101) with 25 unreported patients (104); also this case series did not distinguish splenectomized from nonsplenectomized patients (104).
Data are adapted from Vesely SK, Perdue JJ, Rizvi MA, et al. Management of adult patients with idiopathic thrombocytopenic purpura after failure of splenectomy. A systematic review. *Ann Intern Med* 2004;140:112–120, plus review of additional case series published through October 2005.

## Management of Immune Thrombocytopenic Purpura During Pregnancy

The greatest concern for ITP during pregnancy comes as delivery approaches and the risks of thrombocytopenia in the newborn infant must be considered. Although published data vary widely on the risk of thrombocytopenia in infants born to mothers with ITP (1), a summary of published case series suggests that there is approximately a 10% risk of having a platelet count of 50,000 per μL and approximately a 4% risk of having a platelet count of less than 20,000 per μL (118,119). The severity of ITP in the mother appears to correlate with the risk for thrombocytopenia in the infant; neonatal thrombocytopenia is more frequent when the mother has had a splenectomy or when her platelet count has been less than 50,000 per μL at some time during the pregnancy (120,121). The occurrence of neonatal thrombocytopenia is similar among siblings (119,121). Current recommendations are to manage the delivery in a conventional manner, with cesarean delivery only for obstetrical indications (1,119,122,123). The critical complication of neonatal intracerebral hemorrhage at birth is very rare (118,120,121). It is important to carefully monitor the infant's platelet counts through the first several days of life, as severe thrombocytopenia and major hemorrhage can develop after delivery (1,120–122,124) related to maturation of splenic function (125,126).

## *References*

1. George JN, Woolf SH, Raskob GE, et al. Idiopathic thromboctyopenic purpura: a practice guideline developed by explicit methods for the American Society of Hematology. *Blood* 1996;88:3–40.
2. British Committee for Standards in Haematology. Guidelines for the investigation and management of idiopathic thrombocytopenic purpura in adults, children and in pregnancy. *Br J Haematol* 2003;120:574–596.
3. Cines DB, Blanchette VS. Immune thrombocytopenic purpura. *N Engl J Med* 2002;346:995–1008.
4. Hedman A, Henter JI, Hedlund I, et al. Prevalence and treatment of chronic idiopathic thrombocytopenic purpura of childhood in Sweden. *Acta Paediatr* 1997;86:226–227.
5. Bolton-Maggs PHB, Moon I. Assessment of UK practice for management of acute childhood idiopathic thrombocytopenic purpura against published guidelines. *Lancet* 1997;350:620–623.
6. Frederiksen H, Schmidt K. The incidence of ITP in adults increases with age. *Blood* 1999;94:909–913.
7. Neylon AJ, Saunders PWG, Howard MR, et al. Clinically significant newly presenting autoimmune thrombocytopenic purpura in adults: a prospective study of a population-based cohort of 245 patients. *Br J Haematol* 2003;122:966–974.
8. Terrell DR, Johnson KR, Vesely SK, et al. Is immune thrombocytopenic purpura less common among black Americans? *Blood* 2005;105:1368–1369.
9. Cortelazzo S, Finazzi G, Buelli M, et al. High risk of severe bleeding in aged patients with chronic idiopathic thrombocytopenic purpura. *Blood* 1991;77:31–33.
10. Stasi R, Stipa E, Masi M, et al. Long-term observation of 208 adults with chronic idiopathic thrombocytopenic purpura. *Am J Med* 1995;98:436–442.
11. Zeller B, Helgestad J, Hellebostad M, et al. Immune thrombocytopenic purpura in childhood in Norway: a prospective, population-based registration. *Pediatr Hematol Oncol* 2000;17:551–558.
12. Harrington WJ, Minnich V, Hollingsworth JW, et al. Demonstration of a thrombocytopenic factor in the blood of patients with thrombocytopenic purpura. *J Lab Clin Med* 1951;38:1.
13. Altman LK. *Black and blue at the flick of a feather. Who goes first?* New York: Random House, 1987:273–282.
14. Shulman NR, Weinrach RS, Libre EP, et al. The role of the reticuloendothelial system in the pathogenesis of idiopathic thrombocytopenic purpura. *Trans Assoc Am Physicians* 1965;78:374–390.
15. Shulman NR, Marder VJ, Weinrach RS. Similarities between known antiplatelet antibodies and the factor responsible for thrombocytopenia in idiopathic purpura. Physiologic, serologic and isotopic studies. *Ann N Y Acad Sci* 1965;124:499–542.
16. Ballem PJ, Segal GM, Stratton JR, et al. Mechanisms of thrombocytopenia in chronic autoimmune thrombocytopenia purpura. Evidence for both impaired platelet production and increased platelet clearance. *J Clin Invest* 1987;80:33–40.
17. Siegel RS, Rae JL, Barth S, et al. Platelet survival and turnover: important factors in predicting response to splenectomy in immune thrombocytopenic purpura. *Am J Hematol* 1989;30:206–212.
18. Stratton JR, Ballem PJ, Gernsheimer T, et al. Platelet destruction in autoimmune thrombocytopenic purpura: kinetics and clearance of indium-111-labeled autologous platelets. *J Nucl Med* 1989;30:629–637.
19. Tomer A, Hanson SR, Harker LA. Autologous platelet kinetics in patients with severe thrombocytopenia: discrimination between disorders of production and destruction. *J Lab Clin Med* 1991;118:546–554.
20. Ballem PJ, Belzberg A, Devine DV, et al. Kinetic studies of the mechanism of thrombocytopenia in patients with human immunodeficiency virus infection. *N Engl J Med* 1992;327:1779–1784.
21. Kappers-Klunne MC, De Haan M, Struijk PC, et al. Serum thrombopoietin levels in relation to disease status in patients with immune thrombocytopenic purpura. *Br J Haematol* 2001;115:1004–1006.
22. Aledort L, Hayward CPM, Chen M-G, et al. Prospective screening of 205 patients with ITP, including diagnosis, serological markers, and the relationship between platelet counts, endogenous thrombopoietin, and circulating antithrombopoietin antibodies. *Am J Hematol* 2004;76:205–213.
23. Houweerzijl EJ, Blom NR, van der Want JJL, et al. Ultrastructural study shows morphologic features of apoptosis and para-apoptosis in megakaryocytes from patients with idiopathic thrombocyotpenic purpura. *Blood* 2004;103:500–506.
24. Takahashi R, Sekine N, Nakatake T. Influence of monoclonal antiplatelet glycoprotein antibodies on *in vitro* human megakaryocyte colony formation and proplatelet formation. *Blood* 1999;93:1951–1958.
25. McMillan R, Wang L, Tomer A, et al. Suppression of *in vitro* megakaryocyte production by antiplatelet autoantibodies from adult patients with chronic ITP. *Blood* 2004;103:1364–1369.
26. Chang M, Nakagawa PA, Williams SA, et al. Immune thrombocytopenic purpura (ITP) plasma and purified ITP monoclonal autoantibodies inhibit megakaryocytopoiesis *in vitro*. *Blood* 2003;102:887–895.
27. Nomura S, Dan K, Hotta T, et al. Effects of pegylated recombinant human megakaryocyte growth and development factor in patients with idiopathic thrombocytopenia purpura. *Blood* 2002;100:728–730.
28. Kuter DJ, Bussel JB, Aledort L, et al. A phase 2 placebo controlled study evaluating the platelet count and safety of weekly dosing with a novel thrombopoietic protein (AMG531) in thrombocytopenic adult patients with immune thrombocytopenic purpura. *Blood* 2004;104:148a–149a.
29. George JN. Platelet immunoglobulin G: its significance for the evaluation of thrombocytopenia and for understanding the origin of alpha-granule proteins. *Blood* 1990;76(5):859–870.
30. George JN, Saucerman S. Platelet IgG, IgA, IgM, and albumin: correlation of platelet and plasma concentrations in normal subjects and in patients with ITP or dysproteinemia. *Blood* 1988;72:362–365.
31. Levin J, Bessman JD. The inverse relation between platelet volume and platelet number. *J Lab Clin Med* 1983;101:295–307.
32. Tavassoli M. Stress platelet: a platelet equivalent of stress reticulocyte. *Blood Cells* 1992;18:295–300.
33. Kelton JG, Powers P, Carter C. A prospective study of the usefulness of the measurement of platelet-associated IgG for the diagnosis of idiopathic thrombocytopenic purpura. *Blood* 1982;60:1050–1053.
34. He R, Reid DM, Jones CE, et al. Spectrum of Ig classes, specificities, and titers of serum antiglycoproteins in chronic idiopathic thrombocytopenic purpura. *Blood* 1994;83:1024–1032.
35. Berchtold P, Wenger M. Autoantibodies against platelet glycoproteins in autoimmune thrombocytopenic purpura: their clinical significance and response to treatment. *Blood* 1993;81:1246–1250.
36. Kosugi S, Tomiyama Y, Honda S, et al. Platelet-associated anti-GPIIb-IIIa autoantibodies in chronic immune thrombocytopenic purpura recognizing epitopes close to the ligand-binding site of glycoprotein (GP) IIb. *Blood* 2001;98:1819–1827.
37. Musaji A, Cormont F, Thirion G, et al. Exacerbation of autoantibody-mediated thrombocytopenic purpura by infection with viruses. *Blood* 2004;104:2102–2106.
38. Solanilla A, Pasquet JM, Viallard JF, et al. Platelet-associated CD154 in immune thrombocytopenic purpura. *Blood* 2005;105:215–218.
39. Lescale KB, Eddleman KA, Cines DB, et al. Antiplatelet antibody testing in thrombocytopenic pregnant women. *Am J Obstet Gynecol* 1996;174:1014–1018.
40. Raife TJ, Olson JD, Lentz SR. Platelet antibody testing in idiopathic thrombocytopenic purpura. *Blood* 1997;89:1112–1113.
41. Kekomaki R, Dawson B, McFarland J, et al. Localization of human platelet autoantigens to the cysteine-rich region of glycoprotein IIIa. *J Clin Invest* 1991;88:847–854.
42. Fujisawa K, O'Toole TE, Tani P, et al. Autoantibodies to the presumptive cytoplasmic domain of platelet glycoprotein IIIa in patients with chronic immune thrombocytopenic purpura. *Blood* 1991;77:2207–2213.
43. Harker LA, Slichter SJ. The bleeding time as a screening test for the evaluation of platelet function. *N Engl J Med* 1972;287:155–159.
44. Balduini CL, Bertolino G, Noris P, et al. Defect of platelet aggregation and adhesion induced by autoantibodies against platelet glycoprotein IIIa. *Thromb Haemost* 1992;68:208–213.
45. Varon D, Gitel SN, Varon N, et al. Immune Bernard Soulier-like syndrome associated with anti-glycoprotein-IX antibody. *Am J Hematol* 1992;41:67–68.
46. Jubelirer SJ, Harpold R. The role of the bone marrow examination in the diagnosis of immune thrombocytopenic purpura: case series and literature review. *Clin Appl Thromb Hemost* 2002;8:73–76.

47. Najean Y, Lecompte T. Chronic pure thrombocytopenia in elderly patients: an aspect of the myelodysplastic syndrome. *Cancer* 1989;64:2506–2510.
48. Menke DM, Colon-Otero G, Cockerill KJ, et al. Refractory thrombocytopenia: a myelodysplastic syndrome that may mimic immune thrombocytopenic purpura. *Am J Clin Pathol* 1992;98:502–510.
49. Kuroda J, Kimura S, Kobayashi Y, et al. Unusual myelodysplastic syndrome with the initial presentation mimicking idiopathic thrombocytopenic purpura. *Acta Haematol* 2002;108:139–143.
50. Payne BA, Pierre RV. Pseudothrombocytopenia: a laboratory artifact with potentially serious consequences. *Mayo Clin Proc* 1984;59:123–125.
51. Savage RA. Pseudoleukocytosis due to EDTA-induced platelet clumping. *Am J Clin Pathol* 1984;81:317–322.
52. Vicari A, Banfi G, Bonini PA. EDTA-dependent pseudothrombocytopaenia: a 12-month epidemiological study. *Scand J Clin Lab Invest* 1988;48:537–542.
53. Garcia Suarez J, Calero MA, Ricard MP, et al. EDTA-dependent pseudothrombocytopenia in ambulatory patients: clinical characteristics and role of new automated cell-counting in its detection. *Am J Hematol* 1992;39:146–147.
54. Sweeney JD, Holme S, Heaton WAL, et al. Pseudothrombocytopenia in plateletpheresis donors. *Transfusion* 1995;35:46–49.
55. Bartels PCM, Schoorl M, Lombarts AJPF. Screening for EDTA-dependent deviations in platelet counts and abnormalities in platelet distribution histograms in pseudothrombocytopenia. *Scand J Clin Lab Invest* 1997;57:629–636.
56. Onder O, Weinstein A, Hoyer LW. Pseudothrombocytopenia caused by platelet agglutinins that are reactive in blood anticoagulated with chelating agents. *Blood* 1980;56:177–182.
57. Bizzaro N. EDTA-dependent pseudothrombocytopenia: a clinical and epidemiological study of 112 cases, with 10-year follow-up. *Am J Hematol* 1995;50:103–109.
58. Hoyt RH, Durie BGM. Pseudothrombocytopenia induced by a monoclonal IgM kappa platelet agglutinin. *Am J Hematol* 1989;31:50–52.
59. Fiorin F, Steffan A, Pradella P, et al. IgG platelet antibodies in EDTA-dependent pseudothrombocytopenia bind to platelet membrane glycoprotein IIb. *Am J Clin Pathol* 1998;110:178–183.
60. Bizzaro N, Goldschmeding R, von dem Borne AEGK. Platelet satellitism is Fcgamma RIII (CD16) receptor-mediated. *Am J Clin Pathol* 1995;103:740–744.
61. Casonato A, Bertomoro A, Pontara E, et al. EDTA dependent pseudothrombocytopenia caused by antibodies against the cytoadhesive receptor of platelet gpIIB-IIIA. *J Clin Pathol* 1994;47:625–630.
62. Kaufman DW, Kelly JP, Johannes CB, et al. Acute thrombocytopenic purpura in relation to the use of drugs. *Blood* 1993;82:2714–2718.
63. George JN, Raskob GE, Shah SR, et al. Drug-induced thrombocytopenia: a systematic review of published case reports. *Ann Intern Med* 1998;129:886–890.
64. Drachman JG. Inherited thrombocytopenia: when a low platelet count does not mean ITP. *Blood* 2004;103:390–398.
65. Burrows RF, Kelton JG. Fetal thrombocytopenia and its relation to maternal thrombocytopenia. *N Engl J Med* 1993;329:1463–1466.
66. Anteby E, Shalev O. Clinical relevance of gestational thrombocytopenia of < 100,000/ml. *Am J Hematol* 1994;47:118–122.
67. Ruggeri M, Schiavotto C, Castaman G, et al. Gestational thrombocytopenia: a prospective study. *Haematologica* 1997;82:341–342.
68. Ajzenberg N, Dreyfus M, Kaplan C, et al. Pregnancy-associated thrombocytopenia revisited: assessment and follow-up of 50 cases. *Blood* 1998;92:4573–4580.
69. Chaplin H, Cohen R, Bloomberg G, et al. Pregnancy and idiopathic autoimmune haemolytic anaemia: a prospective study during 6 months gestation and 3 months post-partum. *Br J Haematol* 1973;24:219–229.
70. Onel K, Bussel JB. Adverse effects of estrogen therapy in a subset of women with ITP. *J Thromb Haemost* 2004;2:670–671.
71. Mosesson MW, Colman RW, Sherry S. Chronic intravascular coagulation syndrome. Report of a case with special studies of an associated plasma cryoprecipitate ("Cryofibrinogen"). *N Engl J Med* 1968;278:815–821.
72. Ghobrial MW, Albornoz MA. Immune thrombocytopenia: a rare presenting manifestation of tuberculosis. *Am J Hematol* 2001;67:139–143.
73. Portielje JEA, Westendorp RGJ, Kluin-Nelemans HC, et al. Morbidity and mortality in adults with idiopathic thrombocytopenic purpura. *Blood* 2001;97:2549–2554.
74. Vesely SK, Perdue JJ, Rizvi MA, et al. Management of adult patients with idiopathic thrombocytopenic purpura after failure of splenectomy. A systematic review. *Ann Intern Med* 2004;140:112–120.
75. Kojouri K, Vesely SK, Terrell DR, et al. Splenectomy for adult patients with idiopathic thrombocytopenic purpura: a systematic literature review to assess long-term platelet count responses, prediction of response, and surgical complications. *Blood* 2004;104:2623–2634.
76. Vianelli N, Valdre L, Fiacchini M, et al. Long-term follow-up of idiopathic thrombocytopenic purpura in 310 patients. *Haematologia* 2001;86:504–509.
77. Cohen YC, Djulbegovic B, Shamai-Lubovitz O, et al. The bleeding risk and natural history of idiopathic thrombocytopenic purpura in patients with persistent low platelet count. *Arch Intern Med* 2000;160:1630–1638.
78. Lacey JV, Penner JA. Management of idiopathic thrombocytopenic purpura in the adult. *Semin Thromb Hemost* 1977;3:160–174.
79. Guthrie TH, Brannan DP, Prisant LM. Idiopathic thrombocytopenic purpura in the older adult patient. *Am J Med Sci* 1988;296:17–21.
80. Bourgeois E, Caulier MT, Delarozee C, et al. Long-term follow-up of chronic autoimmune thrombocytopenic purpura refractory to splenectomy: a prospective analysis. *Br J Haematol* 2003;120:1079–1088.
81. McMillan R, Durette C. Long-term outcomes in adults with chronic ITP after splenectomy failure. *Blood* 2004;104:956–960.
82. Apostolidis J, Tsandekidi M, Kousiafes D, et al. Short-course corticosteroid-induced pulmonary and apparent cerebral aspergillosis in a patient with idiopathic thrombocytopenic purpura. *Blood* 2001;98:2875–2877.
83. McVay PA, Toy PTCY. Lack of increased bleeding after liver biopsy in patients with mild hemostatic abnormalities. *Am J Clin Pathol* 1990;94:747–753.
84. Gernsheimer T, Stratton J, Ballem PJ, et al. Mechanisms of response to treatment in autoimmune thrombocytopenic purpura. *N Engl J Med* 1989;320:974–980.
85. Cheng Y, Wong RSM, Soo YOY, et al. Initial treatment of immune thrombocytopenic purpura with high-dose dexamethasone. *N Engl J Med* 2003;349:831–836.
86. van Staa TP, Leufkens HGM, Cooper C. The epidemiology of corticosteroid-induced osteoporosis: a meta-analysis. *Osteoporos Int* 2002;13:777–787.
87. Jacobs P, Wood L, Novitzky N. Intravenous gammaglobulin has no advantages over oral corticosteroids as primary therapy for adults with immune thrombocytopenia: a prospective randomized clinical trial. *Am J Med* 1994;97:55–59.
88. George JN, Raskob GE, Vesely SK, et al. Initial management of immune thrombocytopenic purpura in adults: a randomized controlled trial comparing intermittent anti-D with routine care. *Am J Hematol* 2003;74:161–169.
89. Doan CA, Bouroncle BA, Wiseman BK. Idiopathic and secondary thrombocytopenic purpura: clinical study and evaluation of 381 cases over a period of 28 years. *Ann Intern Med* 1960;53:861–876.
90. Schilling RF. Estimating the risk for sepsis after splenectomy in hereditary spherocytosis. *Ann Intern Med* 1995;122:187–188.
91. Centers for Disease Control and Prevention. Recommendations of the Advisory Committee on Immunization Practices: use of vaccines and immune globulins in persons with altered immunocompetence. *Morb Mortal Wkly Rep* 1993;42:1–18.
92. Robinette CD, Fraumeni JF. Splenectomy and subsequent mortality in veterans of the 1939-1945 war. *Lancet* 1977;2:127–129.
93. Schilling RF. Spherocytosis, splenectomy, strokes, and heart attacks. *Lancet* 1997;350:1677–1678.
94. Hoeper MM, Niedermeyer J, Hoffmeyer F, et al. Pulmonary hypertension after splenectomy? *Ann Intern Med* 1999;130:506–509.
95. Drachman JG, Jarvik GP, Mehaffey MG. Autosomal dominant thrombocytopenia: incomplete megakaryocyte differentiation and linkage to human chromosome 10. *Blood* 2000;96:118–125.
96. Perotta A, Sunneberg TA, Scott J, et al. Rituxan in the treatment of chronic idiopathic thrombocytopenic purpura (ITP). *Blood* 1999;94:14a.
97. Grossi A, Santini V, Longo G, et al. Treatment with anti-CD 20 antibodies of patients with autoimmune thrombocytopenia with or without haemolytic anemia; worsening in hemoglobin level. *Blood* 2000;96:253a.
98. Saleh MN, Gutheil J, Moore M, et al. A pilot study of the anti-CD20 monoclonal antibody rituximab in patients with refractory immune thrombocytopenia. *Semin Oncol* 2000;27(6S12):99–103.
99. Stasi R, Pagano A, Stipa E, et al. Rituximab chimeric anti-CD20 monoclonal antibody treatment for adults with chronic idiopathic thrombocytopenic purpura. *Blood* 2001;98:952–957.
100. Giagounidis AA, Anhuf J, Schneider P, et al. Treatment of relapsed idiopathic thrombocytopenic purpura with the anti-CD20 monoclonal antibody rituximab: a pilot study. *Eur J Haematol* 2002;69:95–100.
101. Stasi R, Stipa E, Forte V, et al. To the editor: variable patterns of response to rituximab treatment in adults with chronic idiopathic thrombocytopenic purpura. *Blood* 2002;99:3872–3873.
102. Zaja F, Vianelli N, Sperotto A, et al. The B-cell compartment as the selective target for the treatment of immune thrombocytopenias. *Haematologia* 2003;88:538–546.
103. Shanafelt TD, Madueme HL, Wolf RC, et al. Rituximab for immune cytopenia in adults: idiopathic thrombocytopenic purpura, autoimmune hemolytic anemia, and Evans syndrome. *Mayo Clin Proc* 2003;78:1340–1346.
104. Cooper N, Stasi R, Cunningham-Rundles S, et al. The efficacy and safety of B-cell depletion with anti-CD20 monoclonal antibody in adults with chronic immune thrombocytopenic purpura. *Br J Haematol* 2004;125:232–239.
105. Provan D, Newland A. Fifty years of idiopathic thrombocytopenic purpura (ITP): management of refractory ITP in adults. *Br J Haematol* 2002;118:933–944.
106. Wandt H, Frank M, Ehninger G, et al. Safety and cost effectiveness of a $10 \times 10^9$/L trigger for prophylactic platelet transfusions compared with the traditional $20 \times 10^9$/L trigger: a prospective comparative trial in 105 patients with acute myeloid leukemia. *Blood* 1998;91:3601–3606.
107. Rebulla P, Finazzi G, Marangoni F, et al. The threshold for prophylactic platelet transfusions in adults with acute myeloid leukemia. *N Engl J Med* 1997;337:1870–1875.
108. Franquet T, Giménez A, Prats R, et al. Thrombotic microangiopathy of pulmonary tumors: a vascular cause of tree-in-bud pattern on CT. *Am J Roentgenol* 2002;179:897–899.

109. Reiner A, Gernsheimer T, Slichter SJ. Pulse cyclophosphamide therapy for refractory autoimmune thrombocytopenic purpura. *Blood* 1995;85: 351–358.

110. George JN, Kojouri K, Perdue JJ, et al. Management of patients with chronic, refractory idiopathic thrombocytopenic purpura. *Semin Hematol* 2000; 37:1–10.

111. Huhn RD, Fogarty PF, Nakamura R, et al. High-dose cyclophosphamide with autologous lymphocyte-depleted peripheral blood stem cell (PBSC) support for treatment of refractory chronic autoimmune thrombocytopenia. *Blood* 2003;101:71–77.

112. Westhoff TH, Jochimsen F, Schmittel A, et al. Fatal hepatitis B virus reactivation by an escape mutant following rituximab therapy. *Blood* 2003; 102:1930.

113. Burton C, Kaczmarski R, Jan-Mohamed R. Interstitial pneumonitis related to rituximab therapy. *N Engl J Med* 2003;348:2690–2691.

114. Voog E, Morschhauser F, Solal-Celigny P. Neutropenia in patients treated with rituximab. *N Engl J Med* 2003;348:2691–2694.

115. Shah C, Grethlein SJ. Case report of rituximab-induced thrombocytopenia. *Am J Hematol* 2004;75:263.

116. Basser RL, O'Flaherty E, Green M, et al. Development of pancytopenia with neutralizing antibodies to thrombopoietin after multicycle chemotherapy supported by megakaryocyte growth and development factor. *Blood* 2002; 99:2599–2602.

117. Broudy VC, Lin NL. AMG531 stimulates megakaryocytopoiesis *in vitro* by binding to Mpl. *Cytokine* 2004;25:52–60.

118. Burrows RF, Kelton JG. Pregnancy in patients with idiopathic thrombocytopenic purpura: assessing the risks for the infant at delivery. *Obstet Gynecol Surv* 1993;48(12):781–788.

119. Webert KE, Mittal R, Sigourin C, et al. A retrospective 11-year analysis of obstetric patients with idiopathic thrombocytopenic purpura. *Blood* 2003; 102:4306–4311.

120. Payne SD, Resnik R, Moore TR, et al. Maternal characteristics and risk of severe neonatal thrombocytopenia and intracranial hemorrhage in pregnancies complicated by autoimmune thrombocytopenia. *Am J Obstet Gynecol* 1997;177:149–155.

121. Valat AS, Caulier MT, Devos P, et al. Relationships between severe neonatal thrombocytopenia and maternal characteristics in pregnancies associated with autoimmune thrombocytopenia. *Br J Haematol* 1998; 103:397–401.

122. Letsky EA, Greaves M. Guidelines on the investigation and management of thrombocytopenia in pregnancy and neonatal alloimmune thrombocytopenia. *Br J Haematol* 1996;95:21–26.

123. Silver RM, Branch DW, Scott JR. Maternal thrombocytopenia in pregnancy: time for a reassessment. *Am J Obstet Gynecol* 1995;173:479–482.

124. Burrows RF, Kelton JG. Low fetal risks in pregnancies associated with idiopathic thrombocytopenic purpura. *Am J Obstet Gynecol* 1990;163: 1147–1150.

125. Holroyde CP, Oski FA, Gardner FH. The "pocked" erythrocyte. Red cell alterations in reticuloendothelial immaturity of the neonate. *N Engl J Med* 1969;281:516–520.

126. Delhommeau F, Cynober T, Schischmanoff PO, et al. Natural history of hereditary spherocytosis during the first year of life. *Blood* 2000;95: 393–397.

# CHAPTER 73 ■ DRUG-INDUCED THROMBOCYTOPENIA

JAMES N. GEORGE, BENG CHONG, AND XIAONING LI

Many drugs can cause thrombocytopenia by many different mechanisms (see Table 73-1). Decreased platelet production due to generalized hematopoietic suppression can be the expected result of dose-dependent toxicity of chemotherapeutic agents or can be caused by an idiosyncratic reaction to a drug, resulting in aplastic anemia. Rarely, drugs can cause selective suppression of platelet production; an example is anagrelide, an important therapeutic agent to control extreme thrombocytosis (Table 73-1) (1–3).

Drugs may also cause thrombocytopenia by increasing platelet destruction. Some drugs, such as protamine sulfate (8), and growth factors such as GM-CSF (9), M-CSF (10), and interleukin 2 (11,12), may act directly on platelets and cause thrombocytopenia by nonimmune mechanisms. Other drugs, notably quinine, can cause either selective thrombocytopenia (14) or severe systemic reactions with multiorgan failure and the clinical signs of thrombotic thrombocytopenic purpura-hemolytic uremic syndrome with accompanying severe thrombocytopenia (13,15).

This chapter focuses on the clinical aspects of drug-induced selective thrombocytopenia due to increased platelet destruction caused by immune mechanisms, the last category listed in Table 73-1. Other etiologies of drug-induced thrombocytopenia are either predictable and apparent, such as the thrombocytopenia following chemotherapeutic agents, or they are rare. The other mechanisms of drug-induced thrombocytopenia are described in recent reviews (16–18). The mechanisms for drug-induced immune-mediated platelet destruction are described in Chapter 29. The most common mechanism is the formation of drug-dependent antibodies against epitopes created by the noncovalent association of drugs with platelet surface proteins. Noncovalent binding may occur by two types of interactions: (a) hydrophobic interactions and (b) specific ligand–receptor interactions, as it occurs with the platelet glycoprotein (GP) IIb/IIIa receptor antagonists (Table 73-1). Many drugs can create epitopes for antibody formation by noncovalent interactions with platelet surface glycoproteins, but among currently and commonly used drugs, quinine and sulfa drugs are more frequently implicated than others (14,19–21). Drugs that react noncovalently with the platelet surface are typically amphipathic and are normally transported in plasma bound to hydrophobic sites on albumin (22,23). Therefore, it is postulated that they react with hydrophobic domains on platelet surface glycoproteins.

## INCIDENCE

The annual incidence of drug-induced thrombocytopenia has been estimated in four studies to be approximately one case per 100,000 population (see Table 73-2). However, because these data are the result of reporting to national surveillance groups or are from hospital records, it is probable that they markedly underestimate the frequency of drug-induced thrombocytopenia. It can be reasonably assumed that many patients are suspected of having drug-induced thrombocytopenia and are not reported, and also that many patients do not require hospitalization. A clue to the underestimate is the frequent misdiagnosis of drug-induced throbocytopenia as immune thrombocytopenic purpura (ITP) (24).

## DIAGNOSIS

The key aspect of patient evaluation is a detailed, explicit history. Patients with unexpected acute, severe, and symptomatic thrombocytopenia must be suspected of having a drug-induced etiology. Patients with quinine-induced thrombocytopenia characteristically present with an abrupt onset of petechial hemorrhages over the lower legs and mucosal bleeding (33). Rarely, patients may also present with more serious or even fatal bleeding, such as intracranial or retroperitoneal hemorrhages (34). Typically, the platelet count is extremely low, often less than $10 \times 10^9$ per L. Thrombocytopenia caused by other drugs may be less severe and less dramatic in its presentation.

Patients with recurrent episodes of acute severe thrombocytopenia must be assumed to have a drug-induced etiology, and the evaluation must be pursued until the etiologic agent is identified. The history must include explicit questions not only for prescription medicines and conventional over-the-counter medicines, but also for herbal remedies (35,36) and for health supplements that may be taken only intermittently. Typically, patients do not report medicines or other remedies that they regulate themselves with and take only occasionally, assuming that their physician is interested only in regularly prescribed medications (37). Quinine, because it may currently be the most common cause of drug-induced thrombocytopenia (14,19–21), must be specifically asked for, not only in medicines but also in quinine and cinchona-containing remedies and quinine-containing beverages such as tonic water and Schweppes Bitter Lemon (37). The amount of quinine required to trigger severe thrombocytopenia is easily achieved by the concentration in these beverages (38–44). Although the US Food and Drug Administration banned over-the-counter marketing of quinine in 1994 and prohibited the indication for nocturnal leg cramps (45), quinine has continued for more than 60 years to be the universal treatment of persons with the very common symptom of leg cramps (46,47). A variety of quinine-containing products are readily available in general merchandise stores and nutrition centers (37).

## TABLE 73-1

### CLASSIFICATION OF DRUG-INDUCED THROMBOCYTOPENIA

Decreased platelet production
- Generalized suppression of hematopoiesis
  - Dose-dependent toxicity (e.g., chemotherapeutic agents)
  - Idiosyncratic aplastic anemia [e.g., anticonvulsants, sulfonamides, nonsteroidal antiinflammatory drugs (4,5)]
- Selective suppression of platelet production [e.g., anagrelide (1–3), valproic acid (6,7)]

Increased platelet destruction
- Nonimmune [e.g., protamine sulfate (8), growth factors (9–12)]
- Immune
  - Drug-induced systemic disorders that include thrombocytopenia [e.g., thrombotic thrombocytopenic purpura-hemolytic uremic syndrome caused by quinine (13)]
  - Drug-induced selective thrombocytopenia
    - Hapten reaction: covalent binding of a drug to a platelet surface antigen to create a drug-dependent epitope (e.g., penicillin)
    - Noncovalent modification of a platelet surface antigen to create a drug-dependent epitope (e.g., quinine, sulfonamides)
    - Naturally occurring antibodies that react with epitopes on glycoprotein (GP) IIb/IIIa that are created by GP IIb/IIIa receptor antagonists

## Thrombocytopenia Caused by Herbal Remedies and Foods

Documentation of thrombocytopenia caused by herbal remedies is uncommon, perhaps because of lack of recognition and also because the composition of herbal remedies may vary and is often undocumented (48). However, clear examples of a definite causal relation exists, such as in reports of patients with recurrent severe thrombocytopenia caused by the traditional Chinese herbal medicine *Jui* (35,36), a commercial name for a herbal tea containing multiple components. Foods may also cause acute and severe thrombocytopenia; this is also either uncommon or uncommonly recognized. One well-documented case report describes recurrent thrombocytopenia caused by tahini (pulped sesame seeds), the principal ingredient of the traditional Middle Eastern food hummus (49).

## Thrombocytopenia Caused by GP IIb/IIIa Receptor Antagonists

Acute thrombocytopenia caused by antithrombotic agents that block fibrinogen binding to GP IIb/IIIa on the platelet surface has important clinical characteristics distinctive from thrombocytopenia induced by other drugs, herbal remedies, and foods (see Table 73-3). In contrast to other drugs that require time for sensitization to form drug-dependent antibodies, acute severe thrombocytopenia may occur immediately following the initial exposure to GP IIb/IIIa receptor antagonists. Therefore, the drug-dependent antibodies must be preexisting, naturally occurring antibodies that recognize the drug-induced epitopes on GP IIb/IIIa or epitopes on the platelet-bound drug itself. Not only is the thrombocytopenia caused by GP IIb/IIIa receptor antagonists distinct because of the occurrence of naturally occurring antibodies, but also the frequency of severe thrombocytopenia caused by these agents is much greater than for any other drug or class of drugs. For example, current clinical trials with abciximab have documented an immediate occurrence of severe thrombocytopenia in 1% of patients (50). Other reports document even higher frequencies with approved intravenous agents, up to 5% (51). With investigative oral agents given continuously for several weeks, the frequency of thrombocytopenia may be as high as 13% (52). Tests have been developed to screen patients for GP IIb/IIIa–receptor antagonist–dependent antiplatelet antibodies before drug administration, and in one study, roxifiban-dependent antibodies were identified in 4% of patients (53). These naturally occurring antibodies may develop because of alterations in GP IIb/IIIa structure induced by reversible platelet aggregation or senescence.

# DOCUMENATION OF A DRUG-INDUCED ETIOLOGY FOR THROMBOCYTOPENIA

## Clinical Evaluation

The initial assessment of a patient with possible drug-induced thrombocytopenia is based on the clinical evidence that the suspected drug caused the thrombocytopenia. Both the strength of the evidence documenting a causal relation and the frequency of published reports contribute to the clinical assessment. Criteria for assessing the strength of clinical evidence associating a drug with thrombocytopenia are presented in Table 73-4 (14). Most clinical evidence comes from individual patient

## TABLE 73-2

### INCIDENCE OF DRUG-INDUCED THROMBOCYTOPENIA

| Country | Years | Method | Annual incidence |
|---|---|---|---|
| Sweden (25–27) | 1966–1970 | Reports to Swedish Adverse Reaction Committee | 1/100,000 |
| Denmark (28–30) | 1968–1991 | Reports to Danish Committee on adverse drug reactions | 1/100,000 |
| USA (31) | 1972–1981 | Hospital records, Puget Sound Group Health Cooperative | 0.6/100,000 |
| USA (32) | 1983–1991 | Hospital records, case–control study | 1.8/100,000 |

## TABLE 73-3

### CONTRASTING CHARACTERISTICS OF THROMBOCYTOPENIA CAUSED BY TYPICAL DRUG-DEPENDENT ANTIBODIES AND ANTIBODIES ASSOCIATED WITH GP IIb/IIIa RECEPTOR ANTAGONISTS

| Characteristics | Typical drug-dependent antibodies | GP IIb/IIIa receptor antagonist–related antibodies |
|---|---|---|
| Drug class | Many, perhaps all drugs (except GP IIb/IIIa receptor antagonists); quinine is the prototype drug | Drugs that inhibit fibrinogen finding to GP IIb/IIIa |
| Frequency | An uncommon adverse reaction for any drug | Common; severe thrombocytopenia may occur in 1% to 5% of administrations |
| | | Frequency is greater with some investigational agents |
| Mechanism | Previous exposure required to cause antibody formation to drug-dependent epitope | May occur immediately with first exposure, caused by naturally occurring drug-dependent antibodies |

data. Group data can also provide firm evidence for drugs as the cause of thrombocytopenia.

The algorithm described in Table 73-4 presents a sequential approach to documenting the causal relation between a drug and thrombocytopenia in an individual patient. The administration of the suspected drug must precede the onset of thrombocytopenia, and the thrombocytopenia must resolve when the drug is stopped. Exceptions to the rule of prompt recovery are α-methydopa– and gold-induced thrombocytopenia, which

## TABLE 73-4

### CLINICAL CRITERIA TO DOCUMENT A DRUG-INDUCED ETIOLOGY FOR THROMBOCYTOPENIA

| | Individual patient data |
|---|---|
| Criteria | Description |
| 1 | Therapy with the candidate drug preceded thrombocytopenia *and* recovery from thrombocytopenia was complete and sustained after therapy with the drug was discontinued |
| 2 | The candidate drug was the only drug used before the onset of thrombocytopenia, *or* other drugs were continued or reintroduced after discontinuation of therapy with the candidate drug with a sustained normal platelet count |
| 3 | Other causes for thrombocytopenia were excluded |
| 4 | Reexposure to the candidate drug resulted in recurrent thrombocytopenia |

| Level of evidence | |
|---|---|
| Definite: | Criteria 1, 2, 3, and 4 met |
| Probable: | Criteria 1, 2, and 3 met |
| Possible: | Criterion 1 met |
| Unlikely: | Criterion 1 not met |

may have a prolonged course. This assessment is often difficult because most patients, especially older patients in whom drug-induced thrombocytopenia is more common (14,25), are taking multiple drugs (54). Any one of these drugs may be considered a possible cause of thrombocytopenia in the patient based on the assessment of their relative risks using published data (see subsequent text). The drugs most likely to have caused thrombocytopenia are then withheld or stopped, and appropriate alternative drugs are started. Subsequent resolution of the thrombocytopenia should indicate that these are potentially the offending drugs and the continuing drugs are not. Common causes of thrombocytopenia other than drugs—such as infections and autoimmune disorders—should be excluded clinically or by laboratory investigations.

The specific drug that caused the thrombocytopenia may then be identified using drug-dependent antibody assays testing the range of drugs the patient was receiving. This approach, termed *in vitro* rechallenge, is safer than *in vivo* rechallenge, which is usually used only as a last resort. Although rechallenging a patient with the suspected drug is the definitive clinical observation that either confirms or excludes the drug-induced etiology, this procedure may have substantial risk and may not always be appropriate. However, when the suspected agent is commonly available and potentially unavoidable, such as acetaminophen, a rechallenge under carefully controlled observation may be an essential part of patient management. This approach is followed only if laboratory testing using drug-dependent antibody assays fails to identify the offending drug or if the antibody assays are not available (see subsequent section, "Laboratory Evaluation").

To better understand the relative risks of the many drugs associated with thrombocytopenia, we have systematically reviewed all English-language published case reports describing drug-induced thrombocytopenia (14,19–21). Through August 2004, 964 articles containing 1,316 patient case reports describing thrombocytopenia related to 281 drugs have been systematically analyzed (14,19–21). The most commonly reported drugs that have been identified as causing thrombocytopenia are listed in Table 73-5. The complete data are accessible at the Web site, http://moon.ouhsc.edu/jgeorge. This Web site provides information on all case reports, describing the demographic and clinical information for each patient and

**TABLE 73-5**

DRUGS DOCUMENTED TO CAUSE THROMBOCYTOPENIA

| Generic name | No. of case reports | Generic name | No. of case reports |
|---|---|---|---|
| Quinidine | 59 | Ethambutol | 2 |
| Quinine | 24 | Ibuprofen | 2 |
| Trimethoprim/sulfamethoxazole | 15 | Indinavir | 2 |
| Gold[a] | 11 | Iopanoic acid[a] | 2 |
| Interferon | 10 | Levamisole[a] | 2 |
| Carbamazepine | 10 | Meclofenamate | 2 |
| Rifampin | 9 | Methicillin[a] | 2 |
| Abciximab c7E3 Fab | 7 | Oxytetracycline | 2 |
| Acetaminophen | 7 | Oxyphenbutazone[a] | 2 |
| Danazol | 7 | Piperacillin | 2 |
| Procainamide | 7 | Roxifiban[a] | 2 |
| Vancomycin | 7 | Simvastatin | 2 |
| Cimetidine | 6 | Sulfapyridine[a] | 2 |
| Eptifibatide | 6 | Sulindac | 2 |
| Methyldopa | 6 | Tamoxifen | 2 |
| Nalidixic acid | 6 | Terbinafine | 2 |
| Chlorpropamide | 5 | Alprenolol[a] | 1 |
| Diclofenac | 5 | Inamrinone | 1 |
| Hydrochlorothiazide | 5 | Atorvastatin | 1 |
| Ranitidine | 5 | Cephalothin[a] | 1 |
| Sulfisoxazole | 5 | Chlorpromazine | 1 |
| Chlorothiazide | 4 | Deferoxamine | 1 |
| Digoxin | 4 | Diazepam | 1 |
| Naproxen | 4 | Diazoxide | 1 |
| Acetazolamide | 3 | Eflornithine | 1 |
| Aminoglutethimide | 3 | Haloperidol | 1 |
| Aminosalicylic acid | 3 | Isoniazid | 1 |
| Amphotericin B | 3 | Lithium | 1 |
| Diatrizoate meglumine | 3 | Mesalamine | 1 |
| Oxprenolol[a] | 3 | Minoxidil | 1 |
| Phenytoin | 3 | Naphazoline | 1 |
| Sulfamethoxypyridazine[a] | 3 | Nitroglycerin | 1 |
| Sulfasalazine | 3 | Novobiocin | 1 |
| Ticlopidine | 3 | Octreotide | 1 |
| Amiodarone | 2 | Pentoxifylline | 1 |
| Ampicillin | 2 | Rituximab | 1 |
| Captopril | 2 | Sulfathiazole[a] | 1 |
| Clidinium bromide/chlordiazepoxide | 2 | Thiothixene | 1 |
| Clopidogrel | 2 | Tirofiban | 1 |
| Diatrizoate meglumine/diatrizoate sodium | 2 | Tolmetin | 1 |

[a]Drugs that are not manufactured in the United States.
The 80 drugs that have been documented to cause thrombocytopenia by patient case reports with definite evidence (that requires recurrence of thrombocytopenia with *in vivo* rechallenge with the drug) or by two or more patient case reports with probable evidence are listed in the order of the decreasing number of patient cases reported. Only drugs that are currently available are listed. Drug availability was determined by the Micromedex (55) and FDA (56) Web sites.

objective assessment of the level of evidence supporting the drug as the etiology for thrombocytopenia.

Although this database is comprehensive and accessible, it has limitations. Case reports reviewed were limited to those describing thrombocytopenia related to drugs approved by national agencies; therefore, thrombocytopenia caused by herbal remedies (35,36) or foods (49) are not included. Furthermore, reports describing thrombocytopenia associated with chemotherapeutic agents were systematically excluded, although some agents, such as oxaliplatin (57–59), can cause acute immune-mediated thrombocytopenia that has been

confirmed by the demonstration of oxaliplatin-dependent antiplatelet antibodies. Children were also excluded from this analysis because the natural history of childhood ITP, with frequent prompt spontaneous remissions, may be indistinguishable from drug-induced thrombocytopenia.

## Laboratory Evaluation

The laboratory tests used to investigate patients with suspected drug-induced thrombocytopenia are described in

**TABLE 73-6**

## LABORATORY TESTS FOR DETECTION OF DRUG-DEPENDENT PLATELET ANTIBODIES

| Assays | Features | Values |
|---|---|---|
| Phase I (developed in 1950–1970) | They measure platelet changes induced by drug-dependent antibodies: platelet aggregation, $^{14}$C-serotonin and granule content release, fixation of complement, platelet lysis, etc. | Low sensitivity and specificity<br>No longer used to measure drug-dependent antibodies except antibodies in heparin-induced thrombocytopenia |
| Phase II (developed in 1970s) PA IgG assays | Three approaches:<br>1. Two-stage competitive inhibition assays<br>2. Direct binding assays<br>3. Total IgG assays<br>They measure platelet-associated IgG but can be designed to measure IgA, IgM, or IgG separately or together<br>Commonly used methods are flow cytometry and ELISA using direct binding assay | High specificity<br>High sensitivity for detection of quinine- and quinidine-dependent antibodies and antibodies related to GP IIb/IIIa inhibitors<br>Sensitivity for detection of other-related antibodies uncertain<br>Can be used to identify the offending drug (*in vitro* rechallenge) |
| Phase III (developed in 1980s) Platelet glycoprotein-specific antibody assays | They detect drug-dependent platelet glycoprotein-specific antibodies<br>Commonly used methods are MACE and MAIPA<br>Because the most common drug-related autoantigens are GP Ib/IX, GP IIb/IIIa, and/or PECAM-1, monoclonal antibodies against these proteins are usually used to capture the autoantigens in these assays | High specificity<br>High sensitivity for detection of quinine- and quinidine-dependent antibodies<br>Sensitivity for detection of other-related antibodies uncertain<br>Can be used to identify the offending drug (*in vitro* rechallenge) |

ELISA, enzyme-linked immunosorbent assays; MACE, modified antigen-capture enzyme-linked immunosorbent assay; MAIPA, monoclonal antibody-specific immobilization of platelet antigens; PECAM-1, platelet endothelial cell adhesion molecule-1; GP, glycoprotein; PA IgC, platelet-associated IgC assays. In all the assays mentioned in the table, the "indirect" test is preferred because (a) after drug withdrawal, the antibody no longer binds to the platelets and is present in the serum/plasma, usually in high titer; and (b) drug-dependent antibody binding can be demonstrated and exploited to increase test specificity and to identify the offending drug.

Table 73-6. Laboratory documentation of drug-dependent antiplatelet antibodies is not possible in all patients because available techniques vary in their sensitivity. The sensitizing agent may be a metabolite of the drug formed *in vivo*, rather than the primary drug, and tests incorporating the primary drug may therefore be negative. Common techniques are flow cytometry (60,61), enzyme-linked immunosorbent assays (ELISA) using immobilized platelet glycoproteins as targets (61,62), and monoclonal antibody-specific immobilization of platelet antigens (MAIPA) assays (63,64). Different assays may have different sensitivities for different patients and different drugs (65) because of low binding affinity of the drug for platelets, low binding affinity of the drug-dependent antibodies to their antigen, or low antigen site density on the platelet surface (65). These issues are described in greater detail in Chapter 29.

### Direct and Indirect Drug-Dependent Antiplatelet Antibody Assays

Platelet antibody assays are divided into either (a) a *direct test* (in which the patient's platelets are used) or (b) an *indirect test* (in which the patient's serum is used), such as the red cell antibody tests (66). A direct test measures antibodies or immunoglobulins (Ig) attached to the patient's platelets. An indirect test measures antibodies or Ig in the patient's serum that bind to normal platelets when they are incubated together (see Fig. 73-1). The indirect test is the assay of choice for

drug-dependent antibodies because after withdrawal of the suspected drug, the antibody can no longer bind to the patient's platelets *in vivo* but usually remains in the patient's serum in high titer. The patient's serum can be tested with each drug that the patient has taken, assessing drug-dependent antibody binding. This allows the identification of the offending drug (*in vitro* rechallenge).

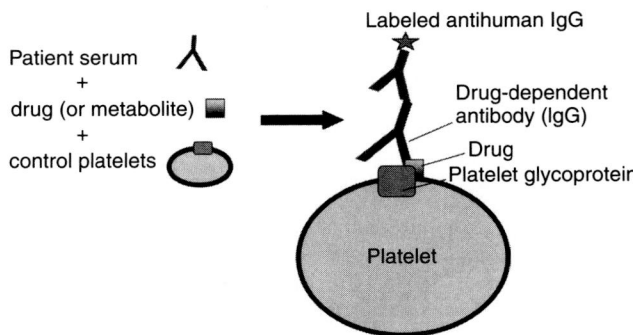

**FIGURE 73-1.** Phase II drug-dependent platelet antibody assay (direct binding assay—indirect test). Patient serum and drug are incubated with normal platelets, and after washing of platelets, the antibody bound to a drug-platelet glycoprotein complex on platelet surface is detected by a secondary antibody (antihuman IgG) labeled with an enzyme (for ELISA, enzyme-linked immunosorbent assays) or a fluorescent (for flow cytometric analysis).

## Types of Drug-Dependent Antiplatelet Antibody Assays

Platelet antibody tests can be divided into three groups: phase I, II, and III assays, depending on the periods in which they were developed.

### Phase I assays

These were developed between 1950 and 1970 (66) and are indirect tests that measure antibody-induced platelet changes such as platelet aggregation and serotonin release when the patient's serum is incubated with normal platelets in the presence of the drug. Most drug-dependent antibodies do not induce these platelet changes. At the same time, there are materials in the serum, such as immune complexes and complement that can induce platelet activation changes and give a false-positive result. These tests have very low sensitivity and specificity and are not currently used for detection of drug-dependent platelet antibodies, except for the investigation of heparin-induced thrombocytopenia.

### Phase II assays

These tests, developed in the 1970s, are known as platelet-associated IgG assays (PA-IgG) (66). Although they usually measure IgG associated with or binding to platelets, they can be designed to measure IgG, IgA, and IgM separately or together. There are three different approaches: (a) two-stage assays such as competitive inhibition assays (66), (b) direct binding (Fig. 73-1), and (c) total PAIgG assays. These assays are notoriously unreliable for measurement of platelet autoantibodies in ITP because of their low specificity (67) due to the presence of nonimmune IgG on platelets in both ITP and nonimmune thrombocytopenias (68). In contrast, these phase II assays are helpful for measurement of the drug-dependent antibodies. We have found them to be sensitive and specific (67), particularly in the detection of quinine- or quinidine-dependent antibodies. Probable reasons for this finding are that (a) drug-dependent antibodies are often present in the patient's serum in high titers, (b) they bind strongly and drug-dependently to platelets, and (c) they can be easily distinguished from other irrelevant serum antibodies, such as anti-HLA antibodies, which bind to platelets drug-independently. The commonly used phase II assays for drug-dependent antibodies are ELISA and flow cytometry (61).

### Phase III assays

These assays, developed in the mid-1980s, detect platelet glycoprotein-specific antibodies (66). Among these are the glycoprotein immobilization assays, such as the modified antigen-capture enzyme-linked immunosorbent assay (MACE) and the MAIPA. In MACE, for example, a glycoprotein-specific monoclonal antibody (e.g., an antibody against GP Ib/IX) is used to capture the platelet antigen in the wells of a microtiter platelet and the antibody in the patient's serum that binds drug-dependently to the target antigen is measured using an enzyme-linked secondary antibody (see Fig. 73-2) (66). In MAIPA, an antimouse IgG coated on the microtiter wells captures a trimolecular complex consisting of a mouse glycoprotein-specific antibody, the platelet antigen, and the patient's serum drug-dependent antibody (69), preformed separately during incubation (see Fig. 73-3) before transfer to the microtiter wells. The drug-dependent antibody is then detected by an enzyme-linked secondary antibody, as in MACE (Fig. 73-2).

In our hands, the MAIPA assay is slightly more sensitive than flow cytometry for detecting drug-dependent antibodies (70). However, the glycoprotein immobilization assays such as MAIPA have one important drawback. Prior knowledge of the antigen of the drug-dependent antibody is required so that an

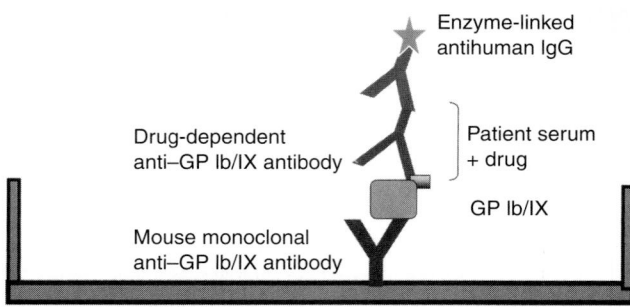

**FIGURE 73-2.** Phase III drug-dependent platelet antibody assay: modified antigen-capture enzyme-linked immunosorbent assay (MACE). In MACE, a monoclonal antibody with specificity for a particular platelet glycoprotein (e.g., GP IX) is bound to the microtiter wells. The antibody captures the glycoprotein from the platelet lysate when it is added to the wells. Drug-glycoprotein complex is formed upon addition of the drug. When the patient's serum is subsequently added, the drug-dependent antibody in the serum binds to the drug/GP IX complex. The drug-dependent antibody is detected by a secondary antihuman Ig antibody labeled with an enzyme.

appropriate antibody can be used to capture the platelet antigen. Fortunately, the epitopes of drug-dependent antibodies, at least those that have been identified, are located on platelet GP Ib/IX (64) and/or GP IIb/IIIa (70), and very occasionally on other glycoproteins such as platelet endothelial cell adhesion molecule-1 (PECAM-1) (63) (see Chapter 29).

In summary, laboratory tests are often helpful in the diagnosis of drug-induced immune thrombocytopenia, particularly quinine-induced thrombocytopenia and thrombocytopenia caused by the GP IIb/IIIa receptor inhibitors. Other drug-induced thrombocytopenias are less well studied, and there are fewer reported experiences in the detection of these antibodies. In laboratory testing for drug-dependent antibodies, the challenges are usually (a) knowing the optimum drug concentration for testing (it often corresponds to the therapeutic plasma concentrations of the drug); (b) obtaining soluble drug

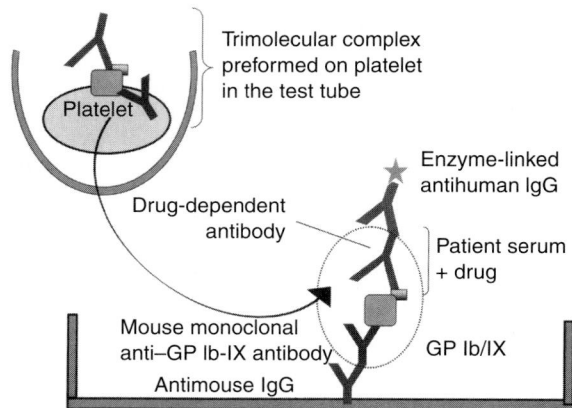

**FIGURE 73-3.** Phase III drug-dependent platelet antibody assay: monoclonal antibodyspecific immobilization of platelet antigens (MAIPA). In the MAIPA assay, the patient serum, drug, platelets, and a monoclonal antibody against the platelet antigen (e.g., GP IX) are incubated in a test tube, resulting in the formation of a trimolecular complex that consists of the monoclonal antibody, the drug/GP IX complex, and the drug-dependent antibody. The platelets are solubilized by triton-X-100, and the platelet lysate containing the trimolecular complex is transferred to the microtiter wells containing an antimouse IgG antibody. This antibody captures the trimolecular complex. The drug-dependent antibody is then detected by an enzyme-linked antihuman IgG antibody.

for testing, because some drugs are difficult to dissolve; (c) obtaining drug metabolites if the antibody does not react with the parent drug; and (d) determining the titer and/or avidity of the antibody, which in some cases may be too low to be detectable by current assays.

# TREATMENT

The only necessary and appropriate treatment is withdrawal of the offending drug, herbal remedy, or food. When the drug is removed, the drug-dependent antibody cannot bind to the platelets although the antibody may persist for a prolonged time in the patient's serum. The exceptions are patients with thrombocytopenia induced by α-methyldopa and gold; in these patients, the antibodies bind to platelets even in the absence of the drug, and the thrombocytopenia persists unless it is effectively treated. Becuase the sudden severe thrombocytopenia caused by a drug can never be clearly distinguished from ITP, steroid treatment (prednisone 1 mg/kg/day) is nearly always given. Intravenous immunoglobulin (IVIG) (0.4 to 1.0 gm per kg for 1 to 2 days) and/or platelet transfusions may also be appropriate for patients with severe thrombocytopenia and overt bleeding. The transfused platelets will be rapidly destroyed, but they may help to form a hemostatic plug at the bleeding site. Furthermore, they may also help to adsorb drug-dependent antibodies from plasma, decreasing the antibody titer and increasing the rate of recovery. The difference between steroid use in a patient with suspected drug-induced thrombocytopenia and its use in patients with suspected ITP is that steroid treatment should be discontinued abruptly as soon as the platelet count recovers in a patient with suspected drug-induced thrombocytopenia. Prompt, sustained recovery of the platelet count following discontinuation of the steroid further supports the clinical diagnosis of drug-induced thrombocytopenia because ITP in adults characteristically has a prolonged course requiring more prolonged immunosuppressive treatment. The exceptions are again the patients with thrombocytopenia induced by α-methyldopa and gold. Their clinical course tends to be more protracted, very similar to that of adult ITP. A longer course of treatment may be necessary in these patients.

## References

1. Solberg LA, Tefferi A, Oles KJ, et al. The effects of anagrelide on human megakaryocytopoiesis. *Br J Haematol* 1997;99:174–180.
2. Oertel MD. Anagrelide a selective thrombocytopenic agent. *Am J Health Syst Pharm* 1998;55:1979–1986.
3. McCune JS, Liles D, Lindley C. Precipitous fall in platelet count with anagrelide: case report and critique of dosing recommendations. *Pharmacotherapy* 1998;17:822–826.
4. Kaufman DW, Kelly JP, Jurgelon JM, et al. Drugs in the aetiology of agranulocytosis and aplastic anaemia. *Eur J Haematol* 1996;60:23–30.
5. Wilholm BE, Emanuelsson S. Drug-related blood dyscrasias in Swedish reporting system. *Eur J Haematol* 1996;60(Suppl.1):42–46.
6. Trannel TJ, Ahmed I, Goebert D. Occurrence of thrombocytopenia in psychiatric patients taking valproate. *Am J Psychiatry* 2001;158:128–130.
7. Kaufman KR, Gerner R. Dose-dependent valproic acid thrombocytopenia in bipolar disorder. *Ann Clin Psychiatry* 1998;10:35–37.
8. Al-Mondhiry H, Pierce W, Basarab R. Protamine-induced thrombocytopenia and leukopenia. *Thromb Haemost* 1985;53:60–64.
9. Tortajada C, Garcia F, Miro JM, et al. Severe thrombocytopenia related to granulocyte-macrophage colony-stimulating factor (rHU-GM-CSF). *Ann Med Interne* 2000;17:671.
10. Baker GR, Levin J. Transient thrombocytopenia produced by administration of macrophage colony-stimulating factor: investigations of the mechanism. *Blood* 1998;91:89–99.
11. Paciucci PA, Mandeli J, Oleksowicz L, et al. Thrombocytopenia during immunotherapy with interleukin-2 by constant infusion. *Am J Med* 1990;89:308–312.
12. Fleischmann JD, Shingleton WB, Gallagher C, et al. Fibrinolysis, thrombocytopenia, and coagulation abnormalities complicating high-dose interleukin-2 immunotherapy. *J Lab Clin Med* 1991;117:76–82.
13. Kojouri K, Vesely SK, George JN. Quinine-associated thrombotic thrombocytopenic purpura-hemolytic uremic syndrome: frequency, clinical features, and long-term outcomes. *Ann Intern Med* 2001;135:1047–1051.
14. George JN, Raskob GE, Shah SR, et al. Drug-induced thrombocytopenia: a systematic review of published case reports. *Ann Intern Med* 1998;129:886–890.
15. Howard MA, Hibbard AB, Terrell DR, et al. Quinine allergy causing acute severe systemic illness: report of four patients manifesting hematologic, renal, and hepatic abnormalities. *Baylor University Medical Proceedings* 2003;16:21–26.
16. Aster RH. Response of thrombocytes to toxic injury. In: Bloom JC, ed. *Toxicology of the hematopoietic system*. St. Louis, MO: Elsevier Science, 1997.
17. Rizvi MA, Shah SR, Raskob GE, et al. Drug-induced thrombocytopenia. *Curr Opin Hematol* 1999;6:349–353.
18. Aster RH. Drug-induced thrombocytopenia. In: Michelson AD, ed. *Platelets*. Amsterdam: Academic Press, 2002:593–606.
19. Rizvi MA, Kojouri K, George JN. Drug-induced thrombocytopenia: an updated systematic review. *Ann Intern Med* 2001;134:346.
20. Hibbard AB, Medina PJ, Vesely SK. Reports of drug-induced thrombocytopenia. *Ann Intern Med* 2003;138:239.
21. Li X, Hunt L, George JN, et al. Drug-induced thrombocytopenia: an updated systematic review, 2004. *Ann Intern Med* 2005:142:474–475.
22. Koch-Weser J, Sellers EM. Binding of drugs to serum albumin (first of two parts). *N Engl J Med* 1976;294:311–316.
23. Koch-Weser J, Sellers EM. Binding of drugs to serum albumin (second of two parts). *N Engl J Med* 1976;294:526–531.
24. Neylon AJ, Saunders PWG, Howard MR, et al. Clinically significant newly presenting autoimmune thrombocytopenic purpura in adults: a prospective study of a population-based cohort of 245 patients. *Br J Haematol* 2003;122:966–974.
25. Bottiger LE, Westerholm B. Thrombocytopenia. I. Etiology and pathogenesis. *Acta Med Scand* 1972;191:535–540.
26. Bottiger LE, Westerholm B. Thrombocytopenia. II. Drug-induced thrombocytopenia. *Acta Med Scand* 1972;191:541–548.
27. Bottiger LE, Bottiger B. Incidence and cause of aplastic anemia, hemolytic anemia, agranulocytosis and thrombocytopenia. *Acta Med Scand* 1981;210:475–479.
28. Pedersen-Bjergaard U, Andersen M, Hansen PB. Thrombocytopenia induced by non-cytotoxic drugs in Denmark 1968-1991. *J Intern Med* 1996;239:509–515.
29. Pedersen-Bjergaard U, Andersen M, Hansen PB. Drug-induced thrombocytopenia: clinical data on 309 cases and the effect of corticosteroid therapy. *Eur J Clin Pharmacol* 1997;52:183–189.
30. Pedersen-Bjergaard U, Anderson M, Hansen PB. Drug-specific characteristics of thrombocytopenia caused by non-cytotoxic drugs. *Eur J Clin Pharmacol* 1998;54:701–706.
31. Danielson DA, Douglas SW III, Herzog P, et al. Drug-induced disorders. *JAMA* 1984;252:3257–3260.
32. Kaufman DW, Kelly JP, Johannes CB, et al. Acute thrombocytopenic purpura in relation to the use of drugs. *Blood* 1993;82:2714–2718.
33. Vipan WH. Quinine as a cause of purpura. *Lancet* 1865;2:37–37.
34. Freiman JP. Fatal quinine-induced thrombocytopenia. *Ann Intern Med* 1990;112:308–309.
35. Azuno Y, Yaga K, Sasayama T, et al. Thrombocytopenia induced by *Jui*, a traditional Chinese herbal medicine. *Lancet* 1999;354:304–305.
36. Ohmori T, Nishii K, Hagihara A, et al. Acute thrombocytopenia induced by *Jui*, a traditional herbal medicine. *J Thromb Haemost* 2004;2:1479–1480.
37. Kojouri K, Perdue JJ, Medina PJ, et al. Occult quinine-induced thrombocytopenia. *Oklahoma State Med J* 2000;93:519–521.
38. Belkin GA. Cocktail purpura: an unusual case of quinine sensitivity. *Ann Intern Med* 1967;66:583.
39. Korbitz BC, Eisner E. Cocktail purpura. Quinine-dependent thrombocytopenia. *Rocky Mt Med J* 1973;70:38–41.
40. Barrett AP, Tversky J, Griffiths CJ. Thrombocytopenia induced by quinine. *Oral Surg Oral Med Oral Pathol* 1983;55:351–354.
41. Wagner GH, Diffey BL, Ive FA. "I'll have mine with a twist of lemon." Quinine photosensitivity from excessive intake of tonic water. *Br J Dermatol* 1994;131:734–735.
42. Brasic JR. Quinine-induced thrombocytopenia in a 64-year-old man who consumed tonic water to relieve nocturnal leg cramps. *Mayo Clin Proc* 2001;76:863–864.
43. Barr E, Douglas JF, Hill CM. Recurrent acute hypersensitivity to quinine. *BMJ* 1990;301:323.
44. Gottschall JL, Elliot W, Lianos E, et al. Quinine-induced immune thrombocytopenia associated with hemolytic uremic syndrome: a new clinical entity. *Blood* 1991;77:306–310.
45. Brinker AD, Beitz J. Spontaneous reports of thrombocytopenia in association with quinine: clinical attributes and timing related to regulatory action. *Am J Hematol* 2002;70:313–317.
46. Moss HK, Herrmann LG. The use of quinine for the relief of "night cramps" in the extremities. *JAMA* 1940;115:1358–1359.
47. Oboler SK, Prochazka AV, Meyer TJ. Leg symptoms in outpatient veterans. *West J Med* 1991;155:256–259.
48. De Smet PAGM. Herbal remedies. *N Engl J Med* 2002;347:2046–2056.
49. Arnold J, Ouwehand WH, Smith G, et al. A young women with petechiae. *Lancet* 1998;352:618.

50. Kastrati A, Mehilli J, Schuhlen H, et al. A clinical trial of abciximab in elective percutaneous coronary intervention after pretreatment with clopidogrel. *N Engl J Med* 2004;350:232–238.

51. Berkowitz SD, Sane DC, Sigmon KN, et al. Occurrence and clinical significance of thrombocytopenia in a population undergoing high-risk percutaneous coronary revascularization. *J Am Coll Cardiol* 1998;32:311–319.

52. Giugliano RP, McCabe CH, Sequeira RF. First report of an intravenous and oral glycoprotein IIb/IIIa inhibitor (RPR 109891) in patients with recent acute coronary syndromes: results of the TIMI 15A and 15B trials. *Am Heart J* 2000;140:81–93.

53. Seiffert D, Stern AM, Ebling W, et al. Prospective testing for drug-dependent antibodies reduces the incidence of thrombocytopenia observed with the small molecule glycoprotein IIb/IIIa antagonist roxifiban: implications for the etiology of thrombocytopenia. *Blood* 2003;101:58–63.

54. Gurwitz JH, Field TS, Harrold LR, et al. Incidence and preventability of adverse drug events among older persons in the ambulatory setting. *JAMA* 2003;289:1107–1116.

55. http://micromedex.ouhsc.edu/mdxcgi/mdxhtml. Accessed February 1, 2005.

56. http://www.accessdata.fda.gov/scripts/cder/drugsatfda/index.cfm. Accessed February 1, 2005.

57. Curtis BR, Kaliszewski J, Blank J, et al. Severe thrombocytopenia caused by high titer IgG oxaliplatin-dependent platelet antibodies. *Blood* 2003;102:538a.

58. Dold FG, Mitchell EP. Sudden-onset thrombocytopenia with oxaliplatin. *Ann Intern Med* 2003;139:E156.

59. Sorbye H, Bruserud Y, Dahl O. Oxaliplatin-induced haematological emergency with an immediate severe thrombocytopenia and haemolysis. *Acta Oncol* 2001;40:882–883.

60. Curtis BR, McFarland JG, Wu G-G, et al. Antibodies in sulfonamide-induced immune thrombocytopenia recognize calcium-dependent epitopes on the glycoprotein IIb/IIIa complex. *Blood* 1994;84:176–183.

61. Visentin GP, Wolfmeyer K, Newman PJ, et al. Detection of drug-dependent, platelet-reactive antibodies by antigen-capture ELISA and flow cytometry. *Transfusion* 1990;30:694–700.

62. Peterson JA, Visentin GP, Newman PJ, et al. A recombinant soluble form of the integrin $a_{IIb}b_3$ (GP IIb-IIIa) assumes an active, ligand-binding conformation and is recognized by GP IIb-IIIa specific monoclonal, allo-, auto-, and drug-dependent platelet antibodies. *Blood* 1998;92:2053–2063.

63. Kroll H, Sun QH, Santoso S. Platelet endothelial cell adhesion molecule-1 (PECAM-1) is a target glycoprotein in drug-induced thrombocytopenia. *Blood* 2000;96:1409–1414.

64. Burgess JK, Lopez JA, Berndt MC, et al. Quinine-dependent antibodies bind a restricted set of epitopes on the glycoprotein Ib-IX complex: characterization of the epitopes. *Blood* 1998;92:2366–2373.

65. Nieminen U, Kekomäki R. Quinidine-induced thrombocytopenic purpura: clinical presentation in relation to drug-dependent and drug-independent platelet antibodies. *Br J Haematol* 1992;80:77–82.

66. Chong BH, Keng TB. Advances in the diagnosis of idiopathic thrombocytopenic purpura. *Semin Hematol* 2000;37:249–260.

67. Brighton T, Evans S, Castaldi PA, et al. Prospective evaluation of the clinical usefulness of an antigen-specific assay (MAIPA) in idiopathic thrombocytopenic purpura and other immune thrombocytopenias. *Blood* 1996;88:194–201.

68. George JN. Platelet immunoglobulin G: its significance for the evaluation of thrombocytopenia and for understanding the origin of alpha-granule proteins. *Blood* 1990;76:859–870.

69. Chong BH, Du X, Berndt MD, et al. Characterization of the binding domains on platelet glycoproteins Ib-IX and IIb/IIIa complexes for the quinine/quinidine-dependent antibodies. *Blood* 1991;77:2190–2199.

70. Asvadi P, Ahmadi Z, Chong BH. Drug-induced thrombocytopenia: localization of the binding site of GP IX-specific quinine-dependent antibodies. *Blood* 2003;102:1670–1677.

# CHAPTER 74 ■ HEMOSTATIC PROBLEMS IN SURGICAL PATIENTS

L. HENRY EDMUNDS, JR.

Bleeding is a major complication of any surgery and a major concern of all surgeons. The discipline of surgery requires the surgeon to be responsible for hemostasis both during and after the operation. All surgeons are trained to control visibly bleeding vessels, but additional skills and information are necessary for successful management of complex operations and multiple trauma victims. Surgical hemostasis now requires knowledge of perioperative coagulation disorders, blood conservation techniques, and the risks and benefits of blood component replacement and transfusion therapy. This chapter outlines a practical approach to the management of bleeding complications related to all surgery, but particularly to cardiac surgery.

## PREOPERATIVE ASSESSMENT

The preoperative evaluation of a patient who requires surgery varies with the type and urgency of the operation. For all patients, a thorough history is the best method to discover clinically significant bleeding states. The history should reveal bleeding related to previous trauma and surgical and dental procedures and also easy bruising or joint or muscle swelling after minor trauma. Positive answers raise the possibility of hereditary or acquired coagulation deficiencies, antibodies to specific coagulation proteins, von Willebrand disease, or platelet disorders. The patient's medication profile may reveal ingestion of inhibitory drugs, such as aspirin, aspirin-containing compounds, warfarin, platelet inhibitors, or injections of standard or low-molecular-weight heparin. The history also may reveal acquired hemorrhagic conditions associated with parenchymal liver disease, renal failure, or myeloproliferative syndromes.

The physical examination should include assessment of a possible bleeding tendency. One may find purpura, which is particularly important if not associated with a known history of trauma. Other findings include petechiae, splenomegaly, hepatomegaly, lymphadenopathy, joint deformities, lack of mobility, palpable collections of blood arising as deep hematomas, and evidence of gastrointestinal (GI) bleeding on digital rectal examination. Discovery of blood in stool is the most effective way to detect occult sources of GI bleeding from esophageal varices, duodenal ulcer, gastritis, diverticulitis, polyps, cancer, and other disorders. Comorbid diseases, such as uremia, cirrhosis, or polycythemia vera, may enhance bleeding from local lesions in the GI tract.

The results of the history and physical examination and the proposed operation determine the selection of preoperative laboratory tests for coagulation disorders and the need for special preoperative or intraoperative therapy. A scheme, modified from that originally proposed by Rappaport, has been suggested (1). If the history and physical examination are not suggestive of a bleeding tendency and relatively minor surgery is planned, no special tests are required. If major surgery is planned and if the history and physical examination are negative for hemostatic deficiencies, a platelet count and activated partial thromboplastin time (aPTT) are recommended. An unexpected low platelet count, particularly in patients with cardiac disorders who have received heparin, raises the possibility of heparin-induced thrombocytopenia (HIT) and the possibility of devastating heparin-induced thrombocytopenia and thrombosis (HITT) if more heparin is given (2). A prolonged aPTT raises the possibility of a circulating anticoagulant or a defect in the intrinsic coagulation system, such as familial factor XI deficiency, that may not be uncovered by a bleeding history.

If the history suggests a hemostatic deficiency or if the patient is undergoing an operation that is frequently complicated by bleeding problems [e.g., cardiac surgery with cardiopulmonary bypass (CPB), central neurosurgery, or prostatectomy], a one-stage prothrombin time (PT), and a thrombin clotting time to screen for deficiency in fibrinogen or fibrin formation is added to the platelet count and aPTT. A prolonged PT suggests deficiency in the extrinsic (tissue factor) and/or common coagulation pathways. A bleeding time test is sometimes added (3), but, because of the wide standard deviation of normal bleeding times, this test has limited value (4). A prolonged aPTT or PT requires a coagulation deficiency workup and consultation with a hematologist is recommended.

If the patient's history, physical examination, and screening tests reveal a hemostatic defect, the specific cause of the defect should be determined before operation, if possible, rather than during or after the procedure. The presence of a positive bleeding history, physical signs of possible hemorrhagic complications, and comorbid conditions or diseases that affect hemostasis are prompts for a more detailed preoperative assessment and the advice of a hematologist.

## COMMON CONDITIONS THAT INCREASE THE LIKELIHOOD OF BLEEDING

Not uncommonly, surgeons must undertake operations in patients with abnormal blood coagulation because of a variety of causes. The severity of perioperative bleeding varies with the magnitude and conduct of the operation, which coagulation protein is deficient, magnitude of the deficiency, and efficacy of replacement therapy. Familial coagulation deficiencies are usually identified by history or screening tests, confirmed by specific laboratory workup, and treated by replacement therapy, which may include purified proteins or specific coagulation factors produced by recombinant technology. Patients with hemophilia A or B may develop IgG antibodies to the deficient coagulation proteins such as FVIII or FIX from chronic replacement therapy. Previous surgery or blood transfusion may trigger antibody formation against factor V. More commonly, antifactor V and antithrombin antibodies are produced by prior surgical use of topical bovine fibrin glue (5,6). Very rarely, antibodies may develop against intrinsic (FXI or FXII), extrinsic (FVII or FX), or common coagulation pathway (FV or prothrombin) proteins or against fibrinogen or fibrin (see Chapter 71). Drug-induced antibodies (quinidine, quinine, some antibiotics) against specific coagulation proteins are uncommon. Patients with fulminant acute hepatitis or severe chronic liver disease may sometimes have abnormal coagulation caused by low concentrations of specific clotting factors produced in the liver. End-stage renal disease may produce mild to moderate thrombocytopenia and platelet dysfunction caused by circulating low molecular weight metabolites (7).

Surgeons also must be aware of a large menu of genetic procoagulant clotting disorders, which increase the likelihood thrombotic and embolic complications. Most of these mutant procoagulant proteins are uncommon causes of clinical disease, but three are not. Factor $V_{Leiden}$ mutation, which prevents active factor V from being degraded by active protein C, is prevalent (2% to 5%) in Northern European whites and the prothrombin 20210 mutation is prevalent (1% to 3%) in Southern Europeans (8). Both mutations increase the risk of venous thrombosis (8). Lupus anticoagulant, a misleading term, and anticardiolipin antibodies against phospholipids occur most commonly, but not exclusively, in patients with autoimmune diseases and may produce thrombotic complications during and after major surgery (9) (see Chapter 112). This abnormality usually is detected by an unexplained prolonged aPTT that is not corrected by infusion of normal plasma.

## Platelet Inhibitors

Aspirin alone or in combination with other drugs is the most commonly used anticoagulant. Aspirin and many nonsteroidal, antiinflammatory drugs irreversibly inhibit platelet cyclooxygense, which partially inhibits platelet function by blocking thromboxane $A_2$ synthesis (10). Aspirin prolongs bleeding times by 1.5 to 2 minutes (11) and partially blocks aggregation (12), but may increase bleeding times further if other, mild hemostatic deficiencies (e.g., von Willebrand disease) are present. Major surgery, including cardiac surgery, in patients with aspirin inhibited platelets may or may not increase perioperative bleeding (12–14). Nearly all patients presenting with acute coronary syndromes receive aspirin as part of their initial therapy, but usually the impact on surgical hemostasis is minor (14). Aspirin-related bleeding is treated by platelet transfusions, because aspirin is cleared from blood in less than 90 minutes (15).

Platelet glycoprotein (GP) IIIa/IIb ($\alpha_{IIb}\beta_3$) receptor antagonists inhibit most platelet functions and prolong bleeding times considerably longer than cyclooxygenase inhibitors (16). Clopidogrel and ticlopidine irreversibly inhibit the platelet (ADP) adenosine diphosphate receptor to prevent platelet adhesion and aggregation and, like aspirin, the duration of inhibition lasts for the life of the platelet, which is approximately 8 days (10). Inhibitory effects of other GP IIb/IIIa receptor antagonists vary from less than 1 hour (eptifibatide) (17) to approximately 48 hours (abciximab) (17). Abciximab (ReoPro) rapidly binds to the platelet receptor and, for the most, part remains bound for the life of the platelet. Platelet inhibitory effects of clopidogrel and ticlopidine last for several days (17). When aspirin is combined with clopidogrel, bleeding complications increase with higher doses of aspirin; therefore, only low-dosage aspirin is recommended for the combination (18). Cilostazol, a cyclic nucleotide phosphodiesterase inhibitor, used in vascular surgery, inhibits platelets within 2 to 4 hours (19). Cardiac surgery soon after administration of short-acting reversible inhibitors (e.g., eptifibatide and tirofiban) does not increase surgical bleeding (20). However, most studies recommend withholding clopidogrel 3 to 5 days before elective major surgery to increase the number of circulating uninhibited platelets (14,21,22).

## Fibrinolytic Drugs

Fibrinolytic drugs are used to lyse blood clots, but tissue-type plasminogen activator (tPA), streptokinase, and urokinase also increase surgical bleeding if operation occurs within 12 hours of the last dose (23). Fibrinolytic drugs reduce fibrinogen concentrations and also mildly impair platelet aggregation (24). If emergency operation is required, cryoprecipitate and/or fresh frozen plasma (FFP) are recommended to replenish fibrinogen. Platelet transfusions are needed to restore full platelet function, especially if a long-acting platelet inhibitor such as clopidogrel or abciximab is circulating in the blood. Antifibrinolytic drugs, ε-amino caproic acid (EACA) or aprotinin, are not recommended for fear of exacerbating the process for which fibrinolytic therapy was prescribed; however, there is little clinical experience.

Fibrinolytic drugs are cautiously recommended for treating thrombotic strokes soon after cardiac or other major surgery. Potential benefits outweigh the risk of causing intracranial hemorrhage or increasing surgical site bleeding (25–27).

## Warfarin

Warfarin is taken daily by millions of Americans to prevent intravascular coagulation and thromboembolic events. For very minor superficial operations (e.g., transvenous pacemaker insertion), it is usually not necessary to reverse warfarin inhibition. For elective major operations, warfarin (also clopidogrel) should be stopped for 3 to 5 days before surgery if the likelihood of a clotting event within that time is small (14). The PT should be checked before operation to be sure most, if not all, of the warfarin effect has been reversed. In patients who cannot safely tolerate interruption of anticoagulation (e.g., mechanical heart valves), intravenous standard heparin is used to maintain anticoagulation until 2 to 3 hours before incision.

Oral vitamin K (2 to 4 mg) usually returns INR (international normalized ratio) PTs of 5.0 or less to the normal value within 24 hours (28). In emergencies, warfarin anticoagulation can be reversed by transfusions of prothrombin complex concentrates, which contain vitamin K–dependent coagulation factors II, VII, IX, and X, or FFP (10 to 20 mL per kg), which also replaces the four deficient vitamin K–dependent coagulation proteins (28). Prothrombin complex concentrates have risk, and intravascular thrombosis has occurred (29). Because of the risk of anaphylaxis (30) or supranormal concentrations of prothrombin (31), intravenous vitamin K (10 mg, IV slowly) should not be given unless bleeding is life-threatening. If replacement therapy, which should be tried first, is not effective, administration of recombinant factor VIIa (41 to 90 $\mu$g per kg, IV) is appropriate in patients with emergency or life-threatening bleeding (32).

## Standard Unfractionated Heparin

Standard, unfractionated heparin does not prevent thrombin formation but inhibits thrombin after it is formed and after most of the enzymes involved in the coagulation cascade have been generated. The drug does not inhibit thrombin directly but acts by catalyzing plasma antithrombin to inhibit thrombin and to a lesser extent factors IXa and Xa (see Chapter 15). Standard heparin does not inhibit thrombin bound in fibrin clots (33). Heparin can be given intravenously, has rapid onset, and is

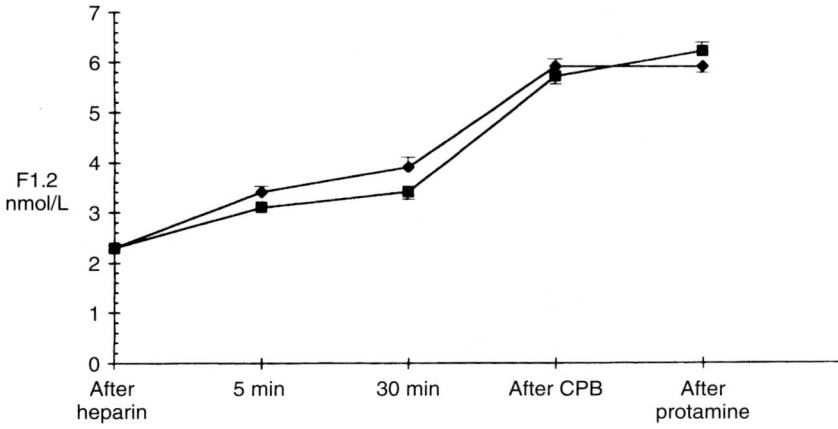

FIGURE 74-1. Plasma prothrombin fragment F1.2 measured after heparin before cardiopulmonary bypass (CPB), after 5 and 30 min during CPB, 5 min after CPB, and 10 min after administration of protamine in two groups of 10 patients (who had open heart surgery). In both groups, full systemic heparin (3 mg per kg) was given. In the experimental group (*squares*), the entire perfusion circuit was coated with covalently bound heparin. Circuits of the control group did not have surface-bound heparin coatings. No significant differences were found between groups. (From Gorman RC, Ziats NP, Rao AK, et al. Surface-bound heparin fails to reduce thrombin formation during clinical cardiopulmonary bypass. *J Thorac Cardiovasc Surg* 1996;111:1, with permission.)

completely reversed by protamine, but the circulating concentration cannot be monitored directly or in real time. Recent data indicates that porcine heparin is less immunogenic than bovine heparin (34). Standard heparin is far from ideal but is reversible and is currently the best anticoagulant for extracorporeal perfusion.

## Cardiopulmonary Bypass

Cardiopulmonary bypass (CPB) is not possible without heparin (35). However, heparin inhibits coagulation at the end of the coagulation cascade; consequently, thrombin is produced and circulates despite doses of heparin that far exceed those used for treatment of other thrombotic disorders (36,37) (see Fig. 74-1). Contact between heparinized blood and both the surgical wound and biomaterials of the perfusion circuit activate platelets, the fibrinolytic system, both the extrinsic and intrinsic coagulation pathways, and the complement (35,38). Most thrombin is generated in the surgical wound, as compared to the perfusion circuit (39–41). At the end of CPB and open heart surgery, platelet counts are typically reduced by 40% to 60%, circulating platelets are dysfunctional, and template bleeding times are approximately twice normal (42,43) (see Fig. 74-2). CPB also activates the fibrinolytic system to produce plasmin (44) (see Fig. 74-3). During CPB and open heart surgery, the concentrations of D-dimer and fibrinopeptide A, fragments of fibrin and fibrinogen, respectively, increase (44). The principal causes of nonsurgical bleeding after open heart surgery are related to heparin, fibrinolysis (44), and loss of platelet numbers and function (42,43).

Although bleeding from unrecognized congenital deficiencies of a soluble coagulation factor may occur, most of these patients are discovered by preoperative screening. CPB dilutes soluble coagulation factors and reduces factors V and VIII to concentrations less than those expected from dilution (45). Nevertheless, bleeding after CPB rarely, if ever, occurs from this cause. Concentrations of soluble coagulation factors required for safe surgical hemostasis are provided in Table 74-1.

Heparin-related causes of bleeding are primarily caused by incomplete neutralization by protamine. Rarely, "heparin rebound"—a term that describes delayed release of bound heparin from the lymphatic system after protamine has been cleared from plasma—causes delayed bleeding. "Heparin resistance" occurs when plasma antithrombin concentrations are deficient from either malnutrition in infants with cyanosis or patients with cachexia or from sustained heparin administration just before operation (46). Anticoagulation and heparin effectiveness are corrected by FFP or recombinant antithrombin.

## Heparin Induced Thrombocytopenia

Heparin induced thrombocytopenia(HIT) is an immune disease related to repeated heparin exposure and mediated by the development of IgG antibodies in some patients to a complex of heparin and platelet factor 4 (PF4) (2,47). The disease affects approximately 2% of all patients undergoing cardiac surgery because of the necessity of heparin and because large amounts of PF4 are produced during cardiopulmonary bypass (42,43,48). In susceptible patients, exposure to heparin stimulates production of transient IgG antibodies to antiheparin-PF4 complexes, which then bind to platelet FcγRIIa receptors (49). These IgG antibodies circulate for 3 to 6 months after heparin exposure (50). Antibody binding to platelet FcγRIIa stimulates platelet aggregation and release of granules to produce thrombocytopenia (HIT) or thrombocytopenia and thrombosis (HITT); however, for unknown reasons, only some patients with antiheparin-PF4 IgG antibodies develop thrombocytopenia (49). HIT is suspected when the platelet count precipitously decreases by 30% to 50% immediately after repeat exposure to heparin (2). Although the

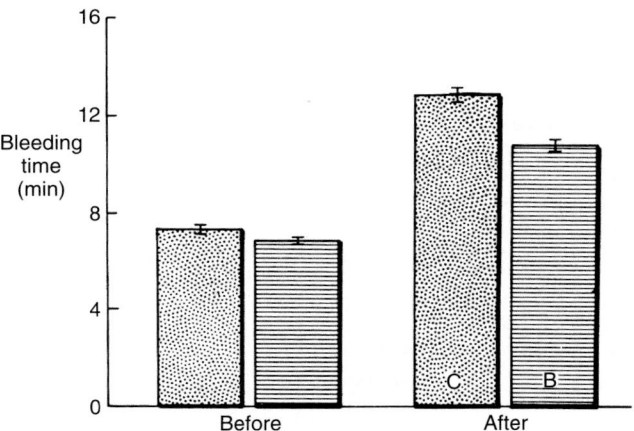

FIGURE 74-1. Mean changes and standard errors in template bleeding times before and after CPB using a bubble oxygenator (*stippled bars*, n = 12) or membrane oxygenator (*hatched bars*, n = 22). Within group P values: B, P <0.05; C, P <0.005. (Reprinted with permission from Edmunds LH Jr, Ellison N, Colman RW, et al. Platelet function during open heart surgery: comparison of the membrane and bubble oxygenators. *J Thorac Cardiovasc Surg* 1982;83:805.)

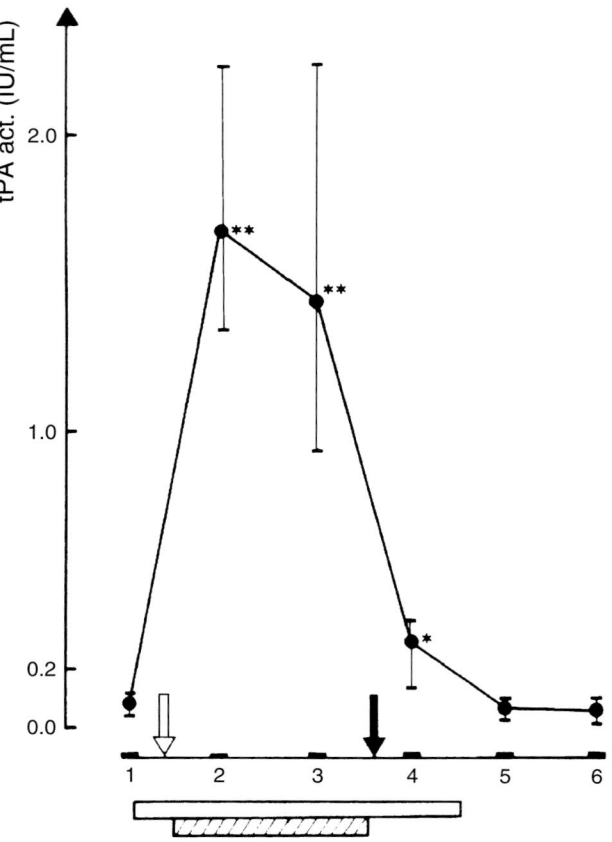

**FIGURE 74-3.** Median concentration and quartiles of free tissue-type plasminogen activator (tPA) in 24 patients undergoing cardiopulmonary bypass and open heart surgery. (From Gram J, Janetzko T, Jespersen J, et al. Enhanced effective fibrinolysis following the neutralization of herparin in open heart surgery increases the risk of postsurgical bleeding. *Thromb Haemost* 1990;63:241, with permission.)

thrombocytopenia rarely causes bleeding, a serotonin release test or enzyme immunoassay to detect the presence of antiheparin-PF4 IgG antibodies (51) is mandatory before any more heparin is given. The combination of three ingredients—unfractionated standard heparin or fractionated low-molecular-weight heparin, PF4, and antiheparin-PF4 IgG antibodies—risks the thrombotic form of HIT: HITT.

Thrombocytopenia and thrombosis caused by massive platelet consumption may produce platelet counts less than 30,000 per $\mu$L, but platelet transfusions are not recommended. Unless plasma antiheparin-PF4 IgG antibodies are removed first, platelet transfusions exacerbate the problem. If serious, nonsurgical bleeding occurs, plasmapheresis is a reasonable option to remove antiheparin-PF4 IgG antibodies, PF4, and heparin before administering platelet transfusions; however, recorded experience is meager (52). HITT causes devastating intravascular thrombosis that produces strokes, myocardial infarction, amputations, and lawsuits (53).

## Low-Molecular-Weight Heparins

Low-molecular-weight heparins (e.g., enoxaparin, fragmin, and fondaparinux) catalyze antithrombin activity, but they primarily inhibit factor Xa (54), which is the enzyme that generates the prothrombinase complex from prothrombin. Low-molecular-weight heparins can be given intravenously; act rapidly; are long-acting (plasma half-life is 4 to 8 hours); are monitored, if necessary, by measuring factor Xa activity; are not adequately reversed by protamine (55); may generate antiplatelet IgG antibodies (HIT and HITT); do not reliably prevent clot formation during CPB; and are associated with excessive postoperative bleeding if used immediately before or during surgery (56,57).

## Bivalirudin

Bivalirudin (Hirulog) is a synthetic, 20–amino acid, reversible, direct thrombin inhibitor that is also effective in fibrin clots (58).

## TABLE 74-1

### COAGULATION FACTORS REQUIRED FOR SAFE SURGICAL HEMOSTASIS

| Factor | *In vivo* half-life | Level required for hemostasis | Storage characteristics | Choice of material for replacement |
|---|---|---|---|---|
| I (fibrinogen) | 3–4 d | 100 mg/100 mL | Stable in plasma at 4°C | Cryoprecipitate (single donor) |
| II (prothrombin) | 2–5 d | 20%–40% | Stable in plasma at 4°C | Frozen plasma, concentrates |
| V | 15–36 h | <25% | Labile except when frozen | Frozen plasma |
| VII | 4–7 h | 10%–20% | Stable in plasma at 4°C | Concentrates, recombinant FVIIa |
| VIII | 9–18 h | Minimum of 30% for major surgery; less for minor procedures | Labile except when frozen | Concentrates [natural (viral inactivated) or recombinant] |
| IX | 20–24 h | 25%–30% | Stable in plasma at 4°C | Concentrates (cryoprecipitate supernatant) |
| X | 32–48 h | 10%–20% | Stable in plasma at 4°C | Frozen plasma, concentrates |
| XI | 40–80 h | 15%–25% | Stable in plasma at 4°C | Stored or frozen plasma, concentrates, supernatant from cryoprecipitate |
| XII | 48–52 h | Deficiency not associated with a bleeding tendency | Stable in plasma at 4°C | Replacement not necessary |
| XIII | 12 d | <5% | Stable in plasma | Stored or frozen plasma, cryoprecipitate |
| von Willebrand | A few hours | 25%–50% | Labile except when frozen | Cryoprecipitate; factor VIII concentrates of intermediate purityless for minor procedures |

The drug has a half-life in plasma of 25 to 36 min (59,60); it is preferably monitored by ecarin clotting time (61) but has been successfully monitored by activated clotting times (ACT) (62,63) or aPTT; it is nontoxic; is essentially nonantigenic; and it has no major side effects except bleeding. The drug acts rapidly, is cleared by proteolysis and the kidneys (64), and has no antidote (60). The drug has been extensively evaluated in patients with acute coronary artery syndromes and is associated with less bleeding than with standard heparin (65). The pharmokinetics of the drug are attractive for use during CPB and open heart surgery (66) (see Fig. 74-4) and the drug has been successfully used in off-pump myocardial revascularization in a series of patients (67). The drug is not approved for CPB, but clinical trials in patients with HIT are underway (68). Drug dosage is under investigation: Initial dosing schedules combine 1.5 mg per kg IV and 50 mg in the pump prime and a continuous infusion at 2.5 to 3.5 mg/kg/hour (2,66,68). Successful anecdotal experience has been reported (62,63,66); however, extensive experience is not available and optimal dosing and the ability to completely suppress F1.2 production are not known.

## Lepirudin

Lepirudin (recombinant hirudin) directly binds and inactivates thrombin, including thrombin within fibrin clots. The drug has a plasma half-life of approximately 80 minutes and is primarily excreted by the kidney (58,69). The duration of anticoagulant activity of lepirudin is inversely proportional to creatinine clearance and is prolonged up to 3 to 5 hours by anesthesia, which reduces renal blood flow (70). Plasma concentrations are monitored by ecarin clotting time or by aPTT (71). Because

aPTT values flatten at high concentrations of lepirudin (>0.6 $\mu$g per mL), a standard curve using pooled plasma is recommended (70). There is no antidote. The major side effect is bleeding, which may be increased by simultaneous administration of fibrinolytic agents. Allergic reactions are minimal.

Lepirudin is approved by the U.S. Food and Drug Administration (FDA) for use during CPB in patients with HIT or HITT and is the most widely used alternative to standard heparin (70,72) (danaproid is no longer available in the United States, although it is elsewhere). For CPB bolus lepirudin (0.25 mg per kg IV plus 0.2 mg per kg in the circuit priming volume) is recommended followed by continuous infusion of 0.5 mg per min (2,68). Lepirudin blood concentrations are maintained at a concentration between 3.5 and 4.5 $\mu$g per mL by measurements of ecarin clotting times every 15 minutes (2,68). In a single case, this concentration suppressed thrombin formation during the first hour of CPB, but supplement bolus doses (6 mg) were needed thereafter to prevent a progressive increase in F1.2 (73).

## Argatroban

Argatroban is a synthetic, low-molecular-weight, reversible, direct thrombin inhibitor derived from L-arginine and avidly binds thrombin even in fibrin clots (74). Given intravenously, the drug acts rapidly, has a half-life in plasma of approximately 45 minutes (75), and is metabolized in the liver. Anticoagulant activity is primarily monitored by aPTT, but when high doses are used, ACT are recommended (74,75). There is no antidote. Bleeding is the only major side effect; no toxic or allergic reactions are known.

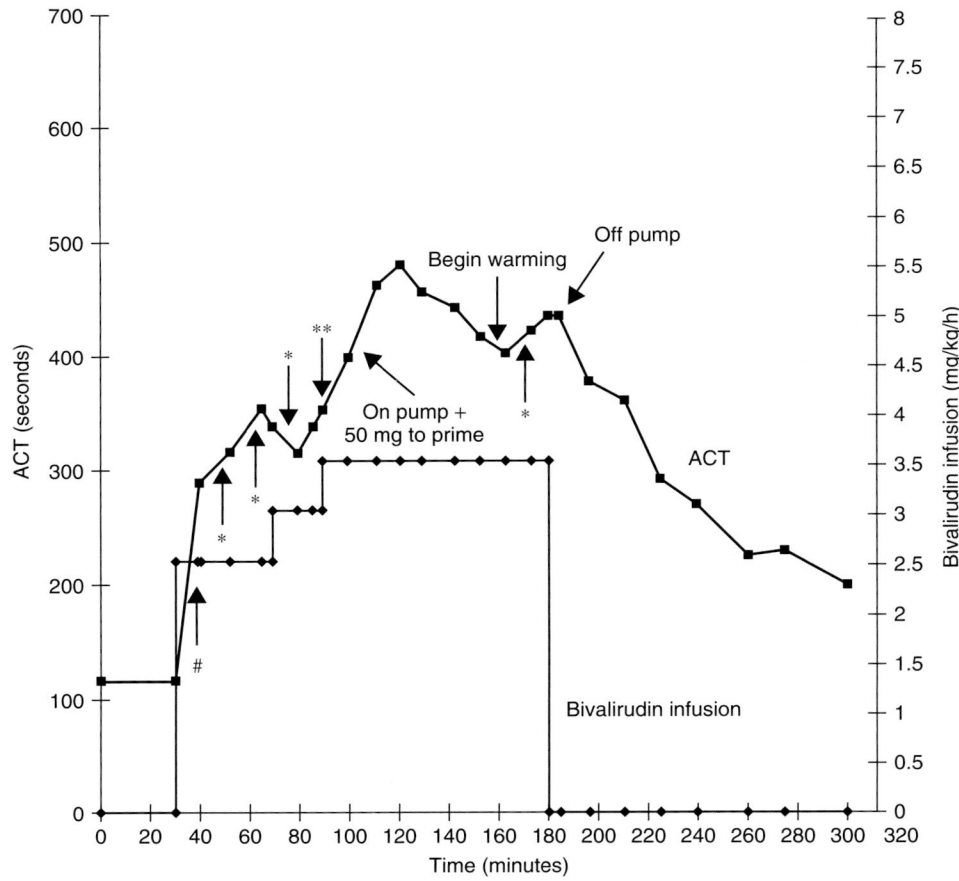

**FIGURE 74-4.** Activated clotting times and bivalirudin infusion protocol during and after myocardial revascularization with cardiopulmonary bypass in a 67-year-old man. (Figure is slightly modified from Clayton SB, Acsell JR, Crumbley AJ III, et al. Cardiopulmonary bypass with bivalirudin in type II heparin induced thrombocytopenia. *Ann Thorac Surg* 2004;78: 2167–2169.)

Argatroban is approved for use in patients with HIT or HITT by the U.S. FDA, but experience during CPB (76,77), left heart bypass (78), and off-pump myocardial revascularization (79) is limited. A bolus dose of 0.1 mg per kg and a continuous infusion of 5 to 10 $\mu$g/kg/minute with occasional bolus doses (2 mg) were used to maintain ACT between 300 and 400 seconds (76,77). In one instance, postoperative bleeding was 3,800 mL in 24 hours (77).

## Disseminated Intravascular Coagulation

Disseminated intravascular coagulation (DIC) is a consumptive coagulopathy that varies in intensity from mild (e.g., CPB) to severe (septic shock). The term *consumptive coagulopathy* describes the simultaneous occurrence of thrombin generation and fibrinolysis with ongoing depletion of coagulation proteins and platelets. Depending on the intensity of stimuli from the causative pathology, DIC combines intravascular coagulation and tissue ischemia with a bleeding diathesis produced by consumption of platelets, soluble coagulation factors, or fibrinolysis (see Chapters 109 and 110).

Simultaneous elevation of F1.2 and D-dimer certifies the consumptive coagulopathy associated with CPB (35), but DIC connotes a more severe and often overwhelming process that is most often triggered by bacterial Gram-positive or Gram-negative septicemia (80). In surgical practice, DIC may complicate severe trauma, particularly if the brain is injured, or complicate postoperative septicemia developing from sources such as intravenous catheters, urinary tract infections, wounds, or pneumonia. The underlying disease—trauma or infection in surgical patients—initiates thrombin generation primarily by the tissue factor pathway. Tissue factor is supplied by cellular tissue factor in injured tissues (41,80,81), by expression of cell-bound tissue factor on monocytes and endothelial cells (82–85), and by elevated concentrations of soluble plasma tissue factor bound to monocytes that are activated by circulating inflammatory cytokines (41,86). Intravascular thrombin stimulates platelet aggregation and granule release, endothelial cell production of tPA, and fibrinolysis (80,87) (see Chapters 109 and 110).

Effective therapy requires control of the initiating cause or causes of the coagulopathy. Except for life-saving transfusions, replacement of blood constituents is usually futile until the etiology of DIC is brought under control (88). Surgery is only undertaken to control the causes of DIC. The least invasive and most rapid operation to alleviate the infection, injury or other cause is best; new incisions are likely to bleed. Preparation for surgery varies and may require heparin or a direct thrombin inhibitor to control thrombin generation and/or FFP, cryoprecipitate, and platelet transfusions to replace consumed procoagulants. Prothrombin concentrates and antifibrinolytic drugs, aprotinin and EACA, are not recommended because of the risk of accelerating intravascular thrombosis and tissue ischemia (29) (see Chapter 107). Emerging therapy includes efforts to suppress inflammatory cytokine production (89) and selective replacement therapy with recombinant antithrombin, recombinant tissue factor pathway inhibitor, and/or recombinant human activated protein C (90,91).

# PREPARATIONS OF STORED BLOOD AND BLOOD PRODUCTS

More than 95% of blood and blood component transfusions are from allogenic donors. Although the nation's blood supply is considered safe and the incidence of transfused disease very low (92,93), costs, availability of blood products, and negative effects and risks of allogenic transfusion (94) have stimulated efforts to define specific indications and "triggers" for transfusion in recent years (95,96). In otherwise healthy, non-bleeding, postoperative patients, blood transfusion is not recommended for hemoglobin concentrations more than 7 g per dL (96,97). The threshold is approximately 8 g per dL for patients with cardiac disorder without myocardial ischemia and 10 g per dL for those with ischemia (92,96). Prophylactic transfusions to replace blood volume or in anticipation of blood loss are not recommended (92). These guidelines do not apply to actively bleeding trauma or surgical patients.

## Whole Blood

Whole blood taken from carefully screened donors is commonly mixed with citrate, phosphate, dextrose, and adenine (CPDA-1; 10:1.4 ratio) or similar anticoagulant preservatives and is further processed into components (98). Citrate chelates calcium to provide anticoagulation, phosphate provides buffer, and dextrose and adenine support ATP (adenine triphosphate) synthesis, which is required to maintain red cell membrane integrity. During storage, 2,3-diphosphoglyceric acid (2-3 DPG) is metabolized and pH progressively decreases from approximately 7.20 as lactate, potassium, ammonia, plasma hemoglobin, cytokines, and other bioactive materials accumulate (94,99). Microparticles are produced from crenated and lyzed red cells, degenerated white cells, aggregated platelets, fibrin filaments, denatured proteins, and lipids (100). Whole blood (approximately 500 mL) contains red cells (hematocrit, 35% to 40%), plasma proteins, white cells ($10^9$ $\mu$L), and approximately 60 mL of the anticoagulant preservative solution. Shelf life is 21 to 35 days (101).

## Fresh Whole Blood

Fresh whole blood stored in heparin or CPDA-1 retains higher concentrations of factors V and VIII if used within a few hours of collection; however, in a randomized trial of pediatric patients undergoing heart surgery, this expensive preparation provided no advantages over the combination of packed cells and FFP (102).

## Packed Red Cells

Packed red cells are produced within 8 hours of donation by centrifugation. The process extends erythrocyte longevity and avoids some of the undesirable products of whole blood storage. Packed cells are prepared by removing 200 to 250 mL of the diluted plasma. The remaining red cells in residual plasma with $10^8$ $\mu$L white cells have a shelf life of 35 days, volume of 250 mL, and a hematocrit between 70% and 80% (101). Before centrifugation, one of several preservative solutions is often added to CPDA-1–preserved whole blood to increase red cell longevity to 42 days. These preparations contain $10^8$ $\mu$L leukocytes, 50% to 60% red cells in a total volume of approximately 350 mL (101). Packed-cell preparations may be washed in 1 to 2 liters of saline to reduce the amounts of plasma proteins, microparticles, and white cells, but washed cells must be used within 24 hours. Packed cells also may be irradiated to prevent graft versus host disease or frozen for long-term storage for up to 10 years (101).

In recent years, adverse effects of stored red cells have received more scrutiny. Red cells stored more than 15 days lose the capacity to transport oxygen and the deformability to pass through capillaries (103). White cells stored with packed cells increase hemolysis and loss of intracellular potassium; release IL-1, IL-8, and tumor necrosis factor (104), and generate neutrophil agonists (105). "Storage lesion" has been implicated in causing increased morbidity (94,106) and perhaps mortality (94,107), although mortality data are not conclusive

(94). Filtration with 20- to 40-$\mu$m pore filters or transfusion of washed or leukocyte-reduced packed red cells can reduce the number of transfused leukocytes and platelets included in packed red cell preparations (104). Leukodepletion of packed cell preparations reduce but do not completely prevent toxic manifestations of "storage lesions" (94,104).

## Fresh Frozen Plasma

Fresh frozen plasma (FFP) is prepared by separation from red cells within 24 hours (preferably within 6 hours) of donation from nonheparinized anticoagulated blood and stored at −18°C or colder for up to 1 year. Frozen plasma is thawed at 30°C to 37°C over 20 to 30 minutes and must be used within 24 hours of thawing. FFP contains 2 to 3 $\mu$g per mL fibrinogen, 60 $\mu$g per mL factor XIII, 5 to 10 $\mu$g per mL von Willebrand factor, and all of the stable coagulation factors, complement proteins, and immunoglobulins, in addition to electrolytes, trace elements, and vitamins (108).

## Cryoprecipitate

Cryoprecipitate is prepared from thawing FFP at 4°C and harvesting the precipitate, which is rich in fibrinogen, factors VIII and XIII, and von Willebrand factor. Cryoprecipitate is diluted in 5 to 10 mL of plasma and refrozen to −18°C for storage up to 1 year (109). Infusions are usually pooled to provide 1 U per 5 kg body weight.

## Platelet Concentrates

Platelet concentrates are prepared from whole blood by low and high spin centrifugation to produce 50 mL containing 55,000 to 70,000 per $\mu$L platelets. Platelet concentrates from five to eight different donors are routinely pooled to produce a single dose of 300,000 to 600,000 per $\mu$L platelets. Platelets are stored at 20°C to 24°C and slightly agitated to prevent aggregation for up to 5 days. Platelet concentrates are prone to bacterial contamination during storage and also express ABO antigens (see subsequent text) (110,111). Platelet ABO matching is seldom done, although mismatches with the recipient plasma may decrease platelet survival (112). Transfused platelets contain small amounts of plasma and leukocytes and have a half-life of approximately 4 days.

# COMPLICATIONS OF TRANFUSION OF ALLOGENIC BLOOD AND BLOOD PRODUCTS

## Mismatch

Fatal hemolytic transfusion reactions caused by ABO incompatibility occur once in every 250,000 to 1 million transfusions and approximately half is a result of human error (92). The incidence of mismatch errors is one in every 14,000 to 18,000 transfusions (110,113). The major red cell antigens that precipitate severe hemolytic reactions in recipients who have incompatible antibodies are ABO group A and B antigens and Rh (D) antigen. More than 250 red cell antigens have been identified (114), but most are not immunogenic or are only weakly so (114). Of the less important antigen groups, anti-K (Kell), anti-Jk$^a$ (Kidd), and anti-Fy$^a$ (Duffy) are the most common causes of severe hemolytic reactions in adults and non-newborns (115), but anti-H in O$_h$ patients and anti-Di$^a$ (Diego) are rare causes (114).

Humans naturally develop A or B antibodies against the antigens that are not expressed on their own red cells and are therefore presensitized against incompatible donor red cells. Antibodies to Rh (D) antigens and hemolytic antigens from the rare groups are produced by sensitization by small amounts of incompatible blood or blood products (e.g., packed cells, FFP or platelets) or by pregnancy in Rh-negative women. A, B, and antigens from the lesser antigen groups produce IgG and IgM antibodies that bind and activate complement to produce severe, life-threatening, intravascular hemolysis. Rh (D) antigens sensitize Rh-negative patients for life, and although the IgG antibody does not bind complement, severe extravascular hemolysis and death may occur. Antibodies to other red cell antigens such as Lewis, MNS, P, Lutheran, E, and C rarely cause serious hemolysis in humans (115,116).

Prior transfusion also can sensitize a recipient to incompatible ABO and Rh red cell antigens and can cause a hemolytic transfusion reaction during subsequent transfusion. Alloantibody screening tests are designed to detect these antibodies during crossmatching (112). Prior sensitization may produce an anamnestic reaction to subsequent exposure and rapid production of anti–red cell antibodies, such as anti-Jk$^a$ (Kidd) (114). An anamnestic response may produce delayed agglutination or hemolysis 3 to 7 days after transfusion. Initial cross-matching may not detect anamnestic antibodies, but a later one does. In some patients, first exposure to small amounts of incompatible red cell antigens may stimulate antibody production that produces very delayed hemolysis of residual transfused cells weeks later (117). Delayed reactions to alloantibodies are generally not severe. However, plasma of "universal donors" (group O, Rh-negative) may contain high titers of anti-A or anti-B antibodies from prior sensitization of the donor. Transfusion of blood from one of these "dangerous universal donors" may cause a severe hemolytic reaction in A, B, and AB recipients.

Anti-A and anti-B are potent hemolysins and can cause rapid intravascular lysis of red cells. Acute (within 24 hours) hemolysis causes severe precordial or flank pain, fever, tachycardia, tachypnea, hypotension, hemoglobinuria, and oliguria. Hemolytic transfusion reactions may produce severe DIC, hypotension, and renal failure. Plasma hemoglobin binds to plasma proteins such as haptoglobin and hemopexin, but when protein-binding capacity is exceeded (150 mg per dL), free hemoglobin and its derivatives precipitate in the renal tubules, particularly if urine is acidic. Plasma hemoglobin does not usually cause oliguria or anuria, but it may do so if complicated by severe hypotension or DIC. Acute ABO/Rh hemolytic reactions occur once in every 6,000 to 33,000 packed cell transfusions and are fatal once in every 0.5 to 1.8 million (118).

Less reactive antibodies, which cause agglutination rather than hemolysis or positive serologic tests, may cause hemolysis within the liver and spleen rather than DIC. When red cells are destroyed more slowly, jaundice and oliguria may be the only overt manifestations, but renal failure can occur.

Mild allergic reactions occur in 1% to 3% of patients receiving large plasma transfusions and 0.3% of those who receive other blood components (119) and may be accompanied by chills, fever, urticaria, pruritus, and erythema. Acute anaphylactic reactions are estimated to occur in one in 20,000 to 50,000 transfusions (117). Most patients respond to antihistamines, although some require epinephrine or corticosteroids.

"Febrile associated transfusion reactions" occur in approximately 0.5% to 2% of recipients (110,120). The incidence is higher with repeated transfusions in susceptible patients and occurs in approximately 18% of patients who receive platelet transfusions (121). The main symptom is fever, which usually occurs with the transfusion and disappears within 1 to 2 hours. The reactions are caused by production of inflammatory cytokines stimulated by agonists in the supernatant plasma (120,122); however, the exact mechanism is still under investigation (120). Leukoreduction of transfused products is not protective (110).

Acute respiratory distress syndrome (ARDS), which can be fatal, may develop within 4 hours of transfusion in one in 5,000 to 8,000 patients who have received transfusions (110,123). Antigens in the donor plasma stimulate recipient neutrophils to increase alveolar-capillary permeability (110). Microscopically, alveoli are filled with a hemorrhagic exudate and varying numbers of granulocytes and macrophages (124).

## Blood-Borne Infections

Currently, the incidence of infection from transfused blood-borne microbes is at record lows in the United States (110). Use of all volunteer donors, better blood conservation techniques, new screening tests, and nucleic acid testing for viral agents have dramatically increased the safety of the nation's blood supply (110). The risk of transmission of human immunodeficiency virus (HIV) and related HIV-2 is so low that rates can only be estimated and approximate one infection in 2 million transfusions (110,125). The risk of transmitting human T-lymphotrophic virus (HTLV-I or II) was reported as one in 640,000 a few years ago (126) and is probably lower now. The risk of hepatitis A infection from transfusion is estimated at one per million U (127). Improved screening tests for hepatitis B and C carriers have reduced the incidence of blood-borne infection to approximately one in 180,000 and 1.6 million transfusions, respectively (110). Hepatitis B remains the highest risk for serious blood-borne viral infection from transfusion in nonimmunosuppressed patients, and a vaccine is available for health care workers.

Cytomegalovirus (CMV), Epstein-Barr virus, and Parvovirus B19 are serious threats to immunosuppressed patients, but not to otherwise healthy individuals, and can be transmitted by leukocytes in red cell transfusions (128). CMV and Epstein-Barr antibodies are nearly ubiquitous in adults and nearly half of adults have antibodies to parvovirus B19. Donors are not always screened for antibodies to these viruses; therefore, screening is essential for transfusions into immunosuppressed patients (110,128). Although the viruses reside in cells, leukocyte reduction is not effective in reducing recipient serocoversion to these and other viral diseases (110).

Platelet transfusions are the greatest risk of transfusion-related infection primarily because platelets are stored at room temperature and concentrates are prepared from five to eight donors. Bacterial contamination occurs in 0.05% to 0.1% of platelet transfusions and may cause severe septicemia and death (110). *Yersinia enterocolitica*–contaminated red cells (approximately 1:1 million U) has been identified as the etiology of a highly lethal septicemia (110).

Very rare and potential infectious agents transmitted by transfusion include brucellosis, West Nile virus, and several parasitic diseases—babesiosis, Chagas disease, leishmaniasis, lyme disease, malaria, syphilis, and toxoplasmosis (110,129,130). Prions have been transmitted by blood transfusion in animals, but no case of Creutzfeldt-Jakob disease or new variant Creutzfeldt-Jakob disease has been reported from transfusion in humans (129). Although many bacterial and parasitic diseases are transmitted by transfusion, the risk of infection in the United States is low and approximately once in 1 million transfusions (131).

## Immune Response

The importance of allogenic blood in suppressing the immune response of the recipient remains controversial (92,110), but there is no conclusive evidence that blood transfusions hasten the recurrence of cancer (110), prolong transplanted organ survival, or increase the risk of wound infections (110,132). Furthermore, leukocyte reduction transfusions have not demonstrated a favorable effect for either cancer recurrence or wound infection (110). Graft versus host disease is a rare event following transfusion of allogenic, competent lymphocytes into an immunosuppressed patient. The reaction is usually fatal (133).

## Massive Transfusion

Massive bleeding (class III or IV hemorrhage, i.e., >30% or 40% of blood volume) (134) triggers massive transfusion, which is generally defined as replacement of one blood volume within 24 hours (99,135). Massive transfusion exposes the patient to additional risks beyond those incurred by transfusing a few units. During surgery, efforts to control bleeding occur simultaneously with massive blood replacement, but in patients with trauma, control of bleeding and replacement are delayed because of transport to a hospital. Rapid replacement of one blood volume with stored blood dilutes the remaining autologous blood to approximately 25% to 30% of the circulating mixture. If two blood volumes are lost and replaced, approximately 10% of the remaining mixture is autologous (99). Transfusion of 1 U of whole blood or packed cells increases the circulating hemoglobin concentration approximately 1 g per dL in nonbleeding adults (136).

Although maintenance of both blood volume and oxygen carrying capacity are essential in patients who are rapidly bleeding, the priority of maintaining blood volume over oxygen carrying capacity is generally recognized (110,132). Acute loss of 30% to 40% of the blood volume in young trauma victims can usually be replaced by crystalloids (132,137,138); however, only 20% of administered crystalloids remain intravascular; therefore three to four times the amount of blood loss must be given (135). In previously healthy patients and those not at increased risk of myocardial or cerebral atherosclerotic occlusive disease, a hemoglobin concentration as low as 6 g per dL is tolerated; lactic acid is produced at lower concentrations (97,139).

Not infrequently, the rate of bleeding and the absolute need to maintain circulating blood volume do not permit full typing of the recipient's erythrocytes, screening for acquired hemolytic antibodies, and cross-matching the recipient's serum against each unit of donor packed red cells (60 to 90 minutes) (135). If the patient's ABO/Rh typing is known, a partial crossmatch between the patient's serum and donor red cells eliminates the risk of serious hemolytic reactions and takes 10 to 15 minutes. If ABO-Rh type is not known, un–cross-matched group O and Rh positive or negative transfusions can be given as an emergency measure until the patient's blood can be typed. Rh-positive blood is avoided, if possible, in young women, who may later become pregnant. If the patient's blood type is accurately known, transfusion of type-specific, un–cross-matched blood produces an antibody reaction in approximately 1% to 2% of transfusions (112).

Massive transfusion produces defects in hemostasis in up to 30% of patients. Dilution reduces the number of circulating platelets and most bleeding abnormalities associated with massive transfusion are caused by platelet deficiencies (140,141). Platelet counts typically fall below 100,000 per $\mu$L after 15 to 20 U of citrated blood and below 50,000 per $\mu$L in 75% of patients who receive more than 20 U (142). Counts remain low for 3 to 5 days (142). More extensive tissue injuries and hypothermia are associated with reduced platelet function, shorter platelet survival, and a more severe consumptive thrombocytopenia (143,144). Prophylactic platelet transfusions in anticipation of bleeding are not recommended (110,132,141); in patients who are bleeding and with platelet counts less than 100,000 per $\mu$L, transfusion is recommended, particularly in patients with trauma or in those with microvascular bleeding, who often have dysfunctional platelets (132,143). One platelet concentrate increases the circulating platelet count by approximately 50,000 to 100,000 per $\mu$L in average-sized adults (132).

Deficiencies in soluble coagulation factors less than the 30% of normal concentrations may occur if only packed cells and platelets are transfused (140); therefore, FFP (10 to 15 mL per kg) is recommended for each blood volume lost and replaced (132,138). Cryoprecipitate is recommended in patients who are bleeding and are subject to massive transfusion, if fibrinogen concentrations are unknown or fall below 80 to 100 mg per dL (132).

Massive transfusion does not cause DIC directly, but massive tissue injury alone or in combination with hemorrhagic shock, poor tissue perfusion, stagnant blood flow, and sepsis may precipitate thrombin formation by the extrinsic coagulation pathway (see preceding text). DIC associated with consumptive coagulopathy and diffuse microvascular bleeding occur in 10% or less of patients who require massive transfusion after injury. Occasionally, patients may develop ARDS (145).

Massive bleeding and transfusion disrupt the coagulation system and often tests of coagulation are out of date when reported. Hemoglobin concentration or hematocrit, platelet count, and fibrinogen concentration are useful markers of deficiencies in packed cells, platelets, and FFP or cryoprecipitate; PT, aPTT are more helpful when bleeding begins to abate. Deficiencies are replaced by the appropriate blood component (132,146). If DIC is suspected, measurements of prothrombin fragment F1.2 and the fibrinolytic marker D-dimer establish the presence or absence of the diagnosis and are recommended if the tests can be done promptly.

Adverse metabolic effects of massive transfusion usually occur in patients who remain poorly perfused, hypotensive, hypothermic, and acidotic from the underlying injury or delay in resuscitation (147). Many of the products causing "storage lesion" are avoided by using packed red cells as opposed to whole blood. Hyperkalemia or hypokalemia, lactate or ammonia accumulation, and citrate toxicity are generally transient and self-correcting if adequate perfusion is restored (148). However, potassium, calcium, and blood gases should be monitored during resuscitation and abnormalities treated until perfusion is adequate. Decreases in 2,3-diphosphoglycerate in stored blood are self-correcting and not a clinical concern (135). Transfused blood and blood components are routinely warmed to ameliorate hypothermia (135).

Whole blood, packed red cells, and platelet concentrates are infused through 18-gauge or larger needles and catheters. A standard blood filter with 170-$\mu$m pores is used for these preparations to remove cellular debris, aggregated proteins, and other particulate matter. More than 90% of microaggregates are removed from washed or frozen red cells (149). Filters are not necessary for FFP or cryoprecipitate.

# BLOOD CONSERVATION

## Asanguinous Intravascular Volume Expanders

Isotonic crystalloid solutions, such as normal saline and Ringer lactate, rapidly equilibrate with the extracellular space, and therefore 3 to 4 mL are required to replace each milliliter of shed blood. Hypertonic solutions (e.g., 300 mEq NaCl) in smaller volumes can be used for this purpose in limited amounts, but these have not been shown to be superior to isotonic crystalloid solutions (150).

Colloid solutions including fresh-frozen plasma, 5% albumin, dextran, hydroxyethyl starch, and gelatin contain proteins or other large molecules and primarily equilibrate with the intravascular space to expand blood volume and maintain plasma oncotic pressure (151). FFP should not be used to expand blood volume, but it is conserved to replace coagulation and other essential plasma proteins (92). Albumin solutions are safe and are less likely to cause allergic reactions and coagulation problems than starch or gelatin solutions (152), but they are expensive. Dextrans are branched polysaccharide macromolecules of varying molecular weight; 40 and 70 kDa are used clinically. Hydroxyethyl starch solutions contain vegetable amylopectin and have a large range of molecular weights up to 450 kDa. Infusion of more than 1 L of nonprotein colloids may temporarily prolong bleeding times and appear to slightly increase blood losses after cardiac surgery (153,154).

## Autologous Blood Donation

Autologous blood donation before elective surgery slightly reduces the already low risks of blood-borne disease (155). Unless the blood is frozen, up to 3 or 4 U can be donated by patients without ischemic heart disease before units become outdated. Predonated autologous transfusions can reduce allogenic transfusions (156), but the practice is both expensive (157) and wasteful; up to half of all stored units are eventually discarded (92).

## Designated Donors

Designated donors do not reduce the risk of blood-borne infections, increase clerical costs and offer donors less protection than anonymous donations (158).

## Autotransfusion

Autotransfusion is a technique in which shed red cells are collected, processed, and reinfused. Autotransfusion is routine during cardiac surgery with CPB; in most operations, heparinized blood is aspirated from the surgical field, filtered to remove particulate matter, and returned directly to the perfusate (159). Wound blood, however, contains high concentrations of thrombin, fibrinolysins, and inflammatory agents (160–162). Increasingly, field blood is collected and washed using a cell saver system before it is returned to the patient as packed red cells (163) (see Fig. 74-5). Cell savers are also used in other operations associated with large blood losses and in the management of some patients with trauma (164). A specialized sucker tip into which a heparin or citrate solution is infused is used to collect the blood. Aspirated blood is filtered through a 40-$\mu$m pore filter, washed with saline solution, and continuously centrifuged to remove plasma and saline. Two percent to 10% of aspirated red cells are lysed by the process, but survival of the remaining red cells is not decreased. The concentrated red cells are resuspended in saline for transfusion as packed, washed red cells. The process requires approximately 10 minutes, is sterile, and removes soluble clotting factors, anticoagulants, white cells, platelets, red cell ghosts, free hemoglobin, lipid emboli, and miscellaneous debris, but it does not sterilize contaminated blood (165).

In massive trauma victims and postoperative cardiac and other surgical patients, blood shed from body cavities may be collected, washed, and reinfused as red cells in the intensive care unit. Potentially contaminated blood (e.g., from the peritoneal cavity after bowel surgery) should not be recycled and great care is necessary to avoid contamination of any collected blood (166). Specially designed hard shell cardiotomy reservoirs containing a 20-$\mu$m pore filter are used. This blood contains a few platelets, is defibrinogenated, and contains higher concentrations of

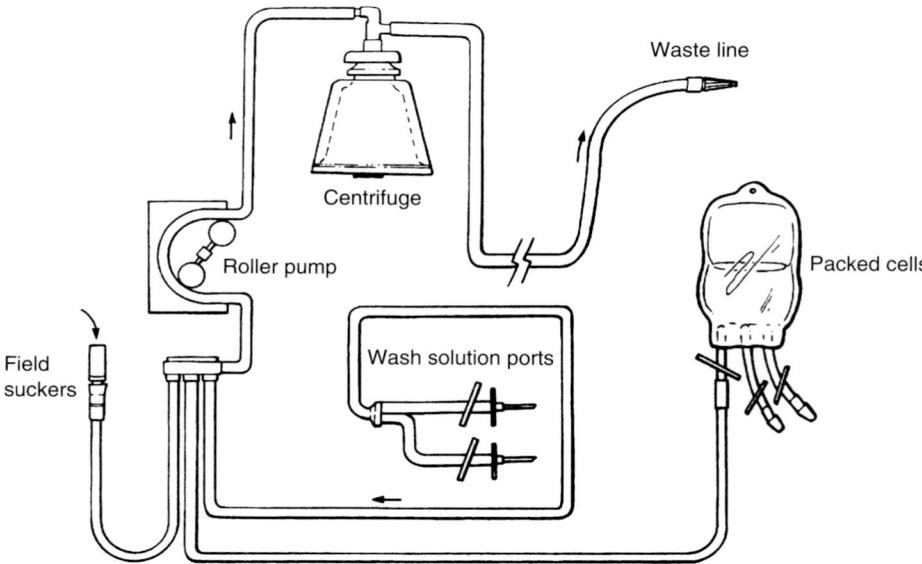

**FIGURE 74-5.** Diagram of a cell-saver system. Blood, before or after systemic heparin, is aspirated from the wound. Dilute heparin is added at the base of the suction catheter by an infusion pump to anticoagulate, aspirated blood. Blood enters near the base of a rotating bell centrifuge to which a saline wash solution is added near the top. During centrifugation, blood and saline are mixed and gradually separated as more blood and saline enter the chamber. As red cells become more concentrated at the bottom of the centrifuge, wash solution is drawn off into a waste bag and discarded. The centrifuge is stopped to remove packed cells from the bottom of the centrifuge chamber. (Reprinted with permission from Edmunds, LH Jr., ed. *Cardiac surgery in the adult.* New York: McGraw-Hill, 1997.)

fibrinopeptide A, fibrin fragments, cardiac enzymes, and inflammatory cytokines than circulating autologous blood or allogenic transfusions (167–169). In patients with a cardiac disorder, autotransfusion does not reduce the amount of mediastinal drainage (162,170,171), but it is safe and does decrease the amount of transfused blood products, particularly if blood losses exceed 500 mL within the first few hours after operation (167,170,171). Red cell survival of autotransfused blood is normal (172). This blood also can be washed prior to reinfusion.

## Blood Sequestration

Blood sequestration is a variation of autologous blood donation and is combined with normovolemic anemia during selected surgical operations. The strategy reduces the need for allogenic blood transfusions and retains platelet function in the donated blood (173). In the operating room, autologous blood is removed, anticoagulated, stored at room temperature, and reinfused at or near the end of the operation. Blood volume is maintained with crystalloid solutions, which dilute the patient's hematocrit to 25% to 30%, and consequently reduce the amount of red cell mass lost during operation. In patients with anemia who are scheduled for elective surgery, the strategy may be combined with administration of erythropoietin and iron to enhance red cell production before the autologous donation (173).

A further refinement involves preparation of autologous platelet-rich plasma (PRP) in the operating room after anesthesia, before CPB. Blood is steadily withdrawn from a venous catheter and processed by centrifugation using a commercially available system (174,175). PRP with some soluble coagulation factors is reinfused after CPB and raises the circulating platelet count and adds functioning platelets during the immediate postoperative period (175). Some reports indicate reduced postoperative bleeding (174,175); others do not (176), but labor and equipment costs limit this practice.

## Antifibrinolytics

Multiple organ trauma, massive transfusion, open heart surgery and occasionally other operations stimulate the fibrinolytic system and production of tPA from endothelial cells (44). The tPA cleaves plasminogen to produce plasmin, which rapidly binds fibrin. To a lesser extent, urokinase, produced from circulating prourokinase by small amounts of kallikrein or plasmin, also cleaves plasminogen to form plasmin (see Chapter 23). Under normal circumstances, plasmin is inactivated by $\alpha_2$-antiplasmin and $\alpha_2$-macroglobulin and does not circulate (see Chapter 23). Lysis of fibrin produces the fragment D-dimer and fibrin degradation products but, most important, increases bleeding.

EACA is an $\omega$-aminocarboxylic acid that blocks the lysine binding sites on plasminogen and tPA and thereby interferes with the ability of these enzymes to bind fibrin. Aprotinin is a serine protease inhibitor that binds plasmin with high affinity and kallikrein with approximately 100-fold less affinity (177). Aprotinin is usually given intravenously and in the priming volume of the perfusion circuit either as a full dose or a half dose. "Full dose" aprotinin comprises an intravenous bolus of 280 mg, an additional 280 mg in the circuit priming volume, and 70 mg per hour thereafter. Both drugs must be given prophylactically; neither is effective after operation (178). There is no difference in reduction of bleeding between full and half doses of aprotinin in adults (179,180), but both doses erroneously increase the activated clotting time, measured to monitor heparin, in celite, but not in kaolin (181,182). Both aprotinin and EACA reduce postoperative blood loss by approximately 40% to 50% in adult patients who have received aspirin preoperatively or have had previous cardiac operations (183–188). Full dose aprotinin also reduces bleeding in infants (189). EACA has fewer side effects, is not allergenic, and is inexpensive (188,190), but it is marginally less effective in reducing postoperative blood loss (183). Aprotinin has a platelet sparing effect (191–193) and in full dose reduces postoperative stroke (187,194) and weakly inhibits kallikrein, which is a major mediator of the inflammatory response to CPB (189,193,195,196).

## Desmopressin

Desmopressin (Desamino-D-arginyl vasopressin, DDAVP) is an analogue of vasopressin that transiently raises plasma concentrations of von Willebrand factor and factor VIII from endogenous sources (197). Desmopressin reduces bleeding times in patients with renal insufficiency (198). The drug is useful in patients with uremia, in patients with mild hemophilia or von

Willebrand disease, or in patients with qualitative platelet disorders who require minor surgery (see Chapter 75). The drug is not effective in reducing bleeding after open heart surgery (188,199–201).

## Erythropoietin

Erythropoietin stimulates red cell production and is used to increase red cell mass before elective surgery in some patients with anemia and in patients with renal failure and with Jehovah's Witnesses (202–204). Erythropoietin therapy is not necessary for healthy patients, whose blood is sequestered during operation (173). The rate of increase in red cell mass varies between patients and is usually effective over a period of weeks (203), but not within days.

In one study of patients who had elective open heart surgery, preoperative erythropoietin and iron treatment increased blood hemoglobin by 1.5 g per dL. When combined with intraoperative blood sequestration and normovolemic anemia, the need for allogenic transfusion was significantly reduced from 53% to 11% of 76 patients (205). Alternative blood conservation strategies, time constraints, and cost considerations compete against the widespread use of erythropoietin in patients undergoing surgery (206).

## Platelet Anesthesia

Platelet anesthesia describes a strategy to prevent platelet activation by temporarily inhibiting platelets during CPB. The concept requires complete inhibition of platelets by a reversible inhibitor that is rapidly removed to restore normal platelet function immediately after CPB. The goal is to achieve a normal bleeding time at the time protamine is given. Several short-acting, reversible platelet inhibitors are available as potential platelet anesthetics (207–209); however, market considerations have preempted a clinical trial.

## Recombinant Factor VIIa

Recombinant factor VIIa (rFVIIa) is an expensive, recombinant protein that is nearly identical with plasma factor VIIa, which is a key protein in the extrinsic coagulation pathway. When complexed with cellular or monocyte or platelet-bound soluble tissue factor, factor X is activated to produce prothrombinase and eventually thrombin. Currently, the drug is approved for patients with factor VIII and IX deficiencies who have antibodies, which limits their response to replacement therapy. The drug has also been used more widely "off label" to control bleeding in a variety of life-threatening medical and surgical emergencies.

Recombinant FVIIa has been reported anecdotally and in small series to dramatically reduce bleeding in patients of massive trauma and in patients undergoing surgery who have had bleeding complications after neurosurgery and cardiac surgery (210–214). In a randomized controlled trial, Freidrickson et al. reported that prophylactic rFVIIa before prostatectomy reduced median blood losses by over 50% (215). An evidence-based consensus conference recommended the use of rFVII in patients with bleeding traumatic head injuries who have been administered anticoagulants; patients with multiple trauma who are receiving massive transfusions (>10 U); and patients undergoing aortic, cardiac, spinal, or hepatic surgery who continue to have severe bleeding after FFP and platelet transfusions (32). Recommended doses are 20 to 40 $\mu$g per kg for nonemergent indications and 41 to 90 $\mu$g per kg for life-threatening emergencies (32). Use of the drug has been associated with some serious thromboembolic events (29,214).

## Oxygen Carrying Solutions

The ideal blood substitute would carry and deliver oxygen to the tissues and remove carbon dioxide; remain in the circulation for weeks or months; not alter plasma oncotic pressure or worsen blood rheology; not be antigenic, toxic, or have undesirable side effects; not contain pathogens; have long storage life; be inexpensive and easy to produce in large quantities; and not interfere with coagulation and laboratory measurements of blood constituents. In early 2005, this product did not exist and no oxygen carrying blood substitutes were available for general use (216), although one hemoglobin derived product may be used for chronic anemia in South Africa (217). Development work has focused on three strategies (218).

Allosteric modification of hemoglobin to improve oxygen delivery to tissues by reducing "p50" of the oxygen–hemoglobin dissociation curve [the oxygen tension (torr) at which hemoglobin is 50% saturated] may incrementally help patients with poor tissue perfusion but may also adversely affect oxygen loading of hemoglobin (219). Drugs to manipulate the hemoglobin–oxygen relation exist and one or more may eventually become an adjunctive therapy for surgical patients with poor tissue perfusion.

Cell-free hemoglobin solutions are derived from human or bovine blood and are conjugated with other molecules to maintain the hemoglobin tetramer that is needed for a workable oxygen saturation curve (p50: 28-37; normal 25-27 torr) and a reasonable half-life in plasma (12–24 hours) (219,220). Cell-free hemoglobin solutions also cause vasoconstriction; oxidative damage; interfere with spectrometric measurements of blood constituents; are limited to 5 to 7 g per dL concentrations (219–222); and produced disappointing results in a prospective, randomized trial of trauma victims (223).

Perfluorocarbon emulsions can dissolve large amounts of oxygen and carbon dioxide (or any gas) and therefore load and off-load both respiratory gases at physiologic gas concentrations. At 0.9 to 1.8 g per kg doses, the highest used in humans, these emulsions cannot bind or deliver as much oxygen or $CO_2$ as red cell or cell-free hemoglobin (219,220,222). Perfluorocarbons are cleared in 24 to 36 hours by the reticuloendothelial cells in the liver and spleen and eventually are exhaled (219). Liver and spleen accumulation and short intravascular residence preclude long-term applications of these chemicals.

# INTRAOPERATIVE MANAGEMENT OF BLEEDING

## Wound Management

Meticulous surgical hemostasis is the cornerstone of any blood conservation program. As the operation progresses, bleeding is carefully stopped by ligature or cautery before proceeding to the next level of dissection. The experienced surgeon's finger is the best hemostatic instrument for unexpected pronounced bleeding until appropriate clamps or sutures can be applied.

During open heart surgery, careful hemostasis before heparin and CPB is as important as hemostasis after administration of protamine. Use of electrocautery or ultrasonic scapel and hemostatic clips greatly speed up the process of dissection and attaining hemostasis (224–226). Use of bone wax to reduce marrow bleeding from sternotomy edges has largely been abandoned because of adverse effects on wound healing, embolization, and increased infection (227,228). Other fibrin sealants to control marrow bleeding have been introduced (229–231), but products that can produce emboli should not be used during cardiac surgery (228,230). During cardiac surgery and operations with large blood loss, all shed blood, except that adsorbed on squeezed sponges and drapes, is usually recovered if not contaminated. Even heavily soaked sponges can be wrung out into a basin and aspirated into the cell saver system to recover red cells.

## Topical Agents

Topical agents are widely used in endoscopic and incisional surgery to reinforce suture lines, provide a fibrin sealant, and control microvascular bleeding from a variety of wounds (232–234). There are several preparations that can be applied by spray or mixed liquids (233–235). Fibrin glue or "sealant" describes a "homemade" mixture of bovine thrombin, calcium, and cryoprecipitate, which contains fibrinogen and factor XIII (236). Commercial "Bioglue" contains bovine serum, albumin, and gluteraldehyde (233,234). Other formulations include fibrinogen, bovine thrombin, calcium, and aprotinin or bovine-derived gelatin and thrombin mixtures (233,234). Gelatin resorcinal formaldehyde (GRF) is not approved by the U.S. FDA but is used outside the United States; adhesive methyl 2-cyanoacrylate is no longer used at all (237).

These tissue adhesives and sealants may be applied by spray, but more frequently they are used with cellulose sponge, oxidized cellulose gauze, or collagen fleece or powder and applied with light pressure to the area of bleeding. These products are often effective for microvascular bleeding in cardiac operations (238), burn debridements, vascular anastomoses, and as a sealant for dural suture lines and parenchymal lung leaks, but they are not a panacea. Glues are also used to obtain lifesaving hemostasis in patients with dissecting aortic aneurysms and aortic resections (239–241), but in some patients GRF [and, in one instance, "Bioglue" (240)] is associated with tissue necrosis and late redissection or pseudoaneurysm formation (240, 242,243). Before using fibrin glue, every effort is made to control surgical bleeding and to replace deficient or dysfunctional coagulation factors including platelets. Some patients who have received topical bovine thrombin in the past develop antibodies to factor V or thrombin (6). On reexposure to bovine thrombin these patients may have late bleeding because of factor V deficiency caused by the antibody (5).

## Intraoperative Tests

If bleeding becomes a problem during operation, a few tests of the coagulation system are helpful. These include the aPTT, PT, and platelet count. If heparin is used, the activated clotting time or various versions of protamine titration tests are useful in neutralizing heparin (244). Heparin anticoagulation and deficiencies of intrinsic pathway coagulation proteins prolong the partial thromboplastin time. Prolonged PTs are associated with deficiencies in the extrinsic coagulation pathway. In patients with active bleeding without obvious surgical sources of bleeding, platelet counts less than 100,000 per $\mu$L and abnormal aPTT or PT times are treated with platelet concentrates and FFP, respectively. If a consumptive coagulopathy is suspected, measurements of prothrombin fragment F1.2 and the fibrinolysis fragment, D-dimer, if available, are highly recommended to establish the diagnosis.

## Delayed Closure

Occasionally, particularly after pediatric cardiac surgery, the chest cannot be closed safely because of compression of the heart, persistent microvascular bleeding, or hemodynamic instability (245–248). In such circumstances, the wound is left open and covered with a rubber dam or silicone membrane sutured or stapled to the skin edges (245–248). In some patients, the bone edges are kept apart by metal or plastic struts to further reduce compression on mediastinal structures (245, 246,248). The wound is closed a few days later when bleeding has stopped and circulatory function has sufficiently improved to permit closure. In newborns and infants, the incidence of delayed closure is approximately 4% to 9% (247,248); in adults, the incidence is approximately less than 2% (245,246). Closure of wound in surviving patients is achieved at a mean of 3 to 4 days (245,246,248), but it may be delayed as long as 2 weeks (247). Wound infections are surprisingly uncommon; a few patients have superficial infections (248); deep infection and poor sternal healing are rare (247).

# POSTOPERATIVE MANAGEMENT

## Monitoring and Initial Tests

Bleeding after most operations is an unusual complication and most often related to delayed bleeding from a vascular suture line, a clipped, ligated or cauterized vessel or from continuous generalized ooze into a hidden body cavity. Unexpected bleeding from these operations is usually recognized by decreases in hematocrit, clinical signs of reduced blood volume, or detection of a hematoma by chest x-ray or magnetic resonance imaging. Management requires prompt restoration of the circulating blood volume, control of the bleeding source, and evacuation of space occupying hematomas. Transfusion of blood or blood products or prompt surgery may or may not be needed.

Two to four percent of patients who have open heart surgery are returned to the operating room for control of postoperative bleeding (249,250). Bleeding protocols are in general use for postoperative cardiac surgical patients (244) and with minor modifications are applicable for many patients with multiorgan system trauma or extensive oncologic or reconstructive operations. If postoperative bleeding is a potential threat, the surgical field is prophylactically drained to provide early detection of bleeding and to remove shed blood. After cardiac surgery, chest tubes are left within the pericardium and mediastinum and are placed on gentle (10 to 20 cm $H_2O$) suction. Attachment to an autotransfusion system (see preceding text) is optional. Patency of the chest tubes is monitored and if any question of blockage arises the tubes are disconnected using sterile precautions and aspirated. The possibility of pericardial tamponade is kept in mind particularly if cardiac output is low or marginally adequate; in this circumstance, bedside echocardiography is strongly recommended and immediate surgical relief may be lifesaving. Hypertension is treated with appropriate vasodilators. If tolerated, airway pressures may be increased to provide mediastinal compression to promote wound clotting (251); however, the effectiveness of this maneuver is disputed (252).

Blood is sent for a postoperative PT, aPTT, and platelet count. In some centers, fibrinogen is also measured. Patients with an elevated PT or fibrinogen concentrations less than 100 mg per dL who are bleeding receive FFP. An elevated aPTT is treated with an additional dose of 25 to 50 mg of protamine. Platelet counts less than 100,000 per $\mu$L are treated with platelet transfusions in patients who are actively bleeding. If ongoing fibrinolysis is suspected, aprotinin or EACA is given empirically.

## Indications for Wound Exploration

Indications for wound exploration may vary from institution to institution; the following represents general guidelines, which are frequently modified by the patient's general condition, competing risks, and availability of personnel, space, and equipment. Bleeding at the rate of 10 mL per kg in the first hour after operation is an indication for prompt wound exploration. If postoperative bleeding during wound closure is anticipated, a platelet count, PT, and aPTT are sent from the operating room. Any deficiencies are corrected as soon as possible. Simultaneously, the circulating blood volume is maintained by appropriate volume expanders or homologous or autologous blood reinfused at the bedside. Cardiac function must be monitored by continuous display of the electrocardiogram, measurements of arterial and central venous pressure, and echocardiography, if cardiac tamponade is suspected. Cardiac output is maintained by appropriate manipulation of preload, afterload, and myocardial contractility.

Persistent bleeding that equals or exceeds 5 mL/kg/hour for each of the next 3 hours or bleeding that totals 20 mL per kg in the first 4 hours after operation are indications for mediastinal exploration after cardiac operations. Bleeding over 5 mg/kg/hour for the first postoperative hour should prompt repeating the platelet count, PT, and aPTT. Postoperative patients with platelet counts less than 100,000 per μL and who have bleeding are treated with one or two doses of pooled platelets. Elevated PTs (INR >1.3) are treated with FFP. Elevated aPTT (>40 seconds) is an indication for additional protamine, after which the aPTT is repeated.

Truly massive bleeding or a sudden increase in the rate of bleeding is justification for opening the wound in the intensive care unit to secure a surgical bleeding point (253,254). Prompt action may save the patient's life if a suture line or tie on a major vessel has failed. If the circulation is not stable or if cardiac tamponade is suspected, immediate reentry also is indicated to control an active bleeding source, if one is present, or to relieve tamponade (253). Immediate hemodynamic improvement with reentry implies some element of cardiac tamponade.

If reoperation for persistent (not massive) bleeding is indicated, an adequate circulation should be established before the patient is shifted to the operating room. The combination of persistent bleeding and low cardiac output is ominous and requires very careful management of cardiac performance, blood volume, and hemostasis simultaneously. This management is often best accomplished in the operating room, where mechanical circulatory assist devices may be available.

Bleeding is the most common postoperative complication following implantation of left ventricular assist devices; it occurs in most patients and is frequently massive (255–258). If possible, a complete assessment of the coagulation system should be made before the device is implanted. Deficiencies are corrected and inhibitors of clotting are either stopped or antidotes arranged for use during operation. During operation, meticulous hemostasis is routine and potential bleeding sites including cannulation ports are often double sutured and reinforced with pledgets. Topical agents, including fibrin glue, are used liberally. High-dose aprotinin is routinely given prophylactically and protamine is monitored closely to assure complete heparin neutralization (258). Many of these patients have a consumptive coagulopathy; therefore, prompt measurement of F1.2 and D-dimer, if available, could provide valuable guidance and reduce blood loss. Often, microvascular bleeding persists, and occasionally the wound must be packed open to manage the hemorrhage until adequate coagulation can be established. Although recombinant factor VIIa has been used (259), this product is also associated with an increased intravascular thrombosis (29,214).

## References

1. Rappaport SI. Preoperative hemostatic evaluation: which tests, if any? *Blood* 1983;61:229.
2. Warkentin TE, Greinacher A. Heparin-induced thrombocytopenia and cardiac surgery. *Ann Thorac Surg* 2003;76:2121–2131.
3. Barber A. The bleeding time as a preoperative screening test. *Am J Med* 1985;78:761.
4. Rodgers RPC, Levin JA. Critical reappraisal of the bleeding time. *Semin Thromb Hemost* 1990;16:1.
5. Cmolik BL, Spero JA, Magovern GJ, et al. Redo cardiac surgery: late bleeding complications from topical thrombin-induced factor V deficiency. *J Thor Cardiovasc Surg* 1993;105:222–227.
6. Fastenau DR, McIntyre JA. Immunochemical analysis of polyspecific antibodies in patients exposed to bovine fibrin sealant. *Ann Thorac Surg* 2000;69:1867–1872.
7. Noris M, Remuzzi G. Uremic bleeding: closing the circle after 30 years of controversies. *Blood* 1999;94:2569–2574.
8. Price DT, Ridker PM. Factor V Leiden mutation and the risks for thromboembolic disease: a clinical perspective. *Ann Intern Med* 1997;127: 895–895.
9. Shapiro SS. The lupus anticoagulant/antiphospholipid syndrome. *Ann Rev Med* 1996;47:533–553.
10. Clarke RJ, Mayo G, Price P, et al. Suppression of thromboxane A2 but not of systemic prostacyclin by controlled-release aspirin. *N Engl J Med* 1991; 325:1137–1141.
11. Amrein PC, Ellman L, Harris WH. Aspirin-induced prolongation of bleeding time and perioperative blood loss. *JAMA* 1981;245:1825.
12. Furukawa K, Ohteki H. Changes in platelet aggregation after suspension of aspirin therapy. *J Thor Cardiovasc Surg* 2004;127:1814–1815.
13. Ferraris VA, Ferraris SP, Joseph O, et al. Aspirin and postoperative bleeding after coronary artery bypass grafting. *Ann Surg* 2002;235: 820–827.
14. Ferraris VA, Ferraris SP, Moliterno DJ, et al. Aspirin and other anti-platelet agents during operative coronary revascularization (Executive summary). *Ann Thorac Surg (In press)*.
15. Pedersen A, Fitzgerald GA. Dose-related kinetics of aspirin. *N Engl J Med* 1984;311:1206–1211.
16. Phillips DR, Charo IF, Parise LV, et al. The platelet membrane glycoprotein IIb/IIIa complex. *Blood* 1988;71:831–843.
17. Cheng DK, Jackevicius CA, Seidelin P, et al. Safety of glycoprotein IIb/IIIa inhibitors in urgent or emergency coronary artery bypass graft surgery. *Can J Cardiol* 2004;20:223–228.
18. Peters RJ, Mehta SR, Fox KA, et al. Effects of aspirin dose when used alone or in combination with clopidogrel in patient with acute coronary syndromes: observations from the Clopidogrel in Unstable angina to prevent Recurrent Events (CURE) study. *Circ* 2003;108:1682–1687.
19. Inoue T, Uchida T, Sakuma M, et al. Cilostazol inhibits leukocyte intergrin Mac-1 leading to a potential reduction in restenosis after coronary stent implantation. *J Am Coll Cardiol* 2004;44:1408–1414.
20. Genoni M, Zeller D, Bertel O, et al. Tirofiban therapy does not increase the risk of hemorrhage after emergency coronary surgery. *J Thorac Cardiovasc Surg* 2001;122:630–632.
21. Genoni M, Tavakoli R, Hofer C, et al. Clopidogrel before urgent coronary artery bypass graft. *J Thorac Cardiovasc Surg* 2003;126:288–289.
22. Ascione R, Ghosh A, Rogers CA, et al. In-hospital patients exposed to clopidogrel prior CABG: a word of caution. *Ann Thorac Surg* 2005;79: 1210–1216.
23. Lee KF, Mandell J, Rankin JS, et al. Immediate versus delayed coronary grafting after streptokinase treatment. *J Thorac Cardiovasc Surg* 1988;95: 216–222.
24. Loscalzo J, Vaughan DE. Tissue plasminogen activator promotes platelet disaggregation in plasma. *J Clin Invest* 1987;79:1749–1749.
25. Chalela JA, Katzan I, Liebeskind DS, et al. Safety of intra-arterial thrombolysis in the postoperative period. *Stroke* 2001;32:1365–1369.
26. Moazami N, Smedira NG, McCarthy PM, et al. Safety and efficacy of intraarterial thrombolysis for perioperative stroke after cardiac operation. *Ann Thorac Surg* 2001;72:1933–1939.
27. Fukuda I, Imazuru T, Osaka M, et al. Thrombolytic therapy for delayed in-hospital stroke after cardiac surgery. *Ann Thorac Surg* 2003;76:1293–1295.
28. Hirsh J, Dalen JE, Anderson DR, et al. Oral anticoagulants: mechanism of action, clinical effectiveness and optimal therapeutic range. *Chest* 1998; 114:445S–469S.
29. Bui JD, Despotis GD, Trulock EP, et al. Fatal thrombosis after administration of activated prothrombin complex concentrates in a patient supported by extracorporeal membrane oxygenation who had received activated recombinant factor VII. *J Thorac Cardiovasc Surg* 2002;124:852–854.
30. Hirsh J, Fuster V. Guide to anticoagulation therapy. Part 2: oral anticoagulants. *Circulation* 1994;89:1469–1480.
31. Whitling AM, Bussey HI, Lyons RM. Comparing different routes and doses of phytonadione for reversing excessive anticoagulation. *Arch Intern Med* 1998;158:2136–2140.
32. Consensus recommendation for off label use of recombinant human factor VIIa therapy. http://www.infoatsabm.org.
33. Weitz JI, Hudoba M, Massel D, et al. Clot-bound thrombin is protected from inhibition by heparin-antithrombin III-independent inhibitors. *J Clin Invest* 1990;86:385–385.
34. Francis JL, Palmer GJ III, Moroose R, et al. Comparison of bovine and porcine heparin in heparin antibody formation following cardiac surgery. *Ann Thorac Surg* 2003;75:17–22.
35. Edmunds LH Jr, Colman RW. Thrombosis and bleeding. In: Cohn LH, Edmunds LH Jr, eds. *Cardiac surgery in the adult*, 2nd ed. New York: McGraw-Hill, 2003:338–348.

36. Boisclair MD, Lane DA, Philippou H, et al. Thrombin production, inactivation and expression during open heart surgery measured by assays for activation fragments including a new ELISA for prothrombin fragment F1+2. *Thromb Haemost* 1993;70:253.

37. Brister SJ, Ofosu FA, Buchanan MR. Thrombin generation during cardiac surgery: is heparin the ideal anticoagulant? *Thromb Haemost* 1993;70:259.

38. Edmunds LH Jr. Cardiopulmonary bypass after fifty years–perspective. *N Engl J Med* 2004;351:1603–1606.

39. Chung JH, Gikakis N, Drake TA, et al. Pericardial blood activates the extrinsic coagulation pathway during clinical cardiopulmonary bypass. *Circulation* 1996;93:2014.

40. Philippou H, Adami A, Davidson SJ, et al. Tissue factor is rapidly elevated in plasma collected from the pericardial cavity during cardiopulmonary bypass. *Thromb Haemost* 2000;84:124–128.

41. Hattori T, Khan MMH, Colman RW, et al. Plasma tissue factor plus activated peripheral mononuclear cells activate factor VII and X in cardiac surgical wounds. *J Am Coll Cardiol* 2005;46:707–713.

42. Edmunds LH Jr, Ellison N, Colman RW, et al. Platelet function during open heart surgery: comparison of the membrane and bubble oxygenators. *J Thorac Cardiovasc Surg* 1982;83:805.

43. Zilla P, Fasol R, Groscurth P, et al. Blood platelets in cardiopulmonary bypass operations. *J Thorac Cardiovasc Surg* 1989;97:379.

44. Gram J, Janetzko T, Jespersen J, et al. Enhanced effective fibrinolysis following the neutralization of herparin in open heart surgery increases the risk of post-surgical bleeding. *Thromb Haemost* 1990;63:241.

45. Harker LA, Malpass TW, Branson HE, et al. Mechanism of abnormal bleeding in patients undergoing cardiopulmonary bypass: acquired transient platelet dysfunction associated with selective alpha granule release. *Blood* 1980;56:824.

46. Dietrich W, Spannagl M, Schramm W, et al. The influence of preoperative anticoagulation on heparin response during cardiopulmonary bypass. *J Thorac Cardiovasc Surg* 1991;102:505–505.

47. Kelton JG, Smith JW, Warkentin TE, et al. Immunoglobulin G from patients with heparin-induced thrombocytopenia binds to a complex of heparin and platelet factor 4. *Blood* 1994;83:3232–3239.

48. Lee DH, Warkentin TE. Frequency of heparin-induced thrombocytopenia. In: Warkentin TE, Greinacher A, eds. *Heparin-induced thrombocytopenia*. New York: Marcel Dekker Inc, 2004:107–148.

49. Denomme GA. The platelet Fc receptor in heparin-induced thrombocytopenia. In: Warkentin TE, Greinacher A, eds. *Heparin-induced thrombocytopenia*. New York: Marcel Dekker Inc, 2004:223–250.

50. Warkentin TE. Clinical picture of heparin-induced thrombocytopenia. In: Warkentin TE, Greinacher A, eds. *Heparin-induced thrombocytopenia*. New York: Marcel Dekker Inc, 2004:53–106.

51. Warkentin TE, Greinacher A. Laboratory testing for heparin-induced thrombocytopenia. In: Warkentin TE, Greinacher A, eds. *Heparin-induced thrombocytopenia*. New York: Marcel Dekker Inc, 2004:271–312.

52. Brady J, Riccio JA, Yumen OH, et al. Plasmapheresis. A therapeutic option in the management of heparin-associated thrombocytopenia and thrombosis. *Am J Clin Pathol* 1991;96:394–397.

53. McIntyre KM, Warkentin TE. Legal aspects of heparin-induced thrombocytopenia: US perspectives. In: Warkentin TE, Greinacher A, eds. *Heparin-induced thrombocytopenia*. New York: Marcel Dekker Inc, 2004:573–585.

54. Weitz JI. Low-molecular-weight heparins. *N Engl J Med* 1997;337:688–698.

55. Gikakis N, Rao AK, Miyamoto S, et al. Enoxaparin suppresses thrombin formation and activity during cardiopulmonary bypass in baboons. *J Thorac Cardiovasc Surg* 1998;116:1043–1051.

56. Robitaille D, Leclerc JR, Laberge R, et al. Cardiopulmonary bypass with a low-molecular-weight heparin fraction (enoxaparin) in a patient with a history of heparin-associated thrombocytopenia. *J Thorac Cardiovasc Surg* 1992;103:597–599.

57. Ganjoo AK, Harlof MG, Johnson WD. Cardiopulmonary bypass for heparin-induced thrombocytopenia: management with a heparin-bonded circuit and enoxaparin. *J Thorac Cardiovasc Surg* 1996;112:1390–1392.

58. Gladwell TD. Bivalirudin: a direct thrombin inhibitor. *Clin Ther* 2002;1:38–58.

59. Parry MA, Maraganore JM, Stone SR. Kinetic mechanism for the interaction of hirulog with thrombin. *Biochemistry* 1994;33:14807–14814.

60. Bartholomew JR. Bivalirudin for the treatment of heparin-induced thrombocytopenia. In: Warkentin TE, Greinacher A, eds. *Heparin-induced thrombocytopenia*. New York: Marcel Dekker Inc, 2004:475–508.

61. Koster A, Chew D, Grundel M, et al. Bivalirudin monitored with ehe ecarin clotting time for anticoagulation during cardiopulmonary bypass. *Anesth Analg* 2003;96:383–386.

62. Vasquez JC, Vichiendilokkul A, Mahmood S, et al. Anticoagulation with bivalirudin during cardiopulmonary bypass in cardiac surgery. *Ann Thorac Surg* 2002;74:2177–2179.

63. Davis Z, Anderson R, Short D, et al. Favorable outcome with bivalirudin anticoagulation during cardiopulmonary bypass. *Ann Thorac Surg* 2003;75:264–265.

64. Robson R, White H, Aylward P, et al. Bivalirudin pharmacokinetics and pharmacodynamics: effect of renal function, dose and gender. *Clin Pharmacol Ther* 2002;71:433–439.

65. Bittl JA, Strony J, Brinker JA, et al. for the Hirulog Angioplasty Study Investigators. Treatment with bivalurin (Hirolog) as compared with heparin during coronary angioplasty for unstable or postinfarction angina. *N Engl J Med* 1995;333:764–769.

66. Clayton SB, Asell JR, Crumbley AJ III, et al. Cardiopulmonary bypass with Bivalirudin in type II heparin-induced thrombocytopenia. *Ann Thorac Surg* 2004;78:2167–2168.

67. Merry AF, Raudkivi P, Middleton NG, et al. Bivalirudin versus heparin and protamine in off-pump coronary artery bypass surgery. *Ann Thorac Surg* 2004;77:925–931.

68. Poetzsch B, Madlener K. Management of cardiopulmonary bypass anticoagulation in patients with heparin-induced thrombocytopenia. In: Warkentin TE, Greinacher A, eds. *Heparin-induced thrombocytopenia*. New York: Marcel Dekker Inc, 2004:531–551.

69. Stringer KA, Lindenfeld J. Hirudins: antithrombin anticoagulants. *Ann Pharmacother* 1992;26:1535–1540.

70. Greinacher A. Lepirudin for the treatment of hepain-induced thrombocytopenia. In: Warkentin TE, Greinacher A, eds. *Heparin-induced thrombocytopenia*. New York: Marcel Dekker Inc, 2004:397–436.

71. Poetzsch B, Madlener K, Seelig C, et al. Monitoring of r-hirudin anticoagulation during cardiopulmonary bypass–assessment of the whole blood ecarin clotting time. *Thromb Haemost* 1997;77:920–925.

72. Koster A, Hansen R, Kuppe H, et al. Recombinant hirudin as an alternative for anticoagulation during cardiopulmonary bypass in patients with heparin-induced thrombocytopenia type II: a 1-year experience in 57 patients. *J Cardiothorac Vasc Anesth* 2000b;14:243–248.

73. Rubens FD, Lavalee G, Ruel MA, et al. Delayed thrombin activity with hirudin anticoagulation during prolonged cardiopulmonary bypass. *Ann Thorac Surg (In press)*.

74. Lewis BE, Hursting MJ. Argatroban therapy in heparin-induced thrombocytopenia. In: Warkentin TE, Greinacher A, eds. *Heparin-induced thrombocytopenia*. New York: Marcel Dekker Inc, 2004:437–474.

75. Swan SK, St.Perer JV, Lanbrecht LJ, et al. Comparison of anticoagulant effects and safety of argatroban and heparin in healthy subjects. *Pharmacotherapy* 2000;20:756–770.

76. Furukawa K, Ohteki H, Hirahara K, et al. The use of argatroban as an anticoagulant for cardiopulmonary bypass in cardiac operations. *J Thorac Cardiovasc Surg* 2001;122:1255–1256.

77. Edwards JT, Hamby JK, Worrall NK. Successful use of argatroban as a heparin substitute during cardiopulmonary bypass: heparin-induced thrombocytopenia in a high-risk cardiac surgical patient. *Ann Thorac Surg* 2003;75:1622–1624.

78. Kawada T, Kitagawa H, Hosan M, et al. Clinical application of argatroban as an alternative anticoagulant for extracorporeal circulation. *Hematol Oncol Clin North Am* 2000;14:445–457.

79. Cannon MA, Butterworth J, Riley RD, et al. Failure of agratroban during off-pump coronary artery surgery. *Ann Thorac Surg* 2004;77:711–713.

80. Levi M, ten Cate H. Disseminated intravascular coagulation. *N Engl J Med* 1999;341:586–592.

81. Osterud B, Flaegstad T. Increased tissue thromboplastin activity in monocytes of patients with meningococcal infection: related to an unfavourable prognosis. *Thromb Haemost* 1983;49:5–7.

82. Nieuwland R, Berchmans RJ, McGregor S, et al. Cellular origin and procoagulant properties of microparticles in meningococcal sepsis. *Blood* 2000;95:77–88.

83. Sabatier F, Roux V, Anfosso F, et al. Interaction of endothelial microparticles with monocytic cells *in vitro* induces tissue factor-dependent procoagulant activity. *Blood* 2002;99:3962–3970.

84. Scholz T, Temmler U, Krause S, et al. Transfer of tissue factor from platelets to monocytes: role of platelet-derived microvesicles and CD62P. *Thromb Haemost* 2002;88:1033–1038.

85. Zillmann A, Luther T, Muller I, et al. Platelet-associated tissue factor contributes to the collagen-triggered activation of blood coagulation. *Biochem Biophys Res Comm* 2001;281:603–609.

86. Phillippou H, Adami A, Davidson SJ, et al. Tissue factor is rapidly elevated in plasma collected from the pericardial cavity during cardiopulmonary bypass. *Thromb Haemost* 2000;84:124–128.

87. Vervloet MG, Thijs LG, Hack CE. Derangements of coagulation and fibrinolysis in critically ill patients with sepsis and septic shock. *Semin Thromb Hemost* 1998;24:33–44.

88. Armand R, Hess JR. Treating coagulopathy in trauma patients. *Transfus Med Rev* 2003;17:223–231.

89. Levi M, de Jonge E, van der Poll T. New treatment strategis for disseminated intravascular coagulation based on current understanding of the pathophysiology. *Ann Med* 2004;36:41–49.

90. Freeman BD, Zehnbauer BA, Buchman TG. A meta-analysis of controlled trials of anticoagulant therapies in patients with sepsis. *Shock* 2003;20:5–9.

91. Bernard G, Vincent J-L, Laterre P-F, et al. Efficacy and safety of recombinant human activated protein C for servere sepsis. *N Engl J Med* 2001;344:699–709.

92. Goodnough LT, Brecher ME, Kanter MH, et al. Transfusion medicine. *N Engl J Med* 1999;340:438–447,525–533.

93. Dzik WH, Corwin H, Goodnough LT, et al. Patient safety and blood transfusion: new solutions. *Transfus Med Rev* 2003;17:169–180.

94. Ho J, Sibbald WJ, Chin-Yee IH. Effects of storage on efficacy of red cell transfusion: when is it not safe? *Crit Care Med* 2003;31:S687–S697.

95. Weil MH. Blood transfusions. *Crit Care Med* 2003;31:2397–2398.

96. Carson JL, Hill S, Carless P, et al. Transfusion triggers: a systematic review of the literature. *Transfus Med Rev* 2002;16:187–199.

97. Hebert PC, Wells G, Blajchman MA, et al. A multicenter, randomized controlled clinical trial of transfusion requirements in critical care. *N Engl J Med* 1999;340:409–417.

98. Allen MB. Component preparation and storage. In: Hillyer CD, Hillyer KL, Strobl FJ et al., eds. *Handbook of transfusion medicine.* San Diego, CA: Academic Press, 2001:19–28.

99. Sohmer PR, Scott RL. Massive transfusion. *Clin Lab Med* 1982;2:21.

100. Solis RT, Gibbs MB. Filtration of the microaggregates in stored blood. *Transfusion* 1972;12:245.

101. Hillyer KL, Hillyer CD. Packed red blood cells and related products. In: Hillyer CD, Hillyer KL, Strobl FJ et al., eds. *Handbook of transfusion medicine.* San Diego, CA: Academic Press, 2001:29–38.

102. Mou SS, Giroir BP, Molitor-Kirsch EA, et al. Fresh whole blood versus reconstituted blood for pump priming in heart surgery in infants. *N Engl J Med* 2004;351:1635–1644.

103. Fitzgerald RD, Martin CM, Dietz GE, et al. Transfusing red blood cells stored in citrate phosphate dextrose adenine-1 for 28 days fails to improve tissue oxygenation in rats. *Crit Care Med* 1997;25:726–732.

104. Shanwell A, Kristiansson M, Remberger M, et al. Generation of cytokines in red cell concentrates during storage is prevented by prestorage white cell reduction. *Transfusion* 1997;37:719–726.

105. Fransen E, Maessen J, Denterer M, et al. Impact of blood transfusions on inflammatory mediator release in patients undergoing cardiac surgery. *Chest* 1999;116:1233–1239.

106. Kopko PM, Marshall CS, MacKenzie BR, et al. Transfusion-related acute lung injury: report of a clinical look-back investigation. *JAMA* 2002;287:1968–1971.

107. Tinmouth A, Chin-Yee IH. The clinical consequences of the red cell storage lesion. *Transfus Med Rev* 2001;15:91–107.

108. Bucur SZ, Hillyer CD. Fresh frozen plasma and related products. In: Hillyer CD, Hillyer KL, Strobl FJ et al., eds. *Handbook of transfusion medicine.* San Diego, CA: Academic Press, 2001:39–46.

109. Bucur SZ, Hillyer CD. Cryoprecipitate and related products. In: Hillyer CD, Hillyer KL, Strobl FJ et al., eds. *Handbook of transfusion medicine.* San Diego, CA: Academic Press, 2001:47–52.

110. Goodnough LT. Risks of blood transfusion. *Crit Care Med* 2003;31:S678–S686.

111. Roback JD, Hillyer CD. Platelets and related products. In: Hillyer CD, Hillyer KL, Strobl FJ et al., eds. *Handbook of transfusion medicine.* San Diego, CA: Academic Press, 2001:53–62.

112. Siegel DL. Pretransfusion compatibility testing. In: Hillyer CD, Hillyer KL, Strobl FJ et al., eds. *Handbook of transfusion medicine.* San Diego, CA: Academic Press, 2001:107–114.

113. Linden JV, Wagner K, Voytovich AE, et al. Transfusion errors in New York State: an analysis of 10 years' experience. *Transfusion* 2001;40:1207–1213.

114. Barclay S. Red blood cell antigens and human blood groups. In: Hillyer CD, Hillyer KL, Strobl FJ et al., eds. *Handbook of transfusion medicine.* San Diego, CA: Academic Press, 2001:91–106.

115. Westhoff CM, Reid ME. Review: the Kell, Duffy and Kidd blood group systems. *Immunohematol* 2004;20:37–49.

116. Oberman HA, Barnes BA, Friedman BA. The risk of abbreviating the major crossmatch in urgent or massive transfusion. *Transfusion* 1978;18:137.

117. Sesok-Pizzini DA. Acute and delayed hemolytic transfusion reactions. In: Hillyer CD, Hillyer KL, Strobl FJ et al., eds. *Handbook of transfusion medicine.* San Diego, CA: Academic Press, 2001:247–252.

118. DeChristopher PJ, Anderson RR. Risks of transfusion and organ and transplantation. Practical concerns that drive practical policies. *Am J Clin Pathol* 1997;107:S2–S7.

119. Sesok-Pizzini DA. Allergic transfusion reactions. In: Hillyer CD, Hillyer KL, Strobl FJ et al., eds. *Handbook of transfusion medicine.* San Diego, CA: Academic Press, 2001:259–261.

120. Eder AF. Febrile nonhemolytic transfusion reactions. In: Hillyer CD, Hillyer KL, Strobl FJ et al., eds. *Handbook of transfusion medicine.* San Diego, CA: Academic Press, 2001:253–258.

121. Chambers LA, Kruskall MS, Pacini DG, et al. Febrile reactions after platelet transfusion: the effect of single vs. multiple donors. *Transfusion* 1990;30:219–221.

122. Heddle NM, Klama L, Singer J, et al. The role of plasma in transfusion reactions. *N Engl J Med* 1994;331:625–628.

123. Wallis JP, Lubenko A, Wells AW, et al. Single hospital experience of TRALI. *Transfusion* 2003;43:1053–1059.

124. Klein HG. Risks of perioperative transfusion. In: Wechsler AS, ed. *Pharmacologic management of perioperative bleeding.* Southampton: CME Network, 1996:1–9.

125. O'Doherty U, Swiggard WJ. HIV and HTLV. In: Hillyer CD, Hillyer KL, Strobl FJ et al., eds. *Handbook of transfusion medicine.* San Diego, CA: Academic Press, 2001:293–299.

126. Schreiber GV, Busch MP, Kleinman SH, et al. The risk of transfusion-transmitted viral infections. *N Engl J Med* 1996;334:1685–1690.

127. Friedman DF. Hepatitis. In: Hillyer CD, Hillyer KL, Strobl FJ et al., eds. *Handbook of transfusion medicine.* San Diego, CA: Academic Press, 2001:275–283.

128. Roback JD. CMV and other herpesviruses. In: Hillyer CD, Hillyer KL, Strobl FJ et al., eds. *Handbook of transfusion medicine.* San Diego, CA: Academic Press, 2001:285–292.

129. Kurtis JD, Strobl FJ. Other transfusion-transmitted infections. In: Hillyer CD, Hillyer KL, Strobl FJ et al., eds. *Handbook of transfusion medicine.* San Diego, CA: Academic Press, 2001:301–306.

130. Armstrong WS, Bashour CA, Smedira NG, et al. A case of fatal West Nile virus meningoencephalitis associated with receipt of blood transfusions after open heart surgery. *Ann Thorac Surg* 2003;76:605–607.

131. Dodd RY. The risk of transfusion-transmitted infection. *N Engl J Med* 1992;327:419–420.

132. Stehling LC, Doherty DC, Faust R, et al. Practice guidelines for blood component therapy. *Anesthesiology* 1996;84:732–747.

133. Anderson KC, Weinstein H. Transfusion-associated graft-versus-host disease. *N Engl J Med* 1990;323:315–321.

134. American College of Surgeons Committee on Trauma. *Advanced trauma life support course manual.* Chicago, IL: American College of Surgeons, 1989.

135. Blackall DP. Approach to actue bleeding and massive transfusion. In: Hillyer CD, Hillyer KL, Strobl FJ et al., eds. *Handbook of transfusion medicine.* San Diego, CA: Academic Press, 2001:189–195.

136. Wiesen AR, Hospenthal DR, Byrd JC, et al. Equilibration of hemoglobin concentration after transfusion in medical inpatients not actively bleeding. *Ann Intern Med* 1994;121:278–280.

137. Rizoli SB. Crystalloids and colloids in trauma resuscitation: a brief overview of the current debate. *J Trauma Inj Infect Crit Care* 2003;54:S82–S88.

138. Shafi S, Kauder DR. Fluid resuscitation and blood replacement in patients with polytrauma. *Clin Orthop Relat Res* 2004;422:37–42.

139. Jan KM, Heldman J, Chien S. Coronary hemodynamics and oxygen utilization after hematocrit variations in hemorrhage. *Am J Physiol* 1980;239:H326–H332.

140. Mannucci PM, Federici AB, Sirchia G. Hemostasis testing during massive blood replacement. *Vox Sang* 1982;42:113.

141. Reed RL, Ciavarella D, Heimbach DM, et al. Prophylactic platelet administration during massive transfusion: A prospective, randomized, double-blind clinical study. *Ann Surg* 1986;203:40–48.

142. Leslie SD, Toy PTCY. Laboratory hemostatic abnormalities in massively transfused patients given PRBCs and crystalloid. *Am J Clin Pathol* 1991;96:770–773.

143. Lim RC, Olcott C, Robinson AJ, et al. Platelet response and coagulation changes following massive blood replacement. *J Trauma* 1973;18:577.

144. Valeri CR, Cassidy G, Khuri S, et al. Hypothermia-induced reversible platelet dysfunction. *Ann Surg* 1987;205:175–181.

145. Collins JA. Pulmonary dysfunction and massive transfusion. *Bibl Haematol* 1980;46:220.

146. Erber WN. Massive blood transfusion in the elective surgical setting. *Transfus Apheresis Sci* 2002;27:83–92.

147. Velmahos GC, Chan L, Chan M, et al. Is there a limit to massive blood transfusion after severe trauma? *Arch Surg* 1998;133:947–952.

148. Wilson RF, Binkley LE, Sabo FM, et al. Electrolyte and acid-base changes with massive blood transfusions. *Ann Surg* 1992;58:535–544.

149. Courcy PA, Brotman S, Dawson B. Letter: massive blood transfusion in acute trauma. *Transfusion* 1983;23:404.

150. Brown MD. Hypertonic versus isotonic crystalloid for fluid resuscitation in critically ill patients. *Ann Emerg Med* 2002;40:113–114.

151. Mazhar R, Samenesco A, Royston D, et al. Cardiopulmonary effects of 7.2% saline solution compared with gelatin infusion in the early postoperative period after coronary artery bypass. *J Thorac Cardiovasc Surg* 1998;115:178–189.

152. Barron ME, Wilkes MM, Navickis RJ. A systematic review of the comparative safety of colloids. *Arch Surg* 2004;139:552–563.

153. Wilkes MM, Navickis RJ, Sibbald WJ. Albumin versus hydroxyethyl starch in cardiopulmonary bypass surgery: a meta-analysis of postoperative bleeding. *Ann Thorac Surg* 2001;72:527–534.

154. De Jonge E, Levi M. Effects of different plasma substitutes on blood coagulation: a comparative review. *Crit Care Med* 2001;29:1261–1267.

155. Lee LY, DeBois WJ, Krieger KH, et al. Transfusion therapy and blood conservation. In: Cohn LH, Edmunds LH Jr, eds. *Cardiac surgery in the adult,* 2nd ed. New York: McGraw-Hill, 2003:389–399.

156. Shibata K, Takamoto S, Kotsuka Y, et al. Effectiveness of combined blood conservation measures in thoracic aortic operations with deep hypothermic circulatory arrest. *Ann Thorac Surg* 2002;73:739–744.

157. Birkmeyer JD, AuBuchon JP, Littenberg B, et al. Cost-effectiveness of preoperative autologous donation in coronary artery bypass grafting. *Ann Thorac Surg* 1994;57:161–169.

158. Cordell RR, Yalon VA, Cigahn-Haskell C, et al. Experience with 11,916 designated donors. *Transfusion* 1986;26:484–486.

159. Hessel EA II, Edmunds LH Jr. Extracorporeal perfusion systems. In: Cohn LH, Edmunds LH Jr, eds. *Cardiac surgery in the adult,* 2nd ed. New York: McGraw-Hill, 2003:317–337.

160. Chung JH, Gikakis N, Drake TA, et al. Pericardial blood activates the extrinsic coagulation pathway during clinical cardiopulmonary bypass. *Circulation* 1996;93:2014–2018.

161. Tabuchi N, de Haan J, Boonstra PW, et al. Activation of fibrinolysis in the pericardial cavity during cardiopulmonary bypass. *J Thorac Cardiovasc Surg* 1993;106:828–833.

162. Bland LA, Villarino ME, Arduino MJ, et al. Bacteriologic and endotoxin analysis of salvaged blood used in autologous transfusions during cardiac operations. *J Thorac Cardiovasc Surg* 1992;103:582.
163. Goodnough LT, Brecher ME. Autologous blood transfusion. *Med Int* 1998; 37:238–245.
164. Smith LA, Barker DE, Burns RP. Autotransfusion utilization in abdominal trauma. *Am Surg* 1997;63:47–49.
165. Kincaid EH, Jones TJ, Stump DA, et al. Processing scavenged blood with a cell saver reduces cerebral lipid microembolization. *Ann Thorac Surg* 2000;70:1296–1300.
166. Andreasen AS, Schmidt H, Jarlov JO, et al. Autologous transfusion of shed mediastinal blood after coronary artery bypass grafting and bacterial contamination. *Ann Thorac Surg* 2001;72:1327–1330.
167. Hartz RS, Smith JA, Green D. Autotransfusion after cardiac operation. *J Thorac Cardiovasc Surg* 1988;96:178.
168. Wahl GW, Feins RH, Alfieres G, et al. Reinfusion of shed blood after coronary operation causes elevation of cardiac enzyme levels. *Ann Thorac Surg* 1992;53:625.
169. Krohn CD, Reikeras O, Aasen AO. Inflammatory cytokines and their receptors in arterial and mixed venous blood before, during and after infusion of drained untreated blood. *Transfus Med* 1999;9:125–130.
170. Morris JJ, Tan YS. Autotransfusion: is there a benefit in a current practice of aggressive blood conservation? *Ann Thorac Surg* 1994;58:502.
171. Robitaille MJ, Perrault LP, Pellerin M, et al. Reinfusion of mediastinal blood after heart surgery. *J Thorac Cardiovasc Surg* 2000;120: 499–504.
172. Schmidt H, Lund JO, Nielson SL. Autotransfused shed mediastinal blood has normal erythrocyte survival. *Ann Thorac Surg* 1996;62:105.
173. Goodnough LT, Monk TG, Andriole GL. Erythropoietin therapy. *N Engl J Med* 1997;336:933–938.
174. Jones JW, McCoy TA, Rawitscher RE, et al. Effects of intraoperative plasmapheresis on blood loss in cardiac surgery. *Ann Thorac Surg* 1990;49:585.
175. DelRossi AJ, Cerniau AC, Vertrees RA, et al. Platelet-rich plasma reduces postoperative blood loss after cardiopulmonary bypass. *J Thorac Cardiovasc Surg* 1990;100:281.
176. Tobe CE, Vocelka C, Sepulvada R, et al. Infusion of autologous platelet rich plasma does not reduce blood loss and product use after coronary artery bypass. *J Thorac Cardiovasc Surg* 1993;105:1007.
177. Gallimore MJ, Fuhrer G, Heller W, et al. Augmentation of kallikrein and plasmin inhibition capacity by aprotinin using a new assay to monitor therapy. *Adv Exp Med Biol* 1989;247B:55–60.
178. Ray MJ, Hales MM, Brown L, et al. Postoperatively administered aprotinin or epsilon aminocaproic acid after cardiopulmonary bypass has limited benefit. *Ann Thorac Surg* 2001;72:521–526.
179. Levy JH, Pifarre R, Schaff HV, et al. A multicenter, double-blind, placebo-controlled trial of aprotinin for reducing blood loss and the requirement for donor-blood transfusion in patients undergoing repeat coronary artery bypass grafting. *Circulation* 1995;92:2236–2244.
180. Speekenbrink RG, Wildevuur CR, Sturk A, et al. Low-dose and high-dose aprotinin improve hemostasis in coronary operations. *J Thorac Cardiovasc Surg* 1996;112:523–530.
181. Hunt BJ, Segal HC, Yacoub M. Guidelines for monitoring heparin by the activated clotting time when aprotinin is used during cardiopulmonary bypass. *J Thorac Cardiovasc Surg* 1992;104:211.
182. Wang J-S, Lin C-Y, Hung W-T, et al. *In vitro* effects of aprotinin on activated clotting time measured with different activators. *J Thorac Cardiovasc Surg* 1992;104:1135–1140.
183. Blauhut B, Klima U, Bettelheim P, et al. Comparison of the effects of aprotinin and tranexamic acid on blood loss and related variables following cardiopulmonary bypass. *J Thorac Cardiovasc Surg* 1994;108:1083–1091.
184. Tabuchi N, Huet RCG, Sturk A, et al. Aprotinin preserves hemostasis in aspirin-treated patients undergoing cardiopulmonary bypass. *Ann Thorac Surg* 1994;58:1036.
185. Speekenbrink RGH, Vonk ABA, Wildevuur CRH, et al. Hemostatic efficacy of dipyridamole, tranexamic acid, and aprotinin in coronary bypass grafting. *Ann Thorac Surg* 1995;59:438.
186. Costello JM, Backer CL, de Hoyos A, et al. Aprotinin reduces operative closure time and blood product use after pediatric bypass. *Ann Thorac Surg* 2003;75:1261–1266.
187. Frumento RJ, O'Malley CMN, Bennett-Guerrero E. Stroke after cardiac surgery: a retrospective analysis of the effect of aprotinin dosing regimens. *Ann Thorac Surg* 2003;75:479–484.
188. Erstad BL. Antifibrinolytic agents and desmopressin as hemostatic agents in cardiac surgery. *Ann Pharmacother* 2001;35:1075–1084.
189. Mossinger H, Dietrich W, Braun SL, et al. High-dose aprotinin reduces activation of hemostasis, allogeneic blood requirement and duration of postoperative ventilation in pediatric cardiac surgery. *Ann Thorac Surg* 2003; 75:430–437.
190. Daily PO, Lampmhere JA, Dembitsky WP, et al. Effect of prophylactic epsilon-aminocaproic acid on blood loss and transfusion requirements in patients undergoing first-time coronary artery bypass grafting. A randomized, prospective, double-blinded trial. *J Thorac Cardiovasc Surg* 1994; 108:99.
191. Lu H, Soria C, Commin PL, et al. Hemostasis in patients undergoing extracorporeal circulation: the effect of aprotinin (Trasylol). *Thromb Haemost* 1991;66:633–637.
192. Wachtfogel YT, Kucich U, Hack CE, et al. Aprotinin inhibits the contact, neutrophil, and platelet activation systems during simulated extracorporeal perfusion. *J Thorac Cardiovasc Surg* 1993;106:1–10.
193. Landis RC, Asimakopoulos G, Poullis M, et al. The antithrombotic and anti-inflammatory mechanisms of action of aprotinin. *Ann Thorac Surg* 2001;72:2169–2175.
194. Hardy JF. Pharmacological strategies for blood conservation in cardiac surgery: erythropoietin and antifibrinolytics. *Can J Anaesth* 2001;48:S24–S31.
195. Wan S, LeClerc J-L, Vincent J-K. Inflammatory response to cardiopulmonary bypass. Mechanisms involved and possible therapeutic strategies. *Chest* 1997;112:676–692.
196. Edmunds LH Jr. The inflammatory response to cardiopulmonary bypass. *Ann Thorac Surg* 1998;66:S12–S16.
197. David JL. Desmopressin and hemostasis. *Regul Pept* 1993;45:311–317.
198. Mannucci PM, Remuzzi G, Pusineri F, et al. Deamino-8-D-arginine vasopressin shortens the bleeding time in uremia. *N Engl J Med* 1983;308:8–12.
199. Levi M, Cromheeche ME, de Jonge E, et al. Pharmacological strategies to decrease excessive blood loss in cardiac surgery: a meta-analysis of clinically relevant endpoints. *Lancet* 1999;354:1940–1947.
200. Orzkisacik E, Islamoglu F, Posacioglu H, et al. Desmopressin usage in elective cardiac surgery. *J Cardiovasc Surg* 2001;42:741–747.
201. Pleym H, Stenseth R, Wahba A, et al. Prophphylactic treatment with desmopressin does not reduce postoperative bleeding after coronary surgery in patients treated with aspirin before surgery. *Anesth Anal* 2004; 98:578–584.
202. Rosengart TK, Helm RC, Klempere J, et al. Combined aprotinin and erythopoietin use for blood conservation: result with Jehovah's witnesses. *Ann Thorac Surg* 1994;58:1397.
203. Hayashi J, Kumon K, Takanashi S, et al. Subcutaneous administration of recombinant human erythropoietin before cardiac surgery: a double-blind, multicenter trial in Japan. *Transfusion* 1994;34:142.
204. Goodnough LT, Rudnick S, Price TH, et al. Increased preoperative collection of autologous blood with recombinant human erythropoietin therapy. *N Engl J Med* 1989;321:1163.
205. Sowade O, Warnke H, Scigalla P, et al. Avoidance of allogeneic blood transfusions by treatment with epoetin beta (recombinant human erythropoietin) in patients undergoing open-heart surgery. *Blood* 1997;89:411–418.
206. Goodnough LT. Erythropoietin therapy versus red cell transfusion. *Curr Opin Hematol* 2001;8:405–410.
207. Hiramatsu Y, Gikakis N, Anderson HL III, et al. Tirofiban provides "platelet anesthesia" during cardiopulmonary bypass in baboons. *J Thorac Cardiovasc Surg* 1996;113:182–193.
208. Suzuki Y, Hillyer P, Miyamoto S, et al. Integrilin® prevents prolonged bleeding times after cardiopulmonary bypass. *Ann Thorac Surg* 1998;66: 373–381.
209. Suzuki Y, Malekan R, Hansen CW III, et al. Platelet anesthesia with nitric oxide with or without eptifibatide during cardiopulmonary bypass in baboons. *J Thorac Cardiovasc Surg* 1999;117:987–993.
210. Goodnough LT, Lublin DM, Zhang L, et al. Transfusion medicine service policies for recombinant factor VIIa administration. *Transfusion* 2004;44: 1325–1331.
211. Park P, Fewel ME, Garton HJ, et al. Recombinant activated factor VII for the rapid correction of coagulopathy in nonhemophiliac neurosurgical patients. *Neurosurgery* 2003;53:34–39.
212. Halkos ME, Levy JH, Chen E, et al. Early experience with activated recombinant factor VII for intractable hemorrhage following cardiovascular surgery. *Ann Thorac Surg (In press)*.
213. Hebertson M. Recombinant activated factor VII in cardiac surgery. *Blood Coagul Fibrinolysis* 2004;15:S31–S32.
214. Raivio P, Suojaranta-Ylinen R, Kuitunen AH. Recombinant factor VIIa in the treatment of post-operative hemorrhage after cardiac surgery. *Ann Thorac Surg* 2005;80:66–71.
215. Friedrich PW, Henny CP, Messelink EJ, et al. Effect of recombinant activated factor VII on perioperative blood loss in patients undergoing retropubic prostatectomy: a double blind, placebo-controlled randomized trial. *Lancet* 2003;361:201–205.
216. Buehler PW, Alayash AI. Toxicities of hemoglobin solutions: in search of in-vitro and in-vivo model systems. *Transfusion* 2004;44:1516–1530.
217. Stokstad E. Not blood simple. *Science* 2002;295:1003.
218. Vandergriff KD. Hemoglobin-based oxygen carriers. *Expert Opin Investig Drugs* 2000;9:1967–1984.
219. Wahr JA. Clinical potential of blood substitutes or oxygen therapeutics during cardiac surgery. *Anesth Clin N Am* 2003;21:553–568.
220. Squires JE. Artificial blood. *Science* 2002;295:1002–1005.
221. Creteur J, Vincent J-L. Hemoglobin solutions. *Crit Care Med* 2003;31: S698–S707.
222. Goodnough LT, Shander A, Brecher ME. Transfusion medicine: looking to the future. *Lancet* 2003;361:161–169.
223. Sloan EP, Koenigsberg M, Gens D, et al. Diaspirin cross-linked hemoglobin (DCL-Hgb) in the treatment of severe traumatic hemorrhagic shock. *JAMA* 1999;282:1857–1864.
224. Ohtsuka T, Wolf RK, Hiratzka LF, et al. Thoracoscopic internal mammary artery harvest for MICABG using the harmonic scapel. *Ann Thorac Surg* 1997;63:S107–S109.
225. Higami T, Yamashita T, Nohara H, et al. Early results of coronary grafting using ultrasonically skeletonized internal thoracic arteries. *Ann Thorac Surg* 2001;71:1224–1228.

226. Luciani N, Anselmi A, Gaudino M, et al. Harmonic scalpel reduces bleeding and postoperative complications in redo cardiac surgery. *Ann Thorac Surg (In press)*.

227. Stahle E, Tammelin A, Bergstrom R, et al. Sternal wound complications–incidence, microbiology and risk factors. *Eur J Cardiothorac Surg* 1997;11:1146–1153.

228. Robicsek F, Masters TN, Littman L, et al. The embolization of bone wax from sternotomy incisions. *Ann Thorac Surg* 1981;31:357–359.

229. Kjaegard HK, Trumbull HR. Bleeding from the sternal marrow can be stopped using vivostat patient-derived fibrin sealant. *Ann Thorac Surg* 2000;69:1173–1175.

230. Robicsek F, Duncan GD, Born GVR, et al. Inherent dangers of simultaneous application of microfibrillar collagen hemostat and blood saving devices. *J Thorac Cardiovasc Surg* 1986;92:766–770.

231. Mair H, Schutz A, Lamm P, et al. Control of bleeding from fragile sternum with a resorbable hemostyptic. *Ann Thorac Surg* 2001;71:759–760.

232. Dunn CJ, Goa KL. Fibrin sealant: a review of its use in surgery and endoscopy. *Drugs* 1999;58:83–86.

233. Albala DM. Fibrin sealants in clinical practice. *Cardiovasc Surg* 2003;11(Suppl. 1):5–11.

234. MacGillivaray TE. Fibrin sealants and glues. *J Card Surg* 2003;18:480–485.

235. Carless PA, Henry DA, Anthong DM. Fibrin sealant use for minimizing peri-operative allogeneic blood transfusion. *Cochrane Database Syst Rev* 2003;2:CD004171.

236. Clark RA. Fibrin glue for wound repair: facts and fancy. *Thromb Haemost* 2003;90:1003–1006.

237. Weissberg D. Surgical glue and necrosis of arterial wall. *Ann Thorac Surg* 2003;75:1063.

238. Oz MC, Cosgrove DM III, Badduke BR et al, The Fusion Matrix Study Group. Controlled clinical trial of a novel hemostatic agent in cardiac surgery. *Ann Thorac Surg* 2000;69:1376–1382.

239. Bachet J, Goudot B, Dreyfus G, et al. A 20-year experience with the GRF glue in acute aortic dissection. *J Card Surg* 1997;12:243–255.

240. Kazui T, Washiyama N, Bashar AH, et al. Role of biologic glue repair of proximal aortic dissection in the development of early and midterm redissection of the aortic root. *Ann Thorac Surg* 2001;72:509–514.

241. Hata M, Shiono M, Sezai A, et al. Type A acute aortic dissection: immediate and mid-term results of emergency aortic replacement with the aid of gelatin resorcin formalin glue. *Ann Thorac Surg* 2004;78:853–857.

242. Bingley JA, Gardner MAH, Stafford EG, et al. Late complications of tissue glues in aortic surgery. *Ann Thorac Surg* 2000;69:1764–1768.

243. Fukunaga S, Kack M, Harringer W, et al. The use of gelatin-resorcine-formalin glue in acute dissection type A. *Eur J Cardiothorac Surg* 1999;15:564–570.

244. Despotis GJ, Skubas NJ, Goodnough LT. Optimal management of bleeding and transfusion in patients undergoing cardiac surgery. *Semin Thorac Cardiovasc Surg* 1999;11:84–104.

245. Anderson CA, Filsoufi F, Aklog L, et al. Liberal use of delayed sternal closure for postcardiotomy hemodynamic instability. *Ann Thorac Surg* 2002;73:1484–1488.

246. Mestres CA, Pomar JL, Acosta M, et al. Delayed sternal closure for life-threatening complications in cardiac operations: an update. *Ann Thorac Surg* 1991;51:773–776.

247. Alexi-Meskishvili V, Weng Y, Uhlemann F, et al. Prolonged open sternotomy after pediatric open heart operation: experience with 113 patients. *Ann Thorac Surg* 1995;59:379–383.

248. Iyer RS, Jacobs JP, de Leval MR, et al. Outcomes after delayed sternal closure in pediatric heart operations: a 10-year experience. *Ann Thorac Surg* 1997;63:489–491.

249. Munoz JJ, Birkmeyer NJO, Dacey LJ, et al. Trends in rates of reexploration for hemorrhage after coronary artery bypass surgery. *Ann Thorac Surg* 1999;68:1321–1325.

250. Barnett SD, Halpin LS, Speir AM, et al. Postoperative complications among octogenarians after cardiovascular surgery. *Ann Thorac Surg* 2003;76:726–731.

251. Helm RE, Rosengart TK, Gomez M, et al. Comprehensive multimodality blood conservation; 100 consecutive CABG operations with transfusion. *Ann Thorac Surg* 1998;65:125–136.

252. Collier B, Kolff J, Devineni R, et al. Prophylactic positive end-expiratory pressure and reduction of postoperative blood loss in open-heart surgery. *Ann Thorac Surg* 2002;74:1191–1194.

253. Fairman RM, Edmunds LH Jr. Emergency thoracotomy in the surgical intensive care unit after open cardiac operation. *Ann Thorac Surg* 1981;32:386–386.

254. McKowen RL, Magovern GJ, Liebler GA, et al. Infectious complications and cost-effectiveness of open resuscitation in the surgical intensive care unit after cardiac surgery. *Ann Thorac Surg* 1985;40:388–392.

255. Livingston ER, Fisher CA, Bibidakis EJ, et al. Increased activation of the coagulation and fibrinloytic systems leads to hemorrhagic complications during left ventricular assist implantation. *Circulation* 1996;94(Suppl. II):II227–II234.

256. Spanier T, Oz M, Levin H, et al. Activation of coagulation and fibrinolytic pathways in patients with left ventricular assist devices. *J Thorac Cardiovasc Surg* 1996;112:1090–1097.

257. Pavie A, Szefner J, Leger P, et al. Preventing, minimizing and managing postoperative bleeding. *Ann Thorac Surg* 1999;68:705–710.

258. Goldstein DJ, Seldomridge JA, Chen JM, et al. Use of aprotinin in LVAD recipients reduces blood loss, blood use and perioperative mortality. *Ann Thorac Surg* 1995;59:1063–1068.

259. Zietkiewicz M, Garlicki M, Domagala J, et al. Successful use of activated recombinant factor VII to control bleeding abnormalities in a patient with a left ventricular assist device. *J Thorac Cardiovasc Surg* 2002;123:384–385.

# CHAPTER 75 ■ OBSTETRIC HEMORRHAGE

PETER W. MARKS

Hemorrhage represents the ultimate manifestation of any one of a number of different pathophysiologic processes in the obstetric patient. It may result from an anatomic defect or be related to medical complications of pregnancy. Alternatively, hemorrhage may be caused by a condition that is coincidentally prevalent in women of childbearing potential rather than specifically associated with pregnancy. This chapter reviews conditions associated with obstetric hemorrhage, as well as those that may raise concern regarding its development during pregnancy and the puerperium.

## ABRUPTIO PLACENTAE

*Abruptio placentae* is the premature separation of the normally implanted placenta from the uterine wall before the delivery of the fetus. In one large epidemiologic survey performed in the United States, the prevalence of this condition was approximately 1% (1). The effect of this condition on the mother and the fetus depends on the severity of the abruption (2). Minor placental abruption may be asymptomatic or be associated with premature labor and cause minimal risk to the infant, whereas major abruption can lead to maternal and/or fetal death. Although the mortality rate from this condition is relatively low, morbidity can be high. Abruptio placentae is associated with an increased rate of caesarean section and an increased use of blood products due to coagulopathy. In fact, placental abruption is the most common cause of abnormal coagulation tests in pregnancy. Hypofibrinogenemia, elevated fibrin degradation products, and decreases in other coagulation factors may be observed.

Vaginal bleeding, uterine irritability manifest as frequent contractions or hypertonus, uterine tenderness, and back pain are the key maternal manifestations of severe abruption. This may be accompanied by fetal distress as evidenced by abnormal fetal heart tones on cardiotocography. Abruption of lesser severity may be more difficult to diagnose. In one series, 22% of individuals with mild to moderate abruption were thought only to be in preterm labor (3). However, the amount of visible vaginal bleeding may bear little relation to the extent of placental separation and the amount of actual blood loss from the circulation.

The coagulopathy of *abruptio placentae* is primarily due to the consumption of fibrinogen and platelets at the placenta–uterus interface (4,5). Fibrinogen levels normally rise significantly during pregnancy to levels that are approximately 50% higher than in nonpregnant women (6). Low fibrinogen levels in a pregnant woman near term are therefore generally indicative of some abnormality. Because fibrinogen levels are not associated with abnormal thrombin times until they are less than approximately 100 mg per dL, direct laboratory assessment of the fibrinogen level can be important in patient assessment.

Delivery of the fetus is the definitive management for abruptio placentae. Vaginal delivery is preferred. This removes the placenta-uterus interface and allows the uterus to contract. In most cases, uterine function is not impaired, and good contraction follows removal of the fetus, placenta, and retroplacental clot. However, postpartum hemorrhage may occur, and patients therefore warrant close monitoring following delivery.

Worsening coagulopathy, severe hemorrhage, or fetal distress may require surgical intervention in some cases of abruptio placentae. Immediate caesarean section should be considered for evidence of fetal distress, because even optimal maternal management is not often associated with fetal recovery. The maternal coagulopathy is usually not overtly manifest when a living fetus is present, and abnormalities tend to resolve spontaneously after delivery. Therefore, administration of blood products is unnecessary in most patients.

If hypofibrinogenemia is detected, fibrinogen can be administered in the form of cryoprecipitate or fresh frozen plasma. The advantage to the latter is that it also provides other clotting factors. One unit of fresh frozen plasma contains approximately 250 to 300 mg of fibrinogen in approximately 200 mL and is generally sufficient to raise the fibrinogen level by 25 to 50 mg per dL (7). If volume expansion is undesirable or contraindicated, the same amount of fibrinogen can be administered in a volume of 15 to 25 mL cryoprecipitate (8). In addition, due to consumption leading to thrombocytopenia, platelet transfusion may be necessary. The use of antifibrinolytic agents such as ε-aminocaproic acid or tranexamic acid have not been shown to improve overall outcome in *abruptio placentae*, although the use of these agents may be considered in certain circumstances (9).

## PLACENTA PREVIA

*Placenta previa* is the term used to describe implantation of the placenta near the internal os of the cervix instead of in the upper segment of the uterus. Painless vaginal bleeding that is characteristic of this condition may be so severe as to require interruption of pregnancy, regardless of fetal maturity. Often, the first bleeding episode ceases, but subsequent episodes provoke delivery of the fetus.

Screening coagulation tests are of limited use in the management of placenta previa, as they are generally normal (10). If the mother is hemodynamically unstable, the fetal cardiotocogram may be abnormal, but it generally normalizes with appropriate management of maternal hemorrhage.

Although placenta previa may require the transfusion of packed red blood cells (RBC) because of hemorrhage, other blood products are less commonly required unless the hemorrhage is particularly severe. Patients should be monitored closely following delivery because placenta previa predisposes to postpartum hemorrhage caused by poor lower uterine contraction, which can even necessitate surgical intervention or hysterectomy in some patients.

## POSTPARTUM HEMORRHAGE

Blood loss after a normal vaginal delivery may exceed 500 mL, particularly if an episiotomy is performed. Caesarean section may lead to additional blood loss. The distinction between normal blood loss and postpartum hemorrhage is that the latter is associated with hemodynamic instability. The major causes of primary postpartum hemorrhage are trauma to the uterus, coagulopathy, and uterine atony (11). Trauma to the uterus should be surgically addressed, and management of coagulopathy is covered later in this chapter.

The goal of management of atonic uterine hemorrhage is to convert the uterus to a tonic state. This involves ensuring that the uterus is empty and using pharmacologic agents to induce uterine contraction, if necessary (12). The placenta should be removed and the uterus explored if placental fragments are suspected. Oxytocin is the most common drug used initially in this setting. A dilute intravenous solution infused at 20 to 30 IU per L of crystalloid at a rate of 125 to 250 mL per hour is frequently preceded by a bolus of 10 IU. In mild cases, consideration may be given to intramuscular administration.

If a response to oxytocin is not obtained, ergot preparations can be used. Ergonovine maleate and methylergonovine can be administered intravenously or intramuscularly at a dose of 0.2 mg every 20 minutes up to three times. Because ergot preparations cause prolonged vasoconstriction, they should be administered with caution in patients with preeclampsia, essential hypertension, heart disease, pheochromocytoma, or thyrotoxicosis. A frequent side effect of the administration of ergot preparations is nausea. Alternatively, 15-methyl-prostaglandin F2$\alpha$ has been reported to have a high response rate in this setting (13). It can be administered intramuscularly or intramyometrially. A dose of 0.25 mg can be repeated as necessary every 1 to 1.5 hours and has a low side-effect profile; however, it has been occasionally associated with arterial oxygen desaturation due to intrapulmonary shunting (14,15).

Failing medical management, surgical intervention may be necessary. Although uterine packing may be performed, it is not always successful (16). Uterine artery ligation or embolization, ovarian artery ligation, internal iliac ligation, or hysterectomy may be necessary (17–20). As a last resort, a few reports indicate the efficacy of recombinant factor VIIa in treating postpartum hemorrhage (21). However, this represents an off-label use of this product, and caution is indicated because of the possibility of thrombotic complications.

# DEAD FETUS SYNDROME

Intrauterine fetal demise can be associated with hypofibrinogenemia in up to 25% to 30% of cases. However, this complication does not usually develop until 4 to 5 weeks after fetal death (22). Improved antenatal care and ultrasonography have therefore reduced the incidence of this finding.

In an individual who is hemodynamically stable, the coagulopathy accompanying fetal demise can sometimes be reversed with a course of heparin prior to induction of labor. A regimen of 1,000 IU per hour for 48 hours may allow the fibrinogen levels to return to normal. Upon normalization of fibrinogen levels, labor may be induced (23).

# THROMBOCYTOPENIA

A decrease in the platelet count is a relatively common finding during pregnancy, occurring in up to 10% of women (24). Fortunately, most decreases are mild and are unassociated with any clinical consequence, representing the potentially physiologic occurrence of gestational thrombocytopenia. When unassociated with other hemostatic defects, platelet counts in the range down to 70,000 per $\mu$L are well tolerated during pregnancy. Below this range, the risk for hemorrhage increases. Burrows and Kelton have reported the causes of low platelet

counts in a large cohort of women representing 15,471 pregnancies (25). There were 1,027 instances of thrombocytopenia. Approximately 74% of cases were attributable to gestational thrombocytopenia, 21% to hypertensive disorders of pregnancy, 4% to immune disorders of pregnancy such as immune thrombocytopenic purpura (ITP), and 2% to a variety of other relatively uncommon disorders, including acute fatty liver of pregnancy, hemolysis, elevated liver function tests, and low platelets (HELLP) syndrome, disseminated intravascular coagulation (DIC), and thrombotic thrombocytopenic purpura (TTP). Diagnostic features helpful in distinguishing the various causes of thrombocytopenia are listed in Table 75-1.

## Gestational Thrombocytopenia

After more serious causes of thrombocytopenia are eliminated from consideration, approximately 6% to 7% of pregnancies are associated with a fall in the platelet count below normal during the second or third trimester to the range of 70,000 to 150,000 per $\mu$L (26). In most of these cases, the decrease is into the range of 100,000 to 150,000 per $\mu$L and is unassociated with any consequence. The etiology for this benign drop in the platelet count may result from effects of the pregnancy on platelet clearance or from hemodilution (27). Because of such effects, there has been the suggestion that the normal range for the platelet count should be considered lower in pregnant women.

Individuals with platelet counts between 70,000 and 100,000 per $\mu$L may have either gestational thrombocytopenia or ITP. The cause of ITP is accelerated clearance of platelets by the reticuloendothelial system due to autoantibodies bound to the platelet membrane. Antiplatelet antibody testing is sometimes performed in an attempt to distinguish gestational thrombocytopenia from ITP. However, antiplatelet antibody testing for the purpose of diagnosing ITP is relatively insensitive and nonspecific during pregnancy (28,29). The distinction may be largely unnecessary for platelet counts in this range because maternal and fetal management is unaffected by confirmation of the diagnosis. Most anesthesiologists decide whether or not to use regional anesthesia on the basis of the platelet count rather than the underlying disorder. In addition, as a precaution against missing neonatal thrombocytopenia in the presence of mild to moderate maternal ITP, consideration should be given to checking the neonatal platelet count when the maternal platelet count is 70,000 to 100,000 per $\mu$L. Cord blood platelet count determination at the time of delivery allows identification of neonates who may be thrombocytopenic due to immunoglobulin G antibodies crossing the placenta in the event that ITP was indeed present in the mother. This facilitates appropriate further monitoring and, if necessary, treatment of these infants.

## Immune Thrombocytopenic Purpura

ITP is difficult to distinguish from gestational thrombocytopenia solely on the basis of the platelet count. In general, however, decreases in the platelet count occurring during the first trimester of pregnancy and decreases in the platelet count to less than 70,000 per $\mu$L any time during pregnancy are more often associated with ITP. A history of autoimmune disease or thrombocytopenia prior to pregnancy also supports the diagnosis of ITP. These features are in contrast to the temporal relation and milder nature of gestational thrombocytopenia.

The need to intervene with therapy for the management of ITP during pregnancy depends on the degree of thrombocytopenia and the proximity to delivery. Women with platelet counts of greater than approximately 30,000 per $\mu$L during the first and second trimesters may simply be monitored if they

**TABLE 75-1**

DISTINGUISHING FEATURES OF CAUSES OF THROMBOCYTOPENIA AND ABNORMAL COAGULATION TESTS IN PREGNANCY

| Diagnosis | Thrombocytopenia[a] | RBC morphology | PT or PTT | Creatinine | ALT/AST |
|---|---|---|---|---|---|
| Gestational | Mild to moderate | Normal | Normal | Normal | Normal |
| ITP | Moderate to severe | Normal | Normal | Normal | Normal |
| Preeclampsia | Mild to moderate | Normal | Normal | Normal | Normal |
| HELLP | Mild to severe | Schistocytes | Normal | Normal | Abnormal |
| TTP | Moderate to severe | Schistocytes | Normal | Variable | Normal |
| HUS | Mild to moderate | Schistocytes | Normal | Abnormal | Normal |
| DIC | None to severe | Schistocytes | Abnormal | Variable | Variable |
| Fatty liver | None to mild | Variable | Abnormal | Normal | Abnormal |
| Factor VIII inhibitor | None | Normal | Abnormal | Normal | Normal |

RBC, red blood cell; PT, prothrombin time; PTT, partial thromboplastin time; ALT, alanine aminotransferase; AST, aspartate aminotransferase; ITP, immune thrombocytopenic purpura; HELLP, hemolysis, elevated liver function tests, and low platelet syndrome; TTP, thrombotic thrombocytopenic purpura; HUS, hemolytic-uremic syndrome; DIC, disseminated intravascular coagulation.
[a]The approximate ranges of the platelet counts correlating to the descriptions of thrombocytopenia are as follows:

| | |
|---|---|
| Mild | 70,000–149,000/$\mu$L |
| Moderate | 30,000–69,000/$\mu$L |
| Severe | <30,000/$\mu$L |

have no evidence of bleeding, as the risk of hemorrhage to both mother and fetus is relatively low (30,31).

Therapy is indicated for platelet counts less than 30,000 per $\mu$L occurring any time during pregnancy to prevent complications. Particularly, during the third trimester, as the delivery date approaches, therapy is generally recommended to increase the platelet count to at least 50,000 to 100,000 per $\mu$L (32). This facilitates hemostasis during delivery and preserves the option of epidural anesthesia. There is debate as to the optimal platelet count for safe epidural anesthesia, with some anesthesiologists accepting platelet counts of greater than 50,000 per $\mu$L and others preferring counts of 70,000 to 100,000 per $\mu$L or more (33,34).

The optimal first-line therapy in patients who are pregnant and who have ITP is controversial (35–37). Oral prednisone, administered initially at approximately 1 mg per kg, then gradually tapered over several weeks, is a convenient therapy and increases the platelet count in most patients. Often, the dose of prednisone can be tapered to 5 to 10 mg daily with maintenance of platelet counts in the range of 50,000 to 100,000 per $\mu$L. However, use of prednisone is associated with hypertension and diabetes during the gestational period. High-dose immunoglobulin therapy (1 to 2 gm per kg) is potentially safer than prednisone and may be administered with similar efficacy (38). However, the effect of immunoglobulin therapy on increasing the platelet count is often transient, so it must be administered on a regular basis every 3 to 6 weeks during pregnancy.

Approximately 10% to 25% of pregnant women with ITP will have thrombocytopenia refractory to treatment with prednisone or immunoglobulin. In such cases, splenectomy may be considered during the second trimester by either traditional or laparoscopic surgery (39,40). Approximately two thirds of women will respond to this procedure (41). The alternatives for pregnant patients who fail to respond to splenectomy are more limited than for nonpregnant patients with ITP. Though intravenous anti-D antibody has been administered with success, its safety in pregnancy is questionable (42). Cytotoxic agents are generally avoided during pregnancy (43). As an alternative, combination treatment with high doses of steroids and immunoglobulin may sometimes prove effective, even when either agent alone was ineffective.

Integral to the management of ITP during pregnancy is planning of the delivery and monitoring of the neonate, since immunoglobulin G antibodies can cross the placenta and cause fetal thrombocytopenia. The subject remains somewhat controversial (44). Two alternative strategies have been advocated, although neither is supported by randomized clinical data, and local practice patterns, rather than clinical data, tend to determine the delivery modality used (45,46). The first strategy is determination of the fetal platelet count by percutaneous umbilical blood sampling (PUBS), an invasive procedure associated with a complication rate of up to 1%, followed by caesarean delivery if the platelet count is less than 50,000 per $\mu$L. The second, based in part on the low occurrence of neonatal thrombocytopenia, is to allow labor to proceed without prior determination of the platelet count. In either case, an umbilical cord blood platelet count should be determined in all infants born to mothers diagnosed with ITP. If the platelet count in the neonate is below normal, it should be monitored for several days. If necessary, treatment should be initiated on the basis of the platelet counts in order to prevent complications, which can include intracranial hemorrhage.

## Preeclampsia and Hemolysis, Elevated Liver Function Tests, and Low Platelets Syndrome

Preeclampsia is a systemic disorder manifest primarily by hypertension and proteinuria that complicates from 2% to 8% of pregnancies during the second or third trimesters. The pathophysiology leading to the low platelet count in preeclampsia is not entirely clear, but may involve platelet activation and increased clearance due to vascular abnormalities (47). Approximately 25% of cases of preeclampsia are accompanied by thrombocytopenia of at least mild severity (48). More severe cases of preeclampsia may be associated with a thrombocytopenia of greater severity. The bleeding time in preeclampsia is sometimes prolonged, and it is unclear whether this reflects the decreased platelet number, abnormal platelet function, increased platelet activation, or some combination of these factors (49). In addition, there may be associated coagulation abnormalities, including decreased antithrombin levels and increased fibrin degradation products or D-dimer levels (50). The prothrombin time (PT) and the partial thromboplastin time (PTT) are generally normal, and elevated values suggest the presence of concomitant DIC.

The thrombocytopenia in mild to moderate preeclampsia generally resolves with delivery of the infant. Prior to delivery, management consists of supportive care, including transfusion of platelets if there is evidence of bleeding or if the platelet count drops to a particularly low level (<30,000 per $\mu$L). Because of the platelet function abnormalities in preeclampsia, some anesthesiologists prefer to use spinal rather than epidural anesthesia during delivery. However, there are few data in the literature to support one approach or the other. There are reports of neonatal thrombocytopenia, particularly in growth-retarded infants born to mothers with preeclampsia; however, the thrombocytopenia may be related to other complications of premature birth (51).

Severe cases of preeclampsia may be associated with the HELLP syndrome. Hemolysis is manifest on the peripheral blood smear as red cell fragmentation (schistocytes), although many patients are not anemic. Presumably due to increased platelet destruction, severe thrombocytopenia (platelets < 30,000 per $\mu$L) occurs in approximately 5% to 10% of patients. HELLP syndrome results from a pathophysiologic process that is distinct from that of DIC or the thrombotic microangiopathies, and it is associated with increased maternal and fetal morbidity and mortality. Variants of HELLP also exist in which the platelet count may be normal or only mildly depressed (52). As in preeclampsia, commonly performed clinical tests of coagulation (PT, PTT, and fibrinogen) are usually normal. If these tests are abnormal, DIC may be present. Although there are no large case series published in the literature, the concomitant presence of HELLP and DIC appears to be associated with even higher rates of morbidity and mortality than that of HELLP syndrome alone (53).

Management of HELLP syndrome consists of stabilizing the patient and transfusing platelets, if necessary, to facilitate delivery. In addition, some have advocated the use of corticosteroids, but routine use is controversial (54). The mode of delivery depends on the clinical status of the patient and fetus, as well as on whether severe thrombocytopenia or other coagulation abnormalities are present. Although HELLP syndrome often resolves soon after delivery, it may also initially develop up to a week postpartum. It therefore warrants consideration in the differential diagnosis of thrombocytopenia in the early postpartum period (55). One small study has suggested that plasmapheresis may be beneficial if HELLP syndrome persists more than 72 hours postpartum (56).

## Thrombotic Thrombocytopenic Purpura/ Hemolytic-Uremic Syndrome

TTP and hemolytic-uremic syndrome are uncommon but serious disorders that complicate approximately one in 25,000 pregnancies (57). Both entities are characterized by microangiopathic hemolytic anemia with a variable extent of thrombocytopenia, often accompanied by renal insufficiency. Clinically, hemolytic-uremic syndrome (HUS) is distinguished from TTP by the presence of fever and/or neurologic changes in the latter. Often, however, distinguishing between the two entities is difficult. Recent developments have helped to elucidate the pathophysiology of TTP. This disorder results from absence of a disintegrin

and metalloprotease with thrombospondin type 1 motif 13 (ADAMTS13), a protease that cleaves von Willebrand factor (58,59). Acquired cases of TTP may be caused by autoantibodies against the protease. The etiology of HUS is less clear at this time but may involve vascular injury (see Chapter 111).

In the absence of complicating factors, neither TTP nor HUS is associated with a prolonged PT or PTT, or with a significantly decreased fibrinogen. Elevated D-dimer levels have been reported in some pregnant patients with TTP or HUS (60). However, D-dimer levels are usually elevated during the second and third trimester of pregnancy (61). Neither TTP nor HUS is typically associated with significant elevations of liver function tests, a distinction between these entities and HELLP syndrome that may otherwise present quite similarly (62). Although criteria for the clinical distinctions exist, sometimes it is impossible to distinguish TTP or HUS from HELLP (63). In these cases, a therapeutic trial of treatment of TTP may be indicated, because there is significant mortality associated with untreated TTP.

The appropriate treatment of TTP is plasma exchange performed daily until the platelet count and the lactate dehydrogenase (LDH) levels normalize (64). If plasma exchange is not immediately available, plasma infusion (approximately 30 mg/kg/day) may be beneficial, although less so than plasmapheresis (65). Packed RBC are administered to maintain an adequate hematocrit. Therapy with prednisone or methylprednisolone (1 to 3 mg/kg/day) is often administered as well, although the benefit of this therapy has not yet been documented in prospective randomized trials (66). Although plasma exchange is less effective in the setting of HUS than in TTP, it may be employed, particularly if the distinction between TTP and HUS cannot be made (38). If plasma exchange is not used, treatment of HUS consists of supportive care and includes dialysis when necessary.

## Heparin-Induced Thrombocytopenia

Not infrequently, pregnant patients require prophylaxis or treatment of venous thromboembolism. Unfractionated heparin and, more recently, low-molecular-weight heparins have been used because of contraindications to warfarin during pregnancy. Interestingly, although heparin-induced thrombocytopenia (HIT) has been reported in pregnant patients, documented HIT is exceedingly rare, particularly in the second or third trimesters (67). Although HIT should certainly be considered in a pregnant patient, other causes of thrombocytopenia (e.g., gestational thrombocytopenia) should also be considered in the differential diagnosis.

# INHERITED COAGULATION DEFECTS

Deficiencies in intrinsic and extrinsic clotting factors are relatively rare in women, because two of the more common deficiencies (factor VIII and IX) are sex-linked recessive traits. On the other hand, deficiencies in factor XI or in von Willebrand factor activity are more common (68,69). Because von Willebrand factor levels generally normalize during labor and delivery in patients with mild to moderate type I von Willebrand disease, delivery is often uncomplicated (70). If bleeding occurs, it generally occurs postpartum, after von Willebrand levels return to baseline levels (71). More severe types of von Willebrand disease (severe type I, moderate to severe type IIA, and type IIB) may require therapy with von Willebrand–containing factor concentrates at the time of delivery and for 1 to 2 weeks afterward to prevent hemorrhage from the uterus as it returns toward normal size (72). Administration of such virally inactivated factor concentrates is preferable to fresh frozen plasma or cryoprecipitate in this setting.

Rare coagulation abnormalities may be associated with excessive mucosal bleeding, including plasminogen activator inhibitor-1 (PAI-1) deficiency (73). In such cases, management with antifibrinolytic agents such as aminocaproic acid may prevent excessive hemorrhage.

# OTHER COAGULATION ABNORMALITIES

Aside from thrombocytopenia and the relatively rare hereditary disorders of coagulation described earlier, disorders resulting in major coagulation abnormalities (manifest as an elevated PT or PTT) are relatively uncommon in pregnancy.

## Acute Fatty Liver of Pregnancy

Acute fatty liver of pregnancy is a disorder of unclear etiology associated with approximately one in 5,000 to 10,000 pregnancies, usually during the third trimester in primiparous individuals (74). It may represent a fulminant variant of preeclampsia (75). Patients present with a variety of symptoms, including right upper quadrant pain, and may have abnormal liver function tests consistent with cholestatic abnormalities. Liver histology demonstrates fatty change in the pericentral areas with minimal inflammatory infiltrate or necrosis (76). In most cases, the PT and/or PTT is abnormal, primarily secondary to decreased vitamin K–dependent coagulation factor synthesis, and fibrinogen may also be decreased, probably secondary to increased fibrinolysis. Mild thrombocytopenia and some red cell fragmentation or acanthocytosis (spur cells) may be seen on the peripheral blood smear.

This complication of pregnancy may progress to hepatic encephalopathy and hepatorenal failure if unaddressed. Treatment consists of delivery as soon as possible and supportive care of the mother and neonate. Plasma containing antithrombin and deficient coagulation factors must be administered to correct coagulation abnormalities. Most often, metabolic derangements correct soon after delivery, and patients are left without sequelae. However, progression of hepatic failure may still occur following delivery, necessitating consideration of liver transplantation (77).

## Disseminated Intravascular Coagulation

DIC, a relatively uncommon complication during pregnancy, may result from several different underlying disease processes. Several of these, such as those relating to infection, are not specific to pregnancy. However, a number of causes are specific to pregnancy or delivery and require prompt recognition, such as the DIC of abruptio placentae or amniotic fluid embolism (78). In the absence of a clear anatomic source from which bleeding is occurring, patients who develop severe hemorrhage following delivery should have coagulation studies performed, including a PT, PTT, and fibrinogen level. Diffuse, heavy postpartum vaginal bleeding or oozing from around intravenous catheter insertion sites can also be an indicator of amniotic fluid embolism. It is associated with a relatively high rate of maternal mortality (16% to 80%, depending on the series) due to hemorrhagic as well as systemic complications (79,80). Since amniotic fluid rapidly leads to defibrination of the plasma, there are severely depressed fibrinogen levels and significant elevations in the PT and PTT. Prompt administration of fresh frozen plasma and cryoprecipitate is indicated. The cryoprecipitate provides a concentrated source of fibrinogen and may help to more rapidly reverse the coagulation abnormalities. Administration of packed RBC is often necessary to replenish blood lost through hemorrhage.

Other causes of DIC should be treated similarly with supportive care. While the underlying cause of DIC is identified and addressed, fresh frozen plasma, packed RBC, and platelets should be administered as required. Serial complete blood counts and coagulation studies assist in the optimal selection of blood products for administration (see Chapter 117).

## Factor VIII Inhibitors

Factor VIII levels rise modestly during pregnancy (41). A rare complication that may occur during the puerperium and for up to several months postpartum is the development of antibody inhibitors to factor VIII, leading to absent or near absent levels of this coagulation factor (81). Patients may present just postpartum with severe hemorrhage or may present months after delivery with excessive bruising, hematomas, mucosal hemorrhage, or life-threatening internal hemorrhage (82). The most marked finding on screening laboratory tests is an elevated PTT. Unless the inhibitor titer is very high, causing interference in the assay, the PT is generally normal. Diagnosis is strongly suggested by an inhibitor screen (mixing study) that is positive and is confirmed by obtaining factor VIII levels, which are reported as a percent of normal, and inhibitor levels, which are measured and reported in Bethesda units (51).

Management of factor VIII inhibitors depends on the setting. If maternal hemorrhage or other major bleeding complications are present in the setting of a high-titer inhibitor (or if therapy is necessary prior to titer determination), treatment with a factor VIII–bypassing concentrate or recombinant human factor VIIa are usually effective (83). In the absence of bleeding complications, observation is reasonable, because these inhibitors often spontaneously resolve without therapy within several months after pregnancy (84). If the inhibitor is of high titer or persists in low titer, immunosuppressive therapy is indicated (85).

# SUMMARY

Obstetric hemorrhage may be caused by anatomic defects or by medical conditions. The distinction between different causes of hemorrhage depends upon the setting, as well as careful consideration of historical features and associated laboratory abnormalities. Although some causes of thrombocytopenia are serious and associated with bleeding complications, most patients with mild to moderate gestational thrombocytopenia or mild ITP and require no therapy to increase the platelet count. Other coagulation abnormalities aside from thrombocytopenia may represent serious underlying pathology and require immediate management.

## References

1. Anath CV, Oyelese Y, Yeo L, et al. Placental abruption in the United States, 1979 through 2001: temporal trends and potential determinants. *Am J Obstet Gynecol* 2005;192:191–198.
2. Abdella TN, Sibai BM, Hayse JM, et al. Perinatal outcome in abruption placentae. *Obstet Gynecol* 1984;63:365–370.
3. Hurd WW, Midovovnik M, Hertzvert V, et al. Selective management of *abruptio placentae*: a prospective study. *Obstet Gynecol* 1983;61:467–473.
4. Pritchard JA, Brekken AL. Clinical and laboratory studies on severe *abruptio placentae*. *Am J Obstet Gynecol* 1967;97:681–700.
5. Hellgren M, Blomback M. Studies of blood coagulation and fibronolysis in pregnancy during delivery and in the puerperium. I. Normal condition. *Gynecol Obstet Invest* 1981;12:141–154.
6. Brenner B. Haemostatic changes in pregnancy. *Thromb Res* 2004;114:409–414.

7. Doyle S, O'Brien P, Murphy K, et al. Coagulation factor content of solvent/detergent plasma compared with fresh frozen plasma. *Blood Coagul Fibrinolysis* 2003;14:283–287.

8. Ness PM, Perkins HA. Cryoprecipitate as a reliable source of fibrinogen replacement. *JAMA* 1979;241:1690–1691.

9. Sher GJ, Stattland BE. *Abruptio placentae* with coagulopathy: a rational basis for management. *Clin Obstet Gynecol* 1985;28:15–23.

10. Wing DA, Paul RH, Millar LK. Usefulness of coagulation studies and blood banking in patients with symptomatic *placentae praevia*. *Am J Perinatol* 1997;4:601–604.

11. McLintock C. Postpartum hemorrhage. *Thomb Res* 2005;115(Suppl. 1):65–68.

12. Roberts WE. Emergency obstetric management of postpartum hemorrhage. *Obstet Gynecol Clin North Am* 1995;22:283–302.

13. Dildy GA III. Postpartum hemorrhage: new management options. *Clin Obstet Gynecol* 2002;45:330–344.

14. Hayash RH, Castillo RN, Noah ML. Management of severe postpartum hemorrhage with a prostaglandin F2α analogue. *Obstet Gynecol* 1984;63:806–808.

15. Hankins GDV, Berryman GK, Scott RT, et al. Maternal arterial desaturation with prostaglandin F2 alpha for uterine atony. *Obstet Gynecol* 1988;72:367–370.

16. Hester JD. Postpartum hemorrhage and reevaluation of uterine packing. *Obstet Gynecol* 1975;45:501–504.

17. O'Leary JA. Uterine artery ligation in the control of postcasearean hemorrhage. *J Reprod Med* 1995;40:189–193.

18. Clark SL, Phelan JP. Surgical control of obstetric hemorrhage. *Contemp Ob Gyn* 1984;24:70–74.

19. Yamashita Y, Harada M, Yamamoto H, et al. Transcatheter arterial embolization of obstetric and gynaecological bleeding: efficacy and clinical outcome. *Br J Radiol* 1994;67:530–534.

20. Clark SL, Yeh SY, Phelan JP, et al. Emergency hysterectomy for the control of obstetric hemorrhage. *Obstet Gynecol* 1984;64:376–380.

21. Segal S, Shemesh IY, Blumenthal R, et al. Treatment of obstetric hemorrhage with recombinant activated factor VII (rVIIa). *Arch Gynecol Obstet* 2003;268:266–267.

22. Pritchard JA. Fetal death *in utero*. *Obstet Gynecol* 1959;14:573–580.

23. Bonnar J. Hemorrhagic disorders during pregnancy. In: Hathaway WE, Bonner J, eds. *Hemostatic disorders of the pregnant woman and newborn infant*. New York: Elsevier Science, 1987:76–103.

24. McCrae KR. Thrombocytopenia in pregnancy: differential diagnosis, pathogenesis, and management. *Blood Rev* 2003;17:7–14.

25. Burrows RF, Kelton JG. Fetal thrombocytopenia and its relationship to maternal thrombocytopenia. *N Engl J Med* 1993;329:1463–1466.

26. Shehata N, Burrows R, Kelton JG. Gestational thrombocytopenia. *Clin Obstet Gynecol* 1999;42:327–334.

27. McCrae KR, Samuels P, Schreiber AD. Pregnancy-associated thrombocytopenia: pathogenesis and management. *Blood* 1992;80:2697–2714.

28. Lescale KB, Eddleman KA, Cines DB, et al. Antiplatelet antibody testing in thrombocytopenic pregnant women. *Am J Obstet Gynecol* 1996;174:1014–1018.

29. Chong BH, Keng TB. Advances in the diagnosis of idiopathic thrombocytopenic purpura. *Semin Hematol* 2000;37:249–260.

30. Webert KE, Mittal R, Sigouin C, et al. A retrospective 11-year analysis of obstetric patients with idiopathic thrombocytopenic purpura. *Blood* 2003;102:4306–4311.

31. Kelton JG. Idiopathic thrombocytopenic purpura complicating pregnancy. *Blood Rev* 2002;16:43–46.

32. Gill KK, Kelton JG. Management of idiopathic thrombocytopenic purpura in pregnancy. *Semin Hematol* 2000;37:275–283.

33. Beilin Y, Zahn J, Comerford M. Safe epidural analgesia in thirty parturients with platelet counts between 69,000 and 98,000 mm(−3). *Anesth Analg* 1997;85:385–388.

34. Kam PC, Thompson SA, Liew AC. Thrombocytopenia in the parturient. *Anaesthesia* 2004;59:255–264.

35. George JN, Woolf SH, Raskob GE, et al. Idiopathic thrombocytopenic purpura: a practice guideline developed by explicit methods for the American Society of Hematology. *Blood* 1996;88:3–40.

36. ACOG Committee on Practice Bulletins. ACOG practice bulletin: thrombocytopenia in pregnancy. *Int J Gynaecol Obstet* 1999;67:117–122.

37. British Committee for Standards in Haematology General Haematology Task Force. Guidelines for the investigation and management of idiopathic thrombocytopenic purpura in adults, children and in pregnancy. *Br J Haematol* 2003;120:574–596.

38. Clark AL, Gall SA. Clinical uses of intravenous immunoglobulin in pregnancy. *Am J Obstet Gynecol* 1997;176:241–253.

39. Gottlieb P, Axelsson O, Bakos O, et al. Splenectomy during pregnancy: an option in the treatment of autoimmune thrombocytopenic purpura. *Br J Obstet Gynaecol* 1999;106:373–375.

40. Anglin BV, Rutherford C, Ramus R, et al. Immune thrombocytopenic purpura during pregnancy: laparoscopic treatment. *J Soc Laparosc Surg* 2001;5:63–67.

41. George J. Idiopathic thrombocytopenic purpura: current issues for pathogenesis, diagnosis, and management in children and adults. *Curr Hematol Rep* 2003;2:381–387.

42. Bussel JB. Splenectomy sparing strategies for the treatment and long term maintenance of chronic idiopathic immune thrombocytopenic purpura. *Semin Hematol* 2000;37:1–3.

43. Cines DB, Blanchette VS. Immune thrombocytopenic purpura. *N Engl J Med* 2002;346:995–1008.

44. Bell JG, Weiner S. Has percutaneous umbilical blood sampling improved the outcome of high-risk pregnancies? *Clin Perinatol* 1993;20:61–80.

45. Cook RL, Miller RC, Katz VL, et al. Immune thrombocytopenic purpura in pregnancy: a reappraisal of management. *Obstet Gynecol* 1991;78:578–583.

46. Peleg D, Hunter SK. Perinatal management of women with immune thrombocytopenic purpura: survey of United States perinatologists. *Am J Obstet Gynecol* 1999;180:645–650.

47. Duley L. Pre-eclampsia and the hypertensive disorders of pregnancy. *Br Med Bull* 2003;67:161–176.

48. Barker P, Callander CC. Coagulation screening before epidural analgesia in pre-eclampsia. *Anaesthesia* 1991;46:64–67.

49. Kelton JG, Hunter DJ, Neame PB. A platelet function defect in preeclampsia. *Obstet Gynecol* 1985;65:107–109.

50. Perry KG Jr, Martin JN Jr. Abnormal hemostasis and coagulopathy in preeclampsia and eclampsia. *Clin Obstet Gynecol* 1992;35:338–350.

51. Burrows RF, Andrew M. Neonatal thrombocytopenia in the hypertensive disorders of pregnancy. *Obstet Gynecol* 1990;76:234–238.

52. Egerman RS, Sibai BM. HELLP syndrome. *Clin Obstet Gynecol* 1999;42:381–389.

53. Tank PD, Nadanwar YS, Mayadeo NM. Outcome of pregnancy with severe liver disease. *Int J Gynaecol Obstet* 2002;76:27–31.

54. Magann EF, Bass D, Chauhan SP, et al. Antepartum corticosteroids: disease stabilization in patients with the syndrome of hemolysis, elevated liver enzymes, and low platelets (HELLP). *Am J Obstet Gynecol* 1994;171:1148–1153.

55. Rath W, Faridi A, Dudenhausen JW. HELLP syndrome. *J Perinat Med* 2000;28:249–260.

56. Martin JN Jr, Files JC, Blake PG, et al. Postpartum plasma exchange for atypical preeclampsia-eclampsia as HELLP (hemolysis, elevated liver enzymes, and low platelets) syndrome. *Am J Obstet Gynecol* 1995;172:1107–1125.

57. Dashe JS, Ramin SM, Cunningham FG. The long-term consequences of thrombotic microangiopathy (thrombotic thrombocytopenic purpura and hemolytic uremic syndrome) in pregnancy. *Obstet Gynecol* 1998;91:662–668.

58. Zheng X, Majerus EM, Sadler JE. ADAMTS13 and TTP. *Curr Opin Hematol* 2002;9:389–394.

59. Moake JL. Thrombotic microangiopathies. *N Engl J Med* 2002;347:589–600.

60. Monteagudo J, Pereira A, Reverter JC, et al. Thrombin generation and fibrinolysis in the thrombotic thrombocytopenic purpura and the hemolytic uremic syndrome. *Thromb Haemost* 1991;66:515–519.

61. Hellgren M. Hemostasis during normal pregnancy and puerperium. *Semin Thromb Hemost* 2003;29:125–130.

62. McMinn JR, George JN. Evaluation of women with clinically suspected thrombotic thrombocytopenic purpura–hemolytic uremic syndrome during pregnancy. *J Clin Apheresis* 2001;16:202–209.

63. Shah NT, Rand JH. Controversies in differentiating thrombotic thrombocytopenic purpura and hemolytic uremic syndrome. *Mt Sinai J Med* 2003;70:344–351.

64. George JN. How I treat patients with thrombotic thrombocytopenic purpura-hemolytic uremic syndrome. *Blood* 2000;96:1223–1229.

65. Rock GA, Shumak KH, Buskard NA, et al. Comparison of plasma exchange with plasma infusion in the treatment of thrombotic thrombocytopenic purpura. Canadian Apheresis Study Group. *N Engl J Med* 1991;325:393–397.

66. Rock G, Porta C, Bobbio-Pallavicini E. Thrombotic thrombocytopenic purpura treatment in the year 2000. *Haematologica* 2000;85:410–419.

67. Fausett MB, Vogtlander M, Lee RM, et al. Heparin-induced thrombocytopenia is rare in pregnancy. *Am J Obstet Gynecol* 2001;185:148–152.

68. Kadir RA, Aledort LM. Obstetrical and gynaecological aspects of a common presenting symptom. *Clin Lab Haematol* 2000;22(Suppl. 1):12–16.

69. Mannucci PM. Treatment of von Willebrand disease. *N Engl J Med* 2004;351:683–694.

70. Sanchez-Luceros A, Meschengiesser SS, Marchese C, et al. Factor VIII and von Willebrand changes during normal pregnancy and the puerperum. *Blood Coagul Fibrinolysis* 2003;14:647–651.

71. Kouides PA. Obstetric and gynaecological aspects of von Willebrand disease. *Best Pract Res Clin Haematol* 2001;14:381–399.

72. Mannucci PM. Treatment of von Willebrand's disease. *N Engl J Med* 2004;351:683–694.

73. Stump DC, Taylor FB Jr, Nesheim ME, et al. Pathologic fibrinolysis as a cause of clinical bleeding. *Semin Thromb Hemost* 1990;16:260–273.

74. Bacq Y. Acute fatty liver of pregnancy. *Semin Perinatol* 1998;22:134–140.

75. Reily CA. Acute fatty liver of pregnancy. *Semin Liver Dis* 1987;7:47–54.

76. Rolfes DB, Ishak KG. Acute fatty liver of pregnancy: a clinicopathologic study of 35 cases. *Hepatology* 1985;5:1149–1158.

77. Strate T, Broering DC, Bloechle C, et al. Orthotopic liver transplantation for complicated HELLP. Case report and review of the literature. *Arch Gynecol Obstet* 2000;264:108–111.

78. Letsky EA. Disseminated intravascular coagulation. *Best Pract Res Clin Obstet Gynaecol* 2001;15:623–644.

79. Locksmith GJ. Amniotic fluid embolism. *Obstet Gynecol Clin North Am* 1999;26:435–444.

80. Tuffnell DJ. Amniotic fluid embolism. *Curr Opin Obstet Gynecol* 2003;15: 119–122.

81. Delgado J, Jimenez-Yuste V, Hernandez-Navarro F, et al. Acquired haemophilia: review and meta-analysis focused on therapy and prognostic factors. *Br J Haematol* 2003;121:21–35.

82. Baudo F, de Cataldo F. Italian Association of Haemophilia Centres (AICE): Register of acquired factor VIII inhibitors (RIIA). Acquired factor VIII inhibitors in pregnancy: data from the Italian haemophilia register relevant to clinical practice. *BJOG* 2003;110(3):311–314.

83. Scharrer I. Recombinant factor VIIa for patients with inhibitors to factor VIII or IX or factor VII deficiency. *Haemophilia* 1999;5:253–259.

84. Michiels JJ. Acquired hemophilia A in women postpartum: clinical manifestations, diagnosis, and treatment. *Clin Appl Thromb Hemost* 2000;6: 82–86.

85. Dykes AC, Walker ID, Lowe GD, et al. Combined prednisone and intravenous immunoglobulin treatment for acquired factor VIII inhibitors: a 2-year review. *Haemophilia* 2001;7:160–163.

# CHAPTER 76 ■

Please note: A finalized version of Chapter 76 (pages 1129 through 1146) was not available at press time for inclusion in the book.

# CHAPTER 77 ■ CLINICAL APPROACH TO THE BLEEDING PATIENT

BARBARA A. KONKLE

The hematologist is often faced with the question of whether a patient has an underlying bleeding disorder. This may be in the setting of unexplained bleeding, either spontaneous or with minor or major trauma or procedures. The hematologist may be asked to evaluate a person's risk of bleeding with an upcoming procedure. The patient under evaluation may have a personal or family history of bleeding or have screening laboratory results that suggest a risk of bleeding. This chapter reviews key points to help determine whether an underlying bleeding disorder is present, first focusing on the history and physical examination. Results of basic screening laboratory testing of a prothrombin time (PT), also expressed as the international normalized ratio (INR), activated partial thromboplastin time (aPTT), and a platelet count are usually available at the time of the evaluation. After discussion of laboratory testing, an approach to patients is divided by clinical presentation and common laboratory findings. Many of the disorders discussed are presented in more detail in other chapters in this text.

Bleeding disorders are classically divided into those of primary or secondary hemostasis. Disorders of primary hemostasis include those that affect initial platelet plug formation: thrombocytopenia, platelet function disorders (thrombocytopathies), and von Willebrand disease (VWD). Disorders of secondary hemostasis involve disorders of fibrin formation. This classically includes the hemophilias, notably factor VIII and IX deficiencies. However, there is considerable overlap in symptomatology. Ecchymoses and oral bleeding are common in the young child with severe factor VIII or IX deficiency, although these are less common in adults with these disorders. In factor XI deficiency, mucosal bleeding symptoms predominate. Also, in the more rare coagulation deficiencies, it appears that mucosal as well as spontaneous and surgery- or trauma-related bleeding is common (1). Mucosal bleeding symptoms are particularly common in severe factor V and factor VII deficiency. On the other hand, spontaneous hemarthroses are highly suggestive of coagulation factor deficiencies and are not seen in disorders of platelet function.

## THE BLEEDING HISTORY

From a detailed personal and family history, the clinician should have a good idea of whether (a) a bleeding disorder is present; (b) the disorder is inherited or acquired; (c) there is a predominance of mucosal bleeding symptoms; or (d) an underlying bleeding disorder has been enhanced by another medical condition or the introduction of medications or dietary supplements.

A history of bleeding is the most important predictor of bleeding risk. In evaluating a patient for a bleeding disorder, a history of at-risk situations should be assessed. Does the patient have a history of spontaneous or trauma- or surgery-induced bleeding? Spontaneous hemarthroses are a hallmark of moderate and severe factor VIII and IX deficiency and rarely of other factor deficiencies. The symptoms of bruising, epistaxis, and menorrhagia may be more difficult to define as abnormal, because these complaints necessarily have a subjective component.

## Easy Bruising and Prolonged Bleeding after Minor Cuts

The development of bruises (ecchymoses) after trauma is normal; however, an exaggerated response to trauma may be an indication of an underlying bleeding disorder. Patients may give a history of large ecchymoses in response to relatively minor trauma. Ecchymoses presenting without known trauma, particularly on the trunk, and especially large ecchymoses (>2 in. in diameter) may be a sign of an underlying bleeding disorder. The sudden development of new or multiple ecchymosis may reflect an acquired underlying medical disorder such as liver disease, thrombocytopenia, or an acquired coagulation factor inhibitor. The introduction of medications or nutritional supplements with platelet inhibitory activity will enhance bruising and bleeding in a patient with an underlying bleeding disorder.

Easy bruising can be a sign of medical conditions in which there is no identifiable coagulopathy or defect of primary hemostasis; instead, the conditions are caused by an abnormality of blood vessels or their supporting tissues. In Ehlers-Danlos syndrome, there may be posttraumatic bleeding and a history of joint hyperextensibility. Cushing syndrome, chronic steroid use, and senile purpura result from changes in skin and subcutaneous tissue, and subcutaneous bleeding occurs in response to minor trauma. The bleeding is more superficial than in ecchymoses. Senile purpura usually occur on sun-damaged skin, most commonly on the hands and forearms, and may result in permanent discoloration.

## Epistaxis

Epistaxis is a common symptom, particularly in children and in dry climates, and may not reflect an underlying bleeding disorder. However, it is the most common symptom in hereditary hemorrhagic telangectasia and in boys with VWD (2,3). Clues that epistaxis is a symptom of an underlying bleeding disorder include lack of seasonal variation and bleeding that requires medical evaluation or treatment, including cauterization.

## Oral Mucosal Bleeding

Bleeding with eruption of primary teeth is seen in children with more severe bleeding disorders, such as moderate and severe hemophilia. It is uncommon in children with mild bleeding disorders. On the other hand, excessive bleeding after molar extractions is a common symptom resulting in diagnosis of patients with milder bleeding disorders. Dental extraction, particularly of molars or premolars, represents a significant hemostatic challenge. The limitations on wound closure imposed by the bony tooth socket and the presence of profibrinolytic enzymes in saliva contribute to difficulties in achieving hemostasis. Bleeding that necessitates a return to the dental surgeon for packing or suturing or that continues for several hours after the operation is suggestive of an underlying bleeding disorder, particularly when such problems recur. Patients with disorders of primary hemostasis have increased bleeding after dental cleaning and other procedures that involve gum manipulation. Gum grafting procedures for periodontal disease can result in considerable bleeding even in patients with mild bleeding disorders.

## Menorrhagia and Postpartum Hemorrhage

Menorrhagia is defined quantitatively as a loss of greater than 80 mL of blood per cycle on the basis of blood loss required to produce iron deficiency anemia (4). A complaint of heavy menses is subjective and has a poor correlation with excessive blood loss. There are, however, predictors of menorrhagia, including bleeding resulting in iron deficiency anemia or a need for blood transfusion, excessive pad or tampon use, menses lasting longer than 8 days, passage of clots, bleeding through protection, or flooding at night (5,6).

Menorrhagia is a common symptom in women with underlying bleeding disorders. In one study where menorrhagia was quantified using a pictorial blood assessment chart, menorrhagia was confirmed in 74%, 59%, and 57% of women with VWD, factor XI deficiency, and in carriers of hemophilia A, respectively (7). VWD is a less common cause of menorrhagia in African Americans, who have a higher normal range of von Willebrand factor (VWF) levels (8). Disorders of platelet function may be more common as an underlying bleeding disorder in African Americans with menorrhagia (9). Women with underlying bleeding disorders are more likely to have other bleeding symptoms, including bleeding after dental extractions, postoperative bleeding, and postpartum bleeding, and are much more likely to have menorrhagia beginning at menarche than are women with menorrhagia due to other causes (10).

Postpartum hemorrhage is a common symptom in women with underlying bleeding disorders. This occurs most commonly in the first 48 hours after delivery but may also be manifest by prolonged or excessive bleeding after discharge from the hospital. Women with a history of postpartum hemorrhage have a high risk of recurrence with subsequent pregnancies (6). Rupture of ovarian cysts with intraabdominal hemorrhage has been reported in women with underlying bleeding disorders.

## Other Mucosal Bleeding

Tonsillectomy is a major hemostatic challenge, as intact hemostatic mechanisms are essential to prevent excessive bleeding from the tonsillar bed. Bleeding may occur early after surgery or after approximately 7 days postoperatively with loss of the eschar at the operative site (11,12). Gastrointestinal (GI) bleeding and hematuria are usually due to underlying pathology and procedures to identify and treat the bleeding site should be undertaken. Recurrent hematuria of unclear

etiology can occur in moderate and severe hemophilia. VWD, particularly types 2 and 3, have been associated with angiodysplasia of the bowel and GI bleeding (13).

## Joint and Muscle Bleeds

Hemarthroses and spontaneous muscle hematomas are characteristic of moderate or severe congenital factor VIII or IX deficiency. It can also be seen in moderate and severe deficiencies of fibrinogen, prothrombin, and factors V, VII, and X (1). Spontaneous hemarthroses occur rarely in other bleeding disorders except for severe VWD, with associated FVIII levels less than 5%. Muscle and soft tissue bleeds are also common in acquired FVIII deficiency.

Bleeding into a joint results in severe pain and swelling, as well as loss of function, but is rarely associated with discoloration from bruising around the joint. The first bleeding episode into a joint is accompanied by considerable swelling, but as bleeding recurs and joint destruction progresses, swelling may be less prominent, but pain and loss of movement may worsen. In patients without a diagnosis of hemophilia, joint bleeding may go unrecognized as such by the patient or family when there is no obvious bruising or ecchymosis. The clinical history, therefore, should specifically include questions about symptoms of severe joint pain and swelling.

## Prohemorrhagic Effects of Medications and Dietary Supplements

Aspirin and other nonsteroidal inflammatory drugs [nonsteroidal antiinflammatory drugs (NSAIDs)] that inhibit cyclooxygenase-1 impair primary hemostasis and may exacerbate bleeding from another cause or even unmask a previously occult mild bleeding disorder such as VWD. NSAID-selective for the cyclooxygenase-2 enzyme has little platelet inhibitory effect and should not enhance or precipitate bleeding (14). All NSAIDs, however, can precipitate GI bleeding, which may be more severe in patients with underlying bleeding disorders. The aspirin effect on platelet function as assessed by aggregometry can persist for up to 7 days, although it has frequently returned to normal by 3 days after the last dose (15). The effect of other NSAIDs is shorter, because the inhibitor effect is reversed when the drug is removed.

Other causes of drug-related bleeding range from the obvious, such as hemorrhage complicating thrombolytic therapy for management of acute myocardial infarction or hemorrhage caused by thrombocytopenia after chemotherapy, to the more diagnostically challenging, such as bleeding secondary to impaired platelet function in subjects on high-dose intravenous penicillin or caused by a combination of a qualitative platelet defect and moderate thrombocytopenia secondary to anticonvulsant therapy with sodium valproate. See Chapter 70 for further discussion of drug-induced qualitative platelet defects. In addition, many drugs have been linked to the development of immune thrombocytopenia.

Many herbal supplements impair hemostatic function (16,17), as shown in Table 77-1. Some have been more convincingly associated with a bleeding risk than others. Fish oil or concentrated omega 3 fatty acid supplements impair platelet function. In fact, diets naturally rich in omega 3 fatty acids can result in a prolonged bleeding time (BT) and abnormal platelet aggregation studies, but the actual associated bleeding risk is unclear. There are conflicting data as to whether vitamin E

## TABLE 77-1

### HERBAL SUPPLEMENTS ASSOCIATED WITH INCREASED BLEEDING

**HERBS WITH POTENTIAL ANTIPLATELET ACTIVITY**
Ginkgo (*Ginkgo bilobae*)
Garlic (*Allium sativum*)
Bilberry (*Vaccinium myrtillus*)
Ginger (*Zingiber officinale*)
Dong quai (*Angelica sinensis*)
Feverfew (*Tanacetum parthenium*)
Asian ginseng (*Panax ginseng*)
American ginseng (*Panax quinquefolius*)
Siberian ginseng/eleuthero (*Eleutherococcus senticosus*)
Tumeric (*Curcuma longa*)
Meadowsweet (*Filipendula ulmaria*)
Willow (*Salix alba*)

**COUMARIN-CONTAINING HERBS**
Motherworth (*Leonurus cardiac*)
Chamomile (*Matricaria recutita, Chamaemelum mobile*)
Horse chestnut (*Aesculus hippocastanum*)
Red clover (*Trifolium pratense*)
Fenugreek (*Trigonella foenum-graecum*)

affects platelet function (18,19). In patients with unexplained bruising or bleeding, it is prudent to review any new medications or supplements and discontinue those that may be associated with bleeding.

## Inherited Versus Acquired Disorders

The history is critical in determining whether a bleeding disorder is likely inherited or acquired. The age at presentation, duration of symptoms, response to previous hemostatic challenges, and family history give a strong indication. The male newborn who presents with umbilical stump bleeding and a family history of hemophilia in a maternal uncle, or an elderly patient with no previous history of excessive bleeding despite surgical challenges who presents with recent onset of massive bruising and forearm compartment syndrome, can easily be ascribed as inherited and acquired, respectively. Diagnostic difficulties arise, however, when a mild familial disorder is present in a patient who previously has not been challenged, because of young age, previous good health, or when the bleeding symptoms are highly variable, as can occur with mild disorders.

The family history may be informative, but can also be misleading. Up to one third of cases of hemophilia A and B arise as a result of recent mutations, and the family history will be negative for abnormal bleeding. Carriers of factor VIII or IX deficiency may or may not have bleeding symptoms, depending on their baseline factor level, which will vary because of random X chromosome inactivation (the Lyon hypothesis) (20). Some carriers will have low enough factor VIII or IX levels to have trauma-induced or, rarely, spontaneous hemorrhage. Because most new mutations causing hemophilia will manifest first in the carrier female (21,22), she may present with symptoms due to a decreased factor VIII level without a diagnosis of hemophilia in the family. Bleeding in patients with FXI deficiency occurs most commonly in those with severe deficiency, although severely affected individuals may be asymptomatic. Most heterozygotes are asymptomatic; however, the relation between the factor XI level and bleeding is not clear-cut (23,24), and some heterozygotes bleed excessively after trauma. VWD is inherited in an autosomal dominant fashion, apart from types 2N and 3, which are recessive. However, family history may not be clear-cut, particularly in type 1, because the clinical manifestations are frequently mild and easily overlooked. In patients with an apparent bleeding disorder, laboratory studies in family members may be helpful in confirming the diagnosis.

## Underlying Systemic Diseases that Cause or Exacerbate a Bleeding Tendency

Acquired bleeding disorders are commonly secondary to, or associated with, systemic disease (see Table 77-2). The clinical evaluation of a patient with a bleeding tendency must therefore include a thorough assessment for evidence of underlying

## TABLE 77-2

### SOME ACQUIRED CAUSES OF BLEEDING

| Disorders of primary hemostasis | Defective coagulation | Fibrinolytic abnormalities | Localized skin bleeding |
|---|---|---|---|
| **THROMBOCYTOPENIC STATES** | Due to anticoagulant drugs | Due to thrombolytic drugs | Senile purpura |
| Immune-mediated destruction | DIC | DIC | Steroid-induced purpura |
| Decreased production | Liver disease | Advanced liver disease | Dermatitis artefacta |
| Sequestration | Vitamin K deficiency | Prostate carcinoma or surgery | Connective tissue disorders |
| Consumption (DIC, TTP) | Coagulation factor inhibitors | Acute promeylocytic leukemia | |
| | Paraproteinemia | Envenomation | |
| **PLATELET DYSFUNCTION** | Amyloidosis | | |
| Due to drugs or supplements | Hypothyroidism | | |
| Paraproteinemia | Massive blood transfusion | | |
| Myeloproliferative disorders | Envenomation | | |
| Uremia | | | |

DIC, disseminated intravascular coagulation; TTP, thrombotic thrombocytopenic purpura.

disease. Bruising or mucosal bleeding may be the presenting complaint in liver disease, severe renal impairment, hypothyroidism, and conditions causing bone marrow failure. Less prevalent disorders, such as paraproteinemias or amyloidosis, occasionally present in this fashion also. In disseminated intravascular coagulation (DIC), presentation may be with symptoms of bleeding and/or microvascular thrombosis, and the underlying trigger for the consumptive coagulopathy is not always immediately obvious (25). A particular example is DIC occurring secondary to an occult malignancy.

## THE PHYSICAL EXAMINATION

The physical examination can provide helpful clues as to the etiology of the bleeding disorder, although many patients with mild bleeding disorders will have normal examinations. Larger ecchymoses (>2 in.), particularly when they occur without apparent trauma or on the trunk, are suggestive of an underlying disorder. Some rare disorders are associated with particular findings on physical exam, such as abnormalities of the forearm in thrombocytopenia with absent radii or defects in skin pigmentation in patients with syndromes associated with platelet granule or storage pool disorders.

Evidence of past joint damage, manifested by abnormal joint appearance and/or a loss of normal range of motion, is suggestive of past hemarthroses. Petechiae are seen in thrombocytopenia, but not in thrombocytopathies. Red to violet blanching telangiectasia on the face, lips, tongue, and/or nasal mucosa can be diagnostic of hereditary hemorrhagic telangiectasia.

## LABORATORY EVALUATION

Careful history taking and clinical examination are essential components in the assessment of bleeding risk. The use of laboratory tests of coagulation and hemostasis cannot substitute for clinical assessment. Indeed, ample evidence exists that screening tests are unhelpful in the prediction of bleeding risk, especially when applied indiscriminately (26–28). The BT is not helpful in predicting surgical bleeding risk (29,30). Although an abnormal PT/INR may reflect liver disease or vitamin K deficiency that had not been previously appreciated, aPTT testing is not helpful in preoperative evaluations in patients with a negative bleeding history. The primary use of coagulation testing should be to confirm the presence and type of bleeding disorder in a patient with a suspicious clinical history. An exception may be the preoperative assessment in infants and young children, in whom the clinical history is less likely to be informative.

The laboratory evaluation is critical in the evaluation of the patient with bleeding. Although there is much interest in developing a global assay of hemostasis, to date there is not one assay that can predict risk of bleeding and thrombosis. The clinician must frequently use the results of several assays combined with the clinical presentation to arrive at a diagnosis or an assessment of bleeding risk.

Because of the nature of coagulation assays, proper sample acquisition and handling is critical to obtaining valid results. In patients with abnormal coagulation assays who have no bleeding history, repeat studies with attention to these factors frequently result in normal values. Most coagulation assays are performed in sodium citrate anticoagulated plasma that is recalcified for the assay. Because the anticoagulant is in liquid solution and needs to be added to blood in proportion to the plasma volume, incorrectly filled or inadequately mixed blood collection tubes will give erroneous results. Vacutainer tubes should be filled to greater than 90% of the recommended fill, which is usually denoted by a line on the tube. An elevated hematocrit

(>55%) can result in a false value because of a decreased plasma-to-anticoagulant ratio. An accurate result is obtained by adjusting the amount of sodium citrate solution added to the blood on the basis of the estimated plasma volume, using the formula:

Na citrate solution (3.2%) to
add (in mL) for total volume          = (100 − hematocrit) (9/495)
(blood + anticoagulant) of 10 mL

## Prothrombin Time

The PT, developed by Quick et al. in 1935, assesses the classic extrinsic coagulation system, including factors I (fibrinogen), II (prothrombin), V, VII, and X (see Fig. 77-1) (31). The PT measures the time for clot formation of the citrated plasma after recalcification and addition of thromboplastin. Thromboplastin is a combination of tissue factor, the membrane receptor for FVII and FVIIa, and phospholipids. The speed of the PT reaction is influenced not only by the plasma concentrations of the extrinsic and common pathway clotting factors but also by the concentration and properties of the tissue factor (32). Tissue factor has been genetically expressed, and human recombinant tissue factor, relipidated with natural and synthetic phospholipids, is now being used in many laboratories (33). The sensitivity to different factor deficiencies and coagulopathies varies by the source of thromboplastin.

The degree of prolongation of the PT is dependent on the thromboplastin in the reaction as well as on the instrument used for the assay. In the past, the use of various thromboplastins and instruments resulted in varying levels of anticoagulation when the PT ratio was used to target warfarin therapy. To adjust for this variability, the overall sensitivity of different thromboplastins to reduction of the vitamin K–dependent clotting factors II, VII, IX, and X in anticoagulated patients is now expressed as the International Sensitivity Index (ISI) (34,35). This is determined by calibrating the thromboplastin against a standard thromboplastin, often a well-characterized secondary WHO International Reference Preparation. An inverse relation exists between ISI and thromboplastin sensitivity. The INR is then determined based on the formula:

$$INR = (PT_{patient}/PT_{normal\ mean})^{ISI}$$

Although the INR was developed to assess anticoagulation due to reduction of vitamin K–dependent coagulation factors, it is helpful in the evaluation of patients with liver disease, particularly when comparing values from testing performed at different laboratories. With use of thromboplastins with a wide range of ISI values in different laboratories, it can be difficult to compare a PT done at one laboratory with that done at another laboratory without using the INR. However, because progressive liver failure is associated with variable changes in

The PT

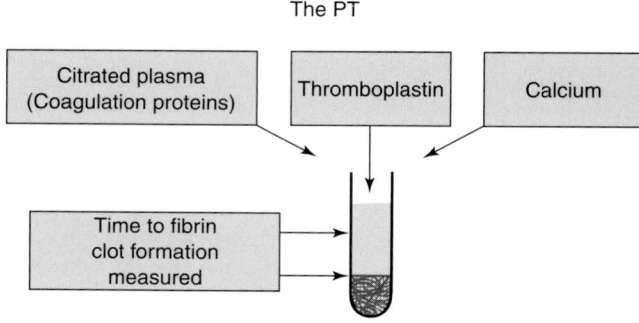

Measures VII, V, X, II, fibrinogen

**FIGURE 77-1.** Elements of the prothrombin time (PT) are shown.

coagulation factors, the degree of prolongation of either the PT or the INR only roughly predicts the bleeding risk (36). The INR is not a reliable measure of warfarin anticoagulation in some patients with lupus anticoagulants (37,38).

## Activated Partial Thromboplastin Time

Like the PT/INR, the aPTT is performed on recalcified citrated plasma (see Fig. 77-2). It assesses the intrinsic and common coagulation pathways. It was originally described as a "partial thromboplastin" time, because the reagents did not induce hemophilic plasma to clot in a normal period of time as do "complete" thromboplastins (39). The aPTT reagent contains phospholipids, derived from either animal or vegetable sources that function as a platelet substitute in the coagulation pathways. The aPTT test system also includes an activator of the intrinsic coagulation system, such as nonparticulate ellagic acid or the particulate activators kaolin, celite, or micronized silica. These provide a large surface area and increase the precision and reproducibility of the test.

The phospholipid composition of different aPTT reagents varies considerably and influences the sensitivity of individual reagents to clotting factor deficiencies and to inhibitors, such as heparin and lupus anticoagulants. Therefore, aPTT results will vary from one laboratory to another, and the normal range in the laboratory where the testing occurs should be used in the interpretation. It has been recommended that the aPTT values correlating with therapeutic heparin anticoagulation should be determined locally by correlating aPTT values with direct measurements of heparin activity (anti-Xa or protamine titration assays) in samples from patients treated with heparin (40). The aPTT reagent will vary in sensitivity to individual factor deficiencies. It usually becomes prolonged, with individual factor deficiencies of 30% to 40%, but the specialized coagulation laboratory should determine the sensitivity of the reagent it is using for each coagulation factor. Reagents vary widely in their sensitivity to lupus anticoagulants (41), and a clue that a prolonged aPTT is due to a lupus anticoagulant can be variable aPTT results on samples with assays performed in different laboratories.

## Mixing Studies

Mixing studies are used to evaluate a prolonged aPTT, or less commonly PT, to distinguish between a factor deficiency and an inhibitor. In this assay, normal plasma and patient plasma are mixed in a 50:50 ratio, and the aPTT or PT is determined immediately after incubation at 37°C and, for varying times, typically 30 minutes, 60 minutes, and/or 120 minutes. With isolated factor deficiencies, the aPTT will correct with mixing and stay corrected with incubation. With aPTT prolongation due to a lupus anticoagulant, the mixing and incubation will show no correction (41). In acquired neutralizing factor antibodies, such as an acquired factor VIII inhibitor, the initial assay may or may not correct immediately after mixing but will prolong or remain prolonged with incubation at 37°C. Failure to correct with mixing can also be caused by the presence of other inhibitors or interfering substances, such as heparin, fibrin split products, and paraproteins.

## Thrombin Clotting Time

Thrombin clotting time (TCT), or simply thrombin time, is a simple test that measures the time for clot formation to occur in citrated plasma after the addition of thrombin (42,43). It therefore reflects the action of thrombin on fibrinogen with the formation of fibrin. During this process, thrombin cleaves the $\alpha$ and $\beta$ chains of fibrinogen at their amino-termini, releasing fibrinopeptides A and B. The residual fibrin monomer of one fibrinogen molecule interacts with others to form polymerized fibrin.

A prolonged TCT is caused by a deficiency or structural abnormality (dysfibrinogenemia) of fibrinogen or by the presence of an inhibitor of the thrombin–fibrinogen reaction. It is abnormal in patients with familial hypofibrinogenemia or dysfibrinogenemia and in patients with acquired manifestations of DIC or advanced hepatic decompensation. Fibrin degradation products also interfere with the assay. The TCT may be prolonged in patients with a monoclonal gammopathy, particularly IgM and IgA isotypes through interference with fibrin polymerization. Clinically, the most important inhibitor causing prolongation of the TCT is unfractionated heparin (44). Low-molecular-weight heparins have a less potent effect on thrombin and exert relatively greater inhibition of factor Xa, with less, if any, effect on the TCT compared to unfractionated heparin.

## Reptilase Time

The snake venom reptilase (from *Bothrops atrox*) induces fibrin clot formation in plasma by a direct action on fibrinogen. In contrast to the action of thrombin, which cleaves fibrinopeptides A and B, reptilase cleaves only fibrinopeptide A (45). Unlike the TCT, the reptilase time is unaffected by heparin and can be used as a quick way to rule out heparin contamination (46). The reptilase time is generally more sensitive to dysfibrinogenemias than is the thrombin time.

## Specific Clotting Factor Assays

Decisions to proceed with specific clotting factor assays will be influenced by the clinical situation and the results of coagulation screening tests. Precise diagnosis and effective management of inherited and acquired coagulation deficiencies necessitate quantitation of the relevant factors. When bleeding is severe, specific assays are often urgently required to guide appropriate therapy. Following factor levels can permit a safe and logical approach to replacement therapy, preventing both undertreatment and overtreatment. In view of important genetic and therapeutic implications, it is essential to distinguish between the classical and acquired forms of hemophilia A and VWD. To avoid misdiagnosis, an abnormal factor VIII assay should trigger assays for VWF antigen and activity to differentiate hemophilia from VWD.

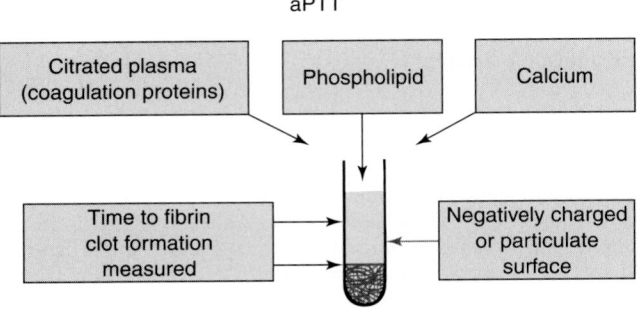

**FIGURE 77-2.** Elements of the activated partial thromboplastin time (aPTT) are shown. Contact factors are factor XII, kininogen, and prekallikrein.

One-stage factor assays are generally used for the quantitation of clotting factors reacting in both the extrinsic and intrinsic coagulation pathways. These are modifications of the aPTT or PT, in which the patient plasma is serially diluted in specific factor-deficient substrate plasma. The concentration of the specific factor in each of the serial dilutions is determined from a standard curve and used to calculate the level of the factor in the undiluted plasma (43). Most laboratories now use automated or semiautomated instruments to perform these assays. An activity level can be assigned only if the values from the serial dilutions fall on a straight line and the line formed by the test plasma is parallel to that of standard normal plasma. Nonparallel plots usually result from an inhibitor in the patient plasma or, occasionally, from an unrecognized deficiency of another factor in the substrate deficient plasma. A two-stage assay, based on the thromboplastin generation test, is infrequently performed. There is increasing use of chromogenic substrates, which mimic the cleavage site on the natural substrate for the clotting factor being tested; release of the chromophore is proportional to factor activity (47).

## The Bethesda Assay for Factor VIII Inhibitor Quantitation

This assay is used to detect the presence of an inhibitor, to quantitate it for therapeutic and comparative purposes, and to follow up response to therapy (48). It is based on the ability of patient plasma to inactive FVIII in normal plasma. In this assay, patient plasma is serially diluted in normal plasma and residual FVIII activity measured after incubation for 2 hours at 37°C using a one-stage assay. The assay is controlled for normal FVIII decay using normal plasma diluted in buffer or FVIII-deficient plasma (Nijmegen modification). Percentage residual factor (corrected for control) is plotted on a logarithmic scale against units of inhibitor on a linear scale (see Fig. 77-3). One unit is the amount of antibody that destroys 0.5 U of factor VIII after incubation at 37°C for 2 hours. This assay can be adapted for inhibitors against other clotting factors, including porcine FVIII.

## von Willebrand Disease Testing

Both immunoassays and functional assays are available for the measurement of VWF in plasma. Antigen level (VWF:Ag) is measured by electroimmunoassay (EIA) or enzyme-linked immunoabsorbent assay (ELISA). In the EIA, antigen–antibody complexes precipitate as a narrow "rocket," the height of which is proportional to the concentration of VWF:Ag. Results obtained by EIA and ELISA are generally comparable, but the latter offers greater precision and sensitivity.

VWF activity is measured by ristocetin cofactor assay (VWF:RCof) or collagen binding assay (CBA) (VWF:CBA) (49,50). Although mutations affecting platelet versus collagen binding to VWF would theoretically result in differences in these assays, in general they provide similar results. Ristocetin is an antibiotic glycopeptide that, when added to platelet-rich plasma containing VWF, results in platelet agglutination. For the ristocetin cofactor assay, ristocetin and formalin-fixed platelets are added to patient and serially diluted control plasma, agglutination assessed by platelet aggregometry, and patient results obtained from a standard curve of the normal control plasma dilutions. An ELISA has been developed to mimic the ristocetin cofactor assay that measures binding of patient VWF to immobilized recombinant platelet GP Ibα fragments in the presence of ristocetin (51). Collagen binding is assessed by ELISA and is dependent on the type of collagen used to coat the plate, but overall this assay has less interlaboratory and

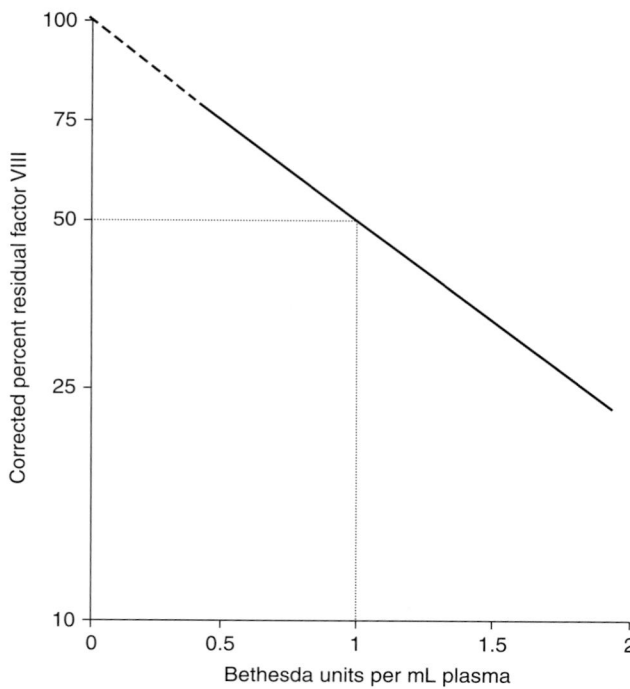

**FIGURE 77-3.** Bethesda assay for FVIII inhibitor quantitation. Relation between corrected residual factor VIII activity and Bethesda titer is shown. If the result is less than 25%, serial dilutions of the patient's plasma are tested until the result is between 25% and 75%. The result is multiplied by the dilution to assign the Bethesda titer. One Bethesda unit is defined by a corrected residual factor VIII of 50% in the assay (*dotted line*).

intralaboratory variation compared to the VWF:RCof assay. There is more variability in results between the functional assays in patients with dysfunctional VWF molecules (VWD types 2A, 2B, 2M) than in patients with quantitative VWF deficiencies (VWD types 1, 3). VWF multimers are visualized by analysis on an unreduced low percentage (1% to 2%) agarose gel.

## Fibrinogen

Fibrinogen is assessed in both quantitative and qualitative assays (52,53). Clottable fibrinogen is determined similarly to the one-stage assay used for other clotting factors using either the TCT (Clauss method) or the PT as the basic assay method. Immunologic methods are used to quantify fibrinogen. A dysfibrinogenemia is diagnosed when the measurement of the total clottable fibrinogen is less than 80% of the immunologic fibrinogen in a sample.

## Factor XIII

Factor XIII deficiency cannot be detected by abnormalities in any of the routine coagulation screening tests. A high index of clinical suspicion is required for its recognition, and when it is suspected, a specific screening test for factor XIII deficiency should be performed. The most commonly used procedure is a clot solubility test, which is based on the fact that non–cross-linked fibrin (due to FXIII deficiency or rarely, inhibitors to FXIII or fibrin) will be soluble in 5M urea, 1% monochloroacetic acid, or 2% acetic acid. Functional and immunologic assays to quantitate FXIII are available (54,55).

## Assessment of Fibrinolysis

Although there are a variety of immunologic, functional, and chromogenic tests for the determination of the components of the fibrinolytic system, they currently have relatively little role in the routine laboratory investigation and diagnosis of a bleeding state. Familial bleeding disorders attributed to excessive fibrinolysis have been reported rarely. These include $\alpha_2$-antiplasmin deficiency (56), in which bleeding occurs because of the proteolytic digestion of procoagulants by plasmin, and deficiency of plasminogen activator inhibitor-1 (PAI-1) (57), the major inhibitor of tissue plasminogen activator (tPA). Both are autosomal recessive in inheritance. Specific testing for these disorders can be obtained through coagulation reference laboratories

Increased fibrinolysis may contribute to bleeding that accompanies acute promyelocytic leukemia, carcinoma of the prostate or with prostatectomy, and end-stage liver disease. The latter is due to lack of clearance of fibrinolytic enzymes by the diseased liver; this increases during the anhepatic phase of liver transplant. Laboratory assessment of increased fibrinolysis is usually limited to measurement of affected factors [fibrinogen, fibrin/fibrinogen degradation products (FDPs), D-dimers], with a goal toward replacement as needed. Enhanced fibrinolysis can be detected by the euglobulin clot lysis time (ECLT), a global test of fibrinolysis (43). In this assay, plasma is treated by dilution to a low ionic strength and acidification to precipitate the euglobulin fraction, containing fibrinogen and plasminogen activators; fibrinolytic inhibitors such as PAI-1 are partially precipitated. The euglobulin fraction is dissolved and the fibrinogen clotted; clot lysis is then timed. The ECLT is dependent on the activity of both tPA and PAI-1 (58). Short lysis times are indicative of increased fibrinolysis.

The measurement of fibrin/FDPs is routine in patients suspected of having DIC. FDP can be measured by latex agglutination using polyclonal antibodies to fibrinogen fragments D and E. A major drawback of this assay is that it is unable to distinguish between fragments of fibrinogen and fibrin. The potential diagnostic value of discriminating between fibrinogenolysis and fibrinolysis led to the development of the D-dimer assay (59). D-dimer is a product formed through digestion of cross-linked fibrin by plasmin, so it is specific for the fragments derived from cross-linked fibrin. Elevated levels of both FDP and D-dimer occur in DIC. Sensitive D-dimer assays can be used in certain clinical situations to assess venous thromboembolism (60).

## Tests of Platelet Function

### Bleeding Time

The skin BT is a test of platelet–vessel wall interactions. The Ivy BT is usually performed in a standardized manner on the forearm (61). The incision on the forearm must be reproducible in length, depth, and direction, which is best achieved using a purpose-built disposable device. Capillary pressure should be standardized through application of a sphygmomanometer cuff to the upper arm, inflated to a pressure of 40 mm Hg, throughout the procedure. Time to cessation of bleeding is measured, and identification of this is aided by removal of blood from the area by applying a filter paper every 15 seconds, taking care not to touch the wound edge. The BT is affected by several factors in addition to operator differences. An inverse linear relation exists between the platelet count and BT, with prolongation of BT from thrombocytopenia alone at platelet counts less than 100,000 per $\mu$L (62). The BT may be prolonged after ingestion of aspirin and other NSAIDs that inhibit cyclooxygenase-1. Like platelet aggregation studies, it may also be affected by other medications and dietary supplements without necessarily reflecting an increased risk of bleeding. A prolonged BT alone does not predict a bleeding risk and therefore has limited value in preoperative screening (30). It may be helpful in evaluating patients with suspected disorders of primary hemostasis, but it may be normal in some disorders of primary hemostasis, including mild type 1 VWD.

### PFA-100

Different methods and instrumentation have been developed to assess platelet and VWF function in an automated assay that may have better reproducibility than the BT. The most widely studied and used is the PFA-100 manufactured by Dade-Behring. In the PFA-100 the time to clot formation (and aperture closure) of anticoagulated whole blood is assessed under flow in a membrane coated with collagen and either adenosine diphosphate (ADP) (C/ADP) or epinephrine (EPI) (C/EPI). The PFA-100 has varying sensitivity to VWD depending on the subtype and VWF levels, particularly as assessed by VWF:CBA, with more severely affected individuals likely to have abnormal values. Favaloro et al. reported a sensitivity of 96.7% (C/EPI) and 76.7% (C/ADP) and a specificity of 69.2% (C/EPI) and 90.6% (C/ADP) for VWD (63). The value of this test as a screening assay for mild VWD, for which the currently used diagnostic assays can be inconclusive, is unclear as false-negative results occur (64,65). The method appears more sensitive and specific for VWD and platelet disorders than is the BT (64,66), but it is not useful as a general screening tool for bleeding risk and will not detect all mild bleeding disorders of primary hemostasis. It has been used to study antiplatelet drug effects; the C/EPI cartridge is particularly sensitive to an aspirin effect (64,67).

### Platelet Aggregometry

Assessment of *ex vivo* platelet function by light transmission aggregometry is useful in the classification of platelet function abnormalities and generally should be performed in patients with a history suggestive of a disorder of primary hemostasis for which there is no obvious cause, such as VWD, thrombocytopenia, use of platelet inhibitory medications, or renal failure. Upon the addition of most aggregating agents, platelets change shape from discs to a more rounded form with pseudopods, resulting in a transient, small decrease in light transmission that is followed by increased light transmission as the platelets aggregate (see Fig. 77-4) (68,69). Aggregating agonists include ADP (0.5 to 10 $\mu$M), EPI (0.05 to 10 $\mu$M), collagen (10 to 50 $\mu$g per mL), arachidonic acid (0.75 to 2.0 $\mu$M), a thromboxane analog such as U46619, and a thrombin receptor-activating peptide (TRAP) such as SFLL-RN. The agglutinating agent ristocetin is also used to investigate VWF and platelet glycoprotein Ib/IX–dependent responses. ADP and EPI are weak agonists compared to collagen or thrombin. Aggregation with these agonists, particularly at low concentrations, will begin with a primary, reversible phase of aggregation, followed by a secondary irreversible phase. The secondary phase is dependent on thromboxane formation and release of granule content. Drugs that inhibit thromboxane formation, such as aspirin, will prevent the secondary phase of aggregation.

The platelet release reaction and platelet granule content can be assessed using lumiaggregometry. The release reaction is studied by measuring the adenosine triphosphate (ATP) released after different agonists are added. The firefly enzyme luciferase produces light proportional to the concentration of ATP, and the light can be quantified in a luminometer (70). Confirmation of $\delta$-platelet storage pool deficiency requires the measurement of platelet nucleotides or an assessment of dense

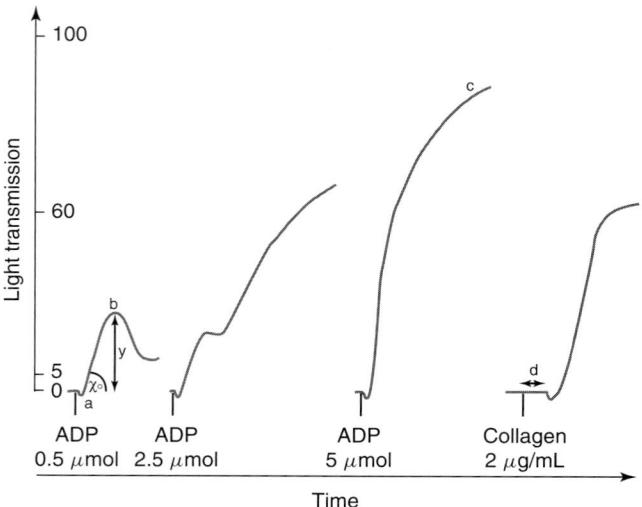

**FIGURE 77-4.** Typical traces obtained during platelet-rich plasma aggregation. *a*, shape change; *b*, primary wave aggregation; *c*, secondary wave aggregation; *d*, lag phase; $\chi°$, angle of ascent of aggregation trace; *y*, height of aggregation trace; ADP, adenosine diphosphate.

body function. Although ADP is not measured directly, an indirect assay is performed by conversion of available ADP to ATP. Total platelet ATP and ADP may also be measured by high-performance liquid chromatography (HPLC). In storage pool disorders, the ratio of ATP to ADP resembles that of the metabolic pool (approximately 8:1) rather than that of the normal platelet pool (approximately 2:1) because this normally includes the relatively ADP-rich storage pool in dense bodies (ratio approximately 2:3) (71).

Dense body function may be assessed by study of radiolabeled serotonin uptake in platelets (72). The proportion of available serotonin that is taken up, as well as released on adding an agonist, is reduced in storage pool disorders. Platelet-granules may also be assessed by electron microscopy, and specific platelet membrane receptors can be assessed by flow cytometry.

Results of platelet-function testing are highly dependent on sample handling and processing. Platelet aggregation studies should be performed within 2 hours of sample collection. Sending samples through a pneumatic tube device will adversely affect platelet aggregation and PFA-100 results (73). For platelet aggregometry, platelet-rich plasma (PRP) must be free of erythrocytes and granulocytes and must not be lipemic because this will interfere with light transmission. Platelet counts should be standardized. If testing is to be delayed for more than 2 hours, storage of whole blood at 4°C (74) or of the PRP under 5% carbon dioxide should be used. Ideally, the patient, rather than the blood sample, should go to the laboratory for on-site testing, to attempt to optimize standardization of the procedure.

# APPROACH TO THE PATIENT: COMBINING CLINICAL PRESENTATION, HISTORY, AND LABORATORY TESTING

In the evaluation of clinical presentation and coagulation testing, several scenarios can occur depending on the presence and type of bleeding symptoms and on which, if any, screening laboratory test results are abnormal. These scenarios are outlined in the following section and are considered in the setting of a normal platelet count, except where noted.

## Patients with Bleeding History, Prolonged Activated Partial Thromboplastin Time, and Prolonged Prothrombin Time

### Inherited Disorders

Inherited deficiencies of the common pathway factors will prolong both the aPTT and, to a greater extent, the PT. Inherited deficiencies of factors I (fibrinogen), II (prothrombin), V, and X are autosomal recessive and are rare. They can present with symptoms of disorders of both primary and secondary hemostasis (1). Dysfibrinogenemias are inherited in an autosomal dominant fashion (75). In addition to a prolonged PT, and less so, aPTT, patients will have a prolonged thrombin time and reptilase time. Total clottable fibrinogen will be less than that determined by immunologic assay. At least one half of patients with dysfibrinogenemias will have no symptoms; approximately one fourth of patients may have bleeding symptoms, usually mild in nature; and occasional patients have venous and/or arterial thrombosis (76). Table 77-3 shows inherited and acquired disorders of patients with bleeding history, prolonged aPTT, and prolonged PT.

### Acquired Disorders

Inhibitors of common pathway factors are infrequently seen. The most common is an inhibitor to factor V resulting from topical bovine thrombin use, which is contaminated with bovine factor V. Cross-reacting antibodies to human factor V can develop (77). Rarely, patients with lupus anticoagulants develop clinically significant prothrombin deficiency. Amyloidosis can produce vitamin K–dependent factor deficiencies, most commonly factor X (78), due to absorption of the factor onto the amyloid fibrils.

**TABLE 77-3**

PATIENT WITH BLEEDING, PROLONGED ACTIVATED PARTIAL THROMBOPLASTIN TIME, AND PROLONGED PROTHROMBIN TIME

**INHERITED**
Deficiencies of factors I (fibrinogen)[a], II, V, or X[b]
Dysfibrinogenemia[a]

**ACQUIRED**
Specific inhibitors of factors V, II, or X
Disseminated intravascular coagulation[a,b,c]
Factor deficiencies due to liver disease[b]
Factor deficiencies due to vitamin K deficiency[b]
Dysfibrinogenemia due to liver disease[a,b]
Paraproteinemia[b]
Amyloidosis
Heparin therapy[d]

---

[a]Thrombin clotting time (TCT) and reptilase time prolonged.
[b]Affects prothrombin time (PT) greater than activated partial thromboplastin time (aPTT) for all.
[c]Often with thrombocytopenia.
[d]Affects aPTT greater than PT.

## Patient with Bleeding History, Prolonged Activated Partial Thromboplastin Time, and Normal Prothrombin Time

### Inherited Disorders

This category includes the classic hemophilias, factor VIII and factor IX deficiency, and factor XI deficiency. Factor VIII deficiency (hemophilia A) and factor IX deficiency (hemophilia B) are indistinguishable in their presentation and symptoms. Factor VIII deficiency is four to five times more common than factor IX deficiency. These disorders are covered more extensively in Chapter 63; however, a few remarks concerning their presentation is worthwhile. Approximately 30% of new cases of hemophilia are due to new mutations. It is therefore not uncommon for patients to present without a family history of hemophilia. Extensive ecchymoses are common in the young child with hemophilia, and initial evaluation of an undiagnosed child with hemophilia or other bleeding disorder may include suspicion of child abuse.

Table 77-4 shows inherited and acquired disorders of patients with bleeding history, prolonged aPTT, and normal PT.

Patients with mild hemophilia may present in adulthood, often with unexplained postoperative bleeding. Carriers of hemophilia A or B may have bleeding symptoms. If levels are decreased, they are usually in the mild hemophilia range (>5%) and may result in postoperative or postpartum bleeding or menorrhagia.

VWD is the most common inherited bleeding disorder. Factor VIII is stabilized by binding to VWF, resulting in a decreased FVIII in the setting of a decreased amount of VWF protein. The aPTT will be prolonged if the FVIII is low enough (usually <35%). Therefore, for many cases of mild VWD, the FVIII will be greater than 35%, so the aPTT will be normal. The FVIII will be 2% to 10% in severe VWD and in patients homozygous for a FVIII-binding mutation (type 2N VWD), and the aPTT will be significantly prolonged.

Patients with factor XI deficiency have variable bleeding symptoms. Even patients with very low FXI levels may have minimal or no excessive bleeding (23). Most patients with values less than 10% are of Ashkenazi Jewish descent. In other populations, severe disease is rare (approximately one per 1,000,000) (79). When bleeding occurs, even in those severely affected, it is less severe than in factor VIII or IX deficiency, spontaneous hemarthroses do not occur, and mucosal bleeding symptoms predominate.

### Acquired Disorders

The most common acquired bleeding disorder with this presentation is due to neutralizing antibodies (inhibitors) to FVIII. Acquired inhibitors to factors IX and XI have rarely been reported. Acquired factor VIII inhibitors occur most commonly in the elderly (mean age 61), but have been reported in children and, notably, can be seen in the postpartum state (80,81). In diagnosing an acquired factor VIII inhibitor, the aPTT will be prolonged, may not correct immediately in a mixing study (see preceding text), and will remain or become prolonged with incubation at 37°C. The presentation of acquired hemophilia differs from inherited hemophilia in that extensive ecchymoses and soft tissue bleeding is common. Depending on the VWF:Ag level, acquired VWD can result in a low FVIII level and therefore a prolonged aPTT. Acquired VWD (or von Willebrand syndrome) is most commonly seen in the setting of lymphoproliferative disorders, but may also be idiopathic or associated with hypothyroidism, valvular disease, myeloproliferative disorders, autoimmune disease, and medications (82,83).

## Patient with Bleeding History, Normal Activated Partial Thromboplastin Time, and Prolonged Prothrombin Time

### Inherited Disorders

Factor VII deficiency is the inherited factor deficiency that classically produces this picture. The level of factor VII needed for hemostasis is probably 10% to 15% (1). The bleeding history is variable and in severe deficiency mucosal symptoms, as well as joint bleeding, may be present. Some patients have thrombosis, particularly in association with treatment (84). Mild factor VII deficiency, not associated with a bleeding risk, may still prolong the PT.

Table 77-5 shows inherited and acquired disorders of patients with bleeding history, normal aPTT, and prolonged PT.

The PT is more sensitive than the aPTT to common pathway factor deficiencies and dysfibrinogenemias, and therefore,

---

**TABLE 77-4**

PATIENTS WITH BLEEDING, PROLONGED ACTIVATED PARTIAL THROMBOPLASTIN TIME, AND NORMAL PROTHROMBIN TIME

**INHERITED**
Deficiencies of factors VIII, IX, or XI
von Willebrand disease[a]

**ACQUIRED**
Specific inhibitors of factors VIII, IX, or XI[b]
Heparin therapy[c]

[a]Due to low factor VIII.
[b]Factor VIII inhibitors are much more common than the others.
[c]Thrombin clotting time (TCT) prolonged, reptilase time normal.

---

**TABLE 77-5**

PATIENTS WITH BLEEDING, NORMAL ACTIVATED PARTIAL THROMBOPLASTIN TIME, AND PROLONGED PROTHROMBIN TIME

**INHERITED**
Factor VII deficiency[a]
Dysfibrinogenemia[b,c]

**ACQUIRED**
Warfarin therapy
Factor deficiencies due to liver disease[d]
Factor deficiencies due to vitamin K deficiency[d]
Dysfibrinogenemia due to liver disease[b,d]
Disseminated intravascular coagulation[d,e]
Paraproteinemia[b]
Specific inhibitor to FVII

[a]Bleeding variable and associated with levels <15%.
[b]Prolonged thrombin clotting time (TCT) and reptilase time.
[c]Bleeding uncommon, when present usually mild.
[d]Activated partial thromboplastin time (aPTT) usually also prolonged when bleeding present.
[e]Often with thrombocytopenia.

patients with mild deficiencies of common pathway factors may have only a prolonged PT, with both the PT and aPTT prolonged in more severe deficiencies. The reptilase time and TCT would be abnormal in quantitative and qualitative abnormalities of fibrinogen.

### Acquired Disorders

The PT is more sensitive to liver disease and vitamin K deficiency than the aPTT because of early decreases in factor VII levels due to its short half-life. Usually, when these are severe enough to cause bleeding, the PTT is also prolonged, although the PT more so. In DIC, the PT may be prolonged with a normal aPTT because of effects on fibrinogen. Again, when associated with bleeding, the aPTT is usually also prolonged, although to a lesser degree than the PT. DIC is often accompanied by thrombocytopenia that increases the bleeding risk. Paraproteins can prolong the PT, usually greater than the aPTT, because of interference with fibrin polymerization (85). This will also result in a prolonged TCT and reptilase time.

## Patients with Bleeding History, Normal Activated Partial Thromboplastin Time, and Normal Prothrombin Time

### Inherited Disorders

As noted previously, patients with VWD types 1 and 2A, 2B, and 2M may have a factor VIII high enough to result in a normal aPTT. Because factor XIII cross-links fibrin, and the PT and aPTT measure fibrin formation, specific assays are needed to diagnose a deficiency of this factor. Also, unless there is significant fibrinogen or fibrin degradation, abnormalities of fibrinolysis will not be detected by PT and aPTT testing. Qualitative disorders of platelet function would be detected only by studies of primary hemostasis, including BT, PFA-100 or similar assay, and tests of platelet aggregometry and release reaction.

Table 77-6 shows inherited and acquired disorders of patients with bleeding history, normal aPTT, and normal PT.

Patients may present with a history compatible with a bleeding disorder, with or without a positive family history, and testing may be completely normal, even with extensive and repeat testing. VWF levels are increased up to three times

over baseline with vigorous exercise, adrenergic stimulation, and inflammatory processes (86,87). VWF levels also vary with menses, with the lowest values early in the follicular phase (88,89). Hormonal therapy has been reported to increase VWF levels, although low-dose combined oral contraceptives may not (89). The timing and setting of VWD testing, particularly repeat testing, should be planned with these factors in mind.

### Acquired Disorders

Drugs or nutritional supplements that interfere with platelet function can precipitate or enhance bleeding symptoms. Acquired inhibitors to factor XIII or fibrin have been reported, albeit rarely (90).

## Patients without Bleeding History, but with Abnormal Coagulation Testing

Abnormal coagulation testing, may be seen in patients without bleeding history, with isolated prolongations of either aPTT or PT or, less commonly, with prolongation of both conditions, as seen in Table 77-7.

### Inherited Disorders

Deficiencies of factors FXII, prekallikrein, and kininogen produce marked prolongation of the aPTT without bleeding symptoms. Because these are deficiencies, mixing studies will result in normal values. Because bleeding symptoms in factor XI deficiency are so variable, and some patients with severe disease may not bleed even with trauma, factor XI deficiency may present with this clinical picture.

An isolated prolonged PT is most commonly seen in factor VII deficiency, particularly when it is mild. Factor VII levels greater than 10% to 15% are usually not associated with bleeding. Patients with levels below this have variable bleeding histories. The PT is more sensitive to dysfibrinogenemias than the aPTT, and as noted previously, many patients with this diagnosis do not have bleeding symptoms; the reptilase time and

---

**TABLE 77-6**

PATIENTS WITH BLEEDING, NORMAL ACTIVATED PARTIAL THROMBOPLASTIN TIME, AND NORMAL PROTHROMBIN TIME

**INHERITED**
Platelet function disorders (thrombocytopathies)
von Willebrand disease
Factor XIII deficiency
$\alpha_2$-Antiplasmin deficiency
Plasminogen activator inhibitor-1 deficiency
Unknown

**ACQUIRED**
Platelet inhibitory drugs
Thrombolytic drugs[a]
von Willebrand syndrome[b]

---
[a]With increasing lysis, will have fibrinogen/fibrin degradation and long prothrombin time (PT), thrombin clotting time (TCT), reptilase time, and possibly long activated partial thromboplastin time (aPTT).
[b]If FVIII decreased.

---

**TABLE 77-7**

PATIENTS WITHOUT BLEEDING, PROLONGED ACTIVATED PARTIAL THROMBOPLASTIN TIME, AND/OR PROLONGED PROTHROMBIN TIME

**INHERITED**
Deficiencies of factor XI,[a] XII, kininogen, or prekallikrein
Dysfibrinogenemia[b,c]
Factor VII deficiency[d]

**ACQUIRED**
Lupus anticoagulants
Heparin therapy[e,f]
Warfarin therapy or vitamin K deficiency[g]
Liver disease[g]
Dysfibrinogenemia[c]
Specific inhibitor of factor V[a]

---
[a]Bleeding symptoms variable.
[b]Greater than 50% of patients will not bleed.
[c]Also with prolonged thrombin clotting time (TCT), reptilase time.
[d]Bleeding variable and seen with level less than 15%.
[e]Activated partial thromboplastin time (aPTT) more prolonged than prothrombin time (PT).
[f]Prolonged TCT, normal reptilase time.
[g]PT more prolonged than aPTT.

TCT would also be prolonged. Most patients with dysfibrino-genemias have no bleeding symptoms.

## ACQUIRED DISORDERS

Lupus anticoagulants (LA) typically prolong the aPTT and not the PT. Most LA result in mild prolongation of the aPTT, but occasionally it can be markedly prolonged, and in that setting the PT is usually also affected. Rarely, LA-associated hypoprothrombinemia can result in prolongation of the PT (91). If severe, it can result in bleeding.

Liver disease and vitamin K deficiency can produce an isolated prolongation of the PT. Early in the course, when factor VII is mostly affected, lack of bleeding symptoms is common. Patients with liver disease may also have an acquired dysfibrinogenemia with or without bleeding symptoms, which will also prolong the TCT and reptilase time.

Patients with factor V inhibitors caused by treatment with topical bovine thrombin may present with a markedly prolonged PT and aPTT, with few or no bleeding symptoms.

## CONCLUSION

Evaluation of the patient with bleeding requires careful attention to history and physical examination. Logical use of screening and specialized coagulation testing, as indicated, will allow diagnosis and appropriate treatment to stop or prevent bleeding.

### *References*

1. Peyvandi F, Duga S, Akhavan S, et al. Rare coagulation deficiencies. *Haemophilia* 2002;8:308–321.
2. Ziv O, Ragni MV. Bleeding manifestations in males with von Willebrand disease. *Haemophilia* 2004;10:162–168.
3. Assar OS, Friedman CM, White RJ. The natural history of epistaxis in hereditary hemorrhagic telangiectasia. *Laryngoscope* 1991;101:977–980.
4. Hallberg L, Hogdahl AM, Nilsson L, et al. Menstrual blood loss—a population study. *Acta Obstet Gynecol Scand* 1996;45:320–351.
5. Lee CA. Women and inherited bleeding disorders: menstrual issues. *Semin Hematol* 1999;36:21–27.
6. Kouides PA, Phatak PD, Burkart P, et al. Gynaecological and obstetrical morbidity in women with type 1 von Willebrand disease: results of a patient survey. *Haemophilia* 2000;6:643–648.
7. Kadir RA, Economides DL, Sabin CA, et al. Assessment of menstrual blood loss and gynaecological problems in patients with inherited bleeding disorders. *Haemophilia* 1999;5:40–48.
8. Miller CH, Haff E, Platt SJ, et al. Measurement of von Willebrand factor activity: relative effects of ABO blood type and race. *J Thromb Haemost* 2003;1:2191–2197.
9. Philipp CS, Dilley A, Miller CH, et al. Platelet functional defects in women with unexplained menorrhagia. *J Thromb Haemost* 2003;1:477–484.
10. Kadir RA, Economides DL, Sabin CA, et al. Frequency of inherited bleeding disorders in women with menorrhagia. *J Thromb Haemost* 1998;351:485–489.
11. Wei JL, Beatty CW, Gustafson RO. Evaluation of post-tonsillectomy hemorrhage and risk factors. *Otolaryngol Head Neck Surg* 2000;123:229–235.
12. Peterson J, Losek JD. Post-tonsillectomy hemorrhage and pediatric emergency care. *Clin Pediatr (Phila)* 2004;43:445–448.
13. Morris ES, Hampton KK, Nesbitt IM, et al. The management of von Willebrand's disease-associated gastrointestinal angiodysplasia. *Blood Coagul Fibrinolysis* 2001;12:143–148.
14. Fitzgerald GA, Patrono C. The coxibs, selective inhibitors of cyclooxygenase −2. *N Engl J Med* 2001;345:433–442.
15. Gibbs NM, Weightman WM, Thackray NM, et al. The effects of recent aspirin ingestion on platelet function in cardiac surgery. *J Cardiothorac Vasc Anesth* 2001;15:55–59.
16. Abebe W. Herbal medication: potential for adverse interactions with analgesic drugs. *J Clin Pharm Ther* 2002;27:391–401.
17. Izzo AA, Ernst E. Interactions between herbal medicines and prescribed drugs. *Drugs* 2001;61:2163–2175.
18. Mabile L, Bruckdorfer KR, Rice-Evans C. Moderate supplementation with natural alpha-tocopherol decreases platelet aggregation and low-density lipoprotein oxidation. *Atherosclerosis* 1999;147:177–185.
19. Morinobu T, Ban R, Yoshikawa S, et al. The safety of high-dose vitamin E supplementation in healthy Japanese males. *J Nutr Sci Vitaminol (Tokyo)* 2002;48:6–9.

20. Miller CH. Genetics of hemophilia and von Willebrand's disease. In: Hilgartner MW, Pochedly C, eds. *Hemophilia in the child and adult.* New York: JB Lippincott Co, 1989:297–345.
21. Ljung R, Kling S, Sjorin E, et al. More than half the sporadic cases of haemophilia A in Sweden are due to a recent mutation. *Acta Paediatr Scand* 1991;80:343–348.
22. Kling S, Ljung R, Sjorin E. Origin of mutation in sporadic cases of haemophilia B. *Eur J Haematol* 1992;48:142–145.
23. Bolton-Maggs PH, Patterson DA, Wensley RT, et al. Definition of the bleeding tendency in factor XI-deficient kindreds—a clinical and laboratory study. *Thromb Haemost* 1995;73:194–202.
24. Ragni MV, Sinha D, Searman F, et al. Comparison of bleeding tendency, factor XI coagulant activity, and factor XI antigen in 25 factor XI deficient kindreds. *Blood* 1985;65:719–724.
25. Levi M. Current understanding of disseminated intravascular coagulation. *Br J Haematol* 2004;124:567–576.
26. Rapaport SI. Preoperative haemostatic evaluation: which tests, if any? *Blood* 1983;61:229–231.
27. Eckman MH, Erban JK, Singh SK, et al. Screening for the risk for bleeding or thrombosis. *Ann Intern Med* 2003;138:W15–W24.
28. Houry S, Georgeac C, Hay J-M, et al. A prospective multicenter evaluation of preoperative hemostatic screening tests. *Am J Surg* 1995;170:19–23.
29. De Caterina R, Lanza M, Manca G, et al. Bleeding time and bleeding; an analysis of the relationship of the bleeding time test with parameters of surgical bleeding. *Blood* 1994;84:3363–3370.
30. Rodgers RPC, Levin J. A critical reappraisal of the bleeding time. *Semin Thromb Hemost* 1990;16:1–20.
31. Quick AJ, Stanley-Brown M, Bancroft FW. A study of the coagulation defect in hemophilia and in jaundice. *Am J Med Sci* 1935;190:501–511.
32. Poller L. Laboratory techniques in thrombosis. In: Jespersen J, Bertina RN, Haverkate F, eds. *E.C.A.T. assay procedures,* 2nd ed. London: Kluwer Academic Publishers, 1999:45–61.
33. Houdijk WPM, van den Besselaar AMHP. International multicenter international sensitivity index (ISI) calibration of a new human tissue factor thromboplastin reagent derived from cultured cells. *J Thromb Haemost* 2004;2:266–270.
34. WHO Expert Committee on Biological Standardization. Guidelines for thromboplastins and plasma used to monitor oral anticoagulant therapy. *World Health Organ Tech Rep Ser* 1999;889:1–111.
35. Hermans J, van den Besselaar AMHP, Loelinger EA, et al. A collaborative calibration study of reference materials for thromboplastins. *Thromb Haemost* 1983;50:712–717.
36. Kovacs MJ, Wong A, MacKinnon K, et al. Assessment of the validity of the INR system for patients with liver impairment. *Thromb Haemost* 1994;71:727–730.
37. Moll S, Ortel TL. Monitoring warfarin therapy in patients with lupus anticoagulants. *Ann Intern Med* 1997;127:177–185.
38. Tripodi A, Chantarangkul V, Clerici M, et al. Laboratory control of oral anticoagulant treatment by the INR system in patients with the antiphospholipid syndrome and lupus anticoagulants. Results of a collaborative study involving nine commercial thromboplastins. *Br J Haematol* 2001;115:672–678.
39. Langdell RD, Wagner RH, Brinkhous KM. Effect of antihemophilic factor on one-stage clotting tests. A presumptive test for hemophilia and a simple one-stage antihemophilic factor assay procedure. *J Lab Clin Med* 1953;41:637–647.
40. Hirsh J, Raschke R. Heparin and low molecular weight heparin: The seventh ACCP conference on antithrombotic and thrombolytic therapy. *Chest* 2004;126:188S–203S.
41. Greaves M, Cohen H, Machin SJ, et al. Guidelines on the investigation and management of the antiphospholipid syndrome. *Br J Haematol* 2000;109:704–715.
42. Jim RTS. A study of the plasma thrombin time. *J Lab Clin Med* 1957;50:45–60.
43. Fritsma GA. Clot-based assays of coagulation. In: Corriveau DM, Fritsma GA, eds. *Hemostasis and thrombosis in the clinical laboratory.* Philadelphia, PA: JB Lippincott Co, 1988:92–127.
44. Penner JA. Experience with a thrombin clotting time assay for measuring heparin activity. *Am J Clin Pathol* 1974;61:645–653.
45. Funk C, Gmur J, Herold R, et al. Reptilase BR-a new reagent in blood coagulation. *Br J Haematol* 1971;21:43–52.
46. Latallo ZS, Teisseyre E. Evaluation of reptilase R and thrombin clotting time in the presence of fibrinogen degradation products and heparin. *Scand J Haematol Suppl* 1971;13:261–266.
47. Walenga JM, Fareed J. Automation and quality control in the coagulation laboratory. *Clin Lab Med* 1994;14:709–728.
48. Sahud MA. Factor VIII inhibitors. Laboratory diagnosis of inhibitors. *Semin Thromb Hemost* 2000;26:195–203.
49. Favaloro EJ, Smith J, Petinos P, et al. Laboratory testing for von Willebrand's disease: an assessment of current diagnostic practice and efficacy by means of a multi-laboratory survey. RCPA Quality Assurance Program (QAP) in Haematology Haemostasis Scientific Advisory Panel. *Thromb Haemost* 1999;82:1276–1282.
50. Favaloro EJ, Henniker A, Facey D, et al. Discrimination of von Willebrand's disease subtypes: direct comparison of von Willebrand factor: collagen binding assay (VWF:CBA) with monoclonal antibody based VWF-capture systems. *Thromb Haemost* 2000;84:541–547.

51. Vanhoorelbeke K, Cauwenberghs N, Vauterin S, et al. A reliable and re-producible ELISA method to measure ristocetin cofactor activity of von Willebrand factor. *Thromb Haemost* 2000;83:107–113.

52. National Committee for Clinical Laboratory Standards NCCLS H30-P. *Proposed guidelines for a standardization procedure for the determination of fibrinogen in biological samples.* Villanova, PA: NCCLS, 1982.

53. Palareti G, Maccaferri M, Manotti C, et al. Fibrinogen assays: a collaborative study of six different methods. CISMEL Comitato Italiano per la Standardizzazione dei Metodi in Ematologia e Laboratorio. *Clin Chem* 1991;37:714–719.

54. Karpati L, Penke B, Katona E, et al. A modified, optimized kinetic photometric assay for the determination of blood coagulation factor XIII activity in plasma. *Clin Chem* 2000;46:1946–1955.

55. Katona E, Haramura G, Karpati L, et al. A simple, quick one-step ELISA assay for the determination of complex plasma factor XIII (A2B2). *Thromb Haemost* 2000;83:268–273.

56. Aoki N, Saito H, Kamiya T, et al. Congenital deficiency of a$_2$-plasmin inhibitor associated with severe hemorrhagic tendency. *J Clin Invest* 1979;63:877–884.

57. Fay WP, Shapiro AD, Shih JL, et al. Brief report: complete deficiency of plasminogen-activator inhibitor type 1 due to a frame-shift mutation. *N Engl J Med* 1992;327:1729–1733.

58. Urano T, Sakakibara K, Rydzewski A, et al. Relationships between euglobulin clot lysis time and the plasma levels of tissue plasminogen activator and plasminogen activator inhibitor. *Thromb Haemost* 1990;63:82–86.

59. Elms MJ, Bunce IH, Bundeson PG, et al. Measurement of crosslinked fibrin degradation products—an immunoassay using monoclonal antibodies. *Thromb Haemost* 1983;50:591–594.

60. Dempfle CE. Use of D-dimer assays in the diagnosis of venous thrombosis. *Semin Thromb Hemost* 2000;26:631–641.

61. Ivy AC, Nelson D, Bucher MS. The standardization of certain factors in the cutaneous "venostasis" bleeding time technique. *J Lab Clin Med* 1941;26:1812–1822.

62. Harker LA, Slichter SJ. The bleeding time as a screening test for evaluation of platelet function. *N Engl J Med* 1972;287:155–159.

63. Favaloro EJ, Kershaw G, Bukuya M, et al. Laboratory diagnosis of von Willebrand disorder and monitoring of DDAVP therapy: efficacy of the PFA-100 and VWF:CBA as combined diagnostic strategies. *Haemophilia* 2001;7:180–189.

64. Harrison P, Robinson M, Liesner R, et al. The PFA-100: a potential rapid screening tool for the assessment of platelet dysfunction. *Clin Lab Haematol* 2002;24:225–232.

65. Konkle BA, Tarng HI. Von Willebrand disease: assessing platelet von Willebrand factor and other variables in patients with presumed type 1 VWD (Abstract). *Blood* 2002;100:1925.

66. Dean JA, Blanchette VS, Carcao MD, et al. von Willebrand disease in a pediatric-based population—comparison of type 2 diagnostic criteria and use of the PFA-100 and a von Willebrand factor/collagen-binding assay. *Thromb Haemost* 2000;84:401–409.

67. Rand ML, Leung R, Packham MA. Platelet function assays. *Transfus Apheresis Sci* 2003;28:307–317.

68. Triplett DA. *Platelet function, laboratory evaluation and clinical application.* Chicago, IL: American Society of Clinical Pathology, 1978.

69. Fritsma GA. Tests of platelet number and function. In: Corriveau DM, Fritsma JB, eds. *Hemostasis and thrombosis in the clinical laboratory.* Philadelphia, PA: JB Lippincott Co, 1988:278–304.

70. White MM, Foust JT, Mauer AM, et al. Assessment of lumiaggregometry for research and clinical laboratories. *Thromb Haemost* 1992;67:572–577.

71. Akkerman JWN, Nieuwenhuis HK, Mommersteeg-Leautaud ME, et al. ATP-ADP compartmentation in storage pool deficient platelets: correlation between grandule-bound ADP and the bleeding time. *Br J Haematol* 1983;55:135–143.

72. David JL, Herion F. Method for measurement of $^{14}$C-HT uptake and release by platelets. In: Mannucci PM, Gorini S, eds. *Platelet functions and thrombosis: a review of methods.* New York: Plenum Publishing, 1972:335.

73. Dyszkiewicz-Korpanty A, Quinton R, Yassine J, et al. The effect of a pneumatic tube transport system on PFA-100 closure time and whole blood aggregation. *J Thromb Haemost* 2004;2:354–356.

74. Choi JW, Pai SH. Influence of storage temperature on the responsiveness of human platelets to agonists. *Ann Clin Lab Sci* 2003;33:79–85.

75. Hayes T. Dysfibrinogenemia and thrombosis. *Arch Pathol Lab Med* 2002;126:1387–1390.

76. Roberts HR, Stinchcombe TE, Gabriel DA. The dysfibrinogenaemias. *Br J Haematol* 2001;114:249–257.

77. Zehdner JL, Leung LL. Development of antibodies to thrombin and factor V with recurrent bleeding in a patient exposed to topical bovine thrombin. *Blood* 1990;76:2011–2016.

78. Choufani EB, Sanchorawala V, Ernst T, et al. Acquired factor X deficiency in patients with amyloid light-chain amyloidosis: incidence, bleeding manifestations, and response to high-dose chemotherapy. *Blood* 2001;97:1885–1887.

79. Asakai R, Chung DW, Davie EW, et al. Factor XI deficiency in Ashkenazi Jews in Israel. *N Engl J Med* 1991;325:153–158.

80. Bossi P, Cabane J, Ninet J, et al. Acquired hemophilia due to factor VIII inhibitors in 34 patients. *Am J Med* 1998;105:400–408.

81. Zakarija A, Green D. Acquired hemophilia: diagnosis and management. *Curr Hematol Rep* 2002;1:27–33.

82. Federici AB, Rand JH, Bucciarelli P, et al. Acquired von Willebrand syndrome: data form an international registry. *Thromb Haemost* 2000;84:345–349.

83. Nitu-Whalley IC, Lee CA. Acquired von Willebrand syndrome—report of 10 cases and review of the literature. *Haemophilia* 1999;4:318–326.

84. Ingerslev J, Kristensen HL. Clinical picture and treatment strategies in factor VII deficiency. *Haemophilia* 1998;4:689–696.

85. Coleman M, Vigliano EM, Weksler ME, et al. Inhibition of fibrin polymerization by lambda myeloma globulins. *Blood* 1972;39:210–223.

86. Rock G, Tittley P, Pipe A. Coagulation factor changes following endurance exercises. *Clin J Sport Med* 1997;7:94–99.

87. van den Burg PJM, Hospers JEH, Mosterd WL, et al. Aging, physical conditioning, and exercise-induced changes in hemostatic factors and reaction products. *J Appl Physiol* 2000;88:1558–1564.

88. Miller CH, Dilley AB, Drews C, et al. Changes in von Willebrand factor and factor VIII levels during the menstrual cycle. *Thromb Haemost* 2002;87:1082–1083.

89. Kadir RA, Economides DL, Sabin CA, et al. Variations in coagulation factors in women: effects of age, ethnicity, menstrual cycle and combined oral contraceptives. *Thromb Haemost* 1999;82:1456–1461.

90. Lorand L. Acquired inhibitors of fibrin stabilization: a class of hemorrhagic disorders of diverse origins. In: Green D, ed. *Anticoagulants: physiologic, pathologic, and pharmacologic.* Boca Raton, FL: CRC Press, 1994:169–191.

91. Triplett DA. Antiphospholipid antibodies. *Arch Pathol Lab Med* 2002;126:1424–1429.

# CHAPTER 78 ■ MANAGEMENT OF ACUTE HEMORRHAGE

THOMAS G. DELOUGHERY

The management of the patient who is acutely bleeding can be a challenge. Often, the physician must make decisions only on the basis of initial impressions, and scant laboratory and historical data. This chapter discusses a general approach to acute bleeding and the basic "tools" for management of these patients, and then discusses a variety of specific situations.

## APPROACH TO THE BLEEDING PATIENT

### Patient Review

Even in the face of an emergency, the physician should try to obtain some history about the patient. A family history of bleeding or bleeding with past surgeries or trauma is evidence for an underlying congenital bleeding disorder. The physician should screen the chart and record any and all medications given to the patient. The physical examination can provide valuable clues. The presence of multiple sites of diffuse bleeding signals the presence of coagulopathy such as disseminated intravascular coagulation (DIC). The appearance of acral skin darkening raises the concern of purpura fulminans. Presence of diffuse, large ecchymoses is the classic presentation of an acquired factor VIII inhibitor.

### Laboratories

The first step in evaluation of the patient with bleeding is to obtain a basic set of coagulation tests. The basic set of a prothrombin time [prothrombin time–international normalized ratio (PT-INR)], activated partial thromboplastin time (aPTT), platelet count, and fibrinogen can be rapidly obtained (1). The sample should be obtained from a peripheral vein: Samples drawn through heparin-containing catheters, even with elaborate maneuvers to prevent contamination, can result in artifactual elevations of the clotting times (2,3). Three patterns of defects can be seen in the PT-INR and aPTT (see Table 78-1). Isolated elevations of the PT-INR are indicative of an isolated factor VII deficiency. In patients who are very sick, low factor VIII levels are common because of third-spacing and increased consumption (4). A marked elevation of the PT-INR out of proportion to the aPTT suggests vitamin K deficiency. Isolated elevation of the aPTT has many causes. Mixing studies can provide information to narrow the list of possible diagnoses. Prolongation of both the PT-INR and aPTT suggests multiple defects or deficiency of factors II, V, or X, and marked prolongation of the PT-INR and aPTT can also be seen with low levels of fibrinogen. Further, coagulation tests are ordered on the basis of the PT-INR and aPTT to better define the defect if the reason for the coagulation deficiency is not apparent by the history.

If the platelet count is low, examination of the blood smear is essential to make sure that pseudothrombocytopenia (5) is not present. Although many processes can cause a moderately low platelet count, the differential diagnosis for isolated profound thrombocytopenia (<10,000 per $\mu$L) is usually limited to immune thrombocytopenia, drug-induced thrombocytopenia, or posttransfusion purpura. Occasionally, thrombotic thrombocytopenic purpura or heparin-induced thrombocytopenia (HIT) (especially with low-molecular-weight heparin) can lower platelet counts significantly, but bleeding is not typical of these conditions (6).

Excessive bleeding has been reported with plasma fibrinogen levels under 50 mg per dL (7). The endpoints of the PT-INR and aPTT are timed to the formation of the fibrin clot. When plasma levels of fibrinogen fall below 80 mg per dL, the clot may be small and not detected by the machine, resulting in a very prolonged PT-INR and aPTT. Low fibrinogen levels reflect either severe liver disease, consumptive coagulopathy, or dilution by infusion of massive amounts of resuscitative fluids.

Some bleeding defects, such as platelet function defects or increases in fibrinolysis, cannot be detected by routine laboratory tests. Performing rapid tests to assess platelet function remains controversial. Bleeding times are difficult to perform and are not predictive of bleeding risk (8,9). Recently, a rapid automatic test for platelet function—the platelet factor analyzer (PFA)100—has been introduced, but there is no data on the use of this rapid test to guide therapy for acute bleeding (10,11). It is also difficult to assess for excessive fibrinolysis. The euglobulin clot lysis time is a screen for fibrinolysis, but it is not standardized and can be difficult to obtain. Thrombelastography is a unique point-of-care laboratory test that examines whole blood thrombus formation and lysis, but it is not widely available and requires experience in interpretation (12).

## NONTRANSFUSION THERAPIES FOR ACUTE BLEEDING

Nonblood product agents for bleeding disorders are shown in Table 78-2.

Several nontransfusion options exist for acute hemorrhage.

### Desmopressin

Desmopressin (1-deamino-8-D-arginine vasopressin) (DDAVP) is a synthetic analog of antidiuretic hormone that raises the levels of both factor VIII and von Willebrand protein several-fold (13). Desmopressin is effective in supporting hemostasis in patients with a wide variety of congenital and acquired bleeding

**TABLE 78-1**

INTERPRETATIONS OF COAGULATION TESTS

**ELEVATED PROTHROMBIN TIME, NORMAL aPTT**
Factor VII deficiency
  Vitamin K deficiency
  Warfarin
  Sepsis

**NORMAL PROTHROMBIN TIME, ELEVATED aPTT**
Isolated factor deficiency (VIII, IX, XI, XII, contact pathway proteins)
Specific factor inhibitor
Heparin
Lupus inhibitor

**ELEVATED PROTHROMBIN TIME, ELEVATED aPTT**
Multiple coagulation factor deficiencies
  Liver disease
  Disseminated intravascular coagulation
Isolated factor X, V, or II deficiency
Factor V inhibitors
High hematocrits (>60%–spurious)
High heparin levels
Severe vitamin K deficiency
Low fibrinogen (<50 mg/dL)
Dysfibrinogemia
Dilutional

aPTT, activated partial thromboplastin time.

**TABLE 78-2**

NONBLOOD PRODUCT AGENTS FOR BLEEDING DISORDERS

**DESMOPRESSIN**
IV: 0.3 $\mu$g/kg over 30 min
Nasal: over 50 kg–one squirt of 150 $\mu$g in each nostril
Under 50 kg–one squirt of 150 $\mu$g total

**AMINOCAPROIC ACID**
IV: 5 g bolus, then 500–1,000 mg/h
Oral: 5 g bolus, then 2 g every 2 h

**TRANEXAMIC ACID**
IV: 10 mg/kg every 6–8 h
Oral: 25 mg/kg every 6–8 h
Conjugated estrogens (uremia)
0.6 mg/kg IV for 5 d

IV, intravenous.

disorders (14–16). However, desmopressin does not reduce blood loss before routine surgery in a healthy patient (17,18).

Desmopressin is available in two forms. The intravenous form is dosed as 0.3 $\mu$g per kg mixed in normal saline and infused over 15 to 30 minutes. It takes 45 minutes after dosing to achieve a full hemostatic effect that can last for 6 to 12 hours. A nasal form of desmopressin (Stimate) is also available (19). The generic desmopressin is dosed for enuresis, not von Willebrand disease (VWD), and contains an inadequate dose that can lead to serious bleeding with surgery.

## Antifibrinolytics

Aminocaproic acid and tranexamic acid are antifibrinolytic agents that block the binding of plasmin to fibrin (see Chapter 79) (20,21). These agents are useful in four situations. The first is in the presence of excessive fibrinolysis, which most often occurs with liver disease but may rarely complicate amyloidosis or rare congenital defects (22–26). Antifibrinolytic agents are also useful as adjunctive therapy for oral or dental procedures in patients with a bleeding diathesis such as hemophilia (27). Antifibrinolytics can prevent blood loss in a variety of surgeries, including heart bypass, liver transplant, and orthopedic surgery (28,29). Finally, in patients with severe thrombocytopenia, the use of antifibrinolytic agents may reduce bleeding (30,31).

These drugs strengthen thrombi and prevent their lysis. In areas of confined bleeding, such as ureteral hemorrhage, use of antifibrinolytic agents may lead to obstruction (32). If the thrombosis fails to pass, interureteral instillation of fibrinolytic agents may be used. In the presence of DIC, where fibrinolysis is a secondary process, the use of antifibrinolytic agents may induce clinical thrombosis (33,34).

As described in the *Physicians' Desk Reference*, a recommended dose of aminocaproic acid is a bolus of 5 g given over 1 hour, followed by a continuous infusion of 1 g per hour for 8

hours intravenously or 5 g orally followed by 2 g every 2 hours for 24 hours, then 4 g every 4 hours for the next 48 hours. The dosing for tranexamic acid is 10 mg per kg IV bolus, followed either by 10 mg per kg IV every 6 to 8 hours or 25 mg per kg every 6 to 8 hours orally.

## Conjugated Estrogens

High doses of conjugated estrogens may ameliorate bleeding in patients with uremia (35–37). The dosing is 0.6 mg/kg/day intravenous or orally for 5 days. The hemostatic effect of estrogens can last for 2 weeks (36). The mechanism of estrogen effectiveness in slowing uremic bleeding is unknown.

## Recombinant Factor VIIa

Recombinant factor VIIa (rVIIa) was originally developed as a "bypass" agent to support hemostasis in hemophiliacs with inhibitors (38,39). Recently, there has been an explosion of information concerning rVIIa use for a wide array of bleeding disorders (39,40), including patients with factor VII and XI deficiency (40,41). The rVIIa also appears useful in patients with Glanzmann thrombasthenia (42–46). One study in patients with prostate cancer showed a significant decrease in blood loss in patients who received one 40 $\mu$g per kg dose preoperatively (47). Small studies in patients undergoing liver surgery have provided conflicting data (48,49).

Increasingly, rVIIa is being used as a "universal hemostatic agent" for patients with uncontrolled bleeding from any mechanism (50). Multiple case reports have shown use of rVIIa for bleeding in patients undergoing cardiac surgery, for obstetrical bleeding, for reversal of anticoagulation, and for trauma-induced bleeding (51–54). Unfortunately, little formal trial data exists to put these anecdotes into perspective.

A general approach for use of rVIIa outside of its approved indication (hemophiliacs with factor VIII or IX inhibitors) is to first ensure that a reasonable attempt has been made to correct coagulation status and that the patient is not in extremis but has a survivable problem (55). Although dosing recommendations vary, a reasonable dose for most situations is 90 $\mu$g per kg (56). If hemostasis is not rapidly obtained, there is little utility in immediately giving a second dose. If the patient rebleeds after 2 to 3 hours, another dose can be given.

In theory, rVIIa-induced coagulation activation would be expected to result in DIC or overwhelming thrombosis. However, thrombotic complications of rVIIa are unusual (57). Patients have been reported to have acute arterial events such as myocardial infarction, but most of these patients were older and had preexistent cardiac risk factors or were receiving simultaneous therapy with activated prothrombin complex concentrates (aPCC). A prudent measure would be to use rVIIa with caution in patients with atherosclerosis or in combination with aPPCs.

# MASSIVE TRANSFUSION THERAPY

Patients who are acutely bleeding can require large amounts of transfusion products. Early data showed high mortality rates with transfusion of more than 20 U of blood (58), but with modern blood banking techniques and improved laboratory testing, this rate has decreased dramatically to survival rates of 43% to 70% in patients transfused with more than 50 U of blood (59–62).

The approach to massive transfusions is to measure the five basic laboratory tests that reflect the fundamental parameters essential for both blood volume and hemostasis:

(a) Hematocrit
(b) Platelet count
(c) Prothrombin time–international normalized ratio
(d) Activated partial thromboplastin time
(e) Fibrinogen level

Replacement therapy is based on these laboratory results and the clinical situation of the patient:

(a) Platelets less than 50,000 to 75,000 per $\mu$L: give platelet concentrates or six to eight packs of single donor platelets
(b) Fibrinogen less than 125 mg per dL: give 10 U of cryoprecipitate
(c) Hematocrit below 30%: give red cells
(d) Protime greater than INR 2.0 and aPTT abnormal: give 2 to 4 U of fresh frozen plasma (FFP)

The transfusion threshold for a low hematocrit depends on the stability of the patient. If the hematocrit is below 30% and the patient is bleeding or is hemodynamically unstable, transfusion of packed red cells is appropriate. Stable patients can tolerate lower hematocrits; an aggressive transfusion policy may even be detrimental (62,63).

If the patient is bleeding, has florid DIC, or has received platelet aggregation inhibitors, then keeping the platelet count above 50,000 per $\mu$L is reasonable. Regarding massive transfusion, existing data show that keeping the platelet count above 50,000 per $\mu$L results in less microvascular bleeding (64,65). The conventional dose of platelets is six to eight platelet concentrates or one plateletpheresis unit.

For a fibrinogen level of less than 100 mg per dL, transfusions of 10 U of cryoprecipitate will increase the plasma fibrinogen level by approximately 100 mg per dL. In certain clinical situations such as brain injuries, hepatic trauma, or ischemic limb reperfusion, severe fibrinolysis may occur, and the use of large amounts of cryoprecipitate can be anticipated.

Patients with an international normalized ratio (INR) greater than 2 and an abnormal aPTT can be given 2 to 4 U of FFP. For an aPTT greater than 1.5 times normal, 2 to 4 U of plasma should be given. Elevation of the aPTT above 1.8 times normal is associated with microvascular bleeding in patients with trauma (7). Patients with marked abnormalities such as an aPTT greater than two times normal may require aggressive therapy with at least 15 to 30 mL per kg (4 to 8 U for an average adult) of plasma (66).

Occasionally, empiric transfusion therapy is required for the patient with severe bleeding. One should start with platelet products because they also provide plasma. In patients likely to also have DIC (i.e., patients with head trauma), administration of 10 U of cryoprecipitate is indicated. For patients who have massive bleeding and are likely to receive 10 or more U of blood, early use of plasma may help preserve coagulation (67). One approach is to thaw and give 2 U of plasma if 6 or more U of un–cross-matched blood is given to a patient who is massively bleeding.

## Complications of Transfusions

Electrolyte abnormalities are unusual even in the patient who receives massive transfusion (68). Platelet concentrates and plasma contain citrate that can chelate calcium. However, the citrate is rapidly metabolized, and it is rare to see clinically significant hypocalcemia. Although empiric calcium replacement is often recommended, one study suggests that this is associated with a worse outcome and should not be done (69). If hypocalcemia is a clinical concern, then levels should be drawn to guide therapy.

Despite that potassium leaks out of stored red cells, even older units of blood contain a total of only 8 mEq per L of potassium, so hyperkalemia is usually not a concern. Stored blood is acidic, with a pH of 6.5 to 6.9, but acidosis attributed solely to transfused blood is rare. Empiric bicarbonate replacement has been associated with severe alkalosis and is not recommended (70,71).

# SPECIFIC SITUATIONS

## Surgical

### Surgical Bleeding

The first discovery of a bleeding diathesis often is during or after surgery, manifest as excessive and diffuse microvascular bleeding during surgery or excessive bleeding presenting hours or days after surgery.

Any disorder of hemostasis may present as surgical bleeding. Many patients with mild congenital bleeding disorders may not have problems until surgery, which may be their first significant hemostatic challenge. The clues of mildly abnormal preoperative coagulation studies may have been dismissed as insignificant by the surgical team (72). Excessive surgical bleeding can be the presenting sign of acquired defects, such as factor VIII inhibitors or drug-induced platelet dysfunction, in older patients.

Excessive bleeding from a primary coagulation defect can result in shock or organ damage, which can then lead to a secondary consumptive coagulopathy that precipitates more bleeding. The presence of multiple secondary coagulation defects can also hinder diagnosis of the primary defect.

The first step when called to see the bleeding surgical patient is to draw the basic set of hemostatic laboratory tests. Any observed coagulation defects should be rapidly corrected. Further therapy depends on the situation. If the patient has received drugs that interfere with platelet function, it is sensible to give a platelet transfusion and desmopressin. If massive diffuse bleeding persists after a prudent attempt at correction, a dose of 90 $\mu$g per kg of rVIIa can be given (53).

Although it is tempting to immediately evaluate the patient for a bleeding diathesis, there are several problems with this. One is the delay in performing and reporting a laboratory result. Second, therapies can obscure the primary hemostatic defect, especially in patients with VWD because von Willebrand factor (VWF) is an acute-phase–reacting protein. Finally, in patients with a secondary coagulopathy, an observed factor deficiency may be caused by the primary problem or may be the consequences of massive bleeding.

There does exist a poorly defined group of patients who have persistent bleeding with surgical procedures but in whom no defect can be found. These patients may have defects that are difficult to test for, such as Quebec platelet syndrome or defects in fibrinolysis (73). Use of antifibrinolytic therapy can be effective as long as untreated DIC is not present.

Blood salvage is frequently used in the bleeding surgical patient to help reduce red cell transfusions, and with the advent of blood washing, coagulopathies are less frequent (74). However, coagulopathy can occur upon fusion of thrombogenic substances (74,75). Patients who receive large amounts of cell-saver blood (>10 to 15 U) should have their coagulation status carefully monitored.

### Coronary Bypass

Cardiac bypass results in very complex and still poorly defined defects in all aspects of hemostasis (76,77). Large amounts of heparin are used for the bypass machine to prevent formation of clots in the filters; levels can reach as high as 5 U per mL. These large doses need to be reversed at the end of surgery to prevent bleeding. Because protamine has a shorter half-life than heparin, patients may rarely experience "heparin rebound" (78). High doses of protamine can lead to coagulation defects or the inhibition of platelet function (79).

Patients who have had multiple transfusions of cell-saver blood or of packed red cells may have dilutional coagulation defects. In the patient with bleeding still on bypass, an infusion of desmopressin is indicated, and given the presumed platelet defect, transfusion of platelets is indicated if the bleeding persists. Patients often respond to empiric transfusions of platelets. In the immediate postoperative state, a thrombin time should be checked to ensure the patient is not experiencing heparin rebound (80,81). If bleeding persists despite attempts at correcting coagulation, one dose of rVIIa is a logical next step (82).

### Liver Transplant

Patients may often require large amounts of blood during liver transplantation. Totals of more than 100 U of red cells and plasma are not unusual in patients who are extremely ill (83,84). Before operation, patients should be screened for baseline coagulations status to identify any unusual defects, although these are not predicative of bleeding with surgery (85). Patients should also undergo a type and screen to identify any unusual red cell alloantibodies. Patients who have had previous abdominal surgery often require extensive dissection of adhesions and aggressive blood support.

Liver transplantation is divided into three phases (84). During the anhepatic phase, the patient is totally dependent on residual coagulation factors and replacement therapy for hemostasis (86). One should anticipate that a "burst" of fibrinolysis will occur when the clamps are released to allow blood flow to the new liver (87). In some patients, a heparinlike inhibitor is also released (88), and nonspecific proteases will augment the coagulopathy (89). If engraftment of the new liver is successful, the coagulation defects will rapidly resolve.

In patients with very severe bleeding, one should assay the euglobulin clot lysis time. Severe fibrinolysis should be treated with antifibrinolytic therapy until the patient is stable (90). If the aPTT remains excessively prolonged and the thrombin time is markedly prolonged, one may assume the presence of a heparinlike substance and attempt to treat with protamine (91). If diffuse bleeding persists, a dose of rVIIa may be reasonable.

Several studies have examined the use of rVIIa in liver transplant, but (48,49,92,93) larger trials are needed to demonstrate both decreased blood loss and safety before routine use can be recommended.

### Trauma

The coagulation defects that occur in patients with trauma are complex in origin (94). The most common etiologies are dilution of hemostatic factors by fluid or blood resuscitation, hypothermia, tissue damage from trauma, and effects of underlying diseases.

After obtaining the basic set of coagulation tests (94–96), red cells and plasma should be empirically infused, if indicated, until results of laboratory tests are back. Because patients with head trauma can develop DIC, therapy with cryoprecipitate and plasma should be considered (97).

Patients with trauma are prone to hypothermia, and this can be a complicating factor in their bleeding (98–101). Hypothermia impairs platelet function, decreases the efficiency of coagulation reactions, and enhances fibrinolysis. Unwarmed packed red cells can lower the body temperature by 0.25°C (102), contributing to the effects on the coagulation system (98,103,104). Hypothermia can be prevented by transfusion of blood through blood warmers and to perform "damage control" surgery to control damaged vessels and oozing sites (105), after which the patient is taken to the intensive care unit (ICU) to be warmed and have coagulation defects corrected.

Preliminary results suggest that rVIIa can decrease blood requirements and may help prevent complications such as respiratory failure (106,107). A sensible approach would be to use rVIIa in a patient in whom microvascular bleeding persists despite attempts at vigorous replacement of blood products using the five basic tests of hemostasis.

## Coagulation Factors

Specific causes of hemorrhage are shown in Table 78-3.

### Acquired von Willebrand Disease

Acquired VWD occurs in lymphomas, myeloproliferative syndromes, myeloma, and monoclonal gammopathies, and with the use of certain drugs (108–111). The most common presentations are diffuse oozing from surgical sites and gastrointestinal bleeding (112). Patients with acquired VWD can present as type 1 (decreased protein) or type 2 (abnormal multimers) disease (113). Levels of factor VIII, ristocetin cofactor activity, and von Willebrand antigen are decreased. Platelet levels of VWF are normal, suggesting depletion of circulating VWF from the plasma. Crossed immunoelectrophoresis is used to differentiate type 1 from type 2 disease.

Patients with acquired VWD have variable responses to therapy (109,114). Desmopressin is effective in many patients with acquired VWD type 1 and 2, but consistent with the antibody-mediated destruction, the magnitude and duration of effect is often reduced (115). In some patients, desmopressin is not effective, which is why all patients should have VWF levels checked with therapy. High-dose immunoglobulin is also effective in reversing acquired VWD by decreasing antibody levels (116). For bleeding patients, high doses of Humate-P are indicated with frequent monitoring of factor VIII levels (117). For patients with very strong inhibitors that factor concentrates cannot overcome, rVIIa may prove useful (118).

### Acquired Factor VIII Inhibitors

Factor VIII deficiency due to autoantibodies is the most frequent acquired coagulation factor deficiency and occurs in patients with autoimmune disease, older patients, and postpartum (119–122). Unlike classic hemophiliacs, these patients often have ecchymoses covering large areas of their body. Patients will have prolonged aPTTs (123), a positive screening test for inhibitors, and a low factor VIII level.

---
**TABLE 78-3**

SPECIFIC CAUSES OF HEMORRHAGE

**ACQUIRED VON WILLEBRAND DISEASE**
Pathology: decreased levels of von Willebrand protein due to autoantibodies or absorption by tumors
Treatment: bleeding: desmopressin, Humate-P, rVIIa
 Autoantibodies: immunoglobulin, steroids
 Absorption: treatment of tumor

**ACQUIRED FACTOR VIII INHIBITORS**
Pathology: decreased level of factor III due to autoantibodies
Treatment: Bleeding: low-titer inhibitor—high-dose factor VIII, high-titer inhibitor—VIIa, prothrombin complex concentrates, porcine factor VIII
 Autoantibody: immunoglobulin, steroids, oral cyclophosphamide, anti-CD20 antibodies

**DISSEMINATED INTRAVASCULAR COAGULATION**
Pathology: excess generation of thrombin
Treatment: factor replacement, protein C concentrates or activated protein C

**LIVER DISEASE**
Pathology: decrease synthesis of coagulation factors, decreased platelet production, enhance fibrinolysis
Treatment: factor replacement, antifibrinolytic therapy, rVIIa

**VIRAL HEMORRHAGIC FEVERS**
Pathology: direct endothelial damage/activation by viruses
Treatment: factor replacement, antiviral therapy, isolation to prevent nosocomial spread

**POSTTRANSFUSION PURPURA**
Pathology: autoimmune destruction of platelets due to anti-PLA$_1$
Treatment: immunoglobulin, plasmapheresis, transfusion of PLA$_1$ negative platelets

**PLATELET REFRACTORINESS**
Pathology: destruction of transfused platelets by anti-HLA antibodies
Treatment: transfusion of HLA-matched platelets

**DRUG-INDUCED THROMBOCYTOPENIA**
Pathology: autoimmune destruction of platelets mediated by antimedication antibody
Treatment: stop offending agent

**UREMIA**
Pathology: uremic toxins affect platelet function
Treatment (short-term): dialysis, desmopressin, transfusion to hematocrit over 30%
Treatment (long-term): conjugated estrogens, use of erythropoietin to maintain hematocrit over 30%

---
rVIIa, recombinant factor VIIa; HLA, human leucocyte antigen.

Therapy is twofold, aimed at correcting the hemostatic defect and at suppressing the inhibitor. For very low-level inhibitors (<5 BU), treatment is directed toward overpowering the inhibitor. With higher-level inhibitors, prothrombin complex concentrates (PCC), at a dose of 75 U per kg twice a day, can be used. The use of these products may be complicated by thrombosis, especially in older patients.

Porcine factor VIII (100 to 150 U per kg) should be reserved for the patient with bleeding because patients can develop antibodies that cross-react with porcine factor VIII and anaphylaxis can occur (124).

Recombinant VIIa is the treatment of choice (94,125). The dose is 90 $\mu$g per kg repeated every 2 to 3 hours until bleeding has stopped. For surgery or life-threatening bleeding, the rVIIa should be "weaned" by decreasing the dose to every 6 hours for several days after 2 to 3 days of every-2-hour therapy.

Patients with factor VIII inhibitors should receive immunosuppression to eliminate the inhibitor. Up to one third of patients may transiently respond to immunoglobulin (1 g per kg a day, for 2 days) (126). Immunosuppression should be started with

prednisone 60 mg per day plus oral cyclophosphamide 100 mg per day (127) continued until inhibitor titers decrease and factor levels increase. If no response is seen after 1 month, then other immunosuppressive therapy can be tried. Patients may respond to rituximab therapy (375 mg/m$^2$/week $\times$ 4) (128).

### Disseminated Intravascular Coagulation

Patients with DIC (see Chapter 109) can present in one of four patterns (129,130):

(a) Asymptomatic—laboratory evidence but no clinical problems
(b) Bleeding caused by combinations of factor depletion, platelet dysfunction, thrombocytopenia, and excessive fibrinolysis (130)
(c) Thrombosis—most often microvascular (renal, cerebral), but venous, arterial, and nonbacterial thrombotic endocarditis have been reported (131)
(d) Purpura fulminans

DIC is best treated by attention to the underlying cause (130, 132–134) and by replacement of coagulation factors. Past concerns about "feeding the fires" have not been shown to be clinically valid (78,135). Heparin therapy is reserved for patients who have thrombosis as a component of their DIC (78, 132,136). Fibrinogen concentrations and heparin levels should be followed up in these patients (137,138).

### Purpura Fulminans

DIC in association with symmetrical limb ecchymosis and necrosis of the skin is seen in two situations (139): primary, after a viral infection (140) beginning with a painful red area on an extremity that rapidly progresses to a black ischemic area, perhaps associated with acquired protein S deficiency (139,141,142), and secondary, most often associated with meningococcal infections and (143–145) postsplenectomy sepsis (146).

Therapy for purpura fulminans is controversial. Primary purpura fulminans, especially those with postvaricella autoimmune protein S deficiency, have responded to plasma infusion titrated to keep the protein S level more than 25% (139). Intravenous immunoglobulin helps to decrease antiprotein S antibodies. Heparin (5 to 8 U/kg/hour) may control DIC and extent of necrosis (132,147).

Patients with secondary purpura fulminans have been treated with plasma infusions, plasmapheresis, and continuous plasma ultrafiltration (147–150). Heparin therapy alone has not been shown to improve survival (151–153). Much attention has been given to replacement of natural anticoagulants such as protein C and antithrombin as therapy for purpura fulminans, but unfortunately, randomized trials using antithrombin have shown mostly negative results (139,142,154–156). Trials using either zymogen protein C concentrates or rAPC (drotrecogin) have shown more promise in controlling the coagulopathy of purpura fulminans and improving outcomes in sepsis (148,157–159). Although bleeding is a concern with use of protein C, most complications occur in patients with platelet counts below 30,000 per $\mu$L or in those who have meningitis (160).

### Liver Disease

Patients with severe liver disease have multiple coagulation defects (161–166) because of deficient synthesis of factors, platelet dysfunction because of the increase in fibrin degradation products (FDPs) (167), and fibrinolysis because of a decrease in plasma levels of fibrinolytic inhibitors and delayed clearance of plasminogen activator tissue-type plasminogen activator (tPA).

Attempting to normalize the INR is often futile and counterproductive (168,169). Because only 5% to 15% of factor VII is needed for hemostasis, isolated minor elevations of the PT-INR (INR less than three) do not require further plasma therapy (170). Overzealous attempts to totally correct the INR are unproductive and will result in volume overload (171).

Abnormal fibrinolysis is an often overlooked cause of bleeding in patients with liver disease (26,172,173), and a trial of antifibrinolytic therapy is warranted (162,174–176).

There is increasing use of rVIIa in patients with liver disease (177,178). Shami reports that the use of 40 $\mu$g per kg of rVIIa before intracranial monitor placement allows successful placement without bleeding or the need for massive plasma infusions (179). There are several reports of use of rVIIa when used as an addition to definitive treatment of bleeding varices (180,181). These reports show decreased bleeding but no influence on survival.

### Viral Hemorrhagic Fevers

Viral hemorrhagic fevers (VHF) are a diverse group of viral infections, including Lassa fever, Rift Valley fever, Ebola, and dengue, that can result in massive bleeding (182–185). The clinical pattern is a febrile illness that proceeds over a few days to shock and diffuse gastrointestinal and mucosal bleeding, with signs of thrombocytopenia and in some cases DIC. Most VHF are associated with leukopenia and hemoconcentration. Therapy is aggressive supportive care of the patients and replacement of coagulation factors. Given the propensity of many of these infections to spread to health care workers, precautions should be taken to prevent nosocomial spread (186).

## Platelet Number and Function

### Posttransfusion Purpura

Patients with this disorder and who lack platelet antigen PLA$_1$ will have the onset of severe thrombocytopenia ($<$10,000 per $\mu$L) 1 to 2 weeks after receiving blood products (187–190). For unknown reasons, exposure to the antigens from the transfusion leads to rapid destruction of the patient's own platelets. The diagnostic clue is thrombocytopenia in patients, typically women, who have received a red cell or platelet blood product in the past 7 to 10 days. Treatment consists of intravenous immunoglobulin (191) and plasmapheresis to remove the offending antibody. If patients with a history of post transfusion purpura (PTP) require further transfusions, only PLA$_1$-negative platelets should be given.

### Bleeding in the Patient with Platelet Refractory

Bleeding in patients who are refractory to platelet transfusion presents a difficult clinical problem (192,193). If patients are demonstrated to have human leukocyte antigen (HLA) antibodies, one can transfuse (HLA)-matched platelets (194). Unfortunately, platelet transfusions are ineffective in 20% to 70% of these patients. Platelets are distributed as HLA-matched if they match even on one HLA locus, but only the three- to four-loci match is effective. Because some loci are difficult to match, effective products may be unavailable. As many as 25% of patients have antiplatelet antibodies in which HLA-matched products will be ineffective. In the patient who is totally refractory to platelet transfusion, consider drugs as an etiology of antiplatelet antibodies (especially vancomycin) (195). Use of antifibrinolytic agents such as epsilon aminocaproic acid or tranexamic acid may decrease the incidence of bleeding. "Platelet drips" consisting of infusing either a platelet concentrate per hour or one plateletpheresis U every 6 hours may be given as a continuous infusion. For life-threatening bleeding, rVIIa may be of use (196). For patients with platelet refractory and with arterial bleeding, the use of angiographic delivery of platelets has been reported to be successful in stopping bleeding (197).

### Thrombocytopenia and Platelet Dysfunction

In patients with a possible drug-induced thrombocytopenia, the standard therapy is to stop the suspect drug (198,199). In a critical review, drugs were implicated in less than 1% of ICU thrombocytopenia (200), and there is an evidence-based list of drugs implicated in drug-induced thrombocytopenia (201). One approach is to stop any drug started in the past 7 days that is strongly associated with thrombocytopenia (202) (Chapter 73). Immunoglobulins, corticosteroids, or intravenous anti-D have been suggested as useful in drug-related thrombocytopenia (203). However, because most patients with thrombocytopenia recover when the agent is cleared from the body, this therapy is probably not necessary and avoids exposing the patients to the risk of therapy.

Acquired abnormalities of platelet function are common, but their clinical significance is controversial (204). Of the many agents that result in impaired platelet performance, only the few reviewed in the subsequent text appear to be of clinical consequence. Many of these proposed abnormalities are reflected only in an increased bleeding time, a test of uncertain clinical value (205). Aspirin is associated with increased bleeding (204), as are ketorolac (206–208), penicillins (209–213), and hydroxyethyl starch, which decrease high molecular forms of VWF and factor VIII, inducing a type 2 defect (214,215).

### Uremia

Before the advent of dialysis, bleeding was a common late complication of uremia (216–219). The defect in uremia is platelet function defect (218); coagulation factors are not affected, and unless other problems are present, the PT-INR/aPTT are not prolonged.

Patients with uremia are prone to vitamin K deficiency, so assessment of the PT-INR is important. The half-life of both unfractionated and low-molecular-weight heparin is increased in renal failure (220,221). Patients usually receive a bolus of heparin with dialysis, and rare patients have a persistently prolonged anticoagulant effect. Low-molecular-weight heparins are cleared in the kidneys, and if the dose is not adjusted, levels can greatly increase above therapeutic levels. Bleeding times are prolonged in renal disease, but there is little correlation between bleeding time and actual bleeding (222).

Multiple treatment options exist for uremic bleeding, including desmopressin, estrogen, and erythropoietin. Patients who are severely uremic and are bleeding may respond to aggressive dialysis (223). Cryoprecipitate is not effective in some patients, and its use exposes the patient to the risk of transfusion-transmitted viral disease (223,224). Desmopressin is effective in patients with uremia, with the bleeding time shortening for at least 4 hours after infusion (218). The reason DDAVP works in uremia is unknown (225).

For chronic bleeding, an infusion of conjugated estrogens, 0.6 mg/kg/day intravenously for 5 days, is effective in reducing bleeding (35,37,226). The onset of action takes up to 1 day but is of long duration, lasting for 2 weeks after the series of infusions (36). For patients with chronic gastrointestinal bleeding from telangiectasias, chronic therapy with oral combinations of estrogen and progesterone may be helpful (227).

Raising the hematocrit above 30% by transfusions or erythropoietin will shorten the bleeding time in some situations (228).

# COMPLICATIONS OF ANTITHROMBOTIC THERAPY

## Antiplatelet Agents

For patients on aspirin with emergency bleeding, platelet transfusions can be given. The half-life of circulating aspirin is short, especially with low-dose therapy, and unless the patient has taken a dose within an hour of the transfusion, the function of the transfused platelets should not be impaired. Desmopressin may reverse aspirin inhibition and is effective for emergency surgery in patients on aspirin therapy who bleed (229–231). Little data exist on specific therapy for bleeding complications in patients on either ticlopidine or clopidogrel. For patients who are severely bleeding, platelet transfusions may be used in an attempt to restore platelet function.

Therapy for bleeding complications seen with glycoprotein (GP) IIb/IIIa inhibitors is guided by the agent received. Most of the infused abciximab binds to the IIb/IIIa with very little found free in the plasma (232,233). Therefore, for abciximab-related bleeding, treatment is to give a platelet transfusion, which leads to redistribution of the abciximab over a wider number of receptors and return of platelet function. Tirofiban

and eptifibatide do not bind as tightly, so platelet transfusion may not fully restore platelet function. *In vitro* studies suggest that the addition of fibrinogen may help restore platelet function (234), so patients with severe bleeding receiving tirofiban or eptifibatide should be transfused with 10 U of cryoprecipitate. Infusion of desmopressin 0.3 $\mu$g per kg may be of benefit (229).

Severe thrombocytopenia has been reported in 0.5% to 7.0% of patients receiving GP IIb/IIIa blockers (229,235, 236), higher in patients previously exposed (233). The onset of the thrombocytopenia is rapid and can occur within 2 to 4 hours (237). Experience with abciximab has shown that infusion of immunoglobulin or steroids is not helpful. The risk of bleeding is higher in patients with thrombocytopenia but, interestingly, so is the risk of ischemic events (236,238, 239).

All patients receiving these agents should have a platelet count checked 2 and 12 hours into therapy. If thrombocytopenia is noted, the blood smear should be reviewed to rule out pseudothrombocytopenia. If the patient has been exposed to heparin in the past 100 days, then heparin-induced thrombocytopenia needs to be considered. For severe thrombocytopenia, the GP IIb/IIIa blockers should be stopped and, if the platelet count is under 20,000 per $\mu$L or the patient is bleeding, a platelet transfusion should be given.

## Warfarin

The key to management of an elevated INR is vitamin K (240,241) (Chapter 119). Both oral and intravenous vitamin K offer considerable advantages over the use of subcutaneous vitamin K or plasma infusion (240–244). Often, only small doses of vitamin K in the range of 0.5 to 3 mg are needed (240,243, 245,246). Intravenous vitamin K, even infused slowly, is associated with a slight risk of anaphylaxis (3:10,000) (247–249). For most situations, the oral route produces reliable results, with an onset of action within 12 hours (243). However, if speedy reversal is needed, then the intravenous route should be used because effects can be seen in as early as 4 hours.

For patients who are not bleeding and with INRs over the therapeutic range but less than 5, one can simply omit or lower the dose. There is a delay of 12 to 36 hours after stopping warfarin before the INR begins to fall (240), so for INRs in the 5 to 10 range, one can hold the next one to two doses and give 1.0 to 2.5 mg of vitamin K orally (250). For INRs of more than 10, one should give 2.5 to 5.0 mg of vitamin K with the expectation that the INR will be lowered in 24 to 48 hours (251–253).

If the patient requires rapid full reversal because of bleeding or need for surgery when the INR is 5 to 10, one can give vitamin K by the intravenous route (240,254) plus FFP. Because one U of plasma raises coagulation factors by only 5% on average, one must give large doses (15 mg per kg or 4 to 5 U) to attempt to correct the INR, and giving this amount of plasma runs the risk of volume overload.

The rate of intracranial hemorrhage occurring in patients on warfarin is 0.2% to 2% per year, with the higher rates being seen in older patients and in patients with higher INRs (240,255,256). These hemorrhages are particularly devastating, with most patients either dying or rendered incapacitated by the bleeding.

Immediate management of bleeding is to rapidly reverse the warfarin effect (257,258). This can be done by giving both vitamin K (10 mg IV slowly over 1 hour) and FFP, or PCC. Clinical data has shown these products (which contain all the vitamin K–dependent clotting factors) result in a more rapid and complete correction of coagulation than does plasma (259–261). Patients in whom intracranial hemorrhages occur should receive prothrombin concentrates such as Konyne or Prophylnine at a dose of 50 U per kg (260,

**TABLE 78-4**

DIRECT THROMBIN INHIBITORS

| Agent formation | Half-life | Renal disease | Liver disease | Antibody |
|---|---|---|---|---|
| Argatroban | 40 min | Not effected | 150 min | No |
| Bivalirudin | 20 min | T1/2 increases to 3.5 h inrenal failure | Not effected | Cross-reacts with antihirudin |
| Hirudin | 40 min | T1/2 increases to 50 h in renal failure | Not effected | Yes |
| Ximelagatran | 2.5–3.5 h | T1/2 increases | Not effected | No |

262–264). There is some recent data showing that the use of rVIIa can reverse warfarin-induced bleeding (265,266).

## Heparin

Standard heparin has a short (30 to 60 minutes) half-life, so in most situations, reversal is not required. Low-molecular-weight heparins have a half-life of several hours, so reversal may be required for serious bleeding soon after drug administration. Protamine is used to reverse heparin and low-molecular-weight heparin (267). The dose for heparin reversal is dependent on timing of the last heparin doses. For immediate reversal (30 minutes or less since the last heparin dose), 1 mg of protamine should be given for every 100 U of heparin; for 30 to 60 minutes after the dose, 0.5 mg of protamine for every 100 U of heparin; and for 60 to 120 minutes, 0.375 mg of protamine for 100 U of heparin (268). The infusion rate of protamine should not exceed 5 mg per minute (268).

Protamine does not fully reverse low-molecular-weight heparin but can neutralize the antithrombin effect (268–270). Owing to the longer half-life of low-molecular-weight heparin, sometimes a second dose of protamine is required. The dose is 1 mg per 100 U of daltaparin or tinzaparin or 1 mg per mg of enoxaparin. If the aPTT is prolonged 4 hours later (reflecting continued thrombin inhibition), one half of the initial dose should be given. Heparanase is a drug in clinical development that can degrade heparin and may be useful for reversing the its anticoagulant effect (271).

Currently, no effective antidote exists for danaparoid, fondaparinux, or idaparinux. Given the prolonged half-life of these agents (26, 18, 72 hours, respectively), severe bleeding represents a major challenge. There is *in vitro* data that rVIIa may reverse the coagulation defect, but the clinical utility of this is unknown (52,272).

## Direct Thrombin Inhibitors

Direct thrombin inhibitors are shown in Table 78-4.

All direct thrombin inhibitors (DTI) (273–275) raise both the INR and aPTT, because thrombin is part of the common pathway of blood coagulation. Clinically, the parenteral DTIs are monitored by the aPTT, usually aiming for a goal of 2 to 2.5 times normal control. In patients with normal renal and hepatic function, the half-life of these agents is short, ranging from 20 minutes to 4 hours for ximelagatran. However, with the exception of argatroban, most DTI are renally cleared and can have dramatic increases in their half-life with renal failure.

No effective reversal agents exist for the DTIs. Anecdotally, rVIIa is useful and could be considered for immediate treatment of life-threatening hemorrhage (276). *In vitro* data suggest that activated prothrombin concentrates at doses of 50 U per kg may also be useful.

Lepirudin poses special issues concerning bleeding risk. The half-life of lepirudin increases with even modest decreases in renal function, and in renal failure the half-life can increase to 50 to 100 hours (277). Therefore, lepirudin should be avoided in patients with any degree of renal insufficiency. Antilepirudin antibodies can be seen in 50% to 80% of patients receiving the agent for more than 5 days, which in some patients can increase the antithrombotic activity of the drug (278). Lepirudin can be removed by hemofiltration using hiflux membranes, with polysulphone being the most efficient (279–281).

## Fibrinolytic Agents

The major complication of thrombolytic therapy is bleeding (Chapter 121). Rates of major bleeding range from 4.6% to 5.94% (232,282). Patients bleed at sites of previous injury because of lysis of previously formed thrombosis or because of underlying vascular problems such as cerebral vascular amyloid (283). The most devastating complication is intracerebral hemorrhage (ICH), which can have a mortality rate of up to 60% (284,285). ICH occurs in approximately 0.4% to 0.8% of patients with acute myocardial infarcts (284,286, 287) and 1% to 2% of patients with pulmonary embolism or deep vein thrombosis (288–290). The highest rates of ICH are seen in patients receiving thrombolytic therapy for stroke, with rates of 3% to 15% (291). Older patients (over 75), smaller patients, patients with previous stoke, patients who are hypertensive, and patients receiving tPA are at higher risk of bleeding (248,284,292,293). Patients will have a low fibrinogen, elevated PT-INR and aPTT caused by destruction of factors V and VIII, and abnormal platelet function and lysis of formed thrombi. Patients in whom severe bleeding occurs after thrombolytic therapy (294) should be infused with cryoprecipitate to replace fibrinogen and factor VIII and platelets. If the patient is having an intracranial hemorrhage, empiric therapy with cryoprecipitate, platelets, and plasma should be given. Although reversal of the fibrinolytic state can be achieved with the use of antifibrinolytic agents, this is rarely required, because the fibrinolytic state, especially with tPA, is short-lived.

## References

1. Goodnight SH, Hathaway WE. Evaluation of bleeding in the hospitalized patient. *Disorders of hemostasis and thrombosis.* New York: McGraw-Hill, 2001:61–69.
2. Alzetani A, Vohra HA, Patel RL. Can we rely on arterial line sampling in performing activated plasma thromboplastin time after cardiac surgery? *Eur J Anaesthesiol* 2004;215:384–388.
3. Newman RS, Fagin AR. Heparin contamination in coagulation testing and a protocol to avoid it and the risk of inappropriate FFP transfusion. *Am J Clin Pathol* 1995;104:447–449.
4. Biron C, Bengler C, Gris JC, et al. Acquired isolated factor VII deficiency during sepsis. *Haemostasis* 1997;272:51–56.

5. Bizzaro N. EDTA-dependent pseudothrombocytopenia: a clinical and epidemiological study of 112 cases, with 10-year follow-up. *Am J Hematol* 1995;502:103–109.

6. Gruel Y, Pouplard C, Nguyen P, et al. Biological and clinical features of low-molecular-weight heparin-induced thrombocytopenia. *Br J Haematol* 2003;121(5):786–792.

7. Ciavarella D, Reed RL, Counts RB, et al. Clotting factor levels and the risk of diffuse microvascular bleeding in the massively transfused patient. *Br J Haematol* 1987;67(3):365–368.

8. Rodgers RPC. A critical reappraisal of the bleeding time. *Semin Thromb Hemost* 1990;16:1–20.

9. Peterson P, Hayes TE, Arkin CF, et al. The preoperative bleeding time test lacks clinical benefit: College of American Pathologists' and American Society of Clinical Pathologists' position article. *Arch Surg* 1998;133(2):134–139.

10. Ortel TL, James AH, Thames EH, et al. Assessment of primary hemostasis by PFA-100 analysis in a tertiary care center. *Thromb Haemost* 2000;84(1):93–97.

11. Cariappa R, Wilhite TR, Parvin CA, et al. Comparison of PFA-100 and bleeding time testing in pediatric patients with suspected hemorrhagic problems. *J Pediatr Hematol Oncol* 2003;25(6):474–479.

12. Whitten CW, Greilich PE. Thromboelastography: past, present, and future.[comment]. [Review] [17 refs]. *Anesthesiology* 2000;92(5):1223–1225.

13. Maloney DG, Grillo-López AJ, Bodkin DJ, et al. IDEC-C2B8: results of a phase I multiple-dose trial in patients with relapsed non-Hodgkin's lymphoma. *J Clin Oncol* 1997;15:3266–3274.

14. Cattaneo M. Desmopressin in the treatment of patients with defects of platelet function. *Haematologica* 2002;87(11):1122–1124.

15. Bauduer F, Bendriss P, Freyburger G, et al. Use of desmopressin for prophylaxis of surgical bleeding in factor XI-deficient patients. *Acta Haematol* 1998;99:52–53.

16. Castaman G, Rodeghiero F. Consistency of responses to separate desmopressin infusions in patients with storage pool disease and isolated prolonged bleeding time. *Thromb Res* 1993;69:407–412.

17. Flordal PA. Use of desmopressin to prevent bleeding in surgery. *Eur J Surg* 1998;164(1):5–11.

18. Cattaneo M, Mannucci PM. Desmopressin and blood loss after cardiac surgery. *Lancet* 1993;342(8874):812.

19. Rose EH, Aledort LM. Nasal spray desmopressin DDAVP for mild hemophilia A and von Willebrand disease. *Ann Intern Med* 1991;114:563–568.

20. Dunn CJ, Goa KL. Tranexamic acid—a review of its use in surgery and other indications. *Drugs* 1999;57:1005–1032.

21. Erstad BL. Antifibrinolytic agents and desmopressin as hemostatic agents in cardiac surgery. [Review] [37 refs]. *Ann Pharmacother* 2001;35(9):1075–1084.

22. Amitrano L, Guardascione MA, Brancaccio V, et al. Coagulation disorders in liver disease. *Semin Liver Dis* 2002;22(1):83–96.

23. Chang JC, Kane KK. Pathologic hyperfibrinolysis associated with amyloidosis: clinical response to epsilon amino caproic acid. *Am J Clin Pathol* 1984;81:382–387.

24. *Med Lett Drugs Ther.* Tranexamic acid. 1987;29:89–90.

25. Schwartz BS, Williams EC, Conlan MG, et al. Epsilon-aminocaproic acid in the treatment of patients with acute promyelocytic leukemia and acquired alpha-2-plasmin inhibitor defiency. *Ann Intern Med* 1986;105:873–877.

26. Takahashi H, Tatewaki W, Wada K, et al. Fibrinolysis and fibrinogenolysis in liver disease. *Am J Hematol* 1990;34:241–245.

27. Small M, Lowe GDO, Douglas JT, et al. Thrombin and plasmin activity in coronary artery disease. *Br Heart J* 1988;60:201–203.

28. Porte RJ, Leebeek FW. Pharmacological strategies to decrease transfusion requirements in patients undergoing surgery. [Review] [138 refs]. *Drugs* 2002;62(15):2193–2211.

29. Jansen AJ, Andreica S, Claeys M, et al. Use of tranexamic acid for an effective blood conservation strategy after total knee arthroplasty. *Br J Anaesth* 1999;83(4):596–601.

30. Chakrabarti S, Varma S, Singh S, et al. Low dose bolus aminocaproic acid: an alternative to platelet transfusion in thrombocytopenia. *Eur J Haematol* 1998;60:313–314.

31. Garewal HS, Durie BG. Antifibrinolytic therapy with aminocaproic acid for the control of bleeding in thrombocytopenic patients. *Scand J Haematol* 1985;35:497–500.

32. Wymenga LF, van der Boon WJ. Obstruction of the renal pelvis due to an insoluble blood clot after epsilon-aminocaproic acid therapy: resolution with intraureteral streptokinase instillations. *J Urol* 1998;159(2):490–492.

33. Gralnick H, Greipp P. Thrombosis with epsilon aminocaproic acid therapy. *Am J Clin Pathol* 1971;56:151.

34. Chatterjee SK, Chakraborty A. Intraocular pressure changes and mountaineering—preliminary observations and possible application. *J Assoc Physicians India* 2001;49:248–252.

35. Heunisch C, Resnick DJ, Vitello JM, et al. Conjugated estrogens for the management of gastrointestinal bleeding secondary to uremia of acute renal failure. *Pharmacotherapy* 1998;18(1):210–217.

36. Vigano G, Gaspari F, Locatelli M, et al. Dose-effect and pharmacokinetics of estrogens given to correct bleeding time in uremia. *Kidney Int* 1988;34(6):853–858.

37. Livio M, Mannucci PM, Vigano G, et al. Conjugated estrogens for the management of bleeding associated with renal failure. *N Engl J Med* 1986;315(12):731–735.

38. Lusher J, Ingerslev J, Roberts H, et al. Clinical experience with recombinant factor VIIa. *Blood Coagul Fibrinolysis* 1998;92:119–128.

39. Hay CR, Negrier C, Ludlam CA. The treatment of bleeding in acquired haemophilia with recombinant factor VIIa: a multicentre study. *Thromb Haemost* 1997;78(6):1463–1467.

40. Di Paola J, Nugent D, Young G. Current therapy for rare factor deficiencies. [Review] [53 refs]. *Haemophilia* 2001;7(Suppl. 1):16–22.

41. Poon MC. Use of recombinant factor VIIa in hereditary bleeding disorders. [Review] [57 refs]. *Curr Opin Hematol* 2001;85:312–318.

42. Poon MC. Management of thrombocytopenic bleeding: is there a role for recombinant coagulation factor VIIa? [Review] [37 refs]. *Curr Hematol Rep* 2003;22:139–147.

43. Caglar K, Cetinkaya A, Aytac S, et al. Use of recombinant factor VIIa for bleeding in children with Glanzmann thrombasthenia. *Pediatr Hematol Oncol* 2003;20(6):435–438.

44. Vidarsson B, Onundarson PT. Recombinant factor VIIa for bleeding in refractory thrombocytopenia. *Thromb Haemost* 2000;83(4):634–635.

45. Bellucci S, Caen J. Molecular basis of Glanzmann's thrombasthenia and current strategies in treatment. *Blood Rev* 2002;16(3):193–202.

46. Almeida AM, Khair K, Hann I, et al. The use of recombinant factor VIIa in children with inherited platelet function disorders. *Br J Haematol* 2003;121(3):477–481.

47. Friederich PW, Henny CP, Messelink EJ, et al. Effect of recombinant activated factor VII on perioperative blood loss in patients undergoing retropubic prostatectomy: a double-blind placebo-controlled randomised trial. *Lancet* 2003;361(9353):201–205.

48. Meijer K, Hendriks HG, De Wolf JT, et al. Recombinant factor VIIa in orthotopic liver transplantation: influence on parameters of coagulation and fibrinolysis. *Blood Coagul Fibrinolysis* 2003;14(2):169–174.

49. Hendriks HG, Meijer K, De Wolf JT, et al. Reduced transfusion requirements by recombinant factor VIIa in orthotopic liver transplantation: a pilot study. *Transplantation* 2001;71(3):402–405.

50. Aledort L. Recombinant factor VIIa Is a pan-hemostatic agent? *Thromb Haemost* 2000;83:637–638.

51. Dutton RP, Hess JR, Scalea TM. Recombinant factor VIIa for control of hemorrhage: early experience in critically ill trauma patients. *J Clin Anesth* 2003;15(3):184–188.

52. Bijsterveld NR, Moons AH, Boekholdt SM, et al. Ability of recombinant factor VIIa to reverse the anticoagulant effect of the pentasaccharide fondaparinux in healthy volunteers. *Circulation* 2002;106(20):2550–2554.

53. Hedner U, Erhardtsen E. Potential role for rFVIIa in transfusion medicine. *Transfusion* 2002;42(1):114–124.

54. Schreiber MA, Holcomb JB, Hedner U, et al. The effect of recombinant factor VIIa on coagulopathic pigs with grade V liver injuries. *J Trauma* 2002;53(2):252–257.

55. Clark AD, Gordon WC, Walker ID, et al. 'Last-ditch' use of recombinant factor VIIa in patients with massive haemorrhage is ineffective. *Vox Sang* 2004;86(2):120–124.

56. Hedner U. Dosing and monitoring NovoSeven treatment. *Haemostasis* 1996;26(Suppl. 1):102–108.

57. Roberts HR, Monroe DM III, Hoffman M. Safety profile of recombinant factor VIIa. *Semin Hematol* 2004;41(1 Suppl. 1):101–108.

58. Wilson RF, Mammen E, Walt AJ. Eight years of experience with massive blood transfusions. *J Trauma Inj Infect Crit Care* 1971;11(4):275–285.

59. Vaslef SN, Knudsen NW, Neligan PJ, et al. Massive transfusion exceeding 50 units of blood products in trauma patients. *J Trauma Inj Infect Crit Care* 2002;53(2):291–295.

60. Hakala P, Hiippala S, Syrjala M, et al. Massive blood transfusion exceeding 50 units of plasma poor red cells or whole blood: the survival rate and the occurrence of leukopenia and acidosis. *Injury* 1999;30(9):619–622.

61. Cinat ME, Wallace WC, Nastanski F, et al. Improved survival following massive transfusion in patients who have undergone trauma. *Arch Surg* 1999;134(9):964–968.

62. Hébert PC, Wells G, Blajchman MA, et al. A multicenter, randomized, controlled clinical trial of transfusion requirements in critical care. *N Engl J Med* 1999;340(6):409–417.

63. Blair SD, Janvrin SB, McCollum CN, et al. Effect of early blood transfusion on gastrointestinal haemorrhage. *Br J Surg* 1986;73(10):783–785.

64. Counts RB, Haisch C, Simon TL, et al. Hemostasis in massively transfused trauma patients. *Ann Surg* 1979;190(1):91–99.

65. Miller RD, Robbins TO, Tong MJ, et al. Coagulation defects associated with massive blood transfusions. *Ann Surg* 1971;174(5):794–801.

66. Chowdhury P, Saayman AG, Paulus U, et al. Efficacy of standard dose and 30 ml/kg fresh frozen plasma in correcting laboratory parameters of haemostasis in critically ill patients. *Br J Haematol* 2004;125(1):69–73.

67. Hirshberg A, Dugas M, Banez EI, et al. Minimizing dilutional coagulopathy in exsanguinating hemorrhage: a computer simulation. *J Trauma Inj Infect Crit Care* 2003;54(3):454–463.

68. Goskowicz R. The complications of massive tranfusion. *Anesth Clin North Am* 1999;174:959–978.

69. Howland WS, Schweizer O, Boyan CP. Massive blood replacement without calcuim administration. *Surg Gynecol Obstet* 1964;159:171–177.

70. Miller RD, Tong MJ, Robbins TO. Effects of massive transfusion of blood on acid-base balance. *JAMA* 1971;216(11):1762–1765.

71. Collins JA. Problems associated with the massive transfusion of stored blood. [Review] [144 refs]. *Surgery* 1974;75(2):274–295.

72. Kitchens CS. Prolonged activated partial thromboplastin time of unknown etiology: a prospective study of 100 consecutive cases referred for consultation. *Am J Hematol* 1988;27(1):38–45.

73. McKay H, Derome F, Haq MA, et al. Bleeding risks associated with inheritance of the quebec platelet disorder. *Blood* 2004;104:159–165.

74. Williamson KR, Taswell HF. Intraoperative blood salvage: a review. [Review] [119 refs]. *Transfusion* 1991;31(7):662–675.

75. Horst HM, Dlugos S, Fath JJ. et al. Coagulopathy and intraoperative blood salvage IBS. *J Trauma Inj Infect Crit Care* 1992;32(5):646–652.

76. Woodman RC, Harker LA. Bleeding complications associated with cardiopulmonary bypass. [Review] [204 refs]. *Blood* 1990;76(9):1680–1697.

77. Bevan DH. Cardiac bypass haemostasis: putting blood throught the mill. *Br J Haematol* 1999;104:208–219.

78. Feinstein DI. Diagnosis and management of disseminated intravascular coagulation: the role of heparin therapy. [Review] [34 refs]. *Blood* 1982;60(2):284–287.

79. DeLaria GA, Tyner JJ, Hayes CL, et al. Heparin-protamine mismatch. A controllable factor in bleeding after open heart surgery. *Arch Surg* 1994;129(9):944–950.

80. Landefeld CS, Rosenblatt MW, Goldman L. Bleeding in outpatients treated with warfarin: relation to the prothrombin time and important remediable lesions. *Am J Med* 1989;87(2):153–159.

81. Butterworth J, Lin YA, Prielipp R, et al. The pharmacokinetics and cardiovascular effects of a single intravenous dose of protamine in normal volunteers. *Anesth Analg* 2002;94(3):514–522.

82. Tanaka KA, Waly AA, Cooper WA, et al. Treatment of excessive bleeding in Jehovah's Witness patients after cardiac surgery with recombinant factor VIIa NovoSeven. *Anesthesiology* 2003;98(6):1513–1515.

83. Donica SK, Roberts LC, Duke PK, et al. Blood transfusion in orthotopic liver transplantation: six-year experience. *Transpl Int* 1992;5(Suppl. 1):S214.

84. Dzik WH. Massive transfusion: lessons from liver transplantation. In: Jefferies LC, Brecher ME, eds. *Massive transfusion*, Bethesda, MD: American Association of Blood Banks, 1994:65–96.

85. Baliga P, Merion RM, Turcotte JG, et al. Preoperative risk factor assessment in liver transplantation. *Surgery* 1992;112:704–711.

86. Bakker CM, Metselaar HJ, Groenland TN, et al. Increased fibrinolysis in orthotopic but not in heterotopic liver transplantation: the role of the anhepatic phase. *Transpl Int* 1992;5(Suppl. 1):S173–S174.

87. Bakker CM, Metselaar HJ, Gomes MJ, et al. Intravascular coagulation in liver transplantation—Is it present or not?—A comparison between orthotopic and heterotopic liver transplantation. *Thromb Haemost* 1993;69:25–28.

88. Kettner SC, Gonano C, Seebach F, et al. Endogenous heparin-like substances significantly impair coagulation in patients undergoing orthotopic liver transplantation. *Anesth Analg* 1998;86(4):691–695.

89. Legnani C, Palareti G, Rodorigo G, et al. Protease activities, as well as plasminogen activators, contribute to the "lytic" state during orthotopic liver transplantation. *Transplantation* 1993;56(3):568–572.

90. Boylan JF, Klinck JR, Sandler AN, et al. Tranexamic acid reduces blood loss, transfusion requirements, and coagulation factor use in primary orthotopic liver transplantation. *Anesthesiology* 1996;85(5):1043–1048.

91. Bayly PJM, Thick M. Reversal of post-reperfusion coagulopathy by protamine sulphate in orthotopic liver transplantation. *Br J Anaesth* 1994;73:840–842.

92. Nonthasoot B, Nivatvongs S. Multiple doses of recombinant factor VIIa in orthotopic liver transplantation: a case report. *Transplant Proc* 2003;35(1):427–428.

93. De Gasperi A, Baudo F, Sciascia A, et al. Recombinanat FVII in orthotopic liver transplantation: a way to reduce blood loss and transfusion requirements? *Haematologica* 2004;88(Suppl. 6):77–78.

94. DeLoughery TG. Coagulation defects in trauma patients: etiology, recognition, and therapy. *Crit Care Clin* 2004;201:13–24.

95. Robb WJ. Massive transfusion in trauma. [Review] [42 refs]. *AACN Clin Issues* 1999;101:69–84.

96. Lynn M, Jeroukhimov I, Klein Y, et al. Updates in the management of severe coagulopathy in trauma patients. [Review] [39 refs]. *Intensive Care Med* 2002;28(Suppl. 2):S241–S247.

97. Goodnight SH, Kenoyer G, Rapaport SI, et al. Defibrination after brain-tissue destruction: a serious complication of head injury. *N Engl J Med* 1974;290(19):1043–1047.

98. Eddy VA, Morris JA Jr, Cullinane DC. Hypothermia, coagulopathy, and acidosis. [Review] [40 refs]. *Surg Clin North Am* 2000;80(3):845–854.

99. Peng RY, Bongard FS. Hypothermia in trauma patients. *J Am Coll Surg* 1999;188(6):685–696.

100. Steinemann S, Shackford SR, Davis JW. Implications of admission hypothermia in trauma patients. *J Trauma Inj Infect Crit Care* 1990;30(2):200–202.

101. Tisherman SA. Hypothermia and injury. *Curr Opin Crit Care* 2004;10(6):512–519.

102. Rajek A, Greif R, Sessler DI, et al. Core cooling by central venous infusion of ice-cold 4 degrees C and 20 degrees C fluid: isolation of core and peripheral thermal compartments. *Anesthesiology* 2000;93(3):629–637.

103. Watts DD, Trask A, Soeken K, et al. Hypothermic coagulopathy in trauma: effect of varying levels of hypothermia on enzyme speed, platelet function, and fibrinolytic activity. *J Trauma Inj Infect Crit Care* 1998;44(5):846–854.

104. Ferrara A, MacArthur JD, Wright HK, et al. Hypothermia and acidosis worsen coagulopathy in the patient requiring massive transfusion. *Am J Surg* 1990;160(5):515–518.

105. Stone HH, Strom PR, Mullins RJ. Management of the major coagulopathy with onset during laparotomy. *Ann Surg* 1983;197(5):532–535.

106. Boffard KD. Recombinant activated factor VII rFVIIa in patients with severe trauma. 6th World Congress on Trauma, Shock, Inflammation and Sepsis. 2004. Ref Type: Abstract

107. Stein DM, Dutton RP. Uses of recombinant factor VIIa in trauma. *Curr Opin Crit Care* 2004;10(6):520–528.

108. Zettervall O, Nilsson IM. Acquired von Willebrand's disease caused by a monoclonal antibody. *Acta Med Scand* 1978;204:521.

109. Tefferi A, Nichols WL. Acquired von Willebrand disease: concise review of occurrence, diagnosis, pathogenesis, and treatment. [Review] [93 refs]. *Am J Med* 1997;103(6):536–540.

110. Jonge Poerink-Stockschlader AB, Dekker I, Risseeuw-Appel IM, et al. Acquired Von Willebrand disease in children with a Wilms' tumor. *Med Pediatr Oncol* 1996;26(4):238–243.

111. Acharya S, Bussel JB. Hematologic toxicity of sodium valproate. [Review] [31 refs]. *J Pediatr Hematol Oncol* 2000;22(1):62–65.

112. Michiels JJ, Budde U, van der PM, et al. Acquired von Willebrand syndromes: clinical features, aetiology, pathophysiology, classification and management. [Review] [148 refs]. *Best Pract Res Clin Haematol* 2001;14(2):401–436.

113. Facon T, Caron C, Courtin P, et al. Acquired type II von Willebrand's disease associated with adrenal cortical carcinoma. *Br J Haematol* 1992;80:488–494.

114. van Genderen PJ, Michiels JJ. Acquired von Willebrand disease. [Review] [54 refs]. *Baillieres Clin Haematol* 1998;11(2):319–330.

115. Federici AB. Therapeutic approaches to acquired von Willebrand syndrome. [Review] [52 refs]. *Expert Opin Investig Drugs* 2000;92:347–354.

116. Delmer A, Horellou MH, Bréchot JM, et al. Acquired von Willebrand disease: correction of hemostatic defect by high-dose intravenous immunoglobulins. *Am J Hematol* 1992;40:151–152.

117. Federici AB, Stabile F, Castaman G, et al. Treatment of acquired von Willebrand syndrome in patients with monoclonal gammopathy of uncertain significance: comparison of three different therapeutic approaches. *Blood* 1998;92(8):2707–2711.

118. Friederich PW, Wever PC, Briet E, et al. Successful treatment with recombinant factor VIIa of therapy-resistant severe bleeding in a patient with acquired von Willebrand disease. *Am J Hematol* 2001;66:292–294.

119. Baudo F, De Cataldo F, Italian Association of Haemophilia Centres AICE. Acquired factor VIII inhibitors in pregnancy: data from the Italian Haemophilia Register relevant to clinical practice. *BJOG* 2003;110(3):311–314.

120. Boggio LN, Green D. Acquired hemophilia. [Review] [99 refs]. *Rev Clin Exp Hematol* 2001;54:389–404.

121. Mostarda G, Caimi TM, Redaelli R, et al. Acquired hemophilia and its treatment. *Haematologica* 2004;88(Suppl. 6):67–71.

122. Delgado J, Jimenez-Yuste V, Hernandez-Navarro F, et al. Acquired haemophilia: review and meta-analysis focused on therapy and prognostic factors. *Br J Haematol* 2003;121(1):21–35.

123. Kessler CM. Acquired factor VIII inhibitors in the nonhemophiliac: Historical perspectives, current therapies, and future approaches. An introduction to factor VIII inhibitors: The detection and quantitation. *Am J Med* 1991;91(Suppl. 5A):5A1S–5A5S.

124. Morrison AE, Ludlam CA, Kessler C. Use of porcine factor VIII in the treatment of patients with acquired hemophilia. *Blood* 1993;81: 1513–1520.

125. Hedner U. Recombinant factor VIIa NovoSeven as a hemostatic agent. [Review] [45 refs]. *Dis Mon* 2003;49(1):39–48.

126. Schwartz RS, Gabriel DA, Aledort LM, et al. A prospective study of treatment of acquired autoimmune factor VIII inhibitors with high-dose intravenous gammaglobulin. *Blood* 1995;86:797–804.

127. Shaffer LG, Phillips MD. Successful treatment of acquired hemophilia with oral immunosuppressive therapy. [see comment] [erratum appears in Ann Intern Med 1998 Feb 15;1284:330]. *Ann Intern Med* 1997;127(3):206–209.

128. Wiestner A, Cho HJ, Asch AS, et al. Rituximab in the treatment of acquired factor VIII inhibitors. [see comment]. *Blood* 2002;100(9):3426–3428.

129. Baker WF Jr. Clinical aspects of disseminated intravascular coagulation: a clinician's point of view. [Review] [635 refs]. *Semin Thromb Hemost* 1989;15(1):1–57.

130. Carey MJ, Rodgers GM. Disseminated intravascular coagulation: clinical and laboratory aspects. *Am J Hematol* 1998;59:65–73.

131. Sharma S, Mayberry JC, DeLoughery TG, et al. Fatal cerebroembolism from nonbacterial thrombotic endocarditis in a trauma patient: case report and review. *Mil Med* 2000;165(1):83–85.

132. De Jonge E, Levi M, Stoutenbeek CP, et al. Current drug treatment strategies for disseminated intravascular coagulation. *Drugs* 1998;55:767–777.

133. Levi M, ten Cate H. Disseminated intravascular coagulation. [Review] [52 refs]. *N Engl J Med* 1999;341(8):586–592.

134. Hoffman JN, Faist E. Coagulation inhibitor replacement during sepsis: useless?. [Review] [44 refs]. *Crit Care Med* 2000;28(9)(Suppl. 1):S74–S76.

135. Rocha E, Paramo JA, Montes R, et al. Acute generalized, widespread bleeding. Diagnosis and management. [Review] [194 refs]. *Haematologica* 1998;83(11):1024–1037.

136. Callander N, Rapaport SI. Trousseau's syndrome. *West J Med* 1993;158 (4):364–371.

137. Brill-Edwards P, Ginsberg JS, Johnston M, et al. Establishing a therapeutic range for heparin therapy [see comments]. *Ann Intern Med* 1993;119(2): 104–109.

138. Olson JD, Arkin CF, Brandt JT, et al. College of American Pathologists Conference XXXI on laboratory monitoring of anticoagulant therapy: laboratory monitoring of unfractionated heparin therapy. [Review] [182 refs]. *Arch Pathol Lab Med* 1998;122(9):782–798.

139. Darmstadt GL. Acute infectious purpura fulminans: pathogenesis and medical management. [Review] [149 refs]. *Pediatr Dermatol* 1998;15(3): 169–183.

140. Spicer TE, Rau JM. Purpura fulminans. [Review] [44 refs]. *Am J Med* 1976; 61(4):566–571.

141. Josephson C, Nuss R, Jacobson L, et al. The varicella-autoantibody syndrome. *Pediatr Res* 2001;50(3):345–352.

142. Smith OP, White B. Infectious purpura fulminans: diagnosis and treatment. [Review] [50 refs]. *Br J Haematol* 1999;104(2):202–207.

143. Gamper G, Oschatz E, Herkner H, et al. Sepsis-associated purpura fulminans in adults. *Wien Klin Wochenschr* 2001;113(3–4):107–112.

144. Ward KM, Celebi JT, Gmyrek R, et al. Acute infectious purpura fulminans associated with asplenism or hyposplenism. *J Am Acad Dermatol* 2002; 47(4):493–496.

145. Childers BJ, Cobanov B. Acute infectious purpura fulminans: a 15-year retrospective review of 28 consecutive cases. *Am Surg* 2003;69(1):86–90.

146. Carpenter CT, Kaiser AB. Purpura fulminans in pneumococcal sepsis: case report and review. [Review] [41 refs]. *Scand J Infect Dis* 1997;29(5): 479–483.

147. Duncan A. New therapies for severe meningococcal disease but better outcomes? [comment] [see comments]. *Lancet* 1997;350(9091):1565–1566.

148. Smith OP, White B, Vaughan D, et al. Use of protein-C concentrate, heparin, and haemodiafiltration in meningococcus-induced purpura fulminans [see comments]. *Lancet* 1997;350(9091):1590–1593.

149. Branson HE, Katz J. A structured approach to the management of purpura fulminans. *J Natl Med Assoc* 1983;75(8):821–825.

150. Nolan J, Sinclair R. Review of management of purpura fulminans and two case reports. *Br J Anaesth* 2001;86(4):581–586.

151. Manios SG, Kanakoudi F, Maniati E. Fulminant meningococcemia. Heparin therapy and survival rate. *Scand J Infect Dis* 1971;32:127–133.

152. Mant MJ, King EG. Severe, acute disseminated intravascular coagulation. A reappraisal of its pathophysiology, clinical significance and therapy based on 47 patients. *Am J Med* 1979;67(4):557–563.

153. Corrigan JJ Jr, Jordan CM Heparin therapy in septicemia with disseminated intravascular coagulation. *N Engl J Med* 1970;283(15):778–782.

154. Giudici D, Baudo F, Palareti G, et al. Antithrombin replacement in patients with sepsis and septic shock. [Review] [54 refs]. *Haematologica* 1999; 84(5):452–460.

155. Fourrier F, Jourdain M, Tournoys A. Clinical trial results with antithrombin III in sepsis. [Review] [27 refs]. *Crit Care Med* 2000;289(Suppl. 9):S43.

156. Levi M, De Jonge E, van der Pool T, et al. Novel approaches to the management of disseminated intravascular coagulation. [Review] [37 refs]. *Crit Care Med* 2000;289(Suppl. 9):S4.

157. Rivard GE, David M, Farrell C, et al. Treatment of purpura fulminans in meningococcemia with protein C concentrate. *J Pediatr* 1995;126:646–652.

158. White B, Livingstone W, Murphy C, et al. An open-label study of the role of adjuvant hemostatic support with protein C replacement therapy in purpura fulminans-associated meningococcemia. *Blood* 2000;96(12): 3719–3724.

159. Aoki N, Matsuda T, Saito H, et al. A comparative double-blind randomized trial of activated protein C and unfractionated heparin in the treatment of disseminated intravascular coagulation. *Int J Hematol* 2002;75(5): 540–547.

160. Taylor FB, Kinasewitz G. Activated protein C in sepsis. *J Thromb Haemost* 2004;25:708–717.

161. DeLoughery TG. Management of bleeding with uremia and liver disease. [Review] [32 refs]. *Curr Opin Hematol* 1999;65:329–333.

162. Carr JM. Hemostatic disorders in liver disease. In: Schiff L, Schiff ER, eds. *Disease of the liver*. Philadelphia, PA: JB Lippincott, 1993:1061–1076.

163. Kelly DA, O'Brien FJ, Hutton RA, et al. The effect of liver disease on factors V, VIII and protein C. *Br J Haematol* 1985;61(3):541–548.

164. Spector I, Corn M. Laboratory assessment of hemostasis. The relation to hemorrhage in liver disease. *Arch Intern Med* 1967;119(6):577–582.

165. Martin TG, Somberg KA, Meng YG, et al. Thrombopoietin levels in patients with cirrhosis before and after orthotopic liver transplantation. *Ann Intern Med* 1997;127(4):285–288.

166. Peck-Radosavljevic M, Zacherl J, Meng YG, et al. Is inadequate thrombopoietin production a major cause of thrombocytopenia in cirrhosis of the liver? [Review] [90 refs]. *J Hepatol* 1997;27(1):127–131.

167. Thorsen LI, Brosstad F, Gogstad G, et al. Competitions between fibrinogen with its degradation products for interactions with the platelet-fibrinogen receptor. *Thromb Res* 1986;44(5):611–623.

168. DeLoughery TG. Management of bleeding with uremia and liver disease. *Curr Opin Hematol* 1999;65:329–333.

169. Youssef WI, Salazar F, Dasarathy S, et al. Role of fresh frozen plasma infusion in correction of coagulopathy of chronic liver disease: a dual phase study. *Am J Gastroenterol* 2003;98(6):1391–1394.

170. Roberts HR, Bingham MD. Other coagulation factor deficiencies. In: Loscalzo JL, Schafer AI, eds. *Thrombosis and Hemorrhage*, Baltimore, MD: Lippincott Williams & Wilkins, 1998:773–800.

171. Elizalde JI, Moitinho E, Garcia-Pagan JC, et al. Effects of increasing blood hemoglobin levels on systemic hemodynamics of acutely anemic cirrhotic patients. *J Hepatol* 1998;29(5):789–795.

172. Mehta AB, McIntyre N. Haematological disorders in liver disease. *Forum (Genova)* 1998;81:8–25.

173. Hu KQ, Yu AS, Tiyyagura L, et al. Hyperfibrinolytic activity in hospitalized cirrhotic patients in a referral liver unit. *Am J Gastroenterol* 2001;96 (5):1581–1586.

174. Palascak JE, Martinez J. Dysfibrinogenemia associated with liver disease. *J Clin Invest* 1977;60(1):89–95.

175. Bolan CD, Alving BM. Pharacologic agents in the management of bleeding disorders. *Transfusion* 1990;30:541–551.

176. Mannucci PM. Hemostatic drugs. [Review] [99 refs]. *N Engl J Med* 1998; 339(4):245–253.

177. Brown JB, Emerick KM, Brown DL, et al. Recombinant factor VIIa improves coagulopathy caused by liver failure. *J Pediatr Gastroenterol Nutr* 2003;37(3):268–272.

178. Caldwell SH, Chang C, Macik BG. Recombinant activated factor VII rFVIIa as a hemostatic agent in liver disease: a break from convention in need of controlled trials. *Hepatology* 2004;39(3):592–598.

179. Shami VM, Caldwell SH, Hespenheide EE, et al. Recombinant activated factor VII for coagulopathy in fulminant hepatic failure compared with conventional therapy. *Liver Transpl* 2003;92:138–143.

180. Romero-Castro R, Jimenez-Saenz M, Pellicer-Bautista F, et al. Recombinant-activated factor VII as hemostatic therapy in eight cases of severe hemorrhage from esophageal varices. *Clin Gastroenterol Hepatol* 2004;21:78–84.

181. Ejlersen E, Melsen T, Ingerslev J, et al. Recombinant activated factor VII rFVIIa acutely normalizes prothrombin time in patients with cirrhosis during bleeding from oesophageal varices. *Scand J Gastroenterol* 2001; 36(10):1081–1085.

182. Barry M. Viral hemmorrhagic fevers. *Hematology* 2000:414–423.

183. Schnittler HJ, Feldmann H. Viral hemorrhagic fever—a vascular disease? [Review] [25 refs]. *Thromb Haemost* 2003;89(6):967–972.

184. Centers for Disease Control and Prevention. Fatal illnesses associated with a new world arenavirus—California, 1999–2000. *MMWR Morb Mortal Wkly Rep* 2000;49(31):709–711.

185. Lupi O, Tyring SK. Tropical dermatology: viral tropical diseases. [Review] [179 refs]. *J Am Acad Dermatol* 2003;49(6):979–1000.

186. Casillas AM, Nyamathi AM, Sosa A, et al. A current review of Ebola virus: pathogenesis, clinical presentation, and diagnostic assessment. [Review] [29 refs]. *Biol Res Nurs* 2003;44:268–275.

187. Mollison PL, Engelfriet CP, Contreras M. Some unfavourable effects of transfusions. In: Mollison PL, Engelfriet CP, Contreras M, eds. *Blood Transfusion in Clinical Medicine*, Oxford: Blackwell Science Ltd, 1997: 487–508.

188. Jenner PW, Holland PV. Diagnosis and managment of transfusion reactions. In: Petz LD, Kleinman S, Swisher SN, et al. eds. *Clinical practice of transfusion medicine*. New York: Chuchill Livingstone, 1996:905–930.

189. Mueller-Eckhardt C. Post-transfusion purpura. *Br J Haematol* 1986;64 (3):419–424.

190. Lubenow N, Eichler P, Albrecht D, et al. Very low platelet counts in post-transfusion purpura falsely diagnosed as heparin-induced thrombocytopenia: report of four cases and review of literature. *Thromb Res* 2000; 100(3):115–125.

191. Mueller-Eckhardt C, Kiefel V. High-dose IgG for post-transfusion purpura-revisited. [Review] [19 refs]. *Blut* 1988;57(4):163–167.

192. Dan ME, Schiffer CA. Strategies for managing refractoriness to platelet transfusions. *Curr Hematol Rep* 2003;22:158–164.

193. Brand A. Alloimmune platelet refractoriness: incidence declines, unsolved problems persist. *Transfusion* 2001;41(6):724–726.

194. Schiffer CA. Diagnosis and management of refractoriness to platelet transfusion. *Blood Rev* 2001;15(4):175–180.

195. Christie DJ, van Buren N, Lennon SS, et al. Vancomycin-dependent antibodies associated with thrombocytopenia and refractoriness to platelet transfusion in patients with leukemia. *Blood* 1990;75(2):518–523.

196. Culligan DJ, Salamat A, Tait J, et al. Use of recombinant factor VIIa in life-threatening bleeding following autologous peripheral blood stem cell transplantation complicated by platelet refractoriness. *Bone Marrow Transplant* 2003;31(12):1183–1184.

197. Madoff DC, Wallace MJ, Lichtiger B, et al. Intraarterial platelet infusion for patients with intractable gastrointestinal hemorrhage and severe refractory thrombocytopenia. *J Vasc Interv Radiol* 2004;15(4): 393–397.

198. DeShazo RD, Kemp SF. Allergic reactions to drugs and biologic agents. [Review] [90 refs]. *JAMA* 1997;278(22):1895–1906.

199. Zondor SD, George JN, Medina PJ. Treatment of drug-induced thrombocytopenia. *Expert Opin Drug Saf* 2002;12:173–180.

200. Bonfiglio MF, Traeger SM, Kier KL, et al. Thrombocytopenia in intensive care patients: a comprehensive analysis of risk factors in 314 patients. *Ann Pharmacother* 1995;29(9):835–842.

201. George JN, Raskob GE, Shah SR, et al. Drug-induced thrombocytopenia: a systematic review of published case reports. *Ann Intern Med* 1998;129: 886–890.

202. Pedersen-Bjergaard U, Andersen M, Hansen PB. Drug-induced thrombocytopenia: clinical data on 309 cases and the effect of corticosteroid therapy. *Eur J Clin Pharmacol* 1997;52(3):183–189.

203. van den Bemt PM, Meyboom RH, Egberts AC. Drug-induced immune thrombocytopenia. *Drug Saf* 2004;27(15):1243–1252.

204. George JN, Shattil SJ. The clinical importance of acquired abnormalities of platelet function [see comments]. [Review] [215 refs]. *N Engl J Med* 1991;324(1):27–39.

205. Lind SE. Prolonged bleeding time. *Am J Med* 1984;77:305–312.

206. Strom BL, Berlin JA, Kinman JL, et al. Parenteral ketorolac and risk of gastrointestinal and operative site bleeding—a postmarketing surveillance study. *JAMA* 1996;275:376–382.

207. Bailey R, Sinha C, Burgess LP. Ketorolac tromethamine and hemorrhage in tonsillectomy: a prospective, randomized, double-blind study. *Laryngoscope* 1997;107(2):166–169.

208. Splinter WM, Rhine EJ, Roberts DW, et al. Preoperative ketorolac increases bleeding after tonsillectomy in children. *Can J Anaesth* 1996;43(6):560–563.

209. Brown CH III, Natelson EA, Bradshaw W, et al. The hemostatic defect produced by carbenicillin. *N Engl J Med* 1974;291(6):265–270.

210. Andrassy K, Weischedel E, Ritz E, et al. Bleeding in uremic patients after carbenicillin. *Thromb Haemost* 1976;36(1):115–126.

211. Wisloff F, Godal HC. Prolonged bleeding time with adequate platelet count in hospital patients. *Scand J Haematol* 1981;27(1):45–50.

212. Brown CH III, Natelson EA, Bradshaw MW, et al. Study of the effects of ticarcillin on blood coagulation and platelet function. *Antimicrob Agents Chemother* 1975;75:652–657.

213. Sattler FR, Weitekamp MR, Ballard JO. Potential for bleeding with the new beta-lactam antibiotics. [Review] [46 refs]. *Ann Intern Med* 1986;105(6):924–931.

214. Treib J, Haass A, Pindur G, et al. Highly substituted hydroxyethyl starch HES200/0.62 leads to Type-I von Willebrand syndrome after repeated administration. *Haemostasis* 1996;26(4):210–213.

215. Sanfelippo MJ, Suberviola PD, Geimer NF. Development of a von Willebrand-like syndrome after prolonged use of hydroxyethyl starch. *Am J Clin Pathol* 1987;88(5):653–655.

216. Livio M, Benigni A, Remuzzi G. Coagulation abnormalities in uremia. *Semin Nephrol* 1985;52:82–90.

217. Rabelink TJ, Zwaginga JJ, Koomans HA, et al. Thrombosis and hemostasis in renal disease. *Kidney Int* 1994;46:287–296.

218. Weigert AL, Schafer AI. Uremic bleeding: pathogenesis and therapy. [Review] [149 refs]. *Am J Med Sci* 1998;316(2):94–104.

219. Sagripanti A, Barsotti G. Bleeding and thrombosis in chronic uremia. *Nephron* 1997;75:125–139.

220. Farooq V, Hegarty J, Chandrasekar T, et al. Serious adverse incidents with the usage of low-molecular-weight heparins in patients with chronic kidney disease. *Am J Kidney Dis* 2004;43(3):531–537.

221. Chow SL, Zammit K, West K, et al. Correlation of antifactor Xa concentrations with renal function in patients on enoxaparin. *J Clin Pharmacol* 2003;43(6):586–590.

222. Rodgers RP, Levin J. A critical reappraisal of the bleeding time. *Semin Thromb Hemost* 1990;16(1):1–20.

223. Andrassy K, Ritz E. Uremia as a cause of bleeding. [Review] [66 refs]. *Am J Nephrol* 1985;5(5):313–319.

224. Triulzi DJ, Blumberg N. Variability in response to cryoprecipitate treatment for hemostatic defects in uremia. *Yale J Biol Med* 1990;63(1):1–7.

225. Mannucci PM. Desmopressin DDAVP in the treatment of bleeding disorders: the first 20 years. *Blood* 1997;90:2515–2521.

226. Liu YK, Kosfeld RE, Marcum SG. Treatment of uraemic bleeding with conjugated oestrogen. *Lancet* 1984;2(8408):887–890.

227. Bronner MH, Pate MB, Cunningham JT, et al. Estrogen-progesterone therapy for bleeding gastrointestinal telangiectasias in chronic renal failure. An uncontrolled trial. *Ann Intern Med* 1986;105(3):371–374.

228. Moia M, Mannucci PM, Vizzotto L, et al. Improvement in the haemostatic defect of uraemia after treatment with recombinant human erythropoietin. *Lancet* 1987;28(570):1227–1229.

229. Reiter RA, Mayr F, Blazicek H, et al. Desmopressin antagonizes the *in vitro* platelet dysfunction induced by GPIIb/IIIa inhibitors and aspirin. *Blood* 2003;102(13):4594–4599.

230. Peter FW, Benkovic C, Muehlberger T, et al. Effects of desmopressin on thrombogenesis in aspirin-induced platelet dysfunction. *Br J Haematol* 2002;117(3):658–663.

231. Flordal PA. Pharmacological prophylaxis of bleeding in surgical patients treated with aspirin. *Eur J Anaesthesiol Suppl* 1997;14:38–41.

232. Schroeder WS, Gandhi PJ. Emergency management of hemorrhagic complications in the era of glycoprotein IIb/IIIa receptor antagonists, clopidogrel, low molecular weight heparin, and third-generation fibrinolytic agents. *Curr Cardiol Rep* 2003;5(4):310–317.

233. Ibbotson T, McGavin JK, Goa KL. Abciximab: an updated review of its therapeutic use in patients with ischaemic heart disease undergoing percutaneous coronary revascularisation. *Drugs* 2003;63(11):1121–1163.

234. Li YF, Spencer FA, Becker RC. Comparative efficacy of fibrinogen and platelet supplementation on the *in vitro* reversibility of competitive glycoprotein IIb/IIIa receptor-directed platelet inhibition. *Am Heart J* 2002;143(4):725–732.

235. Voutilainen S, Lakka TA, Hamelahti P, et al. Plasma total homocysteine concentration and the risk of acute coronary events: the Kuopio Ischaemic Heart Disease Risk Factor Study. *J Intern Med* 2000;248(3):217–222.

236. McClure MW, Berkowitz SD, Sparapani R, et al. Clinical significance of thrombocytopenia during a non-ST-elevation acute coronary syndrome - the platelet glycoprotein IIb IIIa in unstable angina: receptor suppression using integrilin therapy PURSUIT trial experience. *Circulation* 1999;99(22):2892–2900.

237. Berkowitz SD, Harrington RA, Rund MM, et al. Acute profound thrombocytopenia after c7E3 Fab abciximab therapy. *Circulation* 1997;95:809–813.

238. Berkowitz SD, Sane DC, Sigmon KN, et al. Occurrence and clinical significance of thrombocytopenia in a population undergoing high-risk percutaneous coronary revascularization. *J Am Coll Cardiol* 1998;32:311–319.

239. Merlini PA, Rossi M, Menozzi A, et al. Thrombocytopenia caused by abciximab or tirofiban and its association with clinical outcome in patients undergoing coronary stenting. *Circulation* 2004;109(18):2203–2206.

240. Makris M, Watson HG. The management of coumarin-induced over-anticoagulation annotation. *Br J Haematol* 2001;114(2):271–280.

241. Taylor CT, Chester EA, Byrd DC, et al. Vitamin K to reverse excessive anticoagulation: a review of the literature. [Review] [31 refs]. *Pharmacotherapy* 1999;19(12):1415–1425.

242. Nee R, Doppenschmidt D, Donovan DJ, et al. Intravenous versus subcutaneous vitamin $K_1$ in reversing excessive oral anticoagulation. *Am J Cardiol* 1999;83(2):286–288.

243. Whiting AM, Bussey HI, Lyons RM. Comparing different routes and doses of phytonadione for reversing excessive anticoagulation. *Arch Intern Med* 1998;158(19):2136–2140.

244. Wilson SE, Watson HG, Crowther MA. Low-dose oral vitamin K therapy for the management of asymptomatic patients with elevated international normalized ratios: a brief review. *CMAJ* 2004;170(5):821–824.

245. Possidente CJ, Howe JG, Cushman M. Evaluation of very low-dose subcutaneous vitamin K during postoperative warfarin therapy. *Pharmacotherapy* 2001;21(3):295–300.

246. Hung A, Singh S, Tait RC. A prospective randomized study to determine the optimal dose of intravenous vitamin K in reversal of over-warfarinization. *Br J Haematol* 2000;109(3):537–539.

247. Riegert-Johnson DL, Volcheck GW. The incidence of anaphylaxis following intravenous phytonadione vitamin K1: a 5-year retrospective review. *Ann Allergy Asthma Immunol* 2002;89(4):400–406.

248. Watson HG, Baglin T, Laidlaw SL, et al. A comparison of the efficacy and rate of response to oral and intravenous Vitamin K in reversal of over-anticoagulation with warfarin. *Br J Haematol* 2001;115(1):145–149.

249. Shields RC, McBane RD, Kuiper JD, et al. Efficacy and safety of intravenous phytonadione vitamin K1 in patients on long-term oral anticoagulant therapy. *Mayo Clin Proc* 2001;76(3):260–266.

250. Crowther MA, Julian J, McCarty D, et al. Treatment of warfarin-associated coagulopathy with oral vitamin K: a randomised controlled trial. *Lancet* 2000;356(9241):1551–1553.

251. Levine MN, Raskob G, Landefeld S, et al. Hemorrhagic complications of anticoagulant treatment. [Review] [138 refs]. *Chest* 1998;114S(Suppl. 5):S523.

252. Penning-van Beest FJ, Rosendaal FR, Grobbee DE, et al. Course of the international Normalized Ratio in response to oral vitamin K1 in patients overanticoagulated with phenprocoumon. *Br J Haematol* 1999;104(2):241–245.

253. Wentzien TH, O'Reilly RA, Kearns PJ. Prospective evaluation of anticoagulant reversal with oral vitamin K1 while continuing warfarin therapy unchanged [see comments]. *Chest* 1998;114(6):1546–1550.

254. Raj G, Kumar R, McKinney WP. Time course of reversal of anticoagulant effect of warfarin by intravenous and subcutaneous phytonadione [erratum appears in Arch Intern Med 2000 Apr 10;1607:986]. *Arch Intern Med* 1999;159(22):2721–2724.

255. Ansell J, Hirsh J, Bussey HI, et al. Managing oral anticoagulant therapy. *Chest* 2001;119:22S–38S.

256. Levine MN, Raskob G, Landefeld S, et al. Hemorrhagic complications of anticoagulant therapy. *Chest* 2001;119:108S–121S.

257. Butler AC, Tait RC. Management of oral anticoagulant-induced intracranial haemorrhage. [Review] [79 refs]. *Blood Rev* 1998;12(1):35–44.

258. Estol CJ, Kase CS. Need for continued use of anticoagulants after intracerebral hemorrhage. *Curr Treat Options Cardiovasc Med* 2003;5(3):201–209.

259. Nitu IC, Perry DJ, Lee CA. Clinical experience with the use of clotting factor concentrates in oral anticoagulation reversal. *Clin Lab Haematol* 1998;20(6):363–367.

260. Cartmill M, Dolan G, Byrne JL, et al. Prothrombin complex concentrate for oral anticoagulant reversal in neurosurgical emergencies. *Br J Neurosurg* 2000;14(5):458–461.

261. Yasaka M, Sakata T, Minematsu K, et al. Correction of INR by prothrombin complex concentrate and vitamin K in patients with warfarin related hemorrhagic complication. *Thromb Res* 2002;108(1):25–30.

262. Taberner DA, Thomson JM, Poller L. Comparison of prothrombin complex concentrate and vitamin K1 in oral anticoagulant reversal. *Br Med J* 1976;2(6027):83–85.

263. Makris M, Greaves M, Phillips WS, et al. Emergency oral anticoagulant reversal: the relative efficacy of infusions of fresh frozen plasma and

clotting factor concentrate on correction of the coagulopathy. *Thromb Haemost* 1997;77(3):477–480.

264. Warkentin TE, Crowther MA. Reversing anticoagulants both old and new. [Review] [98 refs]. *Can J Anaesth* 2002;49(6):S11–S25.

265. Deveras RA, Kessler CM. Reversal of warfarin-induced excessive anticoagulation with recombinant human factor VIIa concentrate. [see comment] [summary for patients in Ann Intern Med. 2002 Dec 3;13711:I41; PMID: 12459002]. *Ann Intern Med* 2002;137(11):884–888.

266. Berntorp E. Recombinant FVIIa in the treatment of warfarin bleeding. [Review] [13 refs]. *Semin Thromb Hemost* 2000;26(4):433–435.

267. Carr JA, Silverman N. The heparin-protamine interaction. A review. *J Cardiovasc Surg (Torino)* 1999;40(5):659–666.

268. Monagle P, Michelson AD, Bovill E, et al. Antithrombotic therapy in children. [Review] [350 refs]. *Chest* 2001;119(Suppl. 1):S370.

269. Holst J, Lindblad B, Bergqvist D, et al. Protamine neutralization of intravenous and subcutaneous low-molecular-weight heparin tinzaparin, Logiparin. An experimental investigation in healthy volunteers. *Blood Coagul Fibrinolysis* 1994;5(5):795–803.

270. Hirsh J, Warkentin TE, Shaughnessy SG, et al. Heparin and low molecular weight heparin. *Chest* 2001;119:64S–94S.

271. Heres EK, Horrow JC, Gravlee GP, et al. A dose-determining trial of heparinase-I Neutralase for heparin neutralization in coronary artery surgery. *Anesth Analg* 2001;93(6):1446–1452 table.

272. Lisman T, Bijsterveld NR, Adelmeijer J, et al. Recombinant factor VIIa reverses the *in vitro* and *ex vivo* anticoagulant and profibrinolytic effects of fondaparinux. *J Thromb Haemost* 2003;1(11):2368–2373.

273. Kaplan KL, Francis CW. Direct thrombin inhibitors. *Semin Hematol* 2002; 39(3):187–196.

274. Weitz JI, Crowther M. Direct thrombin inhibitors. *Thromb Res* 2002; 106(3):V275–V284.

275. Gustafsson D. Oral direct thrombin inhibitors in clinical development. *J Intern Med* 2003;254(4):322–334.

276. Elg M, Carlsson S, Gustafsson D. Effect of activated prothrombin complex concentrate or recombinant factor VIIa on the bleeding time and thrombus formation during anticoagulation with a direct thrombin inhibitor. *Thromb Res* 2001;101(3):145–157.

277. Greinacher A, Lubenow N. Recombinant hirudin in clinical practice: focus on lepirudin. *Circulation* 2001;103(10):1479–1484.

278. Eichler P, Friesen HJ, Lubenow N, et al. Antihirudin antibodies in patients with heparin-induced thrombocytopenia treated with lepirudin: incidence, effects on aPTT, and clinical relevance. *Blood* 2000;96(7):2373–2378.

279. Fischer KG. Hirudin in renal insufficiency. [Review] [56 refs]. *Semin Thromb Hemost* 2002;28(5):467–482.

280. Bauersachs RM, Lindhoff-Last E, Ehrly AM, et al. Treatment of hirudin overdosage in a patient with chronic renal failure. *Thromb Haemost* 1999; 81(2):323–324.

281. Frank RD, Farber H, Stefanidis I, et al. Hirudin elimination by hemofiltration: a comparative *in vitro* study of different membranes. *Kidney Int Suppl* 1999;72:S41–S45.

282. Van de WF, Barron HV, Armstrong PW, et al. Incidence and predictors of bleeding events after fibrinolytic therapy with fibrin-specific agents: a comparison of TNK-tPA and rt-PA. *Eur Heart J* 2001;22(24):2253–2261.

283. Sloan MA, Price TR, Petito CK, et al. Clinical features and pathogenesis of intracerebral hemorrhage after rt-PA and heparin therapy for acute myocardial infarction: the thrombolysis in myocardial Infarction TIMI II pilot and randomized clinical trial combined experience. *Neurology* 1995; 45:649–658.

284. Gurwitz JH, Gore JM, Goldberg RJ, et al. Risk for intracranial hemorrhage after tissue plasminogen activator treatment for acute myocardial infarction. *Ann Intern Med* 1998;129:597–604.

285. Sloan MA, Sila CA, Mahaffey KW, et al. Prediction of 30-day mortality among patients with thrombolysis-related intracranial hemorrhage. *Circulation* 1998;98(14):1376–1382.

286. Van der Put NMJ, Eskes TKAB, Blom HJ. Is the common 677C → T mutation in the methylenetetrahydrofolate reductase gene a risk factor for neural tube defects? A meta-analysis. *Q J Med* 1997;90:111–115.

287. Brass LM, Lichtman JH, Wang Y, et al. Intracranial hemorrhage associated with thrombolytic therapy for elderly patients with acute myocardial infarction: results from the Cooperative Cardiovascular Project. *Stroke* 2000;31(8):1802–1811.

288. Patel SC, Mody A. Cerebral hemorrhagic complications of thrombolytic therapy. *Prog Cardiovasc Dis* 1999;42(3):217–233.

289. Dalen JE, Alpert JS, Hirsh J. Thrombolytic therapy for pulmonary embolism - Is it effective? Is it safe? When is it indicated. *Arch Intern Med* 1997;157:2550–2556.

290. Mikkola KM, Patel SR, Parker JA, et al. Increasing age is a major risk factor for hemorrhagic complications after pulmonary embolism thrombolysis. *Am Heart J* 1997;134:69–72.

291. Graham GD. Tissue plasminogen activator for acute ischemic stroke in clinical practice: a meta-analysis of safety data. *Stroke* 2003;34(12): 2847–2850.

292. Donat F, Duret JP, Santoni A, et al. The pharmacokinetics of fondaparinux sodium in healthy volunteers. *Clin Pharmacokinet* 2002;41(Suppl. 2): 1–9.

293. Mehta SR, Eikelboom JW, Yusuf S. Risk of intracranial haemorrhage with bolus versus infusion thrombolytic therapy: a meta-analysis.[comment]. *Lancet* 2000;356(9228):449–454.

294. Sane DC, Califf RM, Topol EJ, et al. Bleeding during thrombolytic therapy for acute myocardial infeaction: mechanism and management. *Ann Intern Med* 1989;111:1010–1022.

# CHAPTER 79 ■ THERAPY WITH ANTIFIBRINOLYTIC AGENTS

DAPHNE STEWART AND VICTOR J. MARDER

The innate mechanism to reestablish hemostasis after a vessel is severed is the formation of a stable platelet–fibrin plug at the site of injury (see Table 79-1). Simultaneously, processes to moderate hemostasis are activated in order to prevent thrombosis in the adjacent lumen, to repair the injury, and subsequently, to reestablish normal blood flow. To a large extent, this moderation is accomplished through fibrinolysis—the localized activation of the plasminogen–plasmin proteolytic enzyme system, which is a finely tuned interaction among endothelial cells, plasma proteins, and the platelets and fibrin fibers of the hemostatic plug. Just as plasma protein inhibitors such as antithrombin III locally contain the hemostatic process by inactivating circulating coagulation enzymes, there are circulating plasma inhibitors of fibrinolysis, such as plasminogen activator inhibitors, $\alpha_2$-plasmin inhibitor, and $\alpha_2$-macroglobulin, which contain the fibrinolytic reaction at the injured site. This complex, local system, balancing hemostatic, fibrinolytic, and inhibitory forces, allows hemostasis and healing to occur without compromising recovery of the injured tissue or perturbing systemic hemostasis.

The fibrinolytic enzyme system is critical in modulating pro- and antihemostatic or antithrombotic forces. Its importance is underscored by the observations that constitutional abnormalities in plasminogen (1–3), plasminogen activators (4) or their release (5), are associated with an increased risk for thrombosis, whereas defects in plasminogen activator inhibitors (6), $\alpha_2$-plasmin inhibitor (7), or impaired clearance rates for native released plasminogen activators, are associated with an increased bleeding risk (see Chapter 18). Perhaps misnamed to imply a specific, limited function, the fibrinolytic enzyme system has a much broader role than the dissolution of fibrin. Beyond binding to fibrin, plasminogen is also bound to the platelet membrane (8), the surface of the endothelium (9), and the interplatelet matrix that forms during the process of aggregation (10). Wherever plasminogen binds, there also are binding sites for native plasminogen activators (11–14). Plasmin formed at these different sites can degrade a variety of substrates other than fibrin, including substrates involved in platelet adhesion [glycoprotein (GP) I (15) and von Willebrand factor (15–17)] platelet aggregation [GP IIb/IIIa complex (18) and fibrinogen (19)], maintenance of a stable platelet aggregate [thrombospondin, fibronectin, fibrinogen, fibrin, histidine-rich glycoprotein (10,19)], and the attachment of platelets and fibrin to the endothelial surface (20). Although the fibrinolytic system has a much broader physiologic role as the body's major endogenous proteolytic enzyme system, this chapter focuses on agents that inhibit the fibrinolytic system to the end of preventing dissolution of fibrin and promoting hemostasis.

Hemostasis is initiated by the formation of complexes between tissue factor (TF) and activated factor VIIa, making up approximately 1% of the circulating factor VII pool (21,22). These complexes may also form extravascularly within interstitial fluid (23,24). TF–VIIa complexes activate factor X and result in thrombin generation on TF-bearing cell surfaces. This generated thrombin activates factors VIII and V, and stimulates platelets to expose phosphatidyl serine, leading to further thrombin generation. The formation of a stable fibrin plug is dependent on a maximal thrombin "burst" (25), which allows for activation of factor XIII and adequate cross-linking of fibrin polymers. Simultaneously, the fibrinolytic potential at the site of the thrombin burst is attenuated by thrombin-mediated activation of the "thrombin-activatable fibrinolytic inhibitor" (TAFI) (26). TAFI is a carboxypeptidase that cleaves plasminogen-binding sites from fibrin strands (27), eliminating the accumulation of plasminogen on the surface of the clot. Additionally, TAFI inhibits the activation of glu-plasminogen to the more fibrin-avid lys-plasminogen during fibrin degradation. Large quantities of thrombin are necessary to effect TAFI activation; however, when thrombomodulin is present, much smaller quantities of thrombin are sufficient. By reduced TAFI generation, any defect that impairs thrombin generation may have a profibrinolytic effect (28).

Hemostasis is balanced by fibrinolysis, mediated by the serine protease enzyme plasmin. Descriptions of the enzymatic conversion of plasminogen to plasmin are presented in Chapters 18 and 23. The inactive plasma precursor molecule plasminogen may be converted to its proteolytic derivative plasmin after a single cleavage of its heavy chain at Arg560–Val561 by (29) plasminogen activators. Once generated, trace amounts of plasmin liberate an amino-terminal 76-residue portion of plasminogen (30), coverting glu-plasminogen to lys-plasminogen and producing a dramatic conformational change. Lys-plasminogen binds more efficiently to fibrin (31), is more sensitive to activator action (32,33) [both for tissue-type plasminogen activator (tPA) (34) and for urokinase-type activator (35)], and promotes further conversion of plasminogen to plasmin (36,37).

Plasminogen binding to fibrin during clot formation promotes easy activation to plasmin by protecting the molecule from inactivation by its natural inhibitors and positioning the molecule for efficient digestion of the fibrin substrate (38). There are important regulating influences in order to prevent an uncontrolled plasma fibrinolytic response to injury. First, plasminogen activation in the fluid phase is much less efficient than when bound to fibrin by its lysine binding sites on the kringle domain of the heavy A chain (39,40). Second, circulating plasminogen activator is inhibited by plasminogen activator inhibitors. Third, $\alpha_2$-antiplasmin rapidly inactivates plasmin in solution by avidly binding to the catalytic pocket in the light B chain (41).

The antifibrinolytic agents are best viewed as prohemostatic drugs that act in two situations. The first is to prevent bleeding caused by excessive local or systemic fibrinolytic activity. Bleeding due to excessive local fibrinolysis in the setting of normal hemostatic mechanisms may be seen in primary menorrhagia.

SCHEMA OF BODY'S HEMOSTATIC RESPONSE TO VASCULAR INJURY AND EFFECT
OF IMBALANCES BETWEEN HEMOSTASIS AND FIBRINOLYSIS

| | Injury incurred | Hemostasis | Fibrinolysis | Effect |
|---|---|---|---|---|
| Physiologic response | Platelet adhesion and aggregation, primary hemostatic plug formation → | Fibrin generation, platelet plug reinforced → | Delayed clot resolution → | No bleeding, vessel patency reestablished |
| Bleeding tendency Abnormal hemostasis, normal fibrinolysis | Delayed hemostatic plug formation OR | Inadequate plug reinforcement → | Normal rate of clot resolution → | Prolonged primary bleeding, late rebleeding |
| Normal hemostasis, excessive fibrinolysis | Normal primary hemostatic plug formation → | Fibrin generation, platelet plug reinforced → | Accelerated fibrinolysis of plug → | Delayed bleeding |

The clinical findings of high liquidity of menstrual blood and prolonged duration of bleeding are secondary to an exaggeration of the physiologic fibrinolytic response (42,43). The second situation is to slow down the physiologic fibrinolysis that follows abnormal hemostasis caused by low or dysfunctional platelets, or a coagulation defect. When hemostasis is impaired, the imbalance created by an abnormally slow rate of hemostasis and a normal rate of fibrinolysis culminates in delayed bleeding. This situation may occur in the setting of a hemophiliac after an injury in which bleeding ceases spontaneously, then recurs 24 to 48 hours later as the result of dissolution of the weakened hemostatic plug (44,45). Because thrombin-dependent inhibition of lysis is impaired, lysis of clots in hemophilic plasma is premature, as reported by Broze and Higuchi (28).

Antifibrinolytic agents may improve hemostasis in a wide variety of bleeding states. Among their most useful properties are their ready distribution throughout the body following oral or intravenous administration and their potent inhibition of plasmin. Unlike 1-deamino-8-D-arginine vasopressin (DDAVP), another useful prohemostatic adjunct, the antifibrinolytic agents are not prone to tachyphylaxis. When used appropriately to diminish an exuberant fibrinolytic response, these agents do not result in an activation of coagulation. As seen in patients treated with ε-aminocaproic acid (EACA) or placebo before, during, and after cardiac surgery, inhibition of fibrinolysis was reflected by a lower D-dimer in the treated patients, whereas levels of thrombin–antithrombin complexes or soluble fibrin were unchanged (46). However, given their ability to inhibit systemic fibrinolysis, these agents also have the potential to be prothrombotic. This complication may be seen in patients with an unrecognized systemic hypercoagulable state such as disseminated intravascular coagulation (DIC), in which removal of the physiologic secondary fibrinolysis could aggravate the primary hypercoagulable state (see Chapter 109). In addition, conversion of a bleeding to a clotting state may occur at primary sites, for example, the formation of ureteral clots following antifibrinolytic treatment of hematuria.

Given the risk of tipping the balance in favor of thrombosis, there are three distinct clinical situations in which antifibrinolytic therapy should be most useful: (i) states of systemic hyperfibrinolysis (e.g., following treatment with plasminogen activators, or states of spontaneous, sustained increases in circulating plasminogen activator or plasmin activity), (ii) in patients with a decreased potential for hemostatic plug formation (e.g., hemophilia), and (iii) localized, uncontrolled bleeding that

shows neither decreased hemostatic plug formation nor increased systemic fibrinolysis (e.g., gastric erosions) (47–50).

# MODE OF ACTION OF ANTIFIBRINOLYTIC AGENTS

## Agents Available for Clinical Use

The antifibrinolytic agents fall into three categories:

1. The natural plasma inhibitors of plasmin and of plasminogen activators (51,52), which are not the subject of this chapter (see Chapters 18 and 19).
2. Aprotinin (Trasylol, or bovine pancreatic trypsin inhibitor, BPTI), a 58-residue polypeptide ($M_r = 6,500$) isolated from bovine lung, parotid gland, and, originally, pancreas (53), is a dose-dependent inhibitor of plasmin (50) and at higher concentrations inhibits other serine proteases such as trypsin, kallikreins, and chymotrypsin (47,49,50). Aprotinin has been studied for its antifibrinolytic effects in a number of bleeding states and is available for clinical use in the United States as an intravenous injection. It is also valuable as a laboratory tool to prevent *in vitro* plasminogen activation or plasmin action after collection of blood specimens, especially in the setting of enhanced fibrinolytic activity.
3. The synthetic lysine analogues, such as *trans-p*-aminomethyl-cyclohexane carboxylic acid (AMCA, or tranexamic acid) and 6-aminohexanoic acid (EACA) are effective fibrinolytic inhibitors (54,55). Okamoto (56,57) is responsible for describing the inhibitory action of these compounds and for systematically assessing many related synthetic compounds.

## Biochemistry

Aprotinin is a nonspecific serine protease inhibitor of the Kunitz family. Its active residue, 15-lysine, binds reversibly to its target's catalytic site and inhibits numerous serine proteases, including trypsin, plasmin, chymotrypsin, kallikrein, elastase, urokinase, and thrombin, over a range of concentrations (50). *In vivo*, it binds directly to plasmin at a lower dose [plasma concentration

137 kallikrein inhibitor units (KIU) per mL], whereas it binds to kallikrein at a higher plasma concentration (>250 KIU per mL). Its inhibition of both the direct fibrinolytic effector enzyme and an early activator of the fibrinolytic cascade makes it an especially effective therapeutic agent. However, given its higher affinity for plasmin, aprotinin's clinical, hemostatic effect is most likely predominantly the result of its plasmin inhibition. Aprotinin binds to plasmin in a manner analogous to plasmin's fibrin substrate, however, unlike plasmin's fibrin substrate, aprotinin is not hydrolyzed. Side chain Lys15 of aprotinin binds to the aspartate side chain in the specificity pocket of plasmin (see Fig. 79-1). In addition, there are many hydrogen bonds between plasmin and aprotinin, as in an antiparallel β-sheet, increasing the stability of the complex. It is an important inhibitor of plasmin in the presence of fibrin clot (51), as well as compounds that reduce plasmin's catalytic activity by binding to its kringle domains (58). Kringle-binding compounds, which interfere with $\alpha_2$-antiplasmin or $\alpha_2$-macroglobulin-mediated plasmin inhibition, do not affect aprotinin's inhibition of plasmin (51). In addition, aprotinin blocks activation of PAR-1 (protease activated receptor-1) on platelets, preventing thrombin-induced platelet aggregation, thought to be particularly important in the platelet

dysfunction acquired during exposure to cardiopulmonary bypass circuits and its associated bleeding (59). Aprotinin inhibits the inflammatory cascade at multiple levels, protects against kallikrein-induced generation of bradykinin, decreases neutrophil degranulation and extravasation at inflammatory sites, decreases expression of proinflammatory glycoproteins (CD11b) on neutrophils, and attenuates complement generation (60,61).

In contrast, the lysine analogs (AMCA and EACA) prevent excessive plasmin formation by occupying plasminogen's lysine-binding site for fibrin and precluding plasminogen localization to the fibrin clot for activation by plasminogen activators. Lysine analogs may interact with fibrin directly, and also bind tPA kringles, interfering with plasminogen activation (51,54). Fibrinolysis is thereby prevented; however, plasmin itself may still be generated. *In vitro*, these aminocarboxylic acids bind to the lysine binding sites of the plasminogen molecule, resulting in a conformational change in plasminogen (52,54,55,65). Under most experimental conditions *in vitro*, plasminogen activation, paradoxically, is accelerated, and binding to plasmin kringles reduces the binding by major plasmin inhibitors $\alpha_2$-antiplasmin and $\alpha_2$-macroglobulin (66,67). Yet, the major action of these

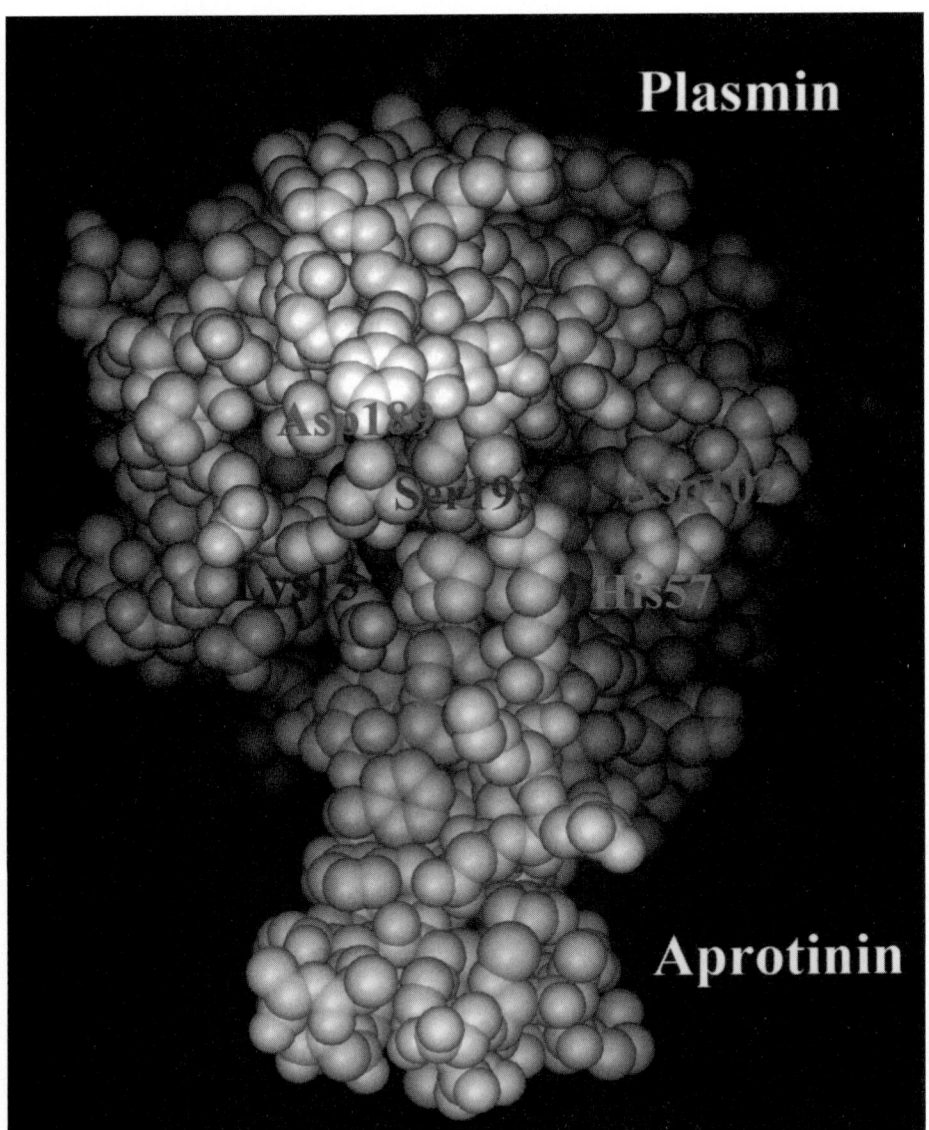

**FIGURE 79-1.** Modeled complex of the interaction between Aprotinin and plasmin's protease domain. The plasmin active site triads residues—His57(603), Asp102(646), and Ser195(741) are shown. Lys15 (shown in *blue*) of aprotinin inserts into the active site of the enzyme, forming a salt bridge with Asp189(736) (shown in *red*) at the base of the active site. The plasmin structure of plasmin is from Wang et al. (62) and that of aprotinin from (63). The model was built using the methodology by Bajaj et al. (64) (see Color Fig. 79-1).

compounds *in vivo* is antifibrinolytic, inhibiting association between plasmin(ogen), tPA, and fibrin (68,69).

The seemingly disparate effects may be explained by the two-step process required for binding of plasminogen to fibrin, as demonstrated schematically in Figure 79-2. Normally, plasminogen is activated by a well-placed proteolytic cleavage that exposes the serine-histidine catalytic site, converting glu-plasminogen to lys-plasminogen. This cleavage promotes binding to a fibrin or fibrinogen substrate (70) by a lock-and-key fit between one or more lysine-binding sites on plasminogen and specific lysine residues of the substrate. Without proper binding, proteolysis cannot proceed. This two-step requirement explains the seeming discrepancy of *in vivo* inhibition (69,71–76) and *in vitro* activation (55,65–78). *In vitro*, EACA and AMCA accelerate plasminogen activation by altering plasminogen's conformation and making it more susceptible to proteolytic action by activators. This is much like the self-accelerating effect produced by the plasmin-mediated conversion of glu-plasminogen to lys-plasminogen. However, lysis of a fibrin substrate is inhibited by the lysine analogs because the same binding phenomenon also blocks functional activity by occupying the lysine-binding site. Therefore, any plasmin molecule that forms, no matter how rapidly, cannot bind effectively to the fibrin substrate, thereby precluding proteolytic action by the serine enzyme site.

EACA and AMCA are structurally similar to lysine and therefore capable of steric inhibition between fibrin(ogen) lysine residues and plasmin(ogen)'s lysine-binding sites. Thorsen was the first to suggest that the antifibrinolytic effect of EACA and AMCA was due to dissociation of lys-plasminogen from fibrin (79), a mechanism later confirmed by Petersen and Suenson (80). The latter showed that the lys-plasminogen binding to fibrin involves the lysine-binding site with the highest affinity for AMCA, probably located on Kringle 1 (81), as supported by

previous studies (82). Subtle differences in the synthetic analogs markedly affect their inhibitory potential, as exemplified by the approximately sixfold to 10-fold higher molar potency of AMCA in comparison with EACA (83) and the ineffectiveness of the *cis* form of AMCA in comparison with the *trans* form (83). Other active analogs of lysine, which have been studied less intensively, include *p*-amino methylbenzoic acid (PAMBA) and 4-amino ethylbicyclo-[2.2.2]-octane-1-carboxylic acid (AMBOCA), which are five- to 10-fold and 100-fold, respectively, more potent than EACA (84). α-N-acetyl-L-lysine methyl ester (NALME) is a lysine analog, which, unlike EACA and AMCA, competitively inhibits plasmin amidase activity (85).

*In vitro* studies of the mechanisms of aprotinin and the lysine analogs demonstrate distinct mechanisms of action, and when tested together at low aprotinin doses, their effects are synergistic (51). However, there has been no clinical study of the combination of antifibrinolytic agents.

## Pharmacology

Aprotinin must be administered parenterally. After drug administration, it is rapidly distributed within the extravascular space. Following its distribution phase, aprotinin's plasma half-life is approximately 150 minutes, and its terminal half-life is 5 to 10 hours. Although aprotinin is filtered in the kidney, it is primarily reabsorbed in the proximal tubules, with only approximately 10% excreted unchanged in the urine. Ultimately, the drug is taken up by tubular endothelium, stored in phagolysosomes, and slowly degraded by lysosomal enzymes (53).

Aprotinin dosing is measured as KIU, or the amount of aprotinin to decrease 2 biologic units of kallikrein activity by 50%. Two dosages have been determined through clinical use during cardiopulmonary bypass operations, known as the *full kallikrein inhibitory* dose, and the *half plasmin inhibitory* dose (50). The full kallikrein dose is a $2 \times 10^6$ KIU loading dose given over 20 to 30 minutes, $2 \times 10^6$ KIU into pump prime volume, followed by continuous infusion of $5 \times 10^5$ KIU per hour, to achieve mean plasma level of 250 KIU per mL. The half plasmin inhibitory dose to achieve plasma levels of 137 KIU per mL consists of $1 \times 10^6$ KIU loading dose over 20 to 30 minutes, $1 \times 10^6$ KIU into pump prime volume, followed by $2.5 \times 10^5$ KIU per hour. Clinically significant decreases in surgical blood loss and transfusion requirements are closely correlated with higher doses, as demonstrated by placebo-controlled trials comparing pump prime only with low- and high-dose regimens in cardiac and orthopedic surgeries (86–89). Because aprotinin is associated with risk for anaphylaxis, a test dose of 10,000 KIU must be given to exclude hypersensitivity at least 10 minutes prior to the loading dose (53).

EACA and AMCA are rapidly absorbed from the gastrointestinal (GI) tract, allowing oral or intravenous administration (90–92). Peak plasma levels are seen 1 to 2 hours after oral dosing. Elimination is primarily via renal excretion and metabolism; approximately 65% of an administered dose is excreted in the urine unchanged, and 10% appears as an inactive metabolite, adipic acid. Approximately 85% of an intravenous dose is cleared within 3 hours, but because EACA penetrates the entire extravascular space, urinary excretion may be detected 12 to 36 hours after an intravenous dose (91).

The recommended dose for EACA has been derived from *in vitro* studies and shown to be effective for the treatment of hyperfibrinolytic states; however, the minimal dose required to inhibit normal or enhanced local fibrinolysis is not known. EACA is usually administered as an intravenous priming dose of 0.1 g per kg over 20 to 30 minutes, followed by a continuous infusion of 0.5 to 1 g per hour or an equivalent intermittent dose

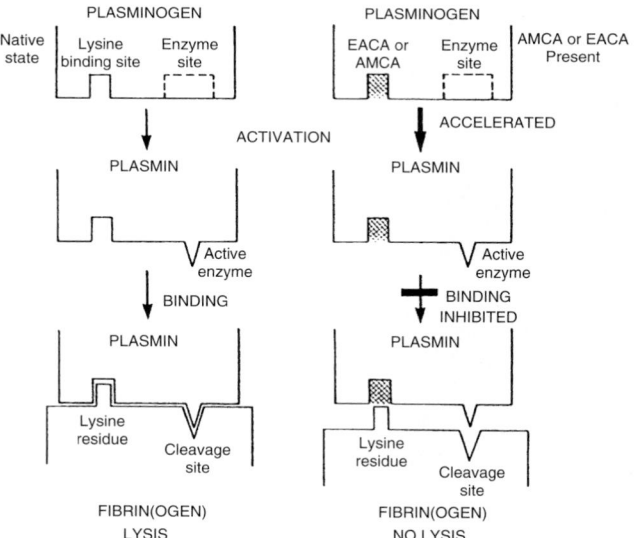

**FIGURE 79-2.** Schematic diagram of the *in vitro* mode of action of synthetic lysine analogs on plasminogen activation and plasmin proteolysis of fibrin(ogen). ε-aminocaproic acid (EACA) and *trans-p*-aminomethyl-cyclohexane carbolyxic acid (AMCA) accelerate plasminogen activation by inducing a conformational change in the molecule; however, they inhibit fibrinolysis by blocking the lysine binding site necessary for the binding of plasmin(ogen) to its substrate. Therefore, even though plasmin may be rapidly formed, it cannot reach the fibrin substrate because its binding site is occupied by the synthetic inhibitor. The accelerated activation as shown in the figure is from the *in vitro* experiments; it remains to be demonstrated *in vivo*.

every 1, 2, or 4 hours, generally until acute bleeding is controlled (75). Alternative oral dosing consists of 5 g the first hour, followed by 1 g per hour until bleeding is controlled. Plasma levels of at least 0.001 M (13 mg per 100 mL) are adequate to inhibit *in vivo* fibrinolysis (69,73,83,93). Urinary concentration is generally 75- to 100-fold higher than plasma (91); therefore, much lower doses may be used to control urinary tract bleeding (3 g EACA per day). As renal clearance approximates endogenous creatinine clearance (90), patients with renal insufficiency should have their doses reduced according to creatinine clearance.

The serum half-life of AMCA is similar to EACA, 1 to 2 hours, and it is also rapidly excreted unchanged in the urine, more than 90% in 24 hours (92,94). Compared with EACA, AMCA is much more potent, inhibiting fibrinolysis at much lower plasma concentrations; therefore, its inhibitory effect lasts for 7 to 8 hours. The oral recommended dose is 25 mg per kg, three times daily. Intravenous infusion is delivered at a dose of 10 mg per kg, three times per day, or if used for surgical prophylaxis of bleeding, 10 mg per kg loading dose followed by continuous infusion of 1 mg/kg/hour. Although studies in aprotinin have demonstrated a clear dose-response curve with regard to reduction in fibrinolytic bleeding, assessment of a dose response among lysine analogs is limited by a lack of randomized, placebo-controlled trials (95). However, pooling data from trials utilizing different dosing schedules is not supportive of a benefit to higher dosing.

## Side Effects and Complications

All of the commercially available antifibrinolytic agents are generally well tolerated, although each is associated with well-known as well as theoretical side effects. Aprotinin, a bovine-derived protein, is associated with hypersensitivity reactions, including skin eruption, pruritus, dyspnea, and fatal anaphylactic shock, in 0.3% to 0.6% of treated patients (95). Although exceedingly rare with first exposure, the incidence of anaphylaxis may be as high as 2.5% upon second exposure, with the incidence in the subgroup undergoing retreatment within 3 to 6 months as high as 5% (96). The incidence of anaphylaxis following retreatment longer than 6 months from first exposure fell to 0.9%. The manufacturer's guidelines strictly advise a pretreatment test dose to exclude those at risk for hypersensitivity. Among those patients requiring cardiac surgery within 6 months of previous treatment with aprotinin, efforts to decrease incidence of anaphylactic shock (pretreatment with antihistamines, steroids, and administration of test dose following opening of sternum to facilitate rapid transition to bypass in case of emergency) have not proven effective. Additional well-known side effects of aprotinin include vasodilation, generally transient and preventable with slow drug administration, and prolongation of the partial thromboplastin time (PTT) and activated clotting time (ACT) due to its inhibition of the intrinsic clotting cascade.

Both EACA and AMCA are associated with nasal stuffiness, conjunctival suffusion, and skin rash, and dose-related GI discomfort, including nausea, vomiting, and diarrhea, occur in 30% of patients treated orally (75,92). EACA treatment has been associated with reported cases of myopathy. A literature review (97) found 33 cases of clinically significant myopathy between 1972 and 1995. The review suggested that this complication was associated with prolonged administration of high doses of EACA (16 to 36 g per day for more than 28 days) and that patients recovered after discontinuing the medication.

The association of antifibrinolytic therapy with the development of thromboembolic events, including acute myocardial infarction and DIC, is still debated. Serious systemic thrombotic complications have been reported following the use of antifibrinolytic therapy, although these complications are unlikely to occur unless there is an ongoing or transient thrombogenic stimulus (e.g., a patient with masked DIC or one with a localized, pathologic lesion as seen in Kasabach-Merritt syndrome, or a patient during surgery with extensive clotting due to tissue trauma with impaired normal breakdown). A small number of case reports of devastating, systemic thrombotic episodes following antifibrinolytic therapy may be found in the literature (97–105) and generally are associated with conditions predisposing to coagulopathy (surgery for prostate carcinoma, septic abortion, acute promyelocytic leukemia, or all-*trans*-retinoic acid therapy). Central venous catheter thrombosis may occur more commonly following antifibrinolytic therapy (106–109), possibly because of the absence of an endothelial lining capable of generating adequate local tPA to counterbalance the effect of antifibrinolytic therapy (97).

In spite of these associations, clinical trials exploring the use of antifibrinolytic therapy for various clinical indications have not borne out an increased risk for systemic thrombotic events. Five studies evaluating cardiac graft patency after cardiopulmonary bypass grafting surgery, comparing aprotinin-treated patients with controls, included more than 1,300 patients and demonstrated no increased rate of graft occlusion among those treated with aprotinin (110–114). In the Cochrane Systematic Review, aprotinin treatment did not affect the incidence of myocardial infarction and may have been associated with a reduction in incidence of stroke following cardiac surgery (115). Also reported by the same database review, there was no association between treatment with AMCA and an increased risk for thromboembolic events.

Further, antifibrinolytic agents do not incite *de novo* venous thrombus formation. A metaanalysis analyzing the use of AMCA in patients undergoing major joint replacement surgeries showed no increased risk of venous thromboses in treated patients (89). A randomized, double-blind study after prostate surgery demonstrated a similar incidence in venous thromboses in EACA-treated patients (16 of 259) and controls (17 of 256) (116). A study of patients treated with EACA during prostatectomy examining the endpoint of incidence of deep vein thrombosis (DVT) using venography failed to demonstrate any increased incidence of DVT versus control (117).

Thrombosis following antifibrinolytic therapy for upper genitourinary bleeding, a situation common in hemophilia and the hemoglobinopathies, occurs when the clot-dissolving action of urokinase is neutralized by the fibrinolytic inhibitor generating lysis-resistant clots in the renal pelvis (118–121). Antifibrinolytic therapy for urinary tract bleeding in the hemophilias is more likely to lead to high-grade urinary tract obstruction than when used in other patients because of the concomitant administration of plasma concentrates that accelerate clotting (122). Such therapy is best reserved for use in cases of excessive, protracted bleeding in those for whom surgical intervention is contemplated. An unusual case of left renal pelvis obstruction in a patient with renal adenocarcinoma treated with EACA for prolonged hematuria resolved successfully after ureteral delivery of low-dose streptokinase (123).

Lysine analogs have been used successfully to treat postpartum hemorrhage and hemorrhage associated with *abruptio placentae*. Because pregnancy depresses the endogenous fibrinolytic system, pregnant women could be suspected to be a high risk for thrombotic complications following use of antifibrinolytic therapy. However, a retrospective analysis of 2,102 pregnant women showed two of 256 AMCA-treated patients versus four of 1,846 matched controls developed thrombotic complications (124), and the authors concluded there was no thrombogenic effect of AMCA in this high-risk group.

# CLINICAL APPLICATION

Table 79-2 provides a summary of the use of antifibrinolytic therapy for bleeding states and their clinical associations.

## Management of Fibrinolytic Hemorrhage

Hemorrhage is promoted by fibrinolysis when there is an improper balance between hemostatic and antihemostatic forces. Indications for antifibrinolytic therapy include hemorrhage in the setting of (a) systemic states of increased fibrinolysis, (b) defective hemostasis in the presence of normally active fibrinolysis, and (c) enhanced local fibrinolysis in the presence of a normal hemostatic mechanism. Additionally, antifibrinolytic therapy has been increasingly employed during elective surgery as hemostatic agents to reduce blood loss and allogeneic transfusion requirements.

### Systemic Hyperfibrin(ogen)olysis

Many pathologic states may generate hyperplasminemia through the release of endothelial stores of plasminogen activator in

## TABLE 79-2

### CLINICAL APPLICATION OF ANTIFIBRINOLYTIC THERAPY

| Bleeding state | Clinical association | Use of antifibrinolytic therapy | Comment |
|---|---|---|---|
| Systemic hyperfibrinolysis | Spontaneous bleeding | Uncommon, because hyperfibrinolytic state usually self-limited | If DIC present, antifibrinolytic therapy is contraindicated |
| | Cardiac surgery/ cardiopulmonary bypass | Prophylactic administration indicated, particularly when high transfusion requirements anticipated, for example, repeat sternotomy, prolonged pump time, preoperative aspirin use | Aprotinin proven in randomized, placebo-controlled trials to decrease perioperative blood loss and red blood cell transfusion requirements; AMCA/EACA reduce blood loss; however, no clear benefit toward reducing transfusion requirements |
| | Liver transplant | Prophylaxis indicated prior to graft reperfusion to control commonly encountered intraoperative "oozing," and reduce overall perioperative bleeding complications and transfusion requirements | Adults with hepatocellular dysfunction more prone to hyperfibrinolytic bleeding state; case reports of thrombotic events suggest use may be best guided by coagulation testing; aprotinin and lysine analogs likely equivalent in efficacy |
| | Therapeutic (e.g., following thrombolysis) | Uncommon, usually unnecessary | Potentially useful if bleeding occurs during or just after therapy |
| | Congenital antiplasmin deficiency | Lysine analogs indicated | Chronic administration controls lifelong bleeding state |
| | Acquired antiplasmin deficiency | Lysine analogs indicated to control acute bleeding | Condition seen with acute promyelocytic leukemia, systemic amyloidosis |
| Defective hemostasis, followed by normal fibrinolysis | Hemophilia, von Willebrand disease | Indicated to control mucosal bleeding and as adjunctive prohemostatic treatment postoperatively | Reduces blood loss and use of factor concentrates after dental extraction, synovectomy, joint replacement; likely useful in all postoperative settings |
| | Chronic anticoagulation | Indicated to prevent interruption of therapeutic anticoagulation during dental extraction | Has potential use in management of minor bleeding complications in chronically anticoagulated patients |
| | Quantitative/Qualitative platelet dysfunction | Indicated for acute bleeding episodes to reduce platelet transfusions | Less effective if platelet count less than $10,000/\mu L$ (inadequate or absent hemostatic plug formation) |
| Enhanced local fibrinolysis | Genitourinary bleeding, upper urinary tract | Indicated for essential hematuria, renal disease postbiopsy, prolonged, spontaneous hematuria in sickle cell disease or hemophilias | Risk for obstructive clot formation in hemophiliacs treated simultaneously with factor replacement; |

*(continued)*

**TABLE 79-2**

CONTINUED

| Bleeding state | Clinical association | Use of antifibrinolytic therapy | Comment |
|---|---|---|---|
| | Lower urinary tract | Indicated for patients undergoing prostatectomy with excessive intraoperative or postoperative bleeding | Studies with lysine analogs demonstrate reduced blood loss, no effect on transfusion rate; no benefit shown for aprotinin |
| | Dysfunctional uterine bleeding | Indicated for treatment of essential menorrhagia or menorrhagia in patients with underlying bleeding disorder | Underlying pathology must be excluded; menorrhagia associated with IUD use or following cervical conization also decreased with lysine analogs |
| | Subarachnoid hemorrhage | Reduces incidence of rebleeding, but currently, antifibrinolytic treatment not indicated | Treatment associated with higher rate of vasospasm and focal ischemic events, negating mortality benefit from decreased rebleeding |
| | Gastrointestinal bleeding<br>Upper: varices, gastritis, ulcers | Indicated to treat acute bleeding episodes | Benefit from decreased rate of rebleeding, need for surgical intervention, and mortality |
| | Lower: inflammatory bowel disease | May reduce blood loss from lesions unresponsive to other therapies | No effect on underlying disease process; increased local fibrinolysis is a variable finding |
| | Traumatic hyphema | Indicated in patients with high risk for bleeding (e.g., aspirin use) | Lysine analogs decrease rate of rebleeding without affecting rate of vision improvement |
| | Mucous membranes | Indicated for recurrent epistaxis; may be useful for excessive bleeding following tonsillectomy | May be given orally, or topically as packing component |
| Blood conservation strategies | Orthopedic surgery | Indicated to reduce blood loss in procedures anticipating high volume blood loss | High-dose aprotinin proven to reduce transfusions in primary or revision arthroplasty and oncologic surgery; prophylactic AMCA reduces transfusion rate in hip or knee arthroplasty |

DIC, disseminated intravascular coagulation; AMCA, *trans-p*-aminomethyl-cyclohexane carboxylic acid; EACA, ε-aminocaproic acid; IUD, intrauterine device.

sufficient quantities to overcome natural inhibitors and convert circulating plasminogen to plasmin (see Chapter 22). Plasmin, in turn, degrades fibrinogen and fibrin, and previously hemostatic sites or newly traumatized sites are prone to bleed. Acute conditions including heat stroke, hypoxia, hypotension, cardiothoracic surgery, and treatment with thrombolytic agents. Chronic diseases (neoplasm, cirrhosis) may be associated with a systemic hyperfibrinolytic, hemorrhagic state characterized by a shortened euglobulin lysis time, elevated levels of plasma tPA, decreased plasminogen and fibrinogen, and elevated fibrinogen degradation products. The short lysis time is an essential feature distinguishing pathologic hyperfibrin(ogen)olysis. The clinical picture may be more complex, however, because cells also contain proteolytic enzymes that may stimulate coagulation, and tissue damage may produce activation of either the coagulation, fibrinolytic, or a combination of both systems. In most cases, enzyme release is of limited duration, and the most essential intervention is management of the underlying condition inducing the tissue damage. If bleeding is considerable, treatment with antifibrinolytic agents should be reserved for hyperfibrinolysis without DIC or for life-threatening bleeding associated with DIC.

Acute, systemic hyperfibrin(ogen)olytic states responding dramatically to EACA have been reported in portal hypertension following bowel surgery, a plasminogen-activator–secreting tumor, and with amyloidosis (125–127). Chronic hyperfibrin(ogen)olysis may exist with some neoplasms and with the more rare congenital $\alpha_2$-antiplasmin deficiency, manifest as a bleeding tendency effectively controlled with chronic antifibrinolytic therapy (128). Acquired $\alpha_2$-antiplasmin deficiency may be seen in acute promyelocytic leukemia systemic amyloidosis, and metastatic adenocarcinoma, and hemorrhagic complications may be successfully controlled by treatment with antifibrinolytic agents (129–132).

Bleeding may accompany treatment with systemic thrombolytic therapy. Because the lysine analogs inhibit plasminogen-activator–mediated fibrinolysis, such agents would be a reasonable antidote for acute bleeding after treatment; however, prospective trials have not been performed.

**Liver Transplantation.** Many coagulation defects are present in the setting of end-stage liver disease, including increased fibrinolytic activity due to impaired hepatic clearance as well as enhanced endothelial release of tissue-plasminogen activator. Orthotopic liver transplantation is associated with still increased fibrinolytic activity related to ischemic insult to the mesenteric vascular bed and release of activators from the transplanted graft associated with the anhepatic and reperfusion phases of transplantation (133). To reduce hemorrhage associated with hyperfibrinolysis, an antifibrinolytic agent is commonly administered just prior to graft reperfusion (134). The central role played by the liver in clearing circulating tPA was demonstrated by Illig et al. in a study of patients undergoing aortic clamping during repair of abdominal aortic aneurysms (135). Patients who underwent supraceliac clamping of the aorta compared to those requiring infrarenal clamping experienced a reversible primary fibrinolytic state manifest by a shortened euglobulin lysis time, increased circulating tPA, and decreased $\alpha_2$-antiplasmin concentration, likely caused by hepatic hypoperfusion. These changes are analogous to what occurs during the anhepatic phase of liver transplantation and demonstrate the importance of impaired tPA clearance in the pathogenesis of hyperfibrinolysis. In the study by Segal et al. (136), patients treated with aprotinin during liver transplantation had a blunted increase in circulating tPA, prolonged euglobulin lysis time, decreased peak D-dimer levels, and increased circulating $\alpha_2$-antiplasmin concentration during the reperfusion phase compared with control subjects, consistent with reduced systemic fibrinolytic activity.

Studies evaluating the efficacy of prophylactic treatment with antifibrinolytic agents in reducing blood loss and transfusion requirements during orthotopic liver transplantation have been performed. The European Multicenter Study on the use of Aprotinin in Liver Transplantation (EMSALT) trial, a randomized, double-blind, placebo-controlled study of 137 patients undergoing liver transplantation, demonstrated lower intraoperative blood loss as well as considerably reduced transfusion requirements in patients treated with aprotinin versus placebo. No differences were seen in 30-day mortality or incidence of thrombotic events (137). A study of low-dose (2 mg/kg/hour), continuous AMCA during transplantation demonstrated decreased laboratory parameters of fibrinolysis but no effect on blood loss or transfusion requirement versus placebo (138). A prospective, placebo-controlled study in 132 patients comparing prophylactic treatment with high-dose AMCA (10 mg/kg/hour) and EACA (16 mg/kg/hour) to placebo demonstrated significantly reduced transfusion requirements for patients treated with AMCA, although not EACA, versus placebo (139). Blinded comparison of AMCA and aprotinin in 127 patients showed no difference in blood loss, transfusion requirements, mortality, or thrombotic events between groups (140).

The use of prophylactic antifibrinolytic agents may not be useful in all clinical situations, and may even lead to adverse events (134,141). Coagulation changes and excessive intraoperative bleeding due to hyperfibrinolysis are less common in children undergoing liver transplant, possibly because most are being treated for cholestatic rather than hepatocellular liver failure (142). Adults with primary biliary cirrhosis have less laboratory evidence of hyperfibrinolysis than patients with cirrhosis due to hepatocellular disease (143). Reports of intracardiac thrombosis and pulmonary embolism during liver transplantation have been published (134), although the association with antifibrinolytic therapy is inconsistent, leading authors to conclude the use of prophylactic antifibrinolytics should be guided by intraoperative coagulation testing (e.g., thromboelastography).

**Cardiac Surgery.** Sternotomy and cardiopulmonary bypass are associated with laboratory findings of hyperfibrinolysis: a shortened clot lysis time, increased tPA activity, and increased plasma D-dimer, and these findings are positively correlated with more serious bleeding complications (144,145). This finding has led to attempts to exploit antifibrinolytic therapies to block these physiologic manifestations of hyperfibrinolysis and thereby minimize perioperative blood product transfusions (146).

As a means to reduce blood loss, the most widely used antifibrinolytic therapy during cardiac surgery is high-dose aprotinin, administered prior to skin incision, into the priming blood volume for the bypass pump, and as a continuous infusion. Its use was first described in 1987 by Royston et al. (147) in 22 patients undergoing repeat open heart surgery randomized to high-dose aprotinin versus placebo. Aprotinin-treated patients had a highly significant eightfold decrease in allogeneic transfusion requirement. In pediatric cardiac surgery, a randomized, double-blind trial of high-dose aprotinin in 60 patients demonstrated decreased perioperative blood loss as well as a significantly reduced proportion of patients requiring blood transfusion support (13% vs. 47%) (148).

Owing to the risk of hypersensitivity associated with aprotinin, the American College of Cardiology and the American Heart Association treatment guidelines recommend use of aprotinin in primary cardiac surgery be reserved for selected patients at high risk for blood loss [e.g., patients older than 65 years, women, history of heart surgery, greater than one diseased vessel, poor left ventricular function, urgent coronary artery bypass grafting (CABG)] (149). However, because trials have shown greater benefit in patients undergoing repeat sternotomy procedures (150,151), aprotinin is routinely recommended in these patients (141). Although less well studied in thoracic surgery, two randomized trials of aprotinin in patients undergoing lung resections who were deemed at high risk for bleeding demonstrated significantly reduced blood loss, need for transfusion, and need for reexploration due to bleeding in the treated group versus placebo (152,153). A randomized, double-blind, placebo-controlled trial of 70 patients undergoing myocardial revascularization by total arterial grafting evaluating high-dose aprotinin in reducing blood loss showed a significantly reduced proportion of patients requiring transfusion (39% vs. 77%) and a significantly lower number of U transfused (0.8 vs. 2.6) (154).

Numerous studies have shown AMCA and EACA given prophylactically during cardiopulmonary bypass procedures are associated with decreased early postoperative blood loss, but evidence for an effect on decreasing transfusion requirements has not been consistently shown (155). EACA was first studied for prophylaxis against excessive blood loss in pediatric patients undergoing repair of congenital defects. McClure et al. evaluated 56 patients, finding lower blood loss over the first 24 hours postoperatively among patients treated with EACA, an effect that was more marked in patients with cyanotic heart disease or on cardiopulmonary bypass for longer than 1 hour (156). The largest trial of EACA prophylaxis, published in 1989, randomized 350 patients undergoing elective cardiac surgery (including revascularization, valve repair, and replacement) to EACA versus placebo. The patients treated with EACA had significantly less postoperative blood loss, lower red blood cell transfusion requirements (2.8 vs. 4.2 U), and less reoperation for bleeding complications (157). There was no increased rate of thrombotic complications such as stroke, myocardial infarction, or graft occlusion. Early reports exploring the use of EACA reported rare adverse events, including DIC unmasked by therapy (99), and significant intracavitary bleeding with the formation of lysis-resistant clots (44,144). Six prospective, randomized, placebo-controlled trials of prophylactic AMCA in pediatric or adult cardiac surgery were published in the 1990s evaluating the benefit of treatment in reducing need for blood product transfusion (158–161). In one trial of 90 patients undergoing primary cardiopulmonary bypass surgery, three groups were randomized: AMCA prior to bypass, AMCA after bypass, and saline placebo. The number of U of transfused blood was significantly less in the AMCA prebypass group versus control (0 vs. 4.5) (162). A larger trial of 210 patients, which randomized patients undergoing primary or repeat sternotomy procedures or valve operations, evaluated prophylactic treatment with high-dose AMCA prior to initiation of bypass versus saline placebo. A significantly smaller proportion of patients treated with AMCA required blood product transfusion support (13% vs. 31%) (163). Importantly, there was no increased incidence of thrombotic events in the treatment group. In the two trials of prophylactic AMCA in pediatric cardiac surgery, one trial of 41 patients undergoing repeat sternotomy treated with high-dose AMCA had significantly decreased transfusion support (160), whereas another study of 85 patients showed decreased blood loss without a difference in transfusion versus placebo (164). As off-pump revascularization procedures are increasingly being performed, a recent trial compared patients scheduled for on-pump ($n = 51$) or off-pump ($n = 51$) procedures randomized to prophylactic treatment with high-dose AMCA or placebo. AMCA treatment reduced perioperative blood loss considerably in both on- and off-pump groups, although the reduction was considerably greater in on-pump procedures; however, no significant effect on transfusion exposure was detected (165).

Trials directly comparing the prophylactic use of aprotinin with the lysine analogs in cardiac surgery have demonstrated approximate equivalence between the two treatment approaches. A metaanalysis of all randomized trials of antifibrinolytic therapies in cardiac surgery analyzed the proportion of patients receiving at least one perioperative allogeneic red blood cell transfusion and found the use of aprotinin and AMCA were associated with a significant decrease in number of patients requiring transfusion, whereas EACA did not demonstrate a significant effect (see Table 79-3) (166). In contrast to AMCA, aprotinin was equally effective in reducing transfusions among patients undergoing primary or repeat sternotomy or those taking aspirin, and it significantly reduced the incidence of resternotomy for bleeding complications (166). A randomized, double-blind, placebo-controlled study of high-dose aprotinin versus EACA in 72 patients undergoing CABG with cardiopulmonary bypass demonstrated decreased perioperative blood loss in both treatment groups compared with placebo; however, there was no effect on the number of patients requiring blood transfusion (167). In a trial of 204 patients undergoing repeat sternotomy with cardiopulmonary bypass randomized to receive high-dose aprotinin versus EACA, there was a considerable decrease in postoperative thoracic drainage in the aprotinin group, but this did not affect the rate of transfusion (151). Two prospective, randomized trials of more than 1,000 patients undergoing primary, elective cardiac

surgery with cardiopulmonary bypass treated with prophylactic high-dose aprotinin versus AMCA demonstrated no difference between groups with regard to postoperative bleeding or transfusion (168,169). A randomized, double-blind study of 80 patients undergoing high-risk cardiac procedures (repeat sternotomy, multiple valve replacements, aortic arch reconstruction) treated prophylactically with aprotinin versus AMCA disclosed no difference in perioperative blood loss or transfusion requirements (170). In a comparison of high-dose aprotinin versus AMCA versus EACA in patients undergoing primary cardiac surgery, there was no difference in blood loss or transfusion requirements between groups treated with AMCA or aprotinin; however, the 68 patients treated with EACA had considerably greater blood loss and a trend toward greater transfusion requirements versus the former (171). Trials comparing antifibrinolytic agents administered postoperatively to treat excessive bleeding have not shown reduced blood loss compared with placebo (172,173).

AMCA and EACA have been directly compared in patients undergoing primary cardiac surgery using cardiopulmonary bypass in three prospective, randomized trials designed to evaluate transfusion requirements. Among 48 randomized patients during primary cardiac surgery, there was no statistical difference in blood loss or transfusion requirements, although there was no placebo-treated group for comparison (141). In a randomized, placebo-controlled trial of 134 patients undergoing primary cardiac bypass surgery, both agents reduced blood loss versus placebo; however, red cell transfusion was similar in all three groups (174). Among pediatric patients, 150 children with congenital cardiac disease undergoing corrective surgery on cardiopulmonary bypass randomized to AMCA, EACA, or placebo control, AMCA and EACA were equally effective in reducing blood loss and transfusion requirements versus placebo (175).

Therefore, prophylactic antifibrinolytic therapy is highly effective at reducing blood loss as well as blood product transfusion requirements in cardiac operations requiring cardiopulmonary bypass as well as off-pump and thoracic procedures. Its use is not hampered by an increased incidence of thrombotic complications. Head-to-head comparisons suggest aprotinin may be slightly superior to the lysine analogs with regard to volume of blood loss but does not show clear superiority with regard to reduction of allogeneic blood product exposure. In a published cost-benefit analysis comparing prophylactic aprotinin to EACA, the use of EACA was more cost-effective with respect to bleeding-related complications

## TABLE 79-3

### METAANALYSIS OF 60 TRIALS OF BLOOD CONSERVATION IN CARDIAC SURGERY

|  | Number of patients | Exposed to allogeneic transfusion | Incidence of reoperation for bleeding | Incidence of perioperative MI |
|---|---|---|---|---|
| Aprotinin (45 trials) | 5,808 | OR, 0.31; $P < 0.0001$ | 1.8% versus 5.2% $P = 0.001$ | OR, 1.12 ($P = 0.48$) |
| AMCA (12 trials) | 882 | OR, 0.50; $P = 0.0009$ | 2.4% versus 2.9% $P = 0.84$ | OR, 0.30 ($P = 0.30$) |
| EACA (3 trials) | 118 | OR, 0.20; $P = 0.07$ |  |  |

MI, myocardial infarction; OR, odds ratio; AMCA, *trans-p*-aminomethyl-cyclohexane carbolyxic acid; EACA, ε-aminocaproic acid.
From Laupacis A, Fergusson D. Drugs to minimize perioperative blood loss in cardiac surgery: metaanalysis using perioperative blood transfusion as the outcome. The International Study of Peri-Operative Transfusion (ISPOT) Investigators. *Anesth Analg* 1997;85:1258.

(151). When choosing to use aprotinin over the synthetic lysine analogs, its high cost and association with severe hypersensitivity reactions should be considered.

## Localized Fibrinolysis with Defective Hemostasis

The formation of a stabilized and solid hemostatic plug is dependent on full thrombin generation because thrombin is necessary for the conversion of fibrinogen into fibrin as well as the activation of factor XIII, factor XI, and TAFI. Studies have demonstrated that most of the thrombin is generated after initial fibrin plug formation (176,177). Thrombin formed after initial clotting inhibits endogenous fibrinolytic mechanisms through activation of factor XIII and factor XI–mediated production of TAFI (26,178). Therefore, any state in which full thrombin generation is impaired, as in hemophilia and other hereditary coagulation disorders, is also associated with impaired antifibrinolytic responses (179,180) and hemostatic plugs, which are highly sensitive to fibrinolytic dissolution.

Antifibrinolytic drugs may help maintain hemostasis in patients with defective coagulation by impairing normal fibrinolysis of nascent hemostatic plugs. Although systematic trials of fibrinolysis inhibitors have been concerned predominantly with hemophiliacs, a similar approach is justified in patients with a variety of congenital or acquired hemostatic defects, as long as precautions regarding local or systemic unmasking of hypercoagulable states are first considered.

**Hemophilia.** Thrombin generation is considerably depressed in hemophilia A and B because autocatalytic feedback activation of thrombin formation caused by explosive prothrombin activation requires factor VIII and factor IX (176,181). Accordingly, fibrin plugs formed in patients with hemophilia are fragile and extremely sensitive to the action of fibrinolytic enzymes. Antifibrinolytic therapy has been used in hemophilia (i) as prophylaxis to prevent hemarthrosis; (ii) for treatment of hematuria; (iii) for treatment of gum bleeding and epistaxis; and (iv) as adjunctive, prohemostatic treatment during and following surgery. In most cases, lysine analogs are used in conjunction with factor concentrates. There is minimal experience with aprotinin in hemophilia (182). Given the propensity in hemophilia toward recurrent, frequent bleeds, aprotinin, with its high risk for hypersensitivity upon repeated use, would be of limited value outside of a major surgical operation.

Hemarthrosis may be effectively treated with small doses of factor VIII or factor IX administered as prophylaxis or early after bleeding begins. A number of studies have evaluated the addition of antifibrinolytic therapy for the purpose of altering the long-term incidence or severity of bleeding episodes. Although some studies have concluded the combination produces an enhanced effect (183,184), the weight of the evidence indicates that EACA and AMCA may be useful for treatment of individual bleeding episodes but are not effective prophylaxes (185–187).

Treatment of hematuria due to bleeding from the upper urinary tract may lead to renal functional impairment or extrarenal obstruction in hemophiliacs treated with factor replacement (188). However, additional risk probably occurs with the use of antifibrinolytic agents because they prevent or retard dissolution of large clots. Residual large clots may lead, in some cases, to frank renal obstruction (120–123). Therefore, upper urinary tract bleeding should be managed conservatively for as long as possible, using factor replacement as indicated and high fluid intake to maintain a low urinary hematocrit and fibrinogen concentration. If bleeding lasts for weeks and requires blood transfusions, or if surgical intervention is considered, then the benefit relative to risk justifies therapy with antifibrinolytic agents.

Mucosal tissue is rich in plasminogen activator, and gum bleeding and epistaxis in patients with hemophilia may be difficult to stop effectively with factor VIII or factor IX concentrates. In oral bleeding not incurred due to dental extraction, the addition of antifibrinolytic agents to cryoprecipitate in 10 patients with hemophilia improved hemostasis (189). Further, a case report describes a patient with acquired factor VIII inhibitor and with recurrent, severe epistaxis, who was successfully treated with oral EACA (190).

Although factor-replacement therapy is effective in providing normal hemostasis after all types of major surgical procedures in hemophiliacs (22), the addition of antifibrinolytic agents reduces the requirement for factor VIII or factor IX administration. This has been clearly demonstrated by the studies of dental extractions in patients with congenital factor VIII or factor IX deficiency by Reid et al. (191), Walsh et al. (192), Forbes et al. (193), and others (194–196). Blood loss was less in EACA- or AMCA-treated patients, and the amount of factor VIII or factor IX concentrate required was reduced by an average of more than 80%. It seems reasonable to suggest that patients with hemophilia undergoing other surgical procedures can be similarly supported by jointly administered antifibrinolytic and factor-replacement therapy, as seen, for example, in synovectomies (197,198). Because a hypercoagulable state may occur secondary to administration of factor IX–rich concentrates (199), their use along with antifibrinolytic agents in patients with factor IX deficiency may present a greater risk of thrombotic complication than does their use in patients with classic hemophilia (factor VIII deficiency) who receive the relatively less prothrombotic factor VIII concentrate. However, the combination of factor IX concentrates and antifibrinolytic therapy studied in patients undergoing hip replacement surgery was not associated with a greater risk for thrombotic events (200).

**Chronic Anticoagulation.** The potential application of antifibrinolytic therapy to prevent excessive bleeding in patients on chronic anticoagulation has been recently explored in an effort to avoid discontinuation of therapeutic anticoagulation around minor procedures. A randomized trial of an AMCA mouthwash after oral surgery in patients on chronic anticoagulation for a prosthetic cardiac valve or vascular prosthesis was effective in reducing the incidence of bleeding episodes as compared to the saline control group (201). AMCA administered as mouthwash four times daily for 7 days efficiently controlled bleeding in patients on oral anticoagulants without alteration in the intensity of their anticoagulant therapy (202,203). A prospective trial of 85 patients on chronic anticoagulation who underwent dental extraction demonstrated AMCA mouthwash used for 2 days postprocedure was as hemostatically effective as a 5-day course (204). Although studies have been limited to oral bleeding situations, these studies suggest a role for antifibrinolytic agents as an adjunct to vitamin K or its analogs in the management of all uncontrollable bleeding episodes in patients on chronic oral anticoagulation. Antifibrinolytic therapy also has been found useful after minor oral surgery and for tonsillectomy in von Willebrand disease (205,206) and as an adjunct to recombinant factor VIIa in patients with inhibitors to factor VIII and uncontrolled bleeding (207), although the latter use is not yet generally applied (208).

**Thrombocytopenic and Thrombocytopathic States.** Because qualitative and quantitive platelet deficiencies lead to fragile hemostatic plugs, antifibrinolytic therapy should be useful in these settings by protecting clots sensitive to dissolution by fibrinolytic enzymes. A hemostatic effect of EACA has been demonstrated in patients with bleeding due to immune thrombocytopenia or thrombocytopenia due to induction chemotherapy for leukemia (209–212) and in Bernard-Soulier (giant platelet) syndrome (213,214) in the control of obstetric bleeding. Some authors advocate the use of EACA in bleeding episodes in platelet-refractory patients following bone marrow transplant (215).

## Normal Hemostasis with Localized Fibrinolysis

Bleeding can result from a localized fibrinolytic effect caused by an imbalance between heightened local lysis and normal hemostasis, as described by Nilsson (43) and Prentice (125). Tissues that are rich in plasminogen activator might be more likely to be affected by such imbalances. The uterus, for example, is especially rich in tissue activator, which increases in concentration during menstrual bleeding (216). Bleeding via this mechanism in specific organs is not a reflection of total content of fibrinolytic enzymes; rather, it relates to the fibrinolytic activity in specific sites as well as modes of release of plasminogen activator. Important sites of heightened fibrinolytic activity include the vascular endothelium; cells that line glands, ducts, tubules, or body spaces (endometrium, meninges, pleura, pericardium, and peritoneum); invasive tumors and cells; and fluids exposed to or draining such sites. In fact, the earliest clinical applications of antifibrinolytic therapies were for bleeding at sites of known, enhanced fibrinolytic activity: prostate, bladder, uterus, and uterine cervix.

**Upper Urinary Tract.** Andersson et al. reported the successful treatment of 13 patients with "essential hematuria" with EACA and AMCA (217). The observations of Immergut and Stevenson (218) and others (219–223) demonstrate that antifibrinolytic therapy for prolonged, spontaneous, upper urinary bleeding in patients with sickle cell disease and sickle cell trait can be dramatically successful. However, there is an increased risk of significant clot formation in the renal collecting system when antifibrinolytic agents are given to patients with hemophilia who are bleeding into the renal pelvis (122). This complication is usually of minor importance, but in a small number of patients the clot is large enough to seriously impair renal function (119,120,224). The abrupt appearance of extrarenal clot formation is recognized by a combination of clearing of blood from the urine, flank pain, a intravenous pyelogram without dye excretion into the ureters and bladder, or a renal ultrasound showing hydroureter or hydronephrosis. Such clots may be treated, as demonstrated by a patient with considerable upper urinary tract bleeding secondary to renal adenocarcinoma who developed acute obstruction after treatment with EACA, which was successfully resolved with intraureteral infusion of urokinase (123). Formation of such clots can be minimized by maintenance of a high urine output before antifibrinolytic therapy to enhance spontaneous passage of clots. Patients with renal disease or posttransplantation who undergo renal biopsy may have severe and protracted hematuria, and several reports of treatment with EACA indicate reasonable success (225–227), even if an arteriovenous fistula has formed (228) or in the presence of moderate renal failure due to allograft rejection.

**Lower Urinary Tract.** Bleeding after prostatectomy is enhanced by urokinase in the urine, which diffuses into the operative site to dissolve newly formed hemostatic plugs (43,44, 48,49,125,217,229–231). Eight randomized trials in the 1960s and 1970s evaluating EACA therapy after prostatectomy demonstrated a significant decrease in blood loss when compared to placebo (230,232–239); a ninth study found similar results with AMCA treatment (240). In these trials, there was a twofold to fivefold reduction in urinary tract blood loss during the postoperative period, but no effect on the volume of intraoperative blood loss. Although the difference was statistically significant, the findings were not so relevant clinically, because the bleeding in control patients rarely prompted transfusion. Thromboembolic side effects of treatment were no greater than those in control groups (214,216–222,224–227) and were not reduced by the concomitant use of prophylactic subcutaneous heparin (241). A prospective, double-blind study of EACA versus placebo administered immediately following prostatectomy in 61 patients failed to demonstrate any effect of EACA on blood loss (239), leading the authors to conclude its use was not warranted. However, trials of postoperative administration of antifibrinolytic agents in cardiac surgery demonstrated no benefit with regard to blood loss (172,173) as opposed to prophylactic administration. A recent trial of prophylactic AMCA in 136 men undergoing elective transurethral resection of the prostate (TURP) demonstrated decreased operative blood loss in the treatment group but did not show an effect on transfusion requirements, which were low in both groups (242).

In addition to their use after prostatic surgery, antifibrinolytic agents have been used to control lower urinary tract bleeding associated with benign prostatic hyperplasia or prostatic carcinoma (75,231). Lower urinary tract obstruction by clot is less risky than excessive bleeding from the prostatic bed, but Smart suggested that EACA- and AMCA-associated clots in the lower urinary tract do pose a problem after prostatectomy (243). Interestingly, although aprotinin is a potent *in vitro* antifibrinolytic agent, it was not beneficial in a single study of lower urinary tract bleeding (244). This may be explained by its *in vivo* metabolism, which results in the renal excretion of inactive degradation products, or it may be explained simply by limits in trial design. In sum, given the lack of efficacy in preventing transfusion, and its associated risks, antifibrinolytic therapy should be reserved for those patients who demonstrate excessive bleeding at time of prostatectomy or immediately afterward, as suggested by Prentice (125).

**Dysfunctional Uterine Bleeding.** Excessive uterine bleeding due to a variety of pathologic causes has been associated with increased local fibrinolytic activity (43). Higher uterine plasminogen activator activity is present during the secretory phase when compared with the proliferation phase of the menstrual cycle (245), and higher mean plasminogen activator levels on the first day of menses are demonstrated in patients with primary menorrhagia than in those with normal menstrual blood loss (246). Further, there are higher plasminogen activator levels in most patients after placement of intrauterine devices (IUD) or cervical conization than were present prior to instrumentation (247). The hemostatic effect of antifibrinolytic therapy in treatment of primary menorrhagia or following IUD placement or conization of the cervix has been demonstrated in double-blind trials, as reviewed by Verstraete and Ogston (47,48).

Treatment of essential menorrhagia, excluding bleeding due to underlying pathology, has been studied by several groups (75,248,249), and the efficacy of antifibrinolytics was clearly demonstrated by Nilsson and Rybo (250) in a double-blind clinical trial. In the latter study, 37 women received EACA or placebo during two successive menstrual cycles, with the menstrual blood loss quantitated for each cycle. Mean blood loss was significantly different: 120 mL for placebo-treated patients and 52 mL for EACA-treated patients. Later studies of EACA and AMCA (251–254) confirmed these data, and reviews generally agree that a considerable reduction in blood loss can be achieved with antifibrinolytic therapy, especially when taken during the first 3 days of menstrual bleeding (43, 125) with a tapered dose until the completion of the menstrual cycle (255). No benefit was seen in women, with bleeding secondary to uterine fibroids, who were treated with AMCA (256). Patients with von Willebrand disease–associated menorrhagia respond to chronic AMCA with reduced blood loss (257). A systematic review published in the Cochrane database in 2000 addressed the use of antifibrinolytics in menorrhagia, concluding on the basis of four trials appropriate for meta-analysis that antifibrinolytic therapy leads to a greater reduction in blood loss than placebo or other medical therapies such as oral progestagens or nonsteroidal antiinflammatory drugs (NSAIDs) (258). Concern for thrombotic complications with chronic use has not been borne out, as evidenced by a case–control trial in Sweden, a country where 1% of women use AMCA for menorrhagia, which did not support increased incidence of thrombosis in AMCA users (259). Despite the strong evidence in favor of antifibrinolytic therapy in primary menorrhagia, gynecologists prefer treatment with surgery (dilatation and curettage) or hormones, including steroids, estrogens, and progesterones, to use of antifibrinolytic agents (260).

Whether increased bleeding secondary to the placement of an IUD (261) is caused by the higher fibrinolytic activity in the endometrium (262) or by edema, inflammation, and necrosis, antifibrinolytic therapy decreases the menstrual blood loss. In an uncontrolled but single-blind study before and after IUD placement, Kasonde and Bonnar noted that menstrual blood loss increased from 43 mL to 82 mL in 28 untreated women, whereas there was a diminshed increase (from 43 mL to only 54 mL) in patients treated with EACA (12 g per day) (263). A double-blind study in 65 women showed a similar increase in blood loss from 36 mL to 65 mL in control patients but no increase (mean of <4 mL) in patients treated with AMCA (264).

The cervix contains a high concentration of plasminogen activator, which contributes to excessive bleeding in some patients after cervical conization. The possible benefits of antifibrinolytic therapy were explored in a double-blind study by Rybo and Westerberg (265). With treatment with AMCA beginning after surgery and continuing for 12 days, quantitative blood loss in the first week was significantly reduced from 79 mL to 23 mL in the treated group. Seven of the 23 women treated with placebo had unexpected severe bleeding after the fifth postoperative day, requiring resuturing of the operative site; this complication was not seen in the AMCA-treated group. Similar findings were reported by Grundsell et al. (266).

Although providers must rule out underlying pathology in patients with menorrhagia or postoperative bleeding (43, 47,71,125), it would not be unreasonable to attempt to control excessive uterine bleeding from any cause in the absence of DIC with antifibrinolytic therapy while the diagnostic work-up is proceeding, and it may be useful as an adjunctive therapy once definitive treatment of the underlying disorder has been instituted.

**Subarachnoid Hemorrhage and Intracranial Surgery.** Another area of interest for the use of antifibrinolytic agents is control of subarachnoid hemorrhage after rupture of an intracranial aneurysm. Because immediate surgery to clip the vessel has been associated with a high mortality, most neurosurgeons prefer to delay this procedure until the cerebral arterial vasospasm that accompanies the acute event and is responsible for progressive neurologic deterioration has subsided; however, such delays are accompanied by a high incidence of rebleeding. Antifibrinolytic agents have been used with mixed results in an attempt to control the latter so that operative intervention may be delayed.

Although cerebral tissue is not generally rich in tPA activity (216), there are localized regions of high activity in the meninges and the choroid plexus (267). The cerebrospinal fluid (CSF) is usually devoid of plasminogen activator activity, but measurable amounts are present in the CSF after cerebral injury such as subarachnoid hemorrhage, intracranial hemorrhage, or even thrombotic occlusive disease (268,269), and its presence is believed to contribute to lysis of fragile intraaneurysmal thrombi by back diffusion or accelerated recanalization from spontaneous thrombolysis. This rebleeding complication occurs in 6% to 20% of the at-risk population (270,271), usually in the first several weeks after the initial episode but most often on the same day as the initial hemorrhage (272,273). Therapy that could diminish rebleeding could reduce the immediate morbidity of the hemorrhage and improve the chance of successful surgery. Both AMCA and EACA cross the blood–brain barrier, the former more rapidly (274). Indirect evidence for the potential benefit of fibrinolytic inhibitors within such thrombi was provided by the animal work of Patterson and Harpel, who showed that aneurysms of the abdominal aorta resisted rupture by increased

aortic pressure when the thrombi are formed in the presence of EACA or AMCA (275).

The data from clinical trials employing antifibrinolytic therapy in the setting of ruptured intracranial aneurysm is conflicting. Although the initial, uncontrolled studies suggested that therapy after subarachnoid hemorrhage was useful in preventing recurrent hemorrhage (274,276–286), controlled trials of EACA or AMCA are discordant (287–293). There are three controlled, randomized studies that failed to show benefit with antifibrinolytic therapy, although these involved small numbers of patients (289–292). These observations, and concern of increased incidence of thromboembolic complications or cerebral vasospasm in treated patients (293–295), led to two large multiinstitutional studies (295,296) designed to provide a sufficient number of patients to evaluate the opposing influences of rebleeding and potentially enhanced cerebral ischemia. The observations of the Cooperative Aneurysm Study reported by Kassel et al. (272,273,295) were based on 672 patients from 16 countries in North America, Europe, Australia, and Asia, but patients were not randomly selected. The rebleeding incidence was 11.7% in 467 patients receiving treatment, compared with 19.4% in 205 patients without such therapy. However, the rate of focal ischemic events was higher in the treatment group (32.4% vs. 22.7%), as was the incidence of hydrocephalus (14% vs. 7%). The incidence of clinical venous thromboembolic complications and the overall mortality rates were not different. The report of Vermeulen et al. (296) comprised 479 patients in four countries of Western Europe and was organized as a randomized, double-blind, placebo-controlled trial. The results were quite similar to those reported by Kassell et al. (295). The overall mortality rates at 3 months were essentially the same for AMCA and placebo (35% vs. 37%). Although the rate of rebleeding was significantly lower in the AMCA group, the incidence of cerebral infarction was higher. Although antifibrinolytics probably decrease rebleeding, they probably do so at the cost of an increase in cerebral ischemia and infarction, leading to an unchanged mortality rate with treatment. In an effort to exploit improved methods to control cerebral vasospasm, Roos et al. undertook a randomized, placebo-controlled trial of AMCA in 462 patients with aneurysmal hemorrhage in which all patients were treated with calcium antagonists to minimize vasospasm. Although AMCA considerably reduced the incidence of rebleeding, there was no effect on primary functional outcome at 3 months (297). Cochrane Systematic Review published in 2003 included nine trials of 1,399 patients and concluded, in spite of an overall reduction in rebleeding, that treatment with antifibrinolytics does not improve outcome. Further trials may not be justified until the mechanism of ischemic complications is better delineated (298).

**Gastrointestinal Tract.** Certain pathologic lesions that cause upper and lower GI bleeding have been associated with increased fibrinolytic activity, either within the tissues themselves or in veins draining the affected organ (299). Six prospective, controlled clinical trials (299–304) used AMCA in patients with upper GI bleeding and demonstrated significant benefit. The study by Cormack et al. conducted in the early 1970s (300), demonstrated treatment with AMCA was superior to placebo in patients with undiagnosed bleeding distal to the esophagogastric junction; presumably, this group of patients hemorrhaged secondary to diffuse gastritis. A fatal outcome, the need for surgery, or continued bleeding that required blood transfusion occurred in seven of 62 AMCA-treated patients, compared with 17 of 63 placebo-treated patients. There was, however, no difference in the failure rate in patients with bleeding secondary to esophageal varices in this study. A prospective, double-blind study comparing AMCA and placebo in 154 patients with upper GI bleeding from verified, benign lesions, demonstrates a significantly decreased need for blood transfusion or surgical intervention (304). In the study by Biggs et al. (301) of 200 randomized patients with acute upper GI hemorrhage, there was a significant difference in the requirement for surgical intervention to control bleeding, occurring in 23 of 97 control patients but in only seven of 103 AMCA-treated patients. Unlike the study by Cormack et al. (300), this study showed benefit in patients with esophageal varices as well as in those with gastric ulcers and gastric erosions. Barer et al. randomly assigned 775 patients with acute upper GI bleeding to AMCA, cimetidine, or placebo (303), and showed a reduced mortality from 13.5% in the control group to approximately 7% in either of the treatment groups. The reason for mortality benefit in the treatment groups is not obvious because AMCA exposure was not associated with a decreased incidence of rebleeding, and cimetidine has no antifibrinolytic effect (305). Metaanalysis of the effect of fibrinolytic inhibitors on mortality from upper GI hemhorrhage included six randomized, controlled trials involving 1,267 patients and concluded a short-term course of AMCA (2 to 7 days) resulted in a 20% to 30% reduction in the rate of rebleeding and a 30% to 40% reduction in mortality (306). Therefore, the benefit of antifibrinolytic therapy for acute upper GI hemorrhage is mediated through a reduction in amount of blood loss (300–302) or a reduction in mortality independent of blood loss (303). To better evaluate the lack of association between incidence of rebleeding and mortality, a recent trial randomized 414 patients presenting with acute, upper GI bleed to treatment with proton pump inhibition, AMCA, both, or placebo at time of presentation, with endoscopy one to four doses later (307). This trial was intended to establish an objective marker of effect of intervention by the presence of blood in stomach following treatment intervention. Among treated patients, there was considerably less blood in the stomach at endoscopy, although there was no evidence for synergy between proton pump inhibition and antifibrinolytics. Although by regression analysis, absence of blood in the stomach was associated with improved outcomes (decreased mortality, decreased need for surgery), the trial was not designed for efficacy analysis. Another upper GI lesion improved by antifibrinolytic therapy is giant hypertrophic gastritis (Ménétrier disease), through a reduction in incidence of rebleeding (308).

Patients with cirrhosis often have indisputable laboratory evidence of a chronic, systemic lytic state, with elevated D-dimer and tPA concentrations in the blood. Although the incidence of bleeding is higher in those patients with more advanced cirrhosis (ascites, variceal size), and with higher circulating D-dimer and tPA (309), clinical efficacy of fibrinolytic inhibitors may be attributable more to inhibition of local fibrinolysis at lesions prone to bleed than to correction of the systemic fibrinolytic state (310). Evidence for this hypothesis is provided by the work of Cox et al. (299), who found a high level of plasmin activity in gastric veins of patients with peptic ulcers when compared to a control population, and by Oka and Tanaka (311), who demonstrated increased fibrinolytic activity in the mucosa of the esophagus and stomach in patients with cirrhosis and upper GI bleeding. AMCA was effective in one reported patient with cirrhosis and bleeding secondary to gastric antral vascular ectasia who failed to respond to portal decompression or β-blockers, yet had more than 1 year without recurrence of hemorrhage after initiation of antifibrinolytic therapy (312). The use of antifibrinolytic therapy in bleeding complicating portal hypertension and cirrhosis deserves further clinical study.

Kwaan et al. (313) and Kondo et al. (308) demonstrated increased amounts of plasminogen activator in the rectal mucosa in a proportion of patients presenting with active ulcerative colitis. However, clinical trials of antifibrinolytic therapy have been unconvincing. Although an uncontrolled study (314) suggested that the bleeding in such patients was controlled with antifibrinolytic therapy, two controlled trials (315,316) give conflicting

results. Alternate approaches, such as the direct administration of an agent by enema, may prove more useful (317,318) if given to those patients with heightened fibrinolytic activity; however, such patients are not readily identifiable, and further trials have not been performed.

**Traumatic Hyphema.** Increased local fibrinolytic activity is present in circumscribed areas of the eye, specifically in the endothelium of the canal of Schlemm, as well as in the ciliary body, the iris, and the proximal scleral vascular plexus (319). This fibrinolytic activity presumably contributes to the maintenance of the patency of the canal of Schlemm and especially to the prevention of obstruction of intraocular fluid drainage and glaucoma and is responsible for the lysis of any clot formed during ocular trauma. On the other hand, such fibrinolytic activity is likely to contribute to the rebleeding that often follows hemostasis from the initial injury by accelerated lysis of the hemostatic plug.

Therapy with antifibrinolytic agents has been attempted as a prophylactic measure against the rebleeding following traumatic hyphema (320,321), which generally occurs in as many as 30% to 40% of patients, approximately 2 to 6 days after the initial injury. A favorable effect of antifibrinolytic therapy in preventing secondary bleeding after traumatic hyphema was reported in a number of studies based on historical controls (320,322–325) and confirmed in three controlled trials (321,326,327). In a recent study of 238 patients, strictly randomized and placebo-controlled, oral AMCA at 75 mg/kg/day decreased the incidence of secondary hemorrhage from 26% in those receiving placebo to only 10% ($P = 0.008$) (328). A similar benefit has been noted in a study of 118 patients in which topical AMCA was as effective as oral AMCA in reducing secondary hemorrhage (2 of 64 vs. 12 of 54 patients receiving placebo) (329). A 5-day course of topical amicar versus placebo decreased the rate of rebleeding in 51 patients presenting with traumatic hyphema, and there was a nonsignificant trend toward more rapid improvement in vision in the treatment group (330). Yet the study by Taboul et al. (331) suggests that the incidence of secondary hemorrhage after traumatic hyphema is quite low in patients without added risk factors such as aspirin ingestion and, therefore, that routine use of EACA (or any antifibrinolytic) is not warranted. Taken together, the data seems to indicate that on balance, antifibrinolytic therapy is a reasonable approach in the prevention of rebleeding following traumatic hyphema, at least in those who do have added risk factors for hemorrhage, such as aspirin exposure.

**Mucous Membranes.** Antifibrinolytic therapy has been studied in patients undergoing tonsillectomy and adenoidectomy (332–334), demonstrating a significant decrease in blood loss when compared with other treatment modalities, although the amount of blood loss may not suffice in recommending such agents for routine use. Treatment might reasonably be attempted in patients with unexplained serious postoperative bleeding that requires unsuturing or packing; in the latter situation, packs impregnated with an antifibrinolytic agent may prove helpful. Related mucous membrane bleeding, specifically epistaxis, can be a bothersome and recurrent problem, and the study by Petruson suggests that therapy for such patients with AMCA can significantly decrease the number and severity of bleeding episodes as well as shorten the hospitalization time (335).

**Cavernous Hemangioma.** Patients with multiple giant hemangiomata (Kasabach-Merritt syndrome) present a clinical dilemma particularly resistant to medical therapies, with progressive enlargement of vascular tumors that often require extensive, dangerous, and sometimes disfiguring surgery. Ongoing consumption of platelets and fibrinogen suggests that thrombi are continually formed and dissolved within the hemangioma. This led Neidhart and Roach (336) and, later, Warrell and Kempin (337) and Ortel et al. (338), to apply the novel approach of inducing *in situ* thrombosis by the administration of EACA, either alone (336) or with concomitant cryoprecipitate infusion (337). Tumor shrinkage, reversion, or improvement of laboratory evidence of consumption and symptomatic improvement in patient and tumor mass were obtained in all cases. A similar approach has been applied successfully in a reversal of a consumption coagulopathy associated with Klippel-Trenaunay-Weber syndrome (339, 340). Variable success has been achieved using antifibrinolytic agents in hereditary hemorrhagic telangiectasia (341), but, as has been noted in an editorial (342), systematic studies are needed to establish this therapy as definitely effective.

## Applications to Reduce Blood Loss

Given their role in promoting hemostasis, antifibrinolytic agents may be useful adjuncts in surgical settings in order to control bleeding and reduce patient exposure to allogeneic blood products. Employing these agents in conjunction with desmopression and other technical approaches, such as hypotensive anesthesia or hypothermia, may reduce hemorrhage during extensive surgical procedures anticipating large volume blood loss and transfusion requirements, or in the treatment of bleeding patients whose beliefs (e.g., Jehovah's Witness) do not permit the use of blood products (343). The mechanism for efficacy would, by definition, rely on a prohemostatic effect in the absence of an underlying coagulation defect. Cochrane systematic review was performed to assess the effect of antifibrinolytic therapy (aprotinin, AMCA, or EACA) on perioperative red blood cell transfusion (344). Analysis demonstrated an absolute reduction in allogeneic blood transfusion following treatment with aprotinin of 20% versus 17% after treatment with AMCA. Far fewer trials of AMCA were analyzed, and even fewer for EACA. The authors concluded the agents may be equivalent, and lack of comparison between agents warrants further study.

### Orthopedic Surgery

On the basis of its hemostatic efficacy in cardiopulmonary bypass surgery, aprotinin has been evaluated in trials to improve hemostasis in subjects with no antecedent history of coagulation disorders undergoing orthopedic surgery. Two placebo-controlled trials evaluated high-dose aprotinin prophylaxis during hip replacement surgery and demonstrated a significantly reduced rate of allogeneic blood transfusion versus placebo-treated patients, without increased incidence of thrombotic events. Janssens et al. evaluated 40 patients treated by 2 million KIU bolus followed by 500,000 KIU per hour infusion as in cardiac surgery and demonstrated a reduction in transfused U from 3.4 U in the placebo group to 1.8 U in the treatment group ($P < 0.001$) (345). Murkin et al. randomized 225 patients undergoing hip replacement surgery to treatment with high-dose versus low-dose aprotinin, or saline placebo, and demonstrated a significantly lower proportion of aprotinin-treated patients required allogeneic blood transfusion (6% vs. 12%) (346). A randomized study of 40 patients undergoing hip replacement surgery who received a single prophylactic injection of aprotinin, 2 million KIU, versus placebo did not demonstrate any benefit to aprotinin treatment in reducing blood loss or blood product exposure (347). There was no increased incidence of symptomatic DVT in the treatment group. To exclude a dose-dependent hemostatic effect, Samama et al. randomized 58 patients undergoing major joint replacement surgery to standard high-dose aprotinin 2 million KIU followed by 500,000 KIU per hour infusion versus higher than standard aprotinin (4 million KIU followed by 1 million KIU per hour infusion) versus placebo, finding decreased transfusion requirements in both aprotinin groups without

dose-response effect (348). Among patients undergoing revision arthroplasty or orthopedic oncologic surgery, deemed at very high risk for large volume blood loss intraoperatively, Jeserschek et al. demonstrated prophylactic treatment with high-dose aprotinin versus placebo significantly reduced the requirement for intraoperative blood transfusion (1.4 U vs. 3.1 U) as well as decreased the mean length of hospital stay (349). Further, aprotinin's safety and efficacy in pediatric patients undergoing spinal fusion surgery was demonstrated in 44 patients enrolled in a prospective, randomized study that found significantly decreased blood loss and transfusion requirements (1.1 U vs. 2.2 U) (87).

The lysine analogs have also been studied as prophylactic agents in orthopedic surgery. Three placebo-controlled trials have demonstrated treatment with AMCA in primary total knee replacement surgery significantly decreases perioperative blood loss and transfusion requirements (350–352). Hiipala et al. randomized 75 patients undergoing total knee replacement under a pneumatic tourniquet and demonstrated a lower proportion of patients required perioperative transfusion as well as a lower mean number of transfused U (1 per patient vs. 3.4 per patient, $P < 0.0001$) (350). In primary total hip arthroplasty, recent randomized, double-blind studies have demonstrated significantly decreased blood loss and transfusion requirements. Husted et al. randomized 40 patients to AMCA, administered as intraoperative bolus followed by infusion for the duration of the procedure, versus placebo, and demonstrated a significant decrease in postoperative blood loss with a decreased proportion of patients receiving transfusions ($P = 0.04$) (353) with no difference between groups in thrombotic events. In the trial by Lemay et al. in primary hip arthroplasty, significantly fewer patients were transfused (6 of 20 vs. 13 of 19) (354). Metaanalysis of trials of prophylactic AMCA in orthopedic surgery evaluated 12 trials and concluded treatment with AMCA significantly reduces total perioperative blood loss and the proportion of patients requiring transfusion [odds ratio (OR), 0.26] (89).

Similarly, such therapy has been used to reduce transfusion requirements by approximately one half in patients undergoing total knee replacement (339,340). Evidence of a hyperfibrinolytic state has not been documented (47), and results do not correlate with laboratory parameters such as D-dimer and tPA levels. Such therapy is paradoxic in the extreme because the risk of thromboembolic complications usually requires anticoagulant therapy as well, but the available literature suggests that thrombotic events are not increased in patients receiving antifibrinolytic therapy.

### Neurosurgery

There have been reported cases of systemic hyperfibrinolysis as a fatal complication of a neurosurgical procedure. One patient has been reported as developing life-threatening perioperative bleeding associated with elevated levels of circulating tPA, who was successfully resuscitated with high-dose aprotinin (344). Because intravenous treatment with the lysine analogs has been associated with a greater risk for cerebral ischemia when used in the treatment of subarachnoid hemorrhage, the lysine analogs have not been tested to improve surgical hemostasis during craniotomy procedures. However, aprotinin has been tested as a prophylactic measure to decrease perioperative bleeding. One hundred patients undergoing craniotomy for a intracranial meningioma or vestibular schwannoma were randomized to low-dose aprotinin versus placebo. Intraoperative blood loss was reduced by 50% in the group treated with aprotinin (1,014 mL to 508 mL, $P = 0.028$), although the trial was not designed to evaluate efficacy in reducing transfusion requirements (355). Further trials should be undertaken in the future to evaluate the potential for transfusion reduction.

## Fibrin Sealants

Fibrin sealants, containing fibrinogen, thrombin, and factor XIII, have been used for decades to enhance local hemostasis and adhesion during all types of surgical procedures. Currently, commercially available fibrin sealants contain coagulation proteins as well as an antifibrinolytic agent, bovine aprotinin, or tranexamic acid to delay fibrinolysis at the site of the product application (356). Antifibrinolytic agents were incorporated into fibrin sealant products after a study demonstrated cells growing along fibrin sealant were more adhesive to the product in the presence of aprotinin (357). Although these agents have been used effectively in uncontrolled trials in hemophiliacs undergoing dental extractions or numerous other surgical procedures, such as hypospadias repair, endonasal surgery, and tracheoesophageal fistula repair (358–361), there are no randomized trials comparing the efficacy of fibrin sealant products with and without antifibrinolytic additives (356). Among children treated with aprotinin containing fibrin sealant during cardiac surgery, 40% exhibited circulating, aprotinin-specific antibody 6 weeks postoperatively, suggesting use of a test dose remains imperative to avoid anaphylaxis even with topical application (362).

## *References*

1. Aoki N, Moroi M, Sakata Y, et al. Abnormal plasminogen. *J Clin Invest* 1978;61:1186.
2. Kazama M, Tahara C, Suzuki Z, et al. Abnormal plasminogen, a case of recurrent thrombosis. *Thromb Res* 1981;21:517.
3. Soria J, Soria C, Bertrand O, et al. Plasminogen Paris I: congenital abnormal plasminogen and its incidence in thrombosis. *Thromb Res* 1983;32:229.
4. Jorgensen M, Mortensen JZ, Madsen AG, et al. A family with reduced plasminogen activator activity in blood associated with recurrent venous thrombosis. *Scand J Haematol* 1982;9:217.
5. Stead NW, Bauer KA, Kinney TR, et al. Venous thrombosis in a family with defective release of vascular plasminogen activator and elevated plasma factor VIII/von Willebrand's factor. *Am J Med* 1983;74:33.
6. Booth NA, Bennett B, Wijngaards G, et al. A new life-long hemorrhagic disorder due to excess plasminogen activator. *Blood* 1983;61:267.
7. Aoki N, Saito H, Kamiya T, et al. Congenital deficiency of alpha-2-plasmin inhibitor associated with severe hemorrhagic tendency. *J Clin Invest* 1979;63:877.
8. Miles LA, Plow EF. Binding and activation of plasminogen on the platelet surface. *J Biol Chem* 1985;260:4303.
9. Hajjar KA, Harpel PC, Jaffe EA, et al. Binding of plasminogen to cultured human endothelial cells. *J Biol Chem* 1986;261:11656.
10. Silverstein RL, Leung LL, Harpel PC, et al. Platelet thrombospondin forms a trimolecular complex with plasminogen and histidine-rich glycoprotein. *J Clin Invest* 1985;75:2065.
11. Hajjar KA, Hamel NM, Harpel PC, et al. Binding of tissue plasminogen activator to cultured human endothelial cells. *J Clin Invest* 1987;80:1712.
12. Loscalzo J, Vaughan DE. The binding of tissue plasminogen activator to platelets. *Thromb Haemost* 1987;58:431a.
13. Jeanneau C, Sultan Y. Tissue plasminogen activator in human megakaryocytes and platelets: immunocytochemical localization, immunoblotting and zymographic analysis. *Thromb Haemost* 1988;59:529.
14. Park S, Harker LA, Marzec UM, et al. Demonstration of single chain urokinase-type plasminogen activator on human platelet membrane. *Blood* 1989;73:1421.
15. Adelman B, Michelson AD, Loscalzo J, et al. Plasmin effect on glycoprotein Ib—von Willebrand factor interactions. *Blood* 1985;65:32.
16. Hamilton KK, Fretto LJ, Grierson DS, et al. Effects of plasmin on von Willebrand factor multimers—degradation *in vitro* and stimulation of release *in vivo*. *J Clin Invest* 1985;76:261.
17. Federici AB, Berkowitz SD, Zimmerman TS, et al. Proteolysis of von Willebrand factor after thrombolytic therapy in patients with acute myocardial infarction. *Blood* 1992;79:38.
18. Stricker RB, Wong D, Shiu DT, et al. Activation of plasminogen by tissue plasminogen activator on normal and thrombasthenic platelets: effects on surface proteins and platelet aggregation. *Blood* 1986;68:275.
19. Loscalzo J, Vaughan DE. Tissue plasminogen activator promotes platelet disaggregation in plasma. *J Clin Invest* 1987;79:1749.
20. Marder VJ, Sherry S. Thrombolytic therapy: current status. *N Engl J Med* 1988;318:1512.
21. Wildgoose P, Nemerson Y, Hansen LL, et al. Measurement of basal levels of factor VIIa in hemophilia A and B patients. *Blood* 1992;80:25.
22. Morrissey JH, Macik BG, Neuenschwander PF, et al. Quantitation of activated factor VII levels in plasma using a tissue factor mutant selectively deficient in promoting factor VII activation. *Blood* 1993;81:734.
23. Rapaport SI, Rao LVM. The tissue factor pathway: how it has become a "prima ballerina." *Thromb Haemost* 1995;74:7.
24. Le DT, Borgs P, Toneff TW, et al. Hemostatic factors in rabbit limb lymph: relationship to mechanisms regulating extravascular coagulation. *Am J Physiol* 1998;274:H769.
25. Blomback B. Fibrinogen structure, activation, polymerization and fibrin gel structure. *Thromb Res* 1994;75:327.
26. Bajzar L, Manuel R, Nesheim E. Purification and characterization of TAFI, a thrombin-activatable fibrinolysis inhibitor. *J Biol Chem* 1995;270:14477.
27. Sakharov DV, Plow EF, Rijken DC. On the mechanism of the antifibrinolytic activity of plasma carboxypeptidase B. *J Biol Chem* 1997;272:14477.
28. Broze GJ Jr, Higuchi DA. Coagulation-dependent inhibition of fibrinolysis: role of carboxypeptidase-U and the premature lysis of clots from hemophilic plasma. *Blood* 1996;88:3815.
29. Robbins KC, Summaria L, Hsieh B, et al. The peptide chains of human plasmin: mechanisms of activation of human plasminogen to plasmin. *J Biol Chem* 1967;242:2333.
30. Rickli EE, Otavsky WI. Release of an N-terminal peptide from human plasminogen during activation with urokinase. *Biochim Biophys Acta* 1973;295:381.
31. Suenson E, Bjerrum P, Holm A, et al. The role of fragment X polymers in the fibrin enhancement of tissue plasminogen activator-catalyzed plasmin formation. *J Biol Chem* 1990;265:22228.
32. Claeys H, Vermylen J. Physicochemical and proenzyme properties of NH2-terminal glutamic acid and NH2-terminal lysine human plasminogen: influence of 6-aminohexanoic acid. *Biochim Biophys Acta* 1974;342:351.
33. Thorsen S, Kok P, Astrup T. Reversible and irreversible alterations of human plasminogen indicated by changes in susceptibility to plasminogen activators and in response to epsilon-aminocaproic acid. *Thromb Diath Haemorrh* 1974;32:325.
34. Hoylaerts M, Rijken DC, Lijnen HR, et al. Kinetics of the activation of plasminogen by human tissue plasminogen activator. Role of fibrin. *J Biol Chem* 1982;257:2912.
35. Christensen U, Müllertz S. Kinetic studies of the urokinase-catalyzed conversion of NH2-terminal lysine plasminogen to plasmin. *Biochim Biophys Acta* 1977;480:275.
36. Wallén P, Wiman B. On the generation of intermediate plasminogen and its significance for activation. In: Reich E, Rifkin DB, Shaw E, eds. *Proteases and biological control*, Cold Spring Harbor, NY: Cold Spring Harbor Laboratory, 1975:291–303.
37. Violand BN, Castellino FJ. Mechanisms of the urokinase-catalyzed activation of human plasminogen. *J Biol Chem* 1976;251:3906.
38. Alkjaersig N, Flectcher AP, Sherry S. The mechanism of clot dissolution by plasmin. *J Clin Invest* 1959;38:1086.
39. Rickli EE, Otavsky WI. A new method of isolation and some properties of heavy chain of human plasmin. *Eur J Biochem* 1975;9:441.
40. Sottrup-Jensen L, Claeys H, Zajdel N, et al. The primary structure of human plasminogen: isolation of two lysine binding fragments and one "mini" plasminogen (MW 38,000) by elastase-catalyzed-specific limited proteolysis. In: Davidson JR, Rowan RM, Samama MM et al., eds. *Progress in chemical fibrinolysis and thrombosis*, Vol. 3. New York: Raven Press, 1978: 191–209.
41. Collen D, DeCock F, Verstraete M. Immunochemical distinction between antiplasmin and alpha-antitrypsin. *Thromb Res* 1975;7:245.
42. Rybo G. Plasminogen activators in the endometrium. II. Clinical aspects. Variations in the concentration of plasminogen activators during the menstrual cycle and its relation to menstrual blood loss. *Acta Obstet Gynecol Scand* 1966;45:429.
43. Nilsson IM. Local fibrinolysis as a mechanism for haemorrhage. *Thromb Diath Haemorrh* 1975;34:623.
44. McNicol GP. Disordered fibrinolytic activity and its control. *Scott Med J* 1962;7:266.
45. Marder VJ, Shulman NR. Major surgery in classical hemophilia using fraction I: experience in twelve operations and review of literature. *Am J Med* 1966;41:56.
46. Slaughter TF, Faghih F, Greenberg CS, et al. The effects of epsilon-aminocaproic acid on fibrinolysis and thrombin generation during cardiac surgery. *Anesth Analg* 1997;85:1221.
47. Verstraete M. Hemostatic drugs. *A critical appraisal*. The Hague: Martinus Nijhoff, 1997:1.
48. Ogston D. *Antifibrinolytic drugs: chemistry, pharmacology and clinical usage.* Chichester: John Wiley & Sons, 1984:1.
49. Verstraete M. Clinical application of inhibitors of fibrinolysis. *Drugs* 1985;29:236.
50. Levy JH, Sypniewski E. Aprotinin: a pharmacologic overview. *Orthopedics* 2004;27:s653.
51. Longstaff C. Studies on the mechanisms of action of aprotinin and tranexamic acid as plasmin inhibitors and antifibrinolytic agents. *Blood Coagul Fibrinolysis* 1994;5:537.
52. Alkjaersig N. Purification and properities of human plasminogen. *Biochem J* 1964;93:171.
53. *Aprotinin (Trasylolol, aprotinin injection) package insert.* West Haven, CT: Bayer Corporation, March 2001.
54. Brockway WJ, Castellino FJ. The mechanism of the inhibition of plasmin by epsilon-aminocaproic acid. *J Biol Chem* 1971;14:4641.
55. Brockway WJ, Castellino FJ. Measurement of the binding of antifibrinolytic amino acids to various plasminogens. *Arch Biochem Biophys* 1972;151:194.

56. Okamoto S. *British Patent Specification No. 770,693*. London: Her Majesty's Stationery Office, 1957.

57. Okamoto S, Hijikata-Okunomiya A, Wanaka K, et al. Enzyme-controlling medicines: introduction. *Semin Thromb Hemost* 1997;23:493.

58. Christensen U. Allosteric effects of some antifibrinolytic amino acid on the catalytic effect of plasmin. *Biochim Biophys Acta* 1978;526:194.

59. Landis RC, Haskard DO, Taylor KM. New anti-inflammatory and platelet-preserving effects of aprotinin. *Ann Thorac Surg* 2001;72:S1808.

60. Asimakopoulos G, Thompson R, Nourshargh S, et al. An anti-inflammatory property of aprotinin detected at the level of leukocyte extravasation. *J Thorac Cardiovasc Surg* 2000;120:361.

61. Himmelfarb J, Holbrook D, McGonagle E. Effects of aprotinin on complement and granulocyte activation during *ex-vivo* hemodialysis. *Am J Kidney Dis* 1994;24:901.

62. Wang X, Lin X, Loy JA, et al. Crystal structure of the catalytic domain of human plasmin complexed with streptokinase. *Science* 1998;281:1662.

63. Schiffer CA, Huber R, Wuthrich K, et al. Simultaneous refinement of the structure of BPTI against NMR data measured in solution and x-ray diffraction data measured in single crystals. *J Mol Biol*. 1994;241:588.

64. Bajaj MS, Birktoft JJ, Steer SA, et al. Structure and biology of tissue factor pathway inhibitor. *Thromb Haemost* 2001;86:959.

65. Abiko Y, Iwamoto M, Tomikawa M. Plasminogen-plasmin system V. A stoichiometric equilibrium complex of plasminogen and a synthetic inhibitor. *Biochim Biophys Acta* 1969;185:424.

66. Longstaff C, Gaffney PJ. Serpin serine protease binding kinetics: $\alpha_2$-antiplasmin as a model inhibitor. *Biochemistry* 1991;30:979.

67. Anonick PK, Gonias SL. Soluble fibrin preparations inhibit reaction of plasmin with $\alpha_2$-antiplasmin macroglobulin. Comparison with alpha-2-antiplasmin and leupeptin. *Biochem J* 1991;275:53.

68. Alkjaersig N, Fletcher AP, Sherry S. ε-aminocaproic acid: an inhibitor of plasminogen activation. *J Biol Chem* 1959;234:832.

69. Sherry S, Fletcher AP, Alkjaersig N, et al. Epsilon-aminocaproic acid: "a potent antifibrinolytic agent." *Trans Assoc Am Physicians* 1959;72:62.

70. Collen D. On the regulation and control of fibrinolysis. *Thromb Haemost* 1980;43:77.

71. Griffin JD, Ellman L. Epsilon-aminocaproic acid (EACA). *Semin Thromb Hemost* 1978;5:27.

72. Sweeney WM. Aminocaproic acid, an inhibitor of fibrinolysis. *Am J Med Sci* 1965;249:576.

73. Niewiarowski S, Wolosowicz N. The *in vivo* effect of epsilon-aminocaproic acid (EACA) on human plasma fibrinolytic system. *Thromb Diath Haemorrh* 1966;15:491.

74. McNicol GP, Doublas AS. Epsilon-aminocaproic acid and other inhibitors of fibrinolysis. *Br Med Bull* 1964;20:233.

75. Nilsson IM, Andersson L, Bjorkman SE. Epsilon-aminocaproic acid (E-ACA) as a therapeutic agent based on 5 years' clinical experience. *Acta Med Scand* 1996;448(Suppl.):1.

76. Bennett B, Ogston D. Natural and drug-induced inhibition of fibrinolysis. *Clin Hematol* 1973;2:135.

77. Wallén P. Activation of plasminogen with urokinase and tissue activator. In: Paoletti R, Sherry S, eds. *Thrombosis and urokinase*. London: Academic Press, 1977;91.

78. Thorsen S, Müllerts S. Rate of activation and electrophoretic mobility of unmodified and partially degraded plasminogen: effects of 6-aminohexanoic acid and related compounds. *Scand J Clin Lab Invest* 1974;34:167.

79. Thorsen S. Differences in the binding to fibrin of native plasminogen and plasminogen modified by proteolytic degradation. Influence of omega-amino carboxylic acids. *Biochim Biophys Acta* 1975;393:55.

80. Petersen LC, Suenson E. Effect of plasminogen and tissue-type plasminogen activator on fibrin gel structure. *Fibrinolysis* 1991;5:51.

81. Lerch PG, Rickli EE, Lergier D, et al. Localisation of individual lysine-binding regions in human plasminogen and investigation on their complex-forming properties. *Eur J Biochem* 1980;107:7.

82. Wiman B, Wallén P. The specific interaction between plasminogen and fibrin. A physiological role of the lysine binding site in plasminogen. *Thromb Res* 1977;1:213.

83. Okamoto S, Oshiba S, Mihara H, et al. Synthetic inhibitors of fibrinolysis: *in vitro* and *in vivo* mode of action. *Ann N Y Acad Sci* 1968;146:414.

84. Westlund LE, Lunden R, Wallén P. Effect of EACA, PAMBA, AMCA and AMBOCA on fibrinolysis induced by streptokinase, urokinase and tissue activator. *Haemostasis* 1982;11:235.

85. Anonick PK, Vasudevan J, Gonias SL. Antifibrinolytic activities of alpha-N-acetyl-L-lysine methy ester, epsilon-aminocaproic acid, and tranexamic acid. Importance of kringle interactions and active site inhibition. *Arterioscler Thromb* 1992;12:708.

86. Dietrich W, Spannagl M, Jochum M. Influence of high dose aprotinin treatment on blood loss and coagulation patterns in patients undergoing myocardial revascularization. *Anesthesiology* 1990;73:1119.

87. Cole JW, Murray DJ, Snider RJ. Aprotinin reduces blood loss during spine surgery in children. *Spine* 2003;28:2482.

88. Urban MK, Beckman J, Gordon M. The efficacy of antifibrinolytics in the reduction of blood loss during complex adult reconstructive surgery. *Spine* 2001;26:1152–1156.

89. Ko HM, Ismail H. Use of intravenous tranexamic acid to reduce allogeneic blood transfusion in total hip and knee arthroplasty: a meta-analysis. *Anaesth Intensive Care* 2003;31:529.

90. *Aminocaproic acid*, 15th ed. Mosby's Drug Consult, 2005.

91. McNicol GP, Fletcher AP, Alkjaersig N, et al. The absorption, distribution and excretion of epsilon-aminocaproic acid following oral or intravenous administration to man. *J Lab Clin Med* 1962;59:15.

92. Andersson L, Nilsson IM, Nilehn JE, et al. Experimental and clinical studies on AMCA, the antifibrinolytically active isomer of p-aminomethylcyclohexane carboxylic acid. *Scand J Haematol* 1965;2:230.

93. Bennett-Guerrero E, Sorhan JG, Canada AT, et al. Epsilon-aminocaproic acid plasma levels during cardiopulmonary bypass. *Anesth Analg* 1997;85:248.

94. Eriksson O, Kjellman H, Pilbrant A, et al. Pharmacokinetics of tranexamic acid after intravenous administration to normal volunteers. *Eur J Clin Pharmacol* 1974;7:375.

95. Royston D. Aprotinin versus lysine analogues: the debate continues. *Ann Thorac Surg* 1998;65:S9.

96. Dietrich W, Spath P, Ebell A, et al. Prevalence of anaphylactic reactions to aprotinin: analysis of 248 reexposures to aprotinin in heart operations. *J Thorac Cardiovasc Surg* 1997;113:194.

97. Seymour BD, Rubinger M. Rhabdomyolysis induced by epsilonaminocaproic acid. *Ann Pharmacother* 1997;31:56.

98. Clarkson AAR, Sage RE, Lawrence JR. Consumption coagulopathy and acute renal failure due to gram-negative septicemia after abortion: complete recovery with heparin therapy. *Ann Intern Med* 1969;70:1191.

99. Gralnick HR, Greipp P. Thrombosis with epsilon-aminocaproic acid therapy. *Am J Clin Pathol* 1971;56:151.

100. Naeye R. Thrombotic state after a hemorrhagic diathesis, a possible complication of therapy with epsilon-aminocaproic acid. *Blood* 1962;19:694.

101. Charytan C, Purtilo D. Glomerular capillary thrombosis and acute renal failure after epsilon-aminocaproic acid therapy. *N Engl J Med* 1969;280:1102.

102. McKay DG, Muller-Berghaus G, Cruse V. Therapeutic implications of disseminated intravascular coagulation. *Am J Cardiol* 1967;20:392.

103. Sharp AAS. Pathological fibrinolysis. *Br Med Bull* 1964;20:245.

104. Gibbon JH, Camishon RC. Problems in hemostasis with extracorporeal apparatus. *Ann N Y Acad Sci* 1964;115:195.

105. Levin MD, Betjes MG, van der Kwast TH, et al. Acute renal cortex necrosis caused by arterial thrombosis during treatment for acute promyelocytic leukemia. *Haematologica* 2003;88:21.

106. Bohrer H, Fleischer F, Lang J, et al. Early formation of thrombin on pulmonary artery catheters in cardiac surgical patients receiving high-dose aprotinin. *J Cardiothorac Anesth* 1990;4:222.

107. Gitter R, Alivizators P, Capehart U, et al. Aprotinin and aortic cannula thrombosis. *J Thorac Cardiovasc Surg* 1996;112:537.

108. MacIomhair M, Lavelle SM. Thrombus weight as a measure of hypercoagulability induced by drugs. *Thromb Haemost* 1979;42:1018.

109. Dentz ME, Slaughter TF, Mark JB. Early thrombus formulation on heparin-bonded pulmonary artery catheters in patients receiving epsilon-aminocaproic acid. *Anesthesiology* 1995;82:583.

110. Bidstrup BP, Harrision J, Royston D, et al. Aprotinin therapy in cardiac operations: a report of use in 41 cardiac centers in the United Kingdom. *Ann Thorac Surg* 1993;55:971.

111. Havel M, Grabenwoger F, Schneider J, et al. Aprotinin does not decrease early graft patency after coronary artery bypass grafting despite reducing postoperative bleeding and use of donated blood. *J Thorac Cardiovasc Surg* 1994;107:807.

112. Lemmer JH, Stanford W, Bonney SL. Aprotinin for coronary bypass operations: efficacy, safety, and influence on early saphenous graft patency. A multicenter, double blind, placebo-controlled study. *J Thorac Cardiovasc Surg* 1994;107:543.

113. Lass M, Welz A, Kochs M, et al. Aprotinin in elective primary bypass surgery: graft patency and clinical efficacy. *Eur J Cardiothorac Surg* 1995;9:206.

114. Kalangos A, Tayyareci G, Pretre R, et al. Influence of aprotinin on early graft thrombosis in patients undergoing myocardial revascularization. *Eur J Cardiothorac Surg* 1994;8:651.

115. Henry DA, Moxey AJ, Carless PA, et al. Anti-fibrinolytic therapy for minimizing perioperative allogenic blood transfusion. *Cochrane Database Syst Rev* 2001;1:CD001886.

116. Vinnicombe J, Shuttleworth KED. Aminocaproic acid in the control of hemorrhage after prostatectomy: safety of aminocaproic acid—a controlled trial. *Lancet* 1966;1:232.

117. Becker J, Borgström S. Incidence of thrombosis associated with epsilon-aminocaproic acid administration and with combined epsilon-aminocaproic acid and subcutaneous heparin therapy. *Acta Chir Scand* 1968;134:343.

118. Keiller DL. Extraordinary bladder clots. *J Urol* 1977;117:43.

119. Stark SN, White JG, Langer J Jr, et al. Epsilon-aminocaproic acid therapy as a cause of intrarenal obstruction in haematuria of haemophiliacs. *Scand J Haematol* 1965;2:99.

120. Hilgartner MW. Intrarenal obstruction in haemophilia. *Lancet* 1966;1:486.

121. van Itterbeek H, Vermylen J, Verstraete M. High obstruction of urine flow as a complication of the treatment with fibrinolysis inhibitors of haematuria in haemophiliacs. *Acta Haematol* 1968;39:237.

122. Pitts TO, Spero JA, Bontempo FA, et al. Acute renal failure due to high-grade obstruction following therapy with epsilon-aminocaproic acid. *Am J Kidney Dis* 1986;8:441.

123. Wymenga LF, van der Boon WJ. Obstruction of the renal pelvis due to an insoluble blood clot after epsilon-aminocaproic acid therapy: resolution with intraureteral streptokinase instillations. *J Urol* 1998;159:490.

124. Lindoff C, Rybo G, Astedt B. Treatment with tranexamic acid during pregnancy, and the risk of thrombo-embolic complications. *Thromb Haemost* 1993;70:238.

125. Prentice CRM. Indications for antifibrinolysis therapy. *Thromb Diath Haemorrh* 1975;34:634.

126. Sane DC, Pizzo SV, Greenberg CS. Elevated urokinase-type plasminogen activator level and bleeding in amyloidosis; case report and literature review. *Am J Hematol* 1989;31:53.

127. Davidson JF, McNicol GP, Frank GL, et al. Plasminogen activator producing tumor. *BMJ* 1969;1:88.

128. Aoki N, Sakata Y, Masuda M, et al. Fibrinolytic states in a patient with congenital deficiency of alpha 2-plasmin inhibitor. *Blood* 1980;55:483.

129. Avvisati G, TenCate JW, Buller HR, et al. Tranexamic acid for control of hemorrhage in acute promyelocytic leukaemia. *Lancet* 1989;2:122.

130. Schwartz BS, Williams EC, Conlan G, et al. Epsilon-aminocaproic acid in the treatment of patients with acute promyelocytic leukemia and acquired alpha 2-plasmin inhibitor deficiency. *Ann Intern Med* 1986;105:873.

131. Williams EC. Plasma alpha 2-antiplasmin activity. Role in the evaluation of and management of fibrinolytic states and other bleeding disorders. *Arch Intern Med* 1989;149:1769.

132. Meijer K, Smid WM, Geerards S, et al. Hyperfibrinogenolysis in disseminated adenocarcinoma. *Blood Coagul Fibrinolysis* 1998;9:279.

133. Kang Y, Lewis JH, Navalgund A, et al. Epsilon-aminocaproic acid for treatment of fibrinolysis during liver transplantation. *Anesthesiology* 1987;66:766.

134. Gologorsky E, deWolf AM, Scott V, et al. Intracardiac thrombus formation and pulmonary thromboembolism immediately after graft reperfusion in 7 patients undergoing liver transplantation. *Liver Transpl* 2001;7:783.

135. Segal HC, Hunt BJ, Cottam S, et al. Fibrinolytic activity during orthotopic liver transplantation with and without aprotinin. *Transplantation* 1994;58:1356.

136. Illig KA, Green RM, Ouriel K, et al. Primary fibrinolysis during supraceliac aortic clamping. *J Vasc Surg* 1997;25:244.

137. Porte RJ, Molenaar IQ, Begliomini B, et al. EMSALT Study Group. Aprotinin and transfusion requirements in orthotopic liver transplantation: a multicenter randomized double blind study. *Lancet* 2000;355:1303.

138. Kaspar M, Ramsay MA, Nguyen AT, et al. Continuous small-dose tranexamic acid reduces fibrinolysis but not transfusion requirements during orthotopic liver transplantation. *Anesth Analg* 1997;85:281.

139. Dalmau A, Sabate A, Acosta F, et al. Tranexamic acid reduces red cell transfusion better than epsilon-amino caproic acid on placebo in liver transplantation. *Anesth Analg* 2000;91:29.

140. Dalmau A, Sabate A, Koo M, et al. The prophylactic use of tranexamic acid and aprotinin in orthotopic liver transplantation: a comparative study. *Liver Transpl* 2004;10:279.

141. Maineri P, Covaia G, Realini M, et al. Comparison between tranexamic acid and epsilon-aminocaproic acid. *Minerva Cardioangiol* 2000;48:155.

142. Kang Y, Borland LM, Picone J, et al. Intraoperative coagulation changes in children undergoing liver transplantation. *Anesthesiology* 1989;71:44.

143. Segal H, Cottam S, Potter D, et al. Coagulation and fibrinolysis in primary biliary cirrhosis compared with other liver disease and during orthotopic liver transplantation. *Hepatology* 1997;25:683.

144. Kevy SV, Glickman RM, Bernhard WF, et al. The pathogenesis and control of the hemorrhagic defect in open heart surgery. *Surg Gynecol Obstet* 1966;123:313.

145. Kucuk O, Kwaan HC, Frederickson J, et al. Increased fibrinolytic activity in patients undergoing cardiopulmonary bypass operation. *Am J Hematol* 1986;23:223.

146. Kojina T, Gando S, Morimoto Y, et al. Systematic elucidation of effects of tranexamic acid on fibrinolysis and bleeding during and after cardiopulmonary bypass surgery. *Thromb Res* 2001;104:307.

147. Royston D, Bidstrup BP, Taylor KM, et al. Effect of aprotinin on need for blood transfusion after repeat open-heart surgery. *Lancet* 1987;2:1289.

148. Mossinger H, Dietrich W, Braun SL, et al. High dose aprotinin reduces activation of hemostasis, allogeneic blood requirement and duration of postoperative ventilation in pediatric cardiac surgery. *Ann Thorac Surg* 2003;75:430.

149. Eagle KA, Guyton RA, Davidoff R. ACC/AHA guidelines for coronary artery bypass graft surgery: a report of the American College of Cardiology/American Heart Association Task Force on Practice Guidelines. *J Am Coll Cardiol* 1999;34:1262.

150. Jamieson WR, Dryden PJ, O'Connor JP, et al. Beneficial effect of both tranexamic acid and aprotinin of blood loss reduction in reoperative valve replacement surgery. *Circulation* 1997;96(Suppl. 9):II96.

151. Bennett-Guerrero E, Sorohan JG, Gurevich ML, et al. Cost benefit and efficacy of aprotinin compared with epsilon-aminocaproic acid in patients having repeated cardiac operations: a randomized, blinded clinical trial. *Anesthesiology* 1997;87:1373.

152. Kyriss T, Wurst H, Friedel G, et al. Reduced blood loss by aprotinin in thoracic surgical operations associated with high risk of bleeding. A placebo-controlled, randomized phase IV study. *Eur J Cardiothorac Surg* 2001;20:38.

153. Bedirhan MA, Turna A, Yagan N, et al. Aprotinin reduces postoperative bleeding and the need for blood products in thoracic surgery: results of a randomized double-blind study. *Eur J Cardiothorac Surg* 2001;20:1122.

154. Taggart DP, Djapardy V, Naik M, et al. A randomized trial of aprotinin on blood loss, blood product requirement, and myocardial injury in total arterial grafting. *J Thorac Cardiovasc Surg* 2003;126:1087.

155. Horrow JC, Hlavacek J, Strong MD, et al. Prophylactic tranexamic acid decreases bleeding after cardiac operations. *J Thorac Cardiovasc Surg* 1990;99:70.

156. McClure PD, Izsak J. The use of epsilon-aminocaproic acid to reduce bleeding during cardiac bypass in children with congenital heart disease. *Anesthesiology* 1974;40:604.

157. Del Rossi AJ, Cernainu AC, Botros J, et al. Prophylactic treatment of postperfusion bleeding using EACA. *Chest* 1989;96:27.

158. Horrow JC, Van Riper DF, Strong MD, et al. Haemostatic effects of tranexamic acid and desmopressin during cardiac surgery. *Circulation* 1991;84:2063.

159. Karski JM, Teasdale SJ, Norman P, et al. Prevention of bleeding after cardiopulmonary bypass with high-dose tranexamic acid. Double-blind, randomized clinical trial. *J Thorac Cardiovasc Surg* 1995;110:835.

160. Reid RW, Zimmerman AA, Laussen PC, et al. The efficacy of tranexamic acid versus placebo in decreasing blood loss in pediatric patients undergoing repeat cardiac surgery. *Anesth Analg* 1997;84:990.

161. Shore-Lesserson L, Reich DL, Vela-Cantos F, et al. Tranexamic acid reduces transfusions and mediastinal drainage in repeat cardiac surgery. *Anesth Analg* 1996;83:18.

162. Brown RS, Thwaites BK, Morgan PD. Tranexamic acid is effective in decreasing postoperative bleeding and transfusions in primary coronary artery bypass operations: a double-blind, randomized, placebo-controlled trial. *Anesth Analg* 1997;85:963.

163. Katsaros D, Petricevic M, Snow NJ, et al. Tranexamic acid reduces postbypass blood use: a double-blinded, prospective, randomized study of 210 patients. *Ann Thorac Surg* 1996;61:1131.

164. Zonis Z, Seear M, Reichert C, et al. The effect of preoperative tranexamic acid on blood loss after cardiac operations in children. *J Thorac Cardiovasc Surg* 1996;111:982.

165. Casati V, Della Valle P, Benussi S, et al. Effects of tranexamic acid on postoperative bleeding and related hematochemical variables in coronary surgery: comparision between on-pump and off-pump techniques. *J Thorac Cardiovasc Surg* 2004;128:83.

166. Laupacis A, Fergusson D. Drugs to minimize perioperative blood loss in cardiac surgery: meta-analysis using perioperative blood transfusion as the outcome. The International Study of Peri-Operative Transfusion (ISPOT) Investigators. *Anesth Analg* 1997;85:1258.

167. Greilich PE, Okada K, Latham P, et al. Aprotinin but not epsilon-aminocaproic acid decreases interleukin-10 after cardiac surgery with extracorporeal circulation: a randomized double-blind, placebo-controlled study in patients receiving aprotinin and epsilon-aminocaproic acid. *Circulation* 2001;104:I265.

168. Casati V, Guzzon D, Oppizzi M, et al. Tranexamic acid compared with high dose aprotinin in primary elective heart operations: effects on perioperative bleeding and allogeneic transfusions. *J Thorac Cardiovasc Surg* 2000;120:520.

169. Hekmat K, Zimmerman T, Kampe S, et al. Impact of tranexamic acid vs. aprotinin on blood loss and transfusion requirements after cardiopulmonary bypass: a prospective, randomized, double-blind trial. *Curr Med Res Opin* 2004;20:121.

170. Wong BI, Mclean RF, Fremes SE, et al. Aprotinin and tranexamic acid for high transfusion risk cardiac surgery. *Ann Thorac Surg* 2000;69:808.

171. Casati V, Guzzon D, Oppizzi M, et al. Hemostatic effects of aprotinin, tranexamic acid, and epsilon-aminocaproic acid in primary cardiac surgery. *Ann Thorac Surg* 1999;68:2252.

172. Ray MJ, Hales MM, Brown L, et al. Postoperatively administered aprotinin or epsilon aminocaproic acid after cardiopulmonary bypass has limited benefit. *Ann Thorac Surg* 2001;72:521.

173. Casati V, Bellotti F, Gerli C, et al. Tranexamic acid administration after cardiac surgery: a prospective, randomized, double-blind, placebo-controlled study. *Anesthesiology* 2001;94:8.

174. Hardy JF, Belisle S, Dupont C, et al. Prophylactic tranexamic acid and epsilon-aminocaproic acid for primary myocardial revascularization. *Ann Thorac Surg* 1998;65:371.

175. Chauhan S, Das SN, Bisoi A, et al. Comparison of epsilon-aminocaproic acid and tranexamic acid in pediatric cardiac surgery. *J Cardiothorac Vasc Anesth* 2004;18:141.

176. Rand MD, Lock JB, van't Veer C, et al. Blood clotting in minimally altered whole blood. *Blood* 1996;88:3432.

177. Béguin S, Keularts I. On the coagulation of platelet-rich plasma. *Haemostasis* 1999;29:50.

178. Greenberg CS, Miraglia CC, Rickles FR, et al. Cleavage of blood coagulation factor XIII and fibrinogen by thrombin during *in vitro* clotting. *J Clin Invest* 1985;75:1463.

179. von dem Borne PAK, Bajzar L, Meijers JCM, et al. Thrombin-mediated activation of factor XI results in a TAFI (thrombin activatable fibrinolysis inhibitor) dependent inhibition of fibrinolysis. *J Clin Invest* 1997;99:2323.

180. Bolton-Maggs PH, Patterson DA, Wensley RT, et al. Definition of the bleeding tendency in factor-XI deficient kindreds: a clinical and laboratory study. *Thromb Haemost* 1995;73:194.

181. Cawthern KM, van't Veer C, Look JB, et al. Blood coagulation in hemophilia A and hemophilia C. *Blood* 1998;91:4581.

182. Villar A, Jimenez-Yuste V, Quintana M, et al. The use of haemostatic drugs in haemophilia: desmopressin and antifibrinolytic agents. *Haemophilia* 2002;8:189.

183. Reid WO, Hodge SM, Cerutti ER. The use of EACA in preventing or reducing hemorrhages in the hemophiliac. *Thromb Diath Haemorrh* 1967;18:179.

184. Rainsford SG, Jouhar AJ, Hall A. Tranexamic acid in the control of spontaneous bleeding in severe haemophilia. *Thromb Diath Haemorrh* 1973;30:272.

185. Gordon AM, McNicol GP, Dubber AH, et al. Clinical trial of epsilon-aminocaproic acid in severe haemophilia. *BMJ* 1965;2:1632.

186. Bennett AE, Ingram GI, Inglish PJ. Antifibrinolytic treatment in haemophilia: a controlled trial of prophylaxis with tranexamic acid. *Br J Haematol* 1973;24:83.

187. Strauss S, Kevy SV, Diamond LK. Ineffectiveness of prophylactic epsilon-aminocaproic acid in severe hemophilia. *N Engl J Med* 1965;273:301.

188. Prentice CRM, Lindsay RM, Barr RD, et al. Renal complications in haemophilia and Christmas disease. *Q J Med* 1971;40:47.

189. Corrigan JJ Jr. Oral bleeding in hemophilia: treatment with epsilon-aminocaproic acid and replacement therapy. *J Pediatr* 1972;80:124.

190. Lalwani RB, Stricker RB. Case report: successful use of antifibrinolytic therapy in acquired factor VIII deficiency. *Am J Med Sci* 1992;303:398.

191. Reid WO, Lucas ON, Francisco J, et al. The use of epsilon-aminocaproic acid in the management of dental extractions in the hemophiliac. *Am J Med Sci* 1964;248:184.

192. Walsh PN, Rizza CR, Matthews JM, et al. Epsilon-aminocaproic acid therapy for dental extractions in haemophilia and Christmas disease: a double-blind controlled trial. *Br J Haematol* 1971;20:463.

193. Forbes CD, Barr RD, Reid G, et al. Tranexamic acid in control of haemorrhage after dental extraction in haemophilia and Christmas disease. *BMJ* 1972;2:311.

194. Sindet-Petersen S, Ingerslev J, Ramström G, et al. Management of oral bleeding in hemophilic patients. *Lancet* 1988;II:566.

195. Björlin G, Nilsson IM. Tooth extractions in hemophiliacs after administration of a single dose of factor VIII or factor IX concentrate supplemented with AMCA. *Oral Surg Oral Med Oral Pathol* 1973;36:482.

196. Djulbegovic B, Marasa M, Pesto A, et al. Safety and efficacy of purified factor IX concentrate and antifibrinolytic agents for dental extractions in hemophilia B. *Am J Hematol* 1996;51:168.

197. Storti E, Ascari E, Turpini R, et al. Epsilon-aminocaproic acid for synovectomy in haemophilic patients. *Acta Haematol* 1972;47:146.

198. Nilsson IM, Hedner U, Ahlberg A, et al. Surgery of hemophiliacs—20 years' experience. *World J Surg* 1977;1:55.

199. Kasper CK, Dietrich SL. Hemophilia and related conditions. In: Conn HF, ed. *Current therapy*. Philadelphia, PA: WB Saunders, 1982:273.

200. Rizza CR. Inhibitors of fibrinolysis in the treatment of haemophiliacs. *J Clin Pathol Suppl (R Coll Pathol)* 1980;14:50.

201. Sindet-Pedersen S, Ramstrom G, Bernard S, et al. Hemostatic effect of tranexamic acid mouthwash in anticoagulant-treated patients undergoing oral surgery. *N Engl J Med* 1989;320:840.

202. Gaspar R, Brenner B, Ardekian L, et al. Use of tranexamic acid mouthwash to prevent postoperative bleeding in oral surgery patients on oral anticoagulant medication. *Quintessence Int* 1997;28:375.

203. Souto JC, Oliver A, Zuazu-Jausoro I, et al. Oral surgery in anticoagulated patients without reducing the dose of oral anticoagulant: a prospective randomized study. *J Oral Maxillofac Surg* 1996;54:27.

204. Carter G, Goss A. Tranexamic acid mouthwash—a prospective randomized study of a 2-day vs. 5-day regimen to prevent post-operative bleeding in anticoagulated patients requiring dental extractions. *Int J Oral Maxillofac Surg* 2003;32:504.

205. Williamson R, Eggleston DJ. DDAVP and EACA used for minor oral surgery in von Willebrand disease. *Aust Dent J* 1988;33:32.

206. Derkay CS, Werner E, Plotnick E. Management of children with von Willebrand disease undergoing adenotonsillectomy. *Am J Otolaryngol* 1996;17:172.

207. Ciavarella N, Schiavoni M, Valenzano E, et al. Use of recombinant factor VIIa (NovoSeven) in the treatment of two patients with type III von Willebrand's disease and an inhibitor against von Willebrand factor. *Haemostasis* 1996;26(Suppl. 1):150. [].

208. Vermylen J, Peerlinck K. Optimal care of inhibitor patients during surgery. *Eur J Haematol Suppl* 1998;63:15.

209. Gardner FH, Helmer RE III. Aminocaproic acid: use in control of hemorrhage in patients with a megakaryocytic thrombocytopenia. *JAMA* 1980;243:35.

210. Gallardo RL, Gardner FH. Aminocaproic acid for bleeding in thrombocytopenic patients. *Tex Med* 1985;81:30.

211. Bartholomew JR, Salgia R, Bell WR. Control of bleeding in patients with immune and nonimmune thrombocytopenia with aminocaproic acid. *Arch Intern Med* 1989;149:1959.

212. Garewal HS, Durie BGM. Antifibrinolytic therapy with aminocaproic acid for the control of bleeding in thrombocytopenic patients. *Scand J Haematol* 1985;35:497.

213. Zwierzina WD, Schmalzl F, Kunz F, et al. Studies in a case of Bernard-Soulier syndrome. *Acta Haematol* 1983;69:195.

214. Peng TC, Kidder TS, Bell WR, et al. Obstetric complications in a patient with Bernard-Soulier syndrome. *Am J Obstet Gynecol* 1991;165:425.

215. Benson K, Fields K, Hiemenz J, et al. The platelet refractory bone marrow transplant patient: prophylaxis and treatment of bleeding. *Semin Oncol* 1993;20(5 Suppl. 6):102.

216. Astrup T. Tissue activators of plasminogen. *Fed Proc* 1966;25:42.

217. Andersson L, Nilsson IM, Colleen S, et al. Role of urokinase and tissue activator in sustaining bleeding and the management thereof with EACA and AMCA. *Ann N Y Acad Sci* 1968;146:642.

218. Immergut MA, Stevenson T. The use of epsilon-aminocaproic acid in the control of hematuria associated with hemoglobinopathies. *J Urol* 1965;93:110.

219. Vega R, Shanberg AM, Malloy TR. The use of epsilon-aminocaproic acid in sickle cell trait hematuria. *J Urol* 1971;105:552.

220. Bilinsky RT, Kandel GL, Rabiner SF. Epsilon-aminocaproic acid therapy of hematuria due to heterozygous sickle cell diseases. *J Urol* 1969;102:93.

221. Black WB, Hatch FE, Acchiardo S. Aminocaproic acid in prolonged hematuria of patients with sicklemia. *Arch Intern Med* 1976;136:678.

222. Mcinnes BK III. The management of hematuria associated with sickle-hemoglobinopathies. *J Urol* 1980;124:171.

223. Ambrus CM, Ambrus JL, Lassman HB, et al. Studies on the mechanism of action of inhibitors of the fibrinolysis system. *Ann N Y Acad Sci* 1968;146:430.

224. Gobbi F. Use and misuse of aminocaproic acid. *Lancet* 1967;1:472.

225. Savdie E, Mahony JF, Storey BG. Control of bleeding after renal biopsy with epsilon-aminocaproic acid. *Br J Urol* 1978;50:8.

226. Haygood TA, Atkins R, Kennedy JA, et al. Aminocaproic acid treatment of prolonged hematuria following renal biopsy. *Arch Intern Med* 1971;127:478.

227. Silverberg DS, Dossetor JB, Eid TC, et al. Arteriovenous fistula and prolonged hematuria after renal biopsy: treatment with epsilon-aminocaproic acid. *Can Med Assoc J* 1974;110:671.

228. Elliott SJ, Salcedo JR. Hematuria after renal allograft biopsy: treatment with aminocaproic acid. *Urology* 1985;26:20.

229. Schmutzler R, Furstenberg H. Fibrinolysis and blood loss after surgery of the prostate and its response to antifibrinolysis. *Dtsch Med Wochenschr* 1966;91:197.

230. McNicol GP, Fletcher AP, Alkjaersig N, et al. The use of epsilon-aminocaproic acid, a potent inhibitor of fibrinolytic activity in the management of post-operative hematuria. *J Urol* 1961;86:829.

231. Andersson L. Antifibriolytic drugs in the treatment of urinary tact haemorrhage. *Prog Surg* 1972;10:76.

232. Andersson L, Nilsson IM. Effect of epsilon-aminocaproic acid (EACA) on fibrinolysis and bleeding conditions in prostatic disease. *Acta Chir Scand* 1961;121:291.

233. Sack E, Spaet TH, Gentile RL, et al. Reduction of post-prostatectomy bleeding by epsilon aminocaproic acid. *N Engl J Med* 1962;266:541.

234. Miller RA, May MW, Henry WF, et al. The prevention of secondary haemorrhage after prostatectomy: the value of antifibrinolytic therapy. *Br J Urol* 1980;52:26.

235. Madsen PO, Strauch AE. The effect of aminocaproic acid on bleeding following transurethral prostatectomy. *J Urol* 1966;96:255.

236. Lawrence ACK, Ward-McQuaid JN, Holdom GL. The effect of epsilon-aminocaproic acid on the blood loss after retropubic prostatectomy. *Br J Urol* 1966;38:308.

237. Kirkman NF. Post prostatectomy hematuria: treatment with epsilon-aminocaproic acid. *Br J Surg* 1967;54:1026.

238. Smart CJ, Turnbull AR, Jenkins JD. The use of furosemide and epsilon-aminocaproic acid in transurethral prostatectomy. *Br J Urol* 1974;46:521.

239. Smith RB, Riach P, Kaufman JJ. Epsilon-aminocaproic acid and the control of postprostatectomy bleeding. A prospective double-blind study. *J Urol* 1974;131:1093.

240. Hedlund PO. Antifibrinolytic therapy with Cyklokapron in connection with prostatectomy. A double-blind study. *Scand J Urol Nephrol* 1969;3:177.

241. Coggins JT, Allen TD. Insoluble fibrin clots within the urinary tract as a consequence of epsilon-aminocaproic acid therapy. *J Urol* 1972;107:647.

242. Ranniko A, Petas A, Taari K. Tranexamic acid in control of primary hemorrhage during transurethral prostatectomy. *Urology* 2004;64:955.

243. Smart CJ. The use of furosemide and epsilon-aminocaproic acid in transurethral prostatectomy. A review after 7 years. *Br J Urol* 1982;54:437.

244. Pearson BS. The effects of trasylol and aminocaproic acid in postprostatectomy hemorrhage. *Br J Urol* 1969;41:620.

245. Albrechtsen OK. The fibrinolytic activity of the human endometrium. *Acta Endocrinol* 1956;23:207.

246. Rybo G. Clinical and experimental studies on menstrual blood loss. *Acta Obstet Gynecol Scand* 1966;45:1.

247. Larsson B, Liedholm P, Syoberg NO, et al. Increased fibrinolytic activity in the endometrium of patients using copper IUD. *Contraception* 1974;9:531.

248. Nilsson IM, Bjorkman SK, Andersson L. Clinical experiences with epsilon-aminocaproic acid (EACA) as an antifibrinolytic agent. *Acta Med Scand* 1961;170:487.

249. Gennser G. Diskussion. *Nord Med* 1964;18:778.

250. Nilsson L, Rybo G. Treatment of menorrhagia with epsilon-aminocaproic acid: a double blind investigation. *Acta Obstet Gynecol Scand* 1965;44:467.

251. Nilsson L, Rybo G. Treatment of menorrhagia with an anti-fibrinolytic agent, tranexamic acid (AMCA): a double blind investigation. *Acta Obstet Gynecol Scand* 1967;46:572.

252. Vermylen J, Vehaegen-Declercq ML, Verstraete M, et al. A double blind study of the effect of tranexamic acid in essential menorrhagia. *Thromb Diath Haemorrh* 1968;20:583.

253. Callender ST, Warner GT. Treatment of menorrhagia with tranexamic acid: a double blind trial. *BMJ* 1970;4:214.

254. Nilsson L, Rybo G. Treatment of menorrhagia. *Am J Obstet Gynecol* 1971; 110:713.

255. Prentice A. Medical management of menorrhagia. *BMJ* 1999;319:1343.

256. Lakhani KP, Marsh MS, Purcell W, et al. Uterine artery blood flow parameters in women with dysfunctional uterine bleeding and uterine fibroids: the effects of tranexamic acid. *Ultrasound Obstet Gynecol* 1998; 11:283.

257. Ong YL, Hull DR, Mayne EE. Menorrhagia in von Willebrand disease successfully treated with single daily dose tranexamic acid. *Haemophilia* 1998;4:63.

258. Lethaby A, Farquhar C, Cooke I. Antifibrinolytics for heavy menstrual bleeding. *Cochrane Database Syst Rev* 2000;4:CD000249.

259. Bentorp E, Follrud C, Lethagen S. No increased risk of venous thrombosis in women taking tranexamic acid. *Thromb Haemost* 2001;86:714.

260. Mishell DR Jr, Fisher HW, Haynes PJ, et al. Menorrhagia: a symposium. *J Reprod Med* 1984;29:763.

261. Guilleband J, Bonnar J, Morehead J, et al. Menstrual blood-loss with intrauterine devices. *Lancet* 1976;1:387.

262. Larson B, Liedholm P, Astedt B. Increased fibrinolytic activity in the endometrium of patients using copper IUD (Gravegard). *Int J Fertil* 1975; 20:77.

263. Kasonde JM, Bonnar J. Aminocaproic acid and menstrual loss in women using intrauterine devices. *BMJ* 1975;4:17.

264. Westrom L, Bengtsson LP. Effect of tranexamic acid (AMCA) in menorrhagia with intrauterine contraceptive devices: a double-blind study. *J Reprod Med* 1970;5:41.

265. Rybo G, Westerberg H. The effect of tranexamic acid (AMCA) on postoperative bleeding after conization. *Acta Obstet Gynecol Scand* 1972;51:347.

266. Grundsell H, Larsson G, Bekessy Z. Use of an antifibrinolytic agent (tranexamic acid) and lateral sutures with laser conization of the cervix. *Obstet Gynecol* 1984;63:573.

267. Takashima S, Koga M, Tanaka K. Fibrinolytic activity of human brain and cerebrospinal fluid. *Br J Exp Pathol* 1969;50:533.

268. Smith RR, Upchurch JJ. Monitoring antifibrinolytic therapy in subarachnoid hemorrhage. *J Neurosurg* 1973;38:339.

269. Tovi D, Nilsson IM. Increased fibrinolytic activity and fibrin degradation products after experimental intracerebral haemorrhage. *Acta Neurol Scand* 1972;48:403.

270. Sahs AL, Perret G, Locksley HB, et al. *Intracranial aneurysms and subarachnoid hemorrhage: a cooperative study.* Philadelphia, PA: JB Lippincott Co, 1969:296.

271. Alvord EC Jr, Loeser JD, Bailey WL, et al. Subarachnoid hemorrhage due to ruptured aneurysms: a simple method of estimating prognosis. *Arch Neurol* 1972;27:273.

272. Kassell NF, Torner JC. Aneurysmal rebleeding: a preliminary report from the cooperative aneurysm study. *Neurosurgery* 1983;13:479.

273. Kassell NF, Haley EC, Torner JC. Antifibrinolytic therapy in the treatment of aneurysmal subarachnoid hemorrhage. *Clin Neurosurg* 1986;33:37.

274. Uihlein A, MacCarty CS, Michenfelder JD, et al. Deep hypothermia and surgical treatment of intracranial aneurysms: a five-year survey. *JAMA* 1966;195:639.

275. Patterson RH Jr, Harpel P. The effect of epsilon-aminocaproic acid and tranexamic acid on thrombus size and strength in a simulated arterial aneurysm. *J Neurosurg* 1971;34:365.

276. Nibbelink DW, Torner JC, Henderson WG. Intracranial aneurysms and subarachnoid hemorrhage. A cooperative study. Antifibrinolytic therapy in recent onset subarachnoid hemorrhage. *Stroke* 1975;6:622.

277. Sengupta RFP, So SC, Villarejo-Ortega FJ. Use of epsilon-aminocaproic acid (EACA) in the preoperative management of ruptured intracranial aneurysms. *J Neurosurg* 1976;44:479.

278. Tovi D, Nilsson IM, Thulin CA. Fibrinolysis and subarachnoid haemorrhage. Inhibitory effect of tranexamic acid. A clinical study. *Acta Neurol Scand* 1972;48:393.

279. Tovi D. The use of antifibrinolytic drugs to prevent early recurrent aneurysmal subarachnoid haemorrhage. *Acta Neurol Scand* 1973;49:163.

280. Mullan S. Conservative management of the recently ruptured aneurysm. *Surg Neurol* 1975;3:27.

281. Mullan S, Dawley J. Antifibrinolytic therapy for intracranial aneurysms. *J Neurosurg* 1968;28:21.

282. Geronemus R, Herz DA, Shulman K. Streptokinase clot lysis time in patients with ruptured intracranial aneurysms. *J Neurosurg* 1974;40:499.

283. Corkill G. Earlier operation and antifibrinolytic therapy in the management of aneurysmal subarachnoid haemorrhage. Review of recent experience in Tasmania. *Med J Aust* 1974;1:468.

284. Post KD, Flamm ES, Goodgold A, et al. Ruptured intracranial aneurysms: case morbidity and mortality. *J Neurosurg* 1977;46:290.

285. Ransohoff J, Goodgold A, Benjamin MI. Preoperative management of patients with ruptured intracranial aneurysms. *J Neurosurg* 1972;36:525.

286. Chowdhary UM, Carey PC, Hussein MM. Prevention of early recurrence of spontaneous subarachnoid haemorrhage by epsilon-aminocaproic acid. *Lancet* 1979;1:741.

287. Maurice-Williams RS. Prolonged antifibrinolysis. An effective nonsurgical treatment for ruptured intracranial aneurysms? *BMJ* 1978;1:945.

288. Nibbelink DW, Sahs AL. Antifibrinolytic therapy and drug-induced hypotension in treatment of ruptured intracranial aneurysms. *Trans Am Neurol Assoc* 1972;97:145.

289. Fodstad H, Liliquist B, Shannong M, et al. Tranexamic acid in the preoperative management of ruptured intracranial aneurysms. *Surg Neurol* 1978;10:9.

290. Girvin JP. The use of antifibrinolytic agents in the preoperative treatment of ruptured intracranial aneurysms. *Trans Am Neurol Assoc* 1973;98:150.

291. van Rossum J, Wintzen AR, Endtz LJ, et al. Effect of tranexamic acid on rebleeding after subarachnoid hemorrhage: a double blind controlled clinical trial. *Ann Neurol* 1977;2:242.

292. Kaste M, Ramsay M. Tranexamic acid in subarachnoid hemorrhage: a double blind study. *Stroke* 1979;10:519.

293. Scott RM, Garrido E. Spontaneous thrombosis of an intracranial aneurysm during treatment with epsilon-aminocaproic acid. *Surg Neurol* 1977;7:21.

294. Sonntag VKH, Stein BH. Arteriopathic complications occurring during treatment of subarachnoid hemorrhage with epsilon-aminocaproic acid. *J Neurosurg* 1974;40:480.

295. Kassell NF, Torner JC, Adams HP Jr. Antifibrinolytic therapy in the acute period following aneurysmal subarachnoid hemorrhage: preliminary observations from the cooperative aneurysm study. *J Neurosurg* 1984;61:225.

296. Vermeulen M, Lindsay KW, Murray GD, et al. Antifibrinolytic treatment in subarachnoid hemorrhage. *N Engl J Med* 1984;311:432.

297. Roos Y, STAR Study Group. Antifibrinolytic treatment in subarachnoid hemorrhage: a randomized, placebo-controlled trial. *Neurology* 2000;54: 77–82.

298. Roos Y, Rinkel G, Vermeulen M, et al. Antifibrinolytic therapy for aneurysmal subarachnoid hemorrhage. *Cochrane Database Syst Rev* 2003;2: CD001245.

299. Cox HT, Poller L, Thomsen JM. Evidence for the release of gastric fibrinolytic activity into peripheral blood. *Gut* 1969;10:404.

300. Cormack F, Jouhar AJ, Chakrabarti RR, et al. Tranexamic acid in upper gastrointestinal hemorrhage. *Lancet* 1973;2:1207.

301. Biggs JC, Hugh TB, Dobbs AJ. Tranexamic acid and upper gastrointestinal haemorrhage—a double-blind trial. *Gut* 1975;17:729.

302. Engqvist A, Bostrom O, Feilitzen VF, et al. Tranexamic acid in massive haemorrhage from the upper gastrointestinal tract: a double-blind study. *Scand J Gastroenterol* 1979;14:839.

303. Barer D, Ogilvie A, Henry D, et al. Cimetidine and tranexamic acid in the treatment of acute upper gastrointestinal tract bleeding. *N Engl J Med* 1983;308:1571.

304. von Holstein CC, Eriksson SB, Kallen R. Tranexamic acid as an aid to reduced blood transfusion requirements in gastric and duodenal bleeding. *Br Med J* 1987;294:7.

305. Jespersen J, Sidelmann J. A comparison of the effects of cimetidine and epsilon-aminocaproic acid on fibrinolysis induced by activators of plasminogen and on fibrin formation. *Thromb Res* 1981;22:287.

306. Henry DA, O'Connell DL. Effects of fibrinolytic inhibitors on mortality from upper gastrointestinal haemorrhage. *BMJ* 1989;298:1142.

307. Hawkey GM, Cole AT, McIntyre AS, et al. Drug treatments in upper gastrointestinal bleeding: value of endoscope findings as surrogate end points. *Gut* 2001;492:372.

308. Kondo M, Ibezaki M, Kato H, et al. Antifibrinolytic therapy of giant hypertrophic gastritis (Ménétrier's disease). *Scand J Gastroenterol* 1978; 13:851.

309. Violl F, Basili S, Ferro D et al., CALC Group. Association between high values of D-dimer and tissue-plasminogen activator activity and first gastrointestinal bleeding in cirrhotic patients. *Thromb Haemost* 1996;76:177.

310. Bergqvist D, Dahlgren S, Hessman Y. Local inhibition of the fibrinolytic system in patients with massive upper gastrointestinal hemorrhage. *Ups J Med Sci* 1980;85:173.

311. Oka K, Tanaka K. Local fibrinolysis of esophagus and stomach as a cause of hemorrhage in liver cirrhosis. *Thromb Res* 1979;14:837.

312. McCormick PA, Ooi H, Crosbie O. Tranexamic acid for severe bleeding gastric antral vascular ectasia in cirrhosis. *Gut* 1998;42:750.

313. Kwaan HJC, Cocco A, Mendeloff AL. Histologic demonstration of plasminogen activation in rectal biopsies from patients with active ulcerative colitis. *J Lab Clin Med* 1964;64:877 (abst).

314. Salter RH, Read AE. Epsilon-aminocaproic acid therapy in ulcerative colitis. *Gut* 1970;11:585.

315. Mowat NA, Douglas AS, Brunt PW, et al. Epsilon-aminocaproic acid therapy in ulcerative colitis. *Am J Dig Dis* 1973;18:939.

316. Hollanders D, Thomson JM, Schofield PF. Tranexamic acid therapy in ulcerative colitis. *Postgrad Med J* 1983;58:87.

317. Kondo M, Hotta T, Takemura K, et al. Treatment of ulcerative colitis by the direct administration of an antifibrinolytic agent as an enema. *Hepatogastroenterology* 1981;28:270.

318. Kondo M, Fukumoto K, Yoshiikawa T, et al. Tissue fibrinolysis in the digestive mucosa. III. Treatment of ulcerative colitis by the direct administration of an antifibrinolytic agent as an enema. *Nippon Shokakibyo Gakkai Zasshi* 1981;3:653.

319. Pandolfi M, Kwaan HC. Fibrinolysis in the anterior segment of the eye. *Arch Ophthalmol* 1967;77:99.

320. Crouch ER Jr, Frenkel M. Aminocaproic acid in the treatment of traumatic hyphema. *Am J Ophthalmol* 1976;81:355.

321. Jerndal T, Frisen M. Tranexamic acid (AMCA) and late hyphaema: a double blind study in cataract surgery. *Acta Ophthalmol (Copenh)* 1976;54:417.

322. Mortensen KK, Sjolie AK. Secondary haemorrhage following traumatic hyphaema: a comparative study of conservative and tranexamic acid treatment. *Acta Ophthalmol (Copenh)* 1978;56:763.

323. Bramsen T. Traumatic hyphaema treated with the antifibrinolytic drug tranexamic acid. *Acta Ophthalmol (Copenh)* 1976;54:250.

324. Missotten L, de Clippeleer L, Van Tornout I, et al. The value of tranexamic acid (Cyklokapron) in the prevention of secondary bleeding, a complication of traumatic hyphema. *Bull Soc Belge Ophtalmol* 1977;179:47.

325. Musitalo RJ, Saari MWS, Aine E, et al. Tranexamic acid in the prevention of secondary hemorrhage after traumatic hyphaema. *Acta Ophthalmol (Copenh)* 1981;59:539.

326. deBustros S, Glaser BM, Mikchels RG, et al. Effect of epsilon-aminocaproic acid on postvitrectomy hemorrhage. *Arch Ophthalmol* 1985;103:219.

327. McGetrick JJ, Jampol LM, Goldberg MF, et al. Aminocaproic acid decreases secondary hemorrhage after traumatic hyphema. *Arch Ophthalmol* 1983;101:1031.

328. Rahmani B, Jahadi HR. Comparison of tranexamic acid and prednisolone in the treatment of traumatic hyphema. A randomized clinical trial. *Ophthalmology* 1999;106:375.

329. Crouch ER Jr, Williams PB, Gray MK, et al. Topical aminocaproic acid in the treatment of traumatic hyphema. *Arch Ophthalmol* 1997;115:1106.

330. Pieramici DJ, Goldberg MF, Melia M, et al. A phase III, multicenter, randomized, placebo-controlled trial of topical aminocaproic acid (Caprogel) in the management of traumatic hyphema. *Ophthalmology* 2003;110:2106.

331. Taboul BK, Jacob JL, Barsoum-Homsy M, et al. Clinical evaluation of aminocaproic acid for managing traumatic hyphema in children. *Ophthalmology* 1995;102:1646.

332. Falbe-Hansen J Jr, Jacobsen B, Lorenzen E. Local application of an antifibrinolytic tonsillectomy. A double blind study. *J Laryngol Otol* 1974;88:565.

333. Verstraete M, Vermylen J, Tyberghein J. Double blind evaluation of the haemostatic effect of adrenochrome monosemicarbazone, conjugated oestrogens, and epsilon-aminocaproic acid after adenotonsillectomy. *Acta Haematol (Basel)* 1968;40:154.

334. Castelli G, Vogt E. Der erfolg mit antifibrinolytisschen behandlung mit tranexamsaure zur reduction der blutverlustes wahrend und nach tonsillektomien. *Schweiz Med Wochenschr* 1977;107:780.

335. Petruson B. Epistaxis: a clinical study with special reference to fibrinolysis. *Acta Otolaryngol Suppl (Stockh)* 1974;317:1.

336. Neidhart JA, Roach RW. Successful treatment of skeletal hemangioma and Kasabach-Merritt syndrome with aminocaproic acid: is fibrinolysis "defensive"? *Am J Med* 1982;73:434.

337. Warrell RP Jr, Kempin SJ. Treatment of severe coagulopathy in the Kasabach-Merritt syndrome with aminocaproic acid and cryoprecipitate. *N Engl J Med* 1985;313:309.

338. Ortel TL, Onorato JJ, Bedrosian CL, et al. Antifibrinolytic therapy in the management of the Kasabach-Merritt syndrome. *Am J Hematol* 1988;29:44.

339. Katsaros D, Grundfest-Broniatowski S. Successful management of visceral Klippel-Trenaunay-Weber syndrome with the antifibrinolytic agent tranexamic acid (Cyclocapron): a case report. *Am Surg* 1998;64:302.

340. Poon MC, Kloiber R, Birdsell DC. Epsilon-aminocaproic acid in the reversal of consumptive coagulopathy with platelet sequestration in a vascular malformation of Klippel-Trenaunay syndrome. *Am J Med* 1989;87:211.

341. Saba HI, Morelli GA, Logrono LA. Treatment of bleeding in hereditary hemorrhagic telangiectasia with aminocaproic acid. *N Engl J Med* 1994;330:1789.

342. Phillips MD. Stopping bleeding in hereditary telangiectasia. *N Engl J Med* 1994;330:1822.

343. Van Hemelen G, Avery CM, Venn PJ, et al. Management of Jehovah's Witness patients undergoing major head and neck surgery. *Head Neck* 1999;21:80.

344. Palmer JD, Francis DA, Roath DS, et al. Hyperfibrinolysis during intracranial surgery: effect of high dose aprotinin. *J Neurol Neurosurg Psychiatry* 1995;58:104.

345. Janssens M, Joris J, David JL, et al. High dose aprotinin reduces blood loss in patients undergoing total hip replacement surgery. *Anesthesiology* 1994;80:23.

346. Murkin JM, Haig GM, Beer KJ, et al. Aprotinin decreases exposure to allogeneic blood during primary unilateral hip replacement. *J Bone Joint Surg Am* 2000;82:675.

347. Harps A, Murphy DB, McCaroll M. The efficacy of single dose aprotinin 2 million KIU in reducing blood loss and its impact on the incidence of deep venous thrombosis in patients undergoing total hip replacement surgery. *J Clin Anesth* 1996;8:357.

348. Samama CM, Langeron O, Rosencher N, et al. Aprotinin versus placebo in major orthopedic surgery: a randomized, double-blinded, dose-ranging study. *Anesth Analg* 2002;95:287.

349. Jeserschek R, Clar H, Aigner C, et al. Reduction of blood loss using high dose aprotinin in major orthopedic surgery: a prospective, double-blind, randomized and placebo-controlled study. *J Bone Joint Surg Br* 2003;85:174.

350. Hiipala ST, Strid LJ, Wennerstrand MI, et al. Tranexamic acid radically decreases blood loss and transfusions associated with total knee arthroplasty. *Anesth Analg* 1997;84:839.

351. Jansen AJ, Andreica S, Claeys M, et al. Use of tranexamic acid for an effective blood conservation strategy after total knee arthroplasty. *Br J Anaesth* 1999;83:596.

352. Veien M, Sorenson JV, Madsen F, et al. Tranexamic acid given intraoperatively reduces blood loss after total knee replacement: a randomized controlled study. *Acta Anaesthesiol Scand* 2002;46:1206.

353. Husted H, Bloud B, Sonne-Holm S, et al. Tranexamic acid reduces blood loss and blood transfusions in primary total hip arthroplasty: a prospective randomized double-blind study in 40 patients. *Acta Orthop Scand* 2003;74:665.

354. Lemay B, Guay J, Cote C, et al. Tranexamic acid reduces the need for allogeneic red blood cell transfusions in patients undergoing total hip replacement. *Can J Anaesth* 2004;51:31.

355. Palmer JD, Francis JL, Pickard JD, et al. The efficacy and safety of aprotinin for hemostasis during intracranial surgery. *J Neurosurg* 2003;98:1208.

356. Busuttill RW. A comparison of antifibrinolytic agents used in hemostatic fibrin sealants. *J Am Coll Surg* 2003;197(6):1021.

357. Alving BM, Weinstein MJ, Finlayson JS. Fibrin sealant: summary of a conference on characteristics and clinical uses. *Transfusion* 1995;35:783.

358. Rakocz M, Mazar A, Varon D. Dental extractions in patients with bleeding disorders. The use of fibrin glue. *Oral Surg Oral Med Oral Pathol* 1993;75:280.

359. Kinahan TJ, Johnson HW. Tisseel in hypospadias repair. *Can J Surg* 1992;35:75.

360. Vaiman M, Eviatar E, Segal S. The use of fibrin glue as hemostatic in endonasal operations: a prospective randomized study. *Rhinology* 2002;40:88.

361. Wiseman NE. Endoscopic closure of recurrent tracheoesophageal fistula using Tisseel. *J Pediatr Surg* 1995;30:1236.

362. Scheule AM, Beierlein W, Wendel HF. Fibrin sealant, aprotinin, and immune response in children undergoing operations for congenital heart disease. *J Thorac Cardiovasc Surg* 1998;115:883.

# CHAPTER 80 ■ TRANSFUSION MEDICINE: PLATELET TRANSFUSION THERAPY, PLASMA, AND PLASMA CONCENTRATES

THOMAS S. KICKLER

## PLATELET TRANSFUSION THERAPY

Methods for the collection and preparation of blood components used in the treatment of coagulation disorders have undergone major changes in the last 2 decades. These changes have included improved methods to collect and store platelets, and new manufacturing processes that permit the isolation and production of a wide variety of specific plasma proteins for transfusion. The development of recombinant technology has dramatically improved the safety of coagulation factor replacement therapy. The potential infectious risks of transfusion, dwindling blood supply, and considerable increases in cost of blood components are all reasons why one must know the indications of transfusion. The purpose of this chapter is to review the properties and clinical indications of platelets, plasma, and coagulation factor concentrates.

### Platelet Preparations

#### Platelet Concentrates and Pheresis Platelets

Platelet transfusions are available as platelet concentrates or as apheresis units (1). The former are prepared from units of whole blood by centrifugation, and the latter are collected by pheresis devices. Platelet concentrates are separated from whole blood by first preparing platelet-rich plasma and then centrifuging the platelets with a second centrifugation. The contents of the platelet concentrates are highly variable depending upon the technique. However, the 50 mL platelet concentrate usually has at least $5.5 \times 10^{10}$ platelets. In Europe, the buffy coat method is the most common method of platelet preparation. This method uses centrifugation to prepare a buffy coat from which platelets are separated by an additional centrifugation. The white cell contamination is approximately $10^8$ per bag using the platelet-rich plasma method of concentration, and is approximately $10^6$ for platelets prepared by the buffy coat method. The relatively lower white blood cells (WBC) content in platelets prepared by the buffy coat method may be advantageous in reducing alloimmunization and febrile transfusion reactions (2).

Pheresis platelets are collected from donors by apheresis technology that permits continuous processing of large volumes of blood and removal of platelets using an automated system. Because a conventional transfusion dose for an adult patient is approximately 6 U of pooled platelets, collection parameters are used to collect this quantity of platelets from a donor. The leukocyte content of a pheresis platelet depends upon the technology used, but most devices have WBC contamination of less than $10^6$ per bag (3).

### Cyropreserved Platelets

Cyropreserved platelets are used in patients who become alloimmunized during induction chemotherapy. Freezing in a cyroprotective agent such as dimethyl sulfoxide permits platelet storage. Platelets are collected during remission, frozen, and subsequently used when necessary. In early studies, the average posttransfusion recovery of cyropreserved platelets was approximately 50%; this was a limiting factor in achieving therapeutic platelet levels. More recently, there has been renewed interest in cyropreserved platelets. New preservative solutions can be added to dimethyl sulfoxide so that there is less damage to the platelets during preparation and freezing (4,5).

### Lyophilized Platelets and Synthetic Platelets

The lyophilization of outdated platelets is one alternative to liquid stored platelets that has been studied. Lyophilized platelets may support hemostasis because lipids that are present in it provide procoagulant activity. This form of platelets has been studied in a phase II trial but not in larger clinical trails (6). A variety of other approaches have been studied, primarily in animal models, including fibrinogen-coated albumin spheres and fibrinogen-coated red cells. Although these studies indicate the usefulness and safety of platelet substitutes in humans, additional studies are needed to substantiate this (7).

### Platelet Storage Lesion

Platelet blood components are licensed for a storage time of 5 days at room temperature. Early studies demonstrated the need to store platelets at room temperature because the storage at 6°C to 10°C led to loss of function and viability. A variety of reasons account for the loss, but one of the most important appears to be an alteration of platelet glycoprotein Ib/IX that leads to platelet clearance by CR3 in the liver, when cold stored platelets are transfused (8). Maintenance of the function and viability of liquid stored platelets is limited to a relatively short period of time because of the storage lesion that develops at room temperature. There has been a great deal of interest in improving the storage condition for platelets to reduce the functional abnormalities that occur during storage. The platelet storage lesion is characterized by an irreversible change in platelet shape from discoid to spherical; the generation of lactic acid from glycolysis, with an associated decrease in pH; the release of cytoplasmic and granule content, a decrease in various *in vitro* measures of platelet function, particularly hypotonic shock response, and adenosine phosphate–induced shape change; and a reduction *in vivo* recovery and survival (2). A variety of storage solutions exist that can now be used to prevent the loss of platelet function and viability (2,8–10).

## Clinical Applications of Platelet Transfusions

### Indications for Platelet Transfusion in the Patient with Thrombocytopenia

Platelet transfusions are given prophylactically or therapeutically in patients with thrombocytopenia. Table 80-1 outlines platelet transfusion guidelines for a variety of clinical situations and considerations for dealing with platelet transfusions on a long-term basis (11–13). There has been considerable interest in defining the lowest safe platelet concentration at which bleeding is unlikely, so that fewer transfusions are given to patients with marrow aplasia. Clinicians have been generally aware that hemorrhage was more common during the most severe stages of thrombocytopenia and that the threshold for prophylactic platelet transfusions has been 20,000 per $\mu$L for many years.

More recently, investigators have shown that a lower transfusion threshold in adult patients with acute leukemia is safe (15–18). These studies have shown that giving prophylactic transfusions only when the platelet count dips below 5,000 per mm$^3$ can decrease platelet utilization with only a small adverse effect on bleeding and with no effect on mortality. It therefore appears that with amegakaryocytic thrombocytopenia, prophylactic transfusions should be given if the count falls below 5,000 per mm$^3$. At values between 5,000 and 10,000 per mm$^3$, one may be able to abstain from transfusing if the patient is stable and if no other conditions make spontaneous bleeding likely. These conditions include blast crisis, anticoagulation with heparin for disseminated intravascular coagulation, drugs that affect platelet function, uremia, and recent invasive procedures, including spinal taps or placement of central venous catheters (17–19).

### Platelet Dosing

Platelet recovery is usually approximately 60% of the number of autologous platelets transfused, but may be as low as 20% to 40% after homologous transfusion in patients with factors affecting platelet recovery. Given the mean number of platelets in 1 U of blood (approximately $0.5 \times 10^{11}$), the calculated platelet increment per platelet unit transfused, is approximately 7,560 to 10,000. The British Committee for Standards in Hematology proposed a formula taking into account the desired platelet increment, the patient's blood volume, and a recovery factor, resulting in recommended platelet doses of approximately $3 \times 10^{11}$ for adults (16,19,20).

Roy et al. compared two platelet doses in children who received a mean of 2.6 and 3.4 U per transfusion. The average 1-hour increments were very small with both doses (18 and $25 \times 10^9$ per L), and the incidence of bleeding was similar;

## TABLE 80-1

### AMERICAN SOCIETY OF CLINICAL PATHOLOGY PLATELET TRANSFUSION GUIDELINES (14)

Platelet products: The benefits of pooled platelets or single-donor platelets are similar; the two products can be used interchangeably; single-donor platelets from selected donors are used when histocompatible platelet transfusion (i.e., HLA-A and HLA-B antigen matched) is needed

**PROPHYLACTIC PLATELET TRANSFUSION THRESHOLDS:**

Acute leukemia: For adult patients a threshold of 10,000/$\mu$L is recommended; transfusion at higher levels may be necessary in the newborn, or in patients with hemorrhage, high fever, hyperleukocytosis, rapid fall in platelet count, or coagulation abnormalities

Hematopoietic cell transplantation: Same as for acute leukemia, with similar exceptions

Chronic stable severe thrombocytopenia: Many patients can be observed without prophylactic transfusion, reserving transfusion for episodes of hemorrhage or during times of active treatment

Solid tumors: Evidence supports the benefit of prophylactic transfusion at a threshold of 10,000/$\mu$L or less; a threshold of 20,000/$\mu$L should be considered for patients receiving aggressive therapy for bladder cancer, as well as for those with demonstrated necrotic tumors

Surgical or invasive procedures: A platelet count of 40 to 50,000/$\mu$L is sufficient to perform major invasive procedures safely, in the absence of associated coagulation abnormalities; certain procedures, such as bone marrow aspiration/biopsy, can be performed safely with counts <20,000/$\mu$L; lumbar puncture in children is safe at platelet counts >10,000/$\mu$L

Prevention of RhD alloimmunization: RhD-negative women of child-bearing potential age should be considered for treatment with either the exclusive use of platelets from RhD-negative donors or cover with anti-D immunoprophylaxis

Prevention of alloimmunization using leukoreduced blood products: It is appropriate to provide leukoreduced blood products to patients with AML from the time of diagnosis to ameliorate the problem of alloantibody-mediated refractoriness to platelet transfusion; currently, this is not indicated in patients with cancer RBCs or treatments that do not produce significant and sustained thrombocytopenia. Universal leukoreduction of blood products would obviate the need for these decisions in individual patients

Diagnosis of refractoriness to platelet transfusion: A CCI of 7,500 is recommended as a definition of a satisfactory response; a rough estimate of CCI of 5,000 is an absolute platelet count increment of 2,000/$\mu$L per U of platelet concentrate given to an average-sized adult; for children, an approximate equivalent is an absolute platelet count increment of 3,500/$\mu$L/m$^2$ transfused U; a diagnosis of refractoriness should be entertained only when at least two consecutive ABO-compatible transfusions, stored <72 h, result in poor increments

Management of refractoriness to platelet transfusion: Patients with alloimmune refractory thrombocytopenia (i.e., poor increments in association with alloantibody detected using lymphocytotoxicity or antiplatelet antibody assays) are best managed with HLA-A and HLA-B antigen–selected donors or from compatible donors identified using platelet cross matching techniques alloimmunized patients do not benefit from unmatched prophylactic platelet transfusions that fail to raise the platelet count such patients should be transfused only for hemorrhagic events

AML, acute myelogenous leukemia; RBC, red blood cells; CCI, corrected count increment; ABO, blood group system; HLA, human leukocyte antigen. From Sacher R, Kickler T, Schiffer CA. Management of platelet transfusion refractoriness. *Arch Pathol Lab Med* 2003;127(4):409–414, with permission.

the lower dose was therefore recommended (17). Norol et al. reported the first prospective comparison of three different doses of platelets (15). The authors eliminated all factors other than the number of platelets transfused that could affect recovery: Platelets were fresh, ABO-compatible, and administered in similar clinical conditions to the same patient; they observed beneficial effects of high platelet doses, in terms of not only higher posttransfusion platelet counts but also longer intervals between transfusions. The larger platelet increments obtained with higher platelet doses increased the transfusion interval from 2 to 4 days.

The longer platelet life span after high doses could be explained by previously reported platelet kinetics in patients with bone marrow hypoplasia. Investigators have proposed the concept of a given platelet requirement to support vascular integrity, with random platelet utilization averaging 18% of overall platelet turnover in healthy individuals; however, this proportion increased rapidly as the platelet count fell below $100 \times 10^9$ per L. Using $^{51}$Cr-labeled platelets, the investigators found that autologous and homologous platelet survival correlated directly with the platelet count, with a reduction in the platelet life span to 3 to 4 days when the count fell below $50 \times 10^9$ per L (20). This observation agreed with that of Norol et al. in patients without clinical factors favoring platelet consumption, of a mean regular daily platelet requirement of $19 \times 10^9$ per L (corresponding to a mean of 31% of circulating platelets). This study therefore supports the concept that when the number of platelets needed for maintenance has been reached, the remaining platelets will continue to circulate, and that the higher the count, the longer the platelets will circulate. This study could also account for the weaker dose–effect relation in patients with clinical factors potentially inducing platelet destruction, independently of platelet numbers and random utilization (15).

## Platelet Transfusion in Specific Disorders

### Consumptive Thrombocytopenias

Thrombocytopenia may develop on the basis of increased consumption. These conditions include increased platelet destruction as seen in autoimmune thrombocytopenia, drug-induced thrombocytopenia, disseminated intravascular coagulation, and thrombotic thrombocytopenia purpura. Thrombocytopenia in these conditions can be quite severe, and profound bleeding and purpura are not uncommon, presenting symptoms in autoimmune or drug-induced thrombocytopenia; therefore, platelet transfusions may be considered necessary in patients who are having catastrophic bleeding. In the immune-mediated thrombocytopenias, the destruction of allogeneic platelets is as likely as that of autologous platelets, and platelets are never the only means to treat this form of thrombocytopenia (21). There has been no documentation of increased morbidity from using platelets in disseminated intravascular coagulation despite some concern that their use may increase the severity of disseminated intravascular coagulation. In thrombotic thrombocytopenic purpura, because of a few clinical reports, the use of platelet transfusions has been said to provoke acute clinical deterioration. There are also a few cases where the patients did receive platelet transfusions without difficulty, but these patients were already undergoing plasma exchange therapy (22).

### Qualitative Platelet Disorders

There are a variety of acquired and congenital qualitative platelet disorders that may lead to bleeding and to the need for platelet transfusion. The most common acquired qualitative platelet abnormalities are either drug-induced or caused by uremia. Other acquired platelet disorders are seen in myeloproliferative disorders, in patients with dysgammaglobulinemias, or because of mechanical assist cardiac devices. Numerous approaches are available to treat bleeding associated with platelet dysfunction. Nonetheless, in acute bleeding, platelet transfusions may be necessary. No specific controlled trials have been conducted to determine what the appropriate platelet dose should be. It has been recommended that for severe bleeding or for extensive surgery at least 10 equivalent platelet equivalents be given, assuming that the patient had no functionally active platelets (23). Aspirin is probably the most common drug affecting platelet function. It has been shown that platelet transfusions can improve the bleeding time in patients taking aspirin if the transfused platelets constitute 10% of the platelet population (24). This observation is especially important in cardiac patients who are receiving prophylactic aspirin or other antiplatelet agents and who require emergency platelet transfusions. A variety of inherited qualitative platelet disorders exist that can be accompanied by severe bleeding, particularly following trauma. These include Glanzmann thrombasthenia and Bernard-Soulier syndrome. Platelet transfusions are effective in these disorders until the patient becomes alloimmunized to human leukocyte antigens (HLA) or to the platelet glycoprotein receptor, IIb/IIIa or Ia/IX complex; when this happens, platelet transfusions are ineffective (25). In this situation, recombinant Factor VIIa has been used successfully (25).

## Platelet Transfusion Refractoriness

Failure to achieve an expected increment to a platelet transfusion is called platelet transfusion refractoriness. Refractoriness may be on an immune basis or nonimmune. The most common cause of immune-mediated platelet transfusion is due to HLA alloantibodies (26,27). Clinically, one can assess the response of a platelet transfusion by measuring the increment in the platelet count over time. The posttransfusion platelet response should be calculated on the basis of the patient's body surface area and should be corrected for the number of platelets transfused. The corrected platelet count increment is calculated using the following formula:

$$\text{Correct count increment} = \frac{(\text{posttransfusion} - \text{pretransfusion increment}) \times \text{body surface area/mm}^2}{\text{number of platelets} \times 10^{11}}$$

In general, a successful corrected count increment should be greater than 7,500 within 1 to 60 minutes of a transfusion, and greater than 4,500 if measured 18 to 24 hours after transfusion.

### Immunologic Basis of Platelet Transfusion Refractoriness

Soon after the introduction of prophylactic platelet transfusion in patients with leukemia or aplastic anemia, it became apparent that serial platelet transfusions resulted in decreasing platelet count increments. These transfusion failures result from the induction of alloantibodies to HLA and other antigens. It is now well recognized that an alloimmune response to HLA-A and -B locus antigens is the major cause of posttransfusion alloimmune transfusion failure (28). Antibodies to the human platelet antigens are only rare causes of platelet transfusion refractoriness. Some patients with blood group O who have high isoagglutin titers to group A or group B antigens present on platelets may also fail to achieve adequate platelet increments because the blood group antigens are also expressed on platelets (29).

## Detection of Antibodies in Platelet Transfusion Refractoriness

Specific identification of alloimmunization can be done by measurement of HLA antibodies using lymphocytotoxicity testing or enzyme-linked immunosorbent assay (ELISA) testing. Serial HLA antibody measurements are helpful in the management of alloimmunized patients. Some patients may have decreases in or a loss of HLA antibody, either permanently or transiently, and can be successfully transfused with platelet concentrates. It should be noted that some patients may have antibodies to HLA Class I and yet not have platelet transfusion failures because some HLA antigens are not well expressed on platelets (30).

## HLA Alloantigens

Understanding the HLA system is important so that compatible platelet transfusions may be selected for alloimmunized patients. Only HLA-A and HLA-B antigens have been shown to be important in causing immune-mediated platelet transfusion refractoriness (31,32). There are two broad types of HLA antibodies produced in response to platelet transfusions. The first type recognizes epitopes unique to a particular HLA allele, referred to as antibodies to private specificities. Antibodies to $A_2$ or $B_{12}$ fall into this group. The second type of HLA antibodies recognize more than one gene product. These antibodies recognize structural similarities between gene products (cross-reactive epitopes) or identical epitopes present on different gene products of different alleles, and are referred to as antibodies to public epitopes. Traditionally, HLA serology has placed the greatest emphasis upon classifying the private antigens. More attention has recently been given to the clinical importance of public HLA specificities. The best known examples of public specificities are Bw4 and Bw6. These antigens are encoded by a diallelic system and are associated with two different groups of HLA-B class I antigens. Other public antigens carried by HLA-B class I antigens have been divided into four cross-reactive groups (CREGs), $B_5$, $B_7$, $B_8$, and $B_{12}$. The observation that the specificity of HLA antibodies in multiply transfused individuals is generally against private epitopes suggests that matching for these public antigens is not necessary (33–35).

## Nonimmune Refractoriness

Platelet transfusions may not result in an increment if the stored platelets are defective; this should be relatively uncommon, given the quality control devoted to producing viable platelets. However, one should not fail to consider freshness of a given platelet transfusion as a cause of a single platelet transfusion failure. Splenomegaly has been shown to be a major cause of platelet transfusion failure. Normally, approximately 30% of a patient's platelet mass is contained within the spleen. With increases in splenic size, up to 90% of circulating platelets can be sequestered in this organ. Characteristically, splenic sequestration is associated with a reduced 1-hour platelet recovery but a normal survival. Studies by several groups have implicated both fever and infection as a cause for decreased platelet survival. One study noted that platelet transfusion requirements were increased by 50% in febrile patients. This may be increased further in patients with major infections; particularly those with disseminated intravascular coagulation. Platelet refractoriness has been reported with a number of medications. Amphotericin, in particular, has been implicated in decreasing platelet recovery and survival. Similarly, vancomycin has been reported to be a major cause of platelet refractoriness, as have antithymocyte globulin, granulocyte-macrophage colony-stimulating factor (GM-CSF), granulocyte colony-stimulating factor (G-CSF), and the interferons (28,36).

---

### TABLE 80-2

#### TWO APPROACHES TO SELECTION OF PLATELETS FOR ALLOIMMUNIZED PATIENTS

(A) Approach A
  (i)   Determine HLA phenotype and ABO type of the recipient
  (ii)  Screen patient's serum for (a) lymphocytotoxic antibody, or (b) antibodies to human platelet antigens (if there is a history of poor response to HLA-identical platelets)
  (iii) Select from the donor pool those units with the most compatible HLA antigens and, if possible, ABO systems

Or

(B) Approach B
  Cross-match available platelet units without regard to patient or donor HLA type (circumvents the need for HLA typing and provides a means of finding compatible platelets when antibodies to human platelet antigens are present); then obtain 10-min and 18–24-h posttransfusion platelet counts, not only to assess transfusion outcome but also to guide the selection of donors for future transfusions

---

## Managing the Alloimmunized Patient

Because alloimmunization to HLA antigens account for most causes of alloimmune platelet transfusion refractoriness, one should select platelets on the basis of HLA matching. Table 80-2 outlines an approach to selecting platelets for an alloimmunized patient. Depending upon the HLA type of an individual, one may have little difficulty in locating platelets that are identical. In some patients with unusual HLA type, such as in some ethnic groups, HLA matching is difficult. Relying only on HLA matching may have shortcomings and in some cases it is overly restrictive, in that some HLA-B loci antigens are not located on platelets. Therefore, in addition to antigen matching there has been a great deal of interest in adopting an approach to red cell compatibility. In this paradigm, one first selects a red cell phenotype that matches the patient's phenotype, and then performs a major crossmatch. This same approach can be used for platelets by also performing a platelet crossmatch. Unlike red cell pretransfusion testing, there are no accepted standards for selecting platelet transfusions in patients with alloantibodies to platelets (37).

## Management of Platelet Transfusion Refractoriness and Bleeding

A variety of approaches have been attempted when no compatible platelets can be found for an alloimmunized patient who is bleeding, or may be undergoing invasive procedures. Therapeutic modalities have included splenectomy, corticosteroids, plasmapheresis, administration of intravenous gammaglobulin, and repeated platelet transfusions. Except for intravenous immunoglobulin, there is little evidence that any of these work (38,39).

Kickler et al. performed a randomized, placebo-controlled clinical trial, investigating the use of intravenous immunoglobulin in patients with alloimmunized thrombocytopenia (38). In this trial, intravenous immunoglobulin was administered at a dosage 400 mg per kg for 5 days. An incompatible platelet transfusion from the same donor was used before and after the patient received study drug or placebo. Seven patients received intravenous immunoglobulin and five received placebo. Although platelet recovery at 1 to 6 hours was satisfactory in five patients after intravenous immunoglobulin treatment, 24-hour survival was not improved in most of these patients. This small study suggests that the kinetics of platelet destruction may be improved by intravenous immunoglobulin to an extent to permit the performance of invasive procedures.

When all conventional methods fail to increase the platelet count to hemostatic levels, the only remaining alternative that has been tried is the continuous transfusion of platelets. It has been proposed that although one does not see an incremental increase in the platelet count, transfused platelets may still exert some effect, permitting platelet plug formation or maintenance of endothelial integrity. These arguments are based on clinical observations and not on clinical trial data.

### Prevention of Alloimmunization

Results of early animal studies showed that depletion of contaminating leukocytes from donor blood components was effective in prevention of alloantibody response to major histocompatibility complex. With the development of highly efficient methods to remove leukocytes from blood products, a large clinical trial was done to study the efficacy of leukocyte removal. In the Trial for the Reduction of Alloimmunization to Platelets (TRAP), 534 patients were studied during an 8-week period for the development of platelet alloantibodies. Forty-five percent of patients in the control group developed HLA antibodies, compared to 18% in the filtered platelet concentrate group and 17% in the filtered apheresis group (40). All the filtered treated platelets were associated with a significant reduction in the development of HLA antibodies and alloimmune platelet refractoriness, compared to the control group. Since this study was done, many institutions have implemented universal leukocyte reduction for all blood products, thereby preventing alloimmunization and reactions caused by white cells.

## Adverse Effects of Platelet Transfusions

Febrile reactions occurring with platelet transfusion are mediated both by donor leukocytes and by cytokine generation and accumulation during the storage of blood components. After transfusion it has been proposed that an interaction between donor leukocytes and recipient antibody leads to interleukin-1 (IL-1) release from donor leukocytes or recipient monocytes. IL-1 produces fever by stimulating prostaglandin $E_2$ ($PGE_2$) production in the hypothalamus. Febrile reactions can be avoided or minimized by reducing the number by one to two logs (90% to 99%) to less than $5 \times 10^8$. The most effective current leukocyte reduction filters four log reduction, leaving residual leukocyte counts less than $5 \times 10^6$, and generally less than $1 \times 10^6$ (41).

### Bacteria Contaminating Platelet Products

Bacterial sepsis is the leading microbial cause of transfusion mortality today in the United States, accounting for 17% of 277 reported transfusion deaths from 1990 to 1998. The sources of bacteria in blood components include contamination from skin organisms at the phlebotomy site due to ineffective disinfection and skin plugs introduced to units during phlebotomy, transient bacteremias in donors, and, rarely, contamination during handling and processing of components (42).

Prevention requires proper screening by the blood collection facility to avoid ill donors, selection of phlebotomy sites with attention to skin hygiene and scarring from prior donations, and scrupulous adherence to effective skin disinfection procedures. Techniques to inactivate pathogens in blood are in

clinical trial but, currently, are unavailable for routine use. Regulatory and accrediting agencies now require that all platelets be tested for bacteria before transfusion.

## PLASMA THERAPY

A variety of plasma products are prepared from whole blood or collected by pheresis of plasma donors. Table 80-3 shows a list of these products along with their properties. Commonly, clinicians are only aware of fresh frozen plasma, whereas in reality, many transfusion services rely primarily on plasma frozen within 24 hours, rather than 8 hours, which is the regulatory definition of fresh frozen plasma. The two services differ slightly in that the plasma frozen within 24 hours has approximately 15% lower levels of factors V and VIII. In the past, transfusion of plasma was used for resuscitation of hypovolemic patients, wound healing, and nutritional supplementation. Now, through education, consensus panels, and careful delineation of the indications plasma by professional organizations, clinicians use plasma solely for replacement therapy where a specific clotting concentrate is not available to treat the bleeding disorder and in patients undergoing repetitive therapeutic plasma exchange, especially in thrombotic thrombocytopenic purpura.

Because plasma can be frozen up to 1 year, some blood centers release the plasma for use when the donor returns at least 112 days later, and the infectious disease tests are found negative for hepatitis B, C, and human immunodeficiency virus (HIV). This form of plasma has been referred to as retested plasma. The 112-day release date was chosen because it exceeds the window period during which virally transmitted diseases can occur despite negative infectious disease testing.

### Indications for Plasma

Table 80-4 lists the indications for plasma transfusions. When plasma was first introduced, it was used as a plasma expander, promoter of improved wound healing, and nutritional support for correcting hypoalbuminea. These transfusion practices are to be strongly discouraged because safer and more effective means are available using nonblood product treatment modalities. However, in the less developed countries of the world, these practices are still common. Crystalloid with dextran is considered a highly effective means for treating hypovolemia. There is no evidence that plasma improves wound healing. Plasma therapy is a very poor method for nutritional support (43–46).

### General Considerations in Plasma Dose and Monitoring

The redundancy in the clotting proteins needs to be emphasized when considering the use of fresh frozen plasma in the surgical patient (47–49). It is well known in patients with hemophilia who have factor VIII levels of 5% to 10% that spontaneous bleeding rarely does occur. When factor VIII levels are increased to 50% activity, effective surgical hemostasis is seen. The goal should therefore be to treat only those patients who have a considerable decrease of coagulant factor activity. The volume of plasma transfused should be sufficient to achieve approximately 30% coagulation factor levels, approximately 10 to 15 mL per kg of body weight. One of the limiting factors in dosing plasma is how well the patient can accommodate the increased plasma volume. In surgery where there is active bleeding, volume overload may not be an issue, whereas in a patient with severe liver disease and requiring a liver biopsy,

## TABLE 80-3

PLASMA PRODUCTS AND THEIR PROPERTIES

| Plasma type | Preparation characteristics | Composition | Comment |
|---|---|---|---|
| Fresh frozen plasma | Separated from whole blood and frozen at −18°C or colder within 8 h of collection | Volume varies between 180 and 300 mL and plasma proteins and all coagulation factors | A 200-mL bag of fresh frozen plasma would contain approximately 200 U of each coagulation factor |
| Plasma frozen within 24 h of collection | Frozen within 24 h of whole blood collection | Levels of factors V and VIII are reduced approximately 15% compared to fresh frozen plasma | |
| Liquid plasma | Liquid plasma is separated no more than 5 d after the expiration date of whole blood | Stable coagulation factors are equivalent to fresh frozen plasma, but the labile factors of V and VIII are significantly reduced | Rarely should this product be used for replacement therapy in massive transfusion or severe liver disease and associated bleeding |
| Cyro-poor plasma | The supernatant plasma after the removal of cryoprecipitate material | Deficient in fibrinogen, factor VIII, and von Willebrand multimers | Has been used in therapeutic pheresis, and in thrombotic thrombocytopenic purpura |
| Cryoprecipitate | Cryoprecipitate is prepared by thawing fresh frozen plasma at 1°C–6°C and recovering the precipitable material and then stored at 18°C or colder for up to 1 yr | Contains more than 150 mg of fibrinogen, more than 80 U of factor VIII, von Willebrand multimers, factor XIII in 15 mL of volume | Used in replacement therapy of hypofibrinogen, in preparation of fibrin sealants used in surgery, and in uremic platelet dysfunction |
| Solvent detergent treated plasma | A pooled plasma product treated with detergent to inactivate lipid envelope viruses | Lacks largest von Willebrand multimers but has other coagulation factors | Used for a few years and, recently, production has been halted |

volume overload is a limiting factor in how much plasma can be given (47,50,51).

## Congenital or Acquired Coagulation Factor Deficiencies

Fresh frozen plasma is indicated for the correction of congenital or acquired coagulation deficiencies, including II, V, VII, X, XI, and XIII deficiencies, in situations with hemorrhage or elective invasive procedures. Adequate hemostasis occurs at factor concentrations of 0.2 to 0.3 U per mL; depending upon the half-life and extent of injury or surgery, additional infusions may be needed.

## Reversal of Warfarin

In the setting of active bleeding, emergency surgery, cardioversion or invasive procedure where there is inadequate time to

## TABLE 80-4

INDICATIONS FOR PLASMA TRANSFUSIONS

Correction of factor deficiencies—factor II, V, VII, X, XI, XIII
Urgent reversal of warfarin
Treatment of hemorrhage following massive blood transfusion
Treatment of hemorrhage in association with liver disease
Treatment of hemorrhage in association with disseminated intravascular coagulation
Treatment of hemorrhage in association with dilutional coagulopathy
Plasma exchange for thrombotic thrombocytopenic purpura

wait for vitamin K reversal, plasma may be given when the international normalized ratio (INR) >1.6. Reversal may require 5 to 8 mL of plasma per kilogram body weight (52).

## Disseminated Intravascular Coagulation

There are varying degrees of disseminated intravascular coagulation, and not all patients have a bleeding diathesis unless sufficient consumption of fibrinogen, clotting factors, and platelets occur. Therefore, therapy should be conducted in relation to the clinical and laboratory findings. In many patients with disseminated intravascular coagulation, severe hypofibrinogenemia may be present. Fresh frozen plasma alone may be insufficient to raise the fibrinogen to hemostatic levels of 100 mg per dL or greater. Fibrinogen is concentrated 15-fold or greater in cryoprecipitate in contrast to fresh frozen plasma. Therefore, cryoprecipitate is the blood component of choice for correcting hypofibrinogenemia. Transfusion of cryoprecipitate in doses of one bag per 5 kg of body weight will increase the fibrinogen levels by 80 mg per dL. Additional doses of cryoprecipitate should be given on the basis of fibrinogen concentration (44,45). Fibrinogen has a half-life of 3 to 5 days. For patients with congenital hypofibrinogenemia needing replacement therapy, transfusions of cryoprecipitate are given on alternate days. In the United States, there are no commercially available fibrinogen concentrates.

## Massive Transfusion

In massive transfusion, there has been a long-standing concept that bleeding can occur in those patients who receive a large volume of blood. A variety of factors may contribute to bleeding in this setting, including transfusion of packed red cells without clotting factors, large volumes of crystalloid leading to clotting factor dilution, and development of concurrent bleeding diathesis from disseminated intravascular coagulation. In general, developing analyses to give blood products is difficult. In the ideal situation, with adequate laboratory resources, monitoring of patients with coagulation testing should guide transfusion therapy. One should note that the thawing of plasma may take up to 1 hour, so that, in some cases, empiric therapy based on clinical judgment may be the best approach in severely hemorrhaging patients (50–52).

## Plasma Derivatives

Plasma derivatives are prepared from pooled plasma products. More recently, the cloning and sequencing of factors VIII and IX along with advances in manufacturing technology have permitted the introduction of recombinant factor concentrates for VII, VIII, and IX (53–56). In the past, plasma products were at a greatly increased risk of disease transmission because of the large number of donations that constituted a single pool. Even a low overall prevalence of infectivity could result in almost all pools being contaminated. The Cohn ethanol fractionation procedure to prepare most plasma derivatives did not alter the infectiveness of viruses. Lyophilization of factor concentrates was introduced in the 1970s, leading to the widespread availability of a stable transfusion product that could be kept without freezing and permitted the introduction of home therapy by many patients with hemophilia. Because of viral contamination, a variety of purification processes and viral inactivation steps are done by detergent and heating. The introduction of viral inactivation and enhanced donor screening, along with the avoidance of paid plasma donors have resulted in highly safe plasma derivatives. Table 80-5 lists the available products, their characteristics, and their properties. The development of recombinant concentrates has provided for the safest possible form of factor replacement.

## Purification Procedures of Plasma

Gel and ion exchange chromatography were used to increase the specific activity of factor VIII preparations to approximately 100 U of factor VIII per mg protein. Polyethylene glycol precipitation followed by affinity chromatography of factor VIII/von Willebrand complex using heparin agarose columns is one method used to obtain relatively high purity concentrate of factor VIII and von Willebrand protein (Alphanate). Other manufacturers employ monoclonal antibodies directed to factor VIII, producing a product of factor VIII that has greater than 3,000 U of factor VIII per mg of protein (Monoclate-P). These affinity chromatography products are referred to as very high purity, in contrast to gel and ion exchange products, which are referred to as high purity (51,52,57,58).

## Viral Inactivation

The introduction of viral inactivation steps was developed in the early 1980s to prevent hepatitis and HIV. Careful longitudinal studies were performed to document the safety of this approach and the pitfalls, namely, the inability to inactivate nonenvelope viruses by detergent (59). Dry heat activation concentrates are those heated at 68°C for 32 to 72 hours, eliminating hepatitis infectivity. Although this approach was partially effective for HIV, it was not at all effective for hepatitis. Prolonged dry heating at 68°C for 144 hours is used for the preparation of Autoplex T (Nabi) and for Proplex T (Baxter). Moist-heated concentrates involve viral inactivation of lyophilized concentrates by heating under pressurized vapor at 60°C for 10 hours. FEIBA (Baxter) is prepared in this manner. Wet-heated concentrates also include Humate-P and Monoclate-P (Centeon). These wet-heated underpressure concentrates do not appear to transmit hepatitis C or HIV. However, there have been reports of parvovirus transmission.

Solvent detergent treatment of concentrates is another approach that is used by some manufacturers in conjunction with chromatographic purification. The solvent detergent disrupts viral lipid membranes. No cases of hepatitis C or B, or HIV have occurred with the use of factor VIII concentrates. Most of the currently available factor concentrates are treated with solvent detergent; these include Profilate SD, Alpha Therapeutic; Koate-HP, Bayer; Hemofil-M, Baxter; and Monarc-M, American Red Cross.

# SPECIALIZED COAGULATION CONCENTRATES

## Recombinant Derived Factor VIII Concentrates

Several recombinant coagulation formulations are available for the treatment of Hemophilia A (55,56,60). After more than 15 years of experience with the rFVIII preparations, we know that the rFVIII preparations are efficacious and safe. All products are manufactured in controlled processes, yielding rFVIII of high purity and activity. ReFacto, the B-region deleted recombinant factor VIII product, is more stable than the natural full-length rFVIII, making production in mammalian cell culture less difficult. It may, however, be less bioactive than the other rFVIII products. In the case of Recombinate, the full-length molecule was stabilized through coexpression of VWF. For Kogenate, the stabilization was accomplished through supplementation of the culture medium with small synthetic compounds as well as through the adjustment of steady state physiologic conditions during perfusion fermentation.

The purification processes are all effective, leading to low impurity levels in the final product. The second-generation products ReFacto and Kogenate Bayer/Kogenate FS are superior from a virus safety perspective because they are not supplemented with human serum albumin but rather contain sucrose-based synthetic formulations. Because mammalian cells theoretically can carry viruses, all rFVIII products are produced under rigorous viral safety programs. Raw materials are controlled, and cell line characterization and viral and microbial contamination tests are carried out for each fermentation run, and the viral clearance or inactivation capacity of the purification process is evaluated. However, because animal albumin– and human albumin–derived additives are still used, the theoretical risk of a virus transmission from biologic source materials remains.

The second-generation products ReFacto and Kogenate Bayer/Kogenate FS have an improved virus safety profile because of their synthetic formulations and the active solvent detergent virus inactivation step taken in the purification process. However, human serum albumin is still required for the culture medium upstream in the manufacturing process. Therefore, third-generation Kogenate and Recombinate product lines that are completely independent of animal and human additives are currently under development. These products will likely represent the final generation of recombinant FVIII products for replacement therapy.

There is only one recombinant factor IX product available for treatment of hemophilia B. Structurally, functionally, and therapeutically, recombinant factor IX is comparable to monoclonal plasma-derived factor IX (54,55). The only observed difference

**TABLE 80-5**

PLASMA DERIVATIVES, CHARACTERISTICS, AND PROPERTIES

**RECOMBINANT FACTOR VIII**

| Product | Generation[a] | Albumin in cell culture | Albumin as stabilizer | Viral inactivation | Comments |
|---|---|---|---|---|---|
| Helixate FS Manufactured by Bayer, distributed by Aventis Behring | 2 | Yes (human albumin) | No (stabilized with sucrose) | Solvent detergent: TNBP/ Polysorbate 80 | Full-length factor VIII molecule, no von Willebrand factor |
| Kogenate FS Manufactured and distributed by Bayer | 2 | Yes (human albumin) | No (stabilized with sucrose) | Solvent detergent: TNBP/ Polysorbate 80 | Full-length factor VIII molecule, no von Willebrand factor |
| Recombinate Manufactured and distributed by Baxter | 1 | Yes (bovine albumin) | Yes | None | Full-length factor VIII molecule, no von Willebrand factor |
| ReFacto Manufactured and distributed by Wyeth | 2 | Yes (human albumin) | No (stabilized with sucrose) | Solvent detergent: TNBP/Triton X 100 | B-domain–deleted factor VIII molecule, no von Willebrand factor |

**PLASMA-DERIVED FACTOR VIII**

| Product | Plasma source | Fractionation | Viral inactivation | Comments |
|---|---|---|---|---|
| Hemofil M Manufactured by Baxter, United States | Paid plasmapheresis donors | Monoclonal antibody affinity and ion exchange chromatography | TNBP/Triton X 100 | Albumin added as stabilizer, no von Willebrand factor |
| Monoclate-P Manufactured by Aventis Behring, United States | Paid plasmapheresis donors | Monoclonal antibody affinity chromatography | Pasteurization at 60°C, 10 h | Albumin added as stabilizer, no von Willebrand factor |

**RECOMBINANT FACTOR IX**

| Product | Generation | Albumin in cell culture | Albumin in stabilizer | Viral inactivation |
|---|---|---|---|---|
| BeneFix Manufactured and distributed by Wyeth | 3 | No | No | Nanofiltration |

**PLASMA-DERIVED FACTOR IX**

| Product | Plasma source | Fractionation | Viral inactivation | Comments |
|---|---|---|---|---|
| Immunine Manufactured by Baxter United States | Paid plasmapheresis donors | Ion exchange and hydrophobic interaction chromatography | Polysorbate 80; vapor heat, 60°C, 10 h at 190 mbar; then 80°C, 1 h at 375 mbar | |
| Mononine Manufactured by Aventis Behring, United States | Paid plasmapheresis donors | Immunoaffinity chromatography | Sodium thiocyanate and ultrafiltration | Albumin added as stabilizer |

**PRODUCTS FOR PATIENTS WITH INHIBITORS**

| Product | Type | Fractionation | Viral inactivation | Comments |
|---|---|---|---|---|
| Novo 7 Manufactured by Novo Nordisk | Recombinant | | None | No albumin added as stabilizer, used in patients with both factors VIII and IX inhibitors |
| FEIBA VH Manufactured by Baxter United States | Plasma-derived; paid plasma-pheresis donors | Surface-activated prothrombin complex concentrates, batch-controlled | Vapor heat, 60°C, 10 h at 190 mbar; then 80°C, 1 h at 375 mbar | Albumin added as stabilizer, used in patients with both factors VIII and IX inhibitors |
| Hyate-C Manufactured by Ipsen, Inc. | Porcine factor VIII | Cryoprecipitation and polyelectrolyte ion exchange chromatography | None; end product cell culture viral screen | Used in patients with factors VIII inhibitors |

*(continued)*

**TABLE 80-5**

CONTINUED

### FACTOR CONCENTRATES TO TREAT VON WILLEBRAND DISEASE

| Product | Type | Fractionation | Viral inactivation | Comments |
|---|---|---|---|---|
| Humate-P<br>Manufactured by<br>Aventis Behring | Plasma-derived | Multiple precipitation | Pasteurization at<br>60°C, 20 h | Albumin added as stabilizer,<br>contains von Willebrand<br>factor |

### PRODUCTS TO TREAT RARE FACTOR DEFICIENCIES

| Product | Type | Fractionation | Viral inactivation | Comments |
|---|---|---|---|---|
| Haemocomplettan<br>Manufactured by<br>Aventis Behring | Plasma-derived | Multiple precipitation | Pasteurization at<br>60°C, 20 h | Used to treat fibrinogen<br>deficiency |
| Clottagen<br>Manufactured by LFB | Plasma-derived,<br>French unpaid<br>donors | | TNBP/<br>polysorbate 80 | Used to treat fibrinogen<br>deficiency |
| Prothromplex-T<br>Manufactured<br>by Baxter | Plasma-derived | Ion exchange adsorption | Vapor heat, 60°C,<br>10 h at 190 mbar;<br>then 80°C, 1 h<br>375 mbar | Contains factors II, VII,<br>IX and X |
| Factor VII concentrate<br>Manufactured<br>by Baxter | Plasma-derived | Ion exchange<br>chromatography | Dry heat,<br>80°C, 72 h | Used to treat factor VII<br>deficiency |
| Factor XI concentrate<br>Manufactured by BPL | Plasma-derived | Affinity heparin sepharose<br>chromatography | Dry heat,<br>80°C, 72 h | Used to treat factor XI<br>deficiency |
| Hemoleven<br>Manufactured by LFB | Plasma-derived | Dialysis, cation exchange<br>chromatography | Solvent/detergeny,<br>15-nm<br>nanofiltration | Used to treat factor XI<br>deficiency |
| Fibrogrammin P<br>Manufactured by<br>Aventis Behring | Plasma-derived | Multiple precipitation | Pasteurization at<br>60°C, 10 h | Used to treat factor XIII<br>deficiency |

TNBP, tri-n-butyl phosphate.
[a]Generation 1: Human or animal albumin as both nutrient in cell culture and as stabilizer in final bottle.
Generation 2: Human albumin as nutrient in cell culture but not as stabilizer in final bottle.
Generation 3: No human or animal albumin either as nutrient in cell culture or as stabilizer in final bottle.

between recombinant and plasma factor IX is the recovery in pharmacokinetic studies, where recombinant factor IX recovery was approximately 72% of that of a plasma factor IX product. This difference is due to minor differences in the posttranslational modification of recombinant factor IX compared to plasma. Clinical studies demonstrate that recombinant factor IX is effective in the treatment of hemophilia B and has the safety profile expected from a product prepared by recombinant technology.

## Concentrates for Treatment of Factor VIII Inhibitors

### Prothrombin Complexes

Anti–Inhibitor Coagulant Complex, Feiba VH, Vapor Heated, is a freeze-dried sterile human plasma fraction with factor VIII inhibitor bypassing activity. *In vitro*, Feiba VH shortens the activated partial thromboplastin time (aPTT) of plasma containing factor VIII inhibitor. Factor VIII inhibitor bypassing activity is expressed in arbitrary units. One IMMUNO unit of activity is defined as that amount of Anti–Inhibitor Coagulant Complex, Feiba VH, Vapor Heated, that shortens the aPTT of high-titer factor VIII inhibitor reference plasma by 50% of the blank. Anti–Inhibitor Coagulant Complex, Feiba VH, Vapor Heated contains factors II, IX, and X, mainly nonactivated, and factor VII, mainly in the activated form. The product contains approximately equal units of factor VIII inhibitor activity and prothrombin complex factors. In addition, 1 to 6 U of factor VIII coagulant antigen (VIII C: Ag) per mL are present. The preparation contains only traces of factors of the kinin-generating system and contains no heparin (55,56).

### Coagulation Factor VIIa (Recombinant)

Factor VII is a serine protease and a vitamin K–dependent coagulation factor. The primary sequence of FVII is similar to other vitamin K–dependent coagulation proteases, and it circulates in blood as a single-chain zymogen of 406 residues. Production of recombinant human factor VIIa requires a mammalian expression system. The gene for human FVII, isolated from chromosome 13, is transfected into a baby hamster kidney (BHK) cell line that secretes FVII into the culture medium in its single chain form. The product is purified with murine monoclonal anti-FVII antibodies and is subjected to treatment with 0.1% Triton X-100 to inactivate enveloped viruses. Subsequent ion exchange chromatography further purifies the product and causes autoactivation, producing an activated form of FVII (60,61).

FVIIa promotes hemostasis by enhancing thrombin generation through direct activation of FX after complexing with tissue factor (TF) at the site of injury. FVIIa by itself does not have proteolytic activity. In healthy individuals, a small amount of thrombin formed by the FVIIa/TF pathway activates FV and FVIII as well as platelets accumulated at the site of injury. The activated platelets then provide negatively charged surfaces for further thrombin generation. The administration of rFVIIa enhances thrombin generation through direct activation of FX independent of FVIII or FIX, on thrombin-activated platelet surfaces, ensuring a full thrombin burst needed for formation of a fully stabilized fibrin plug. NovoSeven may also directly activate platelets at the site of injury.

rFVIIa is approved by the U.S. Food and Drug Administration (FDA) for treatment of bleeding episodes in patients with hemophilia A or B when inhibitors to these factors are present. Currently, the safety and efficacy of rFVIIa is being investigated in a number of trials designed to establish the efficacy of rFVIIa as a rescue treatment in episodes of severe life-threatening bleeding, stem cell transplantation, intracerebral hemorrhage, and trauma. Several case reports in the literature support the use of rFVIIa in patients who have bleeding but do not have hemophilia and in patients with thrombocytopenia, but no formal randomized trials have been presented and the drug is not licensed for these indications (61). In Europe, FVIIa is approved for use in alloimmunized patients with Glanzmann thrombasthenia, who are bleeding and need therapy to stop bleeding.

### Porcine Factor VIII Transfusion Guidelines

Hyate-C is a highly purified porcine antihemophilic factor VIII derived from pooled porcine plasma and containing minimal amounts of porcine von Willebrand factor. The product is not virally attenuated; however, the source plasma is extensively screened by cell culture and polymerase chain reaction (PCR) techniques for porcine parvovirus and other viruses. It has not been shown to transmit any known viral diseases.

Porcine factor VIII is indicated for the treatment of patients with congenital hemophilia A who are bleeding or undergoing surgery, in the presence of demonstrated moderate or high-titer inhibitors. Porcine factor VIII may be considered for the primary treatment of acquired hemophilia A with inhibitor autoantibodies. Porcine factor VIII shows low-level cross-reactivity with human factor VIII (approximately 15%). Patients with extremely high inhibitor levels to human factor VIII [>50 Bethesda units (BU)] should have their inhibitors directly measured against porcine factor VIII. Porcine factor VIII has not been shown to be effective when antiporcine factor VIII titers are greater than 20 BU. Porcine factor VIII is contraindicated in patients who have had prior anaphylactic responses to this product (62).

Porcine factor VIII is produced from pooled porcine plasma and carries the risk of porcine viral contamination. To date, no evidence of such transmission has been documented. Allergic reactions, including anaphylactic responses, have been documented to porcine factor VIII. Immune responses to porcine factor VIII may cross-react with human factor VIII, leading to an anamnestic response. Acute thrombocytopenia has rarely been reported with porcine factor VIII therapy.

### Activated Protein C (Drotrecogin α-Activated)

Drotrecogin α (activated) is a recombinant form of human activated protein C (APC) that is manufactured as an inactive zymogen, and is enzymatically activated by cleavage with thrombin and then purified using monoclonal antibodies (63–65). APC exerts an anticoagulant effect, along with its cofactor protein S, by inactivating factors Va and VIIIa, two critical procoagulants that lead to thrombin formation. Thrombin binds to thrombomodulin on endothelial cells at, and adjacent to, the site of vascular injury, which stimulated the coagulation process. Thrombomodulin serves as a cofactor for the conversion of protein C, present in the plasma, by thrombin to activated protein C. APC also inhibits tumor necrosis factor production by monocytes, blocks leukocyte adhesion to selectins, and limits thrombin-induced microvascular damage (65).

APC is approved by the FDA for use in severe sepsis, on the basis of the finding that it decreased mortality and the development of DIC (disseminated intravascular coagulation) in high-risk patients (defined by APACHE II scores >25) by approximately 20%. Although there are documented instances of familial protein C deficiency, the only approved indication, currently, is the acquisition of deficiency in the presence of severe sepsis. APC therapy increases the risk of bleeding and is contraindicated in patients with active internal bleeding, recent spinal or cranial surgery or trauma, presence of an epidural catheter, or an intracranial neoplasm or mass lesion (65).

### Antithrombin

Antithrombin concentrate is a sterile lyophilized preparation of human antithrombin isolated from pooled plasma by a modification of the Cohn fractionation technique (66,67). Viral attenuation is achieved by heat treatment at 60°C for at least 10 hours. It has not been shown to transmit viral infections. Antithrombin is thought to serve as a control mechanism on low-level coagulation activation in the circulation: It inhibits thrombin, factor Xa, and other serine proteases much more efficiently in plasma than when those factors are bound to platelets or fibrin.

Antithrombin is FDA approved for use in the treatment of patients with hereditary antithrombin deficiency as prophylaxis against thrombosis following surgery or obstetric procedures, and for therapeutic use when such patients have thrombosis. Without adequate levels of antithrombin, heparin is much less effective. Debate continues about the use of antithrombin concentrates in patients with "acquired" antithrombin deficiency, such as in cases of sepsis and DIC, or in those with relative heparin resistance during surgery and extracorporeal circulation; it is not approved for pediatric use. Replacement therapy is designed to achieve levels of 120% following infusion, with subsequent doses (60% of the loading dose) administered empirically to keep levels between 70% and 120%. In stable antithrombin-deficient patients, the normal half-life of infused antithrombin is between 60 and 90 hours after an initial half-disappearance time of 22 hours. In acute DIC, the half-life is usually half that of stable patients, and may be as short as 4 hours. Dosage should be determined on an individual basis depending on the pretherapy plasma antithrombin level, in order to increase the plasma antithrombin level to that normally found in human plasma (100%). Incremental *in vivo* recovery of 1.4% per IU per kg administered is expected.

## References

1. Goodnough LT. Platelet transfusion therapy. *J Clin Apheresis* 2001;16:43–48.
2. Gulliksson H, AuBuchon JP, Vesterinen M, et al. Additive solutions for the storage of platelets for transfusion. *Transfus Med* 2000;10:257–264.
3. Heddle NH, Blajchman MA, Meyer RM, et al. A randomized controlled trial comparing the frequency of acute reactions to plasma-removed platelets and prestorage WBC-reduced platelets. *Transfusion* 2002;42:556–566.
4. Perseghin P, Dassi M. Safety and usefulness of autologous cryopreserved platelets. *Lancet* 2002;360:1985–1986.
5. Wautier JL. Safety and usefulness of autologous cryopreserved platelets. *Lancet* 2002;360:1985.
6. Fischer TH, Merricks EP, Russell KE, et al. Intracellular function in rehydrated lyophilized platelets. *Br J Haematol* 2000;111:167–174.

7.  Blajchman MA. Substitutes and alternatives to platelet transfusions in thrombocytopenic patients. *J Thromb Haemost* 2003;1:1637–1641.

8.  Hoffmeister KM, Felbinger TW, Falet H, et al. The clearance mechanism of chilled blood platelets. *Cell* 2003;112:87–97.

9.  Vasconcelos E, Figueiredo AC, Seghatchian J. Quality of platelet concentrates derived by platelet rich plasma, buffy coat and apheresis. *Transfus Apheresis Sci* 2003;29(1):13–16.

10. Gulliksson H. Additive solutions for the storage of platelets for transfusion. *Transfus Med* 2000;10:257–264.

11. Schiffer CA, Anderson KC, Bennett CL, et al. Platelet transfusion for patients with cancer: clinical practice guidelines of the american society of clinical oncology. *J Clin Oncol* 2001;19:1519–1538.

12. Schiffer CA. Diagnosis and management of refractoriness to platelet transfusion. *Blood Rev* 2001;15(4):175–180.

13. Freireich EJ. Supportive care for patients with blood disorders. *Br J Haematol* 2000;111(1):68–77.

14. Sacher R, Kickler T, Schiffer CA. Management of platelet transfusion refractoriness. *Arch Pathol Lab Med* 2003;127(4):409–414.

15. Norol F, Bierling F, Roudot-Thoraval F, et al. Platelet transfusion: a dose-response study. *Blood* 1998;92(4):1448–1453.

16. British Committee for Standards in Haematology. Blood transfusion task force. *Br J Hematology* 2003;122:10–23.

17. Roy AJ, Jaffe N, Djerassi I. Prophylactic platelet transfusions in children with acute leukemia: a dose response study. *Transfusion* 1973;13:283–290.

18. Klumpp TR, Herman JH, Gaughan JP, et al. Clinical consequences of alterations in platelet transfusion dose: a prospective, randomized, double-blind trial. *Transfusion* 1999;39:674–681.

19. Schlossberg HR, Herman JH. Platelet dosing. *Transfus Apheresis Sci* 2003;28(3):221–226.

20. Davis KB, Slichter SJ, Corash L. Corrected count increment and percent platelet recovery as measures of posttransfusion platelet response: problems and a solution. *Transfusion* 1999;39(6):586–592.

21. Rosse WF. Clinical management of adult ITP prior to splenectomy: a perspective. *Blood Rev* 2002;16(1):47–49.

22. Rubia J, de la G, Plume F, et al. Platelet transfusion and thrombotic thrombocytopenic purpura. *Transfusion* 2002;42(10):1384–1385.

23. Kao AK, Walsh P. Qualitative platelet disorders. *Clin Haematol* 1983;12: 201–238.

24. Bashein G, Nessly ML, Rice AL, et al. Preoperative aspirin therapy and reoperation for bleeding after coronary artery bypass surgery. *Arch Intern Med* 1991;151:89–93.

25. Poon MC, D'Oiron R, Hann I, et al. Use of recombinant factor VIIa (NovoSeven) in patients with Glanzmann thrombasthenia. *Semin Hematol* 2001;38(4 Suppl. 12):21–25.

26. Kickler TS, Kennedy SD, Braine HG. Alloimmunization to platelet specific antigens on glycoprotein IIB-IIIA and IB/IX in multitransfused thrombocytopenic patients. *Transfusion* 1990;30:622.

27. Kickler TS. The challenge of platelet alloimmunization. *Transfus Med Rev* 1990;4:8–18.

28. Lee EJ, Schiffer CA. Serial measurement of lymphocytotoxic antibody and response to non-matched platelet transfusions in alloimmunized patients. *Blood* 1987;70:1727.

29. Lozano M, Cid J. The clinical implications of platelet transfusions associated with ABO or Rh(D) incompatibility. *Transfus Med Rev* 2003;17(1):57–68.

30. Kao KJ, Scornik JC, Small S. Enzyme linked immunoassay for anti-HLA antibodies- an alternative to panel studies by lymphocytotoxicity. *Transplantation* 1993;55:192–196.

31. Duquesnoy RJ. HLAMatchmaker: a molecularly based algorithm for histocompatibility determination. I. Description of the algorithm. *Hum Immunol* 2002;63(5):339–352.

32. Duquesnoy RJ. HLA humoral allosensitization. Clinical significance of humoral allosensitization of HLA antigens. In: Lee J, ed. *The first HLA symposium. proceedings first red cross international workshop.* New York: Springer-Verlag, 1990:27.

33. McElligott MN, Menitove JE, Duquesnoy RJ, et al. Effect of HLA Bw4/Bw6 compatibility on platelet transfusion response of refractory thrombocytopenic patients. *Blood* 1982;59:971.

34. Rodey GE, Park M, Fuller T, et al. Analysis of sera that define public or cross-reactive HLA class I epitopes. In: Dupont B, ed. *Immunobiology of HLA,* Vol 1. Basel: Springer Verlag, 1989:288.

35. Rodey GE. Class I antigens: HLA-A, -B, -C and cross reactive groups. In: Moulds J, Fawcett KJ, Garner RJ, eds. *Scientific and technical aspects of the major histocompatibility complex.* Arlington, VA: American Association of Blood Banks, 1989:23.

36. Inverardi D, Bocchio C, Rossi L, et al. Clinical, immunologic, and technical factors affecting recovery of platelet count after platelet transfusion. *Haematologica* 2002;87(8):893–894.

37. Kickler TH. Pretransfusion testing for platelet transfusions. *Transfusion* 2000;40(12):1425–1426.

38. Kickler TS, Braine HG, Piantadosi S, et al. A randomized placebo controlled trial of intravenous gammaglobulin in alloimmunized thrombocytopenic patients. *Blood* 1990;75:313–316.

39. Lee EJ, Norris D, Schiffer CA. Intravenous immune globulin for patients alloimmunized to random donor platelet transfusions. *Transfusion* 1987;27:245–250.

40. TRAP Study Group. Trial for the reduction of platelet alloimmunization. *N Engl J Med* 1997;337:1861.

41. Heddle NM, Klama LN, Griffith R, et al. A prospective study to identify the risk factors associated with acute reactions to platelet and red cell transfusion. *Transfusion* 1993;33:794–797.

42. Braine HG, Kickler TS, Char ache P, et al. Bacterial sepsis secondary to platelet transfusion; an adverse effect of extended storage. *Transfusion* 1986;26:391–394.

43. American Society of Anesthesiologists Task Force on Blood Component Therapy. Practice guidelines for blood component therapy. *Anesthesiology* 1996;84:732–747.

44. Fresh Frozen Plasma. Indication and risks. *NIH consensus statement,* Bethesda, MD: National Institutes of Health, 1984.

45. Practice Guidelines for Blood Component Therapy. Task force of the american society of anesthesiologists. *Anesthesiology* 1996;84:498–501.

46. Practice Parameter for the use of FFP, Cryoprecipitate, and Platelets. Task force of the american college of american pathologists. *JAMA* 1994;271: 777–781.

47. Roberts HR, Monroe DM, Escobar MA. Current concepts of hemostasis: implications for therapy. *Anesthesiology* 2004;100:722–730.

48. Leslie SD, Toy PTCY. Laboratory hemostatic abnormalities in massively transfused patients given red blood cells and crystalloid. *Am J Clin Pathol* 1991;96:770–773.

49. Counts RB, Haisch C, Simon TL, et al. Hemostasis in massively transfused trauma patients. *Ann Surg* 1979;190:91–99.

50. Lodge JP. Hemostasis in liver resection surgery. *Semin Hematol* 2004;41: 70–75.

51. Hoyt DB. A clinical review of bleeding dilemmas in trauma. *Semin Hematol* 2004;41:40–43.

52. Abshire T, Kenet G. Recombinant factor VIIa: review of efficacy, dosing regimens and safety in patients with congenital and acquired factor VIII or IX inhibitors. *J Thromb Haemost* 2004;2:899–909.

53. Acharya SS, Coughlin A, DiMichele DM. Rare bleeding disorder registry: deficiencies of factors II, V, VII, X, XIII fibrinogen and dysfibrinogenemias. *Journal of Thrombosis and Haemostasis* 2004;2:248–256.

54. Lusher JM. Congenital disorders of clotting proteins and their management. In: Simon T, Dzik S, Snyder EL et al., eds. *Rossi's principles of transfusion medicine,* 3rd ed. Philadelphia, PA: Lippincott, Williams and Williams, 2002:448–462.

55. Manco-Johnson MJ, Riske B, Kasper CK. Advances in care of children with hemophilia. *Seminars in thrombosis and hemostasis* 2003;29:585–594.

56. Manco-Johnson MJ. Introduction: hemophilia treatment today. *Seminars in Hematology* 2003;40:1–2.

57. Mannucci PM. Hemophilia: treatment options in the twenty-first century. *Journal of Thrombosis and Haemostasis* 2003;1:1349–1355.

58. Mariani G, Dinucci GD, Arcieri P. Immunopurified clotting factor concentrates. *Nouvelle Revue Francaise D Hematologie* 1994;36:S61–S65.

59. Horowitz B, Bonomo R, Prince AM, et al. Solvent/detergent-treated plasma: a virus-inactivated substitute for fresh frozen plasma. *Blood* 1992;79: 826–831.

60. Hedner U, Erhardtsen E. Potential role of rFVIIa in transfusion medicine. *Transfusion* 2002;42:114–124.

61. Hedner U. Recombinant coagulation factor VIIa: from the concept to clinical application in hemophilia treatment in 2000. *Seminars in Thrombosis and Hemostasis* 2000;26:363–366.

62. Brettler DB, Forsberg AD, Levine PH, et al. The use of porcine factor VIII concentrate (Hyate:C) in the treatment of patients with inhibitor antibodies to factor VIII: a multicenter US experience. *Arch Intern Med* 1989; 149:1381–1385.

63. Gerson WT, Dickerman JD, Bovill EG, et al. Severe acquired protein C deficiency in purpura fulminans associated with DIC: treatment with protein C concentrate. *Pediatrics* 1993;91:418.

64. Kraus M. The anticoagulant potential of the protein C system in hereditary and acquired thrombophilia: pathomechanisms and new tools for assessing its clinical relevance. *Sem Thromb Hemost* 2004;1–10.

65. Bernard GR, Vincent JL, Laterre PF. Efficacy and safety of recombinant human activated protein C for severe sepsis. *N Engl J Med* 2001;344: 699–799.

66. Menache D, Grossman BJ, Jackson CM. Antithrombin III: physiology, deficiency and replacement therapy. *Transfusion* 1992;32:580.

67. Bucur SC, Levy JH, Despotis GJ, et al. Uses of antithrombin III concentrates in congenital and acquired deficiency states. *Transfusion* 1998; 38:481.

# CHAPTER 81 ■ NEW APPROACHES FOR THE THERAPY OF BLEEDING DISORDERS, INCLUDING GENE THERAPY

GILBERT C. WHITE II AND HAROLD R. ROBERTS

Better understanding of the molecular mechanisms of blood coagulation and the structure and function of blood clotting factors, along with advances in recombinant DNA technology have placed us on the threshold of remarkable new approaches to the treatment of bleeding disorders. Gene therapy is the most visible of these new approaches, but mechanisms now exist to actually make coagulation factors that are better than the native proteins. Some of these new approaches are the subject of this chapter.

## HISTORICAL PERSPECTIVE

The treatment of bleeding disorders has traditionally been through the use of fresh frozen plasma or plasma-derived coagulation factor preparations. The first of these coagulation factor preparations was cryoprecipitate, which was developed by Judith Graham Pool in 1964. Cryoprecipitate was enriched in factor VIII, as well as fibrinogen, von Willebrand factor and fibronectin, and for the first time provided a method of increasing factor VIII levels with less volume overload. Later came other coagulation factor preparations, including glycine-precipitated purified factor VIII and barium sulfate purified prothrombin complex concentrates containing factors II, VII, IX, and X. These were produced commercially and revolutionized the treatment of hemophilia A and B, leading to home treatment. The prothrombin complex concentrates were also effective in the treatment of patients with coagulation factor inhibitors, allowing treatment of these individuals for the first time. The mechanism of action was uncertain, but activated clotting factors in the concentrates were thought to "bypass" the inhibitor block in the coagulation cascade. Although these crude plasma-derived concentrates changed the treatment of hemophilia, they contained blood-borne viruses that were transmitted to hemophiliacs. By the early and middle 1970s, hepatitis B and a new non-A, non-B form of hepatitis, later renamed hepatitis C, were becoming epidemic in the hemophilic population. Even worse, human immunodeficiency virus (HIV)/acquired immunodeficiency syndrome (AIDS) appeared in the hemophilic population in the early 1980s and eventually led to the untimely death of thousands of patients with hemophilia. In response to these blood-borne infections, the academic-industry complex developed physical and chemical methods for inactivating hepatitis, HIV, and other blood-borne viruses, used monoclonal antibodies to factors VIII and IX to generate antibody affinity-purified ultrapure forms of both factors, and developed recombinant DNA techniques for producing factors VIII and IX, resulting in synthetic forms of both factors that were essentially free of blood-borne contaminants. As a result of these and other advances, current products used to treat hemophilia are the safest ever developed.

Despite their safety, the current products have some drawbacks. They are expensive, require intravenous administration, and must be administered frequently because of the short biologic half-life of the normal coagulation factor proteins. For the average hemophiliac, who might bleed as many as 50 times a year or more, the cost of replacement therapy with current products can be as much as $50,000 per year. Prophylaxis, the treatment to prevent bleeding and the damage to joint and tissues, would require treatment two to three times a week or 100 to 150 times a year, with costs in excess of $50,000 and considerable damage to veins from frequent venipuncture. Using available technologies to make clotting factors that are cheaper, last longer after infusion into patients, or could be administered by alternative routes (including oral) would be advantageous. Gene therapy is another approach that has received considerable attention. This chapter reviews these new approaches to the treatment of bleeding disorders. The focus of the chapter is primarily on hemophilia A, but the concepts can be applied broadly to all bleeding disorders.

## GENE THERAPY APPROACHES

Gene therapy is literally the use of genes, DNA or RNA, as treatment of a particular condition or disorder. In most cases, it is the proteins produced from the genes that have the intended effect in gene therapy, although DNA itself can have effects. For monogenic disorders like hemophilia or cystic fibrosis, the intent of gene therapy is curative. The aim is to use normal genes to express enough normal protein to correct the abnormality. For complex multigenic disorders, such as atherosclerosis, diabetes, or cancer, the aim of gene therapy is modification of the disease process. The goal might be to express a protein or gene that is toxic to a cancer cell or inhibits smooth muscle proliferation in atherosclerosis. One of the great promises of gene therapy is the ability to cure monogenic disorders such as hemophilia.

The origins of gene therapy lie in the remarkable advances in recombinant DNA technology that occurred in the middle and latter half of the last century. The ability to isolate and manipulate DNA, and the development and use of viral and nonviral plasmid vectors to introduce DNA into cells where the DNA products could be expressed were critical developments. In one of the early reports using direct injection of DNA into cell nuclei, Jaenisch and Mintz reported injecting SV40 DNA into mouse blastocysts and finding SV40 gene sequences in the animals developing from the blastocysts (1). The notion of using viruses as vectors to introduce new genetic information into cells evolved very quickly. By 1979, several laboratories were employing the SV40 virus, using viral promoter, splicing, and polyadenylation sequences in plasmid vectors to introduce β-globin sequences into cells and drive transgene expression (2–4). Retroviruses, which are adept at gaining entry into cells and inserting their genetic material into the host genome, soon followed. Defective retroviruses in which the malignant transforming gene region was eliminated, were shown to retain the ability to transduce cells (5–7). The first gene transfer experiments in humans were carried out by Cline in 1980 in two subjects with severe $\beta$ thalassemia (8). Nucleated cells, obtained by bone marrow aspiration, were transfected *in vitro* using a pBR vector containing a herpes simplex virus thymidine kinase (*HSVtk*) marker gene, and then returned to the subject intravenously. HSVtk sequences were detected at low levels 1 to 2 weeks after transfection and lasted 3 months in one subject and 9 months in the second.

Hemophilia A is a monogenic disorder which, like sickle cell disease, cystic fibrosis, and muscular dystrophy, has historically been considered as an attractive target for treatment using gene transfer approaches. Primary prophylaxis studies in which clotting factor concentrates have been administered to maintain low levels of factor VIII have shown that near-continuous correction of the clotting factor defect prevents bleeding in unaffected joints and delays progression in diseased joints (9–11). Logically, more continuous levels of factor VIII, as might be anticipated with gene therapy, provide the rationale for the enthusiasm for this approach in hemophilia A.

Other aspects of hemophilia A add to its attractiveness as a candidate disorder for gene transfer (see Table 81-1). As a monogenic disorder, correction of the factor VIII defect should correct the phenotype. Furthermore, unlike monogenic inborn errors of metabolism, levels of factor VIII are not regulated in any way and do not require feedback or other control as, for example, insulin requires regulation by blood glucose levels. Another important feature is that complete correction of the factor VIII level is not absolutely necessary in hemophilia for gene transfer to be effective. For example, an increase in plasma levels of factor VIII by even as little as 1% to 2% could have a beneficial effect, especially in patients with severe hemophilia. Persistence of expression after gene transfer might also have beneficial effects. Given the biological half-life for current plasma products of approximately 12 hours, expression of factor VIII for even a month would change patients' lives. Factor VIII message is detected in a number of tissues (12), but as long as the factor VIII that is expressed after gene transfer is processed correctly and has access to blood, it does not matter where the protein is produced. There is no current evidence that synthesis of factor VIII in tissues outside its site of normal synthesis is detrimental to that tissue. Therefore, it is not necessary to target the factor VIII to a particular tissue or to its tissue of natural synthesis. In addition, factor VIII is a secreted protein that would be expected to gain easy access to blood. The gene for factor VIII is well characterized and, based on homology modeling, much is known about the structure of the factor VIII

protein and the function of the various structural domains (13). A crystal structure of the C2-domain of factor VIII is available (14). Good clinical and laboratory parameters of efficacy are available. Large and small animal models of hemophilia are available for preclinical trials (15,16). Finally, safe and effective treatments for hemophilia currently exist, and so subjects can make appropriate decisions about participation in clinical trials without the pressure engendered by the lack of adequate treatment.

## Gene Transfer Vectors[1]

### Viral Vectors

Viruses have evolved highly efficient mechanisms for entering human cells and using the DNA/RNA replication machinery of the cell to produce viral products (17). By replacing viral coding sequences with genes of particular interest (for example, the cDNA for factor VIII) one can use viruses as agents to introduce the gene into cells where they use the cellular machinery to produce therapeutic quantities of the protein. The obvious advantage of viruses as vectors is their native ability to get into cells; the general disadvantage is their toxicity.

**Retrovirus Vectors.** Retroviruses are enveloped RNA viruses that use reverse transcriptase to convert virion RNA into double-stranded DNA; the DNA is subsequently integrated into the genome of the cell. The surface of the retrovirus consists of a lipid bilayer with protruding membrane proteins, GP41 and GP120, both encoded by the *env* gene. The tropism of the virus, that is the host cell that is targeted by the virus, is determined by these surface proteins. For example, for HIV-1, GP120 mediates the interaction of HIV-1 with CD4 lymphocytes. For gene therapy vectors, it is common to replace the retroviral *env* gene with other sequences that change the tropism of the vector. This can be done to either target a particular tissue or cell or to broaden the tropism of the vector to increase the number of cells that are transduced. Two sequences that are frequently used to broaden the tropism of retrovirus vectors are the amphotropic envelope gene of murine leukemia viruses, which is able to interact with a widely expressed phosphate transporter on human cells, and the glycoprotein of vesicular stomatitis virus (VSV-G), which interacts with a ubiquitous receptor on cells. Retroviral vector production is through a three-part packaging system, consisting of a genome vector that contains the packaging signal and the cDNA of interest, an expression vector that contains the pseudotyped envelope glycoprotein, and an expression vector that expresses the viral *gag* and *pol* genes. These are assembled into vector particles in a packaging cell. The retroviral packaging systems in current use appear safe and are designed to prevent the generation of replication-competent virus. In addition, sufficient modifications are made in the viral sequence to minimize the possibility of homologous recombination with retroviral sequences in target cells. Self-inactivating ("sin") vectors are ones in which the long-terminal repeats (LTRs) have been removed to prevent activation of downstream cellular genes.

Vectors derived from the Moloney murine leukemia virus (MoMLV) were the first retroviral vectors used for gene transfer. MoMLV has a 9-kb cDNA expression cassette and is therefore able to accept the entire 7.1-kb factor VIII cDNA or

---

## TABLE 81-1

### HEMOPHILIA AS A TARGET FOR GENE TRANSFER

Monogenic disorders; correction of factors VIII or IX will correct the phenotype

Complete correction of factors VIII or IX is not required; any level of factor VIII will have a clinical effect

Production of factors VIII or IX can occur in any tissue that has access to blood

The genes for factors VIII and IX are well characterized and protein structure is understood

Large and small animal models of hemophilia A and B exist

Safe and effective treatments for hemophilia A and B exist

---

[1]Sections of text on gene transfer vectors and phase I gene transfer trials in hemophilia A and B have also been used by G. C. White in the *Textbook of Hemophilia*, eds. Lee, C., Berntorp, E. and Hoots, W. K., Blackwell Publishing, Oxford, UK.

1.9-kb factor IX cDNA. Although MoMLV can be produced in large quantities and is able to efficiently gain entry into cells, it only transduces dividing cells (18), a disadvantage for many tissues such as liver where the rate of cell replication is low. Strategies for inducing cell division in the liver using partial hepatectomy (19,20), chemical injury (21), or hepatocyte growth factor (22–25) have been proposed to increase retrovirus-mediated transduction.

More recently, vectors derived from lentiviruses, including HIV-1, have been developed (26,27). Members of this family of retroviruses include feline immunodeficiency virus (FIV), simian immunodeficiency virus (SIV), and equine infectious anemia virus (EIAV) (28–30). Like MoMLV, lentiviral vectors have a 9-kb cDNA expression cassette. These vectors retain some of the attractive features of the Moloney-based retroviral vectors, such as stable integration into the host chromosome and targeted cellular uptake through coat proteins, and they are able to infect nondividing and dividing cells (26,31). More recent observations provide greater understanding of the mechanisms of nuclear import by lentiviruses and may lead to improvements in cell transduction. During reverse transcription (RT) of HIV-1, a three-stranded DNA flap is formed which is composed of the central polypurine tract (cPPT) from the *pol* gene and central termination sequences (CTS). This flap functions as a cis-acting element to enhance nuclear import and improve gene transduction in nondividing cells (32–35). Other cis-acting DNA elements that enhance transgene expression, perhaps through a mechanism like the DNA flap, have been identified, including the matrix attachment region from immunoglobulin $\kappa$ (36) or from $\beta$ interferon (37,38).

Although retroviral integration is not sequence-specific, there is increasing evidence that it is also not completely random. The ability of retroviruses to successfully replicate themselves depends on integration of the viral DNA into transcriptionally active areas of the host cell chromosome. Integration into silent areas would prevent expression of viral proteins and inhibit replication. Studies to map the site of retrovirus integration demonstrate that active genes are preferential integration targets, especially genes that are activated by infection of the cell by the retrovirus (39,40). Regional hotspots also exist (39). Whether the predilection for active genes results from increased chromatin accessibility, locally bound transcription factors, or some other influence is not clear.

Retroviruses insert their DNA into the host chromosome and are therefore termed *integrating vectors*. Because of their integrating properties, insertional mutagenesis is a concern with retroviruses. Integration of retroviral sequences near protooncogenes has been known to be capable of activating their expression, contributing to tumorigenesis in animal models (41,42). A recent report of T-cell leukemia in two subjects with X-linked severe combined immunodeficiency syndrome treated by retrovirus-mediated gene transfer (43) shows that insertional mutagenesis occurs in man. The two subjects were among 10 receiving *ex vivo* retrovirus-mediated gene transfer into autologous CD34$^+$ bone marrow cells. Approximately 3 years after treatment, the subjects developed acute T-cell lymphocytic leukemia. The leukemic T cells showed evidence for retroviral insertion near the LMO2 proto-oncogene promoter. Because of the survival advantage that the cells expressing the retroviral $\gamma$c-transgene had over the normal T cells, it has been suggested that the insertional mutation in the LMO2 promoter region results in uncontrolled clonal expansion of the corrected T cells, initially correcting the severe combined immunodeficiency and then resulting in T-cell leukemia.

**Adenovirus Vectors.** Adenoviruses are linear, double-stranded DNA viruses that infect a wide variety of human cells, both dividing and nondividing, including lung, liver, heart, and brain. The 36-kb viral genome consists of a number of early and late genes. Transcription and translation of the early genes

modulates cell function to facilitate replication of the viral DNA, whereas the late genes are involved in the structural aspects of viral replication. The icosahedral adenoviral capsid is composed of three major components: the hexon, penton base, and knobbed fiber. Viral entry into cells is accomplished through an initial high-affinity interaction between the knobbed fiber (44,45) and a widely expressed, 46-kDa coxsackie-adenovirus receptor (CAR) on the surface of cells (46). After the initial interaction with CAR, entry of the virus into the cell proceeds through clathrin-mediated endocytosis, by an interaction between the penton base and $\alpha_V\beta_3$ and $\alpha_V\beta_5$ integrins on the cell surface. Disruption of the viral capsid occurs in the endocytic vesicle and the viral genome enters the nucleus through nuclear pores. In the nucleus, the adenoviral genome does not integrate into the chromosomes of the host cell, functioning instead from an extrachromosomal or episomal template.

Adenoviral vectors characteristically elicit an intense inflammatory response. This is due in part to capsid proteins, which provoke a brisk humoral and cellular immune response (47). At the same time, adenovirus (Ad) is designed to evade the immune response that it elicits (48,49). Products of the *E1A* gene interfere with nuclear factor $\kappa$B, NF$\kappa$B, which is a key regulator of the innate antiviral response by cells. Products of the *E3* gene are also known to subvert the host immune response. Other gene products play a role, as well. One of the goals in the generation of adenoviral vectors is to retain the high degree of efficiency that these vectors have with respect to cell infection while moderating or eliminating the inflammation that they cause. First-generation adenoviral vectors were deleted in E1 and E3, removing some of the primary mediators of the immune response while increasing the expression cassette to 6.5 kb. The E2 genes were removed in the second-generation vectors and, in recent vectors, all of the viral coding sequences have been removed, rendering the vector "gutless" (50,51). Although preclinical studies indicate that removing these proteins may reduce the cellular immune response (52–54), there is also evidence that the virion shell alone elicits substantial cellular responses (55).

There are at least 47 different adenoviral serotypes, each immunologically distinct. The development of an immune response to one vector serotype generally precludes readministration of that vector. Adenoviral vectors for gene transfer are primarily Ad2 or Ad5.

The only death that was directly attributable to a gene transfer trial occurred with an adenoviral vector in an 18-year old subject with ornithine transcarbamylase (OTC) deficiency (56). The second-generation vector used in this study was based on human Ad5 and was deleted in E1 and E4. Following administration of the vector in the right hepatic artery, altered mental status and jaundice were noted 18 hours later, and the ensuing clinical course was marked by a systemic inflammatory response syndrome with high levels of interleukin-6 (IL-6) and IL-10, biochemically detectable disseminated intravascular coagulation, and multiple organ system failure, leading to death 98 hours following gene transfer. The story of Jessie Gelsinger has been well-chronicled in the news media (57).

### Adeno-Associated Virus Vectors

Adeno-associated viruses (AAV) are small, nonenveloped, single stranded DNA viruses, which require helper virus to facilitate efficient replication. In the absence of helper-virus mediated replication, the wild-type virus persists in the host cell in a latent state. The 4.7-kb genome of AAV consists of two inverted terminal repeats (ITRs) and two open reading frames that code for the rep and cap proteins. There are four rep proteins that function in regulating AAV replication and three cap proteins that form the protein coat of the virus. AAV stably integrates into the host genome at the AAVS1 region of chromosome 19q13.3-qter (58). Two of the *rep* gene products, rep68 and rep78, are believed to direct integration to the AAVS1 site on chromosome 19 (59). Nine different AAV serotypes have been identified, AAV1 to 9, each with distinct tissue tropism (60). AAV8 targets primarily liver, whereas AAV1 and AAV7 transduce muscle with high efficiency. The cellular receptor for AAV2, the serotype most commonly used for gene transfer studies, is heparan sulfate, a glycosaminoglycan that is variably present on the surface of most cells (61). Slow-twitch (slow myosin-expressing) skeletal muscle fibers have higher concentrations of heparan sulfate proteoglycan on their surface and are better transduced by AAV2 than fast-twitch fibers (62). Interestingly, AAVS1, the site of integration, is closely linked to the slow skeletal troponin $T$ gene, TNNT1 (63), raising an interesting correlate with the preference of AAV for slow myofibers. The integrin $\alpha_V\beta_5$ and fibroblast growth factor receptor 1 are coreceptors for AAV2 (64,65).

Typical AAV gene transfer vectors have been derived from AAV2. The ITRs are retained but the rest (96%) of the viral genome has been removed, including the *rep* gene. As a result, AAV vectors currently in general use are unable to integrate into the host chromosome in a site-specific manner, and persistence as integrated sequences appears to be a low-frequency event, if it occurs at all. Efforts to quantify *in vivo* integration in skeletal muscle and liver suggest that at least 99.5% (skeletal muscle) or at least 90% (liver) of persisting AAV vector DNA was episomal, present in large concatemers (66,67).

The AAV expression cassette is approximately 5 kb, too small to accommodate the whole factor VIII cDNA but large enough to accommodate the factor IX cDNA. Several groups have separately packaged factor VIII light and heavy chain sequences under the control of minimal transcriptional regulatory elements into AAV vectors and demonstrated expression *in vivo* after coinfection (68–71).

AAV are not associated with any known disease and are not pathogenic (72). On the basis of this nonpathogenicity, the toxicity associated with AAV has been expected to be low. In preclinical studies, AAV has been well tolerated with no effects on hematopoiesis, liver function, or other organs. Reports of late tumors in mice treated with AAV vectors (73) have not been confirmed and the chromosomal breaks that have been observed in cells following AAV integration (74) are of uncertain significance, especially because integration by AAV vectors lacking the *rep* gene is infrequent. However, in liver-directed human trials in hemophilia B, transient liver enzyme abnormalities have been reported and were associated with loss of transgene expression (75).

### Plasmid Vectors

Nonviral approaches for delivering therapeutic genes as naked plasmid DNA are attractive because plasmid DNA is relatively simple and inexpensive to produce, does not engender cell-mediated immune responses, and does not result in humoral immune responses against the DNA vehicle that would limit the opportunity for repeated delivery. Until recently, most plasmid DNA applications have resulted in short-lived (days to weeks) transgene expression. Recent attempts to use electrical (76) or hydrodynamic (77) approaches to augment target cell uptake of plasmid DNA have resulted in expression of clotting factors lasting months after delivery. By rapidly treating mice through the tail vein with factor VIII expression sequences under the control of transcriptional regulatory elements optimized for liver expression, in large fluid volumes, supraphysiologic factor VIII levels were obtained (77). Immune responses that are species independent have been reported (78). Despite the attractive features of nonviral approaches, current technical limitations reduce the likelihood of human use in the near future.

### Chimeraplasty

Cells contain DNA repair mechanisms that can detect and replace incorrect nucleotides that occur during the process of DNA replication. Kmiec et al. have used these natural mismatch repair mechanisms to develop a strategy for repair of small mutations (79,80). The overall approach is to employ a chemically stable chimeraplast, a double-stranded DNA-RNA chimeric oligonucleotide that contains the correct DNA sequence, to drive a nucleotide exchange reaction using the natural DNA repair mechanisms of the cell. The oligonucleotide is typically 70 to 80 nucleotides in length and is designed with a homologous targeting sequence comprised of a complementary DNA region flanked by RNA residues (the chimeric strand), an all-DNA second strand, thymidine hairpin caps, and a double-stranded guanine and cytosine (GC) clamp region. The double-hairpin configuration of the chimeraplast reduces nuclease digestion and the concatenation of double-stranded molecules that occurs in mammalian cells and thereby facilitates the stability of the molecule. Because of the sequence complementarity with the genomic target, the chimeraplast aligns in perfect register with the target DNA except for the designed single base pair mismatch, which is recognized and corrected by harnessing the cell's endogenous DNA repair system.

Chimeraplasty can be used to repair single nucleotide mutations or even several nucleotide deletions, but would not be applicable to larger defects or to the common inversion mutations that account for a large number of cases of hemophilia A. This approach has been used both *in vitro* and *in vivo* to effect single nucleotide changes in genes, including inducing a hemophilic mutation in the liver of a mouse (81). There are more than 600 different single base substitutions leading to hemophilia A, with all 26 exons affected and more than 400 substitutions leading to hemophilia B with all 8 exons affected, so that a large library of specific factor VIII or factor IX chimeroplasts would be required to treat the population. Nevertheless, it is attractive to view chimeroplasty as a true "gene cure," rather than gene replacement.

### Spliceosome-Mediated Pre-mRNA Transsplicing

Another specific repair mechanism that may be especially applicable to the common inversion mutations that cause approximately 30% of hemophilia A is an approach termed *spliceosome-mediated mRNA transsplicing* (82). This method is used to repair messenger RNA, rather than DNA. In the final steps of transcription, the introns are removed and exons are spliced together to form mature, functional mRNA. The site of splicing is directed by 30 to 40 nucleotides at each end of the intron that form consensus binding sites for the spliceosome, a large ribonucleoprotein complex composed of small nuclear ribonucleoprotein particles (snRNPs) that catalyze the splicing reaction. Spliceosome-mediated pre-mRNA transsplicing takes advantage of this normal cellular process to effect RNA repair. The method involves synthesis of a pretranssplicing molecule (PTM) that contains the corrected mRNA fused to a 30 to 40 nucleotide sequence that targets a specific pre-mRNA. The PTM binds to the pre-mRNA, allowing specific transsplicing of the corrected mRNA through normal mechanisms.

Chao et al. used a transsplicing approach to correct the hemophilic defect in factor VIII knockout mice (83). The repair PTM consisted of a 125-nucleotide binding domain that was complementary to intron 15 of the gene, a spacer sequence, and a strong 3' splice acceptor site, linked to exons 16 to 26 for the mouse factor VIII cDNA. Correctly transspliced factor VIII was detectable genetically and functionally in the treated mice, with up to 17% factor VIII activity observed. It was estimated that conservatively between 1.6% and 6.3% of mutant transcripts were being repaired.

## Enhanced Translational "Read through"

In prokaryotes and eukaryotes, aminoglycoside antibiotics cause ribosomes to read through stop codons during translation (84,85). As a result, these antibiotics can suppress nonsense genotypes, increasing expression of the full-length protein and partially restoring the normal phenotype. In tissue culture cells, restoration of gene expression to as much as 20% of wild-type levels has been observed after aminoglycoside treatment (84). Clinical trials of gentamicin in cystic fibrosis showed that translational "read through" could be obtained in patients who were both homozygous and heterozygous for stop mutations with a reduction in basal potential difference in nasal mucosa and an increase in response to chloride-free isoproterenol solution (86). Approximately 9% of hemophilia A and hemophilia B mutations are nonsense mutations that might respond to aminoglycoside treatment. Several small preliminary studies have examined the responses to aminoglycoside antibiotics in patients with hemophilia A and B and nonsense mutations with inconsistent results (87,88).[2]

## Phase I Gene Transfer Trials in Hemophilia A and B[3]

Before gene transfer trials can be carried out in humans, clinical grade vectors—viral, plasmid, or naked DNA—must undergo rigorous testing. Vectors driving expression of factor VIII or factor IX are first tested in tissue culture systems, then in small animal models, usually mice, in large animal models, usually dogs or monkeys, and in factor VIII– or factor IX–deficient models, usually knockout mice and/or hemophilic dogs. These studies test the safety and efficacy of the vectors. Current U.S. National Institutes of Health (NIH), U.S. Food and Drug Administration (FDA), and the European Agency for the Evaluation of Medicinal Products (EMEA) regulations for gene transfer trials are available at http://www4.od.nih.gov/oba/rac/guidelines/guidance.html, at http://www.fda.gov/cber/genetherapy/gtpubs.htm under guidance, and at http://www.emea.eu.int/index/indexh1.htm, respectively. Safety must be rigorously demonstrated before initiating human trials.

Clinical trials have been performed in hemophilia A and B (see Table 81-2) (89–93).

### Chinese Trial in Hemophilia B

The initial clinical trial in hemophilia was undertaken at Fudan University in China in 1991 (89). This was a phase I trial in hemophilia B using *ex vivo* retrovirus-mediated gene transfer in autologous skin fibroblasts (94). Two vectors were used: XL-IX, a Moloney murine leukemia virus-based vector containing human factor IX cDNA under control of the retroviral LTR, and N2CMV-IX, a Moloney-based vector containing human factor IX cDNA under control of the CMV promoter.

Two brothers with moderately severe hemophilia B, ages 9 and 13, were studied. Baseline factor IX activity and antigen levels were 2%. Skin fibroblasts obtained by biopsy and maintained in culture were transduced with XL-IX or N2CMV-IX. Following demonstration of *in vitro* synthesis of factor IX, the resulting HBSF-IX cells were injected subcutaneously into multiple sites in the wall of the abdomen and the back at approximately monthly intervals. A total of 6.6 to 11 × 10^8 cells were injected. No treatment-related side effects were observed. An increase in factor IX was observed in both subjects, as early

as 15 to 20 days after the first set of injections. Although the pretreatment variation in factor IX levels was not reported, plasma factor IX antigen and activity following treatment was increased to more than twofold in both subjects and was reported to persist for more than 420 days. There was also a reduced tendency to bleed. One subject received an additional set of injections of HBSF-IX cells at 16 months after factor IX levels had diminished and demonstrated another increase in factor IX levels in response to the injections.

### Transkaryotic Therapy Inc. Trial in Hemophilia A

In overall design, this trial employed an *ex vivo* approach (95), similar to that employed in the initial Chinese trial in hemophilia B, except that the TKT trial used a nonviral, plasmid vector rather than a viral vector and the target disorder was hemophilia A rather than hemophilia B. The plasmid used for the TKT trial contained the cDNA for the B-domain deleted form of human factor VIII under control of the CMV promoter.

A total of 12 subjects, ranging in age from 19 to 71 years, were studied, nine in a dose-escalation trial, and three in a comparison of sites of intraperitoneal injection. Seven of the twelve were HIV-seropositive without AIDS and all were hepatitis C virus (HCV)-seropositive with stable liver function. Dermal fibroblasts obtained from the subjects by excisional skin biopsy were electroporated with the plasmid containing the B-domain deleted human factor VIII cDNA. Fibroblasts expressing the factor VIII gene were clonally expanded, characterized for the stability of the integrated gene sequences and production of factor VIII, and administered by laparoscopic intraperitoneal injection, either into the fat of the greater omentum, or into the fibrofatty tissue that bound the lesser omentum. Laparoscopy was performed under general anesthesia. A total of 100, 400, or 800 million autologous clonal cells were injected in three cohorts of three subjects per cohort. Follow-up was up to 24 months. There were no serious adverse events related to the study material, the skin biopsy, or the intraperitoneal injection. No inhibitors to factor VIII were reported. Seven of the 12 subjects demonstrated a decreased bleeding frequency and/or factor VIII use following cell transfer, with low levels of factor VIII detected transiently in plasma, up to 1% to 2% of normal, with a maximum of 4%. Injection of cells into the lesser omentum appeared to be less effective than injection into the greater omentum. The first six subjects in this study were reported by Roth et al. (90).

### Chiron Trial in Hemophilia A

The Chiron study was designed as a phase I, open-label, multi-institution, single-dose, dose-escalation trial in volunteers with severe hemophilia A using a replication-deficient Moloney murine leukemia virus (MoMLV) derived vector to deliver B-domain deleted human factor VIII cDNA [hFVIII(V)]. The vector was complement resistant and employed a human packaging cell line system with reduced homology between the retroviral vector and the packaging components, thereby allowing production of high-titer virus production without the generation of replication-competent retrovirus (96). Expression of the B-domain deleted factor VIII was driven by the retroviral LTRs.

The study was undertaken in subjects over the age of 18 with severe hemophilia A and no inhibitor. Subjects could be HIV seropositive or seronegative, but were required to have stable CD4 counts over 400 per mm^3 and were excluded if taking reverse transcriptase inhibitors because of their effect on RT of the [hFVIII(V)]. Five doses, 2.2 × 10^7, 9.2 × 10^7, 2.2 × 10^8, 4.4 × 10^8, and 8.8 × 10^8 transduction units per kg, were administered in divided daily doses by peripheral vein injection. A total of 13 subjects were enrolled, three at each of the first four doses and one at the highest dose (91). The mean age of the 13 subjects was 37.5 years, with a range of 18 to 55 years. Two subjects dropped out of the study for personal reasons. The

---

[2]Sommer, S, unpublished data.
[3]Sections of text on gene transfer vectors and phase I gene transfer trials in hemophilia A and B have also been used by G. C. White in the *Textbook of Hemophilia*, eds. Lee, C., Berntorp, E. and Hoots, W. K., Blackwell Publishing, Oxford, UK.

**TABLE 81-2**

GENE THERAPY FOR HEMOPHILIA CLINICAL TRIAL SUMMARY

| | Subject | Age | Dose | Inhibitor | Semen PCR | Peak factor[a] |
|---|---|---|---|---|---|---|
| **Chinese study—hemophilia B (89)** | 1 | 9 | $11 \times 10^8$ cells | No | Unk | 5.92% |
| *ex vivo* transduction | 2 | 13 | $6.6 \times 10^8$ cells | No | Unk | 4.13% |
| **TKT study—hemophilia A (90)** | 1 | Unk | $1 \times 10^8$ cells | No | Neg | <0.8% |
| *ex vivo* transfection | 2 | Unk | $1 \times 10^8$ cells | No | Neg | <0.8% |
| | 3 | Unk | $1 \times 10^8$ cells | No | Neg | 2.0% |
| | 4 | Unk | $4 \times 10^8$ cells | No | Neg | <0.8% |
| | 5 | Unk | $4 \times 10^8$ cells | No | Neg | 1.0% |
| | 6 | Unk | $4 \times 10^8$ cells | No | Neg | 4.0% |
| | 7 | Unk | $4 \times 10^8$ cells | No | Neg | <0.8% |
| | 8 | Unk | $4 \times 10^8$ cells | No | Neg | <0.8% |
| | 9 | Unk | $4 \times 10^8$ cells | No | Neg | <0.8% |
| | 10 | Unk | $8 \times 10^8$ cells | No | Neg | <0.8% |
| | 11 | Unk | $8 \times 10^8$ cells | No | Neg | 1.1% |
| | 12 | Unk | $8 \times 10^8$ cells | No | Neg | 1.0% |
| **Chiron study—hemophilia A (91)** | 2–1 | 50 | $2.8 \times 10^7$ TU/kg | No | Neg | 1.8% |
| retrovirus | 5–1 | 33 | $2.8 \times 10^7$ TU/kg | No | Neg | 6.6% |
| | 5–2 | 30 | $2.8 \times 10^7$ TU/kg | No | Neg | 3.0% |
| | 3–1 | 51 | $9.2 \times 10^7$ TU/kg | No | Neg | 1.7% |
| | 3–2 | 55 | $9.2 \times 10^7$ TU/kg | No | Neg | 1.3% |
| | 5–3 | 50 | $9.2 \times 10^7$ TU/kg | No | Neg | 6.2% |
| | 2–2 | 20 | $2.2 \times 10^8$ TU/kg | No | Neg | 1.1% |
| | 3–3 | 43 | $2.2 \times 10^8$ TU/kg | No | Neg | <0.1% |
| | 5–4 | 18 | $2.2 \times 10^8$ TU/kg | No | Neg | 2.6% |
| | 1–1 | 52 | $4.4 \times 10^8$ TU/kg | No | Pos | <0.1% |
| | 5–5 | 48 | $4.4 \times 10^8$ TU/kg | No | Neg | 1.4% |
| | 5–6 | 18 | $4.4 \times 10^8$ TU/kg | No | Neg | 4.4% |
| | 5–7 | 20 | $8.8 \times 10^8$ TU/kg | No | Neg | 2.1% |
| **Avigen study—hemophilia B (92)** | 1 | 38 | $2 \times 10^{11}$ vg/kg | No | Neg | 3.7% |
| muscle-directed AAV | 2 | 23 | $2 \times 10^{11}$ vg/kg | No | Neg | 0.8% |
| | 3 | 67 | $2 \times 10^{11}$ vg/kg | No | Neg | <0.3% |
| | 4 | 29 | $6 \times 10^{11}$ vg/kg | No | Neg | <0.1% |
| | 5 | 44 | $6 \times 10^{11}$ vg/kg | No | Neg | <0.1% |
| | 6 | 43 | $6 \times 10^{11}$ vg/kg | No | Neg | 1% |
| | 7 | 38 | $1.8 \times 10^{12}$ vg/kg | No | Neg | <0.1% |
| | 8 | 30 | $1.8 \times 10^{12}$ vg/kg | No | Neg | <0.1% |
| **Genstar study—hemophilia A** "gutless" adenovirus | 1 | 23 | $4.3 \times 10^{10}$ vg/kg | No | Unk | N/A |
| **Avigen study—hemophilia B (93)** | 1 | 63 | $2 \times 10^{11}$ vg/kg | No | Pos | <0.1% |
| liver-directed AAV | 2 | 49 | $2 \times 10^{11}$ vg/kg | No | Pos | <0.1% |
| | 3 | 20 | $1 \times 10^{12}$ vg/kg | No | Unk | <0.1% |
| | 4 | 22 | $1 \times 10^{12}$ vg/kg | No | Unk | <0.1% |
| | 5 | 31 | $5 \times 10^{12}$ vg/kg | No | Unk | 11.8% |
| | 6 | 28 | $5 \times 10^{12}$ vg/kg | No | Unk | 3% |
| | 7 | 20 | $1 \times 10^{12}$ vg/kg | No | Unk | <0.1% |

PCR, polymerase chain reaction; AAV, adeno-associated virus; TU, transduction units; vg, vector genomes; Unk, unknown.
[a]Peak factor levels. In the Chiron study, this was defined as the highest level observed in those individuals who demonstrated levels >1% on at least two occasions, 5 or more days after infusion of exogenous factor.

infusion of [hFVIII(V)] was well tolerated, with no serious adverse events. There was no acceleration of chronic HIV or HCV disease and all tests for replication-competent retrovirus (RCR) were negative. No FVIII inhibitor activity was detected in any subject. Although no subject had sustained levels greater than 1%, six patients showed FVIII levels of more than 1% on at least two occasions, 5 or more days after infusion of exogenous FVIII. Most elevated levels were in the range of 1.0% to 1.8%, although isolated levels of 2.3%, 3.0%, 4.3%, and 6.2% were reported for three subjects. Elevated levels of factor VIII were

detected as early as 8 days following treatment. Peripheral blood mononuclear cells (PBMC) demonstrated the presence of vector gene sequences by polymerase chain reaction (PCR) testing to 6 months in all 10 subjects tested and to 1 year in three of four subjects tested. All of the four subjects tested at 1 year were in the two lowest dose groups, indicating long-term persistence of vector sequences even at the lowest dose. Pharmacokinetic examination following the infusion of exogenous FVIII 13 weeks after vector infusion showed a statistically increased half-life (T1/2) and area under the curve (AUC) compared to prestudy values. Bleeding frequency was decreased in six subjects compared to historical rates.

A single, transient, low-level positive signal was detected in a single semen sample from one subject at week 9; no other unusual events or complications were observed.

### Avigen Trial in Hemophilia B

The Avigen trial was a prospective, multiinstitution, single-dose, dose-escalation, phase I trial to examine the safety of an adeno-associated virus vector to deliver human factor IX to skeletal muscle in subjects with severe hemophilia B. Coagulin-B, the recombinant AAV produced by Avigen which was used in the study, was derived from serotype AAV-2.

A total of seven subjects were enrolled in the trial, three at $2 \times 10^{11}$, three at $5 \times 10^{11}$, and one at $2 \times 10^{12}$ vg per kg (92,97). Vector was administered under general anesthesia through ultrasound-guided injections in the *vastus lateralis* muscle of the leg. The number of injections ranged from 10 to 72, depending on the dose administered. Muscle biopsies performed 8 to 12 weeks after vector administration showed immunohistochemical evidence for factor IX in the extracellular space in a pattern similar to that observed in preclinical studies. There was no muscle injury or inflammation. Although subjects had detectable pretreatment titers of neutralizing antibodies against AAV that were as high as 1:1000, gene transfer and expression was demonstrated in each subject by Southern blot on DNA extracted from muscle and by RT-PCR. No antibodies against factor IX were detected. Although there was evidence for transient dissemination of virus in serum, saliva, and urine, there were no detectable vector sequences in semen at any time. One subject developed thrombocytopenia after vector administration, but the individual had a history of thrombocytopenia. No other toxicity was observed. Increased plasma levels of factor IX were observed on multiple occasions beginning approximately 8 weeks after vector administration in one subject with CRM (cross-reacting material) positive severe hemophilia B receiving $2 \times 10^{11}$ vg per kg. The highest level was 1.6% at week 10 and increased levels were detected up to at least 22 weeks. A second subject had levels up to 0.8%. Both subjects had reduced requirement for replacement factor.

### Genstar Trial in Hemophilia A

The aim of the Genstar trial was to examine the safety of MaxAdFVIII, a "gutless" adenovirus vector derived from Ad5 (98). The vector was devoid of all viral genes except essential cis-elements and carried a 27-kb expression cassette that contained the full-length factor VIII cDNA under the control of the human 12.5-kb albumin promoter.

The Genstar trial was designed as a phase I, multiinstitutional, single-dose, dose-escalation study in subjects with severe hemophilia A with normal liver function. One subject was enrolled in the trial. Infusion of MaxAdFVIII in that subject was associated with high fevers at the time of injection. There was an approximately 50% decrease in platelet count, starting posttreatment day 1 with a return to normal by day 7, and a 10-fold increase in alanine aminotransferase (ALT) starting on posttreatment day 2 and returning to normal by approximately day 20. The reduction in platelet count and increase in liver enzymes constituted serious adverse events and the trial was placed on hold by the FDA while further analyses were performed. The trial was reopened at a fivefold lower dose, but no further patients were enrolled and the study has been discontinued.

### Avigen Liver-Directed Trial in Hemophilia B

A second, liver-directed Avigen trial has been performed. The AAV vector used in this trial was similar to that used in the initial muscle trial but contained the $\alpha_1$-antitrypsin promoter and apolipoprotein E-enhancer/hepatic control locus region to drive liver-specific factor IX expression. Vector was injected directly in the liver through a hepatic artery approach.

The trial was a phase I, single-dose, dose-escalation study to examine the safety of liver-directed AAV-AAT-FIX in severe hemophilia B (99). A total of seven subjects were enrolled, ranging in age from 20 to 63 years. Three cohorts of two patients each received doses of $2 \times 10^{11}$, $1 \times 10^{12}$, or $5 \times 10^{12}$ vg per kg by injection directly into the liver via cannulation of the hepatic artery. The liver-directed injections were well tolerated. Two subjects at the highest dose achieved significant increases in factor IX level, one to 11.8% and the second to 3%. However, expression in both subjects was transient and the loss of expression was accompanied in the subject with the highest expression level by significant liver enzyme abnormalities starting approximately 3 weeks after vector administration (75,93). A third subject treated with $1 \times 10^{12}$ vg per kg also developed transient asymptomatic transaminitis. T-cell immune responses to two conserved AAV-2 capsid peptides were identified in this subject. Because of the grade 3 liver toxicity and the lack of persistent effect, the trial was discontinued.

No inhibitors to factor IX were detected. The first two subjects developed PCR-positive signals in sperm. Both subjects cleared vector signal over time and all subsequent subjects were advised to use contraception until the semen was negative.

## NEW APPROACHES TO THE SYNTHESIS OF COAGULATION FACTOR CONCENTRATES

Despite intense interest in gene transfer approaches, coagulation factor concentrates continue to be the mainstay of treatment in hemophilia and other bleeding disorders. In the developed world, approximately 70% of patients with hemophilia are treated with recombinant concentrates, either factor VIII, factor IX, or factor VIIa. The commercial synthesis of these factors has not changed substantially because the initial products were introduced in 1990, although the promise of recombinant technology has always been the ability to use it to make better products. With increasing knowledge of the three-dimensional structure of coagulation proteins and better correlates between structure and the function of these molecules, it becomes more feasible to use recombinant technology to make proteins that have improved function. Some of the current directions in developing improved coagulation factor proteins are described here.

Current recombinant clotting factor concentrates are synthesized in well-characterized mammalian cells such as Chinese hamster ovary (CHO) and baby hamster kidney (BHK) cells. The proteins synthesized in these cells are fully active and are identical with purified plasma-derived proteins in their ability to participate in blood coagulation. However, there are minor differences between recombinant and plasma proteins that are due in part to differences in the posttranslational modifications that take place in tissue culture cells compared to human cells. All three plasma proteins contain complex N- and O-linked carbohydrates. In the recombinant proteins, the carbohydrates are attached normally, but the complex structure of the N-linked carbohydrates in the recombinant proteins differs from that in the native molecules. Although the carbohydrate changes do not appear to affect the function of the recombinant molecules, it is possible that other unknown functions may be affected. Plasma factor VIII contains six sulfated tyrosine residues at positions 346, 718, 719, 723, 1,664, and 1,680 (100) and these appear to be present and fully modified in recombinant factor VIII. Plasma factors IX and VIIa each contain 12 $\gamma$-carboxylated glutamic acid (Gla) residues in the amino-terminal portion of the molecule that are important for binding of the proteins to phospholipid surfaces and therefore for the coagulant activity of the proteins. Recombinant factor IX is less than fully $\gamma$-carboxylated, with approximately 60% of the recombinant molecules containing 12 Gla residues, 35% containing 11 Gla residues, and 5% containing 10 Gla residues (101,102). The less than fully modified proteins demonstrated a specific clotting activity that was indistinguishable from the fully modified form. Plasma factor IX contains a single $\beta$-hydroxylated aspartic acid residue, which appears to be comparably modified in recombinant and plasma factor IX. In addition, factor IX contains a sulfated tyrosine at amino acid 155 and a phosphorylated serine at amino acid 158 in the activation domain that appear to be important for the distribution of the protein in the circulation. In plasma factor IX, these two residues are fully modified. In recombinant factor IX, Ser158 is not phosphorylated, and Tyr158 is only 15% sulfated.

## Synthesis of Properly Modified Proteins

One major area for improvement in the production of recombinant clotting factor proteins is better control of the post-translational modification of proteins to more closely approximate plasma proteins. For example, the recent identification of the genes for vitamin K carboxylase and vitamin K epoxidase/reductase (103–105) potentially permit better control of the carboxylation process during the tissue culture synthesis of the vitamin K–dependent proteins. More importantly, full sulfation of Tyr155 and phosphorylation of Ser158 in the activation domain of factor IX would be expected to improve the recovery of factor IX and have a beneficial effect in the treatment of hemophilia B. Because changes in the conditions of synthesis or structure of recombinant coagulation factors require extensive preclinical and clinical testing to compare the new product with the old before the changes can be approved by the FDA, the cost of modification can be very high. As a result, the improvement in molecular function must be considerable to make the cost worthwhile.

Active forms of factors VIII and IX have been synthesized in transgenic livestock (106–109). Velander et al. showed that the factor VIII and IX produced in mammary epithelium is catalytically active and can be easily purified from endogenous milk proteins. Expressed under control of the whey acidic protein or $\beta$-lactoglobulin promoter, factor VIII or IX concentration in bovine or porcine milk is over 10-fold to 200-fold higher than in plasma (107). The porcine mammary gland has been shown to carry out the posttranslational processing necessary for full biologic activity and normal half-life in the human circulation. The advantage of the transgenic approach in milk is the large volume of protein that can be produced and the ease of purification because of the small number of endogenous proteins. In addition, it has been suggested that the large amount of protein that can be produced from transgenic animals makes alternative delivery methods, including oral methods, feasible.

## Super-Molecules

One of the promises of recombinant technology is the ability to make proteins that have enhanced functions. In the case of coagulation factors, this might be increased coagulant activity, or an increased half-life in the circulation, or reduced immunogenicity. As the structure and function of clotting factors become better defined, it may be possible to synthesize coagulation factor molecules that are actually better than the native proteins. Early attempts to make such molecules are underway.

### Coagulation Factors with Improved Coagulant Function

Proteins with increased coagulation factor activity have been achieved by a number of laboratories. In some cases, this has been accomplished by an actual improvement in the catalytic efficiency of the molecule. For example, the catalytic efficiency of factor IX was increased by the replacement of selected sequences in the catalytic domain of factor IX with the corresponding sequences from factor X (110). Substitution of selected sequences from the catalytic domain of factor X for the corresponding sequences in the catalytic domain of factor IX resulted in a 56-fold increase in the amidolytic activity of factor IX. There was no significant change in inhibition by $p$-aminobenzoic acid (PABA), an S1 pocket–directed reversible inhibitor of serine proteases, demonstrating that the integrity of the active site was unchanged. Chang et al. showed that the apparent activity of factor IX could also be enhanced by replacing the epidermal growth factor (EGF)-1 domain of factor IX with the corresponding domain from factor VII (111). The increased factor IX activity was demonstrated both in vitro and in a canine model. The EGF-1 substitution increased the rate but not the extent of factor Xa generation, suggesting that the EGF-1 domain of factor VII was more efficient in promoting assembly of the tenase complex. Although the immunogenicity of the chimeric factor IX-VII molecule was not examined in the canine model, the substitution of whole domains is likely to preserve the tertiary structure of the domain and therefore be less immunogenic than the substitution of individual amino acids.

Although factor VIII does not have intrinsic protease activity, the cofactor activity of factor VIII in generating tenase activity can be similarly enhanced. Voorberg et al. reported that substitution of the factor VIII sequences that direct thrombin cleavage to a site between the A2 and A3 domains with sequences that direct thrombin cleavage of heparin cofactor II, increased factor VIII cofactor activity (112). The increased factor VIII activity is believed to result from improved cleavage at a critical site in thrombin-induced activation of factor VIII.

### Factors with Increased Survival

Another approach to generating improved forms of factor VIII has been to synthesize molecules that have prolonged activity in the circulation. Factor VIII circulates as an inactive procofactor that must be activated by thrombin to participate in the activation of factor X. Factor VIII is then rapidly inactivated by either spontaneous dissociation of the A1 and A2 domains or by further proteolytic cleavage by activated protein C. A critical event in the inactivation of factor VIII is the dissociation of the A2 domain from the light chain and A1 domain (see Chapter 8). The A2 domain exists in a metal-ion complex with the other domains and either falls apart spontaneously or during cleavage by activated protein C. By linking the A2 domain to the light chain, the activity of factor VIII can be considerably prolonged in vitro. Pipe and Kaufman replaced the thrombin cleavage site between the A2 and A3 domains of B-domain deleted factor VIII with a noncleavable spacer so the A2 domain remains covalently linked to the light chain after activation (113). The result was the generation of an inactivation-resistant form of factor VIII. Using a similar rationale, Gale and Pellequer engineered factor VIII to create disulfide links between the A2 and A3 domain (114). In both cases, the inactivation-resistant factor VIII showed persistence for up to 40 minutes after activation, a marked increase compared with native factor VIII. The rapid inactivation of factor VIII activity under normal physiologic conditions suggests that there may be biologic advantages to limiting the presence of activated factor VIII in the circulation. Persistence of activated factor VIII might lead to more generalized generation of thrombin and an increased risk of thromboembolism. Modifications of factor VIII that increase its activity—either by decreasing the inactivation of activated factor VIII or by increasing the intrinsic catalytic activity of the protein—must be examined carefully in *in vivo* models before clinical trials proceed in humans.

Interfering with the interaction of factor VIII with receptors involved in the clearance of clotting factors from the circulation constitutes another method to prolong the survival of factor VIII in the circulation. The advantage of this approach is that one does not have to worry about the effect of increased circulation of an activated clotting factor. The low density lipoprotein–related protein (LRP) receptor, a hepatic protein that has been implicated in the clearance of low density lipoproteins and other proteins from the circulation, has been shown to interact with and bind factor VIII through cysteine-rich low density lipoprotein receptor class A repeats in the LRP extracellular domain (115,116) (see Chapter 8). Heparin sulfate proteoglycans may also participate in the clearance of factor VIII by LRP. Conditions that inhibit the interaction of factor VIII with LRP prolong the survival of factor VIII in hemophilic mice (117).

### Immunologically Altered Proteins

Inhibitors in hemophilia A are a common and serious complication that renders normal therapy with replacement factor VIII ineffective. Forms of factor VIII that evade or prevent an immune response would be advantageous for patients with inhibitors. One approach to generate antigenically altered factor VIII, based on the observation that porcine factor VIII is able to substitute for human factor VIII in coagulation, but is poorly recognized by antibodies to the human protein, has been to engineer chimeras of human and porcine factor VIII (118,119). The substitution of porcine sequences, either entire domains or selected sequences, into human factor VIII significantly reduced recognition of the molecule by inhibitor antibodies while preserving participation in thrombin generation *in vitro*. Nevertheless, although the porcine/human hybrids were not well recognized by established human inhibitor antibodies, it remains to be determined whether the hybrid molecules are immunogenic themselves. Porcine factor VIII is variably immunogenic in humans and the hybrid sequences might be capable of generating an immune response in some individuals. Despite this, the concept of genetically engineering factor VIII to reduce antigenicity would seem to be a viable approach as we learn more about inhibitor epitopes and the three-dimensional structure of factor VIII. The critical question with this approach is whether we can understand the antigenicity and immunogenicity of proteins well enough to engineer molecules that lack both.

### Improved Synthesis of Coagulation Factors

Another area for improvement is in the efficiency of protein synthesis in mammalian cells. The endoplasmic reticulum (ER) is a major site for the folding and assembly of secretory proteins such as factor VIII and factor IX [see Fig. 81-1A (120)]. Proteins destined for the cell surface are cotranslationally translocated into the lumen of the ER where the proteins undergo various posttranslational modifications and proper folding (120,121). These reactions and the orderly movement of proteins through the ER and the Golgi apparatus are facilitated by enzymes and molecular chaperones present in the various compartments of the ER and Golgi. Two homologous protein chaperones that regulate transport of improperly folded

glycoproteins through the ER are calnexin, a conserved integral ER membrane protein, and calreticulin, an ER lumenal protein. Calnexin and calreticulin associate transiently and selectively with newly synthesized glycoproteins in the early stages of folding and are thought to promote the interaction of misfolded proteins with disulfide isomerases that enhance proper folding (122). The oxidizing environment of the ER facilitates the action of these disulfide isomerases to catalyze and monitor disulfide bond formation in an ordered manner. Prolonged association of calnexin or calreticulin is observed when proteins are misfolded or unable to oligomerize. The calnexin or calreticulin recognition motifs are at least partially determined by the structure of asparagine-linked oligosaccharides. Another resident ER protein, immunoglobulin binding protein (BiP)/glucose-regulated protein (GRP78), uses energy from adenosine triphosphate (ATP) hydrolysis to promote folding and prevent aggregation of protein in the ER (123). Feedback mechanisms exist in the ER that also promote proper folding. There is an unfolded protein response (UPR) that senses excess unfolded protein in the ER and generates signals to the nucleus to up-regulate chaperone proteins such as calnexin, calreticulin, and BiP to increase proper folding (120). Amino-terminal fragment (ATF)6, IRE1, and protein kinaselike ER kinase (PERK) are three proteins in the ER that signal to bZip transcription regulators in the nucleus to synthesize new chaperone proteins.

The synthesis of factor VIII has been studied intensely. At a molecular level, glucosylation controls FVIII transit through the ER-Golgi (Fig. 81-1B). In the ER, factor VIII undergoes N-linked glycosylation. After translocation into the lumen of the ER, a core unit of 14 saccharides (GlcNAc2Man9Glc3) is added to targeted Asp residues. The terminal-glucoses are trimmed, first by glucosidase I, which cleaves the first glucose, and then by glucosidase II, which cleaves the second and third glucoses. If the protein is properly folded, the deglucosylated protein is able to interact with the ER-Golgi intermediate compartment (ERGIC53)/multiple coagulation factor deficiency 2 (MCFD2) complex, probably through the terminal mannose groups on the proteins, and factor VIII is transferred through the intermediate compartment to the Golgi apparatus (124). If the protein is not folded properly, it is recognized by a UDP-glucose: glycoprotein glucosyl-transferase (UGGT), which transfers a single glucose to the high mannose containing side chains. The activity of the UGGT to add this single glucose is stimulated by the unfolded protein although the sensing mechanism is uncertain. The monoglucosylated protein interacts with calnexin and calreticulin, which direct the interaction of factor VIII with ERp57, a protein disulfide isomerase that stimulates disulfide bond formation, leading to increased protein folding. The protein then undergoes another cycle of deglucosylation by glucosidase I/II, interaction with UGGT, interaction with calnexin and calreticulin, and disulfide bond formation. Once the protein is properly folded, it is no longer recognized by UGGT and is not glucosylated. The high mannose protein is then able to interact with ERGIC53, a mannose binding cargo protein in the intermediate compartment that transfers the protein to the Golgi apparatus. The interaction with ERGIC53 is facilitated by MCFD2, a calcium binding protein that forms a complex with ERGIC53 (125). In the Golgi, the mannose groups are trimmed to a core of GlcNAc2Man5, knocking off ERGIC53, which recycles to the ER to transport more protein to the Golgi. If, despite maximal folding, the protein remains misfolded, it is removed from the ER. This degradative pathway is through a transport protein called sec 61 to the 20S proteasome and is facilitated by BiP.

The synthesis of factor VIII, in particular, is inefficient compared with factor IX, factor VII, or even factor V, which is highly homologous with factor VIII. Studies by Kaufman, Pipe et al. (121) have shown some of the reasons for the inefficient

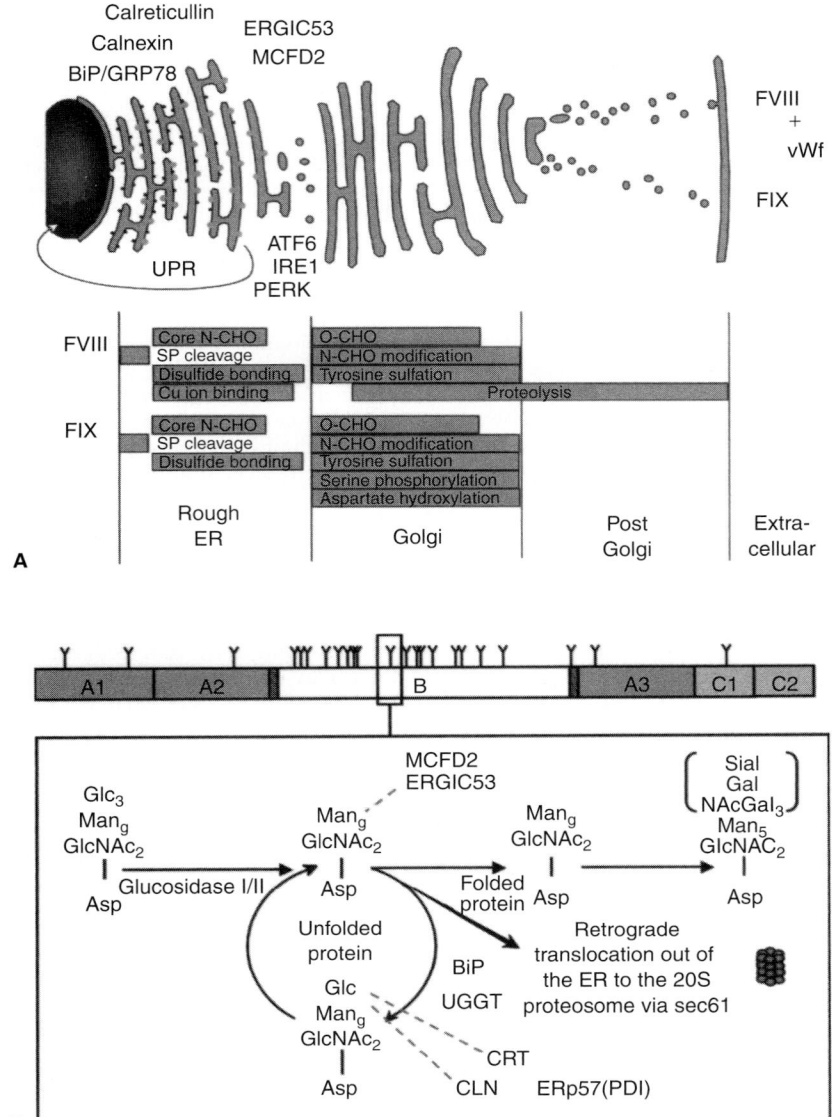

**FIGURE 81-1.** Cellular biosynthesis and assembly of factor VIII and IX. Secretory proteins like factors VIII and IX undergo complex intracellular processing. **Panel A:** Factors VIII and IX are cotranslationally translocated into the lumen of the endoplasmic reticulum (ER) where they undergo various modifications and folding. After cleavage of the signal peptide, factor VIII and factor IX undergo specific posttranslational modifications. Copper atoms are bound to factor VIII in the rough ER. Protein folding begins and disulfide bonds are formed, providing stability to the tertiary structure of the protein. These changes are monitored by chaperone proteins, calnexin, calreticulin, and BiP/GRP78, which provide "quality control" to the folding process. The presence of unfolded protein in the ER leads to an integrated signaling response that transmits information from the ER to the nucleus to affect protein synthesis. ATF6, IRE1, and PERK are ER transmembrane proteins that initiate transduction of the unfolded protein response. Also in the ER, N-linked carbohydrates are added to target asparagine residues, a process that is thought to be critical to the monitoring process by chaperone proteins. Once the protein is properly folded, it can bind to the ERGIC53/MCFD2 complex and transit to the Golgi apparatus. In the Golgi, the N-linked carbohydrates are modified, O-linked carbohydrates are added and target tyrosine residues are sulfated. Like factor VIII, factor IX undergoes extensive posttranslational processing in the ER and Golgi, but the secretion of factor IX is more efficient than that of factor VIII and there does not appear to be the same critical monitoring of factor IX structure that occurs for factor VIII. In particular, the ERGIC53/MCFD2 complex is not involved in factor IX movement through the ER-Golgi. **Panel B:** The folding cycle for factor VIII. The N-linked carbohydrates in factor VIII play an important role in proper folding of the protein in the ER. Following the addition of carbohydrates, the terminal-glucose residues are sequentially removed by glucosidases. A UGGT in the ER senses improperly folded proteins by an unknown process and is activated by the unfolded protein to transfer glucose to the carbohydrate. Calnexin and calreticulin bind to the monoglucosylated protein, leading to an interaction with ERp57, a protein disulfide isomerase that stimulates disulfide bond formation. The protein undergoes another cycle of deglucosidation and, if still improperly folded, interaction with UGGT, monoglucosylation, binding to calnexin and calreticulin, and disulfide bond formation. Once properly folded, the factor VIII binds to the ERGIC53/MCFD2 complex to transit to the Golgi. Conversely, if the protein fails to fold properly, it is eventually translocated out of the ER through an ATP-dependent interaction with BiP. (Adapted from Kaufman RJ. Orchestrating the unfolded protein response in health and disease. *J Clin Invest* 2002;110:1389–1398.)

production of factor VIII. First, factor VIII secretion from cells is affected by its interaction with the chaperone protein BiP/GRP78 and subsequent ATP-dependent release. The requirement of ATP hydrolysis by BiP/GRP78 is unique for factor VIII and is not required for release of factor V. Binding of factor VIII to BiP/GRP78 occurs through Phe309 in the A1 domain and mutation of this residue results in improved factor VIII secretion efficiency (126). Interestingly, Phe309 is adjacent to Cys310, which is a site of copper binding in factor VIII (see Chapter 8). It has been suggested that binding of copper to factor VIII stabilizes the factor VIII structure and BiP/GRP78 may monitor this stability. Second, the B-domain of factor VIII is important for efficient secretion. The B-domain deleted form of factor VIII is 10 times less efficiently secreted than full-length factor VIII. The important sequences in the B-domain for this are the amino-terminal 226 amino acids of the B-domain, which contain six asparagine-linked glycosylation sites. Mutation of these asparagines residues to glutamine reduces the efficiency of factor VIII secretion, perhaps by reducing the interaction of factor VIII with ERGIC53/MCFD2 (127).

The increased understanding of the transport of secretory proteins like factor VIII through the ER and Golgi will have its greatest application in the synthesis of recombinant proteins for clinical use, not as a method for treatment of hemophiliacs, although methods of increasing protein production in mild hemophilia might be useful. In the manufacture of recombinant clotting factor proteins, any enhancement in the amount of protein synthesized per cell would reduce the cost of production and result in cheaper products for patients, allowing more frequent treatment and prevention of bleeding.

# SUMMARY

The treatment of hemophilia and other bleeding disorders is on the threshold of a new era. Clinical trials of gene transfer approaches have been started and although none has resulted in dramatic effects, continued advances in the field promise to impact hemophilia in the future. Current understanding of the structure and function of factors VIII, IX, VII, and other clotting factors also promise to lead to the development of new and better proteins. We are at a point in time where we can truly consider the possibility of making proteins that are potentially better than those that exist in nature. However, the pursuit of making such molecules must be done carefully, and with circumspection.

## *References*

1. Jaenisch R, Mintz B. Simian virus 40 DNA sequences in DNA of healthy adult mice derived from preimplantation blastocysts injected with viral DNA. *Proc Natl Acad Sci U S A* 1974;71:1250–1254.
2. Mulligan RC, Howard BH, Berg P. Synthesis of rabbit beta-globin in cultured monkey kidney cells following infection with a SV40 beta-globin recombinant genome. *Nature* 1979;277:108–114.
3. Hamer DH, Leder P. Expression of the chromosomal mouse Beta$_{maj}$-globin gene cloned in SV40. *Nature* 1979;281:35–40.
4. Hamer DH, Leder P. SV40 recombinants carrying a functional RNA splice junction and polyadenylation site from the chromosomal mouse beta$_{maj}$ globin gene. *Cell* 1979;17:737–747.
5. Shimotohno K, Temin HM. Formation of infectious progeny virus after insertion of herpes simplex thymidine kinase gene into DNA of an avian retrovirus. *Cell* 1981;26:67–77.
6. Tabin CJ, Hoffmann JW, Goff SP, et al. Adaptation of a retrovirus as a eucaryotic vector transmitting the herpes simplex virus thymidine kinase gene. *Mol Cell Biol* 1982;2:426–436.
7. Mann R, Mulligan RC, Baltimore D. Construction of a retrovirus packaging mutant and its use to produce helper-free defective retrovirus. *Cell* 1983;33:153–159.
8. Cline MJ. Perspectives for gene therapy: inserting new genetic information into mammalian cells by physical techniques and viral vectors. *Pharmacol Ther* 1985;29:69–92.
9. Ahlberg Å. Haemophilia in Sweden. VII. Incidence, treatment and prophylaxis of arthropathy and other musculoskeletal manifestations of haemophilia A and B. *Acta Orthop Scand* 1965;77(Suppl. 1):3–132.
10. Nilsson I-M, Berntorp E, Lofqvist T, et al. Twenty-five years' experience of prophylactic treatment of severe hemophilia A and B. *J Intern Med* 1992;232:25–32.
11. Manco-Johnson MJ. Update on treatment regimens: prophylaxis versus on-demand therapy. *Semin Hematol* 2003;40(Suppl. 3):3–9.
12. Wion KL, Kelly D, Summerfield JA, et al. Distribution of factor VIII mRNA and antigen in human liver and other tissues. *Nature* 1985;317:726–729.
13. Fuentes-Prior P, Fujikawa K, Pratt KP. New insights into binding interfaces of coagulation factors V and VIII and their homologues lessons from high resolution crystal structures. *Curr Protein Pept Sci* 2002;3:313–339.
14. Pratt KP, Shen BW, Takeshima K, et al. Structure of the C2 domain of human factor VIII at 1.5 A resolution. *Nature* 1999;402:439–442.
15. Graham JB, Buckwalter JA, Hartley LJ, et al. Canine hemophilia. Observations on the course, the clotting anomaly, and the effect of blood transfusions. *J Exp Med* 1949;90:97–111.
16. Bi L, Lawler AM, Antonarakis SE, et al. Targeted disruption of the mouse factor VIII gene produces a model of haemophilia A. *Nat Genet* 1995;10:119–121.
17. Kay MA, Glorioso JC, Naldini L. Viral vectors for gene therapy: the art of turning infectious agents into vehicles of therapeutics. *Nat Med* 2001;7:33–40.
18. Miller DG, Adam MA, Miller AD. Gene transfer by retrovirus vectors occurs only in cells that are actively replicating at the time of infection. *Mol Cell Biol* 1990;10:4239–4242.
19. Rettinger SD, Ponder KP, Saylors RL, et al. In vivo hepatocyte transduction with retrovirus during in-flow occlusion. *J Surg Res* 1993;54: 418–425.
20. Kay MA, Rothenberg S, Landen CN, et al. In vivo gene therapy of hemophilia B: sustained partial correction in factor IX-deficient dogs. *Science* 1993;262:117–119.
21. Kaleko M, Garcia JV, Miller AD. Persistent gene expression after retroviral gene transfer into liver cells in vivo. *Hum Gene Ther* 1991;2:27–32.
22. Pages JC, Loux N, Bellusci S, et al. Hepatocyte growth factor expressed by a retrovirus-producing cell line enhances retroviral transduction of primary hepatocytes: implications for in vivo gene transfer. *Biochem Biophys Res Commun* 1996;222:726–731.
23. Nguyen TH, Pages JC, Farge D, et al. Amphotropic retroviral vectors displaying hepatocyte growth factor-envelope fusion proteins improve transduction efficiency of primary hepatocytes. *Hum Gene Ther* 1998;9:2469–2479.
24. Gao C, Jokerst R, Gondipalli P, et al. Intramuscular injection of an adenoviral vector expressing hepatocyte growth factor facilitates hepatic transduction with a retroviral vector in mice. *Hum Gene Ther* 1999; 10: 911–922.
25. Xu L, Gao C, Sands MS, et al. Neonatal or hepatocyte growth factor-potentiated adult gene therapy with a retroviral vector results in therapeutic levels of canine factor IX for hemophilia B. *Blood* 2003;101:3924–3932.
26. Naldini L, Blomer U, Gallay P, et al. In vivo gene delivery and stable transduction of nondividing cells by a lentiviral vector. *Science* 1996;272:263–267.
27. Naldini L. In vivo gene delivery by lentiviral vectors. *Thromb Haemost* 1999;82:552–554.
28. Olsen JC. Gene transfer vectors derived from equine infectious anemia virus. *Gene Ther* 1998;5:1481–1487.
29. Poeschla EM, Wong-Staal F, Looney DJ. Efficient transduction of nondividing human cells by feline immunodeficiency virus lentiviral vectors. *Nat Med* 1998;4:354–357.
30. Curran MA, Kaiser SM, Achacoso PL, et al. Efficient transduction of non-dividing cells by optimized feline immunodeficiency virus vectors. *Mol Ther* 2000;1:31–38.
31. Russell DW, Miller AD. Foamy virus vectors. *J Virol* 1996;70:217–222.
32. Zennou V, Petit C, Guetard D, et al. HIV-1 genome nuclear import is mediated by a central DNA flap. *Cell* 2000;101:173–185.
33. Follenzi A, Ailles LE, Bakovic S, et al. Gene transfer by lentiviral vectors is limited by nuclear translocation and rescued by HIV-1 pol sequences. *Nat Genet* 2000;25:217–222.
34. Zennou V, Serguera C, Sarkis C, et al. The HIV-1 DNA flap stimulates HIV vector-mediated cell transduction in the brain. *Nat Biotechnol* 2001;19:446–450.
35. Follenzi A, Sabatino G, Lombardo A, et al. Efficient gene delivery and targeted expression to hepatocytes in vivo by improved lentiviral vectors. *Hum Gene Ther* 2002;13:243–260.
36. Park F, Kay MA. Modified HIV-1 based lentiviral vectors have an effect on viral transduction efficiency and gene expression in vitro and in vivo. *Mol Ther* 2001;4:164–173.
37. Agarwal M, Austin TW, Morel F, et al. Scaffold attachment region-mediated enhancement of retroviral vector expression in primary T cells. *J Virol* 1998;72:3720–3728.
38. Dang Q, Auten J, Plavec I. Human beta interferon scaffold attachment region inhibits de novo methylation and confers long-term, copy number-dependent expression to a retroviral vector. *J Virol* 2000;74:2671–2678.
39. Schroder AR, Shinn P, Chen H, et al. HIV-1 integration in the human genome favors active genes and local hotspots. *Cell* 2002;110:521–529.

40. Wu X, Li Y, Crise B, et al. Transcription start regions in the human genome are favored targets for MLV integration. *Science* 2003;300: 1749–1751.

41. Coffin JM, Hughes SH, Varmus HE. *Retroviruses.* Cold Spring Harbor, NY: Cold Spring Harbor Laboratory Press, 1997.

42. Li Z, Dullmann J, Schiedlmeier B, et al. Murine leukemia induced by retroviral gene marking. *Science* 2002;296:497.

43. Hacein-Bey-Abina S, Von Kalle C, Schmidt M, et al. LMO2-associated clonal T cell proliferation in two patients after gene therapy for SCID-X1. *Science* 2003;302:415–419.

44. Kirby I, Davison E, Beavil AJ, et al. Mutations in the DG loop of adenovirus type 5 fiber knob protein abolish high-affinity binding to its cellular receptor CAR. *J Virol* 1999;73:9508–9514.

45. Kirby I, Davison E, Beavil AJ, et al. Identification of contact residues and definition of the CAR-binding site of adenovirus type 5 fiber protein. *J Virol* 2000;74:2804–2813.

46. Bergelson JM, Cunningham JA, Droguett G, et al. Isolation of a common receptor for Coxsackie B viruses and adenoviruses 2 and 5. *Science* 1997; 275:1320–1323.

47. Schnell MA, Zhang Y, Tazelaar J, et al. Activation of innate immunity in nonhuman primates following intraportal administration of adenoviral vectors. *Mol Ther* 2001;3:708–722.

48. Burgert HG, Ruzsics Z, Obermeier S, et al. Subversion of host defense mechanisms by adenoviruses. *Curr Top Microbiol Immunol* 2002;269: 273–318.

49. Schaack J, Bennett ML, Colbert JD, et al. E1A and E1B proteins inhibit inflammation induced by adenovirus. *Proc Natl Acad Sci U S A* 2004;19:19.

50. Kochanek S, Clemens PR, Mitani K, et al. A new adenoviral vector: replacement of all viral coding sequences with 28 kb of DNA independently expressing both full-length dystrophin and beta-galactosidase. *Proc Natl Acad Sci U S A* 1996;93:5731–5736.

51. Morsy MA, Gu M, Motzel S, et al. An adenoviral vector deleted for all viral coding sequences results in enhanced safety and extended expression of a leptin transgene. *Proc Natl Acad Sci U S A* 1998;95:7866–7871.

52. Morral N, Parks RJ, Zhou H, et al. High doses of a helper-dependent adenoviral vector yield supraphysiological levels of alpha1-antitrypsin with negligible toxicity. *Hum Gene Ther* 1998;9:2709–2716.

53. O'Neal WK, Zhou H, Morral N, et al. Toxicity associated with repeated administration of first-generation adenovirus vectors does not occur with a helper-dependent vector. *Mol Med* 2000;6:179–195.

54. Balague C, Zhou J, Dai Y, et al. Sustained high-level expression of full-length human factor VIII and restoration of clotting activity in hemophilic mice using a minimal adenovirus vector. *Blood* 2000;95:820–828.

55. Stilwell JL, McCarty DM, Negishi A, et al. Development and characterization of novel empty adenovirus capsids and their impact on cellular gene expression. *J Virol* 2003;77:12881–12885.

56. Raper SE, Chirmule N, Lee FS, et al. Fatal systemic inflammatory response syndrome in a ornithine transcarbamylase deficient patient following adenoviral gene transfer. *Mol Genet Metab* 2003;80:148–158.

57. Weiss R, Nelson D. *Teen dies undergoing experimental gene therapy.* Washington, DC: The Washington Post, 1999:A01.

58. Kotin RM, Menninger JC, Ward DC, et al. Mapping and direct visualization of a region-specific viral DNA integration site on chromosome 19q13-qter. *Genomics* 1991;10:831–834.

59. Weitzman MD, Kyostio SR, Kotin RM, et al. Adeno-associated virus (AAV) rep proteins mediate complex formation between AAV DNA and its integration site in human DNA. *Proc Natl Acad Sci U S A* 1994;91: 5808–5812.

60. Gao GP, Alvira MR, Wang L, et al. Novel adeno-associated viruses from rhesus monkeys as vectors for human gene therapy. *Proc Natl Acad Sci U S A* 2002;99:11854–11859.

61. Summerford C, Samulski RJ. Membrane-associated heparan sulfate proteoglycan is a receptor for adeno-associated virus type 2 virions. *J Virol* 1998;72:1438–1445.

62. Pruchnic R, Cao B, Peterson ZQ, et al. The use of adeno-associated virus to circumvent the maturation-dependent viral transduction of muscle fibers. *Hum Gene Ther* 2000;11:521–536.

63. Dutheil N, Shi F, Dupressoir T, et al. Adeno-associated virus site-specifically integrates into a muscle- specific DNA region. *Proc Natl Acad Sci U S A* 2000;97:4862–4866.

64. Summerford C, Bartlett JS, Samulski RJ. AlphaVbeta5 integrin: a co-receptor for adeno-associated virus type 2 infection. *Nat Med* 1999;5:78–82.

65. Qing K, Mah C, Hansen J, et al. Human fibroblast growth factor receptor 1 is a co-receptor for infection by adeno-associated virus 2. *Nat Med* 1999;5: 71–77.

66. Nakai H, Yant SR, Storm TA, et al. Extrachromosomal recombinant adeno-associated virus vector genomes are primarily responsible for stable liver transduction in vivo. *J Virol* 2001;75:6969–6976.

67. Schnepp BC, Clark KR, Klemanski DL, et al. Genetic fate of recombinant adeno-associated virus vector genomes in muscle. *J Virol* 2003;77: 3495–3504.

68. Chao H, Sun L, Bruce A, et al. Expression of human factor VIII by splicing between dimerized AAV vectors. *Mol Ther* 2002;5:716–722.

69. Mah C, Sarkar R, Zolotukhin I, et al. Dual vectors expressing murine factor VIII result in sustained correction of hemophilia A mice. *Hum Gene Ther* 2003;14:143–152.

70. Scallan CD, Liu T, Parker AE, et al. Phenotypic correction of a mouse model of hemophilia A using AAV2 vectors encoding the heavy and light chains of FVIII. *Blood* 2003;102:3919–3926.

71. Sarkar R, Tetreault R, Gao G, et al. Total correction of hemophilia A mice with canine FVIII using an AAV 8 serotype. *Blood* 2004;103:1253–1260.

72. Monahan PE, Jooss K, Sands MS. Safety of adeno-associated virus gene therapy vectors: a current evaluation. *Expert Opin Drug Saf* 2002;1: 79–91.

73. Donsante A, Vogler C, Muzyczka N, et al. Observed incidence of tumorigenesis in long-term rodent studies of rAAV vectors. *Gene Ther* 2001;8: 1343–1346.

74. Miller DG, Rutledge EA, Russell DW. Chromosomal effects of adeno-associated virus vector integration. *Nat Genet* 2002;30:147–148.

75. High KA, Manno CS, Sabatino DE, et al. Immune responses to AAV and to factor IX in a phase I study of AAV-mediated liver-directed gene transfer for hemophilia B. *Blood* 2003;102:532a.

76. Fewell JG, MacLaughlin F, Mehta V, et al. Gene therapy for the treatment of hemophilia B using PINC-formulated plasmid delivered to muscle with electroporation. *Mol Ther* 2001;3:574–583.

77. Miao CH, Ye X, Thompson AR. High-level factor VIII gene expression *in vivo* achieved by nonviral liver-specific gene therapy vectors. *Hum Gene Ther* 2003;14:1297–1305.

78. Ye P, Thompson AR, Sarkar R, et al. Naked DNA transfer of factor VIII induced transgene-specific, species-independent immune response in hemophilia A mice. *Mol Ther* 2004;10:117–126.

79. Kmiec EB. Targeted gene repair. *Gene Ther* 1999;6:1–3.

80. Kmiec EB. Targeted gene repair–in the arena. *J Clin Invest* 2003; 112: 632–636.

81. Kren BT, Bandyopadhyay P, Steer CJ. In vivo site-directed mutagenesis of the factor IX gene by chimeric RNA/DNA oligonucleotides. *Nat Med* 1998;4:285–290.

82. Puttaraju M, Jamison SF, Mansfield SG, et al. Spliceosome-mediated RNA trans-splicing as a tool for gene therapy. *Nat Biotechnol* 1999;17:246–252.

83. Chao H, Mansfield SG, Bartel RC, et al. Phenotype correction of hemophilia A mice by spliceosome-mediated RNA trans-splicing. *Nat Med* 2003;9: 1015–1019.

84. Burke JF, Mogg AE. Suppression of a nonsense mutation in mammalian cells in vivo by the aminoglycoside antibiotics G-418 and paromomycin. *Nucleic Acids Res* 1985;13:6265–6272.

85. Martin R, Mogg AE, Heywood LA, et al. Aminoglycoside suppression at UAG, UAA and UGA codons in Escherichia coli and human tissue culture cells. *Mol Gen Genet* 1989;217:411–418.

86. Wilschanski M, Yahav Y, Yaacov Y, et al. Gentamicin-induced correction of CFTR function in patients with cystic fibrosis and CFTR stop mutations. *N Engl J Med* 2003;349:1433–1441.

87. Srivastava A, Viswabandya A, Baidya S, et al. Administration of gentamicin does not increase factor levels in severe hemophilia B due to premature termination codons. *J Thromb Haemost* 2003;(Suppl. 1):CD043.

88. James PD, Raut S, Rivard GE, et al. Aminoglycoside suppression of nonsense mutations in severe hemophilia. *Blood* 2005; (in press).

89. Qiu X, Lu D, Zhou J, et al. Implantation of autologous skin fibroblast genetically modified to secrete clotting factor IX partially corrects the hemorrhagic tendencies in two hemophilia B patients. *Chin Med J* 1996;109: 832–839.

90. Roth DA, Tawa NE Jr, O'Brien JM, et al. Nonviral transfer of the gene encoding coagulation factor VIII in patients with severe hemophilia A. *N Engl J Med* 2001;344:1735–1742.

91. Powell JS, Ragni MV, White GC II, et al. Phase 1 trial of FVIII gene transfer for severe hemophilia A using a retroviral construct administered by peripheral intravenous infusion. *Blood* 2003;102:2038–2045.

92. Manno CS, Chew AJ, Hutchison S, et al. AAV-mediated factor IX gene transfer to skeletal muscle in patients with severe hemophilia B. *Blood* 2003;101:2963–2972.

93. High KA, Tigges M, Manno CS, et al. Human immune responses to AAV-2 capsid may limit duration of expression in liver-directed gene transfer in humans with hemophilia B. *Blood* 2004;104:121a.

94. Hsueh JL. Clinical protocol of human gene transfer for hemophilia B. *Hum Gene Ther* 1992;3:543–552.

95. Selden RF, Skoskiewicz MJ, Howie KB, et al. Implantation of genetically engineered fibroblasts into mice: implications for gene therapy. *Science* 1987;236:714–718.

96. DePolo NJ, Harkleroad CE, Bodner M, et al. The resistance of retroviral vectors produced from human cells to serum inactivation *in vivo* and *in vitro* is primate species dependent. *J Virol* 1999;73:6708–6714.

97. Kay MA, Manno CS, Ragni MV, et al. Evidence for gene transfer and expression of factor IX in haemophilia B patients treated with an AAV vector. *Nat Genet* 2000;24:257–261.

98. Zhang WW, Josephs SF, Zhou J, et al. Development and application of a minimal-adenoviral vector system for gene therapy of hemophilia A. *Thromb Haemost* 1999;82:562–571.

99. Nakai H, Ohashi K, Arruda V, et al. A proposed rAAV-liver directed clinical trial for hemophilia B. *Blood* 2000;96:798a.

100. Michnick DA, Pittman DD, Wise RJ, et al. Identification of individual tyrosine sulfation sites within factor VIII required for optimal activity and efficient thrombin cleavage. *J Biol Chem* 1994;269:20095–20102.

101. White GC II, Beebe A, Nielsen B. Recombinant factor IX. *Thromb Haemost* 1997;78:261–265.

102. Bond M, Jankowski M, Patel H, et al. Biochemical characterization of recombinant factor IX. *Semin Hematol* 1998;35:11–17.

103. Wu SM, Cheung WF, Frazier D, et al. Cloning and expression of the cDNA for human gamma-glutamyl carboxylase. *Science* 1991; 254: 1634–1636.

104. Rost S, Fregin A, Ivaskevicius V, et al. Mutations in VKORC1 cause warfarin resistance and multiple coagulation factor deficiency type 2. *Nature* 2004;427:537–541.

105. Li T, Chang CY, Jin DY, et al. Identification of the gene for vitamin K epoxide reductase. *Nature* 2004;427:541–544.

106. Schnieke AE, Kind AJ, Ritchie WA, et al. Human factor IX transgenic sheep produced by transfer of nuclei from transfected fetal fibroblasts. *Science* 1997;278:2130–2133.

107. Paleyanda RK, Velander WH, Lee TK, et al. Transgenic pigs produce functional human factor VIII in milk. *Nat Biotechnol* 1997;15:971–975.

108. Niemann H, Halter R, Carnwath JW, et al. Expression of human blood clotting factor VIII in the mammary gland of transgenic sheep. *Transgenic Res* 1999;8:237–247.

109. Van Cott KE, Butler SP, Russell CG, et al. Transgenic pigs as bioreactors: a comparison of gamma-carboxylation of glutamic acid in recombinant human protein C and factor IX by the mammary gland. *Genet Anal* 1999;15:155–160.

110. Hopfner KP, Brandstetter H, Karcher A, et al. Converting blood coagulation factor IXa into factor Xa: dramatic increase in amidolytic activity identifies important active site determinants. *EMBO J* 1997; 16: 6626–6635.

111. Chang JY, Monroe DM, Stafford DW, et al. Replacing the first epidermal growth factor-like domain of factor IX with that of factor VII enhances activity *in vitro* and in canine hemophilia B. *J Clin Invest* 1997;100: 886–892.

112. Voorberg J, van Stempvoort G, Bos JM, et al. Enhanced thrombin sensitivity of a factor VIII-heparin cofactor II hybrid. *J Biol Chem* 1996;271: 20985–20988.

113. Pipe SW, Kaufman RJ. Characterization of a genetically engineered inactivation-resistant coagulation factor VIIIa. *Proc Natl Acad Sci U S A* 1997;94: 11851–11856.

114. Gale AJ, Pellequer JL. An engineered interdomain disulfide bond stabilizes human blood coagulation factor VIIIa. *J Thromb Haemost* 2003;1: 1966–1971.

115. Lenting PJ, Neels JG, van den Berg BM, et al. The light chain of factor VIII comprises a binding site for low density lipoprotein receptor-related protein. *J Biol Chem* 1999;274:23734–23739.

116. Saenko EL, Yakhyaev AV, Mikhailenko I, et al. Role of the low density lipoprotein-related protein receptor in mediation of factor VIII catabolism. *J Biol Chem* 1999;274:37685–37692.

117. Bovenschen N, Herz J, Grimbergen JM, et al. Elevated plasma factor VIII in a mouse model of low density lipoprotein receptor-related protein deficiency. *Blood* 2003;101:3933–3939.

118. Barrow RT, Healey JF, Gailani D, et al. Reduction of the antigenicity of factor VIII toward complex inhibitory antibody plasmas using multiply-substituted hybrid human/porcine factor VIII molecules. *Blood* 2000;95: 564–568.

119. Parker ET, Healey JF, Barrow RT, et al. Reduction of the inhibitory antibody response to human factor VIII in hemophilia A mice by mutagenesis of the A2 domain B-cell epitope. *Blood* 2004;104:704–710.

120. Kaufman RJ. Orchestrating the unfolded protein response in health and disease. *J Clin Invest* 2002;110:1389–1398.

121. Kaufman RJ, Pipe SW, Tagliavacca L, et al. Biosynthesis, assembly and secretion of coagulation factor VIII. *Blood Coagul Fibrinolysis* 1997;8 (Suppl. 2):S3–14.

122. Pipe SW, Morris JA, Shah J, et al. Differential interaction of coagulation factor VIII and factor V with protein chaperones calnexin and calreticulin. *J Biol Chem* 1998;273:8537–8544.

123. Morris JA, Dorner AJ, Edwards CA, et al. Immunoglobulin binding protein (BiP) function is required to protect cells from endoplasmic reticulum stress but is not required for the secretion of selective proteins. *J Biol Chem* 1997; 272:4327–4334.

124. Cunningham MA, Pipe SW, Zhang B, et al. LMAN1 is a molecular chaperone for the secretion of coagulation factor VIII. *J Thromb Haemost* 2003;1: 2360–2367.

125. Zhang B, Cunningham MA, Nichols WC, et al. Bleeding due to disruption of a cargo-specific ER-to-Golgi transport complex. *Nat Genet* 2003;34: 220–225.

126. Swaroop M, Moussalli M, Pipe SW, et al. Mutagenesis of a potential immunoglobulin-binding protein-binding site enhances secretion of coagulation factor VIII. *J Biol Chem* 1997;272:24121–24124.

127. Miao HZ, Sirachainan N, Palmer L, et al. Bioengineering of coagulation factor VIII for improved secretion. *Blood* 2004;103:3412–3419.

# CHAPTER 82 ■ OVERVIEW OF VENOUS THROMBOEMBOLISM

**HENRI BOUNAMEAUX**

Although thrombosis can affect any venous circulation, this section on "Venous Thromboembolic Disorders" deals mainly with thrombotic events that occur in the deep veins of the leg, arm, and pelvis, and their complications: early pulmonary embolism (PE), late postthrombotic syndrome (PTS), and chronic thromboembolic pulmonary hypertension. Chapter 86, however, covers thromboses occurring in less common sites, including upper limbs, a location that is increasingly affected (1).

The present overview pursues two aims: first, introducing the section, and second, focusing on some contemporary controversies in the field.

## EPIDEMIOLOGY AND NATURAL HISTORY

PE, the source of which is predominantly located in a thrombosis of the deep veins of the legs, [deep vein thrombosis (DVT)], is a major health concern: The third cause of mortality by cardiovascular disease after coronary artery disease and stroke, it remains a leading cause of death in the puerperium and the postoperative period in western countries. In addition, late sequelae of DVT may produce disabling leg symptoms in a substantial proportion of patients, including venous ulcers in some of them, resulting in a considerable economic burden, and also chronic thromboembolic pulmonary hypertension in few of them (see Chapter 92).

Venous thromboembolism (VTE) is mostly a disease in elderly persons with a slightly predominant proportion of men over women, except during the childbearing years of women (see Chapter 84). It is also a recurrent disease, with one third of patients developing recurrence within 10 years, the risk of recurrence being highest within the first 6 to 12 months of the incident event, in men compared to women (2), and following idiopathic (unprovoked) compared to secondary (provoked) event.

The possibility for blood clots formed in the venous circulation to traverse the interatrial heart septum through a persistent aperture called patent foramen ovale (PFO) and to produce systemic embolization—the so-called paradoxical embolism—potentially causing stroke, myocardial infarction, or peripheral occlusive events, has been increasingly recognized in the last decade (see Chapter 93). Because small venous thrombi can produce devastating consequences in the arterial tree, the source of the paradoxic events is often not found in the veins. Approximately 30% of the population has a PFO, and a small proportion of them are at particular risk of paradoxical embolization, such as a large aperture or an associated septal aneurysm. Although the decision to close the PFO, surgically or by endovascular approach, is easy in symptomatic patients, it is more difficult in the more numerous asymptomatic individuals.

Independent risk factors for DVT and PE include surgery, trauma, hospital or nursing home confinement, active malignancy, central vein catheterization (or transvenous pacemaker), prior DVT, PE or superficial thrombophlebitis, varicose veins, and extremity paresis. Among these factors, cancer takes a special place (see Chapter 85). Indeed, all pathogenic factors of VTE described by Trousseau in the 19th century are at play in patients with malignant disease, and thromboembolic complications usually signal a short life expectancy. In addition, treatment may be more complicated, with an increased risk of bleeding and a resistance to oral anticoagulants in some patients. Thromboprophylaxis must be aggressive in patients with cancer, but more data is needed on long-term prevention in patients who receive radiation and chemotherapy and in patients with central vein catheters.

Additional risk factors include pregnancy, puerperium, and use of oral hormone therapy (contraceptives or substitution therapy). In recent years, there has been a dramatic drop in the use of hormone therapy because of the publication of large, randomized, controlled trials that convincingly demonstrated an increased incidence of cardiovascular events, both venous and arterial. Although some advantages of long-term hormone therapy were seen, it was deemed that the overall risks of the therapy outweighed benefits (see Chapter 84).

As underlined by Rosendaal in an authoritative review (3), thrombosis is a multicausal disease with many common biologic risk factors in the general population, such as factor $V_{Leiden}$, prothrombin 20210A, high concentrations of factor VIII, and increased homocysteinemia, which quite frequently occur together in one individual. The acquired risk factors also affect many persons, and so a combination of risk factors in one person is not rare. Indeed, multiple risk factors are a prerequisite for thrombosis to develop. Thrombosis is a disease in which genetic and acquired risk factors interact dynamically. A time-dependent model that incorporates interaction of risk factors is valuable to explain why thrombosis occurs in one person at a specific time (see Fig. 82-1). Theoretically, such a model could help the clinician to provide individual risk estimates and set tailored guidelines for prophylaxis.

## DIAGNOSIS AND RISK STRATIFICATION

During the last 2 decades, the approach to diagnosing DVT and PE has changed in several major ways. Most importantly, that these two conditions are manifestations of a single entity, VTE, has now been integrated in the diagnostic strategies. In addition, novel, noninvasive diagnostic tools such as venous compression ultrasonography (CUS), D-dimer (DD) measurement, and spiral or helical computed tomography (hCT) scan are now available

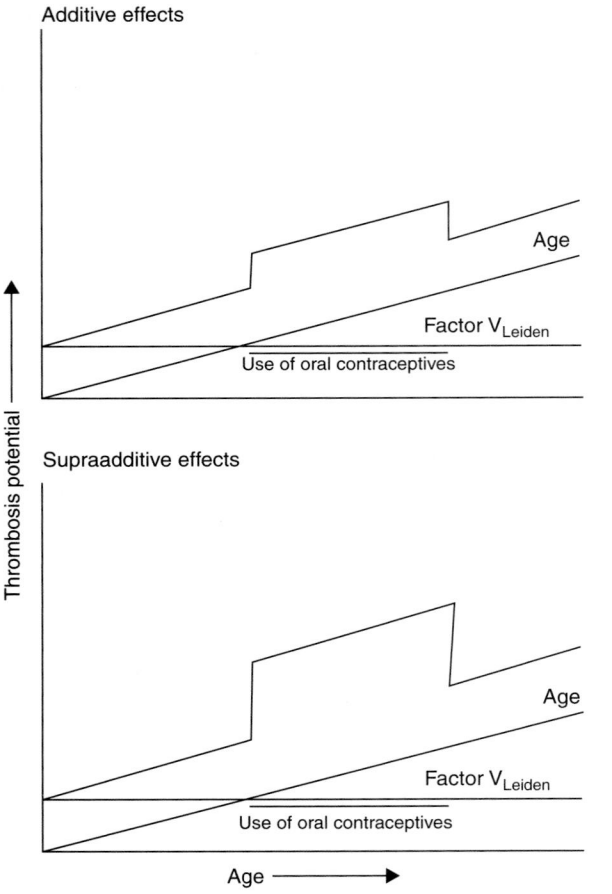

**Figure 82-1.** Models of thrombosis risk with different interactions between factor V$_{Leiden}$ and use of oral contraceptive. **Top:** the thrombosis potentials add to form the resultant potential. **Bottom:** effect of the combination is supraadditive. (Reprinted with permission from Elsevier, and Rosendaal FR. Venous thrombosis: a multicausal disease. *Lancet* 1999;353:1167–1173.)

and have drastically reduced the need for invasive tools such as phlebography and pulmonary angiography (see Chapter 87). Finally, the appropriate approach to the diagnosis of VTE differs depending on the nature of the clinical setting: clinical suspicion of a first episode of DVT or PE, clinical suspicion of a recurrent episode of DVT or PE, and screening of asymptomatic DVT or PE in high-risk patients or in patients participating in clinical trials on prophylaxis or therapy for VTE.

Most validated diagnostic strategies in individuals clinically suspected of DVT or PE include some form of clinical assessment that can be established implicitly or explicitly by means of clinical decision rules or scores. A combination of clear-cut variables and of softer implicit judgment has been shown to be the most optimal tool at this stage (4), but attempts to achieve a fully objective score without resorting to implicit criteria or arterial blood gases are still ongoing. Recently, the Geneva group reported an important and independent association with the diagnosis of PE for eight objective simple clinical variables (points): age more than 65 years (1 point); previous DVT or PE (3 points); surgery or fracture within 1 month (2 points); active malignancy (2 points); unilateral lower limb pain (3 points); hemoptysis (2 points); heart rate 75 to 94 beats per minute (3 points), 95 beats per minute or more (5 points); and pain on lower limb deep vein palpation and unilateral edema (4 points). The predictive accuracy of the score was similar in the derivation set and

in an external validation set. In the latter set, the prevalence of PE was 7.9% in the low probability category (0 to 3 points), 28.5% in the intermediate probability category (4 to 10 points), and 73.7% in the high clinical probability patients (11 points or more) (5).

Because clinically overt VTE encompasses a wide clinical spectrum, from small, distal DVT to large, life-threatening PE, with widely diverging prognosis, and because management may differ depending upon this prognosis, risk stratification belongs now to the diagnostic process, especially for PE (see Chapter 88). It includes clinical variables, cardiac biomarkers, electrocardiography, and chest CT scan. The clinical evaluation was long restricted to the sole appreciation of the hemodynamic instability (i.e., shock or systolic hypotension <100 mm Hg) that defines the massive form of PE. This evaluation has been refined thanks to a clinical prognostic score (6) that was recently validated externally (7). The score contains the following items: cancer, systolic blood pressure less than 100 mm Hg (2 points each), heart failure, previous DVT, partial arterial oxygen pressure less than 8 kDa (or 60 mm Hg), and DVT shown by ultrasonography (1 point each). A score of 2 or less was associated with a good prognosis (5% risk of complication at 3 months); a score above 2 predicted a 27.5% risk of complication. Although echocardiography cannot be used for diagnostic purpose in hemodynamically stable patients, because of lack of sensitivity, it can be used to confirm or exclude right ventricular dysfunction (RVD). This characteristic has been found in several registries and retrospective studies to correlate with mortality in patients with PE. It now defines a subgroup among patients with nonmassive PE, those with RVD. Cardiac troponins might have similar performance and may require less resource than echocardiography (see Chapter 88). Regardless, identifying a subgroup at poorer prognosis is meaningful only if it changes patient management (see subsequent text), which is not established at this stage. On the basis of our present knowledge, a poorer clinical prognostic score does not mandate a prolonged duration of anticoagulant treatment, nor do elevated cardiac biomarkers or RVD necessitate thrombolytic therapy.

# TREATMENT

Major advances have been made in the initial and long-term (also called secondary prevention) treatment of VTE (see Chapter 89). Today, most episodes of DVT and an increasing proportion of episodes of PE can be managed in an outpatient setting. This was made possible by the advent of low-molecular-weight heparin (LMWH) fractions that progressively replaced unfractionated heparin (UFH). The new fractions have definite practical advantages (essentially, once-daily subcutaneous administration compared to cumbersome continuous infusion) and one disadvantage (clearance through the kidney, requiring caution in case of renal insufficiency). A common disadvantage of UFH and LMWH lies in the risk of inducing heparin-induced thrombocytopenia (HIT). Although this complication is 10 times less frequent with LMWH, platelet count must be closely monitored with both substances. A further refinement of LMWH, fondaparinux, the synthetic pentasaccharide and the smallest component of natural heparin able to bind antithrombin and to specifically inhibit activated factor X, has not been associated with HIT and might replace LMWH, at least in some indications in which it exhibited superior benefit-to-risk ratio.

Recently, a new oral anticoagulant with a completely different mechanism of action compared to that of the traditional vitamin K antagonists (VKA), ximelagatran, acts as a synthetic, direct thrombin inhibitor. The substance might theoretically replace both heparins and VKA. Conveniently, it is administered as a fixed dose, without the need for dose adjustment with coagulation tests. Unfortunately, it produces elevated transaminases in approximately 10% of patients, especially when used for prolonged periods of time, such as for treatment (8) or secondary prevention (9) of DVT or prevention of systemic embolism associated with atrial fibrillation. With long-term administration, up to one in 2,000 patients might develop liver failure. There is also an indication that it could cause heart attack, which led the FDA to reject it until more data are available on these aspects. The European regulatory agency, however, has registered its short-term prophylactic use in major orthopedic surgery.

Usually, the current treatment of acute VTE consists of a short course of subcutaneous LMWH overlapped and followed by VKA for a more or less prolonged period of time and with an intensity of anticoagulation corresponding to an international normalized ratio (INR) of 2 to 3, that can be reduced to 1.5 to 2 after 3 to 12 months. However, the latter attitude remains controversial (see subsequent text).

Thrombolytic treatment of DVT has been largely abandoned (10) except in the rare cases of limited proximal (read: iliac) thrombosis, especially if associated with some form of external compression, the Cockett syndrome. The treatment is then often applied locally, and the underlying lesion treated with venous angioplasty and stenting.

In massive PE, which implies hemodynamic compromise, systemic thrombolysis is the treatment of choice although reduction in mortality was never convincingly proven. In rare cases, surgical or endovascular thrombectomy may be preferred (see Chapter 91), depending upon the grade of emergency and local expertise. For approximately 15 years, it has been suggested that patients with nonmassive PE and RVD who exhibit a poorer prognosis (11) might benefit from thrombolysis, a controversial issue (see Chapter 90) that was not really settled by the randomized controlled study by Konstantinides et al. (12).

# PREVENTION

Surgery is a well-established transient risk factor for VTE. Specific preventive measures have been adopted on the basis of evidence for both the efficacy of the measure for the particular intervention and the safety of the measure with respect to the particular patient (see Chapter 94). Studies over the last three decades have convincingly demonstrated the efficacy of pharmacologic prophylaxis and the rarity of induced perioperative bleeding. The surgery at highest risk is without any doubt major orthopedic surgery, which includes hip and knee arthroplasty and hip fracture (see Chapter 95). In all types of surgery, the thromboembolic risk extends beyond hospital stay. Following hip arthroplasty, it has been demonstrated that prolonging the usual prophylactic week to 4 to 5 weeks with LMWH is associated with a substantial decrease of postoperative thromboembolic events. For all these situations, guidelines are regularly updated and are largely followed up by surgeons (13).

In acutely ill patients hospitalized in medical wards, evidence is accumulating (14) (see Chapter 96), but guidelines remain less precise, and field surveys suggest that different institutions behave quite variably in deciding which medical patients should or should not be given prophylaxis (15).

Although LMWH have progressively replaced UFH in almost all prophylactic indications, new compounds are coming into the market, especially fondaparinux in the area of major orthopedic surgery, and several other compounds are undergoing intensive clinical testing. Finally, in the rare patients in whom pharmacologic prophylaxis is contraindicated, usually because of an excessive bleeding risk, mechanical measures can be used, but they are probably less effective than anticoagulant prophylaxis.

# SOME CONTEMPORARY CONTROVERSIES IN THE FIELD

VTE is probably one of the fields in medicine that possesses the most evidence-based corpus of knowledge. Nevertheless, there are still several controversial issues in the area. The following sections briefly discuss (i) treatment and subsequent diagnosis of distal vein thrombosis; (ii) use of hCT scan for diagnosis of PE; (iii) duration and intensity of long-term anticoagulant treatment (so-called secondary prevention) of VTE; and (iv) endpoints in clinical trials on VTE prophylaxis.

## Diagnosis and Treatment of Distal Deep Vein Thrombosis

Symptomatic lower limbs DVT may be *proximal* (from and including the popliteal vein or upwards) or *distal* (below the popliteal veins), an important distinction because the embolic potential of proximal vein thrombosis is definitely higher than that of distal DVT. The need for diagnosing distal DVT strongly depends upon the evidence for treating this condition. Although the Seventh Consensus Conference of the American College of Chest Physicians (ACCP) (16) recommends anticoagulant treatment of symptomatic DVT, both proximal and distal, the evidence supporting this strong recommendation (grade 1A, the strongest recommendation possible) in the latter case is limited to a single clinical study published in the mid-1980s (17): after an initial short course of heparin, 51 patients with calf-vein thrombosis were randomized to receive warfarin ($n = 23$) or no warfarin ($n = 28$). Diagnosis of recurrence was suspected on serial isotope tests and physical examination and, in case of suspicion, confirmed by venography. During the first 3 months, eight patients in the nonwarfarin group experienced recurrence compared with zero in the warfarin group, a statistically significant difference. The study had a small sample size, was not double-blind, and used diagnostic criteria for recurrence that are, at best, doubtful.

In contemporary diagnostic studies of DVT in symptomatic outpatients using CUS limited to the proximal veins, the 3-month thromboembolic risk in patients in whom the test was negative would have been, had the repeat CUS not been performed, approximately 2% in the serial CUS series (18) because of the very low prevalence of proximal DVT at 1 week in patients with an initially negative CUS (this is assuming that all patients in whom a DVT was shown by the repeat CUS would have had a thromboembolic event during the 3-month follow-up if left untreated). For comparison, the 3-month thromboembolic risk in patients with clinically suspected DVT who had a negative venogram was found to be as high as 1.9% [95% confidence interval (CI), 0.4 to 5.4].

Complete examination of the leg deep vein system is associated with a 3-month thromboembolic risk that is approximately 1.5% lower than for the CUS limited to the proximal veins. However, almost half of the DVTs diagnosed in those recent series resorting on complete examination of the lower limb veins were distal; such an approach entails a substantial risk of overdiagnosis and overtreatment that may outweigh the apparent small difference in terms of 3-month thromboembolic risk. In addition, the exam protocols that include a study of the distal veins are quite cumbersome and require more specialized skills.

The observation of a low 3-month thromboembolic risk in patients with a negative CUS of the proximal veins (approximately 1% in management studies) questions the need for diagnosing distal DVT. Indeed, detecting clots in the posterior tibial or peroneal veins or even in calf muscle veins may be double-edged:

On one hand, the potential of reducing the 3-month thromboembolic risk is limited (because it is already quite low), and on the other hand, the risk of false-positive findings and subsequent unnecessary anticoagulant treatment in patients who could be left untreated is quite high.

Interestingly, Gottlieb et al. (19) randomized more than 500 patients clinically suspected of DVT to undergo routine complete US of the calf veins or selective exam in the area of calf symptoms if present. The rate of isolated calf DVT detected was very low and similar in the two groups (1.3% and 1.5%, respectively), and the 3-month thromboembolic risk was less than 1% with no difference between the groups. Again, these findings question the pertinence of the systematic complete calf veins examination, especially in view of a positive predictive value of at best 50% if we assume a specificity of distal CUS of 99% (quite an optimistic assumption) in a population with such a low prevalence of the disease.

As long as convincing hard data on the need for treating isolated distal DVT are not available, CUS should probably be limited to the proximal veins in clinically suspected DVT (18), except perhaps in patients with a high clinical probability in whom a lower rate of false-positive CUS may be anticipated. Strategies with a so-called complete CUS are associated with a high risk of overdiagnosis and hence potentially dangerous overtreatment without obvious clinical benefit. Admittedly, this opinion is not shared by all experts in the field.

## Use of Helical Computed Tomography Scan for Diagnosing Pulmonary Embolism: The Story of a Near Miss

The use of hCT scan for diagnosing PE is a story of a near miss (20). The history of the rapid uptake of hCT scan in the field of PE diagnosis (21,22) is fascinating. In 2000, two systematic reviews (23,24) looking back at 10 years of research on the use of CT scan in suspected PE underlined the vastly different performances recorded by individual studies, with sensitivity of hCT scan ranging from 53% to 100% and specificity from 81% to 100%. The authors attributed those differences to patient selection, nonstandardized image acquisition protocols, and poor methodology. Yet, already at that time, in most European and some US centers, hCT scan had at least complemented and sometimes completely replaced ventilation-perfusion lung scintigraphy in the diagnostic work-up, as recommended by, among others, the British Thoracic Society (25). Meanwhile, two clinical studies had reported a sensitivity of single-detector hCT scan of approximately 70% only (26,27).

How can we explain this apparent paradox? In a series by Dutch investigators (28), the risk of venous thromboembolic events was low during the 3-month follow-up in patients with either a negative single-detector CT scan or a CT scan negative for PE, but showing evidence of an alternative diagnosis explaining the patient's symptoms. In patients with a negative CT scan and no evidence of an alternative diagnosis, the 3-month event rate was one per 248 [0.4%; 95% CI, 0.1 to 1.8]. Those patients also underwent serial lower limb CUS to enhance the detection rate of the overall diagnostic strategy, but only two deep venous thromboses were found in patients with a negative CT scan. Hence, even if serial ultrasound had not been performed, the 3-month thromboembolic risk would still have been only 1.2% (95% CI, 1.2 to 3.0), in keeping with the results of similar outcome studies. Two other recent outcome studies have shown an acceptably low 3-month thromboembolic risk in patients left untreated on the basis of the combination of a negative, mainly single-detector hCT scan and the absence of deep venous thrombosis on lower limb venous CUS in patients with a nonhigh clinical probability of PE (29,30). In those series, it is not possible to derive what that risk might have been if only helical CT scan

had been used, because all patients with a negative helical CT scan and a deep venous thrombosis were treated by anticoagulants. However, in a validation study by the Geneva group, combining venous ultrasonography with hCT scan improved the overall sensitivity to only 80%. Therefore, the only explanation for the satisfactory ability of single-detector helical CT scan to rule out PE in outcome studies, despite its poor sensitivity in validation series that compare its performance to accepted diagnostic standards, is that the small peripheral emboli that are preferentially missed by that type of CT scan are clinically irrelevant.

What lessons can we draw from what has probably been a "near miss" in the validation of a new diagnostic technology for a frequent clinical problem (a "near miss" in the aviation jargon is a catastrophe that did not occur but for which nearly all the ingredients were present)? In the case of CT scan, the ingredients were lack of rigor, attraction to a new and easily available imaging technique, and pressure from constantly evolving technology. Büller et al. (31) proposed the following steps for developing a new diagnostic test: (a) elaboration and standardization of the technical aspects of a new test corresponding to a phase I study in therapeutic investigations; (b) comparison of the new test's characteristics with an accepted diagnostic criterion (the previously *gold standard*) to define its sensitivity and specificity in studies adhering to rigorous methodologic criteria (phase II); and (c) validation of the new test in real-life setting outcome studies in which the test is used for clinical decision making and the outcomes are compared with those of patients managed according to the reference diagnostic test (phase III). The first study by van Strijen et al. is a phase II study, and it is ironic that it is being published more than a year after the corresponding phase III outcome study by the same group, pointing out that its sobering message was possibly somewhat frowned upon by the medical community, always enthusiastic to endorse new technology and especially so when the pictures are beautiful. Moreover, most clinicians prefer using a less extensively validated technology if it is available in their institution rather than transferring a patient to another facility. It is therefore not surprising that the most rapid uptake of hCT scan for suspected PE occurred in countries with limited access to ventilation-perfusion scintigraphy. Finally, how can we rigorously follow the validation steps described earlier when the technology changes as rapidly as it did for hCT scan in the last 15 years? In that short period, we have migrated from single-detector machines with 5-mm reconstructions to 4-detector and 16-detector scanners allowing 1-mm reconstructions with shorter image acquisition time, and more evolutions are yet to come. The tension between enthusiastic discoverers and conservative scientists will always exist, but true progress stems only from the resolution of that tension by high-quality studies, not from its negation; clearly, more rigor is required.

In summary, hCT scan is certainly becoming the cornerstone for investigating patients with suspected PE. But caution is still warranted, and we should remind ourselves that the only diagnostic criterion validated in outcome studies for safely ruling out PE combines a negative hCT scan, the absence of proximal deep venous thrombosis, and a nonhigh clinical probability of PE (32). As a matter of fact, one large-scale multicenter study using multidetector hCT scan (33) strongly suggests that using that type of CT scan as a standalone test is probably acceptable but should still be submitted to a specifically designed outcome study.

## Duration and Intensity of Anticoagulant Long-Term Treatment

The duration of anticoagulant treatment following a venous thromboembolic episode has always been a matter of debate, with recommended durations following a first episode varying between 3 months and 1 year, depending upon the weight given to the respective risks of recurrence and bleeding induced by the treatment. Because VTE is a recurrent disease, anticoagulation should ideally last forever. However, the risk of recurrence diminishes with time, and the risk of bleeding, after an initial peak, is rather constant over time. Therefore, there must be some time-point for which the bleeding risk exceeds the protective effect of the treatment, which should then be stopped. This risk-benefit analysis should be performed for each individual, and Dutch authors have provided us with a mathematical model that balances these two opposite risks and should allow a more tailored treatment duration (34). In most cases, the duration will be 3 to 12 months.

However, even if reduced, the risk of recurrence persists beyond that limit, and some clinicians were prescribing oral anticoagulant treatment for longer (indefinite) periods of time, but at a reduced intensity, with a view toward achieving some antithrombotic effect (even if diminished) and a reduced bleeding risk. Recently, Ridker et al. were able to demonstrate the validity of this empirical practice. In the Prevention of Recurrent Venous Thromboembolism (PREVENT) study (35), 508 patients have been followed-up for up to 4.3 years (mean, 2.1). Of 253 patients randomly assigned to placebo, 37 experienced recurrent VTE (7.2 per 100 person-years), as compared with 14 of 255 patients assigned to low-intensity warfarin (targeted INR 1.5 to 2.0) (2.6 per 100 person-years), a risk reduction of 64% (hazard ratio, 0.36 [95% CI, 0.19 to 0.67]; $P$ <0.001). Major hemorrhage occurred in two patients assigned to placebo and five assigned to low-intensity warfarin ($P$ = 0.25). Eight patients in the placebo group and four in the group assigned to low-intensity warfarin died ($P$ = 0.26). Low-intensity warfarin was thereby associated with a 48% reduction in the composite endpoint of recurrent VTE, major hemorrhage, or death.

Shortly after the PREVENT study, the Extended Low-intensity Anticoagulation for Thromboembolism Investigators (ELATE) study (36) reported on a total of 738 individuals with VTE who had completed at least 3 months of conventional-intensity warfarin before randomization. During follow-up, the mean INR in the low-intensity group (targeted INR 1.5 to 1.9) was 1.8, and the mean INR in the conventional-intensity group (targeted INR 2 to 3) was 2.4. The mean duration of anticoagulant treatment in the ELATE trial was 2.1 years, almost identical to that in the PREVENT trial.

As could have been anticipated, there were fewer recurrent VTE events in the conventional-intensity warfarin group (0.7 events per 100 person-years) compared with the low-intensity warfarin group (1.9 events per 100 person-years), a statistically

significant difference ($P$ = 0.03) such that the hazard ratio for recurrent events in association with low-intensity warfarin was 2.8 (95% CI, 1.1, 7.0). There were 16 deaths in the low-intensity group and eight deaths in the conventional-intensity group (hazard ratio, 2.1; 95% CI, 0.9, 4.8). Therefore, in terms of the endpoint of recurrent events prevented, the conventional-intensity warfarin regimen tested in ELATE provided additive benefit compared with the low-intensity warfarin regimen used in PREVENT. The magnitude of this benefit is represented in Figure 82-2, which directly compares the PREVENT and ELATE outcome data for rates of recurrent VTE (37).

However, both PREVENT and ELATE were underpowered to test formally for any true differences in hemorrhagic complication rates between the two study arms. Fully unexpectedly, bleeding rates were nonsignificantly higher in the low-intensity warfarin group within ELATE than in the conventional-intensity warfarin group, so the hazard ratio for any bleeding episode was 1.3 (95% CI, 0.8, 2.1) and the hazard ratio for major bleeds was 1.2 (95% CI, 0.4, 3.0). Although neither of these differences was statistically significant, the data did not conform to the ELATE investigators' *a priori* assumptions that there would be increased hemorrhage among those allocated to higher levels of anticoagulation. Therefore, as stated by Ridker in an in-depth commentary (37), "If one chooses to interpret the ELATE data in isolation from all other knowledge regarding warfarin therapy, full-intensity warfarin might well be misconstrued as being safer than low-intensity warfarin and therefore appear to have a superior overall benefit-to-risk ratio." However, as shown in Figure 82-3, the annual hemorrhage rates for the conventional-intensity warfarin group within the ELATE trial are substantially lower than rates observed in all prior trials. Moreover, these bleeding rates for conventional-intensity warfarin are substantially lower than all published registries in outpatient settings where less careful monitoring and a broader range of patients are being treated. A balanced interpretation of ELATE, therefore, is that long-term conventional-intensity warfarin may provide further benefit over low-intensity warfarin in preventing recurrent events, but that the magnitude of this added effect is modest for most patients and must be carefully considered within the context of known bleeding rates for conventional-intensity warfarin observed in usual practice settings.

In practice, after an initial course of 3 to 12 months of conventional-intensity warfarin, depending upon the individual situation, the option of prolonging the treatment with low-intensity warfarin may be useful at least in select patients at higher risk of bleeding. However, this suggestion is contrary to the Seventh ACCP Consensus guidelines that recommend

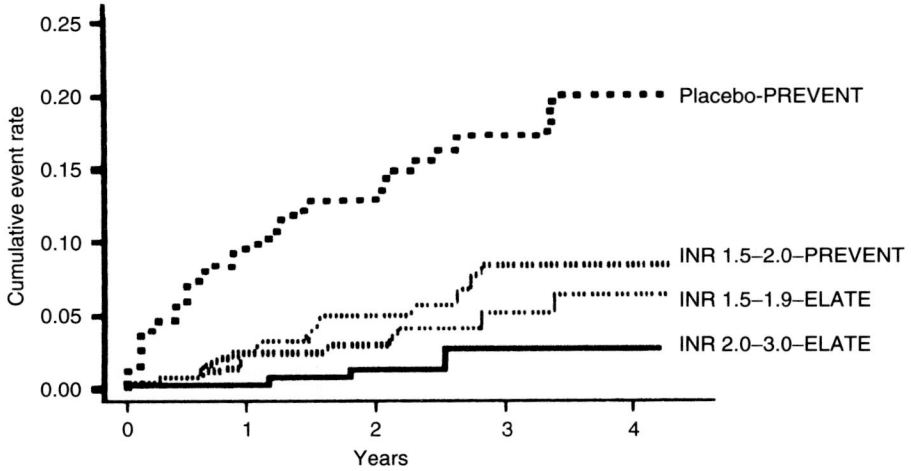

**FIGURE 82-2.** Cumulative rate of thromboembolic recurrence in the Prevention of Recurrent Venous Thromboembolism (PREVENT) and Extended Low-intensity Anticoagulation for Thromboembolism Investigators (ELATE) studies. INR, international normalized ratio. (Reproduced from Ridker PM. Long-term low-dose warfarin use is effective in the prevention of recurrent venous thromboembolism: yes. *J Thromb Haemost* 2004;2:1034–1037, with permission.)

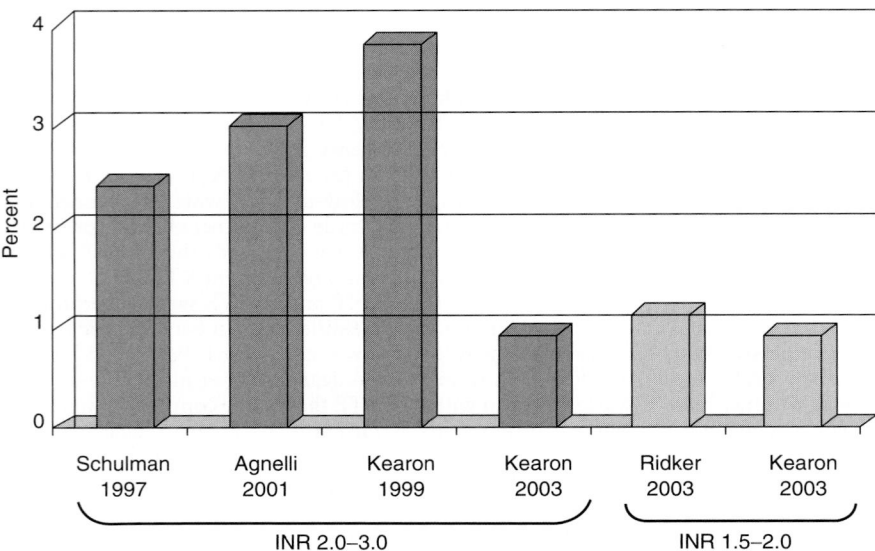

FIGURE 82-3. Annual rate of major bleeding in recent large trials on warfarin treatment of venous thromboembolism. INR, international normalized ratio. (Reproduced from Ridker PM. Long-term low-dose warfarin use is effective in the prevention of recurrent venous thromboembolism: yes. *J Thromb Haemost* 2004;2:1034–1037, with permission.)

against low-intensity warfarin with a highly debatable 1A statement grading (16).

## Endpoints in Clinical Trials on Venous Thromboembolism

Ideally, the endpoint of thromboprophylactic trials should be quite frequent, reliably measurable, and clinically relevant. Because the ultimate aim of thrombosis prevention is to avoid death, mortality is a potential candidate. Fortunately, however, it is rare in this setting, which would result in the need for studying very large patient populations. Furthermore, overall postoperative mortality is influenced by factors not related to VTE. This "background noise" reduces the specificity of the study intervention and amplifies the sample size required to demonstrate its efficacy. An alternative to the endpoint "death" would be "death due to VTE," but this endpoint has a limited diagnostic accuracy because PE is not always diagnosed before death and because autopsy rates are steadily decreasing in most countries. On the other hand, studies targeting clinically overt events carry the disadvantages of low sensitivity and specificity of clinical signs of VTE and the need for large numbers of patients due to the lower number of events. For all these reasons, the endpoint "postoperative phlebographic DVT" has been used. It is, however, almost invariably asymptomatic, which led to questioning its clinical relevance. Moreover, using a surrogate such as phlebography may only be valid if we assume first that fatal PE can occur only as a consequence of a lower limb "phlebographic" DVT, and second, that the prevention's entire effect on the undisputed true clinical outcome of fatal PE is mediated through its effect on the surrogate (38). Although these two assumptions are likely to be true, definitive proof is lacking.

The risk of postoperative VTE following major surgery extends beyond hospital stay, but prevention is usually stopped after 7 to 10 days or, at the latest, at the time of hospital discharge. Therefore, the proportion of after-discharge PE was found to be at least 25% in a large survey on more than 19,000 patients who underwent general surgery (39). The hypothesis of the efficacy of prolonging pharmacologic prophylaxis with LMWH for up to 5 weeks following surgery has been tested in five studies of patients undergoing total hip replacement (THR) using phlebography as endpoint (40–44). All these studies convincingly demonstrated a statistically significant, more than 40% reduction (from 29.0% to 17.5%) of total *phlebographic* DVT in the group of patients given LMWH beyond hospital discharge compared to those given placebo, and in the largest one, statistical significance was also reached for the reduction of proximal DVT (7). A metaanalysis has recently extended these findings by demonstrating that the overall risk reduction for the *symptomatic* events in these five trials and in one additional study that used a clinical endpoint with confirmatory phlebography was 50% (from 3.3% with extended thromboprophylaxis to 1.6% with placebo) (45). These findings clearly suggest a continuum from asymptomatic DVT to fatal PE through symptomatic DVT, asymptomatic PE, and symptomatic PE (46). By contrast, four large cohort studies and one randomized study of patients who underwent THR and were followed-up for 4 to 5 weeks after discharge, and in whom prophylaxis had been stopped at discharge, suggest that the risk of clinically overt VTE during follow-up is low (<2% symptomatic events in more 3,700 patients) in such patients provided LMWH or warfarin was administered during the 9 to 15 days of hospital stay (47–49). In the latter studies, objective diagnostic confirmation was obtained only in patients with clinical symptoms or signs of DVT or PE, a policy that raises the issues of what is symptomatic and what is clinically relevant.

Pain, swelling, and cyanosis are cardinal symptoms of DVT; their sensitivity and specificity averages 50%. Furthermore, as far as patients who underwent THR in the previous weeks are concerned, the specificity of these clinical signs and symptoms might be further reduced because at least some form of pain or swelling is likely to be present in most of these patients. Dyspnea, chest pain, and death are typical symptoms of PE. Although death is clinically relevant and poses no diagnostic problem, dyspnea and chest pain are highly nonspecific and quite frequent symptoms in elderly patients, especially in the postoperative period. These soft definitions of signs and symptoms of VTE raise the question of arbitrary screening, preferentially in more plaintive patients or by more anxious doctors, the so-called referral or diagnostic bias. This reduced accuracy and validity of clinically overt events as study endpoints primarily affect the generalizability or external validity of the study results. On the other hand, the internal validity of the comparison of different interventions would not be affected as long as the study design is methodologically sound.

Fortunately, death is too rare an event following surgery, even following THR, to be a useful endpoint in efficacy trials. On the other hand, is a painful calf-vein thrombosis more clinically relevant than an asymptomatic iliac-vein obstruction? Or, is a small peripheral PE with pleuritic chest pain more relevant and dangerous than a painless central embolus? Here, we have to go back to the goal of thromboprophylaxis, which is primarily to prevent fatal PE without inducing too many side effects, and secondarily, to prevent late PTS and also chronic thromboembolic pulmonary hypertension. In this respect, everybody will agree that both fatal PE and severe PTS are very unlikely to occur in the absence of (venographic) DVT (see Fig. 82-4), as evidenced from the event-free follow-up of patients undergoing THR who had no venographically verified DVT at discharge (50).

Because eradication of postoperative, asymptomatic, venographic DVT would ultimately prevent PE, and especially fatal PE, the clinical relevance of this endpoint is obvious. At least, this surrogate endpoint could be used in a first approach while testing the efficacy of a new prophylactic modality. If the tested intervention does not reduce the incidence of postoperative venographic DVT, it is unlikely to prevent fatal PE. Provided this endpoint is well defined, including a minimal size (thereby excluding, for example, very small thrombi in calf muscle veins), is reproducible, and adjudicated centrally by experienced experts, it may be of great value in phase II thromboprophylactic trials.

In summary, *symptomatic* does not necessarily mean *clinically relevant*: A clinical endpoint may be without clinical relevance, whereas an asymptomatic endpoint may be clinically highly relevant. In thromboprophylactic trials, venographic DVT—a surrogate—correlates with clinically relevant symptomatic events and can be assessed more reliably. Ultrasonography can be used as an alternative to venography for proximal DVT. Finally, hemorrhage should not be forgotten as an essential part of the net effect of thrombosis prophylaxis. A drug reducing venographic DVT at the cost of increasing clinically major bleeding has no future in our armamentarium.

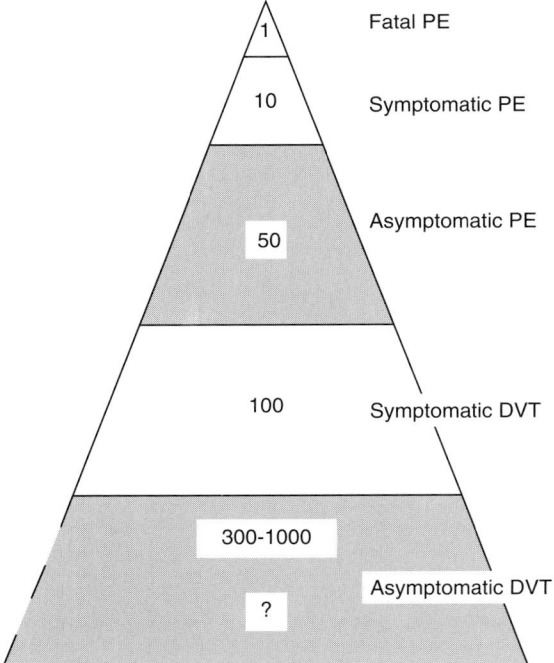

**FIGURE 82-4.** Tentative representation of the spectrum of postoperative venous thromboembolism from asymptomatic "phlebographic" deep vein thrombosis (DVT) to fatal pulmonary embolism (PE).

# CONCLUSION

Venous thromboembolic disorders encompass a wide spectrum of conditions with various severity and prognostic implications. Technical improvements and development of validated algorithms have rendered diagnostic work-ups easier, almost totally noninvasive, and safer, mainly thanks to plasma DD measurement (to rule out the disease in selected patients with suspected VTE), CUS for suspected DVT, and multislice helical CT scan for suspected PE. In spite of these advances, the field faces several challenges for the future. One challenge is establishing which conditions need to be treated with anticoagulant drugs, a question that pertains essentially to distal or muscle vein thrombosis and isolated subsegmental PE. Its answer will have consequences for diagnostic algorithms. Another challenge must address the need for a refined prognostic stratification of PE patients and its potential therapeutic implications. Finally, several new, orally active anticoagulant compounds, such as direct antithrombin or antifactor Xa agents, are presently being tested in clinical studies. Should their promises be fulfilled, our antithrombotic armamentarium could be profoundly modified in the near future. However, the way is long from the clinical trials, diagnostic or therapeutic, to the patient management, and repeat efforts of continuous medical education will be necessary to translate valid study results into true clinical progresses for most patients with suspected or confirmed VTE.

## References

1. Joffe HV, Kucher N, Tapson VF, et al. Deep Vein Thrombosis (DVT) FREE Steering Committee. Upper-extremity deep vein thrombosis: a prospective registry of 592 patients. *Circulation* 2004;110:1605–1611.
2. Kyrle PA, Minar E, Bialonczyk C, et al. The risk of recurrent venous thromboembolism in men and women. *N Engl J Med* 2004;350:2558–2563.
3. Rosendaal FR. Venous thrombosis: a multicausal disease. *Lancet* 1999;353:1167–1173.
4. Chagnon I, Bounameaux H, Aujesky D, et al. Prediction of pulmonary embolism in emergency patients: The revised Geneva score. Ann Intern Med 2005 (in press).
5. Le Gal G, Righini M, Roy PM, et al. Prediction of pulmonary embolism in emergency patients: The revised Geneva score. *Ann Intern* Med 2005 (in press).
6. Wicki J, Perrier A, Perneger TV, et al. Predicting adverse outcome in patients with acute pulmonary embolism: a risk score. *Thromb Haemost* 2000;84:548–552.
7. Nendaz MR, Bandelier P, Aujesky D, et al. Validation of a risk score identifying patients with acute pulmonary embolism who are at low risk of clinical adverse outcome. *Thromb Haemost* 2004;91:1232–1236.
8. Fiessinger JN, Huisman MV, Davidson BL, et al. Ginsberg JS for the THRIVE Treatment Study Investigators. Ximelagatran versus low-molecular-weight heparin and warfarin for the treatment of deep-vein thrombosis. A randomized controlled trial. *JAMA* 2005;293:681–689.
9. Schulman S, Wahlander K, Lundstrom T, et al. THRIVE III Investigators. Secondary prevention of venous thromboembolism with the oral direct thrombin inhibitor ximelagatran. *N Engl J Med* 2003;349:1713–1721.
10. Wells PS, Forster AJ. Thrombolysis in deep vein thrombosis: is there still an indication? *Thromb Haemost* 2001;86:499–508.
11. Schoepf UJ, Kucher N, Kipfmueller F, et al. Right ventricular enlargement on chest computed tomography: a predictor of early death in acute pulmonary embolism. *Circulation* 2004;110:3276–3280.
12. Konstantinides S, Geibel A, Heusel G, et al. Management strategies and prognosis of pulmonary embolism-3 trial investigators. Heparin plus alteplase compared with heparin alone in patients with submassive pulmonary embolism. *N Engl J Med* 2002;347:1143–1150.
13. Geerts WH, Pine GF, Heit JA, et al. Prevention of venous thromboembolism. The seventh ACCP conference on antithrombotic and thrombolytic therapy. *Chest* 2004;126:338S–400S.
14. Goldhaber SZ, Turpie AGG. Prevention of venous thromboembolism among hospitalized patients. *Circulation* 2005;111:e1–e3.
15. Chopard P, Dörffler-Melly J, Hess U, et al. Venous thromboembolism prophylaxis in acutely ill medical patients: definite need for improvement. *J Intern Med* 2005;257:352–357.
16. Büller HR, Agnelli G, Hull RD, et al. Antithrombotic therapy for venous thromboembolic disease: the seventh ACCP conference on antithrombotic and thrombolytic therapy. *Chest* 2004;126:401S–428S.

17. Lagerstedt CI, Fagher BO, Olsson CG, et al. Need for long-term anticoagulant treatment in symptomatic calf-vein thrombosis. *Lancet* 1985;326:515–518.
18. Bounameaux H, Righini M, Perrier A. Diagnosing deep vein thrombosis: the case for compression ultrasonography limited to the proximal veins. *J Thromb Haemost* 2004;2:2260–2261.
19. Gottlieb RH, Voci SL, Syed L, et al. Randomized prospective study comparing routine versus selective use of sonography of the complete calf in patients with suspected deep venous thrombosis. *AJR Am J Roentgenol* 2003;180:241–245.
20. Perrier A, Bounameaux H. Validation of helical computed tomography for suspected pulmonary embolism: a near-miss? *J Thromb Haemost* 2004;3:14–16.
21. Wittram C, Meehan MJ, Halpern EF, et al. Trends in thoracic radiology over a decade at a large academic medical center. *J Thorac Imaging* 2004;19:164–170.
22. Stein PD, Kayali F, Olson RE. Trends in the use of diagnostic imaging in patients hospitalized with acute pulmonary embolism. *Am J Cardiol* 2004;93:1316–1317.
23. Mullins MD, Becker DM, Hagspiel KD, et al. The role of spiral volumetric computed tomography in the diagnosis of pulmonary embolism. *Arch Intern Med* 2000;160:293–298.
24. Rathbun SW, Raskob GE, Whitsett TL. Sensitivity and specificity of helical computed tomography in the diagnosis of pulmonary embolism: a systematic review. *Ann Intern Med* 2000;132:227–232.
25. British Thoracic Society Standards of Care Committee Pulmonary Embolism Guideline Development Group. British Thoracic Society guidelines for the management of suspected acute pulmonary embolism. *Thorax* 2003; 58:470–483.
26. Perrier A, Howarth N, Didier D, et al. Performances of helical computed tomography in unselected outpatients with suspected pulmonary embolism. *Ann Intern Med* 2001;135:88–97.
27. van Strijen MJL, de Monye W, Kieft GJ, et al. Accuracy of single detector spiral CT in the diagnosis of pulmonary embolism: a prospective multicenter cohort study of consecutive patients with abnormal perfusion scintigraphy. *J Thromb Haemost* 2004;3:17–25.
28. Van Strijen MJ, De Monye W, Schiereck J, et al. Single-detector helical computed tomography as the primary diagnostic test in suspected pulmonary embolism: a multicenter clinical management study of 510 patients. *Ann Intern Med* 2003;138:307–314.
29. Perrier A, Roy PM, Aujesky D, et al. Diagnosing pulmonary embolism in outpatients with clinical assessment, D-dimer measurement, venous ultrasound, and helical computed tomography: a multicenter management study. *Am J Med* 2004;116:291–299.
30. Musset D, Parent F, Meyer G, et al. Diagnostic strategy for patients with suspected pulmonary embolism: a prospective multicentre outcome study. *Lancet* 2002;360:1914–1920.
31. Buller HR, Lensing AW, Hirsh J, et al. Deep vein thrombosis: new noninvasive diagnostic tests. *Thromb Haemost* 1991;66:133–137.
32. Kamphuisen PW, Agnelli G. Spiral computed tomography is the first-line chest imaging test for acute pulmonary embolism: no. *J Thromb Haemost* 2005;3:11–13.
33. Perrier A, Roy PM, Sanchez O, et al. Performance of multi-detector row computed tomography in outpatients with suspected pulmonary embolism. *N Engl J Med* 2005 ;352:1760–1768.
34. Vink R, Kraaijenhagen RA, Levi M, et al. Individualized duration of oral anticoagulant therapy for deep vein thrombosis based on a decision model. *J Thromb Haemost* 2003;1:2523–2530.
35. Ridker PM, Goldhaber SZ, Danielson E, et al. Long-term, low-intensity warfarin for the prevention of recurrent venous thromboembolism: a randomized. Double-blind, placebo-controlled trial. *N Engl J Med* 2003; 348:1425–1434.
36. Kearon C, Ginsberg JS, Kovacs MJ, et al. Extended Low-Intensity Anticoagulation for Thrombo-Embolism Investigators. Comparison of low-intensity warfarin therapy with conventional-intensity warfarin therapy for long-term prevention of recurrent venous thromboembolism. *N Engl J Med* 2003; 349:631–639. "http://www.blackwell-synergy.com/na102/home/ACS/upublisher/synergy/journals/entities/2013.gif" \* .
37. Ridker PM. Long-term low-dose warfarin use is effective in the prevention of recurrent venous thromboembolism: yes. *J Thromb Haemost* 2004; 2:1034–1037.
38. Fleming TR, DeMets DL. Surrogate end points in clinical trials: are we being misled? *Ann Intern Med* 1996;125:605–613.
39. Huber O, Bounameaux H, Borst F, et al. Postoperative pulmonary embolism after hospital discharge: an underestimated risk. *Arch Surg* 1992;127:310–313.
40. Planes A, Vochelle N, Darmon JY, et al. Risk of deep-vein thrombosis after hospital discharge in patients having undergone total hip replacement: double-blind randomised comparison of enoxaparin versus placebo. *Lancet* 1996;348:224–228.
41. Bergqvist D, Benoni G, Bjorgell O, et al. Low-molecular-weight heparin (enoxaparin) as prophylaxis against thromboembolism after total hip replacement. *N Engl J Med* 1996;335:696–700.
42. Dahl OE, Andreassen G, Aspelin T, et al. Prolonged thromboprophylaxis following hip replacement surgery – results of a double-blind, prospective, randomised, placebo-controlled study with dalteparin (Fragmin). *Thromb Haemost* 1997;77:26–31.
43. Lassen MR, Borris LC, Anderson BS, et al. Efficacy and safety of prolonged thromboprophylaxis with a low molecular weight heparin (dalteparin) after total hip arthroplasty - The Danish Proplonged Prophylaxis (DaPP) Study. *Thromb Res* 1998;89:281–287.
44. Hull RD, Pineo GF, Francis C, et al. Low-molecular-weight heparin prophylaxis using dalteparin extended out-of-hospital vs. In-hospital warfarin/out-of hospital placebo in hip arthroplasty patients: a double-blind.,randomized comparison. North-American Fragmin Trial Investigators. *Arch Intern Med* 2000;160:2208–2215.
45. Cohen AT, Bailey CS, Alikhan R, et al. Extended thromboprophylaxis with low molecular weight heparin reduces symptomatic venous thromboembolism following lower limb arthroplasty. *Thromb Haemost* 2001;85:940–941.
46. Bounameaux H. Integrating pharmacologic and mechanical prophylaxis. *Thromb Haemost* 1999;82:931–937.
47. Robinson KS, Anderson DR, Gross M, et al. Ultrasonographic screening before hospital discharge for deep venous thrombosis after arthroplasty: the post-arthroplasty screening study. A randomized controlled trial. *Ann Intern Med* 1997;127:439–445.
48. Leclerc JR, Gent M, Hirsh J, et al. The incidence of symptomatic venous thromboembolism during and after prophylaxis with enoxaparin: a multi-institutional cohort study of patients who underwent hip or knee arthroplasty. *Arch Intern Med* 1998;158:873–878.
49. Heit JA, Elliott CG, Trowbridge AA, et al. Ardeparin sodium for extended out-of hospital prophylaxis against venous thromboembolism after total hip or knee replacement. *Ann Intern Med* 2000;132:853–861.
50. Ricotta S, Iorio A, Parise P, et al. post discharge clinically overt venous thromboembolism in orthopaedic surgery patients with negative venography - an overview analysis. *Thromb Haemost* 1996;76:887–892.

# CHAPTER 83 ■ EPIDEMIOLOGY OF VENOUS THROMBOEMBOLISM

JOHN A. HEIT

Thrombosis can affect virtually any venous circulation. This chapter focuses on the epidemiology of common deep vein thrombosis (DVT) of the leg, arm, or pelvis, and its complication (i.e., pulmonary embolism). Venous thromboembolism is now recognized as a complex (multifactorial) disease involving both environmental exposures (e.g., clinical risk factors) and genetic and environmental interactions. Most epidemiologic studies to date have addressed populations of primarily European origin, and the data discussed in this chapter mainly relate to these populations. Where available, data from populations originating from other continents are presented. This chapter also focuses on population-based studies of venous thromboembolism incidence, survival, recurrence, complications, and risk factors. Keeping the caveat about racial composition in mind, it is data from these populations that will be most generalizable to the individual patients of the reader.

## INCIDENCE OF DEEP VEIN THROMBOSIS AND PULMONARY EMBOLISM

The average annual incidence rate of venous thromboembolism (age- and sex-adjusted to the population of whites in the United States in 2000) is 121.5 per 100,000 person-years (1). The incidence is similar or higher among African Americans and is lower among Asian Americans and Native Americans (2–4), underscoring the role of heritability in the etiology of venous thromboembolism. Using the age- and sex-specific incidence rates for the 5-year period, 1991 to 1995, projected to the population of whites in the United States in 2000, at least 260,000 new cases of venous thromboembolism occur annually among whites in the United States. If incidence rates among African Americans are similar, then 27,000 additional incident cases occur annually among African Americans.

Venous thromboembolism is predominantly a disease of older age (1,5). In the absence of a central venous catheter (6) or thrombophilia (7), venous thromboembolism is rare before late adolescence (1,8). The age- and sex-adjusted venous thromboembolism incidence rate for individuals of 15 years or older is 149 per 100,000 population (1). Incidence rates increase markedly with age for both men and women (see Fig. 83-1) and for both DVT and pulmonary embolism (see Fig. 83-2). The overall age-adjusted incidence rate is higher for men (i.e., 130 per 100,000) than for women (i.e., 110 per 100,000; male:female sex ratio is 1.2:1). Incidence rates are higher in women during the childbearing years, whereas incidence rates after the age of 45 years are generally higher in

men. Pulmonary embolism accounts for an increasing proportion of venous thromboembolism with increasing age for both genders.

## SURVIVAL AFTER DEEP VEIN THROMBOSIS AND PULMONARY EMBOLISM

Overall, survival after venous thromboembolism is worse than expected, and survival after pulmonary embolism is much worse than after DVT alone (see Table 83-1) (9–11). The risk of early death among patients with pulmonary embolism is 18-fold higher compared to patients with DVT alone (9). Pulmonary embolism is an independent predictor of reduced survival for up to 3 months after onset. For approximately one fourth of patients with pulmonary embolism, the initial clinical presentation is sudden death. Independent predictors of reduced early survival after venous thromboembolism include increasing age, male gender, lower body mass index, confinement to a hospital or a nursing home at the onset of venous thromboembolism, congestive heart failure, chronic lung disease, serious neurologic disease, and active malignancy (9,10). Additional clinical predictors of poor early survival after pulmonary embolism include syncope and arterial hypotension (12). Evidence of right ventricular failure based on clinical examination, plasma markers (e.g., cardiac troponin T and brain natriuretic peptide) (13,14), or echocardiography (10,15,16) predicts poor survival among patients with normotensive pulmonary embolism. Aggressive anticoagulation therapy, and possibly thrombolytic therapy in select cases, should be given to patients with pulmonary embolism having these characteristics (17,18). Survival over time may be improving for those patients with pulmonary embolism living sufficiently long to be diagnosed and treated (9,19,20).

## VENOUS THROMBOEMBOLISM RECURRENCE

Venous thromboembolism recurs frequently; approximately 30% of patients develop recurrence over a period of 10 years (21). The hazard of recurrence varies with the time since the incident event and is highest within the first 6 to 12 months but never falls to zero (see Table 83-2 and Fig. 83-3). Whereas active therapeutic anticoagulation is effective in preventing recurrence (22–24), the duration of anticoagulation does not affect the risk of recurrence after it is stopped (22–28). These data suggest that venous thromboembolism is a chronic disease with episodic recurrence (21,29–31). Independent predictors of recurrence include increasing patient age and body mass index, neurologic disease with extremity paresis, and active

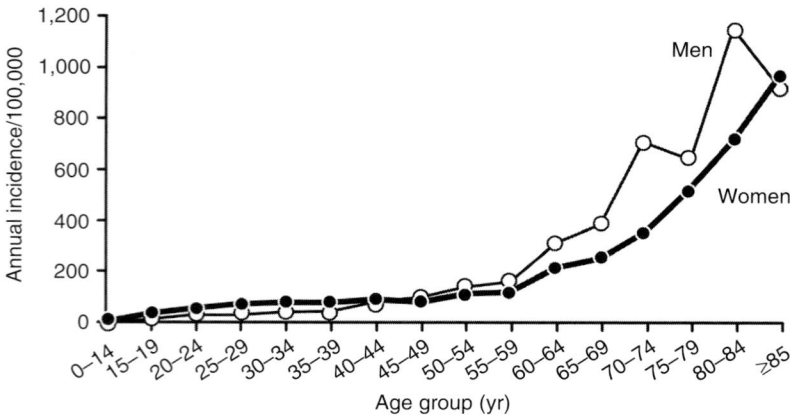

**FIGURE 83-1.** Annual incidence of venous thromboembolism by age and gender. (From Silverstein MD, Heit JA, Mohr DN, et al. Trends in the incidence of deep vein thrombosis and pulmonary embolism: a 25-year population-based study. *Arch Intern Med* 1998; 158:585–593, with permission.)

malignancy (see Table 83-3) (21,29,30,32). Additional predictors include "idiopathic" venous thromboembolism (24–26,33), a lupus anticoagulant or antiphospholipid antibody (23,34), antithrombin, protein C or protein S deficiency (35), and, possibly, persistent residual DVT (36). Prolonged secondary prophylaxis with anticoagulation therapy should be considered for patients with these characteristics.

It is of equal importance that several baseline characteristics either predict a reduced risk of recurrence or are not predictive of recurrence (21,25,29,32,33). For women, pregnancy or the postpartum state, oral contraceptive use, and gynecologic surgery are associated with a reduced risk of recurrence (21). Recent surgery, trauma, or fracture either have no effect (21) or predict a reduced risk of recurrence (32). Additional characteristics having no significant effect on the recurrence risk include recent immobilization, hormone or tamoxifen therapy, and failed prophylaxis (21). For the patients with any of these characteristics, and for patients with isolated calf vein thrombosis, a shorter duration of oral anticoagulation therapy is likely to be adequate (25,26). Although the incident event type (deep vein thrombosis alone vs. pulmonary embolism) is not a predictor of recurrence, patients with recurrence are significantly more likely to recur with the same event type as the incident event type (37,38). Because the 7-day case fatality rate is significantly higher for recurrent pulmonary embolism (34%) compared to recurrent DVT alone (4%) (38), prolonged anticoagulation should be considered for incident pulmonary embolism, especially for patients with chronically reduced cardiopulmonary functional reserve.

# COMPLICATIONS OF VENOUS THROMBOEMBOLISM: VENOUS STASIS SYNDROME AND VENOUS ULCER

The major complications of venous thromboembolism are venous stasis syndrome (i.e., dependent leg swelling and pain, and stasis dermatitis) and venous ulcer. The 20-year cumulative incidence of venous stasis syndrome after venous thromboembolism and after proximal DVT are approximately 25% and 40%, respectively (32,39,40). Risk factors for venous stasis syndrome include the venous thromboembolism event type (DVT) and location (proximal DVT). The 20-year cumulative incidence of venous ulcer is 3.7% (39). The risk for venous ulcer is increased 30% per decade of age at the incident venous thromboembolism (39). Venous thromboembolism accounts for approximately 11% of all venous stasis syndrome occurring in the community (41). Given the pain, impairment, and high costs associated with these complications (42,43), prevention of venous stasis syndrome is of paramount importance. However, the efficacy of graduated compression stockings for prevention or therapy of venous stasis syndrome is uncertain (44,45).

## TABLE 83-1

### SURVIVAL (%) AFTER DEEP VEIN THROMBOSIS VERSUS PULMONARY EMBOLISM

| Time | Deep vein thrombosis alone | Pulmonary embolism |
|---|---|---|
| 0 d | 97.0 | 76.5 |
| 7 d | 96.2 | 71.1 |
| 14 d | 95.7 | 68.7 |
| 30 d | 94.5 | 66.8 |
| 90 d | 91.9 | 62.8 |
| 1 yr | 85.4 | 57.4 |
| 2 yr | 81.4 | 53.6 |
| 5 yr | 72.6 | 47.4 |
| 8 yr | 65.2 | 41.5 |

From Heit JA, Silverstein MD, Mohr DN, et al. Predictors of survival after deep vein thrombosis and pulmonary embolism: a population-based cohort study. *Arch Intern Med* 1999;159: 445–453, with permission.

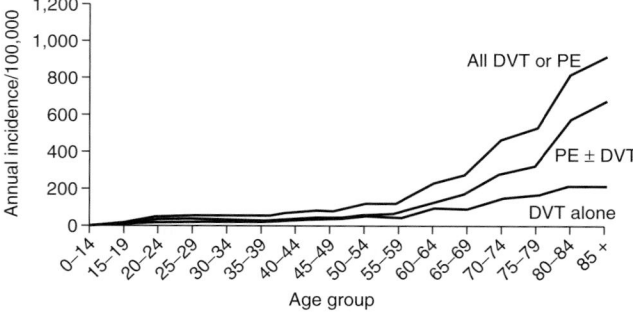

**FIGURE 83-2.** Annual incidence of all venous thromboembolism, deep vein thrombosis (DVT) alone, and pulmonary embolism (PE) with or without deep vein thrombosis (PE ± DVT) by age. (From Silverstein MD, Heit JA, Mohr DN, et al. Trends in the incidence of deep vein thrombosis and pulmonary embolism: a 25-year population-based study. *Arch Intern Med* 1998;158:585–593, with permission.)

## TABLE 83-2

### CUMULATIVE INCIDENCE AND HAZARD OF VENOUS THROMBOEMBOLISM RECURRENCE

| Time to recurrence | Venous thromboembolism recurrence | |
|---|---|---|
| | Cumulative recurrence (%) | Hazard of recurrence [per 1,000 person-days (±SD)] |
| 0 d | 0.0 | 0 |
| 7 d | 1.6 | 170 (30) |
| 30 d | 5.2 | 130 (20) |
| 90 d | 8.3 | 30 (5) |
| 180 d | 10.1 | 20 (4) |
| 1 yr | 12.9 | 20 (2) |
| 2 yr | 16.6 | 10 (1) |
| 5 yr | 22.8 | 6 (1) |
| 10 yr | 30.4 | 5 (1) |

SD, standard deviation.
From Heit JA, Mohr DN, Silverstein MD, et al. Predictors of recurrence after deep vein thrombosis and pulmonary embolism: a population-based cohort study. *Arch Intern Med* 2000;160:761–768, with permission.

## TABLE 83-3

### INDEPENDENT PREDICTORS OF VENOUS THROMBOEMBOLISM RECURRENCE

| Characteristics | Hazard ratio | 95% CI |
|---|---|---|
| Age[a] | 1.17 | 1.11–1.24 |
| Body mass index[b] | 1.24 | 1.04–1.47 |
| Neurologic disease with extremity paresis | 1.87 | 1.28–2.73 |
| Active malignancy | | |
| Malignancy with chemotherapy | 4.24 | 2.58–6.95 |
| Malignancy without chemotherapy | 2.21 | 1.60–3.06 |

CI, confidence interval.
[a]Per decade increase in age.
[b]Per 10 kg/m² increase in body mass index.
From Heit JA, Mohr DN, Silverstein MD, et al. Predictors of recurrence after deep vein thrombosis and pulmonary embolism: a population-based cohort study. *Arch Intern Med* 2000;160:761–768, with permission.

# RISK FACTORS FOR VENOUS THROMBOEMBOLISM

The occurrence of venous thromboembolism must be reduced to improve survival, avoid recurrence, prevent complications, and reduce health care costs. However, the incidence of venous thromboembolism has remained virtually unchanged since about 1980 (see Fig. 83-4) (1,46), possibly reflecting an increase in the population at risk (e.g., an increase in the average population age), exposure of the population to more or new risk factors [e.g., an increase in surgical procedures (47)], inadequate identification of all high-risk populations, underutilization of appropriate prophylaxis (48–51), or prophylaxis failure (52,53).

Persons at risk for venous thromboembolism must be identified in order to provide appropriate prophylaxis. Independent risk factors for venous thromboembolism include surgery, trauma, confinement to hospital or nursing home, active malignant neoplasm with or without concurrent chemotherapy, central vein catheterization or transvenous pacemaker, prior superficial vein thrombosis, varicose veins, and neurologic disease with extremity paresis; patients with chronic liver disease have a reduced risk (see Table 83-4) (54). Compared to residents in the community, hospitalized residents have a more than 150-fold increased incidence of acute venous thromboembolism (46). Hospitalization and nursing home residence together account for approximately 60% of incident venous thromboembolism events occurring in the community (55). Therefore, hospital confinement provides an important opportunity to considerably reduce the incidence of venous thromboembolism. Notably, hospitalization for medical illness and hospitalization for surgery account for almost equal proportions of venous thromboembolism (22% and 24%, respectively), emphasizing the need to provide prophylaxis to both these risk groups. Nursing home residence independently accounts for more than one tenth of all venous thromboembolism disease in the community (55).

The risk among patients who have undergone surgery can be further stratified on the basis of patient age, type of surgery, and the presence of active cancer (56,57). The incidence of postoperative venous thromboembolism is increased for surgery patients that are 65 years of age or older (58). High-risk surgical procedures include neurosurgery; major orthopedic surgery of the leg; thoracic, abdominal, or pelvic surgery for malignancy; renal transplantation; and cardiovascular surgery. Obesity (51,53,59) and poor physical status, according to the American Society of

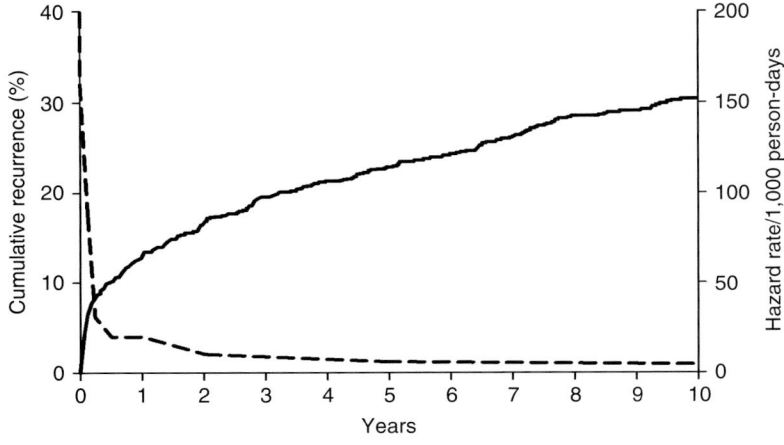

**FIGURE 83-3.** Cumulative incidence of the first venous thromboembolism recurrence (*solid line*), and the hazard of first recurrence per 1,000 person-days (*dashed line*). (From Heit JA, Mohr DN, Silverstein MD, et al. Predictors of recurrence after deep vein thrombosis and pulmonary embolism: a population-based cohort study. *Arch Intern Med* 2000;160:761–768, with permission.)

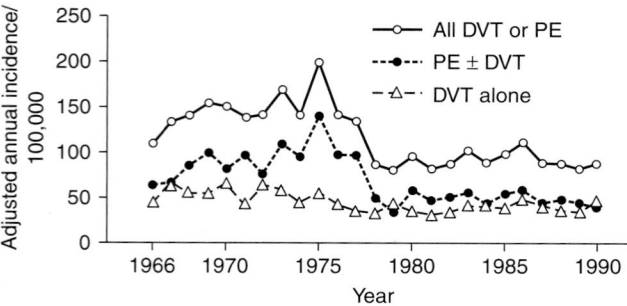

**FIGURE 83-4.** Age- and sex-adjusted annual incidence of all venous thromboembolism, deep vein thrombosis (DVT) alone, and pulmonary embolism (PE) with or without deep vein thrombosis (PE ± DVT). (From Heit JA, Mohr DN, Silverstein MD, et al. Predictors of recurrence after deep vein thrombosis and pulmonary embolism: a population-based cohort study. *Arch Intern Med* 2000;160:761–768, with permission.)

Anesthesiologists (51), are risk factors for venous thromboembolism after total hip arthroplasty. The risk from surgery may be less with neuraxial (i.e., spinal or epidural) anesthesia than with general anesthesia (60).

Active cancer accounts for approximately 20% of incident venous thromboembolism events occurring in the community (55). The risk appears to be higher for patients with malignant brain tumors and with cancer of the ovary, pancreas, colon, stomach, lung, and kidney (61). Patients with cancer, receiving immunosuppressive or cytotoxic chemotherapy, are at an even higher risk for venous thromboembolism (Table 83-4) (46), including therapy with L-asparaginase (62,63), thalidomide (64), or tamoxifen (65). A routine examination for occult malignancy is warranted for patients presenting with idiopathic venous thromboembolism, especially among patients in whom venous thromboembolism recurs (66).

A central venous catheter or transvenous pacemaker now accounts for 9% of incident venous thromboembolism occurring

## TABLE 83-4

### INDEPENDENT RISK FACTORS FOR DEEP VEIN THROMBOSIS OR PULMONARY EMBOLISM

| Baseline characteristics | Odds ratio | 95% CI |
|---|---|---|
| Institutionalization with or without recent surgery | | |
| Institutionalization without recent surgery | 7.98 | 4.49–14.18 |
| Institutionalization with recent surgery | 21.72 | 9.44–49.93 |
| Trauma | 12.69 | 4.06–39.66 |
| Malignancy without chemotherapy | 4.05 | 1.93–8.52 |
| Malignancy with chemotherapy | 6.53 | 2.11–20.23 |
| Prior central venous catheter or transvenous pacemaker | 5.55 | 1.57–19.58 |
| Prior superficial vein thrombosis | 4.32 | 1.76–10.61 |
| Neurologic disease with extremity paresis | 3.04 | 1.25–7.38 |
| Serious liver disease | 0.10 | 0.01–0.71 |

CI, confidence interval.
From Heit JA, Silverstein MD, Mohr DN, et al. Risk factors for deep vein thrombosis and pulmonary embolism: a population-based case-control study. *Arch Intern Med* 2000;160:809–815, with permission.

in the community (55). Central venous access by femoral vein catheters is associated with a higher incidence of venous thrombosis than with subclavian vein catheterization (67). Prior superficial vein thrombosis is an independent risk factor for subsequent deep vein thrombosis or pulmonary embolism remote from the episode of superficial thrombophlebitis (54). The risk of DVT imparted by varicose veins is uncertain and appears to vary with patient age (54,68,69). Long-haul (>6-hour) air travel is associated with a slightly increased risk for venous thromboembolism that is preventable with elastic stockings (70). Coenzyme A reductase inhibitor (statin) therapy may provide a 20% to 50% risk reduction for venous thromboembolism (71,72). However, the risk associated with atherosclerosis, or other risk factors for atherosclerosis, remains uncertain (73–75). Body mass index, current or past tobacco smoking, chronic obstructive pulmonary disease, and renal failure are not independent risk factors for venous thromboembolism (54,70,71). The risk associated with congestive heart failure, independent of hospitalization, is low (54,56,70,71).

Among women, additional risk factors for venous thromboembolism include oral contraceptive use (56,76,77), hormone replacement therapy (71,77,78), pregnancy and the postpartum period (56,77,79), and therapy with the selective estrogen receptor modulator, raloxifene. First- and third-generation oral contraceptives convey higher risk than second-generation oral contraceptives (80–85). Hormone replacement therapy is associated with a twofold to fourfold increased risk of venous thrombosis (71,78). Approximately 1 in 2,000 women will develop venous thrombosis during pregnancy (79,86). The risk during the postpartum period is approximately fourfold higher than the risk during pregnancy. Prior superficial vein thrombosis is an independent risk factor for venous thrombosis during pregnancy or postpartum (87).

Other conditions associated with venous thromboembolism include heparin-induced thrombocytopenia, myeloproliferative disorders (especially polycythemia rubra vera and essential thrombocythemia), intravascular coagulation and fibrinolysis/disseminated intravascular coagulation (ICF/DIC), nephrotic syndrome, paroxysmal nocturnal hemoglobinuria, thromboangiitis obliterans (Buerger disease), thrombotic thrombocytopenic purpura, Behcet syndrome, systemic lupus erythematosis, inflammatory bowel disease, Wegeners granulomatosis, homocystinuria, and possibly, hyperhomocysteinemia (88,89).

# THE GENETIC EPIDEMIOLOGY OF VENOUS THROMBOEMBOLISM

Recent family-based studies indicate that venous thromboembolism is highly heritable and follows a complex mode of inheritance involving environmental interaction (90–92). Inherited reductions in plasma natural anticoagulants (e.g., antithrombin, protein C, or protein S) have long been recognized as being uncommon but potent risk factors for venous thromboembolism (93–95). More recent discoveries of impaired downregulation of the procoagulant system (e.g., activated protein C resistance and Factor V$_{Leiden}$) (96–102), and increased plasma concentrations of procoagulant factors [e.g., factors I (fibrinogen), II (prothrombin), VIII, IX, and XI] (103–110), have added new paradigms to the list of inherited or acquired disorders predisposing to thrombosis (thrombophilia). Prospective cohort studies indicate that patients with venous thromboembolism have increased basal fibrin formation (111,112). These plasma hemostasis-related factors or markers of coagulation activation both correlate with increased thrombotic risk and are highly heritable (113–118). These inherited thrombophilias interact with such clinical risk factors (e.g., environmental exposures) as oral contraceptives (85,119,120), pregnancy (121–123), hormone therapy (124), and surgery (52,125) to increase the risk of incident venous thromboembolism. Similarly, genetic interaction increases the risk of incident (126–130) and recurrent venous thromboembolism (35,131–137). Although the clinical utility of diagnostic testing for an inherited or acquired thrombophilia remains controversial (33,106,138,139), such studies hold the potential for further stratifying individual patients into high and low risk for incident and recurrent venous thromboembolism, targeting primary and secondary prophylaxis to those who would benefit most, and, ultimately, reducing the occurrence of venous thromboembolism.

# ACKNOWLEDGMENTS

Funded, in part, by grants from the National Institutes of Health (HL 60279, HL 66216) and Centers for Disease Control and Prevention (TS326), U.S. Public Health Service; and by Mayo Foundation.

## References

1. Silverstein MD, Heit JA, Mohr DN, et al. Trends in the incidence of deep vein thrombosis and pulmonary embolism: a 25-year population-based study. *Arch Intern Med* 1998;158:585–593.
2. White RH, Zhou H, Romano PS. Incidence of idiopathic deep venous thrombosis and secondary thromboembolism among ethnic groups in California. *Ann Intern Med* 1998;128:737–740.
3. Klatsky AL, Armstrong MA, Poggi J. Risk of pulmonary embolism and/or deep venous thrombosis in Asian-Americans. *Am J Cardiol* 2000;85(11):1334–1337.
4. Hooper WC, Holman RC, Heit JA, et al. Venous thromboembolism hospitalizations among American Indians and Alaska natives. *Thromb Res* 2002;108(5–6):273–278.
5. Anderson FA Jr, Wheeler HB, Goldberg RJ, et al. The Worchester DVT Study. A population-based perspective of the hospital incidence and case-fatality rates of deep vein thrombosis and pulmonary embolism. *Arch Intern Med* 1991;151:933–938.
6. Massicote MP, Dix D, Monagle P, et al. Central venous catheter related thrombosis in children: analysis of the Canadian registry of venous thromboembolic complications. *J Pediatr* 1998;133:770–776.
7. Tormene D, Simioni P, Prandoni P, et al. The incidence of venous thromboembolism in thrombophilic children: a prospective cohort study. *Blood* 2002;100(7):2403–2405.
8. van Ommen CH, Heijboer H, Büller HR, et al. Venous thromboembolism in childhood: a prospective two-year registry in the Netherlands. *J Pediatr* 2001;139:676–681.
9. Heit JA, Silverstein MD, Mohr DN, et al. Predictors of survival after deep vein thrombosis and pulmonary embolism: a population-based cohort study. *Arch Intern Med* 1999;159:445–453.
10. Goldhaber SZ, Visani L, De Rosa M, ICOPER. Acute pulmonary embolism: clinical outcomes in the International Cooperative Pulmonary Embolism Registry (ICOPER). *Lancet* 1999;353:1386–1389.
11. Janata K, Holzer M, Domanovits H, et al. Mortality of patients with pulmonary embolism. *Wien Klin Wochenschr* 2002;114(17–18):766–772.
12. Konstantinides S, Geibel A, Olschewski M, et al. Association between thrombolytic treatment and the prognosis of hemodynamically stable patients with major pulmonary embolism: results of a multicenter registry. *Circulation* 1997;96:882–888.
13. Pruszczyk P, Bochowicz A, Torbicki A, et al. Cardiac troponin T monitoring identifies high-risk group of normotensive patients with acute pulmonary embolism. *Chest* 2003;123:1947–1952.
14. Kucher N, Printzen G, Doernhoefer T, et al. Low pro-brain natriuretic peptide levels predict benign clinical outcome in acute pulmonary embolism. *Circulation* 2003;107(12):1576–1578.
15. Kasper W, Konstantinides S, Geibel A, et al. Prognostic significance of right ventricular afterload stress detected by echocardiography in patients with clinically suspected pulmonary embolism. *Heart* 1997;77:346–349.
16. Grifoni S, Olivotto I, Cecchini P, et al. Short-term clinical outcome of patients with acute pulmonary embolism, normal blood pressure, and echocardiographic right ventricular dysfunction. *Circulation* 2000;101:2817–2822.
17. Agnelli G, Becattini C, Kirschstein T. Thrombolysis vs. heparin in the treatment of pulmonary embolism: a clinical outcome-based meta-analysis. *Arch Inter Med* 2002;162(22):2537–2541.
18. Konstantinides S, Geibel A, Heusel G, et al. Heparin plus alteplase compared with heparin alone in patients with submassive pulmonary embolism. *N Engl J Med* 2002;347:1143–1150.
19. Janke RM, McGovern PG, Folsom AR. Mortality, hospital discharges, and case fatality for pulmonary embolism in the twin cities: 1980–1995. *J Clin Epidemiol* 2000;53(1):103–109.

20. Horlander KT, Mannino DM, Leeper KV. Pulmonary embolism mortality in the United States, 1979–1998: an analysis using multiple-cause mortality data. *Arch Intern Med* 2003;163(14):1711–1717.
21. Heit JA, Mohr DN, Silverstein MD, et al. Predictors of recurrence after deep vein thrombosis and pulmonary embolism: a population-based cohort study. *Arch Intern Med* 2000;160:761–768.
22. Schulman S, Granqvist S, Holmstrom M, et al. The Duration of Anticoagulation Trial Study Group. The duration of oral anticoagulant therapy after a second episode of venous thromboembolism. *N Engl J Med* 1997;336:393–398.
23. Kearon C, Gent M, Hirsh J, et al. A comparison of three months of anticoagulation with extended anticoagulation for a first episode of idiopathic venous thromboembolism. *N Engl J Med* 1999;340(12):901–907.
24. Agnelli G, Prandoni P, Santamaria MG, et al. Three months versus one year of oral anticoagulant therapy for idiopathic deep venous thrombosis. *N Engl J Med* 2001;345:165–169.
25. Schulman S, Rhedin A-S, Lindmarker P, et al. A comparison of six weeks with six months of oral anticoagulant therapy after a first episode of venous thromboembolism. *N Engl J Med* 1995;332:1661–1665.
26. Pinede L, Ninet J, Duhaut P, et al. Comparison of 3 and 6 months of oral anticoagulant therapy after a first episode of proximal deep vein thrombosis or pulmonary embolism and comparison of 6 and 12 weeks of therapy after isolated calf deep vein thrombosis. *Circulation* 2001;103:2453–2460.
27. Agnelli G, Prandoni P, Becattini C, et al. Extended oral anticoagulant therapy after a first episode of pulmonary embolism. *Ann Intern Med* 2003;139:19–25.
28. van Dongen CJJ, Vink R, Hutten BA, et al. The incidence of recurrent venous thromboembolism after treatment with vitamin K antagonists in relation to time since first event; a meta-analysis. *Arch Intern Med* 2003;163:1285–1293.
29. Hansson P-O, Sörbo J, Eriksson H. Recurrent venous thromboembolism after deep vein thrombosis. *Arch Intern Med* 2000;160:769–774.
30. Prandoni P, Lensing AWA, Piccioli A, et al. Recurrent venous thromboembolism and bleeding complications during anticoagulant treatment in patients with cancer and venous thrombosis. *Blood* 2002;100:3484–3488.
31. Kyrle PA, Eichinger S. The risk of recurrent venous thromboembolism: the Austrian study on recurrent venous thromboembolism. *Wien Klin Wochenschr* 2003;115(13–14):471–474.
32. Prandoni P, Lensing AW, Cogo A, et al. The long-term clinical course of acute deep venous thrombosis. *Ann Intern Med* 1996;125:1–7.
33. Baglin T, Luddington R, Brown K, et al. Incidence of recurrent venous thromboembolism in relation to clinical and thrombophilic risk factors: prospective cohort study. *Lancet* 2003;362(9383):523–526.
34. Schulman S, Svenungsson E, Granqvist S, Duration of Anticoagulation Study Group. Anticardiolipin antibodies predict early recurrence of thromboembolism and death among patients with venous thromboembolism following anticoagulant therapy. *Am J Med* 1998;104:332–338.
35. van den Belt AGM, Sanson B-J, Simioni P, et al. Recurrence of venous thromboembolism in patients with familial thrombophilia. *Arch Inter Med* 1997;157:227–232.
36. Prandoni P, Lensing AW, Prins MH, et al. Residual venous thrombosis as a predictive factor of recurrent venous thromboembolism. *Ann Intern Med* 2002;137(12):955–960.
37. Murin S, Romano PS, White RH. Comparison of outcomes after hospitalization for deep venous thrombosis or pulmonary embolism. *Thromb Haemost* 2002;88:407–414.
38. Heit JA, Farmer SA, Petterson TM, et al. Venous thromboembolism event type (PE ± DVT vs. DVT alone) predicts recurrence type and survival. *Blood* 2002;100(11):149a (abstract# 560).
39. Mohr DN, Silverstein MD, Heit JA, et al. The venous stasis syndrome after deep venous thromboembolism or pulmonary embolism: a population-based study. *Mayo Clin Proc* 2000;75:1249–1256.
40. Beyth RJ, Cohen AM, Landefeld CS. Long-term outcomes of deep-vein thrombosis. *Arch Intern Med* 1995;155:1031–1037.
41. Heit JA, Rooke TW, Silverstein MD, et al. Trends in the incidence of venous stasis syndrome and venous ulcer: a 25-year population-based study. *J Vasc Surg* 2001;33:1022–1027.
42. Bergqvist D, Jendteg S, Johansen L, et al. Cost of long-term complications of deep venous thrombosis of the lower extremities: an analysis of a defined patient population in Sweden. *Ann Intern Med* 1997;126:454–457.
43. Criqui MH, Jamosmos M, Fronek A, et al. Chronic venous disease in an ethnically diverse population: the San Diego population study. *Am J Epidemiol* 2003;158(5):448–456.
44. Brandjes DPM, Büller HR, Heijboer H, et al. Randomized trial of effect of compression stockings in patients with symptomatic proximal-vein thrombosis. *Lancet* 1997;349:759–762.
45. Kahn SR, Azoulay L, Hirsch A, et al. Effect of graduated elastic compression stockings on leg symptoms and signs during exercise in patients with deep venous thrombosis: a randomized cross-over trial. *J Thromb Haemost* 2003;1(3):494–499.
46. Heit JA, Melton LJI, Lohse CM, et al. Incidence of venous thromboembolism in hospitalized patients versus community residents. *Mayo Clin Proc* 2001;76:1102–1110.
47. Madhok R, Lewallen DG, Wallrichs SL, et al. Trends in the utilization of primary total hip arthroplasty, 1969 through 1990: a population-based study in Olmsted county, Minnesota. *Mayo Clin Proc* 1993;68:11–18.

48. Anderson FA Jr, Wheeler HB, Goldberg RJ, et al. Physician practices in the prevention of venous thromboembolism. *Ann Intern Med* 1991;115: 591–595.

49. Bratzler DW, Raskob GE, Murray CK, et al. Underuse of venous thromboembolism prophylaxis for general surgery patients in the community. *Arch Intern Med* 1998;158:1909–1912.

50. Mantilla CB, Horlocker TT, Schroeder DR, et al. Risk factors for clinically relevant pulmonary embolism and deep venous thrombosis in patients undergoing primary hip or knee arthroplasty. *Anesthesiology* 2003;99(3): 552–560.

51. Goldhaber SZ, Tapson VF, DVT FREE Steering Committee. A prospective registry of 5,451 patients with ultrasound-confirmed deep vein thrombosis. *Am J Cardiol* 2004;93(2):259–262.

52. Lowe GD, Haverkate F, Thompson SG, et al. Prediction of deep vein thrombosis after elective hip replacement surgery by preoperative clinical and haemostatic variables: the ECAT DVT study. European concerted action on thrombosis. *Thromb Haemost* 1999;81(6):879–886.

53. Anderson FA Jr, Hirsh J, White K, et al. Hip and knee registry investigators. Temporal trends in prevention of venous thromboembolism following primary total hip or knee arthroplasty 1996–2001: findings from the hip and knee registry. *Chest* 2003;124(Suppl. 6):349S–356S.

54. Heit JA, Silverstein MD, Mohr DN, et al. Risk factors for deep vein thrombosis and pulmonary embolism: a population-based case-control study. *Arch Intern Med* 2000;160:809–815.

55. Heit JA, O'Fallon WM, Petterson TM, et al. Relative impact of risk factors for deep vein thrombosis and pulmonary embolism: a population-based study. *Arch Intern Med* 2002;162:1245–1248.

56. Samama M-M for the Sirius Study Group. An epidemiologic study of risk factors for deep vein thrombosis in medical outpatients. *Arch Intern Med* 2000;160:3415–3420.

57. Geerts WH, Pineo GF, Heit JA, et al. Prevention of venous thromboembolism. 7th ACCP consensus conference on antithrombotic therapy. *Chest* 2004;126(Suppl):338S–400S.

58. White RH, Zhou H, Romano PS. Incidence of symptomatic venous thromboembolism after different elective or urgent surgical procedures. *Thromb Haemost* 2003;90:446–455.

59. White RH, Gettner S, Newman JM, et al. Predictors of rehospitalization for symptomatic venous thromboembolism after total hip arthroplasty. *N Engl J Med* 2000;343:1758–1764.

60. Sharrock NE, Haas SB, Hargett MJ, et al. Effects of epidural anesthesia on the incidence of deep vein thrombosis after total knee replacement. *J Bone Joint Surg* 1991;73A:502–506.

61. Levitan N, Dowlati A, Remick SC, et al. Rates of initial and recurrent thromboembolic disease among patients with malignancy versus those without malignancy. *Medicine (Baltimore)* 1999;78:285–291.

62. Kucek O, Kwaan HC, Gunnak W, et al. Thromboembolic complications associated with L-asparaginase therapy. *Cancer* 1985;55:702.

63. Liebman HA, Wada JK, Patch MJ, et al. Depression of functional and antigenic plasma antithrombin III due to therapy with L-asparaginase. *Cancer* 1982;50:451.

64. Zangari M, Anaissie E, Barlogie B, et al. Increased risk of deep-vein thrombosis in patients with multiple myeloma receiving thalidomide and chemotherapy. *Blood* 2001;98:1614–1615.

65. Meier CR, Jick H. Tamoxifen and the risk of idiopathic venous thromboembolism. *Br J Pharmacol* 1998;45:608–612.

66. Hettiarachchi RJ, Lok J, Prins MH, et al. Undiagnosed malignancy in patients with deep vein thrombosis: incidence, risk indicators, and diagnosis. *Cancer* 1998;83(1):180–185.

67. Merrer J, De Jonghe B, Lefrant J-Y, et al. Complications of femoral and subclavian venous catheterization in critically ill patients: a randomized controlled trial. *JAMA* 2001;286:700–707.

68. Goldhaber SZ, Savage DD, Garrison RJ, et al. Risk factors for pulmonary embolism: the Framingham study. *Am J Med* 1983;74:1023–1028.

69. Cogo A, Bernadi E, Prandoni P, et al. Acquired risk factors for deep-vein thrombosis in symptomatic outpatients. *Arch Intern Med* 1994;154: 164–168.

70. Dalen J. Economy class syndrome; too much flying or too much sitting? *Arch Intern Med* 2003;163:2674.

71. Grady D, Wenger NK, Herrington D, et al. Postmenopausal hormone therapy increases risk for venous thromboembolic disease. *Ann Intern Med* 2000;132:689–696.

72. Ray JG, Mamdani M, Tsuyuki RT, et al. Use of statins and the subsequent development of deep vein thrombosis. *Arch Intern Med* 2001;161: 1405–1410.

73. Prandoni P, Bilora F, Marchiori A, et al. An association between atherosclerosis and venous thrombosis. *N Engl J Med* 2003;348(15):1435–1441.

74. Marcucci R, Liotta AA, Cellai AP, et al. Increased plasma levels of lipoprotein(a) and the risk of idiopathic and recurrent venous thromboembolism. *Am J Med* 2003;115(8):601–605.

75. Tsai AW, Cushman M, Rosamond WD, et al. Cardiovascular risk factors and venous thromboembolism incidence. *Arch Intern Med* 2002;162: 1182–1189.

76. Chasan-Taber L, Stampfer MJ. Epidemiology of oral contraceptives and cardiovascular disease. *Ann Intern Med* 1998;128:467–467.

77. Rosendaal FR. Risk factors for venous thrombotic disease. *Thromb Haemost* 1999;82:610–619.

78. Grady D, Furberg C. Venous thromboembolic events associates with hormone replacement therapy. *JAMA* 1997;278:477.

79. Kierkegaard A. Incidence and diagnosis of deep vein thrombosis associated with pregnancy. *Acta Obstet Gynecol Scand* 1983;62:239–243.

80. World Health Organization. Venous thromboembolic disease and combined oral contraceptives: results of international multicentre case-control study. World Health Organization collaborative study of cardiovascular disease and steroid hormone contraception. *Lancet* 1995;346:1575–1582.

81. Gerstman BB, Piper JM, Tomita DK, et al. Oral contraceptive estrogen dose and the risk of deep venous thromboembolitic disease. *Am J Epidemiol* 1991;133:32–37.

82. Böttiger LE, Boman G, Eklund G, et al. Oral contraceptives and thromboembolic disease: effects of lowering oestrogen content. *Lancet* 1989;8178: 1097–1101.

83. Bloemenkamp KW, Rosendaal FR, Büller HR, et al. Risk of venous thrombosis with use of current low-dose oral contraceptives is not explained by diagnostic suspicion and referral bias. *Arch Intern Med* 1999;159:65–70.

84. Bloemenkamp KWM, Rosendaal FR, Helmerhorst FM, et al. Enhancement by factor V leiden mutation of risk of deep-vein thrombosis associated with oral contraceptives containing a third-generation progestagen. *Lancet* 1995;346:1593–1596.

85. Kemmeren JM, Algra A, Grobbee DE. Third generation oral contraceptives and risk of venous thrombosis: meta-analysis. *BMJ* 2001;323:131–134.

86. McColl MD, Ramsay JE, Tait RC, et al. Risk factors for pregnancy associated venous thromboembolism. *Thromb Haemost* 1997;78:1183–1188.

87. Danilenko-Dixon DR, Heit JA, Watkins T, et al. Risk factors for deep vein thrombosis and pulmonary embolism during pregnancy or the postpartum period: a population-based case-control study. *Am J Obstet Gynecol* 2001;184:104–110.

88. Key NS, McGlennen RC. Hyperhomocyst(e)inemia and thrombophilia. *Arch Pathol Lab Med* 2002;126:1367–1375.

89. Tsai AW, Cushman M, Tsai MH, et al. Serum homocysteine, thermolabile variant of methylene tetrahydrofolate reductase (MTHFR), and venous thromboembolism: Longitudinal Investigation of Thromboembolism Etiology (LITE). *Am J Hematol* 2003;72:192–200.

90. Souto J, Almasy L, Borrell M, et al. Genetic susceptibility to thrombosis and its relationship to physiological risk factors: the GAIT study. Genetic analysis of idiopathic thrombophilia. *Am J Hum Genet* 2000;67(6): 1452–1459.

91. Larsen TB, Sorensen HT, Skytthe A, et al. Major genetic susceptibility for venous thromboembolism in men: a study of Danish twins. *Epidemiology* 2003;14(3):328–332.

92. Heit JA, Phelps MA, Ward SA, et al. Familial segregation of venous thromboembolism. *J Thromb Haemost* 2004;2:731–736.

93. Heijboer H, Brandjes DPM, Büller HR, et al. Deficiencies of coagulation-inhibiting and fibrinolytic proteins in outpatients with deep-vein thrombosis. *N Engl J Med* 1990;323:1512–1516.

94. Sanson B-J, Simioni P, Tormene D, et al. The incidence of venous thromboembolism in asymptomatic carriers of a deficiency of antithrombin, protein C, or protein S: a prospective cohort study. *Blood* 1999;94:3702–3706.

95. Folsom AR, Aleksic N, Wang N, et al. Protein C, antithrombin, and venous thromboembolism incidence; a prospective population-based study. *Arterioscler Thromb Vasc Biol* 2002;22:1018–1022.

96. Dahlbäck B, Carlsson M, Svensson PR. Familial thrombophilia due to a previously unrecognized mechanism characterized by poor anticoagulant response to activated protein C: prediction of a cofactor to activated protein C. *Proc Natl Acad Sci U S A* 1993;90:1004–1008.

97. Bertina R, Koeleman B, Koster T, et al. Mutation in blood coagulation factor V associated with resistance to activated protein C. *Nature* 1994; 369:64–67.

98. Koster T, Rosendaal FR, de Ronde H, et al. Venous thrombosis due to poor anticoagulant response to activated protein C: leiden thrombophilia study. *Lancet* 1993;342:1503–1506.

99. Ridker PM, Hennekens CH, Lindpainter K, et al. Mutation in the gene coding for coagulation factor V and the risk of myocardial infarction, stroke, and venous thrombosis in apparently healthy men. *N Engl J Med* 1995;332:912–917.

100. Rosendaal FR, Koster T, Vandebroucke JP, et al. High risk of thrombosis in patients homozygous for factor V leiden (activated protein C resistance). *Blood* 1995;85:1504–1508.

101. Folsom AR, Cushman M, Tsai MY, et al. A prospective study of venous thromboembolism in relation to factor V leiden and related factors. *Blood* 2002;88:2720–2725.

102. Juul K, Tybjærg-Hansen A, Schnohr P, et al. Factor V leiden and the risk for venous thromboembolism in the adult danish population. *Ann Intern Med* 2004;140:330–337.

103. Koster T, Rosendaal FR, Reitsma PH, et al. Factor VII and fibrinogen levels as risk factors for venous thrombosis. *Thromb Haemost* 1994;71: 719–722.

104. van Hylckama Vlieg A, Rosendaal FR. High levels of fibrinogen are associated with the risk of deep venous thrombosis mainly in the elderly. *J Thromb Haemost* 2003;1(12):2677–2678.

105. Poort SR, Rosendaal FR, Reitsma PH, et al. A common genetic variation in the 3'-untranslated region of the prothrombin gene is associated with elevated plasma prothrombin levels and an increase in venous thrombosis. *Blood* 1996;88:3698–3703.

106. McGlennen RC, Key NS. Clinical and laboratory management of the prothrombin G20210A mutations. *Arch Pathol Lab Med* 2002;126: 1319–1325.

107. Folsom AR, Cushman M, Tsai MY, et al. Prospective study of the G20210A polymorphism in the prothrombin gene, plasma prothrombin concentration, and incidence of venous thromboembolism. *Am J Hematol* 2002;71:285–290.

108. Koster T, Blann AD, Briët E, et al. Role of clotting factor VIII in effect of von Willebrand factor on occurrence of deep-vein thrombosis. *Lancet* 1995;345:152–155.

109. van Hylckama Vlieg A, van der Linden IK, Bertina RM, et al. High levels of factor IX increase the risk of venous thrombosis. *Blood* 2000;95: 3678–3682.

110. Meijers JCM, Tekelenburg WLH, Bouma BN, et al. High levels of coagulation factor XI as a risk factor for venous thrombosis. *N Engl J Med* 2000;342:696–701.

111. Folsom AR, Cushman M, Heckbert SR, et al. Prospective study of fibrinolytic markers and venous thromboembolism. *J Clin Epidemiol* 2003; 56:598–603.

112. Cushman M, Folsom AR, Wang L, et al. Fragmin fragment D-dimer and the risk of future venous thrombosis. *Blood* 2003;101:1243–1248.

113. Souto J, Almasy L, Borrell M, et al. Genetic determinants of hemostasis phenotypes in Spanish families. *Circulation* 2000;101(13):1546–1551.

114. de Lange M, Snieder H, Ariëns RA, et al. The genetics of haemostasis: a twin study. *Lancet* 2001;357(9250):101–105.

115. Ariëns R, de Lange M, Snieder H, et al. Activation markers of coagulation and fibrinolysis in twins: heritability of the prethrombotic state. *Lancet* 2002;359:667–671.

116. Rosendaal FR, Bovill EG. Heritability of clotting factors and the revival of the prothrombotic state. *Lancet* 2002;359(9307):638–639.

117. Soria J, Almasy L, Souto J, et al. Linkage analysis demonstrates that the prothrombin G20210A mutation jointly influences plasma prothrombin levels and risk of thrombosis. *Blood* 2000;95(9):2780–2785.

118. Gehring NH, Frede U, Neu-Yilik G, et al. Increased efficiency of mRNA 3′ end formation: a new genetic mechanism contributory to hereditary thrombophilia. *Nat Genet* 2001;28:389–392.

119. Vandenbroucke JP, Koster T, Briet E, et al. Increased risk of venous thrombosis in oral-contraceptive users who are carriers of factor V leiden mutation. *Lancet* 1994;344:1453–1457.

120. Middeldorp S, Meinardi JR, Koopman MMW, et al. A prospective study of asymptomatic carriers of the factor V leiden mutation to determine the incidence of venous thromboembolism. *Ann Intern Med* 2001;135: 322–327.

121. Friederich PW, Sanson B-J, Simioni P, et al. Frequency of pregnancy-related venous thromboembolism in anticoagulant factor-deficient women: implications for prophylaxis. *Ann Intern Med* 1996;125:955–960.

122. Gerhardt A, Scharf RE, Beckmann MW, et al. Prothrombin and factor V mutations in women with a history of thrombosis during pregnancy and the puerperium. *N Engl J Med* 2000;342:374–380.

123. Martinelli I, De Stefano V, Taioli E, et al. Inherited thrombophilia and first venous thromboembolism during pregnancy and puerperium. *Thromb Haemost* 2002;87(5):791–795.

124. Rosendaal FR, Vessey MP, Rumley A. Hormonal replacement therapy, prothrombotic mutations and the risk of venous thrombosis. *Br J Haematol* 2002;116:851–854.

125. Lindahl TL, Lundahl TH, Nilsson L, et al. APC-resistance is a risk factor for postoperative thromboembolism in elective replacement of the hip or knee—a prospective study. *Thromb Haemost* 1999;81:18–21.

126. van Boven HA, Reitsma PH, Rosendaal FR, et al. Factor V leiden (FV R506Q) in families with inherited antithrombin deficiency. *Thromb Haemost* 1996;75:417–421.

127. Koeleman B, Reitsma P, Allaart C, et al. Activated protein C as an additional risk factor for thrombosis in protein C-deficient families. *Blood* 1994;84:1031–1035.

128. Gandrille S, Greengard JS, Alhenc-Gelas M, et al. Incidence of activated protein C resistance caused by the ARG 506 GLN mutation in factor V in 113 unrelated symptomatic protein C-deficient patients: the French network on the behalf of INSERM. *Blood* 1995;86:219–224.

129. Zöller B, Berntsdotter A, Garcia de Frutos P, et al. Resistance to activated protein C as an additional genetic risk factor in hereditary deficiency of protein S. *Blood* 1995;85:3518–3523.

130. Libourel EJ, Bank I, Meinardi JR, et al. Co-segregation of thrombophilic disorders in factor V leiden carriers; the contributions of factor VIII, factor XI, thrombin activatable fibrinolysis inhibitor and lipoprotein(a) to the absolute risk of venous thromboembolism. *Haematologica* 2002;87: 1068–1073.

131. Lindmarker P, Schulman S, Sten-Linder M, et al. The risk of recurrent venous thromboembolism in carriers and non-carriers of the G1691A allele in the coagulation factor V gene and the G20210a allele in the prothrombin gene. *Thromb Haemost* 1999;81(5):684–689.

132. De Stefano V, Martinelli I, Mannucci PM, et al. The risk of recurrent deep venous thrombosis among heterozygous carriers of both factor V leiden and the G20210A prothrombin mutation. *N Engl J Med* 1999;341: 801–808.

133. Eichinger S, Weltermann A, Mannhalter C, et al. The risk of recurrent venous thromboembolism in heterozygous carriers of factor V leiden and a first spontaneous venous thromboembolism. *Arch Intern Med* 2002; 162(20):2357–2360.

134. Meinardi JR, Middeldorp S, de Kam PJ, et al. The incidence of recurrent venous thromboembolism in carriers of factor V leiden is related to concomitant thrombophilic disorders. *Br J Haematol* 2002;116:625–631.

135. Kyrle PA, Minar E, Hirschl M, et al. High plasma levels of factor VIII and the risk of recurrent venous thromboembolism. *N Engl J Med* 2000;343: 457–462.

136. Weltermann A, Eichinger S, Bialonczyk C, et al. The risk of recurrent venous thromboembolism among patients with high factor IX levels. *J Thromb Haemost* 2003;1(1):28–32.

137. Eichinger S, Minar E, Bialonczyk C, et al. D-dimer levels and risk of recurrent venous thromboembolism. *JAMA* 2003;290(8):1071–1074.

138. Bauer KA. The thrombophilias, well-defined risk factors with uncertain therapeutic implications. *Ann Intern Med* 2001;135:367–373.

139. Press RD, Bauer KA, Kujovich JL, et al. Clinical utility of factor V leiden (R506Q) testing for the diagnosis and management of thromboembolic disorders. *Arch Pathol Lab Med* 2002;126:1304–1318.

# CHAPTER 84 ■ WOMEN'S HEALTH AND VENOUS THROMBOEMBOLISM

AGNES Y. Y. LEE

Venous thromboembolism (VTE) is the most frequent vascular disease in young women. In women aged 20 to 49 years, the estimated incidence of venous thromboembolism is two to five per 100,000 woman-years (1,2). The most common acquired conditions associated with thrombotic events in young women are those involving hormonal exposure, including oral contraceptive use, hormonal replacement therapy, and pregnancy.

## ORAL CONTRACEPTIVES

More than 100 million women worldwide use oral contraceptives (3); when used properly, they are highly effective in preventing pregnancy, with fewer than one per 100 women using the oral contraceptives becoming pregnant per year (4). In addition to this benefit, oral contraceptive use is also reported to provide protection against ovarian and endometrial cancer and to reduce the severity of acne and dysfunctional uterine bleeding (5). However, these products are also associated with definite and serious adverse effects, including vascular complications such as myocardial infarction, ischemic stroke, and venous thromboembolism, as well as possible increased risks of breast, cervical, and colorectal cancer (5). Despite numerous epidemiologic and clinical studies that have been conducted since the introduction of these drugs in 1960, definitive data on the exact risks of some of these complications are still lacking. Some of the reasons for the uncertainty include biologic differences between preparations, changes in formulation (including drug, dose, and mode of delivery) over time, and imprecise understanding of the mechanisms of action. In addition, inherent methodologic limitations of observational studies and differences among studies in screening and selection of patients, and in the tests and the criteria used for making a diagnosis of adverse outcomes further add to the discrepancy.

Also, the classification of oral contraceptives according to "generation" has been confusing and may contribute to the uncertainty and controversy about the relative safety of different agents (6). Although the term has been used most commonly for identifying the timing of the introduction of a product, it has also been used to indicate the introduction of the particular progestin component into the market or the structure of the carbon ring from which the progestin is derived (i.e., estrane, gonane, or pregnane). For example, norgestimate-containing oral contraceptives have been classified as second-generation products in some studies and as third-generation in others because although norgestimate-containing agents are considered as third-generation oral contraceptives according to their chronological introduction, the pharmacologic action of norgestimate is predominantly due to its metabolite levonorgestrel, which is a second-generation product. Currently, four generations of products are commercially available (see Table 84-1).

## Combination Pills and Venous Thromboembolism

The increased risk of venous thromboembolism, including pulmonary embolism and deep vein thrombosis, was first reported shortly after the introduction of oral contraceptives (7). This complication and other vascular complications were linked to the high doses of estrogen and progestins contained in these early products, and, consequently, these adverse effects prompted the development of low-dose formulations (8,9). These low-estrogen contraceptives are associated with minimal changes in laboratory hemostatic markers and, therefore, were considered to have a lower risk of venous thromboembolism (10). Furthermore, because the effects of combination oral contraceptives on cardiovascular risk factors such as lipid levels and glucose tolerance are dependent on the type of progestins, formulations with different progestins that had more favorable metabolic profiles were developed in an effort to reduce arterial vascular complications. The low-estrogen combination oral contraceptives now available contain 20 to 50 $\mu$g of ethinylestradiol (about one third to one fifth of the estrogen content of the original agents) and one of the several progestins in doses that are about one tenth of the first-generation products.

The risk of venous thromboembolism is unequivocally elevated in current users of low-estrogen combination oral contraceptives (3,11–22). On the basis of published clinical data, the risk in women using first- or second-generation products containing lynestrenol, norethindrone, norethindrone acetate, ethynodiol diacetate, or levonorgestrel is increased threefold to fourfold as compared with the risk in nonusers. In absolute terms, roughly three to four per 10,000 users of second-generation oral contraceptives will experience a first episode of venous thromboembolic event annually, compared with a baseline incidence of five to 10 cases per 100,000 women of reproductive age (13,16,17). In contrast to the known interactions between oral contraceptive usage and smoking, as well as contraceptive usage and old age, that increase the risk of arterial vascular events such as myocardial infarction and stroke (23–25), it is uncertain whether smoking influences the risk of venous thromboembolism in oral contraceptive users (26,27). Obesity, on the other hand, appears to have a synergistic effect with oral contraceptives for both arterial and venous vascular disease (11,27,28). The elevated risk for venous thromboembolism is persistent for the duration of use and does not persist beyond the discontinuation of oral contraceptives (29,30). The risk is highest during the first year of use (22,31,32), suggesting that some women, likely those with thrombophilia, are particularly predisposed to developing venous thromboembolism.

Following the publication of several large epidemiologic studies in 1995 that reported that women who used oral contraceptives containing desogestrel or gestodene have a higher

## TABLE 84-1

TYPES OF PROGESTIN IN COMBINATION
ESTROGEN–PROGESTIN ORAL CONTRACEPTIVES

| Time of market introduction | Generation | Progestin contained in combination contraceptives |
|---|---|---|
| Before 1973 | First | Chlormadinone acetate<br>Dimethisterone<br>Ethynodiol acetate<br>Ethynodiol diacetate<br>Medroxyprogesterone acetate<br>Norethindrone<br>Norethindrone acetate<br>Norethisterone<br>Norethynodrel<br>Norgestrel<br>Lynestrenol |
| 1973–1989 | Second | Levonorgestrel<br>Norgestrione |
| 1990–2000 | Third | Desogestrel<br>Gestodene<br>Norgestimate |
| After 2000 | Fourth | Cyproterone<br>Drospirenone |

risk of venous thromboembolism than women who used oral contraceptives containing levonorgestrel (11–14), there has been much debate about the relative risk of venous thromboembolism between second- and third-generation oral contraceptives. Although a few of the subsequent studies did not find a difference between these classes of oral contraceptives (16,33–35), most studies reported that users of third-generation oral contraceptives have a 1.3-fold to fourfold higher risk of venous thromboembolism than the users of second-generation oral contraceptives or a sixfold to ninefold higher risk than the nonusers (12–15,18,22,32,36). This finding of a higher risk has been suggested by some to be the result of confounding, "attrition of susceptibles" and other methodologic limitations and biases that are inherent in observational studies (35,37–39), but others argue this increase in risk is real (30,40,41). The most recent metaanalyses have concluded that use of low-estrogen oral contraceptives containing desogestrel or gestodene (i.e., progestins contained in third-generation products) increases the risk of venous thromboembolism by a factor of 1.7 compared to the formulations containing the second-generation progestin levonorgestrel (42,43). It remains uncertain whether differences in the induced changes in hemostatic markers and coagulation activity explain the higher risk of venous thrombosis observed in women using third-generation agents compared with the women using second-generation ones.

Although true differences may exist in thrombotic risk among commercially available products, rigorous direct comparisons of these agents have not been performed in large, randomized trials to establish equivalence or to demonstrate whether any specific product is superior in efficacy or safety over others. On the basis of the balance of evidence to date, the increased annual incidence of venous thromboembolism related to third-generation oral contraceptive use is approximately 10 to 15 cases per 100,000 women and the number of excess deaths is approximately five to 10 per million women (13,42,44). Given that both second- and third-generation oral contraceptives are equally effective in preventing pregnancy, it seems reasonable to avoid formulations with desogestrel or

gestodene as first choice agents, particularly in patients who have other risk factors for venous thromboembolism. Furthermore, there appears to be no real benefit with third-generation products because their theoretical advantage of a lower risk of arterial vascular complications compared with levonorgestrel has not been confirmed in the clinical setting (45,46).

Controversy over the risk of venous thromboembolism also exists for newer generations of combined estrogen–progesterone agents (47–49). Cyproterone is a progestin with strong androgenic properties and is indicated for the treatment of hirsutism or acne when used in combination with ethinylestradiol. This combination product is also effective for contraception, but it should not be prescribed only for its contraceptive properties, as indicated in the product monograph. Cyproterone alone in high doses is also used for treatment of prostate cancer (50). Case–control data have suggested that cyproterone combined with estrogen is associated with a twofold to fourfold risk of venous thromboembolism compared with combined oral contraceptives containing levonorgestrel (51–53). However, other studies, including a metaanalysis of the published literature, have not shown an excess risk of venous thromboembolism among women using cyproterone combined with ethinylestradiol compared with conventional oral contraceptive users (11,27,54,55). For the recently introduced ethinylestradiol–drospirenone combination pills, clinical experience is very limited and evidence for an increased risk of thrombosis has come from case reports only (47,56,57). Therefore, until more information is available, it remains uncertain whether combined oral contraceptives containing cyproterone or drospirenone differ from traditional combined agents in the risk for venous thromboembolism. Similarly, there is insufficient data on the safety of the recently available transdermal combination products with respect to the risk of venous thromboembolism. This mode of delivery appears to improve compliance and to minimize the peaks and troughs of hormone concentrations associated with daily oral administration (58,59). The efficacy and safety of these patches appear to be comparable to oral agents in small clinical trials to date, but it is possible that the avoidance of a first-pass effect through the hepatic circulation will reduce the thrombogenecity of contraceptive patches as compared with oral agents. This theoretical advantage remains to be confirmed in large clinical trials.

Overall, given the risk of pregnancy and its potential complications, combination low-estrogen oral contraceptives are associated with an overall health benefit to young women who wish to prevent pregnancy and who do not have major vascular risk factors (see Table 84-2) (6). In women with a history of ischemic heart disease, stroke, or venous thromboembolism, however, combination estrogen–progestin oral contraceptives should be avoided, and alternative birth control methods should be used. Women with risk factors for any of these vascular conditions, such as cigarette smoking and obesity, should also be strongly discouraged from using hormonal forms of contraception.

## Progestin-Only Contraceptives

Progestin-only contraceptives are less popular for contraception than combined agents because they are less effective in preventing pregnancy and are associated with irregular bleeding (60). However, progestin-only pills, implants, and injectables are considered to be safer than combination formulations with respect to the risk of venous thromboembolism because laboratory studies have demonstrated minimal or no activation of coagulation by these agents (61–67). Recent experiments also have shown that levonorgestrel and desogestrel have differential antithrombotic effects, which counteract the

**TABLE 84-2**

AGE-SPECIFIC ESTIMATE OF THE EXCESS RATES OF MYOCARDIAL INFARCTION, ISCHEMIC STROKE, AND VENOUS THROMBOEMBOLISM ATTRIBUTED TO THE USE OF LOW-ESTROGEN ORAL CONTRACEPTIVES AND PREGNANCY-RELATED MORTALITY

| Variable | Age | | |
|---|---|---|---|
| | 20–30 yr | 30–34 yr | 40–44 yr |
| No. of excess cases of myocardial infarction and ischemic stroke attributed to oral contraceptives use (per 100,000 woman-years of use) | | | |
|    Among nonsmokers | 0.4 | 0.6 | 2 |
|    Among smokers | 1 | 2 | 20 |
|    Among women with hypertension | 4 | 7 | 29 |
| No. of pregnancy-related deaths (per 100,000 live births) | 10 | 12 | 45 |
| No. of excess cases of venous thromboembolism attributable to oral contraceptive use (per 100,000 woman-years of use) | | | |
|    With norethindrone, norethindrone acetate, levonorgestrel, or ethynodiol diacetate | 6 | 9 | 12 |
|    With desogestrel or gestodene | 16 | 23 | 30 |

From Petitti DB. Clinical practice. Combination estrogen-progestin oral contraceptives. *N Engl J Med* 2003;349(15):1443–1450, with permission.

prothrombotic influence of the estrogen component in second- and third-generation combined oral contraceptives (68). Furthermore, case–control studies have shown no difference in the risk of venous thromboembolism in women using progestin-only oral or injectable contraceptives compared with nonusers (69,70). Consequently, some experts recommend progestin-only pills or injections for women who wish to use hormonal contraceptives and have an increased risk of venous thromboembolism, such as those who are carriers of factor $V_{Leiden}$ mutation (61,71,72). Nonetheless, the true risk of venous thromboembolism with progestin-only contraceptives has not been established because most of the clinical studies are not large enough to have the statistical power to detect small differences.

## Mechanisms of Hypercoagulability

The pathogenic mechanisms responsible for the prothrombotic state induced by hormone contraceptives are not understood but have been largely attributed to the estrogen component of these agents. Although changes in the levels of coagulant factors, anticoagulant proteins, and fibrinolytic markers following the introduction of oral contraceptives are well documented, it remains difficult to explain the observed increased risk of venous thromboembolism when such changes are typically minor and the levels of markers usually remain within the normal range during oral contraceptive use (61,73–77).

Increases in the levels of prothrombin, factor VII, factor VIII, factor X, fibrinogen, and prothrombin fragment 1 + 2 have been documented in women who are using oral contraceptives. Higher elevations of prothrombin and factor VII levels are reported in women taking preparations containing desogestrel than in those taking formulations with levonorgestrel (76). In contrast, factor V levels have been reported to decrease during the use of oral contraceptives (76). Because factor V also exhibits anticoagulant activity by acting as a cofactor in the inactivation of activated factor VIII by activated protein C (78,79), a decrease in factor V level may

contribute to the thrombotic effects of oral contraceptives. This decrease in concentration may be also one of the mechanisms of acquired resistance to activated protein C that develops in women using oral contraceptives. Because acquired resistance to protein C should have a similar hemostatic effect as factor $V_{Leiden}$, it is likely an important mechanism in the thrombotic potential of oral contraceptives (80,81). Studies have also suggested that third-generation formulations are associated with a greater acquired resistance to protein C than second-generation products (82–84); however, there is some debate about the validity of the measurements (85).

Current evidence suggests that overall fibrinolytic activity is unchanged during oral contraceptive use. Enhancement of fibrinolytic activity, as reflected by changes in the levels of plasminogen, tissue plasminogen activator, plasminogen activator inhibitor type 1 (PAI-1), plasmin–antiplasmin complexes, and D-dimer appears to be balanced by downregulation of fibrinolysis by the increased activation of thrombin-activated fibrinolysis inhibitor (TAFI) (75,86). The effects of contraceptives on fibrinolytic parameters also appears to be largely independent of the type of progestagen (86).

Recently, differential changes in the proteins involved in the protein C anticoagulant pathway were shown to contribute to the difference in thrombotic effects between the second- and third-generation oral contraceptives (68,74,81–83). Compared with levonorgestrel, desogestrel-containing oral contraceptive significantly decreased protein S level and increased activated protein C resistance. Therefore, it appears that in combined oral contraceptives, progestagens counteract the thrombotic effect of the estrogen component and desogestrel is less antithrombotic than levonorgestrel. This effect was most pronounced in carriers of factor $V_{Leiden}$ (68).

## Thrombophilia and Oral Contraceptive

It is well established that inherited thrombophilia is associated with increased risk of venous thromboembolism. However, reliable estimates are not available about the risk of a first venous thrombosis in asymptomatic women with inherited thrombophilia who use oral contraceptives (87). Also, there are no reliable data on the risk of recurrent thrombosis in users with inherited thrombophilia who have a personal history of venous thrombosis. According to case–control studies, the risk of a first episode of venous thrombosis among women with inherited thrombophilia who are users of oral contraceptives is approximately 20- to 30-fold higher than among nonusers with thrombophilia and users without thrombophilia (88,89). Women with inherited thrombophilia also tend to develop venous thromboembolism within the first year of use (31), highlighting their predisposition to thrombotic events when additional risk factors are present.

The low prevalence of natural anticoagulant deficiencies (i.e., antithrombin, protein C, and protein S) has made it difficult to determine the exact risk of venous thromboembolism in affected women who use oral contraceptives, but multiple case reports and family studies have indicated that the risk is particularly high in these women (90–92). More data are available for the risk of venous thromboembolism in users of oral contraceptives who have the factor $V_{Leiden}$ mutation. The Leiden Thrombophilia Study (LETS) was the first population-based case–control study to report on this interaction (19). This study found that whereas the risk of venous thromboembolism is fourfold higher in users than in nonusers of oral contraceptives who do not have factor $V_{Leiden}$ mutation, and the risk is eightfold higher in heterozygous carriers of factor $V_{Leiden}$ mutation who do not use oral contraceptives, the risk of venous thromboembolism is 35-fold higher in heterozygous carriers of factor $V_{Leiden}$ who use second-generation oral contraceptives (19). These findings suggest that there is a synergistic or multiplicative interaction between these conditions. Further studies have confirmed the synergistic effect although the risk estimates vary to a small extent (88,89,93,94). For current users of oral contraceptives who are homozygous for factor $V_{Leiden}$ or are double heterozygous for combined defects, the risk is estimated to be 80-fold higher (89,95). In an analysis of data from case–control studies, the pooled odds ratio for venous thromboembolism has been found to be 10.3 among users of oral contraceptives who are heterozygous or homozygous carriers of factor $V_{Leiden}$, as compared with 2.3 among users who are not carriers (96). Accordingly, given the average incidence of venous thromboembolism among women of reproductive age who do not use oral contraceptives is approximately five per 100,000 per year (13,16,17), the number of women per year who would have a thromboembolic event if they were using oral contraceptives (number needed to harm) is 2,222 for carriers of factor $V_{Leiden}$ and 20,000 for noncarriers (71). Recent studies have also shown that reduced sensitivity to activated protein C in the absence of factor $V_{Leiden}$ also interacts synergistically with oral contraceptives to increase the risk of venous thrombosis (97).

For users of oral contraceptive with the prothrombin gene mutation, the risk of venous thromboembolism is increased by 20-fold compared with nonusers and noncarriers (89,98–100). An elevated risk has also been observed in oral contraceptive users who have elevated prothrombin levels but who are not carriers of the mutation (101).

Despite the increased risk of venous thromboembolism in women with thrombophilic defects, routine screening for thrombophilia is not indicated in those who are considering oral contraceptive use. On the basis of the estimated incidence of venous thrombosis and the case fatality rate of a thrombotic event, approximately 400,000 women must be screened in order to detect 20,000 factor $V_{Leiden}$ carriers, all of whom would need to be denied oral contraception in order to prevent one death (102); an even greater number of patients would have to be screened and denied the use of pills for the other thrombophilic defects with lower prevalence. Moreover, the presence of an inherited thrombophilia does not absolutely predict the presence of thrombosis and the absence of an identifiable molecular or biochemical thrombophilic state does not provide absolute protection against thrombosis. Cost-effectiveness analyses also have concluded that universal screening is not warranted (103,104). Finally, the psychosocial, medical, insurance, and legal consequences of knowing one has genetic thrombophilic defect also argue against unselected thrombophilia screening.

## Management of Venous Thromboembolism Associated with Oral Contraceptive Use

Standard therapy is recommended for the treatment of venous thromboembolism associated with oral contraceptive use. Usually, heparin is started at the time of diagnosis along with a vitamin K antagonist for secondary prophylaxis. Unfractionated or low-molecular-weight heparin is given for a minimum of 5 days and until the international normalized ratio (INR) has reached therapeutic levels (105). Warfarin, the most common coumarin agent used in the United States, is usually given for a minimum of 3 months, during which laboratory monitoring of the INR is required to maintain a therapeutic target level between 2.0 and 3.0. Because oral contraceptives are considered a transient or temporary risk factor for venous thromboembolism, a longer duration of anticoagulant therapy may not be necessary if hormonal contraception is discontinued. Although it has been shown that extended therapy with an anticoagulant will reduce the risk of recurrent venous thromboembolism in patients with idiopathic thrombosis (106–108), it is unclear whether these studies included women who had developed thrombosis while taking oral contraceptives. Also, it is unknown whether the risk of recurrent venous thromboembolism outweighs the potential harm of extended anticoagulation, particularly in this patient group in whom the risk of teratogenicity secondary to warfarin must be considered. Longer duration of anticoagulant therapy may be indicated in patients with larger thrombus burdens (e.g., extensive iliofemoral thrombosis) or pulmonary embolism, but studies have not been performed to identify the optimal duration of anticoagulant therapy in these patients.

Although oral contraceptives should be discontinued following the diagnosis of venous thromboembolism, it is important for the patient to use an alternative form of reliable contraception while on warfarin because of the teratogenicity of vitamin K antagonists (109,110). Ideally, nonhormonal forms of contraception should be used. However, for patients who choose to, or have no option but to, remain on hormonal forms of contraception, it is important to maintain the INR in the mid to high therapeutic range in order to avoid subtherapeutic levels. Switching to a progestin-only preparation may also be considered because they have less effect on hemostatic markers (72), but there is insufficient evidence to support that these agents are associated with a lower risk of recurrent venous thromboembolism compared with combined oral contraceptives.

# HORMONE THERAPY

Natural menopause occurs when ovarian hormone secretion of endogenous estrogens and progesterone diminishes. As a result, menopausal symptoms largely reflect the effects of estrogen deficiency, including vasomotor flushes, vaginal dryness, and urinary symptoms. Postmenopausal women are also at a higher risk for osteoporosis and coronary heart disease compared to age-matched women who are not menopausal. Consequently, it has been assumed that treatment with exogenous forms of ovarian steroid hormones will eliminate or at least diminish menopausal symptoms, as well as protect aging women against vascular disease and accelerated bone loss. Although the simplicity of this hypothesis is very attractive and constructively valid, the complexity and our limited understanding of the physiology of estrogens and progestins, particularly at the target cellular level, have produced confusing results and false conclusions from clinical studies of hormone therapy (111–113).

Hormonal therapy has been in common use for more than 30 years. By 1995, approximately 38% of postmenopausal women in the United States were taking some form of hormonal regimen (114). The most frequently prescribed regimen in North America is continuous oral conjugated equine estrogen (CEE) with or without a progestin component. Transdermal and subcutaneous formulations are also available. In addition to providing amelioration of menopausal symptoms, these estrogen–progestin products were found to provide protection against coronary heart disease and osteoporosis in observational studies (115–117) and, therefore, were thought to offer overall health benefits to all postmenopausal women (118). Compelling findings from animal models and hormone-induced changes in hemostatic markers from laboratory studies also supported these results. Physicians in general had largely accepted this favorable profile and were consequently treating many of their postmenopausal women with hormonal therapy on a long-term basis for the prevention of coronary heart disease and osteoporosis, rather than on a short-term basis for the amelioration of menopausal symptoms.

However, recent large-scale randomized clinical trials, the Heart and Estrogen/progestins Replacement Study (HERS and HERS II) (119,120) and the Women's Health Initiative (WHI) (121,122), have raised serious concerns about the true risks and benefits of hormonal therapy. These well-designed, placebo-controlled trials demonstrated that hormone therapy is associated with an increased risk for cardiovascular disease in women taking continuous estrogen and combined regimens. In the HERS trial, postmenopausal women with established coronary heart disease were randomized to receive combined therapy (i.e., CEE plus medroxyprogesterone acetate) or placebo (119). The results showed an increased incidence in coronary heart disease and nonfatal myocardial infarction during the first year of the trial. The WHI comprised two large, randomized, placebo-controlled trials designed to evaluate the cardiac and vascular effects of combined estrogen-progestin in postmenopausal women and estrogen-only therapy in those who had undergone hysterectomy (121,122). Both components were terminated prematurely because the overall health risk was found to outweigh the benefits of treatment. The estrogen–progestin versus placebo trial, which involved more than 16,000 women, was stopped in 2002 when increased incidence of breast cancer and cardiovascular complications (coronary heart disease, stroke, and venous thromboembolism) were observed (see Table 84-3) (121). In the estrogen-only versus placebo trial, almost 11,000 women were enrolled when it was discontinued in March 2004 owing to a small increase in the risk of stroke (see Table 84-4) (122). In contrast to the estrogen–progestin trial, no increase in breast cancer or coronary heart disease was observed. Although a risk reduction was seen for fractures in both trials, it was deemed that the overall risks of hormonal therapy outweighed the benefits. Consequently, there has been a dramatic drop in the use of hormone therapy since the publication of these studies (123), and it has been recommended that clinicians stop prescribing hormone therapy for long-term use (refer to the NIH Web site: www.nhlbi.nih.gov/whi/) (121). International trials studying other potential benefits of hormone therapy (e.g., cognitive function and quality of life) are ongoing currently (124).

It is uncertain why the HERS and WHI trials have provided the opposite conclusion compared with previous observational studies about the cardiovascular effects of hormone therapy. Methodologic limitation of cohort studies is likely

only one of the reasons (125). Other possibilities include differences in patient population and selection (including the "healthy user" bias) (126) and in duration of estrogen deficiency. In addition, it is important to keep in mind that the absolute risks of arterial and venous vascular effects, as well as other metabolic influences, are likely dependent upon the specific steroid, dose, route and sequence of administration such that the results of the HERS and WHI studies might not be generalized broadly from the specific regimens tested in these trials to potential effects of other treatment protocols. However, further studies are required to address this issue (127).

## TABLE 84-3

RESULTS FROM THE WOMEN'S HEALTH INITIATIVE: CONJUGATED EQUINE ESTROGEN AND MEDROXYPROGESTERONE (CEE/P) VERSUS PLACEBO IN POSTMENOPAUSAL WOMEN

| Outcomes | HR | 95% CI | Attributable risk/ 10,000 person-yrs with CEE/P |
|---|---|---|---|
| Coronary heart disease | 1.29 | 1.02–1.63 | 7 more |
| Stroke | 1.41 | 1.07–1.85 | 8 more |
| Venous thromboembolism | 2.11 | 1.58–2.82 | 18 more |
| Pulmonary embolism | 2.13 | 1.39–3.25 | 8 more |
| Invasive breast cancer | 1.26 | 1.00–1.59 | 8 more |
| Colorectal cancer | 0.63 | 0.43–0.92 | 6 fewer |
| Hip fracture | 0.66 | 0.45–0.98 | 5 fewer |

CEE/P, conjugated equine estrogen and medroxyprogesterone; HR, hazard ratio; CI, confidence interval.
Rossouw JE, Anderson GL, Prentice RL, et al. Risks and benefits of estrogen plus progestin in healthy postmenopausal women: principal results from the women's health initiative randomized controlled trial. *JAMA* 2002;288(3):321–333.

## TABLE 84-4

RESULTS FROM THE WOMEN'S HEALTH INITIATIVE: CONJUGATED EQUINE ESTROGEN (CEE) VERSUS PLACEBO IN POSTMENOPAUSAL WOMEN WITH HYSTERECTOMY

| Outcomes | HR | 95% CI | Absolute risk difference/ 10,000 person-yrs with CEE |
|---|---|---|---|
| Coronary heart disease | 0.91 | 0.75–1.12 | 5 fewer |
| Stroke | 1.39 | 1.10–1.77 | 12 more |
| Venous thromboembolism | 1.34 | 0.87–2.06 | 7 more |
| Invasive breast cancer | 0.77 | 0.59–1.01 | 7 fewer |
| Colorectal cancer | 1.08 | 0.75–1.55 | No difference |
| Hip fracture | 0.61 | 0.41–0.91 | 6 fewer |

CEE, conjugated equine estrogen; HR, hazard ratio; CI, confidence interval.
Anderson GL, Limacher M, Assaf AR, et al. Effects of conjugated equine estrogen in postmenopausal women with hysterectomy: the women's health initiative randomized controlled trial. *JAMA* 2004;291(14):1701–1712.

## Hormone Therapy and Venous Thromboembolism

One of the common vascular complications of hormone therapy is venous thromboembolism. On the basis of observational studies, the risk estimates associated with CEE with or without progestins range from 1.7-fold to 3.5-fold (128–131). Although some studies have not found an increased risk of venous thromboembolism associated with hormonal therapy (132), the recent HERS trial found a statistically significant threefold higher risk (relative hazard, 2.66; 95% CI, 1.41 to 5.04; $P = 0.003$) of a first episode of deep vein thrombosis and pulmonary embolism in postmenopausal women with established coronary disease who were randomized to receive 0.625 mg of conjugated estrogen and 2.5 mg of medroxyprogesterone compared to those receiving placebo (119). Confirmed venous thromboembolic events occurred in 34 women in the hormone group (6.3 per 1,000 woman-years) versus 12 women in the placebo group (2.2 per 1,000 woman-years) during 4 years of follow-up. The risk remained elevated throughout the follow-up period but appeared highest during the first year of use. Extended follow-up of the participants in the HERS study (HERS II) show a continued elevated risk of venous thromboembolism, although the relative hazard was lower between 4 and 6 years of therapy, with the value being 1.4 (95% CI, 0.64 to 3.05) (120). Similarly, the WHI found an absolute excess risk of eight more episodes of pulmonary embolism per 10,000 women taking CEE and medroxyprogesterone (121). The risk of venous thromboembolism was twofold higher in women taking hormone therapy, with 34 per 10,000 person-years in the hormone group versus 16 per 10,000 person-years in the placebo group developing symptomatic thrombotic events (hazard ratio, 2.11; 95% CI, 1.58 to 2.82). As found in the HERS/HERS II studies, the increased risk continues throughout the period of hormone use but appears to diminish over time. In postmenopausal women who had undergone hysterectomy who were taking conjugated estrogen, the WHI found seven more episodes of pulmonary embolism per 10,000 women, although the relative hazard was not statistically significant (hazard ratio, 1.34; 95% CI, 0.87 to 2.06) after an average of 6.8 years of follow-up (122).

## Selective Estrogen Receptor Modulators

As the term suggests, selective estrogen receptor modulators (SERM) are estrogenlike compounds having selective estrogen effects that depend on the specific interaction between the ligand and receptors among different cell types (113). The prototype agent of this class of drugs is tamoxifen, which functions as an estrogen antagonist in the breast but as an agonist in bone and the uterus (133). Like estrogen, tamoxifen is associated with an increased risk of venous thromboembolism. On the basis of data from randomized controlled trials in women receiving adjuvant therapy for breast cancer, tamoxifen increases the risk of venous thrombosis by approximately threefold to fourfold (134,135). This risk is higher in postmenopausal women and in those who are also receiving combination chemotherapy (136–140). With tamoxifen, the incidence of venous thromboembolism is approximately 1% to 2% in women with early stage disease and may be up to 10% in those with advanced disease who are also receiving chemotherapy (134–138). Of note, cases of superficial thrombophlebitis were also considered as a thrombotic event in these studies. The National Surgical Adjuvant Breast and Bowel Project P-1 Study (141) and the International Breast Cancer Intervention Study (IBIS-1) (142) also demonstrated that tamoxifen increases the risk of venous thromboembolism

by twofold in healthy women who have a high risk for developing breast cancer. In these studies, the absolute risk of venous thrombosis was 0.2% per year on tamoxifen and 0.1% per year on placebo. The thrombotic risk associated with tamoxifen will likely have less clinical impact in the future because an alternative is now available for treatment of hormone-sensitive breast cancer. Aromatase inhibitors, which were shown recently to be more effective than tamoxifen (143,144) and which improve disease-free survival (145) in postmenopausal women with estrogen receptor–positive breast cancer, are associated with approximately 50% of the risk of venous thromboembolism at less than 1% per year (143–145). Although there is still limited clinical experience with these agents, they are likely to replace tamoxifen in several treatment settings, especially in women with a history of venous thromboembolism.

Raloxifene is an SERM recommended for prevention of osteoporosis. According to the Multiple Outcomes of Raloxifene Evaluation (MORE) trial (146), in which 7,700 postmenopausal women were randomized to receive raloxifene or placebo, raloxifene-treated patients were three times more likely to develop venous thromboembolism (relative risk, 3.1; 95% CI, 1.5 to 6.2), with an incidence of 1% after 40 months of follow-up. Consequently, raloxifene, similar to hormone therapy, is relatively contraindicated for the treatment of osteoporosis in women with a prior history of venous thromboembolism.

## Mechanisms of Hypercoagulability

Changes in coagulation and hemostatic markers are well documented in postmenopausal women on oral estrogen or combined hormone therapy. The results, however, have been inconsistent among studies, most of which are small and included selected patients (147). As a result, the mechanisms of hypercoagulability remain poorly understood. Previously, a reduction in PAI-1 levels had been interpreted as a marker of enhanced fibrinolysis and had been used to explain the cardioprotective effects of hormone therapy (148,149). On the basis of the results of the HERS and WHI studies, it is likely that such a change is reflective of the hypercoagulable state induced by hormones rather than of a protective mechanism for arterial disease. Increases in prothrombin fragment 1 + 2 and fibrinopeptide A, indicating increased thrombin generation, have also been reported with hormone therapy (150,151). In addition, hormone-induced suppression of antithrombin, protein S, and tissue factor pathway inhibitor levels might contribute to the hypercoagulable state (151–153). Furthermore, hormone therapy has been found to increase resistance to activated protein C (or increase the normalized activated protein C sensitivity ratio) (154–156) as well as C-reactive protein (157). Although recent studies have found that transdermal estrogen preparations are associated with no or minimal changes in coagulation activation markers or C-reactive protein (153,155–158), it remains uncertain whether they are associated with a lower risk of thrombosis compared to traditional oral agents. Well-designed laboratory studies are needed to investigate the thrombogenic mechanisms of hormone therapy.

## Thrombophilia and Hormone Therapy

Observational studies have provided evidence that women with thrombophilia have a particularly high risk of venous thromboembolism when exposed to hormone therapy (159–161). In the Oxford hospital-based case–control study of 77 women with a first episode of venous thrombosis, those who had factor

$V_{Leiden}$ or prothrombin 20210A gene mutation and those who used hormone therapy had a 15-fold increased risk (odds ratio, 15.5; 95% CI, 3.1 to 77) compared with controls (159). The risk was highest during the first year of hormone use. This observation is consistent with a nested case–control study from the HERS trial, which found that women with factor $V_{Leiden}$ who were randomized to hormone therapy had a 14-fold risk of venous thrombosis (odds ratio, 14.1; 95% CI, 2.7 to 72.4) compared to women without the mutation who were taking placebo. This finding corresponds to an estimated absolute incidence of venous thromboembolism of 15.4 per 1,000 person-years compared with 2.0 per 1,000 person-years (160). These results are not surprising given the synergistic interaction observed between oral contraceptive use and thrombophilia (87).

## Management of Venous Thromboembolism and Hormone Therapy

With the current knowledge of the risks of hormone therapy from the HERS and WHI trials, it is anticipated that fewer women will be exposed to hormone therapy and, consequently, the incidence of venous thromboembolism associated with hormone therapy will diminish. In women who still opt for therapy to control severe menopausal symptoms, those with a history of venous thromboembolism should be strongly discouraged because of the marked increase in the risk of recurrent thrombosis (162), in addition to the other adverse effects observed in the WHI studies. In these women, transdermal forms of hormone therapy have been suggested to be a reasonable alternative to traditional oral agents on the basis of the differences in pharmacology of these products. Because transdermal preparations avoid the supraphysiologic concentrations of estrogen that is delivered to the liver with oral formulations, the hemostatic and metabolic consequences that can lead to arterial and venous thrombotic events are attenuated (113,153,155–158). Whether these differences in laboratory parameters translate to a lower risk of clinical events for transdermal therapy, however, remains uncertain, and the safety and efficacy of different hormonal therapies have not been directly compared in large clinical trials (127).

In women who develop acute venous thromboembolism in the setting of hormone therapy, standard treatment with heparin followed by vitamin K antagonist is recommended. Patients should be treated with anticoagulant therapy for a minimum of 3 months and hormone therapy should be discontinued. The risk of recurrence is likely to be slightly above background if the patient receives adequate anticoagulant therapy and future hormone exposure is avoided. Limited but methodologically sound data do suggest that women with previous venous thromboembolism have an increased risk of recurrent thrombosis on subsequent hormone therapy at 8.5% per year, as compared with 1.1% per year in placebo controls (162).

# PREGNANCY AND PUERPERIUM

## Incidence and Risk Factors

Pregnancy is an independent risk factor for deep vein thrombosis and pulmonary embolism and is associated with a five-fold to sixfold higher risk of venous thromboembolism than age-matched nonpregnant women (163,164). Approximately one in 1,000 deliveries are complicated by pregnancy-associated venous thrombosis, and one in 1,000 women develop thrombosis in the postpartum period, making venous thromboembolic disease the leading cause of morbidity and mortality during pregnancy and puerperium (165). However, the exact risk of venous thromboembolism in an individual pregnant woman also depends on other risk factors, including age (older than 35 years), weight [body mass index (BMI) >29 kg per m$^2$], parity (four or more pregnancies), mode of delivery (cesarean), and presence of any inherited thrombophilia or a personal or family history of venous thromboembolism (see Table 84-5) (165–170). Although these are commonly accepted risk factors for venous thromboembolism in pregnancy, supportive evidence is weak and sparse. Almost 90% of thrombosis

---

**TABLE 84-5**

### COMMON RISK FACTORS FOR VENOUS THROMBOEMBOLISM IN PREGNANCY

| Patient factors | Pregnancy/Obstetric factors |
|---|---|
| Age more than 35 years | Ovarian hyperstimulation |
| Obesity (BMI >29 kg/m$^2$) in early pregnancy | Cesarean section, particularly as an emergency in labor |
| Thrombophilia | Complicated vaginal delivery |
| Past history of VTE (especially if idiopathic or thrombophilia associated) | Major obstetric hemorrhage |
| Gross varicose veins | Multiparity (four or more deliveries) |
| Significant current medical problems (e.g., nephritic syndrome) | Hyperemesis gravidarum |
| Current infection or inflammatory process (e.g., active inflammatory bowel disease or urinary tract infection) | Preeclampsia |
| Immobility (e.g., bed rest or lower limb fracture) | |
| Paraplegia | |
| Recent long-distance travel | |
| Dehydration | |
| Intravenous drug abuse | |

BMI, body mass index; VTE, venous thromboembolism.

occurs in the left leg, possibly because during pregnancy the left iliac vein is compressed by the overlying right iliac and ovarian arteries only on the left side of the pelvis (171,172). This anatomical arrangement may also explain the higher incidence of iliofemoral thrombosis during pregnancy compared with that in the nonpregnant patients, but the exact cause is unknown (166).

## Mechanisms of Hypercoagulability

Hypercoagulability in pregnancy is attributed to hemostatic changes that lead to activation of coagulation, a gravid uterus, and vessel wall changes that enhance venous stasis, as well as mechanical trauma to pelvic vessels during delivery which results in endothelial damage (165,166,173). Furthermore, inherited thrombophilia appears to play a more prominent role in pregnancy-associated venous thromboembolism and in recurrent fetal loss than in other clinical situations (174,175).

Activation of coagulation during pregnancy is well documented. The levels of multiple coagulant factors are elevated, including factor XII, factor X, factor IX, factor VIII, factor VII, factor V, von Willebrand antigen, and ristocetin cofactor. Fibrinogen level is particularly heightened and is doubled by term (176–178). These changes enhance thrombin generation, as indicated by high levels of prothrombin fragment 1 + 2, thrombin–antithrombin complex, fibrinopeptide A, and D-dimer (179,180), and are reflected by shortening of the prothrombin time and partial thromboplastin time (181). Also, platelets are activated as measured by platelet factor 4 levels (182), but the platelet count may decrease moderately, particularly during the third trimester when benign gestational thrombocytopenia develops as a result of increased consumption of platelets in the uteroplacental unit and expansion of the maternal plasma volume (183). Pregnant women also develop a suppression of the natural anticoagulant pathways, as indicated by an acquired resistance to activated protein C (184), a decrease in free protein S levels (178), as well as increases in the levels of thrombomodulin (185) and tissue factor pathway inhibitor (186). Enhanced inhibition of fibrinolysis occurs as a result of markedly increased levels of PAI-1 from endothelial cells and PAI-2 from the placenta (177,184,187,188). TAFI increases moderately during pregnancy but D-dimer levels also increases progressively with each trimester (189), suggesting that fibrin formation is elevated during pregnancy and that fibrinolysis is not shut down.

Venous stasis occurs by the end of the first trimester because of enlargement of vessel diameter and reduced flow (190–192). This is followed by a gradual and progressive reduction in venous flow to approximately 50% of normal flow by 25 to 29 weeks gestation, reaching a nadir at 36 weeks (193). Flow then returns to normal by 6 weeks after delivery (168). These vascular changes are presumed to be due to hormonal influence but the exact physiology remains unclear.

Endothelial damage of pelvic vessels is also thought to contribute to the hypercoagulability in pregnancy. However, there is little evidence, if any, to support this. During normal pregnancy, injury to the pelvic vessels should be minimal. In the puerperium, venous thromboembolism may occur as a result of vessel damage from the trauma of vaginal delivery or caesarean section. It has also been suggested that the risk of venous thromboembolism is higher in emergency than in elective cesarean cases (165).

## Thrombophilia and Venous Thromboembolism in Pregnancy

Approximately 50% of all episodes of venous thromboembolism in pregnancy occur in women with hereditary thrombophilia (194) and this is proportionally higher than in other clinical situations, likely because women of reproductive age have few other risk factors for thrombosis.

The risk of venous thromboembolism in pregnant women with inherited thrombophilia varies depending on the type of abnormality and the presence of other risk factors; however, reliable data on the true incidence is not available because most of the studies have been small and retrospective and have used selected populations. On the basis of retrospective studies in symptomatic kindreds, it has been estimated that the incidence of venous thromboembolism during pregnancy is 32% to 44% in those with antithrombin deficiency, 3% to 10% for protein C deficiency and 0% to 6% for protein S deficiency, and 14% for factor $V_{Leiden}$ deficiency (195–197). However, these incidences may be overestimates because these studies targeted women in symptomatic families, who may have a higher risk of venous thromboembolism for other reasons. Other retrospective and case–control studies have estimated the incidence of thrombosis during pregnancy and puerperium have ranged from 0.2% to 36% among carriers of antithrombin deficiency, 0.1% to 0.9% for those with protein C deficiency, 0.1% to 0.2% among carriers of factor $V_{Leiden}$, and 0.3% to 0.5% in carriers of prothrombin gene mutation (170,198,199).

In a case–control study of 119 women with a first episode of venous thromboembolism during pregnancy, Gerhardt et al. found that factor $V_{Leiden}$ was present in 43.7% of these women and prothrombin mutation was found in 16.9% (198). The relative risk for thrombosis in pregnancy after adjusting for other variables was 6.9 (95% CI, 3.3 to 15.2) for heterozygous carriers of factor $V_{Leiden}$, 9.5 (95% CI, 2.1 to 66.7) for heterozygous carriers of prothrombin mutation, 10.4 (95% CI, 2.2 to 62.5) for those with antithrombin deficiency, and 2.2 (95% CI, 0.8 to 6.1) for those with protein C deficiency (198). In another case–control study, Martinelli et al. reported the relative risk of thrombosis was 10.6 (95% CI, 5.6 to 20.4) for heterozygous carriers of factor $V_{Leiden}$, 2.9 (95% CI, 1.0 to 8.6) for heterozygous carriers of prothrombin mutation, and 13.1 (95% CI, 5.0 to 34.2) for those with antithrombin, protein C, or protein S deficiency (200). In general, the risk of venous thromboembolism in these affected women is even higher in the postpartum period, but reliable estimates are not available (195, 196,201).

## Management of Venous Thromboembolism in Pregnancy

### Screening for Thrombophilia

Despite the heightened risk of venous thromboembolism in women with congenital thrombophilia, there is no evidence to support routine screening of all pregnant women for these defects (169,194,199). There is also no evidence or consensus on the need for screening in women with a family history of thrombosis or thrombophilia but who have no personal history of venous thromboembolism. However, there is expert consensus that screening is reasonable in pregnant women who have had documented venous thromboembolism so that antepartum and postpartum prophylaxis could be offered if a thrombophilic condition is detected (see Table 84-6) (194,202,203). Whether screening and subsequent intervention will significantly reduce the risk of recurrent thrombosis and, most importantly, fatal pulmonary embolism, has not been studied.

### Prophylaxis in High-Risk Patients

Evidence is lacking on which to base recommendations for thromboprophylaxis during pregnancy and early postpartum period (204). Current guidelines are largely based on expert

## TABLE 84-6

THROMBOPHILIA TESTING IN PREGNANT WOMEN WITH A PREVIOUS HISTORY OF VENOUS THROMBOEMBOLISM

Antithrombin deficiency
Protein C deficiency
Protein S deficiency
Activated protein C resistance (factor $V_{Leiden}$ testing if positive)
Prothrombin G20210A mutation
Lupus anticoagulant

opinion, and the available data have come from small clinical trials. Therefore, not surprisingly, the role of antepartum prophylaxis in women with a previous history of venous thromboembolism remains controversial. Although these women are considered to have an increased risk for venous thromboembolism during pregnancy, accurate risk estimates of recurrent thrombosis in these women are not available. Retrospective studies have reported recurrence rates of 11% to 12% per year (205,206). The most reliable data come from a prospective cohort study by Brill-Edwards et al. (202). In this study that followed 125 pregnant women who had a single previous episode of venous thromboembolism and no known thrombophilia, 2.4% of them (4.0% per patient-year of follow-up) experienced antepartum recurrence of venous thromboembolism. These events occurred exclusively in the 51 women who tested positive for thrombophilia or had a previous episode of idiopathic thrombosis, thereby corresponding to a recurrence risk of 5.9% (95% CI, 1.2% to 16.2%). In contrast, none of the 44 women (95% CI, 0.0% to 8.0%) without thrombophilia and whose previous episode of venous thromboembolism was secondary to a transient risk factor had recurrent thrombosis. On the basis of these results, the investigators concluded that the risk of recurrent antepartum venous thromboembolism is low and that routine antepartum prophylaxis is not warranted. However, they recommended thrombophilia testing for women with previous venous thromboembolism so that those testing positive could be offered a choice of heparin prophylaxis or clinical follow-up.

Other experts also concur that routine prophylaxis antepartum is not warranted in all pregnant women with a history of thrombosis (169,199,203), but others do recommend prophylaxis throughout pregnancy for these women (207). Clearly, further studies are needed to help tailor prophylaxis in patients with previous episode of venous thrombosis. On the basis of the evidence to date, my approach for prophylaxis is outlined in Table 84-7. Briefly, thrombophilia testing is not necessary in women with a history of unprovoked or recurrent thromboembolism, or thrombosis that occurred during hormone exposure, because prophylaxis is recommended. Women who had a thrombotic event that was secondary to a transient major risk factor should be offered thrombophilia testing because the recommendation for prophylaxis depends on the outcome of the tests. Prophylaxis may be appropriate in certain settings in women without a history of venous thromboembolism but with known underlying thrombophilia. Others have proposed different recommendations (169,199,207). In all cases, it is of utmost importance to discuss the known risks and benefits with each woman so that management is individualized on the basis of an informed decision and her personal values.

Studies have not been performed to evaluate the need for prophylaxis in women with thrombophilia who do not have a personal history of venous thromboembolism. Extrapolating from the results from the study of Brill-Edwards et al., routine prophylaxis is likely not indicated because the risk of a first episode of thrombosis in these asymptomatic women is likely less than 5%.

All women with a history of venous thromboembolism, independent of their thrombophilia status, should receive at least 6 weeks of postpartum prophylaxis because the risk of thrombosis is highest and the risks associated with anticoagulant use are low for mother and neonate during this period (203,208).

### Treatment of Acute Venous Thromboembolism

Unfractionated and low-molecular-weight heparins, heparinoids, and coumarin derivatives have been evaluated and used for prevention and treatment of venous thromboembolism in pregnant women (209). Direct thrombin inhibitors and fondaparinux are able to cross the placenta and have not been evaluated. The

## TABLE 84-7

RECOMMENDATIONS FOR PROPHYLAXIS IN WOMEN DURING PREGNANCY AND PUERPERIUM

| Previous VTE | Thrombophilia status[a] | Antepartum prophylaxis | Postpartum prophylaxis |
|---|---|---|---|
| Unprovoked or recurrent | Positive | Yes | Yes |
| | Negative | Yes, especially if family history is positive for VTE | Yes |
| Secondary to hormone exposure | Positive | Yes | Yes |
| | Negative | Yes, only if family history is positive for VTE | Yes |
| Secondary to major risk factor | Positive | Consider prophylaxis if antithrombin deficiency or double heterozygosity | Yes |
| | Negative | No | Yes |
| None | Positive | Consider prophylaxis if antithrombin deficiency or double heterozygosity | Consider prophylaxis if antithrombin deficiency or double heterozygosity |
| | Negative | No | No |

VTE, venous thromboembolism.
[a]Including deficiency of antithrombin, protein C, or protein S, factor $V_{Leiden}$, prothrombin G20210A mutation, and lupus anticoagulant.

major concerns about the use of anticoagulant therapy are efficacy of the regimens, maternal and fetal risks, and management around the time of delivery.

Large clinical studies are not available to document the efficacy of heparins for the acute treatment of venous thromboembolism in pregnancy. However, on the basis of prospective cohort studies in pregnant women and vast clinical experience in nonpregnant patients, it can be assumed that unfractionated and low-molecular-weight heparins are efficacious and safe for maternal use (209). Low-molecular-weight heparins are preferred over unfractionated heparin for treatment because their pharmacokinetic properties allow them to be given as once-daily injections with weight-adjusted dosing. It is also associated with a lower risk of osteoporosis and heparin-induced thrombocytopenia compared with unfractionated heparin (210). Like unfractionated heparin, low-molecular-weight heparins also do not cross the placenta. Coumarin derivatives, on the other hand, do cross the placenta and can cause fetal nasal hypoplasia and/or stippled epiphyses if exposure occurs during 6 to 12 weeks of gestation and is associated with central nervous system abnormalities with exposure at any time during the pregnancy (109,110). Hence, low-molecular-weight heparin is the preferred anticoagulant for treatment of venous thromboembolism in pregnant women (209).

What remains uncertain, however, is the optimal dosing schedule of low-molecular-weight heparins in women who are pregnant because these patients are routinely excluded from clinical trials and pharmacoloic studies. Consequently, the pharmacokinetic and pharmacodynamic properties of these agents in pregnancy are largely unknown and they may be influenced by physiologic changes during gestation, such as maternal weight gain and the volume of distribution of low-molecular-weight heparins. A recent study found that anti–factor Xa levels in women receiving prophylactic doses of a low-molecular-weight heparin are significantly lower near term (211), thereby suggesting that dose adjustments during pregnancy may be indicated in order to provide sufficient anticoagulant effects. When laboratory testing of anti–factor Xa levels is readily accessible, blood samples should be drawn at 4 hours after the morning dose of low-molecular-weight heparin at every 1 to 3 months of gestation. The dose should be adjusted to achieve an anti–factor Xa level of 0.5 to 1.2 U per mL for twice-daily dosing and approximately 1.0 to 2.0 U per mL for once-daily injections (203,209). It should be noted, however, that clinical evidence supporting a need for anti–factor Xa monitoring in pregnant women is lacking. Furthermore, there is a paucity of data to show a strong correlation between anti–factor Xa levels and efficacy and safety, even for the general, nonpregnant population (212). If laboratory monitoring is not available, then weight-adjusted doses of low-molecular-weight heparin should be used. Clinical trials are needed to compare these different approaches. For those who choose to use unfractionated heparin, the drug must be given as twice-daily injections and the mid-interval activated partial thromboplastin time (aPTT) must be monitored every 1 to 2 weeks to ensure maintenance of therapeutic levels.

### Peripartum and Postpartum Management of Venous Thromboembolism

Women receiving anticoagulant therapy during pregnancy should undergo planned, elective induction of labor and heparin should be stopped 24 hours prior to induction in order to avoid excessive bleeding during delivery. If spontaneous labor occurs while the mother is fully anticoagulated, then an anti–factor Xa level for low-molecular-weight heparin or an aPTT for unfractionated heparin should be checked. Elevated levels should be corrected with protamine sulfate and epidurals should be avoided if an anticoagulant effect is detectable.

Postpartum anticoagulant therapy can be initiated within 12 hours after an uneventful delivery starting with heparin and followed by a coumarin. Management is comparable to the nonpregnancy setting, and warfarin can be safely given in nursing mothers because a clinical anticoagulant effect is not detectable in breast milk (213). Anticoagulation should be continued for a minimum of 4 weeks after delivery and total treatment should be given for no less than 3 months from the time of diagnosis.

# THROMBOPHILIA AND POOR FETAL OUTCOME

The association between thrombophilia and poor fetal outcome is now well documented (214). Both congenital and acquired types of thrombophilia are found to be overrepresented in cases with recurrent first- and second-trimester miscarriages, intrauterine fetal death, intrauterine growth retardation (IUGR), placental abruption, or preeclampsia. Because these disorders are associated with thrombotic complications of the placental vasculature, it is biologically plausible that thrombophilia is a potential mechanism contributing to the pathophysiology of these conditions (215,216).

## Thrombophilia and Fetal Loss

Approximately 30% of women experience at least one fetal loss and approximately 5% of women of reproductive age experience recurrent fetal loss (217). Although a small number of cases are due to identifiable anatomic, chromosomal, endocrinologic, or immunologic problems in the mother or the fetus, compelling evidence has emerged in the last few years that thrombotic problems underlie a substantial proportion of fetal losses.

On the basis of available evidence from case–control and retrospective cohort studies, women who have a deficiency of antithrombin, protein C, or protein S have a twofold to fivefold risk of spontaneous pregnancy loss compared to women without these defects (218,219). Although there are inconsistencies between studies, available data also suggest that factor $V_{Leiden}$ is associated with a twofold to fourfold risk of fetal loss, particularly in the second or third trimester (219–222). Also, fetuses with factor $V_{Leiden}$ genotype are more susceptible to spontaneous abortion because of placental infarction (223,224). In one case–control study, factor $V_{Leiden}$ was found in 48% of women with more than three consecutive first- or second-trimester miscarriages (225), and a Swedish study showed that 28% of women who are primary habitual aborters have factor $V_{Leiden}$ mutation, as compared with 3% of controls (226). Activated protein C resistance in the absence of factor $V_{Leiden}$ has also been reported to be associated with pregnancy loss (225,227). There are conflicting data on whether other mutations such as prothrombin gene mutation and the methylenetetrahydrofolate reductase C677T mutation are also associated with a higher risk of fetal wastage (217,228,229). However, women with combined defects or those who are homozygous carriers appear to have the highest risk for fetal loss (219,228,230).

Acquired hypercoagulable conditions such as hyperhomocysteinemia and antiphospholipid antibody syndrome are also associated with recurrent fetal loss. In a metaanalysis of 10 case–control studies, Nelen et al. reported a threefold to fourfold increased risk of recurrent fetal loss in women with hyperhomocysteinemia (231). Presence of an anticardiolipin antibody or lupus anticoagulant is also a frequent finding in women with recurrent miscarriages. Approximately 15% of affected women will test positive for these markers, as compared with 3% in unselected women without a history of pregnancy complications (232). The reduced expression of Annexin V, a natural anticoagulant found on placental tissue, has been implicated as the pathogenic mechanism in women with antiphospholipid antibody syndrome (233). More recently, circulating procoagulant microparticles has been reported in approximately 50% of women with unexplained pregnancy losses (234). These microparticles are able to participate in thrombin generation by serving as a catalytic surface for the assembly of tenase and prothrombinase complexes and activating platelets (235,236). It has been suggested that these prothrombotic microparticles may target placental tissue and render it vulnerable to thrombosis but the exact source and role of microparticles remain unclear (175,237).

## Thrombophilia and Obstetrical Vascular Complications

Thrombophilia also appears to have a role in vascular disorders of the placenta, including preeclampsia, abruption, and intrauterine growth restriction. In a case–control study by Kupferminc et al., an eightfold higher prevalence of inherited or acquired thrombophilia (including deficiency of antithrombin, protein C or protein S, factor $V_{Leiden}$, prothrombin gene G20210A mutation, anticardiolipin antibodies, or homozygosity for methylenetetrahydrofolate reductase C677T mutation) was found in women with pregnancy-related vascular complications compared with women with normal pregnancies (238). For those with deficiency of antithrombin, protein C, or protein S, the odds ratio was 9.7, whereas for those with factor $V_{Leiden}$, the odds ratio was 3.7. This estimate is consistent with other observational studies (239–241). A recent systematic review also reported a significant association between preeclampsia and carriers of factor $V_{Leiden}$, prothrombin G21210A mutation, MTHFR C677T homozygosity, and protein C and protein S deficiency, as well as a positive association between abruption and stillbirth with factor $V_{Leiden}$ and anticardiolipin antibodies (242). However, this review is inconsistent with the results of a large, population-based study that did not find an association between preeclampsia and factor $V_{Leiden}$, prothrombin G21210A, or MTHFR C677T in 404 women with a history of preeclampsia compared with controls (243). A large case–control study in 965 newborns also failed to find an increased risk of IUGR among mothers with factor $V_{Leiden}$, prothrombin G20210, or MTHFR C677T (244). The reasons for these discrepant findings are unclear but may reflect differences in diagnostic criteria, small sample size of most studies, patient selection and bias. Further investigations are warranted to clarify the risk of obstetrical vascular complications in association with thrombophilia.

## Management of Thrombophilia and Poor Fetal Outcome

### Screening for Thrombophilia

Currently, there is no data to suggest that screening for thrombophilia in women with recurrent first-trimester fetal loss is justified, but testing has become accepted practice in patients with recurrent pregnancy loss, including a second-trimester miscarriage, a history of an intrauterine death, or women with recurrent intrauterine growth retardation or severe preeclampsia (175,245). Such women testing positive for a thrombophilic defect are often offered antithrombotic therapy although such an approach is not based on evidence from large clinical trials.

### Therapeutic Options

The use of low, fixed-dose, once-daily low-molecular-weight heparin is now common practice to improve fetal outcome in women with recurrent pregnancy loss and gestational vascular complications. However, strong evidence showing efficacy and safety of antithrombotic therapy in these clinical scenarios is lacking because most of the data are from small, uncontrolled series. A small randomized trial by Rai et al. first demonstrated the efficacy of low-dose aspirin and unfractionated heparin 5,000 U twice daily over aspirin alone in improving the live birth rate in 90 women with antiphospholipid antibodies and recurrent miscarriages (246). Since then, empiric therapy with heparins has been used in most women with recurrent pregnancy failures, regardless of the underlying cause. A recent collaborative study in 486 gestations suggested that low-molecular-weight heparin is safe and was associated with a successful pregnancy outcome in 89% of the gestations in women with previous history of preeclampsia (247). A live birth rate of 75% was also reported in 50 women treated with enoxaparin 40 mg once or 40 mg twice daily who have documented heritable thrombophilia and recurrent pregnancy loss, and a historic live birth rate of 20% (248). In this small randomized trial (LIVE-ENOX), no difference in the proportion of live births and no major bleeding complications were observed between the two enoxaparin doses. Although these results are encouraging, there was no concurrent control group to demonstrate efficacy and the sample size was small. Larger clinical trials are needed to establish the efficacy and safety of anticoagulant therapy in this setting and determine the optimal dosage and regimen needed. The use of unfractionated heparin in this setting is largely of historic interest given its higher risk of heparin-induced thrombocytopenia and osteoporosis compared with low-molecular-weight heparin, and the need for twice daily, large-volume injections.

The benefit of aspirin in patients with thrombophilia and gestational vascular complications also remains uncertain. In many women with antiphospholipid antibody syndrome and in those with combined thrombophilia, aspirin is taken along with low-molecular-weight heparin. The efficacy and safety of aspirin alone and in combination with low-molecular-weight heparin require investigation.

# ACKNOWLEDGMENT

Dr. Lee is a recipient of a New Investigator Award from the Canadian Institutes of Health Research/Rx & D Research Program.

## *References*

1. Anderson FA Jr, Wheeler HB, Goldberg RJ, et al. The Worcester DVT Study. A population-based perspective of the hospital incidence and case-fatality rates of deep vein thrombosis and pulmonary embolism. *Arch Intern Med* 1991;151(5):933–938.
2. Nordstrom M, Lindblad B, Bergqvist D, et al. A prospective study of the incidence of deep-vein thrombosis within a defined urban population. *J Intern Med* 1992;232:155–160.
3. WHO Scientific Group. Cardiovascular disease and steroid hormone contraception: report of a WHO Scientific Group. *WHO Tech Rep Ser* 2004; 877:1–89.
4. Fu H, Darroch JE, Haas T et al. National Survey of Family Growth. Contraceptive failure rates: new estimates from the 1995. *Fam Plann Perspect* 1999;31(2):56–63.
5. Burkman R, Schlesselman JJ, Zieman M. Safety concerns and health benefits associated with oral contraception. *Am J Obstet Gynecol* 2004; 190(Suppl. 4):S5–S22.
6. Petitti DB. Clinical practice. Combination estrogen-progestin oral contraceptives. *N Engl J Med* 2003;349(15):1443–1450.
7. Jordan WM. Pulmonary embolism. *Lancet* 1961;2:1146–1147.
8. Vandenbroucke JP, Rosing J, Bloemenkamp KW, et al. Oral contraceptives and the risk of venous thrombosis. *N Engl J Med* 2001;344(20):1527–1535.
9. Rosendaal FR, van HV, Tanis BC, et al. Estrogens, progestogens and thrombosis. *J Thromb Haemost* 2003;1(7):1371–1380.
10. Winkler UH. Blood coagulation and oral contraceptives. A critical review. *Contraception* 1998;57(3):203–209.

11. World Health Organization Collaborative Study of Cardiovascular Disease and Steroid Hormone Contraception. Venous thromboembolic disease and combined oral contraceptives: results of international multicentre case-control study [see comments]. *Lancet* 1995;346(8990):1575–1582.

12. World Health Organization Collaborative Study of Cardiovascular Disease and Steroid Hormone Contraception. Effect of different progestagens in low oestrogen oral contraceptives on venous thromboembolic disease. *Lancet* 1995;346(8990):1582–1588.

13. Jick H, Jick SS, Gurewich V, et al. Risk of idiopathic cardiovascular death and nonfatal venous thromboembolism in women using oral contraceptives with differing progestagen components [see comments]. *Lancet* 1995;346(8990):1589–1593.

14. Bloemenkamp KW, Rosendaal FR, Helmerhorst FM, et al. Enhancement by factor V Leiden mutation of risk of deep-vein thrombosis associated with oral contraceptives containing a third-generation progestagen [see comments]. *Lancet* 1995;346(8990):1593–1596.

15. Spitzer WO, Lewis MA, Heinemann LA et al, Transnational Research Group on Oral Contraceptives and the Health of Young Women. Third generation oral contraceptives and risk of venous thromboembolic disorders: an international case-control study [see comments]. *BMJ* 1996; 312(7023):83–88.

16. Farmer RD, Lawrenson RA, Thompson CR, et al. Population-based study of risk of venous thromboembolism associated with various oral contraceptives. *Lancet* 1997;349(9045):83–88.

17. Hannaford PC, Owen-Smith V. Using epidemiological data to guide clinical practice: review of studies on cardiovascular disease and use of combined oral contraceptives. *BMJ* 1998;316(7136):984–987.

18. Lidegaard O, Edstrom B, Kreiner S. Oral contraceptives and venous thromboembolism. A case-control study. *Contraception* 1998;57(5):291–301.

19. Vandenbroucke JP, Koster T, Briet E, et al. Increased risk of venous thrombosis in oral-contraceptive users who are carriers of factor V Leiden mutation. *Lancet* 1994;344(8935):1453–1457.

20. Bloemenkamp KW, Rosendaal FR, Buller HR, et al. Risk of venous thrombosis with use of current low-dose oral contraceptives is not explained by diagnostic suspicion and referral bias. *Arch Intern Med* 1999; 159(1):65–70.

21. Parkin L, Skegg DC, Wilson M, et al. Oral contraceptives and fatal pulmonary embolism. *Lancet* 2000;355(9221):2133–2134.

22. Lidegaard O, Edstrom B, Kreiner S. Oral contraceptives and venous thromboembolism: a five-year national case-control study. *Contraception* 2002; 65(3):187–196.

23. Tanis BC, van den Bosch MA, Kemmeren JM, et al. Oral contraceptives and the risk of myocardial infarction. *N Engl J Med* 2001;345(25):1787–1793.

24. WHO Collaborative Study of Cardiovascular Disease and Steroid Hormone Contraception. Acute myocardial infarction and combined oral contraceptives: results of an international multicentre case-control study. *Lancet* 1997;349(9060):1202–1209.

25. Kemmeren JM, Tanis BC, van den Bosch MA, et al. Risk of Arterial Thrombosis in Relation to Oral Contraceptives (RATIO) Study: oral contraceptives and the risk of ischemic stroke. *Stroke* 2002;33(5):1202–1208.

26. Carter CJ. The natural history and epidemiology of venous thrombosis. *Prog Cardiovasc Dis* 1994;36(6):423–438.

27. Farmer RD, Lawrenson RA, Todd JC, et al. A comparison of the risks of venous thromboembolic disease in association with different combined oral contraceptives. *Br J Clin Pharmacol* 2000;49(6):580–590.

28. Abdollahi M, Cushman M, Rosendaal FR. Obesity: risk of venous thrombosis and the interaction with coagulation factor levels and oral contraceptive use. *Thromb Haemost* 2003;89(3):493–498.

29. Stampfer MJ, Willett WC, Colditz GA, et al. Past use of oral contraceptives and cardiovascular disease: a meta-analysis in the context of the Nurses' Health Study. *Am J Obstet Gynecol* 1990;163(1 Pt 2):285–291.

30. Hannaford P. Cardiovascular events associated with different combined oral contraceptives: a review of current data. *Drug Saf* 2000;22(5):361–371.

31. Bloemenkamp KW, Rosendaal FR, Helmerhorst FM, et al. Higher risk of venous thrombosis during early use of oral contraceptives in women with inherited clotting defects. *Arch Intern Med* 2000;160(1):49–52.

32. Herings RM, Urquhart J, Leufkens HG. Venous thromboembolism among new users of different oral contraceptives. *Lancet* 1999;354(9173):127–128.

33. Lewis MA, MacRae KD, Kuhl-Habichl D, et al. The differential risk of oral contraceptives: the impact of full exposure history. *Hum Reprod* 1999;14(6):1493–1499.

34. Suissa S, Blais L, Spitzer WO, et al. First-time use of newer oral contraceptives and the risk of venous thromboembolism. *Contraception* 1997; 56(3):141–146.

35. Lewis MA, Heinemann LA, MacRae KD et al. The Transnational Research Group on Oral Contraceptives and the Health of Young Women. The increased risk of venous thromboembolism and the use of third generation progestagens: role of bias in observational research. *Contraception* 1996;54(1):5–13.

36. Burnhill MS. The use of a large-scale surveillance system in planned parenthood federation of America clinics to monitor cardiovascular events in users of combination oral contraceptives. *Int J Fertil Womens Med* 1999; 44(1):19–30.

37. Farmer RD, Lawrenson RA. Oral contraceptives and venous thromboembolic disease: the findings from database studies in the United Kingdom and Germany. *Am J Obstet Gynecol* 1998;179(3 Pt 2):S78–S86.

38. Farmer RD, Williams TJ, Simpson EL, et al. Effect of 1995 pill scare on rates of venous thromboembolism among women taking combined oral contraceptives: analysis of general practice research database. *BMJ* 2000; 321(7259):477–479.

39. Spitzer WO. Bias versus causality: interpreting recent evidence of oral contraceptive studies. *Am J Obstet Gynecol* 1998;179(3 Pt 2):S43–S50.

40. Walker AM. Newer oral contraceptives and the risk of venous thromboembolism. *Contraception* 1998;57(3):169–181.

41. O'Brien PA. The third generation oral contraceptive controversy. The evidence shows they are less safe than second generation pills. *BMJ* 1999; 319(7213):795–796.

42. Hennessy S, Berlin JA, Kinman JL, et al. Risk of venous thromboembolism from oral contraceptives containing gestodene and desogestrel versus levonorgestrel: a meta-analysis and formal sensitivity analysis. *Contraception* 2001;64(2):125–133.

43. Kemmeren JM, Algra A, Grobbee DE. Third generation oral contraceptives and risk of venous thrombosis: meta-analysis. *BMJ* 2001;323(7305): 131–134.

44. Vandenbroucke JP, Bloemenkamp KW, Helmerhorst FM, et al. Mortality from venous thromboembolism and myocardial infarction in young women in the Netherlands. *Lancet* 1996;348(9024):401–402.

45. Dunn N, Thorogood M, Faragher B, et al. Oral contraceptives and myocardial infarction: results of the MICA case-control study. *BMJ* 1999; 318(7198):1579–1583.

46. Heinemann LA, Lewis MA, Thorogood M, et al. Case-control study of oral contraceptives and risk of thromboembolic stroke: results from International Study on Oral Contraceptives and Health of Young Women. *BMJ* 1997;315(7121):1502–1504.

47. Shulman LP, Goldzieher JW. The truth about oral contraceptives and venous thromboembolism. *J Reprod Med* 2003;48(Suppl. 11):930–938.

48. Mishell DR Jr. State of the art in hormonal contraception: an overview. *Am J Obstet Gynecol* 2004;190(Suppl. 4):S1–S4.

49. Burkman RT. The transdermal contraceptive system. *Am J Obstet Gynecol* 2004;190(Suppl. 4):S49–S53.

50. Goldenberg SL, Bruchovsky N. Use of cyproterone acetate in prostate cancer. *Urol Clin North Am* 1991;18(1):111–122.

51. Seaman HE, de Vries CS, Farmer RD. The risk of venous thromboembolism in women prescribed cyproterone acetate in combination with ethinyl estradiol: a nested cohort analysis and case-control study. *Hum Reprod* 2003;18(3):522–526.

52. Vasilakis-Scaramozza C, Jick H. Risk of venous thromboembolism with cyproterone or levonorgestrel contraceptives. *Lancet* 2001;358(9291): 1427–1429.

53. Farmer RD, Lawrenson RA, Todd JC, et al. Oral contraceptives and venous thromboembolic disease. Analyses of the UK general practice research database and the UK Mediplus database. *Hum Reprod Update* 1999;5(6):688–706.

54. Lidegaard O. Absolute and attributable risk of venous thromboembolism in women on combined cyproterone acetate and ethinylestradiol. *J Obstet Gynaecol Can* 2003;25(7):575–577.

55. Spitzer WO. Cyproterone acetate with ethinylestradiol as a risk factor for venous thromboembolism: an epidemiological evaluation. *J Obstet Gynaecol Can* 2003;25(12):1011–1018.

56. van Grootheest K, Vrieling T. Thromboembolism associated with the new contraceptive Yasmin. *BMJ* 2003;326(7383):257.

57. Vaya A, Mira Y, Ferrando F, et al. Transient ischaemic attack associated with the new contraceptive Yasmin. *Thromb Res* 2003;112(1–2):121.

58. Dittrich R, Parker L, Rosen JB, et al. Transdermal contraception: evaluation of three transdermal norelgestromin/ethinyl estradiol doses in a randomized, multicenter, dose-response study. *Am J Obstet Gynecol* 2002; 186(1):15–20.

59. Plourd DM, Rayburn WF. New contraceptive methods. *J Reprod Med* 2003;48(9):665–671.

60. Apgar BS, Greenberg G. Using progestins in clinical practice. *Am Fam Physician* 2000;62(8):1839–1850.

61. Winkler UH, Howie H, Buhler K, et al. A randomized controlled double-blind study of the effects on hemostasis of two progestogen-only pills containing 75 microgram desogestrel or 30 microgram levonorgestrel. *Contraception* 1998;57(6):385–392.

62. Singh K, Viegas OA, Koh SC, et al. Effect of long-term use of norplant implants on haemostatic function. *Contraception* 1992;45(3):203–219.

63. Shaaban MM, Elwan SI, el Kabsh MY, et al. Effect of levonorgestrel contraceptive implants, norplant, on blood coagulation. *Contraception* 1984; 30(5):421–430.

64. Schindler AE. Differential effects of progestins on hemostasis. *Maturitas* 2003;46(Suppl. 1):S31–S37.

65. Kaunitz AM. Injectable contraception. New and existing options. *Obstet Gynecol Clin North Am* 2000;27(4):741–780.

66. Rosano GM, Vitale C, Silvestri A, et al. Metabolic and vascular effect of progestins in post-menopausal women. Implications for cardioprotection. *Maturitas* 2003;46(Suppl. 1):S17–S29.

67. Egberg N, van Beek A, Gunnervik C, et al. Effects on the hemostatic system and liver function in relation to implanon and norplant. A prospective randomized clinical trial. *Contraception* 1998;58(2):93–98.

68. Kemmeren JM, Algra A, Meijers JC, et al. Effect of second- and third-generation oral contraceptives on the protein C system in the absence or

presence of the factor V Leiden mutation: a randomized trial. *Blood* 2004; 103(3): 927–933.

69. World Health Organization Collaborative Study of Cardiovascular Disease and Steroid Hormone Contraception. Cardiovascular disease and use of oral and injectable progestogen-only contraceptives and combined injectable contraceptives. Results of an international, multicenter, case-control study. *Contraception* 1998;57(5):315–324.

70. Vasilakis C, Jick H, Mar Melero-Montes M. Risk of idiopathic venous thromboembolism in users of progestagens alone. *Lancet* 1999; 354(9190): 1610–1611.

71. Petitti DB. Combined estrogen-progestin oral contraceptives. *N Engl J Med* 2004;350:307–308.

72. Frederiksen MC. Depot medroxyprogesterone acetate contraception in women with medical problems. *J Reprod Med* 1996;41(Suppl. 5):414–418.

73. Kluft C, Lansink M. Effect of oral contraceptives on haemostasis variables. *Thromb Haemost* 1997;78(1):315–326.

74. Tans G, Curvers J, Middeldorp S, et al. A randomized cross-over study on the effects of levonorgestrel- and desogestrel-containing oral contraceptives on the anticoagulant pathways. *Thromb Haemost* 2000;84(1):15–21.

75. Meijers JC, Middeldorp S, Tekelenburg W, et al. Increased fibrinolytic activity during use of oral contraceptives is counteracted by an enhanced factor XI-independent down regulation of fibrinolysis: a randomized cross-over study of two low-dose oral contraceptives. *Thromb Haemost* 2000;84(1):9–14.

76. Middeldorp S, Meijers JC, van den Ende AE, et al. Effects on coagulation of levonorgestrel- and desogestrel-containing low dose oral contraceptives: a cross-over study. *Thromb Haemost* 2000;84(1):4–8.

77. Samsioe G. Coagulation and anticoagulation effects of contraceptive steroids. *Am J Obstet Gynecol* 1994;170(5 Pt 2):1523–1527.

78. Shen L, Dahlback B. Factor V and protein S as synergistic cofactors to activated protein C in degradation of factor VIIIa. *J Biol Chem* 1994; 269(23):18735–18738.

79. Varadi K, Rosing J, Tans G, et al. Factor V enhances the cofactor function of protein S in the APC-mediated inactivation of factor VIII: influence of the factor VR506Q mutation. *Thromb Haemost* 1996;76(2):208–214.

80. Olivieri O, Friso S, Manzato F, et al. Resistance to activated protein C in healthy women taking oral contraceptives. *Br J Haematol* 1995;91(2): 465–470.

81. Osterud B, Robertsen R, Asvang GB, et al. Resistance to activated protein C is reduced in women using oral contraceptives. *Blood Coagul Fibrinolysis* 1994;5(5):853–854.

82. Rosing J, Tans G, Nicolaes GA, et al. Oral contraceptives and venous thrombosis: different sensitivities to activated protein C in women using second- and third-generation oral contraceptives. *Br J Haematol* 1997; 97(1):233–238.

83. Rosing J, Middeldorp S, Curvers J, et al. Low-dose oral contraceptives and acquired resistance to activated protein C: a randomised cross-over study. *Lancet* 1999;354(9195):2036–2040.

84. Alhenc-Gelas M, Plu-Bureau G, Guillonneau S, et al. Impact of progestagens on activated protein C (APC) resistance among users of oral contraceptives. *J Thromb Haemost* 2004;2(9):1594–1600.

85. Bates SM, Ginsberg JS, Straus SE, et al. Criteria for evaluating evidence that laboratory abnormalities are associated with the development of venous thromboembolism. *CMAJ* 2000;163(8):1016–1021.

86. Kemmeren JM, Algra A, Meijers JC, et al. Effect of second- and third-generation oral contraceptives on fibrinolysis in the absence or presence of the factor V Leiden mutation. *Blood Coagul Fibrinolysis* 2002;13(5): 373–381.

87. Mac Gillavry MR, Prins MH. Oral contraceptives and inherited thrombophilia: a gene-environment interaction with a risk of venous thrombosis? *Semin Thromb Hemost* 2003;29(2):219–226.

88. Andersen BS, Olsen J, Nielsen GL, et al. Third generation oral contraceptives and heritable thrombophilia as risk factors of non-fatal venous thromboembolism. *Thromb Haemost* 1998;79(1):28–31.

89. Legnani C, Palareti G, Guazzaloca G, et al. Venous thromboembolism in young women; role of thrombophilic mutations and oral contraceptive use. *Eur Heart J* 2002;23(12):984–990.

90. Pabinger I, Kyrle PA, Heistinger M, et al. The risk of thromboembolism in asymptomatic patients with protein C and protein S deficiency: a prospective cohort study. *Thromb Haemost* 1994;71(4):441–445.

91. Simioni P, Sanson BJ, Prandoni P, et al. Incidence of venous thromboembolism in families with inherited thrombophilia. *Thromb Haemost* 1999; 81(2):198–202.

92. Girolami A, Simioni P, Girolami B, et al. The role of drugs, particularly oral contraceptives, in triggering thrombosis in congenital defects of coagulation inhibitors: a study of six patients. *Blood Coagul Fibrinolysis* 1991; 2(5):673–678.

93. Spannagl M, Heinemann LA, Schramm W. Are factor V Leiden carriers who use oral contraceptives at extreme risk for venous thromboembolism? *Eur J Contracept Reprod Health Care* 2000;5(2):105–112.

94. Hellgren M, Svensson PJ, Dahlback B. Resistance to activated protein C as a basis for venous thromboembolism associated with pregnancy and oral contraceptives. *Am J Obstet Gynecol* 1995;173(1):210–213.

95. Rosendaal FR, Koster T, Vandenbroucke JP, et al. High risk of thrombosis in patients homozygous for factor V Leiden (activated protein C resistance). *Blood* 1995;85(6):1504–1508.

96. Emmerich J, Rosendaal FR, Cattaneo M, et al. Study Group for Pooled-Analysis in Venous Thromboembolism. Combined effect of factor V Leiden and prothrombin 20210A on the risk of venous thromboembolism—pooled analysis of 8 case-control studies including 2310 cases and 3204 controls. *Thromb Haemost* 2001;86(3):809–816.

97. Legnani C, Cini M, Cosmi B, et al. Oral contraceptive use in women with poor anticoagulant response to activated protein C but not carrying the factor V Leiden mutation increases the risk of venous thrombosis. *Thromb Haemost* 2004;91(4):712–718.

98. Martinelli I, Taioli E, Bucciarelli P, et al. Interaction between the G20210A mutation of the prothrombin gene and oral contraceptive use in deep vein thrombosis. *Arterioscler Thromb Vasc Biol* 1999;19(3):700–703.

99. Aznar J, Vaya A, Estelles A, et al. Risk of venous thrombosis in carriers of the prothrombin G20210A variant and factor V Leiden and their interaction with oral contraceptives. *Haematologica* 2000;85(12):1271–1276.

100. Santamaria A, Mateo J, Oliver A, et al. Risk of thrombosis associated with oral contraceptives of women from 97 families with inherited thrombophilia: high risk of thrombosis in carriers of the G20210A mutation of the prothrombin gene. *Haematologica* 2001;86(9):965–971.

101. Legnani C, Cosmi B, Valdre L, et al. Venous thromboembolism, oral contraceptives and high prothrombin levels. *J Thromb Haemost* 2003;1(1): 112–117.

102. Vandenbroucke JP, van der Meer FJ, Helmerhorst FM, et al. Factor V Leiden: should we screen oral contraceptive users and pregnant women? *BMJ* 1996;313(7065):1127–1130.

103. Creinin MD, Lisman R, Strickler RC. Screening for factor V Leiden mutation before prescribing combination oral contraceptives. *Fertil Steril* 1999; 72(4):646–651.

104. Palareti G, Legnani C, Frascaro M, et al. Screening for activated protein C resistance before oral contraceptive treatment: a pilot study. *Contraception* 1999;59(5):293–299.

105. Hyers TM, Agnelli G, Hull RD, et al. Antithrombotic therapy for venous thromboembolic disease. *Chest* 2001;119(Suppl. 1):176S–193S.

106. Ridker PM, Goldhaber SZ, Danielson E, et al. Long-term, low-intensity warfarin therapy for the prevention of recurrent venous thromboembolism. *N Engl J Med* 2003;348(15):1425–1434.

107. Kearon C, Ginsberg JS, Kovacs MJ, et al. Comparison of low-intensity warfarin therapy with conventional-intensity warfarin therapy for long-term prevention of recurrent venous thromboembolism. *N Engl J Med* 2003;349(7):631–639.

108. Schulman S, Wahlander K, Lundstrom T, et al. Secondary prevention of venous thromboembolism with the oral direct thrombin inhibitor ximelagatran. *N Engl J Med* 2003;349(18):1713–1721.

109. Hall JG, Pauli RM, Wilson KM. Maternal and fetal sequelae of anticoagulation during pregnancy. *Am J Med* 1980;68(1):122–140.

110. Iturbe-Alessio I, Fonseca MC, Mutchinik O, et al. Risks of anticoagulant therapy in pregnant women with artificial heart valves. *N Engl J Med* 1986;315(22):1390–1393.

111. Kopernik G, Shoham Z. Tools for making correct decisions regarding hormone therapy. Part II. Organ response and clinical applications. *Fertil Steril* 2004;81(6):1458–1477.

112. Shoham Z, Kopernik G. Tools for making correct decisions regarding hormone therapy. Part I: background and drugs. *Fertil Steril* 2004;81(6): 1447–1457.

113. Turgeon JL, McDonnell DP, Martin KA, et al. Hormone therapy: physiological complexity belies therapeutic simplicity. *Science* 2004;304(5675): 1269–1273.

114. Keating NL, Cleary PD, Rossi AS, et al. Use of hormone replacement therapy by postmenopausal women in the United States. *Ann Intern Med* 1999;130(7):545–553.

115. Psaty BM, Heckbert SR, Atkins D, et al. The risk of myocardial infarction associated with the combined use of estrogens and progestins in postmenopausal women. *Arch Intern Med* 1994;154(12):1333–1339.

116. Grady D, Rubin SM, Petitti DB, et al. Hormone therapy to prevent disease and prolong life in postmenopausal women. *Ann Intern Med* 1992; 117(12):1016–1037.

117. Grodstein F, Stampfer MJ, Manson JE, et al. Postmenopausal estrogen and progestin use and the risk of cardiovascular disease. *N Engl J Med* 1996;335(7):453–461.

118. Col NF, Eckman MH, Karas RH, et al. Patient-specific decisions about hormone replacement therapy in postmenopausal women. *JAMA* 1997; 277(14):1140–1147.

119. Hulley S, Grady D, Bush T, et al. Heart and Estrogen/progestin Replacement Study (HERS) Research Group. Randomized trial of estrogen plus progestin for secondary prevention of coronary heart disease in postmenopausal women. *JAMA* 1998;280(7):605–613.

120. Hulley S, Furberg C, Barrett-Connor E, et al. Noncardiovascular disease outcomes during 6.8 years of hormone therapy: Heart and Estrogen/progestin Replacement Study follow-up (HERS II). *JAMA* 2002;288(1):58–66.

121. Rossouw JE, Anderson GL, Prentice RL, et al. Risks and benefits of estrogen plus progestin in healthy postmenopausal women: principal results from the women's health initiative randomized controlled trial. *JAMA* 2002;288(3):321–333.

122. Anderson GL, Limacher M, Assaf AR, et al. Effects of conjugated equine estrogen in postmenopausal women with hysterectomy: the women's health initiative randomized controlled trial. *JAMA* 2004;291(14):1701–1712.

123. Haas JS, Kaplan CP, Gerstenberger EP, et al. Changes in the use of postmenopausal hormone therapy after the publication of clinical trial results. *Ann Intern Med* 2004;140(3):184–188.

124. Beral V, Banks E, Reeves G. Evidence from randomised trials on the long-term effects of hormone replacement therapy. *Lancet* 2002;360(9337):942–944.

125. Col NF, Pauker SG. The discrepancy between observational studies and randomized trials of menopausal hormone therapy: did expectations shape experience? *Ann Intern Med* 2003;139(11):923–929.

126. Nabulsi AA, Folsom AR, White A, et al. The Atherosclerosis Risk in Communities Study Investigators. Association of hormone-replacement therapy with various cardiovascular risk factors in postmenopausal women [see comments]. *N Engl J Med* 1993;328(15):1069–1075.

127. Warren MP. A comparative review of the risks and benefits of hormone replacement therapy regimens. *Am J Obstet Gynecol* 2004;190(4): 1141–1167.

128. Jick H, Derby LE, Myers MW, et al. Risk of hospital admission for idiopathic venous thromboembolism among users of postmenopausal oestrogens [see comments]. *Lancet* 1996;348(9033):981–983.

129. Daly E, Vessey MP, Hawkins MM, et al. Risk of venous thromboembolism in users of hormone replacement therapy [see comments]. *Lancet* 1996;348(9033):977–980.

130. Grodstein F, Stampfer MJ, Goldhaber SZ, et al. Prospective study of exogenous hormones and risk of pulmonary embolism in women [see comments]. *Lancet* 1996;348(9033):983–987.

131. Gutthann SP, Rodriguez LAG, Castellsague J, et al. Hormone replacement therapy and risk of venous thromboembolism: population based case-control study. *BMJ* 1997;314(7083):796–800.

132. The Postmenopausal Estrogen/Progestin Interventions (PEPI) Trial. The Writing Group for the PEPI Trial. Effects of estrogen or estrogen/progestin regimens on heart disease risk factors in postmenopausal women. *JAMA* 1995;273(3):199–208.

133. Love RR. Tamoxifen therapy in primary breast cancer: biology, efficacy, and side effects. *J Clin Oncol* 1989;7(6):803–815.

134. Fisher B, Dignam J, Wolmark N, et al. Tamoxifen in treatment of intraductal breast cancer: National Surgical Adjuvant Breast and Bowel Project B-24 randomised controlled trial [see comments]. *Lancet* 1999;353(9169):1993–2000.

135. Fisher B, Costantino J, Redmond C, et al. A randomized clinical trial evaluating tamoxifen in the treatment of patients with node-negative breast cancer who have estrogen-receptor-positive tumors. *N Engl J Med* 1989;320(8):479–484.

136. Pritchard KI, Paterson AH, Paul NA, et al. National Cancer Institute of Canada Clinical Trials Group Breast Cancer Site Group. Increased thromboembolic complications with concurrent tamoxifen and chemotherapy in a randomized trial of adjuvant therapy for women with breast cancer. *J Clin Oncol* 1996;14(10):2731–2737.

137. Clahsen PC, van de Velde CJ, Julien JP, et al. Thromboembolic complications after perioperative chemotherapy in women with early breast cancer: a European Organization for Research and Treatment of Cancer Breast Cancer Cooperative Group study. *J Clin Oncol* 1994;12(6):1266–1271.

138. Saphner T, Tormey DC, Gray R. Venous and arterial thrombosis in patients who received adjuvant therapy for breast cancer. *J Clin Oncol* 1991;9(2):286–294.

139. Levine MN, Gent M, Hirsh J, et al. The thrombogenic effect of anticancer drug therapy in women with stage II breast cancer. *N Engl J Med* 1988;318(7):404–407.

140. Fisher B, Redmond C, Legault-Poisson S, et al. Postoperative chemotherapy and tamoxifen compared with tamoxifen alone in the treatment of positive-node breast cancer patients aged 50 years and older with tumors responsive to tamoxifen: results from the National Surgical Adjuvant Breast and Bowel Project B-16 [see comments]. *J Clin Oncol* 1990;8(6):1005–1018.

141. Fisher B, Costantino JP, Wickerham DL, et al. Tamoxifen for prevention of breast cancer: report of the National Surgical Adjuvant Breast and Bowel Project P-1 Study [see comments]. *J Natl Cancer Inst* 1998;90(18):1371–1388.

142. IBIS Investigators. First results from the International Breast Cancer Intervention Study (IBIS-I): a randomised prevention trial. *Lancet* 2002;360(9336):817–824.

143. Bonneterre J, Buzdar A, Nabholtz JM, et al. Anastrozole is superior to tamoxifen as first-line therapy in hormone receptor positive advanced breast carcinoma. *Cancer* 2001;92(9):2247–2258.

144. ATAC Trial. Anastrozole alone or in combination with tamoxifen versus tamoxifen alone for adjuvant treatment of postmenopausal women with early breast cancer: first results of the ATAC randomised trial. *Lancet* 2002;359(9324):2131–2139.

145. Goss PE, Ingle JN, Martino S, et al. A randomized trial of letrozole in postmenopausal women after five years of tamoxifen therapy for early-stage breast cancer. *N Engl J Med* 2003;349(19):1793–1802.

146. Ettinger B, Black DM, Mitlak BH et al, Multiple Outcomes of Raloxifene Evaluation (MORE) Investigators. Reduction of vertebral fracture risk in postmenopausal women with osteoporosis treated with raloxifene: results from a 3-year randomized clinical trial. *JAMA* 1999;282(7):637–645.

147. Douketis JD, Gordon M, Johnston M, et al. The effects of hormone replacement therapy on thrombin generation, fibrinolysis inhibition, and resistance to activated protein C: prospective cohort study and review of literature. *Thromb Res* 2000;99(1):25–34.

148. Gebara OC, Mittleman MA, Sutherland P, et al. Association between increased estrogen status and increased fibrinolytic potential in the Framingham Offspring Study. *Circulation* 1995;91(7):1952–1958.

149. Koh KK, Mincemoyer R, Bui MN, et al. Effects of hormone-replacement therapy on fibrinolysis in postmenopausal women. *N Engl J Med* 1997;336(10):683–690.

150. van Wersch JW, Ubachs JM, van den EA, et al. The effect of two regimens of hormone replacement therapy on the haemostatic profile in postmenopausal women. *Eur J Clin Chem Clin Biochem* 1994;32(6):449–453.

151. Caine YG, Bauer KA, Barzegar S, et al. Coagulation activation following estrogen administration to postmenopausal women. *Thromb Haemost* 1992;68(4):392–395.

152. Dahm A, van HV, Bendz B, et al. Low levels of tissue factor pathway inhibitor (TFPI) increase the risk of venous thrombosis. *Blood* 2003; 101(11):4387–4392.

153. Kroon UB, Silfverstolpe G, Tengborn L. The effects of transdermal estradiol and oral conjugated estrogens on haemostasis variables. *Thromb Haemost* 1994;71(4):420–423.

154. Post MS, Rosing J, van der Mooren MJ, et al. Increased resistance to activated protein C after short-term oral hormone replacement therapy in healthy post-menopausal women. *Br J Haematol* 2002;119(4):1017–1023.

155. Lowe GD, Upton MN, Rumley A, et al. Different effects of oral and transdermal hormone replacement therapies on factor IX, APC resistance, t-PA, PAI and C-reactive protein—a cross-sectional population survey. *Thromb Haemost* 2001;86(2):550–556.

156. Post MS, Christella M, Thomassen LG, et al. Effect of oral and transdermal estrogen replacement therapy on hemostatic variables associated with venous thrombosis: a randomized, placebo-controlled study in postmenopausal women. *Arterioscler Thromb Vasc Biol* 2003;23(6):1116–1121.

157. Lacut K, Oger E, Le Gal G, et al. Differential effects of oral and transdermal postmenopausal estrogen replacement therapies on C-reactive protein. *Thromb Haemost* 2003;90(1):124–131.

158. Vehkavaara S, Silveira A, Hakala-Ala-Pietila T, et al. Effects of oral and transdermal estrogen replacement therapy on markers of coagulation, fibrinolysis, inflammation and serum lipids and lipoproteins in postmenopausal women. *Thromb Haemost* 2001;85(4):619–625.

159. Rosendaal FR, Vessey M, Rumley A, et al. Hormonal replacement therapy, prothrombotic mutations and the risk of venous thrombosis. *Br J Haematol* 2002;116(4):851–854.

160. Herrington DM, Vittinghoff E, Howard TD, et al. Factor V Leiden, hormone replacement therapy, and risk of venous thromboembolic events in women with coronary disease. *Arterioscler Thromb Vasc Biol* 2002;22(6):1012–1017.

161. Lowe G, Woodward M, Vessey M, et al. Thrombotic variables and risk of idiopathic venous thromboembolism in women aged 45-64 years. relationships to hormone replacement therapy. *Thromb Haemost* 2000;83(4):530–535.

162. Hoibraaten E, Qvigstad E, Arnesen H, et al. Increased risk of recurrent venous thromboembolism during hormone replacement therapy—results of the randomized, double-blind, placebo-controlled estrogen in venous thromboembolism trial (EVTET). *Thromb Haemost* 2000;84(6):961–967.

163. Kierkegaard A. Incidence and diagnosis of deep vein thrombosis associated with pregnancy. *Acta Obstet Gynecol Scand* 1983;62(3):239–243.

164. Treffers PE, Huidekoper BL, Weenink GH, et al. Epidemiological observations of thrombo-embolic disease during pregnancy and in the puerperium, in 56,022 women. *Int J Gynaecol Obstet* 1983;21(4):327–331.

165. Greer IA. Thrombosis in pregnancy: maternal and fetal issues. *Lancet* 1999;353(9160):1258–1265.

166. Greer IA. Epidemiology, risk factors and prophylaxis of venous thromboembolism in obstetrics and gynaecology. *Baillieres Clin Obstet Gynaecol* 1997;11(3):403–430.

167. McColl MD, Walker ID, Greer IA. Risk factors for venous thromboembolism in pregnancy. *Curr Opin Pulm Med* 1999;5(4):227–232.

168. Macklon NS, Greer IA. The deep venous system in the puerperium: an ultrasound study. *Br J Obstet Gynaecol* 1997;104(2):198–200.

169. Greer IA. Prevention of venous thromboembolism in pregnancy. *Best Pract Res Clin Haematol* 2003;16(2):261–278.

170. McColl MD, Ramsay JE, Tait RC, et al. Risk factors for pregnancy associated venous thromboembolism. *Thromb Haemost* 1997;78(4):1183–1188.

171. Ginsberg JS, Brill-Edwards P, Burrows RF, et al. Venous thrombosis during pregnancy: leg and trimester of presentation. *Thromb Haemost* 1992;67(5):519–520.

172. Cockett FB, Thomas ML, Negus D. Iliac vein compression.—Its relation to iliofemoral thrombosis and the post-thrombotic syndrome. *Br Med J* 1967;2(543):14–19.

173. Hellgren M. Hemostasis during normal pregnancy and puerperium. *Semin Thromb Hemost* 2003;29(2):125–130.

174. Greer IA. The challenge of thrombophilia in maternal-fetal medicine. *N Engl J Med* 2000;342(6):424–425.

175. Greer IA. Thrombophilia: implications for pregnancy outcome. *Thromb Res* 2003;109(2–3):73–81.

176. Stirling Y, Woolf L, North WR, et al. Haemostasis in normal pregnancy. *Thromb Haemost* 1984;52(2):176–182.

177. Hellgren M, Blomback M. Studies on blood coagulation and fibrinolysis in pregnancy, during delivery and in the puerperium. I. Normal condition. *Gynecol Obstet Invest* 1981;12(3):141–154.

178. Clark P, Brennand J, Conkie JA, et al. Activated protein C sensitivity, protein C, protein S and coagulation in normal pregnancy. *Thromb Haemost* 1998;79(6):1166–1170.

179. Eichinger S, Weltermann A, Philipp K, et al. Prospective evaluation of hemostatic system activation and thrombin potential in healthy pregnant women with and without factor V Leiden. *Thromb Haemost* 1999;82(4):1232–1236.

180. Sattar N, Greer IA, Rumley A, et al. A longitudinal study of the relationships between haemostatic, lipid, and oestradiol changes during normal human pregnancy. *Thromb Haemost* 1999;81(1):71–75.

181. Cerneca F, Ricci G, Simeone R, et al. Coagulation and fibrinolysis changes in normal pregnancy. Increased levels of procoagulants and reduced levels of inhibitors during pregnancy induce a hypercoagulable state, combined with a reactive fibrinolysis. *Eur J Obstet Gynecol Reprod Biol* 1997;73(1):31–36.

182. Ayhan A, Akkok E, Urman B, et al. Beta-thromboglobulin and platelet factor 4 levels in pregnancy and preeclampsia. *Gynecol Obstet Invest* 1990;30(1):12–14.

183. Burrows RF, Kelton JG. Thrombocytopenia at delivery: a prospective survey of 6715 deliveries. *Am J Obstet Gynecol* 1990;162(3):731–734.

184. Kjellberg U, Andersson NE, Rosen S, et al. APC resistance and other haemostatic variables during pregnancy and puerperium. *Thromb Haemost* 1999;81(4):527–531.

185. de Moerloose P, Mermillod N, Amiral J, et al. Thrombomodulin levels during normal pregnancy, at delivery and in the postpartum: comparison with tissue-type plasminogen activator and plasminogen activator inhibitor-1. *Thromb Haemost* 1998;79(3):554–556.

186. Bellart J, Gilabert R, Fontcuberta J, et al. Coagulation and fibrinolysis parameters in normal pregnancy and in gestational diabetes. *Am J Perinatol* 1998;15(8):479–486.

187. Nakashima A, Kobayashi T, Terao T. Fibrinolysis during normal pregnancy and severe preeclampsia relationships between plasma levels of plasminogen activators and inhibitors. *Gynecol Obstet Invest* 1996;42(2):95–101.

188. Bellart J, Gilabert R, Fontcuberta J, et al. Fibrinolysis changes in normal pregnancy. *J Perinat Med* 1997;25(4):368–372.

189. Ballegeer V, Mombaerts P, Declerck PJ, et al. Fibrinolytic response to venous occlusion and fibrin fragment D-dimer levels in normal and complicated pregnancy. *Thromb Haemost* 1987;58(4):1030–1032.

190. Cordts PR, Gawley TS. Anatomic and physiologic changes in lower extremity venous hemodynamics associated with pregnancy. *J Vasc Surg* 1996;24(5):763–767.

191. Palmgren J, Kirkinen P. Venous circulation in the maternal lower limb: a Doppler study with the Valsalva maneuver. *Ultrasound Obstet Gynecol* 1996;8(2):93–97.

192. Rabhi Y, Charras-Arthapignet C, Gris JC, et al. Lower limb vein enlargement and spontaneous blood flow echogenicity are normal sonographic findings during pregnancy. *J Clin Ultrasound* 2000;28(8):407–413.

193. Macklon NS, Greer IA, Bowman AW. An ultrasound study of gestational and postural changes in the deep venous system of the leg in pregnancy. *Br J Obstet Gynaecol* 1997;104(2):191–197.

194. Greer IA. Inherited thrombophilia and venous thromboembolism. *Best Pract Res Clin Obstet Gynaecol* 2003;17(3):413–425.

195. Conard J, Horellou MH, Van Dreden P, et al. Thrombosis and pregnancy in congenital deficiencies in AT III, protein C or protein S: study of 78 women. *Thromb Haemost* 1990;63(2):319–320.

196. Pabinger I, Schneider B, Gesellschaft fur Thrombose- und Hamostaseforschung (GTH) Study Group on Natural Inhibitors. Thrombotic risk in hereditary antithrombin III, protein C, or protein S deficiency. A cooperative, retrospective study. *Arterioscler Thromb Vasc Biol* 1996;16(2):742–748.

197. Bokarewa MI, Bremme K, Blomback M. Arg506-Gln mutation in factor V and risk of thrombosis during pregnancy. *Br J Haematol* 1996;92(2):473–478.

198. Gerhardt A, Scharf RE, Beckmann MW, et al. Prothrombin and factor V mutations in women with a history of thrombosis during pregnancy and the puerperium [see comments]. *N Engl J Med* 2000;342(6):374–380.

199. Zotz RB, Gerhardt A, Scharf RE. Prediction, prevention, and treatment of venous thromboembolic disease in pregnancy. *Semin Thromb Hemost* 2003;29(2):143–154.

200. Martinelli I, De SV, Taioli E, et al. Inherited thrombophilia and first venous thromboembolism during pregnancy and puerperium. *Thromb Haemost* 2002;87(5):791–795.

201. De Stefano V, Mastrangelo S, Paciaroni K, et al. Thrombotic risk during pregnancy and puerperium in women with APC-resistance—effective subcutaneous heparin prophylaxis in a pregnant patient. *Thromb Haemost* 1995;74(2):793–794.

202. Brill-Edwards P, Ginsberg JS, Gent M, et al. Safety of withholding heparin in pregnant women with a history of venous thromboembolism. *N Engl J Med* 2000;343(20):1439–1444.

203. Bates SM, Ginsberg JS. How we manage venous thromboembolism during pregnancy. *Blood* 2002;100(10):3470–3478.

204. Gates S, Brocklehurst P, Davis LJ. Prophylaxis for venous thromboembolic disease in pregnancy and the early postnatal period. *Cochrane Database Syst Rev* 2002;2:CD001689.

205. Pabinger I, Grafenhofer H, Kyrle PA, et al. Temporary increase in the risk for recurrence during pregnancy in women with a history of venous thromboembolism. *Blood* 2002;100(3):1060–1062.

206. Tengborn L, Bergqvist D, Matzsch T, et al. Recurrent thromboembolism in pregnancy and puerperium. Is there a need for thromboprophylaxis? *Am J Obstet Gynecol* 1989;160(1):90–94.

207. Conard J, Horellou MH, Samama MM. Inherited thrombophilia and gestational venous thromboembolism. *Semin Thromb Hemost* 2003;29(2):131–142.

208. Greer IA, Thomson AJ. Management of venous thromboembolism in pregnancy. *Best Pract Res Clin Obstet Gynaecol* 2001;15(4):583–603.

209. Bates SM, Greer IA, Hirsh J, et al. Use of antithrombotic agents during pregnancy: the Seventh ACCP conference on antithrombotic and thrombolytic therapy. *Chest* 2004;126(Suppl. 3):627S–644S.

210. Weitz JI. Low-molecular-weight heparins [published erratum appears in N Engl J Med 1997 Nov 20;337(21):1567] [see comments]. *N Engl J Med* 1997;337(10):688–698.

211. Sephton V, Farquharson RG, Topping J, et al. A longitudinal study of maternal dose response to low molecular weight heparin in pregnancy. *Obstet Gynecol* 2003;101(6):1307–1311.

212. Bounameaux H, de Moerloose P. Is laboratory monitoring of low-molecular-weight heparin therapy necessary? No. *J Thromb Haemost* 2004;2(4):551–554.

213. McKenna R, Cole ER, Vasan U. Is warfarin sodium contraindicated in the lactating mother? *J Pediatr* 1983;103(2):325–327.

214. Brenner B. Thrombophilia and fetal loss. *Semin Thromb Hemost* 2003;29(2):165–170.

215. Gris JC, Quere I, Monpeyroux F, et al. Case-control study of the frequency of thrombophilic disorders in couples with late fetal loss and no thrombotic antecedent—the Nimes Obstetricians and Haematologists Study5 (NOHA5). *Thromb Haemost* 1999;81(6):891–899.

216. Mousa HA, Alfirevic1 Z. Do placental lesions reflect thrombophilia state in women with adverse pregnancy outcome? *Hum Reprod* 2000;15(8):1830–1833.

217. Brenner B, Sarig G, Weiner Z, et al. Thrombophilic polymorphisms are common in women with fetal loss without apparent cause. *Thromb Haemost* 1999;82(1):6–9.

218. Sanson BJ, Friederich PW, Simioni P, et al. The risk of abortion and stillbirth in antithrombin-, protein C-, and protein S-deficient women. *Thromb Haemost* 1996;75(3):387–388.

219. Preston FE, Rosendaal FR, Walker ID, et al. Increased fetal loss in women with heritable thrombophilia. *Lancet* 1996;348(9032):913–916.

220. Grandone E, Margaglione M, Colaizzo D, et al. Factor V Leiden is associated with repeated and recurrent unexplained fetal losses. *Thromb Haemost* 1997;77(5):822–824.

221. Ridker PM, Miletich JP, Buring JE, et al. Factor V Leiden mutation as a risk factor for recurrent pregnancy loss. *Ann Intern Med* 1998;128(12 Pt 1):1000–1003.

222. Rai R, Regan L, Hadley E, et al. Second-trimester pregnancy loss is associated with activated C resistance. *Br J Haematol* 1996;92(2):489–490.

223. Dizon-Townson DS, Meline L, Nelson LM, et al. Fetal carriers of the factor V Leiden mutation are prone to miscarriage and placental infarction. *Am J Obstet Gynecol* 1997;177(2):402–405.

224. Rai RS, Regan L, Chitolie A, et al. Placental thrombosis and second trimester miscarriage in association with activated protein C resistance. *Br J Obstet Gynaecol* 1996;103(8):842–844.

225. Brenner B, Mandel H, Lanir N, et al. Activated protein C resistance can be associated with recurrent fetal loss. *Br J Haematol* 1997;97(3):551–554.

226. Wramsby ML, Sten-Linder M, Bremme K. Primary habitual abortions are associated with high frequency of factor V Leiden mutation. *Fertil Steril* 2000;74(5):987–991.

227. Tal J, Schliamser LM, Leibovitz Z, et al. A possible role for activated protein C resistance in patients with first and second trimester pregnancy failure. *Hum Reprod* 1999;14(6):1624–1627.

228. Sarig G, Younis JS, Hoffman R, et al. Thrombophilia is common in women with idiopathic pregnancy loss and is associated with late pregnancy wastage. *Fertil Steril* 2002;77(2):342–347.

229. Martinelli I, Taioli E, Cetin I, et al. Mutations in coagulation factors in women with unexplained late fetal loss. *N Engl J Med* 2000;343(14):1015–1018.

230. Meinardi JR, Middeldorp S, de Kam PJ, et al. Increased risk for fetal loss in carriers of the factor V Leiden mutation. *Ann Intern Med* 1999;130(9):736–739.

231. Nelen WL, Blom HJ, Steegers EA, et al. Hyperhomocysteinemia and recurrent early pregnancy loss: a meta-analysis. *Fertil Steril* 2000;74(6):1196–1199.

232. Rai RS, Clifford K, Cohen H, et al. High prospective fetal loss rate in untreated pregnancies of women with recurrent miscarriage and antiphospholipid antibodies. *Hum Reprod* 1995;10(12):3301–3304.

233. Rand JH, Wu XX, Andree HA, et al. Pregnancy loss in the antiphospholipid-antibody syndrome—a possible thrombogenic mechanism. *N Engl J Med* 1997;337(3):154–160.

234. Laude I, Rongieres-Bertrand C, Boyer-Neumann C, et al. Circulating procoagulant microparticles in women with unexplained pregnancy loss: a new insight. *Thromb Haemost* 2001;85(1):18–21.

235. Sims PJ, Faioni EM, Wiedmer T, et al. Complement proteins C5b-9 cause release of membrane vesicles from the platelet surface that are enriched in the membrane receptor for coagulation factor Va and express prothrombinase activity. *J Biol Chem* 1988;263(34):18205–18212.

236. Barry OP, Pratico D, Lawson JA, et al. Transcellular activation of platelets and endothelial cells by bioactive lipids in platelet microparticles. *J Clin Invest* 1997;99(9):2118–2127.

237. Greer IA. Procoagulant microparticles: new insights and opportunities in pregnancy loss? *Thromb Haemost* 2001;85(1):3–4.

238. Kupferminc MJ, Eldor A, Steinman N, et al. Increased frequency of genetic thrombophilia in women with complications of pregnancy. *N Engl J Med* 1999;340(1):9–13.

239. Dizon-Townson DS, Nelson LM, Easton K, et al. The factor V Leiden mutation may predispose women to severe preeclampsia. *Am J Obstet Gynecol* 1996;175(4 Pt 1):902–905.

240. Grandone E, Margaglione M, Colaizzo D, et al. Factor V Leiden, C > T MTHFR polymorphism and genetic susceptibility to preeclampsia. *Thromb Haemost* 1997;77(6):1052–1054.

241. Lindqvist PG, Svensson PJ, Dahlback B, et al. Factor V Q506 mutation (activated protein C resistance) associated with reduced intrapartum blood loss—a possible evolutionary selection mechanism. *Thromb Haemost* 1998;79(1):69–73.

242. Alfirevic Z, Roberts D, Martlew V. How strong is the association between maternal thrombophilia and adverse pregnancy outcome? A systematic review. *Eur J Obstet Gynecol Reprod Biol* 2002;101(1):6–14.

243. Morrison ER, Miedzybrodzka ZH, Campbell DM, et al. Prothrombotic genotypes are not associated with pre-eclampsia and gestational hypertension: results from a large population-based study and systematic review. *Thromb Haemost* 2002;87(5):779–785.

244. Infante-Rivard C, Rivard GE, Yotov WV, et al. Absence of association of thrombophilia polymorphisms with intrauterine growth restriction. *N Engl J Med* 2002;347(1):19–25.

245. Brenner B. Clinical management of thrombophilia-related placental vascular complications. *Blood* 2004;103(11):4003–4009.

246. Rai R, Cohen H, Dave M, et al. Randomised controlled trial of aspirin and aspirin plus heparin in pregnant women with recurrent miscarriage associated with phospholipid antibodies (or antiphospholipid antibodies). *BMJ* 1997;314(7076):253–257.

247. Sanson BJ, Lensing AW, Prins MH, et al. Safety of low-molecular-weight heparin in pregnancy: a systematic review. *Thromb Haemost* 1999;81(5):668–672.

248. Brenner B, Hoffman R, Blumenfeld Z, et al. Gestational outcome in thrombophilic women with recurrent pregnancy loss treated by enoxaparin. *Thromb Haemost* 2000;83(5):693–697.

# CHAPTER 85 ■ CANCER AND THROMBOSIS

MARK N. LEVINE, AGNES Y. Y. LEE, AND AJAY K. KAKKAR

For many years, it has been recognized that venous thromboembolism (VTE) is a common occurrence in patients with malignant disease. Compared to other groups of patients with VTE, the cancer population is unique because the pathogenesis of thrombosis differs, the frequency of VTE is greater, and the clinical management required is more complex. In recent years, much progress has been made in scientific research and clinical care as they relate to thrombosis in the patient with cancer. In this chapter, the following topics will be considered: pathogenesis of thrombosis in cancer, epidemiologic aspects of thrombosis and cancer, prevention of thrombosis in the surgical and medical patient with cancer, treatment of acute VTE, and the antineoplastic effect of antithrombotic therapy.

## THE PATHOGENESIS OF THROMBOSIS IN CANCER

In 1865, Professor Armand Trousseau first reported on the association between cancer and thrombosis (1). The pathogenic mechanisms of thrombosis in the patient with cancer involve a complex interaction between the tumor cell, the patient, and the hemostatic system. Virchow described three classic mechanisms that play a role in thrombogenesis: stasis, activation of blood coagulation, and vascular injury (2). All three are at play in patients with malignant disease. *Stasis*: Patients with cancer are often immobile and bedridden as a result of their cancer or complications of cancer (e.g., infection, surgery, pain crisis). Also, extrinsic venous compression from tumor masses and lymphadenopathy can lead to stasis. *Blood coagulation*: Tumor cells can produce procoagulant molecules that activate coagulation either directly or indirectly by initiating an inflammatory response. The two best-characterized procoagulants associated with tumor cells are tissue factor (TF) (3) and cancer procoagulant (CP) (4). Tumors, through expression of the procoagulant molecule TF, are capable of activating blood coagulation; the systemic manifestation of which is clinical thromboembolic disease. The human TF molecule is a single-chain 263–amino acid, 47-kDa transmembrane glycoprotein (5). It acts as both a surface receptor and cofactor for activated coagulation protease factor VII (FVIIa). Upon binding of factor VIIa to TF, blood coagulation is initiated with downstream generation of activated coagulation serine proteases, factor Xa, and factor IIa (thrombin). CP is a cysteine protease that directly activates factor X and functions in the absence of factor VII. At present, TF appears to play a more important role in the pathogenesis of clinical thrombosis than does CP. Studies have examined whether the presence of hereditary thrombophilia, for example, factor $V_{Leiden}$ contributes to thrombosis in patients with cancer with some studies reporting an association (6–8) and others not (9). *Vascular injury*: Extrinsic factors such as surgery, chemotherapy drugs, and vascular access catheters can all damage the vessel wall. The mechanism of chemotherapy-induced thrombosis is unclear but likely to be multifactorial. In one study, low levels of protein C and protein S were observed in patients with breast cancer receiving cyclophosphamide, methotrexate, and fluorouracil (FU) chemotherapy (10). It is likely that chemotherapy causes endothelial cell damage or change (11). Thrombosis has been reported in patients receiving tamoxifen for breast cancer (12). The mechanism is presumably due to its estrogen agonist effect.

## EPIDEMIOLOGY

### Incidence of Thrombosis in Patients with Malignancy

The incidence of thrombosis in patients with cancer can be gleaned from several different sources. Large epidemiologic studies specifically examining the incidence of VTE in patients with cancer are lacking. In one population-based study, the incidence of a first episode of deep vein thrombosis (DVT) or pulmonary embolism (PE) was recorded in Olmsted County, Minnesota, from 1966 to 1990 (13). During this period, the overall age and sex-adjusted annual incidence of VTE was 117 per 100,000. A dramatic rise in the incidence rates occurred among patients older than 65 years, with rates almost doubling for each subsequent decade of age. This study population was composed of both patients with cancer and patients who did not have cancer. The observed incidence rates may represent a very conservative estimate of the incidence of VTE in a cancer population. In a nested case–control study of 625 patients with a first episode of VTE from this database, risk factors for thrombosis were examined (14). Malignancy was associated with an odds ratio of 6.5 for the occurrence of VTE.

In another population-based study, Levitan et al. examined the diagnosis at hospital discharge of more than 7,000 Medicare patients (>65 years of age) admitted to hospital with a diagnosis of both malignancy and DVT or PE (15). The ratio of the number of patients with a particular type of cancer who had VTE to the number of patients with that type of malignancy, provided an estimate of which cancers were most likely to lead to thrombosis. The highest rates were found with cancer of the ovary (120 per 10,000 patients), brain tumors (117 per 10,000 patients), and cancer of the pancreas (110 per 10,000 patients).

Although VTE has been reported in up to 30% of patients with cancer at autopsy (16), the optimal study design for determining the true incidence of clinical VTE in patients with cancer is a prospective cohort study. The best evidence on the incidence of thrombosis in a particular cancer type comes from clinical trials of systemic therapy in women with early breast cancer. Such rates are described in Table 85-1. The rate of thrombosis over a 5-year period in women with axillary

**TABLE 85-1**

INCIDENCE OF THROMBOSIS IN EARLY STAGE BREAST CANCER

| Study | Treatment | No. of patients | % of patients with thrombosis |
|---|---|---|---|
| **NODE-NEGATIVE** | | | |
| Fisher 1989 (17) | T | 1,318 | 0.9 |
| | Placebo | 1,326 | 0.15 |
| Fisher 1997 (18) | CMFT | 768 | 4.2 |
| | T | 771 | 0.8 |
| | | | |
| **NODE-POSITIVE** | | | |
| Levine 1988 (21) | CMFVP | 102 | 8.8 |
| | CMFVP + AT | 103 | 4.9 |
| Pritchard 1996 (12) | CMF + T | 353 | 9.6 |
| | T | 352 | 1.4 |
| Clahsen 1994 (22) | Perioperative FAC | 1,292 | 2.1 |
| | No Rx | 1,332 | 0.8 |
| Rivkin 1994 (23) | CMFVP + T | 303 | 3.6 |
| | CMFVP | 300 | 1.3 |
| | T | 295 | 0 |
| Fisher 1990 (24) | ACT | 383 | 3.1 |
| | T | 367 | 1.6 |
| Weiss 1981 (25) | CMFVP | 143 | 6.3 |
| | CMF | 144 | 3.5 |

A, adriamycin; C, cyclophosphamide; F, fluorouracil; M, methotrexate; P, prednisone; T, tamoxifen; V, vincristine; Rx, treatment.

node-negative breast cancer on tamoxifen is approximately 0.9% (17,18). Although it was recognized that tamoxifen was thrombogenic in women with breast cancer, the results of the Breast Cancer Prevention Trial conducted by the National Surgical Breast and Bowel Project (NSABP) provided an opportunity to estimate the thrombogenic effect of tamoxifen alone (19). In this trial, healthy women at risk for developing breast cancer were randomized to either tamoxifen or placebo for 5 years. There was an increased risk of DVT in the tamoxifen group compared to placebo: 0.13% per year versus 0.084% per year. The corresponding rates for PE were 0.069% and 0.023%, respectively. In this trial, the highest rates of thrombosis associated with the use of tamoxifen were observed in women older than 50 years. In this trial, there was an increased risk of stroke with tamoxifen but no increase in myocardial infarction. Clinicians are often faced with the scenario of a patient with a past history of VTE who develops breast cancer and requires therapy with a hormonal agent. On the basis of the results of a recent trial, an aromatase inhibitor that has a much lower risk of thrombosis than tamoxifen can be used (20).

The rates of thrombosis in women with node-positive breast cancer on chemotherapy ranged between 1% and 9%, with the highest rates of thrombosis observed in postmenopausal women (12,21,22,24–26). In these trials, chemotherapy plus tamoxifen increased the risk of thrombosis over chemotherapy alone. The rates of thrombosis in women with metastatic breast cancer vary. In a case series reported by Goodnough, the rate of thrombosis in patients receiving chemotherapy for metastatic breast cancer was 17.5% (27). However, in a randomized trial reported by Levine et al., the rate was 4.5% (28). Recent trials evaluating aromatase inhibitors in women with advanced breast cancer report thrombosis rates of approximately 2% to 4% (20,29).

The incidence of thrombosis in other patient groups is limited. Data from the available studies are presented in Table 85-2. Another group of patients that has emerged to be at high risk

for thrombosis are patients with brain tumors who are on extended follow-up. In a review by Marras et al. (30), rates of symptomatic VTE as high as 18% per year were reported in one study (31). Weijl et al. reported that 8.4% of 179 patients with germ cell tumors who received platinum-based chemotherapy developed thromboembolism (32). Reported rates of thromboembolism in other solid tumors include: 4.4% per year in patients with lung cancer (33), 10.6% in women with advanced ovarian cancer receiving chemotherapy (34), 17% in men with prostate cancer receiving chemotherapy (35), and 3% in women with carcinoma of the cervix receiving concurrent chemotherapy and radiation (36). In the latter study, erythropoietin increased the thrombotic risk to 23%. There is emerging evidence that erythropoietin increases the thrombotic risk. In another study in women with advanced cervix cancer receiving radiation, cisplatin chemotherapy, and erythropoietin, the rate of thrombosis was 13% (37). A randomized trial which evaluated erythropoietin in women with advanced breast cancer was stopped early when four of 14 (28.5%) patients in the erythropoietin arm developed thrombosis compared to none in 13 women in the control arm (38). It is interesting that most trials in patients with colorectal cancer receiving chemotherapy have not reported on rates of thrombosis. The explanation for this is unclear, but it is possible that this is due to underreporting (39). A careful audit of early deaths in a randomized trial of irinotecan, 5-FU, and leucovorin versus 5-FU plus leucovorin as adjuvant therapy in colon cancer noted an excess of vascular deaths (arterial and venous) in the former arm, 1.9% versus 0.6%, respectively (40). In a trial of irinotecan plus 5-FU/leucovorin versus 5-FU/leucovorin in patients with metastatic colorectal cancer there was a statistically significant increased rate of thromboembolic events in patients receiving the three-drug regimen versus 5-FU/leucovorin, 5% versus less than 1%, respectively (39). Thrombosis rates of 5% to 10% have been reported in patients with Hodgkin or non-Hodgkin lymphoma

## TABLE 85-2

INCIDENCE OF THROMBOSIS IN DIFFERENT TUMORS

| Study | Tumor[a] | Patient no. | Thrombosis (%) |
|---|---|---|---|
| Brandes et al. (31) | Malignant glioma | 75 | 24.0 |
| Weijl et al. (32) | Germ cell | 179 | 8.4 |
| Blom et al. (33) | Lung | 537 | 4.4 |
| Solit et al. (35) | Prostate | 30 | 17.0 |
| von Tempelhoff (34) | Ovarian | 47 | 10.6 |
| Wun et al. (36) | Cervix (cisplatin, radiation, erythropoietin) | 75 | 22.6 |
| Wun et al. (36) | Cervix (cisplatin, radiation) | 72 | 2.7 |
| Lavey et al. (37) | Cervix (cisplatin, radiation, erythropoietin) | 53 | 13 |
| Ottinger (41) | Non-Hodgkin lymphoma | 593 | 6.6 |
| Clarke (53) | Non-Hodgkin lymphoma | 85 | 4.7 |
| DeStefano (43) | Leukemia | 379 | 6.3 |

[a]Patients with advanced cancer receiving chemotherapy.

receiving chemotherapy (41,42), and a rate of 6.3% in adult patients with acute leukemia (43). In this study, the highest rate was in patients with promyelocytic leukemia. Finally, interest in the thrombogenicity of anticancer agents has been rekindled among medical oncologists because of the unexpectedly high rate of VTE in patients with cancer receiving novel anticancer agents aimed at specific molecular targets in the cancer cell, for example, antivascular endothelial growth factor (VEGF), antiepidermal growth factor receptor, and thalidomide (44–50) (see Table 85-3). In a recent cohort study in patients with myeloma, the cumulative risk of thrombosis over 12 months was 15% in patients on chemotherapy alone and 35% in patients on chemotherapy and thalidomide (51). In a randomized phase II trial, 104 patients with metastatic colorectal cancer were randomized to 5-FU plus leucovorin, 5-FU plus leucovorin plus high-dose bevacizumab. Seven of 67 (10.4%) patients who received bevacizumab compared to one of 35 (2.9%) control patients experienced thrombosis (50). There was also an increase in bleeding associated with the bevacizumab. In a second trial, 813 patients with metastatic colorectal cancer receive irinotecan, 5-FU and leucovorin or the same drugs plus bevacizumab (52). The incidence of thrombosis (arterial and venous) was 16.2% versus 19.4% (not statistically significantly different).

## Prognosis of Patients with Cancer and Venous Thrombotic Event

Patients with cancer who develop VTE have a short life expectancy. In a population-based study reported by Heit et al., the presence of cancer was an independent predictor of worse survival in patients presenting with acute venous thrombosis (14). In the study by Sorensen et al., patients with cancer and VTE had a worse survival than those with cancer without VTE (54) (see Fig. 85-1). Similarly, in the study by Levitan et al., the mortality rate for patients with VTE and malignant disease was substantially increased compared to those with malignant disease alone (15).

## The Association Between Venous Thrombotic Event and Occult Cancer

Patients who present with idiopathic DVT have an increased risk of subsequently developing cancer compared to patients with secondary DVT and to patients with symptoms of DVT, but who are not found to have DVT (55).

## TABLE 85-3

INCIDENCE OF THROMBOSIS WITH TARGETTED ANTICANCER AGENTS

| Study | Tumor | Patient no. | Thrombosis (%) |
|---|---|---|---|
| Zangari et al. (51) | *Myeloma:* | | |
| | Chemotherapy plus thalidomide | 87 | 35 |
| | Chemotherapy | 134 | 15 |
| Kabbinavar et al. (50) | *Colorectal cancer:* | | |
| | 5-FU + L | 36 | 2.9 |
| | 5-FU + L + bevacizumab (5 mg/kg) | 35 | 14.2 |
| | 5-FU + L + bevacizumab (10 mg/kg) | 33 | 6.2 |
| Hurwitz et al. (52) | 5-FU + L | 411 | 16.2 |
| | 5-FU + L + bevacizumab | 402 | 19.4 |

5-FU, 5-fluorouracil; L, leucovorin.

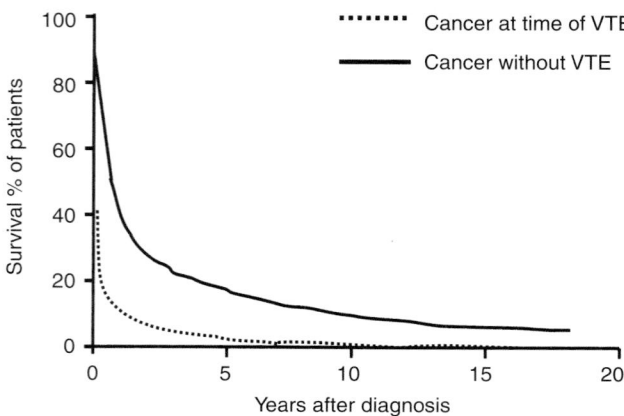

FIGURE 85-1. Survival with venous thrombotic event and cancer. VTE, venous thromboembolism. [Reproduced with permission from Sorensen HT, Mellemkjaer L, Olsen JH, et al. Prognosis of cancers associated with venous thromboembolism. *N Engl J Med* 2000; 343(25):1846–1850.]

In a population-based study conducted in Sweden for patients hospitalized between 1965 and 1983, Baron et al. calculated the standardized incidence ratios (SIRs) for cancer in patients with VTE (56). The SIR at 1 year following the diagnosis of VTE was 4.4. In a study using a similar database linkage strategy among Danish hospital and cancer registries for the years 1977 to 1992, Sorensen et al. found the SIR at 1 year to be 2.3 for VTE (57). Finally, Schulman and Lindmarker used the Swedish cancer registry to determine the incidence of subsequent cancer diagnosis in patients from a trial on the duration of anticoagulant therapy (58). The SIR for the development of cancer was approximately 4 in the first year after an idiopathic thromboembolic event. The cumulative probability of cancer over 6 years of follow-up in those subjects categorized as having idiopathic VTE was 17%, compared to 5% in patients with secondary VTE.

On the basis of the reported association between VTE and occult cancer, it has been suggested that patients presenting with idiopathic thrombosis should undergo extensive investigations for an underlying cancer. There has been much discussion concerning this issue because the potential benefit of screening for occult malignancy must be weighed against potential harms such as procedure-related morbidity, the psychological burden of a false-positive test, and the cost of screening procedures. In addition, an important methodologic consideration in establishing the effectiveness of a screening test is that there needs to be effective therapy with curative potential. Otherwise by discovering a cancer that is "incurable" early, a patient is basically given extra time of disease, a so-called lead-time bias. To date, data to support the efficacy of screening for the following cancers have been established: breast, cervix, and possibly colon.

A small randomized trial evaluating extensive screening versus no screening in patients presenting with idiopathic VTE has been conducted (59). The battery of tests used in the extensively screened group included ultrasonography and computed tomography of the abdomen and pelvis, a hemoccult test, gastroscopy, colonoscopy, sputum cytology, mammography, a pelvic examination, a prostate examination, and tumor markers. Thirteen of the 99 patients in the extensively screened group had cancers detected initially compared to none of the 102 patients in the control group. However, 10 patients in the control group and one in the screened group developed cancer during the 2-year follow-up period. There was no statistically significant difference detected in cancer-related mortality in the two groups, 3.9% versus 2%, respectively.

Given such results, it is premature to recommend extensive screening in patients who present with idiopathic VTE. Often a complete history, physical examination, chest x-ray, and rectal examination can provide a clue as to the presence of an underlying cancer. This approach is supported by the retrospective cohort study reported by Cornuz (60).

# PREVENTION OF THROMBOSIS IN CANCER

## Surgical Prophylaxis

Patients with cancer undergoing surgery are at increased risk for postoperative thrombosis compared to patients who do not have cancer (61). Clinical trials have demonstrated the efficacy of subcutaneous unfractionated heparin (UFH) in preventing DVT and PE in patients undergoing major surgery (62,63). In these studies, many of the patients had cancer (62). Mismetti et al. have conducted a metaanalysis of trials that compared a low-molecular-weight heparin (LMWH) to UFH in high-risk major surgery (64). In the analysis of the eight trials that included patients undergoing surgery for cancer, no differences in asymptomatic DVT, clinical PE, death, and major bleeding were detected between LMWH and UFH. The results of these studies provide evidence that once daily LMWH is as safe and effective as several injections of UFH per day for the prevention of postoperative DVT in patients with cancer. The once per day injection is attractive because of the comfort for patients and convenience for medical staff, and the lower risk of drug error. In a recent subgroup analysis of over 6,000 patients with malignant disease receiving perioperative UFH or LMWH, compared to 17,000 patients without malignancy, fatal PE was three times as common in patients with cancer than in surgical patients who did not have cancer despite use of prophylaxis (65).

In a study of over 2,000 patients undergoing laparotomy for cancer, the hypothesis that a higher dose of LMWH would be associated with a low incidence of postoperative thromboembolic complications in patients with cancer was tested. In this trial, in the patients undergoing operation for malignant disease, increasing the dose of the LMWH dalteparin sodium from 2,500 IU once daily to 5,000 IU once daily was associated with a reduction in the frequency of postoperative DVT from 14.9% to 8.5% (66). In the patients with cancer in this trial, there was no significant increase in bleeding complications associated with increasing the dose of LMWH. For patients without malignant disease, although there was a reduction in the frequency of postoperative DVT with the higher dose of LMWH, this was associated with a significant increase in perioperative bleeding complications (66).

In recent years, a number of trials have shown that venographic DVT can be reduced with extended out-of-hospital prophylaxis with LMWH in patients undergoing major joint replacement surgery. A metaanalysis of these trials has suggested that the rate of clinical DVT after hip replacement is also reduced with the longer treatment (67). On the basis of the results of these trials and the notion that the risk of VTE extends beyond the immediate postoperative period in patients undergoing cancer surgery, Bergqvist et al. studied extended prophylaxis in cancer surgery. In the ENOXACAN (Enoxaparin in Cancer) II Study, patients undergoing surgery for abdominal malignancy received 1 week of enoxaparin and then were randomized to enoxaparin or placebo for another 21 days (68). Bilateral venography was performed at the end of treatment. There was a statistically significant reduction in DVT from 12% with placebo to 4.8% with extended prophylaxis. These results are supported by the data from a trial by

Rasmussen et al. in which patients undergoing general surgery received regular postoperative prophylaxis or extended prophylaxis with dalteparin LMWH (69). There was a reduction in venographically detected clot with extended therapy.

Extended prophylaxis in cancer surgery is potentially an important advance in the care of patients with cancer undergoing surgery. However, further research is required to show that continuing anticoagulant therapy beyond hospitalization will also reduce the risk of clinically important VTE.

# Prophylaxis in the Medical Patient with Cancer

There are two main clinical situations when considering the prevention of VTE in the medical patient with cancer. The first involves the ambulatory patient who is receiving chemotherapy or radiation. The second is the patient who is bedridden for prolonged periods of time.

There is very little data available on the primary prevention of thrombosis in ambulatory patients with cancer. In one study, Levine et al. showed that low dose warfarin is effective in reducing the rate of thrombosis during chemotherapy (28). In a double-blind randomized trial, 311 patients with metastatic breast cancer were given either very low-dose warfarin [1 mg for 6 weeks followed by an adjusted dose to a target international normalized ratio (INR) of 1.3 to 1.9] or placebo while they were receiving chemotherapy. The average duration of therapy was 6 months. There was an 85% risk reduction in the rate of thromboembolism, which was statistically significant. There was no increase in bleeding. Despite this study, oncologists do not routinely use prophylaxis in patients with cancer receiving chemotherapy with oral anticoagulants. The most likely reasons are the concern for bleeding and the logistics of laboratory monitoring and dose adjustment. An alternative is to reserve prophylaxis for high-risk situations (e.g., previous history of VTE or a pelvic mass causing poor venous drainage from the lower limbs).

Patients with cancer who are bedridden are at risk for thrombosis. This occurs in the setting of a patient with cancer who is hospitalized with an acute complication related to their cancer (e.g., pain crisis, infection, or hypercalcemia). There are also situations when patients with advanced cancer are admitted to hospital for palliative care. Low dose UFH and LMWH have been found to be effective in patients hospitalized with acute medical illnesses (70,71). It would seem reasonable therefore that patients with advanced malignancy who are bedridden should receive prophylaxis with either low dose UFH or LMWH.

# Central Vein Catheter Thrombosis

Thrombosis associated with central vein catheters can be particularly problematic in the patient with cancer. Until recently, there were only two small randomized trials evaluating primary prevention in patients with catheters. Two studies, one with warfarin (1 mg per day) and the second with LMWH (dalteparin 2,500 IU daily), had demonstrated significant reductions in catheter thrombosis (72,73) (see Table 85-4). In these trials, many of the thrombotic events were asymptomatic. Despite the results of these trials, there is substantial variation in the use of antithrombotic prophylaxis; some physicians use it (often 1 mg of warfarin), whereas others do not. Although it was originally felt that 1 mg of warfarin did not prolong the prothrombin time, a recent study in patients with colorectal cancer receiving infusional 5-FU showed that INR can be substantially prolonged (74). Recently, the results of three randomized trials in patients with central vein catheters were reported (Table 85-3). In the trial by Reichardt et al., patients with cancer were randomized to dalteparin (5,000 IU once daily) or placebo (75). Screening ultrasonography was done at the end of the study. The rates of thrombosis were very low in both groups, approximately 3%. In the trial by Couban et al., patients with cancer received 1 mg of warfarin or placebo (76). No difference was detected in symptomatic thrombosis and the rates were low in both groups, approximately 4%. In the most recent trial, reported by Verso et al., patients with cancer were randomized to enoxaparin LMWH or placebo (77). Patients underwent venography. The rate of venography-detected thrombosis was 18% in the placebo group and 14% in the LMWH group. This difference was not statistically significant. The rates of symptomatic thrombosis were low in both groups, 3.1% versus 1%, respectively. A recent cohort study also reported low rates of thrombosis in patients with cancer with central vein catheters (78). The reason for the observed low rates of thrombosis in these trials is unclear. One possible explanation is that newer generations of catheters and improved catheter care have reduced the rates of associated thrombosis. Clearly, further research is required. At this juncture, the weight of the evidence would not support the use of antithrombotic prophylaxis in such patients.

## TABLE 85-4

### CENTRAL VEIN CATHETER THROMBOSIS

| Study | Treatment | Patient no. | Thrombosis (%) | P |
|---|---|---|---|---|
| Bern et al. (72)[a] | Warfarin 1 mg | 40 | 10 | <0.001 |
| | Control | 42 | 37 | |
| Monreal et al. (73)[a] | Dalteparin 2,500 IU | 16 | 6 | 0.002 |
| | Control | 13 | 62 | |
| Reichardt et al. (75)[b] | Dalteparin 5,000 IU | 294 | 2.7 | NS |
| | Placebo | 145 | 3.4 | |
| Couban et al. (76) | Warfarin 1 mg | 130 | 4.6 | NS |
| | Placebo | 125 | 4 | |
| Verso et al. (77)[a] | Enoxaparin | 155 | 14 | NS |
| | Placebo | 155 | 18 | |

IU, international units; NS, not significant.
[a]Screening venography.
[b]Screening upper limb ultrasound.

# TREATMENT OF VENOUS THROMBOEMBOLISM

Treatment of patients with cancer with VTE is difficult because these patients have an increased risk of recurrent VTE and anticoagulant-induced bleeding compared to patients who do not have cancer (79,80). In addition, many patients with cancer have a compromised quality of life and the occurrence of thrombosis has an additional negative impact on their quality of life. Furthermore, patients with cancer who develop VTE have an increased mortality compared to patients with cancer without VTE (54).

## Risk of Recurrence and Bleeding

Hutten et al. performed a retrospective analysis of the rates of recurrent thrombosis and bleeding for patients who received at least 3 months of oral anticoagulant therapy in two large randomized clinical trials that compared LMWH with UFH for the initial therapy for acute VTE (79). The incidence of recurrent thrombosis in patients with cancer was 27.1 per 100 patient-years versus 9 per 100 patient-years in those without cancer, $P = 0.003$. The risk of bleeding was approximately six times higher in patients with cancer (13.3 per 100 patient-years) than in patients without cancer (2.1 per 100 patient-years), ($P = 0.002$).

More recently, Prandoni et al. reported on the outcomes of anticoagulant treatment in a cohort of 842 patients who received initial UFH or LMWH followed by oral anticoagulants for acute VTE (80). The 12-month cumulative incidence of recurrent thromboembolism in the 181 patients with cancer was 20.7% versus 6.8% in patients without cancer, for a hazard ratio of 3.2. The 12-month cumulative incidence of major bleeding was 12.4% in patients with cancer compared to 4.9% in patients without cancer, for a hazard ratio of 2.2. Recurrence and bleeding were both related to the cancer severity and occurred predominantly during the first month of anticoagulant therapy. The incidence of recurrent VTE also directly correlates with the intensity of the INR, but the risk of major bleeding appears to be independent of the anticoagulant effect.

## Initial Treatment of Venous Thromboembolism

On the basis of the results of numerous randomized controlled trials, LMWH has replaced UFH as the first-line treatment in most patients with acute VTE. Large metaanalyses of these clinical trials have shown that weight-adjusted subcutaneous LMWH is safer and probably more effective than UFH administered by continuous intravenous infusion and monitored by the activated partial thromboplastin time (aPTT) (81–84). Despite the observed efficacy and safety of LMWH in these trials, it should be noted that only approximately 20% of patients in these studies had cancer. Nonetheless, it would seem reasonable to generalize the results of these trials to the patients with cancer with acute VTE. In terms of optimizing treatment, the use of LMWH avoids intravenous administration of anticoagulant therapy and the need for laboratory monitoring, thereby improving the quality of life of the patient.

One of the controversial areas in the initial treatment of acute VTE is the dosing regimen. Merli et al. compared UFH with once-a-day enoxaparin and with twice-a-day enoxaparin (85). In the subgroup of patients with cancer, there was a suggestion that the rate of recurrent thromboembolism was twofold higher in the patients who received the once-a-day dose. Other LMWHs, such as dalteparin, use a once-a-day dosing regimen. Patients with cancer, with established VTE, have a higher rate of recurrent VTE than patients without cancer even when treated with LMWH. It is conceivable that better antithrombotic efficacy might be achieved in the patient with cancer with VTE with a twice-a-day dosing regimen, but this requires future research.

There have been three clinical trials that demonstrated that patients with acute proximal DVT could be treated safely at home with subcutaneous LMWH without admission to hospital (86–88). In these trials, some of the patients were treated entirely at home and some were admitted to hospital for a short while and then discharged home early. In these trials, there were approximately 400 patients with cancer who received either LMWH or UFH. The rate of recurrent VTE in patients with cancer at 3 months was approximately 10% in both treatment arms. Additional cohort studies have shown that approximately 80% of unselected outpatients with newly diagnosed DVT can be treated entirely at home, and up to 50% of these patients had cancer (89,90). Hence, use of LMWH at home in the patient with cancer with acute VTE is recommended because of the substantial positive impact on quality of life. Clearly, some patients with acute VTE will require hospitalization because of symptoms and other complications related to their cancer. If patients are to be treated at home, they must be reliable and compliant, and have a good support system.

In contrast to DVT, there are relatively few trials that have compared LMWH with UFH in patients with acute PE. Simonneau et al. compared the LMWH tinzaparin with IV UFH in hospitalized patients with PE, and no difference was detected in recurrent VTE and bleeding between treatment groups (91). In the trial performed by the Columbus investigators, which found no difference in these outcomes between the LMWH, reviparin, and UFH, most patients were treated at home and 27% of all patients had PE (88). In these two trials, 10% and 23% of patients had cancer, respectively. Finally, in a prospective cohort study, Kovacs et al. treated 108 patients with PE as outpatients with the LMWH, dalteparin; 22% had cancer (92). The rate of recurrent thrombosis was 5.6%, and major bleeding occurred in 2.9% of the patients. Hence, on the basis of this evidence and the large experience with LMWHs in DVT, it seems reasonable to manage acute PE patients, who are hemodynamically stable, by treating them with outpatient LMWH. However, in patients with acute PE who are hemodynamically unstable, the use of iv UFH can be considered, because such patients were excluded from the clinical trials that compared LMWH with UFH.

There has been a tendency in some institutions to insert inferior vena caval (IVC) filters in patients with cancer with acute VTE because of the concern for anticoagulant-associated bleeding, particularly with periods of thrombocytopenia during chemotherapy. The use of IVC filters will reduce the short-term risk of PE, but is associated with an increased risk long term of recurrent DVT, despite concurrent oral anticoagulant therapy (93). Therefore, the use of an IVC filter in a patient with cancer presenting with acute VTE is not recommended. Filters should be reserved for patients who are actively bleeding and cannot receive anticoagulant therapy and for patients who develop multiple episodes of recurrent thromboembolism despite therapeutic LMWH.

There are recent reports on retrievable IVC filters that could potentially be useful in a patient who presents with acute VTE and is actively bleeding (94). In such patients, a filter can be inserted and then removed within 7 to 10 days if the bleeding has stopped and is well controlled. This would avoid the long-term potential complications of IVC filters. However, the results of additional studies on patients with cancer are required.

## Long-Term Anticoagulant Therapy

Long-term anticoagulant therapy using coumarin derivatives is required to prevent recurrent thrombosis. An oral anticoagulant such as warfarin is commenced on the first or second day

## TABLE 85-5

### LONG-TERM TREATMENT WITH LOW-MOLECULAR-WEIGHT HEPARIN

| Study | Treatment | Patient no. | Recurrent VTE (%) | Bleeding major (%) |
|---|---|---|---|---|
| Meyer et al. (103) | Enoxaparin 1.5 mg/kg for 3 mo | 67 | 3[a] | 16.9[a] |
|  | Warfarin INR 2.0–3.0 for 3 mo | 71 | 4.2 | 7.5 |
| Lee (104) | Dalteparin 200 IU/kg daily for 1 mo, followed by 75%–80% of this dose for 5 mo | 336 | 8[b] | 5.6[c] |
|  | Warfarin or acenocoumarol at target INR 2.5 | 336 | 16 | 3.6 |

VTE, venous thromboembolism; INR, international normalized ratio.
[a]$P$ value for composite endpoint of VTE and bleeding, 0.09.
[b]$P$ value for recurrent VTE, 0.0017.
[c]$P = 0.27.$

of treatment and the aim is to achieve an INR of between 2.0 and 3.0. Warfarin therapy is particularly complicated in the patient with cancer for a number of reasons. It is often difficult to maintain the INR within the therapeutic range because patients with cancer have anorexia and vomiting. In addition, drug interactions (e.g., chemotherapy and antibiotics) can influence the anticoagulant effect of vitamin K–dependent anticoagulants. Often it is necessary to interrupt oral anticoagulant therapy because of thrombocytopenia and procedures such as thoracentesis and abdominal paracentesis. This requires reversal of the anticoagulant effect with vitamin K. Subsequently, it takes several days to achieve the targeted therapeutic range after reintroduction of warfarin. Finally, frequent blood sampling is required for the INR and venous access can often be difficult in the patient with cancer.

There are certain features of long-term anticoagulant therapy with LMWH that are attractive for the patient with cancer. LMWH does not require laboratory monitoring and can be administered subcutaneously once or twice daily, based on body weight. There is the clinical experience that LMWH can be effective in warfarin failure (95). Finally, based on preclinical data and metaanalyses, there is the potential for less bleeding. There have been a number of trials that have compared long-term oral anticoagulant therapy with long-term LMWH (96–102). These trials were relatively small in size and had very few patients with cancer. No definitive conclusions can be drawn from these trials concerning long-term treatment with LMWH in the patient with cancer.

Several recent randomized trials, however, have provided new information concerning the long-term treatment of patients with cancer with VTE (see Table 85-5). In the trial reported by Meyer et al., patients with cancer with acute VTE were randomized to 3 months of enoxaparin or warfarin at a targetted INR of 2.0 to 3.0 (103). The primary outcome measure was a composite outcome consisting of major bleeding and recurrent VTE. In the 71 patients who received warfarin, the outcome event rate was 21% compared to 10.5% in the 67 patients who received LMWH, $P = 0.09$. This observed difference was mainly as a result of the rates of major bleeding in the two groups; 16.9% in warfarin patients versus 7.5% in the LMWH patients. Recently, Lee et al. reported the results of the CLOT (randomized comparison of low-molecular-weight heparin versus oral anticoagulant therapy for the prevention of recurrent venous

thromboembolism in patients with cancer) trial in which patients with cancer with acute VTE and/or PE were randomized to long-term dalteparin versus long-term oral anticoagulant therapy (104). Over the 6-month study period, 27 of 336 patients in the dalteparin group compared with 53 of 336 patients in the oral anticoagulant group experienced recurrent VTE. The probability of VTE at 6 months was reduced from 17.4% in the oral anticoagulant group to 8.8% in the dalteparin group, hazard ratio, 0.48; $P = 0.002$ (see Fig. 85-2). No statistically significant difference was detected in major bleeding between groups, 3.6% and 5.6%, respectively. The rate of any bleeding (major plus minor) was 18.5% in the oral anticoagulant group compared to 13.6% in the dalteparin group, $P = 0.09$. On the basis of the results of these trials, long-term therapy with LMWH is an important advance in the management of patients with cancer with acute VTE. It substantially reduces the rate of recurrent VTE without an increase in bleeding, thereby improving the quality of life of the patient with cancer. The use of long-term LMWH also simplifies the management of such patients. It avoids the need for laboratory monitoring which is advantageous for both the patient and physician. If a patient requires

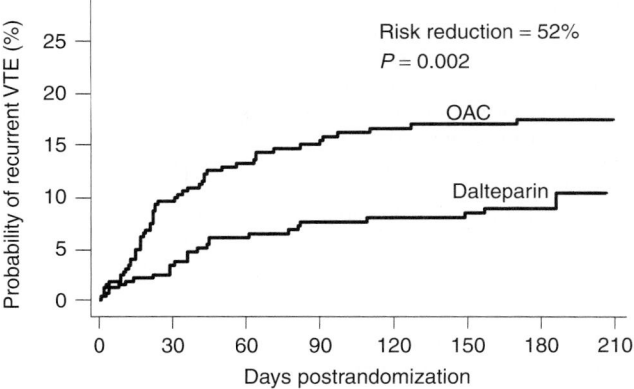

**FIGURE 85-2.** Recurrent venous thrombotic event. (Reproduced with permission from Lee AY, Levine MN, Baker RI, et al. Low-molecular-weight heparin versus a coumarin for prevention of recurrent venous thromboembolism in patients with cancer. *N Engl J Med* 2003;349: 146–153.)

an urgent procedure, the LMWH is just stopped; it is not necessary to reverse the anticoagulant effect.

In general, the duration of long-term treatment of VTE is based on a patient's risk of recurrent thrombosis and bleeding. In patients with malignancy, the risk of recurrent thrombosis depends on the usual thrombotic risk factors (e.g., surgery, bed rest), as well as factors specific to cancer, such as stage or activity of the cancer and the use of chemotherapy and hormonal agents. There are no trials evaluating the duration of anticoagulant therapy in patients with cancer with VTE and data have to be extrapolated from trials of patients with idiopathic thrombosis (105–107).

Currently, the recommendation from American College of Chest Physicians (ACCP) for patients with cancer who experience an acute thromboembolic event is to treat them for a minimum of 12 months with anticoagulant therapy (108). However, as inpatients without cancer, the exact duration of therapy should be tailored individually. In patients with metastatic disease, anticoagulant therapy should be continued indefinitely or until a contraindication to anticoagulation develops. In those who have active but not metastatic disease, anticoagulant therapy should be given for at least 6 months and as long as there is any evidence of cancer or while the patient is receiving chemotherapy. In patients with cancer who have no evidence of active cancer and who developed the thrombotic event in association with a strong risk factor such as surgery, a minimum of 3 months of anticoagulant treatment is probably reasonable, especially if there are relative contraindications for continuing anticoagulation.

# ANTINEOPLASTIC EFFECT OF ANTICOAGULANTS

## Pathophysiology

Over the years, there has been much laboratory research on the effect of the hemostatic system on tumor biology, for example, tumor growth and metastases. A detailed discussion of these data is beyond the scope of this chapter. However, we will briefly consider some of these results as a background to the clinical discussion.

TF activity is dependent upon its expression in conjunction with a suitable lipid surface that can be provided by a variety of tumor cells (109). TF is seldom expressed in normal epithelial tissue, but is expressed as a result of malignant transformation. For example, TF is expressed in ductal epithelium of pancreatic adenocarcinoma (110) and a number of other tumors. TF expression not only correlates with the degree of histologic dedifferentiation in a number of solid tumors but it also appears to alter tumor cell phenotypic behavior. For instance, overexpression of TF using techniques of gene transfer, results in both enhanced tumor cell invasion *in vitro* and primary tumor growth *in vivo* in experimental animal models (111), as well as enhanced metastatic potential in such *in vivo* models (112). Interestingly, in experiments where the effects of TF gene expression on the constitutive expression of potential proangiogenic and antiangiogenic genes has been studied, overexpression of TF appears to be associated with a switch in angiogenic balance toward a more proangiogenic phenotype with upregulation of vascular endothelial growth factor (VEGF) and downregulation of the antiangiogenic thrombospondin (TSP) (113). Other cellular biological manifestations of procoagulant expression are dependent upon signalling of TF upon binding to its extracellular ligand FVIIa. These include stimulation of the interaction of TF cytoplasmic tail with actin-binding protein 280 (ABP-280), with subsequent reorganization of intracellular actin filaments (114). Similar TF:FVIIa interactions on the surface of SW979 pancreatic

adenocarcinoma cells (a high constitutive expressor of TF) *in vitro* result in the upregulation of expression of urokinase plasminogen activator receptor (uPAR) gene, which results in the production of the proteolytic enzyme, plasmin, capable of extracellular proteolysis and matrix degradation. This mechanism may promote tumor cell invasion and endothelial cell invasion toward the tumor as part of the process of angiogenesis (115).

The downstream-activated coagulation proteases also appear to have direct biological effects on tumor cell behavior. Factor Xa appears to be able to induce signalling events in vascular endothelial cells (116) potentially mediated through protease activated receptor 2 (PAR-2), and in HeLa cells by a PAR-1–dependent mechanism, resulting in expression of the angiogenesis-promoting genes Cyr-61 and connective tissue growth factor (CTGF) (117). Thrombin, ultimately generated as a result of the conversion of prothrombin by the prothrombinase complex, interacts with PAR-1 that is expressed on a number of epithelial-derived tumor cell lines. Indeed, PAR-1 appears to be preferentially expressed in highly metastatic cell lines (118). The binding of thrombin to its receptor has a number of cellular effects in cancer, including upregulation of TF expression and enhanced procoagulant activity in colon adenocarcinoma cell lines (119), enhanced expression of urokinase plasminogen activator (uPA) in prostatic carcinoma (120), and enhanced invasive potential of breast carcinoma cells (121). Thrombin also up regulates expression of the VEGF receptor on endothelial cells (122).

Clearly, local peritumor activation of coagulation may have important effects in the biology of cancer, and interference with this activation by antithrombotic agents may alter tumor biology.

## Clinical Studies

The antineoplastic effects of anticoagulants have been studied in a number of clinical trials. In 1984, a large Veterans Administration (VA) Cooperative Trial reported a survival advantage in patients with small cell lung cancer who were randomized to receive warfarin in addition to multiagent chemotherapy as compared to chemotherapy alone (123). Two subsequent randomized trials were carried out in patients with small cell lung cancer evaluating warfarin, and the results were inconclusive (124,125). A trial of low-dose warfarin versus placebo to prevent VTE in women with metastatic breast cancer failed to detect an improvement in survival in women who received warfarin (28). Another trial, which compared a short course of LMWH with UFH for the prevention of postoperative thromboembolism in patients with breast and pelvic malignancies, showed a significantly improved 2-year survival in the patients who received the LMWH (126). Lebeau et al. randomized patients with small cell lung cancer to receive chemotherapy plus adjusted dose UFH for 5 weeks or chemotherapy alone (127). There was a statistically significant improvement in survival with the heparin. Interest in the potential for antithrombotics to impact on survival waned until a number of metaanalyses of trials of LMWH versus UFH for the initial treatment of acute VTE demonstrated a reduction in mortality in favor of LMWH (82,128–130). The observed reduction was due to the effect in the subgroup of patients with cancer. In these trials, the difference was not explained by a reduction in fatal PE. However, none of these trials were designed with survival as the primary outcome.

There are basic science studies that have shown that LMWH can have an effect on angiogenesis, apoptosis, and tumor cell invasion (131–134). Recently, a number of randomized trials have examined the effect of LMWH on the survival of patients with cancer (see Table 85-6). Kakkar et al. recently reported the results of a trial that was specifically designed to test the effect of LMWH on survival in patients with cancer (135). Three hundred and eighty-five patients with advanced solid

### TABLE 85-6

### TRIALS OF LOW-MOLECULAR-WEIGHT HEPARIN AND EFFECT ON SURVIVAL

| Study | Treatment | Patient no. | Results (1-year survival) |
|---|---|---|---|
| Kakkar (135) | Dalteparin 5,000 IU for up to 12 mo | 190 | 46%[a] |
| | Placebo | 184 | 41% |
| Lee (136) | *No metastases* | | |
| | Dalteparin 200 IU/kg for 1 mo followed by 75–80% dose for 5 mo | 75 | 36%[b] |
| | Warfarin acenocoumarol (INR 2.5) | 75 | 20% |
| | *Metastases* | | |
| | Dalteparin 200 IU/kg for 1 mo followed by 75%—80% dose for 5 mo | 221 | 72% |
| | Warfarin acenocoumarol (INR 2.5) | 231 | 69% |
| Klerk (137) | Nadroparin for 6 wk <50Kg 3,800 IU 50–70 kg 5,700 IU >70 kg 7,600 IU | 148 | 39%[c] |
| | Placebo | 154 | 27% |
| Altinbas (138) | Dalteparin 5,000 IU for 18 wk | 42 | 51.3%[d] |
| | Control | 42 | 29.5% |

IU, international units; INR, international normalized ratio.
[a]$P = 0.19$.
[b]$P = 0.03$.
[c]$P = 0.02$.
[d]$P = 0.01$.

tumors were randomized to the LMWH dalteparin or placebo for up to 1 year. No difference was detected in survival at 1 year. However, in a subgroup analysis of patients with good prognosis, there was a statistically significant improvement in survival in favor of the LMWH. In the CLOT trial, no difference was detected in 12-month survival between patients who received LMWH and oral anticoagulant therapy (136). However, in an exploratory subgroup analysis defined *a priori*, the treatment effect on survival was compared between patients with metastatic and those with nonmetastatic cancer. Among patients without metastatic disease, the probability of death at 12 months was 20% in the dalteparin group, as compared with 36% in the oral anticoagulant group (hazard ratio, 0.50; $P = 0.03$). In patients with metastatic disease, no difference in mortality between groups was observed, 72% and 69%, respectively ($P = 0.46$) (see Fig. 85-3). In the Malignancy

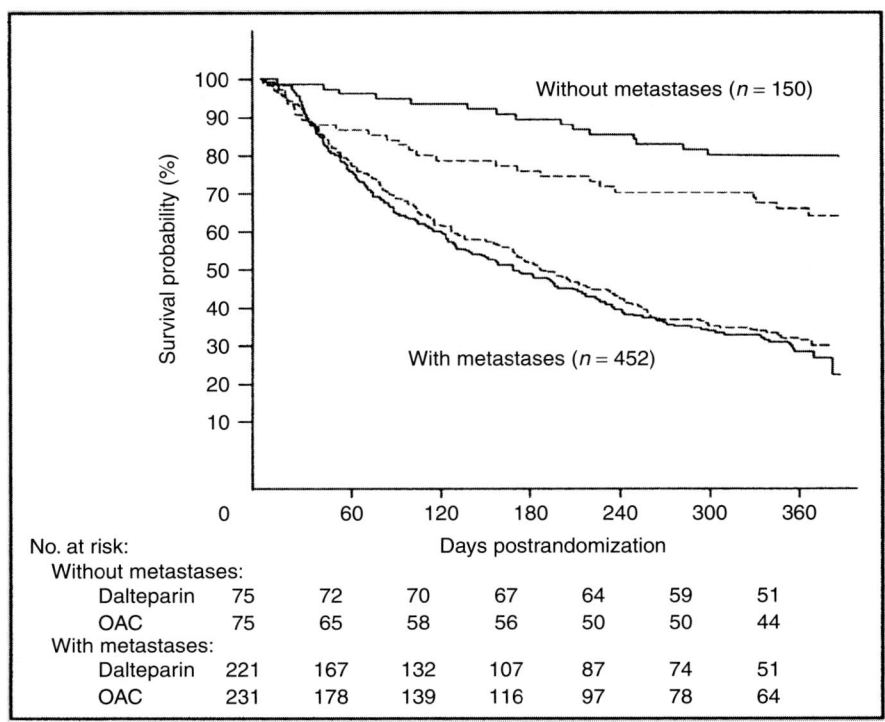

| No. at risk: | | | | | | | |
|---|---|---|---|---|---|---|---|
| Without metastases: | | | | | | | |
| Dalteparin | 75 | 72 | 70 | 67 | 64 | 59 | 51 |
| OAC | 75 | 65 | 58 | 56 | 50 | 50 | 44 |
| With metastases: | | | | | | | |
| Dalteparin | 221 | 167 | 132 | 107 | 87 | 74 | 51 |
| OAC | 231 | 178 | 139 | 116 | 97 | 78 | 64 |

**FIGURE 85-3.** Low-molecular-weight heparin (LMWH) and effect on survival. [Reproduced with permission from Lee AY, Rickles FR, Julian JA, et al. Randomized comparison of LMWH and coumarin derivatives on the survival of patients with cancer and venous thromboembolism. *J Clin Oncol* 2005; 23(10):2123–2129.]

Advanced Low-molecular-weight heparin Trial (MALT), 148 patients with locally advanced or metastatic cancer were randomized to 6 weeks of nadroparin or placebo (137). The survival at 12 months for the LMWH patients was 39% versus 27% in the control group, hazard ratio, 0.75; $P = 0.02$. Finally, in another recent trial, patients with small cell lung cancer were randomized to chemotherapy plus dalteparin for 18 weeks or chemotherapy alone (138). The overall tumor response to treatment was 70% with LMWH compared to 43% without. The median survival was 13 months with LMWH compared to 8 months without; this difference was statistically significant. The results of these trials are encouraging, and further trials evaluating the antineoplastic effect of LMWH are warranted.

# CONCLUSION

In recent years, there has been renewed enthusiasm in the area of thrombosis and cancer that has led to much new research. LMWH administered once daily is effective, safe, and convenient in patients with cancer undergoing surgery. However, there are still some forms of cancer surgery in which clinicians are reluctant to use pharmacologic prophylaxis because of the concern of bleeding, and further research is required. In some patients with cancer undergoing surgery, extended prophylaxis may be beneficial. There is clearly a need for more information on long-term prophylaxis in medical patients with cancer who receive radiation and chemotherapy and in patients with central vein catheters. Some of these patients are clearly at increased risk for thrombosis. The challenge however, is to identify those at highest risk who could benefit from primary prevention. There have been many advances in the management of patients with cancer with acute VTE. Subcutaneous LMWH has replaced intravenous UFH for the initial treatment of VTE and in many instances patients can be treated at home. The use of long-term LMWH instead of oral anticoagulants can substantially reduce the risk of recurrent VTE in this high-risk group of patients, without increased bleeding. A number of novel agents that target specific coagulation proteases are currently undergoing investigation for both the prevention and treatment of VTE (139). Such agents could potentially improve thrombosis management in patients with cancer. Finally, the results of recent clinical trials have supported the concept that antithrombotic therapy can actually have an antineoplastic effect.

## References

1. Trousseau A. Phlegmasia alba dolens. *Clinique Medicale de l'Hotel-Dieu de Paris* 1865;3:654–712.
2. Virchow R. Phlogose und thrombose in GeraBsystem. In: Virchow R, ed. *Gesammette abhandlungen zur wissenchaftichen medicin.* Frankfurt: Von Meidinger Sohn, 1856:458–636.
3. Ruf W. Molecular regulation of blood clotting in tumor biology. *Haemostasis* 2001;31(Suppl. 1):5–7.
4. Gale AJ, Gordon SG. Update on tumor cell procoagulant factors. *Acta Haematol* 2001;106(1-2):25–32.
5. Bazan JF. Structural design and molecular evolution of a cytokine receptor superfamily. *Proc Natl Acad Sci U S A* 1990;87:6934–6938.
6. Mandala M, Curigliano G, Bucciarelli P, et al. Factor V Leiden and G20210A prothrombin mutation and the risk of subclavian vein thrombosis in patients with breast cancer and a central venous catheter. *Ann Intern Med* 2004;15:590–593.
7. Van Rooden CJ, Rosendaal FR, Meinders AE, et al. The contribution of factor V Leiden and prothrombin G20210A mutation to the risk of central venous catheter-related thrombosis. *Haematologica* 2004;89:201–206.
8. Fijnheer R, Paijmans B, Verdonck LF, et al. Factor V Leiden in central venous catheter-associated thrombosis. *Br J Haematol* 2002;118:267–270.
9. Sifontes MT, Nuss R, Hunger SP, et al. The factor V Leiden mutation in children with cancer and thrombosis. *Br J Haematol* 1997;96:474–489.
10. Rogers JS, Murgo AJ, Fontana JA, et al. Chemotherapy for breast cancer decreases plasma protein C and protein S. *J Clin Oncol* 1988;6(2):276–281.
11. Bertomeu MC, Gallo S, Lauri D, et al. Chemotherapy enhances endothelial cell reactivity to platelets. *Clin Exp Metastasis* 1990;8(6):511–518.
12. Pritchard KI, Paterson AH, Paul NA, et al. National Cancer Institute of Canada Clinical Trials Group Breast Cancer Site Group. Increased thromboembolic complications with concurrent tamoxifen and chemotherapy in a randomized trial of adjuvant therapy for women with breast cancer. *J Clin Oncol* 1996;14(10):2731–2737.
13. Silverstein MD, Heit JA, Mohr DN, et al. Trends in the incidence of deep vein thrombosis and pulmonary embolism: a 25-year population-based study. *Arch Intern Med* 1998;158(6):585–593.
14. Heit JA, Silverstein MD, Mohr DN, et al. Predictors of survival after deep vein thrombosis and pulmonary embolism: a population-based, cohort study. *Arch Intern Med* 1999;159(5):445–453.
15. Levitan N, Dowlati A, Remick SC, et al. Rates of initial and recurrent thromboembolic disease among patients with malignancy versus those without malignancy. Risk analysis using Medicare claims data. *Medicine (Baltimore)* 1999;78(5):285–291.
16. Shen VS, Pollak EW. Fatal pulmonary embolism in cancer patients: is heparin prophylaxis justified? *South Med J* 1980;73(7):841–843.
17. Fisher B, Costantino J, Redmond C, et al. A randomized clinical trial evaluating tamoxifen in the treatment of patients with node-negative breast cancer who have estrogen-receptor-positive tumors. *N Engl J Med* 1989;320(8):479–484.
18. Fisher B, Dignam J, Wolmark N, et al. Tamoxifen and chemotherapy for lymph node-negative, estrogen receptor-positive breast cancer. *J Natl Cancer Inst* 1997;89(22):1673–1682.
19. Fisher B, Costantino JP, Wickerham DL, et al. Tamoxifen for prevention of breast cancer: report of the National Surgical Adjuvant Breast and Bowel Project P-1 Study. *J Natl Cancer Inst* 1998;90(18):1371–1388.
20. The ATAC Group. Anastrozole alone or in combination with tamoxifen versus tamoxifen alone for adjuvant treatment of postmenopausal women with early breast cancer: first results of the ATAC randomised trial. *Lancet* 2002;359:2131–2139.
21. Levine MN, Gent M, Hirsh J, et al. The thrombogenic effect of anticancer drug therapy in women with stage II breast cancer. *N Engl J Med* 1988;318(7):404–407.
22. Clahsen PC, van de Velde CJ, Julien JP, et al. Thromboembolic complications after perioperative chemotherapy in women with early breast cancer: a European Organization for Research and Treatment of Cancer Breast Cancer Cooperative Group Study. *J Clin Oncol* 1994;12(6):1266–1271.
23. Rivkin SE, Greens, Metch B, et al. Adjuvant CMFVP versus tamoxifen versus concurrent CMFVP and tamoxifen for postmenopausal, node-positive, and estrogen receptor-positive breast cancer patients: a Southwest Oncology Group Study. *J Clin Oncol* 1994;12:2078–2085.
24. Fisher B, Redmond C, Legault-Poisson S, et al. Postoperative chemotherapy and tamoxifen compared with tamoxifen alone in the treatment of positive-node breast cancer patients aged 50 years and older with tumors responsive to tamoxifen: results from the National Surgical Adjuvant Breast and Bowel Project B-16. *J Clin Oncol* 1990;8(6):1005–1018.
25. Weiss RB, Tormey DC, Holland JF, et al. Venous thrombosis during multimodal treatment of primary breast carcinoma. *Cancer Treat Rep* 1981;65(7-8):677–679.
26. Saphner T, Tormey DC, Gray R. Venous and arterial thrombosis in patients who received adjuvant therapy for breast cancer. *J Clin Oncol* 1991;9(2):286–294.
27. Goodnough LT, Saito H, Manni A, et al. Increased incidence of thromboembolism in stage IV breast cancer patients treated with a five-drug chemotherapy regimen. A study of 159 patients. *Cancer* 1984;54(7):1264–1268.
28. Levine M, Hirsh J, Gent M, et al. Double-blind randomised trial of a very-low-dose warfarin for prevention of thromboembolism in stage IV breast cancer. *Lancet* 1994;343(8902):886–889.
29. Bonneterre J, Thurlimann B, Robertson JFR, et al. Anastrozole versus tamoxifen as first-line therapy for advanced breast cancer in 668 postmenopausal women: results of the tamoxifen or arimidex randomized group efficacy and tolerability study. *J Clin Oncol* 2000;22:3748–3757.
30. Marras LC, Geerts WH, Perry JR. The risk of venous thromboembolism is increased throughout the course of malignant glioma: an evidence-based review. *Cancer* 2000;89(3):640–646.
31. Brandes AA, Scelzi E, Salmistrato E, et al. Incidence and risk of thromboembolism during treatment of high grade gliomas: a prospective study. *Eur J Cancer* 1997;33:1592–1596.
32. Weijl NI, Rutten MF, Zwinderman AH, et al. Thromboembolic events during chemotherapy for germ cell cancer: a cohort study and review of the literature. *J Clin Oncol* 2000;18(10):2169–2178.
33. Blom JW, Osanto S, Rosendaal FR. The risk of a venous thrombotic event in lung cancer patients: higher risk for adenocarcinoma than squamous cell carcinoma. *J Thromb Haemost* 2004;2(10):1760–1765.
34. von Tempelhoff GF, Dietrich M, Niemann F, et al. Blood coagulation and thrombosis in patients with ovarian malignancy. *Thromb Haemost* 1997;77(3):456–461.
35. Solit DB, Morris M, Slovin S, et al. Clinical experience with intravenous estramustine phosphate, paclitaxel, and carboplatin in patients with castrate, metastatic prostate adenocarcinoma. *Cancer* 2003;98:1842–1848.

36. Wun T, Law L, Harvey D, et al. Increased incidence of symptomatic venous thrombosis in patients with cervical carcinoma treated with concurrent chemotherapy, radiation and erythropoeitin. *Cancer* 2003;98:1514–1520.

37. Lavey RS, Liu PY, Greer BE, et al. Recombinant human erythropoietin as an adjunct to radiation therapy and cisplatin for Stage IIB-IVA carcinoma of the cervix: a Southwest Oncology Group Study. *Gynecol Oncol* 2004; 95:145–151.

38. Rosenzweig MQ, Bender CM, Lucke JP, et al. The decision to prematurely terminate a trial of R-HuEPO due to thrombotic events. *J Pain Symptom Manage* 2004;27:185–190.

39. Bleiberg H, Di Leo A, Rothenberg ML, et al. Mortality associated with irinotecan plus bolus fluorouracil/leucovorin. *J Clin Oncol* 2002;20(4): 1145–1146.

40. Rothenberg ML, Meropol NJ, Poplin EA, et al. Mortality associated with irinotecan plus bolus fluorouracil/leucovorin: summary findings of an independent panel. *J Clin Oncol* 2001;19(18):3801–3807.

41. Ottinger H, Belka C, Kozole G, et al. Deep venous thrombosis and pulmonary artery embolism in high-grade non Hodgkin's lymphoma: incidence, causes and prognostic relevance. *Eur J Haematol* 1995;54(3):186–194.

42. Seifter EJ, Young RC, Longo DL. Deep venous thrombosis during therapy for Hodgkin's disease. *Cancer Treat Rep* 1985;69(9):1011–1013.

43. DeStefano V, Sora F, Rossi E. The risk of thrombosis in patients with acute leukemia: ocurrence of thrombosis at diagnosis and during treatment. *J Thromb Haemost* 2005;3:1985–1992.

44. Marx GM, Steer CB, Harper P, et al. Unexpected serious toxicity with chemotherapy and antiangiogenic combinations: time to take stock! *J Clin Oncol* 2002;20:1446–1448.

45. Zangari M, Anaissie E, Barlogie B, et al. Increased risk of deep-vein thrombosis in patients with multiple myeloma receiving thalidomide and chemotherapy. *Blood* 2001;98:1614–1615.

46. Osman K, Comenzo R, Rajkumar SV. Deep venous thrombosis and thalidomide therapy for multiple myeloma. *N Engl J Med* 2001;344:1951–1952.

47. Urbauer E, Kaufmann H, Nosslinger T, et al. Thromboembolic events during treatment with thalidomide. *Blood* 2002;99:4247–4248.

48. Kuenen BC, Rosen L, Smit EF. Dose-finding and pharmacokinetic study of cisplatin, gemcitabine and SU5416 in patients with solid tumors. *J Clin Oncol* 2002;20:1657–1667.

49. Cropp GF, Hannah AL. SU5416, a molecularly targeted novel anti-angiogenic drug: clinical pharmacokinetics and safety review. *Clin Cancer Res* 2002;6:95.

50. Kabbinavar F, Hurwitz HI, Fehrenbacher L, et al. Phase II, randomized trial comparing bevacizumab plus fluorouracil (FU)/leucovorin (LV) with FU/LV alone in patients with metastatic colorectal cancer. *J Clin Oncol* 2003;21(1): 60–65.

51. Zangari M, Barlogie B, Anaissie E, et al. Deep vein thrombosis in patients with multiple myeloma treated with thalidomide and chemotherapy: effects of prophylactic and therapeutic anticoagulation. *Br J Cancer* 2004; 126:715–721.

52. Hurwitz H, Fehrenbacher L, Novotny W, et al. Bevacizumab plus irinotecan, fluorouracil, and leucovorin for metastatic colorectal cancer. *N Engl J Med* 2004;350:2335–2342.

53. Clarke CS, Otridge BW, Carney DN. Thromboembolism. A complication of weekly chemotherapy in the treatment of non-Hodgkin's lymphoma. *Cancer* 1990;66:2027–2030.

54. Sorensen HT, Mellemkjaer L, Olsen JH, et al. Prognosis of cancers associated with venous thromboembolism. *N Engl J Med* 2000;343(25): 1846–1850.

55. Hettiarachchi RJ, Lok J, Prins MH, et al. Undiagnosed malignancy in patients with deep vein thrombosis: incidence, risk indicators, and diagnosis. *Cancer* 1998;83(1):180–185.

56. Baron JA, Gridley G, Weiderpass E, et al. Venous thromboembolism and cancer. *Lancet* 1998;351:1077–1080.

57. Sorensen HT, Mellemkjaer L, Steffensen FH, et al. The risk of a diagnosis of cancer after primary deep venous thrombosis or pulmonary embolism. *N Engl J Med* 1998;338(17):1169–1173.

58. Schulman S, Lindmarker P. Duration of Anticoagulation Trial. Incidence of cancer after prophylaxis with warfarin against recurrent venous thromboembolism. *N Engl J Med* 2000;342(26):1953–1958.

59. Piccioli A, Lensing AWA, Prins MH, et al. Extensive screening for occult malignant disease in idiopathic venous thromboembolism: a prospective clinical trial. *J Thromb Haemost* 2004;2:884–889.

60. Cornuz J, Pearson SD, Creager MA, et al. Importance of findings on the initial evaluation for cancer in patients with symptomatic idiopathic deep venous thrombosis. *Ann Intern Med* 1996;125(10):785–794.

61. Kakkar VV, Howe CT, Nicolaides AN, et al. Deep vein thrombosis of the leg. Is there a "high risk" group? *Am J Surg* 1970;120(4):527–530.

62. Kakkar AK, Williamson RC. Prevention of venous thromboembolism in cancer patients. *Semin Thromb Hemost* 1999;25(2):239–243.

63. Prevention of fatal postoperative pulmonary embolism by low doses of heparin. An international multicentre trial. *Lancet* 1975;2:45–51.

64. Mismetti P, Laporte S, Darmon JY, et al. Meta-analysis of low molecular weight heparin in the prevention of venous thromboembolism in general surgery. *Br J Surg* 2001;88:913–930.

65. Kakkar AK, Haas S, Wolf H, et al. Evaluation of perioperative fatal pulmonary embolism and death in cancer surgical patients: the MC-4 cancer substudy. *Thromb Haemost* (in press).

66. Bergqvist D, Burmark US, Flordal PA, et al. Low molecular weight heparin started before surgery as prophylaxis against deep vein thrombosis: 2500 versus 5000 XaI units in 2070 patients. *Br J Surg* 1995;82(4):496–501.

67. Hull R, Pineo G, Stein PD. Extended out-of-hospital low molecular weight heparin prophylaxis against deep vein thrombosis in patients after elective hip arthroplasty. *Ann Intern Med* 2001;135:858–869.

68. Bergqvist D, Agnelli G, Cohen AT, et al. Duration of prophylaxis against venous thromboembolism with enoxaparin after surgery for cancer. *N Engl J Med* 2002;346:975–980.

69. Rasmussen MS, Wille-Jorgensen P, Jorgensen LN, et al. Prolonged thromboprophylaxis with low molecular weight heparin (dalteparin) after major abdominal surgery: the FAME Study. *J Thromb Haemost* 2003;1(Suppl. 1): CD ROM.OC 399.

70. Geerts WH, Heit JA, Clagett GP, et al. Prevention of venous thromboembolism. *Chest* 2001;119(Suppl. 1):132S–175S.

71. Samama MM, Cohen AT, Darmon JY et al., Prophylaxis in Medical Patients with Enoxaparin Study Group. A comparison of enoxaparin with placebo for the prevention of venous thromboembolism in acutely ill medical patients. *N Engl J Med* 1999;341(11):793–800.

72. Bern MM, Lokich JJ, Wallach SR, et al. A randomized prospective trial. Very low doses of warfarin can prevent thrombosis in central venous catheters. *Ann Intern Med* 1990;112(6):423–428.

73. Monreal M, Alastrue A, Rull M, et al. Upper extremity deep venous thrombosis in cancer patients with venous access devices—prophylaxis with a low molecular weight heparin (Fragmin). *Thromb Haemost* 1996;75(2): 251–253.

74. Masci G, Magagnoli M, Zucali PA, et al. Minidose warfarin prophylaxis for catheter-associated thrombosis in cancer patients: can it be safely associated with fluorouracil-based chemotherapy? *J Clin Oncol* 2003;21(4):736–739.

75. Reichardt P, Kretzschmar A, Biakhov M, et al. A Phase III double-blind, placebo-controlled study evaluating the efficacy and safety of daily low-molecular-weight heparin (dalteparin sodium, fragmin) in preventing catheter-related complications in cancer patients with central venous catheters. *Proc Annu Meet Am Soc Clin Oncol* 2002;21:1474 (Abstract).

76. Couban S, Goodyear M, Burnell M, et al. Randomized placebo-controlled study of low-dose warfarin for the prevention of symptomatic central venous catheter-associated thrombosis in patient with cancer. *J Clin Oncol* 2005;23:4063–4069.

77. Verso M, Agnelli G, Bertoglio S, et al. Enoxaparin for the prevention of venous thromboembolism associated with central vein catheter: a double-blind, placebo-controlled, randomized study in cancer patients. *J Clin Oncol* 2005;23:4051–4062.

78. Walshe LJ, Malak SF, Eagan J, et al. Complication rates among cancer patients with peripherally inserted central catheters. *J Clin Oncol* 2002;20: 3276–3281.

79. Hutten BA, Prins MH, Gent M, et al. Incidence of recurrent thromboembolic and bleeding complications among patients with venous thromboembolism in relation to both malignancy and achieved international normalized ratio: a retrospective analysis. *J Clin Oncol* 2000;18(17):3078–3083.

80. Prandoni P, Lensing AWA, Piccioli A, et al. Recurrent venous thromboembolism and bleeding complications during anticoagulant treatment in patients with cancer and venous thrombosis. *Blood* 2002;100:3484–3488.

81. Hettiarachchi RJ, Prins MH, Lensing AW, et al. Low molecular weight heparin versus unfractionated heparin in the initial treatment of venous thromboembolism. *Curr Opin Pulm Med* 1998;4(4):220–225.

82. Gould MK, Dembitzer AD, Doyle RL, et al. Low-molecular-weight heparins compared with unfractionated heparin for treatment of acute deep venous thrombosis. A meta-analysis of randomized, controlled trials. *Ann Intern Med* 1999;130(10):800–809.

83. Dolovich LR, Ginsberg JS, Douketis JD, et al. A meta-analysis comparing low-molecular-weight heparins with unfractionated heparin in the treatment of venous thromboembolism: examining some unanswered questions regarding location of treatment, product type, and dosing frequency. *Arch Intern Med* 2000;160(2):181–188.

84. van Den Belt AG, Prins MH, Lensing AW, et al. Fixed dose subcutaneous low molecular weight heparins versus adjusted dose unfractionated heparin for venous thromboembolism. *Cochrane Database Syst Rev* 2000; (2):CD001100.

85. Merli G, Spiro TE, Olsson CG, et al. Subcutaneous enoxaparin once or twice daily compared with intravenous unfractionated heparin for treatment of venous thromboembolic disease. *Ann Intern Med* 2001;134(3):191–202.

86. Levine M, Gent M, Hirsh J, et al. A comparison of low-molecular-weight heparin administered primarily at home with unfractionated heparin administered in the hospital for proximal deep-vein thrombosis. *N Engl J Med* 1996;334(11):677–681.

87. Koopman MM, Prandoni P, Piovella F et al., The Tasman Study Group. Treatment of venous thrombosis with intravenous unfractionated heparin administered in the hospital as compared with subcutaneous low-molecular-weight heparin administered at home. *N Engl J Med* 1996; 334(11):682–687.

88. The Columbus Investigators. Low-molecular-weight heparin in the treatment of patients with venous thromboembolism. *N Engl J Med* 1997;337 (10): 657–662.

89. Harrison L, McGinnis J, Crowther M, et al. Assessment of outpatient treatment of deep-vein thrombosis with low-molecular-weight heparin. *Arch Intern Med* 1998;158(18):2001–2003.

90. Wells PS, Kovacs MJ, Bormanis J, et al. Expanding eligibility for outpatient treatment of deep venous thrombosis and pulmonary embolism with low-molecular-weight heparin: a comparison of patient self-injection with homecare injection. *Arch Intern Med* 1998;158(16):1809–1812.

91. Simonneau G, Sors H, Charbonnier B, et al. A comparison of low-molecular-weight heparin with unfractionated heparin for acute pulmonary embolism. The THESEE Study Group. Tinzaparine ou Heparine Standard: Evaluations dans l'Embolie Pulmonaire. *N Engl J Med* 1997;337(10):663–669.

92. Kovacs MJ, Anderson D, Morrow B, et al. Outpatient treatment of pulmonary embolism with dalteparin. *Thromb Haemost* 2000;83(2):209–211.

93. Decousus H, Leizorovicz A, Parent F et al., Prevention du Risque d'Embolie Pulmonaire par Interruption Cave Study Group A clinical trial of vena caval filters in the prevention of pulmonary embolism in patients with proximal deep-vein thrombosis. *N Engl J Med* 1998;338(7):409–415.

94. Millward SF, Oliva VL, Bell SD, et al. Gunther tulip retrievable venacava filter: results from the registry of the Canadian Interventional Radiology Association. *J Vasc Interv Radiol* 2001;12:1053–1058.

95. Luk C, Wells PS, Anderson D, et al. Extended outpatient therapy with low molecular weight heparin for the treatment of recurrent venous thromboembolism despite warfarin therapy. *Am J Med* 2001;111:270–273.

96. Pini M, Aiello S, Manotti C, et al. Low molecular weight heparin versus warfarin in the prevention of recurrences after deep vein thrombosis. *Thromb Haemost* 1994;72(2):191–197.

97. Das SK, Cohen AT, Edmondson RA, et al. Low-molecular-weight heparin versus warfarin for prevention of recurrent venous thromboembolism: a randomized trial. *World J Surg* 1996;20(5):521–526.

98. Lopaciuk S, Bielska-Falda H, Noszczyk W, et al. Low molecular weight heparin versus acenocoumarol in the secondary prophylaxis of deep vein thrombosis. *Thromb Haemost* 1999;81(1):26–31.

99. Gonzalez-Fajardo JA, Arreba E, Castrodeza J, et al. Venographic comparison of subcutaneous low-molecular weight heparin with oral anticoagulant therapy in the long-term treatment of deep venous thrombosis. *J Vasc Surg* 1999;30(2):283–292.

100. Veiga F, Escriba A, Maluenda MP, et al. Low molecular weight heparin (enoxaparin) versus oral anticoagulant therapy (acenocoumarol) in the long-term treatment of deep venous thrombosis in the elderly: a randomized trial. *Thromb Haemost* 2000;84(4):559–564.

101. Hull R, Pineo G, Mah A. Long-term low molecular weight heparin treatment versus oral anticoagulant therapy for proximal deep vein thrombosis [abstract]. *Blood* 2000;96:449 (Abstract).

102. Lorio A, Guercini F, Pini M. Low molecular weight heparin for the long-term treatment of symptomatic venous thromboembolism: meta-analysis of the randomized comparisons with oral anticoagulants. *J Thromb Haemost* 2003;1:1906–1913.

103. Meyer G, Marjanovic Z, Valcke J, et al. Comparison of low-molecular-weight heparin and warfarin for the secondary prevention of venous thromboembolism in patients with cancer. *Arch Intern Med* 2002;162:1729–1735.

104. Lee AY, Levine MN, Baker RI, et al. Low molecular weight heparin versus a coumarin for prevention of recurrent venous thromboembolism in patients with cancer. *N Engl J Med* 2003;349:146–153.

105. Agnelli G, Prandoni P, Santamaria MG et al., Warfarin Optimal Duration Italian Trial Investigators. Three months versus one year of oral anticoagulant therapy for idiopathic deep venous thrombosis. *N Engl J Med* 2001;345(3):165–169.

106. Kearon C, Gent M, Hirsh J, et al. A comparison of three months of anticoagulation with extended anticoagulation for a first episode of idiopathic venous thromboembolism. *N Engl J Med* 1999;340(12):901–907.

107. Schulman S, Rhedin AS, Lindmarker P et al., Duration of Anticoagulation Trial Study Group A comparison of six weeks with six months of oral anticoagulant therapy after a first episode of venous thromboembolism. *N Engl J Med* 1995;332(25):1661–1665.

108. Hyers TM, Agnelli G, Hull RD, et al. Antithrombotic therapy for venous thromboembolic disease. *Chest* 2001;119(Suppl.1):176S–193S.

109. Van de Water L, Tracy PB, Aronson D, et al. Tumour cell generation of thrombin via functional prothrombinase assembly. *Cancer Res* 1985;45:5521–5525.

110. Kakkar AK, Lemoine NR, Scully MF, et al. Tissue factor expression correlates with histological grade in human pancreatic cancer. *Br J Surg* 1995;82:1101–1104.

111. Kakkar AK, Chingwangwatanakul V, Lemoine NR, et al. Role of tissue factor expression on tumour cell invasion and growth of experimental pancreatic adenocarcinoma. *Br J Surg* 1999;86:890–894.

112. Mueller BM, Reisfeld RA, Edgington TS, et al. Expression of tissue factor by melanoma cells promotes efficient hematogenous metastasis. *Proc Natl Acad Sci U S A* 1992;89:11832–11836.

113. Zhang Y, Deng Y, Luther T, et al. Tissue factor controls the balance of angiogenic and antiangiogenic properties of tumor cells in mice. *J Clin Invest* 1994;94:1320–1327.

114. Ott I, Fischer EG, Miyagi Y, et al. A role for tissue factor in cell adhesion and migration mediated by interaction with actin-binding protein 280. *J Cell Biol* 1998;140:1241–1253.

115. Taniguchi T, Kakkar AK, Tuddenham EG, et al. Enhanced expression of urokinase receptor induced through the tissue factor-factor VIIa pathway in human pancreatic cancer. *Cancer Res* 1998;58:4461–4467.

116. Bono F, Schaeffer P, Herault JP, et al. Factor Xa activates endothelial cells by a receptor cascade between EPR-1 and PAR-2. *Arterioscler Thromb Vasc Biol* 2000;20(11):107–112.

117. Riewald M, Kravechenko VV, Petrovan RJ, et al. Gene induction by coagulation factor Xa is mediated by activation of protease-activated receptor 1. *Blood* 2001;97:3109–3116.

118. Even-Ram S, Uziely B, Cohen P, et al. Thrombin receptor overexpression in malignant and physiological invasion processes. *Nat Med* 1998;4(8):909–914.

119. Tanimoto K, Parmley TH, Parham GB, et al. Heparin, a cell surface serine protease identified in hepatoma cells, is overexpressed in ovarian cancer. *Cancer Res* 1997;57:2884–2887.

120. Yoshida E, Verrusio EN, Mihara H, et al. Enhancement of the expression of urokinase-type plasminogen activator from PC-3 human prostate cancer cells by thrombin. *Cancer Res* 1994;54:3300–3304.

121. Even-Ram S, Maoz M, Pokroy E, et al. Tumor cell invasion is promoted by activation of protease activated receptor-1 in cooperation with the alpha vbeta 5 integrin. *J Biol Chem* 2001;276:10952–10962.

122. Zucker S, Conner C, DiMassmo BI, et al. Thrombin induces the activation of progelatinase A in vascular endothelial cells. *J Biol Chem* 1995;270:23730–23738.

123. Zacharski LR, Henderson WG, Rickles FR, et al. Effect of warfarin anticoagulation on survival in carcinoma of the lung, colon, head and neck, and prostate. Final report of VA Cooperative Study #75. *Cancer* 1984;53(10):2046–2052.

124. Chahinian AP, Propert KJ, Ware JH, et al. A randomized trial of anticoagulation with warfarin and of alternating chemotherapy in extensive small-cell lung cancer by the Cancer and Leukemia Group B. *J Clin Oncol* 1989;7(8):993–1002.

125. Maurer LH, Herndon JE, Hollis DR, et al. Randomized trial of chemotherapy and radiation therapy with or without warfarin for limited-stage small-cell lung cancer: a Cancer and Leukemia Group B study. *J Clin Oncol* 1997;15(11):3378–3387.

126. Von Tempelhoff GF, Harenberg J, Niemann F, et al. Effect of low molecular weight heparin (Certoparin) versus unfractionated heparin on cancer survival following breast and pelvic cancer surgery: A prospective randomized double-blind trial. *Int J Oncol* 2000;16(4):815–824.

127. Lebeau B, Chastang C, Brechot JM et al., "Petites Cellules" Group Subcutaneous heparin treatment increases survival in small cell lung cancer. *Cancer* 1994;74(1):38–45.

128. Lensing AW, Prins MH, Davidson BL, et al. Treatment of deep venous thrombosis with low-molecular-weight heparins. A meta-analysis. *Arch Intern Med* 1995;155(6):601–607.

129. Siragusa S, Cosmi B, Piovella F, et al. Low-molecular-weight heparins and unfractionated heparin in the treatment of patients with acute venous thromboembolism: results of a meta-analysis. *Am J Med* 1996; 100(3):269–277.

130. Hettiarachchi RJ, Smorenburg SM, Ginsberg J, et al. Do heparins do more than just treat thrombosis? The influence of heparins on cancer spread. *Thromb Haemost* 1999;82(2):947–952.

131. Nash GF, Walsh DC, Kakkar AK. The role of the coagulation system in tumour angiogenesis. *Lancet* 2001;2:608–613.

132. Norrby K. Heparin and angiogenesis: a low-molecular-weight fraction inhibits and a high-molecular-weight fraction stimulates angiogenesis systemically. *Haemostasis* 1993;23(Suppl. 1):141–149.

133. Folkman J, Langer R, Linhardt RJ, et al. Angiogenesis inhibition and tumor regression caused by heparin or a heparin fragment in the presence of cortisone. *Science* 1983;221(4612):719–725.

134. Zacharski LR, Loynes JT. The heparins and cancer. *Curr Opin Pulm Med* 2002;8:379–382.

135. Kakkar AJ, Levine MN, Kadziola Z, et al. Low molecular weight heparin, therapy with Dalteparin, and survival in advanced cancer: the fragmin advanced malignancy outcome study (FAMOUS). *J Clin Oncol* 2004;22(10):1944–1948.

136. Lee AY, Rickles FR, Julian JA, et al. Randomized comparison of low molecular weight heparin and coumarin derivatives on the survival of patients with cancer and venous thromboembolism. *J Clin Oncol* 2005;23(10):2123–2129.

137. Klerk CP, Smorenburg SM, Otten HM, et al. The effect of low molecular weight heparin on survival in patients with advanced malignancy. *J Clin Oncol.* 2005;23(10):2130–2135.

138. Altinbas M, Coskun HS, Er O, et al. A randomized clinical trial of combination chemotherapy with and without low-molecular-weight heparin in small cell lung cancer. *J Thromb Haemost* 2004;2:1266–1271.

139. Hirsh J, Weitz JI. New antithrombotic agents. *Lancet* 1999;353(9162):1431–1436.

# CHAPTER 86 ■ VENOUS THROMBOSIS IN UNUSUAL SITES

Venous thromboembolism (VTE) typically presents with lower extremity deep vein thrombosis (DVT) or pulmonary embolism (PE) (1,2). Thrombosis in other deep veins, such as the cerebral, subclavian, mesenteric, renal, and pelvic veins, is much less common and may be a clue to an underlying thrombophilia (3). Patients with VTE in these unusual sites have distinct risk factors, signs and symptoms, diagnostic evaluations, and treatment considerations compared to patients with traditional lower extremity DVT or PE (4,5). Axillary or subclavian DVT due to anatomical defects of the thoracic inlet is probably best treated with thrombolysis, surgical correction, and anticoagulation (6–8). Mesenteric vein thrombosis, which is usually caused by inherited or acquired thrombophilia, often presents with vague signs and symptoms not suggestive of thrombosis, and may require prompt resection of necrotic bowel (9). Therefore, VTE in unusual sites should alert the physician to the need for specialized diagnostic tests, therapeutic approaches, and family studies.

# PART I
# Upper Extremity Deep Vein Thrombosis

*Hylton V. Joffe*

Upper extremity deep vein thrombosis (UEDVT), which most commonly refers to thrombosis of the axillary or subclavian veins, has become increasingly common with widespread use of central venous catheters for chemotherapy, dialysis, parenteral nutrition, and bone marrow transplantation (10,11). Historically, UEDVT was considered a benign and self-limited condition (12–14). However, recent studies have demonstrated that UEDVT may have significant complications, including PE, loss of vascular access, the superior vena cava (SVC) syndrome, and long-term arm pain and swelling (15,16).

## ANATOMY

The deep venous system begins at the axillary vein (AV), which is the upward continuation of the basilic vein (see Fig. 86-1). The AV starts at the lower border of the teres major and latissimus dorsi tendons and extends to the outer border of the first rib where it becomes the subclavian vein. The subclavian vein joins the internal jugular vein (IJV) at the inner end of the clavicle to form the brachiocephalic vein (BCV), which merges with the contralateral BCV to form the SVC (17).

The subclavian artery and vein pass under the clavicle and subclavius muscle, and over the first rib. The subclavian artery travels between the anterior and middle scalene muscles, whereas the subclavian vein passes in front of the anterior scalene muscle. The brachial plexus is superior and posterior to the subclavian artery and anterior to the middle scalene muscle. The brachial plexus, subclavian artery, and subclavian vein comprise the neurovascular bundle. Compression of this bundle as it exits the thoracic inlet causes the thoracic outlet syndrome and predisposes to UEDVT (18).

## ETIOLOGY

*Primary UEDVT* refers either to idiopathic disease or to Paget-Schroetter syndrome and occurs in approximately two cases per 100,000 persons per year (19,20). Idiopathic UEDVT has no identifiable precipitant but may be associated with occult neoplasms, especially lung cancer and lymphomas (21,22). Paget-Schroetter syndrome refers to spontaneous UEDVT following strenuous activity, such as pole-vaulting, boxing, baseball pitching, weight lifting, or rowing in young and otherwise healthy individuals (20,23). In this setting, repeated injury to the intimal lining of the upper extremity veins activates prothrombotic mechanisms, eventually causing clinical thrombosis (23). These patients sometimes have coexisting conditions that cause mechanical compression of the vasculature, including the thoracic outlet syndrome, rib anomalies, long transverse processes of the cervical spine, or musculofascial bands (see Fig. 86-2) (6,18,24,25).

*Secondary UEDVT* develops in patients with underlying comorbidities, including cancer (21,26,27), pacemakers (28,29), and central venous catheters (11,30–34) and accounts for most cases of UEDVT (see Table 86-1). Patients with central venous catheters constitute up to one fourth of cases of UEDVT (11, 30,35). Thrombotic risk may be higher with polyvinyl chloride catheters compared to silicone catheters (31). A prospective registry of 5,451 patients with ultrasonography-confirmed DVT demonstrated that an indwelling central venous catheter within the preceding 30 days was the most important independent predictor of UEDVT (compared to lower extremity DVT), increasing the odds of UEDVT approximately 10-fold (33). These catheters also predispose to UEDVT in patients with heparin-induced thrombocytopenia (34). Likely explanations for catheter-associated UEDVT include venous stasis and vessel wall injury (30,36), and the toxic effect of infusate on the vein (27,37,38). Catheter tips should be positioned in the proximal SVC or at the junction between the SVC and right atrium, where blood flow is most rapid (11,30,32,39). Venous thrombosis and stenosis frequently develop because of permanent transvenous pacemaker implantation, although most patients are asymptomatic (28,29). Independent predictors of these venous lesions include previous transvenous temporary leads and a left ventricular ejection fraction of 40% or less (29). Several conventional risk factors for lower extremity DVT, such as surgery, advancing age, and obesity, do not predispose to noncatheter associated UEDVT (33). Rather, independent predictors of this condition include younger age, normal body weight, and hospitalization. A personal history of VTE is also less frequent in patients with non–catheter-associated UEDVT (33).

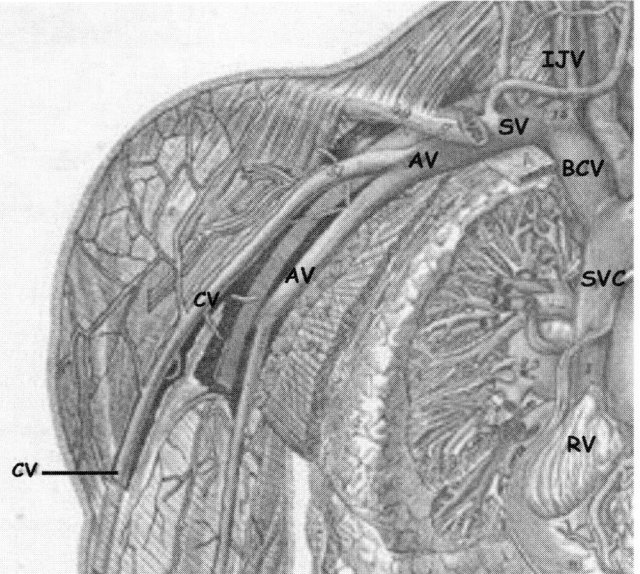

**FIGURE 86-1.** Veins of the upper extremity. The axillary vein (*AV*) extends to the outer border of the first rib where it becomes the subclavian vein (*SV*). The subclavian vein joins the internal jugular vein (*IJV*) at the inner end of the clavicle to form the brachiocephalic vein (*BCV*), which merges with the contralateral BCV to form the superior vena cava (*SVC*). [Copyright protected material used with permission of the authors and the University of Iowa's Virtual Hospital, www.vh.org. Bergman RA, et al. Atlas of Human Anatomy in Cross Section. (Web document). The University of Iowa: Virtual Hospital, 1995:(2001). http://www.vh.org/adult/provider/anatomy/atlasofanatomy/plate19/0 4overview_m.html.]

## CLINICAL PRESENTATION

Patients with UEDVT have a wide spectrum of presentation, ranging from no symptoms to catastrophic SVC syndrome, characterized by facial edema, blurred vision, head fullness, vertigo, and dyspnea (16,40). A coexisting thoracic outlet syndrome may injure the brachial plexus and cause radiation of pain down

### RISK FACTORS FOR UPPER EXTREMITY DEEP VEIN THROMBOSIS

**PRIMARY UPPER EXTREMITY DEEP VEIN THROMBOSIS**
Strenuous activity of the upper extremity (Paget-Schroetter syndrome)
Thoracic outlet syndrome
Idiopathic

**SECONDARY UPPER EXTREMITY DEEP VEIN THROMBOSIS**
Central venous catheters, including the Swan-Ganz catheter
Cancer (perhaps more prevalent in lung neoplasms and lymphoma)
Pacemakers
Implantable cardioverter-defibrillator
Fibrosing mediastinitis
Heparin-induced thrombocytopenia
Ovarian hyperstimulation syndrome
Cocaine abuse
Amyloidosis

the medial aspect of the arm into the fourth and fifth fingers (18). The usual symptoms of UEDVT are extremity edema, discomfort, and erythema (16), but features usually associated with PE, including dyspnea, chest pain, and cough may occasionally be present (33).

Findings on physical examination may include fever, sinus tachycardia, arm and hand edema, supraclavicular fullness, jugular venous distension, upper extremity cyanosis, a palpable tender cord, dilated cutaneous collateral veins over the chest or upper arm, and a completely or partially occluded central venous catheter (16,40–42). Low-grade fever may be present, but high fever is likely due to another cause, such as septic thrombophlebitis, coexisting infection, or underlying neoplasm (43, 44). Sinus tachycardia suggests compensation for reduced venous return to the heart and may occur in the setting of PE (45).

If thoracic outlet syndrome is suspected, the examiner should palpate the supraclavicular fossa for brachial plexus tenderness

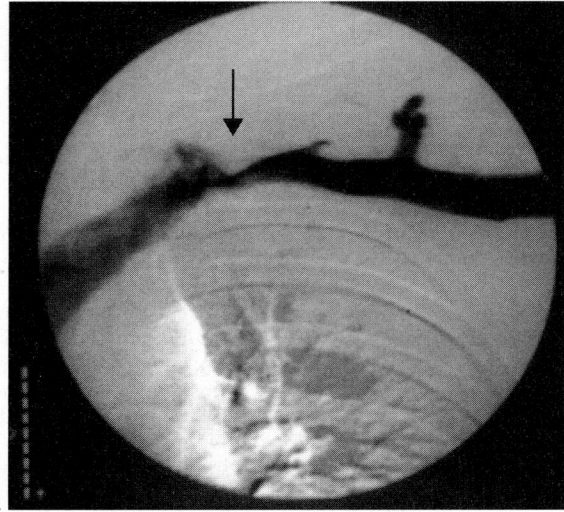
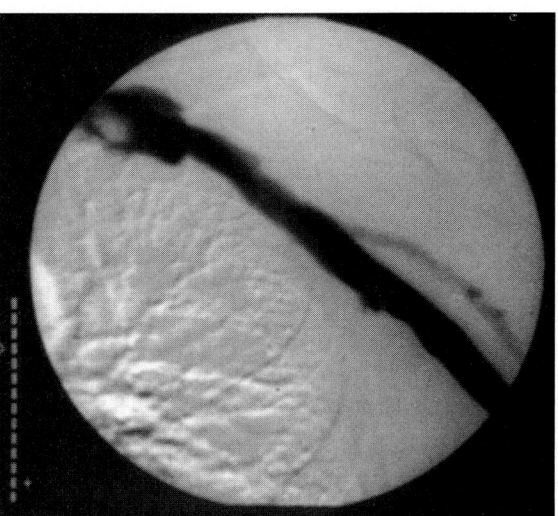

**FIGURE 86-2.** Venogram showing intermittent compression (*arrow*) of the left axillary-subclavian vein with arm abduction. [Adapted with permission from Joffe HV, Goldhaber SZ. Upper extremity deep vein thrombosis. *Circulation* 2002;106(14):1874–1880.]

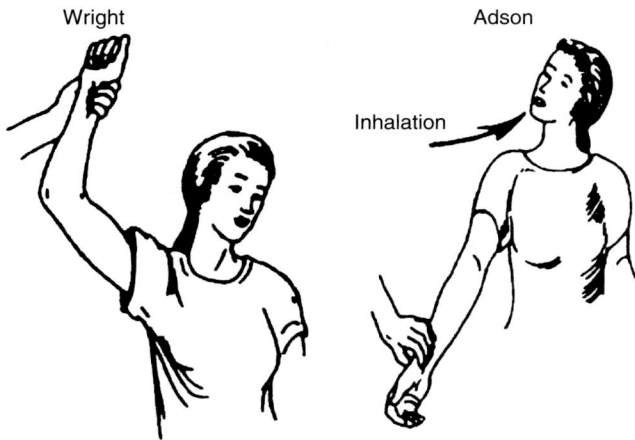

Wright    Adson

Inhalation

**FIGURE 86-3.** Wright and Adson maneuvers. Wright maneuver (**left**) tests for reproduction of symptoms and weakening of the radial pulse when the patient's shoulder is abducted and the humerus is externally rotated. Adson maneuver (**right**) is positive if there is weakening of the radial pulse with deep inspiration when the patient's arm and head are extended and the head is rotated toward the same side. (Adapted from reference Gelberman RH, ed. *Operative nerve repair and reconstruction*. Philadelphia, PA: JB Lippincott Co, 1991:1178, page 1178; illustration by Elizabeth Roselius reproduced with permission.)

and perform provocative tests, such as Wright and Adson maneuvers (see Fig. 86-3) (18,46,47). The Wright test attempts to reproduce symptoms and causes weakening of the radial pulse when the patient's shoulder is abducted and the humerus is externally rotated (18). For the Adson test, the examiner extends the patient's arm on the affected side while the patient extends the neck and rotates the head toward the same side. Weakening of the radial pulse with deep inspiration suggests compression of the subclavian artery (18).

## DIAGNOSIS

Muscle injury, superficial vein thrombosis, lymphedema, and neoplastic compression of the vasculature frequently mimic UEDVT (16). Therefore, the diagnosis of UEDVT cannot be made solely on the basis of the history and physical examination, but must be confirmed with objective testing.

*Duplex ultrasonography* is recommended as the initial test for diagnosing UEDVT because it is noninvasive and has good sensitivity and specificity for jugular, distal subclavian, and axillary UEDVT (16,48–53). However, acoustic shadowing from the clavicle and sternum limits the reliability of this technique for assessing thrombosis in the brachiocephalic and proximal subclavian veins (49,50).

*Contrast venography* provides excellent characterization of the venous anatomy (54) but has several important drawbacks, including technical difficulty cannulating the vein in an edematous arm, use of an iodinated contrast agent, and radiation exposure (see Table 86-2) (55). The contrast agent may cause renal injury, allergic reactions, including urticaria, bronchospasm, and anaphylaxis, or local extravasation and chemical phlebitis (55,56). Acetylcysteine and adequate hydration may reduce nephrotoxicity in patients with abnormal renal function (57). Although iodinated (contrast is rated pregnancy class B and radiation exposure from venography confers minimal risk to the fetus) concerns over teratogenicity limit the use of venography during pregnancy (58). Despite these disadvantages, venography may be required to confirm or exclude the diagnosis of UEDVT when there is high suspicion for thrombosis despite a negative or inconclusive ultrasonography study (48). Venography is also required before interventions, including catheter-directed thrombolysis and angioplasty, and is used to assess the response to these treatments (7,8,59–61).

*Magnetic resonance angiography* (MRA) correlates extremely well with venography and provides a more complete evaluation of blood flow, contralateral vessels, and the SVC and the brachiocephalic vessels (62–67). Therefore, MRA is an excellent noninvasive alternative when venography is contraindicated or technically impossible (see Fig. 86-4).

## TREATMENT

*Anticoagulation* is the cornerstone of therapy for DVT at any site (68), reducing thrombus propagation and maintaining patency of venous collaterals (11). Usually, intravenous unfractionated heparin (UFH) is promptly started at the time of diagnosis unless there is an absolute contraindication to anticoagulation. Low-molecular-weight heparin (LMWH) is a safe and effective alternative and may reduce the duration of hospitalization (69). Typically, heparin is used as a "bridge" to warfarin therapy, which is continued for a minimum of 3 months with a goal international normalized ratio (INR) of 2.0 to 3.0 (12,41). A

**TABLE 86-2**

ADVANTAGES AND DISADVANTAGES OF IMAGING MODALITIES USED TO DIAGNOSE UPPER EXTREMITY DEEP VEIN THROMBOSIS

|  | Advantages | Disadvantages |
|---|---|---|
| **ULTRASONOGRAPHY** | 1. Inexpensive<br>2. Noninvasive<br>3. Reproducible | 1. May fail to detect central thrombus that is directly below the clavicle or sternum |
| **CT SCAN** | 1. May detect central thrombus<br>2. May detect the presence of extrinsic vessel compression | 1. Contrast dye<br>2. Not fully validated |
| **MAGNETIC RESONANCE IMAGING** | 1. Accurately detects central thrombus<br>2. Provides detailed evaluation of collaterals and blood flow | 1. Limited availability<br>2. Claustrophobia<br>3. Not suitable for some patients with implanted metal |

CT, computerized tomography.
Adapted with permission from Joffe HV, Goldhaber SZ. Upper-extremity deep vein thrombosis. *Circulation* 2002;106(14):1874–1880.

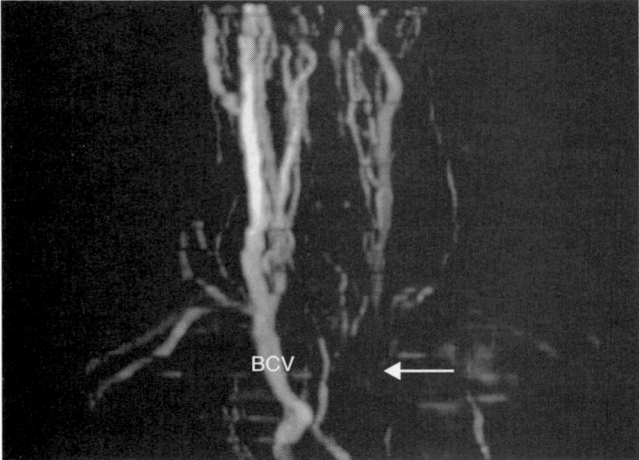

**FIGURE 86-4.** Magnetic resonance angiography demonstrating left brachiocephalic vein thrombosis (BVC) (*arrow*). [Adapted with permission from Joffe HV, Goldhaber SZ. Upper-extremity deep vein thrombosis. *Circulation* 2002;106(14):1874–1880.]

longer duration of anticoagulation is probably appropriate if there is an underlying hypercoagulable state (45,70,71).

*Thrombolysis.* Several case series of UEDVT catheter-directed thrombolysis in carefully selected patients have reported excellent outcomes with only minor bleeding complications, such as occasional hematomas or oozing at catheter sites (8,59,60,72). Although these small studies are underpowered to assess the risk of intracranial or gastrointestinal hemorrhage, the frequency of these serious events is probably similar to that of catheter-directed thrombolysis of lower extremity DVT (73–75).

The best thrombolysis candidates are young, otherwise healthy patients with primary UEDVT because these individuals may have significant long-term morbidity if treated only with conventional anticoagulation (7,76–78). Other appropriate candidates for thrombolysis include patients with symptomatic SVC syndrome and those who require preservation of a mandatory central venous catheter (60,79–81). Catheter-directed recombinant tissue-type plasminogen activator (tPA) may be administered as a continuous infusion of 1 to 2 mg per hour, for at least 8 hours, and serial venography is used to assess treatment response (see Fig. 86-5). Percutaneous mechanical thrombectomy with devices such as the AngioJet (Possis Medical Inc; Minneapolis, Minnesota) can be used to rapidly extract large quantities of thrombus with the goal of reducing the dose and duration of thrombolytic therapy (82).

Unlike conventional anticoagulation, thrombolysis restores venous patency early, which minimizes injury to the vessel endothelium and reduces the risk of long-term complications, including the morbid postthrombotic syndrome (41,76). Contraindications to thrombolysis include active bleeding, a history of hemorrhagic stroke, surgery within the preceding 10 days, neurosurgery within the last 2 months, and hypersensitivity to the thrombolytic agent.

Several thrombolytic agents have been used to treat DVT. Urokinase is effective (59,60,81,83,84) but is no longer manufactured. Streptokinase has also been used successfully (85–88), but may be ineffective if previously administered. tPA is a popular choice in the United States (89). Catheter-directed thrombolysis is preferred over systemic thrombolysis because local delivery of therapy achieves higher rates of complete clot resolution with lower doses of medication (60,61,90,91). Heparin is usually given concurrently to prevent peri-catheter thrombus formation (41). Thrombolysis is most effective when used within several weeks of the onset of symptoms before progressive thrombus organization (60,61,79,84).

*Surgery.* Although thrombolysis may successfully restore vessel patency, persistent vein compression may predispose to recurrent thrombosis and long-term morbidity (8,41). Therefore, after successful thrombolysis for primary UEDVT, most vascular surgeons recommend early assessment for vein compression followed by prompt surgical correction, which typically includes resection of bone or lysis of dense, perivascular adhesions (8,15,41,82,92–96). Persistent structures after surgery should be treated with venoplasty and possibly vein stenting (97,98). This multimodal approach successfully achieves long-term vessel patency (6–8,77,98–101). Although surgical thrombectomy restores venous patency, this technique of treatment is considered as a last resort because it is invasive, requires general anesthesia, and may be complicated by pneumothorax and brachial plexus damage (41). Conservative therapy rather than prompt surgical intervention may be preferable for patients with the thoracic outlet syndrome, because physical therapy, weight loss, and nonsteroidal antiinflammatory medications may avert the need for surgery (18).

*SVC filters* may protect against clinical PE but there is limited data about their safety and efficacy (102,103). There is concern that the benefits of SVC filters may be outweighed by their risks, including filter migration, dislodgment, fracture, and precipitation of the SVC syndrome. Potential candidates for SVC filter placement include patients with UEDVT, with

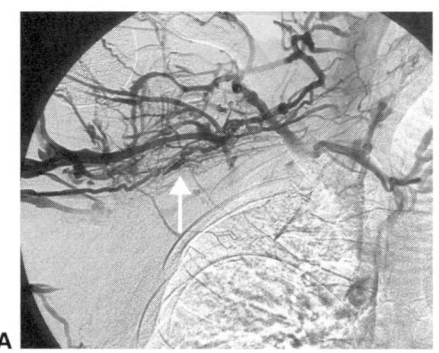
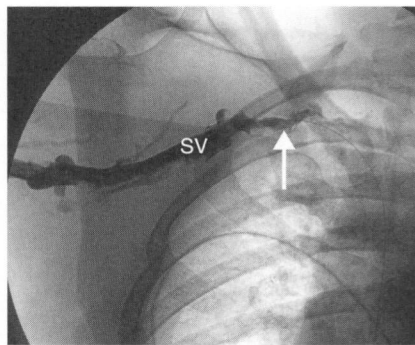
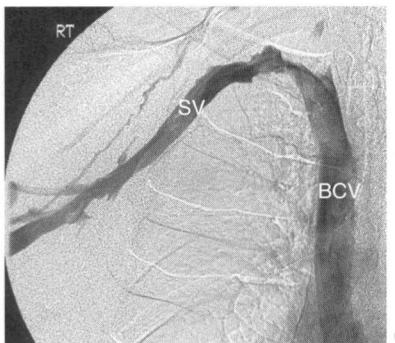

**FIGURE 86-5.** Multimodal therapy for upper extremity deep vein thrombosis: 51-year-old weight lifter complaining of right arm pain. Initial venogram (**A**) shows occluded right axillary and subclavian veins with flow through collateral vessels (*arrow*). After percutaneous thrombectomy (**B**), there is persistent occlusion of the proximal subclavian vein (*arrow*). After thrombolysis (**C**), the subclavian vein (*SV*) is fully patent with flow into the brachiocephalic vein (*BCV*). [Adapted with permission from Joffe HV, Goldhaber SZ. Upper-extremity deep vein thrombosis. *Circulation* 2002;106(14):1874–1880.]

## TABLE 86-3

**EFFECT OF PROPHYLAXIS ON THE INCIDENCE OF UPPER EXTREMITY DEEP VEIN THROMBOSIS IN PATIENTS WITH CANCER AND AN INSERTED CENTRAL VENOUS CATHETER**

| Reference | Prophylactic agent | Duration of observation | Prophylaxis withheld | Prophylaxis given | Risk reduction | Investigation |
|---|---|---|---|---|---|---|
| Bern et al. (104) | 1 mg warfarin daily | 90 d | 37.5% | 9.5% | 75% | Venography |
| Boraks et al. (105) | 1 mg warfarin daily | Catheter duration | 13% | 5% | 62% | Venography or ultrasonography |
| Monreal et al. (106) | 2,500 IU dalteparin | 90 d | 62% | 6% | 90% | Venography |

absolute contraindications to anticoagulation, or those who develop PE despite adequate anticoagulation.

*Prophylaxis.* Patients with cancer and an inserted central venous catheter probably benefit from pharmacologic prophylaxis (see Table 86-3). In two studies, minidose warfarin (1 mg daily) reduced the incidence of UEDVT (104,105). The LMWH dalteparin is an appropriate alternative when patients have comorbidities that substantially increase sensitivity to warfarin, including malnutrition, liver dysfunction, or broad-spectrum antibiotics. In one study (106), there were no bleeding complications from dalteparin, even for patients on chemotherapy with bone marrow suppression. In a head-to-head comparison, low-dose warfarin and LMWH had comparable risk-benefit ratios for UEDVT prophylaxis in patients with cancer and an inserted central venous catheter (107).

It is unclear whether pharmacologic prophylaxis protects against catheter-associated UEDVT in patients without cancer (108,109). Adding heparin to parenteral nutrition does not significantly reduce the risk of catheter-associated UEDVT, but these studies are small and underpowered (108). These limited data may explain why pharmacologic prophylaxis of catheter-associated UEDVT is not commonly used in the United States. In the DVT registry database (33), less than one fourth of patients with catheter-associated UEDVT and no obvious contraindication to anticoagulation were receiving prophylaxis at the time of diagnosis. Furthermore, one fourth of the patients with UEDVT who had an inserted central venous catheter, and who received pharmacologic prophylaxis within 30 days of diagnosis, were given subcutaneous UFH, which, unlike low-dose warfarin (104,105) or LMWH (106), does not reduce the risk of UEDVT.

## COMPLICATIONS

UEDVT may cause significant morbidity (13,14,16). PE is present in up to one third of patients with UEDVT, although fatal PE arising from UEDVT is uncommon (16,110–112). PE may occur during removal of a central venous catheter because fibrin sheaths may peel off, break loose, and embolize (40). Therapeutic heparinization for at least 24 hours before removal of the catheter is a reasonable approach.

Other complications include loss of vascular access, SVC syndrome, septic thrombophlebitis, brachial plexopathy, and thoracic duct obstruction (15,113). The postthrombotic syndrome, secondary to venous hypertension from outflow obstruction and valvular injury, can lead to incapacitating limb pain and swelling (114). This syndrome probably occurs to some degree in most patients treated only with conventional anticoagulation, and may be less likely to occur following multimodal therapy (7,76–78,115,116). Therefore, aggressive treatment, including thrombolysis, may be most suitable for patients with primary UEDVT who are usually young and otherwise healthy, and more likely to be bothered by the postthrombotic syndrome than are patients with chronic medical conditions. Patients with secondary UEDVT have very high short-term mortality rates compared with patients with lower extremity DVT (117), most of them dying from underlying medical problems.

### Thrombophilia

Several observational studies have evaluated the prevalence of inherited and acquired thrombophilia in patients with UEDVT (see Table 86-4) (3,16,118–123). Antithrombin III, protein C, and

## TABLE 86-4

**PREVALENCE (%) OF ACQUIRED AND INHERITED THROMBOPHILIA IN PATIENTS WITH UPPER EXTREMITY DEEP VEIN THROMBOSIS**

| Study | FVL | Prothrombin gene mutation | Hyper homocysteinemia | APLA | ATIII def | Protein S deficiency | Protein C deficiency |
|---|---|---|---|---|---|---|---|
| Bombeli (3) | 25 | 7 | Not tested | Not tested | 1 | 2 | 2 |
| Ellis (118) | 50 | Not tested | Not tested | 22[a] | Not tested | Not tested | Not tested |
| Heron (119) | 10.6 | 0 | Not tested | 22 | 0 | 4.3 | 0 |
| Leebeek (120) | 4.9 | 0 | Not tested | 26.8 | 2.4 | 0 | 0 |
| Martinelli (121) | 8.3 | Not tested | 5.6 | 0 | 0 | 0 | 0 |
| Prandoni (16) | 7.4 | Not tested | Not tested | 3.7 | 3.7 | 3.7 | 7.4 |
| Ruggeri (122) | 3.7 | Not tested | Not tested | 14.8 | 0 | 0 | 3.7 |
| Vaya (123) | 3.8 | 11.4 | Not tested | 7.6[a] | 0 | 0 | 0 |

FVL, factor V$_{Leiden}$; APLA, antiphospholipid antibodies; ATIII Def, antithrombin III deficiency.
[a]Anticardiolipin antibodies.
Adapted with permission from Joffe HV, Goldhaber SZ. Upper-extremity deep vein thrombosis. *Circulation* 2002;106(14):1874–1880.

protein S deficiencies are seldom present in these patients, and the prevalence of factor $V_{Leiden}$, antiphospholipid antibodies and anticardiolipin antibodies varies widely so their role in UEDVT is inconclusive. This inconsistency between studies may be partially attributed to differences in the number of patients studied, types of coagulation tests used, and inclusion of all or only the patients with primary UEDVT.

# PART II
# Cranial and Abdominal Venous Thrombosis
*Victor J. Marder*

One of the hallmarks of thrombophilia is venous thrombosis in unusual sites, such as those of the central nervous system or abdominal cavity. Venous thromboembolic disease usually involves peripheral veins of the limbs, even in patients with hereditary predispositions. However, the existence of a homozygous or doubly heterozygous hereditary predisposition, or the combination of a thrombophilic mutation plus an administered drug, or a particularly oriented illness alone can induce thrombosis at an unusual site. A diagnostic difficulty may be present, because symptoms of venous thrombosis, which are not of the extremities, are often vague or may mimic symptoms of nonthrombotic pathology. Venous thrombi in these locations result from an interaction of acquired insults on a backdrop of congenital abnormalities, compounded to some degree by organ-specific pathology. Examples of special note would be cerebral sinus thrombosis in patients with the G20210A prothrombin mutation, aggressive antiphospholipid syndrome that induces multiorgan disease and multivessel thrombosis, or a myeloproliferative syndrome with predilection for abdominal venous thrombosis. This section describes the unusual sites of venous thrombosis other than the upper extremity that should be considered as potential manifestations of hereditary or acquired thrombophilia. Whatever the cause of a given venous occlusion, aggressive anticoagulation, or regional thrombolytic therapy often can be applied safely to correct venous hypertension and organ dysfunction.

# CEREBRAL VEINS AND DURAL SINUSES

## Anatomy and Pathogenesis

Cerebral venous thrombosis includes thrombosis of the veins and dural sinuses of the brain (124,125). Most often, thrombosis involves the superior sagittal sinus (see Fig. 86-6), which occupies the superior border of the falx cerebri, draining posteriorly into a "confluence of sinuses," then coursing mostly into one of the transverse sinuses, following the sigmoid sinus as it becomes continuous with the IJV. In the preantibiotic era, cerebral venous thrombosis was associated with chronic suppurant infections of the inner ear and skull, but most cases today have no identifiable cause or are associated with head trauma, oral contraceptive (OC) usage, pregnancy or the puerperium, cachexia, dehydration, local malignancy, arteriovenous malformations, or other causes of generalized hypercoagulability. Cerebral venous thrombosis is a well-recognized manifestation of the inherited and acquired thrombophilias, complicating virtually all of the known causes (126–129). Of note is the danger of cerebral vein thrombosis in patients with a hereditary predisposition who have been prescribed OC agents (130) and in patients with paroxysmal nocturnal hemoglobinuria, antiphospholipid syndrome and myeloproliferative disorders (see Chapter 108) (131–134). Following thrombus formation in a venous sinus, increased venous pressure leads to cerebral edema and even hemorrhage (see Fig. 86-7), a process that may progress to the development of large and/or multiple venous infarctions, which cross the normal boundaries of arterial supply (135).

## Clinical Aspects

The diagnosis is often difficult to make because the clinical features may be nonspecific and are often insidious in onset (124, 125,135). Headache, secondary to increased intracranial pressure, occurs in most cases, and in combination with papilledema and the absence of focal neurologic signs, the syndrome can simulate that of a brain tumor ("pseudotumor cerebri")

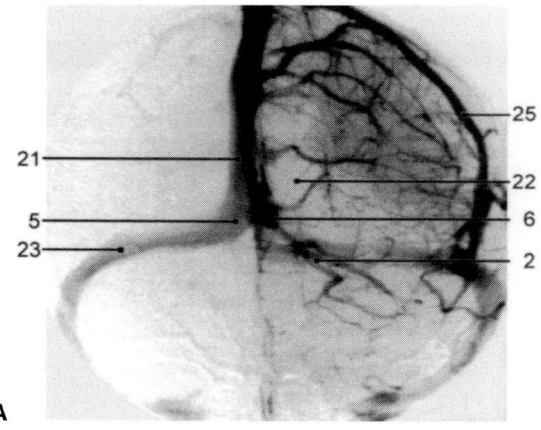
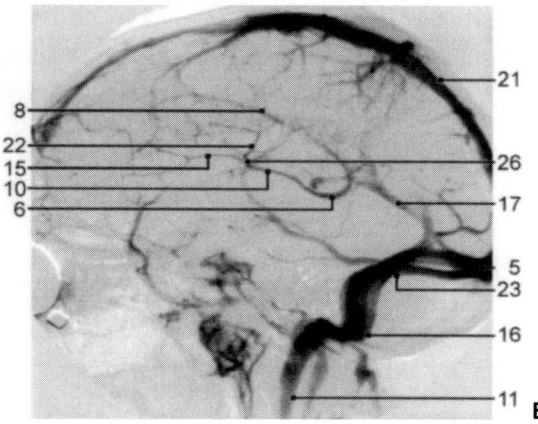

**FIGURE 86-6.** Venous phase of carotid angiography in the anteroposterior (**left panel**) and lateral (**right panel**) projections. The superior sagittal sinus (*21*), confluence of sinuses (*5*), transverse sinus (*23*), sigmoid sinus (*16*), and internal jugular vein (IJV) (*11*) are as indicated. [Reproduced with permission from the Encyclopedia of Medical Imaging (Medcyclopaedia).]

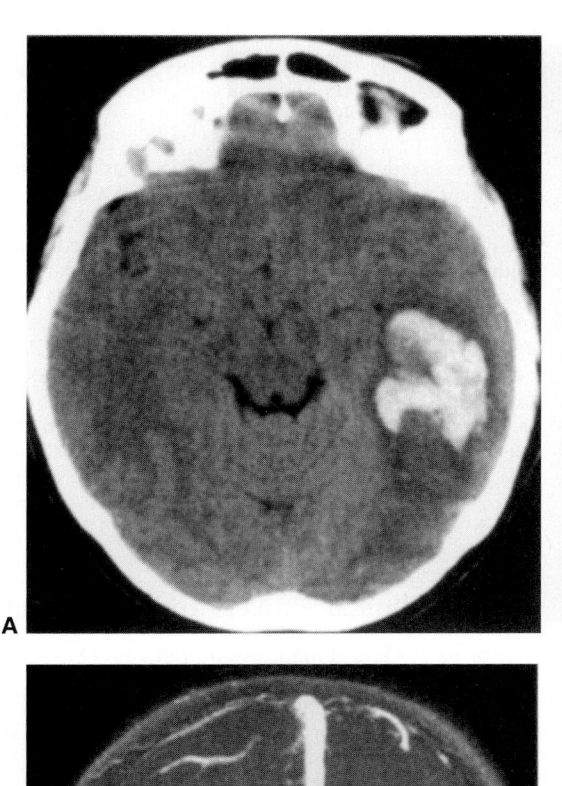

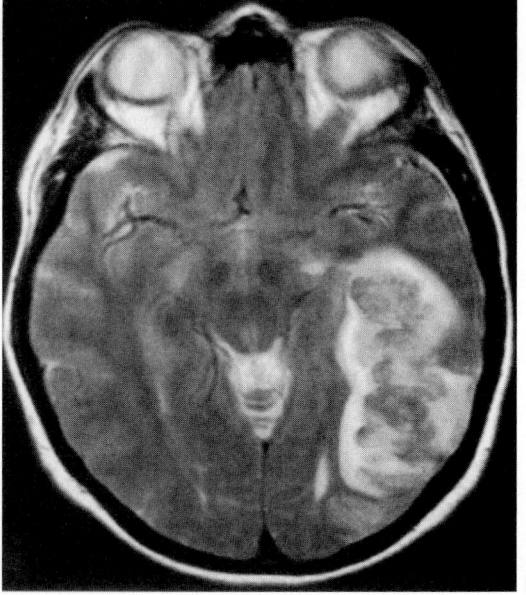

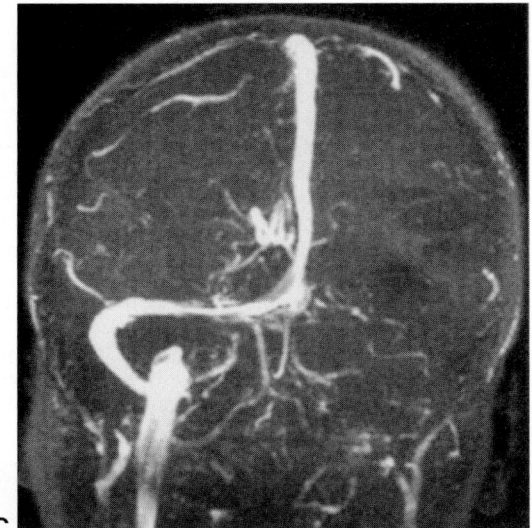

FIGURE 86-7. Intracerebral venous sinus thrombosis. (**A**) shows an axial computerized tomography (CT) scan with hemorrhagic infarction of the left temporal lobe. (**B**) shows the MR, T2-weighted axial image, with an isointense area of recent hemorrhage and a hyperintense area surrounding the infarcted edematous zone. (**C**) shows an angiographic MR study with occlusion of the left transverse sinus, the sigmoid sinus, and the internal jugular vein. [Reproduced with permission from the Encyclopedia of Medical Imaging (Medcyclopaedia).]

(136,137). Nausea, vomiting, and mental confusion develop over hours to days, followed in the most severe cases by stupor and coma, but focal sensory or motor loss are unusual, and the cerebrospinal fluid and the electroencephalogram may show only nonspecific findings. Fever will usually accompany sinusitis or other infection that leads to direct extension of the process into a contiguous (e.g., cavernous) sinus. Diagnosis is most accurately established by magnetic resonance imaging (MRI) studies (125,138–140), which have documented the important contribution of "cytotoxic edema" in the pathogenesis of cerebral venous infarction (141).

## Treatment

The principles of management of cerebral venous or sinus thrombosis are to aggressively treat an identifiable underlying cause such as infection (142), and to initiate anticoagulant or, in select cases, regional thrombolytic therapy, taking care to balance the presence of cerebral hemorrhage with the thrombotic insult.

## Heparin

Controlled studies of anticoagulant therapy are limited: one in 1991 that compared UFH with placebo in 20 patients and one in 1999 that compared LMWH (nadroparin), with placebo in 60 patients (143,144). Using an adjusted-dose intravenous UFH regimen, eight of 10 treated patients had complete clinical recovery at 3 months, compared with one of 10 who received placebo. A retrospective comparison of an additional 43 patients with intracerebral hemorrhage secondary to sinus thrombosis showed complete recovery in 14 patients and mortality in four (15%), compared with three recoveries and nine deaths (69%) in a similar (but uncontrolled) patient group that was not treated with UFH (143). Retrospective observation of 37 patients treated with UFH showed recanalization at discharge in 60% and an "excellent" functional outcome in 89% of patients at 3 months (145). A group of 15 children with cerebral sinus thrombosis who received anticoagulant therapy showed no clinical recurrence and there was complete angiographic resolution in 60% of them, without hemorrhagic complication (146).

LMWH has been randomized against placebo for 3 weeks' treatment in a blinded manner, followed by 3 months of coumadin therapy for all patients (144). Results at 3 weeks showed poor outcome in both groups (20% vs. 24% for placebo) and a nonsignificant trend that favored LMWH at 12 weeks (13% vs. 21% for placebo). Treatment with LMWH was safe with regard to recurrent or new intracranial hemorrhage, but any strong conclusion about efficacy must be tempered by the nonsignificant difference between groups. A 1-year follow-up evaluation of 47 patients showed a disappointing number of patients with cognitive impairment (35%), and the authors further concluded that the outcome was not significantly influenced by treatment (147). Using the Cochrane Database, the same group of authors concluded (148) that anticoagulant treatment "appeared to be safe" and was associated with a reduction in the pooled risk of death (0.33) or dependency (0.46), but that such trends were not statistically significant. A similar conclusion in favor of anticoagulant use has been proposed for children, namely, that no data to prove efficacy exists, but the long-term sequelae (death or neurologic deficit in 50% of children), warrants empiric anticoagulation (149). Clinical outcome of treatment has been summarized for 624 adults in 21 countries, 520 (83%) of whom received anticoagulation therapy (150). The prognosis was better than reported earlier (147), with 356 (57%) having no residue of the illness and 30% with minor or mild impairment.

The accumulated evidence certainly warrants serious consideration of anticoagulant treatment in patients with cerebral sinus thrombosis, even in those patients with demonstrable intracerebral hemorrhage.

### Thrombolytic Therapy

There are numerous reports (151–160) on the use of thrombolytic therapy, usually by regional administration, and so this approach can no longer be considered as unduly risky in a seriously ill patient, and one report used this approach in the face of documented intracranial hemorrhage (161). However, a Cochrane Database review found no randomized, controlled trial of thrombolytic therapy that evaluated efficacy or safety (162). Still, a search of the literature found 169 patients with cerebral sinus thrombosis who received a plasminogen activator (urokinase in 76%), administered regionally into the thrombus in 88% of cases (163). The aggregate experience showed death in nine cases (5%), adverse outcome (dependency) in 7% and intracranial hemorrhage with clinical deterioration in 5%. Without a comparison group, no conclusion about outcome can be drawn about the efficacy or safety of thrombolytic intervention; so for now, this treatment should be applied only after careful consideration of the anticipated prognosis and risk of hemorrhagic complication.

# CENTRAL RETINAL VEIN THROMBOSIS

## Pathogenesis

Central retinal vein thrombosis (CRVO) occurs against a backdrop of the systemic vascular complex of diabetes mellitus, hypertension, and atherosclerosis, and this clinical event has an unclear relation to thrombophilia. CRVO is reported in patients with inherited thrombophilia due to the prothrombin 20210 G/A mutation (164), familial hyperhomocysteinemia (165), the MTHFR mutation (166), and activated protein C resistance (167–169). In one survey of patients with retinal vein occlusion, the factor V R506Q mutation ($V_{Leiden}$) was present in 10 of 35 (29%) pastients with CRVO, similar to that observed

in patients with DVT (40 of 209, 19%) (170), but another retrospective study failed to show this relation (171). The same survey found no preponderance of protein C or protein S deficiency, or lupus inhibitor (170).

Other studies note CRVO as a potential complication of the antiphospholipid syndrome (172,173), in association with external forces, such as trauma, increased intravascular pressure, and ocular pressure from tumor or hemorrhage (174). A recent meta-analysis of 614 patients with CRVO showed a significantly higher homocysteine level and lower serum folate level in comparison with those in 762 controls, but no increased prevalence of the MTHFR genotype (172). Correlations of elevated homocysteine and plasminogen activator inhibitor-1 (PAI-1) and an association with positive antiphospholipid antibody have been highlighted in review articles (173,174,175). Thrombosis has occurred in hematologic diseases with the common denominator of hyperviscosity, including hyperleukocytosis, dysproteinemia, erythrocytosis, hemoglobinopathy, and cryofibrinogenemia (176), and case reports mention association (probably coincidental) with hepatitis C and lung cancer (177,178).

## Clinical Aspects and Treatment

The primary clinical manifestation of CRVO is painless loss of visual acuity, the acuteness and severity of which depends upon the degree of venous occlusion and whether the central (see Fig. 86-8) or a branch vessel is involved. The natural history of the disorder, assessed in 725 patients by the Central Vein Occlusion Study Group, indicates that 15% (81 of 547) of "eyes" with perfusion evolve to ischemia at 4 months, 34% by 3 years, and that the strongest predictor of visual acuity at 3 years is visual acuity at the onset of disease (179). Attempts to alter the course of illness have utilized hemodilution, with both negative and positive effect (180,181), laser photocoagulation without benefit over placebo for visual acuity at 3 months or with protection in some eyes against neovascularization (182,183), rheologic agents with a suggestion of positive results in preliminary studies (184,185), thrombolytic therapy with unconvincing results (186–188), or even surgical decompression (of a branch occlusion) in an uncontrolled trial (189).

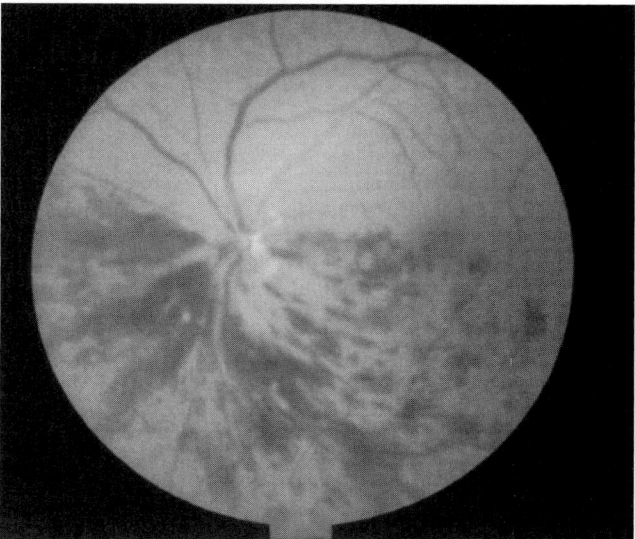

**FIGURE 86-8.** Funduscopic examination of the retina, showing central retinal vein occlusion. Widespread hemorrhages primarily over the inferior aspect of the retina, with venous engorgement and papilledema. (Reproduced with permission, John A. Moran Eye Center, University of Utah. http://insight.med.utah.edu/opatharch/images/retina/22222.jpg.)

The indistinct time of onset of vascular obstruction and the variable nature of retinal edema, hemorrhage, and ischemia makes a trial of therapy difficult to interpret. It is not possible to suggest a single modality of treatment of CRVO, because of the paucity of meaningful studies, although careful prophylactic anticoagulation therapy should be considered for patients at risk of recurrent or progressive thrombotic disease.

# PORTAL/MESENTERIC VEIN THROMBOSIS

## Predispositions

Symptoms of portal/mesenteric vein thrombosis are vague and nonspecific (190–192). Nonlocalized, colicky pain that is severe and out of proportion to physical findings, is nearly universal. Nausea with or without vomiting is seen in half the cases, as is anorexia, but ileus is absent until the condition evolves after days or weeks into a surgical abdomen, the harbinger of bowel infarction (193). Portal vein thrombosis is not usually recognized in the acute-phase and may present clinically as progressive splenomegaly and ascites without evidence of worsening hepatic function. The stool is often guaiac-positive, but laboratory findings are nonspecific, with mild hemoconcentration and a moderate neutrophilia. Blood-tinged ascites signifies bowel infarction as a late manifestation.

Conditions that predispose to portal/mesenteric venous thrombosis include 1% to 5% of patients with inflammatory bowel disease (194,195), cirrhosis and portal hypertension (196), intraabdominal neoplasm (especially carcinoma of the pancreas), intraabdominal infection (especially spontaneous bacterial peritonitis), and blunt or penetrating trauma (including abdominal surgery) (197). Local conditions may be especially prevalent with organ removal as, for example, after splenectomy, in which the incidence has been reported to be 7% (4 of 60) (198), and after liver transplantation, which carries a prevalence of 8% to 26% (199,200). Although not common, portal vein thrombosis has been noted after umbilical vein catheterization (201) and gastric bypass surgery (202).

A substantial portion of patients with "primary" portal/mesenteric venous thrombosis have an underlying thrombophilic condition (203), and it has been reported with deficiencies of antithrombin, protein C, or protein S; mutations of prothrombin G20210A, MTHFR genotype TT677, and factor $V_{Leiden}$; with acquired diseases such as paroxysmal nocturnal hemoglobinuria, antiphospholipid syndrome, and myeloproliferative disorders; and as a complication of factor IX concentrate use and estrogen administration (190,204–215). There does seem to be a real increased prevalence of the prothrombin mutation (40% vs. 5% in controls) (216), but some questions exist about the involvement of the factor $V_{Leiden}$ mutation in this condition (217,218). The important impact of the myeloproliferative disorders on portal/mesenteric venous thrombosis is discussed in Chapter 116.

## Diagnosis and Management

Plain abdominal x-rays and barium contrast studies are nonspecific and are of little assistance in the diagnosis (219). Pseudoobstruction of the colon may be present (220). The bowel wall may be thick, edematous, and dark, but not frankly gangrenous; veins are engorged but arteries are patent, and ischemia is not as clearly demarcated as with arterial occlusion. The bowel may appear dark and purplish on endoscopy, and microscopically, there is extensive hyperemia and hemorrhage (221).

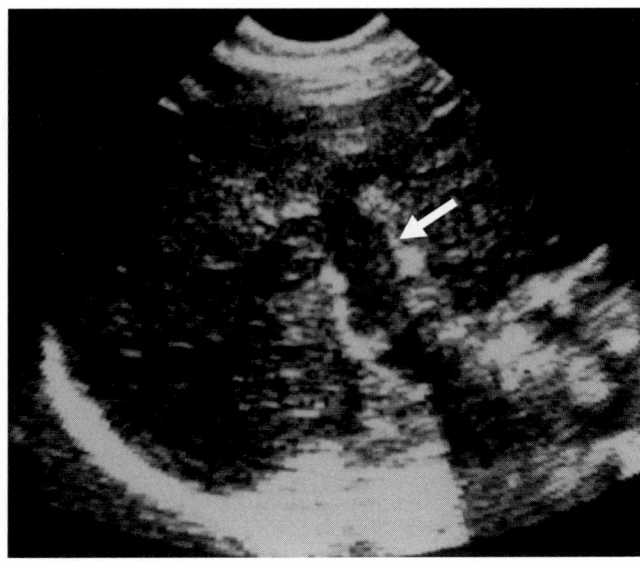

**FIGURE 86-9.** Ultrasonography image of abdomen showing portal vein thrombus. Echogenic structure in the portal vein (*arrow*), with dilation of a portal vein branch in the right lobe of the liver. [Reproduced with permission from the Encyclopedia of Medical Imaging (Medcyclopaedia).]

Noninvasive imaging studies using ultrasonography (see Fig. 86-9), MRI, or CT scan with contrast, are reliable for confirming the diagnosis (222–224). Since the advent of readily available diagnostic tools, there has been a shift in emphasis from primary surgical correction to management with anticoagulation. Two retrospective surveys emphasize this transition as of 1995, and reinforce a conservative approach to begin with, using surgery for evident cases of bowel infarction, necrosis, and potential perforation (225,226). Early noninvasive diagnosis has allowed more efficient treatment, decreasing the mortality from 90% for untreated patients, and 30% to 50% primarily for surgery-treated patients (191,193,227), to more favorable outcomes of 90% or better survival (226).

Medical treatment includes heparin anticoagulation aimed at control of the thrombotic process (225,226), although a role for mechanical thrombectomy or early vascular grafting has been advocated in patients after orthotopic liver transplant (200). In patients with unusual problems with heparin usage, direct antithrombin agents such as argatroban or hirudin are reasonable options (228,229), and gradual vascular recanalization is to be expected in patients who are appropriately treated with anticoagulation (230). Under proper imaging guidance, rapid lysis of thrombus can be achieved by regional thrombolytic administration (231–241), even in the neonatal period (242).

*Splenic vein thrombosis* is rarely recognized at the time of the acute event (243). Typically, the thrombosed vein is discovered during an evaluation of vague abdominal pain with isolated splenomegaly but without ascites or significant hepatic dysfunction, or in relation to pancreatic disease (inflammatory, malignant, or traumatic) (244,245). Splenic vein thrombosis has been reported after "noninvasive" laparoscopic splenectomy (246) and is associated with the same acquired disorders that predispose to portal/mesenteric venous thrombosis (247,248). Portal and splenic vein thrombosis occasionally complicate the nephrotic syndrome, as does renal vein thrombosis, which is a known risk in this condition (249). Anticoagulant therapy for the acute thrombosis may not be indicated, unless a significant thrombophilic process is discovered, but invasive approaches of splenic artery embolism (250) or vascular stenting (251) may be needed for complicating bleeding varices.

# HEPATIC VEIN THROMBOSIS

## Clinical Presentation

In classic hepatic venous outflow obstruction (Budd-Chiari syndrome), the major hepatic veins or the inferior vena cava (IVC) are occluded. Symptoms may be acute and fulminant, with sudden abdominal pain, enlarging liver, rapid development of massive ascites, and mortality risk of up to 67% (252,253). More often the course is chronic and insidious, leading variably to intractable ascites, hepatic insufficiency, and gastrointestinal bleeding due to varices (252–256). The process may develop so rapidly that liver function tests may be normal or near normal at presentation. Common to all presentations is an absence of hepatic venous flow (257).

Hepatic vein thrombosis is associated with a variety of conditions. Toxins such as alkaloids found in senecio beans, comfrey tea ("bush tea"), and high-dosage alkylating agents can thrombose or fibrose the smallest hepatic veins (258–260). Other conditions include hepatocellular carcinoma, renal neoplasm, trauma, intraabdominal infection, pregnancy, OC use, inflammatory bowel disease, and Behçet disease (254,261–263).

Many cases are associated with hematologic disease, including deficiency of antithrombin (264) and heparin-induced thrombocytopenia (265), but especially with paroxysmal nocturnal hemoglobinuria, antiphospholipid syndrome and myeloproliferative syndromes (211,212,264,266–268). There is evidence for a significant contribution of the factor $V_{Leiden}$ mutation, which occurred in 23% (seven of 32 patients) (217) and was reported in an impressive series of six cases (269). "Congenital webs" have been noted in the hepatic veins (254,270) and are generally considered as contributory to the disease (see Fig. 86-10). However, studies show the webs to constitute "organized thrombi of varying ages" and fibrous and recanalized material (271). Therefore, in some cases at

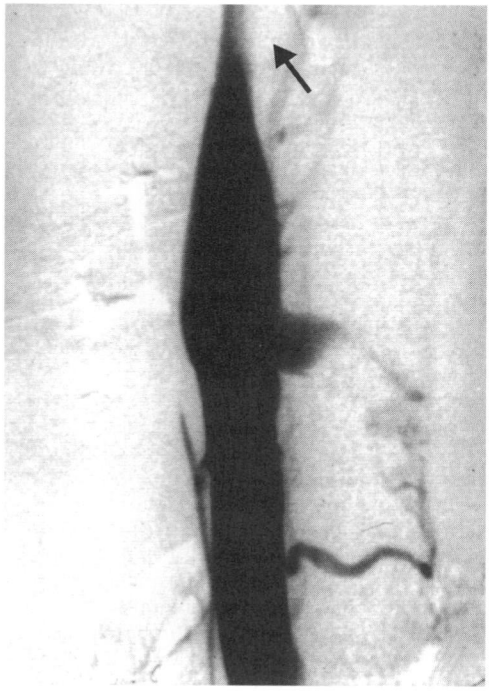

**FIGURE 86-10.** Inferior vena cavography. There is narrowing and occlusion (*arrow*) of the inferior vena cava at the level of the confluence of the hepatic veins caused by an endoluminal "web." [Reproduced with permission from the Encyclopedia of Medical Imaging (Medcyclopaedia).]

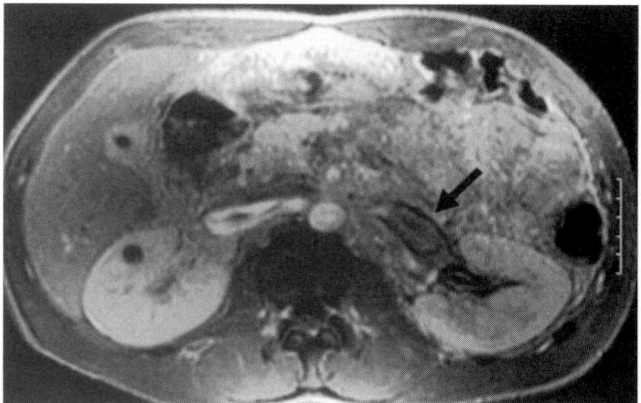

**FIGURE 86-11.** Renal vein thrombosis. Axial contrast-enhanced T1-weighted magnetic resonance image section demonstrating thrombosis of the left renal vein (*arrow*). [Reproduced with permission from the Encyclopedia of Medical Imaging (Medcyclopaedia).]

least, the "webs" represent a sequelae of thrombi rather than congenital malformations, prevalent especially in Asia, and presenting as a more gradual obstructive illness than does acute thrombosis of the hepatic veins (272,273).

Hepatic venography is sensitive and specific for advanced Budd-Chiari syndrome but may be negative in the early stages of the process. Ultrasonography, computed tomography with contrast, and especially MRI provide impressive documentation of pathology (274–276), including clear demonstration of caudate lobe hypertrophy, which results from its direct drainage into the IVC.

## Treatment

Therapy should be early and aggressive, and experience with regional thrombolytic therapy is striking enough to have demonstrated adequate safety and reasonable likelihood for success under dire clinical circumstances (277–281). In addition to or following a thrombolysis attempt, transjugular intrahepatic portosystemic shunt (TIPSS) placement is applied widely to patients with Budd-Chiari syndrome, as a less invasive means of achieving hepatic vein to portal vein anastomosis than with surgical side-to-side portocaval shunting (282). The procedure may improve vascular flow (283) and symptomatic aspects, but encephalopathy may worsen, restenosis may occur, and long-term anticoagulation is still required (284–286). Hepatic transplantation is indicated for patients with hepatic decompensation and can be lifesaving in select cases (287–289).

# RENAL VEIN THROMBOSIS

Renal vein thrombosis is associated with acute illness and severe dehydration in the neonate and may also occur acutely in the adult; however, the more common form in the adult is a chronic presentation caused by the nephrotic syndrome, usually secondary to membranous glomerulonephritis (290,291). Acute renal vein thrombosis (see Fig. 86-11) presents with a triad of flank pain, hematuria, and sudden deterioration of renal function, whereas the chronic form is usually asymptomatic and often undetected until sought by appropriate diagnostic tests (292,293).

The nephrotic syndrome not only predisposes to renal vein thrombosis, but also to extension into the IVC (see Fig. 86-12) and to lower extremity DVT, pulmonary embolism (290,294), and to involvement of the splenic/mesenteric/portal vein system (249,251). Several factors may contribute to the thrombotic

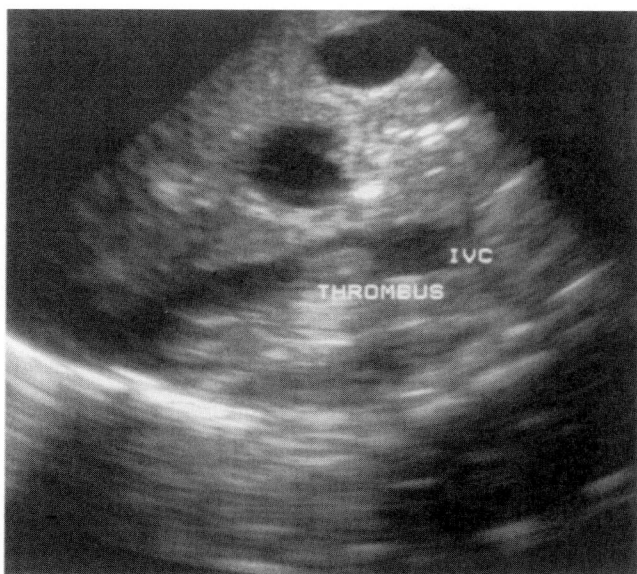

**FIGURE 86-12.** Abdominal ultrasonography of inferior vena cava (*IVC*). A renal vein thrombus has extended into the IVC. [Reproduced with permission from the Encyclopedia of Medical Imaging (Medcyclopaedia).]

tendency, including reduced plasma levels of antithrombin, caused by excessive urinary loss of the protein, and reduced levels of free protein S, perhaps secondary to an increase in C4b-BP (295).

Renal vein thrombosis occurs in patients with inherited thrombophilias, such as deficiency of antithrombin or protein C, or the factor $V_{Leiden}$ mutation (296–298), and with acquired illnesses such as sickle cell disease, paroxysmal nocturnal hemoglobinuria, antiphospholipid syndrome, and Behçet disease (133,299–302). Renal vein thrombosis also may follow renal transplantation, as reflected by a 4% rate of postgraft thrombosis (seven out of 176 transplants), of which five grafts were lost (303). Renal grafts that are threatened by vascular thrombosis can be salvaged by thrombolytic treatment (303–305). Patients with acute renal vein thrombosis are usually treated with anticoagulants, but fibrinolytic therapy has now been used in many patients by regional and systemic routes (306–310), including to a neonate (311).

## PELVIC VEIN THROMBOSIS

Pelvic vein thrombosis, as a distinct entity unassociated with extension of DVT from the lower extremities, occurs in and around the uterine adnexa and complicates 0.1% or fewer of all deliveries, perhaps as many as 1% of patients with pelvic infection (312). Ovarian venous thrombosis is considered to be a form of septic thrombophlebitis (313,314), usually on the right side, and because fever and pain may be present, appendicitis is the differential diagnosis. When limited to the ovarian vein, treatment with antibiotics alone may be all that is required, but if thrombosis also involves the iliac system, heparin treatment is required (314).

## SUPERFICIAL VEIN THROMBOSIS

Superficial vein thrombosis usually occurs in a localized and self-limited form, but a certain proportion of patients (5% to 9%) also have DVT (315,316). Most notable of these superficial vein thrombi are those that involve the greater saphenous

vein, 10% of which are associated with pulmonary embolization. The presence of factor $V_{Leiden}$, the prothrombin G20210A mutation, and protein C, protein S, or antithrombin deficiency can all significantly elevate the odds ratio for formation of superficial vein thrombosis (317–319).

In a retroprospective assessment of 427 hospitalized patients with symptomatic "isolated" superficial vein thrombosis, 19 (4.4%) developed a DVT or pulmonary embolism, the single important predictive factor being severe chronic venous insufficiency (320). Treatment of superficial vein thrombosis has been assessed in two randomized prospective trials, one of which showed a trend (not significant) for decreased incidence of DVT after 12 days of LMWH therapy (1% vs. 3.6% for placebo, $P = 0.37$) (321). The second study, of 60 patients with greater saphenous vein thrombosis, showed fewer symptomatic or asymptomatic DVT or pulmonary embolic events at 6 months using high-dose heparin (3.3% vs. 20% for LMWH, $P = 0.05$) (322). An appropriate management approach would be to make certain that DVT is not already present in a patient with superficial vein thrombosis, and then to tailor the anticoagulant approach on the basis of clinical findings, including the degree of involvement of the greater saphenous vein and the presence of concomitant thrombophilic conditions.

## References

1. Goldhaber SZ, Tapson VF. A prospective registry of 5,451 patients with ultrasound-confirmed deep vein thrombosis. *Am J Cardiol* 2004;93(2): 259–262.
2. Silverstein MD, Heit JA, Mohr DN, et al. Trends in the incidence of deep vein thrombosis and pulmonary embolism: a 25-year population-based study. *Arch Intern Med* 1998;158(6):585–593.
3. Bombeli T, Basic A, Fehr J. Prevalence of hereditary thrombophilia in patients with thrombosis in different venous systems. *Am J Hematol* 2002; 70(2):126–132.
4. Ludemann P, Nabavi DG, Junker R, et al. Factor V Leiden mutation is a risk factor for cerebral venous thrombosis: a case-control study of 55 patients. *Stroke* 1998;29(12):2507–2510.
5. Martinelli I, Sacchi E, Landi G, et al. High risk of cerebral-vein thrombosis in carriers of a prothrombin-gene mutation and in users of oral contraceptives. *N Engl J Med* 1998;338(25):1793–1797.
6. Kunkel JM, Machleder HI. Treatment of Paget-Schroetter syndrome. A staged, multidisciplinary approach. *Arch Surg* 1989;124(10):1153–1157.
7. Adelman MA, Stone DH, Riles TS, et al. A multidisciplinary approach to the treatment of Paget-Schroetter syndrome. *Ann Vasc Surg* 1997;11(2): 149–154.
8. Machleder HI. Evaluation of a new treatment strategy for Paget-Schroetter syndrome: spontaneous thrombosis of the axillary-subclavian vein. *J Vasc Surg* 1993;17(2):305–315; discussion 316–307.
9. Kumar S, Sarr MG, Kamath PS. Mesenteric venous thrombosis. *N Engl J Med* 2001;345(23):1683–1688.
10. Joffe HV, Goldhaber SZ. Upper-extremity deep vein thrombosis. *Circulation* 2002;106(14):1874–1880.
11. Horattas MC, Wright DJ, Fenton AH, et al. Changing concepts of deep venous thrombosis of the upper extremity—report of a series and review of the literature. *Surgery* 1988;104(3):561–567.
12. Ameli FM, Minas T, Weiss M, et al. Consequences of "conservative" conventional management of axillary vein thrombosis. *Can J Surg* 1987;30(3): 167–169.
13. Tilney ML, Griffiths HJ, Edwards EA. Natural history of major venous thrombosis of the upper extremity. *Arch Surg* 1970;101(6):792–796.
14. Swinton NW Jr, Edgett JW Jr, Hall RJ. Primary subclavian-axillary vein thrombosis. *Circulation* 1968;38(4):737–745.
15. Becker DM, Philbrick JT, Walker FB IV. Axillary and subclavian venous thrombosis. Prognosis and treatment. *Arch Intern Med* 1991;151(10): 1934–1943.
16. Prandoni P, Polistena P, Bernardi E, et al. Upper-extremity deep vein thrombosis. Risk factors, diagnosis, and complications. *Arch Intern Med* 1997; 157(1):57–62.
17. Gray H, Pick TP, Howden R. *Anatomy, descriptive and surgical*, 1901 ed. Philadelphia, PA: Running Press, 1974.
18. Parziale JR, Akelman E, Weiss AP, et al. Thoracic outlet syndrome. *Am J Orthop (Chatham, NJ)* 2000;29(5):353–360.
19. Lindblad B, Tengborn L, Bergqvist D. Deep vein thrombosis of the axillary-subclavian veins: epidemiologic data, effects of different types of treatment and late sequelae. *Eur J Vasc Surg* 1988;2(3):161–165.
20. Hughes ESR. Venous obstruction in the upper extremity. *Br J Surg* 1949; 36:155–163.

21. Girolami A, Prandoni P, Zanon E, et al. Venous thromboses of upper limbs are more frequently associated with occult cancer as compared with those of lower limbs. *Blood Coagul Fibrinolysis* 1999;10(8):455–457.

22. Mason BA. Axillary-subclavian vein occlusion in patients with lung neoplasms. *Cancer* 1981;48(8):1886–1889.

23. Zell L, Kindermann W, Marschall F, et al. Paget-Schroetter syndrome in sports activities—case study and literature review. *Angiology* 2001;52(5):337–342.

24. Makhoul RG, Machleder HI. Developmental anomalies at the thoracic outlet: an analysis of 200 consecutive cases. *J Vasc Surg* 1992;16(4):534–542; discussion 542–535.

25. Roos DB. Congenital anomalies associated with thoracic outlet syndrome. Anatomy, symptoms, diagnosis, and treatment. *Am J Surg* 1976;132(6):771–778.

26. Anderson AJ, Krasnow SH, Boyer MW, et al. Thrombosis: the major Hickman catheter complication in patients with solid tumor. *Chest* 1989;95(1):71–75.

27. Lokich JJ, Becker B. Subclavian vein thrombosis in patients treated with infusion chemotherapy for advanced malignancy. *Cancer* 1983;52(9):1586–1589.

28. Stoney WS, Addlestone RB, Alford WC Jr, et al. The incidence of venous thrombosis following long-term transvenous pacing. *Ann Thorac Surg* 1976;22:166–170.

29. Da Costa SS, Scalabrini Neto A, Costa R, et al. Incidence and risk factors of upper extremity deep vein lesions after permanent transvenous pacemaker implant: a 6-month follow-up prospective study. *Pacing Clin Electrophysiol* 2002;25:1301–1306.

30. Eastridge BJ, Lefor AT. Complications of indwelling venous access devices in cancer patients. *J Clin Oncol* 1995;13:233–238.

31. Bozzetti F, Scarpa D, Terno G, et al. Subclavian venous thrombosis due to indwelling catheters: a prospective study on 52 patients. *JPEN J Parenter Enteral Nutr* 1983;7:560–562.

32. Luciani A, Clement O, Halimi P, et al. Catheter-related upper extremity deep venous thrombosis in cancer patients: a prospective study based on Doppler US. *Radiology* 2001;220:655–660.

33. Joffe HV, Kucher N, Tapson VF et al. DVT FREE Steering Committee. Upper-extremity deep vein thrombosis: a prospective registry of 592 patients. *Circulation* 2004;110:1605–1611.

34. Hong AP, Cook DJ, Sigouin CS, et al. Central venous catheters and upper-extremity deep-vein thrombosis complicating immune heparin-induced thrombocytopenia. *Blood* 2003;101:3049–3051.

35. Martin C, Viviand X, Saux P, et al. Upper-extremity deep vein thrombosis after central venous catheterization via the axillary vein. *Crit Care Med* 1999;27(12):2626–2629.

36. Ross AH, Griffith CD, Anderson JR, et al. Thromboembolic complications with silicone elastomer subclavian catheters. *JPEN J Parenter Enteral Nutr* 1982;6(1):61–63.

37. Baglin TP, Boughton BJ. Central venous thrombosis due to bolus injections of antileukaemic chemotherapy. *Br J Haematol* 1986;63(3):606–607.

38. Valerio D, Hussey JK, Smith FW. Central vein thrombosis associated with intravenous feeding—a prospective study. *JPEN J Parenter Enteral Nutr* 1981;5(3):240–242.

39. Kearns PJ, Coleman S, Wehner JH. Complications of long arm-catheters: a randomized trial of central vs peripheral tip location. *JPEN J Parenter Enteral Nutr* 1996;20(1):20–24.

40. Mayo DJ. Catheter-related thrombosis. *J Intraven Nurs* 2001;24:S13–S24.

41. Hicken GJ, Ameli FM. Management of subclavian-axillary vein thrombosis: a review. *Can J Surg* 1998;41(1):13–25.

42. Rochester JR, Beard JD. Acute management of subclavian vein thrombosis. *Br J Surg* 1995;82(4):433–434.

43. Chirinos JA, Lichtstein DM, Garcia J, et al. The evolution of Lemierre syndrome: report of 2 cases and review of the literature. *Medicine (Baltimore)* 2002;81(6):458–465.

44. Stein PD, Afzal A, Henry JW, et al. Fever in acute pulmonary embolism. *Chest* 2000;117(1):39–42.

45. Kumasaka N, Sakuma M, Shirato K. Clinical features and predictors of in-hospital mortality in patients with acute and chronic pulmonary thromboembolism. *Intern Med* 2000;39(12):1038–1043.

46. Gillard J, Perez-Cousin M, Hachulla E, et al. Diagnosing thoracic outlet syndrome: contribution of provocative tests, ultrasonography, electrophysiology, and helical computed tomography in 48 patients. *Joint Bone Spine* 2001;68(5):416–424.

47. Gelberman RH, ed. *Operative nerve repair and reconstruction.* Philadelphia, PA: JB Lippincott Co, 1991:1178.

48. Baarslag HJ, van Beek EJ, Koopman MM, et al. Prospective study of color duplex ultrasonography compared with contrast venography in patients suspected of having deep venous thrombosis of the upper extremities. *Ann Intern Med* 2002;136(12):865–872.

49. Knudson GJ, Wiedmeyer DA, Erickson SJ, et al. Color Doppler sonographic imaging in the assessment of upper-extremity deep venous thrombosis. *AJR Am J Roentgenol* 1990;154(2):399–403.

50. Haire WD, Lynch TG, Lund GB, et al. Limitations of magnetic resonance imaging and ultrasound-directed (duplex) scanning in the diagnosis of subclavian vein thrombosis. *J Vasc Surg* 1991;13(3):391–397.

51. Hubsch PJ, Stiglbauer RL, Schwaighofer BW, et al. Internal jugular and subclavian vein thrombosis caused by central venous catheters. Evaluation using Doppler blood flow imaging. *J Ultrasound Med* 1988;7(11):629–636.

52. Baxter GM, Kincaid W, Jeffrey RF, et al. Comparison of colour Doppler ultrasound with venography in the diagnosis of axillary and subclavian vein thrombosis. *Br J Radiol* 1991;64(765):777–781.

53. Mustafa BO, Rathbun SW, Whitsett TL, et al. Sensitivity and specificity of ultrasonography in the diagnosis of upper extremity deep vein thrombosis: a systematic review. *Arch Intern Med* 2002;162(4):401–404.

54. Stanford W, Jolles H, Ell S, et al. Superior vena cava obstruction: a venographic classification. *AJR Am J Roentgenol* 1987;148(2):259–262.

55. Redman HC. Deep venous thrombosis: is contrast venography still the diagnostic "gold standard"? *Radiology* 1988;168(1):277–278.

56. Lensing AW, Prandoni P, Buller HR, et al. Lower extremity venography with iohexol: results and complications. *Radiology* 1990;177(2):503–505.

57. Tepel M, van der Giet M, Schwarzfeld C, et al. Prevention of radiographic-contrast-agent-induced reductions in renal function by acetylcysteine. *N Engl J Med* 2000;343(3):180–184.

58. Toglia MR, Weg JG. Venous thromboembolism during pregnancy. *N Engl J Med* 1996;335(2):108–114.

59. Seigel EL, Jew AC, Delcore R, et al. Thrombolytic therapy for catheter-related thrombosis. *Am J Surg* 1993;166(6):716–718.

60. Fraschini G, Jadeja J, Lawson M, et al. Local infusion of urokinase for the lysis of thrombosis associated with permanent central venous catheters in cancer patients. *J Clin Oncol* 1987;5(4):672–678.

61. Chang R, Horne MK III, Mayo DJ, et al. Pulse-spray treatment of subclavian and jugular venous thrombi with recombinant tissue plasminogen activator. *J Vasc Interv Radiol* 1996;7(6):845–851.

62. Hartnell GG, Hughes LA, Finn JP, et al. Magnetic resonance angiography of the central chest veins. A new gold standard? *Chest* 1995;107(4):1053–1057.

63. Dymarkowski S, Bosmans H, Marchal G, et al. Three-dimensional MR angiography in the evaluation of thoracic outlet syndrome. *AJR Am J Roentgenol* 1999;173(4):1005–1008.

64. Hansen ME, Spritzer CE, Sostman HD. Assessing the patency of mediastinal and thoracic inlet veins: value of MR imaging. *AJR Am J Roentgenol* 1990;155(6):1177–1182.

65. Thornton MJ, Ryan R, Varghese JC, et al. A three-dimensional gadolinium-enhanced MR venography technique for imaging central veins. *AJR Am J Roentgenol* 1999;173(4):999–1003.

66. Rose SC, Gomes AS, Yoon HC. MR angiography for mapping potential central venous access sites in patients with advanced venous occlusive disease. *AJR Am J Roentgenol* 1996;166(5):1181–1187.

67. Fielding JR, Nagel JS, Pomeroy O. Upper extremity DVT. Correlation of MR and nuclear medicine flow imaging. *Clin Imaging* 1997;21(4):260–263.

68. Hyers TM, Agnelli G, Hull RD, et al. Antithrombotic therapy for venous thromboembolic disease. *Chest* 2001;119(Suppl. 1):176S–193S.

69. Savage KJ, Wells PS, Schulz V, et al. Outpatient use of low molecular weight heparin (Dalteparin) for the treatment of deep vein thrombosis of the upper extremity. *Thromb Haemost* 1999;82(3):1008–1010.

70. Bauer KA. The thrombophilias: well-defined risk factors with uncertain therapeutic implications. *Ann Intern Med* 2001;135(5):367–373.

71. Ridker PM, Goldhaber SZ, Glynn RJ. Low-intensity versus conventional-intensity warfarin for prevention of recurrent venous thromboembolism. *N Engl J Med* 2003;349(22):2164–2167.

72. Beygui RE, Olcott C IV, Dalman RL. Subclavian vein thrombosis: outcome analysis based on etiology and modality of treatment. *Ann Vasc Surg* 1997;11(3):247–255.

73. Bjarnason H, Kruse JR, Asinger DA, et al. Iliofemoral deep venous thrombosis: safety and efficacy outcome during 5 years of catheter-directed thrombolytic therapy. *J Vasc Interv Radiol* 1997;8(3):405–418.

74. Mewissen MW, Seabrook GR, Meissner MH, et al. Catheter-directed thrombolysis for lower extremity deep venous thrombosis: report of a national multicenter registry. *Radiology* 1999;211(1):39–49.

75. Martin M. Results of the PHLEFI study (phlebothrombosis-fibrinolytic therapy): a prospective, multicenter study of the fate of 1498 patients receiving fibrinolytic therapy for deep vein thrombosis. *Int J Angiol* 1998;7(1):68–76.

76. Aburahma AF, Sadler DL, Robinson PA. Axillary subclavian vein thrombosis. Changing patterns of etiology, diagnostic, and therapeutic modalities. *Am Surg* 1991;57(2):101–107.

77. Kreienberg PB, Chang BB, Darling RC III, et al. Long-term results in patients treated with thrombolysis, thoracic inlet decompression, and subclavian vein stenting for Paget-Schroetter syndrome. *J Vasc Surg* 2001;33 (Suppl. 2):S100–S105.

78. Donayre CE, White GH, Mehringer SM, et al. Pathogenesis determines late morbidity of axillosubclavian vein thrombosis. *Am J Surg* 1986;152 (2):179–184.

79. Gray BH, Olin JW, Graor RA, et al. Safety and efficacy of thrombolytic therapy for superior vena cava syndrome. *Chest* 1991;99(1):54–59.

80. Greenberg S, Kosinski R, Daniels J. Treatment of superior vena cava thrombosis with recombinant tissue type plasminogen activator. *Chest* 1991;99(5):1298–1301.

81. Haire WD, Lieberman RP, Lund GB, et al. Obstructed central venous catheters. Restoring function with a 12-hour infusion of low-dose urokinase. *Cancer* 1990;66(11):2279–2285.

82. Kasirajan K, Gray B, Ouriel K. Percutaneous AngioJet thrombectomy in the management of extensive deep venous thrombosis. *J Vasc Interv Radiol* 2001;12(2):179–185.

83. Goldhaber SZ, Polak JF, Feldstein ML, et al. Efficacy and safety of repeated boluses of urokinase in the treatment of deep venous thrombosis. *Am J Cardiol* 1994;73(1):75–79.

84. Zimmermann R, Morl H, Harenberg J, et al. Urokinase therapy of sub-clavian-axillary vein thrombosis. *Klin Wochenschr* 1981;59(15):851–856.

85. Huey H, Morris DC, Nichols DM, et al. Low-dose streptokinase thrombolysis of axillary-subclavian vein thrombosis. *Cardiovasc Intervent Radiol* 1987;10(2):92–95.

86. Steed DL, Teodori MF, Peitzman AB, et al. Streptokinase in the treatment of subclavian vein thrombosis. *J Vasc Surg* 1986;4(1):28–32.

87. Druy EM, Trout HH III, Giordano JM, et al. Lytic therapy in the treatment of axillary and subclavian vein thrombosis. *J Vasc Surg* 1985;2(6):821–827.

88. Wilson JJ, Zahn CA, Newman H. Fibrinolytic therapy for idiopathic sub-clavian-axillary vein thrombosis. *Am J Surg* 1990;159(2):208–210; discussion 201–210.

89. Semba CP, Bakal CW, Calis KA, et al. Alteplase as an alternative to urokinase. Advisory Panel on Catheter-Directed Thrombolytic Therapy. *J Vasc Interv Radiol* 2000;11(3):279–287.

90. Kalman PG, Lindsay TF, Clarke K, et al. Management of upper extremity central venous obstruction using interventional radiology. *Ann Vasc Surg* 1998;12(3):202–206.

91. Sheeran SR, Hallisey MJ, Murphy TP, et al. Local thrombolytic therapy as part of a multidisciplinary approach to acute axillosubclavian vein thrombosis (Paget-Schroetter syndrome). *J Vasc Interv Radiol* 1997;8(2):253–260.

92. Thompson RW, Schneider PA, Nelken NA, et al. Circumferential venolysis and paraclavicular thoracic outlet decompression for "effort thrombosis" of the subclavian vein. *J Vasc Surg* 1992;16(5):723–732.

93. Lee MC, Grassi CJ, Belkin M, et al. Early operative intervention after thrombolytic therapy for primary subclavian vein thrombosis: an effective treatment approach. *J Vasc Surg* 1998;27(6):1101–1107; discussion 1107–1108.

94. Azakie A, McElhinney DB, Thompson RW, et al. Surgical management of subclavian-vein effort thrombosis as a result of thoracic outlet compression. *J Vasc Surg* 1998;28(5):777–786.

95. Lee WA, Hill BB, Harris EJ Jr, et al. Surgical intervention is not required for all patients with subclavian vein thrombosis. *J Vasc Surg* 2000;32(1):57–67.

96. Strange-Vognsen HH, Hauch O, Andersen J, et al. Resection of the first rib, following deep arm vein thrombolysis in patients with thoracic outlet syndrome. *J Cardiovasc Surg (Torino)* 1989;30(3):430–433.

97. Oderich GS, Treiman GS, Schneider P, et al. Stent placement for treatment of central and peripheral venous obstruction: a long-term multi-institutional experience. *J Vasc Surg* 2000;32(4):760–769.

98. Hall LD, Murray JD, Boswell GE. Venous stent placement as an adjunct to the staged, multimodal treatment of Paget-Schroetter syndrome. *J Vasc Interv Radiol* 1995;6(4):565–569; discussion 569–570.

99. Sharafuddin MJ, Sun S, Hoballah JJ. Endovascular management of venous thrombotic diseases of the upper torso and extremities. *J Vasc Interv Radiol* 2002;13(10):975–990.

100. Coletta JM, Murray JD, Reeves TR, et al. Vascular thoracic outlet syndrome: successful outcomes with multimodal therapy. *Cardiovasc Surg* 2001;9(1):11–15.

101. Malcynski J, O'Donnell TF Jr, Mackey WC, et al. Long-term results of treatment for axillary subclavian vein thrombosis. *Can J Surg* 1993;36(4):365–371.

102. Ascher E, Hingorani A, Tsemekhin B, et al. Lessons learned from a 6-year clinical experience with superior vena cava Greenfield filters. *J Vasc Surg* 2000;32(5):881–887.

103. Spence LD, Gironta MG, Malde HM, et al. Acute upper extremity deep venous thrombosis: safety and effectiveness of superior vena caval filters. *Radiology* 1999;210(1):53–58.

104. Bern MM, Lokich JJ, Wallach SR, et al. Very low doses of warfarin can prevent thrombosis in central venous catheters. A randomized prospective trial. *Ann Intern Med* 1990;112(6):423–428.

105. Boraks P, Seale J, Price J, et al. Prevention of central venous catheter associated thrombosis using minidose warfarin in patients with haematological malignancies. *Br J Haematol* 1998;101(3):483–486.

106. Monreal M, Alastrue A, Rull M, et al. Upper extremity deep venous thrombosis in cancer patients with venous access devices—prophylaxis with a low molecular weight heparin (Fragmin). *Thromb Haemost* 1996;75(2):251–253.

107. Mismetti P, Mille D, Laporte S, et al. Low-molecular-weight heparin (nadroparin) and very low doses of warfarin in the prevention of upper extremity thrombosis in cancer patients with indwelling long-term central venous catheters: a pilot randomized trial. *Haematologica* 2003;88(1):67–73.

108. Klerk CP, Smorenburg SM, Buller HR. Thrombosis prophylaxis in patient populations with a central venous catheter: a systematic review. *Archives of Internal Medicine.* 2003;163(16):1913–1921.

109. Bern MM, Bothe A, Jr., Bistrian B, Champagne CD, Keane MS, Blackburn GL. Prophylaxis against central vein thrombosis with low-dose warfarin. *Surgery.* Feb 1986;99(2):216–221.

110. Monreal M, Lafoz E, Ruiz J, Valls R, Alastrue A. Upper-extremity deep venous thrombosis and pulmonary embolism. A prospective study. *Chest* 1991;99(2):280–283.

111. Monreal M, Raventos A, Lerma R, et al. Pulmonary embolism in patients with upper extremity DVT associated to venous central lines—a prospective study. *Thrombosis & Haemostasis.* 1994;72(4):548–550.

112. Harley DP, White RA, Nelson RJ, et al. Pulmonary embolism secondary to venous thrombosis of the arm. *American Journal of Surgery.* 1984;147(2):221–224.

113. Whigham CJ, Greenbaum MC, Fisher RG, et al. Incidence and management of catheter occlusion in implantable arm ports: results in 391 patients. *J Vasc Interv Radiol.* Jun 1999;10(6):767–774.

114. Machleder HI. Effort thrombosis of the axillosubclavian vein: a disabling vascular disorder. *Compr Ther.* May 1991;17(5):18–24.

115. AbuRahma AF, Robinson PA. Effort subclavian vein thrombosis: evolution of management. *Journal of Endovascular Therapy: An Official Journal of the International Society of Endovascular Specialists.* 2000;7(4):302–308.

116. Kerr TM, Lutter KS, Moeller DM, et al. Upper extremity venous thrombosis diagnosed by duplex scanning. *Am J Surg.* Aug 1990;160(2):202–206.

117. Hingorani A, Ascher E, Lorenson E, et al. Upper extremity deep venous thrombosis and its impact on morbidity and mortality rates in a hospital-based population. *J Vasc Surg* 1997;26(5):853–860.

118. Ellis MH, Manor Y, Witz M. Risk factors and management of patients with upper limb deep vein thrombosis. *Chest* 2000;117(1):43–46.

119. Heron E, Lozinguez O, Alhenc-Gelas M, et al. Hypercoagulable states in primary upper-extremity deep vein thrombosis. *Arch Intern Med* 2000;160(3):382–386.

120. Leebeek FW, Stadhouders NA, van Stein D, et al. Hypercoagulability states in upper-extremity deep venous thrombosis. *Am J Hematol* 2001;67(1):15–19.

121. Martinelli I, Cattaneo M, Panzeri D, et al. Risk factors for deep venous thrombosis of the upper extremities. *Ann Intern Med* 1997;126(9):707–711.

122. Ruggeri M, Castaman G, Tosetto A, et al. Low prevalence of thrombophilic coagulation defects in patients with deep vein thrombosis of the upper limbs. *Blood Coagul Fibrinolysis* 1997;8(3):191–194.

123. Vaya A, Mira Y, Mateo J, et al. Prothrombin G20210A mutation and oral contraceptive use increase upper-extremity deep vein thrombotic risk. *Thromb Haemost* 2003;89(3):452–457.

124. Srinivasan K. Cerebral venous and arterial thrombosis in pregnancy and puerperium: a study of 135 patients. *Angiology* 1983;34:731.

125. Ameri A, Bousser M-G. Cerebral venous thrombosis. *Neurol Clin* 1992;10:87.

126. Brenner B, Fishman A, Goldsher D, et al. Cerebral thrombosis in a newborn with a congenital deficiency of antithrombin III. *Am J Hematol* 1988;27:209.

127. Vieregge P, Schwieder G, Kompf D. Cerebral venous thrombosis in hereditary protein C deficiency. *J Neurol Neurosurg Psychiatry* 1989;52:135.

128. Koelman JH, Bakker CM, Plandsoen WC, et al. Hereditary protein S deficiency presenting with cerebral sinus thrombosis in an adolescent girl. *J Neurol* 1992;239:105.

129. Deschiens MA, Conard J, Horellou MH, et al. Coagulation studies, factor V Leiden, and anticardiolipin antibodies in 40 cases of cerebral venous thrombosis. *Stroke* 1996;27:1724.

130. Martinelli I, Sacchi E, Landi G, et al. High risk of cerebral-vein thrombosis in carriers of a prothrombin-gene mutation and in users of oral contraceptives. *N Engl J Med* 1998;338:1793.

131. Moreb J, Kitchens CS. Acquired functional protein S deficiency, cerebral venous thrombosis, and coumarin skin necrosis in association with antiphospholipid syndrome: report of two cases. *Am J Med* 1989;98:207.

132. Levine SR, Kieran S, Puzio K, et al. Cerebral venous thrombosis with lupus anticoagulants: report of two cases. *Stroke* 1987;18:801.

133. Forman K, Sokol RJ, Hewitt S, et al. Paroxysmal nocturnal haemoglobinuria: a clinicopathological study of 26 cases. *Acta Haematol (Basel)* 1984;71:217.

134. Haan J, Caekebeke JFV, Van Der Meer FJM, et al. Cerebral venous thrombosis as presenting sign of myeloproliferative disorders. *J Neurol Neurosurg Psychiatry* 1988;51:1219.

135. May-Malone LJ. Severe headache for 5 weeks. *BUMC Proc* 2003;16:347–348.

136. Gates PC, Barnett HJM. Venous disease: cortical veins and sinuses. In Barnett HJM, Stein BM, Mohr JP, et al., eds. *Stroke: Pathophysiology, diagnosis, and management.* New York: Churchill Livingstone, 1986.

137. Parnass SM, Goodwin JA, Patel DV, et al. Dural sinus thrombosis: a mechanism for pseudotumor cerebri in systemic lupus erythematosus. *J Rheumatol* 1987;14:152.

138. Huang HK, Aberle DR, Lufkin R, et al. Advances in medical imaging. *Ann Intern Med* 1990;112:203.

139. Connor SE, Jarosz JM. Magnetic resonance imaging of cerebral venous sinus thrombosis. *Clin Radiol* 2002;57:449–461.

140. Kirchhof K, Welzel T, Jansen O, et al. More reliable noninvasive visualization of the cerebral veins and dural sinuses: comparison of three MR angiographic techniques. *Radiology* 2002;224:804–810.

141. Forbes KPN, Pipe JG, Heiserman JE. Evidence for cytotoxic edema in the pathogenesis of cerebral venous infarction. *AJNR Am J Neuroradiol* 2001;22:450–455.

142. Bousser MG, Chiras J, Bories J, et al. Cerebral venous thrombosis: a review of 38 cases. *Stroke* 1985;16:199.

143. Einhaupl KM, Villringer A, Meister W, et al. Heparin treatment in sinus venous thrombosis. *Lancet* 1991;338:597–600.

144. De Bruijn SF, Stam J. Randomized, placebo-controlled trial of anticoagulant treatment with low-molecular-weight heparin for cerebral sinus thrombosis. *Stroke* 1999;30:484–488.

145. Stolz E, Trittmacher S, Rahimi A, et al. Influence of recanalization on outcome in dural sinus thrombosis: a prospective study. *Stroke* 2004;35: 544–547.

146. Johnson MC, Parkerson N, Ward S, et al. Pediatric sinovenous thrombosis. *J Pediatr Hematol Oncol* 2003;25:312–315.

147. De Bruijn SF, Budde M, Teunisse S, et al. Long-term outcome of cognition and functional health after cerebral venous sinus thrombosis. *Neurology* 2000;54:1687–1689.

148. Stam J, De Bruijn SF, DeVeber G. Anticoagulation for cerebral sinus thrombosis. *Cochrane Database Syst Rev* 2002;(4):CD002005.

149. Shroff M, deVeber G. Sinovenous thrombosis in children. *Neuroimaging Clin N Am* 2003;13:115–138.

150. Ferro JM, Canhao P, Stam J, et al. ISCVT Investigators. Prognosis of cerebral vein and dural sinus thrombosis: results of the International Study on Cerebral Vein and Dural Sinus Thrombosis (ISCVT). *Stroke* 2004;35: 664–670.

151. Khoo KB, Long FL, Tuck RR, et al. Cerebral venous sinus thrombosis associated with the primary antiphospholipid syndrome: resolution with local thrombolytic therapy. *Med J Aust* 1995;162:30.

152. Horowitz M, Purdy P, Unwin H, et al. Treatment of dural sinus thrombosis using selective catheterization and urokinase. *Ann Neurol* 1995;38:58.

153. Smith AG, Cornblath WT, Deveikis JP. Local thrombolytic therapy in deep cerebral venous thrombosis. *Neurology* 1997;48:1613.

154. Spearman MP, Jungreis CA, Wehner JJ, et al. Endovascular thrombolysis in deep cerebral venous thrombosis. *AJNR Am J Neuroradiol* 1997;18:502.

155. Aoki N, Uchinuno H, Tanikawa T, et al. Superior sagittal sinus thrombosis treated with combined local thrombolytic and systemic anticoagulation therapy. *Acta Neurochir (Wien)* 1997;139:332.

156. D'Alise MD, Fichtel F, Horowitz M. Sagittal sinus thrombosis following minor head injury treated with continuous urokinase infusion. *Surg Neurol* 1998;49:430.

157. Ekseth K, Bostrom S, Vegfors M. Reversibility of severe sagittal sinus thrombosis with open surgical thrombectomy combined with local infusion of tissue plasminogen activator: technical case report. *Neurosurgery* 1998;43:960.

158. Philips MF, Bagley LJ, Sinson GP, et al. Endovascular thrombolysis for symptomatic cerebral venous thrombosis. *J Neurosurg* 1999;90:65.

159. Kuether TA, O'Neill O, Nesbit GM, et al. Endovascular treatment of traumatic dural sinus thrombosis: case report. *Neurosurgery* 1998;42: 1163–1166.

160. Yamini B, Loch Macdonald R, Rosenblum J. Treatment of deep cerebral venous thrombosis by local infusion of tissue plasminogen activator. *Surg Neurol* 2001;55:340–346.

161. Rael JR, Orrison WW Jr, Baldwin N, et al. Direct thrombolysis of superior sagittal sinus thrombosis with coexisting intracranial hemorrhage. *AJNR Am J Neuroradiol* 1997;18:1238.

162. Ciccone A, Canhao P, Falcao F, et al. Thrombolysis for cerebral vein and dural sinus thrombosis. *Cochrane Database Syst Rev* 2004;(1):CD003693.

163. Canhao P, Falcao F, Ferro JM. Thrombolytics for cerebral sinus thrombosis: a systematic review. *Cerebrovasc Dis* 2003;15:159–166.

164. Incorvaia C, Lamberti G, Parmeggiani F, et al. Idiopathic central retinal vein occlusion in a thrombophilic patient with heterozygous 20210 G/A prothrombin genotype. *Am J Ophthalmol* 1999;128:247.

165. Biousse V, Newman NJ, Sternberg P Jr. Retinal vein occlusion and transient monocular visual loss associated with hyperhomocysteinemia. *Am J Ophthalmol* 1997;124:257.

166. Loewenstein A, Winder A, Goldstein M, et al. Bilateral retinal vein occlusion associated with 5,10-methylenetetrahydrofolate reductase mutation. *Am J Ophthalmol* 1997;124:840.

167. Larsson J, Olafsdottir E, Bauer B. Activated protein C resistance in young adults with central retinal vein occlusion. *Br J Ophthalmol* 1996;80:200.

168. Larson J, Sellman A, Bauer B. Activated protein C resistance in patients with central retinal vein occlusion. *Br J Ophthalmol* 1997;81:832.

169. Dhote R, Bachmeyer C, Horellou MH, et al. Central retinal vein thrombosis associated with resistance to activated protein C. *Am J Ophthalmol* 1995;120:388.

170. Greiner K, Hafner G, Dick B, et al. Retinal vascular occlusion and deficiencies in the protein C pathway. *Am J Ophthalmol* 1999;128:69.

171. Linna T, Ylikorkala A, Kontula K, et al. Prevalence of factor V Leiden in young adults with retinal vein occlusion. *Thromb Haemost* 1997;77: 212–224.

172. Cahill MT, Stinnett SS, Fekrat S. Meta-analysis of plasma homocysteine, serum folate, serum vitamin B(12), and thermolabile MTHFR genotypes as risk factors for retinal vascular occlusive disease. *Am J Ophthalmol* 2003;136:1136–1150.

173. Prisco D, Marcucci R. Retinal vein thrombosis: risk factors, pathogenesis and therapeutic approach. *Pathophysiol Haemost Thromb* 2002;32: 308–311.

174. Fegan CD. Central retinal vein occlusion and thrombophilia. *Eye* 2002; 16:98–106.

175. Lahey JM, Kearney JJ, Tune M. Hypercoagulable states and central retinal vein occlusion. *Curr Opin Pulm Med* 2003;9:385–392.

176. Scimeca GH, Magargal LE, Jaeger EA, et al. Medical conditions and retinal vein obstruction. *Pa Med* 1985;88:50.

177. Nadir A, Amin A, Chalisa N, et al. Retinal vein thrombosis associated with chronic hepatitis C: a case series and review of the literature. *J Viral Hepat* 2000;7:466–470.

178. Ronchetto F. Occlusion of a branch of the central retinal vein as a manifestation of hypercoagulability in a patient with lung cancer. A possible paraneoplastic event. *Recenti Prog Med* 1994;85:108–112.

179. The Central Vein Occlusion Study Group. Natural history and clinical management of central retinal vein occlusion. *Arch Ophthalmol* 1997;115: 486–491.

180. Luckie AP, Wroblewski JJ, Hamilton P, et al. A randomised prospective study of outpatient haemodilution for central retinal vein obstruction. *Aust N Z J Ophthalmol* 1996;24:223–232.

181. Chen HC, Wiek J, Gupta A, et al. Effect of isovolaemic haemodilution on visual outcome in branch retinal vein occlusion. *Br J Ophthalmol* 1998; 82:162–167.

182. Battaglia Parodi M, Saviano S, Bergamini L, et al. Grid laser treatment of macular edema in macular branch retinal vein occlusion. *Doc Ophthalmol* 1999;97:427–431.

183. The Central Vein Occlusion Study Group. A randomized clinical trial of early panretinal photocoagulation for ischemic central vein occlusion. *Ophthalmology* 1995;102:1434–1444.

184. Glacet-Bernard A, Coscas G, Chabanel A, et al. A randomized, double-masked study on the treatment of retinal vein occlusion with troxerutin. *Am J Ophthalmol* 1994;118:421–429.

185. De Sanctis MT, Cesarone MR, Belcaro G, et al. Treatment of retinal vein thrombosis with pentoxifylline: a controlled, randomized trial. *Angiology* 2002;53(Suppl. 1):S35–S38.

186. Elman MJ. Thrombolytic therapy for central retinal vein occlusion: results of a pilot study. *Trans Am Ophthalmol Soc* 1996;94:471.

187. Costen MT, Donaldson WB, Olson JA. Acute central retinal vein occlusion successfully treated with intravenous thrombolysis. *Br J Ophthalmol* 1999;83:1196.

188. Hattenbach LO, Wellermann G, Steinkamp GW, et al. Visual outcome after treatment with low-dose recombinant tissue plasminogen activator or hemodilution in ischemic central retinal vein occlusion. *Ophthalmologica* 1999; 213:360–366.

189. Opremcak EM, Bruce RA. Surgical decompression of branch retinal vein occlusion via arteriovenous crossing sheathotomy: a prospective review of 15 cases. *Retina* 1999;19:1–5.

190. Harward TR, Green D, Bergan JJ, et al. Mesenteric venous thrombosis. *J Vasc Surg* 1989;9:328.

191. Abdu RA, Zakhour BJ, Dallis DJ. Mesenteric venous thrombosis, 1911 to 1984. *Surgery* 1987;101:383.

192. Clavien PA, Huber O, Rohner A. Venous mesenteric ischaemia: conservative or surgical treatment? *Lancet* 1989;2:48.

193. Clavien PA, Durig M, Harder F. Venous mesenteric infarction: a particular entity. *Br J Surg* 1988;75:252.

194. Fichera A, Cicchiello LA, Mendelson DS, et al. Superior mesenteric vein thrombosis after colectomy for inflammatory bowel disease: a not uncommon cause of postoperative acute abdominal pain. *Dis Colon Rectum* 2003;46:643–648.

195. Hatoum OA, Spinelli KS, Abu-Hajir M, et al. Mesenteric venous thrombosis in inflammatory bowel disease. *J Clin Gastroenterol* 2005;39:27–31.

196. Grendell JH, Ockner RK. Mesenteric venous thrombosis. *Gastroenterology* 1982;82:358.

197. Triger DR. Extrahepatic portal venous obstruction. *Gut* 1987;28:1193.

198. Chaffanjon PC, Brichon PY, Ranchoup Y, et al. Portal vein thrombosis following splenectomy for hematologic disease: prospective study with Doppler color flow imaging. *World J Surg* 1998;22:1082.

199. Gayowski TJ, Marino IR, Doyle HR, et al. A high incidence of native portal vein thrombosis in veterans undergoing liver transplantation. *J Surg Res* 1996;60:333.

200. Yerdel MA, Gunson B, Mirza D, et al. Portal vein thrombosis in adults undergoing liver transplantation: risk factors, screening, management, and outcome. *Transplantation* 2000;69:1873–1881.

201. Schwartz DS, Gettner PA, Konstantin MM, et al. Umbilical venous catheterization and the risk of portal vein thrombosis. *J Pediatr* 1997; 131:760.

202. Sonpal IM, Patterson L, Schreiber H, et al. Mesenteric venous thrombosis after gastric bypass. *Obes Surg* 2004;14:419–421.

203. Kitchens CS. Evolution of our understanding of the pathophysiology of primary mesenteric venous thrombosis. *Am J Surg* 1992;163:346.

204. Broekmans AQW, van Rooyen W, Westerveld BD, et al. Mesenteric vein thrombosis as presenting manifestation of hereditary protein S deficiency. *Gastroenterology* 1987;92:240.

205. Umpleby HC. Thrombosis of the superior mesenteric vein. *Br J Surg* 1987; 74:694.

206. Dale BM, Naujalis J, Barber S. Congenital antithrombin III deficiency with mesenteric venous thrombosis: functional and immunological estimations. *Pathology* 1984;16:424.

207. Vellenga E, Mulder NH, Gips CH, et al. Vascular problems in paroxysmal nocturnal haemoglobinuria: a report of two cases. *Blut* 1982;45:261.

208. Hoyle M, Kennedy A, Prior AL, et al. Small bowel ischaemia and infarction in young women taking oral contraceptives and progestational agents. *Br J Surg* 1977;64:533.

209. Bergenfeldt M, Svensson PJ, Borgstrom A. Mesenteric vein thrombosis due to factor V Leiden gene mutation. *Br J Surg* 1999;86:1059.

210. Balian A, Veyradier A, Naveau S, et al. Prothrombin 20210G/A mutation in two patients wth mesenteric ischemia. *Dig Dis Sci* 1999;44:1910.

211. Asherson RA, Khamashta MA, Ordi–Ros J, et al. The "primary" antiphospholipid syndrome: major clinical and serological features. *Medicine* 1989; 68:366.

212. Peytremann R, Rhodes RS, Hartmann RC. Thrombosis in paroxysmal nocturnal hemoglobinuria with particular reference to progressive diffuse hepatic venous thrombosis. *Ser Haematol* 1972;3:115.

213. Valla D, Casadevall N, Huisse MG, et al. Etiology of portal vein thrombosis in adults: a prospective evaluation of primary myeloproliferative disorders. *Gastroenterology* 1988;94:1063.

214. Friederich P, Putensen C, Stuber F. Prothrombin gene G20210A mutation and elevated anticardiolipin antibodies in a patient with combined portal-mesenteric vein thrombosis. *Intensive Care Med* 2000;26:1571–1574.

215. Amitrano L, Brancaccio V, Guardascione MA, et al. High prevalence of thrombophilic genotypes in patients with acute mesenteric vein thrombosis. *Am J Gastroenterol* 2001;96:146–149.

216. Chamouard P, Pencreach E, Maloisel F, et al. Frequent factor II G20210A mutation in idiopathic portal vein thrombosis. *Gastroenterology* 1999; 116:144.

217. Mahmoud AE, Elias E, Beauchamp N, et al. Prevalence of the factor V Leiden mutation in hepatic and portal vein thrombosis. *Gut* 1997;40:798.

218. Seixas CA, Hessel G, Ribeiro CC, et al. Factor V Leiden is not common in children with portal vein thrombosis. *Thromb Haemost* 1997;77:258.

219. Font VE, Hermann RE, Longworth DL. Chronic mesenteric venous thrombosis: difficult diagnosis and therapy. *Cleve Clin J Med* 1989;56:823.

220. Roman RJ, Loeb PM. Massive colonic dilatation as initial presentation of mesenteric vein thrombosis. *Dig Dis Sci* 1987;32:323.

221. Jabbari M, Cherry R, Goresky CA. The endoscopic diagnosis of mesenteric venous thrombosis. *Gastrointest Endosc* 1985;31:405.

222. Subramanyam BR, Balthazar EJ, Lefleur RS, et al. Portal vein thrombosis: correlative analysis of sonography, CT, and angiography. *Am J Gastroenterol* 1984;79:773.

223. Matos C, Van Gansbeke D, Zalcman M, et al. Mesenteric vein thrombosis: early CT and US diagnosis and conservative management. *Gastrointest Radiol* 1986;11:322.

224. Bradbury MS, Kavanagh PV, Bechtold RE, et al. Mesenteric venous thrombosis: diagnosis and noninvasive imaging. *Radiographics* 2002;22: 527–541.

225. Brunaud L, Antunes L, Collinet-Adler S, et al. Acute mesenteric venous thrombosis: case for nonoperative management. *J Vasc Surg* 2001;34: 673–679.

226. Zhang J, Duan ZQ, Song QB, et al. Acute mesenteric venous thrombosis: a better outcome achieved through improved imaging techniques and a changed policy of clinical management. *Eur J Vasc Endovasc Surg* 2004; 28:329–334.

227. Rhee RY, Gloviczki P, Mendonca CT, et al. Mesenteric venous thrombosis: still a lethal disease in the 1990s. *J Vasc Surg* 1994;20:688–697.

228. Gordon MB, Beckman JA. Successful anticoagulation with hirudin in a patient with mesenteric venous thrombosis and multiple coagulation abnormalities. *Vasc Med* 2000;5:159–162.

229. Dager WE, Gosselin RC, Owings JT. Argatroban therapy for antithrombin deficiency and mesenteric thrombosis: case report and review of the literature. *Pharmacotherapy* 2004;24:653–659.

230. Condat B, Pessione F, Helene Denninger M, et al. Recent portal or mesenteric venous thrombosis: increased recognition and frequent recanalization on anticoagulant therapy. *Hepatology* 2000;32:466–470.

231. Bilbao JI, Rodriguez CJ, Longo J, et al. Portal thrombosis: percutaneous transhepatic treatment with urokinase—a case report. *Gastrointest Radiol* 1989;14:326.

232. Bizollon T, Bissuel F, Detry L, et al. Fibrinolytic therapy for portal vein thrombosis. *Lancet* 1991;337:1416.

233. Suzuki S, Nakamura S, Baba S, et al. Portal vein thrombosis after splenectomy successfully treated by an enormous dosage of fibrinolytic agent in a short period: report of two cases. *Surg Today* 1992;22:464.

234. Dahm JB, Riebeling VJ. The thrombolysis of a septic portal vein thrombosis with ultrahigh-dosage streptokinase. *Dtsch Med Wochenschr* 1993; 118:582.

235. Haskal ZJ, Naji A. Treatment of portal vein thrombosis after liver transplantation with percutaneous thrombolysis and stent placement. *J Vasc Interv Radiol* 1993;4:789.

236. Jager D, Huppe D, Weber A, et al. Portal vein thrombosis in protein C deficiency: successful fibrinolytic therapy with ultra-high dose streptokinase. *Med Klin* 1994;89:453.

237. Blum U, Haag K, Rossle M, et al. Noncavernomatous portal vein thrombosis in hepatic cirrhosis: treatment with transjugular intrahepatic portosystemic shunt and local thrombolysis. *Radiology* 1995;195:153.

238. Cherukuri R, Haskal ZJ, Naji A, et al. Percutaneous thrombolysis and stent placement for the treatment of portal vein thrombosis after liver transplantation: long-term follow-up. *Transplantation* 1998;65:1124.

239. Ludwig DJ, Hauptmann E, Rosoff L Jr, et al. Mesenteric and portal vein thrombosis in a young patient with protein S deficiency treated with urokinase via the superior mesenteric artery. *J Vasc Surg* 1999; 30:551.

240. Kaplan JL, Weintraub SL, Hunt JP, et al. Treatment of superior mesenteric and portal vein thrombosis with direct thrombolytic infusion via an operatively placed mesenteric catheter. *Am Surg* 2004;70:600–604.

241. Schafer C, Zundler J, Bode JC. Thrombolytic therapy in patients with portal vein thrombosis: case report and review of the literature. *Eur J Gastroenterol Hepatol* 2000;12:1141–1145.

242. Rehan VK, Cronin CM, Bowman JM. Neonatal portal vein thrombosis successfully treated by regional streptokinase infusion. *Eur J Pediatr* 1994; 153:456.

243. Moosa AR, Gadd MA. Isolated splenic vein thrombosis. *World J Surg* 1985;9:384.

244. Belli AM, Jennings CM, Nakielny RA. Splenic and portal venous thrombosis: a vascular complication of pancreatic disease demonstrated on computed tomography. *Clin Radiol* 1990;41:13.

245. Lewis JD, Faigel DO, Morris JB, et al. Splenic vein thrombosis secondary to focal pancreatitis diagnosed by endoscopic ultrasonography. *J Clin Gastroenterol* 1998;26:54.

246. Brink JS, Brown AK, Palmer BA, et al. Portal vein thrombosis after laparoscopy-assisted splenectomy and cholecystectomy. *J Pediatr Surg* 2003; 38:644–647.

247. Lee JJ, Kim HJ, Chung IJ, et al. Portal, mesenteric, and splenic vein thromboses after splenectomy in a patient with chronic myeloid leukemia variant with thrombocythemic onset. *Am J Hematol* 1999;61:212.

248. Teofili L, DeStefano V, Leone G, et al. Hematologic causes of venous thrombosis in young people: high incidence of myeloproliferative disorder as underlying disease in patients with splenic venous thrombosis. *Thromb Haemost* 1992;67:297.

249. Etoh Y, Ohsawa I, Fujita T, et al. Nephrotic syndrome with portal, splenic and renal vein thrombosis. A case report. *Nephron* 2002;92:680–684.

250. McDermott VG, England RE, Newman GE. Case report: bleeding gastric varices secondary to splenic vein thrombosis successfully treated by splenic artery embolization. *Br J Radiol* 1995;68:928–930.

251. Stein M, Link DP. Symptomatic spleno-mesenteric-portal venous thrombosis: recanalization and reconstruction with endovascular stents. *J Vasc Interv Radiol* 1999;10:363–371.

252. Valla D, Dhumeaux D, Babany G, et al. Hepatic vein thrombosis in paroxysmal nocturnal hemoglobinuria: a spectrum from asymptomatic occlusion of hepatic venules to fatal Budd-Chiari syndrome. *Gastroenterology* 1987;93:569.

253. Maddrey WC. Hepatic vein thrombosis (Budd-Chiari syndrome). *Hepatology* 1984;4:44S.

254. Mitchell MC, Boitnott JK, Kaufman S, et al. Budd-Chiari syndrome: etiology, diagnosis and management. *Medicine* 1982;61:199.

255. Hartmann RC, Luther AB, Jenkins DE Jr, et al. Fulminant hepatic venous thrombosis (Budd-Chiari syndrome) in paroxysmal nocturnal hemoglobinuria: definition of a medical emergency. *Johns Hopkins Med J* 1980; 146:247.

256. Olzinski AT, Sanyal AJ. Treating Budd-Chiari syndrome: making rational choices from a myriad of options. *J Clin Gastroenterol* 2000;30:155–161.

257. Noone TC, Semelka RC, Siegelman ES, et al. Budd-Chiari syndrome: spectrum of appearances of acute, subacute, and chronic disease with magnetic resonance imaging. *J Magn Reson Imaging* 2000;11:44–50.

258. Bach N, Thung SN, Schaffner F. Comfrey herb tea-induced hepatic veno-occlusive disease. *Am J Med* 1989;87:97.

259. Feugen M. Fatal veno-occlusive disease of the liver associated with herbal tea consumption and radiation. *Aust N Z J Med* 1984;14:61.

260. Rollins BJ. Hepatic veno-occlusive disease. *Am J Med* 1986;81:297.

261. Orloff LA, Orloff MJ. Budd-Chiari syndrome caused by Behçet's disease: treatment by side-to-side portacaval shunt. *J Am Coll Surg* 1999;188: 396–407.

262. Lewis JH, Tice HL, Zimmerman HJ. Budd-Chiari syndrome associated with oral contraceptive steroids: review of treatment of 47 cases. *Dig Dis Sci* 1983;28:673.

263. Praderio L, Dagna L, Longhi P, et al. Budd-Chiari syndrome in a patient with ulcerative colitis: association with anticardiolipin antibodies. *J Clin Gastroenterol* 2000;30:203–204.

264. Thaler F, Lechner K. Antithrombin III deficiency and thromboembolism. *Clin Haematol* 1981;10:369.

265. Theuerkauf I, Lickfett L, Harbrecht U, et al. Segmental hepatic vein thrombosis associated with heparin-induced thrombocytopenia II. *Virchows Arch* 2000;436:88.

266. Gentil-Kocher S, Bernard O, Brunelle F, et al. Budd-Chiari syndrome in children: report of 22 cases. *J Pediatr* 1988;113:30.

267. Asherson RA, Cervera R. Unusual manifestations of the antiphospholipid syndrome. *Clin Rev Allergy Immunol* 2003;25:61–78.

268. De Stefano V, Teofili L, Leone G, et al. Spontaneous erythroid colony formation as the clue to an underlying myeloproliferative disorder in patients with Budd-Chiari syndrome or portal vein thrombosis. *Semin Thromb Hemost* 1997;23:411–418.

269. Hoffman R, Nimer A, Lanir N, et al. Budd-Chiari syndrome associated with factor V Leiden mutation: a report of 6 patients. *Liver Transpl Surg* 1999;5:96.

270. Kakizaki K, Yamauchi H. Hepatic venous obstruction by a membranous web. *N Engl J Med* 1996;334:1237.

271. Kage M, Arakawa M, Kojiro M, et al. Histopathology of membranous obstruction of the inferior vena cava in the Budd Chiari syndrome. *Gastroenterology* 1992;102:2081.

272. Okuda K. Membranous obstruction of the inferior vena cava (obliterative hepatocavopathy, Okuda). *J Gastroenterol Hepatol* 2001;16: 1179–1183.

273. Rickes S, Csepregi A. Hepatobiliary and pancreatic: Budd-Chiari syndrome. *J Gastroenterol Hepatol* 2004;19:828.

274. Gupta S, Barter S, Phillips GWL, et al. Comparison of ultrasonography, CT, and 99mTc liver scan in the diagnosis of Budd-Chiari syndrome. *Gut* 1987;28:242.

275. Lin J, Xiao-Hai C, Zhou K-R, et al. Budd-Chiari syndrome: diagnosis with three-dimensional contrast-enhanced magnetic resonance angiography. *World J Gastroenterol* 2003;9:2317–2321.

276. Erden A, Erden I, Yurdaydin C, et al. Hepatic outflow obstruction: enhancement patterns of the liver on MR angiography. *Eur J Radiol* 2003;48:203–208.

277. Leebeek FW, Lameris JS, van Buuren HR, et al. Budd-Chiari syndrome, portal vein and mesenteric vein thrombosis in a patient hyomozygous for factor V Leiden mutation treated by TIPS and thrombolysis. *Br J Haematol* 1988;102:929.

278. Frawley KJ, MacKechnie SG, Taylor KM. Thrombolytic therapy in paroxysmal nocturnal haemoglobinuria complicated by hepatic vein thrombosis. *Australas Radiol* 1993;37:396.

279. Frank JW, Kamath PS, Stanson AW. Budd-Chiari syndrome: early intervention with angioplasty and thrombolytic therapy. *Mayo Clin Proc* 1994;69:877.

280. Patel NH, Bradshaw B, Meissner MH, et al. Posttraumatic Budd-Chiari syndrome treated with thrombolytic therapy and angioplasty. *J Trauma* 1996;40:294.

281. Sawamura R, Fernandes MI, Galvao LC, et al. Report of two cases of children with Budd-Chiari syndrome successfully treated with streptokinase. *Arq Gastroenterol* 1996;33:179.

282. Sanyal AJ. The use and misuse of transjugular intrahepatic portasystemic shunts. *Curr Gastroenterol Rep* 2000;2:61–71.

283. Middleton WD, Teefey SA, Darcy MD. Doppler evaluation of transjugular intrahepatic portosystemic shunts. *Ultrasound Q* 2003;19:56–70.

284. Klein AS, Molmenti EP. Surgical treatment of Budd-Chiari syndrome. *Liver Transpl* 2003;9:891–896.

285. Boyer TD. Transjugular intrahepatic portosystemic shunt: current status. *Gastroenterology* 2003;124:1700–1710.

286. van Buuren HR, ter Borg PC. Transjugular intrahepatic portosystemic shunt (TIPS): indications and long-term patency. *Scand J Gastroenterol* 2003;38(Suppl. 239):100–104.

287. Henderson JM, Warren WD, Millikan WJ Jr, et al. Surgical options, hematologic evaluation, and pathologic changes in Budd-Chiari syndrome. *Am J Surg* 1990;159:41.

288. Halff G, Todo S, Tzakis AG, et al. Liver transplantation for the Budd-Chiari syndrome. *Ann Surg* 1990;211:43.

289. Averhaus W, Ullerich H, Menzel J, et al. Budd-Chiari syndrome in a patient with factor V Leiden: successful treatment by TIPSS placement followed by a liver transplantation. *Z Gastroenterol* 1999;37:277.

290. Llach F. Hypercoagulability, renal vein thrombosis, and other thrombotic complications of nephrotic syndrome. *Kidney Int* 1985;28:429.

291. Keating MA, Althausen AF. The clinical spectrum of renal vein thrombosis. *J Urol* 1985;133:938.

292. Mahmoud EI. Acute renal vein thrombosis in adults. *Int Urol Nephrol* 1986;18:243.

293. Velasquez FF, Garcia PN, Ruiz MN. Idiopathic nephrotic syndrome of the adult with asymptomatic thrombosis of the renal vein. *Am J Nephrol* 1988;8:457.

294. Laville M, Aquilera D, Maillet J, et al. The prognosis of renal vein thrombosis: a re-evaluation of 27 cases. *Nephrol Dial Transplant* 1988;3:247.

295. Vigano-D'Angelo S, D'Angelo A, Kaufman DE Jr, et al. Protein S deficiency occurs in the nephrotic syndrome. *Ann Intern Med* 1987;107:42.

296. Rogers PC, Silva MP, Carter JE, et al. Renal vein thrombosis and response to therapy in a newborn due to protein C deficiency. *Eur J Pediatr* 1989;149:124.

297. Melissari E, Kakkar VV. Congenital severe protein C deficiency in adults. *Br J Haematol* 1989;72:222.

298. Withrich RP. Factor V Leiden mutation: potential thrombogenic role in renal vein, dialysis graft and transplant vascular thrombosis. *Curr Opin Nephrol Hypertens* 2001;10:409–414.

299. Mintz G, Acevedo-Vazauez E, Gutierrez-Espinosa G, et al. Renal vein thrombosis and inferior vena cava thrombosis in systemic lupus erythematosus: frequency and risk factors. *Arthritis Rheum* 1984;27:539.

300. Glueck HI, Kant KS, Weiss MA, et al. Thrombosis in systemic lupus erythematosus: relations to the presence of circulating anticoagulants. *Arch Intern Med* 1985;145:1389.

301. Nzerue CM, Hewan-Lowe K, Pierangeli S, et al. "Black swan in the kidney": renal involvement in the antiphospholipid syndrome. *Kidney Int* 2002;62:733–744.

302. Akpolat T, Akkoyunlu M, Akpolat I, et al. Renal Behçet's disease: a cumulative analysis. *Semin Arthritis Rheum* 2002;31:317–337.

303. Ismail H, Kalicinski P, Drewniak T, et al. Primary vascular thrombosis after renal transplantation in children. *Pediatr Transplant* 1997;1:43.

304. Schwieger J, Reiss R, Cohen JL, et al. Acute renal allograft dysfunction in the setting of deep venous thrombosis: a case of successful urokinase thrombolysis and a review of the literature. *Am J Kidney Dis* 1993;22:345.

305. Lee G, Watson CW, Mammen KJ, et al. Successful selective thrombolysis of a spontaneous transplant renal vein thrombosis. *BJU Int* 1999;83:869.

306. Rowe JM, Rasmussen RL, Mader SL, et al. Successful thrombolytic therapy in two patients with renal vein thrombosis. *Am J Med* 1984;77:1111.

307. Crowley JP, Matarese RA, Ouevedo SE, et al. Fibrinolytic therapy for bilateral renal vein thrombosis. *Arch Intern Med* 1984;144:159.

308. Modrall JG, Teitelbaum GP, Diaz-Luna H, et al. Local thrombolysis in a renal allograft threatened by renal vein thrombosis. *Transplantation* 1993;56:1011.

309. Markowitz GS, Brignol F, Burns FR, et al. Renal vein thrombosis treated with thrombolytic therapy: case report and brief review. *Am J Kidney Dis* 1995;25:801.

310. Morrissey EC, McDonald BR, Rabetoy GM. Resolution of proteinuria secondary to bilateral renal vein thrombosis after treatment with systemic thrombolytic therapy. *Am J Kidney Dis* 1997;29:615.

311. Duncan BW, Adzick NS, Longaker MT, et al. In utero arterial embolism from renal vein thrombosis with successful postnatal thrombolytic therapy. *J Pediatr Surg* 1991;26:741.

312. Duff P, Gibbs RS. Pelvic vein thrombophlebitis: diagnostic dilemma and therapeutic challenge. *Obstet Gynecol Surv* 1983;38:365.

313. Munsick RA, Gillanders LA. A review of the syndrome of puerperal ovarian vein thrombophlebitis. *Obstet Gynecol Surv* 1981;36:57.

314. Brown CE, Lowe TW, Cunningham FG, et al. Puerperal pelvic thrombophlebitis: impact on diagnosis and treatment using x-ray CT and MRI. *Obstet Gynecol* 1986;68:789.

315. Bounameaux H, Reber-Wasem MA. Superficial thrombophlebitis and deep vein thrombosis: a controversial association. *Arch Intern Med* 1997;157:1822.

316. Blumenberg RM, Barton E, Gelfand ML, et al. Occult deep venous thrombosis complicating thrombophlebitis. *J Vasc Surg* 1998;27:338.

317. Hanson JN, Ascher E, DePippo P, et al. Saphenous vein thrombophlebitis (SVT): a deceptively benign disease. *J Vasc Surg* 1998;27:677.

318. de Moerloose P, Wutschert R, Heinzmann M, et al. Superficial vein thrombosis of lower limbs: influence of factor V Leiden, factor II G20210A and overweight. *Thromb Haemost* 1998;80:239.

319. Martinelli I, Cattaneo M, Taioli E, et al. Genetic risk factors for superficial vein thrombosis. *Thromb Haemost* 1999;82:1215.

320. Quenet S, Laporte S, Decousus H, et al. Factors predictive of venous thrombotic complications in patients with isolated superficial vein thrombosis. *J Vasc Surg* 2003;38:944–949.

321. Superficial Thrombophlebitis Treated By Enoxaparin Study Group. A pilot randomized double-blind comparison of a low-molecular-weight heparin, a nonsteroidal anti-inflammatory agent, and placebo in the treatment of superficial vein thrombosis. *Arch Intern Med* 2003;163:1657–1663.

322. Marchiori A, Verlato F, Sabbion P, et al. High versus low doses of unfractionated heparin for the treatment of superficial thrombophlebitis of the leg. A prospective, controlled, randomized study. *Haematologica* 2002;87:523–527.

# CHAPTER 87 ■ DIAGNOSIS OF VENOUS THROMBOEMBOLISM

HENRI BOUNAMEAUX AND ARNAUD PERRIER

Pulmonary embolism (PE), the source of which is predominantly located in a thrombosis of the deep veins of the legs [deep vein thrombosis (DVT)], is a major health concern—it is the third cause of mortality by cardiovascular disease after coronary artery disease and stroke. In Western countries, DVT remains a leading cause of death in the puerperium and the postoperative period. In addition, late sequelae of DVT may produce disabling leg symptoms in a substantial proportion of patients, including venous ulcers in a few of them, resulting in considerable economic burden.

During the last 2 decades, the approach to diagnosing DVT and PE has changed in several major ways. First, it has been recognized that these two conditions are manifestations of a single entity, venous thromboembolism (VTE). Second, novel noninvasive diagnostic tools such as venous compression ultrasonography (CUS), D-dimer (DD) measurement, and spiral (or helical) computerized tomography (s-CT) scan have become available, which have drastically reduced the need for invasive tools such as phlebography and pulmonary angiography. Third, the clinical index of suspicion has progressively become lower, thereby resulting in most (80% or even more) patients with suspected VTE not having the disease (see Fig. 87-1). Fourth, efficient, mainly noninvasive, strategies have been validated in large-scale outcome studies, and more attention has been paid to their cost implications (1).

Finally, the appropriate approach to the diagnosis of VTE differs depending on the nature of the clinical setting—clinical suspicion of a first episode of DVT or PE, clinical suspicion of a recurrent episode of DVT or PE, and screening of asymptomatic DVT or PE in high-risk patients or in patients participating in clinical trials on prophylaxis or therapy for VTE.

## DEFINITIONS

DVT is defined as the presence of a thrombus in the deep vein system. Although DVT may occur in all veins (lower and upper limbs, or renal, mesenteric, splenic, portal, or cerebral veins), it mainly affects the deep veins of the lower limbs (see Fig. 87-2). DVT must be distinguished from superficial thrombophlebitis, a definitely more benign condition that is rarely associated with DVT (2) and that usually does not require anticoagulant therapy. In general, thrombi arise in the calf veins (i.e., peroneal and posterior tibial veins, and very rarely, anterior tibial veins) and may progress proximally, the so-called ascending thrombosis. In some cases (i.e., pregnancy, Cockett syndrome, and tumor), DVT may develop proximally (e.g. in the common or external iliac vein) and progress distally, the so-called descending thrombosis.

DVT of the lower limbs may be *proximal* (from and including the popliteal vein or upwards) or *distal* (below the popliteal veins), an important distinction because the embolic

potential of proximal vein thrombosis is definitely higher than that of distal vein thrombosis.

DVT can be *symptomatic* or *asymptomatic*. Asymptomatic thromboses occur more frequently in bedridden patients, especially in the postoperative period, because symptoms (mainly pain and swelling) that are essentially caused by venous stasis are usually more prominent in patients who are in the upright position than in those who are bedridden.

Traditionally, PE was classified as *massive* or *nonmassive,* but this classification is ambiguous because it could refer to the clinical presentation of PE accompanied by shock, or at least systemic hypotension, or to the radiologic extent (usually more than 50% amputation of the pulmonary vasculature) of the emboli. Moreover, this classification does not account for those patients who have no systemic hypotension but present with echographically detected right ventricular dysfunction secondary to PE. Therefore, in this chapter, we classify PE into three categories (3):

- Massive PE: PE provoking shock or cardiorespiratory arrest (5% of cases)
- Submassive PE: PE provoking right ventricular strain despite normal systemic blood pressure (30% of cases)
- Nonmassive PE: PE associated with normal systemic blood pressure and normal right ventricular function (65% of cases).

## CLINICAL PRESENTATION

Symptoms of DVT are nonspecific and insensitive (4,5). Many nonthrombotic conditions can produce symptoms similar to those encountered in DVT, such as muscle strain, direct twisting injury to the leg and hematoma, Baker popliteal cyst, cellulitis, and postthrombotic syndrome. In clinically suspected patients, most signs and symptoms are present in similar frequency in patients who have and in those who do not have the disease (see Table 87-1), which precludes any definitive clinical diagnosis of DVT. Moreover, they are not sensitive because many thrombi are nonobstructive and are not associated with venous stasis or with significant inflammation of the vessel wall or perivascular tissue.

Like DVT, PE cannot be diagnosed on a sole clinical basis because of the lack of sensitivity and specificity of clinical signs and symptoms (6) (Table 87-1). PE presents as one of the following three clinical presentations: dyspnea with or without pleuritic pain (65% of cases); isolated dyspnea, usually acute but sometimes slowly progressive (20%); or syncope or shock (less than 10%). In exceptional cases, PE may be found during the investigation of a radiologic infiltrate. These clinical presentations correspond to three syndromes of different pathology and variable severity (7): pulmonary infarction, isolated dyspnea, and shock.

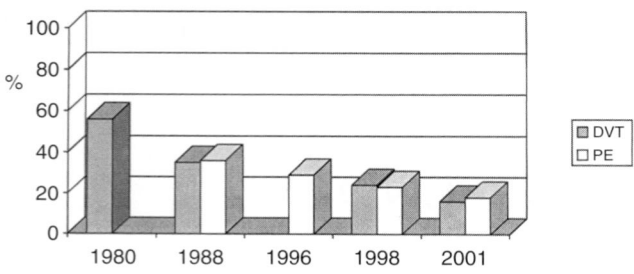

**FIGURE 87-1.** Evolution over time of the prevalence of DVT and PE among clinically suspected patients. (From database of the Geneva Angiology Unit.)

## Pulmonary Infarction

The clinical hallmark of pulmonary infarction is pleuritic pain caused by irritation of the visceral pleura and, more rarely, by hemoptysis. The syndrome is caused by peripheral emboli. Although the syndrome is usually coined as "pulmonary infarction," the histopathologic correlate is in fact an alveolar hemorrhage probably provoked by the efflux of blood from the high-pressure bronchial circulation in the segment obstructed by

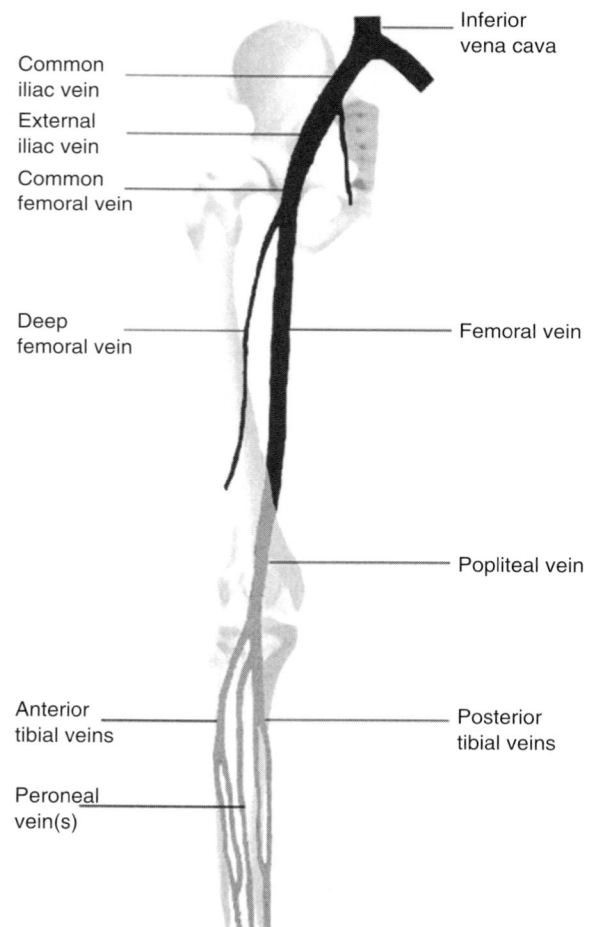

**FIGURE 87-2.** Anatomy of the deep veins of the lower limb. Note that the femoral vein was previously named "superficial femoral vein," a potentially dangerous misnomer because this vein belongs to the deep vein system.

**TABLE 87-1**

### INACCURACY OF ISOLATED CLINICAL SYMPTOMS AND SIGNS IN PATIENTS SUSPECTED OF DEEP VEIN THROMBOSIS OR PULMONARY EMBOLISM

| Symptoms of DVT | Patients with DVT (%) | Patients without DVT (%) |
|---|---|---|
| Pain | 75 | 80 |
| Tenderness | 78 | 66 |
| Homan sign | 40 | 45 |
| Unilateral leg swelling | 45 | 37 |
| Superficial venous dilation | 25 | 19 |

| Symptoms of PE | Patients with PE (%) | Patients without PE (%) |
|---|---|---|
| Dyspnea | 32 | 35 |
| Pleuretic pain | 53 | 57 |
| Cough | 6 | 15 |
| Leg edema | 32 | 26 |
| Calf pain | 38 | 20 |
| Hemoptysis | 34 | 22 |

DVT, deep vein thrombosis; PE, pulmonary embolism.

the embolus (8). The classic radiologic picture is a wedge-shaped pleural-based infiltrate that affects approximately 20% of patients (9). Other common chest x-ray anomalies include platelike atelectasis and pleural effusion. Tachycardia and dyspnea are less frequent in this clinical syndrome, reflecting the peripheral character and lesser hemodynamic repercussions of such pulmonary emboli (7).

## Isolated Dyspnea

The absence of pleuritic pain in this syndrome is probably due to the more proximal embolization of the pulmonary vasculature. Patients may complain of retrosternal chest pain that is oppressive in character, evoking the differential diagnosis of angina. In fact, such pain probably reflects true myocardial ischemia caused by increased right ventricular wall tension and reduced right coronary artery flow. Tachycardia, although more frequent, is still present in only 45% of patients (7). The electrocardiogram is rarely normal, but its anomalies are often nonspecific. Although dyspnea is usually of abrupt or rapid onset, in some patients it may progress over several days.

## Shock

Syncope and/or shock are the clinical manifestations of massive PE causing acute severe pulmonary hypertension and right ventricular failure. Shock is usually caused by large central clots. Although suggestive of PE in patients with obvious risk factors such as recent surgery, syncope may be a misleading presentation (10). Suspected massive PE with shock is a distinct situation requiring a specific diagnostic approach detailed in the section, "Massive Pulmonary Embolism."

# DIAGNOSTIC GOLD STANDARDS

Ascending phlebography is still considered the diagnostic standard for diagnosing DVT, but it is invasive, costly, and not devoid of risk. The procedure consists of the injection of an iodinated contrast dye in a superficial foot vein with sequential radiograms of the leg in order to follow the dynamic course of the contrast in the veins. Tourniquets can be used to force the dye into the deep veins, but their use is controversial. The documentation is adequate when images are obtained in different views, and a filling defect surrounded by contrast is characteristic for a fresh thrombus (see Fig. 87-3). Ascending phlebography is still used as the only accepted surrogate endpoint in thromboprophylactic trials for efficacy assessment of new drugs. It can be used for quantification of the thrombotic burden, for example, by means of the Marder score (11). In clinically suspected individuals, however, it has been largely replaced by CUS, mainly because it does not confer diagnostic certainty. Indeed, according to Hull et al. (12), the 3-month thromboembolic

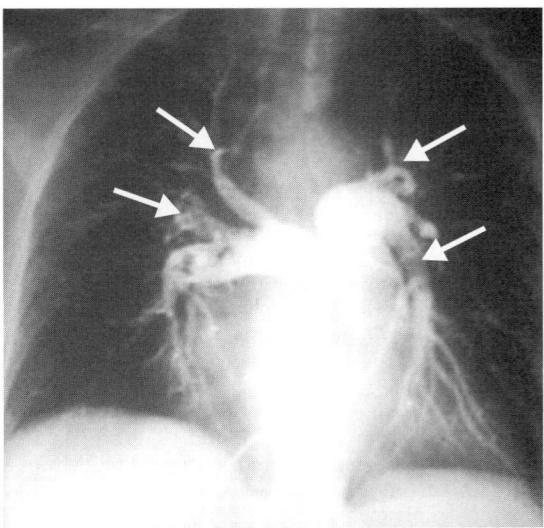

FIGURE 87-4. Pulmonary angiogram showing filling defects in the left superior lobar artery and in all the right lobar arteries (*arrows*). The only well-perfused arteries are the left (with a partially occluding thrombus) and right inferior lobar artery.

risk was 1.9% [95% confidence interval (CI), 0.4 to 5.4] in a series of 160 patients who were clinically suspected of DVT and were left untreated following a phlebogram that was considered normal.

Although it is considered the standard criterion for diagnosing PE, pulmonary angiography is difficult to interpret, with frequent disagreement occurring even between expert readers (13), more often about the absence of PE (17% of angiograms) than about its presence (8% of angiograms) (14). Moreover, the 3-month thromboembolic risk in patients left untreated after an angiogram that was considered normal was 1.7% (95% CI, 1.0 to 2.7) in a recent systematic review pooling the results of eight series including a total of 1,050 patients (15,16). This test is also costly, invasive, and not devoid of hazards. Thus the mortality due to pulmonary angiography was 0.2% (95% CI, 0 to 0.3) in a pooled analysis of five series regrouping a total of 5,696 patients (16). However, the rare deaths attributable to pulmonary angiography occurred in very sick patients with hemodynamic compromise or acute respiratory failure. Nevertheless, pulmonary angiography provides excellent anatomic views of the arterial vasculature of the lungs (see Fig. 87-4) and allows quantification of the embolic burden quite precisely, for example, by means of the Miller index (17).

The two gold standards are no longer used routinely in patients with a clinical suspicion of DVT or PE. Nevertheless, they still have a role in patients in whom the clinical likelihood of an acute thromboembolic event is high and in whom noninvasive tests have remained inconclusive. Although valid, the change in clinical preference will probably result in decreasing expertise among radiologists performing these examinations, which may decrease their accuracy in the future and further restrict the role of these examinations.

## HISTORIC DIAGNOSTIC TOOLS

Venous occlusion plethysmography and continuous wave Doppler flow examination are only used in anecdotal situations nowadays, whereas electrocardiogram, arterial blood gases, and chest x-ray are now part of the so-called prior clinical probability assessment in clinically suspected PE (see section, "Clinical Probability Assessment").

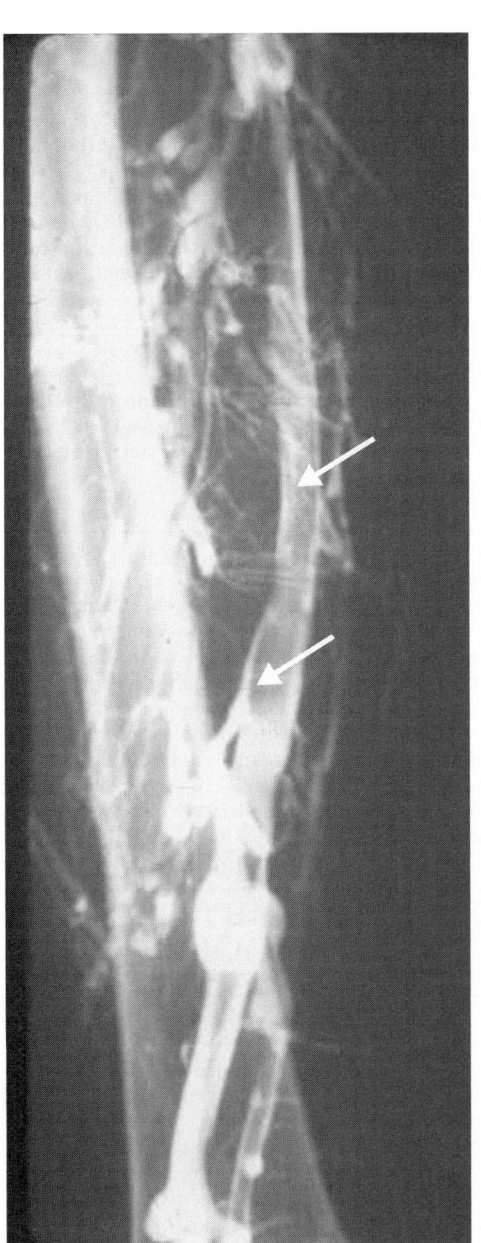

FIGURE 87-3. Phlebogram showing a filling defect (*arrows*) in the femoral vein, surrounded by contrast dye, characteristic for a fresh thrombus.

## Plethysmography

Venous occlusion plethysmography using the impedance or the strain gauge technique has been used in the 1970s and 1980s for noninvasive diagnosis of DVT, either alone or in combination with continuous wave Doppler (18). This noninvasive technique detects volume changes in the leg. Its principle is based on changes in blood volume in the calf produced by inflation and deflation of a pneumatic cuff at 50 to 60 mm Hg, which result in changes in electrical resistance (impedance technique) or in the length of a mercury or indium strain gauge, which is in turn translated electrically. These changes are reduced in patients with thrombosis of the proximal veins. Using serial impedance plethysmography, the Amsterdam group, in a landmark prospective outcome study, demonstrated (19) that none of the 289 patients (68% of the initial population) whose plethysmograms were normal on days 1, 2, 5, and 10 died of VTE or presented with clinically suspected and confirmed PE. Moreover, all patients with an abnormal plethysmogram underwent phlebography, which confirmed DVT in 92%. Overall, the sensitivity and specificity of impedance plethysmography for proximal vein thrombosis are approximately 92% and 95%, respectively. Consistent with this mitigated performance, a computerized impedance plethysmography device failed to accurately separate the patients with proximal DVT from those without DVT in a series of 381 consecutive clinically suspected patients. This failure resulted in 10 thromboembolic events (including four fatal PE) among the patients in whom DVT had been ruled out by impedance plethysmography (20). In a subsequent study, Ginsberg et al. reassessed the performance of impedance plethysmography in a series of 132 patients and found a sensitivity of only 65%, which they attributed to the referral of an increasing proportion of patients with less severe symptoms to their center (21). Such patients have smaller, nonocclusive thrombi that are less likely to yield abnormal plethysmographic findings.

Photoplethysmography is a technique that uses the absorption property of light by hemoglobin in the red cells. Digital plethysmography is assisted by a microprocessor and is easy to perform (22), but there has been no proper assessment of its performance so far.

## Continuous Wave Doppler and Measurement of the Venous Stop Flow Pressure

Lack of respiratory variation of the venous Doppler has been considered suggestive of DVT. However, this sign is nonspecific because it may also be caused by increased flow, for example, in inflammatory conditions (lymphangitis, erysipela, cellulitis). Moreover, it is operator dependent and requires considerable skill and experience to perform reliably. In order to increase specificity and interobserver agreement, a simple semiquantitative technique (23,24) has been proposed to distinguish continuous (nonrespiratory modulated) venous flow resulting from increased flow (e.g., inflammation) from continuous flow secondary to increased pressure resulting from an obstacle (thrombosis). With this improved technique, continuous wave Doppler had a sensitivity of 83% and a specificity of 62%. By combining Doppler with strain gauge venous occlusion plethysmography, sensitivity was improved to 96% but specificity was only 51% (18).

## 125I Fibrinogen Uptake Test

This test is based on the detection of the accumulation of fibrinogen in a growing thrombus, by an external count of radioactivity over well-defined locations in order to detect localized peaks of radioactivity as compared with the adjacent or contralateral locus. The test has been mainly used as a screening method in the frame of thromboprophylactic studies. It has been abandoned because of the fear of transmission of viral particles by the fibrinogen that was obtained from blood donors. In addition, its accuracy is far from ideal: In a study on 255 patients who underwent bilateral phlebography following hip fracture (25), the sensitivity of radioactive fibrinogen scanning was found to be as low as 44% for the nonoperated leg and 50% for calf vein thrombosis, and the predictive value of a negative result was approximately 90%. This poor performance was confirmed by a systematic assessment of all pertinent studies (26), calling into question the validity of the many studies evaluating prophylactic agents for venous thrombosis that used leg scanning as the only test for the assessment of efficacy.

## Electrocardiogram

The electrocardiogram (ECG) is usually normal in small peripheral PE. Larger PE may induce modifications such as large P waves in leads II, III, and aVF and the $S_1Q_3T$ pattern or ST segment depression in leads $V_1$ to $V_4$. A right bundle branch block or right axis deviation is also possible, when observed in a patient with a suggestive clinical presentation and risk factors for venous thromboembolism abnormalities (27).

## Arterial Blood Gases

Hypocapnia and hypoxemia are frequent in PE. However, approximately 20% of patients with proved PE have a normal arterial oxygen pressure and alveoloarterial oxygen gradient (28,29).

## Chest Radiograph

The most frequent anomalies of the chest radiograph are cardiomegaly, pleural effusion, platelike atelectasis, and elevated hemidiaphragm (9,30). The presence of these anomalies increases the probability of PE, although modestly. Pulmonary artery enlargement and oligemia are rare and nonspecific. The typical infiltrate of so-called pulmonary infarction has already been discussed. Nevertheless, in a patient with suspected PE, the chest radiograph remains extremely useful for differential diagnosis with conditions such as left ventricular failure, pneumonia, or pneumothorax.

# CONTEMPORARY DIAGNOSTIC TOOLS

## Clinical Probability Assessment

Sensitivity and specificity of clinical symptoms, signs, and abnormalities of blood gases, chest radiograph, and electrocardiogram in suspected DVT or PE are low when considered singly. Nevertheless, clinicians can combine these findings effectively either implicitly or by prediction rules in order to classify patients according to their probability of having the disease, the so-called prior clinical probability.

For suspected DVT, the Wells score (31,32) has gained relatively wide acceptance in spite of its partial subjectivity (see Table 87-2). This score is probably not more accurate than the simple implicit evaluation (33); however, it is easier to

## TABLE 87-2

### DESCRIPTION OF THE WELLS SCORE FOR PATIENTS WITH CLINICALLY SUSPECTED DEEP VEIN THROMBOSIS

| Wells clinical prediction score for DVT | Points |
|---|---|
| Cancer | +1 |
| Paralysis or recent immobilization | +1 |
| Bedridden >3 d, or surgery/trauma <4 wk | +1 |
| Pain on palpation of the deep veins | +1 |
| Edema of thigh and calf | +1 |
| Pitting edema (symptomatic side only) | +1 |
| Dilated superficial veins (symptomatic side only) | +1 |
| Alternative diagnosis at least as likely as DVT | −2 |
| Clinical probability | |
| Low | ≤0 |
| Intermediate | 1–2 |
| High | ≥3 |

DVT, deep vein thrombosis.

teach to junior physicians and allows the discussion of occasional disagreements among experienced clinicians on explicit grounds. Nevertheless, both the implicit assessment and the explicit Wells score allow a useful categorization of patients into low, intermediate, or high clinical probability groups in which the prevalence of DVT is approximately 5%, 20%, and 80%, respectively.

For suspected PE, two scores (see Table 87-3) have recently been proposed (34,35) and externally validated (36). The Wells score (34) includes a subjective item (likelihood of an alternative diagnosis), whereas the Geneva score is entirely objective but has the disadvantage of requiring blood gases analysis (35). As shown in Figure 87-5, these two scores have very similar performances but do not perform better than implicit judgment (14,37,38). Again, however, they have the advantage of explicitness and are useful educational tools. Allowing the clinician to override the totally objective Geneva score notably provides a statistically significant additional, although small, gain in performance (36). All these means of assessing clinical likelihood of DVT and PE allow a fairly accurate classification of patients into three categories corresponding to a prevalence of the disease: 6% to 10% (low clinical probability), 21% to 30% (intermediate clinical probability), and 63% to 78% (high clinical probability) (see Table 87-4) (14,31–37,39–45). Most patients with suspected DVT or PE have a low or intermediate clinical probability of having the disease. Those with a low probability of PE or a low to intermediate probability of DVT can usually be investigated by entirely noninvasive algorithms.

## Fibrin D-Dimer Measurement

DD is a degradation product of crosslinked fibrin and its levels increase in the plasma of patients with acute VTE (46). DD, when assayed by a quantitative enzyme-linked immunoassay (ELISA) or by some automated turbidimetric assays, has been shown to be highly sensitive (>98%) in acute DVT or PE, usually at a cutoff value of 500 $\mu$g per L. Hence, a DD level less than this value reasonably rules out acute VTE, at least in patients with low or intermediate clinical probability. Table 87-5 summarizes the pooled analysis of the published literature on most commercially available rapid DD tests (47). Tests vary

## TABLE 87-3

### DESCRIPTION OF TWO EXTERNALLY VALIDATED SCORES IN PATIENTS WITH CLINICALLY SUSPECTED PULMONARY EMBOLISM

| Geneva prediction score for PE | Points | Wells clinical prediction score for PE | Points |
|---|---|---|---|
| Previous PE or DVT | +2 | Previous PE or DVT | +1.5 |
| Heart rate >100/min | +1 | Heart rate >100/min | +1.5 |
| Recent surgery | +3 | Recent surgery or immobilization | +1.5 |
| Age | | Clinical signs of DVT | +3 |
| 60–79 yr | +1 | Alternative diagnosis less likely than PE | +3 |
| ≥80 yr | +2 | Hemoptysis | +1 |
| PaCO$_2$ | | Cancer | +1 |
| <4.8 kPa (36 mm Hg) | +2 | | |
| 4.8–5.19 kPa (36–38.9 mm Hg) | +1 | | |
| PaO$_2$ | | | |
| <6.5 kPa (48.7 mm Hg) | +4 | | |
| 6.5–7.99 kPa (48.7–59.9 mm Hg) | +3 | | |
| 8–9.49 kPa (60–71.2 mm Hg) | +2 | | |
| 9.5–10.99 kPa 71.3–82.4 mm Hg) | +1 | | |
| Atelectasis | +1 | | |
| Elevated hemidiaphragm | +1 | | |
| Clinical probability | | Clinical probability | |
| Low | 0–4 | Low | 0–1 |
| Intermediate | 5–8 | Intermediate | 2–6 |
| High | ≥9 | High | ≥7 |

DVT, deep vein thrombosis; PE, pulmonary embolism.

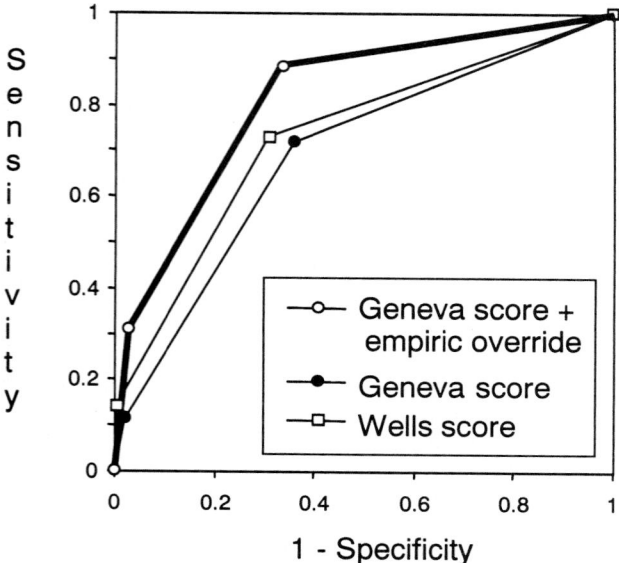

**FIGURE 87-5.** Comparison by receiver-operating characteristics (ROC) curve analysis of the Wells score (*open squares*) and the Geneva score (*filled circles*) for clinical assessment of patients with clinically suspected PE. The *bold line* indicates the result obtained when the Geneva score could be overridden by the clinician's empirical judgment, which typically occurs in approximately 20% of the cases. (From Chagnon I, Bounameaux H, Aujesky D, et al. Comparison of two clinical prediction rules and implicit assessment for suspected pulmonary embolism. *Am J Med* 2002;113:269–275, with permission.)

with respect to several characteristics, including assay technique (e.g., ELISA, latex, or automated turbidimetric tests), specificity of monoclonal antibodies used, calibrators, and quantitative or semiquantitative results. It is therefore not surprising that results may be heterogeneous. For clinical purpose, tests that were studied in sufficiently large patient populations and those that were validated in outcome studies should be used (48).

Although DD is very specific for fibrin, the specificity of fibrin for VTE is poor because fibrin is produced in a wide variety of conditions such as cancer, inflammation, infection, or necrosis (49). Hence, a DD level of more than 500 $\mu$g per L has a poor positive predictive value for VTE and cannot reliably confirm the disease. Whole-blood agglutination assays have a lower sensitivity (approximately 85%) and must be combined with a low (not intermediate or high) clinical probability in order to safely rule out VTE (50). Specificity of DD is lower in geriatric patients (9% in patients older than 80 years) suspected of having a PE (51) and in inpatients experiencing suspected PE during their hospital stay (52). Hence, DD measurement is unlikely to be very useful in those populations. Although rapid single-batch ELISA DD tests have proved to be safe and effective in ruling out VTE in management studies (33), their theoretical negative predictive value is lower in patients with a high clinical probability of PE despite their very high sensitivity. Moreover, a DD level less than the cutoff value appears to be rare in such patients—in a series of 918 patients (33), 101 patients had a high clinical probability of VTE, of whom only 10 had a normal DD level. Similarly, in a pooled series of 1,409 patients with suspected PE, only 13 had a negative DD test out of the 121 patients with a high clinical probability, leaving an upper limit of the 95% confidence interval for the 3-month thromboembolic risk as high as 21% (53).

In summary, highly sensitive DD assays allow elimination of DVT and PE in outpatients with a low or intermediate clinical probability of PE, whereas whole-blood agglutination tests only rule out the disease in patients with a low clinical probability. Finally, DD is unlikely to be useful in geriatric patients or in hospitalized patients with suspected VTE.

## Venous Compression Ultrasonography

In studies using phlebography as the gold standard, lower limb venous CUS, an entirely noninvasive test, has a sensitivity of 97% (95% CI, 96% to 98%) and a specificity of 98% for symptomatic proximal DVT (54). It has become the cornerstone of DVT diagnosis in clinically suspected individuals (55–57). The single, well-validated, diagnostic criterion for DVT on CUS is absence of full compressibility of the deep vein when applying pressure through the ultrasound probe (see Fig. 87-6). Intraluminal venous ultrasonography has been reported to have variable accuracy, and neither the changes in venous diameter during Valsalva maneuver nor the assessment of Doppler flow have been found to improve diagnostic accuracy for DVT (57). The extensiveness of the examination (particularly, including or excluding calf veins in the diagnostic procedure) is heavily debated among experts and will be discussed in the next paragraph. In a patient with clinically suspected PE, finding a DVT (at least a proximal one) by CUS is sufficient evidence to warrant anticoagulant treatment without performing further lung imaging. CUS shows a DVT in approximately 50% of patients with proven PE (33,58). The position of CUS in the diagnostic sequence for suspected PE is still a matter of debate. When performed after only a lung scan in patients with a nondiagnostic result, the diagnostic yield of CUS is quite low (4% to 10%) (59). In contrast, given a 20% to 30% prevalence of PE in the suspected population, CUS performed before lung scan may allow confirmation of the disease in 10% to 15% of all outpatients suspected of the disease (33,58).

The observation of a low 3-month thromboembolic risk in patients with a negative CUS of the proximal veins [approximately 1% in management studies (31,33,60,61)] challenges the need for diagnosing the so-called distal DVT, at least in non–high clinical probability patients. Indeed, in such patients, detecting clots in the posterior tibial or peroneal veins or even in calf muscle veins may be double edged: On one hand, the potential for reducing the 3-month thromboembolic risk is limited (because it is already quite low), and on the other hand, the risk of false-positive findings and subsequent unnecessary anticoagulant treatment in patients who could be left untreated, is quite high. Nevertheless, two recent large series suggest that complete examination of the leg deep vein system without any other examination is safe and effective in managing patients with clinically suspected DVT (62,63): Elias et al. (62) examined 623 patients of whom 401 (64.4%) were declared without DVT and were followed-up for 3 months with a low thromboembolic risk of 0.5% (95% CI, 0.1% to 1.8%). However, among the 204 patients with DVT, 92 (45%) were distal and most of them would not have been treated (and submitted to the hazards of anticoagulant treatment) with a similarly low 3-month thromboembolic risk if only a proximal CUS had been performed. Schellong et al. (63) reported a similar 3-month thromboembolic risk of 0.3% in a series of 1,646 patients of whom 275 were positive for DVT but, again, 154 (56%) of the cases of DVT were distal, suggesting a risk of overdiagnosis and overtreatment. Table 87-6 offers a comparison of the results obtained with the simplified or complete lower limbs venous ultrasonography. In addition, the examination protocols that study both proximal and distal veins are quite cumbersome and require

## TABLE 87-4

**ACCURACY OF IMPLICIT (OR EMPIRICAL) AND EXPLICIT (OR SCORE) CLINICAL PROBABILITY ASSESSMENT OF DEEP VEIN THROMBOSIS AND PULMONARY EMBOLISM**

| Study | Instrument | All | Prevalence of VTE according to clinical probability, % (n/n) | | |
|---|---|---|---|---|---|
| | | | Low | Intermediate | High |
| **DVT—IMPLICIT ASSESSMENT** | | | | | |
| Perrier 1999 (33) | Implicit | 23% (111/474) | 2% (3/129) | 19% (56/291) | 96% (52/54) |
| Cornuz 2002 (39) | Implicit | 29% (82/278) | 13% (11/86) | 24% (30/127) | 63% (41/65) |
| *All* | | *26% (189/752)* | *7% (14/215)* | *21% (86/418)* | *78% (93/119)* |
| **DVT—EXPLICIT ASSESSMENT** | | | | | |
| Wells 1995 (32) | Wells score (derivation) | 26% (135/529) | 5% (16/301) | 33% (47/143) | 85% (72/85) |
| Wells 1997 (31) | Wells score (validation) | 16% (95/593) | 3% (10/329) | 17% (32/193) | 75% (53/71) |
| Miron 2000 (40) | Wells score (validation) | 21% (57/270) | 3% (4/125) | 19% (19/99) | 74% (34/46) |
| Shields 2002 (41) | Wells score (validation) | 17% (17/102) | 2% (1/41) | 14% (6/44) | 59% (10/17) |
| Cornuz 2002 (39) | Wells score (validation) | 29% (82/278) | 13% (14/109) | 30% (36/121) | 67% (32/48) |
| Anderson 2003 (42) | Wells score (validation) | 18% (195/1,075) | 4% (20/448) | 19% (80/426) | 47% (95/201) |
| Kraaijenhagen 2002 (43) | Wells score (validation) | 25% (433/1,726) | 8% (70/880) | 27% (135/501) | 66% (228/345) |
| Kilroy 2003 (44) | Wells score (validation) | 15% (43/296) | 6% (12/187) | 24% (23/94) | 53% (8/15) |
| *All* | | *22% (1,057/4,869)* | *6% 147(2,420)* | *23% (378/1,621)* | *64% (532/828)* |
| **PE—IMPLICIT ASSESSMENT** | | | | | |
| PIOPED 1990 (14) | Implicit | 28% (252/887) | 9% (21/228) | 30% (170/569) | 68% (61/90) |
| Wicki 2001 (35) | Implicit | 27% (268/985) | 9% (33/368) | 33% (173/523) | 66% (62/94) |
| Musset 2002 (37) | Implicit | 35% (360/1,041) | 12% (28/231) | 26% (138/525) | 68% (194/285) |
| *All* | | *30% (880/2,913)* | *10% (82/827)* | *30% (481/1,617)* | *68% (317/469)* |
| **PE—EXPLICIT ASSESSMENT** | | | | | |
| Wells 2000 (34) | Wells score (derivation) | 17% (165/972) | 4% (14/392) | 21% (105/511) | 67% (46/69) |
| Wells 2001 (45) | Wells score (validation) | 9% (86/930) | 1% (7/527) | 16% (55/339) | 38% (24/64) |
| Chagnon 2002 (36) | Wells score (validation) | 26% (71/277) | 12% (19/162) | 40% (42/104) | 91% (10/11) |
| Wicki 2001 (35) | Geneva score (derivation) | 27% (266/986) | 10% (49/486) | 38% (166/437) | 81% (51/63) |
| Chagnon 2002 (36) | Geneva score (validation) | 26% (71/277) | 13% (20/152) | 38% (43/113) | 67% (8/12) |
| *All* | | *19% (659/3,442)* | *6% (109/1,719)* | *27% (411/1,504)* | *63% (139/219)* |

VTE, venous thromboembolism; DVT, deep vein thrombosis; PE, pulmonary embolism.

more specialized skills. Gottlieb et al. (64) randomized more than 500 patients clinically suspected of DVT to undergo routine complete ultrasonography of the calf veins or selective examination in the area of calf for symptoms, if any are present. Interestingly, the rate of isolated calf DVT detected was very low and similar in the two groups (1.3%, and 1.5%, respectively), and the 3-month thromboembolic risk was less than 1%, with no difference between the groups. Again, these findings challenge the pertinence of the systematic complete calf veins examination, especially in view of a positive predictive value of 50% at best for a positive finding (if we assume that the specificity of the examination is 99%, quite an optimistic assumption indeed) in a population with such a low prevalence of the disease (65).

## Ventilation–Perfusion Lung Scintigraphy

Perfusion lung scintigraphy is a noninvasive technique allowing the visualization of pulmonary perfusion through intravenous injection of albumin macroaggregates labeled by Technetium 99m. The macroaggregates are trapped in approximately 0.1% of the pulmonary capillary vessels and may be imaged by a γ-camera. Pulmonary hypoperfusion is not highly specific for an embolus because any disease that narrows the airways or fills the alveoli with fluid will result in hypoxic pulmonary vasoconstriction, a protective mechanism designed to minimize the shunt effect caused by poorly ventilated alveolar units. A perfusion defect corresponding to a segment or a large part of a segment is a more specific indication for PE. The addition of

## TABLE 87-5

**PERFORMANCE OF MOST COMMERCIALLY AVAILABLE RAPID D-DIMER TESTS FOR DIAGNOSING VENOUS THROMBOEMBOLISM (POOLED ANALYSIS FROM THE PUBLISHED LITERATURE)**

| Test (Producer) | *n* (nVTE) | Sensitivity % | Specificity (95% CI) |
|---|---|---|---|
| **ELISA TESTS** | | | |
| VIDAS DD (bioMérieux)[a] | 3575 (809) | 99 (98–100) | 44 (42–45) |
| Instant IA[b] (Stago) | 1549 (686) | 92 (89–94) | 54 (50–58) |
| Nycocard[b] (Nycomed) | 938 (337) | 92 (89–95) | 45 (41–49) |
| **LATEX[b] OR AUTOMATED TURBIDIMETRIC TESTS** | | | |
| SimpliRED[b] (Agen)[a] | 2303 (567) | 85 (82–88) | 69 (66–71) |
| Liatest (Stago) | 1113 (370) | 95 (92–97) | 39 (36–43) |
| MDA (Organon Tecnika) | 642 (133) | 96 (91–99) | 46 (41–51) |
| Minutex[b] (Biopool) | 565 (264) | 89 (84–93) | 58 (52–64) |
| DDPlus (Dade Behring) | 481 (154) | 96 (91–99) | 46 (40–51) |
| Tinaquant (Boehringer Mannheim)[a] | 286 (162) | 99 (96–100) | 40 (31–49) |
| Turbiquant (Dade Behring) | 183 (19) | 89 (67–99) | 57 (49–64) |
| LPIA D-Dimer (Mitsubishi) | 87 (42) | 95 (89–100) | 69 (55–84) |
| Nephelotex (Biopool) | 87 (42) | 98 (93–100) | 65 (62–89) |

CI, confidence interval; VTE, venous thromboembolism; ELISA, enzyme-linked immunoassay; DD, D-dimer; n, the number of patients included in the study; nVTE, the number of patients diagnosed with VTE. Results are almost identical for suspected deep vein thrombosis and for suspected pulmonary embolism.
[a]Outcome studies available.
[b]Semiquantitative test.
From Bounameaux H, Perrier A. D-dimer in the diagnosis of venous thromboembolism. In: Dalen JE, ed. *Venous thromboembolism.* New York: Marcel Dekker Inc, 2003:133–148, with permission.

ventilation scintigraphy (by Xenon 133, Krypton 81m, or aerosolized Technetium 99m) further increases specificity, a so-called mismatched defect (perfusion defect with normal ventilation) usually representing PE (66). The interpretation of lung scan has long been based on the criteria validated in the landmark Prospective Investigation On Pulmonary Embolism Diagnosis (PIOPED) study (14), and the interpretations have been subsequently revised (67,68). More recently, it has been greatly simplified and lung scan results are now classified into three categories: normal, high probability, and nondiagnostic. Classification of a lung scintigram into the high-probability category requires two or more mismatched segmental defects or, if only one is present, the addition of two large mismatched subsegmental defects according to the revised PIOPED criteria (67,68). The presence of one or more mismatched segmental defects or two or more large mismatched subsegmental defects

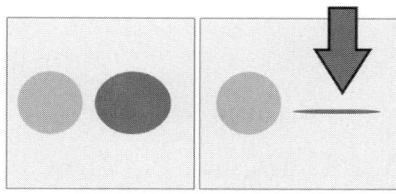

**A**

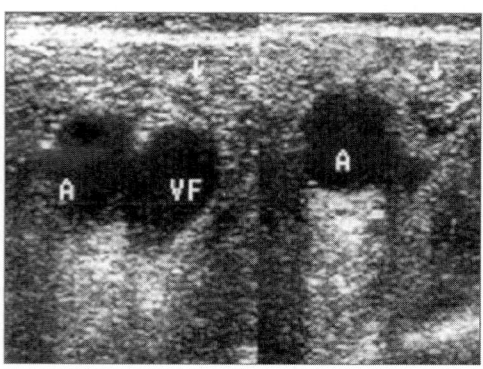

**B**

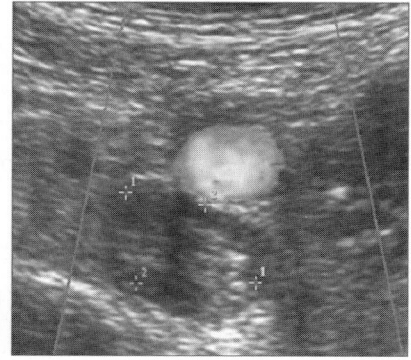

**C**

FIGURE 87-6. Ultrasonogram showing from the left to right, the adjacent femoral artery (*A*) and vein (*VF*), the full compressibility of the vein by the transducer, characteristic of the absence of thrombosis, and the incompressibility of the vein by the transducer, characteristic of the presence of an occluding thrombus. This procedure is called compression ultrasonography (CUS).

## TABLE 87-6

### PERFORMANCE AND SAFETY OF VARIOUS DIAGNOSTIC STRATEGIES FOR DEEP VEIN THROMBOSIS

| | Patients (n) | Prevalence of DVT (%) | Proportion of distal DVTs (%) | Number of CUS performed per 100 patients (n) | 3-month thromboembolic risk (%) (95% CI)[a] |
|---|---|---|---|---|---|
| **PROXIMAL CUS ONLY** | | | | | |
| Cogo et al. (61) | 1,702 | 24 | — | 176 | 0.7 (0.3–1.2) |
| Bernardi et al. (60) | 946 | 28 | — | 109 | 0.4 (0–0.9) |
| Wells et al. (31) | 593 | 16 | — | 128 | 0.6 (0.1–1.8) |
| Perrier et al. (33) | 474 | 24 | — | 73 | 2.6 (0.2–4.9) |
| Kraaijenhagen et al. (43) | 1,756 | 22 | — | 121 | 0.7 (0.3–1.6) |
| **PROXIMAL AND DISTAL CUS** | | | | | |
| Elias et al. (62) | 623 | 36 | 45 | 100 | 0.5 (0.1–1.8) |
| Schellong et al. (63) | 1,646 | 17 | 56 | 100 | 0.3 (0.1–0.8) |

DVT, deep vein thrombosis; CUS, compression ultrasonography.
[a]During 3-month follow-up in patients left untreated.

suffices for the Canadian classification (59) but these differences of interpretation appear to be of little clinical consequence. The high negative predictive value of a normal lung scan has been confirmed by several studies, including the initial study by Hull (69), and has been recognized as a valid criterion for eliminating PE. The positive predictive value of a high-probability scan is approximately 90%, and most clinicians consider such a result to confirm PE. Recent evidence suggests that the ventilation scan may be validly replaced by chest x-ray with an overall agreement of 88% and a positive predictive value of 86% for a scintigraphic mismatch (70).

The proportion of diagnostic ventilation–perfusion (V/Q) lung scans (i.e., in the normal or high probability range) was only 41% in the study by Wells et al. (59) and was 48% in the pooled Geneva experience (38). Hence, two large series have attempted to combine clinical probability with lung scan to increase diagnostic yield of V/Q lung scans. A recent analysis of suspected PE in the emergency ward (38) showed that the 3-month thromboembolic risk was very low (1.7%, 95% CI, 0.4 to 4.9) in 175 suspected patients with PE who are not treated on the grounds of a low empiric clinical probability and a nondiagnostic lung scan, provided lower limb venous CUS did not show a proximal DVT. This combination was found in 21% of patients, who, therefore, did not undergo an angiogram. Similarly, Wells et al. (59) withheld anticoagulant treatment in 702 of 1,239 (57%) patients who had a nondiagnostic scan, a low or intermediate clinical probability of PE, and normal serial CUS and the 3-month thromboembolic risk was only 0.5% (95% CI, 0.1 to 1.3).

Whether a baseline lung scan should be systematically performed in patients with suspected PE and a proximal DVT shown by CUS remains controversial. Recurrent PE is quite a rare event in treated patients, and the interpretation of a lung scan performed for a suspected recurrence is not always straightforward. In our experience, a baseline lung scan is rarely useful and is unlikely to be cost-effective (see specific section on recurrent VTE in subsequent text).

## Spiral Computerized Tomography Scan

The rapid acquisition of high contrast images by spiral (also called helical) computerized tomography (CT) scanning allows an adequate visualization of the pulmonary arteries up to

at least the segmental level (71) (see Fig. 87-7). Two systematic overviews (72,73) on the performance of single-detector spiral CT scan in suspected cases of PE reported wide variations about both CT scan sensitivity (53% to 100%) and specificity (73% to 100%). Variations in image acquisition protocols, selection bias, and flaws in the design of the older studies may partly account for these differences. Two clinical studies (74,75) have shed new light on the performance of spiral CT scan. They included a wide spectrum of patients with suspected PE; the diagnostic criteria for PE were appropriate and both spiral CT scan and reference diagnostic tests were read in a blinded fashion. Both studies report a sensitivity of approximately 70% and a specificity of 90%. As in previous series, spiral CT scan was technically inadequate in 5% to 8% of patients because of motion artifacts or insufficient opacification of the pulmonary vessels.

Sensitivity of CT scan is higher in central pulmonary emboli than in segmental and subsegmental arteries. Multidetector CT scan (76), which allows both a thinner collimation (1- to 2-mm collimation) and a better definition without increasing image acquisition time, will likely improve sensitivity. To what extent this will be at the expense of specificity remains to be evaluated. Indeed, in the Geneva series, the positive

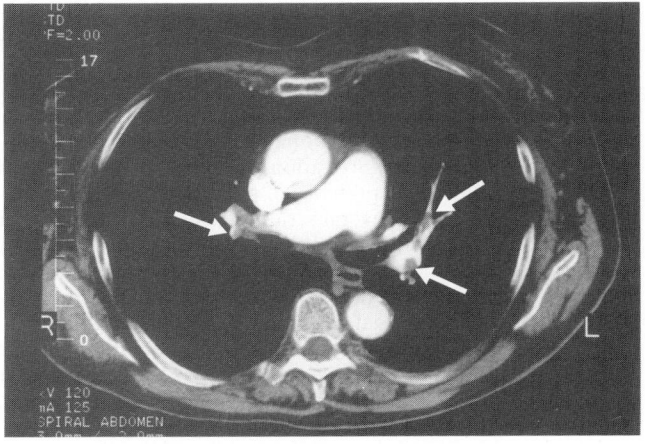

**FIGURE 87-7.** Spiral computerized tomography (CT) scan showing filling defects in the right pulmonary artery and in several segments of the left pulmonary artery tree (*arrows*).

predictive value of spiral CT scan decreased from 100% and 85% at the main pulmonary and lobar artery level, respectively, to 62% at the segmental level, demonstrating that specificity of CT scan also depends on the vascular level. In a recent multicenter French study (37) performed with single-detector CT scan, the prevalence of isolated subsegmental PE was only 3%, and only three of 12 such results were confirmed by pulmonary angiography. Moreover, the clinical importance of isolated segmental and subsegmental emboli is widely debated, and patients with no DVT, a negative CT scan, and a low or intermediate clinical probability of PE who are left untreated may have a very low thromboembolic risk (37,58), as discussed in the section, "Sequential Diagnostic Strategies for Suspected Pulmonary Embolism."

In summary, a spiral CT scan showing a thrombus up to the segmental level can be taken as adequate evidence of PE, whereas the necessity to treat isolated subsegmental thrombi in a patient without a DVT is unclear. A negative spiral CT scan alone does not rule out PE. Finally, the probability of PE is very low in patients with a low or intermediate clinical probability, no proximal DVT, and a negative spiral CT scan. The performance of second-generation "multidetector" spiral CT scan has not been studied specifically so far but enhanced sensitivity can be anticipated at the possible cost of reduced specificity.

Some groups proposed a combined spiral CT scan phlebography of lower limbs and abdominal veins together with CT scan angiography of the pulmonary arteries, allowing a complete examination of VTE in one session (77–79). Although appealing at first glance, the examination is costly and results in greater irradiation of the patient. Moreover, patients with suspected PE in whom a DVT is found by CUS do not require a CT scan at all and are thus spared the irradiation, contrast dye administration, inconvenience, and costs of CT scan. More experience is needed before any recommendation can be made about this combined technique.

## Echocardiography

Doppler echocardiography has several uses in suspected PE, and it may play a role in risk stratification. In a small subset of patients with PE [4% in a recent registry (80)], transthoracic echocardiography allows direct visualization of the clot in the right heart chambers or in the right main pulmonary artery. Direct imaging of part of the left main pulmonary artery requires transesophageal echocardiography. However, transesophageal echocardiography is uncomfortable for patients, and its sensitivity in suspected PE does not appear to be significantly higher than that of transthoracic echocardiography (81,82). In fact, the most frequent echocardiographic manifestations of PE are indirect and reflect the hemodynamic changes caused by an acute increase in pulmonary arterial resistance and pulmonary hypertension.

Pulmonary arterial pressure may be estimated in most patients by the tricuspid regurgitation velocity. A cutoff value of 2.7 m per second for the presence of pulmonary arterial hypertension was adopted in several series. Signs of right ventricular strain include dilation of the right ventricle, right ventricular hypokinesis, and, in severe cases, paradoxical motion of the interventricular septum. Several echocardiographic measurements have been proposed to quantify right ventricular dilation, of which the most standardized is the ratio of right ventricle to left ventricle diameter. However, a visual estimate by an experienced observer appears to be just as accurate (83). A particular pattern of right ventricular hypokinesis characterized by hypokinesis of the mid–free wall and preservation of apex motion ("McConnell sign") appear to be quite specific for acute as opposed to chronic pulmonary hypertension (84). Conversely, right ventricular hypertrophy and pulmonary artery

pressures greater than 60 mm Hg suggest chronic pulmonary hypertension. The sensitivity of these signs, which are often combined, lies between 40% and 70% in clinically suspected PE, and their specificity is approximately 90%, provided the patient does not have another disease causing chronic pulmonary hypertension. Echocardiography is the first-line test in suspected massive PE (see section, "Sequential Diagnostic Strategies for Suspected Pulmonary Embolism"). Indeed, in patients with shock, it is extremely effective for differential diagnosis of tamponade and cardiogenic shock. Moreover, absence of pulmonary hypertension and/or right ventricular dilation and hypokinesis in that situation renders it unlikely that PE is the cause of the shock.

In patients with suspected nonmassive PE, echocardiography may also represent a useful tool (83) for prognostic stratification of patients (see subsequent text and Chapter 88).

## Magnetic Resonance Pulmonary Angiography

Magnetic resonance (MR) pulmonary angiography is only a second-line diagnostic tool because of its higher cost, limited availability, and other logistic constraints (85–89). Limitations on spatial resolution and breath-holding make evaluation of the pulmonary vascular tree difficult, even at the level of segmental arteries. As the technology improves and becomes more widely available, MR imaging may play a greater role in the evaluation of patients with suspected venous thromboembolic disease.

# PROGNOSTIC MARKERS

Prognostic tools in patients with established PE include a clinical prediction rule (90), echocardiography (80,91,92), and the measurement of plasma troponin (93–95) or brain natriuretic peptide (BNP) levels (96–99). However, the predictive value of those instruments has not been compared and the impact of risk stratification of patients with nonmassive PE on treatment remains to be established.

## Clinical Scoring

Logistic regression was used to predict death, recurrent thromboembolic event, and/or major bleeding during the 3-month period that followed the initial diagnosis of PE among 296 consecutive patients (90). Thirty patients (10.1%) experienced one or more adverse events during that period: 25 died, 10 had a recurrent event, and five experienced major bleeding. Factors associated with an adverse outcome in multivariate analysis are displayed in Table 87-7. A score of 2 or less best identified patients at low risk of adverse outcome, that is, 2.2%, compared to 26.1% in the patients with a score of 3 or more. The low-risk group represented two thirds of the initial population. The score exhibited similar results in an external validation performed retrospectively on another sample of patients from three centers (100). Therefore, this simple risk score based on easily available variables can accurately identify patients with PE who are at low risk of an adverse outcome, which might be used to select those patients eligible for outpatient care.

## Echocardiography

Echocardiography has emerged as a potentially interesting tool for risk stratification in acute PE (91,92). In a large international registry, right ventricular dysfunction was suggested as an independent predictor of early death in patients with acute PE (80).

**TABLE 87-7**

DESCRIPTION OF A CLINICAL PROGNOSTIC SCORE
IN PATIENTS WITH PULMONARY EMBOLISM

| Geneva clinical prognostic score | Points |
|---|---|
| Cancer | +2 |
| Heart failure | +1 |
| Previous venous thromboembolism | +1 |
| Systolic blood pressure <100 mm Hg | +1 |
| PaO$_2$ <8 kPa | +1 |
| DVT shown by CUS | +1 |
| Prognosis | |
|   At low risk of poor outcome (2%) | <3 |
|   At high risk of poor outcome (25%) | ≥3 |

DVT, deep vein thrombolism; CUS, compression ultrasonography.
From Wicki J, Perrier A, Perneger TV, et al. Predicting adverse
outcome in patients with acute pulmonary embolism: a risk score.
*Thromb Haemost* 2000;84:548–552, with permission.

## Cardiac Biomarkers Such as Troponins and Brain Natriuretic Peptide

Cardiac troponins are the most sensitive and specific markers
of myocardial cell damage (101). Their prognostic role is well
established in patients with acute myocardial infarction as
well as in critically ill patients without acute coronary syndromes (102). In patients with acute PE, troponin levels correlated well with the extent of right ventricular dysfunction
(97), probably reflecting myocardial ischemia and microin-
farction because of alterations in oxygen supply and IN demand of the failing right ventricle.

The natriuretic peptides usually reflect congestive heart failure. Although atrial natriuretic peptides originate mainly from
atrial tissue, brain BNP is produced to a larger degree from
ventricular myocardial cells. Similar to cardiac troponins, elevations in BNP levels are associated with right ventricular dysfunction in acute PE (93,103).

Both troponins and BNP are accurate in identifying patients at low risk for developing PE and have a high negative
predictive value (98% or more) for in-hospital death (104).
Their utility in clinical daily practice, however, remains to be
established in large outcome studies.

# PRINCIPLES OF VALIDATION OF DIAGNOSTIC TESTS OR STRATEGIES

Systematic evaluation of a new diagnostic test or strategy in
suspected cases of VTE (105) should include the following
four steps: (a) technical description of the method; (b) systematic comparison with a diagnostic standard to establish
the critical cutoff concentration in tests with continuous values such as DD (using receiver-operating characteristics curve
analysis) and to establish the values of sensitivity and specificity of the test for VTE; (c) use of the test in so-called management trials in which anticoagulation is withheld in
patients with a diagnostic criterion ruling out VTE; a systematic 3-month follow-up allows detection of delayed events
and establishment of the safety of the test; (d) cost-effectiveness
analyses comparing the "new" strategy with other management policies.

# SEQUENTIAL DIAGNOSTIC STRATEGIES FOR SUSPECTED DEEP VEIN THROMBOSIS

Several noninvasive strategies have been reported to have a
high sensitivity for diagnosing DVT (1). Some strategies rely
on serial proximal CUS of proximal veins (common femoral,
superficial femoral, and popliteal veins). The rationale for repeating CUS after 1 week in patients in whom it was initially
negative is the detection of the rare proximal extension of the
distal DVTs that were not searched for. Because the yield of
repeat CUS after 1 week is very low (31,60,61,65), CUS has
been combined with a clinical prediction rule and/or DD
measurement to lower the number of necessary repeat compression sonograms (31,33,60,106). In another strategy (61),
single CUS was restricted to patients with a DD concentration greater than a critical cutoff level (500 μg per L), thereby
avoiding approximately 30% of CUS examinations. All these
strategies are associated with a low (approximately 2% or
less) 3-month thromboembolic risk, which is similar to that
observed in suspected patients left untreated following a normal phlebogram (12). In a randomized study, Wells et al.
compared the clinical outcome in 530 patients who underwent CUS (control group) and in 566 patients who underwent DD testing followed by CUS, unless the DD test was
negative and the patient was considered at low clinical probability (107). The 3-month thromboembolic risk among patients in whom the initial diagnostic strategy had ruled out
DVT was 0.4% in the DD group, compared with 1.4% in the
control group. The difference did not reach statistical significance, but the use of DD resulted in a statistically significant
reduction in the use of CUS because 39% of patients did not
require ultrasound imaging.

As mentioned earlier in the section on CUS, this observation challenges the need for diagnosing so-called distal DVT,
at least in non–high clinical probability patients. Figure 87-8
displays the strategy that appeared to be most cost-effective in
a formal cost-effectiveness analysis (108) (see section, "Cost-
Effectiveness of the Diagnostic Strategies in Suspected Deep
Vein Thrombosis and/or Pulmonary Embolism").

# SEQUENTIAL DIAGNOSTIC STRATEGIES FOR SUSPECTED PULMONARY EMBOLISM

## Nonmassive Pulmonary Embolism

One noninvasive strategy has been shown to be highly sensitive
for diagnosing PE. The strategy relies on assessing prior clinical
probability, either empirically or using a prediction rule, and
on the use of V/Q lung scanning. It uses CUS at an early stage
of the diagnostic workup, given that diagnosing DVT in a patient clinically suspected of PE warrants anticoagulant therapy.
The strategy starts with measuring DD and withholding anticoagulants in patients with a concentration less than the cutoff
level (33). Notably, the strategy is associated with a very low
(<1%) 3-month thromboembolic risk, similar to that associated with a normal lung perfusion scan (69) or a negative
pulmonary angiogram (15). The issue of whether a DD concentration less than the cutoff level detected using a highly sensitive assay rules out PE even in patients with a high clinical
probability remains controversial, and a conservative approach
might be appropriate in such patients (53,109). Recently, spiral
chest CT scan has been added to the diagnostic arsenal, but the
sensitivity of the single-detector technique was recently found

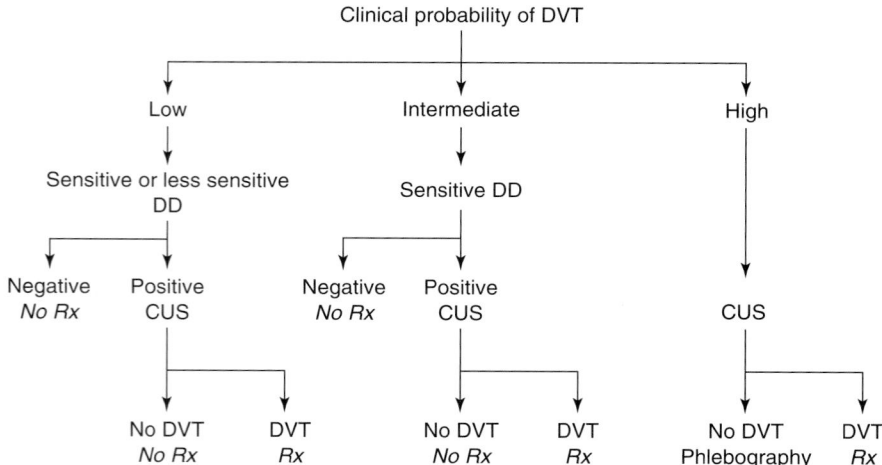

**FIGURE 87-8.** Algorithm for the diagnostic workup of suspected deep vein thrombosis. Sensitive D-dimer (DD) assay means at least 95% sensitivity for the presence of pulmonary embolism (PE). CUS, lower limb venous compression ultrasonography; DVT, deep vein thrombosis; V/Q, ventilation–perfusion; Rx, anticoagulant treatment.

to be only 70%, which precludes its use as the sole diagnostic test. Its implementation in a sequential approach (to replace V/Q lung scanning) has been studied in two recently reported management studies (37,58). In both studies, the requirement for pulmonary angiography was less than 2%, and the 3-month thromboembolic risk was also less than 2%. Table 87-8 displays the performance of the various diagnostic tests, and Figures 87-9 and 87-10 show two validated strategies that appeared to be cost-effective in a formal cost-effectiveness analysis (110) (see section, "Cost-Effectiveness of the Diagnostic Strategies in Suspected Deep Vein Thrombosis and/or Pulmonary Embolism"). The strategy including spiral CT scan (Fig. 87-10) is cost-effective, albeit less so than the one using V/Q lung scintigraphy but it includes a more widely available diagnostic tool. Note that to rule out PE, the combination of a negative lower limb CUS and a negative chest CT scan was required in patients with a low or intermediate clinical probability of PE, and that V/Q scintigraphy and/or pulmonary angiography was required in high-probability patients with a negative noninvasive workup. In addition, Figure 87-11 illustrates the advantage of measuring DD and performing CUS of

the proximal veins of the lower limbs as initial steps of the diagnostic sequence in suspected PE. Overall, this procedure avoids further lung imaging in 50% of patients (in fact, two of three patients younger than 50, one of two younger than 80, and one of three older than 80) (51). However, this view has been challenged by the recently demonstrated higher sensitivity of multidetector spiral CT scan compared to single-detector spiral CT scan, resulting in sufficient safety of a negative test result to rule out PE without combining it with a lower limb CUS (111). The issue of cost and availability of this tool would then become crucial in deciding whether the examination should be preceded by DD, CUS, both, or none.

Table 87-9 summarizes the diagnostic criteria that are presently accepted to confirm or eliminate PE, according to the prior clinical probability. In Table 87-10, the safety of some of those criteria for ruling out PE is presented for the 3-month thromboembolic risk.

Because there is no convincing evidence so far that patients with submassive PE should receive thrombolytic therapy, systematic echocardiographic screening of patients with nonmassive PE is not indicated. Indeed, in the single randomized trial

## TABLE 87-8

PERFORMANCES OF DIAGNOSTIC TESTS FOR NONMASSIVE PULMONARY EMBOLISM

| Test (references) | Sensitivity (%) | Specificity (%) | Likelihood ratio | |
| --- | --- | --- | --- | --- |
| | | | Positive result | Negative result |
| Pulmonary angiography (14,112) | 97 | 98 | 48 | 0.03 |
| V/Q lung scan | | | | |
| Normal (14,59,113,114) | 99 | — | 0.02 | — |
| Nondiagnostic (14) | — | — | 0.9 | — |
| High probability (14) | — | 91 | — | 14 |
| Plasma DD | | | | |
| Rapid ELISA (33,115) | 99 | 41 | 1.7 | 0.02 |
| Immunoturbidimetric (116,117) | 98 | 40 | 1.6 | 0.05 |
| Whole-blood agglutination (45,50) | 85 | 68 | 2.7 | 0.2 |
| Lower limb CUS (54,59,118,119) | 50 | 97 | 17 | 0.5 |
| Spiral CT scan (74,75) | 69 | 89 | 6.3 | 0.3 |
| Echocardiography (81,120–123) | 60 | 90 | 6.0 | 0.4 |

DD, D-dimer; ELISA, enzyme-linked immunoassay; V/Q, ventilation–perfusion; CUS, compression ultrasonography; CT, computerized tomography.

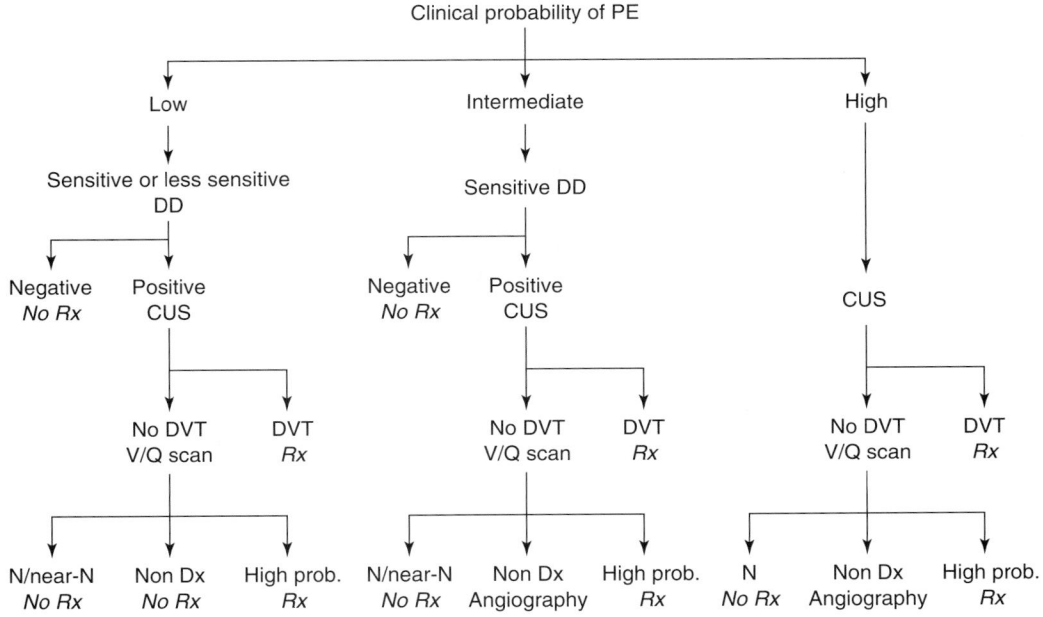

**FIGURE 87-9.** Algorithm for the diagnostic workup of suspected nonmassive pulmonary embolism on the basis of lung scintigraphy. Preliminary evidence suggests that angiography may be substituted by helical computerized tomography (CT) scan. Sensitive D dimmer (DD) assay means at least 95% sensitive for the presence of pulmonary embolism (PE). CUS, lower limb venous compression ultrasonography; DVT, deep vein thrombosis; V/Q, ventilation–perfusion; Rx, anticoagulant treatment.

comparing alteplase and heparin to heparin alone in patients with submassive PE (126), the mortality was similar in both groups and the only difference favoring thrombolysis was more frequent clinical deterioration in the heparin arm necessitating secondary salvage thrombolysis.

## Massive Pulmonary Embolism

Patients with suspected massive PE have a very high mortality rate and require emergent thrombolytic or surgical treatment in the event PE is confirmed. The clinical presentation requires a differential diagnosis that includes other causes of shock such as pericardial tamponade or myocardial infarction. The clot burden is usually high in massive PE, and the diagnostic yield of any imaging study, whether lung scan or spiral CT scan, is likely to be high. Therefore, the logical initial test in such patients is transthoracic echocardiography. An ECG showing signs of acute pulmonary hypertension and right ventricular strain in a patient with shock, normal left ventricular contractility, and absence of pericardial effusion is a very strong argument in favor of massive PE. In fact, most clinicians would readily begin thrombolytic

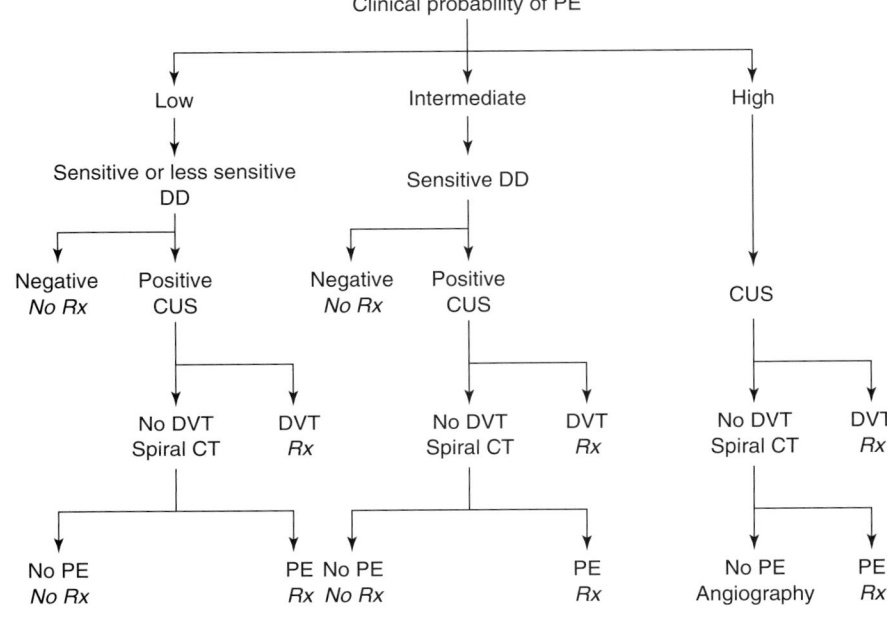

**FIGURE 87-10.** Algorithm for the diagnostic workup of suspected nonmassive pulmonary embolism (PE) based on helical computerized tomography (CT) scan. CUS, lower limb venous compression ultrasonography; DVT, deep vein thrombosis; V/Q, ventilation–perfusion; Rx, anticoagulant treatment.

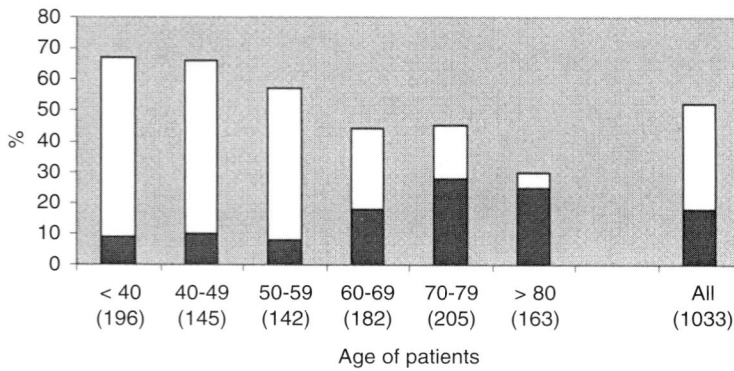

**FIGURE 87-11.** Relative contribution of a positive compression ultrasonography (CUS) (showing a proximal DVT, *black bar*) and negative D-dimer (DD) measurement (<500 μg per L, *white bar*) as initial diagnostic steps in suspected PE according to the patient's age. Figures within brackets indicate the number of patients. (From Righini M, Goehring C, Bounameaux H, et al. Effects of age on the performance of common diagnostic tests for pulmonary embolism. *Am J Med* 2000;109:357–361, with permission.)

treatment in such a highly unstable patient without awaiting further diagnostic information. On the other hand, in a patient temporarily stabilized by vasopressors (such as dopamine or norepinephrine), confirmation may be sought by either lung scan or spiral CT scan, whichever is the most rapidly available. Angiography should be avoided whenever possible because it carries the highest risk in this patient population (127) and increases the risk of a major bleed at the puncture site because of thrombolytic treatment (128). The outcome of leg venous CUS has not been studied systematically in this situation, but data collected in patients with nonmassive PE but a high clot burden on V/Q lung scan suggest that it may be associated with a 20% to 30% false-negative rate (129). Figure 87-12 summarizes the proposed diagnostic algorithm.

## TABLE 87-9

ACCEPTABLE DIAGNOSTIC CRITERIA FOR DIAGNOSING PULMONARY EMBOLISM ACCORDING TO CLINICAL PROBABILITY

| Diagnostic criterion | Clinical probability of pulmonary embolism | | |
|---|---|---|---|
| | Low | Intermediate | High |
| **ABSENCE OF PULMONARY EMBOLISM** | | | |
| Normal pulmonary angiogram | Yes | Yes | Yes |
| Normal lung scan | Yes | Yes | Yes |
| Plasma ELISA DD level <500 μg/L[a] | Yes | Yes | Yo |
| Nondiagnostic lung scan and negative proximal CUS | Yes | No | No |
| Normal spiral CT scan and negative proximal CUS[b] | Yes | Yes | No |
| Normal spiral CT scan alone | No | No | No |
| **PULMONARY EMBOLISM** | | | |
| Pulmonary angiogram showing PE | Yes | Yes | Yes |
| High-probability lung scan | Yes[c] | Yes | Yes |
| Proximal US showing a DVT | Yes | Yes | Yes |
| Spiral CT scan showing PE | Yes[c] | Yes | Yes |

CUS, proximal lower limb venous ultrasonography; CT, computerized tomography; PE, pulmonary embolism; DVT, deep vein thrombosis; ELISA, enzyme-linked immunoassay; DD, D-dimer.
[a]Or highly sensitive immunoturbidimetric assay.
[b]Preliminary evidence.
[c]Lower positive predictive value in that clinical probability subgroup.

# COST-EFFECTIVENESS OF THE DIAGNOSTIC STRATEGIES IN SUSPECTED DEEP VEIN THROMBOSIS AND/OR PULMONARY EMBOLISM

Several diagnostic strategies have demonstrated their efficacy and safety. Their implementation in daily clinical practice will be triggered mainly by the availability of the techniques and the expertise present in each institution. However, the cost issue may also play a role, and decision makers might recommend the implementation of one or the other strategy on an economic basis. Moreover, third-party payers may also limit their reimbursement at the level of the most cost-effective strategy.

## Cost-Effectiveness of Diagnostic Strategies in Suspected Deep Vein Thrombosis

In a formal cost-effectiveness analysis, using a decision-analysis model based on four contemporary diagnostic strategies for clinically suspected DVT (108), we considered costs per patient, 3-month mortality, number of lives saved per 1,000 patients, and incremental costs per life and per year of life saved. Under baseline conditions (prevalence of DVT, 24%), the effectiveness of all strategies was similar (4.2 to 4.4 lives saved per 1,000 patients managed). The most expensive strategy was serial CUS (second ultrasonography on day 7 in all patients with a normal first ultrasonography). Performing a second ultrasonography only in patients with an elevated DD level reduced costs. Taking clinical probability into account (serial ultrasonography only in patients with an intermediate clinical probability of DVT) yielded further savings. DD as a first test, followed by a single CUS only in case of an abnormal DD level, and by phlebography only in patients with a normal CUS and a high clinical probability of DVT (Fig. 87-3), was the cheapest, and, therefore, the most cost-effective option. This strategy allowed a 15% reduction in incremental costs compared to the most expensive algorithm.

## Cost-Effectiveness of Diagnostic Strategies in Suspected Nonmassive Pulmonary Embolism

In the setting of clinically suspected PE, we also performed a formal decision analysis to evaluate the cost-effectiveness of various strategies including spiral CT scan in order to determine the most cost-effective schemes for each clinical probability of PE (110). Other tests included DD, lower limb venous

**TABLE 87-10**

THREE-MONTH THROMBOEMBOLIC RISK IN PATIENTS LEFT UNTREATED
ACCORDING TO VARIOUS DIAGNOSTIC CRITERIA FOR RULING OUT
PULMONARY EMBOLISM

| Diagnostic criterion | Patients (n) | 3-month thromboembolic risk (%) (95% CI) | References |
|---|---|---|---|
| Normal pulmonary angiogram | 1,050 | 1.7 (1.0–2.7) | 15,59,69,113,124 |
| Normal lung scan | 1,031 | 0.7 (0.3–1.4) | 59,69,113,124 |
| Plasma ELISA DD level <500 µg/L and low to intermediate clinical probability of PE | 1,643 | 0 (0–0.7) | 33,58,125 |
| Nondiagnostic lung scan and negative proximal US and low clinical probability of PE | 864 | 2.3 (1.5–3.5) | 38,59 |
| Normal spiral CT scan and negative proximal US and low or intermediate clinical probability of PE | 975 | 1.7 (1.1–2.8) | 37,58 |

ELISA, enzyme-linked immunoassay; DD, D-dimer; PE, pulmonary embolism; US, ultrasonography;
CT, computerized tomography; CI, confidence interval.

CUS, V/Q scan, and angiography. Outcome measures were 3-month survival and costs per 1,000 patients managed. Baseline sensitivity of CT scan was 70%, corresponding to the performance of single-detector CT scan, and this figure was raised in sensitivity analysis to account for the expected higher sensitivity of newer multidetector CT scanners. All strategies were compared to a reference strategy consisting of V/Q scan in all patients followed by an angiogram when nondiagnostic (*V/Q scan ± angiography*, $2,596,100 for 1,000 patients managed). The highest cost savings were obtained by a scheme in which patients with a low clinical probability of PE would be managed with DD, ultrasonography, and V/Q scan, angiography being performed in patients with an intermediate or high probability (*DD-CUS-V/Q scan ± angiography*, $1,995,900). A similar strategy in which V/Q scan was replaced by CT scan (*DD-CUS-CT ± angiography*, $2,365,700) was less cost saving. Replacing angiography entirely (DD, ultrasound, and CT scan irrespective of the clinical probability of PE) would be moderately cost saving ($2,150,600) but requires a sensitivity

of spiral CT scan in the multidetector range. Finally, single-detector spiral CT scan as a single test is not effective and costlier than combinations with DD and ultrasound. Using multidetector CT scan would increase effectiveness but not decrease costs. In summary, single-detector spiral CT scan as a single test is not cost-effective. In contrast, algorithms combining clinical assessment, DD, and lower limb ultrasonography to either V/Q scan or single-detector spiral CT scan are highly cost-effective, provided an angiogram is performed in patients with an intermediate or high clinical probability of PE. Using multidetector CT scan combined with DD and ultrasonography might allow foregoing angiography in all clinical probability subgroups. Admittedly, such analyses are only valid under certain conditions. However, overall, the ranking of strategies for PE was not affected by any variation within the range of values that were defined before performing the analysis, at least for the following variables: prevalence of PE in clinical probability categories and diagnostic performance of the various tests used.

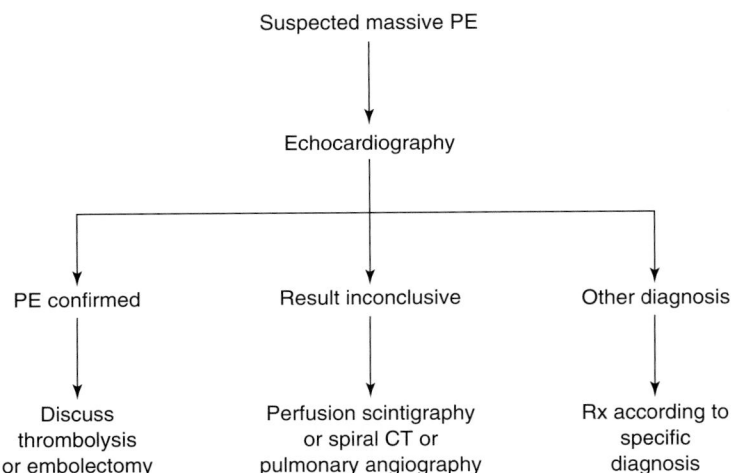

FIGURE 87-12. Algorithm for the diagnostic workup of suspected massive pulmonary embolism (PE). CT, computerized tomography; Rx, treatment.

# SPECIAL SITUATIONS

## Suspected Recurrent Deep Vein Thrombosis or Pulmonary Embolism

Diagnosis of recurrent DVT is difficult because acute thrombi cannot be easily distinguished from old thrombi, unless the suspected recurrent event occurs in a location that is different from that of the initial event. Because initially abnormal plethysmography results return to normal in 90% of patients at 1 year, recurrent DVT in symptomatic patients might be inferred from an abnormal plethysmographic result at least 1 year after the previous event but such an inference has a positive predictive value of only 80% (130). Alternatively, repeated measurements of the diameter of the common femoral and popliteal veins have been proposed as a tool to discriminate new from old thrombi (131). The vein diameter has to be measured under compression with the transducer and compared with earlier measurements. Patients with stable or diminished vein diameters can be considered as free of recurrence. The predictive value of a stable or improved diameter to rule out recurrence was 90% (95% CI, 77% to 97%). In a prospective study of 205 consecutive patients, the policy of withholding anticoagulant treatment in patients clinically suspected of recurrent DVT in whom CUS showed stable or improved vein diameters was found to be safe (132). The main limitation of this method is the need for iterative vein diameter measurements in patients with DVT, which is costly and resource demanding. Moreover, it does not account for the possibility that asymptomatic events may have occurred between two measurements. In selected cases, phlebography may be the only solution, the presence of an intraluminal defect in at least two views proving the recurrence.

Diagnosis of recurrent PE is also challenging. It can only be confirmed if new emboli can be detected in locations that were previously documented as free of thrombi. For this reason, some opinion leaders strongly advise performing lung imaging in all patients with PE, including patients with proximal DVT and respiratory signs and symptoms, in whom the diagnosis could be made without lung imaging. But again, this suggestion does not account for the eventuality that asymptomatic emboli may have occurred between the two imaging procedures. In selected cases, pulmonary angiography may be required to settle the case. Diagnostic criteria for recurrent events are presented in Table 87-11.

Recurrent VTE will be readily ruled out by a DD measurement if the concentration is less than the diagnostic cutoff, but, at best, this will occur in one third of patients when

---

**TABLE 87-11**

### CRITERIA FOR DIAGNOSING RECURRENT VENOUS THROMBOEMBOLISM

**RECURRENT DEEP VEIN THROMBOSIS**
Noncompressibility of a previously compressible venous segment
Increase of at least 4 mm in the diameter of the residual thrombus
New filling defect on a phlebogram

**RECURRENT PULMONARY EMBOLISM**
New thrombus on spiral computed tomography
New mismatsched defect on a ventilation–perfusion lung scintigraphy
New defect on a pulmonary angiogram

---

ELISA methods or automated turbidimetric assays are used. In the other cases, the diagnosis will rely upon the subjective combination of clinical findings and imaging modalities, a situation that is far from satisfying.

## Suspected Venous Thromboembolism in Pregnancy

Pregnancy constitutes an additional challenge in case of suspected DVT or PE. Hemodynamic changes interfere with the interpretation of tests for DVT, and tests using ionizing radiation may theoretically harm the fetus. Widely used noninvasive initial tests such as DD measurement or CUS are of limited value because of a reduced specificity (DD) (133) (see Fig. 87-13) or sensitivity (CUS). Nevertheless, a DD concentration less than the diagnostic cutoff value rules out VTE.

Many clinicians advocate using phlebography but it is suboptimal under these conditions. The examination should, however, be performed only if CUS has not demonstrated the presence of DVT. Alternatively, magnetic resonance imaging (MRI) may be used (134) although the experience with this modality is scarce and it lacks accessibility in many countries. As a potential advantage, MRI may diagnose isolated iliac DVT, a condition that is more common during pregnancy, in addition to femoropopliteal DVT, and it is not associated with radiation exposure.

In suspected PE, objective testing is mandatory, and the previously described diagnostic strategy for nonpregnant women should be applied. If DD is greater than the diagnostic cutoff

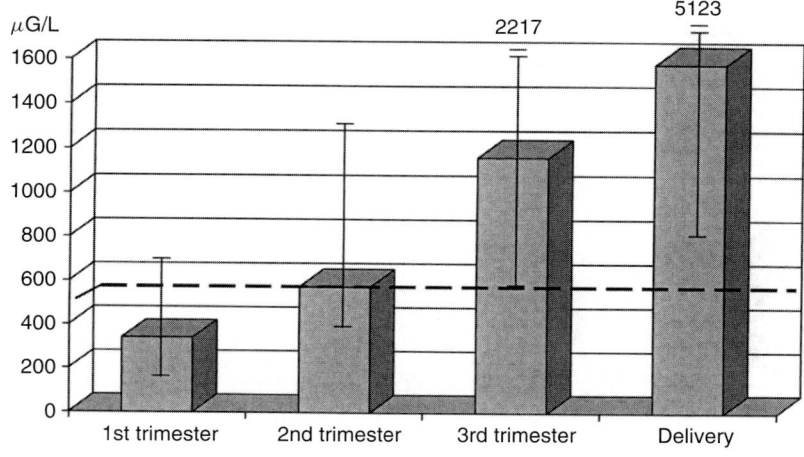

**FIGURE 87-13.** Median D-dimer (DD) concentration during pregnancy and after delivery. The *vertical bars* represent the fifth and ninety-fifth percentiles of the distribution, and the *dashed line* indicates the diagnostic cutoff less than which venous thromboembolism can be ruled out (90). (Derived from Chabloz P, Reber G, Boehlen F, et al. TAFI antigen and D-dimer levels during normal pregnancy and at delivery. *Br J Haematol* 2001;115:150–152.)

and if no DVT is diagnosed on CUS, imaging should be performed. Because of the minimal radiation of V/Q lung scan, this examination may be preferred to spiral CT scan, although recent data suggest that CT scan may not deliver higher radiation doses to the fetus than V/Q lung scintigraphy (135). Another reason to resort primarily to V/Q lung scanning is that it is the only imaging modality that has been assessed in an outcome study, although retrospectively. Chan et al. reviewed the outcomes of 120 pregnant patients with suspected PE in Ontario for more than 10 years: 75% of them had a normal V/Q scan ruling out PE, and none had an event during the remaining pregnancy (136). In fact, whenever possible, in this category of young women, perfusion scan alone should be performed and if perfusion is normal, PE is excluded. In case of abnormal perfusion, ventilation imaging should be performed to categorize the lung scan result as high probability or nondiagnostic lung scan. In the latter case, spiral CT scan should then be performed unless *a priori* clinical probability was low. Most experts concur that the diagnosis should be confirmed before labeling a pregnant woman as having PE. Indeed, the risk of anticoagulant treatment throughout pregnancy and the weight of carrying that label for young women of childbearing age far outweigh the minimal risk of irradiation to the fetus (137,138).

## Screening Asymptomatic Patients at High Risk of Deep Vein Thrombosis

Screening patients at high risk of DVT is mainly done in the context of thromboprophylactic trials testing the efficacy of new prophylactic drugs or strategies, especially in the postoperative period. In that situation, phlebographically diagnosed DVT is the most commonly employed endpoint. There is a good basis for this policy (139): asymptomatic distal DVT is probably the only causal pathway leading to proximal DVT and PE, and the reduction of adverse clinical events is owing to the effect of antithrombotic drugs on those asymptomatic events. In the case of phlebographically diagnosed DVT, fatal PE is unlikely to occur if all phlebographically diagnosed asymptomatic thrombi are prevented. Hence, asymptomatic distal DVT may be considered as a valid surrogate endpoint to clinical events in such trials. Some investigators have advocated the use of phlebography only in symptomatic patients but using nonspecific and insensitive symptoms such as leg pain or swelling, especially following total hip or knee arthroplasty, does not appear very promising. Other screening techniques such as thermography could not confirm initial expectations.

It has been shown that screening to detect and treat postoperative DVT following major orthopedic surgery is not cost-effective, compared to systematic prolongation of prophylaxis for four weeks in a decision-analysis model (140).

## CONCLUSION AND PERSPECTIVES

In summary, diagnosing VTE depends upon several, mainly noninvasive, diagnostic tools that must be used sequentially. Validated diagnostic algorithms for suspected DVT/PE should be implemented in all institutions that depend upon local availability and expertise, and they must also take into account the cost issues. With the development of potentially more sensitive diagnostic tests such as multidetector spiral CT scan, and possibly MR pulmonary angiography, or calf veins ultrasonography, physicians will have to face the risk of overdiagnosis and, hence overtreatment, with its associated iatrogenic risk. Indeed, one of the important lessons of the last 10 years' outcome studies is that not all thrombi need to be treated.

Therefore, the true issue in the near future will no longer be just to detect clots but to identify patients who must really be treated by anticoagulants, which may turn out to be more complicated.

## *References*

1. Perrier A, Bounameaux H. Cost-effective diagnosis of deep vein thrombosis and pulmonary embolism. *Thromb Haemost* 2001;86:475–487.
2. Bounameaux H, Reber-Wasem MA. Superficial thrombophlebitis and deep vein thrombosis. A controversial association. *Arch Intern Med* 1997; 157:1822–1824.
3. Guidelines on diagnosis and management of acute pulmonary embolism. Task Force on Pulmonary Embolism, European Society of Cardiology. *Eur Heart J* 2000;21:1301–1336.
4. Haeger K. Problems of acute deep venous thrombosis. I. The interpretation of signs and symptoms. *Angiology* 1969;20:219–223.
5. McLachlin J, Richards T, Paterson JC. An evaluation of clinical signs in the diagnosis of venous thrombosis. *Arch Surg* 1962;85:738–744.
6. Hildner FJ, Ormond RS. Accuracy of the clinical diagnosis of pulmonary embolism. *JAMA* 1967;202:115–118.
7. Stein PD, Henry JW. Clinical characteristics of patients with acute pulmonary embolism stratified according to their presenting syndromes. *Chest* 1997;112:974–979.
8. Dalen JE, Haffajee CI, Alpert JS, et al. Pulmonary embolism, pulmonary hemorrhage, pulmonary infarction. *N Engl J Med* 1977;296:1431–1435.
9. Elliott CG, Goldhaber SZ, Visani L, et al. Chest radiographs in acute pulmonary embolism. Results from the international cooperative pulmonary embolism registry. *Chest* 2000;118:33–38.
10. Thames MD, Alpert JS, Dalen JE. Syncope in patients with pulmonary embolism. *JAMA* 1977;238:2509–2511.
11. Marder VJ, Soulen RL, Atichartakarn V, et al. Quantitative venographic assessment of deep vein thrombosis in the evaluation of streptokinase and heparin therapy. *J Lab Clin Med* 1977;89:1018–1029.
12. Hull R, Hirsh J, Sackett DL. Clinical validity of a negative venogram in patients with clinically suspected venous thrombosis. *Circulation* 1981; 64:622–625.
13. van Beek EJ, Bakker AJ, Reekers JA. Pulmonary embolism: interobserver agreement in the interpretation of conventional angiographic and DSA images in patients with nondiagnostic lung scan results. *Radiology* 1996; 198:721–724.
14. The PIOPED Investigators. Value of the ventilation-perfusion scan in acute pulmonary embolism. *JAMA* 1990;263:2753–2759.
15. van Beek EJ, Brouwerst EM, Song B, et al. Clinical validity of a normal pulmonary angiogram in patients with suspected pulmonary embolism—a critical review. *Clin Radiol* 2001;56:838–842.
16. Perrier A, Bounameaux H. Acute pulmonary embolism: diagnosis. In: Peacock AJ, Rubin LJ, eds. *Pulmonary Circulation*. London: Arnold, 2004.
17. Miller GA, Sutton GC, Kerr IH, et al. Comparison of streptokinase and heparin in treatment of isolated acute massive pulmonary embolism. *Br Med J* 1971;2:681–684.
18. Bounameaux H, Krahenbuhl B, Vukanovic S. Diagnosis of deep vein thrombosis by combination of Doppler ultrasound flow examination and strain gauge plethysmography. An alternative to venography only in particular conditions despite improved accuracy of the Doppler method. *Thromb Haemost* 1982;47:141–144.
19. Huisman MV, Buller HR, ten Cate JW, et al. The Amsterdam General Practitioner Study. Serial impedance plethysmography for suspected deep venous thrombosis in outpatients. *N Engl J Med* 1986;314:823–828.
20. Prandoni P, Lensing AW, Buller HR, et al. Failure of computerized impedance plethysmography in the diagnostic management of patients with clinically suspected deep-vein thrombosis. *Thromb Haemost* 1991;65: 233–236.
21. Ginsberg JS, Wells PS, Hirsh J, et al. Reevaluation of the sensitivity of impedance plethysmography for the detection of proximal deep vein thrombosis. *Arch Intern Med* 1994;154:1930–1933.
22. Tan YK, da Silva AF. Digital photoplethysmography in the diagnosis of suspected lower limb DVT: is it useful? *Eur J Vasc Endovasc Surg* 1999; 18:71–79.
23. Simon CA, Krahenbuhl B. Venous stop-flow pressure: a simple and noninvasive technique for diagnosing deep-vein thrombosis. *Lancet* 1977;2: 1008–1009.
24. Lensing AW, Levi MM, Buller HR, et al. Diagnosis of deep-vein thrombosis using an objective Doppler method. *Ann Intern Med* 1990;113:9–13.
25. Fauno P, Suomalainen O, Bergqvist D, et al. The use of fibrinogen uptake test in screening for deep vein thrombosis in patients with hip fracture. *Thromb Res* 1990;60:185–190.
26. Lensing AW, Hirsh J. 125I-fibrinogen leg scanning: reassessment of its role for the diagnosis of venous thrombosis in post-operative patients. *Thromb Haemost* 1993;69:2–7.
27. Rodger M, Makropoulos D, Turek M, et al. Diagnostic value of the electrocardiogram in suspected pulmonary embolism [in process citation]. *Am J Cardiol* 2000;86:807–809, A10.

28. Stein PD, Goldhaber SZ, Henry JW. Alveolar-arterial oxygen gradient in the assessment of acute pulmonary embolism. *Chest* 1995;107:139–143.

29. Rodger MA, Carrier M, Jones GN, et al. Diagnostic value of arterial blood gas measurement in suspected pulmonary embolism. *Am J Respir Crit Care Med* 2000;162:2105–2108.

30. Stein PD, Terrin ML, Hales CA, et al. Clinical, laboratory, roentgenographic, and electrocardiographic findings in patients with acute pulmonary embolism and no pre-existing cardiac or pulmonary disease. *Chest* 1991;100:598–603.

31. Wells PS, Anderson DR, Bormanis J, et al. Value of assessment of pretest probability of deep-vein thrombosis in clinical management. *Lancet* 1997;350:1795–1798.

32. Wells PS, Hirsh J, Anderson DR, et al. Accuracy of clinical assessment of deep-vein thrombosis. *Lancet* 1995;345:1326–1330.

33. Perrier A, Desmarais S, Miron MJ, et al. Non-invasive diagnosis of venous thromboembolism in outpatients. *Lancet* 1999;353:190–195.

34. Wells PS, Anderson DR, Rodger M, et al. Derivation of a simple clinical model to categorize patients probability of pulmonary embolism: increasing the models utility with the SimpliRED D-dimer. *Thromb Haemost* 2000;83:416–420.

35. Wicki J, Perneger TV, Junod A, et al. Assessing clinical probability of pulmonary embolism in the emergency ward: a simple score. *Arch Intern Med* 2001;161:92–97.

36. Chagnon I, Bounameaux H, Aujesky D, et al. Comparison of two clinical prediction rules and implicit assessment for suspected pulmonary embolism. *Am J Med* 2002;113:269–275.

37. Musset D, Parent F, Meyer G, et al. Diagnostic strategy for patients with suspected pulmonary embolism: a prospective multicentre outcome study. *Lancet* 2002;360:1914–1920.

38. Perrier A, Miron MJ, Desmarais S, et al. Using clinical evaluation and lung scan to rule out suspected pulmonary embolism: Is it a valid option in patients with normal results of lower-limb venous compression ultrasonography? *Arch Intern Med* 2000;160:512–516.

39. Cornuz J, Ghali WA, Hayoz D, et al. Clinical prediction of deep venous thrombosis using two risk assessment methods in combination with rapid quantitative D-dimer testing. *Am J Med* 2002;112:198–203.

40. Miron MJ, Perrier A, Bounameaux H. Clinical assessment of suspected deep vein thrombosis: comparison between a score and empirical assessment. *J Intern Med* 2000;247:249–254.

41. Shields GP, Turnipseed S, Panacek EA, et al. Validation of the Canadian clinical probability model for acute venous thrombosis. *Acad Emerg Med* 2002;9:561–566.

42. Anderson DR, Kovacs MJ, Kovacs G, et al. Combined use of clinical assessment and D-dimer to improve the management of patients presenting to the emergency department with suspected deep vein thrombosis (the EDITED Study). *J Thromb Haemost* 2003;1:645–651.

43. Kraaijenhagen RA, Piovella F, Bernardi E, et al. Simplification of the diagnostic management of suspected deep vein thrombosis. *Arch Intern Med* 2002;162:907–911.

44. Kilroy DA, Ireland S, Reid P, et al. Emergency department investigation of deep vein thrombosis. *Emerg Med J* 2003;20:29–32.

45. Wells PS, Anderson DR, Rodger M, et al. Excluding pulmonary embolism at the bedside without diagnostic imaging: management of patients with suspected pulmonary embolism presenting to the emergency department by using a simple clinical model and d-dimer. *Ann Intern Med* 2001;135:98–107.

46. Bounameaux H, de Moerloose P, Perrier A, et al. D-dimer testing in suspected venous thromboembolism: an update. *QJM* 1997;90:437–442.

47. Bounameaux H, Perrier A. D-dimer in the diagnosis of venous thromboembolism. In: Dalen JE, ed. *Venous thromboembolism.* New York: Marcel Dekker Inc, 2003:133–148.

48. Stein PD, Hull RD, Patel KC, et al. D-dimer for the exclusion of acute venous thrombosis and pulmonary embolism: a systematic review. *Ann Intern Med* 2004;140:589–602.

49. Raimondi P, Bongard O, de Moerloose P, et al. D-dimer plasma concentration in various clinical conditions: implications for the use of this test in the diagnostic approach of venous thromboembolism. *Thromb Res* 1993;69:125–130.

50. Ginsberg JS, Wells PS, Kearon C, et al. Sensitivity and specificity of a rapid whole-blood assay for D-dimer in the diagnosis of pulmonary embolism. *Ann Intern Med* 1998;129:1006–1011.

51. Righini M, Goehring C, Bounameaux H, et al. Effects of age on the performance of common diagnostic tests for pulmonary embolism. *Am J Med* 2000;109:357–361.

52. Miron MJ, Perrier A, Bounameaux H, et al. Contribution of noninvasive evaluation to the diagnosis of pulmonary embolism in hospitalized patients. *Eur Respir J* 1999;13:1365–1370.

53. Righini M, Aujesky D, Roy PM, et al. Clinical usefulness of D-dimer according to clinical probability in outpatients with suspected pulmonary embolism. *Arch Intern Med* 2004;164:2483–2487.

54. Kearon C, Ginsberg JS, Hirsh J. The role of venous ultrasonography in the diagnosis of suspected deep venous thrombosis and pulmonary embolism. *Ann Intern Med* 1998;129:1044–1049.

55. The diagnostic approach to acute venous thromboembolism. Clinical practice guideline. *Am J Respir Crit Care Med* 1999;160:1043–1066.

56. Keeling DM, Mackie IJ, Moody A, et al. The diagnosis of deep vein thrombosis in symptomatic outpatients and the potential for clinical assessment

57. Kearon C, Julian JA, Math M, et al. Noninvasive diagnosis of deep venous thrombosis. *Ann Intern Med* 1998;128:663–677.

58. Perrier A, Roy PM, Aujesky D, et al. Diagnosing pulmonary embolism with clinical assessment, D-dimer, venous ultrasound and helical computed tomography: a multicenter management study. *Am J Med* 2004;116:291–299.

59. Wells PS, Ginsberg JS, Anderson DR, et al. Use of a clinical model for safe management of patients with suspected pulmonary embolism. *Ann Intern Med* 1998;129:997–1005.

60. Bernardi E, Prandoni P, Lensing AW et al, The Multicentre Italian D-dimer Ultrasound Study Investigators Group. D-dimer testing as an adjunct to ultrasonography in patients with clinically suspected deep vein thrombosis: prospective cohort study. *BMJ* 1998;317:p1037–p1040.

61. Cogo A, Lensing AWA, Koopman MMW, et al. Compression ultrasonography for diagnostic management of patients with clinically suspectged deep vein thrombosis: prospective cohort study. *BMJ* 1998;316:17–20.

62. Elias A, Mallard L, Elias M, et al. A single complete ultrasound investigation of the venous network for the diagnostic management of patients with a clinically suspected first episode of deep venous thrombosis of the lower limbs. *Thromb Haemost* 2003;89:221–227.

63. Schellong SM, Schwarz T, Halbritter K, et al. Complete compression ultrasonography of the leg veins as a single test for the diagnosis of deep vein thrombosis. *Thromb Haemost* 2003;89:228–234.

64. Gottlieb RH, Voci SL, Syed L, et al. Randomized prospective study comparing routine versus selective use of sonography of the complete calf in patients with suspected deep venous thrombosis. *AJR Am J Roentgenol* 2003;180:241–245.

65. Bounameaux H, Perrier A. Compression ultrasonography for diagnosing deep vein thrombosis. Repeat testing is unjustified. *BMJ* 1998;316:1534–1535.

66. Alderson PO, Martin EC. Pulmonary embolism: diagnosis with multiple imaging modalities. *Radiology* 1987;164:297–312.

67. Gottschalk A, Sostman HD, Coleman RE, et al. Ventilation-perfusion scintigraphy in the PIOPED study. Part II. Evaluation of scintigraphic criteria and interpretations. *J Nucl Med* 1993;34:1119–1126.

68. Sostman HD, Coleman RE, De Long DM, et al. Evaluation of revised criteria for ventilation-perfusion scintigraphy in patients with suspected pulmonary embolism. *Radiology* 1994;193:p103–p107.

69. Hull RD, Raskob GE, Coates G, et al. Clinical validity of a normal perfusion lung scan in patients with suspected pulmonary embolism. *Chest* 1990;97:23–26.

70. de Groot MR, Turkstra F, van Marwijk Kooy M, et al. Value of chest X-ray combined with perfusion scan versus ventilation/perfusion scan in acute pulmonary embolism. *Thromb Haemost* 2000;83:412–415.

71. Rémy-Jardin M, Rémy J, Wattinne L, et al. Central pulmonary tromboembolism: diagnosis with spiral volumetric CT with the single-breath-holds technique. Comparison with pulmonary angiography. *Radiology* 1992;185:381–387.

72. Rathbun SW, Raskob GE, Whitsett TL. Sensitivity and specificity of helical computed tomography in the diagnosis of pulmonary embolism: a systematic review. *Ann Intern Med* 2000;132:227–232.

73. Mullins MD, Becker DM, Hagspiel KD, et al. The role of spiral volumetric computed tomography in the diagnosis of pulmonary embolism. *Arch Intern Med* 2000;160:293–298.

74. Perrier A, Howarth N, Didier D, et al. Performances of helical computed tomography in unselected outpatients with suspected pulmonary embolism. *Ann Intern Med* 2001;135:88–97.

75. van Strijen MJL, de Monye W, Kieft GJ et al, The ANTELOPE Study Group. Accuracy of spiral CT in the diagnosis of pulmonary embolism: a prospective multicenter cohort study of consecutive patients. *Thromb Haemost* 2001;86 OC154.

76. Ghaye B, Szapiro D, Mastora I, et al. Peripheral pulmonary arteries: how far in the lung does multi-detector row spiral CT allow analysis? *Radiology* 2001;219:629–636.

77. Yankelevitz DF, Gamsu G, Shah A, et al. Optimization of combined CT pulmonary angiography with lower extremity CT venography. *AJR Am J Roentgenol* 2000;174:67–69.

78. Garg K, Kemp JL, Wojcik D, et al. Thromboembolic disease: comparison of combined CT pulmonary angiography and venography with bilateral leg sonography in 70 patients. *AJR Am J Roentgenol* 2000;175:997–1001.

79. Loud PA, Grossman ZD, Klippenstein DL, et al. Combined CT venography and pulmonary angiography: a new diagnostic technique for suspected thromboembolic disease. *AJR Am J Roentgenol* 1998;170:951–954.

80. Goldhaber SZ, Visani L, De Rosa M. Acute pulmonary embolism: clinical outcomes in the International Cooperative Pulmonary Embolism Registry (ICOPER). *Lancet* 1999;353:1386–1389.

81. Steiner P, Lund GK, Debatin JF, et al. Acute pulmonary embolism: value of transthoracic and transesophageal echocardiography in comparison with helical CT. *AJR Am J Roentgenol* 1996;167:931–936.

82. Pruszczyk P, Torbicki A, Pacho R, et al. Noninvasive diagnosis of suspected severe pulmonary embolism: transesophageal echocardiography vs. spiral CT. *Chest* 1997;112:722–728.

83. Goldhaber SZ. Echocardiography in the management of pulmonary embolism. *Ann Intern Med* 2002;136:691–700.

84. McConnell MV, Solomon SD, Rayan ME, et al. Regional right ventricular dysfunction detected by echocardiography in acute pulmonary embolism. *Am J Cardiol* 1996;78:469–473.

85. Kanne JP, Lalani TA. Role of computed tomography and magnetic resonance imaging for deep venous thrombosis and pulmonary embolism. *Circulation* 2004;109:I15–I21.

86. Stein PD, Woodard PK, Hull RD, et al. Gadolinium-enhanced magnetic resonance angiography for detection of acute pulmonary embolism: an in-depth review. *Chest* 2003;124:2324–2328.

87. Haage P, Piroth W, Krombach G, et al. Pulmonary embolism: comparison of angiography with spiral computed tomography, magnetic resonance angiography, and real-time magnetic resonance imaging. *Am J Respir Crit Care Med* 2003;167:729–734.

88. Oudkerk M, van Beek EJ, Wielopolski P, et al. Comparison of contrast-enhanced magnetic resonance angiography and conventional pulmonary angiography for the diagnosis of pulmonary embolism: a prospective study. *Lancet* 2002;359:1643–1647.

89. Meaney JF, Weg JG, Chenevert TL, et al. Diagnosis of pulmonary embolism with magnetic resonance angiography. *N Engl J Med* 1997;336:1422–1427.

90. Wicki J, Perrier A, Perneger TV, et al. Predicting adverse outcome in patients with acute pulmonary embolism: a risk score. *Thromb Haemost* 2000;84:548–552.

91. Grifoni S, Olivotto I, Cecchini P, et al. Short-term clinical outcome of patients with acute pulmonary embolism, normal blood pressure, and echocardiographic right ventricular dysfunction. *Circulation* 2000;101:2817–2822.

92. Kasper W, Konstantinides S, Geibel A, et al. Prognostic significance of right ventricular afterload stress detected by echocardiography in patients with clinically suspected pulmonary embolism. *Heart* 1997;77:346–349.

93. Douketis JD, Crowther MA, Stanton EB, et al. Elevated cardiac troponin levels in patients with submassive pulmonary embolism. *Arch Intern Med* 2002;162:79–81.

94. Janata K, Holzer M, Laggner AN, et al. Cardiac troponin T in the severity assessment of patients with pulmonary embolism: cohort study. *BMJ* 2003;326:312–313.

95. Pruszczyk P, Bochowicz A, Torbicki A, et al. Cardiac troponin T monitoring identifies high-risk group of normotensive patients with acute pulmonary embolism. *Chest* 2003;123:1947–1952.

96. Kruger S, Graf J, Merx MW, et al. Brain natriuretic peptide predicts right heart failure in patients with acute pulmonary embolism. *Am Heart J* 2004;147:60–65.

97. Kucher N, Printzen G, Goldhaber SZ. Prognostic role of brain natriuretic peptide in acute pulmonary embolism. *Circulation* 2003;107:2545–2547.

98. ten Wolde M, Tulevski II, Mulder JW, et al. Brain natriuretic peptide as a predictor of adverse outcome in patients with pulmonary embolism. *Circulation* 2003;107:2082–2084.

99. Pruszczyk P, Kostrubiec M, Bochowicz A, et al. N-terminal pro-brain natriuretic peptide in patients with acute pulmonary embolism. *Eur Respir J* 2003;22:649–653.

100. Nendaz MR, Bandelier P, Aujesky D, et al. Validation of a risk score identifying patients with acute pulmonary embolism who are at low risk of clinical adverse outcome. *Thromb Haemost* 2004;91:1232–1236.

101. Alpert JS, Thygesen K, Antman E, et al. Myocardial infarction redefined—a consensus document of The Joint European Society of Cardiology/American College of Cardiology Committee for the redefinition of myocardial infarction. *J Am Coll Cardiol* 2000;36:959–969.

102. Ammann P, Maggiorini M, Bertel O, et al. Troponin as a risk factor for mortality in critically ill patients without acute coronary syndromes. *J Am Coll Cardiol* 2003;41:2004–2009.

103. Meyer T, Binder L, Hruska N, et al. Cardiac troponin I elevation in acute pulmonary embolism is associated with right ventricular dysfunction [in process citation]. *J Am Coll Cardiol* 2000;36:1632–1636.

104. Kucher N, Goldhaber SZ. Cardiac biomarkers for risk stratification of patients with acute pulmonary embolism. *Circulation* 2003;108:2191–2194.

105. Buller HR, Lensing AW, Hirsh J, et al. Deep vein thrombosis: new noninvasive diagnostic tests. *Thromb Haemost* 1991;66:133–137.

106. Tick LW, Ton E, van Voorthuizen T, et al. Practical diagnostic management of patients with clinically suspected deep vein thrombosis by clinical probability test, compression ultrasonography, and D-dimer test. *Am J Med* 2002;113:630–635.

107. Wells PS, Anderson DR, Rodger M, et al. Evaluation of D-dimer in the diagnosis of suspected deep-vein thrombosis. *N Engl J Med* 2003;349:1227–1235.

108. Perone N, Bounameaux H, Perrier A. Comparison of four strategies for diagnosing deep vein thrombosis: a cost-effectiveness analysis. *Am J Med* 2001;110:33–40.

109. British Thoracic Society Standards of Care Committee Pulmonary Embolism Guideline Development Group. British Thoracic Society guidelines for the management of suspected acute pulmonary embolism. *Thorax* 2003;58:470–483.

110. Perrier A, Nendaz MR, Sarasin FP, et al. Cost-effectiveness of diagnostic strategies for suspected pulmonary embolism including helical computed tomography. *Am J Respir Crit Care Med* 2003;167:39–44.

111. Perrier A, Roy PM, Sanchez O, et al. Multidetector-row computed tomography in suspected pulmonary embolism. *N Engl J Med* 2005;352:1760–1768.

112. Carson JL, Kelley MA, Duff A, et al. The clinical course of pulmonary embolism. *N Engl J Med* 1992;326:1240–1245.

113. Kipper MS, Moser KM, Kortman KE, et al. Longterm follow-up of patients with suspected pulmonary embolism and a normal lung scan. *Chest* 1982;82:411–415.

114. Hull RD, Raskob GE, Ginsberg JS, et al. A noninvasive strategy for the treatment of patients with suspected pulmonary embolism. *Arch Intern Med* 1994;154:289–297.

115. de Moerloose P, Desmarais S, Bounameaux H, et al. Contribution of a new, rapid, individual and quantitative automated D-dimer ELISA to exclude pulmonary embolism. *Thromb Haemost* 1996;75:11–13.

116. Oger E, Leroyer C, Bressollette L, et al. Evaluation of a new, rapid, and quantitative D-Dimer test in patients with suspected pulmonary embolism. *Am J Respir Crit Care Med* 1998;158:65–70.

117. Bates SM, Grand'Maison A, Johnston M, et al. A latex D-dimer reliably excludes venous thromboembolism. *Arch Intern Med* 2001;161:447–453.

118. Turkstra F, Kuijer PMM, van Beek EJR, et al. Diagnostic utility of ultrasonography of leg veins in patients suspected of having pulmonary embolism. *Ann Intern Med* 1997;126:775–781.

119. Perrier A, Bounameaux H. Ultrasonography of leg veins in patients suspected of having pulmonary embolism. *Ann Intern Med* 1998;128:243.

120. Perrier A, Tamm C, Unger PF, et al. Diagnostic accuracy of doppler-echocardiography in unselected patients with suspected pulmonary embolism. *Int J Cardiol* 1998;65:101–109.

121. Jackson RE, Rudoni RR, Hauser AM, et al. Prospective evaluation of two-dimensional transthoracic echocardiography in emergency department patients with suspected pulmonary embolism [in process citation]. *Acad Emerg Med* 2000;7:994–998.

122. Nazeyrollas P, Metz D, Chapoutot L, et al. Diagnostic accuracy of echocardiography-Doppler in acute pulmonary embolism. *Int J Cardiol* 1995;47:273–280.

123. Miniati M, Monti S, Pratali L, et al. Value of transthoracic echocardiography in the diagnosis of pulmonary embolism: results of a prospective study in unselected patients. *Am J Med* 2001;110:528–535.

124. van Beek EJR, Kuyer PMM, Schenk BS, et al. A normal perfusion lung scan in patients with clinically suspected pulmonary embolism. Frequency and clinical validity. *Chest* 1995;108:170–173.

125. Kruip MJ, Slob MJ, Schijen JH, et al. Use of a clinical decision rule in combination with D-dimer concentration in diagnostic workup of patients with suspected pulmonary embolism: a prospective management study. *Arch Intern Med* 2002;162:1631–1635.

126. Konstantinides S, Geibel A, Heusel G, et al. Heparin plus alteplase compared with heparin alone in patients with submassive pulmonary embolism. *N Engl J Med* 2002;347:1143–1150.

127. Stein PD, Athanasoulis C, Alavi A, et al. Complications and validity of pulmonary angiography in acute pulmonary embolism. *Circulation* 1992;85:462–468.

128. Meyer G, Gisselbrecht M, Diehl JL, et al. Incidence and predictors of major hemorrhagic complications from thrombolytic therapy in patients with massive pulmonary embolism. *Am J Med* 1998;105:472–477.

129. Galle C, Papazyan JP, Miron MJ, et al. Prediction of pulmonary embolism extent by clinical findings, D-dimer level and deep vein thrombosis shown by ultrasound. *Thromb Haemost* 2001;86:1156–1160.

130. Huisman MV, Buller HR, ten Cate JW. Utility of impedance plethysmography in the diagnosis of recurrent deep-vein thrombosis. *Arch Intern Med* 1988;148:681–683.

131. Prandoni P, Cogo A, Bernardi E, et al. A simple ultrasound approach for detection of recurrent proximal-vein thrombosis. *Circulation* 1993;88:1730–1735.

132. Prandoni P, Lensing AW, Bernardi E, et al. The diagnostic value of compression ultrasonography in patients with suspected recurrent deep vein thrombosis. *Thromb Haemost* 2002;88:402–406.

133. Chabloz P, Reber G, Boehlen F, et al. TAFI antigen and D-dimer levels during normal pregnancy and at delivery. *Br J Haematol* 2001;115:150–152.

134. Fraser DG, Moody AR, Morgan PS, et al. Diagnosis of lower-limb deep venous thrombosis: a prospective blinded study of magnetic resonance direct thrombus imaging. *Ann Intern Med* 2002;136:89–98.

135. Winer-Muram HT, Boone JM, Brown HL, et al. Pulmonary embolism in pregnant patients: fetal radiation dose with helical CT. *Radiology* 2002;224:487–492.

136. Chan WS, Ray JG, Murray S, et al. Suspected pulmonary embolism in pregnancy; clinical presentation, results of lung scanning, and subsequent maternal and pediatric outcomes. *Arch Intern Med* 2002;162:1170–1175.

137. Ginsberg JS, Hirsh J, Turner DC, et al. Risks to the fetus of anticoagulant therapy during pregnancy. *Thromb Haemost* 1989;61:p197–p203.

138. Ginsberg JS, Hirsh J, Rainbow AJ, et al. Risks to the fetus of radiologic procedures used in the diagnosis of maternal venous thromboembolic disease. *Thromb Haemost* 1989;61:189–196.

139. Fleming TR, DeMets DL. Surrogate end points in clinical trials: are we being misled? *Ann Intern Med* 1996;125:605–613.

140. Sarasin FP, Bounameaux H. Antithrombotic strategy after total hip replacement. A cost-effectiveness analysis comparing prolonged oral anticoagulants with screening for deep vein thrombosis. *Arch Intern Med* 1996;156:1661–1668.

# CHAPTER 88 ■ RISK STRATIFICATION IN PATIENTS WITH PULMONARY EMBOLISM

NILS KUCHER AND SAMUEL Z. GOLDHABER

Acute pulmonary embolism (PE) spans a wide spectrum of acuity, with varying early and long-term clinical outcomes. Therefore, risk stratification is paramount in selecting the appropriate management strategy.

Overall mortality in patients with PE is higher than that in patients with acute myocardial infarction, exceeding 10% at 30 days and 16% at 3 months (1,2). Within 30 days, the most common cause of death is right ventricular failure, and most deaths beyond 30 days are attributed to underlying chronic disease, including cancer, congestive heart failure, or chronic lung disease (3).

With therapeutic levels of anticoagulation, most patients will likely have an uneventful clinical course. Some patients, however, suffer rapid clinical deterioration, including death from right ventricular failure or from the need for cardiopulmonary resuscitation, mechanical ventilation, administration of pressors for systolic arterial hypotension, rescue thrombolysis, or surgical embolectomy.

Contemporary PE risk stratification tools are (a) the clinical evaluation, (b) cardiac biomarkers, (c) 12-lead electrocardiography, (d) echocardiography, and (e) chest computed tomography (CT).

## THE CLASSICAL APPROACH

The classical approach to assess risk in a patient with PE has relied primarily on systemic arterial pressure. Patients with systolic blood pressure less than 90 mm Hg were started on catecholamines or vasopressors. If this technique failed to raise the systolic blood pressure more than 90 mm Hg or if clinical signs of cardiogenic shock worsened, thrombolysis or open surgical embolectomy was considered. This strategy may potentially delay implementation of aggressive therapy. Consequently, patients had often passed the point of "no return," with irreversible cardiogenic shock and multisystem organ failure.

Contemporary risk stratification focuses on early detection of those patients who are at increased risk for adverse clinical events while the systemic arterial pressure is preserved, prior to the development of cardiogenic shock (1).

## CLINICAL EVALUATION

Profound dyspnea, cyanosis, and syncope usually indicate hemodynamically significant PE. The clinical examination often shows signs of acute right ventricular dysfunction, including tachycardia, a low arterial blood pressure, distended neck veins, an accentuated pulmonic component of the second heart sound, or a tricuspid regurgitation murmur. Conversely, pleuritic chest pain usually indicates anatomically smaller PE, often accompanied by subsegmental pulmonary infarction.

Comorbidities increase the risk of adverse clinical events, even in the presence of anatomically small PE. In the International Cooperative Pulmonary Embolism registry (ICOPER) (2), advanced age, congestive heart failure, cancer, or chronic lung disease were identified as independent predictors of a 3-month mortality, with an approximately twofold increase in the risk of death.

The Geneva Prognostic Index is a clinical risk assessment tool based mainly on the findings from the past medical history and the clinical examinations (4) (see Table 88-1). This index was used to identify low-risk patients who were managed successfully as outpatients. Risk stratification was performed using a clinical score with a maximum of 8 points. The score had to be less than or equal to 2 to qualify for treatment as outpatients. During a 3-month follow-up, none of the 43 patients died, and there was no major bleeding. One of the 43 outpatients had an objectively confirmed deep venous thrombosis (DVT) during follow-up. In conclusion, this study showed that carefully selected patients with PE at low risk for right ventricular failure and recurrent venous thromboembolism (VTE) can be treated safely only as outpatients.

## ELECTROCARDIOGRAPHY

The 12-lead electrocardiogram (ECG) helps exclude acute ST elevation myocardial infarction (5). In 1935, McGinn and White described the well-known $S_1 Q_3 T_3$ type as a common finding among patients with acute PE (6). Unfortunately, approximately 25% of the patients with acute PE have a normal ECG without signs of right ventricular strain (7–14). Although the ECG is neither sensitive nor specific for the diagnosis of PE (15), signs of right ventricular strain (see Table 88-2) can help raise the suspicion for PE.

The ECG also helps identify patients with PE who are at increased risk for developing adverse clinical outcomes. T wave inversion in the anterior precordial leads $V_2$ and $V_3$ and the pseudoinfarction pattern, Qr in $V_1$ (see Fig. 88-1), usually indicate right ventricular dilation and dysfunction (11,16). Right ventricular strain on the ECG was shown to correlate with the extent of lung scan abnormalities and with hemodynamic measurements obtained from right heart catheterization (17). Patients with right ventricular strain often present with elevated cardiac biomarker levels, including cardiac troponins and natriuretic peptides, suggesting that ECG signs correlate with the extent of right ventricular dilation and dysfunction (16). Furthermore, both T-wave inversions and the pseudoinfarction pattern in the precordial leads were found to predict adverse clinical outcomes, including death, cardiopulmonary resuscitation, mechanical ventilation, and the administration of pressors or thrombolysis (16). The pseudoinfarction pattern is occasionally seen in the right-sided precordial leads $V_{R1}$–$V_{R4}$ (18).

1299

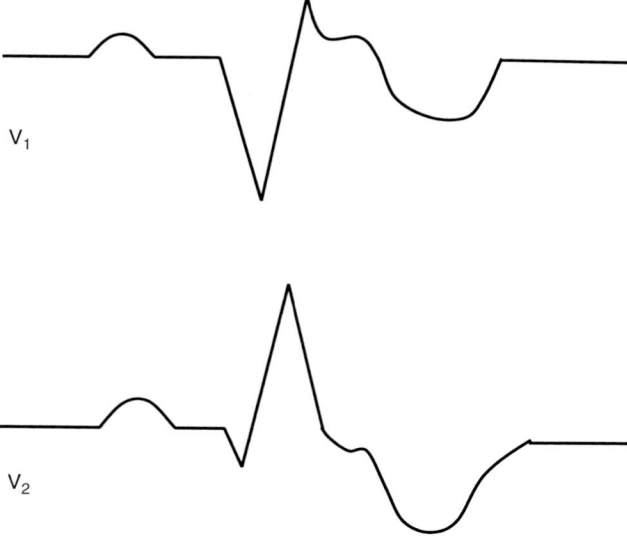

**FIGURE 88-1.** From the electrocardiographic sign of right ventricular strain, the pseudoinfarction pattern, Qr in $V_1$ (**upper panel**), and T-wave inversion in $V_2$ or $V_3$ (**lower panel**) correlate with right ventricular dysfunction and predict adverse clinical outcomes in acute pulmonary embolism (PE).

# ECHOCARDIOGRAPHY

Transthoracic echocardiography cannot be recommended to diagnose PE in hemodynamically stable patients because it is normal in approximately 50% of the patients with suspected acute PE (19–21). Echocardiography aims to confirm or exclude right ventricular dysfunction. Occasionally, centrally located emboli may be seen with the transthoracic approach. The transesophageal approach may be used to diagnose emboli in the main pulmonary artery, the right and left main pulmonary artery, but not in lobar and segmental branches (22). Bedside echocardiography is helpful in patients with suspected acute PE and hemodynamic instability because potentially life-saving measures, including thrombolysis or surgical embolectomy, can be initiated without necessarily obtaining time-consuming imaging tests to confirm the diagnosis (see Fig. 88-2) (23). Echocardiography also helps diagnose conditions that mimic acute PE but which are treated very differently, such as acute myocardial infarction, aortic dissection, or pericardial tamponade.

Transthoracic echocardiography is an important tool for risk stratification because right ventricular dysfunction on the echocardiogram is a powerful and independent predictor of mortality (21,24). From a prognostic point of view, echocardiography helps to classify PE into three groups: nonmassive PE (i.e., no right ventricular dysfunction), submassive PE (i.e., right ventricular dysfunction and a preserved arterial pressure >90 mm Hg), and massive PE (i.e., right ventricular dysfunction and cardiogenic shock or an arterial pressure <90 mm Hg). In 1,112 patients from the ICOPER, right ventricular hypokinesis on the echocardiogram predicted a 3-month mortality in all three PE categories, with early separation of the Kaplan–Meier survival curves (Fig. 88-3). Three-month survival rates were 87.7% (95% CI, 84.8% to 90.0%) for nonmassive

PE, 84.5% (95% CI, 80.6% to 88.2%) for submassive PE, and 66.4% (95% CI, 56.2% to 74.7%) for massive PE.

Right ventricular dysfunction is diagnosed in the presence of: (a) right ventricular dilatation, defined as a right ventricular to left ventricular end-diastolic dimension ratio greater than 0.6 in the parasternal long-axis view or a ratio greater than 0.9 in the four-chamber view, (b) right ventricular systolic free wall hypokinesis, or (c) systolic pulmonary arterial hypertension, defined as a tricuspid regurgitant velocity greater than 2.6 m per second (see Table 88-3) (19). Indirect signs of right ventricular pressure overload are a flattened interventricular septum, paradoxical systolic motion of the interventricular septum toward the left ventricle, or a dilated inferior vena cava with reduced respiratory variability.

Echocardiography in the setting of acute PE is also useful to diagnose a patent foramen ovale or an atrial septal defect. A patent foramen ovale identifies patients at risk for paradoxical embolism and stroke. In one study of patients with acute PE (26), the presence of a patent foramen ovale was as strong a

**TABLE 88-2**

### ELECTROCARDIOGRAPHIC RISK ASSESSMENT IN ACUTE PULMONARY EMBOLISM

Sinus tachycardia >100 bpm
Complete or incomplete right bundle branch block
$S_1$ $Q_3$ $T_3$
T wave inversion in $V_2$, $V_3$
ST segment depression
Qr in $V_1$ (pseudoinfarction pattern)
ST segment elevation, especially in $V_1$
Shift of QRS transition to $V_5$
Low limb lead voltage

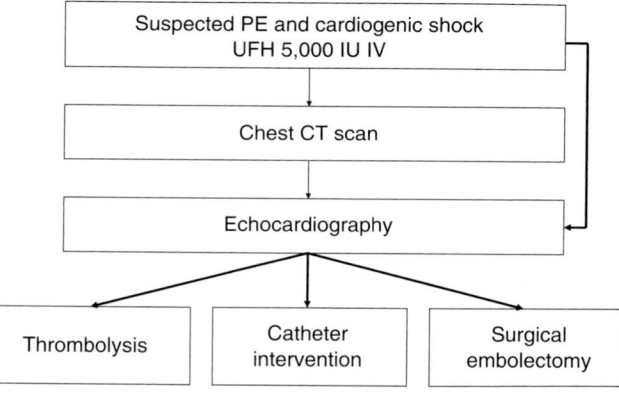

**FIGURE 88-2.** In patients with suspected massive pulmonary embolism (PE) and cardiogenic shock, the decision to obtain a chest computed tomogram (CT) or ventilation perfusion scan may delay the initiation of reperfusion therapy. In the presence of severe right ventricular dysfunction on the bedside echocardiogram, reperfusion therapy may be initiated without delay (see text). UFH, unfractionated heparin.

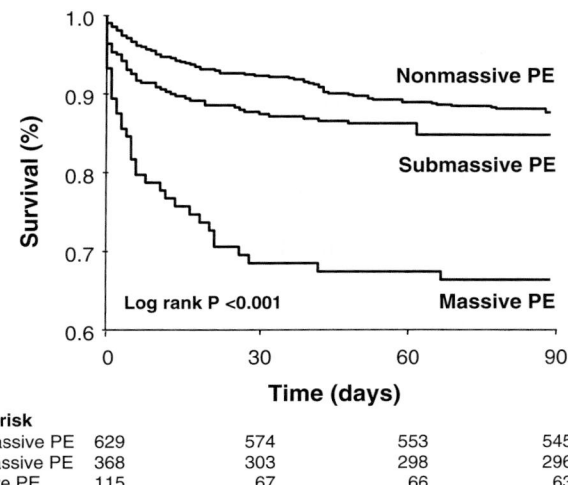

No. at risk

| | | | | |
|---|---|---|---|---|
| Nonmassive PE | 629 | 574 | 553 | 545 |
| Submassive PE | 368 | 303 | 298 | 296 |
| Massive PE | 115 | 67 | 66 | 63 |

FIGURE 88-3. Kaplan–Meier survival curves in 629 patients with nonmassive pulmonary embolism (PE), 368 patients with submassive PE, and 115 patients with massive PE from the International Cooperative Pulmonary Embolism registry (ICOPER).

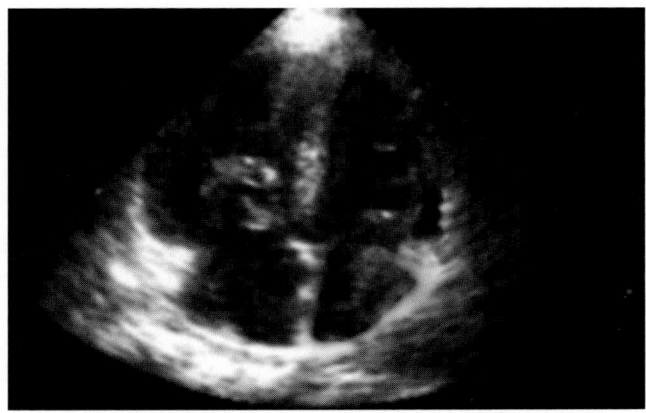

FIGURE 88-4. Apical four-chamber view from a patient with massive pulmonary embolism (PE) obtained from a bedside echocardiogram. Note the presence of right ventricular dilation, with a right-to-left ventricular diameter ratio >0.9 and the presence of a free-floating right ventricular thrombus.

predictor of mortality as arterial hypotension. In patients with recurrent PE and paradoxical embolism, percutaneous closure of the patent foramen ovale and placement of an inferior vena cava filter prevented recurrent thromboembolic events (27). Further studies are required to investigate the long-term efficacy and safety of this approach.

In patients with acute PE, free-floating right heart thrombi (see Fig. 88-4) increases the risk for adverse clinical events (24). In ICOPER, the overall mortality rate at 14 days (21% vs. 11%) and at 3 months (29% vs. 16%) was higher in patients with right heart thrombi than patients without it. The increase in early mortality was observed almost entirely within the subgroup of patients treated with heparin alone (23.5% vs. 8%), despite similar clinical severity at presentation.

Echocardiographic findings at the time of PE diagnosis also confer predictive information about the risk of developing chronic thromboembolic pulmonary hypertension. An estimated systolic pulmonary artery pressure of greater than 50 mm Hg at the time of PE diagnosis was associated with persistent pulmonary hypertension at 1 year (28). In a longitudinal study of patients with acute PE, the cumulative incidence of chronic thromboembolic pulmonary hypertension was 3.1% at 1 year (Table 88-4) (29). In this study, prior and idiopathic PE, younger age, or a large perfusion defect increased the risk of developing chronic thromboembolic pulmonary hypertension during the ensuing 2 years. Echocardiographic follow-up performed 6 weeks after the diagnosis can identify patients with persistent pulmonary hypertension and may be of value in planning the long-term care of these patients. Patients with persistent symptoms and chronic thromboembolic hypertension may benefit from surgical thromboendarterectomy with insertion of a vena cava filter (30–32), percutaneous interventional therapy with stent placement (33,34), or long-term vasodilator treatment (35).

## TABLE 88-3

### ECHOCARDIOGRAPHIC RISK ASSESSMENT IN ACUTE PULMONARY EMBOLISM

| Finding | Comment |
|---|---|
| Right ventricular dilation | Right-to-left ventricular diameter ratio >0.6 in parasternal long axis view, or >0.9 in apical four-chamber view |
| Right atrial dilation with bulging of the interatrial septum toward the left atrium | Indirect sign of increased central venous pressure |
| Reduced respiratory variability of dilated inferior vena cava | Subcostal view, diameter >2 cm with <50% respiratory variability; indirect sign of increased central venous pressure |
| Pulmonary artery dilation | Main artery >2.5 cm in parasternal short axis view, indirect sign of pulmonary hypertension |
| Flattening or paradoxical motion of interventricular septum | Indirect sign of pulmonary hypertension |
| Tricuspid regurgitation jet velocity >2.6 m/s | Direct evidence of pulmonary hypertension |
| Right ventricular systolic hypokinesis | Apical or subcostal four-chamber view, qualitative assessment |
| Right ventricular regional systolic wall motion abnormalities (25) | Hypokinesis of the free wall but preserved apical kinesis |
| Right ventricular hypertrophy | End-diastolic free-wall >5 mm, sign of chronic pulmonary hypertension |
| Pulmonary artery thrombi | Rarely seen with transthoracic approach |
| Right ventricular or atrial thrombi | Usually free floating |
| Patent foramen ovale; atrial septal defect | Color duplex or echocontrast study |

TABLE 88-4

CUMULATIVE INCIDENCE OF SYMPTOMATIC CHRONIC THROMBOEMBOLIC PULMONARY HYPERTENSION AFTER AN ACUTE EPISODE OF PULMONARY EMBOLISM

| Follow-up | Incidence (%) | 95% CI |
|---|---|---|
| 6 mo | 1.0 | 0.0–2.4 |
| 1 yr | 3.1 | 0.7–5.5 |
| 2 yr | 3.8 | 1.1–6.5 |

CI, confidence interval.
From Pengo V, Lensing AW, Prins MH, et al. Incidence of chronic thromboembolic pulmonary hypertension after pulmonary embolism. *N Engl J Med* 2004;350:2257–2264, with permission.

A limitation of echocardiography is its restricted availability on a 24-hour basis 365 days per year as well as its cost. Although sophisticated software techniques exist in quantifying right ventricular performance on the echocardiogram (36), right ventricular dysfunction in routine clinical practice is usually assessed on a qualitative basis. The lack of a clear definition for right ventricular dysfunction on the echocardiogram is problematic (37). Another difficulty is occasional poor imaging quality of the right ventricle, particularly in patients with obesity or chronic lung disease. In the latter case, the transoesophageal approach may be used to image the right ventricle.

## CARDIAC BIOMARKERS

Cardiac troponins I and T as well as NT-pro–brain natriuretic peptide (NT-proBNP) and brain natriuretic peptide (BNP) have emerged as promising tools for risk stratification (38).

Cardiac troponins are sensitive and specific markers of myocardial injury (39,40). Elevations of troponin levels in patients with PE are brief and subtle compared to patients with acute coronary syndrome (41). In acute PE, troponin levels correlate with the extent of right ventricular dysfunction (42–46). At the time of diagnosis, a few patients with PE have negative troponin test results, but the values may show an increase several hours later. Myocardial ischemia due to alterations in oxygen supply and demand of the failing right ventricle plays a major role in the pathogenesis of troponin level elevation (see Fig. 88-5) (47). Increased troponin levels in patients with acute PE were reported in the absence of angiographic coronary artery disease (46,48). In autopsy studies, acute transmural right ventricular myocardial infarction following massive PE has been reported in the absence of coronary artery disease

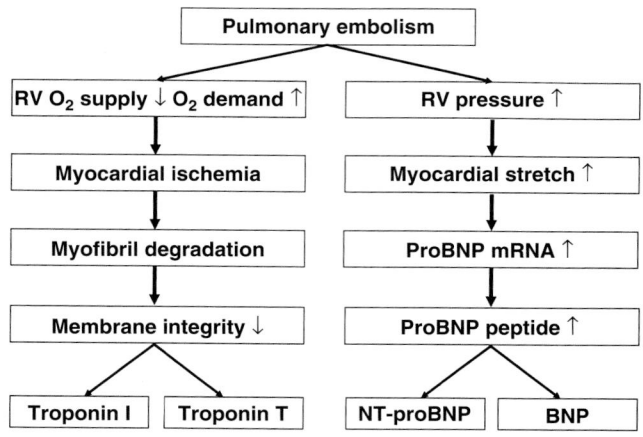

FIGURE 88-5. Mechanism of cardiac biomarker release from cardiac myocytes in acute pulmonary embolism (PE) (see text). O$_2$, oxygen; RV, right ventricular; NT-proBNP, NT-pro–brain natriuretic peptide; mRNA, messenger ribonucleic acid.

(49–52). In some patients with massive PE, a transient elevation of creatine kinase (CK) or of the CK-MB isoenzyme fraction because of right ventricular infarction was observed (50). Elevated serum myoglobin levels may be detectable in some patients with PE before release of cardiac troponin (53,54).

The natriuretic peptides are useful diagnostic and prognostic markers for patients with congestive heart failure (55–60). The stimulus for BNP synthesis and secretion is cardiomyocyte stretch (Fig. 88-5) (61). The intact 108–amino acid prohormone (proBNP), the biologically active BNP (32 amino acids, plasma half-life 20 minutes), and the amino-terminal part of the prohormone NT-proBNP (76 amino acids, plasma half-life 60 to 120 minutes) can be measured with commercially available assays. Prohormone in normal ventricular myocytes is not stored to a considerable amount. Therefore, it takes a few hours for the plasma natriuretic peptides levels to increase after the onset of acute cardiomyocyte stretch (61). This increase in peptide levels involves myocardial BNP messenger ribonucleic acid (mRNA) synthesis, prohormone synthesis, and plasma release. Elevations in BNP and NT-proBNP levels are associated with right ventricular dysfunction in acute PE (38,62–67).

Natriuretic peptide levels are also increased in patients with primary pulmonary hypertension, chronic thromboembolic pulmonary hypertension, and chronic lung disease (64,68–70).

Troponins and natriuretic peptides are similarly accurate in identifying patients who are at low risk for developing PE. The negative predictive value (NPV) for in-hospital death exceeds 97% for the biomarker assays (see Table 88-5). The cutoff levels

TABLE 88-5

CARDIAC BIOMARKERS AND IN-HOSPITAL MORTALITY IN PATIENTS WITH PULMONARY EMBOLISM

| Biomarker | Assay | Cutoff level | NPV % | PPV % |
|---|---|---|---|---|
| cTnI | Centaur, Bayer (42) | 0.07 ng/mL | 98 | 14 |
| CTnT | Elecsys, Roche (42) | 0.04 ng/mL | 97 | 12 |
| CTnT | TropT, Roche (46) | 0.10 ng/mL | 97 | 44 |
| CTnT | Elecsys, Roche (44) | 0.09 ng/mL | 99 | 34 |
| CTnT | Elecsys, Roche (45) | 0.01 ng/mL | 100 | 25 |
| BNP | Shionoria, CIS (66) | 21.7 pmol/L | 99 | 17 |
| BNP | Triage, Biosite (63) | 50 pg/mL | 100 | 12 |
| NT-proBNP | Elecsys, Roche (62) | 500 pg/mL | 100 | 12 |

NPV, negative predictive value; PPV, positive predictive value.

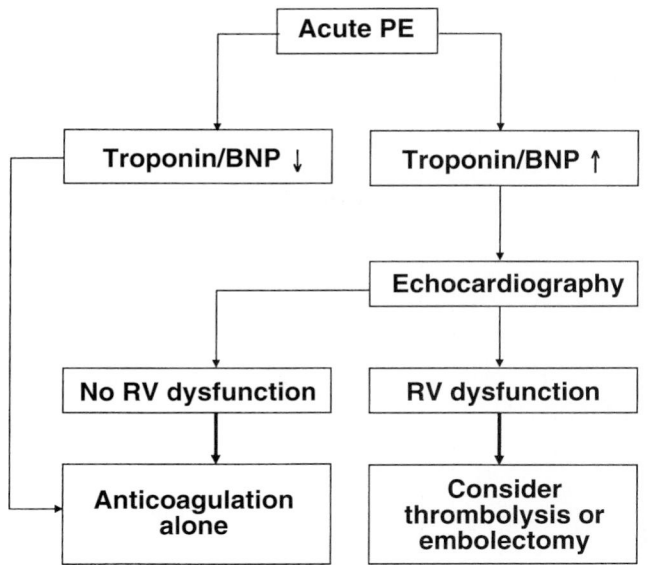

FIGURE 88-6. Suggested strategy for risk stratifying patients with acute pulmonary embolism (PE) (see text). BNP, brain natriuretic peptide; RV, right ventricular.

for cardiac troponins usually are the lower detection limits reported by the manufacturer. The cutoff level for the BNP Triage assay for predicting an uneventful clinical course in patients with PE is lower (<50 pg per mL) than the "congestive heart failure" cutoff level (90 pg per mL).

Considering that BNP synthesis and plasma release is an active neurohormonal process requiring several hours after the onset of myocardial stretch, an initially negative BNP test result in a symptomatic patient with PE with a short duration of symptoms should be interpreted with caution.

In patients with PE with increased cardiac biomarker levels, further risk stratification with echocardiography is warranted because of limited specificity of the assays for predicting right ventricular dysfunction (see Fig. 88-6). In patients with biomarker levels below the assay-specific cutoff limit, echocardiography will likely not add prognostic information.

# CONTRAST-ENHANCED MULTIDETECTOR ROW COMPUTED TOMOGRAPHY

Contrast-enhanced chest CT scan is increasingly utilized as the first-line PE imaging test and is available around the clock at most institutions (71–76). With newer generation scanners, standardized cardiac views are easily obtained in almost all patients who undergo contrast-enhanced chest CT scan (72). Most contemporary CT scanners allow online two-dimensional reconstruction of standardized cardiac views, with direct measurement of ventricular dimensions. The cardiac four-chamber view is obtained by (a) craniocaudal rotation of the viewport in the coronal CT view and (b) tilting the viewport in the axial CT view until both ventricles are fully depicted (Fig. 88-7). In the reconstructed 4-CH view, right ventricular dimensions ($RV_D$) and left ventricular dimensions ($LV_D$) are then measured by identifying the maximal distance between the ventricular endocardium and the interventricular septum, perpendicular to the long axis of the heart. Right ventricular enlargement is defined as $RV_D/LV_D$ value greater than 0.9.

In 63 patients with acute PE, the presence of right ventricular enlargement on the reconstructed four-chamber view by CT scan correlated with the determination of the presence of right ventricular dysfunction on echocardiogram (77). In another study of 25 patients with acute PE, CT scan signs of right ventricular pressure overload were closely correlated with echocardiographic signs of right ventricular dysfunction

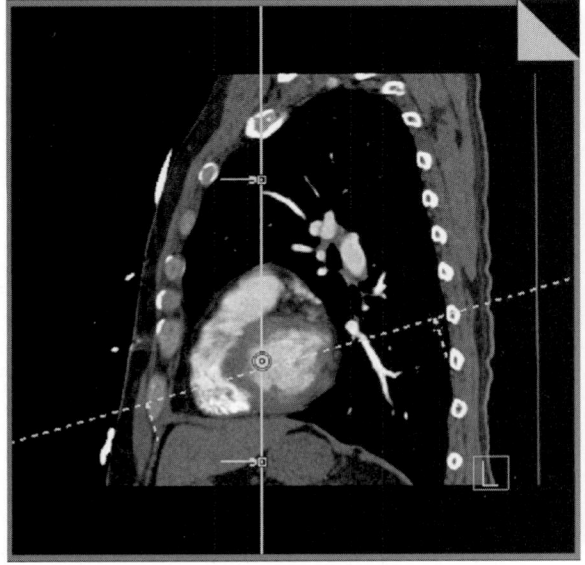

**A**

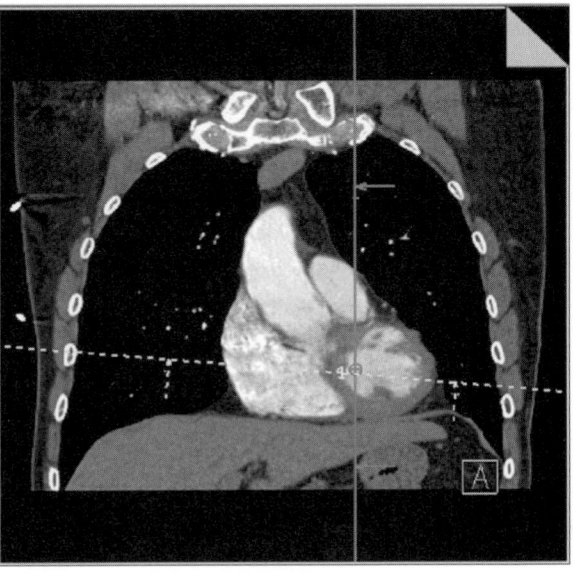

**B**

FIGURE 88-7. Multiplanar reconstruction of the four-chamber (4-CH) view of the computerized tomography (CT) scan with measurement of right and left ventricular dimensions. In the sagittal view (**A**), the viewport (*dashed line*) is rotated counterclockwise to obtain a craniocaudal axis. After tilting the viewport (*dashed line*) slightly clockwise in the coronal view (**B**), the 4-CH view (**C**) is obtained. Measurement of right and left ventricular dimensions in the reconstructed 4-CH view is shown in (**D**) (see text).

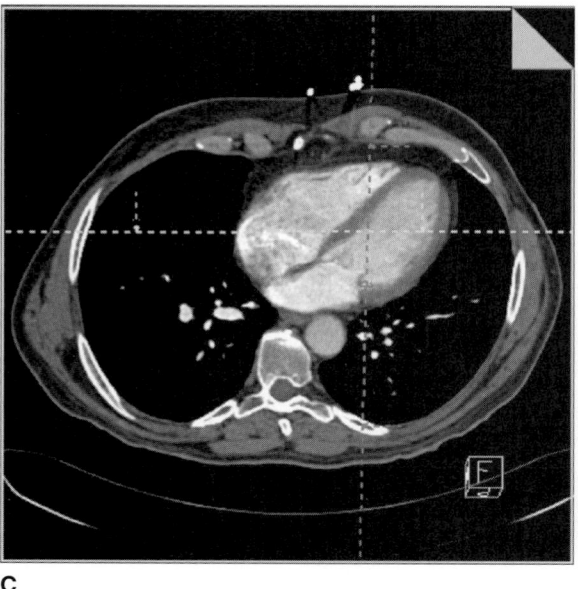

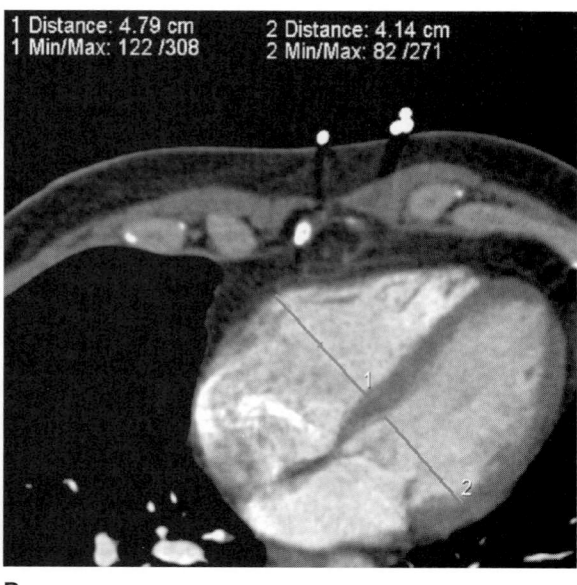

**FIGURE 88-7.** Continued.

(78). In 79 patients with PE, CT scan signs of right ventricular dysfunction correlated with clinical severity (79).

Right ventricular enlargement on chest CT scan helps identify patients at risk of death from right ventricular failure. In a study of 431 consecutive patients with acute PE, right ventricular enlargement on the reconstructed four-chamber view of the CT scan was an independent predictor of 30-day mortality (hazard ratio, 5.2; 95% CI; 1.6 to 16.4) after adjustment for important patient characteristics (80). Among patients who died within 30 days, 43 (78.2%) had RV enlargement (see Fig. 88-8). Prospective management studies are needed to investigate whether cardiac measurements on reconstructed CT scan 4-CH views should guide treatment decisions in patients with acute PE.

# FUTURE RESEARCH PERSPECTIVES

According to the European Task Force Guidelines on Pulmonary Embolism (81), risk stratification in patients with PE is mandatory and is of paramount importance for selecting the appropriate therapy. However, the role of reperfusion therapy, including thrombolysis, catheter interventions, or surgical embolectomy is not well defined, particularly for patients with submassive PE.

Future research activities are warranted for identifying patients with PE who may benefit from early aggressive intervention. Patients with submassive PE who present with elevated cardiac biomarker levels and right ventricular dysfunction may have a survival benefit with early initiation of reperfusion therapy or embolectomy. However, this hypothesis has to be confirmed or rejected by conducting large randomized controlled trials.

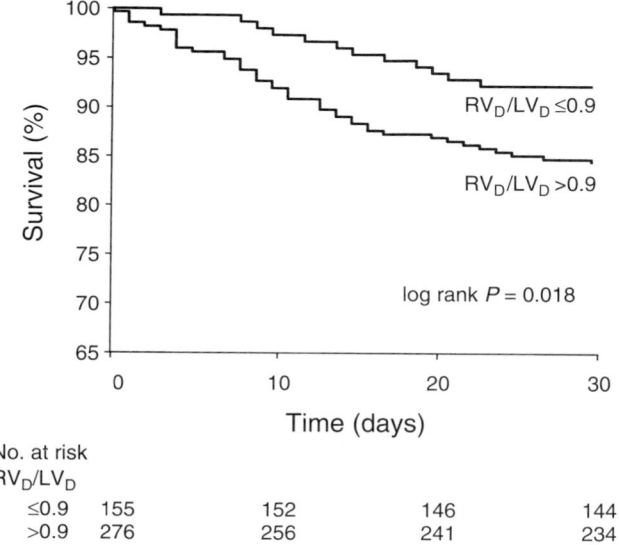

**FIGURE 88-8.** Kaplan-Meier survival curves in 155 patients with and 276 patients without right ventricular enlargement on reconstructed four-chamber views of a computerized tomography (CT) scan. $RV_D/LV_D$, right-to-left ventricular dimension ratio.

## References

1. Goldhaber SZ, Elliott CG. Acute pulmonary embolism: part II: risk stratification, treatment, and prevention. *Circulation* 2003;108:2834–2838.
2. Goldhaber SZ, Visani L, De Rosa M. Acute pulmonary embolism: clinical outcomes in the international cooperative pulmonary embolism registry (ICOPER). *Lancet* 1999;353:1386–1389.
3. Goldhaber SZ. Pulmonary embolism. *Lancet* 2004;363:1295–1305.
4. Wicki J, Perrier A, Perneger TV, et al. Predicting adverse outcome in patients with acute pulmonary embolism: a risk score. *Thromb Haemost* 2000;84:548–552.
5. Ullman E, Brady WJ, Perron AD, et al. Electrocardiographic manifestations of pulmonary embolism. *Am J Emerg Med* 2001;19:514–519.
6. Mc Ginn S, White PD. Acute cor pulmonale resulting from pulmonary embolism. Its clinical recognition. *JAMA* 1935;104:1473–1480.
7. Moccia JM. Using the ECG to identify pulmonary embolism. *Dimens Crit Care Nurs* 2000;19:27–31.
8. Punukollu G, Gowda RM, Khan IA, et al. QT interval prolongation with global T-wave inversion: a novel ECG finding in acute pulmonary embolism. *Ann Noninvasive Electrocardiol* 2004;9:94–98.
9. Petruzzelli S, Palla A, Giuntini C. Limitations of ECG in diagnosing pulmonary embolism. *Chest* 1998;113:559.
10. Daniel KR, Courtney DM, Kline JA. Assessment of cardiac stress from massive pulmonary embolism with 12-lead ECG. *Chest* 2001;120: 474–481.

11. Ferrari E, Imbert A, Chevalier T, et al. The ECG in pulmonary embolism. Predictive value of negative T waves in precordial leads–80 case reports. *Chest* 1997;111:537–543.

12. Chung DK, Chung EK. ECG findings in pulmonary embolism. *W V Med J* 1972;68:71–72.

13. Dune H, Pernow B, Rigner KG. The ECG pattern in pulmonary embolism. *Acta Med Scand* 1960;168:397–404.

14. Mazuch J, Kukura A, Pavlik V, et al. Effect of massive embolism of the pulmonary artery on haemodynamics and respiration, capnography, ECG, acid-base balance and blood clotting in dogs. *Cas Lek Cesk* 1975;114:651–655.

15. Cutforth RH, Oram S. The electrocardiogram in pulmonary embolism. *Br Heart J* 1958;20:41–60.

16. Kucher N, Walpoth N, Wustmann K, et al. QR in V1 – an ECG sign associated with right ventricular strain and adverse clinical outcome in pulmonary embolism. *Eur Heart J* 2003;24:1113–1119.

17. Stein PD, Dalen JE, McIntyre KM, et al. The electrocardiogram in acute pulmonary embolism. *Prog Cardiovasc Dis* 1975;17:247–257.

18. Akula R, Hasan SP, Alhassen M, et al. Right-sided EKG in pulmonary embolism. *J Natl Med Assoc* 2003;95:714–717.

19. Goldhaber SZ. Echocardiography in the management of pulmonary embolism. *Ann Intern Med* 2002;136:691–700.

20. Nazeyrollas P, Metz D, Jolly D, et al. Use of transthoracic doppler echocardiography combined with clinical and electrocardiographic data to predict acute pulmonary embolism. *Eur Heart J* 1996;17:779–786.

21. Ribeiro A, Lindmarker P, Juhlin-Dannfelt A, et al. Echocardiography doppler in pulmonary embolism: right ventricular dysfunction as a predictor of mortality rate. *Am Heart J* 1997;134:479–487.

22. Pruszczyk P, Torbicki A, Kuch-Wocial A, et al. Diagnostic value of transoesophageal echocardiography in suspected haemodynamically significant pulmonary embolism. *Heart* 2001;85:628–634.

23. Kucher N, Luder CM, Dornhofer T, et al. Novel management strategy for patients with suspected pulmonary embolism. *Eur Heart J* 2003;24:366–376.

24. Torbicki A, Galie N, Covezzoli A, et al. Right heart thrombi in pulmonary embolism: results from the international cooperative pulmonary embolism registry. *J Am Coll Cardiol* 2003;41:2245–2251.

25. McConnell MV, Solomon SD, Rayan ME, et al. Regional right ventricular dysfunction detected by echocardiography in acute pulmonary embolism. *Am J Cardiol* 1996;78:469–473.

26. Konstantinides S, Geibel A, Kasper W, et al. Patent foramen ovale is an important predictor of adverse outcome in patients with major pulmonary embolism. *Circulation* 1998;97:1946–1951.

27. Donti A, Giardini A, Formigari R, et al. Treatment of recurrent stroke and pulmonary thromboembolism with percutaneous closure of a patent foramen ovale and placement of inferior vena cava filter. *Catheter Cardiovasc Interv* 2003;58:413–415.

28. Ribeiro A, Lindmarker P, Johnsson H, et al. Pulmonary embolism: one-year follow-up with echocardiography doppler and five-year survival analysis. *Circulation* 1999;99:1325–1330.

29. Pengo V, Lensing AW, Prins MH, et al. Incidence of chronic thromboembolic pulmonary hypertension after pulmonary embolism. *N Engl J Med* 2004;350:2257–2264.

30. Fedullo PF, Auger WR, Channick RN, et al. Chronic thromboembolic pulmonary hypertension. *Clin Chest Med* 2001;22:561–581.

31. Fedullo PF, Auger WR, Channick RN, et al. Chronic thromboembolic pulmonary hypertension. *Clin Chest Med* 1995;16:353–374.

32. Jamieson SW, Kapelanski DP, Sakakibara N, et al. Pulmonary endarterectomy: experience and lessons learned in 1,500 cases. *Ann Thorac Surg* 2003;76:1457–1462.

33. Feinstein JA, Goldhaber SZ, Lock JE, et al. Balloon pulmonary angioplasty for treatment of chronic thromboembolic pulmonary hypertension. *Circulation* 2001;103:10–13.

34. Pitton MB, Herber S, Mayer E, et al. Pulmonary balloon angioplasty of chronic thromboembolic pulmonary hypertension (CTEPH) in surgically inaccessible cases. *Rofo Fortschr Geb Rontgenstr Neuen Bildgeb Verfahr* 2003;175:631–634.

35. Bresser P, Fedullo PF, Auger WR, et al. Continuous intravenous epoprostenol for chronic thromboembolic pulmonary hypertension. *Eur Respir J* 2004;23:595–600.

36. Nass N, McConnell MV, Goldhaber SZ, et al. Recovery of regional right ventricular function after thrombolysis for pulmonary embolism. *Am J Cardiol* 1999;83:804–806.

37. ten Wolde M, Sohne M, Quak E, et al. Prognostic value of echocardiographically assessed right ventricular dysfunction in patients with pulmonary embolism. *Arch Intern Med* 2004;164:1685–1689.

38. Kucher N, Goldhaber SZ. Cardiac biomarkers for risk stratification of patients with acute pulmonary embolism. *Circulation* 2003;108:2191–2194.

39. Alpert JS, Thygesen K, Antman E, et al. Myocardial infarction redefined—a consensus document of The Joint European Society of Cardiology/American College of Cardiology Committee for the redefinition of myocardial infarction. *J Am Coll Cardiol* 2000;36:959–969.

40. Wu AH, Feng YJ, Moore R, et al. Characterization of cardiac troponin subunit release into serum after acute myocardial infarction and comparison of assays for troponin T and I. American association for clinical chemistry subcommittee on cTnI standardization. *Clin Chem* 1998;44:1198–1208.

41. Muller-Bardorff M, Weidtmann B, Giannitsis E, et al. Release kinetics of cardiac troponin T in survivors of confirmed severe pulmonary embolism. *Clin Chem* 2002;48:673–675.

42. Konstantinides S, Geibel A, Olschewski M, et al. Importance of cardiac troponins I and T in risk stratification of patients with acute pulmonary embolism. *Circulation* 2002;106:1263–1268.

43. Kucher N, Wallmann D, Carone A, et al. Incremental prognostic value of troponin I and echocardiography in patients with acute pulmonary embolism. *Eur Heart J* 2003;24:1651–1656.

44. Janata K, Holzer M, Laggner AN, et al. Cardiac troponin T in the severity assessment of patients with pulmonary embolism: cohort study. *BMJ* 2003;326:312–313.

45. Pruszczyk P, Bochowicz A, Torbicki A, et al. Cardiac troponin T monitoring identifies high-risk group of normotensive patients with acute pulmonary embolism. *Chest* 2003;123:1947–1952.

46. Giannitsis E, Muller-Bardorff M, Kurowski V, et al. Independent prognostic value of cardiac troponin T in patients with confirmed pulmonary embolism. *Circulation* 2000;102:211–217.

47. Meyer T, Binder L, Hruska N, et al. Cardiac troponin I elevation in acute pulmonary embolism is associated with right ventricular dysfunction. *J Am Coll Cardiol* 2000;36:1632–1636.

48. Ammann P, Maggiorini M, Bertel O, et al. Troponin as a risk factor for mortality in critically ill patients without acute coronary syndromes. *J Am Coll Cardiol* 2003;41:2004–2009.

49. Jerjes Sanchez C, Gutierrez-Fajardo P, Ramirez-Rivera A, et al. Acute infarct of the right ventricle secondary to a massive pulmonary thromboembolism. *Arch Inst Cardiol Mex* 1995;65:65–73.

50. Adams JE, Siegel BA, Goldstein JA, et al. Elevations of CK-MB following pulmonary embolism. A manifestation of occult right ventricular infarction. *Chest* 1992;101:1203–1206.

51. Andrade de la Cal FJ, Aguado Borruey JM, Narvaez Bermcjo JM, et al. Pulmonary embolism and occult right ventricular infarction. *Chest* 1994;105:1617.

52. Coma-Canella I, Gamallo C, Martinez Onsurbe P, et al. Acute right ventricular infarction secondary to massive pulmonary embolism. *Eur Heart J* 1988;9:534–540.

53. Bochowicz A, Kostrubiec M, Pruszczyk P. Serum myoglobin in pulmonary embolism. *Circulation* 2004;109:e194.

54. Pruszczyk P, Bochowicz A, Kostrubiec M, et al. Myoglobin stratifies short-term risk in acute major pulmonary embolism. *Clin Chim Acta* 2003;338:53–56.

55. Maisel AS, Krishnaswamy P, Nowak RM, et al. Rapid measurement of B-type natriuretic peptide in the emergency diagnosis of heart failure. *N Engl J Med* 2002;347:161–167.

56. Maisel AS, McCord J, Nowak RM, et al. Bedside B-Type natriuretic peptide in the emergency diagnosis of heart failure with reduced or preserved ejection fraction. Results from the breathing not properly multinational study. *J Am Coll Cardiol* 2003;41:2010–2017.

57. Talwar S, Squire IB, Davies JE, et al. Plasma N-terminal pro-brain natriuretic peptide and the ECG in the assessment of left-ventricular systolic dysfunction in a high risk population. *Eur Heart J* 1999;20:1736–1744.

58. Richards AM, Nicholls MG, Yandle TG, et al. Plasma N-terminal pro-brain natriuretic peptide and adrenomedullin: new neurohormonal predictors of left ventricular function and prognosis after myocardial infarction. *Circulation* 1998;97:1921–1929.

59. Hammerer-Lercher A, Neubauer E, Muller S, et al. Head-to-head comparison of N-terminal pro-brain natriuretic peptide, brain natriuretic peptide and N-terminal pro-atrial natriuretic peptide in diagnosing left ventricular dysfunction. *Clin Chim Acta* 2001;310:193–197.

60. Dao Q, Krishnaswamy P, Nowak RM, et al. Utility of B-type natriuretic peptide (BNP) in the diagnosis of CHF in an urgent care setting. *J Am Coll Cardiol* 2001;37:379–385.

61. Hama N, Itoh H, Shirakami G, et al. Rapid ventricular induction of brain natriuretic peptide gene expression in experimental acute myocardial infarction. *Circulation* 1995;92:1558–1564.

62. Kucher N, Printzen G, Doernhoefer T, et al. Low pro-brain natriuretic peptide levels predict benign clinical outcome in acute pulmonary embolism. *Circulation* 2003;107:1576–1578.

63. Kucher N, Printzen G, Goldhaber SZ. Prognostic role of brain natriuretic peptide in acute pulmonary embolism. *Circulation* 2003;107:2545–2547.

64. Nagaya N, Nishikimi T, Okano Y, et al. Plasma brain natriuretic peptide levels increase in proportion to the extent of right ventricular dysfunction in pulmonary hypertension. *J Am Coll Cardiol* 1998;31:202–208.

65. Pruszczyk P, Kostrubiec M, Bochowicz A, et al. N-terminal pro-brain natriuretic peptide in patients with acute pulmonary embolism. *Eur Respir J* 2003;22:649–653.

66. ten Wolde M, Tulevski II, Mulder JW, et al. Brain natriuretic peptide as a predictor of adverse outcome in patients with pulmonary embolism. *Circulation* 2003;107:2082–2084.

67. Tulevski II, Hirsch A, Sanson BJ, et al. Increased brain natriuretic peptide as a marker for right ventricular dysfunction in acute pulmonary embolism. *Thromb Haemost* 2001;86:1193–1196.

68. Bando M, Ishii Y, Sugiyama Y, et al. Elevated plasma brain natriuretic peptide levels in chronic respiratory failure with cor pulmonale. *Respir Med* 1999;93:507–514.

69. Nagaya N, Nishikimi T, Uematsu M, et al. Plasma brain natriuretic peptide as a prognostic indicator in patients with primary pulmonary hypertension. *Circulation* 2000;102:865–870.

70. Tulevski II, Groenink M, van Der Wall EE, et al. Increased brain and atrial natriuretic peptides in patients with chronic right ventricular pressure overload: correlation between plasma neurohormones and right ventricular dysfunction. *Heart* 2001;86:27–30.

71. Schoepf UJ, Costello P. CT angiography for diagnosis of pulmonary embolism: state of the art. *Radiology* 2004;230:329–337.

72. Schoepf UJ, Goldhaber SZ, Costello P. Spiral computed tomography for acute pulmonary embolism. *Circulation* 2004;109:2160–2167.

73. Schoepf UJ, Holzknecht N, Helmberger TK, et al. Subsegmental pulmonary emboli: improved detection with thin-collimation multidetector row spiral CT. *Radiology* 2002;222:483–490.

74. Schoepf UJ, Costello P. Multidetector-row CT imaging of pulmonary embolism. *Semin Roentgenol* 2003;38:106–114.

75. Schoepf UJ, Becker CR, Hofmann LK, et al. Multislice CT angiography. *Eur Radiol* 2003;13:1946–1961.

76. Lomis NN, Yoon HC, Moran AG, et al. Clinical outcomes of patients after a negative spiral CT pulmonary arteriogram in the evaluation of acute pulmonary embolism. *J Vasc Interv Radiol* 1999;10:707–712.

77. Quiroz R, Kucher N, Schoepf UJ, et al. Right ventricular enlargement on chest computed tomography: prognostic role in acute pulmonary embolism. *Circulation* 2004;109:2401–2404.

78. Collomb D, Paramelle PJ, Calaque O, et al. Severity assessment of acute pulmonary embolism: evaluation using helical CT. *Eur Radiol* 2003;13: 1508–1514.

79. Reid JH, Murchison JT. Acute right ventricular dilatation: a new helical CT sign of massive pulmonary embolism. *Clin Radiol* 1998;53:694–698.

80. Schoepf UJ, Kucher N, Kipfmueller F, et al. Right ventricular enlargement on chest CT: a predictor of early death in acute pulmonary embolism. *Circulation* 2004;110:3276–3280.

81. Guidelines on Diagnosis and Management of Acute Pulmonary Embolism. Task force on pulmonary embolism, European society of cardiology. *Eur Heart J* 2000;21:1301–1336.

# CHAPTER 89 ■ TREATMENT OF VENOUS THROMBOEMBOLISM

PETER W. MARKS

The last decade has witnessed major advances in the management of venous thromboembolic disease (1). Today, most episodes of deep vein thrombosis (DVT) and some cases of pulmonary embolism (PE) can be managed in the outpatient setting (2,3). The identification of prevalent genetic predispositions toward thrombosis (e.g., factor $V_{Leiden}$, prothrombin G20210A gene mutation) and results of clinical trials examining the potential benefits of long-term anticoagulation have provoked reexamination of the optimal duration of therapy (4,5). This chapter focuses primarily on the anticoagulant management of venous thromboembolism (VTE), concentrating on clinical data supporting the nature and duration of therapy administered. Detailed reviews on the diagnosis of VTE and on individual anticoagulants are provided in Chapters 87 and 116, respectively.

## ANTICOAGULANT MANAGEMENT OF DEEP VEIN THROMBOSIS/PULMONARY EMBOLISM

Three phases of anticoagulant management can be described for documented DVT or uncomplicated PE (see Fig. 89-1). These encompass the acute, subacute, and long-term management of VTE. In some instances, therapy is complete after the subacute phase, whereas in others, long-term therapy appears to be indicated. Although the same anticoagulant could potentially be used throughout for management, the description of different phases facilitates discussion of the different practical considerations involved in patient care.

### Acute Management

Once the diagnosis of proximal DVT or uncomplicated PE is confirmed, unless there is a contraindication to anticoagulation, such as active bleeding, severe thrombocytopenia, or recent neurosurgery, the standard of care is immediate treatment with an agent that rapidly produces antithrombotic effect in order to prevent further clot propagation. Unfractionated heparin (UFH) was for many years essentially the only parenteral agent available for this purpose; however, with the introduction of the low-molecular-weight heparins (LMWHs) and fondaparinux, a variety of alternatives now exist (see Table 89-1).

UFH is an effective anticoagulant in the setting of acute VTE (6). When intravenous UFH is used, an appropriate bolus dose should be followed by a weight-based continuous infusion to achieve a partial thromboplastin time (PTT) between 1.5 and 2.5 times control (7). Because of variability in PTT reagents, more reproducible anticoagulation may be achieved when UFH is administered to an antifactor Xa level between 0.3 and 0.7 U per mL. Knowledge of the correlation between the PTT and the antifactor Xa level obtained at a given laboratory facilitates use of the PTT, which is less expensive and more readily available. Alternatively, bolus dose subcutaneous UFH appears to be equally effective in the management of VTE when it is dosed in a sufficiently aggressive manner to prolong the PTT to a similar extent as intravenously administered heparin. The Galilei investigators compared subcutaneous bolus dose UFH to an LMWH in 720 patients with VTE, including noncritically ill patients with PE and patients with recurrent VTE (8). Recurrence rates (approximately 4%), bleeding complications (approximately 1%), and overall mortality (3.3%) were similar between the two groups. In addition, although several earlier studies with LMWHs suggested that these agents were superior to UFH, more recent studies show less of a difference between the two treatments, possibly because of improvements in nomogram-based dosing of UFH (9).

Although effective and inexpensive, there are several disadvantages to UFH for the acute management of VTE. In general, patients require hospitalization for 4 to 5 days because of the need for frequent monitoring of the PTT, regardless of whether the intravenous or subcutaneous route is utilized. Even when compared in an inpatient setting to the use of LMWH, UFH is associated with longer duration hospital stays (10). More significantly, heparin-induced thrombocytopenia (HIT) occurs in approximately 5% of treated patients, depending on the clinical setting (11). Despite appropriate treatment, this complication is associated with a high rate of morbidity and mortality.

Nonetheless, in certain settings, such as when rapid reversal of anticoagulation is potentially necessary (e.g., because of a high risk for bleeding or because of impending invasive procedures), UFH may be the anticoagulant agent of choice. Among parenteral anticoagulants for use in the acute setting, it remains the only agent that is fully reversible with protamine (12).

LMWHs are now routinely used in the management of DVT and/or PE (dalteparin, enoxaparin, and tinzaparin among others). Although differences in the various preparations of LMWH clearly exist, they are all similar in efficacy when used appropriately in the management of VTE.

A number of studies have demonstrated the anticoagulant equivalence of various LMWH preparations to UFH for the acute management of DVT or uncomplicated PE (13–15). Some of these studies have even shown the superiority of LMWH to UFH in this setting. However, this is likely related to the delay that often exists in achieving therapeutic anticoagulant levels with UFH rather than to intrinsic anticoagulant superiority of LMWH over UFH.

Depending on the particular LMWH, once- or twice-daily subcutaneous administration of these agents based on a fixed dose per kg without monitoring is appropriate for both DVT and uncomplicated PE. This approach facilitates management of most patients who present with proximal DVT in the

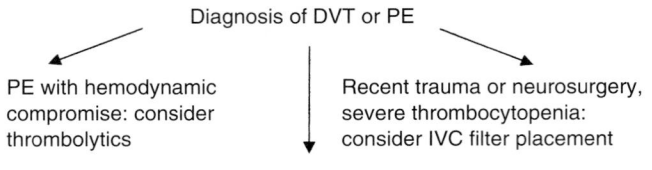

Diagnosis of DVT or PE

PE with hemodynamic compromise: consider thrombolytics

Recent trauma or neurosurgery, severe thrombocytopenia: consider IVC filter placement

**Acute phase**
- Assess for history of HIT
- Iinitiate anticoagulant therapy with LMWH or with fondaparinux
- Consider use of UFH if interventional procedures are planned or rapid reversal may be necessary

**Sub-acute phase**
- Initiation of therapy with warfarin
- Consider continued use of LMWH in specific circumstances: for example, patients with underlying malignancy
- Consider use of compression stockings

**Chronic phase**
- Assess indications for prolonged anticoagulation
  - Hereditary risk factors
  - Malignancy
  - Idiopathic VTE
- Consider use of either low-intensity warfarin (INR 1.5 to 2.0) or standard intensity warfarin (2.0 to 2.5)

**FIGURE 89-1.** The management of venous thromboembolism can be divided into acute, subacute, and chronic phases. For some patients, management may be complete after the subacute phase. DVT, deep vein thrombosis; PE, pulmonary embolism; IVC, inferior vena cava; HIT, heparin-induced thrombocytopenia; LMWH, low-molecular-weight heparin; UFH, unfractionated heparin; VTE, venous thromboembolism; INR, international normalized ratio.

outpatient setting. In addition, clinical trials have demonstrated the safe treatment of uncomplicated PE in the outpatient setting with LMWHs (16). There is some controversy as to whether twice-daily administration of LMWH is somewhat more effective than once-daily administration. In a clinical trial with arms comparing the administration of enoxaparin once or twice daily to UFH, there was a nonstatistically significant trend toward increased efficacy with twice-daily administration (13). In the absence of larger definitive trials, some clinicians who treat DVT with an LMWH preparation once daily treat patients with PE twice-daily.

Although associated with an approximately 10-fold lower incidence of HIT in previously heparin-naïve patients, LMWHs are still associated with this complication of therapy (17). Patients recently diagnosed with HIT have a high likelihood (approximately 50%) of having antibodies that will cross-react with LMWH. In addition, these agents are cleared through the kidney, so they must be administered with caution to patients with renal insufficiency (18). When administered to patients with considerable renal insufficiency (glomerular filtration rate of less than 30 to 45 mL per minute), monitoring of anti-Xa

levels (aiming for 0.6 to 1.0 U per mL in the case of enoxaparin) is advisable. Although the general use of antifactor Xa levels to monitor patients receiving LMWH is an area of controversy, the need for such monitoring in renal insufficiency is acknowledged (19–22). Finally, because they are only partially reversible with protamine, LMWHs should be used cautiously in patients with a high risk of bleeding.

Despite a few potential drawbacks, the introduction of the LMWHs has dramatically altered the management of VTE. Diagnoses that formerly required hospitalization are now managed entirely in the outpatient setting. A number of studies in diverse populations have demonstrated that the outpatient administration of LMWH for the management of DVT is safe and cost effective (23). Further studies are in progress to confirm a similar benefit for PE.

Recently, fondaparinux, a synthetic anticoagulant mimicking the portion of heparin that binds to factor Xa, was approved in the United States when combined with warfarin for the management of DVT (inpatient or outpatient) and PE (inpatient) (24,25). Studies supporting this indication were performed by the Methodologies and Technologies for Industrial Strength Systems Engineering (MATISSE) investigators who examined daily subcutaneous fondaparinux for the management of the acute phase of DVT and PE during the transition to warfarin anticoagulation (26). Most patients in the trial weighed between 50 and 100 kg and received fondaparinux 7.5 mg subcutaneously daily. More than 2,000 patients were involved in each of the two trials, one for DVT and one for PE, that demonstrated the equivalence of fondaparinux to LMWH and to UFH, respectively.

Because fondaparinux is cleared through the kidney, it must be used with caution in patients with major renal impairment. It can be monitored using anti-Xa levels, provided the laboratory has produced the correct calibration curve. Even more so than the LMWHs, it is not reversible by protamine, so it should be used cautiously in patients with a high risk of hemorrhage. In addition, because of its relatively long half-life, careful consideration of the potential need for invasive diagnostic procedures before administration of fondaparinux is essential.

A major benefit does result from the small size of fondaparinux: It does not appear to be associated with HIT, and, therefore, its use has the potential to eliminate the morbidity and mortality from this condition (27). Further studies are necessary, however, to confirm that this agent may routinely be used in patients with a history of HIT.

Although they are still investigational agents with potential safety concerns (elevations in liver function tests of unclear etiology), it is possible that an oral direct thrombin inhibitor such as dabigatran etexilate will eventually be approved for use (28–30).

Once therapeutic levels of anticoagulation are obtained, it is reasonable for patients with uncomplicated DVT to begin ambulation. One clinical trial using LMWH has suggested that early ambulation is associated with more rapid resolution of pain and swelling from DVT without an increased risk of PE (31). Such an approach is also supported by a number of ambulatory trials examining the use of LMWH. The data are less clear in patients with DVT and PE, in whom there is a suggestion from clinical trials that 48 to 72 hours of bed rest may perhaps be beneficial (32).

## Subacute Management

Irrespective of the initial anticoagulant used, a large number of trials have documented the benefit of extended duration anticoagulation for at least 3 months in the management of VTE. Studies examining the optimal duration of this subacute phase of anticoagulation are discussed in the subsequent text. For patients with identifiable transient risk factors associated with the

**TABLE 89-1**

### ADVANTAGES AND DISADVANTAGES OF ANTICOAGULANTS FOR USE IN THE ACUTE SETTING

| Agent | Advantages | Disadvantages |
|---|---|---|
| UFH | ■ Well-established agent for the treatment of acute VTE<br>■ Relatively short half-life (advantageous if procedures are required)<br>■ Most experience in combination with thrombolytic agents<br>■ Fully reversible with protamine | ■ Generally requires hospitalization for 4–5 d<br>■ Significant incidence of HIT, dependent on setting<br>■ Higher cost in comparison to outpatient management with LMWH or fondaparinux |
| LMWH | ■ Demonstrated efficacy similar to UFH in this setting<br>■ Does not require monitoring in patients with normal renal function<br>■ Facilitates outpatient management of many cases of VTE | ■ Incidence of HIT still present (although reduced in comparison to UFH)<br>■ Monitoring may be required in patients with impaired renal function (anti-Xa levels)<br>■ In the event of bleeding, only partially reversible with protamine (consider recombinant human factor VIIa, other measures) |
| Fondaparinux | ■ Demonstrated efficacy similar to UFH in this setting<br>■ Does not require monitoring in patients with normal renal function<br>■ Facilitates outpatient management of many cases of VTE<br>■ Does not appear to be associated with the development of HIT | ■ Monitoring may be required in patients with impaired renal function (anti-Xa levels)<br>■ In the event of bleeding not reversible with protamine (consider recombinant human factor VIIa, other measures) |

UFH, unfractionated heparin; LMWH, low-molecular-weight heparin; HIT, heparin-induced thrombocytopenia; VTE, venous thromboembolism.

occurrence of VTE, this may represent the full extent of the duration of anticoagulation. Examples of such risk factors include recent surgical procedures, immobility, and medications such as oral contraceptives. However, for other patients, such as those with idiopathic VTE or VTE in the setting of hereditary risk factors, serious consideration should be given to the benefits and risks of chronic anticoagulation.

In the most widely used and traditional approach, warfarin or another coumarin derivative is started around the time that therapy with the acute anticoagulant is initiated (be it UFH, LMWH, or fondaparinux; see Table 89-2). A period of 4 to 5 days of overlap is then required to achieve adequate antithrombotic effect of warfarin. Recent studies have indicated that with rare exception (such as recurrent VTE while on antithrombotic therapy), anticoagulation to an international normalized ratio (INR) of 2.0 to 3.0 is an appropriate intensity for all patients with VTE. This includes those with lupus anticoagulants or anticardiolipin antibodies, which previously were thought to merit higher-intensity therapy (33).

Some debate exists as to the optimal warfarin regimen for use in the initiation of anticoagulation. A starting dose of 5 mg daily for most patients was found in one study to lead to effective anticoagulation while minimizing hemorrhagic complications (34). However, a nomogram-based approach using a 10-mg initial dose of warfarin with LMWH recently was found to most reproducibly reach the target range within 5 days of therapy, without an excessive risk of bleeding (35). Whatever the approach, if warfarin is used as the subacute anticoagulant, the parenteral agent should not be discontinued until the INR is therapeutic and 4 to 5 days have elapsed.

LMWHs have also been investigated for use in the subacute setting for prolonged anticoagulation (36,37). LMWH given either once or twice daily is effective for the extended therapy for DVT, particularly in patients who cannot be effectively maintained on a therapeutic dose of warfarin in particular

settings. For example, the recurrence of wide variation in superatherapeutic INR values caused by chemotherapy-related toxicities such as diarrhea can be avoided using this approach. One trial by Beckman et al. also demonstrated the feasibility and possible benefit (in terms of a decreased recurrence rate) of extended therapy with LMWH for uncomplicated PE (38). In addition, in a population of patients with cancer, Lee et al. and the Clinical Leaders of Thrombosis (CLOT) investigators compared extended therapy for VTE with dalteparin to a coumarin. This trial included randomization of 211 patients with PE with or without accompanying DVT. Dalteparin was found to be superior to coumarin in preventing recurrence, without an excess risk of bleeding (39).

A few large studies have examined the optimal duration of anticoagulation in the subacute setting (40–42). These studies have demonstrated that a duration of therapy for less than 6 weeks is associated with a higher risk of VTE recurrence. In addition, one study demonstrated that a duration of therapy for 1 year versus 3 months was not associated with a considerable decrease in relapses once anticoagulation was discontinued (43). In the absence of large studies comparing 3 to 6 months of regular intensity anticoagulation in the subacute phase of VTE, some practitioners elect to recommend anticoagulation to patients with DVT for 3 months and to patients with PE for 6 months. This distinction is perhaps more important for those individuals for whom chronic anticoagulation is not being considered (e.g., those individuals with transient hypercoagulable risk factors such as recent surgery or casting).

Although it has not yet been formally studied in a large trial, fondaparinux should be effective for use in the subacute setting, much in the same way as LMWH. In addition, use of oral direct thrombin inhibitors in development may obviate the need for discussion of different anticoagulants for use in the acute, subacute, and chronic settings. The availability of

**TABLE 89-2**

ADVANTAGES AND DISADVANTAGES OF ANTICOAGULANTS FOR USE IN THE SUBACUTE SETTING

| Agent | Advantages | Disadvantages |
|-------|-----------|---------------|
| Warfarin | ■ Well-established standard of care for the reduction of recurrent VTE in this setting<br>■ Large body of evidence documenting well-defined potential complications of use<br>■ In the event of bleeding, readily reversible with vitamin K (h) or fresh frozen plasma (immediate)<br>■ Relatively low-cost | ■ Higher risk of recurrent VTE in certain settings (e.g., patients with cancer)<br>■ Higher risk of hemorrhagic complications in certain populations (e.g., patients with cancer)<br>■ Requires regular monitoring and dose adjustment as necessary |
| LMWH | ■ Appears to be very effective for reducing recurrent VTE in this setting<br>■ Does not require monitoring in patients with normal renal function | ■ Requires subcutaneous injection<br>■ Monitoring may be required in patients with impaired renal function (anti-Xa levels)<br>■ Risk of HIT still possible<br>■ In the event of bleeding, only partially reversible with protamine (consider recombinant human factor VIIa, other measures)<br>■ Higher cost than warfarin |
| Fondaparinux | ■ Appears to be very effective for reducing recurrent VTE in this setting<br>■ Does not require monitoring in patients with normal renal function | ■ Monitoring may be required in patients with impaired renal function (anti-Xa levels)<br>■ In the event of bleeding not reversible with protamine (consider recombinant human factor VIIa, other measures)<br>■ Higher cost than warfarin |

VTE, venous thromboembolism; LMWH, low-molecular-weight heparin; HIT, heparin-induced thrombocytopenia.

such oral agents will almost certainly lead to further evolution in the management of VTE in the years ahead.

Much of the controversy on the choice of therapeutic agent, duration, and intensity of anticoagulation originates from the concomitant associated bleeding risk. As it turns out, the acute and subacute phases of therapy for VTE are the periods during which the highest incidence of serious bleeding complications occur, at least when warfarin is used as an anticoagulant. Koo et al. determined that excessive anticoagulation with warfarin was associated with increased mortality in a cohort of hospitalized patients, suggesting the importance of appropriate control of the intensity of anticoagulation (44). In addition, a metaanalysis by Linkins et al. demonstrated an intracranial hemorrhage (ICH) rate of 1.15 per 100 patient-years and a 13.4% case-fatality rate during the first 3 months of anticoagulation compared to an ICH rate of 0.65 per 100 patient-years and a 9.1% case-fatality rate after that time (45). Whether the increased risk during the first 3 months in this study represents exposure of preexisting hemostatic defects, initial difficulty in appropriately titrating anticoagulation, or a combination of these and other factors can only be speculated at this time.

## Chronic Management

Administration of long-term anticoagulant therapy was once reserved for patients with recurrent VTE or those diagnosed with thrombophilic conditions that clearly placed them at high risk for recurrence (e.g., antithrombin deficiency, antiphospholipid antibody syndrome). More recently, however, two important trials have suggested that the benefits of long-term

anticoagulation may extend to a much wider population: patients with idiopathic VTE (46).

In the prevention of recurrent venous thromboembolism (PREVENT) trial, Ridker et al. demonstrated a significant reduction in the recurrence rate of VTE in patients treated with low-intensity (INR 1.5 to 2.0) anticoagulation after an initial 3-month period of therapeutic anticoagulation (47). In a rigorously controlled trial involving 506 patients with a mean of 2.1 years of follow-up, there was a 76% reduction in recurrent VTE in patients maintained on low-intensity anticoagulation versus placebo. This benefit extended across subgroups of patients with and without hereditary thrombophilia. There was no statistically significant increase in the risk of major bleeding in the group that received warfarin. With this low-intensity approach, monitoring of the INR was only required every 2 months. At least one report has specifically documented patient preference for this approach over conventional monitoring every 2 to 4 weeks (48).

The approach taken in the extended low-intensity anticoagulation for thromboembolism (ELATE) trial of Kearon et al. was to compare long-term low-intensity anticoagulation with standard intensity anticoagulation. In this trial involving 738 patients with a mean of 2.4 years of follow-up, standard intensity anticoagulation was found to be superior to low-intensity therapy (49). The recurrence rate was 0.7 per 100 person-years versus 1.9 per 100 person-years, respectively. Note that the recurrence rate on low-intensity therapy was similar to the rate of 2.6 per 100 person-years in patients on this arm of the PREVENT trial. Bleeding complications in the two arms of the trial were similar.

There has been controversy about the interpretation and applicability of these two trials to individual patients (50,51).

## TABLE 89-3

ADVANTAGES AND DISADVANTAGES OF ANTICOAGULANTS FOR USE IN THE LONG-TERM SETTING

| Agent | Advantages | Disadvantages |
|---|---|---|
| Warfarin (low intensity) | ■ Reduces rate of recurrent VTE<br>■ Low rate of serious bleeding complications<br>■ Less frequent monitoring required (every 2 mo)<br>■ In the event of bleeding, readily reversible with vitamin K (h) or fresh frozen plasma (immediate) | ■ Reduction in rate of VTE many be less than with standard intensity therapy<br>■ Increased risk of nonserious bleeding complications<br>■ Still requires some monitoring |
| Warfarin (standard intensity) | ■ Reduces rate of recurrent VTE even further than low-intensity therapy<br>■ Low rate of serious bleeding complications<br>■ In the event of bleeding, readily reversible with vitamin K (h) or fresh frozen plasma (immediate) | ■ Serious bleeding complications may be more of an issue in large populations (data not yet available)<br>■ Requires at least monthly monitoring of therapy |
| LMWH | ■ May be more effective than warfarin in certain settings (e.g., patients with cancer)<br>■ Does not require monitoring in patients with normal renal function | ■ Requires subcutaneous injection<br>■ Monitoring may be required in patients with impaired renal function (anti-Xa levels)<br>■ Although less so than for UFH, long-term use associated with osteoporosis<br>■ Risk of HIT still possible<br>■ In the event of bleeding, only partially reversible with protamine (consider recombinant human factor VIIa, other measures)<br>■ Higher cost than warfarin |
| Fondaparinux | ■ May be more effective than warfarin in certain settings (e.g., patients with cancer)<br>■ Does not require monitoring in patients with normal renal function<br>■ No apparent risk of HIT<br>■ Although no long-term data, less likely to be associated with osteoporosis | ■ Requires subcutaneous injection<br>■ No data available on long-term use<br>■ Monitoring may be required in patients with impaired renal function (anti-Xa levels)<br>■ In the event of bleeding not reversible with protamine (consider recombinant human factor VIIa, other measures)<br>■ Higher cost than warfarin |

LMWH, low-molecular-weight heparin; HIT, heparin-induced thrombocytopenia; VTE, venous thromboembolism.

However, rather than contradicting one another, these trials both support the concept that long-term anticoagulation may benefit certain populations (see Table 89-3). Other trials have also demonstrated a benefit of long-term anticoagulation in patients with VTE (52,53). Although higher intensity therapy may be associated with a greater reduction in recurrence rate, it also appears to be associated with increased patient inconvenience (48). Unless larger studies are performed, it will be difficult to determine if there are actually small but significant differences in rates of bleeding complications between the two approaches.

Use of laboratory testing may provide additional insight into the need for chronic anticoagulation. Elevated D-dimer levels following cessation of anticoagulation have been associated with an increased risk of recurrence, particularly in patients with congenital thrombophilia (54,55). In pediatric patients, factor VIII levels above 150 IU and D-dimer levels greater than 500 ng per mL at diagnosis, or one of these abnormalities after 3 to 6 months of standard anticoagulation, were predictive of poor outcome (lack of thrombus resolution, recurrent thrombosis, or the postphlebitic syndrome) (56). However, no prospective data exist on the use of anticoagulation for prevention of recurrence in the setting of elevated D-dimer or factor VIII levels (57).

It is reasonable to offer long-term anticoagulation to patients after an episode of idiopathic VTE or after a first episode of unprovoked VTE in the setting of hereditary thrombophilia. Some of the factors that might be considered in the risk-to-benefit analysis include the potential for hemorrhagic complications, the hereditary context, whether repeated events have occurred, and whether an underlying malignancy is present.

Individualized discussion of the potential benefits and risks may help patients to choose among the options. In addition, risk assessment models have been developed (58). Both approaches involving long-term anticoagulation (low intensity and standard intensity) offer increased protection against recurrence, although likely with some increase in hemorrhagic risk. Patient acceptance of long-term anticoagulation may ultimately depend not only on the perceived risk of continued anticoagulation but also on the severity of the initial episode of VTE.

One final consideration in the chronic management of lower extremity DVT is the use of elastic compression stockings to try to reduce the rate or extent of postphlebitic syndrome (lower extremity swelling and erythema following an episode of DVT). Up to 50% of patients may be affected by some swelling of the limb as a result of prior DVT, particularly in the setting of recurrent events in a given limb. Although patients with symptomatic swelling following lower extremity DVT have often been prescribed elastic compression stockings, there are few data supporting their efficacy. One randomized trial examined the utility of the routine use of elastic compression stockings in patients after the initial diagnosis of lower extremity DVT. This study by Prandoni et al., involving 90 patients in each arm, demonstrated a 50% reduction in postthrombotic sequalae after 2 years (59). The routine use of elastic compression stockings for all patients, however, must be balanced against their inconvenience. Aside from difficulty in getting into elastic compression stockings (which can be addressed with proper fitting and training in appropriate application techniques), many patients find these stockings cosmetically unappealing or uncomfortable, particularly in warmer climates. Further clinical trials may identify risk factors that are indicative of the potential benefit from elastic compression stockings.

## CALF VEIN THROMBOSIS

Not infrequently, lower extremity discomfort or swelling is attributable to DVT occurring below the knee. Vital literature has been published on the optimal monitoring for progression to proximal vein DVT, which may occur in up to approximately 20% of cases. Although patients with incidentally discovered asymptomatic calf vein thrombosis may be followed serially for progression, patients with symptomatic calf vein thrombosis should receive systemic anticoagulation similar to patients with proximal DVT (60). Data suggest that 6 weeks of anticoagulation may be sufficient in this setting (61). A randomized open-label trial by Pinede et al. that included 197 patients with isolated calf vein thrombosis demonstrated the equivalence of 6 and 12 weeks of oral anticoagulant therapy (62).

## UPPER EXTREMITY DEEP VEIN THROMBOSIS

Although commonly associated with intravascular devices (for which prophylactic anticoagulation may reduce the rate of occurrence), up to 20% of upper extremity DVT occurs spontaneously (63). Prospective registry data of Joffe et al. examining the etiology of upper extremity DVT suggest that aside from the association with intravascular device placement, other risk factors, including younger age and leaner body mass, may be different from those for lower extremity DVT (64).

Irrespective of etiology and contrary to some beliefs, DVT in the upper extremities is associated with a significant risk of PE if untreated (65). Therefore, aggressive management is indicated once the diagnosis is confirmed. In the past, venography was the reference standard for documenting upper extremity VTE; however, noninvasive techniques such as vascular ultrasound and magnetic resonance imaging are now increasingly employed (66). Alternatively, in the presence of indwelling central venous catheters, nuclear medicine flow studies may be used for this purpose.

Whatever the method employed for diagnosis, the initial therapy remains the same: full dose anticoagulation. In the absence of large, well-controlled clinical trials, there is some debate as to the duration of anticoagulation for upper extremity DVT. When DVT occurs in the presence of intravascular devices that are subsequently removed, a 3-month course of anticoagulation is reasonable. If an attempt is made to manage DVT without removal of the indwelling device (which is successful approximately 25% to 50% of the time),

anticoagulation should continue for the duration of placement of the device because the risk of progression or recurrence is otherwise high. Reasoning by analogy, idiopathic spontaneous upper extremity DVT may warrant prolonged anticoagulation with either low-intensity or full-intensity anticoagulation, as for lower extremity DVT, if the benefit-to-risk ratio is felt to be acceptable.

## SUPERFICIAL THROMBOPHLEBITIS

Thrombosis of superficial veins can create considerable discomfort for patients. In addition, migratory or recurrent superficial thrombophlebitis carries a significant association with underlying malignancy, as originally described by Trousseau (Trousseau syndrome). Once the possibility of concomitant DVT is ruled out, several different approaches to management may be taken (67). No single approach has yet been demonstrated to be superior to others in a large, well-controlled randomized trial.

Elevation, application of warm compresses, and administration of nonsteroidal antiinflammatory drugs (NSAIDs) have been used for symptomatic relief. Management with prophylactic dose LMWH for 1 month in combination with elastic compression stockings has been also been advocated by Decousus et al. (68). In relation to this, one randomized trial demonstrated that LMWH or NSAIDs are superior to placebo in the treatment of superficial thrombophlebitis (69). In the absence of additional data, it is reasonable to treat limited episodes conservatively with topical measures and NSAIDs, and to treat patients with more extensive episodes with LMWH. Patients who are found to have malignancies may also be candidates for LMWH if the benefit-to-risk ratio is reasonable.

## SPECIAL SITUATIONS

### Use of Vena Caval Filters

Over the last several decades, a variety of refinements have been made to intravascular devices designed for placement in the inferior vena cava in order to prevent PE from DVT. The design of the Greenfield filter has been refined in an effort to prevent small clots from escaping capture. In addition, retrievable devices have been developed (70). The design and use of vena caval filters is covered in detail in Chapter 91.

Despite technical advances in the design and placement of vena caval filters and the publication of small case series with individual devices, controversy exists about when and how these devices should be employed (71,72). This controversy is significant because there is some indication that placement of vena caval filters may be associated with increased morbidity and mortality when compared to treatment with standard anticoagulation, although it is somewhat difficult to distinguish whether the increase is the result of the treatment modality used or of associated comorbid illness. For example, data from a registry in Spain involving more than approximately 4,000 patients reported a 2% rate of placement of vena caval filters and a 12.5% death rate in these individuals (73). It is clear that, absent administration of systemic anticoagulation, DVT may progress after filter placement, leading to significant local complications such as swelling and discomfort.

Because there are no data from large, well-controlled clinical trials, general guidelines for the placement of these devices in VTE can be surmised from smaller studies. In general, placement of vena caval filters should be reserved for patients in whom clear contraindications to systemic anticoagulation exist. The most notable indications are those individuals who have undergone neurosurgery within the recent past (< 2 weeks), those with significant recent intracerebral hemorrhage, and those who are actively bleeding (74). There may also be a role for temporary filters in critically ill surgical patients who need to undergo additional procedures (75).

When vena caval filters are placed in patients with contraindications to anticoagulation, careful consideration should be given to the timing of the initiation of systemic anticoagulation. In general, systemic anticoagulation should be administered as soon as possible after the hemorrhagic risk has declined because it minimizes both proximal and distal complications (vena caval thrombosis, progression of lower extremity DVT). It is important to remember that placement of an intravascular device alone may lead to further thrombotic complications and does nothing to interrupt the local propagation of DVT.

## Thrombolysis and Thrombectomy

The use of thrombolytic agents in the management of VTE makes logical sense; however, except in the case of massive PE with hemodynamic compromise, a clear benefit for the routine use of these agents in DVT or PE has yet to be demonstrated (76–78). The use of thrombolytic agents in VTE is covered in detail in Chapter 90, and the complication of pulmonary hypertension resulting from VTE is covered in Chapter 92.

A number of trials and metaanalyses have not demonstrated a clear benefit for systemic thrombolysis in PE without hemodynamic compromise, although there is indication that it may reduce the development of subsequent pulmonary hypertension. A major issue is that the benefit of thrombolytic agents must be balanced by the accompanying increased risk of ICH (79). In addition, the use of catheter-directed thrombolysis in adults with DVT has not yet been clearly shown to reduce long-term postthrombotic complications (80). Catheter-directed thrombolysis is, however, increasingly being used in the pediatric population (81).

Transvenous catheter embolectomy and surgical thrombectomy remain alternatives in patients with massive PE, and there are case reports describing success with these methods of management (82,83). If an experienced surgical team is available, surgical thrombectomy is a particularly reasonable approach when there is a contraindication to thrombolysis in the presence of large clots.

## Malignancy

Cancer is associated with a considerable increase in the risk of DVT and PE. In fact, certain malignancies, such as glioblastoma multiforme, are associated with rates of VTE in excess of 25% (84). Underuse of appropriate prophylactic measures and insufficient treatment of thrombotic episodes, in terms of either anticoagulation intensity or duration, may contribute to the morbidity from VTE in patients with cancer (85).

A variety of factors combine to produce higher VTE risk in patients with cancer, including compression or invasion of venous structures by tumors, humoral factors secreted by tumors, alterations in the levels of procoagulant and anticoagulant factors, and indwelling vascular access devices. In addition to the increased incidence of VTE in patients with malignancy, there is also an increased rate of anticoagulant failure or recurrence associated with standard therapy (heparin or LMWH followed by warfarin), as well as increased risk of hemorrhage associated particularly with certain types of malignancy or locations of metastases (brain) (86). Finally, patients with cancer

often have poor or variable oral intake and are on concomitant medications, making it difficult to maintain a therapeutic level of anticoagulation with warfarin. This has led to the investigation of novel treatment strategies.

Several recent trials have investigated anticoagulation with LMWH in patients with cancer and with VTE. Meyer et al. compared anticoagulation with standard intensity warfarin to therapeutic doses of LMWH (enoxaparin) in a 3-month trial involving randomization of 138 patients. The composite outcome measure of major bleeding and recurrent VTE in those receiving enoxaparin was half that of those receiving warfarin (10.5% vs. 21%) (87). Most of this difference was due to a reduction in major bleeding events. The CLOT trial, lasting 6 months, involved randomization of 672 patients to warfarin or LMWH (dalteparin). In this trial, it was observed that the risk of recurrence on dalteparin was half that of those receiving warfarin (8.8% vs. 17.4%) (39).

Summarizing these and other data on the use of LMWH in malignancy, it appears that these agents reduce the risk of recurrent VTE with an improved margin of safety. Use of LMWH may also have antineoplastic effects, although these are still controversial and under investigation (88). Issues surrounding thrombosis in patients with cancer are covered in further detail in Chapter 85.

## Pregnancy

Pregnancy and the immediate postpartum period confer a heightened risk for VTE (89). Once diagnosed, appropriate management of DVT or PE in this population includes full dose anticoagulation lasting until at least 4 to 6 weeks after delivery, with a brief interruption during the peripartum period (90). Complicating the administration of anticoagulation to this population is the fact that coumarin derivatives such as warfarin are teratogenic when administered during the first trimester of pregnancy. There is also some evidence that it may increase fetal bleeding (91,92). For this reason, in the United States, its use is generally avoided entirely during pregnancy; however, in some regions of the world, it is considered an acceptable anticoagulant during the second and third trimesters.

In lieu of coumarin derivatives, adjusted-dose subcutaneous UFH (which does not cross the placenta) has been used effectively in the past for the treatment of VTE throughout pregnancy (93). However, its administration is cumbersome, often requiring three injections a day, and its use has been associated with the development of some degree of osteoporosis, even when administered only for a number of months.

More recently, LMWHs (which also do not cross the placenta) have been demonstrated to be safe and effective when administered for the treatment of VTE during pregnancy (94,95). Although they are more expensive than UFH, when administered during pregnancy, LMWHs have been associated with a decreased incidence of bleeding, and they likely reduce the rate of the development of osteoporosis. However, changes in body weight and drug clearance during pregnancy can affect the antifactor Xa levels achieved. There is some controversy regarding the optimal management of LMWH in patients who are pregnant. One study has demonstrated that adequate antifactor Xa levels may be achieved with adjustment of dose for change in weight (96). Alternatively, Ginsberg and Bates have suggested that optimal dosing of LMWH in pregnancy be based on antifactor Xa levels (97). These are checked monthly 4 to 6 hours after the morning dose, and the dose is adjusted to achieve an antifactor Xa level of 1.0 to 2.0 U per mL for once-daily dosing or 0.5 to 1.2 U per mL for twice-daily dosing. Checking antifactor Xa levels as suggested by this approach may help to assure both safety and efficacy in this setting.

Clinical trials examining fondaparinux did not include patients who were pregnant. Although *in vitro* data suggested that fondaparinux does not cross the placenta, there has been one small case series reporting transplacental passage (98). Until further data are available, use of fondaparinux during pregnancy is not recommended unless no other therapeutic alternatives exist.

# COMPLICATIONS OF THERAPY FOR VENOUS THROMBOEMBOLISM

## Hemorrhage

Recent clinical data highlight issues regarding the potential benefits versus the hemorrhagic risks of anticoagulation, particularly in the case of the recent clinical trials indicating the potential benefit of long-term anticoagulation for idiopathic VTE. The hemorrhagic complications of anticoagulant therapy in general and their management are covered in detail in Chapter 119.

Before initiation of anticoagulation in any patient, consideration should be given to potential bleeding risks such as active gastrointestinal bleeding and ICH. The potential need for invasive diagnostic or surgical procedures should also be addressed because alternative modes of anticoagulation other than standard practice may be optimal (e.g., maintenance on heparin or LMWH rather than initiation and transition to warfarin). Evidence suggests that the highest risk of bleeding complications, particularly ICH, occurs during the first 3 months of therapy in patients treated with warfarin (45). Heightened vigilance for such complications is therefore indicated during this period. In addition, there is some evidence that maintenance of anticoagulation within the therapeutic range may decrease the morbidity or mortality from hemorrhagic events in anticoagulated patients. In this regard, specialized anticoagulation clinics familiar with the intricacies of patient management, including appropriate education and monitoring, may lead to improved outcomes (99).

## Heparin-Induced Thrombocytopenia

The use of UFH is associated with an approximately 5% incidence of HIT (100). The actual frequency of this complication depends on several factors, including the heparin preparation used (bovine has a higher rate than porcine) and the clinical setting (medical vs. specific types of surgical procedures). In contrast, the incidence of HIT is about an order of magnitude lower when LMWH is used. Because a significant percentage of cases of HIT are associated with severe thrombotic complications, identification of this complication is critical. The management of HIT is covered in detail in Chapter 114.

The platelet count should initially be monitored at least every few days in patients on therapy with UFH. Patients receiving LMWH as a bridge to warfarin should have a platelet count checked on or about day 5 of LMWH. In either case, identification of a 50% drop in the platelet count should trigger consideration of the possibility of HIT. Because most laboratory assays for HIT lack sufficient sensitivity or specificity, the diagnosis of HIT remains mainly a clinical one. In this regard, Warkentin has proposed a clinical scoring system for estimating the pretest probability of HIT on the basis of the severity of the thrombocytopenia, the timing of onset, the presence or absence of thrombosis, and whether or not other potential causes of thrombocytopenia are present (101). If the differential diagnosis includes HIT, heparin or LMWH should be discontinued, and an alternative anticoagulant (such as a direct thrombin inhibitor) should be initiated at least until the platelet count normalizes.

It appears that the pentasaccharide anticoagulant fondaparinux may not be associated with HIT. If confirmed, this might indicate an additional advantage of this agent over LMWH.

## Osteoporosis

Long-term therapy with UFH is associated with osteoporosis and potentially with an increased susceptibility to fractures. Heparin binds to calcium and results in its mobilization from bone. This complication has been most apparent in pregnancy and in cases of thrombophilia treated for several months with this agent. LMWH appears to be associated with a lower incidence of osteoporosis, and this may be one of its advantages when used in the long-term setting (102). The incidence of osteoporosis with fondaparinux is not yet known, but on theoretical grounds, there may be even less of a concern with this agent.

## Warfarin-Induced Skin Necrosis

Initiation of warfarin therapy in the absence of heparin or another anticoagulant is rarely associated with the occurrence of skin necrosis because of thrombosis of small vessels within several days after initiating anticoagulation (103). The vitamin K–dependent anticoagulants protein C and protein S have short half-lives, and their levels drop rapidly with the initiation of warfarin therapy. Patients with protein C or protein S deficiency are therefore particularly susceptible to this complication (104). The best method to avoid this complication when using warfarin for the therapy for VTE is to use another anticoagulant when necessary as a bridge to effective anticoagulation. This is indicated in the setting of acute VTE because effective antithrombotic effect with initiation of warfarin requires 4 to 5 days, and this is essentially irrespective of the prolongation of the prothrombin time. However, when patients are anticoagulated for chronic conditions such as atrial fibrillation, in which the time to achievement of therapeutic anticoagulation is not critical, such bridging is not considered necessary (105).

## Anticoagulant Failure

Despite maintenance of therapeutic levels of anticoagulation, some patients develop recurrent episodes of VTE. This is particularly true for patients with indwelling vascular devices and those with malignancy. In such cases, consideration may be given to several different strategies, although none is based on randomized clinical data. For those patients anticoagulated with warfarin at standard intensity (INR 2.0 to 3.0), the intensity of anticoagulation may be increased to an INR of 2.5 to 3.5. Unfortunately, in clinical practice, this may be inadequate, in which case the administration of LMWH may be considered.

A small number of patients will subsequently appear to have recurrence while receiving LMWH at standard doses. Antifactor Xa levels should be obtained in these individuals because sometimes standard dosing results in inadequate anticoagulant levels. If anti-factor Xa levels are documented to be in the low therapeutic range during the period of a recurrence, consideration may be given to increasing the intensity of therapy for LMWH with close monitoring.

# SUMMARY

VTE remains a major cause of morbidity and mortality. However, there have been major advances, including the development and application of strategies that allow safe and effective outpatient management of many patients using LMWH as a bridge to warfarin therapy. Novel oral anticoagulants may replace warfarin as the standard for oral therapy. The concept of long-term anticoagulation after idiopathic VTE will likely see significant application in the coming years. These advances will decrease the burden of illness from VTE.

## *References*

1. Bates SM, Ginsberg JS. Treatment of deep-vein thrombosis. *N Engl J Med* 2004;351:268–277.
2. Heit JA. Current management of acute symptomatic deep vein thrombosis. *Am J Cardiovasc Drugs* 2001;1:45–50.
3. McRae SJ, Ginsberg JS. Initial treatment of venous thromboembolism. *Circulation* 2004;110(9 Suppl. 1):I3–I9.
4. Perry SL, Ortel TL. Clinical and laboratory evaluation of thrombophilia. *Clin Chest Med* 2003;24:153–170.
5. Seligsohn U, Lubetsky A. Genetic susceptibility to venous thrombosis. *N Engl J Med* 2001;344:1222–1231.
6. Brandjes DPM, Heijboer H, Buller HR, et al. Acenocoumarol and heparin compared with acenocoumarol alone in the initial treatment of proximal-vein thrombosis. *N Engl J Med* 1992;327:1485–1489.
7. Hirsh J, Raschke R. Heparin and low-molecular-weight heparin: the Seventh ACCP Conference on Antithrombotic and Thrombolytic Therapy. *Chest* 2004;126(Suppl. 3):188S–203S.
8. Prandoni P, Carnovali M, Marchiori A, Galilei Investigators. Subcutaneous adjusted-dose unfractionated heparin vs fixed-dose low-molecular-weight heparin in the initial treatment of venous thromboembolism. *Arch Intern Med* 2004;24:1077–1083.
9. Krishnan JA, Segal JB, Streiff MB, et al. Treatment of venous thromboembolism with low-molecular weight heparin: a synthesis of the evidence published in systematic literature reviews. *Respir Med* 2004;98:376–386.
10. Dunn A, Bioh D, Beran M, et al. Effect of intravenous heparin administration on duration of hospitalization. *Mayo Clin Proc* 2004;79:159–163.
11. Powers PJ, Kelton JG, Carter CJ. Studies of the frequency of heparin-associated thrombocytopenia. *Thromb Res* 1984;33:439–443.
12. Warkentin TE, Crowther MA. Reversing anticoagulants old and new. *Can J Anaesth* 2002;49:S11–S25.
13. Merli G, Spiro TE, Olsson CG. Subcutaneous enoxaparin once or twice daily compared with intravenous unfractionated heparin for treatment of venous thromboembolic disease. *Ann Intern Med* 2001;134:191–202.
14. Nutescu EA, Shapiro NL, Feinstein H, et al. Tinzaparin: considerations for use in clinical practice. *Ann Pharmacother* 2003;37:1831–1840.
15. Quinlan DJ, McQuillan A, Eikelboom JW. Low-molecular-weight heparin compared with intravenous unfractionated heparin for treatment of pulmonary embolism: a meta-analysis of randomized, controlled trials. *Ann Intern Med* 2004;140:175–183.
16. Kovacs MJ, Anderson D, Morrow B, et al. Outpatient treatment of pulmonary embolism with dalteparin. *Thromb Haemost* 2002;83:209–211.
17. Warkentin TE, Levine MN, Hirsh J, et al. Heparin-induced thrombocytopenia in patients treated with low-molecular-weight heparin or unfractionated heparin. *N Engl J Med* 1995;332:543–548.
18. Schulman S. Unresolved issues in anticoagulant therapy. *J Thromb Haemost* 2003;1:1464–1470.
19. Harenberg J. Is laboratory monitoring of low-molecular-weight heparin therapy necessary? Yes. *J Thromb Haemost* 2004;2:547–550.
20. Bounameaux H, de Moerloose P. Is laboratory monitoring of low-molecular-weight heparin therapy necessary? No. *J Thromb Haemost* 2004;2:551–554.
21. Kearon C. Laboratory monitoring of low-molecular-weight heparin therapy. *J Thromb Haemost* 2004;2:1006–1007.
22. Fiessinger JN. Laboratory monitoring of low-molecular-weight heparin therapy. *J Thromb Haemost* 2004;2:1007.
23. Segal JB, Bolger DT, Jenckes MW, et al. Outpatient therapy with low molecular weight heparin for the treatment of venous thromboembolism: a review of efficacy safety, and costs. *Am J Med* 2003;115:298–308.
24. O'Shaughnessy DF. Current perspectives on the treatment of venous thromboembolism: need for effective, safe and convenient new antithrombotic drugs. *Int J Clin Pract* 2004;58:227–284.
25. Turpie AG, Eriksson BI, Lassen MR, et al. Fondaparinux, the first selective Xa inhibitor. *Curr Opin Hematol* 2003;10:327–332.
26. Büller HR, Davidson BL, Decousus H, et al. Fondaparinux or enoxaparin for the initial treatment of symptomatic deep venous thrombosis. *Ann Intern Med* 2004;140:867–873.
27. Savi P, Chong BH, Greinacher A, et al. Effect of fondaparinux on platelet activation in the presence of heparin-dependent antibodies. A blinded comparative multicenter study with unfractionated heparin. *Blood* 2005;105:139–144.
28. Crowther MA, Weitz JI. Ximelagatran: the first oral direct thrombin inhibitor. *Expert Opin Investig Drugs* 2004;13:403–413.
29. Eriksson BI, Dahl OE, Ahnfelt L, et al. Dose escalating safety study of a new oral direct thrombin inhibitor, dabigatran etexilate in patients undergoing total hip replacement: BISTRO I. *J Thromb Haemost* 2004;2: 1573–1580.
30. McCullough PA, Dorrell KA, Sandberg KR, et al. Ximelagatran: a novel direct thrombin inhibitor for long-term anticoagulation. *Rev Cardiovasc Med* 2004;5:99–103.
31. Partsch H, Blattler W. Compression and walking versus bed rest in the treatment of proximal deep venous thrombosis with low molecular weight heparin. *J Vasc Surg* 2000;32:861–869.
32. Kiser TS, Stefans VA. Pulmonary embolism in rehabilitation patients: relation to time before return to physical therapy after diagnosis of deep vein thrombosis. *Arch Phys Med Rehabil* 1997;78:942–945.
33. Crowther MA, Ginsberg JS, Julian J, et al. A comparison of two intensities of warfarin for the prevention of recurrent thrombosis in patients with the antiphospholipid antibody syndrome. *N Engl J Med* 2003;349: 1133–1138.
34. Crowther MA, Ginsberg JS, Kearon C, et al. A randomized trial comparing 5-mg and 10-mg warfarin doses. *Arch Intern Med* 1999;159:46–48.
35. Kovacs MJ, Rodger M, Anderson DR, et al. Comparison of 10-mg and 5-mg warfarin initiation nomograms together with low-molecular-weight heparin for outpatient treatment of acute venous thromboembolism. A randomized double-blind, controlled trial. *Ann Intern Med* 2003;138:714–719.
36. Iorio A, Guercini F, Pini M. Low molecular-weight heparin for the long-term treatment of symptomatic venous thromboembolism: meta-analysis of the randomized comparisons with oral anticoagulants. *J Thromb Haemost* 2003;1:1906–1913.
37. Kakkar VV, Gebska M, Kadziola Z, et al. Low-molecular-weight heparin in the acute and long-term treatment of deep vein thrombosis. *Thromb Haemost* 2003;89:674–680.
38. Beckman JA, Dunn K, Sasahara AA, et al. Enoxaparin monotherapy without oral anticoagulation to treat acute symptomatic pulmonary embolism. *Thromb Haemost* 2003;89:953–958.
39. Lee AY, Levine MN, Baker RI, et al. Low-molecular-weight heparin versus a coumarin for the prevention of recurrent venous VTE in cancer patients. *N Engl J Med* 2003;349:146–153.
40. Prins MN, Hutten BA, Koopman MMW, et al. Long-term treatment of venous thromboembolic disease. *Thromb Haemost* 1999;82:892–898.
41. Schulman S, Rhedin AS, Lindmarker P, et al. A comparison of six weeks with six months of oral anticoagulant therapy after a first episode of venous thromboembolism. *N Engl J Med* 1995;332:1661–1665.
42. Kearon C, Gent M, Hirsh J, et al. A comparison of three months of anticoagulation with extended anti-coagulation for a first episode of idiopathic venous thromboembolism. *N Engl J Med* 1999;340:901–906.
43. Agnelli G, Prandoni P, Santamaria MG et al. Warfarin Optimal Duration Italian Trial Investigators. Three months versus one year of oral anticoagulant therapy for idiopathic deep venous thrombosis. *N Engl J Med* 2001; 345:165–169.
44. Koo S, Kucher N, Nguyen PL, et al. The effect of excessive anticoagulation on mortality and morbidity in hospitalized patients with anticoagulant-related major hemorrhage. *Arch Intern Med* 2004;164:1557–1560.
45. Linkins LA, Choi PT, Douketis JD. Clinical impact of bleeding in patients taking oral anticoagulant therapy for venous thromboembolism: a meta-analysis. *Ann Intern Med* 2003;139:893–900.
46. Frazee LA, Chomo DL. Duration of anticoagulation therapy after initial idiopathic venous thromboembolism. *Ann Pharmacother* 2003;37: 1489–1496.
47. Ridker PM, Goldhaber SZ, Danielson E, et al. Long-term low-intensity warfarin therapy for the prevention of recurrent venous thromboembolism. *N Engl J Med* 2003;348:1425–1434.
48. Svensson P, Sodermark A, Schulman S. Experiences of a low-intensity anticoagulation regimen for extended secondary prevention of venous thromboembolism. *Hematol J* 2002;3:311–314.
49. Kearon C, Ginsberg JS, Kovacs MJ, et al. Comparison of low-intensity warfarin therapy with conventional-intensity warfarin therapy for long-term prevention of recurrent venous thromboembolism. *N Engl J Med* 2003;349:631–639.
50. Ridker PM. Long-term low-dose warfarin use is effective in the prevention of recurrent venous thromboembolism: yes. *J Thromb Haemost* 2004;2: 1034–1037.
51. Agnelli G. Long-term low-dose warfarin use is effective in the prevention of recurrent venous thromboembolism: no. *J Thromb Haemost* 2004;2: 1038–1040.
52. Agnelli G, Prandoni P, Becattini C, et al. Extended oral anticoagulant therapy after a first episode of pulmonary embolism. *Ann Intern Med* 2003; 139:19–25.
53. Schulman S, Wahlander K, Lundstrom T, et al. Secondary prevention of venous thromboembolism with the oral direct thrombin inhibitor ximelagatran. *N Engl J Med* 2003;349:1713–1721.
54. Eichinger S, Minar E, Bialonczyk C, et al. D-dimer levels and risk of recurrent venous thromboembolism. *JAMA* 2003;290:1071–1074.

55. Palareti G, Legnani C, Cosmi B, et al. Predictive value of D-dimer test for recurrent venous thromboembolism after anticoagulation withdrawal in subjects with a previous idiopathic event and and in carriers of congenital thrombophilia. *Circulation* 2003;108:313–318.

56. Goldenberg NA, Knapp-Clevenger R, Manco-Johnson MJ, for the Mountain States Regional Thrombophilia Group. Elevated plasma factor VIII and D-dimer levels as predictors of poor outcomes of thrombosis in children. *N Engl J Med* 2004;351:1081–1088.

57. Palareti G, Cosmi B. Predicting the risk of recurrence of venous thromboembolism. *Curr Opin Hematol* 2004;11:192–197.

58. Vink R, Kraaijenhagen RA, Levi M, et al. Individualized duration of oral anticoagulant therapy for deep vein thrombosis based on a decision model. *J Thromb Haemost* 2003;1:2523–2530.

59. Prandoni P, Lensing AWA, Prins MH, et al. Below-knee elastic compression stockings to prevent the post-thrombotic syndrome. *Ann Intern Med* 2004;141:249–256.

60. Büller HR, Agnelli G, Hull RD, et al. Antithrombotic therapy for venous thromboembolic disease: the Seventh ACCP Conference on Antithrombotic and Thrombolytic Therapy. *Chest* 2004;126:401S–428S.

61. Astermark J, Bjorgell O, Linden E, et al. Low recurrence rate after deep calf-vein thrombosis with 6 weeks of oral anticoagulation. *Intern Med* 1998;244:79–82.

62. Pinede L, Ninet J, Duhaut P, et al. Comparison of 3 and 6 months of oral anticoagulant therapy after a first episode of proximal deep vein thrombosis or pulmonary embolism and comparison of 6 and 12 weeks of therapy after isolated calf deep vein thrombosis. *Circulation* 2001;103:2453–2460.

63. Bernardi E, Piccioli A, Marchiori A, et al. Upper extremity deep vein thrombosis: risk factors, diagnosis, and management. *Semin Vasc Med* 2001; 1:105–110.

64. Joffe HV, Kucher N, Tapson VF, et al. Upper-extremity deep vein thrombosis: a prospective registry of 592 patients. *Circulation* 2004;110: 1605–1611.

65. Joffe HV, Goldhaber SZ. Upper-extremity deep vein thrombosis. *Circulation* 2002;106:1874–1880.

66. Baarslag HJ, Koopman MM, Reekers JA, et al. Diagnosis and management of deep vein thrombosis of the upper extremity: a review. *Eur Radiol* 2004;14:1263–1274.

67. Quenet S, Laporte S, Decousus H, et al. Factors predictive of venous thrombotic complications in patients with isolated superficial vein thrombosis. *J Vasc Surg* 2003;38:944–949.

68. Decousus H, Epinat M, Guillot K, et al. Superficial vein thrombosis: risk factors, diagnosis, and treatment. *Curr Opin Pulm Med* 2003;9:393–397.

69. Superficial Thrombophlebitis Treated by Enoxaparin Study Group. A pilot randomized double-blind comparison of a low-molecular weight heparin, a non-steroidal anti-inflammatory agent, and placebo in the treatment of superficial vein thrombosis. *Arch Intern Med* 2003;163:1657–1663.

70. Jacobs DG, Sing RF. The role of vena caval filters in the management of venous thromboembolism. *Am Surg* 2003;69:635–642.

71. Girard P, Stern JB, Parent F. Medical literature and vena caval filters: so far so weak. *Chest* 2002;122:963–967.

72. Streiff MB. Vena caval filters: a review for intensive care specialists. *J Intensive Care Med* 2003;18:105–107.

73. Arcelus JI, Caprini JA, Monreal M, et al. The management and outcome of acute venous thromboembolism: a prospective registry including 4011 patients. *J Vasc Surg* 2003;38:916–922.

74. Kelly J, Hunt BJ, Lewis RR, et al. Anticoagulation or inferior vena cava filter placement for patients with intracerebral hemorrhage developing venous thromboembolism? *Stroke* 2003;34:2999–3005.

75. Offner PJ, Hawkes A, Madayag R, et al. The role of temporary inferior vena caval filters in critically ill surgical patients. *Arch Surg* 2003;138:591–594.

76. Jerjes-Sanchez C, Ramirez-Rivera A, De Lourdes Garcia M, et al. Streptokinase and heparin versus heparin alone in massive pulmonary embolism. *J Thromb Thrombolysis* 1995;2:227–229.

77. Arcasoy SM, Vachani A. Local and systemic thrombolytic therapy for acute venous thromboembolism. *Clin Chest Med* 2003;24:73–91.

78. Goldhaber SZ. Thrombolysis in pulmonary embolism: a debatable indication. *Thromb Haemost* 2001;86:444–451.

79. Goldhaber SZ, Bounameaux H. Thrombolytic therapy in pulmonary embolism. *Semin Vasc Med* 2001;1:213–220.

80. Meissner MH. Thrombolytic therapy for acute deep vein thrombosis and the venous registry. *Rev Cardiovasc Med* 2002;3(Suppl. 2):S53–S60.

81. Ronghe MD, Halsey C, Goulden NJ. Anticoagulation therapy in children. *Paediatr Drugs* 2003;5:803–820.

82. Meyer G, Koning R, Sors H. Transvenous catheter embolectomy. *Semin Vasc Med* 2001;1:247–252.

83. Augustinos P, Ouriel K. Invasive approaches to treatment of venous thromboembolism. *Circulation* 2004;110(9 Suppl. 1):I27–I34.

84. Wen PY, Marks PW. Medical management of patients with brain tumors. *Curr Opin Oncol* 2002;14:299–307.

85. Wong JE. Are patients with cancer receiving adequate treatment for thrombosis? Results from FRONTLINE. *Cancer Treat Rev* 2003;29 (Suppl. 2):11–13.

86. Prandoni P, Lensing AW, Piccioli A, et al. Recurrent venous thromboembolism and bleeding complications during anticoagulant treatment in patients with cancer and venous thrombosis. *Blood* 2002;100:3484–3488.

87. Meyer G, Marjanovic Z, Valcke J, et al. Comparison of low-molecular-weight heparin and warfarin for the secondary prevention of venous thromboembolism in patients with cancer: a randomized controlled study. *Arch Intern Med* 2002;162:1729–1735.

88. Kakkar AK, Levine MN, Kadziola Z, et al. Low molecular weight heparin, therapy with dalteparin, and survival in advanced cancer: the fragmin advanced malignancy outcome study (FAMOUS). *J Clin Oncol* 2004; 22:1944–1948.

89. Pabinger I, Grafenhofer H. Pregnancy-associated thrombosis. *Wien Klin Wochenschr* 2003;115:482–484.

90. Bates SM, Ginsberg JS. How we manage venous thromboembolism during pregnancy. *Blood* 2002;100:3470–3478.

91. Hall JG, Pauli RM, Wilson KM. Maternal and fetal sequalae of anticoagulants during pregnancy. *Am J Med* 1980;68:122–140.

92. Ginsberg JS, Hirsh J, Turner C, et al. Risks to the fetus of anticoagulant therapy during pregnancy. *Thromb Haemost* 1989;61:197–203.

93. Hommes DW, Bura A, Mazzolai L, et al. Subcutaneous heparin administration in the initial treatment of deep venous thrombosis. A meta-analysis. *Ann Intern Med* 1992;116:279.

94. Jacobsen AF, Qvigstad E, Sandset PM. Low molecular weight heparin (dalteparin) for the treatment of venous thromboembolism in pregnancy. *BJOG* 2003;110:139–144.

95. Rodie VA, Thomson AJ, Stewart FM, et al. Low molecular weight heparin for the treatment of venous thromboembolism in pregnancy: a case series. *BJOG* 2002;109:1020–1024.

96. Crowther MA, Spitzer K, Julian J, et al. Pharmacokinetic profile of a low-molecular weight heparin (reviparin) in pregnant patients. A prospective cohort study. *Thromb Res* 2000;98:133–138.

97. Ginsberg JS, Bates SM. Management of venous thromboembolism during pregnancy. *J Thromb Haemost* 2003;1:1435–1442.

98. Dempfle CEH. Mild transplacental passage of fondaparinux. *N Engl J Med* 2004;350:1914–1915.

99. Ansell JE. Optimizing the efficacy and safety of oral anticoagulant therapy: high-quality dose management, anticoagulation clinics, and patient self-management. *Semin Vasc Med* 2003;3:261–270.

100. Chong BH. Heparin induced thrombocytopenia. *J Thromb Haemost* 2003;1:1471–1478.

101. Warkentin TE. Heparin-induced thrombocytopenia: diagnosis and management. *Circulation* 2004;110:e454–e458.

102. Pettilä V, Leinonen P, Markkola A, et al. Postpartum bone mineral density in women treated for thromboprophylaxis with unfractionated heparin or low-molecular-weight heparin. *Thromb Haemost* 2002;87:182–186.

103. Chan YC, Valenti D, Mansfield AO, et al. Warfarin-induced skin necrosis. *Br J Surg* 2000;87:266–272.

104. Eby CS. Warfarin-induced skin necrosis. *Hematol Oncol Clin North Am* 1993;7:1291–1300.

105. Singer DE, Albers GW, Dalen JE, et al. Antithrombotic therapy in atrial fibrillation: the Seventh ACCP Conference on Antithrombotic and Thrombolytic Therapy. *Chest* 2004;126:429S–456S.

# CHAPTER 90 ■ THROMBOLYSIS IN VENOUS THROMBOEMBOLIC DISEASE

STAVROS KONSTANTINIDES AND VICTOR J. MARDER

## PULMONARY EMBOLISM

As described in a recent position statement (1), more than 30 years have passed since the first reports on the use of thrombolytic agents in acute pulmonary embolism (PE). During this time, clinical observations and randomized trials consistently demonstrated the favorable effects of thrombolysis on angiographic, hemodynamic, and scintigraphic parameters of patients with acute PE. However, this evidence has not been translated into a wide clinical acceptance of thrombolytic agents by the clinicians caring for patients with acute PE. In particular, opposition to the use of thrombolysis in patients who are hemodynamically stable and with PE continues to be strong and its arguments quite convincing because they are based on the critical review and interpretation (2–5) of randomized trials. The review of the literature indeed suggests that (a) the hemodynamic benefits of thrombolytic agents compared to heparin anticoagulation alone may be short-lasting; (b) thrombolysis is a potentially life-threatening treatment because of its relatively high bleeding risk; and (c) with the exception of massive PE resulting in cardiogenic shock, thrombolytic therapy for PE does not appear to reduce in-hospital or long-term mortality compared to heparin alone. However, when each one of these important aspects is revisited in the light of recent data, it can be recognized that we have made important steps toward a consensus about the indications for thrombolysis in PE.

### Efficacy of Plasminogen Activators Compared to Heparin

In 1971, Miller et al. observed that streptokinase (SK) infusion for more than 72 hours resulted in a considerable reduction of systolic pulmonary artery pressure, total pulmonary resistance, and the angiographic index of PE severity (6). In comparison, conventional heparin anticoagulation had no appreciable effect on these parameters during the first 3 days. The hemodynamic benefits of thrombolysis were subsequently confirmed in 11 controlled randomized trials that compared various regimens of SK, urokinase (UK), or recombinant tissue-type plasminogen activator (rtPA) (alteplase) with heparin alone (see Table 90-1) (7–18). Most of these trials were small, with patient populations between 8 and 53, and only three included more than 100 patients (7,16,18). Overall, a significant reduction in the extent of thrombotic pulmonary vascular obstruction and pulmonary artery pressure could be achieved promptly (usually within 2 hours) in patients who received thrombolytics (see Fig. 90-1), but not in those treated with heparin alone. The main *clinical* findings of the

thrombolysis trials performed in patients with PE were recently reviewed in an updated metaanalysis (5). The efficacy of thrombolysis (compared to heparin alone) in reducing mortality or PE recurrence was calculated from the pooled data of these studies and is shown in Figure 90-2.

The Urokinase Pulmonary Embolism Trial (UPET), published in 1973, enrolled 160 patients and, with the exception of the Management Strategy and Prognosis of Pulmonary Embolism Study (MAPPET)-3 study published in 2002, was the largest randomized thrombolysis trial in patients with PE. In UPET, urokinase (bolus injection followed by infusion over 24 hours) was superior to heparin alone in resolving pulmonary artery thrombi (7). In some patients, this effect appeared to result in clinical stabilization and reversal of cardiogenic shock. However, during the 2-week follow-up period, overall mortality was not significantly different (7.3% in the urokinase vs. 9.0% in the heparin group), although more deaths in the heparin group were due to the PE, whereas more patients in the UK group died of a bleeding complication; further, the incidence of recurrent PE was only slightly reduced (17.1% vs. 23.1%). Because of these seemingly disappointing results, UPET has been cited as proof that thrombolysis is generally not indicated in acute PE.

In 1993, Goldhaber et al. compared alteplase (100 mg infusion over 2 hours) to heparin alone (16) in 101 patients, using echocardiographic indicators of right ventricular pressure overload and dysfunction to evaluate PE severity. Pathognomonic echocardiographic findings were present in 54% of the patients, but the study did not exclude patients with a normally functioning right ventricle. There was rapid improvement of right ventricular function, as assessed by 24-hour echocardiographic follow-up, and the absence of PE recurrence in the alteplase group, but thrombolysis had no effect on survival, possibly owing to the low (2%) overall in-hospital mortality.

The recently published MAPPET-3 compared alteplase or placebo with concomitant heparin in 256 patients who were hemodynamically stable, but who had evidence of pulmonary hypertension on right heart catheterization and/or right ventricular dysfunction on echocardiography (18). The combined primary endpoint was in-hospital death or need for escalation of treatment, defined as catecholamine administration, secondary (emergency) thrombolysis, endotracheal intubation, cardiopulmonary resuscitation, or emergency surgical embolectomy or catheter thrombus fragmentation. Alteplase reduced the incidence of the primary endpoint from 25% to 11% ($P = 0.006$). Although in-hospital mortality was not considerably different between the alteplase and the heparin-only group, the results suggested that early treatment with alteplase may improve the *clinical* course of selected stable patients with acute PE, and particularly that it reduces the risk of clinical deterioration requiring emergency escalation of treatment (see Fig. 90-3).

**TABLE 90-1**

RANDOMIZED TRIALS COMPARING THROMBOLYSIS WITH HEPARIN ALONE IN PULMONARY EMBOLISM

| Study/Author | Year | N | Inclusion criteria Treatment groups (N) | Diagnosis of PE | Severity assessment | Follow-up (days) | Primary endpoints groups |
|---|---|---|---|---|---|---|---|
| UPET (7) | 1973 | 160 | UK (82), heparin (78) | Angiogram, lung scan | — | 14 | Angiographic reperfusion, hemodynamic (PAP) |
| Tibbutt et al. (8) | 1974 | 30 | SK i.p. (13), heparin (17) | Angiogram | Massive PE | 3 | Angiographic reperfusion |
| Ly et al. (9) | 1978 | 25 | SK (14), heparin (11) | Angiogram | >1 Lobar branch | 10 | Angiographic reperfusion |
| Dotter et al. (10) | 1979 | 31 | SK (15), heparin (16) | Angiogram | ≥1 Lobar branch | 2–5 | Angiographic reperfusion |
| Marini et al. (11) | 1988 | 30 | UK (20), heparin (10) | Angiogram, lung scan | >9 Nonperfused segments | 7 | Lung scan reperfusion |
| PIOPED (12,13) | 1990 | 13 | rtPA (9), heparin (4) | Angiogram, lung scan | >1 Lobar or >2 segmental branches | 7 | Hemodynamic (PAP) |
| Levine et al. (14) | 1990 | 58 | rtPA (33), heparin (25) | Angiogram, lung scan | — | 10 | Lung scan reperfusion |
| PAIMS-2 (15) | 1992 | 36 | rtPA (20), heparin (16) | Angiogram | Miller score >11 | 7 | Angiographic reperfusion, hemodynamic (PAP) |
| Goldhaber et al. (16) | 1993 | 101 | rtPA (46) heparin (55) | Angiogram, lung scan, echo | — | 14 | Echocardiographic (RV function) |
| Jerjes-Sanchez et al. (17) | 1995 | 8 | SK (4), heparin (4) | Angiogram | >9 Nonperfused segments or >9 segments plus RV dysfunction | 3 | Lung scan reperfusion |
| MAPPET-3 (18) | 2002 | 256 | rtPA (118), heparin (138) | Echo, lung scan, CT scan | RV dysfunction | 30 | Clinical (mortality, complications) |

PE, pulmonary embolism; UPET, Urokinase Pulmonary Embolism Trial; UK, urokinase; PAP, pulmonary artery pressure; SK, streptokinase; i.p., administration into the pulmonary artery; PIOPED, Prospective Investigation of Pulmonary Embolism Diagnosis; rtPA, recombinant tissue-type plasminogen activator; PAIMS, Plasminogen Activator Italian Multicenter Study; RV, right ventricular; MAPPET, Management Strategy and Prognosis of Pulmonary Embolism Study; CT, computerized tomography.

Thrombolysis rapidly improves the hemodynamics of patients with acute PE, but its advantages over heparin treatment may be short-lived. Dalen et al. suggested that heparin anticoagulation reverses pulmonary artery hypertension in most patients, although this may require 3 weeks or longer (19). Konstantinides et al. showed a substantial reduction of pulmonary artery pressure and total pulmonary resistance combined with an increase in cardiac output within the first 12 hours after alteplase but not heparin (20). Patients given alteplase also had rapid normalization of the diameter of the right and the left ventricle as assessed by echocardiography. By the end of the first week, however, no difference existed between the two treatment groups in the overall change in the right or left heart chamber dimensions, or the incidence of right ventricular dilation and paradoxical septal wall motion. Therefore, a critical issue is whether the relatively short period of time (1 week or even less) during which the hemodynamic parameters return to normal in patients treated with thrombolytic agents, but not in those who receive heparin alone, can affect the prognosis of PE substantially enough to justify the potential risks of thrombolytic treatment.

## Relative Efficacy of Different Plasminogen Activators

Short-term improvement of angiographic findings, the lung scan, and pulmonary arterial pressure is obtained to an approximately equal degree with tissue-type plasminogen activator (tPA), UK, or SK-plus heparin compared to treatment with heparin alone (21). The greatest benefit is obtained if treatment is initiated within 48 hours of symptom onset (9), but some acceleration of response can be seen in patients treated for up to 2 weeks (22). Studies comparing UK and SK documented equal efficacy for both agents when infused for more than 12 or 24 hours (9,23). When administered for more than 2 hours, tPA achieves more rapid thrombolysis than does a 24-hour infusion of UK (24,25). However, large

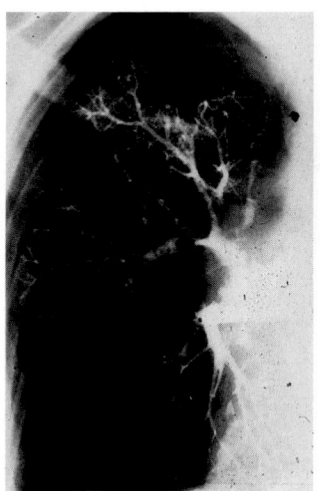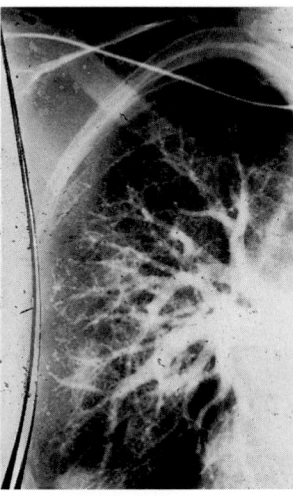

**FIGURE 90-1.** Pulmonary angiography performed before (**left**) and after (**right**) a 12-hour course of intravenous urokinase (UK) therapy. Pretreatment pattern demonstrates filling defects of the right main pulmonary artery as well as occlusion of lobar branches. The post-treatment angiogram showed virtually none of the embolic material.

dosages of tPA and UK administered in an equivalent manner for more than 2 hours produced equal angiographic improvement (26). Similarly, a short infusion of SK (1.5 million U over 2 hours) compared with a 2-hour infusion of alteplase in 66 patients with acute massive PE showed a greater efficacy of alteplase in decreasing pulmonary resistance at the first hour, but equal effects at 2 hours (27). These data suggest that a short course of SK and, by extrapolation, essentially all plasminogen activators, will be equally effective in patients with PE. Similar results were obtained with double bolus reteplase (two injections 30 minutes apart), which showed

equivalent decreases in pulmonary resistance and pulmonary artery pressure compared to tPA administered for more than 2 hours (28). Of note, attempts at short courses of tPA therapy (50 to 100 mg over 10 to 15 minutes) have proved to be no better than the 2-hour regimen (29). Finally, in one trial that compared intravenous (systemic) versus intrapulmonary artery (regional) administration of plasminogen activator (alteplase as bolus plus 2-hour infusion of 50 mg total dose), there was no difference in angiographic outcome (30).

## Bleeding Complications

The risk of life-threatening or disabling hemorrhage associated with thrombolysis is reason for concern. The pooled data from all major thrombolysis trials conducted since 1973 yield a 13% rate of major bleeding complications and a 1.8% rate of intracranial and/or fatal hemorrhage (see Table 90-2), higher than the intracranial hemorrhage rate after thrombolytic treatment of acute myocardial infarction (0.5% to 1.0%) (21,35). On the other hand, data from retrospective cohort studies and registries show an incidence of major bleeding events as high as 36% and that of intracranial/fatal hemorrhage of 4% (Table 90-2). It can be argued that registry data are more realistic (and therefore more alarming) in relation to the true risks of thrombolytic treatment because they reflect everyday clinical practice. However, clinicians may decide to use a thrombolytic agent despite the presence of contraindications, as happened in up to 40% of the patients treated with thrombolytics in the MAPPET registry (36). In any case, the results of both registries and randomized trials highlight the critical importance of carefully defining the indications for thrombolysis in acute PE, particularly in patients who appear hemodynamically stable at presentation. Moreover, the potential for bleeding should discourage the routine use of invasive procedures (e.g., conventional pulmonary angiography) in patients who will receive a thrombolytic agent (37,40).

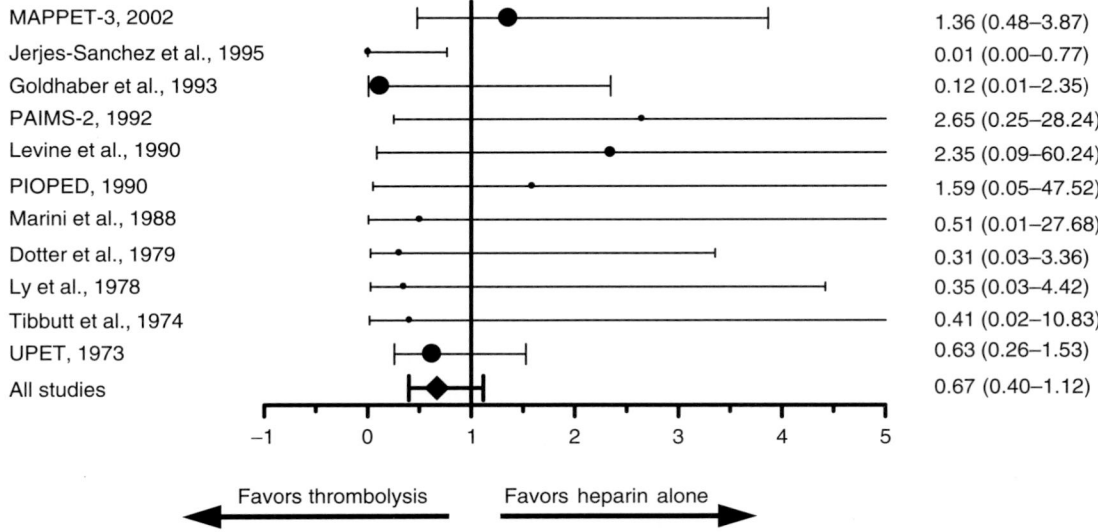

| | |
|---|---|
| MAPPET-3, 2002 | 1.36 (0.48–3.87) |
| Jerjes-Sanchez et al., 1995 | 0.01 (0.00–0.77) |
| Goldhaber et al., 1993 | 0.12 (0.01–2.35) |
| PAIMS-2, 1992 | 2.65 (0.25–28.24) |
| Levine et al., 1990 | 2.35 (0.09–60.24) |
| PIOPED, 1990 | 1.59 (0.05–47.52) |
| Marini et al., 1988 | 0.51 (0.01–27.68) |
| Dotter et al., 1979 | 0.31 (0.03–3.36) |
| Ly et al., 1978 | 0.35 (0.03–4.42) |
| Tibbutt et al., 1974 | 0.41 (0.02–10.83) |
| UPET, 1973 | 0.63 (0.26–1.53) |
| All studies | 0.67 (0.40–1.12) |

Favors thrombolysis ← → Favors heparin alone

**FIGURE 90-2.** The relative risk of death or recurrent pulmonary embolism (PE) with the corresponding 95% confidence interval (CI) in the randomized thrombolysis trials presented in Table 90-1. The size of the black circles corresponds to the size of the trials, only three of which included more than 100 patients (7,16,18). The results suggest an insignificant tendency toward improved recurrence-free survival in patients treated with thrombolytic agents rather than heparin alone. (Reproduced from Wan S, Quinlan DJ, Agnelli G, et al. Thrombolysis compared with heparin for the initial treatment of pulmonary embolism: a meta-analysis of the randomized controlled trials. *Circulation* 2004;110:744–749, with permission.)

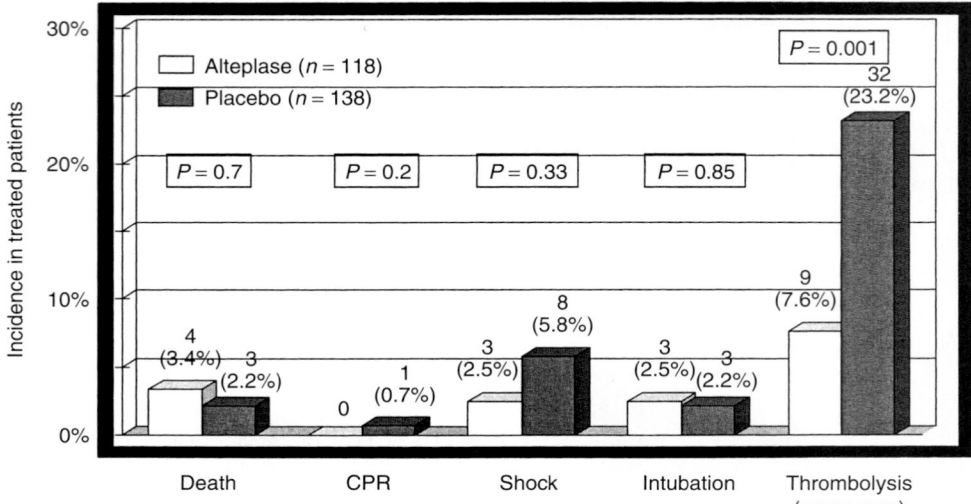

**FIGURE 90-3.** Analysis of the primary endpoint "death or escalation of treatment" in the Management Strategies and Prognosis of Pulmonary Embolism-3 trial (MAPPET). The incidence of the primary endpoint was considerably lower in patients treated with heparin plus alteplase compared to those who received heparin plus placebo (11.0% vs. 24.6%; *P* = 0.006) (18). However, the difference was due to the decrease (from 23.2% to 7.6%) in the need for secondary thrombolysis (cross-over) rather than to a decreased mortality. These results support, but do not prove, the favorable effects of thrombolysis on the clinical course of patients with submassive pulmonary embolism (PE).

## TABLE 90-2

### BLEEDING COMPLICATIONS ASSOCIATED WITH THROMBOLYTIC TREATMENT OF PULMONARY EMBOLISM

| Study/Author (Year) | Study design | Thrombolytic agent | Bleeding episodes (thrombolysis group) | |
|---|---|---|---|---|
| | | | Major bleeding (n/N) | Intracranial/ Fatal bleeding (n/N) |
| UPET (1973) (7) | Prospective, randomized | UK (vs. heparin) | 37/82 | 1/82 |
| USPET (1974) (23) | Prospective, randomized | UK versus SK (no heparin group) | 32/113 12/54 | 0/113 0/54 |
| Goldhaber et al. (1988) (24) | Prospective, randomized | rtPA (2 h) versus UK (24 h) | 1/45 | 0/45 |
| Verstraete et al. (1988) (30) | Prospective, randomized | Intravenous versus intraarterial rtPA | 5/34 | 1/34 |
| Levine (1990) (14) | Prospective, randomized | rtPA (vs. heparin) | 0/33 | 0/33 |
| PAIMS-2 (1992) (15) | Prospective, randomized | rtPA versus heparin | 4/20 | 2/20 |
| Meyer et al. (1992) (25) | Prospective, randomized | rtPA versus UK (noheparin group) | 7/34 8/29 | 1/34 1/29 |
| Goldhaber et al. (1992) (26) | Prospective, randomized | rtPA (2 h) versus UK (2 h) | 16/90 | 1/90 |
| Sors et al. (1994) (31) | Prospective, randomized | rtPA 2 regimens (no heparin group) | 0/53 | 0/53 |
| Kanter and Goldhaber (1997) (32) | Metaanalysis from 5 studies (16,24,26,33,34) | rtPA versus UK (or vs. heparin) | — | 6/312 |
| MAPPET-3 (2002) (18) | Prospective, randomized | rtPA (vs. heparin) | 1/118 | 0/118 |
| **OVERALL (PROSPECTIVE TRIALS)** | | | **91/685 (13%)** | **12/685 (1.8%)** |
| MAPPET (1997) (36) | Registry (prospective) | Various | 37/169 | 2/169 |
| Meyer et al. (1998) (37) | Retrospective | rtPA | 33/132 | 2/132 |
| ICOPER (1999) (38) | Registry (prospective) | Various | 66/304 | 9/304 |
| Hamel et al. (2001) (39) | Registry (retrospective) | various | 6/64 | 3/64 |
| **OVERALL (REGISTRIES/RETROSPECTIVES)** | | | **142/399 (36%)** | **16/399 (4.0%)** |

n, number of patients with major and intracranial/fatal bleeding, respectively; N, number of all patients treated with thrombolytic agents in the study; UPET, Urokinase Pulmonary Embolism Trial; UK, urokinase; USPET, Urokinase-Streptokinase Pulmonary Embolism Trial; SK, streptokinase; rtPA, recombinant tissue-type plasminogen activator; PAIMS, Plasminogen Activator Italian Multicenter Study; MAPPET, Management Strategy and Prognosis of Pulmonary Embolism Study; ICOPER, International Cooperative Pulmonary Embolism Registry.

## The Need for Risk Stratification

### Variable Prognosis

Although PE has been associated with an "unacceptably high" mortality (41), the literature does not overall appear to support this notion. Some studies, which included patients with fulminant PE, did report high mortality rates of 30% or more (36,42,43), but a study performed by the British Thoracic Society to define the optimal duration of anticoagulation in patients with venous thromboembolism reported a mortality of only 1% in the acute-phase of the disease (44). Similarly, the clinical arm of the Prospective Investigation of Pulmonary Embolism Diagnosis (PIOPED) study (13) found that, although overall in-hospital mortality was as high as 9.5% in the study population, death was directly related to the venous thromboembolic event in only 2.5% of the patients. Age and underlying disease were the most important prognostic indicators in the PIOPED series and it was therefore argued that PE is "an unusual cause of death" (45). If this assumption is correct, patients with acute PE would be expected to benefit little, if at all, from thrombolytic treatment in terms of survival. In fact, this appears to be the case in the randomized thrombolysis trials presented in Table 90-1 and Figure 90-2. However, the strict diagnostic criteria and the invasive, time-consuming imaging procedures required to confirm PE in these trials may have precluded the enrollment of patients who are critically ill and unstable. Selection of a low-risk patient population also occurs in clinical practice, in which the patients who are able to undergo diagnostic workup for PE are those who have a more favorable outcome (36). Therefore, patients with acute PE comprise a heterogeneous population whose prognosis needs to be stratified rather than globally determined in order to understand and investigate the potential benefit of thrombolytic therapy.

### Overt Right Ventricular Failure and Hemodynamic Instability in Massive Pulmonary Embolism

McIntyre and Sasahara (46,47) helped establish right ventricular pressure overload and dysfunction as crucial events in the pathophysiology of acute PE. Elevation of pulmonary artery pressure occurs in 60% to 70% of the patients after venous thromboembolism, and its magnitude correlates with the extent and severity of thromboembolic obstruction. In addition, vasoconstrictive factors released from the thrombus, and from the pulmonary vasculature as a reaction to hypoxia, increase pulmonary vascular resistance. Right ventricular dilation and hypokinesis as a response to pressure overload may initiate a vicious cycle of increased myocardial oxygen demand, myocardial ischemia or infarction, left ventricular preload reduction, and inability to maintain the cardiac index and arterial pressure, leading to cardiogenic shock (48). Overt right ventricular failure with hemodynamic instability and cardiogenic shock as a result of *massive* PE are associated with a particularly poor prognosis and mortality rates of up to 65% in the acute-phase (36). As a result, there is consensus (49), even in the absence of large randomized trials (5,17,42), that these patients should be treated urgently with thrombolytic agents or receive some other acute intervention such as emergency surgical embolectomy or catheter fragmentation of centrally located pulmonary emboli.

### Imaging Methods for Detecting Right Ventricular Dysfunction

Risk assessment is most effective if right ventricular dysfunction can be recognized and treated *before* it leads to refractory arterial hypotension and shock. Therefore, attention currently focuses on the subset of patients with acute *submassive* PE. By

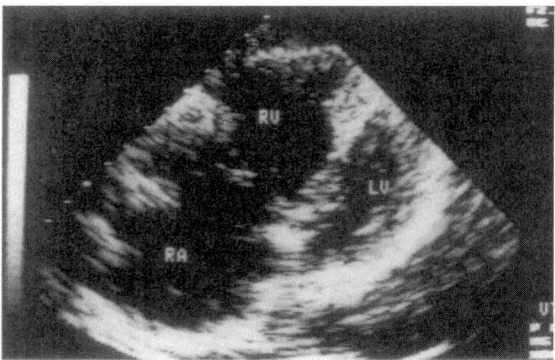

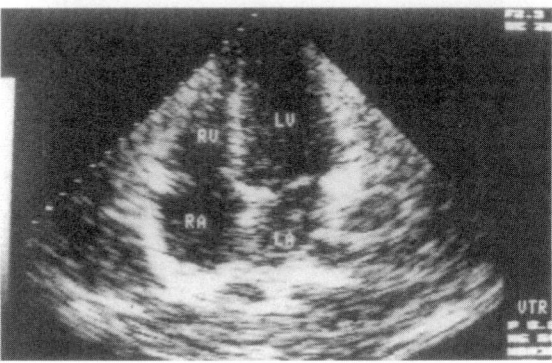

**FIGURE 90-4.** Bedside echocardiography for the assessment of right ventricular dysfunction and response to thrombolytic treatment. **Upper panel:** Massive enlargement of the right ventricle (RV) and right atrium (RA) is shown from the apical view, causing compression of the left ventricle (LV) and left atrium (LA), respectively. The arrows indicate a possible thrombus (TH) in the right ventricular apex. **Lower panel:** Follow-up echocardiography a few hours after thrombolytic treatment shows normal dimensions of the cardiac cavities. (Reproduced from Kasper W, Meinertz T, Henkel B, et al. Echocardiographic findings in patients with proved pulmonary embolism. *Am Heart J* 1986;112:1284–1290, with permission.)

reliably detecting acute right ventricular enlargement and hypokinesis (see Fig. 90-4), leftward septal shift, and pulmonary hypertension (see Table 90-3) (50–54), bedside tranthoracic echocardiography is now established as a powerful tool for diagnosis of right ventricular dysfunction and therefore for risk stratification of PE (50–55). Evidence of right ventricular dysfunction on the echocardiogram predicts a relatively poor in-hospital outcome (mortality between 12% and 23%), even in the presence of normal arterial blood pressure on admission (see Fig. 90-5) (56–59). On the other hand, acute mortality is negligible if cardiac ultrasound reveals the normal function of the right ventricle. In addition to arterial hypotension and shock as independent predictors of mortality in the acute-phase, the significant impact of an abnormal echocardiogram on clinical outcome was confirmed in a large multinational registry of 2,454 consecutive patients with PE (38), and in a prospective registry of 1,001 patients (60). Furthermore, multivariate analysis of the patients who were hemodynamically stable but had an abnormal echocardiogram, that is, right ventricular dysfunction, at presentation, suggested a significant reduction of mortality as a result of early thrombolytic treatment (61).

Limitations of cardiac ultrasound include, apart from the need for an experienced echocardiographer on a round-the-clock basis, the poor quality of tranthoracic imaging which may yield inconclusive findings in some individuals. Reconstructed 4-chamber views of the heart on chest CT scan may, according to recent data, reliably detect right ventricular

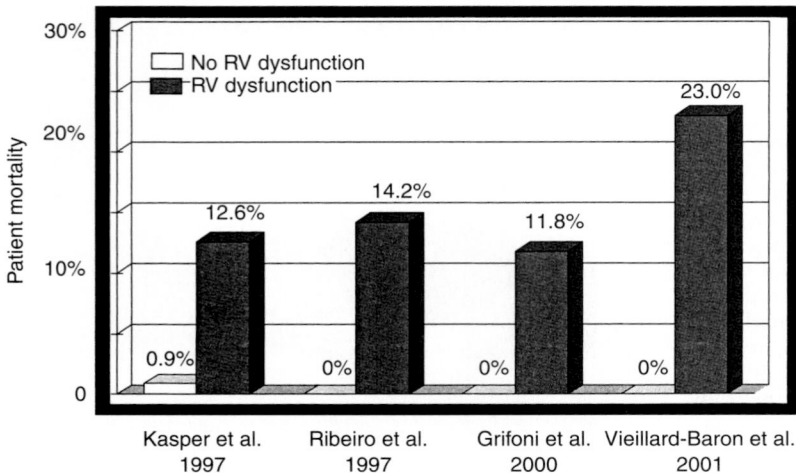

FIGURE 90-5. Overview of four echocardiographic studies of 811 patients with acute pulmonary embolism (PE) (56–59). Although the authors did not use identical criteria for diagnosing right ventricular dysfunction by cardiac ultrasound, all studies reported excellent in-hospital survival rates in patients who presented without right ventricular dysfunction as opposed to those with an abnormal echocardiogram on admission. These results were confirmed by two large prospective registries (36,38). RV, right ventricle.

enlargement due to PE and predict early death (62,63). Therefore, chest CT scan may become a reasonable alternative to echocardiography for diagnosing right ventricular dysfunction (apart from confirmation of PE itself) in institutions with newer-generation, multidetector-row scanners.

Despite the ample evidence supporting the value of cardiac ultrasound in the management of acute PE, only one prospective randomized trial has used echocardiography to assess clinical benefit from thrombolytic treatment in patients with submassive PE (18). In that study, the incidence of the combined primary endpoint (in-hospital mortality or treatment escalation) was considerably lower in patients treated with heparin plus alteplase compared to those who received heparin plus placebo (11.0% vs. 24.6%). However, mortality was low in both treatment groups, and the overall reduction in the need for treatment escalation was driven by the decrease (from 23.2% to 7.6%) in secondary thrombolysis (cross-over; Fig. 90-3). Not surprisingly, this latter finding has been viewed with scepticism by some authors (2,64). Therefore, a larger study using a contemporary inclusion algorithm and a prognostically more relevant combined endpoint (e.g., death or cardiogenic shock) is needed before a definitive statement can be made regarding the favorable effects of thrombolysis on patients with PE who appear clinically stable but have evidence of right ventricular dysfunction at presentation.

## TABLE 90-3

### ECHOCARDIOGRAPHIC INDICATORS OF RIGHT VENTRICULAR DYSFUNCTION

Right ventricular dilation[a]
Right ventricular free wall hypokinesis (global or regional hypocontractility)
Paradoxical septal motion
Pulmonary artery hypertension detected by Doppler flow velocity of tricuspid regurgitant jet
Patent foramen ovale (risk of paradoxical embolism)

[a]Right ventricular dilation is usually defined as right ventricular end-diastolic diameter >30 mm measured from the parasternal short-axis view, or a right ventricle appearing larger than the left ventricle from the apical or subcostal four-chamber view; slight variations of this definition were used by other authors (59).

## Prognostic Importance of Cardiac Biomarkers

Cardiac biomarkers, particularly troponins and natriuretic peptides, which are successfully employed in the diagnostic workup of patients with acute chest pain (65) and dyspnea (66,67), are promising emerging tools for risk stratification of PE. Elevated cardiac troponin I or T levels are encountered in 11% to 50% of patients with acute PE, correlate with echocardiographically detected right ventricular dysfunction, and predict in-hospital mortality or a complicated course (see Fig. 90-6) (68–72). In particular, the negative predictive value of cardiac troponins in patients with confirmed PE is 90% to 99%, implying that a negative troponin I or T test virtually rules out the possibility of an adverse outcome. Brain natriuretic peptide (BNP) and N-terminal (NT)-proBNP levels possess an equal (or even higher) prognostic sensitivity which approaches 100% (73–77). For example, in a population of 124 consecutive patients with proved PE, it was found that a cutoff level of 1,000 pg per mL for NT-proBNP had a high negative predictive value for an adverse outcome, whereas, on the other hand, patients with NT-proBNP 5,000 pg per mL or more, were at high risk for early death or major complications during the hospital stay (78). Taken together, these observations support the hypothesis that

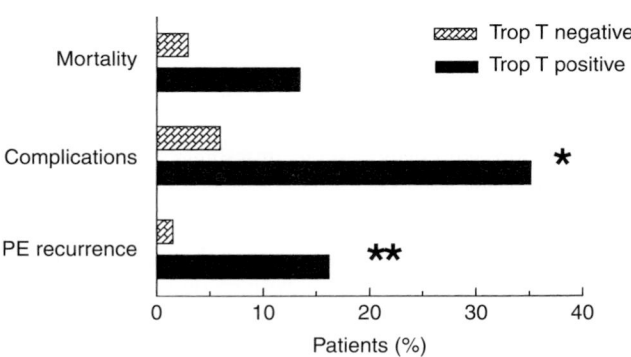

FIGURE 90-6. Higher incidence of mortality, a complicated in-hospital course, and pulmonary embolism (PE) recurrence in patients with cardiac troponin T elevation (defined as troponin T levels ≥0.04 ng/mL) on admission: results of the Management Strategies and Prognosis of Pulmonary Embolism trial (MAPPET)-2 study. *P = 0.02; **P = 0.005. (From Konstantinides S, Geibel A, Olschewski M, et al. Importance of cardiac troponins I and T in risk stratification of patients with acute pulmonary embolism. *Circulation* 2002;106:1263–1268, with permission.)

cardiac biomarkers and echocardiography may complement each other to identify high-risk patients with acute PE (79). For example, the indication for thrombolytic treatment could be rejected in patients with a negative troponin test, or with natriuretic peptide levels below the cutoff values defined in each clinical laboratory, whereas clinically stable patients with elevated biomarkers should undergo echocardiography or chest CT scan and be considered as candidates for thrombolysis if they have evidence of right ventricular dysfunction. Of course, this concept needs to be tested and validated in a randomized therapeutic trial before being implemented in clinical practice.

## Implications of Risk Stratification for Thrombolysis versus Heparin Alone in Pulmonary Embolism

The following management principles can be recommended for patients with clinically suspected PE. Apart from the usual baseline diagnostic tests such as electrocardiogram (ECG), chest x-ray, and D-dimer assay, a screening tool may include cardiac troponin and/or natriuretic peptide tests. Patients who are hemodynamically stable with low clinical probability for venous thromboembolism and a negative D-dimer test can be discharged without further diagnostic workup for PE (80,81). On the other hand, patients who appear critically ill at presentation and those with proved PE and elevated cardiac biomarkers merit a bedside echocardiogram, which provides rapid evaluation of possible right ventricular dysfunction. If this assumption is confirmed, the diagnosis of *submassive or massive* PE is a virtual certainty. Heparin anticoagulation should be initiated promptly, and close monitoring of the patient in an intensive care unit is mandatory. Thrombolytic treatment should be considered, especially at the first signs of hemodynamic instability. If there are absolute contraindications to thrombolysis, or if thrombolysis does not prevent clinical deterioration, mechanical relief by surgical embolectomy or catheter fragmentation is warranted, preceded by emergency pulmonary angiography. Emergency surgical embolectomy may also be indicated if mobile thrombi are found in the proximal pulmonary artery or the right heart cavities, or if they are trapped in the foramen ovale, although evidence suggests that thrombolysis may be a reasonable and safe alternative in such cases (82).

Stable patients with proven PE but with a normal echocardiogram, and particularly those who also have normal troponin or low natriuretic peptide levels, constitute a low-risk group. In these cases, heparin anticoagulation suffices, because emphasis is placed on the treatment of deep vein thrombosis (DVT) and the effective prevention of PE recurrence.

# DEEP VEIN THROMBOSIS

Considering that systemic thrombolytic treatment is indicated for massive PE and probably for submassive PE with right ventricular dysfunction, but not for most patients with non–life-threatening or subclinical disease, it is not surprising that most patients with DVT are managed with an anticoagulant rather than a thrombolytic agent. Consideration of the heightened risk of bleeding incurred by plasminogen activators in comparison with heparin further dampens the enthusiasm for the more potent thrombolytic approach. Yet, thrombosis of the proximal veins of the lower extremity causes significant acute symptoms, the potential for serious PE, and a tangible risk of the postthrombotic syndrome (PTS). Therefore, this subgroup of patients with extensive proximal DVT merits consideration for thrombolytic therapy (81). Additionally, thrombosis of mesenteric veins, upper extremity venous thrombosis, and

cerebral sinus thrombosis represent special circumstances of significant clinical risk, and may benefit from more rapid resolution of vein obstruction by thrombolysis. However, questions (82–84) about the short-term venographic clearance of thrombus, the role of catheter-directed delivery of agent and adjunctive revascularization approaches, and the long-term effects of either the systemic or the regional approach on the PTS remain.

## Systemic (Intravenous) Administration of Plasminogen Activator

There is no question that plasminogen activators mediate lysis of venous thrombi in patients with relatively acute symptoms of 7 days or less, more rapidly and completely than does heparin anticoagulation (85–93). Table 90-4 shows the pooled results of eight randomized trials that compared intravenous infusion of SK or tPA with heparin, using posttreatment versus pretreatment venographic data to assess venous thrombus burden. A marked thrombolytic response (see Fig. 90-7) was attained in 45% of patients treated with SK or tPA, compared with only 10% of patients receiving heparin alone, and twice as many patients treated with heparin had no lysis (78% vs. 38%) (94). This difference is highly significant for reduction in thrombus size using thrombolytic agents ($\chi^2$ for combined results $P <0.000001$). Further, some patients, perhaps up to 10% of those with acute and ongoing thrombosis, have thrombus extension despite ongoing heparin infusion (95), probably the result of inefficient neutralization of thrombus-bound thrombin by the heparin–antithrombin complex (96).

The incidence of bleeding was significantly higher among patients treated with thrombolytics (24.2%) than among patients treated with heparin (11%, relative increase 2.2; $P <0.002$). Major bleeding was observed more often with thrombolytic therapy (13.2% vs. 3.5% using heparin, relative increase 3.8; $P <0.004$). With treatment intervals of up to 7 days, the period of hemorrhagic risk can be prolonged and the incidence of intracranial hemorrhage approaches 1% (97).

The risk of PTS has been clearly linked to prior thrombosis of major deep veins of the lower extremity (98), and even to thrombosis isolated to the calf veins (99), with a cumulative incidence of 27% during the 20 years after the acute event, including 3.7% of patients developing venous stasis ulcers (100). The results of randomized trials of patients with proximal DVT suggest that the incidence of PTS is reduced if complete thrombolysis is achieved, from approximately 40% to 10% (90–92,101–103). Cochrane analysis notes that overall, there is "significantly less PTS in those receiving thrombolysis [risk ratio (RR), 0.66; 95% CI, 0.47 to 0.94], and that

### TABLE 90-4

PLASMINOGEN ACTIVATOR VERSUS HEPARIN FOR TREATMENT OF PROXIMAL LOWER EXTREMITY DEEP VEIN THROMBOSIS

| Agent | Lysis | | Bleeding | |
|---|---|---|---|---|
| | Marked | Moderate | None | Major |
| Plasminogen activator | 45% | 18% | 38% | 13% |
| Unfractionated heparin | 10% | 12% | 78% | 4% |

From Turpie AGG, Levine MN, Hirsh J, et al. Tissue plasminogen activator (rt-PA) vs. heparin in deep vein thrombosis: results of a randomized trial. *Chest* 1990;97(Suppl. 4):172S–175S.

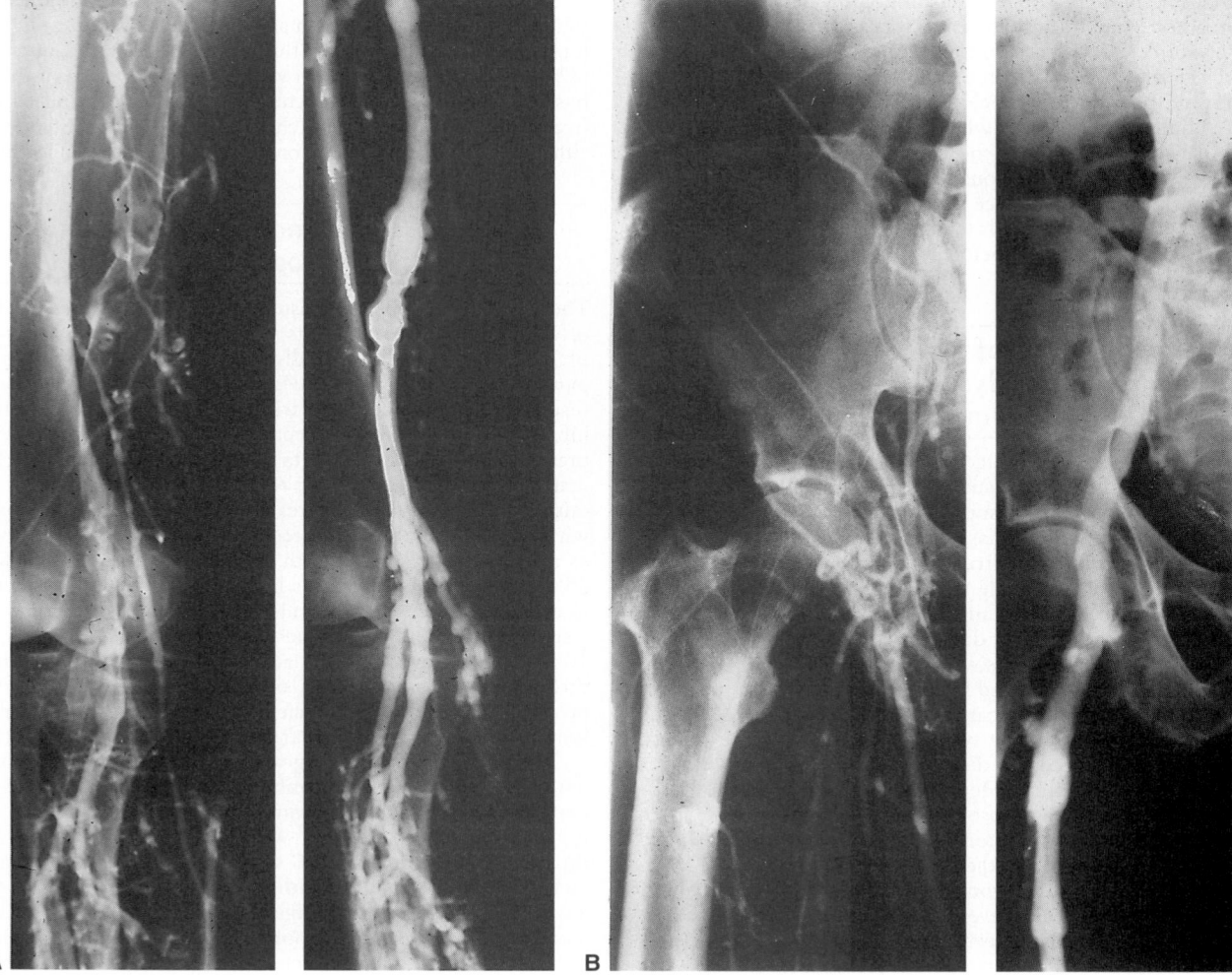

**FIGURE 90-7.** Venograms of left lower extremity before (**left**) and after (**right**) a short (12-hour) course of urokinase (UK) administered intravenously. Thrombotic occlusion of the entire deep venous system of the calf, popliteal area, and iliofemoral veins is apparent prior to treatment, including filling defects in the valves of the superficial femoral veins. The thrombi were completely lysed, as shown by filling of the entire vascular system, including the valve pockets, with contrast material.

leg ulceration is reduced, although the data are limited by small numbers (RR, 0.53; 95% CI, 0.12 to 2.43)" (85). Presumably, the desired clinical result depends upon rapid clot lysis, maintenance of venous valve leaflet function, and prevention of venous hypertension and poor viability of subcutaneous tissues. This is a meritorious outcome when considering the debilitating nature of chronic edema and the risk of recurrent ulcerations that can require hospitalization. Although not life-threatening, this complication of DVT considerably affects the patient's quality of life.

Therefore, thrombolytic treatment of proximal DVT induces more rapid lysis of offending thrombus than does heparin, probably dissolves coincidental PEs that accompany the process, and reduces the occurrence of severe or symptomatic PTS. Still, intravenous plasminogen activator therapy is used infrequently for DVT. The explanation is a reasonable emphasis by the clinician on clinical outcome rather than a radiologic or physiologic result. Although most patients with significant DVT may have venous duplex evidence of obstruction and/or reflux (104), only a few develop severe PTS. Although very few patients dissolve thrombus with heparin anticoagulation alone, rarely does a patient develop a clinically important PE

despite heparin treatment. Because a lethal outcome is rare, careful attention is paid to the risk of hemorrhage, which is considerably greater than that with heparin alone. The relatively benign course of DVT treated with heparin usually convinces the clinician to reserve plasminogen activator only for the patient with proximal thrombus and without risk factors for serious bleeding.

## Catheter-Oriented (Regional) Therapy

Since the mid-1990s, a more aggressive approach to plasminogen activator delivery has used regional perfusion by catheter directly into the venous thrombus. Impressive recanalization rates have been attained, and in anecdotal cases, substantial benefit occurs even in patients with "old" thrombi, that is, in patients with symptoms of more than 4 weeks (105–108). It is likely that such thrombi are resistant to systemic thrombolysis because of inadequate delivery of activator to a fully occluded vessel, a situation that can be overcome by direct catheter delivery of agent to an actually dissolvable thrombus.

## TABLE 90-5

### REGIONAL (CATHETER-DIRECTED) REVASCULARIZATION OF DEEP VEIN THROMBOSIS

| Author | Study type | No. of patients (limbs) | Lytic agent | Vascular patency | | Bleeding | | Stent placed | Mech. device |
|---|---|---|---|---|---|---|---|---|---|
| | | | | Marked | Mod. | Major | Total | | |
| Semba and Dake (108) | Trial | 21 (27) | UK | 72% | 20% | — | — | 52% | |
| Grossman (111) | Review | 263 | | 84% | | | | | |
| Mewissen[a] et al. (112) | Registry | 287 (303) | UK | 83% | 17% | 11% | | 34% | |
| Sugimoto[b] (113) | Retrospective | 89 (93) | tPA, UK | 86%–89% | | 2% | 12% | ? | |
| Grunwald and Hofmann (114) | Retrospective | 74 (82) | UK | 71% | 26% | | | ? | |
| | | | tPA | 66% | 31% | 3%–8% | 10%–17% | | |
| | | | Reteplase | 50% | 50% | | | | |
| Castaneda et al. (115) | Trial | 25[c] | Reteplase | 92% | | 4% | | 52% | |
| Vedantham et al. (116) | Trial | 18 (25) | Reteplase | 83% | | 6% | | ? | 100% |

UK, urokinase; tPA, tissue-type plasminogen activator; ?, not known.
[a]Mewissen: one intracranial hemorrhage (0.4%).
[b]Sugimoto: includes results of both DVT and peripheral arterial occlusion.
[c]Castaneda: of the 25, 14 were lower extremity deep vein thrombosis (DVT), seven upper extremity DVT and four vena caval thrombosis.

The venographic results of this approach have been consistently impressive in relation to the proportion of vessels that show either lysis of thrombus or flow restoration (see Table 90-5). Success is consistently 70% or greater, as shown in one of the first reports of a small study in 21 patients (27 limbs) (106), and often reported as 90% and greater, using all of the tested activators, including UK, tPA, and reteplase (109–114). However, this regional approach is not limited to delivery of the thrombolytic agent, but rather is a mode for a three-pronged therapy, namely, activator infusion, stent placement, and mechanical fragmentation (see Fig. 90-8). Generally, approximately half of the limbs, vessels are treated by stent placement and/or mechanical fragmentation in addition to the initial thrombolytic infusion, the latter usually lasting about 1 day or longer. In the report by Vandantham et al. (116), all patients were treated by mechanical fragmentation in addition to reteplase. This approach is effective for recanalization of thrombosed veins, but precludes a simple comparison with systemic (intravenous) infusion of activator; it is not possible to derive a meaningful understanding of their relative *thrombolytic* success rates with the data that is available.

All of the studies of catheter-delivered therapy have been either unblended or retrospective, so a determination of the risk of major hemorrhage relative to systemic therapy may

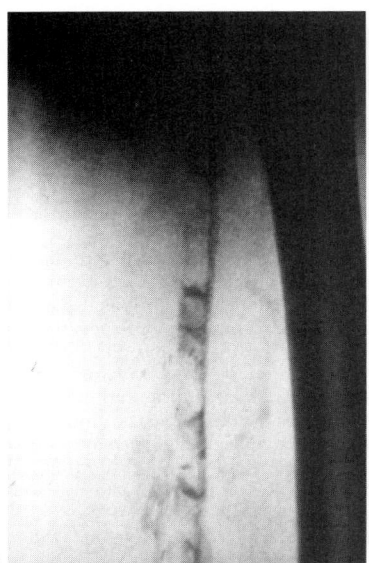
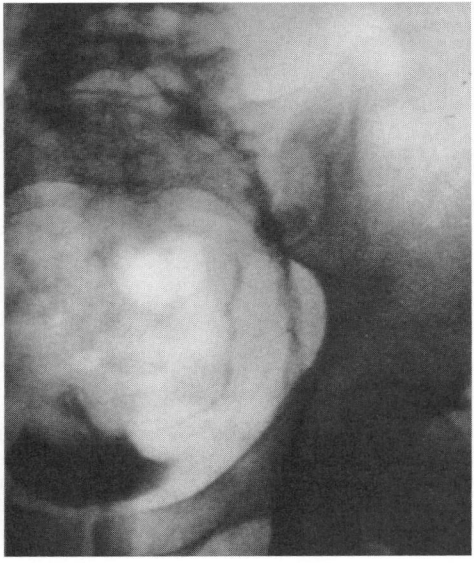

A

FIGURE 90-8. Activator infusion, stent placement, and mechanical fragmentation.

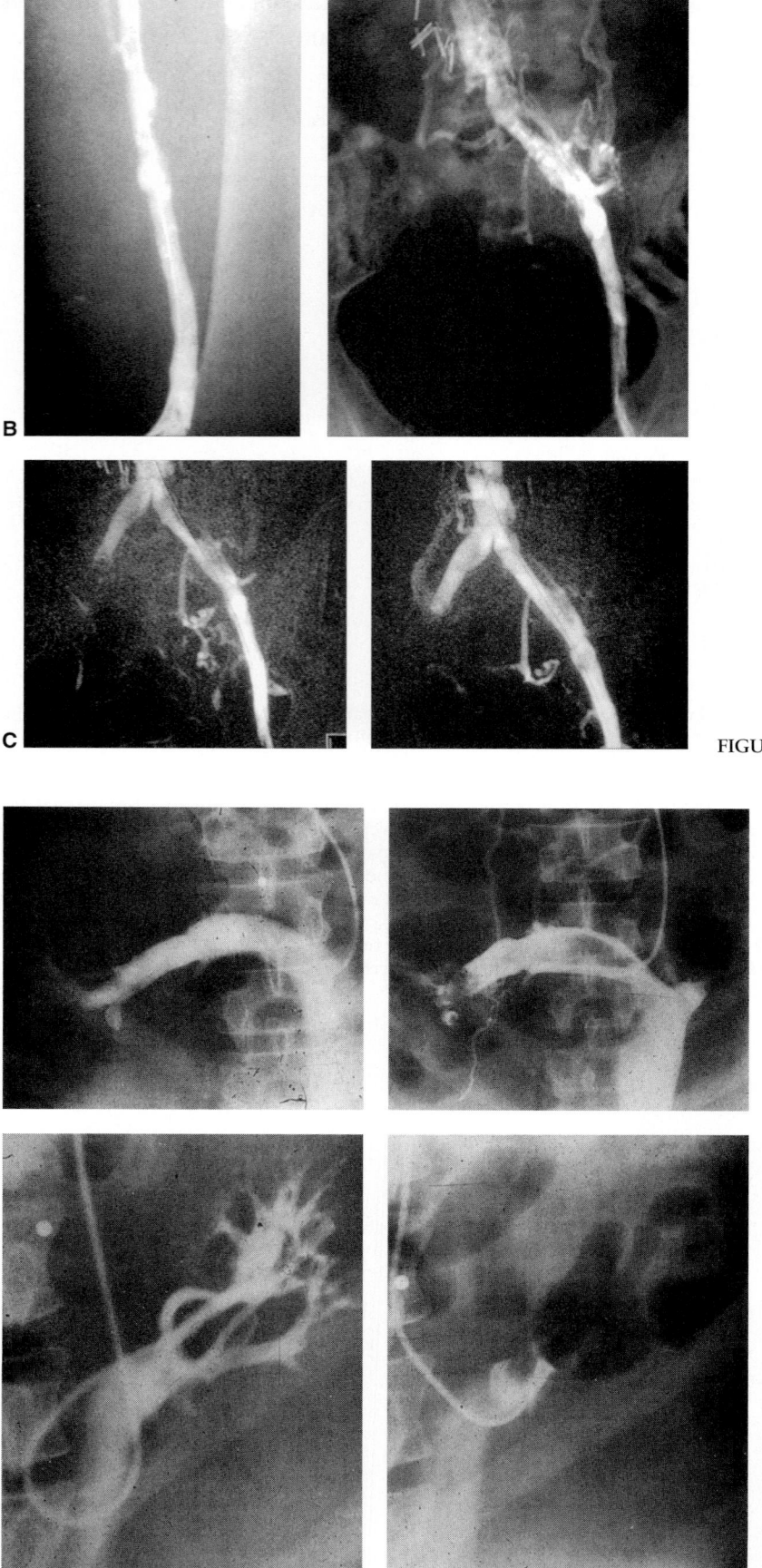

**FIGURE 90-8.** Continued.

**FIGURE 90-9.** Renal venograms before and after thrombolytic therapy for bilateral renal vein thrombosis. The filling defect in the proximal portion of the right renal vein completely obstructs the vessel distally (**top left**); lysis of the thrombus and distal filling is shown after systemic streptokinase (SK) therapy (**top right**). A large thrombus occupies the entire length of the left renal vein (**bottom left**), and this thrombus is completely dissolved after regional infusion of SK and urokinase (UK) (**bottom right**). (From Rowe JM, Rasmussen RL, Mader SL, et al. Successful thrombolytic therapy in two patients with renal vein thrombosis. *Am J Med* 1984;77: 1111–1114, with permission.)

not be possible. In general, the rate of intracranial hemorrhage has been low, cited as only 0.1% by Grunwald and Hofman (112) among "741 limbs" treated with UK, tPA, reteplase, or tenecteplase. This is considerably less than the published experience using intravenous thrombolytic, either long-term for DVT or short-term for acute myocardial infarction, and lower than reported for regional infusions for peripheral arterial occlusions (82,115). Plasminogen activator does circulate even with regional infusion, and intracranial hemorrhage has occurred during catheter infusion of thrombolytic (110), so a much larger experience will be needed to determine if the risk of serious bleeding is indeed less using this approach.

There is a suggestion that venous hypertension and the PTS may be effectively treated by the three-pronged regional approach, perhaps to a greater degree than is attained with systemic thrombolysis. In a small trial of 32 patients, blinded evaluation concluded that valvular competence was better preserved (44% vs. 13%, $P = 0.049$), and venous reflux was present in fewer patients (44% vs. 81%, $P = 0.03$) (116). A quality-of-life survey of 98 patients showed better functioning and fewer postthrombotic symptoms than was the case for patients treated with heparin alone (117). To some degree, any advantage in vein competence might seem to be incongruous for patients subjected to mechanical fragmentation devices, given the evidence of arterial vascular endothelial and medial damage that could predispose to inflammatory or procoagulant reaction (118).

For venous thrombosis at sites other than the lower extremities, the trial data suggest that equally impressive results can be attained in some patients with upper extremity venous thrombosis (113,119–122), although long-term benefit may be impacted by an aggressive underlying cause such as malignancy. Mesenteric and renal venous thrombi (see Fig. 90-9) are also amenable to regional infusion of activator, and cerebral sinus thrombosis may merit this therapeutic approach.

## References

1. Konstantinides S. Thrombolysis in submassive pulmonary embolism? Yes. *J Thromb Haemost* 2003;1:1127–1129.
2. Dalen JE. Thrombolysis in submassive pulmonary embolism? No. *J Thromb Haemost* 2003;1:1130–1132.
3. Dalen JE. The uncertain role of thrombolytic therapy in the treatment of pulmonary embolism. *Arch Intern Med* 2002;162:2521–2523.
4. Dalen JE, Alpert JS, Hirsch J. Thrombolytic therapy for pulmonary embolism: is it effective? Is it safe? When is it indicated? *Arch Intern Med* 1997;157:2550–2556.
5. Wan S, Quinlan DJ, Agnelli G, et al. Thrombolysis compared with heparin for the initial treatment of pulmonary embolism: a meta-analysis of the randomized controlled trials. *Circulation* 2004;110:744–749.
6. Miller GA, Sutton GC, Kerr IH, et al. Comparison of streptokinase and heparin in treatment of isolated acute massive pulmonary embolism. *Br Heart J* 1971;33:616.
7. The Urokinase Pulmonary Embolism Trial. A national cooperative study. *Circulation* 1973;47(Suppl. II):1–108.
8. Tibbutt DA, Davies JA, Anderson JA, et al. Comparison by controlled clinical trial of streptokinase and heparin in treatment of life-threatening pulmonary embolism. *Br Med J* 1974;1:343–347.
9. Ly B, Arnesen H, Eie H, et al. A controlled clinical trial of streptokinase and heparin in the treatment of major pulmonary embolism. *Acta Med Scand* 1978;203:465–470.
10. Dotter CT, Seamon AJ, Rosch J, et al. Streptokinase and heparin in the treatment of pulmonary embolism: a randomized comparison. *Vasc Surg* 1979;13:42–52.
11. Marini C, Di Ricco G, Rossi G, et al. Fibrinolytic effects of urokinase and heparin in acute pulmonary embolism: a randomized clinical trial. *Respiration* 1988;54:162–173.
12. PIOPED Investigators. Tissue plasminogen activator for the treatment of acute pulmonary embolism. A collaborative study by the PIOPED Investigators. *Chest* 1990;97:528–533.
13. The PIOPED Investigators. Value of the ventilation/perfusion scan in acute pulmonary embolism. Results of the Prospective Investigation Of Pulmonary Embolism Diagnosis (PIOPED). *JAMA* 1990;263:2753–2759.
14. Levine M, Hirsh J, Weitz J, et al. A randomized trial of a single bolus dosage regimen of recombinant tissue plasminogen activator in patients with acute pulmonary embolism. *Chest* 1990;98:1473–1479.
15. Dalla-Volta S, Palla A, Santolicandro A, et al. PAIMS 2: alteplase combined with heparin versus heparin in the treatment of acute pulmonary embolism. Plasminogen Activator Italian Multicenter Study 2. *J Am Coll Cardiol* 1992;20:520–526.
16. Goldhaber SZ, Haire WD, Feldstein ML, et al. Alteplase versus heparin in acute pulmonary embolism: randomised trial assessing right-ventricular function and pulmonary perfusion. *Lancet* 1993;341:507–511.
17. Jerjes-Sanchez C, Ramírez-Rivera A, de Lourdes G, et al. Streptokinase and heparin versus heparin alone in massive pulmonary embolism: a randomized controlled trial. *J Thromb Thrombolysis* 1995;2:227–229.
18. Konstantinides S, Geibel A, Heusel G, et al. Heparin plus alteplase compared with heparin alone in patients with submassive pulmonary embolism. *N Engl J Med* 2002;347:1143–1150.
19. Dalen JE, Banas JS Jr, Brooks HL, et al. Resolution rate of acute pulmonary embolism in man. *N Engl J Med* 1969;280:1194–1199.
20. Konstantinides S, Tiede N, Geibel A, et al. Comparison of alteplase versus heparin for resolution of major pulmonary embolism. *Am J Cardiol* 1998; 82:966–970.
21. Marder VJ, Stewart D. Towards safer thrombolytic therapy. *Semin Hematol* 2002;39:206–216.
22. Daniels LB, Parker JA, Patel SR, et al. Relation of duration of symptoms with response to thrombolytic therapy in pulmonary embolism. *Am J Cardiol* 1997;80:184–188.
23. Urokinase-Streptokinase Embolism Trial. Phase 2 results. A cooperative study. *JAMA* 1974;229:1606–1613.
24. Goldhaber SZ, Kessler CM, Heit J, et al. Randomised controlled trial of recombinant tissue plasminogen activator versus urokinase in the treatment of acute pulmonary embolism. *Lancet* 1988;2:293–298.
25. Meyer G, Sors H, Charbonnier B, et al. Effects of intravenous urokinase versus alteplase on total pulmonary resistance in acute massive pulmonary embolism: a European multicenter double-blind trial. The European Cooperative Study Group for Pulmonary Embolism. *J Am Coll Cardiol* 1992;19:239–245.
26. Goldhaber SZ, Kessler CM, Heit JA, et al. Recombinant tissue-type plasminogen activator versus a novel dosing regimen of urokinase in acute pulmonary embolism: a randomized controlled multicenter trial. *J Am Coll Cardiol* 1992;20:24–30.
27. Meneveau N, Schiele F, Metz D, et al. Comparative efficacy of a two-hour regimen of streptokinase versus alteplase in acute massive pulmonary embolism: immediate clinical and hemodynamic outcome and one-year follow-up. *J Am Coll Cardiol* 1998;31:1057–1063.
28. Tebbe U, Graf A, Kamke W, et al. Hemodynamic effects of double bolus reteplase versus alteplase infusion in massive pulmonary embolism. *Am Heart J* 1999;138:39–44.
29. Goldhaber SZ, Feldstein ML, Sors H. Two trials of reduced bolus alteplase in the treatment of pulmonary embolism. An overview. *Chest* 1994; 106:725–726.
30. Verstraete M, Miller GAH, Bounameaux H, et al. Intravenous and intrapulmonary recombinant tissue-type plasminogen activator in the treatment of acute massive pulmonary embolism. *Circulation* 1988;77:353–360.
31. Sors H, Pacouret G, Azarian R, et al. Hemodynamic effects of bolus vs 2-h infusion of alteplase in acute massive pulmonary embolism. A randomized controlled multicenter trial. *Chest* 1994;106:712–717.
32. Kanter DS, Mikkola KM, Patel SR, et al. Thrombolytic therapy for pulmonary embolism. Frequency of intracranial hemorrhage and associated risk factors [comment]. *Chest* 1997;111:1241–1245.
33. Goldhaber SZ, Agnelli G, Levine MN. Reduced dose bolus alteplase vs conventional alteplase infusion for pulmonary embolism thrombolysis. An international multicenter randomized trial. The Bolus Alteplase Pulmonary Embolism Group. *Chest* 1994;106:718–724.
34. Goldhaber SZ, Vaughan DE, Markis JE, et al. Acute pulmonary embolism treated with tissue plasminogen activator. *Lancet* 1986;2:886–889.
35. Levine MN, Goldhaber SZ, Gore JM, et al. Hemorrhagic complications of thrombolytic therapy in the treatment of myocardial infarction and venous thromboembolism. *Chest* 1995;108:291S–301S.
36. Kasper W, Konstantinides S, Geibel A, et al. Management strategies and determinants of outcome in acute major pulmonary embolism: results of a multicenter registry. *J Am Coll Cardiol* 1997;30:1165–1171.
37. Meyer G, Gisselbrecht M, Diehl JL, et al. Incidence and predictors of major hemorrhagic complications from thrombolytic therapy in patients with massive pulmonary embolism. *Am J Med* 1998;105:472–477.
38. Goldhaber SZ, Visani L, De Rosa M. Acute pulmonary embolism: clinical outcomes in the International Cooperative Pulmonary Embolism Registry (ICOPER). *Lancet* 1999;353:1386–1389.
39. Hamel E, Pacouret G, Vincentelli D, et al. Thrombolysis or heparin therapy in massive pulmonary embolism with right ventricular dilation: results from a 128-patient monocenter registry. *Chest* 2001;120:120–125.
40. Stein PD, Hull RD, Raskob G. Risks for major bleeding from thrombolytic therapy in patients with acute pulmonary embolism. Consideration of noninvasive management [see comments]. *Ann Intern Med* 1994;121: 313–317.
41. Moser KM. Venous thromboembolism. *Am Rev Respir Dis* 1990;141: 235–249.

42. Gulba DC, Schmid C, Borst HG, et al. Medical compared with surgical treatment for massive pulmonary embolism. *Lancet* 1994;343:576–577.

43. Alpert JS, Smith R, Carlson J, et al. Mortality in patients treated for pulmonary embolism. *JAMA* 1976;236:1477–1480.

44. Research Committee of the British Thoracic Society. Optimum duration of anticoagulation for deep-vein thrombosis and pulmonary embolism. *Lancet* 1992;340:873–876.

45. Carson JL, Kelley MA, Duff A, et al. The clinical course of pulmonary embolism. *N Engl J Med* 1992;326:1240–1245.

46. McIntyre KM, Sasahara AA. Determinants of right ventricular function and hemodynamics after pulmonary embolism. *Chest* 1974;65:534–543.

47. McIntyre KM, Sasahara AA. The hemodynamic response to pulmonary embolism in patients without prior cardiopulmonary disease. *Am J Cardiol* 1971;28:288–294.

48. Lualdi JC, Goldhaber SZ. Right ventricular dysfunction after acute pulmonary embolism: pathophysiologic factors, detection, and therapeutic implications. *Am Heart J* 1995;130:1276–1282.

49. Task Force on Pulmonary Embolism, European Society of Cardiology. Guidelines on diagnosis and management of acute pulmonary embolism. *Eur Heart J* 2000;21:1301–1336.

50. Come PC, Kim D, Parker JA, et al. Early reversal of right ventricular dysfunction in patients with acute pulmonary embolism after treatment with intravenous tissue plasminogen activator. *J Am Coll Cardiol* 1987;10: 971–978.

51. Jardin F, Dubourg O, Gueret P, et al. Quantitative two-dimensional echocardiography in massive pulmonary embolism: emphasis on ventricular interdependence and leftward septal displacement. *J Am Coll Cardiol* 1987;10:1201–1206.

52. Kasper W, Meinertz T, Henkel B, et al. Echocardiographic findings in patients with proved pulmonary embolism. *Am Heart J* 1986;112:1284–1290.

53. Cheriex EC, Sreeram N, Eussen YF, et al. Cross sectional Doppler echocardiography as the initial technique for the diagnosis of acute pulmonary embolism. *Br Heart J* 1994;72:52–57.

54. Konstantinides S, Geibel A, Kasper W, et al. Patent foramen ovale is an important predictor of adverse outcome in patients with major pulmonary embolism. *Circulation* 1998;97:1946–1951.

55. Goldhaber SZ. Echocardiography in the management of pulmonary embolism. *Ann Intern Med* 2002;136:691–700.

56. Kasper W, Konstantinides S, Geibel A, et al. Prognostic significance of right ventricular afterload stress detected by echocardiography in patients with clinically suspected pulmonary embolism. *Heart* 1997;77: 346–349.

57. Ribeiro A, Lindmarker P, Juhlin-Dannfelt A, et al. Echocardiography Doppler in pulmonary embolism: right ventricular dysfunction as a predictor of mortality rate. *Am Heart J* 1997;134:479–487.

58. Grifoni S, Olivotto I, Cecchini P, et al. Short-term clinical outcome of patients with acute pulmonary embolism, normal blood pressure, and echocardiographic right ventricular dysfunction. *Circulation* 2000;101: 2817–2822.

59. Vieillard-Baron A, Page B, Augarde R, et al. Acute cor pulmonale in massive pulmonary embolism: incidence, echocardiographic pattern, clinical implications and recovery rate. *Intensive Care Med* 2001;27:1481–1486.

60. Geibel A, Zehender M, Kasper W, et al. Prognostic value of ECG, clinical and echocardiographic parameters in pulmonary embolism. *Eur Respir J* 2005;25:843–848.

61. Konstantinides S, Geibel A, Olschewski M, et al. Association between thrombolytic treatment and the prognosis of hemodynamically stable patients with major pulmonary embolism: results of a multicenter registry. *Circulation* 1997;96:882–888.

62. Quiroz R, Kucher N, Schoepf UJ, et al. Right ventricular enlargement on chest computed tomography: prognostic role in acute pulmonary embolism. *Circulation* 2004;109:2401–2404.

63. Schoepf UJ, Kucher N, Kipfmueller F, et al. Right ventricular enlargement on chest computed tomography: a predictor of early death in acute pulmonary embolism. *Circulation* 2004;110:3276–3280.

64. Goldhaber SZ. Thrombolysis for pulmonary embolism. *N Engl J Med* 2002;347:1131–1132.

65. Hamm CW, Goldmann BU, Heeschen C, et al. Emergency room triage of patients with acute chest pain by means of rapid testing for cardiac troponin T or troponin I. *N Engl J Med* 1997;337:1648–1653.

66. Maisel AS, Krishnaswamy P, Nowak RM, et al. Rapid measurement of B-type natriuretic peptide in the emergency diagnosis of heart failure. *N Engl J Med* 2002;347:161–167.

67. McCullough PA, Nowak RM, McCord J, et al. B-type natriuretic peptide and clinical judgment in emergency diagnosis of heart failure: analysis from Breathing Not Properly (BNP) Multinational Study. *Circulation* 2002;106:416–422.

68. Giannitsis E, Muller-Bardorff M, Kurowski V, et al. Independent prognostic value of cardiac troponin T in patients with confirmed pulmonary embolism. *Circulation* 2000;102:211–217.

69. Douketis JD, Crowther MA, Stanton EB, et al. Elevated cardiac troponin levels in patients with submassive pulmonary embolism. *Arch Intern Med* 2002;162:79–81.

70. Konstantinides S, Geibel A, Olschewski M, et al. Importance of cardiac troponins I and T in risk stratification of patients with acute pulmonary embolism. *Circulation* 2002;106:1263–1268.

71. Janata K, Holzer M, Laggner AN, et al. Cardiac troponin T in the severity assessment of patients with pulmonary embolism: cohort study. *BMJ* 2003;326:312–313.

72. Pruszczyk P, Bochowicz A, Torbicki A, et al. Cardiac troponin T monitoring identifies high-risk group of normotensive patients with acute pulmonary embolism. *Chest* 2003;123:1947–1952.

73. Kucher N, Printzen G, Doernhoefer T, et al. Low pro-brain natriuretic peptide levels predict benign clinical outcome in acute pulmonary embolism. *Circulation* 2003;107:1576–1578.

74. Kucher N, Printzen G, Goldhaber SZ. Prognostic role of brain natriuretic peptide in acute pulmonary embolism. *Circulation* 2003;107:2545–2547.

75. Pruszczyk P, Kostrubiec M, Bochowicz A, et al. N-terminal pro-brain natriuretic peptide in patients with acute pulmonary embolism. *Eur Respir J* 2003;22:649–653.

76. ten Wolde M, Tulevski II, Mulder JW, et al. Brain natriuretic peptide as a predictor of adverse outcome in patients with pulmonary embolism. *Circulation* 2003;107:2082–2084.

77. Krüger S, Graf J, Merx MW, et al. Brain natriuretic peptide predicts right heart failure in patients with acute pulmonary embolism. *Am Heart J* 2004; 147:60–65.

78. Binder L, Pieske B, Olschewski M, et al. N-terminal pro-BNP testing combined with echocardiography for risk stratification of acute pulmonary embolism. *Circulation* 2005; (in press).

79. Kucher N, Goldhaber SZ. Cardiac biomarkers for risk stratification of patients with acute pulmonary embolism. *Circulation* 2003;108:2191–2194.

80. Wells PS, Anderson DR, Rodger M, et al. Excluding pulmonary embolism at the bedside without diagnostic imaging: management of patients with suspected pulmonary embolism presenting to the emergency department by using a simple clinical model and d-dimer. *Ann Intern Med* 2001;135: 98–107.

81. Wells PS, Anderson DR, Rodger M, et al. Evaluation of D-dimer in the diagnosis of suspected deep-vein thrombosis. *N Engl J Med* 2003;349: 1227–1235.

82. Chartier L, Bera J, Delomez M, et al. Free-floating thrombi in the right heart: diagnosis, management, and prognostic indexes in 38 consecutive patients. *Circulation* 1999;99:2779–2783.

83. Hirsh J, Hoak J. Management of deep vein thrombosis and pulmonary embolism. A statement for healthcare professionals. *Circulation* 1996;93: 2212.

84. Marder VJ. Thrombolytic therapy: 2001. *Blood Rev* 2001;15:143–157.

85. Wells PS, Forster AJ. Thrombolysis in deep vein thrombosis: is there still an indication? *Thromb Haemost* 2001;86:499–508.

86. Arcasoy SM, Vachani A. Local and systemic thrombolytic therapy for acute venous thromboembolism. *Clin Chest Med* 2003;24:73–91.

87. Watson L, Armon M. Thrombolysis for acute deep vein thrombosis. *Cochrane Database Syst Rev* 2004;18:CD002783.

88. Robertson BR, Nilsson IM, Nylander G. Value of streptokinase and heparin treatment of acute DVT. *Acta Chir Scand* 1968;134:203.

89. Kakkar VV, Flanc C, Howe CT, et al. Treatment of DVT: a trial of heparin, streptokinase and arvin. *Br Med J* 1969;1:806.

90. Robertson BR, Nilsson IM, Nylander G. Thrombolytic effect of streptokinase as evaluated by phlebography of deep venous thrombi of the leg. *Acta Chir Scand* 1970;136:173.

91. Tsapogas MJ, Peabody RA, Wu KT, et al. Controlled study of thrombolytic therapy in DVT. *Surgery* 1973;74:973.

92. Elliot MS, Immelman EJ, Benatar JSR, et al. A comparative randomized trial of heparin versus streptokinase in the treatment of acute proximal venous thrombosis. An interim report of a prospective trial. *Br J Surg* 1979; 66:838.

93. Goldhaber SZ, Meyerovitz MF, Green D, et al. Randomized controlled trial of tissue plasminogen activator in proximal DVT. *Am J Med* 1990;88:235.

94. Turpie AGG, Levine MN, Hirsh J, et al. Tissue plasminogen activator (rt-PA) vs. heparin in deep vein thrombosis: results of a randomized trial. *Chest* 1990;97(Suppl. 4):172S–175S.

95. Porter J, Seaman AJ, Common HC, et al. Comparison of heparin and streptokinase in the treatment of venous thrombosis. *Am Surg* 1975;41:511.

96. Hirsh J, Salzman EW, Marder VJ. Treatment of venous thromboembolism. In: Colman RW, Hirsh J, Marder VJ, et al., eds. *Hemostasis and thrombosis: basic principles and clinical practice*, 3rd ed. Philadelphia, PA: JB Lippincott Co, 1994:1346–1366.

97. Marder VJ, Soulen RL, Atichartakarn V, et al. Quantitative venographic assessment of DVT in the evaluation of streptokinase and heparin therapy. *J Lab Clin Med* 1977;89:1018–1029.

98. Weitz JI, Hudoba M, Massel D, et al. Clot-bound thrombin is protected from inhibition by heparin-antithrombin III but is susceptible to inactivation by antithrombin III-independent inhibitors. *J Clin Invest* 1990;86:385–391.

99. Thrombolytic therapy in thrombosis. A National Institutes of Health consensus development conference. *Ann Intern Med* 1980;93:141.

100. Corrigan TP, Kakkar VV. Early changes in the post-phlebitic limb, their clinical significance. *Br J Surg* 1973;60:808–813.

101. Schulman S, Granqvist S, Juhlin-Dannfelt A, et al. Long-term sequelae of calf vein thrombosis treated with heparin or low-dose streptokinase. *Acta Med Scand* 1986;219:349–357.

102. Mohr DN, Silverstein MD, Heit JA, et al. The venous stasis syndrome after deep venous thrombosis or pulmonary embolism: a population-based study. *Mayo Clin Proc* 2000;75:1249–1256.

103. Goldhaber SZ, Buring JE, Lipnick RJ, et al. Pooled analyses of randomized trials of streptokinase and heparin in phlebographically documented acute deep venous thrombosis. *Am J Med* 1984;76:393–397.

104. Markel A, Manzo RA, Strandness DE. The potential role of thrombolytic therapy in venous thormbosis. *Arch Intern Med* 1992;152:1265–1267.

105. O' Meara JJ, McNutt RA, Evans AT, et al. A decision analysis of streptokinase plus heparin as compared with heparin alone for deep-vein thrombosis. *N Engl J Med* 1994;330:1864–1869.

106. Johnson BF, Manzo RA, Bergelin RO, et al. Relationship between changes in the deep venous sytem and the development of the prostthrombotic syndrome after an acute episode of lower limb deep vein thrombosis: a one-to six-year follow-up. *J Vasc Surg* 1995;21:307.

107. Comerota AJ, Aldridge SC, Cohen G, et al. A strategy of aggressive regional therapy for acute iliofemoral venous thrombosis with contemporary venous thrombectomy or catheter-directed thrombolysis. *J Vasc Surg* 1994;20:244.

108. Semba CP, Dake MD. Iliofemoral deep venous thrombosis: aggressive therapy with catheter-directed thrombolysis. *Radiology* 1994;191:487–494.

109. Vehaeghe R, Stockx L, Locroix H, et al. Catheter-directed lysis of iliofemoral vein thrombosis with use of rt-PA. *Eur Radiol* 1997;7:996.

110. Bjarnason H, Kruse JR, Azinger DA, et al. Iliofemoral deep vein thrombosis: safety and efficacy outcome during 5 years of catheter-directed thrombolytic therapy. *J Vasc Interv Radiol* 1997;8:405.

111. Grossman C, McPherson S. Safety and efficacy of catheter-directed thrombolysis for iliofemoral venous thrombosis. *Am J Roentgenol* 1999;211:39–49.

112. Mewissen MW, Seabrook GR, Meissner MH, et al. Catheter-directed thrombolysis for lower extremity deep venous thrombosis: report of a national multicenter registry. *Radiology* 1999;211:39.

113. Sugimoto K, Hofmann LV, Razavi MK, et al. The safety, efficacy, and pharmacoeconomics of low-dose alteplase compared with urokinase for catheter-directed thrombolysis of arterial and venous occlusions. *J Vasc Surg* 2003;38:411–412.

114. Grunwald MR, Hofmann LV. Comparison of urokinase, alteplase and reteplase for catheter-directed thrombolysis of deep venous thrombosis. *J Vasc Interv Radiol* 2004;15:347–352.

115. Castaneda F, Li R, Young K, et al. Catheter-directed thrombolysis in deep venous thrombosis with use of reteplase: immediate results and complications from a pilot study. *J Vasc Interv Radiol* 2002;13:577–580.

116. Vedantham S, Vesely TM, Sicard GA, et al. Pharmacomechanical thrombolysis and early stent placement for iliofemoral deep vein thrombosis. *J Vasc Interv Radiol* 2004;15:565–574.

117. Ouriel K, Veith FJ, Sasahara AA, for the Thrombolysis or Peripheral Arterial Surgery (TOPAS) Investigators. A comparison of recombinant urokinase with vascular surgery as intial treatment for acute arterial occlusion of the legs. *N Engl J Med* 1998;338:1105.

118. Laiho MK, Oinonen A, Sugano N, et al. Preservation of venous valve function after catheter-directed and systemic thrombolysis for deep venous thrombosis. *Eur J Vasc Endovasc Surg* 2004;28:391–396.

119. Comerota AJ, Throm RC, Mathias SD, et al. Catheter-directed thrombolysis for iliofemoral deep venous thrombosis improves health-related quality of life. *J Vasc Surg* 2000;32:130–137.

120. Casteneda F, Li R, Patel J, et al. Comparison of three mechanical thrombus removal devices in thrombosed canine iliac arteries. *Radiology* 2001;219:153–156.

121. Sakakibara Y, Shigeta O, Ishikawa S, et al. Upper extremity vein thrombosis: etiologic categories, precipitating causes, and management. *Angiology* 1999;50:547–553.

122. Prandoni P, Bernardi E. Upper extremity deep vein thrombosis. *Curr Opin Pulm Med* 1999;5:222–226.

123. Rowe JM, Rasmussen RL, Mader SL, et al. Successful thrombolytic therapy in two patients with renal vein thrombosis. *Am J Med* 1984;77:1111–1114.

# CHAPTER 91 ■ MECHANICAL DEVICES AND EMBOLECTOMY

LAZAR J. GREENFIELD

Mechanical approaches to the management of pulmonary thromboembolism have been used for both treatment and prophylaxis. Operative treatment on cardiopulmonary bypass has been reserved for emergency cases following massive pulmonary embolism (PE) when survival was in doubt (1,2), except for rare cases of chronic pulmonary hypertension that were felt to be amenable to pulmonary thromboendarterectomy (3). For the patient with acute massive PE who is in shock and who is refractory to medical management, embolectomy on cardiopulmonary bypass can be performed with reasonably successful outcomes. However, the magnitude of the procedure carries a significant mortality rate and has prompted a number of less-invasive approaches, including a technique for catheter pulmonary embolectomy (4).

## OPEN PULMONARY EMBOLECTOMY

Pulmonary embolectomy on cardiopulmonary bypass was the natural outgrowth from extracorporeal circulation because external bypass was originally developed to support patients with right heart failure from massive pulmonary embolism. However, a patient with hypotension is not an optimal candidate for general anesthesia and sternotomy, so the operative approach often includes preliminary cannulation of the femoral vessels under local anesthesia to allow for partial circulatory support prior to the open procedure. Candidates for the surgery are usually hypotensive patients who have failed to respond to thrombolytic or mechanical catheter techniques, or who have sustained cardiac arrest and are actively being resuscitated. Once the patient is safely on bypass, the operative procedure usually consists of opening the pulmonary artery for manual extraction of emboli using forceps, balloon catheters, irrigation, and manual massage of the lungs. Emboli that have been in place for several days become adherent to the pulmonary artery and are much more difficult to remove safely. There is a high incidence of complication reported in most series, including right ventricular dysfunction and adult respiratory distress syndrome with or without lethal pulmonary hemorrhage. Reported hospital mortality rates typically exceed 30% (5,6), but some recent reports indicate mortality rates in small series of 8% to 11% (7,8). There has even been a report of a successful embolectomy off-pump using minimally invasive techniques (9).

## CATHETER PULMONARY EMBOLECTOMY

The technique of catheter embolectomy utilizes a cup device attached to the end of a steerable catheter that can be positioned in proximity to the embolus under a fluoroscope. The device can be inserted under local anesthesia through a venotomy in the jugular or femoral vein. Once the position of the cup is confirmed to be adjacent to the embolus by injecting a contrast material, syringe suction can be applied to the catheter to aspirate the end of the embolus into the cup where it is held in position by sustained syringe vacuum (see Fig. 91-1). The entire catheter is then withdrawn with the trailing embolus. The procedure can be repeated as many times as is necessary to restore sufficient pulmonary perfusion to allow vasopressors to be discontinued.

## Indications for Catheter Pulmonary Embolectomy

A number of grading systems for the severity of pulmonary embolism have been developed on the basis of the extent or distribution of emboli within the pulmonary artery on arteriography. The limitation of this approach is that patients vary in cardiac and pulmonary reserve and comorbidities, making physiologic changes more reliable in predicting outcome. The sudden onset of severe dyspnea, cyanosis, and elevated central venous pressure (CVP) with systemic hypotension requires active measures to establish the diagnosis of pulmonary embolism. The most ominous change is in the cardiac output with systemic hypotension refractory to resuscitation. A grading scale (see Table 91-1) that can be used to stratify patients acutely has been developed. Patients with massive embolism have been considered appropriate candidates for catheter embolectomy because of their limited likelihood of survival (2). Early favorable experience encouraged us to extend the indications to include immunocompromised patients with major PE requiring mechanical ventilation because restoration of pulmonary blood flow facilitated weaning from the ventilator (10).

## Results of Catheter Embolectomy

Effectiveness of the embolectomy procedure was judged by increased cardiac output, weaning from inotropic or vasopressor agents, and restoration of hemodynamic stability. In most patients, there appears to be a critical threshold of pulmonary vascular obstruction beyond which effective cardiac output is not possible. This threshold can be recognized during sequential removal of emboli when there is a sudden increase in systemic blood pressure with improved mental status. Mean pulmonary artery pressure can be readily measured and usually declines toward 20 mm Hg as cardiac output increases and as heart rate declines. Repeat echocardiography may also demonstrate improved right ventricular function and reduction in size.

Appropriate patient selection is important to limit morbidity, especially for patients with chronic rather than acute pulmonary hypertension. These patients can be identified by the

1331

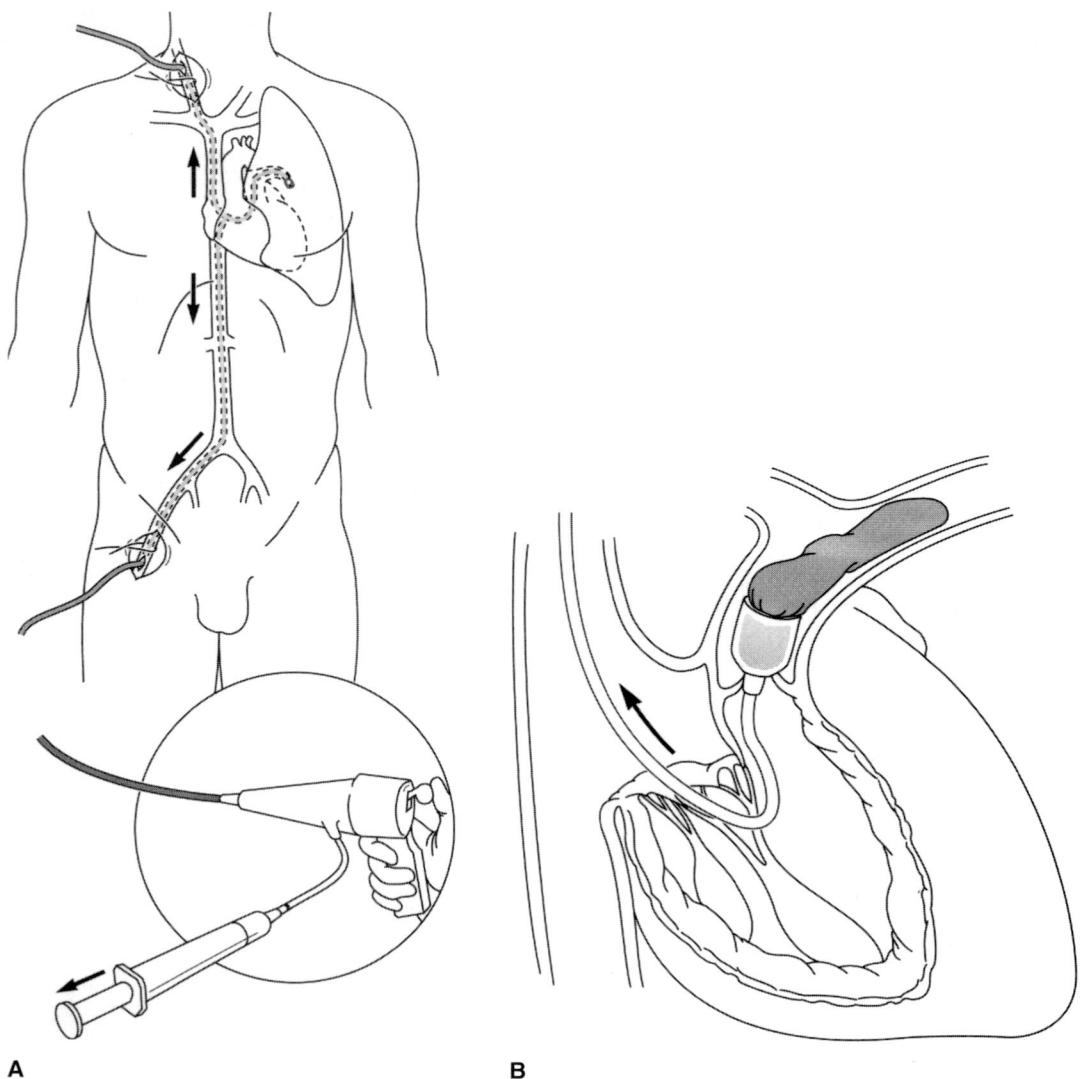

**A**          **B**

FIGURE 91-1. Access for pulmonary embolectomy can be obtained under local anesthesia from the right jugular vein or the femoral vein. The steerable cup-catheter then is positioned under a fluoroscope in proximity to the embolus. Syringe suction is applied to capture the embolus within the cup, which is then withdrawn while syringe suction is maintained. (From Greenfield LJ. Venous thrombosis and pulmonary embolism. *Surgery: Scientific principles and practice*, 2nd ed. Philadelphia, PA: Lippincott, Williams & Wilkins, 1997, with permission.)

presence of mean pulmonary artery pressures in the 40 mm Hg range, which exceeds the limits of a normal right ventricle and usually indicates ventricular hypertrophy from recurrent PE. It is usually not possible to remove chronic thrombus because of adherence to the pulmonary artery wall, and such changes may be observed as early as 72 hours following the initial episode.

In the initial cohort of 46 patients selected for catheter embolectomy, the 30-day mortality was 30%, with a long-term mortality of 46%. The most common cause of death was cardiac arrest during the procedure, which occurred in 6 out of 14 patients. The cardiac arrest was often associated with the injection of bolus contrast material into the pulmonary artery early in the procedure. Results were improved by hand injection of smaller quantities of contrast into select vessels. Two procedural deaths related to the

catheter were also eliminated by change from a metal to a plastic cup. Subsequent mortality was related to heart failure, myocardial infarction, or respiratory decompensation. With improved technology, the technique of catheter embolectomy in patients with major and massive embolism resulted in a 30-day survival rate of 70% (10). However, the requirement for open access to the jugular or femoral vein to perform the procedure limited its applicability to surgeons who were familiar with the technique. The potentially wider applicability of percutaneous techniques made them much more attractive for emergency situations, and the reported experience with these approaches has recently been reviewed (11). None of the approaches have been approved by the U.S. Food and Drug Administration (FDA), and the procedure remains under clinical investigation and is reserved for emergency situations.

**TABLE 91-1**

STRATIFICATION OF PULMONARY EMBOLISM

| Category | Signs and symptoms | PA gases | Occlusion (%) | Hemodynamics |
|---|---|---|---|---|
| Minor | Anxiety Hyperventilation | $PaO_2$ <80 mm Hg $PaCO_2$ <35 mm Hg | 20–30 | Tachycardia |
| Major | Dyspnea | $PaO_2$ <65 mm Hg | 30–50 | CVP elevated; PA pressure >20 mm Hg; responds to resuscitation |
| Massive | Collapse Dyspnea | $PaCO_2$ <30 mm Hg $PaO_2$ <50 mm Hg | >50 | CVP elevated; PA pressure >25 mm Hg; requires pressors, inotropic agents |
| Chronic | Shock Dyspnea | $PaCO_2$ <30 mm Hg $PaO_2$ <70 mm Hg | >50 | CVP elevated; PA pressure >40 mm Hg; fixed low cardiac output |
| | Syncope | $PaCO_2$ 30–40 mm Hg | | |

PA, pulmonary arterial pressure; CVP, central venous pressure.

# PERCUTANEOUS TECHNIQUES FOR PULMONARY EMBOLISM

The mechanisms of action of percutaneous catheter systems include fragmentation, maceration, and aspiration. In general, the success of this approach is based on the greater cross-sectional area of the distal pulmonary vascular bed, which can accommodate fragmented thrombotic material. With improved pulmonary artery blood flow, cardiac output improves, and the greater surface area of thrombus exposed can facilitate the effectiveness of lytic therapy as well. Similarly, the effectiveness of the fragmentation devices can be improved by pretreatment with lytic agents to soften the thrombus, making the two approaches complementary rather than competitive. Balloon angioplasty has also been used to fragment emboli alone or in combination with pharmacologic thrombolysis (12).

## Rotational Catheters

The Kensey device (Dow Corning) was the prototypical rotating-cam catheter, driven at speeds up to 100,000 rpm and originally designed for arterial atherectomy (13). The device created a vortex at the tip that could be used for pulmonary embolectomy experimentally in animals, but no human series has been reported. In arterial use, it was associated with complications of perforation and intimal dissection.

## Jet Vortex Catheters

The Hydrolyser catheter (Cordis Corporation, Warren, New Jersey) is a double-lumen system with the smaller jet component directed at the larger aspirating lumen through a curved metal tube (14). The high-velocity injection creates a Venturi effect, causing fragmentation and aspiration of adjacent thrombi (see Fig. 91-2). The Hydrolyser catheter, as a 7-Fr catheter, can be passed over a guide wire from the jugular vein to selected sites in the pulmonary artery. Only limited clinical experience has been reported suggesting more effectiveness in distal pulmonary arteries than proximal, and only with fresh thrombus (15). The Oasis catheter (Boston Scientific, Natick, Massachusetts) is a similar Venturi-effect device, but has three lumens that allow

simultaneous use of the guide wire, injection, and aspiration portals (16) (see Fig. 91-3). Both of these devices will need increases in size and power to achieve consistently effective pulmonary embolectomy.

The Venturi effect is also used in the double-lumen design of the AngioJet catheter (Possis), but its use of metal tubing for the injection system allows for a high-velocity jet through a curved metal ring directed to the aspirating main lumen. This catheter can be inserted over a guide wire and is available in diameters from 4 to 6 Fr (17) (see Fig. 91-4). Favorable results have been reported in both experimental and clinical studies, but the high-pressure system results in large infusions of saline and similar aspiration of larger volumes of blood (18). This system has also been associated with fatal complications such as pulmonary artery disruption (19). When used in combination with thrombolytic therapy in 10 of 17 patients treated, there were two deaths and a favorable response in 15 patients (20). This therapy can also create small channels in more mature thrombi, thereby improving pulmonary blood flow.

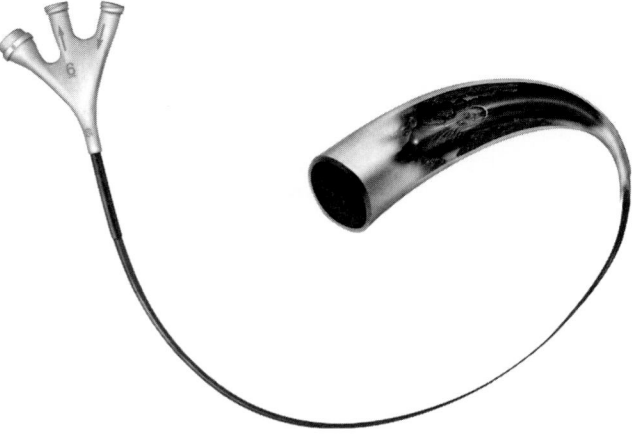

**FIGURE 91-2.** The Hyrolyser catheter (Cordis Corporation, Warren, NJ) uses a high-velocity injection tube to produce a Venturi effect to fragment and aspirate adjacent thrombus. (Manufacturer image, used with permission, © Cordis Corporation, 2004.)

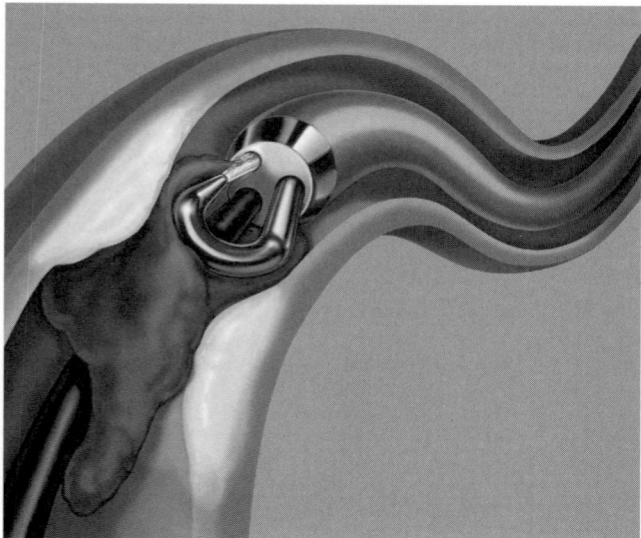

FIGURE 91-3. The Oasis catheter (Boston Scientific) also uses the Venturi effect from high-velocity injection, but also has a third lumen for simultaneous use of a guide wire. (Manufacturer image, used with permission.)

## Impeller Catheter Devices

Another method of thrombofragmentation involves use of a small impeller mounted in the center of a basket device and driven by a wire connected to an external electric motor capable of achieving up to 100,000 rpm (Cook Incorporated, Bloomington, Indiana). The impeller creates a vortex that can pull thrombus into the basket where it is fragmented into small particles. The vessel wall is protected by the basket, as demonstrated in both animal and clinical reports (21).

The thrombolizer and modified impeller catheters are similar in concept. The thrombolizer consists of a rotating 5-Fr catheter within an outer 8-Fr catheter. Longitudinal slits in the end of the inner catheter allow the tip to respond to the centrifugal force of

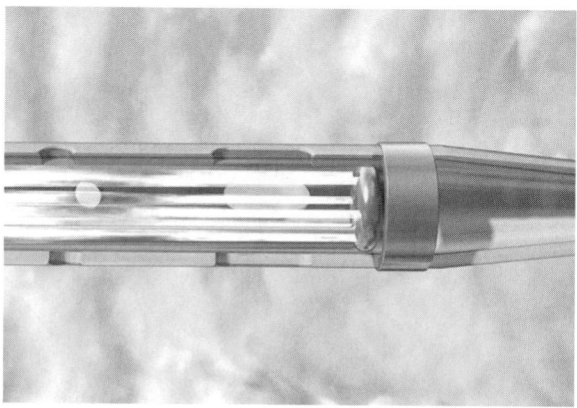

FIGURE 91-4. The Angiojet catheter (6F Xpeedior, Possis Medical, Minneapolis, Minnesota) is a double-lumen catheter that aspirates and macerates thrombus by means of the same high-velocity jet described previously. The aspirated material flows into a collection bag. (Manufacturer image, used with permission, courtesy of Possis Medical, Inc.)

rotation by changing into a basket shape, causing fragmentation of the thrombi. However, the basket is not protected and can come in contact with the vessel wall. Only animal studies have been reported, and these studies suggest that some tissue injury has occurred with evidence of periarterial and peribronchial hemorrhage (21).

The modified impeller device has an 8-Fr outer Teflon catheter with slits in the wall, allowing it to self-expand to 10-mm diameter, and a rotating 5-Fr inner catheter with slits, allowing it to expand to 5-mm diameter when rotating at speeds up to 100,000 rpm. This feature creates an effective vortex and thrombus fragmentation. The device has also been tested in animals, but not clinically (16).

## Rotatable Pigtail Catheter

This is a customized pigtail 5-Fr high-torque catheter (Cook Incorporated) that has a radiopaque tip and 10 side holes for contrast medium injection (see Fig. 91-5). A distal side hole allows the catheter to be placed over a guide wire, and then the pigtail end can be rotated manually or by an electric motor to fragment the thrombus. Effectiveness of this approach has been demonstrated both experimentally and in clinical studies (22) where a 70% success rate was reported in a series of 10 patients. These patients also received thrombolytic therapy with

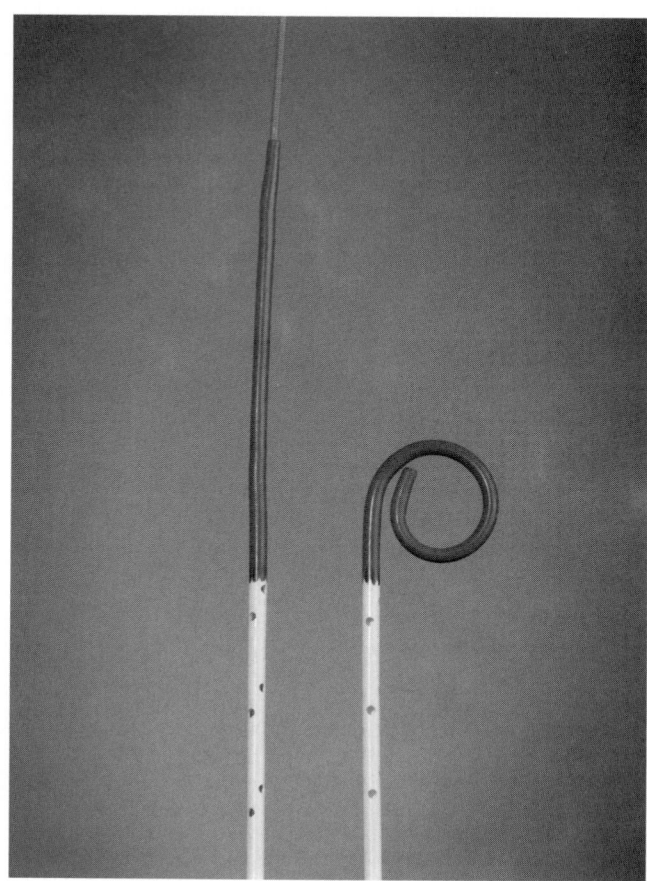

FIGURE 91-5. The pigtail rotary catheter (Cook Incorporated) can be inserted over a guide wire, and then rotated manually or by an electric motor to fragment adjacent thrombus. (Manufacturer image, used with permission.)

recombinant tissue plasma activator (rtPA) and a more recent update of the experience in 20 patients showed a mortality rate of 20%, with 33% recanalization by catheter alone and further improvement with lytic therapy (11).

## Arrow-Trerotola Device

This percutaneous rotational catheter was designed for thrombectomy in dialysis grafts but has been modified for treatment of PE in an animal model. This catheter utilizes a low-speed basket at 3,000 rpm to scrape the wall of the vessel while fragmenting the thrombus (see Fig. 91-6). The nitinol wire basket expands from 9 to 15 mm diameter in a 5-Fr catheter that can be passed over a guide wire. In the experimental study, there was some evidence of intimal injury to the pulmonary artery, but no disruption (23). Use of the device has been reported in one case with marginal improvement (24).

## Amplatz/EV3 Device

The Amplatz/EV3 is also an impeller device within a metal tip housing attached to an 8-Fr polyurethane catheter. Additional side ports behind the impeller allow for recirculation and for further fragmentation of thrombus particles (see Fig. 91-7). An air turbine is used to achieve 150,000 rpm, and saline is infused into the catheter for cooling of the drive shaft. An additional side port on the catheter allows contrast medium injection for visualization of emboli during the procedure. The catheter system is positioned through a 10-Fr guiding catheter

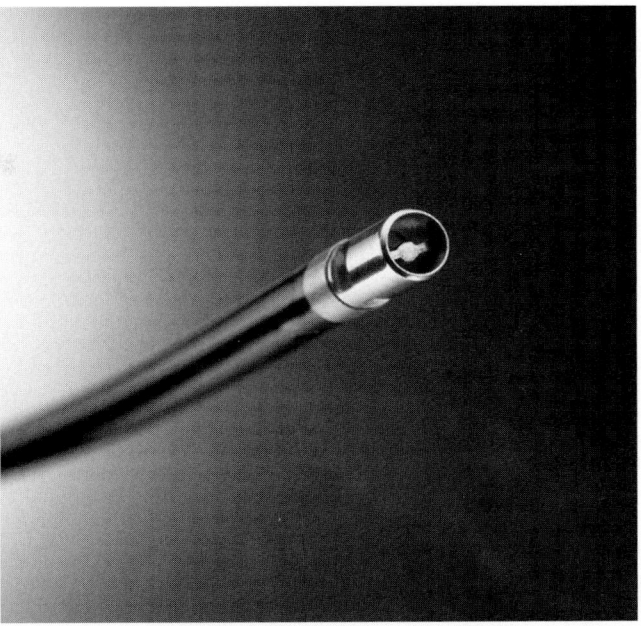

FIGURE 91-7. The Amplatz/Helix thrombectomy catheter (EV3) has an encapsulated rotating impeller powered by compressed air or nitrogen that recirculates and macerates thrombus. (Manufacturer image, used with permission.)

that is placed into the thrombus. Preliminary clinical experience with the device has been favorable, although it is associated with transient hemolysis (25).

## Lang Thrombectomy Device

The Lang thrombectomy suction catheter system is composed of available catheters of varied size. A 16-Fr sheath is used to introduce a 14-Fr Ultratane catheter (Cook Incorporated), which is advanced over a 6-Fr guiding catheter and guide wire. The suction catheter is used to aspirate and propel the thrombus distally, assisted by manipulation of the guiding catheter. It is difficult to interpret the reported experience because it is small and includes treatment with a pigtail catheter, balloon catheter, and urokinase (26).

## Experimental Catheter Systems

A combination aspiration/maceration thrombectomy catheter has been developed by Amplatz (Plymouth, Minnesota) and consists an electrically powered basket rotating at 5,000 rpm inside of a window basket at the tip a 9-Fr double-lumen catheter. Manual suction is applied to aspirate thrombus into the window for maceration and removal. Application of the device in the pulmonary artery in an animal model was limited by the ability to orient the side window and by the age of the thrombus (27).

The Rotarex catheter (Straub Medical, Wangs, Switzerland) is an 8-Fr catheter containing a motor-driven stainless steel spiral moving a steel cylinder with slits, inside which is another cylinder with slits attached to the shaft of the catheter. The spinning cylinder (40,000 to 60,000 rpm) creates negative pressure to aspirate the thrombus and to macerate it where it is transported by the spiral to a port for removal. The cylinder has been found to be capable of removing obstructing thrombus in the

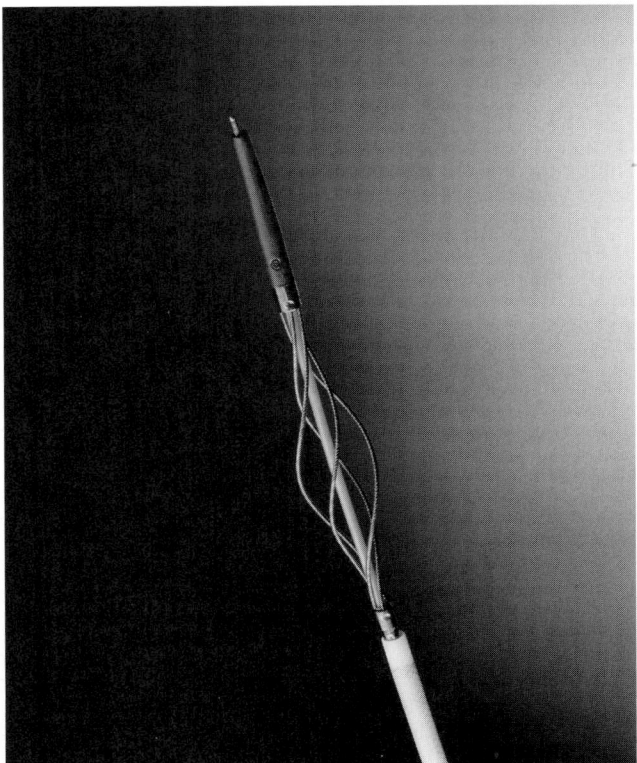

FIGURE 91-6. This rotational catheter (Arrow International, Reading, Pennsylvania) uses a nitinol wire basket at 3,000 rpm to scrape the wall of the vessel and fragment the thrombus. (Manufacturer image, used with permission, Arrow International, Inc.)

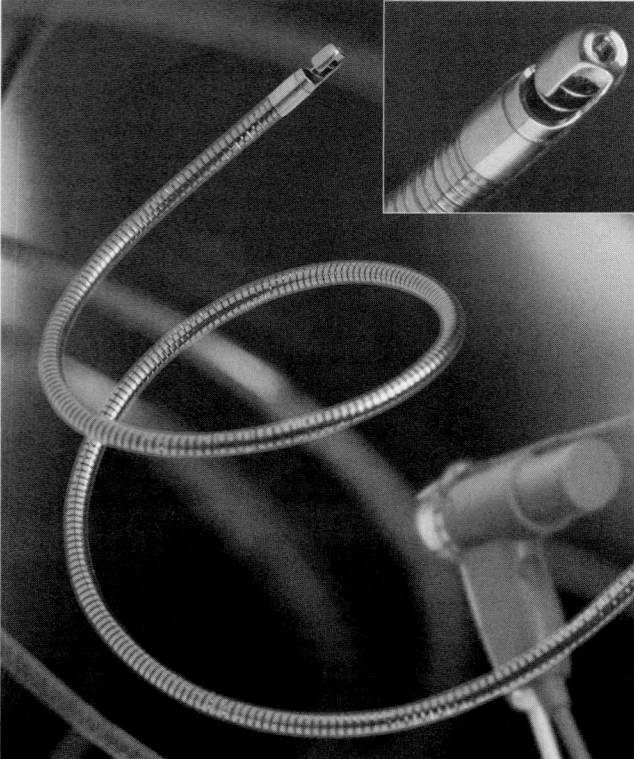

**FIGURE 91-8.** The Aspirex pulmonary embolism thrombectomy catheter (Straub Medical) is shown with an L-shaped suction port (*inset*), internal spiral coil and a guide wire port at the tip. (Manufacturer image, used with permission.)

arterial circulation of an animal model and in an *in vitro* system (28). The Rotarex catheter is not currently available in the United States nor is it recommended for use in the central circulation.

## Aspirex Thrombectomy Catheter

A newer suction catheter system, the Aspirex pulmonary embolism catheter (Straub Medical), has been developed by Kucher et al., which uses wire guidance for catheters 6 to 14 mm in diameter. There is an L-shaped port at the catheter tip within which is a powered spiral coil rotating at 32,500 rpm (see Fig. 91-8). The device has been found effective in experimental *in vitro* and *in vivo* studies in pigs but may require blood replacement for the volumes removed. Clinical studies are being planned. (Findings by Kucher N, Windecker S, Banz Y, et al. Novel catheter thrombectomy device for acute pulmonary embolism. Unpublished data, 2004.)

# STENT USE IN THE PULMONARY ARTERY

For patients in a critical condition with right heart failure and cor pulmonale, the placement of a pulmonary artery stent may be of value. Case reports of the use of both Wallstents (Boston Scientific) (29) and Gianturco Z (Cook Incorporated) stents (30) suggest a beneficial effect in patients who had failed to respond to all other treatment. However, the long-term fate of stents in the thin-walled pulmonary arteries is unknown, and their use in these circumstances should be reserved for life-saving emergencies.

# EXTRACORPOREAL LIFE SUPPORT FOR MASSIVE PULMONARY EMBOLISM

Because the original motivation to develop a heart–lung machine came from Gibbon's experience with a fatal outcome from pulmonary embolism in a young woman, it is logical to consider it as a form of potential management of the disorder. Unfortunately, until recently, it was not possible to support a patient on an extracorporeal circuit for a prolonged period. Advances in the technique of extracorporeal support have now made it possible to extend the use of venoarterial and venovenous bypass for days, making survival possible for patients with reversible pulmonary disorders. A recent report of the use of extracorporeal life support (ECLS) in a series of 15 patients has renewed interest in this approach for patients with massive PE. (Findings by Swaniker F, Hemmila M, Lynch W, et al. Extracorporeal life support for massive pulmonary embolism: Gibbon fulfilled. Unpublished data, 2002.) All the patients were on vasoactive drugs and were acidotic and hypoxic at the time of institution of support. Twelve of 15 patients were in shock despite treatment, and 9 out of 15 patients were in cardiac arrest. Most of the patients were placed on venoarterial bypass (i.e., 13 patients), and the average duration of support for survivors was 5 ± 3 days. Emboli resolved with anticoagulation in 8 out of 11 survivors, and 3 out of 11 survivors underwent operative pulmonary embolectomy. Overall survival rate was 73%, whereas a comparable group of 15 patients referred for ECLS for massive PE, but in whom it was not utilized, had a survival rate of 7% only. For institutions where this modality is available, this support may increase the chances for survival in patients with persistent hypotension from massive PE.

# EXPERIMENTAL APPROACHES TO PULMONARY EMBOLISM

Some experimental approaches to restoring patency to thrombosed vascular grafts, such as thrombolytic brushes, have been demonstrated to cause vessel wall injury, and are not likely to be utilized in arteries or veins. Other approaches such as the use of high-energy acoustic waves as a minilithotriptor may have more promise, when used either alone or in combination with lytic therapy (31). The principle is based on the ability of a transducer to convert electrical signals to ultrasonic motion of a probe, producing cavitation in the area. Preliminary studies suggest that the resulting particulate size is small and that there is minimal vessel wall damage, but clinical trials to date have been limited to thrombosed hemodialysis grafts.

# PREVENTION OF RECURRENT PULMONARY EMBOLISM

Patients who have sustained pulmonary embolism, but who cannot be anticoagulated or who have failed anticoagulant therapy and have had recurrent embolism, are candidates for mechanical protection by placement of a vena caval filter. The most extensive long-term experience is with the Greenfield vena caval filters that have been utilized since 1972. This device provides protection from recurrent embolism in 96% of patients on a long-term basis and retains vena caval patency in 97% of them (32). The advent of percutaneous techniques for filter insertion in the 1980s led to a number of alternative filter designs that have similar effectiveness in

## TABLE 91-2

### SUMMARY OF THE MOST RECENTLY PUBLISHED OUTCOME STUDIES OF MARKETED VENA CAVAL FILTERS

| Source | Greenfield SGF 24F (Greenfield and Proctor, 1995) | Greenfield TGF-MH (Greenfield et al.,1994) | Vena Tech (Crochet et al., 1993) | Bird's Nest (Lord and Benn,1994) | Simon Nitinol (McCOWAN et al., 1992) |
|---|---|---|---|---|---|
| No. placed | 642 | 173 | 142 | 61 | 20 |
| No. monitored | 246 | 113 | 137 | 37 | 16 |
| Recurrent PE (%) | 4 | 4 | 4 | 5 | 0 |
| Caval patency | 96 | 99 | 70 | 97 | 75 |
| Filter patency (%) | 96 | 99 | NR | 95 | NR |
| Insertion-site DVT (%) | 1 | 2 | 8 | NR | NR |
| Migration (%) | NR | 7 | 18 | 0 | 6 |
| Penetration (%) | NR | <1 | 0 | NR | 31 |
| Follow-up period (yr) | 20 | 4 | 6 | 3.5 | 2 |
| Follow-up tests | AP and lateral radiographs Duplex ultrasonography Venacavography | AP and lateral radiographs Duplex ultrasonography Venacavography | AP radiograph Duplex ultrasonography Venacavography | AP radiograph Duplex ultrasonography | AP radiograph Duplex ultrasonography Venacavography |

SGF, stainless steel Greenfield filter; TGF-MH, titanium Greenfield filter with modified hook; PE, pulmonary embolism; NR, not reported; DVT, deep vein thrombosis; AP, anteroposterior.
From Greenfield LJ, Proctor MC. Indications and techniques of inferior vena cava interruption. In: Gloviczki P, Yao JST, eds. *Handbook of venous disorders: Guidelines of the American Venous Forum* 2001. London: Chapman & Hall, 2001:314, with permission.

preventing recurrent embolism in short-term follow-up, but have a higher rate of vena caval occlusion (see Table 91-2). This effect is thought to result from more complexity of design, more disturbance of caval blood flow patterns, and more metal surface area (33). There has also been concern about a report of a higher rate of recurrent deep vein thrombosis (DVT) in patients with vena caval filters on the basis of a 2-year follow-up of patients in a multicenter study of combined heparin and filter treatment (34). The 8-year follow-up in this series, however, did not substantiate the association (35), and other observations confirmed the principle that anticoagulation can be discontinued once the treatment of the underlying DVT is completed. For cone-shaped wire–constructed filters, long-term anticoagulation is not necessary and has not been associated with either a reduction in recurrent DVT or an improvement in the patency of the vena cava (36). Favorable long-term experience with the Greenfield filter has allowed it to be placed above the renal veins (for specific indications) (37) and in the superior vena cava. Most available filter devices work well to trap emboli, but because they differ in long-term patency rates of the vena cava, there has been interest in temporary filter placement (38).

The theoretical appeal of a temporary filter must be tempered by the awareness that the period of risk of PE in patients with venous thrombosis cannot be predicted, that the efficacy of temporary filters in comparison to permanent has not been established; that complication rates of temporary filters in reported series are comparable to permanent filters, if not increased; that patient cost is increased with unknown risk of a second procedure to remove the device; and that the risk of permanent Greenfield filters followed in excess of 20 years decreases with the passage of time. The late filter occlusion rate is 2%, and the only mechanical wear has been isolated limb fracture in 0.01%, with no clinical consequences (39).

## References

1. Doerge HC, Schoendube FA, Loeser H, et al. Pulmonary embolectomy: review of a 15-year experience and role in the age of thrombolytic therapy. *Eur J Cardiothorac Surg* 1996;10:952–957.
2. Lishan A, Christopher SW, Byrne JG, et al. Acute pulmonary embolectomy: a contemporary approach. *Circ J Am Heart Assoc* 2002;105:1416–1419.
3. Jamieson SW, Kapelanski DP. Pulmonary endarterectomy. *Curr Probl Surg* 2003;37:165–252.
4. Greenfield LJ, Kimmell GO, McCurdy WC. Transvenous removal of pulmonary emboli by vacuum-cup catheter technique. *J Surg Res* 1969;9: 347–352.
5. Uilmann M, Hemmer W, Hannekum A. The urgent pulmonary embolectomy: mechanical resuscitation in the operating theatre determines the outcome. *Cardiovasc Surg* 1999;47:5–8.
6. Meyer G, Tamisier D, Sors H, et al. Pulmonary embolectomy: a 20-year experience at one center. *Ann Thorac Surg* 1991;51:232–236.
7. Yalamanchili K, Fleischer AG, Lehrman SG, et al. Open pulmonary embolectomy for treatment of major pulmonary embolism. *Ann Thorac Surg* 2004;77(3):819–823.
8. Aklog L, Williams CS, Byrne JG, et al. Acute pulmonary embolectomy: a contemporary approach. *Circulation* 2002;105:1416–1419.
9. Ashrafian H, Kumar P, Athanasiou T, et al. Minimally invasive off-pump pulmonary embolectomy. *Cardiovasc Surg* 2003;11(6):471–473.
10. Greenfield LJ, Proctor MC, Williams DM, et al. Long-term experience with transvenous catheter pulmonary embolectomy. *J Vasc Surg* 1993; 18(3):450–458.
11. Uflacker R. Interventional therapy for pulmonary embolism. *J Vasc Interv Radiol* 2001;12(2):147–164.
12. Fava M, Loyola S, Flores P, et al. Mechanical fragmentation and pharmacologic thrombolysis in massive pulmonary embolism. *J Vasc Interv Radiol* 1997;8:261–266.
13. Stein PD, Sabbah HN, Basha MA, et al. Mechanical disruption of pulmonary emboli in dogs with a flexible rotating-tip catheter (Kensey Catheter). *Chest* 1990;98:994–998.
14. Reekers J, Kromhout J, van der Wall K. Catheter for percutaneous thrombectomy: first clinical experience. *Radiology* 1993;188:871–874.
15. Michalis LK, Tsetis DK, Rees MR. Case report: percutaneous removal of pulmonary artery thrombus in a patient with massive pulmonary embolism using the hydrolyser catheter: the first human experience. *Clin Radiol* 1997; 52:158–161.

16. Sharafuddin MIA, Hicks ME. Current status of percutaneous mechanical thrombectomy. Part I: general principles. *J Vasc Interv Radiol* 1997;8: 911–921.

17. Voigtlander T, Rupprecht HJ, Nowak B, et al. Clinical application of a new rheolytic thrombectomy catheter system for massive pulmonary embolism. *Catheter Cardiovasc Interv* 1999;47:91–96.

18. Koning R, Cribier A, Gerber L, et al. A new treatment for severe pulmonary embolism. *Circ J Am Heart Assoc* 1997;96:2498–2500.

19. Biederer J, Schoene A, Reuter M, et al. Suspected pulmonary artery disruption after transvenous pulmonary embolectomy using hydrodynamic thrombectomy device. *J Endovasc Ther* 2003;10:99–110.

20. Zeni PT Jr., Blank BG, Peeler DW. Use of rheolytic thrombectomy in treatment of acute massive pulmonary embolism. *J Vasc Interv Radiol* 2003;14:1511–1515.

21. Schmitz-Rode T, Adam G, Kilbingr M, et al. Fragmentation of pulmonary emboli: *in vivo* experimental evaluation of 2 high-speed rotating catheters. *Cardiovasc Intervent Radiol* 1996;19:165–169.

22. Schmitz-Rode T, Janssens U, Schild HH, et al. Fragmentation of massive pulmonary embolism using a pigtail rotation catheter. *Chest* 1998;114: 1427–1436.

23. Brown DB, Cardella JF, Wilson RP, et al. Evaluation of a modified Arrow-Trerotola percutaneous thrombolytic device for treatment of acute pulmonary embolus in a canine model. *J Vasc Interv Radiol* 1999;10: 733–740.

24. Rocek M, Peregrin J, Velimsky T. Mechanical thrombectomy of massive pulmonary embolism using an Arrow-Trerotola percutaneous thrombolytic device. *Eur Radiol* 1998;8:1683–1685.

25. Uflacker R, Stange C, Vujic I. Massive pulmonary embolism: preliminary results of treatment with the Amplatz thrombectomy device. *J Vasc Interv Radiol* 1996;7:519–528.

26. Lang EV, Barnhart WH, Walton DL, et al. Percutaneous pulmonary thrombectomy. *J Vasc Interv Radiol* 1997;8:427–432.

27. Sharafuddin MIA, Hicks ME. Current status of percutaneous mechanical thrombectomy. Part II: devices and mechanisms of action. *J Vasc Interv Radiol* 1998;9:15–31.

28. Schmitt HE, Jager KA, Jacob AL, et al. A new rotational thrombectomy catheter: system design and first clinical experience. *Cardiovasc Intervent Radiol* 1999;22:504–509.

29. Haskal ZJ, Soulen MC, Huetti EA, et al. Life-threatening pulmonary emboli and cor pulmonale: treatment with percutaneous pulmonary artery stent placement. *Radiology* 1994;191:473–475.

30. Koizumi J, Kusano S, Akima T, et al. Emergent Z stent placement for treatment of cor pulmonale due to pulmonary emboli after failed lytic treatment: technical considerations. *Cardiovasc Intervent Radiol* 1998; 21:254–255.

31. Haskal ZJ. Mechanical thrombectomy devices for the treatment of peripheral arterial occlusions. *Rev Cardiovasc Med* 2002;3(Suppl. 2): S45–S52.

32. Proctor MC, Greenfield LJ. Thirty year Greenfield filter experience: are temporary filters needed? Paper presented at: Annual Meeting International Society of Cardiovascular Surgery, Maui, HI, Mar. 23, 2004.

33. Leask RL, Johnston KW, Ojha M. *In vitro* hemodynamic evaluation of a simon-nitinol vena cava filter: possible explanation of IVC occlusion. *J Vasc Interv Radiol* 2001;12(5):613–618.

34. Decousus H, Leizorovicz A, Parent F, et al. A clinical trial of vena caval filters in the prevention of pulmonary embolism in patients with proximal deep vein thrombosis. *N Engl J Med* 1998;338:409–415.

35. Decousus H. Eight year followup of a randomized trial investigating vena caval filters in patients presenting a proximal DVT: the PREPRIC trial. *J Thromb Haemost* 2003;1(Suppl. 1):OC440.

36. Greenfield LJ, Proctor MC. Recurrent thromboembolism in patients with vena cava filters. *J Vasc Surg* 2001;33(3):510–514.

37. Greenfield LJ, Proctor MC. Suprarenal filter placement. *J Vasc Surg* 1998; 28(3):432–438.

38. Offner PJ, Hawkes A, Madayag R, et al. The role of temporary inferior vena cava filters in critically ill surgical patients. *Arch Surg* 2003;138(6): 591–594.

39. Greenfield LJ, Proctor MC. Twenty year experience with the Greenfield filter. *Cardiovasc Surg* 1995;3(2):199–205.

# CHAPTER 92 ■ CHRONIC THROMBOEMBOLIC PULMONARY HYPERTENSION

IRENE M. LANG AND WALTER KLEPETKO

Chronic thromboembolic pulmonary hypertension (CTEPH) is an enigmatic disorder characterized by a failure to resolve extensive pulmonary thromboemboli, leading to severe pulmonary hypertension. Although CTEPH is believed to be a thromboembolic disease, the classical risk factors for venous thromboembolism are absent. The present review provides an update on the current knowledge of pathophysiology, diagnosis, and therapy of CTEPH.

## DEFINITION

CTEPH is believed to result from single or recurrent pulmonary thromboemboli arising from sites of venous thrombosis. CTEPH after a diagnosis of acute pulmonary embolism has been considered rare. A recent review has estimated CTEPH to occur in 0.1% to 0.5% of acute nonfatal pulmonary thromboemboli (1). The natural history of pulmonary thromboemboli is to undergo total resolution, or resolution leaving minimal residua, with restoration of normal pulmonary hemodynamics within 30 days in more than 90% of patients. Repeated catheterizations after acute pulmonary embolism have led to the observation that right heart pressures return to near-normal values in most patients within 10 to 21 days. However, echocardiographic data have indicated that there are more patients with significant persistent pulmonary hypertension after an acute pulmonary embolism than previously reported (2). Recently, Pengo et al. have observed a cumulative incidence of 3.8% of CTEPH as the result of a careful prospective multicenter cohort study with a median observation period of almost 8 years (3). Nevertheless, in large prospective series of patients with venous thromboembolism (4), cases of CTEPH are rare (unpublished observation).

Although CTEPH is understood as a rare outlier disease in the spectrum of venous thromboembolism (see Fig. 92-1), the disease does not share important characteristics of venous thromboembolism, that is, thrombophilic risk factors (5,6) or evidence of deep vein thrombosis (DVT) in the course of the disease, which has led to alternative pathophysiologic theories (7). However, histology shows a striking similarity between organized deep venous thrombi and CTEPH vascular obstructions (see Fig. 92-2).

## PATHOPHYSIOLOGY

### Natural History

The initial thromboembolic event is asymptomatic in most patients with CTEPH (1). For example, 90 of 142 consecutive patients with CTEPH (63%) who were followed at our institution have not experienced symptomatic venous thromboembolism (unpublished data). Therefore, the true incidence of CTEPH may be even higher than what is found in a cohort of patients with symptomatic venous thromboembolism (3). Thromboemboli in patients with CTEPH fail to resolve, and these clots form endothelialized fibrotic obstructions of the pulmonary vascular bed, including the major branches. There is a striking difference in the macroscopic appearance of the thromboembolic material harvested during PEA and the acute pulmonary emboli retrieved during open surgical embolectomy. CTEPH thrombi comprise mostly whitish, organized tissues tightly attached to the pulmonary arterial medial layer, replacing the normal intima (Fig. 92-1, right inset). In contrast, pulmonary emboli are red fragile thrombi that adhere loosely to the pulmonary arterial wall (Fig. 92-1, second-to-right inset). Whereas the initial major vessel red thrombi transform into whitish adherent masses of granulation tissue, high pulmonary vascular resistance (PVR) and slow flow through multiple irregular vascular channels lined with dysfunctional endothelium cause further apposition of fresh red thrombus. Dyspnea on exertion develops after a period of months to years without any clinical symptoms. While clinical deterioration parallels the loss of right ventricular functional capacity, additional changes occur in the pulmonary vascular bed. These changes are histologically indistinguishable from pulmonary vascular lesions found in any other kind of pulmonary vascular hypertension (8) and contribute to a further increase in PVR. The magnitude of these "secondary" changes determines normalization of pressures after successful PEA.

### Pulmonary Hemodynamics

As PVR rises, left ventricular diastolic function deteriorates because of interventricular interdependence and diastolic forward movement of the ventricular septum (9,10). In contrast to acute right ventricular pressure rise, pericardial constriction does not appear to play a role in this process (11). Because of segmental underperfusion, alveolar dead space increases. Finally, right ventricular failure ensues. Hypoxemia becomes exaggerated by a combination of factors including a decline in cardiac output with a fall in mixed venous oxygen saturation, worsening of ventilation–perfusion relations, reopening of the foramen ovale, and development of small pulmonary arteriovenous fistulas in the lungs.

Right ventricular impairment is reversible with decrease of PVR (12). Unilateral disease is rare (13) with unpredictable postoperative outcome. Hemodynamics at rest may be normal in this group of patients.

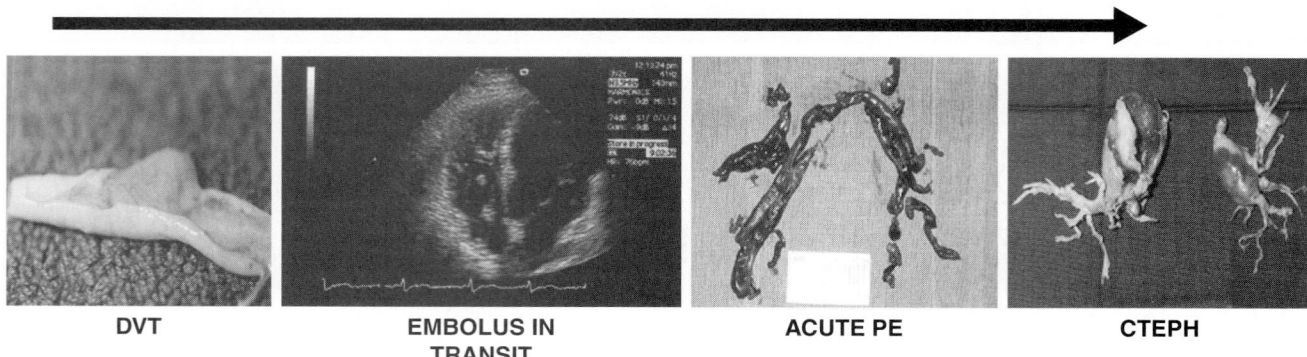

**DVT**          **EMBOLUS IN**          **ACUTE PE**          **CTEPH**
                      **TRANSIT**

**FIGURE 92-1.** Spectrum of venous thromboembolism. The *arrow* illustrates the directionality of venous thromboemboli following venous blood flow from the peripheral venous bed, with the pulmonary arteries as the ultimate landing zone (see Color Fig. 92-1).

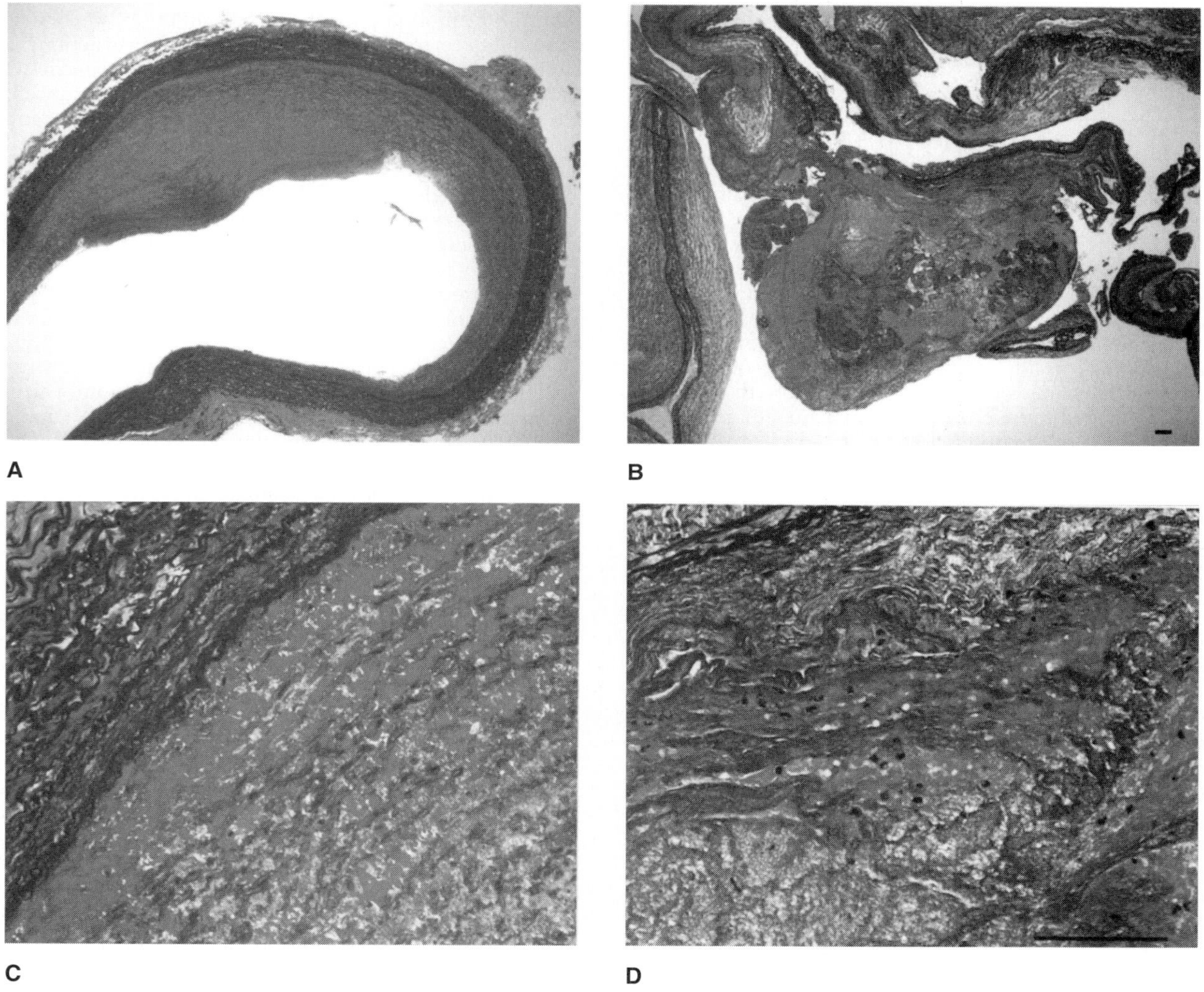

**A**          **B**

**C**          **D**

**FIGURE 92-2.** Trichrome stain of a representative deep venous thrombus (**A** and **C**) and a pulmonary arterial thrombus (**B** and **D**) harvested at pulmonary thromboendarterectomy (PEA). The modified trichrome stain identifies elastic fibers as *black*, collagen as *green*, fibrin as *red*, erythrocytes as *orange-yellow*, and nuclei as *blue-black*. Panels (**A**) and (**C**) show a representative example of a partly organized deep vein thrombus, with panel (**C**) (200-fold) representing a higher magnification of panel (**A**) (40-fold). Panels (**B**) and (**D**) show a representative chronic thromboembolic pulmonary hypertension (CTEPH) thrombus, with panel (**D**) representing a higher magnification of panel (**B**) (200-fold vs. 40-fold). Scale bars represent 100 $\mu$m (see Color Fig. 92-2).

## Coagulation and Fibrinolysis

CTEPH does not share important characteristics of venous thromboembolism [i.e., traditional risk factors involving the coagulation system (1) or systematic evidence of deep venous thrombosis]; this has led to the speculation that CTEPH is not a thromboembolic disease. No abnormalities of coagulation and fibrinolysis have been identified in patients with CTEPH (14,15). Recent data suggest that lupus anticoagulant (LAC), high levels of anticardiolipin, and anti-β2-glycoprotein I antibodies are associated with CTEPH (16). Approximately 10% of patients demonstrate LAC, and there exists a significant association with heparin-induced thrombocytopenia (17). Several studies have demonstrated no increased prevalence of the factor $V_{Leiden}$ mutation in CTEPH (6), but a 10% to 20% frequency of anticardiolipin antibodies (5) has been reported. Combined thrombophilic defects are rare (18).

A recent study has shown that an elevated level of factor VIII greater than 230 IU per dL was more prevalent in patients with CTEPH (39%, $n = 122$) than in patients with PAH (20%, $P = 0.042$, $n = 88$) and controls (5%, $P <0.0001$, $n = 82$) (19). The prevalence of factor VIII levels greater than 150 IU per dL was 87% in patients with CTEPH, 56% in patients with nonthromboembolic pulmonary hypertension, and 13% in controls. Factor VIII ($233 \pm 83$ IU per dL) and VWF:Ag (von Willebrand factor antigen) ($261 \pm 130$ IU per dL) plasma levels were higher in patients with CTEPH than in patients with nonthromboembolic pulmonary hypertension (factor VIII: $158 \pm 61$ IU per dL, $P <0.0001$; VWF:Ag: $204 \pm 107$ IU per dL, $P <0.05$) and controls (factor VIII: $123 \pm 40$ IU per dL, $P <0.05$; VWF:Ag: $132 \pm 48$ IU per dL, $P <0.05$) after adjusting for the covariates, age and sex. These data were confirmed by antigen measurements. The calculated theoretical odds ratio for the development of CTEPH was 13.6 for subjects with plasma factor VIII levels greater than 200 IU per dL. The plasma level of factor VIII was not correlated with any hemodynamic variable. Mean factor VIII ($212 \pm 94$ IU per dL) and VWF:Ag ($213 \pm 81$ IU per dL) levels were statistically unchanged 1 year after surgery when compared with preoperative values (factor VIII: $226 \pm 88$ IU per dL, VWF:Ag: $271 \pm 162$ IU per dL). In contrast to reports from patients with nonthromboembolic pulmonary hypertension (20), HMW (high molecular weight) multimers were preserved in preoperative and postoperative plasma samples of patients presenting with CTEPH, and multimeric distribution did not differ from healthy control samples assayed in parallel. VWF-cleaving protease activity that is responsible for multimeric distribution was within the normal range ($117\% \pm 48\%$) and was unchanged after surgery ($131\% \pm 28\%$, $P = 0.39$).

## Chronic Thromboembolic Pulmonary Hypertension and Associated Conditions

Most patients with CTEPH were found to have a history of deep venous thrombosis when carefully questioned. Venous thromboembolism can be documented in 61% of patients, and evidence for recurrence is present in approximately 34% (unpublished data). Still, a large group of patients lack signs of prior DVT at the time of diagnosis (14).

Case reports have suggested a link between chronic thromboembolism and prior splenectomy (21–23), ventriculoatrial (VA) shunt for the treatment of hydrocephalus (24–30), or chronic inflammatory conditions (31).

Apart from these observations, association of CTEPH with pacemaker leads, sickle cell disease (32), hereditary stomatocytosis (33), and Klippel-Trenaunay-Weber syndrome (34) have been described.

## Genetics of Chronic Thromboembolic Pulmonary Hypertension

Because of the finding of elevated levels of VWF in patients with CTEPH and the fact that blood group oligosaccharide structures on the VWF molecule account for the clearance and plasma levels of the factor VIII/VWF complex (35), the blood group distribution among patients with CTEPH was analyzed. Blood groups non-0 were more prevalent in patients with CTEPH (82%) than in patients with PAH (56%, $P <0.05$), or in the Middle European population (approximately 60%). Despite this suggestion of a genetic predisposition, evidence is lacking that CTEPH occurs in a familial pattern. Nevertheless, no mutation of the BMPRII (bone morphogenic protein receptor II) gene has yet been identified in a patient with CTEPH.

## Animal Models

The difficulty of inducing CTEPH by repeated release of preformed clots from the inferior vena cava of mongrel dogs (36) was explained by analyzing biochemical factors contributing to increased vascular fibrinolytic activity in these animals (37). It was found that high plasma levels of urokinase plasminogen activator (uPA) activity are present in this species (38). Furthermore, uPA is associated with canine platelets and mediates rapid clot lysis.

## Cell Biology of Pulmonary Artery and Pulmonary Arterial Thromboemboli— Molecular Dissection of the Vascular Remodeling Associated with Acute Pulmonary Thromboembolism

Under the assumption that CTEPH thrombi result from the embolization of thrombi to the pulmonary vasculature, we designed experiments to understand the regulation of fibrinolytic genes in the first hours after a fatal pulmonary embolism. Because previous data suggest that the balance between plasminogen activators (PAs) and type 1 plasminogen activator inhibitor (PAI-1) plays a role in regulating cell migration within the extracellular matrix, we investigated the expression of these molecules by immunohistochemical and *in situ* hybridization analysis of pulmonary artery specimens from patients suffering fatal pulmonary embolism. The data were compared with the expression of these molecules in both the noninvolved pulmonary arteries and organ donor pulmonary arteries of the patients. Regions of initial organization and vascular remodeling were identified by a modified trichrome stain and by the presence of proliferating cell nuclear antigen (PCNA), a cell cycle molecule used as a marker of proliferation. Staining for tissue-type PA antigen was low to undetectable in endothelial cells directly in contact with the fibrin–platelet thromboembolus and in areas in which the endothelial cell lining was replaced by cell growth into the thrombus. uPA expression was detected in mononuclear cells within the thrombus in the initial phase of thromboembolism and within cells migrating into the thrombus during the later stages of organization. PAI-1 expression was elevated in the monolayer of endothelial cells underlying the fresh fibrin–platelet thromboembolus and in a PCNA-positive cell population present between the pulmonary arterial intima and the thromboembolus that represents early organization. Increased expression of PAI-1 may play a role in inhibiting proteolysis and in fostering the localization of the acute fibrin–platelet thrombus to the vascular wall, which is followed by the upregulation of uPA in migrating cells during the reorganization process.

Recent research has focused on local gene expression within pulmonary arterial thromboemboli and pulmonary arteries from patients with CTEPH. By a candidate gene approach utilizing *in situ* techniques, increased expression of PAI-1 was found in small thrombus neovessels, thereby potentially promoting small-vessel thrombosis and thrombus growth from within (39). On the other hand, elevated PAI-1 gene expression was also identified at a specific stage in the natural course of organization of acute pulmonary thromboemboli (40). This analysis of patterns of gene expression during the vascular remodeling that is associated with the organization of acute pulmonary thromboemboli has shed new light on the events leading to restoration of normal pulmonary blood flow after venous thromboembolism. One hypothesis emerging from these studies is that, by a mechanism yet to be defined, deep venous thrombi undergo extensive organization in the vascular compartment of the deep femoral and pelvic veins. When such thrombi are embolized, even well-functioning mechanisms of fibrinolysis and thrombolysis do not suffice to remove these organized materials, thereby leading to CTEPH. In other studies, the expression of a potent inhibitor of factor IXa and factor XIa [i.e., protease nexin-2 (PN2)/amyloid $\beta$-protein precursor (A $\beta$ PP)] was demonstrated in the organized vascular occlusions harvested from patients with this disease (41). Clot vessel hemorrhage is a feature of CTEPH thrombus histology, and it is speculated to be a powerful stimulator for angiogenesis. In fact, recent studies have correlated the pulmonary expression of angiogenetic molecules with CTEPH severity (42).

---

### Expression of Angiogenic Growth Factors Within Chronic Nonresolving Pulmonary Thromboemboli—Defining Basic Mechanisms Involved in the Remodeling of Atherosclerotic Tissues and Chronic Pulmonary Thromboemboli

To test the hypothesis that mechanisms of vascular remodeling as observed in systemic arteries are underlying the chronic expansion of nonresolving pulmonary thromboemboli, a gene expression–analysis approach was taken. Although a clear distinction between predominantly proliferative and regressive lesions can be made in coronary artery lesions, growth patterns varied within a single chronic thromboembolus. Most cells were undergoing apoptosis by morphology and positive immunoreactivity with a TUNEL (terminal deoxynucleotidyl transferase–mediated dUTP-biotin end labeling of fragmented DNA) stain. In addition, areas with numerous PCNA-positive cells were found, colocalizing with neovessels and stellate smooth muscle cells that were morphologically similar to neointimal smooth muscle cells of coronary plaques. Second, candidate angiogenic growth factors were analyzed by immunohistochemistry. Intense immunoreactivities for bFGF (basic fibroblast growth factor) and platelet-derived endothelial cell growth factor were detected. Vast extracellular deposits of a protein cross-reacting with monospecific antibodies directed against transforming growth factor (TGF) $\beta1$–3 protein were identified. Because lipoprotein (a) can interfere with the colocalization of plasmin activity and hence the activation of TGF-$\beta$, we extended our analysis of growth factors to include this molecule. Extracellular deposits of lipoprotein (a) were present around vascular lumen in thromboembolic specimens. In contrast, vascular endothelial cell growth factor protein was

confined to few cells within the thromboemboli. *In situ* hybridization analysis demonstrated bFGF in endothelial cells, whereas TGF-$\beta$ and platelet-derived endothelial cell growth factor expression was localized in smooth muscle cells. The data indicate that organization of nonresolving pulmonary thromboemboli is regulated by a diverse set of growth factors predominantly expressed by vascular smooth muscle cells.

# DIAGNOSIS

## Clinical Presentation

Exertional dyspnea is the leading complaint in patients with CTEPH. The key to diagnosis is to consider CTEPH in patients complaining of exertional dyspnea in the presence of a normal lung function.

## Physical Findings

In the absence of right ventricular failure, clinical findings are minimal. Tricuspid regurgitation and pulmonary flow murmurs are often the only findings.

## Differential Diagnosis

Accurate diagnosis of CTEPH requires experienced centers (43). *Primary pulmonary hypertension* (PPH) must be ruled out. The terminology "primary" denotes idiopathic pulmonary hypertension, and includes pulmonary hypertension of unknown cause, and pulmonary hypertension associated with known causes such as appetite suppressants, human immunovirus (HIV), portal hypertension, and congenital heart disease. Prevalence in women (men : women = 1:4), familial occurrence, past intake of appetite suppressant drugs, a normal or patchy nonsegmentally abnormal ventilation/perfusion scan, and vascular pruning on the angiogram suggest PPH. However, forms of CTEPH where thrombus is located mainly in the peripheral pulmonary vasculature (type IV CTEPH, Fig. 92-9), and PPH with thrombi in the major pulmonary arteries, complicate the diagnosis and the nomenclature (44).

Further differential diagnoses to be excluded are fibrosing mediastinitis, pulmonary arterial tumor or tumor invasion of the pulmonary arteries, tumor embolism (45), or pulmonary arteritis (46) [e.g., giant cell arteritis (47)]. Because of excessive bronchopulmonary anastomoses (48), vascular transformation of mediastinal lymph nodes may occur (49).

In the moderately symptomatic patient, left ventricular diastolic dysfunction with oxygen desaturation during exercise is frequently observed and must be considered as a differential diagnosis.

## Electrocardiogram

The electrocardiogram (ECG) may show evidence of chronic right ventricular hypertrophy, an indirect sign of advanced pulmonary vascular disease. Abnormal P waves are tall-peaked in leads II and aVF, and in the midprecordium. Right axis deviation, monophasic R waves in $V_1$ and deep S waves in $V_6$ are observed. Sinus tachycardia is a malignant sign of right heart failure, along with persistently negative precordial T waves that indicate right ventricular strain. Initially, T waves may rapidly reverse, reflecting intermittent right ventricular ischemia. Atrial fibrillation may result in major hemodynamic compromise. Compression of the left main coronary artery may result from dilatation of the proximal pulmonary arteries (50).

## Pulmonary Function Test and Blood Gas Analysis

Pulmonary function tests are usually within normal limits. Approximately 20% of patients have "a restrictive defect" because of parenchymal scarring (51). The diffusion capacity of carbon monoxide (D$_{LCO}$) can be impaired for the same reason, but does not reflect the degree of vascular obstruction. Although it may be reduced, a normal D$_{LCO}$ does not exclude the diagnosis of CTEPH. Normalization of D$_{LCO}$ in the course of the disease probably reflects the extensive bronchial arterial collateral flow, which may exceed 10% of cardiac output in these patients. Arterial blood gas studies at rest and with exercise are important for patient evaluation. A decline in arterial P$O_2$ and widening of the alveolar–arterial oxygen difference is common during exercise, even with normal resting blood gases.

## Chest X-ray

Lung fields are clear. On closer inspection, areas of hypoperfusion may be seen. The hilar structures may be prominent and may be interpreted as lymphomas. In extreme cases a reduction in vascular size may suggest agenesis of the pulmonary artery(ies). In some patients, cavitary lesions form newly at areas of old infarctions, any time in the course of the disease.

## Ventilation and Perfusion Scans

In CTEPH, a segmentally positive ventilation and perfusion (V/Q) scan is diagnostic (see Fig. 92-3). In the absence of at least one segmental defect, the diagnosis CTEPH cannot be made. However, the severity of V/Q mismatches underestimates the severity of vascular occlusions (52). Although CTEPH is a vascular disorder, ventilation scanning is recommended.

Postoperatively, "reverse" V/Q scan patterns are observed because of a vascular steal of blood flow from the nonatherectomized segments (53).

## Exercise Stress Test

Exercise stress test with arterial blood gas analysis is important for patients with normal values of resting pulmonary pressures and suspicion of unilateral disease. Frequently, desaturation with exercise is the first objective finding in patients who present early in their course. Classic cardiac stress testing without measurement of arterial partial pressure of oxygen saturations usually yields negative results. Exercise echocardiography may unravel CTEPH when screening patients at risk.

## Echocardiography

Transthoracic echocardiography is a very helpful tool for the diagnosis of CTEPH. Although the exact measurement of right ventricular dimensions is difficult, interventricular septal motion, right ventricular cavity dimensions, thickness of the right ventricular free wall, and the velocity of tricuspid regurgitation help establish the diagnosis of pulmonary hypertension. In our experience, approximately 20% of patients with CTEPH (usually young patients) present with normal or near-normal right ventricular cavity dimensions.

Perfusion scan

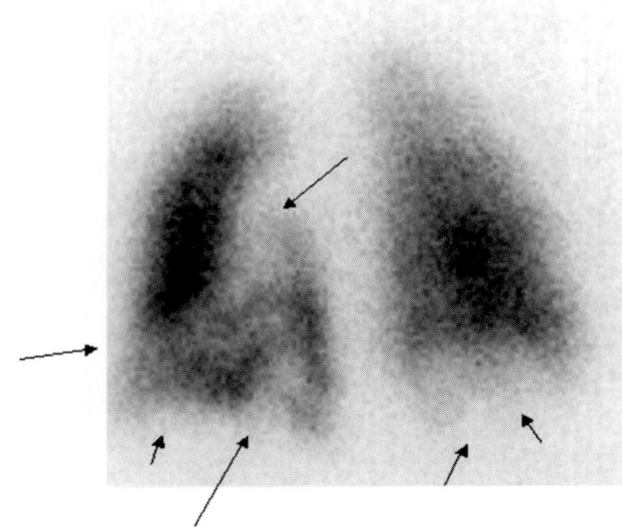

**FIGURE 92-3.** Example of a perfusion scintigram of a patient with chronic thromboembolic pulmonary hypertension. The corresponding ventilation scan was normal. The perfusion scan shows multiple segmental, triangular, mismatched defects. An anteroposterior view is shown.

Transesophageal echocardiography is helpful for the diagnosis of patent or a functionally patent foramen ovale and thereby helps to explain severe hypoxemia in some patients. Furthermore, in 40% of patients, proximal pulmonary arterial thrombus can be seen. Unfortunately, wall irregularities, scars, and bands in the pulmonary artery cannot be visualized with this technique. In most patients, these signs are the only proximal indicators of thromboembolic disease and can presently only be demonstrated by angioscopy.

## Computerized Tomography

Spiral computerized tomography (CT) scan with contrast agent is a valuable and indispensable diagnostic procedure for the diagnosis of CTEPH. However, because of limits in resolution beyond segmental arteries, distal vascular occlusions are not seen. In these instances and in all other cases, a mosaic perfusion pattern reflecting perfusion inequalities offers important diagnostic clues. Recently, modern CT scan technologies (e.g., 16–64 row multislice CT scans) have revolutionized imaging in CTEPH with images that approach the quality of pulmonary angiography (see Figs. 92-4 and 92-5) (54).

## Lung Biopsy

Because of a lack in specific pathologic changes in CTEPH, lung biopsy cannot provide differential diagnostic clues.

## Right Heart Catheterization

Right heart catheterization should be performed in any case of suspected pulmonary hypertension. The assessment of pulmonary artery systolic, diastolic, and mean pressures; pulmonary capillary wedge pressure; cardiac output; and oxygen saturations are important for the calculation of shunts and PVR. Central venous saturation and cardiac output are important prognostic parameters.

## CTEPH TYPE II

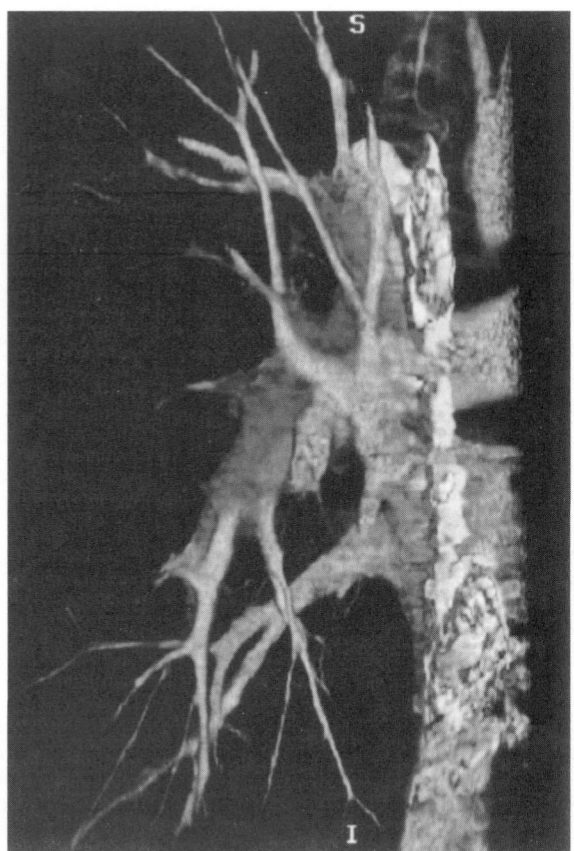 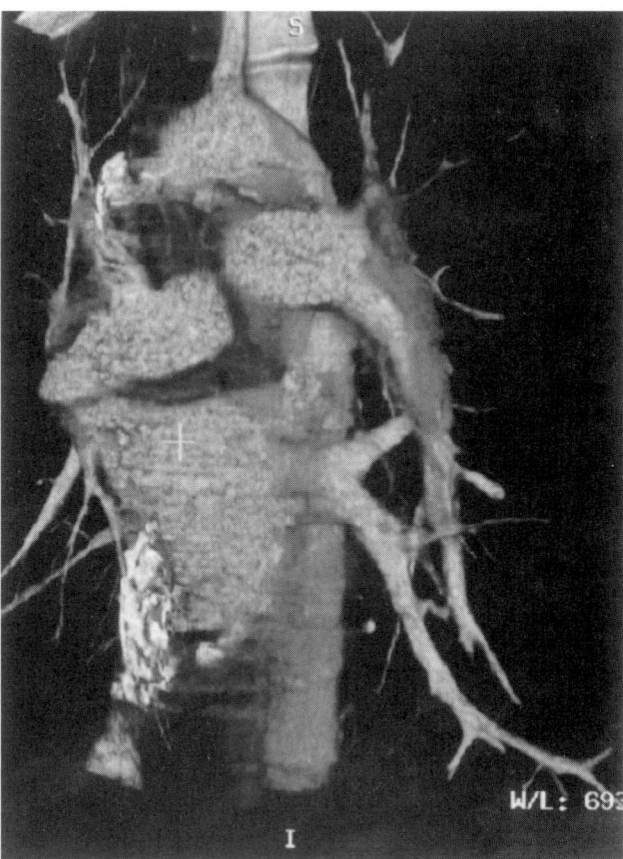

**FIGURE 92-4.** Representative computerized tomography images of a patient with type II chronic thromboembolic pulmonary hypertension (CTEPH). The 3-D rendering demonstrates thrombus in *red*. Pulmonary arteries and veins are imaged at the same time (see Color Fig. 92-4).

Although pulmonary arterial hypertension tends to involve the small muscular vessels, the primary site of vasculopathy in CTEPH are the large elastic pulmonary arteries. Concomitant small-vessel arteriopathy is also often present to varying degrees in CTEPH (8). In these patients, pulmonary hypertension persists despite removal of proximal material. Persistent pulmonary hypertension after PEA remains a significant problem and is associated with increased morbidity and mortality. More than one third of perioperative deaths and nearly half of long-term deaths have been attributed to persistent pulmonary hypertension (55,56). The current standard preoperative evaluation does not accurately detect the presence or assess the degree of small-vessel involvement in patients with CTEPH, nor is it suited to predict postoperative hemodynamic outcome. Fesler et al. have described a sophisticated pulmonary artery occlusion technique to estimate pulmonary capillary wedge pressure for approximating pressure in the precapillary small pulmonary arteries preoperatively (occlusion pressure; Poccl) (57). With Poccl, the pulmonary arterial resistance can be partitioned into large arterial (upstream) and small arterial plus venous (downstream) components (58). Kim et al. showed that a higher upstream resistance (Rup) was observed in patients with CTEPH who have predominantly proximal (large-vessel) disease, whereas patients with CTEPH with a Rup less than 60% demonstrated statistically significant concomitant small-vessel disease, had the highest postoperative total pulmonary resistance index (TPRi) and mean pulmonary artery

pressure (mPpa) values, and exhibited more frequent perioperative deaths (59).

## Pulmonary Angiography

Pulmonary angiography usually completes the diagnostic sequence; in general, it is an indispensable examination. Experience over the last decade has indicated that pulmonary angiography can be carried out safely in any patient with pulmonary hypertension when a rigorous protocol is followed (60). Venous access may be from arm, neck, or femoral vein if cavography is performed first to rule out vena caval thrombosis. Usually, diagnostic right heart catheterization is carried out prior to angiography. Selective injection of nonionic contrast agent and minimizing the amount of contrast help ensure that hemodynamic compromise does not occur. The pulmonary angiographic findings suggestive of chronic thromboembolic disease include "pouching" defects, webs, or bands, intimal irregularities, abrupt vascular narrowing, and complete vascular obstruction (see Fig. 92-6) (61). When bands, webs, and vessel cutoffs are observed, the procedure is concluded with the insertion of a vena caval filter when thromboembolism originating from the deep leg veins and pelvic veins is likely. Several centers are starting to abandon routine caval filter placement because of the uncertainty of the thromboembolic nature of the disease.

## CTEPH TYPE IV

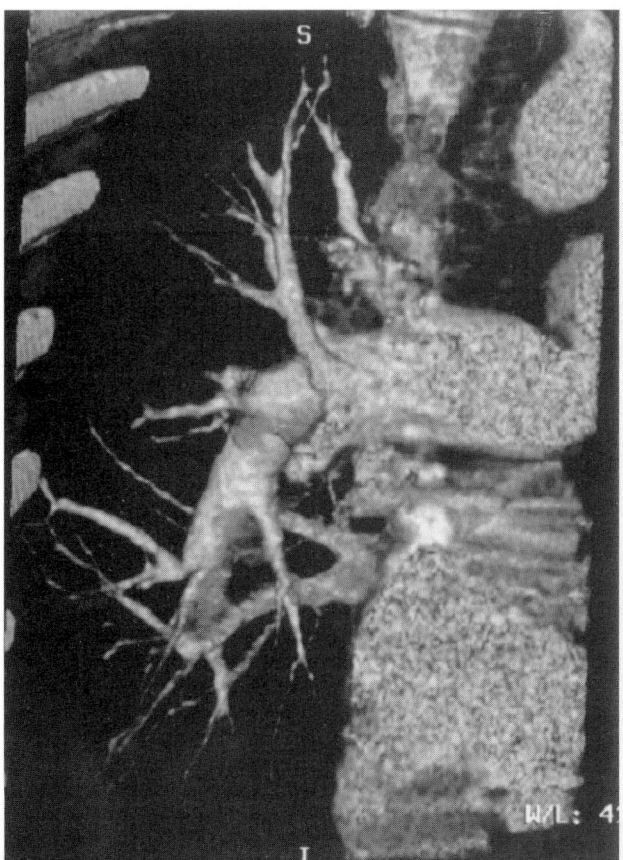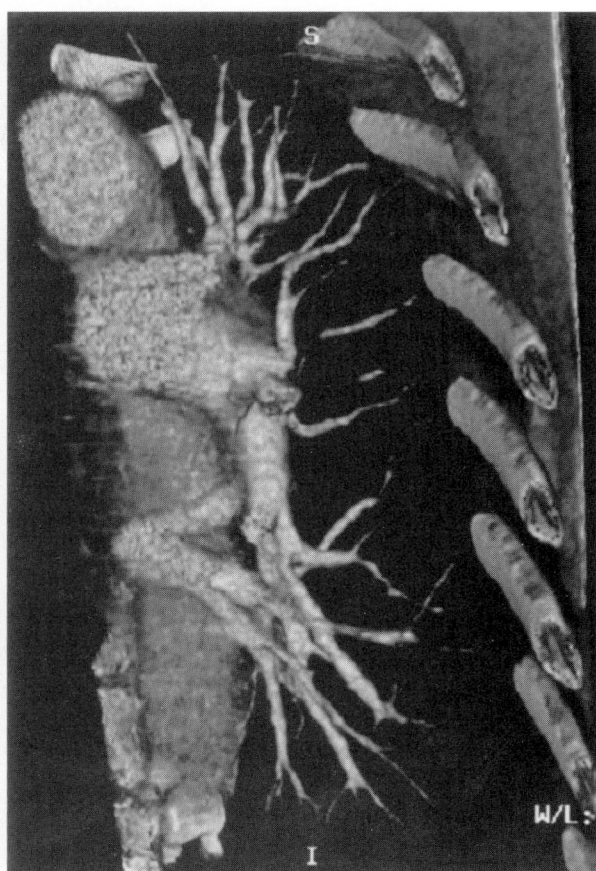

**FIGURE 92-5.** Representative computerized tomographic images of a patient with type IV chronic thromboembolic pulmonary hypertension (CTEPH) (see Color Fig. 92-5).

The choice of the angiographic technique, that is, conventional versus digital subtraction pulmonary angiography, is at the operator's discretion.

### Risk Stratification

Preoperative parameters can be utilized to assess postoperative mortality and hemodynamic improvement after PEA. Patient age and the relation between hemodynamic severity of pulmonary hypertension and distality of vascular occlusions determine hospital mortality. In a multivariate analysis, age ($P = 0.1$), right atrial pressure ($P = 0.002$), and female sex ($P = 0.007$) were the risk factors for minimal hemodynamic improvement (62). Recently, it was reported that fractional pulse pressure (pulmonary arterial pulse pressure/mPpa) was higher in CTEPH than in PPH and that fractional pulse pressure in PEA survivors ($1.26 \pm 0.21$) was higher than that in nonsurvivors ($1.06 \pm 0.16$; $P = 0.03$), and the value was statistically significant. Fractional pulse pressure is an important predictor for mortality in patients with PVR greater than 1,100 dynes sec per cm$^5$ (63). These data are in accord with recent data reporting poor outcome in patients with predominantly distal vascular obstructions (59).

The prognosis of not operated patients with CTEPH is determined by hemodynamics, coexistence of COPD, and the degree of exercise intolerance (64).

## TREATMENT

### Pulmonary Thromboendarterectomy

The surgical treatment of CTEPH was first described in 1965 (65). Pulmonary thromboendarterectomy (unfortunately abbreviated as "PEA" at the 2003 Venice WHO meeting on pulmonary hypertension, thereby competing with the abbreviation for pulseless electrical activity) is a standardized procedure today, representing a classical bilateral endarterectomy where the thrombus and the adjacent medial layer are carefully dissected with dedicated surgical instruments (Fig. 92-7) (56,66,67). The procedure is the treatment of choice for CTEPH (68,69). In contrast to acute embolectomy (70,71), PEA is not a thrombectomy but an endarterectomy, and a major challenge for the surgeon. To prevent bronchial arterial backflow into the operating field, dissections are performed under cardiopulmonary bypass with repeated periods of circulatory arrest, and the patient is cooled to 20°C (72,73). Complete endarterectomy of the pulmonary vascular bed (Fig. 92-8), extending far into the segmental arteries, is the goal. Depending on the location of thrombus, an operative classification has been proposed (Fig. 92-9) (74). Criteria for PEA are surgically accessible pulmonary thrombus (thrombi visible at least at the origin of the segmental arteries, types I to III), a resting PVR of

Successful PEA in a patient with unilateral CTEPH

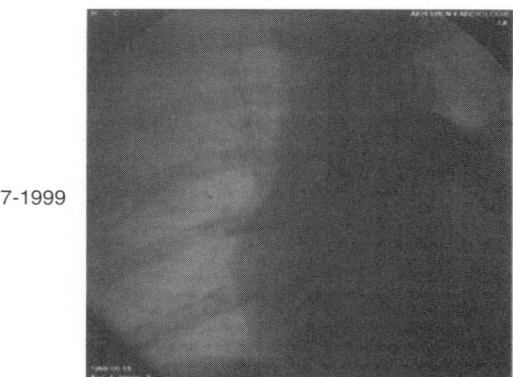

7-1999

3-2002

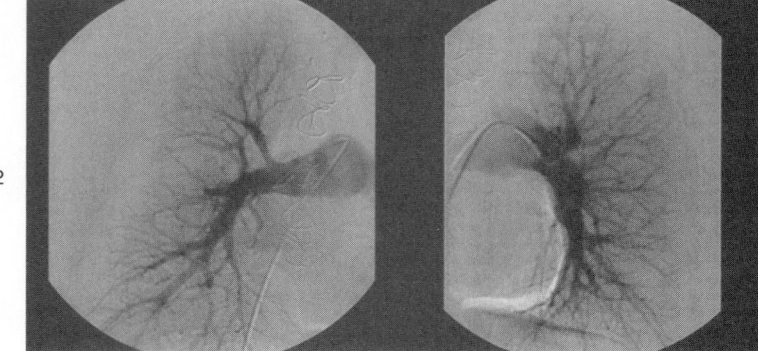

**FIGURE 92-6.** Example of sequential pulmonary angiograms of a patient with unilateral chronic thromboembolic pulmonary hypertension (CTEPH). The **upper** panel demonstrates a cine-angiogram showing total obstruction of the right pulmonary artery. The lower panel shows a follow-up digital angiogram 2 years after successful unilateral pulmonary thromboendarterectomy (PEA).

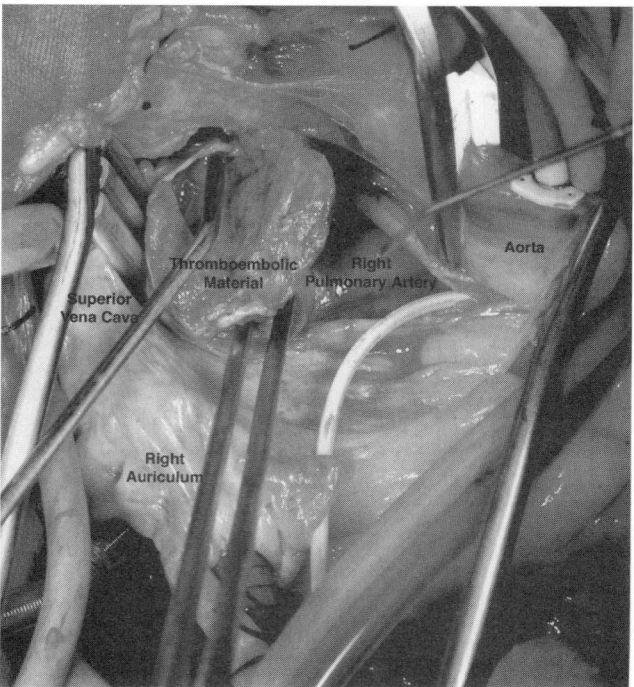

**FIGURE 92-7.** The typical operative field of surgical pulmonary thromboendarterectomy shows a lengthwise incised pulmonary artery with a sizeable thrombus being removed (see Color Fig. 92-7).

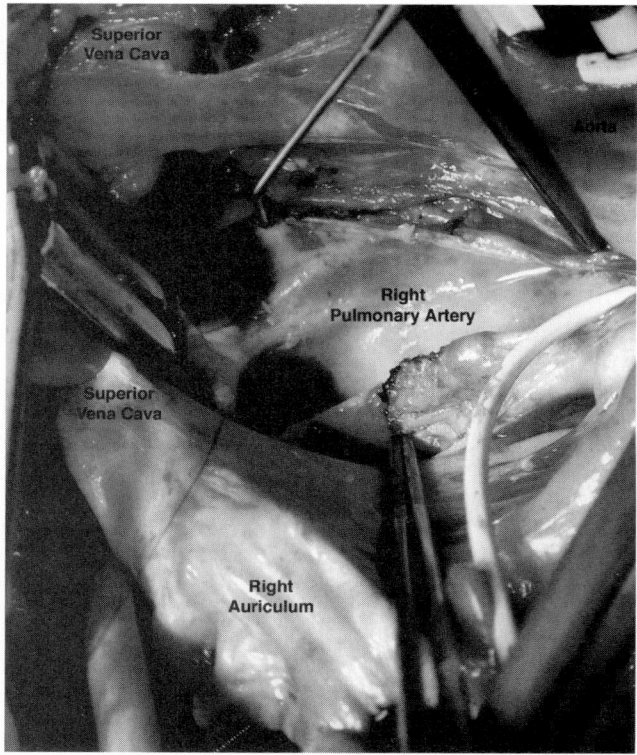

**FIGURE 92-8.** At the end of surgical pulmonary thromboendarterectomy, a new inner surface of the pulmonary artery is created that is devoid of fibrotic thrombus tissue. The most relevant anatomical structures are labeled in the photomicrograph (see Color Fig. 92-8).

## CTEPH classification

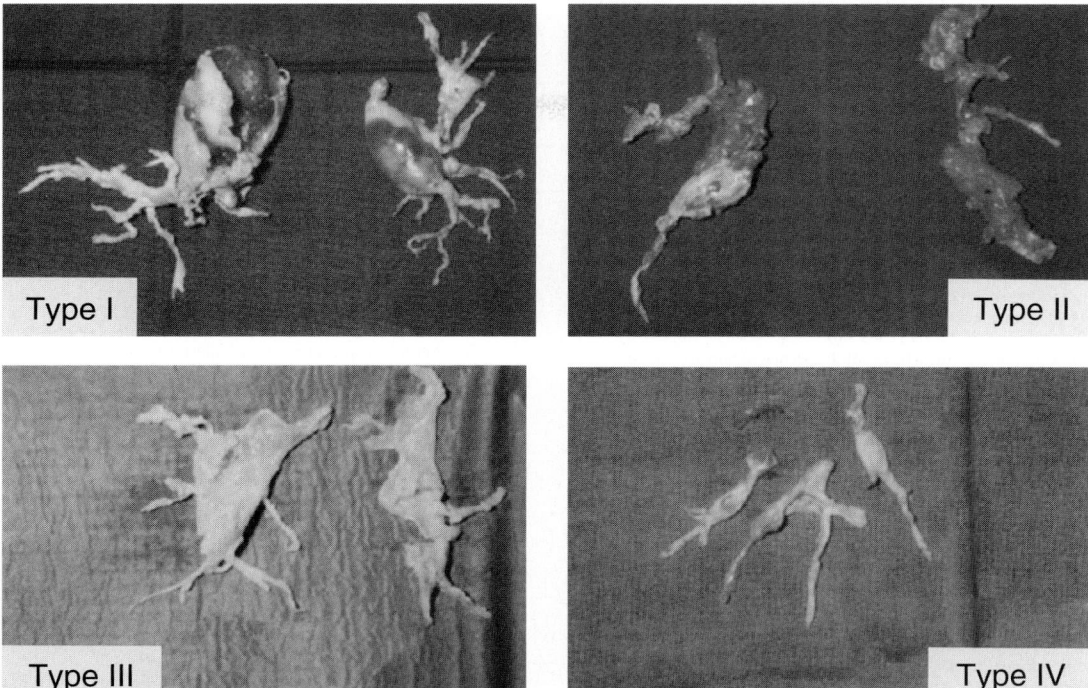

**FIGURE 92-9.** Surgical classification of chronic thromboembolic pulmonary hypertension. Most patients (roughly two thirds) present with type II disease. Type IV disease does not yield any thrombus at surgery in most cases. In the example that is shown, small amounts of thrombus were recovered (see Color Fig. 92-9).

greater than 300 dynes sec per cm$^5$, or an inadequate pressure rise under exertion. Meticulous postoperative care is required. A 24-hour mechanical ventilation period and fluid restriction are designed to prevent reperfusion pulmonary edema (75). This life-threatening complication of PEA is an acute lung injury pattern resulting from perfusion of a dysfunctional capillary bed in a chronically underperfused lung segment. A pharmacologic approach has blocked selectin mediated adhesion of neutrophils to the endothelium with Cylexin (CY-1503) and has demonstrated a decreased incidence of reperfusion injury, however without decreasing the total number of days on mechanical ventilation (76).

For a small subset of patients who present with concomitant coronary or valvular disease, combined surgical treatments are required (77). Tricuspid regurgitation, even of severe grades, usually does not require additional valve surgery because it disappears when pulmonary pressures normalize (78).

## Outcome

Patient age, hemodynamics and clinical status, location of thrombus, and comorbidity determine postoperative outcome (79). Thrombus localization is a clear determinant of operative outcome (Fig. 92-2) (74). Distal location of pulmonary thromboemboli doubles operative risk. Perioperative mortality is also dependent on the surgeon's experience and postoperative care, and it varies from 4% to 25% (56,73,80–82). Currently, the most experienced PEA center is the University of California at San Diego where more than 1,800 operations

have been performed, with a mortality rate as low as 4% in uncomplicated cases. Other than warfarin, patients do not usually require specific postoperative medication. Favorable results have been reported with perioperative use of NO (83). Recurrent thromboembolism is rare. Why some patients (approximately 10%) do not experience hemodynamic improvement despite removal of significant amounts of thrombus remains unexplained.

## Other Treatments

There is room for medical therapy of CTEPH in patients who appear too ill to undergo surgery immediately and in those who do not improve after successful PEA. Furthermore, despite great progress in surgical technique, there are patients who are inoperable. Conventional therapy consists of diuretics, digitalis, anticoagulation, caval filters, chronic oxygen therapy, and low-dose calcium antagonists. Recent reports suggest a benefit of preoperative vasodilator therapy and a benefit of postoperative inhaled Iloprost (84–86). Successful oral therapy with sildenafil has been reported (87), while treatment with endothelin receptor blockers is under investigation.

Prostaglandins or endothelin receptor antagonists are not known to improve hemodynamic status or survival in CTEPH and should be considered investigational. Lung transplantation is an established treatment for patients who are not candidates for PEA and who deteriorate under medical therapy (88). Balloon pulmonary angioplasty in a few experienced centers has been reported to be a treatment option for severely ill patients who are inoperable (89).

# ACKNOWLEDGMENT

This research was supported by the Austrian fellowship grant FWF P13834-MED (to IML), the Österreichischer Selbsthilfeverein Lungenhochdruck and the Ludwig Boltzmann Institute for Cardiovascular Research.

## *References*

1. Fedullo PF, Auger WR, Kerr KM, et al. Chronic thromboembolic pulmonary hypertension. *N Engl J Med* 2001;345:1465–1472.
2. Ribeiro A, Lindmarker P, Johnsson H, et al. Pulmonary embolism: one-year follow-up with echocardiography doppler and five-year survival analysis. *Circulation* 1999;99:1325–1330.
3. Pengo V, Lensing AWA, Prins MH, et al. Incidence of chronic thromboembolic pulmonary hypertension after pulmonary embolism. *N Engl J Med* 2004;350:2257–2264.
4. Kyrle PA, Eichinger S. The risk of recurrent venous thromboembolism: the Austrian Study on recurrent venous thromboembolism. *Wien Klin Wochenschr* 2003;115:471–474.
5. Wolf M, Boyer-Neumann C, Parent F, et al. Thrombotic risk factors in pulmonary hypertension. *Eur Respir J* 2000;15:395–399.
6. Lang IM, Klepetko W, Pabinger I. No increased prevalence of the factor V Leiden mutation in chronic major vessel thromboembolic pulmonary hypertension (CTEPH). *Thromb Haemost* 1996;76:476–477.
7. Egermayer P, Peacock AJ. Is pulmonary embolism a common cause of chronic pulmonary hypertension? Limitations of the embolic hypothesis. *Eur Respir J* 2000;15:440–448.
8. Moser KM, Bloor CM. Pulmonary vascular lesions occurring in patients with chronic major vessel thromboembolic pulmonary hypertension. *Chest* 1993;103:685–692.
9. Mahmud E, Raisinghani A, Hassankhani A, et al. Correlation of left ventricular diastolic filling characteristics with right ventricular overload and pulmonary artery pressure in chronic thromboembolic pulmonary hypertension. *J Am Coll Cardiol* 2002;40:318–324.
10. Menzel T, Wagner S, Kramm T, et al. Pathophysiology of impaired right and left ventricular function in chronic embolic pulmonary hypertension: changes after pulmonary thromboendarterectomy. *Chest* 2000;118:897–903.
11. Blanchard DG, Dittrich HC. An Intraoperative Transesophageal Echocardiographic Study. Pericardial adaptation in severe chronic pulmonary hypertension. *Circulation* 1992;85:1414–1422.
12. Dittrich HC, Chow LC, Nicod PH. Early improvement in left ventricular diastolic function after relief of chronic right ventricular pressure overload. *Circulation* 1989;80:823–830.
13. Hirsch AM, Moser KM, Auger WR, et al. Unilateral pulmonary artery thrombotic occlusion: is distal arteriopathy a consequence? *Am J Respir Crit Care Med* 1996;154:491–496.
14. Moser KM, Auger WR, Fedullo PF. Chronic major-vessel thromboembolic pulmonary hypertension. *Circulation* 1990;81:1735–1743.
15. Olman MA, Marsh JJ, Lang IM, et al. Endogenous fibrinolytic system in chronic large-vessel thromboembolic pulmonary hypertension. *Circulation* 1992;86:1241–1248.
16. Martinuzzo ME, Pombo G, Forastiero RR, et al. Lupus anticoagulant, high levels of anticardiolipin, and anti-beta2-glycoprotein I antibodies are associated with chronic thromboembolic pulmonary hypertension. *J Rheumatol* 1998;25:1313–1319.
17. Auger WR, Permpikul P, Moser KM. Lupus anticoagulant, heparin use, and thrombocytopenia in patients with chronic thromboembolic pulmonary hypertension: a preliminary report. *Am J Med* 1995;99:392–396.
18. Laczika K, Lang IM, Quehenberger P, et al. Unilateral chronic thromboembolic pulmonary disease associated with combined inherited thrombophilia. *Chest* 2002;121:286–289.
19. Bonderman D, Turecek PL, Jakowitsch J, et al. High prevalence of elevated clotting factor VIII in chronic thromboembolic pulmonary hypertension. *Thromb Haemost* 2003;90:372–376.
20. Veyradier A, Nishikubo T, Humbert M, et al. Improvement of von Willebrand factor proteolysis after prostacyclin infusion in severe pulmonary arterial hypertension. *Circulation* 2000;102:2460–2462.
21. Cappellini MD, Robbiolo L, Bottasso BM, et al. Venous thromboembolism and hypercoagulability in splenectomized patients with thalassaemia intermedia. *Br J Haematol* 2000;111:467–473.
22. Stewart GW, Amess JA, Eber SW, et al. Thrombo-embolic disease after splenectomy for hereditary stomatocytosis. *Br J Haematol* 1996;93:303–310.
23. Chou R, DeLoughery TG. Recurrent thromboembolic disease following splenectomy for pyruvate kinase deficiency. *Am J Hematol* 2001;67:197–199.
24. Favara BE, Paul RN. Thromboembolism and cor pulmonale complicating ventriculovenous shunt. *Jama* 1967;199:668–671.
25. Unnithan RR, Bahuleyan CG, Sambasivan M, et al. Ventriculo-atrial shunt producing pulmonary hypertension. *J Assoc Physicians India* 1984;32:1000–1001.
26. Trowitzsch E, Ostrejz M, Evers D, et al. Echocardiographic proof of pulmonary hypertension with irreversible increased resistance in the pulmonary circulation as a complication after placement of a ventriculo-atrial shunt for internal hydrocephalus. *Eur J Pediatr Surg* 1992;2:361–364.
27. Haasnoot K, van Vught AJ. Pulmonary hypertension complicating a ventriculo-atrial shunt. *Eur J Pediatr* 1992;151:748–750.
28. Drucker MH, Vanek VW, Franco AA, et al. Thromboembolic complications of ventriculoatrial shunts. *Surg Neurol* 1984;22:444–448.
29. Pascual JM, Prakash UB. Development of pulmonary hypertension after placement of a ventriculoatrial shunt. *Mayo Clin Proc* 1993;68:1177–1182.
30. Rao PS, Molthan ME, Lipow HW. Cor pulmonale as a complication of ventriculoatrial shunts. Case report. *J Neurosurg* 1970;33:221–225.
31. Ralston DR, St John RC. Progressive shortness of breath in a 50-year-old man with ulcerative colitis. *Chest* 1996;110:1608–1610.
32. Yung GL, Channick RN, Fedullo PF, et al. Successful pulmonary thromboendarterectomy in two patients with sickle cell disease. *Am J Respir Crit Care Med* 1998;157:1690–1693.
33. Murali B, Drain A, Seller D, et al. Pulmonary thromboendarterectomy in a case of hereditary stomatocytosis. *Br J Anaesth* 2003;91:739–741.
34. Walder B, Kapelanski DP, Auger WR, et al. Successful pulmonary thromboendarterectomy in a patient with Klippel-Trenaunay syndrome. *Chest* 2000;117:1520–1522.
35. Kamphuisen PW, Eikenboom JC, Bertina RM. Elevated factor VIII levels and the risk of thrombosis. *Arterioscler Thromb Vasc Biol* 2001;21:731–738.
36. Marsh JJ, Konopka RG, Lang IM, et al. Suppression of thrombolysis in a canine model of pulmonary embolism. *Circulation* 1994;90:3091–3097.
37. Lang IM, Marsh JJ, Olman MA, et al. Parallel analysis of tissue-type plasminogen activator and type 1 plasminogen activator inhibitor in plasma and endothelial cells derived from patients with chronic pulmonary thromboemboli. *Circulation* 1994;90:706–712.
38. Lang IM, Marsh JJ, Konopka RG, et al. Factors contributing to increased vascular fibrinolytic activity in mongrel dogs. *Circulation* 1993;87:1990–2000.
39. Lang IM, Marsh JJ, Olman MA, et al. Expression of type 1 plasminogen activator inhibitor in chronic pulmonary thromboemboli. *Circulation* 1994;89:2715–2721.
40. Lang IM, Moser KM, Schleef RR. Elevated expression of urokinase-like plasminogen activator and plasminogen activator inhibitor type 1 during the vascular remodeling associated with pulmonary thromboembolism. *Arterioscler Thromb Vasc Biol* 1998;18:808–815.
41. Lang IM, Moser KM, Schleef RR. Expression of kunitz protease inhibitor—containing forms of amyloid beta-protein precursor within vascular thrombi. *Circulation* 1996;94:2728–2734.
42. Thistlethwaite PA, Lee SH, Du LL, et al. Human angiopoietin gene expression is a marker for severity of pulmonary hypertension in patients undergoing pulmonary thromboendarterectomy. *J Thorac Cardiovasc Surg* 2001;122:65–73.
43. Auger WR, Channick RN, Kerr KM, et al. Evaluation of patients with suspected chronic thromboembolic pulmonary hypertension. *Semin Thorac Cardiovasc Surg* 1999;11:179–190.
44. Moser KM, Fedullo PF, Finkbeiner WE, et al. Do patients with primary pulmonary hypertension develop extensive central thrombi? *Circulation* 1995;91:741–745.
45. Paw P, Jamieson SW. Pulmonary thromboendarterectomy for the treatment of pulmonary embolism caused by renal cell carcinoma. *J Thorac Cardiovasc Surg* 1997;114:295–297.
46. Kerr KM, Auger WR, Fedullo PF, et al. Large vessel pulmonary arteritis mimicking chronic thromboembolic disease. *Am J Respir Crit Care Med* 1995;152:367–373.
47. Brister SJ, Wilson-Yang K, Lobo FV, et al. Pulmonary thromboendarterectomy in a patient with giant cell arteritis. *Ann Thorac Surg* 2002;73:1977–1979.
48. Ley S, Kreitner KF, Morgenstern I, et al. Bronchopulmonary shunts in patients with chronic thromboembolic pulmonary hypertension: evaluation with helical CT and MR imaging. *AJR Am J Roentgenol* 2002;179:1209–1215.
49. Meysman M, Diltoer M, Raeve HD, et al. Chronic thromboembolic pulmonary hypertension and vascular transformation of the lymph node sinuses. *Eur Respir J* 1997;10:1191–1193.
50. Bonderman D, Fleischmann D, Prokop M, et al. Images in cardiovascular medicine. Left main coronary artery compression by the pulmonary trunk in pulmonary hypertension. *Circulation* 2002;105:265.
51. Morris TA, Auger WR, Ysrael MZ, et al. Parenchymal scarring is associated with restrictive spirometric defects in patients with chronic thromboembolic pulmonary hypertension. *Chest* 1996;110:399–403.
52. Ryan KL, Fedullo PF, Davis GB, et al. Perfusion scan findings understate the severity of angiographic and hemodynamic compromise in chronic thromboembolic pulmonary hypertension. *Chest* 1988;93:1180–1185.
53. Olman MA, Auger WR, Fedullo PF, et al. Pulmonary vascular steal in chronic thromboembolic pulmonary hypertension. *Chest* 1990;98:1430–1434.

54. Fleischmann D, Scholten C, Klepetko W, et al. Three-dimensional visualization of pulmonary thromboemboli in chronic thromboembolic pulmonary hypertension with multiple detector-row spiral computed tomography. *Circulation* 2001;103:2993.

55. Archibald CJ, Auger WR, Fedullo PF, et al. Long-term outcome after pulmonary thromboendarterectomy. *Am J Respir Crit Care Med* 1999;160:523–528.

56. Jamieson SW, Nomura K. Indications for and the results of pulmonary thromboendarterectomy for thromboembolic pulmonary hypertension. *Semin Vasc Surg* 2000;13:236–244.

57. Fesler P, Pagnamenta A, Vachiery JL, et al. Single arterial occlusion to locate resistance in patients with pulmonary hypertension. *Eur Respir J* 2003;21:31–36.

58. Hakim TS, Michel RP, Chang HK. Partitioning of pulmonary vascular resistance in dogs by arterial and venous occlusion. *J Appl Physiol* 1982;52:710–715.

59. Kim NH, Fesler P, Channick RN, et al. Preoperative partitioning of pulmonary vascular resistance correlates with early outcome after thromboendarterectomy for chronic thromboembolic pulmonary hypertension. *Circulation* 2004;109:18–22, Epub 2003 Dec 29.

60. Nicod P, Peterson K, Levine M, et al. Pulmonary angiography in severe chronic pulmonary hypertension. *Ann Intern Med* 1987;107:565–568.

61. Auger WR, Fedullo PF, Moser KM, et al. Chronic major-vessel thromboembolic pulmonary artery obstruction: appearance at angiography. *Radiology* 1992;182:393–398.

62. Tscholl D, Langer F, Wendler O, et al. Pulmonary thromboendarterectomy—risk factors for early survival and hemodynamic improvement. *Eur J Cardiothorac Surg* 2001;19:771–776.

63. Tanabe N, Okada O, Abe Y, et al. The influence of fractional pulse pressure on the outcome of pulmonary thromboendarterectomy. *Eur Respir J* 2001;17:653–659.

64. Lewczuk J, Piszko P, Jagas J, et al. Prognostic factors in medically treated patients with chronic pulmonary embolism. *Chest* 2001;119:818–823.

65. Moser KM, Houk VN, Jones RC, et al. Chronic, massive thrombotic obstruction of the pulmonary arteries. Analysis of four operated cases. *Circulation* 1965;32:377–385.

66. Jamieson SW. Pulmonary thromboendarterectomy [editorial]. *Heart* 1998;79:118–120.

67. Daily PO, Dembitsky WP, Daily RP. Dissectors for pulmonary thromboendarterectomy. *Ann Thorac Surg* 1991;51:842–843.

68. Moser KM, Braunwald NS. Successful surgical intervention in severe chronic thromboembolic pulmonary hypertension. *Chest* 1973;64:29–35.

69. Zoia MC, D'Armini AM, Beccaria M, et al. Mid term effects of pulmonary thromboendarterectomy on clinical and cardiopulmonary function status. *Thorax* 2002;57:608–612.

70. Ando M, Takamoto S, Kawaguchi A, et al. Review of results after surgery for pulmonary embolism. *Nippon Kyobu Geka Gakkai Zasshi* 1996;44:505–510.

71. Aklog L, Williams CS, Byrne JG, et al. Acute pulmonary embolectomy: a contemporary approach. *Circulation* 2002;105:1416–1419.

72. Daily PO, Kinney TB. Optimizing myocardial hypothermia: II. Cooling jacket modifications and clinical results. *Ann Thorac Surg* 1991;51:284–289.

73. Jamieson SW, Kapelanski DP, Sakakibara N, et al. Pulmonary endarterectomy: experience and lessons learned in 1,500 cases. *Ann Thorac Surg* 2003;76:1457–1462; discussion 1462–1464.

74. Thistlethwaite PA, Mo M, Madani MM, et al. Operative classification of thromboembolic disease determines outcome after pulmonary endarterectomy. *J Thorac Cardiovasc Surg* 2002;124:1203–1211.

75. Levinson RM, Shure D, Moser KM. Reperfusion pulmonary edema after pulmonary artery thromboendarterectomy. *Am Rev Respir Dis* 1986;134:1241–1245.

76. Kerr KM, Auger WR, Marsh JJ, et al. The use of cylexin (CY-1503) in prevention of reperfusion lung injury in patients undergoing pulmonary thromboendarterectomy. *Am J Respir Crit Care Med* 2000;162:14–20.

77. Thistlethwaite PA, Auger WR, Madani MM, et al. Pulmonary thromboendarterectomy combined with other cardiac operations: indications, surgical approach, and outcome. *Chest* 2003;123:319–320.

78. Thistlethwaite PA, Jamieson SW. Tricuspid valvular disease in the patient with chronic pulmonary thromboembolic disease. *Curr Opin Cardiol* 2003;18:111–116.

79. Hartz RS, Byrne JG, Levitsky S, et al. Predictors of mortality in pulmonary thromboendarterectomy. *Ann Thorac Surg* 1996;62:1255–1259; discussion 1259–1260.

80. Klepetko W, Moritz A, Burghuber OC, et al. [Chronic thromboembolic pulmonary hypertension and its treatment with pulmonary thrombendarterectomy]. *Wien Klin Wochenschr* 1995;107:396–402.

81. Dartevelle P, Fadel E, Chapelier A, et al. Pulmonary thromboendarterectomy with video-angioscopy and circulatory arrest: an alternative to cardiopulmonary transplantation and post-embolism pulmonary artery hypertension. *Chirurgie* 1998;123:32–40.

82. Klepetko W, Mayer E, Sandoval J, et al. Interventional and surgical modalities of treatment for pulmonary arterial hypertension. *J Am Coll Cardiol* 2004;(12 Suppl. S):73S–80S.

83. Imanaka H, Miyano H, Takeuchi M, et al. Effects of nitric oxide inhalation after pulmonary thromboendarterectomy for chronic pulmonary thromboembolism. *Chest* 2000;118:39–46.

84. Kerr KM, Rubin LJ. Epoprostenol therapy as a bridge to pulmonary thromboendarterectomy for chronic thromboembolic pulmonary hypertension. *Chest* 2003;123:319–320.

85. Nagaya N, Sasaki N, Ando M, et al. Prostacyclin therapy before pulmonary thromboendarterectomy in patients with chronic thromboembolic pulmonary hypertension. *Chest* 2003;123:338–343.

86. Kramm T, Eberle B, Krummenauer F, et al. Inhaled iloprost in patients with chronic thromboembolic pulmonary hypertension: effects before and after pulmonary thromboendarterectomy. *Ann Thorac Surg* 2003;76:711–718.

87. Ghofrani HA, Schermuly RT, Rose F, et al. Sildenafil for long-term treatment of nonoperable chronic thromboembolic pulmonary hypertension. *Am J Respir Crit Care Med* 2003;167(8):1139–1141. Epub 2003.

88. Pereszlenyi A, Lang G, Steltzer H, et al. Bilateral lung transplantation with intra and postoperatively prolonged ECMO support in patients with pulmonary hypertension. *Eur J Cardiothorac Surg* 2002;21:858–863.

89. Feinstein JA, Goldhaber SZ, Lock JE, et al. Balloon pulmonary angioplasty for treatment of chronic thromboembolic pulmonary hypertension. *Circulation* 2001;103:10–13.

# CHAPTER 93 ■ PARADOXICAL EMBOLISM

THURAIA NAGEH, STEPHAN WINDECKER, AND BERNHARD MEIER

Venous thrombus, air, or fat can traverse a patent foramen ovale (PFO), a persistent aperture in the interatrial septum, and embolize from the right side to the left side of the heart, potentially leading to stroke, transient ischemic attack (TIA), myocardial infarction, or peripheral embolic occlusive events. The first description of this phenomenon was by Connheim in 1877 (1). He described a stroke in the presence of a PFO in a young woman. Zahn coined the term "paradoxical" embolism in 1885 to describe migratory thrombus through a PFO into the systemic circulation (2). Since then, there has been a dramatic increase in awareness, documentation, and appreciation of the clinical importance of paradoxical emboli.

The confirmation of paradoxical emboli through a PFO is a diagnostic challenge. The documentation of a thrombus crossing the PFO is rarely possible (see Fig. 93-1). The diagnosis of paradoxical embolism is essentially done by exclusion, based on three presumptive criteria: (a) the presence of a right-to-left shunt, (b) the absence of a left-sided thromboembolic source, and (c) the detection of venous thrombosis, thrombus in the right side of the heart, or pulmonary embolism. By definition, paradoxical embolism remains an option even if the latter two criteria are not met.

PFOs are increasingly recognized as mediators of paradoxical embolism (3–5), with a transient (release phase following a Valsalva maneuver during coughing, defecation, etc.) or permanent pressure gradient with a right-to-left shunt. Several studies have established a strong association between the presence of PFO and cryptogenic stroke in adults younger than 55 years (6–10), but this relation is less well defined in older age groups (8,9,11). The absolute risk of paradoxical embolism through a PFO is higher in older individuals because of the prevalence of venous thrombosis increasing with age. Yet, other reasons for stroke (the most important manifestation of paradoxical embolism) are even more common; this diminishes the relative importance of a PFO in the final decades of life.

In addition to stroke, paradoxical embolism can have peripheral sequelae with end-organ ischemia, presenting as acute retinal, cardiac, hepatic, renal, abdominal, or limb ischemia. Thrombotic peripheral emboli are the most commonly reported types, but air and fat emboli have also been described in individual case reports. Air embolism through a PFO can occur as a rare complication of central venous catheters, of vascular access for hemodialysis, or in the course of general, neurologic, or orthopedic surgery. Moreover, paradoxical fat embolism has been described following bone fractures or orthopedic surgery.

## PARADOXICAL EMBOLISM AND STROKE

The incidence of stroke in the United States is estimated at 730,000 cases annually, with a mortality rate of 27%, thereby constituting the third leading cause of death after heart disease and cancer, respectively (12). Stroke is the leading cause of serious morbidity in the United States and all other industrialized societies, accounting for more than $50 billion in lost productivity and total health care costs (13). The risk of recurrence of stroke after a first event has been estimated at 9% to 13% at 1 year and 20% to 30% at 5 years (14,15).

The etiology of stroke can be either hemorrhagic or ischemic. However, up to 40% of ischemic strokes in young adults have no clearly definable cause and are therefore termed "cryptogenic" (16–19). Cryptogenic strokes form 64% of all strokes in patients younger than 55 years (10). There have been a number of reports of a high prevalence of PFOs in patients presenting with clinically and radiologically confirmed TIAs and strokes. An estimated 60,000 to 110,000 events per year are thought to be secondary to paradoxical emboli by a PFO in the United States (15,20).

Lechat et al. and Webster et al. initially described the association between PFO and cryptogenic stroke *in vivo* (6,7). This link has been confirmed in numerous case–control studies as well as metaanalyses. Although the PFO is widely accepted as an independent risk factor for a first cerebrovascular event and paradoxical embolism has been suggested as the most likely stroke mechanism in these patients, its role in recurrent embolic stroke has not been elucidated.

This phenomenon summarizes a complex sequence of events. First, an occult thrombus is formed somewhere in the venous system from where it dislodges to reach the right heart chambers. Predisposing intracardiac structures, such as the Chiari network or a prominent Eustachian valve, direct the dislodged thrombus towards the atrial septum rather than the right ventricle. Under conditions of increased pressure in the right atrium (e.g., pulmonary embolism, Valsalva maneuver, etc.), the one-way PFO flap valve may open widely to allow thrombus embolization into the left atrium. From there, the thrombus travels through the left ventricle gaining free access to the systemic circulation to manifest as arterial embolic occlusion.

Notwithstanding, paradoxical embolism is by no means confined to the brain but may affect any other arterial bed. When the thrombus enters the arterial tree, it must be large enough to occlude an end artery and persist long enough to result in tissue necrosis. Clinically, the most devastating consequence of paradoxical embolism arises from cerebral (stroke) and coronary (myocardial infarction) embolizations.

Although a cause–effect relation remains hypothetical, several lines of evidence support the concept of PFO-mediated paradoxical embolism. First, thrombus trapped within the PFO has been documented and provides pathophysiologic evidence for a causal relation. Second, larger PFO size has been associated with a higher recurrence rate, suggesting a "dose-response" relation. Third, the higher frequency of deep venous thrombosis in patients with stroke and PFO supports the concept of thrombi crossing the PFO to cause paradoxical embolism. Fourth, the SPARC (Stroke Prevention: Assessment of Risk in a Community) study suggested paradoxical embolism as the principal mechanism of stroke in patients with PFO and associated atrial sepal aneurysm, whereas atrial septal aneurysm without

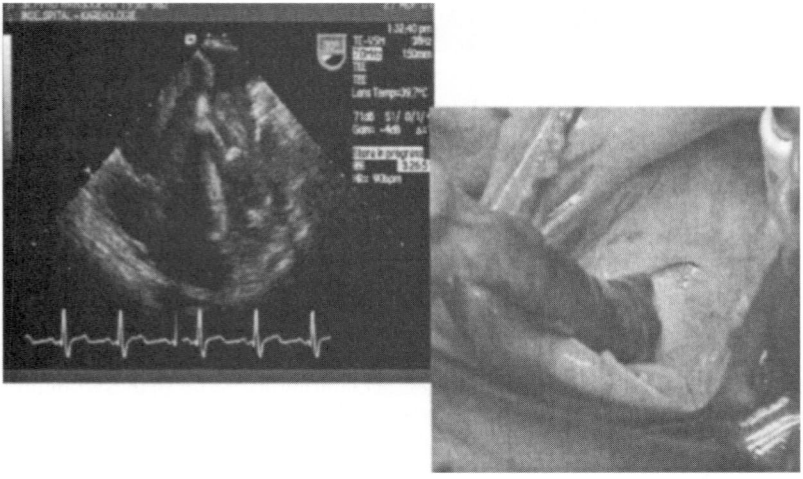

FIGURE 93-1. "Caught in the act"—right atrial thrombus straddling a patent foramen ovale (PFO), transesophageal echocardiography (TEE) appearance (**left**), and intraoperative aspect (**right**).

PFO (absence of right-to-left shunt) has been shown to portend no particular risk of recurrent cerebrovascular events (16).

# PREDISPOSING CLINICAL ASSOCIATIONS WITH PARADOXICAL EMBOLISM

## Patent Foramen Ovale/Atrial Septal Aneurysm

The atrial septum is formed by two overlapping embryological structures, the fibrous septum primum on the anatomical left and the muscular septum secundum on the right (see Fig. 93-2). The foramen ovale is an aperture in the inferoposterior aspect of the septum secundum, with the septum primum serving as a one-way valve allowing for a physiologic right-to-left shunt during *in utero* development. The postnatal increase in left atrial pressures with the establishment of a pulmonary circulation results in functional closure of the foramen ovale by apposition of the septa, followed by anatomic closure over the ensuing months. However, autopsy series have revealed that fusion of the septa fails to occur in 17% to 35% of adults, resulting in a PFO in approximately one in four people, which represents the commonest cardiac congenital abnormality. Clinical studies using transesophageal echocardiography (TEE) have estimated the prevalence of PFO at approximately 30% in the healthy adult population (21,22).

The prevalence of PFO appears to decline in older age groups from 34% during the first three decades, to 24% for the fourth to eighth decade, and to 20% in the ninth decade and beyond (23). This decline suggests spontaneous late closure of PFOs but may also reflect selective mortality. There does not appear to be a difference in prevalence among men and women and PFO size can range from very small (i.e., probe patent) to large (i.e., pencil patent, or involving nearly the entire septum in case of a floppy interatrial septum), with a mean diameter of 5 mm (23).

Atrial septal aneurysm describes a congenital abnormality of the atrial septum primum, characterized by a redundant muscular membrane in the region of the fossa ovalis. Reports of the prevalence of atrial septal aneurysms vary from 1% to 2% in autopsy and TEE studies (24–27). The echocardiographic diagnosis of an atrial septal aneurysm is based on the diameter of its base exceeding 15 mm and on the excursion of the interatrial septum amounting to at least 10 mm in total amplitude. Atrial septal aneurysms are rarely found as isolated (probably innocent) entities (28) but tend to be associated with PFOs in 50% to 85% of cases, implying that the atrial septal aneurysm impedes closure of the foramen after birth.

Atrial septal dysmorphogenesis, manifesting as a frequent association of PFO and atrial septal aneurysm, has recently been correlated with a heterozygous mutation of the cardiac homeodomain transcription factor Nkx2-5 in mice (29). This observation suggests that the frequency of PFOs may be a function of genetic factors, with PFOs representing an index of septal dysmorphogenesis encompassing other congenital defects such as atrial septal aneurysms and atrial and ventricular septal defects. Table 93-1 summarizes the association between PFO and atrial septal aneurysm with stroke in young adults.

PFOs are not detectable at clinical examination. Their diagnosis requires one or more of the following investigative modalities.

### Transthoracic Echocardiography

Transthoracic echocardiography (TTE) is the typical initial diagnostic tool in coincidentally identified PFOs. The technique is

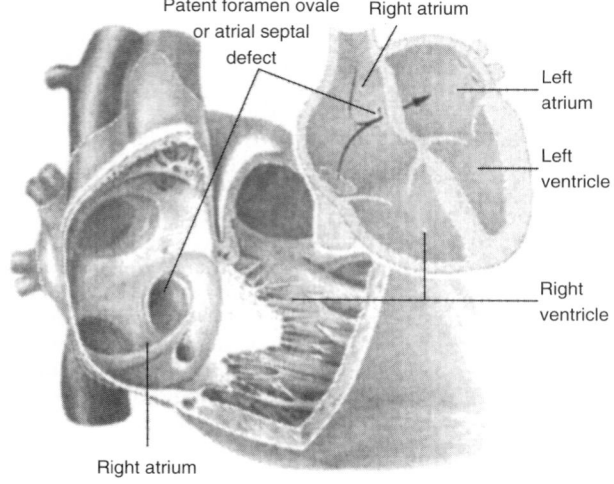

Patent foramen ovale or atrial septal defect — Right atrium — Left atrium — Left ventricle — Right ventricle — Right atrium

FIGURE 93-2. Anatomy of the patent foramen ovale.

**TABLE 93-1**

ASSOCIATION OF PATENT FORAMEN OVALE AND ATRIAL SEPTAL ANEURYSM WITH STROKE IN YOUNG ADULTS (<55 YEARS)

| | Odds ratio (95% CI) | | |
| --- | --- | --- | --- |
| | PFO | Aneurysm | PFO + Aneurysm |
| Stroke versus nonstroke controls | 3 (2–4) | 6 (3–15) | 16 (3–86) |
| Cryptogenic stroke versus known cause | 6 (4–10) | 7 (2–31) | 17 (2–133) |
| Cryptogenic stroke versus nonstroke controls | 5 (3–8) | 19 (3–150) | 24 (3–185) |

CI, confidence interval; PFO, patent foramen ovale.
From Overell JR, Bone I, Lees KR. Interatrial septal abnormalities and stroke: a meta-analysis of case-control studies. *Neurology* 2000;55:1172–1179, with permission.

simple, inexpensive, and noninvasive but has its limitations in patients with inadequate acoustic windows, resulting in relatively poor images of insufficient resolution. Notwithstanding, atrial septal aneurysms can often be well documented with TTE, which led to the initial misconception that they are an independent source of cerebral embolism. In fact, the real culprit, the associated PFO, just went undetected. "Indirect" signs of a PFO can sometimes be demonstrated by color Doppler mapping or a bubble test after a Valsalva maneuver as described in subsequent paragraphs.

### Transesophageal Echocardiography

Multiplane TEE with contrast and Valsalva maneuver is generally considered the most sensitive and specific method for the noninvasive detection of PFOs and represents the diagnostic "gold standard." The technique provides high-resolution images of the interatrial septum and allows for accurate sizing of the separation between septum primum and secundum, the definition of anatomic boundaries of the PFO, and the demonstration of a right-to-left shunt by either color flow mapping or contrast bubble injection. It is important to inject the contrast medium into a peripheral vein (ideally a leg vein) immediately at the end of a sustained Valsalva maneuver. During Valsalva maneuver, both atria stay underfilled secondary to the high intrathoracic pressure. At the end of Valsalva maneuver, the right atrium fills up immediately with blood, primarily from the lower part of the body, while the left atrium stays volume-depleted for a few more seconds until the blood tide has passed through the lungs; this engenders a transient right-to-left shunt in case of a PFO.

The shunt may be semiquantitatively assessed by the amount of bubbles seen on a still frame, having crossed from the right to the left atrium after intravenous injection of agitated saline [grade 0, none; grade 1, minimal (one to five bubbles); grade 2, moderate (six to 20 bubbles); grade 3, severe (>20 bubbles)] (7). TEE enables the identification of an associated atrial septal aneurysm and allows for reliable exclusion of other potential intracardiac sources of embolism. TEE can also be used as an imaging tool to guide device deployment during percutaneous PFO or atrial septal defects (ASD) closure.

### Transcranial Contrast Doppler Ultrasonography

Transcranial contrast Doppler (TCD) ultrasonography provides another noninvasive modality to obtain indirect proof of the presence of PFO. The technique is based on the detection of an intravenously injected contrast agent passing through intracranial arteries (e.g., middle cerebral artery), which are insonated through the temporal bone windows. The echocardiographic contrast agents (with microbubbles) used are unable to pass the pulmonary capillary bed. Injected into a peripheral vein, they are detectable by TCD in the cerebral circulation only if a right to left shunt exists (see Fig. 93-3) (30). In experienced hands, the sensitivity and specificity of TCD approach, and that of TEE approach, and the quantification of right-to-left shunts using provocative (i.e., Valsalva) maneuvers may be more easily accomplished with less patient discomfort. Moreover, TCD allows for the detection of extracardiac shunts, which can also be a pathway for paradoxical embolism (31).

### Intracardiac Echocardiography

Intracardiac echocardiography (ICE) is not practically used for diagnostic purposes and is, therefore, outside the scope of this review. However, ICE can play a role in guiding percutaneous closure of PFOs and ASDs.

### Right Heart Catheterization

This invasive technique can also be used to diagnose PFOs, with contrast medium injection (see Fig. 93-4) or catheter or guide wire passage of the defect from the right to the left atrium.

## Deep Venous Thrombosis

The pelvic and deep lower limb veins form an important potential thromboembolic source. Autopsy studies suggest isolated pelvic veins or inferior vena cava thrombus in 22% of patients with paradoxical emboli with an identifiable source (2), and a number of studies have described pelvic and lower limb deep vein thrombosis (DVT) in patients with cryptogenic stroke and PFO (32–35). The PELVIS (Paradoxical Embolism from Large Veins in Ischemic Stroke) study assessed young (<60 years) patients presenting with ischemic strokes and found a higher prevalence of both PFOs and pelvic DVTs in patients with cryptogenic compared with those with strokes of determined origin (36). Some studies have reported a 4% to 10% association between DVT and strokes in patients with PFO (37,38).

Before    After

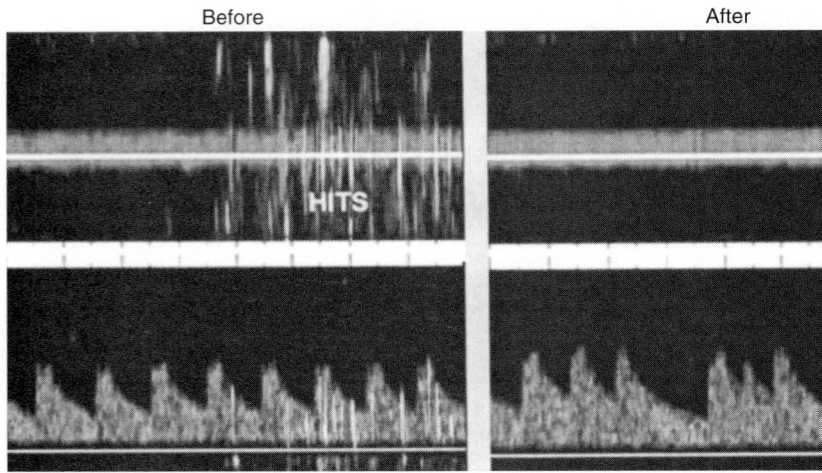

FIGURE 93-3. Transcranial contrast Doppler ultrasonography with bubble test after Valsalva maneuver of a cerebral artery in a 55-year-old man immediately before (**left**) and after (**right**) percutaneous patent foramen ovale (PFO) occlusion with an Amplatzer device. The paradoxically embolized bubbles produce high-intensity transient signals (*HITS*) before closure that are completely absent after closure.

Noninvasive tests such as duplex scanning and plethysmography of lower limb/pelvic veins have limited sensitivities and specificities (39,40). The sensitivity of radionuclide scanning is marginally higher, but this technique is restricted to specialized centers. Invasive diagnostic methods such as contrast venography, either alone or in combination with computerized tomography scan (spiral-CT scan) or magnetic resonance imaging (MRI), have a higher detection rate (41,42).

All techniques are limited by a relatively low yield, and the presence of a predisposing venous thrombus is often very difficult to establish in clinical practice. A comprehensive workup, using multiple imaging methods, may increase the detection rate. Fifty percent of thromboses were reported to be clinically "silent" in a large autopsy study (43). The thrombus may have already dissipated, embolized, or recanalized, and any residual clot may be too small to be detected even by the most sensitive methods. The thrombosis may be localized in veins other than those in the legs (e.g., subclavian, splenic, hepatic, mesenteric, parauterine, paraprostatic, or hemorrhoidal veins). Additionally, the venous thrombus may be a consequence rather than a cause of arterial embolism, especially in patients who are paralyzed with a stroke. Therefore, it is generally accepted that the inability to detect venous thrombus does not preclude the diagnosis of paradoxical embolism.

## Hypercoagulable Disorders

Several reports have described hypercoagulability in patients with ischemic strokes and PFO (44–46). Disorders such as elevated lipoprotein (a), hyperhomocysteinemia, and dysfibrigonemia are primarily associated with arterial thrombosis (47–49). Elevated factor VIII levels; prothrombin gene G202010A mutation; factor $V_{Leiden}$ (with activated protein C resistance); and protein C, protein S, and antithrombin III deficiencies are associated with venous thrombosis (50). A comprehensive coagulability screening of patients presenting with stroke/TIAs should include assessment of D-dimer levels; thrombin, prothrombin, and partial thromboplastin times; fibrinogen level; kaolin/silica clotting time; factors V, VII, and VIII concentration; and antithrombin III, protein C and S, lupus anticoagulant, anticardiolipin IgG and IgM, lipoprotein (a), and homocysteine levels.

Finding such coagulation anomalies does not acquit a possibly coexisting PFO. Rather, these anomalies may enhance the danger of a PFO and heighten the importance of its closure.

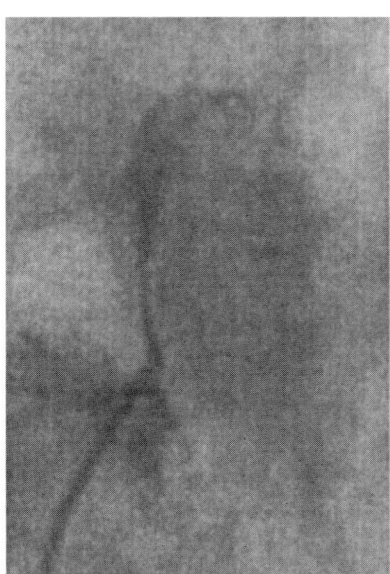
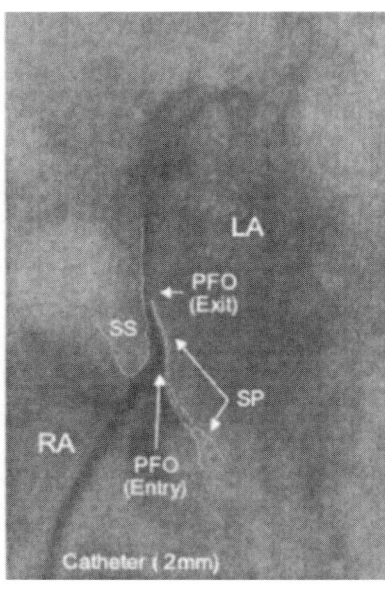

FIGURE 93-4. Documentation of a patent foramen ovale (*PFO*) by right atrial (*RA*) contrast medium injection. LA, left atrium; SP, septum primum; SS, septum secundum.

**TABLE 93-2**

DIAGONASTIC WORKUP OF PARADOXIAL EMBOLISM

| Essential | Recommended | Optional |
|---|---|---|
| **CENTRAL NERVOUS SYSTEM** | | |
| CT scan | MRI | Cerebral artery bubble test |
| Carotid Doppler ultrasonography | | |
| | | |
| **HEART/LUNG** | | |
| TEE | TTE | Right heart catheterization |
| 12-lead ECG | TCD | Perfusion lung scan |
| | | |
| **BLOOD** | | |
| D-dimers; prothrombin, thrombin, | Fibrinogen, factor | Homocysteine, |
| partial thromboplastin time; | VII, factor VIII | lipoprotein (a) |
| factor V; ATIII; protein C and S; | | |
| lupus anticoagulant/anticardiolipin | | |
| IgG and IgM | | |
| | | |
| **PELVIC/LOWER LIMBS** | | |
| Contrast venography ± CT/MRI | Radionuclide | Duplex vein scans, |
| | scintigraphy | plethysmography |

CT, computerized tomography; ECG, electrocardiogram; MRI, magnetic resonance imaging; ATIII, antithrombin III; TEE, transesophageal echocardiography; Ig, immunoglobulin; TCD, transcranial Doppler ultrasound.

## Associated Atrial Arrhythmias

A relatively small study of patients younger than 55 years with ischemic cryptogenic stroke and TEE evidence of atrial septal aneurysm or PFO, investigated whether paroxysmal atrial arrhythmias resulting from abnormal atrial septal anatomy could be an underlying cause of thromboembolic stroke (51). All patients underwent electrophysiologic studies for inducible sustained atrial fibrillation. Patients with atrial septal abnormalities were found to have a significantly higher inducibility than those without such abnormalities [58% vs. 25%, odds ratio (OR), 4; 95% confidence interval (CI), 1 to 13; $P <0.02$]. Despite this study suggesting a role of transient atrial arrhythmias in patients with cryptogenic stroke, the clinical relevance of this association needs to be confirmed.

Table 93-2 summarizes the diagnostic workup for patients suspected of having paradoxical embolism.

# OTHER DISEASE MANIFESTATIONS ASSOCIATED WITH PATENT FORAMEN OVALE

Apart from the association with stroke/TIA, the PFO has also been etiologically linked with decompression illness in divers (52), with migraine with aura (53,54), and with the platypnea-orthodeoxia syndrome (55).

Decompression illness in divers results from regional nitrogen and oxygen gas formation in predominantly fat-containing tissues and from arterial gas embolism. Both conditions can produce ischemic brain lesions. Gas passage from the venous to the arterial circulation can occur because of either pulmonary barotraumas or intravascular shunting. There is an increasingly well-recognized association between decompression illness in divers and the presence of PFO, and correlation with the PFO size (56).

The role of PFO in cases of migraine complicated by aura is a subject of controversy. PFO-mediated paradoxical embolisms of particulate matter, certain triggering substances, or changes in arterial oxygenation have all been implicated in migraine attacks with aura. A higher prevalence of right-to-left shunt was observed in patients with migraine with aura compared to healthy controls. Studies have suggested symptomatic improvement in patients with migrainous headaches following percutaneous shunt closure (53,54).

The platypnea-orthodeoxia syndrome is a rare clinical entity comprising breathlessness related to oxygen desaturation induced by the upright position and relieved by recumbency. The most common etiologic association is with an interatrial right-to-left shunt through a PFO, and the condition can be cured by percutaneous or surgical PFO closure (PC) (55).

Furthermore, paradoxical embolism can be facilitated in cases of PFO associated with increased right-sided pressures as a consequence of primary or secondary pulmonary hypertension and in right ventricular infarction. In fact, paradoxical embolism is often preceded by pulmonary embolism, which, by raising the pressure in the right ventricle and atrium, favors the passage of subsequent emboli from the right side to the left side of the heart. An increased risk of death and thromboembolic complications has been reported in patients with major pulmonary embolism in the presence of PFO (21).

# THERAPEUTIC CONSIDERATIONS

There are a broad range of treatment options with considerable variation in associated risk and cost. These options consist of antiplatelet agents, oral anticoagulants, or percutaneous and surgical closure of the PFO.

## Medical Treatment

Medical therapy for neurologic events secondary to paradoxical embolism comprises either antiplatelet agents (principally acetylsalicylic acid at a dose of 250 to 500 mg per day) or oral anticoagulation [target international normalized ratio (INR) 2 to 3]. The reported annual rates of stroke/TIA recurrence with medical therapy ranges from 0% to 20% (57–64).

A large prospective study by Mas et al. (28) reported on the clinical outcome of 581 patients, younger than 55 years (mean age 42 years), with cryptogenic stroke who were treated with acetylsalicylic acid 300 mg per day and followed up for up to 4 years. At 4 years, they reported a risk of recurrent stroke or TIA of 5.6% in patients with PFO alone, 19.2% in patients with both PFO and atrial septal aneurysm, 0% in patients with atrial septal aneurysm alone, and 6.2% in patients without atrial septal abnormality. The authors concluded that patients with both PFO and atrial septal aneurysm are at substantial risk of recurrence, requiring additional preventive strategies beyond treatment with acetylsalicylic acid alone, whereas patients with PFO alone are at low risk of recurrence comparable to those patients without atrial septal abnormality. Hence, the study confirmed that a large PFO, rather than the associated atrial septal aneurysm, was responsible for recurrences.

The Warfarin in Aspirin Recurrent Stroke Study (WARSS) randomized patients aged 30 to 85 years with a recent ischemic stroke to either acetylsalicylic acid (325 mg) or warfarin (INR 1.4 to 2.8) and found no difference in recurrence of ischemic neurologic events or death at 2 years (65). The achieved mean INR in this series was 2.0, and this could have been inadequate to demonstrate a statistically significant difference between the two treatment groups.

A prospective subgroup analysis, the PFO in Cryptogenic Stroke Study (PICSS), also found no statistically significant difference in the rate of recurrence of stroke/TIA or death in patients treated with acetylsalicylic acid or warfarin (66). It was reported that the presence of PFO did not have an adverse impact on recurrent cerebrovascular events regardless of PFO size and presence of an atrial septal aneurysm. However, only 42%

of patients included in this study had a cryptogenic stroke as opposed to stroke of known etiology (large vessels 11%, lacunar 39%, other determined cause 4%, and conflicting mechanism 4%). Therefore, it is not surprising that PFO was only an "innocent bystander" in most of these patients. Notwithstanding, the investigators were able to reproduce the prevalence of large PFOs in patients with cryptogenic stroke compared with controls of known stroke cause. The recurrent stroke and death rates at 2 years were 9.5% and 17.9% for patients with cryptogenic stroke with PFO receiving warfarin or acetylsalicylic acid, respectively [relative risk (RR), 0.52; 95% CI, 0.16 to 1.67; $P = 0.3$]. Although not statistically significant, these rates correspond to a 48% event reduction in favor of warfarin and contrast with the event rates of 16.5% and 13.2% for patients treated with warfarin or acetylsalicylic acid, respectively, in the entire PICSS cohort of patients with PFO. However, a similar 49% reduction in favor of warfarin was observed in patients with cryptogenic stroke without PFO, implying a PFO-independent but possibly anticoagulation-responsive stroke mechanism.

Table 93-3 summarizes the results of published studies of medical treatment for secondary prevention of stroke recurrence in the presence of PFO.

## Surgical Patent Foramen Ovale Closure

Limited data describe surgical PFO closure as a safe and effective means of treatment, with reported ischemic neurologic event annual recurrence rates of 0% to 19.5% (67–70). However, these figures may be distorted by limited and selected enrollment, as well as by the single-center nature of these case series. Table 93-4 summarizes the results of published studies on surgical PFO closure for the secondary prevention of stroke recurrence.

### TABLE 93-3

**MEDICAL TREATMENT FOR SECONDARY PREVENTION OF STROKE RECURRENCE WITH PARADOXIAL EMBOLISM**

| Study (yr) | Patients (*n*) | Follow-up (mo) | Annual CVA recurrence (%) | Annual TIA and CVA recurrence (%) |
|---|---|---|---|---|
| Comess et al. (1994) (62) | 33 | 12 | — | 16 |
| Hanna et al. (1994) (59) | 13 | 41 | 0 | — |
| Mas and Zuber (1995) (58) | 132 | 22 | 1.2 | 3.4 |
| Bogousslavsky et al. (1996) (61) | 140 | 36 | 1.9 | 3.8 |
| Cujec et al. (1999) (63) | 52 | 12 | — | 12 |
| De Castro et al. (2000) (60) | 86 | 36 | 0.7 | 2.4 |
| Mas et al. (2001) (28) | 571 | 48 | 1.1 | 1.6 |
| Nedeltchev et al. (2002) (64) | 159 | 29 | 1.8 | 5.5 |
| Homma et al. (2002) (66) | 203 | 24 | 4.6 | 10.4 |

CVA, cerebrovascular accident; TIA, transient ischemic attack.

## TABLE 93-4

**SURGICAL PFO CLOSURE FOR SECONDARY PREVENTION OF STROKE RECURRENCE**

| Study (yr) | Patients (*n*) | Follow-up (mo) | Annual CVA recurrence (%) | Annual TIA and CVA recurrence (%) |
|---|---|---|---|---|
| Devuyst et al. (1996) (70) | 30 | 24 | 0 | 0 |
| Homma et al. (1997) (67) | 28 | 19 | 3.6 | 19.5 |
| Ruchat et al. (1997) (68) | 32 | 22 | 0 | 0 |
| Dearani et al. (1999) (69) | 91 | 48 | 0 | 4.3 |

CVA, cerebrovascular accident; TIA, transient ischemic attack.

## Percutaneous Patent Foramen Ovale Closure

Percutaneous closure of a PFO was first performed in 1989, after experience had been gained with percutaneous closure of ASD. The technique was initially advocated for the prevention of recurrent strokes by Bridges et al. (71). Since then, there have been a number of reports on safety, feasibility, and recurrence of thromboembolic events with the use of various closure devices (see Table 93-5).

Braun et al. (77) reported a 100% implantation success in 276 consecutive patients undergoing percutaneous closure of PFO associated with a thromboembolic event. Transient ST segment elevation occurred in 1.8% and TIA in 0.8%. At 15 months follow-up, there were no recurrent strokes or peripheral emboli, and only 1.7% of patients experienced a repeat TIA.

Martin et al. (78) also reported 100% success in implantation of percutaneous PFO occluder devices in 110 consecutive patients, with device migration (requiring surgical intervention)

## TABLE 93-5

**PERCUTANEOUS PFO CLOSURE SAFETY AND FEASIBILITY**

| Study (yr) | Patients (*n*) | Device | Success (%) | Complications (%) | Closure[a] (%) |
|---|---|---|---|---|---|
| Bridges et al. (1992) (71) | 36 | Clamshell | 100 | 3 | 82[b,c] |
| Ende et al. (1996) (72) | 10 | Buttoned | 90 | 10 | 60[c] |
| Hung (2000) (73) | 63 | Clamshell CardioSeal Buttoned | 100 | (Not reported) | 86[a] |
| Windecker et al. (2000) (74) | 80 | Buttoned Amplatzer Angel Wings CardioSeal PFO Star | 98 | 10 | 73[c] |
| Wahl et al. (2001) (75) | 152 | Buttoned Amplatzer Angel Wings CardioSeal PFO Star | 99 | 6 | 80[c] |
| Bruch et al. (2002) (76) | 66 | Amplatzer PFO Star CardioSeal Starflex | 100 | 0 | 100[b,c] |
| Braun et al. (2002) (77) | 276 | PFO Star | 100 | 4 | 96[c] |
| Martin et al. (2002) (78) | 110 | Buttoned CardioSeal | 100 | 5 | 51[c] |
| Khositseth et al. (2004) (79) | 103 | Amplatzer | 100 | 7 | 93[b,c] |

PFO, patent foramen ovale.
[a]Immediate.
[b]At transthoracic echocardiography follow-up.
[c]At transesophageal echocardiography follow-up.

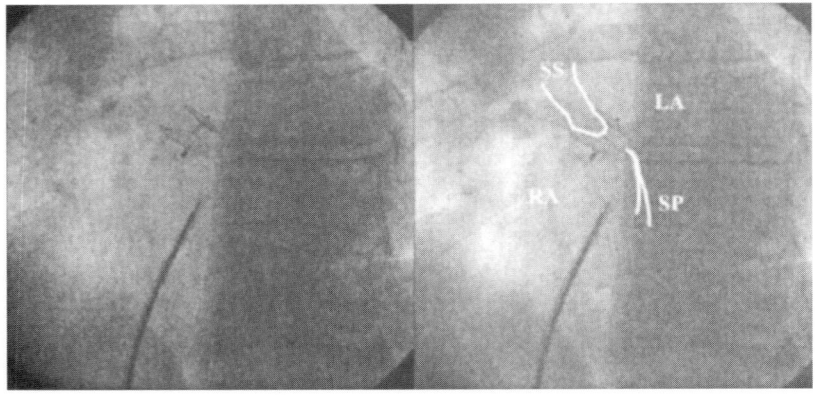

FIGURE 93-5. Percutaneous patent foramen ovale (PFO) closure using an Amplatzer PFO Occluder Device (left cranial oblique view). The **right** and **left** discs of the device deployed are connected by a thin waist across the PFO. LA, left atrium; RA, right atrium; SP, septum primum; SS, septum secundum.

in one patient (0.9%) and one case of cardiac tamponade treated with percutaneous drainage. These patients received acetylsalicylic acid 325 mg daily or clopidogrel 75 mg daily or ticlopidine 250 mg twice a day following device implantation. Two-year follow-up revealed one fatal stroke (0.9%) and one case of recurrent TIA, in addition to four patients (3.6%) requiring reintervention for device malalignment or significant considerable residual shunt.

More recently, Khositseth et al. (79) published their data for 103 consecutive patients undergoing 100% successful percutaneous device deployment in patients with PFO or ASD with presumed paradoxical embolism. All patients received warfarin and acetylsalicylic acid or clopidogrel for 3 months after closure, and acetylsalicylic acid or clopidogrel for a further 3 months. Patients with hypercoagulable states were maintained on warfarin and acetylsalicylic acid or clopidogrel for 6 months after closure. One case of device embolization (successfully retrieved) was reported, in addition to two cases of atrial fibrillation, three of vessel injury, and one of profound sinus node dysfunction. Their average annual recurrence for thromboembolic events was 3.6% at 23 months follow-up.

In our own experience, device implantation was successful in 98% of 80 cases, with an actuarial annual risk of recurrence of 2.5% for TIA, 0% for stroke, and 0.9% for peripheral emboli (combined endpoint 3.4%) in more than 5 years of follow up. Acetylsalicylic acid 100 mg was used for the first 6 months after device closure. We found that a postprocedural transseptal right-to-left shunt was a predictor of recurrent paradoxical embolism with a relative risk of 4 (95% CI, 1 to 18; $P = 0.03$). The risk of recurrent embolic events in patients with both atrial septal aneurysm and PFO was not significantly higher when compared with patients with PFO only. The risk of recurrence was highest during the first year after closure, with no further events beyond 2 years (74).

In contrast to the earlier devices initially developed for closure of secundum ASDs, the dedicated PFO closure devices have a lower risk of embolization and a higher closure potential (with complete closure reported in >95% of patients). Figure 93-5 illustrates an example of percutaneous PFO closure using the Amplatzer PFO Occluder. The technique can be performed under local anesthesia in less than 15 minutes with the possibility for the patient to return to normal physical activities as early as a few hours later. The risk of the intervention is small and the rate of complete and permanent closure of the PFO is greater than 90%. Potential complications arising from percutaneous device closure of PFO include device embolization, air embolism, tamponade, retroperitoneal hematoma (inadvertent femoral artery puncture during venous access), and thrombus formation on the

occluder device. The incidence of thrombus formation on ASD or PFO closure devices was reportedly low (<7%) in a large prospective study, with most thrombi resolving uneventfully with anticoagulation (80,81). There was a significantly different propensity for thrombosis among the devices compared.

# COMPARISON OF MEDICAL TREATMENT WITH PERCUTANEOUS CLOSURE OF PATENT FORAMEN OVALE

Comparisons between medical therapy and percutaneous PFO closure for secondary prevention of stroke/TIAs have been reported in a case–control study (82) and in a metaanalysis of observational studies of medical treatment and percutaneous PFO closure (83).

In our experience of 311 patients with cryptogenic stroke and PFO, 150 patients underwent percutaneous PFO closure, using a variety of closure devices, and 161 patients were treated medically (81 with antiplatelet agents and 80 with oral anticoagulation). We found a trend of higher actuarial freedom from recurrence of stroke/TIA for more than 4 years with device closure (see Fig. 93-6). In patients with more than one cerebrovascular event at baseline and those with complete occlusion

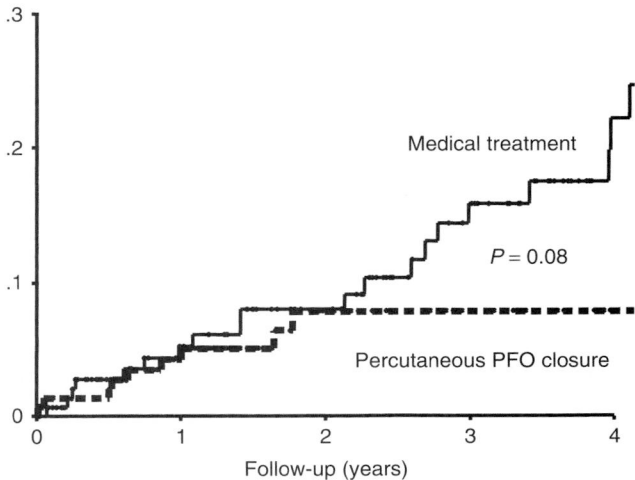

FIGURE 93-6. Recurrence of stroke/transient ischemic attack (TIA) following percutaneous patent foramen ovale (PFO) closure (150 patients) compared with medical therapy (161 patients).

of PFO, there was a significantly lower risk for recurrent stroke/TIA after device closure than with medical treatment (7% vs. 33%; $P = 0.01$; 95% CI, 0.1 to 0.8; and 7% vs. 22%; $P = 0.04$; 95% CI, 0.1 to 1.0, respectively) (82).

In a recent systematic review of the relative benefits of percutaneous PFO closure compared with medical treatment, Khairy et al. (83) reported a protective effect of percutaneous PFO closure compared with medical treatment on stroke/TIA recurrence (annual incidence 2% vs. 5%; RR, 0.4; 95% CI, 0.2 to 0.6; $P <0.0001$). At 1 year follow-up, one of every 23 patients undergoing percutaneous PFO closure was prevented from recurrent stroke/TIA compared with medical treatment.

The randomized PFO Closure (PC) study has enrolled approximately 250 patients by summer 2005. Three other randomized trials, CLOSURE-1, RESPECT, and CARDIA are in their recruiting phases. Until the outcomes of these trials are known, there are no data to conclusively support PFO closure for paradoxical embolism. Percutaneous PFO closure remains feasible, but should be restricted to patients who are carefully selected and who are fully informed. Surgical treatment of PFO has been largely abandoned in favor of catheter-based closure. This was compelled by the ease and efficiency of the percutaneous technique and the fact that a surgical intervention could still be used in case of a failed percutaneous attempt. Incidentally, this latter strategy was never necessary in more than 500 consecutive cases at our center.

# CONCLUSIONS

Approximately 20% to 40% of ischemic strokes are cryptogenic, with substantial evidence indicating paradoxical embolism as the responsible stroke mechanism. There is currently no consensus as to the optimal therapy for patients with PFO and paradoxical embolism (84). Long-term results of medical therapy to prevent recurrent strokes have been somewhat disappointing. Percutaneous closure has been shown to be safe and feasible, with high procedural success rates and is less invasive than the surgical approach. Until the results of randomized controlled trials are available, percutaneous closure of PFOs in patients with paradoxical embolism represents an attractive, but investigational, treatment option.

## *References*

1. Connheim J. *Thrombose und embolie: vorlesung über allgemeine pathologie.* Berlin: Hirschwald, 1877:134.
2. Johnson BI. Paradoxical embolism. *J Clin Pathol* 1951;4:316–332.
3. Falk V, Walther T, Krankenberg H, et al. Trapped thrombus in a patent foramen ovale. *Thorac Cardiovasc Surg* 1997;45:90–92.
4. Caes FL, van Belleghem YV, Missault LH, et al. Surgical treatment of impending paradoxical embolism through patent foramen ovale. *Ann Thorac Surg* 1995;59:1559–1561.
5. Pell AC, Hughes D, Keating J, et al. Brief report: fulminating fat embolism syndrome caused by paradoxical embolism through a patent foramen ovale. *N Engl J Med* 1993;329:926–929.
6. Lechat P, Mas JL, Lascault G, et al. Prevalence of patent foramen ovale in patients with stroke. *N Engl J Med* 1988;318:1148–1152.
7. Webster MW, Chancellor AM, Smith HJ, et al. Patent foramen ovale in young stroke patients. *Lancet* 1988;2:11–12.
8. Hausmann D, Mugge A, Becht I, et al. Diagnosis of patent foramen ovale by transesophageal echo and association with cerebral and peripheral embolic events. *Am J Cardiol* 1992;70:668–672.
9. Di Tullio M, Sacco RL, Gopal A, et al. Patent foramen ovale as a risk factor for cryptogenic stroke. *Ann Intern Med* 1992;117:461–465.
10. Cabanes L, Mas JL, Cohen A, et al. Atrial septal aneurysm and patent foramen ovale as risk factors for cryptogenic stroke in patients less than 55 years of age: a study using transesophageal echocardiography. *Stroke* 1993;24:1865–1873.
11. de Belder MA, Tourikis L, Leech G, et al. Risk of patent foramen ovale for thromboembolic events in all age groups. *Am J Cardiol* 1992;69: 1316–1320.
12. Broderick J, Brott T, Kothari R, et al. The Greater Cincinnati/Northern Kentucky Stroke Study: preliminary first-ever and total incidence rates of stroke among blacks. *Stroke* 1998;29:415–421.
13. Goldstein LB, Adams R, Becker K, et al. Primary prevention of ischemic stroke: a statement for healthcare professionals from The Stroke Council of the American Heart Association. *Circulation* 2001;103:163–182.
14. Burn J, Dennis M, Bamford J, et al. Long-term risk of recurrent stroke after a first-ever stroke. The Oxfordshire community stroke project. *Stroke* 1994;25:333–337.
15. Sacco RL, Shi T, Zamanillo MC, et al. Predictors of mortality and recurrence after hospitalized cerebral infarction in an urban community: the Northern Manhattan Stroke Study. *Neurology* 1994;44:626–634.
16. Meissner I, Whisnant JP, Khandheria BK, et al. Prevalence of potential risk factors for stroke assessed by transesophageal echocardiography and carotid ultrasonography: the SPARC study. Stroke prevention: assessment of risk in a community. *Mayo Clin Proc* 1999;74:862–869.
17. Bogousslavsky J, Van Melle G, Regli F. The lausanne stroke registry: analysis of 1,000 consecutive patients with first stroke. *Stroke* 1988;19:1083–1092.
18. Sacco RL, Ellenberg JH, Mohr JP, et al. Infarcts of undetermined cause: the NINCDS Stroke Data Bank. *Ann Neurol* 1989;25:382–390.
19. Hart RG, Miller VT. Cerebral infarction in young adults: a practical approach. *Stroke* 1983;14:110–114.
20. Overell JR, Bone I, Lees KR. Interatrial septal abnormalities and stroke: a meta-analysis of case-control studies. *Neurology* 2000;55:1172–1179.
21. Konstantinides S, Geibel A, Kasper W, et al. Patent foramen ovale is an important predictor adverse outcome in patients with major pulmonary embolism. *Circulation* 1998;97:1946–1951.
22. Royden J, Caplan LR, Come PC, et al. Cerebral emboli of paradoxical origin. *Ann Neurol* 1983;13:314–319.
23. Hagen PT, Scholz DG, Edwards WD. Incidence and size of patent foramen ovale during the first 10 decades of life: an autopsy study of 965 normal hearts. *Mayo Clin Proc* 1984;59:17–20.
24. Windecker S, Meier B. Patent foramen ovale and atrial septal aneurysm: when and how should they be treated? *ACC Curr J Rev* 2002;11:97–101.
25. Hanley PC, Tajik AJ, Hynes JK, et al. Diagnosis and classification of atrial septal aneurysm by two-dimensional echocardiography: report of 80 consecutive cases. *J Am Coll Cardiol* 1985;6:1370–1382.
26. Pearson AC, Nagelhout D, Castello R, et al. Atrial septal aneurysm and stroke: a transesophageal echocardiographic study. *J Am Coll Cardiol* 1991;18:1223–1229.
27. Agmon Y, Khandheria BK, Meissner I, et al. Frequency of atrial septal aneurysms in patients with cerebral ischemic events. *Circulation* 1999;99: 1942–1944.
28. Mas JL, Arquizan C, Lamy C et al, Patent Foramen Ovale and Atrial Septal Aneurysm Study Group. Recurrent cerebrovascular events associated with patent foramen ovale, atrial septal aneurysm, or both. *N Engl J Med* 2001;345:1740–1746.
29. Biben C, Weber R, Kesteven S, et al. Cardiac septal and valvular dysmorphogenesis in mice heterozygous for mutations in the homeobox gene Nkx2-5. *Circ Res* 2000;87:833–834.
30. Droste DW, Lakemeier S, Wichter T, et al. Optimizing the technique of contrast transcranial ultrasound in the detection of right-to-left shunts. *Stroke* 2002;33:2211–226.
31. Yeung M, Khan KA, Antecol DH, et al. Transcranial doppler ultrasonography and transesophageal echocardiography in the investigation of pulmonary arteriovenous malformation in a patient with hereditary hemorrhagic telangiectasia presenting with stroke. *Stroke* 1995;26: 1941–1944.
32. Cramer SC, Rordorf G, Kaufmann JA, et al. Clinically occult pelvic-vein thrombosis in cryptogenic stroke. *Lancet* 1998;351:1927–1928.
33. Greer DM, Buonnano FS. Cerebral infarction in conjunction with patent foramen ovale and May-Thurner syndrome. *J Neuroimaging* 2001;11: 432–434.
34. Cramer SC, Maki JH, Waitches GM, et al. Paradoxical emboli from calf and pelvic veins in cryptogenic stroke. *J Neuroimaging* 2003;13:218–223.
35. Stollberger C, Slany J, Schuster I, et al. The prevalence of deep venous thrombosis in patients with suspected paradoxical embolism. *Ann Intern Med* 1993;119:461–465.
36. Cramer SC, Rordorf G, Maki JH, et al. Increased pelvic vein thrombi in cryptogenic stroke. Results of the paradoxical emboli from large veins in ischemic stroke (PELVIS) study. *Stroke* 2004;35:46–50.
37. Ranoux D, Cohen A, Cabanes L, et al. Patent foramen ovale: is stroke due to paradoxical embolism? *Stroke* 1993;24:31–34.
38. Lethen H, Flachskampf FA, Schneider R, et al. Frequency of deep vein thrombosis in patients with patent foramen ovale and ischemic stroke or transient ischemic attack. *Am J Cardiol* 1997;80:1066–1069.
39. Kearon C, Julian JA, Math M, et al. Non-invasive diagnosis of deep venous thrombosis. *Ann Intern Med* 1998;128:663–677.
40. Dorfman GS, Cronan JJ. Venous ultrasonography. *Radiol Clin North Am* 1992;30:879–893.
41. Spritzer CE, Arata MA, Freed KS. Isolated pelvic deep venous thrombosis: relative frequency as detected with MR imaging. *Radiology* 2001;219: 521–525.
42. Fraser DG, Moody AR, Morgan PS, et al. Diagnosis of lower-limb deep venous thrombosis: a prospective blinded study of magnetic resonance direct thrombus imaging. *Ann Intern Med* 2002;136:89–98.

43. Sevitt S, Gallagher N. Venous thrombosis and pulmonary embolism. A clinico-pathological study in injured and burned patients. *Br J Surg* 1961;48:457–489.

44. Bezzi G, Bolzani W, Compagnoni V, et al. Factor V leiden mutation and patent foramen ovale in ischemic stroke. *Neurol Sci* 2002;23:229–231.

45. Karttunen V, Hiltunen L, Rasi V, et al. Factor V Leiden and prothrombin gene mutation may predispose to paradoxical embolism in subjects with patent foramen ovale. *Blood Coagul Fibrinolysis* 2003;14:261–268.

46. Dodge SM, Hassell K, Anderson A, et al. Antiphospholipid antibodies are common in patients referred for percutaneous patent foramen ovale closure. *Catheter Cardiovasc Interv* 2004;61:123–127.

47. Milionis HJ, Winder AF, Mikhailidis DP. Lipoprotein (a) and stroke. *J Clin Pathol* 2000;53:487–496.

48. van Beynum IM, Smeitink JAM, den Heijer M, et al. Hyperhomocysteine-mia: a risk factor for ischemic stroke in children. *Circulation* 1999;99:2070–2072.

49. Coté HCF, Lord ST, Pratt KP. Gamma-chain dysfibrinogenemias: molecular structure-function relationships of naturally occurring mutations in the g chain of human fibrinogen. *Blood* 1998;92:2195–2212.

50. Thomas RH. Hypercoagulability syndromes. *Arch Intern Med* 2001;161:2433–2439.

51. Berthet K, Lavergen T, Cohen A, et al. Significant association of atrial vulnerability with atrial septal abnormalities in young patients with ischaemic stroke of unknown cause. *Stroke* 2000;31:398–403.

52. Schwerzmann M, Seiler C, Lipp E, et al. Relation between directly detected patent foramen ovale and ischemic brain lesions in sport divers. *Ann Intern Med* 2001;134:21–24.

53. Schwerzmann M, Wiher S, Nedletchev K, et al. Percutaneous closure of patent foramen ovale reduces the frequency of migraine attacks. *Neurology* 2004;62:1399–1401.

54. Wilmshurst PT, Nightingale S, Walsh KP, et al. Effect on migraine of closure of cardiac right-to-left shunts to prevent recurrence of decompression illness or stroke or for hemodynamic reasons. *Lancet* 2000;356:1658–1651.

55. Seward JB, Hayes DL, Smith HC, et al. Platypnea-orthodeoxia: clinical profile, diagnostic workup, management, and report of seven cases. *Mayo Clin Proc* 1984;59:221–231.

56. Torti SR, Billinger M, Schwerzmann M, et al. Risk of decompression illness among 230 divers in relation to the presence and size of patent foramen ovale. *Eur Heart J* 2004;25:1014–1020.

57. Meier B, Lock JE. Contemporary management of patent foramen ovale. *Circulation* 2003;107:5–9.

58. Mas JL, Zuber M, French Study Group on Patent Foramen Ovale and Atrial Septal Aneurysm. Recurrent cerebrovascular events in patients with patent foramen ovale, atrial septal aneurysm, or both and cryptogenic stoke or transient ischemic attack. *Am Heart J* 1995;130:1083–1088.

59. Hanna JP, Sun JP, Furlan AJ, et al. Patent foramen ovale and brain infarct. Echocardiographic predictors, recurrence, and prevention. *Stroke* 1994;25:782–786.

60. De Castro S, Cartoni D, Fiorelli M, et al. Morphological and functional characteristics of patent foramen ovale and their embolic implications. *Stroke* 2000;31:2407–2413.

61. Bogoussslavsky J, Garazi S, Jeanrenaud X et al, Lausanne Stroke with Paradoxical Embolism Study Group. Stroke recurrence in patients with patent foramen ovale: the Lausanne Study. *Neurology* 1996;46:1301–1305.

62. Comess KA, DeRook Fa, Beach KW, et al. Transesophageal echocardiography and carotid ultrasound in patients with cerebral ischemia: prevalence of findings and recurrent stroke risk. *J Am Coll Cardiol* 1994;23:1598–1603.

63. Cujec B, Mainra R, Johnson DH. Prevention of recurrent cerebral ischemic events in patients with patent foramen ovale and cryptogenic strokes or transient ischemic attacks. *Can J Cardiol* 1999;15:57–64.

64. Nedeltchev K, Arnold M, Wahl A, et al. Outcome of patients with cryptogenic stroke and patent foramen ovale. *J Neurol Neurosurg Psychiatry* 2002;72:347–350.

65. Mohr JP, Thompson JL, Lazar RM et al, Warfarin-Aspirin Recurrent Stroke Study Group. A comparison of warfarin and aspirin for the prevention of recurrent ischemic stroke. *N Engl J Med* 2001;345:1740–1751.

66. Homma S, Sacco RL, Di Tullio et al, PFO in Cryptogenic Stroke Study (PICSS) Investigators. Effect of medical treatment in stroke patients with patent foramen ovale: patent foramen ovale in Cryptogenic Stroke Study. *Circulation* 2002;105:2625–2631.

67. Homma S, Di Tullio MR, Sacco RL, et al. Surgical closure of patent foramen ovale in cryptogenic stroke patients. *Stroke* 1997;28:2376–2331.

68. Ruchat P, Bogousslavsky J, Hurni M, et al. Systematic surgical closure of patent foramen ovale in selected patients with cerebrovascular events due to paradoxical embolism. Early results of a preliminary study. *Eur J Cardiothorac Surg* 1997;11:824–827.

69. Dearani JA, Ugurlu BS, Dainelson GK, et al. Surgical patent foramen ovale closure for prevention of paradoxical embolism-related cerebrovascular ischemic events. *Circulation* 1999;100:171–175.

70. Devuyst G, Bogousslavsky J, Ruchat P, et al. Prognosis after stroke followed by surgical closure of patent foramen ovale: a prospective follow-up study with brain MRI and simultaneous transesophogeal and transcranial doppler ultrasound. *Neurology* 1996;47:1162–1166.

71. Bridges ND, Hellebrand W, Latson L, et al. Transcatheter closure of patent foramen ovale after presumed paradoxical embolism. *Circulation* 1992;86:1902–1908.

72. Ende DJ, Chopra PS, Rao PS. Transcatheter closure of atrial septal defect or patent foramen ovale with the buttoned device for prevention of recurrence of paradoxical embolism. *Am J Cardiol* 1996;78:233–236.

73. Hung J, Landzberg MJ, Jenkins KJ, et al. Closure of patent foramen ovale for paradoxical emboli: intermediate-risk of recurrent neurological events following transcatheter device placement. *J Am Coll Cardiol* 2000;35:1311–1316.

74. Windecker S, Wahl A, Chatterjee T, et al. Percutaneous closure of patent foramen ovale in patients with paradoxical embolism: long term risk of recurrent thromboembolic events. *Circulation* 2000;101:893–898.

75. Wahl A, Meier B, Haxel B, et al. Prognosis after percutaneous closure of patent foramen ovale for paradoxical embolism. *Neurology* 2001;57:1330–1332.

76. Bruch L, Parsi A, Grad MO, et al. Transcatheter closure of interatrial communications for secondary prevention of paradoxical embolism: single-center experience. *Circulation* 2002;105:2845–2848.

77. Braun MV, Fassbender D, Schoen SP, et al. Transcatheter closure of patent foramen ovale in patients with cerebral ischemia. *J Am Coll Cardiol* 2002;39:2019–2025.

78. Martin F, Sanchez PL, Doherty E, et al. Percutaneous transcatheter closure of patent foramen ovale in patients with paradoxical embolism. *Circulation* 2002;106:1121–1126.

79. Khositseth A, Cabalka AK, Sweeney JP, et al. Transcatheter amplatzer device closure of atrial septal defect and patent foramen ovale in patients with presumed paradoxical embolism. *Mayo Clin Proc* 2004;79:15–20.

80. Kromsdorf U, Ostermayer S, Billinger K, et al. Incidence and clinical course of thrombus formation in atrial septal defects and patent foramen ovale closure devices in 1000 consecutive patients. *J Am Coll Cardiol* 2004;43:302–309.

81. Anzai H, Child J, Natterson B, et al. Incidence of thrombus formation on the CardioSEAL and the amplatzer interatrial closure devices. *Am J Cardiol* 2004;93:426–431.

82. Windecker S, Wahl A, Nedeltchev K, et al. Comparison of medical treatment with percutaneous closure of patent foramen ovale in patients with cryptogenic stroke. *J Am Coll Cardiol* 2004;44:750–758.

83. Khairy P, Landzberg MJ. Systematic review and analysis of transcatheter closure versus medical therapy for patent foramen ovale. *Ann Intern Med* 2003;139:753–760.

84. Messe SR, Silverman IE, Kizer JR, et al. Practice parameter: recurrent stroke with patent foramen ovale and atrial septal aneurysm: report of the Quality Standards Subcommittee of the American Academy of Neurology. *Neurology* 2004;62:1042–1050.

# CHAPTER 94 ■ PREVENTION OF VENOUS THROMBOEMBOLISM IN GENERAL SURGERY

AJAY K. KAKKAR

Venous thromboembolic disease frequently complicates the course of patients undergoing a variety of surgical interventions. Indeed, it was in the determination of the frequency of thrombosis in general surgical patients using the $I^{125}$ labelled fibrinogen leg scanning that Kakkar et al. in 1969 (1) were able to describe the natural history of postoperative deep vein thrombosis (DVT). The understanding of the natural history of this disease, and, subsequently, risk factors associated with its occurrence in surgical patients, as well as its wider epidemiology have allowed the development of strategies to both identify patient populations at risk for the development of venous thromboembolism (VTE) in the perioperative period, and quantify that risk, thereby providing methods for prophylaxis against venous thromboembolic episodes.

Beyond recognition that thrombosis commonly occurs in surgical populations has been the establishment of evidence that demonstrates the adverse consequences if thromboembolic disease is not prevented. Not only would patients have symptomatic DVT or pulmonary embolism (PE) but they may also experience, as a first manifestation of their thrombosis, a fatal PE (2). Approximately 80% of patients who develop pulmonary emboli will have no evidence of peripheral venous thrombosis before their presentation with PE (3). Because PE is frequently fatal even if diagnosed and treated in hospital (4), strategies based on a policy of treating massive PE or DVT as a way of preventing death from fatal PE expose surgical patients to an unacceptable risk of fatal thromboembolic complications. Beyond the consequences for the patient, in terms of their acute thrombotic episode, are the longer-term implications beyond the requirement for initial treatment. In the intermediate term, there is the need for prolonged anticoagulant therapy for treatment of a thrombotic episode. This treatment is frequently associated with serious, if not fatal bleeding complications (5). Furthermore, patients who develop an acute thrombosis, despite treatment with anticoagulants, are at greater risk for the development of recurrent thromboembolism, which in some cases may be fatal (6). Beyond this intermediate risk, patients with either symptomatic or asymptomatic DVT or PE are at greater risk for the development of the postphlebitic syndrome, the symptoms of which include leg swelling, varicose veins, venous ulceration, and other trophic skin changes, which are disabling and have an impact on the patient's quality of life (7).

## RISK OF VENOUS THROMBOEMBOLIC DISEASE IN GENERAL SURGICAL PROCEDURES

More than 3 decades of research have identified risk factors associated with the development of postoperative venous thromboembolic disease in general surgical patients. Most important among these are advancing age, previous history of venous thromboembolic disease, long periods of immobility, malignant disease, obesity, use of estrogen-containing oral contraception or hormone replacement therapy, and the type of surgical intervention (8,9). The way these risk factors interact in an individual patient to create a specific risk for the development of thrombosis is unpredictable. Therefore, although it would be possible to assign an individual surgical patient a score about his or her risk for the development of thromboembolic episodes in the perioperative period, the use of such risk assessment models has not been fully validated. A second approach on which decisions about thromboprophylaxis can be made is to define specific surgical risk groups in whom decisions about the use of thromboprophylaxis can be made (10).

## CLINICAL TRIALS IN VENOUS THROMBOEMBOLISM: CONSIDERATIONS ABOUT EFFICACY AND SAFETY

The adoption of any specific measure for the prevention of venous thromboembolic disease in surgical patients must be based on evidence for both the efficacy of a particular intervention with regard to preventing thrombosis in patients at differing risks for the development of this complication, and the safety of the intervention, in particular for pharmacologic methods of prophylaxis, this being the rate of the bleeding complications associated with anticoagulant therapy.

In terms of assessing the efficacy of any given method of thromboprophylaxis, a number of different efficacy endpoints have been identified. Clearly, the most important endpoint is that of the prevention of fatal PE (11). Although this complication is rare, and trials designed with this endpoint are the most challenging, landmark studies in the field of thrombosis research have used autopsy to prove fatal PE as a primary clinical trial endpoint (11). The prevention of fatal PE is the most important reason for the use of thromboprophylaxis. Demonstration that an individual method of prophylaxis is able to reduce the frequency of PE provides strong confirmation of its utility and relevance in routine clinical practice for the given patient population.

Beyond the endpoint of fatal PE, symptomatic venous thromboembolic disease, whether it be PE or DVT, represents an important clinical complication which occurs more frequently than that of fatal PE. The use of this clinical endpoint, objectively confirmed using appropriate diagnostic tests, also represents a clinically important endpoint in trials assessing the efficacy of various thromboprophylactic strategies (12–14).

However, most of thromboembolic disease is asymptomatic. Therefore, methods which screen for asymptomatic DVT have the advantage that because this endpoint is more frequent in surgical patients than that of either symptomatic thrombosis or fatal PE, fewer numbers of patients are required in clinical trials that use this endpoint to compare various methods of thromboprophylaxis than those that use symptomatic or fatal VTE. Studies using either fibrinogen leg scanning or more recently venography for the detection of asymptomatic DVT have provided the foundations of our understanding of the efficacy of various methods for preventing DVT in surgical patients. These studies form the basis of many of the guidelines on the use of antithrombotic therapy in the perioperative period (10,15–17). It is essential, however, when using such surrogate endpoints as venographically proven DVT as the basis for assessing an antithrombotic intervention in the prevention of thromboembolic disease, that the consistency of the natural history of the thrombotic episode between the asymptomatic DVT and the potential fatal PE has been defined for the population in question. It is also essential that the antithrombotic intervention does not change that natural history, thereby potentially providing an erroneous result by the use of this surrogate endpoint.

Beyond measures of efficacy for any individual antithrombotic strategy are issues of safety (18). Indeed, it is this balance between the efficacy in preventing a thromboembolic episode versus considerations of an adverse safety impact in perioperative bleeding complications that must be addressed in the use of any antithrombotic agent. This balance must be considered in the specific clinical setting in which the patients find themselves because the potential risk for the development of thrombosis or bleeding complications is dependent upon the individual clinical scenario (type and site of operation, patient comorbidities, concomitant medication).

Studies over the last 3 decades have established that pharmacologic prophylaxis is not only effective in preventing thrombosis, but is infrequently associated with any increase in perioperative bleeding complications. Therefore, the balance between efficacy and safety for routine pharmacologic thromboprophylaxis demonstrates a most desirable benefit risk ratio and has the additional benefits of proven cost efficacy which provide an economic rationale for routine protection against thromboembolic disease in moderate and high-risk general surgical populations.

# METHODS OF PROPHYLAXIS

## Mechanical Methods of Prophylaxis

Mechanical methods of prophylaxis are designed either to eliminate stasis or to interrupt thrombus progression from the deep venous system to the pulmonary circulation.

None of the currently available mechanical methods of thromboprophylaxis have been as extensively investigated as the pharmacologic methods (10). Of those available methods, one of the most popular is graduated compression stockings. These stockings apply a decreasing pressure from ankle to thigh across the lower limb, reducing the venous cross-sectional area thereby enhancing venous flow, and reducing stasis. Beyond the use of graduated compression stockings are mechanical methods that increase pulsatile flow such as pneumatic calf compression, electrical calf stimulation, and venous foot pumps. All these methods enhance venous flow and can be used intraoperatively and in the postoperative period, although after surgery they are cumbersome and may be difficult to use to maximum effect. Another approach is either venous ligation (19) or insertion of inferior vena cava filters to interrupt the transition of thrombus

from the venous system to pulmonary circulation. There have been no randomized trials which have evaluated inferior vena cava filters for primary prophylaxis in surgical patients. In patients with established DVT, filters have been shown to be effective in reducing the frequency of PE initially, but in the longer term, have been associated with an excess of venous thromboembolic events (20).

## Pharmacologic Methods of Prophylaxis

A more popular approach to the prevention of VTE in the perioperative period has been the use of pharmacologic methods.

### Aspirin

Aspirin and other antiplatelet drugs have become the mainstay of antithrombotic therapy for patients with atherosclerosis. Aspirin is highly effective in the prevention of arterial thrombotic episodes in patients with established vascular disease. Aspirin's mechanism action is through the inhibition of prostaglandin G-H synthetase and therefore a resultant loss of platelet cyclooxygenase activity (21).

Interestingly, although aspirin has been shown to be effective in the prevention of arterial thromboembolic events, its role in the prevention of venous thrombosis remains controversial. Studies which have evaluated its use in the prevention of venous thromboembolic disease have often been of limited size and attended by important methodologic flaws which make their interpretation very difficult (22,23). When compared to studies utilizing other methods of thromboprophylaxis, those studies undertaken with aspirin do not justify its routine use, as a sole agent, for VTE prevention in medium- or high-risk surgical patients.

### Dextrans

The polysaccharide Dextrans have been evaluated as a potential thromboprophylactic agent (24). Their mode of action appears to be that of hemodilution, combined with an inhibitory effect on fibrin polymerization, and an enhancement of fibrinolysis with some antiplatelet effect. They must be given intravenously, and run the risk of severe anaphylactic reaction and volume overload. They are, therefore, not routinely used for thromboprophylaxis in most centers.

### Unfractionated Heparin

Low-dose unfractionated heparin has, for many years, been the mainstay of thromboprophylaxis in general surgical patients (9,25). Indeed, it is through the evaluation of this agent that so much of our understanding of the natural history of venous thromboembolic disease in surgical patients has been generated. Unfractionated heparin binds and potentiates the activity of circulating antithrombin with the resultant inhibition of activated clotting factors X and II (Thrombin). The agent can be given in a fixed dose of 5,000 anti-Xa U subcutaneously, commenced preoperatively, and continued in the postoperative period without the need for monitoring of anticoagulant activity.

### Low-Molecular-Weight Heparin

Low-molecular-weight heparins, are derived from unfractionated heparin through depolymerization (26). A variety of different low-molecular-weight heparins are available for clinical practice. Each of these has a different molecular weight and a different ratio of anti-Xa to anti-IIa inhibitory activity. The mechanism of action of low-molecular-weight heparins is the same as that of unfractionated heparin, that is, the potentiation of antithrombin activity and the ability to release tissue factor pathway inhibitor therefore being able to inhibit TF:VIIa activity. Low-molecular-weight heparins achieve a lesser degree of inhibition of thrombin activity when compared to unfractionated heparin, but a greater inhibition of factor Xa activity. Advantages of the low-molecular-weight heparins include a longer plasma half-life, the ability to dose once or twice daily subcutaneously without need for dose monitoring, a limited effect on platelet activation, and a reduced incidence of heparin-induced thrombocytopenia (27) and osteoporosis.

## Fondaparinux

Recently, the first of a new class of agents has become available for clinical practice, namely the indirect selective inhibitors of activated factor X. The pentasaccharide (fondaparinux) has a short five-saccharide sequence which is able to bind antithrombin and potentiate its inhibition of activated factor X. The molecular length is not sufficiently long to bind and inhibit thrombin. This agent has primarily been evaluated in the prevention of thromboembolic disease in patients with orthopaedic disorders, or those undergoing high-risk hip or knee replacement procedures (28–31), or treatment of DVT and PE (32).

A single study has been undertaken to evaluate its use in the prevention of thromboembolic disease in general surgical patients (33). This study compared fondaparinux in a dose of 2.5 mg once daily with the low-molecular-weight heparin dalteparin sodium in a dose of 5,000 U once daily. There were no significant differences in efficacy or safety between fondaparinux and the low-molecular-weight heparin.

## Direct Thrombin Inhibitors

Another interesting class of antithrombotic agents are the direct thrombin inhibitors. These agents, either naturally occurring or synthetic, are able to directly bind and inhibit thrombin. Amongst such agents are hirudin, bivalirudin, argatroban, and melagatran–ximelagatran. Most of these agents require parenteral administration apart from ximelagatran which is a pro drug and orally bioavailable; it undergoes metabolic conversion *in vivo*.

These agents are primarily being evaluated in either prophylaxis against thromboembolic disease in high-risk patients with orthopaedic disorders undergoing joint arthroplasty (34–36), or as a rescue antithrombotic strategy in patients with heparin-induced thrombocytopenia.

## INTERPRETING DATA FROM CLINICAL TRIALS WHICH HAVE ASSESSED ANTITHROMBOTIC AGENTS FOR THROMBOPROPHYLAXIS IN SURGICAL PATIENTS

Thromboprophylaxis in surgical patients represents a major challenge. Thrombosis is a common postoperative complication and may result in fatal PE or the late sequelae of chronic and potentially debilitating postthrombotic syndrome. However, surgical trauma makes patients prone to perioperative bleeding complications even without antithrombotic drugs; in the presence of such therapy, bleeding complications may be increased and adversely affect surgical outcome. Therefore, thromboprophylaxis in the perioperative period is a delicate balance between efficacy (in terms of preventing VTE) and safety (in terms of not inducing excessive bleeding complications) with the use of pharmacologic agents.

In assessing the potential value of a given antithrombotic agent, it is essential that trials use appropriate endpoints not only for the assessment of efficacy but also for the assessment of any potential adverse events, especially bleeding complications.

To this end, an important trial endpoint is that of a reduction in fatal PE associated with prophylaxis strategies (11). However, confirmation of PE requires autopsy and only a few antithrombotic agents have been assessed to the extent that there is a clear demonstration that their use is associated with a significant reduction in fatal PE, in well-designed randomized clinical trials (11,37). However, when metaanalyses are undertaken of methodologically sound clinical trials in which PE has been included as one of the endpoints in the study, then a number of agents, on this basis, have been shown to possess antithrombotic efficacy.

Beyond the endpoint of fatal PE is the clinical endpoint of symptomatic VTE, whether it is DVT or PE, confirmed by objective diagnostic strategies. Although fewer patients are required in these studies than in the larger mortality endpoint, in fatal PE trials, patient numbers are still considerable.

As an alternative strategy, asymptomatic endpoints using screening with sensitive tests that are able to diagnose DVT such as fibrinogen scanning or venography (or ultrasound, such as the dalteparin-PREVENT Trial in *Circulation* in 2004), have been adopted. These trials are clinically relevant because asymptomatic thrombosis will predict both symptomatic DVT and potentially fatal PE (25,38,39).

When considering safety endpoints in clinical trials, consistent assessment of bleeding in surgical patients is difficult. Bleeding in the perioperative period is determined not only by factors inherent to the patient, but also by the nature and extent of operation, the experience of the surgeon undertaking the procedure, and any other concomitant drug therapy. These factors interact in an unpredictable way with the administration of any particular antithrombotic therapy in the intraoperative and postoperative periods. Because bleeding is an expected complication of operation, blood loss *per se,* both intraoperatively and in the early postoperative period, and consequent requirement for transfusion are difficult surrogate markers for assessment of bleeding risk for an antithrombotic agent in the perioperative setting. This situation is contrary to that seen, for instance, in patients who are receiving antithrombotic therapy for treatment of established thrombosis where bleeding would not be expected (40). Wound hematoma and bleeding at the operation site, although potentially expected in a normal surgical procedure, may increase in frequency as a result of antithrombotic therapy. Such differences are important to identify because their occurrence outside the controlled setting of a clinical trial may have important adverse consequences.

Few perioperative pharmacologic prophylaxis trials have used endpoints which assess the potential impact of excessive bleeding on surgical outcome (41). However, such endpoints, which include the need for reoperation secondary to bleeding, the need for surgical evacuation of wound haematomas, or consequences of bleeding which result in either anastomotic dehiscence, wound dehiscence, or arthroplasty joint sepsis may represent more important endpoints in "real world" clinical practice.

However, when looking across the board at the results of clinical trials that have assessed antithrombotic agents in the perioperative period, it is clear that routine antithrombotic therapy with unfractionated or low-molecular-weight heparin is not associated with a significant adverse impact in bleeding on surgical outcome in the general surgical population.

# GENERAL SURGERY

## Frequency of Thromboembolic Events

The rate of thrombosis reported in patients without prophylaxis undergoing general surgical procedures ranges between 15% and 30%, with rates of PE of approximately 0.08% (1,9,11,25,42) (see Table 94-1). Some believe that these historic rates of thrombosis overestimate the magnitude of the current problem in surgical practice. It is indeed true that earlier mobilization, shorter length of hospital stay, improved anaesthetic techniques, greater attention to a reduction in perioperative sepsis through antibiotic prophylaxis, and greater use of thromboprophylaxis itself have had an important impact on reducing the frequency of postoperative DVT in general surgical patients. However, against this is the clear trend for surgical procedures to be undertaken in very sick patients, who spend greater periods of time severely immobilized in the intensive care unit, and that procedures are now undertaken in older patients and in a greater number of patients with malignant disease. Therefore, in an era when studies using control or placebo against novel antithrombotic agents in surgical practice are no longer ethically justified, it is not possible to know the current rate of thromboembolic disease in patients who do not receive any form of thromboprophylaxis. Nevertheless, it would be wrong to assume that VTE is no longer a serious complication in contemporary surgical patients (43).

Methods for prophylaxis against VTE in general surgical patients include general measures and specific interventions with antithrombotic strategies. General measures include careful history-taking to assess thrombosis risk, and in particular to identify important risk factors such as increasing age, obesity, the presence of malignancy, and a previous history of venous thromboembolic disease (44,45) (see Table 94-2). Careful attention to the prevention of perioperative sepsis, fluid balance, and early mobilization also play an important role in the reduction of thrombosis risk. Patients undergoing surgical intervention who are on either the oral contraceptive pill or hormone replacement therapy should also have this therapy discontinued before operative intervention.

The two most popular methods for the prevention of thromboembolic disease in general surgical patients are either low-dose-unfractionated heparin or low-molecular-weight heparin. Indeed, the highest quality of evidence in terms of both efficacy

## TABLE 94-2

### RISK FACTORS FOR VENOUS THROMBOEMBOLISM IN SURGICAL PATIENTS

|  | Severity |
|---|---|
| **RISK FACTORS** | |
| Age | Moderate |
| Obesity | Mild |
| Ethnicity | Mild |
| Immobilization | Moderate |
| Previous VTE | Severe |
| Estrogen therapy | Mild |
| Inherited thrombophilia | Severe |
| Malignancy | Moderate |
| Heparin-induced thrombocytopenia | Severe |
| **SURGICAL FACTORS** | |
| Orthopaedic surgery | Severe |
| Tourniquet application | Moderate |
| General anaesthesia >30 min | Moderate |
| Venous catheterization | Moderate |
| Major trauma | Severe |
| Paralysis | Moderation |

Cancer chemotherapy, antiphospholipid antibodies, and hyperhomocysteinemia, all recognized risk factors for venous thromboembolism (VTE) in nonsurgical patients, are also likely to increase the risk of postoperative VTE.

and safety with regard to thromboprophylaxis in the perioperative period are available with these two agents.

The International Multicentre trial published in 1975 randomized 4,121 patients older than 40 years undergoing major surgical intervention to a control group or to receive low-dose unfractionated heparin in a dose of 5,000 U commenced 1 to 2 hours before operation and continued three times daily in the postoperative period until the patient was fully mobile (11). The primary endpoint in this study was autopsy-proven fatal PE. Approximately 70% of patients in this study who died underwent autopsy. The trial demonstrated a considerable reduction in the frequency of fatal PE (16 patients in the control group vs. two in the lose-dose-heparin group) and provided the first evidence that heparin-based thromboprophylaxis not only prevented DVT, but was also able to reduce the frequency of

## TABLE 94-1

### RISK STRATIFICATION FOR POSTOPERATIVE VENOUS THROMBOEMBOLISM AND FREQUENCY OF VENOUS THROMBOEMBOLISM WITHOUT PROPHYLAXIS

|  | Venographic DVT | | Pulmonary embolism | |
|---|---|---|---|---|
|  | Calf | Proximal | Symptomatic | Fatal |
| Low risk: <40 yr and uncomplicated surgery and no additional risk factors | 2% | 0.4% | 0.2% | <0.01% |
| Moderate risk: >40 yr of prolonged/complicated surgery or additional "minor" risk factors | 20% | 5% | 2% | 0.5% |
| High risk: major surgery for malignancy or previous VTE or knee/hip surgery of heparin-induced thrombocytopenia | 50% | 15% | 5% | 2% |

DVT, deep vein thrombosis; VTE, venous thromboembolism.

fatal PE and to have a significant impact on improving surgical outcome. The International Multicentre trial hailed the modern era of thromboprophylaxis and has formed the basis of recommendations for thromboprophylaxis adopted throughout the world. It initiated interest in further improvement of such strategies with the objective of reducing the incidence of perioperative bleeding complications, manifest by an increase in wound hematoma rates associated with low-dose prophylactic heparin therapy.

Numerous studies have assessed the use of low-dose unfractionated heparin with endpoints including PE, symptomatic venous thromboembolic disease, and asymptomatic DVT (25). These studies all confirm that when compared to control groups, low-dose-heparin therapy is associated with more than 60% reduction in the frequency of both DVT and symptomatic thromboembolic disease (25).

The striking feature of low-dose-heparin prophylaxis is the associated reduction in perioperative mortality, with the frequency of PE-associated mortality falling from eight per 1,000 to one per 1,000 operated patients, thereby profoundly impacting surgical outcome. However, concerns about potential bleeding complications as manifest by wound haematoma formation, drove the quest for the development of safer antithrombotic agents in surgical practice (11,25).

As a result, the low-molecular-weight heparins were developed. Low-molecular-weight heparin has been extensively investigated (41,42,46–50) since the first report of its use for the thromboprophylaxis in man in general surgical patients by Kakkar et al. in 1982 (51). In this study, patients were randomized to receive one of two doses of a low-molecular-weight heparin. The endpoint of the study was to assess the overall frequency of thrombosis and safety. The study confirmed that low-molecular-weight heparin given in a fixed dose was capable of providing thromboprophylatic efficacy and was safe.

A recent metaanalysis has reviewed studies which have randomized more than 44,000 general surgical patients in trials comparing low-molecular-weight against low-dose unfractionated heparin (42). In this metaanalysis, both agents, low-molecular-weight and low-dose heparin, provided equal efficacy and safety. The advantage of low-molecular-weight heparin is that it can be administered once daily, whereas low-dose unfractionated heparin requires twice or three times daily administration to achieve antithrombotic efficacy in surgical patients. Low-molecular-weight heparins have broadly replaced low-dose unfractionated heparins for thromboprophylaxis in general surgical patients.

The selective inhibitor of factor Xa, fondaparinux, has also been evaluated in patients undergoing abdominal surgery (33). In a single trial of approximately 3,000 general surgical patients, most of whom underwent operation for malignant disease, there was no substantial difference in either efficacy of thromboprophylaxis or bleeding complications in patients who received fondaparinux commenced postoperatively with low-molecular-weight heparin (dalteparin) commenced preoperatively.

## Mechanical Methods of Prophylaxis

Mechanical methods of prophylaxis have been assessed in general surgical patients (52). Although they have no risk of bleeding complications, few trials of methodologic quality have evaluated their efficacy. In particular, no trials have demonstrated that mechanical methods of thromboprophylaxis, alone, are able to reduce the frequency of fatal PE in general surgical patients.

The use of graduated compression stockings alone is not advocated, although recent analyses suggested a 50% reduction in the rate of DVT with their use compared to control (53,54).

However, when used in combination with low-dose unfractionated heparin, they appear to be of benefit. Studies have demonstrated a 75% reduction in the rate of DVT identified among patients using both low-dose unfractionated heparin and graduated compression stockings compared to those who received low-dose unfractionated heparin alone (54). There is no evidence that mechanical prophylaxis alone can reduce the frequency of PE. In addition, graduated compression stockings which are used inappropriately may cause a tourniquet effect on the lower limb, which may be associated with a potential enhanced risk of thromboembolic disease (55).

Intermittent pneumatic calf compression has been assessed for the prevention of DVT in general surgical patients (56,57). It is not possible, however, on the basis of the small studies which have been undertaken to assess this technique, to make recommendations about its routine use. Results of these trials either suggest a similar efficacy to low-dose unfractionated heparin or no definite thromboprophylactic effect for the use of intermittent pneumatic calf compression alone. In a large randomized trial of more than 2,000 cardiac surgical patients, the combination of pneumatic calf compression with low-dose unfractionated heparin reduced the rate of symptomatic PE to 1.5% from 4.0% compared with low-dose unfractionated heparin alone (58).

## Laparoscopic Surgery

Laparoscopic surgery represents a major advance in general surgical practice, providing opportunities for reducing surgical trauma, patient discomfort associated with intraabdominal and pelvic surgical procedures, and hospital length of stay. The problem of venous thromboembolic disease has not been extensively investigated in patients undergoing minimal access surgical procedures (59). From the point of view of the pathogenesis of venous thromboembolic disease, minimal access surgical procedures such as cholecystectomy are associated with varying reports of activation of blood coagulation ranging from only minimal (60–62) to the same degree of coagulopathy as observed with open cholecystectomy (63,64). Often, laparoscopic procedures may take longer than the open surgical procedure and during operation, both the pneumoperitoneum and the reverse Trendelenburg position used in operations such as cholecystectomy or fundoplication result in profound venous stasis of the lower limbs (65). Laparoscopic surgical procedures appear to be associated with a shorter hospital stay and, therefore, a potentially more rapid postoperative mobilization. The outcome of patients once discharged from hospital in terms of their mobility after laparoscopic procedures, compared to those who remain in hospital, has not been extensively investigated (59).

A number of surveys have determined current surgical practice of thromboprophylaxis after laparoscopic cholecystectomy and reported rates of thromboembolic complications. In a UK study of 417 surgeons, 91% reported never having encountered a thromboembolic episode after laparoscopic cholecystectomy (66). Most surgeons use low-dose unfractionated heparin in these patients. In a similar study undertaken in Denmark, 80% of surveyed surgical departments reported no problems with postoperative VTE in patients undergoing laparoscopic cholecystectomy (67).

Beyond these surveys, there have been a few studies using objective screening techniques, which have attempted to determine the rates of thromboembolic disease associated with various laparoscopic procedures. In a small study, with the screening endpoint of contrast venography 6 to 10 days after operation, no DVT was identified in 25 patients who underwent laparoscopic cholecystectomy without thromboprophylaxis (68). Similarly, low rates of thromboembolic disease in the absence of thromboprophylaxis have been identified in a series of laparoscopic surgical patients screened with lower limb Duplex ultrasonography (69,70).

Registries of surgical outcome also indicate a low frequency of thromboembolic complications in laparoscopic procedures. In a North American analysis of more than 100,000 laparoscopic cholecystectomies, the rate of symptomatic VTE was 0.2% up to 3 months after operation (71). Similar findings were identified in a further literature review including more than 150,000 laparoscopic cholecystectomies where various thromboprophylactic strategies were used, and where the rates of DVT, PE, and fatal PE were 0.03%, 0.06%, and 0.02%, respectively (72). Finally, the Swedish registry of laparoscopic cholecystectomy reported a rate of VTE of 0.2% in more than 11,000 cases (73).

As a consequence of these very low reported rates of thromboembolic disease, there have been only a limited number of randomized trials that have determined the potential benefit of routine thromboprophylaxis in minimal access surgical patients. In one study, patients were randomized to either placebo or to the low-molecular-weight heparin dalteparin sodium in a dose of 2,500 U once daily for up to 10 days after operation. There was no evidence of DVT screened venographically in either group of patients (68). In a second trial, graduated compression stockings alone were compared to graduated compression stockings plus the low-molecular-weight heparin, reviparin sodium. The screening endpoint was venous ultrasound 5 to 7 days after operation, with a thrombosis rate below 1%.

## Cancer Surgery

Cancer is an important risk factor for the development of venous thromboembolic disease (9,42) (see also Chapter 85). The frequency of thromboembolic complications in patients undergoing major operation for cancer is about twice that of patients undergoing the equivalent operation without malignant disease (9,74,75). In general, low-dose unfractionated heparin (11,25) and low-molecular-weight heparin (42) have been validated for the prevention of thromboembolic disease in patients undergoing major abdominal or pelvic procedures for cancer. In a recent posthoc subgroup analysis of more than 6,000 patients with malignant disease receiving perioperative unfractionated or low-molecular-weight heparin, compared to 17,000 patients without malignancy, fatal PE was three times as common in patients with cancer than in surgical patients without cancer, despite use of prophylaxis (75).

In a study of more than 2,000 patients undergoing laparotomy for cancer, the hypothesis that a higher dose of low-molecular-weight heparin would be associated with a lower incidence of postoperative thromboembolic complications in patients with cancer was tested. In this trial, in two thirds of patients undergoing operation for malignant disease, increasing the dose of the low-molecular-weight heparin dalteparin sodium from 2,500 U once daily to 5,000 U once daily was associated with a reduction in the frequency of postoperative DVT from 14.9% to 8.5%. In patients with cancer in this trial, there was no significant increase in bleeding complications associated with increase in the dose of low-molecular-weight heparin. For one third of the patients without malignant disease, although there was a reduction in the frequency of postoperative DVT with the higher dose of low-molecular-weight heparin, this was associated with increased perioperative bleeding complications (76).

Beyond the intensity of perioperative antithrombotic therapy has been the suggestion that prolonging the duration of postoperative prophylaxis into the postdischarge period might be associated with a lower frequency of late thromboembolic complications in patients with malignant disease. This hypothesis has been tested in two recent randomized clinical trials (76,77). Patients undergoing laparotomy for cancer were randomized to either 1 week of in-hospital prophylaxis or 4 weeks of in-hospital and postdischarge prophylaxis with the low-molecular-weight heparin, enoxaparin, 40 mg once daily. Prolonged prophylaxis was associated with a reduction in the frequency of postoperative DVT as screened by venography at the end of the 4-week treatment period (76). A similar study including patients with and without malignant disease demonstrated the benefit of prolonged thromboprophylaxis in cancer surgical patients with the low-molecular-weight heparin, dalteparin sodium, 5,000 U once daily for up to 4 weeks (77). These data suggest that for certain surgical patients with cancer at high risk for the development of postoperative DVT, prolonged thromboprophylaxis may be indicated, although no definite recommendations about routine use for postdischarge prophylaxis can be made on the basis of currently available studies.

## SUMMARY

VTE remains an important potential complication in patients undergoing major general surgical procedures and operation for malignant disease. Routine pharmacologic thromboprophylaxis with low-dose unfractionated heparin or low-molecular-weight heparin has been validated both in terms of safety and efficacy with or without the combination of mechanical methods and should be considered for all such patients.

## References

1. Kakkar VV, Howe CT, Flanc C, et al. Natural history of postoperative deep vein thrombosis. *Lancet* 1969;2:230–233.
2. Lindblad B, Eriksson A, Bergqvist D. Autopsy-verified pulmonary embolism in a surgical department: analysis of the period from 1951 to 1968. *Br J Surg* 1991;78:849–852.
3. Stein PD, Henry JW. Prevalence of acute pulmonary embolism among patients in a general hospital and at autopsy. *Chest* 1995;108:978–981.
4. Goldhaber SZ, Visni L, De Rosa M. Acute pulmonary embolism: clinical outcomes in the International Cooperative Pulmonary Embolism Registry (ICOPER). *Lancet* 1999;353:1386–1389.
5. Kearon C. Natural history of venous thromboembolism. *Circulation* 2003; 107:I22–I30.
6. Prandoni P, Lensing AW, Cogo A, et al. The long-term clinical course of acute deep venous thrombosis. *Ann Intern Med* 1996;125:1–7.
7. Kakkar VV, Lawrence D. Hemodynamic and clinical assessment after therapy for acute deep vein thrombosis. *Am J Surg* 1985;150:54.
8. Anderson FA, Spencer FA. Risk factors for venous thromboembolism. *Circulation* 2003;107:I9–I16.
9. Kakkar VV, Howe CT, Nicolaides AN, et al. Deep vein thrombosis of the leg: is there a "high risk" group? *Am J Surg* 1970;120:527–530.
10. Geerts W, Pineo GF, Heit JA, et al. Prevention of venous thromboembolism. *Chest* 2004;126:338S–400S.
11. International Multicentre Trial. Prevention of fatal pulmonary embolism by low doses of heparin. *Lancet* 1975;2:45–51.
12. Nurmohamed MT, Rosendaal FR, Buller HR, et al. Low molecular weight heparin versus standard heparin in general and orthopaedic surgery: a meta-analysis. *Lancet* 1992;340:152–156.
13. Koch A, Bouges S, Ziegler S, et al. Low molecular weight heparin and unfractionated heparin in thrombosis prophylaxis after major surgical intervention: update of previous meta-analyses. *Br J Surg* 1997;84:750–759.
14. Leizorovicz A, Haugh MC, Chapius F-R, et al. Low molecular weight heparin in prevention of perioperative thrombosis. *Br Med J* 1992;305: 913–920.
15. Second Thromboembolic Risk Factors (THRiFT II) Consensus Group. Risk of prophylaxis for venous thromboembolism in hospital patients. *Phlebology* 1998;13:87–97.
16. Scottish Intercollegiate Guidelines Network (SIGN). Prophylaxis of venous thromboembolism: a national clinical guideline. Edinburgh 2002 (SIGN publication no. 62) 2002. Available from http://www.sign.ac.uk.
17. Nicolaides AN, Bergqvist D, Hull RD, et al. Prevention of venous thromboembolism: international consensus statement. *Int Angiol* 1997;16:3–38.
18. Landefeld CS, Beyth RJ. Anticoagulant-related bleeding: clinical epidemiology, prediction and prevention. *Am J Med* 1993;95:315–328.
19. Bergqvist D. The role of vena caval interruption in patients with venous thromboembolism. *Prog Cardiovasc Dis* 1994;37:25–37.
20. Decousus H, Leizorovicz A, Parent F, et al. A clinical trial of vena caval filters in the prevention of pulmonary embolism in patients with proximal deep vein thrombosis. *N Engl J Med* 1998;338:409–415.

21. Patrono C. Aspirin as an antiplatelet drug. *N Engl J Med* 1994;330: 1287–1294.
22. Antiplatelet Trialists Collaboration. Collaborative overview of randomised trials of antiplatelet therapy III: reduction in venous thrombosis and pulmonary embolism by antiplatelet prophylaxis among surgical and medical patients. *Br Med J* 1994;308:235–246.
23. Prevention of pulmonary embolism and deep vein thrombosis with low dose aspirin: Pulmonary Embolism Prevention (PEP) trial. *Lancet* 2000; 355:1295–1302.
24. Clagett GP, Reisch JS. Prevention of venous thromboembolism in general surgical patients: results of meta-analysis. *Ann Surg* 1988;208(2):227–240.
25. Collins R, Scrimgeour A, Yusuf S, et al. Reduction in fatal pulmonary embolism and venous thrombosis by perioperative administration of subcutaneous heparin. Overview of results of randomized trials in general, orthopaedic and urologic surgery. *N Engl J Med* 1988;318:1162–1173.
26. Weitz J. Low molecular weight heparins. *N Engl J Med* 1997;337(10): 688–698.
27. Warkentin TE, Levine MN, Hirsh J, et al. Heparin-induced thrombocytopenia in patients treated with low molecular weight heparin or unfractionated heparin. *N Engl J Ned* 1995;332:1330–1335.
28. Lassen MR, Bauer KA, Eriksson BI, et al. Efficacy and safety of enoxaparin versus unfractionated heparin for prevention of deep venous thrombosis after elective knee arthroplasty. *Clin Orthop* 1995;321:19–27.
29. Turpie AGG, Bauer KA, Eriksson BI, et al. Postoperative fondaparinux versus postoperative enoxaparin for prevention of venous thromboembolism after elective hip replacement surgery: a randomized double-blind trial. *Lancet* 2002;359:1721–1726.
30. Bauer KA, Eriksson BI, Lassen MR, et al. Fondaparinux compared with enoxaparin for the prevention of venous thromboembolism after elective major knee surgery. *N Engl J Med* 2001;345:1305–1310.
31. Eriksson BI, Bauer KA, Lassen MR, et al. Fondaparinux compared with enoxaparin for the prevention of venous thromboembolism after hip fracture surgery. *N Engl J Med* 2001;345:1298–1304.
32. Buller HR, Davidson BE, Deconsus H, et al. Subcutaneous fondaparinux versus intravenous unfractionated heparin to the initial treatment of pulmonary embolism. *N Engl J Med* 2003;349:1695–1702.
33. Agnelli G, Bergqvist D, Cohen A, et al. Randomized double-blind study to compare the efficacy and safety of postoperative fondaparinux (Arixtra®) and preoperative dalteparin in the prevention of venous thromboembolism after high-risk abdominal surgery: the PEGASUS study [abstract]. *Blood* 2003;102:15a.
34. Erikkson BI, Bergqvist D, Kalebo P, et al. Ximelagatran and melagatran compared with dalteparin for prevention of venous thromboembolism after total hip or knee replacement: the METHRO II randomized trial. *Lancet* 2002;360:1441–1447.
35. Eriksson BI, Wille-Jorgensen P, Kalebo P, et al. A comparison of recombinant hirudin with a low molecular weight heparin to prevent thromboembolic complications after total hip replacement. *N Engl J Med* 1997;337: 1329–1335.
36. Colwell CW, Berkowitz SD, Davidson BL, et al. Comparison of ximelagatran, an oral direct thrombin inhibitor, with enoxaparin for the prevention of venous thromboembolism following total hip replacement. A randomized double-blind study. *J Thromb Haemost* 2003;1:2119–2130.
37. Haas SK, Wolf H, Encke A, et al. Prevention of fatal postoperative pulmonary embolism by low molecular weight heparin–a double blind comparison of certoparin and unfractionated heparin [abstract]. *Thromb Haemost* 1999;82(Suppl.1):491.
38. Eikelboom JW, Quinlan DJ, Douketis JD. Extended duration prophylaxis against venous thromboembolism after total hip or knee replacement: a meta analysis of the randomized trials. *Lancet* 2001;358:9–15.
39. Cohen AT, Bailey CS, Alikhan R, et al. Extended thromboprophylaxis with low molecular weight heparin reduces symptomatic venous thromboembolism following lower limb arthroplasty—a meta-analysis. *Thromb Haemost* 2001;85:940–941.
40. Levine MN, Raskob G, Beyth RJ, et al. Hemorrhagic complications of anticoagulant treatment. *Chest* 2004;126:287S–310S.
41. Kakkar VV, Cohen AT, Edmondson RA, et al. Low molecular weight versus standard heparin for prevention of venous thromboembolism after major abdominal surgery. *Lancet* 1993;341:259–265.
42. Mismetti P, Laporte S, Darmon JY, et al. Meta-analysis of low molecular weight heparin in the prevention of venous thromboembolism in general surgery. *Br J Surg* 2001;88:913–930.
43. Goldhaber SZ, Savage DD, Garison RJ, et al. Risk factors for pulmonary embolism: the Farningham study. *Am J Med* 1983;74:1023–1028.
44. Nicolaides A, Irving D, Pretzell M, et al. The risk of deep vein thrombosis in surgical patients. *Br J Surg* 1973;60:312.
45. Flordal PA, Bergqvist D, Burmark US, et al. Risk factors for major thromboembolism and bleeding tendency after elective general surgical operations. *Eur J Surg* 1996;162:783–789.
46. Nurmohamed MT, Verhaeghe R, Haas S, et al. A comparative trial of low molecular weight heparin (enoxaparin) versus standard heparin for the prophylaxis of postoperative deep vein thrombosis in general surgery. *Am J Surg* 1995;169:567–571.
47. Kakkar VV, Murray WJ. Efficacy and safety of low molecular weight heparin (CY216) in preventing postoperative venous thromboembolism: a cooperative study. *Br J Surg* 1985;72:786–791.
48. Bergqvist S, Burmark US, Frisell J, et al. Low molecular weight heparin once daily compared with conventional low dose heparin twice daily. A prospective double-blind multicentre trial on prevention of postoperative thrombosis. *Br J Surg* 1986;73:204–208.
49. Bergqvist D, Matzsch T, Burmark US, et al. Low molecular weight heparin given the evening before surgery compared with conventional lose dose heparin in prevention of thrombosis. *Br J Surg* 1988;75:888–891.
50. Samama MM, Bernard P, Bonnardot JP, et al. Low molecular weight heparin compared with unfractionated heparin in prevention of postoperative thrombosis. *Br J Surg* 1988;75:128–131.
51. Kakkar VV, Djazaeri B, Fok J, et al. Low molecular weight heparin and prevention of postoperative deep vein thrombosis. *Br Med J* 1982;284:375.
52. Clagett GP, Reisch JS. Prevention of venous thromboembolism in general surgical patients. Results of meta-analysis. *Ann Surg* 1988;208:227–240.
53. Agu O, Hamilton G, Baker D. Graduated compression stockings in the prevention of venous thromboembolism. *Br J Surg* 999;86:992–1004.
54. Amarigiri SV, Lees TA. *Elastic compression stockings for prevention of deep vein thrombosis. (Cochrane review)*. Oxford: The Cochrane Library, 2001 Issue 1, Update Software 2001.
55. Comerota AJ, Katz ML, White JV. Why does prophylaxis with external pneumatic compression for deep vein thrombosis fail? *Am J Surg* 1992;164: 265–268.
56. Nicolaides AN, Miles C, Hoare M, et al. Intermittent sequential pneumatic compression of the legs and thromboembolism-deterrent stockings in the prevention of postoperative deep vein thrombosis. *Surgery* 1983;94: 21–25.
57. Scurr JH, Coleridge-Smith PD, Hasty JH. Regimen for improved effectiveness of intermittent pneumatic compression in deep vein thrombosis prophylaxis. *Surgery* 1987;102:816–820.
58. Ramos R, Salem BI, De Pawlikowski MP, et al. The efficacy of pneumatic compression stockings in the prevention of pulmonary embolism after cardiac surgery. *Chest* 1996;109:82–85.
59. Zacharoulis D, Kakkar AK. Venous thromboembolism in laparoscopic surgery. *Curr Opin Pulm Med* 2003;9:356–361.
60. Caprini JA, Arcelus JI, Laubach M, et al. Postoperative hypercoagulability and deep vein thrombosis after laparoscopic cholecystectomy. *Surg Endosc* 1995;9:304–309.
61. Dabrowiecki S, Rosc D, Jurkowski P. The influence of laparoscopic cholecystectomy on perioperative blood clotting and fibrinolysis. *Blood Coagul Fibrinolysis* 1997;8:1–5.
62. Rahr HB, Fabrin K, Larsen JF, et al. Coagulation and fibrinolysis during laparoscopic cholecystectomy. *Thromb Res* 1999;93:121–127.
63. Dexter SP, Griffith JP, Grant PJ, et al. Activation of coagulation and fibrinolysis in open and laparoscopic cholecystectomy. *Surg Endosc* 1996;10: 1069–1074.
64. Vander Velpen G, Penninckx F, Kerremans R, et al. Interleukin-6 and coagulation fibrinolysis fluctuations after laparoscopic and conventional cholecystectomy. *Surg Endosc* 1994;8:1216–1220.
65. Jorgensen JO, Lalak NJ, North L, et al. Venous stasis during laparoscopic cholecystectomy. *Surg Laparosc Endosc* 1994;4:128–133.
66. Bradbury AW, Chan YC, Darzi A, et al. Thromboembolism prophylaxis during laparoscopic cholecystectomy. *Br J Surg* 1997;84:962–964.
67. Tvedskov TF, Rasmussen MS, Willie-Jorgensen P. Survey of the use of thromboprophylaxis in laparoscopic surgery in Denmark. *Br J Surg* 2001; 88:1413–1416.
68. Bounmeaux H, Didier D, Polat O, et al. Antithrombotic prophylaxis in patients undergoing laparoscopic cholecystectomy. *Thromb Res* 1997;86: 271–273.
69. Baca I, Schneider B, Kohler T, et al. Prevention of venous thromboembolism in patients undergoing minimally invasive surgery with a short-term hospital stay: results of a multicentre, prospective, randomised, controlled clinical trial with a low molecular weight heparin. *Chirurg* 1997;68:1275–1280.
70. Wazz G, Branicki F, Taji H, et al. Influence of pneumoperitoneum on the deep venous system during laparoscopy. *J Soc Laparosc Surg* 2004;4: 291–295.
71. White RH, Zhou H, Romano PS. Incidence of symptomatic venous thromboembolism after different elective or urgent surgical procedures. *Thromb Haemost* 2003;90:446–455.
72. Lindberg F, Bergqvist D, Rasmussen I. Incidence of thromboembolic complications after laparoscopic cholecystectomy: review of the literature. *Surg Laprosc Endosc* 1997;7:324–331.
73. Hjelmqvist B. Complications of laparoscopic cholecystectomy as recorded in the Swedish laparoscopic registry. *Eur J Surg* 2000;585:18–21.
74. Kakkar AK, Williamson RCN. Prevention of venous thromboembolism in cancer patients. *Semin Thromb Haemost* 1999;25:239–243.
75. Kakkar AK, Haas S, Walsh D, et al. Prevention of perioperative venous thromboembolism: outcome after cancer and non-cancer surgery [abstract]. *Thromb Haemost* 2001;86(Suppl. 1):OC1732.
76. Bergqvist D, Agnelli G, Cohen AT, et al. Duration of prophylaxis against venous thromboembolism with enoxaparin after surgery for cancer. *N Engl J Med* 2002;346:975–980.
77. Rasmussen MS. Preventing thromboembolic complications in cancer patients after surgery: a role for prolonged trhomboprophylaxis. *Cancer Treat Rev* 2002;28:141–144.

# CHAPTER 95 ■ PREVENTION OF VENOUS THROMBOEMBOLISM IN ORTHOPEDIC SURGERY

GIANCARLO AGNELLI

## EPIDEMIOLOGY OF VENOUS THROMBOEMBOLISM AFTER ORTHOPEDIC SURGERY

Orthopedic surgery is associated with a high risk for venous thromboembolism (VTE) (1,2). This is particularly the case for major orthopedic surgery, which includes elective hip and knee replacement and surgery for hip fracture.

In patients undergoing major orthopedic surgery without antithrombotic prophylaxis, the prevalence of deep vein thrombosis (DVT) and proximal DVT, as shown by venography, is as high as 60% and 30%, respectively (see Table 95-1) (3–35). The rate of venography-detected DVT is higher after knee replacement than after hip replacement, but patients undergoing hip replacement have higher rates of proximal DVT than patients undergoing knee replacement (1). Patients undergoing surgery for hip fracture have a particularly high incidence of pulmonary embolism (PE), probably because they are older than patients undergoing elective hip or knee replacement and more often have an associated comorbidity (4,11,16,34–40). The delay commonly occurring between fracture and surgery and the resulting prolonged immobilization could also be responsible for the high incidence of PE in patients with hip fracture.

In patients undergoing major orthopedic surgery, routinely performed lung scan shows findings that are compatible with PE in a proportion of patients as high as 28% (19,26). Fatal PE has been reported to occur in approximately 0.2% of the patients undergoing elective hip replacement and to be in the range of 1.4% to 7.5% within 3 months after surgery for hip fracture (5,41–43). PE was found to be the cause of death in 14% of patients who died after surgery for hip fracture (44).

In patients undergoing major orthopedic surgery, clinically overt VTE occurs in approximately 1.5% to 2.5% of patients (6,20,45–49) and remains high even in patients receiving prophylaxis (50). Most of the clinically overt thromboembolic episodes occur after hospital discharge (6,50–52), and VTE is the commonest cause for readmission to hospital following major orthopedic surgery (53). It is unclear whether patients with late-occurring clinically overt thrombosis already have, at discharge, an asymptomatic thrombus that becomes symptomatic thereafter, or whether the thrombus actually develops after discharge. Both explanations are plausible. In those patients who have an asymptomatic DVT at discharge, discontinuation of prophylaxis may facilitate the extension of thrombosis, thereby making the disease clinically overt (54). A study reported a high incidence of VTE over the subsequent 3 weeks in patients who underwent elective hip replacement and had a negative venography at discharge, thereby suggesting that in many patients, late-occurring thrombosis develops after hospital discharge (55).

The use of antithrombotic agents for the prophylaxis of VTE following hip and knee replacement and surgery for hip fracture has been assessed in a number of clinical studies, and reliable recommendations on the optimal approach can be made. Limited data are currently available concerning knee arthroscopic surgery, elective spine surgery, and injuries of the lower extremity. Furthermore, some issues, such as the optimal timing of initiation of prophylaxis, its optimal duration, and the role of noninvasive screening for DVT before hospital discharge, remain controversial.

## PREVENTION OF VENOUS THROMBOEMBOLISM IN ELECTIVE HIP REPLACEMENT

Primary prophylaxis is recommended for all patients undergoing elective hip replacement unless they have a clear contraindication to the use of an antithrombotic agent.

A number of antithrombotic agents have been evaluated for the prophylaxis of VTE in patients undergoing elective hip replacement (see Table 95-2). Metaanalyses have shown that aspirin (56) and fixed low-dose unfractionated heparin (57) are superior to placebo or no prophylaxis; however, both agents are less effective than alternative prophylactic regimens (58–65). Aspirin should not be used as the only prophylactic agent after elective hip replacement. Fixed low-dose unfractionated heparin has a limited efficacy in this clinical setting. Unfractionated heparin is safe and effective when the dosage is adjusted in the postoperative period to maintain the activated partial thromboplastin time around the upper range of normal, but this regimen is impractical for routine clinical practice (60,66–68).

Adjusted-dose oral vitamin K antagonists are effective and safe for the prevention of VTE in patients undergoing elective hip replacement and continue to be the prophylactic approach that is most commonly followed in the United States (69–74). In Europe, vitamin K antagonists are rarely used and other forms of prophylaxis are preferred. Need for frequent monitoring and dose adjustment, as well as interactions with other drugs, are the main limitations of vitamin K antagonists. If vitamin K antagonists are used, they should be administered in doses sufficient to prolong the international normalized ratio (INR) to a target of 2.5 (range 2.0 to 3.0). The initial dose of vitamin K antagonists should be given either the evening before surgery or the evening after surgery. The target range for the INR is usually not reached until at least the third postoperative day (49,75–77).

## TABLE 95-1

### VENOUS THROMBOEMBOLISM PREVALENCE AFTER MAJOR ORTHOPEDIC SURGERY IN ABSENCE OF PROPHYLAXIS

| | DVT (%) | | PE (%) | |
|---|---|---|---|---|
| | Total | Proximal | Total | Fatal |
| Hip arthroplasty | 42–57 | 18–36 | 0.9–28 | 0.1–2.0 |
| Knee arthroplasty | 41–85 | 5–22 | 1.5–10 | 0.1–1.7 |
| Hip fracture surgery | 46–60 | 23–30 | 3–11 | 2.5–7.5 |

DVT, deep vein thrombosis; PE, pulmonary embolism.
DVT rates are based on the results of clinical studies that used venography to assess the prevalence of thrombosis.
Modified from Geerts WH, Pineo GF, Heit JA, et al. Prevention of venous thromboembolism. The seventh ACCP Conference on Antithrombotic and Thrombolytic Therapy. *Chest* 2004;126:338S–400S.

Low-molecular-weight heparins (LMWHs) have been extensively evaluated in patients undergoing elective hip replacement and are the preferred form of prophylaxis in Europe. LMWHs are more efficacious than low-dose unfractionated heparin (7,61,78–81) or adjusted-dose unfractionated heparin (66,67). The relative value of LMWHs and vitamin K antagonists in the prevention of VTE in patients undergoing hip replacement is less clear. No difference was found in three clinical trials in which LMWHs were compared with adjusted-dose warfarin (75,82,83). In a fourth trial, the LMWH dalteparin, started preoperatively, was significantly more effective than vitamin K antagonists (76), but it was associated with a significantly higher rate of bleeding complications, mainly at the surgical site. A subsequent study compared dalteparin, started at half the usual daily dose either less than 2 hours before surgery or within 4 hours after surgery, with warfarin started postoperatively (84). In this study, dalteparin was associated with a significant reduction in the risk of both total and proximal DVT, as seen at venography, and with a lower incidence of symptomatic, objectively confirmed VTE. Pooling the results of the five clinical studies in which LMWHs were compared with adjusted-dose warfarin, the respective rates of DVT were 13.7% and 20.7%, a statistically significant difference (75,76,82–84). The proximal DVT rates were 4.8% and 3.4%, respectively. Pooled rates of major bleeding were 3.3% and 5.3% in patients receiving vitamin K antagonists and LMWH, respectively. Therefore, LMWHs are more potent in preventing DVT but cause more major bleeding than vitamin K antagonists.

In a clinical outcome–based, open trial, more than 3,000 patients undergoing hip replacement were randomized to receive prophylaxis with either the LMWH enoxaparin, 30 mg twice a day started postoperatively, or warfarin, dose-adjusted for an INR of 2.0 to 3.0 (25). The in-hospital incidence of clinically overt, objectively confirmed VTE was 0.3% and 1.1%, respectively, in the enoxaparin and vitamin K antagonists groups, a statistically significant difference. Major bleeding occurred in 1.2% of the patients receiving enoxaparin and in 0.5% of patients receiving warfarin, a difference that was almost statistically significant.

The synthetic pentasaccharide fondaparinux has been compared with the LMWH enoxaparin for the prevention of VTE in patients undergoing hip replacement in two large clinical trials (85,86). In the study performed in Europe, 2,309 patients were randomized to fondaparinux, given subcutaneously at the dose of 2.5 mg once daily starting 4 to 8 hours after surgery, or enoxaparin, 40 mg given once daily starting 12 hours before surgery (85). The overall rate of VTE was 4% and 9% for fondaparinux and enoxaparin, respectively, a statistically significant difference. Fondaparinux was associated with a statistically significant reduction in the rate of proximal DVT that was 1% in patients receiving this agent and 2% in patients receiving enoxaparin. In the study performed in the United States that included 2,275 patients, the same fondaparinux regimen used in the European study was compared to enoxaparin, given at the dose of 30 mg twice a day starting 12 to 24 hours after surgery (86). Neither the overall rate of VTE,

## TABLE 95-2

### PREVENTION OF DEEP VEIN THROMBOSIS AFTER TOTAL HIP REPLACEMENT

| Prophylaxis regimen | No. of trials | Combined enrollment | Total DVT | | Proximal DVT | |
|---|---|---|---|---|---|---|
| | | | Prevalence % (95% CI) | RRR % | Prevalence % (95% CI) | RRR% |
| Placebo/control | 11 | 598 | 54.8 (51–59) | — | 26.6 (23–31) | — |
| GCS | 5 | 318 | 41.5 (36–47) | 24 | 26.4 (22–32) | 0 |
| Aspirin | 5 | 429 | 41.7 (37–47) | 24 | 11.4 (8–16) | 57 |
| Low-dose heparin | 11 | 1,097 | 19.2 (26–32) | 47 | 18.5 (16–21) | 31 |
| Warfarin | 12 | 1,793 | 22.3 (20–24) | 59 | 5.2 (4–6) | 81 |
| IPC | 7 | 423 | 20.3 (17–24) | 63 | 13.7 (11–17) | 49 |
| Recombinant hirudin | 3 | 1,172 | 16.3 (14–19) | 70 | 4.1 (3–5) | 85 |
| LMWH | 31 | 8,655 | 15.4 (15–16) | 72 | 4.9 (4–5) | 82 |

CI, confidence interval; DVT, deep vein thrombosis; GCS, graduated compression stockings; IPC, intermittent pneumatic compression; LMWH, low-molecular-weight heparin; RRR, relative risk reduction.

which was 6% in comparison with 8%, nor proximal DVT, 2% in comparison to 1%, differed significantly between the two groups. Following the study protocol, the first postoperative dose of fondaparinux was given approximately 6 hours after surgery, and enoxaparin was started approximately 18 hours after surgery. Both trials showed a nonsignificant increase in bleeding with fondaparinux.

These data indicate that the LMWHs and likely fondaparinux, by indirect comparison, are more effective than vitamin K antagonists in preventing VTE in patients undergoing major orthopedic surgery. There is a slight increase in surgical site bleeding with these more effective forms of prophylaxis. The higher efficacy and bleeding risks are likely attributable to the more rapid onset of anticoagulant activity with LMWH and fondaparinux compared to the vitamin K antagonists.

Randomized clinical trials in the prevention of VTE in patients undergoing elective hip replacement have found that recombinant hirudin, a direct thrombin inhibitor, given subcutaneously at the dose of 15 mg twice a day beginning just before surgery, is more effective than low-dose unfractionated heparin (63,64) or LMWH (87). No differences in bleeding were observed. Hirudin is not currently available for this indication.

Several nonpharmacologic methods have been evaluated for the prophylaxis of VTE in patients undergoing hip replacement. These include graduated compression stockings (17,20,88–91), intermittent pneumatic compression (8,9,92–96), and pneumatic foot pump (90,97). The risk reduction conferred by the nonpharmacologic methods of prophylaxis is uncertain but probably lower than that provided by the anticoagulant-based prophylaxis strategies. This seems to be particularly true for proximal DVT (1,9,91,95). The evidence for the efficacy of foot pump is limited and essentially based on two studies with reduced sample size and methodologic limitations (90,97).

Spinal or epidural anesthesia is associated with a significant reduction in the incidence of postoperative DVT in patients undergoing elective hip replacement in the absence of prophylaxis (98,99). However, regional anesthesia without pharmacologic prophylaxis is largely suboptimal because it is associated with an unacceptably high risk of VTE.

Multimodal prophylaxis is commonly used in major orthopedic surgery, but the evidence in favor of this approach is limited. Epidural anesthesia has been combined with intermittent pneumatic compression and aspirin (100), as well as aspirin with graduated compression stockings or intermittent pneumatic compression (101). Although it is plausible to expect an advantage from multimodal prophylaxis, additional data are required before calling this approach superior to more simple and less expensive alternatives.

# PREVENTION OF VENOUS THROMBOEMBOLISM IN ELECTIVE KNEE REPLACEMENT

The prophylactic measures used in elective knee replacement are similar to those used in patients undergoing elective hip replacement. However, some prophylaxis measures used successfully in patients undergoing elective hip replacement seem to be less effective in patients undergoing elective knee replacement (see Table 95-3). In particular, the risk reduction conferred by the use of LMWH versus the vitamin K antagonists is greater in patients undergoing knee replacement than in those undergoing hip replacement. Low-dose unfractionated heparin (102,103) and aspirin (10,12,27,58,104,105) are not recommended for the prevention of VTE in patients undergoing elective knee replacement because of their limited efficacy.

Adjusted-dose vitamin K antagonists have been evaluated in a number of randomized clinical trials that used routine venography to measure the incidence of DVT (10,75,82,83,94,106–112). In patients receiving vitamin K antagonists for 10 days after surgery, the rate of venography-detected DVT ranges between 25% and 50%, and the rate of symptomatic VTE in the 3 months after surgery is approximately 1% (113,114).

LMWHs are effective and safe when used to prevent VTE in patients undergoing elective knee replacement (6,29,30,75,82,83,103,107–109,115,116). Combining the results of the six studies that compared different LMWHs with vitamin K antagonists for the prevention of VTE in patients undergoing elective knee replacement, the pooled rate of DVT is 48% in patients receiving vitamin K antagonists and 33% in patients receiving LMWHs (75,82,83,107–109). The respective rates of proximal DVT are 10.4% and 7.1%. In two of these studies, a higher risk of bleeding was observed in patients receiving LMWH, but this increased risk was limited to minor bleeding (82,109). Two formal metaanalyses have confirmed the superior efficacy of LMWH over both fixed low-dose unfractionated heparin and vitamin K antagonists in reducing venography-detected DVT, without showing an increased risk in bleeding (117,118). Cost analyses of prophylaxis with warfarin or LMWH resulted in

---

**TABLE 95-3**

PREVENTION OF DEEP VEIN THROMBOSIS AFTER TOTAL KNEE REPLACEMENT SURGERY

| Prophylaxis regimen | No. of trials | Combined enrollment | Total DVT Prevalence % (95% CI) | RRR % | Proximal DVT Prevalence % (95% CI) | RRR% |
|---|---|---|---|---|---|---|
| Placebo/control | 6 | 199 | 64.3 (57–71) | — | 15.3 (10–23) | — |
| GCS | 2 | 145 | 60.7 (52–69) | 6 | 16.6 (11–24) | — |
| Aspirin | 5 | 416 | 54.6 (50–59) | 15 | 8.9 (6–12) | 42 |
| VFP | 5 | 271 | 46.9 (41–53) | 27 | 3.0 (1–6) | 80 |
| Warfarin | 10 | 1,501 | 44.2 (42–47) | 31 | 9.2 (8–11) | 40 |
| Low-dose heparin | 2 | 236 | 43.2 (37–50) | 33 | 11.4 (8–16) | 26 |
| LMWH | 18 | 2,776 | 33.5 (32–35) | 48 | 5.3 (4–6) | 65 |
| IPC | 4 | 110 | 28.2 (20–38) | 56 | 7.3 (3–14) | 52 |

CI, confidence interval; DVT, deep vein thrombosis; GCS, graduated compression stockings; IPC, intermittent pneumatic compression; LMWH, low-molecular-weight heparin; VFP, venous foot pump; RRR, relative risk reduction.

conflicting results possibly because of the difficulty in assessing the indirect cost associated with the administration of warfarin (119–123).

In a double-blind study of patients undergoing elective major knee surgery, fondaparinux, given subcutaneously at a dose of 2.5 mg once daily starting 6 hours after surgery, was compared to enoxaparin, 30 mg twice a day starting 12 to 24 hours after surgery. The rates of venography-detected DVT were 12.5% in patients receiving fondaparinux and 27.8% in patients receiving enoxaparin, a statistically significant difference. The rate of proximal DVT was halved in patients receiving fondaparinux, from 5.4% to 2.4%. Major bleeding was significantly more common in the fondaparinux group (2.1% vs. 0.2%). Some of the patients included in this study received fondaparinux before 6 hours after surgery, and in these patients, major bleeding was significantly more common than in patients who received fondaparinux 6 hours or more after surgery (124).

Nonpharmacologic methods of prophylaxis are commonly used in patients undergoing knee replacement. However, data about the efficacy and safety of these methods are limited in comparison with those available with LMWH and warfarin. In patients undergoing total knee replacement, the results of four studies with a small sample size indicate that intermittent pneumatic compression devices may provide effective prophylaxis (94,104,105,125). These devices are most effective when applied either preoperatively or immediately postoperatively and used continuously at least until the patient is fully ambulatory. Poor compliance, improper use of the devices, patient intolerance, and the inability to continue prophylaxis after hospital discharge limit the utility of intermittent pneumatic compression. Intermittent pneumatic compression may be useful as an in-hospital adjunct to anticoagulant-based prophylaxis in the presence of multiple risk factors for postoperative VTE, although combined prophylaxis using intermittent pneumatic compression and either LMWH or adjusted-dose vitamin K antagonists has not been properly evaluated in studies with adequate design.

## PREVENTION OF VENOUS THROMBOEMBOLISM IN HIP FRACTURE SURGERY

Routine prophylaxis for VTE should be provided to all patients undergoing surgery for hip fracture unless firmly contraindicated. Unfortunately, less information is available concerning the optimal prophylaxis in patients undergoing hip fracture surgery in comparison with elective hip and knee replacements (see Table 95-4).

The role of aspirin for prophylaxis of VTE is particularly controversial in patients undergoing surgery for hip fracture. A metaanalysis suggested that aspirin and other antiplatelet agents are effective in preventing postoperative VTE (56). In the Pulmonary Embolism Prevention (PEP) Trial, 13,356 patients with hip fracture were randomized to receive either 160 mg of aspirin or placebo. Aspirin was started before surgery and was continued for 35 days thereafter (58). Additional prophylaxis with graduated elastic stockings, LMWHs, or fixed low-dose unfractionated heparin was used in approximately one quarter of patients. Aspirin was associated with a statistically significant absolute risk reduction of 0.4% of fatal PE and clinically overt DVT. Surprisingly, neither myocardial infarction nor stroke was reduced by aspirin, as was the case for mortality from any cause. In the aspirin-treated patients, a significant increase in wound-related and gastrointestinal bleeding and increased need for blood transfusion were observed. No difference was observed between aspirin and placebo in 3,424 patients with hip fracture who also received a LMWH for combined prophylaxis.

A recent overview showed that both fixed low-dose unfractionated heparin and LMWH are effective in the prophylaxis against VTE in patients with hip fracture without increasing the risk of bleeding (126). This review was unable to determine the superiority of one agent over the other.

Low-dose unfractionated heparin was compared with the LMWH dalteparin in a randomized study of approximately 60 patients that used routine venography to screen DVT (127). In this study, unfractionated heparin of 5,000 U given three times a day was more efficacious than dalteparin given at the dose of 5,000 U once daily.

LMWHs were evaluated for prevention of VTE in patients with hip fracture in five studies, four of which were of a small sample size (40,127–129). The single placebo-controlled clinical trial did not demonstrate a significant benefit from LMWH (40). No clinical trials have directly compared LMWH and vitamin K antagonists in patients undergoing surgery for hip fracture. No excessive bleeding seems to be associated with the use of LMWH in comparison with placebo (40) or unfractionated heparin (127).

Prophylaxis with vitamin K antagonists is effective and safe in patients undergoing surgery for hip fracture. Warfarin

## TABLE 95-4

### PREVENTION OF DEEP VEIN THROMBOSIS AFTER HIP FRACTURE SURGERY

| Prophylaxis regimen | No. of trials | Combined enrollment | Total DVT Prevalence % (95% CI) | RRR % | Proximal DVT Prevalence % (95% CI) | RRR% |
|---|---|---|---|---|---|---|
| Placebo/control | 8 | 364 | 50 (45–56) | — | 27 (22–32) | — |
| GCS | 1 | 23 | 39 (20–61) | 22 | 17 (5–39) | 35 |
| Aspirin | 3 | 204 | 39 (32–46) | 23 | 13 (8–19) | 53 |
| Low-dose heparin | 1 | 30 | 20 (8–39) | 60 | 17 (6–35) | 38 |
| Warfarin | 3 | 126 | 20 (13–28) | 61 | 9 (4–19) | 66 |
| LMWH | 5 | 887 | 18 (15–21) | 65 | 6 (4–8) | 78 |

CI, confidence interval; DVT, deep vein thrombosis; GCS, graduated compression stockings; LMWH, low-molecular-weight heparin; RRR, relative risk reduction.

started postoperatively (target INR 2.0 to 2.7) was found to be more effective than aspirin, given at the dose of 650 mg twice daily, or no prophylaxis. The respective rates of DVT were 20%, 41%, and 46%, and those of proximal DVT were 9%, 11%, and 30%. Bleeding rates were similar in the three groups. The pooled results from three studies comparing adjusted-dose vitamin K antagonists with no prophylaxis show a 61% RRR for DVT and a 66% reduction for proximal DVT (11,36,37). The reported bleeding rates observed with vitamin K antagonists ranged from 0% to 47% (11,36,37); no difference in bleeding compared with placebo was observed in the largest of these studies (11).

Fondaparinux has been compared with enoxaparin for the prevention of VTE in patients undergoing surgery for hip fracture (130). In this study, 1,711 patients were randomized to receive either enoxaparin, 40 mg once daily starting 12 to 24 hours postoperatively, or fondaparinux, 2.5 mg once daily starting 4 to 8 hours after surgery. Enoxaparin and fondaparinux were administered preoperatively in 26% and 11% of patients, respectively. By postoperative day 11, fondaparinux reduced the rate of VTE from 19.1% to 8.3% and that of proximal DVT from 4.3% to 0.9%. Both differences were statistically significant. Major bleeding was observed in 2.2% of patients in both groups.

A delay often occurs between hip fracture and hospital admission. A further delay may occur between hospital admission and surgery. This delay increases the risk of VTE in patients with hip fracture, because DVT may develop between the time of injury and surgery (131–134). If surgery is likely to be delayed, prophylaxis probably should be started during the preoperative period with the use of a short-acting anticoagulant, such as unfractionated heparin or LMWH.

There is no sufficient data to support the use of nonpharmacologic prophylaxis alone to prevent DVT in patients with hip fracture (126). No studies have compared nonpharmacologic prophylaxis with other methods of prophylaxis in patients undergoing surgery for hip fracture using contrast venography to detect DVT. Intermittent pneumatic compression has been shown to be effective in a single study in comparison with no prophylaxis (135). Data on the efficacy and safety of graduated compression stockings remain insufficient to establish them as a reliable alternative to pharmacologic prophylaxis (58,136).

## PREVENTION OF VENOUS THROMBOEMBOLISM IN ELECTIVE SPINE SURGERY

The incidence of VTE in patients undergoing elective spine surgery remains poorly defined and influenced by the associated risk factors in the individual patient (11,58). The incidence of venography-detected DVT in the absence of prophylaxis is approximately 18% (137–139). An incidence of symptomatic DVT of 3.7% and of PE of 2.2% was found in an overview that included patients undergoing lumbar spinal fusions (140). Age and surgery of the lumbar, more than cervical spine, seem to be independent predictors for VTE (139).

Information concerning the prophylaxis for VTE in patients undergoing spinal surgery is limited.

Low-dose unfractionated heparin was found to be more effective than no prophylaxis in a small study in patients undergoing laminectomy (141). Enoxaparin was also shown to be of promising efficacy in two small trials (142,143).

Intermittent pneumatic compression was found to be effective compared to no prophylaxis in an observational study of patients undergoing elective spinal surgery (137).

## PREVENTION OF VENOUS THROMBOEMBOLISM IN LOWER EXTREMITY INJURY

Injuries of the lower extremities include fractures of below-knee bones, injuries of ligaments and cartilages of the knee and ankle, and rupture of the Achilles tendon. These injuries are managed surgically or by using plaster casts or braces. Risk factors for VTE following lower extremity injury include advanced age (144–147), bone fractures rather than soft tissue injuries alone (148), and obesity (147).

In patients with fractures of the lower extremity not receiving any prophylaxis, the incidence of DVT screened by venography ranged between 19% and 45%, with an incidence of proximal DVT of approximately 5% (148–151).

The role of pharmacologic prophylaxis in patients with fractures of the lower extremity remains undefined (see Table 95-5).

## TABLE 95-5

PREVENTION OF VENOUS THROMBOEMBOLISM IN PATIENTS WITH ISOLATED LOWER EXTREMITY INJURIES[a]

| | Patients | Diagnostic test | Interventions Control | Interventions Experimental | DVT, n/N (%) Control | DVT, n/N (%) Experimental |
|---|---|---|---|---|---|---|
| Kujath (148), 1993 | Leg injuries managed with plaster casts | DUS when cast removed | No prophylaxis | Nadroparin ~3,000 U daily | 21/127 (17) | 6/126 (5) |
| Kock (146), 1995 | Leg injuries managed with plaster casts | DUS when cast removed | No prophylaxis | Certoparin 3,000 U daily | 7/163 (4) | 0/176 |
| Lassen (149), 2002 | Below-knee fractures | Venography ≥5 wk | Placebo | Reviparin 1,750 U daily | 29/159 (18) | 14/134 (10) |
| | Achilles tendon repair | | | | 6/28 (21) | 3/48 (6) |
| Jorgensen (152), 2002 | Below-knee fractures | Venography ≥5 wk | No prophylaxis | Tinzaparin 3,500 U daily | 10/77 (13) | 8/73 (11) |
| | Tendon ruptures | | | | 6/21 (29) | 2/20 (10) |

DUS, duplex ultrasonography; DVT, deep vein thrombosis.
[a]Randomized clinical trials with routine screening using an objective outcome.

The LMWHs nadroparin and certoparin, at the dose of approximately 3,000 U once daily, have been found to be more effective than no prophylaxis in outpatients with plaster casts without increasing the rate of bleeding complications (146,152). In two venography studies, patients with injuries of the lower extremities were randomized to either no prophylaxis or LMWH (149,152). In the first trial, 440 patients with fracture of the lower extremities or Achilles tendon rupture were randomized to placebo or to the LMWH reviparin, 1,750 U once a day for at least 5 weeks (149). Reviparin significantly reduced the rate of DVT from 19% to 9%. The corresponding rates of proximal DVT were 5% and 2%. Major bleeding was observed in less than 1% of patients in both groups. In the second trial, tinzaparin, at the dose of 3,500 U, was compared with no prophylaxis in 300 patients with lower extremity injuries managed with plaster casts (152). DVT was found in 17% of the control patients and in 10% of those who received tinzaparin. LMWH did not significantly reduce the risk of DVT in patients with fractures in either of these two trials.

# CONTROVERSIAL ISSUES IN THE PREVENTION OF VENOUS THROMBOEMBOLISM IN ORTHOPEDIC SURGERY

## Prevention of Venous Thromboembolism after Knee Arthroscopy

Arthroscopy of the knee and arthroscopic assisted knee surgery, including meniscectomy, synovectomy, and reconstruction of the cruciate ligaments, are among the most common orthopedic procedures. Available information about the risks of VTE associated with arthroscopy is controversial (see Table 95-6) (153, 154). In a large series of 8,791 knee arthroscopies, the rate of symptomatic VTE was found to be less than 0.15%, and no fatal PE occurred (155). Even lower figures were found in another series of 8,500 patients undergoing arthroscopy for various reasons (156). More recently, a rate of 0.6% of clinically overt, objectively confirmed DVT was found in a series of 1,355 patients undergoing diagnostic knee arthroscopy without prophylaxis (47). The rate of asymptomatic DVT detected by mandatory testing ranges from 3% to 18% (28). Risk factors for VTE in patients undergoing arthroscopy are unclear. Therapeutic arthroscopy seems to be associated with a higher risk of VTE

than diagnostic arthroscopy; the duration of the tourniquet use is a risk factor in patients undergoing arthroscopy (157,158).

The evidence for the use of prophylaxis in patients undergoing knee arthroscopy is limited. In one trial, patients were randomized to receive either no prophylaxis or the LMWH reviparin, at the dose of 1,750 U once daily for 7 to 10 days (159). Among the 239 patients with adequate compression ultrasonography, DVT was found in 4% of control patients and in 1% of patients who received reviparin. In a second trial, 130 patients undergoing either diagnostic or therapeutic arthroscopy were randomized to receive either no prophylaxis or once-daily dalteparin for up to 30 days (160). Dalteparin significantly reduced from 16% to 2% the rate of DVT, as shown by ultrasonography. There were no cases of proximal DVT. No excess of bleeding was observed in patients who received LMWH in these two studies (159,161).

## The Optimal Initiation Time for Pharmacologic Prophylaxis

Two important issues should be considered about the timing of prophylaxis in major orthopedic surgery. The first relates to preoperative versus postoperative initiation of prophylaxis, and the second relates to how early after surgery anticoagulant prophylaxis should be started (162).

In Europe, LMWH is generally started 10 to 12 hours before surgery. In the United States, prophylaxis with LMWH usually begins 12 to 24 hours after surgery. Two reviews have provided conflicting results about the relative value of preoperative and postoperative start of prophylaxis (150,163).

This controversial issue has been addressed in a study performed in patients undergoing hip replacement. In this three-arm study, patients were randomized to preoperative dalteparin, 2,500 U started 1 hour before surgery, followed by a second dose of 2,500 U given about 7 hours after surgery, and then 5,000 U once daily; or postoperative dalteparin, 2,500 U subcutaneously started about 7 hours after surgery, and then 5,000 U once daily; or postoperative adjusted-dose warfarin (84,151). The rate of overall DVT observed in the warfarin recipients was 24% and was significantly higher than with either dalteparin regimen. The rates of total DVT in patients receiving dalteparin preoperatively and postoperatively were 10.7% and 13.1%, respectively. The rate of major bleeding was significantly higher in patients randomized to preoperative dalteparin than to warfarin, but no increased risk of bleeding was found when postoperative dalteparin was compared to warfarin.

## TABLE 95-6

### PROSPECTIVE STUDIES OF DEEP VEIN THROMBOSIS RATES AFTER KNEE ARTHROSCOPY[a]

|  | Method of diagnosis | When screened after surgery | No. | DVT, no. (%) | Proximal DVT, no. (%) |
|---|---|---|---|---|---|
| Stringer (28), 1989 | Venography | 7–10 d | 48 | 2 (4) | 0 |
| Durica, 1997 | Venography | 10–14 d | 161 | 5 (3) | 2 (1) |
| Demers (157), 1998 | Venography | 1 wk | 184 | 33 (18) | 9 (5) |
| Williams, 1993 | DUS | 7–14 d | 85 | 3 (4) | 0 |
| Cullison, 1996 | DUS | 2–3 d | 67 | NR | 1 (1) |
| Jaureguito (158), 1999 | DUS | 5–10 d | 239 | 5 (2) | 0–1 |
| Delis, 2001 | DUS | ≤1 wk | 102 | 8 (8) | 0 |
| Wirth (159), 2001 | DUS | 7–10 d | 111 | 5 (5) | 2 (2) |
| Michot (160), 2002 | DUS | 12 and 30 d | 63 | 10 (16) | 0 |

DVT, deep vein thrombosis; DUS, duplex ultrasonography.
[a]Routine screening for DVT in patients undergoing knee arthroscopy in absence of prophylaxis.

A systematic review concluded that starting LMWH prophylaxis postoperatively provided comparable protection to preoperative initiation of LMWH (164). A second systematic review showed that the advantage of LMWH over warfarin in patients undergoing hip replacement is seen only when LMWH is initiated in close proximity to surgery (either <2 hours before or 6 to 8 hours after surgery) (165). However, starting LMWH just before surgery was associated with an increased risk of major bleeding. A systematic review also concluded that LMWH administered shortly before surgery is more effective than after surgery, but this benefit is offset by an increased risk of bleeding (166).

## Predischarge Screening for Deep Vein Thrombosis

Routine screening for asymptomatic DVT has been promoted to prevent the occurrence of late thrombosis and to avoid extension of antithrombotic prophylaxis in patients who underwent major orthopedic surgery (166). Routine screening for asymptomatic DVT using Doppler ultrasonography was not found to be clinically effective in three large studies (6,113,167). Only 0.15% of the patients who underwent major orthopedic surgery and received in-hospital prophylaxis with LMWH were found to have asymptomatic DVT at predischarge ultrasonography (6). In a different study, patients who have undergone major orthopedic surgery were randomized to receive predischarge compression ultrasonography or sham compression ultrasonography (113). Active compression ultrasonography detected DVT in 2.5% of patients but was not associated with a reduced risk of late occurring symptomatic VTE. These findings were confirmed in a third trial in which patients who have undergone major surgery received LMWH prophylaxis for 10 days and were then randomized either to continue LMWH for another 3 weeks or to have predischarge screening with compression ultrasonography (167). Compression ultrasonography did not reduce the incidence of symptomatic VTE on subsequent 3-month follow-up, leading to the conclusion that routine predischarge screening is not warranted.

## The Optimal Duration of Prophylaxis

The optimal duration of antithrombotic prophylaxis after major orthopedic surgery has been a matter of debate (168). There is evidence that the risk of VTE persists for at least 4 weeks after hip replacement (47,50,52,161,169–174), Indeed, approximately three quarters of symptomatic DVT occur after hospital discharge (50). The rate of VTE occurring after hospital discharge is higher in patients undergoing hip replacement than in those undergoing knee replacement. Risk factors for rehospitalization for symptomatic VTE include a body mass index of 25 kg per m (2) or greater, history of prior VTE, and age older than 85 years (124). Early ambulation before the second postoperative day and the use of mechanical and pharmacologic prophylaxis after discharge are protective factors against VTE.

Three systematic reviews found that postdischarge prophylaxis reduced VTE and was safe (51,175,176). No excess of bleeding was observed in patients receiving extended prophylaxis, thereby suggesting that in patients undergoing major orthopedic surgery, the risk–benefit ratio favors use of extended prophylaxis. The benefit of extending prophylaxis is higher in patients undergoing hip replacement than in those undergoing knee replacement (175). In a metaanalysis restricted to patients undergoing elective hip replacement, the rates of symptomatic VTE among patients who received in-hospital LMWH and those who were given postdischarge LMWH, were 2.7% and 1.1%, respectively, corresponding to an absolute risk reduction of 1.6% [95% confidence intervals (CI), 0.2 to 3.3; number needed to treat (NNT) = 64] (177). The absolute risk reduction for symptomatic PE was 0.4% (95% CI, 0.3 to 1.4; NNT = 278) and for fatal PE, 0.1% (95% CI, 0.1 to 0.3; NNT = 1,093).

Six randomized placebo-controlled studies have evaluated extended prophylaxis with LMWH for up to 35 days in patients who underwent elective hip replacement and completed in-hospital prophylaxis with either LMWH (enoxaparin or dalteparin) or warfarin (55,151,173,178,179). In all the studies, extended prophylaxis was more effective than prophylaxis limited to the hospital stay. A systematic review of these six trials demonstrated a significant decrease in both total and proximal DVT with extended LMWH, as well as reduced risk of symptomatic VTE (180). The rates of out-of-hospital symptomatic VTE were 4.2% with in-hospital prophylaxis and 1.4% with extended prophylaxis (relative risk = 0.36; P <0.001; NNT = 36). In another randomized clinical trial that compared in-hospital use of LMWH and LMWH continued after discharge, extended prophylaxis did not prevent additional symptomatic VTE (48).

A clinical trial showed the benefit of postdischarge prophylaxis with vitamin K antagonists in patients undergoing hip surgery in terms of both efficacy and safety (181). In another trial, patients undergoing hip replacement were randomized either to the LMWH reviparin, at the dose of 4,200 U once daily, or to prophylaxis with vitamin K antagonists (target INR 2 to 3). Both treatments were given for 6 weeks (182). Objectively confirmed, symptomatic thrombosis occurred in 2.3% of patients receiving reviparin and in 3.3% of those given vitamin K antagonists. The rate of major bleeding was significantly higher in patients receiving vitamin K antagonists.

In a study of knee replacement, extending prophylaxis with LMWH for 4 weeks did not significantly reduce the rate of objectively screened DVT and of readmission for VTE in comparison to in-hospital prophylaxis (178).

The clinical benefit of extending antithrombotic prophylaxis has also been assessed in patients undergoing surgery for hip fracture. In a cohort study, enoxaparin was associated with a relative low rate of VTE but also with bleeding complications. In a more recent double-blind study, all patients with hip fracture received fondaparinux, at the dose of 2.5 mg once daily for approximately 7 days, and were then randomized in a double-blind fashion to continue fondaparinux for 3 additional weeks or to receive placebo for an additional 3 weeks (130). At the end of the study, venography showed DVT in 1.4% of the patients receiving extended prophylaxis and in 35.0% of the patients receiving placebo (RRR, 96%; P <0.001). The respective rates of symptomatic VTE were 0.3% and 2.7% (RRR, 89%; P = 0.02). Bleeding rates were not significantly different in patients receiving fondaparinux or placebo for extended prophylaxis.

Some economic studies suggested that extended, postdischarge prophylaxis may be cost-effective in comparison with in-hospital prophylaxis (123,183–185).

On the basis of the available data, extended prophylaxis up to 28 to 35 days is recommended for patients undergoing major orthopedic surgery, particularly for those at high risk for VTE. Further studies are needed to define who is at high risk; however, a history of VTE, obesity, prolonged immobilization, advanced age, or cancer have all been shown to predispose to VTE after major orthopedic surgery (174,180). Congestive heart failure, chronic obstructive pulmonary disease, and female gender are additional risk factors for postoperative VTE (174,186,187).

LMWH and vitamin K antagonists (INR target 2.5, range 2.0 to 3.0) are the agents of choice for extended prophylaxis in elective major orthopedic surgery, although vitamin K antagonists are less extensively evaluated. Fondaparinux is recommended for extended prophylaxis following hip fracture.

LMWH or vitamin K antagonists may also be effective for extended prophylaxis of VTE in patients with hip fracture, although prolonged use of these agents has not been properly evaluated in these patients.

## References

1. Geerts WH, Pineo GF, Heit JA, et al. Prevention of venous thromboembolism. The seventh ACCP Conference on Antithrombotic and Thrombolytic Therapy. *Chest* 2004;126:338S–400S.
2. NIH Consensus Conference. Prevention of venous thrombosis and pulmonary embolism. *JAMA* 1986;256:744–749.
3. Scottish Intercollegiate Guidelines Network (SIGN). Prophylaxis of venous thromboembolism: a national clinical guideline. Edinburgh: SIGN Publication o. 62, Scottish Intercollegiate Guidelines Network, 2002: Available from http://www.sign.ac.uk.
4. Todd CJ, Freeman CJ, Camilleri-Ferrante C, et al. Differences in mortality after fracture of hip: the East Anglian audit. *BMJ* 1995;310:904–908.
5. Fender D, Harper WM, Thompson JR, et al. Mortality and fatal pulmonary embolism after primary total hip replacement: results from a regional hip register. *J Bone Joint Surg* 1997;79-B:896–899.
6. Leclerc JR, Gent M, Hirsh J, et al. The incidence of symptomatic venous thromboembolism during and after prophylaxis with enoxaparin: a multi-institutional cohort study of patients who underwent hip or knee arthroplasty. *Arch Intern Med* 1998;158:873–878.
7. Freedman KB, Brookenthal KR, Fitzgerald RH, et al. A meta-analysis of thromboembolic prophylaxis following elective total hip arthroplasty. *J Bone Joint Surg* 2000;82-A:929–938.
8. Hull RD, Raskob GE, Gent M, et al. Effectiveness of intermittent pneumatic leg compression for preventing deep vein thrombosis after total hip replacement. *JAMA* 1990;263:2313–2317.
9. Gallus A, Raman K, Darby T. Venous thrombosis after elective hip replacement—the influence of preventive intermittent calf compression and of surgical technique. *Br J Surg* 1983;70:17–19.
10. Lotke PA, Palevsky H, Keenan AM, et al. Aspirin and warfarin for thromboembolic disease after total joint arthroplasty. *Clin Orthop* 1996;324: 251–258.
11. Powers PJ, Gent M, Jay RM, et al. A randomized trial of less intense postoperative warfarin or aspirin therapy in the prevention of venous thromboembolism after surgery for fractured hip. *Arch Intern Med* 1989;149: 771–774.
12. Westrich GH, Sculco TP. Prophylaxis against deep venous thrombosis after total knee arthroplasty: pneumatic planter compression and aspirin compared with aspirin alone. *J Bone Joint Surg* 1996;78-A:826–834.
13. Leandri P, Rossignol G, Gautier J-R, et al. Radical retropubic prostatectomy: morbidity and quality of life. Experience with 620 consecutive cases. *J Urol* 1992;147:883–887.
14. Turpie AGG, Levine MN, Hirsh J, et al. A randomized controlled trial of a low-molecular-weight heparin (enoxaparin) to prevent deep-vein thrombosis in patients underoging elective hip surgery. *N Engl J Med* 1986; 315: 925–929.
15. Beisaw NE, Comerota AJ, Groth HE, et al. Dihydroergotamine/heparin in the prevention of deep-vein thrombosis after total hip replacement: a controlled, prospective randomized multicenter trial. *J Bone Joint Surg* 1988; 70-A:2–10.
16. Haake DA, Berkman SA. Venous thromboembolic disease after hip surgery: risk factors, prophylaxis, and diagnosis. *Clin Orthop* 1989;242: 212–231.
17. Lassen MR, Borris LC, Christiansen HM, et al. Prevention of thromboembolism in 190 hip arthroplasties: comparison of LMW heparin and placebo. *Acta Orthop Scand* 1991;62:33–38.
18. Hoek JA, Nurmohamed MT, Hamelynck KJ, et al. Prevention of deep vein thrombosis following total hip replacement by low molecular weight heparinoid. *Thromb Haemost* 1992;67:28–32.
19. Eriksson BI, Kalebo P, Anthmyr BA, et al. Prevention of deep-vein thrombosis and pulmonary embolism after total hip or knee replacement: a meta-analysis fo prospective studies investigating symptomatic outcomes. *J Bone Joint Surg* 1991;73-A:484–493.
20. Warwick D, Bannister GC, Glew D, et al. Perioperative low-molecular-weight heparin: is it effective and safe? *J Bone Joint Surg* 1995;77-B:715–719.
21. Mahomed NN, Barrett JA, Latz JN, et al. Rates and outcomes of primary and revision total hip replacement in the United States Medicare population. *J Bone Joint Surg* 2003;85-A:27–32.
22. Phillips CB, Barrett JA, Losina E, et al. Incidence rates of dislocation, pulmonary embolism, and deep infection during the first six months after elective total hip replacement. *J Bone Joint Surg* 2003;85-A:20–26.
23. Mohr DN, Silverstein MD, Ilstrup DM, et al. Venous thromboembolism associated with hip and knee arthroplasty: current prophylactic practices and outcomes. *Mayo Clin Proc* 1992;67:861–870.
24. Murray DW, Britton AR, Bulstrode CJK. Thromboprophylaxis and death after total hip replacement. *J Bone Joint Surg* 1996;78-B:863–870.
25. Colwell CW, Collis DK, Paulson R, et al. Comparison of enoxaparin and warfarin for the prevention of venous thromboembolic disease after total hip arthroplasty: evaluation during hospitalization and three months after discharge. *J Bone Joint Surg* 1999;81-A:932–940.
26. Stulberg BN, Insall JN, Williams GW, et al. Deep-vein thrombosis following total knee replacement: an analysis of six hundred and thirty-eight arthroplasties. *J Bone Joint Surg* 1984;66-A:194–201.
27. Lynch AF, Bourne RB, Rorabeck CH, et al. Deep-vein thrombosis and continuous passive motion after total knee arthroplasty. *J Bone Joint Surg* 1988;70-A:11–14.
28. Stringer MD, Steadman CA, Hedges AR, et al. Deep vein thrombosis after elective knee surgery: an incidence study in 312 patients. *J Bone Joint Surg* 1989;71-B:492–497.
29. Leclerc JR, Geerts WH, Desjardins L, et al. Prevention of deep vein thrombosis after major knee surgery—a randomized, double-blind trial comparing a low molecular weight heparin fragment [enoxaparin] to placebo. *Thromb Haemost* 1992;67:417–423.
30. Levine MN, Gent M, Hirsh J, et al. Ardeparin (low-molecular-weight heparin) vs graduated compression stockings for the prevention of venous thromboembolism: a randomized trial in patients undergoing knee surgery. *Arch Intern Med* 1996;156:851–856.
31. Warwick D, Harrison J, Whitehouse S. A randomised comparison of a foot pump and low-molecular-weight heparin in the prevention of deep-vein thrombosis after total knee replacement. *J Bone Joint Surg* 2002; 84-B:344–350.
32. Khaw FM, Moran CG, Pinder IM, et al. The incidence of fatal pulmonary embolism after knee replacement with no prophylactic anticoagulation. *J Bone Joint Surg* 1993;75-B:940–941.
33. Ansari S, Warwick D, Ackroyd CE, et al. Incidence of fatal pulmonary embolism after 1,390 knee arthroplasties without routine prophylactic anticoagulation, except in high-risk cases. *J Arthroplasty* 1997;12:599–602.
34. Snook GA, Chrisman OD, Wilson TC. Thromboembolism after surgical treatment of hip fractures. *Clin Orthop* 1981;155:21–24.
35. Agnelli G, Cosmi B, DiFilippo P, et al. A randomised, double-blind, placebo-controlled trial of dermatan sulphate for prevention of deep vein thrombosis in hip fracture. *Thromb Haemost* 1992;67:203–208.
36. Borgstrom S, Greitz T, van der Linden W, et al. Anticoagulant prophylaxis of venous thrombosis in patients with fractured neck of the femur: a controlled clinical trial using venous phlebography. *Acta Chir Scand* 1965;129:500–508.
37. Hamilton HW, Crawford JS, Gardiner JH, et al. Venous thrombosis in patients with fracture of the upper end of the femur: a phlebographic study of the effect of prophylactic anticoagulation. *J Bone Joint Surg* 1970;52-B:268–289.
38. Lowe GD, Campbell AF, Meek DR, et al. Subcutaneous ancrod in prevention of deep-vein thrombosis after operation for fractured neck of femur. *Lancet* 1978;2:698–700.
39. Rogers PH, Walsh PN, Marder VJ, et al. Controlled trial of low-dose heparin and sulfinpyrazone to prevent venous thromboembolism after operation on the hip. *J Bone Joint Surg* 1978;60-A:758–762.
40. Jorgensen PS, Strandberg C, Willie-Jorgensen P, et al. Early preoperative thromboprophylaxis with Klexane® in hip fracture surgery: a placebo-controlled study. *Clin Appl Thromb Hemost* 1998;4:140–142.
41. Warwick D, Williams MH, Bannister GC. Death and thromboembolic disease after total hip replacement: a series of 1162 cases with no routine chemical prophylaxis. *J Bone Joint Surg* 1995;77-B:6–10.
42. Gillespie W, Murray D, Gregg PJ, et al. Risks and benefits of prophylaxis against venous thromboembolism in orthopaedic surgery. *J Bone Joint Surg* 2000;82-B:475–479.
43. Wroblewski BM, Siney PD, Fleming PA. Fatal pulmonary embolism after total hip arthroplasty: diurnal variations. *Orthopedics* 1998; 21:1269–1271.
44. Perez JV, Warwick DJ, Case CP, et al. Death after proximal femoral fracture: an autopsy study. *Injury* 1995;26:237–240.
45. White RH, Zhou H, Romano PS. Incidence of symptomatic venous thromboembolism after different elective or urgent surgical procedures. *Thromb Haemost* 2003;90:446–455.
46. Warwick DJ, Whitehouse S. Sympotomatic venous thromboembolism after total knee replacement. *J Bone Joint Surg* 1997;78-B:780–786.
47. Dahl OE, Gudmundsen TE, Haukeland L. Late occurring clinical deep vein thrombosis in joint-operated patients. *Acta Orthop Scand* 2000;71: 47–50.
48. Heit JA, Elliott CG, Trowbridge AA, et al. Ardeparin sodium for extended out-of-hospital prophylaxis against venous thromboembolism after total hip or knee replacement: a randomized, double-blind, placebo-controlled trial. *Ann Intern Med* 2000;132:853–861.
49. Anderson DR, Wilson SJ, Blundell J, et al. Comparison of a nomogram and physician-adjusted dosage of warfarin for prophylaxis against deep-vein thrombosis after arthroplasty. *J Bone Joint Surg* 2002;84-A: 1992–1997.
50. White RH, Romano PS, Zhou H, et al. Incidence and time course of thromboembolic outcomes following total hip or knee arthroplasty. *Arch Intern Med* 1998;158:1525–1531.
51. Douketis JD, Eikelboom JW, Quinlan DJ, et al. Short-duration prophylaxis against venous thromboembolism after total hip or knee replacement: a meta-analysis of prospective studies investigating symptomatic outcomes. *Arch Intern Med* 2002;162:1465–1471.

52. Pellegrini VD, Clement D, Lush-Ehmann C, et al. Natural history of thromboembolic disease after total hip arthroplasty. *Clin Orthop* 1996; 333:27–40.

53. Seagroatt V, Tan HS, Goldacre M. Elective total hip replacement: incidence, emergency readmission rate, and postoperative mortality. *BMJ* 1991;303:1431–1435.

54. Maynard MJ, Sculco TP, Ghelman B. Progression and regression of deep vein thrombosis after total knee arthroplasty. *Clin Orthop* 1991;273: 125–130.

55. Planes A, Vochelle N, Darmon JY, et al. Risk of deep-venous thrombosis after hospital discharge in patients having undergone total hip replacement: double-blind randomised comparison of enoxaparin versus placebo. *Lancet* 1996;348:224–228.

56. Antiplatelet Trialists' Collaboration. Collaborative metaanalysis of randomised trials of antiplatelet therapy for prevention of death, myocardial infarction and stroke in high-risk patients. *BMJ* 2002;324:71–86.

57. Collins R, Scrimgeour A, Yusuf S, et al. Reduction in fatal pulmonary embolism and venous thrombosis by perioperative administration of subcutaneous heparin. Overview of results of randomized trials in general, orthopedic, and urologic surgery. *N Engl J Med* 1988;318:1162–1173.

58. Pulmonary Embolism Prevention (PEP) Trial Collaborative Group. Prevention of pulmonary embolism and deep vein thrombosis with low dose aspirin: Pulmonary Embolism Prevention (PEP) Trial. *Lancet* 2000;355: 1295–1302.

59. Harris WH, Salzman EW, Athansoulis C, et al. Comparison of warfarin, low-molecular-weight dextran, aspirin, and subcutaneous heparin in prevention of venous thrombombolism following total hip replacement. *J Bone Joint Surg* 1974;56-A:1552–1562.

60. Leyvraz PF, Richard J, Bachmann F, et al. Adjusted versus fixed-dose subcutaneous heparin in the prevention of deep-vein thrombosis after total hip replacement. *N Engl J Med* 1983;309:954–958.

61. Planes A, Vochelle N, Mazas F, et al. Prevention of postoperative venous thrombosis: a randomized trial comparing unfractionated heparin with low molecular weight heparin in patients undergoing total hip replacement. *Thromb Haemost* 1988;60:407–410.

62. Anderson DR, O'Brien BJ, Levine MN, et al. Efficacy and cost of low-molecular-weight heparin for the prevention of deep vein thrombosis after total hip arthroplasty. *Ann Intern Med* 1993;119:1105–1112.

63. Eriksson BI, Ekman S, Kalebo P, et al. Prevention of deep-vein thrombosis after total hip replacement: direct thrombin inhibition with recombinant hirudin, CGP 39393. *Lancet* 1996;347:635–639.

64. Eriksson BI, Ekman S, Lindbratt S, et al. Prevention of thromboembolism with use of recombinant hirudin: results of a double-blind, multicenter trial comparing the efficacy of desirudin (Revasc) with that of unfractionated heparin in patients having a total hip replacement. *J Bone Joint Surg* 1997;79-A:326–333.

65. Kakkar VV, Howes J, Sharma V, et al. A comparative, double-blind, randomised trial of a new second generation LMWH (bemiparin) and UFH in the prevention of post-operative venous thromboembolism. *Thromb Haemost* 2000;83:523–529.

66. Dechavanne M, Ville D, Berruyer M, et al. Randomized trial of a low-molecular-weight heparin (Kabi 2165) versus adjusted-dose subcutaneous standard heparin in the prophylaxis of deep-vein thrombosis after elective hip surgery. *Haemostasis* 1989;19:5–12.

67. Leyvraz PF, Bachmann F, Hoek J, et al. Prevention of deep vein thrombosis after hip replacement: randomised comparison between unfractionated heparin and low molecular weight heparin. *BMJ* 1991;303: 543–548.

68. Rader CP, Kramer C, Konig A, et al. Low-molecular-weight heparin and partial thromboplastin time-adjusted unfractionated heparin in thromboprophylaxis after total knee and total hip arthroplasty. *J Arthroplasty* 1998;13:180–185.

69. Amstutz HC, Friscia DA, Dorey F, et al. Warfarin prophylaxis to prevent mortality from pulmonary embolism after total hip replacement. *J Bone Joint Surg* 1989;71-A:321–326.

70. Paiement GD, Wessinger SJ, Hughes R, et al. Routine use of adjusted low-dose warfarin to prevent venous thromboembolism after total hip replacement. *J Bone Joint Surg* 1993;75-A:893–898.

71. Janku GV, Paiement GD, Green HD. Prevention of thromboembolism in orthopaedics in the United States. *Clin Orthop* 1996;325:313–321.

72. Lieberman JR, Wollaeger J, Dorey F, et al. The efficacy of prophylaxis with low-dose warfarin for prevention of pulmonary embolism following total hip arthroplasty. *J Bone Joint Surg* 1997;79-A:319–325.

73. Gross M, Anderson DR, Nagpal S, et al. Venous thromboembolism prophylaxis after total hip or knee arthroplasty: a survey of Canadian orthopedic surgeons. *Can J Surg* 1999;42:457–461.

74. Mesko JW, Brand RA, Iorio RA, et al. Venous thromboembolic disease management patterns in total hip arthroplasty and total knee arthroplasty patients: a survey of the AAHKS membership. *J Arthroplasty* 2001;16: 679–688.

75. RD Heparin Arthroplasty Group. RD heparin compared with warfarin for prevention of venous thromboembolic disease following total hip or knee arthroplasty. *J Bone Joint Surg* 1994;76-A:1174–1185.

76. Francis CW, Pellegrini VD, Totterman S, et al. Prevention of deep-vein thrombosis after total hip arthroplasty: comparison of warfarin and dalteparin. *J Bone Joint Surg* 1997;79-A:1365–1372.

77. Caprini JA, Arcelus JI, Motykie G, et al. The influence of oral anticoagulation therapy on deep vein thrombosis rates four weeks after total hip replacement. *J Vasc Surg* 1999;30(5):813–820.

78. Nurmohamed MT, Rosendaal FR, Buller HR, et al. Low-molecular-weight heparin versus standard heparin in general and orthopaedic surgery: a meta-analysis. *Lancet* 1992;340:152–156.

79. Koch A, Ziegler S, Breitschwerdt H, et al. Low molecular weight heparin and unfractionated heparin in thrombosis prophylaxis: meta-analysis based on original patient data. *Thromb Res* 2001;102:295–309.

80. German Hip Arthroplasty Trial Group (GHAT). Prevention of deep vein thrombosis with low molecular-weight heparin in patients undergoing total hip replacement: a randomized trial. *Arch Orthop Trauma Surg* 1992;111:110–120.

81. Colwell CW, Spiro TE, Trowbridge AA, et al. Use of enoxaparin, a low-molecular-weight heparin, and unfractionated heparin for the prevention of deep venous thrombosis after elective hip replacement: a clinical trial comparing efficacy and safety. *J Bone Joint Surg* 1994;76-A:3–14.

82. Hull R, Raskob GE, Pineo G, et al. A comparison of subcutaneous low-molecular-weight heparin with warfarin sodium for prophylaxis against deep-vein thrombosis after hip or knee implantation. *N Engl J Med* 1993;329:1370–1376.

83. Hamulyak K, Lensing AWA, van der Meer J, et al. Subcutaneous low-molecular weight heparin or oral anticoagulants for the prevention of deep-vein thrombosis in elective hip and knee replacement? *Thromb Haemost* 1995;74:1428–1431.

84. Hull RD, Pineo GF, Francis C, et al. Low-molecular-weight heparin prophylaxis using dalteparin in close proximity to surgery vs warfarin in hip arthroplasty patients: a double-blind, randomized comparison. *Arch Intern Med* 2000;160:2199–2207.

85. Lassen MR, Bauer KA, Eriksson BI, et al. Postoperative fondaparinux versus preoperative enoxaparin for prevention of venous thromboembolism in elective hip-replacement surgery: a randomised double-blind comparison. *Lancet* 2002;359:1715–1720.

86. Turpie AGG, Bauer KA, Eriksson BI, et al. Postoperative fondaparinux versus postoperative enoxaparin for prevention of venous thromboembolism after elective hip-replacement surgery: a randomised double-blind trial. *Lancet* 2002;359:1721–1726.

87. Eriksson BI, Wille-Jorgensen P, Kalebo P, et al. A comparison of recombinant hirudin with a low-molecular-weight heparin to prevent thromboembolic complications after total hip replacement. *N Engl J Med* 1997;337: 1329–1335.

88. Barnes RW, Brand RA, Clarke W, et al. Efficacy of graded-compression antiembolism stockings in patients undergoing total hip arthroplasty. *Clin Orthop* 1978;132:61–67.

89. Nilsen DWT, Naesss-Andresen KF, Kierulf P, et al. Graded pressure stockings in prevention of deep vein thrombosis following total hip replacement. *Acta Chir Scand* 1984;150:531–534.

90. Fordyce MJF, Ling RSM. A venous foot pump reduces thrombosis after total hip replacement. *J Bone Joint Surg* 1992;74-B:45–49.

91. Samama CM, Clergue F, Barre J, et al. Low molecular weight heparin associated with spinal anaesthesia and gradual compression stockings in total hip replacment surgery. *Br J Anaesth* 1997;78:660–665.

92. Paiement G, Wessinger SJ, Waltman AC, et al. Low-dose warfarin versus external pneumatic compression for prophylaxis against venous thromboembolism following total hip replacement. *J Arthroplasty* 1987;2: 23–26.

93. Bailey JP, Kruger MP, Solano FX, et al. Prospective randomized trial of sequential compression devices vs low-dose warfarin for deep venous thrombosis prophylaxis in total hip arthroplasty. *J Arthroplasty* 1991;6 (Suppl.):S29–S35.

94. Kaempffe FA, Lifeso RM, Meinking C. Intermittent pneumatic compression versus Coumadin: prevention of deep vein thrombosis in low-extremity total joint arthroplasty. *Clin Orthop* 1991;269:89–97.

95. Francis CW, Pellegrini VD, Marder VJ, et al. Comparison of warfarin and external pneumatic compression in prevention of venous thrombosis after total hip replacement. *JAMA* 1992;267:2911–2915.

96. Norgren L, Austrell C, Brummer R, et al. Low incidence of deep vein thrombosis after total hip replacement: an interim analysis of patients on low molecular weight heparin vs sequential gradient compression prophylaxis. *Int Angiol* 1996;15(Suppl. 1):11–14.

97. Warwick D, Harrison J, Glew D, et al. Comparison of the use of a foot pump with the use of low-molecular-weight heparin for the prevention of deep-vein thrombosis after total hip replacement. *J Bone Joint Surg* 1998; 80-A:1158–1166.

98. Prins MH, Hirsh J. A comparison of general anesthesia and regional anesthesia as a risk factor for deep vein thrombosis following hip surgery: a critical review. *Thromb Haemost* 1990;64:497–500.

99. Eriksson BI, Ekman S, Baur M, et al. Regional block anaesthesia versus general anaesthesia. Are different antithrombotic drugs equally effective in patients undergoing hip replacement? Retrospective analysis of 2354 patients undergoing hip replacement receiving either recombinant hirudin, unfractionated heparin or enoxaparin [abstract]. *Thromb Haemost* 1997; 77(Suppl.):487–488.

100. Ryan MG, Westrich GH, Potter HG, et al. Effect of mechanical compression on the prevalence of proximal deep venous thrombosis as assessed by magnetic resonance venography. *J Bone Joint Surg* 2002;84-A: 1998–2004.

101. Sarmiento A, Goswani ADK. Thromboembolic prophylaxis with use of aspirin, exercise, and graded elastic stockings or intermittent compression devices in patients managed with total hip arthroplasty. *J Bone Joint Surg* 1999;81-A:339–346.

102. Colwell CW, Spiro TE, Trowbridge AA, et al. Efficacy and safety of enoxaparin versus unfractionated heparin for prevention of deep venous thrombosis after elective knee arthroplasty. *Clin Orthop* 1995;321:19–27.

103. Fauno P, Suomalainen O, Rehnberg V, et al. Prophylaxis for the prevention of venous thromboembolism after total knee arthroplasty: a comparison between unfractionated and low-molecular-weight heparin. *J Bone Joint Surg* 1994;76-A:1814–1818.

104. McKenna R, Galante J, Bachmann F, et al. Prevention of venous thromboembolism after total knee replacement by high-dose aspirin or intermittent calf and thigh compression. *BMJ* 1980;280:514–517.

105. Haas SB, Insall JN, Scuderi GR, et al. Pneumatic sequential-compression boots compared with aspirin prophylaxis of deep-vein thrombosis after total knee arthroplasty. *J Bone Joint Surg* 1990;72-A:27–31.

106. Francis CW, Pellegrini VD, Leibert KM, et al. Comparison of two warfarin regimens in the prevention of venous thrombosis following total knee replacment. *Thromb Haemost* 1996;75:706–711.

107. Leclerc JR, Geerts WH, Desjardins L, et al. Prevention of venous thromboembolism after knee arthroplasty: a randomized, double-blind trial comparing enoxaparin with warfarin. *Ann Intern Med* 1996;124:619–626.

108. Heit JA, Berkowitz SD, Bona R, et al. Efficacy and safety of low molecular weight heparin (ardeparin sodium) compared to warfarin for the prevention of venous thromboembolism after total knee replacement surgery: a doube-blind, dose-ranging study. *Thromb Haemost* 1997;77:32–38.

109. Fitzgerald RH, Spiro TE, Trowbridge AA, et al. Prevention of venous thromboembolic disease following primary total knee arthroplasty: a randomized, multicenter, open-label, parallel-group comparison of enoxaparin and warfarin. *J Bone Joint Surg* 2001;83-A:900–906.

110. Francis CW, Davidson BL, Berkowitz SD, et al. Ximelagatran versus warfarin for the prevention of venous thromboembolism after total knee arthroplasty: a randomized, double-blind trial. *Ann Intern Med* 2002; 137:648–655.

111. Colwell CW, Berkowitz SD, Comp PC, et al. Randomized, double-blind comparison of ximelagatran, an oral direct thrombin inhibitor, and warfarin to prevent venous thromboembolism (VTE) after total knee replacement (TKR): EXULT B. [abstract]. *Blood* 2003;102:14a.

112. Francis CW, Berkowitz SD, Comp PC, et al. Comparison of ximelagatran with warfarin for the prevention of venous thromboembolism after total knee replacement. *N Engl J Med* 2003;349:1703–1712.

113. Robinson KS, Anderson DR, Gross M, et al. Ultrasonographic screening before hospital discharge for deep venous thrombosis after arthroplasty: the post-arthroplasty screening study. A randomized, controlled trial. *Ann Intern Med* 1997;127:439–445.

114. Lieberman JR, Sung R, Dorey F, et al. Low-dose warfarin prophylaxis to prevent symptomatic pulmonary embolism after total knee arthroplasty. *J Arthroplasty* 1997;12:180–184.

115. Heit JA, Colwell CW, Francis CW, et al. Comparison of the oral direct thrombin inhibitor ximelagatran with enoxaparin as prophylaxis against venous thromboembolism after total knee replacement: a phase 2 dose-finding study. *Arch Intern Med* 2001;161:2215–2221.

116. Navarro-Quilis A, Castellet E, Rocha E, et al. Efficacy and safety of bemiparin compared with enoxaparin in the prevention of venous thromboembolism after total knee arthroplasty: a randomized, double-blind clinical trial. *J Thromb Haemost* 2003;1:425–432.

117. Howard AW, Aaron SD. Low molecular weight heparin decreases proximal and distal deep venous thrombosis following total knee arthroplasty: a meta-analysis of randomized trials. *Thromb Haemost* 1998;79:902–906.

118. Brookenthal KR, Freedman KB, Lotke PA, et al. A meta-analysis of thromboembolic prophylaxis in total knee arthroplasty. *J Arthroplasty* 2001;16:293–300.

119. Menzin J, Colditz GA, Regan MM, et al. Cost-effectiveness of enoxaparin vs low-dose warfarin in the prevention of deep-vein thrombosis after total hip replacement surgery. *Arch Intern Med* 1995;155:757–764.

120. Saltiel E, Shane R. Evaluation costs of a pharmacist-run thromboprophylaxis program. *Formulary* 1996;31:276–290.

121. Hull RD, Raskob GE, Pineo GF, et al. Subcutaneous low-molecular-weight heparin vs warfarin for prophylaxis of deep vein thrombosis after hip or knee implantation: an economic perspective. *Arch Intern Med* 1997;157:298–303.

122. Hawkins DW, Langley PC, Krueger KP. A pharmacoeconomic assessment of enoxaparin and warfarin as prophylaxis for deep vein thrombosis in patients undergoing knee replacement surgery. *Clin Ther* 1998;20: 182–195.

123. Friedman RJ, Dunsworth GA. Cost analyses of extended prophylaxis with enoxaparin after hip arthroplasty. *Clin Orthop* 2000;370:171–182.

124. Turpie AGG, Bauer KA, Eriksson BI, et al. Fondaparinux vs enoxaparin for the prevention of venous thromboembolism in major orthopedic surgery: a meta-analysis of 4 randomized double-blind studies. *Arch Intern Med* 2002;162:1833–1840.

125. Hull RD, Delmore TJ, Hirsh J, et al. Effectiveness of intermittent pulsatile elastic stockings for the prevention of calf and thigh vein thrombosis in patients undergoing elective knee surgery. *Thromb Res* 1979;16:37–45.

126. Handoll HH, Farrar MJ, McBirnie J, et al. Heparin, low molecular weight heparin and physical methods for preventing deep vein thrombosis and pulmonary embolism following surgery for hip fractures. (Cochrane Review). *The Cochrane Library*, Issue 1. Oxford: Update Software, 2003.

127. Monreal M, Lafoz E, Navarro A, et al. A prospective double-blind trial of a low molecular weight heparin once daily compared with conventional low-dose heparin three times daily to prevent pulmonary embolism and venous thrombosis in patients with hip fracture. *J Trauma* 1989;29:873–875.

128. Barsotti J, Gruel Y, Rosset P, et al. Comparative double-blind study of two dosage regimens low-molecular weight heparin in elderly patients with a fracture of the neck of the femur. *J Orthop Trauma* 1990;4:371–375.

129. TIFDED Study Group. Thromboprophylaxis in hip fracture surgery: a pilot study comparing danaparoid, enoxaparin and dalteparin. *Haemostasis* 1999;29:310–317.

130. Eriksson BI, Bauer KA, Lassen MR, et al. Fondaparinux compared with enoxaparin for the prevention of venous thromboembolism after hip-fracture surgery. *N Engl J Med* 2001;345:1298–1304.

131. Hefley WF, Nelson CL, Puskarich-May CL. Effect of delayed admission to the hospital on the preoperative prevalence of deep-vein thrombosis associated with fractures about the hip. *J Bone Joint Surg* 1996;78-A:581–583.

132. Roberts TS, Nelson CL, Barnes CL, et al. The preoperative prevalence and postoperative incidence of thromboembolism in patients with hip fractures treated with dextran prophylaxis. *Clin Orthop* 1990;255:198–203.

133. Girasole GJ, Cuomo F, Denton JR, et al. Diagnosis of deep vein thrombosis in elderly hip-fracture patients by using the duplex scanning technique. *Orthop Rev* 1994;23:411–416.

134. Williams WE, Wisniewski TF. Pre-operative anticoagulant prophylaxis in elderly patients with proximal femur fractures [abstract]. *J Bone Joint Surg* 1994;76-B:79.

135. Fisher CG, Blachut PA, Salvian AJ, et al. Effectiveness of leg compression devices for the prevention of thromboembolic disease in orthopaedic trauma patients: a prospective, randomized study of compression alone versus no prophylaxis. *J Orthop Trauma* 1995;9:1–7.

136. Moskovitz PA, Ellenberg SS, Feffer HL, et al. Low-dose heparin for prevention of venous thromboembolism in total hip arthroplasty and surgical repair of hip fractures. *J Bone Joint Surg* 1978;60-A:1065–1070.

137. Tetzlaff JE, Yoon HJ, O'Hara J, et al. Influence of anesthetic technique on the incidence of deep venous thrombosis after elective lumbar spine surgery [abstract]. *Reg Anesth Pain Med* 1994;19(Suppl. ):28.

138. Fujita T, Kostuik JP, Huckell CB, et al. Complications of spinal fusion in adult patients more than 60 years of age. *Orthop Clin North Am* 1998; 29:669–678.

139. Oda T, Fuji T, Kato Y, et al. Deep venous thrombosis after posterior spinal surgery. *Spine* 2000;25:2962–2967.

140. Turner JA, Ersek M, Herron L, et al. Patient outcomes after lumbar spinal fusions. *JAMA* 1992;268:907–911.

141. Gallus AS, Hirsh J, O'Brien SE, et al. Prevention of venous thrombosis with small, subcutaneous doses of heparin. *JAMA* 1976;235:1980–1982.

142. Macouillard G, Castagnera L, Claverie JP, et al. Prevention of deep venous thrombosis in spinal surgery: comparison of intermittent sequential pneumatic compression versus low molecular weight heparin [abstract]. *Thromb Haemost* 1993;69:646.

143. Macouillard G, Castagnera L, Claverie JP, et al. Comparative efficacy of two dosages of a low molecular weight heparin for prevention of deep venous thrombosis in spinal surgery [abstract]. *Thromb Haemost* 1995; 73:979.

144. Hjelmstedt A, Bergvall U. Incidence of thrombosis in patients with tibial fractures: a phlebographic study. *Acta Chir Scand* 1968;134:209–218.

145. Abelseth G, Buckley RE, Pineo GE, et al. Incidence of deep-vein thrombosis in patients with fractures of the lower extremity distal to the hip. *J Orthop Trauma* 1996;10:230–235.

146. Kock HJ, Schmit-Neuerburg KP, Hanke J, et al. Thromboprophylaxis with low-molecular-weight heparin in outpatients with plaster-cast immobilization of the leg. *Lancet* 1995;346:459–461.

147. Spannagel U, Kujath P. Low molecular weight heparin for the prevention of thromboembolism in outpatients immobilized by plaster cast. *Semin Thromb Hemost* 1993;19(Suppl. 1):131–141.

148. Kujath P, Spannagel U, Habscheid W. Incidence and prophylaxis of deep venous thrombosis in outpatients with injury of the lower limb. *Haemostasis* 1993;23(Suppl. 1):20–26.

149. Lassen MR, Borris LC, Nakov RL. Use of the low-molecular-weight heparin reviparin to prevent deep-vein thrombosis after leg injury requiring immobilization. *N Engl J Med* 2002;347:726–730; (correspondence 2003; 2348:1062).

150. Hull RD, Brant RF, Pineo GF, et al. Preoperative vs postoperative initiation of low-molecular-weight heparin prophylaxis against venous thromboembolism in patients undergoing elective hip replacement. *Arch Intern Med* 1999;159:137–141.

151. Hull RD, Pineo GF, Francis C, et al. Low-molecular-weight heparin prophylaxis using dalteparin extended out-of-hospital vs in-hospital warfarin/out-of-hospital placebo in hip arthroplasty patients: a double-blind, randomized comparison. *Arch Intern Med* 2000;160:2208–2215.

152. Jorgensen PS, Warming T, Hansen K, et al. Low molecular weight heparin (Innohep) as thromboprophylaxis in outpatients with a plaster cast: a venografic controlled study. *Thromb Res* 2002;105:477–480.

153. Bergqvist D, Lowe G. Venous thromboembolism in patients undergoing laparoscopic and arthroscopic surgery and in leg casts. *Arch Intern Med* 2002;162:2173–2176.

154. Hoppener MR, Ettema HB, Kraaijenhagen RA, et al. Day-care or short-stay surgery and venous thromboembolism. *J Thromb Haemost* 2003; 1:863–865.

155. Small NC. Complications in arthroscopic surgery performed by experienced arthroscopists. *Arthroscopy* 1988;4:215–221.

156. Bamford DJ, Paul AS, Noble J, et al. Avoidable complications of arthroscopic surgery. *J R Coll Surg Edinb* 1993;38:92–95.

157. Demers C, Marcoux S, Ginsberg JS, et al. Incidence of venographically proved deep vein thrombosis after knee arthroscopy. *Arch Intern Med* 1998;158:47–50.

158. Jaureguito JW, Greenwald AE, Wilcox JF, et al. The incidence of deep venous thrombosis after arthroscopic knee surgery. *Am J Sports Med* 1999; 27:707–710.

159. Wirth T, Schneider B, Misselwitz F, et al. Prevention of venous thromboembolism after knee arthroscopy with low-molecular weight heparin (reviparin): results of a randomized controlled trial. *Arthroscopy* 2001; 17:393–399.

160. Sikorski JM, Hampson WG, Staddon GE. The natural history and aetiology of deep vein thrombosis after total hip replacement. *J Bone Joint Surg* 1981;63-B:171–177.

161. Michot M, Conen D, Holtz D, et al. Prevention of deep-vein thrombosis in ambulatory arthroscopic knee surgery: a randomized trial of prophylaxis with low-molecular weight heparin. *Arthroscopy* 2002;18:257–263.

162. Raskob GE, Hirsh J. Controversies in timing of the first dose of anticoagulant prophylaxis against venous thromboembolism after major orthopedic surgery. *Chest* 2003;124(Suppl. 6):379S–385S.

163. Kearon C, Hirsh J. Starting prophylaxis for venous thromboembolism postoperatively. *Arch Intern Med* 1995;155:366–372.

164. Strebel N, Prins M, Agnelli G, et al. Preoperative or postoperative start of prophylaxis for venous thromboembolism with low-molecular-weight heparin in elective hip surgery? *Arch Intern Med* 2002;162:1451–1456.

165. Hull RD, Pineo GF, Stein PD, et al. Timing of initial administration of low-molecular-weight heparin prophylaxis against deep vein thrombosis in patients following elective hip arthroplasty: a systematic review. *Arch Intern Med* 2001;161:1952–1960.

166. Berry DJ. Surveillance for venous thromboembolic disease after total knee arthroplasty. *Clin Orthop* 2001;392:257–266.

167. Schmidt B, Michler R, Klein M, et al. Ultrasound screening for distal vein thrombosis is not beneficial after major orthopedic surgery. A randomized controlled trial. *Thromb Haemost* 2003;90:949–954.

168. Kearon C. Duration of venous thromboembolism prophylaxis after surgery. *Chest* 2003;124(Suppl. 6):386S–392S.

169. Dahl OE, Aspelin T, Arnesen H, et al. Increased activation of coagulation and formation of late deep venous thrombosis following discontinuation of thromboprophylaxis after hip replacement surgery. *Thromb Res* 1995; 80:299–306.

170. Arnesen H, Dahl OE, Aspelin T, et al. Sustained prothrombotic profile after hip replacement surgery: the influence of prolonged prophylaxis with dalteparin. *J Thromb Haemost* 2003;1:971–975.

171. Lotke PA, Steinberg ME, Ecker ML. Significance of deep venous thrombosis in the lower extremity after total joint arthroplasty. *Clin Orthop* 1994;229:25–30.

172. Trowbridge A, Boese CK, Woodruff B, et al. Incidence of posthospitalization proximal deep venous thrombosis after total hip arthroplasty: a pilot study. *Clin Orthop* 1994;299:203–208.

173. Bergqvist D, Benoni G, Bjorgell O, et al. Low-molecular-weight heparin (enoxaparin) as prophylaxis against venous thromboembolism after total hip replacement. *N Engl Med* 1996;335:696–700.

174. White RH, Gettner S, Newman JM, et al. Predictors of rehospitalization for symptomatic venous thromboembolism after total hip arthroplasty. *N Engl J Med* 2000;343:1758–1764.

175. Eikelboom JW, Quinlan DJ, Douketis JD. Extended-duration prophylaxis against venous thromboembolism after total hip or knee replacement: a meta-analysis of the randomised trials. *Lancet* 2001;358:9–15.

176. Cohen AT, Bailey CS, Alikhan R, et al. Extended thromboprophylaxis with low molecular weight heparin reduces symptomatic venous thromboembolism following lower limb arthroplasty—a meta-analysis. *Thromb Haemost* 2001;85:940–941.

177. O'Donnell M, Linkins LA, Kearon C, et al. Reduction of out-of-hospital symptomatic venous thromboembolism by extended thromboprophylaxis with low-molecular-weight heparin following elective hip arthroplasty: a systematic review. *Arch Intern Med* 2003;163:1362–1366.

178. Lassen MR, Borris LC, Anderson BS, et al. Efficacy and safety of prolonged thromboprophylaxis with a low molecular weight heparin (dalteparin) after total hip arthroplasty—the Danish Prolonged Prophylaxis (DaPP) Study. *Thromb Res* 1998;89:281–287.

179. Comp PC, Spiro TE, Friedman RJ, et al. Prolonged enoxaparin therapy to prevent venous thromboembolism after primary hip or knee replacement. *J Bone Joint Surg* 2001;83-A:336–345.

180. Hull RD, Pineo GF, Stein PD, et al. Extended out-of-hospital low-molecular-weight heparin prophylaxis against deep venous thrombosis in patients after elective hip arthroplasty: a systematic review. *Ann Intern Med* 2001;135: 858–869.

181. Prandoni P, Bruchi O, Sabbion P, et al. Prolonged thromboprophylaxis with oral anticoagulants after total hip arthroplasty: a prospective controlled randomized study. *Arch Intern Med* 2002;162:1966–1971.

182. Samama CM, Vray M, Barre J, et al. Extended venous thromboembolism prophylaxis after total hip replacement: a comparison of low-molecular-weight heparin with oral anticoagulant. *Arch Intern Med* 2002;162: 2191–2196.

183. Bergqvist D, Jonsson B. Cost-effectiveness of prolonged administration of a low molecular weight heparin for the prevention of deep venous thrombosis following total hip replacement. *Value Health* 1999;2:288–294.

184. Davies LM, Richardson GA, Cohen AT. Economic evaluation of enoxaparin as postdischarge prophylaxis for deep vein thrombosis (DVT) in elective hip surgery. *Value Health* 2000;3:397–406.

185. Dahl OE, Pleil AM. Investment in prolonged thromboprophylaxis with dalteparin improves clinical outcomes after hip replacement. *J Thromb Haemost* 2003;1:896–906.

186. Cogo A, Bernardi E, Prandoni P, et al. Acquired risk factors for deep-vein thrombosis in symptomatic outpatients. *Arch Intern Med* 1994;154: 164–168.

187. Samama MM. An epidemiologic study of risk factors for deep vein thrombosis in medical outpatients: the Sirius study. *Arch Intern Med* 2000;160: 3415–3420.

# CHAPTER 96 ■ VENOUS THROMBOPROPHYLAXIS IN MEDICAL PATIENTS

ALAIN LEIZOROVICZ AND PATRICK MISMETTI

Venous thromboembolism (VTE) remains a major cause of morbidity and mortality in patients who are hospitalized (1–7).

Despite the availability of effective treatment of deep vein thrombosis (DVT) and pulmonary embolism (PE), clinically overt VTE increases morbidity and cost, and may lead to an increase in preventable death (8). Therefore, thromboprophylaxis has been advocated in high-risk patients.

Venous thromboprophylaxis is widely practiced in surgical patients, but, in contrast, many medical patients still do not receive it despite recommendations and guidelines (9–11). There is a need for a constant reappraisal of the burden of VTE in medical patients and of the evidence from prophylactic randomized studies.

## THE IMPORTANCE OF VENOUS THROMBOEMBOLISM

In the United States and in Europe, VTE is frequent and is associated with a high risk of death. It has been estimated that more than 200,000 cases of VTE occur each year in the United States, corresponding to an incidence of one per 10,007 population.

Over the last few years, the incidence and prognosis of VTE appear stable. Although prophylaxis may have been applied to an increasing number of patients, other factors may account for the observed trend (12). Old age is a major determinant of the risk of VTE and of its secondary complications, and there is an increased number of older individuals in the population. The development of noninvasive and reliable methods for the diagnosis of DVT and PE has facilitated its recognition. Widespread imaging is increasing the apparent incidence of VTE.

In addition to age, population studies have also identified other major risk factors for VTE, including obesity, chronic heart failure, chronic lung diseases, malignancy, ischemic stroke, birth control pills, and hormone therapy. In many countries, these factors are increasing as the population grows. The prevalence of risk factors such as heart failure or malignancy will increase because of the availability of treatments that effectively increase life expectancy.

Factors associated with institutionalization (current or recent hospitalization or nursing home residence) account for 59% of cases of VTE in a community with equal attributable risk for surgical and medical illnesses (13). Medical patients who are hospitalized are at particular risk of developing VTE and its complications because of the combination of chronic risk factors (e.g., age, heart failure, and prior VTE) and an acute, transient increased risk associated with conditions leading to the hospitalization [e.g., aggravation of heart failure or pulmonary failure, infectious disease, stroke, or acute myocardial infarction (MI)]. These acute medical conditions are each independent risk factors for VTE (12,13) and often a cause of prolonged immobilization, which is also an independent risk factor (see Table 96-1).

Outpatients are also at a risk of VTE. The same chronic and triggering risk factors in medical patients who are hospitalized have been identified in a general population of outpatients (14).

## ISSUES IN THE ACCEPTANCE OF THROMBOPROPHYLAXIS STUDIES

Surveys show that many medical patients who may benefit from thromboprophylaxis do not receive it (15,16). Some claim that they do not use thromboprophylaxis in medical patients because clinically relevant benefits have not been demonstrated. However, there is now solid evidence to endorse prophylaxis in patients who are hospitalized with medical illness.

### Asymptomatic Deep Vein Thrombosis as Primary Endpoint in Prophylactic Studies

The main endpoint used in most prophylactic clinical trials in medical, as well as in surgical patients, is a DVT (in most cases asymptomatic) diagnosed by imaging (e.g., venography or ultrasonography). Asymptomatic DVT has been used as a surrogate endpoint for symptomatic DVT and PE, which constitute the burden of VTE described in epidemiologic studies. Although there is no perfect surrogate endpoint (17), asymptomatic DVT (combined with symptomatic events) has been adopted in most prophylactic studies as the main endpoint. Most thromboprophylactic anticoagulants have been approved by health authorities on the basis of this endpoint. In metaanalyses of placebo-controlled studies, there are good correlations between the incidence of asymptomatic DVT and that of symptomatic PE, and between the reduction of asymptomatic DVT and that of PE. However, in studies comparing unfractionated heparins (UFH) and low-molecular-weight heparins (LMWH), the reduction of PE cannot be predicted as accurately by the reduction of asymptomatic DVT, mainly because of the wide confidence interval (CI) around the estimate of the reduction of PE. Furthermore, intriguing discrepant results were found in metaanalysis reviewing studies comparing

TABLE 96-1

INDEPENDENT RISK FACTORS FOR VTE

**ACUTE MEDICAL ILLNESS**
Stroke
Myocardial infarction
Illness requiring intensive care
Other acute illnesses requiring immobilization for at
    least 3 d

**CLINICAL RISK FACTORS**
Previous PE or DVT
Cancer
Congestive heart failure
Chronic obstructive pulmonary disease
Diabetes mellitus
Inflammatory bowel disease
Antipsychotic drug use
Chronic indwelling central venous catheter
Permanent pacemaker
Active collagen vascular disorders
Internal cardiac defibrillator
Stroke with limb paresis
Nursing-home confinement or current or repeated hospital
    admission
Varicose veins
HRT
Obesity
Anticancer treatments

**THROMBOPHILIA**
Factor $V_{Leiden}$ mutation
Prothrombin gene mutation
Hyperhomocysteinaemia (including mutation in
    methylenetetrahydrofolate reductase)
Antiphospholipid antibody syndrome
Deficiency of antithrombin III, protein C, or protein S
High concentrations of factor VIII or XI
Increased lipoprotein (a) levels

PE, pulmonary embolism; DVT, deep vein thrombosis; HRT, hormone
replacement therapy.

LMWH and UFH in surgical patients: The relative risks of
LMWH versus UFH were 0.92 (95% CI, 0.80–1.05) for total
DVT and 0.66 (95% CI, 0.45–0.97) for PE. Therefore, the
small beneficial effect for total DVT did not accurately predict
the larger beneficial effect for preventing PE (18).

To overcome the limitation of using all (including *isolated
calf*) asymptomatic DVT as the main endpoint, recent studies
have used only asymptomatic *proximal* DVT as the major
component of their primary endpoint: Proximal DVT correlates more closely than isolated calf DVT with the risk of PE
and death.

## Venography or Ultrasonography to Assess Asymptomatic Deep Vein Thrombosis

Venography was used in most studies to evaluate the primary
endpoint. However, in a recent study (19), the major component of the primary endpoint, asymptomatic proximal DVT,
was assessed by systematic screening with CUS (compression
ultrasound). There is now evidence that the technique of CUS
is at least as reliable as venography for the diagnosis of asymptomatic proximal DVT (20). CUS is more practical because it has
almost no contraindication, thereby improving compliance, and

it is now accepted as a diagnostic method for the evaluation of
proximal DVT in prophylaxis studies by drug agencies (21).
In addition, dynamic CUS examinations can be fully video-
taped and be read centrally by a core lab (19–22) as is done
with venograms in other studies.

## REVIEW OF EVIDENCE FOR THROMBOPROPHYLAXIS IN MEDICAL PATIENTS

There are two types of populations of patients at risk of VTE:
those with a permanent, moderate, or high risk, such as patients with permanent restricted mobility or patients with a
chronic evolving cancer, and those with a transient risk of
VTE triggered by an acute event. There are two approaches
for defining the study populations of prophylaxis studies: by
disease or condition, and by global risk (23).

## Prophylaxis in Medical Patients at Permanent Risk for Venous Thromboembolism

Patients living in a nursing home with limited mobility or those
needing long-term hospitalization for chronic conditions, such
as paraplegia or the need for permanent respiratory assistance,
may be candidates for prophylaxis. However, the real long-
term risk of VTE among these patients is not well known, and
no studies have been performed to evaluate the benefit of prophylaxis with the appropriate length of treatment.

Patients with cancer are at a risk of VTE not only because
of their disease but also because anticancer drugs and central
venous lines for anticancer treatments are risk factors. A clinically overt VTE may be the occasion for diagnosing a previously unknown cancer. The prognosis of VTE is more severe
in patients with cancer than in patients without cancer (24).

Clinical trials have been conducted to evaluate the benefit
of long-term anticoagulation in patients with cancer, not only
to prevent VTE but also to improve survival. In a placebo-
controlled study designed to show a reduction in mortality in
patients with cancer without VTE, there was a nonsignificant
trend toward lower mortality in the LMWH group compared
with the placebo group (25). Interaction between cancer and
VTE may depend on the type of cancer and its treatment.
These encouraging preliminary findings warrant further investigation.

## Prophylaxis in Medical Patients with Acute Disease at High Risk of Venous Thromboembolism

Patients hospitalized for acute MI are at high risk of VTE. In a
metaanalysis (26) reviewing placebo-controlled studies of antithrombotic drugs, the rate of PE in the placebo group was 3.9%.

Prevention of recurrent MI rather than prevention of VTE is
the primary therapeutic objective in patients with acute MI.
For this objective, patients with acute MI already receive combinations of high doses of antithrombotic treatments, including fibrinolytics, antiplatelet agents [e.g., aspirin, clopidogrel,
and glycoprotein (GP) IIb/IIIa antagonists] and full-dose heparin. Heparin confers incremental benefit in addition to other
antithrombotic treatment for the prevention of VTE (26).

Patients with acute hemiplegic stroke have an incidence of
DVT of approximately 50% within 2 weeks in the absence of
prophylaxis. Pulmonary emboli are frequent in patients who
have a stroke; 13% to 25% of early deaths from stroke have
been attributed to PE, most often between the second and

fourth weeks (27). Aspirin given as soon as the diagnosis of ischemic stroke is confirmed can reduce the risk of recurrent stroke, improve survival, and help prevent PE (one incidence of PE avoided for 1,000 patients treated) (28,29).

Unfractionated heparin, LMWH, and heparinoids have been evaluated in patients who have acute stroke. Although anticoagulants did not improve survival, LMWH was shown to reduce the risk of PE by 66% [odds ratio (OR), 0.34; 95% CI, 0.17 to 0.69] and DVT by 73% (OR, 0.27; 95% CI, 0.08 to 0.96). However, there was increased risk of major bleeding (OR, 2.17; 95% 1.10 to 4.28) (30). A review of studies, comparing UFH and LMWH, or heparinoids, which included five trials involving 705 patients, showed a statistically significant reduction of DVT in favor of LMWH (OR, 0.52; 95% CI, 0.56 to 0.79) (31).

Admission to a medical intensive care unit is associated with a high risk of VTE (32,33). Four studies of VTE prophylaxis in this setting have been published: two comparing UFH versus control (34,35) (with 119 and 791 patients, respectively), one comparing an LMWH versus placebo (223 patients) (36), and one comparing an LMWH versus UFH (325 patients) (37). An approximate, yet statistically significant, 50% decrease in asymptomatic DVT was observed with UFH (34,35) or LMWH (36) versus placebo, whereas there was no statistically significant difference between LMWH and UFH (37). The latter study had a patient population with respiratory failure requiring mechanical ventilation. Other preventive measures such as mechanical prevention and/or early mobilization of the lower limbs are now more often applied in this setting (38).

## Prophylaxis in Other Medical Patients

There is a diversity of other acute medical conditions that may increase the risk of VTE. Thromboprophylaxis was evaluated in a number of trials, which included a broader spectrum of patients. Eligibility for these studies was mainly driven by the patient's global risk of developing VTE.

### Mechanical Prevention

There were a few randomized studies performed in a limited number of patients, mainly surgical patients and patients with neurologic disorders, to evaluate graduated compression stockings and intermittent pneumatic compression. The meta-analysis (39) of the studies performed in the absence of other prophylactic treatments showed an OR of 0.34 (95% CI, 0.25 to 0.46), favoring compression stockings over control for the reduction of asymptomatic DVT. In other studies evaluating compression stockings in patients receiving pharmacologic prophylaxis, compression stockings conferred additional benefit on prevention of DVT, with an OR of 0.24 (95% CI, 0.15 to 0.37). There are limitations for the application of these studies in medical patients. To our knowledge, no randomized clinical trials have evaluated mechanical methods of prophylaxis in general medical patients. All the studies were small, with an open design, and were therefore subject to bias in the outcome—asymptomatic total DVT. None of the two meta-analyses, let alone individual studies, were powerful enough to demonstrate a beneficial effect on the reduction of PE. These methods have not been properly compared with more established prophylactic treatments such as anticoagulant treatment and cannot be regarded as an alternative for anticoagulants in patients who could receive them. However, because of their safety, the use of mechanical prophylaxis could be recommended in medical patients with risk factors for VTE in whom there is a strict contraindication to prophylaxis with anticoagulants or in patients already receiving anticoagulant for a potential additive benefit.

### Antiplatelet Agents

Antiplatelet agents, aspirin in particular, may have some benefit in preventing VTE (40,41), but only eight randomized studies, with less than 600 patients, have compared antiplatelet agents versus no prophylaxis in medical patients. A metaanalysis of these clinical trials has shown a statistically nonsignificant 47% ± 17% odds reduction in asymptomatic DVT with antiplatelet agents (39 out of 261 patients vs. 61 out of 266 patients), whereas there was no effect on the bleeding risk (major event rate of <1% in the two groups) (40).

### Heparin and Low-Molecular-Weight Heparin

A metaanalysis of 15,095 patients concluded that, in medical patients who are hospitalized, heparin showed a statistically significant reduction in the risk of asymptomatic DVT by 56% (relative risk, 0.44; 95% CI, 0.29 to 0.64; $P < 0.001$) and the risk of PE by 52% (relative risk, 0.48; 95% CI, 0.34 to 0.68; $P < 0.001$) (42). There was a nonsignificant ($P = 0.08$) adverse trend for major bleeding and a neutral effect for total mortality (see Fig. 96-1). There were limitations for the interpretation of the results of the metaanalysis such as the heterogeneity of the different studied populations and the relative small number of patients in most of them. Moreover, the baseline risk of asymptomatic DVT was quite low [approximately 17% (42)].

The two largest studies, which recruited 2,474 patients (43) and 11,693 patients (44), respectively, were designed primarily as mortality studies, but could not demonstrate a reduction in total mortality or in fatal PE. Furthermore, the open design and the lack of concealment of the randomization (patients had a choice not to accept the result of the treatment allocation) of that study could have led to biases in the reporting of total PE, the only secondary endpoint for which a reduction was observed.

These limitations may have been seen strong enough to hamper the implementation of VTE prophylaxis in many hospitals where a typical prescription rate of less than 60% could be observed in patients in whom a prophylaxis may be recommended (45). Three contemporary placebo-controlled studies have been designed with more solid methodology to evaluate the benefit of thromboprophylaxis in acutely ill medical patients (22,46,47). The three studies included patients hospitalized for acute medical illness requiring temporary immobilization and sufficient VTE risk factors, to ensure a moderate level of VTE risk (see Table 96-2). Higher-risk patients, such as patients with acute stroke or acute MI, were not eligible. MEDENOX (46) (prophylaxis in MEDical patients with ENOXaparin study) randomized 1,102 patients in three arms (enoxaparin 40 mg, enoxaparin 20 mg, and placebo). PREVENT (22)

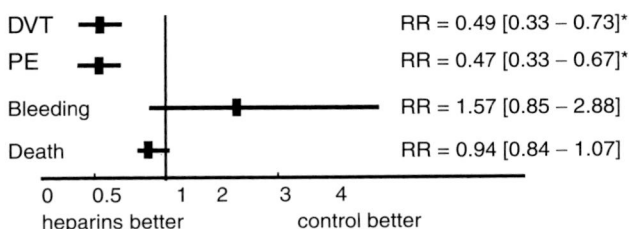

*P <0.001

**FIGURE 96-1.** Metaanalysis of trials comparing unfractionated heparin (UFH) or low-molecular-weight heparin (LMWH) to control in acutely ill medical patients (seven trials, 15,095 patients). DVT, deep venous thrombosis; PE, pulmonary embolism; RR, relative risk. (From Mismetti P, Laporte-Simitsidis S, Tardy B, et al. Prevention of venous thromboembolism in internal medicine with unfractionated or low-molecular-weight heparins: a meta-analysis of randomised clinical trials. *Thromb Haemost* 2000;83:14–19, with permission.)

## MAIN DESIGN FEATURES OF MEDENOX, PREVENT, AND ARTEMIS

| MEDENOX | PREVENT | ARTEMIS |
|---|---|---|
| **TREATMENTS** | **TREATMENTS** | **TREATMENTS** |
| Enoxaparin 40 mg, Enoxaparin 20 mg, placebo q.i.d. 14 d | Dalteparin 5,000 IU, placebo q.i.d. 14 d | Fondaparinux 2.5 mg, placebo q.i.d. 14 d |
| **ELIGIBILITY CRITERIA** | **ELIGIBILITY CRITERIA** | **ELIGIBILITY CRITERIA** |
| Age ≥40 yr | Age ≥40 yr | Age ≥60 yr and expected bed rest ≥4 d |
| Expected hospital stay ≥6 d | Expected hospital stay ≥4 d Recent | and congestive heart failure (NYHA |
| Recent immobilization (≤3 d) and | immobilization (≤3 d) and CHF | class III/IV) or acute or chronic lung |
| CHF (NYHA III/IV) or acute | (NYHA III/IV) or acute respiratory | disease or acute infectious or |
| respiratory illness or infection or | illness or infection or bone/joint or | inflammatory disease; no other risk |
| bone/joint or inflamed bowel if ≥1 | inflamed bowel if ≥1 added risk for | factor analysis required |
| added risk for VTE (i.e., >75 yr; | VTE (i.e., >75 yr; cancer, previous | |
| cancer, previous VTE, obesity, | VTE, obesity, varicose veins, hormones, | |
| varicose veins, hormones, or chronic | or chronic heart or lung failure) | |
| heart or lung failure) | | |
| **PRIMARY EFFICACY** | **PRIMARY EFFICACY** | **PRIMARY EFFICACY** |
| At d 14 | At d 21 | At d 14 |
| ■ Distal and proximal | ■ Proximal ultrasonographic DVT | ■ Distal and proximal |
| ■ Venographic DVT | ■ Symptomatic VTE | ■ Venographic DVT |
| ■ Symptomatic VTE | ■ Fatal PE | ■ Symptomatic VTE |
| ■ Fatal PE | ■ Sudden death | ■ Fatal PE |
| **SAFETY** | **SAFETY** | **SAFETY** |
| ■ Major bleeding | ■ Major bleeding | ■ Major bleeding |
| ■ Death at d 90 | ■ Death at d 90 | ■ Death at d 90 |

VTE, venous thromboembolism; DVT, deep vein thrombosis; PE, pulmonary embolism; CHF, congestive heart failure; NYHA, New York Heart Association.

(Prospective Evaluation of Dalteparin Efficacy for Prevention of VTE in Immobilized Patients Trial) recruited 3,681 patients (dalteparin 5,000 IU vs. placebo). This sample size was tailored to look primarily at proximal asymptomatic DVT or symptomatic VTE. ARTEMIS (47) (ARixtra for ThromboEmbolism Prevention in a Medical Indications Study) recruited 849 patients (fondaparinux 2.5 mg vs. placebo).

Patient characteristics differed among these studies. The total mortality rate in the placebo group of MEDENOX, 14%

at 3 months, was more than double the rate of approximately 6% in PREVENT and 6% in ARTEMIS (see Table 96-3). However, the incidence of asymptomatic proximal DVT at 2 to 3 weeks was similar in all three studies.

The three studies showed consistent efficacy results for enoxaparin, dalteparin, and fondaparinux—a reduction of VTE in the range of 50%. The relative risks for each study are: MEDENOX: 0.37 (95% CI, 0.22 to 0.63), PREVENT: 0.55 (95% CI, 0.38 to 0.80), and ARTEMIS: 0.53 (95% CI, 0.31 to 0.92). The overall estimate of the relative risk from these three trials is 0.50 (95% CI, 0.38 to 0.66).

When looking at the reduction of asymptomatic proximal DVT or symptomatic VTE in the three studies, there is again a consistent approximate 50% reduction in favor of the prophylaxis (see Table 96-4).

In all three trials, the active pharmacologic prophylaxis was given for a maximum of 14 days. Despite this short duration, the beneficial effect persisted at 3 months in MEDENOX

## CHARACTERISTICS OF PATIENTS IN THE PLACEBO GROUPS OF MEDENOX, PREVENT, AND ARTEMIS

| | MEDENOX | PREVENT | ARTEMIS |
|---|---|---|---|
| **BASELINE CHARACTERISTICS** | | | |
| Age | 73 | 68 | 74 |
| Male | 50.0% | 48.0% | 44.0% |
| Prior VTE | 9.5% | 4.7% | 5.0% |
| Cancer | 14.3% | 5.1% | 15.8% |
| **REASONS FOR HOSPITALIZATION** | | | |
| Heart failure | 34% | 51% | 37% |
| Respiratory failure | 55% | 31% | 43% |
| Sepsis | 53% | 38% | 50% |
| **TOTAL DEATH** | | | |
| End of follow-up | 14% (d 90) | 6% (d 90) | 6% (d 30) |

VTE, venous thromboembolism.

## PROXIMAL DEEP VEIN THROMBOSIS OR SYMPTOMATIC VENOUS THROMBOEMBOLISM AT DAYS 14 TO 21 IN MEDENOX, PREVENT, AND ARTEMIS

| MEDENOX | PREVENT | ARTEMIS |
|---|---|---|
| Enoxaparin 2.1% | Dalteparin 2.6% | Fondaparinux 1.5% |
| Placebo 6.6% | Placebo 5.0% | Placebo 3.4% |
| P = 0.037 | P = 0.002 | P = 0.085 |

and PREVENT and at 1 month in ARTEMIS. In all three studies, major bleeding in the treated groups remained very low (<1%).

These newer studies confirm the efficacy of heparins, mainly LMWHs and fondaparinux, in reducing the risk of VTE without increasing major bleeding.

# APPLICATION OF THROMBOPROPHYLAXIS IN MEDICAL PATIENTS: FROM RANDOMIZED STUDIES TO REAL LIFE

One alleged limitation was that patients enrolled in the studies did not represent real-life patients. In fact, requiring risk assessment in the selection of patients in the latest studies, rather than a specific disease, makes the results more applicable to all patients who present with similar levels of risk. Subgroup analyses trials have confirmed that the proportional risk reduction in favor of prophylaxis applies to almost all subgroups of patients (48). Patients receiving antiplatelet treatment, for example, for coronary disease, benefit from the addition of heparin or LMWH (49). Similarly, the use of mechanical prevention, such as compression stockings (39), seems to be additive to pharmacologic thromboprophylaxis

## There Remain Some Questions That Need Further Evaluation

*Should outpatients at risk of VTE be given thromboprophylaxis?* There is still a substantial number of VTE occurring outside the hospital, and risk factors in outpatients are the same as in patients who are hospitalized. The benefit and feasibility of outpatient prophylactic, as well as curative treatment with anticoagulants, has long been established for a variety of indications. Many patients at risk for VTE remain in nursing homes and may well benefit from thromboprophylaxis. Additionally, patients treated at home with similar diseases and risk factors as those evaluated in hospital studies should probably benefit from thromboprophylaxis. However, the risk-to-benefit ratio should be carefully considered in these patients who may be less compliant.

It has been reported that long haul air travelers have a risk of developing VTE but the evidence is still controversial and possibly only passengers of very long flights (>10 hours) may be at a considerably higher risk (50). However, the absolute risk of VTE is very small in this population. Of a total of 135.29 million consecutive passengers arriving at Charles de Gaulle Airport (France), 56 had confirmed PE (51). Although the risk of PE was three times higher in passengers traveling more than 10,000 km than in those traveling less than 5,000 km, the absolute risk of PE in the highest risk group was 4.8 per million. Clinical trials have shown that both compression stockings and LMWH could potentially reduce the rate of asymptomatic DVT (52–56). However, these are small open design trials, and the clinical relevance of systematic preventive treatment needs to be confirmed by much larger studies.

*For how long should treatment be given?* Typically, in the clinical trials performed so far, UFH and LMWH prophylaxis did not exceed 2 weeks. Although most of the VTE that occur after an acute medical event are observed within the first 2 weeks, some patients may still be at risk beyond that period. Ongoing and future studies will determine whether extended prophylaxis confers additional benefit.

# CONCLUSIONS

VTE remains a public health burden. The results of recent, well-conducted clinical trials reinforce the evidence-based recommendations for more systematic assessment of global risk of VTE in medical patients and for the wider use of thromboprophylaxis.

## References

1. Anderson FA Jr, Wheeler HB, Goldberg RJ et al, The Worcester DVT Study. A population-based perspective of the hospital incidence and case-fatality rates of deep vein thrombosis and pulmonary embolism. *Arch Intern Med* 1991;151:933–938.
2. Dalen JE. Pulmonary embolism: what have we learned since virchow: natural history, pathophysiology, and diagnosis. *Chest* 2002;122:1440–1456.
3. Goldhaber SZ, Visani L, De Rosa M. Acute pulmonary embolism: clinical outcomes in the international cooperative pulmonary embolism registry (ICOPER). *Lancet* 1999;353:1386–1389.
4. Oger E, EPI-GETBP Study Group. Incidence of venous thromboembolism: a community-based study in Western France. Groupe d'Etude de la thrombose de bretagne occidentale. *Thromb Haemost* 2000;83:657–660.
5. Silverstein MD, Heit JA, Mohr DN, et al. Trends in the incidence of deep vein thrombosis and pulmonary embolism: a 25-year population-based study. *Arch Intern Med* 1998;158:585–593.
6. Goldhaber SZ, Elliott CG. Acute pulmonary embolism: part I: epidemiology, pathophysiology, and diagnosis. *Circulation* 2003;108:2726–2729.
7. Goldhaber SZ. Pulmonary embolism. *Lancet* 2004;363:1295–1305.
8. Heit JA, Silverstein MD, Mohr DN, et al. The epidemiology of venous thromboembolism in the community. *Thromb Haemost* 2001;86:452–463.
9. THRIFT Consensus Group. Risk of and prophylaxis for venous thromboembolism in hospital patients. *BMJ* 1992;305:567–574.
10. Geerts WH, Heit JA, Clagett GP, et al. Prevention of venous thromboembolism. *Chest* 2001;119(Suppl. 1):132S–175S.
11. Goldhaber SZ, Dunn K, MacDougall RC. New onset of venous thromboembolism among hospitalized patients at birgham and women's hospital is caused more often by prophylaxis failure than by withholding treatment. *Chest* 2000;118:1664–1684.
12. Kearon C. Epidemiology of venous thromboembolism. *Semin Vasc Med* 2001;1:7–25.
13. Heit JA, O'Fallon WM, Petterson TM, et al. Relative impact of risk factors for deep vein thrombosis and pulmonary embolism: a population-based study. *Arch Intern Med* 2002;162:1245–1248.
14. Samama MM. An epidemiologic study of risk factors for deep vein thrombosis in medical outpatients: the sirius study. *Arch Intern Med* 2000;160:3415–3420.
15. Arnold DM, Kahn S, Shrier I. Missed opportunities for prevention of venous thromboembolism an evaluation of the use of thromboprophylaxis guidelines. *Chest* 2001;120:1965.
16. Goldhaber SZ, Tapson VF. DVT FREE steering committee a prospective registry of 5,451 patients with ultrasound-confirmed deep vein thrombosis. *Am J Cardiol* 2004;15:93259–93262.
17. Fleming TR, DeMets D. Surrogate end points in clinical trials: are we being misled? *Ann Intern Med* 1996;125:605–613.
18. Koch A, Ziegle S, Breitschwerdt H, et al. Low molecular weight heparin and unfractionated heparin in thrombosis prophylaxis: meta-analysis based on original patient data. *Thromb Res* 2001;102:295–309.
19. Vaitkus PT, Leizorovicz A, Goldhaber SZ, et al. Rationale and design of a clinical trial of a low-molecular-weight heparin in preventing clinically important venous thromboembolism in medical patients: the prospective evaluation of dalteparin efficacy for prevention of venous thromboembolism in immobilized patients trial (the PREVENT study). *Vasc Med* 2002;7:269–273.
20. Kassai B, Boissel JP, Cucherat M, et al. A systematic review of the accuracy of ultra sound in the diagnostic of deep venous thrombosisin asymptomatic patients. *Thromb Haemost* 2004;91:655–666.
21. Leizorovicz A, Kassai B, Becker F, et al. The assessment of deep vein thromboses for therapeutic trials. *Angiology* 2003;54:19–24.
22. Leizorovicz A, Cohen AT, Turpie AGG et al, PREVENT Medical Thromboprophylaxis Study Group. A randomized, placebo-controlled trial of dalteparin for the prevention of venous thromboembolism in acutely Ill medical patients. *Circulation* 2004;110:874–879.
23. Cohen AT. Venous thromboembolism disease management of the non surgical moderate and high risk patient. *Semin Hematol* 2000;37:19–22.
24. Piccioli A, Prandoni P, Goldhaber SZ. Epidemiologic characteristics, management, and outcome of deep venous thrombosis in a tertiary-care hospital: the brigham and women's hospital DVT registry. *Am Heart J* 1996;132:1010–1014.
25. Kakkar A. An expanding role for antithrombotic therapy in cancer patients. *Cancer Treat Rev* 2003;29:23–26.
26. Collins R, MacMahon S, Flather M, et al. Clinical effects of anticoagulant therapy in suspected acute myocardial infarction: systematic overview of randomised trials. *BMJ* 1996;313:652–659.

27. Kelly J, Rudd A, Lewis R, et al. Venous thromboembolism after acute stroke. *Stroke* 2001;32:262–267.

28. International Stroke Trial Collaborative Group. The international stroke trial (IST): a randomised trial of aspirin, subcutaneous heparin, both, or neither among 19435 patients with acute ischaemic stroke. *Lancet* 1997;349:1569–1581.

29. Gubitz G, Sandercock P, Counsell C. Antiplatelet therapy for acute ischaemic stroke. *Cochrane Database Syst Rev* 2003;2:CD000029.

30. Bath PMW, Iddenden R, Bath FJ. Low-molecular-weight heparins and heparinoids in acute ischemic stroke a meta-analysis of randomized controlled trials. *Stroke* 2000;31:1770–1778.

31. Counsell C, Sandercock P. Low-molecular-weight heparins or heparinoids versus standard unfractionated heparin for acute ischaemic stroke. *Cochrane Database Syst Rev* 2000;2:CD000119.

32. Hirsch DR, Ingenito EP, Goldhaber SZ. Prevalence of deep venous thrombosis among patients in medical intensive care. *JAMA* 1995;274: 335–337.

33. Cook D, McMullin J, Hodder R et al, Canadian ICU Directors Group. Prevention and diagnosis of venous thromboembolism in critically ill patients: a canadian survey. *Crit Care* 2001;5:336–342.

34. Cade JF. High risk of the critically ill for venous thromboembolism. *Crit Care Med* 1982;10:448–450.

35. Kapoor M, Kupfer YY, Tessler S. Subcutaneous heparin prophylaxis significantly reduces the incidence of venous thromboembolic events in the critically ill [abstract]. *Crit Care Med* 1999;27(Suppl.):A69.

36. Fraisse F, Holzapfel L, Couland JM et al, Association of Non-University Affiliated Intensive Care Specialist Physicians of France. Nadroparin in the prevention of deep vein thrombosis in acute decompensated COPD. *Am Rev Resp Crit Care Med* 2000;161:1109–1114.

37. Goldhaber SZ, Kett DH, Cusumano CJ, et al. Low molecular weight heparin versus minidose unfractionated heparin for prophylaxis against venous thromboembolism in medical intensive care unit patients: a randomized controlled trial [abstract]. *J Am Coll Cardiol* 2000;35(Suppl.):325A.

38. Lacherade J, Cook D, Heyland D et al, French and Canadian ICU Directors Groups. Prevention of venous thromboembolism in critically ill medical patients: a franco-canadian cross-sectional study. *J Crit Care* 2003; 18:228–237.

39. Amarigiri SV, Lees TA. Elastic compression stockings for prevention of deep vein thrombosis. *Cochrane Database Syst Rev* 2000;3:CD001484.

40. APT group. Collaborative overview of randomised trials of antiplatelet therapy—III: reduction in venous thrombosis and pulmonary embolism by antiplatelet prophylaxis among surgical and medical patients. *BMJ* 1994;308:235–246.

41. Pulmonary Embolism Prevention (PEP). Trial collaborative group prevention of pulmonary embolism and deep vein thrombosis with low dose aspirin: Pulmonary Embolism Prevention (PEP) trial. *Lancet* 2000;355: 1295–1302.

42. Mismetti P, Laporte-Simitsidis S, Tardy B, et al. Prevention of venous thromboembolism in internal medicine with unfractionated or low-molecular-weight heparins: a meta-analysis of randomised clinical trials. *Thromb Haemost* 2000;83:14–19.

43. Bergmann JF, Caulin C. Heparin prophylaxis in bedridden patients. *Lancet* 1996;348:205–206.

44. Gardlund B, Heparin Prophylaxis Study Group. Randomised, controlled trial of low-dose heparin for prevention of fatal pulmonary embolism in patients with infectious diseases. *Lancet* 1996;347:1357–1361.

45. Anderson FA, Decousus H, Bergman JF et al, IMPROVE Investigators. A multinational observational cohort study in hospitalized medical patients of practices in prevention of venous thromboembolism and clinical outcomes: findings of the international medical prevention registry on venous thromboembolism (IMPROVE). International Society on Thrombosis and Haemostasis (ISTH) XIX Congres and 49th Annual SSC Meeting, 2003, Birmingham, UK *J Thromb Haemost* 2003;(Suppl.):1438.

46. Samama MM, Cohen AT, Darmon JY et al, Prophylaxis in Medical Patients with Enoxaparin Study Group. A comparison of enoxaparin with placebo for the prevention of venous thromboembolism in acutely ill medical patients. *NEJM* 1999;11:793–800.

47. Cohen AT, Gallus AS, Lassen MR, et al. Fondaparinux vs placebo for the prevention of venous thromboembolism in acutely ill medical patients (ARTEMIS). Program and abstracts of the XIX Congress of the international society on thrombosis and haemostasis, Birmingham, AL, July 12–18, 2003, P2406.

48. Alikhan R, Cohen AT, Combe S, et al. Prevention of venous thromboembolism in medical patients with enoxaparin: a subgroup analysis of the MEDENOX study. *Blood Coagul Fibrinolysis* 2003;4:341–346.

49. Leizorovicz A, Cohen AT, Turpie AGG et al, PREVENT Medical Thromboprophylaxis Study Group. Efficacy and safety of combining dalteparin with aspirin in preventing venous thromboembolism in medical patients. *Blood* ASH Meeting Abstracts, 2003;102:1153.

50. Ten Wolde M, Kraaijenhagen RA, Schiereck J, et al. Travel and the risk of symptomatic venous thromboembolism. *Thromb Haemost* 2003;89: 499–505.

51. Lapostolle FK, Surget V, Borron SW, et al. Severe pulmonary embolism associated with air travel. *N Engl J Med* 2001;345:779–783.

52. Belcaro G, Geroulakos G, Nicolaides AN, et al. Venous thromboembolism from air travel: the LONFLIT study. *Angiology* 2001;52: 369–374.

53. Scurr JH, Machin SJ, Bailey-King S, et al. Frequency and prevention of symptomless deep-vein thrombosis in long-haul flights: a randomised trial. *Lancet* 2001;357:1485–1489.

54. Cesarone MR, Belcaro G, Nicolaides AN, et al. Venous thrombosis from air travel: the LONFLIT3 study. Prevention with aspirin vs low-molecular-weight heparin (LMWH) in high-risk subjects: a randomized trial. *Angiology* 2002;53:1–6.

55. Belcaro G, Cesarone MR, Shah SSG, et al. Prevention of edema, flight microangiopathy and venous thrombosis in long flights with elastic stockings. A randomized trial: the LONFLIT 4 concorde edema-SSL study. *Angiology* 2002;53:635–645.

56. Belcaro G, Cesarone MR, Nicolaides AN, et al. Prevention of venous thrombosis with elastic stockings during long-haul flights: the LONFLIT 5 JAP study. *Clin Appl Thromb Hemost* 2003;9:197–201.

# CHAPTER 97 ■ ACUTE CORONARY SYNDROMES

ELI V. GELFAND AND CHRISTOPHER P. CANNON

Current estimates are that 1.68 million patients with acute coronary syndromes (ACS) are admitted each year to hospitals in the United States (1). Of these, one fourth of patients present with acute myocardial infarction (MI) associated with electrocardiographic ST segment elevation (STEMI), whereas three fourths of them, or approximately 1.3 million patients, have non–ST elevation acute coronary syndrome (NSTEACS) (1). MI is most commonly caused by acute total occlusion of a coronary artery, and, therefore, urgent reperfusion is the mainstay of therapy, whereas NSTEACS is usually associated with a nonocclusive thrombus (2). Among patients with NSTEACS, between 40% and 60% will have evidence of myocardial necrosis with elevated troponin, and are therefore diagnosed with a non–ST elevation myocardial infarction (NSTEMI). Patients without evidence of myocardial necrosis are diagnosed with unstable angina (UA) (3,4).

## PATHOPHYSIOLOGY

The pathophysiology of ACS can be divided into four phases: (a) the development of the atherosclerotic plaque; (b) rupture of an unstable, or vulnerable, plaque; (c) the acute ischemic event; and (d) the long-term risk of recurrent coronary events that remains after the acute event. The acute event usually involves thrombus formation at the site of a ruptured atherosclerotic plaque and is the clinical manifestation of a generalized and progressive vascular disease, currently referred to as *atherothrombosis*. This new term has emerged in place of atherosclerosis because it illustrates the pathophysiology of the disease more fully—where there is both progression of the atheroma (e.g., cholesterol plaque development) and disruption of the plaque with superimposed thrombosis. Inflammation plays a major role in making a plaque more unstable: Inflammatory cells release cytokines, which in turn augment the release of matrix metalloproteinases, which then contribute to the rupture of the fibrous cap and the initiation of thrombosis. Separately, inflammation can decrease the synthesis of collagen, thereby weakening the plaque further and increasing the chance of rupture.

There are five principal pathophysiologic processes that may contribute to the development of an acute atherothrombotic event (see Fig. 97-1). These include (a) erosion or rupture of a vulnerable plaque, (b) dynamic obstruction of a coronary artery [such as spasm of a major epicardial coronary vessel in variant (Prinzmetal) angina or constriction of small muscular coronary arteries], (c) progressive mechanical obstruction, (d) inflammation and/or infection, and (e) secondary unstable angina (UA), related to oxygen supply–demand mismatch (e.g., anemia, hypotension, tachycardia, or systemic infection). Individual patients may have several of these processes coexisting as the cause of their episode of ACS.

## THROMBOSIS

Thrombosis plays a central role in the pathogenesis of ACS; this is supported by the presence of thrombi at the site of a ruptured coronary plaque at autopsy (5), in atherectomy specimens from patients with UA (6), and on angioscopy and angiography of patients with UA (7,8). Indirect evidence of ongoing thrombosis in ACS is provided by the elevation in levels of markers of platelet activation and fibrin formation (9–11). Finally, marked improvement in the clinical outcome of patients with ACS is achieved with specific antithrombotic therapy with aspirin (12), heparin (unfractionated or low-molecular-weight) (13–15), platelet glycoprotein (GP) IIb/IIIa inhibitors (16–18), and clopidogrel (19).

### Role of Platelets in Acute Coronary Syndrome

Platelets play a central role in the transformation of a stable atherosclerotic plaque into an unstable lesion. When an atherosclerotic plaque ruptures, collagen and tissue factors are exposed to blood. The first step in the platelet cascade is adhesion through the interaction of the GP Ib receptor with von Willebrand factor. The adhesion is followed by platelet activation, which encompasses a shape change of the platelet, degranulation of the $\alpha$-granules and dense granules with release of thromboxane $A_2$ ($TxA_2$), serotonin, and other platelet aggregatory and chemoattractant agents; and expression of GP IIb/IIIa receptors on the platelet surface with the activation of the receptor such that it can bind fibrinogen. Finally, there is platelet aggregation, that is, the formation of the platelet plug. Fibrinogen binds to the activated GP IIb/IIIa receptors of two platelets and thereby creates a growing platelet aggregate. Because of the central role of the platelets in the pathophysiology of ACS, antiplatelet therapy is one of the cornerstones of therapy and is directed at decreasing the formation of $TxA_2$ (aspirin), inhibiting the adenosine diphosphate (ADP) receptor pathway of platelet activation (ticlopidine and clopidogrel) (20), and directly inhibiting platelet aggregation (GP IIb/IIIa inhibitors).

### Plasma Coagulation System in Acute Coronary Syndrome

Concurrently with formation of the platelet aggregate, the plasma coagulation system is activated. Rupture of the atherosclerotic plaque and release of Tissue Factor activate factor X, converting it to factor Xa, which in turn generates thrombin (factor IIa). Thrombin converts fibrinogen to fibrin in the final common pathway for clot formation, stimulates platelet aggregation, and activates factor XIII, thereby cross-linking and stabilizing the fibrin clot. In the course of spontaneous,

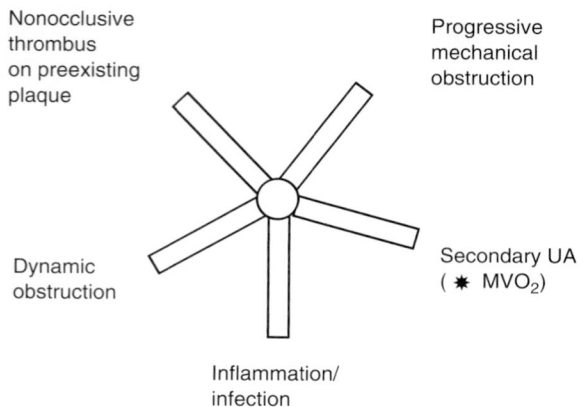

Nonocclusive
thrombus
on preexisting
plaque

Progressive
mechanical
obstruction

Dynamic
obstruction

Secondary UA
( ✳ MVO$_2$)

Inflammation/
infection

**FIGURE 97-1.** The Braunwald model of five pathophysiologic mechanisms of non–ST elevation acute coronary syndrome (NSTEACS). [From Braunwald, E. Unstable angina: an etiologic approach to management. *Circulation* 1998;98(21):2219–2222, with permission.]

mechanical, or pharmacologic thrombolysis, newly exposed thrombin molecules can form a nidus for recurrent thrombosis, which may manifest clinically as coronary reocclusion and reinfarction. Accordingly, pharmacologic inhibition of thrombin and factor Xa plays an important part of the therapy for ACS.

## Coronary Vasoconstriction

Dynamic coronary obstruction can occur at the level of the major epicardial coronary arteries (21), as well as small intramural coronary resistance vessels (22). The most common setting for coronary vasoconstriction is in the region of atherosclerotic plaques. Coronary vasoconstriction may occur because of local vasoconstrictors released from platelets, serotonin, and TxA$_2$, as well as the local vasoconstrictors present within the thrombus, such as thrombin. In *Prinzmetal (variant) angina*, there is an intense focal spasm of a segment of a coronary artery. Arteries with no atherosclerosis or with mild nonobstructive atheromata may be affected by the spasm. Small intramural arteries are affected by vasoconstriction in *microcirculatory angina*, where coronary flow is slow despite lack of epicardial stenoses. Adrenergic stimuli, cold exposure, cocaine (23), or profound mental stress (24) can also cause coronary vasoconstriction.

## Progressive Mechanical Obstruction

The fourth etiology of ACS is progressive narrowing of a coronary lumen, which was most commonly seen in the setting of restenosis following percutaneous coronary intervention (PCI), prior to the widespread use of drug-eluting stents. Angiographic and atherectomy studies have demonstrated that many patients without previous intracoronary procedures have also shown progressive luminal narrowing of the culprit vessel in the period preceding the onset of ACS that is related to rapid cellular proliferation (25).

## Secondary Unstable Angina

This form of UA is caused by profound imbalances in myocardial oxygen supply and demand. Patients with secondary UA usually have significant coronary stenoses, which may cause either exertional symptoms (chronic stable angina) or no symptoms at all (26–28). The causes of myocardial oxygen

supply–demand mismatch include conditions that cause increased oxygen demand, such as tachycardia (supraventricular or ventricular), systemic infection with fever, thyrotoxicosis, hyperadrenergic states, and elevations of left ventricular afterload such as hypertension or aortic stenosis, or those that cause impaired oxygen delivery, such as anemia, hypoxemia, or systemic hypotension. Secondary UA may have a worse prognosis than primary UA (27).

## ST Segment Elevation Myocardial Infarction

In acute STEMI, an occlusive thrombus is composed of platelets, fibrin, erythrocytes, and leukocytes. Platelet activation induces release of specific mediators including TxA$_2$, serotonin (5-HT), ADP, platelet activating factor (PAF), thrombin, Tissue Factor, and oxygen-derived free radicals. The presence of these mediators in conjunction with the paucity of prostacyclin (PGI$_2$), endogenous tissue-type plasminogen activator (tPA), and endothelial nitric oxide (NO) at sites of local vascular injury promotes platelet aggregation and obstruction of the narrowed coronary lumen. On the surface of the activated platelet, the coagulation cascade is propagated, leading to the deposition of thrombin and fibrin, thus obstructing arterial blood flow and leading to myocardial necrosis.

Epicardial coronary arteries and the coronary microcirculation play equally crucial roles in the pathophysiology of STEMI. Cycles of occlusion and reperfusion of the occluded artery, mediated by the variation in vasomotor tone and by the balance of endogenous thrombolytic and procoagulant factors, make the process of thrombotic occlusion of an epicardial coronary artery a dynamic one. Microvascular obstruction can occur due to embolization of platelet and platelet–thrombin aggregates (spontaneous or induced by pharmacologic or mechanical reperfusion), microvascular spasm, and *in situ* leukocyte plugging. Even among patients with successful reperfusion of the occluded epicardial artery, microvascular obstruction, as measured by the TIMI myocardial perfusion (TMP) grade is associated with adverse clinical outcome (29). Therefore, the coronary microcirculation has emerged as an important target for therapies in STEMI.

## Clinical Presentation

Patients with an ACS present with pain from angina pectoris typically while at rest. Stable angina is characterized by a poorly localized chest or arm discomfort (frequently described as pressure rather than pain), which is associated with physical exertion or emotional stress, and is relieved within 5 to 15 minutes by rest and/or nitroglycerin. In contrast, unstable angina is defined as angina pectoris with at least one of three features: (a) occurring at rest (or with light exertion), usually lasting at least 20 minutes, unless interrupted by nitroglycerin; (b) being severe and described as frank pain, and of recent onset, that is within 1 month; (c) occurring with a crescendo pattern, that is more severe, prolonged, or frequent than during previous occurrences (30). If patients with a background of unstable anginal symptoms exhibit serum biomarker evidence of myocardial necrosis [elevated creatine kinase (CK)-MB fraction, and/or cardiac troponin (cTn) I or T], a diagnosis of NSTEMI is given. In contrast, patients with STEMI typically present with a single prolonged (>30 minutes) episode of chest pain, or a stuttering series of chest pain episodes at rest, and have evidence of ST segment elevation on the electrocardiogram (ECG). The physical examination may be unremarkable or may corroborate the diagnosis of cardiac ischemia. Signs that suggest that ACS involves a larger fraction of the left ventricle include evidence of low cardiac output, such as diaphoresis, pale cool skin, and sinus tachycardia, and elevated filling pressures such as third or fourth heart sound and basilar rales on lung examination. If the infarction is large, the severity of left ventricular dysfunction may cause systemic hypotension. Right ventricular infarction is a distinct entity, usually caused by an acute occlusion of the proximal right coronary artery, and commonly occurs in association with the infarction of the inferior left ventricular wall. Physical signs of right ventricular infarction include hypotension and elevation of jugular venous pressure, in concert with the relative paucity of signs of left ventricular failure.

# PATHOPHYSIOLOGY OF RECURRENT ISCHEMIA FOLLOWING ACUTE CORONARY SYNDROME

Studies of coronary anatomy in patients with ACS using angiography (31–33), intravascular coronary ultrasonography (34), and angioscopy (35) have shown multiple "vulnerable" plaques in addition to the culprit lesion. Presence of such multifocal lesions likely underlies much of the pathophysiology of the recurrent ischemia after the primary event. As aggressive interventional approaches aimed at the culprit lesion continue to be perfected, the remaining plaques, which may or may not have unstable features on angiographic examination, continue to be responsible for recurrent ischemia. An important link between a more diffuse coronary artery disease and recurrent cardiac events in the months to years following ACS is inflammation. In one study, the percentage of patients with more than one active plaque on angiography was related to an increasing baseline C-reactive protein (CRP) level (34).

# MEDICAL THERAPY

## Treatment Goals

The treatment objectives for patients with ACS include *immediate* reperfusion in patients with STEMI, and stabilizing and "passivating" the acute coronary lesion, treatment of residual ischemia, and long-term secondary prevention in all patients. *Reperfusion* in patients with STEMI is achieved either with intravenous thrombolytic therapy or with PCI. Adjunctive *antithrombotic therapy* uses both *antiplatelet* and *antithrombin* medications. Aspirin, clopidogrel, unfractionated or low-molecular-weight heparin (LWMH), direct thrombin inhibitors (DTI), and GP IIb/IIIa inhibitors are used to prevent further thrombosis and to allow endogenous thrombolysis to dissolve the thrombus. *Antiplatelet therapy* is continued on a long-term basis to reduce the risk of developing recurrent thrombosis and to prevent progression to complete occlusion of the coronary artery. *Antiischemic therapies*, with agents such as β-blockers, nitrates, and angiotensin-converting enzyme (ACE) inhibitors, are used primarily to reduce myocardial oxygen demand and also appear to be effective in preventing plaque rupture, as shown in clinical event prevention with β-blockers and ACE inhibition. *Coronary revascularization* is routinely used to treat the severe stenosis of a culprit lesion, thereby preventing the thrombus from progressing and causing recurrent ischemia. Following the acute event, the treatment focus shifts to secondary prevention, and *aggressive treatment of atherosclerotic risk factors* such as hypercholesterolemia and hypertension, and cessation of smoking is undertaken. This treatment contributes to the stabilization of the cholesterol-laden plaque and to the healing of the endothelium.

## General Measures

Patients with STEMI are routinely admitted to the coronary care units after pharmacologic or mechanical reperfusion has taken place, whereas those with NSTEACS can usually be managed on telemetry units. Reliable intravenous access, continuous ECG monitoring, and rapid availability of bedside cardioverters–defibrillators are essential.

## Nitrates

Nitroglycerin is an excellent antiischemic agent, which increases myocardial oxygen supply and decreases myocardial oxygen demand. The former effects are produced through reliable endothelium-independent coronary vasodilation, and the latter effects are produced through venodilation and reduction of left ventricular preload and wall stress. Nitroglycerin can be given sublingually, as a buccal spray, or as an intravenous infusion. Tolerance to nitroglycerin develops rapidly but can be largely avoided by providing regular 8- to 10-hour nitrate-free intervals. Contraindications to nitrate use include hypotension, as well as use of PDE-5 antagonists within 24 hours [sildenafil (Viagra) and vardenafil (Levitra)] to 48 hours [tadalafil (Cialis)] (36). Nitrates should also not be used in patients with right ventricular infarction, where the decrease in preload may lead to life-threatening hypotension.

As was shown in the GISSI-3 (Gruppo Italiano per lo Studio della Streptochinasi nell'Infarto Miocardico) and ISIS-4 (Fourth International Study of Infarct Survival) trials, nitrates have a neutral effect on mortality in MI (37,38). Therefore, the goal of nitrate therapy is relief from pain; chronic nitrate therapy can usually be discontinued in the long-term management of patients after ACS, with the primary therapy remaining aspirin, clopidogrel, β-blockers, and lipid-lowering agents.

## β-Blockers

In trials conducted in the prethrombolytic area, in which patients with both STEMI and NSTEMI were included, β-blockers were shown to reduce infarct size, reinfarction, and mortality (39). Several placebo-controlled trials in NSTEACS have shown the benefit of β-blockade in reducing progression to MI and/or recurrent ischemia (40–42).

Therefore, β-blockers are recommended for all patients with ACS who do not have contraindications to β-blockade, such as history of severe bronchospasm, bradycardia, second- or third-degree atrioventricular (AV) block, persistent hypotension, previously known systolic dysfunction with acute pulmonary edema, or cardiogenic shock. Patients with a reduced ejection fraction, and chronic compensated congestive heart failure (CHF) exhibit a decreased mortality rate with β-blockade, and such therapy should not be withheld in this population.

## Calcium Channel Blockers

Calcium antagonists have vasodilatory effects and decreased blood pressure, and some also slow heart rate (e.g., verapamil and diltiazem). They may be used in patients who have persistent or recurrent symptoms after treatment with full dose of nitrates and β-blockers or in patients with bronchospasm, where β-blockers cannot be used.

Diltiazem was shown to be superior to placebo in reducing recurrent MI both in patients with non–Q-wave MI (44), and in patients following thrombolytic therapy for STEMI (45, 46). In a slightly lower-risk ACS population studied in the Danish Verapamil Infarction Trial (DAVIT) II, where nearly half of the patients did not have a confirmed MI, verapamil tended to reduce recurrent MI or death (47). However, meta-analyses have not found any beneficial effect of the calcium channel blockade in reducing mortality or subsequent infarction (48,49). Moreover, in patients with acute MI with left ventricular dysfunction or CHF, a harmful effect of diltiazem was observed (50). Likewise, short-acting nifedipine, which does not lower heart rate (instead causing reflex *tachycardia*), has been shown to be harmful in patients with acute MI when administered without a β-blocker (51). On the other hand, amlodipine (52) or felodipine (53) may be safely used in patients with ACS with left ventricular dysfunction.

In summary, calcium antagonists should be used in patients with ACS only if needed for recurrent ischemia despite β-blockade or in patients in whom β-blockade is contraindicated; diltiazem should be avoided in patients with left ventricular dysfunction and/or CHF, and therapy with short-acting nifedipine should best be avoided altogether.

## Angiotensin-Converting Enzyme Inhibitors

In STEMI, benefits of early ACE inhibition are considerable. In the GISSI-3 (37) trial, early initiation of lisinopril was associated with a 12% mortality reduction, and, in ISIS-4 (38), captopril therapy resulted in a 7% mortality reduction. Benefits were more pronounced in patients with anterior MI. In patients with left ventricular (LV) dysfunction, the benefits are even more substantial: Oral ACE inhibition reduced mortality by 20% to 30% in Survival and Ventricular Enlargement (SAVE) (54), Trandolapril Cardiac Evaluation (TRACE) (55), and Acute Infarction Ramipril Efficacy (AIRE) (56) trials. A significant benefit of ACE inhibition is seen in the first few days after the MI.

Data for *acute treatment* in NSTEACS is more controversial. Three large trials showed a 0.5% absolute reduction in mortality with early ACE inhibition in patients with acute MI (37,38,57). However, no benefit was observed in patients without ST elevation in the ISIS-4 study. Therefore, ACE inhibition in the short term does not appear to confer any benefit for patients with NSTEACS.

Two large randomized controlled trials recently demonstrated benefits of *long-term* ACE inhibition in a broad population of patients at risk for coronary artery disease, also including those without any current evidence of atherosclerosis (58,59).

On the basis of these data, the current indications for ACE inhibitors in ACS include treatment within 24 hours for patients with anterior STEMI, CHF, or less than 40% LV ejection fraction immediately following MI or during recovery period. However, all patients post-ACS should probably be considered for long-term ACE inhibition.

Whereas ACE inhibitors block most of the production of angiotensin (AT) II in the human heart, other ACE-independent pathways exist that convert AT I to AT II. Angiotensin receptor blockers (ARB) offer more complete protection against AT II by directly blocking the type 1 AT II receptor. Recent data from the Valsartan in Acute Myocardial Infarction Trial (VALIANT) demonstrated that among more than 14,000 patients with LV dysfunction or heart failure after acute MI, mortality rate for valsartan was equal to that for captopril after a median follow-up of 24.7 months (60). Notably, although providing a more complete renin–angiotensin–aldosterone system (RAAS) blockade, the *combination* of valsartan with captopril led to an increase in the rate of adverse events without improving overall survival (60). At this time, given the established benefits of ACE inhibitors after MI, and their comparatively low cost, ARBs should be reserved for those patients who are intolerant to ACE inhibitors.

Aldosterone is another component of the RAAS that potentially contributes to the development of adverse ventricular remodeling after MI by promoting cardiac fibrosis. Blockade of aldosterone receptors with spironolactone and related compounds has been used for diuresis and for the treatment of patients with advanced heart failure. A new-generation aldosterone receptor blocker, eplerenone, has been studied in the Infarction Heart Failure and Survival Study (EPHESUS) of over 6,600 patients with acute myocardial infarction (AMI) complicated by left ventricular dysfunction and heart failure. Patients were randomized to receive eplerenone or placebo in addition to standard therapy, which could include reperfusion, aspirin, lipid-lowering drugs, ACE inhibitors, ARBs, and β-blockers. Patients treated with eplerenone for a mean of 7.3 days (3 to 14 days) achieved a 15% reduction in total mortality and a 17% reduction in cardiovascular mortality, driven mainly by a 21% reduction in sudden cardiac death (61). The results of EPHESUS suggest that aldosterone blockade may be an important addition to the current therapy for patients with AMI. Further trials will more precisely define the population that benefits from aldosterone blockade after an MI because it is possible that even patients with normal left ventricular EF should be given these agents. In addition, it remains to be seen whether the mortality reduction seen in EPHESUS is specific to eplerenone or is expected with a less specific aldosterone blocker, such as spironolactone.

## Lipid-Lowering Therapy

Long-term lipid-lowering therapy, especially with 3-hydroxy-3-methyl-glutaryl coenzyme A (HMG-CoA) reductase inhibitors (statins), has been shown to be beneficial in patients following ACS (62–64). In the landmark 4S trial, simvastatin reduced mortality by 30% and coronary deaths by 42% in patients with hypercholesterolemia and with a history of ACS (62). Recurrent MI and the need for coronary revascularization were also decreased by 37% (62,65).

The National Cholesterol Education Panel (NCEP) recommends treatment with diet and drug therapy if the low density lipoprotein (LDL) value is greater than 100 mg per dL, with a goal of reducing LDL value to less than 100 mg per dL (66). A recent update to these guidelines established the category of very high-risk patients, including those with recent ACS, and recommended an LDL goal of less than 70 mg per dL for this population.

Several pilot studies and recent observational studies have sought to determine whether there is a clinical benefit of *early* initiation of statin therapy in ACS (67–70). A large randomized Myocardial Ischaemia Reduction with Aggressive Cholesterol Lowering (MIRACL) trial found that a 4-month course of high-dose atorvastatin reduced the incidence of cardiovascular death, nonfatal MI, resuscitated sudden cardiac death, or urgent rehospitalization for recurrent ischemia by 16%. In a second, longer-term Aggrastat to Zocor (A to Z) [Thrombolysis in Myocardial Infarction (TIMI 21)] trial, there was likewise a trend toward reduction of cardiovascular events with early aggressive simvastatin treatment (71).

The Pravastatin or Atorvastatin Evaluation and Infection Therapy—Thrombolysis in Myocardial Infarction (PROVE IT-TIMI) 22 trial evaluated the role of intensive lipid-lowering therapy (atorvastatin 80 mg per day) as compared to standard lipid-lowering therapy (pravastatin 40 mg per day) in patients with ACS. Treatment with standard therapy achieved a median LDL value of 95 mg per dL while intensive therapy lowered LDL to a median value of 62 mg per dL. The risk of death, MI, UA, revascularization, or stroke was reduced by 16% with intensive therapy, setting the stage for updated NCEP recommendations. Therefore, patients with ACS should be discharged on high-dose statin therapy.

# Antithrombotic Therapy in Acute Coronary Syndrome

## Aspirin

Aspirin permanently acetylates cyclooxygenase (COX)-1, thereby blocking the production of $TxA_2$ by the platelet. By attenuating the release of $TxA_2$, which normally acts to stimulate other platelets, aspirin decreases overall platelet aggregation at the site of thrombosis. The inhibition of COX-1 by aspirin is permanent, therefore, the antiplatelet effects last for the lifetime of the platelets (7 to 10 days).

In acute STEMI, treatment with aspirin is lifesaving. The large ISIS-2 trial demonstrated a significant 23% reduction in 5-week cardiovascular mortality with aspirin (160 mg per day) (72). These benefits translated into 2.4 cardiovascular deaths being prevented for every 100 patients treated and were equivalent to the treatment effect of streptokinase in the same trial. When aspirin was added to thrombolysis with streptokinase, the 5-week cardiovascular mortality was reduced by 42%. In a more recent metaanalysis of antiplatelet therapy in 15 trials of acute MI, treatment with aspirin was associated with a 30% reduction in 1-month mortality, and an absolute benefit of prevention of 3.8 cardiovascular events for every 100 patients treated (73).

Beneficial effects of aspirin in NSTEACS have been demonstrated in several trials as well, with greater than 50% reduction in the risk of death or MI (12,74). The benefit is seen as early as the first day of treatment (74). Because aspirin has a dramatic effect in reducing adverse clinical events both early and late in the course of treatment of ACS, it remains a primary therapy for these patients.

The optimal dosage of aspirin during the acute phase of ACS appears to be at least 160 mg per day, based on the mortality benefit in ISIS-2 (72). For long-term treatment, a dose of 75 to 81 mg per day is equally effective as compared to the higher dosage and appears safer in the rate of bleeding (75,76).

Aspirin resistance is a phenomenon reported in 5% to 8% of patients during chronic therapy with the drug (77–79), and is not dose dependent. It manifests as minimal change in the degree of platelet aggregation with aspirin treatment. These patients tend to have a higher risk of recurrent cardiac events (78,79). In one study, outcome at 5 years was correlated with the amount of thromboxane metabolites in urine (77). Higher event rates were seen as the amount of thromboxane metabolites rose (77). Ongoing research is attempting to characterize whether true aspirin resistance exists or whether there could be an inadequate blockade of this pathway.

Absolute contraindications for aspirin therapy are few, and include documented aspirin allergy (e.g., bronchoconstriction), active bleeding, or a known platelet disorder. For patients with mild gastrointestinal symptoms, such as nonulcer dyspepsia, in response to aspirin therapy, it is usually safe to continue such therapy, at least in the short term. Options for patients with true aspirin allergy include use of clopidogrel (see subsequent text) (30) or aspirin desensitization in an intensive care unit setting.

## Clopidogrel and Ticlopidine

Clopidogrel and ticlopidine are both thienopyridine derivatives that inhibit platelet aggregation and increase bleeding time by inhibiting ADP action on platelet receptors (20). They achieve their action by blocking the binding of ADP to the $P_2Y_{12}$ component of the ADP receptor (20). In addition to inhibiting the ADP-induced platelet activation and subsequent aggregation, blockade of the ADP appears to decrease platelet activation by von Willebrand factor and other factors (80). For this reason, inhibition of this receptor appears to have a broader effect in attenuating platelet activation than just inhibition of ADP-induced aggregation.

Ticlopidine, the first of the two currently available ADP receptor blockers, has been compared to placebo (without aspirin) in a randomized trial of 652 patients with NSTEACS and was found to produce a significant 46% reduction in vascular death or nonfatal MI (81). In combination with aspirin, ticlopidine is effective in the prevention of thrombosis and recurrent ischemic events in patients undergoing coronary stent implantation (82). The downside of ticlopidine therapy is the complication of neutropenia and thrombocytopenia (approximately 1% of patients). A less frequent but potentially life-threatening complication is thrombotic thrombocytopenic purpura (TTP), which can be fatal in 25% to 40% of cases (83,84). Therefore, patients on chronic ticlopidine therapy require frequent monitoring of complete blood count.

Clopidogrel is currently the most commonly used ADP antagonist and is its use associated with the incidence of neutropenia and TTP similar to that of aspirin (19,85,86). When added to aspirin, clopidogrel is as effective as ticlopidine in preventing stent thrombosis (87–89). Dual antiplatelet therapy with clopidogrel and aspirin in non–ST elevation ACS was addressed in a large Clopidogrel in Unstable Angina to Prevent Recurrent Events (CURE) trial (90), and in the related Percutaneous Cornoray Intervention-CURE (PCI-CURE) study (19,91). In CURE, patients with NSTEACS were randomized to receive aspirin alone, or aspirin plus clopidogrel, in addition to other standard treatments. The primary endpoint of cardiovascular death, MI, or stroke through follow-up (mean: 9 months, maximum: 1 year) was reduced by 20%, from 11.4% to 9.3%. Benefit of dual antiplatelet therapy continued up to 1 year (90). PCI-CURE studied the subset of patients enrolled in CURE who underwent percutaneous revascularization. Pretreatment with clopidogrel reduced the primary endpoint from 6.4% for placebo to 4.5% for clopidogrel—a 30% relative reduction. The endpoint of cardiovascular death or MI was reduced from 4.4% to 2.9%—a 34% risk reduction (91).

In the Clopidogrel for Recurrent of Events During Observation (CREDO) trial, early pretreatment with clopidogrel before PCI was studied. Approximately two thirds of the patients in the trial had ACS. A 31% relative risk reduction was seen at 30 days and 1 year with clopidogrel pretreatment (91).

In summary, the results of PCI-CURE and CREDO trials support preprocedural loading as well as long-term therapy with clopidogrel in patients scheduled or expected to undergo PCI. Pretreatment at least 6 hours prior to the procedure ensures optimal platelet inhibition. The significant benefits of clopidogrel pretreatment are seen with or without the concomitant use of GP IIb/IIIa inhibitors.

In ACS, clopidogrel should be used as an initial loading dose of 300 mg, followed by 75 mg daily. Whereas initiation of a dose of 75 mg daily without the load achieves the target level of platelet inhibition after 3 to 5 days; the loading dose of 300 mg achieves effective platelet inhibition within 4 to 6 hours (92,93). The use of a 600 mg loading dose has been shown to achieve steady state level of platelet inhibition after just 2 hours (94). In the Intracoronary Stenting with Antithrombotic Regimen-Rapid Early Action for Coronary Treatment (ISAR-REACT) study, 2,159 patients received a 600 mg loading dose 2 to 3 hours prior to PCI and were randomized to a GP IIb/IIIa inhibitor abciximab and reduced-dose heparin versus placebo and standard-dose heparin. There was no significant difference in the outcome at 30 days between the groups (95). This indirectly suggests that the achievement of effective levels of platelet inhibition with clopidogrel pre-PCI is effective in reducing events.

Similar to aspirin, "clopidogrel resistance" has been identified in several studies (96–98). Currently available assays preclude precise determination of the cause of the low response to clopidogrel or the differences between inherent patient-to-patient variability in platelet aggregation and the isolated "failure" of the drug. Nevertheless, although no large study has been able to assess whether there are any clinical consequences of clopidogrel resistance, these issues have fueled interest in development of newer drugs in this class that might achieve higher levels of platelet inhibition (20).

Clopidogrel has been added to fibrinolytic therapy with heparin and aspirin in pilot studies, but larger trials are studying whether this agent could improve the outcome with an acceptable safety profile.

### Heparin

Anticoagulation with unfractionated heparin (UFH) is a cornerstone in the therapy for patients with NSTEACS, partly because of several randomized trials that found lower rates of death or MI in patients treated with UFH plus aspirin compared with aspirin alone (12,74,99,100). A metaanalysis showed a 33% relative risk reduction in death or MI at 2 to 12 weeks follow-up when comparing UFH plus aspirin versus aspirin alone, although this reduction was not statistically significant (13).

There is limited data from randomized controlled clinical trials about the use of intravenous UFH in STEMI. However, its use as an adjunctive therapy to primary reperfusion is widespread and routine. The main role of heparin as an adjunctive agent is to decrease reocclusion following the administration of a fibrin-specific lytic agent. Although no difference in infarct-related artery (IRA) patency is seen at 90 minutes, patency is higher between 18 hours and 5 days in patients receiving intravenous heparin, suggesting that the benefit of heparin is a result of decreased reocclusion rather than enhanced thrombolysis. Concomitant anticoagulation with UFH is recommended during thrombolysis with fibrin-specific agents [alteplase (tPA), reteplase (rPA), tenecteplase (TNK)]. Following administration of nonfibrin specific agents, such as streptokinase or anistreplase [anisoylated plasminogen streptokinase activator complex (APSAC)], the role of UFH is less clear. Patients treated with streptokinase and intravenous or subcutaneous heparin in the Global Utilization of Streptokinase and Tissue Plasminogen Activator for Occluded Coronary Arteries (GUSTO)-I trial had similar IRA patency at 90 minutes and 24 hours, but those receiving intravenous UFH had significantly higher patency at 5 to 7 days (84% vs. 72%) (101). However, overall mortality and the rate of clinical reinfarction were the same between these two groups. Therefore, intravenous heparin may be considered optional in streptokinase-treated patients.

There is inherent heterogeneity in the anticoagulant effects of UFH (102) because of its neutralization by circulating plasma factors and proteins released by activated platelets (103). In the clinical setting, frequent monitoring of the anticoagulant response using activated partial thromboplastin time (aPTT) is recommended, with titrations made according to a standardized nomogram (see Table 97-1). The latter minimizes the variability in the dosing and improves the achievement of a target aPTT (104,105).

The level of anticoagulation that constitutes the optimal therapeutic range has not been firmly established. Small studies have suggested that lower aPTT values may be associated with an increased incidence of recurrent ischemic events (106–108). On the other hand, higher aPTT values are associated with an increased risk of hemorrhage (108). The lowest rate of bleeding and mortality in patients with STEMI treated with thrombolysis therapy was observed when the 12-hour aPTT was between

**TABLE 97-1**

### STANDARDIZED NOMOGRAM FOR TITRATION OF HEPARIN

| aPTT (s) | Change | IV infusion (U/kg/h) |
|----------|--------|----------------------|
| <35 | 70 U/kg bolus | +3 |
| 35–49 | 35 U/kg bolus | +2 |
| 50–70 | 0 | 0 |
| 71–90 | 0 | −2 |
| >100 | Hold infusion for 30 min | −3 |

aPTT, activated partial thromboplastin time.
From Becker RC, Ball SP, Eisenberg P, et al. A randomized, multicenter trial of weight-adjusted intravenous heparin dose titrations and point-of-care coagulation monitoring in hospitalized patients with active thromboembolic disease. Antithrombotic Therapy Consortium Investigators. *Am Heart J* 1999;137:59–71, with permission.

50 and 70 seconds (108). It has also become apparent that the dose of intravenous heparin is an important risk factor for the development of intracranial hemorrhage (ICH) after thrombolysis in patients with STEMI. Hence, the American College of Cardiology (ACC)/American Heart Association (AHA) guidelines recommend that a reduced dose of UFH be given with tPA, rPA, or TNK: a bolus of 60 U per kg (maximum 4,000 U) and an infusion of 12 U/kg/hour (maximum 1,000 U per hour).

### Low-Molecular-Weight Heparins

Low-molecular-weight heparins (LMWHs) have become an increasingly important tool in the pharmacologic arsenal for treatment of ACS. These compounds have increased ratios of anti-Xa to anti-IIa activity, compared to UFH—either 2:1 (dalteparin) or 3:1 (enoxaparin or nadroparin). Greater inhibition of factor Xa is likely to be responsible for the greater anticoagulant potency of LMWH over UFH. Likewise, excellent bioavailability and reproducible anticoagulant response of LMWH allow for subcutaneous administration without monitoring of the coagulation system (see Table 97-2). Although this is an advantage in patients with non–ST elevation ACS, the long half-life of LMWH is a potential disadvantage early in the course of STEMI when patients are being considered for thrombolytic therapy or primary PCI.

In STEMI, LMWHs have been studied in combination with thrombolytic therapy and mechanical reperfusion. The Assessment of the Safety and Efficacy of a New Thrombolytic Regimen (ASSENT)-3 trial compared enoxaparin to UFH when combined with full-dose TNK among 6,095 patients with STEMI (109). Patients treated with TNK plus enoxaparin had a significantly lower incidence of mortality, in-hospital reinfarction, or refractory ischemia at 30 days compared with patients treated with TNK plus UFH (11.4% vs. 15.4%) (109). The rate of ICH was similar between the two treatment arms. Results similar to ASSENT-3 were observed in the ENTIRE (Enoxaparin and TNK-tPA with or without PG IIb/IIIa Inhibitor as Reperfusion strategy in ST elevation MI) trial (110). Despite the promising results of ENTIRE-TIMI 23 and ASSENT 3, it is still too early to recommend that enoxaparin be considered as a replacement for UFH in pharmacologic reperfusion strategies for STEMI. This is in part due to an increased risk of stroke and ICH seen with enoxaparin plus TNK in the ASSENT-3 PLUS trial, where this strategy was tested in the prehospital setting (111). The increased risk of stroke and ICH was seen solely in the older age population (>75 years). In an attempt to further define the role of enoxaparin in pharmacologic reperfusion, the Enoxaparin and

TABLE 97-2

ADVANTAGES OF LOW-MOLECULAR-WEIGHT HEPARIN OVER UNFRACTIONATED HEPARIN IN TREATMENT OF ACUTE CORNARY SYNDROME

| | UFH | LMWH | Advantage of LMWH |
|---|---|---|---|
| Anti-Xa:Anti-IIa activity | 1:1 | ≈2–3.8:1 | |
| Plasma protein binding | Significant | Minimal | Higher bioavailability |
| Endothelial binding | Significant | Minimal | |
| Inhibition of fibrin-bound thrombin | No | Yes | |
| Neutralization by platelet factor 4 | Significant | Minimal | Higher potency |
| Release of tissue factor pathway inhibitor | Minimal | Significant | |
| Inhibition of platelet-bound factor Xa | Minimal | Significant | |
| Inhibition of platelet function | More | Less | Less bleeding |
| Thrombocytopenia | 1%–2% | Rare | |
| Bioavailability | ≈30% | 90%–95% | |
| Route of administration | IV | Sc | Easier to administer |
| Need for aPTT monitoring | Yes | No | |

UFH, unfractionated heparin; LMWH, low-molecular-weight heparin; aPTT, activated partial thromboplastin time; IV, intravenous; Sc, subcutaneous.

Thrombolysis Reperfusion for Acute Myocardial Infarction Trial (EXTRACT-TIMI 25) is being conducted. The dose of enoxaparin in EXTRACT-TIMI 25 has been reduced for patients over the age of 75.

In NSTEACS, the role of LMWH is much better defined. There have been several trials comparing LMWH to placebo or UFH in NSTEACS (see Table 97-3) and one trial comparing two different LMWHs. In a systematic review of six major trials comparing enoxaparin to UFH in NSTEACS, enoxaparin was found to be more effective in preventing death or MI, although bleeding rates were not different between the two drugs (112).

In comparisons of LMWHs versus UFH, benefits have not been seen across the entire compound class. In trials to date, no significant difference was observed between dalteparin (117) or nadroparin and UFH (117,119).

On the other hand, with enoxaparin, three trials have found a significant benefit over UFH. In ESSENCE (14) and TIMI 11B (15), enoxaparin was shown to confer a significant 20% reduction in death, MI and/or recurrent ischemia compared with UFH. Higher-risk patients with NSTEACS derive greater relative benefit from enoxaparin (over UFH) than lower-risk patients. In both ESSENCE and TIMI 11B, benefits of enoxaparin were limited to patients with ST segment deviation (14,15). In the TIMI 11B troponin substudy, among patients who were CK-MB negative, those with elevations of troponin I derived a significantly greater benefit from enoxaparin than from UFH, compared with those with negative troponins (120). Similarly, using the TIMI risk score, the benefit of enoxaparin over UFH was seen among patients with a score of 3 or higher.

The rates of catheterization and PCI in the early enoxaparin trials were lower than what is seen in current practice (e.g., only 13% to 17% of patients underwent PCI in ESSENCE). Consequently, recent investigations focused on higher-risk patients with NSTEACS undergoing treatment with GP IIb/IIIa inhibitors and early angiography/PCI. In particular, SYNERGY was a large trial comparing enoxaparin with UFH in patients undergoing treatment with frequent use of GP IIb/IIIa inhibitors

and an early invasive therapy (116). The trial was designed to show noninferiority of enoxaparin to UFH in preventing death or MI at 30 days, and enoxaparin met the noninferiority criteria at the expense of modest increase in bleeding. In A to Z, noninferiority criteria were met, without a significant increase in bleeding, but benefit was seen in patients managed conservatively (121).

These data suggest that enoxaparin has a particular benefit in NSTEACS, and unless new trials with other LMWHs demonstrate a benefit over UFH, enoxaparin is the LMWH (and antithrombin) of choice in NSTEACS.

Use of enoxaparin is not recommended in patients with moderate or severe renal impairment (serum creatinine level >2.5 mg per dL or creatinine clearance <30 ml per min). Morbidly obese patients (>130 kg) may have unpredictable total body distribution of enoxaparin, and thereby may be at risk for inadequate anticoagulation. Therefore, monitoring of anti-Xa activity ("anti-Xa level") may be desirable in these patients, as well as in geraitric patients and in those with *mild* renal insufficiency. In such cases, goal anti-Xa levels are 0.6 to 1.8 IU per mL. A point-of-care assay has recently become available and is increasingly being used in the catheterization labs for patients undergoing PCI (122,123).

Because one of the proposed advantages of LMWH over UFH is its more potent inhibition of factor Xa, research is progressing with testing of pure inhibitors of factor Xa. One agent is fondaparinux, a synthetic pentasaccharide, which has been found to be more effective than enoxaparin in the prevention of deep vein thrombosis (124), and it is currently being tested in NSTEACS and STEMI.

## Direct Thrombin Inhibitors

DTI have undergone extensive evaluation in ACS. Several DTIs, including desirudin, lepirudin, and bivalirudin, have been tested in the context of NSTEMI, STEMI, and elective or urgent PCI.

TABLE 97-3

TRIALS OF LOW-MOLECULAR-WEIGHT HEPARIN VERSUS UNFRACTIONATED HEPARIN FOR TREATMENT OF NON–ST ELEVATION ACUTE CORNARY

| Trial | Treatment | *n* | Major results |
|-------|-----------|-----|---------------|
| ESSENCE (14) | Enoxaparin versus UFH for 2–8 d | 3,171 | 16% relative reduction in rate of death, MI or angina at 14 d with enoxaparin (16.6% vs. 19.8%); similar rate of major bleeding (6.5% vs. 7.0%) |
| TIMI 11B (15) | Enoxaparin versus UFH for up to 43 d | 3,910 | 12% relative reduction in rate of death/MI/urgent revascularization by d 43 with enoxaparin (17.3% vs. 19.7%); benefit persisted out to 1 yr; rate of major hemorrhage higher with enoxaparin (2.9% vs. 1.5%) |
| ACUTE II (113) | Enoxaparin versus UFH for 24–96 h in patients receiving tirofiban | 525 | Similar incidence of major bleeding at 30 d; similar mortality at 30 d; less refractory ischemia and rehospitalization for unstable angina with enoxaparin (0.6% vs. 4.3% and 1.6% vs. 7.1%, respectively) |
| INTERACT (114) | Enoxaparin versus UFH in patients receiving eptifibatide | 746 | Lower incidence of major bleeding at 96 h with enoxaparin (1.8% vs. 4.6%); lower incidence of death or MI at 30 d with enoxaparin (5.0% vs. 9.0%) |
| A-to-Z (115) | Enoxaparin versus UFH in patients receiving tirofiban (crossover allowed from LMWH to UFH in the catheterization lab) | 3,987 | Enoxaparin noninferior to UFH in reducing death, MI, or refractory ischemia (8.4% vs. 9.4%) |
| SYNERGY (116) | Enoxaparin versus UFH in patients treated with early invasive strategy | 10,027 | Similar rates of death or MI at 30 d (enoxaparin *noninferior* to UFH); more major bleeding (by TIMI criteria) with enoxaparin (9.1% vs. 7.6%) |
| FRIC (117) | Dalteparin versus UFH for 6 d (phase I); low-dose dalteparin versus placebo for 45 d (phase II) | 1,482 | No difference in death, MI or recurrent angina in phase I (9.3% dalteparin vs. 7.6% UFH), or phase II (composite endpoint 12.3% in both arms) |
| FRISC II (118) | Dalteparin versus placebo for 90 d | 2,267 | Significant reduction in death/MI with dalteparin at 30 d (3.1% vs. 5.9%), but not significant after 6 mo (38.4% vs. 39.9%) |
| FRAXIS (119) | Nadroparin for 6 d versus nadroparine for 14 d versus UFH | 3,468 | Similar incidence of CV death/MI/recurrent angina/ recurrent unstable angina at 14 d in all three groups (17.8% vs. 20.0% vs. 18.1%) |

UFH, unfractionated heparin; MI, myocardial infarction; LMWH, low-molecular-weight heparin; CV, cardiovascular system.

Desirudin was tested in a heterogeneous ACS population (both patients with NSTEMI and STEMI were included) enrolled in the GUSTO IIb trial. There was no difference in mortality between patients receiving desirudin and UFH, but the 30-day rate of death or MI tended to be lower (8.9% vs. 9.8%, P = 0.06). There was a statistically significant, albeit small, reduction in recurrent infarction with desirudin (5.4% vs. 6.3%, P = 0.04) (125). The Organization to Assess Strategies for Ischemic Syndromes (OASIS)-2 trial (126) compared recombinant hirudin—lepirudin—with UFH and found a trend toward decreased rate of death or MI at 7 days with lepirudin compared to heparin but significantly more major hemorrhage requiring transfusion. However, a metaanalysis of bivalirudin trials, which included 1,071 patients with ACS, showed that safety with bivalirudin was superior to that with heparin, with 59% less major bleeding (127). Importantly, most of the data on the use of DTIs in NSTEACS predates the widespread use of GP IIb/IIIa inhibitors, and a trial comparing DTIs with heparin plus GP IIb/IIIa inhibitor combination in ACS is ongoing. Bivalirudin has been tested during urgent PCI for unstable or postinfarct angina and has been found to have a trend toward a superior outcome versus UFH (128) and a similar outcome to the combination of UFH plus a GP IIb/IIIa inhibitor (129). In the latter trial, less than half of the patients were characterized as having NSTEACS. Therefore, the efficacy of bivalirudin has not fully been evaluated in NSTEACS, but a large trial is currently underway.

In STEMI, DTI have also undergone extensive evaluation. In the TIMI 9B trial, hirudin reduced the rate of recurrent MI following thrombolytic therapy; however, there was no difference in the composite primary endpoint, death, MI, or severe CHF at 30 days (130). In the GUSTO IIb trial, which enrolled patients across the full spectrum of ACS, there was a statistically significant reduction in reinfarction (5.4% vs. 6.3%, P = 0.04) but only a statistically insignificant trend toward reduction in death or MI at 30 days (8.9% vs. 9.8%, P = 0.06) (131). Bivalirudin was evaluated in the large HERO (Hirulog and Early Reperfusion/Occlusion)-2 thrombolytic trial of patients with STEMI receiving streptokinase (132). No difference between bivalirudin and UFH was observed in the rate of death at 30 days, but there was a 30% reduction in the incidence of new MI in the bivalirudin group at 96 hours, a benefit that was maintained up to 30 days. In the bivalirudin group, there was a significant excess of moderate bleeding and a similar trend for excess severe bleeding (0.7% vs. 0.5%, P = 0.07). In summary, multiple trial data do not currently support DTIs as a replacement for UFH in patients with STEMI treated with thrombolysis.

## Oral Anticoagulation in Acute Coronary Syndrome

The rationale for oral anticoagulation with warfarin following ACS is that prolonged treatment might extend the benefit of early anticoagulation with an antithrombin agent such as UFH or LMWH and attenuate the small apparent increase in recurrent thrombosis following cessation of heparin treatment. The initial large trials—OASIS-2 (133), Combination Hemotherapy and Mortality Prevention (CHAMP) (134), and Coumarin Aspirin Reinfarction Study (CARS) (135)—compared a combination therapy of low-dose warfarin plus aspirin to aspirin alone and failed to demonstrate any difference in mortality or recurrent MI. In addition, there was a higher rate of major hemorrhage among patients on warfarin therapy in the CHAMP trial (134). Three subsequent trials in ACS patients, however, demonstrated that if a sufficient degree of anticoagulation was achieved, a benefit can be observed with the combination of aspirin plus warfarin as compared with aspirin alone (136–139). In the largest of these trials, during an average of 4 years of follow-up, the incidence of death, MI, or stroke occurred in 20.0% of patients receiving aspirin, in 16.7% of patients receiving warfarin ($P = 0.03$), and in 15.0% of patients receiving warfarin and aspirin ($P = 0.001$). The international normalized ratio (INR) goal for the aspirin plus warfarin group was 2.0 to 2.5, indicating full anticoagulation. Rates of major bleeding were 0.62% per treatment-year in both groups receiving warfarin and 0.17% in patients receiving aspirin alone, and the odds ratio was 3.64 ($P <0.001$). Therefore, the combination of aspirin plus warfarin appears to be more effective than aspirin alone for long-term secondary prevention, but results in a significant increase in the risk of major bleeding.

Given the similar benefit seen with the dual platelet inhibition with clopidogrel plus aspirin, and the lack of the need to monitor the INR, as well as the frequent use of PCI and stenting in the patient population where benefit of clopidogrel is well established, the clinical use of aspirin plus warfarin is limited. Currently, such approach should be taken in patients with another indication for warfarin therapy, such as chronic atrial fibrillation or severe left ventricular dysfunction who are at a high risk for systemic embolization (140). The combination of all three agents has not been tested to date in a clinical trial setting, but might result in excessive bleeding risk during long-term therapy. In patients with atrial fibrillation who have ACS and in whom a stent is placed, low-dose aspirin, clopidogrel for 1 to 6 months (depending on the type of stent) and well-monitored, long-term warfarin is generally used.

## Glycoprotein IIb/IIIa Inhibitors

The GP IIb/IIIa receptor inhibitors are a potent class of antiplatelet drugs that act by blocking the final common pathway of platelet aggregation, that is, fibrinogen-mediated crosslinkage of platelets. Three agents are now available for use in ACS, as well as during PCI: abciximab, eptifibatide, and tirofiban. Of these, abciximab is only approved in patients with ACS who are treated with invasive strategy (i.e., PCI). Abciximab is a Fab fragment of a monoclonal antibody to the GP IIb/IIIa receptor. Eptifibatide, a synthetic peptide, and tirofiban, a nonpeptide molecule, are small-molecule antagonists of the GP IIb/IIIa receptor, whose structure mimics the Arg-Gly-Asp sequence, responsible for binding of fibrinogen to the receptor.

### Glycoprotein IIb/IIIa Inhibitors in Non–ST Elevation Acute Coronary Syndrome

For patients with NSTEACS, several trials have shown benefits of IIb/IIIa inhibition, whether the management strategy is predominantly medical (17), early invasive (141), or both (16,18,142). Therapy with tirofiban plus heparin and aspirin was compared to heparin plus aspirin in the Platelet Receptor Inhibition for Ischemic Syndrome Management in Patients Limited by Unstable Signs and Symptoms (PRISM-PLUS) trial and was found to significantly reduce the rate of death, MI, or refractory ischemia at 7 days (18). Eptifibatide significantly reduced the rate of death or MI at 30 days in the Platelet Glycoprotein IIb/IIIa in Unstable Angina Receptor Suppression Using Integrin Therapy (PURSUIT) trial (16). GP IIb/IIIa inhibitors have been observed to lead to more complete resolution of intracoronary thrombus and improved coronary flow compared with aspirin and heparin alone (143,144). This supports earlier administration of the drug relative to the onset of pain (i.e., within the first 6 to 12 hours) (145). Abciximab is currently approved only for *early invasive* management of NSTEACS because the GUSTO-IV ACS trial found no benefit and a higher early mortality with the use of abciximab in high-risk NSTEACS patients for whom an early conservative strategy (initial medical management) was planned (146). The proposed explanation for these unexpected results was that levels of inhibition of platelet aggregation were low at the dose of abciximab tested in the trial.

### Risk Stratification in Non–ST Elevation Acute Coronary Syndrome to Target Glycoprotein IIb/IIIa Inhibitor Therapy

Inhibition of GP IIb/IIIa receptors appears to primarily benefit higher-risk patients with NSTEACS. In the early trials, it was observed that the subgroup of patients with significant ST segment deviations (depression or transient elevations) had a two to three times greater absolute benefit as compared with patients without ST changes (18). In a metaanalysis, patients with diabetes and with NSTEACS were found to have a 26% reduction in mortality with GP IIb/IIIa inhibition, as compared with no reduction in mortality in patients without diabetes (147). Substudies of the CAPTURE (148), PRISM (149), and other (150,151) trials using baseline cardiac biomarkers (mostly troponin) have found that the benefit of GP IIb/IIIa inhibition appears to be greatest in patients with elevated levels of markers. Analogous findings were seen using the TIMI risk score to identify high-risk patients who benefit from GP IIb/IIIa inhibition (152). These subgroups have a higher thrombus burden at coronary angiography (153,154) and, therefore, are at a higher risk for microvascular embolization (155).

In summary, patients with NSTEACS and high-risk features, such as recurrent ischemia, CHF, elevated troponin, significant ST segment changes, history of prior coronary revascularization, or TIMI Risk Score of 3 or more, should be treated with GP IIb/IIIa inhibitors, and plans should be made for early invasive strategy.

### Glycoprotein IIb/IIIa Inhibition and Nonemergent Percutaneous Coronary Intervention

Trials of GP IIb/IIIa inhibitors have generally demonstrated a greater reduction in cardiovascular events in patients undergoing PCI than in the general NSTEACS patient population (156,157). A metaanalysis found that most of the benefit in the NSTEACS trials was seen in those who had early PCI [or Coronary Artery Bypass Graft Surgery (CABG)] (158). However, the proportion of benefit that was achieved before the PCI procedure with the so-called upstream GP IIa/IIIb inhibition was not specifically addressed. In a pooled analysis of three trials, PRISM-PLUS, PURSUIT, and CAPTURE involving 12,296 patients, there was a 34% relative reduction in occurrence of death or MI during a period of first 24 hours of medical management only (3.8% vs. 2.5%). This benefit continued up to the time of PCI (159) and is likely due to the reduction of the ongoing thrombosis, and stabilization of preexisting thrombus, which then reduces thrombotic periprocedural complications. Patients undergoing CABG also derive benefit from the upstream treatment with GP IIb/IIIa inhibition (160).

It, therefore, appears that there is a significant benefit of GP IIb/IIIa inhibition in patients undergoing medical treatment, as well as in those undergoing PCI and CABG.

### Glycoprotein IIb/IIIa Inhibitors as Adjuncts to Primary Percutaneous Coronary Intervention

As discussed above, GP IIb/IIIa inhibitors are useful as adjuncts to elective and urgent PCI. Because of their effectiveness in these settings, GP IIb/IIIa inhibitors were also evaluated in patients undergoing mechanical and pharmacologic reperfusion. The ADMIRAL trial demonstrated that addition of abciximab to standard therapy before primary PCI with stenting improved outcomes in patients with STEMI. In this trial, the group receiving abciximab had higher procedural success rates, decreased rates of reocclusion, better epicardial blood flow, and a markedly lower rate of clinical adverse events (161). To date, the largest study of GP IIb/IIIa inhibitors during primary PCI was the CADILLAC (Controlled Abciximab and Device Investigation to Lower Late Angioplasty Complications) study, in which 2,082 patients with STEMI were randomly assigned in a $2 \times 2$ factorial design to primary percutaneous transluminal coronary angioplasty (PTCA) alone, primary PTCA + abciximab, stenting alone, or stenting + abciximab. The composite endpoint of death, reinfarction, revascularization, or disabling stroke at 6 months occurred in 20% of patients in the primary PTCA group, 16.5% in the primary PTCA + abciximab group, 11.5% in the stenting alone group, and 10.2% in the stenting plus abciximab group ($P <0.001$) (162). These results suggested that the combination of abciximab and stenting leads to a small but significant reduction in the need for repeat revascularization at 6 months, and that stenting is preferred to PTCA as the primary mechanical reperfusion strategy.

### Safety of GP IIb/IIIa Inhibitors

Use of GP IIa/IIIb blockers is associated with a slightly higher rate of major hemorrhage: 2.4% versus 1.4% for placebo in one metaanalysis of patients with NSTEACS (142). Small-molecule GP IIb/IIIa inhibitors (eptifibatide or tirofiban) should be used with discretion in patients with renal insufficiency because these inhibitors are renally cleared. In patients with creatinine clearance less than 50 mL per minute, the infusion of tirofiban must be reduced by 50%, and use of half-dose infusion of eptifibatide is recommended for patients with creatinine levels between 2.0 and 4.0 mg per dL. The use of eptifibatide is discouraged in patients with creatinine levels more than 4.0 mg per dL. On the other hand, abciximab may be used in patients with renal insufficiency, including in those on hemodialysis.

The most important side effect of GP IIb/IIIa inhibitor therapy besides bleeding is clinically significant thrombocytopenia, the incidence of which ranges from 0.2% to approximately 2% in clinical trials. Thrombocytopenia is associated with increased bleeding and, infrequently, recurrent thrombotic events (163,164). For this reason, routine measurement of platelet count is indicated before initiation of GP IIb/IIIa therapy, 6 to 8 hours later, and daily thereafter until the infusion is terminated. Treatment of GP IIb/IIIa inhibitor-induced thrombocytopenia includes cessation of the infusion and close observation for bleeding complications. Platelet transfusions are reserved for profound thrombocytopenia (platelet count <10,000 per mm$^3$) or clinically significant bleeding.

### Oral GP IIb/IIIa Inhibition

Despite the impressive benefits of intravenous GP IIb/IIIa blockade across a wide spectrum of atherothrombotic events, five large clinical trials failed to show any benefit of prolonged oral IIb/IIIa inhibition (75,165–168). On the contrary,

a significant 35% increase in mortality was seen across the trials. Lower levels of platelet inhibition than those seen with intravenous agents (169), as well as unmasking and shedding of the proinflammatory and prothrombotic CD40 ligand (170,171), may account for these untoward effects of oral GP IIb/IIIa blockers. Some of the oral agents may have intrinsic proaggregatory effects (172,173).

## Pharmacologic Reperfusion: Thrombolysis

### Thrombolytic Therapy for ST Segment Elevation

Thrombolytic therapy is one of the two critical therapies for acute STEMI; the other is primary PCI. Time is of utmost importance with either strategy. Patients who are treated with thrombolysis within 1 hour from the onset of chest pain have an approximately 50% reduction in mortality, whereas those presenting more than 12 hours after the onset of symptoms do not derive significant benefit from thrombolytic therapy.

Thrombolysis has been shown to reduce mortality in several large placebo-controlled trials using streptokinase, APSAC and tPA. These benefits persist through at least 10 years of follow-up. The Fibrinolytic Therapy Trialists' overview of all the major placebo-controlled studies showed a 2.6% absolute reduction in mortality for patients with STEMI treated within the first 12 hours after the onset of symptoms (174). Patients presenting with new left bundle branch block and a strong clinical history for acute MI also derive a substantial benefit from thrombolysis. Patients with non–ST elevation ACS, however, do not benefit from thrombolysis and indeed may be harmed (see subsequent text).

### Guidelines for Thrombolytic Therapy

Thrombolytic therapy is indicated for patients presenting within 12 hours of symptom onset if they have ST segment elevation, or new left bundle branch block, or ST depressions in leads $V_1$ to $V_3$ indicative of a true posterior MI, provided they have no contraindications to thrombolytic therapy (see Table 97-4). Patients should not be treated if the time to treatment is more than 24

---

**TABLE 97-4**

CONTRAINDICATIONS TO THROMBOLYTIC THERAPY

**ABSOLUTE CONTRAINDICATIONS**
- Hemorrhagic stroke at any time
- Other stroke within preceding 12 mo
- Known intracranial neoplasm, AV malformation, or aneurysm of the cranial vessel
- Active gastrointestinal bleeding
- Suspected aortic dissection
- Trauma or major surgery within preceding 2–4 wk
- Pregnancy

**RELATIVE CONTRAINDICATIONS**
- Blood pressure >180/110 mm Hg at presentation
- Nonhemorrhagic stroke >1 yr earlier
- Cardiopulmonary resuscitation >10 min, especially with rib fractures
- Active peptic ulcer disease
- Chronic anticoagulation with warfarin

AV, arteriovenous.

hours or if they present only with ST segment depression (other than those felt to represent an acute true posterior MI).

## Comparison of Different Thrombolytic Agents

All of the currently available thrombolytic agents activate plasminogen, converting a single-chain plasminogen molecule to the double-chain plasmin, which has potent intrinsic thrombolytic activity. Streptokinase, a nonenzymatic protein produced by $\beta$-hemolytic streptococci, was used in the initial trials of thrombolytic therapy for STEMI. Both GISSI (175) and ISIS-2 (72) trials demonstrated that the administration of streptokinase for evolving MI-reduced mortality when compared to the then standard (no reperfusion) therapy. More fibrin-specific thrombolytic agents such as tPA were first studied on a large scale in the TIMI trial, which demonstrated infarct-related artery patency in nearly twice as many patients randomized to tPA versus streptokinase therapy (176). Four different thrombolytic regimens were directly compared in the GUSTO trial. It showed that among regimens of "accelerated" or "front-loaded" tPA and concomitant intravenous heparin, streptokinase with intravenous heparin, streptokinase with subcutaneous heparin, and a combination of tPA and streptokinase with intravenous heparin, the accelerated tPA plus heparin regimen achieved the highest 90-minute IRA patency and was associated with a highly significant 14% reduction in mortality. When comparing the net clinical benefit (death or disabling stroke) between the different regimens, tPA was clearly superior compared to the other regimens (nine fewer deaths or disabling strokes per 1,000 patients treated with tPA). Other complications of acute MI were also less frequent with tPA, including CHF, cardiogenic shock, arrhythmias, and allergic reactions.

Despite impressive reduction in mortality and in nonfatal complications of acute STEMI, traditional thrombolytic regimens still fail to induce early and sustained reperfusion in nearly half the patients. Additionally, reocclusion occurs in another 5% (in-hospital) and up to 30% of patients by 3 months, frequently leading to recurrent MI. Therefore, subsequent efforts have concentrated on the development of new thrombolytics, as well as combination reperfusion strategies, using adjunctive antiplatelet therapy.

rPA and TNK have been synthesized by molecular modification of the recombinant tissue plasminogen activator, and have longer plasma half-lives that allow a single or double bolus administration regimen instead of an infusion. However, although the newer agents are certainly easier to administer than tPA (which may improve door-to-needle time), phase III trials failed to demonstrate significant improvements in 30-day mortality rates over tPA.

## Combination Thrombolysis with Reduced-Dose Lytics and Glycoprotein IIb/IIIa Inhibitors

Preclinical studies have suggested that the use of GP IIb/IIIa receptor inhibitors with thrombolytic agents accelerates reperfusion and reduces the risk of acute reocclusion. Because of the concern for excessive bleeding with the combination of full-dose thrombolytic and a potent intravenous antiplatelet agent, *reduced-dose* tPA plus abciximab was evaluated in the phase II TIMI 14 trial. The rate of TIMI 3 flow was significantly higher at both 60 and 90 minutes in patients receiving half-dose tPA and abciximab, compared to those receiving full-dose tPA only (77% and 72%, respectively) (177). In addition, ST segment resolution was improved, even among those with TIMI grade 3 flow (69% for combination therapy vs. 44% for tPA alone), suggesting an additional benefit of combination therapy on improving microvascular perfusion (178). Subsequent trials demonstrated only a nonsignificant trend toward increased TIMI 3 flow

with half-dose rPA (179) and TNK (110,180), combined with GP IIb/IIIa inhibitors.

Clinical endpoints with combination reperfusion therapy have been examined more recently in the GUSTO-V and AS-SENT-3 trials. In GUSTO-V, more than 16,000 patients with STEMI were randomized to therapy with full-dose rPA and heparin or a combination of half-dose rPA, abciximab, and reduced-dose heparin (181). The combination regimen reduced rates of reinfarction and emergent PCI within 7 days, but this did not translate into improved 1-year mortality (181). Moreover, at 30 days, the primary endpoint of death from any cause was not significantly different between the rPA group and the combined rPA and abciximab group. The overall rates of ICH were similar in the two treatment groups, but non-ICH bleeding, transfusions, and thrombocytopenia were higher in the combination therapy arm. In patients older than 75 years, the rate of both ICH and other major bleeding was higher with combination therapy.

The ASSENT-3 trial findings confirmed the results of GUSTO-V in STEMI by demonstrating lack of significant reduction in mortality, as well as higher rates of bleeding complications with a combination regimen of half-dose TNK plus abciximab.

In summary, large randomized trials with relevant clinical endpoints have shown that the strategy of combining GP IIb/IIIa inhibitors with reduced doses of thrombolytics is not superior to thrombolytic monotherapy. Currently, these regimens are not recommended outside of a clinical trial setting and are *contraindicated* in older patients because of an unacceptably high risk of bleeding.

## Thrombolytic Therapy for Non–ST Elevation Acute Coronary Syndrome

Thrombolysis is contraindicated in patients with NSTEACS. The TIMI-IIIB trial showed that thrombolytic therapy with tPA in NSTEACS was associated with more fatal and nonfatal MI compared to heparin alone and with a higher rate of ICH (182). The TIMI-IIIB results are supported by a metaanalysis of the previous small trials of thrombolytic therapy in NSTEACS, in which no benefit of thrombolytic therapy was observed (183).

The proposed mechanism for adverse effect of thrombolysis in NSTEACS is the previously discussed prothrombotic and proaggregatory effects of thrombolysis. The prothrombotic forces in NSTEACS potentially lead to total occlusion of a previously patent culprit vessel. In contrast, in STEMI, the culprit artery is usually already occluded and can only improve with thrombolysis.

## Limitations of Thrombolytic Therapy

1. *Incomplete reperfusion*
   Contemporary thrombolytic regimens achieve IRA patency in approximately 80% of patients but complete reperfusion (TIMI grade 3 flow) in only 50% to 60% of cases. Incomplete reperfusion in STEMI is associated with a poor prognosis. Additionally, following successful thrombolysis, 10% to 30% of patients suffer reocclusion of the IRA and experience reinfarction in the following 3 months which is associated with a twofold to threefold increase in mortality (184).

2. *Missed opportunities for reperfusion*
   In spite of widespread availability of thrombolytic agents, a significant number of patients presenting with STEMI do not receive such therapy (185). A disproportionate number of patients are eligible for receiving thrombolytic therapy, including women, the elderly, and those with a history of prior MI, multivessel coronary

disease, or CHF. Although, as shown in the preceding text, the relative risks of reperfusion therapy are greater in older patients, it is clear that this population derives the same, if not greater, benefits from thrombolysis as the younger patients do (186).

3. *Complications of thrombolysis*
ICH is the most devastating of the complications, is fatal in most patients affected and causes a virtually universal disability in survivors. In major clinical trials, ICH has occurred in 0.6% to 1.4% of patients receiving thrombolytic therapy, with the elderly women and those with low body weight being at higher risk.

Allergic reactions, including anaphylaxis, occur with administration of thrombolytics, and are most notable with streptokinase. Readministration of streptokinase to patients should be avoided for at least 4 years, and probably indefinitely, because of a high prevalence of neutralizing antibodies, and because there is a substantial risk for anaphylaxis upon reexposure to these drugs.

## Mechanical Reperfusion

### Percutaneous Coronary Intervention in ST Segment Elevation—Primary Percutaneous Coronary Intervention

The preferred contemporary method of achieving coronary reperfusion in the appropriately skilled facility is the use of immediate or "primary" PCI.

Many randomized controlled trials have compared pharmacologic and mechanical reperfusion during STEMI. A metaanalysis of the 23 such trials found that primary PCI was superior to thrombolytic therapy in reducing mortality, nonfatal reinfarction, stroke, and the combined endpoint of death, nonfatal reinfarction, and stroke (187). The benefits of PCI in reducing mortality and recurrent MI were particularly striking.

At this time, only 20% to 25% of hospitals have primary PCI capabilities. Therefore, hospitals that do *not* have PCI capabilities can either treat patients with STEMI with immediate thrombolysis, or emergently transfer them to a site where PCI can be performed. Recent clinical trials have evaluated as to which strategy is superior in such a situation. The DANAMI-2 (DANish trial in Acute Myocardial Infarction 2) (188), PRAGUE-2 (Primary Angioplasty in patients transferred from General community hospitals to specialized PTCA Units with or without Emergency thrombolysis) (189) and Air PAMI (Air Primary Angioplasty in Myocardial Infarction) (190) trials show a benefit for catheter-based reperfusion over on-site thrombolytic therapy with respect to the combined endpoint of death, reinfarction, or stroke. All three trials had a similar rate of adverse events in the PCI group (8% to 8.5%) and in the thrombolytic assigned group (13.5% to 15%), and demonstrated a 40% to 50% reduction of the combined endpoint.

In summary, whereas thrombolysis is more widely available, is simple to give, and produces results that are independent of operator experience, primary PCI in experienced hands is associated with less recurrent infarction and ischemia, lower short-term mortality, and less stroke and ICH than thrombolysis. PCI also results in higher early IRA patency rate and reduced residual stenosis, as compared with thrombolysis. The current ACC/AHA guidelines (see Table 97-5) recommend invasive strategy with PCI if a timely intervention can be performed, that is—if "door-to-balloon" time is less than 90 minutes, or if the delay to PCI as compared to on-site thrombolysis is less than 1 hour. Primary PCI is also generally preferred for patients in cardiogenic shock, those with contraindications to thrombolysis,

**TABLE 97-5**

**CHOICE OF REPERFUSION STRATEGY IN ST SEGMENT ELEVATION**

**FIBRINOLYSIS IS GENERALLY PREFERRED IF:**
- Early presentation (3 h or less from symptom onset and delay to invasive strategy: see subsequent text)
- Invasive strategy is not an option
Catheterization laboratory occupied/not available
Vascular access difficulties
Lack of access to a skilled PCI laboratory
- Delay to invasive strategy
Prolonged transport
(Door-to-balloon)—(door-to-needle) time is >1 h
Medical contact-to-balloon or door-to-balloon time is >90 min

**AN INVASIVE STRATEGY IS GENERALLY PREFERRED IF:**
- Skilled PCI laboratory available with surgical backup
Medical contact–to-balloon or door-to-balloon time <90 min
(Door-to-balloon)—(door-to-needle) is <1 h
- High risk from STEMI
Cardiogenic shock
Killip class ≥3
- Contraindications to fibrinolysis, including increased risk of bleeding and ICH
- Late presentation
Symptom onset was more than 3 h ago
- Diagnosis of STEMI is in doubt

PCI, percutaneous coronary intervention; STEMI, ST segment elevation myocardial infarction; ICH, intracranial hemorrhage.

and those in whom thrombolysis is unlikely to produce meaningful benefit (e.g., symptom onset is >3 hours before presentation).

### Intracoronary Stenting

Intracoronary stents have been shown early to reduce the risk of early reocclusion and restenosis when used for elective PCI, and subsequent trials have shown similar benefits, as well as a trend for decreased mortality at 6 months in STEMI (162). Primary stenting is now the preferred modality of percutaneous intervention for STEMI.

Recently, stents coated with antiproliferative agents have been introduced: These drug-eluting stents dramatically reduce rates of in-stent restenosis compared with traditional bare-metal stents in patients undergoing routine PCI. Within a short period, it is likely that drug-eluting stents will replace bare-metal stents in primary PCI.

### Routine Percutaneous Coronary Intervention after Successful Thrombolytic Therapy

TIMI 2B evaluated a *delayed* invasive versus conservative (catheterization and PTCA for spontaneous or inducible ischemia only) strategy following tPA administration. No differences in death or MI were seen between the two strategies through 3 years of follow-up, despite the fact that revascularization rates were twice as high in the invasive arm. The current AHA/ACC guideline recommendation is to reserve cardiac catheterization after *successful* thrombolytic therapy to patients with spontaneous or inducible ischemia, or those with significantly reduced left ventricular function (with "viable" myocardium). Of note, however, more recent observational studies have shown a lower rate of mortality in patients undergoing routine PCI after thrombolysis versus those managed conservatively (184). The recent GRACIA (Grupo de Análisis de la Cardiopatía Isquémica Aguda) randomized trial of 500 patients confirmed the benefit with significantly lower mortality at 1 year with routine PCI following thrombolysis as compared with standard care (192). Therefore, it may be reasonable to perform catheterization in other high-risk patients who may benefit from revascularization, including those with prior MI and those with significant ventricular arrhythmias.

### Rescue Percutaneous Coronary Intervention

As mentioned previously, following administration of thrombolytic therapy, the IRA remains occluded in approximately 20% of patients, and coronary blood flow is abnormal in another 20% to 30% of patients. In such patients, urgent PCI following thrombolysis, or so-called rescue PCI, is frequently performed. Data to support rescue PCI in patients with persistent infarct artery occlusion are limited. Nevertheless, most moderate-to-high risk patients with persistent ST segment elevations and ongoing chest pain 90 to 120 minutes after the administration of thrombolytic therapy should probably undergo urgent angiography and PCI.

### Facilitated Percutaneous Coronary Intervention

Facilitated PCI refers to administration of pharmacologic reperfusion regimen en route to the cardiac catheterization laboratory for *primary* PCI. Justification for facilitated PCI has been provided by the observation that patients with STEMI who arrive in the catheterization laboratory with a patent IRA prior to PCI are at an extremely low risk for mortality. It has been shown before that thrombolytics and GP IIb/IIIa inhibitors, or their combination, increase the probability of early reperfusion (see preceding text). Finally, it is known that initially successful thrombolysis, but *not* primary PCI, is associated with significant rates of reocclusion

and reinfarction. Hence, administration of a pharmacologic reperfusion regimen *prior* to primary PCI may increase the probability of reperfusion prior to PCI, thereby "facilitating" an excellent long-term result of PCI.

In a recent small Bavarian Reperfusion Alternatives Evaluation (BRAVE) trial (193), patients with STEMI were randomized to receive the combination of half-dose rPA plus abciximab, or abciximab alone prior to undergoing primary PCI. Patients who received combination therapy had higher coronary patency rates at the time of initial angiography than those treated with abciximab alone (40% vs. 18%), but the angiographic benefits did not translate into smaller infarct size, as measured by nuclear scintigraphy. In addition, bleeding rates were significantly higher in the combination thrombolytic plus GP IIb/IIIa inhibitor group than in the monotherapy group. Other trials, including TIMI 14 (194), Glycoprotein Receptor Antagonist Patency Evaluation (GRAPE) (195), and TIrofiban Given in the Emergency Room before Primary Angioplasty (TIGER PA) (196) have supported the notion that GP IIb/IIIa inhibitors alone may be the best facilitation strategy before PCI because they improve patency rates prior to primary PCI, do not increase the rate of ICH, and may improve microvascular perfusion after PCI (197).

## Revascularization in Non–ST Elevation Acute Coronary Syndrome: Invasive Versus Conservative Strategy

An overall treatment plan for NSTEACS involves stabilization of a ruptured plaque, prevention of recurrent thrombosis with intensive antiplatelet and antithrombin therapy, and treatment of ongoing ischemia. Following initial therapy, two principal strategies are employed: invasive strategy involving routine cardiac catheterization, with revascularization if feasible, and a conservative strategy where angiography and revascularization are reserved for patients who have evidence of recurrent ischemia either at rest or on provocative testing. Several adequately sized clinical trials have so far compared invasive and conservative strategies in patients with NSTEACS (17,83,118, 198–202). All trials except for VANQWISH (Veterans Affairs Non-Q-Wave Infarction Strategies in Hospitals) (198) demonstrated an advantage to early invasive therapy in patients at moderate or high risk of death, MI, or CHF. In fact, data from the ISAR-COOL (Intracoronary Stenting with Antithrombotic Regimen Cooling-off) study recently found a benefit of an *immediate* invasive strategy with an average time to catheterization of 2 hours, compared with a delayed invasive strategy (average time to catheterization 4 days) (202). An added benefit of an early invasive strategy is its cost-effectiveness: $13,000 to $17,000 per life year saved, even in low-risk patients (203).

As shown in the preceding text, it is clear that unlike STEMI, where the primary goal is always immediate reperfusion, the choice of strategy in NSTEACS depends on an individual patient's risk of major adverse cardiac events. In general, high-risk features in NSTEACS include recurrent ischemia, marked ST segment deviations, elevated levels of cardiac biomarkers, heart failure, or ventricular arrhythmia (see Table 97-6). There are several convenient risk assessment tools in NSTEACS, the most widely utilized of which is the TIMI Risk Score (see Table 97-7). In the TIMI 11B trial, the risk of death, MI, or severe ischemia was found to increase proportional to a higher TIMI risk score (TRS), from less than 5% for patients with TRS 0 to 1, to greater than 40% for those with TRS 6 to 7 (204). In addition to providing the means for assessing the patient's short-term risk of adverse events, the TIMI risk score defines benefit from specific interventions in NSTEACS. Patients with a high TIMI risk score

## TABLE 97-6

### INDICATORS OF INCREASED RISK IN PATIENTS WITH NON–ST ELEVATION ACUTE CORONARY SYNDROME

1. Recurrent ischemia at rest or with minimal activity, despite intensive antiischemic therapy
2. Elevated serum troponin level
3. New ST segment depression or T-wave inversion
4. Recurrent ischemia with heart failure symptoms, an $S_3$ gallop, pulmonary edema, rales, or new mitral regurgitation
5. High-risk findings on noninvasive stress testing
6. LV ejection fraction <40%
7. Hemodynamic instability or angina at rest accompanied by hypotension
8. Sustained ventricular tachycardia
9. Percutaneous intervention within 6 mo
10. Prior coronary artery bypass graft surgery

LV, left ventricular.

($\geq$3) benefit from GP IIb/IIIA blockers (vs. placebo), LMWH (vs. UFH), and invasive (vs. conservative) management strategy.

# LONG-TERM SECONDARY PREVENTION AFTER ACUTE CORONARY SYNDROME

Diagnosis of ACS is commonly perceived by patients as a "life-changing" event, and physicians and staff have an opportunity to provide teaching, as well as to optimize the medical regimen for long-term treatment (205). Discussion of risk-factor modification is crucial, and, for an individual patient, the discussion may include the importance of smoking cessation, achieving optimal weight, daily exercise, following appropriate diet, good blood pressure control, tight control of hyperglycemia in diabetics, and lipid level management.

## TABLE 97-7

### THROMBOLYSIS IN MYOCARDIAL INFARCTION RISK SCORE FOR UNSTABLE ANGINA NON–ST ELEVATION MYOCARDIAL INFARCTION

| | Points |
|---|---|
| ■ Age ≥65 yr | 1 |
| ■ Documented pilor coronary artery stenosis >50% | |
| ■ Three or more conventional cardiac risk factors (e.g., age, sex, family history, hyperlipidomia, diabetes, smoking, hypertension, and obesity) | 1 |
| ■ Use of aspirin in the preceding 24 h | 1 |
| ■ Two or more anginal events in the preceding 24 h | 1 |
| ■ ST segment deviation (transient elevation or persistent depression) | 1 |
| ■ Increased cardiac biomarkers | 1 |
| Risk score 5 total points | 0–7 |

From Antman EM, Cohen M, Bernink PJ, et al. The TIMI Risk Score for unstable angina\non–ST elevation MI: a method for prognostication and therapeutic decision making. *JAMA* 2000:284:835–842, with permission.

Five general classes of drugs have been shown in large randomized clinical trials to improve outcomes following ACS and are now recommended for long-term treatment. Each agent may contribute to long-term clinical stability in different ways: HMG-CoA reductase inhibitors (statins) (206,207), Tonkin 2000#641, and ACE inhibitors (59,208,209) may facilitate plaque stabilization, $\beta$-blockers are indicated for antiischemic therapy (39,210), and the combination of aspirin and clopidogrel administered for at least 1 year has also been shown to be beneficial (86,211) and decreases the severity of any thrombosis in case of plaque rupture.

## References

1. American Heart Association. Heart and stroke statistical update: American Heart Association 2004 (*in press*). Available at http://www.americanheart.org/presenter.jhtml?identifier=3000090. Accessed on July 7, 2005.
2. The TIMI IIIA Investigators. Early effects of tissue-type plasminogen activator added to conventional therapy on the culprit lesion in patients presenting with ischemic cardiac pain at rest. Results of the Thrombolysis in Myocardial Ischemia (TIMI IIIA) Trial. *Circulation* 1993;87:38–52.
3. Cannon CP, Weintraub WS, Demopoulos LA, et al. Comparison of early invasive and conservative strategies in patients with unstable coronary syndromes treated with the glycoprotein IIb/IIIa inhibitor tirofiban. *N Engl J Med* 2001;344(25):1879–1887.
4. Fox KA, Goodman SG, Klein W, et al. Management of acute coronary syndromes. Variations in practice and outcome; findings from the Global Registry of Acute Coronary Events (GRACE). *Eur Heart J* 2002;23(15):1177–1189.
5. Davies MJ. The composition of coronary-artery plaques. *N Engl J Med* 1997;336:1312–1314.
6. Harrington RA, Califf RM, Holmes DR Jr, et al. Is all unstable angina the same? Insights from the Coronary Angioplasty Versus Excisional Atherectomy Trial (CAVEAT-I). *Am Heart J* 1999;137(2):227–233.
7. Silva JA, White CJ, Collins TJ, et al. Morphologic comparison of atherosclerotic lesions in native coronary arteries and saphenous vein grafts with intracoronary angioscopy in patients with unstable angina. *Am Heart J* 1998;136(1):156–163.
8. Nesto RW, Waxman S, Mittleman MA, et al. Angioscopy of culprit coronary lesions in unstable angina pectoris and correlation of clinical presentation with plaque morphology. *Am J Cardiol* 1998;81(2):225–228.
9. Kennon S, Price CP, Mills PG, et al. The central role of platelet activation in determining the severity of acute coronary syndromes. *Heart* 2003;89(10):1253–1254.
10. Serebruany VL, Glassman AH, Malinin AI, et al. Enhanced platelet/endothelial activation in depressed patients with acute coronary syndromes: evidence from recent clinical trials. *Blood Coagul Fibrinolysis* 2003;14(6):563–567.
11. Merlini PA, Ardissino D, Bauer KA, et al. Persistent thrombin generation during heparin therapy in patients with acute coronary syndromes. *Arterioscler Thromb Vasc Biol* 1997;17(7):1325–1330.

12. Theroux P, Ouimet H, McCans J, et al. Aspirin, heparin or both to treat unstable angina. *N Engl J Med* 1988;319:1105–1111.

13. Oler A, Whooley MA, Oler J, et al. Adding heparin to aspirin reduces the incidence of myocardial infarction and death in patients with unstable angina. A meta-analysis. *JAMA* 1996;276:811–815.

14. Cohen M, Demers C, Gurfinkel EP, et al. A comparison of low-molecular-weight heparin with unfractionated heparin for unstable coronary artery disease. *N Engl J Med* 1997;337:447–452.

15. Antman EM, McCabe CH, Gurfinkel EP, et al. Enoxaparin prevents death and cardiac ischemic events in unstable angina/non-Q-wave myocardial infarction: results of the Thrombolysis In Myocardial Infarction (TIMI) 11B trial. *Circulation* 1999;100(15):1593–1601.

16. The PURSUIT Trial Investigators. Inhibition of platelet glycoprotein IIb/IIIa with eptifibatide in patients with acute coronary syndromes. *N Engl J Med* 1998;339:436–443.

17. The Platelet Receptor Inhibition for Ischemic Syndrome Management (PRISM) Study Investigators. A comparison of aspirin plus tirofiban with aspirin plus heparin for unstable angina. *N Engl J Med* 1998;338:1498–1505.

18. The Platelet Receptor Inhibition for Ischemic Syndrome Management in Patients Limited by Unstable Signs and Symptoms (PRISM-PLUS) Trial Investigators. Inhibition of the platelet glycoprotein IIb/IIIa receptor with tirofiban in unstable angina and non-Q-wave myocardial infarction. *N Engl J Med* 1998;338:1488–1497.

19. Clopidogrel in Unstable Angina to Prevent Recurrent Events Trial Investigators. Effects of clopidogrel in addition to aspirin in patients with acute coronary syndromes without ST-segment elevation. *N Engl J Med* 2001;345:494–502.

20. Storey RF, Newby LJ, Heptinstall S. Effects of P2Y(1) and P2Y(12) receptor antagonists on platelet aggregation induced by different agonists in human whole blood. *Platelets* 2001;12(7):443–447.

21. Prinzmetal M, Kennamer R, Merliss R, et al. A variant form of angina pectoris. *Am J Med* 1959;27:375–375.

22. Bottcher M, Botker HE, Sonne H, et al. Endothelium-dependent and -independent perfusion reserve and the effect of L-arginine on myocardial perfusion in patients with syndrome X. *Circulation* 1999;99(14):1795–1801.

23. Pitts WR, Lange RA, Cigarroa JE, et al. Cocaine-induced myocardial ischemia and infarction: pathophysiology, recognition, and management. *Prog Cardiovasc Dis* 1997;40(1):65–76.

24. Strike PC, Steptoe A. Systematic review of mental stress-induced myocardial ischaemia. *Eur Heart J* 2003;24(8):690–703.

25. Kaski JC. Rapid coronary artery disease progression and angiographic stenosis morphology. *Ital Heart J* 2000;1(1):21–25.

26. Braunwald E. Unstable angina: a classification. *Circulation* 1989;80:410–414.

27. Scirica BM, Cannon CP, McCabe CH, et al. Prognosis in the thrombolysis in myocardial ischemia III registry according to the braunwald unstable angina pectoris classification. *Am J Cardiol* 2002;90:821–826.

28. Hamm CW, Braunwald E. A classification of unstable angina – revisited. *Circulation* 2000;102:118–122.

29. Angeja BG, Gibson CM, Chin R, et al. Predictors of door-to-balloon delay in primary angioplasty. *Am J Cardiol* 2002;89(10):1156–1161.

30. Braunwald E, Antman EM, Beasley JW, et al. ACC/AHA guideline update for the management of patients with unstable angina and non-ST-segment elevation myocardial infarction-2002: summary article: a report of the American College of Cardiology/American Heart Association Task Force on Practice Guidelines (Committee on the Management of Patients with Unstable Angina). *Circulation* 2002;106(14):1893–1900.

31. Kerensky RA, Wade M, Deedwania P, et al. Revisiting the culprit lesion in non-Q-wave myocardial infarction. Results from the VANQWISH trial angiographic core laboratory. *J Am Coll Cardiol* 2002;39(9):1456–1463.

32. Goldstein JA, Demetriou D, Grines CL, et al. Multiple complex coronary plaques in patients with acute myocardial infarction. *N Engl J Med* 2000;343(13):915–922.

33. Rioufol G, Finet G, Ginon I, et al. Multiple atherosclerotic plaque rupture in acute coronary syndrome: a three-vessel intravascular ultrasound study. *Circulation* 2002;106(7):804–808.

34. Zairis MN, Papadaki OA, Manousakis SJ, et al. C-reactive protein and multiple complex coronary artery plaques in patients with primary unstable angina. *Atherosclerosis* 2002;164(2):355–359.

35. Asakura M, Ueda Y, Yamaguchi O, et al. Extensive development of vulnerable plaques as a pan-coronary process in patients with myocardial infarction: an angioscopic study. *J Am Coll Cardiol* 2001;37(5):1284–1288.

36. Cheitlin MD, Hutter AM Jr, Brindis RG et al, American College of Cardiology/American Heart Association. ACC/AHA expert consensus document. Use of sildenafil (Viagra) in patients with cardiovascular disease. *J Am Coll Cardiol* 1999;33(1):273–282.

37. Gruppo Italiano per lo Studio della Sopravvivenza nell'Infarto Miocardico. GISSI-3: effect of lisinopril and trasdermal glyceryl trinitrate singly and together on 6-week mortality and ventricular function after acute myocardial infarction. *Lancet* 1994;343:1115–1122.

38. ISIS-4 Collaborative Group. ISIS-4: randomized factorial trial assessing early oral captopril, oral mononitrate, and intravenous magnesium sulphate in 58,050 patients with suspected acute myocardial infarction. *Lancet* 1995;345:669–685.

39. Yusuf S, Peto R, Lewis J, et al. Beta-blockade during and after myocardial infarction: an overview of the randomized trials. *Prog Cardiovasc Dis* 1985;27:335–371.

40. Gottlieb SO, Weisfeldt ML, Ouyang P, et al. Effect of the addition of propranolol to therapy with nifedepine for unstable angina: a randomized, double-blind, placebo-controlled trial. *Circulation* 1986;73:331–337.

41. The Holland Interuniversity Nifedipine/Metoprolol Trial (HINT) Research Group. Early treatment of unstable angina in the coronary care unit: a randomised, double blind, placebo controlled comparison of recurrent ischaemia in patients treated with nifedipine or metoprolol or both. *Br Heart J* 1986;56(5):400–413.

42. Theroux P, Taeymans Y, Morissette D, et al. A randomized study comparing propranolol and diltiazem in the treatment of unstable angina. *J Am Coll Cardiol* 1985;5(3):717–722.

43. Foody JM, Farrell MH, Krumholz HM. Beta-blocker therapy in heart failure: scientific review. *JAMA* 2002;287(7):883–889.

44. Gibson RS, Boden WE, Theroux P, et al. Diltiazem and reinfarction in patients with non-Q wave myocardial infarction. Results of a double-blind, randomized, multicenter trial. *N Engl J Med* 1986;315:423–429.

45. Theroux P, Gregoire J, Chin C, et al. Intravenous diltiazem in acute myocardial infarction. Diltiazem as adjunctive therapy to activase (DATA) trial. *J Am Coll Cardiol* 1998;32(3):620–628.

46. Boden WE, van Gilst WH, Scheldewaert RG, et al. Diltiazem in acute myocardial infarction treated with thrombolytic agents: a randomised placebo-controlled trial. Incomplete Infarction Trial of European Research Collaborators Evaluating Prognosis post-Thrombolysis (INTERCEPT). *Lancet* 2000;355(9217):1751–1756.

47. The Danish Study Group on Verapamil in Myocardial Infarction. Effect of verapamil on mortality and major events after acute infarction (The Danish Verapamil Infarction Trial II-DAVIT II). *Am J Cardiol* 1990;66:779.

48. Yusuf S, Wittes J, Friedman L. Overview of results of randomized clinical trials in heart disease. II. Unstable angina, heart failure, primary prevention with aspirin and risk factor reduction. *JAMA* 1988;260:2259–2263.

49. Hennekens CH, Albert CM, Godfried SL, et al. Adjunctive drug therapy of acute myocardial infarction–evidence from clinical trials. *N Engl J Med* 1996;335:1660–1667.

50. The Multicenter Diltiazem Postinfarction Trial Research Group. The effect of diltiazem on mortality and reinfarction after myocardial infarction. *N Engl J Med* 1988;319:385–392.

51. Wilcox RG, Hampton JR, Banks DC, et al. Trial of early nifedepine in acute myocardial infarction: the TRENT study. *BMJ* 1986;293:1204–1208.

52. Packer M, O'Connor CM, Ghali JK, et al. Effect of amlodipine on morbidity and mortality in severe chronic heart failure. *N Engl J Med* 1996;335(15):1107–1114.

53. Cohn JN, Ziesche S, Smith R et al, Vasodilator-Heart Failure Trial (V-HeFT) Study Group. Effect of the calcium antagonist felodipine as supplementary vasodilator therapy in patients with chronic heart failure treated with enalapril: V-HeFT III. *Circulation* 1997;96(3):856–863.

54. Pfeffer MA, Braunwald E, Moye LA, et al. Effect of captopril on mortality and morbidity in patients with left ventricular dysfunction after myocardial infarction. *N Engl J Med* 1992;327:669–677.

55. Kober L, Torp-Pedersen C, Carlsen JE et al, Trandolapril Cardiac Evaluation (TRACE) Study Group. A clinical trial of the angiotensin-converting-enzyme inhibitor trandolapril in patients with left ventricular dysfunction after myocardial infarction. *N Engl J Med* 1995;333(25):1670–1676.

56. The Acute Infarction Ramipril Efficacy (AIRE) Study Investigators. Effect of ramipril on mortality and morbidity of survivors of acute myocardial infarction with clinical evidence of heart failure. *Lancet* 1993;342:821–828.

57. Chinese Cardiac Study Collaborative Group. Oral captopril versus placebo among 13,634 patients with suspected myocardial infarction: interim report from the Chinese Cardiac Study(CCS-1). *Lancet* 1995;345:686–687.

58. Yusuf S, Sleight P, Pogue J, et al. Effects of an angiotensin-converting-enzyme inhibitor, ramipril, on cardiovascular events in high-risk patients. *N Engl J Med* 2000;342(3):145–153; [published erratum appears in *N Engl J Med* 2000;342(10):748].

59. Fox KM. Efficacy of perindopril in reduction of cardiovascular events among patients with stable coronary artery disease: randomised, double-blind, placebo-controlled, multicentre trial (the EUROPA study). *Lancet* 2003;362(9386):782–788.

60. Pfeffer MA, McMurray JJ, Velazquez EJ, et al. Valsartan, captopril, or both in myocardial infarction complicated by heart failure, left ventricular dysfunction, or both. *N Engl J Med* 2003;349(20):1893–1906.

61. Pitt B, Remme W, Zannad F, et al. Eplerenone, a selective aldosterone blocker, in patients with left ventricular dysfunction after myocardial infarction. *N Engl J Med* 2003;348(14):1309–1321.

62. Scandinavian Simvastatin Survival Study Group. Randomised trial of cholesterol lowering in 4444 patients with coronary heart disease: the Scandinavian Simvastatin Survival Study (4S). *Lancet* 1994;344:1383–1389.

63. The Long-Term Intervention with Pravastatin in Ischaemic Disease (LIPID) Study Group. Prevention of cardiovascular events and death with pravastatin in patients with coronary heart disease and a broad range of initial cholesterol levels. *N Engl J Med* 1998;339(19):1349–1357.

64. Heart Protection Study Collaborative Group. MRC/BHF Heart Protection Study of antioxidant vitamin supplementation in 20,536 high-risk individuals: a randomised placebo-controlled trial. *Lancet* 2002;360(9326):23–33.

65. Pedersen TR, Kjekshus J, Berg K et al, Results of the Scandinavian Simvastatin Survival Study. Cholesterol lowering and the use of healthcare resources. *Circulation* 1996;93:1796–1802.

66. Grundy SM, et al. Executive Summary of The Third Report of The National Cholesterol Education Program (NCEP) Expert Panel on Detection,

Evaluation, And Treatment of High Blood Cholesterol In Adults (Adult Treatment Panel III). *JAMA* 2001;285(19):2486–2497.

67. Arntz HR, Agrawal R, Wunderlich W, et al. Beneficial effects of pravastatin (+/−colestyramine/niacin) initiated immediately after a coronary event (the randomized Lipid-Coronary Artery Disease [L-CAD] Study). *Am J Cardiol* 2000;86(12):1293–1298.

68. Liem AH, van Boven AJ, Veeger NJ, et al. Effect of fluvastatin on ischaemia following acute myocardial infarction: a randomized trial. *Eur Heart J* 2002;23(24):1931–1937.

69. Aronow HD, Topol EJ, Roe MT, et al. Effect of lipid-lowering therapy on early mortality after acute coronary syndromes: an observational study. *Lancet* 2001;357(9262):1063–1068.

70. Stenestrand U, Wallentin L. Early statin treatment following acute myocardial infarction and 1-year survival. *JAMA* 2001;285(4):430–436.

71. De Lemos JA, Blazing MA, Wiviott SD, et al. Early intensive vs a delayed conservative simvastatin strategy in patients with acute coronary syndromes: phase Z of the A to Z trial. *JAMA* 2004;292:1307–1316.

72. ISIS-2 (Second International Study of Infarct Survival) Collaborative Group. Randomised trial of intravenous streptokinase, oral aspirin, both, or neither among 17,187 cases of suspected acute myocardial infarction: ISIS-2. *Lancet* 1988;2:349–360.

73. Antithrombotic Trialists' Collaboration. Collaborative meta-analysis of randomised trials of antiplatelet therapy for prevention of death, myocardial infarction, and stroke in high risk patients. *BMJ* 2002;324(7329):71–86.

74. The RISC Group. Risk of myocardial infarction and death during treatment with low dose aspirin and intravenous heparin in men with unstable coronary artery disease. *Lancet* 1990;336:827–830.

75. Topol EJ, Easton D, Harrington RA, et al. Randomized, double-blind, placebo-controlled, international trial of the oral IIb/IIIa antagonist lotrafiban in coronary and cerebrovascular disease. *Circulation* 2003;108(4):399–406.

76. Peters RJ, Mehta SR, Fox KA, et al. Effects of aspirin dose when used alone or in combination with clopidogrel in patients with acute coronary syndromes: observations from the Clopidogrel in Unstable angina to prevent Recurrent Events (CURE) study. *Circulation* 2003;108:1682–1687.

77. Eikelboom JW, Hirsh J, Weitz JI, et al. Aspirin-resistant thromboxane biosynthesis and the risk of myocardial infarction, stroke, or cardiovascular death in patients at high risk for cardiovascular events. *Circulation* 2002;105(14):1650–1655.

78. Gum PA, Kottke-Marchant K, Welsh PA, et al. A prospective, blinded determination of the natural history of aspirin resistance among stable patients with cardiovascular disease. *J Am Coll Cardiol* 2003;41(6):961–965.

79. Gum PA, Kottke-Marchant K, Poggio ED, et al. Profile and prevalence of aspirin resistance in patients with cardiovascular disease. *Am J Cardiol* 2001;88(3):230–235.

80. Goto S, Tamura N, Eto K, et al. Functional significance of adenosine 5′-diphosphate receptor (P2Y(12)) in platelet activation initiated by binding of von willebrand factor to platelet GP ibalpha induced by conditions of high shear rate. *Circulation* 2002;105(21):2531–2536.

81. Balsano F, Rizzon P, Violi F, et al. Antiplatelet treatment with ticlopidine in unstable angina: a controlled multicenter clinical trial. *Circulation* 1990;82:17–26.

82. Leon MB, Baim DS, Popma JJ et al, Stent Anticoagulation Restenosis Study Investigators. A clinical trial comparing three antithrombotic-drug regimens after coronary-artery stenting. *N Engl J Med* 1998;339(23):1665–1671.

83. Bennett CL, Weinberg PD, Rozenberg-Ben-Dror K, et al. Thrombotic thrombocytopenic purpura associated with ticlopidine. A review of 60 cases. *Ann Intern Med* 1998;128(7):541–544.

84. Steinhubl SR, Tan WA, Foody JM, et al, EPISTENT Investigators. Incidence and clinical course of thrombotic thrombocytopenic purpura due to ticlopidine following coronary stenting. *JAMA* 1999;281(9):806–810.

85. CAPRIE Steering Committee. A randomised, blinded, trial of clopidogrel versus aspirin in patients at risk of ischaemic events (CAPRIE). *Lancet* 1996;348:1329–1339.

86. Steinhubl SR, Berger PB, Mann JT III, et al. Early and sustained dual oral antiplatelet therapy following percutaneous coronary intervention: a randomized controlled trial. *JAMA* 2002;288(19):2411–2420.

87. Bertrand ME, Rupprecht HJ, Urban P et al, CLASSICS Investigators. Double-blind study of the safety of clopidogrel with and without a loading dose in combination with aspirin compared with ticlopidine in combination with aspirin after coronary stenting: the clopidogrel aspirin stent international cooperative study (CLASSICS). *Circulation* 2000;102: 624–629.

88. Taniuchi M, Kurz HI, Lasala JM. Randomized comparison of ticlopidine and clopidogrel after intracoronary stent implantation in a broad patient population. *Circulation* 2001;104(5):539–543.

89. Bhatt DL, Bertrand ME, Berger PB, et al. Meta-analysis of randomized and registry comparisons of ticlopidine with clopidogrel after stenting. *J Am Coll Cardiol* 2002;39(1):9–14.

90. Yusuf S, Zhao F, Mehta SR, et al. Effects of clopidogrel in addition to aspirin in patients with acute coronary syndromes without ST-segment elevation. *N Engl J Med* 2001;345(7):494–502.

91. Mehta SR, Yusuf S, Peters RJ, et al. Effects of pretreatment with clopidogrel and aspirin followed by long-term therapy in patients undergoing percutaneous coronary intervention: the PCI-CURE study. *Lancet* 2001; 358(9281):527–533.

92. Helft G, Osende JI, Worthley SG, et al. Acute antithrombotic effect of a front-loaded regimen of clopidogrel in patients with atherosclerosis on aspirin. *Arterioscler Thromb Vasc Biol* 2000;20(10):2316–2321.

93. Savcic M, Hauert J, Bachmann F, et al. Clopidogrel loading dose regimens: kinetic profile of pharmacodynamic response in healthy subjects. *Semin Thromb Hemost* 1999;25(Suppl. 2):15–19.

94. Muller I, Seyfarth M, Rudiger S, et al. Effect of a high loading dose of clopidogrel on platelet function in patients undergoing coronary stent placement. *Heart* 2001;85(1):92–93.

95. Neumann F *Intracoronary stenting and antithrombotic regimen rapid early action for coronary treatment (ISAR REACT).* Chicago, IL: American College of Cardiology Scientific Sessions, 2003.

96. Muller I, Besta F, Schulz C, et al. Prevalence of clopidogrel non-responders among patients with stable angina pectoris scheduled for elective coronary stent placement. *Thromb Haemost* 2003;89(5):783–787.

97. Jaremo P, Lindahl TL, Fransson SG, et al. Individual variations of platelet inhibition after loading doses of clopidogrel. *J Intern Med* 2002;252(3):233–238.

98. Gurbel PA, Bliden KP, Hiatt BL, et al. Clopidogrel for coronary stenting: response variability, drug resistance, and the effect of pretreatment platelet reactivity. *Circulation* 2003;107(23):2908–2913.

99. Theroux P, Waters D, Qiu S, et al. Aspirin versus heparin to prevent myocardial infarction during the acute phase of unstable angina. *Circulation* 1993;88:2045–2048.

100. Cohen M, Adams PC, Parry G, et al. Combination antithrombotic therapy in unstable rest angina and non-Q-wave infarction in nonprior aspirin users. Primary end points analysis from the ATACS trial. *Circulation* 1994;89:81–88.

101. Califf RM, White HD, Van der Werf F, et al. One-year results from the Global Utilization of Streptokinase and TPA for occluded coronary arteries (GUSTO-I) trial. *Circulation* 1996;94:1233–1238.

102. Young E, Prins M, Levine MN, et al. Heparin binding to plasma proteins, an important mechanism for heparin resistance. *Thromb Haemost* 1992;67:639–643.

103. Hirsh J, Anand SS, Halperin JL, et al. Guide to anticoagulant therapy: heparin: a statement for healthcare professionals from the American Heart Association. *Circulation* 2001;103(24):2994–3018.

104. Cruikshank MK, Levine MN, Hirsh J, et al. A standard nomogram for the management of heparin therapy. *Arch Intern Med* 1991;151:333–337.

105. Flaker GC, Bartolozzi J, Davis V, et al. Use of a standardized nomogram to achieve therapeutic anticoagulation after thrombolytic therapy in myocardial infarction. *Arch Intern Med* 1994;154:1492–1496.

106. Anand SS, Yusuf S, Pogue J, et al. Relationship of activated partial thromboplastin time to coronary events and bleeding in patients with acute coronary syndromes who receive heparin. *Circulation* 2003;107(23):2884–2888.

107. Tracy RP, Kleiman NS, Thompson B, et al. Relation of coagulation parameters to patency and recurrent ischemia in the Thrombolysis in Myocardial Infarction (TIMI) phase II trial. *Am Heart J* 1998;135:29–37.

108. Granger CB, Hirsh J, Califf RM, et al. Activated partial thromboplastin time and outcome after thrombolytic therapy for acute myocardial infarction: results from the GUSTO-I trial. *Circulation* 1996;93:870–878.

109. The Assessment of the Safety and Efficacy of a New Thrombolytic regimen (ASSENT) 3 investigators. Efficacy and safety of tenecteplase in combination with enoxaparin, abciximab, or unfractionated heparin: the ASSENT-3 randomised trial in acute myocardial infarction. *Lancet* 2001; 358(9282):605–613.

110. Antman EM, Louwerenburg HW, Baars HF, et al. Enoxaparin as adjunctive antithrombin therapy for ST-elevation myocardial infarction: results of the ENTIRE-thrombolysis in myocardial infarction (TIMI) 23 trial. *Circulation* 2002;105(14):1642–1649.

111. Wallentin L, Goldstein P, Armstrong PW, et al. Efficacy and safety of tenecteplase in combination with the low-molecular-weight enoxaparin or unfractionated heparin in the prehospital setting: the Assessment of the Safety and Efficacy of a New Thrombolytic Regimen (ASSENT)-3 PLUS randomized trial in acute myocardial infarction. *Circulation* 2003;108(2):135–142.

112. Petersen JL, Mahaffey KW, Hasselblad V, et al. Efficacy and bleeding complications among patients randomized to enoxaparin or unfractionated heparin for antithrombin therapy in non-ST-Segment elevation acute coronary syndromes: a systematic overview. *JAMA* 2004;292(1):89–96.

113. Cohen M, Theroux P, Borzak S, et al. Randomized double-blind safety study of enoxaparin versus unfractionated heparin in patients with non-ST-segment elevation acute coronary syndromes treated with tirofiban and aspirin: the ACUTE II study. The Antithrombotic Combination Using Tirofiban and Enoxaparin. *Am Heart J* 2002;144(3):470–477.

114. Goodman SG, Fitchett D, Armstrong PW, et al. Randomized evaluation of the safety and efficacy of enoxaparin versus unfractionated heparin in high-risk patients with non-ST-segment elevation acute coronary syndromes receiving the glycoprotein IIb/IIIa inhibitor eptifibatide. *Circulation* 2003;107:238–244.

115. Blazing MA. *The A-to-Z trial: results of the A-phase, investigating combined use of low-molecular-weight heparin with the glycoprotein IIb/IIIa inhibitor tirofiban.* Chicago, IL: American College of Cardiology Scientific Sessions, 2003.

116. Ferguson JJ, Califf RM, Antman EM, et al. Enoxaparin vs unfractionated heparin in high-risk patients with non-ST-segment elevation acute coronary syndromes managed with an intended early invasive strategy: primary results of the SYNERGY randomized trial. *JAMA* 2004;292(1):45–54.

117. Klein W, Buchwald A, Hillis SE, et al. Comparison of low-molecular-weight heparin with unfractionated heparin acutely and with placebo for

6 weeks in the management of unstable coronary artery disease. Fragmin in Unstable Coronary Artery Disease Study (FRIC). *Circulation* 1997; 96:61–68.

118. FRagmin and Fast Revascularisation during InStability in Coronary Artery Disease Investigators. Invasive compared with non-invasive treatment in unstable coronary artery disease: FRISC II prospective randomised multicentre study. *Lancet* 1999;354(9180):708–715.

119. The FRAX.I.S. Study Group. Comparison of two treatment durations (6 days and 14 days) of a LMWH with a 6-day treatment of unfractionated heparin in the initial management of unstable angina or non-Q wave myocardial infarction: FRAX.I.S. (FRAxiparine in Ischaemic Syndrome). *Eur Heart J* 1999;20(21):1553–1562.

120. Morrow DA, Antman EM, Tanasijevic M, et al. Cardiac troponin I for stratification of early outcomes and the efficacy of enoxaparin in unstable angina: a TIMI 11B substudy. *J Am Coll Cardiol* 2000;36:1812–1817.

121. Blazing MA, de Lemos JA, White HD, et al. Safety and efficacy of enoxaparin vs unfractionated heparin in patients with non-ST-segment elevation acute coronary syndromes who receive tirofiban and aspirin: a randomized controlled trial. *JAMA* 2004;292(1):55–64.

122. Moliterno DJ, Hermiller JB, Kereiakes DJ et al, Results of the Evaluating Enoxaparin Clotting Times (ELECT) Study. A novel point-of-care enoxaparin monitor for use during percutaneous coronary intervention. *J Am Coll Cardiol* 2003;42(6):1132–1139.

123. Saw J, Kereiakes DJ, Mahaffey KW, et al. Evaluation of a novel point-of-care enoxaparin monitor with central laboratory anti-Xa levels. *Thromb Res* 2003;112(5-6):301–306.

124. Eriksson BI, Bauer KA, Lassen MR, et al. Fondaparinux compared with enoxaparin for the prevention of venous thromboembolism after hip-fracture surgery. *N Engl J Med* 2001;345(18):1298–1304.

125. The Global Use of Strategies to Open Occluded Coronary Arteries (GUSTO) IIb Investigators. A comparison of recombinant hirudin with heparin for the treatment of acute coronary syndromes. *N Engl J Med* 1996;335:775–782.

126. Organisation to Assess Strategies for Ischemic Syndromes (OASIS-2) Investigators. Effects of recombinant hirudin (lepirudin) compared with heparin on death, myocardial infarction, refractory angina, and revascularisation procedures in patients with acute myocardial ischaemia without ST elevation: a randomised trial. *Lancet* 1999;353(9151):429–438.

127. Kong DF, Topol EJ, Bittl JA, et al. Clinical outcomes of bivalirudin for ischemic heart disease. *Circulation* 1999;100(20):2049–2053.

128. Bittl JA, Strony J, Brinker JA, et al. Treatment with bivalirudin (Hirulog) as compared with heparin during coronary angioplasty for unstable or post-infarction angina. *N Engl J Med* 1995;333:764–769.

129. Lincoff AM, Bittl JA, Harrington RA, et al. Bivalirudin and provisional glycoprotein IIb/IIIa blockade compared with heparin and planned glycoprotein IIb/IIIa blockade during percutaneous coronary intervention: REPLACE-2 randomized trial. *JAMA* 2003;289(7):853–863.

130. Antman EM, TIMI 9B Investigators. Hirudin in acute myocardial infarction: Thrombolysis and Thrombin Inhibition in Myocardial Infarction (TIMI) 9B trial. *Circulation* 1996;94:911–921.

131. The Global Use of Strategies to Open Occluded Coronary Arteries (GUSTO) IIb Investigators. A comparison of recombinant hirudin with heparin for the treatment of acute coronary syndromes. *N Engl J Med* 1996;335(11):775–782.

132. White H. Thrombin-specific anticoagulation with bivalirudin versus heparin in patients receiving fibrinolytic therapy for acute myocardial infarction: the HERO-2 randomised trial. *Lancet* 2001;358(9296):1855–1863.

133. The Organization to Assess Strategies for Ischemic Syndromes (OASIS) Investigators. Effects of long-term, moderate-intensity oral anticoagulation in addition to aspirin in unstable angina. *J Am Coll Cardiol* 2001; 37(2):475–484.

134. Fiore LD, Ezekowitz MD, Brophy MT, et al. Department of veterans affairs cooperative studies program clinical trial comparing combined warfarin and aspirin with aspirin alone in survivors of acute myocardial infarction: primary results of the CHAMP study. *Circulation* 2002;105(5):557–563.

135. Coumarin Aspirin Reinfarction Study (CARS) Investigators. Randomised double-blind trial of fixed low-dose warfarin with aspirin after myocardial infarction. *Lancet* 1997;350:389–396.

136. Anand SS, Yusuf S, OASIS Investigators. Randomized trial of oral anticoagulation therapy in patient with acute ischemic syndromes without ST elevation: importance of good compliance. *J Am Coll Cardiol* 1999;33 (Suppl. A):396A.

137. van Es RF, Jonker JJ, Verheugt FW, et al. Aspirin and coumadin after acute coronary syndromes (the ASPECT-2 study): a randomised controlled trial. *Lancet* 2002;360(9327):109–113.

138. Hurlen M, Abdelnoor M, Smith P, et al. Warfarin, aspirin, or both after myocardial infarction. *N Engl J Med* 2002;347(13):969–974.

139. Brouwer MA, van den Bergh PJ, Aengevaeren WR, et al. Aspirin plus coumarin versus aspirin alone in the prevention of reocclusion after fibrinolysis for acute myocardial infarction: results of the Antithrombotics in the Prevention of Reocclusion In Coronary Thrombolysis (APRICOT)-2 Trial. *Circulation* 2002;106(6):659–665.

140. Loh E, Sutton MS, Wun CC, et al. Ventricular dysfunction and the risk of stroke after myocardial infarction. *N Engl J Med* 1997;336:251–257.

141. The CAPTURE Investigators. Randomised placebo-controlled trial of abciximab before and during coronary intervention in refractory unstable angina: the CAPTURE study. *Lancet* 1997;349:1429–1435; [published erratum appears in *Lancet* 1997;350:744].

142. Boersma E, Harrington RA, Moliterno DJ, et al. Platelet glycoprotein IIb/IIIa inhibitors in acute coronary syndromes: a meta-analysis of all major randomised clinical trials. *Lancet* 2002;359:189–198.

143. van den Brand M, Laarman GJ, Steg PG, et al. Assessment of coronary angiograms prior to and after treatment with abciximab, and the outcome of angioplasty in refractory unstable angina patients. Angiographic results from the CAPTURE trial. *Eur Heart J* 1999;20(21):1572–1578.

144. Zhao X-Q, Theroux P, Snapinn SM et al, PRISM-PLUS Investigators. Intracoronary thrombus and platelet glycoprotein IIb/IIIa receptor blockade with tirofiban in unstable angina or non-Q-wave myocardial infarction. Angiographic results from the PRISM-PLUS trial (Platelet Receptor Inhibition for Ischemic Syndrome Management in Patients Limited by Unstable Signs and Symptoms). *Circulation* 1999;100: 1609–1615.

145. Bhatt DL, Topol EJ. Current role of platelet glycoprotein IIb/IIIa inhibitors in acute coronary syndromes. *JAMA* 2000;284(12):1549–1558.

146. The GUSTO IV-ACS Investigators. Effect of glycoprotein IIb/IIIa receptor blocker abciximab on outcome in patients with acute coronary syndromes without early coronary revascularisation: the GUSTO IV-ACS randomised trial. *Lancet* 2001;357(9272):1915–1924.

147. Roffi M, Chew DP, Mukherjee D, et al. Platelet glycoprotein IIb/IIIa inhibitors reduce mortality in diabetic patients with non-ST-segment-elevation acute coronary syndromes. *Circulation* 2001;104(23):2767–2771.

148. Hamm CW, Heeschen C, Goldmann B, et al. Benefit of abciximab in patients with refractory unstable angina in relation to serum troponin T levels. *N Engl J Med* 1999;340(21):1623–1629.

149. Heeschen C, Hamm CW, Goldmann B, et al. Troponin concentrations for stratification of patients with acute coronary syndromes in relation to therapeutic efficacy of tirofiban. *Lancet* 1999;354(9192):1757–1762.

150. Newby LK, Ohman EM, Christenson RH, et al. Benefit of glycoprotein IIb/IIIa inhibition in patients with acute coronary syndromes and troponin t-positive status: the PARAGON-B troponin T substudy. *Circulation* 2001;103(24):2891–2896.

151. Januzzi JL, Chai CU, Sabatine MS, et al. Elevation in serum troponin I predicts the benefit of tirofiban. *J Thromb Thrombolysis* 2001;11:211–215.

152. Morrow DA, Antman EM, Snapinn SM, et al. An integrated clinical approach to predicting the benefit of tirofiban in non-ST elevation acute coronary syndromes: application of the TIMI risk score for UA/NSTEMI in PRISM-PLUS. *Eur Heart J* 2002;23:223–229.

153. Wong GC, Morrow DA, Murphy S, et al. Elevations in troponin T and I are associated with abnormal tissue level perfusion: A TACTICS-TIMI 18 substudy. *Circulation* 2002;106(2):202–207.

154. Heeschen C, van Den Brand MJ, Hamm CW, et al. Angiographic findings in patients with refractory unstable angina according to troponin T status. *Circulation* 1999;100(14):1509–1514.

155. Topol EJ, Yadav JS. Recognition of the importance of embolization in atherosclerotic vascular disease. *Circulation* 2000;101(5):570–580.

156. The ESPRIT Investigators. Novel dosing regimen of eptifibatide in planned coronary stent implantation (ESPRIT): a randomised, placebo-controlled trial. *Lancet* 2000;356(9247):2037–2044.

157. The EPISTENT Investigators. Randomised placebo-controlled and balloon-angioplasty-controlled trail to assess the safety of coronary stenting with use of platelet glycoprotein-IIb/IIIa blockade. *Lancet* 1998;352:87–92.

158. Roffi M, Chew D, Mukherjee D, et al. Platelet glycoprotein IIb/IIIa inhibition in acute coronary syndromes. Gradient of benefit related to the revascularization strategy. *Eur Heart J* 2002;23(18):1441.

159. Boersma E, Akkerhuis KM, Theroux P, et al. Platelet glycoprotein IIb/IIIa receptor inhibition in non-ST-elevation acute coronary syndromes: early benefit during medical treatment only, with additional protection during percutaneous coronary intervention. *Circulation* 1999;100(20):2045–2048.

160. Marso SP, Bhatt DL, Roe MT, et al. Enhanced efficacy of eptifibatide administration in patients with acute coronary syndrome requiring in-hospital coronary artery bypass grafting. *Circulation* 2000;102(24):2952–2958.

161. Montalescot G, Barragan P, Wittenberg O, et al. Platelet glycoprotein IIb/IIIa inhibition with coronary stenting for acute myocardial infarction. *N Engl J Med* 2001;344(25):1895–1903.

162. Stone GW, Grines CL, Cox DA, et al. Comparison of angioplasty with stenting, with or without abciximab, in acute myocardial infarction. *N Engl J Med* 2002;346(13):957–966.

163. Berkowitz SD, Sane DC, Sigmon KN et al, Evaluation of c7E3 for the Prevention of Ischemic Complications (EPIC) Study Group. Occurrence and clinical significance of thrombocytopenia in a population undergoing high-risk percutaneous coronary revascularization. *J Am Coll Cardiol* 1998;32(2):311–319.

164. Mahaffey KW, Harrington RA, Simoons ML, et al. Stroke in patients with acute coronary syndromes: incidence and outcomes in the Platelet glycoprotein IIb/IIIa in Unstable angina Receptor suppression using integrilin therapy (PURSUIT). *Circulation* 1999;99(18):2371–2377.

165. O'Neill WW, Serruys P, Knudtson M, et al. Long-term treatment with a platelet glycoprotein-receptor antagonist after pecutaneous coronary revascularization. *N Engl J Med* 2000;342:1316–1324.

166. Cannon CP, McCabe CH, Wilcox RG, et al. Oral glycoprotein IIb/IIIa inhibition with orbofiban in patients with unstable coronary syndromes (OPUS-TIMI 16) trial. *Circulation* 2000;102:149–156.

167. The SYMPHONY Investigators. Comparison of sibrafiban with aspirin for prevention of cardiovascular events after acute coronary syndromes: a randomised trial. *Lancet* 2000;355(9201):337–345.

168. Second Symphony Investigators. Randomized trial of aspirin, sibrafiban, or both for secondary prevention after acute coronary syndromes. *Circulation* 2001;103(13):1727–1733.

169. Cannon CP, McCabe CH, Borzak S, et al. A randomized trial of an oral platelet glycoprotein IIb/IIIa antagonist, sibrafiban, in patients after an acute coronary syndrome: results of the TIMI 12 trial. *Circulation* 1998; 97:340–349.

170. Nannizzi-Alaimo L, Alves VL, Phillips DR. Inhibitory effects of glycoprotein IIb/IIIa antagonists and aspirin on the release of soluble CD40 ligand during platelet stimulation. *Circulation* 2003;107(8):1123–1128.

171. Andre P, Nannizzi-Alaimo L, Prasad SK, et al. Platelet-derived CD40L: the switch-hitting player of cardiovascular disease. *Circulation* 2002; 106(8):896–899.

172. Peter K, Schwarz M, Ylanne J, et al. Induction of fibrinogen binding and platelet aggregation as a potential intrinsic property of various glycoprotein IIb/IIIa ($\alpha_{IIb}\beta_3$) inhibitors. *Blood* 1998;92:3240–3249.

173. Serrano CV Jr, Nicolau JC, Venturinelli M, et al. Role of oral blockade of platelet glycoprotein IIb/IIIa on neutrophil-platelet interactions in patients with acute coronary syndromes. *Cardiovasc Drugs Ther* 2003;17: 129–132.

174. Fibrinolytic Therapy Trialists' (FTT) Collaborative Group. Indications for fibrinolytic therapy in suspected acute myocardial infarction: collaborative overview of early mortality and major morbidity results from all randomised trials of more than 1000 patients. *Lancet* 1994;343(8893):311–322.

175. Gruppo Italiano per lo Studio della Streptochinasi nell'Infarto Miocardico (GISSI). Effectiveness of intravenous thrombolytic treatment in acute myocardial infarction. *Lancet* 1986;1:397–402.

176. TIMI Study Group. The Thrombolysis in Myocardial Infarction (TIMI) Trial; Phase I findings. *N Engl J Med* 1985;312:932–936.

177. Antman EM, Cohen M, Radley D, et al. Assessment of the treatment effect of enoxaparin for unstable angina/non-Q-wave myocardial infarction: TIMI 11B-ESSENCE meta-analysis. *Circulation* 1999;100:1602–1608.

178. de Lemos JA, Antman EM, Gibson CM, et al. Abciximab improves both epicardial flow and myocardial reperfusion in ST-elevation myocardial infarction: observations from the TIMI 14 trial. *Circulation* 2000;101: 239–243.

179. Hermann HC, Moliterno DJ, Bode C, et al. Combination abciximab and reduced-dose reteplase facilitates early PCI in acute MI: results from the SPEED trial. *Circulation* 1999;100(Suppl. I):I–188.

180. Giugliano RP, Roe MT, Harrington RA, et al. Combination reperfusion therapy with eptifibatide and reduced-dose tenecteplase for ST-elevation myocardial infarction: results of the integrilin and tenecteplase in acute myocardial infarction (INTEGRITI) phase II angiographic trial. *J Am Coll Cardiol* 2003;41(8):1251–1260.

181. Topol EJ. Reperfusion therapy for acute myocardial infarction with fibrinolytic therapy or combination reduced fibrinolytic therapy and platelet glycoprotein IIb/IIIa inhibition: the GUSTO V randomised trial. *Lancet* 2001;357(9272):1905–1914.

182. The TIMI IIIB Investigators. Effects of tissue plasminogen activator and a comparison of early invasive and conservative strategies in unstable angina and non-Q-wave myocardial infarction: results of the TIMI IIIB trial. *Circulation* 1994;89:1545–1556.

183. Braunwald E, Mark DB, Jones RH, et al. *Unstable angina: diagnosis and management*, Clinical Practice Guideline Number 10. Rockville, MD: Agency for Health Care Policy and Research and the National Heart, Lung, and Blood Institute, Public Health Service, U.S. Department of Health and Human Services, 1994.

184. Gibson CM, Karha J, Murphy SA, et al. Early and long-term clinical outcomes associated with reinfarction following fibrinolytic administration in the Thrombolysis in Myocardial Infarction trials. *J Am Coll Cardiol* 2003;42(1):7–16.

185. Eagle KA, Goodman SG, Avezum A, et al. Practice variation and missed opportunities for reperfusion in ST-segment-elevation myocardial infarction: findings from the Global Registry of Acute Coronary Events (GRACE). *Lancet* 2002;359(9304):373–377.

186. Berger AK, Schulman KA, Gersh BJ, et al. Primary coronary angioplasty vs thrombolysis for the management of acute myocardial infarction in elderly patients. *JAMA* 1999;282(4):341–348.

187. Keeley EC, Boura JA, Grines CL. Primary angioplasty versus intravenous thrombolytic therapy for acute myocardial infarction: a quantitative review of 23 randomised trials. *Lancet* 2003;361(9351):13–20.

188. Andersen HR, Nielsen TT, Rasmussen K, et al. A comparison of coronary angioplasty with fibrinolytic therapy in acute myocardial infarction. *N Engl J Med* 2003;349(8):733–742.

189. Widimsky P, Budesinsky T, Vorac D, et al. Long distance transport for primary angioplasty vs immediate thrombolysis in acute myocardial infarction. Final results of the randomized national multicentre trial—PRAGUE-2. *Eur Heart J* 2003;24(1):94–104.

190. Grines CL, Westerhausen DR Jr, Grines LL, et al. A randomized trial of transfer for primary angioplasty versus on-site thrombolysis in patients with high-risk myocardial infarction: the air primary angioplasty in myocardial Infarction study. *J Am Coll Cardiol* 2002;39(11):1713–1719.

191. Antman EM, Anbe DT, Armstrong PW, et al. ACC/AHA guidelines for the management of patients with ST-elevation myocardial infarction—executive summary: a report of the American College of Cardiology/American Heart Association Task Force on Practice Guidelines (Writing Committee to Revise the 1999 Guidelines for the Management of Patients With Acute Myocardial Infarction).*Circulation* 2004;110(5):588–636.

192. Fernandez-Aviles F, Alonso JJ, Castro-Beiras A, et al. Routine invasive strategy within 24 hours of thrombolysis versus ischaemia-guided conservative approach for acute myocardial infarction with ST-segment elevation (GRACIA-1): a randomised controlled trial. *Lancet* 2004;364(9439): 1045–1053.

193. Kastrati A, Mehilli J, Schlotterbeck K, et al. Early administration of reteplase plus abciximab vs abciximab alone in patients with acute myocardial infarction referred for percutaneous coronary intervention: a randomized controlled trial. *JAMA* 2004;291(8):947–954.

194. Antman EM, Giugliano RP, Gibson CM et al, The TIMI 14 Investigators. Abciximab facilitates the rate and extent of thrombolysis: results of the thrombolysis in myocardial infarction (TIMI) 14 trial. *Circulation* 1999; 99(21):2720–2732.

195. van den Merkhof LF, Zijlstra F, Olsson H et al, Results of the Glycoprotein Receptor Antagonist Patency Evaluation (GRAPE) Pilot Study. Abciximab in the treatment of acute myocardial infarction eligible for primary percutaneous transluminal coronary angioplasty. *J Am Coll Cardiol* 1999;33(6):1528–1532.

196. Lee DP, Herity NA, Hiatt BL, et al. Adjunctive platelet glycoprotein IIb/IIIa receptor inhibition with tirofiban before primary angioplasty improves angiographic outcomes: results of the TIrofiban Given in the Emergency Room before Primary Angioplasty (TIGER-PA) pilot trial. *Circulation* 2003;107(11):1497–1501.

197. Montalescot G, Borentain M, Payot L, et al. Early vs late administration of glycoprotein IIb/IIIa inhibitors in primary percutaneous coronary intervention of acute ST-segment elevation myocardial infarction: a meta-analysis. *JAMA* 2004;292(3):362–366.

198. Boden WE, O'Rourke RA, Crawford MH, et al. Outcomes in patients with acute non-Q-wave myocardial infarction randomly assigned to an invasive as compared with a conservative strategy. *N Engl J Med* 1998;338: 1785–1792.

199. McCullough PA, O'Neill WW, Graham M, et al. A prospective randomized trial of triage angiography in acute coronary syndromes ineligible for thrombolytic therapy. Results of the medicine versus angiography in thrombolytic exclusion (MATE) trial. *J Am Coll Cardiol* 1998;32(3): 596–605.

200. Spacek R, Widimsky P, Straka Z et al, The VINO Study. Value of first day angiography/angioplasty in evolving non-ST segment elevation myocardial infarction: an open multicenter randomized trial. *Eur Heart J* 2002; 23(3):230–238.

201. Fox KA, Poole-Wilson PA, Henderson RA, et al. Interventional versus conservative treatment for patients with unstable angina or non-ST-elevation myocardial infarction: the British Heart Foundation RITA 3 randomised trial. Randomized intervention trial of unstable angina. *Lancet* 2002; 360(9335):743–751.

202. Harrington RA. Antithrombotic therapy and the invasive cardiac catheterization management strategy: the intracoronary stenting with antithrombotic regimen cooling-off trial. *Curr Cardiol Rep* 2004;6(4):271.

203. Mahoney EM, Jurkovitz CT, Chu H, et al. Cost and Cost-Effectiveness of an Early Invasive versus Conservative Strategy for the Treatment of Unstable Angina and non-ST Elevation Myocardial Infarction. *JAMA* 2002;288(15):1851–1858.

204. Antman EM, Cohen M, Bernink PJ, et al. The TIMI risk score for unstable angina/non-ST elevation MI: a method for prognostication and therapeutic decision making. *JAMA* 2000;284:835–842.

205. Fonarow GC. In-hospital initiation of statins: taking advantage of the "teachable moment." *Cleve Clin J Med* 2003;70(6):502, 4–6.

206. Heart Protection Study Collaborative Group. MRC/BHF heart protection study of cholesterol lowering with simvastatin in 20 536 high-risk individuals: a randomised placebo controlled trial. *Lancet* 2002;360:7–22.

207. Schwartz GG, Olsson AG, Ezekowitz MD, et al. Effects of atorvastatin on early recurrent ischemic events in acute coronary syndromes: the MIRACL study: a randomized controlled trial. *JAMA* 2001;285(13):1711–1718.

208. Rutherford JD, Pfeffer MA, Moye LA, et al. Effects of captopril on ischemic events after myocardial infarction. Results of the survival and ventricular enlargement trial. *Circulation* 1994;90:1731–1738.

209. Heart Outcomes Prevention Evaluation Study Investigators. Effects of ramipril on cardiovascular and microvascular outcomes in people with diabetes mellitus: results of the HOPE study and MICRO-HOPE substudy. *Lancet* 2000;355(9200):253–259.

210. Shivkumar K, Schultz L, Goldstein S, et al. Effects of propanolol in patients entered in the beta-blocker heart attack trial with their first myocardial infarction and persistent electrocardiographic ST-segment depression. *Am Heart J* 1998;135(2 Pt 1):261–267.

211. Yusuf S, Mehta SR, Zhao F, et al. Early and late effects of clopidogrel in patients with acute coronary syndromes. *Circulation* 2003;107(7):966–972.

# CHAPTER 98 ■ ANTITHROMBOTIC THERAPY FOR PERCUTANEOUS CORONARY INTERVENTION

GREGORY R. GIUGLIANO, AMIR LOTFI, AND DANIEL I. SIMON

Percutaneous coronary intervention (PCI) is performed in approximately 1 million patients yearly in the United States and has supplanted coronary artery bypass graft (CABG) as the primary revascularization strategy in patients with ischemic heart disease. Over the last quarter century, steady advances in PCI have included breakthroughs in device technology [e.g., drug-eluting stents (DES), rheolytic thrombectomy, and embolic protection devices], and refinements in adjunctive pharmacology [e.g., glycoprotein IIb/IIIa (GP IIb/IIIa) inhibitors, and thienopyridine class of adenosine 5′-diphosphate (ADP) receptor blockers] have led to striking improvements in procedural success, safety, and durability (see Fig. 98-1). Major adverse cardiovascular events (MACE) as a result of acute ischemic complications, including death, myocardial infarction (MI), and the need for urgent revascularization, occur in less than 7% of even higher risk interventions. Restenosis, the major long-term limitation of balloon angioplasty and bare metal stenting that led to repeat revascularization procedures in 20% to 30% of patients within 6 to 8 months, has been reduced to less than 5% with DES. These improved clinical outcomes are the direct result of a multitude of prospective, randomized clinical trials. This chapter focuses on evidence-based recommendations for antithrombotic therapy during PCI based on clinical presentation (see Tables 98-1 and 98-2).

## ASPIRIN

### Aspirin: Mechanism of Action

Acetylsalicylic acid (ASA) is one of the most valuable medications used in cardiovascular medicine today. ASA exerts its effect primarily by interfering with the biosynthesis of cyclic prostanoids [e.g., thromboxane $A_2$ ($TxA_2$) and prostacyclin]. Prostanoids are generated by the enzymatically catalyzed oxidation of arachidonic acid. By irreversibly inhibiting cyclooxygenase (COX), ASA blocks platelet synthesis of $TxA_2$, a humoral mediator which promotes platelet aggregation (1). ASA may also inhibit thrombosis by acetylation of guanosine triphosphate (GTP) binding proteins, thrombin receptors, and prothrombin (2).

### Acetylsalicylic Acid: Pharmacology/Pharmacokinetics

ASA results in a measurable inhibition of platelet function within 60 minutes because of its rapid absorption in the upper gastrointestinal tract (3). The plasma half-life of ASA is 20 minutes

and peak plasma levels occur 30 to 40 minutes after ingestion. Ingestion of enteric-coated ASA delays absorption with peak plasma levels at 3 to 4 hours (4).

The optimal dose of ASA for the primary or secondary prevention of cardiovascular disease or during PCI is not firmly established. Well-designed randomized trials have shown that ASA is an effective antithrombotic agent when used in dosages ranging between 50 and 100 mg per day, and there is a suggestion that it is effective in dosages as low as 30 mg per day. ASA in an oral dosage of 75 mg per day was shown to be effective in reducing the risk of myocardial infarction and death from unstable angina (5) and chronic stable angina (6). When given in combination with other anticoagulant (warfarin) or antiplatelet (thienopyridines) agents, the ASA dose should be lowered to 80 to 100 mg on the basis of a *post hoc* analysis of data from the Clopidogrel in Unstable angina to prevent Recurrent Events (CURE) study in which similar efficacy, but less major bleeding was seen in the low-dose (<100 mg) ASA group (7). The results of biochemical studies on its mechanism of action, the lack of dose-response relation in clinical studies evaluating its antithrombotic effects, and the dose dependence of its side effects all support the use of low-dose ASA. It is of clinical importance that the concomitant use of nonsteroidal antiinflammatory drugs (NSAIDs) may inhibit the clinical benefits of ASA (8), possibly secondary to the fact that ASA and NSAIDs compete for a common docking site on COX-1 (9). For patients using NSAIDs intermittently, a dose of ASA taken immediately before a single NSAID dose may counteract this inhibition. However, if NSAIDs are taken regularly, the effect of ASA on platelets is inhibited and is not overcome by the preadministration of ASA (10).

### Aspirin in Coronary Artery Disease and Percutaneous Coronary Intervention

ASA is a cornerstone treatment of coronary artery disease. There are four randomized trials demonstrating beneficial effects of ASA in patients with unstable angina and non–ST segment elevation myocardial infraction (NSTEMI), with approximately 50% reductions in the risk of death or MI (5,11–13). The Swedish angina pectoris ASA trial, in which 2,035 patients were allocated to receive 75 mg ASA daily or placebo (6), showed that ASA therapy led to considerable reductions in death and MI among patients with unstable angina (46% reduction), among those undergoing coronary angioplasty (53% reduction), and in those with stable angina (33% reduction).

In the setting of acute ST segment elevation myocardial infarction (STEMI), ASA was found to decrease the rate of angiographic reocclusion by more than 50% in a metaanalysis of

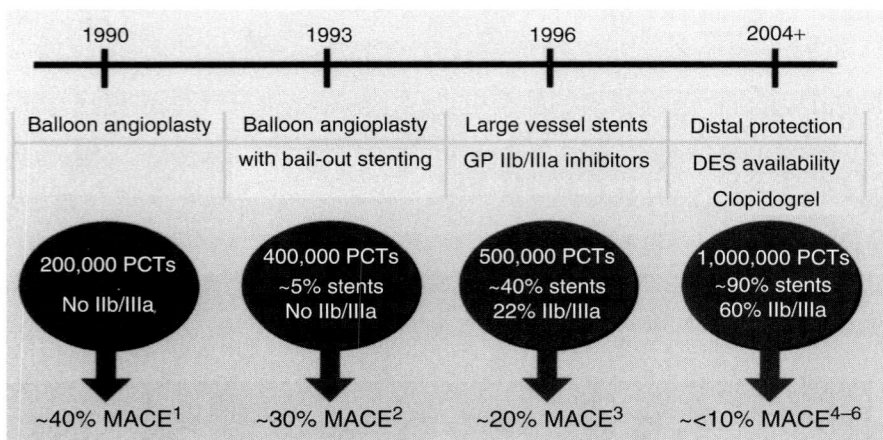

**FIGURE 98-1.** Evolution of percutaneous coronary intervention (PCI) techniques and adjunctive pharmacologic therapy improved patient outcomes over time. MACE = 30-day death, myocardial infarction, urgent target vessel revascularization. DES, diethylstilbestrol. References: [1]EPIC, *N Eng J Med* 1994;330:956–961; [2]IMPACT *Lancet* 1997;349:1422–1428; [3]EPISTENT *Lancet* 1998;352:7–92; [4]TARGET *N Eng J Med* 2001;344:1888–1894; [5]Sirius *N Eng J Med* 2003;349:1315–1323; [6]Taxus IV *N Eng J Med* 2004;350:221–231.

---

**TABLE 98-1**

## ANTITHROMBOTIC REGIMENS FROM RANDOMIZED CLINICAL TRIALS STRATIFIED BY CLINICAL PRESENTATION

| Clinical presentation | % Patients ACC/NCDR $n = 158,367$ | UFH + IIb/IIIa inhibitor | Bivalirudin | LMWH ± IIb/IIIa inhibitor | UFH + clopidogrel |
|---|---|---|---|---|---|
| STEMI | 13.9% | RAPPORT | HORIZON (pending) | None | None |
| | | ISAR-2 ADMIRAL CADILLAC TITAN–TIMI 34 (enrolling) | | | |
| NSTEMI | 14.6% | CAPTURE PRISM/PRISM–PLUS | BAT ACUITY (enrolling) | INTERACT A–Z | ISAR–REACT-2 |
| | | PURSUIT PARAGON A/B | | SYNERGY CRUISE | |
| UA | 38.4% | CAPTURE PRISM/PRISM–PLUS | BAT ACUITY (enrolling) | INTERACT A–Z | ISAR–REACT-2 |
| | | PURSUIT PARAGON A/B | | SYNERGY | |
| Elective PCI or low-risk ACS | 33.1% | EPILOG EPISTENT ESPRIT | REPLACE-2 | CRUISE | ISAR–REACT |

ACC, American College of Cardiology; UFH, unfractionated heparin; LMWH, low-molecular-weight heparin; STEMI, ST segment elevation myocardial infraction; RAPPORT, ReoPro and Primary PTCA Organization and Randomized Trial; ISAR, Intracoronary Stenting with Antithrombotic Regimen; TIMI, Thrombolysis in Myocardial Infarction; NSTEMI, non–ST segment elevation myocardial infraction; CAPTURE, C73 Antiplatelet Therapy in Unstable Refractory angina; PRISM-PLUS, Platelet Receptor Inhibition in Ischemic Syndrome Management in Patients Limited by Unstable Signs and Symptoms; BAT, Bivalirudin Angioplasty Trial; INTERACT, Integrilin and Enoxaparin Randomized Assessment of Acute Coronary Syndrome Treatment; A–Z, Aggrastat to Zocor; PURSUIT, Platelet GP IIb/IIIa in Unstable Angina: Receptor Suppression Using Integrilin Therapy; PARAGON, Platelet IIb/IIIa Antagonist for the Reduction of Acute Coronary Syndrome Events in a Global Organization Network; SYNERGY, Superior Yield of the New strategy of Enoxaparin Revascularization Glycoprotein IIb/IIIa inhibitors; PCI, percutaneous coronary intervention; ACS, acute coronary syndrome; EPILOG, Evaluation in PTCA to Improve Long-term Outcome with abciximab GP IIb/IIIa blockade; EPISTENT, Evaluation of Platelet GP IIb/IIIa Inhibitor for Stenting; ESPIRIT, Enhanced Suppression of Platelet Receptor GP IIb/IIIa using Integrilin Therapy; REPLACE, Randomized Evaluation in PCI Linking Angiomax to Reduced Clinical Events; CRUISE, Coronary Revascularization Using Integrilin and Single Bolus Enoxaparin.

## TABLE 98-2

**ANTITHROMBOTIC REGIMENS FOR PERCUTANEOUS CORONARY INTERVENTION**

Aspirin, 81–325 mg at least 2 h prior to PCI
UFH using weight-adjusted dosing:
50–70 U/kg bolus (+GP IIb/IIIa) with ACT target 200–250 s
70–100 U/kg bolus (−GP IIb/IIIa) with ACT target 250–350 s
Bivalirudin 0.75 mg/kg bolus followed by 1.75 mg/kg/h
   infusion during PCI only
LMWH (enoxaparin)
0.5–0.75 mg/kg IV (+GP IIb/IIIa)
1.0 mg/kg IV (−GP IIb/IIIa)
Eptifibatide, 180 $\mu$/kg bolus × 2 (10 min apart) followed by
   2 $\mu$/kg/min infusion × 18 h post–PCI
Abciximab, 0.25 mg/kg IV bolus followed by
   0.125 $\mu$/kg/min infusion × 12 h post–PCI
Clopidogrel, 300–600 mg load, 75 mg daily
Ticlopidine, 500 mg load, 250 mg twice daily

PCI, percutaneous coronary intervention; UFH, unfractionated heparin; GP, glycoprotein; ACT, activated clotting time; LMWH, low-molecular-weight heparin.

32 angiographic trials (14). The Second International Study of Infarct Survival (ISIS-2) (15) is a landmark trial demonstrating the clinical benefit of ASA in STEMI. In this trial, 17,187 patients presenting within 24 hours of the onset of STEMI were randomized to receive intravenous streptokinase, 162.5 mg of ASA daily for 30 days, both, or neither. The patients receiving ASA therapy alone had a significant 23% reduction in vascular mortality and an approximately 50% reduction in the risk of nonfatal reinfarction and nonfatal stroke at the end of 5 weeks. This beneficial effect of aspirin occurred irrespective of whether heparin was given and occurred independently, albeit additively to the beneficial effect of streptokinase. Five studies examined the use of ASA in the primary prevention of cardiovascular disease. Among the 55,580 randomized patients (11,466 women), ASA was associated with a statistically significant 32% reduction in the risk of a first MI and significant 15% reduction in the risk of all-important vascular events (16).

ASA is recommended for patients who undergo CABG (17,18). CABG with saphenous vein grafts is associated with a 5% to 15% graft occlusion rate during the first postoperative month (19,20). When given in the immediate postoperative period, ASA decreases the rate of early thrombotic graft occlusion by approximately 50%, and continued ASA therapy for 1 year further decreases occlusive events (19,20). Although there does not appear to be an additional benefit of ASA in relation to long-term graft patency after 1 year of therapy (21), continued ASA therapy is required for secondary prevention of atherothrombotic events.

The benefits of ASA in reducing cardiovascular death, MI, and stroke in patients with CAD (22) has led to the near universal use of this medication for patients undergoing PCI. PCI with balloon angioplasty or intracoronary stenting results in local vascular trauma, with endothelial denudation and platelet and fibrin deposition, leading to a 3.5% to 8.6% risk of abrupt vessel closure or subacute thrombosis (23–25). The initial studies involving ASA in PCI included combined antiplatelet regimens with dipyridamole or ticlopidine. The combination of ASA and dipyridamole was shown to reduce the incidence of periprocedural MI during PCI by 77% compared to patients receiving placebo when administered 24 hours before angioplasty and continued for 4 to 7 months (26). Dipyridamole was shown to

provide no additional benefit beyond that conveyed by ASA alone during elective angioplasty (27). ASA has been shown to be effective in patients undergoing intracoronary stent placement, especially in combination with ticlopidine or clopidogrel (28–30). However, ASA does not reduce the rate of restenosis in patients undergoing angioplasty (26,31).

## Adverse Effects of Aspirin

In the Antithrombotic Trialists' Collaboration metaanalysis (22), the proportional increase in risk of a major extracranial bleed with antiplatelet therapy was approximately 60% [odds ratio (OR), 1.6, 1.4 to 1.8]. The proportional increase in fatal bleeds was not significantly different from that for nonfatal bleeds; however, only the excess of nonfatal bleeds was significant (1). In one small study, ASA (75 to 325 mg per day) was associated with considerable decrease in creatinine clearance, and decrease in uric acid excretion after 2 weeks of therapy in elderly patients (32).

## Aspirin Resistance

Several studies have suggested that a significant proportion of patients may not respond to ASA (33). This concept of ASA "nonresponsiveness" or "resistance" is based on variable definitions, including, among others, inability to protect against thrombotic complications, failure to cause prolongation of bleeding time, failure to inhibit platelet aggregation, or failure to inhibit platelet TxA$_2$ production. ASA resistance has been observed in 5% to 60% of patients (34–43). The precise mechanism of ASA resistance is unknown, but is likely multifactorial, including a host of cellular, clinical, and genetic factors (see Fig. 98-2) (44). Some patients may be able to generate TxA$_2$ despite usual therapeutic doses of ASA and therefore fail to benefit from ASA treatment (45). Higher doses of ASA than currently used may be required in some patients to overcome this resistance (46,47).

There is emerging clinical evidence that ASA resistance is associated with an increased risk of MACE. Using a variety of definitions of ASA resistance, five studies in patients with coronary, peripheral, and/or cerebrovascular disease have reported 1.8 to 10-fold increased risk of thrombotic events (35,40,43,48,49). Using a bedside point-of-care device, Wang et al. (50) reported the incidence of ASA nonresponsiveness (as assessed by the Ultegra Rapid Platelet Function Assay-ASA) in a prospective multicenter registry to be 23%, and determined a history of coronary artery disease to be associated with twice the odds of being a nonresponder [OR, 2.01; 95% confidence intervals (CI), 1.189 to 3.411; $P = 0.0009$]. This bedside assay is a quantitative test developed to aid in detecting platelet dysfunction caused by aspirin ingestion in citrated whole blood. ASA nonresponsiveness detected by this method appears to have important clinical implications in the PCI setting with a significant increased risk of periprocedural myocardial infarction in ASA nonresponsive compared to ASA sensitive patients (see Fig. 98-3) (51). Although the mechanism(s) of ASA resistance remain to be established, and additional outcome data are needed to confirm the link between ASA resistance and adverse cardiovascular outcomes, there is increasing evidence that monitoring and tailoring antiplatelet therapy in the individual patient may help optimize clinical outcomes.

## Aspirin-Allergic Patients

Allergic reactions to ASA include generalized urticaria, maculopapular rash, asthma, angioedema, and anaphylaxis. ASA

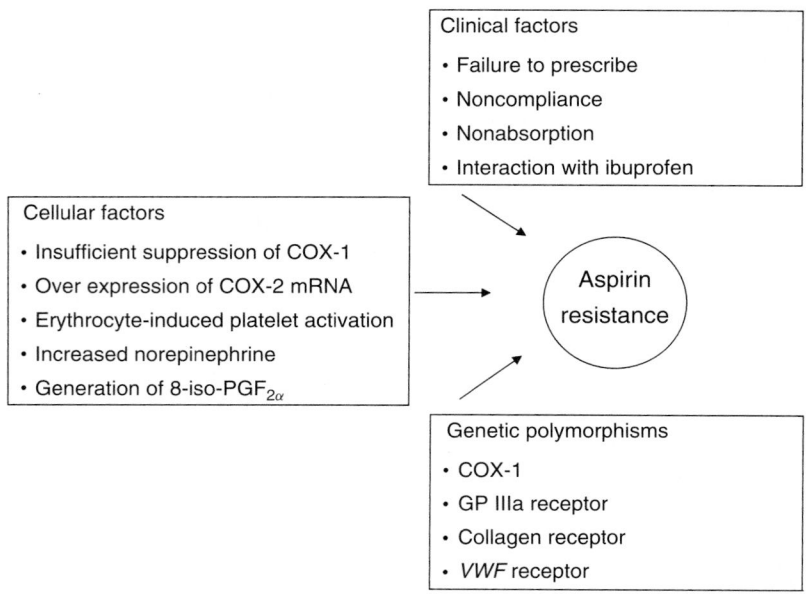

**FIGURE 98-2.** Possible mechanisms of acetylsalicylic acid resistance. COX, cyclooxygenase; GP, glycoprotein; VWF, von Willebrand factor. (Reprinted from Bhatt DL. Aspirin resistance: more than just a laboratory curiosity. *J Am Coll Cardiol* 2004;43:1127–1129.)

allergic patients with coronary disease undergoing PCI may be treated with a thienopyridine (e.g., clopidogrel) alone or in combination with cilostazol. Cilostazol, however, is contraindicated in patients with congestive heart failure. Some interventional cardiologists favor ASA desensitization using escalating doses of oral ASA challenge before known coronary interventions. This can be done safely and likely reduces the ischemic complications of PCI without ASA pretreatment (52–54).

## Recommendations for the Use of Acetylsalicylic Acid in Patients Undergoing Percutaneous Coronary Intervention

- For patients undergoing PCI, pretreatment with ASA, 75 to 325 mg is recommended (Grade 1A) (55).
- ASA, 75 to 162 mg per day is recommended for long-term treatment after PCI (Grade 1A) (55).

- For long-term treatment after PCI in patients who receive antithrombotic agents such as clopidogrel or warfarin, a lower-dose ASA, 75 to 100 mg per day is recommended (Grade 1C+) (55).

## THIENOPYRIDINES

### Thienopyridines: Mechanism of Action

The thienopyridine derivatives selectively and irreversibly inhibit the $P2Y_{12}$ ADP receptor, which plays a critical signaling role in orchestrating platelet activation and aggregation (56–58). Ticlopidine and clopidogrel both inhibit ADP-induced platelet activation (56,57,59,60) and, when given in combination with ASA, thienopyridines inhibit platelet aggregation to a greater extent than either agent alone (61).

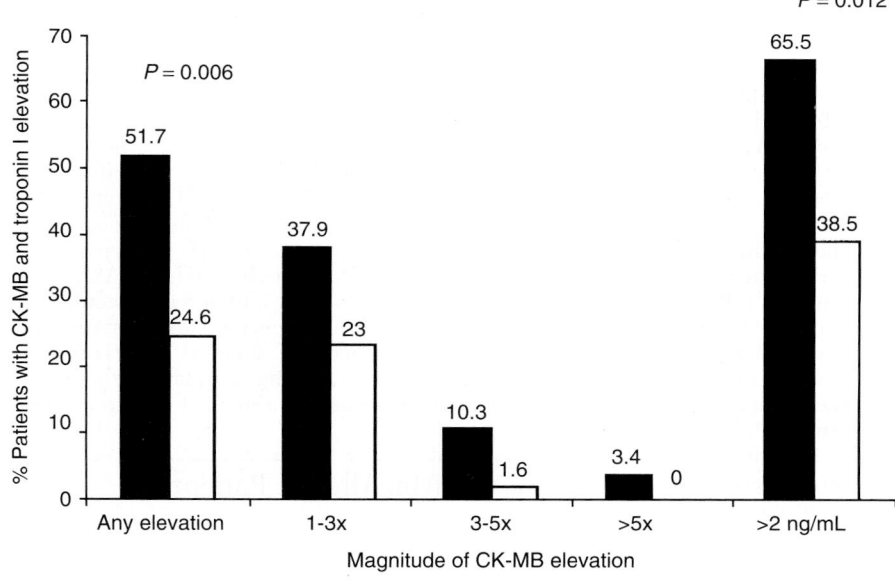

**FIGURE 98-3.** Incidence and magnitude of creatine kinase-myocardial band (CK-MB) and troponin I (TnI) elevation in aspirin-resistant (*black*) and aspirin-sensitive (*white*) patients after percutaneous coronary intervention (PCI). (Reprinted from Chen WH, Lee PY, Ng W, et al. Aspirin resistance is associated with a high incidence of myonecrosis after non-urgent percutaneous coronary intervention despite clopidogrel pretreatment. *J Am Coll Cardiol* 2004;43:1122–1126.)

## Thienopyridines: Pharmacodynamics/Pharmacokinetics

Clopidogrel differs structurally from ticlopidine with the addition of a carboxymethyl group. Ticlopidine and clopidogrel are inactive *in vitro* and are metabolized by hepatic cytochrome P-450-3A4 to produce active metabolites (62,63). Clopidogrel is six times more potent than ticlopidine and does not share any common metabolites with ticlopidine (64). The inhibition of platelet aggregation by ticlopidine and clopidogrel is concentration-dependent and significant inhibition is present after 2 to 3 days of therapy with ticlopidine 500 mg per day or clopidogrel 75 mg per day (65). Both ticlopidine and clopidogrel are irreversible inhibitors of platelet function that cannot be reversed by platelet transfusion. Platelet function recovers in 5 to 7 days after the discontinuation of clopidogrel therapy in healthy volunteers (66). Pretreatment with clopidogrel before PCI improves 30-day outcomes compared to those not pretreated (67–69), reducing death and MI by approximately 39% (69). To achieve the pretreatment benefit of early clopidogrel, patients must be treated for at least more than 6 hours, and likely more than 12 hours before PCI (68). Use of a 600-mg clopidogrel load may allow one to reduce the pretreatment period to as short as 2 hours before PCI (70). High-dose loading of clopidogrel pre-PCI is appealing, but carries an increased risk of bleeding in those patients who subsequently require CABG.

## Clopidogrel versus Ticlopidine

Four randomized clinical trials (71–74) have directly compared ticlopidine and clopidogrel in combination with ASA after stenting. Three (71,72,74) trials demonstrated that clopidogrel and ticlopidine have comparable efficacy in relation to cardiac events after stenting. However, the safety and tolerability of clopidogrel was superior to that of ticlopidine. A metaanalysis demonstrated that clopidogrel was associated with a significant reduction in the incidence of major adverse cardiac events (OR, 0.50; $P = 0.001$) and mortality (OR, 0.43; $P = 0.001$) compared with ticlopidine (75). One randomized trial demonstrated the superiority of ticlopidine over clopidogrel in stented patients in relation to the combined endpoint of death or MI (hazard ratio, 0.45; $P = 0.005$) (73). Ticlopidine has been virtually abandoned in the United States because of its increased risk of neutropenia.

## Thienopyridines in Percutaneous Coronary Intervention

The early experience with coronary stenting was notable for unacceptably high rates of subacute stent thrombosis, occurring

in 3% to 5% of patients and associated with myocardial infarction, need for urgent CABG, and/or death (57,76–78). Aggressive anticoagulation regimens (including intravenous heparin and dextran, warfarin, ASA, and dipyridamole) to minimize the risk of stent thrombosis led to frequent bleeding complications and prolonged hospitalizations (23,79–81).

Several studies have demonstrated a dramatic, approximately fivefold reduction in acute and subacute stent thrombosis when ASA in combination with a thienopyridine was used post-PCI compared with either ASA alone, warfarin, heparin, or long-term LMWH (29,82–86) (see Fig. 98-4).

The CURE study randomized 12,562 patients who presented within 24 hours of symptoms to receive clopidogrel 300-mg bolus, followed by 75 mg daily and ASA versus ASA and placebo (87). There was a significant reduction (9.3% vs. 11.4%, relative risk reduction 20%, $P < 0.001$) in the primary endpoint (death from cardiovascular cause, nonfatal myocardial infarction, or stroke) in the group receiving clopidogrel. The benefit with clopidogrel was noted early (within 24 hours of treatment), was sustained at 1-year, and observed in all patients with acute coronary syndromes (ACS) irrespective of their level of risk (88).

In a prespecified substudy (67) of CURE, patients ($n = 2,658$) who underwent PCI and were randomized to clopidogrel had a 31% relative risk reduction (RRR) in death and myocardial infarction compared to placebo-treated PCI patients. Furthermore, long-term (9 to 12 months) compared to short-term (4 weeks) clopidogrel therapy post-PCI was associated with a 31% lower rate of cardiovascular death, MI, or revascularization ($P = 0.03$).

The clopidogrel to reduce events during observation (CREDO) trial (68) extended the benefits of clopidogrel pretreatment and long-term therapy to a more stable population undergoing stenting. These patients were randomly assigned to receive a 300-mg clopidogrel loading dose or placebo, 3 to 24 hours before PCI, followed by clopidogrel 75 mg daily for 28 days post-PCI. Patients loaded with clopidogrel were continued on active drug from day 28 through 12 months and those patients in the control group received placebo. There was a significant 27% ($P = 0.02$) reduction in death, myocardial infarction, or stroke in patients receiving clopidogrel, suggesting that clopidogrel therapy in addition to ASA should be continued for a minimum of 9 months post-PCI.

In CURE, there was a significant increase in major bleeding in those receiving clopidogrel compared to placebo (3.7% vs. 2.7%, $P = 0.001$), and this was most notable in those patients requiring CABG (87). In contrast, CREDO showed only a trend toward more Thrombolysis in Myocardial Infarction (TIMI) major bleeding with clopidogrel compared to placebo (8.8% vs. 6.7%, $P = 0.07$), and no excess bleeds among patients undergoing CABG (68). These findings have led to the recommendation to delay elective CABG for 5 days after stopping clopidogrel. In addition, some clinicians prefer to

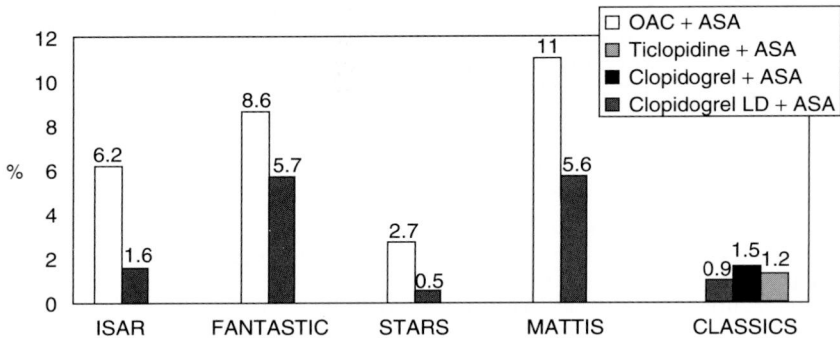

**FIGURE 98-4.** Comparison of MACE rates (%) in CLASSICS with those of ISAR, FANTASTIC, STARS, and MATTIS trials. OAC, oral anticoagulants; ASA, acetylsalicylic acid (aspirin); LD, loading dose. [Reprinted from Bertrand ME, Rupprecht HJ, Urban P, et al. Double-blind study of the safety of clopidogrel with and without a loading dose in combination with aspirin compared with ticlopidine in combination with aspirin after coronary stenting: the clopidogrel aspirin stent international cooperative study (CLASSICS). *Circulation* 2000; 102:624–629.]

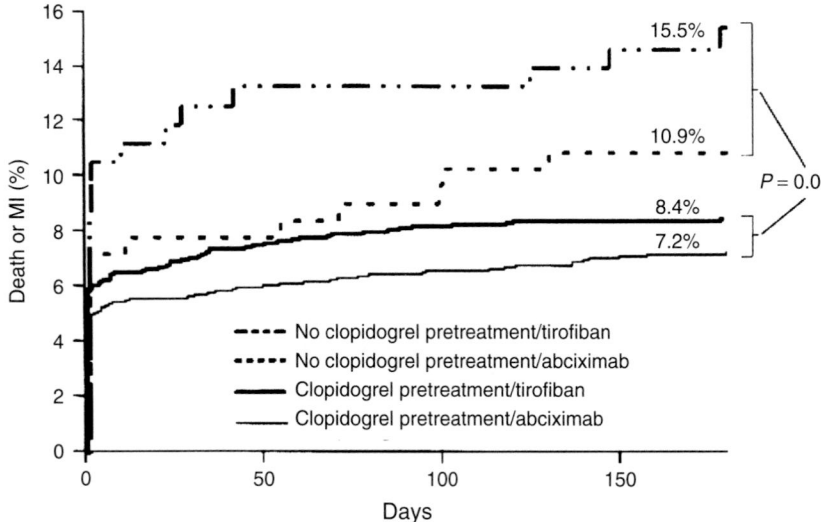

FIGURE 98-5. Pretreatment with clopidogrel in the TARGET study demonstrated a significant reduction in death or myocardial infarction (MI) irrespective of glycoprotein (GP) IIb/IIIa inhibitor therapy. [Reprinted from Chan AW, Moliterno DJ, Berger PB, et al. Triple antiplatelet therapy during percutaneous coronary intervention is associated with improved outcomes including one-year survival: results from the Do Tirofiban and ReoPro Give Similar Efficacy Outcome Trial (TARGET). *J Am Coll Cardiol* 2003;42:1188–1195.]

avoid preloading of clopidogrel in UA/NSTEMI patients until after the coronary anatomy is identified and the need for CABG excluded. However, it is important to emphasize that the risk-benefit of pretreatment needs to be established for each individual patient, recognizing the consistent and substantial benefit of clopidogrel pretreatment in reducing the risk of death and myocardial infarction (see Fig. 98-5), and estimating the likelihood of CABG given the fact that revascularization by PCI is more likely than CABG. Importantly, in PCI-CURE (67), there was no significant difference in major bleeding between the groups at 30 days (1.4% vs. 1.6%, $P = 0.69$) nor at the end of follow-up (2.5% vs. 2.7%, $P = 0.64$). The episodes of minor bleeding were greater in the clopidogrel group than the placebo group at the end of follow-up (2.1% vs. 3.5%, $P = 0.03$).

Although long-term (9 to 12 months) clopidogrel treatment post-PCI has been widely adopted and supported by clinicians (89,90) at this time on the basis of PCI-CURE and CREDO results, the clinical efficacy and cost-effectiveness of this approach has recently been questioned (91–93). A formal cost-effectiveness analysis (94) of clopidogrel treatment in addition to ASA as secondary prevention in all patients with coronary heart disease demonstrated that the widespread use of clopidogrel in this manner is not cost-effective. However, there are currently no formal cost-effectiveness analyses available that assess long-term clopidogrel use in patients post-PCI. Therefore, until further data becomes available, treatment duration of clopidogrel post-PCI is based on the PCI-CURE and CREDO dosing regimens.

# THIENOPYRIDINES AND BRACHYTHERAPY

Intracoronary brachytherapy using either a $\beta$- or $\gamma$-radiation source has been used to treat in-stent restenosis. However, this treatment has been associated with late stent thrombosis, particularly when a new stent is implanted at the time of radiation therapy. It is thought that radiation therapy leads to delayed healing and reendothelialization of the stented vessel, and therefore to a higher risk of thrombotic complication. For this reason, extended use of clopidogrel was evaluated and shown to reduce the incidence of late stent thrombosis when continued for at least 6 months following brachytherapy (95–97).

## Thienopyridines and Drug-Eluting Stents

Although altered and delayed vascular repair potentially increases the risk of stent thrombosis following placement of a sirolimus- or paclitaxel-eluting stent, no increase in subacute stent thrombosis has been observed across the five large randomized DES trials to date with extended dual antiplatelet therapy (98–102). On the basis of these studies, recommendations for prolonged thienopyridine use post-PCI with DES have emerged to include a minimum of 2 to 3 months of therapy with sirolimus-eluting stents (101,102) and 6 months of therapy with paclitaxel-eluting stents (98,99).

## Noncardiac Surgery Following Percutaneous Coronary Intervention

Nonemergent surgery should be postponed until adequate "passivation" of the coronary vessel and stented segment occurs. In a series of 207 patients who underwent noncardiac surgery shortly after PCI, 4% died, or there was an occurrence of MI, or development of stent thrombosis (103). All of these complications occurred in patients undergoing surgery within 6 weeks of stent placement, and no events occurred in those patients undergoing surgery between 7 to 9 weeks post-PCI. Therefore, noncardiac surgery should be delayed ideally for a minimum of 6 weeks postbare metal stent placement. In the era of DES, this delay should be extended to 2 to 6 months depending on the type of stent. Antiplatelet therapy with ASA and clopidogrel should be continued in the preoperative, perioperative, and postoperative setting whenever possible. If the surgical bleeding risk is substantial, clopidogrel may be discontinued 6 weeks postbare metal stent, 2 to 3 months post-sirolimus-eluting stent, and 6 months postpaclitaxel-eluting stent. If urgent surgery is required before the minimum recommended treatment duration of poststenting, the risk of surgical bleeding on therapy versus the increased risk of thrombotic complications of the therapy must be individually addressed on a case-by-case basis.

## Adverse Events

Diarrhea, nausea, and vomiting are common with ticlopidine and occur in 30% to 50% of recipients (104). Skin rash occurs

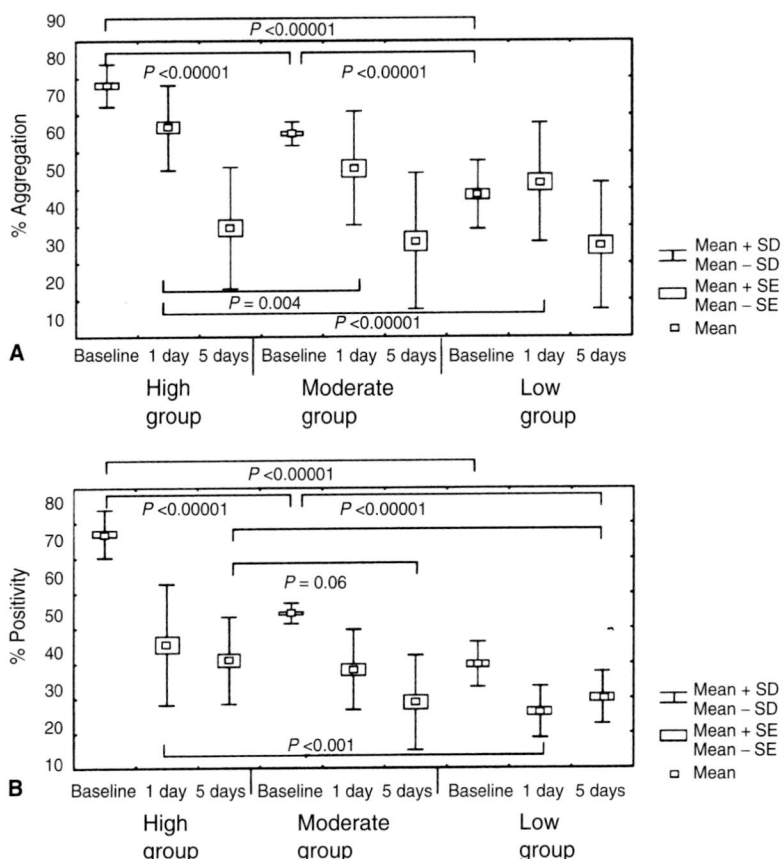

**FIGURE 98-6.** Clopidogrel nonresponsiveness. **A:** Adenosine 5′ diphosphate (ADP)-induced platelet aggregation (5 μmol per L ADP) in high-, moderate-, and low-reactivity groups at baseline and at 1 and 5 days after clopidogrel therapy. High-reactivity patients were defined as pretreatment percent aggregation >70%; moderate, 60% to 70%; and low, <60%. **B:** Stimulated P selectin expression in high-, moderate-, and low-reactivity groups at baseline and at 1 and 5 days after clopidogrel therapy. High-reactivity patients were defined as pretreatment percent positivity >50%; moderate, 40% to 50%; and low, <40%. SD, standard deviation; SE, standard error. (Reprinted from Gurbel PA, Bliden KP, Hiatt BL, et al. Clopidogrel for coronary stenting: response variability, drug resistance, and the effect of pretreatment platelet reactivity. *Circulation* 2003;107: 2908–2913.)

rarely (105). Neutropenia is a serious side effect and the incidence associated with ticlopidine is 1.3% to 2.1% (106) compared with 0.10% (86) with clopidogrel. Neutropenia can be severe (<450 neutrophils per mm$^3$ in 0.9% of patients treated with ticlopidine) and has resulted in death (107). In the Clopidogrel versus Aspirin in Patients of Ischemic Events (CAPRIE) trial, the neutrophil count fell below 450 neutrophils per mm$^3$ for five (0.05%) and four (0.04%) patients in the clopidogrel and ASA groups, respectively. With ticlopidine, most cases develop within the first 3 months of therapy and initially may be clinically silent. Complete blood counts should be performed every 2 weeks during the first 3 months of therapy (108). Bone marrow aplasia and thrombotic thrombocytopenia purpura (TTP) have been reported with ticlopidine (109–111). The estimated incidence of ticlopidine-associated TTP is 1 per 1,600 to 5,000 patients treated (64,112). The incidence of TTP with clopidogrel is lower (110). Ticlopidine had been reported to increase serum cholesterol levels by an average of 9% (113), but no change was associated with clopidogrel in the CAPRIE trial. Although hematologic complications may occur with clopidogrel (e.g., hemolytic uremic syndrome and thrombotic thrombocytopenic purpura), they appear to be rare (114).

## Thienopyridines: Drug Interactions

Ticlopidine has been shown to affect the metabolism of some medications. Doses of cyclosporine may need to be increased (115). The doses of theophylline, carbamazepine, and phenytoin may need to be reduced when these drugs are used with ticlopidine (116–118). The clearance of ticlopidine is reduced by 50% with concomitant cimetidine use (119).

Interindividual variability in platelet inhibition by clopidogrel and the occurrence of "clopidogrel resistance" has been documented by several groups (see Fig. 98-6) (120–123). Recent observations suggest that hepatic cytochrome P-450-3A4 metabolic activity contributes significantly to the phenomenon of clopidogrel resistance (123). Among healthy volunteers, 22% were found to be nonresponders and 32% were low responders based on light transmission aggregometry (LTA). One report in patients ($n = 60$) presenting with STEMI has recently shown that those patients in the lowest quartile of clopidogrel responsiveness (<20% inhibition to ADP-induced platelet aggregation) had a 40% risk of recurrent atherothrombotic events at 6 months compared to 0% risk in the two highest quartiles (124). Bedside, point-of-care testing for clopidogrel is presently under evaluation by the FDA.

## Recommendations for the Use of Thienopyridines in Patients Undergoing Percutaneous Coronary Intervention

- For patients who undergo stent placement, the combination of ASA and a thienopyridine derivative (ticlopidine or clopidogrel) is recommended over systemic anticoagulation therapy (Grade 1A) (55).
- Clopidogrel is recommended over ticlopidine (Grade 1A) (55).
- A loading dose of 300 mg of clopidogrel at least 6 hours before planned PCI is recommended (Grade 1B). If clopidogrel is started less than 6 hours before planned PCI, a 600-mg loading dose of clopidogrel is recommended (Grade 2C) (55).

- If ticlopidine is administered, a loading dose of 500 mg at least 6 hours before planned PCI is recommended (Grade 2C) (55).
- For PCI patients who cannot tolerate ASA, the loading dose of clopidogrel (300 mg) or ticlopidine (500 mg) should be administered at least 24 hours before planned PCI (Grade 2C) (55).
- After PCI with a bare metal stent, in addition to ASA, clopidogrel (75 mg per day) is recommended for at least 9 to 12 months (Grade 1A). If ticlopidine is used in place of clopidogrel, ticlopidine should be administered for 2 weeks in addition to ASA after placement of a bare metal stent (Grade 1B) (55).
- After PCI with a sirolimus-eluting stent, clopidogrel (75 mg per day) is recommended for 2 to 3 months minimum in addition to ASA (Grade 1C+). After PCI with a paclitaxel-eluting stent, clopidogrel (75 mg per day) is recommended to a minimum of 6 months in addition to ASA (55).

## UNFRACTIONATED HEPARIN

Unfractionated heparin (UFH) is the most commonly used anticoagulant during PCI. Although UFH is administered to limit acute ischemic events, its use is based on observational data. Activated clotting time (ACT) monitoring in the cardiac catheterization laboratory guides heparin dosing during PCI because the required level of anticoagulation is beyond the range that can be measured using the activated partial thromboplastin time (aPTT) (125,126). Hemochron and HemoTec devices are commonly used to measure the ACT and the Hemochron ACT generally exceeds the HemoTec ACT by up to 30% (127), although considerable variability exists (125). At least two studies have retrospectively related ACT values to clinical outcomes after PCI (128,129). A third retrospective analysis of data from 5,216 patients receiving heparin during PCI suggested that ischemic complications at 7 days were 34% lower with a Hemochron ACT in the range of 350 to 375 seconds than they were with an ACT between 171 and 295 seconds ($P = 0.001$) (130). Although ischemic complications were reduced at higher levels of ACT, this was at the cost of progressively increased bleeding from 8.6% at ACTs less than 350 seconds to 12.4% at ACTs 350 to 375 seconds. A substantial increase in bleeding events was observed when ACT values exceeded 400 seconds (130). Importantly, these studies were performed in patients who were given heparin without adjunctive GP IIb/IIIa inhibitors that require lower ACT targets (see the subsequent text).

The dosing regimen for heparin was evaluated in two small randomized trials comparing empiric and weight-adjusted heparin dosing. Both approaches showed comparable results (131,132). On the basis of these data, heparin is given in doses of 70 to 100 IU per kg and a target Hemochron ACT between 250 and 350 seconds is advocated in the absence of adjunctive GP IIb/IIIa inhibition. In contrast, a target Hemochron ACT of 200 to 250 seconds is advocated when heparin (bolus dose of UFH 40 to 60 IU per kg) is given in conjunction with a GP IIb/IIIa inhibitor. Removal of the femoral sheath should be delayed until the ACT is between 150 and 180 seconds (see Table 98-3).

Routine use of intravenous heparin after PCI is no longer used because several randomized studies have showed that prolonged heparin infusions do not reduce ischemic complications and are associated with a higher rate of bleeding at the catheter insertion site (133,134).

Recently, minimal doses (≤1,000 U) of UFH with abciximab were proven to be safe and efficacious in a low-risk population undergoing PCI (135). The mean ACT for patients during PCI was 168 seconds and there were no major adverse clinical events during the 24 hours after PCI.

Despite the wealth of knowledge and experience with UFH during PCI, UFH has several limitations (see Table 98-4), providing the impetus for alternative antithrombin approaches, including low-molecular-weight heparin (LMWH) and direct antithrombins.

## TABLE 98-3

### MANAGEMENT OF ANTITHROMBOTIC/ANTIPLATELET THERAPIES POSTPERCUTANEOUS CORONARY INTERVENTION

| | Sheath removal | When to stop for patients who require CABG | Reversal agents for bleeding complications | Thrombocytopenia (etiology) |
|---|---|---|---|---|
| UFH | Once ACT <150 –180 s | 4–6 h prior | Protamine 1–1.5 mg IV per 100 U heparin | HIT occurs more commonly with prolong infusions (~1% incidence) |
| LMWH | 8 h after last dose | >8 h prior | 1 mg for each mg of drug—this will reverse approximately 50% of the drug | HIT possible, but less frequent |
| Eptifibatide or Tirofiban | Based on antithrombin used | 4–6 h prior | Stop infusion | Immunologic origin, discontinue therapy and do not readminister |
| Abciximab | Based on antithrombin used | 12 h prior | Transfuse platelets | Immunologic origin with antibody development—discontinue therapy and do not readminister |
| Bivalirudin | 2 h post-PCI | 2 h prior | Stop infusion | None |
| Clopidogrel | N/A | 5 d prior | None | Rare |

CABG, coronary artery bypass graft; UFH, unfractionated heparin; ACT, activated clotting time; HIT, heparin-induced thrombocytopenia; LMWH, low-molecular-weight heparin; PCI, percutaneous intervention.

TABLE 98-4

## TABLE 98-4

### LIMITATIONS OF UNFRACTIONATED HEPARIN

| Properties of unfractionated heparin | Pharmacologic consequences | Clinical consequences |
|---|---|---|
| **THROMBIN-DEPENDENT PROPERTIES** | | |
| Nonspecific protein binding | Less drug binding to thrombin | Variable anticoagulation levels requiring frequent monitoring |
| | Sensitivity to inactivation by PF4 and histidine-rich glycoprotein | |
| Short plasma half-life | Poor bioavailability with single dose | IV infusion required |
| Depletion of TFPI | ↓ attenuation of TF/FVIIa complex | Rebound hypercoagulability |
| Relative inability to inhibit fibrin-bound thrombin | ↑ thrombin generation following clot lysis in presence of therapeutic UFH levels | Rebound thrombosis during and post-UFH therapy |
| Requires a cofactor (AT III) to optimally bind thrombin | ↓↓ thrombin-inhibition if AT III not available | Cannot be used in patients with AT III deficiency |
| **THROMBIN-INDEPENDENT PROPERTIES** | | |
| ↑ binding to platelets | ↑ immunogenicity<br>↑ platelet activation and adhesion | ↑ potential for bleeding, HITTS, or thrombosis |
| Inability to blunt the increase | ↑ VWF levels | ↑ potential for thrombosis |
| Primarily excreted renally | ↓ clearance, ↑ levels in patients with renal insufficiency | ↑ potential for bleeding in patients with renal insufficiency |

PF, platelet factor; TFPI, tissue factor pathway inhibitor; TF, tissue factor; UFH, unfractionated heparin; HITTS, heparin-induced thrombocytopenia-thrombosis syndrome; VWF, von Willebrand factor.

## Recommendations for the Use of Unfractionated Heparin in Patients Undergoing Percutaneous Coronary Intervention

■ In patients receiving a GP IIb/IIIa inhibitor, a UFH bolus of 50 to 70 IU per kg to achieve a target Hemochron ACT greater than 200 seconds is recommended (Grade 1C) (55).

■ In patients not receiving a GP IIb/IIIa inhibitor, a UFH dose sufficient to produce a Hemochron ACT of 250 to 350 seconds is recommended (Grade 1C+). A weight-adjusted UFH bolus of 60 to 100 IU per kg is recommended (Grade 2C) (55).

■ Following uncomplicated PCI, routine postprocedural infusion of UFH is not recommended (Grade 1A) (55).

# LOW-MOLECULAR-WEIGHT HEPARINS

LMWHs are fragments of UFH produced by controlled enzymatic or chemical depolymerization processes that yield chains with a mean molecular weight of approximately 5,000 Da. LMWHs exert their anticoagulant effect by activating antithrombin. Binding of the pentasaccharide sequence to antithrombin causes a conformational change in antithrombin that accelerates its interaction with thrombin and activated factor X (factor Xa) by approximately 1,000 times (136).

Although many different LMWH preparations have been developed, only two (enoxaparin, dalteparin) have been widely studied in patients with ACSs (see Table 98-5). Enoxaparin has a mean molecular weight of 4,200 Da with anti-Xa:anti-IIa ratio of 3:8, and dalteparin has a mean molecular weight of 6,000 Da with anti-Xa: anti-IIa ratio of 2:7 (136). Both drugs

are administered in a weight-based fashion subcutaneously in their maintenance dosing.

Seven large randomized trials have directly compared UFH to either dalteparin (137); nadroparin (138), or enoxaparin (139–143) in patients with unstable coronary syndromes. In the FRagmin In unstable Coronary artery disease (FRIC) study, 1,482 patients with UA/NSTEMI received open-label dalteparin (120 IU per kg subcutaneously twice a day) or UFH for 6 days (137). At day 6 and until day 45, patients were randomized a second time to double-blind administration of dalteparin (120 IU per kg once a day) or placebo. During the first part of the study, the risk of death, MI, or recurrent angina was similar with dalteparin (9.3% vs. 7.65%, $P = 0.33$), the risk of death or MI was similar (3.9% vs. 3.6%, $P = 0.8$), and the risk of death alone tended to occur more frequently with dalteparin (1.5% vs. 0.4% with UFH, $P = 0.057$). Between days 6 and 45, the rates of death, MI, and recurrence of angina were comparable between the active treatment and placebo groups (144).

The FRAXiparine in Ischemic Syndrome (FRAXIS) trial had three parallel arms and compared the LMWH nadroparin administered for 6 or 14 days with control treatment with UFH (138). Three thousand, four hundred and sixty-eight patients with UA or NSTEMI were enrolled. The composite outcome of death, MI, or refractory angina occurred at 14 days in 18.1% of patients in the UFH group, 17.8% of patients treated with nadroparin for 6 days, and 20.0% of patients treated with nadroparin for 14 days; the values at 3 months were 22.2%, 22.3%, and 26.2% of patients, respectively, ($P < 0.03$ for the comparison of 14-day nadroparin therapy with UFH therapy). Trends to more frequent death, and to more frequent death or MI were observed at all-time points in nadroparin-treated patients (144).

The Efficacy and Safety of Subcutaneous Enoxaparin in Non–Q-Wave Coronary Events (ESSENCE) trial compared enoxaparin (1 mg per kg twice daily subcutaneous administration) with standard UFH (5,000 U bolus), followed by an infusion

**TABLE 98-5**

TRIALS WITH LOW-MOLECULAR-WEIGHT HEPARIN IN PERCUTANEOUS CORONARY INTERVENTION

| Trial (no. of patients) | Therapy | Efficacy | Timing | Event rate % | | | Major bleeding % | | |
|---|---|---|---|---|---|---|---|---|---|
| | | | | LMWH | Control | Abs diff | LMWH | Control | Abs diff |
| REDUCE (306) | Reviparin | D, MI, R | 30 wk | 33.3 | 32 | 1.3 | 2.3 | 2.6 | −0.3 |
| Rabah (30) | Enox | TIMI 3 flow | Post-PCI | 97 | 93 | 4 | 3.3 | 0 | 3.3 |
| | | RI events | 30 d | 0 | 10 | −10 | | | |
| Choussat (242) | Enox | D, MI, UR | 30 d | 2.5 | 0 | — | 0.4 | — | — |
| PEPCI (40) | Enox | D, MI, UR | 30 d | 5.4 | — | — | 0 | — | — |
| NICE 1 (828) | Enox | D, MI, UR | 30 d | 7.7 | — | — | 1.1 | — | — |
| Collet (132) | Enox | D, MI | 30 d | 3.0 | — | — | 0.8 | — | — |
| ESSENCE[a]/ TIMI 11B[a] (431) | Enox | D, MI | 43 d | 3.3 | 5.9 | −2.6 (P = 0.06) | 5.4 | 6.2 | −0.8 |
| FRISC II (1222) (Invasive) | Any LMWH | D, MI | 6 mo | 9.4 | — | — | 1.6 | — | — |
| NICE 4 (818) | Enox, Abx | D, MI, UR | 30 d | 6.8 | — | — | 0.4 | — | — |
| Kereiakes (103) | Dalt, Abx | D, MI, UR | Discharge | 11.1[d] 17.1[e] | — — | — — | 3.7[d] 2.6[e] | — — | — — |
| NICE 3[b] (283) | Enox, Any GP | D, MI, RI | 30 d | 11.3[f] | — | — | 1.4[f] | — | — |
| ACUTE II (315) | Enox, Tiro | D, MI, UR | Discharge | 9.2 | 9.0 | 0.2 | 0.3 | 1.0 | −0.7 |
| GUSTO IV (646) (Dalteparin[c]) | Dalt, Abx | D, MI | 30 d | 9.6 | 8.5 | 1.1 | 1.2 | 0.5 | 0.5 |
| INTERACT (380) | Enox, Ept | D, MI | 30 d | 10.1 | 11.8 | −1.7 | 1.8 | 4.6 | −2.8 (P = 0.03) |
| CRUISE (129) | Enox, Ept | D, MI, UR | 48 h | 8.5 | 7.6 | 0.9 | 2.5 | 1.6 | 0.9 |
| A to Z | Enox, tiro | D, MI, RI | 30 d | 8.4 | 9.4 | 1.0 | 0.9 | 0.4 | 0.5 |
| SYNERGY | Enox, any | D, MI | 30 d | 14 | 14.5 | 0.5 | 9.1 | 7.6 | 1.5 |

Enox, enoxaparin; Tiro, tirofiban; GP, abciximab, eptifibatide, or tirofiban; Dalt, dalteparin; Abx, abciximab; Ept, eptifibatide; RI, recurrent ischemia; REDUCE, Reduction of Restenosis after PTCA Early Administration of Reviparin in a Double-blind Unfractionated Heparin and Placebo-controlled Evaluation; PEPCI, Pharmacokinetic Study of Enoxaparin in Patients Undergoing Coronary Intervention; NICE, National Investigators Collaborating on Enoxaparin; ESSENCE, Efficacy and Safety of Subcutaneous Enoxaparin in Unstable Angina and Non–Q-Wave MI; TIMI, Thrombolysis in Myocardial Infarction; FRISC, Fragmin and Fast Revascularization During Instability in Coronary Artery Disease; CRUISE, Coronary Revascularization Using Integrilin and Single Bolus Enoxaparin; INTERACT, Integrilin and Enoxaparin Randomized Assessment of Acute Coronary Syndrome Treatment; A to Z, Aggrastat to Zocor; SYNERGY, Superior Yield of the New strategy of Enoxaparin Revascularization & Glycoprotein IIb/IIIa inhibitors; D, death; MI, myocardial infarction; R, revascularization; RI, recurrent ischemic; UR, urgent revascularization.
[a]Among patients who received enoxaparin and underwent PCI during the index admission.
[b]Cohort of patients undergoing PCI.
[c]Dalteparin substudy.
[d]Data observed with 40 IU/kg dalteparin IV.
[e]Data observed with 60 IU/kg dalteparin IV.
[f]Pooled data across all 3 GP IIb/IIIa inhibitors.

titrated to an aPTT of 55 to 86 seconds, administered for 48 hours to 8 days (median duration in both groups of 2.6 days) (139). With UFH, only 46% of patients reached the target aPTT within 12 to 24 hours. The composite outcome of death, MI, or recurrent angina was reduced by 16.2% at 14 days with enoxaparin (19.8% UFH vs. 16.6% enoxaparin, P = 0.019) and by 19% at 30 days (23.3% vs. 19.8%, P = 0.017). The rates of death were unaffected, whereas there were trends to reductions in the rates of death and MI by 29% (P = 0.06) at 14 days and by 26% (P = 0.08) at 30 days. Similarly, the TIMI 11B trial randomized 3,910 patients with UA/NSTEMI to enoxaparin (30 mg IV initial bolus immediately followed by subcutaneous injections of 1 mg per kg every 12 hours) or UFH (70 U per kg bolus followed by an infusion of 15 U/kg/hour titrated to a target aPTT 1.5 to 2.5 times control) (140). The acute-phase therapy was followed by an outpatient phase, during which enoxaparin or placebo for patients who were initially randomized to UFH was administered in a double-blind manner twice a day. Enoxaparin was administered for a median of 4.6 days, and UFH was administered for a median of 3 days. The composite endpoint of death, MI, or need for an urgent revascularization was reduced at 8 days from 14.5% to 12.4% (P = 0.048), and at 43 days from 19.6% to 17.3%

(P = 0.048). The rates of death or MI were reduced from 6.9% to 5.7% (P = 0.114) at 14 days and from 8.9% to 7.9% (P = 0.276) at 43 days. No incremental benefit was observed with outpatient treatment, whereas the risk of major bleeding was significantly greater during the outpatient treatment. The risk of minor bleeding was also increased both in and out of hospital with enoxaparin (144).

The Integrilin and Enoxaparin Randomized Assessment of Acute Coronary Syndrome Treatment (INTERACT) study randomized 746 patients with high-risk ACS to receive eptifibatide plus either enoxaparin (1 mg per kg twice daily subcutaneously for 48 hours), or weight-adjusted UFH for 48 hours (143). Cardiac catheterization and coronary revascularization were performed at the discretion of the investigator [63% (n = 573) of patients underwent angiography, 28.5% (n = 224) underwent PCI]. The primary safety endpoint was the incidence of major non–CABG-related bleeding at 96 hours. Compared with UFH, enoxaparin significantly reduced the rate of non–CABG-related major bleeding: 3.8% versus 1.1% at 48 hours (P = 0.014) and 4.6% versus 1.8% at 96 hours (P = 0.03), respectively. The rate of the secondary endpoint, death or MI, was significantly lower in the enoxaparin group than in the UFH group (5% vs. 9%, respectively; P = 0.03).

Recurrent ischemia, determined by continuous electrocardiographic monitoring, was significantly lower in the enoxaparin group compared with the UFH group, both during the initial 48 hours (14.3% vs. 25.4%; $P = 0.0002$) and from 48 to 96 hours following study entry (12.7% vs. 25.9%; $P < 0.0001$).

In the Aggrastat to Zocor (A to Z) study, 3,987 high-risk ACS patients were randomized to enoxaparin (1 mg per kg twice daily subcutaneously) plus tirofiban versus weight-adjusted UFH plus tirofiban (141). Treatment was given for a maximum of 120 hours, but could be stopped or switched at any time at the treating physician's discretion. The primary endpoint of death/MI/refractory ischemia was not significant between the groups (enoxaparin 8.4% vs. UFH 9.4%, $P = 0.23$), and this finding fulfilled the prespecified requirements necessary to show noninferiority of enoxaparin to UFH. TIMI major bleeding was similar between the groups (enoxaparin group 0.9% vs. 0.4% UFH group, $P = NS$).

In Superior Yield of the New strategy of Enoxaparin Revascularization & Glycoprotein (SYNERGY) trial IIb/IIIa inhibitors, 10,027 high-risk ACS patients were randomized to enoxaparin (1 mg per kg twice daily subcutaneously) or UFH (60 U per kg bolus followed by 12 U/kg/hour infusion) with a goal of early invasive therapy (142). The primary endpoint of death and MI was 14% in the enoxaparin group versus 14.5% in the UFH group ($P = 0.396$). TIMI major bleeding was significantly higher in the enoxaparin group versus the UFH group (9.1% vs. 7.6%, $P = 0.008$, respectively), but there was no difference in the rate of packed red blood cell transfusion (17% vs. 16%, $P = 0.155$, respectively). Overall, SYNERGY demonstrated that enoxaparin was statistically not inferior to UFH in preventing ischemic events in high-risk ACS patients treated with an early aggressive invasive management (92% underwent angiography to define coronary anatomy) and revascularization strategy (approximately 47% PCI, 19% CABG); however, there were significantly higher rates of bleeding with enoxaparin (see Table 98-6). The final analysis of SYNERGY

shows that cross-over therapy and protocol violations contributed adversely to bleeding complications. It is important to note that steady-state anticoagulation without intravenous bolus of enoxaparin (0.3 mg per kg) requires 3 subcutaneous doses. Because many interventional cardiologists favor rapid triage to the cardiac catheterization laboratory in STEMI (door-to-balloon <90 minutes), and increasingly in US/NSTEMI as well [door-to-cath lab <6 hours based on the results of Intracoronary Stenting with Antithrombotic Regimen Cooling-off (ISAR-COOL) (145)], intravenous UFH is likely to remain the anticoagulant of choice at the present time.

Therefore, three (139,140,143) randomized ACS trials with enoxaparin have shown a benefit over UFH, whereas two (141,142) studies demonstrated the noninferiority of enoxaparin to UFH. Either neutral or negative trends were shown with either dalteparin or nadroparin in comparison to UFH. Although these heterogeneous results may be explained by different populations, study designs, various heparin dose regimens, properties of the various LMWHs (more specifically different molecular weights and antifactor Xa/antifactor IIa ratios), or other unrecognized influences, these data suggest a potential difference between LMWHs and serve as the basis for the ACC/American Heart Association (AHA) recommendations (144).

LMWHs are alternative anticoagulants to UFH in the PCI setting. Given the benefit shown with upstream use of enoxaparin versus UFH in ACS patients (139,140,146,147) and ACC/AHA guidelines (144) recommending enoxaparin over UFH (Class IIa) in ACS, the use of enoxaparin in PCI has been considered. Difficulties associated with monitoring the anticoagulation intensity of enoxaparin during PCI have led to empiric dosing algorithms and consensus statements guiding its use on the basis of pharmacokinetic data and registry data (148). In general, if the last dose of enoxaparin was less than 8 hours before PCI, no additional UFH or LMWH is needed. If the last dose of enoxaparin was given between 8 to 12 hours before PCI, a 0.3 mg per kg

## TABLE 98-6

### IN-HOSPITAL BLEEDING[a]

| | No./Total (%) | | |
|---|---|---|---|
| | **Enoxaparin** | **Unfractionated heparin** | **_P_ value** |
| GUSTO severe | 136/4993 (2.7) | 109/4983 (2.2) | .08 |
| TIMI major[b] | 453/4993 (9.1) | 379/4984 (7.6) | .008 |
| CABG-related | 338/4993 (6.8) | 295/4984 (5.9) | .08 |
| Non–CABG-related | 119/4993 (2.4) | 87/4984 (1.8) | .03 |
| TIMI minor | 611/4885 (12.5) | 603/4888 (12.3) | .80 |
| Decrease in hemoglobin and/or hematocrit[c] | 743/4874 (15.2) | 611/4882 (12.5) | <.001 |
| Any transfusion | 850/4993 (17.0) | 796/4985 (16.0) | .16 |
| Lowest platelet count, $\times 10^3/\mu L$ | | | |
| ≥100 | 4393/4675 (94.0) | 4424/4697 (94.2) | |
| >50 to <100 | 250/4675 (5.3) | 250/4697 (5.3) | |
| >20 to ≤50 | 22/4675 (0.5) | 16/4697 (0.3) | .67 |
| ≤20 | 10/4675 (0.2) | 7/4697 (0.1) | |

CABG, coronary artery bypass graft; GUSTO, global utilization of streptokinase and tPA for occluded arteries; TIMI, thrombolysis in myocardial infarction.

[a]GUSTO severe bleeding was defined as intracranial hemorrhage or if bleeding results in hemodynamic compromise. TIMI major bleeding was defined as at least a 5 g/dL decrease in hemoglobin, at least a 15% decrease in hematocrit, or intracranial bleeding. TIMI minor bleeding was noted if it was associated with gastrointestinal or genitourinary bleeding, with an absolute decrease in hemoglobin of 4 g/dL or more, or decrease in hematocrit of at least 12%.

[b]Associated with clinical bleed.

[c]At least a 5 g/dL decrease in hemoglobin or at least a 15% decrease in hematocrit not associated with an overt bleeding event.

From Theroux P, Ouimet H, McCans J, et al. Aspirin, heparin, or both to treat acute unstable angina. _N Engl J Med_ 1988;319:1105–1111, with permission.

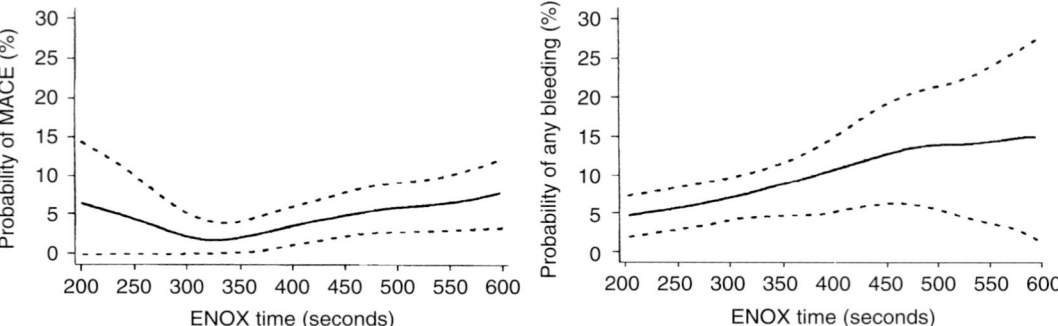

**FIGURE 98-7.** A novel point-of-care enoxaparin monitor for use during percutaneous coronary intervention (PCI): Results of the Evaluating Enoxaparin Clotting Times (ELECT) Study. Kernel smoothing regression and 95% confidence interval (CI) lines assessing the occurrence of major adverse cardiac events (MACE) over the range of procedural ENOX times. For display purposes, several ENOX values less than 200 were truncated at 200 and several greater than 600 were truncated at 600. ENOX, enoxaparin. [Reprinted from Moliterno D, Hermiller J, Kereiakes D, et al. A novel point-of-care enoxaparin monitor for use during percutaneous coronary intervention. Results of the Evaluating Enoxaparin Clotting Times (ELECT) Study. *J Am Coll Cardiol* 2003;42:1132–1139.]

bolus of intravenous enoxaparin should be given before PCI. If the last dose of enoxaparin was administered more than 12 hours before PCI, conventional anticoagulation therapy with UFH is warranted. Alternatively, 0.75 to 1.0 mg per kg bolus of intravenous enoxaparin without GP IIb/IIIa inhibitors and 0.5 to 0.75 mg per kg bolus of intravenous enoxaparin with GP IIb/IIIa could be used at the time of the intervention. A rapid, point-of-care assay designed for estimating the anticoagulant activity of enoxaparin has been developed (enoxaparin clotting time, ECT), and evaluated in a clinical trial to define optimal range of anticoagulation with respect to efficacy and safety outcomes (see Fig. 98-7) (149). The trial investigators proposed guidelines for ECT target (260 to 450 seconds) before PCI and for sheath removal (ECT <180 seconds). Anti-Xa testing was performed in parallel and suggested that the optimal anti-Xa range was 0.8 to 2.2 IU per mL.

The safety and efficacy of enoxaparin compared to UFH in the PCI setting has been evaluated in ACS patients undergoing invasive therapy in SYNERGY (142), INTERACT (143) and A to Z (141) as described in the preceding text. In the Coronary Revascularization Using Integrilin and Single Bolus Enoxaparin (CRUISE) study, 261 patients undergoing elective or emergent PCI were randomized to either eptifibatide plus enoxaparin, or eptifibatide plus UFH (150). The primary endpoint of the study, the bleeding index (change in hemoglobin corrected for blood transfusions), was 0.8 in the patients randomized to enoxaparin and 1.1 in patients randomized to UFH (P = 0.15). The rate of vascular access site complications was 9.3% in the enoxaparin arm versus 9.8% in the UFH arm (P = NS). There were no substantial differences in the composite of death, myocardial infarction, or urgent target vessel revascularization (TVR) at 30 days (enoxaparin 8.5% vs. UFH 7.6%, P = NS). CRUISE demonstrated comparable safety and efficacy of enoxaparin to UFH during PCI in a randomized controlled study.

In summary, enoxaparin appears to be equally effective as UFH during PCI in preventing MACE. The largest study to date (142) demonstrated that, in high-risk patients with ACS who are managed with an early aggressive management strategy including high rates of early coronary angiography, clopidogrel, and GP IIb/IIIa inhibitors, enoxaparin was not inferior to UFH in preventing death and nonfatal infarction at 30 days, but was associated with an excess of 15 per 1,000 major bleeds (Table 98-6). The most important additional finding was that switching between antithrombotics during the same hospitalization increased the risk of bleeding.

## Recommendations for the Use of Low-Molecular-Weight Heparin in Patients Undergoing Percutaneous Coronary Intervention

In patients who have received LMWH prior to PCI, the administration of additional anticoagulant therapy is dependent on the timing of the last dose of LMWH (Grade 1C). If the last dose of enoxaparin is administered less than 8 hours before PCI, no additional anticoagulant therapy is recommended (Grade 2C). If the last dose of enoxaparin is administered between 8 to 12 hours before PCI, a 0.3 mg per kg bolus of IV enoxaparin at the time of PCI is recommended (Grade 2C). If the last enoxaparin dose is administered more than 12 hours before PCI, conventional anticoagulation therapy during PCI is recommended (Grade 2C) (55).

# DIRECT THROMBIN INHIBITORS

The direct thrombin inhibitors (DTI) hirudin, bivalirudin, and argatroban have been used during PCI in lieu of the combination of UFH (151–153) and GP IIb/IIIa platelet antagonist. Of these agents, bivalirudin has been the most extensively studied (152,154,155). DTIs offer a number of theoretical advantages over UFH including activity against fibrin-bound thrombin, less nonspecific protein binding, direct action without a cofactor, absence of known inhibitors, and less platelet binding. These benefits ultimately result in more effective and reliable thrombin inhibition, less platelet activation, less thrombocytopenia, and a more predictable pharmacokinetic profile obviating the need to measure ACTs. Although the anticoagulant effect of bivalirudin dissipates quickly, owing to its short half-life of 25 minutes, there is no rapid reversal agent available in the event of life-threatening bleeding. Furthermore, in patients with severe impairment of renal function, the half-life may be increased significantly. Following PCI with bivalirudin, sheath removal should be delayed for 2 hours in patients with normal renal function, and up to 8 hours in patients on dialysis.

The Bivalirudin Angioplasty Trial (BAT) randomized 4,098 high-risk patients with ACS undergoing PCI to high-dose heparin bolus (175 IU per kg bolus followed by a 15 IU/kg/hour infusion for 18 to 24 hours) or to bivalirudin (1 mg per kg bolus followed by an infusion of 2.5 mg/kg/hour for 4 hours, reduced to 0.2 mg/kg/hour for the next 14 to 20 hours). Bleeding complications were reduced with bivalirudin, and ischemic complications were lower in the subset of patients with postinfarction angina. Reanalysis of this data using a contemporary combined endpoint of death, MI, or repeat revascularization showed a significant reduction in this endpoint with bivalirudin compared to UFH (6.2% vs. 7.9%, $P = 0.039$, respectively) (155).

The Randomized Evaluation in PCI Linking Angiomax to Reduced Clinical Events (REPLACE-2) trial assigned 6,010 patients undergoing PCI to intravenous bivalirudin (0.75 mg per kg bolus plus 1.75 mg/kg/hour infusion for the duration of PCI) with provisional GP IIb/IIIa inhibition, or heparin (65 U per kg bolus) with planned GP IIb/IIIa inhibition (abciximab or eptifibatide) (153). "Planned" GP IIb/IIIa inhibition was defined as the addition of a GP IIb/IIIa inhibitor to all cases randomized to the UFH arm. "Provisional" GP IIb/IIIa inhibition was defined as the addition of GP IIb/IIIa inhibitor during the procedure at the discretion of the operator secondary to procedural or angiographic complications (e.g., dissection, side-branch occlusion, thrombus formation). The primary composite endpoint was a 30-day incidence of death, MI, urgent repeat revascularization, or in-hospital major bleeding, and occurred among 9.2% of patients in the bivalirudin group and 10.0% of patients in the heparin plus GP IIb/IIIa group (OR, 0.92; 95% CI, 0.77 to 1.08; $P = 0.32$). The secondary composite endpoint of death, MI, or urgent revascularization occurred in 7.6% of patients in the bivalirudin group versus 7.1% of patients in the heparin plus GP IIb/IIIa group (OR, 1.09; 95% CI, 0.90 to 1.32; $P = 0.40$). Bivalirudin with provisional GP IIb/IIIa blockade was statistically not inferior to heparin plus planned GP IIb/IIIa blockade and, by historical comparisons, statistically superior to heparin alone in suppressing acute ischemic endpoints with less associated bleeding (see Fig. 98-8, Table 98-7). In-hospital major bleeding rates were significantly reduced by bivalirudin (2.4% vs. 4.1%; $P < 0.001$). It is important to note, however, that heparin dosing in this trial resulted in higher ACTs (317 seconds, interquartile range 263 to 373 seconds) than reported in prior GP IIb/IIIa trials and may have contributed to the excess bleeding complication in patients assigned to treatment with UFH and GP IIb/IIIa inhibitors. Although bivalirudin is FDA approved for use during PCI, based on the dosing from BAT (155), the lower dosing regimen of bivalirudin in REPLACE-2 has not received FDA approval, making firm recommendations about its use unclear at the present time. However, the use of bivalirudin may be particularly useful in patients with conditions associated with increased bleeding risk (e.g., old age, renal insufficiency, bleeding disorders, and immediate postoperative state) because it allows the GP IIb/IIIa inhibitor to be avoided. It is now recognized that 5% of patients who received prolonged intravenous UFH develop heparin-induced thrombocytopenia (HIT). On the basis of the large clinical experience with bivalirudin in REPLACE-2, bivalirudin is likely to become the anticoagulant of choice in patients undergoing PCI with a known prior history of HIT (151,156–158). Clinical trials evaluating the use of bivalirudin in STEMI and NSTEMI-UA are currently underway.

## Recommendations for the Use of Direct Thrombin Inhibitors in Patients Undergoing Percutaneous Coronary Intervention

■ For patients undergoing PCI who are not treated with a GP IIb/IIIa inhibitor or UFH, bivalirudin (0.75 mg per kg bolus followed by an infusion of 1.75 mg/kg/hour for the duration of PCI) during PCI is recommended (Grade 1A) (55).

■ In PCI patients who are at low risk for complications, bivalirudin with provisional use of GP IIb/IIIa inhibitors as an alternative to UFH with planned GP IIb/IIIa inhibition is recommended (Grade 1B) (55).

■ In PCI patients who are at high risk for bleeding, bivalirudin over UFH as an adjunct to GP IIb/IIIa inhibitors is recommended (Grade 1B) (55).

# INTRAVENOUS GLYCOPROTEIN IIb/IIIa INHIBITORS

## Glycoprotein IIb/IIIa Inhibitors: Mechanism of Action

The central role of platelets in the pathogenesis of acute coronary syndromes and the acute ischemic complications associated with PCI have emerged from experimental and clinical studies (159,160). Platelet GP IIb/IIIa receptors mediate the "final common pathway" of platelet aggregation by binding fibrinogen and other adhesive proteins that bridge adjacent platelets and have, therefore, served as a primary focus of pharmacologic antiplatelet strategies. Three parenteral agents—abciximab (ReoPro), eptifibatide (Integrilin), and tirofiban (Aggrastat)—are currently approved for clinical use by the United States FDA.

Abciximab is a humanized Fab fragment engineered from murine monoclonal antibody 7E3 directed against GP IIb/IIIa (161). Unlike the small-molecule agents, abciximab interacts with the GP IIb/IIIa receptor at sites distinct from the ligand-binding RGD sequence site, and exerts its inhibitory effect noncompetitively (162). The antibody has unique pharmacokinetics, with most of the drug cleared from plasma within 26 minutes, but much slower clearance from the body with a functional half-life up to 7 days (163). Because of the high affinity of abciximab for GP IIb/IIIa, the number of abciximab molecules bound to platelets is considerably higher than the free plasma pool of the drug for the duration of treatment. Platelet-associated abciximab can be detected for more than 14 days after the infusion is stopped (164). With an average period of platelet circulation of approximately 7 days, it appears that abciximab molecules can freely dissociate and reassociate with GP IIb/IIIa as the turnover of platelets in the circulation continues, thereby prolonging the "biological" half-life of the drug (165).

The design of the cyclic heptapeptide eptifibatide is based on barbourin, a 73-amino acid peptide isolated from the venom of the Southeastern pygmy rattlesnake *Sistrurus m. barbouri* (166). Plasma concentration of eptifibatide is proportional to the administered dose for a range of bolus and infusion doses. With the recommended double bolus (180 $\mu$g per kg bolus followed 10 minutes later by 180 $\mu$g/kg/second bolus) and infusion (2 $\mu$g/kg/minute) regimen, peak plasma levels are established shortly after the bolus doses, and slightly lower concentration is subsequently maintained throughout the infusion period; plasma concentration decreases rapidly after the infusion is discontinued. Approximately, 25% of eptifibatide molecules in plasma are protein-bound, leaving the remaining 75% to constitute the pool of pharmacologically active drug (167). Eptifibatide has an elimination half-life of 2.5 hours, with most of the drug eliminated through renal mechanisms (165). A lower infusion dose (1 $\mu$g/kg/minute) of eptifibatide is recommended in patients with creatinine clearance less than 50 mL per minute. Substantial recovery of platelet aggregation is apparent within

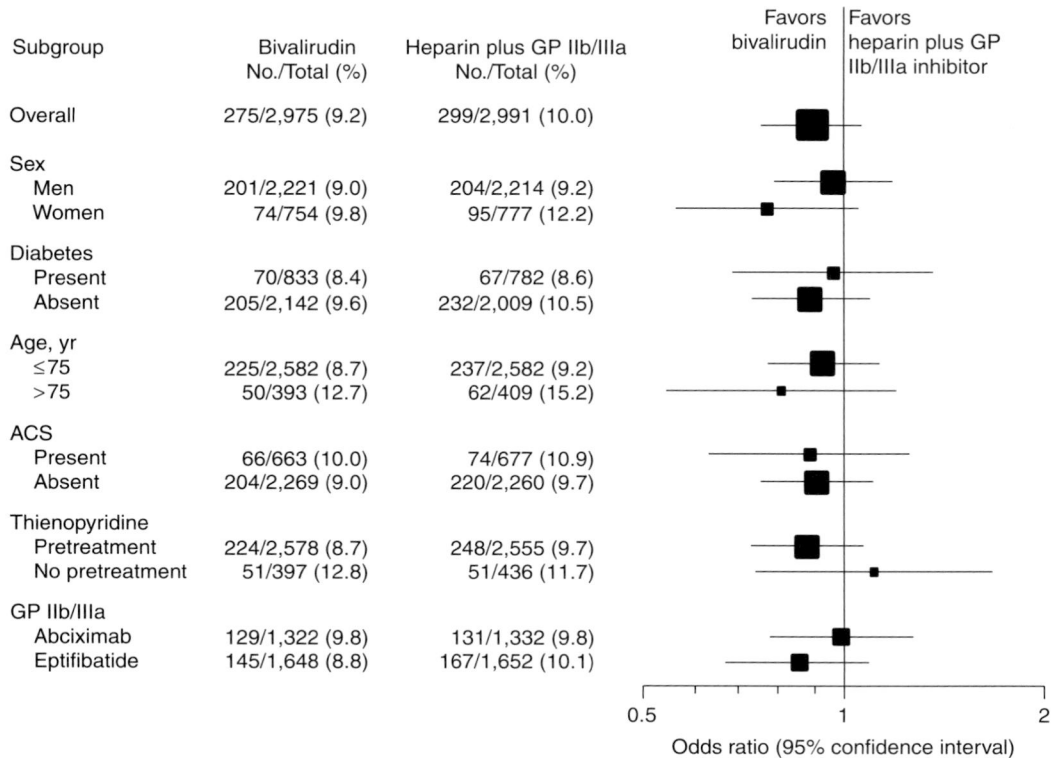

**FIGURE 98-8.** Primary endpoint results and subgroup analysis of the REPLACE-2 trial. Primary endpoint and subgroups by treatment assignment ACS indicates, defined as unstable angina within preceding 48 hours or myocardial infarction (MI) within the prior 7 days. The size of the data markers are approximately proportional to the size of the subgroup. (Reprinted from Lincoff AM, Bittl JA, Harrington RA, et al. Bivalirudin and provisional glycoprotein IIb/IIIa blockade compared with heparin and planned glycoprotein IIb/IIIa blockade during percutaneous coronary intervention: REPLACE-2 randomized trial. *JAMA* 2003;289:853–863.)

**TABLE 98-7**

PRIMARY ENDPOINT COMPONENTS BY 30 DAYS[a]

| Variables | Heparin plus glycoprotein IIb/IIIa | Bivalirudin | P value |
|---|---|---|---|
| Quadruple composite (death, MI, urgent revascularization, or major bleeding) | 299/2991 (10.0)[b] | 275/2975 (9.2) | 0.32 |
| Triple composite (death, MI, or urgent revascularization) | 211/2990 (7.1) | 227/2975 (7.6) | 0.40 |
| Death | 12/3000 (0.4) | 7/2986 (0.2) | 0.26 |
| MI | 185/2990 (6.2) | 207/2975 (7.0) | 0.23 |
| Q-wave MI | 13/2990 (0.4) | 12/2975 (0.4) | 0.43[b] |
| Non–Q-wave MI | 172/2990 (5.8) | 195/2975 (6.6) | |
| CK-MB <3 × control | 3/2987 (0.1) | 3/2971 (0.1) | 0.41 |
| CK-MB >3 to 5 × control | 6/2987 (2.5) | 70/2971 (2.4) | |
| CK-MB >5 to 10 × control | 52/2987 (1.7) | 72/2971 (2.4) | |
| CK-MB >10 × control | 38/2987 (1.3) | 43/2971 (1.4) | |
| Urgent revascularization | 42/2990 (1.4) | 35/2975 (1.2) | 0.44 |
| Urgent percutaneous revascularization | 27/2990 (0.9) | 22/2975 (0.7) | 0.49 |
| Urgent surgical revascularization | 16/2990 (0.5) | 14/2975 (0.5) | 0.73 |
| Major bleeding | 123/3008 (4.1)[c] | 71/2993 (2.4)[b] | <.001 |

MI, myocardial infarction; CK-MB, creatine kinase-myocardial band isoenzyme.
[a]Values are expressed as number/total (percentage). Denominators are corrected for missing values or follow-up of less than 25 days.
[b]Complete data were available for 2,990, but bleeding data were available for 1 additional patient who reached the endpoint of the quadruple composite.
[c]P value for trends in MI type or CK-MB elevation.

4 hours of completion of infusion, whereas bleeding times returns to baseline within 1 hour (167).

Tirofiban, a peptidometic inhibitor, occupies the binding pocket on GP IIb/IIIa and thereby competitively inhibits platelet aggregation mediated by fibrinogen or von Willebrand factor (168). The stoichiometry of both eptifibatide and tirofiban is greater than 100 molecules of drug per GP IIb/IIIa receptor needed to achieve full platelet inhibition. This compares with a stoichiometry of 1.5 molecules of abciximab for each receptor (165). Like eptifibatide, substantial recovery of platelet aggregation is apparent within 4 hours of completion of infusion (167).

## Glycoprotein IIb/IIIa: Pharmacodynamics and Optimal Dosing with Glycoprotein IIb/IIIa Inhibitors

Both preclinical and clinical pharmacodynamic studies have set the range of greater than 80% inhibition of platelet aggregation by LTA as the target for clinically effective antiplatelet activity (161,167,169). The level of platelet inhibition varies among the three GP IIb/IIIa inhibitors following the recommended bolus and infusions (170). In general, the bolus and infusion regimen of abciximab and the double bolus and infusion regimen of eptifibatide are associated with rapid and profound inhibition of platelet function (69,170,171). Several studies have documented that the FDA-approved bolus and infusion regimen for tirofiban achieves suboptimal levels of platelet inhibition for up to 4 to 6 hours that likely accounted for inferior clinical results in the PCI setting (69). The degree of platelet inhibition appears central to the efficacy of GP IIb/IIIa inhibitors, achieving greater than 95% platelet inhibition 10 minutes after the bolus in patients undergoing PCI was associated with a 55% reduction in MACE compared to those patients with less than 95% platelet inhibition (172).

## Initial Trial Experience with Glycoprotein IIb/IIIa Inhibitor

The landmark trial demonstrating efficacy of GP IIb/IIIa inhibition in the PCI setting was the evaluation of IIb/IIIa platelet receptor antagonist 7E3 in Preventing Ischemic Complications (EPIC) trial (169). In this study, high-risk patients undergoing balloon angioplasty were randomized to abciximab bolus and infusion versus abciximab bolus alone versus placebo. The group treated with abciximab bolus and infusion had a 35% lower rate of death, MI, or unplanned urgent revascularization at 30 days compared to the placebo group (8.3% vs. 12.8%, P = 0.008). No substantial benefit with abciximab bolus alone was observed, suggesting that shorter duration of platelet inhibition was insufficient to favorably affect clinical outcomes. A considerable reduction in the primary endpoint with abciximab was also observed at 6 months and 3 years (173,174). Major bleeding complications occurred in an unacceptably high proportion of patients treated with abciximab compared to placebo (major bleeding 14% vs. 7%, transfusion 15% vs. 7%, respectively). Interventional cardiologists embarked on a series of procedural modifications, including performing frontwall arterial access only, reducing arterial sheath size from 8F to 6F, reducing heparin dosing to target ACT 200 to 250 seconds rather than greater than 300 seconds, removing sheaths as soon as possible (ACT <180 seconds) rather than overnight, and abandoning the use of routine venous sheaths, that successfully reduced major bleeding complications to less than 1% to 1.5% in future trials.

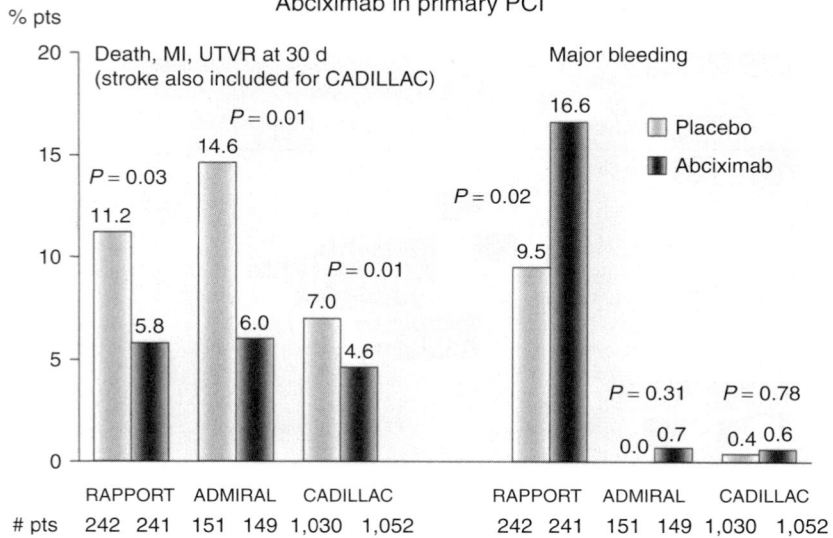

**FIGURE 98-9.** Summary of the randomized clinical trials comparing abciximab versus placebo in patients undergoing primary percutaneous coronary intervention (PCI) for ST segment elevation myocardial infarction (STEMI). RAPPORT (181); ISAR-2 (145); ADMIRAL (182); CADILLAC (90).

## Glycoprotein IIb/IIIa Inhibitors in Patients Undergoing Percutaneous Coronary Intervention

GP IIb/IIIa inhibitors have been rigorously studied through randomized controlled trials in a variety of clinical scenarios. The benefit of adjunctive GP IIb/IIIa inhibition during PCI has been shown in patients with stable coronary artery disease (175–177), unstable angina/NSTEMI (178–180), and STEMI (181–185) (see Fig. 98-9, Table 98-8). A significant reduction in MACE has been shown in all patients undergoing PCI who are treated with GP IIb/IIIa inhibitors irrespective of their level of risk. However, the benefit seen with upstream use of GP IIb/IIIa inhibitors is greatest in patients with high-risk features (178,179).

## Glycoprotein IIb/IIIa Inhibitors and Mortality

GP IIb/IIIa inhibitors have been shown to reduce major adverse cardiac events (death, MI, and urgent revascularization) by 35% to 50% in patients undergoing PCI (186). Although no single study demonstrated a significant reduction in mortality alone with GP IIb/IIIa inhibitors, metaanalysis suggests that these agents as a class reduce death by 20% to 30% (187) (see Fig. 98-10, and see Table 98-9). Another metaanalysis of 12 abciximab trials ($n = 20{,}186$ patients) demonstrated a significant reduction in 30-day mortality with abciximab (OR, 0.73; 95% CI, 0.55 to 0.96; $P = 0.024$) (see Fig. 98-11) (188). The mechanism by which GP IIb/IIIa inhibitors reduce long-term mortality is unclear and cannot be explained solely by its ability to reduce peri procedural death or myocardial infarction. Investigators have postulated that antithrombotic therapy may also be associated with significant antiinflammatory properties that may favorably influence the course of atherothrombotic disease (189,190).

## Head-to-Head Trials

Pharmacodynamic studies verify that the three approved GP IIb/IIIa antagonists have nonequivalent effects on platelet function (171, 191–193). Most of these studies measured platelet aggregation on blood samples collected in both citrate and D-phenylalanyl-L-prolyl-L-arginine chloromethylketone-anticoagulated tubes using standard LTA (LTA). The overall results of these studies suggest that the FDA-approved dosing regimens for abciximab and eptifibatide result in profound platelet inhibition (>80%) within 10 minutes of the bolus. In contrast, the dosing regimens for tirofiban in PRISM-PLUS (0.4 $\mu$/kg/minute load over 30 minutes followed by an infusion of 0.1 $\mu$/kg/minute for 12 to 24 hours thereafter) and in the Tirofiban and ReoPro Give Similar Efficacy Trial (194) (TARGET) (10 $\mu$ per kg bolus followed by an infusion of 0.15 $\mu$/kg/minutes for 18 to 24 hours post-PCI) lead to inadequate platelet inhibition (60% to 80%) up to 3 to 6 hours after the bolus, leading some investigators to recommend that the bolus dose for tirofiban may need to be increased 2.5-fold to threefold (195). The clinical relevance of these pharmacodynamic observations was tested in TARGET, which randomized 5,308 points to tirofiban or abciximab before undergoing percutaneous coronary revascularization with the intent to perform stenting (194). The primary endpoint was a composite of death, nonfatal MI, or urgent at 30 days. The primary endpoint (6.0% vs. 7.6%, $P = 0.038$) as well as the incidence of MI (5.4% vs. 6.9%, $P = 0.04$) were significantly lower in the abciximab group compared to the tirofiban group, respectively. There was no significant difference in the rate of major bleeding between the two groups; however, the incidence of minor bleeding and thrombocytopenia was significantly greater in the abciximab group.

## Facilitated Percutaneous Coronary Intervention with Half-Dose Thrombolytic Therapy and Glycoprotein IIb/IIIa Combination

Effective and rapid reperfusion of the infarct-related coronary artery is the critical goal in the treatment of acute MI. The optimal pharmacologic strategy for bridging between admission and performance of PCI in a patient with acute MI has not been defined. Although several drugs or combinations of drugs may meet the requirements for effective facilitated PCI, comparative evidence and clinical efficacy of the optimal regimen is lacking. Several studies (196–200) have been performed to assess the safety and efficacy of combination therapy using half-dose thrombolytic therapy and various GP IIb/IIIa inhibitors pre-PCI to improve baseline angiographic patency of the infarct-related artery. Each of these trials has demonstrated improved early patency of the infarct-related artery compared to full-dose thrombolytic therapy alone.

**TABLE 98-8**

RANDOMIZED TRIALS OF GP IIB/IIIA INHIBITORS DURING PERCUTANEOUS CORONARY INTERVENTION

| Trials | N | Randomization groups | Endpoint | Events (%) | P value | Conclusion |
|---|---|---|---|---|---|---|
| **ELECTIVE** | | | | | | |
| EPISTENT (175) | 2,399 | UFH + stent | 30-d MACE | 10.8 | <0.001[a] | abc + UFH superior to UFH alone |
| | | UFH + abc + stent | | 5.3 | | |
| | | UFH + abc + poba | | 6.9 | | |
| ESPIRIT (177) | 2,064 | UFH | 48 h MACE + bailout | 10.5 | 0.0017 | ept + UFH superior to UFH alone |
| | | UFH + ept | | 6.6 | | |
| **UNSTABLE ANGINA/NSTEMI** | | | | | | |
| CAPTURE (180) | 1,265 | UFH | MACE | 15.9 | 0.012 | abc superior to UFH alone |
| | | UFH + abc | | 11.3 | | |
| PRISM-PLUS (179) | 1,915 | UFH | 7-d death/MI or recurrent ischemia | 17.9 | 0.004 | tir + UFH superior to UFH alone. tir alone harmful |
| | | UFH + tir | | 12.9 | | |
| | | Tir alone | | stopped early | | |
| PURSUIT (178) | 10,948 | UFH | 30-d death or MI | 16.7 | 0.01 | ept + UFH superior to UFH alone |
| | | UFH + ept | | 11.6 | | |
| **STEMI** | | | | | | |
| RAPPORT (181) | 483 | UFH | 30-d MACE[b] | 11.2 | 0.03 | abc + UFH superior to UFH alone |
| | | UFH + abc | | 5.8 | | |
| ADMIRAL (182) | 300 | UFH | 30-d MACE | 14.6 | 0.01 | abc + UFH superior to UFH alone |
| | | UFH + abc | | 6.0 | | |
| CADILLAC (183) | 2,082 | UFH + poba | 6 mo MACE + CVA | 20 | <0.001[c] | Stent superior to poba regardless of abc use |
| | | UFH + stent | | 11.5 | 0.03[d] | |
| | | UFH + abc + poba | | 16.5 | 0.004[e] | |
| | | UFH + abc + stent | | 10.2 | | |
| TIGER-PA (184) | 100 | UFH | TIMI 3-flow | 32 | 0.007 | Tir + UFH yields better TIMI flow rates |
| | | UFH + tir | | 10 | | |
| On-TIME (185) | 507 | UFH + early tir | TIMI 2–3 flow | 34 | 0.04 | Early administration of tir superior to initiation in cath lab |
| | | UFH + cath lab tir | 43 | | | |

UFH, unfractionated heparin; abc, abciximab; poba, plain old balloon angioplasty; ept, eptifibatide; tir, tirofiban; EPISTENT, Evaluation of Platelet GP IIb/IIIa Inhibitor for Stenting; MACE, major adverse cardiovascular events; ESPRIT, Enhanced Suppression of Platelet Receptor GP IIb/IIIa using Integrilin Therapy; CAPTURE, C73 Antiplatelet Therapy in Unstable Refractory Angina; PRISM-PLUS, Platelet Receptor Inhibition in Ischemic Syndrome Management in Patients Limited by Unstable Signs and Symptoms; PURSUIT, Platelet G IIb/IIIa in Unstable Angina: Receptor Suppression Using Integrilin Therapy; RAPPORT, ReoPro and Primary PTCA Organization and Randomized Trial; CVA, cerebrovascular accident; TIMI, Thrombolysis in Myocardial Infarction.

[a]P <0.001 for the comparison of UFH + abc + stent versus UFH + stent.

[b]In RAPPORT, the primary endpoint was 6-month (MACE + any revascularization) although 30-day MACE was a prespecified endpoint and is listed here for comparison purposes.

[c]P <0.001 for the comparison of UFH + poba versus UFH + stent.

[c]P <0.001 for the comparison of UFH + poba versus UFH + abc + stent.

[d]P = 0.03 for the comparison of UFH + stent versus UFH + abc + poba.

[e]P = 0.004 for the comparison of UFH + abc + poba versus UFH + abc + stent.

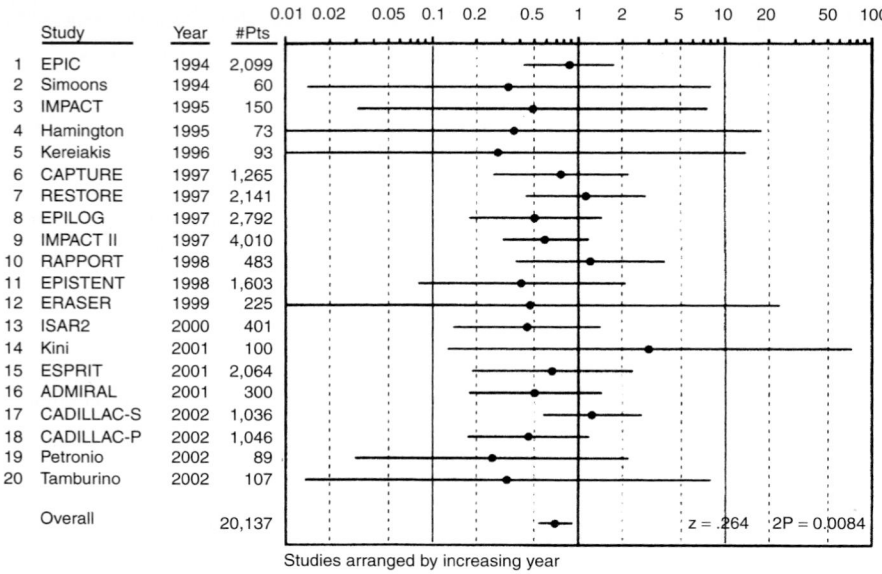

**A**

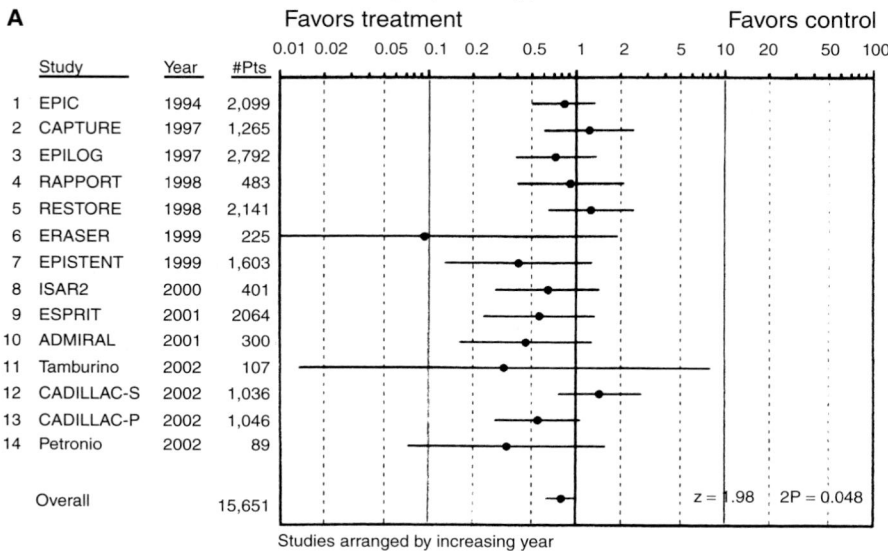

**B**

FIGURE 98-10. Metaanalysis of glycoprotein (GP) IIb/IIIa inhibitors and mortality reduction. Mortality at 30-day (A) and 6-month (B) follow-up. Risk ratios and 95% confidence intervals (CI) are shown for each study and for the random effects summary. P, PTCA; S, stenting. (Reprinted from Karvouni E, Katritsis DG, Ioannidis JP. Intravenous glycoprotein IIb/IIIa receptor antagonists reduce mortality after percutaneous coronary interventions. *J Am Coll Cardiol* 2003;41: 26–32.)

## TABLE 98-9

### OUTCOMES OF PATIENTS RECEIVING GLYCOPROTEIN IIB/IIIA INHIBITORS

| Outcome | No. of studies (n) | Total events/patients (%) | | RR (95% CI) |
| | | Active treatment | Control arm | |
|---|---|---|---|---|
| MI (30 d) | 20 (20,137) | 537/11,676 (4.6) | 585/8,461 (6.9) | 0.63 (0.56–0.70) |
| MI (6 mo) | 13 (15,250) | 481/8,485 (5.7) | 550/6,765 (8.1) | 0.67 (0.60–0.76) |
| Composite[a] (30 d) | 20 (20,137) | 926/11,676 (7.9) | 978/8,461 (11.6) | 0.65 (0.59–0.72) |
| Composite[a] (6 mo) | 13 (15,250) | 1,817/8,485 (21.4) | 1,624/6,765 (24.0) | 0.85 (0.80–0.90) |
| Major bleeding | 20 (20,137) | 531/11,676 (4.6) | 273/8,461 (3.2) | 1.26 (1.09–1.46) |
| Hemorrhagic stroke[b] | 18 (19,612) | 14/11,373 (0.1) | 10/8,239 (0.1) | 0.89 (0.46–1.72) |

CI, confidence intervals; RR, risk ratio, based on fixed effects calculations.
[a]The composite outcome includes death, myocardial infarction (MI), or revascularization. For the last component, we used any target vessel revascularization, except for studies where this was not a trial outcome, in which case, urgent or all revascularizations were counted.
[b]The ADMIRAL and ERASER trials provided no data on hemorrhagic stroke. There was no statistically significant heterogeneity, and random effects estimates were very similar (data not shown), except for the composite outcome at 30 days (P = 0.04 for heterogeneity, random effects RR, 0.66 [95% CI, 0.57–0.75]) and major bleeding (P = 0.08 for heterogeneity, random effects RR, 1.19 [95% CI, 0.96–1.48]).
From Karvouni E, Katritsis DG, Ioannidis JP. Intravenous glycoprotein IIb/IIIa receptor antagonists reduce mortality after percutaneous coronary interventions. *J Am Coll Cardiol* 2003;41:26–32.

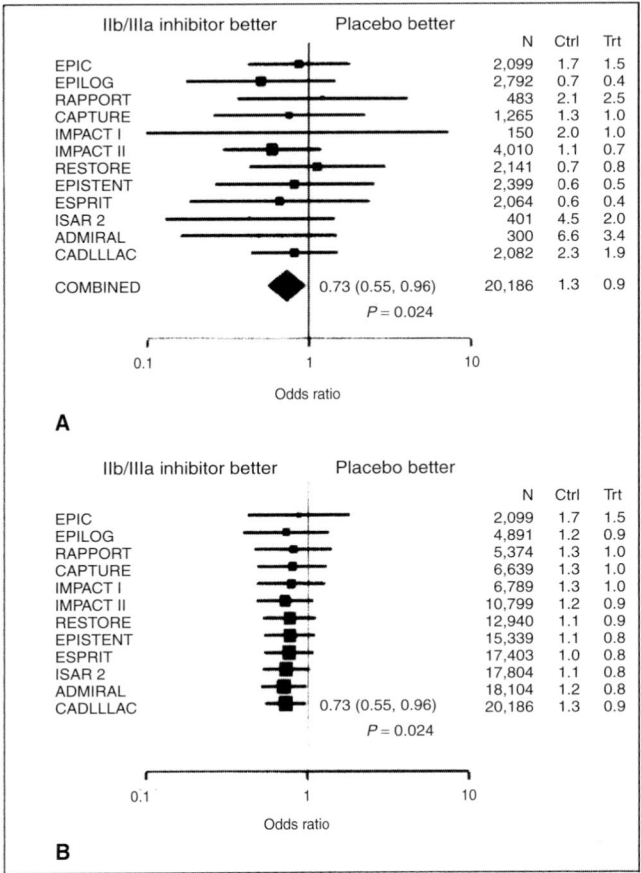

**FIGURE 98-11.** Risk of death at 30 days after randomization to a GP IIb/IIIa inhibitor (vs. placebo) in a standard metaanalysis (A) and a cumulative metaanalysis (B). Odds ratios (*squares*) and 95% confidence intervals (CI) (bars) are shown for each study and for the combined trials (*diamond*). Event rates (A) and cumulative event rates (B) are listed for the control (Ctrl) and treatment (Trt) arms in each study. CAPTURE, C73 AntiPlatelet Therapy in Unstable Refractory angina; EPIC, Evaluation of c73 for Prevention of Ischemic Complications; EPILOG, Evaluation in PTCA to Improve Long-term Outcome with abciximab GP IIb/IIIa blockade; EPISTENT, Evaluation of Platelet GP IIb/IIIa Inhibitor for Stenting; ESPRIT, Enhanced Suppression of Platelet Receptor GP IIb/IIIa using Integrilin Therapy; IMPACT, Integrilin to Minimize Platelet Aggregation and Coronary Thrombosis; ISAR, Intracoronary Stenting and Antithrombotic Regimen; RAPPORT, ReoPro and Primary PTCA Organization and Randomized Trial; RESTORE, Randomized Efficacy Study of Tirofiban for Outcomes and Restenosis. (Reprinted from Kong D, Hasselblad V, Harrington R, et al. Metaanalysis of survival with platelet glycoprotein IIb/IIIa antagonists for percutaneous coronary interventions. *Am J Cardiol* 2003; 92:651–655.)

However, this benefit may be at the expense of increased major bleeding (197,199). Improvement of hard clinical endpoints using this combination has yet to be shown and one study (200) of reteplase plus abciximab versus abciximab alone demonstrated no significant difference in final infarct size using technetium $^{99m}$Tc sestemibi. The Facilitated Intervention with Enhanced Reperfusion Speed to Stop Events (FINESSE) (196) study has been designed to test the hypothesis that facilitated PCI would be more effective than primary PCI. FINESSE is currently randomizing approximately 3,000 patients with STEMI undergoing primary PCI to receive either upstream abciximab, upstream half-dose reteplase plus abciximab, or abciximab at the time of PCI. The primary endpoint is a 90-day composite of all-cause mortality or complications of MI.

## Oral Glycoprotein IIb/IIIa Inhibitors

There have been six phase III trials conducted with oral GP IIb/IIIa receptor inhibitors (e.g., sibrafiban, orbofiban, xemilofiban), all with no improvement in outcome (201–208). Metaanalysis of these trials further demonstrated an increased bleeding risk and increased mortality in patients treated with oral GP IIb/IIIa inhibitors (209). One of the possible explanations for the poor outcomes and increased mortality in these trials was the patient-to-patient variability in the level of platelet inhibition over time (210). Another potential mechanism is that partial-agonist properties of oral IIb/IIIa inhibitors enhance platelet activation, especially at times when the serum drug levels are low, leaving more GP IIb/IIIa receptors available for binding fibrinogen. Proinflammatory effects have also been cited as another explanation for the unanticipated adverse events with oral GP IIb/IIIa inhibitors in these studies (211). Although oral GP IIb/IIIa inhibitors have no currently approved clinical uses, future study of these agents is ongoing and will evaluate higher doses, longer duration of therapy, and use in conjunction with other antiplatelet therapies.

## Glycoprotein IIb/IIIa and Thrombocytopenia

In a metaanalysis of eight clinical trials, abciximab increased the incidence of mild thrombocytopenia (>50,000 <90,000 to 100,000) compared to placebo group (4.2% vs. 2.0%, $P$ <0.001; OR, 2.13) (212). Eptifibatide or tirofiban with heparin did not increase mild thrombocytopenia compared with placebo with heparin (OR, 0.99). Small-molecule IIb/IIIa inhibitors did not cause a significant excess of thrombocytopenia in either PCI or ACS trials. Patients receiving abciximab with heparin had more than twice the frequency of severe thrombocytopenia (defined as >20,000 and <50,000) than those receiving placebo with heparin (1.0% vs. 0.4%, $P$ = 0.01; OR, 2.48). Eptifibatide or tirofiban with heparin did not cause a significant excess of severe thrombocytopenia compared with placebo with heparin (0.3% vs. 0.2%, $P$ = 0.16). ACS trials tended to report higher incidence of thrombocytopenia compared to PCI trials, perhaps because of longer heparin infusions–producing HIT (212).

Although uncommon, severe and profound (<20,000) thrombocytopenia require immediate cessation of GP IIb/IIIa therapy. An algorithm for evaluation of these patients has been proposed (see Figs. 98-12 and 98-13) (213). Pseudothrombocytopenia due to platelet clumping and HIT needs to be ruled out. The platelet count usually returns to normal within 48 to 72 hours in most cases. Severe and profound thrombocytopenia from GP IIb/IIIa receptor inhibitors are infrequent, more commonly associated with abciximab use. Irrespective of etiology, thrombocytopenia in patients undergoing PCI is associated with more ischemic events, bleeding complications, and transfusions (214).

The mechanism(s) of thrombocytopenia are unknown. The platelet count falls within hours of GP IIb/IIIa administration. Readministration of abciximab, but not the small-molecule inhibitors (eptifibatide and tirofiban), is associated with a slight increased risk of recurrent thrombocytopenia (215).

## Recommendations for the Use of Glycoprotein IIb/IIIa Inhibitors in Patients Undergoing Percutaneous Coronary Intervention

- For all patients undergoing PCI, particularly those undergoing primary PCI, or those with refractory UA or other

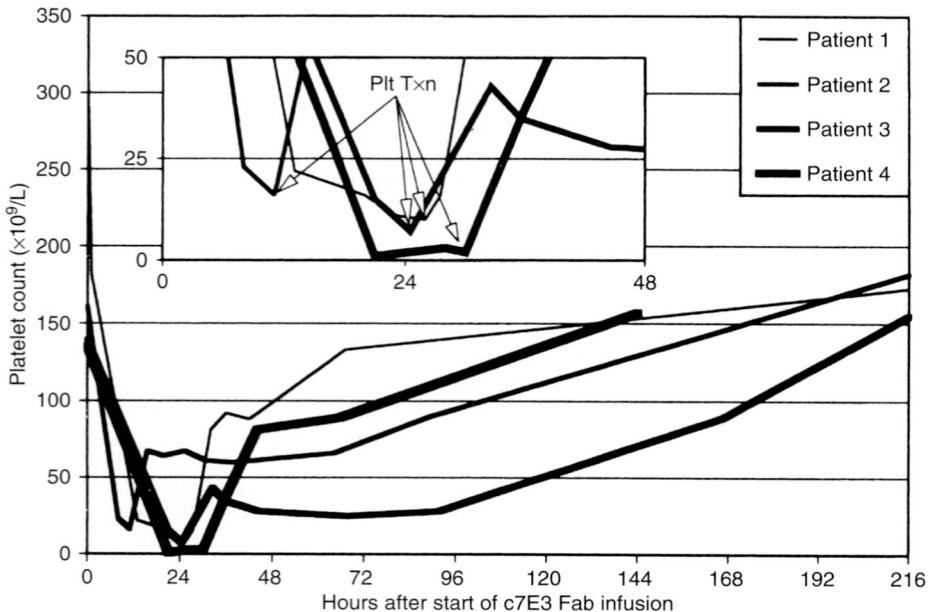

**FIGURE 98-12.** Time course of thrombocytopenia following administration of abciximab. Platelet counts before and during therapy and after recovery in four patients who developed acute profound thrombocytopenia after receiving c7E3 Fab bolus plus infusion. The inset focuses on the platelet counts during the first 48 hours and notes the first platelet transfusion (Plt Txn) given. [Reprinted from Berkowitz SD, Harrington RA, Rund MM, et al. Acute profound thrombocytopenia after c7E3 Fab (abciximab) therapy. *Circulation* 1997;95:809–813.]

high-risk features, use of a GP IIb/IIIa inhibitor (abciximab or eptifibatide) in addition to an antithrombin (UFH or enoxaparin) is recommended (Grade 1A) (55).

- Administration of abciximab as a 0.25 mg per kg bolus followed by a 12-hour infusion at a rate of 10 μcg per minute is recommended (Grade 1A). Administration of eptifibatide as a double bolus (each of 180 μcg per kg administered 10 minutes apart) followed by an 18-hour infusion of 2.0 μ/kg/minute is recommended (Grade 1A) (55).
- In patients undergoing PCI for STEMI, abciximab is recommended over eptifibatide (Grade 1B) (55).
- In patients undergoing PCI, the use of tirofiban as an alternative to abciximab is not recommended (Grade 1A) (55).
- For patients with NSTEMI/UA who are designated as moderate-to-high risk based on TIMI risk score, upstream use of a GP IIb/IIIa inhibitor (either eptifibatide or tirofiban) should be started as soon as possible based on PCI (Grade 1A) (55).
- In NSTEMI/UA patients who receive upstream treatment with tirofiban, PCI should be deferred for at least 4 hours after initiating the tirofiban infusion (Grade 2C) (55).
- With planned PCI in NSTEMI/UA patients with an elevated troponin level, abciximab should be started within 24 hours before PCI (Grade 1A) (55).
- Abciximab should not be administrated in patients in whom PCI is not planned (55,144).

## MECHANICAL APPROACHES

Antithrombotic therapies during PCI also include mechanical devices which exclude atherosclerotic plaque and thrombus (i.e., stents), actively remove preexisting thrombus (thrombectomy devices), or prevent thrombus and/or plaque embolization with embolic protection devices.

### Percutaneous Coronary Intervention for STEMI and UA/NSTEMI

All patients with STEMI should be rapidly assessed for treatment with fibrinolysis or primary PCI with balloon angioplasty

and/or stenting. The goal of early recanalization therapy is to salvage ischemic but viable myocardium, thereby preserving left ventricular (LV) function. More than 23 head-to-head randomized trials have randomly assigned approximately 8,000 thrombolytic-eligible patients with STEMI to primary PCI (balloon angioplasty or stenting) or thrombolytic therapy. Recent overview of these trials showed that primary PCI was better than thrombolytic therapy at reducing short-term death (7% vs. 9%, $P = 0.0002$), nonfatal reinfarction (3% vs. 7%, $P < 0.0001$), stroke (1% vs. 2%, $P = 0.0004$), and the combined endpoint of death, nonfatal reinfarction, and stroke (8% vs. 14%, $P < 0.0001$) (see Fig. 98-14) (216). The results seen with primary PCI remained better than those with thrombolytic therapy during long-term follow-up, and were independent of the type of thrombolytic agent used and whether or not the patient was transferred for primary PCI. This overview suggests that for every 1,000 patients treated with primary angioplasty rather than thrombolytic therapy, an additional 20 lives are saved, 43 reinfarctions are prevented, 10 fewer strokes occurred, and 13 intracranial hemorrhages are prevented. Myocardial salvage is greater with PCI, and primary PCI gives better results than thrombolytic therapy even in community hospitals without on-site surgical backup (217). Most importantly, primary PCI reduces death, recurrent MI, or stroke compared with front-loaded tPA (14.2% vs. 8.5%, $P < 0.002$) even if patients must be transferred by ambulance for up to 3 hours to reach an interventional center (218).

An invasive approach defining the coronary anatomy with an eye toward revascularization is also recommended for all higher-risk patients with US/NSTEMI on the basis of two clinical trials (219,220) showing a significant reduction in MACE compared to conservative therapy. These include patients with refractory ischemia, positive cardiac markers, ST segment depression, hemodynamic instability, signs of left ventricular dysfunction, or history of revascularization within 6 months. On the basis of clinical trial evidence (219,220), all patients with NSTEMI should proceed to the cardiac catheterization laboratory after a period of medical stabilization for delineation of coronary anatomy and revascularization by PCI or CABG. Although guidelines have recommended cardiac catheterization within 48 hours of presentation, a recent study has suggested significant clinical benefit of an early (<6 hours) invasive strategy compared to delayed cardiac catheterization (72 to 120 hours) after medical stabilization (145).

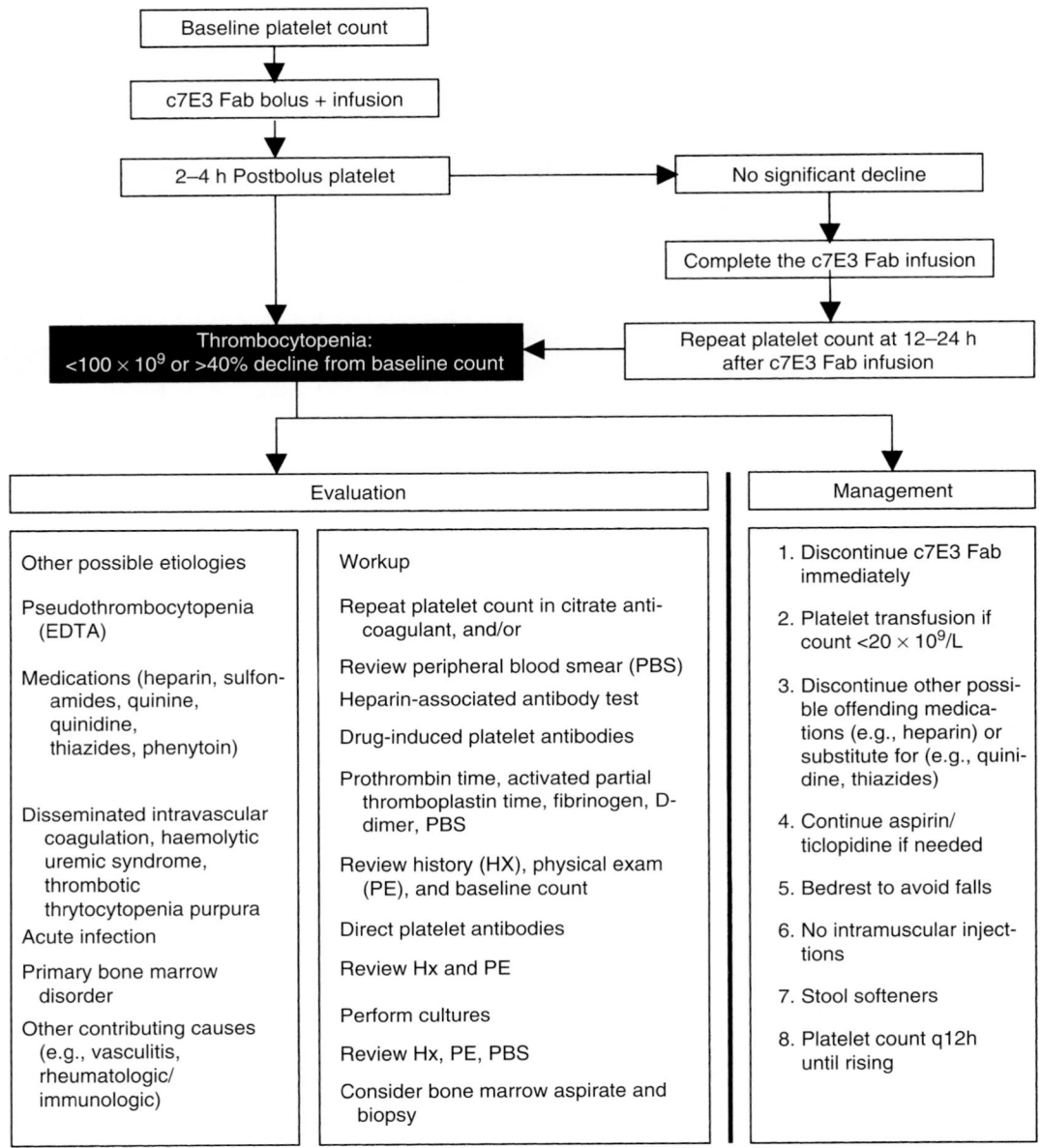

**FIGURE 98-13.** Platelet monitoring algorithm, thrombocytopenia workup, and treatment strategies for patients receiving abciximab. Evaluation and management of thrombocytopenia with c7E3 Fab therapy. ANA, antinuclear antibody; EDTA, ethylene diamine tetraacetic acid. [Reprinted from Berkowitz SD, Harrington RA, Rund MM, et al. Acute profound thrombocytopenia after C7E3 Fab (abciximab) therapy. *Circulation* 1997;95:809–813.]

## Thrombectomy Devices

The treatment of intracoronary thrombus visible by angiography has included various strategies including intracoronary thrombolytics (221,222), intracoronary GP IIb/IIIa inhibitors (223), balloon angioplasty, mechanical extraction and atherectomy devices (224–226), and ultrasonic thrombolysis (227, 228). The Possis Angiojet is a catheter-based system that uses high-velocity water jets to produce a vacuum for thrombus aspiration and extraction, termed *rheolytic thrombectomy*. A trial comparing rheolytic thrombectomy with intragraft or coronary urokinase for coronary and vein graft thrombus, (Vein Graft AngioJet Study (VeGAS 2) in a total of 349 patients demonstrated superior efficacy with reduced bleeding in those treated with thrombectomy compared to urokinase

(229). Rheolytic thrombectomy is a reasonable option for the treatment of angiographically visible thrombus in saphenous vein grafts and native coronary arteries. Use of this device in patients with acute myocardial infarction was studied in a large-scale, prospective, multicenter, randomized clinical trial, but failed to demonstrate a substantial reduction in myocardial infarct size with the routine use of rheolytic thrombectomy (230).

## Embolic Protection Devices

Percutaneous intervention within saphenous vein bypass grafts results in a high (approximately 20%) risk of MACE, driven by post-PCI myocardial infarction and reduced anterograde flow (the no-reflow phenomenon) (231–234). This

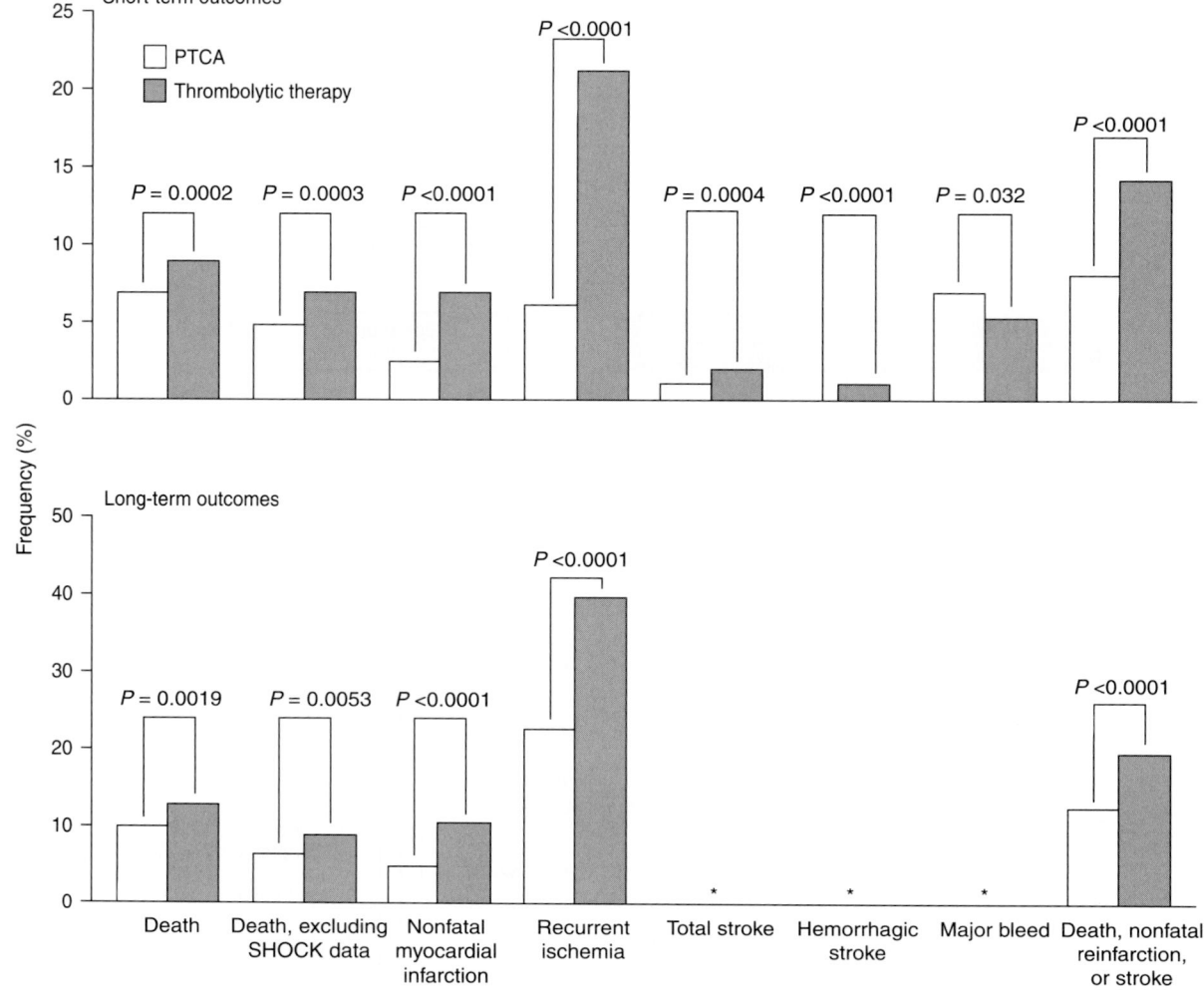

**FIGURE 98-14.** Primary angioplasty versus intravenous thrombolytic therapy for acute myocardial infarction: a quantitative review of 23 randomized trials. Primary PTCA is more effective than thrombolytic therapy for the treatment of STEMI. (Reprinted from Keeley EC, Boura JA, Grines CL. Primary angioplasty versus intravenous thrombolytic therapy for acute myocardial infarction: a quantitative review of 23 randomized trials. *Lancet* 2003;361:13–20.)

increased risk has been attributed to distal embolization of atherosclerotic debris which occurs consistently during PCI of saphenous vein grafts, with recovery of such debris in more than 95% of cases when using embolic protection devices (235). The Saphenous vein graft Angioplasty Free of Emboli Randomized (SAFER) trial (236) demonstrated a 42% reduction in MACE (primarily peri procedural myocardial infarction) and a 60% reduction in no-reflow seen when saphenous vein graft PCI was performed using the Medtronic GuardWire balloon occlusion and aspiration system compared with no embolic protection. Similar clinical benefits are also seen with a filter rather than balloon occlusion device (237). The potential advantage of a filter-based embolic protection device compared to balloon occlusion is the ability to maintain anterograde flow during the PCI. However, this theoretical advantage did not translate into clinical superiority of a filter over balloon occlusion (237). Multiple other embolic protection devices, including proximal protection systems that provide side-branch protection, are currently under clinical investigation at this time.

Additional interest in enhancing microvascular flow by preventing distal embolization in the setting of acute myocardial infarction was investigated recently in the Enhance Myocardial Efficacy and Removal by Aspiration of Liberated Debris (EMERALD) trial (238). In EMERALD, patients with STEMI were randomized to undergo primary angioplasty over a standard guidewire or with the Medtronic GuardWire embolic protection device. Preliminary results, available only in abstract form, demonstrated no considerable advantage to GuardWire distal protection over conventional guidewire use for patients with acute myocardial infarction (238).

There are no formal guideline recommendations for the use of these specialized devices during PCI. The following recommendations are based on general consensus of the aforementioned randomized trials:

1. Embolic protection devices are recommended for PCI within saphenous vein grafts unless contraindicated on the basis of anatomical location.
2. PCI with embolic protection is not superior to PCI alone for STEMI.

3. Rheolytic thrombectomy is recommended for use in bulky thrombus-containing lesions in saphenous vein grafts and native coronary vessels.

# RESTENOSIS PREVENTION

Restenosis is defined as the combination of neointimal hyperplasia with smooth muscle cells and vessel wall remodeling. Although the advent of coronary stents has reduced the incidence of restenosis compared with balloon angioplasty, this problem is still seen in 20% to 30% of cases following bare metal stenting. Systemic approaches, including a variety of antiplatelet agents (26,239–245), antithrombin inhibitors (e.g., UFH, LMWH, and DTIs) (133,246–250), GP IIb/IIIa inhibitors (251), and warfarin (252,253) have uniformly failed. One systemic drug, cilostazol, a platelet phosphodiesterase inhibitor, has shown promise in a large, prospective randomized trial (254). Patients undergoing bare metal stenting were treated with a 6-month course of cilostazol 100 mg bid plus ASA and clopidogrel or placebo plus ASA and clopidogrel. Angiographic restenosis was reduced by 39.5% in the cilostazol-treated group.

Restenosis therapies are now focused on local drug–delivery approaches using DES that target the inflammatory and proliferative phases of this wound healinglike response to vascular injury. Five large-scale randomized trials using either sirolimus-eluting or paclitaxel-eluting stents have demonstrated dramatic and consistent reductions (approximately 75% to 90%) in angiographic and clinical restenosis (98–102). It is estimated that DES are currently used in more than 70% of PCI procedures in the United States. Potential problems with DES such as late restenosis, allergic reactions, and increased rates of stent thrombosis have been postulated. However, no single randomized DES trial and the largest analysis of published randomized DES trials have not substantiated any of these concerns (255).

# FUTURE THERAPIES AND DIRECTIONS

Antithrombotic regimens for PCI have reduced the rate of acute ischemic complications to less than 7% even in high-risk interventions. Newer approaches under active clinical investigation include targeting tissue factor (256), factor Xa (257), and platelet adhesion. Large megatrials are evaluating the optimal combinations of antiplatelet and antithrombin agents in US/NSTEMI. Finally, personalized medicine approaches incorporating genetic and clinical factors may be necessary to optimize clinical benefit.

## *References*

1. Awtry EH, Loscalzo J. Aspirin. *Circulation* 2000;101:1206–1218.
2. Szczeklik A. Thrombin generation in myocardial infarction and hypercholesterolemia: effects of aspirin. *Thromb Haemost* 1995;74:77–80.
3. Patrono C, Coller B, Dalen JE, et al. Platelet-active drugs: the relationships among dose, effectiveness, and side effects. *Chest* 1998;114:470S–488S.
4. Latini R, Cerletti C, de Gaetano G, et al. Comparative bioavailability of aspirin from buffered, enteric-coated and plain preparations. *Int J Clin Pharmacol Ther Toxicol* 1986;24:313–318.
5. The RISC Group. Risk of myocardial infarction and death during treatment with low dose aspirin and intravenous heparin in men with unstable coronary artery disease. *Lancet* 1990;336:827–830.
6. Juul-Moller S, Edvardsson N, Jahnmatz B, et al. The Swedish Angina Pectoris Aspirin Trial (SAPAT) Group. Double-blind trial of aspirin in primary prevention of myocardial infarction in patients with stable chronic angina pectoris. *Lancet* 1992;340:1421–1425.
7. Peters R, Mehta S, Fox K, et al. Effects of aspirin dose when used alone or in combination with clopidogrel in patients with acute coronary syndromes: observations from the Clopidogrel in Unstable angina to prevent Recurrent Events (CURE) study. *Circulation* 2003;108:1682–1687.
8. Kurth T, Glynn RJ, Walker AM, et al. Inhibition of clinical benefits of aspirin on first myocardial infarction by nonsteroidal antiinflammatory drugs. *Circulation* 2003;108:1191–1195.
9. Loll PJ, Picot D, Garavito RM. The structural basis of aspirin activity inferred from the crystal structure of inactivated prostaglandin H2 synthase. *Nat Struct Biol* 1995;2:637–643.
10. Catella-Lawson F, Reilly MP, Kapoor SC, et al. Cyclooxygenase inhibitors and the antiplatelet effects of aspirin. *N Engl J Med* 2001;345:1809–1817.
11. Lewis HD Jr, Davis JW, Archibald DG, et al. Protective effects of aspirin against acute myocardial infarction and death in men with unstable angina. Results of a Veterans Administration Cooperative Study. *N Engl J Med* 1983;309:396–403.
12. Cairns JA, Gent M, Singer J, et al. Aspirin, sulfinpyrazone, or both in unstable angina. Results of a Canadian multicenter trial. *N Engl J Med* 1985;313:1369–1375.
13. Theroux P, Ouimet H, McCans J, et al. Aspirin, heparin, or both to treat acute unstable angina. *N Engl J Med* 1988;319:1105–1111.
14. Roux S, Christeller S, Ludin E. Effects of aspirin on coronary reocclusion and recurrent ischemia after thrombolysis: a meta-analysis. *J Am Coll Cardiol* 1992;19:671–677.
15. Randomized trial of intravenous streptokinase, oral aspirin, both, or neither among 17,187 cases of suspected acute myocardial infarction: ISIS-2. ISIS-2 (Second International Study of Infarct Survival) Collaborative Group. *J Am Coll Cardiol* 1988;12:3A–13A.
16. Eidelman RS, Hebert PR, Weisman SM, et al. An update on aspirin in the primary prevention of cardiovascular disease. *Arch Intern Med* 2003;163:2006–2010.
17. FDA Talk Paper: FDA approves new prescribed uses for aspirin. Vol. 1998: United States Food and Drug Administration, U.S Department of Health and Human Services, 1998. 1998.
18. Antiplatelet Trialists' Collaboration. Collaborative overview of randomised trials of antiplatelet therapy—II: maintenance of vascular graft or arterial patency by antiplatelet therapy. *BMJ* 1994;308:159–168.
19. Gavaghan TP, Gebski V, Baron DW. Immediate postoperative aspirin improves vein graft patency early and late after coronary artery bypass graft surgery. A placebo-controlled, randomized study. *Circulation* 1991;83:1526–1533.
20. Goldman S, Copeland J, Moritz T, et al. Improvement in early saphenous vein graft patency after coronary artery bypass surgery with antiplatelet therapy: results of a Veterans Administration Cooperative Study. *Circulation* 1988;77:1324–1332.
21. Goldman S, Copeland J, Moritz T, et al. Long-term graft patency (3 years) after coronary artery surgery. Effects of aspirin: results of a VA Cooperative study. *Circulation* 1994;89:1138–1143.
22. Antithrombotic Trialists' Collaboration. Collaborative meta-analysis of randomised trials of antiplatelet therapy for prevention of death, myocardial infarction, and stroke in high risk patients. *BMJ* 2002;324:71–86.
23. Serruys PW, de Jaegere P, Kiemeneij F, et al. A comparison of balloon-expandable-stent implantation with balloon angioplasty in patients with coronary artery disease. *N Engl J Med* 1994;331:489–495.
24. de Feyter P, van den Brand M, Jaarman G, et al. Acute coronary artery occlusion during and after percutaneous transluminal coronary angioplasty: frequency, prediction, clinical course, management and follow-up. *Circulation* 1991;83:927–936.
25. Baim DS, Carrozza JP Jr. Stent thrombosis. Closing in on the best preventive treatment. *Circulation* 1997;95:1098–1100.
26. Schwartz L, Bourassa MG, Lesperance J, et al. Aspirin and dipyridamole in the prevention of restenosis after percutaneous transluminal coronary angioplasty. *N Engl J Med* 1988;318:1714–1719.
27. Lembo NJ, Black A, Roubin G, et al. Effect of pretreatment with aspirin versus aspirin plus dipyridamole on frequency and type of acute complications of percutaneous transluminal coronary angioplasty. *Am J Cardiol* 1990;65:422–426.
28. Goods CM, al-Shaibi KF, Liu MW, et al. Comparison of aspirin alone versus aspirin plus ticlopidine after coronary artery stenting. *Am J Cardiol* 1996;78:1042–1044.
29. Leon M, Baim D, Popma J, et al. Stent Anticoagulation Restenosis Study Investigators. A clinical trial comparing three antithrombotic-drug regimens after coronary-artery stenting. *N Engl J Med* 1998;339:1665–1671.
30. Stephens NG, Ludman PF, Petch MC, et al. Changing from intensive anticoagulation to treatment with aspirin alone for coronary stents: the experience of one centre in the United Kingdom. *Heart* 1996;76:238–242.
31. Taylor R, Gibbons F, Cope G, et al. Effects of low-dose aspirin on restenosis after coronary angioplasty. *Am J Cardiol* 1991;68:874–878.
32. Segal R, Lubart E, Leibovitz A, et al. Early and late effects of low-dose aspirin on renal function in elderly patients. *Am J Med* 2003;115:462–466.
33. Howard PA. Aspirin resistance. *Ann Pharmacother* 2002;36:1620–1624.
34. Gum PA, Kottke-Marchant K, Poggio ED, et al. Profile and prevalence of aspirin resistance in patients with cardiovascular disease. *Am J Cardiol* 2001;88:230–235.
35. Gum PA, Kottke-Marchant K, Welsh PA, et al. A prospective, blinded determination of the natural history of aspirin resistance among stable patients with cardiovascular disease. *J Am Coll Cardiol* 2003;41:961–965.

36. Grotemeyer KH. Effects of acetylsalicylic acid in stroke patients. Evidence of nonresponders in a subpopulation of treated patients. *Thromb Res* 1991; 63:587–593.

37. Tohgi H, Konno S, Tamura K, et al. Effects of low-to-high doses of aspirin on platelet aggregability and metabolites of thromboxane A2 and prostacyclin. *Stroke* 1992;23:1400–1403.

38. Helgason CM, Tortorice KL, Winkler SR, et al. Aspirin response and failure in cerebral infarction. *Stroke* 1993;24:345–350.

39. Pappas JM, Westengard JC, Bull BS. Population variability in the effect of aspirin on platelet function. Implications for clinical trials and therapy. *Arch Pathol Lab Med* 1994;118:801–804.

40. Mueller MR, Salat A, Stangl P, et al. Variable platelet response to low-dose ASA and the risk of limb deterioration in patients submitted to peripheral arterial angioplasty. *Thromb Haemost* 1997;78:1003–1007.

41. Hurlen M, Seljeflot I, Arnesen H. The effect of different antithrombotic regimens on platelet aggregation after myocardial infarction. *Scand Cardiovasc J* 1998;32:233–237.

42. Grotemeyer KH. The platelet-reactivity-test—a useful "by-product" of the blood-sampling procedure? *Thromb Res* 1991;61:423–431.

43. Grotemeyer KH, Scharafinski HW, Husstedt IW. Two-year follow-up of aspirin responder and aspirin non responder. A pilot-study including 180 post-stroke patients. *Thromb Res* 1993;71:397–403.

44. Bhatt DL. Aspirin resistance: more than just a laboratory curiosity. *J Am Coll Cardiol* 2004;43:1127–1129.

45. Vejar M, Fragasso G, Hackett D, et al. Dissociation of platelet activation and spontaneous myocardial ischemia in unstable angina. *Thromb Haemost* 1990;63:163–168.

46. Patrono C. Prevention of myocardial infarction and stroke by aspirin: different mechanisms? Different dosage? *Thromb Res* 1998;92:S7–12.

47. Dyken ML, Barnett HJ, Easton JD, et al. Low-dose aspirin and stroke. "It ain't necessarily so". *Stroke* 1992;23:1395–1399.

48. Eikelboom JW, Hirsh J, Weitz JI, et al. Aspirin-resistant thromboxane biosynthesis and the risk of myocardial infarction, stroke, or cardiovascular death in patients at high risk for cardiovascular events. *Circulation* 2002; 105:1650–1655.

49. Grundmann K, Jaschonek K, Kleine B, et al. Aspirin non-responder status in patients with recurrent cerebral ischemic attacks. *J Neurol* 2003;250: 63–66.

50. Wang J, Aucoin-Barry D, Manuelian D, et al. Incidence of aspirin nonresponsiveness using the Ultegra Rapid Platelet Function Assay-ASA. *Am J Cardiol* 2003;92:1492–1494.

51. Chen WH, Lee PY, Ng W, et al. Aspirin resistance is associated with a high incidence of myonecrosis after non-urgent percutaneous coronary intervention despite clopidogrel pretreatment. *J Am Coll Cardiol* 2004;43: 1122–1126.

52. Wong J, Nagy C, Krinzman S, et al. Rapid oral challenge-desensitization for patients with aspirin-related urticaria-angioedema. *J Allergy Clin Immunol* 2000;105:997–1001.

53. Wilson S, Rihal C, Bell M, et al. Timing of coronary stent thrombosis in patients treated with ticlopidine and aspirin. *Am J Cardiol* 1999;83: 1006–1011.

54. Schaefer O, Gore J. Aspirin sensitivity: the role for aspirin challenge and desensitization in postmyocardial infarction patients. *Cardiology* 1999;91: 8–13.

55. Popma J, Berger PB, Ohman EM, et al. Antithrombotic therapy during percutaneous coronary intervention. The 7th ACCP Consensus Conference on Antithrombotic and Thrombolytic Therapy. *Chest* 2004;126: 576S–599S.

56. Hollopeter G, Jantzen H, Vincent D, et al. Identification of the platelet ADP receptor targeted by antithrombotic drugs. *Nature* 2001;409: 202–207.

57. Sharis P, Cannon C, Loscalzo J. The antiplatelet effects of ticlopidine and clopidogrel. *Ann Intern Med* 1998;129:394–405.

58. Andre P, Delaney SM, LaRocca T, et al. P2Y12 regulates platelet adhesion/activation, thrombus growth, and thrombus stability in injured arteries. *J Clin Invest* 2003;112:398–406.

59. Feliste R, Delebassee D, Simon MF, et al. Broad spectrum anti-platelet activity of ticlopidine and PCR 4099 involves the suppression of the effects of released ADP. *Thromb Res* 1987;48:403–415.

60. Schafer AI. Antiplatelet therapy. *Am J Med* 1996;101:199–209.

61. Herbert J, Bono F, Herault J, et al. Effector protease receptor 1 mediates the mitogenic activity of factor Xa for vascular smooth muscle cells *in vitro* and *in vivo*. *J Clin Invest* 1998;101:993–1000.

62. Gachet C, Stierle A, Cazenave JP, et al. The thienopyridine PCR 4099 selectively inhibits ADP-induced platelet aggregation and fibrinogen binding without modifying the membrane glycoprotein IIb-IIIa complex in rat and in man. *Biochem Pharmacol* 1990;40:229–238.

63. Gachet C. ADP receptors of platelets and their inhibition. *Thromb Haemost* 2001;86:222–232.

64. Steinhubl S, Tan W, Foody J, et al. Incidence and clinical course of thrombotic thrombocytopenic purpura due to ticlopidine following coronary stenting. EPISTENT Investigators. Evaluation of Platelet IIb/IIIa Inhibitor for Stenting. *JAMA* 1999;281:806–810.

65. Coukell AJ, Markham A. Clopidogrel. *Drugs* 1997;54:745–750; discussion 751.

66. Weber AA, Braun M, Hohlfeld T, et al. Recovery of platelet function after discontinuation of clopidogrel treatment in healthy volunteers. *Br J Clin Pharmacol* 2001;52:333–336.

67. Mehta SR, Yusuf S, Peters RJ, et al. Effects of pretreatment with clopidogrel and aspirin followed by long-term therapy in patients undergoing percutaneous coronary intervention: the PCI-CURE study. *Lancet* 2001;358: 527–533.

68. Steinhubl SR, Berger PB, Mann JT III, et al. Early and sustained dual oral antiplatelet therapy following percutaneous coronary intervention: a randomized controlled trial. *JAMA* 2002;288:2411–2420.

69. Kabbani S, Aggarwal A, Terrien E, et al. Suboptimal early inhibition of platelets by treatment with tirofiban and implications for coronary interventions. *Am J Cardiol* 2002;89:647–650.

70. Kastrati A, Mehilli J, Schuhlen H, et al. A clinical trial of abciximab in elective percutaneous coronary intervention after pretreatment with clopidogrel. *N Engl J Med* 2004;350:232–238.

71. Taniuchi M, Kurz HI, Lasala JM. Randomized comparison of ticlopidine and clopidogrel after intracoronary stent implantation in a broad patient population. *Circulation* 2001;104:539–543.

72. Muller C, Buttner HJ, Petersen J, et al. A randomized comparison of clopidogrel and aspirin versus ticlopidine and aspirin after the placement of coronary-artery stents. *Circulation* 2000;101:590–593.

73. Mueller C, Roskamm H, Neumann F, et al. A randomized comparison of clopidogrel and aspirin versus ticlopidine and aspirin after the placement of coronary artery stents. *J Am Coll Cardiol* 2003;41:969–973.

74. Bertrand ME, Rupprecht HJ, Urban P, et al. Double-blind study of the safety of clopidogrel with and without a loading dose in combination with aspirin compared with ticlopidine in combination with aspirin after coronary stenting: the clopidogrel aspirin stent international cooperative study (CLASSICS). *Circulation* 2000;102:624–629.

75. Bhatt D, Marso S, Hirsch A, et al. Amplified benefit of clopidogrel versus aspirin in patients with diabetes mellitus. *Am J Cardiol* 2002;90:625–628.

76. Moussa I, Di Mario C, Reimers B, et al. Subacute stent thrombosis in the era of intravascular ultrasound-guided coronary stenting without anticoagulation: frequency, predictors and clinical outcome. *J Am Coll Cardiol* 1997;29:6–12.

77. Mak KH, Belli G, Ellis SG, et al. Subacute stent thrombosis: evolving issues and current concepts. *J Am Coll Cardiol* 1996;27:494–503.

78. Hasdai D, Garratt KN, Holmes DR, et al. Coronary angioplasty and intracoronary thrombolysis are of limited efficacy in resolving early intracoronary stent thrombosis. *J Am Coll Cardiol* 1996;28:361–367.

79. Schatz RA, Baim DS, Leon M, et al. Clinical experience with the Palmaz-Schatz coronary stent. Initial results of a multicenter study. *Circulation* 1991;83:148–161.

80. More RS, Chauhan A. Antiplatelet rather than anticoagulant therapy with coronary stenting. *Lancet* 1997;349:146–147.

81. Fischman DL, Leon MB, Baim DS et al., Stent Restenosis Study Investigators. A randomized comparison of coronary-stent placement and balloon angioplasty in the treatment of coronary artery disease. *N Engl J Med* 1994;331:p496–p501.

82. Karrillon GJ, Morice MC, Benveniste E, et al. Intracoronary stent implantation without ultrasound guidance and with replacement of conventional anticoagulation by antiplatelet therapy. 30-day clinical outcome of the French Multicenter Registry. *Circulation* 1996;94:1519–1527.

83. Urban P, Macaya C, Rupprecht H, et al. Randomized evaluation of anticoagulation versus antiplatelet therapy after coronary stent implantation in high-risk patients: the multicenter aspirin and ticlopidine trial after intracoronary stenting (MATTIS). *Circulation* 1998;98:2126–2132.

84. Bertrand M, Legrand V, Boland J, et al. Randomized multicenter comparison of conventional anticoagulation versus antiplatelet therapy in unplanned and elective coronary stenting. The full anticoagulation versus aspirin and ticlopidine (FANTASTIC) study. *Circulation* 1998;98:1597–1603.

85. Schomig A, Neumann FJ, Kastrati A, et al. A randomized comparison of antiplatelet and anticoagulant therapy after the placement of coronary-artery stents. *N Engl J Med* 1996;334:p1084–p1089.

86. Schuhlen H, Kastrati A, Pache J, et al. Sustained benefit over four years from an initial combined antiplatelet regimen after coronary stent placement in the ISAR trial. Intracoronary Stenting and Antithrombotic Regimen. *Am J Cardiol* 2001;87:397–400.

87. Yusuf S, Zhao F, Mehta SR, et al. Effects of clopidogrel in addition to aspirin in patients with acute coronary syndromes without ST-segment elevation. *N Engl J Med* 2001;345:494–502.

88. Budaj A, Yusuf S, Mehta SR, et al. Benefit of clopidogrel in patients with acute coronary syndromes without ST-segment elevation in various risk groups. *Circulation* 2002;106:1622–1626.

89. Lange RA, Hillis LD. Antiplatelet therapy for ischemic heart disease. *N Engl J Med* 2004;350:277–280.

90. Tcheng JE, Campbell ME. Platelet inhibition strategies in percutaneous coronary intervention: competition or coopetition? *J Am Coll Cardiol* 2003; 42:1196–1198.

91. Steimle AE. Antiplatelet therapy for ischemic heart disease. *N Engl J Med* 2004;350:2101–2102; author reply 2101–2102.

92. Rozenman Y. For how long should treatment with clopidogrel be continued after coronary stent implantation? *J Am Coll Cardiol* 2004;43:1331; author reply 1331–1332.

93. Eriksson P. Long-term clopidogrel therapy after percutaneous coronary intervention in PCI-CURE and CREDO: the "Emperor's New Clothes" revisited. *Eur Heart J* 2004;25:720–722.

94. Gaspoz JM, Coxson PG, Goldman PA, et al. Cost effectiveness of aspirin, clopidogrel, or both for secondary prevention of coronary heart disease. *N Engl J Med* 2002;346:1800–1806.

95. Waksman R, Ajani A, Pinnow E, et al. Twelve versus six months of clopidogrel to reduce major cardiac events in patients undergoing gamma-radiation therapy for in-stent restenosis: Washington Radiation for In-Stent restenosis Trial (WRIST) 12 versus WRIST PLUS. *Circulation* 2002;106:776–778.

96. Waksman R, Ajani A, White R, et al. Prolonged antiplatelet therapy to prevent late thrombosis after intracoronary gamma-radiation in patients with in-stent restenosis: Washington Radiation for In-Stent Restenosis Trial plus 6 months of clopidogrel (WRIST PLUS). *Circulation* 2001;103:2332–2335.

97. Waksman R, Bhargava B, Mintz GS, et al. Late total occlusion after intracoronary brachytherapy for patients with in-stent restenosis. *J Am Coll Cardiol* 2000;36:65–68.

98. Colombo A, Drzewiecki J, Banning A, et al. Randomized study to assess the effectiveness of slow- and moderate-release polymer-based Paclitaxel-eluting stents for coronary artery lesions [In Process Citation]. *Circulation* 2003;108:788–794.

99. Stone G, Ellis S, Cox D, et al. A polymer-based, paclitaxel-eluting stent in patients with coronary artery disease [In Process Citation]. *N Engl J Med* 2004;350:221–231.

100. Schofer J, Schluter M, Gershlick A, et al. Sirolimus-eluting stents for treatment of patients with long atherosclerotic lesions in small coronary arteries: double-blind, randomised controlled trial (E-SIRIUS). *Lancet* 2003;362:1093–1099.

101. Moses J, Leon M, Popma J, et al. Sirolimus-eluting stents versus standard stents in patients with stenosis in a native coronary artery. *N Engl J Med* 2003;349:1315–1323.

102. Morice M, Serruys P, Sousa J, et al. A randomized comparison of a sirolimus-eluting stent with a standard stent for coronary revascularization. *N Engl J Med* 2002;346:1773–1780.

103. Wilson S, Fasseas P, Orford J, et al. Clinical outcome of patients undergoing non-cardiac surgery in the two months following coronary stenting. *J Am Coll Cardiol* 2003;42:234–240.

104. Quinn MJ, Fitzgerald DJ. Ticlopidine and clopidogrel. *Circulation* 1999;100:1667–1672.

105. Whetsel TR, Bell DM. Rash in patients receiving ticlopidine after intracoronary stent placement. *Pharmacotherapy* 1999;19:228–231.

106. Gent M, Blakely JA, Easton JD, et al. The Canadian American Ticlopidine Study (CATS) in thromboembolic stroke. *Lancet* 1989;1:1215–1220.

107. Gill S, Majumdar S, Brown NE, et al. Ticlopidine-associated pancytopenia: implications of an acetylsalicylic acid alternative. *Can J Cardiol* 1997;13:909–913.

108. Love BB, Biller J, Gent M. Adverse haematological effects of ticlopidine. Prevention, recognition and management. *Drug Saf* 1998;19:89–98.

109. Page Y, Tardy B, Seni F, et al. Thrombotic thrombocytopenic purpura related to ticlopidine. *Lancet* 1991;337:774–776.

110. Bennett CL, Weinberg PD, Rozenberg-Ben-Dror K, et al. Thrombotic thrombocytopenic purpura associated with ticlopidine. A review of 60 cases. *Ann Intern Med* 1998;128:541–544.

111. Bellavance A. Efficacy of ticlopidine and aspirin for prevention of reversible cerebrovascular ischemic events. The Ticlopidine Aspirin Stroke Study. *Stroke* 1993;24:1452–1457.

112. Bennett CL, Kiss JE, Weinberg PD, et al. Thrombotic thrombocytopenic purpura after stenting and ticlopidine. *Lancet* 1998;352:1036–1037.

113. Yim HB, Lieu PK, Choo PW. Ticlopidine induced cholestatic jaundice. *Singapore Med J* 1997;38:132–133.

114. Moy B, Wang J, Raffel G, et al. Hemolytic uremic syndrome associated with clopidogrel: a case report. *Arch Intern Med* 2000;160:1370–1372.

115. Boissonnat P, de Lorgeril M, Perroux V, et al. A drug interaction study between ticlopidine and cyclosporin in heart transplant recipients. *Eur J Clin Pharmacol* 1997;53:39–45.

116. Colli A, Buccino G, Cocciolo M, et al. Ticlopidine-theophylline interaction. *Clin Pharmacol Ther* 1987;41:358–362.

117. Donahue SR, Flockhart DA, Abernethy DR, et al. Ticlopidine inhibition of phenytoin metabolism mediated by potent inhibition of CYP2C19. *Clin Pharmacol Ther* 1997;62:572–577.

118. Brown RI, Cooper TG. Ticlopidine-carbamazepine interaction in a coronary stent patient. *Can J Cardiol* 1997;13:853–854.

119. Shah J, Fratis A, Ellis D, et al. Effect of food and antacid on absorption of orally administered ticlopidine hydrochloride. *J Clin Pharmacol* 1990;30:733–736.

120. Gurbel PA, Bliden KP, Hiatt BL, et al. Clopidogrel for coronary stenting: response variability, drug resistance, and the effect of pretreatment platelet reactivity. *Circulation* 2003;107:2908–2913.

121. Muller I, Besta F, Schulz C, et al. Prevalence of clopidogrel non-responders among patients with stable angina pectoris scheduled for elective coronary stent placement. *Thromb Haemost* 2003;89:783–787.

122. Soffer D, Moussa I, Harjai KJ, et al. Impact of angina class on inhibition of platelet aggregation following clopidogrel loading in patients undergoing coronary intervention: do we need more aggressive dosing regimens in unstable angina? *Catheter Cardiovasc Interv* 2003;59:21–25.

123. Lau WC, Gurbel PA, Watkins PB, et al. Contribution of hepatic cytochrome P450 3A4 metabolic activity to the phenomenon of clopidogrel resistance. *Circulation* 2004;109:166–171.

124. Matetzky S, Shenkman B, Guetta V, et al. Clopidogrel resistance is associated with increased risk of recurrent atherothrombotic events in patients with acute myocardial infarction. *Circulation* 2004;109:3171–3175.

125. Bowers J, Ferguson J. The use of activated clotting times to monitor heparin therapy during and after interventional procedures. *Clin Cardiol* 1994;17:357–361.

126. Dougherty K, Gaos C, Bush H, et al. Activated clotting times and activated partial thromboplastin times in patients undergoing coronary angioplasty who receive bolus doses of heparin. *Cathet Cardiovasc Diagn* 1992;26:260–263.

127. Avendano A, Ferguson JJ. Comparison of Hemochron and HemoTec activated coagulation time target values during percutaneous transluminal coronary angioplasty. *J Am Coll Cardiol* 1994;23:907–910.

128. Ferguson J, Dougherty K, Gaos C, et al. Relation between procedural activated clotting time and outcome after percutaneous transluminal coronary angioplasty. *J Am Coll Cardiol* 1994;23:1061–1065.

129. Narins CR, Hillegass WB Jr, Nelson CL, et al. Relation between activated clotting time during angioplasty and abrupt closure. *Circulation* 1996;93:667–671.

130. Chew D, Bhatt D, Lincoff A, et al. Defining the optimal activated clotting time during percutaneous coronary intervention: aggregate results from 6 randomized, controlled trials. *Circulation* 2001;103:961–966.

131. Koch KT, Piek JJ, de Winter RJ, et al. Early ambulation after coronary angioplasty and stenting with six French guiding catheters and low-dose heparin. *Am J Cardiol* 1997;80:1084–1086.

132. Boccara A, Benamer H, Juliard J, et al. A randomized trial of a fixed high dose versus a low weight adjusted low dose of intravenous heparin during coronary angioplasty. *Eur Heart J* 1997;18:631–635.

133. Ellis S, Roubin G, Wilentz J, et al. Effect of 18- to 24-hour heparin administration for prevention of restenosis after uncomplicated coronary angioplasty. *Am Heart J* 1989;117:777–782.

134. Friedman HZ, Cragg DR, Glazier SM, et al. Randomized prospective evaluation of prolonged versus abbreviated intravenous heparin therapy after coronary angioplasty. *J Am Coll Cardiol* 1994;24:1214–1219.

135. Denardo SJ, Davis KE, Reid PR, et al. Efficacy and safety of minimal dose (< or = 1,000 units) unfractionated heparin with abciximab in percutaneous coronary intervention. *Am J Cardiol* 2003;91:1–5.

136. Weitz JI. Low-molecular-weight heparins. *N Engl J Med* 1997;337:688–698.

137. Klein LW, Schaer GL, Calvin JE, et al. Does low individual operator coronary interventional procedural volume correlate with worse institutional procedural outcome? *J Am Coll Cardiol* 1997;30:870–877.

138. FRAXIS Study Group. Comparison of two treatment durations (6 days and 14 days) of a low molecular weight heparin with a 6-day treatment of unfractionated heparin in the initial management of unstable angina or non-Q wave myocardial infarction: FRAX.I.S. (FRAxiparine in Ischaemic Syndrome). *Eur Heart J* 1999;20:1553–1562.

139. Cohen M, Demers C, Gurfinkel E, et al. A comparison of low-molecular-weight heparin with unfractionated heparin for unstable coronary artery disease. *N Engl J Med* 1997;337:447–452.

140. Antman EM, McCabe CH, Gurfinkel EP, et al. Enoxaparin prevents death and cardiac ischemic events in unstable angina/non-Q-wave myocardial infarction. Results of the thrombolysis in myocardial infarction (TIMI) 11B trial. *Circulation* 1999;100:1593–1601.

141. de Lemos JA, Blazing MA, Wiviott SD, et al. Enoxaparin versus unfractionated heparin in patients treated with tirofiban, aspirin and an early conservative initial management strategy: results from the A phase of the A-to-Z trial. *Eur Heart J* 2004;25:1688–1694.

142. Ferguson JJ, Califf RM, Antman EM, et al. Enoxaparin vs. unfractionated heparin in high-risk patients with non-ST-segment elevation acute coronary syndromes managed with an intended early invasive strategy: primary results of the SYNERGY randomized trial. *JAMA* 2004;292:45–54.

143. Goodman SG, Fitchett D, Armstrong PW, et al. Randomized evaluation of the safety and efficacy of enoxaparin versus unfractionated heparin in high-risk patients with non-ST-segment elevation acute coronary syndromes receiving the glycoprotein IIb/IIIa inhibitor eptifibatide. *Circulation* 2003;107:238–244.

144. Braunwald E, Antman E, Beasley J, et al. ACC/AHA 2002 guideline update for the management of patients with unstable angina and non-ST-segment elevation myocardial infarction—summary article: a report of the American College of Cardiology/American Heart Association task force on practice guidelines (Committee on the Management of Patients With Unstable Angina). *J Am Coll Cardiol* 2002;40:1366–1374.

145. Neumann FJ, Kastrati A, Pogatsa-Murray G, et al. Evaluation of prolonged antithrombotic pretreatment ("cooling-off" strategy) before intervention in patients with unstable coronary syndromes: a randomized controlled trial. *JAMA* 2003;290:1593–1599.

146. Antman EM, Cohen M, McCabe C, et al. Enoxaparin is superior to unfractionated heparin for preventing clinical events at 1-year follow-up of TIMI 11B and ESSENCE. *Eur Heart J* 2002;23:308–314.

147. Antman EM, Cohen M, Radley D, et al. Assessment of the treatment effect of enoxaparin for unstable angina/non-Q-wave myocardial infarction. TIMI 11B-ESSENCE meta-analysis. *Circulation* 1999;100:1602–1608.

148. Kereiakes DJ, Montalescot G, Antman EM, et al. Low-molecular-weight heparin therapy for non-ST-elevation acute coronary syndromes and during percutaneous coronary intervention: an expert consensus. *Am Heart J* 2002;144:615–624.

149. Moliterno D, Hermiller J, Kereiakes D, et al. A novel point-of-care enoxaparin monitor for use during percutaneous coronary intervention. Results of the Evaluating Enoxaparin Clotting Times (ELECT) Study. *J Am Coll Cardiol* 2003;42:1132–1139.

150. Bhatt D, Lee B, Casterella P, et al. Safety of concomitant therapy with eptifibatide and enoxaparin in patients undergoing percutaneous coronary intervention: results of the Coronary Revascularization Using Integrilin and Single bolus Enoxaparin Study. *J Am Coll Cardiol* 2003;41:20–25.

151. Lewis B, Matthai W, Cohen M, et al. Argatroban anticoagulation during percutaneous coronary intervention in patients with heparin-induced thrombocytopenia. *Catheter Cardiovasc Interv* 2002;57:177–184.

152. Lincoff A, Kleiman N, Kottke-Marchant K, et al. Bivalirudin with planned or provisional abciximab versus low-dose heparin and abciximab during percutaneous coronary revascularization: results of the Comparison of Abciximab Complications with Hirulog for Ischemic Events Trial (CACHET). *Am Heart J* 2002;143:847–853.

153. Lincoff AM, Bittl JA, Harrington RA, et al. Bivalirudin and provisional glycoprotein IIb/IIIa blockade compared with heparin and planned glycoprotein IIb/IIIa blockade during percutaneous coronary intervention: RE-PLACE-2 randomized trial. *JAMA* 2003;289:853–863.

154. Bittl JA, Strony J, Brinker JA, et al. Treatment with bivalirudin (Hirulog) as compared with heparin during coronary angioplasty for unstable or postinfarction angina. Hirulog Angioplasty Study Investigators. *N Engl J Med* 1995;333:764–769.

155. Bittl J, Chaitman B, Feit F, et al. Bivalirudin versus heparin during coronary angioplasty for unstable or postinfarction angina: Final report reanalysis of the Bivalirudin Angioplasty Study. *Am Heart J* 2001;142:952–959.

156. Mahaffey K, Lewis B, Wildermann N, et al. The Anticoagulant Therapy with Bivalirudin to Assist in the Performance of Percutaneous Coronary Intervention in Patients with Heparin-Induced Thrombocytopenia (ATBAT) Study: main results [In Process Citation]. *J Invasive Cardiol* 2003;15:611–616.

157. Lubenow N, Greinacher A. Management of patients with heparin-induced thrombocytopenia: focus on recombinant hirudin. *J Thromb Thrombolysis* 2000;10(Suppl. 1):47–57.

158. Manfredi J, Wall R, Sane D, et al. Lepirudin as a safe alternative for effective anticoagulation in patients with known heparin-induced thrombocytopenia undergoing percutaneous coronary intervention: case reports. *Catheter Cardiovasc Interv* 2001;52:468–472.

159. Fuster V, Fallon JT, Nemerson Y. Coronary thrombosis. *Lancet* 1996;348(Suppl. 1):s7–s10.

160. Lefkovits J, Plow EF, Topol EJ. Platelet glycoportein IIb/IIIa receptors in cardiovascular medicine. *N Engl J Med* 1995;332:1553–1559.

161. Coller BS. A new murine monoclonal antibody reports an activation-dependent change in the conformation and/or microenvironment of the platelet glycoprotein IIb/IIIa complex. *J Clin Invest* 1985;76:101–108.

162. Topol EJ, Byzova TV, Plow EF. Platelet GPIIb-IIIa blockers. *Lancet* 1999;353:227–231.

163. Kleiman NS, Raizner AE, Jordan R, et al. Differential inhibition of platelet aggregation induced by adenosine diphosphate or a thrombin receptor-activating peptide in patients treated with bolus chimeric 7E3 Fab: implications for inhibition of the internal pool of GPIIb/IIIa receptors. *J Am Coll Cardiol* 1995;26:1665–1671.

164. Mascelli MA, Lance ET, Damaraju L, et al. Pharmacodynamic profile of short-term abciximab treatment demonstrates prolonged platelet inhibition with gradual recovery from GP IIb/IIIa receptor blockade. *Circulation* 1998;97:1680–1688.

165. Topol EJ, Topol EJ. *Acute coronary syndrome*, 2nd ed. New York: Marcel Dekker, 2001:419–445.

166. Scarborough RM, Rose JW, Hsu MA, et al. Barbourin. A GPIIb-IIIa-specific integrin antagonist from the venom of Sistrurus m. barbouri. *J Biol Chem* 1991;266:9359–9362.

167. Kleiman NS. Pharmacokinetics and pharmacodynamics of glycoprotein IIb-IIIa inhibitors. *Am Heart J* 1999;138:263–275.

168. Deckelbaum LI, Sax FL, Tirofiban WG. *A non-peptide inhibitor of the platelet glycoprotein IIb/IIIa receptor*. New York: Marcel Dekker, 1997:355–365.

169. The EPIC Investigators. Use of a monoclonal antibody directed against the platelet glycoprotein IIb/IIIa receptor in high-risk coronary angioplasty. *N Engl J Med* 1994;330:956–961.

170. Kereiakes DJ, Broderick TM, Roth EM, et al. Time course, magnitude, and consistency of platelet inhibition by abciximab, tirofiban, or eptifibatide in patients with unstable angina pectoris undergoing percutaneous coronary intervention. *Am J Cardiol* 1999;84:391–395.

171. Simon DI, Liu CB, Ganz P, et al. A comparative study of light transmission aggregometry and automated bedside platelet function assays in patients undergoing percutaneous coronary intervention and receiving abciximab, eptifibatide, or tirofiban. *Catheter Cardiovasc Interv* 2001;52:425–432.

172. Steinhubl SR. Assessing the optimal level of platelet inhibition with GPIIb/IIIa inhibitors in patients undergoing coronary intervention. Rationale and design of the GOLD study. *J Thromb Thrombolysis* 2000;9:199–205.

173. Topol EJ, Ferguson JJ, Weisman HF, et al. Long-term protection from myocardial ischemic events in a randomized trial of brief integrin beta3 blockade with percutaneous coronary intervention. EPIC Investigator Group. Evaluation of Platelet IIb/IIIa Inhibition for Prevention of Ischemic Complication. *JAMA* 1997;278:479–484.

174. Topol EJ, Califf RM, Weisman HF, et al. The EPIC Investigators. Randomised trial of coronary intervention with antibody against platelet IIb/IIIa integrin for reduction of clinical restenosis: results at six months. *Lancet* 1994;343:881–886.

175. Randomised placebo-controlled and balloon-angioplasty-controlled trial to assess safety of coronary stenting with use of platelet glycoprotein-IIb/IIIa blockade. The EPISTENT Investigators. Evaluation of Platelet IIb/IIIa Inhibitor for Stenting. *Lancet* 1998;352:87–92.

176. Tcheng J. Enhanced Supression of the Platelet IIb/IIIa Receptor with Integrilin Therapy (ESPRIT) trial. *J Am Coll Cardiol* 2000;35:44A.

177. ESPRIT Investigators. Enhanced Suppression of the Platelet IIb/IIIa Receptor with Integrilin Therapy. Novel dosing regimen of eptifibatide in planned coronary stent implantation (ESPRIT): a randomised, placebo-controlled trial. *Lancet* 2000;356:2037–2044.

178. Inhibition of platelet glycoprotein IIb/IIIa with eptifibatide in patients with acute coronary syndromes. The PURSUIT Trial Investigators. Platelet Glycoprotein IIb/IIIa in Unstable Angina: Receptor Suppression Using Integrilin Therapy. *N Engl J Med* 1998;339:436–443.

179. Inhibition of the platelet glycoprotein IIb/IIIa receptor with tirofiban in unstable angina and non-Q-wave myocardial infarction. Platelet Receptor Inhibition in Ischemic Syndrome Management in Patients Limited by Unstable Signs and Symptoms (PRISM-PLUS) Study Investigators. *N Engl J Med* 1998;338:1488–1497.

180. Randomised placebo-controlled trial of abciximab before and during coronary intervention in refractory unstable angina: the CAPTURE Study. *Lancet* 1997;349:1429–1435.

181. Brener SJ, Barr LA, Burchenal JE, et al. Randomized, placebo-controlled trial of platelet glycoprotein IIb/IIIa blockade with primary angioplasty for acute myocardial infarction. ReoPro and Primary PTCA Organization and Randomized Trial (RAPPORT) Investigators. *Circulation* 1998;98:734–741.

182. Montalescot G, Barragan P, Wittenberg O, et al. Platelet glycoprotein IIb/IIIa inhibition with coronary stenting for acute myocardial infarction. *N Engl J Med* 2001;344:1895–1903.

183. Stone GW, Grines CL, Cox DA, et al. Comparison of angioplasty with stenting, with or without abciximab, in acute myocardial infarction. *N Engl J Med* 2002;346:957–966.

184. Lee DP, Herity NA, Hiatt BL, et al. Adjunctive platelet glycoprotein IIb/IIIa receptor inhibition with tirofiban before primary angioplasty improves angiographic outcomes: results of the TIrofiban Given in the Emergency Room before Primary Angioplasty (TIGER-PA) pilot trial. *Circulation* 2003;107:1497–1501.

185. Van't Hof AW, Ernst N, De Boer MJ, et al. Facilitation of primary coronary angioplasty by early start of a glycoprotein 2b/3a inhibitor: results of the ongoing tirofiban in myocardial infarction evaluation (On-TIME) trial. *Eur Heart J* 2004;25:837–846.

186. Boersma E, Akkerhuis KM, Theroux P, et al. Platelet glycoprotein IIb/IIIa receptor inhibition in non-ST-elevation acute coronary syndromes: early benefit during medical treatment only, with additional protection during percutaneous coronary intervention. *Circulation* 1999;100:2045–2048.

187. Karvouni E, Katritsis DG, Ioannidis JP. Intravenous glycoprotein IIb/IIIa receptor antagonists reduce mortality after percutaneous coronary interventions. *J Am Coll Cardiol* 2003;41:26–32.

188. Kong D, Hasselblad V, Harrington R, et al. Meta-analysis of survival with platelet glycoprotein IIb/IIIa antagonists for percutaneous coronary interventions. *Am J Cardiol* 2003;92:651–655.

189. Welt FG, Rogers SD, Zhang X, et al. GP IIb/IIIa inhibition with eptifibatide lowers levels of soluble CD40L and RANTES after percutaneous coronary intervention. *Catheter Cardiovasc Interv* 2004;61:185–189.

190. Lincoff AM, Kereiakes DJ, Mascelli MA, et al. Abciximab suppresses the rise in levels of circulating inflammatory markers after percutaneous coronary revascularization. *Circulation* 2001;104:163–167.

191. Batchelor W, Tolleson T, Huang Y, et al. Randomized COMparison of platelet inhibition with abciximab, tiRofiban and eptifibatide during percutaneous coronary intervention in acute coronary syndromes: the COMPARE trial. Comparison Of Measurements of Platelet aggregation with Aggrastat, Reopro, and Eptifibatide. *Circulation* 2002;106:1470–1476.

192. Jennings LK, Jacoski MV, White MM. The pharmacodynamics of parenteral glycoprotein IIb/IIIa inhibitors. *J Interv Cardiol* 2002;15:45–60.

193. Tcheng JE, Talley JD, O'Shea JC, et al. Clinical pharmacology of higher dose eptifibatide in percutaneous coronary intervention (the PRIDE study). *Am J Cardiol* 2001;88:1097–1102.

194. Topol E, Moliterno D, Herrmann H, et al. Comparison of two platelet glycoprotein IIb/IIIa inhibitors, tirofiban and abciximab, for the prevention of ischemic events with percutaneous coronary revascularization. *N Engl J Med* 2001;344:1888–1894.

195. Schneider DJ, Herrmann HC, Lakkis N, et al. Increased concentrations of tirofiban in blood and their correlation with inhibition of platelet aggregation after greater bolus doses of tirofiban. *Am J Cardiol* 2003;91: 334–336.

196. Ellis SG, Armstrong P, Betriu A, et al. Facilitated percutaneous coronary intervention versus primary percutaneous coronary intervention: design and rationale of the Facilitated Intervention with Enhanced Reperfusion Speed to Stop Events (FINESSE) trial. *Am Heart J* 2004;147:E16.

197. Strategies for Patency Enhancement in the Emergency Department (SPEED) Group. Trial of abciximab with and without low-dose reteplase for acute myocardial infarction. *Circulation* 2000;101:2788–2794.

198. Antman EM, Giugliano RP, Gibson CM, et al. Abciximab facilitates the rate and extent of thrombolysis: results of the thrombolysis in myocardial infarction (TIMI) 14 trial. The TIMI 14 Investigators. *Circulation* 1999;99: 2720–2732.

199. Giugliano R, Roe M, Harrington R, et al. Combination reperfusion therapy with eptifibatide and reduced-dose tenecteplase for ST-elevation myocardial infarction: results of the integrilin and tenecteplase in acute myocardial infarction (INTEGRITI) Phase II Angiographic Trial. *J Am Coll Cardiol* 2003;41:1251–1260.

200. Kastrati A, Mehilli J, Schlotterbeck K, et al. Early administration of reteplase plus abciximab vs. abciximab alone in patients with acute myocardial infarction referred for percutaneous coronary intervention: a randomized controlled trial. *JAMA* 2004;291:947–954.

201. Mousa SA, Khurana S, Forsythe MS. Comparative *in vitro* efficacy of different platelet glycoprotein IIb/IIIa antagonists on platelet-mediated clot strength induced by tissue factor with use of thromboelastography: differentiation among glycoprotein IIb/IIIa antagonists. *Arterioscler Thromb Vasc Biol* 2000;20:1162–1167.

202. Topol EJ, Easton JD, Amarenco P, et al. Design of the blockade of the glycoprotein IIb/IIIa receptor to avoid vascular occlusion (BRAVO) trial. *Am Heart J* 2000;139:927–933.

203. O'Neill WW, Serruys P, Knudtson M, et al. Long-term treatment with a platelet glycoprotein-receptor antagonist after percutaneous coronary revascularization. EXCITE Trial Investigators. Evaluation of Oral Xemilofiban in Controlling Thrombotic Events. *N Engl J Med* 2000;342: 1316–1324.

204. Cannon CP, McCabe CH, Wilcox RG, et al. Oral glycoprotein IIb/IIIa inhibition with orbofiban in patients with unstable coronary syndromes (OPUS-TIMI 16) trial. *Circulation* 2000;102:149–156.

205. Comparison of sibrafiban with aspirin for prevention of cardiovascular events after acute coronary syndromes: a randomised trial. The SYMPHONY Investigators. Sibrafiban versus Aspirin to Yield Maximum Protection from Ischemic Heart Events Post-acute Coronary Syndromes. *Lancet* 2000;355:337–345.

206. Randomized trial of aspirin, sibrafiban, or both for secondary prevention after acute coronary syndromes. *Circulation* 2001;103:1727–1733.

207. Cannon CP. Oral platelet glycoprotein IIb/IIIa receptor inhibitors—part II. *Clin Cardiol* 2003;26:401–406.

208. Cannon CP. Oral platelet glycoprotein IIb/IIIa receptor inhibitors—Part I. *Clin Cardiol* 2003;26:358–364.

209. Newby LK, Califf RM, White HD, et al. The failure of orally administered glycoprotein IIb/IIIa inhibitors to prevent recurrent cardiac events. *Am J Med* 2002;112:647–658.

210. Sy SK, Levenstadt AL. A perspective on the toxicological mechanisms possibly contributing to the failure of oral glycoprotein IIb/IIIa antagonists in the clinic. *Am J Cardiovasc Drugs* 2004;4:1–10.

211. Quinn MJ, Plow EF, Topol EJ. Platelet glycoprotein IIb/IIIa inhibitors: recognition of a two-edged sword? *Circulation* 2002;106:379–385.

212. Dasgupta H, Blankenship JC, Wood GC, et al. Thrombocytopenia complicating treatment with intravenous glycoprotein IIb/IIIa receptor inhibitors: a pooled analysis. *Am Heart J* 2000;140:206–211.

213. Berkowitz SD, Harrington RA, Rund MM, et al. Acute profound thrombocytopenia after C7E3 Fab (abciximab) therapy. *Circulation* 1997;95: 809–813.

214. Merlini PA, Rossi M, Menozzi A, et al. Thrombocytopenia caused by abciximab or tirofiban and its association with clinical outcome in patients undergoing coronary stenting. *Circulation* 2004;109:2203–2206.

215. Tcheng JE, Kereiakes DJ, Lincoff AM, et al. Abciximab readministration: results of the ReoPro Readministration Registry. *Circulation* 2001;104: 870–875.

216. Keeley EC, Boura JA, Grines CL. Primary angioplasty versus intravenous thrombolytic therapy for acute myocardial infarction: a quantitative review of 23 randomized trials. *Lancet* 2003;361:13–20.

217. Aversano T, Aversano LT, Passamani E, et al. Thrombolytic therapy vs primary percutaneous coronary intervention for myocardial infarction in patients presenting to hospitals without on-site cardiac surgery: a randomized controlled trial. *JAMA* 2002;287:1943–1951.

218. Van de Werf F, Ardissino D, Betriu A, et al. Management of acute myocardial infarction in patients presenting with ST-segment elevation. *Eur Heart J* 2003;24:28–66.

219. Cannon C, Weintraub W, Demopoulos L, et al. Comparison of early invasive and conservative strategies in patients with unstable coronary syndromes treated with the glycoprotein IIb/IIIa inhibitor tirofiban. *N Engl J Med* 2001;344:1879–1887.

220. Invasive compared with non-invasive treatment in unstable coronary-artery disease: FRISC II prospective randomised multicentre study. FRagmin and Fast Revascularisation during InStability in Coronary artery disease Investigators. *Lancet* 1999;354:708–715.

221. Hartmann JR, McKeever LS, O'Neill WW, et al. Recanalization of Chronically Occluded Aortocoronary Saphenous Vein Bypass Grafts With Long-Term, Low Dose Direct Infusion of Urokinase (ROBUST): a serial trial. *J Am Coll Cardiol* 1996;27:60–66.

222. Hartmann JR. Urokinase recanalization of chronically occluded aortocoronary vein grafts. *Coron Artery Dis* 1996;7:641–648.

223. Muhlestein JB, Karagounis LA, Treehan S, et al. "Rescue" utilization of abciximab for the dissolution of coronary thrombus developing as a complication of coronary angioplasty. *J Am Coll Cardiol* 1997;30:1729–1734.

224. Stone GW, Cox DA, Babb J, et al. Prospective, randomized evaluation of thrombectomy prior to percutaneous intervention in diseased saphenous vein grafts and thrombus-containing coronary arteries. *J Am Coll Cardiol* 2003;42:2007–2013.

225. Lefkovits J, Holmes DR, Califf RM, et al. Predictors and sequelae of distal embolization during saphenous vein graft intervention from the CAVEAT-II trial. Coronary Angioplasty Versus Excisional Atherectomy Trial. *Circulation* 1995;92:734–740.

226. Dooris M, Hoffmann M, Glazier S, et al. Comparative results of transluminal extraction atherectomy in saphenous vein graft lesions with and without thrombus. *J Am Coll Cardiol* 1995;25:1700.

227. Singh M, Rosenschein U, Ho K, et al. Treatment of saphenous vein bypass grafts with ultrasound thrombolysis: a randomized study (ATLAS). *Circulation* 2003;107:2331–2336.

228. Rosenschein U, Roth A, Rassin T, et al. Analysis of coronary ultrasound thrombolysis endpoints in acute myocardial infarction (ACUTE trial). Results of the feasibility phase. *Circulation* 1997;95:1411–1416.

229. Kuntz R, Baim D, Cohen D, et al. A trial comparing rheolytic thrombectomy with intracoronary urokinase for coronary and vein graft thrombus (the Vein Graft AngioJet Study [VeGAS 2]). *Am J Cardiol* 2002;89: 326–330.

230. Ali A. *AngioJet Rheolytic Thrombectomy in Patients Undergoing Primary Angioplasty for Acute Myocardial Infarction (AiMI) study TCT.* Washington, DC, 2004.

231. Hong MK, Mehran R, Dangas G, et al. Creatine kinase-MB enzyme elevation following successful saphenous vein graft intervention is associated with late mortality. *Circulation* 1999;100:2400–2405.

232. Waksman R, Douglas JJ, Scott NA, et al. Distal embolization is common after directional atherectomy in coronary arteries and saphenous vein grafts. *Am Heart J* 1995;129:430–435.

233. Waksman R, Ghazzal ZM, Baim DS, et al. Myocardial infarction as a complication of new interventional devices. *Am J Cardiol* 1996;78:751–756.

234. Waksman R, Weintraub WS, Ghazzal Z, et al. Short- and long-term outcome of narrowed saphenous vein bypass graft: a comparison of Palmaz-Schatz stent, directional coronary atherectomy, and balloon angioplasty. *Am Heart J* 1997;134:274–281.

235. Grube E, Gerckens U, Yeung A, et al. Prevention of distal embolization during coronary angioplasty in saphenous vein grafts and native vessels using porous filter protection. *Circulation* 2001;104:2436–2441.

236. Baim D, Wahr D, George B, et al. Randomized trial of a distal embolic protection device during percutaneous intervention of saphenous vein aorto-coronary bypass grafts. *Circulation* 2002;105:1285–1290.

237. Stone GW, Rogers C, Hermiller J, et al. Randomized comparison of distal protection with a filter-based catheter and a balloon occlusion and aspiration system during percutaneous intervention of diseased saphenous vein aorto-coronary bypass grafts. *Circulation* 2003;108:548–553.

238. Stone GW, Webb J, Cox DA, et al. Distal microcirculatory protection during percutaneous coronary intervention in acute ST-segment elevation myocardial infarction: a randomized controlled trial. *JAMA* 2005;293: 1063–1072.

239. Darius H, Nixdorff U, Zander J, et al. Effects of ciprostene on restenosis rate during therapeutic transluminal coronary angioplasty. *Agents Actions Suppl* 1992;37:305–311.

240. Serruys P, Rutsch W, Heyndrickx G, et al. Prevention of restenosis after percutaneous transluminal coronary angioplasty with thromboxane A2-receptor blockade. A randomized, double-blind, placebo-controlled trial. *Circulation* 1991;84:1568–1580.

241. Serruys P, Klein W, Tijssen J, et al. Evaluation of ketanserin in the prevention of restenosis after percutaneous transluminal coronary angioplasty. A Multicenter randomized double-blind placebo-controlled trial. *Circulation* 1993;88:1588–1601.

242. Savage M, Goldberg S, Macdonald R, et al. Multi-hospital Eastern Atlantic restenosis trial II: A placebo-controlled trial of thromboxane blockade in the prevention of restenosis following coronary angioplasty. *Am Heart J* 1991;122:1239–1244.

243. Fujita M, Mizuno K, Ho M, et al. Sarpogrelate treatment reduces restenosis after coronary stenting. *Am Heart J* 2003;145:E16.

244. Knudtson ML, Flintoft VF, Roth DL, et al. Effect of short-term prostacyclin administration on restenosis after percutaneous transluminal coronary angioplasty. *J Am Coll Cardiol* 1990;15:691–697.

245. Gershlick A, Spriggins D, Davies S, et al. Failure of epoprostenol (prostacyclin, PGI2) to inhibit platelet aggregation and to prevent restenosis after

coronary angioplasty: results of a randomised placebo controlled trial. *Br Heart J* 1994;71:7–15.

246. Karsch KR, Preisack MB, Baildon R, et al. Low molecular weight heparin (reviparin) in percutaneous transluminal coronary angioplasty. Results of a randomized, double-blind, unfractionated heparin and placebo-controlled, multicenter trial (REDUCE trial). Reduction of Restenosis After PTCA, Early Administration of Reviparin in a Double-Blind Unfractionated Heparin and Placebo-Controlled Evaluation. *J Am Coll Cardiol* 1996;28:1437–1443.

247. Burchenal JE, Marks DS, Tift Mann J, et al. Effect of direct thrombin inhibition with Bivalirudin (Hirulog) on restenosis after coronary angioplasty. *Am J Cardiol* 1998;82:511–515.

248. Serruys PW, Herrman JP, Simon R, et al. A comparison of hirudin with heparin in the prevention of restenosis after coronary angioplasty. Helvetica Investigators. *N Engl J Med* 1995;333:757–763.

249. Lablanche JM, McFadden EP, Meneveau N, et al. Effect of nadroparin, a low-molecular-weight heparin, on clinical and angiographic restenosis after coronary balloon angioplasty: the FACT study. Fraxiparine Angioplastie Coronaire Transluminale. *Circulation* 1997;96:3396–3402.

250. Brack MJ, Ray S, Chauhan A, et al. The Subcutaneous Heparin and Angioplasty Restenosis Prevention (SHARP) trial. Results of a multicenter randomized trial investigating the effects of high dose unfractionated heparin on angiographic restenosis and clinical outcome. *J Am Coll Cardiol* 1995;26:947–954.

251. Roffi M, Moliterno D, Meier B, et al. Impact of different platelet glycoprotein IIb/IIIa receptor inhibitors among diabetic patients undergoing percutaneous coronary intervention: do Tirofiban and ReoPro Give Similar Efficacy Outcomes Trial (TARGET) 1-year follow-up. *Circulation* 2002;105:2730–2736.

252. Kastrati A, Schuhlen H, Hausleiter J, et al. Restenosis after coronary stent placement and randomization to a 4-week combined antiplatelet or anticoagulant therapy: six-month angiographic follow-up of the Intracoronary Stenting and Antithrombotic Regimen (ISAR) Trial. *Circulation* 1997;96:462–467.

253. ten Berg J, Kelder J, Suttorp M, et al. A randomized trial assessing the effect of coumarins started before coronary angioplasty on restenosis: results of the 6-month angiographic substudy of the Balloon Angioplasty and Anticoagulation Study (BAAS). *Am Heart J* 2003;145:58–65.

254. Douglas JS, Weintraub WS, Holmes D. Rationale and design of the randomized, multicenter, cilostazol for RESTenosis (CREST) trial. *Clin Cardiol* 2003;26:451–454.

255. Babapulle MN, Joseph L, Belisle P, et al. A hierarchical Bayesian meta-analysis of randomised clinical trials of drug-eluting stents. *Lancet* 2004; 364:583–591.

256. Moons AH, Peters RJ, Bijsterveld NR, et al. Recombinant nematode anticoagulant protein c2, an inhibitor of the tissue factor/factor VIIa complex, in patients undergoing elective coronary angioplasty. *J Am Coll Cardiol* 2003;41:2147–2153.

257. Wong NN. Fondaparinux: a synthetic selective factor-Xa inhibitor. *Heart Dis* 2003;5:295–302.

# CHAPTER 99 ■ CORONARY BYPASS GRAFTING AND CARDIAC SURGERY

PETER W. MARKS

Cardiothoracic surgery requiring extracorporeal circulation poses one of the greatest challenges in the hematologic management of patients. There is a delicate balance between the maintenance of hemostasis and the prevention of thrombosis. A variety of factors related to the patient, to the procedure, and to perioperative management can significantly affect the outcome (1). Postoperative bleeding, sometimes requiring surgical reexploration, remains a major cause of morbidity and mortality in this setting (2,3). In addition, coagulation abnormalities may persist for a few months after cardiopulmonary bypass (4). Over the last decade, a number of reports have appeared in the literature that have suggested improved techniques for the management of patients. This chapter reviews the issues applicable to the optimal hematologic management of patients undergoing procedures involving cardiopulmonary bypass.

## PREOPERATIVE ISSUES

### Risk Assessment for Bleeding and Thrombosis

Identifying patients with increased risk for bleeding complications before surgery allows the institution of appropriate prophylactic measures for prevention. Historical factors are important. For example, patients undergoing reoperative cardiac surgical procedures are generally at a higher risk for bleeding complications due to the presence of adhesions and scarring (5).

As for general surgery, the preoperative assessment of individuals for hereditary or acquired hemostatic disorders is indicated in candidates for cardiac surgery (6). A personal history of excessive bleeding, of excessive blood loss, or of the need for blood transfusion with prior surgical procedures, and a family history of a bleeding diathesis should be sought. A thorough review of prescribed medications, over-the-counter medications, and supplements should be performed because quite a number of drugs and even supplements (e.g., *Ginkgo biloba*) can have adverse effects on the hemostatic system (7). In addition, a detailed history of the recent use of antithrombotic agents is important. Patients who have undergone invasive cardiac procedures earlier deserve special attention because a history of relevant adverse effects of anticoagulation, such as heparin-induced thrombocytopenia (HIT), may be elicited from the patient or found in prior medical records.

Although there is some controversy about the utility of coagulation test screening before general surgery, in the context of cardiac surgery, preoperative laboratory tests should generally include a complete blood count, prothrombin time (PT), and partial thromboplastin time (PTT) (8,9). In the absence of the concomitant administration of anticoagulants, any abnormalities in the PT or PTT should be further investigated before surgery. Aside from the detection of hereditary bleeding diatheses, identification of acquired conditions such as the presence of lupus anticoagulants is relevant because the latter can affect the performance of laboratory assays for monitoring anticoagulation and requires special approaches for intraoperative management (10,11). Performance of a bleeding time is not routinely recommended because it is not adequately predictive of bleeding complications and is often modestly prolonged in patients who have been receiving antiplatelet agents recently (12).

Routine testing for common hereditary hypercoagulable states prior to cardiac surgery is not indicated at this time, although there is some controversy in the literature. There have been some reports of thrombotic events in carriers of factor $V_{Leiden}$ who were treated with aprotinin or antifibrinolytic agents (13,14). However, another trial in a population of young children undergoing cardiac surgery for congential heart disease demonstrated no apparent effect of factor $V_{Leiden}$ on thrombotic events (15). One small trial examining patients' heterozygous for factor $V_{Leiden}$ even demonstrated an apparently protective effect of this trait on blood loss (16). Larger prospective studies are needed to define more clearly the effect of hypercoagulable risk factors such as factor $V_{Leiden}$ and the prothrombin G20210A gene mutation on the outcome of cardiac surgery.

### Preoperative Antithrombotic Agents

Frequently, patients undergoing cardiovascular procedures receive antiplatelet agents or other anticoagulants agents prior to surgery. Use of aspirin in the days before the cardiac surgery may be associated with greater blood loss at the time of surgery or postoperatively but has not clearly been associated with an increased need for blood transfusion or with adverse outcomes (17–19). In one randomized controlled trial examining patients on aspirin until the day before the surgery, treatment with desmopressin (ddAVP) after administration of protamine sulfate did not reduce the amount of postoperative bleeding (20). Other antiplatelet agents may have more considerable effects. There is at least one report in the literature in which the use of adenosine 5′-diphosphate (ADP) receptor antagonists was associated with increased chest tube drainage (21). Because clopidigrel, like aspirin, has an irreversible effect on platelet function, discontinuation of this drug at least 7 days before surgery is necessary to allow for significant platelet recovery.

Increasingly, patients may have received glycoprotein IIb/IIIa antagonists (e.g., abciximab) before surgery. In the case of abciximab, which has a prolonged effect, careful consideration should be given to the timing of the surgery. If emergent surgery is necessary soon after the administration of abciximab, the literature suggests that careful heparin monitoring at the time of bypass and early platelet transfusion may reduce excess bleeding (22).

Warfarin is usually discontinued 4 to 5 days before the surgery, to allow normalization of the international normalized ratio (INR) to 1.2 or less (23). However, data from one retrospective trial suggested that normalization of the INR is not required before surgery; INR values in the midtherapeutic range at the time of cardiac surgery were not associated with any excessive bleeding (24).

In patients for whom continuous anticoagulation is indicated (such as those with metallic prosthetic valves), the use of low-molecular-weight heparin (LMWH) may be considered as an outpatient bridge until the time of the surgical procedure. However, one study suggests that administration of dalteparin within the 12 hours prior to cardiac surgery is associated with greater blood loss and transfusion requirements (25). A potential compromise is to use LMWH until 24 hours prior to surgery, and then to switch to the administration of unfractionated heparin.

If patients have received heparin either immediately prior to or in the months preceding bypass surgery, records should be reviewed to determine whether there was any significant (>50%) reduction in the platelet count. Such a decrease might be suggestive of HIT and would warrant consideration of alternative strategies for perioperative anticoagulation (26). Additionally, a certain percentage of patients who have received heparin in the days prior to the cardiac surgery will be found to be relatively resistant to the large doses of heparin given at the time of cardiac bypass (27). The mechanism for this resistance, long thought to be associated with a deficiency of antithrombin III (ATIII), has recently been questioned (28).

## Optimization of Hematologic Parameters

There is some evidence that hematocrit values of 30% or greater are associated with a decreased incidence of perioperative blood loss (29). The postulated mechanism for the effect is that the platelet pool is marginalized to a greater extent in the circulation, allowing for more effective hemostasis. As an alternative to blood transfusion, preoperative administration of erythropoietin may be considered in patients when cardiac surgery is planned, although it has not been demonstrated to be cost effective (30). Although preoperative administration of erythropoietin is an unapproved use in the setting of cardiac surgery, it is particularly appropriate in the case of Jehovah's Witnesses who refuse blood product administration but may be willing to accept this therapy (31). In patients who are iron replete, adequate hematocrit responses generally occur within a few weeks, depending on the regimen administered. Although not uncommonly employed in clinical practice, data available at this time do not clearly support the cost-effectiveness of autologous blood donation or cell-saving devices in the setting of cardiac surgery (32).

# OPERATIVE ISSUES

## Anticoagulation

In contrast to other arenas, in which the use of alternative parenteral agents for anticoagulation is increasing (e.g., LMWH), unfractionated heparin remains the standard for cardiac bypass; a number of reasons account for this: (a) the extent of anticoagulation required for cardiac surgical procedures has been well defined, (b) unfractionated heparin is readily reversed completely with protamine sulfate, and (c) both anticoagulation and reversal can be titrated using either the activated clotting time (ACT) or heparin levels determined in the surgical suite.

Heparin has also been used for the coating of the extracorporeal bypass circuit, in an effort to decrease its thrombogenic properties. Approaches using heparin-coated cardiopulmonary bypass circuits to facilitate reduced-dose anticoagulation during surgery are being explored. Although further trials are necessary, there is some evidence that the use of the technique using heparin-coated cardiopulmonary bypass circuits may have several benefits, including decreasing postoperative blood loss (33).

Because it facilitates more accurate titration of the extent of anticoagulation, heparin levels are now used with increasing frequency. Heparin level–based dosing appears to decrease thrombin generation, decrease fibrinolysis, and decrease neutrophil activation when compared to ACT-based dosing (34). However, the clinical benefits on blood loss are yet to be demonstrated in clinical trials. The use of the heparin assay for dosing may also facilitate the maintenance of higher levels of anticoagulation and the management of heparin resistance. Patients who have received heparin in the days before surgery may demonstrate such heparin resistance, and these patients may require doses of heparin up to double the dose that is normally required for initiation of bypass. In some cases, the degree of heparin resistance is significant enough that consideration may be given to the administration of antithrombin in the form of either fresh frozen plasma (FFP) or commercially available plasma-derived concentrate. The administration of plasma-derived ATIII concentrate has been shown to lead to significant increases in the ACT (35). However, the relation of this response to preoperative ATIII levels is not entirely clear; the preoperative ATIII level in some responders is already within the normal range. In the absence of data suggesting other beneficial effects of this agent, the use of ATIII is somewhat controversial.

Following surgery, appropriate reversal of heparin anticoagulation is important because when unbound to heparin, protamine can have an adverse effect on platelet function (36). Although not yet documented in prospective clinical trials, careful calculation of the individualized dose of protamine to be administered, or heparin–protamine titration using a laboratory instrument in the surgical suite, may minimize excessive bleeding (37).

A history of HIT presents special management challenges. Although a variety of alternative anticoagulants are available, including hirulog analogues such as lepirudin and argatroban, these direct thrombin inhibitors are not reversible. In addition, there is limited experience with each of these agents in the setting of bypass surgery. In particular, because appropriate parameters for monitoring remain to be well established, inappropriate anticoagulation, and, particularly, excessive anticoagulation, is possible (38,39).

A reasonable approach to the management of cardiac bypass surgery in patients with a history of heparin-induced thrombocytopenia has been suggested by Wartenkin (see Fig. 99-1) (40). As antibody titers tend to decline with time, patients with a history of HIT should be retested before surgery for the presence of the antibody using a heparin-PF4 enzyme-linked immunosorbent assay (ELISA) or using other sensitive methodology. If antibodies are not detected, it is reasonable to proceed with bypass using heparin in the standard manner. However, if anticoagulation is necessary pre- or postoperatively, an alternative anticoagulant (e.g., a direct thrombin inhibitor) should be administered instead of heparin. The management of patients who are positive for heparin antibodies just prior to surgery presents a greater challenge (41). A variety of approaches have been explored, including one-time exposure to heparin, as noted in preceding text; use of the alternative anticoagulants lepirudin or argatroban; treatment with GP IIb/IIIa antagonists in conjunction with heparin at the time of bypass; treatment with

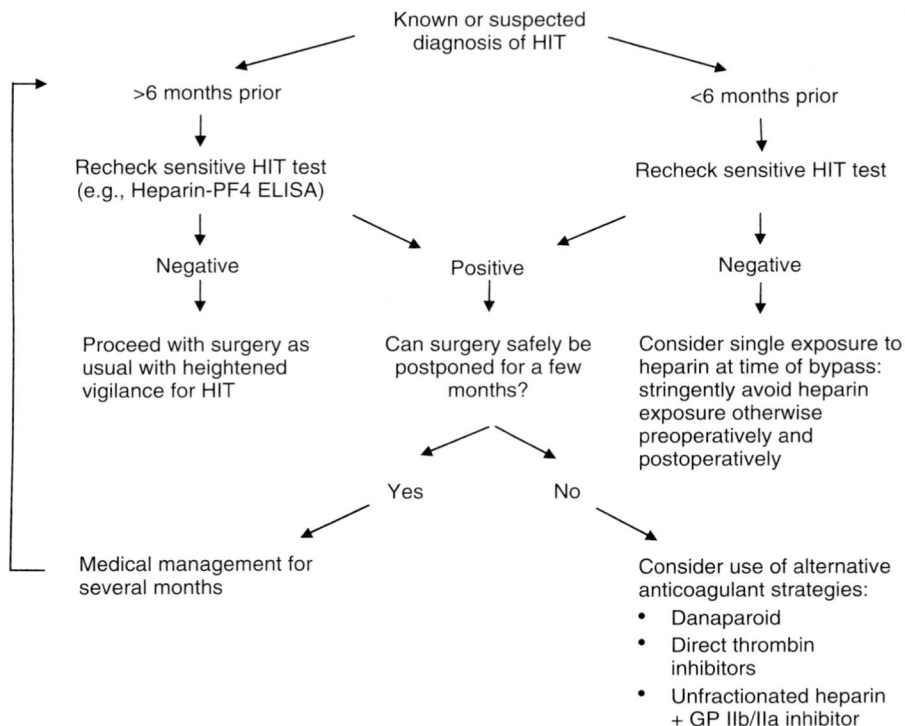

**FIGURE 99-1.** An algorithm for the management of heparin-induced thrombocytopenia in the setting of cardiac surgery. HIT, heparin-induced thrombocytopenia; ELISA, enzyme-linked immunosorbent assay; GP, glycoprotein.

prostacyclin analogs (iloprost); and immune modulation (e.g., γ globulin administration, and plasmapheresis) (42). A number of challenges exist when using alternative strategies for anticoagulation. These strategies include the fact that the optimal dosing and monitoring strategy for providing sufficient anticoagulation without excessive hemorrhage is yet to be identified for lepirudin or argatroban (43). Many cardiac surgery teams, therefore, continue to prefer the use of heparin, if at all possible, for the reasons already cited in the preceding text (i.e., reversibility, ease of monitoring, and wealth of experience).

Patients with lupus anticoagulants deserve special attention because these can sometimes interfere with accurate determination of the ACT and/or the heparin assay. Such cases may warrant preoperative evaluation to assess whether this is the case. In some instances, calculation and administration of the appropriate weight-based dose of heparin may be necessary.

Despite therapeutic anticoagulation at the time of bypass surgery with heparin or other agents, thrombotic complications can still occur even in the absence of complicating factors such as HIT. For this reason, efforts are being made to optimize anticoagulant regimens, as well as to decrease the thrombogenicity of the materials used in the bypass circuit that come in contact with the blood.

## Hemostatic Agents

A number of randomized clinical trials have examined maneuvers to decrease perioperative blood loss in the setting of cardiac surgery. Data are most convincing for the serine protease inhibitor aprotinin and for the antifibrinolytic agents α-aminocaproic acid (Amicar) and tranexamic acid (see Table 99-1) (44–47).

Originally tested as an agent to reduce complement activation in cardiac surgery, aprotinin is the only hemostatic agent specifically labeled for the reduction of bleeding in the setting of cardiac surgery (48). Aprotinin inhibits the action of a number of factors in the clotting cascade, and it, therefore, should be noted that aprotinin increases the ACT and prolongs the activated partial thromboplastin time (aPTT) to a variable extent, depending on the laboratory reagent utilized (49). Several randomized clinical trials have demonstrated that aprotinin reduces blood loss by 30% to 40% and thereby decreases the need for blood transfusion. In the setting of pediatric cardiac surgery, the use of high-dose aprotinin at 30,000 kallikrein inhibitory unit per kg (KIU per kg), with a fixed 500,000 KIU bolus added to prime the pump, has also been associated with reduced time on mechanical ventilation (50).

Although it possesses a reasonable safety profile, and is not associated with increased thrombotic complications, the use of aprotinin has occasionally been associated with transient renal insufficiency, and rarely with renal failure. For use in decreasing perioperative blood loss, regimens have generally employed a 2,000,000 KIU dose and a 500,000 KIU per hour continuous infusion during surgery. Alternatively, rather than giving a continuous infusion during surgery, some perfusionists simply prime the bypass pump with 500,000 KIU. One clinical trial demonstrated that half the standard dose can potentially be as effective as full-dose aprotinin and suggested that this dose might reduce the risk for complications (51). However, a larger confirmatory trial is required. There is also one small randomized trial reported in the literature suggesting that aprotinin applied topically to the surgical site may be as effective as when systemically administered (52). The advantage to this approach of using aprotinin, if confirmed in further studies, might be to reduce systemic complications.

In the absence of additional large randomized trials in uncomplicated cardiac surgery, the decision to use aprotinin for patients at low risk for hemorrhagic complications (i.e., no prior bleeding history and no prior cardiac surgery) rests largely with the surgical team's individual experience. Routine

## TABLE 99-1

HEMOSTATIC AGENTS WITH DOCUMENTED EFFICIANCY IN THE SETTING OF CARDIAC SURGERY

| Drug | Mechanism of action | Half-life (h) | Route of elimination | Standard dosing regimen (adults) |
|------|---------------------|---------------|----------------------|----------------------------------|
| Aprotinin | Serine protease inhibitor | 2 | Renal | Loading: $2 \times 10^6$ KIU bolus<br>Maintenance: $5 \times 10^5$ KIU/h |
| Tranexamic acid | Competitive inhibitor of plasminogen/plasmin binding | 2 | Renal | Loading: 10 mg/kg bolus<br>Maintenance: 1.0 mg/kg/h |
| ε-aminocaproic acid | Competitive inhibitor of plasminogen/plasmin binding | 2 | Renal | Loading: 150 mg/kg bolus<br>Maintenance: 15 mg/kg/h |

KIU, kallikrein inhibitory unit.

use of aprotinin in these cases may decrease blood loss. At this time, for patients at high risk of hemorrhagic complications (i.e., with prior bleeding history and reoperations), aprotinin should be administered at standard doses (i.e., 2,000,000 KIU bolus and a 500,000 KIU per hour continuous infusion) during surgery.

Tranexamic acid and ε-aminocaproic acid (Amicar) are lysine analogues that bind to plasmin and inhibit fibrinolysis. Both have similar properties, although tranexamic acid is about seven times more potent and has a longer half-life than ε-aminocaproic acid, and there are more data available from clinical trials examining tranexamic acid (53). These trials have demonstrated that when started at the time of surgery and when continued through the procedure, tranexamic and ε-aminocaproic acids are approximately as effective as aprotinin in decreasing bleeding and in the need for blood product transfusion without an increased risk for thrombosis (54). ε-Aminocaproic acid regimens vary, but clinical trials have used a 150 mg per kg intravenous bolus before surgery, followed by 15 mg/kg/hour. For tranexamic acid, regimens have used a 10 mg per kg intravenous bolus before surgery, and then 1 mg/kg/hour during the procedure. The benefit in using tranexamic acid to lessen bleeding seems to be reduced if it is started postoperatively and it is possible that this might also apply to ε-aminocaproic acid. Most likely because of the theoretical concerns for thrombotic complications, combinations of aprotinin and ε-aminocaproic acid or tranexamic acid have not been examined in clinical trials.

Several other hemostatic agents have been investigated for the reduction of bleeding, including desmopressin (ddAVP) and epoprostenol (prostacyclin). However, similar reductions in blood loss due to use of aprotinin and the antifibrinolytic amino acids have not been demonstrated, particularly for ddAVP, which has been examined in a number of trials (55, 56). In addition, each of these agents has potentially significant side effects (i.e., hyponatremia for ddAVP and hypotension for epoprostenol).

The use of platelet concentrates and/or FFP may be necessary during surgery because of consumption in the bypass circuit. Cardiac reoperations, in particular, are more prolonged and are associated with a higher risk for complications, and tend to require considerably more blood products, including packed cells, platelets, and FFP (57). Maintaining an intraoperative hematocrit of approximately 30% may act like a hemostatic agent by facilitating platelet margination. Therefore, it is somewhat of a paradox that transfusion of packed red blood cells may actually help decrease blood loss. In general, patients undergoing uncomplicated cardiac surgery should have at least two units of packed red blood cells typed, cross-matched,

and ready at the time of surgery. For reoperations or more complicated procedures (such as valve replacements) at least 4 U should be reserved.

There has been some concern about transfusion of the residual cardiopulmonary bypass volume, in terms of its effect on coagulation parameters and hemostasis. Data from one trial demonstrated that, despite laboratory measures of impaired hemostasis, transfusion of cell saver–processed volume was not associated with an increased need for the transfusion of FFP or platelets, and this practice may significantly decrease the need for allogeneic transfusion (58,59).

## Management of Excessive Intraoperative Bleeding

Distinguishing local surgical bleeding from medical bleeding intraoperatively after protamine neutralization of heparin, can be challenging, but is integral to the initiation of the appropriate therapy. Careful review of the operative field should be performed, and overall assessment of the patient should be undertaken. Signs such as oozing from line sites suggest a systemic process. Rapid results of a complete blood count (CBC), PT, PTT, and fibrinogen testing performed at the first sign of difficulty in achieving hemostasis can facilitate diagnosis and can guide appropriate therapy (60,61). This is the case even if empiric therapy is initiated in the interval pending results.

Topical measures, such as thrombin preparations and fibrin sealants, can be applied locally to achieve local hemostasis at the surgical site. The use of bovine-derived thrombin for achieving local hemostasis has now been replaced by human thrombin because application of bovine thrombin (which contains trace amounts of other clotting proteins) is occasionally associated with antibody inhibitor formation to human factor V, leading to bleeding complications (62).

Particularly in the setting of reoperation or during prolonged bypass times, empiric administration of platelets may be indicated because platelet number can decline drastically as a result of intraoperative activation and consumption. If a decline in platelets is noted on the CBC, platelet transfusion should be initiated for counts less than 50,000 to 75,000 per μL. In the setting of an elevated PTT and/or PT, administration of FFP may be indicated because it provides the full complement of clotting factors. Although the data is not extensive, there is no evidence that prophylactic administration of FFP perioperatively is of any benefit in decreasing blood loss in the absence of abnormal coagulation parameters (63). Use of cryoprecipitate in addition to FFP in settings of an elevated PT and/or PTT should be reserved for cases in which the fibrinogen level is particularly low (<100 to 150 mg per dL) because this product mainly contains fibrinogen, factor VIII, von Willebrand factor, and factor XIII.

Recently, use of recombinant human activated factor VIIa (rhVIIa) has been applied to obtaining surgical hemostasis. A few small trials suggest that this agent may be beneficial in the setting of diffuse bleeding without incurring a significant thrombotic risk in both children and in adult patients. In this setting, it may considerably decrease the need for reexploration (64). In children, 30 to 60 $\mu$g per kg have been administered every 2 hours for up to four doses, with monitoring of the response by chest tube drainage (65). In addition, there is evidence that rhVIIa may decrease blood loss in patients at high risk of hemorrhage when given after bypass and the administration of protamine. However, additional randomized trials examining the use of rhVIIa in the setting of cardiac surgery are necessary and are in progress (66). At this time, the use of this agent should be reserved for more severe episodes of bleeding or for prophylaxis in certain high-risk cases, in which the benefit to risk ratio is carefully considered.

# POSTOPERATIVE ISSUES

## Anticoagulation

Depending on the nature of the procedure (e.g., coronary artery bypass and prosthetic mechanical valve replacement), antiplatelet agents and/or anticoagulants are frequently used postoperatively in patients undergoing cardiac surgery to prevent thrombotic complications. Complications can arise from their use, including hemorrhage and HIT/thrombosis syndrome in patients treated with antiplatelet agents.

Antiplatelet agents are routinely administered after coronary artery bypass surgery. Aspirin is often administered in the first days postoperatively. Although aspirin is likely to confer some increase in postoperative bleeding, its administration is an accepted practice because of the potential relative benefits in preventing graft occlusion. In a large randomized clinical trial involving over 5,000 patients, the use of aspirin within 48 hours of coronary bypass surgery was associated with a statistically significant reduction both in mortality (1.3% vs. 4%) and ischemic complications (67). The addition of clopidogrel to aspirin postoperatively may provide further benefits. In one large randomized, placebo-controlled trial, the use of clopidogrel was associated both with clinical benefit and with an acceptable increased risk for major hemorrhage (approximately 1%) (68).

Patients undergoing cardiac surgery with bioprosthesis placement often receive anticoagulation with warfarin for approximately 3 months postoperatively, to give time for an endothelial layer to form over the valve (69,70). These patients often have warfarin initiated postoperatively without concomitant heparin. At the other end of the spectrum, patients with mechanical prosthetic valves require anticoagulation to relatively high intensity with warfarin (INR 3.0 to 3.5). These patients do require bridging to warfarin with an anticoagulant such as heparin that is immediately effective. In this setting, the use of LMWH as a bridging agent may be equally effective as unfractionated heparin and can result in a reduced duration of stay in the hospital (71).

## Postoperative Development of Heparin-Induced Thrombocytopenia

Even in the absence of other reasons, many patients undergoing cardiac surgery receive heparin postoperatively, either in the form of heparin flushes or in the form of unfractionated LMWH for prophylaxis against deep vein thrombosis (DVT). Because of the temporal relation between the time when patients have received heparin preoperatively or intraoperatively and the time when they are reexposed postoperatively, they are at a higher than average risk of the development of HIT and heparin-induced thrombocytopenia-thrombosis syndrome (HITTS).

Distinction of HIT from other postoperative causes of thrombocytopenia, such as disseminated intravascular coagulation (DIC) or sepsis, can often be challenging, yet crucial, because missing the diagnosis can lead to disastrous consequences. Assays for heparin-PF4 antibodies are insufficiently reliable for making the diagnosis of HIT and a single negative result does not rule out HIT. For this reason it is crucial to proceed according to the clinical scenario (see Fig. 99-2). All heparin products, including flushes, should be discontinued at once, and therapy with an alternative parenteral anticoagulant, such as a direct thrombin inhibitor, should be initiated. Platelet transfusion is contraindicated in HIT and can theoretically be associated with the instigation of major complications, such as stroke or loss of limbs. Similarly, warfarin should not be administered because it can rapidly decrease levels of the natural anticoagulants Protein C and S leading to thrombotic complications. Although the optimal duration of anticoagulation for HIT has yet to be determined by well-controlled clinical trials, available data suggest that anticoagulation at least can be continued until the platelet count recovers. With the existence of alternative options to heparin, and considering the potential consequences of a missed diagnosis, the threshold for initiating therapy for HITTS should be low.

## Other Thrombotic–Embolic Complications

Cardiac surgery is associated with a variety of other thrombotic–embolic complications, including DVT, pulmonary embolism, and stroke. Because of the high rate of postoperative venous thromboembolism (20% of patients develop DVT), all patients should be considered as candidates for appropriate DVT prophylaxis. According to one review by Goldhaber and Schoepf, prophylactic unfractionated heparin (5,000 U b.i.d.) is reasonable in low-risk patients, whereas high-risk candidates should receive a more aggressive regimen of unfractionated heparin, or else should be treated with low-molecular weight heparin (72). Should they occur, DVT and pulmonary embolism can for the most part be treated as for any patient undergoing surgery who is experiencing these events. In some instances, because these events are detected early owing to the patients being already hospitalized, surgical embolectomy may be indicated (73).

Preventing embolic phenomena such as stroke relies on optimal application of protocols for anticoagulation; for instance, appropriately intense anticoagulation after valve replacement surgery. Patients who have undergone such surgery should be instructed about the necessity of appropriate anticoagulation, as well as its potential hemorrhagic side effects.

## Postoperative Hemorrhagic Complications

Not infrequently, patients develop bleeding complications postoperatively. As in the intraoperative setting, distinguishing surgical from medical causes of bleeding can be challenging. Patients with chest tube output that exceeds 1L or chest tube output that continues at a rate of more than 100 mL per hour for several hours postoperatively in the absence of major coagulopathy may be considered as candidates for surgical reexploration.

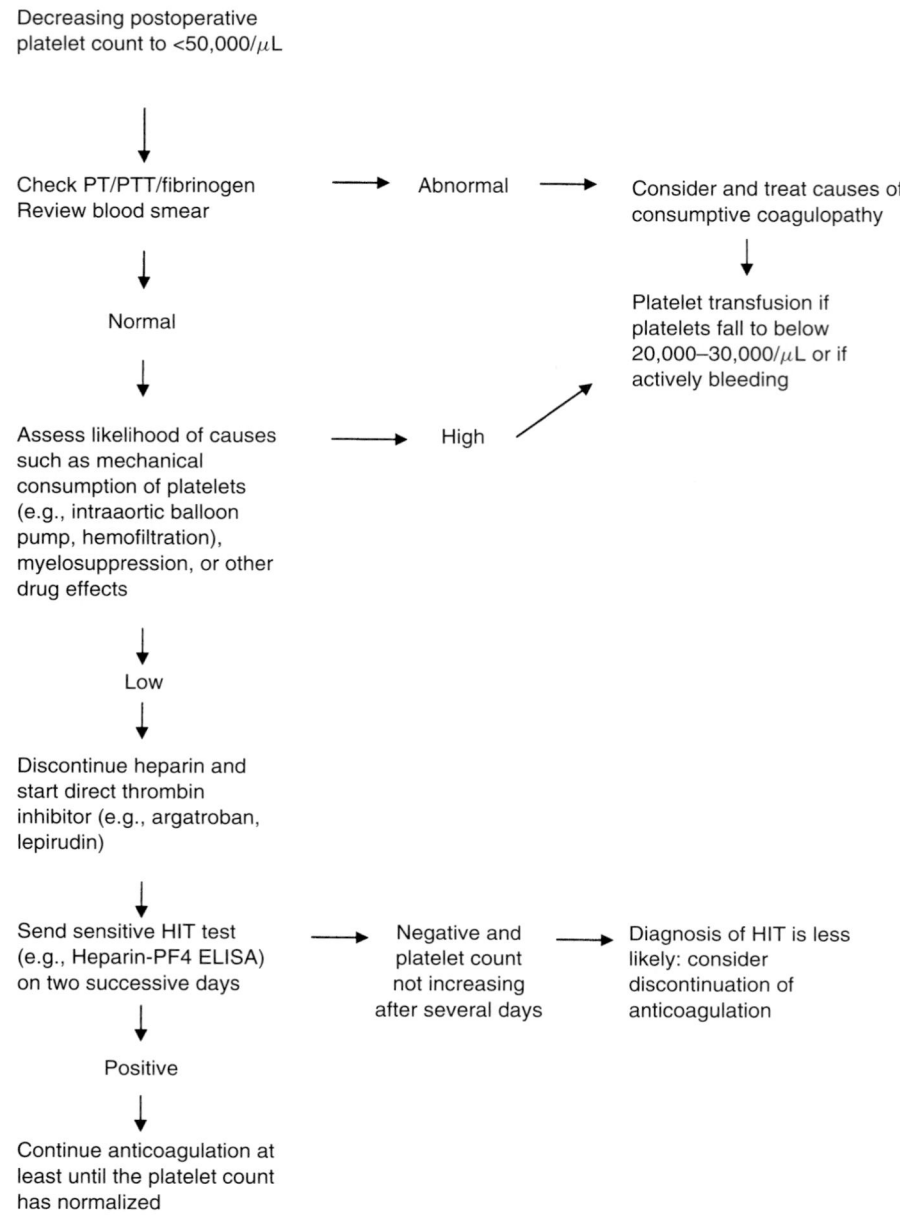

Decreasing postoperative
platelet count to <50,000/$\mu$L

Check PT/PTT/fibrinogen → Abnormal → Consider and treat causes of
Review blood smear                    consumptive coagulopathy

Normal                          Platelet transfusion if
                                platelets fall to below
                                20,000–30,000/$\mu$L or if
                                actively bleeding

Assess likelihood of causes → High
such as mechanical
consumption of platelets
(e.g., intraaortic balloon
pump, hemofiltration),
myelosuppression, or other
drug effects

Low

Discontinue heparin and
start direct thrombin
inhibitor (e.g., argatroban,
lepirudin)

Send sensitive HIT test → Negative and → Diagnosis of HIT is less
(e.g., Heparin-PF4 ELISA)   platelet count   likely: consider
on two successive days      not increasing   discontinuation of
                            after several days   anticoagulation

Positive

Continue anticoagulation at
least until the platelet count
has normalized

**FIGURE 99-2.** A practical algorithm for the evaluation and management of thrombocytopenia after cardiopulmonary bypass surgery. PT, prothrombin time; PTT, partial thromboplastin time; HIT, heparin-induced thrombocytopenia; ELISA, enzyme-linked immunosorbent assay.

The need to rapidly distinguish patients with coagulation abnormalities requiring correction from patients without such abnormalities who may have bleeding on the basis of a surgically correctable defect is clear; the former benefit from the administration of hemostatic agents, whereas the latter require reexploration in the surgical suite. Because of the long turn-around times for coagulation tests, and, particularly, for assays of platelet function, point-of-care testing has been advocated in the setting of cardiac surgery (74).

Because it may be reflective of the contribution of platelets and coagulation factors, and because it can be performed near the bedside, thromboelastography (TEG) has been explored for the evaluation of coagulopathy in the setting of cardiac surgery. Studies have not shown a high positive predictive value (PPV) for this test; however, the negative predictive value (NPV) for an underlying hemostatic defect is significantly higher (PPV of approximately 40% vs. NPV of approximately 80%) (75). Re-

sults from one small prospective randomized trial suggest that TEG can reduce the requirement for blood product transfusion in cardiac surgery; however, additional confirmatory studies are required (76).

If excessive bleeding is suspected on a medical basis, all drugs with potential anticoagulant effects should be withdrawn if possible, and the platelet count, PT, PTT, and fibrinogen should be reviewed. Transfusion of FFP and platelets based on the results of coagulation tests, rather than on an empiric basis, may be associated with a reduction in the number of products administered.

When significant coagulopathy is present, its cause should be determined and, in general, it should be corrected. Postoperative thrombocytopenia is common because of consumption during bypass or because of the use of intraaortic balloon pumps (IABP) perioperatively, which are associated with a 11% incidence of thrombocytopenia (77). In the absence of devices such as an IABP, thrombocytopenia should resolve within 24 to 48 hours of surgery. Persistent thrombocytopenia should trigger an evaluation for the etiology. Common causes in this setting include medication effects (antibiotics, heparin), myelosuppression due to concomitant infection, and consumption due to DIC. Elevated levels of PT and/or PTT in coagulation tests (PT and/or PTT) may be related to insufficient clotting factor synthesis (hepatic dysfunction) or to consumption due to DIC. Rarely, a hereditary hemostatic deficit, such as mild factor VIII or factor XI deficiency, will be detected postoperatively. If such a defect is suspected on the basis of family history, specific factor assays should be obtained to confirm the diagnosis and to guide further therapy with clotting factor concentrates or FFP.

Often, no apparent cause for excessive postoperative bleeding can be identified. Although clinical judgment for each individual situation is necessary, some general guidelines exist for the correction of coagulopathy. The platelet count should be maintained over 50,000 per $\mu$L, provided that there are no contraindications to platelet transfusion, such as significant suspicion of heparin-induced thrombocytopenia. If such a suspicion exists, it is reasonable to withhold platelet transfusion, pending further investigation. FFP should be administered if depletion of clotting factors is suspected on the basis of an elevated PT and PTT. Administration of cryoprecipitate should be reserved for situations in which fibrinogen levels are particularly low and administration of volume is an issue (4 U of FFP provide approximately the same amount of fibrinogen as one 10-U cryoprecipitate bag).

Although there are few data available in the literature to support postoperative use of antifibrinolytic agents, these may be utilized in the setting of ongoing bleeding in case of normal or near normal values of the PT and PTT tests; such bleeding is potentially due to platelet dysfunction. However, these agents are contraindicated in the presence of DIC. If no effect is seen after 24 hours of administration, it is unlikely that clinical benefit will be achieved, and alternatives should be considered. Recombinant human activated factor VII (rhVIIa, Novoseven) has been administered in a few cases of excessive postoperative bleeding. Few data are available to support its use in this setting, and given the potential thrombotic complications, rhVIIa should be used cautiously only when other interventions have failed.

# SUMMARY

Surgery involving use of cardiopulmonary bypass is associated with a relatively high incidence of hemostatic abnormalities because of the delicate balance that must be achieved between preventing thrombosis and maintaining hemostasis. Careful preoperative evaluation of patients can help identify those at a higher risk for complications. Measures to minimize operative blood loss include optimization of hematologic parameters and use of antifibrinolytic agents. A number of causes may produce postoperative bleeding. Because no single approach is broadly applicable for the management of all situations, a thoughtful approach to the evaluation and the management of the individual patient is required.

## References

1. Harker LA. Bleeding after cardiopulmonary surgery. N Engl J Med 1986;314:1446–1448.
2. Dacey LJ, Munoz JJ, Baribeau YR et al, Northern New England Cardiovascular Disease Study Group. Reexploration for hemorrhage following coronary artery bypass grafting: incidence and risk factors. Arch Surg 1998;133:442–447.
3. McKusker K, Lee S. Post cardiopulmonary bypass bleeding: an introductory review. J Extra Corpor Technol 1999;31:23–36.
4. Parolari A, Colli S, Mussoni L, et al. Coagulation and fibrinolytic markers in a two-month follow-up of coronary bypass surgery. J Thorac Cardiovasc Surg 2003;125:336–343.
5. Smith CR. Management of bleeding complication in redo cardiac operations. Ann Thorac Surg 1998;65:S2–S8.
6. Messmore HL Jr, Godwin J. Medical assessment of bleeding in the surgical patient. Med Clin North Am 1994;78:625–634.
7. Ang-Lee MK, Moss J, Yuan CS. Herbal medicines and perioperative care. JAMA 2001;286:208–216.
8. Baker R. Pre-operative hemostatic assessment and management. Transfus Apheresis Sci 2002;27:45–53.
9. Eckman MH, Erban JK, Singh SK, et al. Screening for the risk of bleeding or thrombosis. Ann Intern Med 2003;138:W15–W24.
10. Ducart AR, Collard EL, Osselaer JC, et al. Management of anticoagulation during cardiopulmonary bypass in a patient with circulating lupus anticoagulant. J Cardiothorac Vasc Anesth 1997;11:878–879.
11. East CJ, Clements F, Mathew J, et al. Antiphospholipid syndrome and cardiac surgery: management of anticoagulation in two patients. Anesth Analg 2000;90:1098–1101.
12. Lind S. The bleeding time does not predict surgical bleeding. Blood 1991;77:2547–2552.
13. Moor E, Silveira A, van't Hooft F, et al. Coagulation factor V (Arg506?Gln) mutation and early saphenous vein graft occlusion after coronary artery bypass grafting. Thromb Haemost 1998;80:220–224.
14. Sweeney JD, Blair AJ, Dupuis MP, et al. Aprotinin, cardiac surgery, and factor V Leiden. Tranfusion 1997;37:1173–1178.
15. Ong BC, Zimmermann AA, Zappulla DC, et al. Prevalence of factor V Leiden in a population of patients with congenital heart disease. Can J Anaesth 1998;45:1176–1180.
16. Donahue BS, Gailani D, Higgins MS, et al. Factor V Leiden protects against blood loss and transfusion after cardiac surgery. Circulation 2003; 107:1003–1008.
17. Schafer AI. Effects of nonsteroidal anti-inflammatory therapy on platelets. Am J Med 1999;106:25S–36S.
18. Reich DL, Patel GC, Vela-Cantos F, et al. Aspirin does not increase homologous blood requirements in elective coronary bypass surgery. Anesth Analg 1994;79:4–8.
19. Moulton MJ, Creswell LL, Mackey ME, et al. Reexploration for bleeding is a risk factor for adverse outcomes after cardiac operations. J Thorac Cardiovasc Surg 1996;111:1037–1046.
20. Pleym H, Stenseth R, Wahba A, et al. Prophylactic treatment with desmopressin does not reduce postoperative bleeding after coronary surgery in patients treated with aspirin before surgery. Anesth Analg 2004;98:578–584.
21. Pothula S, Sanchala VT, Nagappala B, et al. The effect of preoperative antiplatelet/anticoagulant prophylaxis on postoperative blood loss in cardiac surgery. Anesth Analg 2004;98:4–10.
22. Silvestry SC, Smith PK. Current status of cardiac surgery in the abciximab-treated patient. Ann Thorac Surg 2000;70(Suppl. 2):S12–S19.
23. Kearon C. Perioperative management of long-term anticoagulation. Semin Thromb Hemost 1998;24(Suppl. 1):77–83.
24. Dietrich W, Dilthey G, Spannagl M, et al. Warfarin pretreatment does not lead to increased bleeding tendency during cardiac surgery. J Cardiothorac Vasc Anesth 1995;9:250–254.
25. Clark SC, Vitale N, Zacharias J, et al. Effect of low molecular weight heparin (fragmin) on bleeding after cardiac surgery. Ann Thorac Surg 2000;69:762–764.
26. Warkentin TE. Heparin-induced thrombocytopenia: pathogenesis and management. Br J Haematol 2003;121:373–374.
27. Staples MH, Dunton RF, Karlson KJ, et al. Heparin resistance after preoperative therapy or intraaortic balloon pumping. Ann Thorac Surg 1994;57:1211–1216.
28. Linden MD, Schneider M, Baker S, et al. Decreased concentration of antithrombin after preoperative heparin does not cause heparin resistance during cardiopulmonary bypass. J Cardiothorac Vasc Anesth 2004;18: 131–135.
29. Liu B, Belboul A, Larsson S, et al. Factors influencing hemostasis and blood transfusion in cardiac surgery. Perfusion 1996;11:131–143.
30. Coyle D, Lee KM, Fergusson DA, et al. Cost effectiveness of epoetin-alpha to augment preoperative autologous blood donation in elective cardiac surgery. Pharmacoeconomics 2000;18:161–171.
31. Goodnough LT, Despotis GJ. Transfusion medicine: support of patients undergoing cardiac surgery. Am J Cardiovasc Drugs 2001;1:337–351.
32. Freischlag JA. Intraoperative blood salvage in vascular surgery – worth the effort? Crit Care 2004;8(Suppl. 2):S53–S56.
33. Ovrum E, Tangen G, Oystese R, et al. Heparin-coated circuits (Duraflo II) with reduced versus full anticoagulation during coronary artery bypass surgery. J Card Surg 2003;18:140–146.
34. Despotis GJ, Joist JH, Hogue CW Jr, et al. More effective suppression of hemostatic system activation in patients undergoing cardiac surgery by heparin dosing based on heparin blood concentrations rather than ACT. Thromb Haemost 1996;76:902–908.
35. Lemmer JH Jr, Despotis GJ. Antithrombin III concentrate to treat heparin resistance in patients undergoing cardiac surgery. J Thorac Cardiovasc Surg 2002;123:213–217.
36. Barstad RM, Stephens RW, Hamers MJ, et al. Protamine sulphate inhibits platelet membrane glycoprotein Ib-von Willebrand factor activity. Thromb Haemost 2000;83:334–337.

37. Shigeta O, Kojima H, Hiramatsu Y, et al. Low-dose protamine based on heparin-protamine titration method reduces platelet dysfunction after cardiopulmonary bypass. *J Thorac Cardiovasc Surg* 1999;118:354–360.

38. Gitlin SD, Deeb GM, Yann C, et al. Intraoperative monitoring of danaparoid sodium anticoagulation during cardiovascular operations. *J Vasc Surg* 1998; 27:568–575.

39. Despotis GJ, Hogue CW, Saleem R, et al. The relationship between hirudin and activated clotting time: implications for patients with heparin-induced thrombocytopenia undergoing cardiac surgery. *Anesth Analg* 2001;93: 28–32.

40. Warkentin TE. Heparin-induced thrombocytopenia: pathogenesis and management. *Br J Haematol* 2003;121:535–555.

41. Warkentin TE, Greinacher A. Heparin-induced thrombocytopenia and cardiac surgery. *Ann Thorac Surg* 2003;76:2121–2131.

42. Palatianos GM, Foroulis CN, Vassili MI, et al. Preoperative detection and management of immune heparin-induced thrombocytopenia in patients undergoing heart surgery with iloprost. *J Thorac Cardiovasc Surg* 2004;127:548–554.

43. Cannon MA, Butterworth J, Riley RD, et al. Failure of argatroban anticoagulation during off-pump coronary artery bypass surgery. *Ann Thorac Surg* 2004;77:711–713.

44. Horrow JC, Van Riper DF, Strong MD, et al. Hemostatic effects of tranexamic acid and desmopressin during cardiac surgery. *Circulation* 1991;84: 2063–2070.

45. Jamieson WR, Dryden PJ, O'Connor JP, et al. Beneficial effect of both tranexamic acid and aprotinin on blood loss reduction in reoperative valve replacement surgery. *Circulation* 1997;96(Suppl. 9):II-96–II-100.

46. Levi M, Cromheecke ME, de Jonge E, et al. Pharmacological strategies to decrease excessive blood loss in cardiac surgery: a meta-analysis of clinically relevant endpoints. *Lancet* 1999;354:1940–1947.

47. Porte RJ, Leebeek FW. Pharmacological strategies to decrease transfusion requirements in patients undergoing surgery. *Drugs* 2002;62:2193–2211.

48. Landis RC, Asimakopoulos G, Poullis M, et al. The antithrombotic and anti-inflammatory mechanisms of action of aprotinin. *Ann Thorac Surg* 2001;72:2169–2175.

49. Francis JL, Howard C. The effect of aprotinin on the response of the activated partial thromboplastin time (APTT) to heparin. *Blood Coagul Fibrinolysis* 1993;4:35–40.

50. Mossinger H, Dietrich W, Braun SL, et al. High-dose aprotinin reduces activation of hemostasis, allogeneic blood requirement, and duration of postoperative ventilation in pediatric cardiac surgery. *Ann Thorac Surg* 2003;75:430–437.

51. Koster A, Huebler S, Merkle F, et al. Heparin-level-based anticoagulation management during cardiopulmonary bypass: a pilot investigation on the effects of a half-dose aprotinin protocol on postoperative blood loss and hemostatic activation and inflammatory response. *Anesth Analg* 2004;98: 285–290.

52. Isgro F, Stanisch O, Kiessling AH, et al. Topical application of aprotinin in cardiac surgery. *Perfusion* 2002;17:347–351.

53. Maineri P, Covaia G, Realini M, et al. Postoperative bleeding after coronary revascularization. Comparison between tranexamic acid and epsilon-aminocaproic acid. *Minerva Cardioangiol* 2000;48:155–160.

54. Armellin G, Casella S, Guzzinati S, et al. Tranexamic acid in aortic valve replacement. *J Cardiothorac Vasc Anesth* 2001;15:331–335.

55. Temeck BK, Bachenheimer LC, Katz NM, et al. Desmopressin acetate in cardiac surgery: a double-blind, randomized study. *South Med J* 1994;87: 611–615.

56. Ozkisacik E, Islamoglu F, Posacioglu H, et al. Desmopressin use in elective cardiac surgery. *J Cardiovasc Surg (Torino)* 2001;42:741–747.

57. Utley JR. Pathophysiology of cardiopulmonary bypass: current issues. *J Card Surg* 1990;5:177–189.

58. Daane CR, Golab HD, Meeder JH, et al. Processing and transfusion of residual cardiopulmonary bypass volume: effects on haemostasis, complement activation, postoperative blood loss and transfusion volume. *Perfusion* 2003;18:115–121.

59. McGill N, O'Shaughnessy D, Pickering R, et al. Mechanical methods of reducing blood transfusion in cardiac surgery: randomized controlled trial. *BMJ* 2002;324:1299.

60. Despotis GJ, Skubas NJ, Goodnough LT. Optimal management of bleeding and transfusion in patients undergoing cardiac surgery. *Semin Thorac Cardiovasc Surg* 1999;11:84–104.

61. Nuttall GA, Oliver WC, Santrach PJ, et al. Efficacy of a simple intraoperative transfusion algorithm for nonerythrocyte component utilization after cardiopulmonary bypass. *Anesthesiology* 2001;94:773–781.

62. Streiff MB, Ness PM. Acquired FV inhibitors: a needless iatrogenic complication of bovine thrombin exposure. *Transfusion* 2002;42:18–26.

63. Casbard AC, Williamson LM, Murphy MF, et al. The role of prophylactic fresh frozen plasma in decreasing blood loss and correcting coagulopathy in cardiac surgery. A systematic review. *Anaesthesia* 2004;59:550–558.

64. Al Douri M, Shafi T, Al Khudairi D, et al. Effect of the administration of recombinant activated factor VII (rVIIa; NovoSeven) in the management of severe uncontrolled bleeding in patients undergoing heart valve replacement surgery. *Blood Coagul Fibrinolysis* 2000;11(Suppl. 1):S121–S127.

65. Pychynska-Pokorska M, Moll JJ, Krajewski W, et al. The use of recombinant coagulation factor VIIa in uncontrolled postoperative bleeding in children undergoing cardiac surgery with cardiopulmonary bypass. *Pediatr Crit Care Med* 2004;5:246–250.

66. Herbertson M. Recombinant activated factor VII in cardiac surgery. *Blood Coagul Fibrinolysis* 2004;15(Suppl. 1):S31–S32.

67. Mangano DT, Multicenter Study of Perioperative Ischemia. Aspirin and mortality from coronary bypass surgery. *N Engl J Med* 2002;347: 1309–1317.

68. Fox KAA, Mehta SR, Peters R et al. Benefits and risks of the combination of clopidogrel and aspirin in patients undergoing surgical revascularization for non-ST elevation acute coronary syndrome: The Clopidogrel in Unstable angina to prevent Recurrent ischemic Events (CURE) trial. *Circulation* 2004;110:1202–1208 (Aug 14 epub).

69. Orszulak TA, Schaff HV, Mullany CJ, et al. Risk of thromboembolism with the aortic Carpentier-Edwards bioprosthesis. *Ann Thorac Surg* 1995; 59:462–468.

70. Stein PD, Alpert JS, Bussey HI, et al. Antithrombotic therapy in patients with mechanical and biological prosthetic heart valves. *Chest* 2001;119: 220S–227S.

71. Fanikos J, Tsilimingras K, Kucher N, et al. Comparison of efficacy, safety, and cost of low-molecular-weight heparin with continuous-infusion unfractionated heparin for initiation of anticoagulation after mechanical prosthetic valve implantation. *Am J Cardiol* 2004;93:247–250.

72. Goldhaber SZ, Schoepf UJ. Pulmonary embolism after coronary artery bypass grafting. *Circulation* 2004;109:2712–2715.

73. Aklog L, Williams CS, Byrne JG, et al. Acute pulmonary embolectomy: a contemporary approach. *Circulation* 2002;105:1416–1419.

74. Prisco D, Paniccia R. Point-of-care testing of hemostasis in cardiac surgery. *Thromb J* 2003;6:1 (epub).

75. Cammerer U, Dietrich W, Rampf T, et al. The predictive value of modified computerized thromboelastography and platelet function analysis for postoperative blood loss in routine cardiac surgery. *Anesth Analg* 2003;96:51–57.

76. Shore-Lesserson L, Manspeizer HE, DePerio M, et al. Thromboelastography-guided transfusion algorithm reduces transfusions in complex cardiac surgery. *Anesth Analg* 1999;88:312–319.

77. Meco M, Gramegna G, Yassini A, et al. Mortality and morbidity from intra-aortic balloon pumps. Risk analysis. *J Cardiovasc Surg (Torino)* 2002;43:17–23.

# CHAPTER 100 ■ MEDICAL THERAPY FOR PERIPHERAL ARTERIAL DISEASE

JAMES J. JANG AND JEFFREY W. OLIN

## BACKGROUND: LIFE, LIMB, AND MORBIDITY IN PATIENTS WITH PERIPHERAL ARTERIAL DISEASE

Peripheral arterial disease (PAD) is a marker of systemic atherosclerosis. The prevalence of PAD is approximately 12% of the adult population, with men being affected slightly more than women (1,2). However, this percentage is dependent on the age of the cohort studied (see Table 100-1). Almost 20% of adults older than 70 years have PAD (3). Findings from a national cross-sectional survey of "PAD awareness, risk, and treatment: New resources for survival" (PARTNERS) found that PAD afflicts 29% of patients who are either as old as 70 years or older, or between 50 and 69 years, who have a 10-pack-year history of smoking or have diabetes (4). Despite the strikingly high prevalence of this disease, especially in older patients, this disease is underdiagnosed because it often presents with atypical symptoms or with no symptoms related to the legs. The PARTNERS study demonstrated that more than 70% of primary care providers whose patients were screened in this study were unaware of the presence of PAD (4). The clinical presentation of PAD may vary from intermittent claudication, atypical leg pain, rest pain, ischemic ulcers, or gangrene to no symptoms at all. Claudication is the typical symptomatic expression of PAD. However, the prevalence of asymptomatic disease is thought to be higher than that of symptomatic PAD, with an estimated ratio of 0.9 to 7.7:1 (5). The Walking and Leg Circulation Study evaluated the symptoms in patients with PAD. Of the 460 patients with PAD, 19.8% had no exertional leg pain, 28.5% had atypical leg pain, 32.6% had classic intermittent claudication, and 19.1% had pain at rest (6). Results from large epidemiologic studies suggest that only 2% to 6% of patients aged 60 years or older are symptomatic with intermittent claudication, despite the high prevalence of PAD in that age-population (7). The Rotterdam Study identified a 19.1% prevalence of PAD in their cohort population; however, intermittent claudication was reported in only 6.3% of patients in the PAD group (8). Similarly, the Edinburgh Artery Study surveyed 1,592 subjects aged 55 to 74 years and identified a 4.5% prevalence of intermittent claudication and an 8.0% prevalence of asymptomatic PAD (9). The results of these studies make it readily apparent that more patients with PAD are asymptomatic or have atypical leg symptoms than those with classic intermittent claudication do.

There are two major consequences of PAD: a decrease in overall well-being and quality of life due to claudication and atypical leg pain, and a markedly increased cardiovascular morbidity and mortality. Treatment should be directed at each of these facets.

PAD is most often diagnosed by an ankle-brachial–index (ABI) less than 0.9. The ABI is the ratio of the ankle systolic pressure to the arm systolic pressure. Using a Doppler ultrasonographic device, the higher systolic pressure measured from either the posterior tibial or the dorsalis pedis artery (in each leg) is compared with the highest brachial artery pressure taken from either arm (see Fig. 100-1). A low ABI has been shown to be an independent predictor of increased mortality (10,12–16). Each 0.1 decrement less than 1.0 in the ABI has been shown to have a significant decrease in survival (10). Patients with an ABI of 0.9 to 1.0 had a mortality of approximately 15% at 6 years, whereas patients with an ABI less than 0.9 had a mortality of almost 25% (10). The incidence of transient ischemic attack (TIA)/stroke and cardiac events was proportional to the decrease in the ABI (11,17). Patients with an ABI less than 0.9 were twice as likely to have a history of myocardial infarction (MI), angina, and congestive heart failure than patients with an ABI of 1.0 to 1.5 (11,17). In fact, men with an ABI less than 0.9 were more than four times likely to have TIAs/strokes than those with an ABI greater than 0.9 (11). From the Framingham Study, mortality in patients with intermittent claudication was two to three times higher than in age- and sex-matched controls with 75% of patients with PAD dying from cardiovascular events (2). In a 15-year review of patients with claudication, more than 66% of mortality was attributable to cardiovascular disease. Interestingly, a history of angina or MI was not predictive of mortality. Instead, a reduced ABI at rest or after exercise, older age, and diabetes were the only significant negative predictors (18). In a 10-year prospective study by Criqui et al. patients with PAD, with and without a history of cardiovascular disease, had significantly increased risk of dying from cardiovascular and coronary heart disease than age-matched controls did (19). The 10-year mortality increased as the severity of PAD increased (see Fig. 100-2). The all-cause mortality was 3.1 times greater and cardiovascular disease mortality was 5.9 times greater in those patients with PAD compared to patients without PAD. The risk of cardiovascular events has been found to be similar between patients with PAD with claudication and those without symptoms (20). In a study of 2,023 middle-aged asymptomatic men without coronary artery disease (CAD), an ABI less than 0.9 was independently associated with higher coronary and cardiovascular mortality in the asymptomatic men than in subjects with a normal ABI (21). The extremely high morbidity and mortality in the PAD population is due to MI and stroke (22,23). Both the Atherosclerosis Risk in Communities (ARIC) and Edinburgh Artery Studies correlated an increased risk of stroke and TIA with increased PAD severity (11,20). The combination of known coronary or cerebrovascular disease with PAD has been shown to increase mortality risk. The Bypass Angioplasty Revascularization Investigation (BARI)

**TABLE 100-1**

PREVALENCE OF PERIPHERAL DISEASE

| Study | Subjects (no.) | Age | ABI | Prevalence (%) | Claudication (%) |
|---|---|---|---|---|---|
| PARTNERS (4) | 6,417 | ≥70 or >50 with DM or tobacco history | ≤0.9 | 29 | 11 |
| Rotterdam (8) | 7,715 | ≥55 | <0.9 | 19 | 6 |
| Edinburgh (9) | 1,592 | 55–74 | <0.9 | 18 | 5 |
| CHS (10) | 5,714 | ≥65 | <0.9 | 13 | 1 |
| ARIC (11) | 15,106 | 45–64 | ≤0.9 | 3 | 1 |

ABI, ankle-brachial index; PARTNERS, Peripheral arterial disease awareness, risk and treatment: new resources for survival; DM, diabetes mellitus; CHS, Cardiovascular Heart Study; ARIC, Atherosclerosis Risk in Communities.

trial demonstrated that patients with multivessel CAD and PAD had a 4.9 times greater relative risk of death compared to those individuals without PAD (24).

## RISK FACTORS

Many of the known risk factors for cerebral and coronary atherosclerosis such as age, sex, tobacco smoking, hypertension, diabetes mellitus, dyslipidemia, and hyperhomocystinemia have been shown to promote atherogenesis in the peripheral arterial system (see Table 100-2). However, smoking and diabetes are the most important risk factors associated with the occurrence of PAD and its progression to critical limb ischemia. In addition to traditional risk factors, C-reactive protein (CRP), an inflammatory biomarker, has been shown to be a strong independent risk factor for future PAD in otherwise healthy patients (25). The addition of CRP to standard lipid screening significantly improves the ability to predict the development of PAD (see Fig. 100-3).

## TREATMENT OF PERIPHERAL ARTERIAL DISEASE

All patients with PAD, including those undergoing percutaneous therapy or surgical revascularization, should receive medical management. The indications for these invasive therapies include lifestyle-interfering claudication, rest pain or ischemic ulceration or gangrene. The types and results of such interventions are beyond the scope of this chapter.

Medical treatment of PAD should be directed toward two major goals: improvement of limb-related complications such as claudication and a decrease in the morbidity and mortality

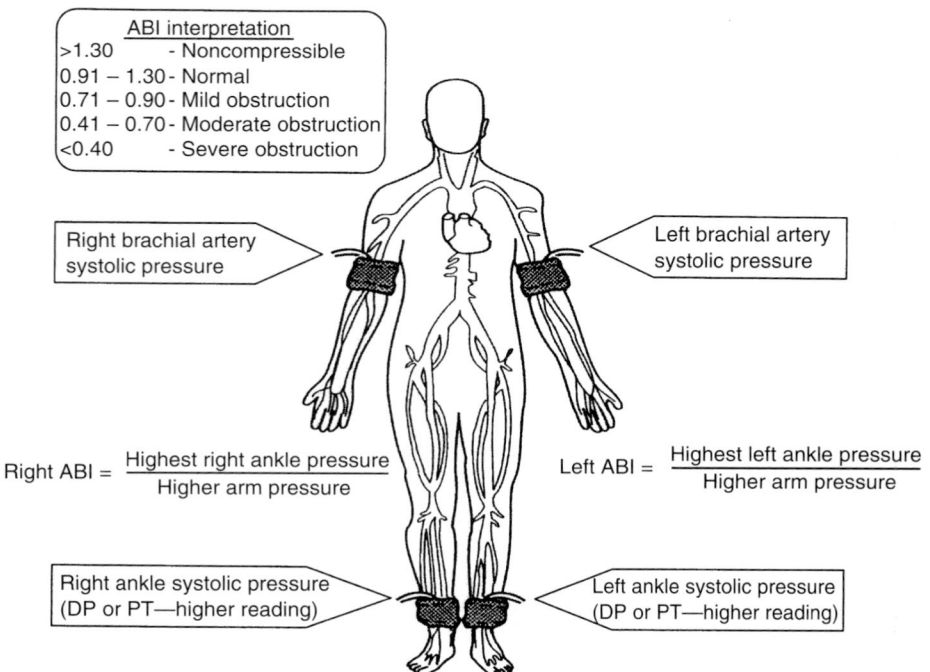

ABI interpretation
>1.30 - Noncompressible
0.91 – 1.30 - Normal
0.71 – 0.90 - Mild obstruction
0.41 – 0.70 - Moderate obstruction
<0.40 - Severe obstruction

Right brachial artery systolic pressure

Left brachial artery systolic pressure

$$Right\ ABI = \frac{Highest\ right\ ankle\ pressure}{Higher\ arm\ pressure}$$

$$Left\ ABI = \frac{Highest\ left\ ankle\ pressure}{Higher\ arm\ pressure}$$

Right ankle systolic pressure (DP or PT—higher reading)

Left ankle systolic pressure (DP or PT—higher reading)

**FIGURE 100-1.** Measurement of ankle-brachial index (ABI). DP, dorsalis pedis; PT, posterior tibeal.

10-year survival curves for patients with symptomatic
or asymptomatic PAD compared with normal subjects

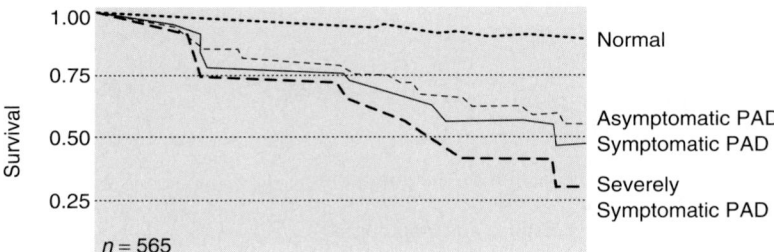

**FIGURE 100-2.** Mortality over a period of 10 years in patients with peripheral arterial disease (PAD). (From Criqui MH, Langer RD, Fronek A, et al. Mortality over a period of 10 years in patients with peripheral arterial disease. *N Engl J Med* 1992;326:381–386, with permission.)

due to MI and stroke (see Table 100-3). It is important that treatment go beyond symptomatic improvement alone, otherwise the patients may feel better but then succumb to a cardiovascular event.

# NON-PHARMACOLOGIC TREATMENTS

## Smoking Cessation

Cigarette smoking has been shown to be the most important independent risk factor for the development of PAD. From the Rotterdam Study, 69% of older patients identified as having PAD had known attributable cardiovascular risk factors. Smoking was the most commonly identified risk factor at 18.1% (26). In the Rotterdam Study, more than 80% of male patients with PAD were found to be current or former smokers (8). In fact, the Edinburgh Artery Study found that cigarette smoking was a stronger predictor of PAD than CAD (27,28). In a case–control study of 1,119 smokers, the total cumulative pack-year smoking history was independently associated with the development of PAD (29). In the Framingham Offspring

| TABLE 100-2 |
| --- |

**PERIPHERAL ARTERIAL DISEASE RISK FACTORS**

- Age
- Gender[a]
- Tobacco smoking
- Hypertension
- Diabetes mellitus
- Dyslipidemia
- Hyperhomocysteinemia
- Increased fibrinogen
- Elevated C-reactive protein

[a]Some studies have shown gender equivalence.

Study, for each 10-pack-year increment in smoking there was 1.3-fold increase in the incidence of PAD (30). In addition, increased pack-years have been associated with increased risk of amputation and peripheral graft occlusion (31,32).

Behavior modification, nicotine replacement therapy, and antidepressants such as bupropion are effective strategies to

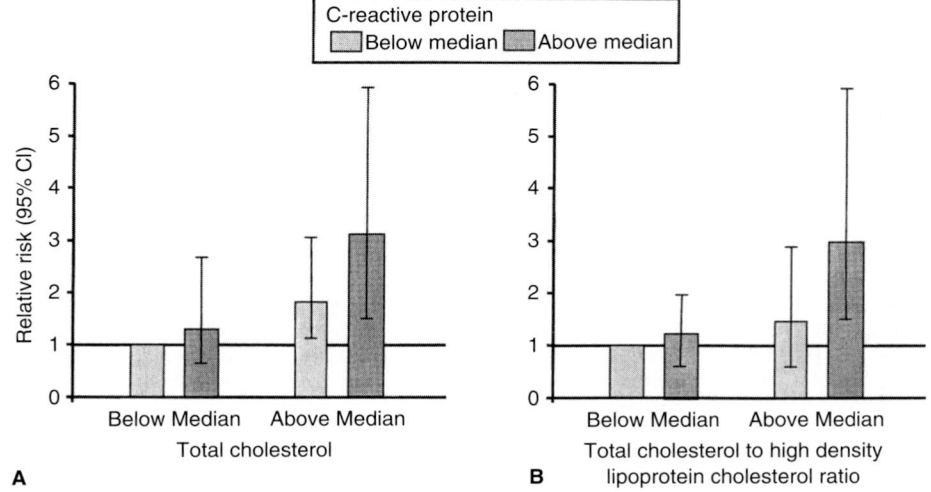

**FIGURE 100-3.** Relative risk of developing peripheral arterial disease among apparently healthy men. **A:** Stratification by baseline levels of total cholesterol and C-reactive protein. **B:** Stratification by baseline levels of total cholesterol–high density lipoprotein cholesterol ratio and C-reactive protein. Relative risks and 95% confidence intervals (CI) were derived from logistic regression models. [From Ridker PM, Stampfer MJ, Rifai N. Novel risk factors for systemic atherosclerosis: A comparison of C-reactive protein, fibrinogen, homocysteine, lipoprotein (a), and standard cholesterol screening as predictors of peripheral arterial disease. *JAMA* 2001;285:2481–2485, with permission.]

**TABLE 100-3**

GOALS IN THE TREATMENT OF PERIPHERAL ARTERIAL DISEASE

| Symptom improvement | Mortality reduction |
|---|---|
| Smoking cessation[a] | Smoking cessation |
| Exercise | Diabetic control ($\pm$) |
| Statins[b] | Lipid lowering |
| Pentoxifylline[a] | Antihypertensive medications (ACE inhibitors and ARBs) |
| Cilostazol | Antiplatelet therapy (aspirin and clopidogrel) |
| Propionyl-L-carnitine | |
| Therapeutic angiogenesis[c] | |
| L-Arginine | |
| Immunomodulation therapy[c] | |

ACE, angiotensin-converting enzyme; ARBs, angiotensin receptor blockers.
[a]Conflicting data on symptom improvement.
[b]Benefit was small in two randomized trials.
[c]Undergoing clinical trials.

achieve smoking cessation (33). Smoking cessation has been shown to decrease mortality, cardiovascular events, and amputation rates (34,35). Patients with intermittent claudication who stopped smoking appear to have twice the survival benefit at 5 years and 10 years compared to patients who continued to smoke (34,36). Although individual studies have demonstrated an improvement in the walking distance in patients who successfully stopped smoking, a recent metaanalysis revealed no significant difference in total walking distance or in resting ABIs on cessation of smoking (37). Because discontinuation of smoking or using tobacco in any form is so important, it is the first item that is discussed with the patient during each visit to the clinic. In a nonjudgmental way, it is important to let the patient know how important this is for their overall cardiovascular health in general and their PAD in particular.

## Exercise Therapy

It is known that patients with an abnormally low ABI have decreased walking ability and impaired functional status (38,39). Using validated questionnaires, it has been demonstrated that the quality of life is markedly diminished in patients with PAD (40). The goal of an exercise-conditioning program is primarily to increase functional capacity and walking ability and also to improve overall cardiovascular health. A supervised exercise program has been shown to be superior to any pharmacologic agent to date, particularly in patients with infrainguinal disease. In patients with iliac disease and claudication, angioplasty and stent implantation may be a first-line therapy. It has been shown that supervised exercise improves pain-free walking, and maximal walking time and distance in patients with intermittent claudication (37,41). Predictors of a successful exercise program include walking to near-maximal pain (and then stopping until the discomfort disappears), for more than 30 minutes per session, for at least three times a week, and for at least 6 months of training (41). Although there is no evidence of benefit in mortality or improvement in the ABI or calf blood flow, the quality of life and functional capacity improve with exercise in patients with PAD (37,42). It has been shown that a structured exercise is superior to home-based exercise programs. However, there is currently no reimbursement for the time and effort needed to successfully implement this type of program.

# PHARMACOLOGIC TREATMENTS TO REDUCE CARDIOVASCULAR MORBIDITY AND MORTALITY

## Hypertension

Elevated blood pressure is a strong predictor for PAD (28,43,44). From the Framingham Study Cohort, hypertension increased the risk of PAD by 2.5-fold to fourfold in men and women, respectively (2). According to the seventh report by the Joint National Committee on Prevention, Detection, Evaluation, and Treatment of High Blood Pressure, PAD is equivalent in risk to ischemic heart disease. These guidelines recommend that any class of antihypertensive drugs may be used with PAD. As such, $\beta$-blockers and angiotensin-converting enzyme (ACE) inhibitors are generally recommended for the cardioprotective effects of both drug classes, especially in patients with PAD and concomitant CAD (45–47). A metaanalysis by Radack and Deck found that $\beta$-blockers do not worsen claudication symptoms and can be used safely in patients with PAD (48). An aggressive antihypertensive approach appears to have clear benefits in patients with PAD. In the Appropriate Blood Pressure Control in Diabetes (ABCD) trial, patients who received intensive hypertension treatment to a blood pressure of 128/75 mm Hg with either an ACE inhibitor (enalapril) or a calcium channel blocker (nisoldipine) had a significant decrease in cardiovascular events compared to those randomized to moderate hypertension treatment to a blood pressure of 137/81 mm Hg (49). Although the patient numbers were small, those in the moderate hypertension control group had a marked increase in cardiovascular mortality as the ABI declined, whereas those in the intensive blood pressure control group had no such response.

Beyond the antihypertensive effects, ACE inhibitors, such as ramipril and perindopril, have been shown to benefit patients who are at high risk for cardiovascular events. On the basis of the Hope Outcomes Prevention Evaluation (HOPE) study, patients with diabetes or with evidence of vascular disease plus one other cardiovascular risk factor who received ramipril had a 22% risk reduction of stroke, MI, and death compared to patients who received a placebo (50). Interestingly, the subgroup of patients with PAD who were treated with ramipril had a 27% relative risk reduction in the primary endpoints compared to the placebo-treated group (51). From the European trial on Reduction Of cardiac events with Perindopril in patients with stable coronary Artery disease (EUROPA) study, 12,218 patients with stable coronary heart disease were randomly assigned to perindopril (8 mg daily) or a placebo (52). After a mean follow-up of 4.2 years, cardiovascular events were significantly decreased in patients treated with perindopril. All predefined subgroups including the 883 patients who had documented peripheral vascular disease benefited from perindopril (52).

Similar to ACE inhibitors, angiotensin receptor blockers (ARBs), have demonstrated cardiovascular benefits beyond its antihypertensive properties. In particular, ARBs have improved endothelial function through increased nitric oxide bioavailability or decreased vascular inflammation (53,54). Patients with high cardiovascular risks, including PAD, are likely to benefit from ARBs. ARBs, such as losartan and candesartan, have clearly shown benefits in morbidity and mortality, either alone or in combination with ACE inhibitors, as demonstrated in the Losaratan Intervention For Endpoint reduction (LIFE) and the Candesartan in Heart Failure Assessment of Reduction in Mortality and Morbidity (CHARM) studies (55,56).

## Diabetes

There is a strong association between diabetes and the risk and progression of claudication. On the basis of the Framingham Study, men and women with diabetes had approximately fourfold to fivefold increased relative risk for the development of intermittent claudication even after adjusting for age, systolic blood pressure, smoking, hypercholesterolemia, and left ventricular hypertrophy (57). The risk of PAD is significantly related to the duration of type 2 diabetes mellitus (58). Additionally, patients with diabetes and intermittent claudication are more likely to progress to rest pain and gangrene than patients witout diabetes with intermittent claudication will (59). Despite the increased mortality and morbidity inflicted by diabetes, intensive glycemic control has not been shown to prevent or deter the progression of macrovascular disease such as PAD in patients with both type 1 and type 2 diabetes (60,61). The Diabetes Control and Complications trial showed a trend toward decreased peripheral vascular events (i.e., claudication, amputation, and arterial events requiring bypass) with intensive diabetic management; however, the results were not statistically significant (60). Similarly, the UK Prospective Diabetes Study (UKPDS) demonstrated that aggressive glucose control produced a nonsignificant risk reduction of MI, stroke, death from PAD, and amputation (61). Although the peripheral arterial benefits of intensive glucose management in patients with diabetes are unclear, aggressive glucose control should still be recommended because of its beneficial effects on microvascular disease complications (i.e., retinopathy and nephropathy) (60,61). The American Diabetes Association recommends a HbA1C goal of less than 7.0% in patients with diabetes (62). In addition, patients with diabetes are at high risk for peripheral sensory neuropathy and for the development of foot ulcers. Careful foot examination and foot care education should be advocated for all patients with diabetes, particularly for those with underlying PAD.

## Dyslipidemia

Dyslipidemia is an important risk factor in PAD. PAD is associated with elevated total cholesterol, triglycerides, and low density lipoprotein (LDL) concentrations and decreased high density lipoprotein (HDL) levels. From the Framingham Heart Study, a fasting cholesterol level greater than 270 mg per dL (7 mmol per L) was associated with a twofold increased incidence of claudication (63). The Edinburgh Artery Study demonstrated that PAD was directly associated with elevated serum cholesterol levels and was inversely related to HDL levels (28). The balance between lipid peroxides and protective HDL levels appears to be critical in the development of PAD. In particular, the development of PAD in young patients (<50 years) is independently associated with elevations in lipid peroxides, specifically oxidized LDL and very low density lipoprotein (VLDL) (64,65). In contrast, low levels of total HDL and HDL subfractions (i.e., HDL2a, HDL2b, and HDL3a) are highly associated with patients with intermittent claudication and PAD (28,30,66,67). According to third report of the National Cholesterol Education Program (NCEP) Expert Panel on Detection, Evaluation, and Treatment of High Blood Cholesterol in Adults [Adult Treatment Panel III (ATP III)], PAD is a coronary heart disease risk equivalent and should have a primary treatment goal of an LDL level less than 100 mg per dL (68). After LDL goal is reached, ATP III recommends that HDL levels be modified but does not specify a target goal for raising HDL. The Veterans Affair High-Density Lipoprotein Cholesterol Intervention Trial (VA-HIT) studied patients with CAD and low HDL concentrations (≤40 mg per dL) and found that treatment with the fibrate medication, gemfibrozil, significantly reduced major cardiovascular events (69). A metaanalysis was performed on lipid-lowering therapy (i.e., cholestyramine, probucol, nicotinic acid, and diet modification) trials in patients with PAD (70). Unfortunately, the analysis demonstrated no significant difference in mortality or nonfatal cardiovascular events. In addition, a recent trial was performed to assess the benefits of a fibrate medication, bezafibrate, in patients with PAD (71). Although there was a reduced incidence of nonfatal coronary events, there was no significant difference in all coronary, stroke, and fatal events (71).

Numerous cardiovascular trials have demonstrated that statin medications play a critical role in primary and secondary cardiovascular prevention. In patients with PAD, two trials have shown a small improvement in claudication symptoms and in walking distance in patients treated with statins (72,73). Independent of cholesterol-lowering effects, the use of statin improved walking distance and speed in patients with PAD (74). In a trial of 354 patients with PAD, atorvastatin (80 mg per day) given for 12 months demonstrated a significant improvement in pain-free walking time (but not in the primary endpoint of peak walking time) compared to placebo, 81 ± 15 seconds versus 39 ± 8 seconds, respectively ($P = 0.025$) (72). In addition, there was no difference in quality of life as measured by several questionnaires. In another study, simvastatin (40 mg per day) given for 6 months to 43 patients with PAD showed an increase in mean pain-free and total walking distance and an improvement in the ABI (73). The effects of statins in both of these studies were small, and although statins should be used to lower cardiovascular risk, these medications should not be a primary treatment of the symptoms of claudication in patients with PAD.

There has been no trial to study exclusively the mortality benefit of statins in patients with PAD. In the Long-Term Intervention with Pravastatin in Ischaemic Disease (LIPID) trial, all patients treated with pravastatin (40 mg per day) had a significant risk reduction of fatal and nonfatal MIs compared to patients treated with placebo. In the LIPID trial, 10% of the patients had a documented history of claudication (75). In a subgroup analysis of the Scandinavian Simvastatin Survival Study (4S), the risk of developing new intermittent claudication or worsening of the existing disease was reduced by 38% in the group treated with simvastatin for 72 months (76). The largest study evaluating the effects of statin use (simvastatin

40 mg daily) in high-risk patients, the Heart Protection Study (HPS), demonstrated a 24% risk reduction in first-time cardiovascular events (77). The subgroup of patients with PAD had similar cardiovascular benefits regardless of prior history of MI or coronary heart disease. Interestingly, the HPS was also the first study to demonstrate a decrease in vascular events regardless of baseline LDL concentrations. Even the subgroup population who had LDL levels less than 100 mg per dL at baseline benefited from statin therapy (77).

## Hyperhomocysteinemia

Hyperhomocysteinemia is strongly associated with the development of PAD. In a number of case–control studies, an elevated plasma homocysteine level was found to be an independent risk factor for the development and progression of coronary and PAD (78–81). The relative risk for atherosclerotic vascular disease (i.e., cardiac, cerebral, and peripheral) was 2.2 times greater with an elevated homocysteine concentration (82). The prevalence of hyperhomocysteinemia in patients with PAD has been reported to be approximately 24% to 45% (83,84). In a recent study determining the incidence of hyperhomocysteinemia in patients with PAD, homocysteine concentrations were elevated in 27% of patients with intermittent claudication and in 50% of patients with rest pain (85). In patients with symptomatic atherosclerotic disease, each 1.0 $\mu$mol per L increase in plasma homocysteine levels resulted in a 3.6% increase in the risk of all-cause death and a 5.6% increase in the risk of cardiovascular death at 3 years (86). A case–control study by Ridker et al. found a nonsignificant elevation in homocysteine levels in subjects who developed symptomatic PAD during a 9-year follow-up (25). Despite the strong association between hyperhomocysteinemia and the incidence and progression of PAD, there have been no studies demonstrating that the treatment to decrease homocysteine concentrations decreases mortality and morbidity in this patient group.

## Antiplatelet Therapy

Antiplatelet agents such as aspirin are indicated for secondary prevention in patients at high-risk for cardiovascular problems. PAD is a marker of systemic atherosclerosis. Before the clinical manifestations of PAD, early stages of atherogenesis appear to be associated with endothelial dysfunction. An impaired endothelium is vulnerable to increased adhesion and activation of leukocytes and platelets (87). Recent studies have shown that platelets from the serum of patients with PAD have increased activation and aggregation (88,89). The Antithrombotic Trialists' Collaboration (ATC), a metaanalysis of randomized antiplatelet therapy trials, concluded that antiplatelet agents reduce all cardiovascular events in high-risk patients (90). In the 9,214 patients with PAD reviewed in the ATC metaanalysis, antiplatelet drugs reduced serious vascular events by 23% (90). A similar reduction was seen in patients with intermittent claudication, and patients undergoing peripheral graft procedures or angioplasty (90).

From the ATC metaanalysis, aspirin doses of 75 to 150 mg daily were found to be as effective as the higher doses (160 to 1,500 mg daily) in preventing serious vascular events (90). In trials comparing aspirin to a placebo, there was no significant difference in major extracranial bleeding in aspirin doses less than 325 mg daily. The odds ratio for major extracranial bleeding was 1.5 and 1.4 among patients taking aspirin at doses of 75 to 150 mg daily and 160 to 325 mg daily, respectively (90). In the US Physicians Health Study, 22,071 apparently healthy men were randomized to aspirin 325 mg on alternate days versus placebo. The healthy men treated with aspirin had a reduced the risk of peripheral artery surgery by 54% (91).

Thienopyridine drugs, such as ticlopidine and clopidogrel, inhibit the activation of platelets by adenosine diphosphate (ADP). Both medications have been investigated as an alternative antiplatelet agent to aspirin in patients with PAD. From the ATC, both drugs demonstrated an efficacy similar to aspirin in reducing vascular events (90).

Ticlopidine has been shown to be effective in reducing vascular events in patients with PAD. The Swedish Ticlopidine Multicentre Study (STIMS) found that ticlopidine administered to 687 patients with intermittent claudication reduced the incidence of fatal and nonfatal MI, stroke, TIA, and the need for peripheral vascular surgery (92,93). Despite promising results, the use of ticlopidine has been limited by the occurrence of neutropenia and thrombotic thrombocytopenic purpura and by the need to take the drug twice a day. Clopidogrel has demonstrated fewer adverse hematologic effects and is administered in a dosage of 75 mg once daily (94,95).

The efficacy of clopidogrel has been directly compared to aspirin in Clopidogrel versus Aspirin in Patients of Ischaemic Events (CAPRIE) trial (96). Of the 19,185 high-risk cardiovascular patients (i.e., recent MI, recent ischemic stroke, and PAD) recruited for the study, 6,452 patients had PAD. The patients were randomized to either clopidogrel (75 mg daily) or aspirin (325 mg daily). After 3 years, there was a 8.7% relative risk reduction in MI, stroke or cardiovascular death in the group assigned to clopidogrel compared to aspirin. The PAD subgroup had the greatest benefit in favor of clopidogrel, with a 23.8% relative risk reduction over aspirin (see Fig. 100-4) (96). This benefit has led some experts to recommend clopidogrel in all patients with PAD to prevent cardiovascular morbidity and mortality. In the Clopidogrel in Unstable Angina to Prevent Recurrent Events (CURE) trial, the addition of clopidogrel to aspirin in patients with non–ST elevation MI confirmed an improved benefit in preventing major cardiovascular events than

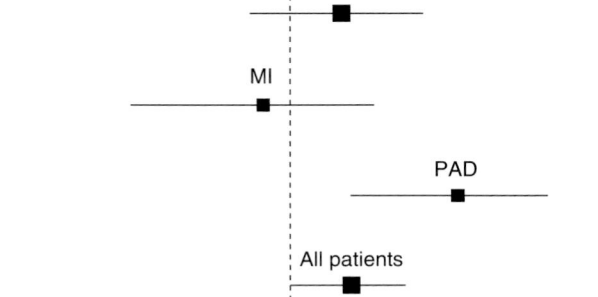

**FIGURE 100-4.** Relative risk reduction and 95% confidence intervals (CI) by disease subgroup in the CAPRIE (Clopidogrel vs. Aspirin in Patients of Ischaemic Events) trial. MI, myocardial infarction; PAD, peripheral arterial disease. [From CAPRIE Steering Committee. A randomised, blinded trial of clopidogrel vs. aspirin in patients at risk of ischaemic events (CAPRIE). *Lancet* 1996;348:1329–1339, with permission.]

that with aspirin alone (97). The combination of clopidogrel and aspirin versus aspirin alone in a high-risk group of patients including those with PAD is currently under way in the Clopidogrel for High Atherothrombotic Risk and Ischemic Stabilization, Management, and Avoidance (CHARISMA) trial.

Oral anticoagulants such as warfarin has been studied as an alternative to antiplatelet therapy in high-risk cardiovascular patients. A recent metaanalysis performed in patients with established CAD found that high-intensity oral anticoagulation, defined as an international normalized ratio (INR) of greater than 2.8, significantly reduced primary outcomes of mortality, MI, and stroke compared to control (98). However, this benefit was associated with a 4.5-fold increase in major bleeding. Moderate- to high-intensity anticoagulation (INR = 2 to 3) was associated with a nonsignificant reduction in cardiovascular death, MI, and stroke compared to that for control but continued to show a significant increase in major bleeding (98).

The utility of oral anticoagulation versus aspirin has not been studied well in patients with PAD. In a trial of 2,690 patients with PAD undergoing infrainguinal grafting, oral anticoagulation (INR = 2.0 to 4.5) was not associated with a reduction in graft occlusion compared to aspirin (99). However, oral anticoagulation did appear to produce a nonsignificant reduction in the composite endpoints of vascular death, MI, stroke, or amputations despite a significant increase in major bleeding (99). Oral anticoagulation has no role in the treatment of patients with claudication. Despite the conflicting data, there are vascular surgeons who routinely use anticoagulation in patients who have undergone bypass surgery of the lower extremity.

## PHARMACOLOGIC TREATMENTS TO IMPROVE CLAUDICATION SYMPTOMS

Only two drugs have been approved by the U.S. Food and Drug Administration (FDA) for the treatment of intermittent claudication—pentoxifylline (Trental) and cilostazol (Pletal). Pentoxifylline is a methylxanthine derivative with hemorheologic properties. The mechanism of pentoxifylline is thought to be through an improvement in red cell and leukocyte flexibility, an inhibition of neutrophil adhesion and activation, a decrease in fibrinogen concentrations, and reduction in blood viscosity (100–102). However, a recent study failed to support this hypothesis in blood samples taken from patients with moderate to severe claudication (103). Two metaanalyses have shown that pentoxifylline increases pain-free and maximal walking distance (37,104). However, the results are conflicting in a number of randomized, double-blind, placebo-controlled trials

(105–107). Porter et al. reported in a study of 128 patients with intermittent claudication that those treated with pentoxifylline (up to 1,200 mg per day) had only a 12% increase in maximum walking distance (105). In a similar study by Gallus et al., patients with claudication treated with pentoxifylline had no difference in claudication distance as compared to patients treated with placebo (106). On the basis of observations from a metaanalysis by Girolami et al., less clinical benefit is observed with pentoxifylline in larger trials of more than 100 subjects with intermittent claudication than in trials with fewer subjects (37). Adverse effects associated with pentoxifylline include abdominal discomfort, nausea, sore throat, and diarrhea (108). The recommended dose is 400 mg three times a day with meals. The beneficial response to pentoxifylline is so small in most patients that the overall data is insufficient to support its widespread use in patients with claudication (95). Its use should be reserved for those patients who cannot take cilostazol, have not responded to an exercise program, are not candidates for revascularization procedures, and are not interested in a clinical trial for one of the newer therapies being tested.

Cilostazol, a phosphodiesterase type 3 inhibitor, has multiple properties that benefit patients with PAD. The mechanism of action for improving claudication is not known, but it does have the following properties: antiplatelet activity, vasodilatory properties, and *in vitro* inhibition of vascular smooth muscle cells. It also moderately increases HDL cholesterol levels and decreases triglyceride levels (109).

Because cilostazol is a phosphodiesterase inhibitor similar to milrinone, it is contraindicated (black box warning) in patients with a history of congestive heart failure or in patients with an ejection fraction less than 40% (110,111). Chronic use of oral milrinone in patients with cardiomyopathy was associated with increased mortality (112). However, the cardiac response to cilostazol has been shown to be significantly less compared to the response to milrinone (113). This dissimilar effect may be attributed to the discovery that milrinone and cilostazol interact with different residues on the phospodiesterase type 3 active sites (114).

In a recently published metaanalysis of eight randomized, double-blind, placebo-controlled trials, cilostazol increased maximal and pain-free walking distances by 50% and 67%, respectively (109). Cilostazol was superior to placebo in most studies performed to date (see Fig. 100-5) (95). Dawson et al. compared the efficacy and safety of cilostazol (100 mg twice a day) to that of pentoxifylline (400 mg three times a day) in patients with intermittent claudication (108). After 24 weeks, cilostazol significantly increased walking distance compared to pentoxifylline and placebo (see Fig. 100-6) (108). It should be noted that there was a progressive increase in walking distance over the 24 weeks of the study. Therefore, patients should be given an adequate trial of at least 4 months before deciding the medication is not working.

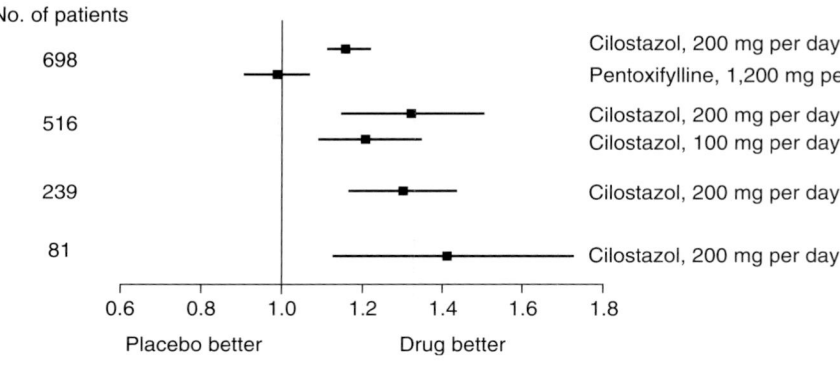

**FIGURE 100-5.** Results of four randomized, placebo-controlled trials of cilostazol for the treatment of claudication. (From Hiatt WR. Medical Treatment of Peripheral Arterial Disease and Claudication. *N Engl J Med* 2001;344:1608–1621, with permission.)

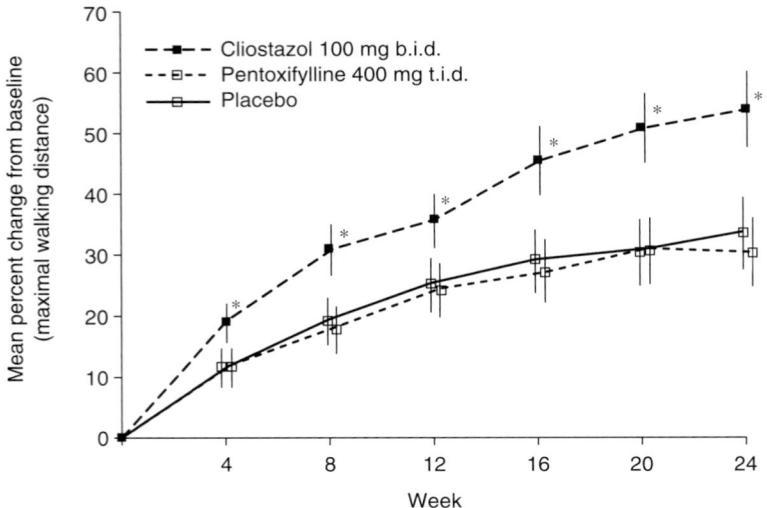

**FIGURE 100-6.** Mean (±95% confidence interval) maximal walking distance by intention-to-treat analysis, using the mean percentage change from baseline. The cilostazol-treated group was significantly different ($P < 0.05$) at each 4-week point, compared with either the pentoxifylline- or placebo-treated groups. There were no significant differences at any time point between the pentoxifylline-treated group and the placebo-treated group. (From Dawson DL, Cutler BS, Hiatt WR, et al. A comparison of cilostazol and pentoxifylline for treating intermittent claudication. *Am J Med* 2000;109:523–530, with permission.)

Despite similar withdrawal rates between cilostazol and pentoxifylline, cilostazol had more minor side effects including headaches, palpitations, dizziness, and diarrhea. Death and serious adverse rates were similar in both groups. The optimal dosage of cilostazol is 100 mg twice a day and it should be given on an empty stomach (30 minutes before or 2 hours after breakfast and dinner). In addition, patients who are taking medications that inhibit cytochrome P-450 isoenzymes CYP3A4 or CYP2C19 (i.e., erythromycin, diltiazem, and omeprazole) should reduce the cilostazol dose to half because of the inhibitory effects on metabolism (110).

## NOVEL THERAPIES FOR CLAUDICATION

There have been a number of novel agents that have been studied for the treatment of claudication. Although showing initial promise, agents such as beraprost, an orally active prostaglandin analog, and AT-1015, a serotonin receptor antagonist, failed to improve treadmill performance or quality-of-life measurements

(115,116). Despite these negative trials, there are several novel treatment modalities that have demonstrated encouraging results (see Table 100-4).

Therapeutic angiogenesis is the concept of growing new blood vessels from existing vessels. Numerous studies have attempted to use this strategy of administering growth factors, to stimulate angiogenesis, and to bypass obstructions in the coronary and peripheral circulation. The Therapeutic Angiogenesis with Recombinant Fibroblast Growth Factor-2 for Intermittent Claudication (TRAFFIC) trial used a single intraarterial infusion of recombinant fibroblast growth factor-2 (rFGF-2) in patients with intermittent claudication (117). At 90 days, patients who received one dose of rFGF-2 had significantly improved peak walking time compared to those who received placebo. A repeat infusion at 30 days had no additional effects. Despite these promising results, the Regional Angiogenesis with Vascular Endothelial growth factor (RAVE) trial showed no difference in peak walking time between patients with PAD who received a single intramuscular administration of vascular endothelial growth factor (VEGF) in an adenovirus vector versus patients who received placebo (118).

## TABLE 100-4

### NOVEL THERAPIES FOR CLAUDICATION

| Treatment modalities | Subjects (no.) | Route of administration | Follow-up | Improvement (peak or pain-free walking time) |
|---|---|---|---|---|
| FGF-2 (117) | 190 | Intraarterial | 90 d | 1.7 min ($P = 0.075$) |
| VEGF (118) | 105 | Intramuscular | 12 wk | None |
| Bone marrow cells (119) | 25 | Intramuscular | 24 wk | 3.5 min ($P = 0.0001$) |
| Del-1 (120)[a] | N/A | N/A | N/A | N/A |
| HIF-1 $\alpha$ (121)[a] | N/A | N/A | N/A | N/A |
| Propionyl-L-carnitine (122) | 155 | Oral | 6 mo | 162 ± 222 ($P < 0.001$) |
| L-Arginine (123) | 41 | Oral | 2 wk | 66% walking distance ($P < 0.04$) |
| Avasimide (124) | 373 | Oral | 52 wk | 0.76 min (NS) |
| IMT (125)[b] | 85 | Intramuscular | 24 wk | 81% walking distance ($P < 0.04$) |

FGF-2, fibroblast growth factor-2; VEGF, vascular endothelial growth factor; Del-1, developmental endothelial locus-1; HIF, hypoxia-inducible factor; IMT, immune modulation therapy.
[a]Studies in progress.
[b]Pivotal study in progress ($n = 500$).

Disparity in these randomized trials could be explained by differences in the angiogenic growth factors, the vehicle used, or the mode of delivery. Recently, a randomized pilot trial examined the efficacy and safety of intramuscular injections of bone marrow-mononuclear cells into the legs of patients with chronic limb ischemia (119). The hypothesis of this study was that injected marrow cells would supply endothelial progenitor cells, angiogenic growth factors, and cytokines to enhance angiogenesis. Twenty-four weeks after implantation, patients with PAD who received bone marrow cells had significantly improved ABI, transcutaneous oximetry and peak walking time compared to controls. Currently, studies evaluating developmental endothelial locus-1 (Del-1) and hypoxia-inducible factor 1 $\alpha$ (HIF-1 $\alpha$) as potential treatments for patients with claudication are or will soon be under way (120,121). The future of therapeutic angiogenesis is certainly challenging but, with continued research, it may find utility in treating patients with PAD refractory to medical and surgical interventions.

Several pharmacologic approaches to the treatment of claudication have shown potential efficacy. Administration of propionyl-L-carnitine, an analog of carnitine, has been shown to increase carnitine levels in the ischemic muscles of patients with PAD (126). An increase in total carnitine content in ischemic muscle reduces lactate production during exercise and improves symptoms. Patients with claudication treated with propionyl-L-carnitine for 6 months had significantly improved walking time and distance, and overall functional ability than patients treated with placebo (122). Brevetti et al. found similar efficacy with propionyl-L-carnitine but only in patients with significant walking impairment (less than 250 m) (127,128). Additionally, a 2-week administration of oral L-arginine, a substrate for nitric oxide, on subjects with intermittent claudication increased pain-free and total walking distance by 66% and 23%, respectively (123). Recently, avasimibe, an inhibitor of acyl coenzyme A-cholesterol acyltransferase (ACAT), given to patients with claudication for 52 weeks revealed a trend toward improved walking distance with a smaller (50 mg) rather than higher (250 or 750 mg) dose of the agent (124).

A new therapeutic technique, immune modulation therapy (IMT), has been evaluated as a treatment of patients with claudication. IMT involves the administration of autologous blood following their *ex vivo* processing by exposure to thermal and oxidative stress (129). IMT is believed to reduce vascular inflammation and inhibit atherosclerotic progression (130,131). A small trial consisting of 70 patients with PAD found that IMT administered to patients with severe walking impairments (<100 m) significantly increased claudication distance at 24 weeks (125). A larger study is currently under way to further understand the effects of IMT in patients with claudication.

# CONCLUSION

PAD is defined as atherosclerosis of the aorta and lower extremity arteries. Not only are patients with PAD significantly impaired in their ability to walk but they also have a high cardiovascular morbidity and mortality usually from MI and stroke. Treatment of patients with PAD should encompass two important aspects: improvement in functional capacity and quality of life, and reduction in cardiovascular morbidity and mortality.

## *References*

1. Criqui MH, Fronek A, Barrett-Connor E, et al. The prevalence of peripheral arterial disease in a defined population. *Circulation* 1985;71: 510–515.

2. Kannel WB, McGee DL. Update on some epidemiologic features of intermittent claudication: the Framingham Study. *J Am Geriatr Soc* 1985;33: 13–18.

3. Regensteiner JG, Hiatt WR. Current medical therapies for patients with peripheral arterial disease: a critical review. *Am J Med* 2002;112:49–57.

4. Hirsch AT, Criqui MH, Treat-Jacobson D, et al. Peripheral arterial disease detection, awareness, and treatment in primary care. *JAMA* 2001;286: 1317–1324.

5. Dormandy J, Heeck L, Vig S. Intermittent claudication: a condition with underrated risks. *Semin Vasc Surg* 1999;12:96–108.

6. McDermott MM, Greenland P, Liu K, et al. The ankle brachial index is associated with leg function and physical activity: the Walking and Leg Circulation Study. *Ann Intern Med* 2002;136:873–883.

7. Dormandy JA, Rutherford RB, TASC Working Group. TransAtlantic Inter-Society Concensus (TASC). Management of Peripheral Arterial Disease (PAD). *J Vasc Surg* 2000;31:S1–S296.

8. Meijer WT, Hoes AW, Rutgers D, et al. Peripheral arterial disease in the elderly: the Rotterdam Study. *Arterioscler Thromb Vasc Biol* 1998;18: 185–192.

9. Fowkes FG, Housley E, Cawood EH, et al. Edinburgh Artery Study: prevalence of asymptomatic and symptomatic peripheral arterial disease in the general population. *Int J Epidemiol* 1991;20:384–392.

10. Newman AB, Shemanski L, Manolio TA et al. The Cardiovascular Health Study Group. Ankle-arm index as a predictor of cardiovascular disease and mortality in the Cardiovascular Health Study. *Arterioscler Thromb Vasc Biol* 1999;19:538–545.

11. Zheng ZJ, Sharrett AR, Chambless LE, et al. Associations of ankle-brachial index with clinical coronary heart disease, stroke and preclinical carotid and popliteal atherosclerosis: the Atherosclerosis Risk In Communities (ARIC) Study. *Atherosclerosis* 1997;131:115–125.

12. Vogt MT, Cauley JA, Newman AB, et al. Decreased ankle/arm blood pressure index and mortality in elderly women. *JAMA* 1993;270:465–469.

13. McKenna M, Wolfson S, Kuller L. The ratio of ankle and arm arterial pressure as an independent predictor of mortality. *Atherosclerosis* 1991; 87:119–128.

14. Criqui MH, Coughlin SS, Fronek A. Noninvasively diagnosed peripheral arterial disease as a predictor of mortality: results from a prospective study. *Circulation* 1985;72:768–773.

15. Newman AB, Tyrrell KS, Kuller LH. Mortality over four years in SHEP participants with a low ankle-arm index. *J Am Geriatr Soc* 1997;45: 1472–1478.

16. Resnick HE, Lindsay RS, McDermott MM, et al. Relationship of high and low ankle brachial index to all-cause and cardiovascular disease mortality: the Strong Heart Study. *Circulation* 2004;109:733–739.

17. Newman AB, Siscovick DS, Manolio TA et al. Cardiovascular Heart Study (CHS) Collaborative Research Group. Ankle-arm index as a marker of atherosclerosis in the Cardiovascular Health Study. *Circulation* 1993; 88:837–845.

18. Muluk SC, Muluk VS, Kelley ME, et al. Outcome events in patients with claudication: a 15-year study in 2777 patients. *J Vasc Surg* 2001;33: 251–257.

19. Criqui MH, Langer RD, Fronek A, et al. Mortality over a period of 10 years in patients with peripheral arterial disease. *N Engl J Med* 1992;326: 381–386.

20. Leng GC, Lee AJ, Fowkes FG, et al. Incidence, natural history and cardiovascular events in symptomatic and asymptomatic peripheral arterial disease in the general population. *Int J Epidemiol* 1996;25:1172–1181.

21. Kornitzer M, Dramaix M, Sobolski J, et al. Ankle/arm pressure index in asymptomatic middle-aged males: an independent predictor of 10-year coronary heart disease mortality. *Angiology* 1995;46:211–219.

22. Criqui MH, Denenberg JO, Langer RD, et al. The epidemiology of peripheral arterial disease: importance of identifying the population at risk. *Vasc Med* 1997;2:221–226.

23. Ness J, Aronow WS. Prevalence of coexistence of coronary artery disease, ischemic stroke, and peripheral arterial disease in older persons, mean age 80 years, in an academic hospital-based geriatrics practice. *J Am Geriatr Soc* 1999;47:1255–1256.

24. Burek KA, Sutton-Tyrrell K, Brooks MM, et al. Prognostic importance of lower extremity arterial disease in patients undergoing coronary revascularization in the Bypass Angioplasty Revascularization Investigation (BARI). *J Am Coll Cardiol* 1999;34:716–721.

25. Ridker PM, Stampfer MJ, Rifai N. Novel risk factors for systemic atherosclerosis: a comparison of C-reactive protein, fibrinogen, homocysteine, lipoprotein(a), and standard cholesterol screening as predictors of peripheral arterial disease. *JAMA* 2001;285:2481–2485.

26. Meijer WT, Grobbee DE, Hunink MG, et al. Determinants of peripheral arterial disease in the elderly: the Rotterdam study. *Arch Intern Med* 2000; 160:2934–2938.

27. Price JF, Mowbray PI, Lee AJ, et al. Relationship between smoking and cardiovascular risk factors in the development of peripheral arterial disease and coronary artery disease: Edinburgh Artery Study. *Eur Heart J* 1999; 20:344–353.

28. Fowkes FG, Housley E, Riemersma RA, et al. Smoking, lipids, glucose intolerance, and blood pressure as risk factors for peripheral atherosclerosis compared with ischemic heart disease in the Edinburgh Artery Study. *Am J Epidemiol* 1992;135:331–340.

29. Powell JT, Edwards RJ, Worrell PC, et al. Risk factors associated with the development of peripheral arterial disease in smokers: a case–control study. *Atherosclerosis* 1997;129:41–48.

30. Murabito JM, Evans JC, Nieto K, et al. Prevalence and clinical correlates of peripheral arterial disease in the Framingham Offspring Study. *Am Heart J* 2002;143:961–965.

31. Stewart CP. The influence of smoking on the level of lower limb amputation. *Prosthet Orthot Int* 1987;11:113–116.

32. Ameli FM, Stein M, Prosser RJ, et al. Effects of cigarette smoking on outcome of femoral popliteal bypass for limb salvage. *J Cardiovasc Surg (Torino)* 1989;30:591–596.

33. Jorenby DE, Leischow SJ, Nides MA, et al. A controlled trial of sustained-release bupropion, a nicotine patch, or both for smoking cessation. *N Engl J Med* 1999;340:685–691.

34. Faulkner KW, House AK, Castleden WM. The effect of cessation of smoking on the accumulative survival rates of patients with symptomatic peripheral vascular disease. *Med J Aust* 1983;1:217–219.

35. Hirsch AT, Treat-Jacobson D, Lando HA, et al. The role of tobacco cessation, antiplatelet and lipid-lowering therapies in the treatment of peripheral arterial disease. *Vasc Med* 1997;2:243–251.

36. Jonason T, Bergstrom R. Cessation of smoking in patients with intermittent claudication. Effects on the risk of peripheral vascular complications, myocardial infarction and mortality. *Acta Med Scand* 1987;221:253–260.

37. Girolami B, Bernardi E, Prins MH, et al. Treatment of intermittent claudication with physical training, smoking cessation, pentoxifylline, or nafronyl: a meta-analysis. *Arch Intern Med* 1999;159:337–345.

38. McDermott MM, Mehta S, Liu K, et al. Leg symptoms, the ankle-brachial index, and walking ability in patients with peripheral arterial disease. *J Gen Intern Med* 1999;14:173–181.

39. Vogt MT, Cauley JA, Kuller LH, et al. Functional status and mobility among elderly women with lower extremity arterial disease: the Study of Osteoporotic Fractures. *J Am Geriatr Soc* 1994;42:923–929.

40. Khaira HS, Hanger R, Shearman CP. Quality of life in patients with intermittent claudication. *Eur J Vasc Endovasc Surg* 1996;11:65–69.

41. Gardner AW, Poehlman ET. Exercise rehabilitation programs for the treatment of claudication pain. A meta-analysis. *JAMA* 1995;274:975–980.

42. Regensteiner JG, Steiner JF, Hiatt WR. Exercise training improves functional status in patients with peripheral arterial disease. *J Vasc Surg* 1996;23:104–115.

43. Vogt MT, Cauley JA, Kuller LH, et al. Prevalence and correlates of lower extremity arterial disease in elderly women. *Am J Epidemiol* 1993;137:559–568.

44. Murabito JM, D'Agostino RB, Silbershatz H, et al. Intermittent claudication. A risk profile from The Framingham Heart Study. *Circulation* 1997;96:44–49.

45. Chobanian AV, Bakris GL, Black HR, et al. The Seventh Report of the Joint National Committee on prevention, detection, evaluation, and treatment of high blood pressure: the JNC 7 report. *JAMA* 2003;289:2560–2572.

46. Hennekens CH, Albert CM, Godfried SL, et al. Adjunctive drug therapy of acute myocardial infarction—evidence from clinical trials. *N Engl J Med* 1996;335:1660–1667.

47. Hiatt WR. Pharmacologic therapy for peripheral arterial disease and claudication. *J Vasc Surg* 2002;36:1283–1291.

48. Radack K, Deck C. Beta-adrenergic blocker therapy does not worsen intermittent claudication in subjects with peripheral arterial disease. A meta-analysis of randomized controlled trials. *Arch Intern Med* 1991;151:1769–1776.

49. Mehler PS, Coll JR, Estacio R, et al. Intensive blood pressure control reduces the rate of cardiovascular events in patients with peripheral arterial disease and type 2 diabetes. *Circulation* 2003;107:753–756.

50. Yusuf S, Sleight P, Pogue J, et al. The Heart Outcomes Prevention Evaluation Study Investigators. Effects of an angiotensin-converting-enzyme inhibitor, ramipril, on cardiovascular events in high-risk patients. *N Engl J Med* 2000;342:145–153.

51. Ostergren J, Sleight P, Dagenais G, et al. Impact of ramipril in patients with evidence of clinical or subclinical peripheral arterial disease. *Eur Heart J* 2004;25:17–24.

52. Fox KM. Efficacy of perindopril in reduction of cardiovascular events among patients with stable coronary artery disease: randomised, double-blind, placebo-controlled, multicentre trial (the EUROPA study). *Lancet* 2003;362:782–788.

53. Navalkar S, Parthasarathy S, Santanam N, et al. Irbesartan, an angiotensin type 1 receptor inhibitor, regulates markers of inflammation in patients with premature atherosclerosis. *J Am Coll Cardiol* 2001;37:440–444.

54. Prasad A, Tupas-Habib T, Schenke WH, et al. Acute and chronic angiotensin-1 receptor antagonism reverses endothelial dysfunction in atherosclerosis. *Circulation* 2000;101:2349–2354.

55. Dahlof B, Devereux RB, Kjeldsen SE, et al. Cardiovascular morbidity and mortality in the Losartan Intervention For Endpoint reduction in hypertension study (LIFE): a randomised trial against atenolol. *Lancet* 2002;359:995–1003.

56. Pfeffer MA, Swedberg K, Granger CB, et al. Effects of candesartan on mortality and morbidity in patients with chronic heart failure: the CHARM-overall programme. *Lancet* 2003;362:759–766.

57. Kannel WB, McGee DL. Diabetes and cardiovascular disease. The Framingham Study. *JAMA* 1979;241:2035–2038.

58. Katsilambros NL, Tsapogas PC, Arvanitis MP, et al. Risk factors for lower extremity arterial disease in non-insulin-dependent diabetic persons. *Diabet Med* 1996;13:243–246.

59. Jonason T, Ringqvist I. Diabetes mellitus and intermittent claudication. Relation between peripheral vascular complications and location of the occlusive atherosclerosis in the legs. *Acta Med Scand* 1985;218:217–221.

60. The Diabetes Control and Complications Trial Research Group. Effect of intensive diabetes management on macrovascular events and risk factors in the Diabetes Control and Complications Trial. *Am J Cardiol* 1995;75:894–903.

61. UK Prospective Diabetes Study (UKPDS) Group. Intensive blood-glucose control with sulphonylureas or insulin compared with conventional treatment and risk of complications in patients with type 2 diabetes (UKPDS 33). *Lancet* 1998;352:837–853.

62. American Diabetes Association. Standards of medical care for patients with diabetes mellitus. *Diabetes Care* 2003;26 Suppl. 1:S33–S50.

63. Kannel WB, Skinner JJ Jr, Schwartz MJ, et al. Intermittent claudication. Incidence in the Framingham Study. *Circulation* 1970;41:875–883.

64. Sanderson KJ, van Rij AM, Wade CR, et al. Lipid peroxidation of circulating low density lipoproteins with age, smoking and in peripheral vascular disease. *Atherosclerosis* 1995;118:45–51.

65. Harris LM, Armstrong D, Browne R, et al. Premature peripheral vascular disease: clinical profile and abnormal lipid peroxidation. *Cardiovasc Surg* 1998;6:188–193.

66. Johansson J, Egberg N, Johnsson H, et al. Serum lipoproteins and hemostatic function in intermittent claudication. *Arterioscler Thromb* 1993;13:1441–1448.

67. Mowat BF, Skinner ER, Wilson HM, et al. Alterations in plasma lipids, lipoproteins and high density lipoprotein subfractions in peripheral arterial disease. *Atherosclerosis* 1997;131:161–166.

68. Expert Panel on Detection, Evaluation, and Treatment of High Blood Cholesterol in Adults. Executive summary of the third report of the National Cholesterol Education Program (NCEP) Expert Panel on Detection, Evaluation, and Treatment of High Blood Cholesterol in Adults (Adult Treatment Panel III). *JAMA* 2001;285:2486–2497.

69. Rubins HB, Robins SJ, Collins D, et al. Veterans Affairs High-Density Lipoprotein Cholesterol Intervention Trial Study Group. Gemfibrozil for the secondary prevention of coronary heart disease in men with low levels of high-density lipoprotein cholesterol. *N Engl J Med* 1999;341:410–418.

70. Leng GC, Price JF, Jepson RG. Lipid-lowering for lower limb atherosclerosis. *Cochrane Database Syst Rev* 2000;2:CD000123.

71. Meade T, Zuhrie R, Cook C, et al. Bezafibrate in men with lower extremity arterial disease: randomised controlled trial. *BMJ* 2002;325:1139.

72. Mohler ER III, Hiatt WR, Creager MA. Cholesterol reduction with atorvastatin improves walking distance in patients with peripheral arterial disease. *Circulation* 2003;108:1481–1486.

73. Mondillo S, Ballo P, Barbati R, et al. Effects of simvastatin on walking performance and symptoms of intermittent claudication in hypercholesterolemic patients with peripheral vascular disease. *Am J Med* 2003;114:359–364.

74. McDermott MM, Guralnik JM, Greenland P, et al. Statin use and leg functioning in patients with and without lower-extremity peripheral arterial disease. *Circulation* 2003;107:757–761.

75. The Long-Term Intervention with Pravastatin in Ischaemic Disease (LIPID) Study Group. Prevention of cardiovascular events and death with pravastatin in patients with coronary heart disease and a broad range of initial cholesterol levels. *N Engl J Med* 1998;339:1349–1357.

76. Pedersen TR, Kjekshus J, Pyorala K, et al. Effect of simvastatin on ischemic signs and symptoms in the Scandinavian Simvastatin Survival Study (4S). *Am J Cardiol* 1998;81:333–335.

77. The Heart Protection Study Collaborative Group. MRC/BHF Heart Protection Study of cholesterol lowering with simvastatin in 20,536 high-risk individuals: a randomised placebo-controlled trial. *Lancet* 2002;360:7–22.

78. Taylor LM Jr, DeFrang RD, Harris EJ Jr, et al. The association of elevated plasma homocyst(e)ine with progression of symptomatic peripheral arterial disease. *J Vasc Surg* 1991;13:128–136.

79. Clarke R, Daly L, Robinson K, et al. Hyperhomocysteinemia: an independent risk factor for vascular disease. *N Engl J Med* 1991;324:1149–1155.

80. Molgaard J, Malinow MR, Lassvik C, et al. Hyperhomocyst(e)inaemia: an independent risk factor for intermittent claudication. *J Intern Med* 1992;231:273–279.

81. Robinson K, Arheart K, Refsum H, et al. European COMAC Group. Low circulating folate and vitamin B6 concentrations: risk factors for stroke, peripheral vascular disease, and coronary artery disease. *Circulation* 1998;97:437–443.

82. Graham IM, Daly LE, Refsum HM, et al. Plasma homocysteine as a risk factor for vascular disease. The European concerted action project. *JAMA* 1997;277:1775–1781.

83. Rassoul F, Richter V, Janke C, et al. Plasma homocysteine and lipoprotein profile in patients with peripheral arterial occlusive disease. *Angiology* 2000;51:189–196.

84. Darius H, Pittrow D, Haberl R, et al. Are elevated homocysteine plasma levels related to peripheral arterial disease? Results from a cross-sectional study of 6880 primary care patients. *Eur J Clin Invest* 2003;33:751–757.

85. Spark JI, Laws P, Fitridge R. The incidence of hyperhomocysteinaemia in vascular patients. *Eur J Vasc Endovasc Surg* 2003;26:558–561.

86. Taylor LM Jr, Moneta GL, Sexton GJ, et al. Prospective blinded study of the relationship between plasma homocysteine and progression of symptomatic peripheral arterial disease. *J Vasc Surg* 1999;29:8–19.

87. Harrison DG. Cellular and molecular mechanisms of endothelial cell dysfunction. *J Clin Invest* 1997;100:2153–2157.

88. Robless PA, Okonko D, Lintott P, et al. Increased platelet aggregation and activation in peripheral arterial disease. *Eur J Vasc Endovasc Surg* 2003;25:16–22.

89. Cassar K, Bachoo P, Ford I, et al. Platelet activation is increased in peripheral arterial disease. *J Vasc Surg* 2003;38:99–103.

90. Gerald F. Collaborative meta-analysis of randomised trials of antiplatelet therapy for prevention of death, myocardial infarction, and stroke in high risk patients. *BMJ* 2002;324:71–86.

91. Goldhaber SZ, Manson JE, Stampfer MJ, et al. Low-dose aspirin and subsequent peripheral arterial surgery in the Physicians' Health Study. *Lancet* 1992;340:143–145.

92. Janzon L, Bergqvist D, Boberg J et al. Results from STIMS, the Swedish Ticlopidine Multicentre Study. Prevention of myocardial infarction and stroke in patients with intermittent claudication; effects of ticlopidine. *J Intern Med* 1990;227:301–308.

93. Bergqvist D, Almgren B, Dickinson JP. Reduction of requirement for leg vascular surgery during long-term treatment of claudicant patients with ticlopidine: results from the Swedish Ticlopidine Multicentre Study (STIMS). *Eur J Vasc Endovasc Surg* 1995;10:69–76.

94. Bennett CL, Connors JM, Carwile JM, et al. Thrombotic thrombocytopenic purpura associated with clopidogrel. *N Engl J Med* 2000;342:1773–1777.

95. Hiatt WR. Medical treatment of peripheral arterial disease and claudication. *N Engl J Med* 2001;344:1608–1621.

96. CAPRIE Steering Committee. A randomised, blinded, trial of clopidogrel versus aspirin in patients at risk of ischaemic events (CAPRIE). *Lancet* 1996;348:1329–1339.

97. Yusuf S, Zhao F, Mehta SR, et al. Effects of clopidogrel in addition to aspirin in patients with acute coronary syndromes without ST-segment elevation. *N Engl J Med* 2001;345:494–502.

98. Anand SS, Yusuf S. Oral anticoagulants in patients with coronary artery disease. *J Am Coll Cardiol* 2003;41:62S–69S.

99. Dutch Bypass Oral Anticoagulants or Aspirin (BOA) Study Group. Efficacy of oral anticoagulants compared with aspirin after infrainguinal bypass surgery (The Dutch Bypass Oral Anticoagulants or Aspirin Study): a randomised trial. *Lancet* 2000;355:346–351.

100. Strano A, Davi G, Avellone G, et al. Double-blind, crossover study of the clinical efficacy and the hemorheological effects of pentoxifylline in patients with occlusive arterial disease of the lower limbs. *Angiology* 1984;35:459–466.

101. Rao KM, Simel DL, Cohen HJ, et al. Effects of pentoxifylline administration on blood viscosity and leukocyte cytoskeletal function in patients with intermittent claudication. *J Lab Clin Med* 1990;115:738–744.

102. Franzini E, Sellak H, Babin-Chevaye C, et al. Effects of pentoxifylline on the adherence of polymorphonuclear neutrophils to oxidant-stimulated human endothelial cells: involvement of cyclic AMP. *J Cardiovasc Pharmacol* 1995;25(Suppl. 2):S92–S95.

103. Dawson DL, Zheng Q, Worthy SA, et al. Failure of pentoxifylline or cilostazol to improve blood and plasma viscosity, fibrinogen, and erythrocyte deformability in claudication. *Angiology* 2002;53:509–520.

104. Hood SC, Moher D, Barber GG. Management of intermittent claudication with pentoxifylline: meta-analysis of randomized controlled trials. *CMAJ* 1996;155:1053–1059.

105. Porter JM, Cutler BS, Lee BY, et al. Pentoxifylline efficacy in the treatment of intermittent claudication: multicenter controlled double-blind trial with objective assessment of chronic occlusive arterial disease patients. *Am Heart J* 1982;104:66–72.

106. Gallus AS, Gleadow F, Dupont P, et al. Intermittent claudication: a double-blind crossover trial of pentoxifylline. *Aust N Z J Med* 1985;15:402–409.

107. De Sanctis MT, Cesarone MR, Belcaro G, et al. Treatment of intermittent claudication with pentoxifylline: a 12-month, randomized trial—walking distance and microcirculation. *Angiology* 2002;53(Suppl. 1):S7–S12.

108. Dawson DL, Cutler BS, Hiatt WR, et al. A comparison of cilostazol and pentoxifylline for treating intermittent claudication. *Am J Med* 2000;109:523–530.

109. Thompson PD, Zimet R, Forbes WP, et al. Meta-analysis of results from eight randomized, placebo-controlled trials on the effect of cilostazol on patients with intermittent claudication. *Am J Cardiol* 2002;90:1314–1319.

110. Olin JW. Management of patients with intermittent claudication. *Int J Clin Pract* 2002;56:687–693.

111. *Physicians' desk reference 2005*, 59th ed. Montvale, NJ: Thompson PDR 2005;07645–1742

112. Packer M, Carver JR, Rodeheffer RJ et al. The PROMISE Study Research Group. Effect of oral milrinone on mortality in severe chronic heart failure. *N Engl J Med* 1991;325:1468–1475.

113. Cone J, Wang S, Tandon N, et al. Comparison of the effects of cilostazol and milrinone on intracellular cAMP levels and cellular function in platelets and cardiac cells. *J Cardiovasc Pharmacol* 1999;34:497–504.

114. Zhang W, Ke H, Colman RW. Identification of interaction sites of cyclic nucleotide phosphodiesterase type 3A with milrinone and cilostazol using molecular modeling and site-directed mutagenesis. *Mol Pharmacol* 2002;62:514–520.

115. Mohler ER III, Hiatt WR, Olin JW, et al. Treatment of intermittent claudication with beraprost sodium, an orally active prostaglandin I2 analogue: a double-blinded, randomized, controlled trial. *J Am Coll Cardiol* 2003;41:1679–1686.

116. Hiatt WR, Hirsch AT, Cooke JP, et al. Randomized trial of AT-1015 for treatment of intermittent claudication. A novel 5-hydroxytryptamine antagonist with no evidence of efficacy. *Vasc Med* 2004;9(1):18:25

117. Lederman RJ, Mendelsohn FO, Anderson RD, et al. Therapeutic angiogenesis with recombinant fibroblast growth factor-2 for intermittent claudication (the TRAFFIC study): a randomised trial. *Lancet* 2002;359:2053–2058.

118. Rajagopalan S, Mohler ER III, Lederman RJ, et al. Regional angiogenesis with vascular endothelial growth factor in peripheral arterial disease: a phase II randomized, double-blind, controlled study of adenoviral delivery of vascular endothelial growth factor 121 in patients with disabling intermittent claudication. *Circulation* 2003;108:1933–1938.

119. Tateishi-Yuyama E, Matsubara H, Murohara T, et al. Therapeutic angiogenesis for patients with limb ischaemia by autologous transplantation of bone-marrow cells: a pilot study and a randomised controlled trial. *Lancet* 2002;360:427–435.

120. Ho HK, Jang JJ, Kaji S, et al. Developmental endothelial locus-1 (Del-1), a novel angiogenic protein: its role in ischemia. *Circulation* 2004;109:1314–1319.

121. Kelly BD, Hackett SF, Hirota K, et al. Cell type-specific regulation of angiogenic growth factor gene expression and induction of angiogenesis in nonischemic tissue by a constitutively active form of hypoxia-inducible factor 1. *Circ Res* 2003;93:1074–1081.

122. Hiatt WR, Regensteiner JG, Creager MA, et al. Propionyl-L-carnitine improves exercise performance and functional status in patients with claudication. *Am J Med* 2001;110:616–622.

123. Maxwell AJ, Anderson BE, Cooke JP. Nutritional therapy for peripheral arterial disease: a double-blind, placebo-controlled, randomized trial of HeartBar. *Vasc Med* 2000;5:11–19.

124. Hiatt WR, Klepack E, Nehler M, et al. Effects of avasimide in claudicants with peripheral arterial disease. *J Am Coll Cardiol* 2004;41 (Suppl. A):304A.

125. McGrath C, Robb R, Lucas AJ, et al. A randomised, double blind, placebo-controlled study to determine the efficacy of immune modulation therapy in the treatment of patients suffering from peripheral arterial occlusive disease with intermittent claudication. *Eur J Vasc Endovasc Surg* 2002;23:381–387.

126. Brevetti G, Perna S, Sabba C, et al. Propionyl-L-carnitine in intermittent claudication: double-blind, placebo-controlled, dose titration, multicenter study. *J Am Coll Cardiol* 1995;26:1411–1416.

127. Brevetti G, Perna S, Sabba C, et al. Effect of propionyl-L-carnitine on quality of life in intermittent claudication. *Am J Cardiol* 1997;79:777–780.

128. Brevetti G, Diehm C, Lambert D. European multicenter study on propionyl-L-carnitine in intermittent claudication. *J Am Coll Cardiol* 1999;34:1618–1624.

129. Bulmer J, Bolton AE, Pockley AG. Effect of combined heat, ozonation and ultraviolet irradiation (VasoCare) on heat shock protein expression by peripheral blood leukocyte populations. *J Biol Regul Homeost Agents* 1997;11:104–110.

130. Babaei S, Stewart DJ, Picard P, et al. Effects of VasoCare therapy on the initiation and progression of atherosclerosis. *Atherosclerosis* 2002;162:45–53.

131. Shivji GM, Suzuki H, Mandel AS, et al. The effect of VAS972 on allergic contact hypersensitivity. *J Cutan Med Surg* 2000;4:132–137.

# CHAPTER 101 ■ SURGERY FOR PERIPHERAL ARTERIAL DISEASE

ANTHONY J. COMEROTA

Peripheral arterial disease (PAD) is precisely defined as any disease of the arteries outside of the cranium and outside of the coronary circulation and aortic arch. The conventional definition of PAD is atherosclerotic disease involving the arteries supplying circulation to the lower extremities. For the purpose of this chapter, the conventional definition is adopted and is its major focus.

The importance of the diagnosis of PAD and its aggressive management with risk factor modification and appropriate pharmacotherapy cannot be overstated. Patients with clinically apparent PAD are at high risk for subsequent cardiovascular ischemic events and death. Furthermore, the prevalence of PAD is increasing, because it is a disease of increasing age. Aging patients are living longer, and a larger proportion of the population is entering the older age strata. The epidemiology of PAD, its risk factors and management, and appropriate pharmacotherapy are well covered in Chapter 100. This chapter reviews the diagnosis of PAD, discusses the implications of acute versus chronic arterial occlusion, reviews operative and percutaneous revascularization procedures, and addresses the pharmacotherapeutic management of patients following revascularization procedures, specifically infrainguinal revascularization. Where appropriate, other disease states are included in the discussion.

## DIAGNOSIS

The symptomatic manifestation of PAD results from arterial stenosis or occlusion leading to a reduction in distal blood flow. Patients with intermittent claudication have no reduction of blood flow at rest; however, their symptoms are the consequence of exercise-induced muscle ischemia resulting from inadequate perfusion to the exercising limb.

Pressure gradients across a stenotic lesion depend upon the peripheral resistance of the outflow bed and the flow velocity across the lesion, as well as the luminal area reduction. This value varies in different arteries (1,2). A critical stenosis occurs with less luminal narrowing in arteries supplying outflow beds with low peripheral resistance, which have higher flow velocities across the lesion, the typical example being the internal carotid artery or a coronary artery versus the superficial femoral artery (SFA), which has a high outflow resistance. Sequential, subcritical stenoses may also reduce pressure and flow because their effects are additive (3). The appropriate management of peripheral arterial occlusive disease depends on its accurate detection and localization of such flow-reducing lesions.

### Clinical Evaluation

Most patients with PAD can be accurately diagnosed with a good history and physical examination. Typical symptoms of intermittent claudication are those of exercise-induced muscle

pain, which occurs with a constant amount of exercise and which is relieved with rest. Symptoms do not vary from day to day because the underlying arterial lesion is fixed. Rest pain due to chronic ischemia of PAD often presents in its early stages as nocturnal pain in the feet and toes after the patient assumes a recumbent position. Patients often awaken during the night and find that by getting up and ambulating, or simply by hanging their foot over the side of the bed, their pain diminishes or is relieved. At this point, any further reduction in perfusion or minor trauma to the extremity will produce an ischemic wound that is unlikely to heal, thereby placing the patient at high risk for limb loss.

Patients with advanced arterial occlusive disease, such as those with ischemic rest pain or ischemic lesions on their feet, do not have enough perfusion to support distal hair growth. Temperature differences are often observed. The fingertips can detect a 1°F temperature difference between extremities or segments of the limb, although temperature change is not specific to arterial occlusive disease.

A pulse deficit is the hallmark of hemodynamically significant arterial disease and provides some localization of the most proximal extent of disease. On occasion, distal pulses may be preserved, and intraobserver variability is high. Palpation of peripheral pulses alone may be associated with a significant degree of both overdiagnosis and underdiagnosis (4). An assessment of arterial Doppler signals is a simple and valuable adjunct to simple palpation of peripheral pulses. A triphasic Doppler signal at the ankle implies the absence of proximal arterial disease; a monophasic signal suggests major proximal obstruction (5).

A more objective measure of distal perfusion is the ankle systolic blood pressure compared to the brachial pressure. This is performed using a Doppler to measure the systolic pressure in the dorsalis pedis and posterior tibial arteries and comparing them to the highest brachial systolic pressure. This generates the ankle-brachial index (ABI). The ABI is useful in comparing groups of patients and in following up individuals over time (6,7). The blood pressure in both arms always should be measured, and the higher of the two systolic pressures should be considered the true systemic systolic pressure and should be used to calculate the ABI. Healthy individuals have a systolic pressure at the ankle equal to or exceeding the brachial systolic pressure (ABI $\geq 1.0$) (8). The ABI tends to be greater than 0.5 in limbs with single-level occlusive disease and less than 0.5 in extremities with multilevel disease (6,9). This parallels the clinical presentation of most patients because most patients with intermittent claudication will have an ABI of 0.5 to 0.9 (10) and single-segment disease. Patients with ischemic rest pain and ischemic necrosis often have ABIs less than 0.4 and have multilevel occlusive disease. When followed up over time, a decrease in ABI is associated with both disease progression and the ultimate need for revascularization (11). Not only is the

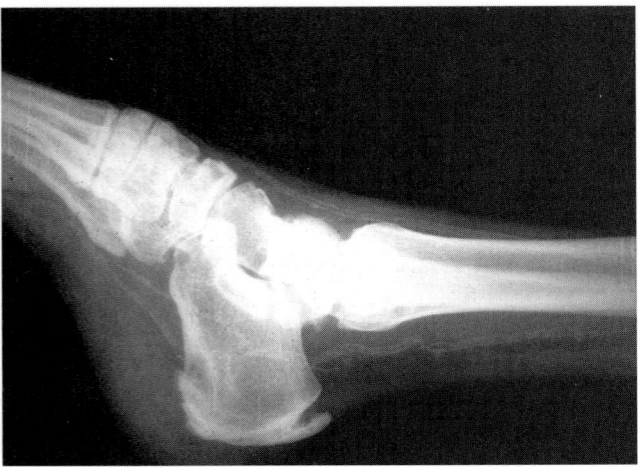

**FIGURE 101-1.** Lower extremity x-ray of the foot in a patient with diabetes presenting with cellulitis due to foot ulceration. Note calcification of the posterior tibial, anterior tibial, dorsalis pedis, and plantar arteries.

ABI important in objectifying the degree of limb ischemia but it is also an important predictor in the long-term outcome of patients. Patients with an ABI less than 0.5 have a reported 7-year mortality rate of 69% compared to 24% for those with an ABI greater than 0.5 (12).

The pressure at the ankle may be artifactually elevated by medial calcification (see Fig. 101-1), commonly seen in patients with diabetes, corticosteroid therapy, renal failure, and renal transplantation (13). Up to 14% of patients with diabetes have incompressible arteries (9). The measurement of toe systolic pressures using 2- to 3-cm toe cuffs and a photosensor to detect systolic pressure may be a better indicator of perfusion pressure in some of these patients. The toe systolic pressure normally is at least 70% of that recorded in the brachial artery (9). However, even digital arteries can be calcified, and pulse volume recordings (PVR) may serve as a semiquantitative indicator of distal perfusion and may help localize the level of disease (see Fig. 101-2). Critical limb ischemia presenting with rest pain or tissue loss is associated with an ankle systolic pressure less than or equal to 50 mm Hg or toe systolic pressures less than or equal to 30 mm Hg (7,13,14). Healing of ischemic skin lesions is unlikely at pressures below these values.

The ABI occasionally may be normal in patients with symptoms of intermittent claudication. When this occurs, repeating these measurements following treadmill exercise hemodynamically unmasks arterial lesions that are insignificant at rest. Exercise lowers peripheral resistance, thereby increasing the pressure gradient across the lesion and its hemodynamic significance. In the absence of arterial disease, the ankle systolic pressure remains stable with moderate exercise. In contrast, ankle systolic pressure decreases and remains depressed for 2 to 20 minutes in limbs with hemodynamically significant stenoses (8,10,15). Limbs with single-segment occlusive disease have more rapid recovery to baseline compared to limbs with multisegment occlusive disease (see Fig. 101-3).

## Arterial Duplex Imaging

Arterial duplex imaging, which combines B-mode ultrasonography with pulsed-wave Doppler, can provide hemodynamic, as well as anatomic, information and has found application in the peripheral arteries (16). Current technology uses color-encoded imaging to identify arterial structures and the pulsed Doppler to characterize velocity changes in areas of stenosis (see Fig. 101-4). Lesions causing a 50% or greater diameter reduction in stenosis are associated with a doubling, or more, increase in peak systolic velocity compared to the preceding segment, loss of flow reversal, and spectral broadening, indicating turbulence (9,17). In comparing duplex to contrast arteriography for the detection of 50% or higher stenosis, pooled estimates from the literature suggest respective sensitivities and specificities of 86% and 97% for aortoiliac stenoses, 80% and 96% for femoropopliteal stenoses, and 83% and 84% for infrageniculate lesions (18). Arterial duplex ultrasound has been used for the initial evaluation of patients who may be candidates for angioplasty, documentation of sources of peripheral emboli, evaluation of nonatherosclerotic causes of claudication, monitoring the course of thrombolytic therapy, and follow-up of arterial revascularization procedures. There also have been reports of revascularization strategies using duplex ultrasonography alone or with selective arteriography (17,19,20).

## Arteriography

Current arteriographic methods take many forms. Arteriographic evaluation of patients is reserved for those in whom a decision has been made to perform a revascularization procedure (see Table 101-1). Imaging of the arterial system is required to appropriately plan the revascularization procedure, be it a percutaneous or open revascularization.

Successful vascular reconstruction requires that the presence, location, and hemodynamic significance of all arterial lesions be accurately defined. Although contrast arteriography remains the gold standard for the anatomic evaluation of peripheral vascular disease, computerized tomographic arteriography (CTA) and magnetic resonance arteriography (MRA) have replaced standard contrast arteriograms in many cases (21). Contrast arteriography is an invasive procedure associated with small but definitive risks of contrast allergy, renal failure, and puncture site complications. Overall complication rates of 2% to 10% and a major complication rate of 0.8% have been reported (22).

Arteriography should be performed only after a decision to proceed with a revascularization procedure following a thorough assessment of the degree of ischemia and acceptance of the potential revascularization procedure by the patient, including potential risk. Therefore, localization of the underlying lesion is required. Often, multiplanar projections are required to accurately assess branch vessels, such as the profunda femoris, as well as the severity of eccentric lesions. The interpretation of the degree of stenosis is associated with substantial interobserver and intraobserver variability. Arteriography provides anatomic rather than physiologic information. The hemodynamic significance of a stenosis, particularly serial stenoses, may be difficult to determine using contrast studies alone. Objective assessment of hemodynamic significance requires measurement of the pressure gradient across a stenosis or multiple lesions. Mean pressure gradients greater than 10 mm Hg are considered hemodynamically significant (5,23,24). In this regard, vasodilators infused into the distal arterial bed may be helpful in identifying hemodynamically significant lesions that may have a minimal gradient at rest because the lower extremity arterial system is a high-resistance outflow bed. The accuracy of visual arteriographic interpretation in comparison to objective pressure measurements for the detection of hemodynamically significant aortoiliac lesions has been reported to be 70% to 74% (25).

The fast acquisition times achieved with spiral computerized tomography (CT) scan permit the demonstration of the peripheral arteries. The limitations, however, include reduced

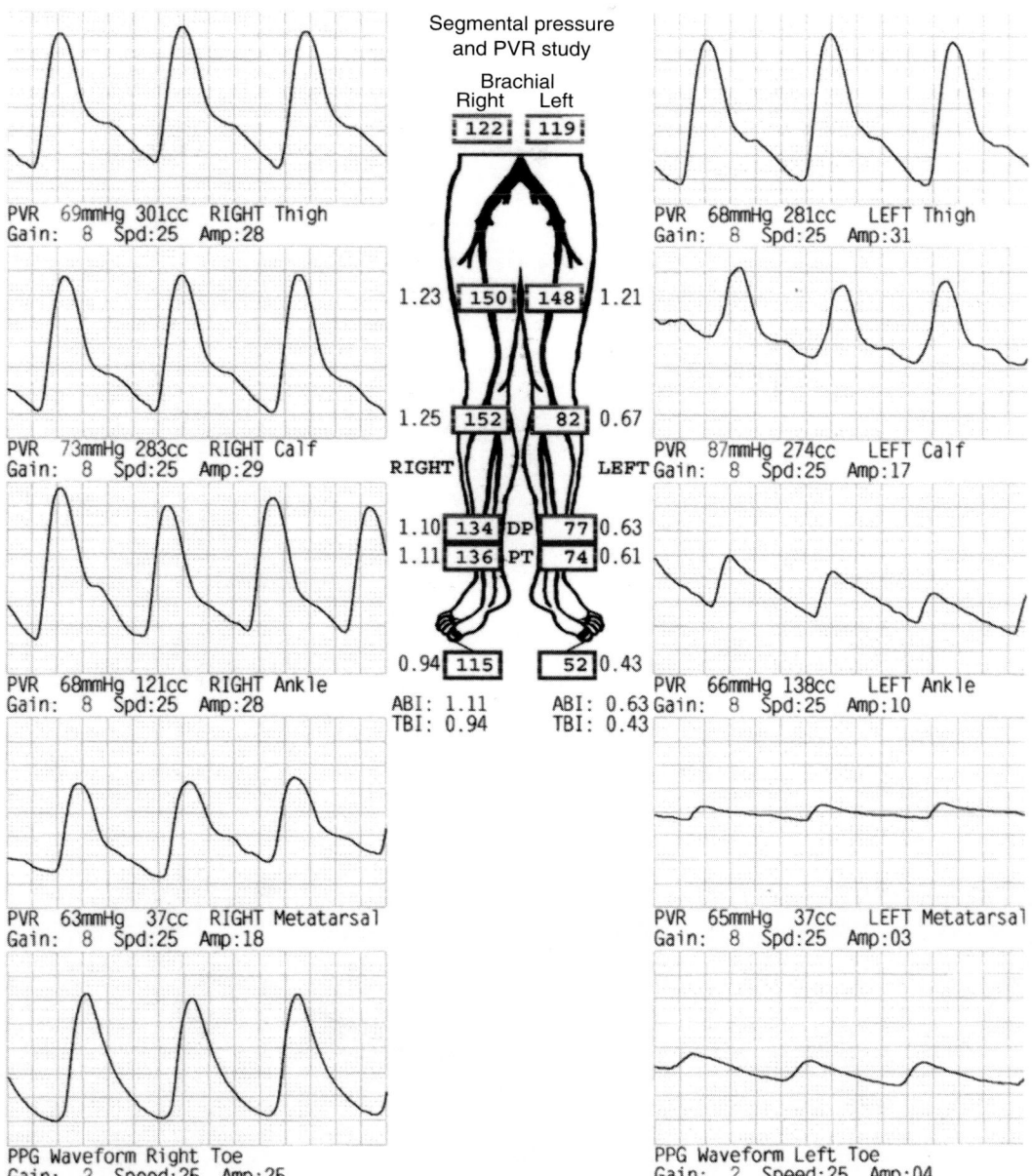

**FIGURE 101-2.** Segmental limb pressures and pulse volume recordings (PVR) in a patient with normal perfusion to the right leg and with superficial femoral arterial disease on the left. Note normal augmentation of the PVR in the calf compared to the thigh in the normal leg with good pulsatile perfusion to the foot and toe, which is associated with normal segmental pressures. In the diseased left leg, there is a marked pressure gradient from the thigh to the calf, as well as marked attenuation of pulsatile perfusion in the calf, foot, and toe. PVRs are especially helpful in evaluating lower limb perfusion in patients with calcified arteries.

spatial resolution, difficulties quantifying calcified stenoses, and the requirement for contrast media.

MRA has enjoyed rapid acceptance in many centers. Using a variety of unenhanced and enhanced techniques offers a useful noninvasive alternative to contrast arteriography (16,26,27). In comparison to contrast arteriography, MRA is noninvasive, requires no intravascular contrast, and may be more cost effective. Furthermore, because MRA depends only on detection of flow rather than the visualization of contrast material that may have to traverse multiple levels of occlusion through collaterals, it has a theoretical advantage of imaging the distal

runoff arteries (28–31). Potential limitations include problems in imaging retrograde flow, overestimation or underestimation of stenoses, and signal loss due to surgical clips (29,30). Agreement between contrast and MRA has been reported in 90% of infrainguinal arterial segments (28). The accuracy of MRA is improved with the use of gadolinium as a nonnephrotoxic contrast agent (16,27,29–31). A combination of time-of-flight imaging of lower leg and foot arteries in addition to gadolinium-enhanced MRA of the more proximal arteries appears to offer the most complete information required for distal revascularization.

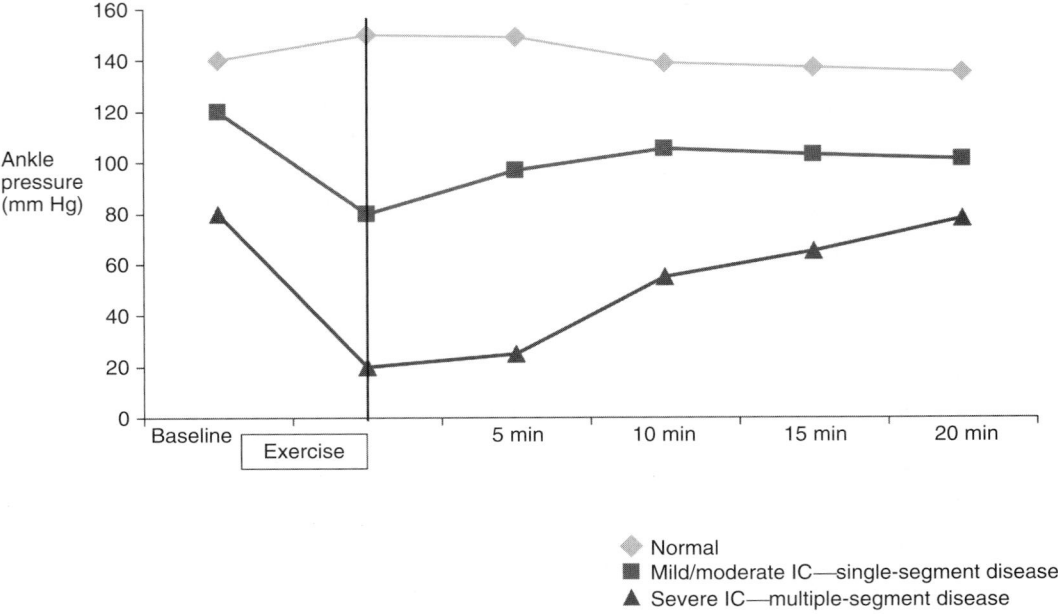

FIGURE 101-3. Treadmill exercise responses in a healthy individual and patients with intermittent claudication (IC). Healthy individuals maintain their distal perfusion pressure with moderate exercise. Patients with mild to moderate IC and single-segment disease drop their pressure; however, it returns to
normal within 5 to 10 minutes. Patients with severe IC associated with multilevel occlusive disease have
a more severe drop in pressure and a prolonged time to return to baseline.

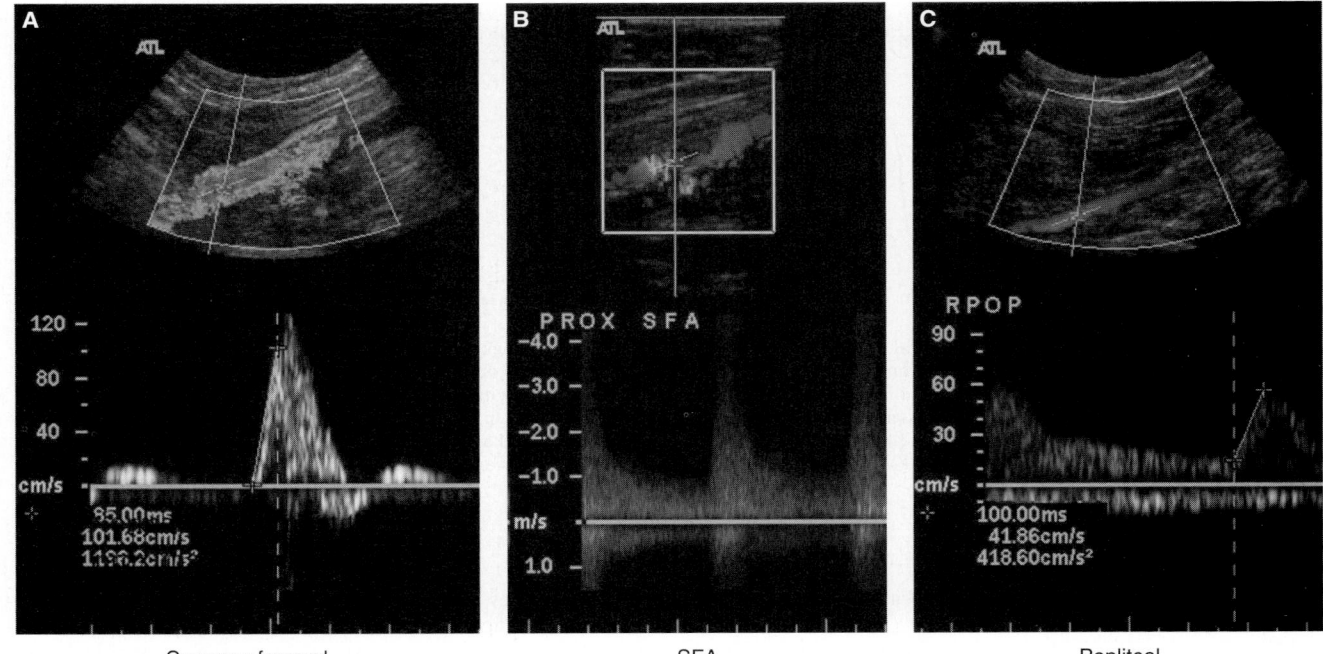

FIGURE 101-4. Arterial duplex in a patient with superficial femoral artery (SFA) stenosis. A: Normal
duplex of the common femoral artery with associated triphasic velocity signal. B: Turbulence and substantially elevated velocity at the site of stenosis in the superficial femoral artery (SFA). C: Attenuated
Doppler signal in the popliteal artery distal to a high-grade SFA stenosis (see Color Fig. 101-4).

## TABLE 101-1

### THE CLINICAL EVALUATION OF PERIPHERAL ARTERIAL DISEASE

| Evaluation | Item | Purpose |
|---|---|---|
| Clinical | History and physical examination/ABI | Diagnosis |
| Noninvasive Resting | Segmental Doppler pressures/PVRs | Quantify disease<br>Objective record<br>Follow-up |
| Provocative | Treadmill exercise/PORH | Refine diagnosis<br>Evaluate physiologic effect of arterial disease<br>Differentiate vascular from nonvascular cause for claudication |
| Invasive | Arteriography<br>Contrast<br>MRA<br>CTA | Plan revascularization |

ABI, ankle-brachial index; PVR, pulse volume recording; PORH, postocclusive reactive hyperemia; MRA, magnetic resonance arteriography; CTA, computerized tomographic arteriography.

# ACUTE ARTERIAL OCCLUSION

## Acute Limb Ischemia

Acute limb ischemia threatens the limb of the young patient and the life and limb of older patients. Clinically, acute limb ischemia classically presents with the "six Ps" of pain, pulselessness, pallor, poikilothermia, parasthesias, and paralysis (32–34). However, the presence of these findings may be variable in an individual patient, influenced by the severity and duration of ischemia. For example, ischemic pain may resolve either as collateral circulation is recruited and the ischemia lessens or as a result of nerve dysfunction as ischemia worsens. Obvious neurologic deficits suggest an advanced state of ischemia, with sensory preceding motor deficits (32,33). Fixed mottling of the skin with muscle necrosis and induration implies an unsalvageable limb.

Despite the obvious clinical findings, a formal system of stratifying acute limb ischemia is required to guide evaluation and management and to define prognosis. Acutely ischemic limbs can be described as viable, threatened, or irreversibly ischemic according to currently accepted reporting standards (7) (see Table 101-2). Threatened limbs are reversibly ischemic and may be salvageable with timely intervention, whereas irreversibly ischemic limbs usually require amputation or are affected by major neuromuscular damage despite successful revascularization.

The degree of ischemia is determined by a number of factors, including the anatomic level of obstruction, the underlying etiology, the adequacy of collateral circulation, the degree of thrombus propagation, and the adequacy of the cardiac output. The peripheral nerves and muscle are most sensitive to hypoxic injury, whereas the skin and subcutaneous tissues may tolerate a longer duration of ischemia (35). Complete cessation of blood flow produced by tourniquet-induced ischemia, which interrupts both axial and collateral perfusion, is associated with histologic evidence of striated muscle injury at 2 hours and extensive necrosis by 6 hours (36–38). Although 6 hours has been historically accepted as the maximum

## TABLE 101-2

### CLASSIFICATION OF ACUTE LIMB ISCHEMIA

| Category | Description/Prognosis | Findings Sensory loss | Muscle weakness | Doppler examination Arterial | Venous |
|---|---|---|---|---|---|
| I. Viable | Not immediately threatened | None | None | Audible | Audible |
| II. Threatened | | | | | |
| a. Marginally | Salvageable if promptly treated | None or minimal (toes) | None | Inaudible | Audible |
| b. Immediately | Salvageable with immediate revascularization | More than toes, associated with rest pain | Mild, moderate | Inaudible | Audible |
| III. Irreversible | Major tissue loss, permanent nerve damage inevitable | Profound, anesthetic | Profound, paralysis (rigor) | Inaudible | Inaudible |

From Rutherford RB, Baker JD, Ernst C, et al. Recommended standards for reports dealing with lower extremity ischemia: revised version. *J Vasc Surg* 1997;26:517–538, with permission.

interval prior to revascularization for acute limb ischemia, the tolerance of skeletal muscle to ischemia is variable because most patients do not have complete cessation of blood flow in both axial and collateral vessels, and acceptable results have been achieved with revascularization after substantially longer periods (39,40). In practice, the degree of ischemia is more important than the absolute duration of ischemia, and patients must be assessed on an individual basis.

### Differential Diagnosis of Acute Limb Ischemia

Acute arterial occlusion may result from an embolus, arterial thrombosis, trauma (iatrogenic or accidental), or spontaneous arterial dissection (see Table 101-3). Excluding trauma, acute upper extremity ischemia is almost always of embolic origin, whereas thrombosis of underlying atherosclerotic lesions is also common in the lower extremities (41). The relative frequencies of embolism versus arterial thrombosis vary widely with referral patterns, the inclusion of vascular graft occlusions, and errors in diagnosis. Depending on these considerations, embolism may account for as few as 8% to over 90% of acutely ischemic limbs (40,42–46). The low frequency of embolic occlusion in recent reports is most likely due to the declining incidence of rheumatic heart disease, more widespread use of anticoagulation in the treatment of myocardial infarction and atrial fibrillation, and an increasing number of patients dependent on arterial grafts for limb viability who are being treated with anticoagulation.

Although many reports include both embolic and thrombotic occlusions, distinction is important because the management and natural history are substantially different (see Table 101-4). Acute embolic occlusions are associated with higher rates of limb salvage (85% vs. 67%) but also higher mortality (20% vs. 8%) than arterial thrombosis (47). Furthermore, embolic occlusions often can be managed with mechanical or pharmacologic removal of the embolus alone, whereas acute thrombosis resulting from underlying arterial occlusive disease requires arterial reconstruction (46–48). Misdiagnosis and inadequate treatment of acute arterial thrombosis with only thrombus extraction has been associated with high rates of limb loss, reoperation, and death (40,41,45).

The absence of atrial fibrillation or recent myocardial infarction, a previous history of claudication, and a reduced ABI in the contralateral limb suggest a diagnosis of thrombosis. Arteriographic findings including evidence of underlying atherosclerosis with well-developed collaterals or signs suggestive of embolism (a meniscus, occlusion at major arterial bifurcations, and multiple sites of occlusion) may further aid in this differentiation (33). However, this distinction may be difficult and some have suggested that a preoperative diagnosis of embolism can be supported only by the presence of atrial fibrillation. The usual risk factors for atherosclerosis have not proven useful in distinguishing thrombosis from embolism because only 40% of patients with thrombosis have a history of claudication (47).

## Arterial Embolism

The peripheral arterial trunks are the site of 84% of embolic occlusions, with the lower extremities affected five to 10 times more frequently than the upper extremities (33,49). Emboli most commonly lodge at bifurcations, typically in the aortoiliac or femoral arteries in association with changes in arterial diameter (50,51). Multiple emboli occur in 12% of initial and 23% of recurrent embolic events (49).

The heart is the source of 75% to 94% of peripheral emboli (34,35,48–51), with atrial fibrillation being present in 43% to 74% of these patients (49–52). However, there has been a shift in associated cardiac diseases from rheumatic to atherosclerotic causes. Although arterial embolization causes complications in fewer than 5% of patients with myocardial infarctions (33), recent myocardial infarction is present in as many as one third of patients with lower extremity emboli (51); however, they are frequently delayed up to 2 weeks or more. Other cardiac sources of emboli include left ventricular aneurysms, mechanical heart valves, valvular vegetations, and intracardiac tumors.

The proportion of acutely ischemic limbs resulting from paradoxical embolization of a venous thrombus to the arterial circulation is unknown but is likely underappreciated. Acute arterial occlusion in the absence of risk factors for cardiac

---

**TABLE 101-3**

DIFFERENTIAL DIAGNOSIS AND ETIOLOGY OF ACUTE LIMB ISCHEMIA

**CONDITIONS MIMICKING ACUTE LIMB ISCHEMIA**
- Heart failure (especially if associated with chronic occlusive disease)
- Acute DVT
- Acute compressive neuropathy

**NONATHEROSCLEROTIC CAUSES OF ACUTE LIMB ISCHEMIA**
- Arterial trauma
- Aortic/arterial dissection
- Arteritis with thrombosis (e.g., giant cell arteritis, thromboangiitis obliterans)
- Spontaneous thrombosis associated with a hypercoagulable state
- Popliteal cyst with thrombosis
- Popliteal entrapment with thrombosis
- Vasospasm with thrombosis (e.g., ergotism)

**CAUSES OF ACUTE LIMB ISCHEMIA IN PATIENTS WITH ATHEROSCLEROSIS**
- Thrombosis of an atherosclerotic stenosed artery
- Thrombosis of an arterial bypass graft
- Embolism from heart, aneurysm, plaque, or critical stenosis upstream (including cholesterol or atherothrombotic emboli secondary to endovascular procedures)
- Thrombosed aneurysm (especially popliteal aneurysm)

DVT, deep vein thrombosis.
Adapted from TASC Working Group. Differential diagnosis of acute limb ischemia. *J Vasc Surg* 2000;31:S138.

## TABLE 101-4

### CHARACTERISTICS OF ACUTE ARTERIAL OCCLUSION: EMBOLIC VERSUS THROMBOTIC ETIOLOGY

| Characteristics of occlusion | Embolic | Thrombotic |
|---|---|---|
| Onset of symptoms | Sudden, rapid | Insidious, slower |
| Prior symptoms | Rare | Frequent |
| Common clinical association | Recent heart disease: arrhythmias, acute MI | PAD |
| Stigmata of PAD | Possible | Common |
| Examination of opposite limb | Often normal | Often abnormal |
| Arteriography | – Crescent/meniscus sign<br>– Multiple sites<br>– Vessel bifurcations | – Blurred demarcations<br>– Prominent collaterals<br>– Atherosclerosis |
| Treatment strategy | Thromboembolectomy or thrombolysis; detect and eliminate (treat) embolic source | Thrombolysis or thrombectomy; must correct or bypass underlying vascular disease |
| Long-term therapy | Anticoagulation (if cardiac source) | Platelet inhibition (add anticoagulation if indicated) |
| Comparative morbidity and mortality | Threat to life, usually cardiac disease | Threat to limb high plus risk of generalized atherosclerosis (coronary, carotid, mesenteric, renal) |

PAD, peripheral arterial disease; MI, myocardial infraction.
Adapted from Comerota AJ, Harada RN. Acute arterial occlusion. In Young JR, Olin JW, Bartholomew JR, eds: *Peripheral vascular diseases*, 2nd ed. St. Louis: Mosby-Year Book, 1996.

emboli in patients with concurrent evidence of deep venous thrombosis or pulmonary embolism should suggest paradoxical embolization. Likewise, acute arterial occlusion in a patient without a history of or without physical findings of vascular or heart disease should stimulate a search for venous thrombosis. Confirmation of the diagnosis requires demonstration of an abnormal communication between the arterial and venous circulations with a right-to-left shunt. A patent foramen ovale, present at autopsy in 11% to 35% of the normal population, accounts for more than 70% of such shunts (53).

The proximal arterial system may be the source of up to 15% of peripheral emboli (51). Proximal aneurysms, accounting for 3% of all cases (48,50,51), are the most common extracardiac source. These may include aortoiliac, femoral, and popliteal aneurysms in the lower extremities. Subclavian aneurysms, commonly associated with thoracic outlet compression, represent a similar source in the upper extremities. The embolic potential of aortic atherosclerotic plaques or thrombi, present at transesophageal echocardiography in 1% to 7% of subjects, has also been recognized (54).

The source of peripheral emboli usually can be documented using a variety of noninvasive tests, most notably echocardiography. In this regard, transesophageal echocardiography is significantly more sensitive than transthoracic techniques in identifying responsible pathology, detecting spontaneous echocontrast suggestive of low flow, and defining abnormalities of the atrial septum (52,53,55). In a small series of patients undergoing both studies, potential embolic sources were identified in eight of 10 patients by transesophageal echocardiography in comparison to only one patient by transthoracic imaging (52). In the absence of a cardiac source, duplex ultrasonography can often be used to localize peripheral aneurysms and paradoxical venous sources. Despite complete evaluation, in up to 20% of patients no source for their lower extremity embolus is identified (34,35,48,49,51).

## Arterial Thrombosis

Arterial thrombosis results from either intrinsic arterial disease or a number of thrombophilic states. Most thrombotic events occur in the setting of atherosclerotic disease with thrombosis following plaque ulceration or intraplaque hemorrhage. Peripheral arterial aneurysms, particularly of the common femoral and popliteal arteries, also may be associated with acute thrombosis. Other nonatherosclerotic etiologies include fibromuscular dysplasia, arterial dissections, adventitial cystic disease, popliteal entrapment, a variety of arteritides, ergot ingestion, intraarterial drug injection, and arterial injury (35,56). Iatrogenic injury is becoming increasingly important, with arterial thrombosis complicating 0.16% of femoral and 6.6% of brachial arteriographic studies, 0.06% to 0.1% of coronary angioplasties, and 1% to 9% of peripheral angioplasty procedures (57,58).

Among the hypercoagulable states, arterial thrombotic events are most often associated with antiphospholipid antibodies (59). Although initially described in association with systemic lupus erythematosis, most cases fail to meet international criteria for the disease but may manifest findings of other rheumatologic diseases (60). Severe complications have been most commonly associated with high levels of immunoglobulin G antiphospholipid antibodies (61). In addition to obstetric complications and deep venous thrombosis, such patients may present with cerebral, visceral, or peripheral arterial occlusions. Recurrent thrombotic events, particularly following surgical or percutaneous intervention, frequently occur in association with antiphospholipid antibodies.

Other thrombophilic conditions also may play a role in arterial thrombosis. Complications of type II heparin-induced thrombocytopenia (HIT) frequently result in arterial thrombosis (62). Increased fibrinogen, von Willebrand factor antigen, tissue plasminogen activator antigen, and factor VII levels have been associated with an increased incidence of acute cardiac events, although their relation to peripheral arterial thrombosis is less well defined (63). In contrast, although both arterial embolization and thrombosis have been occasionally reported in association with protein C, protein S, and antithrombin deficiency (64), the inheritable thrombophilias have been most strongly associated with venous thromboses. The factor $V_{Leiden}$ mutation has not been associated with an increased risk of acute arterial events (63).

## Pathophysiology of Acute Limb Ischemia

The pathophysiology of acute limb ischemia has been well described. Distal arterial spasm, which initially prevents thrombus propagation, is postulated to be the first response to acute arterial occlusion (35,38,65). Propagation of thrombus into the distal circulation follows resolution of this spasm. If distal thrombosis extends beyond the limits of mechanical extraction, relief of the proximal obstruction may fail to restore distal flow. In experimental arterial occlusion, arterial resistance increases at 6 hours in association with thrombosis of small muscular arteries and veins (66). Not only is such distal thrombus difficult to extract using conventional mechanical techniques but endothelial and perivascular swelling also further impede the restoration of microcirculatory flow, resulting in the impaired reflow (no-reflow) phenomenon occurring after relief of proximal obstruction (67).

Inadequate oxygen delivery and depletion of cellular energy stores initiate the ischemia reperfusion syndrome (56).

Subsequent reperfusion of the limb is associated with increased microvascular permeability, extravasation of macromolecules, and the release of enzymes, procoagulants, potassium, myoglobin, and thrombi formed in the static venous system into the systemic circulation (35,68,69). Cellular injury, mediated by oxygen-derived free radicals, may continue even after perfusion is reestablished (56,69). Free radicals alter the adhesion properties of the endothelial surface, with adhesion and subsequent migration of leukocytes producing more free radicals, enzymes, and cytokines such as tumor necrosis factor-$\alpha$ and interleukin-1 (56). Severe manifestations of acidosis, hyperkalemia, myoglobinuria, and azotemia, termed the *myo-nephropathic-metabolic syndrome*, may occur in up to 8% of patients (36). Fibrin-platelet aggregates in the venous effluent from the limb, as well as humoral factors released from the ischemic vascular bed, have also been associated with pathologic pulmonary changes (36,38,66,70).

## Blue Toe Syndrome

Atherothrombotic microembolism warrants separate consideration as the pathophysiology and outcome differs from that of acute lower extremity ischemia (7). Such patients may present with acute focal ischemia of the digits, good perfusion to the remainder of the foot, and minimal clinical evidence of occlusive disease (see Fig. 101-5). The proximal arterial system is patent, as are the arteries distal to the lesion, and the foot is otherwise well perfused. Peripheral pulses may be intact and the ABI may be reduced or normal, depending on the degree of arterial narrowing of the culprit lesion (9). Emboli may consist of either atheromatous material or fibrin and platelet thrombi (71), with sources including arterial aneurysms and atheromatous plaques of the aortoiliac or femoropopliteal arteries (33,72,73). The natural history of these lesions includes

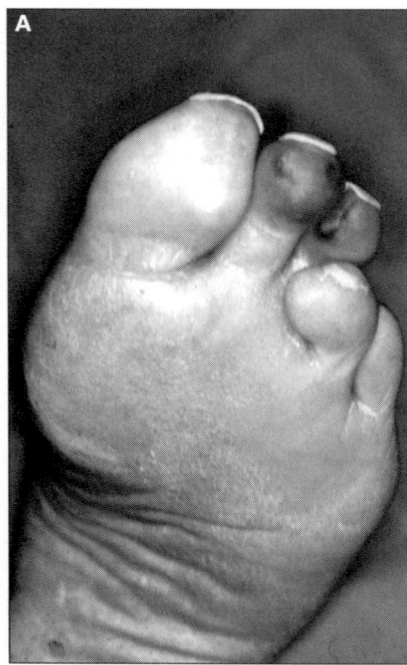
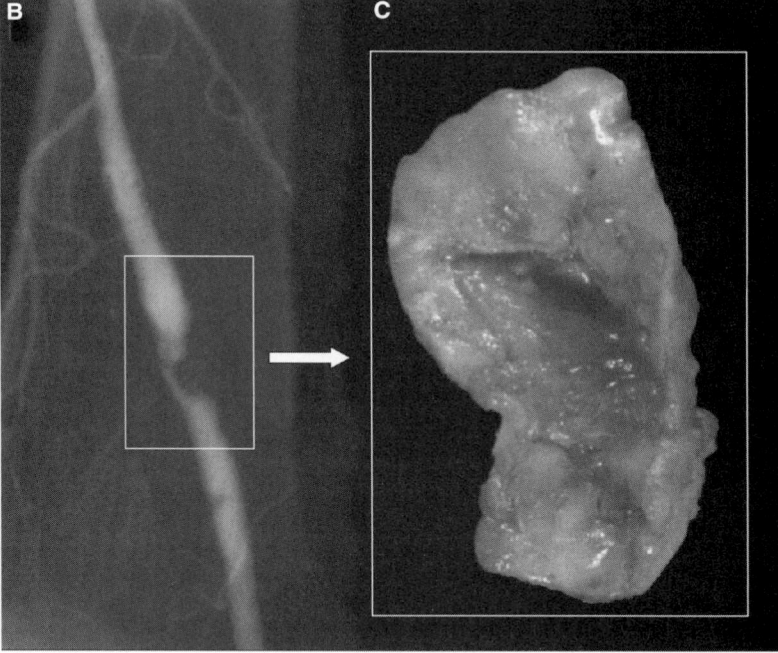

**FIGURE 101-5.** Blue toe syndrome associated with a focal superficial femoral artery (SFA) lesion. **A:** Patient presenting with painful ischemic toes but an otherwise well-perfused foot. The ABI was 0.7. **B:** Arteriogram demonstrates the culprit lesion in the SFA. **C:** Endarterectomy specimen showing ulceration and laminated platelet-fibrin thrombus on the plaque (see Color Fig. 101-5).

repeated episodes of microembolization, eventually threatening viability of the entire foot (72,73). The effectiveness of anticoagulants and antiplatelet agents in preventing recurrent episodes is questionable (73), and surgical or endovascular correction of such lesions should be considered.

## Management of Acute Limb Ischemia

Management options for acute lower extremity ischemia include immediate amputation, early anticoagulation with interval revascularization if required, urgent revascularization, and thrombolytic therapy followed by endovascular or surgical treatment of the underlying stenotic lesions. All patients with acute limb ischemia, except those with aortic dissection, should have heparin administered as soon as feasible. Initial anticoagulation serves to prevent thrombus propagation into the distal arterial branches and to minimize the impact of retained thrombus and intimal trauma following balloon embolectomy (45,65). Experimentally, heparin has been shown to reduce the endothelial cell dysfunction associated with ischemia reperfusion injury (56). Perhaps more important, anticoagulation reduces the incidence of recurrent thromboembolism, which occurs in 6% to 13% of patients (34,43), by approximately 75% (74). Regardless of subsequent treatment, case series have reported higher limb salvage and lower mortality rates in patients treated with anticoagulants (50,75). Good surgical results were obtained in 80% of adequately anticoagulated patients in comparison to 48% of inadequately anticoagulated patients, with corresponding mortality rates of 5% and 26% (75).

Although associated with wound complications in up to 20% of patients (43,75), anticoagulation should be continued into the postoperative period (43,45). Except for those with a correctable embolic source, such as an arterial aneurysm, long-term anticoagulation is appropriate for most patients with peripheral emboli.

Other pharmacologic adjuncts may also have a role in acute limb ischemia. Intravenous mannitol may reduce cellular edema, assist in maintaining microcirculatory flow, and promote osmotic diuresis in patients with myoglobinuria (33,43,67). Furthermore, mannitol may reduce ischemic muscle injury and improve contractile function after revascularization (39). Alkalization of the urine may be of some benefit by reducing the formation of pigment casts within the renal tubules (69).

Although early high-dose heparin anticoagulation followed by delayed revascularization of viable limbs has been advocated by some (65), early amputation of irreversibly ischemic limbs and surgical or thrombolytic reperfusion of threatened limbs is the most widely practiced approach. The need for preoperative diagnostic tests depends upon the clinical presentation, which includes the cardiac and pulse examination, the degree of ischemia, and urgency of the need for revascularization (76). Preoperative arteriography is appropriate for limbs with nonembolic occlusion and those that are not in imminent jeopardy, whereas immediate surgical intervention should be considered in those with severe ischemia due to embolic occlusion, especially those with no femoral pulse in the ischemic leg (and a normal contralateral examination). Arteriography is particularly helpful in patients with a preceding history of claudication or rest pain in whom more complex reconstructive procedures can be anticipated. In series of largely thrombotic occlusions, early operative intervention has been associated with limb salvage rates as high as 87% (42). For embolic occlusions, limb salvage has been achieved in 89% of surgically treated patients in comparison to 77% of nonoperated patients (50). However, patient selection and good clinical judgment remain important, and for good outcomes, initial nonoperative management may be appropriate in the poor-risk patient with a viable extremity.

Embolic occlusions can often be managed with balloon catheter embolectomy, allowing even aortoiliac emboli to be removed from a femoral approach under local anesthesia if necessary. This approach has been associated with a 35% reduction in the amputation rate and a 50% reduction in mortality (49). Thrombotic occlusions arising from underlying arterial lesions often require arterial reconstruction. Intraoperative thrombolytic therapy has a role in the setting of thromboembolectomy for acute limb ischemia and potential distal vascular thrombosis (77). A distal bolus injection has been shown to be a safe adjunct associated with thrombin breakdown without fibrinogen depletion (78). The presence of flow may enhance the effectiveness of intraoperative thrombolysis with a 30-minute continuous infusion being more effective than a bolus injection (39), although likely to be associated with an increased risk of bleeding. The use of intraoperative and postoperative thrombolytic therapy has been reported to increase limb salvage from 90% to 98% (76). Monitoring of compartment pressures and fasciotomy should be used judiciously to prevent further muscle necrosis.

Acute arterial occlusion has been historically associated with a 40% to 81% rate of limb salvage and mortality rates exceeding 25% (35,65). The high mortality has been attributed to surgical stress, underlying cardiac disease, associated pulmonary and peripheral emboli, ongoing limb ischemia, and metabolic derangements accompanying restoration of blood flow. More than half of the deaths following peripheral emboli are due to cardiac causes, with pulmonary embolism being the second leading cause (34,68). Persistent limb ischemia takes a considerable toll in increased mortality in addition to limb loss (41). Developments such as the balloon embolectomy catheter and better management of coronary artery disease have been associated with improvements in both limb salvage and mortality rates. More recent reviews show reduced mortality rates of 15% to 19% and improved limb salvage rates of 82% to 90% (79). However, long-term survival remains low: only 51% at 36 months and less than 30% at 5 years (42,80). Associated myocardial infarction (41,51), underlying malignancy (41), and simultaneous emboli to the carotid or visceral circulation (49) have been particularly associated with a poor outcome.

### Catheter-Directed Thrombolysis

Catheter-directed intrathrombus infusion of plasminogen activators has been used as an alternative to surgery for acute lower extremity ischemia with more gratifying results than observed with systemic infusion (81). The ability to pass a guidewire through and embed a catheter into the occlusion are independent predictors of lytic success (82). Catheter-directed infusion has the advantages of increasing plasmin activity within the thrombus, thereby reducing interaction with circulating plasmin inhibitors and reducing the required dose of thrombolytic agent (83,84). These techniques also provide arterial access for adjunctive procedures such as balloon angioplasty (and stenting) of an underlying culprit lesion.

Catheter-based, intraarterial thrombolysis has been used for embolic and thrombotic arterial occlusions in native arteries and bypass grafts and in both acute and chronic settings. In most situations, thrombolytic therapy is an adjunct to definitive surgical or endovascular treatment, serving to eliminate the thrombus and unmask underlying arterial or graft lesions, observed in 65% to 70% of patients, most of whom can be treated percutaneously, thereby reducing the magnitude of subsequent procedures (79,83,85). Acute upper extremity arterial occlusions are an exception, with only 17% of successful lytic infusions requiring further intervention (82).

Three clinical trials (83–85) have compared patients randomized to thrombolytic treatment or surgical intervention. Ouriel et al. (84) randomized 114 patients with acute limb ischemia of less than 7 days duration to urokinase (UK) or surgical intervention. At 1 year, the cumulative risk of amputation (18%) was identical in the two groups, whereas thrombolysis was associated with a significant 62% reduction in mortality. Thrombolysis was equally effective in those with embolic and thrombotic occlusions, although the survival benefit was greater for embolic occlusions. The Thrombolysis or Peripheral Arterial Surgery (TOPAS) investigators (86) randomized 213 patients with acute lower extremity ischemia secondary to native arterial or bypass graft occlusion of less than 14 days duration to a variable dose of recombinant urokinase (rUK) or surgery. Among patients treated with rUK, surgical operations were avoided in 46% of patients and the magnitude of such procedures was reduced in 50% of cases. Survival and amputation-free survival at 12 months were similar in the rUK and surgical groups. These results have been confirmed in a trial of 544 patients with ischemia less than 14 days duration randomized to the optimal rUK regimen or surgery (85). Amputation-free survival was similar in the two groups. There was a trend toward a higher amputation-free survival among those randomized to surgery and significantly more bleeding in those randomized to rUK. Among patients treated with rUK, thrombus resolution and clinical outcome were somewhat better for acute bypass graft thrombosis than for native arterial occlusion. For thrombi longer than 30 cm, *post hoc* analysis further suggested that 1-year amputation-free survival was better following thrombolytic treatment, potentially because of lack of suitable outflow for a surgical procedure. In contrast, shorter occlusions fared better with surgery (87).

The Surgery versus Thrombolysis for Ischemia of the Lower Extremity (STILE) trial (83) randomized 393 patients with nonembolic lower extremity ischemia of less than 6 months duration to catheter-directed thrombolysis with either UK or recombinant tissue plasminogen activator (rt-PA) or optimal surgical revascularization. Overall, a significantly higher percentage of patients assigned to thrombolysis had treatment failure defined as recurrent or ongoing ischemia (54% vs. 26%) at 30 days. Most patients participating in the STILE trial had chronic ischemia. Because a worse thrombolytic outcome was associated with a longer duration of ischemia, the results in the chronic ischemia group drove the overall observations of the trial, establishing that chronic arterial occlusion is not well treated with catheter-directed thrombolysis. Subsequent analysis, however, offered important insight. Patients presenting with acute ischemia (≤14 days) and randomized to thrombolysis had significantly better limb salvage (89% vs. 70%) and amputation-free survival. This occurred predominantly because of the favorable outcomes in patients with acute graft occlusion (88). As in other trials, catheter-directed thrombolysis was effective in reducing the magnitude of subsequent surgical procedures. Further, 1-year follow-up also has been reported for patients presenting with native arterial occlusions (89). At 1 year, surgery was associated with substantially lower rates of recurrent ischemia and major amputation, although mortality was equal in both groups. However, an interesting observation was made in patients with diabetes with infrainguinal native artery occlusion. Although those randomized to surgery had better limb outcomes, patients receiving catheter-directed thrombolysis had significantly better survival at 1 year (92% vs. 68%). This fits with the observations of Ouriel et al. (84) and the randomized intraoperative UK study of Comerota et al. (78), in which significant reductions in mortality were also observed in patients randomized to lytic therapy. These compelling observations from randomized trials suggest that there is a "systemic benefit" of lytic therapy in patients with advanced arterial occlusive disease, which has not been adequately investigated.

Although none of the trials have been definitive, they have provided insight into potential uses of these agents. The outcomes of catheter-directed thrombolysis appear to be independent of the agent used (UK, rUK, rt-PA), although lysis with rt-PA is more rapid (83,90). Bleeding complications, most of which were minor, occurred in 5% to 20% of patients. Collectively, these trials suggest that thrombolysis has the greatest advantage in acute bypass graft occlusions (88), with initial success rates tending to be better for prosthetic than vein grafts (82). However, long-term patency tends to be better in vein grafts that have a correctable lesion than in prosthetic grafts. Thrombolysis of an acutely occluded graft reduces the complexity of the subsequently required surgical intervention. Patients with chronic ischemic symptoms and those with native arterial occlusions tend to be associated with poorer thrombolytic results than operative revascularization. Surgical revascularization remains the procedure of choice for nonembolic native arterial and chronic graft occlusions (88,89).

# CHRONIC ARTERIAL OCCLUSIVE DISEASE

## Manifestations of Chronic Arterial Occlusive Disease

The signs and symptoms of chronic arterial occlusive disease reflect the severity of distal ischemia, which in turn depends on the degree of stenosis, the number of levels of the arterial system involved, and the adequacy of the collateral circulation. Many patients with lower extremity occlusive disease and compensatory collateral flow have no symptoms. Symptomatic manifestations progress from those that occur only with the increased metabolic demands of exercise (intermittent claudication) to those that occur at rest (ischemic rest pain and tissue necrosis). Categories of chronic limb ischemia are shown in Table 101-5. Single-level occlusion is usually associated with intermittent claudication, whereas multilevel disease is associated with more advanced ischemia. Before the advent of modern vascular reconstruction, presenting complaints among those with peripheral arterial occlusion included claudication in 73%, ischemic rest pain in 16%, and tissue loss in 11% of patients (91). In light of changes in diagnosis of disease and management of risk factors, such observations are of historical interest only.

Intermittent claudication accompanies mild to moderate degrees of ischemia and occurs when the nutrient blood flow below a stenosis or occlusion, although satisfactory at rest, is inadequate to meet the increased metabolic demands of the exercising lower extremity muscles. It is characterized by pain, discomfort, or weakness that affects specific muscle groups, occurs only with exercise, and is relieved by rest (7,10,92). Classic intermittent claudication can be characterized as exercise-induced muscle ischemia causing pain. Such pain is typically localized to the calf muscles but may affect other muscular groups, including the buttocks, hips, or thighs, in the presence of proximal aortoiliac occlusive disease. Typically, the symptomatic muscle groups are located one segment below the arterial occlusive disease. Important differentiating features of intermittent claudication include the consistency of the walk–pain–rest cycle over time, the worsening of symptoms with increased pace or when walking up an incline, and consistent relief within minutes after discontinuing exercise. These features are useful in differentiating vascular claudication from nonvascular etiologies ("pseudoclaudication") due to degenerative hip disease, lumbar disc disease, spinal stenosis, or neuropathy (10,93,94). Features including the onset of symptoms while sitting or standing, a variable cycle of walk–pain–rest, and relief only by sitting or lying down suggest another etiology of lower extremity symptoms.

The prognosis of the limb for patients with intermittent claudication is good with risk factor modification, exercise,

## TABLE 101-5

CATEGORIES OF CHRONIC LIMB ISCHEMIA

| Grade | Category | Clinical description | Objective criteria |
|-------|----------|---------------------|--------------------|
| I | 1 | Mild claudication | Completes treadmill exercise[a] and AP after exercise >50 mm Hg but at least 20 mm Hg lower than resting value |
| | 2 | Moderate claudication | Between categories 1 and 3 |
| | 3 | Severe claudication | Cannot complete standard treadmill exercise[a] and AP after exercise <50 mm Hg |
| II | 4 | Ischemic rest pain | Resting AP <40 mm Hg, flat or barely pulsatile ankle, or metatarsal PVR; TP <30 mm Hg |
| III | 5 | Minor tissue loss— nonhealing ulcer, focal gangrene with diffuse pedal ischemia | Resting AP <60 mm Hg, flat or barely pulsatile ankle, or metatarsal PVR; TP <40 mm Hg |
| | 6 | Major tissue loss— extending above TM level, functional foot no longer salvageable | Same as category 5 |

AP, ankle pressure; PVR, pulse volume recording; TM, transmetatarsal; TP, toe pressure.
Note: Grades II and III, categories 4, 5, and 6, are included in the term *chronic critical ischemia.*
[a]Five minutes at 2 mph on a 12% incline.
From Rutherford RB, Baker JD, Ernst C, et al. Recommended standards for reports dealing with lower extremity ischemia: revised version. *J Vasc Surg* 1997;26:517–538, with permission.

and appropriate pharmacotherapy. Only a few of the limbs progress to tissue loss or amputation (95). In evaluating the natural history of intermittent claudication, McDaniel and Cronenwett (96) found that claudication symptoms remained stable or improved in 55% of patients, became worse in 16%, worsened to a point requiring revascularization in 25%, and culminated in amputation in 4% of patients followed up for 5 years. These authors appear to have studied a cohort of patients with more advanced occlusive disease than other investigators. The risk of limb loss among patients with claudication has varied from 2% to 8% during 2 to 8 years of follow-up (95–99). Among patients without diabetes, progression of claudication to rest pain is correlated with smoking, low initial ABI, and the presence of multiple arterial stenoses (99). Patients with diabetes are at least five times more likely to develop critical limb ischemia than those without diabetes and are more likely to require amputation once critical ischemia develops (100).

More important, 5-year mortality among patients with claudication approaches 30%, with most deaths resulting from associated coronary artery disease (12,95–99). The prevalence of ischemic heart disease is two to four times greater than in the general population (101). Respective 10-year mortality rates of 47% and 43% in men and women with claudication are 2.2 and 4.1 times greater than among patients without claudication (102). Several other studies have confirmed the risk of dying within 5 years to be two to three times higher than age- and sex-matched populations. The ABI is among the most important predictors of death in this population and mortality is substantially higher in patients with diabetes and with claudication who continue to smoke (96,97).

More advanced degrees of ischemia are associated with pain at rest and the development of tissue loss. Ischemic rest pain typically occurs in the toes and forefoot, is usually worse at night, and is characteristically exacerbated by elevation and relieved with dependency of the limb (103). Rest pain implies that blood flow is inadequate to meet the basal metabolic demands of the tissue and is associated with ankle pressures below 40 mm Hg and toe pressures below 30 mm Hg (7). Somewhat higher pressures are required for ulcer healing, commonly defined as an ankle pressure of 60 mm Hg or toe pressure of 40 mm Hg.

In contrast to intermittent claudication, the development of rest pain or tissue loss is a threat to limb viability. Given the diffuse nature of atherosclerotic disease in these patients, their prognosis is less favorable than for patients with claudication. Three years following revascularization, 26% of patients will have undergone an amputation and 25% will have died (100). Others have reported the 5-year survival of patients undergoing revascularization for limb salvage to be only 30% in comparison to 67% for patients operated on for claudication (104). Furthermore, objectively measured quality of life scores among those with critical limb ischemia approach those of seriously ill patients with cancer(105).

Patients with premature atherosclerosis, defined as being younger than 50 years, constitute a special population with a high prevalence of metabolic and coagulation abnormalities. Vascular disease is particularly virulent in this group, with a high incidence of graft failure, amputation, and death (59, 106,107). Multiple level disease is present in up to 87% of such patients and up to 27% ultimately require amputation (106). Lipoprotein (a) [Lp(a)] levels are more closely associated with the risk of premature atherosclerosis than other lipid variables (59), with concentrations greater than 30 mg per dL carrying a twofold to threefold increased risk of cardiovascular disease. The deleterious effects of Lp(a) are thought to be mediated either by competitive inhibition of endothelial plasminogen binding or by excess cholesterol deposition at sites of arterial injury. Some (108,109) have reported elevated plasma homocysteine levels and elevated antiphospholipid antibodies (59) in this population.

## Differential Diagnosis of Lower Extremity Ischemia

Although atherosclerosis is the most common cause of arterial occlusive disease, several less common conditions also result in lower extremity ischemia. Because these entities have differing risk factors, natural histories, and treatment, they require special consideration. Buerger disease (thrombangiitis obliterans) is a segmental, inflammatory occlusive disease typically affecting small and medium caliber arteries and veins. Although infrequent in the United States, the disorder is a common cause of limb ischemia in the Middle and Far East. Among patients with peripheral vascular disease, Buerger disease accounts for 0.75% of cases in North America, 3.3% of patients in Eastern Europe, and 16.6% of cases in Japan (110,111). Clinical criteria for the diagnosis include a history of cigarette smoking, infrapopliteal occlusive lesions, onset prior to age 50 years, evidence of upper extremity involvement, or migratory thrombophlebitis in the absence of atherosclerotic risk factors other than smoking (112). Exclusion of autoimmune arteritides and hypercoagulable states is also important (110,111). The effects of passive smoking are unknown, but essentially all patients with Buerger disease have a history of smoking, which is closely correlated with disease progression and remission (112–114). Although men have historically accounted for over 98% of cases, an increasing prevalence of women has been noted (110,115).

Buerger disease typically presents with symptoms of rest pain or distal tissue loss. Claudication, if present, classically involves the instep of the foot rather than the calf because of the infrapopliteal distribution of arterial occlusion (110). Although characterized by infrapopliteal occlusive disease, upper extremity involvement is frequent and proximal lower extremity arterial disease has occasionally been reported (111). The clinical diagnosis is supported by nonspecific arteriographic findings that include segmental tapering or abrupt occlusion of the infrapopliteal arteries with corkscrew collaterals and a corrugated appearance of patent arterial segments (111–113).

The inflammatory changes of Buerger disease are present in both arteries and veins; early pathologic findings include fibrous intimal thickening with microabscess formation and a neutrophillic infiltrate of both the occluding thrombus and vessel wall. Late findings include thrombus organization with a predominantly mononuclear infiltrate including multinucleated giant cells (114,116). Vessel wall necrosis, characteristic of the true arteritides, is conspicuously absent (110,111).

Despite its association with smoking, the cause of Buerger disease remains enigmatic. A relation to some human lymphocyte antigen (HLA) determinants has been noted, and circulating immune complexes have been reported (114). A variety of coagulation abnormalities, including increased UK release, decreased plasminogen activator inhibitor-1 release, and an increased platelet response to serotonin, have also been demonstrated (114). Regardless of the mechanism, the treatment of Buerger disease requires absolute abstinence from tobacco. Management adjuncts have included antiplatelet agents, hemorrheological drugs, prostaglandins, sympathectomy, and arterial reconstruction in rare cases when feasible (110–116). Despite these measures, major lower extremity amputation ultimately is required in up to 30% of patients.

Aneurysms of the popliteal artery, defined as an arterial diameter greater than 2 cm or greater than 1.5 times normal, may be associated with both acute and chronic limb ischemia. Most popliteal aneurysms arise from arterial dilating disorders often associated with atherosclerosis, with trauma, infection, and popliteal entrapment being rare causes (117). Aneurysms of the popliteal artery are second in frequency only to those involving the abdominal aorta, are bilateral in approximately 50% of

patients, and are associated with aortic aneurysms in 32% to 37% of patients (118,119). Although rupture is a rare complication (120), acute thrombosis may result in limb-threatening ischemia, whereas chronic thrombosis and distal embolization may lead to blue toe syndrome, progressive occlusion of the tibial-peroneal arteries, and chronic limb ischemia. In reviewing 1,673 patients with 2,445 popliteal aneurysms, Dawson et al. (119) reported a mean thromboembolic complication rate of 35% and a mean amputation rate of 25%. By life table analysis, the cumulative incidence of complications increases from 24% at 1 year to 68% at 5 years (121).

Symptomatic popliteal aneurysms require operative repair, usually consisting of a saphenous vein bypass graft with proximal and distal ligation of the aneurysm. If compression symptoms (nerve or vein) exist, the aneurysm should be decompressed at the time of bypass. Because the tibial outflow bed is an important determinant of outcome, intraarterial thrombolytic therapy may be a useful adjunct in patients with acute thromboembolic occlusion of the tibial-peroneal arteries (122,123). Although routine surgical management of asymptomatic aneurysms has been questioned (124), most authorities agree that the risk of complications warrants surgical rather than expectant management (117,119,120). Assuming the patient has autogenous vein for reconstruction and is a reasonable operative risk, surgical repair substantially minimizes the risk to the limb and reduces the risk of postoperative complications following emergent repair, which is reported as high as 36% (117). The 6% 1-year and 49% 10-year incidence of new aortic or peripheral aneurysms requires that all patients receive lifelong follow-up (121).

Ischemic symptoms, particularly claudication, in the young patient should raise the suspicion of adventitial cystic disease or popliteal entrapment syndrome. Although the etiology remains unclear, adventitial cystic disease likely results from the developmental inclusion of mucin-secreting cells within the arterial wall (125). The subsequent development of an adventitial cyst narrows or occludes the arterial lumen. It is hypothesized that this occurs as the fetal axial arteries are involuting and new nonaxial arteries are forming from plexiform networks in close proximity to the condensing mesenchyme of adjacent joints (126). Most symptomatic patients present with intermittent claudication. Although the popliteal artery is most frequently involved, disease of the iliofemoral, brachial, radial, and ulnar arteries, as well as the venous system, has been reported (126,127). This is classically associated with either a scimitar sign or hourglass narrowing of the artery at arteriography and is treated either by cyst excision with arterial preservation or more effectively with arterial resection and interposition vein grafting.

The popliteal entrapment syndromes result from an aberrant relation between the popliteal artery and gastrocnemius or popliteus muscles and are bilateral in 25% of cases. Several classification systems have been proposed, with medial deviation of the popliteal artery around a normally positioned medial head of the gastrocnemius being the most common variant (125). Although most descriptions have included an abnormal relation between the medial head of the gastrocnemius and the popliteal artery, arterial compression in an otherwise normal popliteal fossa has also been described in athletic individuals (128). Such compression is demonstrated by loss of peripheral pulses and arteriographic or ultrasound evidence of medial arterial deviation and compression on passive dorsiflexion or active plantarflexion of the foot. The repetitive trauma of compression may culminate in focal arterial disease and thrombosis, poststenotic dilatation and aneurysm formation, or distal embolization (129).

Although heterogeneous, the arteritides are collectively characterized by inflammatory destruction of the vascular wall. Such inflammation may be localized to an arterial segment or be a consequence of systemic disease. Among these, Takayasu arteritis typically involves the aorta and brachiocephalic arteries but may occasionally affect the arteries of the lower limb (130). The disease is characterized histologically by transmural granulomatous inflammation with disruption of the medial elastic lamina.

---

## Treatment of Chronic Arterial Occlusive Disease

The goals in treating peripheral arterial occlusive disease include reducing the morbidity of associated cardiovascular and cerebrovascular disease, improving walking distance, preventing limb loss, slowing the progression of atherosclerosis, and restoring perfusion in patients with disabling intermittent claudication and critical limb ischemia. Mild symptoms generally require no intervention but should be managed with lifestyle and risk factor modification. Relative indications for intervention include disabling claudication that impacts the patient's lifestyle or ability to work in a patient who accepts the potential complications of the proposed procedure. The development of rest pain or tissue loss demands that revascularization be considered in most patients. Intermittent claudication is patient-dependent because the functional limitations of equivalent degrees of claudication may be substantially different in a young, employed patient than in a retiree. Although symptoms may not substantially limit the retiree, as many as 40% of patients younger than 55 years with claudication are unable to work (107). Depending on the severity of manifestations, distribution of disease, and comorbid medical problems, management options must include smoking cessation and an exercise program in addition to various pharmacologic adjuncts, percutaneous transluminal angioplasty (PTA), and operative revascularization.

### Operative Revascularization

As suggested by the reasonably benign natural history of intermittent claudication and the acceptable results of medical management, the role of surgical or endovascular intervention in the treatment of intermittent claudication remains limited. However, surgical reconstruction should be considered in the patient whose employment or lifestyle is substantially limited. Despite the favorable response to nonoperative therapy, randomized trials suggest significantly larger increases in symptom-free and maximal walking distance after surgical reconstruction (98). Among 75 patients with intermittent claudication randomized to bypass, bypass with physical training, or physical training alone, symptom-free walking distance improved to 600 m or more in 30%, 55%, and 5% of patients, respectively, and maximal walking distance improved to 600 m or more in 45%, 70%, and 30%. Outcome analysis that is based upon quality of life assessment is limited, although early data suggest a greater utility for suprainguinal than infrainguinal reconstruction in the management of intermittent claudication (131).

The role of vascular reconstruction in the critically ischemic limb with rest pain or tissue loss is well established (132). Although most such patients have multiple comorbid medical conditions, the risks associated with modern vascular reconstruction are often less than those associated with primary amputation. Population-based studies suggest that in comparison with primary amputation, revascularization of a critically ischemic limb is less expensive, has lower mortality, increased long-term survival rate, and shorter duration of hospitalization, and results in fewer patients requiring long-term institutional care (100,132,133). As might be anticipated, quality of life in patients with critical limb ischemia has also been noted to improve after arterial reconstruction for critical limb ischemia, but not after major amputation (105). Amputation is clearly associated with deterioration in quality of life (134), and young atherosclerotic amputees may fare as poorly as the elderly. Therefore, there are few medical contraindications to revascularization for

limb salvage other than the nonambulatory patient for whom salvage confers no advantage over amputation.

An appreciation of the distribution of disease is critical in planning surgical reconstruction of the ischemic limb. Atherosclerotic disease of the lower extremities is segmental, tending to occur at arterial bifurcations and in areas of posterior fixation or acute angulation, and is often bilateral (135). The segmental predilection of disease, the well-characterized patterns of collateral circulation, and the reconstructive options available allow division of atherosclerotic lesions of the lower extremities into those affecting the aortoiliac, femoropopliteal, and infrapopliteal arterial segments. The SFA, particularly at the adductor hiatus, is the most common site of symptomatic disease (15). The distribution of atherosclerosis in patients with diabetes differs in several respects, tending to involve the profunda femoris, popliteal, and tibial arteries with relative sparing of the aorta and iliac arteries (136).

Surgical revascularization demands attention to several basic principles. Successful reconstruction requires unobstructed arterial inflow with outflow adequate to maintain patency and provide effective distal perfusion. In the presence of multilevel disease, typical in patients considered for revascularization, the most proximal lesion must be addressed prior to distal reconstruction. A combination of percutaneous and surgical techniques can often be used to meet these requirements, especially if the proximal lesion is segmental and stenotic. The choice of operation is dictated by the arteriographic findings.

Options for surgical reconstruction include endarterectomy or bypass of an obstructed segment using an autogenous or a prosthetic conduit. Endarterectomy is suitable for focal atherosclerotic lesions and involves removal of the plaque using a naturally occurring plane, usually the external elastic lamina (Fig. 101-5). This technique relies on atherosclerosis being localized to the intima and inner media, sparing the outer media and adventitia. Endarterectomy is not suitable for extensive lesions, for which bypass is more appropriate. For bypass procedures, the choice of conduit is determined both by the anatomic distribution of disease and the availability of autogenous vein.

Aortoiliac disease may be focal or diffuse, with or without associated infrainguinal disease. Localized disease is less common, accounting for only 10% of surgical candidates, has an equal sex distribution, and includes patients who are characteristically younger with a high prevalence of type IV hyperlipidemia (93). Diffuse aortoiliac disease is more common, with multilevel disease being the most common pattern. Although aortoiliac endarterectomy is suitable for patients with localized disease and is a reasonable option with iliofemoral disease in men and in women with large arteries, these procedures largely have been replaced by balloon angioplasty and stenting. More extensive disease of the aortoiliac segment is treated with bypass techniques, which most frequently involve prosthetic graft conduits placed between the infrarenal aorta and femoral arteries, although extraanatomic approaches using axillary–bifemoral or femoral–femoral grafts may be appropriate for the high-risk patient, those treated for aortic graft infection, and in patients considered to have a "hostile abdomen." Extraanatomic grafts are tunneled subcutaneously through remote tissue planes, avoiding the requirement for transcavitary abdominal or retroperitoneal exposure. Aortoiliac reconstruction is associated with mortality rates as low as 1% to 2% in experienced centers treating reasonable risk patients, with 5-year patency rates of 85% to 90% (93,137). The results of extraanatomic grafts are less favorable, although patency has improved with the development of externally supported prosthetic grafts. Unilateral iliofemoral reconstruction is an excellent procedure when the ipsilateral common or external iliac artery can be used for inflow. It is associated with minimal operative morbidity and has 72% to 90% 4-year patency rates (138).

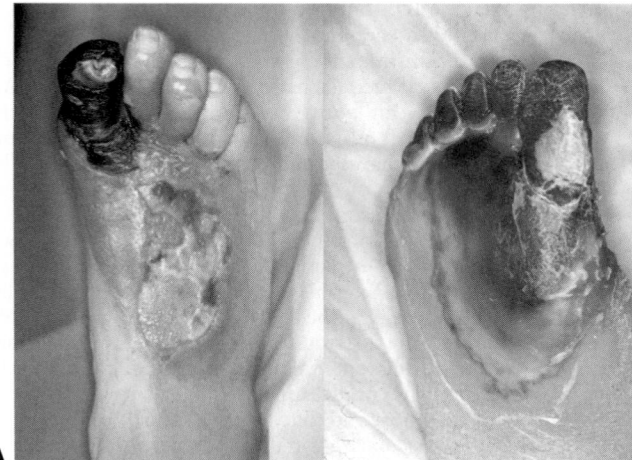
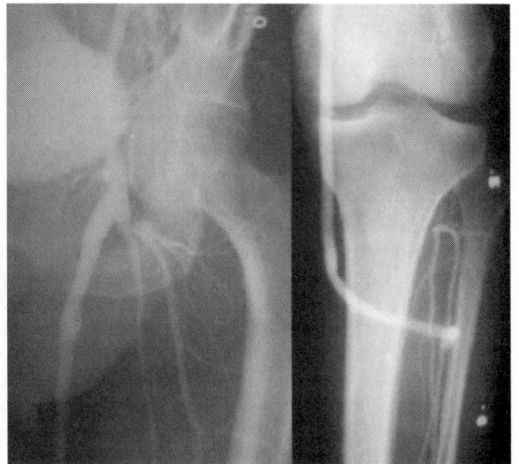

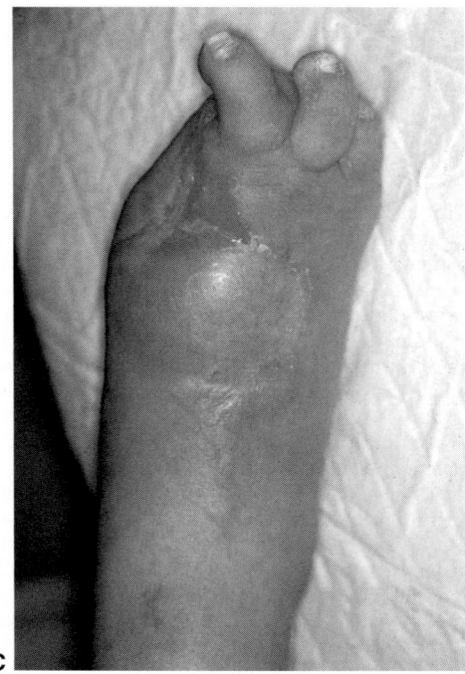

**FIGURE 101-6.** Femoral–tibial bypass for critical limb ischemia. Advanced gangrenous changes of a patient's foot due to multilevel infrainguinal arterial occlusive disease with poor profunda collateral flow (photo taken 5 days following revascularization; note pink foot with demarcation developing between healthy tissue and necrotic tissue) (**A**). **B:** Completion arteriogram shows a patent femoral–anterior tibial bypass using autogenous vein with the *in situ* technique. **C:** Clinical outcome following revascularization and eventual amputation of necrotic toes; patient ambulates normally with shoe prosthesis (see Color Fig. 101-6).

Patency rates for femoral–femoral bypasses range from 40% to 80% and axillofemoral bypasses from 30% to 70% at 5 years. Outcome depends on patient selection, quality of inflow and outflow, size of conduit, and postoperative management.

Although endarterectomy may be appropriate for focal lesions of the common femoral or profunda femoris arteries, infrainguinal occlusive disease is most often treated with bypass grafts to the popliteal or tibial arteries (see Fig. 101-6). Graft patency rates for infrainguinal reconstruction depend on the type of conduit. If prosthetic grafts are used, the site of distal anastomosis significantly impacts patency, decreasing substantially the more distal the anastomosis. For femoropopliteal bypass grafting, the most often used conduits include the great saphenous vein and prosthetic grafts such as expanded polytetrafluoroethylene (PTFE), Dacron, or umbilical vein. The

most favorable results have been achieved using the great saphenous vein, with 5-year primary patency rates as high as 88% for bypasses to the popliteal artery (104). Even in the above-knee popliteal position, randomized trial results have shown significantly better 5-year patency rates with autogenous vein (76%) compared to PTFE (52%) (139). A prior randomized trial demonstrated a similar difference, although because of the small number of patients, the benefit of autogenous vein did not quite reach statistical significance (140). Other studies have documented inferior 3- to 5-year patencies for PTFE (40% to 50%) in comparison to autologous vein (60% to 80%) in the above-knee popliteal position (141). Decision analysis suggests that in comparison to a prosthetic conduit, initial use of autogenous vein in above-knee femoropopliteal bypass is associated with higher amputation-free survival and

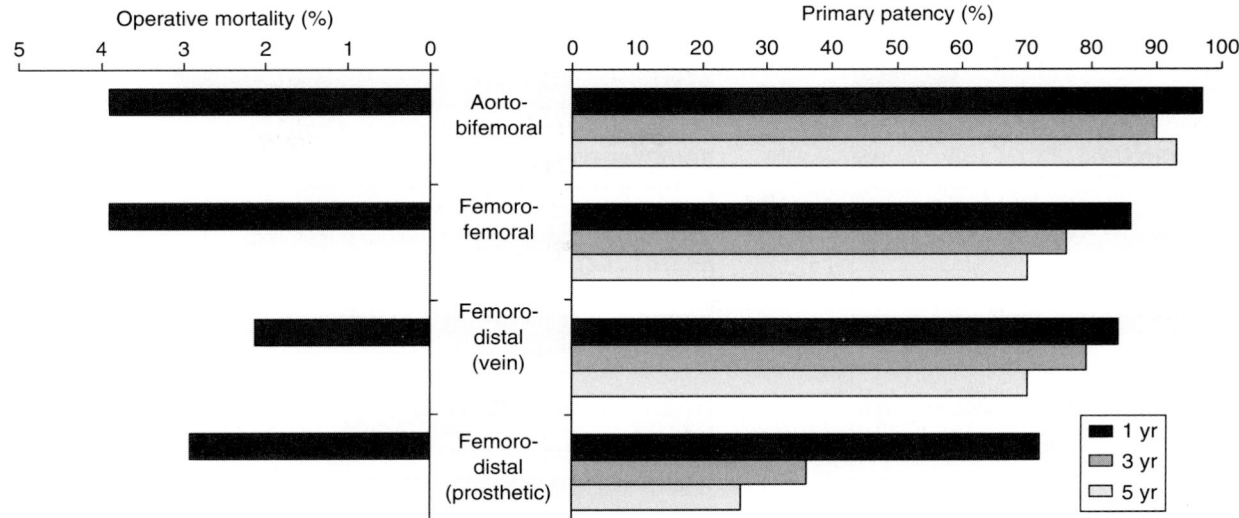

**FIGURE 101-7.** Cumulative results of surgical treatment of peripheral arterial disease (PAD) by level of reconstruction and conduit. Only studies with greater than 50% of patients treated with critical limb ischemia are included. Adapted from TASC Working Group. Management of peripheral arterial disease (PAD). *J Vasc Surg* 2000;31:S138. Used with permission.

lower requirements for subsequent operation (141). Limb salvage rates always exceed patency rates because an ischemic lesion may remain healed despite graft occlusion. Limb salvage is greater than 90% for autogenous femoropopliteal grafts. Prosthetic conduits are significantly less suitable for reconstruction below the knee, with diminished 2-year patency rates for both below-knee popliteal (64% vs. 76%) and infrapopliteal (30% vs. 76%) bypasses in comparison to saphenous vein (140). The results for infrapopliteal saphenous vein grafts are only modestly worse than femoropopliteal reconstruction, with 4-year patency rates of 65% and limb salvage rates of 83% (142). Operative mortality after femoropopliteal bypass grafting has been reported to be 1% to 3%, with myocardial infarction being the most common cause of operative death (104,141) (see Fig. 101-7).

Despite the excellent results achieved by major centers, many opportunities exist to improve outcome and several approaches have been reported to increase the early and late patency of infrainguinal bypass grafts. Early postoperative failures, which account for less than 5% of graft occlusions, are largely due to technical problems with the reconstruction or poor patient selection (140,142). However, hypercoagulability also has been associated with a substantially increased risk of both early and late graft failure (106). Donaldson (143) found a variety of congenital or acquired hypercoagulable conditions in 14% of vascular surgical patients. Early graft occlusion occurred in 3 of 14 (27%) hypercoagulable patients undergoing reconstruction. Others (144) have noted hypercoagulable abnormalities in 35% of patients tested preoperatively, such abnormalities being three times more common among those sustaining graft occlusion within 1 year. Thrombophilic states were significantly more common in those sustaining an occlusion within 1 month (92%) than in those patients with later graft failure (25%). Among acquired hypercoagulable conditions, HIT and antiphospholipid antibodies are among the most common, occurring in association with 32% of occluded grafts but only 7% of patent grafts (143). The lupus anticoagulant has been particularly associated with early reconstruction failures (145), being seven times more common among those with graft occlusion and having

a positive predictive value of 67% for graft failure (144). Although the factor $V_{Leiden}$ mutation is primarily associated with venous thrombosis and has a prevalence among patients with arterial disease similar to control populations, it appears to be associated with an increased risk of late graft failure (143). At 47 months, graft failure has been noted in 60% of patients with resistance to activated protein C (factor $V_{Leiden}$) in comparison to 24% of patients without the marker (146). Anticoagulation is recommended for patients with known hypercoagulable abnormalities undergoing vascular reconstruction (144,145).

General anesthesia also has been associated with markers of hypercoagulability (147), with higher rates of cardiac complications, and with early graft failure compared to epidural anesthesia.

The long-term benefits of most revascularization procedures, whether endovascular or surgical, are limited by restenosis, which is most often due to intimal hyperplasia. Lower extremity bypass grafts are complicated by restenosis in 25% to 30% of cases (148). Late graft occlusion is less dependent on technical factors, with intimal hyperplasia being the most common cause of failure between 3 and 24 months postoperatively. Platelets play an important role in this process. Intimal hyperplasia results from the migration of smooth muscle cells into the intima with subsequent proliferation and elaboration of extracellular matrix (149–151). Migrating smooth muscle cells continue to express a synthetic phenotype for approximately 2 months after angioplasty injury (150). Graft patency beyond 2 years is influenced by progressive atherosclerosis (149).

Pharmacologic approaches to prevent restenosis have been most extensively investigated following coronary angioplasty and, with the exception of drug-eluting stents, few have proven clinically effective (148,150).

### Percutaneous Revascularization

Percutaneous procedures for PAD have become an increasingly important option as technology has advanced. The basic procedure of percutaneous intervention remains balloon dilation of the diseased vessel. The mechanism of balloon dilation

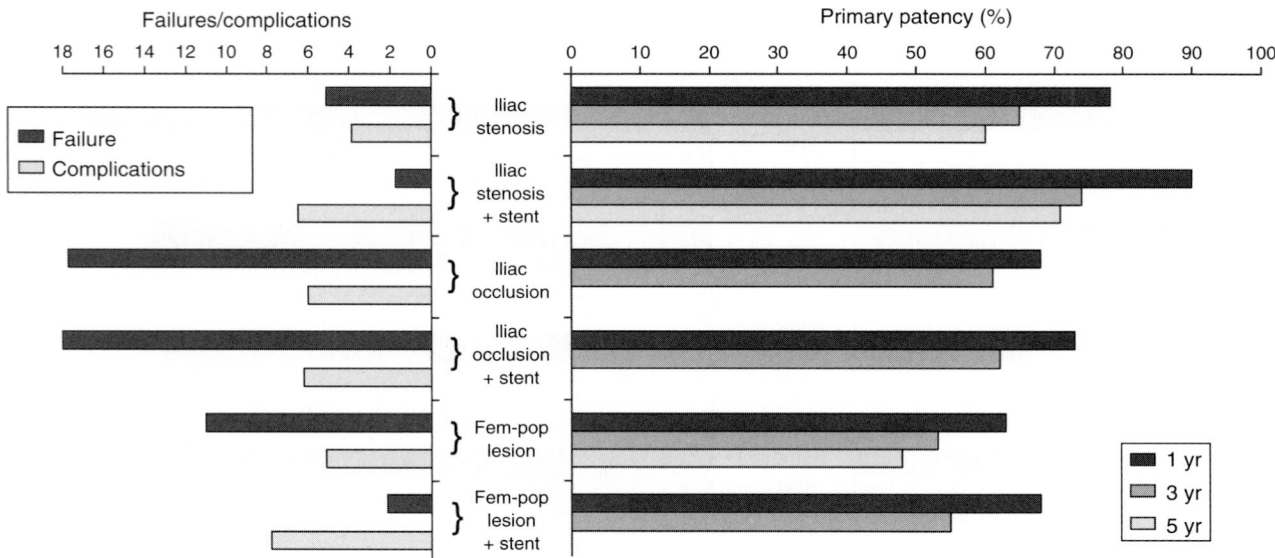

**FIGURE 101-8.** Cumulative results of endovascular treatment of peripheral arterial disease (PAD) by level. Most patients were treated for intermittent claudication. Adapted from TASC Working Group. Management of peripheral arterial disease (PAD). *J Vasc Surg* 2000;31:S138. Used with permission.

is well characterized and is associated with plaque fracture and medial dissection of the diseased arterial wall. The plaque is not simply compacted. In general, endovascular techniques are effective for lesser degrees of disease with milder symptoms, and operative reconstruction is more effective for extensive, limb-threatening disease. Patients who benefit from percutaneous procedures are most frequently afflicted with intermittent claudication, have a stenosis versus an occlusion, and have short-segment disease. Most patients who are offered operative revascularization have long-segment, often multisegment occlusive disease with more severe ischemia (see Fig. 101-8).

The utility and success of percutaneous procedures often depends upon the size of the artery and level of disease. Focal disease of the distal abdominal aorta and common iliac arteries appears to be well treated with aortoiliac PTA. The technical and initial clinical success rates of PTA of iliac stenoses in most series reported exceeds 90% and for focal iliac lesions approaches 100%. The technical success rates for iliac occlusions drop to approximately 85%; however, once an iliac artery occlusion has been successfully recanalized, the patency rate does not appear to be different from that following treatment of a stenosis (152–155). However, complications tend to be higher after PTA and stenting of occlusions (6%) than after treatment of stenotic lesions (3.6%) (156). Long-term patency rates in patients with intermittent claudication are approximately 80% at 12 months and 60% at 5 years.

An important question regarding the percutaneous management of common iliac artery disease was addressed by the Dutch iliac stent trial (23). These investigators compared primary stent placement versus primary balloon angioplasty followed by selective stenting. The indication for stenting in the "selective stenting" cohort was a pressure gradient of 10 mm Hg or more following PTA. Two-hundred and eighty-six patients were studied in this trial, and technical success was achieved in 279 (97.5%). At 2 years, the clinical success rates were 78% in the stent group versus 76% in the selective stent group. The hemodynamic success rate, as determined by the ABI, was 85% in both groups. Patency rates as determined by arterial duplex

were 71% in the primary stent versus 70% in the PTA plus stent group. This study demonstrates that selective stenting offers equivalent effectiveness and much less cost than primary stenting in the management of focal iliac artery occlusive disease in patients with intermittent claudication. Unfortunately, this information has escaped the attention of most interventionalists, and primary stenting appears to be the rule today rather than primary angioplasty with selective stenting.

The level of involvement of iliac artery disease and the patient's gender have a considerable impact on outcome. In a study of 189 patients undergoing iliac angioplasty and stenting, Timaran et al. (157) demonstrated a significant reduction in primary stent patency in the external iliac arteries compared to common iliac artery lesions. These investigators also demonstrated significantly reduced patencies in women compared to men. In their stratified analysis, women with external iliac artery stents had 1-year patencies of 61%, 3-year patencies of 47%, and a 5-year patency of only 23%.

Percutaneous recanalization of the femoropopliteal and infrapopliteal arteries has not enjoyed the same success rates as the iliac arteries. A review of the literature during the past 15 years reveals a relatively consistent observation that the primary patencies of SFA PTA at 1, 3, and 5 years are approximately 60%, 50%, and 45%, respectively (156). This is oversimplified because individual risk factors such as lesion length, occlusion versus stenosis, quality of outflow, medical comorbidities, and adjunctive pharmacotherapy all influence an individual patient's outcome.

The relative role of stenting in the femoropopliteal and infrapopliteal arteries is under active investigation. A randomized trial of PTA alone compared with PTA and stenting (using a Palmaz stent) was performed by Cejna et al. (158). The early success rate was better in the stented patients (98.7%) than in those with PTA alone (87.1%). However, at 6, 12, and 24 months, there was no difference between the two groups. The primary patency rates for stented patients were 86%, 63%, and 58% versus 79%, 64%, and 53% in the PTA patients at the 6-, 12-, and 24-month time points, respectively. Therefore, enthusiasm for stenting the femoropopliteal segment has been dampened. Although the procedural success rate appeared improved, overall results were no different from those for primary angioplasty.

A new enthusiasm for stenting has arisen with the observation that stent materials may affect vessel patency, and nitinol appears better suited for the endovascular application because of its improved hemocompatibility as compared to stainless steel (159). Preliminary observations in a limited clinical experience with the new generation of nitinol stents used in the femoropopliteal segment appear encouraging. Three reports have documented favorable patency results. Two have reported 12- and 18-month patency rates of 86% and 85%, respectively (160,161), and a third documented a 3-year primary patency rate of 76% (162). It should be kept in mind that these results were obtained treating relatively short lesions (≤4.5 cm) in each of the three studies.

Although it was anticipated that covered stents would do at least as well as prosthetic infrainguinal bypasses, experiences with balloon-mounted PTFE stent-grafts and Dacron-covered stents have been disappointing, each showing a 1-year primary patency rate of 29% and 23%, respectively (163,164) (Fig. 101-8).

A technique gaining increasing popularity is subintimal angioplasty of femoropopliteal and infrapopliteal occlusions (165–168). This technique involves the penetration of the plaque by the guidewire and advancing the guidewire distally through the media of the blood vessel wall. Reentry into the lumen below the occlusion is the key to success (see Fig. 101-9). Subsequent balloon angioplasty of the extraluminal channel often results in an adequate lumen and satisfactory flow through the treated segment. Interestingly, there appears to be no significant difference in the ability to recanalize a short- or a long-segment occlusion. Reentry into the distal lumen appears to be the major limiting factor of this procedure. Many reports involve patients with limb-threatening ischemia and, as such, cannot be directly compared to standard transluminal balloon angioplasty and/or stenting. Nydahl et al. (167) reported their results of subintimal angioplasty of infrapopliteal occlusions in 28 critically ischemic limbs. The 12-month patency was 56%, and the limb salvage rate was 85%.

Drug-eluting stents have generated significant enthusiasm for the management of patients with coronary artery disease. Although a large number of therapeutic agents have been tested in animal models, predominantly to prevent neointimal hyperplasia, few have been used in humans. Sirolimus is a potent immunosuppressive agent generally used for the management of renal transplant rejection. It functions by diffusing into smooth muscle cells and binding to intracellular receptor proteins which inhibit signal transduction kinase complexes, resulting in inhibition of cellular proliferation by inducing cell cycle arrest in the late G1 phase. Sirolimus bonded to stents demonstrated reduction of intimal thickening in animal models of vascular injury (169). Human trials have demonstrated significant reduction of in-stent restenosis at 6 months when used for coronary artery disease (170,171).

There is limited experience with drug-eluting stents in the peripheral arterial circulation, specifically the infrainguinal arterial system. The Sirocco study randomized 36 patients with SFA lesions (median length 85 mm) to treatment with the sirolimus-coated shape memory alloy recoverable technology (SMART) stent (Cordis) or a bare SMART stent (172). Although there was a reduction of restenosis in the sirolimus-eluting SMART stents, the 6-month results did not reach significance. Owing to the variability of disease distribution and multiple other factors affecting the success rates of intervention in the infrainguinal arterial system, there appears to be relatively little enthusiasm from the manufacturers in pursuing the use of drug-eluting stents in

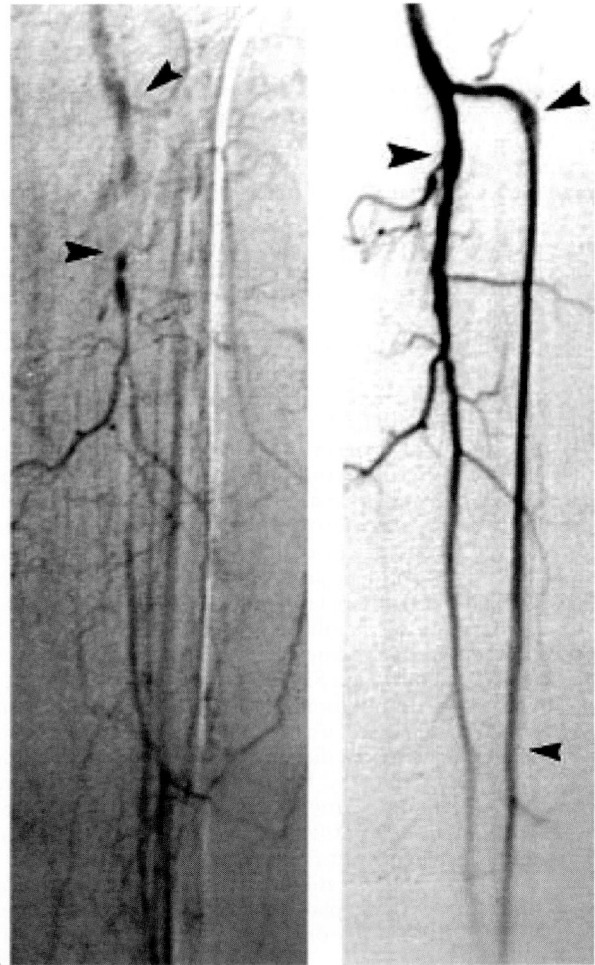

**FIGURE 101-9. A:** Arteriogram of a patient with ischemic rest pain and a chronic, nonhealing ischemic ulcer. Autogenous vein was not available for operative revascularization. A subintimal angioplasty was performed with excellent reperfusion (**B**), relief of rest pain, and healing of the ischemic ulcer.

the peripheral vascular bed compared to the coronary circulation. Other techniques, such as brachytherapy, cryoplasty, cutting balloon technology, and eximer laser angioplasty, are also being used. Most of these techniques are reported in anecdotal fashion. Proper application may yield patient benefit; however, generalizations regarding the efficacy of these techniques cannot be stated.

Pharmacotherapeutic adjuncts have been used to improve the durability of endovascular procedures. Platelet inhibition has been accepted as an important basic treatment for all patients. Combined platelet inhibition with aspirin (ASA) and clopidogrel is used frequently because of its efficacy observed following percutaneous coronary intervention (173). Long-term anticoagulation has not been shown to be beneficial. Platelet glycoprotein IIb/IIIa receptor blockers have been shown to be beneficial for acute coronary intervention (174,175), although their role in preventing restenosis after vascular intervention is unknown. There is increasing enthusiasm for the use of direct thrombin inhibitors such as bivalirudin in addition to or in place of heparin during endovascular procedures (176,177). This potentially important adjunct requires further study.

## Pharmacotherapy Following Infrainguinal Surgical Revascularization

Vascular surgeons have pushed the technical limits of revascularization procedures. Using magnification, autogenous material, ultrafine sutures, and improved techniques of dissection, most technical hurdles of revascularization have been overcome. However, the important question remains: Following a technically successful bypass, can anything more be done to preserve patency? Although this remains an area of some controversy, there is increasing consensus regarding appropriate pharmacotherapy before, during, and following infrainguinal revascularization.

The most recent Alliance for Cervical Cancer Prevention (ACCP) guidelines recommend platelet inhibition for all patients undergoing femoropopliteal prosthetic bypass grafts (178). In a randomized trial, Goldman et al. (179) found that patients treated with aspirin plus dipyridamole had significantly less platelet deposition on prosthetic grafts. That patients having saphenous vein bypass had very little platelet deposition, even in the control group, is a tribute to the value and decreased thrombogenicity of autogenous reconstruction. Reduced early platelet deposition translates into better patency, as demonstrated by Green et al. (180) when they showed that platelet inhibition significantly improved the patency of prosthetic femoral above-knee popliteal bypass grafts compared to placebo. Although Kohler et al. (181) failed to show benefit with platelet inhibition versus placebo in patients undergoing infrainguinal reconstruction, their patients randomized to platelet inhibition did not receive their medications until 5 days postoperatively. Clyne et al. (182) demonstrated the importance of preoperative dosing by showing once again that platelet inhibition improved the patency rates in prosthetic infrainguinal bypass grafts.

In a different subset of patients, Findlay et al. (183) demonstrated that preoperative platelet inhibition significantly reduced platelet deposition on carotid endarterectomy sites compared to placebo. The importance of preoperative administration of platelet inhibitors is illustrated by these prospective studies.

The intraoperative use of dextran-40, a high-molecular-weight polysaccharide with antifactor V and VIII, antiplatelet, and rheolytic effects, was shown to decrease early graft failure in patients undergoing difficult lower extremity bypasses (184). Patients undergoing prosthetic bypasses showed improved patency, whereas those undergoing autogenous bypass had inherently high patency rates and failed to show benefit (184,185).

A prospective blinded trial demonstrated that the adenosine diphosphate (ADP)-receptor blocker ticlopidine was significantly better than placebo in prolonging the 24-month patency of lower extremity saphenous vein bypass grafts (186). Unfortunately, data are not available comparing ADP-receptor blockers to aspirin, a cyclooxygenase inhibitor.

A large metaanalysis of 1,219 patients from 11 studies, performed by the Antiplatelet Trialists' Collaborative (187), demonstrated a 38% odds reduction of graft occlusion if patients received platelet inhibition. The observations from multiple trials have demonstrated that preoperative dosing of platelet inhibitors is important because they reduce platelet deposition on prosthetic grafts and sites of arteries with endothelial disruption. There appears to be particular benefit in patients having prosthetic revascularization, although similar benefit in patients undergoing saphenous vein bypass was observed with ticlopidine.

A somewhat more controversial topic is the use of anticoagulation following lower extremity bypasses. Kretschmer et al. (188) reported their initial observations in 88 patients undergoing saphenous vein femoropopliteal bypass who were randomized to received warfarin or placebo. In a median follow-up of 30 months, there were significantly better patency rates in patients receiving warfarin. A 10-year follow-up study of 130 patients demonstrated significantly better patency rates, limb salvage, and survival of patients receiving warfarin compared to controls (189).

A number of investigators have studied the comparison of anticoagulation versus platelet inhibition in patients undergoing femoropopliteal bypass. Edmondson et al. (190) randomized patients to 3 months of therapy with aspirin and dipyridamole versus fragmin 2,500 International Units (IU) daily for 3 months. Patency at 12 months was significantly greater in patients receiving low-molecular-weight heparin. Interestingly, the benefit was observed in patients undergoing limb salvage procedure versus those operated for claudication.

Several investigators have studied aspirin alone versus the combination of warfarin plus aspirin in patients undergoing lower extremity bypasses. In a single-center study, Sarac et al. (191) randomized patients undergoing lower extremity saphenous vein bypass to aspirin 325 mg plus warfarin [international normalized ratio (INR) 2.0 to 3.0] versus aspiring 325 mg alone. The 3-year patency rate and limb salvage rate was significantly better in patients randomized to warfarin plus aspirin versus aspirin alone. As might be expected, the postoperative hematoma rate was significantly higher in patients receiving the combination of warfarin plus aspirin (32% vs. 3.7%; $P = 0.004$).

Tangelder et al. (192) performed a metaanalysis of aspirin and anticoagulation to prevent graft occlusion. As a result of existing data, and as a prelude to a large randomized trial, they concluded that platelet inhibition and oral anticoagulants reduce the risk of graft occlusion. Platelet inhibition versus placebo had a relative risk reduction of 22%, oral anticoagulation versus placebo a relative risk reduction of 44%, and oral anticoagulation plus aspirin versus aspirin alone a relative risk reduction of 62%. Shortly thereafter, the Dutch bypass oral anticoagulants or aspirin study was published (193). This was a large prospective multicenter trial of 2,690 patients undergoing infrainguinal bypass procedures, 58% with autogenous vein and 42% with a prosthetic bypass. Although patients were randomized to either aspirin (80 mg daily) or warfarin (INR 3.0 to 4.5) *preoperatively*, treatment was not started until 5 days *postoperatively*; consequently, the benefit of preoperative and intraoperative treatment was lost. The primary outcome was graft occlusion. The primary outcome at 21 months (mean) showed no difference between the treatment groups. However, it is emphasized that the treatment began 5 days postoperatively.

Secondary outcomes in this large trial demonstrated a significant interaction of graft material on outcome and treatment effect ($P = 0.002$). Vein grafts had significantly better patency rates than prosthetic grafts. As previously observed, anticoagulants improved the patency rates of vein grafts and aspirin improved the patency rates of prosthetic grafts.

Jackson et al. (194) randomized 402 patients undergoing femoropopliteal bypass grafts, 233 with PTFE and 169 with vein. The patients were randomized to warfarin (INR 1.4 to 2.8) plus aspirin (325 mg per day) versus aspirin (325 mg per day) alone. The endpoints were patency and the grade of ischemia following occlusion of the bypass. The resulting patency rates are categorized by graft type and treatment in Figure 101-10. They demonstrated vein bypasses had significantly better patency rates than prosthetic and that most patients who thrombosed were receiving aspirin alone compared to warfarin plus ASA. Additionally, 50% of all patients with occluded PTFE bypasses performed for intermittent claudication developed critical ischemia at the time of bypass graft occlusion compared to 0% of vein grafts. The combination

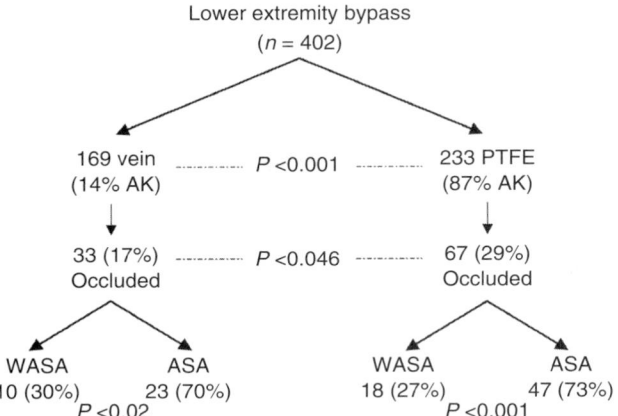

Lower extremity bypass
(*n* = 402)

169 vein          ------ *P* <0.001 ------          233 PTFE
(14% AK)                                            (87% AK)

33 (17%)          ------ *P* <0.046 ------          67 (29%)
Occluded                                            Occluded

WASA        ASA                          WASA        ASA
10 (30%)    23 (70%)                      18 (27%)    47 (73%)
    *P* <0.02                                 *P* <0.001

**FIGURE 101-10.** Outcomes of femoral–popliteal bypasses randomized to aspirin versus warfarin plus aspirin. Of the occluded vein bypasses, 30% were treated with warfarin plus aspirin (WASA) and 70% treated with aspirin alone (*P* <0.02). In the occluded polytetrafluorethylene (PTFE) bypass patients, 27% were treated with WASA and 73% with aspirin alone (*P* <0.001). ASA, aspirin.

of warfarin plus aspirin protected PTFE-grafted patients from severe ischemia at the time of occlusion (20% vs. 50%; *P* <0.05).

In summary, preoperative platelet inhibition is important because it reduces platelet deposition on prosthetic bypasses and areas of arterial wall injury, which results in improved patency of prosthetic bypass grafts. Intraoperative dextran is beneficial, especially in difficult infrainguinal bypasses. Combined platelet inhibition with aspirin and clopidogrel is being used with increased frequency by vascular surgeons due to the observed benefits following coronary intervention (PCI-cure); however, specific data regarding improved patency following lower extremity bypass are lacking.

Anticoagulation with warfarin combined with aspirin improves the patency of both prosthetic and vein bypasses. Improved patency of saphenous grafts with the platelet ADP-receptor blocker ticlopidine was found in one prospective study, suggesting that there may be a difference in outcome

between platelet inhibitors, depending on their mechanism of action. Unfortunately, to date there are no data available evaluating clopidogrel, either alone or in combination with aspirin. Low-molecular-weight heparin also improves patency; however, its cost, risk of osteoporosis, and need for injection makes this an unrealistic form of long-term therapy.

## SUMMARY

Although less frequent than symptomatic coronary or cerebrovascular disease, lower extremity ischemia is a significant cause of cardiovascular morbidity. Appropriate management of patients with arterial occlusive disease depends upon it being diagnosed and then defining the degree and duration of ischemia based on clinical evaluation, which includes the noninvasive determination of lower extremity perfusion. Although contrast arteriography remains the standard for evaluation of patients requiring intervention, more sophisticated noninvasive modalities such as duplex ultrasonography and MRA have an increasingly important role. Limb salvage in patients with acute limb ischemia depends upon prompt recognition of the degree of ischemia, early anticoagulation, and prompt surgical or thrombolytic reperfusion of threatened limbs.

An appreciation of the natural history of chronic peripheral arterial occlusive disease, as well as an understanding of the limitations of all existing interventions, is critical in the management of chronic limb ischemia. Mild symptoms of chronic ischemia, such as claudication, often can be managed with exercise and appropriate risk factor modification. Surgical reconstruction remains the gold standard for more advanced ischemia, although a variety of alternative interventions such as balloon angioplasty, stenting, and thrombolytic therapy are available.

Endovascular techniques are becoming more effective; however, complications and short-term failures occur. Therefore, these interventions should be judiciously offered to patients (see Fig. 101-11). Pharmacologic adjuncts are appropriate in selected patients, although the durability of all interventions remains limited by restenosis and progressive atherosclerosis. Further advances in vascular reconstruction await an improved understanding of these phenomena and pharmacologic control of the vascular injury response

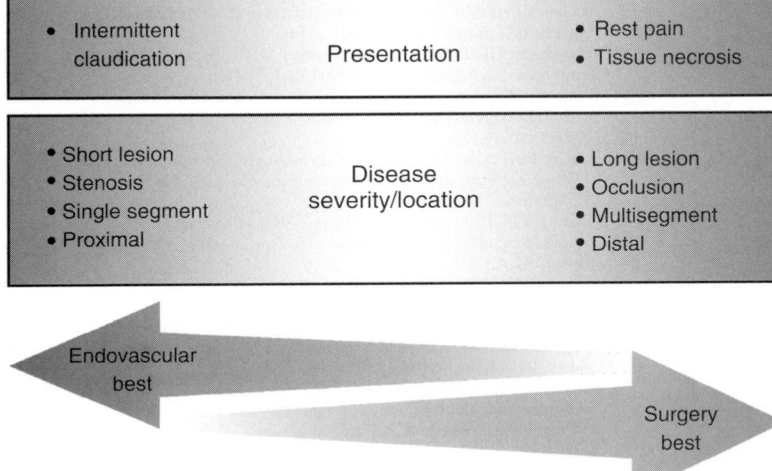

Management of peripheral arterial disease

- Intermittent claudication    Presentation    - Rest pain
                                               - Tissue necrosis

- Short lesion                 Disease         - Long lesion
- Stenosis                     severity/location - Occlusion
- Single segment                               - Multisegment
- Proximal                                     - Distal

Endovascular best

Surgery best

**FIGURE 101-11.** Schematic diagram of the relative roles of endovascular and surgical reconstruction for peripheral arterial disease (PAD).

at the cellular level. Unfortunately, despite improvements in the management of lower extremity ischemia, long-term prognosis for patients remains poor due to their large burden of systemic atherosclerosis.

# ACKNOWLEDGMENTS

Grateful appreciation to Marilyn Gravett for her editorial assistance and Victor Cantu for computer graphics.

## *References*

1. May AG, Van De Berg L, DeWeese JA, et al. Critical arterial stenosis. *Surgery* 1963;54:250–259.
2. May AG, De Weese JA, ROB CG. Hemodynamic effects of arterial stenosis. *Surgery* 1963;53:513–524.
3. Sumner DS. Essential hemodynamic principles. In: Rutherford RB, ed. *Vascular surgery*. Philadelphia, PA: WB Saunders, 2000:73–119.
4. Lundin M, Wiksten JP, Perakyla T, et al. Distal pulse palpation: is it reliable? *World J Surg* 1999;23:252–255.
5. Strandness DE Jr. Traditional methods of patient evaluation. In: Strandness DE Jr, ed. *Duplex scanning in vascular disorders*. New York: Raven Press, 1990.
6. Carter SA. Clinical measurement of systolic pressures in limbs with arterial occlusive disease. *JAMA* 1969;207:1869–1874.
7. Rutherford RB, Baker JD, Ernst C, et al. Recommended standards for reports dealing with lower extremity ischemia: revised version. *J Vasc Surg* 1997;26:517–538.
8. Sumner DS, Strandness DE Jr. The relationship between calf blood flow and ankle blood pressure in patients with intermittent claudication. *Surgery* 1969;65:763–771.
9. Strandness DE Jr. Peripheral arterial system. In: Strandness DE Jr, ed. *Duplex scanning in vascular disorders*. New York: Raven Press, 1990.
10. Kempczinski RF. The differential diagnosis of intermittent claudication. *Practical Cardiol* 1981;7:53.
11. Cronenwett JL, Warner KG, Zelenock GB, et al. Intermittent claudication. Current results of nonoperative management. *Arch Surg* 1984;119: 430–436.
12. O'Riordain DS, O'Donnell JA. Realistic expectations for the patient with intermittent claudication. *Br J Surg* 1991;78:861–863.
13. Carter SA. Role of pressure measurements. In: Bernstein E, ed. *Vascular diagnosis*, 4th ed. St. Louis, MO: Mosby, 1993:486.
14. Second European Consensus Document on Chronic Critical Leg Ischemia. *Circulation* 1991;84:IV1–IV26.
15. Mannick JA. Current concepts in diagnostic methods. Evaluation of chronic lower-extremity ischemia. *N Engl J Med* 1983;309:841–843.
16. Reimer P, Landwehr P. Non-invasive vascular imaging of peripheral vessels. *Eur Radiol* 1998;8:858–872.
17. Ligush J Jr, Reavis SW, Preisser JS, et al. Duplex ultrasound scanning defines operative strategies for patients with limb-threatening ischemia. *J Vasc Surg* 1998;28:482–490.
18. Koelemay MJ, den HD, Prins MH, et al. Diagnosis of arterial disease of the lower extremities with duplex ultrasonography. *Br J Surg* 1996; 83: 404–409.
19. Schneider PA, Ogawa DY. Is routine preoperative aortoiliac arteriography necessary in the treatment of lower extremity ischemia? *J Vasc Surg* 1998; 28:28–34.
20. Ascer E, Pollina RM, Gennaro M, et al. Noninvasive predictors of patency for infrapopliteal PTFE bypasses with combined arteriovenous fistula and vein interposition technique. *Am J Surg* 1995;170:103–105.
21. Huber TS, Back MR, Ballinger RJ, et al. Utility of magnetic resonance arteriography for distal lower extremity revascularization. *J Vasc Surg* 1997;26:415–423.
22. Waugh JR, Sacharias N. Arteriographic complications in the DSA era. *Radiology* 1992;182:243–246.
23. Tetteroo E, Haaring C, van der GY et al. Dutch Iliac Stent Trial Study Group. Intraarterial pressure gradients after randomized angioplasty or stenting of iliac artery lesions. *Cardiovasc Intervent Radiol* 1996;19: 411–417.
24. Tetteroo E, van Engelen AD, Spithoven JH et al. Dutch Iliac Stent Trial Study Group. Stent placement after iliac angioplasty: comparison of hemodynamic and angiographic criteria. *Radiology* 1996;201:155–159.
25. Thiele BL, Strandness DE Jr. Accuracy of angiographic quantification of peripheral atherosclerosis. *Prog Cardiovasc Dis* 1983;26:223–236.
26. Velazquez OC, Baum RA, Carpenter JP. Magnetic resonance imaging and angiography. In: Rutherford RB, ed. *Vascular surgery*. Philadelphia, PA: WB Saunders, 2000:269–285.
27. Gilfeather M, Holland GA, Siegelman ES, et al. Gadolinium-enhanced ultrafast three-dimensional spoiled gradient-echo MR imaging of the abdominal aorta and visceral and iliac vessels. *Radiographics* 1997;17: 423–432.
28. Hoch JR, Tullis MJ, Kennell TW, et al. Use of magnetic resonance angiography for the preoperative evaluation of patients with infrainguinal arterial occlusive disease. *J Vasc Surg* 1996;23:792–800.
29. Schild HH, Kuhl CK. Contrast-enhanced magnetic resonance angiography. Potential applications and pitfalls in magnetic resonance angiography-guided therapy: a review. *Invest Radiol* 1998;33:524–527.
30. Velazquez OC, Baum RA, Carpenter JP. Magnetic resonance angiography of lower-extremity arterial disease. *Surg Clin North Am* 1998; 78: 519–537.
31. Earls JP, Patel NH, Smith PA, et al. Gadolinium-enhanced three-dimensional MR angiography of the aorta and peripheral arteries: evaluation of a multistation examination using two gadopentetate dimeglumine infusions. *AJR Am J Roentgenol* 1998;171:599–604.
32. Schneider FA, Comerota AJ. Acute arterial occlusion. In: Merli GJ, Weitz HH, Carabasi RA, eds. *Peripheral vascular disorders: management in primary care*. Philadelphia, PA: WB Saunders, 2004:81–93.
33. Brewster DC. Acute peripheral arterial occlusion. *Cardiol Clin* 1991;9: 497–513.
34. Thompson JE, Sigler L, Raut PS, et al. Arterial embolectomy: a 20 year experience with 163 cases. *Surgery* 1970;67:212–220.
35. Lusby RJ, Wylie EJ. Acute lower limb ischemia: pathogenesis and management. *World J Surg* 1983;7:340–386.
36. Haimovici H. Metabolic complications of acute arterial occlusions. *J Cardiovasc Surg (Torino)* 1979;20:349–357.
37. Mullick S. The tourniquet in operations upon the extremities. *Surg Gynecol Obstet* 1978;146:821–826.
38. Blaisdell FW. The reperfusion syndrome. *Microcirc Endothelium Lymphatics* 1989;5:127–141.
39. Quinones-Baldrich WJ. Surgical management of acute limb ischemia: intraoperative considerations. *Semin Vasc Surg* 1992;5:42.
40. Field T, Littooy FN, Baker WH. Immediate and long-term outcome of acute arterial occlusion of the extremities. The effect of added vascular reconstruction. *Arch Surg* 1982;117:1156–1160.
41. Jivegard L, Holm J, Schersten T. The outcome in arterial thrombosis misdiagnosed as arterial embolism. *Acta Chir Scand* 1986;152:251–256.
42. Yeager RA, Moneta GL, Taylor LM Jr, et al. Surgical management of severe acute lower extremity ischemia. *J Vasc Surg* 1992;15:385–391.
43. Tawes RL Jr, Harris EJ, Brown WH, et al. Arterial thromboembolism. A 20-year perspective. *Arch Surg* 1985;120:595–599.
44. Jivegard L, Holm J, Bergqvist D, et al. Acute lower limb ischemia: failure of anticoagulant treatment to improve one-month results of arterial thromboembolectomy. A prospective randomized multi-center study. *Surgery* 1991;109:610–616.
45. Tawes RL Jr, Beare JP, Scribner RG, et al. Value of postoperative heparin therapy in peripheral arterial thromboembolism. *Am J Surg* 1983; 146: 213–215.
46. Dale WA. Differential management of acute peripheral arterial ischemia. *J Vasc Surg* 1984;1:269–278.
47. Cambria RP, Abbott WM. Acute arterial thrombosis of the lower extremity. Its natural history contrasted with arterial embolism. *Arch Surg* 1984; 119:784–787.
48. McPhail NV, Fratesi SJ, Barber GG, et al. Management of acute thromboembolic limb ischemia. *Surgery* 1983;93:381–385.
49. Elliott JP Jr, Hageman JH, Szilagyi E, et al. Arterial embolization: problems of source, multiplicity, recurrence, and delayed treatment. *Surgery* 1980;88:833–845.
50. Abbott WM, Maloney RD, McCabe CC, et al. Arterial embolism: a 44 year perspective. *Am J Surg* 1982;143:460–464.
51. Satiani B, Evans WE. Immediate prognosis and five year survival after arterial embolectomy following myocardial infarction. *Surg Gynecol Obstet* 1980;150:41–44.
52. Lagattolla NR, Burnand KG, Stewart A. Role of transoesophageal echocardiography in determining the source of peripheral arterial embolism. *Br J Surg* 1995;82:1651–1654.
53. Meacham RR III, Headley AS, Bronze MS, et al. Impending paradoxical embolism. *Arch Intern Med* 1998;158:438–448.
54. Pasierski T, Jasek S, Firek B, et al. Resolution of an aortic mobile mass with anticoagulation without evidence of arterial embolism. *Clin Cardiol* 1996;19:151–152.
55. Herity NA, Dalzell GW. Venous thrombosis causing arterial embolization to the same limb through a patent foramen ovale. *Clin Cardiol* 1997; 20: 893–896.
56. Duran WN, Takenaka H, Hobson RW. Microvascular pathophysiology of skeletal muscle ischemia-reperfusion. *Semin Vasc Surg* 1998;11: 203–214.
57. Katz SG, Kohl RD. Angiographic catheter induced arterial occlusion. *J Am Coll Surg* 1994;178:439–442.
58. Oweida SW, Roubin GS, Smith RB III, et al. Postcatheterization vascular complications associated with percutaneous transluminal coronary angioplasty. *J Vasc Surg* 1990;12:310–315.
59. Valentine RJ, Kaplan HS, Green R, et al. Lipoprotein (a), homocysteine, and hypercoagulable states in young men with premature peripheral atherosclerosis: a prospective, controlled analysis. *J Vasc Surg* 1996;23: 53–61 discussion.
60. Hughes GR. The antiphospholipid syndrome: ten years on. *Lancet* 1993; 342:341–344.

61. Insko EK, Haskal ZJ. Antiphospholipid syndrome: patterns of life-threatening and severe recurrent vascular complications. *Radiology* 1997; 202: 319–326.

62. Ey FS. Hypercoagulability in vascular surgery patients. *Ann Vasc Surg* 1992;6:313–319.

63. Thomas DP, Roberts HR. Hypercoagulability in venous and arterial thrombosis. *Ann Intern Med* 1997;126:638–644.

64. Coller BS, Owen J, Jesty J, et al. Deficiency of plasma protein S, protein C, or antithrombin III and arterial thrombosis. *Arteriosclerosis* 1987;7: 456–462.

65. Blaisdell FW, Steele M, Allen RE. Management of acute lower extremity arterial ischemia due to embolism and thrombosis. *Surgery* 1978;84: 822–834.

66. Dunant JH, Edwards WS. Small vessel occlusion in the extremity after various periods of arterial obstruction: an experimental study. *Surgery* 1973;73:240–245.

67. Jamison RL. The role of cellular swelling in the pathogenesis of organ ischemia. *West J Med* 1974;120:205.

68. Stallone RJ, Blaisdell FW, Cafferata HT, et al. Analysis of morbidity and mortality from arterial embolectomy. *Surgery* 1969;65:207–217.

69. Perry MO, Fantini G. Ischemia: profile of an enemy. Reperfusion injury of skeletal muscle. *J Vasc Surg* 1987;6:231–234.

70. Stallone RJ, Lim RC Jr, Blaisdell FW. Pathogenesis of the pulmonary changes following ischemia of the lower extremities. *Ann Thorac Surg* 1969;7:539–549.

71. Fisher DF Jr, Clagett GP, Brigham RA, et al. Dilemmas in dealing with the blue toe syndrome: aortic versus peripheral source. *Am J Surg* 1984;148: 836–839.

72. Karmody AM, Powers SR, Monaco VJ, et al. "Blue toe" syndrome. An indication for limb salvage surgery. *Arch Surg* 1976;111:1263–1268.

73. Kempczinski RF. Lower-extremity arterial emboli from ulcerating atherosclerotic plaques. *JAMA* 1979;241:807–810.

74. Jackson MR, Clagett GP. Antithrombotic therapy in peripheral arterial occlusive disease. *Chest* 1998;114:666S–682S.

75. Holm J, Schersten T. Anticoagulant treatment during and after embolectomy. *Acta Chir Scand* 1972;138:683–687.

76. Wyffels PL, DeBord JR, Marshall S, et al. Increased limb salvage with intraoperative and postoperative ankle level urokinase infusion in acute lower extremity ischemia. *J Vasc Surg* 1992;15:771–778.

77. Comerota AJ, White JV, Grosh JD. Intraoperative intra-arterial thrombolytic therapy for salvage of limbs in patients with distal intra arterial thrombosis. *Surg Gynecol Obstet* 1989;169:283–289.

78. Comerota AJ, Rao AK, Throm RC, et al. A prospective, randomized, blinded, and placebo-controlled trial of intraoperative intra-arterial urokinase infusion during lower extremity revascularization. Regional and systemic effects. *Ann Surg* 1993;218:534–541.

79. Diffin DC, Kandarpa K. Assessment of peripheral intraarterial thrombolysis versus surgical revascularization in acute lower-limb ischemia: a review of limb-salvage and mortality statistics. *J Vasc Interv Radiol* 1996;7: 57–63.

80. Jivegard L, Holm J, Schersten T. Acute limb ischemia due to arterial embolism or thrombosis: influence of limb ischemia versus pre-existing cardiac disease on postoperative mortality rate. *J Cardiovasc Surg (Torino)* 1988;29:32–36.

81. Berridge DC, Gregson RH, Hopkinson BR, et al. Randomized trial of intra-arterial recombinant tissue plasminogen activator, intravenous recombinant tissue plasminogen activator and intra-arterial streptokinase in peripheral arterial thrombolysis. *Br J Surg* 1991;78:988–995.

82. Shortell CK, Ouriel K. Thrombolysis in acute peripheral arterial occlusion: predictors of immediate success. *Ann Vasc Surg* 1994;8:59–65.

83. The STILE Investigators. Results of a prospective randomized trial evaluating surgery versus thrombolysis for ischemia of the lower extremity. The STILE trial. *Ann Surg* 1994;220:251–266.

84. Ouriel K, Shortell CK, DeWeese JA, et al. A comparison of thrombolytic therapy with operative revascularization in the initial treatment of acute peripheral arterial ischemia. *J Vasc Surg* 1994;19:1021–1030.

85. Ouriel K, Veith FJ, Sasahara AA, Thrombolysis or Peripheral Arterial Surgery (TOPAS) Investigators. A comparison of recombinant urokinase with vascular surgery as initial treatment for acute arterial occlusion of the legs. *N Engl J Med* 1998;338:1105–1111.

86. Ouriel K, Veith FJ, Sasahara AA, TOPAS Investigators. Thrombolysis or peripheral arterial surgery: phase I results. *J Vasc Surg* 1996;23:64–73.

87. Ouriel K, Veith FJ. Acute lower limb ischemia: determinants of outcome. *Surgery* 1998;124:336–341.

88. Comerota AJ, Weaver FA, Hosking JD, et al. Results of a prospective, randomized trial of surgery versus thrombolysis for occluded lower extremity bypass grafts. *Am J Surg* 1996;172:105–112.

89. Weaver FA, Comerota AJ, Youngblood M, et al. Surgical revascularization versus thrombolysis for nonembolic lower extremity native artery occlusions: results of a prospective randomized trial. *J Vasc Surg* 1996;24: 513–521.

90. Weaver FA, Toms C. The practical implications of recent trials comparing thrombolytic therapy with surgery for lower extremity ischemia. *Semin Vasc Surg* 1997;10:49–54.

91. Juergens JL, Barker NW, Hines EA Jr. Arteriosclerosis obliterans: review of 520 cases with special reference to pathogenic and prognostic factors. *Circulation* 1960;21:188–195.

92. Leng GC, Fowkes FG. The Edinburgh Claudication Questionnaire: an improved version of the WHO/Rose Questionnaire for use in epidemiological surveys. *J Clin Epidemiol* 1992;45:1101–1109.

93. Brewster DC. Clinical and anatomical considerations for surgery in aortoiliac disease and results of surgical treatment. *Circulation* 1991;83:I42–I52.

94. Goodreau JJ, Creasy JK, Flanigan P, et al. Rational approach to the differentiation of vascular and neurogenic claudication. *Surgery* 1978; 84:749–757.

95. Weitz JI, Byrne J, Clagett GP, et al. Diagnosis and treatment of chronic arterial insufficiency of the lower extremities: a critical review. *Circulation* 1996;94:3026–3049.

96. McDaniel M, Cronenwett JL. Natural history of intermittent claudication. In: Porter JM, Taylor LM, eds. *Basic data underlying clinical decision making in vascular surgery*. St. Louis, MO: Quality Medical Publishing, 1994.

97. McDermott MM, McCarthy W. Intermittent claudication. The natural history. *Surg Clin North Am* 1995;75:581–591.

98. Lundgren F, Dahllof AG, Lundholm K, et al. Intermittent claudication—surgical reconstruction or physical training? A prospective randomized trial of treatment efficiency. *Ann Surg* 1989;209:346–355.

99. Jonason T, Ringqvist I. Factors of prognostic importance for subsequent rest pain in patients with intermittent claudication. *Acta Med Scand* 1985; 218:27–33.

100. Tyrrell MR, Wolfe JH, Joint Vascular Research Group. Critical leg ischaemia: an appraisal of clinical definitions. *Br J Surg* 1993;80:177–180.

101. Fowkes FG. Epidemiology of atherosclerotic arterial disease in the lower limbs. *Eur J Vasc Surg* 1988;2:283–291.

102. Kannel WB, McGee DL. Update on some epidemiologic features of intermittent claudication: the Framingham Study. *J Am Geriatr Soc* 1985;33:13–18.

103. Cranley JJ. Ischemic rest pain. *Arch Surg* 1969;98:187–188.

104. Taylor LM, Porter JM Jr. Clinical and anatomic considerations for surgery in femoropopliteal disease and the results of surgery. *Circulation* 1991; 83:I63–I69.

105. Albers M, Fratezi AC, De LN. Assessment of quality of life of patients with severe ischemia as a result of infrainguinal arterial occlusive disease. *J Vasc Surg* 1992;16:54–59.

106. Levy PJ, Hornung CA, Haynes JL, et al. Lower extremity ischemia in adults younger than forty years of age: a community-wide survey of premature atherosclerotic arterial disease. *J Vasc Surg* 1994;19:873–881.

107. Olsen PS, Gustafsen J, Rasmussen L, et al. Long-term results after arterial surgery for arteriosclerosis of the lower limbs in young adults. *Eur J Vasc Surg* 1988;2:15–18.

108. van den BM, Stehouwer CD, Bierdrager E, et al. Plasma homocysteine and severity of atherosclerosis in young patients with lower-limb atherosclerotic disease. *Arterioscler Thromb Vasc Biol* 1996;16:165–171.

109. Bergmark C, Mansoor MA, Swedenborg J, et al. Hyperhomocysteinemia in patients operated for lower extremity ischaemia below the age of 50—effect of smoking and extent of disease. *Eur J Vasc Surg* 1993;7:391–396.

110. Mills JL, Porter JM. Buerger's disease: a review and update. *Semin Vasc Surg* 1993;6:14–23.

111. Olin JW. Thromboangiitis obliterans (Buerger's disease). *N Engl J Med* 2000;343:864–869.

112. Shionoya S. Buerger's disease: diagnosis and management. *Cardiovasc Surg* 1993;1:207–214.

113. Lau H, Cheng SW. Buerger's disease in Hong Kong: a review of 89 cases. *Aust N Z J Surg* 1997;67:264–269.

114. Aqel MB, Olin JW. Thromboangiitis obliterans (Buerger's disease). *Vasc Med* 1997;2:61–66.

115. Cutler DA, Runge MS. 86 years of Buerger's disease—what have we learned? *Am J Med Sci* 1995;309:74–75.

116. Tanaka K. Pathology and pathogenesis of Buerger's disease. *Int J Cardiol* 1998;66(Suppl. 1):S237–S242.

117. Halliday AW, Taylor PR, Wolfe JH, et al. The management of popliteal aneurysm: the importance of early surgical repair. *Ann R Coll Surg Engl* 1991;73:253–257.

118. Quraishy MS, Giddings AE. Treatment of asymptomatic popliteal aneurysm: protection at a price. *Br J Surg* 1992;79:731–732.

119. Dawson I, Sie RB, van Bockel JH. Atherosclerotic popliteal aneurysm. *Br J Surg* 1997;84:293–299.

120. Gawenda M, Sorgatz S, Walter M, et al. Rupture as the exceptional complication of popliteal aneurysm. *Eur J Surg* 1997;163:69–71.

121. Dawson I, Sie R, van Baalen JM, et al. Asymptomatic popliteal aneurysm: elective operation versus conservative follow-up. *Br J Surg* 1994;81: 1504–1507.

122. Ramesh S, Michaels JA, Galland RB. Popliteal aneurysm: morphology and management. *Br J Surg* 1993;80:1531–1533.

123. Elsey JK, Rosenthal D. The use of adjunctive thrombolytic therapy in the management of acute popliteal aneurysm thrombosis. *Am Surg* 1994;60: 942–945.

124. Bowyer RC, Cawthorn SJ, Walker WJ, et al. Conservative management of asymptomatic popliteal aneurysm. *Br J Surg* 1990;77:1132–1135.

125. Cohn SL, Taylor WC. Vascular problems of the lower extremity in athletes. *Clin Sports Med* 1990;9:449–470.

126. Levien LJ, Benn CA. Adventitial cystic disease: a unifying hypothesis. *J Vasc Surg* 1998;28:193–205.

127. Paty PS, Kaufman JL, Koslow AR, et al. Adventitial cystic disease of the femoral vein: a case report and review of the literature. *J Vasc Surg* 1992; 15:214–217.

128. Deshpande A, Denton M. Functional popliteal entrapment syndrome. *Aust N Z J Surg* 1998;68:660–663.

129. Haddad M, Barral X, Boissier C, et al. The embolic type of popliteal entrapment syndrome. *Vasa* 1990;19:63–67.

130. Parums DV. The arteritides. *Histopathology* 1994;25:1–20.

131. Troeng T, Bergqvist D, Janzon L, et al. The choice of strategy in the treatment of intermittent claudication—a decision tree approach. *Eur J Vasc Surg* 1993;7:438–443.

132. The Vascular Surgical Society of Great Britain and Ireland. Critical limb ischaemia: management and outcome. Report of a national survey. *Eur J Vasc Endovasc Surg* 1995;10:108–113.

133. Ouriel K, Fiore WM, Geary JE. Limb-threatening ischemia in the medically compromised patient: amputation or revascularization? *Surgery* 1988; 104:667–672.

134. Tangelder MJ, McDonnel J, Van Busschbach JJ et al. Dutch Bypass Oral Anticoagulants or Aspirin (BOA) Study Group. Quality of life after infrainguinal bypass grafting surgery. *J Vasc Surg* 1999;29:913–919.

135. Skinner JA, Cohen AT. Amputation for premature peripheral atherosclerosis: do young patients do better? *Lancet* 1996;348:1396.

136. Kempczinski RF, Bernhard VM. Management of chronic ischemia of the lower extremities: introduction and general considerations. In: Rutherford RB, ed. *Vascular surgery*, 3rd ed. Philadelphia, PA: WB Saunders, 1989: 643.

137. McDaniel MD, Macdonald PD, Haver RA, et al. Published results of surgery for aortoiliac occlusive disease. *Ann Vasc Surg* 1997;11:425–441.

138. Belkin M. Aortoiliac occlusive disease. In: Moore WS, ed. *Vascular surgery: a comprehensive review*. Philadelphia, PA: WB Saunders, 2002:508–521.

139. Klinkert P, Schepers A, Burger DH, et al. Vein versus polytetrafluoroethylene in above-knee femoropopliteal bypass grafting: five-year results of a randomized controlled trial. *J Vasc Surg* 2003;37:149–155.

140. Veith FJ, Gupta SK, Ascer E, et al. Six-year prospective multicenter randomized comparison of autologous saphenous vein and expanded polytetrafluoroethylene grafts in infrainguinal arterial reconstructions. *J Vasc Surg* 1986;3:104–114.

141. Illig KA, Green RM. Prosthetic above-knee femoropopliteal bypass. *Semin Vasc Surg* 1999;12:38–45.

142. Dalman RL, Taylor LM Jr. Basic data related to infrainguinal revascularization procedures. *Ann Vasc Surg* 1990;4:309–312.

143. Donaldson MC. Evaluation of patients with suspected hypercoagulability: what tests to order. *Semin Vasc Surg* 1996;9:277–283.

144. Ray SA, Rowley MR, Bevan DH, et al. Hypercoagulable abnormalities and postoperative failure of arterial reconstruction. *Eur J Vasc Endovasc Surg* 1997;13:363–370.

145. Eldrup-Jorgensen J, Brace L, Flanigan DP, et al. Lupus-like anticoagulants and lower extremity arterial occlusive disease. *Circulation* 1989;80: III54–III58.

146. Ouriel K, Green RM, DeWeese JA, et al. Activated protein C resistance: prevalence and implications in peripheral vascular disease. *J Vasc Surg* 1996;23:46–51 discussion.

147. Tuman KJ, McCarthy RJ, March RJ, et al. Effects of epidural anesthesia and analgesia on coagulation and outcome after major vascular surgery. *Anesth Analg* 1991;73:696–704.

148. Chan P. Prospects for prevention of graft stenosis and angioplasty restenosis. *Eur J Vasc Endovasc Surg* 1997;13:429–431.

149. Davies MG, Hagen PO. Pathophysiology of vein graft failure: a review. *Eur J Vasc Endovasc Surg* 1995;9:7–18.

150. Bauters C, Meurice T, Hamon M, et al. Mechanisms and prevention of restenosis: from experimental models to clinical practice. *Cardiovasc Res* 1996;31:835–846.

151. Herrman JP, Hermans WR, Vos J, et al. Pharmacological approaches to the prevention of restenosis following angioplasty. The search for the Holy Grail? (Part I). *Drugs* 1993;46:18–52.

152. Tegtmeyer CJ, Hartwell GD, Selby JB, et al. Results and complications of angioplasty in aortoiliac disease. *Circulation* 1991;83:I53–I60.

153. Jeans WD, Armstrong S, Cole SE, et al. Fate of patients undergoing transluminal angioplasty for lower-limb ischemia. *Radiology* 1990;177:559–564.

154. Johnston KW. Iliac arteries: reanalysis of results of balloon angioplasty. *Radiology* 1993;186:207–212.

155. Gupta AK, Ravimandalam K, Rao VR, et al. Total occlusion of iliac arteries: results of balloon angioplasty. *Cardiovasc Intervent Radiol* 1993;16: 165–177.

156. Dormandy JA, Rutherford RB. TASC Working Group. TransAtlantic Inter-Society Consensus (TASC). Management of peripheral arterial disease (PAD). *J Vasc Surg* 2000;31:S1–S296.

157. Timaran CH, Stevens SL, Freeman MB, et al. External iliac and common iliac artery angioplasty and stenting in men and women. *J Vasc Surg* 2001; 34:440–446.

158. Cejna M, Thurnher S, Illiasch H, et al. PTA versus Palmaz stent placement in femoropopliteal artery obstructions: a multicenter prospective randomized study. *J Vasc Interv Radiol* 2001;12:23–31.

159. Thierry B, Merhi Y, Bilodeau L, et al. Nitinol versus stainless steel stents: acute thrombogenicity study in an *ex vivo* porcine model. *Biomaterials* 2002;23:2997–3005.

160. Henry M, Amor M, Beyar R, et al. Clinical experience with a new nitinol self-expanding stent in peripheral arteries. *J Endovasc Surg* 1996;3: 369–379.

161. Jahnke T, Voshage G, Muller-Hulsbeck S, et al. Endovascular placement of self-expanding nitinol coil stents for the treatment of femoropopliteal obstructive disease. *J Vasc Interv Radiol* 2002;13:257–266.

162. Lugmayr HF, Holzer H, Kastner M, et al. Treatment of complex arteriosclerotic lesions with nitinol stents in the superficial femoral and popliteal arteries: a midterm follow-up. *Radiology* 2002;222:37–43.

163. Kessel DO, Wijesinghe LD, Robertson I, et al. Endovascular stent-grafts for superficial femoral artery disease: results of 1-year follow-up. *J Vasc Interv Radiol* 1999;10:289–296.

164. Ahmadi R, Schillinger M, Maca T, et al. Femoropopliteal arteries: immediate and long-term results with a Dacron-covered stent-graft. *Radiology* 2002;223:345–350.

165. Ingle H, Nasim A, Bolia A, et al. Subintimal angioplasty of isolated infragenicular vessels in lower limb ischemia: long-term results. *J Endovasc Ther* 2002;9:411–416.

166. Vraux H, Hammer F, Verhelst R, et al. Subintimal angioplasty of tibial vessel occlusions in the treatment of critical limb ischaemia: mid-term results. *Eur J Vasc Endovasc Surg* 2000;20:441–446.

167. Nydahl S, Hartshorne T, Bell PR, et al. Subintimal angioplasty of infrapopliteal occlusions in critically ischaemic limbs. *Eur J Vasc Endovasc Surg* 1997;14:212–216.

168. Loftus IM, Hayes PD, Bell PR. Subintimal angioplasty in lower limb ischaemia. *J Cardiovasc Surg (Torino)* 2004;45:217–229.

169. Gallo R, Padurean A, Jayaraman T, et al. Inhibition of intimal thickening after balloon angioplasty in porcine coronary arteries by targeting regulators of the cell cycle. *Circulation* 1999;99:2164–2170.

170. Sousa JE, Costa MA, Abizaid A, et al. Lack of neointimal proliferation after implantation of sirolimus-coated stents in human coronary arteries: a quantitative coronary angiography and three-dimensional intravascular ultrasound study. *Circulation* 2001;103:192–195.

171. Serruys PW, Degertekin M, Tanabe K, et al. Intravascular ultrasound findings in the multicenter, randomized, double-blind RAVEL (RAndomized study with the sirolimus-eluting VElocity balloon-expandable stent in the treatment of patients with *de novo* native coronary artery Lesions) trial. *Circulation* 2002;106:798–803.

172. Duda SH, Pusich B, Richter G, et al. Sirolimus-eluting stents for the treatment of obstructive superficial femoral artery disease: six-month results. *Circulation* 2002;106:1505–1509.

173. Steinhubl SR, Berger PB, Mann JT III, et al. Early and sustained dual oral antiplatelet therapy following percutaneous coronary intervention: a randomized controlled trial. *JAMA* 2002;288:2411–2420.

174. Lefkovits J, Topol EJ. Pharmacological approaches for the prevention of restenosis after percutaneous coronary intervention. *Prog Cardiovasc Dis* 1997;40:141–158.

175. Topol EJ, Califf RM, Weisman HF et al. The EPIC Investigators. Randomised trial of coronary intervention with antibody against platelet IIb/IIIa integrin for reduction of clinical restenosis: results at six months. *Lancet* 1994;343:881–886.

176. Lincoff AM, Bittl JA, Harrington RA, et al. Bivalirudin and provisional glycoprotein IIb/IIIa blockade compared with heparin and planned glycoprotein IIb/IIIa blockade during percutaneous coronary intervention: REPLACE-2 randomized trial. *JAMA* 2003;289:853–863.

177. Lincoff AM, Bittl JA, Kleiman NS, et al. Comparison of bivalirudin versus heparin during percutaneous coronary intervention (the Randomized Evaluation of PCI Linking Angiomax to Reduced Clinical Events [REPLACE]-1 trial). *Am J Cardiol* 2004;93:1092–1096.

178. Clagett GP, Sobel M, Jackson MR, et al. Antithrombotic therapy in peripheral arterial occlusive disease: the Seventh ACCP Conference on Antithrombotic and Thrombolytic Therapy. *Chest* 2004;126:609S–626S.

179. Goldman MD, Simpson D, Hawker RJ, et al. Aspirin and dipyridamole reduce platelet deposition on prosthetic femoro-popliteal grafts in man. *Ann Surg* 1983;198:713–716.

180. Green RM, Abbott WM, Matsumoto T, et al. Prosthetic above-knee femoropopliteal bypass grafting: five-year results of a randomized trial. *J Vasc Surg* 2000;31:417–425.

181. Kohler TR, Kaufman JL, Kacoyanis G, et al. Effect of aspirin and dipyridamole on the patency of lower extremity bypass grafts. *Surgery* 1984;96: 462–466.

182. Clyne CA, Archer TJ, Atuhaire LK, et al. Random control trial of a short course of aspirin and dipyridamole (Persantin) for femorodistal grafts. *Br J Surg* 1987;74:246–248.

183. Findlay JM, Lougheed WM, Gentili F, et al. Effect of perioperative platelet inhibition on postcarotid endarterectomy mural thrombus formation. Results of a prospective randomized controlled trial using aspirin and dipyridamole in humans. *J Neurosurg* 1985;63:693–698.

184. Rutherford RB, Jones DN, Bergentz SE, et al. The efficacy of dextran 40 in preventing early postoperative thrombosis following difficult lower extremity bypass. *J Vasc Surg* 1984;1:765–773.

185. Katz SG, Kohl RD. Does dextran 40 improve the early patency of autogenous infrainguinal bypass grafts? *J Vasc Surg* 1998;28:23–26.

186. Becquemin JP. Effect of ticlopidine on the long-term patency of saphenous-vein bypass grafts in the legs. Etude de la Ticlopidine apres Pontage Femoro-Poplite and the Association Universitaire de Recherche en Chirurgie. *N Engl J Med* 1997;337:1726–1731.

187. Antiplatelet Trialists' Collaboration. Collaborative overview of randomised trials of antiplatelet therapy—III: Reduction in venous thrombosis and

pulmonary embolism by antiplatelet prophylaxis among surgical and medical patients. *BMJ* 1994;308:235–246.

188. Kretschmer G, Wenzl E, Piza F, et al. The influence of anticoagulant treatment on the probability of function in femoropopliteal vein bypass surgery: analysis of a clinical series (1970 to 1985) and interim evaluation of a controlled clinical trial. *Surgery* 1987;102:453–459.

189. Kretschmer G, Herbst F, Prager M, et al. A decade of oral anticoagulant treatment to maintain autologous vein grafts for femoropopliteal atherosclerosis. *Arch Surg* 1992;127:1112–1115.

190. Edmondson RA, Cohen AT, Das SK, et al. Low-molecular weight heparin versus aspirin and dipyridamole after femoropopliteal bypass grafting. *Lancet* 1994;344:914–918.

191. Sarac TP, Huber TS, Back MR, et al. Warfarin improves the outcome of infrainguinal vein bypass grafting at high risk for failure. *J Vasc Surg* 1998;28:446–457.

192. Tangelder MJ, Lawson JA, Algra A, et al. Systematic review of randomized controlled trials of aspirin and oral anticoagulants in the prevention of graft occlusion and ischemic events after infrainguinal bypass surgery. *J Vasc Surg* 1999;30:701–709.

193. Algra A, Tangelder MJ, Lawson JA et al. Dutch Bypass Oral anticoagulants or Aspirin Study Group. Interpretation of Dutch BOA trial. *Lancet* 2000;355:1186–1187.

194. Jackson MR, Johnson WC, Williford WO, et al. The effect of anticoagulation therapy and graft selection on the ischemic consequences of femoropopliteal bypass graft occlusion: results from a multicenter randomized clinical trial. *J Vasc Surg* 2002;35:292–298.

# CHAPTER 102 ■ PREVENTION AND TREATMENT OF ACUTE STROKE

GREGORY J. DEL ZOPPO

## PREVENTION AND TREATMENT OF ACUTE STROKE

Stroke is a syndrome of fixed or transient neurologic deficits that result from atherothrombotic events, thromboembolism, subarachnoid hemorrhage, intracerebral hemorrhage, lacunae, and other potential causes (see Table 102-1) (1,2). Atherothrombotic stroke refers to cerebral arterial occlusions due to either *in situ* arterial thrombosis or artery-to-artery emboli from intracranial arteries or from the principal extracranial supply, including the internal carotid artery (ICA), the aortic arch, and the vertebral-basilar (VB) artery system.

Platelet-fibrin thrombi arise on arteriosclerotic lesions in the extracranial portion of the ICA (i.e., at the flow divider) or in the aortic arch, and can embolize downstream, predominantly into the middle cerebral artery (MCA) and anterior cerebral arterial (ACA) territories. A similar process can send emboli from atheromata at the subclavian-vertebral artery junctions into the basilar artery. Cardiac sources of emboli originate from the left ventricular mural thrombi formed during myocardial ischemia (infarction) (MI) or other injury; from atrial thrombi formed in association with (nonvalvular) atrial fibrillation (AF); from valvular injury; from prosthetic valves, or in association with patent foramen ovale (PFO) and atrial septal aneurysm. Less common than atherothrombotic stroke, thrombosis of small, penetrating cerebral arteries leads to lipohyalinosis and formation of lacunae (3).

Studies employing angiography in the acute setting of stroke have shown a high frequency of atherothrombotic or thromboembolic arterial occlusions in patients who present within 6 hours of onset of carotid artery territory ischemic symptoms (see Fig. 102-1) (4–7).

## NATURAL HISTORY OF CEREBRAL ATHEROTHROMBOTIC AND THROMBOEMBOLIC DISEASE

Carotid territory transient ischemic attacks (TIAs) are often accompanied by subsequent strokes or other cardiovascular diseases. Completed stroke has been reported in 40% to 75% of individuals with one or more TIAs (11,12), with a prevalence of approximately 30% per year (11,12). Among individuals with a premonitory TIA, approximately 50% may have a stroke within the first year (13). Stroke-related death and cardiac death occur in 28% and 37% of TIA individuals, respectively, indicating that cardiovascular mortality is statistically significant in the population of patients with stroke (13). More recent evaluations, which have included data from placebo groups in large trials of antithrombotic efficacy,

suggest a lower mortality. For example, the combined outcome events of stroke, MI, and death occurred in 14% of individuals treated with placebo for more than 2 years in the UK-TIA (United Kingdom transient ischemic attack) Study Group Trial (14). Approximately 64% of individuals with TIAs showed evidence of cerebral infarction in their initial computerized tomography (CT) scan (15).

Patients presenting with a stroke are at risk for recurrence, often within the same vascular territory. The 5-year cumulative incidence of secondary stroke was 42% among men in one prospective follow-up study. A separate study noted a 32% 7-year cumulative incidence for recurrent stroke (16). Again, the highest recurrence of stroke is within the first year following the initial event.

Stroke-related mortality during the first 7 days after ictus was examined prospectively by Silver et al. (17) Cerebral edema from large, hemispheric ischemic lesions led to transtentorial herniation and death in 78% of 46 patients who died in that interval. This is consistent with the number of fatal events (82%) in one retrospective pathology study (18). Generally, however, mortality is not considered to be the primary outcome in current acute stroke intervention trials because of its low incidence and multifactorial basis.

Improvements in neurologic outcome are commonly observed among patients who survive a stroke. Both neurologic presentation and outcome depend on stroke subtype (19). Patients with lacunar strokes fare better than those patients with thromboembolic events. The conditions under which stroke occurs can alter the outcome. It has been recently appreciated, both clinically and experimentally, that female patients have a better 1-year survival and lower infarct volume than male patients, although the reasons are unclear (20–22). Experience from 2-hour statin intervention trials for prevention of MI have demonstrated a significant reduction in stroke incidence in patients treated with HMG-CoA reductase inhibitors (23–27). Although, epidemiologic studies have not established cholesterol levels as a risk-factor for ischemic stroke (28), in both situations, the mechanisms of protection are unknown and are under active study (estrogens and statins).

## HEMOSTASIS AND CEREBROVASCULAR ISCHEMIA

Thrombosis and thromboembolism play a central role in focal cerebral ischemia, as suggested by clinical, angiographic, and laboratory observations. The findings of migrating thromboemboli in the retinal artery and refractile bodies in patients with focal cerebral ischemia (29–31), and of thrombi in cortical arteries during cerebral ischemia and on affected carotid arteries support a pathogenic role for these thrombotic events (32,33).

Select acute angiographic studies have documented cerebrovascular occlusions in individuals with focal ischemia. In

**TABLE 102-1**

ETIOLOGY OF FOCAL CEREBRAL ISCHEMIA

| Source | Frequency |
|---|---|
| **ISCHEMIC STROKE** | |
| Atherothrombotic events | 40%–57% |
| Thromboembolism | 16%–23% |
| Lacunae | 14% |
| **HEMORRHAGIC STROKE** | |
| Intracerebral hemorrhage | 4%–18% |
| Subarachnoid hemorrhage | 10%–19% |

three prospective studies, symptomatic occlusion of a brain-supplying artery within the carotid territory was documented in 81% of patients within 8 hours of symptom onset (5–7). Separate angiographic studies have shown arterial occlusions in 59% of patients at 24 hours and in 41% at 1 week after symptom onset in patients with focal cerebral ischemia (4,8). Furthermore, these angiographic studies support the view that large-artery events in the carotid territory are primarily thrombotic or embolic in origin. Basilar arterial ischemia results from *in situ* thrombosis on atheromata in the basilar or vertebral arteries or from emboli from more proximal sources (34). Atherosclerosis of brain-supplying arteries is a thrombophilic state (see Fig. 102-2).

Indirect evidence for the involvement of thrombi in cerebrovascular ischemia has resulted from observation of platelet, coagulation, and fibrinolytic system activation in patients with

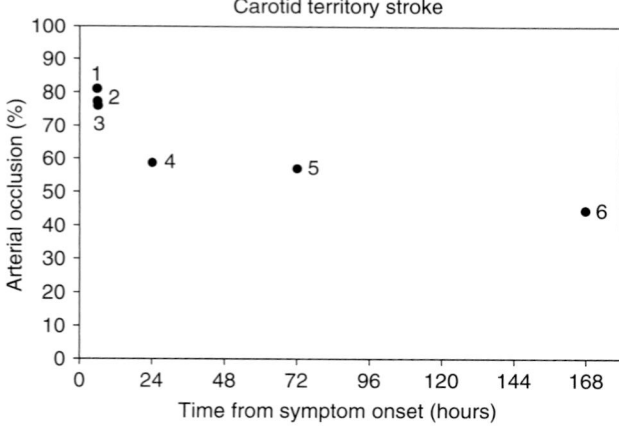

**FIGURE 102-1.** Series of angiography-based studies from separate trials demonstrating the frequency of carotid artery territory obstruction accompanying symptomatic ischemic stroke. Data points 1 to 6 are derived from citations (4,5,7–10) in order. (From Solis OJ, Roberson GR, Taveras JM, et al. Cerebral angiography in acute cerebral infarction. *Rev Interam Radiol* 1977; 2:19–25; Fieschi C, Argentino C, Lenzi GL, et al. Clinical and instrumental evaluation of patients with ischemic stroke within the first six hours. *J Neurol Sci* 1989;91:311–321; del Zoppo GJ, Higashida RT, Furlan AJ, et al. PROACT: a phase II randomized trial of recombinant pro-urokinase by direct arterial delivery in acute middle cerebral artery stroke. *Stroke* 1998; 29:4–11; Irino T, Taneda M, Minami T. Angiographic manifestations in post-recanalized cerebral infarction. *Neurology* 1977; 27:471–475; del Zoppo GJ, Poeck K, Pessin MS, et al. Recombinant tissue plasminogen activator in acute thrombotic and embolic stroke. *Ann Neurol* 1992; 32:78–86; Fieschi C, Bozzao L. Transient embolic occlusion of the middle cerebral and internal carotid arteries in cerebral apoplexy. *J Neurol Neurosurg Psychiatry* 1969;32:236–240, with permission.)

thrombotic stroke or TIAs (35–39). Platelet activation, spontaneous platelet aggregation, and circulating platelet aggregates have been reported in patients with recent atherothrombotic and thromboembolic cerebral ischemia (35,38–45). Experimental studies confirm the deposition of fibrin and activated platelets in microvessels of the ischemic regions shortly after MCA occlusion (46–51). These observations implicate the local activation of hemostasis in the ischemic microvascular bed.

The direct and indirect evidence that platelet activation, acceleration of coagulation, and thrombosis underlie most ischemic strokes supports the use of antithrombotic agents in the management of cerebrovascular ischemia. Antiplatelet agents play a role in the reduction of TIAs and ischemic strokes associated with thromboemboli of atherosclerotic origin. Anticoagulants are employed for prevention of cardiogenic emboli, arising in the setting of nonvalvular AF, ventricular dysfunction, or valvular injury or prosthesis. Both approaches have been combined, but neither has been used in acute treatment of thrombotic stroke. Plasminogen activators are currently used to reduce injury or to improve clinical outcome within 3 to 6 hours of symptom onset, in the absence of detectable cerebral hemorrhage.

# HEMORRHAGIC TRANSFORMATION IN CEREBRAL ISCHEMIA

Hemorrhage accounts for approximately 10% to 15% of all strokes (1,6,7,9,52–58). Normal platelet function appears necessary to maintain the integrity of the cerebrovascular beds and to prevent clinically detectable hemorrhage. Hemorrhage in the ischemic territory can increase with the use of antithrombotic agents (59). Increases in the incidence of symptomatic intracerebral hemorrhage were observed with aspirin [acetylsalicylic acid (ASA)] in the UK-TIA Study, the International Stroke Trial (IST), and the European Stroke Prevention Study-2 (ESPS-2) trial (54,55,60). An increased risk of intracerebral hemorrhage is related to advanced age (>75 years), the intensity of anticoagulation, and the concomitant use of antithrombotics (59).

Hemorrhagic transformation of the ischemic lesion occurs normally during thromboembolic stroke and is classified as hemorrhagic infarction (HI), parenchymal hematoma (PH), or both (see Fig. 102-3). HI refers to petechial or confluent petechial hemorrhage in the area of ischemic injury, typically involving cortical or basal ganglia gray matter (61–64). HI has been shown to occur in 50% to 70% of individuals in postmortem studies (61,63,65), in 10% to 43% of nonanticoagulated individuals with acute cerebral infarction in CT scan–based studies (66,67), in 37.5% of patients with cardiogenic cerebral embolism, but in only 1.9% of patients with carotid territory thrombosis (68). Petechial hemorrhage can result from ischemia-related degradation of the microvessel basal lamina matrix components (69,70).

PH is a homogeneous mass of blood (coagulum) that can displace brain tissue. It is most often the cause of symptomatic hemorrhage. Many reports of PH in patients with cerebral embolism are associated with anticoagulant treatment (71,72). In addition, PH can result from the rupture of small penetrating arteries (see Fig. 102-4).

# ANTITHROMBOTIC APPROACHES TO CEREBRAL ISCHEMIA

Plasminogen activators have been used to limit the consequences of recent transient or fixed neurologic deficits in the

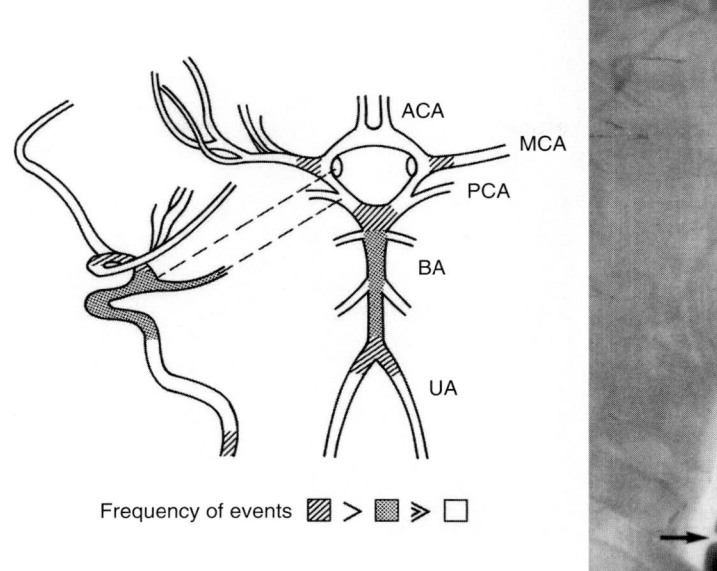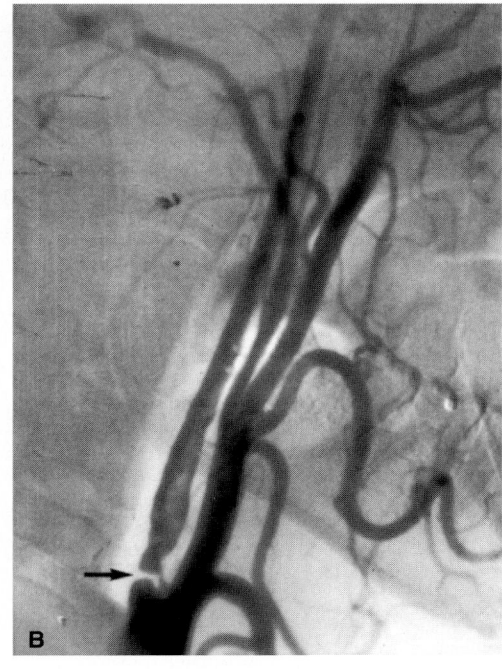

**FIGURE 102-2.** Atherosclerosis as a source of thrombotic and embolic obstruction of arterial circuits in the central nervous system (CNS). **A:** Predilection sites for atheromata in brain-supplying arteries. **B:** Example of severe (99%) stenosis of the internal carotid artery in patient with transient ischemic attacks (TIAs) (*arrow*), ACA, anterior cerebral artery; MCA, middle cerebral artery, PCA, posterior cerebral artery; BA, basilar artery; UA, uncal artery.

acute-phase. Antiplatelet agents and anticoagulants have also been used as prophylaxis against recurrence of the ischemia (i.e., secondary prevention). In addition, anticoagulants have been used for treatment of sinus venous thrombosis and for prevention of thromboembolic events originating in the setting of AF, acute MI, or cardiac valve injury.

# TRANSIENT CEREBRAL ISCHEMIA (TRANSIENT ISCHEMIC ATTACKS)

Because TIAs and ischemic strokes [e.g., transient monocular blindness (amaurosis fugax)] (73–75) can often be manifestations of ongoing activation of platelets and coagulation and of vascular injury in arteries supplying the brain, antiplatelet agents have been applied with benefit (4–8,29,31,39,45,70,76).

## Antiplatelet Agents

### Aspirin (Acetylsalicylic Acid)

In ischemic cerebrovascular disease, ASA can reduce the incidence of TIAs and subsequent ischemic strokes. Despite a number of prospective evaluations of ASA, a small number of well-conducted level I studies support the efficacy of ASA in the carotid artery territory (see Table 102-2).

The Aspirin in Transient Ischemic Attacks (AITIA) study, which randomized patients with a 3-month history of TIAs and who were not considered candidates for carotid endarterectomy to ASA (1,300 mg per day) or to placebo, demonstrated a reduction in stroke and vascular death at 6 months with ASA exposure (77). There was a considerable decrease in the combined outcomes of recurrent TIAs, cerebral/retinal infarction, and death among those receiving ASA, but no reduction by life-table analysis at the 24-month follow-up and no reduction in stroke

incidence. In the Canadian Cooperative Study Group trial, patients with a history of TIAs were randomized to ASA (1,300 mg per day), sulfinpyrazone (800 mg per day), and the combination ASA/sulfinpyrazone, or placebo (78). Patients who received ASA had a significant decrease in the incidence of stroke and death compared to sulfinpyrazone or placebo (78). The risk reduction for stroke and death with ASA was most significant for men. Among patients with a history of TIAs in the double-blind "AICLA" trial who were randomized to ASA (990 mg per day), the combination of ASA (990 mg per day) with dipyridamole (225 mg per day), or placebo, those patients who received ASA or the combination demonstrated a reduced incidence of stroke, MI, and death compared to patients who received placebo (80). Efficacy in the combined outcome seemed to be associated with an ASA dose range of 990 to 1,300 mg per day.

However, those ASA doses were associated with considerable side effects. This was confirmed by the UK-TIA aspirin trial which randomized 2,435 individuals with TIAs or minor ischemic stroke to "high-dose" ASA (1,200 mg per day), "low-dose" ASA (300 mg per day), or placebo (14). The 4-year incidence of nonfatal MI, nonfatal major stroke, and death was significantly reduced by 18% in a dose-dependent manner in patients who received ASA. But, gastrointestinal side effects were more common with the high-dose regimen, and excess mortality was attributed to intracranial hemorrhage in the ASA-treated groups. In a separate study, a decrease in major hemorrhagic events, including fatal intracerebral hemorrhage, was associated with lower ASA doses (30 mg per day vs. 283 mg per day) (81).

The Swedish Aspirin Low-Dose Trial (SALT) Collaborative Group reported an 18% reduction in risk of stroke and death among TIA patients who started ASA (75 mg per day) within 1 to 4 months of their initial symptoms compared to patients who received placebo (82). A 16% to 20% reduction in the risk of stroke, frequent TIAs, and MI was also observed.

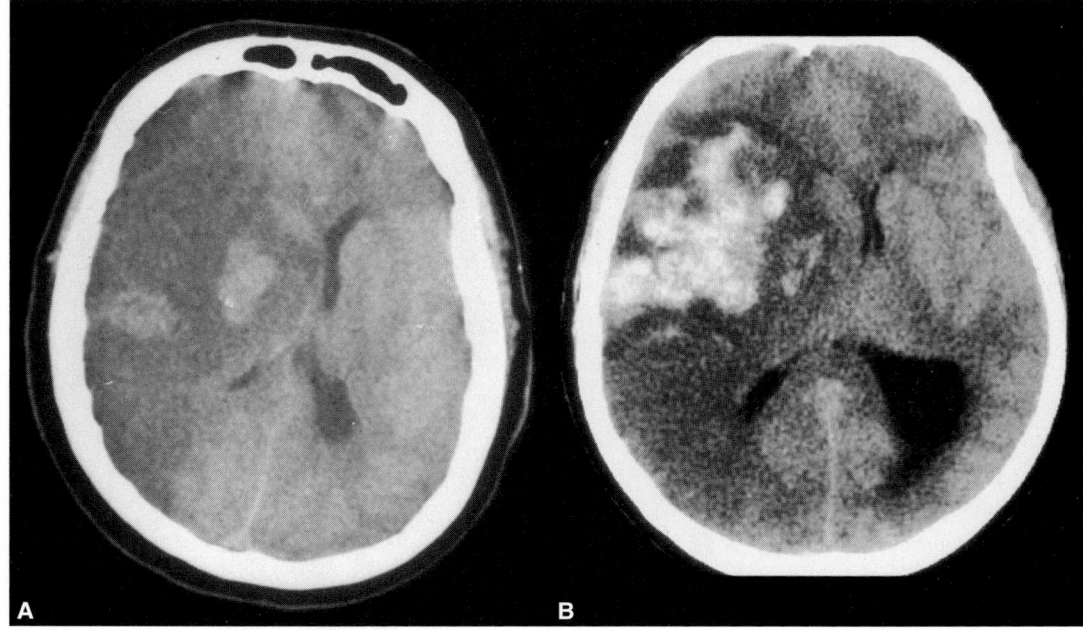

**FIGURE 102-3.** Hemorrhagic transformation. **A:** Hemorrhagic infarction typified by regions of conflu-ent petechiae 24 hours after middle cerebral artery occlusion. Note midline shift due to tissue swelling. **B:** Parenchymal hemorrhage marked by coagulum displacing midline structures and compressing ventri-cle. (Image in panel **A:** From von Kummer R, Bozzao L, Manelf C. *Early CT diagnosis of hemispheric brain infarction.* Berlin: Springer Verlag, 1995:1, with permission.)

The results of these trials, and metaanalyses of all clinical series, suggest that even low doses of ASA benefit early stroke and vascular mortality in patients with a history of TIAs or minor ischemic events.

### Combination Aspirin/Dipyridamole

Clinical use of the combination of ASA with dipyridamole has been based upon positive interactions between the agents in both preclinical experiments and in clinical platelet survival studies (87–90). The efficacy of this combination, however,

has been challenged (88,89). Dipyridamole (400–800 mg per day) alone did not affect the incidence of stroke or related mortality compared with placebo in one limited double-blind, level I randomized trial (91).

The European Stroke Prevention Study (ESPS) Group demonstrated a 33% reduction in risk of stroke and death with ASA (975 mg per day) and dipyridamole (225 mg per day) compared to placebo (83). The three-arm "AICLA" study also demonstrated the benefits from the combination of ASA with dipyridamole over placebo (but no difference with ASA alone) for patients with TIAs when the outcome events of

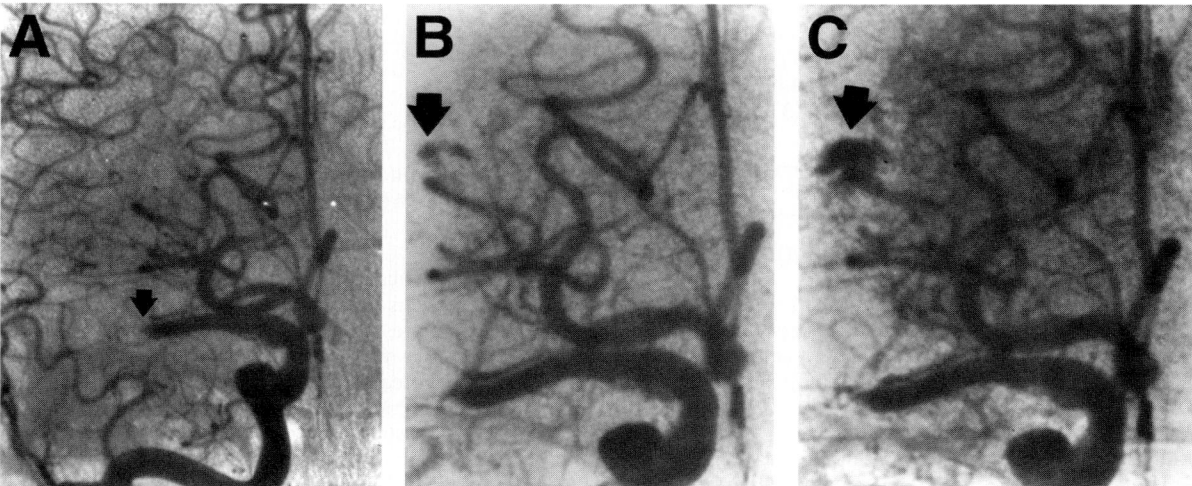

**FIGURE 102-4.** Evolution of parenchymal hemorrhage following intravenous infusion of recombinant tissue-type plasminogen activator (rtPA). *Arrows* indicate evolving hemorrhage. **A:** Obstruction of prox-imal middle cerebral artery (MCA) (M1 segment). **B, C:** During systemic rtPA infusion, following par-tial recanalization of the MCA, progressive extravasation from a distal lenticulostriatal artery was noted. A large parenchymal hematoma with ventricular extension results (see Fig. 102-3). (From the col-lection of M. Pessin, with permission.)

## TABLE 102-2

### TRANSIENT ISCHEMIC ATTACKS (±STROKE): ANTIPLATELET AGENTS

| Study | Agent | Dose (per day) | Patients ($n$) | Stroke ($n$) | Mortality ($n$) |
|---|---|---|---|---|---|
| AITIA Study (77) | ASA | 1,300 mg | 88 | 10 | 3 |
| | Placebo | — | 90 | 12 | 7 |
| Canadian Cooperative Study Group (78) | ASA/placebo 1 | 1,300 mg/— | 144 | 22 | 4 |
| | Sulfinpyrazone/ placebo 2 | 800 mg/— | 156 | | |
| | | | | 29 | 9 |
| | ASA/sulfinpyrazone | 1,300 mg/800 mg | 146 | 14 | 6 |
| | Placebo 1/placebo 2 | —/— | 139 | 20 | 10 |
| Danish Cooperative Study (79) | ASA | 1,000 mg | 101 | 18 | 7 |
| | Placebo | — | 102 | 11 | 7 |
| AICLA (80) | ASA/dipyridamole | 990 mg/225 mg | 202 | 18 | 8 |
| | ASA | 990 mg | 198 | 17 | 10 |
| | Placebo | — | 204 | 31 | 7 |
| UK-TIA Study Group (14) | ASA | 1,200 mg | 815 | 66 | 111 |
| | ASA | 300 mg | 806 | 68 | 106 |
| | Placebo | — | 814 | 88 | 122 |
| Dutch TIA Trial Study Group (81) | ASA | 283 mg | 1,576 | 109 | 151 |
| | ASA | 30 mg | 1,555 | 90 | 160 |
| SALT (82) | ASA | 75 mg | 676 | 93 | 61 |
| | Placebo | — | 684 | 112 | 69 |
| European Stroke Prevention Study Group (83) | ASA/dipyridamole | 975 mg/225 mg | 1,250 | 114 | 108 |
| | Placebo | — | 1,250 | 184 | 156 |
| American–Canadian Cooperative Study Group (84) | ASA/dipyridamole | 1,300 mg/300 mg | 448 | 53 | 46 |
| | ASA | 1,300 mg | 442 | 60 | 38 |
| Matius–Guiu et al. (85) | ASA/dipyridamole | 50 mg/300 mg | 115 | 3 | 2 |
| | Dipyridamole | 400 mg | 71 | 3 | 3 |
| European stroke Prevention Study-2 (60) | ASA/dipyridamole[a] | 400 mg/50 mg | 1,650 | 157 | 285 |
| | Dipyridamole[a] | 400 mg | 1,654 | 211 | 288 |
| | ASA | 50 mg | 1,649 | 206 | 282 |
| | Placebo | — | 1,649 | 250 | 202 |
| Hass et al. (86) | Ticlopidine | 500 mg | 1,529 | 172 | 175 |
| | ASA | 1,300 mg | 1,540 | 212 | 196 |

ASA, aspirin (acetylsalicylic acid); UK-TIA, United Kingdom Transient Ischemic Attack; AITIA, Aspirin in Transient Ischemic Attacks; TIA, transient ischemic attacks; SALT, Swedish Aspirin Low-Dose Trial.
[a]Extended-release dipyridamole.

stroke, MI, and mortality were combined (80). However, there was no difference in stroke or mortality between combination of ASA (1,300 mg per day) and dipyridamole (300 mg per day) and ASA alone in the American–Canadian Cooperative Study Group Study (84).

On the basis of experimental evidence suggesting that sustained release of dipyridamole could produce elevated plasma adenosine levels, the relative efficacy of the fixed combination of low dose ASA (50 mg per day) and sustained release dipyridamole (400 mg per day) was tested in the European Stroke Prevention Study-2 (ESPS-2) against sustained release of dipyridamole, ASA, or placebo. At a 2-year follow-up, low-dose ASA alone and dipyridamole alone [relative risk reduction (RRR) for stroke, 15.8% and 17.7%, respectively] and the combination (RRR, 36.7%) were found to be superior to placebo in limiting stroke, death, or both for individuals with a history of TIAs or recent stroke (60,92).

### Adenosine Diphosphate Receptor Antagonists

Thienopyridines irreversibly block the adenosine diphosphate (ADP) platelet receptor $P2Y_{12}$ and inhibit other downstream events, thereby blocking platelet activation. Ticlopidine has found benefit in patients with TIA/minor stroke (86), and in prevention of secondary stroke (see subsequent text). Ticlopidine (500 mg per day) was associated with a statistically significant 12% reduction in the risk of stroke and death from any cause over ASA (1,300 mg per day), and a 21% reduction in the risk of secondary outcomes of stroke and stroke-related death following transient ischemic symptoms. Reversible leukopenia occurred in 0.8% of patients taking ticlopidine, whereas gastrointestinal symptoms were more common in patients receiving ASA. Intracerebral hemorrhage occurred equally in both groups. Because of concerns about the frequency of thrombotic thrombocytoperic purpura (TTP), ticlopidine has been supplanted by the related thienopyridine clopidogrel.

### Sulfinpyrazone

The Canadian Cooperative Study Group compared ASA, the uricosuric agent sulfinpyrazone (800 mg per day), and placebo but found no significant difference in the incidence of stroke and mortality between sulfinpyrazone and placebo over 2.2 years (78). Sulfinpyrazone (800 mg per day) and placebo were also tested in a double-blind, crossover trial (93). A nonsignificant reduction in TIAs and in stroke and mortality at 4-month follow-up was recorded in patients receiving sulfinpyrazone. Another level I study comparing sulfinpyrazone (800 mg per day) and

ASA (1,000 mg per day) in individuals with TIAs concluded that there was a higher incidence of stroke, MI, and vascular death in the sulfinpyrazone cohort at 11-month follow-up (94). It has been concluded that sulfinpyrazone plays no role in ischemic stroke.

In summary, ASA reduces the risk of stroke, MI, and mortality in individuals with a history of TIAs or minor stroke. This risk reduction is obviously not dose-dependent. The fixed combination of low-dose ASA/sustained-release dipyridamole also produces a substantial risk reduction. Ticlopidine was more effective than ASA in preventing stroke and mortality after TIAs in one study but is seldom used now because of unwanted side effects. When used alone, dipyridamole and sulfinpyrazone have little demonstrated benefit.

## Anticoagulation

Changes in plasma thrombin concentration and FDP levels following ischemic stroke have been reported that suggest that interruption of coagulation may be beneficial. In the 1960s and 1970s, clinical experience with anticoagulation in patients with TIAs or minor stroke was limited (95–98). Uncontrolled reports suggested that heparin could decrease the incidence of basilar artery TIAs (99,100). Fisher observed a transient reduction in the incidence of TIAs in 97% (of 29) patients treated with anticoagulants, with TIAs returning in 60% of those in whom anticoagulation was discontinued (101). Two studies reported that long-term anticoagulation decreased the incidence of strokes and/or vascular death among patients with recent TIAs (102,103); a third separate study showed that despite a decrease in TIA frequency, there was no decrease in the incidence of stroke or vascular death (104). Two other studies failed to show superiority of anticoagulation over its comparator for the incidence of stroke or death (105,106). In a small trial of phenindione sponsored by the Medical Research Council (MRC), patients with TIA receiving fixed "low-dose" oral anticoagulation had a lower incidence of vascular events, stroke, and death than those patients receiving an adjusted "high-dose" regimen (107). Only the Cerebral Embolism Study Group trial indicated a benefit from immediate anticoagulation for cardiogenic embolism (108).

There have been few controlled prospective randomized level I studies. The Warfarin-Aspirin Recurrent Stroke Study (WARSS) found no difference in outcome between TIA and patients with stroke treated with oral anticoagulation under tight control compared to patients treated with ASA (109). There was no increase in intracerebral hemorrhage in the anticoagulated group, most probably because of the rigid control of the international normalized ratio (INR) (109).

The randomized European/Australian Stroke Prevention in Reversible Ischaemia Trial (ESPRIT) group is examining the impact of oral anticoagulation (INR = 2.0 to 3.0), the combination of ASA (30 to 375 mg per day) and dipyridamole (400 mg per day), or ASA alone on the outcomes of vascular death, nonfatal stroke, nonfatal MI, or major hemorrhage on patients with a TIA or minor ischemic stroke (110). A recent interim-safety analysis for intracerebral hemorrhage has indicated that the incidence of these events was acceptable.

Older patients have an age-related increased risk of intracerebral hemorrhage when treated with oral anticoagulants which inhibit vitamin K activity (111). With careful monitoring and dose adjustment, this risk can be reduced (109). However, earlier trials have demonstrated an increase in intracerebral hemorrhage (112,113). The Stroke Prevention in Reversible Ischemic Trial (SPIRIT) was terminated because of an unacceptably high incidence of intracranial hemorrhage in the group at a high target INR of 3.0 to 4.5.

In summary, excluding individuals with AF or cardiac valvular prostheses, the results of various small studies do not conclusively support a role for anticoagulation in patients with TIA or minor stroke, considering the risk of hemorrhage. The risk of intracerebral hemorrhage is increased for patients receiving oral anticoagulants at INRs in excess of 3.0 to 4.5.

## Plasminogen Activators

There is no basis for the use of fibrinolytic agents in patients with TIAs or cerebral ischemic episodes. The excessive use of plasminogen activators after symptom onset does not necessarily exclude treatment of individuals with TIAs.

# STROKE-IN-PROGRESSION

Progressive deterioration following ischemic stroke has been viewed by some as a separate clinical entity. Symptom progression could result from (a) anterograde extension of in situ thrombus to occlude critical arterial branches or from (b) recurrent embolism. The role of anticoagulation in patients with stroke-in-progression, however, remains unsettled, in large part, because of the difficulty in defining what constitutes "progression" at entry, and uncertainties about the pathogenesis of "evolving stroke." Early studies also reveal methodologic weaknesses and conflicting outcomes of this diagnosis (114–116). As noted earlier, deterioration following ischemic stroke may be because of edema, tissue swelling, or hemorrhage (117).

The Trial of Org 10172 in Acute Stroke Treatment (TOAST) was the only level I prospective randomized study of anticoagulation for stroke-in-evolution. However, entry was opened to all patients with hemispheric stroke symptoms for up to 24 hours (118). In this study, there was no advantage of the heparinoid, danaparoid, over placebo in disability indices, neurologic status, or mortality although a short-lived reduction in stroke incidence was seen (118,118–120). The occurrence of intracerebral hemorrhage of a serious nature was significantly more frequent in patients who received danaparoid than in patients receiving placebo (14 of 646 vs. four of 635 patients) (121). But, danaparoid displayed a considerable advantage for prevention of deep venous thrombosis (DVT). Therefore, stroke-in-progression is no longer identified as a separate entity for which a specific treatment is required.

# COMPLETED STROKE

Prospective CT scan and magnetic resonance imaging (MRI) (122–124) have confirmed the experimental observation that the ischemic lesion stabilizes, as an infarct, by 24 hours after occlusion of the supply artery (125,126). These congruent findings suggest that antithrombotic interventions beyond 24 to 72 hours after symptom onset are unlikely to have a beneficial impact on the initial ischemic stroke. Following a signal (first-time) ischemic stroke, the rate of subsequent focal cerebral ischemic events, MI, death, or vascular-related death is 10% to 12% per year (127–129). Therefore, antithrombotic agents can reduce the incidence of second ischemic events after completed stroke (secondary prevention).

## Antiplatelet Agents

Two metaanalyses suggest benefit from antiplatelet agents in patients with TIAs or first stroke (121,130). When considered with TIAs, ASA or ticlopidine can significantly decrease the

## TABLE 102-3

### COMPLETED STROKE: ANTIPLATELET AGENTS

| Study | Agent | Dose (per day) | Patients (n) | Stroke (n) | Mortality (n) |
|---|---|---|---|---|---|
| Swedish Cooperative | ASA | 1,500 mg | 253 | 32 | 34 |
| Study (128) | Placebo | | 252 | 32 | 37 |
| Gent et al. (129) | Suloctidil | 600 mg | 218 | 29[a] | 13[a] |
| | Placebo | | 220 | 28[a] | 25[a] |
| Blakeley (131) | Sulfinpyrazone | 800 mg | 145 | — | 25 |
| | Placebo | | 145 | — | 28 |
| Canadian–American | Ticlopidine | 500 mg | 525 | 54 | 30[a] |
| Ticlopidine Study (127) | Placebo | | 528 | 89 | 38[a] |
| CAPRIE (132)[b] | Clopidogrel | 75 mg | 3,233 | 315 | — |
| | ASA | 325 mg | 3,198 | 338 | — |
| IST (54) | ASA[c] | 300 mg | 9,720 | 362[d] | 872 |
| | no ASA[c] | — | 9,715 | 452[d] | 909 |
| CAST (133) | ASA | 160 mg | 10,554 | 335 | 343 |
| | no ASA | — | 10,552 | 351 | 398 |

ASA, aspirin; CAPRIE, Clopidogrel versus Aspirin in Individuals at Risk of Ischemic Events; IST, International Stroke Trial; CAST, Chinese Acute Stroke Trial.
[a]Eligible events only, excluding events >28 days after study-drug was permanently discontinued.
[b]Stroke subgroup.
[c]Factorial design (include heparin ± ASA).
[d]14-day outcomes.

risk of second cerebral ischemic events (see Table 102-3). As noted in preceding text, the combination of ASA and sustained-release dipyridamole considerably reduces the incidence of second stroke and/or death in patients presenting with a history of TIAs or stroke compared to ASA or dipyridamole alone (92).

The IST randomized 19,435 patients with presumed ischemic stroke within 48 hours of symptom onset to placebo, ASA (300 mg per day) alone, subcutaneous heparin (low dose, 10,000 IU per day; or medium dose, 25,000 IU per day), or both ASA and heparin for 14 days in a 3 × 2 factorial design (54). ASA was associated with an overall statistically significant reduction in total recurrent ischemic strokes within 14 days (P <0.001) and also a significant 0.1% increase in symptomatic intracranial hemorrhage. At 6 months, a modest decrease in the risk of death or dependency was seen. The Chinese Acute Stroke Trial (CAST) demonstrated similar outcomes (134). Together, the IST and CAST trials demonstrated that ASA is associated with a small reduction in the incidence of recurrent stroke and mortality in the first weeks after signal stroke but that the effect did not persist.

Ticlopidine (500 mg per day) was found to be superior to placebo in reducing the risk of second stroke, MI, and vascular mortality compared to placebo when patients were entered into the trial within 1 to 16 weeks following a signal thromboembolic stroke (127). Side effects related to ticlopidine, consisting of reversible leukopenia, diarrhea, or rash occurred in 8% of the treated patients.

Concerns about the side effects of ticlopidine prompted a study of the efficacy of the related thienopyridine derivative clopidogrel. The Clopidogrel versus Aspirin in Individuals at Risk of Ischemic Events (CAPRIE) study, a prospective, randomized, double-blind level I comparison of clopidogrel (75 mg per day) against ASA (325 mg per day) in patients presenting with ischemic stroke (including lacunar disease), MI less than 35 days old, or symptomatic atherosclerotic peripheral arterial disease (PAD), demonstrated a statistically significant 8.7% reduction in the risk of the combined outcomes of ischemic stroke, MI, or vascular-related death compared to ASA with clopidogrel (132). The overall benefit associated with

clopidogrel was driven by the outcome for PAD, but there did not appear to be an independent significant difference in outcome in the stroke cohort. Because of the near equivalent frequency of intracranial hemorrhage (clopidogrel = 0.33% vs. ASA = 0.47%), and clinically significant neutropenia, clopidogrel is now often being substituted for ticlopidine for secondary prevention. The Management of Atherothrombosis with Clopidogrel in high-risk patients (MATCH) trial compared the efficacy of clopidogrel/ASA to clopidogrel alone for ischemic events including stroke. No difference was seen in outcome between the two groups, although the ASA-containing combination was associated with a higher incidence of intracranial hemorrhage. Full assessment of the study awaits publication of the data. More recently, a prospective comparison of clopidogrel to the combination of ASA and sustained-release dipyridamole (with or without a proprietary angiotensin receptor blocker), the Prevention Regimen for Effectively avoiding Second Strokes (PRoFESS) study, has been initiated for nonsuperiority of first recurrent stroke in a 2 × 2 factorial design.

The novel antiplatelet agents sulfinpyrazone (131) and suloctidil (129) failed to demonstrate benefit over placebo in separate modest-sized trials. Neither agent is used in stroke management.

The value of the glycoprotein IIb/IIIa (integrin $\alpha_{IIb}\beta_3$) antagonist abciximab given within 24 hours of the onset of ischemic stroke has been examined in a phase II study (135). No significant improvement in outcome efficacy or increased risk of intracerebral hemorrhage was seen in 74 patients at the doses tested (135). This observation is in contrast to published experimental studies with polypeptide or organic molecule integrin $\alpha_{IIb}\beta_3$ inhibitors in experimental models of middle cerebral artery occlusion (MCA:O) (47,51).

Because of the effects on stroke outcome in patients with TIAs, ASA is recommended for secondary prevention. Ticlopidine produces a considerable reduction in subsequent stroke, MI, or vascular-related death over ASA in individuals with an initial completed stroke. On the basis of its similar mode of action to ticlopidine, clopidogrel has been substituted in practice. Current ACCP (American College of Chest Physicians) recommendations for secondary prevention in noncardioembolic ischemic stroke are management with ASA (50–325 mg per day), ASA/sustained-release dipyridamole, or clopidogrel (75 mg per day).

## Anticoagulants

The evidence that heparin or long-term oral anticoagulation benefits patients with presumed atherothrombotic "completed" stroke is sparse. Early randomized, controlled trials and uncontrolled studies of oral anticoagulation have given the impression that anticoagulant therapy does not prevent second stroke events in patients with an initial TIA or stroke (105,136–140). Subsequent studies have not altered the overall impression that anticoagulant therapy does not prevent second stroke events in patients with an initial TIA or stroke.

IST and CAST were conducted on the premise that proper use of subcutaneous unfractionated heparin should not be associated with an increase in intracerebral hemorrhage and may therefore be safe in the treatment of presumed primary atherothrombotic stroke (54,55,134). In IST, low-dose heparin (5,000 IU or 10,000 IU) was associated with a significant reduction in recurrent stroke over placebo (54,55,134). However, the significant increase in symptomatic intracerebral hemorrhage nullified the benefits of heparin on recurrent stroke. It is uncertain why hemorrhagic complications were so prominent in that study.

Low-molecular-weight heparins (LMWHs) have been tested with the intent to alter the outcome of first-ever stroke, usually not before 24 hours after symptom onset (see Table 102-4). In the Fraxiparin in Stroke Study (FISS), patients were randomized to subcutaneous "high-dose" nadroparin (8,200 IU of anti–factor Xa per day), "low-dose" nadroparin (4,100 IU per day), or placebo for 10 days beginning within 48 hours after onset of stroke (141). A significant dose-dependent reduction in 6-month mortality and dependence was observed favoring the nadroparin arm. FISS-bis, a follow-on trial of nadroparin in stroke, compared similar doses, but demonstrated no difference in combined outcome or mortality (unpublished). In HAEST (heparin in acute embolic stroke trial), the LMWH dalteparin produced no significant improvement in favorable

outcome compared to placebo when both were delivered early following the onset of stroke (142). No difference in detectable intracerebral hemorrhage was observed. The effect of certoparin on ischemic stroke outcome was examined in a level II dose-finding trial. No significant difference in outcome was detected among dose steps ranging from 3,000 U to 16,000 U per day (143). A modest increase in the number of patients with symptomatic hemorrhage was seen at the high dose. Among heparinoids, there was no sustained benefit from danaparoid after stroke in TOAST (118).

With the intent to determine whether oral anticoagulation could be superior to antiplatelet treatment (e.g., ASA), the Warfarin-Aspirin Recurrent Stroke Study (WARSS) found no differential benefit of warfarin or ASA on the frequency of secondary cerebral ischemic events in patients presenting within 30 days of the signal stroke (109). Warfarin was not associated with an increase in intracerebral hemorrhage, probably because of the tight monitoring of the INR. ESPRIT, an ongoing trial, compares therapeutic oral anticoagulation with combination ASA/dipyridamole, or ASA alone (110).

At present, there is no evidence of an advantage to the use of anticoagulants for completed stroke (144,145). However, none of those studies instituted anticoagulants in the acute-phase.

## Plasminogen Activators

Early experience with plasminogen activators in patients with completed stroke failed to demonstrate efficacy when symptomatic improvement and death were the primary outcomes. Level I clinical trials evaluating intravenous infusion of thrombolytic agents in completed stroke were inconclusive. Fletcher et al. observed no benefit in 31 patients treated with urokinase plasminogen activator (uPA) within 10 to 12 hours of symptom onset but observed a troublesome incidence of symptomatic intracranial hemorrhage and related mortality (146). Consequently, there resulted a general contraindication to the use of plasminogen activators in individuals with stroke (147). The long interval to treatment after onset of stroke and the possibility that the stroke was caused by undiagnosed hemorrhage in the absence of the availability of scanning technologies, are

---

**TABLE 102-4**

COMPLETED STROKE: ANTICOAGULATION

| Study | Agent | Dose (per day) | Patients (n) | Stroke (n) | Mortality (n) |
|---|---|---|---|---|---|
| FISS (141) | Nadroparin[a] | 8,200 aFXa | 100 | — | 45[a] |
| | Nadroparin[a] | 4,100 aFXa | 101 | — | 53[a] |
| | Placebo | — | 105 | — | 68[a] |
| FISS-bis | Nadroparin[a] | 172 aFXa/kg | 245 | — | 145[a] |
| | Nadroparin[a] | 86 aFXa/kg | 272 | — | 156[a] |
| | Placebo | — | 250 | — | 142[a] |
| HAEST (142) | Dalteparin | 200 IU/kg | 224 | 19[b] | 148[a] |
| | ASA | 160 mg | 225 | 17[b] | 146[a] |
| TOPAS (143) | Certoparin | 16,000 aFXa | 97 | 13[c] | 12 |
| | Certoparin | 10,000 aFXa | 103 | 10[c] | 7 |
| | Certoparin | 6,000 aFXa | 102 | 6[c] | 7 |
| | Certoparin | 3,000 aFXa | 98 | 11[c] | 4 |

aFXa, antifactor Xa activity; FISS, Fraxiparin in Stroke Study; HAEST, Heparin in Acute Embolic Stroke Trial; TOPAS, Therapy of Patients with Acute Stroke.
[a]Death or dependency at latest follow-up.
[b]At 14 days.
[c]Including transient ischemic attacks (TIAs).

common concerns with these early studies. A group of prospective, randomized, controlled low-dose studies of intravenous urokinase (uPA) or tissue plasminogen activator (tPA) in patients with stable focal neurologic deficits of less than 5 days duration demonstrated no difference in clinical outcome or in the incidence of symptomatic intracerebral hemorrhage (148–151).

# ACUTE INTERVENTIONS IN ISCHEMIC STROKE

A major change in the approach to ischemic stroke followed the proposal that plasminogen activators should be applied acutely (within 6 to 8 hours) after symptom onset (152). Experimental studies support the concept of metastable, potentially reversible zones of neuron and tissue injury in the ischemic vascular territory supplied by the occluded cerebral artery (153,154). The contributions of local vascular anatomy and collateral vascular protection to tissue perfusion, as well as the predominantly thrombotic basis for focal cerebral ischemia, underlie attempts to achieve early recanalization with plasminogen activators.

Acute intervention with plasminogen activators in patients selected by strict CT scan and by clinical criteria is associated with evidence of benefit (6,56). In contrast, although experimental studies have suggested that acute interventions with antiplatelet agents and anticoagulants could increase vascular patency and decrease injury, no clinical studies of acute intervention in ischemic stroke patients with either class have been pursued.

## Systemic Infusion of Plasminogen Activators

Recanalization of ICA occlusions by plasminogen activities is infrequent (0% to 25%) (6,6,148,149,155,156), but partial or complete arterial recanalization has been reported in 34% to 59% of patients with carotid artery territory occlusions who were treated within 6 to 8 hours of symptom onset (6,155–157). Mori et al. demonstrated, in a randomized controlled trial, that patients treated with 20 or 30 MIU of recombinant tissue-type plasminogen activator (rtPA) (duteplase) had improved recanalization and considerable clinical improvement at 30 days compared to patients treated

with placebo (155). Patients demonstrating early recanalization had better neurologic outcome than those patients not exhibiting recanalization. In these studies, detectable hemorrhagic transformation occurred in 29% to 53% of treated individuals (6,155–157), which was similar to natural history (65) (see section, "Hemorrhagic Transformation in Cerebral Ischemia"). Recanalization of vertebral or basilar artery occlusions with rtPA has been reported (156,157).

Three symptom-based, randomized, controlled trials of acute intravenous administration of streptokinase (SK) in patients with ischemic stroke were terminated because of excessive early mortality and symptomatic intracranial hemorrhage in the SK treatment groups (158–160). No preparatory dose-finding studies were performed in any of the trials (161,162). In the Multicentre Acute Stroke Trial-Italy (MAST-I) trial, the combination of ASA with SK produced excessive early case fatality. The outcome of the trial has not been explained, and the potential utility of SK in central nervous system (CNS) ischemia has not been pursued further.

rtPA (alteplase) is approved for intravenous use within 3 hours of symptom onset under strict patient-selection criteria (see Table 102-5). This is based upon the results of a two-part, level I, placebo-controlled outcome study (6). In part 1, there was no difference in neurologic status at 24 hours between the rtPA (0.9 mg per kg) and placebo-treated groups according to the National Institutes of Health Stroke Scale (NIHSS) score. In part 2, at 3 months posttreatment, rtPA recipients displayed a statistically significant 11% to 13% absolute improvement over placebo in Barthel index, modified Rankin scale (mRS) score, Glasgow outcome scale score, and NIHSS for evidence of no or minimal disability/deficit. The frequency of symptomatic hemorrhage was significantly greater among patients treated with rtPA (6.4%) than those patients who received placebo (0.6%). Mortality was unchanged, but intracerebral hemorrhage contributed to death. In follow-up, the outcome benefits in that population were sustained at 12 months and were most apparent in moderately severe strokes (163). Independent postlicensing use of rtPA in general practice has confirmed the original experience (164). Benefit was associated with age less than 75 years and absence of "early signs" of ischemic injury (164).

Three other phase III prospective randomized safety and efficacy studies of intravenous rtPA (alteplase) broaden the data, as shown in preceding table. The European Cooperative Acute

---

**TABLE 102-5**

ACUTE STROKE: PLASMINOGEN ACTIVATORS

| Study[a] | Agent | Patients (n) | Δ(T-0)[b] (h) | Clinical improvement (%) | Hemorrhage | | | |
|---|---|---|---|---|---|---|---|---|
| | | | | | nil | HI | PH | % |
| NINDS (part 1) (6) | rtPA | 144 | ≤1.5, ≤3.0 | 1.2[c] | — | — | 13 | 5.6 |
| | C | 147 | | | — | — | 3 | 0.0 |
| NINDS (part 2) (6) | rtPA | 168 | ≤1.5, ≤3.0 | 50[d] 31[e] | — | — | 21 | 7.1 |
| | C | 165 | | 38[d] 20[e] | — | — | 8 | 2.1 |
| ECASS (56) | rtPA | 313 | <6.0 | 35.9 | 179 | 72 | 62 | 19.8 |
| | C | 307 | | 29.3 | 184 | 93 | 30 | 6.5 |
| ECASS-2 (165) | rtPA | 409 | <6.0 | 40.3[d] | 217 | 142 | 48 | 11.8 |
| | C | 391 | | 36.6[d] | 233 | 141 | 12 | 3.1 |

C, control; HI, hemorrhagic infarction; PH, parenchymatous hematoma; rtPA, recombinant tissue-type plasminogen activator; SK, streptokinase; NINDS, National Institute of Neurologic Disorders and Stroke; ECASS, European Cooperative Acute Stroke Study.
[a]Randomized studies without vascular diagnosis.
[b]Time from symptom onset to treatment.
[c]Relative risk reduction.
[d]Modified Rankin scale (mRS) score 0 and 1.
[e]National Institutes of Health Stroke Scale (NIHSS).

Stroke Study (ECASS) compared intravenous infusion rtPA (1.1 mg per kg to a maximum of 100 mg) to placebo in patients within 6 hours of symptom onset of ischemic stroke. No significant difference was observed between the two groups for 90-day disability outcome (56). A *post hoc* analysis of the "target population" suggested an 11% to 12% absolute improvement over placebo in mRS 0 and 1 (no or minimal disability) in the rtPA–treated group. However, a significantly higher proportion of patients who received rtPA (6.1%) had intracerebral hemorrhage causing neurologic deterioration or death (PH2) than patients who received placebo (2.6%). A subgroup of patients with evidence of ischemia on the entry CT scan displayed increased mortality, which was further increased by treatment with rtPA. ECASS-II, the follow-on, randomized double-blind nonangiographic study, required a careful review of the baseline CT scans for "early signs of ischemia" for exclusion of those patients with ischemia (165,166). The patients were treated within 6 hours of symptom onset, and 40.3% of patients who received rtPA had a favorable outcome (mRS = 0 or 1). Severe symptomatic parenchymal hemorrhage (PH2) was significantly more frequent in the rtPA group (11.7%) than in the placebo group (3.1%).

In contrast, the uncompleted Alteplase Thrombolysis for Acute Noninterventional Therapy in Ischemic Stroke (AT-LANTIS) trial did not support early use of rtPA (167). Viewed together, the results of the ECASS and NINDS (National Institute of Neurologic Disorders and Stroke) studies indicate the enormous importance of individual patient selection in reducing the hemorrhagic risk accompanying the use of plasminogen activators in acute stroke (6,56,57). A recent pooled analysis of the NINDS, ECASS, and ATLANTIS studies indicated that the baseline-adjusted 3-month mortality was not different up to 4 to 5 hours after stroke onset with rtPA exposure (168). Today, rtPA is available for treatment of ischemic stroke in appropriately selected patients within 3 hours of the onset of symptoms in North America and certain other countries.

The studies of intravenous rtPA have underscored major contributors to the risk of intracerebral hemorrhage risk in ischemic stroke as well. These include excessive time from symptom onset to treatment, low body mass, diastolic hypertension, older age, and the use of rtPA (9,169,170). The appearance of "early signs of ischemia," marked by low attenuation and/or sulcal effacement on the initial CT scan, is associated with an increased risk of death and hemorrhage (56,170–173).

## Direct Local Infusion of Plasminogen Activators

Angiographically controlled intraarterial infusion allows delivery of higher local concentrations of plasminogen activators to the thrombus, and the definition of both vascular anatomy and outcome. Refinements of flow-directed and guide wire-directed catheter techniques pioneered by Zeumer et al., and catheter systems for the acute delivery of thrombolytic agents in the cerebral circulation have broadened the experience with local delivery (174), although the approach remains experimental (see Fig. 102-5). Among larger series, recanalization of symptomatic carotid artery territory occlusions has approached 46% to 90% of symptomatic patients treated with intraarterial infusion of SK or uPA within 8 hours (175–177). Detectable hemorrhagic transformation in the ischemia territory occurred in 18% to 33% of treated patients (see Table 102-6) (175–177).

Vertebrobasilar artery territory ischemia can produce considerable disability (180,181). Nenci et al. first demonstrated benefits after local intraarterial treatment of symptomatic

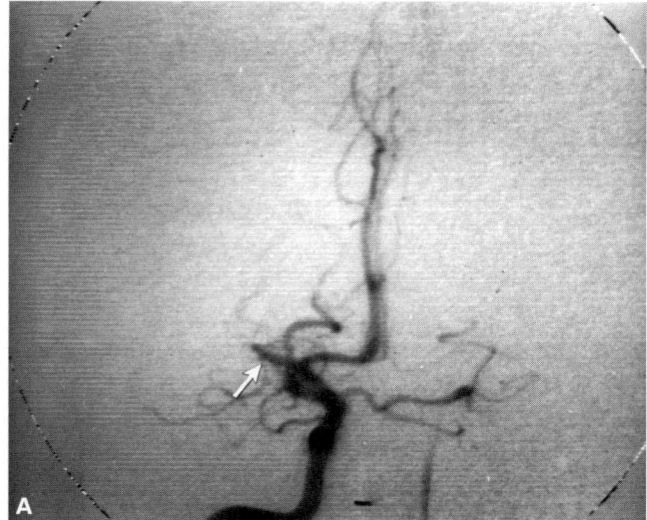
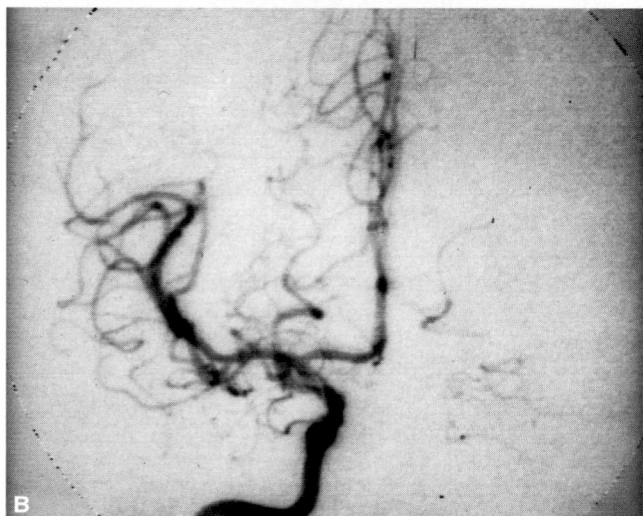

FIGURE 102-5. Recanalization of proximal middle cerebral artery (MCA) occlusion. **A:** Obstruction of the proximal MCA (M1 segment). Arrow indicates the site of thrombotic occlusion of the M1 segment. **B:** Relief of flow obstruction by direct intra-arterial urokinase infusion, with return of downstream arterial patency. (Angiograms courtesy of H. Zeumer.)

basilar thrombosis (182). One retrospective comparison of the clinical outcome in 43 patients who received intraarterial uPA or SK with 22 patients who received conventional therapy (i.e., heparin) suggested a considerable survival benefit in those demonstrating recanalization (who received the fibrinolytic agent) (183). Clinically significant hemorrhagic transformation occurred in four individuals treated with uPA or SK. Subsequent reports have supported recanalization efficacy with these agents (174,177,184).

The Prourokinase in Acute Cerebral Thromboembolism (PROACT) study was the first randomized double-blinded placebo-controlled examination of plasminogen activators by intraarterial infusion (7). In this phase II study, direct arterial infusion recombinant scuPA (rscuPA, rpro-UK) at a dose of 6 mg or placebo were tested for recanalization of M1 and M2 MCA occlusions and safety outcomes (7). Overall, rscuPA produced a significant increase in MCA recanalization and in hemorrhagic transformation. The increases in recanalization and hemorrhage were heparin dependent. The

**TABLE 102-6**

ACUTE STROKE: PLASMINOGEN ACTIVATORS

| Study[a] | Agent | Patients (n) | $\Delta$(T-0)[b] (h) | Recanalization (%) | Hemorrhage (%) |
|---|---|---|---|---|---|
| **CAROTID TERRITORY: INTRAARTERIAL DELIVERY** | | | | | |
| del Zoppo et al. (176) | SK/uPA | 20 | 1–24 | 90.0 | 20.0 |
| Mori et al. (175) | uPA | 22 | 0.82–7 | 45.5 | 18.2 |
| Matsumoto and Satoh (177) | uPA | 40 | 1–24 | 60.0 | 32.5 |
| PROACT (7) | scuPA/h | 26 | <6.0 | 57.7 | 42.3 |
| | C/h | 14 | <6.0 | 14.3 | 7.1 |
| PROACT-2 (178) | scuPA/h | 121 | <6.0 | 65.7 | 10.2 |
| | —/h (iv) | 59 | <6.0 | 18.0 | 1.9 |
| **CAROTID TERRITORY: INTRAVENOUS DELIVERY** | | | | | |
| Yamaguchi (156) | rtPA | 52 | <6.0 | 38.5 | 28.6 |
| von Kummer et al. (157) | rtPA | 22 | <6.0 | 59.1 | 36.4 |
| del Zoppo et al. (9) | rtPA | 93 (104)[c] | <8.0 | 34.4[c] | 30.8 |
| Mori et al. (155) | rtPA | 19 | <6.0 | 47.4 | 52.6 |
| | C | 12 | | 16.7 | 41.7 |
| Yamaguchi (179) | rtPA | 47 (51)[c] | <6.0 | 21.3 | 47.1 |
| | C | 46 (47)[c] | | 4.4 | 46.8 |

C, control; h, heparin; rtPA, recombinant tissue-type plasminogen activator; scuPA, single-chain urokinase plasminogen activator; SK, streptokinase; PROACT, Pro-urokinase in Acute Cerebral Thromboembolism.
[a] Studies employing angiography.
[b] Time from symptom onset to treatment.
[c] ( ) refers to the total number of patients treated in intention-to-treat.

follow-on open study, PROACT-2, randomized patients with symptomatic proximal MCA occlusions to recombinant scuPA (9 mg) or to placebo for recanalization and for 3-month disability outcome (178). Both groups also received heparin. Recanalization was significantly greater with recombinant scuPA (65.7%) compared to no intervention (18.0%), as was the frequency of symptomatic intracerebral hemorrhage. Whereas the proportion of patients with no or minimal disability (measured as mRS = 0 to 1) was not significantly different between the two groups, rscuPA was associated with an improvement in outcome measured as mRS = 0 to 2. No further exploration of rscuPA has ensued, and it is not available for clinical use.

## Defibrinogenating Agents

Fibrinogen in plasma can be degraded by certain snake venoms (185). Reduction of fibrinogen to 100 mg per dL by the defibrinating agent ancrod in patients with acute ischemic stroke has been considered to be safe (186). According to prespecified covariate-adjusted analyses (taking into account baseline stroke severity), favorable outcome was more frequent in the ancrod-treated group (42.2%) than in the placebo-treated group (34.4%) in the Stroke Treatment with Ancrod Trial (STAT) (186,187). Intracranial hemorrhage was moderately more frequent in the ancrod group. The novel design of STAT has demonstrated that careful intervention with this agent could produce a favorable benefit–risk profile. In the European Stroke Treatment with Ancrod Trial (ESTAT), no advantage to ancrod was observed (188). However, differences in study design and patient recruitment with STAT were observed (188). The development of ancrod for the acute treatment of ischemic stroke has continued.

# CAROTID ARTERY ATHEROTHROMBOTIC DISEASE

Atherosclerosis produces a thrombophilic state. The carotid artery bifurcation as well as other large-artery branch points are predilection sites for atheroma formation and are sources of embolic cholesterol and thrombi in the downstream cerebral hemispheres (Fig. 102-2). End arterectomy of the extracranial portion of the carotid artery can resolve the local vascular flow abnormalities, but cerebral ischemic symptoms can recur.

TIAs and minor strokes are products of carotid artery atherosclerosis. Although a major source of thromboemboli, 20% to 45% of strokes are unrelated to carotid artery stenosis (e.g., lacunes) (189). The North American Symptomatic Carotid Endarterectomy Trial (NASCET) and the MRC European Carotid Surgery Trial (ECST) demonstrated significant survival benefit and symptomatic relief from endarterectomy over medical (i.e., antiplatelet agent) therapy for carotid stenoses of 70 to 99% (190,191). Both trials were undertaken to resolve concerns arising from liberal use of this procedure in individuals with TIAs and to establish the role of surgical management. The benefits in reduction of ipsilateral stroke also accrue for endarterectomy of symptomatic stenosis of intermediate extent (50% to 69%) but depend on the balance of surgical risk (192).

The surgical management of asymptomatic carotid artery stenosis has been controversial. The multicenter comparison of carotid endarterectomy with optimal medical management [including antiplatelet agents (ASA)] in 444 men with asymptomatic carotid artery stenosis by the Veterans Affairs Cooperative Study Group demonstrated a statistically significant reduction in combined ipsilateral ischemic neurologic events in the surgical group (8.0% vs. 20.6%, P <0.001 ) (193). The frequency of ipsilateral stroke was 4.7% in the surgical group, and 9.4% in the medical group; however, there was no difference in stroke and stroke-related mortality at 30 days. ACAS prompted examination of local single center experiences with surgical treatment of asymptomatic carotid lesions, and a metaanalyses (194–196). Although benefit could be reproduced, postoperative mortality was a major variable (196). Overall, experience has indicated that benefit from carotid endarterectomy for asymptomatic lesions was modest at best, with no difference between medical management or surgery for perioperative mortality or stroke, although selected patients may benefit (196). Hence, carotid endarterectomy would be expected to benefit a select subset of asymptomatic patients and would depend upon the frequency of surgical complications.

Antiplatelet agents are adjuncts to carotid endarterectomy which lower the incidence of embolic stroke and death or decrease the incidence of carotid restenosis after carotid endarterectomy. In one prospective double-blind, placebo-controlled trial ASA (1,300 mg per day) given within 5 days of carotid endarterectomy, reduced the incidence of stroke or death at 6 months (197). In a separate trial, ASA (50 to 100 mg per day) 1 to 12 weeks after carotid endarterectomy had no appreciable effect on strokes, MI, or vascular death (198). Following a retrospective analysis of experience with ASA (1,500 mg per day) (199), a prospective comparison of presurgical ASA (1,000 mg per day) or no treatment was undertaken (200). Survival was extended in the ASA-treated group, although cerebral events occurred equally in both.

Although there are currently no results of level I trials to support any recommendation for specific adjunctive antiplatelet therapy after endarterectomy, current practice is to continue patients undergoing endarterectomy on ASA (81 to 325 mg per day) after the procedure. There is little information regarding a role for anticoagulants after endarterectomy, and fibrinolytic agents are contraindicated.

# CEREBRAL EMBOLISM FROM A CARDIAC SOURCE

Emboli from cardiac structures can cause focal cerebral ischemia. These sources include mural thrombi associated with left ventricular dyskinesia (e.g., after MI), prosthetic valves, rheumatic valvular vegetations, and thromboemboli arising during AF. Because of the thrombotic nature of most cardioembolic events, the role for anticoagulation has been suggested in both primary and secondary prevention.

## Cardioembolic Stroke Following Myocardial Infarction

The incidence of systemic thromboembolism, including stroke, after MI varies from 1% to 3% per year, but may be as high as 3.7% during the first month after MI (i.e., the acute-phase) (201–206). Antiplatelet agents could be effective in decreasing the incidence of post-MI cerebral events. However, evidence is scant. The CAPRIE study suggested that clopidogrel could reduce the combined events of second MI, stroke, or peripheral artery disease following an initial MI, although the benefit for MI was not significant (132).

Anticoagulation during the acute in-hospital phase and in the chronic posthospitalization phase has been shown to reduce the number of cerebrovascular events (201–207). Secondary prevention trials designed to determine the incidence of recurrent MI as the main outcome event have also examined the effect of long-term anticoagulation on stroke incidence.

Level II trials suggested a trend in favor of a reduction in post-MI stroke incidence. In the Veterans Administration Cooperative Study, however, there was no reduction in stroke incidence 1 to 5 years after MI for patients randomized to long-term anticoagulation within 21 days of their MI (201). The trend favoring anticoagulation for stroke was mirrored by an overall reduction in the combined outcomes of stroke, second MI, and death. A similar trend was seen in two subsequent trials and appeared independent of the type of oral anticoagulant (203,204). The Sixty Plus Reinfarction Study randomized patients older than 60 years who had MI to oral anticoagulation or placebo (205). At 2-year follow-up, anticoagulation was associated with a trend toward a lower stroke incidence.

Those studies also demonstrated an increased incidence of serious hemorrhages, which contributed to morbidity or death in the anticoagulated group (201,203–205). In the GAAT and the Sixty Plus Reinfarction studies, the number of serious anticoagulation-associated hemorrhages, including intracerebral events, was considered to be excessive. In the latter, seven intracranial hemorrhages occurred in the anticoagulated group, compared to one in the placebo group, although fatal intracranial events were equal. Approximately 72% of the anticoagulated patients had an INR of 2.7 to 4.5 (205).

Two level I placebo-controlled trials demonstrated a significant reduction in stroke incidence with anticoagulation (202,206). The Warfarin Reinfarction Study (WARIS) also reported a considerable decrease in the incidence of cerebrovascular events in patients who received warfarin (206). In both trials, hemorrhage was more common in the active treatment group. In WARIS, the target INR was 2.8 to 4.8, considered high by current measures. A randomized three-armed open trial (WARIS-II) of warfarin (INR = 2.8 to 4.2), warfarin and ASA (75 mg per day), or ASA (160 mg per day) alone in patients with MI for the combined outcomes of death, nonfatal reinfarction, and cerebral stroke is underway (208).

Three trials of anticoagulation during the acute in-hospital phase of MI demonstrated a decreased incidence of stroke (209–211). In a single-blind test which randomized patients to heparin/warfarin or placebo post-MI, anticoagulation was associated with a significant decrease in strokes (210). A second study demonstrated a trend in favor of heparin and oral anticoagulation (209). Both studies however, demonstrated no change in the combined outcomes of stroke, second MI, and death. A separate level I MRC-sponsored trial randomized patients to heparin/adjusted high-dose pheninidione or heparin/fixed low-dose pheninidione for 28 days within 14 days of acute MI. A significant decrease in the incidence of systemic embolism with the high-dose group was seen although there was no difference in recurrent MI or death (211). Both the incidence and severity of hemorrhagic complications were quite low. This experience suggests that cerebrovascular ischemic events during the early post-MI period can be reduced with anticoagulation.

In summary, long-term anticoagulation can decrease the number of cerebrovascular events after recovery from MI. In practice, however, concerns about the higher incidence of serious hemorrhagic events, including intracerebral hemorrhage has limited routine use of anticoagulants.

## Cardioembolic Stroke in Atrial Fibrillation

The pathogenesis of stroke and the role of antithrombotic regimens in individuals with nonrheumatic AF have been reviewed (212). In a retrospective study, Sage et al. indicated that the risk of cerebral infarction after an episode of nonvalvular AF can be 20% per year, with a mortality rate from the initial infarct of 38% per year (213). This is in accordance with the experience of Hart et al., who reported a 34.8% incidence of symptomatic embolism (13% cerebral) in individuals not undergoing immediate anticoagulation (214). These, and other data, have suggested the need for prospective clinical trials (see Table 102-7).

The AFASAK (Atrial Fibrillation, Aspirin, Anticoagulation) study openly randomized patients with nonrheumatic, nonvalvular AF to warfarin, ASA (75 mg per day), or placebo (215). At the 2-year follow-up, a significant decrease in cerebral embolic events was apparent in the warfarin group. Hemorrhagic complications were significantly more common in the warfarin group than in the ASA or placebo groups. Two additional trials of primary stroke prevention support this experience (216,217). The Stroke Prevention in Atrial Fibrillation (SPAF) study randomized patients with AF to warfarin, ASA, or placebo (group 1) if they were eligible for warfarin, or to ASA or placebo (group 2, double-blind) if they were not eligible for warfarin (216). SPAF-I was terminated when the warfarin and ASA arms of group 1 demonstrated a statistically significant combined 81% risk reduction in ischemic stroke and systemic embolism. The relative benefit of warfarin over ASA was not reported, but 10.9% of patients randomly assigned to warfarin were withdrawn because of drug intolerance. The Boston Area Anticoagulation Trial for Atrial Fibrillation (BAATAF) trial openly randomized individuals with nonrheumatic AF to long-term, low-dose warfarin or to no therapy (217). A statistically significant risk reduction of 86% for stroke and death favored the warfarin group. The number of fatal hemorrhages in the warfarin and no-therapy groups was identical. In 1990, results of the AFASAK and SPAF studies led to early termination of the Canadian Atrial Fibrillation Anticoagulation (CAFA) Study (218). In that trial, the warfarin group had a 44.8% risk reduction in ischemic stroke and systemic thromboembolism.

Concerns that the risk of intracranial hemorrhage could be associated with warfarin-fueled approaches using ASA (219) or low-dose oral anticoagulation (220). The SPAF-II trial examined the relative efficacies of warfarin and ASA in individuals with nonvalvular AF (219). That study prospectively stratified patients into two age cohorts: those 75 years or older, and those younger than 75 years. A modest, but not statistically significant, reduction in ischemic stroke events was associated with warfarin over ASA. There was a significantly greater frequency of major hemorrhagic events with warfarin in the older cohort than in the younger cohort, however. The low overall annual thromboembolic event rate was a concern. Nonsignificant differences between the ASA treatment and control arms of the AFASAK study, the European Atrial Fibrillation Trial (EAFT), and ESPS-2 were observed in patients with nonvalvular AF (118,215,221). ASA was associated with a statistically significant 21% relative risk reduction in annual stroke events in an individual patient combined analysis of AFASAK, EAFT, and SPAF-I (222). That conclusion was supported by a broader metaanalysis (223). Heterogeneity in the results could not be excluded (224).

More recently, to test the relative efficacy of antiplatelet strategies to standard anticoagulation, the Atrial Fibrillation Clopidogrel Focal with Irbesartan for prevention of Vascular Events (ACTIVE) trial compared the combination ASA and clopidogrel against warfarin for prevention of vascular events including stroke in patients with a high risk for AF. This study compares clopidogrel/ASA with warfarin (ACTIVE-W) and with ASA alone (ACTIVE-A), and the angiotensin II receptor blocker irbesartan versus placebo in a factorial design. The trial is ongoing.

Age greater than 80 years, intensity of anticoagulation, and prolonged prothrombin time from the therapeutic range are all contributors to increased risk of bleeding (225). The SPAF-III

## TABLE 102-7

### ATRIAL FIBRILLATION (NONVALVULAR): ANTIPLATELET AGENTS/ANTICOAGULANTS

| Study | Agent | Dose (per day) | Patients (*n*) | Stroke (*n*) | Mortality (*n*) |
|---|---|---|---|---|---|
| AFASAK (215) | Warfarin | INR = 2.8–4.2 | 335 | 5 | — |
| | ASA | 75 mg | 336 | 17(3) | — |
| | Placebo | | 336 | 19(2) | — |
| SPAF (216) | 1. Warfarin/ASA | INR = 2.0–3.5/ | 393 | 7 | 14 |
| | Placebo | 325 mg | 195 | 17(1) | 8 |
| | 2. ASA | 325 mg | 517 | 18(1) | 31 |
| | Placebo | | 528 | 34(4) | 39 |
| BAATAF (217) | Warfarin | INR = 1.5–2.7 | 212 | 2 | 11 |
| | Placebo | | 208 | — | 26 |
| CAFA (218) | Warfarin | INR = 2.0–3.0 | 187 | 4(1) | 7 |
| | Placebo | | 191 | 9(2) | 6 |
| SPAF II (219) | Warfarin[b] | INR = 2.0–4.5 | 358 | 13(1) | 36 |
| | ASA | 325 mg | 357 | 19(2) | 41 |
| | Warfarin[c] | INR = 2.0–4.5 | 197 | 13(1) | 26 |
| | ASA | 325 mg | 188 | 18(0) | 24 |
| SPAF III (220) | Warfarin | INR = 2.0–3.0 | 523 | 11(0) | 35 |
| | Warfarin | INR = 1.2–1.5 | 521 | 43(1) | 42 |

ASA, aspirin; INR, international normalized ratio; AFASAK, Atrial Fibrillation, Aspirin, Anticoagulation; SPAF, Stroke Prevention in Atrial Fibrillation; BAATAF, Boston Area Anticoagulation Trial for Atrial Fibrillation; CAFA, Canadian Atrial Fibrillation Anticoagulation.
[a]Numbers in parentheses indicate systemic embolic events.
[b]Patients ≤75 yr.
[c]Patients >75 yr.

trial addressed the integrity of anticoagulation (220). Patients were randomized either to adjusted-dose warfarin to maintain an INR of between 2.0 and 3.0, or to low-intensity warfarin with ASA (325 mg per day) to maintain an INR of between 1.2 and 1.5. SPAF-III was terminated when the annual disabling stroke rate of the combination therapy exceeded that of adjusted-dose warfarin (5.6% vs. 1.7%, respectively). When cumulative event rates were calculated, a nearly significant difference ($P = 0.07$) favoring warfarin seemed to support the results of previous studies (Table 102-7). The results of SPAF-III led to the early termination of the AFASAK-2 study of patients with moderate risk (226,227). A recent review of published data indicates that anticoagulation is superior to antiplatelet agents for the reduction of nonfatal stroke risk (228). In one retrospective study, the odds ratios for ischemic stroke incidence among patients with nonvalvular AF treated with warfarin was significantly less among those with INR greater than or equal to 2.0 compared to INR less than 2.0 (229). Hence, in this population oral anticoagulation to an INR greater than or equal to 2.0 decreases the frequency of stroke, its severity, and the risk of demise. These findings are consistent with the results of prospective trials. A recent review of published data indicates that anticoagulation is superior to antiplatelet agents for the reduction of nonfatal stroke risk (221).

Recently it was found that the oral factor Xa inhibitor ximelagatran was not inferior ($\pm2.5\%$) to warfarin in preventing systemic embolic events in patients with nonvalvular AF (230,231). In SPORTIF III warfarin generated a nonsignificant decrease in stroke incidence compared to ximelagatran (230,231). At the time of this writing, ximelagatran is not available for clinical use.

Information from secondary prevention trials involving patients with AF who present with a signal stroke is limited. In an open trial of anticoagulation in patients with stroke and nonvalvular AF, Lodder et al. found no difference in the incidence of second stroke or death at a mean follow-up of 2.25 years (232). Death from serious hemorrhage occurred in six of the 70 anticoagulated patients (18.6%). The Cerebral Embolism Study Group performed a randomized, open trial of immediate versus delayed anticoagulation patients with AF and cardioembolic strokes for the principal outcome event of recurrent embolism (108). Anticoagulation was initiated immediately after a signal stroke or 10 days after the first stroke. In that small series, two patients in the delayed treatment group had second embolic events. This limited experience, suggests caution in the use of anticoagulants in secondary prevention of recurrent cerebral embolism in AF.

In summary, the results of randomized, controlled trials of individuals with nonvalvular AF support the use of oral anticoagulation to reduce the incidence of embolic stroke (233). For patients with a high risk to AF (with a prior TIA/stroke or systemic embolus, history of hypertension, poor left ventricular function, age >75 years, rheumatic mitral valve disease, or a prosthetic valve) the recommended therapy is adjusted-dose warfarin anticoagulation at a target INR of 2.5 (range 2.0 to 3.0) rather than ASA (234).

# VALVULAR CARDIOVASCULAR DISEASE

Rheumatic valvular disease, mechanical or xenograft prosthetic cardiac valves, and calcified mitral annuli generate thromboemboli. Clinically detectable systemic embolism from untreated rheumatic mitral stenosis and mitral insufficiency occurs with a 3.7% and 1.9% yearly incidence, respectively. Recurrent embolism occurs frequently within 6 to 12 months after the signal embolism (235–237). The risk of cerebral embolism is greatly increased by concurrent AF (236,238,239).

And, the incidence of systemic embolism is greater for mechanical devices than for xenograft prostheses. Adjunctive antithrombotic strategies offer protection against thromboembolic complications of valve prostheses (238,239). But the use of xenograft prostheses has significantly altered the antithrombotic approach to prophylaxis.

## Mechanical Prosthetic Cardiac Valves

The incidence of cardiac source thromboembolic events depends upon the type of mechanical valves, their location, and the age of the patient. Although the data is incomplete, the rate of systemic embolic events (per year) appears greatest with caged disk or ball valves (2.5%), in excess of tilting disk (0.7%) or bileaflet (0.5%) valves (240). Generally, thromboembolic risk is higher for mechanical valves in the mitral position than in the aortic position (241), perhaps in part because of the association of AF (242,243). Finally, the incidence of systemic thromboembolisms is greatest in the elderly ($\geq70$ years) (240).

The use of oral anticoagulants has generally reduced the incidence of embolic events. Although individual series vary, and few prospective controlled studies have been undertaken, the higher incidence of emboli with caged devices suggests the need for increases of anticoagulation intensity. In one study of complications with bileaflet aortic valves, a greater reduction in thromboembolic rate was seen with an approximate INR = 2.5 to 3.5 (244). In one review of a number of series, that range of anticoagulation appeared efficacious (245). For valves in the aortic position (bileaflet and tilting variety) anticoagulation to a target INR of 2.5 (range 2.0 to 3.0) is recommended, and for valves in the mitral position the target INR of 3.0 (range 2.5 to 3.5) is recommended (241).

The addition of antiplatelet agents can increase the protection afforded by oral anticoagulation, but may increase the risk of hemorrhagic complications. Two level I studies demonstrated reduced thromboembolic risk in patients receiving combination anticoagulation with ASA over anticoagulation alone (246,247). The rate of systemic thromboembolic or vascular death was significantly reduced by addition of ASA (100 mg per day) to oral anticoagulation at INR 3.0 to 4.5 (248,249). ASA doses of 500 to 1,000 mg per day reduced the number of cerebral embolic and systemic embolic events considerably, although the hemorrhagic risk was dose-dependent (247). In view of the gastrointestinal side effects of ASA-containing regimens, addition of dipyridamole to oral anticoagulation has been successfully tested in patients with mechanical prosthetic cardiac valves (239). Whereas those studies suggested no increase in hemorrhage, the general experience supported an increase in major hemorrhage with this regimen.

Dipyridamole (400 mg per day) with warfarin considerably reduced thromboembolism or death compared to warfarin and placebo (250,251). The combination of dipyridamole with oral anticoagulation (INR 2.0 to 2.5) was associated with a low thromboembolic rate in a separate study (without a control arm) (252). In an open study of patients with mechanical prostheses, dipyridamole (400 mg per day) and warfarin were superior to warfarin and ASA (500 mg per day) (253), and major hemorrhagic complications were considerably fewer with the addition of dipyridamole.

The possibility that low dose ASA might also further reduce embolic events in patients with heart valve replacement already managed with warfarin was tested by Turpie et al. (254). In an open prospective trial, patients randomized to 100 mg per day ASA or 650 mg per day ASA (both receiving warfarin adjusted to a target INR of 2.0 to 3.0) showed no statistically significant difference with respect to systemic embolism, vascular death, or total death. However, the rate of hemorrhagic events in the high dose ASA group (13.4 vs.

7.9 events per 100 patient-years) significantly exceeded that of the low dose group. On this basis low dose ASA is often added to warfarin. However, metaanalysis of trials combining dipyridamole with oral anticoagulation indicated a decrease in fatal and nonfatal thromboemboli (255,256). Overall, dipyridamole further reduced the incidence of valvular thromboembolism.

## Xenograft Cardiac Valves

Systemic thromboembolic events occurred in 4% of patients with bioprostheses at 3 years who are in sinus rhythm and in 16% of patients with AF (257,258). The greatest risk of thromboembolism occured during the first 3 months after placement of the bioprosthesis (259,260). A lower frequency of major embolic events was seen in patients with porcine biosynthetic valves receiving anticoagulation for 6 to 12 weeks in one study (258). There was no difference in incidence of systemic emboli in patients with xenograft prostheses randomized to oral anticoagulation at an INR of 2.0 to 2.25 or at an INR of 2.5 to 4.0 (standard anticoagulation) for the first 3 postoperative months, although, clinically significant hemorrhagic events were more frequent in the group receiving standard anticoagulation (261).

The benefit of antiplatelet agents has been evaluated in several level III studies (262–264). Those studies implied that warfarin or ASA (1,000 or 500 mg per day) produced similar risk reduction in patients in sinus rhythm. Patients with mitral valve bioprostheses who received 500 mg ASA every two days were less likely to have embolic events than those who received 1,000 mg per day (264). However, this conclusion has not been rigorously tested. Accepted clinical practice required anticoagulation for the initial 3 months following placement of the bioprosthesis.

# THROMBOTIC EVENTS ASSOCIATED WITH CENTRAL NERVOUS SYSTEM INJURY

## Deep Venous Thrombosis

DVT can complicate the early course of recovery from stroke (265). Heparinoids and low-molecular-weight heparins have been tested as alternatives to prophylactic unfractionated heparin. Early experience with prophylactic use of two low-molecular-weight heparin preparations, however, was mixed (266–268). Twice-daily subcutaneous treatment with one preparation was associated with considerably reduced frequency of DVT (268). Turpie et al. demonstrated an advantage of twice-daily subcutaneous administration of a low-molecular-weight heparinoid over subcutaneous heparin in decreasing the incidence of DVT (269). In the TOAST trial, danaparoid produced a considerable reduction in the frequency of poststroke DVT, compared to placebo (119,120,270–272).

Hence, prophylactic use of anticoagulants to decrease venous thromboembolism is encouraged for patients having stroke.

## Sagittal Sinus Thrombosis

Cortical vein thrombosis can accompany local inflammation, thrombophilic states (including anticardiolipin or antiphospholipid antibodies), or pregnancy, or it can be idiopathic. Although thrombolytic agents have been employed unusually, anticoagulation is the treatment of choice. Petechial hemorrhage is a common finding with sagittal sinus thrombosis.

## Retinal Vascular Thrombosis

Retinal arterial occlusions are commonly related to carotid artery stenosis (273). In one series, approximately 40% of patients with retinal vein thrombosis had evidence of circulating anticardiolipin antibodies (274). Fibrinolytic agents have been used successfully in patients with retinal artery and retinal vein occlusion (275). Partial recovery of form vision was possible in some patients with acute retinal artery occlusion (276,277). Antiplatelet agents or anticoagulants have been used in patients with cerebral retinal thrombosis before neovascularization (278). To date, these approaches have not been tested prospectively.

# CONCLUSIONS

Atherothrombosis and thromboembolism which lead to acute cerebrovascular disease can be accompanied by activation of the coagulation system and platelets. Antithrombotic agents can preserve or reconstitute vascular patency and thereby minimize permanent injury from focal cerebral ischemia. Both patient selection and the subtype of stroke are relevant to benefit from treatment.

Plasminogen activators can increase the probability of minimal disability or no abnormality in selected patients with acute cerebral ischemia. Intravenous infusion of rtPA has displayed this activity. Recanalization of symptomatic, documented carotid territory occlusions and vertebrobasilar arterial occlusions has been achieved by local intraarterial PA delivery. But, recent studies have underscored the need for careful individual selection, because fatal hemorrhage is a consistent risk.

Antiplatelet agents can reduce risk in individuals with a history of recent TIAs for the combined outcomes of subsequent stroke, MI, and mortality. For secondary prevention of recurrent stroke in patients presenting with a stable, recent focal cerebral deficit, ASA/dipyridamole produces additional benefits. Thienopyridines have been associated with risk reduction in second ischemic events. When TIAs are associated with carotid artery stenosis of 70% to 99%, carotid endarterectomy and ASA are superior to ASA alone in preventing subsequent stroke and stroke-related mortality.

Patients with AF without a valvular abnormality benefit from long-term anticoagulation with or without an antiplatelet agent. Anticoagulation can reduce the risk of systemic and cerebral embolism in individuals with a signal MI, nonvalvular (i.e., nonrheumatic) AF, mechanical valve prosthesis, and xenograft bioprosthesis (for the initial 3 months after placement). Early use of heparin in individuals with sinus venous thrombosis may produce clinical improvement.

### References

1. Mohr JP, Caplan LR, Melski JW, et al. The Harvard cooperative stroke registry: a prospective registry of patients hospitalized with stroke. *Neurology* 1978;28:754–762.
2. Mohr JP, Barnett HJM. Classification of ischemic strokes. In: Barnett HJM, Stein BM, Mohr JP, et al., eds. *Stroke: pathophysiology, diagnosis and management*, Vol. 1. New York: Churchill Livingstone, 1986: 281–291.
3. Fisher CM. The arterial lesions underlying lacunes. *Acta Neuropathol (Berl)* 1969;12:1–15.
4. Solis OJ, Roberson GR, Taveras JM, et al. Cerebral angiography in acute cerebral infarction. *Rev Interam Radiol* 1977;2:19–25.
5. Fieschi C, Argentino C, Lenzi GL, et al. Clinical and instrumental evaluation of patients with ischemic stroke within the first six hours. *J Neurol Sci* 1989;91:311–321.
6. The National Institutes of Neurological Disorders and Stroke rt-PA Stroke Study Group. Tissue plasminogen activator for acute ischemic stroke. *N Engl J Med* 1995;333:1581–1587.

7. del Zoppo GJ, Higashida RT, Furlan AJ, et al. PROACT: a phase II randomized trial of recombinant pro-urokinase by direct arterial delivery in acute middle cerebral artery stroke. *Stroke* 1998;29:4–11.

8. Irino T, Taneda M, Minami T. Angiographic manifestations in post-recanalized cerebral infarction. *Neurology* 1977;27:471–475.

9. del Zoppo GJ, Poeck K, Pessin MS, et al. Recombinant tissue plasminogen activator in acute thrombotic and embolic stroke. *Ann Neurol* 1992;32: 78–86.

10. Fieschi C, Bozzao L. Transient embolic occlusion of the middle cerebral and internal carotid arteries in cerebral apoplexy. *J Neurol Neurosurg Psychiatry* 1969;32:236–240.

11. Marshall J. The natural history of transient ischemic cerebrovascular attacks. *Q J Med* 1964;33:309–324.

12. Wolf PA, Kannel WB, McGee DL, et al. Duration of atrial fibrillation and imminence of stroke: the Framingham Study. *Stroke* 1983;14:664–667.

13. Whisnant JP, Matsumoto N, Elveback LR. Transient cerebral ischemic attacks in a community, rochester, minnesota, 1955 through 1969. *Mayo Clin Proc* 1973;48:194–198.

14. UK-TIA Study Group. United Kingdom Transient Ischemic Attack (UK-TIA) aspirin trial: interim results. *Br Med J* 1988;296:316–320.

15. Caplan LR. Are terms such as completed stroke or RIND of continued usefulness? *Stroke* 1983;14:431–433.

16. Schmidt EV, Smirnov VE, Ryabova VS. Results of the seven-year prospective study of stroke patients. *Stroke* 1988;19:942–949.

17. Silver FL, Norris JLO, Lewis AJ, et al. Early mortality following stroke: a prospective review. *Stroke* 1984;15:492–496.

18. Shaw C-M, Alvord EC Jr, Berry RG. Swelling of the brain following ischemic infarction with arterial occlusion. *Arch Neurol* 1959;1:161–177.

19. Wityk RJ, Pessin MS, Kaplan RF, et al. Serial assessment of acute stroke using the NIH stroke scale. *Stroke* 1994;25:362–365.

20. Holroyd-Leduc JM, Kapral MK, Austin PC, et al. Sex differences and similarities in the management and outcome of stroke patients. *Stroke* 2000; 31:1833–1837.

21. Hurn PD. Estrogen as a neuroprotectant in stroke. *J Cereb Blood Flow Metab* 2000;20:631–652.

22. McCullough LD, Alkayed NJ, Traystman RJ, et al. Postischemic estrogen reduces hypoperfusion and secondary ischemia after experimental stroke. *Stroke* 2001;32:796–802.

23. Scandinavian Simvastatin Survival Study Group. Randomised trial of cholesterol lowering in 4,444 patients with coronary heart disease: the Scandinavian Simvastatin Survival Study (4S). *Lancet* 1994;344:1383–1389.

24. Byington RP, Davis BR, Plehn JF, et al. Reduction of stroke events with pravastatin: the Prospective Pravastatin Pooling (PPP) project. *Circulation* 2001;103:387–392.

25. Heart Protection Study Collaborative Group. MRC/BHF Heart Protection Study of cholesterol lowering with simvastatin in 20,536 high-risk individuals: a randomised placebo-controlled trial. *Lancet* 2002;360:7–22.

26. Saver PS, Dahlof B, Poulter NR, et al. Prevention of coronary and stroke events with atorvastatin in hypertensive patients who have average or lower than average cholesterol concentrations, in the Anglo-Scandinavian Cardiac Outcomes Trial—Lipid Lowering Arm (ASCIT-LLA): a multicentre randomised controlled trial. *Lancet* 2003;361:1149–1158.

27. Amarenco P, Lavallee P, Touboul PJ. Statins and stroke prevention. *Cerebrovasc Dis* 2004;17:81–88.

28. Bowman TS, Sesso HD, Ma J, et al. Cholesterol and the risk of ischemic stroke. *Stroke* 2003;34:2930–2934.

29. Denny-Brown D. Recurrent cerebrovascular episodes. *Arch Neurol* 1960; 2:194–210.

30. Russell RWR. Atheromatous retinal embolism. *Lancet* 1963;2: 1354–1356.

31. Hollenhorst RW. Vascular status of patients who have cholesterol emboli in the retina. *Am J Ophthalmol* 1966;77:1159–1165.

32. Barnett HJM. The pathophysiology of transient cerebral ischemic attacks: therapy with platelet antiaggregants. *Med Clin North Am* 1979;63: 649–679.

33. Marshall J. *The management of cerebrovascular diseases*. Oxford: Blackwell Scientific Publications, 1976.

34. DeWood MA, Spores J, Notske R, et al. Prevalence of total coronary occlusion during the early hours of transmural myocardial infarction. *N Engl J Med* 1980;303:897–902.

35. Dougherty JH, Levy DE, Weksler BB. Platelet activation in acute cerebral ischemia. *Lancet* 1977;3:821–824.

36. Mettinger KL, Nyman D, Kjellin K-G, et al. Factor VIII related antigen, anti-thrombin III, spontaneous platelet aggregation and plasminogen activator in ischemic cerebrovascular disease. *J Neurol Sci* 1979;41:31–38.

37. de Boer AC, Turpie AG, Butt RW, et al. Plasma beta thromboglobulin and serum fragment E in acute partial stroke. *Br J Haematol* 1982;50: 327–334.

38. Cella G, Zahavi J, de Haas HA, et al. β-thromboglobulin, platelet production time, and platelet function in vascular disease. *Br J Haematol* 1979; 43:127–136.

39. Feinberg WM, Bruck DC, Ring ME, et al. Hemostatic markers in acute stroke. *Stroke* 1989;20:592–597.

40. van Kooten F, Ciabattoni G, Patrono C, et al. Evidence for episodic platelet activation in acute ischemic stroke. *Stroke* 1994;25:278–281.

41. Feinberg WM, Pearce LA, Hart RG, et al. Markers of thrombin and platelet activity in patients with atrial fibrillation: correlation with stroke

among 1531 participants in the stroke prevention in atrial fibrillation III study. *Stroke* 1999;30:2547–2553.

42. Fisher M, Zipser R. Increased excretion of immunoreactive thromboxane B2 in cerebral ischemia. *Stroke* 1985;16:10–14.

43. van Kooten F, Ciabattoni G, Koudstaal PJ, et al. Increased platelet activation in the chronic phase after cerebral ischemia and intracerebral hemorrhage. *Stroke* 1999;30:546–549.

44. Shah AB, Beamer N, Coull BM. Enhanced *in vivo* platelet activation in subtypes of ischemic stroke. *Stroke* 1985;16:643–647.

45. Iwamoto T, Kubo H, Takasaki M. Platelet activation in the cerebral circulation in different subtypes of ischemic stroke and Binswanger's disease. *Stroke* 1995;26:52–56.

46. del Zoppo GJ, Copeland BR, Harker LA, et al. Experimental acute thrombotic stroke in baboons. *Stroke* 1986;17:1254–1265.

47. Abumiya T, Fitridge R, Mazur C, et al. Integrin $\alpha_{IIb}\beta_3$ inhibitor preserves microvascular patency in experimental acute focal cerebral ischemia. *Stroke* 2000;31:1402–1410.

48. del Zoppo GJ, Schmid-Schönbein GW, Mori E, et al. Polymorphonuclear leukocytes occlude capillaries following middle cerebral artery occlusion and reperfusion in baboons. *Stroke* 1991;22:1276–1284.

49. Garcia JH, Liu KF, Yoshida Y, et al. Influx of leukocytes and platelets in an evolving brain infarct (Wistar rat). *Am J Pathol* 1994;144:188–199.

50. Okada Y, Copeland BR, Fitridge R, et al. Fibrin contributes to microvascular obstructions and parenchymal changes during early focal cerebral ischemia and reperfusion. *Stroke* 1994;25:1847–1854.

51. Choudri TF, Hoh BL, Zerwes HG, et al. Reduced microvascular thrombosis and improved outcome in acute murine stroke by inhibiting GP IIb/IIIa receptor-mediated platelet aggregation. ***J Clin Invest*** 1998;102:1301–1310.

52. Bogousslavsky J, Van Melle G, Regli F. The lausanne stroke registry: analysis of 1,000 consecutive patients with first stroke. *Stroke* 1988;19: 1083–1092.

53. Foulkes MA, Wolf PA, Price TR, et al. The stroke data bank: design, methods, and baseline characteristics. *Stroke* 1988;19:547–554.

54. International Stroke Trial Collaborative Group. The International Stroke Trial (IST): a randomised trial of aspirin, subcutaneous heparin, both, or neither among 19,435 patients with acute ischaemic stroke. *Lancet* 1997; 349:1569–1681.

55. Chen ZM, Sandercock P, Pan HC, et al. Indications for early aspirin use in acute ischemic stroke: a combined analysis of 40,000 randomized patients from the chinese acute stroke trial and the international stroke trial. On behalf of the CAST and IST collaborative groups. *Stroke* 2000;31: 1240–1249.

56. Hacke W, Kaste M, Fieschi C, et al. The European Cooperative Acute Stroke Study (ECASS). Intravenous thrombolysis with recombinant tissue plasminogen activator for acute hemispheric stroke. *JAMA* 1995;274:1017–1025.

57. del Zoppo GJ. Acute stroke—On the threshold of a therapy? (Editorial). *N Engl J Med* 1995;333:1632–1633.

58. Albers GW, Amarenco P, Easton JD, et al. Antithrombotic and thrombolytic therapy for ischemic stroke. *Chest* 2001;119:300S–320S.

59. Levine MN, Raskob G, Landefeld S, et al. Hemorrhagic complications of anticoagulant treatment. *Chest* 2001;119:108S–121S.

60. Diener H, Cunha L, Forbes C et al. European Stroke Prevention Study 2. Dipyridamole and acetylsalicylic acid in the secondary prevention of stroke. *J Neurol Sci* 1996;143:1–13.

61. Fisher CM, Adams RD. Observations on brain embolism with special reference to hemorrhage infarction. In: Furlan AJ, ed. *The heart and stroke. Exploring mutual cerebrovascular and cardiovascular issues*. New York: Springer-Verlag, 1987:17–36.

62. Fisher M, Adams RD. Observations on brain embolism with special reference to the mechanism of hemorrhagic infarction. *Neuropathol Exp Neurol* 1951;10:92–94.

63. Jörgensen L, Torvik A. Ischaemic cerebrovascular diseases in an autopsy series. Part 2. Prevalence, location, pathogenesis, and clinical course of cerebral infarcts. *J Neurol Sci* 1969;9:285–320.

64. Kwa VI, Franke CL, Verbeeten B Jr., et al. Amsterdam Vascular medicine Group. Silent intracerebral microhemorrhages in patients with ischemic stroke. *Ann Neurol* 1998;44:372–377.

65. Fisher CM, Adams RD. Observations on brain embolism with special reference to the mechanism of hemorrhagic infarction. *J Neuropathol Exp Neurol* 1951;10:92–94.

66. Okada Y, Yamaguchi T, Minematsu K, et al. Hemorrhagic transformation in cerebral embolism. *Stroke* 1989;20:598–603.

67. Hornig CR, Dorndorf W, Agnoli AL. Hemorrhagic cerebral infarction: a prospective study. *Stroke* 1986;17:179–185.

68. Yamaguchi T, Minematsu K, Choki J, et al. Clinical and neuroradiological analysis of thrombotic and embolic cerebral infarction. *Jpn Circ J* 1984; 48:50–58.

69. Hamann GF, Okada Y, Fitridge R, et al. Microvascular basal lamina antigens disappear during cerebral ischemia and reperfusion. *Stroke* 1995;26: 2120–2126.

70. Hamann GF, Okada Y, del Zoppo GJ. Hemorrhagic transformation and microvascular integrity during focal cerebral ischemia/reperfusion. *J Cereb Blood Flow Metab* 1996;16:1373–1378.

71. Cerebral Embolism Study Group. Immediate anticoagulation of embolic stroke: brain hemorrhage and management options. *Stroke* 1984;15: 779–789.

72. Babikian VL, Kase CS, Pessin MS, et al. Intracerebral hemorrhage in stroke patients anticoagulated with heparin. *Stroke* 1989;29:1500–1503.

73. Mundall J, Quintero P, von Kaulla KN, et al. Transient monocular blindness and increased platelet aggregability treated with aspirin. *Neurology* 1972;22:280–285.

74. Harrison MJG, Marshall J, Meadows JC, et al. Effect of aspirin in amaurosis fugax. *Lancet* 1971;2:743–744.

75. Dyken ML, Kolar OJ, Jones FH. Differences in the occurrence of carotid transient ischemic attacks associated with antiplatelet aggregation therapy. *Stroke* 1973;4:732–736.

76. Russell RWR. Observations on the retinal blood vessels in monocular blindness. *Lancet* 1961;2:1422–1428.

77. Fields WS, Lemak NA, Frankowski RF, et al. Controlled trial of aspirin in cerebral ischemia. *Stroke* 1977;8:301–314.

78. The Canadian Cooperative Study Group. A randomized trial of aspirin and sulfinpyrazone in threatened stroke. *N Engl J Med* 1978;299:53–59.

79. Sorenson PS, Pedersen H, Marquardsen J, et al. A Danish Cooperative Study. Acetylsalicylic acid in the prevention of stroke in patients with reversible cerebral ischemic attacks. *Stroke* 1983;14:15–22.

80. Bousser MG, Eschwege E, Haguenau M, et al. "AICLA" controlled trial of aspirin and dipyridamole in the secondary prevention of athero-thrombotic cerebral ischemia. *Stroke* 1983;14:5–14.

81. The Dutch TIA Trial Study Group. A comparison of two doses of aspirin (30 mg vs. 283 mg a day) in patients after a transient ischemic attack or minor ischemic stroke. *N Engl J Med* 1991;325:1261–1266.

82. The SALT Collaborative Group. Swedish Aspirin Low-Dose Trial (SALT) of 75 mg aspirin as secondary prophylaxis after cerebrovascular ischemic events. *Lancet* 1991;338:1345–1349.

83. European Stroke Prevention Study Group. The European Stroke Prevention Study (ESPS) principal end-points. *Lancet* 1987;2:1351–1354.

84. American-Canadian Cooperative Study Group. Persantine aspirin trial in cerebral ischemia. Part II. Endpoint results. *Stroke* 1985;16:406–415.

85. Matias-Guiu J, Davalos A, Pico M, et al. Low-dose acetylsalicylic acid (ASA) plus dipyridamole versus dipyridamole alone in the prevention of stroke in patients with reversible ischemic attacks. *Acta Neurol Scand* 1987;76:413–421.

86. Hass WK, Easton JD, Adams HP Jr, et al. A randomized trial comparing ticlopidine hydrochloride with aspirin for prevention of stroke in high-risk patients. *N Engl J Med* 1989;321:501–507.

87. Harker LA. Antiplatelet drugs in the management of patients with thrombotic disorders. *Semin Thromb Hemost* 1986;12:134–155.

88. Fitzgerald GA. Dipyridamole. *N Engl J Med* 1987;316:1247–1257.

89. Fitzgerald GA. Dipyridamole. *N Engl J Med* 1987;317:1734–1736.

90. Harker LA, Slichter SJ. Arterial and venous thromboembolism. *Diath Haemorrh* 1974;31:188–203.

91. Acheson J, Danta G, Hutchinson EC. Controlled trial of dipyridamole in cerebral vascular disease. *Br Med J* 1969;1:614–615.

92. ESPS-2 Working Group. Second European Stroke Prevention Study. *J Neurol* 1992;239:299–301.

93. Roden S, Low-Beer T, Carmalt M, et al. Transient cerebral ischemic attacks—management and prognosis. *Postgrad Med J* 1981;57:275–278.

94. Candelise L, Landi G, Perrone P, et al. A randomized trial of aspirin and sulfinpyrazone in patients with TIA. *Stroke* 1982;13:175–179.

95. Estol CJ, Pessin MS. Anticoagulation: Is there still a role in atherothrombotic stroke? *Stroke* 1990;21:820–824.

96. Jones S. Anticoagulant therapy in cerebrovascular disease: review and meta-analysis. *Stroke* 1988;19:1043–1048.

97. Fazekas JF, Alman RW, Sullivan JF. Vertebrobasilar insufficiency. *Arch Neurol* 1963;8:115–120.

98. Olsson JE, Müller R, Benneli S. Long-term anticoagulant therapy for transient ischemic attacks and minor strokes with minimum residuum. *Stroke* 1976;7:444–451.

99. Campbell MH. Basilar artery syndrome. *Can Med Assoc J* 1953;69:314–315.

100. Millikan CH, Siekert RG, Shick RM. Studies in cerebrovascular disease: III. The use of anticoagulant drugs in the treatment of insufficiency or thrombosis within the basilar arterial system. *Mayo Clin Proc* 1955;30:116–126.

101. Fisher CM. The use of anticoagulants in cerebral thrombosis. *Neurology* 1958;8:311–332.

102. Siekert RG, Whisnant JP, Millikan CH. Surgical and anticoagulant therapy of occlusive cerebrovascular disease. *Ann Intern Med* 1963;58:637–641.

103. Friedman GD, Wilson WS, Mosier JM, et al. Transient ischemic attacks in a community. *JAMA* 1969;210:1428–1434.

104. Toole JF, Janeway R, Choi K, et al. Transient ischemic attacks due to atherosclerosis. A prospective study of 160 patients. *Arch Neurol* 1975;32:5–12.

105. Baker RN, Broward JA, Fang HC, et al. Anticoagulant therapy in cerebral infarction. *Neurology* 1962;12:823–835.

106. Baker RN, Schwartz WS, Rose AS. Transient ischemic attacks. *Neurology* 1966;16:841–847.

107. Pearce JMS, Gubbay SS, Walton JN. Long-term anticoagulant therapy in transient cerebral ischemic attacks. *Lancet* 1965;1:6–9.

108. Cerebral Embolism Study Group. Immediate anticoagulation of embolic stroke: a randomized trial. *Stroke* 1983;14:668–676.

109. Albers GW. Antithrombotic agents in cerebral ischemia. *Am J Cardiol* 1995;75(6):34B–38B.

110. De Schryver EL. European/Australian Stroke Prevention in Reversible Ischaemia Trial (ESPRIT) Group. Design of ESPRIT: an international randomized trial for secondary prevention after non-disabling cerebral ischaemia of arterial origin. *Cerebrovasc Dis* 2000;10:147–150.

111. Walker AM, Jick H. Predictors of bleeding during heparin therapy. *JAMA* 1980;244:1209–1212.

112. Dahinden C, Galanos C, Fehr J. Granulocyte activation by endotoxin. *J Immunol* 1983;130:857–862.

113. Moggio RA, Hammond GL, Stansel HL Jr, et al. Incidence of emboli with cloth-covered starr-edwards value without anticoagulation and with varying forms of anticoagulation. *J Thorac Cardiovasc Surg* 1978;75:296–299.

114. Millikan CH. Anticoagulant therapy in cerebrovascular disease. In: Millikan CH, Siekert RG, Whisnant JP, eds. *Cerebral vascular diseases.* New York: Grune & Stratton, 1965:183.

115. Carter AB. Anticoagulant treatment in progressing stroke. *Br Med J* 1961;2:70–73.

116. Marshall J, Shaw DA. Anticoagulant therapy in acute cerebrovascular accidents: a controlled trial. *Lancet* 1960;1:995–998.

117. Toni D, Fiorelli M, Gentile M, et al. Progressing neurological deficit secondary to acute ischemic stroke. A study on predicability, pathogenesis, and prognosis. *Arch Neurol* 1995;52:670–675.

118. The Publications Committee for the Trial of ORG 10172 in Acute Stroke Treatment (TOAST) Investigators. Low molecular weight heparinoid, ORG 10172 (danaparoid), and outcome after acute ischemic stroke: a randomized controlled trial. *JAMA* 1998;279:1265–1272.

119. Adams HP Jr, Bendixen BH, Leira E, et al. Antithrombotic treatment of ischemic stroke among patients with occlusion or severe stenosis of the internal carotid artery. *Neurology* 1999;53:122–125.

120. Hassaballa H, Gorelick PB, West CP, et al. Ischemic stroke outcome. *Neurology* 2001;57:691–697.

121. Gubitz G, Sandercock P, Counsell C. Antiplatelet therapy for acute ischaemic stroke. *Cochrane Database Syst Rev* (computer file) 2000:CD000029.

122. Baron JC, von Kummer R, del Zoppo GJ. Treatment of acute ischemic stroke. Challenging the concept of a rigid and universal time window (Editorial). *Stroke* 1995;26:2219–2221.

123. von Kummer R, Meyding-Lamade U, Forsting M, et al. Sensitivity and prognostic value of early CT in occlusion of the middle cerebral artery trunk. *AJNR Am J Neuroradiol* 1994;15:9–15.

124. Warach S, Gaa J, Siewert B, et al. Acute human stroke studied by whole brain echo planar diffusion-weighted magnetic resonance imaging. *Ann Neurol* 1995;37:231–241.

125. Garcia JH, Liu K-F, Ho K-L. Neuronal necrosis after middle cerebral artery occlusion in Wistar rats progresses at different time intervals in the caudoputamen and the cortex. *Stroke* 1995;26:636–643.

126. Tagaya M, Liu K-F, Copeland B, et al. DNA scission after focal brain ischemia: temporal differences in two species. *Stroke* 1997;28:1245–1254.

127. Gent M, Blakely JA, Easton JD, et al. The Canadian-American Ticlopidine Study (CATS) in thromboembolic stroke. *Lancet* 1989;1:1215–1220.

128. Britton M, Helmers C, Samuelsson K. A Swedish Cooperative Study. High-dose acetylsalicylic acid after cerebral infarction. *Stroke* 1987;18:325–334.

129. Gent M, Blakeley JA, Hachinski V, et al. A secondary prevention, randomized trial of suloctidil in patients with a recent history of thromboembolic stroke. *Stroke* 1985;16:416–424.

130. Fisher M, Sandler R, Weiner JM. Delayed cerebral ischemia following arteriography. *Stroke* 1985;16:431–434.

131. Blakeley JA. A prospective trial of sulfinpyrazone and survival after thrombotic stroke. *Thromb Haemost* 1979;42:382.

132. CAPRIE Steering Committee. A randomised, blinded, trial of clopidogrel versus aspirin in patients at risk of ischaemic events (CAPRIE). *Lancet* 1996;348:1329–1339.

133. CAST (Chinese Acute Stroke Trial) Collaborative Group. CAST: a randomised placebo-controlled trial of early aspirin use in 20,000 patients with acute ischaemic stroke. *Lancet* 1997;349:1641–1649.

134. Chen ZM, Xie JX, Peto R, et al. on behalf of the CAST Collaborative Group. Chinese Acute Stroke Trial (CAST): Rationale, design and progress. *Cerebrovasc Dis* 1996;6:23.

135. The Abciximab in Ischemic Stroke Investigators. Abciximab in acute ischemic stroke: a randomized, double-blind, placebo-controlled, dose-escalation study. *Stroke* 2000;31:601–609.

136. Fisher CM. Anticoagulant therapy in cerebral thrombosis and cerebral embolism: a national cooperative study, interim report. *Neurology* 1961;11:119–131.

137. Hill AB, Marshall J, Shaw DA. Cerebrovascular disease: trial of long-term anticoagulant therapy. *Br Med J* 1962;2:1003–1006.

138. McDowell F, McDevitt E. Treatment of the completed stroke with long-term anticoagulant. Six and one-half years' experience. In: Siekert RH, Whisnant JR, eds. *Cerebral vascular diseases, fourth princeton conference.* New York: Grune & Stratton, 1965:185–199.

139. Enger E, Boyesen S. Long-term anticoagulant therapy in patients with cerebral infarction: a controlled clinical study. *Acta Med Scand* 1965;179(Suppl.):1–61.

140. Baker RN. An evaluation of anticoagulant therapy in the treatment of cerebrovascular disease: Report of the Veterans Administration Cooperative Study of Atherosclerosis, Neurology Section. *Neurology* 1961;11: 132–138.

141. Kay R, Wong KA, Yu YL, et al. Low-molecular weight heparin in the treatment of acute ischemic stroke. *N Engl J Med* 1995;333:1588–1593.

142. Berge E, Abdelnoor M, Nakstad PH, Sandset PM, on behalf of the HAEST Study Group. Low molecular-weight heparin versus aspirin in patients with acute ischemic stroke and atrial fibrillation: a double-blind randomised study. *Lancet* 2000;355:1205–1210.

143. Diener HC, Ringelstein EB, von Kummer R, et al. Treatment of acute ischemic stroke with the low-molecular-weight heparin certoparin. *Stroke* 2001;32:22–29.

144. Liu M, Counsell C, Sandercock P. Anticoagulants for preventing recurrence following ischaemic stroke or transient ischaemic attack. *Cochrane Database Syst Rev* 2000;(2):CD000248.

145. Gubitz G, Counsell C, Sandercock P, et al. Anticoagulants for acute ischaemic stroke. *Cochrane Database Syst Rev* 2000;2:CD000024.

146. Fletcher AP, Alkjaersig N, Lewis M, et al. A pilot study of urokinase therapy in cerebral infarction. *Stroke* 1976;7:135–142.

147. NIH Consensus Conference. Thrombolytic therapy in treatment. *Br Med J* 1980;280:1585–1587.

148. Atarashi J, Otomo E, Araki G, et al. Clinical utility of urokinase in the treatment of acute stage of cerebral thrombosis: Multi-center double-blind study in comparison with placebo. *Clin Eval* 1985;13:659–709.

149. Otomo E, Araki G, Itoh E, et al. Clinical efficacy of urokinase in the treatment of cerebral thrombosis. *Clin Eval* 1985;13:711–751.

150. Abe T, Terashi A, Tohgi H, et al. Clinical efficacy of intravenous administration of SM-9527 (t-PA) in cerebral thrombosis. *Clin Eval* 1990;18: 39–69.

151. Otomo E, Tohgi H, Hirai S, et al. Clinical efficacy of AK-124 (tissue plasminogen activator) in the treatment of cerebral thrombosis: study by means of multi-center double blind comparison with urokinase. *Yakuri To Chiryo* 1988;16:3775–3821.

152. del Zoppo GJ, Zeumer H, Harker L. Thrombolytic therapy in stroke: possibilities and hazards. *Stroke* 1986;17:595–609.

153. Astrup J, Siesjö BK, Symon L. Thresholds in cerebral ischemia – the ischemic penumbra. *Stroke* 1981;12(6):723–725.

154. Baron JC. Perfusion thresholds in human cerebral ischemia: historical perspective and therapeutic implications. *Cerebrovascular Disease* 2001; 11(Suppl. 1):2–8.

155. Mori E, Yoneda Y, Tabuchi M, et al. Intravenous recombinant tissue plasminogen activator in acute carotid artery territory stroke. *Neurology* 1992;42:976–982.

156. Yamaguchi T. Intravenous rt-PA in acute embolic stroke. In: Hacke W, del Zoppo GJ, Hirschberg M, eds. *Thrombolytic therapy in acute ischemic stroke*. Heidelberg: Springer-Verlag, 1991:168–174.

157. von Kummer R, Forsting M, Sartor K. Intravenous recombinant tissue plasminogen activator in acute stroke. In: Hacke W, del Zoppo GJ, Hirschberg M, eds. *Thrombolytic therapy in acute ischemic stroke*. Heidelberg: Springer-Verlag, 1991:161–167.

158. Hommel M, Boissel JP, Cornu C, et al. Termination of trial of streptokinase in severe acute ischemic stroke. *Lancet* 1995;345:578–579.

159. Donnan GA, Davis SM, Chambers BR, et al. Trials of streptokinase in severe acute ischaemic stroke. *Lancet* 1995;345:578–579.

160. Multicentre Acute Stroke Trial-Italy (MAST-I) Group. Randomised controlled trial of streptokinase, aspirin, and combination of both in treatment of acute ischaemic stroke. *Lancet* 1995;346:1509–1514.

161. Gruppo Italiano Per Lo Studio Della Streptochinasi Nell'Infarto Miocardico (GISSI). Effectiveness of intravenous thrombolytic treatment in acute myocardial infarction. *Lancet* 1986;1:397–401.

162. Gruppo Italiano Per Lo Studio Della Streptochinasi Nell'Infarto Miocardico (GISSI). GISSI-2: a factorial randomized trial of alteplase versus streptokinase and heparin versus no heparin among 12,490 patients with acute myocardial infarction. *Lancet* 1990;336:65–71.

163. Kwiatkowski TG, Libman RB, Frankel M, et al. National Institute of Neurological Disorders and Stroke Recombinant Tissue Plasminogen Activator Stroke Study Group. Effects of tissue plasminogen activator for acute ischemic stroke at one year. *N Engl J Med* 1999;340:1781–1787.

164. Albers GW, Bates VE, Clark WM, et al. Intravenous tissue-type plasminogen activator for treatment of acute stroke: the Standard Treatment with Alteplase to Reverse Stroke (STARS) Study. *JAMA* 2000;283: 1145–1150.

165. Hacke W, Kaste M, Fieschi C, et al. Randomised double-blind placebo-controlled trial of thrombolytic therapy with intravenous alteplase in acute ischaemic stroke (ECASS II). *Lancet* 1998;352:1245–1251.

166. von Kummer R, Allen KL, Holle R, et al. Acute stroke: usefulness of early CT findings before thrombolytic therapy. *Radiology* 1997;205:327–333.

167. Clark WM, Wissman S, Albers GW, et al. Recombinant tissue-type plasminogen activator (Alteplase) for ischemic stroke 3 to 5 hours after symptom onset. The ATLANTIS Study: a randomized controlled trial. Alteplase Thrombolysis for Actue Noninterventional Therapy in Ischemic Stroke. *JAMA* 1999;282:2019–2026.

168. The ATLANTIS, ECASS, and NINDS rt-PA Study Group Investigators. Association of outcome with early stroke treatment: pooled analysis of ATLANTIS, ECASS, and NINDS rt-PA stroke trials. *Lancet* 2004;363: 768–774.

169. Levy DE, Brott TG, Haley EC Jr, et al. Factors related to intracranial hematoma formation in patients receiving tissue-type plasminogen activator for acute ischemic stroke. *Stroke* 1994;25:291–297.

170. Larrue V, von Kummer R, del Zoppo GJ, et al. Hemorrhagic transformation in acute ischemic stroke: potential contributing factors in the European Cooperative Acute Stroke Study. *Stroke* 1997;28:957–960.

171. Larrue V, von Kummer RR, Muller A, et al. Risk factors for severe hemorrhagic transformation in ischemic stroke patients treated with recombinant tissue plasminogen activator: a secondary analysis of the European-Australiasian Acute Stroke Study (ECASS II). *Stroke* 2001;32(2):438–441.

172. Dubey N, Bakshi R, Wasay M, et al. Early computed tomography hypodensity predicts hemorrhage after intravenous tissue plasminogen activator in acute ischemic stroke. *J Neuroimaging* 2001;11:184–188.

173. Kalafut MA, Schriger DL, Saver JL, et al. Detection of early CT signs of >1/3 middle cerebral artery infarctions: interrater reliability and sensitivity of CT interpretation by physicians involved in acute stroke care. *Stroke* 2000;31:1667–1671.

174. Zeumer H, Freitag HJ, Grzyka U, et al. Local intra-arterial fibrinolysis in acute vertebrobasilar occlusion. Technical developments and recent results. *Neuroradiology* 1989;31:336–340.

175. Mori E, Tabuchi M, Yoshida T, et al. Intracarotid urokinase with thromboembolic occlusion of the middle cerebral artery. *Stroke* 1988;19: 802–812.

176. del Zoppo GJ, Ferbert A, Otis S, et al. Local intra-arterial fibrinolytic therapy in acute carotid territory stroke: a Pilot Study. *Stroke* 1988;19: 307–313.

177. Matsumoto K, Satoh K. Topical intraarterial urokinase infusion for acute stroke. In: Hacke W, del Zoppo GJ, Hirschberg M, eds. *Thrombolytic therapy in acute ischemic stroke*. Heidelberg: Springer-Verlag, 1991: 207–212.

178. Furlan A, Higashida R, Wechsler L, et al. Intra-arterial prourokinase for acute ischemic stroke. The PROACT II study a randomized controlled trial. *JAMA* 1999;282:2003–2011.

179. Yamaguchi T. Intravenous tissue plasminogen activator in acute thromboembolic stroke: a placebo-controlled, double-blind trial. In: del Zoppo GJ, Mori E, Hacke W, eds. *Thrombolytic therapy in acute ischemic stroke II*. Heidelberg: Springer-Verlag, 1993:59–65.

180. Caplan L. "Top of the basilar" syndrome: selected clinical aspects. *Neurology* 1980;30:72–79.

181. Archer CT, Horenstein S. Basilar artery occlusion. Clinical and radiological correlation. *Stroke* 1977;8:383–387.

182. Nenci GG, Gresele P, Taramelli M, et al. Thrombolytic therapy for thromboembolism of vertebrobasilar artery. *Angiology* 1983;34:561–571.

183. Hacke W, Zeumer H, Ferbert A, et al. Intra-arterial thrombolytic therapy improves outcome in patients with acute vertebrobasilar occlusive disease. *Stroke* 1988;19:1216–1222.

184. Mobius E, Berg-Dammer E, Kuhne D. Local thrombolytic therapy in acute basilar artery occlusion. In: Hacke W, del Zoppo GJ, Hirschberg M, eds. *Thrombolytic therapy in acute ischemic stroke*. Berlin: Springer-Verlag, 1991:213–215.

185. Bells WR Jr. Defibrinogenating enzymes. *Drugs* 2001;54(Suppl. 3):18–30.

186. The Ancrod Stroke Study Investigators. Ancrod for the treatment of acute ischemic brain infarction. *Stroke* 1994;25:1755–1759.

187. Sherman DG, Atkinson RP, Chippendale T, et al. Intravenous ancrod for treatment of acute ischemic stroke: the STAT study: a randomized controlled trial. Stroke Treatment with Ancrod Trial. *JAMA* 2000;283: 2395–2403.

188. Orgogozo JM, Verstraete M, Kay R, et al. Outcomes of ancrod in acute ischemic stroke. Independent Data and Safety Monitoring Board for ESTAT. Steering Committee for ESTAT. European Stroke Treatment with Ancrod Trial. *JAMA* 2000;284:1926–1927.

189. Barnett HJ, Gunton RW, Eliasziw M, et al. Causes and severity of ischemic stroke in patients with internal carotid artery stenosis. *JAMA* 2000;283(11):1429–1436.

190. Northern American Symptomatic Carotid Endarterectomy Trial Collaborators. Beneficial effect of carotid endarterectomy in symptomatic patients with high-grade carotid stenosis. *N Engl J Med* 1991;325:445–453.

191. European Carotid Surgery Trialists' Collaborative Group. MRC European Carotid Surgery Trial: interim results for symptomatic patients with severe (70-99%) or with mild (0-29%) carotid stenosis. *Lancet* 1991;337: 1235–1243.

192. Barnett HJM, Taylor DW, Eliasziw M, et al. Benefit of carotid endarterectomy in patients with symptomatic moderate or severe stenosis. *N Engl J Med* 1998;339:1415–1425.

193. Hobson RW, Weiss DG, Fields WS, et al. The Veterans Affairs Cooperative Study Group. Efficacy of carotid endarterectomy for asymptomatic carotid stenosis. *N Engl J Med* 1993;328(4):221–227.

194. Rockman CB, Riles TS, Lamparello PJ, et al. Natural history and management of the asymptomatic, moderately stenotic internal carotid artery. *J Vasc Surg* 1997;25(3):423–431.

195. Benavente O, Moher D, Pham B. Carotid endarterectomy for asymptomatic carotid stenosis: a meta-analysis. *BMJ* 1998;317(7171):1477–1480.

196. Chambers BR, You RX, Donnan GA. Carotid endarterectomy for asymptomatic carotid stenosis. *Cochrane Database Syst Rev* 2000;(2): CD001923.

197. Fields WS, Lemak NA, Frankowski RF, et al. Controlled trial of aspirin in cerebral ischemia. Surgical Group. *Stroke* 1978;9:309–319.

198. Boysen G, Sorensen PS, Juhler M, et al. Danish very low dose aspirin after carotid endarterectomy trial. *Stroke* 1988;19:1211–1215.

199. Kretschmer G, Pratschner T, Prager M, et al. Antiplatelet treatment prolongs survival after carotid bifurcation endarterectomy. *Ann Surg* 1990;211:317–322.

200. Pratschner T, Kretschmeter G, Prager M, et al. Antiplatelet therapy following carotid bifurcation endarerectomy. Evaluation of a controlled clinical trial. Prognostic significance of histologic plaque examination on behalf of survival. *Eur J Vasc Surg* 1990;4:285–289.

201. Cooperative Study. Long-term anticoagulant therapy after myocardial infarction. *JAMA* 1965;193:929–934.

202. Harvald B, Hilden T, Lund E. Long-term anticoagulant therapy after myocardial infarction. *Lancet* 1962;2:626–630.

203. Loeliger EA, Hensen A, Kroes F, et al. A double blind trial of long-term anticoagulant treatment after myocardial infarction. *Acta Med Scand* 1967;182:549–567.

204. Breddin K, Loew D, Lechner K, et al. The German-Austrian aspirin trial: a comparison of acetylsalicyclic acid, placebo, and phenprocoumon in secondary prevention of myocardial infarction. *Circulation* 1980; 62(Suppl.):V63–V72.

205. Sixty-Plus Reinfarction Study Research Group. A double-blind trial to assess long-term anticoagulant therapy in elderly patients after myocardial infarction. *Lancet* 1980;2:989–994.

206. Smith P, Arnesen H, Holme I. The effect of warfarin on mortality and reinfarction after myocardial infarction. *N Engl J Med* 1990;323: 147–152.

207. Breddin K, Loew D, Lechner K, et al. Secondary prevention of myocardial infarction: a comparison of acetylsalicylic acid, placebo, and phenprocoumen. *Haemostasis* 1980;9:325–344.

208. Hurlen M, Smith P, Arnesen H. The WARIS-II (Warfarin-Aspirin Reinfarction Study) Design. Effects of warfarin, aspirin and the two combined, on mortality and thromboembolic morbidity after mycardial infarction. *Scand Cardiovasc J* 2000;34:168–171.

209. Drapkin RL, Gee TS, Dowling MD, et al. Prophylactic heparin therapy in acute promyelocytic leukemia. *Cancer* 1978;41:2484.

210. Veterans Administration Hospital Investigators. Anticoagulants in acute myocardial infarction. Results of a cooperative clinical trial. *JAMA* 1973;225:724–729.

211. Medical Research Council. Assessment of short-term anticoagulant administration after cardiac infarction. *Br Med J* 1969;8:335–342.

212. Cairns JA, Connolly SJ. Nonrheumatic atrial fibrillation. Risk of stroke and role of antithrombotic therapy. *Circulation* 1991;84:469–481.

213. Sage JL, Van Uitert RL. Recurrent stroke in patients with atrial fibrillation and nonvalvular heart disease. *Stroke* 1983;14:537–540.

214. Hart RG, Coull BM, Hart D. Early recurrent embolism associated with nonvalvular atrial fibrillation: a retrospective study. *Stroke* 1983;14: 688–693.

215. Petersen P, Boysen G, Godtfredsen J, et al. The Copenhagen AFASAK Study. Placebo-controlled randomized trial of warfarin and aspirin to prevention of thromboembolic complications in chronic atrial fibrillation. *Lancet* 1989;1:175–179.

216. Stroke Prevention in Atrial Fibrillation Study Group Investigators. Preliminary report of the Stroke Prevention in Atrial Fibrillation Study. *N Engl J Med* 1990;322:863–868.

217. The Boston Area Anticoagulation Trial/Atrial Fibrillation Investigators. The effect of low-dose warfarin on the risk of stroke in patients with non-rheumatic atrial fibrillation. *N Engl J Med* 1990;323:1505–1511.

218. Connolly SJ, Laupacis A, Gent M, et al. Canadian Atrial Fibrillation Anticoagulation (CAFA) study. *J Am Coll Cardiol* 1991;18:349–355.

219. Stroke Prevention in Atrial Fibrillation Investigators. Warfarin versus aspirin for prevention of thromboembolism in atrial fibrillation: Stroke Prevention in Atrial Fibrillation II Study. *Lancet* 1994;343:687–691.

220. Stroke Prevention in Atrial Fibrillation Investigators. Adjusted-dose warfarin versus low-intensity, fixed-dose warfarin plus aspirin for high-risk patients with atrial fibrillation: stroke prevention in atrial fibrillation III randomised clinical trial. *Lancet* 1996;348:633–638.

221. EAFT European Atrial Fibrillation Trial Study Group. Secondary prevention in non-rheumatic atrial fibrillation after transient ischaemic attack or minor stroke. *Lancet* 1993;342:1255–1262.

222. Atrial Fibrillation Investigators. The efficacy of aspirin in patients with atrial fibrillation: analysis of pooled data from three randomized trials. *Arch Intern Med* 1997;157:1237–1240.

223. Hart RG, Benavente O, McBride R, et al. Antithrombotic therapy to prevent stroke in patients with atrial fibrillation: a meta-analysis. *Ann Intern Med* 1999;131:492–501.

224. Segal JB, McNamara RL, Miller MR, et al. Prevention of thromboembolism in atrial fibrillation: a meta-analysis of trials of anticoagulants and antiplatelet drugs. *J Gen Intern Med* 2000;15:56–67.

225. Fihn SD, Callahan CM, Martin DC, et al. The risk for and severity of bleeding complications in elderly patients treated with warfarin. *Ann Intern Med* 1996;124:970–979.

226. Gullov AL, Koefoed BG, Petersen P, et al. Fixed mini-dose warfarin and aspirin alone and in combination with adjusted-dose warfarin for stroke prevention in atrial fibrillation: Second Copenhagen Atrial Fibrillation, Aspirin, and Anticoagulation Study (the AFASAK-2 Study). *Arch Intern Med* 1998;158:1513–1521.

227. Gullov AL, Koefoed BG, Petersen P. Bleeding during warfarin and asirin therapy in patients with atrial fibrillation: the AFASAK-2 study. *Arch Intern Med* 1999;159:1322–1328.

228. Taylor FC, Cohen H, Ebrahim S. Systematic review of long term anticoagulation or antiplatet treatment in patients with non-rheumatic atrial fibrillation. *Br Med J* 2001;322:321–326.

229. Hylek E, Go A, Chang Y, et al. Effect of intensity of oral anticoagulation on stroke severity and mortality in atrial fibrillation. *N Engl J Med* 2004; 11:1019–1026.

230. Halperin JL. Executive steering committee SIaVSI. Ximelagatran compared with warfarin for prevention of thromboembolism in patients withnonvalvular atrial fibrillation: rationale, objectives, and design of a pair of clinical studies and baseline patient characteristics (SPORTIF III and V). *Am Heart J* 2004;146:431–438.

231. Olsson SB, Executive Steering Committee on behalf of the SPORTIFF III Investigators. Stroke prevention with the oral direct thrombin inhibitor ximelagatran compared with warfarin in patients with non-valvular atrial fibrillation (SPORTIF III): randomised controlled trial. *Lancet* 2003;362: 1691–1698.

232. Lodder J, Dennis MS, Van-Raak L, et al. Cooperative study on the value of long-term anticoagulation in patients with stroke and non-rheumatic atrial fibrillation. *Br Med J* 1988;296:1435–1438.

233. Benavente O, Hart R, Koudstaal P, et al. Oral anticoagulants for preventing stroke in patients with non-valvular atrial fibrillation and no previous history of stroke or transient ischemic attacks. *Cochrane Database Syst Rev* 2000;2:CD001927.

234. Albers GW, Dalen JE, Laupacis A, et al. Antithrombotic therapy in atrial fibrillation. *Chest* 2001;119:194S–206S.

235. Coulshed N, Epstein EJ, McKendrick CS, et al. Systemic embolism in mitral valve disease. *Br Med J* 1970;32:26–34.

236. Szekely P. Systemic embolism and anticoagulant prophylaxis in rheumatic heart disease. *Br Med J* 1964;1:1209–1212.

237. Daley R, Mattingly TW, Holt CI, et al. Systemic arterial embolism in rheumatic heart disease. *Am Heart J* 1981;42:566–581.

238. Levine HJ, Pauker SG, Salzman EW. Antithrombotic therapy in valvular heart disease. *Chest* 1989;95:98S–106S.

239. Stein PD, Kantrowitz A. Antithrombotic therapy in mechanical and biological prosthetic heart valves and saphenous vein bypass grafts. *Chest* 1989;95:107S–117S.

240. Cannegieter SC, von Schacky C, Rosendaal FR. Optimal oral anticoagulant therapy in patients with mechanical heart valves. *N Engl J Med* 1995; 333:1504–1505.

241. Stein PD, Alpert JS, Bussey HI, et al. Antithrombotic therapy in patients with mechanical and biological prosthetic heart valves. *Chest* 2001;119: 220S–227S.

242. Horstkotte D, Schulte H, Bircks W, et al. Unexpected findings concerning thromboembolic complications and anticoagulation after complete 10 year follow up of patients with St. Jude Medical Prostheses. *J Heart Valve Dis* 1993;2:291–301.

243. Horstkotte D, Scharf RE, Schultheiss HP. Intracardiac thrombosis: patient-related and device-related factors. *J Heart Valve Dis* 1995;4: 114–120.

244. Horstkotte D, Schulte HD, Bircks W, et al. Lower intensity anticoagulation therapy results in lower complication rates with the St. Jude Medical Prosthesis. *J Thorac Cardiovasc Surg* 1994;107:1136–1145.

245. Stein PD, Grandison D, Hua TA, et al. Therapeutic level of oral anticoagulation with warfarin in patients with mechanical prosthetic heart valves: review of literature and recommendations based on international normalized ratio. *Postgrad Med J* 1994;70:S72–S83.

246. Dale J, Myhre E, Storstein O, et al. Prevention of arterial thromboembolism with acetylsalicylic acid. A controlled clinical study in patients with aortic ball valves. *Am Heart J* 1977;94:101–111.

247. Altman R, Boullon F, Rouvier J, et al. Aspirin and prophylaxis of thromboembolic complications in patients with substitute heart valves. *J Thorac Cardiovasc Surg* 1976;72:127–129.

248. Turpie AGG, Gent M, Laupacis A, et al. Comparison of aspirin with placebo in patients treated with warfarin after heart-valve replacement. *N Engl J Med* 1993;329:524–529.

249. Meschengieser SS, Fondevila CG, Frontroth J, et al. Low-intensity oral anticoagulation plus low-dose aspirin versus high-intensity oral anticoagulation alone: a randomized trial in patients with mechanical prosthetic heart valves. *J Thorac Cardiovasc Surg* 1997;113:910–916.

250. Sullivan JM, Harken DE, Gorlin R. Effect of dipyridamole on the incidence of arterial emboli after cardiac valve replacement. *Circulation* 1969;39/40:I–149–I–153.

251. Sullivan JM, Harken DE, Gorlin R. Pharmacologic control of thromboembolic complications of cardiac valve replacement. *N Engl J Med* 1971;284:1391–1394.

252. Kontozis L, Skudicky D, Hopley MJ, et al. Long-term follow-up of St. Jude Medical prosthesis in a young rheumatic population using low-level warfarin anticoagulation: an analysis of the temporal distribution of causes of death. *Am J Cardiol* 1998;81:736–739.

253. Chesebro JH, Fuster V, Elveback LR, et al. Trial of combined warfarin plus dipyridamole or aspirin therapy in prosthetic heart valve replacement: danger of aspirin compared with dipyridamole. *Am J Cardiol* 1983; 51:1537–1541.

254. Altman R, Rouvier J, Gurfinkel E, et al. Comparison of high-dose with low-dose aspirin in patients with mechanical heart valve replacement treated with oral anticoagulant. *Circulation* 1996;94:2113–2116.

255. Pouleur H, Buyse M. Effects of dipyridamole in combination with antico-agulant therapy on survival and thromboembolic events in patients with prosthetic heart valves: a meta-analysis of the randomized trials. *J Thorac Cardiovasc Surg* 1995;110:463–472.

256. Massel D, Little SH. Risks and benefits of adding anti-platelet therapy to warfarin among patients with prosthetic heart valves: a meta-anaylsis. *J Am Coll Cardiol* 2001;37:569–578.

257. Cohn LH, Allred EN, DiSesa VJ, et al. Early and late risk of aortic valve replacement. A 12-year concomitant comparison of the porcine bioprosthetic and tilting disc prosthetic aortic valves. *J Thorac Cardiovasc Surg* 1984;88:695–705.

258. Williams JB, Karp RB, Kirklin JW, et al. Considerations in selection and management of patients undergoing valve replacement with gluteraldehyde-fixed porcine bioprostheses. *Ann Thorac Surg* 1980;30:247–258.

259. Oyer PE, Stinson EB, Griepp RB, et al. Valve replacement with the Starr-Edwards and Hancock prostheses. Comparative analysis of late morbidity and mortality. *Ann Surg* 1977;186:301–309.

260. Ionescu MI, Smith DR, Hasan SS, et al. Clinical durability of the pericardial xenograft valve: ten years experience with mitral replacement. *Ann Thorac Surg* 1982;34:265–277.

261. Turpie AGG, Gunstensen J, Hirsh J, et al. Randomized comparison of two intensities of oral anticoagulant therapy after tissue heart valve placement. *Lancet* 1988;1:1242–1245.

262. Kelton JG. Antiplatelet agents: rationale and results. *Clin Haematol* 1983;12:311–354.

263. NuZez L, Aguado MG, Celemin D, et al. Aspirin or coumadin as the drug of choice for valve replacement with porcine bioprosthesis. *Ann Thorac Surg* 1982;33:355–358.

264. NuZez L, Aguado MG, Larrea JL, et al. Prevention of thromboembolism using aspirin after mitral valve replacement with porcine bioprosthesis. *Ann Thorac Surg* 1984;37:84–87.

265. Oczkowski WJ, Ginsberg JS, Shin A, et al. Venous thromboembolism in patients undergoing rehabilitation for stroke. *Arch Phys Med Rehabil* 1992;73:712–716.

266. Sandset PM, Dahl T, Stiris M, et al. A double-blind and randomized placebo-controlled trial of low molecular weight heparin once daily to prevent deep-vein thrombosis in acute ischemic stroke. *Semin Thromb Hemost* 1990;16:25–33.

267. Elias A, Milandre L, Lagrange G, et al. Prevention des thromboses veineuses profondes des membres inferieurs par une fraction d'heparine de tres bas poids moleculaire (CY 222) chez des patients porteurs d'une hemiplegie secondaire a un infarctus cerebral: etude pilote randomisee (30 patients). *Rev Med Interne* 1990;11:95–98.

268. Prins MH, Gelsema R, Sing AK, et al. Prophylaxis of deep vein thrombosis with a low-molecular-weight heparin (Kabi 2165/Frgamin) in stroke patients. *Haemostasis* 1989;19:245–250.

269. Turpie AG, Gent M, Cote R, et al. A Randomized, Double-blind Study. A low-molecular weight heparinoid compared with unfractionated heparin in the prevention of deep vein thrombosis in patients with acute ischemic stroke. *Ann Intern Med* 1992;117:353–357.

270. Adams HP Jr, Woolson RF, Biller J, et al. Studies of Org 10172 in patients with acute ischemic stroke. *Haemostasis* 1992;22:99–103.

271. Madden KP, Karanjia PN, Adams HP Jr., et al. The TOAST Investigators. Accuracy of initial stroke subtype diagnosis in the TOAST study. *Neurology* 1995;45:1975–1979.

272. Davis PH, Clarke WR, Bendixen BH, et al. Silent cerebral infarction in patients enrolled in the TOAST study. *Neurology* 1996;46:942–948.

273. Anderson DC, Kappelle LJ, Eliasziw M, et al. Occurrence of hemispheric and retinal ischemia in atrial fibrillation compared with carotid stenosis. *Stroke* 2002;33(8):1963–1967.

274. Bashshur ZF, Taher A, Masri AF, et al. Anticardiolipin antibodies in patients with retinal vein occlusion and no risk factors: a prospective study. *Retina* 2003;23(4):486–490.

275. Kwaan HC. Thromboembolic disorders of the eye. In: Comerota AC, ed. *Thrombolytic therapy*. Orlando, FL: Grune & Stratton, 1988:153–163.

276. Freitag H-J, Zeumer H, Knospe V. Acute central retinal artery occlusion and the role of thrombolysis. In: del Zoppo GJ, Mori E, Hacke W, eds. *Thrombolytic therapy in acute ischemic stroke II*. Heidelberg: Springer-Verlag, 1993:103–105.

277. Schmidt D, Schumacher M, Wakhloo AK. Microcatheter urokinase infusion in central retinal artery occlusion. *Am J Ophthalmol* 1992;113:429–434.

278. Prisco D, Marcucci R. Retinal vein thrombosis: risk factors, pathogenesis and therapeutic approach. *Pathophysiol Haemost Thromb* 2002;32(5-6):308–311.

# CHAPTER 103 ■ INTERDISCIPLINARY MANAGEMENT OF ACUTE STROKE

JEFFREY L. SAVER, CHELSEA S. KIDWELL, AND NEIL A. MARTIN

## EPIDEMIOLOGY

### Incidence

Stroke is a common, crippling, and a deadly disease, the third leading cause of death, and the leading cause of adult disability in the Western world. More than 750,000 symptomatic, nonfatal strokes, more than 160,000 fatal strokes, and more than 11 million silent strokes occur each year in the United States (1–3). Ischemic cerebral infarction accounts for 80% to 85% of all strokes, while approximately 10% are intracerebral hemorrhages, and approximately 7% are subarachnoid hemorrhages (see Table 103-1) (4).

### Acute Mortality and Morbidity

Stroke is frequently fatal, accounting for 10% of all deaths worldwide. The 1-month mortality after subarachnoid hemorrhage is 25% to 55%, after intracerebral hemorrhage is 25% to 64%, and after ischemic stroke is 8% to 20% (5). In ischemic stroke, 30-day mortality varies by stroke subtype, with cardioembolic stroke and strokes of undetermined cause producing higher fatality rates than lacunar strokes and large vessel atherothromboembolic strokes.

When not fatal, stroke is often disabling. Currently, there are more than 4.5 million survivors of symptomatic stroke in the United States (6). More than 70% of stroke survivors are unable to return fully to their prior occupations (7). Thirty-one percent of stroke survivors require assistance with activities of daily living, 20% need help in walking, and 16% are chronically institutionalized (7). The financial toll exacted by stroke is immense—more than $40 billion is spent annually in the United States. The personal toll, on affected patients and families, is even greater. Approximately one half of older Americans consider a major stroke as a fate worse than death (8).

## ACUTE ISCHEMIC STROKE

### Pathophysiology

Cerebral ischemia occurs when disruption in cerebral blood flow (CBF) deprives the tissue of the nutrients required for normal cell function and homeostasis. Within minutes of an ischemic insult, a core region of tissue experiences profound blood flow reduction and becomes irreversibly injured even if blood flow is rapidly restored. However, surrounding this core is a zone of moderate blood flow reduction and ischemic tissue that may still be rescued for several hours or more from symptom onset. This zone has been called the ischemic penumbra and constitutes the target of acute stroke therapy. A variety of definitions have been proposed to demarcate the ischemic penumbra. A straightforward operational approach is to define the penumbra as the zone of tissue that is at risk of infarction, but still salvageable if adequate blood flow is restored.

Changes in CBF result in a continuum of metabolic and ionic disturbances that occur in a predictable order (9). Studies in animal models of focal stroke suggest that, as blood flow declines, inhibition of protein synthesis begins at values that are mildly below normal (40 to 50 mL/100 g/minute), followed by anaerobic glycolysis (35 mL/100 g/minute), loss of synaptic transmission (20 mL/100 g/minute), and finally anoxic depolarization of cell membranes (15 mL/100 g/minute) (10). These observations in stroke animal models have been supported by human positron emission tomography (PET) studies. Regional CBF below 12 mL/100 g/minute results in tissue necrosis, whereas only transient deficits occur when CBF remains above 22 mL/100 g/minute (11). Tissue with CBF between 12 and 22 mL/100 g/minute represents the ischemic penumbra, an area of stunned parenchyma surrounding the ischemic core, which has the potential for recovery, but only if reperfusion is rapidly established.

In addition to the magnitude of blood flow reduction, the length of time that cells are ischemic also determines viability. Numerous studies indicate the threshold for metabolic and ionic disturbance increases as the duration of ischemia increases (10). For example, studies have shown that during the first 2 hours of vascular occlusion, the threshold for irreversible suppression of spontaneous neuronal unit activity rises from 5 to 12 mL/100 g/minute (12). Other studies have shown that when ischemia lasts only for a few hours, brain tissue is able to survive flows as low as 12 mL/100 g/minute. However, if the ischemia is permanent, brain necrosis occurs in regions with flows as high as 24 mL/100 g/minute (10). Therefore, the viability of the ischemic area is in flux in the first few hours after stroke onset, its fate determined by the extent and duration of impaired blood flow. However, this dynamic period of potential reversibility is evanescent. Studies in a large number of rodent and nonhuman primate stroke models demonstrate that substantial volumes of neuronal tissue can be salvaged by reperfusion only within the first several hours of ischemia onset (13).

A variety of underlying vascular lesions produce acute brain ischemia. Large hospital-based registries suggest that 25% to 40% of acute ischemic strokes are due to large artery atherothrombosis, 25% to 35% are due to cardioembolism, 10% to 30% are due to intrinsic disease of small penetrating arteries (microatheromatosis and lipohyalinosis), 10% to 15% are due to diverse other causes (hypercoagulable state, dissection, migraine, vasculitis, etc.), 10% to 20% are cryptogenic, and 2% to 5% are borderzone infarcts due to global cerebral hypoperfusion. Cerebral angiography will demonstrate a large vessel occlusion that is an appropriate target for recanalization therapies in 80% of acute ischemic strokes.

TABLE 103-1

FREQUENCIES OF DIFFERENT VASCULAR
MECHANISMS OF STROKE

| Stroke subtype | Proportion % |
| --- | --- |
| Ischemic | 85 |
| Large-vessel atherothromboembolic | 35 |
| Cardioembolic | 25 |
| Small vessel (lacunar) | 20 |
| Other | 5 |
| Hemorrhagic | 15 |
| Intracerebral hemorrhage | 10 |
| Subarachnoid hemorrhage | 5 |

Data are approximations based on large population-based and registry studies.
© UCLA Stroke Program, reprinted with permission.

# WORKUP OF THE PATIENT WITH ACUTE ISCHEMIC STROKE

The goals of the evaluation of a patient with acute ischemic stroke are to (a) determine if an immediate complication is likely, (b) confirm that ischemic stroke, and not a mimic, is the cause of the focal deficit, (c) assess the reversibility of the pathology, (d) obtain clues to the likely vascular mechanism and etiology, and (e) institute appropriate treatment.

## History

Establishing the time of stroke onset accurately is of utmost importance. When onset cannot be specified precisely, the ischemia duration clock is started from the time the patient was last known to be well. This convention applies to patients who awake with their deficits, who are found down and uncommunicative, or who simply are unable to clearly communicate when their deficit started.

Other essential history questions focus on ruling out stroke mimics (e.g., seizures, intoxications, head trauma, complicated migraine headaches, and acute systemic infections), and provisionally characterizing the stroke mechanism. The presence of cervical trauma and neck pain may point toward a diagnosis of dissection. Headaches and nausea raise the possibility of intracerebral hemorrhage or brainstem infarction. The tempo of deficit onset is ascertained. Registry studies suggest that strokes with maximum disability at onset, but without headache, are most often found to be embolic, either cardiac, or artery-to-artery, whereas those with a fluctuating course are more likely due to thrombosis (14,15). A history of multiple prior transient ischemic attacks (TIAs) in the same circulation suggests an atherothrombotic mechanism. A steadily expanding deficit over 5 to 20 minutes is typical of intracerebral hemorrhage.

Inquiring about previous medical conditions also sheds light on the stroke mechanism. Patients with cardiac disease including arrhythmia, valvular disease, ventricular aneurysm, patent foramen ovale, and congestive heart failure are prone to cardioembolic events. A history of hypertension, coronary artery disease, tobacco use, diabetes, or claudication is associated with large-vessel atherothrombosis. Hypertension, and to a lesser degree, tobacco use and diabetes, are often seen in lacunar infarcts.

## Physical Examination

The goals of the initial examination are to determine patient level of consciousness, stroke severity, stroke localization, and stroke etiology (9,16). Careful neurovascular examination includes auscultating the heart for the presence of gallops, murmurs, or dysrhythmias. The peripheral vascular system is interrogated by palpating the radial, femoral, and pedal pulses to determine strength and regularity. The carotid artery is palpated and the neck auscultated for bruits. The fundoscopic examination provides a unique opportunity to visualize blood vessels directly. Signs of internal carotid artery disease include cholesterol crystals, retinal infarctions, and venous stasis retinopathy. Unexplained fever or nuchal rigidity raise the possibility of other diagnoses such as meningitis or other infection, or subarachnoid hemorrhage. Coma is extremely uncommon in acute ischemic stroke, and suggests intracerebral or subarachnoid hemorrhage, or metabolic and other nonstroke processes.

The neurologic examination includes screening of mental state, including tests of aphasia and neglect, cranial nerve evaluation including visual field and ocular motility testing, motor, coordination, sensory, reflex, and gait examination. The pattern of findings permits localization to the anterior or posterior circulations and their subdivisions. Decision making in acute stroke care requires being able to recognize cardinal stroke syndromes rapidly. In the acute setting, examiners should not dwell in the arcana of neurologic semiology. The ability to recognize broad clinical patterns comprising seven key stroke syndromes suffices for all but the most unusual cases. These seven syndromes reflect ischemic strokes localized in dominant cerebral hemisphere, nondominant cerebral hemisphere, brainstem, cerebellum, and lacunar (penetrating small vessel) distributions, and primary intracerebral and subarachnoid hemorrhages (see Table 103-2).

Use of a formalized examination scale permits quantification of stroke severity. In widest use is the National Institutes of Health (NIH) Stroke Scale, which has been incorporated into the formal guidelines for thrombolytic therapy decision-making (17).

## Laboratory Evaluation

Table 103-3 lists the recommended tests that should be conducted on all patients with stroke on an emergent basis. The frequent coexistence of heart disease with ischemic stroke mandates concern in all patients for acute myocardial infarction, congestive heart failure, arrhythmias, and sudden death, dictating the need for cardiac enzymes, electrocardiography, and chest radiograph. The possibility of early aspiration and pneumonitis also supports chest radiography. Cardiac monitoring should be maintained continuously, throughout the first 24 hours to detect potentially lethal arrhythmias, and to capture episodes of atrial fibrillation. Glucose measurement is essential as hypo and hyperglycemia may mimic or exacerbate stroke deficits. Electrolyte and renal dysfunction may also exacerbate stroke impairments. Tests of blood cell counts, platelet count, and the clotting system identify coagulation abnormalities that may have contributed to the acute stroke and this will influence urgent management. Table 103-4 lists selected tests to be considered in patients with suspected hypercoagulable states as a cause of ischemic stroke.

## TABLE 103-2

### SEVEN KEY STROKE SYNDROMES

| Syndrome | Symptoms |
|---|---|
| Left (dominant)<br>  hemisphere | Right hemiparesis<br>Right hemisensory loss<br>Right visual field defect<br>Left gaze preference<br>Aphasia |
| Right (nondominant)<br>  hemisphere | Left hemiparesis<br>Left hemisensory loss<br>Left visual field deficit<br>Right gaze preference<br>Neglect for left hemispace |
| Brainstem | Hemiparesis or quadriparesis<br>Unilateral or bilateral sensory loss<br>Crossed signs (deficits on one side of face and other side<br>  of body)<br>Dysconjugate gaze or gaze palsy, nystagmus<br>Dysarthria or dysphagia<br>Vertigo, nausea, vomiting<br>Decreased level of consciousness |
| Cerebellum | Truncal/gait ataxia<br>Limb ataxia<br>Nystagmus |
| Lacunar (small vessel) | |
|   Pure motor hemiparesis | Contralateral face, arm, and leg weakness |
|   Pure sensory stroke | Face, arm, and leg numbness, paresthesias or pain |
|   Sensorimotor stroke | Contralateral face, arm, and leg weakness and<br>  hypoesthesia |
|   Clumsy hand/dysarthria | Dysarthria, dysphagia, facial weakness, tongue deviation,<br>  clumsy hand |
|   Ataxic hemiparesis | Ataxia and contralateral weakness |
| Intracerebral hemorrhage | One of the above focal syndromes, plus<br>Headache<br>Neck pain, stiffness<br>Nausea, vomiting<br>Decreased level of consciousness |
| Subarachnoid hemorrhage | Abrupt headache at onset<br>Neck stiffness, pain<br>Decreased level of consciousness<br>Cranial nerve abnormalities |

© UCLA Stroke Program, reprinted with permission.

## Neuroimaging

As therapeutic options for treatment of acute stroke evolve, neuroimaging strategies are assuming an increasingly important role in the initial evaluation and management of patients. Both acute and long-term treatment decisions for patients with stroke are optimally guided by neuroimaging information about tissue status (i.e., size, location, vascular distribution, and degree of reversibility of ischemic injury, as well as presence of hemorrhage), vessel status (i.e., site and severity of stenosis and occlusions), and cerebral perfusion (size, location, and severity of hypoperfusion). All patients with suspected ischemic stroke should undergo imaging of the brain parenchyma and of the cervicocephalic vasculature. In addition, cerebral perfusion imaging is often useful in the acute setting.

Two general multimodal imaging strategies are emerging in the evaluation of the patient with acute ischemic stroke, one employing magnetic resonance (MR), and one employing computerized tomography (CT) scan (see Figs. 103-1 and

103-2). With acquisition times of only 10 to 20 minutes, both permit the distinction of infarct from hemorrhage, delineation of the already irreversibly infarcted tissue, delineation of salvageable penumbral tissue, and identification of the site of vascular occlusions. The resulting multidimensional portrayal of the ischemic process permits selection of acute stroke interventions tailored to the specific pathophysiologic events under way in each individual patient.

### Brain Parenchymal Imaging

**Noncontrast Computerized Tomography Scan.** Noncontrast head CT scan is routinely employed as the initial imaging study in patients with suspected acute ischemic stroke. CT scan is used as a screening tool to exclude hemorrhage and other nonischemic causes of acute neurologic deficits (e.g., tumor, infection), and has the advantages of being rapid and inexpensive with widespread availability. With the advent of intravenous tissue-type plasminogen activator (IV tPA), there has been growing interest in employing CT scan to identify early infarct signs (hyperdense

## TABLE 103-3

### LABORATORY EVALUATION FOR PATIENTS WITH ACUTE ISCHEMIC STROKE

**INITIAL TESTS FOR ALL PATIENTS**
Electrocardiogram and initiation of continuous cardiac monitoring
Chest x-ray
Complete blood count
Platelet count
Prothrombin time
Partial thromboplastin time
Electrolytes
Blood glucose
Troponin or CK/MB
Blood urea nitrogen/creatinine
Pulse oximetry

**ADDITIONAL TESTS IN SELECT PATIENTS**
Lateral cervical spine x-ray (if trauma is suspected)
Lumbar puncture (if subarachnoid hemorrhage is suspected and CT scan is negative)
Electroencephalogram (if seizure is suspected)
Pregnancy test (in women of child-bearing age)
Liver function tests (if altered level of consciousness)
Troponin or CK/MB (if myocardial infarction is suspected)
Arterial blood gas (if hypoxia is suspected)
Urine toxicology (if substance abuse is suspected)
Blood cultures and erythrocyte sedimentation rate (if endocarditis or other infection is suspected)

CK, creatin kinase; MB, myoglobin; CT, computerized tomography.
© UCLA Stroke Program, reprinted with permission.

## TABLE 103-4

### HYPERCOAGULABLE STATE EVALUATION IN ACUTE ISCHEMIC STROKE

**CEREBRAL ARTERIAL THROMBOSIS**
DRVVT (Lupus anticoagulant)
Anticardiolipin antibody
$\beta_2$ Glycoprotein 1 antibodies
Homocysteine

**CEREBRAL VENOUS THROMBOSIS OR PARADOXICAL CEREBRAL EMBOLISM**
Protein C functional activity
Protein S functional activity
Activated protein C resistance (factor $V_{Leiden}$ if abnormal)
Antithrombin III
DRVVT (Lupus anticoagulant)
Anticardiolipin antibody
$\beta_2$ Glycoprotein 1 antibodies
Homocysteine
Prothrombin gene mutation
Factor VIII level
Fibrinogen

DRVVT, dilute Russell viper venom time.
© UCLA Stroke Program, reprinted with permission.

MCA sign, loss of gray–white differentiation, hypodensity, and sulcal effacement—Figure 103-3). These signs may be seen in up to 82% of patients within 6 hours from symptom onset (18). Pathophysiologic studies suggest that parenchymal CT scan shows early infarct signs representing early cytotoxic edema, and that they are only rarely reversible. Several studies have demonstrated that the presence of early infarct signs is associated with a poorer outcome (19,20).

**Magnetic Resonance Imaging.** Within the first few hours of ischemia onset, standard magnetic resonance imaging (MRI) sequences (T1-weighted, T2-weighted, and proton density weighted) are relatively insensitive to ischemia, showing abnormalities in less than 50% of cases (21). The earliest changes, seen as increased signal on T2-weighted and fluid attenuated inversion recovery (FLAIR) sequences, are due to a net increase in overall tissue water content primarily due to *vasogenic edema*—a process which takes several hours to develop to levels visible on MR. Although the preponderance of ischemic lesions are

evident on both CT scan and conventional MRI by 24 hours, standard MRI is superior to CT scan in identifying posterior fossa and subcortical lesions.

Hyperacute parenchymal blood can be reliably detected employing gradient recalled echo (GRE), or echo-planar susceptibility-weighted MR imaging (22). Large, multicenter studies have prospectively validated that MR is at least equally accurate to CT scan in distinguishing acute intracerebral hemorrhage from acute ischemic stroke (23,24).

**Diffusion-Weighted Imaging.** Diffusion-weighted imaging (DWI) allows visualization of regions of ischemia within minutes of symptom onset (25). During ischemia, there is decreased free-water diffusion in the brain tissue, related to the flux of water from the extracellular to intracellular space leading to early *cytotoxic edema*. This impaired water motion causes an increased (bright) signal on DWI sequences. The decrease in diffusion can be quantitatively measured on the apparent diffusion coefficient (ADC) maps, with darker areas representing decreased diffusion. The increase in signal on DWI may persist for several weeks or longer partially due to a T2 effect. The ADC, however, returns to normal or supranormal levels within 7 to 10 days from ischemia onset (26). Early reperfusion, as from thrombolytic therapy, may reverse cytotoxic edema and normalize DWI images (27,28).

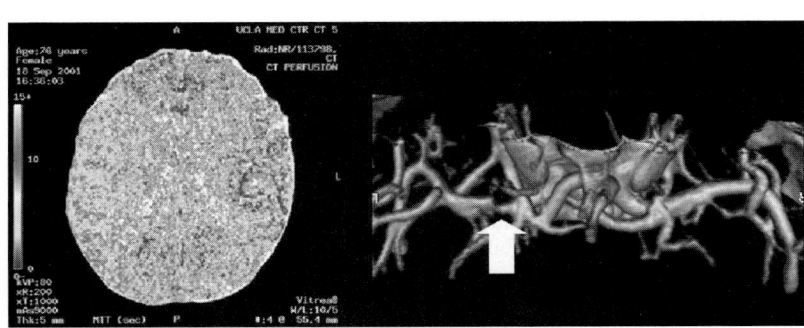

**FIGURE 103-1.** The multimodal computerized tomography (CT) scan strategy in acute stroke neuroimaging. Perfusion CT scan (**left image**) mean transit time (MTT) image shows reduced regional perfusion throughout the right middle cerebral artery (MCA) territory, worse posteriorly. CT scan angiogram (**right image**) demonstrates severe stenosis of the right MCA trunk (*arrow*). (© UCLA Stroke Program, reprinted with permission.)

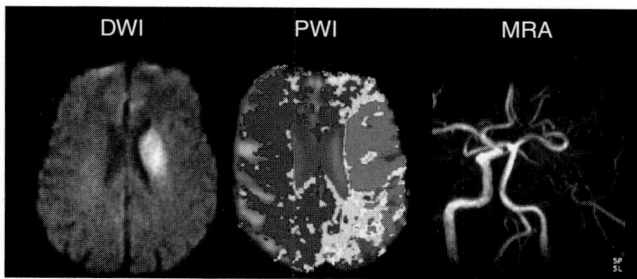

FIGURE 103-2. The multimodal magnetic resonance (MR) strategy in acute stroke neuroimaging. **Left image** is diffusion-weighted sequence showing early diffusion injury (hyperintensity) in the deep left periventricular white matter. **Middle image** is perfusion-weighted magnetic resonance (MR) showing reduced perfusion, throughout the middle cerebral artery (MCA) territory. The large extent of the perfusion than diffusion lesion (perfusion-diffusion mismatch) suggests a large volume of potentially salvageable penumbral tissue. The **right image** is MR angiogram showing absence of signal from the left internal carotid and left middle cerebral arteries. (© UCLA Stroke Program, reprinted with permission.)

Diffusion imaging allows early identification of lesion size, lesion age, neuroanatomic site, and vascular territory involved (29–31). DWI has a high degree of sensitivity (95% to 100%) and specificity (95% to 100%) for acute ischemia, even at very early time points (32–34). DWI hyperintensities may occasionally be seen in diverse other cerebral disorders, including status epilepticus, tumors, Jakob-Creutzfeld disease, and hyperthermia. Examination of the T2-weighted and ADC sequences generally allows these entities to be differentiated from acute ischemia. Numerous studies have shown that initial diffusion lesion volume correlates well with final infarct volume, as well as neurologic and functional outcomes in patients with stroke (30,35,36).

A distinctive advantage of DWI is its ability to distinguish acute from chronic ischemia, allowing new lesions to be identified in patients even when these are near or within areas of prior ischemic injury (29,37,38). Another important insight into stroke pathophysiology offered by diffusion MR, is the frequent visualization of multiple acute lesions in different vascular territories in patients who have only one clinically symptomatic acute insult, providing evidence of an embolic stroke mechanism (39).

### Cerebral Perfusion Imaging

**Perfusion Computerized Tomography.** Perfusion CT scan assesses regional CBF in the acute stroke setting. The technique uses rapid CT scanning to track the first pass of a bolus of contrast material delivered intravenously. Perfusion CT scan identifies regions of irreversible infarction by visualizing areas of vascular collapse [markedly reduced cerebral blood volume (CBV)], and identifies penumbral zones as regions with reduced CBF but not yet vascular collapse (CBF–CBV mismatch) (40). Perfusion CT scan has the advantage of rapid data acquisition and rapid postprocessing and can be performed in conjunction with the baseline head CT scan and CT angiography scans.

**Magnetic Resonance Perfusion Imaging.** Perfusion-weighted imaging (PWI) is most commonly performed by the rapid injection of an intravenous paramagnetic contrast agent. The temporal passage of the contrast agent through contiguous slices of brain tissue is tracked with a sequence of rapid MR scans. This signal intensity information is then used to derive a concentration time curve. Perfusion measures that can be derived from this technique include mean transit time (MTT), relative CBV (rCBV), and relative CBF (rCBF). Baseline MR perfusion lesion volumes correlate well with the final infarct volume, as well as neurologic and functional outcome, and in fact correlate somewhat better than the baseline diffusion lesion volumes (36). Perfusion lesion volume likely identifies all tissue at risk of infarction if vessel recanalization does not occur, whereas diffusion imaging identifies the only tissue that has already sustained advanced bioenergetic failure.

Combined perfusion and diffusion MR imaging permits identification of the ischemic penumbra. A good approximation of the penumbral zone is the region of diffusion–perfusion mismatch, evidencing perfusion but not diffusion abnormality. In these tissues, blood flow is reduced, but advanced tissue bioenergetic failure, resulting in cytotoxic edema, has not yet developed. The natural history of diffusion MR abnormalities is to grow over time into the mismatch zone (41,42), suggesting gradual failure of the ischemic penumbra as it is incorporated into the infarct core. However, the region of diffusion abnormality does not precisely correlate with the infarct core, as animal and human studies show that diffusion abnormalities can be partially reversed with early reperfusion (27,43,44). These observations suggest that early after ischemia onset, the penumbra likely includes not only regions of diffusion/perfusion mismatch, but also portions of the region of diffusion abnormality.

### Cervicocephalic Vessel Imaging

A wide variety of imaging techniques are now available to assess the status of large and medium caliber cervicocephalic vessels in acute stroke.

**Computerized Tomographic Angiography.** Helical computerized tomographic angiography (CTA) is performed by rapid

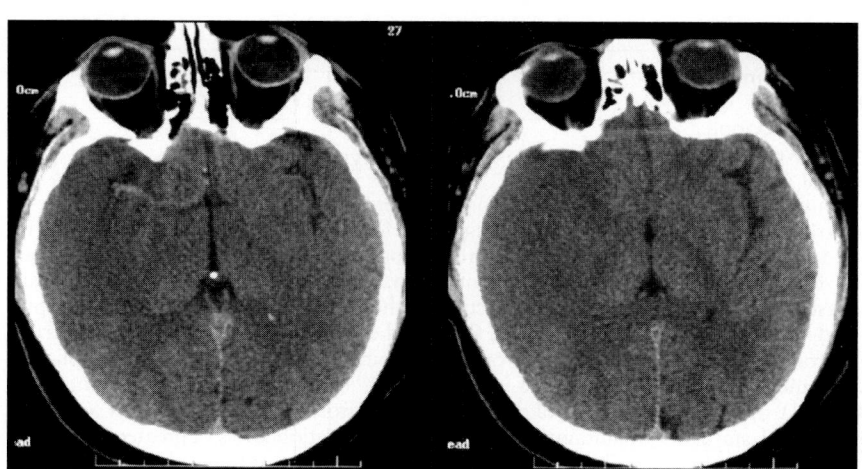

FIGURE 103-3. Early infarct signs on noncontrast computerized tomography (CT) scan. **Left image** shows hyperdensity of the right middle cerebral artery [hyperdense middle cerebral artery (MCA) sign] indicating acute thrombus. Both images show hypodensity and loss of gray–white cortical ribbon in the right temporal lobe. **Right image** shows loss of sulcal markings indicating edema in the right temporal lobe. (© UCLA Stroke Program, reprinted with permission.)

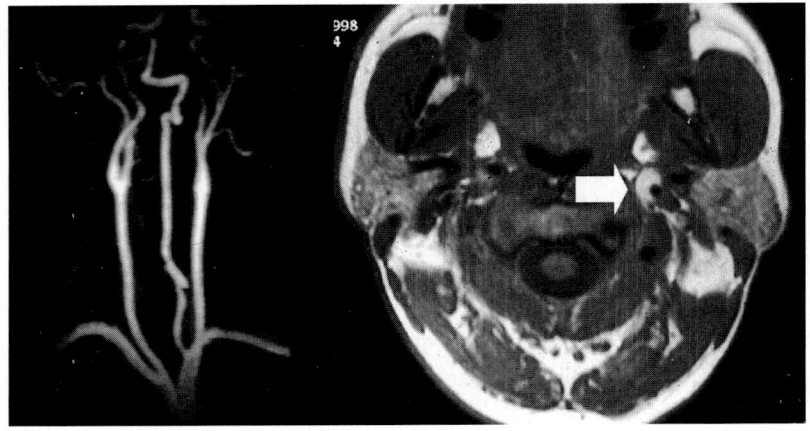

**FIGURE 103-4.** Patient with simultaneous dissection of four cervicocerebral vessels. Contrast enhanced magnetic resonance (MR) angiogram (**left** side of figure) demonstrates dissecting aneurysm in proximal left vertebral artery, narrowed, irregular right vertebral artery from origin upward, and tapering stenoses in both internal carotid arteries distally. Axial T1 MR image (**right** side of figure) shows pathognomonic crescent sign (*arrow*) with stenotic lumen (small flow void) and surrounding crescent of high signal indicating intramural hematoma. (© UCLA Stroke Program, reprinted with permission.)

administration of an intravenous contrast agent followed by data acquisition over the time of passage of the bolus within large vessels of the target vascular system. The method relies on continuous scanning as the patient is moved through the x-ray beam, allowing for volumetric rather than conventional tomographic data acquisition. In addition to acquisition of axial cuts, image postprocessing permits the data to be visualized using multiplanar reformatting, surface or 3D volume-rendering, and maximum intensity projection (MIP) techniques (45).

Helical CTA rapidly and noninvasively evaluates the neurovasculature for patients with suspected cerebrovascular disease, providing important information about the presence and site of vessel occlusions or stenoses in both the intracranial and extracranial circulations (46). Disadvantages of CTA include requirement for intravenous contrast dosing, use of ionizing radiation, and simultaneous arterial and venous phase imaging.

**Magnetic Resonance Angiography.** Magnetic resonance angiography (MRA) is a highly useful technique for noninvasive screening of supraaortic vessels. When compared to digital subtraction angiography for detection of cervical and intracranial stenoses, sensitivity and specificity range from 70% to 100% in various studies (47). In the intracranial vasculature, MRA is useful in identifying acute proximal large vessel occlusions, but is not able to reliably identify distal or branch occlusions. Combined with data from DWI, MRA substantially improves acute diagnosis of stroke mechanism (31).

Time-of-flight MRA techniques employ information from flowing blood within vessels, rather than vessel structure, to construct images. Advantages are rapid acquisition and non-necessity of administration of contrast. Disadvantages are susceptibility to flow artifacts, including in-plane flow saturation, susceptibility to turbulent or complex flow, flowlike effects from adjacent short T1 substances, such as thrombus and fat, and a tendency to overestimate the degree of stenosis. Contrast enhanced MRA techniques that employ gadolinium contrast to outline vascular structures provide more reliable images of the thoracocervical vasculature (see Fig. 103-4).

**Ultrasound Procedures.** Carotid and transcranial Doppler (TCD) ultrasound techniques offer another noninvasive method to assess the neurovasculature acutely. Ultrasound studies of the carotid bifurcation are a well-established noninvasive test in the diagnosis of stroke. A full carotid ultrasonography battery includes continuous wave Doppler measurement of blood velocity, B-mode imaging of vessel anatomy, and color-flow imaging of flow direction and lumen caliber. Carotid ultrasound visualizes only the proximal cervical carotid arteries and very limited segments of the cervical vertebral arteries. TCD ultrasound employs a low frequency probe to penetrate the skull and interrogate the major basal intracranial arteries (48). TCD offers a practical, noninvasive assessment of intracranial vessel status that provides early diagnostic and prognostic information in

patients with acute stroke (49). In addition, TCD can be used to monitor cerebral hemodynamic status and response to recanalization therapy (50). Ultrasound procedures have the advantages of being performed at the bedside in a timely fashion. The costs are minimal and patient cooperation is not essential. Disadvantages of ultrasound include being highly operator dependent and having difficulty in distinguishing high-grade stenosis from complete occlusion.

**Catheter Angiography.** Digital subtraction angiography remains the gold standard imaging modality to assess vessel anatomy and pathology while providing important collateral flow information. Although the 0.5% to 1% permanent neurologic complication risk makes other noninvasive vessel-imaging techniques, such as CTA and MRA, very attractive, it is likely that catheter angiography will continue to play an important role in stroke evaluation. Advantages include better visualization of medium and small vessels than with noninvasive techniques, and the ability to proceed directly to an endovascular intervention after diagnostic imaging. Catheter angiography can detect arterial dissection with high sensitivity and can define the route, and to some degree, the adequacy of collateral circulation. It remains the only way to confidently make a diagnosis of diseases affecting small caliber vessels such as vasculitis. It is also often of help in the rapidly deteriorating patient, the patient with conflicting or unrevealing noninvasive vascular imaging, the patient with suspected dissection, and the young patient with stroke. Disadvantages include periprocedural risks of stroke, exposure to iodinated contrast with nephrotoxicity and potential for allergic response, and lack of round-the-clock availability outside of large medical centers.

# MEDICAL THERAPY FOR ACUTE ISCHEMIC STROKE

## Early Supportive Therapy

### Oxygenation

Systemic oxygen desaturation will exacerbate and extend brain injury originating from focal cerebral hypoxia. Patients with acute stroke are at risk for respiratory compromise owing to aspiration, hypoventilation, upper airway obstruction, atelectasis, or rarely a reduction in the ventilatory drive or neurogenic pulmonary edema. One third of patients with acute ischemic stroke exhibit overt or silent aspiration (51). Pneumonia complicates acute stroke in 5% to 12% of patients (52). All patients with acute stroke should be monitored for hypoxia with a goal of maintaining serum oxygen saturation levels of greater than 95%. If this cannot be achieved in room air, supplemental oxygen should be used. No clinical trial evidence supports the routine use of supplemental oxygen for patients with adequate blood oxygen saturation when breathing room air (16,53). If ventilatory assistance is required to achieve adequate oxygenation, or if the upper airway is threatened because of obtundation or laryngeal dysfunction, endotracheal intubation and mechanical ventilation should proceed with dispatch.

### Blood Pressure Management

The treatment of hypertension in the acute stroke patient has long been the subject of debate. Although it is well known that chronic hypertension is an independent risk factor for the occurrence of ischemic stroke, lowering elevated blood pressure during an episode of cerebral ischemia has the potential to extend the area of hypoperfusion.

Elevated blood pressures occur naturally in the first few hours of ischemic stroke, for a variety of reasons, including response to stress, full bladder, pain, underlying hypertension, physiologic compensation for hypoxia, and increased intracranial pressure (ICP). Untreated, pressures will usually spontaneously decline substantially within 24 hours of onset, and return to the patient's likely baseline in 4 to 7 days (54).

In the normal brain, to ensure adequate oxygenation, CBF is maintained at a constant level over a wide range of systemic perfusion pressures through cerebrovascular autoregulation. When systemic blood pressure rises, cerebral arterioles constrict, increasing vascular resistance, and net CBF remains unchanged. In contrast, a drop in blood pressure results in dilatation of cerebral arterioles to reduce resistance and avoid a fall in blood flow. Patients who have a background history of hypertension will have chronically shifted their autoregulatory range upward, so that CBF declines at a higher mean arterial pressure than in normotensives.

Autoregulation is impaired in the ischemic field of patients with acute ischemic stroke. The cerebrovascular endothelium in these regions is itself experiencing ischemia and loses the ability to respond fully to autoregulatory signals. As a consequence, in the ischemic field, CBF varies directly with systemic blood pressure (55). Reducing the systemic blood pressure may diminish blood flow to the ischemic penumbra and promote extension of the infarct. On the other hand, although it makes sense to prevent precipitous drops in blood pressure in patients with stroke, it is also possible that markedly elevated blood pressures could cause further damage by promoting edema formation, increasing the risk of hemorrhagic transformation, and exacerbating vascular damage.

Conversely, the strategy of actively raising the blood pressure in all patients with ischemic stroke has also not directly been tested in major clinical trials. Indirect observations from randomized clinical trials of hemodilution (sometimes associated with volume expansion and blood pressure elevation) suggest that many elderly patients with stroke and with coexisting cardiac morbidities do not tolerate induced hypertension well, and congestive heart failure, myocardial infarction, and other complications of therapy negate possible gains in cerebral perfusion. In select patients carefully managed in the intensive care unit, induced hypertension with phenylephrine has been shown to improve cerebral perfusion and possibly influence the clinical course favorably (56).

On the basis of these data, it is recommended that antihypertensive therapy should be withheld in the first few hours after ischemic stroke onset, unless blood pressure is in the hypertensive encephalopathy range on two consecutive measurements at least 5 minutes apart, with systolic blood pressure (SBP) above 220 mm Hg or mean arterial pressure greater than 130 mm Hg (16,57). This recommendation is modified if a patient has a concurrent condition that independently requires moderation of blood pressure, including acute myocardial infarction, aortic dissection, acute renal failure due to accelerated hypertension, or early hemorrhagic transformation of cerebral infarct. In these circumstances, a compromise must be struck between the need to maintain systemic blood pressure to maximize cerebral perfusion and the need to lower blood pressure to avoid extension of visceral injury. Another exceptional case is in the first 24 hours after thrombolytic therapy administration, when, to minimize the risk of cerebral hemorrhagic transformation, the SBP should be maintained at less than 180 mm Hg and diastolic blood pressure (DBP) at less than 105 mm Hg.

The choice of antihypertensive medications must take into account the effect of drugs on the cerebrovascular, as well as the systemic circulation (55). Nitroglycerin, sodium nitroprusside, calcium channel blockers, and hydralazine are cerebral venodilators that increase CBV and may thereby increase intracerebral pressure, and impair autoregulation. In contrast, $\alpha$ and $\beta$-adrenergic blockers, ganglion blockers, and angiotensin-converting enzyme inhibitors have little effect on CBV. Parenteral agents that allow rapid, controlled titration to target pressures are often useful in the hyperacute setting, and include nicardipine, nitroprusside, enalapril, and labetalol. Regimens for management of blood pressure in patients who are both thrombolytic and nonthrombolytic adapted from the National Institute of Neurological Disorders and Stroke (NINDS)-tPA trialists approach are shown in Table 103-5 (58).

Hypotension is uncommon in ischemic stroke, but when present, vigorous treatment is warranted. First, a treatable cause such as decreased volume status (e.g., dehydration or hemorrhage), pump failure (e.g., arrhythmia, myocardial infarction, or congestive heart failure), or decreased peripheral vascular resistance (e.g., sepsis) should be sought and corrected, if identified. If the pressure falls below 90/60 mm Hg, or if blood pressure is in low normal range and collateral insufficiency appears to be producing stroke progression, colloid solutions, hypervolemic therapy, and vasopressor agents should be administered. Often in these circumstances, central venous or Swan-Ganz monitoring should be employed because coexisting cardiac disease is common in the elderly ischemic stroke population. Raising blood pressure to the patient's baseline level is a reasonable initial target.

### Fluid Management

Most strokes occur in the elderly, in whom fluid and electrolyte disturbance are liable to occur. Decades ago it was common to restrict fluid intake in patients with acute ischemic stroke because of concern about cerebral edema. However, diminished fluid input decreases intravascular volume, promoting collateral failure, and increases blood viscosity, promoting recurrent arterial and venous thrombosis. Patients with ischemic stroke are often dehydrated upon hospital arrival. Large cohort studies have demonstrated that only 10% to 20% of patients with ischemic stroke develop edema that produces clinical deterioration. Edema generally peaks 3 to 5 days after stroke onset and is essentially never a concern in the first few hours post ictus.

Careful management of fluids is mandatory in patients with acute cerebral ischemia. Because of the frequency of aspiration, oral feedings should be avoided or minimized in the first few hours. All patients with acute stroke require an intravenous access line. Although cerebral edema is rarely a concern in the acute setting, hypotonic intravenous fluids are best avoided. Most patients should receive normal saline at full maintenance volume, with infusion rates of 75 to 125 mL per hour to maintain intravascular volume and optimize brain perfusion (9,16).

### Glucose Management

Hyperglycemia is the most common metabolic derangement in acute ischemic stroke. Many patients have a background

## BLOOD PRESSURE MANAGEMENT ALGORITHMS FOR PATIENTS WITH ACUTE ISCHEMIC STROKE

**FOR PATIENTS NOT TREATED WITH THROMBOLYSIS**
Monitor BP q 15 min for 1 h after ER arrival
    Then q1h × 3 for 3 h
    Then q2h × 2 for 4 h
    Then q4h × 4 for 16 h
For SBP >220 mm Hg or DBP 120–140 mm Hg on two
  readings 5–10 min apart
    Give labetolol 10 mg IV every 1–2 min
    May repeat or double every 10–20 min, up to 150 mg
    If response is not satisfactory, use IV
        Nicardipine, initiate at 5 mg/h, increase as needed
          by 2.5 mg/h every 5 min to max of 15 mg/h, or
          nitroprusside 0.5–10 μg/kg/min
    Monitor BP at least every 15 min
    Observe for hypotension
For DBP >140 mm Hg
    Nicardipine, initiate at 5 mg/h, increase as needed
      by 2.5 mg/h every 5 min to max of 15 mg/h, or
      nitroprusside 0.5–10 μg/kg/min
    Monitor BP at least every 15 min
    Observe for hypotension

**FOR PATIENTS TREATED WITH THROMBOLYTICS**
Monitor BP q 15 min for 2 h after initiation of tPA
    Then q 30 min × 12 for 6 h
    Then q 60 min × 16 for 16 h
For SBP >230 mm Hg or DBP 121–140 mm Hg on
  two readings 5–10 min apart
    Give labetolol 10 mg IV every 1–2 min
    May repeat or double every 10–20 min, up to 150 mg
    If response is not satisfactory, use IV
        Nicardipine, initiate at 5 mg/h, increase as needed by
          2.5 mg/h every 5 min to max of 15 mg/h, or
          nitroprusside 0.5–10 μg/kg/min
    Monitor BP at least every 15 min
    Observe for hypotension
For SBP 180–230 mm Hg and/or DBP 105–120 mm Hg
    Give labetolol 10 mg IV
    May be repeated or doubled every 10–20 min, up to 1,500 mg
For DBP >140 mm Hg
    Nicardipine, initiate at 5 mg/h, increase as needed by
      2.5 mg/h every 5 min to max of 15 mg/h, or
      nitroprusside 0.5–10 μg/kg/min
    Monitor BP at least every 15 min
    Observe for hypotension

BP, blood pressure; SBP, systolic blood pressure; IV, intravenous; DBP, diastolic blood pressure; tPA, tissue plasminogen activator.
© UCLA Stroke Program, reprinted with permission.

history of diabetes that predisposes them to their stroke. Even in patients without diabetes, the physiologic stress of stroke frequently evokes a systemic sympathetic nervous system response that elevates blood sugar acutely.

Studies in animal models of focal and global ischemia have suggested that acute hyperglycemia may increase infarct size. Deprivation of oxygen forces ischemic neuronal tissues to convert from aerobic to anaerobic metabolism. In ischemic regions, serum glucose is metabolized to lactate by anaerobic glycolysis. The greater the glucose level in the blood entering an ischemic neuronal field, the greater is the resulting lactic acidosis. Lactic acid is neurotoxic. Consequently, avoidance of

hyperglycemia in the acute stage might improve stroke outcome. However, overaggressive lowering of serum glucose levels to produce symptomatic hypoglycemia may also adversely affect patient course.

Several large observational studies have demonstrated that elevated blood glucose in patients at admission with acute ischemic stroke correlates with poor outcome (59). However, it has not been demonstrated whether this association reflects a direct adverse effect of hyperglycemia upon outcome, or an epiphenomenon of severe initial brain injury producing a secondary rise in blood sugar. In patients undergoing intravenous thrombolysis, acute hyperglycemia is a risk factor for hemorrhagic transformation (60).

Although definitive studies are pending, current basic science and clinical observations suggest that hyperglycemia should be treated promptly in acute stroke. Aiming to maintain a glucose level of less than 200 mg per dL is a reasonable strategy (9). A sliding subcutaneous (SQ) insulin scale is most often employed for this purpose. Randomized trials are investigating whether continuous intravenous insulin infusions would be even more beneficial; currently, insulin infusion with or without concomitant glucose infusions is an additional reasonable management strategy. In patients with profound hyperglycemia, glucose reduction should be limited to 75 to 100 mg per dL per hour to reduce the risk of osmotic injury to the brain (61). Dextrose containing intravenous solutions in general should be avoided in the first several hours after stroke onset, except in symptomatic hypoglycemia.

## Temperature Management

Hyperthermia markedly worsens ischemic and traumatic brain injury in animal models (62). Several mechanisms have been proposed to explain the deleterious effects of hyperthermia. Enhanced release of neurotransmitters, increased numbers of potentially damaging ischemic depolarizations in the focal ischemic penumbra, impaired recovery of energy metabolism, enhanced inhibition of protein kinases, and worsening of cytoskeletal proteolysis have all been implicated. A few large acute ischemic stroke cohort studies have found hyperthermia on admission to be an independent risk factor for poor outcome from acute ischemic stroke. These observations are intriguing, but they cannot exclude the possibility that early hyperthermia is a consequence of severe stroke, rather than a promoter of increased injury. Induced hypothermia is a promising neuroprotective strategy in human stroke. Conventional hypothermic therapy, however, requires intubation and paralysis of musculature to prevent shivering, steps which may pose risk to patients, especially those with milder strokes. Emerging approaches to delivery of hypothermic therapy include placement of indwelling cooling catheters in the inferior vena cava to more rapidly achieve whole body temperature reduction. With this approach, the need to paralyze and intubate can often be avoided, by inhibiting the shivering response through warming the skin surface with blankets and administering antishivering agents, including meperidine and/or buspirone. Large-scale interventional trials are needed to determine whether systemic or selective cerebral hypothermic treatment can improve stroke outcome. A strategy of maintaining normothermia by administering prophylactic, standing order antipyretics, such as acetaminophen, for the first 24 to 72 hours after stroke onset has shown promise in pilot trials, but is likely to have only mild effects on clinical outcomes (63).

Patients with acute stroke and fever should be investigated for a source of infection and treated. In addition, the fever should be reduced promptly with antipyretics and cooling blankets if necessary.

## Intravenous Fibrinolytic Therapy

### Tissue-Type Plasminogen Activator

Fibrinolytic agents activate plasminogen to form plasmin, which actively digests fibrin strands. The fibrinolytic agents that have been most extensively investigated in ischemic stroke are recombinant tPA and streptokinase. The tPA is a serine protease endogenously released in human tissues from vascular endothelium. Unlike urokinase and streptokinase, tPA preferentially activates plasminogen that is bound to fibrin. It has been proposed that this specificity results in fibrinolysis somewhat confined to localized thrombus, minimizing systemic fibrinolytic activation. Streptokinase is a protein synthesized by streptococci that complexes with and activates both circulating plasminogen and bound plasminogen.

By promoting early recanalization of occluded vessels and early reperfusion of ischemic fields, pharmacologic thrombolysis has the potential to salvage penumbral neuronal tissue. However, by exposing injured brain to lytic agents, thrombolytic therapy also increases the risk of hemorrhagic transformation of infarct with worsening of clinical deficit. Only large-scale clinical trials can determine whether, and when, intravenous thrombolytic therapy confers overall benefit (or harm) in acute ischemic stroke.

Nine large-scale clinical trials of intravenous fibrinolytic therapy have been completed. Trial features and results are summarized in Table 103-6.

The findings of the two NINDS-tPA trials provided the foundation for Food and Drug Administration (FDA) approval of ischemic stroke as an added indication for tPA (64). Patients were enrolled within 3 hours of stroke onset (half of them within 90 minutes of onset) and the total dose administered was 0.9 mg per kg. The only CT scan exclusion criterion was hemorrhage; enrollment of patients with early signs of infarction was permitted.

In trial 1, the primary endpoint was a measure of early drug effect, the percentage of patients who improved by 4 points or more at 24 hours on a neurologic deficit scale, and the NIH Stroke Scale. Trial 1 enrolled 291 patients. In the tPA group, 47% of patients improved by the 4 point threshold versus 39% of the placebo group, a difference that did not reach statistical significance ($P = 0.21$). Other measures of early activity were positive. For example, both the control and the tPA groups had a National Institutes of Health Stroke Scale (NIHSS) score of 14 upon admission. At 24 hours, the tPA group's neurologic deficit score had improved to 8 versus 12 in the placebo group, a statistically significant group difference ($P < 0.02$) (65). Also, 3-month secondary endpoints were positive, including statistically significant differences in Barthel, Rankin, and NIHSS scores.

Trial 2 was similar to trial 1 in all design and dose regimen respects, differing only in the prespecified primary endpoint. This consisted of a global statistic combining 3-month scores on the Barthel, Rankin, and NIHSS scales, and the Glasgow Outcome Scale. A total of 333 patients were enrolled. The primary endpoint and each of its component outcome measures were significantly favorable for the tPA arm. For example, no or minimal disability on the Barthel Index was present in 50% of the tPA group versus 38% of the placebo group. No or minimal residual neurologic deficits measured on the NIHSS was present in 31% of the tPA group versus 20% of the placebo group. The absolute risk difference of 12% in the Barthel outcome translates into a number needed to treat of 8.3, that is, for every 8.3 patients treated with IV tPA, one more patient will have no or minimal disability at 3 months. Patients at all degrees of initial stroke severity and with all stroke subtypes, including large vessel atherothrombotic, small vessel

lacunar, and cardioembolic, all appeared to benefit from tPA in subgroup analysis. Safety data in the NINDS-tPA trials demonstrated a 10-fold increased incidence of symptomatic intracerebral hemorrhage with tPA, 6.4% versus 0.6%. However, no difference was noted in overall 3-month mortality, 17% in the tPA group versus 21% with placebo, because deaths from herniation and systemic medical complications of large cerebral infarcts in the placebo group was more than the offset deaths from intracerebral hemorrhage in the tPA group.

In multifactorial analysis, two variables independently predicted the development of symptomatic hemorrhage with tPA therapy in the combined NINDS-tPA trials. Early signs of mass effect, hypodensity, and edema on the pretreatment CT scan increased the risk of symptomatic hemorrhage 7.8-fold, and severe neurologic deficit at baseline (NIHSS >20) increased the risk 1.8-fold (64). For this reason, some authorities have recommended caution or avoidance of tPA in patients with these features. However, both patients with early hypodensity on CT scan and patients with baseline NIHSS greater than 20 tended to fare better if assigned to thrombolytic therapy (65). The overall prognosis is guarded for both sets of patients, who have evidence of severe ischemia at the time of therapeutic decision making. For example, of those patients with an NIHSS greater than 20, 10% of the tPA group had a favorable outcome compared to 4% of the control group. An analysis of the combined trial populations, analyzing 26 patient variables with 90% power to detect an influence on treatment response, found no single variable or combination of variables that identified nonresponders to therapy, suggesting a generalized efficacy of tPA for patients who met trial inclusion and exclusion criteria (66).

Four other large IV tPA trials have demonstrated convergent results with the initial pivotal NINDS-tPA trials. A pooled analysis of individual patient date from all 6 large intravenous tPA trials conducted through 2004 showed a dramatic benefit of therapy when administered within 90 minutes of onset [odds ratio (OR) for favorable outcome of 2.8], moderate benefit when administered between 91 to 180 minutes (OR of 1.5), a suggestion of likely modest benefit between 181 to 270 minutes (OR of 1.4), and no substantial benefit when administered beyond 271 minutes (67). In the less than 3-hour period, among every 100 patients treated with IV tPA, approximately 32 will benefit and 3 will be harmed as a result (68).

Important additional information regarding the use of IV tPA comes from observations in a large cohort of patients treated in actual clinical practice after marketing. For example, among 960 patients treated according to FDA-approved criteria, symptomatic hemorrhages occurred in only 6%. However, in 57 patients in whom treatment deviated from FDA-approved criteria, symptomatic hemorrhages occurred in 10.7% (69). These data suggest that strict adherence to FDA-approved criteria is required to maximize the safety of therapy.

Substantial clinical trial evidence supports the use of IV tPA in patients who meet the inclusion and exclusion criteria of the NINDS-tPA trials. Patients are candidates for thrombolysis if they have an acute neurologic deficit thought to be caused by cerebral ischemia that is potentially disabling, if their CT scan shows no hemorrhage, and if therapy can be started within 3 hours of symptom onset. A detailed protocol for tPA administration, including a checklist for determining eligibility, is provided in Table 103-7 (57). As with any potentially harmful treatment, the risks and benefits of thrombolytic therapy must be discussed with the patient and/or the patient's representative, or two physicians' consent must be obtained if no legally authorized representive is available. tPA is administered at a dose of 0.9 mg per kg with a maximum dose of 90 mg. Ten percent of the total dose is given as a bolus over 1 to 2 minutes and the remainder is infused over 1 hour. Anticoagulants and

**TABLE 103-6**

CLINICAL TRIALS OF INTRAVENOUS THROMBOLYTICS IN ACUTE ISCHEMIC STROKE

| Trial | Agent | Dose (% of MI dose) | Time window (mean time) | Ischemic stroke type | Sample size | Hematoma/symptomatic Hemorrhage (%) | | Good outcome[a] | |
|---|---|---|---|---|---|---|---|---|---|
| | | | | | | Drug | Placebo | Drug | Placebo |
| NINDS Trial 1 | tPA | 75 | <3 h (≈2.2 h) | All | 291 | 6 | 0 | 47 | 27 |
| NINDS Trial 2 | tPA | 75 | <3 h (≈2.2 h) | All | 333 | 7 | 1 | 39 | 26 |
| ECASS I | tPA | 85 | <6 h (4.4 h) | Mod-sev MCA | 620 | 20 | 7 | 36 | 29 |
| ECASS II | tPA | 75 | <6 h (NA) | Mod-sev MCA | 800 | 8.8 | 3.4 | 40 | 37 |
| ATLANTIS | tPA | 75 | 3–5 h (4.4 h) | All | 613 | 6.7 | 1.3 | 42 | 40 |
| MAST-E | SK | 100 | <6 h (4.6 h) | Mod-sev MCA | 310 | 21 | 3 | 20 | 18 |
| MAST-I | SK | 100 | <6 h (NA) | All | 622 | 8 | 1 | 37 | 35 |
| ASK | SK | 100 | <4 h (3.5 h) | All | 340 | 13 | 2 | 34 | 35 |

ASK, Australian Streptokinase Trial; ATLANTIS, alteplase Thrombolysis for Acute Noninterventional Therapy in Ischemic Stroke; ECASS, European Cooperative Acute Stroke Study; MAST-E, Multicenter Acute Stroke Trial–Europe; MAST-I, Multicenter Acute Stroke Trial–Italy; MCA, middle cerebral artery; MI, myocardial infarction; NA, not available; NINDS, National Institute of Neurologic Diseases and Stroke; tPA, tissue-type plasminogen activator; SK, streptokinase.

[a]Good outcome measures: NINDS Trials 1 and 2, ATLANTIS, Rankin disability score <2; ECASS I and II, MAST-E, and MAST-I, Rankin <3; ASK, Barthel Index 95–100.

© UCLA Stroke Program, reprinted with permission.

**TABLE 103-7**

### ALGORITHM FOR INTRAVENOUS FIBRINOLYTIC THERAPY

#### INCLUSION CRITERIA
1. Ischemic stroke with a defined onset of <3 h from time tPA is to be started
   *Ascertain last time patient known to be awake and deficit-free*
2. Potentially functionally impairing neurologic deficit
   *Neurologic deficit > minimal weakness, isolated ataxia, isolated sensory, or isolated dysarthria*
3. CT scan shows no evidence of intracranial hemorrhage
   *If early signs of new major hemisphere infarct are present, (e.g., edema, mass effect, sulcal effacement) reassess time of onset; the presence of these CT scan findings may be associated with an increased risk of hemorrhage*

#### EXCLUSION CRITERIA
**History**
1. Stroke or serious head trauma within last 3 mo
2. Major surgery or serious trauma within last 14 d
3. History of intracranial hemorrhage, AVM, or aneurysm
4. GI or urinary tract hemorrhage within previous 21 d
5. Arterial puncture at a noncompressible site *or* lumbar puncture within previous 7 d

**Clinical**
6. Rapidly improving neurologic signs or minor symptoms
7. SBP >185 mm Hg *or* diastolic blood pressure >110 mm Hg *or* aggressive (IV) treatment required to reduce patient's blood pressure to specified limits
8. Seizure at onset
9. Symptoms suggestive of subarachnoid hemorrhage
10. Recent myocardial infarction-induced pericarditis

**Laboratory**
11. Patient taking anticoagulants *or* PT >15 s (INR > 1.7)
12. Patient received heparin within 48 h preceding stroke onset AND has an elevated PTT
13. Platelet count <100,000 per mm$^3$
14. Glucose concentration <50 mg/dL (2.7 mmol/L) *or* >400 mg/dL (22.2 mmol/L)
15. Women with a positive pregnancy test
    *Discuss the risks and benefits of thrombolytic therapy with the patient and family (if possible) and document the discussion in the medical record*

#### BEFORE ADMINISTERING TPA
1. Review checklist to confirm inclusion and exclusion critera
2. Confirm patient is not spontaneously improving

#### TREATMENT AND MANAGEMENT
1. tPA 0.9 mg/kg total or maximum 90 mg
2. Administer 10% of tPA dose as a bolus
3. Administer remaining 90% of tPA as a constant infusion over 1 h
4. *Do not* give anticoagulants for 24 h from start of tPA administration
5. *Do not* give antiplatelet agents for 24 h from start of tPA administration
6. Admit to intensive care unit *or* acute stroke unit
7. Maintain SBP *under* 180 mm Hg and diastolic blood pressure *under* 115 mm Hg
8. Restrict central venous line placement *or* arterial puncture for 24 h
9. *Do not* insert indwelling bladder catheter for >30 min after tPA administration
10. *Avoid* insertion of nasogastric tube for 24 h after tPA administration

tPA, tissue-type plasminogen activator; CT scan, computerized tomography scan; AVM, arteriovenous malformation; INR, international normalized ratio; PT, prothrombin time; PTT, partial-thromboplastin time.
© UCLA Stroke Program, reprinted with permission.

antiplatelet agents are not to be administered within the first 24 hours following thrombolytic treatment.

After infusion, close monitoring of blood pressure and neurologic status is mandatory, and is best carried out in a neurologic intensive care unit or stroke unit. Neurologic deterioration, new onset headache, acute hypertension, nausea, or vomiting may be signs of intracranial hemorrhage (ICH) and must be investigated immediately. An acute rise in blood pressure may be the first indication of intracerebral hemorrhage. If the patient is still receiving tPA, the infusion should be discontinued and a CT scan obtained immediately. A stat PT, partial-thromboplastin time (PTT), platelet count, and fibrinogen level should be sent. If the CT scan shows hemorrhage, then the laboratory results should be evaluated for abnormalities and corrected with fibrinogen, cryoprecipitate, and/or platelets. A neurosurgic consultation may be warranted for hematoma evacuation or intervention to relieve increased ICP. If the guidelines for intravenous tPA are rigorously adhered to, this therapy is effective in treating patients with acute ischemic stroke (70,71).

### Additional Intravenous Fibrinolytic Agents

Three randomized, placebo-controlled trials of intravenous streptokinase were conducted in the mid-1990s, and these trials showed no clear benefit, with significant risk of major hemorrhage and only minimal beneficial trends in final outcome, likely owing to the late time window permitted for patient entry and the high dose of streptokinase employed.

Among newer generation fibrinolytics, desmetoplase and tenecteplase have shown greatest promise in preliminary, phase II, human stroke trials. Desmetoplase, the fibrinolytic agent isolated from the saliva of the vampire bat, showed safety and a suggestive signal of efficacy when administered 3 to 9 hours after stroke onset in patients selected for late therapy by the presence of perfusion–diffusion mismatch on MR imaging. Tenecteplase, a genetic modification of tPA with potentially favorable half-life and bleeding avoidance properties, showed low bleeding propensity and a favorable signal of efficacy when administered in lieu of tPA within 3 hours of stroke onset.

### Intraarterial Fibrinolysis

Intraarterial fibrinolysis possesses several theoretical advantages over intravenous fibrinolysis. Higher concentrations of fibrinolytic agent are delivered to the clot, increasing the likelihood of recanalization. Conversely, lower concentrations of fibrinobolytic agent escape into the systemic circulation, potentially decreasing the risk of systemic hemorrhagic complications. Gentle mechanical disruption may be employed to potentiate the pharmacologic thrombolytic intervention. The diagnostic angiogram that immediately precedes intervention provides precise information regarding stroke pathophysiology that is not available from noninvasive testing. The time at which recanalization is achieved is known with certainty, and supportive therapy such as fluid and blood pressure management can immediately be adjusted for a reopened rather than occluded vessel.

These benefits must be weighed against several theoretical disadvantages of intraarterial fibrinolysis versus intravenous fibrinolysis. Start of fibrinolytic therapy is substantially delayed by the need to move the patient to an angiography suite, prep the patient for the procedure, mobilize the interventional team, and catheterize the involved vessel. In controlled trials, the time delay from completion of CT scan to catheter on clot and start of fibrinolyitc infusion has generally ranged from 70 to 120 minutes. Intraarterial therapy requires manipulation of a catheter in the ischemic bed and injured vessels, possibly increasing the risk of cerebral hemorrhage. Intraarterial treatment is both labor- and capital-intensive, and it requires highly experienced interventionalists. Consequently, it is likely,

even if beneficial, to remain an intervention confined to tertiary stroke critical care centers.

Numerous case series, small phase II trials, and one completed phase III trial evaluating intraarterial (IA) fibrinolysis suggest the effectiveness of this treatment strategy. In the phase III trial of IA thrombolysis, the Prolyse in Acute Cerebral Thromboembolism II [Prolyse in Acute Cerebral Thromboembolism (PROACT) II] trial, patients within 6 hours of symptom onset with symptomatic M1 or M2 MCA occlusions were randomized to receive direct intraarterial infusion of 9 mg recombinant prourokinase (pro-UK) for 120 minutes plus systemic heparin, or systemic heparin alone (72). From a total of 474 patients who had angiography for symptoms suggestive of MCA occlusion, 180 had M1 or M2 segment MCA thrombi and met all other eligibility criteria. Median time from symptom onset to initiation of IA pro-UK infusion was 5.3 hours.

The prespecified primary outcome in PROACT II, a good to excellent score on the modified Rankin scale (mRS) of handicap (mRS $\leq$2) was achieved by 40% of pro-UK patients versus 25% of control patients. This difference, although substantial in magnitude, achieved only marginal statistical significance as a result of the small sample size ($P = 0.043$). Recanalization rates, 2 hours after initiation of infusion, were increased markedly in the pro-UK group. Partial or full recanalization [Thrombolysis in Myocardial Infarction (TIMI) grade 2 or 3] was achieved in 66% of pro-UK patients versus only 18% of control patients. Full recanalization (TIMI 3), however, was infrequent even in the pro-UK group (19% in the pro-UK group vs. 2% in the control group). Intracerebral hemorrhage rates at 36 hours were increased for the pro-UK group, both for all hemorrhages [46% vs. 16% (control)] and for symptomatic hemorrhages [10% vs. 2% (control)]; however, no difference in overall mortality between the two treatment groups was observed.

The positive results from PROACT II were not sufficient to win FDA approval for intraarterial prourokinase, given the small trial size and absence of a confirmatory trial. Nonetheless, intraarterial fibrinolysis administered up to 6 hours after onset in anterior circulation ischemic stroke, and up to 12 to 24 hours after onset in vertebrobasilar ischemic stroke is a frequently pursued treatment option at tertiary centers (see Fig. 103-5).

### Combined Intravenous and Intraarterial Fibrinolysis

Combined intravenous and intraarterial fibrinolysis strategies have evolved as an attempt to combine the advantages of rapid start of treatment of intravenous therapy and the eventual more definitive recanalization of intraarterial therapy. Intravenous fibrinolytic strategy is begun immediately upon completion of CT scan, within 3 hours of symptom onset. Simultaneously,

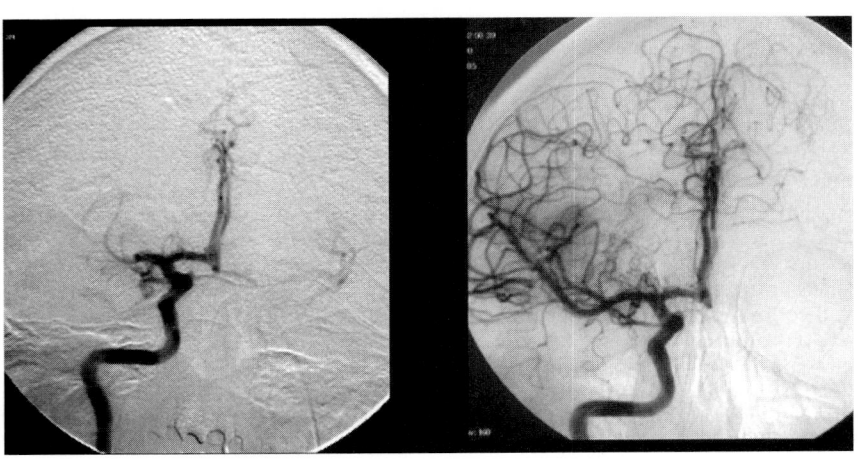

**FIGURE 103-5.** Thrombolytic recanalization. Patient presents with left hemiparesis, hemisensory deficit, hemianopia, and hemineglect and initial angiogram demonstrates right middle cerebral artery (MCA) trunk occlusion (**left** image). Intraarterial thrombolysis with tissue-type plasminogen activator (tPA) is performed. End of procedure angiogram (**right** image) shows full recanalization of MCA and good filling of distal Sylvian MCA branches. (© UCLA Stroke Program, reprinted with permission.)

the patient is transported to the angiography suite and catheterization begun. When the catheter arrives on clot, intravenous infusion is ended (or it has ended earlier after reaching a pre-specified maximal dose) and intraarterial infusion begun.

The feasibility and safety of combined intravenous/intraarterial tPA therapy has been investigated in the Emergency Management of Stroke (EMS) Bridging Trial and the Interventional Management of Stroke Trial (73,74). These studies have demonstrated that combined therapy is feasible, yields good recanalization rates, and appears to have acceptable hemorrhagic adverse event rates. Larger, definitive trials comparing combined intravenous/intraarterial thrombolysis with pure intravenous and pure intraarterial strategies are needed.

## Acute Antiplatelet Therapy

Antiplatelet agents are of potential benefit in acute ischemic stroke by reducing the formation of "white thrombi," platelet, and fibrin aggregates that form in fast-moving arterial streams upon damaged endothelial surfaces. Antiplatelet therapy may discourage propagation of the initial thrombus to block additional vessels and recurrent embolization. However, antiplatelet therapy may also increase the risk of hemorrhagic transformation of an infarct. Several clinical trials have examined the use of antiplatelet therapy in the setting of acute ischemic stroke.

### Aspirin

Two megatrials examined the efficacy of aspirin therapy within 48 hours of ischemic stroke onset. The Chinese Acute Stroke Trial (CAST) enrolled 21,106 patients within 48 hours of stroke onset and randomized patients to 160 mg of aspirin a day or placebo (75). Treatment was administered daily for 4 weeks. Ninety-seven percent of the patients completed the 4 weeks of medication, whether they remained hospitalized for 4 weeks, or discharged before that time. The primary endpoints for the study were death from any cause during the first 4 weeks following stroke, and death or dependence at discharge. Secondary endpoints included fatal or nonfatal recurrent stroke and death or nonfatal stroke within 4 weeks. Study results for the primary endpoint demonstrated a considerable reduction in death at 4 weeks from 3.9% in the control group to 3.3% in the aspirin group. Secondary analyses demonstrated modest, but statistically significant reductions with aspirin in recurrent ischemic strokes at 4 weeks and 4-week mortality.

The International Stroke Trial (IST) employed a $3 \times 2$ factorial design to investigate whether aspirin, low dose unfractionated heparin, high dose unfractionated heparin, or a combination of aspirin and unfractionated heparin are safe and efficacious in the treatment of ischemic stroke (76). There were 19,435 patients enrolled within 48 hours of symptom onset with an average time to randomization of 19 hours. Sixteen percent of patients were enrolled with 6 hours of symptom onset. Subjects were randomized to one of the 6 following groups: unfractionated heparin 5,000 IU SQ b.i.d., unfractionated heparin 12,500 IU SQ b.i.d., aspirin 300 mg q.d, aspirin 300 mg q.d. + unfractionated heparin 5,000 IU SQ b.i.d., aspirin 300 mg q.d. + unfractionated heparin 12,500 IU SQ b.i.d., or avoid aspirin and unfractionated heparin. Subjects were treated for 14 days or until time of discharge. The average duration of treatment was 11 days with the main reason for early discontinuation being hospital discharge. The primary outcomes for the study were death within 14 days and death or dependency at 6 months.

Aspirin-treated patients had significantly fewer recurrent ischemic strokes with no significant increase in hemorrhagic strokes within 14 days. The recurrent ischemic stroke rate declined from 3.9% to 2.8% with aspirin therapy. A nonsignificant decrease in mortality within 14 days was observed. At 6 months there was a nonsignificant trend toward a smaller percentage of the aspirin group being dead or dependent, 62.2% versus 63.5%.

A metaanalysis combining the results in of 40,397 randomized subjects from the IST, CAST, and one additional small trial demonstrates the following statistically significant effects of aspirin: Early recurrent ischemic stroke is reduced from 3.2% to 2.4%, symptomatic hemorrhagic transformation is increased from 0.8% to 1.0%, and overall death or nonfatal stroke at 6 months is reduced from 9.1% to 8.2%. These findings indicate that aspirin confers a statistically significant, but biologically quite small, benefit upon patients with acute ischemic stroke. Use of aspirin in the first weeks after onset yields a reduction of nine deaths or recurrent strokes per 1,000 patients treated. Therefore, the number needed to treat with aspirin to prevent one death or recurrent stroke in the first few weeks is 111. It is unclear from these trials as to what, if any, degree this small treatment effect of aspirin reflects beneficial actions in the first hours after stroke onset, versus prevention of secondary stroke on subsequent days.

These data support the use of aspirin in the first two weeks after ischemic stroke onset and provide some support for the use of aspirin at a dose of 160 to 325 mg in the first few hours. All patients not receiving thrombolytic or anticoagulant therapy should be treated with aspirin, unless there is a history of hypersensitivity to aspirin, active peptic ulcer disease, recent gastrointestinal (GI) bleeding, or other contraindication. To promote rapid therapeutic effect, patients able to take pills orally should be instructed to chew the aspirin tablet before swallowing. Patients unable to swallow safely should receive therapy either by nasogastric tube or rectal suppository.

### Additional Antiplatelet Agents

Other oral antiplatelet agents have not been systematically investigated in the acute stroke setting. Ticlopidine takes 4 to 5 days to reach maximal effectiveness at standard dosing, limiting its theoretical utility in the first few hours. Loading doses of clopidogrel (300 to 375 mg), are well tolerated, yield rapid onset of antiplatelet effect, and have been shown to be beneficial in acute coronary syndromes (77). Loading dose clopidogrel has not been systematically investigated in acute ischemic stroke, but constitute an attractive strategy in the acute ischemic stroke patient who is intolerant of aspirin.

Trials of intravenous glycoprotein 2A3B platelet antagonists in acute ischemic stroke are underway in acute ischemic stroke. Further advanced are studies of abciximab. In a phase II trial, 400 patients within 6 hours of ischemic stroke received a 0.25 mg per kg bolus followed by a 0.125 mg/kg/minute infusion for 12 hours or matched placebo (78). Safety was acceptable, with a 3.6% rate of symptomatic intracerebral hemorrhage. Efficacy trends suggested a potential beneficial effect, with excellent clinical outcome attained in 49% of treated patients versus 40% of control patients.

## Acute Anticoagulation

Large-scale trials have failed to validate the traditional therapeutic practice of administering anticoagulation therapy liberally in acute ischemic stroke. It had been hypothesized that anticoagulation may prevent recurrent embolism from cardiac and arterial sites, retard clot propagation to distal vessel branches, avert thrombotic progression to occlusion of a stenotic lesion, and reduce microthombi formation in the distal microcirculation. Conversely, acute anticoagulation may increase the risk of hemorrhagic transformation. More than 22 trials enrolling more than 24,000 patients have now been performed testing anticoagulation in acute ischemic stroke, and no net benefit has been identified (79).

## Unfractionated Heparin

Unfractionated heparin was initially tested in several small clinical trials, some in the pre-CT scan era when some enrolled patients may have had hemorrhage present on entry. A meta-analysis of all trials of acute anticoagulation (chiefly with unfractionated heparin) reported through 1993 identified 10 trials enrolling a total of only 1,047 patients. Across all studies of ischemic stroke, acute anticoagulation showed a nonsignificant trend toward reduction in the odds of death.

The IST examined the effects of aspirin, SQ unfractionated heparin, and a combination of these two drugs in patients with ischemic stroke who presented within 48 hours of stroke onset (76). As noted in the preceding text, subjects were randomized to 6 treatment arms in a 3 × 2 factorial design, including high SQ dose, low SQ dose, and avoid unfractionated heparin arms. Treatment was continued for 14 days or until the time of discharge and the average duration of treatment was 11 days.

Patients treated with unfractionated heparin had significantly fewer recurrent ischemic strokes within 14 days (2.9% vs. 3.8%), but this benefit was offset by a similar increase in hemorrhagic strokes (1.2% vs. 0.4%). Treatment groups showed no difference in the incidence of death and disability at 6 months. No net benefit of acute anticoagulation was seen when analysis was confined to the subgroup of 3,169 patients who had atrial fibrillation and likely cardioembolic stroke. Considering each of the six treatment group subarms across the entire trial population, there was a trend of best outcome in patients assigned to aspirin plus low dose unfractionated heparin daily.

The results of the IST argue against a policy of fixed, high dose, subcutaneously administered unfractionated heparin for all patients with acute ischemic stroke. Whether these findings are generalizable to the more common US practice of adjusted-dose, intravenous unfractionated heparin for select patients is uncertain. Avoiding acute treatment of patients with risk factors for hemorrhagic transformation might improve the benefit–risk ratio. Large series have suggested that large infarct size, severely elevated blood pressures, and older age increase the risk of hemorrhage (80).

At present, clinical trial data do not suggest major net benefit or harm of intravenous, dose-adjusted unfractionated heparin in acute ischemic stroke. Because aspirin and tPA are of proven benefit, these agents should in general be preferred over acute anticoagulation except in select situations(81).

### Low-Molecular-Weight Heparins and Heparinoids

Several double-blinded, placebo-controlled trials of low-molecular-weight heparins (LMWHs) in acute ischemic stroke have been performed. The first trial, studying nadroparin, found a benefit (82). These promising results, however, were not replicated in a second larger confirmatory trial of nadroparin (83). A trial of tinzaparin also demonstrated no advantage of acute LMWH over control given acutely (84). Another prospective trial compared the LMWH dalteparin with aspirin given within 30 hours of atrial fibrillation-associated stroke. There were no statistically significant differences between treatment groups in death and physical dependency at 3 months (85).

Perhaps the most detailed information about the effect of novel anticoagulants in acute ischemic stroke comes from a trial of a heparinoid in acute ischemic stroke, the Trial of Org 10172 in Acute Stroke Treatment (TOAST) (86). This randomized, double-blind trial compared danaparoid to placebo for 7 days in 1,281 patients enrolled within 24 hours of stroke onset. Danaparoid was administered by continuous intravenous infusion, dose-adjusted by laboratory monitoring of factor Xa. On the primary outcome measure of favorable Barthel activities of daily living score at 3 months, no difference between the treatment groups was observed. Subgroup analysis did suggest

a beneficial effect in patients with large-vessel (primarily carotid) atherothrombotic stroke mechanisms, with very favorable 3-month outcomes in 43.3% of the danaparoid group versus 29.1% of the placebo group. No benefit was detected at all in patients with cardioembolic and lacunar stroke mechanisms.

It is instructive to consider event rates observed in the control arms in recent trials of anticoagulant therapy. In the TOAST trial, progression/recurrence of infarct was observed in only 1.3% of placebo patients over the first 7 days, despite the absence of antiplatelet or anticoagulant therapy. In the cardioembolic TOAST placebo subgroup, recurrent infarct occurred in only 1.6% of patients not receiving anticoagulant therapy. Similarly, in patients with atrial fibrillation enrolled in the IST and assigned to the avoid aspirin and avoid unfractioanted heparin arm, recurrent infarct occurred in only 1.1% of patients over 14 days. These observations suggest that with modern fluid management and general supportive care, progression or recurrence of infarct occurs very infrequently in patients with acute ischemic stroke even in the absence of antithrombotic therapy. As a result, opportunities for anticoagulation therapy to be beneficial are circumscribed.

Clinical trial data provide no firm evidence of net benefit or net harm of LMWHs or heparinoids in acute ischemic stroke. Therefore, no firm recommendation can be given, and their use remains at the discretion of the treating physician. The TOAST trial suggests that patients with large-vessel atherothrombotic stroke may benefit from heparinoid treatment, but this subgroup analysis requires prospective confirmation in a new trial. The risk–benefit ratio of these agents may be improved by avoiding their use in the first 5 to 7 days in patients with large cerebral infarcts (e.g., those involving >3 cm of tissue in longest dimension). In patients with subacute stroke requiring bridging parenteral anticoagulation to long-term warfarin, one cohort study has suggested that LMWHs, used both in hospital and on an outpatient basis, may be safer and more cost-effective than intravenous unfractionated heparin (87).

## Direct Thrombin Inhibitors

The direct thrombin inhibitor, argatroban, has been studied in two small phase II stroke trials, in the United States and Japan. In the US trial, 171 patients with ischemic stroke within 12 hours of stroke onset were randomized to placebo, a low-dose argotroban tier (1 $\mu$g/kg/min), or a high-dose argotroban tier (100 $\mu$g per kg bolus, then 3 $\mu$g/kg/minute) (88). Although not statistically significant, unfavorable trends were noted with regard to symptomatic intracerebral hemorrhage (5.1% in high-dose tier, 3.4% in low-dose tier, 0% in placebo), without strong signals of potential efficacy in averting stroke progression or improving final outcome.

## Combination Fibrinolytic and Antithrombotic Therapies

Facilitating fibrinolysis by combining a fibrinolytic agent with an antiplatelet or anticoagulant agent is being investigated in acute ischemic stroke. NIH-funded phase II studies are exploring the safety of tPA combined with the G2b3a antagonist eptifibatideand and tPA combined with the direct thrombin inhibitor argatroban. Given the greater propensity of the brain to bleed than the heart, it is uncertain if a combination regimen can be identified that yields benefits of increased vessel recanalization without offsetting adverse effects of increased hemorrhagic complications. The strategy of enhancing tPA activity by the simultaneous administration of externally applied ultrasound has shown promise in early clinical trials.

## Acute Mechanical Endovascular Recanalization Techniques

Mechanical endovascular recanalization techniques are promising emerging strategies in the treatment of acute ischemic stroke (89,90). These techniques may be categorized as endovascular strategies that (a) snare, (b) displace, (c) aspirate, or (d) obliterate the occluding thrombus.

Ensnaring and physically removing a clot from the cerebral vasculature is a highly promising strategy in acute ischemic stroke therapy. In a multicenter safety and feasibility study of the Multimedia European Research Conferencing Integration (MERCI) clot retrieval coil device, recanalization was achieved in 54% of patients, with a low rate of device-related complications (91).

Successful application of primary angioplasty and stenting (displacing the clot to the periphery of the occluded lumen) has been reported in several case series. This technique appears especially promising when the target occlusion consists of an underlying *in situ* atherosclerotic plaque with supervening thrombus (89). The underlying atherosclerotic lesion permits angioplasty-mediated vessel dissection to proceed relatively, safely, and effectively. However, appropriate intracranial *in situ* atherosclerotic lesions are infrequent in Western populations, although common in Asian countries. In Western populations, the vascular target lesion is more often an embolus that has landed in a relatively normal recipient artery in the cerebral circulation from a cardiac or cervical arterial source, and these appear less responsive to angioplasty techniques.

Endovascular techniques that employ high vacuum pressures or laser energy to obliterate and aspirate thrombi have shown mixed results in early studies, with damage to delicate cerebral vessels limiting the energies that can be applied and the recanalization rates that can be achieved (89,92).

Early experience with this wide range of mechanical thrombolysis devices suggests the following three fundamental principles that will shape future endovascular thrombolytic therapies. First, cerebral vessels and endothelial surfaces are mechanically fragile. The amplitude of mechanical energies delivered to break up thrombi will be limited by the need to protect the endothelial surface and vessel wall integrity. Second, combined mechanical and pharmacologic therapy will often be required. Mechanical devices currently are too bulky to pass into distal vessels and often generate fragments of proximal clots that embolize distally in the course of their attack on the initial occlusion. Cleanup of intraarterial fibrinolysis directed at distal residua might often be a consideration in patients treated with mechanical devices. Third, composition of clots matters. Emboli composed wholly of thrombus and landing in relatively normal vessels pose different engineering and pharmacologic challenges than *in situ* atherosclerotic lesions with supervening thrombus. Different tailored approaches chosen from a range of mechanical and pharmacologic options will likely be required to achieve optimum recanalization rates.

# INTRACEREBRAL HEMORRHAGE

Intracerebral hemorrhage typically presents with focal symptoms reflecting the site of hemorrhage, and generalized symptoms reflecting raised ICP as a result of the sudden appearance of a new mass lesion. The generalized symptoms include headache, nausea, vomiting, stupor, and coma. The focal symptoms usually steadily worsen over 10 to 25 minutes as the hematoma initially expands. Leading signs are contralateral hemiparesis and hemisensory loss for ganglionic hemorrhages, contralateral sensory loss, oculomotor deficits, and early stupor for thalamic hemorrhages, aphasia or hemineglect accompanying contralateral sensorimotor deficits for lobar hemorrhages, and ataxia and gait difficulty for cerebellar hemorrhages.

The most common etiology is a bleeding-prone, small-vessel angiopathy, related to hypertension and aging. Hypertension is present in 50% to 70% of all cases. Cerebral amyloid angiopathy accounts for approximately 10% of all cases and up to 30% of lobar hemorrhages, and is a leading consideration in elderly individuals. Rupture of arteriovenous malformation (AVM) and saccular aneurysms accounts for 5% to 13%, and are a leading consideration in younger patients. Overt coagulopathies are the fourth most common cause, present in 5% to 6%, including both spontaneous bleeding disorders and iatrogenic (anticoagulant and thrombolytic therapy) disorders. Warfarin-associated hemorrhages have twice the fatality rate as non–warfarin associated hemorrhages (93).

Blood pressure control is critical to management. Excessive arterial pressure may result in extension of the initial hemorrhage and the promotion of vasogenic edema (9,14,26). It has been suggested that overaggressive blood pressure lowering, particularly in patients with chronic hypertension who have upwardly shifted autoregulatory curves, may result in cerebral hypoperfusion and extension of the perifocal ischemic injury. However, recent studies have suggested that perihematomal ischemic injury is infrequent in ICH. Recent guidelines recommend a therapeutic target of a SBP of 140 to 160 mm Hg, with a mean arterial pressure of 100 to 130 mm Hg.

Serial imaging studies have demonstrated that hematoma growth occurs in up to 38% of patients with ICH initially scanned within 3 hours of onset and in 16% scanned between 3 and 6 hours, even in the absence of coagulopathy. On the basis of these observations, it has been suggested that ultraearly hemostatic therapy given in the emergency setting might reduce ICH expansion and improve outcome. Among candidates for this indication, a particularly promising agent is recombinant activated factor VIIa, which promotes local hemostasis at sites of vascular injury in both coagulopathic and healthy patients (94). In a trial comparing 3 dose tiers of recombinant activated factor VIIa with placebo among 200 patients with ICH within 4 hours of onset, all treatment doses reduced hematoma expansion by approximately half (from approximately 30% to approximately 15%), with favorable trends in mortality and functional outcome.

Management of intracranial mass effect, hydrocephalus, and incipient herniation is critical in the care of the patient with ICH. Ventriculostomy should be undertaken for progressive hydrocephalus. ICP should be titrated to maintain a cerebral perfusion pressure of 80 to 100 mm Hg (65).

The decision for surgical treatment of an intracerebral hemorrhage remains somewhat controversial (13,33–35). Most authorities recommend that patients with small hemorrhages (<10 mL) or with minimal neurologic deficits should be managed medically, because the outcome is generally good without surgery. Patients with a Glasgow Coma Scale of 4 or less should be managed medically, because virtually all of these patients die or their outcome is poor. Intracerebral hemorrhages that are associated with an aneurysm or a vascular malformation should be removed at the time of resection of the underlying ruptured vascular lesion. Patients with moderate- or large-size lobar hemorrhages who are deteriorating clinically should have surgical treatment, because mass effect is simply and effectively relieved by hematoma evacuation. Patients with cerebellar hemorrhages larger than 3 cm in diameter, or those who have evidence of brainstem compression, despite adequate ventricular drainage, should have surgical evacuation of the hematoma (17). Evacuation of basal ganglia and thalamic hemorrhages by standard craniotomy did not improve outcome in a large, international clinical trial. However, new, minimally invasive evacuation techniques, including fibrinolytic-assisted aspiration of hematomas through burr hole incisions, show some promise.

# SUBARACHNOID HEMORRHAGE

## Prevention of Rebleeding

Recurrent hemorrhage from a ruptured aneurysm has been an important cause of death and disability in patients who have survived the initial rupture. Rebleeding may occur in approximately 15% to 20% of patients during the first 2 weeks after hemorrhage if the aneurysm is not treated; the first 24 to 48 hours after rupture appears to be the period with the highest risk (36). It has become clear that occlusion of the ruptured aneurysm is the preferred method for avoiding aneurysm rebleeding. In the past, the aneurysm was obliterated acutely only in those patients who were medically and neurologically stable enough to undergo early surgical clipping (38). With the advent of definitive endovascular techniques (primarily the Guglielmi detachable coil) for acute obliteration of a ruptured aneurysm, early treatment of virtually all ruptured intracranial aneurysms can now be accomplished (27). Early surgical clipping may be pursued for patients who are not profoundly compromised by medical complications or cerebral swelling and for aneurysms that are unsuitable for embolization (those with a wide neck). Endovascular therapy is chosen for patients with brain swelling caused by a severe subarachnoid hemorrhage (SAH) or those with significant medical infirmities or advanced age. This strategy of immediate treatment (within 24 hours of admission) of all patients with ruptured intracranial aneurysms has largely eliminated rehemorrhage as a major problem (44).

## Vasospasm

Vasospasm (cerebral arterial spasm) is one of the most frequent causes of morbidity and mortality in patients with SAH. Vasospasm occurs 4 to 10 days after SAH and results in ischemic neurologic deficit in 20% to 30% of patients (38,40,42).

Nimodipine is a standard element of therapy for patients at risk of vasospasm (4). The benefits of this cerebroselective calcium channel blocker are likely mediated to a greater degree by neuroprotective effects in permitting neurons to tolerate ischemic, than by antispasm vessel effects. The current recommendation is that nimodipine, in a dosage of 60 mg every 4 hours for 21 days, be administered to patients with ruptured intracranial aneurysms as soon as possible after admission (40). Nimodipine administration may cause arterial hypotension, and in these patients, we generally split the dosage and administer 30 mg every 2 hours.

Without attentive fluid management, CBF measurements demonstrate a gradual decline in cerebral perfusion during the first week after subarachnoid hemorrhage (50,69). In addition to vasospasm, a reduction in circulating blood volume (of multifactorial origin) appears to explain this decline in CBF. It is now recognized that this post-SAH hypovolemia interacts with vasospasm (39) to increase the risk of ischemic neurologic deficit. Volume repletion, even modest hypervolemia, is now considered to be a key component of management to prevent symptomatic vasospasm. Patients are given a full maintenance dose of crystalloid in combination with colloid (usually 5% albumin) (40). Therapy is modified in patients with compromised

cardiac function or signs of pulmonary edema. When these measurements are available, the central venous pressure is maintained at a range of 5 to 8 mm Hg, and the pulmonary capillary wedge pressure is maintained at the range of 12 to 15 mm Hg.

If vasospasm develops, more aggressive hypervolemic–hypertensive therapy is undertaken. When cerebral autoregulation is disturbed, as is the case with vasospasm, treatment with induced arterial hypertension results in an increase in CBF (71). The initial therapeutic goal of volume expansion is a central venous pressure of approximately 8 to 10 mm Hg or a pulmonary artery wedge pressure of approximately 15 mm Hg. These physiologic targets are modified in each individual to maximize cardiac output (39,45). If the aneurysm has been completely occluded by clipping or endovascular coiling, pressors are employed to raise the SBP to the range of 170 to 200 mm Hg. In patients with very severe vasospasm, the blood pressure may occasionally be raised to as high as 220 mm Hg. If, however, a patient has an unclipped intracranial aneurysm, the degree of hypertensive treatment is limited to below 170 mm Hg systolic.

Approximately 40% of patients with vasospasm-induced neurologic deficits fail to respond favorably to aggressive hypervolemic-hypertensive therapy (5). During the last several years, balloon dilation angioplasty has been used for the treatment of severe vasospasm refractory to intensive hypertensive–hypervolemic therapy (16,19,22). This endovascular technique uses a microballoon catheter to effect mechanical dilation of areas of severe intracranial arterial narrowing. This intervention has been used successfully in patients with delayed ischemic deficits refractory to aggressive hypovolemic hemodilution with arterial hypertension. This form of treatment has been reported to stabilize successfully and to improve 60% to 70% of patients with refractory vasospasm. The mechanical dilation of the spastic vessels appears to be long-lasting; followup TCD studies generally do not demonstrate a recurrence of the spasm.

This form of treatment is not without complications. There have been reports of fatal arterial rupture during balloon angioplasty and reports of distal embolization after the procedure (22). Because delayed intracerebral hemorrhage caused by reperfusion of infarcted areas has been reported, only patients whose pretreatment CT scans do not demonstrate evidence of infarction are considered for angioplasty.

Because only the proximal basal intracranial arteries are large enough to be suitable for balloon dilation angioplasty, intraarterial papaverine infusion has been used for the treatment of distal arterial spasm (40). Papaverine is a powerful vasodilator, and resolution of significant distal vasospasm has been demonstrated with the use of this agent. The intraarterial papaverine infusion requires selected microcatheterization of the distal internal carotid artery or proximal anterior, middle, or posterior cerebral arteries. This form of vasospasm treatment appears not to be as durable as mechanical angioplasty. TCD ultrasound studies have demonstrated recurrent vasospasm after papaverine infusion in as little as 24 hours after therapy. The short-lived action of intraarterial papaverine therapy often necessitates retreatment of these patients.

Hydrocephalus, which occurs in approximately 20% of patients with ruptured intracranial aneurysms, may occur acutely, subacutely, or in a delayed fashion (29,30). Acute hydrocephalus is generally found in poor-grade patients who have had a severe, high-volume SAH. If the patient has a significant depression in the level of consciousness, and, certainly if the patient is deteriorating, ventriculostomy insertion is indicated. Although it is important to provide ventricular decompression and relief of intracranial hypertension, one must be cautious not to lower precipitously the ICP. This has been associated, in some patients, with recurrent aneurysm rupture. It is advisable to limit cerebrospinal fluid (CSF) drainage so as not to lower ICP below 15 to 20 mm Hg.

# REHABILITATION OF ISCHEMIC STROKE

## Mechanisms of Recovery and Rehabilitative Therapies

Most functional recovery following a stroke occurs in the first 3 to 6 months, with lesser degrees of improvement up to 18 months or more (95). Data from the Framingham Study showed that 80% of long-term stroke survivors regain independence in ambulation and 66% independence in activities of daily living. Fundamental mechanisms of recovery include: (a) recovery of neuronal excitability by stunned parenchyma, (b) activity in partially spared pathways, (c) unmasking and dormant parallel pathways, (d) alteration in neuronal networks to recruit cells that are not ordinarily involved in an activity, (e) synaptic sprouting, (f) remyelination, (g) axonal and dendritic regeneration, (h) repopulation from neural stem cell progenitors, and (i) alternate behavioral strategies (96). Important prognostic factors for recovery include severity of initial neurologic impairment, age, and available family and social support systems. Neurorehabilitation using a multidisciplinary team approach increase the likelihood attaining functional independence.

Initial measures that help prevent development of medical complications of stroke include deep venous thrombosis prophylaxis, appropriate evaluation of swallowing function and nutrition, and early mobility. Physical, occupational, and speech therapy should be initiated during the acute hospitalization period for most patients and continued through the subacute to chronic period as needed.

## Neurotransplantation

Cell transplantation is a promising approach to restore function in patients with chronic disabilities due to stroke. Basic science studies have demonstrated that cells derived from a variety of precursor or progenitor cells can develop the capacity to function as mature neuronal cells, expressing neurotransmitters and forming synapses. Studies in animal models of focal ischemia have suggested that cell transplantation is feasible in ischemic stroke and can improve long-term functional outcome (97). Clinical trials are currently underway to test the efficacy of these techniques in humans (98).

# CONCLUSION

Our concepts of the pathophysiology and treatment of stroke have changed dramatically, over the last 20 years. In acute cerebral ischemia, basic science and clinical studies have emphasized the importance of rapid intervention to restore blood flow and prevent permanent ischemic damage. With the recent development of effective thrombolytic acute stroke therapy, the era of therapeutic nihilism is at an end. Stroke is now recognized as an eminently treatable medical emergency, and every minute counts when caring for a patient with acute stroke. In addition to these dramatic advances in acute ischemic stroke therapy, tremendous progress has occurred in stroke prevention. Clinical trial–validated treatments to prevent ischemic stroke are numerous, and could avert more than three fourths of all strokes if widely applied. Care according to the principles outlined in this chapter will help to reduce the personal, familial, and societal burden of this devastating disease.

## References

1. Williams GR. Incidence and characteristics of total stroke in the United States. *BMC Neurol* 2001;1(1):2.
2. Broderick J, Miller R, Khoury J, et al. Incidence rates of stroke for blacks and whites: preliminary results from the Greater Cincinnati/Northern Kentucky Stroke Study. *Stroke* 2001;32:320.
3. Leary M, Saver J. Incidence of silent stroke in the United States. *Stroke* 2001;32:363.
4. Rosamond W, Folsom A, Chambless L, et al. Stroke incidence and survival among middle-aged adults: 9-year follow-up of the Atherosclerosis Risk in Communities (ARIC) Cohort. *Stroke* 1999;30:736–743.
5. Rundek T, Sacco RL. Outcome following stroke. In: Mohr JP, Choi DW, Grotta JC et al., eds. *Stroke: pathophysiology, diagnosis, and management*, 4th ed. Philadelphia, PA: Churchill Livingstone, 2004:35–57.
6. *2001 Heart and Stroke Statistical Update*. Dallas, TX: American Heart Association, 2000.
7. *1999 Heart and Stroke Statistical Update*. Dallas, TX: American Heart Association, 1998.
8. Samsa G, Matchar D, Goldstein L, et al. Utilities for major stroke: results from a survey of preferences among persons at increased risk for stroke. *Am Heart J* 1998;136:703–713.
9. Kalafut MA, Saver JL. The acute stroke patient: the first six hours. In: Cohen SN, ed. *Management of ischemic stroke*. New York: McGraw-Hill, 2000:17–52.
10. Hossmann KA. Viability thresholds and the penumbra of focal ischemia. *Ann Neurol* 1994;36(4):557–565.
11. Heiss WD, Huber M, Fink GR, et al. Progressive derangement of periinfarct viable tissue in ischemic stroke. *J Cereb Blood Flow Metab* 1992; 12(2):193–203.
12. Heiss WD, Graf R, Wienhard K, et al. Dynamic penumbra demonstrated by sequential multitracer PET after middle cerebral artery occlusion in cats. *J Cereb Blood Flow Metab* 1994;14(6):892–902.
13. Zivin JA. Factors determining the therapeutic window for stroke. *Neurology* 1998;50:559–603.
14. Foulkes MA, Wolf PA, Price TR, et al. The Stroke Data Bank: design, methods, and baseline characteristics. *Stroke* 1988;19(5):547–554.
15. Caplan LR, Hier DB, D'Cruz I. Cerebral embolism in the Michael Reese Stroke Registry. *Stroke* 1983;14(4):530–536.
16. Adams HP Jr, Adams RJ, Brott T, et al. Guidelines for the early management of patients with ischemic stroke: a scientific statement from the Stroke Council of the American Stroke Association. *Stroke* 2003;34(4):1056–1083.
17. Brott T, Adams HP Jr, Olinger CP, et al. Measurements of acute cerebral infarction: a clinical examination scale. *Stroke* 1989;20(7):864–870.
18. von Kummer R, Nolte PN, Schnittger H, et al. Detectability of cerebral hemisphere ischaemic infarcts by CT within 6 h of stroke. *Neuroradiology* 1996;38(1):31–33.
19. von Kummer R, Allen KL, Holle R, et al. Acute stroke: usefulness of early CT findings before thrombolytic therapy. *Radiology* 1997;205(2):327–333.
20. Hacke W, Kaste M, Fieschi C, et al. Intravenous thrombolysis with recombinant tissue plasminogen activator for acute hemispheric stroke. The European Cooperative Acute Stroke Study (ECASS). *JAMA* 1995; 274(13): 1017–1025.
21. Mohr JP, Biller J, Hilal SK, et al. Magnetic resonance versus computed tomographic imaging in acute stroke. *Stroke* 1995;26(5):807–812.
22. Kidwell CS, Saver JL, Mattiello J, et al. Diffusion-perfusion MR evaluation of perihematomal injury in hyperacute intracerebral hemorrhage. *Neurology* 2001;57(9):1611–1617.
23. Kidwell CS, Chalela JA, Saver JL, et al. Hemorrhage early MRI evaluation (HEME) study: preliminary results of a multicenter trial of neuroimaging in patients with acute stroke symptoms within 6 hours of onset (abstract). *Stroke* 2003;34:239.
24. Schellinger PD, Fiebach JB, Gass A, et al. Accuracy of stroke MRI in hyperacute intracerebral hemorrhage <6 hours: a prospective standardized blinded multicenter study. *Stroke* 2003;34:239.
25. Baird AE, Warach S. Magnetic resonance imaging of acute stroke. *J Cereb Blood Flow Metab* 1998;18(6):583–609.
26. Schlaug G, Siewert B, Benfield A, et al. Time course of the apparent diffusion coefficient (ADC) abnormality in human stroke. *Neurology* 1997; 49(1):113–119.
27. Kidwell CS, Saver JL, Mattiello J, et al. Thrombolytic reversal of acute human cerebral ischemic injury shown by diffusion/perfusion magnetic resonance imaging. *Ann Neurol* 2000;47(4):462–469.
28. Kidwell CS, Saver JL, Starkman S, et al. Late secondary ischemic injury in patients receiving intraarterial thrombolysis. *Ann Neurol* 2002;52(6): 698–703.
29. Lutsep HL, Albers GW, DeCrespigny A, et al. Clinical utility of diffusion-weighted magnetic resonance imaging in the assessment of ischemic stroke. *Ann Neurol* 1997;41(5):574–580.
30. Barber PA, Darby DG, Desmond PM, et al. Prediction of stroke outcome with echoplanar perfusion and diffusion-weighted MRI. *Neurology* 1998; 51(2):418–426.
31. Lee LJ, Kidwell CS, Alger J, et al. Impact on stroke subtype diagnosis of early diffusion-weighted magnetic resonance imaging and magnetic resonance angiography. *Stroke* 2000;31(5):1081–1089.

32. Lövblad KO, Laubach HJ, Baird AE, et al. Clinical experience with diffusion-weighted MR in patients with acute stroke. *AJNR Am J Neuroradiol* 1998;19(6):1061–1066.

33. Ay H, Buonanno FS, Rordorf G, et al. Normal diffusion-weighted MRI during stroke-like deficits. *Neurology* 1999;52(9):1784–1792.

34. Gonzalez RG, Schaefer PW, Buonanno FS, et al. Diffusion-weighted MR imaging: diagnostic accuracy in patients imaged within 6 hours of stroke symptom onset. *Radiology* 1999;210(1):155–162.

35. Lovblad KO, Baird AE, Schlaug G, et al. Ischemic lesion volumes in acute stroke by diffusion-weighted magnetic resonance imaging correlate with clinical outcome. *Ann Neurol* 1997;42(2):164–170.

36. Tong DC, Yenari MA, Albers GW, et al. Correlation of perfusion- and diffusion-weighted MRI with NIHSS score in acute (<6.5 hour) ischemic stroke. *Neurology* 1998;50(4):864–870.

37. Schonewille WJ, Tuhrim S, Singer MB, et al. Diffusion-weighted MRI in acute lacunar syndromes: a clinical-radiological correlation study. *Stroke* 1999;30:2066–2069.

38. Fitzek C, Tintera J, Müller-Forell W, et al. Differentiation of recent and old cerebral infarcts by diffusion-weighted MRI. *Neuroradiology* 1998;40(12):778–782.

39. Baird AE, Lovblad KO, Schlaug G, et al. Multiple acute stroke syndrome: marker of embolic disease? *Neurology* 2000;54(3):674–678.

40. Wintermark M, Reichhart M, Thiran JP, et al. Prognostic accuracy of cerebral blood flow measurement by perfusion computed tomography, at the time of emergency room admission, in acute stroke patients. *Ann Neurol* 2002;51(4):417–432.

41. Neumann-Haefelin T, Wittsack HJ, Wenserski F, et al. Diffusion- and perfusion-weighted MRI. The DWI/PWI mismatch region in acute stroke. *Stroke* 1999;30(8):1591–1597.

42. Sorensen AG, Copen WA, Ostergaard L, et al. Hyperacute stroke: simultaneous measurement of relative cerebral blood volume, relative cerebral blood flow, and mean tissue transit time. *Radiology* 1999;210(2):519–527.

43. Kidwell CS, Alger JR, Saver JL. Beyond mismatch: evolving paradigms in imaging the ischemic penumbra with multimodal magnetic resonance imaging. *Stroke* 2003;34(11):2729–2735.

44. Hasegawa Y, Fisher M, Latour LL, et al. MRI diffusion mapping of reversible and irreversible ischemic injury in focal brain ischemia. *Neurology* 1994;44(8):1484–1490.

45. Villablanca JP, Martin N, Jahan R, et al. Volume-rendered helical computerized tomography angiography in the detection and characterization of intracranial aneurysms. *J Neurosurg* 2000;93(2):254–264.

46. Leclerc X, Gauvrit JY, Pruvo JP. Usefulness of CT angiography with volume rendering after carotid angioplasty and stenting. *AJR Am J Roentgenol* 2000;174(3):820–822.

47. Leclerc X, Gauvrit JY, Nicol L, et al. Contrast-enhanced MR angiography of the craniocervical vessels: a review. *Neuroradiology* 1999;41(12):867–874.

48. Saver JL, Feldmann E. The basic transcranial Doppler examination: technique and anatomy. In: Babikian VL, Wechsler L, eds. *Transcranial Doppler sonography: clinical and research applications*, Philadelphia, PA: BC Decker, 1992:11–28.

49. Toni D, Fiorelli M, Zanette EM, et al. Early spontaneous improvement and deterioration of ischemic stroke patients. A serial study with transcranial Doppler ultrasonography. *Stroke* 1998;29(6):1144–1148.

50. Sloan MA, Alexandrov AV, Tegeler CH, et al. Assessment: transcranial Doppler ultrasonography: report of the Therapeutics and Technology Assessment Subcommittee of the American Academy of Neurology. *Neurology* 2004;62(9):1468–1481.

51. Daniels SK, Brailey K, Priestly DH, et al. Aspiration in patients with acute stroke. *Arch Phys Med Rehabil* 1998;79(1):14–19.

52. Aslanyan S, Weir CJ, Diener HC, et al. Pneumonia and urinary tract infection after acute ischaemic stroke: a tertiary analysis of the GAIN International trial. *Eur J Neurol* 2004;11(1):49–53.

53. Ronning OM, Guldvog B. Should stroke victims routinely receive supplemental oxygen? A quasi randomized controlled trial. *Stroke* 1999;30(10):2033–2037.

54. Carlberg B, Asplun DK, Hagg E. Course of blood pressure in different subsets of patients after acute stroke. *Cerebrovasc Dis* 1991;1:281–287.

55. Powers WJ. Acute hypertension after stroke: the scientific basis for treatment decisions [editorial]. *Neurology* 1993;43(3 Pt 1):461–467.

56. Hillis AE, Ulatowski JA, Barker PB, et al. A pilot randomized trial of induced blood pressure elevation: effects on function and focal perfusion in acute and subacute stroke. *Cerebrovasc Dis* 2003;16(3):236–246.

57. Saver JL, Starkman S. State of the art medical management of acute ischemic stroke. *J Stroke Cerebrovasc Dis* 1997;4:189–194.

58. Brott T, Lu M, Kothari R, et al. Hypertension and its treatment in the NINDS rt-PA Stroke Trial. *Stroke* 1998;29(8):1504–1509.

59. Baird TA, Parsons MW, Phanh T, et al. Persistent poststroke hyperglycemia is independently associated with infarct expansion and worse clinical outcome. *Stroke* 2003;34(9):2208–2214.

60. Tanne D, Kasner SE, Demchuk AM, et al. Markers of increased risk of intracerebral hemorrhage after intravenous recombinant tissue plasminogen activator therapy for acute ischemic stroke in clinical practice: the Multicenter rt-PA Stroke Survey. *Circulation* 2002;105(14):1679–1685.

61. Wass CT, Lanier WL. Glucose modulation of ischemic brain injury: review and clinical recommendations. *Mayo Clin Proc* 1996;71(8):801–812.

62. Ginsberg MD, Busto R. Combating hyperthermia in acute stroke: a significant clinical concern. *Stroke* 1998;29(2):529–534.

63. Kasner SE, Wein T, Piriyawat P, et al. Acetaminophen for altering body temperature in acute stroke: a randomized clinical trial. *Stroke* 2002;33(1):130–134.

64. The National Institute of Neurological Disorders and Stroke rt-PA Stroke Study Group. Tissue plasminogen activator for acute ischemic stroke. *N Engl J Med* 1995;333(24):1581–1587.

65. Haley EC Jr, Lewandowski C, Tilley BC. Myths regarding the NINDS rt-PA stroke trial: setting the record straight. *Ann Emerg Med* 1997;30(5):676–682.

66. The NINDS t-PA Stroke Trial Study Group. Generalized efficacy of t-PA for acute stroke. Subgroup analysis of the NINDS t-PA stroke trial. *Stroke* 1997;28(11):2119–2125.

67. Hacke W, Donnan G, Fieschi C, et al. Association of outcome with early stroke treatment: pooled analysis of ATLANTIS, ECASS, and NINDS rt-PA stroke trials. *Lancet* 2004;363(9411):768–774.

68. Saver JL. Number needed to treat estimates incorporating effects over the entire range of clinical outcomes: novel derivation method and application to thrombolytic therapy for acute stroke. *Arch Neurol* 2004;61:1066–1070.

69. Tanne D, Bates VE, Verro P, et al. Initial clinical experience with IV tissue plasminogen activator for acute ischemic stroke: a multicenter survey. The t-PA Stroke Survey Group. *Neurology* 1999;53(2):424–427.

70. Katzan IL, Hammer MD, Furlan AJ, et al. Quality improvement and tissue-type plasminogen activator for acute ischemic stroke: a Cleveland update. *Stroke* 2003;34(3):799–800.

71. Graham GD. Tissue plasminogen activator for acute ischemic stroke in clinical practice: a meta-analysis of safety data. *Stroke* 2003;34(12):2847–2850.

72. Furlan A, Higashida R, Wechsler L, et al. Intra-arterial prourokinase for acute ischemic stroke. The PROACT II study: a randomized controlled trial. Prolyse in Acute Cerebral Thromboembolism. *JAMA* 1999;282(21):2003–2011.

73. Lewandowski CA, Frankel M, Tomsick TA, et al. Combined intravenous and intra-arterial r-TPA versus intra-arterial therapy of acute ischemic stroke: Emergency Management of Stroke (EMS) Bridging Trial. *Stroke* 1999;30(12):2598–2605.

74. Combined intravenous and intra-arterial recanalization for acute ischemic stroke: the Interventional Management of Stroke Study. *Stroke* 2004;35(4):904–911.

75. CAST (Chinese Acute Stroke Trial) Collaborative Group. CAST: randomised placebo-controlled trial of early aspirin use in 20,000 patients with acute ischaemic stroke. *Lancet* 1997;349(9066):1641–1649.

76. International Stroke Trial Collaborative Group. The International Stroke Trial (IST): a randomised trial of aspirin, subcutaneous heparin, both, or neither among 19435 patients with acute ischaemic stroke. *Lancet* 1997;349(9065):1569–1581.

77. Yusuf S, Mehta SR, Zhao F, et al. Early and late effects of clopidogrel in patients with acute coronary syndromes. *Circulation* 2003;107(7):966–972.

78. AbeESTT Investigators. Effects of abciximab for acute ischemic stroke: final results of Abciximab in Emergent Stroke Treatment Trial (AbESTT) (abstract). *Stroke* 2003;34:253.

79. Gubitz G, Counsell C, Sandercock P, et al. Anticoagulants for acute ischaemic stroke. *Cochrane Database Syst Rev* 2000;2.

80. Chamorro A, Vila N, Saiz A, et al. Early anticoagulation after large cerebral embolic infarction: a safety study. *Neurology* 1995;45(5):861–865.

81. Coull BM, Williams LS, Goldstein LB, et al. Anticoagulants and antiplatelet agents in acute ischemic stroke: report of the Joint Stroke Guideline Development Committee of the American Academy of Neurology and the American Stroke Association (a division of the American Heart Association). *Stroke* 2002;33(7):1934–1942.

82. Kay R, Wong KS, Yu YL, et al. Low-molecular-weight heparin for the treatment of acute ischemic stroke. *N Engl J Med* 1995;333:1588–1593.

83. Hommel M. Fraxiparine in ischemic stroke study. *Cerebrovasc Dis* 1998;8(suppl. 4):19A.

84. Bath PM, Lindenstrom E, Boysen G, et al. Tinzaparin in acute ischaemic stroke (TAIST): a randomised aspirin-controlled trial. *Lancet* 2001;358(9283):702–710.

85. Berge E, Abdelnoor M, Nakstad PH, et al. Low molecular-weight heparin versus aspirin in patients with acute ischaemic stroke and atrial fibrillation: a double-blind randomised study. HAEST Study Group. Heparin in Acute Embolic Stroke Trial. *Lancet* 2000;355(9211):1205–1210.

86. The Publications Committee for the Trial of ORG 10172 in Acute Stroke Treatment (TOAST) Investigators. Low molecular weight heparinoid, ORG 10172 (danaparoid), and outcome after acute ischemic stroke: a randomized controlled trial. *JAMA* 1998;279(16):1265–1272.

87. Kalafut MA, Gandhi R, Kidwell CS, et al. Safety and cost of low-molecular-weight heparin as bridging anticoagulant therapy in subacute cerebral ischemia. *Stroke* 2000;31(11):2563–2568.

88. LaMonte MP. ARGIS-1 investigators. Results of ARGIS-1: Argatroban injection in acute ischemic stroke. *Stroke* 2003;34:246.

89. Leary MC, Saver JL, Gobin YP, et al. Beyond tissue plasminogen activator: mechanical intervention in acute stroke. *Ann Emerg Med* 2003;41:838–846.

90. Nesbit GM, Luh G, Tien R, et al. New and future endovascular treatment strategies for acute ischemic stroke. *J Vasc Interv Radiol* 2004;15(1Pt2):S103–S110.

91. Starkman S, the MERCI Investigators. Results of the combined MERCI I-II (Mechanical Embolus Removal in Cerebral Ischemia) Trials. *Stroke* 2004; 35:A240.
92. Berlis A, Lutsep H, Barnwell S, et al. Mechanical thrombolysis in acute ischemic stroke with endovascular photoacoustic recanalization. *Stroke* 2004;35(5):1112–1116.
93. Rosand J, Eckman MH, Knudsen KA, et al. The effect of warfarin and intensity of anticoagulation on outcome of intracerebral hemorrhage. *Arch Intern Med* 2004;164(8):880–884.
94. Mayer SA. Ultra-early hemostatic therapy for intracerebral hemorrhage. *Stroke* 2003;34(1):224–229.
95. Jorgensen HS, Nakayama H, Raaschou HO, et al. Stroke. Neurologic and functional recovery the Copenhagen Stroke Study. *Phys Med Rehabil Clin N Am* 1999;10(4):887–906.
96. Dobkin BH. *The clinical science of neurologic rehabilitation*, 2nd ed. New York: Oxford University Press, 2003.
97. Harvey RL, Chopp M. The therapeutic effects of cellular therapy for functional recovery after brain injury. *Phys Med Rehabil Clin N Am* 2003; 14(Suppl. 1):S143–S151.
98. Kondziolka D, Wechsler L, Goldstein S, et al. Transplantation of cultured human neuronal cells for patients with stroke. *Neurology* 2000;55(4): 565–569.

# CHAPTER 104 ■ ANTITHROMBOTIC THERAPY FOR PATIENTS WITH ATRIAL FIBRILLATION

BRUCE J. DARROW AND JONATHAN L. HALPERIN

Atrial fibrillation (AF) is the most common cardiac rhythm disturbance and an important independent risk factor for ischemic stroke. AF affects approximately 2.5 million individuals in the United States (1,2) and millions more worldwide. Prevalence is greater in men than in women (1,3–5) and increases with age, rising rapidly beyond the sixth decade to approximately 10% in those older than 80 years (see Fig. 104-1) (2–6). The median age of patients with AF is approximately 72 years. As the population ages, the number of individuals with AF is likely to increase substantially in the coming decades (2).

## PATTERNS OF ATRIAL FIBRILLATION

Guidelines issued conjointly by the American College of Cardiology, the American Heart Association, and the European Society of Cardiology suggest classification of AF as either paroxysmal, persistent, or permanent based on the duration of episodes of the arrhythmia (7). *Paroxysmal* AF may occur once or multiple times, but by definition, episodes terminate without intervention. *Persistent* AF does not convert to normal sinus rhythm (NSR) without cardioversion (either pharmacological or electrical), but NSR can be restored, at least temporarily. *Permanent* AF is refractory and does not convert to NSR even if cardioversion is attempted. Either paroxysmal or persistent AF may occur as a single episode or be recurrent.

### Risk of Stroke Associated with Nonvalvular Atrial Fibrillation

As a result of disorganized electrical stimulation of atrial systole, the fibrillating atria become passive conduits of blood traveling from the venous systems to the ventricles. Impaired atrial emptying leads to stasis and increases the risk of thrombus formation, particularly in the left-atrial appendage (LAA) (8). The factors that promote embolism of cardiogenic thrombi and subsequent ischemic events (including stroke and peripheral arterial occlusion) are incompletely understood (9,10). In addition to cardiogenic embolism, patients with AF commonly have other cardiovascular disease states, such as hypertension and atherosclerosis, which raise the risk of cerebrovascular ischemic events.

Approximately 15% of all strokes are attributed to AF (11). The rate of ischemic stroke among patients with AF not treated with antithrombotic therapy averages to 4.5% per year (12,13),

approximately fivefold greater than in age- and gender-matched individuals with NSR. The risk of stroke attributable to AF rose from 1.5% in the age group 50 to 59 years to 23.5% in the age group 80 to 89 years in the Framingham Heart Study (14). Because the prevalence of AF and the risk of stroke are both related to age, the problem of stroke prevention is amplified among the elderly; AF is the most common cause of stroke in women older than 75 years (15).

### Valvular Heart Disease

Patients with AF and rheumatic mitral valve disease or prosthetic heart valves (mechanical or biological) have been historically considered at high risk for stroke (10) and were excluded from most randomized trials of antithrombotic therapy because of the perceived need for anticoagulation. Hence, available empirical data pertain mainly to patients with nonvalvular AF. Management of patients with AF associated with mitral stenosis or prosthetic heart valves is beyond the scope of this chapter.

### Atrial Flutter

Sustained atrial flutter is uncommon because the rhythm typically either degenerates to AF or spontaneously reverts to NSR. Patients with persistent atrial flutter may have periods of AF, and vice versa. There are scant data from longitudinal studies assessing the thromboembolic risk associated with isolated, sustained atrial flutter. Echo-Doppler examinations of patients with atrial flutter demonstrate more organized atrial mechanical function and greater LAA flow velocities than are typical of patients with AF (16). Despite this functional distinction, intraatrial thrombus has been documented in a significant percentage of patients with atrial flutter (6,17). In a transesophageal echocardiographic (TEE) study before cardioversion, 25% of patients with atrial flutter of slightly longer than 6 months' mean duration had spontaneous echo contrast, and 7% had LAA thrombus (18). In patients with prior cerebral ischemic events, the prevalence of intraatrial thrombus associated with atrial flutter was even higher (19). A retrospective study of 100 patients with persistent atrial flutter found a higher than anticipated risk of stroke (20). Although the role of anticoagulant therapy for patients with atrial flutter has not been evaluated in clinical trials, current treatment guidelines recommend that decisions regarding antithrombotic therapy follow the same risk-stratification schemes that apply to patients with AF.

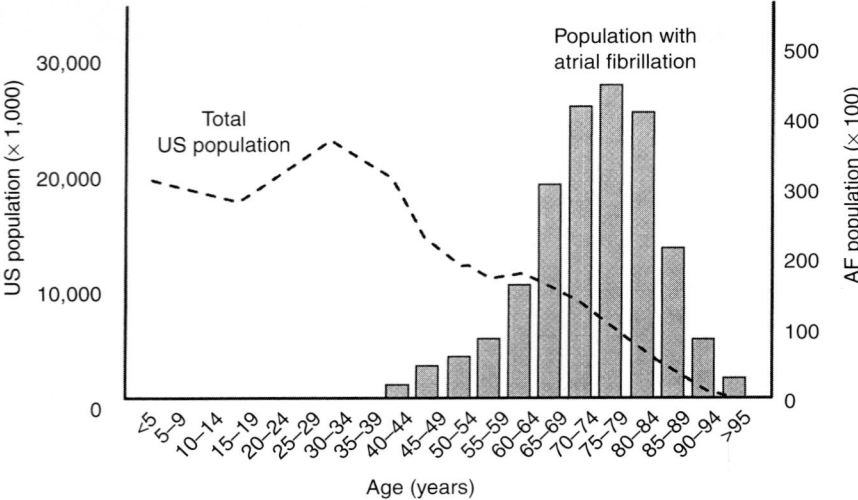

**FIGURE 104-1.** Age distribution of the population of the United States and of patients with atrial fibrillation. The increasing average age of the population is anticipated to double the prevalence of atrial fibrillation over the next two generations. (Adapted from Feinberg WM, Blackshear JL, Laupacis A, et al. Prevalence, age distribution, and gender of patients with atrial fibrillation: analysis and implications. *Arch Intern Med* 1995;155:468–473.)

# STROKE RISK STRATIFICATION OF PATIENTS WITH ATRIAL FIBRILLATION

A combined analysis of untreated control groups in five primary prevention trials found that the stroke rate was more than 8% per year in patients with AF who were older than 75 years and had one additional clinical risk factor. For patients at any age with a history of thromboembolism, the annual risk of stroke was 12% (12,21). Three-year stroke rates in elderly nursing home patients who were not anticoagulated exceeded 50% (22).

Risk factors that increase the probability of stroke among patients with AF not treated with anticoagulants have been determined from randomized trials of antithrombotic therapy (21–26). The most commonly cited risk-stratification strategies were generated from pooled analyses of five trials by the Atrial Fibrillation Investigators (AFI) (12) and from the Stroke Prevention in Atrial Fibrillation (SPAF) cohorts (23,26). The AFI group (12) found the following independent risk factors: age (RR, 1.4 per decade), prior stroke or transient ischemic attack (TIA) (RR, 2.5), history of hypertension (RR, 1.6), and diabetes mellitus (RR, 1.7). Analysis of 854 patients assigned to aspirin from the first two SPAF trials (27) identified three independent risk factors for stroke: women older than 75 years (RR, 3.7), systolic hypertension greater than 160 mm Hg (RR, 2.2), and impaired left ventricular function defined as recent (within 3 months) congestive heart failure or fractional shortening less than 0.25 by M-mode echocardiography (RR, 1.8). Extending analysis to include 2,012 patients allocated to the aspirin or combination therapy arms of the SPAF I–III studies (28) identified five characteristics significantly associated with an increased risk of stroke: age (RR, 1.8 per decade); female gender (RR, 1.6), prior thromboembolism (RR, 2.9), history of hypertension (RR, 2.0), and systolic blood pressure greater than 160 mm Hg (RR, 2.3).

Although prior stroke or TIA, older age, and hypertension were identified as risk factors for stroke in patients with AF in both the AFI- and SPAF-based risk-stratification schemes, there is a differential impact of age in the AFI and SPAF risk-stratification schemes. The AFI scheme classifies all patients with AF as old as or older than 65 years to be at high risk, whereas the SPAF criteria classify women as old as or younger than 75 years and men of any age without other risk factors to be at low risk. Uncertainty about the risk in either gender aged 65 to 75 years and in men at any age without other risk factors applies to approximately 20% of the population with nonvalvular AF (29).

The main clinical risk factors are presented in Table 104-1. In addition, a modified scale, CHADS-2 (congestive heart failure, hypertension, age, diabetes, and stroke), which integrates elements from the AFI and SPAF schemes, was evaluated in 1,733 Medicare beneficiaries with nonvalvular AF aged 65 to 95 years, discharged from hospital off warfarin (30). This index is based on a point system in which a history of stroke or TIA is given two points and age greater than 75 years, history of hypertension, diabetes, or recent congestive heart failure are each given one point. Stroke rates within each risk category differ across the risk schemes, with low rates in the low-risk categories for all schemes but considerable variation in those classified as moderate-to-high risk, as well as in the proportion of subjects in each category.

These clinical trials included patients with chronic persistent (including both persistent and permanent AF) (7) and, less commonly, paroxysmal AF. For the purpose of determining the stroke risk of patients with AF, the distinction between paroxysmal, persistent, and permanent AF is immaterial. Although

---

**TABLE 104-1**

CLINICAL RISK FACTORS FOR STROKE AND SYSTEMIC EMBOLISM IN PATIENTS WITH ATRIAL FIBRILLATION

**HIGH RISK FACTORS**
History of stroke or TIA
Hypertension
Reduced LV function
Age >75 yr
Thyrotoxicosis
Mitral stenosis
Prosthetic heart valve

**MODERATE RISK FACTORS**
Age 65–75 yr
Diabetes mellitus
Coronary artery disease

TIA, transient ischemic attack; LV, left ventricle.
Adapted from Singer DE, Albers GW, Dalen JE, et al. Long-term antithrombotic therapy for chronic atrial fibrillation or atrial flutter: Anticoagulants and antiplatelet agents. In Seventh ACCP Consensus Conference on Antithrombotic Therapy: Antithrombotic Therapy in Atrial Fibrillation. American College of Chest Physicians. *Chest* (Suppl) 2004;126:429S–456S.

patients with paroxysmal AF typically have an overall risk of stroke below that of patients with persistent or permanent AF, they are often younger and have fewer associated stroke risk factors other than AF (31,32). Accordingly, the pattern of AF was not a significant predictor of stroke risk in multivariate analyses of prospectively followed cohorts (12,33). Current recommendations for anticoagulation do not distinguish between patients according to the pattern of AF (7).

## Echocardiographic Markers of Stroke Risk

Although left atrial size and left ventricular systolic function can be assessed by transthoracic echocardiography, TEE is necessary to consistently visualize abnormalities of the LAA and aortic arch linked with thromboembolism. This approach is not only used as an adjunct to elective cardioversion (see subsequent text) but is also employed in patients with persistent AF (34,35). Visible thrombus and dense spontaneous echo contrast (a marker of blood stasis) in the left atrium, and particularly in the LAA, is associated with a twofold to fourfold increased risk of stroke (7,8). In the SPAF III study, patients with atheromatous plaques in the thoracic segments of the aorta that have complex features (mobility, pedunculation, ulceration, or thickness >4 mm) had high stroke rates. Because many of these abnormalities were observed in the descending aorta beyond the origins of the cerebral vessels, the association with stroke may reflect either associated cerebrovascular disease or the pathogenic role of risk factors such as hypertension that are common both to atherosclerosis and to conditions of atrial stasis in patients with AF (35).

## Other Potential Stroke Risk Factors in Atrial Fibrillation

Other characteristics that may augment stroke risk stratification based on clinical and echocardiographic features include genetic polymorphisms, abnormalities of hemostatic and thrombotic factors, platelet activation and aggregation pathways, and endothelial dysfunction (36,37). None have yet proven sufficiently robust for routine clinical use. Thyrotoxicosis is a poorly understood risk factor for stroke among patients with AF, because patients with thyrotoxicosis were largely excluded from the randomized trials of antithrombotic therapy. AF develops in 10% to 15% of patients with hyperthyroidism, and thyrotoxicosis is evident in 2% to 5% of patients with AF (38). A high frequency of stroke and systemic embolism has been reported in several (39–43) but not all studies (44). The association may be mediated partly by coexisting congestive heart failure.

## Patient Preferences and Decision Analyses

In addition to clinical risk stratification, patient perspectives and preferences should be incorporated into the selection of antithrombotic therapy. Patient and physician perspectives often differ, with patients generally placing more value on prevention of stroke than on avoidance of hemorrhage, compared with physicians (45). In fact, many patients fear a stroke of even moderate severity more than they fear death (46,47). To evaluate the net projected benefit or harm associated with different treatment strategies, decision analysis models combine the absolute risks associated with patient characteristics, estimates of treatment efficacy and safety, and assigned values (utilities) of related health states (e.g., taking warfarin, occurance of a major stroke). In general, these analyses have supported the net benefit of anticoagulation with oral vitamin K antagonists for patients with AF

at moderate to high risk for stroke but low risk of bleeding, but the thresholds and criteria for risk stratification vary across studies, and more refined estimates are needed (48,49).

# PHARMACOLOGIC THERAPY FOR PREVENTION OF THROMBOEMBOLISM IN PATIENTS WITH ATRIAL FIBRILLATION

## Oral Anticoagulant Therapy with a Vitamin K Antagonist

Several randomized trials have demonstrated the efficacy of adjusted-dose warfarin for prevention of ischemic stroke in patients with AF with relative risk reductions (RRR) of 47% to 86% versus placebo. Results from these trials are summarized in Figure 104-2. The Atrial Fibrillation Aspirin and Anticoagulation Trial (AFASAK)-1 trial showed a statistically significant 48% RRR with warfarin treatment group [approximate international normalized ratio (INR), 2.8 to 4.2] compared with aspirin (75 mg daily) for prevention of stroke and systemic embolism (50). The adjusted-dose warfarin (target INR, 2.5 to 4.0) arm of the European Atrial Fibrillation Trial (EAFT), which enrolled patients with AF who had recently had a minor ischemic stroke (defined as grade 3 or less on the modified Rankin functional scale), had RRR of 40% [95% confidence interval (CI), 0.41 to 0.87; P = 0.008] compared with aspirin

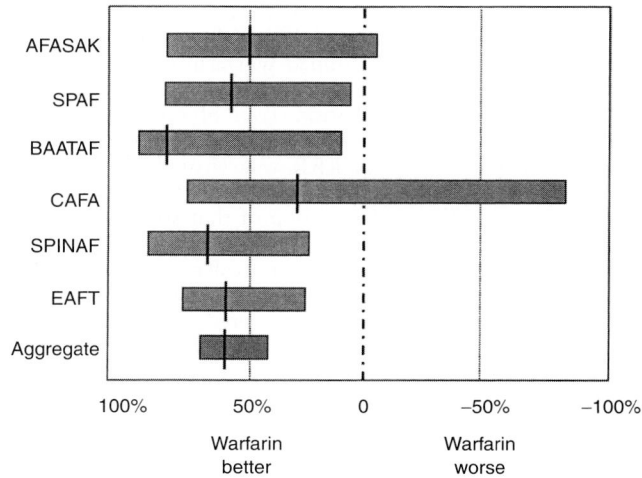

FIGURE 104-2. Stroke risk reductions with warfarin compared to control (placebo or no treatment) in patients with nonvalvular atrial fibrillation. The first five trials listed mainly involved primary prevention, whereas the last was confined to patients with prior nondisabling stroke or transient ischemic attack. Values shown were obtained according to intention-to-treat analysis. AFASAK denotes the Atrial Fibrillation, Aspirin and Anticoagulation Trial (50); SPAF, the Stroke Prevention in Atrial Fibrillation Trial (51); BAATAF, the Boston Area Anticoagulation Trial for Atrial Fibrillation (52); CAFA, the Canadian Atrial Fibrillation Anticoagulation Trial (53); SPINAF, the Veterans Administration Stroke Prevention in Atrial Fibrillation trial (54); and EAFT, the European Atrial Fibrillation Trial (21). (Adapted from Hart RG, Halperin JL. Atrial fibrillation and stroke: concepts and controversies. *Stroke.* 2001;32:803.)

(300 mg daily). The risk reduction for the composite endpoint was driven by a statistically significant RRR of 62% for all strokes (95% CI, 0.23 to 0.64; $P$ <0.001) (21).

In a pooled analysis, adjusted-dose warfarin reduced the risk of stroke by about two thirds versus control (25,38). The magnitude of benefit associated with warfarin was fairly consistent among trials despite variations in design and the intensity of anticoagulation. Compared with aspirin, adjusted-dose warfarin reduces the overall risk of stroke by 36% (CI, 14% to 52%) and ischemic stroke by 46% (CI, 27% to 60%) (28). The discrepancy is driven largely by the results of the SPAF-II trial (mean INR 2.6) in an older patient cohort than those who were enrolled in many other studies (55). The risk of intracranial bleeding among patients receiving adjusted-dose warfarin was substantially increased in this study among patients older than 75 years of age. Exclusion of SPAF-II data from the metaanalysis revealed a 49% reduction in the risk of all stroke for adjusted-dose warfarin compared with aspirin (95% CI, 26% to 65%) (28). Anticoagulation lowered all-cause mortality rate by 33% (95% CI, 9% to 51%) and the combined outcome of stroke, systemic embolism, and death by 48% (95% CI, 34% to 60%) (12).

In most instances, AF had been present for many months to years. Each of these trials was terminated early because of the large effect of antithrombotic therapy (most often warfarin) for prevention of ischemic stroke and systemic embolism. The Canadian Atrial Fibrillation Anticoagulation (CAFA) trial stopped because of the superiority of anticoagulation in other trials (53). By intention-to-treat analysis, the pooled data revealed reduction in annual stroke rate from 4.5% among patients in the control arms to 1.4% for those assigned to adjusted-dose warfarin. The efficacy of warfarin was consistent across studies with an overall RRR of 68% (95% CI, 50% to 79%) (12). The absolute risk-reduction implies prevention of 31 ischemic strokes for every 1,000 patients treated each year (or 32 patients needed-to-treat [number needed to treat (NNT)] for 1 year to prevent a single stroke event) (12).

The efficacy of anticoagulation with warfarin was consistent across all patient subgroups and for preventing strokes of all degrees of severity. Most strokes in the warfarin arms involved patients who had stopped warfarin or in whom the INR or prothrombin time ratio fell below the target range. In the European Atrial Fibrillation Trial of secondary stroke prevention (EAFT), which enrolled only patients with a TIA or recent minor stroke, the RRR was virtually identical, although the absolute risk of stroke was higher; the annual stroke rate was 12% in the control group of that study versus 4% in anticoagulated patients (RRR 66%; 95% CI, 43% to 80%; $P$ <0.001; NNT=13) (21). In short, evidence for the efficacy of anticoagulation in patients with AF is strong and consistent, based on several adequately powered, randomized trials.

In these trials, anticoagulation proved relatively safe when the upper limit of the INR target range was less than 3.0, but whether comparable safety can be reliably achieved in less carefully selected patients outside the rubric of clinical research protocols is a persistent controversy. Pooled analysis of the first five primary prevention trials reported a 1.0% per year rate of major bleeding in control patients versus 1.3% in those treated with warfarin. Intracranial hemorrhage is the only hemorrhagic complication of anticoagulation that regularly produces deficits more severe than the ischemic strokes that such therapy is intended to prevent, and the rate of intracranial hemorrhage was 0.1% per year in the control groups versus 0.3% in anticoagulated patients (12). In the SPAF-II study (55), intracranial hemorrhage was more frequent, with seven such bleeds among 385 patients aged more than 75 years (1.8% per year), compared with 0.8% in aspirin-treated patients and 0.3% per year among those older than 75 years in other primary prevention trials (56). The

reasons for the higher rate of intracranial hemorrhage in elderly patients in the SPAF-II study is uncertain, but the patients were older, on average, than in other AF trials, and the target intensity of anticoagulation was relatively high (upper INR limit approximately 4.5) (57). No intracranial hemorrhages were identified in the EAFT secondary prevention study (mean patient age 71 years), but brain imaging was not performed in all patients with stroke (21,58). The rate was 0.5% per year in the adjusted-dose warfarin arm of the SPAF-III study (57) of high-risk patients (mean age 71 years; mean INR 2.4) versus 0.9% per year in those assigned to a combination of aspirin (325 mg per day) plus low-dose warfarin (1 to 3 mg per day, INR 1.2 to 1.5).

One reason why intracranial hemorrhages occurred at a low rate in the individual randomized trials may have been the exclusion of patients considered at high risk of bleeding. Even when aggregated, these trials contribute less to understanding the determinants of intracranial hemorrhage than do large observational studies, which show a correlation with the intensity of warfarin anticoagulation (INR >4.0) (59,60), although most such bleeds occur in anticoagulated patients with INR values below 4.0. Intracranial hemorrhage is more common in patients with prior ischemic stroke and, as it does for ischemic stroke, the risk of hemorrhage increases with age (59).

## Efficacy of Aspirin

Evidence that aspirin is effective for prevention of thromboembolism in patients with nonvalvular AF is considerably weaker than that supporting the use of warfarin. Metaanalysis of five controlled studies (21,50,51,61–64) found a 22% (95% CI, 2% to 38%) reduction in stroke rates (25). Four of these trials were placebo-controlled (64), and aspirin dose ranged from 50 to 325 mg daily. A patient-level metaanalysis of data from the placebo-controlled AFASAK-1, SPAF-I, and EAFT trials estimated that the RRR was a marginally significant 21% (95% CI, 0% to 38%) (65). The SPAF-I trial, which found a significant 42% RRR, had two randomized cohorts, one consisting of patients eligible for randomization to warfarin and the other of those deemed ineligible on the basis of age, physician's judgment, or patient's refusal. In warfarin-eligible cases, the RRR afforded by aspirin was striking (94%), whereas the RRR in the ineligible cohort was just 8% [not significant (NS)], similar to findings in the AFASAK-1 and EAFT studies. In other studies involving patients with AF, the efficacy of aspirin for prevention of thromboembolism was negligible or inconsistent (61,62,64,66). Aspirin may be more efficacious for patients with AF and hypertension and diabetes (65) and for preventing non-cardioembolic rather than cardioembolic ischemic strokes (67). Cardioembolic strokes are, on average, more disabling than noncardioembolic strokes (68). Aspirin appears to prevent nondisabling more than disabling strokes (25); therefore, the greater the risk of disabling cardioembolic stroke in a population of patients with AF, the less protection afforded by aspirin (68).

The risk reduction afforded by oral vitamin K antagonist therapy is considerably greater than that of aspirin in trials that compared the two therapies (21,50,55,63,69). Metaanalysis of six studies found an RRR of 46% (95 CI, 27% to 60%) with adjusted-dose oral anticoagulation compared with aspirin for ischemic stroke and 36% (95% CI, 14% to 52%) for all (ischemic plus hemorrhagic) stroke (25). The hazard ratio for major bleeding associated with anticoagulation was 1.7 (95% CI, 1.2% to 2.4%) (70). Hence, treatment of 1,000 patients with AF with adjusted-dose oral anticoagulation instead of aspirin for 1 year would cause nine additional major bleeds while avoiding 23 ischemic strokes.

## Alternative Regimens: Other Platelet-Inhibitor Agents and Lower-Intensity Anticoagulation

A randomized trial comparing adjusted-dose warfarin with the platelet inhibitor indobufen found no significant difference between the two groups in the rate of the combined endpoint of stroke, myocardial infarction, pulmonary embolism, or vascular death (12% with indobufen group vs. 10% with warfarin; $P = 0.47$) (71). Major bleeding episodes occurred in none of the patients treated with indobufen and in 0.9% of those treated with warfarin.

Trials of very low-intensity anticoagulation with or without aspirin have generally not identified a suitable alternative to adjusted-dose warfarin for prevention of thromboembolism in patients with AF. Metaanalysis of three studies (63,69,72) that compared fixed, low-dose warfarin (1.25 mg daily) with adjusted-dose warfarin (INR, 2.0 to 3.0) found the RRR 38% (95% CI, 20% to 68%; statistically insignificant) favoring more intensive dosing (25). Aspirin may augment protection against ischemic coronary events but raises the risk of hemorrhage in anticoagulated patients, and both the incremental coronary benefit and hemorrhagic risk of adding aspirin to oral anticoagulation seem modest. The SPAF-III trial compared a combination of warfarin (targeting INR initially to 1.2 to 1.5 with a maximum daily dose of 3 mg) plus aspirin (325 mg daily) with adjusted-dose warfarin (target INR, 2.0 to 3.0). The trial was terminated early because of a higher rate of ischemic stroke and systemic embolism in patients taking the combination therapy (7.9% per year) than in those assigned to conventional warfarin (1.9% per year) (57). There was no significant difference in rates of major hemorrhage between the two regimens, and no significant advantage was identified in coronary outcomes because of the relatively low frequency of such events.

Two trials involving patients with AF evaluated anticoagulation in higher intensities combined with platelet-inhibitor agents. The Fluindione Fibrillation Auriculaire Aspirin et Contraste Spontane (FFAACS) study, in which the oral anticoagulant fluindione (target INR, 2.0 to 2.6) was given alone or in combination with aspirin (100 mg per day) to patients at high risk of stroke, was terminated because of excessive hemorrhage in the combination therapy arm after less than 1 year (mean follow-up of 157 patients) (73). In the National Study for Prevention of Embolism in Atrial Fibrillation (NASPEAF) study, a high-risk group of patients with AF and either rheumatic mitral stenosis or prior thromboembolism ($n = 495$) were randomized to anticoagulation with an oral vitamin K antagonist (target INR, 1.4 to 2.4) combined with the platelet cyclooxygenase inhibitor triflusal (600 mg daily) or to anticoagulation alone (INR, 2 to 3). Lower-risk patients with nonvalvular AF and age above 60 years, hypertension, or heart failure ($n = 714$) were randomized to triflusal alone, anticoagulation alone (INR, 2.0 to 3.0), or the combination of triflusal plus low-intensity anticoagulation (INR, 1.25 to 2.0) (74). The primary endpoint was a composite of thromboembolism and cardiovascular death other than that due to myocardial infarction. The combination therapy was associated with a significantly lower rate of primary events than anticoagulation alone in both types of patients. The achieved INR values were closer than intended in the anticoagulation and combination therapy groups, and differences in primary outcome cluster were largely due to nonthromboembolic events. In the patients without rheumatic valvular disease or prior thromboembolism, the outcome was better with anticoagulation than with triflusal alone. Rates of severe bleeding were not significantly different in the combination therapy arm than with anticoagulation alone.

## Direct Thrombin Inhibitors

Despite their unequivocal efficacy against ischemic stroke in patients with AF, the narrow therapeutic margin of oral vitamin K antagonists and interactions with numerous drugs and foods require frequent INR testing and dose adjustments. The quest for safer, more convenient alternatives has been particularly active and productive in recent years.

Because of its central role in thrombogenesis, thrombin (factor IIa) represents an attractive target for specific inhibition. Binding to the active site of thrombin, direct thrombin inhibitors prevent cleavage of fibrinogen and factors V, VIII, XI, and XIII. Orally administered ximelagatran (AstraZeneca) is a prodrug converted after absorption to the active direct thrombin inhibitor melagatran. The compound has stable pharmacokinetics independent of the hepatic P450 enzyme system and a low potential for food (75) or drug (76) interactions. Ximelagatran compared favorably with low-molecular-weight heparin and with adjusted-dose warfarin for prevention of venous thromboembolism (77–80), and with warfarin for treatment of deep vein thrombosis (78).

Two large, long-term phase III studies, SPORTIF (Stroke Prevention using the ORal Direct Thrombin Inhibitor Ximelagatran in Patients with Atrial Fibrillation) III and V, with a combined patient population of 7,329 patients, compared ximelagatran with warfarin for prevention of stroke and systemic embolism in patients with AF (81,82,83). Eligibility was based on current clinical indications for anticoagulation. Ximelagatran was administered in a fixed oral dose of 36 mg twice daily without routine coagulation monitoring or dose titration, and warfarin dose was adjusted to target INR 2.0 to 3.0 according to a design based on noninferiority (84) within a prespecified absolute margin of 2.0% per year for the difference in rates of all stroke (ischemic or hemorrhagic) or systemic embolism (primary events) (83,85). SPORTIF-III was an open-label study in 23 countries in Europe, Asia, and Australasia involving 3,407 patients; SPORTIF-V, which involved 3,922 patients in the United States, followed the same protocol except that treatment was double blind. The mean age of randomized patients was 70 years. There was a history of stroke or TIA in approximately one fourth, hypertension in more than two thirds, and heart failure or left ventricular systolic dysfunction in more than one third of patients. Approximately 75% of the patients had more than one risk factor for thromboembolism.

Among warfarin-assigned patients, the mean INR was 2.5 across all measurements, and INR values fell within the target range during 66% and 68% of exposure in SPORTIF-III and SPORTIF-V, respectively (81,82). After 4,941 patient-years of exposure in SPORTIF-III and a mean follow-up of 17 months per patient, the annual rate of primary events was 2.3% in the warfarin group and 1.6% in the ximelagatran group ($P = NS$) (81). In SPORTIF-V, the mean exposure was 20 months, and the primary event rates were 1.2% per year in the warfarin group and 1.6% per year in the ximelagatran group ($P = NS$) (82). Results from both trials are shown in Figure 104-3. The primary analysis of each trial confirmed noninferiority and when the results of both trials were pooled (a prespecified analysis), the number of events in patients assigned to each treatment were almost identical.

In the SPORTIF trials, there was no significant difference between the two treatment groups in rates of hemorrhagic stroke, fatal bleeding, or other major bleeding (defined as a decrease in hemoglobin of 2 g per dL, requiring transfusion, or involving a critical anatomical site). When minor bleeding was included, however, the rate was significantly lower in patients assigned to ximelagatran than to warfarin. The principal

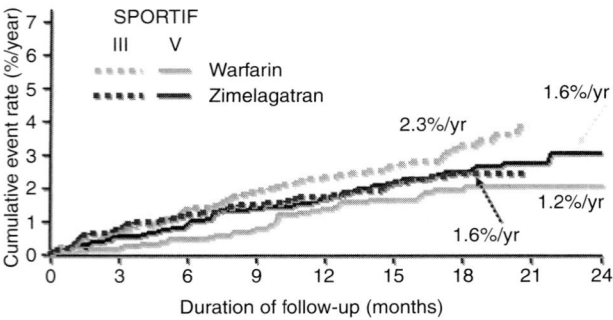

**FIGURE 104-3.** Main results of Stroke Prevention using the ORal Direct Thrombin Inhibitor Ximelagatran in Patients with Atrial Fibrillation (SPORTIF) III and V trials. Rates of stroke and systemic embolism with adjusted-dose warfarin [international normalized ratio (INR) 2 to 3] and fixed-dose oral ximelagatran (36 mg twice daily) according to intention-to-treat analysis. (Adapted from The Executive Steering Committee on behalf of the SPORTIF III Investigators. Stroke prevention using the oral direct thrombin inhibitor ximelagatran compared with warfarin in patients with nonvalvular atrial fibrillation: The SPORTIF III trial. *Lancet* 2003;362:1691–1698; Albers GW, Diener HC, Frison L, et al. The Executive Steering Committee on behalf of the SPORTIF V Investigators. Ximelagatran vs. warfarin for stroke prevention in patients with nonvalvular atrial fibrillation: The SPORTIF V randomized trial. 2005; *JAMA* 293: 690–698.)

toxicity of ximelagatran was elevation of serum transaminase enzyme levels, which exceeded three times the upper limit of normal in approximately 6% of patients, typically 2 to 6 months after initiating treatment; these levels generally returned toward baseline either spontaneously or upon cessation of treatment.

Ximelagatran has not been approved for clinical use in the US at the time of this writing and has not been incorporated into published recommendations for patient management. From the SPORTIF trials, however, it seems reasonable to conclude that in high-risk patients with nonvalvular AF, direct thrombin inhibition represents a promising future treatment option, offering efficacy against thromboembolism comparable to carefully adjusted warfarin (INR 2.0 to 3.0) without the need for coagulation monitoring or dose adjustment and with no increase (perhaps a slight decrease) in bleeding complications. The cause of elevated liver enzyme levels in some patients exposed to ximelagatran remains incompletely understood and will probably require surveillance of liver function during the early months of treatment. Other oral direct thrombin inhibitors are also under development.

## Potential Future Therapies

The synthetic pentasaccharide factor Xa antagonist idraparinux (Sanofi-Organon 34006) is currently being used in trials of thromboembolism prevention in patients with AF. Idraparinux is a novel synthetic pentasaccharide with a structure that mimics the antithrombin-binding site of heparin (86,87). As with fondiparinux, the action of idraparinux is mediated by its interaction with antithrombin. The idraparinux/antithrombin complex binds irreversibly to factor Xa, which is thereby inactivated (88). Because of its long half-life (approximately 80 hours), idraparinux can be administered as a once-weekly subcutaneous injection. In a phase II trial comparing weekly idraparinux and daily warfarin therapy for secondary prevention of deep venous thrombosis (PERSIST), short-term therapy (12 weeks) with idraparinux was noninferior to warfarin in terms of overall safety and efficacy (87). The phase III Atrial fibrillation trial of Monitored Adjusted Dose vitamin K antagonist

comparing Efficacy and safety with Unadjusted San Org 34006 (AMADEUS) trial, a multicenter study comparing idraparinux with warfarin in patients with AF and risk factors for thromboembolism was recently terminated, and additional research will be needed to avoid excess bleeding with the investigational agent.

Although monotherapy with aspirin is of marginal benefit, there is hope that a combination of aspirin and clopidogrel will be a safe and effective strategy for prevention of thromboembolic events in patients with AF. Clopidogrel, which blocks platelet aggregation through inhibition of adenosine diphosphate-dependent pathways (89), has reduced the incidence of ischemic events in studies enrolling patients with atherosclerosis, either in combination with aspirin (90) or instead of aspirin (91). The ACTIVE (Atrial fibrillation Clopidogrel Trial with Irbesartan for prevention of Vascular Events) is currently investigating the benefit of clopidogrel in patients with AF.

Other molecules under development for this indication include antagonists of the initial phase of tissue factor activation of factor VII and agents that stimulate fibrinolysis. Evaluation of each will require large trials because available active comparators (e.g., warfarin) are highly effective, resulting in low event rates.

## Inhibitors of the Renin-Angiotensin System

Although these medications have no apparent effect on coagulation pathways, there is an emerging consensus that angiotensin converting enzyme (ACE) inhibitors and angiotensin-receptor blockers (ARB) may decrease the risk of thromboembolism associated AF and perhaps reduce the prevalence of the arrhythmia itself. Analysis of the Studies Of Left Ventricular Dysfunction (SOLVD) trial involving patients with left ventricular dysfunction treated with enalapril or placebo found an RRR more than 75% in the enalapril group (92). In a small randomized trial of 154 patients treated with amiodarone to prevent recurrent AF, adjunctive treatment with the ARB irbesartan significantly reduced the rate of recurrent AF (93). A recent multicenter prospective registry of patients following coronary bypass surgery found that postoperative use of ACE inhibitors decreased the incidence of AF, whereas withdrawal of ACE inhibitor therapy imparted greater risk (94). The mechanism of action of these agents appears related to their ability to decrease expression of specific kinases; in both dog (95) and human studies (96), there is an association between increased phosphorylation targets of the renin-angiotensin system in fibrillating atria. Furthermore, effective control of hypertension may strike directly at a major mediator of AF-related stroke.

# NONPHARMACOLOGIC THERAPY FOR PREVENTION OF THROMBOEMBOLISM IN PATIENTS WITH ATRIAL FIBRILLATION

## Rate Versus Rhythm Control of Atrial Fibrillation

Until recently, most physicians favored cardioversion and a strategy of rhythm control over rate control for patients with AF of recent onset, presuming that restoration and maintenance of NSR would avoid the adverse hemodynamic consequences of AF and reduce the risk of thromboembolism. Two randomized studies, the Atrial Fibrillation Follow-up Investigation of

Rhythm Management (AFFIRM) (97) and the comparison of Rate Control and Rhythm Control in Patients with Recurrent Persistent atrial fibrillation (RACE) (98) trials, demonstrated that the frequency of ischemic events was equal regardless of whether a rate control or rhythm control strategy was followed, and most of these events occurred after warfarin had been stopped or when the INR fell below the therapeutic range. The largest trial, AFFIRM, enrolled 4,060 patients with recurrent AF (97). Subjects were older than 65 years or had other risk factors for stroke or death without contraindications to anticoagulation. All were initially anticoagulated, but warfarin was often withdrawn from those in the rhythm control arm who maintained NSR. After a mean follow-up of 3.5 years, 35% of patients in the rate control group were in NSR, compared to 63% of those in the rhythm control group. More than 85% of patients in the rate control arm were treated with warfarin, compared to 70% in the rhythm control arm. All-cause mortality (the primary endpoint) was not reduced by rhythm control (26.7% in the rhythm control group versus 25.9% in the rate control group, $P = 0.08$). There was a trend toward a higher incidence of ischemic stroke with the rhythm control strategy (7.1% vs. 5.5%, $P = 0.79$).

The RACE trial enrolled 522 patients with recurrent AF or atrial flutter of less than 1 year duration undergoing cardioversion on one or two occasions over a period of 2 years, randomized to rate control or to rhythm control strategies (98). The primary outcome was a composite of death from cardiovascular causes, heart failure, thromboembolism, bleeding, pacemaker implantation, and severe adverse drug effects. After 2.3 years follow-up, there was a trend toward a lower incidence of the primary endpoint with rate control than with rhythm control (17.2% vs. 22.6%, hazard ratio, 0.73; 90% CI, 0.53 to 1.01). There was no difference in cardiovascular mortality (6.8% vs. 7%) and a trend toward more nonfatal endpoints among patients in the rhythm control arm. The results were marred, however, by some imbalance between arms in the prevalence of hypertension.

In the Pharmacological Intervention in Atrial Fibrillation (PIAF) trial (99), 252 patients with AF of 7 to 360 days duration were randomly assigned to rate control using diltiazem or rhythm control using amiodarone. All were given anticoagulation with oral vitamin K antagonists for the duration of the study. After 1 year, there was no difference in the quality of life between the two groups; patients in the rhythm control group had better exercise tolerance but required hospitalization more often.

Although both rate and rhythm control approaches are reasonable clinical options, the foregoing findings support continuation of anticoagulation in high-risk patients even after NSR is restored following spontaneous, pharmacologic, or direct-current cardioversion. One reason for the failure of rhythm control to reduce thromboembolism is that AF recurs in 40% to 60% of patients by 1 year following initially successful cardioversion, even when antiarrhythmic drug therapy is employed (100,101). Many of these episodes of recurrent AF are paroxysmal and asymptomatic (102). Another potential explanation for the prevalence of ischemic events following apparently successful cardioversion is that patients with AF typically have associated cardiovascular disease states such as atherosclerosis and hypertension that are both implicated as causes of stroke and responsive to anticoagulant therapy.

## The Maze Operation and Radiofrequency Pulmonary Vein Isolation

A cardiac surgical operation known as the Maze procedure involves creation of scars in the interior surface of the atria to interrupt reentrant circuits and thereby maintain NSR; concurrently, the LAA is either amputated or closed by suture (103). In the hands of experienced operators, the long-term success of a Maze procedure in preventing recurrent AF exceeds 90% (104), and this combination of rhythm control and obliteration of the LAA may reduce the risk of thromboembolism, although no controlled studies have been conducted. In a series of 306 patients followed up to 11.5 years, there were two perioperative strokes and one later stroke, corresponding to an annual risk well below 1%, comparable to that reported by other investigators (29,105,106). Although the original procedure was scalpel-based, modifications using intraoperative delivery of radiofrequency, microwave, or cryoablation energy have been described (107). Because patients and physicians are reluctant to embrace major surgery as a strategy for management of AF, the Maze procedure has been restricted most commonly to adjunctive use during other cardiac surgical procedures, such as coronary bypass or valve repair or replacement operations, although less invasive options are under investigation (108).

An alternative treatment involves catheter-based radiofrequency ablation of intraatrial pathways that participate in the initiation or perpetuation of AF. On the basis of the observation that regions in the left atrium proximate to the insertions of the four pulmonary veins are a common site of earliest activation of atrial ectopic beats that engender AF, radiofrequency encirclement and electrical isolation of the pulmonary veins has become an accepted form of catheter-based treatment (109). A nonrandomized, multicenter, prospective study of 79 patients documented freedom from recurrent AF in 84% over follow-up of approximately 1 year (110), but larger studies are needed to adequately address the safety and efficacy of this procedure.

Similarly, no adequate studies have yet been published that specifically assess the risk of thromboembolism in patients who have undergone radiofrequency pulmonary vein isolation. Although some patients undergoing this procedure or the Maze operation may be poor candidates for long-term anticoagulation, there is presently a dearth of evidence to support withdrawal of anticoagulation following either procedure. In the absence of consensus recommendations or trial-based conclusions, it seems prudent to treat such patients in a fashion similar to those undergoing apparently successful cardioversion of AF, basing the duration of anticoagulation on the patient's intrinsic risk of thromboembolism and the likelihood of asymptomatic recurrence.

## Left-Atrial Appendage Closure

Because the LAA has been implicated as an important source of thrombus formation in patients with nonvalvular AF (111), closure or obliteration of the appendage offers a theoretical alternative to anticoagulation for prevention of embolism. One technique designed to accomplish this without open-chest surgery involves catheter-based delivery of a device for percutaneous LAA occlusion [percutaneous left-atrial appendage transcatheter occlusion (PLAATO)] (112). The device, a self-expanding membrane-covered nitinol cage, is deployed at the ostium of the LAA by a catheter introduced through a peripheral vein and transseptal atrial puncture (see Fig. 104-4). Other investigational approaches include obliteration of the LAA under thoracoscopic guidance (113) and deployment of meshlike devices in the carotid arteries to divert embolic material away from the brain. These approaches are currently confined primarily to patients with contraindications to chronic anticoagulation with warfarin, but their use might eventually be extended to a wider array of patients (114).

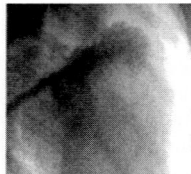
LAA angiography

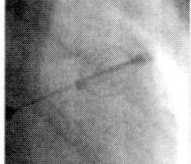
Transcatheter
deployment

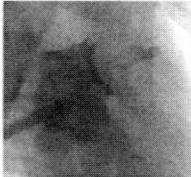
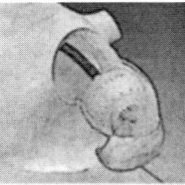
LAA occlusion

**FIGURE 104-4.** Investigational percutaneous device for occlusion of the ostium of the left-atrial appendage (LAA) for prevention of thromboembolism in patients who may be poor candidates for chronic anticoagulation or those in whom antithrombotic therapy has been inadequately effective. The device, designated percutaneous left-atrial appendage transcatheter occlusion (PLAATO) has entered clinical trials in Europe. (Adapted from Ostermayer S, Reschke M, Billinger K, et al. Percutaneous closure of the left atrial appendage. *J Interven Cardiol* 2003;16:553–556.)

# ROLE OF ANTICOAGULATION IN PATIENTS UNDERGOING CARDIOVERSION

Systemic embolism is the most serious complication when restoration of NSR occurs by external or internal direct-current, pharmacologic, or spontaneous cardioversion of AF. Evidence favoring the efficacy of anticoagulation based on observational studies (115–119) has prevented trials comparing anticoagulation to no therapy. In the prospective cohort study of Bjerkelund and Orning (120), cardioversion without anticoagulation was associated with a 5.3% incidence of clinical thromboembolism versus 0.8% in patients selected for treatment with a vitamin K antagonist. Most ischemic events are presumed to result from embolism of thrombus that forms within the left atrium or LAA (121), because atrial mechanical dysfunction may persist or worsen, leading to a prothrombotic state (122–125). Most published guidelines recommend anticoagulation with adjusted-dose warfarin (INR, 2.0 to 3.0) for 3 to 4 weeks before and after elective cardioversion of patients with AF (126,127). Serial TEE studies have demonstrated resolution of thrombus after 1 month of warfarin in most patients with AF of recent onset (8,16,128). However, it is likely that thrombi persist in a significant minority (129). In addition, a month of anticoagulation may enhance thrombus organization and adherence to the atrial endocardial surface, thereby reducing the subsequent risk of embolism.

Most information on cardioversion-related thromboembolism is based on electrical cardioversion but, while data bearing on embolism following pharmacologic or spontaneous cardioversion are limited, anticoagulation in a similar manner is recommended regardless of the method of conversion. In the prospective Assessment of Cardioversion Using Transesophageal Echocardiography (ACUTE) trial (130), the incidence of clinical thromboembolism after treatment with warfarin (INR, 2.0 to 3.0) for 3 weeks before cardioversion was 0.5% in 603 patients. During the conventional treatment phase of the Ludwigshafen Observational Cardioversion study (129),

357 patients undergoing successful DC cardioversion had a 0.8% incidence of neurologic events.

Following restoration of normal atrial electrical activity on the surface electrocardiogram (ECG) after cardioversion, the mechanical contraction of the left atrium may remain dysfunctional for 2 to 4 weeks (131–133). Delayed atrial recovery appears related to the duration of AF before cardioversion (134,135). Hence, anticoagulation should be continued for 1 month following cardioversion. In addition to prophylaxis against thrombus formation pending recovery of atrial mechanical function, warfarin has prophylactic value against thromboembolism in the event of recurrent AF. The duration of anticoagulation following apparently successful cardioversion should be proportionate to the patient-specific intrinsic risk of thromboembolism and to the likelihood of asymptomatic recurrence of AF. Recommendations for the use of anticoagulants in patients undergoing cardioversion have been proposed by the American College of Chest Physicians (ACCP) and are summarized in Table 104-2.

## Transesophageal Echocardiography-Guided Cardioversion

The accuracy of TEE for detection of thrombus in the left atrium and LAA and the association of this finding with the risk of thromboembolism following cardioversion (8,136) offers an opportunity to perform cardioversion earlier in patients in whom no thrombus is found. In several studies (8,16,125,128, 130,133), observed rates of thromboembolism were similar to those associated with standard therapy for 3 to 4 weeks of anticoagulation before elective cardioversion, with the advantages of an earlier recovery of atrial mechanical function, ease of anticoagulation management, elimination of the need for readmission for elective cardioversion, and potential cost-effectiveness (137). Limitations of the TEE approach include patient discomfort, rare procedural complications, and limited availability at some centers. Despite the absence of left-atrial appendage thrombi on precardioversion TEE, stroke has been described among patients who did not receive anticoagulation at the time of TEE or continued anticoagulation during the pericardioversion period through a full month after cardioversion (138–141). Furthermore, anticoagulation with heparin and/or warfarin is necessary at the time of TEE and cardioversion to prevent thrombus formation during or following cardioversion.

The ACUTE trial enrolled 1,222 patients with AF for whom elective electrical cardioversion was planned to compare the conventional versus the TEE-guided approach (7). In the TEE-guided arm, five ischemic neurologic events occurred among 619 subjects versus three events among 603 in the conventional arm (P = NS). Most of the adverse events in the TEE-guided group were associated with recurrent AF and subtherapeutic anticoagulation intensity (INR <2.0). Many of the patients in the conventional management arm converted to NSR spontaneously during the month of anticoagulation before scheduled cardioversion. In general, cardioversion occurred earlier in the TEE-guided group, but there was no difference in the prevalence of NSR by 8 weeks following randomization. In other smaller (nonrandomized) studies of patients in whom the duration of AF was less than 3 weeks, however, the rate of recurrent AF was lower and the likelihood of NSR at 1 year was greater among subjects undergoing TEE-guided cardioversion (142).

## Cardioversion for Atrial Fibrillation of Recent Onset

When AF is known to have been present for less than 48 hours, cardioversion is commonly performed without either

**TABLE 104-2**

RECOMMENDATIONS FOR ANTICOAGULATION OF PATIENTS UNDERGOING
CARDIOVERSION OF ATRIAL FIBRILLATION OR FLUTTER

| Clinical situation | Recommendation |
| --- | --- |
| AF of >48 h or unknown duration; pharmacologic or electrical cardioversion | Oral vitamin K antagonist, such as warfarin (INR, 2.0–3.0), for 3 wk before elective cardioversion and for at least 4 wk after successful cardioversion, regardless of risk factor status; continuation of anticoagulation beyond 4 wk is based on whether the patient has experienced more than one episode of AF and on stroke risk stratification |
| Alternative TEE-guided approach | Intravenous unfractionated heparin (PTT twice the control value [50–70 s]) or warfarin for >5 d (INR, 2.0–3.0) at the time of cardioversion. If no thrombus is visualized on screening multiplane TEE and cardioversion is successful, then warfarin (INR 2.0–3.0) should be continued for at least 4 wk, regardless of risk factor status; continued anticoagulation beyond 4 wk is based on whether there is a history of recurrent AF and on intrinsic thromboembolic risk; when thrombus is identified, cardioversion should be postponed and anticoagulation continued indefinitely, repeating TEE before any subsequent cardioversion attempt |
| AF of presumed duration <48 h in the absence of contraindications to anticoagulation | Intravenous heparin (PTT twice control) or subcutaneous low-molecular-weight heparin (in the dose used for treatment of acute venous thrombosis) during the pericardioversion period; following cardioversion, anticoagulation is based on a history of recurrent AF and risk stratification |
| Emergency cardioversion, when the TEE-guided approach is not feasible | Intravenous unfractionated heparin (target PTT twice control) followed by 4 wk of warfarin (INR, 2.0–3.0) if NSR is restored and persists following cardioversion, continuation of anticoagulation thereafter is based on whether the patient has experienced recurrent AF and on risk stratification |
| Recurrent or paroxysmal AF | Antithrombotic therapy beyond the 4-wk period after cardioversion is based on stroke-risk stratification, regardless of whether cardioversion has successfully restored persistent sinus rhythm |
| Atrial flutter | Same recommendations as for patients with AF |

AF, atrial fibrillation; INR, international normalized ratio; TEE, transesophageal echocardiography; PTT, partial thromboplastin time; NSR, normal sinus rhythm.
Adapted from Singer DE, Albers GW, Dalen JE, et al. Long-term antithrombotic therapy for chronic atrial fibrillation or atrial flutter: Anticoagulants and antiplatelet agents. In Seventh ACCP Consensus Conference on Antithrombotic Therapy: Antithrombotic Therapy in Atrial Fibrillation. American College of Chest Physicians. *Chest* (Suppl) 2004;126:429S–456S.

prolonged antecedent anticoagulation or TEE examination. In a study of 357 patients with symptomatic AF for less than 48 hours (143), 250 converted spontaneously and 107 underwent pharmacologic or electrical cardioversion without prolonged anticoagulation or TEE before cardioversion. The rate of clinical thromboembolism was less than 1%. In another retrospective study of 258 patients undergoing cardioversion for AF of less than 2 days duration, one ischemic event occurred among 198 patients not given anticoagulation before or following cardioversion (0.5%) versus none among 60 patients treated with anticoagulation (144). Given the limitations of

these studies, heparin is generally recommended immediately before and during cardioversion and warfarin for 4 weeks following cardioversion of patients with AF of known recent onset (<48 hours duration). For high-risk patients, it seems prudent either to perform TEE or delay cardioversion for a month to allow prior anticoagulant treatment. When emergency cardioversion is necessary to terminate AF associated with a rapid ventricular response causing angina, heart failure, hypotension, or syncope, heparin is generally recommended at the time of cardioversion followed by oral anticoagulant therapy for at least 4 weeks.

## *References*

1. Go AS, Hylek EM, Phillips KA, et al. Prevalence of diagnosed atrial fibrillation in adults: national implications for rhythm management and stroke prevention: the AnTicoagulation and Risk Factors in Atrial Fibrillation (ATRIA) Study. *JAMA* 2001;285:2370–2375.

2. Feinberg WM, Blackshear JL, Laupacis A, et al. Prevalence, age distribution, and gender of patients with atrial fibrillation: analysis and implications. *Arch Intern Med* 1995;155:468–473.

3. Lake FR, Cullen KJ, de Klerk NH, et al. Atrial fibrillation and mortality in an elderly population. *Aust N Z J Med* 1989;19:321–326.

4. Phillips SJ, Whisnant JP, O'Fallon WM, et al. Prevalence of cardiovascular disease and diabetes mellitus in residents of Rochester, Minnesota. *Mayo Clin Proc* 1990;65:344–359.

5. Furberg CD, Psaty BM, Manolio TA, et al. Prevalence of atrial fibrillation in elderly subjects (the Cardiovascular Health Study). *Am J Cardiol* 1994; 74:236–241.

6. Corrado G, Sgalambro A, Mantero A, et al. Thromboembolic risk in atrial flutter. The FLASIEC (FLutter Atriale Societa Italiana di Ecografia Cardiovascolare) multicentre study. *Eur Heart J* 2001;22:1042–1051.

7. Fuster V, Rydén LE, Asinger RW, et al. ACC/AHA/ESC guidelines for the management of patients with atrial fibrillation: executive summary. A report of the American College of Cardiology/American Heart Association Task Force on Practice Guidelines and the European Society of Cardiology Committee for Practice Guidelines and Policy Conferences (Committee to Develop Guidelines for the Management of Patients with Atrial Fibrillation) Developed in Collaboration with the North American Society of Pacing and Electrophysiology. *Circulation* 2001;104:2118–2150.

8. Collins LJ, Silverman DI, Douglas PS, et al. Cardioversion of nonrheumatic atrial fibrillation. Reduced thromboembolic complications with 4 weeks of precardioversion anticoagulation are related to atrial thrombus resolution. *Circulation* 1995;92:160–163.

9. Bogousslavsky J, Van Melle G, Regli F, et al. Pathogenesis of anterior circulation stroke in patients with nonvalvular atrial fibrillation. *Neurology* 1990;40:1046–1050.

10. Szekely P. Systemic embolism and anticoagulant prophylaxis in rheumatic heart disease. *BMJ* 1964;1:209–212.

11. Cerebral Embolism Task Force. Cardiogenic brain embolism: the second report of the Cerebral Embolism Task Force. *Arch Neurol* 1989; 46: 727–743.

12. Atrial Fibrillation Investigators. Risk factors for stroke and efficacy of antithrombotic therapy in atrial fibrillation. Analysis of pooled data from five randomized controlled trials. *Arch Intern Med* 1994;154: 1449–1457.

13. Wolf PA, Abbott RD, Kannel WB. Atrial fibrillation: a major contributor to stroke in the elderly. The Framingham Study. *Arch Intern Med* 1987; 147: 1561–1564.

14. Wolf PA, Abbott RD, Kannel WB. Atrial fibrillation as an independent risk factor for stroke: the Framingham Study. *Stroke* 1991;22:983–988.

15. Hart RG, Halperin JL. Atrial fibrillation and stroke: revisiting the dilemmas. *Stroke* 1994;25:1337–1341.

16. Grimm RA, Stewart WJ, Arheart KL, et al. Left atrial appendage "stunning" after electrical cardioversion of atrial flutter: an attenuated response compared with atrial fibrillation as the mechanism for lower susceptibility to thromboembolic events. *J Am Coll Cardiol* 1997;29:582–589.

17. Schmidt H, von der Recke G, Illien S, et al. Prevalence of left atrial chamber and appendage thrombi in patients with atrial flutter and its clinical significance. *J Am Coll Cardiol* 2001;38:778–784.

18. Weiss R, Marcovitz P, Knight BP, et al. Acute changes in spontaneous echo contrast and atrial function after cardioversion of persistent atrial flutter. *Am J Cardiol* 1998;82:1052–1055.

19. Bikkina M, Alpert MA, Mulekar M, et al. Prevalence of intraatrial thrombus in patients with atrial flutter. *Am J Cardiol* 1995;76:186–189.

20. Lanzarotti CJ, Olshansky B. Thromboembolism in chronic atrial flutter: is the risk underestimated? *J Am Coll Cardiol* 1997;30:1506–1511.

21. EAFT (European Atrial Fibrillation Trial) Study Group. Secondary prevention in non-rheumatic atrial fibrillation after transient ischaemic attack or minor stroke. *Lancet* 1993;342:1255–1262.

22. Aronow WS, Ahn C, Kronzon I, et al. Incidence of new thromboembolic stroke in persons 62 years and older with chronic atrial fibrillation treated with warfarin versus aspirin. *J Am Geriatr Soc* 1999;47:366–368.

23. SPAFIII Writing Committee for the Stroke Prevention in Atrial Fibrillation Investigators. Patients with nonvalvular atrial fibrillation at low risk of stroke during treatment with aspirin. *JAMA* 1998;279:1273–1277.

24. Atrial Fibrillation Investigators. Echocardiographic predictors of stroke in patients with atrial fibrillation. *Arch Intern Med* 1998;158:1316–1320.

25. Hart RG, Benavente O, McBride R, et al. Antithrombotic therapy to prevent stroke in patients with atrial fibrillation: a meta-analysis. *Ann Intern Med* 1999;131:492–501.

26. Stroke Prevention in Atrial Fibrillation Investigators. Predictors of thromboembolism in atrial fibrillation: I. Clinical features of patients at risk. The Stroke Prevention in Atrial Fibrillation Study. *Ann Intern Med* 1992;116:1–5.

27. Stroke Prevention in Atrial Fibrillation Investigators. Risk factors for thromboembolism during aspirin therapy in patients with atrial fibrillation: the Stroke Prevention in Atrial Fibrillation Study. *J Stroke Cerebrovasc Dis* 1995;5:147–157.

28. Hart RG, Pearce LA, McBride R, et al. Factors associated with ischemic stroke during aspirin therapy in atrial fibrillation: analysis of 2012 participants in the SPAF I-III clinical trials. The Stroke Prevention in Atrial Fibrillation (SPAF) Investigators. *Stroke* 1999;30:1223–1229.

29. Pearce LA, Hart RG, Halperin, JL. Assessment of three schemes for stratifying stroke risk in patients with nonvalvular atrial fibrillation. *Am J Med* 2000;109:45–51.

30. Gage BF, Waterman AD, Shannon W, et al. Validation of clinical classification schemes for predicting stroke: results from the national registry of atrial fibrillation. *JAMA* 2001;285:2864–2870.

31. Petersen P. Thromboembolic complications in atrial fibrillation. *Stroke* 1990;21:4–13.

32. Brand FN, Abbott RD, Kanle WB, et al. Characteristics and prognosis of lone atrial fibrillation: 30 year follow-up in the Framingham Study. *JAMA* 1985;254:3449–3453.

33. Hart R, Pearce L, Miller V, et al. Cardioembolic versus noncardioemblic strokes in atrial fibrillation: frequency and effect of antithrombotic agents in the stroke prevention in atrial fibrillation studies. *Cerebrovasc Dis* 2000; 10:39–43.

34. Stollberger C, Chnupa P, Kronik G, et al. Transesophageal echocardiography to assess embolic risk in patients with atrial fibrillation. *Ann Intern Med* 1998;128:630–638.

35. Stroke Prevention in Atrial Fibrillation Investigators Committee on Echocardiography. Transesophageal echocardiographic correlates of thromboembolism in high-risk patients with nonvalvular atrial fibrillation. *Ann Intern Med* 1998; 128:639–647.

36. Feinberg WM, Kronmal R, Newman AB, et al. Stroke risk in an elderly population with atrial fibrillation. *J Gen Intern Med* 1999;14:56–59.

37. Conway DS, Pearce LA, Chin BS, et al. Plasma von Willebrand factor and soluble p-selectin as indices of endothelial damage and platelet activation in 1321 patients with nonvalvular atrial fibrillation: relationship to stroke risk factors. *Circulation* 2002;106:1962–1967.

38. Singer DE, Albers GW, Dalen JE, Go AS, et al. Long-term Antithrombotic Therapy for Chronic Atrial Fibrillation or Atrial Flutter: Anticoagulants and Antiplatelet Agents. In Seventh ACCP Consensus Conference on Antithrombotic Therapy: Antithrombotic Therapy in Atrial Fibrillation. American College of Chest Physicians. *Chest* (Suppl) 2004;126:429S–456S.

39. Presti CF, Hart RG. Thyrotoxicosis, atrial fibrillation, and embolism, revisted. *Am Heart J* 1989;117:976–977.

40. Staffurth JS, Gibberd MC, Fui SN. Arterial embolism in thyrotoxicosis with atrial fibrillation. *BMJ* 1977;2:688–690.

41. Yuen RW, Gutteridge DH, Thompson PL, et al. Embolism in thyrotoxic atrial fibrillation. *Med J Aust* 1979;1:630–631.

42. Hurley DM, Hunter AN, Hewett MJ, et al. Atrial fibrillation and arterial embolism in hyperthyroidism. *Aust N Z J Med* 1981;11:391–393.

43. Bar-Sela S, Ehrenfeld M, Eliakim M. Arterial embolism in thyrotoxicosis with atrial fibrillation. *Arch Intern Med* 1981;141:1191–1192.

44. Petersen P, Hansen JM. Stroke in thyrotoxicosis with atrial fibrillation. *Stroke* 1988;19:15–18.

45. Devereaux PJ, Anderson DR, Gardner MJ, et al. Differences between perspectives of physicians and patients on anticoagulation in patients with atrial fibrillation. *BMJ* 2001;323:1–7.

46. Gage BF, Cardinalli AB, Owens DK. The effect of stroke and stroke prophylaxis with aspirin or warfarin on quality of life. *Arch Intern Med* 1996; 156: 1829–1836.

47. Solomon NA, Glick HA, Russo CJ, et al. Patient preferences for stroke outcomes. *Stroke* 1994;25:1721–1725.

48. Eckman MH, Levine HJ, Salem DN, et al. Making decisions about antithrombotic therapy in heart disease: decision analytic and cost-effectiveness issues. *Chest* 1998;114(Suppl. 5):699s–714s.

49. Man-Son-Hing M, Laupacis A, O'Connor AM, et al. A patient decision aid regarding antithrombotic therapy for stroke prevention in atrial fibrillation: a randomized controlled trial. *JAMA* 1999;282:737–743.

50. Petersen P, Boysen G, Godtfredsen J, et al. Placebo-controlled, randomised trial of warfarin and aspirin for prevention of thromboembolic complications in chronic atrial fibrillation: the Copenhagen AFASAK study. *Lancet* 1989;1:175–179.

51. Stroke Prevention in Atrial Fibrillation Investigators. Stroke prevention in atrial fibrillation study: final results. *Circulation* 1991;84:527–539.

52. The effect of low-dose warfarin on the risk of stroke in patients with nonrheumatic atrial fibrillation. The Boston Area Anticoagulation Trial for Atrial Fibrillation Investigators. *N Engl J Med* 1990;323:1505–1511.

53. Connolly SJ, Laupacis A, Gent M, Roberts RS, Cairns JA, Joyner C. Canadian Atrial Fibrillation Anticoagulation (CAFA) Study. *J Am Coll Cardiol* 1991;18:349–355.

54. Ezekowitz MD, Bridgers SL, James KE, et al. Warfarin in the prevention of stroke associated with nonrheumatic atrial fibrillation. Veterans Affairs Stroke Prevention in Nonrheumatic Atrial Fibrillation Investigators. *N Engl J Med* 1992;327:1406–1412.

55. Stroke Prevention in Atrial Fibrillation Investigators. Warfarin compared to aspirin for prevention of thromboembolism in atrial fibrillation: results of the Stroke Prevention in Atrial Fibrillation II Study. *Lancet* 1994;343: 687–691.

56. Connolly SJ. Stroke prevention in atrial fibrillation II study [letter]. *Lancet* 1994;343:1509.

57. Miller VT, Pearce L, Feinberg WM, et al. Differential effect of aspirin versus warfarin on clinical stroke types in patients with atrial fibrillation. Stroke Prevention in Atrial Fibrillation Investigators. *Neurology* 1996;46: 238–240.

58. European Atrial Fibrillation Trial Study Group. Optimal oral anticoagulant therapy in patients with nonrheumatic atrial fibrillation and recent cerebral ischemia. *N Engl J Med* 1995;333:5–10.

59. Hylek E, Skates S, Sheehan M, et al. An analysis of the lowest effective intensity of prophylactic anticoagulation for patients with nonrheumatic atrial fibrillation. *N Engl J Med* 1996;335:540–546.

60. Cannegieter SC, Rosendaal FR, Wintzen AR, et al. Optimal oral anticoagulant therapy in patients with mechanical heart valves: the Leiden artificial valve and anticoagulation study. *N Engl J Med* 1995;333:11–17.

61. Diener HC, Cunha L, Forbes C, et al. European stroke prevention study 2: dipyridamole and acetylsalicylic acid in the prevention of stroke. *J Neurol Sci* 1996;143:1–13.

62. Diener HC, Lowenthal A. Letter to the editor. *J Neurol Sci* 1997;153:112.

63. Gullov AL, Koefoed BG, Petersen P, et al. Fixed mini-dose warfarin and aspirin alone and in combination versus adjusted-dose warfarin for stroke prevention in atrial fibrillation: Second Copenhagen Atrial Fibrillation, Aspirin, and Anticoagulation Study. *Arch Intern Med* 1998;158:1513–1521.

64. Posada IS, Barriales V. Alternate-day dosing of aspirin in atrial fibrillation. LASAF Pilot Study Group. *Am Heart J* 1999;138:137–143.

65. Atrial Fibrillation Investigators. The efficacy of aspirin in patients with atrial fibrillation. Analysis of pooled data from 3 randomized trials. *Arch Intern Med* 1997:157:1237–1240.

66. Singer DE, Hughes RA, Gress DR. The effect of aspirin on the risk of stroke in patients with nonrheumatic atrial fibrillation. *Am Heart J* 1992;124: 1567–1573.

67. Miller VT, Rothrock J, Pearce LA, et al. Ischemic stroke in patients with atrial fibrillation: effect of aspirin according to stroke mechanism. *Neurology* 1993;43:32–36.

68. Hart RG, Pearce L, Miller VT, et al. Cardioembolic vs. noncardioembolic strokes in atrial fibrillation: frequency and effect of antithrombotic agents in the stroke prevention in atrial fibrillation studies. *Cerebrovasc Dis* 2000;10:39–43.

69. Hellemons BS, Langenberg M, Lodder J, et al. Primary prevention of arterial thromboembolism in non-rheumatic atrial fibrillation in primary care: randomised controlled trial comparing two intensities of coumarin with aspirin. *BMJ* 1999;319:958–964.

70. Van Walraven C, Hart RG, Singer DE, et al. Oral anticoagulants vs aspirin in nonvalvular atrial fibrillation: an individual patient meta-analysis. *JAMA* 2002;288:2441–2448.

71. Morocutti C, Amabile G, Fattapposta F, et al. Indobufen versus warfarin in the secondary prevention of major vascular events in nonrheumatic atrial fibrillation. *Stroke* 1997;28:1015–1021.

72. Pengo V, Zasso A, Barbero F, et al. Effectiveness of fixed minidose warfarin in the prevention of thromboembolism and vascular death in nonrheumatic atrial fibrillation. *Am J Cardiol* 1998;82:433–437.

73. Lechat P, Lardoux H, Mallet A, et al. Anticoagulant (fluindione)-aspirin combination in patients with high-risk atrial fibrillation. A randomized trial (Fluindione, Fibrillation Auriculaire, Aspirin et Contraste Spontane; FFAACS). *Cerebrovasc Dis* 2001;12:245–252.

74. Perez Gomez F, Lourenzo PI, Companion J, et al. Platelet aggregation in different antithrombotic regimens. Possible proaggregant effect of low level oral anticoagulation. *Rev Port Cardiol* 2002;21:541–551.

75. Eriksson H, Eriksson UG, Frison L, et al. Pharmacokinetics and pharmacodynamics of melagatran, a novel synthetic LMW thrombin inhibitor, in patients with acute DVT. *Thromb Haemost* 1999;81:358–363.

76. Eriksson-Lepkowska M, Thuresson A, Johansson S, et al. The effect of the oral direct thrombin inhibitor ximelagatran on the pharmacokinetics of P450-metabolized drugs, in healthy male volunteers. *Blood* 2001;98:89b.

77. Eriksson BI, Agnelli G, Cohen AT, et al. Direct thrombin inhibitor melagatran followed by oral ximelagatran in comparison with enoxaparin for prevention of venous thromboembolism after total hip or knee replacement. *Thromb Haemost* 2003; 89:288–296.

78. Eriksson BI, Bergqvist D, Kalebo P, et al. Ximelagatran and melagatran compared with dalteparin for prevention of venous thromboembolism after total hip or knee replacement: the METHRO II randomised trial. *Lancet* 2002;360:1441–1447

79. Heit JA, Colwell C, Francis CW, et al. Comparison of the oral direct thrombin inhibitor ximelagatran with enoxaparin as prophylaxis against venous thromboembolism after total knee replacement: a phase 2 dose-finding study. *Arch Intern Med* 2001;161:2215–2221.

80. Francis CW, Davidson B, Berkowitz SD, et al. Ximelagatran versus warfarin for the prevention of venous thromboembolism after total knee arthroplasty. A randomized, double-blind trial. *Ann Intern Med* 2002; 137: 648–655.

81. The Executive Steering Committee on behalf of the SPORTIF III Investigators. Stroke prevention using the oral direct thrombin inhibitor ximelagatran compared with warfarin in patients with nonvalvular atrial fibrillation: The SPORTIF III trial. *Lancet* 2003;362:1691–1698.

82. Albers GW, Diener HC, Frison L, et al. The Executive Steering Committee on behalf of the SPORTIF V Investigators. Ximelagatran vs. warfarin for stroke prevention in patients with nonvalvular atrial fibrillation: The SPORTIF V randomized trial. 2005; *JAMA* 293:690–698.

83. Halperin JL, and the Executive Steering Committee (ESC) on behalf of the SPORTIF III and V Study Investigators. Ximelagatran compared with warfarin for the prevention of thromboembolism in patients with nonvalvular atrial fibrillation: rationale, objectives and design of a pair of clinical trials and baseline patient characteristics (SPORTIF III and V). *Am Heart J* 2003;146:431–438.

84. Ebbutt AF, Frith L. Practical issues in equivalence trials. *Stat Med* 1998;17: 1691–1701.

85. Gomberg-Maitland M, Frison L, Halperin JL. Active-control clinical trials to establish equivalence or noninferiority: methodological and statistical concepts linked to quality. *Am Heart J* 2003;146:398–403.

86. Herbert JM, Herault JP, Bernat A, et al. Biochemical and pharmacological properties of SANORG 34006, a potent and long-acting synthetic pentasaccharide. *Blood* 1998;91:4197–4205.

87. PERSIST Investigators. A novel long-acting synthetic factor Xa inhibitor (SanOrg34006) to replace warfarin for secondary prevention in deep vein thrombosis. A phase II evaluation. *J Thromb Haemost* 2004;2:47–53.

88. Koopman MM, Buller HR. Short- and long-acting synthetic pentasaccharides. *J Intern Med* 2003;254:335–342.

89. Gachet C, Stierle A, Cazenave JP, et al. The thienopyridine PCR 4099 selectively inhibits ADP-induced platelet aggregation and fibrinogen binding without modifying the membrane glycoprotein IIb-IIIa complex in rat and in man. *Biochem Pharmacol* 1990;40:229–238.

90. Yusuf S, Zhao F, Mehta SR, et al. Clopidogrel in Unstable Angina to Prevent Recurrent Events Trial Investigators. Effects of clopidogrel in addition to aspirin in patients with acute coronary syndromes without ST-segment elevation. *N Engl J Med* 2001;345:494–502.

91. CAPRIE Steering Committee. A randomised, blinded, trial of clopidogrel versus aspirin in patients at risk of ischaemic events (CAPRIE). *Lancet* 1996;348:1329–1339.

92. Vermes E, Tardif JC, Bourassa MG, et al. Enalapril decreases the incidence of atrial fibrillation in patients with left ventricular dysfunction: insight from the Studies Of Left Ventricular Dysfunction (SOLVD) trials. *Circulation* 2003;107:2926–2931.

93. Madrid AH, Bueno MG, Rebollo JM, et al. Use of irbesartan to maintain sinus rhythm in patients with long-lasting persistent atrial fibrillation: a prospective and randomized study. *Circulation* 2002;106:331–336.

94. Mathew JP, Fontes ML, Tudor IC, et al. A multicenter risk index for atrial fibrillation after cardiac surgery. *JAMA* 2004;291:1720–1729.

95. Ansell J, Hirsh J, Dalen J, et al. Managing oral anticoagulant therapy. *Chest* 2001;119:22S–38S.

96. Goette A, Staack T, Rocken C, et al. Increased expression of extracellular signal-regulated kinase and angiotensin-converting enzyme in human atria during atrial fibrillation. *J Am Coll Cardiol* 2000;35:1669–1677.

97. AFFIRM Investigators. A comparison of rate control and rhythm control in patients with atrial fibrillation. *N Engl J Med* 2002;347: 1825–1833.

98. Van Gelder IC, Hagens VE, Bosker HA, et al. A comparison of rate control and rhythm control in patients with recurrent persistent atrial fibrillation. *N Engl J Med* 2002;347:1834–1840.

99. Hohnloser SH, Kuck KH, Lilienthal J. Rhythm or rate control in atrial fibrillation—Pharmacological Intervention in Atrial Fibrillation (PIAF): a randomised trial. *Lancet* 2000;356:1789–1794.

100. Zarembski DG, Nolan PE Jr, Slack MK, et al. Treatment of resistant atrial fibrillation. A meta-analysis comparing amiodarone and flecainide. *Arch Intern Med* 1995;155:1885–1891.

101. Antonielli E, Pizzuti A, Palinkas A, et al. Clinical value of left atrial appendage flow for prediction of long-term sinus rhythm maintenance in patients with nonvalvular atrial fibrillation. *J Am Coll Cardiol* 2002;39: 1443–1449.

102. Page RL, Wilkinson WE, Clair WK, et al. Asymptomatic arrhythmias in patients with symptomatic paroxysmal atrial fibrillation and paroxysmal supraventricular tachycardia. *Circulation* 1994;89:224–227.

103. Cox JL, Schuessler RB, D'Agostino HJ Jr, et al. The surgical treatment of atrial fibrillation. III. Development of a definitive surgical procedure. *J Thorac Cardiovasc Surg* 1991;101:569–583.

104. Plumb VJ, Windecker S, Epstein AE, et al. Nonpharmacologic therapy of atrial fibrillation and atrial flutter. *Am J Geriatr Cardiol* 1998;7:21–26.

105. Cox JL, Ad N, Palazzo T. Impact of the maze procedure on the stroke rate in patients with atrial fibrillation. *J Thorac Cardiovasc Surg* 1999;118: 833–840.

106. Handa N, Schaff HV, Morris JJ, et al. Outcome of valve repair and the Cox maze procedure for mitral regurgitation and associated atrial fibrillation. *J Thorac Cardiovasc Surg* 1999;118:628–635.

107. Gillinov AM, McCarthy PM, Marrouche N, et al. Contemporary surgical treatment for atrial fibrillation. *Pacing Clin Electrophysiol* 2003;26: 1641–1644.

108. Garrido MJ, Williams M, Argenziano M. Minimally invasive surgery for atrial fibrillation. *J Card Surg* 2004;19:216–220.

109. Haissaguerre M, Jais P, Shah DC, et al. Spontaneous initiation of atrial fibrillation by ectopic beats originating in the pulmonary veins. *N Engl J Med* 1998;339:659–666.

110. Stabile G, Bertaglia E, Senatore G, et al. Feasibility of pulmonary vein ostia radiofrequency ablation in patients with atrial fibrillation: a multicenter study (CACAF Pilot Study). *Pacing Clin Electrophysiol* 2003;26: 284–287.

111. Blackshear JL, Odell JA. Appendage obliteration to reduce stroke in cardiac surgical patients with atrial fibrillation. *Ann Thorac Surg* 1996;61: 755–759.

112. Ostermayer SH, Reisman M, Kramer PH, et al. Percutaneous left atrial appendage transcatheter occlusion (PLAATO system) to prevent stroke in high-risk patients with non-rheumatic atrial fibrillation: results from the international multi-center feasibility trials. *J Am Coll Cardiol* 2005;46:9–14.

113. Blackshear JL, Johnson WD, Odell JA, et al. Thoracoscopic extracardiac obliteration of the left atrial appendage for stroke risk reduction in atrial fibrillation. *J Am Coll Cardiol* 2003;42:1249–1252.

114. Halperin JL, Gomberg-Maitland M. Obliteration of the left atrial appendage for prevention of thromboembolism. *J Am Coll Cardiol* 2003; 42: 1259–1261.

115. Morris JJ Jr, Peter RH, McIntosh HD. Electrical cardioversion of atrial fibrillation: immediate and long-term results and selection of patients. *Ann Intern Med* 1966;65:216–231.

116. Arnold AZ, Mick M, Mazurek RP, et al. Role of prophylactic anticoagulation for direct current cardioversion in patients with atrial fibrillation or atrial flutter. *J Am Coll Cardiol* 1992;19:851–855.

117. Lown B. Electrical reversion of cardiac arrhythmias. *Br Heart J* 1967; 29: 469–489.

118. Resnekov L, McDonald L. Complication in 220 patients with cardiac dysrhythmias treated by phased DC schock and indications for electroconversion. *Br Heart J* 1967;29:926–936.

119. McCarthy C, Varghese PJ, Barritt DW. Prognosis of atrial arrhythmais treated by electrical countershock therapy. A three-year follow-up. *Br Heart J* 1969;31:496–500.

120. Bjerkelund CJ, Orning OM. The efficacy of anticoagulant therapy in preventing embolism related to DC electrical conversion of atrial fibrillation. *Am J Cardiol* 1969;23:208–216.

121. Berger M, Schweitzer P. Timing of thromboembolic events after electrical cardioversion of atrial fibrillation or flutter: a retrospective analysis. *Am J Cardiol* 1998;82:1545–1547, A8.

122. Grimm RA, Stewart WJ, Maloney JD, et al. Impact of electrical cardioversion of atrial fibrillation on left atrial appendage function and spontaneous echo contrast: characterization by simultaneous transesophageal echocardiography. *J Am Coll Cardiol* 1993;22:1359–1366.

123. Omran H, Jung W, Rabahieh R, et al. Left atrial chamber and appendage function after internal cardioversion: a prospective and serial transesophageal echocardiographic study. *J Am Coll Cardiol* 1997;29:131–138.

124. Grimm R, Leung D, Black I, et al. Left atrial appendage "stunning" after spontaneous conversion of atrial fibrillation demonstrated by transesophageal Doppler echocardiography. *Am Heart J* 1995;130:174–176.

125. Stoddard M, Dawkins P, Prince C, et al. Left atrial appendage thrombus is not uncommon in patients with acute atrial fibrillation and a recent embolic event: a transesophageal echocardiographic study. *J Am Coll Cardiol* 1995;25:452–459.

126. DeSilva RA, Graboys TB, Podrid PJ, et al. Cardioversion and defibrillation. *Am Heart J* 1980;100:881–895.

127. Mancini GB, Goldberger AL. Cardioversion of atrial fibrillation: consideration of embolization, anticoagulation, prophylactic pacemaker and long-term success. *Am Heart J* 1982;104:617–621.

128. Corrado G, Tadeo G, Beretta S, et al. Atrial thrombi resolution after prolonged anticoagulation in patients with atrial fibrillation. *Chest* 1999;115: 140–143.

129. Seidl K, Rameken M, Drogemuller A, et al. Embolic events in patients with atrial fibrillation and effective anticoagulation: value of transesophageal echocardiography to guide direct-current cardioversion. Final results of the Ludwigshafen Observational Cardioversion Study. *J Am Coll Cardiol* 2002;39:1436–1442.

130. Klein AL, Grimm RA, Murray RD, et al. Use of transesophageal echocardiography to guide cardioversion in patients with atrial fibrillation. *N Engl J Med* 2001;344:1411–1420.

131. Manning WJ, Leeman DE, Gotch PJ, et al. Pulsed Doppler evaluation of atrial mechanical function after electrical cardioversion of atrial fibrillation. *J Am Coll Cardiol* 1989;13:617–623.

132. O'Neill PG, Puleo PR, Bolli R, et al. Return of atrial mechanical function following electrical conversion of atrial dysrhythmias. *Am Heart J* 1990; 120:353–359.

133. Manning WJ, Silverman DI, Gordon SP, et al. Cardioversion from atrial fibrillation without prolonged anticoagulation with use of transesophageal echocardiography to exclude the presence of atrial thrombi. *N Engl J Med* 1993;328:750–755.

134. Shapiro EP, Effron MB, Lima S. Transient atrial dysfunction after conversion of chronic atrial fibrillation to sinus rhythm. *Am J Cardiol* 1988;62: 1202–1207.

135. Manning WJ, Silverman DI, Katz SE. Impaired left atrial mechanical function after cardioversion: relationship to the duration of atrial fibrillation. *J Am Coll Cardiol* 1994;23:1535–1540.

136. Fatkin D, Scalia G, Jacobs N, et al. Accuracy of biplane transesophageal echocardiography in detecting left atrial thrombus. *Am J Cardiol* 1996; 77:321–323.

137. Seto TB, Taira DA, Tsevat J, et al. Cost-effectiveness of transesophageal echocardiographic-guided cardioversion: a decision analytic model for patients admitted to the hospital with atrial fibrillation. *J Am Coll Cardiol* 1997;29:122–130.

138. Salka S, Saeian K, Sagar KB. Cerebral thromboembolization after cardioversion of atrial fibrillation in patients without transesophageal echocardiographic findings of left atrial thrombus. *Am Heart J* 1993;126:722–724.

139. Black IW, Chesterman CN, Hopkins AP, et al. Hematologic correlates of left atrial spontaneous echo contrast and thromboembolism in nonvalvular atrial fibrillation. *J Am Coll Cardiol* 1993;21:451–457.

140. Black IW, Fatkin D, Sagar KB, et al. Exclusion of atrial thrombus by transesophageal echocardiography does not preclude embolism after cardioversion of atrial fibrillation. A multicenter study [see comments]. *Circulation* 1994;89:2509–2513.

141. Moreyra E, Finkelhor RS, Cebul RD. Limitations of transesophageal echocardiography in the risk assessment of patients before nonanticoagulated cardioversion from atrial fibrillation and flutter: an analysis of pooled trials. *Am Heart J* 1995;129:71–75.

142. Weigner MJ, Thomas LR, Patel U, et al. Transesophageal-echocardiography-facilitated early cardioversion from atrial fibrillation: short-term safety and impact on maintenance of sinus rhythm at 1 year. *Am J Med* 2001; 110:694–702.

143. Weigner MJ, Caulfield TA, Danias PG, et al. Risk for clinical thromboembolism associated with conversion to sinus rhythm in patients with atrial fibrillation lasting less than 48 hours. *Ann Intern Med* 1997;126:615–620.

144. Gallagher MM, Hennessy BJ, Edvardsson N. Embolic complications of direct current cardioversion of atrial arrhythmias: association with low intensity of anticoagulation at the time of cardioversion. *J Am Coll Cardiol* 2002;40:926–933.

# CHAPTER 105 ■ ADVANCED CARDIOMYOPATHY AND SURGERY

JONATHAN M. CHEN, ANN MARIE SCHMIDT, AND ERIC A. ROSE

Congestive heart failure (CHF) affects more than 4 million people in the United States today and accounts for nearly 250,000 deaths annually. Cardiomyopathy secondary to left ventricular dysfunction currently represents its most common etiology (1). In the setting of severe cardiomyopathy with a significantly depressed left ventricular ejection fraction (LVEF), areas of rheologic stasis within the ventricle, endothelial abnormalities, and the procoagulant state associated with cardiomyopathy all contribute to the potential for thrombus formation and subsequent embolization. One surgical alternative to medical therapy, transplantation, ameliorates these processes, and thereby obviates the need for anticoagulation. The other, left ventricular assist device (LVAD) implantation, does not necessarily alter these phenomena, and may in fact potentiate the procoagulant state.

However, unlike other multicenter, prospective randomized trials of medical therapy for CHF [e.g., angiotensin converting enzyme (ACE) or β-blocker therapy], no comparable data exists to provide specific guidelines about the use of anticoagulants for patients with a depressed LVEF. Instead, most have relied upon substudies of other major clinical trials to guide their practice. In particular, the trials of greatest utility include those about mortality in heart failure, thromboembolic risk in heart failure [with and without atrial fibrillation (Afib)], thromboembolic risk in the postinfarction state, and thromboembolic risk with intracardiac thrombus.

We will review (a) the pathophysiology of thrombotic risk in cardiomyopathy, (b) the data from the clinical trials previously described, (c) novel agents for future anticoagulation, (d) anticoagulation in the setting of LVAD insertion, and (e) our recommendations for anticoagulation both in the setting of CHF and in the setting of LVAD therapy for end-stage cardiomyopathy.

# THROMBOTIC RISK IN CARDIOMYOPATHY

Patients with cardiomyopathy and poor LVEF are at a risk for arterial and venous thrombosis. The components of Virchow's triad have been implicated in these processes (see Fig. 105-1): dilated ventricles with poor function can generate regions of turbulent flow and stasis, endothelial dysfunction as a consequence of coronary atherosclerosis and vasodilatory failure are common in end-stage cardiomyopathy, and several investigations have demonstrated patients with cardiomyopathy to be hypercoagulable.

Regional areas of myocardial dyskinesis commonly form in the setting of myocardial infarction, most notably at the apex and along the septum of the left ventricle (2). A particularly pronounced example of this is represented by ventricular aneurysm formation in which a large area of dyskinesis (often with paradoxical motion) and stasis forms, representing a nidus for thrombosis. In autopsy studies, the frequency of left ventricular (LV) thrombus in patients with ventricular aneurysms has been estimated to range between 14% and 68%, a finding in keeping with anecdotal observation at surgical aneurysmectomy (3,4). Stagnant blood additionally can often be visualized echocardiographically as "smoke" in dilated atria or ventricles, and represents a finding of particular concern even in the absence of mural thrombus. Indeed, patients with other "low-flow" states, such as mitral stenosis and Afib have additionally demonstrated hypercoaguability (5,6).

Endothelial dysfunction in heart failure is most often attributed to advanced atherosclerosis (for those with ischemic cardiomyopathy). However, even in the setting of idiopathic dilated cardiomyopathy, abnormal vasodilatory function has been demonstrated. Alternatively, the impaired release of endothelium-derived nitric oxide in response to stimuli has been hypothesized by some to contribute not only to increased peripheral vasoconstriction, but also to monocyte and platelet adhesion (7,8). Markers of endothelial dysfunction and damage, such as von Willebrand factor (VWF), have also been demonstrated to be abnormal in the heart failure state (9,10).

Several investigators have demonstrated considerable abnormalities in coagulation to be present in patients with cardiomyopathy and heart failure (see Table 105-1). Mehta et al. reported circulating platelet aggregates to be increased in the setting of heart failure (11). Jafri evaluated 70 patients prospectively and compared them to controls and to a matched cohort of patients with coronary artery disease. In their study, those with heart failure additionally demonstrated increased levels of β-thromboglobulin (β-TG), Thrombin-Antithrombin III (TAT), and D-dimer compared with control patients. When compared with patients with coronary artery disease, those with heart failure had elevated levels of D-dimer and evidence of platelet activation (see Table 105-2) (12).

In contrast, Ikeda et al. have asserted that thrombin activity, and not platelet activity, is particularly enhanced in the setting of heart failure (13). Their study, comparing patients with heart failure and with normal controls elucidated elevated levels of fibrinopeptide A and TAT (both of which correlated with LV end-diastolic volume and diminished LV fractional shortening), and comparable levels of platelet factor 4 PF 4, β-TG, and plasmin–$\alpha_2$-plasmin inhibitor complex (PAP) in patients with heart failure when compared with controls. Relatedly, Gibbs et al. demonstrated elevated levels of hemorheological indices in heart failure recipients who demonstrated improvement with treatment with ACE inhibitors (but not with β–blockers) (14). Hoffmeister similarly reported plasma viscosity in patients with CHF to be negatively correlated with LVEF (15).

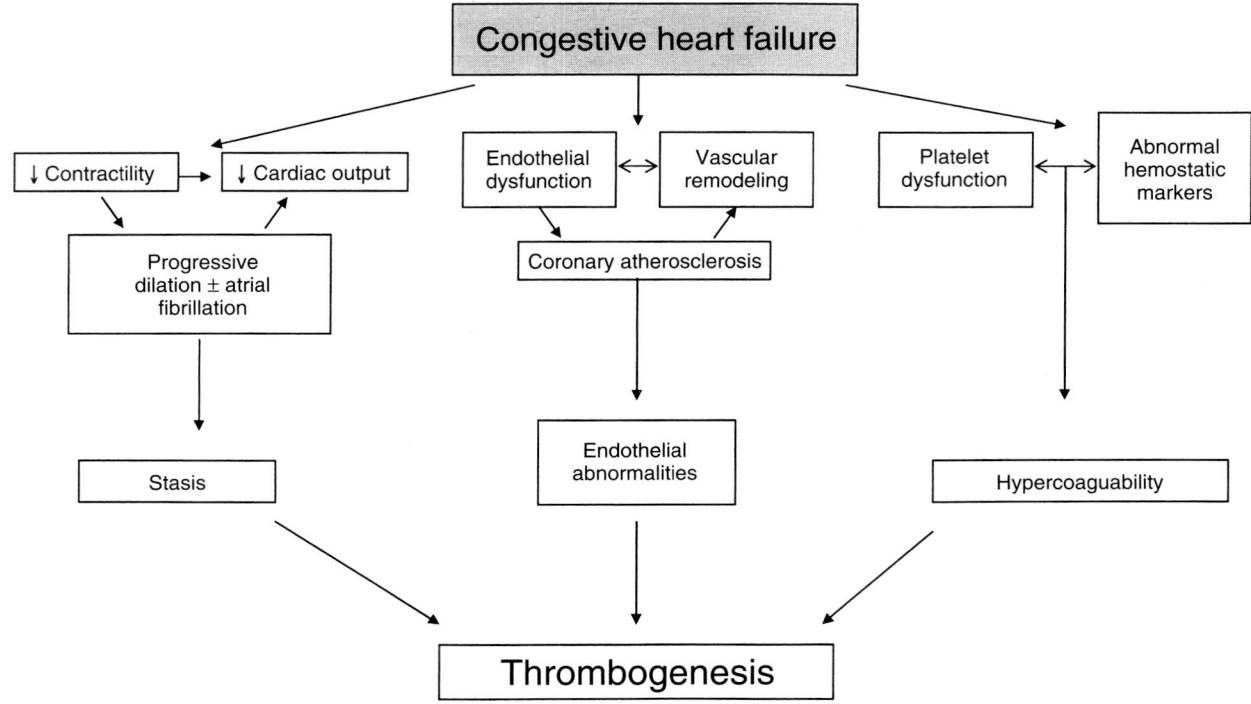

**FIGURE 105-1.** Cascade of pathophysiology in heart failure leading to thrombogenesis. [Modified from Sirajuddin RA, Miller AB, Geraci SA. Anticoagulation in patients with dilated cardiomyopathy and sinus rhythm: a critical literature review. *J Cardiac Failure* 2002;8(1):48–53.]

# INFERENCES FROM CLINICAL TRIALS

## What Is the Risk of Embolic Events with Atrial Fibrillation and a Reduced Left Ventricular Ejection Fraction?

Advanced cardiomyopathy is commonly associated with Afib, and has been identified as an independent risk factor for thromboembolism in all patients with Afib (16,17). Warfarin anticoagulation has been demonstrated in metaanalysis reviews to lower the thromboembolic risk substantially in those patients with Afib, with a relative risk reduction of 68% (19). Stroke prevention trials targeting patients with Afib at a higher risk for embolic events demonstrated superior prophylaxis for those achieving an INR of 2.0 to 3.0, with "heart failure" defined as an LV fractional shortening less than 25% (LVEF <50%) (20).

## What Is the Risk of Embolic Events and Mortality with a Reduced Left Ventricular Ejection Fraction?

The reported incidence of thromboembolism in the setting of heart failure varies substantially. Although historical autopsy

## TABLE 105-1

### STUDIES OF HYPERCOAGUABILITY IN CARDIOMYOPATHY AND HEART FAILURE

| Study | Platelet aggregates | PF4 | β-TG | TAT | D-dimer | PαP | Fibrinopeptide | VWF | Fibrinogen | P selectin |
|---|---|---|---|---|---|---|---|---|---|---|
| Mehta (11) | ↑ | — | — | — | — | — | | | | |
| Jafri (12) | — | Same | ↑ | ↑ | ↑ | — | Same | | | |
| Sbarouni (9) | — | — | ↑ | — | ↑ | — | | | | |
| Lip (10) | — | — | — | — | ↑ | — | — | ↑ | ↑ | |
| Ikeda (13) | — | Same | Same | ↑ | — | Same | ↑ | | | |
| Yamamoto (18) | | Same | Same | ↑ | | Same | ↑ | | | |
| Gibbs (14) | | | | | | | | ↑ | ↑ | ↑ |

PF4, platelet factor 4; β-TG, β-thromboglobulin; TAT, thrombin-antithrombin III complex; PαP, plasmin–α₂-plasmin inhibitor complex; VWF, von Willebrand factor.
From Jafri SM, Ozawa T, Mammen E, et al. Platelet function, thrombin and fibrinolytic activity in patients with heart failure. *Eur Heart J* 1993;14:205–212, with permission.

## TABLE 105-2

### RELATION OF ACTIVATION OF PLATELETS AND COAGULATION SYSTEM TO SEVERITY OF HEART FAILURE

| | | Heart failure | | | |
|---|---|---|---|---|---|
| | Normal | EF >35% | EF <35% | PNE <400 pg/mL | PNE >400 pg/mL |
| | (*n* = 36) | (*n* = 12) | (*n* = 53) | (*n* = 17) | (*n* = 50) |
| **PLATELET FUNCTION** | | | | | |
| β-Thromboglobulin (IU/mL) | 50.2 ± 59.1 | 68 ± 62.4 | 93.7 ± 6.7[a] | 75.3 ± 63.7 | 94.6 ± 62.4[a] |
| **COAGULATION** | | | | | |
| TAT (μg/L) | 2.3 ± 0.6 | 2.7 ± 0.9 | 4.9 ± 4.7[a] | 2.8 ± 1.3 | 5.2 ± 4.8[ab] |
| D-dimer (ng/mL) | 191.1 ± 143.9 | 332 ± 197[a] | 520 ± 448[a] | 269 ± 210 | 586 ± 483[ab] |

EF, ejection fraction; PNE, plasma norepinephrine level; TAT, thrombin-antithrombin III complex.
[a]$P$ <0.05 versus normal.
[b]$P$ <0.05 within heart failure groups.
From Jafri SM, Ozawa T, Mammen E, et al. Platelet function, thrombin and fibrinolytic activity in patients with heart failure. *Eur Heart J* 1993;14:205–212, with permission.

series have reported an incidence as high as 37% to 50% in those with CHF, more recent reports have suggested that the risk of thromboembolism may be as low as 1% to 3% per year for those in sinus rhythm (see Table 105-3) (21–30). Fuster et al. reported an 18% overall prevalence of arterial thromboembolism and an event rate of 3.5 per 100 patient-years in their classic review of 104 patients with idiopathic dilated cardiomyopathy (31). A later study by Katz in 264 patients with a mean LVEF of 27% reported 1.7 cerebral embolic events per 100 patient-years, and a statistically higher mortality and thromboembolic risk in those with LV thrombus (32). These findings were substantiated later by Natterson in 224 patients awaiting transplantation, in whom 3% (3.2 per 100 patient-years) had an arterial embolic episode during the follow-up period (33).

Several postinfarction studies, including the Warfarin Reinfarction Study (WARIS) and Anticoagulants in the Secondary Prevention of Events in Coronary Thrombosis (ASPECT) trials demonstrated a substantial reduction in stroke and mortality in those patients treated with warfarin (INR 2.8 to 4.8) when compared with placebo controls. Although compelling, it must be recalled that these data represent findings in studies of postinfarction patients whose LVEF was not reported (34,35).

The Survival and Ventricular Enlargement (SAVE) trial evaluated the postinfarction of patients with an LVEF less than 40% and demonstrated the stroke risk to be inversely proportional to the ejection fraction (EF); this risk was reduced by both warfarin and aspirin therapy (25). Risk stratification on the basis of LVEF demonstrated those with an LVEF less than 28% to have a twofold increased risk of stroke.

Two large heart failure trials, the Studies of Left Ventricular Dysfunction (SOLVD) and the Vasodilator Heart Failure Trials (V-HEFT I and II), have both been referenced for their conflicting results about anticoagulation in heart failure. In a retrospective analysis of treatment and prevention arms, SOLVD patients (whose LVEF was <35%) were demonstrated to have a significant reduction in all-cause mortality (thought

## TABLE 105-3

### RATES OF STROKE IN HEART FAILURE TREATMENT STUDIES

| Study | NYHA class (median) | LVEF | Stroke rate/yr | Antithrombotics | Afib |
|---|---|---|---|---|---|
| SOLVD (24) | 1.7 | 27% | 1.3% | 63% | 0% |
| SAVE (25) | 1.0 | 31% | 1.5% | 87% | 10% |
| V-HEFT I (26) | 2 or 3 | 30% | 2.0% | 37% | 16% |
| V-HEFT II (26) | 2 or 3 | 29% | 1.9% | 68% | 13% |
| PROMISE (27) | 3.4 | 21% | 3.5% | 81% | N/A |
| Katz (32) | 2.5 | 27% | 1.7% | 49% | 13% |
| Cioffi (28) | 2.7 | 23% | 2.0% | 67% | 16% |
| CONCENSUS (29) | 4.0 | N/A | 2.4% | 26% | 42% |

NYHA class, New York Heart Association Functional Class; LVEF, left ventricular ejection fraction; Afib, atrial fibrillation; SOLVD, Studies of Left Ventricular Dysfunction; SAVE, Survival and Ventricular Enlargement; V-HEFT, Vasodilator Heart Failure Trials; PROMISE, Prospective Randomized Milrinone Survival Evaluation; N/A, not available; CONCENSUS, Cooperative North Scandinavian Enalapril Survival Study.
From Pullicino PM, Halperin JL, Thompson JLP. Stroke in patients with heart failure and reduced left ventricular ejection fraction. *Neurology* 2000;54:288–294, with permission.

**TABLE 105-4**

INCIDENCE AND RELATIVE RISK OF THROMBOEMBOLIC EVENTS BY GENDER AND LEFT VENTRICULAR EJECTION FRACTION IN STUDIES OF LEFT VENTRICULAR DYSFUNCTION

| Left ventricular ejection fraction | No (%) | Incidence | Relative risk (95% confidence interval) |
| --- | --- | --- | --- |
| **MEN (n = 5,457)** | | | |
| ≥30% | 1,892 (35) | 1.70 | 1.00 |
| 21%–30% | 2,590 (47) | 1.83 | 1.08 (0.83–1.41) |
| 11%–20% | 928 (17) | 2.01 | 1.21 (0.86–1.70) |
| ≤10% | 47 (1) | 1.96 | 1.21 (0.30–4.92) |
| **WOMEN (n = 921)** | | | |
| ≥30% | 335 (36) | 1.78 | 1.00 |
| 21%–30% | 422 (46) | 2.41 | 1.35 (0.74–2.47) |
| 11%–20% | 154 (17) | 3.80 | 2.17 (1.10–4.30) |
| ≤10% | 10 (1) | 4.20 | 2.43 (0.32–18.26) |

From Dries DL, Rosenberg YD, Waclawiw MA, et al. Ejection fraction and risk of thromboembolic events in patients with systolic dysfunction and sinus rhythm: evidence for gender differences in studies of left ventricular dysfunction trials. *J Am Coll cardiol* 1997;29:1074–1080, with permission.

primarily to be due to a reduction in cardiovascular mortality) attributed to warfarin therapy (36). Of particular interest was the finding that the relative risk of thromboembolic events was substantially higher among women when compared with men in SOLVD (see Table 105-4) (24).

In contrast, analysis of V-HEFT patients (whose mean LVEF was 29% to 30%) not only failed to show any benefit to anticoagulation in the prevention of thromboembolic events, but also failed to demonstrate an association between Afib and thromboembolic events (26). However, patients with a lower LVEF and lower peak exercise oxygen consumption had a higher risk of stroke. Notably, neither of these trials was designed specifically to evaluate the relative benefits of anticoagulation, nor did either employ a uniform method (or target INR) of anticoagulation.

## What Is the Risk of Embolic Events with Intracardiac Thrombus?

Whereas the presence of an LV thrombus in a patient who has suffered a recent, large myocardial infarction likely increases the thromboembolic risk, the significance of mural thrombi in the setting of chronic heart failure remains less clear. The incidence of mural thrombus after acute anterior myocardial infarction has been documented to range between 21% and 41% (37). Several longitudinal studies have failed to demonstrate a consistent resolution in thrombus as evidenced by echocardiography; however, these studies have suggested protection against stroke for those managed with chronic anticoagulation (38–45). Furthermore, because the sensitivity of echocardiography may not be sufficient to reliably predict systemic embolism in patients with dilated cardiomyopathy and an intracavitary thrombus, often the treatment of such patients is largely empirical (42,43). The American College of Cardiology/American Heart Association guidelines recommend long-term anticoagulation for those with LV thrombus complicating an acute myocardial infarction, a stance supported by metaanalysis of mural thrombus thromboembolic risk after acute myocardial infarction (46,47). Indeed, consistent data support the notion that the appearance of a mobile or protuberant mural thrombus conveys the highest

risk of thromboembolism (and therefore, that such patients with this characteristic should be anticoagulated) (48–50).

# NOVEL AGENTS FOR FUTURE ANTICOAGULATION IN HEART SURGERY

All open-heart surgery requires cardiopulmonary bypass (CPB) to support the circulation and allow for a stable, bloodless operative field. Because of the intense thrombotic response of blood to the extracorporeal circuit of CPB, full-dose heparinization is required to prevent thrombus in the circuit. However, even with protamine reversal, prior heparinization naturally contributes to postoperative coagulopathy, in particular for those with end-stage cardiomyopathy, whose passive hepatic congestion may lead to reduced synthetic function so as to impair normal production of coagulation factors. Cardiac surgery therefore presents a unique platform to study the interaction of intrinsic and extrinsic pathways of coagulation, for while intravascular anticoagulation (for CPB) is required, extravascular hemostasis is valued. In this regard, substantial interest has been expressed toward a more targeted approach to anticoagulation during open-heart surgery.

In CPB, the surfaces of the extracorporeal circuit provide a substrate for activation of the intrinsic (contact) pathway. In normal hemostasis, the contact/intrinsic pathway does not have a significant role. Therefore, inhibition of this pathway would not be expected to cause excessive bleeding because tissue wounds express abundant tissue factor (TF) constitutively in the interstitial and subcutaneous tissues. Once a tissue wound is created, TF may bind factor VIIa and lead to activation of factor X; direct activation of factor X by factor VIIa-TF constitutes the hemostatic response (51,52). It is for this reason that a nearly certain consequence of effective blockade of factor VIIa or TF would be blockade of the hemostatic response and, therefore, a bleeding diathesis.

In the absence of CPB or extracorporeal circuitry, studies by Bauer et al. have demonstrated that factor IX is activated *in vivo* by the TF mechanism and, in homeostasis, factor IXa generation results mainly from the TF mechanism rather than the intrinsic pathway mechanism (53). In homeostasis, in the absence of triggering events, levels of TF are low. However, during CPB, TF generation is magnified because the sternotomy (and pericardiotomy) itself causes TF expression from cells in the intravascular space and TF release from the extravascular space. Further, during CPB, circulating monocytes adhere to the extracorporeal circuit and become activated, and they themselves express TF and thereby trigger the procoagulant mechanism by the TF pathway (54).

Therefore, factor IX/IXa has been targeted as a novel means to render protection against intravascular and circuitry thrombosis in CPB, where blocking the participation of IX/IXa in both the intrinsic pathway and (low) TF-mediated initiation of the procoagulant pathway allows preservation of hemostasis in the extravascular space (i.e., the surgical wound). Because the extravascular pathway (i.e., high TF) of coagulation remains intact, excessive bleeding is not expected to occur because effective extravascular clotting should persist without pharmacologic challenge (see Fig. 105-2).

We first tested these concepts in animal models using active site-blocked factor IXa or so-called IXai. In vivo, IXai was shown to prevent intravascular thrombus formation in the coronary vasculature without inhibiting extravascular coagulation in a canine thrombosis model (55). The critical test of this concept was undertaken in animal models of CPB with sternotomy and pericardiotomy. In dog and baboon models of CPB, the sole use of IXai resulted in circuit patency without intravascular thrombosis in the face of significantly diminished intraoperative blood loss compared with heparin-treated animals (56,57). These studies supported the premise that blockade of this pathway would inhibit pathologic clotting over the extracorporeal circuit and, in parallel, prevent bleeding at sites of high TF, such as tissue wounds.

A drawback of IXai as a therapeutic agent, however, is the extensive number of steps required for its preparation, including such phases as activation of factor IX, inactivation of IXa using dansyl-glu-gly-arg chloromethylketone, and dialysis of the resultant material to remove all traces of this reagent. In this context, novel approaches to the blockade of factor IX/IXa have been reported, including SB249417, a fully humanized inhibitory antifactor IXa monoclonal antibody that specifically interferes with both factor IX activation and IXa activity toward its substrate factor X. This agent was studied in phase I blinded, randomized, and placebo-controlled clinical trials in 26 healthy volunteers. Five different dosing levels were employed; a decline

in factor IX activity during the infusion was observed, thereby confirming the target of the antibody and the potential utility in human subjects (58). In addition to SB249417, a human antibody [F(ab′)2 fragment] that binds the gamma-carboxyglutamic acid domain of factor IX/IXa has also been generated and is denoted as 10C12 (59). Viewed together, these studies using two different monoclonal antibodies directed against factor IX/IXa affirm the rationale behind factor IX/IXa as a target novel antithrombotic agent that may be useful in human subjects.

In an additional strategy to target factor IXa, a nucleic acid–based combinatorial library containing 1,014 species was screened for species capable of binding factor IXa with high affinity. Upon multiple screening steps, an RNA aptamer was identified that bound factor IXa with the highest affinity. An aptamer is an oligonucleotide that exhibits high binding activity for specific target molecules, such as proteins, enzymes, antibodies, peptides, and small molecules. Termed 9.3t, this agent, and an inactive mutant (termed 9.3tM) were tested for specificity and for efficacy in in vitro assays. Compared to factors VIIa, Xa, XIa, and activated protein C, 9.3t exhibited at least a 5,000-greater-fold specificity for factor IXa (60). Further, in vitro studies using human plasma showed that these agents were potent anticoagulants in clotting assays such as the activated partial thromboplastin time, and that oligonucleotides complementary to aptamer 9.3t were generated as antidotes to the anticoagulant in human plasma.

## ANTICOAGULATION AND LEFT VENTRICULAR ASSIST DEVICES

Evidence suggests that after cessation of CPB, gradual resolution of the prothrombotic stimulus occurs. In contrast, subjects undergoing CPB for placement of LVADs experience a sustained trigger to activation of procoagulant pathways, likely due to the direct presence of the LVAD. Multiple different devices are in various phases of clinical trials, or are formally approved for use at this time; the experience with these devices is varied (61). Certain LVADs, such as the Thoratec HeartMate, a pulsatile device with a low thrombogenic surface, do not require obligate anticoagulation in all subjects; all other pulsatile and axial flow devices require systemic anticoagulation and, often, concomitant antiplatelet therapy (61).

Hampton and Verrier summarized the findings obtained from the most commonly used LVADs (see Table 105-5); these authors found that early postoperative bleeding and late thromboembolic events are two of the main complications of LVADs (62). Reoperation for postoperative hemorrhage may occur in up to 20% to 40% of patients after LVAD placement, and late symptomatic thromboembolic events may occur with the same frequency (63–65). Hampton and Verrier noted that as the manufacturers fully recognize that the contact of blood with foreign surfaces is inevitably thrombogenic, their efforts to use textured surfaces to generate a so-called *pseudoneointima* have reduced—but not completely eliminated—thromboembolism (65). These authors also indicate that the tendency toward early hemorrhage in LVAD placement is compounded by changes in coagulation/platelets and hemodilution that occur obligatorily with CPB (61).

Himmelreich et al. followed 12 bridging patients from LVAD placement through transplantation for 51 days (66). They observed decreased levels of factors XI, XII, and prekallikrein within 15 days of LVAD placement, consistent with the hypothesis that activation of the intrinsic pathway of coagulation is triggered by the LVAD. Further, levels of PAP were elevated, indicating generation of plasmin through the intrinsic fibrinolytic

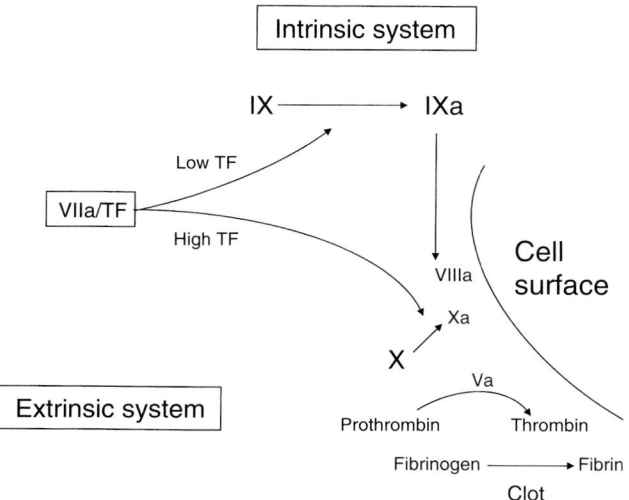

**FIGURE 105-2.** Divergent role of factor IX in the procoagulant response in the setting of low (intrinsic system) or high (extrinsic system) levels of tissue factor (TF).

**TABLE 105-5**

COMMONLY USED VENTRICULAR ASSIST DEVICES AND THEIR CHARACTERISTICS

| Manufacturer | Device type | Duration of support | Anticoagulation | Neointimal lining |
|---|---|---|---|---|
| Thoratec Heartmate | LVAD | Medium to long-term | None or ASA | Yes |
| Novacor | LVAD | Medium to long-term | Warfarin | No |
| Abiomed BVS | Uni or BiVAD | Short-term | Heparin | No |
| Thoratec BiVAD | Uni or BiVAD | Medium to long-term | Warfarin | No |
| MicroMed Debakey | LVAD (Axial flow) | Medium to long-term | ASA, Dipyridamole, Warfarin[a] | No |
| Thoratec Heartmate II | LVAD (Axial flow) | Medium to long-term | ASA, Dipyridamole, Warfarin | No |
| Abiocor | TAH | Long-term | Warfarin | No |

LVAD, left ventricular assist device; ASA, aspirin; Uni, univentricular; BiVAD, biventricular assist device; TAH, total artificial heart.
[a]May also require clopidrogel if hypercoagulable.

pathway induced by contact activation. Beginning in the third operative week, factors XI, XII, and prekallikrein levels began to increase but PAP levels remained elevated; levels of TAT, PF4, and β-TG remained elevated throughout the postoperative period, suggesting ongoing thrombin generation and platelet activation (66).

Wang et al. reported that elevated levels of D-dimers persisted (indicating ongoing fibrinolysis) in patients with LVAD correlating with a 16% incidence of early hemorrhage requiring reoperation (67). Livingston et al. sought to separate the contributions of CPB and subsequent LVAD to the overall hemostatic abnormalities observed in the long-standing LVAD recipient (68). They studied 8 subjects undergoing CPB (coronary artery bypass grafting) and 7 subjects undergoing CPB and LVAD placement with the Thoratec HeartMate device. Patterns of intraoperative platelet adhesion and activation were not statistically different in coronary artery bypass grafting CABG control and LVAD groups. However, in the immediate postoperative period, there was a significant increase in PF4 and β-TG levels in LVAD recipients compared with CABG controls. Consistent with the notion of sustained activation of procoagulant pathways in LVAD subjects, compared with CABG controls (TAT, 26 ± 8 μg per L and F1.2, 4 ± 1 nmol per L), there was a marked increase in TAT levels in LVAD subjects 2 hours after surgery (TAT, 380 ± 112 μg per L and F1.2 23 ± 4 nmol per L). A sharp rise in fibrinopeptide A level was also observed 20 minutes after LVAD initiation (CABG 8 ± 4 ng per mL and LVAD, 235 ± 63 ng per mL), and concomitant increases in PAP levels and D-dimers levels were noted (PAP: CABG, 987 ± 129 μg per L and LVAD: 3,456 ± 721 μg per L; D-Dimer: CABG, 1,678 ± 416 ng per mL and LVAD, 15,243 ± 4,682 ng per mL).

Koster et al. compared the alterations in coagulation observed in subjects with the pulsatile Novacor LVAD and the axial flow MicroMed DeBakey LVAD, both of which require long-term anticoagulation (69). Subjects were investigated for a 6-week period following device implantation. Levels of β-TG, PF4, factor XIIa, TAT complexes, and D-dimers were elevated in both groups. Only levels of PAP were elevated selectively in the MicroMed DeBakey LVAD group. Prior to LVAD implantation, anticoagulation was achieved using unfractionated heparin to an activated thromboplastin time (aPTT) of 40 to 60 seconds. During surgery, anticoagulation was also achieved using unfractionated heparin [aprotinin was also administered (kallikrein inhibitor) during CPB]. After termination of CPB, unfractionated heparin activity was reversed using protamine; at 6 to 12 hours after surgery, heparin was restarted (target activated clotting time, 160 to 180 seconds). After removal of all drainage tubing, anticoagulation

was switched to warfarin and aspirin/dipyridamole was initiated. Therefore, elevation of products of platelet activation and procoagulant pathways persisted despite anticoagulation.

We demonstrated that LVAD subjects (Thoratec Heart-Mate) displayed sustained activation of prothrombotic pathways after LVAD implantation that lasted long after CPB. Further, when compared with subjects without LVADs and in class IV heart failure, substantial increases in activation of procoagulant mechanisms were observed (70,71). Work from other labs has confirmed that the Thoratec HeartMate LVAD recipients display a coagulopathy thought in part to be due to the thromboresistant surface (72,73). Indeed, we and others have reported sustained activation of prothrombotic and fibrinolytic pathways using this LVAD (in the absence of anticoagulation) and the generation of a chronic disseminated intravascular coagulation (DIC)-like picture (70,71).

Other device types more often demonstrate problems related to thrombosis and thromboembolization as demonstrated clinically, or subclinically by Doppler ultrasonography (72,73). In addition to standard protocols with unfractionated heparinization and warfarin, clinical use of novel anticoagulants for LVAD recipients have also been reported, in particular in the setting of heparin-induced thrombocytopenia (74,75).

These considerations underscore the problems that long-term use of LVAD may impart to the coagulation system. Therefore, optimization of thrombotic and bleeding diatheses in LVAD subjects will require extensive elucidation of the time- and site-dependent factors by which LVADs activate and sustain the procoagulant response. As noted by Goldstein and Beauford, the necessity for transfusion and blood product replacement therapy in LVAD subjects carries many risks, including immunosuppression, nosocomial infection, pulmonary insufficiency, and allosensitization (the latter a significant problem for later heart transplantation) (76–79).

In this context, it is likely that intrinsic pathway antagonists, such as inhibitors of factor IX/IXa may represent a rational, safe, and effective strategy for long-term therapy in subjects with LVADs to prevent device-triggered activation of the procoagulant mechanism. Sustained activation of the intrinsic pathway in LVAD subjects is likely to underlie the long-term stress on the hemostatic pathways that may lead to a wide range of clotting disorders, such as consumptive coagulopathy, DIC, and, ultimately, bleeding. Therefore, optimization of strategies to prevent both thrombosis and bleeding in LVAD subjects may hold the key to the long-term safe use of these devices in subjects with end-stage heart failure.

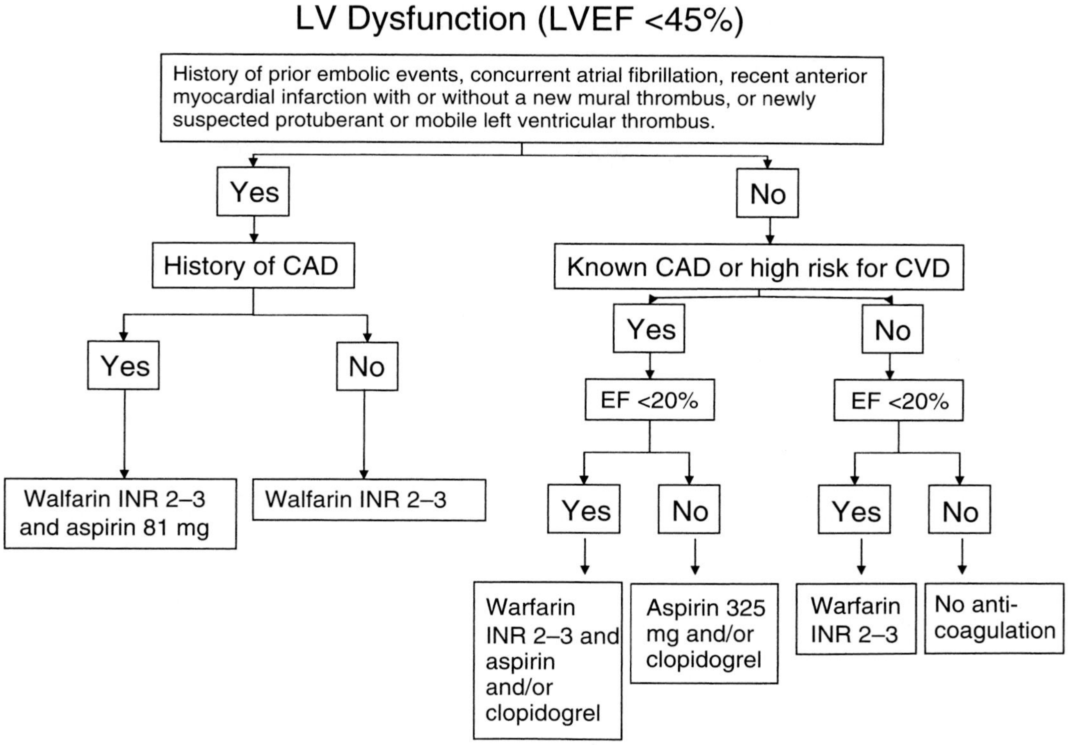

## LV Dysfunction (LVEF <45%)

History of prior embolic events, concurrent atrial fibrillation, recent anterior myocardial infarction with or without a new mural thrombus, or newly suspected protuberant or mobile left ventricular thrombus.

**Yes** → History of CAD
- Yes → Walfarin INR 2–3 and aspirin 81 mg
- No → Walfarin INR 2–3

**No** → Known CAD or high risk for CVD
- Yes → EF <20%
  - Yes → Warfarin INR 2–3 and aspirin and/or clopidogrel
  - No → Aspirin 325 mg and/or clopidogrel
- No → EF <20%
  - Yes → Warfarin INR 2–3
  - No → No anti-coagulation

**FIGURE 105-3.** Anticoagulation strategy for patients with a diminished cardiac ejection fraction. LV, left ventricular; INR, international normalized ratio; CAD, coronary artery disease; CVD, cerebral vascular dysfunction; EF, ejection fraction. [From Pulerwitz T, Rabbani LE, Pinney SP. A rationale for the use of anticoagulation in heart failure management. *J Thromb Thrombolysis* 2004;17(2):87–93, with permission.]

Because there currently exists no right ventricular or biventricular assist devices (e.g., RVADs, BiVADs) that do not require long-term anticoagulation (heparin or warfarin), the issues of related bleeding complications are only more magnified in recipients of these devices.

## RECOMMENDATIONS

The heart failure patient with atrial fibrillation or a significant intracardiac thrombus with the echocardiographic stigmata of potential embolism warrants long-term anticoagulation. All LVAD recipients, other than those with the Heartmate device, require full unfractionated heparinization or warfarin therapy, often in conjunction with aspirin, dipyridamole, or clopidogrel as prophylaxis against pump thrombosis.

However, as Pulerwitz has suggested, while the benefits of anticoagulation may be low for the heart failure patient in sinus rhythm without intracardiac thrombus, clinicians are still often motivated to prescribe anticoagulant therapy because the individual benefit of preventing a major disabling embolic event is high for a given patient (80). The assertion of these investigators (see Fig. 105-3) is to reserve warfarin therapy for those patients in sinus rhythm only when the EF is less than 20%, based upon a notion that at this level of systolic impairment, the chance of experiencing a devastating cerebrovascular event is great enough to outweigh the bleeding risk with anticoagulation.

The possibility of obtaining widely applicable recommendations from large prospective, randomized trials may be small, owing to the resistance of clinicians to part with strongly held individual beliefs with regard to anticoagulation (81). Here, the suggestion for composite registries to help document the use and outcome of anticoagulation in dilated cardiomyopathy is well heeded. It is our hope that novel anticoagulant availability in the near future may also impact favorably on the overall morbidity of anticoagulation in this difficult cohort of patients with a high risk.

### References

1. Massie BM, Shah NB. Evolving trends in the epidemiologic factors of heart failure: rationale for preventive strategies and comprehensive disease management. *Am Heart J* 1997;133:703–712.
2. Yokota Y, Kawanishi H, Hayakawa M, et al. Cardiac thrombus in dilated cardiomyopathy. Relationship between left ventricular pathophysiology and left ventricular thrombus. *Jpn Heart J* 1989;30:1–11.
3. Nixon JV. Left ventricular mural thrombus. *Arch Int Med* 1983;143:1567–1571.
4. Simpson MT, Oberman A, Kouchoukos NT, et al. Prevalence of mural thrombi and systemic embolization with left ventricular aneurysm. *Chest* 1980;77(4):463–469.
5. Yashaka M, Miyataka K, Metani M, et al. Intracardiac mobile thrombus and D-dimer fragment of fibrin in patients with mitral stenosis. *Br Heart J* 1991;62:22–25.
6. Kumangai K, Fukunami M, Ohmori M, et al. Increased intravascular clotting in patients with chronic atria fibrillation. *J Am Coll Cardiol* 1990;16:377–380.
7. Kubo SH, Rectoe TS, Bank AJ, et al. Endothelium-dependent vasodilation is attenuated in patients with heart failure. *Circulation* 1001;84:1589–1596.
8. Lip GYH, Gibbs CR. Does heart failure confer a hypercoaguable state? Virchow's triad revisited. *J Am Coll Cardiol* 1993;33:1424–1426.
9. Sbarouni E, Bradshaw A, Andreotti F, et al. Relationship between hemostatit abnormalities and neuroendocrine activity in heart failure. *Am Heart J* 1994;127:607–612.
10. Lip GYH, Lowe GDO, Metcalf MJ, et al. Effects of warfarin therapy on plasma fibrinogen, von willebrand factor and fibrin d-dimer in left ventricular dysfunction secondary to coronary artery disease and without aneurysms. *Am J Cardiol* 1995;76:453–458.

11. Mehta J, Mehta P. Platelet function studies in heart disease. Enhanced platelet aggregate formation in congestive heart failure. *Circulation* 1979;60:497–503.

12. Jafri SM, Ozawa T, Mammen E, et al. Platelet function, thrombin and fibrinolytic activity in patients with heart failure. *Eur Heart J* 1993;14:205–212.

13. Ikeda U, Yamamoto K, Shimada K. Biochemical markers of coagulation activation in mitral stenosis, atrial fibrillation and cardiomyopathy. *Clin Cardiol* 1997;20:7–10.

14. Gibbs CR, Blann AD, Watson RDS, et al. Abnormalities of hemorheological, endothelial, and platelet function in patients with chronic heart failure in sinus rhythm. *Circulation* 2001;103:1746–1751.

15. Hoffmeister A, Hetzel J, Sander S, et al. Plasma viscosity and fibrinogen in relation to haemodynamic findings in chronic congestive heart failure. *Eur J Heart Fail* 1999;1:293–295.

16. Kannel WB, Abbott RD, Savage DD, et al. Epidemiologic features of chronic atrial fibrillation: The Framingham Study. *N Engl J Med* 1982;306:1018–1022.

17. The Stroke Prevention I Atrial Fibrillation Investigators. Predictors of thromboembolism in atrial fibrillation I. Clinical features of patients at risk. *Ann Int Med* 1992;116:1–5.

18. Yamamoto K, Ikeda U, Furuhashi K, et al. The coagulation system is activated in idiopathic cardiomyopathy. *J Am Coll Cardiol* 1995;25:1634–1640.

19. Atrial Fibrillation Investigators. Risk factors for stroke and efficacy of antithrombotic therapy in atrial fibrillation: analysis of pooled data from five randomized controlled trials. *Arch Int Med* 1994;154:1449–1457.

20. Stroke Prevention in Atrial Fibrillation Investigators. Adjusted-dose warfarin versus low-intensity, fixed-dose warfarin plus aspirin for high-risk patients with atrial fibrillation: stroke prevention in atrial fibrillation III randomized clinical trial. *Lancet* 1996;348:633–638.

21. Spodick DH, Littman D. Idiopathic myocardial hypertrophy. *Am J Cardiol* 1958;1:610–623.

22. Roberts WC, Siegal RJ, McManus BM. Idiopathic dilated cardiomyopathy: analysis of 152 necropsy patients. *Am J Cardiol* 1987;60:1340–1355.

23. Katz SD. Left ventricular thrombus and the incidence of thromboembolism in patients with congestive heart failure: can clinical factors identify patients at increased risk? *J Cardiovasc Risk* 1995;2:97–102.

24. Dries DL, Rosenberg YD, Waclawiw MA, et al. Ejection fraction and risk of thromboembolic events in patients with systolic dysfunction and sinus rhythm: evidence for gender differences in studies of left ventricular dysfunction trials. *J Am Coll cardiol* 1997;29:1074–1080.

25. Loh E, Sutton MSJ, Wun CCC, et al. Ventricular dysfunction and the risk of stroke after myocardial infarction. *N Engl J Med* 1997;336:251–257.

26. Dunkman WB, Johnson Gr, Carson PE, et al. Incidence of thromboembolic events in congestive heart failure. *Circulation* 1993;87(suppl. VI):VI94–VI101.

27. Falk RH, Pollak A, Tandon PK, et al. PROMISE Investigators. The effect of warfarin on prevalence of stroke in patients with severe heart failure. *J Am Coll Cardiol* 1993;21:218A.

28. Cioffi G, Pozzoli M, Fornie G, et al. Systemic thromboembolism in chronic heart failure. *Eur Heart J* 1996;17:1381–1389.

29. The CONCENSUS Trial Study Group. Effects of enalapril on mortality in severe congestive heart failure. *N Engl J Med* 1987;316:1429–1435.

30. Pullicino PM, Halperin JL, Thompson JLP. Stroke in patients with heart failure and reduced left ventricular ejection fraction. *Neurology* 2000;54:288–294.

31. Fuster V, Gersh BJ, Guiliani ER, et al. The natural history of idiopathic dilated cardiomyopathy. *Am J Cardiol* 1981;47:525–531.

32. Katz SD, Marantz PR, Biasucci L, et al. Low incidence of stroke in patients with heart failure: a prospective study. *Am Heart J* 1993;126:141–146.

33. Natterson PD, Stevenson WG, Saxon LA, et al. Risk of arterial embolization in 224 patients awaiting heart transplantation. *Am Heart J* 1995;129:564–570.

34. Smith P, Arnesen H, Holme I. The effect of warfarin on mortality and reinfarction after myocardial infarction. *N Engl J Med* 1990;323:137–152.

35. Anticoagulants in the Secondary Prevention of Events in Coronary Thrombosis (ASPECT) Research Group. Effect of long-term oral anticoagulant treatment on mortality and cardiovascular morbidity after myocardial infarction. *Lancet* 1994;343:499–503.

36. Al-Khadra AS, Salem DN, Rand WM, et al. Warfarin anticoagulation and survival: a cohort analysis from the studies of left ventricular dysfunction. *J Am Coll Cardiol* 1998;31:749–753.

37. Wilensky RL, Jung SC. Thromboembolism in patients with degreased left ventricular function: incidence, risk and treatment. *J Cardiovasc Risk* 1995;2:91–96.

38. Tobin R, Slutsky RA, Higgins CB. Serial echocardiograms in patients with congestive cardiomyopathies: lack of evidence for thrombus formation. *Clin Cardiol* 1984;7:99–101.

39. Falk RH, Foster E, Coats MH. Ventricular thrombi and thromboembolism in dilated cardiomyopathy: a prospective follow-up study. *Am Heart J* 1992;123:136–142.

40. Gottdiener JS, Gay JA, VanVoorhees L, et al. Frequency and embolic potential of left ventricular thrombus in dilated cardiomyopathy: assessment by 2-dimensional echocardiography. *Am J Cardiol* 1983;52:1281–1285.

41. Meltzer RS, Visser CA, Fuster V. Intracardiac thrombi and systemic embolization. *Ann Int Med* 1986;104:689–698.

42. Ciaccheri M, Castelli G, Cecchi F, et al. Lack of correlation between intracavitary thrombosis detected by cross sectional echocardiography and systemic emboli in patients with dilated cardiomyopathy. *Br Heart J* 1989;62:26–29.

43. Reeder GS, Lengyel M, Tajik AJ, et al. Mural thrombus in left ventricular aneurysm. *Mayo Clin Proc* 1981;56:77–81.

44. Weinreich DJ, Burke JF, Pauletto FJ. Left ventricular mural thrombi complicating acute myocardial infarction. *Ann Int Med* 1984;100:789–794.

45. Johannessen KA, Nordrehaug JE, von der Lippe G. Left ventricular thrombi after short-term high-dose anticoagulants in acute myocardial infarction. *Eur Heart J* 1987;8:975–980.

46. Ryan TJ, Antman EM, Brooks NH, et al. A Report of the American College of Cardiology/American Heart Association Task Force on Practice Guidelines. 1999 update: ACC/AHA guidelines for the management of patients with acute myocardial infarction. *J Am Coll Cardiol* 1999;34:890–911.

47. Vaitkus PT, Barnathan ES. Embolic potential, prevention and management of mural thrombus complicating anterior myocardial infarction: a meta-analysis. *J Am Coll Cardiol* 1993;22:1004–1009.

48. Visser CA, Kan G, Meltzer Rs, et al. Embolic potential of left ventricular thrombus after myocardial infarction: a two-dimensional echocardiographic study of 119 patients. *J Am Coll Cardiol* 1985;5:1276–1280.

49. Haugland JM, Asinger RW, Mikell FL, et al. Embolic potential of left ventricular thrombi detected by two-dimensional echocardiography. *Circulation* 1984;70:588–598.

50. Jugdutt BI, Sivaram CA. Prospective two-dimensional echocardiographic evaluation of left ventricular thrombus and embolism after acute myocardial infarction. *J Am Coll Cardiol* 1989;13:554–564.

51. Weiss HJ, Turitto VT, Baumgartner HR, et al. Evidence for the presence of tissue factor activity on subendothelium. *Blood* 1989;73:968–975.

52. Wilcox JN, Smith KM, Schwartz SM, et al. Localization of tissue factor in the normal vessel wall and in the atherosclerotic plaque. *Proc Natl Acad Sci U S A* 1989;86:2839–2843.

53. Bauer KA, Kass BL, ten Cate H, et al. Factor IX is activated *in vivo* by the tissue factor mechanism. *Blood* 1990;76:731–736.

54. Kappelmeyer J, Bernabei A, Edmunds LH Jr, et al. Tissue factor is expressed on monocytes during stimulated extracorporeal circulation. *Circ Res* 1993;72:1075–1081.

55. Benedict CR, Ryan J, Wolitzky B, et al. Active site-blocked factor IXa prevents intravascular thrombus formation in the coronary vasculature without inhibiting extravascular coagulation in a canine thrombosis model. *J Clin Invest* 1991;88:1760–1765.

56. Spanier TB, Oz MC, Minanov OP, et al. Heparinless cardiopulmonary bypass with active site-blocked factor IXa: a preliminary study on the dog. *J Thorac Cardiovasc Surg* 1998;115:1179–1188.

57. Spanier TB, Chen JM, Oz MC, et al. Selective anticoagulation with active site blocked factor IXa suggests separate roles for intrinsic and extrinsic coagulation pathways in cardiopulmonary bypass. *J Thorac Cardiovasc Surg* 1998;116:860–869.

58. Chow FS, Benincosa LJ, Sheth SB, et al. Pharmacokinetic and pharmacodynamic modeling of humanized anti-factor IX antibody (SB 249417) in humans. *Clin Pharmacol Ther* 2002;71:235–245.

59. Refino CJ, Himber J, Burcklen L, et al. A human antibody that binds to the gamma-carboxyglutamic acid domain of factor IX is a potent antithrombotic *in vivo*. *Thromb Haemost* 1999;82:1188–1195.

60. Rusconi CP, Scardino E, Layzer J, et al. RNA aptamers as reversible antagonists of coagulation factor IXa. *Nature* 2002;419:90–94.

61. Deng MC, Naka Y. Mechanical circulatory support devices—state of the art. Heart Fail Monit 2002;4:120–128.

62. Hampton CR, Verrier ED. Systemic consequences of ventricular assist devices: alterations of coagulation, immune function, inflammation and the neuroendocrine system. *Artif Organs* 2002;26:902–908.

63. Kasirajan V, McCarthy PM, Hoercher KJ, et al. Clinical experience with long-term use of implantable left ventricular assist devices: indications, implantation, and outcomes. *Semin Thorac Cardiovasc Surg* 2000;12:229–237.

64. Moazami N, Roberts K, Argenziano M, et al. Asymptomatic microembolism in patients with long-term ventricular assist support. *ASAIO J* 1997;43:177–180.

65. Portner PM, Jansen PGM, Oyer PE, et al. Improved outcomes with an implantable left ventricular assist system: a multicenter study. *Ann Thorac Surg* 2001;71:205–209.

66. Himmelreich G, Ullmann H, Riess H, et al. Pathophysiologic role of contact activation in bleeding followed by thromboembolic complications after implantation of left ventricular assist device. *ASAIO J* 1995;41:M790–M794.

67. Wang IW, Kottke-Marchant K, Vargo RL, et al. Hemostatic profiles of HeartMate ventricular assist device recipients. *ASAIO J* 1995;41:M782–M787.

68. Livingston ER, Fisher CA, Bibidakis EJ, et al. Increased activation of the coagulation and fibrinolytic systems leads to hemorrhagic complications during left ventricular assist implantation. *Circulation* 1996;94(Suppl. II):227–234.

69. Koster A, Loebe M, Hansen R, et al. Alterations in coagulation after implantation of a pulsatile Novacor LVAD and the axial flow MicroMed De-Bakey LVAD. *Ann Thorac Surg* 2000;70:533–537.

70. Spanier T, Oz M, Levin H, et al. Activation of coagulation and fibrinolytic pathways in patients with left ventricular assist devices. *J Thorac Cardiovasc Surg* 1996;112:1090–1097.

71. Spanier TB, Chen JM, Oz MC, et al. Time-dependent cellular population of textured-surface left ventricular assist devices contributes to the development of a biphasic systemic procoagulant response. *J Thorac Cardiovasc Surg* 1999;118:404–413.

72. Schmid C, Weyand M, Nabavi DG, et al. Cerebral and systemic embolization during left ventricular support with the Novacor N100 device. *Ann Thorac Surg* 1998;65:1703–1710.

73. Nabavi DG, Stockmann J, Schmid C, et al. Doppler microembolic load predicts risk of thromboembolic complications in Novacor patients. *J Thorac Cardiovasc Surg* 2003;126:160–167.

74. Takahama T, Kanai F, Onishi K. Anticoagulation during use of a left ventricular assist device. *ASAIO J* 2000;46(3):354–357.

75. Christansen S, Jahn UR, Meyer J, et al. Anticoagulative management of patients requiring left ventricular assist device implantation and suffering from heparin-induced thrombocytopenia type II. *Ann Thorac Surg* 2000;69:774–777.

76. Slater JP, Rose EA, Levin HR, et al. Low thromboembolic risk without anticoagulation using advanced design left ventricular assist devices. *Ann Thorac Surg* 1996;62:1321–1327.

77. Rose EA, Levin HR, Oz MC, et al. Artificial circulatory support with texture interior surfaces: a counterintuitive approach to minimize thromboembolism. *Circulation* 1994;90:II87–II89.

78. Goldstein DJ, Beauford RB. Left ventricular assist devices and bleeding: adding insult to injury. *Ann Thorac Surg* 2003;75:S42–S47.

79. Massie BM, Krol WF, Ammon SE, et al. The warfarin and antiplatelet therapy in heart failure trial (WATCH): rationale, design and baseline patient characteristics. *J Card Fail* 2004;10(2):101–112.

80. Pulerwitz T, Rabbani LE, Pinney SP. A rationale for the use of anticoagulation in heart failure management. *J Thromb Thrombolysis* 2004;17(2):87–93.

81. Koniaris LS, Goldhaber SZ. Anticoagulation in dilated cardiomyopathy. *J Am Coll Cardiol* 1998;31:745–748.

# CHAPTER 106 ■ VALVULAR HEART DISEASE

KENNETH L. BAUGHMAN

This chapter reviews anticoagulation related to native valve disease (rheumatic valvular disease, mitral valve prolapse (MVP), ischemic mitral regurgitation, mitral annular calcification, and aortic valve stenosis and sclerosis), diseases of the aortic arch, and infective endocarditis. The chapter also reviews anticoagulation of prosthetic heart valves, including prosthetic heart valve endocarditis and thrombosis. Finally, other thrombophilias and their influence on cardiac valve disease and embolic risk are addressed. Inherent in this evaluation is the risk of systemic embolization, which often results in devastating cerebral vascular dysfunction, with the risk of bleeding as a result of systemic anticoagulation.

## RHEUMATIC MITRAL STENOSIS OR REGURGITATION

Patients with rheumatic mitral valve disease have a 20% lifetime risk of clinically detectable systemic embolization (1,2). Szekely (3) estimated the incidence of systemic symptomatic embolization to be 1.5% per year in this population. However, the risk may increase up to sevenfold for patients in atrial fibrillation. Systemic embolization may be the first manifestation of rheumatic heart disease (1). Patients who experience one embolization have a lifetime risk of recurrence of up to 65%, two thirds of which occur in the first year after the initial event. Other risk factors for embolization include increasing age, increased left atrial size, atrial arrhythmias, and thrombophilias, including abnormalities of platelet function and survival (4–8). Patients with increased platelet factor 4 and β-thromboglobulin levels, as well as those patients with decreased platelet survival, are more susceptible to systemic embolization.

Systemic anticoagulation with warfarin can reduce the risk of recurrent embolization to 3.4% per year compared to 9.6% per year without systemic anticoagulation (3). Patients with atrial fibrillation with systemic anticoagulation can reduce their risk of systemic embolization to 0.7% per year compared to 5.5% per year of anticoagulation (9).

Transesophageal echocardiographic assessment before electrical cardioversion or valvuloplasty has allowed for the assessment of the efficacy of warfarin on preformed left atrial clot. Six months of systemic anticoagulation in patients with documented left atrial thrombi studied by transesophageal echocardiography (TEE) demonstrated a disappearance in clot in 24% and an average reduction in clot size of 24% was seen in 75% of the patients (10). Those who were more likely to resolve had less severe congestive heart failure, a left atrial clot size of less than 1.6 cm², absence of left atrial spontaneous echo contrast, and an adequate international normalized ratio (INR) of 2.5 or greater during the 6 months of treatment. Long-term follow-up studies (4) have demonstrated that in those patients whose left atrial thrombi resolve, the average time for resolution was 5 months.

Although there has been no randomized trial of anticoagulation, the current recommendations are that patients with rheumatic heart disease, with or without complicating atrial fibrillation, should be systemically anticoagulated unless there are contraindications such as increased risk of bleeding, participation in contact sports, frequent trauma, or an inability to control the level of anticoagulation because of patient or social factors.

## MITRAL VALVE PROLAPSE

MVP occurs because of myxomatous degeneration of the mitral valve leaflets and chordae tendeniae. These defects result in billowing of the redundant valve tissue in systole, which may lead to mitral regurgitation, ruptured chordae tendeniae, or atrial arrhythmias. Mitral valve prolapse may be present in as many as 6% of women and 4% of men (11). Pathologic cardiac findings include endocardial disruption and fibrin deposits on denuded surfaces of the valve, mural thrombus at the junction of the prolapsed leaflet in the atrial wall, or fibrinous endocarditis (12,13).

In a case–control study, Barnett et al. (14) found that in 60 patients younger than 45 years who had experienced a transient ischemic attack (TIA) or stroke, there was a 40% prevalence of MVP compared with a 6.8% prevalence in 60 age-matched controls, and a 5.7% prevalence in 42 patients with stroke, older than 45 years. MVP quickly became suspect in every individual of young age presenting with a TIA or stroke (15).

It was subsequently shown that the survival in patients with MVP who are asymptomatic or minimally symptomatic was similar to an age-matched cohort in follow-up extending to more than 6 years (16). Only patients with redundant mitral valve leaflets had significant complications, including infective endocarditis or cerebral embolization. A larger study of 456 patients (17) demonstrated that systolic displacement of one or both leaflets, mitral valve thickening, and redundancy identified a group more likely to have a stroke (7.5%) compared to those with "nonclassical" findings (5.8%).

Ultimately, a definitive case–control study was performed assessing 213 consecutive patients younger than 45 years with a TIA or ischemic stroke (see Table 106-1) (12). These patients underwent complete neurologic and echocardiographic evaluation to demonstrate the prevalence of MVP compared to 263 control patients without heart disease referred for assessment of left ventricular function. The risk of cerebral vascular accident (CVA) in the MVP group was 1.9% compared to 2.7% in the control group. MVP explained only 2 out of 71 (2.8%) of the cerebral vascular events without another obvious etiology. The crude odds ratio of the association of MVP with a CVA in this population was 0.7, and after age and gender adjustment, was only 0.59.

**TABLE 106-1**

RISK OF TRANSIENT ISCHEMIC ATTACK CEREBRAL VASCULAR ACCIDENT
IN MITRAL VALVE PROLAPSE

| Variable | All case patients (n = 213) | Case patients with no definite cause of stroke or TIA (n = 71) | Controls (n = 263) |
|---|---|---|---|
| Age—yr | 32.5 ± 12.0 | 34.6 ± 11.0 | 25.7 ± 12.5 |
| Mitral-valve prolapse—no. (%) | 4 (1.9) | 2 (2.8) | 7 (2.7) |
| Odds ratio (95% CI)[a] | 0.70 (0.15–2.80) | 1.06 (0.11–5.73) | |
| P value | 0.80 | 1.0 | |

TIA, transient ischemic attack; CI, confidence interval.
Plus–minus values are means ±SD.
[a]The crude odds ratios are for the odds of prolapse in the case patients as compared with the controls.
From Gilon D, Buonanno FS, Joffe MM, et al. Lack of evidence of an association between mitral-valve prolapse and stroke in young patients. *N Engl J Med* 1999;341:8–13, with permission.

Although, MVP is an exceedingly common finding in men and women, only those with valve redundancy, thickening, and prolapse into the left atrium in systole are at risk for embolization. MVP appears to be an infrequent cause of cryptogenic cerebral vascular events. Only those patients with stroke of unknown etiology with classical MVP should be considered for anticoagulation. Antiplatelet therapy should be initiated and systemic warfarin reserved for those who fail antiplatelet therapy alone.

## ISCHEMIC MITRAL REGURGITATION

Coronary artery disease may cause mitral valve dysfunction by several mechanisms. Transient papillary muscle insufficiency may result from diminished perfusion of the single artery supplying the anterolateral or posteromedial papillary muscle. Infarction of the papillary muscle may cause permanent mitral regurgitation affecting either the anterior or posterior mitral valve leaflet, depending on the papillary head damaged. Prolonged ischemia to the papillary muscle or mechanical strain caused by the failing papillary muscle's inability to maintain coaptation of the mitral leaflets may result in rupture of chordae tendeniae or the papillary head and secondary severe mitral regurgitation. Diffuse damage to the left ventricular myocardium (ischemic cardiomyopathy) may cause lateral displacement of the papillary muscles associated with a spherical ventricular shape and secondary mitral regurgitation. Any of these conditions may be associated with an increase in left ventricular end-diastolic and left atrial pressure, which may predispose to left atrial enlargement and atrial fibrillation. Patients with ischemic mitral regurgitation, particularly those with associated atrial arrhythmias, have the same high risk for systemic embolization as patients with rheumatic mitral regurgitation. There are few distinguishing features that differentiate those patients likely to have systemic embolization from those who do not have systemic embolization (18). Therefore, patients with ischemic mitral regurgitation, particularly those with atrial arrhythmias, congestive heart failure, or left atrial enlargement, should be considered for systemic warfarin.

## MITRAL ANNULAR CALCIFICATION

Calcification of the mitral annulus was first described in 1908 and has been associated with complete heart block, coronary artery disease, congestive heart failure, and infective endocarditis (19). The risks for the development of mitral annular calcification are similar to those for cardiovascular disease and include age, hypertension, hyperlipidemia, diabetes, and obesity. Some have suggested that mitral annular calcification may be a marker for systemic atherosclerosis.

The Framingham Heart Study (19) found an association between mitral annular calcification and cardiovascular morbidity and mortality in 16-year follow-up, with a hazard ratio of 1.6 for cardiovascular death (see Fig. 106-1) (19). For each 1 mm increase in mitral annular calcification, the risk of cardiovascular disease, cardiovascular death, and all-cause death increased by 10% (19). The same group of investigators demonstrated in an 8-year follow-up that patients with mitral annular calcification (10.3% of men and 15.8% of women) had a relative risk of stroke of 2.1. There was a continuous relation between the degree of mitral annular calcification and CVA. Each millimeter of mitral annular calcification increased the relative risk of stroke by 1.24. A twofold risk of CVA persisted even after patients with coronary disease and congestive heart failure were excluded. Other investigators have demonstrated an association of mitral annular calcification with aortic atheroma; both are predictors of increased cardiovascular mortality (20,21). Patients with aortic plaque and mitral annular calcification have a 16-fold higher risk of death because of CVA than age- and sex-matched controls.

Therefore, mitral annular calcification, easily demonstrated by transthoracic echocardiography, is a risk factor for systemic atherosclerosis, particularly for aortic atheroma. Although mitral annular calcification may be associated with systemic embolization and infective endocarditis, it is much more likely that its association with aortic atheroma and diffuse vascular disease accounts for the increased incidence of embolic phenomena. There are no trials evaluating systemic antiplatelet or anticoagulant therapies in mitral annular calcification. Aggressive treatment of atherosclerotic risk factors should be considered, including antiplatelet therapy.

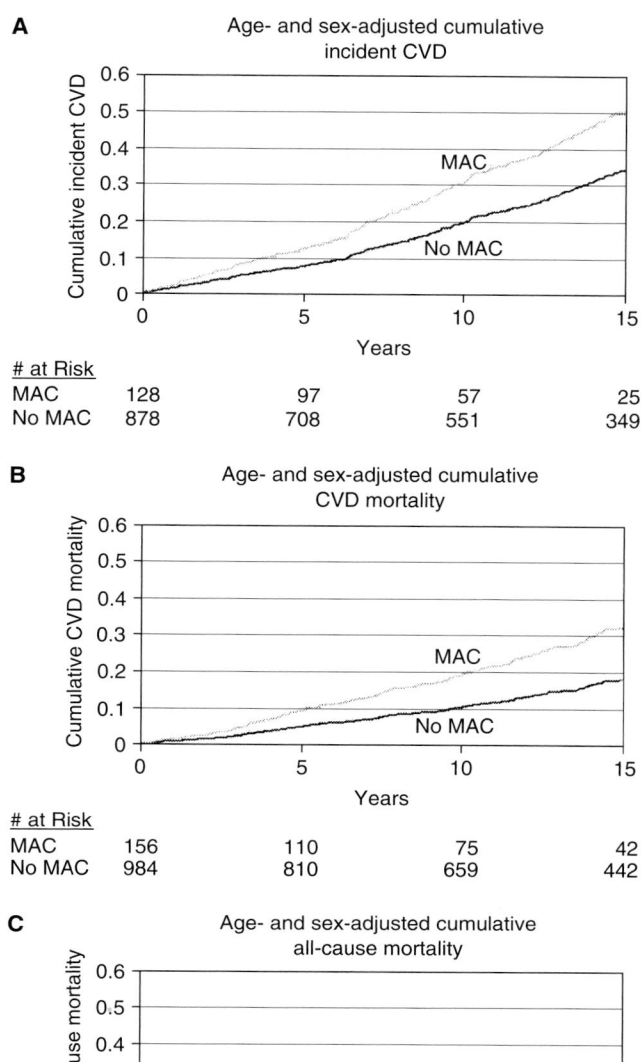

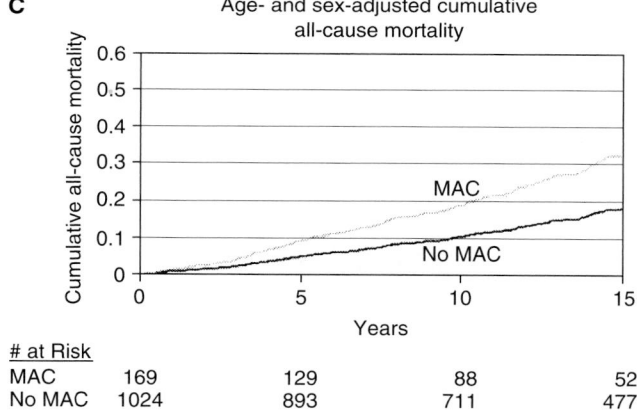

**FIGURE 106-1.** Cardiovascular risks of mitral annular calcification. MAC, mitral annular calcification; CVD, cerebral vascular dysfunction. (From Fox CS, Vasan RS, Parise H, et al. Mitral annular calcification predicts cardiovascular morbidity and mortality: the Framingham Heart Study. *Circulation* 2003;107:1492–1496, with permission.)

## AORTIC ARCH DISEASE

The aortic arch is increasingly being recognized as a potential source for thromboembolic complications. Amarenco et al. (22) evaluated 250 consecutive patients with CVAs and compared their transesophageal echocardiographic findings with 250 controls who were older than 60 years undergoing TEE for other reasons (see Table 106-2) (22). Atherosclerotic plaques greater than 4 mm were found in 14.4% of the patients with stroke and

only in 2% of the controls. After adjustments for atherosclerotic risk factors, the odds ratio for an ischemic stroke with greater than 4 mm of plaque demonstrated by TEE was 9.1. Plaques greater than 4 mm were found in 28.2% of patients without another cause for CVAs, compared to only 8.1% of the population who had a cerebral vascular event and a likely cause. Patients with aortic plaque, compared with controls, are statistically more likely to have history of hypertension, hypercholesterolemia, smoking, and mitral annular calcification (21). Similarly, patients with aortic arch atherosclerosis are statistically more likely to have a CVA, die of a CVA, or die of cardiovascular complications (21). Preliminary evidence (23,24) suggests that oral anticoagulation, as opposed to antiplatelet therapy, is effective in preventing cerebral vascular events in this high-risk population. Ferrari et al. (23) found that patients treated with only antiplatelet agents had a higher mortality rate (relative risk 7.1) than those patients treated with oral anticoagulation. Dressler et al. (24) also demonstrated the increased risk of mobile aortic atheroma when not treated with oral anticoagulants resulted in a 27% incidence in cerebrovascular events compared with 0% incidence for those receiving oral anticoagulants.

No prospective randomized trials have been performed evaluating the influence of statins on the risk of stroke or other embolic phenomenon. Tunick et al. (25) performed a matched-pair analysis of 519 patients with thoracic aortic plaque to address the influence of statins, warfarin, or antiplatelet agents. In this analysis, statins reduced the absolute risk of stroke by 17%, and the relative risk by 59%. The odds ratio for embolic event was 0.3 in patients treated with statin therapy and 0.7 for those patients treated with warfarin. Statins express pleiotrophic effects including vascular wall vasodilatation through the influence of endothelial nitric oxide synthase, and plaque stabilization through suppression of inflammatory markers including proinflammatory cytokines, vascular adhesion molecules, and matrix metalloproteins (26,27). On the basis of the 26% relative risk reduction for stroke in patients with coronary artery disease treated with statins (28), the Stroke AHA Counsel (29) has recommended that "the vast majority of patients with a history of ischemic stroke or transient ischemic attack could benefit from statin use." Patients with coronary artery disease, TIAs, or previous cerebral vascular events should likely be treated with statin therapy. Although there are no prospective trials to support treatment of patients with thoracic atherosclerosis, it would be difficult to ignore this systemic atherosclerosis risk factor as a target for primary and secondary prevention.

Therefore, although there are no prospective randomized trials, patients with large aortic atheroma, particularly those larger than 4 mm and/or mobile, should be considered at high risk for systemic embolization. Antiplatelet or oral anticoagulant treatment, as well as modification of atherosclerotic risk factors, is strongly encouraged.

Fanikos (30) has demonstrated that patients treated with low-molecular-weight heparin had a shorter length of stay and decreased postoperative costs compared with control subjects treated with unfractionated heparin. Patients discharged on combination of low-molecular-weight heparin and warfarin must be managed carefully in the outpatient department because of the potential for excess anticoagulation and coagulation related complications in association with perioperative inflammation in the pericardium or thoracic cavities that may predispose to bleeding in these sites.

## AORTIC VALVE SCLEROSIS AND STENOSIS

Otto et al. (31) performed a population-based prospective echocardiographic study of more than 5,600 men and women

**TABLE 106-2**

RISK OF CEREBRAL VASCULAR ACCIDENT WITH AORTIC ATHEROMA

| Plaque thickness (mm) | % of patients (no.) | | Crude OR (95% CI) | Adjusted OR (95% CI)[a] | P value |
| | Case patients (n = 250) | Controls (n = 250) | | | |
|---|---|---|---|---|---|
| <1[b] | 39.6 (99) | 75.6 (189) | 1 | 1 | |
| 1–1.9 | 11.2 (28) | 6.4 (16) | 3.3 (1.7–6.5) | 4.4 (2.1–8.9) | <0.001 |
| 2–2.9 | 22.4 (56) | 10.4 (26) | 4.1 (2.4–7.0) | 5.0 (2.7–9.0) | <0.001 |
| 3–3.9 | 12.4 (31) | 5.6 (14) | 4.2 (2.2–8.3) | 3.4 (1.5–7.4) | <0.001 |
| ≥4 | 14.4 (36) | 2.0 (5) | 13.8 (5.2–36.1) | 9.1 (3.3–25.2) | <0.001 |

OR, odds ratio; CI, confidence interval.
The adjusted risk associated with plaques 1 to 3.9 mm thick was 4.4 (95% CI, 2.8 to 6.8).
[a]After adjustment for age, sex, hypertension, smoking status, serum cholesterol level, diabetes, previous myocardial infarction, and atrial fibriliation.
[b]Reference category.
From Amarenco P, Cohen A, Tzourio C, et al. Atherosclerotic disease of the aortic arch and the risk of ischemic stroke. N Engl J Med 1994;331:1474–1479, with permission.

older than 65 years, demonstrating that 29% of this population had aortic sclerosis and 2% had aortic stenosis (see Table 106-3) (31). Compared with the group who had neither (70%), those with aortic sclerosis had a relative risk of cardiovascular death of 1.66 after adjustment for gender and age, and a relative risk of myocardial infarction of 1.4. The risk of all-cause death and cardiovascular death were doubled in those patients with aortic sclerosis. Therefore, aortic sclerosis is common in the older patients and is associated with approximately a 50% increase in cardiovascular death and myocardial infarction even without valvular significant obstruction. The risk factors for the development and progression of aortic sclerosis include age, gender, lipid abnormalities, hypertension, tobacco use, and decreased height. Boon (32) specifically evaluated the risk for CVA in 1,815 patients with aortic valve calcification with or without stenosis, compared with 562 controls. In long-term follow-up, the risk of CVA was not associated with aortic valve calcification (sclerosis or stenosis). Adler (33) found aortic valve calcification to be an independent predictor of severe carotid atherosclerosis and suggested that aortic sclerosis, mitral annular calcification, and carotid narrowing are all markers of systemic atherosclerosis.

Autopsy studies have demonstrated that up to 19% of patients with aortic valve calcification have silent emboli, usually to the heart or kidneys (34). Nevertheless, aortic valve calcification and stenosis do not appear to be frequent causes of symptomatic embolic phenomenon. Finding aortic sclerosis should prompt an assessment for other atherosclerotic disease, including mitral annular calcification, carotid atherosclerosis, and aortic arch atheroma. Each of these three findings may be associated with cerebral vascular events and may respond to antiplatelet or anticoagulant treatment. Because of the association

**TABLE 106-3**

CARDIOVASCULAR SYSTEM RISKS OF AORTIC SCLEROSIS

| Event | Normal aortic valves (n = 3919) | Aortic sclerosis (n = 1610); number (percent) | Aortic stenosis (n = 92) | P value for trend |
|---|---|---|---|---|
| Death from any cause | 583 (14.9) | 353 (21.9)[a] | 38 (41.3)[a] | <0.001 |
| Death from cardio-vascular causes | 238 (6.1) | 162 (10.1)[a] | 18 (19.6)[a] | <0.001 |
| Myocardial infarction[b] | 217 (6.0) | 123 (8.6)[c] | 9 (11.3)[c] | <0.001 |
| Angina[b] | 358 (11.0) | 160 (13.0) | 17 (24.3)[a] | 0.001 |
| Congestive heart failure[b] | 337 (8.9) | 192 (12.6)[a] | 21 (24.7)[a] | <0.001 |
| Stroke[b] | 238 (6.3) | 122 (8.0)[d] | 10 (11.6)[d] | 0.003 |

[a]P <0.001 for the comparison with the group with normal aortic valves.
[b]The rates were calculated for subjects at risk for new events.
[c]P <0.01 for the comparison with the group with normal aortic valves.
[d]P = 0.02 for the comparison with the group with normal aortic valves.
From Otto CM, Lind BK, Kitzman DW, et al. Association of aortic-valve sclerosis with cardiovascular mortality and morbidity in the elderly. N Engl J Med 1999;341:142–147, with permission.

with aortic sclerosis with other atherosclerotic markers, consideration should be given to treatment with aggressive risk factor modification, particularly with statins.

# PREGNANCY

Pregnancy is a prothrombotic state because of stasis, venous pressure elevation, increased fibrinogen activity, and decreased protein S activity. Management of anticoagulation during pregnancy is complicated by the potential for increased risk of bleeding, miscarriages, and warfarin-induced embryopathy. All forms of systemic anticoagulation have the potential to increase the risk for spontaneous abortion due to uteroplacental bleeding. In addition, warfarin crosses the placenta and can produce nasal hypoplasia and/or stippled epiphyses when embryos are exposed at 6 to 12 weeks of development. In addition, warfarin may cause neonatal infant hemorrhage because it enters the fetal circulation. Less commonly, exposure to warfarin in the second and third trimester may cause anomalies such as mental retardation, hydrocephalous, polydactyly, cleft lip and palate, and congenital heart abnormalities including left ventricular hypoplasia (35). The risk of warfarin-related complication is from 1.6% to 10% if embryopathy and manifestations of the "broader warfarin syndrome" are included (34,35).

There are several options for chronic anticoagulation available to pregnant women, including heparin or low-molecular-weight heparin in the first trimester followed by oral anticoagulation, or heparin or low-molecular-weight heparin throughout (36,37) (see Table 106-4). Heparin use is associated with the potential to develop osteopenia, heparin-induced thrombocytopenia, as well as the fetal and maternal hemorrhage. Low-molecular-weight heparin has greater bioavailability and a lower incidence of heparin-induced thrombocytopenia and osteoporosis than unfractionated heparin. If patients are treated with oral anticoagulation during the second trimester, conversion to unfractionated or low-molecular-weight heparin must occur during the third trimester.

Anticoagulation during pregnancy is particularly problematic for women with prosthetic heart valve replacements. Women with mechanical valves or biological valves who remain in atrial fibrillation are at a high risk for systemic embolization and must be managed with continuous anticoagulation. Chan et al. (38) reviewed the maternal and fetal risks with varying forms of systemic anticoagulation throughout pregnancy. Overall, the maternal mortality was 2.5%, and there was a 2.5% risk of major bleeding, usually associated with delivery. The risk of spontaneous abortion was virtually identical with each form of systemic anticoagulation (approximately 25%). Congenital defects were found in 6.4% of women exposed to oral anticoagulation throughout, but this risk was virtually eliminated by initiating heparin before 6 weeks of pregnancy, or by use of heparin throughout the pregnancy. Fetal loss rates were high, approximately 35%, and did not vary significantly with the form of anticoagulation used.

Low-molecular-weight heparin has been proposed as a preferred substitute for unfractionated heparin in this population (39,40). The experience with low-molecular-weight heparin is limited (41). In one series, of 14 pregnancies in 11 women treated with enoxaparin at a dose of 1 mg per kg twice per day as well as aspirin, nine live births, three miscarriages, two terminations and one mother with valve thrombosis were reported. Prior reports in 10 pregnant women recorded valve thrombosis in two (39). Sanson et al. (40) evaluated reports of the use of low-molecular-weight heparin in complicated pregnancies. These included patients with antiphospholipid antibody, prior fetal loss, preeclampisa, or other serious conditions, with poor pregnancy outcomes. Adverse results in pregnancy included conceptus death, fetal congenital malformation, premature birth, or poor neonatal outcome. In women without comorbid conditions (196 patients), only 3.1% experienced an adverse outcome, similar to that in the general population. With comorbid conditions (290 patients), 13.4% experienced an adverse outcome. In prior reports (39), the levels of anti-Xa were likely inadequate in patients who experienced valve thrombosis.

Several lessons are evident from these data. Pregnancy is associated with a dramatic increase in thrombosis and thromboembolic complications. Regardless of the anticoagulation regimen chosen, patients must be followed up closely to ensure that full systemic anticoagulation is achieved. This follow-up will require at least weekly analysis of INR for warfarin, activated partial thromboplastin time (aPTT) for unfractionated heparin, and anti-Xa for low-molecular-weight heparin. Doses of anticoagulation will likely change in view of alterations in weight and thrombogenicity during the pregnancy. Patients on warfarin should be maintained at a target INR of 2.0 to 3.0. Patients receiving intravenous or subcutaneous unfractionated heparin should be maintained at approximately two times control aPTT. Patients with low-molecular-weight heparin should have factor Xa levels of 0.5 to 1.1 IU per mL. Periods of transition from warfarin to unfractionated or low-molecular-weight heparin are most vulnerable to thromboembolic events. Because of the high risk for thrombosis in predisposed patients, the addition of aspirin to the medical regimen must be considered. Because of the medicolegal risks associated with warfarin embryopathy, congenital abnormalities, or fetal hemorrhage,

---

| TABLE 106-4 |
| --- |
| **PREGNANT PATIENT WITH MECHANICAL HEART VALVES** |

- Aggressive adjusted dose of unfractionated heparin given q12h subcutaneously throughout pregnancy; midinterval (6 h after last dose) aPTT maintained at greater than two times control levels or anti-Xa heparin level maintained at 0.35 to 0.70 IU/mL
- Low-molecular-weight heparin throughout pregnancy dosage suggested according to weight as necessary to maintain a 4-h postinjection anti-Xa heparin level of 1.0 IU/mL
- Unfractionated or low-molecular weight heparin as above until the 13th week: Change to warfarin until the middle of the third trimester, then restart unfractionated heparin or low-molecular-weight heparin until delivery

aPTT, activated partial thromboplastin time.
From Hung L, Rahimtoola SH. Prosthetic heart valves and pregnancy. *Circulation* 2003;107:1240–1246, with permission.

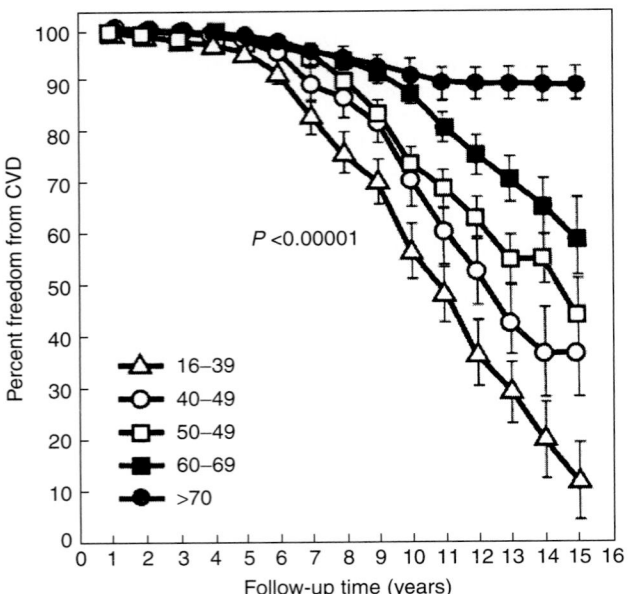

**FIGURE 106-2.** Valvular degeneration in young women with biologic valves. CVD, cerebral vascular dysfunction. (From Hung L, Rahimtoola SH. Prosthetic heart valves and pregnancy. *Circulation* 2003; 107:1240–1246, with permission.)

virtually all patients in the United States take heparin or low-molecular-weight heparin throughout the course of their pregnancy.

Women with biological valves are potentially at risk for structural valve deterioration during or shortly after pregnancy. This is biologically plausible on the basis of increased metabolic activity and dramatically increased hemodynamic burden associated with pregnancy. Some studies, however, have demonstrated that pregnancy is not associated with a greater loss of biological valves (see Fig. 106-2) (37). Mechanical valves do not demonstrate increased structural valve deterioration during pregnancy but do pose an increased risk for thromboembolic complications, including systemic embolization and valve thrombosis (42).

Women with aortic regurgitation or mitral regurgitation usually tolerate pregnancy reasonably well, compared with those women with aortic or mitral stenosis. Women contemplating valve replacement and subsequent pregnancies need to evaluate carefully the risks of thromboembolic complications with mechanical valves compared with the potential for structural valve deterioration of bioprosthetic valves.

The use of homografts (37) diminishes the potential risk for thromboembolic or structural valvular deterioration complications in the aortic valve, but unfortunately, the prosthetic material in the pulmonary circuit may still be at risk for obstruction or deterioration.

## INFECTIVE ENDOCARDITIS AND PROSTHETIC VALVE ENDOCARDITIS

Effective antibiotic therapy has reduced the incidence of systemic embolization associated with infective endocarditis from 70% to 97%, to 12% to 40% (43–49). Prosthetic valve endocarditis is an increasing problem and may occur early (within 60 days) or late following valve implantation. Early infections are due to operative or hematogenous exposure of the valve to

bacterial pathogens. Late endocarditis results from bacteria or other pathogens adhering to platelet fibrin thrombi on the valve or its associated sewing structure. Surgical series (50,51) demonstrate a risk for infective endocarditis on prosthetic valve of approximately 3% in the first year and 5% in long-term follow-up. There appears to be no difference in the risk whether the valve is bioprosthetic or mechanical. Early infections are usually caused by coagulase-negative *Staphylococcus* at a greater frequency than by Gram-negative bacteria, *Enterococcus*, or fungus. Late prosthetic valve endocarditis shares the same bacteriology as infective endocarditis on native valves, with streptococci and staphylococci being more common than *Enterococcus* and Gram-negative organisms.

The diagnosis of the infectious endocarditis is made utilizing clinical criteria and echocardiography. The Duke (52) criteria include a positive blood culture or echocardiogram as major determinates and appropriate clinical predisposition, fever, vascular or neurologic phenomenon, suggestive echocardiogram, or suggestive microbiology as minor determinates. Utilizing these criteria, a diagnosis of definite, possible, or rejected endocarditis can usually be made. Multiple studies (53–55) demonstrate that TEE is more sensitive and specific than transthoracic studies in diagnosing prosthetic and native valve endocarditis. TEE has a sensitivity of approximately 85% and a specificity of approximately 95%. In addition, TEE is superior in demonstrating prosthetic valve complications including vegetations, abscess formation, perivalvular dehiscence, and areas of valvular or prevalvular regurgitation.

The major thromboembolic complications related to native valve and prosthetic valve endocarditis are cerebral vascular events (56) which are increased in the presence of vegetations and may increase further with greater vegetation size. Patients who experience thromboembolic complications and who are taking anticoagulants are at increased risk for intracerebral hemorrhage. Patients with infective endocarditis requiring long-term warfarin usually switch to taking unfractionated heparin for at least 48 hours after any neurologic event, until it is clear that the event is not complicated by an intracerebral bleed. Anticoagulation does not reduce the risk of systemic embolization in patients with vegetations, and may increase the potential for central nervous system bleeding should an embolic event occur.

Patients with prosthetic valve endocarditis often require surgical intervention and excision of the valve (57). Criteria for valvular surgery include persistent evidence of systemic infection despite antibiotics and perivalvular complications, such as heart block, abscess formation, or dehiscence. Operative mortality with endocarditis surgery is often high (58) and is complicated by the need for an appropriate replacement prosthesis. Allografts are occasionally used and appear to have a 5-year actuarial survival of approximately 53%.

## NONBACTERIAL THROMBOTIC ENDOCARDITIS

Systemic embolization is present in approximately 40% of patients (59) with nonbacterial thrombotic endocarditis. This form of valve abnormality is associated with debilitating systemic diseases or malignancy. Although any valve can be affected, the aortic and mitral valves are most frequently involved. The "undersurface" of the left-sided valves display degeneration of valve collagen (59), often associated with coagulopathy and small vegetations. The diagnosis is difficult because a murmur is usually absent, and blood cultures reveal no growth despite systemic embolization.

Nonbacterial thrombotic endocarditis must be differentiated from valve excrescences, which are present in approximately 40% of healthy individuals and in individuals with suspected cardioembolism (60). Excrescences are thin, elongated structures seen near the edges of leaflet closure (60).

Nonbacterial thrombotic endocarditis with embolization should be treated with heparin, and not with warfarin. Improvement will occur only by correcting the underlying medical illness.

## OTHERS

Some other thrombophilias, systemic illnesses, or structural abnormalities may be associated with cardioembolism. Systemic lupus erythematosus, antiphospholipid antibody syndrome, and papillary fibroelastoma are three such examples.

Using TEE for evaluation (61), more than 50% of patients with this connective tissue disorder had mitral abnormalities including mitral valve thickening and regurgitation. The degree of involvement appeared to correlate with the severity of the lupus erythematosus. Twenty-two percent of this population had cerebral vascular events, peripheral embolization, congestive heart failure, infective endocarditis, or required valve placement. The valvular abnormalities were felt to be due to autoimmune or antiphospholipid antibodies or a hypercoaguable state associated with this disorder.

The antiphospholipid antibody syndrome includes the association of anticardiolipin antibodies with a history of arterial or venous thrombosis and/or recurrent fetal loss. It may be associated with valve disease, thrombocytopenia, or *livedo reticularis* (62). Antiphospholipid antibodies may appear transiently, and the syndrome should not be diagnosed unless antibodies persist for at least 3 to 6 months. Antiphospholipid antibodies may alter clotting times and decrease platelet concentration (62), which may cause difficulties during perioperative anticoagulation management or valve thrombosis. Antiphospholipid antibody syndrome associated with valvular disease increases the risk of thromboembolic complications (63). Patients with the antiphospholipid syndrome who have valvular disease and symptoms, a history of arterial occlusive disease, or cardiac thrombi should be treated with oral anticoagulants. Those patients without these findings should be treated with antiplatelet agents (64).

Papillary fibroelastomas are small nonneoplastic intercardiac tumors (60,65) found in approximately 1.3% of patients studied by TEE for a source for cardioembolism. These mobile excrescences appear on the atrial side of atrioventricular valves and on the ventricular surface of the outflow valves. These small, nonmalignant tumors may be associated with cardioembolic events. Anticoagulants reduce the risk of clot-related emboli but not those due to tumor fragments. Occasionally, these growths must be removed surgically (65).

## ANTICOAGULATION IN CARDIOMYOPATHY

Patients with heart failure have decreased blood flow, increased plasma and blood viscosity, increased plasma levels of fibrinopeptide A, $\beta$ thromboglobulin, D-dimer, and von Willebrand factor (66–68). The incidence of cardioembolic phenomenon in patients with cardiomyopathy varies substantially from 1.4 to 4.2 per 100 patient-years (69,70). Because of this wide variation in frequency of both cardioembolic and thromboembolic complications, candidates for systemic anticoagulation must be chosen carefully. All patients with congestive heart failure and atrial fibrillation should be treated with warfarin unless there is a strong contraindication (71).

Two observational studies suggest there may be some benefit to chronic warfarin. A subset analysis of the Studies Of Left Ventricular Dysfunction (SOLVD) population (72), who had left ventricular dysfunction, demonstrated reduced risk of all-cause mortality in patients treated with warfarin. The benefit appeared to be in reduction of death or hospitalization for heart failure and was not influenced by symptoms, medical treatment, gender, atrial fibrillation, ejection fraction, age, or severity of heart dysfunction. In addition, the SAVE (Survival And Ventricular Enlargement) trial demonstrates that for every 5% decrease in the left ventricular ejection fraction, there was an 18% increase in the risk of CVAs. There appeared to be an 81% decrease in the CVA risk for those on warfarin (73).

Two randomized prospective trials have failed to demonstrate significant benefit to systemic warfarin, but were unable to meet their recruitment goals. The WASH (warfarin and aspirin and heart failure) study was able to recruit only 279 of a proposed 6,000 patients with cardiomyopathy treated with warfarin, aspirin, or placebo. At the completion of the trial there was no difference in death, nonfatal myocardial infarction, or cerebral vascular events in the three arms of the trial (74).

The Warfarin and Antiplatelet Therapy in Heart Failure (WATCH) trial randomized patients with systolic congestive heart failure and normal sinus rhythm to warfarin, aspirin, or clopidogrel. Eligibility required normal sinus rhythm and an ejection fraction less than 35%. At 3 years, only 1,587 of the proposed 4,500 patients had been enrolled. There was no difference in the primary endpoint; however, there was a 31% decrease in hospitalizations in the warfarin group (75). The WARCEF (warfarin vs. aspirin in reduced cardiac ejection fraction) trial is currently attempting to recruit 2,860 patients with normal sinus rhythm and ejection fraction below 30% to determine whether there is a benefit to chronic warfarin.

For now, the question of which of the patients with heart failure in normal sinus rhythm should receive warfarin remains unanswered. Patients with increased predisposition to pulmonary or systemic embolization characterized by persistent congestive heart failure symptoms, decreased physical activity, large right or left atrium, previous embolization, or markedly depressed ejection fractions should be considered for indefinite duration anticoagulation with warfarin, target INR of 2.0 to 3.0.

## ANTICOAGULATION OF LEFT VENTRICULAR ASSIST DEVICES

Left ventricular assist devices vary in their degree of thrombogenicity, primarily due to the materials utilized to line the pumping chambers and the potential for platelet or fibrin deposition. Patients who remain in atrial fibrillation will require systemic anticoagulation regardless of the device chosen.

Patients who receive left ventricular assist device therapy with the Thoratec HeartMate require only antiplatelet agent therapy and can avoid the risks of systemic warfarin. Patients with the Novocor World Heart, and patients with extracorporial biventricular support, and current models of total artificial heart (Texas Heart and Abiocor), require full systemic anticoagulation.

## WITHDRAWAL OF ANTICOAGULATION BEFORE NONCARDIAC SURGERY

Occasionally, patients on systemic anticoagulation require withdrawal to safely perform invasive noncardiac surgical intervention. Large series of patients with prosthetic valves have had their warfarin discontinued without apparent thromboembolic complication (76). There are, nonetheless, some high-risk populations who require intravenous unfractionated heparin or low-molecular-weight heparin "bridging" to help them through the surgical intervention. Those at high risk include patients who have had recent embolism or thrombophlebitis, have persistent congestive heart failure, remain in atrial fibrillation, or have had a prior systemic embolization.

Discontinuation of warfarin 4 days before surgery will usually allow the INR to be less than 1.5, a level at which surgery can be performed safely. Warfarin initiated after surgery will usually raise the INR to 2.0 within 3 days (77). Surgery does not increase the risk of arterial embolization but does increase the risk of venous thromboembolic complications. The risk to the patient from cardioembolic complications is obviously much greater: 20% of arterial emboli are fatal and 40% result in a serious disability (77). By comparison, only 3% of major bleeds are fatal (77). The use of unfractionated heparin does increase the risk for gastrointestinal and operative site bleeding (78).

## INITIAL DOSING OF WARFARIN

Certain populations of patients are sensitive to warfarin including the older patients, patients with intrinsic liver disease or hepatic congestion from congestive heart failure, patients consuming drugs that potentiate the action of warfarin, and patients after cardiac surgery (79). Patients after cardiac surgery have a low albumin level and appear to require less warfarin to achieve therapeutic INR levels early postoperatively (80).

Patients with protein C or protein S deficiency may develop skin necrosis when initiated on warfarin therapy. Although this is an unusual complication, it is devastating.

## ANTICOAGULATION ISSUES AND PROSTHETIC HEART VALVES

Patients requiring replacement of a native heart valve have several options for prosthetic heart valve replacement. These include:

1. autograft—utilizing the patient's own valve to replace a defective valve such as use of the pulmonic valve to replace a defective aortic valve
2. homograft—utilization of preserved human valves from postmortem recovery
3. biologic valves constructed of living tissue including porcine valves or valves constructed of bovine pericardial tissue
4. mechanical valves constructed of artificial material.

The potential for thromboembolic complications increases with use of mechanical prosthetic heart valves (see Table 106-5) (11). Mechanical valves vary in their thrombogenicity. Bileaflet valves (St. Jude Medical) are less thrombogenic than tilting disk valves (Bjork Shiley), and both are less thrombogenic than ball and cage valves (Starr-Edwards). Unless other risk factors are present which require systemic anticoagulation, autografts, homografts, and biologic valves do not require long-term anticoagulation but have a higher rate of valve structure deterioration. Mechanical valves have a very low rate of valve structure deterioration but require systemic anticoagulation and therefore have a higher risk of bleeding. Currently, approximately 60,000 valves are replaced in the United States per year (81). The anticipation is that a mechanical valve will last for a "lifetime" whereas 30% of biologic and 10% to 20% of homografts valves will fail within 10 to 15 years (81).

Patients receiving autografts, homografts, and biologic valves are treated with antiplatelet agents. Oral anticoagulants are recommended for 3 months after surgical intervention to allow endothelialzation of the valve and valve-sewing ring. Patients with atrial fibrillation, congestive heart failure, or other indications for systemic oral anticoagulation are continued on warfarin as indicated by their underlying disease state.

There have been no prospective randomized trials of oral anticoagulation in patients following mechanical heart valve replacement. Myers et al. (82) evaluated the need for systemic anticoagulation in 785 patients receiving the St. Jude Medical prosthesis. The rate of thromboembolic complication was 2.6% per patient-year on warfarin, 9.2% per patient-year on antiplatelet agents, and 15.6% per patient-year on no anticoagulants. Randomized analysis of three mechanical valves (Bjork Shiley, Edwards Duromedic, or Medtronic Hall) demonstrated no difference in the rate of anticoagulation related hemorrhage but showed a difference in the rate of thromboembolic complications, with the Medtronic Hall valve at 5.4% per patient-year compared with the Edwards Duromedics and Bjork Shiley at 1.3% and 1.2% per patient-year, respectively (83). Trials comparing bleeding and thromboembolic complications between mechanical and bioprosthetic valves (84–86) have demonstrated no significant difference in thromboembolic complications (approximately 2.5% to 3.5% per patient-year). However, bleeding rates are higher in patients with the mechanical heart valve (due to the use of oral anticoagulants), whereas valve failure rates are higher in patients with bioprosthetic valves. In a 12-year comparison of Bjork Shiley and bioprosthetic valves by Bloomfield et al. (85), the rate of bleeding requiring hospitalization or transfusion was 18.6% in the Bjork Shiley mechanical valve group compared with 7.1% in the Hancock or Carpentier Edwards bioprosthesis group. Thromboembolic complications occurred in 21.1% and 24.6%, respectively, whereas 37% of the bioprosthesis required reoperation compared with only 8.5% of those with the Bjork Shiley prosthesis. The risk of structural valvular deterioration of bioprosthetic valves is considerably lessened in the population older than 65 years, making this valve more attractive for the older patient requiring prosthetic heart valve replacement, particularly as this population may be at higher risk for postoperative anticoagulation related bleeding (86,87).

A number of studies have reported the risk of thromboembolic complications and bleeding in patients with varying mechanical prostheses. These include St. Jude Medical prosthesis (88,89), CarboMedics (90), Medtronic Hall (91), Starr Edwards (92–94), and biologic valves including Carpentier Edwards porcine bioprosthesis (95,96), Hancock bioprosthesis (97), and Ionescu-Shiley porcine versus pericardial valves (98). A prospective randomized trial of three bileaflet valves (ATS, CarboMedics, and St. Jude Medical) demonstrated no difference in thromboembolic complications, death, or need for reoperation (99). These data demonstrate thromboembolic risk in the bileaflet prosthesis of 0.5% per year, 0.7% per year in the tilting disk series, and 2.5% per year in the caged ball prosthesis (see Fig. 106-3) (100). Bioprostheses have a thromboembolic risk varying between 0.2 and 2.6% per year without oral anticoagulation (100).

Investigators have attempted to define a scoring system to quantitate the patient's risk for thromboembolic complications and bleeding (101,102). Thromboembolic risks include prior thromboembolic events, history of malignancy, postoperative infections, hypertension, accompanying bypass graft surgery, diabetes, and increased levels of fibrinogen. Bleeding is more likely in individuals older than 65 years, those with a prior history of gastrointestinal bleeding, patients with cerebral vascular events, or with a considerable number of comorbid conditions.

Butchart et al. (103) demonstrated that better anticoagulant control improved survival after prosthetic valve replacement. In nearly 1,500 patients receiving Medtronic Hall mechanical prosthesis, the rate of death correlated directly with the number of INR values outside the target range of 2.0 to 3.5. The rate of death in the first decile of anticoagulant variability was 2.7% and in the tenth decile, 14.6%. Cannegieter et al. (104)

**TABLE 106-5**

ANTITHROMBOTIC THERAPY IN VALVULAR HEART DISEASE

| Concomitant condition | Recommendation |
|---|---|
| **RHEUMATIC MITRAL VALVE DISEASE (MITRAL STENOSIS AND/OR MITRAL REGURGITATION)** | |
| History of systemic embolism or presence of risk factors for systemic embolization or chronic atrial fibrillation recommendation | Long-term warfarin (range INR 2 to 3) |
| Normal sinus rhythm: left atrial diameter >5.5 | Consider long-term warfarin therapy (range 2 to 3) |
| Recurrent systemic embolization, despite adequate warfarin therapy | Increase INR (range 2.5 to 3.5) or add aspirin 80 to 100 mg/d; for patients unable to take aspirin, add dipyridamole 400 mg/d, ticlopidine 250 mg b.i.d., or clopidogrel 75mg/d |
| **MITRAL VALVE PROLAPSE** | |
| No systemic embolization, unexplained TIA or atrial fibrillation recommendation; no antithromboembolic therapy; documented unexplained TIA | Long-term low-dose aspirin therapy (160 to 325 mg/d) |
| Documented systemic embolism or recurrent TIA, despite aspirin therapy or chronic atrial fibrillation | Long-term warfarin (range 2 to 3) |
| **MITRAL ANNULAR CALCIFICATION** | |
| Systemic embolism, not documented to be calcific or atrial fibrillation | Long-term warfarin therapy (range 2 to 3) |
| **NON-RHEUMATIC MITRAL REGURGITATION** | |
| Atrial fibrillation or history of systemic embolism | Long-term anticoagulation |
| **AORTIC VALVE AND AORTIC ARCH DISORDERS** | |
| Mobile aortic atheroma and aortic plaque >4-mm measured by TEE | Warfarin therapy |
| No other indication for other anticoagulation | Long-term warfarin therapy is not recommended |
| **INFECTIVE ENDOCARDITIS** | |
| Mechanical prosthetic valve | Continued long-term warfarin therapy unless specific contraindication exists |
| **NONBACTERIAL THROMBOTIC ENDOCARDITIS** | |
| Systemic embolization or PE | Heparin therapy |
| Disseminative cancer, or debilitating disease, with aseptic vegetation seen on echocardiography | Heparin therapy |
| **MECHANICAL PROSTHETIC HEART VALUES** | |
| St. Jude Medical bileaflet aortic valve left atrium of normal size | Warfarin therapy long-term (range 2 to 3) |
| CarboMedics bileaflet aortic value or Medtronic Hall tilting disk aortic valve; left atrium and normal size; normal sinus rhythm | Warfarin (range 2 to 3) |
| Tilting disk valve or bileaflet mechanical valve in mitral position; or bileaflet mechanical valve in aortic position and atrial fibrillation; caged ball or caged disk valve recommendation | Warfarin goal 2.5 to 3.5 or goal 2 to 3 plus aspirin 80 to 100 mg/d |
| **BIOPROSTHETIC HEART VALVES** | |
| Valve in mitral position | Oral anticoagulation for 3 mo after valve insertion |
| Valve in aortic position | Oral anticoagulation for 3 mo after valve insertion (INR range 2 to 3) |
| Atrial fibrillation | Long-term anticoagulation therapy (INR range 2 to 3) |
| Evidence of left atrial thrombus after surgery | Long-term anticoagulatant therapy (INR range 2 to 3) |
| Permanent pacemaker | Anticoagulation (INR range 2 to 3) |
| History of systemic embolization | Oral anticoagulation for 3 to 12 mo (INR range 2 to 3) |
| Normal sinus rhythm | Long-term aspirin therapy (80 mg/d) |

INR, international normalized ratio; TIA, transient ischemic attack; TEE, transesophageal echocardiography; PE, pericardial effusion.
From Salem DN, Daudelin HD, Levine HJ, et al. Antithrombotic therapy in valvular heart disease. *Chest* 2001;119:207S–219S, with permission.

evaluated 1,608 patients after mechanical heart valve replacement to determine the optimal level of oral anticoagulant. Assessing the number of events per INR level per patient-year at that INR level, they concluded that the optimal INR was 2.5 to 4.9. Recognizing the amount of time "out of range," they established the ideal target INR of 3.0 to 4.0. Horstkotte (105) evaluated the risk of bleeding in 600 patients with the St. Jude Medical prosthesis treated with oral anticoagulants.

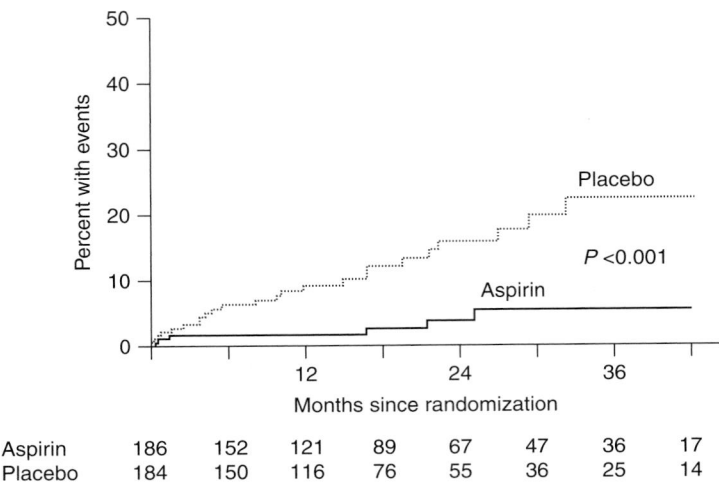

| Aspirin | 186 | 152 | 121 | 89 | 67 | 47 | 36 | 17 |
| Placebo | 184 | 150 | 116 | 76 | 55 | 36 | 25 | 14 |

**FIGURE 106-3.** Aspirin and warfarin. (From Turpie AG, Gent M, Laupacis A, et al. A comparison of aspirin with placebo in patients treated with warfarin after heart-valve replacement. *N Engl J Med* 1993;329:524–529, with permission).

The risk of bleeding with an INR of 4.0 to 6.0 compared with target range of 1.75 to 2.5 was 1.15% versus 0.24% per patient-year in the aortic position and 2.09% compared with 0.72% for mitral valve replacement. There appeared to be no significant change in thromboembolic complications within this INR range.

To lower the risk of thromboembolic complications, investigators have attempted to add antiplatelet agents to oral anticoagulants. Turpie added aspirin 100 mg to warfarin at a target INR of 3.0 to 4.5 in 370 patients with mechanical valves or tissue valves with atrial fibrillation or prior evidence of thromboembolic events. In this prospective randomized analysis, the addition of aspirin reduced major embolic events and death to 1.9% compared with 8.5% per year in the placebo group. Bleeding occurred in 35% of the oral anticoagulant and aspirin population compared with 22% in the placebo group, and the relative risk of major bleeding was increased by 27%. Altman et al. (100,106) evaluated two different levels of INR (2 to 2.9 and 3 to 4.5) in patients receiving aspirin 330 mg and dipyridomole 75 mg twice per day. The risk of thromboembolic complications in the lower INR group was 1.92 per 100 patients-years compared with 4.94 in the group with an INR of 3 to 4.5. Bleeding occurred at a rate of 3.8 per 100 patient-years in the INR group of 2 to 2.9 and 24.7 per 100 patient-years in the INR group of 3 to 4.5. Two different metaanalyses (107,108) concluded that the addition of antiplatelet agents to oral anticoagulants reduced the thromboembolic complication to an odds ratio of 0.33 to 0.41 and total mortality to an odds ratio of 0.49 to 0.60. The rate of major bleeding, however, was increased (odds ratio of 1.5 to 1.65).

Therefore, homografts, allografts, and biological valves do not require long-term oral anticoagulation unless patients are predisposed to thromboembolic complications by features other than the valve itself. Oral anticoagulants are necessary for all patients with mechanical heart valves. The level of INR which is targeted depends on the thrombogenicity of the valve or valves inserted. The addition of antiplatelet agents reduces the risk of thromboembolic complications and mortality but increases the risk of major bleeding. Patients immediately after surgery may be treated with unfractionated heparin or low-molecular-weight heparin (109) if the risk for thromboembolic complications is exceedingly high and justifies the use of systemic anticoagulation early after open-heart surgery.

Homografts and allografts (110–114) have a very low risk of thromboembolic complications, but do have from structural valve deterioration at a rate somewhat less than that for biologic prosthesis.

# VALVE THROMBOSIS

Mechanical prostheses may become obstructed from valve thrombosis or pannus formation. Patients with thrombosis tend to have a shorter duration between insertion of the valve to malfunction, a shorter duration of symptoms, a low level at target anticoagulant therapy, and distinctive features by TEE including larger size (2.8 vs. 1.2 cm) and soft mass–like appearance (92% vs. 29%) (115). Pannus is composed of collagen and elastic fibrous tissue with endothelial cells, chronic inflammatory cells, and myofibroblasts (116). The pannus originates in the neointima and the periannular region of the left ventricular septum and can invade the functional apparatus of the mechanical valve.

As with infective endocarditis, TEE dramatically enhances the ability to diagnose pannus versus valve thrombosis (117, 118). Similarly, echocardiography can be utilized to judge the success of thrombolytic therapy by measuring the change in transvalvular gradient with treatment.

Patients with mechanical valve thrombosis can be treated with unfractionated heparin, streptokinase, urokinase, tissue-type plasminogen activator (tPA), or surgery. Patients with minimal symptoms, low transvalvular gradients, and small thrombi may be treated with unfractionated heparin and higher dose oral anticoagulants with or without the addition of antiplatelet agents. Those who fail to improve can receive more aggressive therapy. Patients with major symptoms of valvular thrombosis, larger thrombotic areas, and higher transvalvular gradients may receive thrombolytic therapy or surgical intervention (119–125). Traditionally, surgical intervention has been the treatment of choice for patients with class III–IV heart failure and significant valvular obstruction (126). At the time of surgery, the valve may be mechanically "declotted" or excised and replaced. The operative mortality is approximately 12% (126) and increases with higher levels of heart failure and preoperative comorbidities.

Thrombolytic therapy is increasingly being utilized in the patient population who could undergo surgery and is the only treatment possible for patients who are too ill to undergo surgical intervention. A number of regimens have been proposed for thrombolytic therapy, including infusions of streptokinase or urokinase, from several hours up to 2 days, in addition to the use of unfractionated heparin. Similarly, TPA has been proposed as a bolus combined with unfractionated heparin, followed by repeat infusions if not improved within 24 hours. After thrombolysis, patients are treated with unfractionated heparin and resumption of oral coagulants until an appropriate INR is reached. In patients who have experienced valve thrombosis, a higher INR level should be used as a target. More frequent follow-up of therapeutic INR levels should be mandated, and consideration should be given to the addition of antiplatelet agents in addition to oral anticoagulants.

With each form of treatment (thrombolytic or surgical), patients are at risk for embolic phenomenon, hemorrhage, or death (119,121,123). Unfortunately, thrombolytic therapy is not uniformly successful, and some patients must still undergo surgical intervention. Similarly, 10% to 20% of those who experience valve thrombosis will have recurrence at a later date and will require repeat thrombolytic or surgical intervention. Clearly, this is a high-risk group who deserve careful follow-up. Approximately 80% of patients treated with thrombolytics will experience a complete response, 10% a partial response, and 10% treatment failure (124).

When TEE is performed routinely soon (day 9) after mechanical mitral valve replacement, nearly 10% of patients have early thrombi (127). Occasionally, those patients with major obstructive features require immediate reoperation. Nonobstructive thrombi are treated with more aggressive anticoagulants in the hope of avoiding intermediate and long-term complications such as embolic events and valve thrombosis.

## References

1. Wood P. *Diseases of the heart and circulation.* Philadelphia, PA: JB Lippincott Co, 1956.
2. Ellis LB, Harken DE. Arterial embolization in relation to mitral valvuloplasty. *Am Heart J* 1961;62:611–620.
3. Szekely P. Systemic embolism and anticoagulant prophylaxis in rheumatic heart disease. *Br Med J* 1964;5392:1209–1212.
4. Kang DH, Song JK, Chae JK, et al. Comparison of outcomes of percutaneous mitral valvuloplasty versus mitral valve replacement after resolution of left atrial appendage thrombi by warfarin therapy. *Am J Cardiol* 1998;81:97–100.
5. Peverill RE, Harris G, Gelman J, et al. Effect of warfarin on regional left atrial coagulation activity in mitral stenosis. *Am J Cardiol* 1997;79:339–343.
6. Tse HF, Lau CP, Cheng G. Relation between mitral regurgitation and platelet activation. *J Am Coll Cardiol* 1997;30:1813–1818.
7. Weily HS, Steele PP, Davies H, et al. Platelet survival in patients with substitute heart valves. *N Engl J Med* 1974;290:534–537.
8. Harker LA, Slichter SJ. Platelet and fibrinogen consumption in man. *N Engl J Med* 1972;287:999–1005.
9. Roy D, Marchand E, Gagne P, et al. Usefulness of anticoagulant therapy in the prevention of embolic complications of atrial fibrillation. *Am Heart J* 1986;112:1039–1043.
10. Silaruks S, Thinkhamrop B, Kiatchoosakun S, et al. Resolution of left atrial thrombus after 6 months of anticoagulation in candidates for percutaneous transvenous mitral commissurotomy. *Ann Intern Med* 2004;140:101–105.
11. Salem DN, Daudelin HD, Levine HJ, et al. Antithrombotic therapy in valvular heart disease. *Chest* 2001;119:207S–219S.
12. Gilon D, Buonanno FS, Joffe MM, et al. Lack of evidence of an association between mitral-valve prolapse and stroke in young patients. *N Engl J Med* 1999;341:8–13.
13. Pomerance A. Ballooning deformity (mucoid degeneration) of atrioventricular valves. *Br Heart J* 1969;31:343–351.
14. Barnett HJ, Boughner DR, Taylor DW, et al. Further evidence relating mitral-valve prolapse to cerebral ischemic events. *N Engl J Med* 1980;302:139–144.
15. Saffro R, Talano JV. Transient ischemic attack associated with mitral systolic clicks. *Arch Intern Med* 1979;139:693–694.
16. Nishimura RA, McGoon MD, Shub C, et al. Echocardiographically documented mitral-valve prolapse. Long-term follow-up of 237 patients. *N Engl J Med* 1985;313:1305–1309.
17. Marks AR, Choong CY, Sanfilippo AJ, et al. Identification of high-risk and low-risk subgroups of patients with mitral-valve prolapse. *N Engl J Med* 1989;320:1031–1036.
18. Dewar HA, Weightman D. A study of embolism in mitral valve disease and atrial fibrillation. *Br Heart J* 1983;49:133–140.
19. Fox CS, Vasan RS, Parise H, et al. Mitral annular calcification predicts cardiovascular morbidity and mortality: the Framingham Heart Study. *Circulation* 2003;107:1492–1496.
20. Adler Y, Vaturi M, Fink N, et al. Association between mitral annulus calcification and aortic atheroma: a prospective transesophageal echocardiographic study. *Atherosclerosis* 2000;152:451–456.
21. Kamensky G, Lisy L, Polak E, et al. Mitral annular calcifications and aortic plaques as predictors of increased cardiovascular mortality. *J Cardiol* 2001;37(Suppl. 1):21–26.
22. Amarenco P, Cohen A, Tzourio C, et al. Atherosclerotic disease of the aortic arch and the risk of ischemic stroke. *N Engl J Med* 1994;331:1474–1479.
23. Ferrari E, Vidal R, Chevallier T, et al. Atherosclerosis of the thoracic aorta and aortic debris as a marker of poor prognosis: benefit of oral anticoagulants. *J Am Coll Cardiol* 1999;33:1317–1322.
24. Dressler FA, Craig WR, Castello R, et al. Mobile aortic atheroma and systemic emboli: efficacy of anticoagulation and influence of plaque morphology on recurrent stroke. *J Am Coll Cardiol* 1998;31:134–138.
25. Tunick PA, Nayar AC, Goodkin GM, et al. Effect of treatment on the incidence of stroke and other emboli in 519 patients with severe thoracic aortic plaque. *Am J Cardiol* 2002;90:1320–1325.
26. Streifler JY. Editorial comment—statins, stroke outcome, and stroke prevention: when should we start treatment? *Stroke* 2004;35:1121–1123.
27. Ridker PM. Inflammatory biomarkers, statins, and the risk of stroke: cracking a clinical conundrum. *Circulation* 2002;105:2583–2585.
28. Corvol JC, Bouzamondo A, Sirol M, et al. Differential effects of lipid-lowering therapies on stroke prevention: a meta-analysis of randomized trials. *Arch Intern Med* 2003;163:669–676.
29. Stroke Council, American Heart Association and American Stroke Association. Statins after ischemic stroke and transient ischemic attack: an advisory statement from the Stroke Council, American Heart Association and American Stroke Association. *Stroke* 2004;35:1023.
30. Fanikos J, Tsilimingras K, Kucher N, et al. Comparison of efficacy, safety, and cost of low-molecular-weight heparin with continuous-infusion unfractionated heparin for initiation of anticoagulation after mechanical prosthetic valve implantation. *Am J Cardiol* 2004;93:247–250.
31. Otto CM, Lind BK, Kitzman DW, et al. Association of aortic-valve sclerosis with cardiovascular mortality and morbidity in the elderly. *N Engl J Med* 1999;341:142–147.
32. Boon A, Lodder J, Cheriex E, et al. Risk of stroke in a cohort of 815 patients with calcification of the aortic valve with or without stenosis. *Stroke* 1996;27:847–851.
33. Adler Y, Levinger U, Koren A, et al. Relation of nonobstructive aortic valve calcium to carotid arterial atherosclerosis. *Am J Cardiol* 2000;86:1102–1105.
34. Holley KE, Bahn RC, McGoon DC, et al. Spontaneous calcific embolization associated with calcific aortic stenosis. *Circulation* 1963;27:197–202.
35. Dyke S, Igic PG. Management of prosthetic heart valve anticoagulation in pregnancy. *ACC Curr J Rev* 2003:17–22.
36. Reimold SC, Rutherford JD. Clinical practice. Valvular heart disease in pregnancy. *N Engl J Med* 2003;349:52–59.
37. Hung L, Rahimtoola SH. Prosthetic heart valves and pregnancy. *Circulation* 2003;107:1240–1246.
38. Chan WS, Anand S, Ginsberg JS. Anticoagulation of pregnant women with mechanical heart valves: a systematic review of the literature. *Arch Intern Med* 2000;160:191–196.
39. Topol EJ, Bosker G, Casele H, et al. Anticoagulation and enoxaparin use in patients with prosthetic heart valves and/or pregnancy. *Clin Cardiol Consens Rep* 2002;3:1–20.
40. Sanson BJ, Lensing AW, Prins MH, et al. Safety of low-molecular-weight heparin in pregnancy: a systematic review. *Thromb Haemost* 1999;81:668–672.
41. Rowan JA, McCowan LM, Raudkivi PJ, et al. Enoxaparin treatment in women with mechanical heart valves during pregnancy. *Am J Obstet Gynecol* 2001;185:633–637.
42. North RA, Sadler L, Stewart AW, et al. Long-term survival and valve-related complications in young women with cardiac valve replacements. *Circulation* 1999;99:2669–2676.
43. Weinstein L. Infective endocarditis. In: Braunwald E. ed. *Heart disease.* Philadelphia, PA: WB Saunders, 1984.
44. Weinstein L. Subacute bacterial endocarditis: a review of 442 patients treated in 14 centers appointed by the penicillin trials committee of the MRC [abstract]. *Q J Med* 1951;20:93.
45. Brunson JG. Coronary embolism in bacterial endocarditis. *Am J Pathol* 1953;29:689–701.
46. Lerner PI, Weinstein L. Infective endocarditis in the antibiotic era. *N Engl J Med* 1966;274:388–393; concl.
47. Pruitt AA, Rubin RH, Karchmer AW, et al. Neurologic complications of bacterial endocarditis. *Medicine (Baltimore)* 1978;57:329–343.
48. Carpenter JL, McAllister CK. Anticoagulation in prosthetic valve endocarditis. *South Med J* 1983;76:1372–1375.
49. Garvey CJ, Neu HC. Infective endocarditis: an evolving disease. *Medicine* 1979;57:105–126.
50. Calderwood SB, Swinski LA, Waternaux CM, et al. Risk factors for the development of prosthetic valve endocarditis. *Circulation* 1985;72:31–37.
51. Rutledge R, Kim BJ, Applebaum RE. Actuarial analysis of the risk of prosthetic valve endocarditis in 1,598 patients with mechanical and bioprosthetic valves. *Arch Surg* 1985;120:469–472.

52. Durack DT, Lukes AS, Bright DK. New criteria for diagnosis of infective endocarditis: utilization of specific echocardiographic findings. Duke endocarditis service. Am J Med 1994;96:200–209.

53. Daniel WG, Mugge A, Martin RP, et al. Improvement in the diagnosis of abscesses associated with endocarditis by transesophageal echocardiography. N Engl J Med 1991;324:795–800.

54. Morguet AJ, Werner GS, Andreas S, et al. Diagnostic value of transesophageal compared with transthoracic echocardiography in suspected prosthetic valve endocarditis. Herz 1995;20:390–398.

55. Daniel WG, Mugge A, Grote J, et al. Comparison of transthoracic and transesophageal echocardiography for detection of abnormalities of prosthetic and bioprosthetic valves in the mitral and aortic positions. Am J Cardiol 1993;71:210–215.

56. Cabell CH, Pond KK, Peterson GE, et al. The risk of stroke and death in patients with aortic and mitral valve endocarditis. Am Heart J 2001;142: 75–80.

57. Lytle BW, Priest BP, Taylor PC, et al. Surgical treatment of prosthetic valve endocarditis. J Thorac Cardiovasc Surg 1996;111:198–207; discussion 207–210.

58. Dearani JA, Orszulak TA, Schaff HV, et al. Results of allograft aortic valve replacement for complex endocarditis. J Thorac Cardiovasc Surg 1997;113:285–291.

59. Lopez JA, Ross RS, Fishbein MC, et al. Nonbacterial thrombotic endocarditis: a review. Am Heart J 1987;113:773–784.

60. Roldan CA, Shively BK, Crawford MH. Valve excrescences: prevalence, evolution and risk for cardioembolism. J Am Coll Cardiol 1997;30: 1308–1314.

61. Roldan CA, Shively BK, Crawford MH. An echocardiographic study of valvular heart disease associated with systemic lupus erythematosus. N Engl J Med 1996;335:1424–1430.

62. Hogan WJ, McBane RD, Santrach PJ, et al. Antiphospholipid syndrome and perioperative hemostatic management of cardiac valvular surgery. Mayo Clin Proc 2000;75:971–976.

63. Bulckaen HG, Puisieux FL, Bulckaen ED, et al. Antiphospholipid antibodies and the risk of thromboembolic events in valvular heart disease. Mayo Clin Proc 2003;78:294–298.

64. Lockshin M, Tenedios F, Petri M, et al. Cardiac disease in the antiphospholipid syndrome: recommendations for treatment. Committee consensus report. Lupus 2003;12:518–523.

65. Yee HC, Nwosu JE, Lii AD, et al. Echocardiographic features of papillary fibroblastoma and their consequences and management. Am J Cardiol 1997;80:811–814.

66. Sbarouni E, Bradshaw A, Andreotti F, et al. Relationship between hemostatic abnormalities and neuroendocrine activity in heart failure. Am Heart J 1994;127:607–612.

67. Jafri SM, Ozawa T, Mammen E, et al. Platelet function, thrombin and fibrinolytic activity in patients with heart failure. Eur Heart J 1993;14: 205–212.

68. Yamamoto K, Ikeda U, Furuhashi K, et al. The coagulation system is activated in idiopathic cardiomyopathy. J Am Coll Cardiol 1995;25: 1634–1640.

69. Fuster V, Gersh BJ, Giuliani ER, et al. The natural history of idiopathic dilated cardiomyopathy. Am J Cardiol 1981;47:525–531.

70. Dunkman WB, Johnson GR, Carson PE et al, The V-HeFT VA Cooperative Studies Group. Incidence of thromboembolic events in congestive heart failure. Circulation 1993;87:V101–VI94.

71. Albers GW, Dalen JE, Laupacis A, et al. Antithrombotic therapy in atrial fibrillation. Chest 2001;119:194S–206S.

72. Al-Khadra AS, Salem DN, Rand WM, et al. Warfarin anticoagulation and survival: a cohort analysis from the studies of left ventricular dysfunction. J Am Coll Cardiol 1998;31:749–753.

73. Loh E, Sutton MS, Wun CC, et al. Ventricular dysfunction and the risk of stroke after myocardial infarction. N Engl J Med 1997;336:251–257.

74. Jones CG, Cleland JG, The Warfarin/Aspirin Study of Heart Failure. Meeting report—the LIDO, HOPE, MOXCON and WASH studies. Heart outcomes prevention evaluation. Eur J Heart Fail 1999;1:425–431.

75. Massie BM, Krol WF, Ammon SE, et al. The Warfarin and Antiplatelet Therapy in Heart Failure trial (WATCH): rationale, design, and baseline patient characteristics. J Card Fail 2004;10:101–112.

76. Tinker JH, Tarhan S. Discontinuing anticoagulant therapy in surgical patients with cardiac valve prostheses. Observations in 180 operations. Jama 1978;239:738–739.

77. Kearon C, Hirsh J. Management of anticoagulation before and after elective surgery. N Engl J Med 1997;336:1506–1511.

78. Katholi RE, Nolan SP, McGuire LB. The management of anticoagulation during noncardiac operations in patients with prosthetic heart valves. A prospective study. Am Heart J 1978;96:163–165.

79. British Society for Haematology. Guidelines on oral anticoagulation: third edition. Br J Haematol 1998;101:374–387.

80. Ageno W, Turpie AG. Exaggerated initial response to warfarin following heart valve replacement. Am J Cardiol 1999;84:905–908.

81. Vongpatanasin W, Hillis LD, Lange RA. Prosthetic heart valves. N Engl J Med 1996;335:407–416.

82. Myers ML, Lawrie GM, Crawford ES, et al. The St. Jude valve prosthesis: analysis of the clinical results in 815 implants and the need for systemic anticoagulation. J Am Coll Cardiol 1989;13:57–62.

83. Kuntze CE, Ebels T, Eijgelaar A, et al. Rates of thromboembolism with three different mechanical heart valve prostheses: randomised study. Lancet 1989;1:514–517.

84. Eberlein UvdEJ, Rein J, et al. Thromboembolic and bleeding complications after mitral valve replacement. Eur J Cardiothorac Surg 1990;4: 605–612.

85. Bloomfield P, Wheatley DJ, Prescott RJ, et al. Twelve-year comparison of a Bjork-Shiley mechanical heart valve with porcine bioprostheses. N Engl J Med 1991;324:573–579.

86. Hammermeister K, Sethi GK, Henderson WG, et al. Outcomes 15 years after valve replacement with a mechanical versus a bioprosthetic valve: final report of the Veterans Affairs randomized trial. J Am Coll Cardiol 2000;36:1152–1158.

87. Masters RG, Semelhago LC, Pipe AL, et al. Are older patients with mechanical heart valves at increased risk? Ann Thorac Surg 1999;68:2169–2172.

88. Khan S, Chaux A, Matloff J, et al. The St. Jude medical valve. Experience with 1,000 cases. J Thorac Cardiovasc Surg 1994;108:1010–1019; discussion 1019–1020.

89. Fernandez J, Laub GW, Adkins MS, et al. Early and late-phase events after valve replacement with the St. Jude medical prosthesis in 1200 patients. J Thorac Cardiovasc Surg 1994;107:394–406; discussion 406–407.

90. Bernal JM, Rabasa JM, Gutierrez-Garcia F, et al. The CarboMedics valve: experience with 1,049 implants. Ann Thorac Surg 1998;65:137–143.

91. Nitter-Hauge S, Abdelnoor M, Svennevig JL. Fifteen-year experience with the Medtronic-Hall valve prosthesis. A follow-up study of 1104 consecutive patients. Circulation 1996;94:II105–II108.

92. Hayashi J, Nakazawa S, Eguchi S, et al. Long-term outcome of patients who received Starr-Edwards valves between 1965 and 1977. Cardiovasc Surg 1996;4:281–287.

93. Godje OL, Fischlein T, Adelhard K, et al. Thirty-year results of Starr-Edwards prostheses in the aortic and mitral position. Ann Thorac Surg 1997;63:613–619.

94. Orszulak TA, Schaff HV, Puga FJ, et al. Event status of the Starr-Edwards aortic valve to 20 years: a benchmark for comparison. Ann Thorac Surg 1997;63:620–626.

95. Jamieson WR, Munro AI, Miyagishima RT, et al. Carpentier-Edwards standard porcine bioprosthesis: clinical performance to seventeen years. Ann Thorac Surg 1995;60:999–1006; discussion 1007.

96. Cosgrove DM, Lytle BW, Taylor PC, et al. The Carpentier-Edwards pericardial aortic valve. Ten-year results. J Thorac Cardiovasc Surg 1995;110: 651–662.

97. Cohn LH, Collins JJ Jr, Rizzo RJ, et al. Twenty-year follow-up of the Hancock modified orifice porcine aortic valve. Ann Thorac Surg 1998;66:S30–S34.

98. Pelletier LC, Carrier M, Leclerc Y, et al. Porcine versus pericardial bioprostheses: a comparison of late results in 1,593 patients. Ann Thorac Surg 1989;47:352–361.

99. Autschbach R, Walther T, Falk V, et al. Prospectively randomized comparison of different mechanical aortic valves. Circulation 2000;102:III1–III4.

100. Turpie AG, Gent M, Laupacis A, et al. A comparison of aspirin with placebo in patients treated with warfarin after heart-valve replacement. N Engl J Med 1993;329:524–529.

101. Butchart EG, Ionescu A, Payne N, et al. A new scoring system to determine thromboembolic risk after heart valve replacement. Circulation 2003;108(Suppl. 1):II68–II74.

102. Beyth RJ, Quinn LM, Landefeld CS. Prospective evaluation of an index for predicting the risk of major bleeding in outpatients treated with warfarin. Am J Med 1998;105:91–99.

103. Butchart EG, Payne N, Li HH, et al. Better anticoagulation control improves survival after valve replacement. J Thorac Cardiovasc Surg 2002;123:715–723.

104. Cannegieter SC, Rosendaal FR, Wintzen AR, et al. Optimal oral anticoagulant therapy in patients with mechanical heart valves. N Engl J Med 1995;333:11–17.

105. Horstkotte D, Schulte HD, Bircks W, et al. Lower intensity anticoagulation therapy results in lower complication rates with the St. Jude medical prosthesis. J Thorac Cardiovasc Surg 1994;107:1136–1145.

106. Altman R, Rouvier J, Gurfinkel E, et al. Comparison of two levels of anticoagulant therapy in patients with substitute heart valves. J Thorac Cardiovasc Surg 1991;101:427–431.

107. Massel D, Little SH. Risks and benefits of adding anti-platelet therapy to warfarin among patients with prosthetic heart valves: a meta-analysis. J Am Coll Cardiol 2001;37:569–578.

108. Cappelleri JC, Fiore LD, Brophy MT, et al. Efficacy and safety of combined anticoagulant and antiplatelet therapy versus anticoagulant monotherapy after mechanical heart-valve replacement: a metaanalysis. Am Heart J 1995;130:547–552.

109. Montalescot G, Polle V, Collet JP, et al. Low molecular weight heparin after mechanical heart valve replacement. Circulation 2000;101:1083–1086.

110. Kirklin JK, Smith D, Novick W, et al. Long-term function of cryopreserved aortic homografts. A ten-year study. J Thorac Cardiovasc Surg 1993;106:154–165; discussion 165–166.

111. Yacoub M, Rasmi NR, Sundt TM, et al. Fourteen-year experience with homovital homografts for aortic valve replacement. J Thorac Cardiovasc Surg 1995;110:186–193; discussion 193–194.

112. Lund O, Chandrasekaran V, Grocott-Mason R, et al. Primary aortic valve replacement with allografts over twenty-five years: valve-related and procedure-related determinants of outcome. *J Thorac Cardiovasc Surg* 1999;117:77–90; discussion 90–91.

113. Palka P, Harrocks S, Lange A, et al. Primary aortic valve replacement with cryopreserved aortic allograft: an echocardiographic follow-up study of 570 patients. *Circulation* 2002;105:61–66.

114. Chambers JC, Somerville J, Stone S, et al. Pulmonary autograft procedure for aortic valve disease: long-term results of the pioneer series. *Circulation* 1997;96:2206–2214.

115. Barbetseas J, Nagueh SF, Pitsavos C, et al. Differentiating thrombus from pannus formation in obstructed mechanical prosthetic valves: an evaluation of clinical, transthoracic and transesophageal echocardiographic parameters. *J Am Coll Cardiol* 1998;32:1410–1417.

116. Teshima H, Hayashida N, Yano H, et al. Obstruction of St Jude medical valves in the aortic position: histology and immunohistochemistry of pannus. *J Thorac Cardiovasc Surg* 2003;126:401–407.

117. Montorsi P, De Bernardi F, Muratori M, et al. Role of cine-fluoroscopy, transthoracic, and transesophageal echocardiography in patients with suspected prosthetic heart valve thrombosis. *Am J Cardiol* 2000;85:58–64.

118. Tong AT, Roudaut R, Ozkan M, et al. Transesophageal echocardiography improves risk assessment of thrombolysis of prosthetic valve thrombosis: results of the international PRO-TEE registry. *J Am Coll Cardiol* 2004;43:77–84.

119. Roudaut R, Lafitte S, Roudaut MF, et al. Fibrinolysis of mechanical prosthetic valve thrombosis: a single-center study of 127 cases. *J Am Coll Cardiol* 2003;41:653–658.

120. Shapira Y, Vaturi M, Hasdai D, et al. The safety and efficacy of repeated courses of tissue-type plasminogen activator in patients with stuck mitral valves who did not fully respond to the initial thrombolytic course. *J Thromb Haemost* 2003;1:725–728.

121. Birdi I, Angelini GD, Bryan AJ. Thrombolytic therapy for left sided prosthetic heart valve thrombosis. *J Heart Valve Dis* 1995;4:154–159.

122. Shapira Y, Herz I, Vaturi M, et al. Thrombolysis is an effective and safe therapy in stuck bileaflet mitral valves in the absence of high-risk thrombi. *J Am Coll Cardiol* 2000;35:1874–1880.

123. Ozkan M, Kaymaz C, Kirma C, et al. Intravenous thrombolytic treatment of mechanical prosthetic valve thrombosis: a study using serial transesophageal echocardiography. *J Am Coll Cardiol* 2000;35:1881–1889.

124. Gupta D, Kothari SS, Bahl VK, et al. Thrombolytic therapy for prosthetic valve thrombosis: short- and long-term results. *Am Heart J* 2000;140:906–916.

125. Lengyel M, Fuster V, Keltai M, et al. Guidelines for management of left-sided prosthetic valve thrombosis: a role for thrombolytic therapy. Consensus conference on prosthetic valve thrombosis. *J Am Coll Cardiol* 1997;30:1521–1526.

126. Deviri E, Sareli P, Wisenbaugh T, et al. Obstruction of mechanical heart valve prostheses: clinical aspects and surgical management. *J Am Coll Cardiol* 1991;17:646–650.

127. Laplace G, Lafitte S, Labeque JN, et al. Clinical significance of early thrombosis after prosthetic mitral valve replacement: a postoperative monocentric study of 680 patients. *J Am Coll Cardiol* 2004;43:1283–1290.

# CHAPTER 107 ■ OVERVIEW OF COMPLEX THROMBOHEMORRHAGIC DISORDERS

THEODORE E. WARKENTIN AND VICTOR J. MARDER

This overview of "complex thrombohemorrhagic disorders" emphasizes their heterogeneous clinical presentation ranging from bleeding to microvascular and macrovascular thrombosis (see Table 107-1). These conditions have in common the potential for clinical presentation without symptoms, with bleeding or thrombotic events, or with simultaneous manifestations of hemorrhage, vascular occlusion, and organ failure. Although this disparate group of disorders has varied and distinct etiologies, they nevertheless can mimic one another. For example, a patient who presents with splenic infarction could have an underlying myeloproliferative disorder (MPD) or infective endocarditis with splenic artery septic emboli. The former diagnosis is suggested by an elevated platelet count, whereas thrombocytopenia suggests sepsis. Consider also the patient with dyspnea and thrombocytopenia beginning 10 days after cardiac surgery for whom the differential diagnosis includes pulmonary embolism (PE) with or without heparin-induced thrombocytopenia (HIT), and acute sepsis. The diagnosis would be clarified once results of blood cultures, radiologic imaging, and serologic testing for HIT antibodies are available.

To add further complexity, these disorders may coexist. For example, patients with antiphospholipid syndrome (APS) occasionally develop thrombotic thrombocytopenic purpura–hemolytic uremic syndrome (TTP–HUS) syndrome (1). Acral (distal extremity) limb necrosis may develop in a patient with HIT and deep vein thrombosis (DVT) who is treated with warfarin and thereby develops a variant of coumarin necrosis, venous limb gangrene (2). Or, consider the occurrence of HIT with a platelet count nadir of $633 \times 10^9$ per L that nonetheless represented a substantial decline from the baseline level of $1,235 \times 10^9$ per L because of preexisting essential thrombocytosis (ET) (3).

The experienced clinician acquires a "feel" for the subtle differences in clinicopathologic profile among these disorders. For example, in TTP–HUS, the presence of red cell fragments (schistocytes), thrombocytopenia, and elevated lactate dehydrogenase (LDH) is usually much more marked than in a patient with disseminated intravascular coagulation (DIC) associated with acute sepsis. Although patients with HIT can have red cell fragments too (4), this is usually present only in the subgroup with more severe thrombocytopenia and overt (decompensated) DIC. Therefore, careful correlation of the laboratory and clinical picture usually points to the correct diagnosis.

## MYELOPROLIFERATIVE DISORDERS

The classic MPD include the clonal stem cell disorders, polycythemia vera (PV), ET, and myelofibrosis with myeloid metaplasia (MMM) (5,6). Unlike the other disorders considered in this section, patients with ET and PV typically have elevated platelet counts. Many patients evince both bleeding and thrombosis; for example, the patient with ET who has increased postoperative bleeding but also an increased risk of thrombotic stroke or myocardial infarction. Prominent microvascular disturbances in MPD include headache, lightheadedness, fleeting visual problems, acral paresthesias, and erythromelalgia (acral erythema, warmth, and pain), the latter a direct result of local platelet injury in vessels of the fingers and feet. Lowering of elevated platelet counts by cytoreductive therapy, paradoxically, can improve bleeding symptoms by correcting acquired von Willebrand syndrome, which results from enhanced platelet–von Willebrand factor (VWF) interactions (7).

## CONSUMPTIVE COAGULOPATHIES

The term "consumptive coagulopathy," or the common term, DIC, does not denote a discrete diagnosis, but rather a heterogeneous group of disorders that have in common increased consumption of coagulation factors and/or platelets (8). Indeed, some of the entities discussed as separate chapters (for e.g., sepsis, TTP–HUS, HIT) represent forms of consumptive coagulopathy. Therefore, consumptive coagulopathies (as with anemia) must not be regarded as a diagnosis, but rather as a clinicopathologic syndrome that begs the question, "what is the underlying diagnosis?"

Systemic activation of hemostasis in pathologic settings can have a wide spectrum of clinical consequences, ranging from no clinical effect, to generalized hemorrhage, to widespread microvascular thrombosis that predisposes to multisystem organ dysfunction and acral necrosis. Bleeding tends to predominate in DIC triggered by trauma, obstetrical complications, or snakebites, whereas DIC caused by HIT or metastatic adenocarcinoma tends to produce macrovascular thrombosis affecting large veins and arteries. Some malignancies, however, produce severe bleeding, such as prostate cancer with DIC and/or hyperfibrinolysis. Microvascular thrombosis often accompanies sepsis, particularly when caused by certain organisms (meningococcus, *Capnocytophaga canimorsus*) that predispose to acral limb necrosis. Contributing causes of thrombosis include severe depletion of protein C, ongoing thrombin production, and reduced limb perfusion secondary to shock (9). To further complicate the myriad clinical features, consumption may be restricted to local processes alone, such as with a vascular malformation, aortic aneurysm, or placental abruption, any of which can cause localized activation of coagulation sufficient to deplete platelets and/or coagulation factors (10).

**TABLE 107-1**

BLEEDING AND THROMBOSIS OF COMPLEX THROMBOHEMORRHAGIC SYNDROMES

| Disorder | Bleeding | Microthrombosis | Macrothrombosis |
|---|---|---|---|
| MPD | Mucocutaneous, CNS, retinal, retroperitoneal, deep tissue, postoperative, aspirin-induced | PV and ET: intracranial (headache, visual disturbances), digital ischemia, erythromelalgia | PV and ET: cerebral artery (transient ischemia or thrombotic stroke), retinal vein occlusion, cerebral sinus thrombosis, coronary (acute MI, coronary syndromes), DVT, PE, mesenteric/portal/hepatic vein thrombosis |
| Consumption coagulopathies (DIC) | Variable, depending on cause | Variable, cerebral (mental status), renal (oliguria), skin (purpura fulminans); limb necrosis (acquired protein C depletion) | Variable, large vein and artery thrombosis with underlying adenocarcinoma or HIT, or with inappropriate use of antifibrinolytic therapy |
| Sepsis | Bleeding associated with thrombocytopenia, elevated PT or aPTT | Variable, organ dysfunction and dermal/acral necrosis | Uncommon unless coexistent heritable thrombophilia (peripheral limb ischemia/necrosis) |
| TTP–HUS | Usually no bleeding, but petechiae and ecchymoses possible with severe thrombocytopenia | Organ dysfunction (CNS, renal) due to arterial platelet-VWF microaggregates | Occasional cerebral artery (thrombotic stroke in children with congenital form) |
| APS | Bleeding uncommon; when present, usually results from associated thrombocytopenia, low factor II, or anticoagulant therapy | Microvascular thrombosis and multiple organ failure in severe cases | Venous thrombosis in unusual sites (upper limb, abdominal, renal, cerebral), PE, coronary artery, cerebral artery (stroke, TIA), retinal ischemia, nonbacterial endocarditis; hemorrhagic adrenal infarction; recurrent fetal loss (placental infarcts) |
| HIT | Bleeding uncommon, except during anticoagulant therapy | Usually associated with coumarin; rarely, overt consumption coagulopathy | DVT and PE, cerebral vein thrombosis, limb artery thrombosis, cerebral (stroke), coronary (acute MI), hemorrhagic adrenal infarction |
| Coumarin-induced necrosis | Early skin necrosis may resemble cutaneous hematoma | Thrombosis of subdermal venules (skin necrosis), venous limb gangrene | Associated large vein thrombosis predisposes to subtending microvascular thrombosis and acral limb necrosis |

MPD, myeloproliferative disorders; CNS, central nervous system; PV, polycythemia vera; ET, essential thrombocytosis; DVT, deep vein thrombosis; MI, myocardial infraction; PE, pulmonary embolism; DIC, disseminated intravascular coagulation; HIT, heparin-induced thrombocytopenia; PT, prothrombin time; aPTT, activated partial thromboplastin time; TTP–HUS, thrombotic thrombocytopenic purpura–hemolytic uremic syndrome; VWF, von Willebrand factor; APS, antiphospholipid syndrome; TIA, transient ischemic attack.

# SEPSIS

Sepsis is a common cause of hemostatic abnormalities. Coagulation testing generally reveals increased fibrin degradation products and thrombocytopenia, with some patients additionally evincing elevation in the prothrombin time (PT) or activated partial thromboplastin time (aPTT), reduced fibrinogen levels, or decreased activity of the coagulation inhibitors, antithrombin and protein C (11). Thrombocytopenia is associated with both increased bleeding risk and mortality (12), as are increases of 1.5 times or more in the global coagulation times (13,14). The association between bacteremia (or fungemia) and thrombocytopenia infers that blood cultures are an appropriate investigation for many patients who

develop thrombocytopenia without apparent cause. Microvascular thrombosis is believed to be at least in part responsible for multiple organ dysfunction (15). The serious clinical sequelae of sepsis and associated DIC are best illustrated by meningococcemia, in which severely affected patients develop multiple organ failure, disseminated purpura (dermal infarction), and acral limb necrosis. In such patients, profound depletion of protein C is largely responsible for the microvascular thrombosis and associated tissue damage (9). Randomized trials of recombinant human activated protein C concentrates show reductions in both mortality (16) and organ failure (17), and patients with overt consumption benefit best from this therapy (18). Large-vessel thrombosis such as DVT occurs less often in sepsis than does microvascular thrombosis.

# THROMBOTIC THROMBOCYTOPENIC PURPURA–HEMOLYTIC UREMIC SYNDROME

The duo of microangiopathic hemolysis (red cell fragmentation) and thrombocytopenia, in the absence of an alternative explanation, constitutes the modern notion of TTP–HUS (19, 20). Many, if not most, patients with "idiopathic" TTP–HUS have autoantibodies that inhibit function of ADAMTS13 (a disintegrin and metalloprotease with thrombospondin 1–like domains) (21). Because ADAMTS13 proteolyzes large multimers of VWF under high shear stress, reduced enzyme activity predisposes patients to formation of platelet–VWF microaggregates in small arterioles (hyaline thrombi) that constitute the pathologic hallmark of TTP–HUS. Associated organ dysfunction can cause neurologic abnormalities, oliguric renal insufficiency, myocardial ischemia, and pancreatitis. The importance of recognizing TTP–HUS relates to its special treatment by plasma exchange with fresh frozen (or cryosupernatant) plasma. This therapy reduces mortality, from greater than 90% as occurred before 1964 to less than 20% today (22). Illnesses strongly resembling TTP–HUS occur with drugs (e.g., quinine, ticlopidine, clopidogrel, mitomycin, cyclosporine), hematopoietic stem cell transplantation, pregnancy and the postpartum period, and autoimmune disorders (e.g., systemic lupus erythematosus, APS, acute scleroderma) (20). Sometimes TTP begins after surgery, a clinical scenario that could mimic sepsis or HIT (23).

Classic HUS refers to a disorder in which oliguric renal failure is predominant, although 15% to 25% of patients develop neurologic abnormalities. HUS usually follows a hemorrhagic colitis that most often is caused by *Escherichia coli* O157:H7 (24). Patients usually are at the extremes of age (i.e., young children and the elderly). Treatment is supportive, although severely affected patients may benefit from plasma exchange.

# ANTIPHOSPHOLIPID SYNDROME

APS is a chronic acquired thrombophilia that is strongly associated with venous and arterial thrombosis. Its *sine qua non* is the presence of autoantibodies that are detected by their effect in prolonging phospholipid-dependent coagulation assays ("lupus anticoagulant") or by immunoassays that detect reactivity against cardiolipin or other phospholipids (25). In actuality, these "antiphospholipid" antibodies are directed against membrane proteins, most often $\beta_2$-glycoprotein 1.

APS is defined as a clinicopathologic syndrome consisting of thrombosis and/or recurrent fetal loss plus the presence of anticardiolipin antibodies and/or lupus anticoagulant, detected on two or more occasions at least 6 weeks apart (25,26). A problem in diagnosis is that nonpathologic antiphospholipid antibodies can be detected in many normal individuals (27) and transiently after infection or use of certain drugs such as procainamide and quinidine (28). Conversely, seronegative antiphospholipid syndrome indicates a patient with acute thrombosis who initially has negative testing for antiphospholipid antibodies that subsequently appear and persist on later testing (29).

Thrombotic events are generally treated as indicated for patients without APS (25), except that the patients with APS with spontaneous thrombosis should receive long-term anticoagulation, certainly for as long as the antibody persists. An additional consideration is that monitoring heparin or warfarin can be complicated by baseline prolongation of the aPTT or PT because of the *in vitro* effects of the antiphospholipid antibodies.

# HEPARIN-INDUCED THROMBOCYTOPENIA

HIT is a clinicopathologic disorder that can be defined as any clinical event best explained by antiplatelet factor 4 (PF4)/heparin antibodies ("HIT antibodies") in a patient who is receiving, or who has recently received, heparin (30,31). The high sensitivity of ELISA-based assays for HIT antibodies means that negative tests virtually rule out the diagnosis. The most common clinical event is thrombocytopenia, which is seen in at least 90% of patients, depending upon the definition of thrombocytopenia. Symptomatic thrombosis that involves large veins and arteries is common in HIT (odds ratio, 20–40:1) (32). Microvascular thrombosis also can occur, usually as a complication of warfarin treatment (2). HIT has a unique transient nature, in contrast to hereditary hypercoagulability states or other acquired severe prothrombotic disorders (e.g., APS, cancer-associated DIC). Indeed, the pathogenic HIT antibodies often become undetectable within a few weeks or months following platelet-count recovery (33). In patients who have a strong indication for heparin, such as needed for cardiac surgery, heparin is usually the best choice despite a history of previous HIT, provided that the antibodies are not detectable at the time of repeat exposure (34).

Another unusual feature of HIT is its well-defined time of onset between 5 and 10 days after the immunizing exposure to heparin (33). Most commonly, heparin causes immunization when given during or immediately before or after a surgical procedure. This suggests that there is an interaction between heparin and perioperative events, such as release of PF4 or inflammatory events, in leading to antibody formation. The characteristic temporal onset, the relatively common occurrence of HIT, and the proven benefit of anticoagulants for preventing or treating thrombosis associated with HIT provide a strong rationale for platelet-count monitoring for this potentially life- and limb-threatening complication of heparin (34).

# COUMARIN NECROSIS

Coumarins are orally active vitamin K antagonists commonly given for long-term anticoagulation. Their anticoagulant effect results from reduction of the vitamin K–dependent procoagulant factors, especially prothrombin (factor II). However, on occasion, the reduction of one or both of the vitamin K–dependent natural anticoagulants—proteins C and S—is sufficiently severe, or occurs in a suitably susceptible patient, to cause microvascular thrombosis and tissue necrosis (35). This pathophysiology reflects the key role of the protein C natural anticoagulant pathway to downregulate thrombin in the microvasculature. Coumarin necrosis generally involves a complex interplay of several factors that conspire to produce a transient disturbance in procoagulant–anticoagulant balance. For example, consider a patient with APS and postpartum DVT, who develops necrosis following high "loading doses" of warfarin and premature discontinuation of heparin (36). The acute DVT and early stopping of heparin may lead to increased procoagulant activity, whereas the high initial warfarin dosing and the (presumably) impaired protein C anticoagulant pathway related to APS creates a "perfect storm" resulting in microvascular thrombosis and skin necrosis.

There are two syndromes of coumarin necrosis: "classic" skin necrosis involving dermal and subdermal tissues, and venous limb gangrene involving acral (distal extremity) necrosis, usually in a limb with DVT (37). As a general rule, skin necrosis often occurs in a patient with chronic impairment of the protein C natural anticoagulant pathway (e.g., congenital deficiency in protein C or protein S, factor V$_{Leiden}$, antiphospholipid antibodies), whereas venous limb gangrene typically occurs in a patient with an acquired hypercoagulability state with prominent platelet activation, such as HIT or cancer-associated consumption coagulopathy (2). However, these distinctions are not absolute: Some patients with HIT develop classic warfarin-induced skin necrosis (38) and factor V$_{Leiden}$ predisposes to venous limb gangrene in a patient receiving warfarin for DVT.

# SUMMARY

Common to all of these disorders is the important role for the clinician to explain and, if possible, treat effectively the combination of bleeding or clotting (sometimes both in the same patient) associated with a wide spectrum of laboratory abnormalities that can involve various coagulation factors, platelet number or function, and even red and white blood cells. The complexity of each underlying condition warrants a careful analysis of cause, manifestation, and pathophysiology, and treatment must be both rational and individualized for each circumstance.

## *References*

1. Amoura Z, Costadoat-Chalumeau N, Veyradier A, et al. Thrombotic thrombocytopenic purpura with severe ADAMTS13 deficiency in two patients with primary antiphospholipid syndrome. *Arthritis Rheum* 2004;50:3260–3264.
2. Warkentin TE, Elavathil LJ, Hayward CPM, et al. The pathogenesis of venous limb gangrene complicating heparin-induced thrombocytopenia. *Ann Intern Med* 1997;127:804–812.
3. Risch L, Pihan H, Zeller C, et al. ET gets HIT—thrombocytotic heparin-induced thrombocytopenia (HIT) in a patient with essential thrombocythemia (ET). *Blood Coagul Fibrinolysis* 2000;11:663–667.
4. Warkentin TE, Poncz M, Cines DB. Heparin-induced thrombocytopenia. In: Young NS, Gerson SL, High KA, eds. *Clinical hematology*. Philadelphia, Pa: Elsevier Science, 2006 (in press).
5. Dameshek W. Some speculations on the myeloproliferative syndromes. *Blood* 1951;6:372–375.
6. Tefferi A, Elliott M. Myeloproliferative disorders and thrombohemorrhagic complications. In: Colman RW, Marder VJ, Clowes AW, et al., eds. *Hemostasis and thrombosis: basic principles and clinical practice*, 5th ed. Philadelphia: Lippincott Williams & Wilkins, 2006.
7. Budde U, van Genderen PJ. Acquired von Willebrand disease in patients with high platelet counts. *Semin Thromb Hemost* 1997;23:425–431.
8. Colman R, Marder VJ. Consumptive thrombohemorrhagic disorders. In: Colman RW, Marder VJ, Clowes AW, et al., eds. *Hemostasis and thrombosis: basic principles and clinical practice*, 5th ed. Philadelphia: Lippincott Williams & Wilkins, 2006.
9. Fijnvandraat K, Derkx B, Peters M, et al. Coagulation activation and tissue necrosis in meningococcal septic shock: severely reduced protein C levels predict a high mortality. *Thromb Haemost* 1995;73:15–20.
10. Rowlands TE, Norfolk D, Homer-Vanniasinkam S. Chronic disseminated intravascular coagulopathy cured by abdominal aortic aneurysm repair. *Cardiovasc Surg* 2000;8:292–294.
11. Levi M, Marder VJ. Coagulation abnormalities in sepsis. In: Colman RW, Marder VJ, Clowes AW, et al., eds. *Hemostasis and thrombosis: basic principles and clinical practice*, 5th ed. Philadelphia: Lippincott Williams & Wilkins, 2006.
12. Strauss R, Wehler M, Mehler K, et al. Thrombocytopenia in patients in the medical intensive care unit: bleeding prevalence, transfusion requirements, and outcome. *Crit Care Med* 2002;30:1765–1771.
13. Chakraverty R, Davidson S, Peggs K, et al. The incidence and cause of coagulopathies in an intensive care population. *Br J Haematol* 1996;93:460–463.
14. MacLeod JB, Lynn M, McKenney MG, et al. Early coagulopathy predicts mortality in trauma. *J Trauma* 2003;55:39–44.
15. Shimamura K, Oka K, Nakazawa M, et al. Distribution patterns of microthrombi in disseminated intravascular coagulation. *Arch Pathol Lab Med* 1983;107:543–547.
16. Bernard GR, Vincent JL, Laterre PF, et al. Efficacy and safety of recombinant human activated protein C for severe sepsis. *N Engl J Med* 2001;344:699–709.
17. Vincent JL, Angus DC, Artigas A, et al. Effects of drotrecogin alfa (activated) on organ dysfunction in the PROWESS trial. *Crit Care Med* 2003;31:834–840.
18. Dhainaut JF, Yan SB, Joyce DE, et al. Treatment effects of drotrecogin alfa (activated) in patients with severe sepsis with or without disseminated intravascular coagulation. *J Thromb Haemost* 2004;2:1924–1933.
19. George JN. How I treat patients with thrombotic thrombocytopenic purpura–hemolytic uremic syndrome. *Blood* 2000;96:1223–1229.
20. George JN, Vesely SK, Lammle B. Thrombotic thrombocytopenic purpura–hemolytic uremic syndrome. In: Colman RW, Marder VJ, Clowes AW, et al., eds. *Hemostasis and thrombosis: basic principles and clinical practice*, 5th ed. Philadelphia: Lippincott Williams & Wilkins, 2006.
21. Moake JL. Thrombotic microangiopathies. *N Engl J Med* 2002;347:589–600.
22. Rock GA, Shumak KH, Buskard NA, et al. Comparison of plasma exchange with plasma infusion in the treatment of thrombotic thrombocytopenic purpura. *N Engl J Med* 1991;325:393–397.
23. Naqvi TA, Baumann MA, Chang JC. Post-operative thrombotic thrombocytopenic purpura: a review. *Int J Clin Pract* 2004;58:169–172.
24. Elliott EJ, Robins-Browne RM, O'Loughlin EV, et al. Nationwide study of haemolytic uraemic syndrome: clinical, microbiological, and epidemiological features. *Arch Dis Child* 2001;85:125–131.
25. Rand JH, Senzel L. Antiphospholipid antibodies and the antiphospholipid syndrome. In: Colman RW, Marder VJ, Clowes AW, et al., eds. *Hemostasis and thrombosis: basic principles and clinical practice*, 5th ed. Philadelphia: Lippincott Williams & Wilkins, 2006.
26. Wilson WA, Gharavi AE, Koike T, et al. International consensus statement on preliminary criteria for definite antiphospholipid syndrome. *Arthritis Rheum* 1999;49:1309–1311.
27. Brey RL, Stallwood CL, McGlasson DL, et al. Antiphospholipid antibodies and stroke in young women. *Stroke* 2002;33:2396–2400.
28. Triplett DA. Many faces of lupus anticoagulants. *Lupus* 1998;7(Suppl. 2):S18–S22.
29. Miret C, Cervera R, Reverter JC, et al. Antiphospholipid syndrome without antiphospholipid antibodies at the time of the thrombotic event: transient "seronegative" antiphospholipid syndrome? *Clin Exp Rheumatol* 1997;15:541–544.
30. Warkentin TE. Heparin-induced thrombocytopenia: pathogenesis and management. *Br J Haematol* 2003;121:535–555.
31. Warkentin TE. Heparin-induced thrombocytopenia. In: Colman RW, Marder VJ, Clowes AW, et al., eds. *Hemostasis and thrombosis: basic principles and clinical practice*, 5th ed. Philadelphia: Lippincott Williams & Wilkins, 2006.
32. Warkentin TE. Management of heparin-induced thrombocytopenia: a critical comparison of lepirudin and argatroban. *Thromb Res* 2003;110:73–82.
33. Warkentin TE, Kelton JG. Temporal aspects of heparin-induced thrombocytopenia. *N Engl J Med* 2001;344:1286–1292.
34. Warkentin TE, Greinacher A. Heparin-induced thrombocytopenia: recognition, treatment, and prevention. The Seventh ACCP Conference on Antithrombotic and Thrombolytic Therapy. *Chest* 2004;126:311S–337S.
35. Warkentin TE. Coumarin-induced skin necrosis and venous limb gangrene. In: Colman RW, Marder VJ, Clowes AW, et al., eds. *Hemostasis and thrombosis: basic principles and clinical practice*, 5th ed. Philadelphia: Lippincott Williams & Wilkins, 2006.
36. Stewart AJ, Penman ID, Cook MK, et al. Warfarin-induced skin necrosis. *Postgrad Med J* 1999;75:233–235.
37. Warkentin TE. Heparin-induced thrombocytopenia: IgG-mediated platelet activation, platelet microparticle generation, and altered procoagulant/anticoagulant balance in the pathogenesis of thrombosis and venous limb gangrene complicating heparin-induced thrombocytopenia. *Transfus Med Rev* 1996;10:249–258.
38. Warkentin TE, Sikov WM, Lillicrap DP. Multicentric warfarin-induced skin necrosis complicating heparin-induced thrombocytopenia. *Am J Hematol* 1999;62:44–48.

# CHAPTER 108 ■ MYELOPROLIFERATIVE DISORDERS AND THROMBOHEMORRHAGIC COMPLICATIONS

AYALEW TEFFERI AND MICHELLE A. ELLIOTT

The term "myeloproliferative disorder" (MPD) was first introduced by Dameshek in 1951 to emphasize the clinicopathologic interrelation between essential thrombocythemia (ET), polycythemia vera (PV), myelofibrosis with myeloid metaplasia (MMM), chronic myeloid leukemia (CML), and erythroleukemia (diGuglielmo syndrome) (1). Between 1967 and 1981, Fialkow et al. showed that the "MPD" was also biologically interrelated on the basis of being clonal stem cell disorders with involvement of both myeloid and lymphoid lineage (2–9). In the interim, several other myeloid entities have been described and shown to display clinicopathologic, as well as biologic attributes that are similar to those of Dameshek's "MPD." In addition, the disease-causing mutations in some of these disorders, such as CML, have been identified (10,11). Accordingly, current classification of MPD recognizes molecularly defined categories, as well as distinguishes "classic" MPD from both "atypical" MPD and myelodysplastic syndrome (MDS). This chapter focuses on the classic MPD that includes ET, PV, and MMM.

## EPIDEMIOLOGY

Incidence figures for ET, PV, and MMM vary across studies but a population-based report from Olmsted county, Minnesota, United States, provided estimates of 2.5, 1.9, and 1.5 per 100,000, respectively (12,13). The corresponding figures for median age at diagnosis were 72, 67, and 70 years. All three MPD are rare in children and there is a slight male predominance in PV and MMM, and female predominance in ET (14–16). A higher disease incidence involving all three MPD has been suggested in persons of Jewish origin (17–21). In general, there is no hard evidence that links any of the MPD with environmental toxins.

### Clinical Features

Currently, most patients with ET are diagnosed incidentally and in an asymptomatic state (22). However, symptoms and signs of disease are usually present when either PV or MMM is diagnosed (23,24). Thrombohemorrhagic manifestations are the most frequent life-threatening events in both PV and ET (see Tables 108-1 and 108-2) and include microvascular disturbances (e.g., headache, lightheadedness, visual symptoms, palpitations, atypical chest pain, acral paresthesias, and erythromyalgia), thrombotic episodes (e.g., stroke, transient ischemic attacks, retinal vein occlusion, cerebrovascular vein thrombosis, myocardial infarctions, angina pectoris, pulmonary embolism, abdominal large vein thrombosis, extremity deep vein thrombosis, and digital ischemia, gangrene), and bleeding complications (e.g., central nervous system, retinal, mucosal, gingival, gastrointestinal, retroperitoneal, cutaneous, deep tissue, postsurgical, aspirin induced) (22,25–27). Bleeding in both PV and ET is exacerbated by the use of aspirin and other nonsteroidal antiinflammatory drugs.

Microvascular symptoms, especially erythromelalgia, are the result of small vessel platelet–endothelium interaction with associated inflammation and transient thrombotic occlusion (28). Erythromelalgia represents acral erythema, warmth, and pain (see Fig. 108-1) (29). Young women with ET may present with recurrent first-trimester miscarriages (30).

Newly diagnosed or untreated patients with PV might display plethora (a red and congested facial complexion), palmar erythema, and sausage-shaped distention of retinal veins. They might also experience symptoms of hyperviscosity that include head fullness, dizziness, flushing, visual disturbances, tinnitus, epistaxis, dyspnea, and increased blood pressure (31–33). Nonvascular symptoms in PV include pruritus and constitutional symptoms including fatigue, malaise, and night sweats. PV-associated pruritus occurs in more than 50% of patients and is usually exacerbated by taking a bath (34). Other symptoms and signs of PV include gout, splenomegaly, and early satiety.

The typical clinical presentation in MMM includes progressive anemia, severe constitutional symptoms, and marked splenomegaly (24). Hepatosplenomegaly in MMM is secondary to extramedullary hematopoiesis (EMH). EMH in MMM may occur in nonhepatosplenic tissue including lymph nodes, pleura (effusion), peritoneum (ascites), lung (interstitial process), and the paraspinal and epidural spaces (spinal cord and nerve root compression). Constitutional symptoms in MMM include profound fatigue, weight loss, night sweats, and low-grade fever. Weight loss in MMM consists of mostly muscle mass wasting. Less frequent disease manifestations include peripheral edema, diarrhea, early satiety, portal hypertension, and splenic infarcts (42,43).

## PATHOGENESIS

### Myeloproliferative Disorders Are Clonal Stem Cell Diseases

As early as the 1970s and 1980s, the use of glucose-6-phosphate dehydrogenase (G-6-PD) isoenzyme analysis has suggested that patients with MPD including ET (9), PV (4), and MMM (7)

**TABLE 108-1**

THROMBOTIC AND HEMORRHAGIC EVENTS REPORTED AT DIAGNOSIS IN ESSENTIAL THROMBOCYTHEMIA AND POLYCYTHEMIA VERA

| Report | n | Platelet count × 10⁹/L mean or median | Without symptoms | Total bleeds (major) | Major thrombosis | MVD | Bleeds and thrombosis |
|---|---|---|---|---|---|---|---|
| **ET** | | | | | | | |
| Bellucci, 1986 (35) | 94 | 1,200 | 67% | 37% (3.2%) | 22% | 43% | 6.4% |
| Fenaux, 1990 (25) | 147 | 1,150 | 36% | 18% (4%) | 18% | 34% | 5% |
| Cortelazzo, 1990 (36) | 100 | 1,135 | 34% | 9% (3%) | 11% | 30% | NA |
| Colombi, 1991 (37) | 103 | 1,200 | 73% | 3.6% (1.9%) | 23.3% | 33% | NA |
| Besses, 1999 (22) | 148 | 898 | 57% | 6.1% (NA) | 25% | 29% | NA |
| Jensen, 2000 (38) | 96 | 1,102 | 52% | 9% (5.2%) | 14% | 23% | NA |
| **PV** | | | | | | | |
| Berk, 1981 (39) | 431 | 532 | NA | 20% (NA) | 13% | NA | NA |
| PVSG, 1995 (40) | 1,213 | NA | NA | NA | 34% | NA | NA |
| Passamonti, 2002 (41) | 163 | 357 | 37% | 3% (NA) | 31% | 24% | NA |

ET, essential thrombocythemia; MVD, microvascular disturbances (erythromelalgia, visual, and sensory disturbances, etc.); NA, not reported; PV, polycythemia vera; PVSG, polycythemia vera study group.

have clonal hematopoiesis that originates at the stem cell level and may involve both myeloid and B lymphoid lineage (44). This early observation has been supported by more recent investigations using X-linked DNA (45,46) and transcript (47) analysis in informative females.

## Myeloproliferative Disorders Are Associated with Bone Marrow Stromal Reaction

Bone marrow histology in MPD, primarily in MMM (48,49), but also to some extent in both PV (50,51) and ET (52–54), displays excess collagen fibrosis, new bone formation, and angiogenesis (53,55–59). Bone marrow fibroblasts in MPD are polyclonal and participate in the altered cellular, as well

as extracellular concentrations of various fibrogenic and angiogenic cytokines (60–63). The latter are believed to derive from clonal megakaryocytes and/or monocytes and include platelet-derived growth factor (PDGF), transforming growth factor-β (TGF-β), basic fibroblast growth factor (bFGF), and vascular endothelial growth factor (VEGF). The current assumption is that these, as well as other cytokines mediate the bone marrow stromal reaction in MPD (60–62). Furthermore, increased tissue levels of pathogenetic cytokines might be promoted by an altered interaction between megakaryocytes and neutrophils that is promoted by increased expression of P selectin by the former (64). Similarly, neutrophil-derived elastase and other enzymes might contribute to the abnormal peripheral blood egress of myeloid progenitors in MMM (65,66).

**TABLE 108-2**

THROMBOTIC AND HEMORRHAGIC EVENTS REPORTED DURING FOLLOW-UP IN ESSENTIAL THROMBOCYTHEMIA AND POLYCYTHEMIA VERA

| Report | n | Total bleeds (major) | Major thrombosis | MVD | Bleeds and thrombosis | Deaths from hemorrhage | Deaths from thrombosis |
|---|---|---|---|---|---|---|---|
| **ET** | | | | | | | |
| Bellucci, 1986 (35) | 94 | 14% (3.2%) | 17% | 17% | 4.3% | 0 | 0 |
| Fenaux, 1990 (25) | 147 | NA (0.7%) | 13.6% | 4.1% | NA | 0 | 25% |
| Cortelazzo, 1990 (36) | 100 | NA (1%) | 20% | NA | 3% | 0 | 100% one pt (IAVT) |
| Colombi, 1991 (37) | 103 | 8.7% (5.8%) | 10.6% | 33% | 1.8% | 0 | 27.3% |
| Besses, 1999 (22) | 148 | 11.5% (4.1%) | 22.3% | 27.7% | NA | 0 | 13.3% |
| Jensen, 2000 (38) | 96 | 13.6% (7.3%) | 16.6% | 16.7% | NA | 3.3% | 16.7% |
| **PV** | | | | | | | |
| Berk, 1981 (39) | 431 | NA | 25% | NA | NA | 7% | 34% |
| PVSG, 1995 (40) | 1,213 | NA | 19% | NA | NA | 3.1% | 29.2% |
| Passamonti, 2002 (41) | 163 | NA (1.8%) | 18.4% | 10% | NA | 6% | 19% |

ET, essential thrombocythemia; MVD, microvascular disturbances (erythromelalgia, visual, and sensory disturbances, etc.); IAVT, intraabdominal venous thrombosis (portal and mesenteric vein); PV, polycythemia vera; NA, not reported; PVSG, polycythemia vera study group.

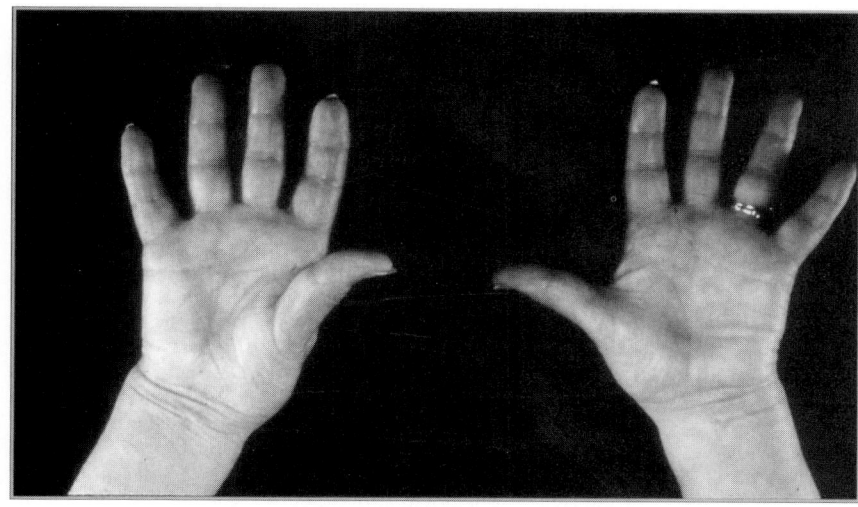

**FIGURE 108-1.** Erythromelalgia represents painful, erythematous discoloration of the hands or toes associated with warmth and burning sensation.

## Myeloproliferative Disorders Are Associated with Endogenous Myeloid Colony Growth

Endogenous (spontaneous, growth factor–independent) *in vitro* erythroid or megakaryocyte colony formation is not seen in either healthy subjects or in reactive myeloproliferation (67). Erythropoietin (EPO)-independent erythroid proliferation is primarily seen in PV (68–70), but is also seen in a proportion of patients with ET (71–74) or MMM (72,75). Furthermore, endogenous colony growth is also manifested by granulocyte (76) and megakaryocyte (77) progenitors. Such growth factor-independence has not been attributed to mutations in ligand receptor (78,79) or receptor-associated signal transducer molecules (80).

## *In Vitro* Myeloid Growth in Myeloproliferative Disorders Is Associated with Growth Factor Hypersensitivity

Growth factor hypersensitivity under *in vitro* conditions has been demonstrated for both PV and ET. Erythroid cells in PV are hypersensitive to a variety of cytokines including insulin-like growth factor (IGF-1) (81), stem cell factor (82), granulocyte-monocyte–colony-stimulating factor (GM-CSF) (83), interleukin-3 (IL-3) (84,85), and thrombopoietin (TPO) (86). A similar growth factor hypersensitivity to IL-3 (87) or TPO (88) has also been suggested in ET. The consistently observed IGF-1 hypersensitivity of erythroid cells in PV has been attributed to alterations in IGF-1–binding proteins (IGF-BP) (89,90). The receptors for both EPO (78,91,92) and TPO (79,93) have been examined in patients with MPD and found to be intact.

## Myeloproliferative Disorders Are Associated with Decreased Megakaryocyte/Platelet Mpl Expression

Decreased megakaryocyte/platelet Mpl expression was first reported in ET (94) and subsequently in PV (95), and other MPD (96,97). In ET, the decreased surface expression of Mpl has been associated with reduced *c-Mpl* transcription (94,98). In PV, the particular defect was traced to a posttranslational hypoglycosylation of the Mpl protein with derailment of membrane localization (99).

## Pathogenesis of Bleeding Diathesis in Myeloproliferative Disorders

Platelet morphology in MPD is variable and includes both small and giant forms (100). These platelets are often hypogranular and on electron microscopy display decreased granular contents involving both $\delta$ (serotonin, adenine nucleotides) and $\alpha$ (platelet-derived growth factor, $\beta$-thromboglobulin, platelet factor 4) specific storage granules (101–106). This acquired storage pool deficiency, as well as altered surface expression of hemostatic molecules are believed to contribute to the prohemorrhagic platelet defects in MPD.

*In vitro* observed hemostatic abnormalities in MPD, include poor platelet aggregation in response to various platelet agonists [i.e., thrombin, adenosine diphosphate (ADP), epinephrine, collagen, thromboxane $A_2$ (TxA2), platelet-activating factor] (107–110), abnormally low intraplatelet levels of adenine nucleotides and serotonin (111), reduced platelet factor X-activating activity (112), defective platelet lipid peroxidation (113), impaired binding to fibrinogen as a result of decreased glycoprotein (GP) IIb/IIIa expression (114), decreased adrenergic receptor expression that could explain the often observed absent epinephrine response and mechanistically involve impaired signal transduction (115,116), and acquired von Willebrand syndrome (AVWS) (117). Similarly, quantitative radiolabeled, as well as flow cytometric studies in PV and ET have revealed decreased expression of platelet GP receptors Ib and IIb/IIIa (114,118,119).

AVWS occurs in more than one third of the patients with MPD and has been associated with a bleeding diathesis (120, 121). Several investigators have established a relation between the platelet count and loss of large von Willebrand factor (VWF) multimers in the plasma of patients with MPD (122–124). The finding that large VWF multimers in plasma decrease progressively at increasing platelet counts of more than $1,000 \times 10^9$ per L is in agreement with epidemiologic studies in ET showing an increased bleeding risk when the platelet count exceeds this level (25,35,125,126). The functional deficiency of MPD-associated acquired von Willebrand disease (AVWD) may not be apparent when measuring VWF:Ag and FVIII levels alone, because these are typically maintained within the normal range (117,127).

The assays used to assess VWF function [collagen-binding activity (VWF:CBA) or ristocetin cofactor activity (VWF:RCoA)] reveal that VWF function declines relative to the VWF:Ag with increasing platelet counts (128–130). This phenomenon is not restricted to MPD, but has also been described among patients with reactive thrombocytosis (122). Therefore, the observed loss of large multimers in ET and PV is likely an effect of the absolute platelet number, rather than an effect of dysfunctional clonal platelets. Further evidence of the importance of platelet number is provided by the observed resolution of the clinical bleeding complications and the AVWD in patients with ET and with PV, following platelet cytoreduction with myelosuppressive therapy or platelet pheresis (117, 122,127,129). Similarly, resolution of reactive thrombocytosis also restores the large multimers and as a result, restores VWF function among affected patients (122).

Studies of patients with ET and PV have demonstrated that the reduction in the levels of large VWF multimers is the result of increased turnover *in vivo* (129). Increased clearance of large VWF multimers in MPD has been proposed by some investigators to be the result of enhanced binding to platelets. However, the binding of VWF to single platelets from patients with either ET or reactive thrombocytosis was not shown to be different from that of normal controls (131). Instead, enhanced proteolytic degradation of VWF is the more likely mechanism (117,132–135). However, the relation between extreme thrombocytosis and decreased large VWF multimers suggests a key role for the number of circulating platelets in mediating this process (122). Platelet excess may facilitate the interaction between platelet surface receptor GPIb and VWF, thereby inducing the appropriate conformational changes in VWF that allows ADAMTS 13 to gain access to its cleavage site.

## Pathogenesis of Thrombotic Diathesis in Myeloproliferative Disorders

Thrombosis is often multifactorial in etiology. The MPD have an inherent predisposition to thrombosis driven by the underlying clonal proliferation, and this risk may be escalated in association with thrombogenic stimuli that contribute to thrombosis in the general population. As such, the role of hereditary and acquired cardiovascular and thrombophilic risk factors have been studied in relation to their contribution to MPD-related vascular complications.

In PV, hematocrit level is the major determinant of thrombosis and the most effective treatment strategy for this has been phlebotomy (136). The relation between thrombosis, hematocrit level, and *in vitro* parameters of blood viscosity and tissue perfusion is complex. For example, although hematocrit has been shown to be the major determinant of whole blood viscosity *in vitro* (137), flow dynamics in blood vessels is different than that predicted by *in vitro* experiments and, in addition, the strong relation between hematocrit and oxygen transport substantially influences *in vivo* blood viscosity (137). For example, *in vivo*, increased hematocrit level is associated with decreased cerebral blood flow rate (138) not because of the change in viscosity but because of arterial oxygen content (139). At low shear rates, which is comparable to flow in large veins, the endothelial displacement of platelets, leukocytes, and other proteins from axial migration of red cells might enhance thrombogenic interaction between endothelial cells and platelets (140). At high shear rates, which is comparable to flow in arterioles and other small vessels, red cell–derived platelet aggregants such as ADP, might contribute to thrombosis.

Although the reduction in hematocrit level by phlebotomy addresses the potentially detrimental, hematocrit-associated conditions (140,141) mentioned in preceding text, it does not abolish the risk of thrombosis in PV. Therefore, factors other than hematocrit (e.g., platelets, leukocytes, endothelial cells, coagulation proteins) might contribute to thrombosis risk in both PV and other MPD. In this context, potentially thrombogenic, qualitative cell defects have been described and include

a diminished response of platelet adenylate cyclase to prostaglandin D2 (a physiologic inhibitor of platelet aggregation) (142), an increased baseline platelet production of TxA2 (a platelet aggregant) (143,144), and abnormal *in vivo* activation of leukocytes (145), endothelial cells (145,146), and platelets (144,146). Furthermore, previous reports of widespread activation in coagulation proteins (145), reduced levels of physiologic anticoagulants (ATIII, proteins C and S) (147, 148), and decreased fibrinolytic activity (149) that may be partly secondary to increased plasma levels of plasminogen activator inhibitor (PAI)-1 (150) suggest a baseline prothrombotic state in these disorders.

Spontaneous platelet activation in MPD has been demonstrated by measurement of plasma and urinary levels of arachidonate metabolites thromboxane $B_2$ ($TxB_2$) and $\alpha$-granule proteins (platelet-derived growth factor, $\beta$-thromboglobulin, platelet factor 4) and accounts for the noted acquired storage pool disorder (102–105). Additional evidence comes from the assessment of platelet surface membrane expression of markers of platelet activation (with monoclonal antibodies to P selectin and the activated fibrinogen receptor, GPIIb/IIIa) by flow cytometry (119). It is possible that this abnormal activation state may be in part because of MPD-specific defects in arachidonic acid metabolism which result in abnormal and sustained spontaneous $TxA_2$ generation in PV and ET (151–153). This observed endogenous $TxA_2$ generation in PV and ET was found to be almost completely suppressible with low-dose aspirin (152,153). Clinically, this effect has been shown to correlate with resolution of microvascular thrombosis (28,154). The pathogenesis of the enhanced $TxA_2$ production in MPD is unknown but may involve preferential shunting of arachidonate to the cyclooxygenase pathway because of concurrent lipoxygenase deficiency (151). However, earlier studies suggested that patients with MPD and with lipoxygenase deficiency might display a hemorrhagic rather than thrombotic phenotype (151).

# DIAGNOSIS AND LABORATORY INVESTIGATION

## Essential Thrombocythemia

A working diagnosis of ET is considered in the presence of persistent nonreactive thrombocytosis and after the diagnostic exclusion of CML, PV, MDS, and MMM (including "cellular phase" MMM) (155–157). Accordingly, one has to first entertain the possibility of reactive thrombocytosis (RT) from various causes (see Table 108-3) during the initial evaluation of all such patients. In this context, patient history and physical examination are crucial and are often adequate to answer the specific question. Additional help is readily available from routine laboratory tests including serum ferritin (to consider the possibility of iron deficiency), peripheral blood smear (to look for Howell-Jolly bodies and other markers of hyposplenism), and C-reactive protein (CRP) or similar acute-phase reactants (to consider the possibility of occult inflammation or malignancy) (158). In addition, rare cases of genetically defined ET (activating mutation of the *c-Mpl* gene) have been described (159) and must be kept in mind while evaluating a patient with either lifelong history of thrombocytosis or a family history of the same (160).

If neither patient history nor the aforementioned laboratory tests suggest RT, a bone marrow examination is indicated to both reinforce the diagnosis of ET (increased megakaryocytes with atypical morphology and cluster formation, see Fig. 108-2) and address the possibility of another chronic myeloid disorder that might mimic ET in its presentation. Morphologic examination of the bone marrow by an experienced clinical pathologist is essential and often adequate to rule out the possibilities of

## TABLE 108-3

### CAUSES OF THROMBOCYTOSIS (161–166)

| Primary thrombocytosis | Reactive thrombocytosis |
|---|---|
| Essential thrombocythemia | Infection |
| Polycythemia vera | Tissue damage |
| Myelofibrosis with myeloid | Chronic inflammation |
| metaplasia (overt) | Malignancy |
| Myelofibrosis with myeloid | Rebound thrombocytosis |
| metaplasia (cellular phase) | Renal disorders |
| Chronic myeloid leukemia | Hemolytic anemia |
| Myelodysplastic syndrome | Postsplenectomy |
| Acute leukemia | Blood loss |

MDS and either overt or cellular phase MMM. Cytogenetic studies and fluorescence *in situ* hybridization (FISH) analysis for *bcr/abl* should accompany bone marrow examination to rule out the possibility of CML (167).

## Polycythemia Vera

The diagnosis of PV should be suspected in the presence of either an increased hemoglobin level (Hb >18 gm per dL in a Caucasian male or the corresponding level in the opposite sex or in the presence of a different ethnic origin) or a PV-associated clinical feature (e.g., pruritus, erythromelalgia, splenomegaly, large-vessel thrombosis, increased leukocytosis or thrombocytosis). In the absence of the above scenario, a repeat complete blood count in 3 months is all that is needed. Otherwise, one should further pursue the diagnosis of PV.

As is the case with ET, PV is currently a diagnosis of exclusion that requires the consideration of other causes of polycythemia including secondary (usually EPO-mediated) and apparent (spurious or relative) polycythemia. Traditionally, this was accomplished through the Polycythemia Vera Study Group (PVSG) criteria, that required the demonstration of an elevated red cell mass (RCM) (168). At present, we seldom use either the PVSG criteria or RCM measurement and instead depend on the clinical presentation, serum erythropoietin (sEPO) level, and bone marrow histology in order to make a working diagnosis of PV (see Fig. 108-3) (23).

Diagnostic workup for suspected PV starts with a determination of sEPO level. In PV, sEPO is usually low, but can be

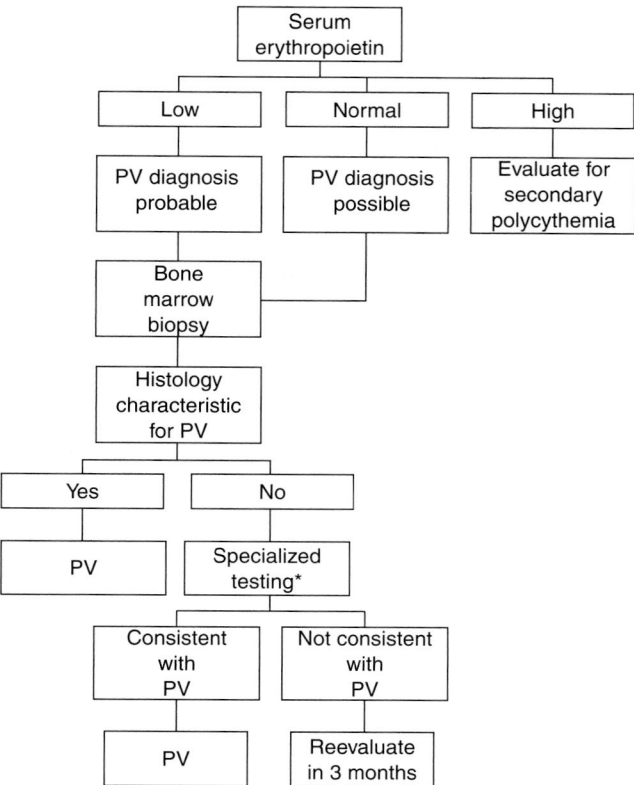

FIGURE 108-3. A practical algorithm for the diagnosis of polycythemia vera (PV). *Specialized testing includes bone marrow immunohistochemistry for the thrombopoietin receptor (c-Mpl), reverse transcriptase-polymerase chain reaction (RT-PCR) for neutrophil expression of polycythemia rubra vera (PRV)-1 gene, and spontaneous erythroid colony assay.

normal (169,170). It is, however, very unlikely to be elevated (169). Therefore, the diagnosis of PV is considered only if the sEPO is low or normal (Fig.108-3). The next step is to perform a bone marrow biopsy to look for morphologic evidence of PV (51). The characteristic histologic features include bone marrow hypercellularity, atypical megakaryocytic hyperplasia and clustering, and decreased bone marrow iron stores.

In more than 90% of the cases, a working diagnosis of PV is made possible on the basis of clinical and bone marrow histologic findings. In the remaining "equivocal" cases, one may need to resort to a specialized test. One such test involves the demonstration of reduced megakaryocyte expression of the TPO receptor (c-Mpl), by standard immunoperoxidase methods (171). Another relatively specific diagnostic test for PV involves the *in vitro* demonstration of EPO-independent erythroid colony formation (172). The most recent addition in the diagnostic armamentarium for PV is a PCR-based assay that shows overexpression of the PRV-1 gene in the peripheral blood neutrophils of patients with PV but not in the case of either secondary or apparent polycythemia (173).

## Myelofibrosis with Myeloid Metaplasia

The first clue to the diagnosis of MMM is a myelophthisic peripheral smear (the presence of nucleated red blood cells, granulocyte precursors, and teardrop-shaped erythrocytes). However, it should be noted that a myelophthisic smear may also be associated with either another myeloid malignancy with bone marrow fibrosis or a nonfibrotic bone marrow infiltrating

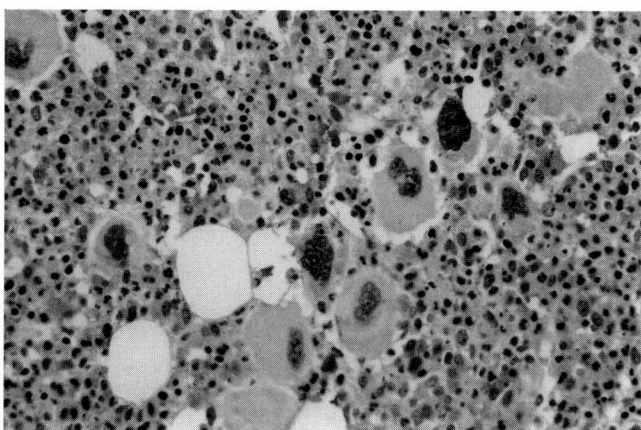

FIGURE 108-2. Megakaryocyte clusters in myeloproliferative disorders.

process including metastatic cancer, granulomatous infection, and lymphoma. Therefore, a careful morphologic evaluation of the bone marrow is necessary before making the diagnosis of MMM and cytogenetic tests, and FISH for *bcr/abl* should always be done to rule out fibrotic CML. Similarly, it is important to know that both MDS and other myeloid entities can be accompanied by bone marrow fibrosis and the input from an experienced clinical pathologist is essential to distinguish these disorders from MMM. Typical MMM is characterized by the presence of dysplastic megakaryocytic hyperplasia, collagen and reticulin fibrosis, osteosclerosis, and intrasinusoidal hematopoiesis. In "cellular phase" MMM, the degree of bone marrow fibrosis may be minimal but splenomegaly, myelophthisis, and increased serum lactate dehydrogenase (LDH) are often present. Recurrent cytogenetic abnormalities are seen in approximately 50% of chemotherapy naïve patients with MMM (174).

## Coagulation and Platelet Function Tests in Myeloproliferative Disorders

Routine coagulation studies, including activated partial thromboplastin time (aPTT), prothrombin time (PT), and fibrinogen are generally normal in both PV and ET. Although AVWS is associated with MPD, unlike the case with congenital VWD, the condition is usually associated with normal factor VIII levels, and therefore will not be detected on the basis of a prolonged aPTT (127). Despite evidence of platelet dysfunction in ET and PV, as assessed by platelet aggregation studies, a prolonged bleeding time is seen only in a few cases (range 7% to 26%) (25,36,37,175). Prolonged bleeding time in MPD has been attributed to an underlying defect in primary hemostasis (primary platelet dysfunction or AVWD), which is exacerbated by aspirin therapy (176).

Platelet aggregation studies are frequently abnormal in MPD (demonstrating either or both hypofunctional and hyperfunction) (25,177,178). In general, platelet hypofunction (decreased aggregation with one or more agonists) is the predominant finding (35). The most commonly reported abnormalities include decreased primary and secondary aggregation patterns to either epinephrine or ADP and decreased response to collagen, in descending order of frequency, with generally normal responses to arachidonic acid (35). In a review of several studies in patients with MPD, decreased aggregation responses to one, two, or all of these agonists were noted in 57%, 39%, and 37%, respectively (175). Unlike the commonly encountered aspirin-type release defect in which the primary wave in response to epinephrine is maintained, but no secondary wave is obtained, complete absence of response to epinephrine is characteristic of MPD (175).

Spontaneous platelet aggregation is another characteristic finding in MPD but has not been correlated with clinical bleeding or thrombosis (25,177). The possibility that whole blood–based platelet aggregation tests might provide a better clinical correlation has been touted but remains to be confirmed by additional studies (179).

# ACQUIRED AND HEREDITARY THROMBOPHILIA AND MYELOPROLIFERATIVE DISORDER

The contribution of well-established risk factors of cardiovascular disease (e.g., hypertension, smoking, hypercholesterolemia, diabetes mellitus) have been assessed in MPD by multiple studies with some conflicting results, possibly reflecting the size of the studies and number of patients with the risk markers of interest

included. On multivariate (hypertension, smoking, hypercholesterolemia, diabetes) analysis, one large retrospective study of patients with ET ($n = 148$) demonstrated only the independent contribution of hypercholesterolemia, and another ($n = 132$), the independent association with smoking only (22,180). The latter finding had been shown in an earlier, smaller ($n = 46$) study (181). However, other large retrospective cohort studies including these variables could not confirm these associations (25,36,38,182).

Over the last 2 decades, there has been a vast expansion in knowledge of hereditary and acquired conditions contributing to thrombosis (183). These include the congenital deficiencies of natural anticoagulants (e.g., antithrombin III, protein C and protein S), genetic mutations (e.g., factor $V_{Leiden}$, prothrombin G20210A, and MTHFR mutations), and acquired conditions (anticardiolipin antibodies and/or lupus anticoagulants). Several recent studies have explored the contribution of these to the occurrence of thrombotic events in MPD. Two prospective studies evaluated patients with ET to determine the allele frequencies factor $V_{Leiden}$, prothrombin G20210A, and MTHFR mutations among those with and without thrombotic complications (184,185). No significant correlation was found in either study, although both were limited by sample size ($n = 43$ and $n = 42$, respectively).

A more recent larger, yet retrospective study of 304 patients with PV ($n = 178$) and ET ($n = 126$), demonstrated a significant difference in the prevalence of the factor $V_{Leiden}$ mutation in patients with (16%), compared to those without (3%), a history of venous thrombotic events (186). No such relation was seen in arterial thrombosis, as would be expected with this mutation (187). This study did not investigate the other common thrombophilic polymorphisms (prothrombin G20210A, MTHFR) or acquired states (antiphospholipid syndrome), known to effect the phenotypic expression of prothrombotic disease (186).

Several studies have confirmed the presence of elevated homocysteine levels among patients with chronic myeloproliferative disorders (188–190). Elevated homocysteine levels may be hereditary (homozygosity for MTHFR mutation) or acquired (folic acid, vitamin $B_{12}$ or $B_6$ deficiencies, renal failure), and is a recognized risk factor for both arterial and venous thrombotic disease (191). However, no association with the homozygosity for the MTHFR mutation could be confirmed in these studies, leading investigators to postulate (and in study confirm) that the acquired increase in homocysteine may be the result of vitamin B deficiencies, possibly related to the persistent hyperproliferative hematopoiesis of these disorders. As for the clinical impact of these observations, an association with arterial thrombotic disease was demonstrated by only one of the aforementioned studies (188), but not by the others (189,190).

Antiphospholipid antibodies [as measured either by a clot-based assay (lupus anticoagulant) or enzyme-linked immunosorbent assay (ELISA)] are established risk factors for both arterial and venous thrombotic disease (192). Several investigators have reported an increased prevalence of antiphospholipid antibodies in ET (193,194). One of these studies suggested an association between the observed antiphospholipid antibodies and thrombosis (193). However, the small sample sizes of patients included and lack of follow-up testing to confirm persistence (and therefore significance) of the detected antibodies precludes any firm conclusions be made of these findings.

# GENERAL MANAGEMENT

## Essential Thrombocythemia

ET is associated with a near-normal life expectancy and, therefore, treatment is never instituted for the purpose of

## TABLE 108-4

### RISK STRATIFICATION IN POLYCYTHEMIA VERA AND ESSENTIAL THROMBOCYTHEMIA

| | |
|---|---|
| Low-risk | Age <60 yr, *and* <br> No history of thrombosis, *and* <br> Platelet count <1.5 million/μL, *and* <br> Absence of cardiovascular risk factors (smoking, hypertension, hyperlipidemia, diabetes) |
| Indeterminate-risk | Neither low-risk nor high-risk |
| High-risk | Age 60 yr or above, *or* <br> A positive history of thrombosis |

improving survival (195). Instead, specific therapy is sought to either alleviate microvascular disturbances or prevent thrombohemorrhagic complications. Microvascular symptoms are often adequately controlled by low-dose aspirin (196). Treatment to prevent vascular events is dictated by the presence or absence of defined risk factors for thrombosis (see Table 108-4) (156). In this context, most investigators consider age 60 years and more, and a history of thrombosis, but not platelet count, as independent risk factors for thrombosis (22,27,35,181). On the other hand, the prognostic relevance of cardiovascular risk factors is debated (27,36,181).

Over the years, remarkably little has been accomplished by way of controlled treatment trials in ET (197). Physicians, therefore, have relied mostly on carefully conducted prospective cohort studies (198), as well as large retrospective studies (22,25,27,36) to guide them in patient management (199,200). Accordingly, it is generally felt that thrombotic events in low-risk patients are too infrequent to justify the long-term use of potentially harmful cytoreductive agents (see Table 108-5). In such patients, the use of low-dose aspirin is encouraged on the basis of the recently demonstrated antithrombotic value in PV (201). The low-risk pregnant patient should not receive any cytoreductive agent, and the use of aspirin is optional and does not influence outcome of pregnancy (202).

In high-risk patients with ET, hydroxyurea is the only cytoreductive agent that has been shown, in a controlled clinical trial setting, to benefit patients by reducing the risk of thrombosis, as opposed to just lowering platelet count (197). In patients with hydroxyurea-associated side effects (e.g., leg ulcers) (203) interferon-α, including the pegylated form, is a reasonable alternative and is the drug of choice during pregnancy (204,205). When both hydroxyurea and interferon-α are not tolerated, other drugs including anagrelide and pipobroman might be considered (see Table 108-6). Once cytoreductive therapy is initiated, the therapeutic goal in terms of platelet count, based on anecdotal evidence of optimal thrombosis control, is less than 400,000 per μL (206,207). There is little evidence to suggest that other drugs are less leukemogenic than hydroxyurea or offer a therapeutic advantage over the same (208–213).

In indeterminate-risk patients with ET (Table 108-4), the use of low-dose aspirin is encouraged in the absence of clinically relevant AVWD (214). The use of platelet-lowering agents, on the other hand, is controversial. However, cytoreductive treatment is appropriate in patients with extreme thrombocytosis that is associated with a bleeding diathesis or aspirin-resistant microvascular symptoms. Table 108-5 outlines a treatment algorithm we currently use for ET.

## Polycythemia Vera

Currently identified risk factors and risk stratification in PV are similar to those of ET (Table 108-4) (32,40). The cornerstone of treatment in PV is phlebotomy (to <45% in men and 42% in women) (40). To date, no other therapy has been shown to offer a survival advantage over treatment with phlebotomy alone (40). However, treatment with phlebotomy alone is associated with a substantial risk of thrombosis in high-risk patients where the concurrent use of myelosuppressive treatment is indicated (40). In the latter instance, the use of chlorambucil or $^{32}$P is contraindicated because of an increased risk of acute leukemia (40) and hydroxyurea is the current drug of choice (215). However, some investigators are concerned about potential leukemogenicity associated with long-term use of hydroxyurea and prefer the use of interferon-α in young patients (216). Similarly, interferon-α is the preferred drug in women of childbearing age. On the basis of the results of a recent randomized treatment trial, low-dose aspirin is recommended in all patients with PV in the absence of contraindications (201). Table 108-7 provides a treatment algorithm for PV. Finally, PV-associated pruritus might be alleviated with the use of a selective-serotonin-reuptake-inhibitor (paroxetine 20 mg per day) (217).

## Myelofibrosis with Myeloid Metaplasia

MMM is also known as idiopathic myelofibrosis and the disease presents either *de novo* [agnogenic myeloid metaplasia (AMM)] or in the setting of either PV (postpolycythemic myeloid

## TABLE 108-5

### TREATMENT ALGORITHM IN ESSENTIAL THROMBOCYTHEMIA

| Risk category | Age <60 yr | Age ≥60 yr | Women of childbearing age |
|---|---|---|---|
| Low-risk | Low-dose aspirin[a] | Not applicable | Low-dose aspirin[a] |
| Indeterminate-risk[b] | Low-dose aspirin[a] | Not applicable | Low-dose aspirin[a] |
| High-risk | Hydroxyurea *and* low-dose aspirin | Hydroxyurea *and* low-dose aspirin | Interferon-α *and* low-dose aspirin |

[a]In the absence of a contraindication including evidence for acquired von Willebrand syndrome, i.e., a von Willebrand antigen/ristocetin cofactor activity ratio of less than 0.7.
[b]The decision to use cytoreductive agents in indeterminate-risk patients should be made on an individual basis (see text for details).

**TABLE 108-6**

CLINICAL PROPERTIES OF PLATELET-LOWERING AGENTS (218–243)

| Drug (class) | Hydroxyurea (myelosuppressive) | Anagrelide (platelet-specific) | Interferon-α (myelosuppressive) | Phosphorous-32 (myelosuppressive) | Pipobroman (myelosuppressive) |
|---|---|---|---|---|---|
| Mechanism of action | Antimetabolite | Unknown | Biologic agent | Radionuclide | Alkylating agent |
| Pharmacology | Half-life ≅ 5 h, renal excretion | Half-life ≅ 1.5 h, renal excretion | Kidney is main site of metabolism | Half-life ≅ 14 d | Insufficient information |
| Starting dose | 500 mg PO b.i.d. | 0.5 mg PO t.i.d. | 5 million U sc t.i.w. | 2.3 mCi/m2 IV | 1 mg/kg/d PO |
| Onset of action | ≅ 3–5 d | ≅ 6–10 d | 1–3 wk | 4–8 wk | ≅ 16 d |
| Frequent side effects | Leucopenia, oral ulcers, anemia, hyperpigmentation, nail discoloration, xerodermia | Headache, palpitations, diarrhea, fluid retention, anemia | Flulike syndrome, fatigue, anorexia, weight loss, lack of ambition, alopecia | Transient mild cytopenia | Nausea, abdominal pain, diarrhea |
| Infrequent side effects | Leg ulcers, nausea, diarrhea, alopecia, skin atrophy | Arrhythmias, light headedness, nausea myalgia, arthritis | Confusion, depression, autoimmune thyroiditis | Prolonged pancytopenia in elderly patients | Leukopenia, thrombocytopenia, hemolysis |
| Rare side effects | Fever, cystitis platelet oscillations | Cardiomyopathy | Pruritis, hyperlipidemia, transaminasemia | Leukemogenic | |
| Cost[a] | Annual = $1,714, for 500 mg t.i.d. dose | Annual = $8,500, for 0.5 mg q.i.d. dose | Annual = $10,500, for 3 million U 5 d/wk | Approximately $1,025 for 4 mCi | Not available in USA |

PO, oral; b.i.d., twice-a-day; t.i.d., thrice-a-day; q.i.d., four times a day; sc, subcutaneous; t.i.w., three times a week; IV, intravenous.
Hydroxyurea (109–117), anagrelide (45,114,118–122), interferon-α (25,35,35–38,44,123–129,129–160,167–182,182–204), phosphorous-32 (35,117,126), pipobroman (113,127–130).
[a] Current cost to patient.

metaplasia, PPMM) or ET (postthrombocythemic myeloid metaplasia, PTMM) at a rate of 10% to 20% after 15 to 20 years of follow-up (40,244). Because of similarities in clinical manifestations and prognosis, PPMM and PTMM are managed similar to AMM. In general, drug therapy has not been shown to prolong survival in MMM and is used to palliate symptoms. Similarly, both splenectomy and involved field irradiation engender a defined palliative role in the treatment of MMM. Allogeneic hematopoietic stem cell transplantation

(AHSCT) has been shown to be both feasible and effective but carries substantial procedure-related mortality and morbidity. As a result, defined risk factors are used to select suitable patients for AHSCT.

Androgen preparations (e.g., oral fluoxymesterone 10 mg two times a day), corticosteroids (e.g., oral prednisone 30 mg per day), and EPO (e.g., 40,000 U subcutaneously once-a-week) are used as first-line therapy for alleviation of anemia (24,245–251). An approximate 30% response rate with median

**TABLE 108-7**

TREATMENT ALGORITHM IN POLYCYTHEMIA VERA

| Risk category | Age < 60 yr | Age ≥60 yr | Women of childbearing age |
|---|---|---|---|
| Low-risk | Phlebotomy and low-dose aspirin[a] | Not applicable | Phlebotomy and low-dose aspirin[a] |
| Indeterminate-risk[b] | Phlebotomy and low-dose aspirin[a] | Not applicable | Phlebotomy and low-dose aspirin[a] |
| High-risk | Phlebotomy + hydroxyurea and low-dose aspirin | Phlebotomy + hydroxyurea and low-dose aspirin | Phlebotomy + interferon-α and low-dose aspirin |

[a] In the absence of a contraindication including evidence for acquired von Willebrand disease, i.e., a von Willebrand antigen/ristocetin cofactor activity ratio of <0.7.
[b] The decision to use cytoreductive agents in indeterminate-risk patients should be made on an individual basis (see text for details).

remission duration of 1 year is expected from the use of one or more of these treatment modalities. Symptomatic splenomegaly is initially treated with hydroxyurea (e.g., starting dose of 500 mg two or three times a day) (252). Splenectomy is indicated in the presence of drug-refractory splenic pain and/or discomfort, high RBC transfusion requirements, and symptomatic portal hypertension (253). The particular procedure provides symptomatic relief for most patients and durable anemia response in 25% of the patients. Splenectomy in MMM carries operative mortality of approximately 9%, and 25% of patients may experience postsplenectomy thrombocytosis and progressive hepatomegaly. Involved field radiation therapy works best for nonhepatosplenic EMH (254,255) but has limited value in controlling symptomatic enlargement of the spleen and liver (256,257).

Thalidomide is now considered an effective drug in MMM. Studies that involved 10 or more patients have demonstrated a response rate of 20% to 62% in anemia, 25% to 80% in thrombocytopenia, and 7% to 30% in splenomegaly (258–263). Information from these studies indicates that low-dose thalidomide (50 mg per day) was as effective as higher doses (200 mg or more per day), and that the addition of prednisone to the lower-dose schedule improves drug tolerance and may enhance the erythropoietic activity of the drug (263,264).

Treatment with AHSCT, either myeloablative (265–267) or reduced-intensity (268,269), is directed at eradicating the mutant MMM clone. The three largest studies about myeloablative AHSCT (both related and matched unrelated) consist of a total 147 patients between them (266,267,270). In general, engraftment was not a problem with more than 80% of patients achieving safe neutrophil counts by day 30 (270). However, transplantation-related death and morbidity were not trivial, resulting in a 5-year survival of only 14% for patients older than 44 years in one study (270) and a 2-year overall survival of 41% in another study (267). In the most favorable of the three studies, 20 of the 56 patients had died within 3 years of the transplantation and the reported incidence of chronic graft versus host disease (CGVHD) was 59% at a median follow-up period of only 2.8 years (266).

In general, transplantation outcome in younger patients was encouraging in all the three studies mentioned earlier with projected 5-year survival rates of more than 60% and clinical, as well as histologic remissions were documented in the surviving patients (266,270). At present, we do not recommend AHSCT, either myeloablative or reduced-intensity conditioning, for the patient whose life expectancy is estimated to exceed 10 years. In contrast, it is reasonable to consider AHSCT in patients younger than 60 years, in whom a survival of less than 5 years can be reliably predicted (271,272).

# MANAGEMENT AND PREVENTION OF THROMBOHEMORRHAGIC COMPLICATIONS

Platelet count reduction to below 1 million per $\mu$L is the most effective means of controlling symptomatic, MPD-associated AVWS, and this is best accomplished by the use of cytoreductive chemotherapy (117,123,176). The main drug of choice for this is hydroxyurea (197). Platelet apheresis for MPD-associated AVWS is indicated when extreme thrombocytosis is accompanied by an urgent need to acutely reduce the platelet count (117,123,176). The procedure has often been employed in the setting of postsplenectomy thrombocytosis because of the associated high risk of hemostatic morbidity (176,273). Because the beneficial effect of platelet pheresis is generally

brief, and repeated procedures are often required, it is recommended that cytoreductive therapy be initiated as soon as possible, to provide long-term control of the platelet count.

Desmopressin, during the treatment of MPD-associated AVWS, has been shown to increase both VWF:Ag and function (117,123,133,176). However, due to the increased VWF proteolysis observed in association with MPD-associated thrombocytosis, the half-life of functional VWF is decreased, rendering the administration of desmopressin generally of a limited value. Furthermore, in view of reports of thrombotic complications (e.g., stroke and myocardial infarction) among patients with increased thrombotic risk (elderly, cardiovascular disease) treated with desmopressin, administration of this agent to patients with MPD may not be prudent (274,275). Similar problems may arise from the administration of VWF-containing plasma products (such as cryoprecipitate or VWF–containing concentrates) (176).

To minimize aspirin-associated bleeding diathesis in MPD, low-dose aspirin (75 to 100 mg per day), is administered with or after a meal and concurrent therapy with a proton-pump inhibitor is considered for patients with gastric symptoms (200). In the presence of extreme thrombocytosis (platelet count greater than $1,000 \times 10^9$ per L), it is recommended that clinically significant AVWS be ruled out before the institution of aspirin therapy. If aspirin therapy is indicated in the particular instance, cytoreduction is necessary to reduce the platelet count to below $800 \times 10^9$ per L, which usually corrects the AVWS, before instituting aspirin therapy.

Thrombotic episodes in patients with MPD are managed in the usual manner with standard dose and schedule of systemic anticoagulant therapy. However, systemic anticoagulation alone is not sufficient and myelosuppressive therapy should be instituted to further reduce the risk of recurrent thrombosis in patients with either PV or ET (40). Because of the potential for increased bleeding risk, especially in patients with MPD (276), long-term warfarin therapy requires close monitoring of both the international normalized ratio (INR), in view of potential drug interactions and dietary influences, and the platelet count to avoid overlooking inadvertent thrombocytopenia caused by excessive myelosuppression. The use of aspirin in combination with oral anticoagulant therapy increases the risk of bleeding. However, no studies have been performed addressing the combined use of these agents in MPD.

Patients with MPD have a higher risk of morbidity and mortality when undergoing surgical procedures. These risks are substantially increased in the setting of splenectomy, a procedure often performed for management of symptomatic splenomegaly due to portal vein thrombosis or MMM (253, 277,278). Splenectomy in MMM typically leads to extreme thrombocytosis postprocedure in the absence of appropriate platelet suppression. In one series of 223 patients undergoing splenectomy for MMM, postoperative thrombocytosis developed in 49 patients (22%) and nine (18%) died as a result of either thrombosis (six patients) or gastrointestinal bleeding (three patients) (253). Therefore, patients with MPD undergoing surgery should first have their disease well controlled (i.e., hematocrit level <45% and platelet count <$400 \times 10^9$ per L), and the prophylactic use of hydroxyurea should be considered before splenectomy.

Daily platelet counts should be performed in the immediate postoperative period. Aspirin therapy should be withheld for at least 1 week before elective surgery, as well as when elective anticoagulation is required perioperatively. Although there are no prospective studies describing the efficacy of prophylactic anticoagulation for patients with MPD, such therapy might be instituted in view of the increased risk of postoperative thrombosis, for patients without known contraindications. However, such patients must be followed closely for the development of hemorrhage. Aspirin can be restarted 24 hours after surgery if no excessive bleeding has occurred or is anticipated by the surgeon. Aspirin can also be restarted 24 hours after stopping heparin prophylaxis in patients where this is prescribed.

# References

1. Dameshek W. Some speculations on the myeloproliferative syndromes. *Blood* 1951;6:372–375.
2. Fialkow PJ, Gartler SM, Yoshida A. Clonal origin of chronic myelocytic leukemia in man. *Proc Natl Acad Sci U S A* 1967;58:1468–1471.
3. Barr RD, Fialkow PJ. Clonal origin of chronic myelocytic leukemia. *N Engl J Med* 1973;289:307–309.
4. Adamson JW, Fialkow PJ, Murphy S, et al. Polycythemia vera: stem-cell and probable clonal origin of the disease. *N Engl J Med* 1976;295:913–916.
5. Fialkow PJ, Jacobson RJ, Papayannopoulou T. Chronic myelocytic leukemia: clonal origin in a stem cell common to the granulocyte, erythrocyte, platelet and monocyte/macrophage. *Am J Med* 1977;63:125–130.
6. Fialkow PJ, Denman AM, Jacobson RJ, et al. Chronic myelocytic leukemia. Origin of some lymphocytes from leukemic stem cells. *J Clin Invest* 1978;62:815–823.
7. Jacobson RJ, Salo A, Fialkow PJ. Agnogenic myeloid metaplasia: a clonal proliferation of hematopoietic stem cells with secondary myelofibrosis. *Blood* 1978;51:189–194.
8. Martin PJ, Najfeld V, Hansen JA, et al. Involvement of the B-lymphoid system in chronic myelogenous leukaemia. *Nature* 1980;287:49–50.
9. Fialkow PJ, Faguet GB, Jacobson RJ, et al. Evidence that essential thrombocythemia is a clonal disorder with origin in a multipotent stem cell. *Blood* 1981;58:916–919.
10. Nowell PC, Hungerford DA. A minute chromosome in human chronic granulocytic leukemia. *J Natl Cancer Inst* 1960;25:85.
11. Cools J, DeAngelo DJ, Gotlib J, et al. A tyrosine kinase created by fusion of the PDGFRA and FIP1L1 genes as a therapeutic target of imatinib in idiopathic hypereosinophilic syndrome. *N Engl J Med* 2003;348: 1201–1214.
12. Mesa RA, Silverstein MN, Jacobsen SJ, et al. Population-based incidence and survival figures in essential thrombocythemia and agnogenic myeloid metaplasia: an Olmsted County study, 1976-1995. *Am J Hematol* 1999;61:10–15.
13. Ania BJ, Suman VJ, Sobell JL, et al. Trends in the incidence of polycythemia vera among Olmsted County, Minnesota residents, 1935-1989. *Am J Hematol* 1994;47:89–93.
14. Hasle H. Incidence of essential thrombocythaemia in children. *Br J Haematol* 2000;110:751.
15. McNally RJ, Rowland D, Roman E, et al. Age and sex distributions of hematological malignancies in the U.K. *Hematol Oncol* 1997;15:173–189.
16. Altura RA, Head DR, Wang WC. Long-term survival of infants with idiopathic myelofibrosis. *Br J Haematol* 2000;109:459–462.
17. Reznikoff P, Foot NC, Bethea JM, et al. Racial and geographic origin by patients suffering from polycythemia vera and pathologic findings in blood vessels and bone marrow. *Trans Assoc Am Physicians* 1934;49:273.
18. Damon A, Holub DA. Host factors in polycythemia vera. *Ann Intern Med* 1958;49:43.
19. Modan B, Kallner H, Zemer D, et al. A note on the increased risk of polycythemia vera in Jews. *Blood* 1971;37:172–176.
20. Chaiter Y, Brenner B, Aghai E, et al. High incidence of myeloproliferative disorders in Ashkenazi Jews in northern Israel. *Leuk Lymphoma* 1992;7:251–255.
21. Najean Y, Rain JD, Billotey C. Epidemiological data in polycythaemia vera: a study of 842 cases. *Hematol Cell Ther* 1998;40:159–165.
22. Besses C, Cervantes F, Pereira A, et al. Major vascular complications in essential thrombocythemia: a study of the predictive factors in a series of 148 patients. *Leukemia* 1999;13:150–154.
23. Tefferi A. Polycythemia vera: a comprehensive review and clinical recommendations. *Mayo Clin Proc* 2003;78:174–194.
24. Tefferi A. Myelofibrosis with myeloid metaplasia. *N Engl J Med* 2000;342:1255–1265.
25. Fenaux P, Simon M, Caulier MT, et al. Clinical course of essential thrombocythemia in 147 cases. *Cancer* 1990;66:549–556.
26. Tefferi A, Fonseca R, Pereira DL, et al. A long-term retrospective study of young women with essential thrombocythemia. *Mayo Clin Proc* 2001;76:22–28.
27. Bazzan M, Tamponi G, Schinco P, et al. Thrombosis-free survival and life expectancy in 187 consecutive patients with essential thrombocythemia. *Ann Hematol* 1999;78:539–543.
28. Michiels JJ, Abels J, Steketee J, et al. Erythromelalgia caused by platelet-mediated arteriolar inflammation and thrombosis in thrombocythemia. *Ann Intern Med* 1985;102:466–471.
29. Davis MD, O'Fallon WM, Rogers RS III, et al. Natural history of erythromelalgia: presentation and outcome in 168 patients. *Arch Dermatol* 2000;136:330–336.
30. Wright CA, Tefferi A. A single institutional experience with 43 pregnancies in essential thrombocythemia. *Eur J Haematol* 2001;66:152–159.
31. Anger B, Haug U, Seidler R, et al. Polycythemia vera. A clinical study of 141 patients. *Blut* 1989;59:493–500.
32. *Ann Intern Med.* Polycythemia vera: the natural history of 1213 patients followed for 20 years. *Gruppo Italiano Studio Policitemia.* 1995;123:656–664
33. Passamonti F, Malabarba L, Orlandi E, et al. Polycythemia vera in young patients: a study on the long-term risk of thrombosis, myelofibrosis and leukemia. *Haematologica* 2003;88:13–18.
34. Diehn F, Tefferi A. Pruritus in polycythaemia vera: prevalence, laboratory correlates and management. *Br J Haematol* 2001;115:619–621.
35. Bellucci S, Janvier M, Tobelem G, et al. Essential thrombocythemias. Clinical evolutionary and biological data. *Cancer* 1986;58:2440–2447.
36. Cortelazzo S, Viero P, Finazzi G, et al. Incidence and risk factors for thrombotic complications in a historical cohort of 100 patients with essential thrombocythemia. *J Clin Oncol* 1990;8:556–562.
37. Colombi M, Radaelli F, Zocchi L, et al. Thrombotic and hemorrhagic complications in essential thrombocythemia. A retrospective study of 103 patients. *Cancer* 1991;67:2926–2930.
38. Jensen MK, de Nully Brown P, Nielsen OJ, et al. Incidence, clinical features and outcome of essential thrombocythaemia in a well defined geographical area. *Eur J Haematol* 2000;65:132–139.
39. Berk PD, Goldberg JD, Silverstein MN, et al. Increased incidence of acute leukemia in polycythemia vera associated with chlorambucil therapy. *N Engl J Med* 1981;304:441–447.
40. Berk PD, Wasserman LR, Fruchtman SM, et al. Treatment of polycythemia vera: a summary of clinical trials conducted by the polycythemia vera study group. In: *Polycyhtemia vera and the myeloproliferative disorders.* Wasserman LR, Berk PD, Berlin NI, eds. Philadelphia, PA: WB Saunders 1995:166–194.
41. Passamonti F, Malabarba L, Orlandi E, et al. Pipobroman is safe and effective treatment for patients with essential thrombocythaemia at high risk of thrombosis. *Br J Haematol* 2002;116:855–861.
42. Wolf BC, Banks PM, Mann RB, et al. Splenic hematopoiesis in polycythemia vera. A morphologic and immunohistologic study. *Am J Clin Pathol* 1988;89:69–75.
43. Jaroch MT, Broughan TA, Hermann RE. The natural history of splenic infarction. *Surgery* 1986;100:743–750.
44. Raskind WH, Jacobson R, Murphy S, et al. Evidence for the involvement of B lymphoid cells in polycythemia vera and essential thrombocythemia. *J Clin Invest* 1985;75:1388–1390.
45. Elkassar N, Hetet G, Briere J, et al. Clonality analysis of hematopoiesis in essential thrombocythemia—advantages of studying T lymphocytes and platelets. *Blood* 1997;89:128–134.
46. Kreipe H, Jaquet K, Felgner J, et al. Clonal granulocytes and bone marrow cells in the cellular phase of agnogenic myeloid metaplasia. *Blood* 1991;78:1814–1817.
47. Prchal JT, Guan YL. A novel clonality assay based on transcriptional analysis of the active X chromosome. *Stem Cells* 1993;11(Suppl. 1):62–65.
48. Tefferi A. The pathogenesis of chronic myeloproliferative diseases. *Int J Hematol* 2001;73:170–176.
49. Mesa RA, Hanson CA, Rajkumar SV, et al. Evaluation and clinical correlations of bone marrow angiogenesis in myelofibrosis with myeloid metaplasia. *Blood* 2000;96:3374–3380.
50. Ellis JT, Peterson P, Geller SA, et al. Studies of the bone marrow in polycythemia vera and the evolution of myelofibrosis and second hematologic malignancies. *Semin Hematol* 1986;23:144–155.
51. Thiele J, Kvasnicka HM, Zankovich R, et al. The value of bone marrow histology in differentiating between early stage polycythemia vera and secondary (reactive) Polycythemias. *Haematologica* 2001;86:368–374.
52. Mesa RA, Hanson CA, Li CY, et al. Diagnostic and prognostic value of bone marrow angiogenesis and megakaryocyte c-Mpl expression in essential thrombocythemia. *Blood* 2002;99:4131–4137.
53. Annaloro C, Lambertenghi Deliliers G, Oriani A, et al. Prognostic significance of bone marrow biopsy in essential thrombocythemia. *Haematologica* 1999;84:17–21.
54. Thiele J, Kvasnicka HM, Zankovich R, et al. Relevance of bone marrow features in the differential diagnosis between essential thrombocythemia and early stage idiopathic myelofibrosis. *Haematologica* 2000; 85:1126–1134.
55. Jensen MK, Holten-Andersen MN, Riisbro R, et al. Elevated plasma levels of TIMP-1 correlate with plasma suPAR/uPA in patients with chronic myeloproliferative disorders. *Eur J Haematol* 2003;71:377–384.
56. Lundberg LG, Lerner R, Sundelin P, et al. Bone marrow in polycythemia vera, chronic myelocytic leukemia, and myelofibrosis has an increased vascularity. *Am J Pathol* 2000;157:15–19.
57. Michiels JJ. Bone marrow histopathology and biological markers as specific clues to the differential diagnosis of essential thrombocythemia, polycythemia vera and prefibrotic or fibrotic agnogenic myeloid metaplasia. *Hematol J* 2004;5:93–102.
58. Panteli K, Zagorianakou N, Bai M, et al. Angiogenesis in chronic myeloproliferative diseases detected by CD34 expression. *Eur J Haematol* 2004;72:410–415.
59. Wrobel T, Mazur G, Surowiak P, et al. Increased expression of vascular endothelial growth factor (VEGF) in bone marrow of patients with myeloproliferative disorders (MPD). *Pathol Oncol Res* 2003;9:170–173.

60. Castro-Malaspina H, Gay RE, Jhanwar SC, et al. Characteristics of bone marrow fibroblast colony-forming cells (CFU-F) and their progeny in patients with myeloproliferative disorders. *Blood* 1982;59:1046–1054.

61. Castro-Malaspina H, Rabellino EM, Yen A, et al. Human megakaryocyte stimulation of proliferation of bone marrow fibroblasts. *Blood* 1981;57: 781–787.

62. Rameshwar P, Denny TN, Stein D, et al. Monocyte adhesion in patients with bone marrow fibrosis is required for the production of fibrogenic cytokines. Potential role for interleukin-1 and TGF-beta. *J Immunol* 1994; 153:2819–2830.

63. Musolino C, Calabro L, Bellomo G, et al. Soluble angiogenic factors: implications for chronic myeloproliferative disorders. *Am J Hematol* 2002; 69:159–163.

64. Schmitt A, Jouault H, Guichard J, et al. Pathologic interaction between megakaryocytes and polymorphonuclear leukocytes in myelofibrosis. *Blood* 2000;96:1342–1347.

65. Pelus LM, Bian H, King AG, et al. Neutrophil-derived MMP-9 mediates synergistic mobilization of hematopoietic stem and progenitor cells by the combination of G-CSF and the chemokines GRObeta/CXCL2 and GRO-betaT/CXCL2delta4. *Blood* 2004;103:110–119.

66. Barosi G, Viarengo G, Pecci A, et al. Diagnostic and clinical relevance of the number of circulating CD34(+) cells in myelofibrosis with myeloid metaplasia. *Blood* 2001;98:3249–3255.

67. Reid CD. The significance of endogenous erythroid colonies (EEC) in haematological disorders. *Blood Rev* 1987;1:133–140.

68. Prchal JF, Axelrad AA. Letter: bone-marrow responses in polycythemia vera. *N Engl J Med* 1974;290:1382.

69. Fisher MJ, Prchal JF, Prchal JT, et al. Anti-erythropoietin (EPO) receptor monoclonal antibodies distinguish EPO-dependent and EPO-independent erythroid progenitors in polycythemia vera. *Blood* 1994;84:1982–1991.

70. Juvonen E, Partanen S, Ikkala E, et al. Megakaryocytic colony formation in polycythaemia vera and secondary erythrocytosis. *Br J Haematol* 1988; 69:441–444.

71. Juvonen E, Ikkala E, Oksanen K, et al. Megakaryocyte and erythroid colony formation in essential thrombocythaemia and reactive thrombocytosis: diagnostic value and correlation to complications. *Br J Haematol* 1993;83:192–197.

72. Juvonen E, Partanen S, Ruutu T. Colony formation by megakaryocytic progenitors in essential thrombocythaemia. *Br J Haematol* 1987;66:161–164.

73. Battegay EJ, Thomssen C, Nissen C, et al. Endogenous megakaryocyte colonies from peripheral blood in precursor cell cultures of patients with myeloproliferative disorders. *Eur J Haematol* 1989;42:321–326.

74. Florensa L, Besses C, Woessner S, et al. Endogenous megakaryocyte and erythroid colony formation from blood in essential thrombocythaemia. *Leukemia* 1995;9:271–273.

75. Lutton JD, Levere RD. Endogenous erythroid colony formation by peripheral blood mononuclear cells from patients with myelofibrosis and polycythemia vera. *Acta Haematol* 1979;62:94–99.

76. Siitonen T, Zheng A, Savolainen ER, et al. Spontaneous granulocyte-macrophage colony growth by peripheral blood mononuclear cells in myeloproliferative disorders. *Leuk Res* 1996;20:187–195.

77. Li Y, Hetet G, Maurer AM, et al. Spontaneous megakaryocyte colony formation in myeloproliferative disorders is not neutralizable by antibodies against IL3, IL6 and GM-CSF. *Br J Haematol* 1994;87:471–476.

78. Hess G, Rose P, Gamm H, et al. Molecular analysis of the erythropoietin receptor system in patients with polycythaemia vera. *Br J Haematol* 1994; 88:794–802.

79. Taksin AL, Couedic JPL, Dusanter-Fourt I, et al. Autonomous megakaryocyte growth in essential thrombocythemia and idiopathic myelofibrosis is not related to a c-mpl mutation or to an autocrine stimulation by Mpl-L. *Blood* 1999;93:125–139.

80. Asimakopoulos FA, Hinshelwood S, Gilbert JGR, et al. The gene encoding hematopoietic cell phosphatase (Shp-1) is structurally and transcriptionally intact in polycythemia vera. *Oncogene* 1997;14:1215–1222.

81. Correa PN, Eskinazi D, Axelrad AA. Circulating erythroid progenitors in polycythemia vera are hypersensitive to insulin-like growth factor-1 *in vitro*: studies in an improved serum-free medium [see comments]. *Blood* 1994;83:99–112.

82. Dai CH, Krantz SB, Green WF, et al. Polycythaemia vera. III. Burst-forming units-erythroid (BFU-E) response to stem cell factor and c-kit receptor expression. *Br J Haematol* 1994;86:12–21.

83. Dai CH, Krantz SB, Dessypris EN, et al. Polycythemia vera. II. Hypersensitivity of bone marrow erythroid, granulocyte-macrophage, and megakaryocyte progenitor cells to interleukin-3 and granulocyte-macrophage colony-stimulating factor. *Blood* 1992;80:891–899.

84. Dai CH, Krantz SB, Means RT Jr, et al. Polycythemia vera blood burst-forming units-erythroid are hypersensitive to interleukin-3. *J Clin Invest* 1991;87:391–396.

85. Montagna C, Massaro P, Morali F, et al. *In vitro* sensitivity of human erythroid progenitors to hemopoietic growth factors: studies on primary and secondary polycythemia. *Haematologica* 1994;79:311–318.

86. Martin JM, Gandhi K, Jackson WR, et al. Hypersensitivity of polycythemia vera megakaryocytic progenitors to thrombopoietin. *Blood* 1996;88:363a.

87. Kobayashi S, Teramura M, Hoshino S, et al. Circulating megakaryocyte progenitors in myeloproliferative disorders are hypersensitive to interleukin-3. *Br J Haematol* 1993;83:539–544.

88. Axelrad AA, Eskinazi D, Correa PN, et al. Hypersensitivity of circulating progenitor cells to megakaryocyte growth and development factor (PEG-rHu MGDF) in essential thrombocythemia. *Blood* 2000;96:3310–3321.

89. Mirza AM, Ezzat S, Axelrad AA. Insulin-like growth factor binding protein-1 is elevated in patients with polycythemia vera and stimulates erythroid burst formation *in vitro*. *Blood* 1997;89:1862–1869.

90. Michl P, Spoettl G, Engelhardt D, et al. Alterations of the insulin-like growth factor system in patients with polycythemia vera. *Mol Cell Endocrinol* 2001;181:189–197.

91. Lecouedic JP, Mitjavila MT, Villeval JL, et al. Missense mutation of the erythropoietin receptor is a rare event in human erythroid malignancies. *Blood* 1996;87:1502–1511.

92. Mittelman M, Gardyn J, Carmel M, et al. Analysis of the erythropoietin receptor gene in patients with myeloproliferative and myelodysplastic syndromes. *Leuk Res* 1996;20:459–466.

93. Harrison CN, Gale RE, Wiestner AC, et al. The activating splice mutation in intron 3 of the thrombopoietin gene is not found in patients with non-familial essential thrombocythaemia. *Br J Haematol* 1998; 102:1341–1343.

94. Horikawa Y, Matsumura I, Hashimoto K, et al. Markedly reduced expression of platelet C-Mpl receptor in essential thrombocythemia. *Blood* 1997;90:4031–4038.

95. Moliterno AR, Hankins WD, Spivak JL. Impaired expression of the thrombopoietin receptor by platelets from patients with polycythemia vera. *N Engl J Med* 1998;338:572–580.

96. Harrison CN, Gale RE, Pezella F, et al. Platelet c-mpl expression is dysregulated in patients with essential thrombocythaemia but this is not of diagnostic value. *Br J Haematol* 1999;107:139–147.

97. Yoon SY, Li CY, Tefferi A. Megakaryocyte c-Mpl expression in chronic myeloproliferative disorders and the myelodysplastic syndrome: immunoperoxidase staining patterns and clinical correlates. *Eur J Haematol* 2000;65:170–174.

98. Li J, Xia Y, Kuter DJ. The platelet thrombopoietin receptor number and function are markedly decreased in patients with essential thrombocythaemia. *Br J Haematol* 2000;111:943–953.

99. Moliterno AR, Spivak JL. Posttranslational processing of the thrombopoietin receptor is impaired in polycythemia vera. *Blood* 1999;94: 2555–2561.

100. Imbert MJ, Pierre R, Thiele J, et al. Essential thrombocythemia. In: Jaffe ES, Harris NL, Stein H, et al., eds. *World Health Organization classification of tumours: pathology and genetics of tumours and lymphoid tissue.* Lyon, France: IARC Press; 2001:39–41

101. Maldonado JE, Pintado T, Pierre RV. Dysplastic platelets and circulating megakaryocytes in chronic myeloproliferative diseases. I. The platelets: ultrastructure and peroxidase reaction. *Blood* 1974;43:797–809.

102. Wehmeier A, Scharf RE, Fricke S, et al. Bleeding and thrombosis in chronic myeloproliferative disorders: relation of platelet disorders to clinical aspects of the disease. *Haemostasis* 1989;19:251–259.

103. Gersuk GM, Carmel R, Pattengale PK. Platelet-derived growth factor concentrations in platelet-poor plasma and urine from patients with myeloproliferative disorders. *Blood* 1989;74:2330–2334.

104. Burstein SA, Malpass TW, Yee E, et al. Platelet factor-4 excretion in myeloproliferative disease: implications for the aetiology of myelofibrosis. *Br J Haematol* 1984;57:383–392.

105. Wehmeier A, Tschope D, Esser J, et al. Circulating activated platelets in myeloproliferative disorders. *Thromb Res* 1991;61:271–278.

106. Gordon N, Thom J, Cole C, et al. Rapid detection of hereditary and acquired platelet storage pool deficiency by flow cytometry. *Br J Haematol* 1995;89:117–123.

107. Berger S, Aledort LM, Gilbert HS, et al. Abnormalities of platelet function in patients with polycythemia vera. *Cancer Res* 1973;33:2683–2687.

108. Weinfeld A, Branehog I, Kutti J. Platelets in the myeloproliferative syndrome. *Clin Haematol* 1975;4:373–392.

109. Ushikubi F, Ishibashi T, Narumiya S, et al. Analysis of the defective signal transduction mechanism through the platelet thromboxane A2 receptor in a patient with polycythemia vera. *Thromb Haemost* 1992;67: 144–146.

110. Le Blanc K, Berg A, Palmblad J, et al. Stimulus-specific defect in platelet aggregation in polycythemia vera. *Eur J Haematol* 1994;53:145–149.

111. Castaldi PA, Berndt MC, Booth W, et al. Evidence for a platelet membrane defect in the myeloproliferative syndromes. *Thromb Res* 1982;27: 601–609.

112. Cortellazzo S, Colucci M, Barbui T, et al. Reduced platelet factor X-activating activity: a possible contribution to bleeding complications in polycythaemia vera and essential thrombocythaemia. *Haemostasis* 1981;10: 37–50.

113. Keenan JP, Wharton J, Shepherd AJ, et al. Defective platelet lipid peroxidation in myeloproliferative disorders: a possible defect of prostaglandin synthesis. *Br J Haematol* 1977;35:275–283.

114. Le Blanc K, Lindahl T, Rosendahl K, et al. Impaired platelet binding of fibrinogen due to a lower number of GPIIB/IIIA receptors in polycythemia vera. *Thromb Res* 1998;91:287–295.

115. Kaywin P, McDonough M, Insel PA, et al. Platelet function in essential thrombocythemia. Decreased epinephrine responsiveness associated with a deficiency of platelet alpha-adrenergic receptors. *N Engl J Med* 1978; 299:505–509.

116. Ushikubi F, Okuma M, Ishibashi T, et al. Deficient elevation of the cytoplasmic calcium ion concentration by epinephrine in epinephrine-insensitive platelets of patients with myeloproliferative disorders. *Am J Hematol* 1990;33:96–100.

117. Budde U, Schaefer G, Mueller N, et al. Acquired von Willebrand's disease in the myeloproliferative syndrome. *Blood* 1984;64:981–985.

118. Mazzucato M, De Marco L, De Angelis V, et al. Platelet membrane abnormalities in myeloproliferative disorders: decrease in glycoproteins Ib and IIb/IIIa complex is associated with deficient receptor function. *Br J Haematol* 1989;73:369–374.

119. Jensen MK, de Nully Brown P, Lund BV, et al. Increased platelet activation and abnormal membrane glycoprotein content and redistribution in myeloproliferative disorders. [see comment]. *Br J Haematol* 2000;110:116–124.

120. Fabris F, Casonato A, Grazia del Ben M, et al. Abnormalities of von Willebrand factor in myeloproliferative disease: a relationship with bleeding diathesis. *Br J Haematol* 1986;63:75–83.

121. Mohri H. Acquired von Willebrand disease in patients with polycythemia rubra vera. *Am J Hematol* 1987;26:135–146.

122. Budde U, Scharf RE, Franke P, et al. Elevated platelet count as a cause of abnormal von Willebrand factor multimer distribution in plasma. *Blood* 1993;82:1749–1757.

123. Budde U, van Genderen PJ. Acquired von Willebrand disease in patients with high platelet counts. *Semin Thromb Hemost* 1997;23:425–431.

124. Sato K. Plasma von Willebrand factor abnormalities in patients with essential thrombocythemia. *Keio J Med* 1988;37:54–71.

125. van Genderen PJ, Michiels JJ. Erythromelalgic, thrombotic and haemorrhagic manifestations of thrombocythaemia. *Presse Med* 1994;23:73–77.

126. Buss DH, Stuart JJ, Lipscomb GE. The incidence of thrombotic and hemorrhagic disorders in association with extreme thrombocytosis: an analysis of 129 cases. *Am J Hematol* 1985;20:365–372.

127. Michiels JJ, Budde U, van der Planken M, et al. Acquired von Willebrand syndromes: clinical features, aetiology, pathophysiology, classification and management. *Baillieres Best Pract Res Clin Haematol* 2001;14:401–436.

128. van Genderen PJ, Budde U, Michiels JJ, et al. The reduction of large von Willebrand factor multimers in plasma in essential thrombocythaemia is related to the platelet count. *Br J Haematol* 1996;93:962–965.

129. van Genderen PJ, Prins FJ, Lucas IS, et al. Decreased half-life time of plasma von Willebrand factor collagen binding activity in essential thrombocythaemia: normalization after cytoreduction of the increased platelet count. *Br J Haematol* 1997;99:832–836.

130. Favaloro EJ. Collagen binding assay for von Willebrand factor (VWF:CBA): detection of von Willebrands Disease (VWD), and discrimination of VWD subtypes, depends on collagen source. *Thromb Haemost* 2000;83:127–135.

131. van Genderen PJ, Leenknegt H. Normal binding of plasma von Willebrand factor to platelets in essential thrombocythemia. *Am J Hematol* 1999;61:153–154.

132. Budde U, Dent JA, Berkowitz SD, et al. Subunit composition of plasma von Willebrand factor in patients with the myeloproliferative syndrome. *Blood* 1986;68:1213–1217.

133. Lopez-Fernandez MF, Lopez-Berges C, Martin R, et al. Abnormal structure of von Willebrand factor in myeloproliferative syndrome is associated to either thrombotic or bleeding diathesis. *Thromb Haemost* 1987; 58:753–757.

134. Tsai HM. Physiologic cleavage of von Willebrand factor by a plasma protease is dependent on its conformation and requires calcium ion. *Blood* 1996;87:4235–4244.

135. Levy GG, Nichols WC, Lian EC, et al. Mutations in a member of the ADAMTS gene family cause thrombotic thrombocytopenic purpura. *Nature* 2001;413:488–494.

136. Chievitz E, Thiede T. Complications and causes of death in polycythemia vera. *Acta Med Scand* 1962;172:513–523.

137. Pearson TC. Hemorheology in the erythrocytoses. *Mt Sinai J Med* 2001;68:182–191.

138. Thomas DJ, du Boulay GH, Marshall J, et al. Cerebral blood flow in polycythemia. *Lancet* 1977;2:161–163.

139. Brown MM, Wade JP, Marshall J. Fundamental importance of arterial oxygen content in the regulation of cerebral blood flow in man. *Brain* 1985;108:81–93.

140. Turitto VT, Weiss HJ. Red blood cells: their dual role in thrombus formation. *Science* 1980;207:541–543.

141. McLachlin AD, McLachlin JA, Jory TA, et al. Venous stasis in the lower extremities. *Ann Surg* 1960;152:678–685.

142. Cooper B, Schafer AI, Puchalsky D, et al. Platelet resistance to prostaglandin D2 in patients with myeloproliferative disorders. *Blood* 1978;52:618–626.

143. Mehta P, Mehta J, Ross M, et al. Decreased platelet aggregation but increased thromboxane A2 generation in polycythemia vera. *Arch Intern Med* 1985;145:1225–1227.

144. Landolfi R, Ciabattoni G, Patrignani P, et al. Increased thromboxane biosynthesis in patients with polycythemia vera: evidence for aspirin-suppressible platelet activation *in vivo*. *Blood* 1992;80:1965–1971.

145. Falanga A, Marchetti M, Evangelista V, et al. Polymorphonuclear leukocyte activation and hemostasis in patients with essential thrombocythemia and polycythemia vera. *Blood* 2000;96:4261–4266.

146. Musolino C, Alonci A, Bellomo G, et al. Myeloproliferative disease: markers of endothelial and platelet status in patients with essential thrombocythemia and polycythemia vera. *Hematology* 2000;4:397–402.

147. Wieczorek I, MacGregor IR, Prescott RJ, et al. The fibrinolytic system and proteins C and S in treated polycythaemia rubra vera. *Blood Coagul Fibrinolysis* 1992;3:823–826.

148. Bucalossi A, Marotta G, Bigazzi C, et al. Reduction of antithrombin III, protein C, and protein S levels and activated protein C resistance in polycythemia vera and essential thrombocythemia patients with thrombosis. *Am J Hematol* 1996;52:14–20.

149. Posan E, Ujj G, Kiss A, et al. Reduced *in vitro* clot lysis and release of more active platelet PAI-1 in polycythemia vera and essential thrombocythemia. *Thromb Res* 1998;90:51–56.

150. Cancelas JA, Garcia-Avello A, Garcia-Frade LJ. High plasma levels of plasminogen activator inhibitor 1 (PAI-1) in polycythemia vera and essential thrombocythemia are associated with thrombosis. *Thromb Res* 1994;75:513–520.

151. Schafer AI. Deficiency of platelet lipoxygenase activity in myeloproliferative disorders. *N Engl J Med* 1982;306:381–386.

152. Landolfi R, Ciabattoni G, Patrignani P, et al. Increased thromboxane biosynthesis in patients with polycythemia vera: evidence for aspirin-suppressible platelet activation *in vivo*. [see comment]. *Blood* 1992;80: 1965–1971.

153. Rocca B, Ciabattoni G, Tartaglione R, et al. Increased thromboxane biosynthesis in essential thrombocythemia. *Thromb Haemost* 1995;74: 1225–1230.

154. Michiels JJ, van Genderen PJ, Jansen PH, et al. Atypical transient ischemic attacks in thrombocythemia of various myeloproliferative disorders. *Leuk Lymphoma* 1996;22(Suppl. 1):65–70.

155. Schafer AI. Thrombocytosis. *N Engl J Med* 2004;350:1211–1219.

156. Tefferi A, Murphy S. Current opinion in essential thrombocythemia: pathogenesis, diagnosis, and management. *Blood Rev* 2001;15:121–131.

157. Murphy S, Peterson P, Iland H, et al. Experience of the polycythemia vera study group with essential thrombocythemia: a final report on diagnostic criteria, survival, and leukemic transition by treatment. [Review] [35 refs]. *Semin Hematol* 1997;34:29–39.

158. Tefferi A, Ho TC, Ahmann GJ, et al. Plasma interleukin-6 and C-reactive protein levels in reactive versus clonal thrombocytosis [see comments]. *Am J Med* 1994;97:374–378.

159. Ding J, Komatsu H, Wakita A, et al. Familial essential thrombocythemia associated with a dominant-positive activating mutation of the c-MPL gene, which encodes for the receptor for thrombopoietin. *Blood* 2004; 103:4198–4200.

160. Florensa L, Besses C, Zamora L, et al. Endogenous erythroid and megakaryocytic circulating progenitors, HUMARA clonality assay, and PRV-1 expression are useful tools for diagnosis of polycythemia vera and essential thrombocythemia. *Blood* 2004;103:2427–2428.

161. Yohannan MD, Higgy KE, al-Mashhadani SA, et al. Thrombocytosis. Etiologic analysis of 663 patients. *Clin Pediatr (Phila)* 1994;33:340–343.

162. Chen HL, Chiou SS, Sheen JM, et al. Thrombocytosis in children at one medical center of southern Taiwan. *Acta Paediatr Taiwan* 1999;40: 309–313.

163. Santhosh-Kumar CR, Yohannan MD, Higgy KE, et al. Thrombocytosis in adults: analysis of 777 patients. *J Intern Med* 1991;229:493–495.

164. Robbins G, Barnard DL. Thrombocytosis and microthrombocytosis: a clinical evaluation of 372 cases. *Acta Haematol* 1983;70:175–182.

165. Buss DH, Cashell AW, O'Connor ML, et al. Occurrence, etiology, and clinical significance of extreme thrombocytosis: a study of 280 cases. *Am J Med* 1994;96:247–253.

166. Chuncharunee S, Archararit N, Ungkanont A, et al. Etiology and incidence of thrombotic and hemorrhagic disorders in Thai patients with extreme thrombocytosis. *J Med Assoc Thai* 2000;83(Suppl. 1):S95–S100.

167. Stoll DB, Peterson P, Exten R, et al. Clinical presentation and natural history of patients with essential thrombocythemia and the Philadelphia chromosome. *Am J Hematol* 1988;27:77–83.

168. Wasserman LR. The management of polycythemia vera. *Br J Haematol* 1971;21:371–376.

169. Messinezy M, Westwood NB, El-Hemaidi I, et al. Serum erythropoietin values in erythrocytoses and in primary thrombocythaemia. *Br J Haematol* 2002;117:47–53.

170. Cotes PM, Dore CJ, Yin JA, et al. Determination of serum immunoreactive erythropoietin in the investigation of erythrocytosis. *N Engl J Med* 1986;315:283–287.

171. Tefferi A, Yoon SY, Li CY. Immunohistochemical staining for megakaryocyte c-mpl may complement morphologic distinction between polycythemia vera and secondary erythrocytosis. *Blood* 2000;96:771–772.

172. Weinberg RS. *In vitro* erythropoiesis in polycythemia vera and other myeloproliferative disorders. [Review] [55 refs]. *Semin Hematol* 1997; 34:64–69.

173. Temerinac S, Klippel S, Strunck E, et al. Cloning of PRV-1, a novel member of the uPAR receptor superfamily, which is overexpressed in polycythemia rubra vera. *Blood* 2000;95:2569–2576.

174. Tefferi A, Mesa RA, Schroeder G, et al. Cytogenetic findings and their clinical relevance in myelofibrosis with myeloid metaplasia. *Br J Haematol* 2001;113:763–771.

175. Schafer AI. Bleeding and thrombosis in the myeloproliferative disorders. *Blood* 1984;64:1–12.

176. van Genderen PJ, Leenknegt H, Michiels JJ. The paradox of bleeding and thrombosis in thrombocythemia: is von Willebrand factor the link? *Semin Thromb Hemost* 1997;23:385–389.

177. Barbui T. Thrombohemorrhagic complications in 101 cases of myeloproliferative disorders: relationship to platelet number and function. *Eur J Cancer Clin Oncol* 1983;19:1593–1599.

178. Wehmeier A, Fricke S, Scharf RE, et al. A prospective study of haemostatic parameters in relation to the clinical course of myeloproliferative disorders. *Eur J Haematol* 1990;45:191–197.

179. Manoharan A, Gemmell R, Brighton T, et al. Thrombosis and bleeding in myeloproliferative disorders: identification of at-risk patients with whole blood platelet aggregation studies. *Br J Haematol* 1999;105:618–625.

180. Jantunen R, Juvonen E, Ikkala E, et al. The predictive value of vascular risk factors and gender for the development of thrombotic complications in essential thrombocythemia. *Ann Hematol* 2001;80:74–78.

181. Watson KV, Key N. Vascular complications of essential thrombocythaemia: a link to cardiovascular risk factors. *Br J Haematol* 1993;83:198–203.

182. van Genderen PJ, Mulder PG, Waleboer M, et al. Prevention and treatment of thrombotic complications in essential thrombocythaemia: efficacy and safety of aspirin. *Br J Haematol* 1997;97:179–184.

183. Van Cott EM, Laposata M, Prins MH. Laboratory evaluation of hypercoagulability with venous or arterial thrombosis. *Arch Pathol Lab Med* 2002;126:1281–1295.

184. Afshar-Kharghan V, Lopez JA, Gray LA, et al. Hemostatic gene polymorphisms and the prevalence of thrombotic complications in polycythemia vera and essential thrombocythemia. *Blood Coagul Fibrinolysis* 2004;15:21–24.

185. Dicato MA, Schroell B, Berchem GJ. V Leiden mutations, prothromin and methylene-tetrahydrofolate reductase are not risk factors for thromboembolic disease in essential thrombocythemia. *Blood* 1999;94:IIIa.

186. Ruggeri M, Gisslinger H, Tosetto A, et al. Factor V Leiden mutation carriership and venous thromboembolism in polycythemia vera and essential thrombocythemia. *Am J Hematol* 2002;71:1–6.

187. Press RD, Bauer KA, Kujovich JL, et al. Clinical utility of factor V leiden (R506Q) testing for the diagnosis and management of thromboembolic disorders. *Arch Pathol Lab Med* 2002;126:1304–1318.

188. Amitrano L, Guardascione MA, Ames PR, et al. Thrombophilic genotypes, natural anticoagulants, and plasma homocysteine in myeloproliferative disorders: relationship with splanchnic vein thrombosis and arterial disease. *Am J Hematol* 2003;72:75–81.

189. Faurschou M, Nielsen OJ, Jensen MK, et al. High prevalence of hyperhomocysteinemia due to marginal deficiency of cobalamin or folate in chronic myeloproliferative disorders. *Am J Hematol* 2000;65:136–140.

190. Gisslinger H, Rodeghiero F, Ruggeri M, et al. Homocysteine levels in polycythaemia vera and essential thrombocythaemia. *Br J Haematol* 1999;105:551–555.

191. Key NS, McGlennen RC. Hyperhomocyst(e)inemia and thrombophilia. *Arch Pathol Lab Med* 2002;126:1367–1375.

192. Galli M, Luciani D, Bertolini G, et al. Lupus anticoagulants are stronger risk factors for thrombosis than anticardiolipin antibodies in the antiphospholipid syndrome: a systematic review of the literature. *Blood* 2003;101:1827–1832.

193. Harrison CN, Donohoe S, Carr P, et al. Patients with essential thrombocythaemia have an increased prevalence of antiphospholipid antibodies which may be associated with thrombosis. *Thromb Haemost* 2002;87:802–807.

194. Jensen MK, de Nully Brown P, Thorsen S, et al. Frequent occurrence of anticardiolipin antibodies, Factor V Leiden mutation, and perturbed endothelial function in chronic myeloproliferative disorders. *Am J Hematol* 2002;69:185–191.

195. Rozman C, Giralt M, Feliu E, et al. Life expectancy of patients with chronic nonleukemic myeloproliferative disorders. *Cancer* 1991;67:2658–2663.

196. McCarthy L, Eichelberger L, Skipworth E, et al. Erythromelalgia due to essential thrombocythemia. *Transfusion* 2002;42:1245.

197. Cortelazzo S, Finazzi G, Ruggeri M, et al. Hydroxyurea for patients with essential thrombocythemia and a high risk of thrombosis. *N Engl J Med* 1995;332:1132–1136.

198. Ruggeri M, Finazzi G, Tosetto A, et al. No treatment for low-risk thrombocythaemia: results from a prospective study. *Br J Haematol* 1998;103:772–777.

199. Tefferi A, Solberg LA, Silverstein MN. A clinical update in polycythemia vera and essential thrombocythemia. *Am J Med* 2000;109:141–149.

200. Barbui T, Barosi G, Grossi A, et al. Practice guidelines for the therapy of essential thrombocythemia. A statement from the Italian Society of Hematology, the Italian Society of Experimental Hematology and the Italian Group for Bone Marrow Transplantation. *Haematologica* 2004;89:215–232.

201. Landolfi R, Marchioli R, Kutti J, et al. Efficacy and safety of low-dose aspirin in polycythemia vera. *N Engl J Med* 2004;350:114–124.

202. Beressi AH, Tefferi A, Silverstein MN, et al. Outcome analysis of 34 pregnancies in women with essential thrombocythemia. *Arch Intern Med* 1995;155:1217–1222.

203. Demircay Z, Comert A, Adiguzel C. Leg ulcers and hydroxyurea: report of three cases with essential thrombocythemia. *Int J Dermatol* 2002;41:872–874.

204. Alvarado Y, Cortes J, Verstovsek S, et al. Pilot study of pegylated interferon-alpha 2b in patients with essential thrombocythemia. *Cancer Chemother Pharmacol* 2003;51:81–86.

205. Elliott MA, Tefferi A. Interferon-alpha therapy in polycythemia vera and essential thrombocythemia. *Semin Thromb Hemost* 1997;23:463.

206. Storen EC, Tefferi A. Long-term use of anagrelide in young patients with essential thrombocythemia. *Blood* 2001;97:863–866.

207. Regev A, Stark P, Blickstein D, et al. Thrombotic complications in essential thrombocythemia with relatively low platelet counts. *Am J Hematol* 1997;56:168–172.

208. Hanft VN, Fruchtman SR, Pickens CV, et al. Acquired DNA mutations associated with *in vivo* hydroxyurea exposure. *Blood* 2000;95:3589–3593.

209. Finazzi G, Ruggeri M, Rodeghiero F, et al. Efficacy and safety of long-term use of hydroxyurea in young patients with essential thrombocythemia and a high risk of thrombosis. *Blood* 2003;101:3749.

210. Randi ML, Fabris F, Girolami A. Second malignancies in patients with essential thrombocythaemia. *Br J Haematol* 2002;116:923–924.

211. Sterkers Y, Preudhomme C, Lai JL, et al. Acute myeloid leukemia and myelodysplastic syndromes following essential thrombocythemia treated with hydroxyurea: high proportion of cases with 17p deletion. *Blood* 1998;91:616–622.

212. Tefferi A. Is hydroxyurea leukemogenic in essential thrombocythemia? *Blood* 1998;92:1459–1460.

213. Bernasconi P, Boni M, Cavigliano PM, et al. Acute myeloid leukemia (AML) having evolved from essential thrombocythemia (ET): distinctive chromosome abnormalities in patients treated with pipobroman or hydroxyurea. *Leukemia* 2002;16:2078–2083.

214. *Br Med J.* Antiplatelet trialist's collaboration collaborative overview of randomised trials of antiplatelet therapy-1. 1994;308:81–106.

215. Fruchtman SM, Mack K, Kaplan ME, et al. From efficacy to safety—a polycythemia vera study group report on hydroxyurea in patients with polycythemia vera. *Semin Hematol* 1997;34:17–23.

216. Silver RT. Treatment of polycythemia vera with recombinant interferon. *Int J Hematol* 2002;76(Suppl. 2):294–295.

217. Tefferi A, Fonseca R. Selective serotonin reuptake inhibitors are effective in the treatment of polycythemia vera-associated pruritus. *Blood* 2002;99:2627.

218. Kennedy BJ, Smith LR, Goltz RW. Skin changes secondary to hydroxyurea therapy. *Arch Dermatol* 1975;111:183–187.

219. Yarbro JW. Mechanism of action of hydroxyurea. *Semin Oncol* 1992;19:1–10.

220. Nguyen TV, Margolis DJ. Hydroxyurea and lower leg ulcers. *Cutis* 1993;52:217–219.

221. Lossos IS, Matzner Y. Hydroxyurea-induced fever: case report and review of the literature. [Review] [6 refs]. *Ann Pharmacother* 1995;29:132–133.

222. Najean Y, Rain JD. Treatment of polycythemia vera—the use of hydroxyurea and pipobroman in 292 patients under the age of 65 years. *Blood* 1997;90:3370–3377.

223. Daoud MS, Pittelkow MR. Hydroxyurea dermopathy: a unique lichenoid eruption complicating long-term therapy with hydroxyurea. *J Am Acad Dermatol* 1997;36:178–182.

224. Best PJ, Daoud MS Pittelkow MR, et al. Hydroxyurea-induced leg ulceration in 14 patients. *Ann Intern Med* 1998;128:29–32.

225. Stevens MR. Hydroxyurea: an overview. *J Biol Regul Homeost Agents* 1999;13:172–175.

226. Tefferi A, Elliott MA, Kao PC, et al. Hydroxyurea-induced marked oscillations of platelet counts in patients with polycythemia vera. *Blood* 2000;96:1582–1584.

227. Silverstein MN, Petitt RM, Solberg LA Jr, et al. Anagrelide: a new drug for treating thrombocytosis. *N Engl J Med* 1988;318:1292–1294.

228. Anagrelide Study Group. Anagrelide, a therapy for thrombocythemic states: experience in 577 patients. *Am J Med* 1992;92:69–76.

229. Mazur EM, Rosmarin AG, Sohl PA, et al. Analysis of the mechanism of anagrelide-induced thrombocytopenia in humans. *Blood* 1992;79:1931–1937.

230. Spencer CM, Brogden RN. Anagrelide. A review of its pharmacodynamic and pharmacokinetic properties, and therapeutic potential in the treatment of thrombocythaemia. *Drugs* 1994;47:809–822.

231. Solberg LA, Tefferi A, Oles KJ, et al. The effects of anagrelide on human megakaryocytopoiesis. *Br J Haematol* 1997;99:174–180.

232. Tefferi A, Silverstein MN, Petitt RM, et al. Anagrelide as a new platelet-lowering agent in essential thrombocythemia: mechanism of action, efficacy, toxicity, current indications. *Semin Thromb Hemost* 1997;23:379.

233. Quesada JR, et al. Clinical toxicity of interferons in cancer patients: a review. *J Clin Oncol* 1986;4:234–243.

234. Gugliotta Lea. *In vivo* and *in vitro* inhibitory effect of alpha-interferon on megakaryocyte colony growth in essential thrombocythemia. *Br J Haematol* 1989;71:177–181.

235. Lengfelder E, Berger U, Hehlmann R. Interferon alpha in the treatment of polycythemia vera [In Process Citation]. *Ann Hematol* 2000;79:103–109.

236. Gilbert HS. Long term treatment of myeloproliferative disease with interferon-alpha-2b—feasibility and efficacy. *Cancer* 1998;83:1205–1213.

237. Arthur K. Radioactive phosphorus in the treatment of polycythaemia. A review of ten years' experience. *Clin Radiol* 1967;18:287–291.

238. Roberts BE, Smith AH. USE of radioactive phosphorus in haematology [Review]. *Blood Rev* 1997;11:146–153.

239. Wagner S, Waxman J, Sikora K. The treatment of essential thrombocythaemia with radioactive phosphorus. *Clin Radiol* 1989;40:190–192.

240. Najman A, Stachowiak J, Parlier Y, et al. Pipobroman therapy of polycythemia vera. *Blood* 1982;59:890–894.

241. *JAMA*. Evaluation of two antineoplastic agents: pipobroman (Vercyte) and thioguanine. 1967;200:619–620.

242. Passamonti F, Brusamolino E, Lazzarino M, et al. Efficacy of pipobroman in the treatment of polycythemia vera: long-term results in 163 patients. *Haematologica* 2000;85:1011–1018.

243. Mazzucconi MG, Francesconi M, Chistolini A, et al. Pipobroman therapy of essential thrombocythemia. *Scand J Haematol* 1986;37:306–309.

244. Cervantes F, Alvarez-Larran A, Talarn C, et al. Myelofibrosis with myeloid metaplasia following essential thrombocythaemia: actuarial probability, presenting characteristics and evolution in a series of 195 patients. *Br J Haematol* 2002;118:786–790.

245. Silverstein MN. *Agnogenic myeloid metaplasia*. Acton, MA: Publishing Science Group, 1975:126.

246. Gardner FH, Nathan DG. Androgens and erythropoiesis. 3. Further evaluation of testosterone treatment of myelofibrosis. *N Engl J Med* 1966;274:420–426.

247. Besa EC, Nowell PC, Geller NL, et al. Analysis of the androgen response of 23 patients with agnogenic myeloid metaplasia: the value of chromosomal studies in predicting response and survival. *Cancer* 1982;49:308–313.

248. Hasselbalch HC, Clausen NT, Jensen BA. Successful treatment of anemia in idiopathic myelofibrosis with recombinant human erythropoietin. *Am J Hematol* 2002;70:92–99.

249. Rodriguez JN, Martino ML, Dieguez JC, et al. rHuEpo for the treatment of anemia in myelofibrosis with myeloid metaplasia. Experience in 6 patients and meta-analytical approach. *Haematologica* 1998;83:616–621.

250. Tefferi A, Silverstein MN. Recombinant human erythropoietin therapy in patients with myelofibrosis with myeloid metaplasia [letter; comment]. *Br J Haematol* 1994;86:893.

251. Aloe Spiriti M, Latagliata R, Avvisati G, et al. Erythropoietin treatment of idiopathic myelofibrosis. *Haematologica* 1993;78:371–373.

252. Lofvenberg E, Wahlin A. Management of polycythaemia vera, essential thrombocythaemia and myelofibrosis with hydroxyurea. *Eur J Haematol* 1988;41:375–381.

253. Tefferi A, Mesa RA, Nagorney DM, et al. Splenectomy in myelofibrosis with myeloid metaplasia: a single-institution experience with 223 patients. *Blood* 2000;95:2226–2233.

254. Steensma DP, Hook CC, Stafford SL, et al. Low-dose, single-fraction, whole-lung radiotherapy for pulmonary hypertension associated with myelofibrosis with myeloid metaplasia. *Br J Haematol* 2002;118:813–816.

255. Koch CA, Li CY, Mesa RA, et al. Nonhepatosplenic extramedullary hematopoiesis: associated diseases, pathology, clinical course, and treatment. *Mayo Clin Proc* 2003;78:1223–1233.

256. Elliott MA, Chen MG, Silverstein MN, et al. Splenic irradiation for symptomatic splenomegaly associated with myelofibrosis with myeloid metaplasia. *Br J Haematol* 1998;103:505–511.

257. Tefferi A, Jimenez T, Gray LA, et al. Radiation therapy for symptomatic hepatomegaly in myelofibrosis with myeloid metaplasia. *Eur J Haematol* 2001;66:37–42.

258. Piccaluga PP, Visani G, Pileri SA, et al. Clinical efficacy and antiangiogenic activity of thalidomide in myelofibrosis with myeloid metaplasia. A pilot study. *Leukemia* 2002;16:1609–1614.

259. Merup M, Kutti J, Birgegard G, et al. Negligible clinical effects of thalidomide in patients with myelofibrosis with myeloid metaplasia. *Med Oncol* 2002;19:79–86.

260. Elliott MA, Mesa RA, Li CY, et al. Thalidomide treatment in myelofibrosis with myeloid metaplasia. *Br J Haematol* 2002;117:288–296.

261. Canepa L, Ballerini F, Varaldo R, et al. Thalidomide in agnogenic and secondary myelofibrosis. *Br J Haematol* 2001;115:313–315.

262. Barosi G, Grossi A, Comotti B, et al. Safety and efficacy of thalidomide in patients with myelofibrosis with myeloid metaplasia. *Br J Haematol* 2001;114:78–83.

263. Marchetti M, Barosi G, Balestri F, et al. Low-dose thalidomide ameliorates cytopenias and splenomegaly in myelofibrosis with myeloid metaplasia: a phase II trial. *J Clin Oncol* 2004;22:424–431.

264. Mesa RA, Steensma DP, Pardanani A, et al. A phase 2 trial of combination low-dose thalidomide and prednisone for the treatment of myelofibrosis with myeloid metaplasia. *Blood* 2003;101:2534–2541.

265. Guardiola P, Anderson JE, Bandini G, et al. Allogeneic stem cell transplantation for agnogenic myeloid metaplasia: a European group for blood and marrow transplantation, Societe Francaise de Greffe de Moelle, Gruppo Italiano per il Trapianto del Midollo Osseo, and Fred Hutchinson Cancer Research Center collaborative study. *Blood* 1999;93:2831–2838.

266. Deeg HJ, Gooley TA, Flowers ME, et al. Allogeneic hematopoietic stem cell transplantation for myelofibrosis. *Blood* 2003;102:3912–3918.

267. Daly A, Song K, Nevill T, et al. Stem cell transplantation for myelofibrosis: a report from two Canadian centers. *Bone Marrow Transplant* 2003;32:35–40.

268. Devine SM, Hoffman R, Verma A, et al. Allogeneic blood cell transplantation following reduced-intensity conditioning is effective therapy for older patients with myelofibrosis with myeloid metaplasia. *Blood* 2002;99:2255–2258.

269. Hessling J, Kroger N, Werner M, et al. Dose-reduced conditioning regimen followed by allogeneic stem cell transplantation in patients with myelofibrosis with myeloid metaplasia. *Br J Haematol* 2002;119:769–772.

270. Guardiola P, Anderson JE, Gluckman E. Myelofibrosis with myeloid metaplasia. *N Engl J Med* 2000;343:659; discussion 659–660.

271. Cervantes F, Barosi G, Demory JL, et al. Myelofibrosis with myeloid metaplasia in young individuals: disease characteristics, prognostic factors and identification of risk groups. *Br J Haematol* 1998;102:684–690.

272. Dupriez B, Morel P, Demory JL, et al. Prognostic factors in agnogenic myeloid metaplasia: a report on 195 cases with a new scoring system. *Blood* 1996;88:1013–1018.

273. Adami R. Therapeutic thrombocytapheresis: a review of 132 patients. *Int J Artif Organs* 1993;5:183–184.

274. Bond L, Bevan D. Myocardial infarction in a patient with hemophilia treated with DDAVP. *N Engl J Med* 1988;318:121.

275. Byrnes JJ, Larcada A, Moake JL. Thrombosis following desmopressin for uremic bleeding. *Am J Hematol* 1988;28:63–65.

276. Brodmann S, Passweg JR, Gratwohl A, et al. Myeloproliferative disorders: complications, survival and causes of death. *Ann Hematol* 2000;79:312–318.

277. Malmaeus J, Akre T, Adami HO, et al. Early postoperative course following elective splenectomy in haematological diseases: a high complication rate in patients with myeloproliferative disorders. *Br J Surg* 1986;73:720–723.

278. Randi ML, Fabris F, Ruzzon E, et al. Splenectomy after portal thrombosis in patients with polycythemia vera and essential thrombocythemia. *Haematologica* 2002;87:1180–1184.

# CHAPTER 109 ■ CONSUMPTIVE THROMBOHEMORRHAGIC DISORDERS

VICTOR J. MARDER, DONALD I. FEINSTEIN, ROBERT W. COLMAN, AND MARCEL LEVI

Known variously as *disseminated intravascular coagulation* (DIC), *defibrination*, or the *consumption coagulopathies*, consumptive thrombohemorrhagic disorders are a heterogeneous group of disorders that can be manifested by the entire range of hemorrhagic and thrombotic pathology. Given that such disorders may be subtle or devastating in clinical presentation and that they are, as McKay (1) aptly describes, "intermediary mechanisms of disease" that can complicate an enormous variety of primary conditions, there is little wonder that confusion often reigns at the bedside of the patient with "positive split products." Also, owing to the complexity of the clinical presentation, the variable and unpredictable course, and the multitude of therapies given to such patients, properly conducted clinical trials are extremely difficult to perform and even to devise. Management, therefore, must rely on case studies precariously applied to the individual patient based on the best understanding of the pathophysiologic mechanisms involved.

We provide a conceptual framework rather than a dogmatic outline for understanding these various clinical states. No single definition or catchword adequately covers all the possible varieties, but we have chosen *consumptive thrombohemorrhagic disorders* because it includes a broad pathologic denominator without placing a limit on the clinical manifestations. Numerous reviews of the subject have presented inventive concepts for pathogenesis and management, and we have benefited from these excellent discussions (1–16).

## HISTORY

More than 100 years ago, Nauyn (17) observed gross intravascular coagulation of animal blood after infusion of hemolyzed erythrocytes, and Foa and Pellacani (18) observed the same phenomenon after injection of a variety of fresh organ extracts. Mellanby (19) recognized that the coagulation defect of DIC produced by snake venoms resulted in hypofibrinogenemia. Penick et al. (20) recognized that thrombocytopenia and decreased levels of factor VIII occurred in experimental DIC and suggested that these might be more sensitive indicators than diminished fibrinogen. McKay (1) correlated the clinical presentations with the pathology. Hardaway (3) emphasized that shock and acidosis occurring in a variety of diseases could initiate clotting with consumption of fibrinogen, platelets, and other coagulation factors. The first use of heparin for DIC was in a case of purpura fulminans described by Little (21). Verstraete et al. (22) reported several other cases of successful heparin use and suggested that this drug might be of more general value. The development of a method for measuring fibrinogen degradation products by Merskey et al. (23) provided a foundation for applying relevant laboratory criteria to the study of these disorders (6).

## INITIATING PATHWAYS

A consumptive thrombohemorrhagic disorder is a pathologic syndrome, the manifestations of which can in large part be regarded as a consequence of excess thrombin formation. Thrombin catalyzes the activation and subsequent consumption of certain coagulant proteins and production of fibrin thrombi. Thrombin also induces the release of tissue-type plasminogen activator (tPA) from the endothelium and is converted to plasmin in the presence of fibrin monomer. This results in secondary fibrinolysis and the generation of fibrin degradation products (FDPs). The manifestations are also influenced by the disease state that triggers the consumptive process. Intravascular coagulation can be triggered by several mechanisms (e.g., endothelial perturbation or injury, monocyte activation, placental abruption, tissue injury, administration of prothrombin complex concentrates, and direct activation of blood coagulation by venoms).

Endothelial injury occurs in disease states (e.g., infections) that specifically injure and perturb the endothelium, with resultant exposure of the blood to prothrombotic influences such as tissue factor (TF), which can initiate coagulation, or collagen, which can promote platelet adherence and aggregation. TF is a single-chain transmembrane glycoprotein that binds factor VII and factor VIIa. When factor VII binds to TF, factor VII becomes a better substrate for either autoactivation or activation by other serine proteases such as factor IXa or Xa. Endothelial cells do not constitutively express TF, but when the endothelium is perturbed by endotoxin, interleukin-1 (IL-1), or tumor necrosis factor (TNF), then TF messenger RNA is induced, resulting in the biosynthesis and expression of TF on the endothelial cell surface. With the acceptance of the primary role of TF, the focus has shifted to endothelial cell adaptive and maladaptive responses (24). Therefore, in addition to the role of TF in initiating and enhancing microvascular thrombosis, TF has been implicated in a variety of nonhemostatic roles, in particular inflammation (25). The TF–factor VIIa complex stimulates the activator nuclear factor $\kappa$B, which in turn stimulates the transcription of TNF-$\alpha$, thereby completing a positive feedback loop by inducing TF synthesis. TNF-$\alpha$ secretion is followed by secretion of other inflammatory cytokines such as IL-1$\beta$ and IL-6, the latter of which is the major stimulator of acute-phase proteins such as C-reactive protein and fibrinogen. C-reactive protein in complex with very low density lipoprotein may allow the spatial and temporal responses characteristic of DIC (26). Endotoxin and the cytokines IL-1 and TNF not only increase TF expression but also increase plasminogen activator inhibitor-1 (PAI-1) synthesis and decrease thrombomodulin expression by endothelial cells, thereby inducing a prothrombotic state by causing hemostatic imbalance (27).

Niemetz (28) has shown that leukocytes (probably monocytes) have coagulant activity after exposure to endotoxin, which activates factor X in the presence of factor VII. Further evidence for the role of TF in (experimental) DIC is the decrease of fibrinogen consumption by an antibody against TF or factor VIIa, although other manifestations of the illness, such as hypotension, are not prevented (29–31). Moreover, treatment with recombinant tissue factor pathway inhibitor (TFPI) resulted in a significant decrease in intensity of experimental DIC and its mortality (32). Animal studies using endotoxin or sepsis models substantiate the initiating role of TF (33,34), whereas the contact phase proteins and intrinsic system are probably unimportant. Although factor XII activation is not the primary factor in triggering DIC, it contributes to pathologic consequences such as vasodilation and hypotension by activation of the kallikrein kinin system (35–37). In pathologic states such as acute promyelocytic leukemia (APL), the malignant cells contain TF (38), and such cells release TF after incubation with endotoxin (39). Peripheral blood monocytes from human subjects with carcinoma express increased TF activity in comparison with those of healthy subjects, and elevated plasma levels of TF are found in patients with acute monocytic leukemia (40).

Solid tumors can express procoagulant molecules, including TF and a "cancer procoagulant" cysteine protease with factor X–activating properties (41,42). Evidence now supports the hypothesis that TF—either as shed vesicles or as expressed on the cell surface—is the major cause of hypercoagulability and DIC in patients with solid tumors (41,42).

Snakebite is the clearest example of how coagulant substances can directly initiate consumption after entering the circulation. *Echis carinatus* venom contains a protease that directly hydrolyzes prothrombin, thereby forming thrombin (43,44). Other snake venoms, such as that of *Crotalus adamanteus*, contain an enzyme that clots fibrinogen directly, without activating platelets, whereas others (e.g., those of timber rattlesnake *Crotalus horridus horridus*) contain one protein that clots fibrinogen and another that activates platelets (45). Envenomation by the Western diamondback rattlesnake (*Crotalus atrox*) may result in a primary fibrinogenolytic state apparently induced through the indirect activation of plasminogen by vascular plasminogen activator released from endothelial and smooth muscle cells by the snake venom (46).

Platelet and red cell injury may accelerate the consumptive process owing to the exposure of acidic phospholipids present on the inner aspect of the cell membrane (47). However, animals that are thrombocytopenic but not leukopenic can still develop endotoxin-induced consumption, implying that platelet injury is the result rather than the cause of the consumption (48). In contrast, neutropenia induced by nitrogen mustard totally inhibits the process (48,49). A transfusion reaction with 150 to 1,000 mL of incompatible blood or acute drug-induced immune hemolysis is associated with profound hypofibrinogenemia and serious bleeding (19,50). However, this reaction is probably the result of antibody–antigen complex formation rather than the effect of hemolysis, given that nonimmune intravascular hemolysis due to fava beans or experimentally induced hemoglobinuria fails to produce consumption (51,52).

Activation of the complement system may modify the consumptive process. Because the concentration of C4 protein is decreased in parallel with a decrease in the concentration of C3 protein (53), the decrease of concentraton of C3 involves the classic pathway (54). In four patients with Rocky Mountain spotted fever, C3 concentration was decreased, although an exact temporal correlation to platelets or fibrinogen was not shown, and in malaria the decrease of concentration of C3 correlated with the severity of the thrombocytopenia (55). Antibody–antigen complex activation of the classic complement pathway in rabbits appears to result in thromboplastin- or thrombin-induced DIC with a decrease in concentration of C3, but the consumption of C3 and C4 proteins may have been associated with, but not necessary for, the induction of consumption (56). If C3 is depleted by cobra venom, endotoxin will still induce consumption in rabbits with concomitant hypotension and leukopenia (57). Moreover, endotoxin-induced consumption was not altered in rabbits that were congenitally deficient in C6 and had defective platelet factor 3 availability (58).

Fibronectin is decreased in patients with DIC, possibly because of cross-linking with fibrin (59). Although a low plasma concentration of fibronectin has been correlated with poor outcome in patients with consumption, transient depletion of fibronectin was noted regularly in patients who recovered from bacterial sepsis, indicating that such a decrease is not necessarily a poor prognostic sign (60).

## ROLE OF THROMBIN

Consumptive processes reflect the multiple actions of thrombin (see Table 109-1). Thrombin proteolytically cleaves fibrinopeptides from fibrinogen to produce fibrin monomers that either combine with fibrinogen to form soluble complexes or polymerize to form fibrin thrombi. Thrombin converts factor XIII to an active transamidase that cross-links fibrin and renders it more resistant to fibrinolysis (61). Fibrin can also be cross-linked to other proteins such as antiplasmin, which also contributes to its plasmin resistance (see Chapter 17).

Thrombin binds to specific platelet receptors at low concentrations and initiates shape change, aggregation, and secretion. Thrombin-stimulated platelets lack both dense granules and α-granules and show functional defects, so even if the platelet count exceeds 100,000 per μL, the bleeding time may be prolonged. The platelet contribution to prothrombin activation is in part due to platelet factor V bound to the platelet surface, which serves as a receptor for factor Xa (62). Thrombin stimulates the platelet to release (from α-granules) platelet factor V, which is then bound to the platelet membrane (63). Thrombin potentiates the coagulation cascade by increasing the activity of factors V and VIII; however, its continued action leads to their degradation by activated protein C (APC). Therefore, thrombin itself accounts for decreases in fibrinogen; platelets; and factors II, V, VIII, and XIII in acute consumption (64). The decrease in other clotting factors, such as factors IX and X, is due to rapid clearance of activated clotting factors *in vivo* (65).

Importantly, thrombin acts at the crossroad of coagulation and inflammation by binding to protease-activated receptors (PARs), a family of transmembrane domain, G protein coupled receptors (66). PARs serve as their own ligand, and proteolytic cleavage by an activated coagulation factor leads to exposure of a neo–amino-terminus that activates the same receptor and initiates transmembrane signaling. PARs 1, 3, and 4 are thrombin receptors, whereas PAR-2 does not bind thrombin but (along with PAR-1) can be activated by the TF–VIIa complex, factor Xa, and trypsin. PARs are localized on endothelial cells, mononuclear cells, platelets, fibroblasts, and smooth muscle cells, and binding of thrombin to these cellular receptors may induce cytokine and growth factor production, thereby promoting the inflammatory response (67).

## ROLE OF COAGULATION INHIBITORS AND FIBRINOLYSIS

Failure of natural inhibitory (anticoagulant) mechanisms, including plasmin, protein C, and protein S, and antithrombin (AT) predisposes to or aggravates hypercoagulable states by allowing fuller expression of thrombin activity (12,68). Therefore,

**TABLE 109-1**

ROLE OF THROMBIN IN THE PATHOGENESIS OF CONSUMPTIVE DISORDERS

| Substrate | Thrombin action |
|---|---|
| Fibrinogen | Cleaves fibrinopeptides, thereby initiating fibrin formation and decreasing plasma fibrinogen concentration |
| Prothrombin (factor II) | Precursor of thrombin that declines owing to conversion to an active enzyme |
| Factors V and VIII | Increases coagulant activity but leads to an unstable derivative with a subsequent decrease in activity |
| Factor XIII | Converts the zymogen to an active enzyme in the presence of calcium, leading to eventual depletion by an unknown mechanism |
| Platelets | Initiates shape change and aggregation, leading to a decrease in circulating platelets; releases dense, $\alpha$-, and lysosomal granules, resulting in acquired storage pool deficiency; contributes to coagulant activity of platelets, including platelet factor 3 |
| TAFI | Activates TAFI to TAFIa, which cleaves plasminogen-binding sites on fibrin, thereby increasing resistance of clots to plasmin-induced fibrinolysis |
| Protease-activated receptor | Binds and cleaves, initiating transmembrane signaling, induces cytokine production and inflammation |

TAFI, thrombin-activatable fibrinolytic inhibitor.

adequate amounts of natural anticoagulants are necessary to dampen or modulate increased procoagulant activity.

Thrombin activity is neutralized by two inhibitory systems, which to different degrees depend on the interaction of plasma proteins with the endothelial surface (68). AT and heparin cofactor II neutralize thrombin slowly by complex formation (see Chapter 13) (69,70). However, such neutralization occurs at markedly accelerated rates in the presence of heparin, albeit at much higher concentrations for heparin cofactor II than for AT (71,72). Heparin exerts its facilitative effect in solution, for example, after administration for therapeutic purposes or as membrane-associated molecules (heparans) that contribute to the antithrombotic properties of the vascular endothelium. In addition, AT neutralizes factor IXa and Xa (73). The protein C–related inhibitor system is dependent *in vivo* on surface-oriented reactions, specifically that of endothelial cells, and acts to facilitate the degradation (inactivation) of factors Va and VIIIa (74–76). In this complex molecular system, thrombin forms a bimolecular complex with the transmembrane protein thrombomodulin, at which point it loses its fibrinogen-clotting, factor XIII–activating, and platelet-stimulating activities (74). However, the thrombin-thrombomodulin complex can convert the inactive plasma precursor, protein C, to an active form (APC). In turn, protein APC in the presence of the facilitating cofactor protein S (77,78) degrades factors Va and VIIIa to inactive forms, thereby negatively influencing the thrombotic tendency. Because of increased utilization and possibly decreased production, AT and protein C levels decrease to a variable degree in patients with DIC.

Venous thrombosis occurs with increased frequency in patients with hereditary deficiency of AT, protein C, and protein S, with unusual instances of complete absence associated with massive and generalized thrombotic phenomena at birth, necessitating long-term treatment with plasma or concentrate replacement infusions (79–82). A deficiency of protein C may be associated with intravascular consumption and skin necrosis associated with warfarin therapy or with purpura fulminans in the newborn (83,84). In both the experimental model of endotoxin-induced DIC and in patients with DIC, the concentrations

of protein C fall, presumably secondary to clearance of a protein C–protein C inhibitor complex formed during the consumptive process (85,86). Warfarin-associated skin necrosis has also been reported in patients with protein S and AT deficiencies (87). The decrease of inhibitors such as AT and protein C has prompted the use of AT or protein C replacement treatment in patients or in experimental animal models of consumption (15,88–92). The possibility has also been raised that such deficiencies of inhibitor may be as much related to decreased hepatic synthesis as to consumption, although this possibility does not preclude the possible benefit of replacement treatment (93).

The role of TFPI has assumed greater significance with the emphasis on TF in the initiation of hemostasis (see Chapter 5). Levels of TFPI in patients with DIC are controversial (29,94). However, the potential role of TFPI in preventing DIC was provided by experiments in rabbits in which pretreatment with anti-TFPI antibody sensitized the animals to more striking laboratory and tissue evidence of DIC (95). Moreover, in an animal model of *Escherichia coli*–induced DIC, recombinant TFPI decreased the coagulopathy and mortality (32), and endothelium-targeted delivery of TFPI inhibited intravascular thrombosis in endotoxin-treated mice (96).

## ROLE OF PLASMIN

Plasmin is a potent proteolytic enzyme capable of digesting fibrin and fibrinogen and other clotting proteins, including factors Va and VIIIa. Thrombin induces the release of tPA from endothelial cells, and tPA activates plasminogen on the fibrin surface and degrades fibrin to soluble peptide products. Therefore, the generation of plasmin tends to minimize the obstructive and ischemic effects of consumption in the microcirculation as well as protect against macrovascular thrombosis. In addition, fibrinolysis may be activated by the contact phase of coagulation (97).

The balance between thrombin and plasmin determines whether the clinical picture is thrombin predominant, characterized by thrombosis, organ ischemia, and bleeding, or plasmin dominant, characterized by bleeding. Increased thrombin generation unbalanced by increased plasmin formation leads to microvascular fibrin deposition, causing organ ischemia and depression of organ dysfunction. If plasmin is formed in sufficient quantities in the circulation, it produces degradation products of fibrinogen, which also inhibit fibrin polymerization (98) and degrades clotting factors V and VIII. In combination with low plasma fibrinogen concentration, low levels of plasma factors V and VIII, and thrombocytopenia, degradation products contribute to bleeding manifestations.

In the microcirculation, plasmin primarily degrades fibrin thrombi. The importance of such secondary (compensatory) fibrinolysis is illustrated by cases in which the fibrinolytic inhibitor ε-aminocaproic acid (EACA) was administered in the face of active fibrin formation, resulting in severe thrombotic complications (99). The plasma inhibitors of fibrinolysis, especially PAI-1, may contribute to the severity of DIC by preventing physiologic fibrinolysis. For example, high levels of PAI-1 correlate with low admission platelet counts in patients with meningococcal sepsis and are associated with a higher mortality (100).

# VARIABLE PRESENTATIONS OF CONSUMPTION

The spectrum of clinical and laboratory presentation is affected by several parameters, as listed in Table 109-2. Herein lies much of the confusion, especially because many cases of so-called DIC are not disseminated, or intravascular, or even related to coagulation. Therefore, it is not surprising that the response to heparin remains problematic, given the possibilities for pathologic states that need not, or cannot, respond to such therapy. These variables determine whether specific therapy for the "consumption" is required, over and above that indicated for the underlying disease or its other complications.

**TABLE 109-2**

**PARAMETERS THAT INFLUENCE THE CLINICAL AND LABORATORY PRESENTATION OF CONSUMPTIVE THROMBOHEMORRHAGIC DISORDERS**

| Parameter | Variation |
|---|---|
| Tempo | Acute versus chronic |
|  | Mild versus severe |
| Location | Localized versus systemic (disseminated) |
|  | Intravascular versus extravascular |
| Pathologic mechanism | Thrombin + increased fibrinolysis |
|  | Thrombin + increased fibrinogenolysis |
|  | Primary fibrinolysis |
|  | Isolated platelet consumption |

When presented with the patient who may have such a disorder, the physician must judge the tempo of the illness, whether the clinical presentation is severe enough to warrant specific therapy, and whether the coagulation disorder is likely to be a self-limiting problem that will wane on therapy for the underlying condition or will gather momentum and assume importance beyond that of the initiating stimulus. If the problem comes to the physician's attention only as the result of a screening laboratory survey, management will depend on whether an abnormal test result is the only reflection of consumption or whether serious clinical manifestations also exist or are likely to develop. In particular, signs of ischemic organ dysfunction, macrovascular thrombosis, excessive bleeding, and fragmentation hemolytic anemia should be sought (see Fig. 109-1).

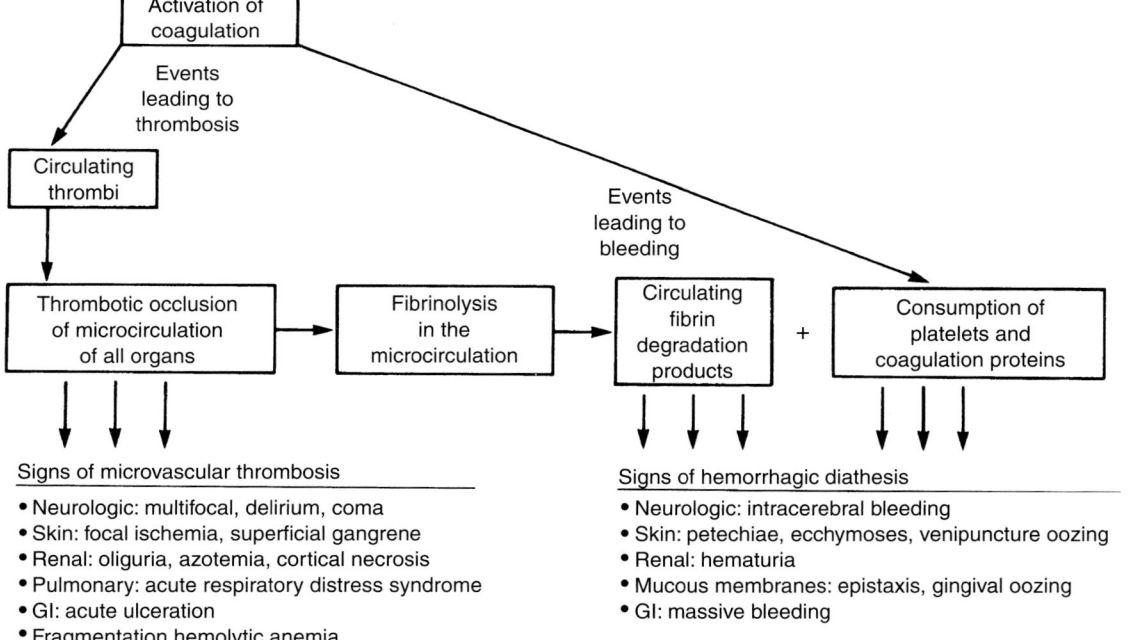

**FIGURE 109-1.** Sequence of events during disseminated intravascular coagulation leading to the clinical appearance of thrombotic and hemorrhagic phenomena. GI, gastrointestinal. (From Marder VJ. Microvascular thrombosis. In: Lichtman MA, ed. *The science and practice of clinical medicine.* Vol 6. New York: Grune & Stratton, 1980:230–234, with permission.)

The underlying disorders encompass all manner of pathologic states and pathophysiologic mechanisms, and their recognition by the physician often provides insight for prognosis. Some have been generally accepted as causes for an extreme form of consumptive thrombohemorrhagic disorder, but there is variability and unpredictability in the degree to which this complication occurs (101–104). Some clinical states may suggest the location of consumption (in an isolated anatomic space rather than disseminated) (105). Infection associated with sepsis, trauma that causes shock, hyperthermia causing tissue necrosis, and other insults are more likely to have disseminated or systemic manifestations. However, anatomically limited lesions may "consume" locally, as with a dissecting aortic aneurysm or giant cavernous hemangioma (106,107). Other disorders may overlap the boundary between such anatomic categories, such as the localized, extravascular (intrauterine) consumption seen in *abruptio placentae*, which is accompanied by the liberation of thromboplastic material into the circulation, causing DIC (108). A recent emphasis considered a continuum of severity, for example, as a localized or compensated process becomes generalized (109), with a goal of defining a nonovert early stage that can be more readily treated.

A judgment must be made as to the pathologic mechanism involved in the consumption. On one hand, the elaboration of thrombin leads to the conversion of fibrinogen to fibrin, whereas the elaboration of plasmin leads to the enzymatic degradation of fibrin and fibrinogen. Thrombin and other active agents, such as bacterial endotoxin or snake venoms, may "consume" (aggregate) platelets and clot fibrinogen, whereas other mechanisms may result in isolated thrombocytopenia without thrombin generation, as in thrombotic thrombocytopenic purpura (TTP) (110) (see Chapter 111).

Given that factors of tempo, location, and pathophysiology can all operate as independent variables superimposed on a variety of underlying disorders, each patient's clinical and laboratory presentation must be individually considered before rational management can be started.

# ACUTE, SEVERE DISSEMINATED INTRAVASCULAR COAGULATION

## Clinical Features

The extreme end of the spectrum is acute, severe DIC of the kind defined as a "pathological syndrome resulting from activation (and consumption) of certain coagulant proteins, formation of thrombin, and production of fibrin thrombi" (9). Although the initial pathologic events are manifested by fibrin deposition in the microcirculation, the patient's initial clinical events usually relate to hemorrhagic manifestations such as mucosal oozing, spontaneous ecchymoses, petechiae, and massive gastrointestinal (GI) blood loss. If the patient has had recent invasive or operative procedures, the incisions will also be vulnerable to excessive bleeding. The latter results from consumption of thrombin-sensitive hemostatic factors, including platelets; fibrinogen; and factors V, VIII, and XIII. Thrombotic occlusive events occur first, as the result of microthrombi of fibrin or platelets that obstruct the microcirculation of organs. These thrombi result from clots that form either in the circulation or *in situ* in arterioles, capillaries, or venules. Circulatory obstruction produces organ hypoperfusion and even ischemia, infarction, and necrosis. The process is disseminated throughout the microcirculation; therefore, all organs are potentially vulnerable. Venous thromboembolism or arterial embolism from nonbacterial endocarditis can occur but are much more common in patients with subacute or chronic DIC, particularly in those patients with malignant disease.

Renal dysfunction in patients with DIC is often multifactorial. The conditions usually associated with DIC frequently are complicated by hypovolemia or hypotension that causes prerenal azotemia, even renal failure due to acute tubular necrosis. Thrombosis of renal afferent arterioles or glomerular capillaries by fibrin thrombi may cause ischemic renal cortical necrosis. The fibrin–platelet clots shown in Figure 109-2 are often not demonstrable at postmortem examination, presumably because of an induced local fibrinolytic response within the occluded vessels.

Cerebral dysfunction is most often manifested as nonspecific changes, such as an altered state of consciousness, convulsions, or coma, rather than by isolated focal lesions. Pathologic lesions affecting cerebral function may also include major vessel occlusion and subarachnoid hemorrhage, as well as multiple cortical and brainstem hemorrhages following microvascular occlusions (111).

Pulmonary function can likewise be affected. Patients may develop adult respiratory distress syndrome (ARDS) owing to endothelial damage, platelet adhesion and activation, and fibrin deposition (112). Although pulmonary hemorrhage is characteristic of DIC (64), ARDS is likely the result of both the underlying disorder and the complicating DIC, for example, after trauma, endotoxic shock, and amniotic fluid embolism (113,114).

GI involvement may produce ulceration in the stomach or duodenum secondary to submucosal necrosis, not infrequently resulting in excessive GI bleeding. When complicated by the hemorrhagic diathesis that follows these thrombotic events (Fig. 109-1), the GI and neurologic pathology is even more difficult to manage. Hemorrhagic necrosis may result in adrenal cortical failure, producing the Waterhouse-Friderichsen syndrome (115). Cellular necrosis around the hepatic central veins may follow shock and hypoxemia or intravascular coagulation (116,117), leading to decreased synthesis of vitamin K–dependent procoagulant and anticoagulant factors.

Fragmentation-type hemolysis (microangiopathy) secondary to fibrin deposition in the microvasculature may contribute to anemia (118). However, overt hemolytic anemia associated with DIC only occurs in 5% to 10% of patients,

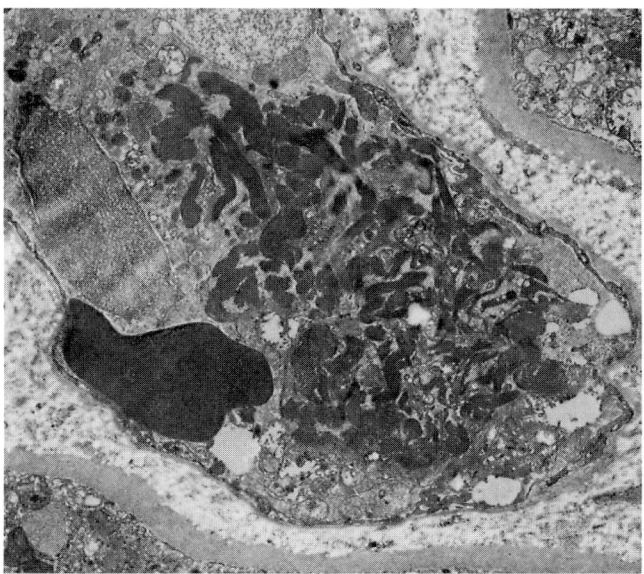

**FIGURE 109-2.** Electron micrograph showing fibrin thrombi in a renal interstitial capillary of a patient with acute disseminated intravascular coagulation. (Courtesy of Dr. Raul Mancilla-Jiminez, General Hospital, Centro Medico Nacional Mexico City.)

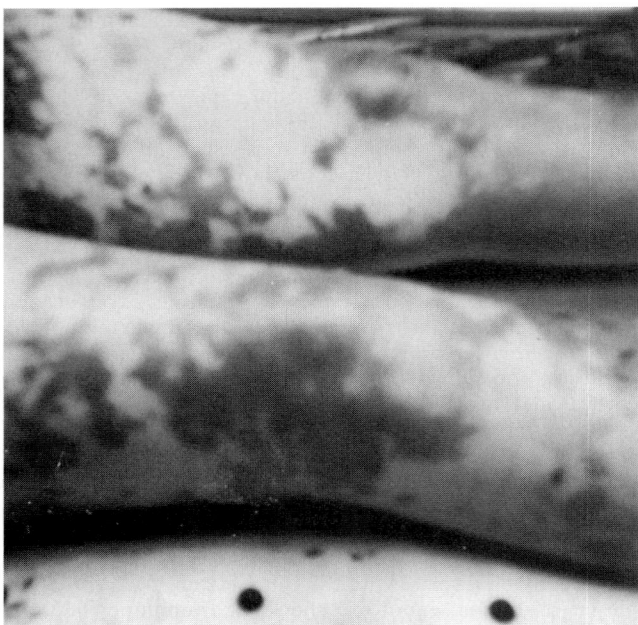

**FIGURE 109-3.** Patient with purpura fulminans, showing the irregular distribution of ischemic and hemorrhagic cutaneous lesions that reflect widespread occlusion of the arteriolar supply to the skin.

and similar morphologic abnormalities occur in many other disorders not associated with fibrin consumption (e.g., TTP).

Dermal ischemia and hemorrhagic skin necrosis may occur in patients with acute DIC (see Fig. 109-3), particularly those associated with severe infection and hypotension. This complication of acute DIC is in contrast to idiopathic purpura fulminans, which typically occurs in young children who may be convalescing from an infection involving the skin and who are *not* acutely infected at the time of the appearance of purpura fulminans (119).

## Disorders Associated with Acute Disseminated Intravascular Coagulation

### Infections

Virtually every type of infectious agent has been implicated in the consumptive thrombohemorrhagic disorders, usually producing mild or severe systemic intravascular coagulation, with consumption of platelets and soluble clotting factors. The most flagrant examples are the Waterhouse-Friderichsen syndrome and purpura fulminans, both of which bear pathologic and histologic similarity to the experimental animal model of consumption, the Shwartzman reaction (120–123). The Waterhouse-Friderichsen syndrome is most commonly seen during fulminant meningococcal sepsis, although other organisms such as *Pneumococcus* may also cause this complication (101–103, 124–128). Widespread intravascular fibrin and platelet thrombi obstruct arterioles, capillaries, and venules of vital organs, especially causing bilateral hemorrhagic necrosis of the adrenals. This type of sepsis is associated with severe shock, which contributes significantly to the high mortality. Although these clinical entities appear to be distinctive syndromes, they can be considered extreme manifestations of acute DIC. Variations in the acuteness of onset and the degree of consumption, perhaps related to the patient's age and health and the type of infectious agent, account for the wide range of clinical manifestations,

including some patients with laboratory abnormalities of consumption but no clinical signs.

Histopathologic evidence of DIC is most often seen in patients with Gram-negative shock who die during the first 24 hours after presentation (103,129,130). Gram-positive bacteria have been less frequently implicated in DIC (103). A significant number of patients with pneumococcal sepsis and DIC have had functional or anatomic asplenia, which probably hinders the clearance of organisms from the circulation and contributes to the consumptive process (127). A particularly aggressive process of DIC and vascular occlusion has been noted in gram-negative bacteremia, leading to progressive gangrenous necrosis and death (see Fig. 109-4) (128). Clostridial organisms have been implicated in the severe DIC of septic abortion, which has a mortality greater than 50% when complicated by shock (131,132).

In patients with severe sepsis and DIC (particularly when associated with shock), certain laboratory parameters have been associated with a poor prognosis, including AT levels lower than 70%, increased PAI-I levels, and decreased factor VIIa levels (133). Decreased levels of the VWF-cleaving protease (ADAMTS13) have been documented in patients with septic shock (134). Although this deficiency could contribute to the process of microvascular platelet thrombus formation, the blood levels were not as strikingly decreased as in patients with TTP (<30% vs. <10%).

Viral diseases such as cytomegalovirus, varicella, variola, rubella, rubeola, and influenza A have also occasionally been associated with a consumptive process (135–137). Laboratory confirmation of DIC is found in more than half of patients with Korean hemorrhagic fever, which is characterized in fatal cases by coagulation necrosis of the renal medulla and pituitary gland (138). Other hemorrhagic fevers plus the Hanta and Ebola viruses are associated with severe bleeding and laboratory evidence of DIC (139). The pathophysiologic mechanisms causing DIC in viral illness are poorly understood but may be due to endothelial damage resulting in a prothrombotic phenotype (15). The severity of dengue hemorrhagic fever has been correlated with shortened fibrinogen survival, thrombocytopenia, prolongation of the partial thromboplastin time (PTT), and increased levels of FDPs (140,141). The thrombocytopenia reported in approximately half the patients with Rocky Mountain spotted fever may reflect intravascular consumption, and, in addition, laboratory evidence of DIC has been associated with a more fulminant clinical course (142,143). Isolated patients with severe *Plasmodium falciparum* malaria complicated by thrombocytopenia and coagulation abnormalities or even by deep vein thrombosis and tissue necrosis may also be examples of DIC complicating the

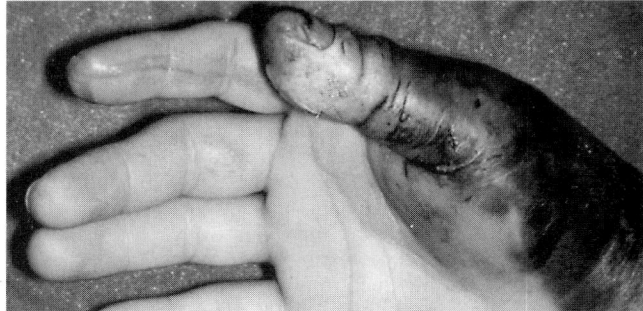

**FIGURE 109-4.** Hemorrhagic necrosis of the thumb and wrist in a patient with polymicrobial bacteremia and purpura fulminans. (From Kusne S, Eibling DE, Yu VL, et al. Gangrenous cellulitis associated with Gram-negative bacilli in pancytopenic patients: dilemma with respect to effective therapy. *Am J Med* 1988;85:490, with permission.)

original infection (144,145). Other organisms such as *Aspergillus*, *Candida*, *Trypanosoma*, and *Mycobacteria* have also been implicated as initiators of consumption, suggesting that virtually any infectious agent can be associated with a consumptive thrombohemorrhagic disorder (146–148).

## Purpura Fulminans

Purpura fulminans is a rare syndrome characterized by dermal vascular thrombosis and progressive hemorrhagic skin necrosis. It occurs in three different clinical settings: (i) in patients with preexisting inherited or acquired disorders of the protein C anticoagulant pathway; (ii) in those with acute infections, usually caused by Gram-negative bacteria; and (iii) in those with neither an abnormality of the protein C pathway nor the presence of acute infection (idiopathic purpura fulminans) (149).

**Idiopathic.** Purpura fulminans was originally described in 1887 (150); Hjort et al. (151) were the first to clearly define its characteristic features:

1. usual occurrence in young children;
2. frequent history of an antecedent "preparatory disease," usually a bacterial or viral infection involving the skin;
3. sudden development during a quiescent convalescent period of progressively enlarging, purplish-black areas of hemorrhagic skin necrosis sharply demarcated from surrounding healthy skin by a narrow red border;
4. histopathologic findings in involved skin of dermal vascular thrombosis and secondary hemorrhagic infarction;
5. usual absence of clinically significant thrombohemorrhagic manifestations in organs other than the skin;
6. association with marked hypofibrinogenemia and thrombocytopenia, all due to acute DIC (151,152).

The most common antecedent illnesses in children are scarlet fever and varicella; in the few cases reported in adults, an antecedent infection is less common (118,149,153,154). The interval between the antecedent illness and the onset of skin necrosis is usually less than 10 days. Most lesions are located on the breasts and the lower half of the body, where the thighs, legs, buttocks, lower abdomen, scrotum, and penis are most commonly involved. This distribution is similar to that seen in protein C– or protein S–deficient heterozygotes with warfarin-induced skin necrosis and in patients with homozygous protein C deficiency. The lesions have irregular areas of blue-black hemorrhagic necrosis surrounded by a thin advancing red border, which fades into uninvolved skin (Fig. 109-3). The lesions are indurated and painful because of bleeding into the necrotic dermis, and hemorrhagic bullae often form in necrotic areas. Necrosis frequently extends deep into the subcutaneous tissue and forms a thick eschar that sloughs. The resulting wound heals slowly by secondary intention, often with severe scarring or contractures. Autoamputation of necrotic extremities and of the male genitalia may occur.

The tendency of idiopathic purpura fulminans to not affect the distal extremities contrasts with the pattern of ascending peripheral gangrene of the distal extremities often seen in sepsis-associated purpura fulminans (155) (Fig. 109-4). This difference reflects the shock and tissue hypoperfusion in acute sepsis, which usually does not occur in idiopathic purpura fulminans.

The pathogenesis of idiopathic purpura fulminans is poorly understood. However, a similar syndrome can be produced in laboratory animals (the local Shwartzman reaction) when the skin of a rabbit is prepared with endotoxin, IL-1, or TNF, and 24 hours later an agent that induces intravascular coagulation is injected intravenously. The prepared skin site undergoes vascular thrombosis and secondary hemorrhagic necrosis similar to that seen in purpura fulminans (123). The antecedent illness in humans (varicella or scarlet fever) is thought to similarly prepare the skin for thrombosis, although the exact mechanism that predisposes the skin to thrombosis and triggers the intravascular coagulation is unknown.

Since 1964, the mortality of idiopathic purpura fulminans has been reduced from 90% to 18% (122,149). This remarkable improvement in survival is the result of more rigorous supportive care, more widespread use of heparin to interrupt the intravascular coagulation process, and vigorous blood and plasma replacement.

**Severe Infection.** Like idiopathic purpura fulminans, sepsis-associated purpura fulminans is much more common in children than in adults (149). Although the *Meningococcus* is the most common organism involved, purpura fulminans has been reported with many different types of Gram-negative and Gram-positive organisms (124,126,154,156–160). The dermal histopathology and the association with intravascular coagulation are similar. However, sepsis-associated purpura fulminans differs in three important ways from idiopathic purpura fulminans:

1. The initial presentation in sepsis-associated purpura fulminans is often that of overwhelming acute infection with hypotension and peripheral hypoperfusion; in contrast, in idiopathic purpura fulminans, the blood pressure is well preserved.
2. The skin necrosis in sepsis-associated purpura fulminans often begins in the distal extremities (see Fig. 109-4), with subsequent proximal progression, or involves the entire body in a patchy distribution (119,161).
3. Thrombohemorrhagic manifestations in other organs are much more common in sepsis-associated purpura fulminans (162).

Therefore, sepsis-associated purpura fulminans is essentially a consequence of acute DIC and hypoperfusion secondary to endotoxemia or exotoxemia. This striking form of purpura fulminans, sometimes termed "symmetrical peripheral gangrene," is strongly associated with DIC, to the extent that it has been called by Molos and Hall as a "cutaneous marker of DIC" (163).

**Protein C or S Deficiency.** Infants who are homozygotes for protein C or S deficiency may be born with severe skin necrosis and intravascular coagulation (hereditary purpura fulminans). Moreover, patients who are heterozygotes for protein C or S deficiency may develop skin necrosis when placed on warfarin therapy (164–166). Protein C or S levels may be low because of liver dysfunction, consumption of these anticoagulants, or, rarely, secondary to an acquired inhibitor (167,168).

## Liver Disease

Complications of acute or chronic liver disease may trigger episodes of acute DIC, most notably in patients with peritoneovenous (LeVeen or Denver) shunts or fatty liver of pregnancy. As reviewed by LeVeen (169), this procedure has a mortality of less than 1% in "uncomplicated cirrhosis," and postoperative coagulopathies can largely be avoided. However, a substantial number of patients develop DIC shortly after shunt placement. Ragni et al. (170) detected DIC in 10 of 11 such patients, and a high incidence of DIC was reported by Rubinstein et al. (171), who found DIC after 14 of 27 shunt procedures and a greater tendency for this complication in patients with cirrhosis.

It is not surprising that these patients develop DIC, because thrombin activity is retained in ascitic fluid, and TF-bearing monocytes and macrophages are probably infused along with the ascitic fluid. The only effective treatment of symptomatic DIC is to discontinue the shunt. AT infusions have been tried but have been unsuccessful (172).

The laboratory changes that accompany fatty liver of pregnancy are compatible with acute DIC. Therefore, Pockros et al. (173) reported abnormalities in four of 10 such patients, with a variable degree of hypofibrinogenemia and thrombocytopenia, a clear-cut elevation of serum fibrinogen degradation products, and a decrease in AT. The cause of the DIC is not clear, but it is usually associated with decreased synthesis of hemostatic factors as seen in patients with liver failure. Early delivery is reasonable in some cases, but this usually does not reverse the underlying hepatic disease or hemostatic laboratory abnormalities for several days. AT levels are frequently very low because of the combination of increased consumption and decreased production. Although it has not been proven, AT replacement therapy may be helpful in curtailing the DIC (174).

In addition to fatty liver of pregnancy, acute DIC may also complicate acute hepatic necrosis and liver failure of different etiologies, including viral hepatitis, toxins, hyperthermia, and drug overdose such as with acetaminophen (175,176).

### Acute Obstetric Complications

Since 1971, when deLee (177) reported a state of "temporary hemophilia" in patients with premature separation of the placenta and a macerated dead fetus, it has been evident that a consumptive thrombohemorrhagic state is observed in a wide range of obstetric complications, including *abruptio placentae*, retained dead fetus, amniotic fluid embolism, saline-induced or septic abortion, and occasionally in toxemia. The site of consumption may be limited to a single extravascular locale (the uterus), disseminated in the blood, or present in both locations; the pathologic mechanism may involve coagulation, fibrinolysis, or both simultaneously; and the broadest range of tempo may occur, from the fulminant onset of an *abruptio placentae* to the chronic, low-grade effects of the retained dead fetus syndrome. An excellent summary of the clinical, pathologic, diagnostic, and therapeutic aspects of such obstetric complications has been prepared by Graeff and Kuhn (178).

Pregnancy is associated with a baseline hypercoagulable state characterized by increased levels of many procoagulant factors, low protein S levels, and reduced fibrinolytic activity (179,180). In the 1- to 4-hour period immediately after uncomplicated single delivery, there is a significant decrease of plasma fibrinogen, a shortening of plasma euglobulin lysis time, and an increase in concentration of fibrinogen degradation products (179). These findings indicate that a "minor degree of physiologic defibrination" is expected under ordinary circumstances and that these changes are similar to, but of less magnitude than, those that occur with *abruptio placentae* or with intrauterine death syndrome.

*Abruptio Placentae.* *Abruptio placentae*, the premature separation of a normally implanted placenta, may occur in the absence of clinical symptoms, in which case the diagnosis becomes apparent only on pathologic examination of the placenta. In contrast, it may be associated with a mild to moderate episode of vaginal bleeding with excessive contraction of the uterus and a significantly increased risk of fetal death, or it may appear as a full-blown picture of generalized bleeding, hemorrhagic shock, severe abdominal pain, and tenderness due to tetanic uterine contraction and fetal death (178). In approximately one third of cases, no bleeding occurs before delivery because the blood is contained within the uterus. The incidence of all degrees of *abruptio placentae* has been variously recorded as somewhat less than 1% of all deliveries, with the severe form occurring in less than 0.2% (181). The process that causes consumption stems from a combination of localized intrauterine hemorrhage and systemic defibrination caused by the release of TF-bearing products from placental tissue or in amniotic fluid (182–184). The organ effects (e.g., compromise of renal function) that may be secondary to DIC respond dramatically after delivery, even with only general support measures, suggesting that hypovolemia secondary to the uterine bleeding is more important than DIC. Although in the classic study by Pritchard and Brekken (180), only 38% of patients had hypofibrinogenemia (<150 mg per dL), most patients had a relatively low fibrinogen for that stage of pregnancy. The degree of placental separation appears to correlate with the extent of fibrin formation and thrombocytopenia, suggesting that local factors are responsible for initiating DIC (185).

*Amniotic Fluid Embolism.* Amniotic fluid embolism was firmly established as a syndrome by the clinical and histopathologic changes described by Steiner and Lushbaugh in 1941 (186). Its incidence has been estimated as 1:8,000 to 1:80,000 live births (187,188), and it is responsible for 10% of maternal deaths in the United States (188,189). Clinically, it is characterized by the sudden onset of severe respiratory distress, cyanosis, profound circulatory shock, and seizures in a multiparous patient during or just after labor (178). The diagnosis can be confirmed antemortem by the demonstration of fetal debris (scales, lanugo, meconium) in the buffy coat, but these abnormalities are neither sensitive nor specific (189). In the National Registry for amniotic fluid embolism (46 patients), cardiac arrest occurred in 87% and mortality was 61%, but only 15% of patients survived neurologically intact (189). Seventy-nine percent of fetuses survived, but only 50% were neurologically unimpaired. In patients who survive the initial episode, excessive bleeding follows in 40% of cases, usually after a latent period of 0.5 to 4 hours, and the great majority have laboratory evidence of consumption (189).

No maternal demographic risk factor (e.g., age, race, parity, obstetric history, route of delivery, and use of oxytocin) predisposed to amniotic fluid embolism except that in 78% of patients, the embolism occurred after spontaneous or artificial rupture of membranes (189). There appears to be no causative link with hypertonic contractions; rather, the contractions may be secondary to entry of amniotic fluid into the maternal circulation. Amniotic fluid may enter the maternal circulation dramatically through a rupture of the uterus, under somewhat less catastrophic circumstances through an abnormal placental placement site through tears in the chorioamniotic membranes, or as part of the *abruptio placentae* syndrome.

Whatever the reason, it appears that the cause of the syndrome is exposure of the maternal circulation to amniotic fluid (190). The administration of homologous meconium preparation in an animal model results in a hemodynamic response similar to that seen in humans (189,191). An anaphylactoid reaction to the fetal material that enters the maternal circulation has been postulated (189), but another explanation is that the amniotic fluid debris mechanically obstructs the pulmonary circulation, resulting in acute cor pulmonale, right-sided congestive heart failure, decreased filling of the left ventricle, decreased cardiac output, profound hypoxemia, and subsequent metabolic disturbances (178,185,192,193). After the initial pulmonary arterial obstructive phenomena, activation of the coagulation system—probably by TF contained in amniotic fluid (194,195)—and severe consumption with intense secondary fibrinolysis and a hemorrhagic disorder follow (178,196,197).

The effectiveness of treatment has not been carefully assessed. Vigorous supportive therapy directed toward gas exchange with mechanical respiratory assistance and fluid and blood replacement to treat severe hypotension are essential. In patients in whom continued entry of amniotic fluid debris may be contributing to further intravascular clotting, heparin is a reasonable adjunct to therapy (198–200). When bleeding is the major manifestation, heparin may make matters worse, especially if adequate replacement therapy for consumed clotting factors has not been achieved (178). In addition to replacement therapy for treatment of dangerous bleeding, fibrinolytic inhibitors may be helpful, but the same precautions regarding their use apply as in other settings of DIC (see subsequent text).

**Saline-Induced Abortion.** Saline-induced abortion during the second trimester of pregnancy has caused laboratory changes of DIC, namely, hypofibrinogenemia, thrombocytopenia, and circulating FDPs (201,202). The mechanism for this mild, acute DIC presumably results from the entry of disintegrated placental tissue into the circulation, resulting in activation of the coagulation system. Systemic manifestations of bleeding or even problems of excessive bleeding with vaginal delivery are unusual. The induced abortion removes the underlying cause of the consumption and is the reason clinical consequences of consumption are uncommon. If excessive bleeding occurs at the time of delivery, deficiencies of fibrinogen and platelets should be corrected.

**Septic Abortion.** In contrast to the relatively mild clinical state of saline-induced abortion, septic abortion heralds the most fulminant type of severe DIC. In a group of more than 6,000 patients who had undergone abortion, 16% were infected, 4% (40) of whom had shock and DIC, leading to death in one half of these seriously affected patients (203). Graeff and Kuhn (178) emphasize that any of a large number of bacterial organisms, both aerobic and anaerobic, may be the inciting agent; a combination of severe hypotension and DIC complicate the clinical picture (204).

Once established, the clinical symptoms, laboratory manifestations, and principles of therapy are as for any severe infection leading to shock, with the added consideration that evacuation of the uterus and sometimes hysterectomy are required to eliminate the infection. These patients can be the most refractory to therapy, and vigorous attention must be paid to proper antibiotic choice, maintenance of blood volume and electrolyte balance, and appropriate replacement of deficient hemostatic factors. The use of heparin in these circumstances is controversial, and there is little evidence of its benefit. As with other circumstances of acute, severe DIC, fibrinolytic inhibitors should be withheld so as not to impair the physiologic fibrinolytic response in the microcirculation of ischemic organs.

**Placenta Accreta.** Placenta accreta (retained placenta) occurs in one of every 1,000 deliveries. A comparison of manual removal of the placenta during the period 1993 to 1997 has been compared with an approach of leaving the placenta *in situ*, during the period 1997 to 2002 (205). There were statistically significant fewer hysterectomies, transfusions, and occurrences of DIC in the latter group of patients, suggesting that leaving the placenta accreta *in situ* was the preferable therapeutic approach.

## Preeclampsia and "Hemolysis, Elevated Liver Enzymes, and a Low Platelet Count" Syndrome

The existence of DIC as a constant feature in patients with preeclampsia or eclampsia is controversial (206–209). Isolated thrombocytopenia or the complete HELLP (*h*emolysis, *el*evated *l*iver enzymes, and a *l*ow *p*latelet count) syndrome may be associated with the typical findings of preeclampsia. In addition, the HELLP syndrome may occur in the absence of any signs of preeclampsia. Although sensitive parameters of thrombin generation (thrombin–AT complexes, D-dimer, etc.) are increased in preeclampsia and HELLP syndrome, the levels of fibrinogen and other clotting factors do not differ from those found during healthy pregnancy (210). Overt intravascular consumption occurs only in few of the cases and is frequently associated with a complicating abruption. The thrombocytopenia is a consistent feature of both syndromes and is probably caused by endothelial perturbation and injury (211).

## Trauma or Massive Tissue Necrosis

DIC complicating severe trauma occurs in several different scenarios, including severe head injury, particularly associated with necrotic brain, massive soft tissue trauma, multiple fractures and fat embolism, gunshot wounds, and extensive burns (212). The cause of DIC in these situations probably stems from exposure of TF to blood. Moreover, these scenarios are complicated by other problems that can aggravate the hemostatic defect, including prolonged hemorrhagic shock itself, the transfusion "washout" syndrome, hepatic dysfunction, and superimposed sepsis.

In a study of 16 patients with head injury who had DIC and came to autopsy within 4 days of injury, Kaufman et al. (213) noted necrosis and bleeding in several organs, most notably the brain and lungs, and microthrombi in the central nervous system, liver, lungs, kidneys, and pancreas. Thrombi were less prevalent with longer delays after injury and before death, attesting to a probable fibrinolytic response in the microcirculation to dissolve these thrombi. Head injury in children is also associated with abnormal clotting tests in 71% of cases, and 32% of such patients have DIC or fibrinolysis; mortality is fourfold greater in the latter patients than in those without DIC (214). The high mortality rate is associated with increased bleeding and laboratory evidence of DIC and has led to the development of scores for prognostic purposes in such patients (214,215).

Many cases of severe trauma are associated with pulmonary dysfunction or ARDS in association with DIC and fibrin deposition in the lung (213,216). ARDS and DIC appear to act cumulatively to result in more severe pulmonary dysfunction. In the study by Bone et al. (217), seven of 30 patients with ARDS and DIC had bleeding, gangrene of the extremities, renal dysfunction, and evidence of microthrombi in the lungs and other organs at autopsy. Of the remaining 23 patients, 12 had thrombocytopenia, and evidence of fibrin deposition limited to the pulmonary vasculature was found in four of five such patients who underwent autopsy. Therefore, in patients with ARDS, overt or subclinical DIC may be seen, but in some patients, isolated thrombocytopenia may be the only hemostatic abnormality. In the latter patients, the platelets appear to be sequestered in the lung, probably owing to damaged endothelial cells.

## Heat Stroke

Heat stroke is frequently complicated by DIC (218–220). This disorder causes rhabdomyolysis and hepatic necrosis, and therefore DIC probably stems from TF released into the circulation from necrotic tissue. In the report by Mustafa et al. (218), 17 of 30 patients had evidence of DIC, and those patients had a higher incidence of bleeding, shock, and mortality. The review by Bouchama and Knochel (221) notes that markers of coagulation activation appear at the onset of the syndrome (thrombin–antithrombin complexes; soluble fibrin; and consumption of the inhibitors protein C, protein S, and antithrombin III). This phase is followed by activation of fibrinolysis (plasmin–antiplasmin complexes, plasminogen consumption, and D-dimers). Therefore, heat stroke may take different forms, some patients having evidence of pathologic fibrinolysis with or without evidence of DIC, others having fibrinolysis so intense that primary fibrinogenolysis is probably superimposed on excessive secondary fibrinolysis.

## Snakebite

The bite of certain snakes, especially vipers and rattlesnakes [e.g., *Daboiat* (Russell), *Bothrops*, *Agkistrodon*, *Echis*, and *Crotalus*] can produce hypofibrinogenemia with or without thrombocytopenia, depending on whether the venom contains enzymes that directly clot fibrinogen (without thrombocytopenia) or indirectly clot by activating factor X or prothrombin and generating thrombin (with thrombocytopenia). Patients with combined hypofibrinogenemia and thrombocytopenia have been exposed to venoms that contain not only procoagulant enzymes but also a platelet aggregating factor (222,223).

Most bites cause striking laboratory abnormalities in all victims but relatively mild clinical disorders in approximately one half of patients (224,225). The symptoms are characterized by local tenderness and swelling, mild bleeding from the wound or from venipunctures, occasional hypotension without shock, and transient mild oliguria. Although some patients have shortened euglobulin lysis times, the syndrome most closely resembles DIC, but with considerable variation in the rate and degree of consumption and in the chronicity of laboratory changes (47,226). Some patients begin to recover spontaneously after 1 to 2 days and are completely normal within 1 week, whereas others demonstrate incoagulable blood without symptoms of hemorrhage for more than 3 weeks (224,227). Active secondary fibrinolysis accounts for the rapid recovery of the presumed renal microcirculatory obstruction. However, the study by Chugh et al. (228) documents more severe illness after viper bites, with 45 of 157 patients having acute renal failure, and death occurring in eight of 10 with bilateral renal necrosis and in four of 23 with "less severe acute tubular lesions."

Treatment in most instances has been conservative, concerned primarily with neutralizing the venom with antivenin; transfusion with platelets and plasma; and maintaining blood volume, blood pressure, and electrolyte balance. Except for the report by Weiss et al. (222), the use of heparin has been unimpressive. Warrell et al. (225) studied 14 patients bitten by *Echis carinatus*, seven of whom were treated primarily with antivenin and seven with antivenin plus heparin; no benefit accrued from the heparin above than that obtained with the antivenin alone, although the dose of heparin may have been too low to have influenced the outcome. However, the generally benign course in humans and the lack of additive beneficial effect of reasonable doses of heparin suggest that the venom procoagulant enzymes may not be inhibitable by AT.

### Acute Hemolysis

Acute hemolysis such as that after the transfusion of 500 mL or more of incompatible blood (major mismatch) can produce a hemorrhagic diathesis characterized by laboratory changes of hypofibrinogenemia and thrombocytopenia (229,230). This pattern is compatible with acute DIC, with variable effects of intravascular thrombi on renal function depending on the acuteness and degree of defibrination and the additional presence of hypovolemia or hypotension (230). However, massive hemolysis (other than that associated with a major mismatch) does not uniformly produce DIC, as Mannucci et al. (231) observed in 28 patients with glucose-6-phosphate dehydrogenase deficiency who were exposed to fava beans. Not only was there no evidence of DIC but the hemolysis also produced elevations in the concentration of fibrinogen and factor VIII, an acute-phase reaction to the stress. Because the tissue macrophages are considered vital in the clearance of the erythrocyte stromal procoagulant material from the circulation, the authors postulated that some insult impairing normal reticuloendothelial system function must coexist during an acute hemolytic episode, thereby predisposing the patient to DIC. Although hypotension, surgery, anesthesia, or sepsis could qualify as significant additional predisposing factors in patients who have been reported to develop DIC after incompatible blood transfusions, it is thought that the severe antigen–antibody reaction that occurs may be the major contributing factor in causing the DIC. The DIC is self-limiting, and in the absence of serious end-organ damage, the patients improve rapidly with supportive measures. Treatment depends on maintenance of blood volume and organ perfusion and on blood replacement with compatible erythrocytes.

# CHRONIC OR SUBACUTE DISSEMINATED INTRAVASCULAR COAGULATION

In contrast to the acutely ill patient with complicated, severe DIC, other patients may have mild or protracted clinical manifestations of consumption or even subclinical disease manifest by only laboratory abnormalities (9,232,233). The clinical picture of subacute to chronic DIC generally occurs in patients with malignancy, in particular with mucin-producing adenocarcinomas and APL. The latter usually is dominated by a hemorrhagic presentation, whereas venous thrombotic manifestations are more common in the former (233). In addition, patients with solid tumors may develop nonbacterial thrombotic endocarditis with systemic arterial embolization and infarction (234). Another cause of subacute to chronic DIC is the retained dead fetus syndrome. These patients have an extremely variable presentation from asymptomatic to mild or moderate skin and mucous membrane bleeding.

In patients with chronic DIC, laboratory manifestations are extremely variable. Some patients have all of the classic abnormalities of thrombocytopenia, hypofibrinogenemia, elevated FDP levels, and prolonged PTT and prothrombin time (PT), whereas other patients have normal results, owing to increased synthesis of proteins such as fibrinogen.

## Clinical Conditions Associated with Subacute or Chronic Disseminated Intravascular Coagulation

### Neoplasia

**Solid Tumors.** Although thrombocytopenia in patients with malignancy is usually secondary to decreased bone marrow production, it can also reflect a more generalized consumptive process with various clinical manifestations, including venous thromboembolic disease, nonbacterial thrombotic valvular endocarditis, bleeding out of proportion to the thrombocytopenia, and microangiopathic hemolytic anemia (233). In addition, an occasional patient with a solid tumor may develop a bleeding disorder as the result of pathologic fibrinogenolysis, either systemically or locally in a tumor mass.

The strong clinical association between solid tumors of visceral origin and thrombohemorrhagic disorders was described vividly by Trousseau in 1865 (234) and has been rediscovered, redefined, and expanded in a profusion of medical literature since then (40,235), perhaps best summarized by the 1977 review by Sack et al. (236). In this group of patients, isolated venous thrombosis occurred in 113 of 182 (62%) patients and "migratory" venous thrombosis in 96 (53%) of the patients (Trousseau syndrome), while a bleeding state existed in only 75 (41%) patients. Microvascular thrombotic occlusive disease is unusual, although the patients uniformly have evidence of intravascular coagulation (i.e., positive assays for fibrinopeptide release or circulating fibrin monomers) (237–240). This probably reflects an effective fibrinolytic response secondary to the low-grade intravascular coagulation.

A unique feature of these chronically ill patients, especially those with mucin-producing carcinoma, is nonbacterial thrombotic endocarditis with systemic embolization and infarction (241). Sack et al. found this in 45 of their 182 patients, and all three clinical reflections of chronic DIC (venous thrombosis, endocarditis, and bleeding) were noted in 12 of their group (236), as well as in single cases reported by others (242).

The pathophysiologic mechanism of DIC in patients with solid tumors is controversial (243). Although a cysteine protease has been described in human carcinoma tissue (244), evidence suggests that TF is the major trigger either expressed on the surface of, or contained in vesicles shed by, the tumor cells (245) or by activating monocytes (possibly activated by tumor antigens or antigen–antibody complexes) with resultant expression of TF on their surface (246,247). In a study of hemostatic parameters in 102 patients with solid tumors (71 had GI tumors), plasma TF was 67% higher and factor VIIa was 46% higher than in healthy controls (248), and in addition, there was an increase in thrombin–AT complexes and prothrombin fragment F1 + 2. Therefore, the data supports the hypothesis that activation of the TF pathway is involved in patients with solid tumors.

Laboratory alterations include thrombocytopenia and hypofibrinogenemia of variable but usually parallel degree, circulating FDPs, and microangiopathic hemolytic anemia. A given patient may show no clinical effects of DIC, in which case laboratory parameters can be monitored to gauge the effect of therapy (236,237,242). In some patients, with or without thrombotic complications, the intravascular coagulation may be relatively well compensated with normal or near-normal fibrinogen, platelet, and clotting factor levels along with elevated D-dimer (8). Presumably, in these patients, increased production of hemostatic factors with slow triggering of intravascular coagulation are present.

Unusual clinical thrombotic states may suggest an occult neoplasm (e.g., recurrence of venous thrombi, multiple limb thrombosis, hemorrhage after reasonable doses of anticoagulation, gangrene secondary to arterial emboli, thrombocytosis, phlegmasia cerulea dolens and venous gangrene, as well as combined thrombosis and bleeding, arterial and venous thromboemboli, or all of these in a single patient) (236,249–254). Patients with carcinoma of the prostate often have hemorrhagic manifestations that dominate the clinical picture, and this could reflect the ability of this tumor to produce fibrinolytic activators as well as procoagulants (236,255). The tendency of some tumor cells to produce such clot-dissolving activity may be reflected by prolonged localized bleeding after biopsy of the tumor (256). Interruption of clinically evident DIC with anticoagulation may provide significant benefit. In the study by Sack et al. (236), 29 of 48 such patients had improvement of hemostatic measurements, and 19 of the patients had recurrent symptoms after heparin was discontinued. Bell et al. (257) described two patients with dramatic major arterial and venous thrombi controlled with heparin, while warfarin therapy is usually ineffective and antiplatelet agents do not suffice for long-term therapy (242). Direct thrombin inhibitors such as hirudin or argatroban are probably more effective than heparin for application to the hospitalized patient, and fondaparinux, low-molecular-weight heparin, or unfractionated heparin are reasonable agents for prolonged (months) outpatient therapy.

**Acute Promyelocytic Leukemia.** APL is characterized by numerous intracytoplasmic inclusions and dense granules in the promyelocytes and a 15-17 chromosomal translocation. It is almost uniformly associated with hemostatic abnormalities (258–260). Although hemorrhagic phenomena predominate, venous as well as arterial thromboembolic complications may occur in up to 5% of such patients, with autopsy evidence of diffuse thrombosis reported in 15% to 25% of patients (261). The majority show a prolonged PT, hypofibrinogenemia, elevated FDP levels, and a shortened fibrinogen half-life, even in patients without clinically identifiable disease (259,261,262). Both TF and fibrinolytic proteases can be demonstrated in promyelocytic subcellular components, but the former predominates in both *in vitro* analyses and clinical presentation (38,263,264).

Urokinase-type plasminogen activator and tPA have been found within APL cells in addition to low plasma PAI and $\alpha_2$-plasmin inhibitor levels (265–269). In addition, nonspecific protease activity stemming from leukocyte elastase can also cause increased fibrinogen catabolism, degrade several clotting factors, and increase fibrinolysis contributing to the process (270,271).

This clinical disorder may present with serious hemorrhagic manifestations due to DIC and fibrin(ogen)olysis, further complicated by severe thrombocytopenia secondary to both the intravascular coagulation and decreased thrombopoiesis. Before the use of all-*trans*-retinoic acid (ATRA), anthracycline-based induction therapy induced complete remission in 50% to 60% of patients, but a significant number died early from intracranial hemorrhage: 16 of 60 (26%) patients died within 2 weeks in the series of Kantarjian et al. (272) and six of seven patients died early (within 5 days) (273–275). The coagulopathy has also been described in patients with chronic myeloid and monocytic leukemia, acute myeloid leukemia, acute lymphoblastic leukemia, and hairy cell leukemia (104,276–279). The syndrome should be distinguished from the thrombotic occlusive disease that results from excessively high white counts in acute or chronic leukemia (280).

Control of the leukemic process determines the patient's ultimate response. A consumptive disorder may be induced or exacerbated by cell lysis during chemotherapy (262), but the coagulopathy associated with APL has dramatically decreased with the introduction of ATRA. The coagulopathy rapidly diminishes over 2 to 6 days with a concomitant decrease in mortality due to bleeding (270). ATRA also dampens the cytokine-induced downregulation of thrombomodulin on endothelial cells, so the net effect of ATRA is to reduce the prothrombotic potential of the endothelium (270,281). In randomized clinical trials comparing ATRA plus chemotherapy to chemotherapy alone, however, no significant difference was noted in hemorrhagic deaths despite that the duration of the coagulopathy was significantly less with ATRA, and ATRA was associated with an increased disease-free and overall survival (282,283).

### Retained Dead Fetus Syndrome

Retained dead fetus syndrome exists if the fibrinogen concentration falls below normal for the stage of pregnancy in the context of intrauterine fetal death. This syndrome is a slowly developing, compensated or low-grade form of DIC. Its incidence increases with longer periods of fetal retention to as much as 35% of patients with a duration of 5 weeks or longer (178,284). Although an occasional patient appears to have an acute primary fibrinolytic response to the dead fetus, the evidence strongly suggests that intravascular coagulation is the sole mechanism for the defibrination in most patients (178,285–288). As expected in patients with slowly developing consumption, the secondary fibrinolytic response keeps pace with the formation of fibrin thrombi, and organ obstruction and ischemia are not part of the clinical picture. The low fibrinogen and platelet counts do not usually cause serious spontaneous bleeding, but the patients are at risk for postpartum hemorrhage if hemostatic defects are not corrected.

As with other obstetric consumptive complications, the essence of treatment is to empty the uterus. However, in the rare instance of a twin pregnancy with a single fetal death and consequent DIC, heparin treatment can reverse DIC and save the second twin (289).

### Liver Disease

A chronic consumptive coagulopathy has been postulated to complicate liver cirrhosis (6,290) on the basis of decreased clearance of activated clotting factors; increased catabolic rate of infused fibrinogen, correction of the shortened fibrinogen half-life by heparin but not by fibrinolytic inhibitors; and increased levels of D-dimers (291), thrombin–AT complexes (292), and fibrinopeptide A (293). Moreover, when AT concentrate is given to patients with severe chronic liver disease, thrombin–AT complexes, prothrombin fragment F1 + 2, plasmin–antiplasmin complexes, and D-dimer levels are decreased (294).

Despite such evidence, a major role for a consumptive thrombohemorrhagic process in patients with liver disease is still controversial. For example, histopathologic changes compatible with DIC are uncommon in patients with liver disease, as reported in an autopsy study showing only four of 184 cases of acute and chronic liver disease with microthrombi in more than one organ (295). However, the absence of fibrin thrombi in patients with chronic liver disease may be a result of a systemic fibrinolytic state in 50% of patients (295). Straub cautioned against simplistic interpretation of the effects of heparin on the half-life of labeled fibrinogen, especially because the changes observed in fibrinogen clearance can be explained by loss of protein into extravascular compartments (ascitic fluid) and increased fibrinolysis, as well as by intravascular coagulation (296). Laboratory abnormalities can be explained by other mechanisms than DIC (e.g., the synthesis of an abnormal fibrinogen with an inherently prolonged thrombin time) (297). Although correction of the coagulation defect may be facilitated in an occasional case by adding heparin therapy to treatment with plasma infusions, no evidence exists that this treatment improves prognosis (175,298). Although the evidence suggests that chronic intravascular coagulation exists in patients with liver cirrhosis, there is scant evidence that it plays a role in the hemostatic defects of cirrhosis.

# LOCALIZED INTRAVASCULAR COAGULATION

Certain disorders are predictably associated with the consumption of platelets and clotting factors in strictly defined, localized anatomic sites. Laboratory studies are frequently characterized by thrombocytopenia, hypofibrinogenemia, and elevated levels of FDPs or D-dimer. Occasionally, the levels may be so low to cause bleeding. However, because the consumption is usually localized, distant microvascular occlusion and organ ischemia do not occur. Two risks of not recognizing the limited disorder are (i) that of inappropriate therapy for a presumed "disseminated" state and (ii) that of failing to recognize the form and location of a potentially reversible underlying disorder. Because management depends more on treatment of the underlying disorder than on correction of the coagulation tests, these are discussed individually according to the clinical state.

## Aortic Aneurysm

Localized consumption of platelets and fibrinogen, which occurs in aortic aneurysms, can produce not only striking laboratory abnormalities but even symptomatic bleeding (232). Although few patients with aneurysm demonstrate overt hemorrhagic manifestations, this complication may be particularly associated with acute extensions and enlargements of the aneurysm (299–303). In some cases, dramatic manifestation of spontaneous bleeding episodes is associated with radiographic evidence of an expanding aneurysmal mass or with the sudden onset of severe pain indicative of dissection. Almost 40% of patients show laboratory evidence of consumption in the form of severe elevation of serum FDP levels (301–303).

Most patients respond to treatment with heparin, showing increases in platelet count and correction of coagulation tests, as well as clinical improvement, but definitive treatment requires surgical or endovascular repair. The severity of the underlying problem is reflected in the death of six of 10 patients in three reports (301,304) and in the series reported by Mulcare et al. (305) describing dramatic perioperative bleeding during surgical repair. Six of these seven patients had renal failure in addition to the prior localized consumption, presumably because of hypotension before and during surgery, but because only three received heparin, its efficacy could not be evaluated. Pretreatment of such patients with heparin and replacement of clotting factors before surgery may reduce the potential of perioperative bleeding complications and organ ischemia.

## Hemangiomas

Kasabach and Merritt (107) first described giant cavernous hemangiomas as a cause of a hemorrhagic diathesis. Primarily a disorder of infants and children, these hemangiomas are usually benign tumors that may enlarge or otherwise evolve into a convoluted mass of vascular channels that sequester and consume platelets and fibrinogen (306). This progression has been clearly demonstrated by physiologic studies in which the half-life of platelets is shortened and radioactive platelets and fibrinogen accumulate in the tumor (307). The concept of local sequestration was first suggested by Good et al. (308) and is compatible with the demonstration of fibrinolytic activity localized to the tumor (309) and the presence of fibrin or platelet thrombi in some but not all cases (309). Although heightened fibrinolytic activity can sometimes be demonstrated in peripheral blood, DIC is not a feature of this illness and distant thrombi in other organs do not occur.

Medical treatment of the tumor is often ineffective, and surgery can be dangerous because of problems in achieving effective hemostasis. Patients are usually managed conservatively, unless cosmetic corrections are needed or symptoms of bleeding result from severe thrombocytopenia and hypofibrinogenemia. These symptoms can be persistent and serious, and their control by treatment of the tumor is unpredictable. The mass can occasionally regress spontaneously, or it may shrink after radiation or laser therapy (306). Antithrombotic treatment with either antiplatelet agents or heparin has been attempted in order to correct the platelet count and fibrinogen level and alleviate bleeding symptoms (310,311). This rationale of first correcting the hemostatic defect by blocking the local consumption has been used in anticipation of, and in preparation for, surgical removal of the tumor under the safety of a normal hemostatic system.

Some patients have had extensive tumor or involvement of vital organs, such that postoperative or spontaneous bleeding from the tumor could not be controlled, leading to death (309). Regression of the tumor may occur by thrombosing the vascular channels by administering a fibrinolytic inhibitor (EACA), either alone or together with infusions of cryoprecipitate (312,313).

## Renal Disease

The presence of FDPs in the urine when absent in the blood indicates that localized consumption has occurred in the kidneys. The most dramatic example is in humoral-antibody–related hyperacute renal allograft rejection, associated with extensive fibrin deposition in the donor kidney arterioles and glomeruli (314,315). The vigorous immunologic reaction activates coagulation locally, mimicking the histologic picture of the

Shwartzman reaction; in unusual cases, systemic consumption occurs as well (316,317).

Braun and Merrill (318) first demonstrated FDPs in the urine of patients with a slower-evolving homograft rejection. All of their patients had urinary degradation products in the first 2 weeks after transplantation regardless of whether subsequent rejection occurred, but the appearance of urinary degradation products after 2 weeks uniformly heralded rejection. Because serum degradation products were absent, their appearance in the urine was best explained by *in situ* degradation of the deposited fibrin by a localized fibrinolytic response, with excretion directly into the draining renal tubular system. These observations have been extended by studying serial samples in patients after renal allotransplantation (319,320). The initial rise of urinary degradation products after transplant can be attributed to perioperative ischemia and the onset of spontaneous renal function, thereby explaining such occurrences in patients whose transplants were not subsequently rejected. Adding heparin anticoagulation may in some cases help control the local fibrin deposition, although the underlying rejection may still be active. Urinary FDPs also may occur in patients with proliferative glomerulonephritis, glomerulonephritis associated with systemic lupus erythematosus, and in association with the nephrotic syndrome (318,319,321).

The hemolytic-uremic syndrome (HUS) (see Chapter 111) is characterized by fragmentation hemolytic anemia and thrombocytopenia associated with renal failure. It often occurs in children after a diarrheal illness (2 to 14 days later) due to *Escherichia coli* 0157:H7 or *Shigella* (322), which produce verocytotoxins that bind with high affinity to receptors expressed with high density on renal glomerular endothelial cells (211). These verocytotoxins are directly cytotoxic to endothelial cells and may cause colonic vascular damage (211,322,323). Although little evidence of overt DIC is seen in these patients, subclinical thrombin generation occurs (324) and thrombi in the renal microvasculature contain both fibrin and platelets (325). Fragmentation hemolysis may be due to microvascular fibrin deposition or secondary to endothelial damage and adherence of red blood cells. Coagulation studies are usually normal except for elevated D-dimer levels. Although heparin, antiplatelet therapy, and fibrinolytic therapy have been used in controlled studies (326–331), the results are no better than with vigorous supportive therapy and hemodialysis (necessary in approximately 50% of patients) (322,332). Plasma exchange produces equivocal results (323). Eighty-five percent of children with this disorder recover completely, 5% to 10% develop chronic renal failure or permanent neurologic injury, and 5% die (322).

In adults (particularly the elderly), HUS may also result from *E. coli* 0157:H7 and *Shigella*, but a similar syndrome may be seen in adult patients with malignant hypertension, TTP, systemic lupus erythematosus, scleroderma, vasculitis, rapidly progressive glomerulonephritis, toxemia of pregnancy, postpartum renal failure, renal failure associated with the use of oral contraceptives, cyclosporine, quinine, and antineoplastic therapy. The morbidity and mortality of the primary HUS in adults is worse than in infants.

# CONSUMPTION RELATED TO ANTITHROMBOTIC OR HEMOSTATIC MEDICATION

## Therapeutic Defibrination

Defibrinating enzymes such as ancrod (Arvin) from *Agkistrodon rhodostoma* and defibrase from *Bothrops atrox* have been purified for therapeutic defibrination and treatment of

patients with venous thromboembolic disease (333–335). The rationale for therapy is that plasma fibrinogen is decreased by conversion to non–cross-linked fibrin, which is in turn lysed without causing any vascular occlusion or organ ischemia, leaving the patient with enough fibrinogen for normal hemostasis but sufficiently decreased to deter propagation of a thrombus. Results show that an antithrombotic state that is as safe and effective as heparin (336).

## Heparin-Induced Thrombocytopenia

Heparin-induced thrombocytopenia (HIT) (see Chapter 114) is a drug-induced immune reaction that causes thrombocytopenia, usually 5 days or more after heparin therapy is started or sooner in the presence of antibody (337). The pathophysiologic mechanism is the induction of antibody to a heparin–platelet factor 4 complex. The antigen–antibody complex activates platelets by binding to the platelet FcγIIa receptor and activates the endothelium by binding to platelet factor 4–proteoglycan complexes. Platelet procoagulant microparticles are released, and platelet aggregation, a variable degree of thrombocytopenia, endothelial cell activation with resultant expression of TF, and venous and/or arterial thrombosis may follow. Multifocal venous and arterial thrombosis may simulate DIC because thrombocytopenia, elevated FDP and D-dimer levels, and hypofibrinogenemia can be present.

## Prothrombin Complex Concentrates

Concentrates of vitamin K–dependent clotting factors are used for the treatment of patients with congenital or acquired deficiencies of prothrombin or factors VII, IX, or X or with acquired inhibitors against factors VIII or IX (338,339). Some preparations contain thrombogenic material in addition to unactivated coagulation factors (340,341), including factors VIIa, IXa, and Xa, and phospholipid, any of which may contribute to thrombotic complications (338,342–344). Patients with liver disease may be especially predisposed, probably as a result of impaired clearance of the activated factors or a decreased plasma concentration of inhibitors. A recombinant preparation of human factor VIIa has shown significant efficacy in patients with inhibitors to factor VIII or IX and in patients with hereditary factor VII deficiency (344,345), although thrombotic events are not avoided (346).

## Coumadin

Other agents or modalities used either in promoting hemostasis or as antithrombotic treatment may induce thrombotic events. Coumarin (see Chapter 115) anticoagulation initiated in patients with partial (heterozygous) deficiency of protein C or protein S may produce the "coumarin necrosis" syndrome or defibrination as the result of a more rapid decrease in the vitamin K–dependent inhibitors than in the vitamin K–dependent coagulation factors (83). In patients with HIT, coumadin-induced thrombosis may result in an exaggerated limb ischemic syndrome (venous gangrene) (347).

# CONSUMPTION IN THE NEONATE

The neonate is susceptible to many of the same pathologic mechanisms leading to consumption as are seen in the adult. Among 201 consecutive autopsies reported by Dairaku et al.

(348), microthrombi were found in 12% of cases, especially involving the lungs but rarely the kidneys. The most prevalent underlying factors in the infant that predisposed to or were associated with these pathologic lesions were hyaline membrane disease (30% of total) and infections (17%), but illness in the mother before or during parturition was the most dominant factor, accounting for 71% of the total. For instance, infants born to mothers with an abruption may experience DIC, and the procoagulant material of the placenta or amniotic fluid that causes intravascular clotting in the mother may also enter the fetal circulation, producing DIC of variable clinical importance. Proper evaluation of newborn hemostasis may be hampered by the age-specific variations in normal values of hemostatic factor assays (see Chapter 76). Special emphasis should be given to the potential clinical manifestations of thrombotic and hemorrhagic disease and not solely to laboratory parameters of DIC (349). Studies of exchange transfusion and plasma and platelet replacement therapy, compared with general support measures, indicate that treatment of the underlying disease is the most important aspect for recovery and that specific therapy for the coagulopathy other than that dictated by common sense does not improve the clinical outcome (350).

In addition to the DIC states that result from other dominant pathologic processes, rare cases of neonatal fulminant DIC may result from the deficiency of coagulation inhibitors, especially protein C (88,351). Such cases are seen in homozygous deficiency states and are variations of the striking thrombotic tendency that is usually manifested as multiple venous thrombi. A relative deficiency of fibrinolytic response in the neonate may reflect a decreased plasma plasminogen concentration, which could contribute to thrombotic occurrences (352). Treatment depends on provision of the missing inhibitor by plasma or purified protein products, complemented by long-term anticoagulant therapy.

# LABORATORY TESTS AND THE DIAGNOSIS OF DISSEMINATED INTRAVASCULAR COAGULATION

Because DIC is associated with a variety of underlying disorders, the laboratory manifestations in a given patient are variable and depend not only on features of DIC but also those due to the underlying disease. In some patients, DIC is of little clinical significance, and the diagnosis is established by laboratory tests, while in other patients, the clinical severity of DIC is striking and obscures the underlying disease. Given this variability, it is not surprising that criteria for the diagnosis of DIC are inadequate. The laboratory criteria are arbitrary, and no consensus exists. For example, because fibrinogen levels increase during normal pregnancy and as an acute-phase reactant in infection, the fibrinogen levels may be normal when DIC complicates pregnancy or infection. Therefore, fibrinogen levels can be normal in up to 57% of patients with DIC (353). In contrast, in DIC complicating severe liver disease, a low fibrinogen level may be caused by decreased synthesis as well as increased consumption. Similar problems may arise using other criteria of DIC, such as thrombocytopenia in the presence of splenomegaly, low protein C in the presence of liver dysfunction, increased factor VIII in the presence of infection, and elevated FDPs in the presence of systemic fibrinolysis.

The most common abnormalities seen in DIC are a low platelet count, elevated D-dimer levels, and decreased fibrinogen concentration. Scoring systems relying on laboratory results alone have been devised to determine prognosis in patients with DIC, but such scores are better directed to organ dysfunction than to laboratory derangement (162,354).

Thrombocytopenia occurs in 98% of patients with DIC; in approximately 50% of these, the count is less than 50,000 per $\mu$L (6). Platelet survival is shortened and is often accompanied by decreased platelet production. In addition, DIC also causes a qualitative defect in platelets that resembles an acquired storage pool defect (355). PT is prolonged in 75% of patients and reflects the decrease in factor V and to a lesser extent in factors II, VII, and X and fibrinogen. Similarly, the activated PTT is prolonged in approximately 60% of patients, primarily reflecting a decrease in the thrombin-sensitive clotting factors V and VIII and fibrinogen. However, both the PTT and PT may be shortened or normal because of the presence of activated clotting factors. The thrombin time may also be prolonged because of fibrinogen depletion or the presence of FDPs that inhibit fibrin polymerization (356). Initial clinical studies indicated that an elevated soluble fibrin concentration almost defined organ failure in DIC (357). Other clinical studies confirmed the high sensitivity for DIC, but also revealed a low specificity (358), and a comparison of soluble fibrin assays showed a wide discordance between results (359).

## Plasmin-Related Changes

The most common tests for global fibrinolytic activity rely on a euglobulin fraction of blood or plasma that contains fibrinogen, plasminogen, and plasminogen activator but not fibrinolytic inhibitors (360–363). Lysis times of normal clotted euglobulin are more than 2 to 4 hours, but with increased amounts of plasminogen activator, the lysis time may be as short as several minutes. Some shortening of the lysis time may result from a low plasma fibrinogen concentration (<100 mg per dL). Fibrin plate lysis performed with the use of fibrinogen measures activator-induced degradation of plasminogen-rich fibrin, but a more sensitive test quantitates the release of radiolabeled soluble products from $^{125}$I-labeled fibrin (364). Plasminogen activator may be quantitated by cleavage of specific chromogenic substrates, S-2322 or S-2288, or in a coupled system in which the plasminogen activator content is measured indirectly by the amount of plasminogen converted to plasmin using the plasmin substrate S-2251 (365). Specific antibodies to activators have allowed immunologic assay of free or inhibitor-bound activator antigen, and a zymographic method uses sulfadiazine silver-polyacrylamide gel electrophoresis to separate proteins by molecular weight and lysis of a fibrin overlay to indicate the location of plasminogen activator (366,367). Measurement of PAI-1 antigen includes both free and plasminogen activator-complexed protein, whereas activity measurements (e.g., by assessment of activator-neutralizing capacity) is better for the functional status of this fibrinolytic inhibitory protein (368,369).

With systemic activation of fibrinolysis, the plasminogen concentration falls below the normal 20 mg per dL (4 to 6 U per mL) as it is converted to plasmin (369,370). Functional assays of plasminogen are based on its conversion to plasmin by an excess of activator; the plasmin is usually quantitated by chromogenic substrate degradation (371). Most plasmin that may be generated in the blood is rapidly inactivated by $\alpha_2$-plasmin inhibitor, and this can be assessed by measuring plasmin–antiplasmin complexes (372,373). The concentration of functional $\alpha_2$-plasmin inhibitor can be measured with the use of the plasmin chromogenic substrate, measuring residual activity after the addition of a known amount of plasmin to the sample (374). The amount of enzyme inhibited is taken as a measure of the $\alpha_2$-plasmin inhibitor content, because the other protease inhibitors in plasma have relatively unimportant short-term effects on plasmin activity. $\alpha_2$-Plasmin inhibitor levels are low in patients with excessive secondary fibrinolysis or with primary fibrinogenolysis.

Because plasmin action on fibrinogen produces FDPs that may be nonclottable, coagulation measurements of fibrinogen may be hampered in patients with consumption coagulopathy (356). A commonly used fibrinogen assay measures thrombin-clottable protein; this assay may be spuriously low in the presence of anticoagulant FDPs, and it does not distinguish between fibrinogen and clottable degradation products such as fragment X (375). The Clauss method of fibrinogen determination relies on the thrombin clotting time of plasma, which is inversely proportional to fibrinogen concentration and may be artifactually prolonged by FDPs or heparin (376).

The clinical laboratory manifestation of fibrinolysis secondary to DIC is usually characterized by a normal euglobulin clot lysis time, because secondary (compensatory) lytic activity is localized to intravascular fibrin, and very little activator circulates. However, in patients with excessive secondary fibrinolysis (approximately 15% of cases of DIC) or in those with simultaneous DIC and primary fibrinogenolysis, clot lysis times are usually short.

## Fibrinogen and Fibrin Degradation Products

A commonly used method for measuring FDPs relies on fibrinogen "antigen" in the serum, essentially detecting nonclottable derivatives (normal, <10 $\mu$g per mL). The most common artifact seen with this assay is caused by incomplete clotting of plasma fibrinogen, usually because of degradation products or heparin, leaving intact fibrinogen in the "serum" and resulting in a spuriously high concentration of "degradation products" (377). Techniques using latex particles coated with antiserum to fibrinogen or degradation products are accurate, sensitive (to 0.5 $\mu$g per mL or less), and rapid and inexpensive enough for both emergency and routine use (378,379). The tanned red cell hemagglutination inhibition immunoassay and the staphylococcal clumping test (380) are no longer in general use. None of the above techniques for measuring serum FDPs distinguishes between those of fibrinogen and cross-linked fibrin, a crucial problem for distinguishing primary fibrinogenolysis from consumption secondary to intravascular coagulation (381). This limitation has led to the development of more specific assays for both fibrinogen and for FDPs, such as an enzyme-linked immunosorbent assay specific for fibrinogen degradation products using two monoclonal antibodies (382), or assays specific for $\beta$15-42 (derived from fibrin) and B$\beta$1-42 (derived from fibrinogen) (383,384).

Because factor XIIIa cross-links thrombi *in vivo*, detection of plasmic degradation products (see Fig. 109-5) of cross-linked fibrin could be a useful marker for identifying fibrin lysis. Reports describe chemical or immunologic extraction of fibrinogen-related antigen from serum followed by electrophoretic separation to identify specific derivatives (385,386), or electrophoresis of plasma or serum in sulfadiazine silver-agarose gels and identification of fibrinogen-related antigen with radiolabeled monospecific antiserum or Western blot (387). These techniques have contributed significantly to understanding pathophysiology but are semiquantitative and not useful for the clinic.

A more clinically useful method for identifying fibrin-specific degradation products relies on recognition of specific neoantigens on FDPs, most especially an assay that detects an epitope related to $\gamma$-chain cross-linking on fragment D-dimer, derived from plasmic degradation of cross-linked fibrin (388,389). However, increased D-dimer concentrations are not specific for consumption coagulopathy, because such concentrations also occur in patients with deep vein thrombosis, pulmonary embolism, or other thromboembolic disorders reflecting physiologic fibrinolysis (390,391), thus the foundation for its use to rule out thrombotic disease.

## Other Markers of Activation of Coagulation

When thrombin acts on fibrinogen, converting it to fibrin monomer, fibrinopeptides A and fibrinopeptide B are released from the amino-termini of the A$\alpha$ and B$\beta$ chains, respectively. Immunoassays for these peptides have been developed, and their levels are elevated in consumption coagulopathies

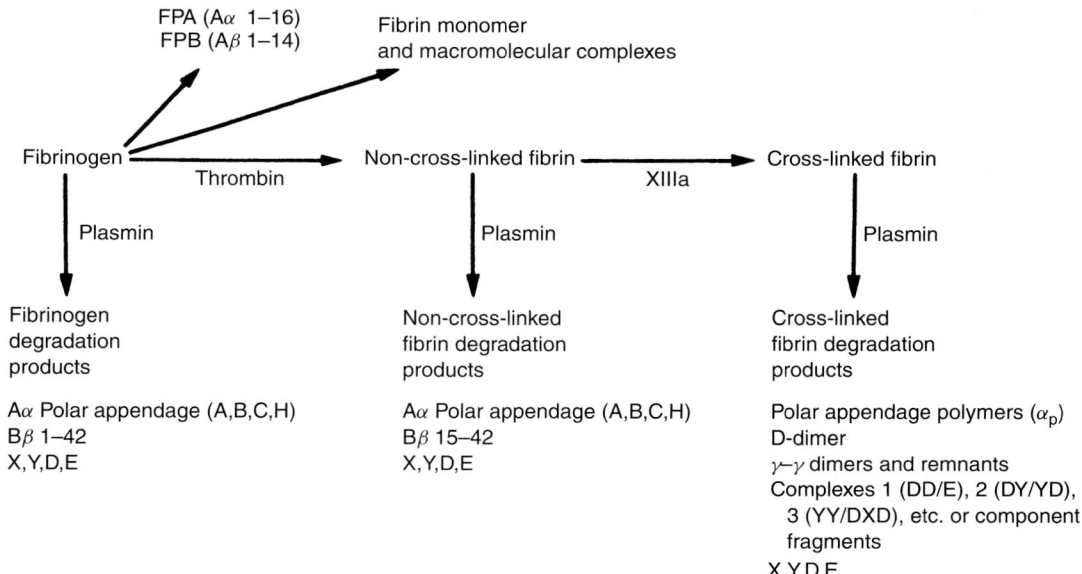

**FIGURE 109-5.** Schematic representation of fibrin formation and degradation showing the derivatives that result from the action of thrombin, factor XIIIa, and plasmin. FPA, fibrinopeptide A; FPB, fibrinopeptide B.

(392,393). Although they are valuable research tools, their clinical value is limited by their sensitivity to artifactual elevation during venipuncture and processing of blood. Several now-outmoded approaches to measuring soluble fibrin have been evaluated, for example, the protamine sulfate or ethanol gelation assays and the fibrin monomer–absorbed red cell agglutination assay (239,394,395). A commercially available assay is based on the principle that fibrin stimulates the activation of plasminogen by tPA, which is then assayed using a chromogenic substrate (396) and an electrophoretic method identifies factor XIIIa–cross-linked fibrin polymers in plasma (397). These assays have value in supporting or confirming a diagnosis of consumption coagulopathy, but results vary between assay (359), thereby limiting clinical application at present.

Other tests are abnormal in patients with DIC, including decreased levels of functional AT, heparin cofactor II, protein C, and protein C inhibitor; increased levels of the activation peptide cleaved from protein C, the prothrombin fragment F1 + 2, β-thromboglobulin, and platelet factor 4; and the detection of thrombin–AT III complexes in plasma (9,10); although not clinically practical, these tests are extremely useful in clinical research.

At present, no single laboratory test can be used to confirm or exclude the diagnosis of DIC, but the combination of a low platelet count and a test for fibrin monomer, low fibrinogen, and elevated FDP or D-dimer levels viewed in the context of the patient's underlying disease appear to be the most helpful clinical laboratory indicators.

## Pathologic (Systemic) Fibrinogenolysis

Spontaneous systemic hyperfibrin(ogen)olysis is an unusual occurrence. Its purest form is illustrated by the changes induced during the therapeutic administration of plasminogen activators such as streptokinase, urokinase, or tPA (see Chapter 121). In this circumstance, plasmin is produced, and susceptible protein substrates such as the fibrin in thrombi and hemostatic plugs, plasma fibrinogen, and factors V and VIII are degraded. The clinical manifestations are those of bleeding that results from the lysis of recently formed hemostatic plugs in the face of clotting factor depletion. The most common disorder associated with systemic fibrinolysis is chronic liver disease. In these patients, systemic fibrinolysis stems from increased circulating plasminogen activator caused by decreased clearance by hepatic cells (398). A rare cause of systemic fibrinolysis is primary

amyloidosis, perhaps secondary to increased plasma urokinase, decreased PAI, and decreased α₂-plasmin inhibitor (399).

Four aspects of the fibrinolytic state are confusing: (i) the same clinical states that cause DIC may also predispose to systemic fibrinolysis; (ii) the major presenting symptoms of both DIC and fibrinolysis are usually hemorrhagic; (iii) high concentrations of fibrinogen and FDPs may circulate in both conditions; and (iv) DIC and fibrin(ogen)olysis may coexist, both having been induced by the same pathologic insult. The best examples of the fourth aspect can be seen in patients with APL or heat stroke, both of which are characterized by DIC and circulating plasminogen activator. In APL, the leukemia cells contain not only TF but also plasminogen activator. As Merskey et al. (4) noted, both DIC and hyperfibrinolysis are characterized by a fibrinolytic response, the distinction being one of the anatomic location. In DIC, the lysis occurs in, and is typically limited to, the microcirculation and is a physiologic response to the deposition of fibrin thrombi. In systemic hyperfibrinogenolysis, plasmin appears in the blood, perhaps as the result of activators released from endothelial or tumor cells.

It may be difficult to distinguish between these possibilities even when abundant laboratory testing is available because virtually all the relevant laboratory assays that reflect DIC can be abnormal in systemic fibrinolysis as well (see Table 109-3). The simplest laboratory characterization of isolated fibrinolysis is a combination of a short clot lysis time without thrombocytopenia. In the absence of any clinical or laboratory indication of thrombosis and the presence of a serious bleeding disorder, therapy with fibrinolytic inhibitors should be considered. However, if the evaluation of the fibrinolytic state is erroneous (e.g., if DIC also exists), then treatment with fibrinolytic inhibitors can be dangerous (400–402).

Many cases that appear to be systemic fibrinolysis are actually either DIC with amplified secondary fibrinolysis or a combination of DIC with systemic fibrinolysis. Therefore, the appropriate therapeutic trial in a patient in whom DIC and systemic fibrinolysis coexist is to first replace deficient hemostatic factors, and if bleeding is not controlled and a significant increment in hemostatic factors is not achieved after transfusion, replacement of deficient factors should be repeated under the cover of both heparin and fibrinolytic inhibitors (403–405).

Fibrinolytic inhibitors have been suggested for routine use in the treatment of systemic fibrinolysis that accompanies extracorporeal bypass cardiac surgery, especially that involving cyanotic heart disease, repeat open heart surgery, and prolonged pump time (see Chapter 74) (406–408). Although the fibrinolytic state can occur during such surgery and excessive

---

**TABLE 109-3**

COMPARISON OF LABORATORY CHANGES THAT OCCUR IN DISSEMINATED INTRAVASCULAR COAGULATION AND SYSTEMIC HYPERFIBRINOLYSIS

| Condition | Fibrinogen | Fibrinogen/Fibrin degradation products | Lysis time | Platelet count | Screening coagulation tests |
|---|---|---|---|---|---|
| DIC | Low | Elevated | Normal | Low | Prolonged |
| Systemic hyperfibrin-(ogen)olysis | Low | Elevated | Short | Normal | Prolonged |
| DIC + systemic hyperfibrin-(ogen)olysis | Low | Elevated | Short | Low | Prolonged |

DIC, disseminated intravascular coagulation.

bleeding may relate to such an abnormality, the use of fibrinolytic inhibitors is still a potential hazard in the unmasking of an unrecognized (subclinical) DIC state. Such primary fibrinolytic states may be the result of short-lived and self-limiting trauma or hypoxia, and therefore do not require treatment with fibrinolytic inhibitors; however, those that accompany chronic illness (e.g., prostatic carcinoma) could require long-term therapy (4).

# CONSUMPTION LIMITED TO PLATELETS

A group of disorders characterized by thrombocytopenia, fragmentation hemolytic anemia, and a variable incidence of renal dysfunction include TTP; HUS; systemic vasculitis; rapidly progressive glomerulonephritis; systemic lupus erythematosus; scleroderma; malignant hypertension of any cause; toxemia of pregnancy and its variant, the HELLP syndrome; postpartum renal failure and renal failure associated with oral contraceptives; cyclosporin; and antineoplastic agents. Because the clinical presentation and laboratory abnormalities may be very similar and the pathophysiologic mechanisms and etiologies are poorly defined, confusion frequently exists when trying to distinguish one from the other.

A major feature of TTP and related disorders is the apparent selective consumption of platelets, usually without accompanying coagulation abnormalities, and the predominance of platelets as the occlusive material in the microvasculature (see Fig. 109-6). Some of these disorders have evidence of endothelial cell damage (110,409,410). Multiple-organ involvement consists primarily of loose platelet aggregates or granular deposits, with minimal regions of interspersed fibrin demonstrable (411). Although thrombocytopenia and fragmentation hemolytic anemia are striking, FDPs are usually not increased, clotting tests are usually normal, and turnover studies indicate

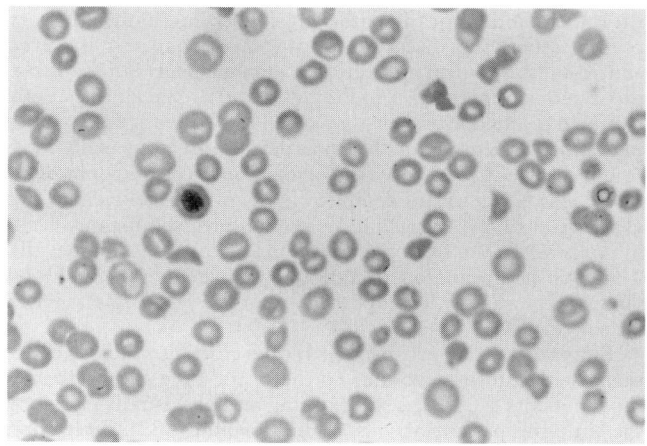

**FIGURE 109-7.** Microangiopathic hemolytic anemia in a patient with thrombotic thrombocytopenia purpura (TTP): A nucleated red blood cell is seen in addition to the schistocytes and other fragmented erythrocytic forms.

that the half-life of platelets is shortened to a much greater extent than fibrinogen, all arguing strongly against significant consumption of fibrinogen (412,413). The ischemic symptoms depend upon the location of platelet thrombi, whereas the hemorrhagic symptoms depend on the severity of the thrombocytopenia. Fragmentation anemia (see Fig. 109-7), elevated lactate dehydrogenase, and elevated levels of indirect bilirubin are part of the hemolytic picture of TTP, but these changes are not specific for TTP.

Lian et al. (414) and Siddiqui and Lian (415) first proposed that pathologic platelet aggregation/agglutination in the plasma is caused by the lack of a normally present immunoglobulin inhibitor or the presence of a platelet-agglutinating protein in the plasma of patients with TTP. Moake et al. (416–418) proposed a process that included "unusually large" VWF multimers and their involvement in the excessive and inappropriate agglutination of platelets. These large multimers appear and disappear in association with remissions and relapses induced by plasma exchanges and splenectomy (419). The unusually large multimeric forms of VWF have a high binding affinity for collagen and platelets and, under high shear stress, bring these components together to cause intravascular platelet aggregation, vessel occlusion, and consumptive thrombocytopenia (322). The unusually large multimers are degraded by a specific protease (ADAMTS13) (420,421), and a deficiency or antibody against this VWF-cleaving protease was found in patients with acute and chronic relapsing TTP (420,422). Untreated, TTP has a mortality as high as 79% (423), and plasma exchange therapy dramatically reduces this mortality (424–427). Plasma infusion and exchange therapy serves to remove an inciting agent or antibody and, at the same time, to infuse the missing protease, thereby correcting the pathology, if only temporarily (426,428). Splenectomy is sometimes effective in refractory cases (419,429,430). Details of therapy and other aspects of TTP are in Chapter 111.

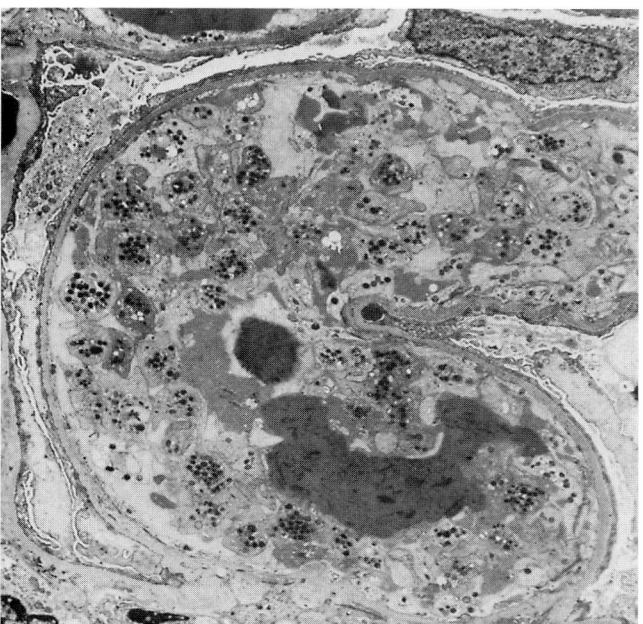

**FIGURE 109-6.** Electron micrograph of a glomerulus obtained by biopsy from a patient with polyarteritis nodosa, showing a thrombus consisting almost exclusively of platelets. Similar lesions are seen in thrombotic thrombocytopenic purpura (TTP). (Courtesy of Dr. Raul Mancilla-Jiminez, General Hospital, Centro Medico Nacional Mexico City.)

# TREATMENT

Because of the tremendous heterogeneity of the underlying disorders causing DIC and the great variability of the manifestations of DIC in a given patient, management is controversial (431). The cornerstone of treatment is prompt, vigorous treatment of the underlying disease and aggressive support measures.

An understanding of the pathophysiology and natural history of the underlying disease and trigger mechanisms involved contributes to logical and rational management. For example, the superb clinical studies of Pritchard and Brekken (180) clearly elucidate the natural history of DIC secondary to *abruptio placentae*. Patients with this disorder almost universally have evidence of DIC and, because of the concealed retroplacental blood loss, a significant degree of hypovolemia. DIC ends with evacuation of the uterus, and patients have significant bleeding only when the fibrinogen level is less than 150 mg per dL. These observations led to rational management with blood volume replacement, prompt delivery, and cryoprecipitate when indicated.

Similarly, serial prospective blood clotting studies in patients with gunshot wounds to the brain have shown that in most patients the DIC is self-limiting and has usually ended by the time the patient arrives at the hospital (432). Therefore, rational management of these patients is to replace fibrinogen with cryoprecipitate and to correct thrombocytopenia with platelet concentrates, particularly if the patient is deemed salvageable and requires débridement (433).

After identifying the cause of DIC and promptly instituting appropriate specific and aggressive supportive therapy for the underlying disease, questions must be asked to determine whether replacement of depleted hemostatic factors is necessary and whether interruption of DIC with heparin should be seriously considered.

**Bleeding.** Does the patient have a low fibrinogen level, low platelet count, or low clotting factor level? If so, is the patient actively bleeding? If the answer to the second question is no and the patient does not require surgery or an invasive procedure, replacement therapy is probably unnecessary. In contrast, if the patient is actively bleeding or requires an invasive procedure, it probably will be necessary to replace the deficient hemostatic factors, which usually means cryoprecipitate, fresh-frozen plasma, and platelet concentrates. The argument that replacement therapy may "fuel the fire" and cause thrombosis in patients with active DIC is theoretically possible, but only on occasion has this been proved to occur (157). However, replacement therapy is most effective in patients with very low levels of platelets and fibrinogen, in whom DIC is self-limiting or concluded. A common problem is the failure to increase the level of hemostatic factors when the patient is bleeding because of ongoing DIC. In these cases, it may be necessary to replace the hemostatic factors under cover of anticoagulant therapy. The effect of replacement therapy should be monitored by platelet and fibrinogen levels 30 to 60 minutes after completing transfusion to determine whether further replacement therapy is necessary.

**Thrombosis.** Does the patient have clinical evidence of fibrin deposition, such as dermal necrosis, oliguria, or confusion? If so, active inhibition of thrombin by anticoagulant therapy is probably indicated. Patients with purpura fulminans, as defined by Hjort et al. (151) and reviewed by Spicer and Rau (122), show a rapid progression of ecchymotic areas of skin to hemorrhagic bullae and hemorrhagic ischemic necrosis, and anticoagulation reduces mortality from 90% to 18% (122,149). A similar clinical picture occurs in patients with bacteremia and sepsis, with patchy hemorrhagic skin lesions progressing symmetric digital gangrene and even gangrene of the extremities (155,163,434). Heparin is indicated but unfortunately is often given after frank gangrene is already present. Therefore, when dermal or acral ischemia is first noted, heparin or other anticoagulant should be given to interrupt the DIC, along with bactericidal antibiotic and aggressive supportive therapy. Although ischemia secondary to DIC has been proposed as a major cause of organ dysfunction, including ARDS and acute renal failure, fibrin deposition per se may not represent the direct cause of these problems

(10,149). ARDS occurs in the absence of DIC, and renal failure in patients with DIC can be due to causes other than renal cortical necrosis (10). Therefore, it is not surprising heparin therapy may not curtail organ damage in a given patient.

## Disorders That May Require Heparin Anticoagulation

### Retained Dead Fetus Syndrome

Retained dead fetus syndrome is defined by the presence of a dead fetus associated with evidence of DIC, which is usually low grade, chronic, and frequently compensated (284,289,307). The major goals of therapy are to deliver the dead fetus and to prevent excessive bleeding at the time of delivery. If the patient presents with hypofibrinogenemia, intravenous heparin is effective in increasing the fibrinogen level to normal before elective delivery (289,307). When a normal fibrinogen level is attained (150 mg per dL), heparin should be discontinued and labor induced. Cryoprecipitates can be infused to increase the fibrinogen level, but they are associated with possible transmission of viral diseases. If the patient presents with hypofibrinogenemia and is already in the process of delivery of a dead fetus, cryoprecipitate alone should be used to prevent excessive bleeding. If the patient presents with a fibrinogen level normal for her stage of pregnancy and is not in labor, the fibrinogen level should be monitored but not supplemented unless a decrease toward 150 mg per dL occurs. In the very rare instance of the intrauterine death of a twin associated with decreasing fibrinogen levels, heparin therapy is effective (289).

### Giant Hemangiomas (Kasabach-Merritt Syndrome)

Giant hemangiomas (Kasabach-Merritt syndrome) (108) are benign childhood tumors that may progressively enlarge and cause localized consumption of platelets and fibrinogen (308–313). Surgical removal can cause massive bleeding and should be avoided in most cases. If the patient requires an elective surgical procedure for reasons other than removal of the tumor, heparin or cryoprecipitate and platelet transfusions can be used before the procedure in an attempt to normalize the platelet count and fibrinogen level. In some patients, the tumor itself has enlarged to such an extent that spontaneous bleeding ensues because of low fibrinogen or platelet levels. In these patients, an attempt to thrombose the vascular channels with selective infusions of EACA with or without cryoprecipitate has led to significant regression of the tumor and control of the localized consumptive process (312,313).

### Aortic Aneurysm

Localized coagulation may occur in the aneurysm, with laboratory evidence of compensated or decompensated intravascular coagulation (299–305,435). In the latter case, the patient may present with spontaneous bleeding or a history of a bleeding tendency associated with minor trauma or invasive procedures (302,303). In patients without an aneurysmal leak who undergo elective surgery, heparin can normalize hemostatic factors before surgical repair (302,304,435). In contrast, patients who have an aneurysmal leak associated with evidence of consumption require emergency surgery; heparin is contraindicated and hemostatic levels of fibrinogen and platelets should be achieved with cryoprecipitate and platelet transfusions, respectively. Patients with symptomatic bleeding require prompt treatment, because significant recent extension has probably occurred. The severity of the underlying condition is reflected in the death of patients due to dramatic perioperative bleeding during surgical repair (301,304,305).

## Solid Tumors

DIC in patients with solid tumors is usually low grade and chronic (236,259,277), but clinical features are tremendously heterogeneous. Patients may present with very serious disease, with excessive bleeding, venous thromboembolism, nonbacterial thrombotic endocarditis with or without arterial thromboembolism, microangiopathic hemolytic anemia, or any combination thereof. In contrast, DIC may be manifested by laboratory abnormalities only with no clinical features. Interruption of clinically evident DIC with anticoagulation may provide significant benefit. In the study by Sack et al. (236), 29 of 48 such patients had improvement of hemostatic measurements and 19 patients had recurrent symptoms after heparin was discontinued. A dramatic report of the fulminant thrombotic tendency of patients with Trousseau syndrome and the critical role of heparin as the effective antithrombotic drug of choice is provided by Bell et al. (257): Two patients had similar courses punctuated by dramatic major arterial and venous thrombi, following shortly after acute DIC states. Heparin controlled the thrombotic process, but both patients died when therapy was discontinued. In these and other cases, warfarin therapy is frequently ineffective, and antiplatelet agents do not suffice for long-term therapy for the prothrombotic state (242). For prolonged outpatient therapy, subcutaneous adjusted-dose, unfractionated, or low-molecular-weight heparin (without monitoring) is effective.

## Acute Promyelocytic Leukemia

APL is often dominated by DIC and hemorrhagic complications (260,436). DIC probably results from the release of procoagulant material (TF and cysteine protease) or procoagulant stimulating activity (IL-1) from the abnormal promyelocytes, and frequently the DIC worsens during induction chemotherapy (without ATRA) (263,436). Fibrinolytic activity is also increased in this disorder owing to cellular urokinase-type plasminogen activator and perhaps leukocyte elastase (38,273,437–440). Because initial induction therapy now includes ATRA, the coagulopathy disappears within 2 to 6 days, and the use of heparin, fibrinolytic therapy, or both is unnecessary. However, if the patient is unresponsive to ATRA, either primarily or in relapse, and chemotherapy is deemed necessary, the use of heparin therapy should be considered as an adjunct to aggressive transfusion therapy. Although most of the previous data strongly suggested that heparin therapy is beneficial in APL, they are nevertheless equivocal (262,272–275,441–443). In studies in which heparin prophylaxis was not used, the incidence of fatal hemorrhage (usually intracerebral) was 16% to 63%; the incidence in studies in which heparin was used was 0% to 44% (262,272–275, 436,442,443). In the report by Goldberg et al. (275), the cumulative incidence of hemorrhagic deaths associated with heparin therapy was 19%, whereas the incidence without heparin was 28% ($P > 0.05$); the complete remission rate using heparin was 63% compared with 54% without heparin ($P > 0.1$). However, in their own series of 25 patients treated with aggressive support measures but without heparin, no hemorrhagic deaths occurred. In another report, consecutive patients given heparin, an antifibrinolytic agent, or supportive therapy only showed an overall remission rate of 62% and no difference in the rate of early hemorrhagic deaths between the three groups (10%) (273). This finding supports the data of Goldberg et al. that heparin is unnecessary, particularly when using aggressive transfusion support.

Although the literature shows fewer hemorrhagic deaths (20.7% vs. 14.6%) in patients treated with heparin, no prospective or well-controlled studies have been reported, and transfusion support varies between trials. Kantarjian et al. (272) attribute the variation in incidence of hemorrhagic deaths to different prognostic factors among the treated patients rather than to the use of heparin. Fatal hemorrhage was associated with thrombocytopenia (<30,000 per $\mu$L), increased blasts and promyelocytes (>1,000 per $\mu$L), age above 50 years, and hemoglobin less than 11 g per dL. The incidence of hemorrhagic deaths in patients who had no more than two risk factors was 5%, compared with 58% in those with more than two risk factors. In the low-risk population, prophylactic heparin was not efficacious (5% vs. 6%); among high-risk patients, a trend toward a decreased incidence of hemorrhagic death was seen (67% vs. 45%).

If heparin is deemed necessary, the dose of heparin is controversial. Many investigators suggest that relatively low doses be given by continuous intravenous infusion (5 to 10 U/kg/hour); others suggest the use of full-dose heparin anticoagulation (15 to 20 U/kg/hour) (272). Full-dose heparinization in the presence of thrombocytopenia and hypofibrinogenemia is dangerous, particularly when the most common cause of death during induction is intracerebral hemorrhage. Therefore, when heparin is used, it should be initiated at a low dose (e.g., 7.5 U/kg/hour), immediately preceded by platelet and cryoprecipitate transfusion so as to achieve a platelet count of 50,000 per $\mu$L and a fibrinogen level of 150 mg per dL. As long as significant platelet and fibrinogen levels can be attained and maintained, the heparin dose need not be increased. Antifibrinolytic therapy has been used without heparin with no significant thrombotic events induced and with similar results to those obtained using heparin or supportive therapy only (273,439).

In summary, DIC associated with APL should be managed with aggressive blood component replacement in an attempt to keep the platelet count greater than 50,000 per $\mu$L and the fibrinogen level greater than 150 mg per dL. If the patient responds to ATRA, the DIC usually subsides rapidly over the first few days and heparin, antifibrinolytic therapy, or both are unnecessary. However, if the patient is resistant to ATRA and requires chemotherapy, aggressive supportive hemostatic replacement therapy may be difficult to achieve. In those patients, the addition of low-dose heparin may help in achieving reasonable platelet and fibrinogen levels. If evidence of systemic fibrinolysis as measured by a low $\alpha_2$-plasmin inhibitor level, a short clot lysis time, or both, is found, EACA can be used either as a simple agent or added to heparin if DIC is also present. Usually after a week of induction chemotherapy, the DIC progressively subsides and heparin, fibrinolytic inhibitor, and cryoprecipitate can be discontinued; platelet transfusions are needed until normal thrombopoiesis returns.

Overt DIC may occur in other types of acute leukemia and is also often associated with the tumor lysis syndrome. Management is the same as for patients with APL, except for the requirements of the underlying disorder.

## When Heparin Is Probably Not Helpful

In most instances of consumption coagulopathy, heparin therapy has not generally proved to be helpful and occasionally has been harmful (444,445). Acute forms of DIC may be either brief or end with prompt treatment of the underlying disease, in which case it is difficult to evaluate the contribution of heparin. Snakebite, heatstroke, rhabdomyolysis, massive head trauma, and acute hemolysis secondary to an incompatible blood transfusion all may result in acute consumption, and the evidence for heparin benefit is mostly from individual case reports, so heparin therapy remains controversial (214,219,225,403,446).

### Septicemia

Colman et al. (9) found a statistically significant improvement in the survival of heparinized septicemic patients (67%) compared with nonheparinized septicemic patients (32%). In contrast, Corrigan's review (447) of patients reported in the literature with septic shock and DIC found no difference in survival between patients receiving (24%) and not receiving (21%) heparin. The major determinant of survival in these patients is probably the presence or absence of shock and not the presence or absence of DIC (448,449). It is prudent to use heparin in patients with evidence of acral or patchy dermal ischemia, venous or arterial thromboembolism, bleeding associated with low platelet and fibrinogen levels, and failure to effect an increase in platelet and fibrinogen levels with aggressive transfusion therapy. Whether renal, hepatic, or pulmonary dysfunction without evidence of generalized fibrin deposition is an indication for heparin therapy remains questionable.

## Complications of Pregnancy

*Abruptio Placentae.* Although renal cortical necrosis with demonstrable intravascular fibrin occurs in a few patients with *abruptio placentae*, the course of the illness is usually favorable when adequate support measures are taken (450). Most important is that blood be given to correct hypovolemia and hypotension, improve renal perfusion, and prevent acute tubular necrosis or renal cortical necrosis. With the use of this therapy alone, vaginal delivery is usually accomplished without hemorrhagic complications, and rapid regeneration of the plasma fibrinogen follows (179,180). If hysterotomy is necessary or episiotomy is performed during vaginal delivery, supplementation with fibrinogen (cryoprecipitate) and platelets is reasonable to provide normal hemostasis. Heparin is contraindicated before surgery, because this could contribute to increased bleeding during vaginal delivery or hysterotomy.

**Amniotic Fluid Embolism.** Amniotic fluid embolism is an acute fulminant catastrophic event that induces pulmonary vascular obstruction. Sudden death follows in as many as 60% of the patients; in the remaining patients, a brief latent period (30 minutes to 4 hours) is followed by evidence of excessive bleeding from venipuncture sites and from the site of placental separation (189). Laboratory studies at this time are consistent not only with DIC but also with fibrinolysis (197,199). Because of its rapid course, the effectiveness of various treatment modalities has not been carefully assessed. Vigorous supportive therapy directed toward gas exchange with mechanical respiratory assistance and fluid and blood replacement to treat severe hypotension are essential. Heparin is a reasonable adjunct to therapy in patients in whom continued entry of amniotic fluid debris may be contributing to further intravascular clotting (198–200). When bleeding becomes the major manifestation, however, the use of heparin may accentuate the bleeding, especially if adequate replacement therapy for consumed clotting factors has not been achieved (178). Intense systemic fibrinolysis may complicate the DIC in amniotic fluid embolism, and fibrinolytic inhibitors may thereby be useful in patients refractory to replacement therapy. However, the same precautions regarding their use apply as in other settings of DIC.

**Saline-Induced Abortion.** During the second trimester, saline-induced abortion often results in mild DIC (201,202). Most of these patients do not have any clinical manifestations, but excessive bleeding sometimes occurs at the time of delivery. If fibrinogen or platelet levels are low, the patients should be transfused appropriately. If the patient has excessive vaginal bleeding and levels of hemostatic factors are normal, the patient's bleeding may be due to retention of fetal products rather than to a systemic hemostatic defect.

**Septic Abortion.** A severe fulminant form of DIC occurs in patients with septic abortion; the mortality rate reaches approximately 50% (178). Severe hypotension and clinical shock

along with endotoxemia contribute to the acute DIC process (204). Once established, the principles of therapy are those noted for any severe infection leading to shock, with the added consideration that evacuation of the uterus and sometimes hysterectomy may be required to eliminate the infection. These patients can be most refractory to therapy, and vigorous attention must be paid to proper antibiotic choice, maintenance of blood volume and electrolyte balance, treatment of shock, and appropriate hemostatic replacement therapy. As with other circumstances of acute, severe DIC, heparin may only be useful in certain circumstances (see preceeding text), but it is difficult to gauge the efficacy of heparin when the patients are dying from septic shock rather than from complications stemming from DIC *per se.*

**Toxemia of Pregnancy and Hemolysis, Elevated Liver Enzymes, and a Low Platelet Count Syndrome.** Although sensitive parameters of thrombin generation are increased in toxemia of pregnancy and patients with the HELLP syndrome and severe toxemia have been observed to have fibrin thrombi in the microvasculature (451–455), overt DIC occurs in only a small number of cases. Therefore, it is not surprising that no significant benefit of heparin therapy in toxemia of pregnancy (or the HELLP syndrome) has been established; in fact, the risk of intracranial bleeding in patients with severe, uncontrolled hypertension makes the use of anticoagulants dangerous (454,456–458). Therapy is directed primarily at controlling the eclamptic state with antihypertensive agents, magnesium sulfate, and rapid termination of the pregnancy. Excellent results with such therapy without the use of heparin have been reported (459). Because significant morbidity and fetal mortality occur in patients with the HELLP syndrome in the absence of signs of preeclampsia, it is important that the syndrome be recognized. Because the syndrome usually reverses approximately 48 hours after delivery, the cornerstone of treatment is delivery of the infant as soon as possible (460). If the syndrome persists beyond 72 to 96 hours, plasmapheresis and exchange with fresh-frozen plasma has been used, albeit with equivocal results (460).

## Liver Disease

Liver disorders that result in hepatic functional failure may be complicated by a variety of hemostatic defects, including decreased synthesis of clotting factors, vitamin K deficiency, thrombocytopenia, a poorly defined qualitative platelet defect, synthesis of an abnormal fibrinogen, and systemic fibrinolysis. Chronic subclinical DIC has been postulated to be an additional problem in these patients, but its existence remains controversial and its detection requires specialized studies (206). Moreover, there is no evidence that heparin therapy will correct the coagulation defect or affect the prognosis (176,461). In contrast to the controversy regarding the presence or absence of chronic subclinical DIC in patients with stable uncomplicated liver failure, most clinicians recognize specific situations in which DIC complicates severe liver disease. Any type of serious infection, particularly one associated with bacteremia, can trigger an episode of DIC. In addition, patients with refractory ascites who undergo peritoneovenous (LeVeen) shunt procedures may develop DIC after shunt placement (169–171). Although AT levels are very low in patients with severe liver failure and shunt-induced DIC, infusions of AT concentrate have not been successful (172).

Acute fatty liver of pregnancy is frequently complicated by DIC, and both the hepatic failure and DIC may persist for a significant period after delivery (173,174,462). The AT level is strikingly decreased, and replacement infusions may modulate the DIC (174).

# Dose and Route of Heparin Administration and Monitoring of Response

The proper dose of heparin and its route of administration—as well as the indications for heparin therapy—are controversial. Although few data exist regarding the dose response in patients with DIC or a direct comparison of routes of administration, the amount of heparin and the route of administration should be tailored to the clinical features and the clinical situation. For example, in patients who have amniotic fluid embolism with acute pulmonary vascular obstruction, it is rational to give an intravenous bolus of 5,000 U of heparin followed by a continuous infusion of 1,000 U per hour to neutralize the anticipated generation of excess thrombin. In contrast, in patients with APL, severe hypofibrinogenemia, and marked thrombocytopenia, a large bolus of full-dose heparin followed by moderate to large doses by continuous intravenous infusion is excessive and could be complicated by a fatal intracerebral hemorrhage. In patients with more chronic DIC, as with the dead fetus syndrome, little rationale exists in most cases to initiate therapy with a maximum dose. A bolus initiating dose is likewise unnecessary, and a moderate starting dose of 15 U/kg/hour by continuous intravenous infusion is reasonable; the subsequent dose is adjusted according to the patient's response.

Because functional AT levels may vary in patients with DIC, effective heparin therapy may require infusions of AT concentrate, although their efficacy has not been proved. Subcutaneous adjusted-dose unfractionated heparin or low-molecular-weight heparin (without monitoring) is efficacious in outpatients with low-grade chronic DIC secondary to solid tumors. Heparin is contraindicated in patients in whom excessive bleeding occurs in a closed space to the degree that it may compromise vital function, as with intracranial, intraspinal, pericardial, or paratracheal bleeding. The activated PTT is often abnormal before heparin is started, so the therapeutic efficacy of heparin in counteracting the effect of activated procoagulant factors is often best monitored by serial measurements of plasma fibrinogen concentration, D-dimer levels, and platelet counts.

# Other Treatment Modalities

## Antithrombin III and Other Thrombin Inhibitors

Replacement of AT in the form of fresh-frozen plasma or AT concentrates with or without heparin should neutralize excess thrombin and dampen or moderate the intravascular coagulation process. This approach should be particularly effective in patients with DIC associated with hepatic failure, because the functional AT level in these patients is frequently extremely low because of the combination of decreased synthesis and increased consumption. Although AT concentrates appear to shorten the length of DIC in some patients with fatty liver of pregnancy, they are not helpful in patients with DIC due to peritoneovenous shunts (173). Low levels of AT occur in patients with severe infection or septic shock, and low levels are poor prognostic signs (133). In the experimental animal models of sepsis and DIC, infusion of AT concentrate results in decreased degree of DIC and mortality, particularly when AT is administered before the induction of sepsis and in very high doses (463). Evidence also suggests that a possible antiinflammatory effect with high doses of AT may contribute to its efficacy in animal models (463,464). The trials of AT concentrate in patients with severe sepsis have been completed. A series of relatively small trials showed a modest reduction in mortality in AT-treated patients (463,465,466), but none of the trials reached statistical significance. A large-scale, multicenter, randomized controlled trial to directly address this issue showed no significant reduction in mortality of patients with sepsis who were treated with AT concentrate (467). Interestingly, *post hoc* subgroup analyses indicated some benefit in patients who did not receive concomitant heparin, but this observation needs prospective validation.

Hirudin and other novel direct thrombin inhibitors have shown efficacy in animal models (96,468) and in experimental lipopolysaccharide (LPS) injections in human volunteers (469), and preliminary observations of coagulation markers have been made in a small group of patients with DIC (469,470), but trials of clinical efficacy in DIC have not yet been performed.

## Activated Protein C

APC, in the presence of protein S as a cofactor, inactivates activated factors V and VIII. In a fascinating and important study by Taylor et al. (471), the infusion of APC along with lethal concentrations of *E. coli* organisms prevented the coagulopathy and lethal effect of *E. coli*. Moreover, inhibiting the system by infusing antibody to protein C along with *E. coli* organisms made the reaction more severe. If in the latter case the effect of the antibody was overwhelmed by the infusion of exogenous APC, the coagulopathy and lethal effects were eliminated. This study suggested that the presence of APC not only served as an anticoagulant but also protected against the lethal effect of endotoxic shock. In addition to the anticoagulant activity of APC, which inactivates factors Va and VIIa, APC administered intravenously to rats given endotoxin reduced the pulmonary vascular injury and hypertension (472), changes that were independent of its anticoagulant effect, perhaps due to a reduction of TNFα production in human monocytes.

In patients with meningococcal sepsis, the severity of the acquired protein C deficiency and the average size of the skin lesions are directly related to a poor clinical outcome (473,474). Protein C concentrate was used in two small trials (19 patients) in children with meningococcal sepsis, shock, DIC, and secondary purpura fulminans with survival in 17 of 19 patients (473,475).

A phase III trial of APC concentrate has now been completed in patients with sepsis, prematurely stopped because of efficacy in reducing mortality (476). All-cause mortality at 28 days after inclusion was 24.7% in the APC group versus 30.8% in the control group (19.4% relative risk reduction). The administration of APC caused an amelioration of DIC, and APC-treated patients had less organ failure (477). Subsequent analysis demonstrates that patients with DIC had a relatively greater benefit of APC treatment than did patients without DIC (478). The relative risk reduction in mortality of patients with sepsis and DIC who received APC was 38%, in comparison with a relative risk reduction of 18% in patients with sepsis without DIC.

## Anticytokine and Antiendotoxin Therapy, and Other Potential Therapy

TNF, a protein secreted by activated macrophages, is an important mediator of the lethal effect of endotoxin. When recombinant TNF is injected into animals, it reproduces many of the same derangements seen with the administration of endotoxin (479). In a study of 79 patients with meningococcal meningitis, TNF was detected in 10 of 11 patients who died but only in eight of 86 survivors (480). Three clinical trials have used a monoclonal antibody to TNF in patients with septic shock (481–483); two showed benefit (482,483), but the more recent trial showed no significant difference in survival, length of shock, and development of organ system failure between patients receiving the antibody or placebo (481).

Because TF is the primary trigger in patients with DIC, TFPI is a possible therapeutic modality in patients with DIC. Although it is clear that TFPI plays an important protective role in animal models of DIC, the level of TFPI is not decreased in patients with DIC (29,95).

### Fibrinolytic Inhibitors

EACA should not be used in most patients with DIC because inhibition of the fibrinolytic system may lead to widespread fibrin deposition in the microcirculation, resulting in ischemic organ dysfunction or failure. In patients with pathologic fibrinogenolysis or in those in whom DIC is associated with excessive fibrinolytic activity, however, EACA may be helpful (436). In addition, in patients with amniotic fluid embolism after the episode of DIC has subsided, the patient may continue to bleed because of intense fibrinolytic activity. In these cases, EACA can be very helpful in controlling excessive bleeding. However, if any doubt remains about the presence of DIC in these cases, heparin should also be used.

It is likely that many cases that appear to be systemic fibrinolysis are actually either DIC with excessive secondary fibrinolysis or a combination of DIC with primary fibrin(ogen)olysis. Such cases illustrate the difficulties presented by the acutely ill, bleeding patient and have led to the approach of assuming that DIC coexists with systemic fibrinolysis in such patients.

Therefore, fibrinolytic inhibitors would be used only if bleeding continues after replacement of deficient hemostatic factors to levels that are sufficient to achieve hemostasis and treatment should not be given without concomitant heparin therapy (403–405).

## Summary of Treatment

Table 109-4 summarizes the general principles of the treatment of DIC. Table 109-5 outlines the indications and contraindications for heparin therapy.

The treatment of DIC is extremely complex because DIC complicates many different disorders and may have a variety of clinical manifestations. In addition, well-controlled studies are lacking regarding various methods of management in relatively homogeneous groups of patients. Therefore, treatment continues to be controversial and probably will remain so. Any careful clinical and laboratory observations in groups of patients with the same underlying disorder are extremely helpful in elucidating the natural history of the process and its effects on the patient, and in clarifying whether certain therapeutic interventions may be helpful. The continued accumulation of careful clinical studies will help in determining the proper management of DIC in patients with the same underlying disorder and in given individual situations.

### TABLE 109-4

#### TREATMENT OF ACUTE, SEVERE DISSEMINATED INTRAVASCULAR COAGULATION

| Modality | Rationale | Details | Expectations |
|---|---|---|---|
| Life-support measures | Self-evident | Fluids, blood, respiratory care, pressors, etc. | Maintain cardiac output, gas exchange, electrolyte balance, etc. |
| Treating the underlying disorder | Correct the cause of DIC | Dependent on the primary diagnosis | Inhibit or block the complicating pathologic mechanism of DIC inparallel with the response (if any) of the disorder |
| Antithrombotic agents | Block microthrombus formation | Heparin by continuous IV infusion, monitor with fibrinogen and platelet levels; continue as long as the predisposing clinical state persists; AT-III concentrate if AT-III level <70% | Prevent fibrin formation; tip the balance within the microcirculation toward physiologic fibrinolysis; allow reperfusion of the skin, kidneys, and brain |
| Transfusion | Reestablish normal hemostatic potential | Infuse platelets and fibrinogen (cryoprecipitate); repeat as indicated by laboratory and clinical observation | Platelet count and fibrinogen should increase significantly; bleeding should diminish and stop during an interval of hours to several days |
| Transfusion + heparin | Restore normal hemostasis if transfusion of hemostatic factors fails to achieve significant increment in factor levels | Infuse platelets and cryoprecipitate 2 h after starting continuous heparin infusion (7.5 U/kg/h); repeat as indicated by laboratory and clinical observation | Platelet count and fibrinogen should increase significantly if consumption is blocked; bleeding should diminish; if bleeding increases, discontinue heparin |
| Fibrinolytic inhibitors | Block excessive fibrinolysis and the accumulation of degradation products in blood; protect hemostatic plugs | For adults, ε-aminocaproic acid: loading dose, 46 g, then 1 g q12h for a limited duration (up to 48 h) | Bleeding ceases rapidly but keeps vascular channels occluded with thrombus; dangerous if the thrombotic process was not previously treated with heparin |

DIC, disseminated intravascular coagulation; IV, intravenous; AT-III, antithrombin III.

## TABLE 109-5

### RECOMMENDED USE OF HEPARIN IN DISSEMINATED INTRAVASCULAR COAGULATION

| Disorder | Treatment approach |
|---|---|
| **INDICATION** | |
| Purpura fulminans | Heparin by continuous infusion |
| Acral or dermal ischemia | Heparin by continuous infusion |
| Venous thromboembolism | Heparin by continuous infusion |
| Bacteremia (associated with dermal ischemia or necrosis) | Heparin by continuous infusion |
| Organ ischemia | Heparin not indicated unless there is evidence of fibrin deposition elsewhere (dermal or acral ischemia) |
| Retained dead fetus syndrome | Heparin IV or cryoprecipitate alone if labor in progress |
| Giant hemangioma | Thrombose with EACA and possibly cryoprecipitate; before elective surgery, heparin, cryoprecipitate (or both), and platelets |
| Aorta aneurysm without rupture | Heparin preceding elective repair |
| Solid tumors | Heparin by continuous infusion; if effective, then adjusted-dose or low-molecular-weight heparin s.c. |
| Promyelocytic leukemia | See section, "Acute Promyelocytic Leukemia" |
| **RELATIVE CONTRAINDICATION** | |
| Aortic aneurysm, leaking | Cryoprecipitate and platelets preceding emergency repair |
| Hemorrhage in a closed space compromising vital function | Heparin a possible option but only with external drainage |
| Septicemia | Heparin only with specific indications; high doses of AT-III concentrate if AT-III level <70% |
| *Abruptio placentae* without significant bleeding | Blood volume replacement, prompt delivery, cryoprecipitate if needed |
| Amniotic fluid embolism | Consider heparin before hemostatic failure; replace hemostatic factors if bleeding is present |
| Saline-induced abortion | Correct excessive bleeding during delivery by replacing fibrinogen and platelets |
| Septic abortion | Consider heparin therapy early in course when DIC is present |
| Severe liver disease with refractory ascites and peritoneo venous shunt | Discontinue shunt |
| Acute fatty liver of pregnancy | AT-III replacement, preferably by concentrate |
| Intracranial gunshot wound or severe brain injury | Cryoprecipitate and platelets |

DIC, disseminated intravascular coagulation; IV, intravenous; EACA, ε-aminocaproic acid; AT-III, antithrombin III.

## *References*

1. McKay DG. *DIC: an intermediary mechanism of disease.* New York: Harper-Hoeber, 1965:493.
2. Rodriguez-Erdmann F. Bleeding due to increased intravascular blood coagulation: hemorrhagic syndromes caused by consumption of blood-clotting factors (consumption-coagulopathies). *N Engl J Med* 1965;273:1370.
3. Hardaway RM. *Syndromes of DIC with special reference to shock and hemorrhage.* Springfield, IL: Charles C Thomas Publisher, 1966.
4. Merskey C, Johnson AJ, Kleiner GJ, et al. The defibrination syndrome: clinical features and laboratory diagnosis. *Br J Haematol* 1967;13:528.
5. Brodsky I, Siegel NH. The diagnosis and treatment of DIC. *Med Clin North Am* 1970;54:555.
6. Colman RW, Robboy SJ, Minna JD. DIC: an approach. *Am J Med* 1972; 52:679.
7. Verstraete M, Vermylen C, Vermylen J, et al. Excessive consumption of blood coagulation components as cause of hemorrhagic diathesis. *Am J Med* 1965;35:899.
8. Owen CA Jr, Bowie EJW. Chronic intravascular coagulation syndromes: a summary. *Mayo Clin Proc* 1974;49:673.
9. Colman RW, Robboy SJ, Minna JD. DIC: a reappraisal. *Annu Rev Med* 1979;30:359.
10. Mant MJ, King EG. Severe acute DIC. *Am J Med* 1979;67:556.
11. Feinstein DI. Diagnosis and management of DIC: the role of heparin therapy. *Blood* 1982;60:288.
12. Schafer AI. The hypercoagulable states. *Ann Intern Med* 1985; 102:814.
13. Kitchens CS. Concept of hypercoagulability: a review of its development, clinical application, and recent progress. *Semin Thromb Hemost* 1985; 11:293.
14. Baker WF Jr. Clinical aspects of DIC: a clinician's point of view. *Semin Thromb Hemost* 1989;15:1.
15. Schuster HP. Disseminated intravascular coagulation syndromes: potential management with antithrombin III concentrates. *Semin Thromb Hemost* 1998;24:1–83.
16. Levi M, ten Cate H. Disseminated intravascular coagulation. *N Engl J Med* 1999;341:586–592.
17. Nauyn B. Unterschungen Ober Blutgerinnung I.M. Lebenden Tiere und Ihre Folgen. *Arch Exp Pathol Pharmakol* 1873;1:1.
18. Foa P, Pellacani P. Sul fermento fibrinogeno: sulle azioni tossiche, escercitate da alcuni organi freschi. *Arch Sci Med (Torino)* 1884;7:113.
19. Mellanby J. The coagulation of blood. Part 2: the actions of snake venoms, peptone, and leech extract. *J Physiol* 1909;38:441.
20. Penick GD, Roberts HR, Webster WB, et al. Hemorrhagic states secondary to intravascular clotting. *Arch Pathol Lab Med* 1958;66:708.

21. Little JR. Purpura fulminans treated successfully with anticoagulation: report of a case. *JAMA* 1959;169:36.
22. Verstraete M, Vermylen C, Vermylen J, et al. Excessive consumption of blood coagulation components as a cause of hemorrhagic diathesis. *Am J Med* 1965;38:899.
23. Merskey C, Kleiner GJ, Johnson AJ. Quantitative estimation of split products of fibrinogen in human serum: relation to diagnosis and treatment. *Blood* 1966;28:1.
24. Aird WC. The role of the endothelium in severe sepsis and multiple organ dysfunction syndrome. *Blood* 2003;101:3765–3777.
25. Morrissey JH. Tissue factor: a key molecule in hemostatic and nonhemostatic systems. *Int J Hematol* 2004;79:103–108.
26. Toh CH, Samis J, Downey C, et al. Biphasic transmittance waveform in the APTT coagulation assay is due to the formation of a Ca(++)-dependent complex of C-reactive protein with very-low-density lipoprotein and is a novel marker of impending disseminated intravascular coagulation. *Blood* 2002;100:2522–2529.
27. Moore KL, Andreoli SP, Esmon NL, et al. Endotoxin enhances tissue factor and suppresses thrombomodulin expression of human vascular endothelium *in vitro*. *J Clin Invest* 1987;79:124.
28. Niemetz J. Coagulant activity of leukocytes: tissue factor activity. *J Clin Invest* 1972;51:307.
29. Warr TA, Rao LV, Rapaport SI. DIC in rabbits induced by administration of endotoxin or tissue factor: effect of anti-tissue factor antibodies and measurement of plasma extrinsic pathway inhibitor activity. *Blood* 1990;75:1481.
30. Taylor FB Jr, Chang A, Ruf W, et al. Lethal *E. coli* septic shock is prevented by blocking tissue factor with monoclonal antibody. *Circ Shock* 1991;33:127.
31. Biemond BJ, ten Cate H, Levi M, et al. Complete inhibition of endotoxin-induced coagulation activation in chimpanzees with a monoclonal fab fragment against factor VII/VIIa. *Thromb Haemost* 1995;73:223.
32. Creasey AA, Chang ACK, Feigen L, et al. Tissue factor pathway inhibitor reduces mortality from *Escherichia coli* septic shock. *J Clin Invest* 1993;91:2850.
33. Warr TA, Rao LHV, Rapaport SI. Disseminated intravascular coagulation. *Blood* 1990;75:1841.
34. Moore HL, Andreoli ST, Esmon NL, et al. Endotoxin enhances tissue factor and suppressed thrombomodulin expression of human vascular endothelium *in vitro*. *J Clin Invest* 1987;79:124.
35. Pixley R, DeLa Cadena R, Page JD, et al. The contact system contributes to hypotension but not disseminated intravascular coagulation in lethal bacteremia. *In vitro* use of a monoclonal anti- factor XII antibody to block contact activation in baboons. *J Clin Invest* 1993;91:61.
36. Mason JW, Colman RW. The role of Hageman factor in DIC induced by septicemia, neoplasia, or liver disease. *Thromb Diath Haemorrh* 1971;26:325.
37. Van Deventer SJH, Büller HR, ten Cate JW, et al. Experimental endotoxemia in humans: analysis of cytokine release and coagulation, fibrinolytic, and complement pathways. *Blood* 1990;76:2520.
38. Gralnick HR, Abrell E. Studies of the procoagulant and fibrinolytic activity of promyelocytes in acute promyelocytic leukaemia. *Br J Haematol* 1973;24:89.
39. Andoh K, Kubota T, Takada M, et al. Tissue factor activity in leukemia cells, with special reference to DIC. *Cancer* 1987;59:748.
40. Rickles FR, Edwards RL. Activation of blood coagulation in cancer: Trousseau's syndrome revisited. *Blood* 1983;62:14.
41. Zacharski LR, Schned AR, Sorenson GD. Occurrence of fibrin and tissue factor antigen in human small cell carcinoma of the lung. *Cancer Res* 1983;43:3963.
42. Donati MB, Falanga A. Pathogenetic mechanisms of thrombosis in malignancy. *Acta Haematol* 2001;106:18–24.
43. Weiss HJ, Phillips LJ, Hopewell W, et al. Heparin therapy in a patient bitten by a saw-scaled viper (*Echis carinatus*), a snake whose venom activates prothrombin. *Am J Med* 1973;54:653.
44. Franza BR, Aronson DL, Finlayson JB. Activation of human prothrombin by procoagulant factor from the venom of *Echis carinatus*. *J Biol Chem* 1975;250:7057.
45. Schmaier AH, Claypool W, Colman RW. Crotalocytin: recognition and purification of a timber rattlesnake platelet aggregating protein. *Blood* 1980;56:1013.
46. Budzynski AZ, Pandya BV, Rubin RN, et al. Fibrinogenolytic afibrinogenemia after envenomation by western diamondback rattlesnake (*Crotalus atrox*). *Blood* 1984;63:1.
47. Evensen SA, Jereminc M. Platelets and the triggering mechanism of intravascular coagulation. *Br J Haematol* 1970;19:33.
48. Lipinski B, Gurewich B. The effect of leukopenia versus thrombocytopenia on endotoxin-induced intravascular coagulation. *Thromb Res* 1976;8:403.
49. Muller-Berghaus G, Eckhardt T. The role of granulocytes in the activation of intravascular coagulation and the precipitation of soluble fibrin by endotoxin. *Blood* 1975;45:631.
50. Weiss HJ, Berger RE, Tice AD, et al. Fatal DIC and hemolytic anemia following stibophen therapy: a study of basic mechanisms. *Am J Med Sci* 1972;264:375.
51. Mannucci PM, Lubina GF, Caocci L, et al. Effect on blood coagulation of massive intravascular haemolysis. *Blood* 1969;33:207.
52. Spector JL, Crosby JI. Coagulation studies during experimental hemoglobinemia in humans. *J Appl Physiol* 1975;38:195.
53. Tomar RH, Kolchins D. Complement and coagulation: serum b1c- b1a in DIC. *Thromb Diath Haemorrh* 1972;27:389.
54. Branson HE, Wyatt DO, Schmer G. Complement consumption in acute DIC without antecedent immunopathology. *Am J Clin Pathol* 1976;66:967.
55. Stichaikul T, Puwasatien P, Karnjanajetanee J, et al. Complement change and DIC in *Plasmodium falciparum* malaria. *Lancet* 1975;1:770.
56. Kalowske S, Howers EL Jr, Margaretten W, et al. Effects of intravascular clotting on the activation of the complement system: the role of the platelet. *Am J Pathol* 1975;78:525.
57. Ulevitch RJ, Cochrane CG, Hemson PG, et al. Mediation systems in bacterial lipopolysaccharide-induced hypotension and DIC. *J Exp Med* 1975;142:1570.
58. Muller-Berghaus G, Lohmann E. The role of complement in endotoxin-induced DIC: studies in congenitally $C_6$-deficient rabbits. *Br J Haematol* 1974;28:403.
59. Sherman LA, Lee J. Fibronectin: blood turnover in normal animals and during intravascular coagulation. *Blood* 1982;60:588.
60. Mosher DF, Williams EM. Fibronectin concentration is decreased in plasma of severely ill patients with DIC. *J Lab Clin Med* 1978;91:729.
61. Gormsen J, Fletcher AP, Alkjaersig M, et al. Enzymatic lysis of plasma clots: the influence of fibrin stabilization on lysis rates. *Biochem Biophys Res Commun* 1967;120:654.
62. Miletich JP, Kane WH, Hofmann SL, et al. Deficiency of factor $X_{a}$- factor $V_a$ binding sites on the platelets of a patient with a bleeding disorder. *Blood* 1979;54:1015.
63. Itteryah TR, Rawala R, Colman RW. Immunochemical studies of bovine platelet factor V. *Fed Proc* 1979;38:811.
64. Minna JD, Robboy SJ, Colman RW. *DIC in man*. Springfield, IL: Charles C Thomas Publisher, 1974.
65. Wessler S. Studies in intravascular coagulation: the pathogenesis of serum-induced venous thrombosis. *J Clin Invest* 1955;34:647.
66. Coughlin SR. Thrombin signalling and protease-activated receptors. *Nature* 2000;407:258–264.
67. Levi M, van der Poll T, Buller HR. Bidirectional relation between inflammation and coagulation. *Circulation* 2004;109:2698–2704.
68. Rosenberg RD, Rosenberg JS. Natural anticoagulant mechanisms. *J Clin Invest* 1984;74:1.
69. Tollefsen DM, Blank MK. Detection of a new heparin-dependent inhibitor of thrombin in human plasma. *J Clin Invest* 1981;68:589.
70. Griffith MJ, Carraway T, White GC, et al. Heparin cofactor activities in a family with hereditary ATIII deficiency: evidence for a second heparin cofactor in human plasma. *Blood* 1983;61:111.
71. Rosenberg RD, Damus PS. The purification and mechanism of action of human antithrombin-heparin cofactor. *J Biol Chem* 1973;248:6490.
72. Briginshaw GF, Shanberge JN. Identification of two distinct heparin cofactors in human plasma: inhibition of thrombin and activated factor X. *Thromb Res* 1974;4:463.
73. Marcum JA, McKenney JB, Rosenberg RD. The acceleration of thrombin-antithrombin complex formation in rat hindquarters via naturally occurring heparin-like molecules bound to the endothelium. *J Clin Invest* 1984;74:341.
74. Esmon C, Owen W. Identification of an endothelial cell cofactor for thrombin-catalyzed activation of protein C. *Proc Natl Acad Sci U S A* 1981;78:2249.
75. Kisiel W, Canfield WM, Ericsson LH, et al. Anticoagulant properties of bovine plasma protein C following activation by thrombin. *Biochemistry* 1977;16:5824.
76. Esmon CT. Protein C: biochemistry, physiology, and clinical implications. *Blood* 1983;62:1155.
77. DiScipio RG, Davie EW. Characterization of protein S, a gamma-carboxyglutamic acid containing protein from bovine and human plasma. *Biochemistry* 1979;18:899.
78. Walker FJ. Protein S and the regulation of activated protein C. *Semin Thromb Hemost* 1984;10:131.
79. Marciniak E, Farley CH, DeSimone PA. Familial thrombosis due to ATIII deficiency. *Blood* 1974;43:219.
80. Broekmans AW, Veltkamp JJ, Bertina RM. Congenital protein C deficiency and venous thromboembolism. *N Engl J Med* 1983;309:340.
81. Schwarz HP, Fischer M, Hopmeier P, et al. Plasma protein S deficiency in familial thrombotic disease. *Blood* 1984;64:1297.
82. Seligsohn U, Berger A, Abend M, et al. Homozygous protein C deficiency manifested by massive venous thrombosis in the newborn. *N Engl J Med* 1984;310:559.
83. McGehee WG, Klotz TA, Epstein DJ, et al. Coumarin necrosis associated with hereditary protein C deficiency. *Ann Intern Med* 1984;101:59.
84. Branson HE, Katz J, Marble R, et al. Inherited protein C deficiency and coumarin-responsive chronic relapsing purpura fulminans in a newborn infant. *Lancet* 1983;2:1165.
85. Madden RM, Ward M, Marlar RA. Protein C activity levels in endotoxin-induced DIC in a dog model. *Thromb Res* 1989;55:297.
86. Marlar RA, Endres-Brooks J, Miller C. Serial studies of protein C and its plasma inhibitor in patients with DIC. *Blood* 1985;66:59.
87. Anderson DR, Brill-Edwards P, Walker I. Warfarin-induced skin necrosis in two patients with protein S deficiency: successful reinstatement of warfarin therapy. *Haemostasis* 1992;22:124.
88. Bauer KA, Rosenberg RD. Thrombin generation in acute promyelocytic leukemia. *Blood* 1984;64:791.

89. Mammen EF, Miyakawa T, Phillips TF, et al. Human antithrombin concentrates and experimental DIC. *Semin Thromb Hemost* 1985;11:373.

90. Emerson TE Jr, Fournel MA, Redens TB, et al. Efficacy of ATIII supplementation in animal models of fulminant *Escherichia coli* endotoxemia or bacteremia. *Am J Med* 1989;87:27S.

91. Gerson WT, Dickerman JD, Bovill EG, et al. Severe acquired protein C deficiency in purpura fulminans associated with disseminated intravascular coagulation: treatment with protein C concentrate. *Pediatrics* 1993; 91:418.

92. Rivard GE, David M, Farrell C, et al. Treatment of purpura fulminans in meningococcemia with protein C concentrate. *J Pediatr* 1995;126:646.

93. Tollefsen DM, Pestka CA. Heparin cofactor II activity in patients with DIC and hepatic failure. *Blood* 1985;66:769.

94. Bajaj MS, Rana SV, Wysolmerski RB, et al. Inhibitor of the factor VIIa–tissue factor complex is reduced in patients with DIC but not in patients with severe hepatocellular disease. *J Clin Invest* 1987;79:1874.

95. Sandset PM, Warn-Cramer BJ, Maki SL, et al. Immunodepletion of extrinsic pathway inhibitor sensitizes rabbits to endotoxin-induced intravascular coagulation and the generalized Shwartzman reaction. *Blood* 1991; 78:1496.

96. Chen D, Giannopoulos K, Shiels PG, et al. Inhibition of intravascular thrombosis in murine endotoxemia by targeted expression of hirudin and tissue factor pathway inhibitor analogs to activated endothelium. *Blood* 2004;104:1344–1349.

97. Colman RW. Activation of plasminogen by human plasma kallikrein. *Biochem Biophys Res Commun* 1969;35:273.

98. Marder VJ, Shulman NR, Carroll WR. High-molecular-weight derivatives of human fibrinogen produced by plasmin: physiochemical and immunological characterization. *J Biol Chem* 1969;244:2111.

99. Ratnoff OD. Epsilon aminocaproic acid—a dangerous weapon. *N Engl J Med* 1969;180:1124.

100. Paramo JA, Fernandez-Diaz FJ, Rocha E. Plasminogen activator inhibitor activity in bacterial infection. *Thromb Haemost* 1988;59:451.

101. Dennis LH, Cohen RJ, Schachner SH, et al. Consumptive coagulopathy in fulminant meningococcemia. *JAMA* 1968;205:182.

102. Corrigan JJ Jr, Ray WL, May N. Changes in the blood coagulation system associated with septicemia. *N Engl J Med* 1968;279:851.

103. Yoshikawa T, Tanaka KR, Guze LB. Infection and DIC. *Medicine (Baltimore)* 1971;50:237.

104. Gralnick HR, Marchesi S, Givelber H. Intravascular coagulation in acute leukemia: clinical and subclinical abnormalities. *Blood* 1972;40:709.

105. McKay DG. Intravascular coagulation: acute and chronic, disseminated and local. *Proc Inst Med Chic* 1972;29:159.

106. Bieger R, Vreeken J, Stibbe J, et al. Arterial aneurysm as a cause of consumption coagulopathy. *N Engl J Med* 1971;285:152.

107. Kasabach HH, Merritt KK. Capillary hemangioma with extensive purpura. *Am J Dis Child* 1940;59:1063.

108. Sutton DM. Intravascular coagulation in abruptio placenta. *Am J Obstet Gynecol* 1971;109:604.

109. Toh CH, Dennis M. Disseminated intravascular coagulation: old disease, new hope. *BMJ* 2003;327:974–977.

110. Moschcowitz E. An acute febrile pleiochromic anemia with hyaline thrombosis of terminal arterioles and capillaries: an undescribed disease. *Arch Intern Med* 1925;36:89.

111. Schwartzman RJ, Hill JB. Neurologic complications of DIC. *Neurology* 1982;32:791.

112. Levi M, Schultz MJ, Rijneveld AW, et al. Bronchoalveolar coagulation and fibrinolysis in endotoxemia and pneumonia. *Crit Care Med* 2003;31: S238–S242.

113. Bone RC, Francis PB, Pierce AK. Disseminated intravascular coagulation with the adult respiratory distress syndrome. *Am J Med* 1976;61:585.

114. Rinaldo JE, Rogers RM. Adult respiratory distress syndrome. Changing concepts of lung injury and repair. *N Engl J Med* 1982;306:900.

115. McGehee WG, Rapaport SI, Hjort PF. Intravascular coagulation in fulminant meningococcemia. *Ann Intern Med* 1967;67:250.

116. Regoeczi E, Brain MC. Organ distribution of fibrin in DIC. *Br J Haematol* 1969;17:73.

117. Robboy SJ, Colman RW, Minna JD. Pathology of DIC: analysis of 26 cases. *Hum Pathol* 1972;3:327.

118. Brain MC, Dacie JV, Hourihane DOB. Microangiopathic haemolytic anaemia: the possible role of vascular lesions in pathogenesis. *Br J Haematol* 1962;8:358.

119. Dick G, Miller EM, Edmondson H. Severe purpura with gangrene of the lower extremity following scarlet fever. *Am J Dis Child* 1934;47:374.

120. Rich AR. A peculiar type of adrenal cortical damage associated with acute infections, and its possible relation to circulatory collapse. *Bull Johns Hopkins Hosp* 1944;74:1.

121. Ferguson JH, Chapman OD. Fulminating meningococcic infections and the so-called Waterhouse-Friderichsen syndrome. *Am J Pathol* 1948; 24:763.

122. Spicer TE, Rau JM. Purpura fulminans. *Am J Med* 1976;61:566.

123. Hjort PF, Rapaport SI. The Shwartzman reaction: pathogenetic mechanisms and clinical manifestations. *Annu Rev Med* 1965;16:135.

124. Evans RW, Glick B, Kimball F, et al. Fatal intravascular consumption coagulopathy in meningococcal sepsis. *Am J Med* 1969;48:910.

125. Gerard P, Moriau M, Bachy A, et al. Meningococcal purpura: report of 19 patients treated with heparin. *J Pediatr* 1973;82:780.

126. Hathaway WE. Heparin therapy in acute meningococcemia. *J Pediatr* 1973; 82:900.

127. Whitaker AN. Infection and the spleen: association between hyposplenism, pneumococcal sepsis, and DIC. *Med J Aust* 1969;1:1213.

128. Kusne S, Eibling DE, Yu VL, et al. Gangrenous cellulitis associated with gram-negative bacilli in pancytopenic patients: dilemma with respect to effective therapy. *Am J Med* 1988;85:490.

129. Rapaport SI, Tatter D, Coeur-Barron N. Pseudomonas septicemia with intravascular clotting leading to the generalized Shwartzman reaction. *N Engl J Med* 1964;271:80.

130. McGovern VJ. The pathophysiology of gram-negative septicaemia. *Pathology* 1972;4:265.

131. Lutz EE. Afibrinogenemia due to postabortal *Clostridium welchii* infection. *Obstet Gynecol* 1962;20:270.

132. Rubenberg ML, Baker LR, McBride JA, et al. Intravascular coagulation in a case of *Clostridium perfringens* septicaemia: treatment by exchange transfusion and heparin. *BMJ* 1967;4:271.

133. Mammen EF. Antithrombin: its physiological importance and role in DIC. *Semin Thromb Hemost* 1998;24:19.

134. Bianchi V, Robles R, Alberio L, et al. Von Willebrand factor-cleaving protease (ADAMTS13) in thrombocytopenic disorders: a severely deficient activity is specific for thrombotic thrombocytopenic purpura. *Blood* 2002; 100:710–713.

135. McKay DG, Margaretten W. DIC in virus disease. *Arch Intern Med* 1967; 120:129.

136. Davison AM, Thomson D, Robson JS. Intravascular coagulation complicating influenza virus A infection. *BMJ* 1973;1:654.

137. Whitaker AN, Bunce I, Graeme ER. DIC and acute renal failure in influenza A2 infection. *Med J Aust* 1974;2:196.

138. Lee M, Lee JS, Kim BK. DIC in Korean hemorrhagic fever. *Bibl Haematol* 1983;49:181.

139. Fisher-Hoch SP. The haemostatic defect in viral haemorrhagic fevers. *Br J Haematol* 1983;55:565.

140. Srichaikul T, Nimmanitaya S, Artchararit N, et al. Fibrinogen metabolism and DIC in dengue hemorrhagic fever. *Am J Trop Med Hyg* 1977;26:525.

141. Funahara Y, Sumarmo WirawanR. Features of DIC in dengue hemorrhagic fever. *Bibl Haematol* 1983;49:201.

142. Schaffner W, McLeod AC, Koenig MG. Thrombocytopenic Rocky Mountain spotted fever. *Arch Intern Med* 1965;116:857.

143. Trigg JW Jr. Hypofibrinogenemia in Rocky Mountain spotted fever: report of a case. *N Engl J Med* 1964;270:1042.

144. Dennis LH, Eichelberger JW, Inman MM, et al. Depletion of coagulation factors in drug-resistant *Plasmodium falciparum* malaria. *Blood* 1967; 29:713.

145. Paar D, Konig E, Fonk I, et al. Cerebral malaria and intravascular coagulation. *BMJ* 1970;4:805.

146. Doughten RM, Pearson HA. DIC associated with *Aspergillus endocarditis*. *J Pediatr* 1968;73:576.

147. Prochazka JV, Lucas RN, Beauchamp CJ, et al. Systemic candidiasis with DIC. *Am J Dis Child* 1971;122:255.

148. Barrett-Connor E, Ugoretz RJ, Braude AI. DIC in trypanosomiasis. *Arch Intern Med* 1973;131:574.

149. Frances RB. Acquired purpura fulminans. *Semin Thromb Hemost* 1990; 16:310.

150. Henoch E. Ueber purpura fulminans. *Berl Klin Wochenschr* 1887;24:8.

151. Hjort PF, Rapaport SI, Jergensen L. Purpura fulminans: report of a case successfully treated with heparin and hydrocortisone and review of 50 cases from the literature. *Scand J Haematol* 1964;1:169.

152. Antley RM, McMillan CW. Sequential coagulation studies in purpura fulminans. *N Engl J Med* 1967;276:1287.

153. Chambers WN, Holyoke JB, Wilson RF. Purpura fulminans: report of two cases following scarlet fever. *N Engl J Med* 1952;247:933.

154. Hall WH. Purpura fulminans with group B b-hemolytic streptococcal endocarditis. *Arch Intern Med* 1965;116:594.

155. Johansen K, Hansen ST Jr. Symmetrical peripheral gangrene (purpura fulminans) complicating pneumococcal sepsis. *Am J Surg* 1993;165:642–645.

156. Fishbein RH. Purpura fulminans: an analysis of the lesion and its treatment. *J Pediatr Surg* 1969;4:320.

157. Wong VK, Hitchcock W, Mason WH. Meningococcal infections in children: a review of 100 cases. *Pediatr Infect Dis J* 1989;8:224.

158. Feigin RD, San Joaquin V, Middelkamp JN. Purpura fulminans associated with *Neisseria catarrhalis* septicemia and meningitis. *Pediatrics* 1969; 44:120.

159. Adner MM, Kauff RE, Sherman JD. Purpura fulminans in a child with pneumococcal septicemia two years after splenectomy. *JAMA* 1970;213:1681.

160. Brazilian Purpuric Fever Study Group. Haemophilus aegyptius bacteraemia in Brazilian purpuric fever. *Lancet* 1987;2:761.

161. Molos MA, Hall JC. Symmetrical peripheral gangrene and DIC. *Arch Dermatol* 1985;121:1057.

162. ACCP/SCCM Consensus Conference Committee. Definitions for sepsis and organ failure and guidelines for the use of innovative therapies in sepsis. *Crit Care Med* 1992;20:864–874.

163. Molos MA, Hall JC. Symmetrical peripheral gangrene and disseminated intravascular coagulation. *Arch Dermatol* 1985;121:1057–1061.

164. Nalbandian RM, Mader IJ, Barrett JL, et al. Petechiae, ecchymoses, and necrosis of skin induced by coumarin congeners. *JAMA* 1965;192:603.

165. Koch-Weser J. Coumarin necrosis. *Ann Intern Med* 1968;68:1365.

166. McGehee WG, Klotz TA, Epstein DJ, et al. Coumarin necrosis associated with hereditary protein C deficiency. *Ann Intern Med* 1984;100:59.

167. Mitchell CA, Rowell JA, Hau L, et al. A fatal thrombotic disorder associated with an acquired inhibitor of protein C. *N Engl J Med* 1987;317:1638.

168. Nguyen P, Reynaud J, Pouzol P, et al. Varicella and thrombotic complications associated with transient protein C and protein S deficiencies in children. *Eur J Pediatr* 1994;153:646–649.

169. LeVeen HH. The LeVeen shunt. *Annu Rev Med* 1985;36:453.

170. Ragni MV, Lewis JH, Spero JA. Ascites-induced LeVeen shunt coagulopathy. *Ann Surg* 1983;198:91.

171. Rubinstein D, McInnes I, Dudley F. Morbidity and mortality after peritoneovenous shunt surgery for refractory ascites. *Gut* 1985;26:1070.

172. Buller HR, ten Cate JW. ATIII infusion in patients undergoing peritoneovenous shunt operation: failure in the prevention of DIC. *Thromb Haemost* 1983;49:128.

173. Pockros PJ, Peters RL, Reynolds TB. Idiopathic fatty liver of pregnancy: findings in 10 cases. *Medicine (Baltimore)* 1984;63:1.

174. Liebman HA, McGehee WG, Patch MJ, et al. Severe depression of ATIII associated with DIC in women with fatty liver of pregnancy. *Ann Intern Med* 1983;98:330.

175. Hillenbrand P, Parbhoo SP, Jedrychowski A, et al. Significance of intravascular coagulation and fibrinolysis in acute hepatic failure. *Gut* 1974;15:83.

176. Gazzard BG, Clark R, Borirakchanyavat V, et al. A controlled trial of heparin therapy in the coagulation defect of paracetamol- induced hepatic necrosis. *Gut* 1974;15:89.

177. deLee JB. A case of fatal hemorrhagic diathesis, with premature detachment of the placenta. *Am J Obstet Gynecol* 1971;44:785.

178. Graeff H, Kuhn W, eds. *Coagulation disorders in obstetrics: pathobiochemistry, pathophysiology, diagnosis, treatment.* Stuttgart: George Thieme Verlag, 1980.

179. Kleiner GJ, Merskey C, Johnson AJ, et al. Defibrination in normal and abnormal parturition. *Br J Haematol* 1970;19:159.

180. Pritchard JA, Brekken AL. Clinical and laboratory studies on severe abruptio placentae. *Am J Obstet Gynecol* 1967;97:681.

181. Bieber GF. Review of 353 cases of premature separation of the placenta. *Am J Obstet Gynecol* 1953;65:257.

182. Beller FK, Epstein MD. Traumatic placental abruption. *Obstet Gynecol* 1966;27:484.

183. Nilsen PA. The mechanism of hypofibrinogenemia in premature separation of the normally implanted placenta. *Acta Obstet Gynecol Scand Suppl* 1963;42(2):96.

184. Page EW, Fulton LD, Glendening MB. The cause of the blood coagulation defect following abruptio placentae. *Am J Obstet Gynecol* 1951;61:1116.

185. Weiner CP. The obstetric patient and disseminated intravascular coagulation. *Clin Perinatol* 1986;13:705–717.

186. Steiner PE, Lushbaugh CC. Maternal pulmonary embolism by amniotic fluid. *JAMA* 1941;117:1245.

187. Russell WS, Jones WN. Amniotic fluid embolism. *Obstet Gynecol* 1965;26:476.

188. Morgan M. Amniotic fluid embolism. *Anaesthesia* 1979;34:20.

189. Clark SL, Hankins GDV, Dudley DA, et al. Amniotic fluid embolism: analysis of the national registry. *Am J Obstet Gynecol* 1995;172:1158.

190. Purdie FR, Nieto JM, Summerson DJ, et al. Rupture of the uterus with DIC. *Ann Emerg Med* 1983;12:174.

191. Hankins CDV, Snyder RR, Clark SL, et al. Acute hemodynamic and respiratory effects of amniotic fluid embolism in the pregnant goat model. *Am J Obstet Gynecol* 1993;168:1113.

192. Agullon A, Andjus T, Grayson A, et al. Amniotic fluid embolism: a review. *Obstet Gynecol Surg* 1962;17:619.

193. Liban E, Raz S. Clinicopathologic study of 14 cases of amniotic fluid embolism. *Am J Clin Pathol* 1969;51:477.

194. Yaffe H, Eldor A, Hornshtein E, et al. Thromboplastic activity in amniotic fluid during pregnancy. *Obstet Gynecol* 1977;50:454.

195. Lang Phillips L, Davidson EC. Procoagulant properties of amniotic fluid. *Am J Obstet Gynecol* 1972;113:911.

196. Ratnoff OD, Vosburgh GJ. Observations on the clotting defect in amniotic fluid embolism. *N Engl J Med* 1952;247:970.

197. Albrechtsen OK, Storm O, Trolle D. Fibrinolytic activity in the circulating blood following amniotic fluid infusion. *Acta Haematol* 1955;14:309.

198. Verstraete M, Vermylen J. Acute and chronic "defibrination" in obstetrical practice. *Thromb Diath Haemorrh* 1968;20:444.

199. Bonnar J. Blood coagulation and fibrinolysis in obstetrics. *Clin Lab Haematol* 1973;2:213.

200. Maki M, Tachita K, Kawasaki Y, et al. Heparin treatment of amniotic fluid embolism. *Tohoku J Exp Med* 1969;97:155.

201. Beller FK, Rosenberg M, Kolker M, et al. Consumptive coagulopathy associated with intra-amniotic infusion of hypertonic salt. *Am J Obstet Gynecol* 1972;112:534.

202. Halbert DR, Buffington JS, Crenshaw C, et al. Consumptive coagulopathy with generalized hemorrhage after hypertonic saline- induced abortion. *Obstet Gynecol* 1972;39:41.

203. Zander J. *Septischer Abort und bakterieller Schock.* Berlin: Springer, 1968.

204. Cavanagh D, Clark PJ, McLeod AGW. Septic shock of endotoxin type: some observations based on the management of 50 patients. *Am J Obstet Gynecol* 1968;102:13.

205. Kayem G, Davy C, Goffinet F, et al. Conservative versus extirpative management in cases of placenta accreta. *Obstet Gynecol* 2004;104:531–536.

206. McKay DG. Chronic intravascular coagulation in normal pregnancy and preeclampsia. *Contrib Nephrol* 1981;25:108.

207. Gibson B, Hunter D, Neame PB, et al. Thrombocytopenia in preeclampsia and eclampsia. *Semin Thromb Hemost* 1982;8:234.

208. Bonnar J, McNicol GP, Douglas AS. Coagulation and fibrinolytic systems in preeclampsia and eclampsia. *BMJ* 1971;2:12.

209. Giles C. Intravascular coagulation in gestational hypertension and preeclampsia: the value of haematological screening tests. *Clin Lab Haematol* 1982;4:351.

210. Kobayashi T, Terao T. Preeclampsia as chronic disseminated intravascular coagulation: study of two parameters: thrombin- antithrombin III complex and D-dimers. *Gynecol Obstet Invest* 1987;24:170.

211. Cines DB, Pollak ES, Buck CA, et al. Endothelial cells in physiology and in the pathophysiology of vascular disorders. *Blood* 1998;91:3527.

212. Ordog GJ, Wasserberger J, Balasubramanium S. Coagulation abnormalities in traumatic shock. *Ann Emerg Med* 1985;14:650.

213. Kaufman HH, Hui KS, Mattson JC, et al. Clinicopathological correlations of DIC in patients with head injury. *Neurosurgery* 1984;15:34.

214. Miner ME, Kaufman HH, Graham SH, et al. DIC fibrinolytic syndrome following head injury in children: frequency and prognostic implications. *J Pediatr* 1982;100:687.

215. Simmons RL, Collins JA, Heisterkamp CA, et al. Coagulation disorders in combat casualties: I. Acute changes after wounding. II. Effect of massive transfusion. III. Post-resuscitation changes. *Ann Surg* 1960;169:455.

216. Modig J, Hedstrand U, Wegenius G. Determinants of early adult respiratory distress syndrome: a retrospective study of 220 patients with major fractures. *Acta Chir Scand* 1985;151:413.

217. Bone RC, Francis PB, Pierce AK. Intravascular coagulation associated with the adult respiratory distress syndrome. *Am J Med* 1976;61:585.

218. Mustafa KY, Omer O, Khogali M, et al. Blood coagulation and fibrinolysis in heat stroke. *Br J Haematol* 1985;61:517.

219. Meikle AW, Graybill JR. Fibrinolysis and hemorrhage in a fatal case of heat stroke. *N Engl J Med* 1967;276:911.

220. Shibolet S, Coll R, Gilat T, et al. Heatstroke: its clinical picture and mechanism in 36 cases. *Q J Med* 1967;36:525.

221. Bouchama A, Knochel JP. Heat stroke. *N Engl J Med* 2002;346:1978–1988.

222. Weiss HJ, Phillips LL, Hopewell WS, et al. Heparin therapy in a patient bitten by a saw-scaled viper (*Echis carinatus*), a snake whose venom activates prothrombin. *Am J Med* 1973;54:653.

223. Hasiba U, Rosenbach LM, Rockwell D, et al. DIC-like syndrome after envenomation by the snake *Crotalus horridus horridus*. *N Engl J Med* 1975;292:505.

224. Fainaru M, Eisenberg S, Manny N, et al. The natural course of defibrination syndrome caused by *Echis colorata* venom in man. *Thromb Diath Haemorrh* 1974;31:420.

225. Warrell DA, Pope HM, Prentice CRM. DIC caused by the carpet viper (*Echis carinatus*): trial of heparin. *Br J Haematol* 1976;33:335.

226. Reid HA. Epsilon-aminocaproic acid and fibrinolysis in viper bite defibrination. *Lancet* 1965;1:5.

227. Reid HA, Chan KE, Thean PC. Prolonged coagulation defect (defibrination syndrome) in Malayan viper bite. *Lancet* 1963;1:621.

228. Chugh KS, Pal Y, Chakravarty RN, et al. Acute renal failure following poisonous snake bite. *Am J Kidney Dis* 1984;4:30.

229. Friesen SR, Harsha WN, McCroskey CH. Massive generalized wound bleeding during operation, with clinical and experimental evidence of blood transfusion reactions. *Surgery* 1952;32:620.

230. Hardaway RM, McKay D, Williams JH. Lower nephron nephrosis (ischemuric nephrosis) with special reference to hemorrhagic diathesis following incompatible blood transfusion reaction. *Am J Surg* 1954;87:41.

231. Mannucci PM, Lobina GF, Caocci L, et al. Effect on blood coagulation of massive intravascular haemolysis. *Blood* 1969;33:207.

232. Straub PW. Chronic intravascular coagulation: clinical spectrum and diagnostic criteria, with special emphasis on metabolism, distribution, and localization of 131I-fibrinogen. *Acta Med Scand Suppl* 1971;526:1.

233. Slichter SJ, Harker LA. Hemostasis in malignancy. *Ann N Y Acad Sci* 1974;230:252.

234. Trousseau A. *Phlegmasia alba dolens: Clinique medicale de l'Hotel-Dieu de Paris*, Vol. 3. London: The New Sydenham Society, 1865:94.

235. Colman RW, Rubin RN. Disseminated intravascular coagulation due to malignancy. *Semin Oncol* 1990;17:172.

236. Sack GH, Levin J, Bell WR. Trousseau's syndrome and other manifestations of chronic disseminated coagulopathy in patients with neoplasms: clinical, pathologic and therapeutic features. *Medicine (Baltimore)* 1977;56:1.

237. Kierulf P, Godal HC. Fibrinaemia and multiple thrombi in pancreatic carcinoma: a case studied with quantitative N-terminal analysis. *Scand J Haematol* 1972;9:370.

238. Nossel HL, Yudelman I, Canfield RE, et al. Measurement of fibrinopeptide A in human blood. *J Clin Invest* 1974;54:43.

239. Breen FA, Tullis JL. Ethanol gelation: a rapid screening test for intravascular coagulation. *Ann Intern Med* 1968;69:1197.

240. Lipinski B, Worowski K. Detection of soluble fibrin monomer complexes in blood by means of protamine sulfate test. *Thromb Diath Haemorrh* 1968;20:44.

241. Rohner RF, Prior JT, Sipple JH. Mucinous malignancies, venous thrombosis and terminal endocarditis with emboli: a syndrome. *Cancer* 1966; 19:1805.

242. Mosesson MW, Colman RW, Sherry S. Chronic intravascular coagulation syndrome: report of a case with special studies of an associated plasma cryoprecipitate ("cryofibrinogen"). *N Engl J Med* 1968;278:815.

243. De Cicco M. The prothrombotic state in cancer: pathogenic mechanisms. *Crit Rev Oncol Hematol* 2004;50:187–196.

244. Gordon SG, Cross BA. A factor X-activating cysteine protease from malignant tissue. *J Clin Invest* 1981;67:1665.

245. Callander NS, Varki N, Rao LVM. Immunohistochemical identification of tissue factor in solid tumors. *Cancer* 1992;70:1194.

246. O'Meara RAQ. Coagulative properties of cancers. *Ir J Med Sci* 1958;3 94:474.

247. Edwards RL, Rickles FR, Cronlund M. Abnormalities of blood coagulation in patients with cancer: mononuclear cell tissue factor generation. *J Lab Clin Med* 1981;98:917.

248. Kakkar AK, DeRuvo N, Chinswangwatanakul V, et al. Extrinsic-pathway activation in cancer with high factor VIIa and tissue factor. *Lancet* 1995; 346:1004.

249. Cooper T, Barker NW. Recurrent venous thrombosis: an early complication of obscure visceral cancer. *Minn Med* 1944;27:31.

250. Fountain JR, Taverner D. Gangrene of three limbs resulting from venous occlusion. *Ann Intern Med* 1956;44:549.

251. Levin J, Conley CL. Thrombocytosis associated with malignant disease. *Arch Intern Med* 1964;114:497.

252. Smith SB, Arkin C. Cryofibrinogenemia: incidence, clinical correlations, and a review of the literature. *Am J Clin Pathol* 1972;58:524.

253. Grant RN, Deddish MR. Phlegmasia cerulea dolens and gangrene. *N Y State J Med* 1952;52:584.

254. Gaillard L. Gangrene humide de pied gauche par thrombose de la veine femorale chez une cancereuse de 27 ans. *Bull Mem Soc Med Hop Paris* 1894;11:315.

255. Tagnon HJ, Whitmore WF Jr, Shulman NR. Fibrinolysis in metastatic cancer of the prostate. *Cancer* 1952;5:9.

256. Davidson JF, McNicol GP, Frank GL, et al. Plasminogen-activator- producing tumour. *BMJ* 1969;1:88.

257. Bell WR, Starksen NF, Tong S, et al. Trousseau's syndrome: devastating coagulopathy in the absence of heparin. *Am J Med* 1985;79:423.

258. Gralnick HR, Tan HK. Acute promyelocytic leukemia: a model for understanding the role of the malignant cell in hemostasis. *Hum Pathol* 1974;5:661.

259. Didisheim P, Trombold JS, Vandervoort RLE, et al. Acute promyelocytic leukemia with fibrinogen and factor V deficiencies. *Blood* 1964;23:717.

260. Rosenthal R. Acute promyelocytic leukemia associated with hypofibrinogenemia. *Blood* 1963;21:495.

261. Gralnick HR, Sultan C. Acute promyelocytic leukaemia: haemorrhagic manifestations and morphologic criteria. *Br J Haematol* 1975;29:373.

262. Daly PA, Schiffer CA, Wiernik PH. Acute promyelocytic leukemia: clinical management of 15 patients. *Am J Hematol* 1980;8:347.

263. Gouault-Heilmann M, Chardon E, Sultan C, et al. The procoagulant factor of leukaemic promyelocytes: demonstration of immunologic cross-reactivity with human brain tissue factor. *Br J Haematol* 1975;30:151.

264. Egbring R, Schmidt W, Fuchs G, et al. Demonstration of granulocytic proteases in plasma of patients with acute leukemia and septicemia with coagulation defects. *Blood* 1977;49:219.

265. Avvisati G, ten Cate JW, Buller HR, et al. Tranexamic acid for control of haemorrhage in acute promyelocytic leukemia. *Lancet* 1989;2:122.

266. Bennett B, Booth NA, Croll A, et al. The bleeding disorder in acute promyelotic leukemia: fibrinolysis due to u-PA rather than defibrination. *Br J Haematol* 1989;71:511.

267. Schwartz BS, Williams EC, Conlan MG, et al. Epsilon-aminocaproic acid in the treatment of patients with acute promyelocytic leukemia and acquired alpha-2-plasmin inhibitor deficiency. *Ann Intern Med* 1986;105:873.

268. Williams EC. Plasma alpha$_2$-antiplasmin activity. Role in the evaluation and management of fibrinolytic states and other bleeding disorders. *Arch Intern Med* 1989;149:1769.

269. Sakata Y, Murakami T, Noro A, et al. The specific activity of plasminogen activator inhibitor-1 in disseminated intravascular coagulation with acute promyelocytic leukemia. *Blood* 1991;77:1949.

270. Barbui T, Finazzi G, Falanga A. The impact of all-*trans*-retinoic acid on the coagulopathy of acute promyelocytic leukemia. *Blood* 1998;91:3093.

271. Falanga A, Iacoviello L, Evangelista V, et al. Loss of blast cell procoagulant activity and improvement of hemostatic variables in patients with acute promyelocytic leukemia given all-*trans*-retinoic acid. *Blood* 1995;86:1072.

272. Kantarjian HM, Keating MJ, Walters RS, et al. Acute promyelocytic leukemia. *Am J Med* 1986;80:789.

273. Rodegiero F, Avrisati G, Castamen G, et al. Early deaths and antihemorrhagic treatments in acute promyelocytic leukemia: a GIMEMA retrospective study in 268 patients. *Blood* 1990;75:2112.

274. Hoyle CF, Swirsky DM, Freedman I, et al. Beneficial effect of heparin in the management of patients with acute promyelocytic leukemia. *Br J Haematol* 1988;68:283.

275. Goldberg MA, Ginsburg D, Mayer RJ, et al. Is heparin administration necessary during induction chemotherapy for patients with acute promyelocytic leukemia? *Blood* 1987;69:187.

276. Gingrich RD, Burns CP. Disseminated coagulopathy in chronic myelomonocytic leukemia. *Cancer* 1979;44:2249.

277. Goodnight SH Jr. Bleeding and intravascular clotting in malignancy: a review. *Ann N Y Acad Sci* 1974;230:271.

278. Baker WG, Bang NU, Nachman RL, et al. Hypofibrinogenemic hemorrhage in acute myelogenous leukemia treated with heparin, with autopsy findings of widespread intravascular clotting. *Ann Intern Med* 1964;61:116.

279. Chorba TL, Orenstein JM, Ney AB, et al. Phenotypic and ultrastructural characterization of a medullary thymocyte acute lymphoblastic leukemia with cellular procoagulant activity. *Cancer* 1985;55:675.

280. McKee LC, Collins RD Jr. Intravascular leukocyte thrombi and aggregates as a cause of morbidity and mortality in leukemia. *Medicine (Baltimore)* 1974;53:463.

281. Ishii H, Horie S, Kizaki K, et al. Retinoic acid counteracts both the down-regulation of thrombomodulin and the induction of tissue factor in cultured human endothelial cells exposed to tumor necrosis factor. *Blood* 1992;80:2556.

282. Fenaux P, LeDeley MC, Castaigne S, et al. Effect of all-*trans*-retinoic acid in newly diagnosed acute promyelocytic leukemia: results of a multicenter randomized trial. *Blood* 1993;82:3241.

283. Tallman MS, Andersen JW, Schiffer CA, et al. A prospective randomized study of all-trans-retinoic acid induction and maintenance therapy for patients with acute promyelocytic leukemia. *N Engl J Med* 1997; 337:1021.

284. Pritchard JA, Ratnoff OD. Studies of fibrinogen and other hemostatic factors in women with intrauterine death and delayed delivery. *Surg Gynecol Obstet* 1955;101:467.

285. Pfeffer RI. Hypofibrinogenemia in the dead fetus syndrome treated with aminocaproic acid. *Am J Obstet Gynecol* 1966;95:1095.

286. Phillips LL, Sciarra JJ. Hypofibrinogenemia with a dead fetus treated with intravenous heparin. *Am J Obstet Gynecol* 1965;92:1161.

287. Gallup DG, Lucas WE. Heparin treatment of consumption coagulopathy associated with intrauterine fetal death. *Obstet Gynecol* 1970;35:690.

288. Talbert LM, Blatt PM. DIC in obstetrics. *Clin Obstet Gynecol* 1979;22:889.

289. Romero R, Duffy TP, Berkowitz RL, et al. Prolongation of a preterm pregnancy complicated by death of a single twin *in utero* and DIC: effects of treatment with heparin. *N Engl J Med* 1984;310:772.

290. Mant MJ, Hirsh J, Pineo GF, et al. Prolonged prothrombin time and partial thromboplastin time in DIC not due to deficiency of factors V and VIII. *Br J Haematol* 1973;24:725.

291. Carr JM, McKinney M, McDonagh J. Diagnosis of DIC: role of D- dimer. *Am J Clin Pathol* 1989;91:280.

292. Paramo JA, Rifon J, Hernandez J, et al. Thrombin activation and increased fibrinolysis in patients with chronic liver disease. *Blood Coagul Fibrinolysis* 1991;2:227.

293. Coccheri S, Mannucci PM, Palaret G, et al. Significance of plasma fibrinopeptide A and high molecular fibrinogen in patients with liver cirrhosis. *Br J Haematol* 1982;52:503.

294. Carmassi F, DeNegri F, Morale M, et al. Antithrombotic and antifibrinolytic effects of antithrombin III replacement in liver cirrhosis. *Lancet* 1997; 349:1069.

295. Oka K, Tanaka K. Intravascular coagulation in autopsy cases with liver diseases. *Thromb Haemost* 1979;42:564.

296. Straub PW. Diffuse intravascular coagulation in liver disease. *Semin Thromb Hemost* 1977;4:29.

297. Palascak JE, Martinez J. Dysfibrinogenemia associated with liver disease. *J Clin Invest* 1977;60:89.

298. Rake MO, Flute PT, Shilkin KTS, et al. Early intensive therapy of intravascular coagulation in acute liver failure. *Lancet* 1971;2:1215.

299. Mannick JA. Diagnosis of ruptured aneurysm of the abdominal aorta. *N Engl J Med* 1967;276:1305.

300. Fine NL, Applebaum J, Elguezabal A, et al. Multiple coagulation defects in association with dissecting aneurysm. *Arch Intern Med* 1967;119:522.

301. ten Cate JW, Timmers H, Becker AE. Coagulopathy in ruptured or dissecting aortic aneurysms. *Am J Med* 1975;59:171.

302. Siebert WT, Natelson EA. Chronic consumption coagulopathy accompanying abdominal aortic aneurysm. *Arch Surg* 1976;111:539.

303. Fisher DR Jr, Yawn DH, Crawford ES. Preoperative DIC associated with aortic aneurysms: a prospective study of 76 cases. *Arch Surg* 1983; 118:1252.

304. Kimoto A, Kawaguchi H, Tadakuma K, et al. Surgical treatment of abdominal aortic aneurysm complicated with chronic disseminated intravascular coagulopathy. *J Cardiovasc Surg (Torino)* 1985;26:280.

305. Mulcare RJ, Royster TS, Weiss HJ, et al. DIC as a complication of abdominal aortic aneurysm repair. *Ann Surg* 1974;180:343.

306. Sutherland DA, Clark H. Hemangioma associated with thrombocytopenia: report of a case and review of the literature. *Am J Med* 1962;33:150.

307. Petit P, Schweisguth O, Contoni A, et al. Les angiomes geants du nourrisson avec thrombopenie. *Arch Pediatr* 1957;14:789.

308. Good TA, Carnazzo SF, Good RA. Thrombocytopenia and giant hemangioma in infants. *Am J Dis Child* 1955;90:260.

309. Inceman S, Tangrin Y. Chronic defibrination syndrome due to a giant hemangioma associated with microangiopathic hemolytic anemia. *Am J Med* 1969;46:997.

310. Rodriguez-Erdmann F, Button L, Murray JE, et al. Kasabach-Merritt syndrome: coagulo-analytical observations. *Am J Med Sci* 1971;261:9.

311. Hagerman LJ, Czapek EE, Donnellan WL. Giant hemangioma with consumption coagulopathy. *J Pediatr* 1975;87:766.

312. Neidhart JA, Roach RW. Successful treatment of skeletal hemangioma and Kasabach-Merritt syndrome with aminocaproic acid: is fibrinolysis "defensive"? *Am J Med* 1982;73:434.

313. Warrell RP Jr, Kempin SJ. Treatment of severe coagulopathy in the Kasabach-Merritt syndrome with aminocaproic acid cryoprecipitate. *N Engl J Med* 1985;313:309.

314. Starzl TE, Lerner RA, Dixon FJ, et al. Shwartzman reaction after human renal homotransplantation. *N Engl J Med* 1968;278:642.

315. Williams CM, Hume DM, Hudson RP Jr, et al. "Hyperacute" renal homograft rejection in man. *N Engl J Med* 1968;279:611.

316. Colman RW, Braun WE, Busch GJ, et al. Coagulation studies in the hyperacute and other forms of renal allograft rejection. *N Engl J Med* 1969; 281:685.

317. Starzl TE, Boehmig HJ, Amemiya H, et al. Clotting changes, including DIC, during rapid renal homograft rejection. *N Engl J Med* 1970; 283:383.

318. Braun WE, Merrill JP. Urine fibrinogen fragments in human renal allografts: a possible mechanism of renal injury. *N Engl J Med* 1968;278:1366.

319. Clarkson AR, Morton JB, Cash JD. Urinary fibrin/fibrinogen degradation products after renal homotransplantation. *Lancet* 1970;2:1220.

320. Scott WL, Francis CW, Knutson DW, et al. Specific identification of urinary fibrinogen, fibrinogen degradation products and crosslinked FDP in renal diseases and following renal allotransplantation. *J Lab Clin Med* 1986;107:534.

321. Clarkson AR, MacDonald MK, Petrie JJB, et al. Serum and urinary fibrin/fibrinogen degradation products in glomerulonephritis. *BMJ* 1971; 3:447.

322. Boyce TG, Swerdlow DL, Griffin PM. Escherichia coli O157:H7 and the hemolytic-uremic syndrome. *N Engl J Med* 1995;333:364.

323. Moake JL. Thrombotic microangiopathies. *N Engl J Med* 2002;347: 589–600.

324. Nevard CHF, Jurdi KM, Lane DA, et al. Activation of coagulation and fibrinolysis in childhood diarrhoea-associated haemolytic uraemic syndrome. *Thromb Haemost* 1997;78:1450.

325. Habib R. Pathology of the hemolytic uraemic syndrome. In: Kaplan BS, Thrompeter RS, Moake JL, eds. *Haemolytic uraemic syndrome and thrombocytopenic purpura.* New York: Marcel Dekker, 1992:315.

326. Lieberman E. Hemolytic-uremic syndrome. *J Pediatr* 1972;80:1.

327. Gilchrist GS, Lieberman E, Ekert H, et al. Heparin therapy in HUS. *Lancet* 1969;1:1123.

328. Thorsen CA, Rossi EC, Green D, et al. The treatment of HUS with inhibitors of platelet function. *Am J Med* 1979;66:711.

329. Kinkaid-Smith P. The modification of the vascular lesions of rejection in cadaveric renal allografts by dipyridamole and anticoagulants. *Lancet* 1969;2:920.

330. Bergstein JM, Edson JR, Michael AF. Fibrinolytic treatment of HUS. *Lancet* 1972;1:448.

331. Stuart J, Winterborn MW, White RHR, et al. Thrombolytic therapy in HUS. *Lancet* 1974;3:217.

332. Vitacco M, Avalos JS, Gianantonio CA. Heparin therapy in HUS. *J Pediatr* 1973;83:271.

333. Reid HA. Therapeutic defibrination by ancrod (Arvin). *Folia Haematol (Leipz)* 1971;95:209.

334. Davies JA, Sharp AA, Merrick MV, et al. Controlled trial of ancrod and heparin in treatment of deep-vein thrombosis of lower limb. *Lancet* 1972;1:113.

335. Bell WR, Pitney WR, Goodwin JF. Therapeutic defibrination in the treatment of thrombotic disease. *Lancet* 1968;1:490.

336. Kakkar VV, Flanc C, Howe CT, et al. Treatment of deep vein thrombosis: a trial of heparin streptokinase and arvin. *BMJ* 1969;1:806.

337. Warkentin TE. Heparin-induced thrombocytopenia: pathogenesis and management. *Br J Haematol* 2003;121:535–555.

338. White GC II, Lundblad RL, Kingdon HS. Prothrombin complex concentrates: preparation, properties, and clinical uses. *Curr Top Hematol* 1979; 2:203.

339. Lusher JM, Shapiro SS, Palascak JE, et al. Efficacy of prothrombin-complex concentrates in hemophiliacs with antibodies to factor VIII. *N Engl J Med* 1980;303:421.

340. Kingdon HS, Lundblad RL, Veltkamp JJ, et al. Potentially thrombogenic materials in factor IX concentrates. *Thromb Diath Haemorrh* 1975; 33:617.

341. Pepper DS, Banhegyi D, Howie A, et al. *In vitro* thrombogenicity tests of factor IX concentrates. *Br J Haematol* 1977;36:573.

342. Hultin MB. Activated clotting factors in factor IX concentrates. *Blood* 1979;54:1028.

343. White GC II, Roberts HR, Kingdon HS, et al. Prothrombin complex concentrates: potentially thrombogenic materials and clues to the mechanism of thrombosis *in vivo. Blood* 1977;49:159.

344. Vermylen J, Schetz J, Sermeraro N, et al. Evidence that "activated" prothrombin concentrates enhance platelet coagulant activity. *Br J Haematol* 1978;38:235.

345. Schmidt ML, Gamerman S, Smith HE, et al. Recombinant activated factor VIIa (rFVIIa) therapy for intracranial hemorrhage in hemophilia A patients with inhibitors. *Am J Hematol* 1994;47:36.

346. Aledort LM. Comparative thrombotic event incidence after infusion of recombinant factor VIIa versus factor VIII inhibitor bypass activity. *J Thromb Haemost* 2004;2:1700–1708.

347. Warkentin TE, Elavathil LJ, Hayward CP, et al. The pathogenesis of venous limb gangrene associated with heparin-induced thrombocytopenia. *Ann Intern Med* 1997;127:804.

348. Dairaku M, Sueishi K, Tanaka K. DIC in newborn infants: prevalence in autopsies and significance as a cause of death. *Pathol Res Pract* 1982; 174:106.

349. Montgomery RR, Marlar RA, Gill JC. Newborn haemostasis. *Clin Haematol* 1985;14:443.

350. Gross SJ, Filston HC, Anderson JC. Controlled study of treatment for DIC in the neonate. *J Pediatr* 1982;100:445.

351. Estelles A, Garcia-Plaza I, Dasi A, et al. Severe inherited "homozygous" protein C deficiency in a newborn infant. *Thromb Haemost* 1984;52:53.

352. Andrew M, Brooker L, Leaker M, et al. Fibrin clot lysis by thrombolytic agents is impaired in newborns due to a low plasminogen concentration. *Thromb Haemost* 1992;68:325.

353. Spero JA, Lewis JH, Hasiba U. DIC: findings in 346 patients. *Thromb Haemost* 1980;43:28.

354. Olson JD, Kaufman HH, Moake J, et al. The incidence and significance of hemostatic abnormalities in patients with head injuries. *Neurosurgery* 1989;24:825.

355. Weiss HJ, Vicic WJ, Lages BA, et al. Isolated deficiency of platelet procoagulant activity. *Am J Med* 1979;67:206.

356. Marder VJ, Shulman NR, Carroll WR. The importance of intermediate degradation products of fibrinogen in fibrinolytic hemorrhage. *Trans Assoc Am Physicians* 1967;80:156.

357. Bredbacka S, Blomback M, Wiman B. Soluble fibrin: a predictor for the development and outcome of multiple organ failure. *Am J Hematol* 1994;46: 289–294.

358. Horan JT, Francis CW. Fibrin degradation products, fibrin monomer and soluble fibrin in disseminated intravascular coagulation. *Semin Thromb Hemost* 2001;27:657–666.

359. McCarron BI, Marder VJ, Francis CW. Reactivity of soluble fibrin assays with plasmic degradation products of fibrin and in patients receiving fibrinolytic therapy. *Thromb Haemost* 1999;82:1722–1729.

360. Johnson AJ, Semar M, Newman J. Estimation of fibrinolytic activity by whole-blood euglobulin clot lysis. In: Tocantins LM, Kazal LA, eds. *Blood coagulation, hemorrhage and thrombosis.* New York: Grune & Stratton, 1964.

361. von Kaulla KN, von Kaulla E. Remarks on the euglobulin lysis time. In: Davidson JF, Samama JF, Desnoyers PC, eds. *Progress in chemical fibrinolysis and thrombolysis.* New York: Raven Press, 1975.

362. Kluft C, Brakman P. Effect on euglobulin fibrinolysis: involvement of $C_1$-inactivator. In: Davidson JF, Samama MM, Desnoyers PC, eds. *Progress in chemical fibrinolysis and thrombolysis.* New York: Raven Press, 1975.

363. Astrup T, Müllertz S. The fibrin plate method for estimating fibrinolytic activity. *Arch Biochem Biophys* 1952;40:346.

364. Moroz LA, Gilmore NJ. A rapid and sensitive 125I-fibrin solid-phase fibrinolytic assay for plasmin. *Blood* 1975;46:543.

365. Shimada H, Mori T, Takada Y, et al. Use of chromogenic substrate S-2251 for determination of plasminogen activator in rat ovaries. *Thromb Haemost* 1981;46:507.

366. Heussen C, Dowdle EB. Electrophoretic analysis of plasminogen activators in polyacrylamide gels containing sodium dodecyl sulfate and copolymerized substrates. *Anal Biochem* 1980;102:196.

367. Rijken DO, Juhan-Vague I, de Cock F, et al. Measurement of human tissue-type plasminogen activator by a two-site immunoradiometric assay. *J Lab Clin Med* 1983;101:274.

368. Juhan-Vague I, Moerman B, DeCock F, et al. Plasma levels of specific inhibitor of tissue-type plasminogen activator (and urokinase) in normal and pathological conditions. *Thromb Res* 1984;33:523.

369. Robbins KC. Plasmin. In: Markwardt F, ed. *Fibrinolytics and antifibrinolytics: handbook of experimental pharmacology,* Vol 46. Heidelberg: Springer-Verlag, 1978.

370. Sasahara AA, Hyers TM, Cole CM, et al. The urokinase pulmonary embolism trial: a national cooperative study. *Circulation* 1973;47(Suppl. 11):33.

371. Knos M, Friberger P. Methods for plasminogen determination in human plasma and for streptokinase standardization. In: Davidson JF, Cepelak V, Samama MM, Desnoyers PC, eds. *Progress in chemical fibrinolysis and thrombolysis,* Vol. 4. Edinburgh: Churchill Livingstone, 1979.

372. Collen D, DeCock F, Cambiaso L, et al. A latex agglutination test for rapid quantitative estimation of the plasmin-antiplasmin complex in human plasma. *Eur J Clin Invest* 1977;7:21.

373. Harpel PC. Alpha$_2$-plasmin inhibitor and alpha$_2$-macroglobulin-plasmin complexes in plasma: quantitation by an enzyme-linked differential antibody immunosorbent assay. *J Clin Invest* 1981;68:46.

374. Teger-Nilsson A-C, Friberger P, Gyzander E. Determination of a new rapid plasma inhibitor in human blood by means of a plasmin specific tripeptide substrate. *Scand J Clin Lab Invest* 1977;37:403.

375. Ratnoff OD, Menzie C. A new method for the determination of fibrinogen in small samples of plasma. *J Lab Clin Med* 1951;37:316.

376. von Clauss A. Gerinnungsphysiologische Schnellmethode zur Bestimmung des fibrinogens. *Acta Haematol* 1957;17:237.

377. Connaghan DG, Francis CW, Ryan DH, et al. Prevalence and clinical implications of heparin-associated false-positive tests for serum fibrin(ogen) degradation products. *Am J Clin Pathol* 1986;86:304.

378. Ferreira HC, Murat LG. An immunological method for demonstrating FDP in serum and its use in the diagnosis of fibrinolytic states. *Br J Haematol* 1963;9:299.

379. Marder VJ, Cruz GO, Schumer BR. Evaluation of a new antifibrinogen-coated latex particle agglutination test in the measurement of serum FDP. *Thromb Haemost* 1977;37:183.

380. Marder VJ, Matchett MO, Sherry S. Detection of serum fibrinogen and FDP: comparison of six techniques using purified products and application in clinical studies. *Am J Med* 1971;51:71.

381. Marder VJ, Budzynski AZ. Degradation products of fibrinogen and crosslinked fibrin: projected clinical applications. *Thromb Diath Haemorrh* 1974;32:49.

382. Koppert PW, Kuipers W, Hoegee-de Nobel B, et al. A quantitative enzyme immunoassay for primary fibrinogenolysis products in plasma. *Thromb Haemost* 1987;57:25.

383. Weitz JI, Koehn JA, Canfield RE, et al. Development of a radioimmunoassay for the fibrinogen-derived peptide B beta 1-42. *Blood* 1986;67:1014.

384. Kudryk B, Robinson D, Netre C, et al. Measurement in human blood of fibrinogen/fibrin fragments containing the B beta 15-42 sequence. *Thromb Res* 1982;25:277.

385. Gaffney PJ. Distinction between fibrinogen and FDP in plasma. *Clin Chim Acta* 1975;65:109.

386. Francis CW, Marder VJ, Martin SE. Detection of circulating cross-linked fibrin derivatives by a heat extraction-SDS gradient gel electrophoretic technique. *Blood* 1979;54:1282.

387. Connaghan DG, Francis CW, Lane DA, et al. Specific identification of fibrin polymers, fibrinogen degradation products, and crosslinked FDP in plasma and serum with a new sensitive technique. *Blood* 1985;65:589.

388. Rylatt DB, Blake AS, Cottis LE, et al. An immunoassay for human D-dimer using monoclonal antibodies. *Thromb Res* 1983;31:767.

389. Whitaker AN, Elms MJ, Masci PP, et al. Measurement of cross-linked fibrin derivatives in plasma: an immunoassay using monoclonal antibodies. *J Clin Pathol* 1984;37:882.

390. Goldhaber SZ, Vaughan DE, Tumeh SS, et al. Utility of cross-linked FDP in the diagnosis of pulmonary embolism. *Am Heart J* 1988;116:505.

391. Bounameaux H, Schneider P-A, Reber G, et al. Measurement of plasma D-dimer for diagnosis of deep venous thrombosis. *Am J Clin Pathol* 1989;91:82.

392. Nossel HL. Radioimmunoassay of fibrinopeptides in relation to intravascular coagulation and thrombosis. *N Engl J Med* 1976;295:428.

393. Cronlund M, Hardin J, Burton J, et al. Fibrinopeptide A in plasma of normal subjects and patients with DIC and systemic lupus erythematosus. *J Clin Invest* 1976;58:142.

394. Niewiarowski S, Gurewich V. Laboratory identification of intravascular coagulation: the serial dilution protamine sulfate test for the detection of fibrin monomer and FDP. *J Lab Clin Med* 1971;77:665.

395. Largo R, Heller V, Straub PW. Detection of soluble intermediates of the fibrinogen-fibrin conversion using erythrocytes coated with fibrin monomers. *Blood* 1976;47:991.

396. Wiman B, Ranby M. Determination of soluble fibrin in plasma by a rapid and quantitative spectrophotometric assay. *Thromb Haemost* 1986;55:189.

397. Francis CW, Connaghan DG, Scott WL, et al. Increased plasma concentration of cross-linked fibrin polymers in acute myocardial infarction. *Circulation* 1987;75:1170.

398. Hersch Sl, Kunelis T, Francis RB Jr. The pathogenesis of accelerated fibrinolysis in liver cirrhosis: a critical role for tissue plasminogen activator inhibitor. *Blood* 1987;69:1315.

399. Liebman HA, Carfagno MK, Weitz IC, et al. Excessive fibrinolysis in amyloidosis associated with elevated plasma single-chain urokinase. *Am J Clin Pathol* 1992;98:534.

400. Naeye RL. Thrombotic state after a hemorrhagic diathesis, a possible complication of therapy with epsilon-aminocaproic acid. *Blood* 1962;19:694.

401. Gralnick HR, Greipp P. Thrombosis with epsilon-aminocaproic acid therapy. *Am J Clin Pathol* 1971;56:151.

402. Bergin JJ. Complications of therapy with epsilon-aminocaproic acid. *Med Clin North Am* 1966;50:1669.

403. Bergin JJ, Crosby WH, Jahnke EJ. Massive bleeding with fibrinolysis: management with heparin and epsilon-aminocaproic acid. *Mil Med* 1966;131:340.

404. Weber MB, Blakeley JA. The hemorrhagic diathesis of heatstroke: a consumption coagulopathy successfully treated with heparin. *Lancet* 1969;1:1190.

405. Stefanini M, Spicer DD. Hemostatic breakdown, fibrinolysis, and acquired hemolytic anemia in a patient with fatal heatstroke: pathogenetic mechanisms. *Am J Clin Pathol* 1971;55:180.

406. Kevy SV, Glickman RM, Bernhard WF, et al. The pathogenesis and control of the hemorrhagic defect in open heart surgery. *Surg Gynecol Obstet* 1966;123:313.

407. McClure PD, Izsak J. The use of epsilon-aminocaproic acid to reduce bleeding during cardiac bypass in children with congenital heart disease. *Anesthesiology* 1974;40:604.

408. Lambert CJ, Marengo-Rowe AJ, Leveson JE, et al. The treatment of postperfusion bleeding using epsilon-aminocaproic acid, cryoprecipitate, fresh-frozen plasma, and protamine sulfate. *Ann Thorac Surg* 1979;28:440.

409. Altschule MD. A rare type of acute thrombocytopenic purpura: widespread formation of platelet thrombi in capillaries. *N Engl J Med* 1942;227:477.

410. Baehr G, Klemperer P, Schifrin A. An acute febrile anemia and thrombocytopenic purpura with diffuse platelet thrombosis of capillaries and arterioles. *Trans Assoc Am Physicians* 1936;51:43.

411. Neame PB, Lechago J, Ling ET, et al. TTP: report of a case with disseminated intravascular platelet aggregation. *Blood* 1973;42:805.

412. Jaffe EA, Nachman RL, Merskey C. TTP: coagulation parameters in 12 patients. *Blood* 1973;42:499.

413. Harker LA, Slichter SJ. Platelet and fibrinogen consumption in man. *N Engl J Med* 1972;287:999.

414. Lian EC-Y, Miu PTK, Siddiqui FA. Inhibition of platelet-aggregating activity in TTP plasma by normal adult immunoglobulin G. *J Clin Invest* 1984;73:548.

415. Siddiqui FA, Lian EC. Novel platelet-agglutinating protein from a TTP plasma. *J Clin Invest* 1985;76:1330.

416. Moake JL, Rudy CK, Troll JH, et al. Unusually large plasma factor VIII: von Willebrand factor multimers in chronic relapsing TTP. *N Engl J Med* 1982;307:1432.

417. Moake JL, Byrnes JJ, Troll JH, et al. Effects of fresh-frozen plasma and its cryosupernatant fraction on von Willebrand factor multimeric forms in chronic relapsing TTP. *Blood* 1985;65:1232.

418. Moake JL, Byrnes JJ, Troll JH, et al. Abnormal VIII: von Willebrand factor patterns in the plasma of patients with HUS. *Blood* 1984;64:592.

419. Rowe JM, Francis CW, Cyran EM, et al. TTP: recovery after splenectomy associated with persistence of abnormally large von Willebrand factor multimers. *Am J Hematol* 1985;20:161.

420. Furlan M, Robles R, Solenthaler M, et al. Acquired deficiency of von Willebrand factor-cleaving protease in a patient with thrombotic thrombocytopenic purpura. *Blood* 1998;91:2839.

421. Furlan M, Robles R, Lämmie B. Partial purification and characterization of a protease from human plasma cleaving von Willebrand factor to fragments produced by *in vivo* proteolysis. *Blood* 1996;87:4223.

422. Furlan M, Robles R, Solenthaler M, et al. Deficient activity of von Willebrand factor-cleaving protease in chronic relapsing thrombotic thrombocytopenic purpura. *Blood* 1997;89:3097.

423. Amorosi EL, Ultmann JE. TTP: report of 16 cases and review of the literature. *Medicine (Baltimore)* 1966;45:139.

424. Byrnes JJ, Khurana M. Treatment of TTP with plasma. *N Engl J Med* 1977;297:1386.

425. Bukowski RM, King JW, Hewlett JS. Plasmapheresis in the treatment of TTP. *Blood* 1977;50:413.

426. Upshaw JD Jr. Congenital deficiency of a factor in normal plasma that reverses microangiopathic hemolysis and thrombocytopenia. *N Engl J Med* 1978;298:1350.

427. Rock GA, Shumak KH, Buskard NA et al, Canadian Apheresis Study Group. Comparison of plasma exchange with plasma infusion in the treatment of thrombotic thrombocytopenic purpura. *N Engl J Med* 1991;325:393.

428. Aster RH. Plasma therapy for TTP: sometimes it works, but why? *N Engl J Med* 1985;312:985.

429. Rodriguez HF, Babb DF, Santiago EP, et al. TTP: remission after splenectomy. *N Engl J Med* 1957;257:983.

430. Bernard RP, Bauman AW, Schwartz SI. Splenectomy for TTP. *Ann Surg* 1969;169:616.

431. Corrigan JJ, Colman RW, Robboy SJ, et al. Management of DIC. In: Inglefinger FJ, Ebert RV, Finland M et al., eds. *Controversies in internal medicine II*. Philadelphia, PA: WB Saunders, 1974.

432. Goodnight SH, Kenoyer G, Patch MJ, et al. Defibrination after brain-tissue destruction. *N Engl J Med* 1974;290:1043.

433. Kaufman HH, Makela ME, Lee KF, et al. Gunshot wounds to the head: a perspective. *Neurosurgery* 1986;18:689.

434. Jacobsen ST, Crawford AH. Amputation following meningococcemia. A sequela to purpura fulminans. *Clin Orthop* 1984;185:214.

435. Thompson RW, Adams DH, Cohen JR, et al. DIC caused by abdominal aortic aneurysm. *J Vasc Surg* 1986;4:184.

436. Bernard J, Weil M, Boiron M, et al. Acute promyelocytic leukemia. Results of treatment with daunorubicin. *Blood* 1973;41:489.

437. Chan TK, Chan GTC, Chan V. Hypofibrinogenemia due to increased fibrinolysis in two patients with acute promyelocytic leukemia. *Aust N Z J Med* 1984;14:245.

438. Booth NA, Bennett B. Plasmin-alpha-antiplasmin complexes in bleeding disorders characterized by primary or secondary fibrinolysis. *Br J Haematol* 1984;56:545.

439. Avrisati G, Buller HR, ten Cate JW, et al. Tranexamic acid for control of haemorrhage in acute promyelocytic leukemia. *Lancet* 1989;2:122.

440. Bennett B, Booth A, Croll A, et al. The bleeding disorder in acute promyelocytic leukemia: fibrinolysis due to u-PA rather than defibrination. *Br J Haematol* 1989;71:511.

441. Gralnick HR, Bagley J, Abrell E. Heparin treatment for the hemorrhagic diathesis of acute promyelocytic leukemia. *Am J Med* 1972;52:167.

442. Drapkin RL, Gee TS, Dowling MD, et al. Prophylactic heparin therapy in acute promyelocytic leukemia. *Cancer* 1978;41:2484.

443. Ruggero D, Baccarani M, Guarine A, et al. Acute promyelocytic leukemia: results of therapy and analysis of 13 cases. *Acta Haematol* 1977; 58:108.

444. Straub PW. A case against heparin therapy of intravascular coagulation. *Thromb Diath Haemorrh* 1974;33:107.

445. Lasch HG, Heene DH. Heparin therapy of DIC. *Thromb Diath Haemorrh* 1975;33:105.

446. McKay DG. Hematologic evidence of DIC in eclampsia. *Obstet Gynecol Surv* 1972;27:399.

447. Corrigan JJ Jr. Heparin therapy in bacterial septicemia. *J Pediatr* 1977; 91:695.

448. Corrigan JJ Jr, Jordan CM, Bennett BB. DIC in septic shock: report of three cases not treated with heparin. *Am J Dis Child* 1973;126:629.

449. Haneberg B, Gutteberg TJ, Moe JP, et al. Heparin for infants and meningococcal septicemia: results of a randomized therapeutic trial. *NIPH Ann* 1983;6:43.

450. Williams TF. Renal cortical necrosis, renal infarction, and hypertension due to renal vascular disease. In: Strauss MB, Welt LG, eds. *Diseases of the kidney*. Boston: Little, Brown & Co, 1963:526.

451. Galton M, Merritt K, Beller FK. Coagulation studies on the peripheral circulation of patients with toxemia of pregnancy: a study for the evaluation of DIC in toxemia. *J Reprod Med* 1971;6:89.

452. Pritchard JA, Cunningham FG, Mason RA. Coagulation changes in eclampsia: their frequency and pathogenesis. *Am J Obstet Gynecol* 1976; 124:855.

453. Vassalli P, Morris RH, McClusky RT. The pathogenic role of fibrin deposition in the glomerular lesions of toxemia of pregnancy. *J Exp Med* 1963;118:467.

454. Beecham JB, Watson WJ, Clapp JF III. Eclampsia, preeclampsia, and DIC. *Obstet Gynecol* 1974;43:576.

455. McKay DG. Clinical significance of the pathology of toxemia of pregnancy. *Circulation* 1964;30(Suppl. II):66.

456. Howie PW, Prentice CRM, Forbes CD. Failure of heparin therapy to affect the clinical courses of severe preeclampsia. *Br J Obstet Gynaecol* 1975;82:711.

457. Brain MC, Kuah K-B, Dixon HG. Heparin treatment of haemolysis and thrombocytopenia in preeclampsia. *J Obstet Gynaecol Br Commonw* 1967;74:702.

458. Butler BC, Taylor HC Sr, Graff S. The relationship of disorders of the blood-clotting mechanism to toxemia of pregnancy and the value of heparin in therapy. *Am J Obstet Gynecol* 1950;60:564.

459. Pritchard JA, Pritchard SA. Standardized treatment of 154 consecutive cases of eclampsia. *Am J Obstet Gynecol* 1975;123:543.

460. Martin JN Jr, Blake PG, Perry KG Jr, et al. The natural history of HELLP syndrome: patterns of disease progression and regression. *Am J Obstet Gynecol* 1991;164:1500.

461. Heene DL. DIC: evaluation of therapeutic approaches. *Semin Thromb Hemost* 1977;3:291.

462. Riely CA, Latham PS, Romero R, et al. Acute fatty liver of pregnancy. *J Intern Med* 1987;106:703.

463. Eisele B, Lamy M. Clinical experience with antithrombin III concentrates in critically ill patients with sepsis and multiple organ failure. *Semin Thromb Hemost* 1998;24:71.

464. Okajima K, Uchida M. The anti-inflammatory properties of antithrombin III: new therapeutic implications. *Semin Thromb Hemost* 1998;24:27.

465. Fourrier F, Chopin C, Huart JJ, et al. Double-blind, placebo-controlled trial of antithrombin III concentrates in septic shock with disseminated intravascular coagulation. *Chest* 1993;104:882–888.

466. Baudo F, Caimi TM, de Cataldo F, et al. Antithrombin III (ATIII) replacement therapy in patients with sepsis and/or postsurgical complications: a controlled double-blind, randomized, multicenter study. *Intensive Care Med* 1998;24:336–342.

467. Warren BL, Eid A, Singer P, et al. Caring for the critically ill patient. High-dose antithrombin III in severe sepsis: a randomized controlled trial. *JAMA* 2001;286:1869–1878.

468. Munoz MC, Montes R, Hermida J, et al. Effect of the administration of recombinant hirudin and/or tissue-plasminogen activator (t-PA) on endotoxin-induced disseminated intravascular coagulation model in rabbits. *Br J Haematol* 1999;105:117–121.

469. Pernerstorfer T, Hollenstein U, Hansen JB, et al. Lepirudin blunts endotoxin-induced coagulation activation. *Blood* 2000;95:1729–1734.

470. Saito M, Asakura H, Jokaji H, et al. Recombinant hirudin for the treatment of disseminated intravascular coagulation in patients with haematological malignancy. *Blood Coagul Fibrinolysis* 1995;6:60–64.

471. Taylor FB, Chang A, Esmon CT, et al. Protein C prevents the coagulopathic and lethal effects of *Escherichia coli* infusion in the baboon. *J Clin Invest* 1987;79:918.

472. Okajima K. Regulation of inflammatory responses by activated protein C: the molecular mechanism(s) and therapeutic implications. *Clin Chem Lab Med* 2004;42:132–141.

473. Smith OP. Protein-C concentrate for meningococcal purpura fulminans. *Lancet* 1998;351:986.

474. Fijinvandraat K, Derkx B, Peters M, et al. Coagulation activation and tissue necrosis in meningococcal septic shock: severely reduced protein C levels predict a high mortality. *Thromb Haemost* 1995;73:15.

475. Smith OP, White B, Vaughan D, et al. Use of protein-C concentrate, heparin, and haemodiafiltration in meningococcus-induced prupura fulminans. *Lancet* 1997;350:1590.

476. Bernard GR, Vincent JL, Laterre PF, et al. Efficacy and safety of recombinant human activated protein C for severe sepsis. *N Engl J Med* 2001; 344:699–709.

477. Vincent JL, Angus DC, Artigas A, et al. Effects of drotrecogin alfa (activated) on organ dysfunction in the PROWESS trial. *Crit Care Med* 2003; 31:834–840.

478. Dhainaut JF, Yan SB, Joyce DE, et al. Treatment effects of drotrecogin alfa (activated) in patients with severe sepsis with or without overt disseminted intravascular coagulation. *J Thromb Haemost* 2004;2:1924–1933.

479. Beutler B, Milsark IW, Cerami AC. Passive immunization against cachectin/tumor necrosis factor protects mice from lethal effect of endotoxin. *Science* 1985;229:869.

480. Waage A, Halstensen A, Espevik T. Association between tumor necrosis factor in serum and fatal outcome in patients with meningococcal disease. *Lancet* 1987;1:355.

481. Abraham E, Anzueto A, Gutierrez G, et al. Double-blind randomised controlled trial of monoclonal antibody to human tumour necrosis factor in treatment of septic shock. *Lancet* 1998;351:929.

482. Abraham E, Wunderink R, Silverman H et al, TNF-alpha MAb Sepsis Study Group. Efficacy and safety of monoclonal antibody to human tumor necrosis factor alpha in patients with sepsis syndrome: a randomized, controlled, double-blind, multicenter clinical trial. *JAMA* 1995;273:934.

483. Cohen J, Carlet J. INTERSEPT: an international, multicenter, placebo-controlled trial of monoclonal antibody to human tumor necrosis factor in patients with sepsis. *Crit Care Med* 1996;24:1431.

# CHAPTER 110 ■ COAGULATION ABNORMALITIES IN SEPSIS

MARCEL LEVI AND VICTOR J. MARDER

Sepsis is a clinical syndrome that is caused by an infection, often associated with bacteremia and characterized by the presence of systemic signs and symptoms of inflammation (1). When sepsis leads to organ failure, the term severe sepsis is used. The incidence of sepsis is estimated to be about 2.5 per 1,000 in the United States and European countries and has shown a rapid 8.7% annual increase over the last 20 years (2). Total in-hospital mortality of sepsis is approximately 20%, whereas severe sepsis is associated with mortality rates of 40% to 50% (3). Treatment of sepsis is focused on adequate antibiotic therapy, source control, and general and specific organ function support.

Almost all patients with sepsis have coagulation abnormalities. These abnormalities range from subtle activation of coagulation that can be detected only by sensitive specialized laboratory assay to a moderate coagulation activation that is detectable by a mild decrease in platelet count and modest prolongation of global clotting times to fulminant disseminated intravascular coagulation (DIC), characterized by simultaneous widespread microvascular thrombosis and profuse bleeding from various sites (4) (see Chapter 109). Patients with sepsis and with severe forms of DIC may present with manifest thromboembolic disease or clinically less apparent microvascular fibrin deposition that causes multiple organ dysfunction (5–8). Alternatively, severe bleeding may be the leading symptom (9), but quite often a patient with DIC has simultaneous thrombosis and bleeding (see Fig. 110-1). Bleeding is caused by consumption and consequent deficiency of coagulation proteins and platelets due to ongoing activation of coagulation (10). In its most severe form, this combination may present as the Waterhouse-Friderichsen syndrome, as seen during fulminant meningococcal septicemia (11).

## INCIDENCE OF COAGULATION ABNORMALITIES IN SEPSIS

Clinically relevant coagulation abnormalities may occur in 50% to 70% of patients with sepsis, whereas approximately 35% of patients will meet the criteria for DIC (1,12). Thrombocytopenia (platelet count $<150 \times 10^9$ per L) occurs in 35% to 50% of critically ill medical patients (13–15), typically manifests during the first 4 days in the intensive care unit (ICU) (16), and correlates with the severity of sepsis (17). The main factors that contribute to thrombocytopenia are impaired platelet production, increased consumption or destruction, sequestration in the spleen, or adhesion to the endothelium. Platelet production is stimulated by high levels of proinflammatory cytokines such as tumor necrosis factor (TNF)-$\alpha$ and interleukin (IL)-6, and by a high concentration

of thrombopoietin (18), but marrow output is limited by marked hemophagocytosis, hypothetically due to high levels of macrophage colony stimulating factor (M-CSF) (19). Platelet consumption is increased due to ongoing thrombin generation and extensive endothelial cell–platelet interaction, which may vary in vascular beds of different organs (20). Abnormal coagulation assays include prolongation of global coagulation times [such as the prothrombin time (PT) or the activated partial thromboplastin time (aPTT)] (14% to 28%) (21,22), increased fibrin-split products (99%) (23–25), and decreased coagulation inhibitors such as antithrombin and protein C (90%) (25,26).

## RELEVANCE OF COAGULATION ABNORMALITIES IN PATIENTS WITH SEPSIS

There is ample evidence that activation of coagulation in concert with inflammatory activation results in microvascular thrombosis and contributes to multiple organ failure in patients with severe sepsis (27). First, autopsy findings include diffuse bleeding, hemorrhagic necrosis, microthrombi in small blood vessels, and thrombi in midsize and larger arteries and veins (28,29). Fibrin deposition in small and midsize vessels was invariably associated with ischemia and necrosis and to clinical dysfunction of organs (30). Second, experimental bacteremia or endotoxemia in animals causes intravascular and extravascular fibrin deposition in kidneys, lungs, liver, and brain, and amelioration of the hemostatic defect improves organ failure and, in some cases, mortality (9,31–35). Finally, DIC is an independent predictor of organ failure and mortality in patients with sepsis (5,36), with death occurring in 43%, as compared with 27% in patients without DIC (37).

Critically ill patients with a platelet count of less than $50 \times 10^9$ per L have a fourfold to fivefold higher risk for bleeding than patients with a higher platelet count (13,15). The risk of intracerebral bleeding in patients with sepsis during intensive care admission is relatively low (0.3% to 0.5%), but 88% of patients with this complication had platelet counts of less than $100 \times 10^9$ per L (38). Regardless of the cause, thrombocytopenia is an independent predictor of ICU mortality (relative risk, 1.9 to 4.2) (13,15,39), and a sustained thrombocytopenia of more than 4 days after ICU admission or a drop in platelet count of greater than 50% during the ICU stay is related to a fourfold to sixfold increase in mortality (13,16). Decreased coagulation factors, as reflected by prolonged global coagulation times (PT or aPTT ratio greater than 1.5), are also predictors of bleeding and mortality in critically ill patients (21,22).

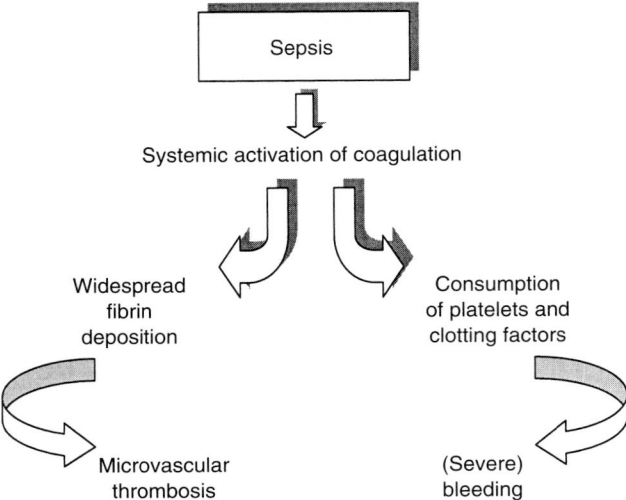

**FIGURE 110-1.** Schematic representation of the coagulopathy in sepsis. Systemic activation of coagulation leads to microvascular thrombosis, contributing to organ dysfunction. Simultaneous loss of platelets and coagulation factors contributes to bleeding risk.

# PATHOGENETIC PATHWAYS IN THE COAGULOPATHY OF SEPSIS

The most important mediators that orchestrate the imbalance of the coagulation system toward a procoagulant state during sepsis are cytokines (40) (see Fig. 110-2). There is extensive cross-talk between these systems, whereby inflammation activates coagulation, and coagulation in turn affects inflammatory activity (41), the consequences of which can have organ-specific manifestations (42).

## Initiation of Coagulation Activation

The principal initiator of thrombin generation in sepsis is tissue factor, not the contact system, as previously postulated (43). Studies of human endotoxemia or cytokinemia show changes indicative of tissue factor/factor VII(a) pathway but not of contact system activation (44,45), and monoclonal antibodies directed against tissue factor or factor VIIa inhibit thrombin generation in endotoxin-challenged chimpanzees and prevent DIC and mortality in baboons infused with *Escherichia coli* (33,46,47).

Tissue factor is a transmembrane 45-kDa protein that is constitutively expressed on a number of cells throughout the body (48) (see Chapter 5). Most of these cells are not in direct contact with blood, such as the adventitial layer of large blood vessels. However, tissue factor contacts blood when the vascular integrity is disrupted or if circulating cells express tissue factor. In sepsis, circulating mononuclear cells, stimulated by proinflammatory cytokines, synthesize and express tissue factor on their surface, which leads to systemic activation of coagulation. However, other than in severe meningococcemia (49), it has proved difficult to demonstrate *ex vivo* tissue factor expression on monocytes of patients with sepsis or of experimental animals systemically exposed to microorganisms. It has been shown, however, that low-dose endotoxemia in healthy subjects results in a 125-fold increase in monocyte tissue factor mRNA levels (50). Tissue factor may also be present on polymorphonuclear cells (51), although it is unlikely that these cells synthesize tissue factor in substantial quantities (52). On the basis of the observation of transfer of tissue factor from leukocytes to activated platelets on a collagen surface in an *ex vivo* perfusion system, it is hypothesized that this "blood-borne" tissue factor is transferred between cells through microparticles derived from activated mononuclear cells (53).

Platelets play a pivotal role in the pathogenesis of coagulation abnormalities in sepsis. Platelets can be activated directly by proinflammatory mediators, such as platelet-activating

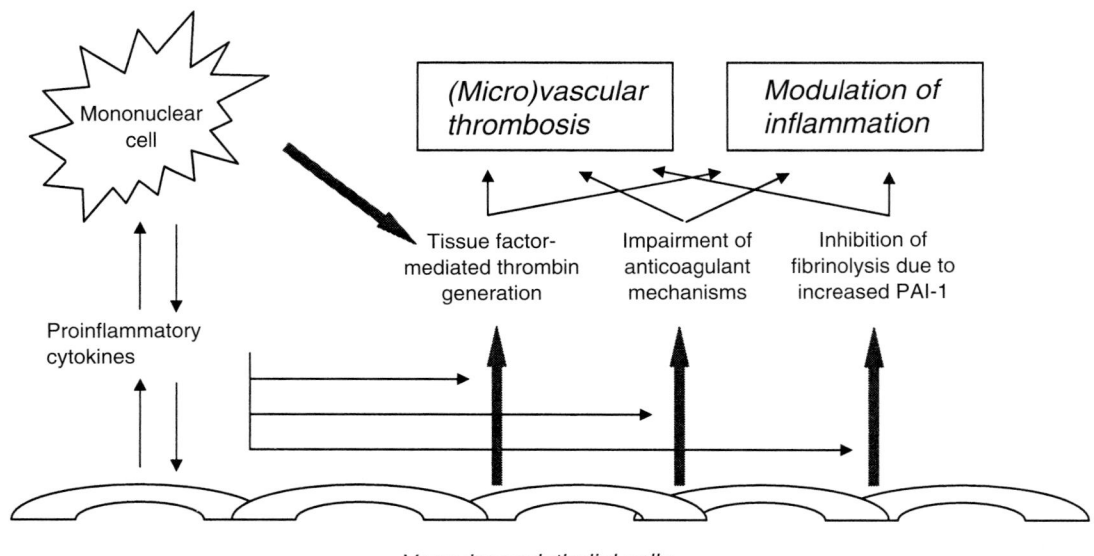

**FIGURE 110-2.** Schematic representation of pathogenetic pathways involved in the activation of coagulation in sepsis. During sepsis, both perturbed endothelial cells and activated mononuclear cells may produce proinflammatory cytokines that mediate coagulation activation by tissue factor expression. Downregulation of physiologic anticoagulant mechanisms and inhibition of fibrinolysis by endothelial cells further promotes intravascular fibrin deposition. PAI-1, plasminogen activator inhibitor-1.

factor (54), and once the thrombin forms, additional platelets are activated. The expression of P selectin on the platelet membrane not only mediates the adherence of platelets to leukocytes and endothelial cells but also enhances the expression of monocyte tissue factor (55), an effect that relies on nuclear factor κ-B (NFκB) activation. P selectin can be shed from the platelet membrane, and soluble P selectin levels have been shown to be increased during systemic inflammation (55).

## The Contact Activation Pathway

Contact system activation can be detected with sensitive assays for complexes of activated contact system factors and their inhibitors (56). However, the contact system is not important for sepsis-related activation of coagulation, as blocking monoclonal antibody against factor XIIa did not affect E. coli–induced coagulation abnormalities in baboons (57). Further, a murine model of streptococcal necrotizing fasciitis showed no coagulopathy or bleeding despite dramatically reduced factor XII and prekallikrein levels (58), and activation of factor XI in endotoxemic humans did not result in contact system activation (59). However, there is evidence that the contact system plays an important role in other pathophysiologic mechanisms, most importantly on the occurrence and severity of shock (57,60–63) and in fibrinolysis and complement activation in septic conditions (64). The mechanism by which the contact system affects blood pressure regulation is most likely dependent on the formation and release of bradykinin and other kinins upon activation of the kallikrein–kinin system.

## Impairment of the Antithrombin, Protein C, and Tissue Factor Pathway Inhibitor Anticoagulant Pathways

Activation of coagulation is regulated by three major anticoagulant pathways: antithrombin, the protein C system, and tissue factor pathway inhibitor (TFPI) (see Chapter 2). During sepsis-induced activation of coagulation, the function of all three pathways can be impaired (see Fig. 110-3).

*Antithrombin* is a serine protease inhibitor and the main inhibitor of thrombin and factor Xa. During severe inflammatory responses, antithrombin levels are markedly decreased due to consumption (as a result of ongoing thrombin generation), impaired synthesis (as a result of a negative acute-phase response), and degradation by elastase from activated neutrophils (65,66). A reduction in glycosaminoglycan availability at the endothelial surface, due to the influence of proinflammatory cytokines on endothelial synthesis, contributes to reduced antithrombin function because glycosaminoglycans act as physiologic heparinlike cofactors of antithrombin. Binding of glycosaminoglycans to antithrombin induces a conformational change at the reactive center of the antithrombin molecule, thereby converting it from a slow to an efficient inhibitor (67). Prospective clinical studies in patients at high risk for sepsis have shown that a marked decrease in levels of antithrombin precedes the clinical manifestation of the infection, which may indicate that antithrombin is involved in the early stages of coagulation activation during sepsis (68).

Endothelial dysfunction is even more important in the impairment of the *protein C* system during inflammation. Under

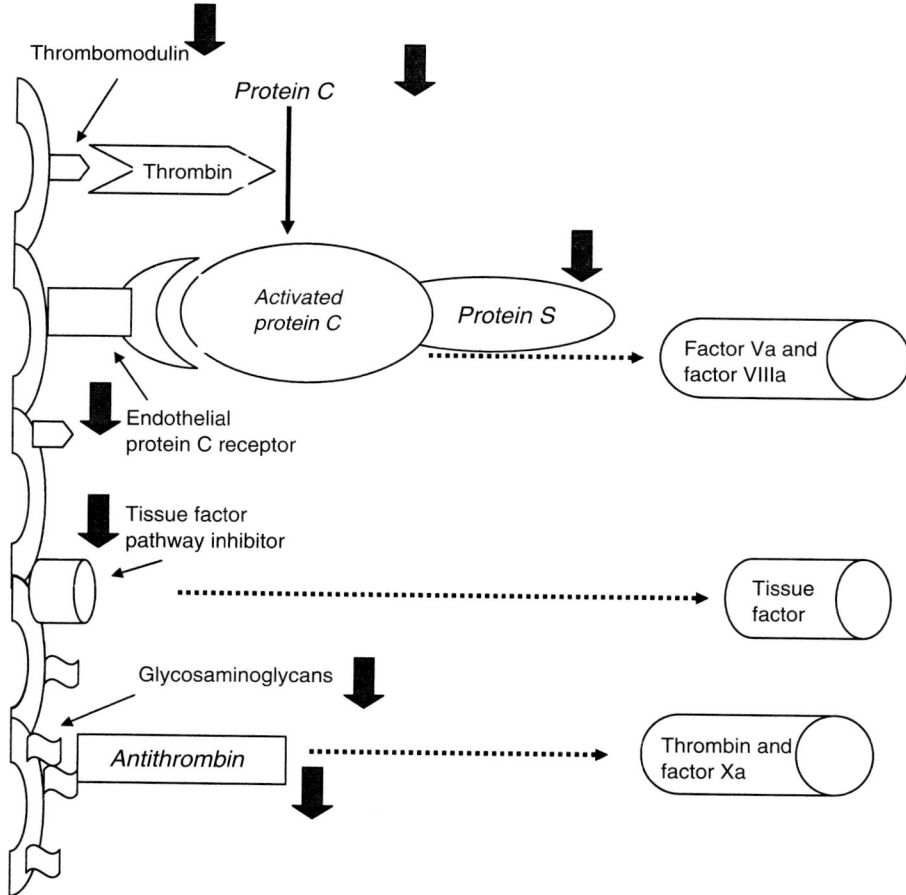

**FIGURE 110-3.** Schematic representation of the three important physiologic anticoagulant mechanisms and their point of impact in the coagulation system. In sepsis, these mechanisms are impaired by various means (*arrows*). The protein C system is dysfunctional because of low levels of zymogen protein C, downregulation of thrombomodulin and the endothelial protein C receptor, and low levels of free protein S caused by acute-phase–induced high levels of its binding protein, C4b-binding protein. There is a relative insufficiency of the endothelial cell–associated tissue factor pathway inhibitor. The antithrombin system is defective due to low levels of antithrombin and impaired glycosaminoglycan expression on perturbed endothelial cells.

physiologic conditions, protein C is activated by the thrombin bound to the endothelial cell thrombomodulin, a membrane protein with a lectinlike domain, six epidermal growth factor (EGF)-like repeats, a transmembrane domain, and a short cytoplasmic tail (69). Thrombin binding to thrombomodulin occurs of the EGF-repeats (70), results in a100-fold increase in the activation of protein C, and blocks the thrombin-mediated conversion of fibrinogen into fibrin and thrombin binding to platelets and inflammatory cells. Thrombomodulin also accelerates the activation of the plasma carboxypeptidase thrombin-activatable fibrinolysis inhibitor (TAFI), an important inhibitor of fibrinolysis (71). Activated protein C regulates coagulation by cleavage of the activated cofactors Va and VIIIa. Protein C binding to endothelial cell protein C receptor (EPCR) results in a fivefold augmentation of the activation of protein C by the thrombomodulin–thrombin complex (72). However, during severe inflammation, such as that occuring in sepsis, protein C concentration is decreased because of impaired synthesis (65) and degradation by neutrophil elastase (73). Further, the protein C system is defective due to downregulation of endothelial thrombomodulin, mediated by the proinflammatory cytokines TNF-α and IL-1β (74), as observed in patients with severe Gram-negative septicemia (75). In that study, histologic analysis of skin biopsies from patients with meningococcal sepsis showed decreased endothelial expression of thrombomodulin in vessels both with and without thrombosis. Low levels of free protein S (the cofactor of activated protein C) may further compromise an adequate function of the protein C system. Increased plasma levels of C4b-binding protein (C4bBP) as a consequence of the acute-phase reaction in inflammatory diseases may result in a relative free protein S deficiency. Although the β chain of C4bBP (which mainly governs the binding to protein S) is not affected during the acute-phase response (76), support from this hypothesis comes from studies showing that infusion of C4bBP increases organ dysfunction and mortality in baboons with sepsis (77). Animal experiments show that compromise of the protein C system results in increased morbidity and mortality, whereas restoring an adequate function of activated protein C improves survival and organ failure (78). Experiments in mice with a one-allele–targeted deletion of the protein C gene have more severe DIC and organ dysfunction and a higher mortality than wild-type littermates (79).

*TFPI* is a complex, multidomain, Kunitz-type protease inhibitor, which binds to the tissue factor–factor VIIa complex and to factor Xa (80). The role of TFPI in the regulation of inflammation-induced coagulation activation is not completely clear. Administration of recombinant TFPI blocks inflammation-induced thrombin generation in humans, and pharmacologic doses of TFPI are capable of preventing mortality during systemic infection and inflammation, suggesting that high concentrations of TFPI can modulate tissue factor–mediated coagulation (31,81). However, the endogenous concentration of TFPI is inadequate for regulating coagulation activation and downstream consequences during systemic inflammation, as has been confirmed in a clinical study of patients with sepsis (82,83).

## Inhibition of Endogenous Fibrinolysis

Experimental models indicate that at the time of maximal activation of coagulation in sepsis, the fibrinolytic system is largely shut off. The acute fibrinolytic response to inflammation is the release of plasminogen activators, particularly tissue-type plasminogen activator (tPA) and urokinase plasminogen activator (uPA), from storage sites in vascular endothelial cells. However, this increase in plasminogen activation and subsequent plasmin generation is counteracted by a delayed but sustained increase in plasminogen activator inhibitor, type 1 (PAI-1) (84,85). The resulting effect on fibrinolysis is complete

inhibition and, as a consequence, inadequate fibrin removal, thereby contributing to microvascular thrombosis. Mice with a deficiency of plasminogen activators have more extensive fibrin deposition in organs when challenged with endotoxin, whereas PAI-1 knockout mice, in contrast to wild-type controls, have no microvascular thrombosis upon endotoxin challenge (86,87). A functional mutation in the PAI-1 gene, the 4G/5G polymorphism, influences the plasma levels of PAI-1 and is linked to clinical outcome of meningococcal septicemia. Patients with the 4G/4G genotype have considerably higher PAI-1 concentrations in plasma and an increased risk of death (88). Further investigations demonstrate that the PAI-1 polymorphism does not influence the risk of contracting meningitis as such, but probably increases the likelihood of developing septic shock from meningococcal infection (89).

## Regulatory Role of Cytokines in the Coagulopathy

Most proinflammatory cytokines activate coagulation *in vitro*. In patients with sepsis, high levels of cytokines are detectable in the circulation, and experimental bacteremia or endotoxemia results in the transient enhancement of serum levels of these cytokines (90). TNF is detectable first, followed by an increase in circulating levels of interleukin-6 (IL-6), and IL 1 (IL-1). Since TNF is the first cytokine to appear in the circulation after infusion of bacteria or endotoxin and to exert potent procoagulant effects *in vitro*, it was initially thought that activation of coagulation was mediated by TNF, a hypothesis that was strengthened by studies in which patients with cancer or healthy human volunteers were injected with purified recombinant TNF (45,91). Following TNF injection, the observed activation of coagulation was virtually identical to endotoxin-induced effects. However, endotoxin-induced increase in TNF can be completely abolished, whereas activation of coagulation is unchanged (92,93), and treatment with an anti-TNF antibody in baboons infused with a lethal dose of *E. coli* had little or no effect on fibrinogen consumption (94). Moreover, clinical studies in patients with sepsis and with an anti-TNF monoclonal antibody did not show a beneficial effect (95). These observations made it necessary to reconsider the role of TNF as principal mediator of endotoxin-induced activation of coagulation. Monoclonal anti–IL-6 antibody results in the complete abrogation of endotoxin-induced activation of coagulation in chimpanzees (96), and studies in patients with cancer receiving recombinant IL-6 indicated that thrombin is generated by this cytokine (97). Therefore, these data suggest that IL-6 rather than TNF is relevant as a mediator for the induction of the procoagulant response in DIC. Although IL-1 is a potent agonist of tissue factor expression *in vitro*, its role has not been clarified *in vivo*. Administration of an IL-1 receptor antagonist partly blocked the procoagulant response in a sepsis model in baboons, and treatment of patients with an IL-1 receptor inhibitor reduced thrombin generation (98–100). However, most of the procoagulant changes after an endotoxin challenge occur well before IL-1 becomes detectable in the circulation, leaving its role in coagulation activation in sepsis unresolved. Infusion of recombinant antiinflammatory human IL-10 completely blocks endotoxin-induced changes in coagulation and fibrinolysis in human volunteers (101), but the relevance of this regulatory role of IL-10 remains to be established.

## Cross-talk Between Coagulation and Inflammation in Sepsis

Coagulation proteases and protease inhibitors interact not only with coagulation protein zymogens, but also with specific cell receptors to induce signaling pathways, interactions that are important in sepsis. Coagulation of whole blood *in vitro* results in IL-1$\beta$ mRNA expression in blood cells (102), and thrombin markedly enhances endotoxin-induced IL-1 activity in culture supernatants of guinea pig macrophages (103). Similarly, clotting blood produces IL-8 *in vitro* (104). Factor Xa, thrombin, and fibrin activate endothelial cells, eliciting the synthesis of IL-6 and/or IL-8 (105,106). The most important mechanisms by which coagulation proteases influence inflammation is by binding to protease-activated receptors (PARs), of which four types (PAR 1 to 4) have been identified, all belonging to the family of transmembrane domain, the G-protein-coupled receptors (107). A peculiar feature of PARs is that they serve as their own ligand. Proteolytic cleavage by an activated coagulation factor leads to exposure of a neo–amino-terminus that activates the same receptor, initiating transmembrane signaling. PARs 1, 3, and 4 are thrombin receptors, whereas PAR-2 is activated by the tissue factor–factor VIIa complex, factor Xa, and trypsin. PAR-1 can also serve as receptor of the tissue factor–factor VIIa complex and factor Xa. PARs are localized on endothelial cells, mononuclear cells, platelets, fibroblasts, and smooth muscle cells (107). Binding of thrombin to its cellular receptor may induce the production of several cytokines and growth factors. Binding of tissue factor–factor VIIa to PAR-2 also results in upregulation of inflammatory responses (production of reactive oxygen species and expression of major histocompatibility complex class II and cell adhesion molecules) in macrophages and affects neutrophil infiltration and proinflammatory cytokine (i.e., TNF-$\alpha$ and IL-1$\beta$) expression (108,109). *In vivo* evidence for a role of coagulation-protease stimulation of inflammation comes from experiments showing that the administration of recombinant factor VIIa to healthy human subjects causes a threefold to fourfold rise in plasma levels of IL-6 and IL-8 (110).

Fibrinogen and fibrin can directly stimulate expression of proinflammatory cytokines (such as TNF-$\alpha$ and IL-1$\beta$) on mononuclear cells and can induce production of chemokines (including IL-8 and MCP-1) by endothelial cells and fibroblasts (111). The effects of fibrin(ogen) on mononuclear cells are at least in part mediated by Toll-like receptor-4, which is also the receptor of endotoxin (112), and fibrinogen-deficient mice show inhibition of macrophage adhesion and less thrombin-mediated cytokine production *in vivo* (111).

There is also cross-talk between physiologic anticoagulant pathways and inflammatory mediators. Antithrombin can act as a mediator of inflammation, for example, by binding to neutrophils and by attenuating cytokine and chemokine receptor expression (113). In addition, the protein C system has an important function in modulating inflammation (69,114). Activated protein C inhibits endotoxin-induced production of TNF-$\alpha$, IL-1$\beta$, IL-6, and IL-8 by cultured monocytes/macrophages (115,116) and abrogates endotoxin-induced cytokine release and leukocyte activation in rats *in vivo* (117). Blocking the protein C pathway by monoclonal antibody in baboons with sepsis exacerbates the inflammatory response (118,119); conversely, administration of activated protein C abrogates inflammatory activity and improves organ function and survival in an experimental *E. coli* sepsis model in baboons (78), and it also improves organ function in models of endotoxin-induced shock and lung and kidney injury in rats (114). Mice with a one-allele-targeted disruption of the protein C gene have a more severe coagulation response to endotoxin and produce higher levels of circulating proinflammatory cytokines (79). The effects of activated protein C on inflammation are likely mediated by the EPCR, which may mediate downstream inflammatory processes (69). Binding of activated protein C to the EPCR affects gene expression profiles of cells by inhibiting endotoxin-induced calcium fluxes and by blocking NF$\kappa$B nuclear translocation, which is a prerequisite for increases in proinflammatory cytokines and adhesion molecules

(120,121). EPCR binding of activated protein C can result in activation of PAR-1 (122). Soluble EPCR, the extracellular domain of the cell-associated EPCR shed from the cell surface by the action of an inducible metalloproteinase (123), can bind to proteinase 3, with the resulting complex binding to the adhesion integrin macrophage 1 antigen (MAC-1) (124). Blocking EPCR with a specific monoclonal antibody aggravates both the coagulation and the inflammatory response to *E. coli* infusion (119). Activated protein C is capable of inhibiting endothelial cell apoptosis, which also seems to be mediated by binding of activated protein C to the EPCR and seems to require PAR-1 (125,126).

Thrombomodulin can also exert significant antiinflammatory activity by enhancing thrombin-induced activation of TAFI (71), which is the primary enzyme responsible for inactivation of complement factor C5a (127). Considering that thrombomodulin is abundantly present in the microcirculation, TAFI-mediated inactivation of C5a should protect against complement-mediated injury. The lectinlike domain of thrombomodulin has a function in inhibiting leukocyte adhesion to activated endothelium (128), and mice with a targeted deletion of the lectin domain display increased leukocyte tissue infiltration after injury caused by endotoxin inhalation.

# DIAGNOSTIC APPROACH TO COAGULATION ABNORMALITIES IN SEPSIS

Thrombocytopenia may be caused by other (sometimes simultaneously occurring) diseases, such as immune thrombocytopenia, medication-induced bone marrow depression, heparin-induced thrombocytopenia, or thrombotic microangiopathies (14,129) (see Table 110-1). It is important to properly diagnose these causes of thrombocytopenia because they may require distinctive treatment strategies (20). Laboratory tests can be helpful in differentiating the coagulopathy in sepsis from various other hemostatic disorders, such as vitamin K deficiency or liver failure. Since such conditions, however, may also occur simultaneously with, for example, DIC, this differentiation is not always simple (130).

## Tests for Intravascular Fibrin Formation and Fibrin Degradation Products

According to the current understanding of sepsis-associated coagulation abnormalities, the determination of soluble fibrin in plasma appears to be crucial (131–134), and clinical studies indicate that a diagnosis of DIC can be made if the concentration is more than a defined threshold (23,131,133,135). Most of the clinical studies show a sensitivity of 90% to 100% for the diagnosis of DIC but a rather low specificity (136) and a wide discordance among various assays (137).

Fibrin degradation products (FDPs) may be detected by specific enzyme-linked immunosorbent assays (ELISAs) or by latex agglutination assays, allowing for rapid and bedside determination (138). None of the available assays discriminates between degradation products of cross-linked fibrin and fibrinogen, a situation that may cause spuriously high results (139,140). The specificity of high levels of FDPs is therefore limited, and many other conditions, such as trauma, recent surgery, inflammation, or venous thromboembolism, are associated with elevated concentration of FDPs. More recently developed tests are aimed at the detection of neoantigens on degraded cross-linked fibrin, one of which detects an epitope related to plasmin-degraded cross-linked $\gamma$ chain, associated with D-dimer formation. These tests better differentiate degradation of cross-linked fibrin from fibrinogen or fibrinogen degradation products (141). D-dimer

**TABLE 110-1**

ROUTINE LABORATORY VALUE ABNORMALITIES IN PATIENTS WITH SEPSIS DUE TO DISSEMINATED INTRAVASCULAR COAGULATION (DIC) OR OTHER CAUSES

| Test | Abormality | Causes other than DIC contributing to test result |
|---|---|---|
| Platelet count | Decreased | Sepsis, impaired production, major blood loss, hypersplenism hematophagocytosis, immune thrombocytopenia, microangiopathy, heparin-induced thrombocytopenia |
| Prothrombin time | Prolonged | Vitamin K deficiency, liver failure, major blood loss |
| aPTT | Prolonged | Liver failure, heparin treatment, major blood loss |
| Fibrin degradation products | Elevated | Surgery, trauma, infection, hematoma |
| Protease inhibitors | Decreased | Liver failure, capillary leakage |

DIC, disseminated intravascular coagulation; aPTT, activated partial thromboplastin time.

levels are high in patients with DIC and these levels also poorly distinguish patients with DIC from patients with venous thromboembolism, recent surgery, or inflammatory conditions (138,142).

## Markers for Thrombin Generation and Coagulation Activation

Activation peptides that are released upon the conversion of a coagulation factor zymogen to an active protease are sensitive markers for coagulation activation. Examples of such markers are prothrombin activation fragment F1+2 and the activation peptides of factors IX and X (143–145). Elevated plasma concentrations of thrombin–antithrombin complexes may reflect the increased generation of thrombin, and thrombin–mediated conversion of fibrinogen to fibrin can be monitored by increased levels of fibrinopeptide A (146,147). The levels of these markers are increased in most patients with sepsis, and their high sensitivity may be helpful in detecting even low-grade disease. Specificity of these markers is probably limited because many other conditions may lead to elevated values, including artifacts attributed to venipuncture alone; these tests are generally limited to specialized coagulation laboratories.

## Platelet Count and Coagulation Factors

The platelet count in sepsis correlates with markers of thrombin generation because thrombin-induced platelet aggregation is to a large part responsible for platelet consumption (129). Since the normal platelet count may vary considerably, a single determination may not be instructive, but a continuous drop in platelet count, determined in patients with sepsis at intervals of about 4 hours, indicates thrombin generation causing intravascular platelet aggregation. Low levels of coagulation factors result from consumption, impaired synthesis, and loss of coagulation proteins, as from massive bleeding (148). Although the value of the measurement of one-stage clotting assays in DIC has been contested due to the presence of activated coagulation factors in plasma, the level of coagulation factors correlates with the severity of DIC (148). Plasma levels of factor VIII are paradoxically increased in most patients with DIC, probably due to release of von Willebrand factor from the endothelium in combination

with acute-phase increase of factor VIII (149). Measurement of fibrinogen levels is not helpful in diagnosing DIC in most cases (10), partly because fibrinogen is an acute-phase reactant and can remain well within the normal range despite ongoing consumption.

Plasma levels of physiologic coagulation inhibitors, such as antithrombin or protein C, are useful indicators of ongoing coagulation activation (36,68). Antithrombin is the principal inhibitor of thrombin and may be readily exhausted during continuous thrombin generation; the plasma level is a good predictor for survival in patients with sepsis and DIC (68). In patients with meningococcal septicemia, very low plasma levels of protein C may play a pivotal role in the pathogenesis of purpura fulminans (150,151), and plasma levels are strong predictors for outcome in patients with DIC (152).

## Diagnostic Management in a Routine Setting

Without a specialized laboratory, the diagnosis of DIC may be made by a combination of platelet count, PT, measurement of fibrinogen, and FDP (130). A scoring system utilizing such simple laboratory tests has been reviewed by the subcommittee on DIC of the International Society on Thrombosis and Haemostasis (153), and a five-step diagnostic algorithm to calculate a DIC score is summarized in Table 110-2, which is based partly on that of the Japanese Ministry of Health and Welfare (154). Tentatively, a score equal to or more than 5 is compatible with DIC, whereas a score of less than 5 may be indicative (but is *not* affirmative) of nonovert DIC. Initial prospective studies show that the sensitivity of the DIC score is 93%, and the specificity is 98% (155), but, importantly, the severity of DIC according to this scoring system is related to the mortality in patients with sepsis (see Fig. 110-4) (37).

# SUPPORTIVE TREATMENT OF COAGULATION ABNORMALITIES IN SEPSIS

The keystone of the treatment of hemostatic abnormalities in patients with sepsis is appropriate antibiotics and control of source of infection. However, in many cases additional treatment is required, aimed at circulatory and respiratory

## TABLE 110-2

### DIAGNOSTIC ALGORITHM FOR THE DIAGNOSIS OF OVERT DISSEMINATED INTRAVASCULAR COAGULATION

1. Risk assessment: Does the patient have an underlying disorder known to be associated with overt DIC?
   If yes, proceed; if no, do not use this algorithm
2. Order global coagulation tests (e.g., platelet count, PT, fibrinogen, soluble fibrin monomers, or fibrin degradation products)
3. Score global coagulation test results:
   - Platelet count (>100 = 0, <100 = 1, <50 = 2)
   - Elevated level of fibrin-related marker (e.g., soluble fibrin monomers/FDPs) (no increase: 0, moderate increase: 2, strong increase: 3)
   - Prolonged prothrombin time (<3 s = 0, >3 but <6 s = 1, >6 s = 2)
   - Fibrinogen level (>1.0 g/L = 0, <1.0 g/L = 1)
4. Calculate score
5. If ≥5: Compatible with overt DIC; repeat scoring daily
   If <5: Suggestive (not affirmative) for nonovert DIC; repeat scoring next 1–2 d

DIC, disseminated intravascular coagulation; PT, prothrombin time; FDPs, fibrin degradation products.

support, replacement of organ function, and management of the coagulation disorder.

## Plasma and Platelet Substitution Therapy

Low levels of platelets and coagulation factors may increase the risk of bleeding. However, plasma or platelet substitution therapy should not be instituted on the basis of laboratory results alone; it is indicated only in patients with active bleeding and in those requiring an invasive procedure, or in those who are otherwise at risk for bleeding complications (156). The suggestion that administration of blood components might "add fuel to the fire" has in fact never been proved in clinical or experimental studies. The presumed efficacy of treatment with plasma, fibrinogen, cryoprecipitate, or platelets is not based on randomized controlled trials but appears to be rational therapy in patients with bleeding or in patients at risk

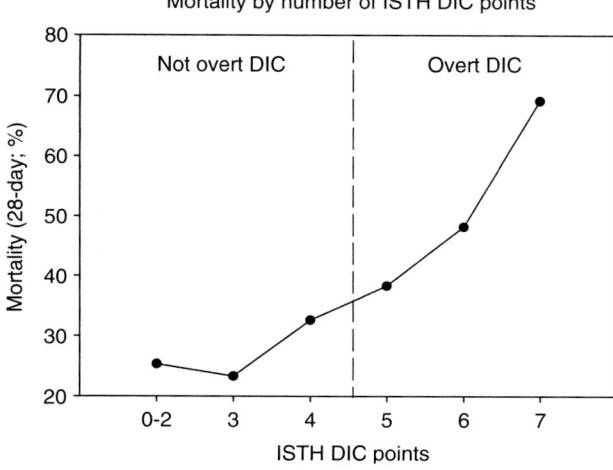

**FIGURE 110-4.** International Society on Thrombosis and Hemostasis (ISTH) disseminated intravascular coagulation (DIC) score relative to 28-day mortality in patients with severe sepsis. [Data were derived from the placebo group (*n* = 840) in the Prowess trial on the efficacy of activated protein C in sepsis [Bernard GR, Vincent JL, Laterre PF, et al. Efficacy and safety of recombinant human activated protein C for severe sepsis. *N Engl J Med* 2001;344(10):699–709].]

for bleeding with a significant depletion of these hemostatic factors (157). It may be necessary to use large volumes of plasma to correct the coagulation defect. Coagulation factor concentrates, such as prothrombin complex concentrate, may overcome this obstacle, but these compounds may lack essential factors, such as factor V. Moreover, the older literature cautions against the use of prothrombin complex concentrates in DIC because it may worsen the coagulopathy due to small traces of activated factors. It is, however, not clear whether this is still relevant for the concentrates that are currently in use. Specific deficiencies in coagulation factors may be corrected by administration of purified coagulation factor concentrates, and fibrinogen (and factor VIII) deficiency can be treated with single-donor cryoprecipitate.

## Anticoagulants

Experimental studies have shown that heparin can at least partly inhibit the activation of coagulation in sepsis (158). Uncontrolled case series in patients with sepsis and DIC have claimed to be successful. However, a beneficial effect of heparin on clinically important outcome events in patients with DIC has never been demonstrated in controlled clinical trials (159). Furthermore, the safety of heparin treatment is debatable in patients with DIC who are prone to bleeding. Therapeutic doses of heparin are indicated in patients with clinically overt thromboembolism or extensive fibrin deposition, such as purpura fulminans or acral ischemia. Patients with sepsis may benefit from prophylaxis to prevent venous thromboembolism, which may not be achieved with standard low-dose subcutaneous heparin (160). Theoretically, the most logical anticoagulant agent to use in DIC is directed against tissue factor activity. Potential agents include recombinant TFPI, inactivated factor VIIa, and recombinant NAPc2, a potent and specific inhibitor of the ternary complex between tissue factor/factor VIIa and factor Xa (161). Phase II trials of recombinant TFPI in patients with sepsis show promising results (162), but a recently completed phase III trial did not show an overall survival benefit in patients who were treated with TFPI (162,163).

## Restoration of Anticoagulant Pathways

In view of the deficient state of physiologic anticoagulant pathways in patients with sepsis, restoration of these natural inhibitors may be a rational approach (164). Because antithrombin is one of the most important physiologic inhibitors of coagulation and is based on successful preclinical results, antithrombin concentrates in patients with DIC have been studied in patients with sepsis, septic shock, or both. All trials show some beneficial effect in terms of improvement of laboratory parameters, shortening of the duration of DIC, or even improvement in organ function (10). In the more recent clinical trials, very high doses of antithrombin concentrate were used to attain supraphysiological plasma levels. Relatively small trials showed a modest reduction in mortality in patients treated with antithrombin (165–167); however, in none of the trials did the effect reach statistical significance. A large-scale, multicenter, randomized controlled trial to directly address this issue showed no significant reduction in mortality of patients with sepsis who were treated with antithrombin concentrate (168). Interestingly, *post hoc* subgroup analyses indicated some benefit in patients who did not receive concomitant heparin, but this observation needs prospective validation.

On the basis of the notion that depression of the protein C system may significantly contribute to the pathophysiology of DIC, supplementation of (activated) protein C is a rational approach (169). A beneficial effect of recombinant human activated protein C was demonstrated in two randomized controlled trials. In a dose-ranging clinical trial, 131 patients with sepsis (170) received activated protein C by continuous infusion at doses ranging from 12 $\mu$g/kg/hour to 30 $\mu$g/kg/hour, or placebo. On the basis of D-dimer plasma levels, the optimal dose of recombinant human-activated protein C was determined to be 24 $\mu$g/kg/hour, and there was a trend toward lower mortality (40% reduction) in patients receiving higher doses. The potential benefit of activated protein C was also shown for duration of mechanical ventilation, shock, and length of ICU stay, as well as for days free of systemic inflammatory response. A subsequent phase III trial of activated protein C concentrate in patients with sepsis was prematurely stopped when efficacy was documented for reducing mortality (25). All-cause mortality at 28 days was 24.7% in the activated protein C group versus 30.8% in the control group [19.4% relative risk reduction (RRR)]. The administration of activated protein C improved coagulation abnormalities and the treated patients had less organ failure (171). Part of the success has been ascribed to a beneficial effect on inflammatory pathways. A recent analysis of this trial demonstrated that patients who classify as having DIC, according to the DIC scoring system of the International Society on Thrombosis and Hemostasis (ISTH) (153), had a relatively greater benefit of activated protein C treatment than did patients who did not have overt DIC (RRR 38% vs. 18%) (37). This study underscores the importance of the coagulation derangement in the pathogenesis of sepsis and the point of impact that restoration of microvascular anticoagulant pathways may provide in the treatment of sepsis. Recombinant human-activated protein C has been licensed in most countries for treatment of patients with *severe sepsis* and two or more organ failures. The most frequently encountered adverse effect of activated protein C is bleeding. In the phase III study in patients with severe sepsis, the incidence of major bleeding (i.e., bleeding reported as a serious adverse event) during the infusion period was 2.4% in the activated protein C group as compared with 1.0% in the control group ($P = 0.02$) (25). During the 28-day study period, the incidence of major bleeding was 3.5% in the activated protein C group and 2.0% in the placebo group ($P = 0.06$). Gastrointestinal bleeding was the most frequently occurring bleeding complication in both groups. Most of the bleeding episodes were procedure-related or occurred in patients with a severely deranged coagulation system [aPTT >120 seconds or PT international normalized ratio (INR) >3.0], whereas spontaneous bleeding was rare. Of note, severe thrombocytopenia

(i.e., platelet count $< 50 \times 10^9$ per L) was an exclusion criterion for the trial, but patients with lower platelet count appeared to have had relatively more benefit of the administration of activated protein C than patients with higher platelet counts. Ongoing studies focus on the concomitant use of heparin in patients who receive activated protein C and the efficacy of activated protein C in patients with less severe sepsis.

---

## *References*

1. Wheeler AP, Bernard GR. Treating patients with severe sepsis. *N Engl J Med* 1999;340:207–214.
2. Martin GS, Mannino DM, Eaton S, et al. The epidemiology of sepsis in the United States from 1979 through 2000. *N Engl J Med* 2003;348: 1546–1554.
3. Angus DC, Linde-Zwirble WT, Lidicker J, et al. Epidemiology of severe sepsis in the United States: analysis of incidence, outcome, and associated costs of care. *Crit Care Med* 2001;29:1303–1310.
4. Levi M, ten Cate H, van der Poll T, et al. Pathogenesis of disseminated intravascular coagulation in sepsis. *JAMA* 1993;270:975–979.
5. Levi M, ten Cate H. Disseminated intravascular coagulation. *N Engl J Med* 1999;341:586–592.
6. Colman RW, Robboy SJ, Minna JD. Disseminated intravascular coagulation: a reappraisal. *Annu Rev Med* 1979;30:359–374.
7. Marder VJ, Feinstein D, Francis C. Consumptive thrombohemorrhagic disorders. In: Colman RW, Hirsh J, Marder VJ et al. eds. *Hemostasis and thrombosis. Basic principles and clinical practice.* Philadelphia, PA: JB Lippincott Co, 2001:1023–1063.
8. Levi M, van Gorp E, ten Cate H. Disseminated intravascular coagulation. In: Handin RI, Lux SE, Stossel TP, eds. *Blood: principles and practice of hematology.* Philadelphia, PA: JB Lippincott Co, 2002.
9. Miller DL, Welty-Wolf K, Carraway MS, et al. Extrinsic coagulation blockade attenuates lung injury and proinflammatory cytokine release after intratracheal lipopolysaccharide. *Am J Respir Cell Mol Biol* 2002;26: 650–658.
10. Levi M, ten Cate H, van der Poll T. Disseminated intravascular coagulation: state of the art. *Thromb Haemost* 1999;82:695–705.
11. Ratnoff OD, Nebehay WG. Multiple coagulative defects in a patient with the Waterhouse-Friderichsen syndrome. *Ann Intern Med* 1962;56:627.
12. Levi M, de Jonge E, van der Poll T. Sepsis and disseminated intravascular coagulation. *J Thromb Thrombolysis* 2003;16:43–47.
13. Vanderschueren S, De Weerdt A, Malbrain M, et al. Thrombocytopenia and prognosis in intensive care. *Crit Care Med* 2000;28:1871–1876.
14. Baughman RP, Lower EE, Flessa HC, et al. Thrombocytopenia in the intensive care unit. *Chest* 1993;104:1243–1247.
15. Strauss R, Wehler M, Mehler K, et al. Thrombocytopenia in patients in the medical intensive care unit: bleeding prevalence, transfusion requirements, and outcome. *Crit Care Med* 2002;30:1765–1771.
16. Akca S, Haji Michael P, de Medonca A, et al. The time course of platelet counts in critically ill patients. *Crit Care Med* 2002;30:753–756.
17. Mavrommatis AC, Theodoridis T, Orfanidou A, et al. Coagulation system and platelets are fully activated in uncomplicated sepsis. *Crit Care Med* 2000;28:451–457.
18. Folman CC, Linthorst GE, van Mourik J, et al. Platelets release thrombopoietin (Tpo) upon activation: another regulatory loop in thrombocytopoiesis? *Thromb Haemost* 2000;83:923–930.
19. Francois B, Trimoreau F, Vignon P, et al. Thrombocytopenia in the sepsis syndrome: role of hemophagocytosis and macrophage colony-stimulating factor. *Am J Med* 1997;103:114–120.
20. Warkentin TE, Aird WC, Rand JH, et al. Platelet-endothelial interactions: sepsis, HIT, and antiphospholipid syndrome. *Hematology (Am Soc Hematol Educ Program)* 2003:497–519.
21. Chakraverty R, Davidson S, Peggs K, et al. The incidence and cause of coagulopathies in an intensive care population. *Br J Haematol* 1996;93: 460–463.
22. MacLeod JB, Lynn M, McKenney MG, et al. Early coagulopathy predicts mortality in trauma. *J Trauma* 2003;55:39–44.
23. Shorr AF, Thomas SJ, Alkins SA, et al. D-dimer correlates with proinflammatory cytokine levels and outcomes in critically ill patients. *Chest* 2002; 121:1262–1268.
24. Owings JT, Gosselin RC, Anderson JT, et al. Practical utility of the D-dimer assay for excluding thromboembolism in severely injured trauma patients. *J Trauma* 2001;51:425–429.
25. Bernard GR, Vincent JL, Laterre PF, et al. Efficacy and safety of recombinant human activated protein C for severe sepsis. *N Engl J Med* 2001; 344(10):699–709.
26. Gando S, Nanzaki S, Sasaki S, et al. Significant correlations between tissue factor and thrombin markers in trauma and septic patients with disseminated intravascular coagulation. *Thromb Haemost* 1998;79:1111–1115.
27. Levi M, Keller TT, van Gorp E, et al. Infection and inflammation and the coagulation system. *Cardiovasc Res* 2003;60:26–39.

28. Robboy SJ, Major MC, Colman RW, et al. Pathology of disseminated intravascular coagulation (DIC). Analysis of 26 cases. *Human Pathol* 1972;3:327–343.

29. Shimamura K, Oka K, Nakazawa M, et al. Distribution patterns of microthrombi in disseminated intravascular coagulation. *Arch Pathol Lab Med* 1983;107:543–547.

30. Coalson JJ. Pathology of sepsis, septic shock, and multiple organ failure. *Perspective on sepsis and septic shock*. Fullerton, CA: Society of Critical Care Medicine, 1986:27–59.

31. Creasey AA, Chang AC, Feigen L, et al. Tissue factor pathway inhibitor reduces mortality from *Escherichia coli* septic shock. *J Clin Invest* 1993; 91:2850–2856.

32. Kessler CM, Tang Z, Jacobs HM, et al. The suprapharmacologic dosing of antithrombin concentrate for *Staphylococcus aureus*-induced disseminated intravascular coagulation in guinea pigs: substantial reduction in mortality and morbidity. *Blood* 1997;89:4393–4401.

33. Taylor FB Jr, Chang A, Ruf W, et al. Lethal *E. coli* septic shock is prevented by blocking tissue factor with monoclonal antibody. *Circ Shock* 1991;33: 127–134.

34. Taylor FB Jr, Chang A, Esmon CT, et al. Protein C prevents the coagulopathic and lethal effects of *Escherichia coli* infusion in the baboon. *J Clin Invest* 1987;79:918–925.

35. Welty-Wolf KE, Carraway MS, Miller DL, et al. Coagulation blockade prevents sepsis-induced respiratory and renal failure in baboons. *Am J Respir Crit Care Med* 2001;164:1988–1996.

36. Fourrier F, Chopin C, Goudemand J, et al. Septic shock, multiple organ failure, and disseminated intravascular coagulation. Compared patterns of antithrombin III, protein C, and protein S deficiencies [see comments]. *Chest* 1992;101:816–823.

37. Dhainaut JF, Yan SB, Joyce DE, et al. Treatment effects of drotrecogin alfa (activated) in patients with severe sepsis with or without overt disseminated intravascular coagulation. *J Thromb Haemost* 2004;2:1924–1933.

38. Oppenheim-Eden A, Glantz L, Eidelman LA, et al. Spontaneous intracerebral hemorrhage in critically ill patients: incidence over six years and associated factors. *Intensive Care Med* 1999;25:63–67.

39. Stephan F, Hollande J, Richard O, et al. Thrombocytopenia in a surgical ICU. *Chest* 1999;115:1363–1370.

40. Levi M, van der Poll T, ten Cate H, et al. The cytokine-mediated imbalance between coagulant and anticoagulant mechanisms in sepsis and endotoxaemia. *Eur J Clin Invest* 1997;27:3–9.

41. Levi M, van der Poll T, Buller HR. The bidirectional relationship between coagulation and inflammation. *Circulation* 2004;109:2698–2704.

42. Aird WC. Vascular bed-specific hemostasis: role of endothelium in sepsis pathogenesis. *Crit Care Med* 2001;29:S28–S34.

43. Kalter ES, Daha MR, ten CJ, et al. Activation and inhibition of Hageman factor-dependent pathways and the complement system in uncomplicated bacteremia or bacterial shock. *J Infect Dis* 1985;151:1019–1027.

44. van DS, Buller HR, ten CJ, et al. Experimental endotoxemia in humans: analysis of cytokine release and coagulation, fibrinolytic, and complement pathways. *Blood* 1990;76:2520–2526.

45. van der Poll T, Buller HR, ten Cate H, et al. Activation of coagulation after administration of tumor necrosis factor to normal subjects. *N Engl J Med* 1990;322:1622–1627.

46. Levi M, ten Cate H, Bauer KA, et al. Inhibition of endotoxin-induced activation of coagulation and fibrinolysis by pentoxifylline or by a monoclonal anti-tissue factor antibody in chimpanzees. *J Clin Invest* 1994;93: 114–120.

47. Biemond BJ, Levi M, ten CH, et al. Complete inhibition of endotoxin-induced coagulation activation in chimpanzees with a monoclonal Fab fragment against factor VII/VIIa. *Thromb Haemost* 1995;73:223–230.

48. Ruf W, Edgington TS. Structural biology of tissue factor, the initiator of thrombogenesis *in vivo*. *FASEB J* 1994;8:385–390.

49. Osterud B, Flaegstad T. Increased tissue thromboplastin activity in monocytes of patients with meningococcal infection: related to an unfavourable prognosis. *Thromb Haemost* 1983;49:5–7.

50. Franco RF, de JE, Dekkers PE, et al. The *in vivo* kinetics of tissue factor messenger RNA expression during human endotoxemia: relationship with activation of coagulation. *Blood* 2000;96:554–559.

51. Giesen PL, Rauch U, Bohrmann B, et al. Blood-borne tissue factor: another view of thrombosis. *Proc Natl Acad Sci U S A* 1999;96:2311–2315.

52. Osterud B, Rao LV, Olsen JO. Induction of tissue factor expression in whole blood—lack of evidence for the presence of tissue factor expression on granulocytes. *Thromb Haemost* 2000;83:861–867.

53. Rauch U, Bonderman D, Bohrmann B, et al. Transfer of tissue factor from leukocytes to platelets is mediated by CD15 and tissue factor. *Blood* 2000;96:170–175.

54. Zimmerman GA, McIntyre TM, Prescott SM, et al. The platelet-activating factor signaling system and its regulators in syndromes of inflammation and thrombosis. *Crit Care Med* 2002;30:S294–S301.

55. Shebuski RJ, Kilgore KS. Role of inflammatory mediators in thrombogenesis. *J Pharmacol Exp Ther* 2002;300:729–735.

56. Nuijens JH, Huijbregts CC, Eerenberg-Belmer AJ, et al. Quantification of plasma factor XIIa-Cl(-)-inhibitor and kallikrein-Cl(-)-inhibitor complexes in sepsis. *Blood* 1988;72:1841–1848.

57. Pixley RA, De LC, Page JD, et al. The contact system contributes to hypotension but not disseminated intravascular coagulation in lethal bacteremia.

58. Sriskandan S, Kemball-Cook G, Moyes D, et al. Contact activation in shock caused by invasive group A *Streptococcus pyogenes*. *Crit Care Med* 2000;28:3684–3691.

59. Minnema MC, Pajkrt D, Wuillemin WA, et al. Activation of clotting factor XI without detectable contact activation in experimental human endotoxemia. *Blood* 1998;92:3294–3301.

60. Colman RW, Schmaier AH. Contact system: a vascular biology modulator with anticoagulant, profibrinolytic, antiadhesive, and proinflammatory attributes. *Blood* 1997;90:3819–3843.

61. Levi M. Keep in contact: the role of the contact system in infection and sepsis. *Crit Care Med* 2000;28:3765–3766.

62. O'Donnell TF Jr, Clowes GH Jr, Talamo RC, et al. Kinin activation in the blood of patients with sepsis. *Surg Gynecol Obstet* 1976;143:539–545.

63. Kaufman N, Page JD, Pixley RA, et al. Alpha 2-macroglobulin-kallikrein complexes detect contact system activation in hereditary angioedema and human sepsis. *Blood* 1991;77:2660–2667.

64. Jansen PM, Pixley RA, Brouwer M, et al. Inhibition of factor XII in septic baboons attenuates the activation of complement and fibrinolytic systems and reduces the release of interleukin-6 and neutrophil elastase. *Blood* 1996;87:2337–2344.

65. Vary TC, Kimball SR. Regulation of hepatic protein synthesis in chronic inflammation and sepsis. *Am J Physiol* 1992;262:C445–C452.

66. Seitz R, Wolf M, Egbring R, et al. The disturbance of hemostasis in septic shock: role of neutrophil elastase and thrombin, effects of antithrombin III and plasma substitution. *Eur J Haematol* 1989;43:22–28.

67. Opal SM, Kessler CM, Roemisch J, et al. Antithrombin, heparin, and heparan sulfate. *Crit Care Med* 2002;30:S325–S331.

68. Mesters RM, Mannucci PM, Coppola R, et al. Factor VIIa and antithrombin III activity during severe sepsis and septic shock in neutropenic patients [see comments]. *Blood* 1996;88:881–886.

69. Esmon CT. New mechanisms for vascular control of inflammation mediated by natural anticoagulant proteins. *J Exp Med* 2002;196:561–564.

70. Zushi M, Gomi K, Yamamoto S, et al. The last three consecutive epidermal growth factor-like structures of human thrombomodulin comprise the minimum functional domain for protein C-activating cofactor activity and anticoagulant activity. *J Biol Chem* 1989;264:10351–10353.

71. Bajzar L, Morser J, Nesheim M. TAFI, or plasma procarboxypeptidase B, couples the coagulation and fibrinolytic cascades through the thrombin-thrombomodulin complex. *J Biol Chem* 1996;271:16603–16608.

72. Taylor FB Jr, Peer GT, Lockhart MS, et al. Endothelial cell protein C receptor plays an important role in protein C activation *in vivo*. *Blood* 2001;97:1685–1688.

73. Eckle I, Seitz R, Egbring R, et al. Protein C degradation *in vitro* by neutrophil elastase. *Biol Chem Hoppe Seyler* 1991;372:1007–1013.

74. Nawroth PP, Stern DM. Modulation of endothelial cell hemostatic properties by tumor necrosis factor. *J Exp Med* 1986;163:740–745.

75. Faust SN, Levin M, Harrison OB, et al. Dysfunction of endothelial protein C activation in severe meningococcal sepsis. *N Engl J Med* 2001;345(6): 408–416.

76. Garcia de Frutos P, Alim RI, Hardig Y, et al. Differential regulation of alpha and beta chains of C4b-binding protein during acute-phase response resulting in stable plasma levels of free anticoagulant protein S. *Blood* 1994;84:815–822.

77. Taylor F, Chang A, Ferrell G, et al. C4b-binding protein exacerbates the host response to *Escherichia coli*. *Blood* 1991;78:357–363.

78. Taylor FB Jr, Dahlback B, Chang AC, et al. Role of free protein S and C4b binding protein in regulating the coagulant response to *Escherichia coli*. *Blood* 1995;86:2642–2652.

79. Levi M, Dorffler-Melly J, Reitsma PH, et al. Aggravation of endotoxin-induced disseminated intravascular coagulation and cytokine activation in heterozygous protein C deficient mice. *Blood* 2003;101:4823–4827.

80. Broze GJ Jr, Girard TJ, Novotny WF, et al. Regulation of coagulation by a multivalent Kunitz-type inhibitor. *Biochemistry* 1990;29:7539–7546.

81. de Jonge E, Dekkers PE, Creasey AA, et al. Tissue factor pathway inhibitor (TFPI) dose-dependently inhibits coagulation activation without influencing the fibrinolytic and cytokine response during human endotoxemia. *Blood* 2000;95:1124–1129.

82. Gando S, Kameue T, Morimoto Y, et al. Tissue factor production not balanced by tissue factor pathway inhibitor in sepsis promotes poor prognosis. *Crit Care Med* 2002;30:1729–1734.

83. Levi M. The imbalance between tissue factor and tissue factor pathway inhibitor in sepsis. *Crit Care Med* 2002;30:1914–1915.

84. van der Poll T, Levi M, Buller HR, et al. Fibrinolytic response to tumor necrosis factor in healthy subjects. *J Exp Med* 1991;174:729–732.

85. Biemond BJ, Levi M, ten CH, et al. Plasminogen activator and plasminogen activator inhibitor I release during experimental endotoxaemia in chimpanzees: effect of interventions in the cytokine and coagulation cascades. *Clin Sci (Colch)* 1995;88:587–594.

86. Yamamoto K, Loskutoff DJ. Fibrin deposition in tissues from endotoxin-treated mice correlates with decreases in the expression of urokinase-type but not tissue-type plasminogen activator. *J Clin Invest* 1996;97: 2440–2451.

87. Pinsky DJ, Liao H, Lawson CA, et al. Coordinated induction of plasminogen activator inhibitor-1 (PAI-1) and inhibition of plasminogen activator

gene expression by hypoxia promotes pulmonary vascular fibrin deposition. *J Clin Invest* 1998;102:919–928.

88. Hermans PW, Hibberd ML, Booy R, et al. 4G/5G promoter polymorphism in the plasminogen-activator-inhibitor-1 gene and outcome of meningococcal disease. Meningococcal research group. *Lancet* 1999;354:556–560.

89. Westendorp RG, Hottenga JJ, Slagboom PE. Variation in plasminogen-activator-inhibitor-1 gene and risk of meningococcal septic shock. *Lancet* 1999;354:561–563.

90. Hack CE, Aarden LA, Thijs LG. Role of cytokines in sepsis. *Adv Immunol* 1997;66:101–195.

91. Bauer KA, ten CH, Barzegar S, et al. Tumor necrosis factor infusions have a procoagulant effect on the hemostatic mechanism of humans. *Blood* 1989;74:165–172.

92. van der Poll T, Levi M, van Deventer SJ, et al. Differential effects of anti-tumor necrosis factor monoclonal antibodies on systemic inflammatory responses in experimental endotoxemia in chimpanzees. *Blood* 1994;83:446–451.

93. van der Poll T, Coyle SM, Levi M, et al. Effect of a recombinant dimeric tumor necrosis factor receptor on inflammatory responses to intravenous endotoxin in normal humans. *Blood* 1997;89:3727–3734.

94. Hinshaw LB, Tekamp-Olson P, Chang AC, et al. Survival of primates in LD100 septic shock following therapy with antibody to tumor necrosis factor (TNF alpha). *Circ Shock* 1990;30:279–292.

95. Abraham E, Wunderink R, Silverman H et al. TNF-alpha MAb Sepsis Study Group. Efficacy and safety of monoclonal antibody to human tumor necrosis factor alpha in patients with sepsis syndrome. A randomized, controlled, double-blind, multicenter clinical trial. *JAMA* 1995;273:934–941.

96. van der Poll T, Levi M, Hack CE, et al. Elimination of interleukin 6 attenuates coagulation activation in experimental endotoxemia in chimpanzees. *J Exp Med* 1994;179:1253–1259.

97. Stouthard JM, Levi M, Hack CE, et al. Interleukin-6 stimulates coagulation, not fibrinolysis, in humans. *Thromb Haemost* 1996;76:738–742.

98. Fischer E, Marano MA, Van Zee KJ, et al. Interleukin-1 receptor blockade improves survival and hemodynamic performance in *Escherichia coli* septic shock, but fails to alter host responses to sublethal endotoxemia. *J Clin Invest* 1992;89:1551–1557.

99. Jansen PM, Boermeester MA, Fischer E, et al. Contribution of interleukin-1 to activation of coagulation and fibrinolysis, neutrophil degranulation, and the release of secretory-type phospholipase A2 in sepsis: studies in nonhuman primates after interleukin-1 alpha administration and during lethal bacteremia. *Blood* 1995;86:1027–1034.

100. Boermeester MA, van LP, Coyle SM, et al. Interleukin-1 blockade attenuates mediator release and dysregulation of the hemostatic mechanism during human sepsis. *Arch Surg* 1995;130:739–748.

101. Pajkrt D, van der Poll T, Levi M, et al. Interleukin-10 inhibits activation of coagulation and fibrinolysis during human endotoxemia. *Blood* 1997;89:2701–2705.

102. Mileno MD, Margolis NH, Clark BD, et al. Coagulation of whole blood stimulates interleukin-1 beta gene expression. *J Infect Dis* 1995;172:308–311.

103. Jones A, Geczy CL. Thrombin and factor Xa enhance the production of interleukin-1. *Immunology* 1990;71:236–241.

104. Johnson K, Choi Y, DeGroot E, et al. Potential mechanisms for a proinflammatory vascular cytokine response to coagulation activation. *J Immunol* 1998;161:5130–5135.

105. Sower LE, Froelich CJ, Carney DH, et al. Thrombin induces IL-6 production in fibroblasts and epithelial cells. Evidence for the involvement of the seven-transmembrane domain (STD) receptor for alpha-thrombin. *J Immunol* 1995;155:895–901.

106. van der Poll T, de Jonge E, Levi M. Regulatory role of cytokines in disseminated intravascular coagulation. *Semin Thromb Hemost* 2001;27:639–651.

107. Coughlin SR. Thrombin signalling and protease-activated receptors. *Nature* 2000;407:258–264.

108. Cunningham MA, Romas P, Hutchinson P, et al. Tissue factor and factor VIIa receptor/ligand interactions induce proinflammatory effects in macrophages. *Blood* 1999;83:3413–3420.

109. Cenac N, Coelho AM, Nguyen C, et al. Induction of intestinal inflammation in mouse by activation of proteinase-activated receptor-2. *Am J Pathol* 2002;161:1903–1915.

110. de Jonge E, Friederich PW, Levi M, et al. Activation of coagulation by administration of recombinant factor VIIa elicits interleukin-6 and interleukin-8 release in healthy human subjects. *Clin Diagn Lab Immunol* 2003;10:495–497.

111. Szaba FM, Smiley ST. Roles for thrombin and fibrin(ogen) in cytokine/chemokine production and macrophage adhesion in vivo. *Blood* 2002;99:1053–1059.

112. Smiley ST, King JA, Hancock WW. Fibrinogen stimulates macrophage chemokine secretion through toll-like receptor 4. *J Immunol* 2001;167:2887–2894.

113. Kaneider NC, Forster E, Mosheimer B, et al. Syndecan-4-dependent signaling in the inhibition of endotoxin-induced endothelial adherence of neutrophils by antithrombin. *Thromb Haemost* 2003;90:1150–1157.

114. Okajima K. Regulation of inflammatory responses by natural anticoagulants. *Immunol Rev* 2001;184:258–274.

115. Grey ST, Tsuchida A, Hau H, et al. Selective inhibitory effects of the anticoagulant activated protein C on the responses of human mononuclear phagocytes to LPS, IFN-gamma, or phorbol ester. *J Immunol* 1994;153:3664–3672.

116. Yuksel M, Okajima K, Uchiba M, et al. Activated protein C inhibits lipopolysaccharide-induced tumor necrosis factor-alpha production by inhibiting activation of both nuclear factor-kappa B and activator protein-1 in human monocytes. *Thromb Haemost* 2002;88:267–273.

117. Murakami K, Okajima K, Uchiba M, et al. Activated protein C attenuates endotoxin-induced pulmonary vascular injury by inhibiting activated leukocytes in rats. *Blood* 1996;87:642–647.

118. Taylor FB Jr. Studies on the inflammatory-coagulant axis in the baboon response to *E. coli*: regulatory roles of proteins C, S, C4bBP and of inhibitors of tissue factor. [Review] [13 refs]. *Prog Clin Biol Res* 1994;388:175–194.

119. Taylor FB Jr, Stearns-Kurosawa DJ, Kurosawa S, et al. The endothelial cell protein C receptor aids in host defense against *Escherichia coli* sepsis. *Blood* 2000;95:1680–1686.

120. White B, Schmidt M, Murphy C, et al. Activated protein C inhibits lipopolysaccharide-induced nuclear translocation of nuclear factor kappaB (NF-kappaB) and tumour necrosis factor alpha (TNF-alpha) production in the THP-1 monocytic cell line. *Br J Haematol* 2000;110:130–134.

121. Hancock WW, Grey ST, Hau L, et al. Binding of activated protein C to a specific receptor on human mononuclear phagocytes inhibits intracellular calcium signaling and monocyte-dependent proliferative responses. *Transplantation* 1995;60:1525–1532.

122. Riewald M, Petrovan RJ, Donner A, et al. Activation of endothelial cell protease activated receptor 1 by the protein C pathway. *Science* 2002;296:1880–1882.

123. Xu J, Qu D, Esmon NL, et al. Metalloproteolytic release of endothelial cell protein C receptor. *J Biol Chem* 2000;275:6038–6044.

124. Kurosawa S, Esmon CT, Stearns-Kurosawa DJ. The soluble endothelial protein C receptor binds to activated neutrophils: involvement of proteinase-3 and CD11b/CD18. *J Immunol* 2000;165:4697–4703.

125. Cheng T, Liu D, Griffin JH, et al. Activated protein C blocks p53-mediated apoptosis in ischemic human brain endothelium and is neuroprotective. *Nat Med* 2003;9:338–342.

126. Mosnier LO, Griffin JH. Inhibition of staurosporine-induced apoptosis of endothelial cells by activated protein C requires protease activated receptor-1 and endothelial cell protein C receptor. *Biochem J* 2003;373(Pt 1):65–70.

127. Campbell W, Okada N, Okada H. Carboxypeptidase R is an inactivator of complement-derived inflammatory peptides and an inhibitor of fibrinolysis. *Immunol Rev* 2001;180:162–167.

128. Conway EM, Van de WM, Pollefeyt S, et al. The lectin-like domain of thrombomodulin confers protection from neutrophil-mediated tissue damage by suppressing adhesion molecule expression via nuclear factor kappaB and mitogen-activated protein kinase pathways. *J Exp Med* 2002;196:565–577.

129. Neame PB, Kelton JG, Walker IR, et al. Thrombocytopenia in septicemia: the role of disseminated intravascular coagulation. *Blood* 1980;56:88–92.

130. Levi M, de Jonge E, Meijers J. The diagnosis of disseminated intravascular coagulation. *Blood Rev* 2002;16:217–223.

131. Dempfle CE, Pfitzner SA, Dollman M, et al. Comparison of immunological and functional assays for measurement of soluble fibrin. *Thromb Haemost* 1995;74:673–679.

132. Bredbacka S, Blomback M, Wiman B. Soluble fibrin: a predictor for the development and outcome of multiple organ failure. *Am J Hematol* 1994;46:289–294.

133. Okajima K, Uchiba M, Murakami K, et al. Determination of plasma soluble fibrin using a new ELISA method in patients with disseminated intravascular coagulation. *Am J Hematol* 1996;51:186–191.

134. McCarron BI, Marder VJ, Kanouse JJ, et al. A soluble fibrin standard: comparable dose-response with immunologic and functional assays. *Thromb Haemost* 1999;82:145–148.

135. Dempfle CE. The use of soluble fibrin in evaluating the acute and chronic hypercoagulable state. *Thromb Haemost* 1999;82:673–683.

136. Horan JT, Francis CW. Fibrin degradation products, fibrin monomer and soluble fibrin in disseminated intravascular coagulation. *Semin Thromb Hemost* 2001;27(6):657–666.

137. McCarron BI, Marder VJ, Francis CW. Reactivity of soluble fibrin assays with plasmic degradation products of fibrin and in patients receiving fibrinolytic therapy. *Thromb Haemost* 1999;82:1722–1729.

138. Carr JM, McKinney M, McDonagh J. Diagnosis of disseminated intravascular coagulation. Role of D-dimer. *Am J Clin Pathol* 1989;91:280–287.

139. Boisclair MD, Ireland H, Lane DA. Assessment of hypercoagulable states by measurement of activation fragments and peptides. *Blood Rev* 1990;4:25–40.

140. Prisco D, Paniccia R, Bonechi F, et al. Evaluation of new methods for the selective measurement of fibrin and fibrinogen degradation products. *Thromb Res* 1989;56:547–551.

141. Shorr AF, Trotta RF, Alkins SA, et al. D-dimer assay predicts mortality in critically ill patients without disseminated intravascular coagulation or venous thromboembolic disease. *Intensive Care Med* 1999;25:207–210.

142. Greenberg CS, Devine DV, McCrae KM. Measurement of plasma fibrin D-dimer levels with the use of a monoclonal antibody coupled to latex beads. *Am J Clin Pathol* 1987;87:94–100.

143. Teitel JM, Bauer KA, Lau HK, et al. Studies of the prothrombin activation pathway utilizing radioimmunoassays for the F2/F1 + 2 fragment and thrombin—antithrombin complex. *Blood* 1982;59:1086–1097.

144. Bauer KA, Kass BL, Ten CH, et al. Detection of factor X activation in humans. *Blood* 1989;74:2007–2015.

145. ten Cate H, Bauer KA, Levi M, et al. The activation of factor X and prothrombin by recombinant factor VIIa *in vivo* is mediated by tissue factor. *J Clin Invest* 1993;92:1207–1212.

146. Takahashi H, Wada K, Niwano H, et al. Comparison of prothrombin fragment 1 + 2 with thrombin-antithrombin III complex in plasma of patients with disseminated intravascular coagulation. *Blood Coagul Fibrinolysis* 1992;3:813–818.

147. Kario K, Matsuo T, Kodama K, et al. Imbalance between thrombin and plasmin activity in disseminated intravascular coagulation. Assessment by the thrombin-antithrombin-III complex/plasmin-alpha-2-antiplasmin complex ratio. *Haemostasis* 1992;22:179–186.

148. Bick RL. Disseminated intravascular coagulation: objective clinical and laboratory diagnosis, treatment, and assessment of therapeutic response. *Semin Thromb Hemost* 1996;22:69–88.

149. Hesselvik JF, Blomback M, Brodin B, et al. Coagulation, fibrinolysis, and kallikrein systems in sepsis: relation to outcome. *Crit Care Med* 1989; 17:724–733.

150. Fijnvandraat K, Derkx B, Peters M, et al. Coagulation activation and tissue necrosis in meningococcal septic shock: severely reduced protein C levels predict a high mortality. *Thromb Haemost* 1995;73:15–20.

151. Wuillemin WA, Fijnvandraat K, Derkx BH, et al. Activation of the intrinsic pathway of coagulation in children with meningococcal septic shock. *Thromb Haemost* 1995;74:1436–1441.

152. Mesters RM, Helterbrand J, Utterback BG, et al. Prognostic value of protein C concentrations in neutropenic patients at high risk of severe septic complications. *Crit Care Med* 2000;28:2209–2216.

153. Taylor FB Jr, Toh CH, Hoots WK, et al. Towards definition, clinical and laboratory criteria, and a scoring system for disseminated intravascular coagulation. *Thromb Haemost* 2001;86:1327–1330.

154. Wada H, Wakita Y, Nakase T, et al. Mie DIC Study Group. Outcome of disseminated intravascular coagulation in relation to the score when treatment was begun. *Thromb Haemost* 1995;74:848–852.

155. Bakhtiari K, Meijers JC, de Jonge E, et al. Prospective validation of the International Society of Thrombosis and Maemostasis scoring system for disseminated intravascular coagulation. *Crit Care Med* 2004;32:2416–2421.

156. Alving BM, Spivak JL, DeLoughery TG. Consultative hematology: hemostasis and transfusion issues in surgery and critical care medicine. In: McArthur JR, Schechter GP, Schrier SL, eds. *Hematology 1998 (The American Society of Hematology Education Program Book)*. Washington: The American Society of Hematology. 1998:320–341.

157. de Jonge E, Levi M, Stoutenbeek CP, et al. Current drug treatment strategies for disseminated intravascular coagulation. *Drugs* 1998;55:767–777.

158. du Toit H, Coetzee AR, Chalton DO. Heparin treatment in thrombin-induced disseminated intravascular coagulation in the baboon. *Crit Care Med* 1991;19:1195–1200.

159. Feinstein DI. Diagnosis and management of disseminated intravascular coagulation: the role of heparin therapy. *Blood* 1982;60:284–287.

160. Dorffler-Melly J, de Jonge E, Pont AC, et al. Bioavailability of subcutaneous low-molecular-weight heparin to patients on vasopressors. *Lancet* 2002;359:849–850.

161. Vlasuk GP, Bergum PW, Bradbury AE, et al. Clinical evaluation of rNAPc2, an inhibitor of the fVIIa/tissue factor coagulation complex. *Am J Cardiol* 1997;80:66S.

162. Abraham E, Reinhart K, Svoboda P, et al. Assessment of the safety of recombinant tissue factor pathway inhibitor in patients with severe sepsis: a multicenter, randomized, placebo-controlled, single-blind, dose escalation study. *Crit Care Med* 2001;29:2081–2089.

163. Abraham E, Reinhart K, Opal S, et al. Efficacy and safety of tifacogin (recombinant tissue factor pathway inhibitor) in severe sepsis: a randomized controlled trial. *JAMA* 2003;290:238–247.

164. de Jonge E, van der Poll T, Kesecioglu J, et al. Anticoagulant factor concentrates in disseminated intravascular coagulation: rationale for use and clinical experience. *Semin Thromb Hemost* 2001;27:667–674.

165. Fourrier F, Chopin C, Huart JJ, et al. Double-blind, placebo-controlled trial of antithrombin III concentrates in septic shock with disseminated intravascular coagulation. *Chest* 1993;104:882–888.

166. Eisele B, Lamy M, Thijs LG, et al. Antithrombin III in patients with severe sepsis. A randomized, placebo-controlled, double-blind, multicenter trial plus a meta-analysis on all randomized, placebo-controlled, double-blind trials with antithrombin III in severe sepsis [see comments]. *Intensive Care Med* 1998;24:663–672.

167. Baudo F, Caimi TM, de CF, et al. Antithrombin III (ATIII) replacement therapy in patients with sepsis and/or postsurgical complications: a controlled double-blind, randomized, multicenter study [see comments]. *Intensive Care Med* 1998;24:336–342.

168. Warren BL, Eid A, Singer P, et al. Caring for the critically ill patient. High-dose antithrombin III in severe sepsis: a randomized controlled trial. *JAMA* 2001;286:1869–1878.

169. Levi M, de Jonge E, van der Poll T. Rationale for restoration of physiological anticoagulant pathways in patients with sepsis and disseminated intravascular coagulation. *Crit Care Med* 2001;29:S90–S94.

170. Bernard GR, Ely EW, Wright TJ, et al. Safety and dose relationship of recombinant human activated protein C for coagulopathy in severe sepsis. *Crit Care Med* 2001;29:2051–2059.

171. Vincent JL, Angus DC, Artigas A, et al. Effects of drotrecogin alfa (activated) on organ dysfunction in the PROWESS trial. *Crit Care Med* 2003;31:834–840.

# CHAPTER 111 ■ THROMBOTIC THROMBOCYTOPENIC PURPURA–HEMOLYTIC UREMIC SYNDROME

JAMES N. GEORGE, SARA K. VESELY, AND BERNHARD LÄMMLE

Thrombotic thrombocytopenic purpura (TTP) (1,2) and the hemolytic uremic syndrome (HUS) (3,4) were described initially as distinct disorders. Although they are distinct in their most typical presentations, TTP in adults with severe acquired ADAMTS13 (A Disintegrin And Metalloprotease with ThromboSpondin 1–like domains) deficiency and typical HUS in children preceded by a prodrome of bloody diarrhea, in many patients this distinction is not apparent. TTP is often said to have more severe neurologic abnormalities and HUS more severe renal failure. However, even among children with typical HUS whose primary abnormality is acute renal failure, 15% to 25% have severe neurologic abnormalities (5–7). Many adult patients have both severe neurologic abnormalities and acute renal failure, or neither (8). Therefore, in adult patients it may be appropriate to consider TTP and HUS as a single clinical syndrome described as TTP–HUS.

Pathologic abnormalities are similar in TTP and HUS; thrombi in terminal arterioles and capillaries are characteristic of both disorders (see Fig. 111-1) (9,10). Furthermore, these pathologic features are not specific for TTP–HUS but are also present in patients with malignant hypertension, scleroderma, antiphospholipid antibody syndrome, acute renal allograft rejection, and severe preeclampsia and the HELLP syndrome (9). Because clinical features of these other conditions may also be similar to TTP–HUS, a definitive diagnosis at the time of initial presentation may not be possible.

The presenting clinical features in adults and outcomes with plasma exchange treatment are not different across the spectrum of idiopathic TTP and HUS (11–13), except that patients presenting with acute renal failure have less risk for relapse and a greater risk for persistent renal failure (8). In young children with typical HUS who present following a prodrome of hemorrhagic colitis, usually caused by *Escherichia coli* (*E. coli*) 0157:H7, supportive care without plasma exchange is the conventional management. However, even in these children, a benefit from plasma exchange treatment for decreasing death and chronic renal failure has been suggested (14). When elderly persons have a syndrome of TTP or HUS following *E. coli* 0157:H7 colitis, mortality is high, similar to other presentations of TTP–HUS in adults, and plasma exchange is the conventional management and appears to be associated with increased survival (15).

The issues of definition and diagnosis of TTP–HUS are even more difficult in our current era of effective treatment. The definition of TTP–HUS has changed since the original descriptions (1,3) and the classic review in 1966 (16), which defined the pentad of clinical features: (a) microangiopathic hemolytic anemia, (b) thrombocytopenia, (c) neurologic symptoms and signs, (d) renal function abnormalities, and (e) fever. In that review (16), the diagnosis of TTP was supported by pathologic demonstration of hyaline thrombi (Fig. 111-1) in 93% of patients; 90% of the patients died. In the last 30 years, the availability of curative plasma exchange treatment (11,17) has created an urgency for establishing the diagnosis, which in turn has resulted in less stringent diagnostic criteria (13). Now only the criteria of thrombocytopenia and microangiopathic hemolytic anemia without another clinically apparent cause are sufficient to establish the diagnosis of TTP–HUS (11,13). Decreased stringency of diagnostic criteria have led inevitably to an increased frequency of diagnosis (18) and therefore to a broader clinical spectrum of disorders for which plasma exchange treatment is considered.

A current classification of presenting clinical features and disease associations is presented in Table 111-1. This classification has value to define patients according to the clinical setting in which they initially present. However, patients in these categories are often not distinct, and also, these disorders have changed over time. Epidemic HUS in young children, typically 2 to 5 years old, is different from the original description of HUS in 1955 (3). Descriptions of what is currently the most common childhood syndrome only began in 1982 with the recognition of preceding hemorrhagic colitis caused by Shiga-toxin-producing *E. coli* (typically *E. coli* 0157:H7) (19–21).

This chapter focuses on TTP–HUS in adults, initially describing adults who present without clinically apparent underlying or associated condition and who are described as idiopathic in Table 111-1. Specific characteristics of the TTP–HUS syndromes that are associated with other conditions and apparent etiologies are discussed in subsequent sections.

## PATHOGENESIS

von Willebrand factor (VWF) abnormalities are central to the pathogenesis of TTP in many patients (22,23). VWF, a multimeric glycoprotein synthesized by endothelial cells and megakaryocytes (see Chapter 46), is secreted by endothelial cells into the plasma, where it is processed into smaller multimers that do not spontaneously interact with circulating platelets. Reactivity with platelets correlates with VWF multimer size, with larger multimers being more reactive. In 1982, Moake et al. observed unusually large VWF multimers in the plasma of patients with chronic relapsing TTP (24), which were comparable in size to the unprocessed VWF found

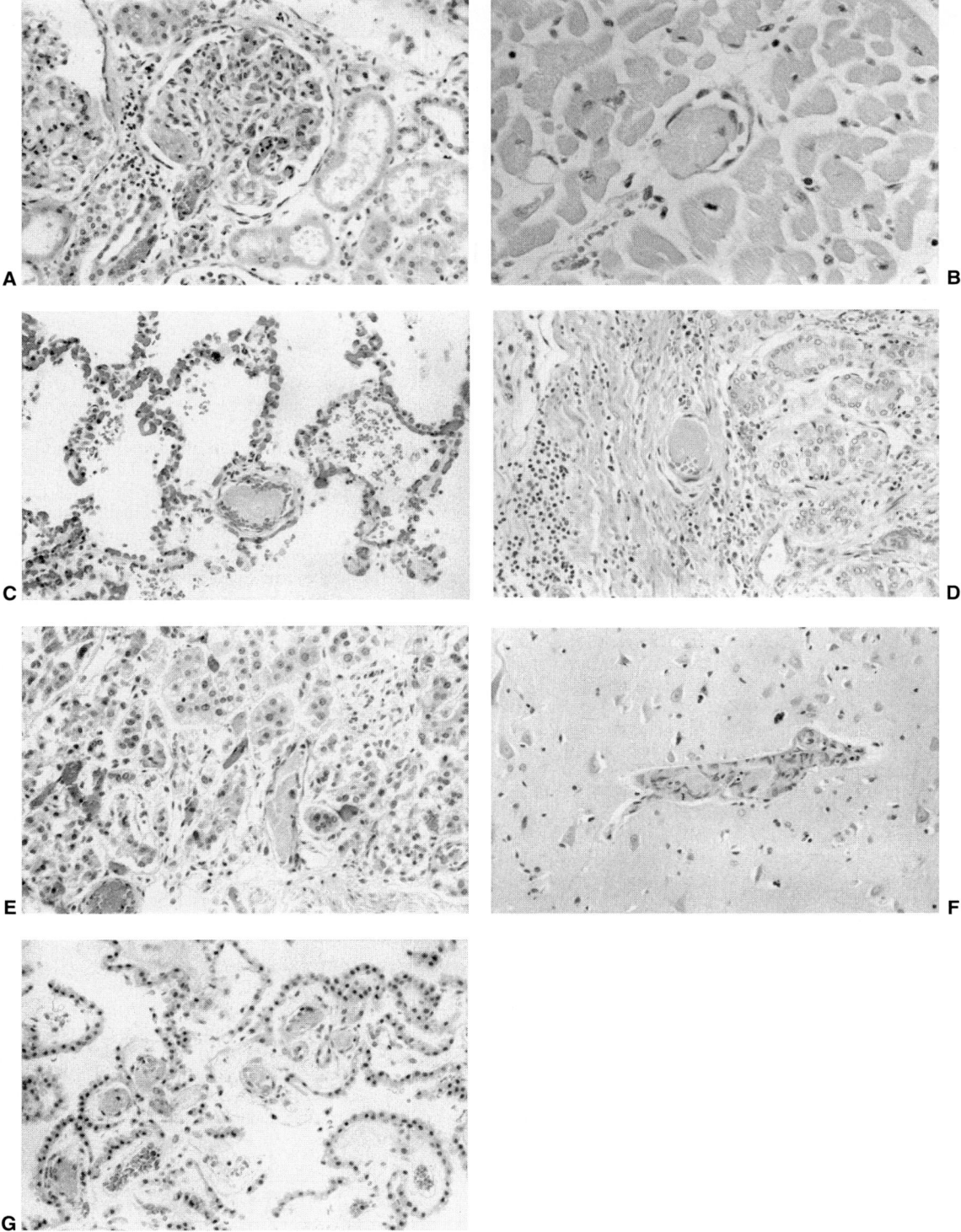

**FIGURE 111-1.** Hyaline thrombi in thrombotic thrombocytopenic purpura (TTP). These autopsy tissue sections are from a 30-year-old previously healthy man, who became ill with 3 days of abdominal pain, nausea, and vomiting followed by severe confusion. TTP was diagnosed on admission to the hospital on May 4, 1999, on the basis of platelet count 11,000/$\mu$L, hematocrit 21%, lactate dehydrogenase (LDH) 2231 U/L, creatinine 1.0 mg per dL, urinalysis with proteinuria and hematuria, but no fever. He received three plasma exchange treatments plus prednisone but died with grand mal seizures and cardiopulmonary arrest, 60 hours after hospital admission. Tissue sections demonstrate: (**A**) kidney afferent arteriole and glomerular capillary thrombi; (**B**) myocardial thrombi; (**C**) pulmonary thrombi; (**D**) gastric submucosal thrombi; (**E**) adrenal thrombi; (**F**) cerebral thrombi; and (**G**) thrombi in the choroid plexus. (Photographs by Zoltan Laszik, M.D., Department of Pathology, University of Oklahoma).

## TABLE 111-1

THROMBOTIC THROMBOCYTOPENIC PURPURA–HEMOLYTIC UREMIC SYNDROME: A CLASSIFICATION OF THE SYNDROMES AND THEIR CLINICAL FEATURES

**CONGENITAL**

| | |
|---|---|
| *ADAMTS13* mutation | Severe congenital ADAMTS13 deficiency; may present as neonatal hemolysis and thrombocytopenia, or may not be apparent until adulthood; plasma infusion is effective treatment; can result in end-stage renal disease |
| *HF1* or *MCP* mutation | Factor H or MCP deficiency; presents in children or adults with hemolysis, thrombocytopenia, and renal insufficiency; plasma infusion is effective treatment; can result in end-stage renal disease |

**ACQUIRED**

| | |
|---|---|
| ADAMTS13 deficiency | Caused by autoantibody; risk factors include female sex, black race, and obesity; acute renal failure rare; may manifest only with hemolysis and thrombocytopenia without neurologic abnormalities; may require immunosuppressive treatment in addition to plasma exchange |
| Shiga-toxin, following *E. coli* 0157:H7 or other Shiga-toxin–producing bacteria | The typical D (diarrhea)$^+$-HUS of children; also occurs in the elderly; may occur sporadically or in outbreaks; usually preceded by bloody diarrhea and manifested by acute renal failure, although some patients maintain normal renal function; severe neurologic abnormalities occur in 15%–25% of children with typical HUS; plasma exchange may be effective, although children traditionally managed only by supportive care and hemodialysis as needed |
| Drug-induced: immune-mediated | Quinine hypersensitivity most common; caused by drug-dependent antibodies to platelets, neutrophils, endothelial cells, and possibly other cells; sudden onset, renal failure predominant; plasma exchange may be effective; cases also reported following ticlopidine, clopidogrel, and other drugs |
| Drug-induced: dose-dependent toxicity | Mitomycin C most commonly reported chemotherapeutic agent, also reports following gemcitabine and pentastatin; cyclosporine A most commonly reported immunosuppressive agent; also reports following tacrolimus; insidious onset, often occurring after treatment has been discontinued; renal failure predominant; efficacy of plasma exchange uncertain |
| Pregnancy | May be a trigger for acute episodes associated with congenital or acquired ADAMTS13 deficiency; obstetric complications of severe preeclampsia/eclampsia and HELLP syndrome may be clinically indistinguishable from TTP–HUS |
| Autoimmune disorders | May be associated with acquired severe ADAMTS13 deficiency; acute flares of SLE, scleroderma, or antiphospholipid antibody syndrome may be indistinguishable from TTP–HUS |
| Allogeneic hematopoietic stem cell transplantation | Clinical features suggesting TTP–HUS are sometimes caused by angioinvasive infections, such as aspergillosis and cytomegalovirus |

ADAMTS13, A Disintegrin And Metalloprotease with ThromboSpondin 1–like domains; MCP, membrane cofactor protein; HUS, hemolytic-uremic syndrome; TTP, thrombotic thrombocytopenic purpura; SLE, systemic lupus erythematosus.

in the supernatant fluid of cultured endothelial cells. These unusually large multimers can directly agglutinate platelets when the VWF structure is altered by the high shear stress (25) that occurs in arterioles (25,26). Microangiopathic hemolysis with red cell fragmentation may result from the turbulence and high shear stress of circulation through partially occluded arterioles.

Enzymatic processing of plasma VWF following endothelial synthesis and secretion may be the result of both reduction of the disulfide bonds that link the VWF dimers (27) and proteolysis of VWF monomers by a metalloprotease, ADAMTS13, present in normal plasma (28–32). Proteolysis of VWF is enhanced by shear stress; therefore, the same physical forces that can change VWF conformation and enhance its reactivity with platelets, also make the VWF molecule vulnerable to proteolysis (33,34). In patients with nonfamilial TTP, autoantibodies that inhibit ADAMTS13 function have been demonstrated in many patients (34,35); in patients with familial TTP, mutations in the *ADAMTS13* gene causing severely deficient protease activity have been demonstrated (31,36–42).

# ETIOLOGIES OF THROMBOTIC THROMBOCYTOPENIC PURPURA AND HEMOLYTIC UREMIC SYNDROME

## Congenital Thrombotic Thrombocytopenic Purpura

Multiple mutations of the *ADAMTS13* gene can cause congenital deficiency of ADAMTS13 activity (31,36–42). Patients are either homozygous or compound heterozygotes. The wide distribution of mutation sites over exons 3 to 29 of the 29 exons (40) suggests a complex interaction between ADAMTS13 and its substrate, VWF, and essential functions for each of the structural elements of ADAMTS13. The clinical features of congenital TTP are extremely variable. Although all identified patients have undetectable ADAMTS13 activity, variation in residual enzyme activity below the threshold of detection, typically less than 3% to 5%, may be important for modifying clinical features (43,44). Some patients have severe microangiopathic hemolysis and hyperbilirubinemia at birth (40,42). In other families, women have been asymptomatic until near term of their first pregnancy and male siblings have remained asymptomatic (43). Although microangiopathic hemolysis and thrombocytopenia are initially predominant, end-stage renal failure may ultimately occur (40,42), consistent with the lack of clinical distinction between TTP and HUS. These patients may also have severe cerebrovascular ischemic events (45).

## Congenital Hemolytic Uremic Syndrome

Mutations of complement regulatory proteins, factor H (46, 47) and membrane cofactor protein (MCP, CD46) (48,49), have been associated with familial disorders described as HUS. Similar to patients with congenital TTP, these patients have microangiopathic hemolysis and thrombocytopenia. Signs of renal involvement have been described in all patients; some patients had minimal abnormalities that were reversible with plasma infusion, whereas others developed end-stage renal failure (48,49).

## Thrombotic Thrombocytopenic Purpura Associated with Acquired ADAMTS13 Deficiency

In patients with acquired TTP, ADAMTS13 deficiency can be caused by inhibitory autoantibodies. The disorder in these patients is therefore similar to other autoimmune disorders. However, different from the legendary experiments that induced severe thrombocytopenia in healthy subjects by infusion of plasma from patients with immune thrombocytopenic purpura (50,51), infusion of TTP plasma into a healthy volunteer caused no abnormalities (52). A study of epitope mapping of ADAMTS13 autoantibodies from 25 patients demonstrated that each autoantibody reacted with the cysteine-rich and spacer domains of ADAMTS13 (53), a domain essential for VWF cleavage (54). Most autoantibodies reacted with multiple domains (53).

Familial TTP may, rarely, be caused by autoantibody inhibition of ADAMTS13 rather than by a defect of the *ADAMTS13* gene, as documented in identical twins (55). This observation may be related to an increased familial risk for autoimmune disorders. Although acquired TTP is rare in children, not all TTP in infants is congenital. A 9-month-old girl

has been described with acquired TTP due to a high-titer inhibitor against ADAMTS13 (56). The recovery of normal ADAMTS13 activity in this infant distinguished her from the possible, but not yet described, occurrence of congenital TTP with an acquired alloantibody inhibitor.

In some patients with apparently acquired TTP and ADAMTS13 deficiency, but no inhibitory autoantibodies, autoantibodies may be present that impair ADAMTS13 function by accelerating clearance from plasma or by impairing binding to the endothelial cell surface (57). This observation is consistent with data suggesting that physiologic cleavage of the ultralarge VWF multimers secreted from endothelial cells occurs on the endothelial cell surface (58).

As in patients with congenital TTP, undetectable ADAMTS13 activity is not always associated with evidence for disease. Patients have been reported who had persistent undetectable ADAMTS13 activity, as well as persistent inhibitor activity, for prolonged periods following complete recovery from all signs and symptoms of TTP (55,59). Therefore, severe ADAMTS13 deficiency may not be a sufficient etiology for TTP but may be a contributing risk factor. The conditions that contribute to the initiation of the acute onset of TTP–HUS may include the risk factors and associated conditions described in the following section.

## Risk Factors and Conditions Associated with Thrombotic Thrombocytopenic Purpura

Similar to other thrombotic and autoimmune disorders, multiple risk factors may contribute to the onset of TTP. Severe ADAMTS13 deficiency is clearly an important risk factor. But similar to systemic lupus erythematosus (SLE) (60), female gender and black race are also important risk factors (8,59). Among patients with acquired TTP and severe ADAMTS13 deficiency, the standardized incidence rate ratios of women to men and blacks to nonblacks were 2.68:1 and 9.29:1, respectively (61). Pregnancy is a condition consistently associated with episodes of both congenital and acquired TTP (43,62). The increased risk for TTP during pregnancy may be related to the decreased ADAMTS13 plasma levels during the third trimester (63), which are more severe when obstetric complications such as HELLP syndrome occur (64). The decreased plasma levels of ADAMTS13 may be related to the increased plasma VWF levels during pregnancy (65), similar to the decreased ADAMTS13 levels that occur after desmopressin-induced increase of VWF levels (66). Inflammatory conditions may also trigger episodes of TTP (67,68), and these episodes may be mediated by inflammatory cytokines, IL-6, IL-8, and TNF-$\alpha$, which can stimulate endothelial cell release of ultralarge VWF multimers and impair proteolysis of VWF by ADAMTS13 (69).

## Shiga-Toxin–Producing *E. coli*

Typical HUS of young children follows acute enteric infection caused by *E. coli* or *Shigella dysenteriae* serotypes that produce Shiga toxin. Enterohemorrhagic strains of *E. coli* (predominantly *E. coli* 0157:H7) that acquired a plasmid containing the Shiga-toxin were first recognized as human pathogens in 1982 (19,20,70); in 1983, the association between Shiga-toxin–producing *E. coli* 0157:H7 and HUS was documented (21). The occurrence of gastrointestinal infections caused by *E. coli* 0157:H7 is increasing dramatically throughout the world (20), but HUS can also follow diarrhea caused by Shiga-toxin–producing *E. coli* serotypes other than 0157:H7 (70). Most outbreaks are traced to undercooked beef; however, contamination of unpasteurized milk, juices, fruits, vegetables, and water from sources located near cattle have all been implicated in outbreaks of colitis (19,20,70,71). The occurrence of colitis in persons consuming infected food is estimated to be 4% to 8% in community outbreaks but was 33% in a nursing-home epidemic, which also included person-to-person transmission (70). Progression of *E. coli* 0157:H7 infection to HUS is estimated to be 2% to 7% in sporadic cases but up to 30% in some epidemics (19,70,72). The peak age of infection is 6 months to 5 years, suggesting that older children and adults may acquire immunity to the Shiga-toxin (19,20,70), but Shiga-toxin–induced TTP–HUS can occur at any age. One mechanism by which the Shiga-toxin of *E. coli* 0157:H7 may cause diffuse endothelial damage is by mediating neutrophil adhesion to endothelial cells with resulting neutrophil activation and secretion of proteases (73).

## Drug Hypersensitivity

TTP–HUS can be an idiosyncratic, acute adverse reaction to a drug, mediated by drug-dependent antibodies to platelets, neutrophils, endothelial cells, and perhaps also other cells (74,75). Recognition of drug-induced TTP–HUS is critical because withdrawal of the offending drug is essential both for recovery and avoidance of recurrence. Quinine is the most common cause of immune-mediated drug-induced TTP–HUS (76). Repeated ingestion of a single quinine tablet or even quinine water (tonic) (77) can cause an immediate recurrence. TTP that is apparently immune-mediated can also occur following ticlopidine and clopidogrel (78–80).

## Drug Toxicity

Toxicity related to the cumulative dose or to high plasma levels of chemotherapeutic or immunosuppressive drugs can cause syndromes identical to TTP–HUS, with predominant renal failure. Mitomycin C is the most commonly associated chemotherapeutic agent (81–85). TTP–HUS has also been reported after gemcitabine (86) and pentostatin (87). Cyclosporine A is the most common immunosuppressive agent associated with TTP–HUS; TTP–HUS has also resulted from tacrolimus toxicity (86). In some patients, the clinical features suggesting TTP–HUS resolve following discontinuation of cyclosporine A and substitution with another immunosuppressive agent. Plasma exchange may be neither effective nor required.

## Hematopoietic Stem Cell Transplantation

Although TTP–HUS is described after allogeneic hematopoietic stem cell transplantation (HSCT) (88–90), reports are difficult to interpret because patients in whom the diagnosis is considered are often critically ill with complications involving multiple organ systems. The lack of clear diagnostic criteria for TTP–HUS has inevitably led to extreme variation in the frequency of its diagnosis (0.5% to 63.6%) following allogeneic HSCT and in reported mortality (0% to 100%) (91). All features of TTP–HUS may be caused by more clearly defined complications of allogeneic HSCT, such as acute graft versus host disease and systemic angioinvasive infections. Nephrotoxicity and neurotoxicity of cyclosporine may also be complicating factors (88). There are no reports of autopsies of patients diagnosed with TTP–HUS after HSCT that have documented systemic microvascular thrombi (91), the diagnostic pathologic feature of TTP (Fig. 111-1) (16). Following HSCT, TTP–HUS is most often diagnosed in patients with the most complications who are at greatest risk for critical complications: patients who have received transplants from matched, unrelated donors and patients who had an HLA antigen–mismatched donor (91,92).

This is consistent with the concept that in most patients, the clinical features suggesting the diagnosis of TTP–HUS are caused by systemic infection (91). Therefore, in contrast to patients with idiopathic TTP–HUS, delay in initiating plasma exchange treatment while alternative etiologies are assessed may be a prudent and appropriate decision.

## Pregnancy

In many case series of TTP–HUS, 10% to 25% of patients are pregnant or in the postpartum period (93). The clinical and pathologic similarity to preeclampsia creates diagnostic difficulty (94). However, the consistent occurrence of acute episodes of TTP triggered by pregnancy in patients with congenital ADAMTS13 deficiency supports an etiologic relation (43,62,93).

## Autoimmune Disorders

An association of TTP–HUS with autoimmune disorders such as SLE has been well described (16). The diagnosis of TTP–HUS in a patient with SLE is complicated because the signs and symptoms of SLE can mimic those of TTP–HUS (95–97). The clinical features of catastrophic antiphospholipid syndrome may also be identical to those of TTP–HUS (98), but patients with primary antiphospholipid syndrome may also have TTP resulting from severe ADAMTS13 deficiency caused by autoantibodies (99). Acute scleroderma can also be clinically (100,101) and pathologically (9,101) indistinguishable from TTP–HUS. Also, patients who have TTP associated with severe ADAMTS13 deficiency have a high frequency of anti-dsDNA autoantibodies, suggesting a risk for subsequently developing SLE (102,103).

# CLINICAL AND LABORATORY FEATURES

Because of the urgent need to initiate plasma exchange treatment, the diagnosis requires only the presence of microangiopathic hemolytic anemia and thrombocytopenia in the absence of another clinically apparent cause (11,13). These minimal diagnostic criteria are confirmed by the presenting features of patients who have TTP associated with severe ADAMTS13 deficiency, many of whom have no neurologic or renal function abnormalities (8,104). Consistent with the severe hemolysis, serum lactate dehydrogenase (LDH) levels are typically very high. However, LDH isoenzyme analysis documents that high serum LDH levels reflect not only hemolysis but also the ischemic injury of multiple organs (105). In three patients who have recovered from TTP associated with severe ADAMTS13 deficiency, subsequent stroke symptoms have been attributed to TTP even in the absence of thrombocytopenia and microangiopathic hemolytic anemia (106,107). The role of TTP in the etiology of the stroke symptoms was postulated because of the presence of severe ADAMTS13 deficiency and apparent response to plasma exchange treatment (106,107).

# TREATMENT

Plasma exchange with fresh frozen plasma replacement has profoundly affected the prognosis of acquired TTP, decreasing the mortality from greater than 90% before 1964 (16) to approximately 4% to 20% in current series (8,11,12,59,108). Plasma exchange may be required for patients with acquired TTP to remove antibodies to ADAMTS13 as well as to replace

ADAMTS13 with the fresh plasma. A randomized, controlled trial has documented the superiority of plasma exchange over plasma infusion (11). Plasma exchange may also benefit some patients with acquired TTP who do not have severe ADAMTS13 deficiency (8,59). In patients with congenital TTP, intermittent plasma infusion to replace ADAMTS13 is sufficient therapy (44,109,110). Observations in patients with congenital ADAMTS13 deficiency have documented that the half-life of ADAMTS13 in plasma is 2 to 3 days, and the minimum plasma activity sufficient to prevent microangiopathic abnormalities is 5% (44,110).

In patients who have acquired ADAMTS13 deficiency and inhibitory autoantibodies, glucocorticoid therapy may be required in addition to plasma exchange to achieve a durable remission (59,111,112). In patients with high titers of autoantibodies to ADAMTS13, more intensive immunosuppression with cyclophosphamide and/or rituximab in addition to glucocorticoids may be required (59,112,113).

## LONG-TERM OUTCOMES

Relapses, defined as recurrences following a complete clinical and hematologic remission on no treatment for more than 1 month (8,114), are increasingly common as more patients are observed for longer periods. Relapses are rare among patients diagnosed with TTP who do not have severe ADAMTS13 deficiency; among patients with severe acquired ADAMTS13 deficiency, the relapse rate is approximately 50% with a median follow-up of 3 years (8,104). Although splenectomy has been reported in small case series to be effective for the prevention of relapses (108,115–117), the importance of these observations is uncertain because most patients who relapse have their initial relapse within the first year, and most patients have only one relapse (104).

## *References*

1. Moschcowitz E. An acute febrile pleiochromic anemia with hyaline thrombosis of the terminal arterioles and capillaries. *Arch Intern Med* 1925;36:89–93.
2. Marcus AJ. Dr. Eli Moschcowitz. In: Kaplan BS, Trompeter RS, Moake JL, eds. *Hemolytic uremic syndrome and thrombotic thrombocytopenic purpura.* New York: Marcel Dekker Inc, 1992:19–27.
3. Gasser C, Gautier E, Steck A, et al. Hamolytisch-uramische syndrome: Bilaterale Nierenrindennekrosen bei akuten erworbenen hamolytischen Anamien. *Schweiz Med Wochenschr* 1955;85:905–909.
4. Gautier E, Siebenmann RE. The birth of the hemolytic uremic syndrome. In: Kaplan BS, Trompeter RS, Moake JL, eds. *Hemolytic uremic syndrome and thrombotic thrombocytopenic purpura.* New York: Marcel Dekker Inc, 1992:1–17.
5. Martin DL, MacDonald KL, White KE, et al. The epidemiology and clinical aspects of the hemolytic uremic syndrome in Minnesota. *N Eng J Med* 1990;323:1161–1167.
6. Elliott EJ, Robins-Browne RM, O'Loughlin EV, et al. Nationwide study of haemolytic uraemic syndrome: clinical, microbiological, and epidemiological features. *Arch Dis Child* 2001;85:125–131.
7. Gerber A, Karch H, Allerberger F, et al. Clinical course and the role of Shiga toxin-producing *Escherichia coli* infection in the hemolytic uremic syndrome in pediatric patients, 1997-2000, in Germany and Austria: a prospective study. *J Infect Dis* 2002;186:493–500.
8. Vesely SK, George JN, Lammle B, et al. ADAMTS13 activity in thrombotic thrombocytopenic purpura-hemolytic uremic syndrome: relation to presenting features and clinical outcomes in a prospective cohort of 142 patients. *Blood* 2003;101:60–68.
9. Laszik Z, Silva F. Hemolytic uremic syndrome, thrombotic thrombocytopenia purpura, and systemic sclerosis (systemic scleroderma). In: Jennett JC, Olson JL, Schwartz MM, et al. eds. *Heptinstall's pathology of the kidney.* Philadelphia, PA: Lippincott Williams & Wilkins, 1998:1003–1057.
10. Hosler GA, Cusumano AM, Hutchins GM. Thrombotic thrombocytopenic purpura and hemolytic uremic syndrome are distinct pathologic entities. A review of 56 autopsy cases. *Arch Pathol Lab Med* 2003;127:834–839.
11. Rock GA, Shumak KH, Buskard NA, et al. Comparison of plasma exchange with plasma infusion in the treatment of thrombotic thrombocytopenic purpura. *N Eng J Med* 1991;325:393–397.
12. Rock G, Shumak K, Kelton J, et al. Thrombotic thrombocytopenic purpura: outcome in 24 patients with renal impairment treated with plasma exchange. *Transfusion* 1992;32:710–714.
13. George JN. How I treat patients with thrombotic thrombocytopenic purpura-hemolytic uremic syndrome. *Blood* 2000;96:1223–1229.
14. Garg AX, Suri RS, Barrowman N, et al. Long-term renal prognosis of diarrhea-associated hemolytic uremic syndrome. A systematic review, meta-analysis, and meta-regression. *JAMA* 2003;290:1360–1370.
15. Dundas S, Murphy J, Soutar RL, et al. Effectiveness of therapeutic plasma exchange in the 1996 Lanarkshire *Escherichia coli* O157:H7 outbreak. *Lancet* 1999;354:1327.
16. Amorosi EL, Ultmann JE. Thrombotic thrombocytopenic purpura: report of 16 cases and review of the literature. *Medicine* 1966;45:139–159.
17. Bukowski RM, King JW, Hewlett JS. Plasmapheresis in the treatment of thrombotic thrombocytopenic purpura. *Blood* 1977;50:413–417.
18. Clark WF, Garg AX, Blake PG, et al. Effect of awareness of a randomized controlled trial on use of experimental therapy. *JAMA* 2003;290:1351–1355.
19. Mead PS, Griffin PM. *Escherichia coli* O157:H7. *Lancet* 1998;352:1207–1212.
20. Boyce TG, Swerdlow DL, Griffin PM. *Escherichia coli* O157:H7 and the hemolytic uremic syndrome. *N Eng J Med* 1995;333:364–368.
21. Karmali MA, Steele BT, Petric M, et al. Sporadic cases of haemolytic-uraemic syndrome associated with faecal cytotoxin and cytotoxin-producing *Escherichia coli* in stools. *Lancet* 1983;1:619–620.
22. Moake JL. Thrombotic microangiopathies. *N Eng J Med* 2002;347:589–600.
23. George JN, Sadler JE, Lammle B. Thrombotic thrombocytopenic purpura. In: Broudy VC, Abkowitz JL, Vose JM, eds. *Hematology.* Washington, DC: American Society of Hematology, 2002:315–334.
24. Moake JL, Rudy CK, Troll JH, et al. Unusually large plasma factor VIII: von Willebrand factor multimers in chronic relapsing thrombotic thrombocytopenic purpura. *N Eng J Med* 1982;307:1432–1435.
25. Moake J. Studies on the pathophysiology of thrombotic thrombocytopenic purpura. *Semin Hematol* 1997;34:83–89.
26. Kroll MH, Hellums JD, McIntire LV, et al. Platelets and shear stress. *Blood* 1996;88:1525–1541.
27. Pimanda JE, Annis DS, Raftery M, et al. The von Willebrand factor-reducing activity of thrombospondin-1 is located in the calcium-binding/C-terminal sequence and requires a free thiol at position 974. *Blood* 2002;100:2832–2838.
28. Furlan M, Robles R, Lammle B. Partial purification and characterization of a protease from human plasma cleaving von Willebrand factor to fragments produced by *in vivo* proteolysis. *Blood* 1996;87:4223–4234.
29. Tsai H-M. Physiologic cleavage of von Willebrand factor by a plasma protease is dependent on its conformation and requires calcium ion. *Blood* 1996;87:4235–4244.
30. Zheng X, Chung D, Takayama TK, et al. Structure of von Willebrand factor-cleaving protease (ADAMTS13), a metalloprotease involved in thrombotic thrombocytopenic purpura. *J Biol Chem* 2001;276:41059–41063.
31. Levy GG, Nichols WC, Lian EC, et al. Mutations in a member of the *ADAMTS* gene family cause thrombotic thrombocytopenic purpura. *Nature* 2001;413:488–494.
32. Plaimauer B, Zimmermann K, Volkel D, et al. Cloning, expression, and functional characterization of the von Willebrand factor-cleaving protease (ADAMTS13). *Blood* 2002;100:3626–3632.
33. Tsai HM, Sussman II, Nagel RL. Shear stress enhances the proteolysis of von Willebrand factor in normal plasma. *Blood* 1994;83:2171–2175.
34. Tsai H-M, Lian ECY. Antibodies to von-Willebrand factor-cleaving protease in acute thrombotic thrombocytopenic purpura. *N Eng J Med* 1998;339:1585–1594.
35. Furlan M, Robles R, Galbusera M, et al. Von Willebrand factor-cleaving protease in thrombotic thrombocytopenic purpura and the hemolytic-uremic syndrome. *N Engl J Med* 1998;339:1578–1584.
36. Kokame K, Matsumoto M, Soejima K, et al. Mutations and common polymorphisms in *ADAMTS13* gene responsible for von Willebrand factor-cleaving protease activity. *Proc Natl Acad Sci U S A* 2002;99:11902–11907.
37. Schneppenheim R, Budde U, Oyen F, et al. Von Willebrand cleaving protease and *ADAMTS13* mucations in childhood TTP. *Blood* 2003;101:1845–1850.
38. Uchida T, Wada H, Mizutani M, et al. Identification of novel mutations in *ADAMTS13* in an adult patient with congenital thrombotic thrombocytopenic purpura. *Blood* 2004;104:2081–2083.
39. Antoine G, Zimmermann K, Plaimauer B, et al. *ADAMTS13* gene defects in two brothers with constitutional thrombotic thrombocytopenic purpura and normalization of von Willebrand factor-cleaving protease activity by recombinant human ADAMTS13. *Br J Haematol* 2003;120:821–824.
40. Matsumoto M, Kokame K, Soejima K, et al. Molecular characterization of *ADAMTS13* gene mutations in Japanese patients with Upshaw-Schulman syndrome. *Blood* 2004;103:1305–1310.
41. Pimanda JE, Maekawa A, Wind T, et al. Congenital thrombotic thrombocytopenic purpura in association with a mutation in the second CUB domain of ADAMTS13. *Blood* 2004;103:627–629.
42. Veyradier A, Lavergne J-M, Ribba A, et al. Ten candidate ADAMTS13 mutations in six French families with congenital thrombotic thrombocytopenic

purpura (Upshaw-Schulman syndrome). *J Thromb Haemost* 2004;2: 424–429.

43. Furlan M, Lammle B. Aetiology and pathogenesis of thrombotic thrombocytopenic purpura and haemolytic uraemic syndrome: the role of von Willebrand factor-cleaving protease. *Best Pract Res Clin Haematol* 2001; 14:437–454.

44. Barbot J, Costa E, Guerra M, et al. Ten years of prophylactic treatment with fresh-frozen plasma in a child with chronic relapsing thrombotic thrombocytopenic purpura as a result of a congenital deficiency of von Willebrand factor-cleaving protease. *Br J Haematol* 2001;113:649–651.

45. Furlan M, Robles R, Solenthaler M, et al. Deficient activity of von Willebrand factor-cleaving protease in chronic relapsing thrombotic thrombocytopenic purpura. *Blood* 1997;89:3097–3103.

46. Landau D, Shalev H, Levy-Finer G, et al. Familial hemolytic uremic syndrome associated with complement factor H deficiency. *J Pediatr* 2001; 138:412–417.

47. Taylor CM. Complement factor H and the haemolytic uraemic syndrome. *Lancet* 2001;358:1200–1202.

48. Noris M, Brioschi S, Caprioli J, et al. Familial haemolytic uraemic syndrome and an MCP mutation. *Lancet* 2003;362:1542–1547.

49. Richards A, Kemp EJ, Liszewski MK, et al. Mutations in human complement regulator, membrane cofactor protein (CD46), predispose to development of familial hemolytic uremic syndrome. *Proc Natl Acad Sci U S A* 2003;100:12966–12971.

50. Harrington WJ, Minnich V, Hollingsworth JW, et al. Demonstration of a thrombocytopenic factor in the blood of patients with thrombocytopenic purpura. *J Lab Clin Med* 1951;38:1.

51. Altman LK. Black and blue at the flick of a feather. *Who goes first?* New York: Random House; 1987:273–282.

52. Brittingham TE, Chaplin H. Attempted passive transfer of thrombotic thrombocytopenic purpura. *Blood* 1957;12:480–182.

53. Klaus C, Plaimauer B, Studt J-D, et al. Epitope mapping of ADAMTS13 autoantibodies in acquired thrombotic thrombocytopenic purpura. *Blood* 2004;103:4514–4519.

54. Soejima K, Matsumoto M, Kokame K, et al. ADAMTS13 cysteine-rich/spacer domains are functionally essential for von Willebrand factor cleavage. *Blood* 2003;102:3232–3237.

55. Studt J-D, Hovinga JK, Radonic R, et al. Familial acquired thrombotic thrombocytopenic purpura: ADAMTS13 inhibitory autoantibodies in identical twins. *Blood* 2004;103:4195–4197.

56. Ashida A, Nakamura H, Yoden A, et al. Successful treatment of a young infant who developed high-titer inhibitors against VWF-cleaving protease (ADAMTS-13): important discrimination from Upshaw-Schulman syndrome. *Am J Hematol* 2002;71:318–322.

57. Scheiflinger F, Knobl P, Trattner B, et al. Nonneutralizing IgM and IgG antibodies to von Willebrand factor-cleaving protease (ADAMTS13) in a patient with thrombotic thrombocytopenic purpura. *Blood* 2003;102:3241–3243.

58. Dong JF, Moake JL, Nolasco L, et al. ADAMTS-13 rapidly cleaves newly secreted ultralarge von Willebrand factor multimers on the endothelial surface under flowing conditions. *Blood* 2002;100:4033–4039.

59. Zheng XL, Kaufman RM, Goodnough LT, et al. Effect of plasma exchange on plasma ADAMTS13 metalloprotease activity, inhibitor level, and clinical outcome in patients with idiopathic and non-idiopathic thrombotic thrombocytopenic purpura. *Blood* 2004;103:4043–4049.

60. McCarty DJ, Manzi S, Medsger TA Jr, et al. Incidence of systemic lupus erythematosus: race and gender differences. *Arthritis Rheum* 1995;38: 1260–1276.

61. Terrell DR, Williams LA, Vesely SK, et al. The incidence of thrombotic thrombocytopenic purpura-hemolytic uremic syndrome: all patients, idiopathic patients, and patients with severe ADAMTS13 deficiency. *J Thromb Haemost* 2005;3:1432–1436.

62. Vesely SK, Li X, McMinn JR, et al. Pregnancy outcomes after recovery from thrombotic thrombocytopenic purpura-hemolytic uremic syndrome. *Transfusion* 2004;44:1149–1158.

63. Mannucci PM, Canciani MT, Forza I, et al. Changes in health and disease of the metalloprotease that cleaves von Willebrand factor. *Blood* 2001;98: 2730–2735.

64. Lattuada A, Rossi E, Calzarossa C, et al. Mild to moderate reduction of a von Willebrand factor cleaving protease (ADAMTS-13) in pregnant women with HELLP microangiopathic syndrome. *Haematologica* 2003; 88:1029–1034.

65. Stirling Y, Woolf L, North WRS, et al. Haemostasis in normal pregnancy. *Thromb Haemost* 1984;52:176–182.

66. Reiter RA, Knobl P, Varadi K, et al. Changes in von Willebrand factor-cleaving protease (ADAMTS13) activity after infusion of desmopressin. *Blood* 2003;101:946–948.

67. Boyer A, Chadda K, Salah A, et al. Thrombotic microangiopathy: an atypical cause of acute renal failure in patients with acute pancreatitis. *Intensive Care Med* 2004;30:1235–1239.

68. Naqvi TA, Baumann MA, Chang JC. Post-operative thrombotic thrombocytopenic purpura: a review. *Int J Clin Pract* 2004;58:169–172.

69. Bernardo A, Ball C, Nolasco L, et al. Effects of inflammatory cytokines on the release and cleavage of the endothelial cell-derived ultralarge von Willebrand factor multimers under flow. *Blood* 2004;104:100–106.

70. Su C, Brandt LJ. *Escherichia coli* O157:H7 infection in humans. *Ann Intern Med* 1995;123:698–714.

71. Slutsker L, Ries AA, Greene KD, et al. *Escherichia coli* O157:H7 diarrhea in the United States: clinical and epidemiologic features. *Ann Intern Med* 1997;126:505–513.

72. Rowe PC, Orrbine E, Lior H, et al. Risk of hemolytic uremic syndrome after sporadic *Escherichia coli* O157:H7 infection: results of a Canadian collaborative study. *J Pediatr* 1998;132:777–782.

73. Morigi M, Micheletti G, Figliuzzi M, et al. Verotoxin-1 promotes leukocyte adhesion to cultured endothelial cells under physiologic flow conditions. *Blood* 1995;86:4553–4558.

74. Gottschall JL, Neahring B, McFarland JG, et al. Quinine-induced immune thrombocytopenia with hemolytic uremic syndrome: clinical and serological findings in nine patients and review of literature. *Am J Hematol* 1994;47:283–289.

75. Stroncek DF, Vercellotti GM, Hammerschmidt DE, et al. Characterization of multiple quinine-dependent antibodies in a patient with episodic hemolytic uremic syndrome and immune agranulocytosis. *Blood* 1992;80: 241–248.

76. Kojouri K, Vesely SK, George JN. Quinine-associated thrombotic thrombocytopenic purpura-hemolytic uremic syndrome: frequency, clinical features, and long-term outcomes. *Ann Intern Med* 2001;135:1047–1051.

77. Gottschall JL, Elliot W, Lianos E, et al. Quinine-induced immune thrombocytopenia associated with hemolytic uremic syndrome: a new clinical entity. *Blood* 1991;77:306–310.

78. Bennett CL, Weinberg PD, Rozenberg-Ben-Dror K, et al. Thrombotic thrombocytopenic purpura associated with ticlopidine – a review of 60 cases. *Ann Intern Med* 1998;128:541–544.

79. Bennett CL, Connors JM, Carwile JM, et al. Thrombotic thrombocytopenic purpura associated with clopidogrel. *N Eng J Med* 2000;342: 1773–1777.

80. Tsai HM, Rice L, Sarode R, et al. Antibody inhibitors to von Willebrand factor metalloproteinase and increased binding of von Willebrand factor to platelets in ticlopidine-associated thrombotic thrombocytopenic purpura. *Ann Intern Med* 2000;132:794–799.

81. Lesesne JB, Rothschild N, Erickson B, et al. Cancer-associated hemolytic-uremic syndrome: analysis of 85 cases from a national registry. *J Clin Oncol* 1989;7:781–789.

82. Murgo AJ. Thrombotic microangiopathy in the cancer patient including those induced by chemotherapeutic agents. *Semin Hematol* 1987;24: 161–177.

83. Loprinzi CL. Mitomycin C-induced pulmonary and renal toxicities. *Wis Med J* 1984;83:16–17.

84. Verwey J, de Vries J, Pinedo HM. Mitomycin C-induced renal toxicity, a dose-dependent side effect? *Eur J Cancer* 1987;23:195–199.

85. Fielding JWL, Fagg SL, Jones BG, et al. An interim report of a prospective, randomized, controlled study of adjuvant chemotherapy in operable gastric cancer: British stomach cancer group. *World J Surg* 1983;7:390–399.

86. Medina PJ, Sipols JM, George JN. Drug-associated thrombotic thrombocytopenic purpura-hemolytic uremic syndrome. *Curr Opin Hematol* 2001; 8:286–293.

87. Leach JW, Pham T, Diamandidis D, et al. Thrombotic thrombocytopenic purpura-hemolytic uremic syndrome (TTP-HUS) following treatment with deoxycoformycin in a patient with cutaneous T cell lymphoma (Sezary Syndrome): a case report. *Am J Hematol* 1999;61:268–270.

88. Pettitt AR, Clark RE. Thrombotic microangiopathy following bone marrow transplantation. *Bone Marrow Transplant* 1994;14:495–504.

89. Zeigler ZR, Shadduck RK, Nemunaitis J, et al. Bone marrow transplant-associated thrombotic microangiopathy: a case series. *Bone Marrow Transplant* 1995;15:247–253.

90. Schriber JR, Herzig GP. Transplantation-associated thrombotic thrombocytopenic purpura and hemolytic uremic syndrome. *Semin Hematol* 1997; 34:126–133.

91. George JN, Li X, McMinn JR, et al. Thrombotic thrombocytopenic purpura-hemolytic uremic syndrome following allogeneic hematopoietic stem cell transplantation: a diagnostic dilemma. *Transfusion* 2004;44:294–304.

92. Roy V, Rizvi MA, Vesely SK, et al. Thrombotic thrombocytopenic purpura-like syndromes following bone marrow transplantation: an analysis of associated conditions and clinical outcomes. *Bone Marrow Transplant* 2001; 27:641–646.

93. George JN. The association of pregnancy with thrombotic thrombocytopenic purpura-hemolytic uremic syndrome. *Curr Opin Hematol* 2003; 10:339–344.

94. McMinn JR, George JN. Evaluation of women with clinically suspected thrombotic thrombocytopenic purpura-hemolytic uremic syndrome during pregnancy. *J Clin Apheresis* 2001;16:202–209.

95. Devinsky O, Petito CK, Alonso DR. Clinical and neuropathological findings in systemic lupus erythematosus: the role of vasculitis, heart emboli, and thrombotic microangiopathy. *Ann Neurol* 1988;23:380–384.

96. Jorfén M, Callejas JL, Formiga F, et al. Fulminant thrombotic thrombocytopenic purpura in systemic lupus erythematosus. *Scand J Rheumatol* 1998; 27:76–77.

97. Jain R, Chartash E, Susin M, et al. Systemic lupus erythematosus complicated by thrombotic microangiopathy. *Semin Arthritis Rheum* 1994;24: 173–182.

98. Asherson RA, Cervera R, Piette JC, et al. Catastrophic antiphospholipid syndrome. Clinical and laboratory features of 50 patients. *Medicine* 1998; 77:195–207.

99. Amoura Z, Costadoat-Chalumeau N, Veyradier A, et al. Thrombotic thrombocytopenic purpura with severe ADAMTS13 deficiency in two patients with primary antiphospholipid syndrome. *Arthritis Rheum* 2004; 50:3260–3264.

100. Miller A, Ryan PFJ, Dowling JP. Vasculitis and thrombotic thrombocytopenic purpura in a patient with limited scleroderma. *J Rheumatol* 1997; 24:598–600.

101. Kapur A, Ballou SP, Renston JP, et al. Recurrent acute scleroderma renal crisis complicated by thrombotic thrombocytopenic purpura. *J Rheumatol* 1997;24:2469–2472.

102. Hunt L, Li X, James JA, et al. Thrombotic thrombocytopenic purpura and systemic lupus erythematosis: distinct but potentially overlapping syndromes. *Blood* 2004;104:245a.

103. Gungor T, Furlan M, Lammle B, et al. Acquired deficiency of von Willebrand factor-cleaving protease in a patient suffering from acute systemic lupus erythematosus. *Rheumatology* 2001;40:940–942.

104. Sadler JE, Moake JL, Miyata T. Recent advances in thrombotic thrombocytopenic purpura. In: Broudy VC, Berliner N, Larson RA, et al. eds. *Hematology.* Washington, DC: American Society of Hematology, 2004: 407–423.

105. Cohen JD, Brecher ME, Bandarenko N. Cellular source of serum lactate dehydrogenase elevation in patients with thrombotic thrombocytopenia purpura. *J Clin Apheresis* 1998;13:16–19.

106. Tsai HM, Shulman K. Rituximab induces remission of cerebral ischemia caused by thrombotic thrombocytopenic purpura. *Eur J Haematol* 2003; 70:183–185.

107. Downes KA, Yomtovian R, Tsai H-M, et al. Relapsed thrombotic thrombocytopenic purpura presenting as an acute cerebrovascular accident. *J Clin Apheresis* 2004;19:86–89.

108. Thompson CE, Damon LE, Ries CA, et al. Thrombotic microangiopathies in the 1980s: clinical features, response to treatment, and the impact of the human immunodeficiency virus epidemic. *Blood* 1992;80:1890–1895.

109. Upshaw JD Jr. Congenital deficiency of a factor in normal plasma that reverses microangiopathic hemolysis and thrombocytopenia. *N Eng J Med* 1978;298:1350–1352.

110. Furlan M, Robles R, Morselli B, et al. Recovery and half-life of von Willebrand factor-cleaving protease after plasma therapy in patients with thrombotic thrombocytopenic purpura. *Thromb Haemost* 1999;81:8–13.

111. Bell WR, Braine HG, Ness PM, et al. Improved survival in thrombotic thrombocytopenic purpura - hemolytic uremic syndrome. *N Eng J Med* 1991;325:398–403.

112. Zheng XL, Pallera AM, Goodnough LT, et al. Remission of chronic thrombotic thrombocytopenic purpura treated with cyclophosphamide and rituximab. *Ann Intern Med* 2003;138:105–108.

113. Tsai HM. High titers of inhibitors of von Willebrand factor-cleaving metalloproteinase in a fatal case of acute thrombotic thrombocytopenic purpura. *Am J Hematol* 2000;65:251–255.

114. George JN, Vesely SK, Terrell DR. The Oklahoma thrombotic thrombocytopenic purpura-hemolytic uremic syndrome (TTP-HUS) registry: a community perspective of patients with clinically diagnosed TTP-HUS. *Semin Hematol* 2004;41:60–67.

115. Cuttner J. Thrombotic thrombocytopenic purpura: a ten-year experience. *Blood* 1980;56:302–306.

116. Crowther MA, Heddle N, Hayward CPM, et al. Splenectomy done during hematologic remission to prevent relapse in patients with thrombotic thrombocytopenic purpura. *Ann Intern Med* 1996;125:294–296.

117. Kremer Hovinga JA, Studt J-D, Demarmels Biasiutti F, et al. Splenectomy in relapsing and plasma-refractory acquired thrombotic thrombocytopenic purpura. *Haematologica* 2004;89:320–324.

# CHAPTER 112 ■ ANTIPHOSPHOLIPID ANTIBODIES AND THE ANTIPHOSPHOLIPID SYNDROME

JACOB H. RAND AND LISA SENZEL

Antiphospholipid antibodies (aPL antibodies) comprise a broad family of autoantibodies that are detected by lupus anticoagulant (LA) tests, by enzyme-linked immunosorbent assays (ELISAs) for anticardiolipin antibodies (aCLs), and by antibodies that recognize other phospholipids and phospholipid-binding proteins (1). Although aPL antibodies were first described more than 50 years ago, the mechanistic relation to clinical events has not been established. Nevertheless, an understanding of the laboratory diagnosis, clinical manifestations, and presumptive biology of these antibodies is important to the clinician for several reasons. First, the aPL syndrome is the most common cause of acquired thrombophilia and is strongly associated with excess cardiovascular morbidity and mortality (2). Second, aPL antibodies are associated with several other clinical manifestations, such as recurrent fetal loss, in which their presence may alter prognosis and therapy. Third, LAs are a common cause of a prolonged partial thromboplastin time (PTT) and are, not infrequently, detected during the course of general medical care or preoperative screening.

## HISTORICAL PERSPECTIVE

The existence of phospholipid-reactive antibodies in human sera was first described in patients with biologic false-positive (BFP) serologic tests for syphilis (3). The antibodies responsible for the BFP syphilis tests recognized cardiolipin within the test reagent. In 1952, Conley and Hartmann published the first description of phospholipid-dependent coagulation inhibitors in two patients with systemic lupus erythematosus (SLE) (4). In 1957, Laurell and Nilsson described an association between a chronic biologically false-positive serologic test for syphilis, a circulating anticoagulant, and recurrent pregnancy loss (5). A paradoxic association between phospholipid-dependent coagulation inhibitors and thrombosis, rather than bleeding, was first recognized by Bowie et al. in 1963 (6), and the term LA was proposed 9 years later by Feinstein and Rapaport on the basis of LA's prevalence in patients with SLE (7). In 1980, an immunoglobulin monoclonal (IgM) antibody displaying LA characteristics was demonstrated to react with anionic phospholipids other than cardiolipin (8). In the early 1980s, immunoassays (9,10) were developed to measure aCL antibodies, and the association of aCL antibodies with thromboembolic events was appreciated (9). In 1990, it became recognized that a subset of these antibodies actually recognized a plasma protein, $\beta_2$-glycoprotein I ($\beta_2$-GP I), in complex with phospholipids (11,12). This observation led to the identification of additional phospholipid-binding protein cofactors recognized by "antiphospholipid" antibodies (13).

## PREVALENCE OF ANTIPHOSPHOLIPID ANTIBODIES

The prevalence of aPL antibodies in the asymptomatic "normal" population has generally been estimated to range from approximately 3% to 10% (14,15). In one group of healthy young women who served as controls in a study, 18.2% had elevated aCL antibodies and 12.8% tested LA-positive (16). aPL antibodies are also common after certain infections and after exposure to specific medications. In most of these settings, the aPL antibodies appear to be distinct from those that are associated with thrombosis. aPL antibodies develop in a substantial fraction of children and adults infected with mycobacteria, malaria, other parasitic organisms, or viruses (17). Medications associated with the development of aPL antibodies include neuroleptics, quinidine, and procainamide (18). The duration of aPL antibodies after infection or discontinuation of drug exposure is not well established, and the risk of thrombosis is variable (19,20). aPL antibodies also occur in patients with autoimmune disorders, most commonly SLE. Although estimates vary, LAs have been identified in 10% to 20% and aCLs in 30% to 50% of the patients with well-established SLE (21). aPL antibodies are also common in patients with Sjögren syndrome, mixed connective tissue disease, rheumatoid arthritis, idiopathic thrombocytopenic purpura (ITP), and other immunologic disorders. aPL antibodies are most frequently detected in individuals with no evidence of another underlying immune disorder. aPL antibodies may be a risk factor for the subsequent development of SLE; one study found that 18% of the patients with SLE were positive for aCL antibodies before SLE diagnosis, and this subset of patients had a more severe clinical course (22). It has been suggested that autoimmune aPL antibodies may arise through molecular mimicry, a concept that is supported by an animal model in which thrombogenic aPL antibodies appeared after immunization with phospholipid-binding viral peptides (23).

Genetic factors may also contribute to the development of aPL antibodies. In some (24,25), but not all, studies (26), the incidence of aCLs among patients with SLE has been higher in patients who are HLA-DR4 or -DR7 positive. Several cases of familial aPL syndrome have been described (27,28). The inheritance pattern of aPL antibodies in such kindreds appears to be autosomal dominant (26).

# LABORATORY DIAGNOSIS OF ANTIPHOSPHOLIPID ANTIBODIES

Two types of assays are used for the detection of aPL antibodies: coagulation assays, in which LAs are detected by their ability to prolong phospholipid-dependent coagulation reactions, and immunoassays, in which aCLs and antibodies against other phospholipids and protein cofactors are detected most commonly by ELISA. LAs and aCLs may occur independently or may coexist in individual patients.

## Lupus Anticoagulants

LAs appear to be heterogeneous in terms of the antigens they recognize (*vide infra*). Variability in the phospholipid composition of coagulation reagents, especially PTT reagents, used by different clinical laboratories, influences the utility of the various LA tests. Of the several assays that are available (see Table 112-1), no single one identifies every LA; as a result, the number of approaches for their detection has proliferated. The Subcommittee on Antiphospholipid Antibodies of the International Society of Thrombosis and Hemostasis has proposed specific criteria in an attempt to standardize the diagnosis of LAs (see Table 112-2) (29). Generally, LAs are suspected when one of several screening assays, most commonly the PTT, is prolonged. A suspected LA is further evaluated using an inhibitor screen (mixing study), in which the PTT of a mixture of the test and normal plasma (NP) is measured. LAs, in contrast to inhibitors that are specific for coagulation factors, usually prolong the clotting time of NP immediately after mixing, but occasionally require incubation. A confirmatory test is then used to establish the phospholipid dependence of the inhibitor effect (Table 112-1) (29). An approach to the diagnosis of LAs is depicted in Figure 112-1.

Several considerations concerning the diagnosis of LAs warrant mention. First, the effect of LAs on phospholipid-dependent coagulation assays depends on the depletion of platelets and platelet fragments from plasma. Second, as with screening assays, the sensitivity and specificity of confirmatory assays also vary. Such technical issues may lead to discrepant results when patients are studied in different laboratories. Third, it follows from the above that a normal PTT is not sufficient to exclude an LA (Fig. 112-1). Hence, if an LA is suspected, an additional screening assay, such as dilute Russell viper venom time or kaolin clotting time, should be performed before the diagnosis is excluded. Finally, the evaluation of a patient with a prolonged PTT must also take into account clinical considerations. A patient in whom the laboratory diagnosis of an LA is equivocal should be evaluated for concurrent deficiencies of or specific inhibitors against coagulation proteins themselves, especially if there are symptoms consistent with a bleeding tendency. These evaluations may be complicated by the propensity of LAs to inhibit the *in vitro* activity of several coagulation factors. The apparent coincidence of inhibitors directed at multiple coagulation factors in a plasma sample is often a clue to the presence of LAs.

## Antiphospholipid Antibody Immunoassays

The first of these to be developed was the aCL (9). These assays were developed as quantitative methods for assessing the biologic false-positive syphilis test. Cardiolipin, the phospholipid used in that test, is actually an intracellular membrane phospholipid. In the aCL ELISA, the amount of binding of IgG– and IgM–aCL is expressed in standardized GPL or MPL units, one unit representing the cardiolipin-binding activity of 1 $\mu$g per mL of affinity-purified aPL antibodies from a reference sera. Binding reflects both the titer and affinity of the antibody. Correlation of aCL levels determined in reference sera by different laboratories has been problematic, particularly when aCLs are measured using different commercial ELISA kits (30).

**TABLE 112-1**

### COMMON SCREENING AND CONFIRMATORY TESTS USED IN THE DIAGNOSIS OF LUPUS ANTICOAGULANTS

| Screening assays | Confirmatory studies |
|---|---|
| Partial thromboplastin time | Platelet neutralization procedure |
|  | Tissue thromboplastin inhibition |
|  | Hexagonal phase phospholipids |
| Dilute Russell viper venom time | DVV confirm platelet neutralization procedure |
| Kaolin clotting time | Platelet vesicles |

Modified from Brandt JT, Triplett DA, Alving B, et al. Criteria for the diagnosis of lupus anticoagulants: an update. *Thromb Haemost* 1995;74:1185–1190.

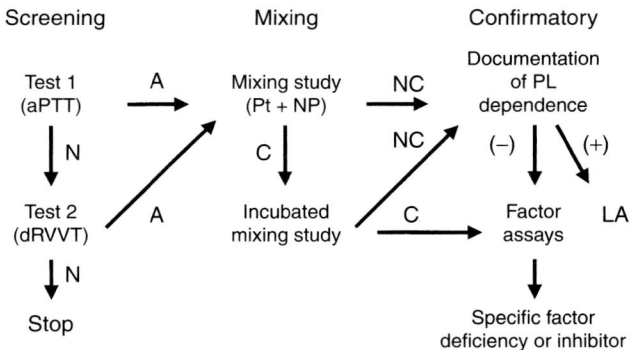

**FIGURE 112-1.** Approach to the diagnosis of a lupus anticoagulant (LA). A, abnormal; aPTT, activated partial thromboplastin time; C, correction; dRVVT, dilute Russell viper venom time; N, normal; NC, no correction; NP, normal plasma; PL, phospholipid; Pt, patient. (Modified from Brandt JT, Triplett DA, Alving B, et al. Criteria for the diagnosis of lupus anticoagulants: an update. *Thromb Haemost* 1995;74:1185–1190.)

# ANTIGENIC SPECIFICITY OF "ANTIPHOSPHOLIPID" ANTIBODIES

## Direct Reactivity with Anionic Phospholipids

Before 1990, it was thought that aPL antibodies recognize determinants within anionic phospholipids themselves. This view was supported by the finding that antibodies apparently reactive with cardiolipin, other anionic phospholipids, and occasionally the zwitterionic phospholipid, phosphatidylethanolamine (but rarely neutral phospholipids), were detected using ELISAs. The composition and physical state of the phospholipid may influence antibody binding. It has been suggested that $\beta$2GP I (see next section) may shift the orientation of some phospholipids from the lamellar to the hexagonal phase.

## Reactivity with $\beta_2$-Glycoprotein I

In 1990, it was discovered that rather than binding directly to phospholipid, many aCLs actually recognized $\beta_2$GP I (also known as lipoprotein ApoH) bound to the cardiolipin used to coat the ELISA plates (11,12). It was subsequently demonstrated that $\beta_2$GP I–dependent aPL antibodies (referred to as anti-$\beta_2$GP I antibodies) occur preferentially in patients with SLE or in those who have experienced aPLA-associated clinical events, whereas antibodies that recognize cardiolipin directly occur more commonly after infection, exposure to medications, or in otherwise healthy individuals. Two explanations for the reactivity of anti-$\beta_2$GP I antibodies with phospholipid-associated $\beta_2$GP I have been proposed. aPL antibodies may recognize a specific conformation of $\beta_2$GP I induced after binding to anionic phospholipid or cell membranes. In support of this is the observation that, although these antibodies do not recognize $\beta_2$GP I bound to standard polystyrene plates, binding occurs after adsorption of the protein to polystyrene that has been modified by irradiation to incorporate carboxyl or reactive oxygen groups (31). An alternative explanation is that anti-$\beta_2$GP I antibodies preferentially recognize phospholipid or modified polystyrene-bound $\beta_2$GP I when the surface concentration is enhanced, which allows bivalent antibody binding to occur (32).

$\beta_2$GP I is a 50-kDa glycoprotein composed of five domains, each containing about 60 amino acids, that bear homology to other members of the complement control protein superfamily (33). The protein is thought to insert into phospholipid bilayers through a hydrophobic cationic segment near the carboxyl terminus of its fifth short chain consensus repeat (SCR) domain. There is convincing evidence that dimerization of the protein, by aPL IgG recognition of epitopes in the other domains, increases the avidity of the antibody–protein complex for membrane phospholipids (33,34).

The physiologic function of $\beta_2$GP I has not yet been established. $\beta_2$GP I has been shown to bind to endothelial cells by annexin II, a protein that also serves as a receptor for plasminogen and tissue plasminogen activator (35). As further described below, it has been proposed that antibody binding to $\beta_2$GP I on the endothelial surface can trigger the increased expression of adhesion molecules on the membrane (36).

## Reactivity of Antiphospholipid Antibodies with Oxidized Low Density Lipoproteins

The oxidation of phospholipids may be necessary for aPL antibody recognition (37,38). The epitopes for some aPL antibodies appear to be adducts of oxidized phospholipid and

protein such as $\beta_2$GP I (39). Therefore, some affinity-purified cardiolipin-binding antibodies in sera from patients with SLE appear to cross-react with oxidized (40) low density lipoproteins (LDL). Elevated levels of the latter antibodies have been proposed to be markers for arterial thrombosis (41); however, there is controversy on this point (42). Patients with SLE, particularly those with aPL antibodies, excrete elevated levels of arachidonic acid oxidation products such as 8-epi-prostaglandin $F_{2\alpha}$ and isoprostane $F_{2\alpha}$ in their urine (43).

## Binding of Antiphospholipid Antibodies to Other Proteins

Additional candidate cofactors and antigenic targets have been identified (44). These include prothrombin (coagulation factor II), coagulation factor V, protein C, protein S, annexin A5, high- and low-molecular-weight kininogens, heparin, and factor VII/VIIa (45). Infrequently, patients may develop a bleeding disorder characterized by prolongation of the prothrombin time or kaolin clotting time and severe hypoprothrombinemia resulting from the accelerated clearance of prothrombin–antibody complexes (46). Hypoprothrombinemia should be suspected in patients with LAs who have bleeding manifestations.

# RELATION BETWEEN ANTIPHOSPHOLIPID ANTIBODY TARGETS AND CLINICAL EVENTS

As mentioned earlier, the diagnosis of the aPL syndrome requires evidence for the presence of antibodies against phospholipids and/or relevant protein cofactors. This is most commonly obtained through immunoassays that detect aCL, antiphosphatidyl serine, anti-$\beta_2$GP I, or antiprothrombin antibodies or through evidence for interference with phospholipid-dependent coagulation assays known as the "lupus anticoagulant" (LA) phenomenon. Laboratory diagnosis of the aPL syndrome in the clinic setting can often be problematic. Research criteria have been developed to identify patients with the "definite" autoimmune aPL syndrome (47) (Table 112-3). It is important for the physician to recognize that these criteria were intended to categorize patients who fit the diagnosis of aPL syndrome with sufficient certainty for clinical research studies; they were not intended to be required criteria for the routine clinical diagnosis of the syndrome. As mentioned earlier, at present, no single test is sufficient for diagnosing this disorder. It is therefore recommended, when the disorder is suspected, that a panel of tests be performed, including syphilis testing, antibodies against cardiolipin, phosphatidyl serine, and $\beta_2$GP I, and coagulation tests for LA.

# IMMUNOASSAYS

## Anticardiolipin Antibody Assays

High levels of aCL antibodies are associated with an increased risk of thrombosis. During a 10-year follow-up on one group of patients who presented with elevated levels of aCL antibodies, approximately 50% of patients who presented with the antibodies, but without clinical manifestations of the syndrome, went on to develop the syndrome (48). Also, the presence of elevated titers of aCL 6 months after an episode of venous thromboembolism was associated with an increased risk of recurrence and of death (2). Women with IgM aCL antibodies, IgG aCL antibodies lower than 20 IgG binding units, or without an LA did not appear to be at risk for the aPL syndrome (49). In contrast,

**TABLE 112-3**

SAPPORO CRITERIA FOR THE CLASSIFICATION OF THE ANTIPHOSPHOLIPID SYNDROME[a]

**CLINICAL CRITERIA**

1. Vascular thrombosis
   a. One or more episodes of arterial, venous, or small-vessel thrombosis in any tissue or organ[b]
2. Pregnancy morbidity
   a. One or more unexplained deaths of a morphologically normal fetus at or beyond the 10th week of gestation, with normal fetal morphology documented by ultrasound or direct examination of the fetus, or
   b. One or more premature births of a morphologically normal neonate at or before the 34th week of gestation because of severe preeclampsia or eclampsia, or severe placental insufficiency, or
3. Three or more unexplained consecutive spontaneous abortions before the 10th week of gestation, with maternal anatomic or hormonal abnormalities and paternal and maternal chromosomal causes excluded

**LABORATORY CRITERIA**

1. Anticardiolipin antibody of immunoglobulin G and/or IgM isotype in blood, present in medium or high titer on two or more occasions at least 6 weeks apart, as measured by a standardized enzyme-linked immunosorbent assay for $\beta_2$-glycoprotein I–dependent anti-cardiolipin antibodies
2. Lupus anticoagulant present in plasma on two or more occasions at least 6 weeks apart, detected according to the guidelines of the International Society of Thrombosis and Haemostasis (Scientific Committee on Lupus Anticoagulants/Phospholipid-Dependent Antibodies), in the following steps:
   a. Prolonged phospholipid-dependent coagulation demonstrated with a screening test (e.g., activated partial thromboplastin time, kaolin clotting time, dilute Russell viper venom time, dilute prothrombin time, Textarin time)
   b. Failure to correct the prolonged coagulation time on the screening test by mixing with normal platelet-poor plasma (i.e., mixing incubation study)
   c. Shortening or correction of the prolonged coagulation time on the screening test by the addition of excess phospholipids
   d. Exclusion of other coagulopathies, as appropriate; definite antiphospholipid antibody syndrome is considered present if at least one of the clinical criteria and one of the laboratory criteria are met

[a]No exclusions other than those contained within the above criteria are needed. Because thrombosis may be multifactorial in patients with the antiphospholipid antibody syndrome, it is recommended that (i) patient populations being studied be assessed for other contributing causes of thrombosis, and (ii) such populations should be stratified according to identifiable or probable risk factors (e.g., age or comorbidities). Specific limits were not placed on the interval between the clinical event and the positive laboratory findings, although it is recommended that information about such intervals be assessed when relevant and that strict definitions of laboratory criteria be followed to exclude an association of antiphospholipid antibody positivity that represents an epiphenomenon to clinical events.
[b]Thrombosis must be confirmed by imaging, Doppler studies, or histopathology, with the exception of superficial venous thrombosis. For histopathologic confirmation, thrombosis should be present without evidence of considerable inflammation in the vessel wall.
Modified from Wilson WA, Gharavi AE, Koike T, et al. International consensus statement on preliminary classification criteria for definite antiphospholipid syndrome. *Arthritis Rheum* 1999;42:1309–1311.

women with an IgG aCL titer greater than 20 binding units or a positive LA were found to be more likely to develop complications (49). Elevated aCL antibodies of IgG or IgM isotype are a significant risk factor for stroke (50). The aPL antibodies are also an independent risk factor for stroke in young women (16). In the Antiphospholipid Antibodies and Stroke Study, 41% of the patients who met the study criteria of having experienced an ischemic stroke within 30 days tested aPL-positive (51).

In a systematic literature review, 15 of 28 studies showed significant associations between aCL antibodies and thrombosis (see Fig. 112-2) (52). In all of the studies, there was a correlation between higher antibody titers and increased odds ratios for thrombosis. Elevated aCL antibodies, whether high- or low-titer,

were significantly associated with both myocardial infarction and cerebral stroke. Only high-titer aCL antibodies were significantly associated with increased risk of deep vein thrombosis.

There have been some reports of patients with elevated IgA aCL antibodies with aPL syndrome. However, the determination of IgA aCL antibodies does not appear to be helpful in diagnosing the aPL syndrome or in explaining thrombotic events or fetal loss because the prevalence of true positivity to IgA ACL is extremely low; for example, in one study of 795 patients, IgA aPL were found in only two patients, both of whom were also positive to IgG aPL (53). In contrast, IgA anti-$\beta_2$GP I antibodies did appear to be significantly associated with thrombosis (54).

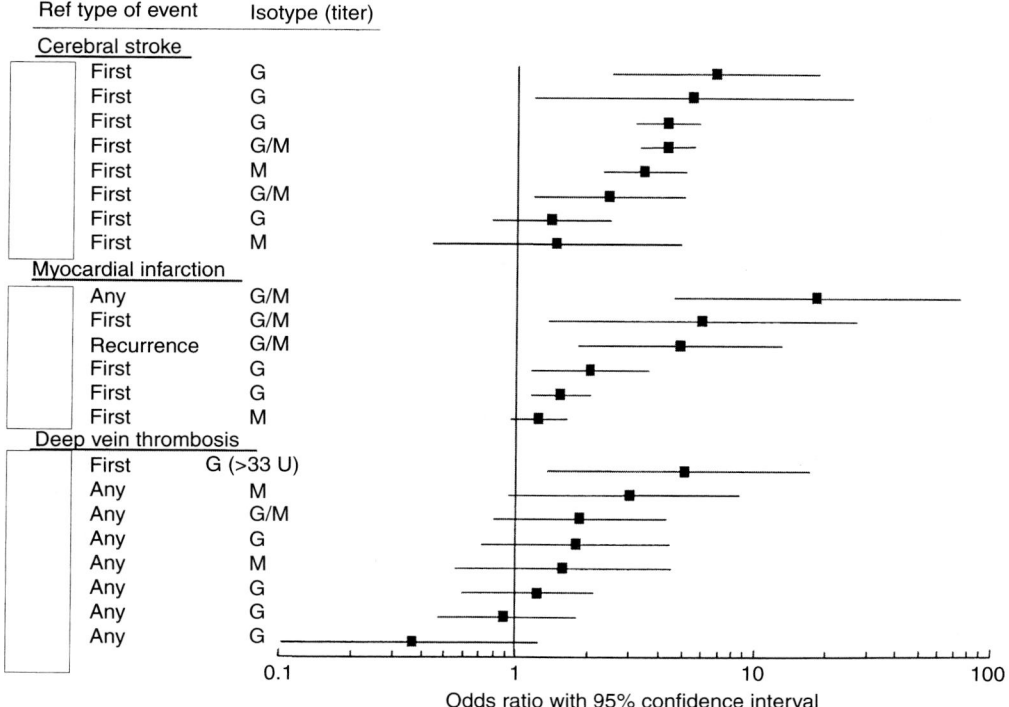

**Odds ratio with 95% confidence interval**

**FIGURE 112-2.** Anticardiolipin antibodies and thrombosis: analysis of 11 cross-sectional, case–control, and ambispective studies on 1,883 cases and 2,469 controls. Odds ratios (OR) with 95% confidence intervals (CI) are grouped according to the site and type of thrombosis and the antibody isotype. [Modified from Galli M, Luciani D, Bertolini G, et al. Lupus anticoagulants are stronger risk factors for thrombosis than anticardiolipin antibodies in the antiphospholipid syndrome: a systematic review of the literature. *Blood* 2003;101(5):1827–1832. Please refer to that article for the references cited in the figure. Copyright American Society of Hematology, used with permission.]

## Antiphosphatidyl Serine Antibody Assay

Cardiolipin is normally present in intracellular membranes and probably does not become exposed to plasma coagulation proteins *in vivo*. It was therefore hypothesized that immunoassays for antibodies against phosphatidyl serine, another anionic phospholipid that is normally present in the inner leaflet of the plasma membrane, and is exposed on syncytialized cells, apoptotic cells, and activated platelets, may be more relevant pathophysiologically. Antibodies to phosphatidyl serine (aPS) may correlate more specifically with aPL syndrome than aCL antibodies, particularly for arterial thrombosis (55,56).

## Assays for Antibodies Against Other Phospholipids

Antibodies against the zwitterionic phospholipid, phosphatidyl ethanolamine, have been associated with thrombosis and with activated protein C (APC) resistance (57). Some studies have suggested that antiphosphatidyl ethanolamine antibodies can occur in the aPL syndrome in the absence of antibodies against cardiolipin or other anionic phospholipids (58). Antiphosphatidylinositol antibodies are prevalent in young patients with cerebral ischemia (59,60). With the apparent heterogeneity of phospholipid antigenic targets, which phospholipids should clinicians utilize for clinical testing? No official recommendations or guidelines have yet been issued by a panel of authorities or regulatory agency regarding this matter. Some investigators have advocated testing for antibodies

against a panel of phospholipids in addition to cardiolipin (58,61–63), whereas others have disagreed (64), and one group recommends that a mixture of anionic and zwitterionic phospholipids be used for testing for antibodies (65).

## Anti-$\beta_2$GPI Antibody Assay

As discussed earlier, $\beta_2$GP I is believed to be the major protein cofactor for the aPL antibodies. ELISAs for anti-$\beta_2$GP I antibodies are considered to be more specific but less sensitive for the aPL syndrome than are aCL assays (66). Although these antibodies are usually present in conjunction with abnormal aCL and aPS antibodies, some patients with the aPL syndrome may present with antibodies to $\beta_2$GP I but without antibodies detectable in standard aPL assays (67,68). Despite their higher specificity for the aPL syndrome (98%), $\beta_2$GP I antibodies cannot be relied upon alone for the diagnosis because of their low sensitivity, which is believed to be approximately 40% to 50% (69,70). Concurrent testing for aCL and aPS antibodies and LA is therefore advised.

In a systematic literature review, 34 of 60 studies, none of them prospective, showed significant associations between anti-$\beta_2$GP I antibodies and thrombosis (see Fig. 112-3) (54). Of the 10 studies that included multivariate analysis, only two confirmed that IgG anti-$\beta_2$GP I antibodies were independent risk factors for venous thrombosis. Anti-$\beta_2$GP I antibodies were more often associated with venous events than arterial events. IgA anti-$\beta_2$GP I antibodies were always significantly associated with thrombosis. Interlaboratory variation has been a major problem with anti-$\beta_2$GP I antibody assays (71).

**A**

**B**

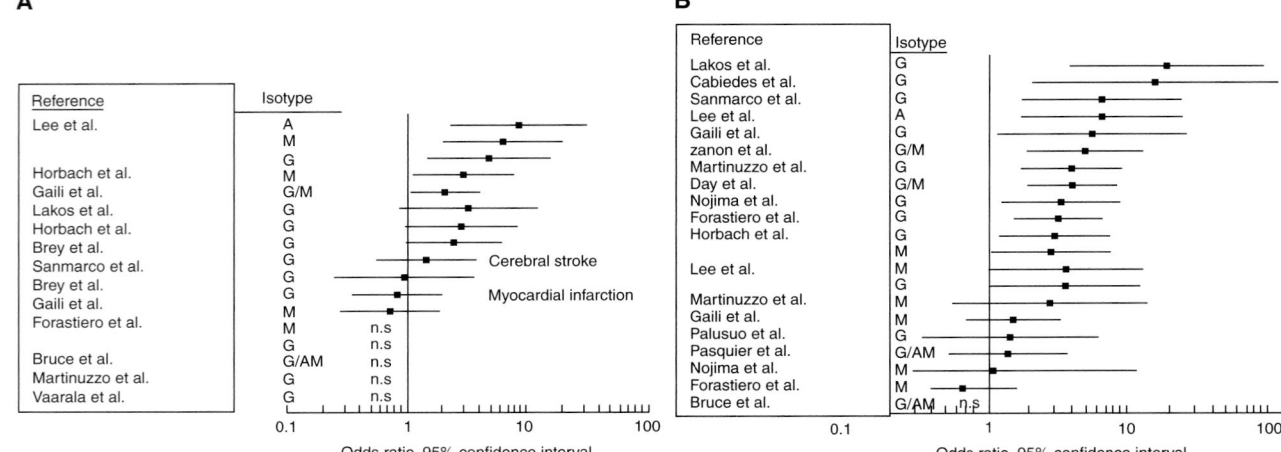

**FIGURE 112-3.** Anti-$\beta_2$-glycoprotein I antibodies and thrombosis: odds ratio (OR) with 95% confidence intervals (CI) grouped according to the type of thrombosis. **A:** Arterial thrombosis **B:** Venous thrombosis. [Modified from Galli M, Luciani D, Bertolini G, et al. Anti-beta 2-glycoprotein I, antiprothrombin antibodies, and the risk of thrombosis in the antiphospholipid syndrome. *Blood* 2003;102(8): 2717–2723. Please refer to that article for details of the references cited in the figure. Copyright American Society of Hematology, used with permission.]

## Antiprothrombin Antibody Assay

Prothrombin is considered to be the second major cofactor for aPL antibodies. In a systematic literature review, 17 of 46 studies showed significant associations between antiprothrombin antibodies and thrombosis (54). Of the eight studies that included multivariate analysis, two confirmed that antiprothrombin antibodies were independent risk factors for thrombosis and three others showed that they added to the risk borne by LA or aCL antibodies.

## Anti-Factor VII/VIIa Antibody Assay

Antibody to factor VII/VIIa was seen in 22 of 33 patients with aPL syndrome (45). The IgM class correlated with arterial thrombosis and the IgG class with venous thrombosis.

# COAGULATION ASSAYS

## Lupus Anticoagulants

The presence of the LA activity is more predictive and more specific for the occurrence of thrombosis or pregnancy loss than the aCL ELISA assays, both in patients with lupus (72) and others. In a metaanalysis of the risk for aPL-associated venous thromboembolism in individuals with aPL antibodies without underlying autoimmune disease or previous thrombosis for a 15-year period, the mean odds ratios were: for aCL antibodies, 1.6; for high titers of aCL, 3.2; and for LA, 11.0 (73). In a systematic literature review, 12 of 12 studies showed significant associations between LA and thrombosis, with odds ratios ranging from 5.7 to 9.4 (52). LA increased the risks of arterial and venous events to the same extent. Figure 112-4 shows the odds ratios for four of these studies. In contrast, only 15 of 28 studies showed significant associations between aCL and thrombosis. In the AntiPhospholipid Antibody Stroke Study (APASS) (51), positivity for both LA and aCL, but not for aCL alone, predicted a higher risk of recurrent thrombo-occlusive events in patients with first ischemic stroke.

# PATHOGENESIS OF THE ANTIPHOSPHOLIPID SYNDROME

The pathogenesis of the aPL syndrome has not been established. The fundamental paradox, demonstrated by the LA phenomenon, is that aPL antibodies prolong clotting times *in vitro*, and yet are associated with apparently increased coagulation *in vivo*. It is currently considered likely that aPL antibodies predispose to thrombosis either by inhibiting cell surface anticoagulant processes or by causing cells that are in the blood or in contact with the blood circulation to acquire a procoagulant phenotype.

## Inhibition of Cellular Anticoagulant Activity by Antiphospholipid Antibodies

The protein C pathway, an important endogenous antithrombotic system, is initiated when thrombin binds to thrombomodulin on endothelial cells. This binding modifies the substrate specificity of thrombin; the enzyme loses its procoagulant specificities and cleaves protein C to APC. In the presence of the free-form of protein S, APC proteolyzes coagulation factors Va and VIIIa. aPL antibodies can interfere with the protein C system by (a) decreasing the activation of protein C by the thrombomodulin–thrombin complex; (b) inhibiting the assembly of the protein C complex; (c) inhibiting the activity of protein C, directly or through its cofactor protein S, and (d) binding to factors Va and VIIIa in a manner that protects them from proteolysis by APC (44). In addition, patients with aPL syndrome have been described to have protein S deficiency (74,75).

Antithrombin-III is a member of the serine protease inhibitors family. The antithrombotic activity of this protein is markedly accelerated by the presence of heparin. *In vivo*, heparan sulfate proteoglycans may exert a thrombomodulatory effect. It has been demonstrated that at least some aPL antibodies cross-react with heparin and heparinoid molecules (which are highly polyanionic) and inhibit the acceleration of antithrombin-III activity (76).

It has been suggested that fibrinolysis may be impaired in the aPL syndrome, because women with the disorder have been described to have elevated plasminogen activator inhibitor-1

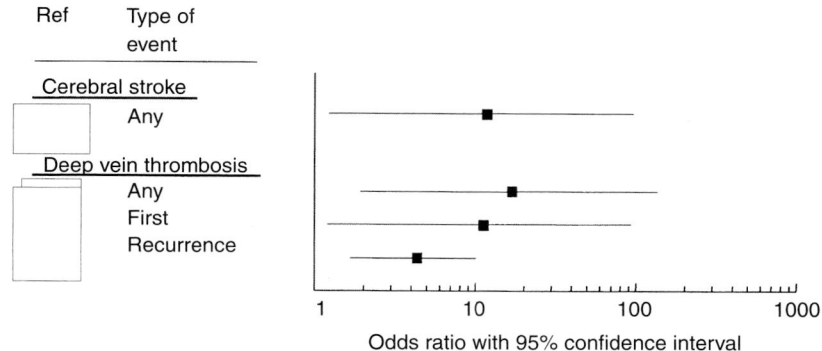

**FIGURE 112-4.** Lupus anticoagulants and thrombosis: analysis of four studies on 226 cases and 447 controls. Odds ratios (OR) with 95% confidence intervals (CI) are grouped according to the site and type of thrombosis and the study design. [Modified from Galli M, Luciani D, Bertolini G, et al. Lupus anticoagulants are stronger risk factors for thrombosis than anticardiolipin antibodies in the antiphospholipid syndrome: a systematic review of the literature. *Blood* 2003;101(5):1827–1832. Please refer to that article for the references cited in the figure. Copyright American Society of Hematology, used with permission.]

levels (74). Fibrinolysis may also be impaired by anti-$\beta_2$GP I–*mediated* inhibition of the autoactivation of factor XII (77) and the ensuing reductions of kallikrein and urokinase. Autoantibodies against tissue factor pathway inhibitor (TFPI) (78) and tissue-type plasminogen activator (tPA) (79) have been reported in the aPL syndrome.

As discussed in the next section, aPL antibodies may also promote thrombosis by disrupting the crystallization of the phospholipid-binding anticoagulant protein annexin A5 on phospholipid bilayers (80). This disruption of the annexin A5 anticoagulant shield exposes thrombogenic phospholipids and accelerates coagulation reactions. It has recently been demonstrated that aPL antibodies from patients with the aPL syndrome inhibit the binding of annexin A5 to phospholipids and also interfere with annexin A5 anticoagulant activity (see Fig. 112-5) (81).

## Induction of Cellular Activation by Antiphospholipid Antibodies

As shown in Table 112-4, aPL antibodies have been shown to recognize, injure, and/or activate cultured vascular endothelial cells (82–85). Cultured endothelial cells incubated with aPL antibodies express increased levels of cell adhesion molecules (86), an effect that may be mediated by $\beta_2$GP I (87) and may increase the adhesion of leukocytes to the vascular wall and promote inflammation and thrombosis. Not all studies have been able, however, to demonstrate such an effect (88). It has also been demonstrated that incubation of cultured endothelial cells with

### TABLE 112-4

**EFFECTS OF ANTIPHOSPHOLIPID ANTIBODIES ON ENDOTHELIAL CELL FUNCTION *IN VITRO***

| Function affected | Reference | Comments |
|---|---|---|
| Adhesion molecule expression | (91,92) | $\beta_2$GP I–dependent |
| Tissue factor expression | (89) | — |
| Endothelial-derived microparticle formation | (93) | Procoagulant activity marker |
| von Willebrand factor release | (94) | — |
| Cytokine release | (36) | Interleukin-1, -6, -8 |
| Production of platelet-activating factor (PAF) | (95) | — |
| Stimulation of platelet adhesion | (96,97) | Attenuated by PAF antagonists |
| Inhibition of migration | (98) | — |
| Induction of apoptosis | (99,100) | Possible association with antiannex in V |
| Inhibition of phospholipase A$_2$ | (101) | — |
| Endothelin-1 release | (102) | |
| Reduction of endothelial-surface annexin A5 | (103) | |

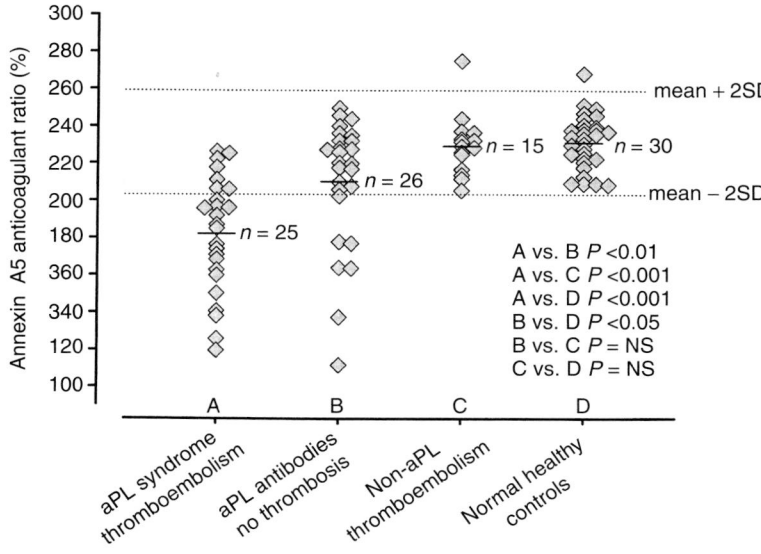

**FIGURE 112-5.** Annexin A5 resistance assays for patient plasma groups. The annexin A5 anticoagulant ratio for the aPL syndrome with thromboembolism group (**A**) was significantly decreased compared with the aPL antibodies without thrombosis history group (**B**), the non-aPL thromboembolism group (**C**), and the healthy control group (**D**). The ratio for the plasmas from the aPL antibodies without thrombosis history group (**B**) also was significantly reduced compared with the healthy control group (**D**). There were no significant differences in annexin A5 anticoagulant ratio for the non-aPL thromboembolism group (**C**) compared with the aPL antibodies without thrombosis history group (**B**) and the healthy control group (**D**). [Copyright American Society for Hematology. Reprinted from Rand JH, Wu XX, Lapinski R, et al. Detection of antibody-mediated reduction of annexin A5 anticoagulant activity in plasmas of patients with the antiphospholipid syndrome. *Blood* 2004;104(9):2783–2790.]

aPL antibodies results in the increased expression of tissue factor (89,90).

The activation of endothelial cells by anti-$\beta_2$GP I is followed by redistribution of nuclear factor $\kappa$B (NF$\kappa$B) from the cytoplasm to the nucleus, a process that is accompanied by increased expression of tissue factor and of the leukocyte adhesion molecules intercellular cell adhesion molecule-1 (ICAM-1), vascular cell adhesion molecule-1 (VCAM-1), and E selectin. Inhibition of the nuclear translocation of NF$\kappa$B abolished the response to these antibodies. In an immortalized human microvascular endothelial cell model, the signaling cascade was shown to involve TRAF6 and MyD88 but not TRAF2 and to show the same kinetics as IL-1 receptor-activated kinase phosphorylation, suggesting an involvement of the toll-like receptor family (104). The procoagulant and proinflammatory effects of anti-$\beta_2$GP I antibodies have been reported to be comparable to those of lipopolysaccharide (LPS), IL-1, and tumor necrosis factor-$\alpha$, and utilize the same signaling cascade as LPS and IL-1, which is depicted in Figure 112-6 (36). The aPL antibody-induced adhesion of leukocytes to endothelium with concurrent thrombosis was confirmed *in vivo* in a murine model of vascular injury, where it was shown to be mediated by ICAM-1, VCAM-1, and P selectin (91). Endothelial-derived microparticles are detectable in normal human blood and are increased in patients with LA (93). Patients with aPL syndrome and arterial thrombosis were found to have significantly increased plasma levels of endothelin-1 (102); the protein is thought to play a role in arterial tone, vasospasm, and thrombotic arterial occlusion. Human monoclonal aCL induced prepro-endothelin-1 mRNA levels significantly more than control monoclonal antibody.

aPL antibodies stimulate the expression of tissue factor by human monocytes and induce degranulation of human neutrophils (105,106). Also, aPL antibodies can stimulate platelet aggregation (107). Circulating activated (CD62-positive) platelets were detected by flow cytometry in the majority of a group of patients with primary aPL syndrome and neurologic disease, suggesting the existence of a relation among activated platelets, aCL, and the neurologic disorders (108). Some studies (109,110), but not others (111,112), have shown that aPL antibodies may alter the balance of eicosanoid synthesis toward prothrombotic moieties, as indicated by the presence of an increased quantity of thromboxane metabolites in the urine of patients with aPL, compared to controls (109,110). Dimers of $\beta_2$GP I, which mimic effects of $\beta_2$GP I–anti$\beta_2$GP I antibody complexes, increase platelet adhesion to collagen and thrombus formation in a flow system; these effects can be abrogated by inhibition of thromboxane synthesis (96).

## Potential Mechanisms Involved in Antiphospholipid Antibody-Associated Fetal Loss

In animal models, aPL antibodies can play a causal role in the development of thrombosis and pregnancy loss. Mice immunized against $\beta_2$GP I develop aPL antibodies and pregnancy wastage (113). Complement activation plays a critical role in this process. Disruption of the alternative pathway by preventing complexation of C3b and factor B led to protection against aPL-induced fetal loss in mice (114).

There is evidence that coagulation mechanisms are activated in pregnant women with the aPL syndrome. Prothrombin activation fragment F1.2, a marker for thrombin generation, is increased in patients who are pregnant, with aPL antibodies and a previous history of pregnancy losses, compared to control healthy non-aPL pregnant women (115). Histologic abnormalities were found in many, but not all, placentas of patients with aPL (116). Studies of placental pathology in patients with aPL antibodies, but without a prior history of fetal loss, showed that approximately half had uteroplacental vascular pathology, about half had evidence of thrombotic occlusion, and approximately one third had chronic villitis and/or decidual plasma cell infiltrates (117,118).

The pregnancy losses in the aPL syndrome may be a consequence of the marked reduction of the placental anticoagulant protein, annexin A5, on the apical membranes of aPL placental syncytiotrophoblasts (119). It has been proposed that the reduction of this protein, which normally coats the interface between the maternal and fetal circulations, may disrupt a constitutive antithrombotic mechanism within the intervillous blood circulation (120,121). This would accelerate coagulation within the maternal side of the maternal–fetal interface.

As described earlier, there is evidence to suggest that annexin A5 plays an antithrombotic role in physiologic conditions. Phosphatidyl serine is present on the apical membranes of syncytialized trophoblasts where it is covered by a binding layer of annexin A5 (120,122,123). Dissociation of annexin A5 from the surface of human placental trophoblasts and human umbilical vein endothelial cells accelerates the coagulation of plasma exposed to those cells (103). Therefore, annexin

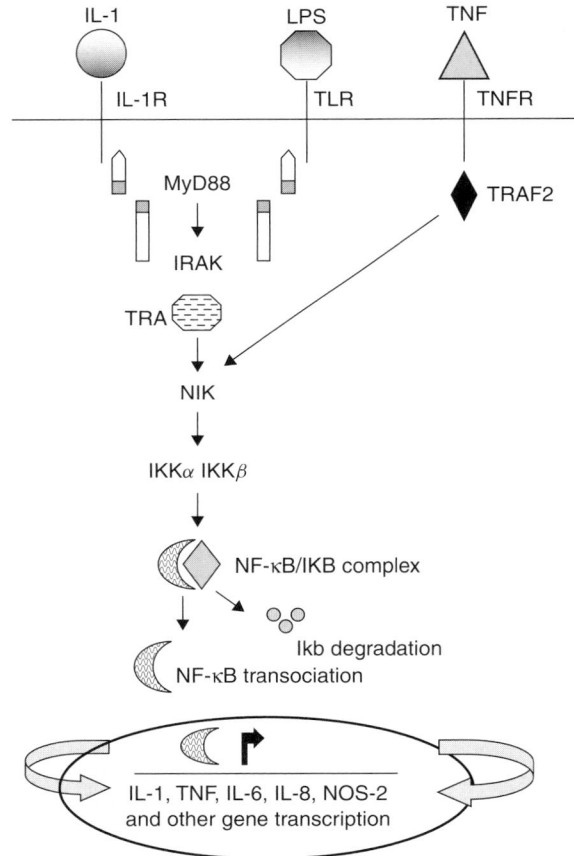

**FIGURE 112-6.** Interleukin-1 (IL-1), lipopolysaccharide (LPS), and tumor necrosis factor (TNF) signaling cascade in endothelial cells. This cascade is also activated by anti-$\beta_2$-glycoprotein I antibodies and may mediate their proinflammatory effects. A key intermediate is nuclear factor $\kappa$B (NF$\kappa$B), which translocates to the nucleus and modulates gene transcription. [Reprinted with permission from *Biomedicine and pharmacotherapy*, Vol 57, pp. 282–286, Copyright 2003; with permission from Elsevier; Raschi E, Testoni C, Borghi MO, et al. Endothelium activation in the anti-phospholipid syndrome. *Biomed pharmacother* 2003;57(7):282–286.]

A5 may play a thrombomodulatory role on the surfaces of cells lining the placental and possibly also the systemic vasculatures. Treatment of pregnant mice with antiannexin A5 antibodies resulted in placental necrosis, fibrosis, and pregnancy loss (121). However, it should be noted that an annexin A5-null mouse has been reported and does not have any apparent disease (124). This discrepancy is not yet understood and may be the result of compensating factors in the transgenic model.

There is a significant reduction of annexin A5 on the apical membranes of human placentas of women with aPL antibodies as compared to placentas of women with uncomplicated term deliveries, non-aPL–related pregnancy losses, and elective pregnancy terminations (103,119). Moreover, IgG fractions from patients with aPL syndrome reduce the quantity of annexin A5 on cultured trophoblasts and endothelial cells and also accelerate the coagulation of plasma exposed to these cells (103).

Although the displacement of annexin A5 occurs via aPL antibodies, some investigators have identified patients with aPL with antibodies that recognize annexin A5 directly (125, 126). Antiannexin A5 antibodies from patients with the aPL syndrome can induce apoptosis in cultured human umbilical vein endothelial cells (99).

# CLINICAL MANIFESTATIONS OF THE ANTIPHOSPHOLIPID SYNDROME

## Systemic Vascular Thrombosis

Patients may present with spontaneous venous and/or arterial thrombosis or embolism in any site of the vasculature. In one study of patients with aPL antibodies and radiologic evidence of thrombosis, 59% had thrombi limited to the venous circulation, 28% had solely arterial thrombi, and 13% had both types of events (127). Deep vein thrombosis of the lower extremities was the most common finding, occurring in about half of the patients; other sites of venous thrombotic events included pulmonary embolism, thoracic veins (superior vena cava, subclavian vein, or jugular vein), and abdominal or pelvic veins (127).

Thrombosis may occur spontaneously or in the presence of a predisposing factor such as estrogen hormone replacement therapy, oral contraceptives, pregnancy, the postpartum state (128,129), vascular stasis, surgery, or trauma. Some patients with venous thrombosis, but generally not with arterial thrombosis (130), also have concurrent genetic thrombophilic conditions such as heterozygosity for the factor $V_{Leiden}$ polymorphism (130–133).

## Stroke and Other Neurologic Conditions

Prospective analysis for the presence of aPL antibodies in patients with stroke, in the APASS, demonstrated that elevated levels of ACL are associated with increased risk for developing stroke but not with subsequent thromboembolic events (134). However, patients who tested positive for both aCL and LA tended to have more subsequent thrombo-occlusive events than patients who tested negative for both (31.7% vs. 24.0%, $P = 0.07$) (51). The aPL syndrome should be suspected in young patients with transient ischemic attacks or stroke, particularly when the usual risk factors for cerebrovascular disease are absent (135). Recurrent cerebrovascular events may lead to multiinfarct dementia (see Fig. 112-7). Some of the patients with aPL presenting with stroke have cerebral infarction due to venous, rather than arterial, occlusion (136). The patients with aPL and with cerebral venous thrombosis tend to be younger and have more extensive involvement of the venous system than aPL-negative patients with this disorder (136).

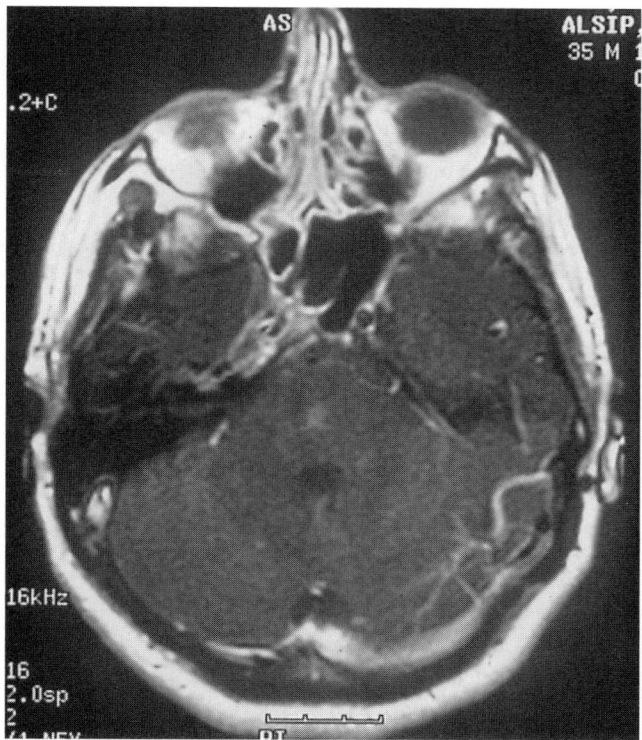

**FIGURE 112-7.** Magnetic resonance imaging (MRI) findings in a patient with aPL antibody–associated cerebrovascular disease. A 35-year-old man with mild systemic lupus erythematosus presented with diffuse supratentorial dysfunction. MRI examination showed, on T2-weighted imaging, diffuse enhancing lesions in gray and white matter, along with infarcts in the medulla with extension into the spinal cord. He subsequently developed axillary thrombosis, and high levels of immunoglobulin IgG and IgM anticardiolipin antibodies were identified. His neurologic status improved dramatically after the institution of heparin and aspirin, 81 mg per day. A repeat MRI study 3 weeks after the institution of therapy showed significant improvement in the ischemic lesions. (Photo courtesy of Dr. Gale A. McCarty, Division of Rheumatology, University of Virginia, Charlottesville, VA.)

Additional neurologic abnormalities that have been associated with aPL antibodies include seizures, chorea, migraines, Guillain-Barrè syndrome, transient global amnesia, dementia, diabetic peripheral neuropathy, and orthostatic hypotension (137). There is a high incidence of elevated aCL antibodies in patients with multiple sclerosis (in one series, 9% had IgG antibodies and 44% had IgM antibodies) (138); however, no clinical distinction has been observed between aPL-positive and aPL-negative patients with multiple sclerosis.

## Catastrophic Antiphospholipid Syndrome

Rare patients present with a *catastrophic* form of the aPL syndrome, which is characterized by severe, widespread vascular occlusions, sometimes leading to death. These patients present with evidence for severe multiorgan ischemia/infarction, usually with concurrent microvascular thrombosis. Patients with catastrophic aPL syndrome can present with massive venous thromboembolism, along with respiratory failure, stroke, abnormal liver enzymes, renal impairment, adrenal insufficiency, and areas of cutaneous infarction. The respiratory failure is usually due to acute respiratory distress syndrome and diffuse alveolar hemorrhage. Laboratory evidence for disseminated intravascular coagulation is frequently present. Reviews of 130 patients with catastrophic aPL syndrome (139,140) showed that most were women with a mean age in the late thirties, but ranging from childhood to old age. Most had either primary aPL syndrome or SLE; a few had other autoimmune conditions, including Sjögren syndrome, scleroderma, and rheumatoid arthritis. Precipitating factors were thought to contribute to the development of catastrophic aPL syndrome in some of the patients; these included infections, drugs (sulfur-containing diuretics, captopril, and oral contraceptives), surgical procedures, and cessation of prior anticoagulant therapy. The patients usually presented with multiple organ failure developing over a very short period of time. Most patients manifested evidence of microangiopathy affecting predominantly small vessels of the kidney, lungs, brain, heart, and liver. Only few of the patients experienced large-vessel occlusions. Death occurred in approximately half of the patients. A remarkable aspect of the catastrophic syndrome is that those patients who survive rarely experience a recurrence. Preliminary catastrophic antiphospholipid antibodies (CAPS) classification criteria and treatment guidelines were presented during the 10th International Congress on aPL (141). Diagnostic criteria include evidence of involvement of at least three organs, systems, and/or tissues; development of manifestations simultaneously or in less than 1 week; histopathologic confirmation of small-vessel occlusion; and laboratory confirmation of the presence of aPL (142).

## Pregnancy Losses, Obstetrical Complications, and Infertility

For a comprehensive review on the association of aPL antibodies with reproductive complications, refer to reference (143). Most studies have estimated the prevalence of aPL antibodies among general obstetric populations at approximately 5% or less; most of these patients are not clinically affected (144). Among obstetrical patients with recurrent fetal losses, approximately 16% to 38% of patients were found to have aPL antibodies.

Women patients with the aPL syndrome often present with a history of recurrent (usually defined as three or more) spontaneous pregnancy losses. Pregnancies occurring in women with aPL antibodies are at considerably increased risk of miscarriage, prematurity, intrauterine growth retardation, and preeclampsia (145). Although pregnancy losses occurring in the middle trimester or later in pregnancy are most striking, it has been estimated that approximately half of the patients experience first-trimester losses. Patients who are pregnant with the aPL syndrome are also more prone to develop deep vein thrombosis during pregnancy or the puerperium. Rarely, patients who are pregnant develop the catastrophic form of the aPL syndrome described earlier (146). The best predictor for pregnancy loss in a patient testing positive for aPL antibodies is not the degree of laboratory abnormality, but simply whether the patient has a history of previous pregnancy loss or thrombosis (147).

There is controversy about whether aPL syndrome is a cause of reproductive failure (i.e., infertility) in patients undergoing *in vitro* fertilization (IVF). Although most studies have reported an increased prevalence of elevated aPL antibodies among women undergoing IVF, prospective studies have not demonstrated that the presence of aPL antibodies considerably affect either the implantation or ongoing pregnancy rates (148). A randomized trial of heparin and aspirin for women with IVF failure and aPL antibodies did not show any improvement in pregnancy or implantation rates (149).

## Cardiac Manifestations

### Coronary Artery Disease

aPL antibodies have been associated with increased susceptibility to coronary artery disease, particularly premature atherosclerosis

(150). Antiprothrombin antibodies were reported to be a predictor of myocardial infarction in middle-aged men, and one study found that the joint effect of antiprothrombin antibodies with other known risk factors were multiplicative (151). Coronary artery disease also appears to be associated with antibodies against oxidized-LDL. The aPL syndrome should be considered in patients who lack the usual risk factors for coronary artery disease or who have evidence for thrombotic or embolic coronary occlusion without angiographic evidence of atherosclerotic disease. The aPL antibodies also appear to be a risk factor for restenosis with recurrent ischemia after percutaneous transluminal coronary angioplasty (152,153).

### Valvular Heart Disease

A significant fraction—approximately 35%—of patients with the primary aPL syndrome have cardiac valvular abnormalities detectable by echocardiography (154). Also, approximately 20% of patients with valvular heart disease have evidence for aPL antibodies compared with approximately 10% of matched controls (155). Valvular abnormalities occur in approximately half of patients with the combination of SLE and aPL antibodies; these abnormalities include leaflet thickening, vegetations, regurgitation, and stenosis (156). The mitral valve is mainly affected, followed by the aortic valve (157). In a prospective follow-up of 89 patients with severe, nonspecific valvular heart disease, thromboembolic events were significantly more frequent in the aPL-positive group than in the aPL-negative group; however, the presence of aPL antibodies was not an independent risk factor for thromboembolic events (158). One study did not find a relation between increased aCL antibodies and valvular abnormalities in patients with SLE, progressive systemic sclerosis, rheumatoid arthritis, and primary aPL syndrome (159).

## Thrombocytopenia

Thrombocytopenia occurs in a large fraction of patients with the aPL syndrome, but is rarely significant enough to cause bleeding complications or to affect anticoagulant therapy (160,161). Most cases appear to be immune-mediated. According to one study, most of the patients with the aPL syndrome and thrombocytopenia were found to have antibodies against the platelet membrane glycoprotein (GP) IIb/IIIa and/or GP Ib/IX complexes (162). However, in another study, no correlation was found between the presence of antibodies against platelet GP IIb/IIIa, GP Ib/IX, and thrombocytopenia, and the eluted platelet antibodies did not have any LA activity (163). Conversely, aPL antibodies and antibodies against platelet membrane glycoprotein were present simultaneously in approximately 70% of patients with immune-mediated thrombocytopenia (164). In a prospective cohort study, 5-year thrombosis-free survival of aPL-positive and aPL-negative ITP patients was 39% and 98%, respectively (165), indicating that thrombocytopenia itself is not protective against thrombosis in these patients.

## Other Organs

Cutaneous thrombi may manifest as livedo reticularis, ulcers, and necrotizing purpura (166). Other, less frequently reported complications of aPL syndrome include arterial occlusion involving the retina (167,168) and extremities (169). Pulmonary involvement may range from acute or recurrent pulmonary emboli to alveolar hemorrhage and acute respiratory distress syndrome (170). Adrenal infarction, hemorrhage, and Addisonian crises have been reported (171). In the kidney, occlusion of the main renal artery or vein, as well as diffuse microvascular occlusion, occasionally accompanied by microangiopathic hemolytic anemia and thrombocytopenia, acute renal failure, posttransplant rejection, and other syndromes, have all been reported in association with aPL antibodies (172–174).

# THERAPY FOR PATIENTS WITH ANTIPHOSPHOLIPID ANTIBODIES

## Thrombosis

For patients presenting with venous thromboembolism, care must be taken to determine whether the patient might have a preexisting LA that can interfere with the monitoring of unfractionated heparin therapy by activated partial thromboplastin time (aPTT). If there is an LA, then the heparin concentration can be estimated with an LA-insensitive aPTT reagent, with a specific heparin assay, or with the activated coagulation time test, which is usually insensitive to LAs. The problem of aPTT monitoring can also be avoided by treating with a low-molecular-weight heparin (LMWH).

Patients who have experienced spontaneous thromboembolism and have evidence for the aPL syndrome should be treated with long-term oral anticoagulant therapy. Prospective studies on the treatment of venous thromboembolism concluded that an international normalized ratio (INR) in the range of 2.0 to 3.0 will prevent recurrences (175,176). A retrospective study of a variety of patients with the aPL syndrome indicated that a higher intensity (INR >3.0) was necessary for preventing recurrences (177). In one retrospective study, six out of 16 patients (37%) followed-up over 6 to 42 months developed deep vein thrombosis (DVT) in spite of oral anticoagulation (INR 1.5-3.0) (178). Another study of secondary aPL syndrome concluded that conventional management of thromboembolic manifestations with heparin and/or oral anticoagulants prevented neither recurrent thromboses nor fatal outcomes (179).

A prospective randomized trial of 114 patients showed no benefit of high-intensity warfarin (INR 3.1 to 4.0) compared to moderate-intensity warfarin (INR 2.0 to 3.0) thromboprophylaxis in patients with aPL antibodies and previous thrombosis (176). Recurrent thromboses were rare in both groups. Most patients were not treated with aspirin. The APASS showed no benefit of warfarin (median INR 1.9) over aspirin for prevention of recurrent thrombo-occlusive events in aPL-positive patients with first ischemic stroke (51); however, most patients in this study had low-positive or moderate aCL IgG titers. The high prevalence of aPL immunoreactivity (41%) in that study suggested that nonspecific immune activation may have caused some of the aPL antibodies. At this time, it is appropriate to conclude that patients with DVTs can be treated with moderate-intensity warfarin, as recommended by the American College of Chest Physicians (180). However, the treatment of patients with arterial events is not resolved. Patients who develop thrombosis in the face of conventional oral anticoagulant therapy should be treated with either higher-intensity therapy or with a form of heparin for the long term; the risk of osteopenia with long-term heparin treatment should be considered.

A high titer of aCL (>30 U/mL) is generally not sufficient to justify prophylactic anticoagulation therapy in asymptomatic patients (178), and the same conclusion can be applied to patients with LAs who have not experienced thrombotic or embolic events. Anticoagulant therapy may be considered for the rare asymptomatic patient who has a convincing family history for thromboembolic complications of the aPL syndrome and has significant laboratory abnormalities, for patients with SLE who have marked aPL laboratory abnormalities, and for patients who also have other reasons for being at increased risk

for thrombosis (severe valvular heart disease and malignancy are examples of such situations) (158).

An important practical consequence of the LA effect is that prothrombin time and INR results overestimate the INRs in occasional patients with the aPL syndrome and LAs treated with warfarin anticoagulant therapy (181). As with the aPTT, there may be differences in the prothrombin time reagent with regard to their sensitivity to LAs, and different LAs vary significantly in their effects on the prothrombin time (182). It has been suggested that alternative tests, such as specific chromogenic coagulation factor assays for vitamin K–dependent proteins or the "prothrombin and proconvertin time," would be useful to confirm the appropriate warfarin effect in these patients (181). However, a multicenter study found that all but one of the commercial thromboplastins in use at nine centers provided acceptable INR values for patients with aPL syndrome with LA (183). Therefore, new thromboplastins should be checked for their responsiveness to LA before being used to monitor oral anticoagulant treatment in patients with the syndrome.

Fibrinolytic treatment has been described in primary aPL syndrome for extensive thrombosis of the common femoral and iliac veins extending to the lower vena cava (184), acute ischemic stroke (185), and acute myocardial infarction (186). Treatment with the antimalarial drug hydroxychloroquine may have an antithrombotic effect in patients with the aPL syndrome and SLE (187,188). The potential effectiveness of this treatment has also been supported by animal studies (189).

Patients with the catastrophic aPL syndrome require aggressive immunosuppressive therapy in the form of high-dose glucocorticoids in addition to anticoagulation. Second-line therapies, including intravenous Ig and/or plasma exchange, are necessary in the absence of a clinical response or in the presence of ongoing thrombosis despite treatment. Third-line treatments include fibrinolytics, cyclophosphamide, and prostacyclin (142).

Experimental therapies of the aPL syndrome include specific antiidiotypic or anti-CD4 antibodies, IL-3, ciprofloxacin or bromocriptine, and bone-marrow transplantation (190). Other new pharmacologic strategies that are under consideration but are unproven at the time of writing include use of statins, ACE inhibitors to inhibit monocyte tissue factor expression, a $\beta_2$GP I–specific B cell toleragen known as LJP 1082, and oral direct thrombin inhibitors such as ximelagatran (106). It is hoped that the Antiphospholipid Syndrome Collaborative Registry (APSCORE), a clinical trial that is recruiting patients at the time of writing, will contribute toward resolving questions regarding the nature, dosage, and duration of treatment of the syndrome.

## Pregnancy Loss

A systematic review of randomized trials on aPL antibody-positive women with recurrent pregnancy loss evaluated 10 trials on 627 women. Three trials on aspirin alone showed no significant reduction in pregnancy loss, whereas heparin plus aspirin (two trials) significantly reduced pregnancy loss compared to aspirin alone. Prednisone plus aspirin (two trials) resulted in a significant increase in prematurity and no significant reduction in pregnancy loss. Intravenous immunoglobulin did not add significant benefit to heparin plus aspirin (one trial), and heparin plus aspirin was superior to prednisone plus aspirin (one trial). High-dose and low-dose heparin did not show significantly different results (one trial) (191).

Women with a history of three or more spontaneous pregnancy losses and evidence of aPL antibodies should be treated with a combination of low-dose aspirin (75 to 81 mg daily) and with prophylactic doses of unfractionated heparin. Treatment should be started as soon as pregnancy is documented and continued until delivery in order to reduce the rate of late complications (143,192). The clearance of both unfractionated and LMWH increases as pregnancy progresses (193), and the dose required to prolong the PTT (or anti-Xa activity, in the case of LMWH) requires continual adjustment. In especially high-risk situations, induction of early delivery may be necessary. Prophylactic doses of heparin (i.e., 5,000 U q12h subcutaneous) should be started approximately 4 to 6 hours after delivery, if considerable bleeding has ceased, and continued until the patient is fully ambulatory. For patients who have experienced systemic thromboembolism, oral anticoagulant therapy is warranted for at least 6 weeks after delivery. For patients who have not had vascular thrombosis or embolism, the duration of postpartum treatment is not known, although many physicians recommend prophylactic treatment for the period of the puerperium. A study using treatment with LMWH produced similar results to unfractionated heparin (194); however, at the time of writing, these drugs have not been approved in the United States by the FDA for use during pregnancy. The potential benefits of LMWH would include once-daily injections; a decreased rate of allergic reactions, including heparin-induced thrombocytopenia; and the possibility of decreased bone loss compared to unfractionated heparins.

Close obstetric surveillance is required for all patients who are pregnant and with aPL antibodies. Doppler analysis of umbilical artery blood flow in these patients should be followed up as a measure of placental perfusion, with reversed or absent flow indicative of a poor fetal outcome, preeclampsia, or intrauterine growth retardation (195).

The presence of aPL antibodies during pregnancy in patients without any prior history for spontaneous pregnancy losses, other attributable pregnancy complications, thrombosis, or embolism warrants close surveillance and possibly prophylaxis. Some prospective studies show that aPL antibodies confer a twofold to threefold increased risk for pregnancy loss in otherwise low-risk pregnancies (196–198), with one study showing an eightfold increased risk (199); other prospective studies show no increased risk (200). The American College of Chest Physicians recommended in 2004 that patients with aPLs and no prior thrombosis or pregnancy loss should be monitored closely and possibly offered mini-dose heparin or LMWH and/or low-dose aspirin (201).

Corticosteroids or intravenous IgG (see subsequent text) should be considered only for patients who are refractory to anticoagulant therapy, who have a severe immune thrombocytopenia or other significant bleeding problem, or have a contraindication to heparin therapy. Treatment with the combination of prednisone and heparin should be avoided, when possible, because of the increased risk of osteopenia and of vertebral fractures (193). A randomized placebo-controlled pilot study evaluated treatment of aPL-positive pregnant women with intravenous Ig (202). All were treated with heparin and low-dose aspirin. No differences were observed in live birth rates or placental insufficiency, and differences in fetal growth restriction were not statistically significant. A metaanalysis failed to demonstrate a benefit of intravenous immunoglobulin in women with unexplained recurrent miscarriages; however, this remains a subject of some controversy (203).

## SUMMARY

The appropriate diagnosis and management of patients with aPL antibodies remains a confusing issue for many clinicians, largely because there is an incomplete understanding of the mechanisms that underlie the pathogenesis of aPL antibody–associated disorders. Although many unanswered questions still remain, empiric but effective diagnostic and management strategies have been developed for patients with aPL antibody–associated disease.

The identification of protein cofactors of aPL antibodies has broadened the scope of research efforts and offers promise for the development of more specific therapies in the future (106).

## References

1. Levine JS, Branch DW, Rauch J. The antiphospholipid syndrome. *N Engl J Med* 2002;346(10):752–763.
2. Schulman S, Svenungsson E, Granqvist S. Anticardiolipin antibodies predict early recurrence of thromboembolism and death among patients with venous thromboembolism following anticoagulant therapy. Duration of Anticoagulation Study Group. *Am J Med* 1998;104(4):332–338.
3. Moore JE, Mohr CF. Biologically false positive serological tests for syphilis: type, incidence, and cause. *J Am Med Assoc* 1952;150:467–473.
4. Conley CL, Hartmann RC. A hemorrhagic disorder caused by circulating anticoagulant in patients with disseminated lupus erythematosus. *J Clin Invest* 1952;31:621.
5. Laurell A, Nilsson I. Hypergammaglobulinemia, circulating anticoagulant and biologic false-positive wassermann reaction. *J Lab Clin Med* 1957;49:694–707.
6. Bowie EJ, Thompson JH Jr, Pascuzzi CA, et al. Thrombosis in systemic lupus erythematosus despite circulating anticoagulants. *J Lab Clin Med* 1963;62:416–430.
7. Feinstein DI, Rapaport SI. Acquired inhibitors of blood coagulation. In: Spaet TH, ed. *Progress in hemostasis and thrombosis*. New York: Grune & Stratton, 1972:75–95.
8. Thiagarajan P, Shapiro SS, De Marco L. Monoclonal immunoglobulin M lambda coagulation inhibitor with phospholipid specificity. Mechanism of a lupus anticoagulant. *J Clin Invest* 1980;66(3):397–405.
9. Harris EN, Gharavi AE, Boey ML, et al. Anticardiolipin antibodies: detection by radioimmunoassay and association with thrombosis in systemic lupus erythematosus. *Lancet* 1983;2(8361):1211–1214.
10. Loizou S, McCrea JD, Rudge AC, et al. Measurement of anti-cardiolipin antibodies by an enzyme-linked immunosorbent assay (ELISA): standardization and quantitation of results. *Clin Exp Immunol* 1985;62(3):738–745.
11. McNeil HP, Simpson RJ, Chesterman CN, et al. Anti-phospholipid antibodies are directed against a complex antigen that includes a lipid-binding inhibitor of coagulation: beta 2-glycoprotein I (apolipoprotein H). *Proc Natl Acad Sci U S A* 1990;87(11):4120–4124.
12. Galli M, Comfurius P, Maassen C, et al. Anticardiolipin antibodies (ACA) directed not to cardiolipin but to a plasma protein cofactor [see comments]. *Lancet* 1990;335(8705):1544–1547.
13. Galli M. Non beta 2-glycoprotein I cofactors for antiphospholipid antibodies. *Lupus* 1996;5(5):388–392.
14. Mateo J, Oliver A, Borrell M, et al. Laboratory evaluation and clinical characteristics of 2,132 consecutive unselected patients with venous thromboembolism—results of the Spanish Multicentric Study on Thrombophilia (EMET-Study). *Thromb Haemost* 1997;77(3):444–451.
15. Jones JV, Eastwood BJ, Jones E, et al. Antiphospholipid antibodies in a healthy population: methods for estimating the distribution. *J Rheumatol* 1995;22(1):55–61.
16. Brey RL, Stallworth CL, McGlasson DL, et al. Antiphospholipid antibodies and stroke in young women. *Stroke* 2002;33(10):2396–2400.
17. Labarca JA, Rabagliati RM, Radrigan FJ, et al. Antiphospholipid syndrome associated with cytomegalovirus infection: case report and review. *Clin Infect Dis* 1997;24(2):197–200.
18. Triplett DA. Many faces of lupus anticoagulants. *Lupus* 1998;7(Suppl. 2):S18–S22.
19. Uthman IW, Gharavi AE. Viral infections and antiphospholipid antibodies. *Semin Arthritis Rheum* 2002;31(4):256–263.
20. Drouvalakis KA, Buchanan RR. Phospholipid specificity of autoimmune and drug induced lupus anticoagulants; association of phosphatidylethanolamine reactivity with thrombosis in autoimmune disease [see comments]. *J Rheumatol* 1998; 25(2):290–295.
21. Sammaritano LR, Gharavi AE, Lockshin MD. Antiphospholipid antibody syndrome: immunologic and clinical aspects. *Semin Arthritis Rheum* 1990; 20(2):81–96.
22. McClain MT, Arbuckle MR, Heinlen LD, et al. The prevalence, onset, and clinical significance of antiphospholipid antibodies prior to diagnosis of systemic lupus erythematosus. *Arthritis Rheum* 2004;50(4):1226–1232.
23. Gharavi AE, Pierangeli SS, Espinola RG, et al. Antiphospholipid antibodies induced in mice by immunization with a cytomegalovirus-derived peptide cause thrombosis and activation of endothelial cells *in vivo*. *Arthritis Rheum* 2002;46(2):545–552.
24. Goldstein R, Moulds JM, Smith CD, et al. MHC studies of the primary antiphospholipid antibody syndrome and of antiphospholipid antibodies in systemic lupus erythematosus. *J Rheumatol* 1996;23(7):1173–1179.
25. Granados J, Vargas AG, Drenkard C, et al. Relationship of anticardiolipin antibodies and antiphospholipid syndrome to HLA-DR7 in Mexican patients with systemic lupus erythematosus (SLE). *Lupus* 1997;6(1):57–62.
26. Goel N, Ortel TL, Bali D, et al. Familial antiphospholipid antibody syndrome: criteria for disease and evidence for autosomal dominant inheritance. *Arthritis Rheum* 1999;42(2):318–327.

27. Hellan M, Kuhnel E, Speiser W, et al. Familial lupus anticoagulant: a case report and review of the literature. *Blood Coagul Fibrinolysis* 1998;9(2):195–200.

28. Cevallos R, Darnige L, Arvieux J, et al. Antiphospholipid and anti-beta 2 glycoprotein I antibodies in monozygotic twin sisters. *J Rheumatol* 1994;21(10):1970–1971.

29. Brandt JT, Triplett DA, Alving B, et al. Criteria for the diagnosis of lupus anticoagulants: an update. On behalf of the Subcommittee on Lupus Anticoagulant/Antiphospholipid Antibody of the Scientific and Standardisation Committee of the ISTH. *Thromb Haemost* 1995;74(4):1185–1190.

30. Reber G, Arvieux J, Comby E, et al. Multicenter evaluation of nine commercial kits for the quantitation of anticardiolipin antibodies. The Working Group on Methodologies in Haemostasis from the GEHT (Groupe d'Etudes sur l'Hemostase et la Thrombose). *Thromb Haemost* 1995;73(3):444–452.

31. Matsuura E, Igarashi Y, Yasuda T, et al. Anticardiolipin antibodies recognize beta 2-glycoprotein I structure altered by interacting with an oxygen modified solid phase surface. *J Exp Med* 1994;179(2):457–462.

32. Roubey RA, Eisenberg RA, Harper MF, et al. "Anticardiolipin" autoantibodies recognize beta 2-glycoprotein I in the absence of phospholipid. Importance of Ag density and bivalent binding. *J Immunol* 1995;154(2):954–960.

33. Bouma B, de Groot PG, van den Elsen JM, et al. Adhesion mechanism of human beta(2)-glycoprotein I to phospholipids based on its crystal structure. *EMBO J* 1999;18(19):5166–5174.

34. Willems GM, Janssen MP, Pelsers MM, et al. Role of divalency in the high-affinity binding of anticardiolipin antibody-beta 2 glycoprotein I complexes to lipid membranes. *Biochemistry* 1996;35(43):13833–13842.

35. Ma K, Simantov R, Zhang JC, et al. High affinity binding of beta 2-glycoprotein I to human endothelial cells is mediated by annexin II. *J Biol Chem* 2000;275(20):15541–15548.

36. Raschi E, Testoni C, Borghi MO, et al. Endothelium activation in the antiphospholipid syndrome. *Biomed Pharmacother* 2003;57(7):282–286.

37. Witztum JL, Horkko S. The role of oxidized LDL in atherogenesis: immunological response and anti-phospholipid antibodies. *Ann N Y Acad Sci* 1997;811:88–96.

38. Horkko S, Miller E, Dudl E, et al. Antiphospholipid antibodies are directed against epitopes of oxidized phospholipids. Recognition of cardiolipin by monoclonal antibodies to epitopes of oxidized low density lipoprotein. *J Clin Invest* 1996;98(3):815–825.

39. Horkko S, Miller E, Branch DW, et al. The epitopes for some antiphospholipid antibodies are adducts of oxidized phospholipid and beta2 glycoprotein 1 (and other proteins). *Proc Natl Acad Sci U S A* 1997;94(19):10356–10361.

40. Vaarala O, Puurunen M, Lukka M, et al. Affinity-purified cardiolipin-binding antibodies show heterogeneity in their binding to oxidized low-density lipoprotein. *Clin Exp Immunol* 1996;104(2):269–274.

41. Amengual O, Atsumi T, Khamashta MA, et al. Autoantibodies against oxidized low-density lipoprotein in antiphospholipid syndrome. *Br J Rheumatol* 1997;36(9):964–968.

42. Romero FI, Amengual O, Atsumi T, et al. Arterial disease in lupus and secondary antiphospholipid syndrome: association with anti-beta2-glycoprotein I antibodies but not with antibodies against oxidized low-density lipoprotein. *Br J Rheumatol* 1998;37(8):883–888.

43. Iuliano L, Pratico D, Ferro D, et al. Enhanced lipid peroxidation in patients positive for antiphospholipid antibodies. *Blood* 1997;90(10):3931–3935.

44. de Groot PG, Horbach DA, Derksen RH. Protein C and other cofactors involved in the binding of antiphospholipid antibodies: relation to the pathogenesis of thrombosis. *Lupus* 1996;5(5):488–493.

45. Bidot CJ, Jy W, Horstman LL, et al. Factor VII/VIIa: a new antigen in the anti-phospholipid antibody syndrome. *Br J Haematol* 2003;120(4):618–626.

46. Galli M, Barbui T. Antiprothrombin antibodies: detection and clinical significance in the antiphospholipid syndrome. *Blood* 1999;93(7):2149–2157.

47. Wilson WA, Gharavi AE, Koike T, et al. International consensus statement on preliminary classification criteria for definite antiphospholipid syndrome: report of an international workshop. *Arthritis Rheum* 1999;2(7):1309–1311.

48. Shah NM, Khamashta MA, Atsumi T, et al. Outcome of patients with anticardiolipin antibodies: a 10 year follow-up of 52 patients. *Lupus* 1998;7(1):3–6.

49. Silver RM, Porter TF, van Leeuween I, et al. Anticardiolipin antibodies: clinical consequences of "low titers". *Obstet Gynecol* 1996;87(4):494–500.

50. Tuhrim S, Rand JH, Wu XX, et al. Elevated anticardiolipin antibody titer is a stroke risk factor in a multiethnic population independent of isotype or degree of positivity. *Stroke* 1999;30(8):1561–1565.

51. Levine SR, Brey RL, Tilley BC, et al. Antiphospholipid antibodies and subsequent thrombo-occlusive events in patients with ischemic stroke. *JAMA* 2004;291(5):576–584.

52. Galli M, Luciani D, Bertolini G, et al. Lupus anticoagulants are stronger risk factors for thrombosis than anticardiolipin antibodies in the antiphospholipid syndrome: a systematic review of the literature. *Blood* 2003;101(5):1827–1832.

53. Selva-O'Callaghan A, Ordi-Ros J, Monegal-Ferran F, et al. IgA anticardiolipin antibodies—relation with other antiphospholipid antibodies and clinical significance. *Thromb Haemost* 1998;79(2):282–285.

54. Galli M, Luciani D, Bertolini G, et al. Anti-beta 2-glycoprotein I, antiprothrombin antibodies, and the risk of thrombosis in the antiphospholipid syndrome. *Blood* 2003;102(8):2717–2723.

55. Audrain MA, El Kouri D, Hamidou MA, et al. Value of autoantibodies to beta(2)-glycoprotein 1 in the diagnosis of antiphospholipid syndrome. *Rheumatology (Oxford)* 2002;41(5):550–553.

56. Lopez LR, Dier KJ, Lopez D, et al. Anti-beta 2-glycoprotein I and antiphosphatidylserine antibodies are predictors of arterial thrombosis in patients with antiphospholipid syndrome. *Am J Clin Pathol* 2004;121(1):142–149.

57. Esmon NL, Smirnov MD, Esmon CT. Lupus anticoagulants and thrombosis: the role of phospholipids. *Haematologica* 1997;82(4):474–477.

58. Berard M, Chantome R, Marcelli A, et al. Antiphosphatidylethanolamine antibodies as the only antiphospholipid antibodies. I. Association with thrombosis and vascular cutaneous diseases. *J Rheumatol* 1996;23(8):1369–1374.

59. Panarelli P, Viola-Magni MP, Albi E. Antiphosphatidylinositol antibody in deep venous thrombosis patients. *Int J Immunopathol Pharmacol* 2003;16(1):61–66.

60. Toschi V, Motta A, Castelli C, et al. High prevalence of antiphosphatidylinositol antibodies in young patients with cerebral ischemia of undetermined cause. *Stroke* 1998;29(9):1759–1764.

61. Rauch J, Janoff AS. Antibodies against phospholipids other than cardiolipin: potential roles for both phospholipid and protein. *Lupus* 1996;5(5):498–502.

62. Yetman DL, Kutteh WH. Antiphospholipid antibody panels and recurrent pregnancy loss: prevalence of anticardiolipin antibodies compared with other antiphospholipid antibodies. *Fertil Steril* 1996;66(4):540–546.

63. de Maistre E, Gobert B, Bene MC, et al. Comparative assessment of phospholipid-binding antibodies indicates limited overlapping. *J Clin Lab Anal* 1996;10(1):6–12.

64. Branch DW, Silver R, Pierangeli S, et al. Antiphospholipid antibodies other than lupus anticoagulant and anticardiolipin antibodies in women with recurrent pregnancy loss, fertile controls, and antiphospholipid syndrome. *Obstet Gynecol* 1997;89(4):549–555.

65. Laroche P, Berard M, Rouquette AM, et al. Advantage of using both anionic and zwitterionic phospholipid antigens for the detection of antiphospholipid antibodies. *Am J Clin Pathol* 1996;106(4):549–554.

66. Amengual O, Atsumi T, Khamashta MA, et al. Specificity of ELISA for antibody to beta 2-glycoprotein I in patients with antiphospholipid syndrome. *Br J Rheumatol* 1996;35(12):1239–1243.

67. Alarcon-Segovia D, Mestanza M, Cabiedes J, et al. The antiphospholipid/cofactor syndromes. II. A variant in patients with systemic lupus erythematosus with antibodies to beta 2-glycoprotein I but no antibodies detectable in standard antiphospholipid assays. *J Rheumatol* 1997;24(8):1545–1551.

68. Cabral AR, Amigo MC, Cabiedes J, et al. The antiphospholipid/cofactor syndromes: a primary variant with antibodies to beta 2-glycoprotein-I but no antibodies detectable in standard antiphospholipid assays. *Am J Med* 1996;101(5):472–481.

69. Sanmarco M, Soler C, Christides C, et al. Prevalence and clinical significance of IgG isotype anti-beta 2-glycoprotein I antibodies in antiphospholipid syndrome: a comparative study with anticardiolipin antibodies. *J Lab Clin Med* 1997;129(5):499–506.

70. Day HM, Thiagarajan P, Ahn C, et al. Autoantibodies to beta2-glycoprotein I in systemic lupus erythematosus and primary antiphospholipid antibody syndrome: clinical correlations in comparison with other antiphospholipid antibody tests. *J Rheumatol* 1998;25(4):667–674.

71. Reber G, Schousboe I, Tincani A, et al. Inter-laboratory variability of anti-beta2-glycoprotein I measurement. A collaborative study in the frame of the European Forum on Antiphospholipid Antibodies Standardization Group. *Thromb Haemost* 2002;88(1):66–73.

72. Somers E, Magder LS, Petri M. Antiphospholipid antibodies and incidence of venous thrombosis in a cohort of patients with systemic lupus erythematosus. *J Rheumatol* 2002;29(12):2531–2536.

73. Wahl DG, Guillemin F, De-Maistre E, et al. Meta-analysis of the risk of venous thrombosis in individuals with antiphospholipid antibodies without underlying autoimmune disease or previous thrombosis. *Lupus* 1998;7(1):15–22.

74. Ames PR, Tommasino C, Iannaccone L, et al. Coagulation activation and fibrinolytic imbalance in subjects with idiopathic antiphospholipid antibodies—a crucial role for acquired free protein S deficiency. *Thromb Haemost* 1996;76(2):190–194.

75. Crowther MA, Johnston M, Weitz J, et al. Free protein S deficiency may be found in patients with antiphospholipid antibodies who do not have systemic lupus erythematosus. *Thromb Haemost* 1996;76(5):689–691.

76. Shibata S, Harpel PC, Gharavi A, et al. Autoantibodies to heparin from patients with antiphospholipid antibody syndrome inhibit formation of antithrombin III-thrombin complexes. *Blood* 1994;83(9):2532–2540.

77. Schousboe I, Rasmussen MS. Synchronized inhibition of the phospholipid mediated autoactivation of factor XII in plasma by beta 2-glycoprotein I and anti-beta 2- glycoprotein I. *Thromb Haemost* 1995;73(5):798–804.

78. Forastiero RR, Martinuzzo ME, Broze GJ. High titers of autoantibodies to tissue factor pathway inhibitor are associated with the antiphospholipid syndrome. *J Thromb Haemost* 2003;1(4):718–724.

79. Cugno M, Cabibbe M, Galli M, et al. Antibodies to tissue-type plasminogen activator (tPA) in patients with antiphospholipid syndrome:

evidence of interaction between the antibodies and the catalytic domain of tPA in 2 patients. *Blood* 2004;103(6):2121–2126.

80. Rand JH, Wu XX, Quinn AS, et al. Human monoclonal antiphospholipid antibodies disrupt the annexin a5 anticoagulant crystal shield on phospholipid bilayers: evidence from atomic force microscopy and functional assay. *Am J Pathol* 2003;163(3):1193–1200.

81. Rand JH, Wu XX, Lapinski R, et al. Detection of antibody-mediated reduction of annexin A5 anticoagulant activity in plasmas of patients with the antiphospholipid syndrome. *Blood* 2004;104(9):2783–2790.

82. Dueymes M, Levy Y, Ziporen L, et al. Do some antiphospholipid antibodies target endothelial cells? *Ann Med Interne (Paris)* 1996;147(Suppl. 1):22–23.

83. Del-Papa N, Raschi E, Catelli L, et al. Endothelial cells as a target for antiphospholipid antibodies: role of anti-beta 2 glycoprotein I antibodies. *Am J Reprod Immunol* 1997;38(3):212–217.

84. Matsuda J, Gotoh M, Gohchi K, et al. Anti-endothelial cell antibodies to the endothelial hybridoma cell line (EAhy926) in systemic lupus erythematosus patients with antiphospholipid antibodies. *Br J Haematol* 1997;97(1):227–232.

85. Navarro M, Cervera R, Teixido M, et al. Antibodies to endothelial cells and to beta 2-glycoprotein I in the antiphospholipid syndrome: prevalence and isotype distribution. *Br J Rheumatol* 1996;35(6):523–528.

86. Simantov R, Lo SK, Gharavi A, et al. Antiphospholipid antibodies activate vascular endothelial cells. *Lupus* 1996;5(5):440–441.

87. Meroni PL, Papa ND, Beltrami B, et al. Modulation of endothelial cell function by antiphospholipid antibodies. *Lupus* 1996;5(5):448–450.

88. Hanly JG, Hong C, Issekutz A. Beta 2-glycoprotein I and anticardiolipin antibody binding to resting and activated cultured human endothelial cells. *J Rheumatol* 1996;23(9):1543–1549.

89. Branch DW, Rodgers GM. Induction of endothelial cell tissue factor activity by sera from patients with antiphospholipid syndrome: a possible mechanism of thrombosis. *Am J Obstet Gynecol* 1993;168(1 Pt 1):206–210.

90. Oosting JD, Derksen RH, Blokzijl L, et al. Antiphospholipid antibody positive sera enhance endothelial cell procoagulant activity—studies in a thrombosis model. *Thromb Haemost* 1992;68(3):278–284.

91. Pierangeli SS, Espinola RG, Liu X, et al. Thrombogenic effects of antiphospholipid antibodies are mediated by intercellular cell adhesion molecule-1, vascular cell adhesion molecule-1, and P-selectin. *Circ Res* 2001;88(2):245–250.

92. Riboldi P, Gerosa M, Raschi E, et al. Endothelium as a target for antiphospholipid antibodies. *Immunobiology* 2003;207:29–36.

93. Combes V, Simon AC, Grau GE, et al. *In vitro* generation of endothelial microparticles and possible prothrombotic activity in patients with lupus anticoagulant. *J Clin Invest* 1999;104(1):93–102.

94. Ames PR, Pyke S, Iannaccone L, et al. Antiphospholipid antibodies, haemostatic variables and thrombosis—a survey of 144 patients. *Thromb Haemost* 1995;73(5):768–773.

95. Silver RK, Adler L, Hickman AR, et al. Anticardiolipin antibody-positive serum enhances endothelial cell platelet-activating factor production. *Am J Obstet Gynecol* 1991;165(6 Pt 1):1748–1752.

96. Lutters BC, Derksen RH, Tekelenburg WL, et al. Dimers of beta 2-glycoprotein I increase platelet deposition to collagen via interaction with phospholipids and the apolipoprotein E receptor 2'. *J Biol Chem* 2003; 278(36):33831–33838.

97. Silver RK, Mullen TA, Caplan MS, et al. Inducible platelet adherence to human umbilical vein endothelium by anticardiolipin antibody-positive sera. *Am J Obstet Gynecol* 1995;173(3 Pt 1):702–707.

98. Lanir N, Zilberman M, Yron I, et al. Reactivity patterns of antiphospholipid antibodies and endothelial cells: effect of antiendothelial antibodies on cell migration. *J Lab Clin Med* 1998;131(6):548–556.

99. Nakamura N, Ban T, Yamaji K, et al. Localization of the apoptosis-inducing activity of lupus anticoagulant in an annexin V-binding antibody subset. *J Clin Invest* 1998;101(9):1951–1959.

100. Bordron A, Dueymes M, Levy Y, et al. The binding of some human antiendothelial cell antibodies induces endothelial cell apoptosis. *J Clin Invest* 1998;101(10):2029–2035.

101. Schorer AE, Duane PG, Woods VL, et al. Some antiphospholipid antibodies inhibit phospholipase A2 activity. *J Lab Clin Med* 1992;120(1): 67–77.

102. Atsumi T, Khamashta MA, Haworth RS, et al. Arterial disease and thrombosis in the antiphospholipid syndrome: a pathogenic role for endothelin 1. *Arthritis Rheum* 1998;41(5):800–807.

103. Rand JH, Wu XX, Andree HA, et al. Pregnancy loss in the antiphospholipid-antibody syndrome—a possible thrombogenic mechanism. *N Engl J Med* 1997;337(3):154–160.

104. Raschi E, Testoni C, Bosisio D, et al. Role of the MyD88 transduction signaling pathway in endothelial activation by antiphospholipid antibodies. *Blood* 2003;101(9):3495–3500.

105. Martini F, Farsi A, Gori AM, et al. Antiphospholipid antibodies (aPL) increase the potential monocyte procoagulant activity in patients with systemic lupus erythematosus. *Lupus* 1996;5(3):206–211.

106. Roubey RA. New approaches to prevention of thrombosis in the antiphospholipid syndrome: hopes, trials, and tribulations. *Arthritis Rheum* 2003;48(11):3004–3008.

107. Lin YL, Wang CT. Activation of human platelets by the rabbit anticardiolipin antibodies. *Blood* 1992;80(12):3135–3143.

108. Emmi L, Bergamini C, Spinelli A, et al. Possible pathogenetic role of activated platelets in the primary antiphospholipid syndrome involving the central nervous system. *Ann N Y Acad Sci* 1997;823:188–200.

109. Lellouche F, Martinuzzo M, Said P, et al. Imbalance of thromboxane/prostacyclin biosynthesis in patients with lupus anticoagulant. *Blood* 1991;78(11):2894–2899.

110. Kaaja R, Julkunen H, Viinikka L, et al. Production of prostacyclin and thromboxane in lupus pregnancies: effect of small dose of aspirin. *Obstet Gynecol* 1993;81(3):327–331.

111. Hasselaar P, Derksen RH, Blokzijl L, et al. Thrombosis associated with antiphospholipid antibodies cannot be explained by effects on endothelial and platelet prostanoid synthesis. *Thromb Haemost* 1988;59(1): 80–85.

112. Schinco PC, Marranca D, Bazzan M, et al. Lupus anticoagulant: interference with *in vivo* prostaglandin production and with platelet sensitivity to prostacyclin. *Scand J Rheumatol* 1992;21(3):124–128.

113. Garcia CO, Kanbour-Shakir A, Tang H, et al. Induction of experimental antiphospholipid antibody syndrome in PL/J mice following immunization with beta 2 GPI. *Am J Reprod Immunol* 1997;37(1):118–124.

114. Thurman JM, Kraus DM, Girardi G, et al. A novel inhibitor of the alternative complement pathway prevents antiphospholipid antibody-induced pregnancy loss in mice. *Mol Immunol* 2005;42(1):87–97.

115. Zangari M, Lockwood CJ, Scher J, et al. Prothrombin activation fragment (F1.2) is increased in pregnant patients with antiphospholipid antibodies. *Thromb Haemost* 1997;85(3):177–183.

116. Locatelli A, Patane L, Ghidini A, et al. Pathology findings in preterm placentas of women with autoantibodies: a case-control study. *J Matern Fetal Neonatal Med* 2002;11(5):339–344.

117. Salafia CM, Cowchock FS. Placental pathology and antiphospholipid antibodies: a descriptive study. *Am J Perinatol* 1997;14(8):435–441.

118. Salafia CM, Parke AL. Placental pathology in systemic lupus erythematosus and phospholipid antibody syndrome. *Rheum Dis Clin North Am* 1997;23(1):85–97.

119. Rand JH, Wu XX, Guller S, et al. Reduction of annexin-V (placental anticoagulant protein-I) on placental villi of women with antiphospholipid antibodies and recurrent spontaneous abortion. *Am J Obstet Gynecol* 1994;171(6):1566–1572.

120. Krikun G, Lockwood CJ, Wu XX, et al. The expression of the placental anticoagulant protein, annexin V, by villous trophoblasts: immunolocalization and *in vitro* regulation. *Placenta* 1994;15(6):601–612.

121. Wang X, Campos B, Kaetzel MA, et al. Annexin V is critical in the maintenance of murine placental integrity. *Am J Obstet Gynecol* 1999;180(4):1008–1016.

122. Lyden TW, Vogt E, Ng AK, et al. Monoclonal antiphospholipid antibody reactivity against human placental trophoblast. *J Reprod Immunol* 1992;22(1):1–14.

123. Vogt E, Ng AK, Rote NS. Antiphosphatidylserine antibody removes annexin-V and facilitates the binding of prothrombin at the surface of a choriocarcinoma model of trophoblast differentiation. *Am J Obstet Gynecol* 1997;177(4):964–972.

124. Brachvogel B, Dikschas J, Moch H, et al. Annexin A5 is not essential for skeletal development. *Mol Cell Biol* 2003;23(8):2907–2913.

125. Matsuda J, Saitoh N, Gohchi K, et al. Anti-annexin V antibody in systemic lupus erythematosus patients with lupus anticoagulant and/or anticardiolipin antibody. *Am J Hematol* 1994;47(1):56–58.

126. Matsuda J, Gotoh M, Saitoh N, et al. Anti-annexin antibody in the sera of patients with habitual fetal loss or preeclampsia. *Thromb Res* 1994;75(1):105–106.

127. Provenzale JM, Ortel TL, Allen NB. Systemic thrombosis in patients with antiphospholipid antibodies: lesion distribution and imaging findings. *AJR Am J Roentgenol* 1998;170(2):285–290.

128. Krnic BS, O'Connor CR, Looney SW, et al. A retrospective review of 61 patients with antiphospholipid syndrome. Analysis of factors influencing recurrent thrombosis. *Arch Intern Med* 1997;157(18):2101–2108.

129. Girolami A, Zanon E, Zanardi S, et al. Thromboembolic disease developing during oral contraceptive therapy in young females with antiphospholipid antibodies. *Blood Coagul Fibrinolysis* 1996;7(4):497–501.

130. Montaruli B, Borchiellini A, Tamponi G, et al. Factor V Arg506 → Gln mutation in patients with antiphospholipid antibodies. *Lupus* 1996;5(4):303–306.

131. Simantov R, Lo SK, Salmon JE, et al. Factor V Leiden increases the risk of thrombosis in patients with antiphospholipid antibodies. *Thromb Res* 1996;84(5):361–365.

132. Schutt M, Kluter H, Hagedorn GM, et al. Familial coexistence of primary antiphospholipid syndrome and factor V Leiden. *Lupus* 1998;7(3):176–182.

133. Brenner B, Vulfsons SL, Lanir N, et al. Coexistence of familial antiphospholipid syndrome and factor V Leiden: impact on thrombotic diathesis. *Br J Haematol* 1996;94(1):166–167.

134. The Antiphospholipid Antibodies and Stroke Study Group (APASS). Anticardiolipin antibodies and the risk of recurrent thrombo-occlusive events and death. *Neurology* 1997;48:91–94.

135. Weingarten K, Filippi C, Barbut D, et al. The neuroimaging features of the cardiolipin antibody syndrome. *Clin Imaging* 1997;21(1):6–12.

136. Carhuapoma JR, Mitsias P, Levine SR. Cerebral venous thrombosis and anticardiolipin antibodies. *Stroke* 1997;28(12):2363–2369.

137. Brey RL, Escalante A. Neurological manifestations of antiphospholipid antibody syndrome. *Lupus* 1998;7(Suppl. 2):S67–S74.

138. Sugiyama Y, Yamamoto T. Characterization of serum anti-phospholipid antibodies in patients with multiple sclerosis. *Tohoku J Exp Med* 1996; 178(3):203–215.

139. Asherson RA. The catastrophic antiphospholipid syndrome, 1998. A review of the clinical features, possible pathogenesis and treatment. *Lupus* 1998;7(Suppl. 2):S55–S62.

140. Asherson RA, Cervera R, Piette JC, et al. Catastrophic antiphospholipid syndrome: clues to the pathogenesis from a series of 80 patients. *Medicine (Baltimore)* 2001;80(6):355–377.

141. Asherson RA, Cervera R, de Groot PG, et al. Catastrophic antiphospholipid syndrome: international consensus statement on classification criteria and treatment guidelines. *Lupus* 2003;12(7):530–534.

142. Erkan D, Cervera R, Asherson RA. Catastrophic antiphospholipid syndrome: where do we stand? *Arthritis Rheum* 2003;48(12):3320–3327.

143. Galli M, Barbui T. Antiphospholipid antibodies and pregnancy. *Best Pract Res Clin Haematol* 2003;16(2):211–225.

144. Lockshin MD. Pregnancy loss and antiphospholipid antibodies. *Lupus* 1998; 7(Suppl. 2): S86–S89.

145. Rai R, Regan L. Obstetric complications of antiphospholipid antibodies. *Curr Opin Obstet Gynecol* 1997;9(6):387–390.

146. Ornstein MH, Rand JH. An association between refractory HELLP syndrome and antiphospholipid antibodies during pregnancy; a report of 2 cases. *J Rheumatol* 1994;21(7):1360–1364.

147. Finazzi G, Brancaccio V, Moia M, et al. Natural history and risk factors for thrombosis in 360 patients with antiphospholipid antibodies: a four-year prospective study from the Italian registry. *Am J Med* 1996;100(5): 530–536.

148. Backos M, Rai R, Regan L. Antiphospholipid antibodies and infertility. *Hum Fertil (Camb)* 2002;5(1):30–34.

149. Stern C, Chamley L, Norris H, et al. A randomized, double-blind, placebo-controlled trial of heparin and aspirin for women with *in vitro* fertilization implantation failure and antiphospholipid or antinuclear antibodies. *Fertil Steril* 2003;80(2):376–383.

150. Vaarala O. Antiphospholipid antibodies and myocardial infarction. *Lupus* 1998;7(Suppl. 2):S132–S134.

151. Vaarala O, Puurunen M, Manttari M, et al. Antibodies to prothrombin imply a risk of myocardial infarction in middle-aged men. *Thromb Haemost* 1996;75(3):456–459.

152. Ludia C, Domenico P, Monia C, et al. Antiphospholipid antibodies: a new risk factor for restenosis after percutaneous transluminal coronary angioplasty? *Autoimmunity* 1998;27(3):141–148.

153. Chambers JD Jr, Haire HD, Deligonul U. Multiple early percutaneous transluminal coronary angioplasty failures related to lupus anticoagulant. *Am Heart J* 1996;132(1 Pt 1):189–190.

154. Niaz A, Butany J. Antiphospholipid antibody syndrome with involvement of a bioprosthetic heart valve. *Can J Cardiol* 1998;14(7):951–954.

155. Bouillanne O, Millaire A, de Groote P, et al. Prevalence and clinical significance of antiphospholipid antibodies in heart valve disease: a case-control study. *Am Heart J* 1996;132(4):790–795.

156. Nesher G, Ilany J, Rosenmann D, et al. Valvular dysfunction in antiphospholipid syndrome: prevalence, clinical features, and treatment. *Semin Arthritis Rheum* 1997;27(1):27–35.

157. Hojnik M, George J, Ziporen L, et al. Heart valve involvement (Libman-Sacks endocarditis) in the antiphospholipid syndrome. *Circulation* 1996; 93(8):1579–1587.

158. Bulckaen HG, Puisieux FL, Bulckaen ED, et al. Antiphospholipid antibodies and the risk of thromboembolic events in valvular heart disease. *Mayo Clin Proc* 2003;78(3):294–298.

159. Gabrielli F, Alcini E, Prima MA, et al. Cardiac involvement in connective tissue diseases and primary antiphospholipid syndrome: echocardiographic assessment and correlation with antiphospholipid antibodies. *Acta Cardiol* 1996;51(5):425–439.

160. Galli M, Finazzi G, Barbui T. Thrombocytopenia in the antiphospholipid syndrome. *Br J Haematol* 1996;93(1):1–5.

161. Cuadrado MJ, Mujic F, Munoz E, et al. Thrombocytopenia in the antiphospholipid syndrome. *Ann Rheum Dis* 1997;56(3):194–196.

162. Macchi L, Rispal P, Clofent SG, et al. Anti-platelet antibodies in patients with systemic lupus erythematosus and the primary antiphospholipid antibody syndrome: their relationship with the observed thrombocytopenia. *Br J Haematol* 1997;98(2):336–341.

163. Panzer S, Gschwandtner ME, Hutter D, et al. Specificities of platelet autoantibodies in patients with lupus anticoagulants in primary antiphospholipid syndrome. *Ann Hematol* 1997;74(5):239–242.

164. Lipp E, von-Felten A, Sax H, et al. Antibodies against platelet glycoproteins and antiphospholipid antibodies in autoimmune thrombocytopenia. *Eur J Haematol* 1998;60(5):283–288.

165. Diz-Kucukkaya R, Hacihanefioglu A, Yenerel M, et al. Antiphospholipid antibodies and antiphospholipid syndrome in patients presenting with immune thrombocytopenic purpura: a prospective cohort study. *Blood* 2001; 98(6):1760–1764.

166. Gibson GE, Su WP, Pittelkow MR. Antiphospholipid syndrome and the skin. *J Am Acad Dermatol* 1997;36(6 Pt 1):970–982.

167. Au A, O'Day J. Review of severe vaso-occlusive retinopathy in systemic lupus erythematosus and the antiphospholipid syndrome: associations, visual outcomes, complications and treatment. *Clin Experiment Ophthalmol* 2004;32(1):87–100.

168. Coniglio M, Platania A, Di Nucci GD, et al. Antiphospholipid-protein antibodies are not an uncommon feature in retinal venous occlusions. *Thromb Res* 1996;83(2):183–188.

169. Lee RW, Taylor LM Jr, Landry GJ, et al. Prospective comparison of infrainguinal bypass grafting in patients with and without antiphospholipid antibodies. *J Vasc Surg* 1996;24(4):524–531.

170. Karmochkine M, Cacoub P, Dorent R, et al. High prevalence of antiphospholipid antibodies in precapillary pulmonary hypertension. *J Rheumatol* 1996;23(2):286–290.

171. Espinosa G, Santos E, Cervera R, et al. Adrenal involvement in the antiphospholipid syndrome: clinical and immunologic characteristics of 86 patients. *Medicine (Baltimore)* 2003;82(2):106–118.

172. Nochy D, Daugas E, Huong DL, et al. Kidney involvement in the antiphospholipid syndrome. *J Autoimmun* 2000;15(2):127–132.

173. Asherson RA, Cervera R. The antiphospholipid syndrome: multiple faces beyond the classical presentation. *Autoimmun Rev* 2003;2(3): 140–151.

174. Fakhouri F, Noel LH, Zuber J, et al. The expanding spectrum of renal diseases associated with antiphospholipid syndrome. *Am J Kidney Dis* 2003; 41(6):1205–1211.

175. Ginsberg JS, Wells PS, Brill Edwards P, et al. Antiphospholipid antibodies and venous thromboembolism. *Blood* 1995;86(10):3685–3691.

176. Crowther MA, Ginsberg JS, Julian J, et al. A comparison of two intensities of warfarin for the prevention of recurrent thrombosis in patients with the antiphospholipid antibody syndrome. *N Engl J Med* 2003;349(12): 1133–1138.

177. Khamashta MA, Cuadrado MJ, Mujic F, et al. The management of thrombosis in the antiphospholipid-antibody syndrome. *N Engl J Med* 1995; 332(15):993–997.

178. Urfer C, Pichler WJ, Helbling A. Antiphospholipid antibodies syndrome: follow-up of patients with a high antiphospholipid antibodies titer. *Schweiz Med Wochenschr* 1996;126(49):2136–2140.

179. Petrovic R, Petrovic M, Novicic SD, et al. Anticardiolipin antibodies and clinical spectrum of antiphospholipid syndrome in patients with systemic lupus erythematosus. *Vojnosanit Pregl* 1998;55(Suppl. 2):23–28.

180. Buller HR, Agnelli G, Hull RD, et al. Antithrombotic therapy for venous thromboembolic disease: the Seventh ACCP Conference on Antithrombotic and Thrombolytic Therapy. *Chest* 2004;126(Suppl. 3):401S–428S.

181. Moll S, Ortel TL. Monitoring warfarin therapy in patients with lupus anticoagulants. *Ann Intern Med* 1997;127(3):177–185.

182. Della VP, Crippa L, Safa O, et al. Potential failure of the International Normalized Ratio (INR) system in the monitoring of oral anticoagulation in patients with lupus anticoagulants. *Ann Med Interne (Paris)* 1996;147 (Suppl. 1):10–14.

183. Tripodi A, Chantarangkul V, Clerici M, et al. Laboratory control of oral anticoagulant treatment by the INR system in patients with the antiphospholipid syndrome and lupus anticoagulant. Results of a collaborative study involving nine commercial thromboplastins. *Br J Haematol* 2001; 115(3):672–678.

184. Camps GM, Guil M, Sanchez LJ, et al. Fibrinolytic treatment in primary antiphospholipid syndrome. *Lupus* 1996;5(6):627–629.

185. Julkunen H, Hedman C, Kauppi M. Thrombolysis for acute ischemic stroke in the primary antiphospholipid syndrome. *J Rheumatol* 1997; 24(1):181–183.

186. Ho YL, Chen MF, Wu CC, et al. Successful treatment of acute myocardial infarction by thrombolytic therapy in a patient with primary antiphospholipid antibody syndrome. *Cardiology* 1996;87(4):354–357.

187. Petri M. Thrombosis and systemic lupus erythematosus: the Hopkins lupus cohort perspective [editorial]. *Scand J Rheumatol* 1996;25(4):191–193.

188. Wallace DJ. The use of chloroquine and hydroxychloroquine for non-infectious conditions other than rheumatoid arthritis or lupus: a critical review. *Lupus* 1996;5(Suppl. 1):S59–S64.

189. Edwards MH, Pierangeli S, Liu X, et al. Hydroxychloroquine reverses thrombogenic properties of antiphospholipid antibodies in mice. *Circulation* 1997;96(12):4380–4384.

190. Krause I, Blank M, Shoenfeld Y. Immunomodulation of experimental APS: lessons from murine models. *Lupus* 1996;5(5):458–462.

191. Empson M, Lassere M, Craig JC, et al. Recurrent pregnancy loss with antiphospholipid antibody: a systematic review of therapeutic trials. *Obstet Gynecol* 2002;99(1):135–144.

192. Rai R. Obstetric management of antiphospholipid syndrome. *J Autoimmun* 2000;15(2):203–207.

193. Cowchock S. Treatment of antiphospholipid syndrome in pregnancy. *Lupus* 1998;7(Suppl. 2):S95–S97.

194. Backos M, Rai R, Baxter N, et al. Pregnancy complications in women with recurrent miscarriage associated with antiphospholipid antibodies treated with low dose aspirin and heparin. *Br J Obstet Gynaecol* 1999; 106(2):102–107.

195. Mascola MA, Repke JT. Obstetric management of the high-risk lupus pregnancy. *Rheum Dis Clin North Am* 1997;23(1):119–132.

196. Lynch A, Marlar R, Murphy J, et al. Antiphospholipid antibodies in predicting adverse pregnancy outcome. A prospective study. *Ann Intern Med* 1994;120(6):470–475.

197. Yasuda M, Takakuwa K, Tokunaga A, et al. Prospective studies of the association between anticardiolipin antibody and outcome of pregnancy. *Obstet Gynecol* 1995;86(4 Pt 1):555–559.

198. Lockwood CJ, Romero R, Feinberg RF, et al. The prevalence and biologic significance of lupus anticoagulant and anticardiolipin antibodies in a general obstetric population. *Am J Obstet Gynecol* 1989;161(2):369–373.

199. Lynch A, Byers T, Emlen W, et al. Association of antibodies to beta2-gly-coprotein 1 with pregnancy loss and pregnancy-induced hypertension: a prospective study in low-risk pregnancy. *Obstet Gynecol* 1999;93(2):193–198.

200. Cowchock S, Reece EA. Do low-risk pregnant women with antiphospholipid antibodies need to be treated? Organizing Group of the Antiphospholipid Antibody Treatment Trial. *Am J Obstet Gynecol* 1997;176(5):1099–1100.

201. Bates SM, Greer IA, Hirsh J, et al. Use of antithrombotic agents during pregnancy: the Seventh ACCP Conference on Antithrombotic and Thrombolytic Therapy. *Chest* 2004;126(Suppl. 3):627S–644S.

202. Branch DW, Peaceman AM, Druzin M, et al. A multicenter, placebo-controlled pilot study of intravenous immune globulin treatment of antiphospholipid syndrome during pregnancy. The Pregnancy Loss Study Group. *Am J Obstet Gynecol* 2000;182(1 Pt 1):122–127.

203. Daya S, Gunby J, Porter F, et al. Critical analysis of intravenous immunoglobulin therapy for recurrent miscarriage. *Hum Reprod Update* 1999;5(5):475–482.

# CHAPTER 113 ■ THROMBOSIS IN INFANCY AND CHILDHOOD

JANNA M. JOURNEYCAKE

Thromboembolic disease in children is being diagnosed at an increasing rate. This is due to more sophisticated diagnostic tools and therapies for chronic, severe, and life-threatening medical conditions in children. Imaging modalities such as computerized tomography (CT) scan and magnetic resonance imaging (MRI) scans provide a superior quality picture than what was two decades ago, and they are more widely available. The care of neonates and children with chronic and life-threatening disease incorporates the use of central venous catheters (CVCs) for rapid and/or continuous administration of fluids, antibiotics, nutritional and blood products, and medications for pressure support or pain, and CVCs are recognized as the primary risk factor for thromboembolic conditions (1–5). We are just beginning to realize the complications of these intensive therapies, including thrombosis, because these children are now surviving their diseases. Over the last 10 years, the index of suspicion for thrombosis has also increased primarily owing to the relatively recent identification and knowledge of inherited predisposition to develop thromboembolic disease or "thrombophilia."

Despite the increased awareness and identification of thromboembolic diseases in childhood, it is still a rare phenomenon when compared with the incidence in adults. Thromboembolic events occur at a rate of 5.3 per 10,000 hospitalized children but appears to be increasing (3,6). This chapter focuses on the differences in the hemostatic systems of infants and children compared to adults. It will explore the etiology and risk factors for thrombosis as well as current diagnosis and treatment guidelines. Finally, long-term complications related to thrombotic events of childhood is discussed.

## DEVELOPMENTAL HEMOSTASIS

Hemostasis is a dynamic process throughout childhood, and is different from that of adults (7–10). Overall, these differences offer a protective advantage to children with hemorrhagic and thrombotic complications. This is demonstrated clearly by the low prevalence of thrombosis seen in children (0.07 per 10,000) compared to adults (2.5 to 5 per 100) (3).

Coagulation factors are produced by the fetal liver by 10 weeks of age (7,8,10,11). At birth, the plasma levels of the vitamin K–dependent coagulation proteins (factor II, VII, IX, and X) and the contact factors are half the adult values and remain approximately 15% lower throughout childhood (7–11). In contrast, the levels of fibrinogen and factors V and VIII are equal to adult values (7–11).

Coagulation inhibitors are also reduced in the plasma at birth (7,10,11). Levels of antithrombin, heparin cofactor, protein C, and protein S are all considerably reduced. The level of antithrombin and heparin cofactor reach adult values during early childhood, but the levels of protein C and S remain lower than adult norms until adolescence (7,10,11). Despite lower antigen level of protein S, its activity is not substantially reduced in infancy because the amount of C4b-binding protein is also lower in infants, therefore, allowing more protein S to be present in the active state (11,12). In contrast to these natural inhibitors, the plasma level of α-2 macroglobulin in infants and children is nearly twice that found in adults (7,10,11).

The abundance of α-2 macroglobulin compensates for the deficiencies of the natural inhibitors of coagulation (e.g., protein C, protein S, and antithrombin). Together, a 25% decrease in thrombin generation and appropriate inhibition of coagulation provide protection against the development of most thromboembolic phenomenon during childhood (10,11).

There are published reference ranges for coagulation tests and for plasma levels of factors and inhibitors of coagulation in healthy preterm and term infants, as well as for children and adolescents (7–10).

Although the overall rate of occurrence of thromboembolic events in children is low, the rate is highest in infants and in adolescents (3,11). In fact, the rate of thrombosis in newborns admitted to intensive care units is as high as 2.4 per 1,000 admissions (4,12). Twelve percent of pediatric thrombosis is diagnosed in the first month of life (13,14). One explanation for this higher prevalence is the reduction in the activity of the fibrinolytic system during these developmental periods (11,15). In the newborn, there is decreased activity of plasminogen and increased concentration of tissue-type plasminogen activator inhibitor (PAI) (11). During puberty, there is also a marked increase in PAI-1 activity and reduced tissue-type plasminogen activator antigen levels (15).

## ETIOLOGY OF THROMBOSIS

For the most part, thrombosis in childhood is a multifactorial event. Less than 10% of events are idiopathic (3,4,16). Generally, children have an underlying medical condition that alters the hemostatic system to induce activation of coagulation and/or to prevent the inhibition of coagulation. Most conditions are related to stimulation of the inflammatory system or to abnormal blood flow. Some of the medical disorders are prematurity, cancer, rheumatologic disease, malabsorption syndromes, renal disease, congenital heart disease, severe infection, trauma, and burns (see Table 113-1). In addition to the hemostatic changes secondary to the underlying illness, many children also have the additional risk factor of a tunneled CVC inserted to facilitate therapy for the underlying illness (2–4,16). CVCs are associated with 65% of blood clots occurring in children and up to 90% in neonates (2). As many as 60% of children will also have an inherited prothrombotic abnormality, but the clinical relevance of isolated thrombophilia is still uncertain (3,13,17).

TABLE 113-1

ACQUIRED RISK FACTORS FOR THROMBOSIS
IN INFANTS AND CHILDREN

Central venous catheters
Infection: sepsis, musculoskeletal infections, head and neck
  infections
Congenital heart disease
Lupus anticoagulant and antiphospholipid antibodies
Trauma
Burns
Malignancy (especially leukemia and brain tumors) and
  associated therapies
Inflammatory diseases: systemic lupus erythematosus,
  inflammatory bowel disease
Renal disease: nephrotic syndrome, renal transplantation
Surgery
Pregnancy
Obesity
Diabetes mellitus
Vascular malformations

# THROMBOSIS IN NEONATES

Although most thrombotic events in newborns are associated with the use of a catheter, other risk factors include dehydration, hypoxia, infection, cardiac disease, maternal diabetes mellitus, and inherited thrombophilias (13,14,18). Neonatal thrombosis presents equally as arterial or venous events and can be categorized as catheter-related or not. The most commonly involved vessels are those where catheters have been inserted (i.e., umbilical artery or vein) (14). The other common areas are the brain, renal vein, and portal vein (13,19).

## Neonatal Stroke

Neonatal stroke, defined as a cerebrovascular event that occurs between 28 weeks gestation and 7 days of age, occurs in four of 1,000 live births (12). It occurs more commonly in men than in women (20). Most infants will present in the newborn period with seizures. However, many children do not present for several months when they are noted to have hemiparesis, early hand preference or seizures (21). Most neonatal stroke occurs in the distribution of the left middle cerebral artery. It is often very difficult to determine whether the stroke occurred *in utero*, at the time of delivery or within the first week. MRI and angiography is the best test to determine the extent of disease (22,23).

There is no standard approach for the evaluation and treatment of a perinatal stroke. However, at the time of diagnosis, it is important to determine whether the thrombotic event was related to an underlying disorder (24,25). Table 113-2 provides a list of conditions that are associated with neonatal stroke (25). The most common disorders are congenital heart disease, blood disorders, coexisting infections such as the TORCH infections (toxoplasmosis, syphilis, herpes, CMV), or systemic bacterial infections. Other rare conditions include metabolic diseases. Obtaining a thorough prenatal and birth history is also important in determining the cause of stroke. Maternal drugs and medical conditions, placental disorders, perinatal asphyxia, and birth trauma have all been associated with neonatal cerebrovascular events. Several studies have demonstrated an association between inherited prothrombotic condition and neonatal stroke (26). In a report of the Childhood Stroke Study Group, 68% of the evaluated patients with stroke had at least one prothrombotic risk factor compared to 24% of a control group (26). However, the Canadian Pediatric

Ischemic Stroke Registry found the presence of a prothrombotic factor in only 38% of patients (4).

Fortunately, the incidence of recurrent stroke is extremely low (i.e., <5%), and as many as 50% of these children will be neurologically healthy by 12 to 18 months of age (27,28). Long-term sequelae such as mild hemiparesis, speech or learning problems, behavioral problems, and seizures are more likely to persist in patients who present outside the newborn period (27,29). Treatment generally involves supportive care alone (24,30). There have been no clinical trials to evaluate the necessity of anticoagulant or antiplatelet therapy for stroke in the newborn (24).

## Cerebral Sinovenous Thrombosis

Cerebral venous thrombosis is seen much more commonly in the neonatal period than in any other age group (27,31). These infants present in a very similar way to infants with neonatal stroke, with seizure being the most common presenting symptom, but decreased level of consciousness, hemiparesis, and cranial nerve palsies are also seen (31). Cerebral venous thrombosis can be diagnosed by CT scan or magnetic resonance venography (MRV) (31). The risk factors for cerebral sinovenous thrombosis (CSVT) are again very similar to those of acute arterial stroke. They include asphyxia and perinatal complications, infection (particularly head and neck infection or bacterial sepsis), dehydration, cardiac disease, CVCs, and inherited coagulation disorders (26,31).

Approximately 40% of neonates have ischemia associated with the cerebral venous thrombosis, which may be a predictor of adverse neurologic outcome (31). In adults with cerebral venous thrombosis, anticoagulant therapy is instituted to prevent neurologic sequelae (32). Treatment of children and especially neonates has been demonstrated to be safe, but its efficacy has not been studied in clinical trials (33–35). The risks and benefits of anticoagulation or thrombolytic therapy needs to be determined on an individual basis, especially in sick neonates.

TABLE 113-2

CONDITIONS ASSOCIATED WITH *IN UTERO*
AND NEONATAL STROKE

**IN UTERO**
Inherited hypercoagulable state in mother
Inherited hypercoagulable state in infant
Autoimmune disease in mother
Prenatal substance abuse
Preeclampsia
Peripartum infection
Placental thrombosis
Hydrops fetalis
Intrauterine growth retardation
Asphyxia
Trauma

**NEONATAL**
Inherited hypercoagulable state
Polycythemia
Cardiac anomalies
Sepsis
Asphyxia
Extracorporeal membrane oxygenation
Catheterization

Adapted from Golomb MR, MacGregor DL, Domi T, et al. Presumed
pre- or perinatal arterial ischemic stroke: risk factors and outcomes.
*Ann Neurol* 2001;50(2):163–168.

## Abdominal Thrombosis

Spontaneous thrombosis is rare in newborns. When it occurs the most common site is the abdomen. Renal, caval, portal, and hepatic vein thrombosis have all been reported (19,36–38). Generally these are associated with birth trauma and asphyxia, sepsis, maternal diabetes, or preeclampsia.

Renal vein thrombosis (RVT) is the most common non-catheter-related thrombotic event and accounts for 10% of all venous occlusion in the newborn period (3,4,19,36,38). Presenting symptoms include hematuria and a flank mass. Occasionally, the infant has evidence of proteinuria, thrombocytopenia, or poor kidney function (19,38). If the thrombus extends into the inferior vena cava (IVC), the infant may present with signs of caval syndrome such as lower extremity swelling and discoloration. The child will usually have a history of dehydration and hypovolemia, or other conditions that will lead to reduced kidney blood flow (i.e., cyanotic heart disease) (19,36).

Ultrasonography is the radiologic test of choice to diagnose RVT because of its lack of side effects and sensitivity for diagnosing enlarged kidneys. Ultrasound can also determine if there is any associated adrenal hemorrhage. Treatment of RVT depends on its extent (38). Unilateral disease can be safely monitored and treated with supportive care. If there is evidence of uremia, extension into the IVC, or bilateral disease anticoagulant therapy should be initiated (35). Thrombolytic therapy should be reserved for infants with the risk of renal failure (35,39).

In newborns, portal vein thrombosis (PVT) is usually related to the insertion of an umbilical venous catheter (4). If it is diagnosed early, the infant will likely have an acute abdomen. However, it is often not appreciated until after collateral vessels have developed and presents as splenomegaly or recurrent gastrointestinal bleeding (40). A late complication of PVT is portal hypertension and variceal hemorrhage (41). Imaging modalities used to diagnose PVT include ultrasound, CT scan, and MRI/magnetic resonance angiography (MRA). Acute PVT can be treated with anticoagulant therapy (35). However, chronic disease may be better treated with thrombectomy or supportive care (41). Varices are treated with sclerotherapy (42).

## Homozygous Protein C or S Deficiency

One of the most severe forms of thrombosis found in the newborn period is the development of purpura fulminans within hours after birth. Skin lesions are found on the extremities, buttocks, abdomen, scrotum, or scalp, and begin as small ecchymotic areas that quickly increase in size. They are purplish/black with bullae and become necrotic within hours. This clinical picture is seen with a congenital homozygous deficiency of protein C, or less commonly protein S (14,43,44). Associated findings include evidence of cerebral or ophthalmic thrombosis that likely occurred before birth (14). Diagnosis must be made promptly as immediate therapy is indicated. Although protein C concentrates have been produced, they are not widely available for use (45). Therefore, the best initial therapy is 10 to 20 mL per kg of fresh frozen plasma (FFP) every 12 hours in order to achieve physiologic levels of protein C to prevent further progression of purpura fulminans (35,43). However, FFP is not virally inactivated, and most neonates will not be able to tolerate the volume necessary for treatment over many weeks until the lesions have resolved. Protein C concentrate is purified from a prothrombin complex concentrate (45). The major problem with long-term therapy for these infants is the need for intravenous access, the cost of therapy, and the availability of the product. There has been one study evaluating the efficacy of activated protein C concentrates in this population (46). Long-term anticoagulation therapy is also initiated at the time of diagnosis (35,47). With protein C replacement and anticoagulation, some infants have fewer episodes of skin necrosis. However, they have a lifetime risk for venous thrombosis and pulmonary embolism (PE) (48).

# THROMBOSIS IN CHILDHOOD AND ADOLESCENCE

Thrombosis in children and adolescence is a multifactorial event caused by both genetic and acquired risk factors (see Tables 113-1 and 113-3). Because children generally have healthier vascular systems than adults, spontaneous thrombotic events are rare. In fact, in most cases of childhood thrombosis, three or four different thrombotic risk factors are identified (3,5,49,50). Beyond the neonatal period, the younger the child, the more precipitating factors are generally found. The use of CVCs constitutes the most common acquired risk factor for thrombosis, and are present in 25% to 75% of cases (49,51).

## Catheter-Related Thrombosis

The prevalence of catheter-related thrombosis is 50% in children with cancer, hemophilia, chronic malnutrition, and other medical conditions (3,52–58). Although most thromboembolic events that present in children who have clinical signs such as extremity swelling, discoloration, and pain occur in association with a CVC, the rate of silent thrombosis is far greater and sometimes identified only by radiographic imaging (51). The "gold standard" test to identify catheter-related deep vein thrombosis (DVT) remains to be contrast venography (55,56,59,60). However, this test is considered by some to be invasive and carries a very small risk of anaphylaxis or renal complications related to the use of contrast medium. Because most CVCs in children are inserted into the veins of the upper extremities and chest, diagnosis of DVT

**TABLE 113-3**

INHERITED RISK FACTORS FOR THROMBOSIS IN INFANTS AND CHILDREN

**HIGH RISK OF THROMBOSIS**
Severe deficiencies of natural anticoagulation proteins
    Protein C, protein S, antithrombin
    Combined genetic mutations
        Heterozygous for both factor $V_{Leiden}$ and prothrombin
          G20210A
        Homozygous for factor $V_{Leiden}$, prothrombin
          G20210A, or MTHFR

**MODERATE RISK OF THROMBOSIS**
Heterozygous for factor $V_{Leiden}$ or prothrombin G20210A
    Risk increases with use of estrogen therapy
Elevated FVIII
Hyperhomocysteinemia
Elevated lipoprotein (a)
Dysfibrinogenemia
Dys/Hypoplasminogenemia

**RISK FACTORS ASSOCIATED WITH THROMBOSIS IN ADULTS, UNCERTAIN CLINICAL SIGNIFICANCE IN CHILDREN**
Increased FIX and FXI
Platelet glycoprotein polymorphisms
PAI-1 polymorphisms

PAI-1, plasminogen activator inhibitor 1.
Adapted from Journeycake JM, Manco-Johnson MJ. Thrombosis during infancy and childhood: what we know and what we do not know. *Hematol Oncol Clin North Am* 2004;18(6):1315–1338, viii–viix.

can be difficult. Doppler ultrasonography (appropriate for screening lower extremities) can miss thrombi in the internal jugular vein (60). Therefore, it is recommended to use both modalities to assess the vessels of the upper venous system. MRV is an appealing alternative because it can image all veins equally (61), but it is sensitive to motion artifact and many young children will require sedation to undergo the study (61,62). Occult DVT (identified only by imaging study) may be associated with other signs and symptoms such as catheter occlusion or malfunction, and catheter-related infection (63–66).

## Medical Conditions and Thrombosis

### Malignancy

Like in adults, cancer in children is one of the primary conditions associated with thromboembolic conditions. Childhood acute lymphoblastic leukemia (ALL) is the most common malignancy. On diagnosis, these children demonstrate activated coagulation by having increased levels of thrombin–antithrombin complexes stimulated by tumor cells (67). However, they also have long-term tunneled CVCs to administer therapy (67–69). Finally, they are universally prescribed chemotherapeutic agents that are caustic to vessel walls and can induce a transient hypercoagulable state (67,70). For example, asparaginase considerably reduces the amount of circulating antithrombin and fibrinogen (70,71). If asparaginase is given along with steroids, particularly prednisone, the risk for thrombosis is potentiated (72). The most common thrombotic event in children with ALL is catheter-related thrombosis, but central nervous system events (e.g., arterial ischemic stroke and cerebral venous thrombosis) are also commonly seen (73). There have been studies to determine whether thrombosis can be prevented in children with ALL by giving antithrombin concentrate or anticoagulants which suggested that this is a reasonable approach, but the studies were underpowered to make definite conclusions (71,74). Current recommendations are not to give prophylactic anticoagulation and to reserve antithrombin replacement during asparaginase therapy for children who have demonstrated the propensity to develop thrombi. Brain tumors are also commonly associated with thrombotic events (75).

### Infection

Thrombosis is seen as a systemic complication or as an invasive local infection. Head and neck infections often trigger CSVT (31). Musculoskeletal infections are now being recognized as a predisposing factor for venous thrombosis as well (76,77).

### Congenital and Acquired Heart Disease

Another condition that is highly associated with thrombotic events is complex congenital heart disease which is associated with both venous and arterial disease (78). Children require cardiac catheterization for diagnosis and treatment, and each procedure carries a risk of arterial thrombosis at the site of catheterization, primarily at the femoral artery. Late complications of femoral artery thrombosis include leg growth retardation (8%) or persistence of arterial occlusion (30%) (79,80). Most cardiac defects are treated by surgery. The Fontan procedure, and its variations, are performed for lesions where a biventricular circulation is not feasible. The systemic circulation is diverted directly to the pulmonary arteries and pumped by a single ventricle. After this procedure, children are at risk of venous (vena caval) and right atrial thrombosis that may involve the Fontan circuit. These thromboembolic complications can obstruct blood flow or embolize into the pulmonary or systemic arterial vessels (81,82). If the pulmonary vessels are obstructed and develop high vascular resistance, then the Fontan circuit is rendered useless (83). The most common site of arterial embolism is the central nervous system (84). Although half of the events can occur within the first 3 months after surgery, thrombi may develop decades later, and so most patients will receive indefinite prophylactic anticoagulation (85,86).

Children with dilated cardiomyopathy or heart conditions that require a mechanical valve are also at risk for embolic events primarily to the central nervous system. Indefinite anticoagulation with either aspirin or oral vitamin K antagonists (VKA) is recommended (35).

Kawasaki disease was first described in 1967 as a syndrome of fever for more than 5 days, with rash, nonexudative conjunctivitis, erythema of oral mucosa, lymphadenopathy, and swelling of the hands and feet. The inflammation can trigger a vasculitis of medium and large arteries, coronary aneurysms, and myocarditis. If initial treatment with intravenous immunoglobulins and antiinflammatory agents is delayed, the incidence of coronary artery aneurysm is 20% to 25% (87). Because these patients are at a risk for thrombosis of the aneurismal vessels and associated infarction, they should receive prophylactic aspirin after the inflammatory phase has subsided (35,88).

## Childhood Stroke

Stroke affects three to 15 per 100,000 children per year. As many as 65% of affected children will have lifelong disabilities such as neurologic defects and seizures, and the risk of a second stroke is 20% (28). Despite therapy, mortality rates as high as 10% have been reported.

There are certain comorbid conditions that are highly correlated with stroke, including congenital or acquired cardiac disease that can cause embolic phenomena and sickle cell anemia (26,89). Numerous systemic disorders can contribute to stroke (e.g., systemic vasculitis, metabolic disease, diabetes, trauma, cancer, lupus anticoagulants and antiphospholipid antibodies, and infection), and inherited prothrombotic states are causative as well (90–93). Although there has been a decline in the incidence of stroke after varicella infection, recent case reports describe a similar syndrome developing after the vaccine (94,95). A rare cause of stroke in childhood is anemia caused by severe iron deficiency (96). Despite the extensive list of potential causes (see Table 113-4), 50% of children with stroke will have no known primary disorder (2).

There is often a delay in the diagnosis of childhood stroke because the signs and symptoms of an acute event can be subtle. Children often have focal neurologic deficits (e.g., cranial nerve palsies, hemiparesis), but more systemic problems such as headache, lethargy, and seizures can occur (24).

There is limited published information about the etiology and outcome of childhood stroke, and very little evidence in the literature about appropriate management and prevention approaches. Most treatment strategies have been extrapolated from the practice in adult medicine and the results of retrospective cohort studies in children. However, there are no large randomized therapeutic trials in childhood stroke. Embolic stroke resulting from cardiac disease or carotid dissection and stroke associated with severe prothrombotic conditions (e.g., congenital homozygous protein C deficiency or antiphospholipid antibody syndrome) appears to benefit from anticoagulation (24). Warfarin, heparin, or more recently, low-molecular-weight heparin (LMWH) has been successful in treating and preventing recurrence of acute stroke in children with these underlying disorders (27,97). Unfortunately, anticoagulation does not improve the outcome better than treatment with antiplatelet agents for strokes of other

## TABLE 113-4

EPIDEMIOLOGY OF CHILDHOOD STROKE

**VASCULAR**
| | |
|---|---|
| Arteriopathy | Transient arteriopathy of childhood |
| | Postvaricella infection/vaccine |
| | Postradiation changes |
| | Moyamoya |
| Vasospastic | Migraine |
| Vasculitis | Systemic lupus |
| | Radiation injury |
| | Infection |
| | Drugs of abuse |
| Trauma | Carotid dissection |

**INTRAVASCULAR**
| | |
|---|---|
| Hematologic | Hemoglobinopathies (sickle cell disease) |
| | Hyperviscosity (polycythemia, leukemia) |
| | Hemolytic/uremic syndrome/thrombotic thrombocytopenia purpura |
| | Severe iron deficiency |
| | Hypercoagulable states (dehydration, antiphospholipid antibodies, pregnancy, medications, systemic disease, and inherited thrombophilia) |
| Metabolic | Mitochondrial myopathy, encephalopathy, lactic acidosis, and stroke (MELAS) |

**EMBOLIC**
Congenital and acquired heart disease
Carotid dissection

etiologies. Although the use of thrombolytic agents within 3 hours of initiation of the signs of stroke can be successful in improving outcomes in adults, its safety and efficacy in children has not been demonstrated. Any use of thrombolytic agents ideally should be in conjunction with a clinical trial to answer questions of dosing, timing, safety, and outcome. Surgical management of stroke and chronic ischemic disease in adults includes carotid stenting and angioplasty. However, these are invasive and potentially risky procedures that have not been well studied in children.

### Deep Venous Thrombosis

The rate of spontaneous thrombosis in children is <4%, but increases in adolescence. DVT of the lower extremities can occur with or without PE. In teenage girls, it is often associated with the recent administration of oral contraceptive pills, with the risk being highest in the first 6 months of therapy (98,99). As with other age groups, older children generally develop thrombotic events only in association with an underlying medical illness. Adolescence is the time when many autoimmune diseases present, such as the development of antiphospholipid antibodies and/or lupus anticoagulant (100). Although these proteins are known to be common and transient in small children, they contribute to thrombosis in teenagers (101).

Thrombosis of the axillary and subclavian venous systems is seen in athletes who participate in activities involving repetitive motion of the arms that leads to an impingement syndrome of the vessels by the rib cage (102). Although surgical removal of the ribs has been advocated to treat and prevent new occurrences, anticoagulation remains the standard of therapy (103,104). More recently, thrombolysis has been shown to improve the long-term outcome of these children (105,106).

### Cerebral Sinovenous Thrombosis

Although most CSVT events will occur in the neonatal period, the complication develops in older children at the rate of 0.67 per 100,000 children per year (31). Most commonly it will occur in conjunction with a deep tissue infection of the head and neck, dehydration, hypoxia, and the use of CVCs (31). More severe neurologic impairment will be seen in the children who present with seizures or have associated venous infarct (31). Anticoagulation is recommended in these patients even when the thrombus is associated with parenchymal hemorrhage, because the accumulation of blood is considered to be a continuation of the coagulation process (27,33,35).

### Pulmonary Embolism

PE is considered a rare event in children, but the incidence is likely underestimated as most cases are not detected until autopsy (3). Because affected children will generally have a concurrent medical condition with symptoms that can mimic those of PE (i.e., dyspnea, chest pain, hypoxia, and fever), physicians do not often have a high index of suspicion for thrombosis. For children without an underlying medical condition, PE can present in an insidious manner. The rate of PE associated with DVT is approximately 25% (107), and children with PE are likely to have a hypercoagulable state identified. In fact, half of the patients with PE will be positive for a lupus anticoagulant (107).

## SCREENING FOR THROMBOPHILIA

There is significant debate about when to screen for inherited thrombophilic conditions, and whether there is a role for screening asymptomatic children (108). Although the rate of thrombosis in preadolescent children with known thrombophilias is rare (109), identifying them at a young age may improve their healthcare by allowing for educational opportunities and prophylaxis against thrombosis in high-risk situations (99,110). However, screening may simply place additional anxiety on a family and child about a problem that is unlikely to affect them until adulthood (111). Finally, there may be problems with insurability. Those opposing the screening of asymptomatic family members state that knowing that a family has a tendency to thrombosis has the same benefits as laboratory screening (111). In addition, many inherited causes of thrombophilia are unknown, and a negative screening test in a child with a significant family history does not guarantee that the child will not develop thrombosis.

Some experts recommend screening symptomatic children for all known thrombophilic conditions. During the acute thrombotic event, there can be transient reductions in the levels of the natural anticoagulant proteins due to consumption or loss (112). Any low level would need to be repeated 3 to 6 months later to confirm a congenital deficiency. Despite the potential for transient deficiency, identifying significantly low protein C or antithrombin levels at the time of diagnosis of an extensive or progressive life-threatening thrombosis would provide an opportunity to replace the factor with protein concentrates or FFP (6). Table 113-5 outlines one approach to testing a symptomatic child for prothrombotic conditions.

## TREATMENT OF THROMBOSIS

Guidelines for the treatment of thromboembolic events in neonates and children have been extrapolated from the experience in adults. Virtually, no clinical trials have been conducted

TABLE 113-5

## APPROACH TO TESTING A CHILD WITH THROMBOSIS FOR A PROTHROMBOTIC STATE

**DURING ACUTE EVENT (BUT BEFORE INITIATION OF WARFARIN)**
Lupus anticoagulant
Antiphospholipid antibodies
FVIII
D-Dimer
Factor V$_{Leiden}$ gene mutation
Prothrombin G20210A mutation
Protein C
Protein S
Antithrombin
Fasting plasma homocysteine (especially for arterial events)

**THREE MONTHS AFTER ACUTE EVENT OR WHEN ANTICOAGULATION THERAPY IS DISCONTINUED**
Repeat tests that were abnormal at diagnosis (not gene tests)
Lipoprotein (a)
Consider: FIX, FIX, PAI-1, plasminogen, fibrinogen studies, and MTHFR mutation

PAI-1, plasminogen activator inhibitor 1.
Adapted from Journeycake JM, Manco-Johnson MJ. Thrombosis during infancy and childhood: what we know and what we do not know. *Hematol Oncol Clin North Am* 2004;18(6):1315–1338, viii–viix.

in children that successfully define optimal duration and dosing. There are, however, published guidelines by the American College of Chest Physicians that are acknowledged by many as reasonable and rational, albeit not necessarily evidence-based (35). Tables 113-6 and 113-7 provide details about treatment, dosing, and monitoring.

## Heparin and Low-Molecular-Weight Heparin

There are several key points to consider when initiating antithrombotic therapy in children. The activity of heparin, more so unfractionated than LMWH, relies on the presence of antithrombin which is often reduced in children (113). Newborns have physiologically low levels of antithrombin, and certain disease states (i.e., sepsis, nephrotic syndrome, and ALL) that are associated with an acquired deficiency (9,11). Antithrombin supplementation may be necessary for these groups especially if they appear to be resistant to heparin therapy or cannot achieve therapeutic levels. Neonates may require higher doses of heparin because the clearance is faster secondary to a large volume of distribution (113–115). The risk of bleeding associated with the use of heparin is 1.5% to 10% (114). Heparin-induced thrombocytopenia is reported occasionally in pediatric patients on unfractionated heparin (UFH) in intensive care, but is rare with LMWH (116,117). Although there are case reports of osteoporosis in children on standard heparin, it has occurred primarily in conjunction with the use of steroids or long-term use (35,118). There is also a theoretical risk of osteoporosis with LMWH use, so children who are treated with LMWH for more than 3 months should be monitored for this complication (119).

LMWH is administered as subcutaneous injection. Many neonates (especially preterm) have minimal subcutaneous tissue thereby making injection impractical. LMWH is considered to be advantageous over both UFH and oral anticoagulants because it has more predictable pharmacokinetics and requires less monitoring (120,121). However, because most LMWH therapy is instituted in children who are critically or chronically ill, monitoring with antifactor Xa levels is still advocated.

TABLE 113-6

## TREATMENT GUIDELINES FOR THROMBOTIC EVENTS

**SYSTEMIC VENOUS THROMBOTIC EVENTS**
Neonates
1. Close observation with radiographic imaging
2. If extensive thrombosis or extension of thrombus treat with UFH or LMWH for 10 d to 3 mo
3. Thrombolytic therapy should be used for thrombosis threatening organs or limbs

Children
1. Begin therapy with UFH or LMWH for 5 to 10 d Continue anticoagulation with LMWH or oral VKA for 3 mo (secondary thrombotic events) or 6 mo (idiopathic events)
2. For children with ongoing risk factors, anticoagulation should continue beyond 3 mo until risk factor is removed

**RENAL VEIN THROMBOSIS**
1. Anticoagulation therapy for children and neonates with unilateral disease invading the IVC

**CEREBRAL SINOVENOUS THROMBOSIS**
Neonates
1. Close observation for neonates with or 5 to 7 d of UFH or LMWH followed by 3 mo anticoagulation therapy

Children
1. 5 to 7 d of UFH or LMWH followed by 3 to 6 mo of anticoagulation, even in the presence of localized hemorrhage

**ARTERIAL ISCHEMIC STROKE**
Neonates
1. Anticoagulation therapy not recommended unless cause determined to be cardioembolic in origin; then treat with anticoagulation with LWMH for 3 mo

Children
1. 5 to 7 d UFH or LMWH until cardioembolic or carotid dissection has been excluded
2. Cardioembolic disease or vascular dissection: treat with 3 to 6 mo of anticoagulation (LMWH or oral VKA) followed by aspirin for 1 yr
3. Nonembolic arterial ischemic stroke: treat with aspirin alone after anticoagulation is discontinued

**CATHETER-RELATED THROMBOSIS**
1. Remove catheter if nonfunctioning or no longer needed after 3 to 5 d of anticoagulation
2. Anticoagulation for 3 mo
3. Prophylactic doses of warfarin or LMWH after the initial 3 mo if catheter remains in place

**PRIMARY PROPHYLAXIS**
CVCs: not indicated
Fontan procedure: aspirin or therapeutic warfarin
Dilated cardiomyopathy: therapeutic warfarin
Mechanical heart valves: therapeutic warfarin

UFH, unfractionated heparin; LMWH, low-molecular-weight heparin; VKA, vitamin K antagonist; IVC, inferior vena cava; CVCs, central venous catheters.
Adapted from Monagle P, Chan A, Massicotte P, et al. Antithrombotic therapy in children: the Seventh ACCP Conference on Antithrombotic and Thrombolytic Therapy. *Chest.* 2004;126(Suppl. 3): 645S–687S.

## TABLE 113-7

### DOSING AND MONITORING OF ANTITHROMBOTIC AGENTS

**UNFRACTIONATED HEPARIN**
Loading dose

|  |  |
|---|---|
|  | 75 U/kg |
| Continuous infusion |  |
| Infants | 28 U/kg/h |
| Children | 15–20 U/kg/h |

Monitor with aPTT every 6 h until therapeutic range is obtained
Therapeutic range is aPTT 2–2.5 times normal range and corresponds to an antifactor Xa level of 0.3–0.7 U/mL

**LOW-MOLECULAR-WEIGHT HEPARIN**
Prophylactic dose

|  |  |
|---|---|
| <2 mo | 0.75 mg/kg every 12 h |
| >2 mo | 0.5 mg/kg every 12 h |
| Therapeutic dose |  |
| <2 mo | 1.5 mg/kg every 12 h |
| >2 mo | 1 mg/kg every 12 h |

Monitor with antifactor Xa 4 to 6 h after a dose
Therapeutic range is 0.5–1.0 U/mL

**WARFARIN**
To achieve an INR of 2.0–3.0

**INITIAL DOSAGE (DAY 1)**
If baseline INR is 1.0–1.3, start with 0.2 mg/kg orally (maximum of 10 mg)
Reduce the dose to 0.1 mg/kg PO (max 5 mg) in patients with liver dysfunction, after a Fontan procedure, or in the presence of other hemorrhagic risk (e.g., hemodialysis)

**ADJUSTING DOSAGE (DAYS 2–5)**

| INR 1.1–1.3 | Repeat initial dose |
|---|---|
| INR 1.4–1.9 | 50% initial dose |
| INR 2.0–3.0 | 50% initial dose |
| INR 3.1–3.5 | 25% initial dose |
| >3.5 | Hold until INR <3.5, restart at 50% less than previous dose |

**MAINTENANCE DOSAGE**

| INR 1.1–1.4 | Increase by 20% |
|---|---|
| INR 1.5–1.9 | Increase by 10% |
| INR 2.0–3.0 | No change |
| INR 3.1–3.5 | Decrease by 10% of dose |
| INR 3.6–4.0 | Decrease dose by 20% |
| INR >4.0 | Hold on dose; check INR daily until <3.5, restart at 20% less than previous dose |

aPTT, activated partial thromboplastin time; INR, international normalized ratio.
Adapted from Monagle P, Chan A, Massicotte P, et al. Antithrombotic therapy in children: the Seventh ACCP Conference on Antithrombotic and Thrombolytic Therapy. *Chest* 2004;126(Suppl. 3):645S–687S.

## Vitamin K Antagonists

Oral VKA or warfarin use is problematic in very young children. First, newborns have reduced values of the vitamin K–dependent proteins (9,11). Infant formulas are supplemented with vitamin K which can cause resistance to VKAs, and if the infants are breastfed, then they are very sensitive to VKAs, because there is a negligible amount of vitamin K in breast milk (35). Second, most infants have inadequate venous access to monitor therapy. Third, monitoring oral anticoagulant therapy is affected by febrile illnesses, dehydration, the concurrent use of antibiotics for common childhood infections, dietary changes, and weight gain (122). The major complication of VKA use is bleeding occurring in 3% to 12 % of patients (123). Reported nonhemorrhagic complications include hair loss, tracheal calcification, and loss of bone density in children who are treated with oral VKAs for more than a year (35). "Point-of-care" whole blood monitors have made regulating therapy more convenient for families because they can test regularly at home (35).

## Alternative Thrombin Inhibitors

The successful use of alternative thrombin inhibitors such as lepirudin, hirudin, argatroban, and danaparoid sodium has been reported in a small number of pediatric cases primarily in the setting of heparin-induced thrombocytopenia (124,125). There are ongoing studies on the use of argatroban and bivalirudin in children.

## Antiplatelet Agents

Aspirin is the most commonly used antiplatelet agent. Indications for long-term aspirin therapy include stroke prevention in patients with congenital heart disease and a history of arterial stroke and Kawasaki disease (35,97,126,127). The dose is generally 1 to 5 mg per kg daily but there is variability in the dose required to inhibit platelet aggregation in children (35). The primary side effects of long-term aspirin therapy is bleeding, but it is rarely seen except in neonates who have slower clearance, patients with concurrent bleeding disorders, or children receiving concurrent anticoagulation therapy (35). There is also theoretical concern for Reye syndrome, but this is not usually seen unless the dose of aspirin is greater than 40 mg per kg, the dose for an antiinflammatory effect (35).

Dipyramidole in doses of 2 to 5 mg per kg is an alternative to aspirin therapy (35). Drugs that selectively inhibit ADP-induced platelet aggregation, such as ticlopidine and clopidogrel have not been studied in children (35). There has been one report ticlopidine, but appropriate doses have not been determined (128).

## Thrombolytic Agents

Three types of thrombolytic agents have previously been used in children, streptokinase, urokinase, and recombinant tissue-type plasminogen activator (rtPA). The lytic agent of choice is rtPA for several reasons. First, rtPA has improved clot lysis in *in vitro* studies than either of the other two agents. Second, streptokinase is associated with anaphylaxis and can have reduced bioavailability after streptococcal infections. Third, recombinant urokinase is currently not available, and the Food and Drug Administration distributed a warning about possible viral transmission associated with the use of native urokinase harvested from fetal kidneys. Finally, rtPA is fibrin specific and potentially has fewer systemic effects.

The use of thrombolytic agents at low doses (1 to 2 mg) has been shown to be safe and effective at restoring patency to occluded CVCs (129,130). Higher systemic doses (0.1 to 0.5 mg/kg/hour continuously for 6 to 12 hours) have been used to treat massive PE, and arterial and extensive venous thrombosis with success rates of 65% to 90% (39,131). Recently,

**TABLE 113-8**

INDICATIONS FOR THROMBOLYTIC THERAPY

Arterial thrombosis that fails to respond to heparin or is
  acutely limb threatening
Superior vena cava syndrome
Large inferior vena cava thrombosis
Bilateral renal vein thrombosis with any degree of renal
  insufficiency
Massive pulmonary embolism
Atrial thrombosis with any degree of cardiac compromise

Adapted from Monagle P, Chan A, Massicotte P, et al. Antithrombotic
therapy in children: the Seventh ACCP Conference on Antithrombotic
and Thrombolytic Therapy. *Chest* 2004;126(Suppl. 3):645S–687S.

investigators have reported the use of lower doses of systemic
tissue-type plasminogen activator (tPA) (0.03 to 0.06 mg/kg/hour)
or urokinase given over a longer duration were shown to be
effective with less bleeding complications than standard dose
tPA (132,133). Important considerations in the use of rtPA are
the need for plasminogen supplementation (using FFP) and concurrent heparin administration. At birth, plasma concentrations
of plasminogen are reduced compared to adults by 50% and
make thrombolytic therapy less effective (9,10). Because tPA
does not inhibit clot propagation or alter hypercoagulability,
heparin at prophylactic doses must be used to prevent recurrent
thrombosis (35).

The major complication of systemic thrombolytic therapy
is bleeding (131). Up to 65% of patients will experience some
degree of hemorrhage, usually oozing of mucous membranes
and at puncture sites, but 10% to 39% will require blood
transfusions (35). The rate of intracranial hemorrhage is 0.4%
to 13.2% with the highest rates found in preterm neonates
(131). The risk of bleeding increases with prolonged administration of rtPA. Children receiving rtPA must be monitored
closely for bleeding, and supplemental blood products (fibrinogen, platelets, packed red blood cells) may be necessary
during treatment. Because of this severe complication, the
current recommendation for tPA at standard doses is for life,
organ or limb-threatening thrombosis such as massive pulmonary emboli, thrombosis of the vena cava, arterial thrombosis, bilateral RVT when there is potential of renal failure,
CSVT with neurologic deficits, and atrial thrombosis (see
Table 113-8) (35). There are currently no recommendations
for its use in the treatment of other DVT or arterial ischemic
stroke, but studies are ongoing. Contraindications for the therapy (e.g., history of stroke, brain tumor, major surgery within
past 10 days, neurosurgery within the last 3 weeks, uncontrolled hypertension, and active major bleeding, or potential
for uncontrolled bleeding) should be balanced against the
risks and benefits of lysing the thrombus on an individual basis.

# LONG-TERM EFFECTS OF CHILDHOOD THROMBOSIS

## Postthrombotic Syndrome

Postthrombotic syndrome(PTS) is a chronic complication of
DVT that is a direct consequence of injury to the venous valves,
with resultant outflow obstruction and ultimately venous hypertension (134). Signs of PTS include skin changes such as
hyperpigmentation, redness, dependent cyanosis, and ulceration. Symptoms are heaviness, pain, swelling, paresthesias, and
cramping (135). The incidence has been reported to be as high

as 65% to 80% in adults with acute DVT involving the upper or
lower extremity, but the rate in children is not as well-defined
(135). Most definitions of PTS reflect findings in patients with
lower extremity DVT and deep venous reflux. Severe PTS in the
legs can limit functional status of the individual, and studies in
adults have demonstrated the benefit of anticoagulation and
compression stockings in its prevention (136–140). It is unknown if these same management practices are necessary or useful after DVT involving the upper extremity. However, there is a
suggestion that use of thrombolytic agents may help prevent PTS
by hastening clot resolution (141). In children, most DVT is associated with CVCs and, therefore, more likely to involve subclavian, jugular or brachiocephalic veins, or the superior vena cava
(i.e., the upper venous system) (3,51). PTS occurs less frequently
after upper extremity DVT, likely due to the reduced effect of
gravity on blood flow. Moreover, the nonspecific criteria for diagnosis of PTS following lower extremity DVT are often difficult
to apply to the arm (9,10). Unfortunately, there is no "gold standard" definition of PTS. However, patients can manifest this
complication weeks or even years after acute DVT (142). In
adults, most patients develop signs and symptoms within 2 years
of diagnosis, but it is not known how long these signs and symptoms can be seen after childhood thromboembolic events (32).

Only recently have investigators attempted to assess the
problem of PTS in children. In 2000, a retrospective review
of the outcome of 405 children on the Canadian Childhood
Thrombophilia Registry reported that 12% had been diagnosed with PTS (3). However, no standard diagnostic criteria were described, nor did the analysis define the rate of
occurrence in the upper versus lower extremities. Other limited evidence of PTS includes case reports of children with
congenital heart and renal disease (36,143). There are also
reports of children born prematurely who manifest signs of
PTS when they reach adolescence (144). More recently,
there was a report on a cohort of 153 children with clinically symptomatic thrombosis, among whom 123 (80%) had
catheter-related DVT, with 62 (40%) involving the upper
extremity (145). A scoring system was used to define PTS
employing change in skin color, varicosities, skin ulceration,
limb circumference discrepancies, collateral vessel formation, tenderness to palpation, and edema. Subjective criteria
included extremity pain/abnormal use, and swelling. Their
scale was a dichotomous measure with any score above 8 indicating severe disease, and scores between 1 and 3 arbitrarily designated as mild disease. The mean score was 2.2 ± 1.3,
yet a diagnosis of PTS was given to 63% (96 of 153) of this
cohort. PTS was considered mild in 80% of the cases, with
the most common finding being "increased" limb circumference (145). However, the mean increase in circumference
compared to the contralateral extremity was not reported,
and the study did not correlate the diagnosis of PTS with
clinical findings. In a recent study of childhood cancer survivors who had CVCs in place during therapy, signs, and
symptoms of PTS were rarely observed (146).

There are still many unanswered questions about the clinical severity and implications of PTS in children, but a recent
report suggested that PTS and recurrence of thrombosis can
be predicted by laboratory studies. Children with elevated levels of both quantitative D-Dimer and factor VIII at the time of
diagnosis and 3 to 6 months later were more likely to have
long-term complications (147). More studies are needed to confirm this association.

# CONCLUSION

Thromboembolic disorders are an increasing problem in children. In response, many pediatric hematologists have instituted specialized thrombosis clinics to monitor anticoagulation

therapy and to determine ongoing prothrombotic risks. Because the implications of vascular injury in a young child are not completely understood, these children need to be followed-up over time. Pediatric hematologists are also challenged to conduct the much needed clinical trials about the best treatment and prevention strategies.

## References

1. van Ommen CH, Heijboer H, van den Dool EJ, et al. Pediatric venous thromboembolic disease in one single center: congenital prothrombotic disorders and the clinical outcome. *J Thromb Haemost* 2003;1(12): 2516–2522.
2. Massicotte MP, Dix D, Monagle P, et al. Central venous catheter related thrombosis in children: analysis of the Canadian registry of venous thromboembolic complications. *J Pediatr* 1998;133(6):770–776.
3. Monagle P, Adams M, Mahoney M, et al. Outcome of pediatric thromboembolic disease: a report from the Canadian childhood thrombophilia registry. *Pediatr Res* 2000;47(6):763–766.
4. Schmidt B, Andrew M. Neonatal thrombosis: report of a prospective Canadian and international registry. *Pediatrics* 1995;96(5 Pt 1):939–943.
5. Kurnik K, Duering C, Bidlingmaier C, et al. Thromboembolism in neonates and infants: impact of underlying diseases, prothrombotic risk factors and treatment modalities. *Thromb Res* 2005;115(Suppl. 1):71–77.
6. Journeycake JM, Manco-Johnson MJ. Thrombosis during infancy and childhood: what we know and what we do not know. *Hematol Oncol Clin North Am* 2004;18(6):1315–1338, viii–viix.
7. Andrew M, Paes B, Johnston M. Development of the hemostatic system in the neonate and young infant. *Am J Pediatr Hematol Oncol* Spring 1990; 12(1):95–104.
8. Andrew M, Paes B, Milner R, et al. Development of the human coagulation system in the healthy premature infant. *Blood* 1988;72(5):1651–1657.
9. Andrew M, Paes B, Milner R, et al. Development of the human coagulation system in the full-term infant. *Blood* 1987;70(1):165–172.
10. Andrew M, Vegh P, Johnston M, et al. Maturation of the hemostatic system during childhood. *Blood* 1992;80(8):1998–2005.
11. Andrew M. Developmental hemostasis: relevance to thromboembolic complications in pediatric patients. *Thromb Haemost* 1995;74(1):415–425.
12. Nowak-Gottl U, Kosch A, Schlegel N. Neonatal thromboembolism. *Semin Thromb Hemost* 2003;29(2):227–234.
13. Nowak-Gottl U, Duering C, Kempf-Bielack B, et al. Thromboembolic diseases in neonates and children. *Pathophysiol Haemost Thromb* 33(5-6): 269–274, 2003-2004 Dec 2003.
14. Greenway A, Massicotte MP, Monagle P. Neonatal thrombosis and its treatment. *Blood Rev* 2004;18(2):75–84.
15. Monagle P, Chan AK, Albisetti M, et al. Fibrinolytic system in adolescents: response to venous occlusion stress tests. *Pediatr Res* 2003; 53(2): 333–337.
16. Richardson MW, Allen GA, Monahan PE. Thrombosis in children: current perspective and distinct challenges. *Thromb Haemost* 2002;88(6): 900–911.
17. Nowak-Gottl U, Junker R, Kreuz W, et al. Risk of recurrent venous thrombosis in children with combined prothrombotic risk factors. *Blood* 2001; 97(4):858–862.
18. Heller C, Nowak-Gottl U. Maternal thrombophilia and neonatal thrombosis. *Best Pract Res Clin Haematol* 2003;16(2):333–345.
19. Kuhle S, Massicotte P, Chan A, et al. A case series of 72 neonates with renal vein thrombosis. Data from the 1-800-NO-CLOTS Registry. *Thromb Haemost* 2004;92(4):729–733.
20. Golomb MR, Dick PT, MacGregor DL, et al. Neonatal arterial ischemic stroke and cerebral sinovenous thrombosis are more commonly diagnosed in boys. *J Child Neurol* 2004;19(7):493–497.
21. Ozduman K, Pober BR, Barnes P, et al. Fetal stroke. *Pediatr Neurol* 2004; 30(3):151–162.
22. Counsell SJ, Rutherford MA, Cowan FM, et al. Magnetic resonance imaging of preterm brain injury. *Arch Dis Child Fetal Neonatal Ed* 2003;88(4): F269–F274.
23. Golomb MR, Dick PT, MacGregor DL, et al. Cranial ultrasonography has a low sensitivity for detecting arterial ischemic stroke in term neonates. *J Child Neurol* 2003;18(2):98–103.
24. deVeber G. Arterial ischemic strokes in infants and children: an overview of current approaches. *Semin Thromb Hemost* 2003;29(6):567–573.
25. Golomb MR, MacGregor DL, Domi T, et al. Presumed pre- or perinatal arterial ischemic stroke: risk factors and outcomes. *Ann Neurol* 2001; 50(2):163–168.
26. deVeber G, Monagle P, Chan A, et al. Prothrombotic disorders in infants and children with cerebral thromboembolism. *Arch Neurol* 1998;55(12): 1539–1543.
27. Lynch JK, Hirtz DG, DeVeber G, et al. Report of the National Institute of Neurological Disorders and Stroke workshop on perinatal and childhood stroke. *Pediatrics* 2002;109(1):116–123.
28. Brankovic-Sreckovic V, Milic-Rasic V, Jovic N, et al. The recurrence risk of ischemic stroke in childhood. *Med Princ Pract* 2004;13(3):153–158.
29. Golomb MR, deVeber GA, MacGregor DL, et al. Independent walking after neonatal arterial ischemic stroke and sinovenous thrombosis. *J Child Neurol* 2003;18(8):530–536.
30. Pavlakis SG, deVeber G. Little folk strokes: current questions. *CNS Spectr* 2004;9(6):418–419.
31. deVeber G, Andrew M, Adams C, et al. Cerebral sinovenous thrombosis in children. *N Engl J Med* 2001;345(6):417–423.
32. Buller HR, Agnelli G, Hull RD, et al. Antithrombotic therapy for venous thromboembolic disease: the Seventh ACCP Conference on Antithrombotic and Thrombolytic Therapy. *Chest* 2004;126(Suppl. 3):401S–428S.
33. deVeber G, Chan A, Monagle P, et al. Anticoagulation therapy in pediatric patients with sinovenous thrombosis: a cohort study. *Arch Neurol* 1998; 55(12):1533–1537.
34. Andrew ME, Monagle P, deVeber G, et al. Thromboembolic disease and antithrombotic therapy in newborns. *Hematology (Am Soc Hematol Educ Program)* 2001;2001:358–374.
35. Monagle P, Chan A, Massicotte P, et al. Antithrombotic therapy in children: the Seventh ACCP Conference on Antithrombotic and Thrombolytic Therapy. *Chest* 2004;126(Suppl. 3):645S–687S.
36. Kosch A, Kuwertz-Broking E, Heller C, et al. Renal venous thrombosis in neonates: prothrombotic risk factors and long-term follow-up. *Blood* 2004; 104(5):1356–1360.
37. Schmidt B, Andrew M. Neonatal thrombotic disease: prevention, diagnosis, and treatment. *J Pediatr* 1988;113(2):407–410.
38. Bokenkamp A, von Kries R, Nowak-Gottl U, et al. Neonatal renal venous thrombosis in Germany between 1992 and 1994: epidemiology, treatment and outcome. *Eur J Pediatr* 2000;159(1-2):44–48.
39. Manco-Johnson MJ, Grabowski EF, Hellgreen M, et al. Recommendations for tPA thrombolysis in children. On behalf of the Scientific Subcommittee on Perinatal and Pediatric Thrombosis of the Scientific and Standardization Committee of the International Society of Thrombosis and Haemostasis. *Thromb Haemost* 2002;88(1):157–158.
40. Gurakan F, Eren M, Kocak N, et al. Extrahepatic portal vein thrombosis in children: etiology and long-term follow-up. *J Clin Gastroenterol* 2004; 38(4):368–372.
41. Losty PD, Lynch MJ, Guiney EJ. Long term outcome after surgery for extrahepatic portal vein thrombosis. *Arch Dis Child* 1994;71(5): 437–440.
42. Karrer FM, Narkewicz MR. Esophageal varices: current management in children. *Semin Pediatr Surg* 1999;8(4):193–201.
43. Greffe BS, Marlar RA, Manco-Johnson MJ. Neonatal protein C: molecular composition and distribution in normal term infants. *Thromb Res* 1989; 56(1):91–98.
44. Nowak-Gottl U, Auberger K, Gobel U, et al. Inherited defects of the protein C anticoagulant system in childhood thrombo-embolism. *Eur J Pediatr* 1996;155(11):921–927.
45. Manco-Johnson M, Nuss R. Protein C concentrate prevents peripartum thrombosis. *Am J Hematol* 1992;40(1):69–70.
46. Manco-Johnson MJ, Knapp-Clevenger R. Activated protein C concentrate reverses purpura fulminans in severe genetic protein C deficiency. *J Pediatr Hematol Oncol* 2004;26(1):25–27.
47. Monagle P, Andrew M, Halton J, et al. Homozygous protein C deficiency: description of a new mutation and successful treatment with low molecular weight heparin. *Thromb Haemost* 1998;79(4):756–761.
48. Manco-Johnson MJ, Abshire TC, Jacobson LJ, et al. Severe neonatal protein C deficiency: prevalence and thrombotic risk. *J Pediatr* 1991;119(5):793–798.
49. Kuhle S, Massicotte P, Chan A, et al. Systemic thromboembolism in children. Data from the 1-800-NO-CLOTS consultation service. *Thromb Haemost* 2004;92(4):722–728.
50. Heller C, Heinecke A, Junker R, et al. Cerebral venous thrombosis in children: a multifactorial origin. *Circulation* 2003;108(11):1362–1367.
51. Journeycake JM, Buchanan GR. Thrombotic complications of central venous catheters in children. *Curr Opin Hematol* 2003;10(5):369–374.
52. Ljung R. Central venous catheters in children with haemophilia. *Blood Rev* 2004;18(2):93–100.
53. Aitken ML, Tonelli MR. Complications of indwelling catheters in cystic fibrosis: a 10-year review. *Chest* 2000;118(6):1598–1602.
54. Barnes C, Newall F, Monagle P. Thromboembolic complications related to indwelling central venous catheters in children with oncological/haematological diseases: a retrospective study of 362 catheters. *Support Care Cancer* 2002;10(3):256–257; author reply 260–251.
55. Journeycake JM, Quinn CT, Miller KL, et al. Catheter-related deep venous thrombosis in children with hemophilia. *Blood* 2001;98(6): 1727–1731.
56. Price VE, Carcao M, Connolly B, et al. A prospective, longitudinal study of central venous catheter-related deep venous thrombosis in boys with hemophilia. *J Thromb Haemost* 2004;2(5):737–742.
57. Timsit JF, Farkas JC, Boyer JM, et al. Central vein catheter-related thrombosis in intensive care patients: incidence, risks factors, and relationship with catheter-related sepsis. *Chest* 1998;114(1):207–213.
58. Andrew M, Marzinotto V, Pencharz P, et al. A cross-sectional study of catheter-related thrombosis in children receiving total parenteral nutrition at home. *J Pediatr* 1995;126(3):358–363.
59. Medeiros D, Miller KL, Rollins NK, et al. Contrast venography in young haemophiliacs with implantable central venous access devices. *Haemophilia* 1998;4(1):10–15.
60. Male C, Chait P, Ginsberg JS, et al. Comparison of venography and ultrasound for the diagnosis of asymptomatic deep vein thrombosis in the

upper body in children: results of the PARKAA study. Prophylactic Antithrombin Replacement in Kids with ALL treated with Asparaginase. *Thromb Haemost* 2002;87(4):593–598.

61. Kaste SC, Gronemeyer SA, Hoffer FA, et al. Pilot study of noninvasive detection of venous occlusions from central venous access devices in children treated for acute lymphoblastic leukemia. *Pediatr Radiol* 1999;29(8):570–574.

62. Baarslag HJ, Van Beek EJ, Reekers JA. Magnetic resonance venography in consecutive patients with suspected deep vein thrombosis of the upper extremity: initial experience. *Acta Radiol* 2004;45(1):38–43.

63. Lordick F, Hentrich M, Decker T, et al. Ultrasound screening for internal jugular vein thrombosis aids the detection of central venous catheter-related infections in patients with haemato-oncological diseases: a prospective observational study. *Br J Haematol* 2003;120(6):1073–1078.

64. van Rooden CJ, Schippers EF, Barge RM, et al. Infectious complications of central venous catheters increase the risk of catheter-related thrombosis in hematology patients: a prospective study. *J Clin Oncol* 2005;23(12): 2655–2660.

65. Pierce CM, Wade A, Mok Q. Heparin-bonded central venous lines reduce thrombotic and infective complications in critically ill children. *Intensive Care Med* 2000;26(7):967–972.

66. Tolar B, Gould JR. The timing and sequence of multiple device-related complications in patients with long-term indwelling Groshong catheters. *Cancer* 1996;78(6):1308–1313.

67. Athale UH, Chan AK. Thrombosis in children with acute lymphoblastic leukemia. Part II. Pathogenesis of thrombosis in children with acute lymphoblastic leukemia: effects of the disease and therapy. *Thromb Res* 2003; 111(4-5):199–212.

68. Schmid L, Walser K, Kessler W, et al. Use of a fully implantable drug delivery system in the treatment of acute leukemias and disseminated lymphomas. *Oncology* 1990;47(6):449–455.

69. Athale UH, Chan AK. Thrombosis in children with acute lymphoblastic leukemia Part III. Pathogenesis of thrombosis in children with acute lymphoblastic leukemia: effects of host environment. *Thromb Res* 2003; 111(6):321–327.

70. Nowak-Gottl U, Heinecke A, von Kries R, et al. Thrombotic events revisited in children with acute lymphoblastic leukemia: impact of concomitant Escherichia coli asparaginase/prednisone administration. *Thromb Res* 2001;103(3):165–172.

71. Mitchell L, Andrew M, Hanna K, et al. Trend to efficacy and safety using antithrombin concentrate in prevention of thrombosis in children receiving l-asparaginase for acute lymphoblastic leukemia. Results of the PAARKA study. *Thromb Haemost* 2003;90(2):235–244.

72. Nowak-Gottl U, Ahlke E, Fleischhack G, et al. Thromboembolic events in children with acute lymphoblastic leukemia (BFM protocols): prednisone versus dexamethasone administration. *Blood* 2003;101(7):2529–2533.

73. Kieslich M, Porto L, Lanfermann H, et al. Cerebrovascular complications of L-asparaginase in the therapy of acute lymphoblastic leukemia. *J Pediatr Hematol Oncol* 2003;25(6):484–487.

74. Mitchell LG, Andrew M, Hanna K, et al. A prospective cohort study determining the prevalence of thrombotic events in children with acute lymphoblastic leukemia and a central venous line who are treated with L-asparaginase: results of the Prophylactic Antithrombin Replacement in Kids with Acute Lymphoblastic Leukemia Treated with Asparaginase (PARKAA) Study. *Cancer* 2003;97(2):508–516.

75. Deitcher SR, Gajjar A, Kun L, et al. Clinically evident venous thromboembolic events in children with brain tumors. *J Pediatr* 2004;145(6): 848–850.

76. Yuksel H, Ozguven AA, Akil I, et al. Septic pulmonary emboli presenting with deep venous thrombosis secondary to acute osteomyelitis. *Pediatr Int* 2004;46(5):621–623.

77. Walsh S, Phillips F. Deep vein thrombosis associated with pediatric musculoskeletal sepsis. *J Pediatr Orthop* 2002;22(3):329–332.

78. Monagle P. Thrombosis in pediatric cardiac patients. *Semin Thromb Hemost* 2003;29(6):547–555.

79. Marcelletti CF, Iorio FS, Abella RF. Late results of extracardiac Fontan repair. *Semin Thorac Cardiovasc Surg Pediatr Card Surg Annu* 1999;2: 131–142.

80. Freedom RM, Hamilton R, Yoo SJ, et al. The Fontan procedure: analysis of cohorts and late complications. *Cardiol Young* 2000;10(4):307–331.

81. Jacobs ML. The Fontan operation, thromboembolism, and anticoagulation: a reappraisal of the single bullet theory. *J Thorac Cardiovasc Surg* 2005; 129(3):491–495.

82. Casolo G, Rega L, Gensini GF. Detection of right atrial and pulmonary artery thrombosis after the Fontan procedure by magnetic resonance imaging. *Heart* 2004;90(7):825.

83. Kammeraad JA, Sreeram N. Acute thrombosis of an extracardiac Fontan conduit. *Heart* 2004;90(1):76.

84. Monagle P, Karl TR. Thromboembolic problems after the Fontan operation. *Semin Thorac Cardiovasc Surg Pediatr Card Surg Annu* 2002;5:36–47.

85. Kaulitz R, Ziemer G, Rauch R, et al. Prophylaxis of thromboembolic complications after the Fontan operation (total cavopulmonary anastomosis). *J Thorac Cardiovasc Surg* 2005;129(3):569–575.

86. Jacobs ML, Pourmoghadam KK, Geary EM, et al. Fontan's operation: is aspirin enough? Is coumadin too much? *Ann Thorac Surg* 2002;73(1):64–68.

87. Durongpisitkul K, Gururaj VJ, Park JM, et al. The prevention of coronary artery aneurysm in Kawasaki disease: a meta-analysis on the efficacy of aspirin and immunoglobulin treatment. *Pediatrics* 1995;96(6):1057– 1061.

88. Newburger JW, Takahashi M, Gerber MA, et al. Diagnosis, treatment, and long-term management of Kawasaki disease: a statement for health professionals from the Committee on Rheumatic Fever, Endocarditis, and Kawasaki Disease, Council on Cardiovascular Disease in the Young, American Heart Association. *Pediatrics* 2004;114(6):1708–1733.

89. DeVeber G. Risk factors for childhood stroke: little folks have different strokes! *Ann Neurol* 2003;53(2):149–150.

90. Barnes C, Newall F, Harvey AS, et al. Thrombophilia interpretation in childhood stroke: a cautionary tale. *J Child Neurol* 2004;19(3):218–219.

91. Young G, Manco-Johnson M, Gill JC, et al. Clinical manifestations of the prothrombin G20210A mutation in children: a pediatric coagulation consortium study. *J Thromb Haemost* 2003;1(5):958–962.

92. Deda G, Icagasioglu D, Caksen H, et al. Combined genetic defects in a child with ischemic stroke: case report. *J Child Neurol* 2002;17(7): 533–534.

93. Levy DM, Massicotte MP, Harvey E, et al. Thromboembolism in paediatric lupus patients. *Lupus* 2003;12(10):741–746.

94. Wirrell E, Hill MD, Jadavji T, et al. Stroke after varicella vaccination. *J Pediatr* 2004;145(6):845–847.

95. Lanthier S, Armstrong D, Domi T, et al. Post-varicella arteriopathy of childhood: natural history of vascular stenosis. *Neurology* 2005;64(4): 660–663.

96. Saxena K, Ranalli M, Khan N, et al. Fatal stroke in a child with severe iron deficiency anemia and multiple hereditary risk factors for thrombosis. *Clin Pediatr (Phila)* 2005;44(2):175–180.

97. deVeber G, Chan A. Aspirin versus low-molecular-weight heparin for ischemic stroke in children: an unanswered question. *Stroke* 2002;33(8): 1947–1948; author reply 1947–1948.

98. Gomes MP, Deitcher SR. Risk of venous thromboembolic disease associated with hormonal contraceptives and hormone replacement therapy: a clinical review. *Arch Intern Med* 2004;164(18):1965–1976.

99. Sass AE, Neufeld EJ. Risk factors for thromboembolism in teens: when should I test? *Curr Opin Pediatr* 2002;14(4):370–378.

100. Casais P, Meschengieser SS, Gennari LC, et al. Morbidity of lupus anticoagulants in children: a single institution experience. *Thromb Res* 2004; 114(4):245–249.

101. Briones M, Abshire T. Lupus anticoagulants in children. *Curr Opin Hematol* 2003;10(5):375–379.

102. Zell L, Kindermann W, Marschall F, et al. Paget-Schroetter syndrome in sports activities—case study and literature review. *Angiology* 2001;52(5): 337–342.

103. Sevestre MA, Kalka C, Irwin WT, et al. Paget-Schroetter syndrome: what to do? *Catheter Cardiovasc Interv* 2003;59(1):71–76.

104. Angle N, Gelabert HA, Farooq MM, et al. Safety and efficacy of early surgical decompression of the thoracic outlet for Paget-Schroetter syndrome. *Ann Vasc Surg* 2001;15(1):37–42.

105. Feugier P, Aleksic I, Salari R, et al. Long-term results of venous revascularization for Paget-Schroetter syndrome in athletes. *Ann Vasc Surg* 2001; 15(2):212–218.

106. Kreienberg PB, Chang BB, Darling RC III, et al. Long-term results in patients treated with thrombolysis, thoracic inlet decompression, and subclavian vein stenting for Paget-Schroetter syndrome. *J Vasc Surg* 2001; 33(Suppl. 2):S100–S105.

107. Babyn PS, Gahunia HK, Massicotte P. Pulmonary thromboembolism in children. *Pediatr Radiol* 2005;35(3):258–274.

108. Sutor AH. Screening children with thrombosis for thrombophilic proteins. Cui bono? *J Thromb Haemost* 2003;1(5):886–888.

109. Tormene D, Simioni P, Prandoni P, et al. The incidence of venous thromboembolism in thrombophilic children: a prospective cohort study. *Blood* 2002;100(7):2403–2405.

110. Mannucci PM. Genetic hypercoagulability: prevention suggests testing family members. *Blood* 2001;98(1):21–22.

111. Green D. Genetic hypercoagulability: screening should be an informed choice. *Blood* 2001;98(1):20.

112. Male C, Mitchell L, Julian J, et al. Acquired activated protein C resistance is associated with lupus anticoagulants and thrombotic events in pediatric patients with systemic lupus erythematosus. *Blood* 1997;97(4):844–849.

113. Andrew M, Marzinotto V, Massicotte P, et al. Heparin therapy in pediatric patients: a prospective cohort study. *Pediatr Res* 1994;35(1):78–83.

114. Andrew M, Schmidt B. Use of heparin in newborn infants. *Semin Thromb Hemost* 1988;14(1):28–32.

115. Vieira A, Berry L, Ofosu F, et al. Heparin sensitivity and resistance in the neonate: an explanation. *Thromb Res* 1991;63(1):85–98.

116. Newall F, Barnes C, Ignjatovic V, et al. Heparin-induced thrombocytopenia in children. *J Paediatr Child Health* 2003;39(4):289–292.

117. Klenner AF, Lubenow N, Raschke R, et al. Heparin-induced thrombocytopenia in children: 12 new cases and review of the literature. *Thromb Haemost* 2004;91(4):719–724.

118. Bussey H, Francis JL. Heparin overview and issues. *Pharmacotherapy* 2004;24(8 Pt 2):103S–107S.

119. Wawrzynska L, Tomkowski WZ, Przedlacki J, et al. Changes in bone density during long-term administration of low-molecular-weight heparins or acenocoumarol for secondary prophylaxis of venous thromboembolism. *Pathophysiol Haemost Thromb* 2003;33(2):64–67.

120. Dix D, Andrew M, Marzinotto V, et al. The use of low molecular weight heparin in pediatric patients: a prospective cohort study. *J Pediatr* 2000; 136(4):439–445.

121. Massicotte P, Julian JA, Marzinotto V, et al. Dose-finding and pharmacokinetic profiles of prophylactic doses of a low molecular weight heparin (reviparin-sodium) in pediatric patients. *Thromb Res* 2003;109(2-3): 93–99.

122. Streif W, Andrew M, Marzinotto V, et al. Analysis of warfarin therapy in pediatric patients: a prospective cohort study of 319 patients. *Blood* 1999; 94(9):3007–3014.

123. Andrew M, Marzinotto V, Brooker LA, et al. Oral anticoagulation therapy in pediatric patients: a prospective study. *Thromb Haemost* 1994;71(3): 265–269.

124. Young G, Yonekawa KE, Nakagawa P, et al. Argatroban as an alternative to heparin in extracorporeal membrane oxygenation circuits. *Perfusion* 2004; 19(5):283–288.

125. Young G. Current and future antithrombotic agents in children. *Expert Rev Cardiovasc Ther* 2004;2(4):523–534.

126. Michelfelder EC, Shim D. Kawasaki disease: current therapeutic perspectives. *Curr Treat Options Cardiovasc Med* 2002;4(4):341–350.

127. Monagle P, Cochrane A, McCrindle B, et al. Thromboembolic complications after fontan procedures—the role of prophylactic anticoagulation. *J Thorac Cardiovasc Surg* 1998;115(3):493–498.

128. O'Brien M, Parness IA, Neufeld EJ, et al. Ticlopidine plus aspirin for coronary thrombosis in Kawasaki disease. *Pediatrics* 2000;105(5):E64.

129. Terrill KR, Lemons RS, Goldsby RE. Safety, dose, and timing of reteplase in treating occluded central venous catheters in children with cancer. *J Pediatr Hematol Oncol* 2003;25(11):864–867.

130. Choi M, Massicotte MP, Marzinotto V, et al. The use of alteplase to restore patency of central venous lines in pediatric patients: a cohort study. *J Pediatr* 2001;139(1):152–156.

131. Gupta AA, Leaker M, Andrew M, et al. Safety and outcomes of thrombolysis with tissue plasminogen activator for treatment of intravascular thrombosis in children. *J Pediatr* 2001;139(5):682–688.

132. Wang M, Hays T, Balasa V, et al. Low-dose tissue plasminogen activator thrombolysis in children. *J Pediatr Hematol Oncol* 2003;25(5):379–386.

133. Pilloud J, Rimensberger PC, Humbert J, et al. Successful local low-dose urokinase treatment of acquired thrombosis early after cardiothoracic surgery. *Pediatr Crit Care Med* 2002;3(4):355–357.

134. Prandoni P, Frulla M, Sartor D, et al. Vein abnormalities and the postthrombotic syndrome. *J Thromb Haemost* 2005;3(2):401–402.

135. Kahn SR, Ginsberg JS. The post-thrombotic syndrome: current knowledge, controversies, and directions for future research. *Blood Rev* 2002;16(3): 155–165.

136. Prandoni P. Elastic stockings, hydroxyethylrutosides or both for the treatment of post-thrombotic syndrome. *Thromb Haemost* 2005;93(1):183–185.

137. Prandoni P, Lensing AW, Prins MH, et al. Below-knee elastic compression stockings to prevent the post-thrombotic syndrome: a randomized, controlled trial. *Ann Intern Med* 2004;141(4):249–256.

138. Kolbach DN, Sandbrink MW, Hamulyak K, et al. Non-pharmaceutical measures for prevention of post-thrombotic syndrome. *Cochrane Database Syst Rev* 2004(1):CD004174.

139. Hudgens SA, Cella D, Caprini CA, et al. Deep vein thrombosis: validation of a patient-reported leg symptom index. *Health Qual Life Outcomes* 2003; 1(1):76.

140. Kahn SR, Azoulay L, Hirsch A, et al. Effect of graduated elastic compression stockings on leg symptoms and signs during exercise in patients with deep venous thrombosis: a randomized cross-over trial. *J Thromb Haemost* 2003; 1(3):494–499.

141. Forster AJ, Wells PS. The rationale and evidence for the treatment of lower-extremity deep venous thrombosis with thrombolytic agents. *Curr Opin Hematol* 2002;9(5):437–442.

142. Ziegler S, Schillinger M, Maca TH, et al. Post-thrombotic syndrome after primary event of deep venous thrombosis 10 to 20 years ago. *Thromb Res* 2001;101(2):23–33.

143. Barnes C, Newall F, Monagle P. Post-thrombotic syndrome. *Arch Dis Child* 2002;86(3):212–214.

144. Hausler M, Hubner D, Delhaas T, et al. Long term complications of inferior vena cava thrombosis. *Arch Dis Child* 2001;85(3):228–233.

145. Kuhle S, Koloshuk B, Marzinotto V, et al. A cross-sectional study evaluating post-thrombotic syndrome in children. *Thromb Res* 2003;111(4-5): 227–233.

146. Journeycake JM, Eshelman DA, Buchanan GR. Post-thrombotic syndrome following central venous catheter use in childhood cancer survivors. *Blood* 2003;102:2031.

147. Goldenberg NA, Knapp-Clevenger R, Manco-Johnson MJ. Elevated plasma factor VIII and D-dimer levels as predictors of poor outcomes of thrombosis in children. *N Engl J Med* 2004;351(11):1081–1088.

# CHAPTER 114 ■ HEPARIN-INDUCED THROMBOCYTOPENIA

THEODORE E. WARKENTIN

Heparin-induced thrombocytopenia (HIT) is an immune-mediated adverse drug reaction caused by heparin-dependent, platelet-activating immunoglobulin (Ig)G antibodies that recognize complexes of platelet factor 4 (PF4) bound to heparin (1). HIT represents a strong, independent risk factor for venous and arterial thrombosis, even in patients at high baseline risk for thrombosis (2).

HIT typically causes thrombosis in large veins and arteries; characteristic platelet-rich, intraarterial "white thrombi" were first described in 1958 (3). However, HIT is also a risk factor for microvascular thrombosis in certain situations, such as in coumarin treatment of deep vein thrombosis (DVT) [i.e., coumarin-associated venous limb gangrene (see Chapter 115)] or severe HIT-associated disseminated intravascular coagulation (DIC) (4,5).

Thrombosis typically occurs in anti-PF4-heparin antibody-positive patients who develop significant declines in platelet count (6–8), pointing to clinically relevant consequences of *in vivo* platelet activation induced by these antibodies. A central role for *in vivo* thrombin generation in HIT (4) provides a rationale for use of anticoagulants that inhibit thrombin or its generation (9).

## DEFINITION AND TERMINOLOGY

HIT can be defined as any clinical event best explained by anti-PF4-heparin antibodies ("HIT antibodies") in a patient who is receiving, or who has recently received, heparin (or another polyanion implicated in this syndrome) (1). Thrombocytopenia is the most common event in HIT and occurs in at least 90% of the patients, depending on the definition of thrombocytopenia. A high proportion (50% to 75%) of patients with HIT develop thrombosis.

A consensus report (9) recommended that the term *heparin-induced thrombocytopenia* should be used to refer to the antibody-mediated disorder. Therefore, HIT can be considered a *clinicopathologic* syndrome in which the diagnosis can be made accurately when one or more *clinical* events (e.g., thrombocytopenia, thrombosis, skin lesions, acute systemic reactions, and decompensated DIC) occur together with laboratory detection of the *pathologic* HIT antibodies. In contrast, it is recommended that the term *nonimmune heparin-associated thrombocytopenia* should be used to describe thrombocytopenia occurring during heparin use that is not associated with HIT antibodies. Often, nonimmune heparin-associated thrombocytopenia (HAT) is due to a comorbid disorder (e.g., perioperative hemodilution and systemic inflammatory response syndrome), although a direct platelet-activating effect of heparin that is not mediated by antibody may occur in some patients (10). Unlike the situation in HIT, the causative role of heparin in nonimmune HAT in a given patient cannot readily be ascertained.

## PATHOGENESIS

Figure 114-1 summarizes the pathogenesis of HIT (11). The central concept is the formation of heparin-dependent IgG immunoglobulin that activates platelets via their FcγIIa receptors (12). It remains controversial whether IgA and IgM antibodies evince pathogenicity (13). The target antigen is a complex of heparin and the positively charged platelet α-granule protein, platelet factor 4 (PF4) (14–17), a member of the CXC subfamily of chemokines. HIT antibodies are directed against one or more sites on PF4 that have been conformationally altered by binding to negatively charged heparin (18–20). This model is consistent with reports that other highly sulfated, nonheparin carbohydrates such as pentosan polysulfate (21) and polysulfated chondroitin sulfate (22) can trigger a prothrombotic syndrome resembling HIT, characterized by antibodies indistinguishable from those generated in HIT. It may also explain why low-molecular-weight heparin (LMWH) is less likely to trigger HIT (6,7), as only heparin molecules of at least 12 saccharides in length bind PF4 so as to induce neoepitope formation (23).

Several factors contribute to the prothrombotic nature of HIT (Fig. 114-1): (a) the potent platelet-activating properties of the HIT antibodies, which also generate procoagulant, platelet-derived microparticles (24); (b) pancellular activation (either directly or indirectly by HIT antibodies) (25), manifesting as tissue factor expression on endothelium (16,26) and monocytes (27), and possibly platelet-leukocyte complexes formation (28); and, (c) neutralization of the heparin anticoagulant effects by PF4.

Women are more likely than men to develop HIT (1.5-fold to threefold increase by odds ratio) (29). However, no HLA association or other genetic risk factor has been identified (30). Although the platelets bearing FcγIIa receptors of the His131 phenotype (approximately 70% of the population) are more readily activated by HIT antibodies of IgG1 subclass (the predominant subclass in HIT) (31,32), no clear association between HIT and Fc receptor genotype has been established (33,34). A strong, albeit indirect, argument against a genetic risk factor is the surprising observation that even patients with a previous history of HIT do not usually regenerate HIT antibodies upon repeat heparin exposure (35,36).

## FREQUENCY

The frequency of HIT is influenced by the type of patient population (surgical > medical > obstetrical), the type of heparin used [bovine unfractionated heparin (UFH) > porcine UFH > porcine low-molecular-weight heparin (LMWH)] and the duration of heparin therapy (the risk begins at day 5 and peaks between days 10 and 14) (37). Accordingly, a high frequency of HIT (5%) occurs in postoperative orthopedic surgery patients receiving UFH for up to 14 days (6,7). In contrast, HIT was not

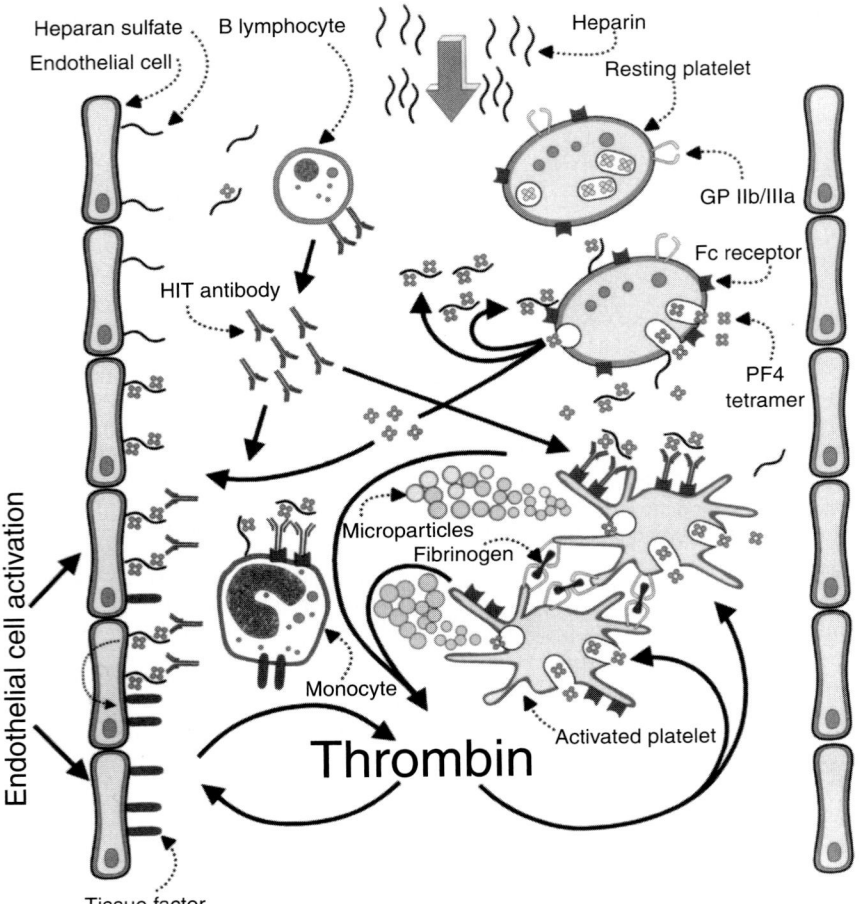

**FIGURE 114-1.** Pathogenesis of heparin-induced thrombocytopenia (HIT). Heparin produces mild platelet activation, resulting in the release of platelet factor 4 (PF4) from platelet α-granules and in the formation of immunogenic PF4/heparin complexes. B lymphocytes generate IgG that recognize the PF4/heparin complexes; the Fc "*tails*" of the IgG bind to platelet FcγII receptors, resulting in Fc receptor clustering and consequent strong platelet activation. Platelet aggregation is mediated by glycoprotein (GP) IIb/IIIa. Platelet-derived microparticles that accelerate thrombin generation are produced. The HIT antibodies also recognize PF4 bound to endothelial heparan sulfate, leading to tissue factor expression on endothelium. HIT antibodies also can activate monocytes. In all, increased thrombin generation results can explain some of the unusual clinical manifestations of HIT (e.g., venous limb gangrene and disseminated intravascular coagulation) and provides a rationale for treatment that reduces thrombin generation. (From Greinacher A, Warkentin TE. Treatment of heparin-induced thrombocytopenia: an overview. In: Warkentin TE, Greinacher A. *Heparin-induced thrombocytopenia*, 3rd ed. New York: Marcel Dekker, Inc., 2004:335–370.)

observed in several large studies in which LMWH was administered for many weeks during pregnancy (38,39). The frequency of occurrence is estimated to be about 1% in patients receiving UFH for treatment of venous thromboembolism or for prevention of HIT in medical patients, and approximately 0.1% to 0.5% in postoperative patients receiving LMWH (37,40). Given the decreasing use of UFH postorthopedic surgery, the most common scenario for HIT today is probably antithrombotic prophylaxis with UFH following cardiac surgery (risk: 2% to 3% if UFH is given for >1 week) (41).

Patient-dependent risk factors influence the type of HIT-associated thrombotic event. For example, venous thrombosis occurs in at least half of postorthopedic surgery patients who develop HIT, with relatively few arterial thrombi observed (6,7). In contrast, arterial thrombosis occurs at least as often as venous thrombosis in postcardiac surgery patients with HIT, suggesting a predisposing role for atherosclerosis (37,42,43). Patients with a central venous catheter who develop HIT have

about a 10% chance of developing symptomatic upper-limb DVT at the catheter site, reflecting the interaction of localized vessel injury with the systemic hypercoagulability of HIT (44).

## CLINICAL PRESENTATION

HIT is a distinct immunohematologic syndrome that usually can be distinguished on clinical grounds from IgG-mediated thrombocytopenia caused by drugs such as quinine/quinidine and sulfa antibiotics.

### Thrombocytopenia

The thrombocytopenia is usually mild to moderate in severity (median platelet count nadir, approximately 50 to 60 × $10^9$ per L) (1,5) (see Fig. 114-2). The platelet count is less

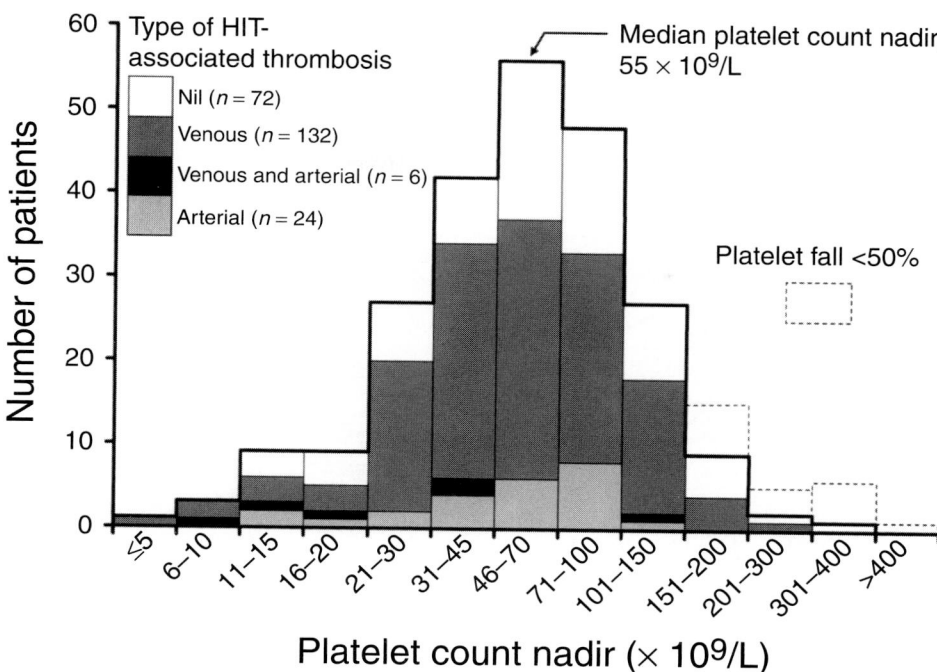

FIGURE 114-2. Platelet count nadirs in heparin-induced thrombocytopenia (HIT). All patients had a 50% or greater fall in the platelet count except in those indicated by the *dotted lines*. Most patients with HIT developed thrombosis, usually venous. The risk of thrombosis in HIT is substantial irrespective of the severity of the thrombocytopenia. (From Warkentin TE. Heparin-induced thrombocytopenia: pathogenesis and management. *Br J Haematol* 2003;116:535–555, with permission.)

than $20 \times 10^9$ per L in only 5% to 10% of patients with HIT; in contrast, severe thrombocytopenia typically occurs in patients with immune thrombocytopenia caused by other drugs (45). Petechiae and ecchymoses are usually absent even in patients with HIT who have severe thrombocytopenia. Thrombosis is common in HIT, irrespective of the severity of the thrombocytopenia, and can occur in patients with a decreased platelet count that may not be lower than $150 \times 10^9$ per L (1,7) (see Fig. 114-3), although studies suggest that the risk and severity of thrombosis increases with the degree of thrombocytopenia (7,8). In postoperative patients, a proportional fall in platelet count ($\geq 50\%$) between postoperative days 4 to 14 is more sensitive (and similarly specific) for HIT than the conventional definition of thrombocytopenia (platelet count fall to $<150 \times 10^9$ per L).

## Timing

Patients with HIT typically develop a platelet count fall between days 5 to 10 of heparin treatment (first day of heparin use = day zero) (35,46). Sometimes, thrombocytopenia can begin earlier in patients who have been exposed previously to heparin. In general, this is observed only in patients whose previous heparin exposure is recent (within the past 3 months), in which case an immediate recurrence of thrombocytopenia can occur on reexposure to heparin (35,46). A true anamnestic immune response, in which previous heparin exposure predisposes to a greater probability of forming more avid (higher-titer, higher-affinity) antibodies, is *not* a feature of HIT. Rarely, HIT can begin several days after all heparin has been stopped (delayed-onset HIT) (47–49). This syndrome is characterized by high-titer HIT antibodies that can activate platelets even in the absence of heparin (47).

## Complications

Table 114-1 lists various complications of HIT by frequency. The strong association between HIT and thrombosis means that this diagnosis should be considered in all patients who develop thrombosis or other unusual events in association with a falling platelet count during, or shortly after stopping, heparin therapy.

*Venous thrombosis* is the most common complication of HIT and includes DVT and pulmonary embolism (1,8,50). Severe headache and acute neurologic sequelae suggests dural sinus (cerebral venous) thrombosis (49). Abdominal or flank pain suggests adrenal hemorrhagic necrosis, which can lead to shock secondary to acute adrenal failure if bilateral. This complication is believed to result from adrenal vein thrombosis and secondary ischemic necrosis of the adrenal glands (5).

*Arterial thrombosis* is relatively common in HIT and most often involves large limb arteries, resulting in acute arterial occlusion with absent pulses (4). Thrombotic stroke, myocardial infarction, or mesenteric artery thrombosis occur less often (5,50).

*Limb ischemia or gangrene* can be categorized as limb ischemia with and without palpable or Doppler-identifiable pulses (see Fig. 114-4) (3,4,51). Absent pulses suggests that the acute limb ischemia is caused by large artery occlusion by platelet-rich "white clots." In contrast, severe limb ischemia with pulses present indicates microvascular thrombosis in HIT and is most commonly caused by treatment of DVT using warfarin (coumarin) (see Chapter 115) (4,52–54). The laboratory hallmark of coumarin-associated venous limb ischemia is a supratherapeutic international normalized ratio (INR) (usually $>3.5$), which is a surrogate marker for severe protein C depletion (in parallel with a severe reduction of factor VII) complicating coumarin therapy for HIT-associated DVT (see Chapter 115). Rarely, venous limb ischemia or necrosis is associated with decompensated DIC in HIT in the absence of coumarin therapy, with or without associated DVT (5), possibly because of acquired natural anticoagulant depletion.

*Classic (nonacral) coumarin-induced skin necrosis* has been reported in patients with HIT (4,55), but this is less common than venous limb gangrene (see Chapter 115).

*Heparin-induced skin lesions* are dermal reactions noted within 24 hours of subcutaneous heparin injection that begin 5 or more days after heparin initiation (56,57). These lesions are associated with HIT antibodies and are otherwise

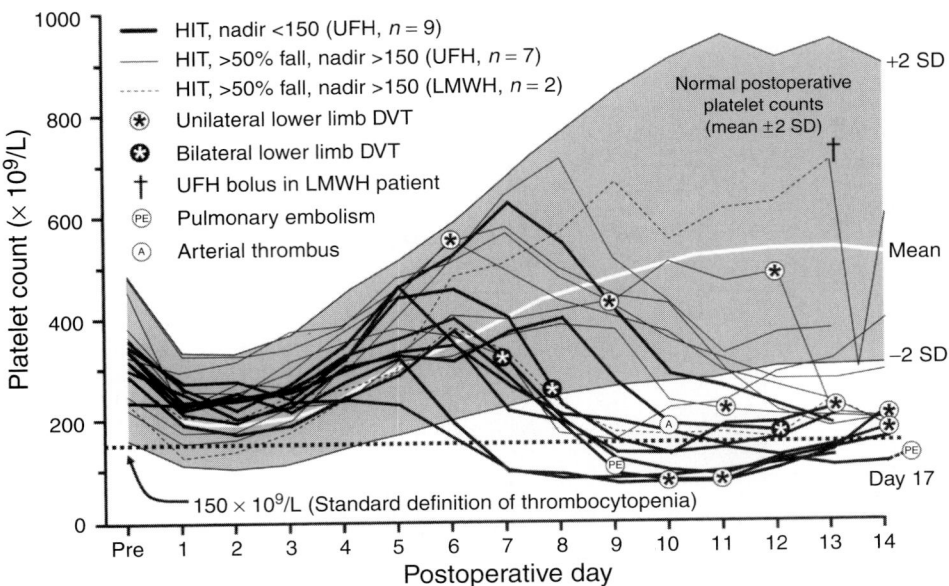

**FIGURE 114-3.** Characteristic timing, severity, and prothrombotic nature of heparin-induced thrombocytopenia (HIT). The *shaded area* indicates the mean [± 2 standard deviation (SD)] platelet count range in the reference population without HIT. There is an immediate postoperative decrease in the platelet count (maximal, days 1 to 3), followed by a rise to levels greater than baseline (maximal, days 11 to 14). Antithrombotic prophylaxis with subcutaneous unfractionated heparin (7,500 U twice daily) or the LMWH, enoxaparin (30 mg twice daily), was begun usually on postoperative day 1. Eighteen patients developed HIT (50% or greater fall in the platelet count from the postoperative peak), with nine evincing a platelet count nadir less than $150 \times 10^9$ per L and nine a platelet count nadir greater than $150 \times 10^9$ per L. The *symbols* indicate thrombotic events, 18 of which occurred in 13 of the 18 patients with HIT. One patient who received enoxaparin developed an abrupt platelet count fall when given a 5,000 U bolus of unfractionated heparin (†). (From Warkentin TE, Levine MN, Hirsh J, et al. Heparin-induced thrombocytopenia in patients treated with low-molecular-weight heparin or unfractionated heparin. *N Engl J Med* 1995;332:1330–1335; Warkentin TE, Roberts RS, Hirsh J, et al. An improved definition of immune heparin-induced thrombocytopenia in postoperative orthopedic patients. *Arch Intern Med* 2003;163:2518–2524, with permission.)

indistinguishable from those associated with thrombocytopenia. Although only about one fourth of patients who develop skin lesions together with HIT antibodies develop thrombocytopenia, those with heparin-induced skin lesions and thrombocytopenia are at particularly high risk for limb arterial thrombosis (58).

Two types of skin lesions are described: painful, red plaques and frank skin necrosis (see Fig. 114-5). Skin grafting may be required for patients with large necrotic lesions. Close clinical observation and monitoring of platelet count should be performed for several days after stopping heparin injections in patients with skin lesions because thrombocytopenia and thrombosis can begin several days later (58).

*Acute systemic reactions* refers to a variety of systemic symptoms and signs that begin within 5 to 30 minutes of receiving an intravenous heparin bolus and are accompanied by an abrupt decrease in platelet count (5,59,60). Clinical features are inflammatory (i.e., fever, chills, and flushing), cardiopulmonary (i.e., hypertension, tachycardia, dyspnea or tachypnea, and cardiac or pulmonary arrest), neurologic (i.e., transient global amnesia and pounding headache), and gastrointestinal (i.e., watery diarrhea).

*Decompensated DIC* refers to an elevated INR; reduced concentration of fibrinogen, red cell fragments, circulating normoblasts; or other laboratory features of severe DIC. Although increased thrombin generation is a universal feature of HIT (as shown by increased levels of thrombin–antithrombin complexes) (4), only 10% to 15% of the patients evince decompensated DIC. These patients may be at an unusually high risk for developing multiple thrombi and/or microvascular thrombosis.

## LABORATORY TESTING

Both activation and antigen assays are useful to support the diagnosis of HIT (61,62). In general, the more abnormal the test result, the greater the likelihood that the patient has HIT (63). HIT antibodies are usually detectable in patient serum or plasma only for a few weeks or months (35), and therefore, acute serum or plasma should be tested.

### Activation Assays

Activation assays exploit the platelet-activating properties of the HIT-IgG antibodies. The characteristic profile of HIT sera is the activation of normal donor platelets using therapeutic heparin concentrations (optimal at 0.1 to 0.3 U per mL) and the inhibition of activation of normal donor platelets at supratherapeutic heparin concentrations (10 to 100 U per mL) (64,65). Washed platelets that have been resuspended in divalent cation-containing buffer respond optimally to HIT antibodies. These features have been incorporated into a gold standard assay, the platelet serotonin release assay (SRA) (64,66), a positive result for which is strongly associated with thrombocytopenia that begins on day 5 or later of heparin treatment (odds ratio, 78; 95% CI, 12 to 819; $P < 0.001$) (6).

Methods to improve quality control in the detection of HIT antibodies include using an Fc receptor-blocking monoclonal antibody to ascertain inhibition of platelet activation by

**TABLE 114-1**

COMPLICATIONS OF HEPARIN-INDUCED THROMBOCYTOPENIA

| Venous thrombosis | Arterial thrombosis | Miscellaneous |
|---|---|---|
| Deep vein thrombosis (50%) | Aortoiliac thrombosis (acute limb ischemia) (5%–15%) | Heparin-induced skin lesions (≈25% of sensitized patients receiving subcutaneous heparin injections) |
| Pulmonary embolism (25%) | Acute thrombotic cerebrovascular accident (5%–10%) | Acute systemic reactions postintravenous heparin bolus (≈25% of sensitized patients who receive a heparin bolus) |
| Warfarin-induced venous limb gangrene (≈10% of HIT patients with DVT treated with warfarin) | Myocardial infarction (3%–5%) | Adrenal hemorrhagic infarction (1%–3%) |
| Rare: Cerebral sinus thrombosis (<3%) | Rare: Thrombosis of upper limb, renal, mesenteric, spinal, other arteries (<3%) | Rare: DIC with hypofibrinogenemia and microvascular thrombosis (<3%) |

HIT, heparin-induced thrombocytopenia; DVT, deep vein thrombosis; DIC, disseminated intravascular coagulation.
Estimated frequencies of the various complications of HIT are taken from several series of patients with serologic support of the diagnosis of HIT.
From Warkentin TE, Levine MN, Hirsh J, et al. Heparin-induced thrombocytopenia in patients treated with low-molecular-weight heparin or unfractionated heparin. *N Engl J Med* 1995;332:1330–1335; Warkentin TE, Roberts RS, Hirsh J, et al. An improved definition of immune heparin-induced thrombocytopenia in postoperative orthopedic patients. *Arch Intern Med* 2003;163:2518–2524; Fabris F, Luzzatto G, Soini B, et al. Risk factors for thrombosis in patients with immune heparin-induced thrombocytopenia. *J Intern Med* 2002;252:149–154; Wallis DE, Workman DL, Lewis BE, et al. Failure of early heparin cessation as treatment for heparin-induced thrombocytopenia. *Am J Med* 1999;106:629–635; Warkentin TE, Kelton JG. A 14-year study of heparin-induced thrombocytopenia. *Am J Med* 1996;101:502–507.

# Three ischemic limb syndromes in HIT

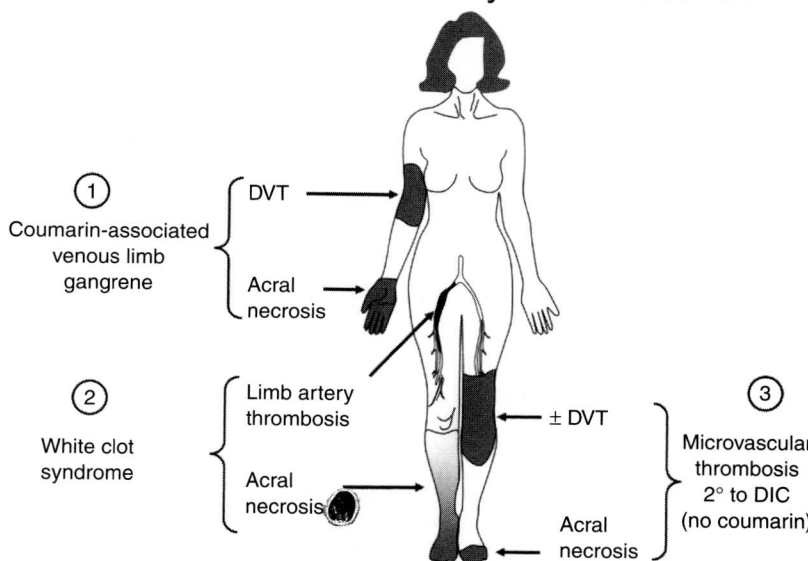

**FIGURE 114-4.** Three ischemic limb syndromes in heparin-induced thrombocytopenia (HIT). The two most common causes of limb loss in HIT are coumarin-induced venous limb gangrene [microvascular thrombosis in a limb affected by deep vein thrombosis (DVT)] and white clot syndrome (occlusion of large limb arteries by platelet-rich white clots). Rarely, microvascular thrombosis (with or without associated DVT) is associated with limb ischemia in the absence of coumarin use. DIC, disseminated intravascular coagulation. (From Warkentin TE. Heparin-induced thrombocytopenia: IgG-mediated platelet activation, platelet microparticle generation, and altered procoagulant/anticoagulant balance in the pathogenesis of thrombosis and venous limb gangrene complicating heparin-induced thrombocytopenia. *Transfus Med Rev* 1996;10:249–258.)

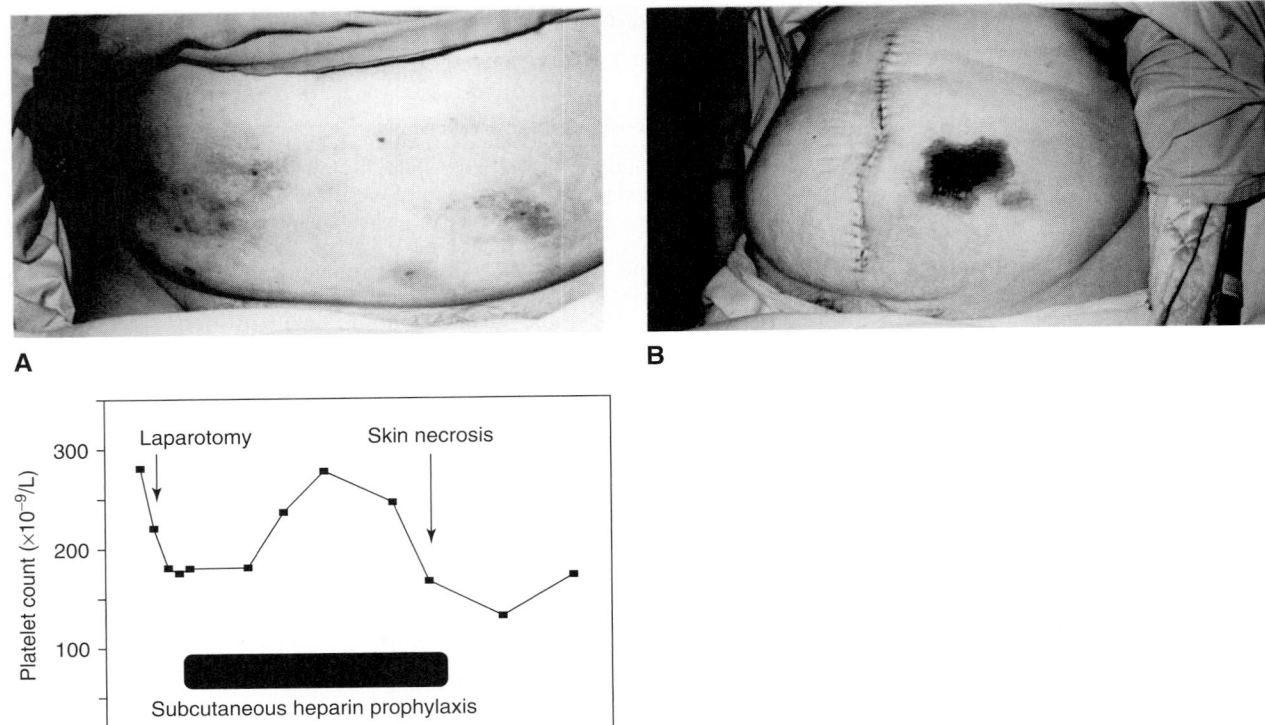

**FIGURE 114-5.** Heparin-induced skin lesions. **A:** Erythematous plaques and (**B**) skin necrosis. The serial platelet counts of the patient with skin necrosis shown in (**B**) is shown in (**C**). Note that only mild thrombocytopenia was observed despite the severe skin necrosis at the heparin injection site (see Color Fig. 114-5). [(**A**) From Warkentin TE. Heparin-induced skin lesions. *Br J Haematol* 1996;92:494–497.]

HIT serum (12) and testing a panel of negative, weak, and strong HIT control sera to confirm that the test platelets selected are adequate to detect HIT antibodies of varying reactivity (66). When performed by experienced technologists, the sensitivity and specificity of washed platelet assays for HIT are greater than 90% (61). Other acceptable platelet activation endpoints include platelet aggregation (67) and flow cytometric detection of platelet-derived microparticles (68).

Conventional platelet aggregation assays using normal donor platelets suspended in citrated plasma have a relatively low sensitivity for HIT (50% to 80%) (69) and are no longer widely used. Specificity also is lower because heparin can produce nonspecific activation of platelets under these test conditions.

## Antigen Assays

Antigen assays using the enzyme immunoassay (EIA) technique have been developed using the PF4-heparin (or PF4-polyanion) target antigen (14,23,69,70). False-negative results arise when HIT antibodies recognize PF4-related chemokines (e.g., interleukin-8 and neutrophil-activating peptide-2) rather than PF4 itself (71,72). Although the PF4-heparin-EIA is more sensitive than the SRA for detecting HIT antibodies, this may not be an advantage because more clinically insignificant antibodies are detected (70,73), resulting in a lower specificity for clinical HIT (63). The nonspecific nature of the negatively charged coantigen of HIT is illustrated by the development of an antigen assay using PF4 complexed to polyvinyl sulfonate,

a negatively charged material devoid of both carbohydrate and sulfate groups (23). Despite the absence of heparin, this assay has high sensitivity for detecting HIT antibodies.

A rapid antigen assay ("particle gel immunoassay") (74) has operating characteristics (sensitivity–specificity trade-offs) intermediate between the commercial EIA and a washed platelet activation assay (75); one study (76) suggests that the utility of this test is enhanced by interpreting the assay results quantitatively (rather than simply as positive or negative).

The concordance between activation and antigen assays is 85% to 90% ($\kappa$, 0.74) (69). For example, sometimes strong but heparin-independent platelet activation is produced by the serum of the patient (i.e., an indeterminate result), in which case, the PF4-heparin EIA is required for diagnosis. If a negative result is obtained using the EIA in a patient strongly suspected as having HIT, a functional assay should be performed because the target antigen could be an antigen other than PF4–heparin complex. In most situations, however, a negative EIA rules out HIT.

## Interpretation of Heparin-Induced Thrombocytopenia Assays

Results of HIT antibody tests must be interpreted in the appropriate clinical context of pretest probability. Further, the magnitude of the HIT antibody test result provides useful diagnostic information. For example, in postcardiac surgery patients (where 50% of the patients develop subclinical HIT antibody seroconversion) (70,73), a strong-positive SRA result (e.g., >90% serotonin release) is associated with a much higher likelihood ratio for clinical HIT than a weak-positive EIA (e.g., optical density of 0.5 to 0.75 absorbance units), approximately 15 to 30 versus only 2 to 3, respectively. Therefore, a non-HIT explanation for thrombocytopenia remains likely in a postcardiac surgery patient with a low pretest probability for HIT whose blood showed a weak-positive EIA.

## TREATMENT

Table 114-2 lists recent consensus conference treatment recommendations for HIT (77). Heparin should be discontinued in all patients strongly suspected of having HIT. However, the risk for subsequent thrombosis ranges from 25% to 50% even after heparin is discontinued in patients with serologically confirmed HIT (1,43,50,78). Further, the risk of sudden thrombotic death is about 5% (1,78). Therefore, heparin should be substituted by an acceptable, rapidly acting, alternative anticoagulant, such as a direct thrombin inhibitor (DTI) (e.g., lepirudin, argatroban, or bivalirudin) or factor Xa inhibitor (e.g., danaparoid or fondaparinux), generally in therapeutic doses, until the platelet count has recovered (77,79,80). In addition, to rule out DVT, duplex ultrasound examination of the lower limbs should be performed prior to discharge in patients strongly suspected or confirmed as having HIT (77).

Two DTIs, lepirudin and argatroban, are approved for management of HIT in the United States. Both agents have relative advantages and disadvantages. Careful drug selection, dosing, and monitoring are important because neither agent has a specific antidote.

## Recombinant Hirudin

Lepirudin (Refludan) is a recombinant hirudin derivative that inhibits thrombin via a high-affinity, noncovalent interaction (81–84). The C-terminal region of this 65–amino acid polypeptide (6,980 Da) binds to thrombin's fibrinogen-binding site (exosite 1), and a highly packed hydrophobic region near the N-terminus (produced by three disulfide bridges) binds to the apolar region of thrombin, thereby blocking the active (catalytic) site of thrombin. Its anticoagulant effect is usually monitored with the activated partial thromboplastin time (aPTT). Lepirudin is renally eliminated, and greatly reduced dosing (if it is used at all) is required in patients with renal failure. Anti-hirudin antibodies are commonly generated in patients treated with lepirudin; in a minority of patients, this can lead paradoxically to a greater anticoagulant effect of lepirudin (85) due to an immune complex-mediated prolonged half-life of active agent. It may be advisable to avoid the initial intravenous bolus to minimize risk of postbolus anaphylaxis (86). Lepirudin is approved in the United States and in the European Union to treat HIT complicated by thrombosis, but the potential for bleeding has prevented approval for other indications, such as acute coronary syndrome. Table 114-3 lists dosing recommendations, including various considerations to reduce the risk of bleeding.

## TABLE 114-2

**TREATMENT OF HEPARIN-INDUCED THROMBOCYTOPENIA: RECOMMENDATIONS$^a$ OF THE SEVENTH AMERICAN COLLEGE OF CHEST PHYSICIANS (ACCP) CONFERENCE ON ANTITHROMBOTIC AND THROMBOLYTIC THERAPY: EVIDENCE-BASED GUIDELINES, 2004**

| Treatment strategy | Recommendation |
| --- | --- |
| Nonheparin anticoagulants for HIT | For patients with strongly suspected (or confirmed) HIT, whether or not complicated by thrombosis, we recommend use of an alternative nonheparin anticoagulant, such as lepirudin (Grade 1C+), argatroban (Grade 1C), bivalirudin (Grade 2C), or danaparoid (Grade 1B) over further UFH or LMWH therapy and over no anticoagulation (with or without vena cava filter). |
| Screening for DVT | For patients with strongly suspected (or confirmed) HIT, whether or not there is clinical evidence of lower limb DVT, we recommend routine ultrasonography of the lower limb veins for investigation of DVT over not performing routine ultrasonography (Grade 1C). |
| Management of direct thrombin inhibitor–vitamin K antagonist overlap | For patients with strongly suspected or confirmed HIT, we recommend *against* the use of vitamin K antagonist (coumarin) therapy until after the platelet count has substantially recovered (e.g., to *at least* $100 \times 10^9$/L, and preferably, $150 \times 10^9$/L); that the vitamin K antagonist be given only during overlapping alternative anticoagulation (minimum, 5-d overlap) and begun with low, maintenance doses (maximum, 5 mg of warfarin; 6 mg of phenprocoumon); that the alternative anticoagulant not be stopped until the platelet count has reached a stable plateau and with at least the last 2 d in the target therapeutic range (all Grade 1C). |
| Reversal of vitamin K antagonist anticoagulation | For patients receiving vitamin K antagonists at the time of diagnosis of HIT, we suggest use of vitamin K (Grade 2C). |
| LMWH for HIT | For patients with strongly suspected HIT, whether or not complicated by thrombosis, we recommend *against* use of LMWH (Grade 1C+). |
| Prophylactic platelet transfusions for HIT | For patients with strongly suspected or confirmed HIT who do not have active bleeding, we suggest that prophylactic platelet transfusions not be given (Grade 2C). |

HIT, heparin-induced thrombocytopenia; DVT, deep vein thrombosis; UFH, unfractionated heparin; LMWH, low-molecular-weight heparin.
$^a$Grading of recommendations: Recommendations are ranked as Grade 1 (risk benefit is clear) and Grade 2 (risk benefit is unclear). Methodologic strength of supporting evidence is ranked as A (randomized clinical trials without important limitations), B (randomized clinical trials with important limitations), C (observational studies), and C+ (no randomized clinical trials but randomized clinical trial data can be unequivocally extrapolated, or there is overwhelming evidence from observational studies).
From Warkentin TE, Greinacher A. Heparin-induced thrombocytopenia: recognition, treatment, and prevention. The Seventh ACCP Conference on Antithrombotic and Thrombolytic Therapy. *Chest* 2004;126(Suppl. 3):311S–337S.

**TABLE 114-3**

LEPIRUDIN FOR TREATMENT OF HEPARIN-INDUCED THROMBOCYTOPENIA

**Standard protocol:** *HIT with thrombosis*: initial bolus, 0.4 mg/kg IV; followed by IV infusion at 0.15 mg/kg/h (target aPTT, 1.5–2.5 × baseline), aPTT adjusted 4 h later and 4 h after any dose adjustment; increase rate by 20% and decrease by 50% if aPTT below or above target range, respectively. *HIT without thrombosis*: no initial bolus; initial infusion rate, 0.1 mg/kg/h, adjusted by aPTT as in preceding text.

| Other dosing considerations | Rationale |
|---|---|
| Laboratory tests to determine standard curve of plasma lepirudin (using normal plasma "spiked" with lepirudin) to aPTT, including low- and high-therapeutic lepirudin levels (0.6–1.4 µg/mL) (83) | Because different aPTT reagents show flattening of the lepirudin–aPTT curve at different lepirudin concentrations, the standard curve is used to determine the lepirudin level beyond which accurate assessment by aPTT is no longer possible |
| Avoid the initial bolus dose, beginning with infusion alone (unless severe thrombosis is present) | Safety enhanced by minimizing risk of postbolus anaphylaxis, with only minor delay (approximately 6 h) in achieving therapeutic anticoagulation |
| In elderly patients (>60 yr), even with normal creatinine levels, begin with lower infusion rate (0.1 mg/kg/h) | Renal function declines with age and may be underestimated by serum creatinine levels; overdosing can occur at 0.15 mg/kg/h (with or without bolus) |
| Repeat aPTT monitoring at 4 h intervals until steady state is obtained | Steady state may not be reached at 4 h, especially if any renal dysfunction is present |
| Monitor aPTT daily while on lepirudin | Antihirudin antibodies can affect lepirudin clearance (either increase or decrease aPTT) |

Dose adjustments in renal insufficiency

| Creatinine clearance (mL/min) | Serum creatinine mg/dL (µmol/L) | Adjusted initial IV infusion rate (% of original dose) (then adjust by aPTT) |
|---|---|---|
| 45–60 | 1.6–2.0 (141–177) | 50 |
| 30–44 | 2.1–3.0 (178–265) | 25 |
| 15–29 | 3.1–6.0 (266–530) | 10 |
| <15 | >6.0 (>530) | 0.005 mg/kg/h body weight |

HIT, heparin-induced thrombocytopenia; IV, intravenous; aPTT, activated partial thromboplastin time.
From Greinacher A. Lepirudin for the treatment of heparin-induced thrombocytopenia. In: Warkentin TE, Greinacher A, eds. *Heparin-induced thrombocytopenia*, 3rd ed. New York: Marcel Dekker Inc, 2004:397–436; Greinacher A. Lepirudin: a bivalent direct thrombin inhibitor for anticoagulation therapy. *Expert Rev Cardiovasc Ther* 2004;2:339–357.

## Argatroban

Argatroban (non-US trademark, Novastan) is a synthetic, small-molecule DTI (527 Da) derivative of arginine (87,88). Argatroban inhibits thrombin [and possibly to a minor extent factor Xa (89)] at therapeutically relevant concentrations. The anticoagulant effect is monitored using the aPTT (usual target: 1.5 to 3.0 times baseline, maximum 100 seconds). Unlike lepirudin, however, argatroban is predominantly metabolized by the liver and, therefore, may be safer in patients with renal failure. Argatroban prolongs the INR to a greater extent than does bivalirudin or lepirudin, complicating the monitoring of overlapping warfarin anticoagulation.

Argatroban is approved in the United States, Canada, and several countries within Europe for treatment of HIT with or without associated thrombosis (87) and also for anticoagulation during percutaneous coronary intervention (PCI) in patients with, or at risk for, HIT (87,90).

## Direct Thrombin Inhibitor–Coumarin Overlap

The risk of warfarin-associated venous limb gangrene (discussed in Chapter 123) remains when warfarin is prematurely started and/or when the DTI is prematurely discontinued in a patient with HIT-associated venous thrombosis and ongoing thrombocytopenia (53,54). Therefore, it is prudent to delay commencing warfarin until the platelet count has substantially recovered (to >100 or, preferably, >150 × 10$^9$ per L) and any clinically manifest thrombosis is improving. Further, there should be at least a 5-day overlap between the DTI and warfarin (with target INR levels achieved for at least the last 2 days), and the DTI should not be stopped until the platelet count has reached a stable plateau. If warfarin has already been initiated when HIT is recognized, vitamin K should be given for two reasons: (a) to reduce the risk of warfarin-induced microvascular thrombosis and (b) to avoid underdosing of DTI because warfarin also prolongs the aPTT (77).

## Other Anticoagulants

*Bivalirudin* (Angiomax) is a hirulog (analog of hirudin) composed of only 20 amino acids (2,180 Da) (82,91,92). Bivalirudin is composed of two subunits: the *C*-terminal dodecapeptide of hirudin and a thrombin active site-binding *N*-terminal tetrapeptide (D-Phe1-Pro2-Arg3-Pro4) bridged by four glycine "spacers." As with hirudin, the *C*-terminus moiety binds to the fibrinogen recognition site of thrombin (exosite 1). This "designer molecule" has several theoretical advantages over hirudin (92), including (a) predominant nonrenal elimination (80% of its degradation is by plasma proteases), (b) a shorter half-life (25 vs >80 minutes), (c) reduced or absent immunogenicity, and (d) minimal prolongation of the INR (greater than lepirudin, but less than argatroban). Favorable results of "off-label" use of bivalirudin for HIT have been reported in uncontrolled studies (92,93), with initial dosing of 0.15 mg/kg/hour and aPTT monitoring (target aPTT 1.5 to 2.5-fold greater than baseline). Bivalirudin is undergoing assessment as an anticoagulant for "on-pump" and "off-pump" cardiac surgery in patients with HIT (41,92).

*Danaparoid sodium* (Orgaran) is a mixture of anticoagulant glycosaminoglycans with predominant anti–factor Xa activity, including low-sulfated heparan sulfate (84%) and dermatan sulfate (12%) (94,95). The anti-Xa/anti-IIa ratio is 22:1 [contrast LMWH, 2 to 4:1, and unfractionated (UF) heparin, 1:1]. Some of these sulfated constituents appear to interact with HIT antibodies, because 10% to 40% of HIT sera will show some degree of *in vitro* cross-reactivity for danaparoid, depending upon the sensitivity of the assay performed. However, *in vitro* cross-reactivity is usually not of clinical significance (96), and treatment with danaparoid should not be delayed to perform *in vitro* cross-reactivity studies. Anticoagulant monitoring of danaparoid is performed by measuring anti–factor Xa activity. However, monitoring is not usually required because the anticoagulant effect is largely predictable when administered on a weight-adjusted basis, and the likelihood of obtaining therapeutic anticoagulant levels is high using an empirically derived standard treatment protocol. Danaparoid can accumulate in renal failure; therefore, the maintenance dose should be reduced in these cases, and anti–factor Xa activity should be closely monitored. No antidote for danaparoid exists. Danaparoid's long half-life and lack of effect on the INR generally make for a smooth transition to warfarin monotherapy, suggesting that the risk of iatrogenic venous limb gangrene during overlapping therapy with danaparoid and coumarin is very low (in contrast to DTI–warfarin overlap). To date, danaparoid is the only therapy for HIT that has been evaluated in a randomized clinical trial (vs. the antiplatelet agent, dextran-70) (97,98). Danaparoid has been withdrawn from the U.S. market (April 2002) but is still available in Canada and Europe.

*Fondaparinux* (Arixtra) is a synthetic, sulfated pentasaccharide that catalyzes antithrombin-mediated inactivation of factor Xa. It does not cross-react with HIT antibodies (99) and, theoretically, should be effective in patients with HIT. However, there is minimal experience using this anticoagulant for HIT (100), and dosing is uncertain. The long half-life (17 hours) and lack of antidote suggest that it is not ideal for a patient who may require invasive procedures.

## PROGNOSIS

Many patients with HIT present with life- or limb-threatening thrombosis (43). Without effective anticoagulation, as many

as 50% of the patients with "isolated HIT" develop thrombosis (6,7,43). Limb amputation occurs in approximately 10% of the patients (78,101). The mortality rate is 15% to 25%, but deaths often reflect comorbidities rather than thrombotic death (78,101).

Table 114-4 lists treatment outcomes of lepirudin and argatroban, assessed in prospective cohort studies (with historic controls), as well as that of danaparoid, which was compared against dextran-70 in a randomized controlled trial (78,97,98,101–105). All three agents appeared to prevent thrombosis in HIT, although an impact on overall mortality and limb loss is less clear. Because these trials were performed before the clinical recognition of the danger of premature coumarin anticoagulation, it is possible that limb loss rates would be improved with measures to minimize this complication (Table 114-2).

## PREVENTION OF HEPARIN-INDUCED THROMBOCYTOPENIA AND ITS COMPLICATIONS

The recent emphasis on substituting heparin with an alternative anticoagulant even in patients with isolated HIT suggests an important role for platelet count monitoring for HIT. Recent consensus conferences (61,77) have adopted the view that the most intense monitoring (at least every other day) should be performed in situations in which HIT is common (>1%), such as in postoperative patients receiving antithrombotic prophylaxis with UFH or treatment of thrombosis with UFH. Less frequent monitoring (two or three times per week) is appropriate if HIT occurs at a frequency of 1/1,000 to 1/100, such as in medical and surgical patients receiving prophylaxis with UFH and LMWH, respectively. Routine monitoring is not recommended in circumstances in which HIT is rare (<1/1,000 in medical or obstetrical patients receiving LMWH). Nevertheless, HIT is frequently recognized only after a new thrombosis has occurred, even when frequent platelet count monitoring is performed (1,28), and there is no proof to date that frequent platelet count monitoring will prevent HIT-associated thrombosis.

Physicians should suspect HIT in any patient who develops new or progressive thrombosis during or shortly after stopping heparin therapy. In 10% to 15% of the patients with HIT, the platelet count nadir is greater than $150 \times 10^9$ per L (Fig. 114-2), although usually a proportional platelet count decline of at least 50% had occurred. Heparin should be discontinued and an alternative management strategy instituted in any patient in whom HIT is a likely diagnosis, even prior to obtaining diagnostic laboratory results.

The frequency of HIT, HIT-associated thrombosis, and HIT–IgG seroconversion is lower in patients treated with LMWH than in those treated with UF heparin (6,7,37). However, LMWH should not be used to treat HIT because HIT antibodies can activate platelets in the presence of LMWH (6,106). Based on the risk of worsening thrombocytopenia or thrombosis in a patient with acute HIT, and the availability of other options, LMWH is contraindicated for the treatment of HIT (77).

## SPECIAL SITUATIONS

Table 114-5 lists treatment recommendations of the ACCP in special situations such as heparin reexposure in patients with previous HIT and PCI (77). For patients with a previous history of HIT who have an important indication for heparin, such as cardiac or vascular surgery, the recommended approach is to use heparin, provided that HIT antibodies are undetectable (77). This is because HIT antibodies

# TABLE 114-4

## HEPARIN-INDUCED THROMBOCYTOPENIA TREATMENT OUTCOMES

| Study, yr (reference) | Regimen | n | Mean days of alternative anticoagulant | % HIT antibody-positive | New thrombosis rate (RRR)[a] | Amputation rate (RRR)[a] | Composite endpoint (RRR)[a] | Major bleed (% per d alternative anticoagulant given)[b] |
|---|---|---|---|---|---|---|---|---|
| **HIT-associated thrombosis** | | | | | | | | |
| HAT-1/2, 2000 (101) | Lep 0.4 mg/kg bolus + 0.15 mg/kg/h | 113 | 13.3 | 100% | 10.1 (63%) | 6.5% (38%) | 21.3% (55%) | 1.4% |
| HAT-3, 2004 (102) | Lep bolus + 0.15 mg/kg/h | 98 | 14 | 100% | 6.1% (78%) | 5.1% (51%) | 21.5% (55%) | 1.5% |
| DMP, 2003 (103) | Lep bolus + 0.15 mg/kg/h | 496 | 12.1 | 77% | 5.2% (NA) | 5.8% (NA) | 21.9% | 0.45% |
| Arg911, 2001 (78) | Arg 2 μg/kg/min | 144 | 5.9 | 65% | 19.4% (35%) | 11.8% (−8%) | 43.8% (22%) | 1.9% |
| Arg915, 2003 (104) | Arg 2 μg/kg/min | 229 | 7.1 | NA | 13.1% (62%) | 14.8% (−36%) | 41.5% (27%) | 0.9% |
| RCT versus dextran, 2001 (97) | Danap bolus + inf 200 U/h | 25 | 6[c] | 83% | 12.0% (77%) | NA | 20.0% (62%) | 0% |
| **Isolated HIT** | | | | | | | | |
| HAT1-3, 2002 (105) | Lep: 0.10 mg/kg/h | 111 | 13.5 | 100% | 2.7% (NA)[d] | 2.7% (NA)[d] | 9.0% (NA)[d] | 1.1%[d] |
| DMP, 2002 (103) | Lep: 0.10 mg/kg/h | 612 | 11 | 66% | 2.1% (NA)[e] | 1.3% (NA)[e] | ≥15.7% | 0.5%[e] |
| Arg911, 2001 (78) | Arg: 2 μg/kg/min | 160 | 5.9 | 65% | 8.1% (64%) | 1.9% (5%) | 25.6% (34%) | 0.6% |
| Arg915, 2003 (104) | Arg: 2 μg/kg/min | 189 | 5.1 | NA | 5.8% (75%) | 4.2% (−45%) | 28.0% (28%) | 1.0% |

Arg, argatroban; DMP, drug monitoring program (postmarketing study); Danap, danaparoid; HAT, heparin-associated thrombocytopenia (prospective lepirudin study); Lep, lepirudin; NA, not available; RCT, randomized controlled trial; RRR, relative risk reduction.

[a]RRR (relative risk reduction, expressed as percent) compared with historical controls (not shown).
[b]Calculated by dividing major bleed rate by number of mean days of alternative anticoagulant given.
[c]Median (data provided by Dr. Harry Magnani, Organon NV).
[d]Data limited to on-treatment observation period.
[e]Data limited to on-treatment observation period + 1 day.
From Warkentin TE, Poncz M, Cines DB. Heparin-induced thrombocytopenia. In: Young NS, Gerson SL, High KA, eds. Clinical hematology. Philadelphia: Elsevier/Mosby, 2006 (in press).

**TABLE 114-5**

TREATMENT OF HEPARIN-INDUCED THROMBOCYTOPENIA: SPECIAL SITUATIONS; RECOMMENDATIONS OF THE SEVENTH AMERICAN COLLEGE OF CHEST PHYSICIANS (ACCP) CONFERENCE ON ANTITHROMBOTIC AND THROMBOLYTIC THERAPY: EVIDENCE-BASED GUIDELINES, 2004

| Clinical situation | Recommendation (Grade of recommendations[a]) |
|---|---|
| Patients with previous HIT undergoing cardiac or vascular surgery | For patients with a history of HIT who are HIT antibody–negative and require cardiac surgery, we recommend the use of UFH over a nonheparin anticoagulant (Grade 1C) (Remark: Preoperative and postoperative anticoagulation, if indicated, should be given with a nonheparin anticoagulant) |
| Patients with acute HIT undergoing cardiac surgery | For patients with acute HIT (thrombocytopenic, HIT antibody–positive) who require cardiac surgery, we recommend one of the following alternative anticoagulant approaches (in descending order of preference): delaying surgery (if possible) until HIT antibodies are negative (Grade 1C); using bivalirudin for intraoperative anticoagulation during cardiopulmonary bypass (if ECT available) (Grade 1C) or during "off-pump" cardiac surgery (Grade 1C+); using lepirudin for intraoperative anticoagulation (if ECT available and patient has normal renal function) (Grade 1C); using UFH plus the antiplatelet agent epoprostenol (if ECT monitoring not available or renal insufficiency precludes lepirudin use) (Grade 2C); using UFH plus the antiplatelet agent, tirofiban (Grade 2C); or using danaparoid for intraoperative anticoagulation (if anti–factor Xa levels are available) (Grade 2C). |
| Patients with subacute HIT undergoing cardiac surgery | For patients with subacute HIT (platelet count recovery, but continuing HIT antibody–positive), we recommend delaying surgery (if possible) until HIT antibodies are negative, then using heparin (Grade 1C); alternatively, we suggest the use of a nonheparin anticoagulant (Grade 2C) |
| PCI | For patients with acute or previous HIT who require cardiac catheterization or PCI, we recommend use of an alternative anticoagulant, such as argatroban (Grade 1C), bivalirudin (Grade 1C), lepirudin (Grade 1C), or danaparoid (Grade 2C) over the use of heparin |

HIT, heparin-induced thrombocytopenia; UFH, unfractionated heparin; ECT, ecarin clotting time; PCI, percutaneous coronary interventions.
[a]See footnote of Table 114-2 for grading of recommendations.
From Warkentin TE, Greinacher A. Heparin-induced thrombocytopenia: recognition, treatment, and prevention. The Seventh ACCP Conference on Antithrombotic and Thrombolytic Therapy. *Chest* 2004;126(Suppl. 3):311S–337S.

are transient (35) and usually decline to nondetectable levels (by SRA) within a few weeks following an episode of HIT, although the antigen assay may persist at low-positive levels for a somewhat longer period. Furthermore, upon heparin reexposure, HIT antibodies are usually not regenerated (36), or if regenerated do not form quickly (minimum of 5 days) (35), thereby safely permitting at least a brief intraoperative reexposure to heparin. It is prudent to use alternative anticoagulants for preoperative and postoperative anticoagulation in this setting. Patients with recent HIT whose platelet count has recovered, but who still have detectable HIT antibodies ("subacute HIT"), should be considered to be at risk for developing rapid-onset HIT upon heparin reexposure unless the activation assay is negative and the antigen assay is only weakly positive (77). Alternative anticoagulant approaches for patients in whom heparin is not judged appropriate (because of acute or very recent HIT with residual antibodies) are listed in Table 114-5 (77).

# ACKNOWLEDGMENTS

Studies (1,2,4–7,9,11,24,25,29,31,35,37,41,42,44,47,49–53,55, 56,58,59,61–63,66,68,70,77,80,81,89,94,96,98,99) described in this chapter were supported by the Heart and Stroke Foundation of Ontario grants #A2449, #T2967, #B3763, #T4502, and #T5207 (from 1993-2006). Dr. Warkentin was supported by a research fellowship (1988-1991) and a research scholarship (1993-1998) from the Heart and Stroke Foundation of Canada.

## References

1. Warkentin TE. Heparin-induced thrombocytopenia: pathogenesis and management. *Br J Haematol* 2003;121:535–555.
2. Warkentin TE. Management of heparin-induced thrombocytopenia: a critical comparison of lepirudin and argatroban. *Thromb Res* 2003;110: 73–82.
3. Weismann RE, Tobin RW. Arterial embolism occurring during systemic heparin therapy. *Arch Surg* 1958;76:219–227.
4. Warkentin TE, Elavathil LJ, Hayward CPM, et al. The pathogenesis of venous limb gangrene associated with heparin-induced thrombocytopenia. *Ann Intern Med* 1997;127:804–812.
5. Warkentin TE. Clinical picture of heparin-induced thrombocytopenia. In: Warkentin TE, Greinacher A, eds. *Heparin-induced thrombocytopenia*, 3rd ed. New York: Marcel Dekker, 2004:53–106.
6. Warkentin TE, Levine MN, Hirsh J, et al. Heparin-induced thrombocytopenia in patients treated with low-molecular-weight heparin or unfractionated heparin. *N Engl J Med* 1995;332:1330–1335.
7. Warkentin TE, Roberts RS, Hirsh J, et al. An improved definition of immune heparin-induced thrombocytopenia in postoperative orthopedic patients. *Arch Intern Med* 2003;163:2518–2524.
8. Fabris F, Luzzatto G, Soini B, et al. Risk factors for thrombosis in patients with immune heparin-induced thrombocytopenia. *J Intern Med* 2002; 252:149–154.
9. Warkentin TE, Chong BH, Greinacher A. Heparin-induced thrombocytopenia: towards consensus. *Thromb Haemost* 1998;79:1–7.
10. Horne MK III. Nonimmune heparin-platelet interactions: implications for the pathogenesis of heparin-induced thrombocytopenia. In: Warkentin TE, Greinacher A, eds. *Heparin-induced thrombocytopenia*, 3rd ed. New York: Marcel Dekker, 2004:149–163.
11. Greinacher A, Warkentin TE. Treatment of heparin-induced thrombocytopenia: an overview. In: Warkentin TE, Greinacher A, eds. *Heparin-induced thrombocytopenia*, 3rd ed. New York: Marcel Dekker, 2004: 335–370.
12. Kelton JG, Sheridan D, Santos A, et al. Heparin-induced thrombocytopenia: laboratory studies. *Blood* 1988;72:925–930.

13. Amiral J, Wolf M, Fischer AM, et al. Pathogenicity of IgA and/or IgM antibodies to heparin–PF4 complexes in patients with heparin-induced thrombocytopenia. *Br J Haematol* 1996;92:954–959.

14. Amiral J, Bridey F, Dreyfus M, et al. Platelet factor 4 complexed to heparin is the target for antibodies generated in heparin-induced thrombocytopenia [letter]. *Thromb Haemost* 1992;68:95–96.

15. Greinacher A, Pötzsch B, Amiral J, et al. Heparin-associated thrombocytopenia: isolation of the antibody and characterization of a multimolecular PF4-heparin complex as the major antigen. *Thromb Haemost* 1994; 71:247–251.

16. Visentin GP, Ford SE, Scott JP, et al. Antibodies from patients with heparin-induced thrombocytopenia/thrombosis are specific for platelet factor 4 complexed with heparin or bound to endothelial cells. *J Clin Invest* 1994;93:81–88.

17. Kelton JG, Smith JW, Warkentin TE, et al. Immunoglobulin G from patients with heparin-induced thrombocytopenia binds to a complex of heparin and platelet factor 4. *Blood* 1994;83:3232–3239.

18. Suh JS, Aster RH, Visentin GP. Antibodies from patients with heparin-induced thrombocytopenia/thrombosis recognize different epitopes on heparin:platelet factor 4. *Blood* 1998;91:916–922.

19. Ziporen L, Li ZQ, Park KS, et al. Defining an antigenic epitope on platelet factor 4 associated with heparin-induced thrombocytopenia. *Blood* 1998; 92:3250–3259.

20. Li ZQ, Liu W, Park KS, et al. Defining a second epitope for heparin-induced thrombocytopenia/thrombosis antibodies using KKO, a murine HIT-like monoclonal antibody. *Blood* 2002;99:1230–1236.

21. Goad KE, Horne MK, Gralnick HR III. Pentosan-induced thrombocytopenia: support for an immune complex mechanism. *Br J Haematol* 1994;88:803–808.

22. Greinacher A, Michels I, Schafer M, et al. Heparin-associated thrombocytopenia in a patient treated with polysulphated chondroitin sulphate: evidence for immunological crossreactivity between heparin and polysulphated glycosaminoglycan. *Br J Haematol* 1992;81:252–254.

23. Visentin GP, Moghaddam M, Beery SE, et al. Heparin is not required for detection of antibodies associated with heparin-induced thormbocytopenia thrombosis. *J Lab Clin Med* 2001;138:22–31.

24. Warkentin TE, Hayward CPM, Boshkov LK, et al. Sera from patients with heparin-induced thrombocytopenia generate platelet-derived microparticles with procoagulant activity: an explanation for the thrombotic complications of heparin-induced thrombocytopenia. *Blood* 1994; 84:3691–3699.

25. Warkentin TE. An overview of the heparin-induced thrombocytopenia syndrome. *Semin Thromb Hemost* 2004;30:273–283.

26. Hartmann W, Greinacher A, Lubenow L, et al. Heparin-induced thrombocytopenia: in-vitro studies on the interaction of HIT-antibodies with endothelial cells [abstract]. Proceedings of the 8th European Symposium on Platelet and Granulocyte Immunobiology, Rust, Austria, May 13-16, 2004, COM06.

27. Pouplard C, Iochmann S, Renard B, et al. Induction of monocyte tissue factor expression by antibodies to heparin-platelet factor 4 complexes developed in heparin-induced thrombocytopenia. *Blood* 2001;97:3300–3302.

28. Khairy M, Lasne D, Brohard-Bohn B, et al. A new approach in the study of the molecular and cellular events implicated in heparin induced thrombocytopenia. Formation of leukocyte-platelet aggregates. *Thromb Haemost* 2001;85:1090–1096.

29. Warkentin TE, Sigouin CS. Gender and risk of immune heparin-induced thrombocytopenia. *Blood* 2002;100(Suppl. 1):17a.

30. Greinacher A, Mueller-Eckhardt G. Heparin-associated thrombocytopenia: no association of immune response with HLA. *Vox Sang* 1993;65:151–153.

31. Denomme GA, Warkentin TE, Horsewood P, et al. Activation of platelets by sera containing IgG1 heparin-dependent antibodies: an explanation for the predominance of the FcγRIIa "low responder" (His$_{131}$) gene in patients with heparin-induced thrombocytopenia. *J Lab Clin Med* 1997;130:278–284.

32. Bachelot-Loza C, Saffroy R, Lasne D, et al. Importance of the FcγRIIa-Arg/His-131 polymorphism in heparin-induced thrombocytopenia diagnosis. *Thromb Haemost* 1998;79:523–528.

33. Carlsson LE, Santoso S, Baurichter G, et al. Heparin-induced thrombocytopenia: new insights into the impact of the FcγRIIa-R-H131 polymorphism. *Blood* 1998;92:1526–1531.

34. Denomme GA. The platelet Fc receptor in heparin-induced thrombocytopenia. In: Warkentin TE, Greinacher A, eds. *Heparin-induced thrombocytopenia*, 3rd ed. New York: Marcel Dekker Inc, 2004:223–250.

35. Warkentin TE, Kelton JG. Temporal aspects of heparin-induced thrombocytopenia. *N Engl J Med* 2001;344:1286–1292.

36. Pötzsch B, Klövekorn WP, Madlener K. Use of heparin during cardiopulmonary bypass in patients with a history of heparin-induced thrombocytopenia [letter]. *N Engl J Med* 2000;343:515.

37. Lee DH, Warkentin TE. Frequency of heparin-induced thrombocytopenia. In: Warkentin TE, Greinacher A, eds. *Heparin-induced thrombocytopenia*, 3rd ed. New York: Marcel Dekker Inc, 2004:107–148.

38. Lepercq J, Conard J, Borel-Derlon A, et al. Venous thromboembolism during pregnancy: a retrospective study of enoxaparin safety in 624 pregnancies. *BJOG* 2001;108:1134–1140.

39. Fausett MB, Vogtlander M, Lee RM, et al. Heparin-induced thrombocytopenia is rare in pregnancy. *Am J Obstet Gynecol* 2001;185:148–152.

40. Girolami B, Prandoni P, Stefani PM, et al. The incidence of heparin-induced thrombocytopenia in hospitalized medical patients treated with subcutaneous unfractionated heparin: a prospective cohort study. *Blood* 2003;101:2955–2959.

41. Warkentin TE, Greinacher A. Heparin-induced thrombocytopenia and cardiac surgery. *Ann Thorac Surg* 2003;76:2121–2131.

42. Boshkov LK, Warkentin TE, Hayward CPM, et al. Heparin-induced thrombocytopenia and thrombosis: clinical and laboratory studies. *Br J Haematol* 1993;84:322–328.

43. Wallis DE, Workman DL, Lewis BE, et al. Failure of early heparin cessation as treatment for heparin-induced thrombocytopenia. *Am J Med* 1999;106:629–635.

44. Hong AP, Cook DJ, Sigouin CS, et al. Central venous catheters and upper-extremity deep-vein thrombosis complicating immune heparin-induced thrombocytopenia. *Blood* 2003;101:3049–3051.

45. Pedersen-Bjergaard U, Andersen M, Hansen PB. Drug-induced thrombocytopenia: clinical data on 309 cases and the effect of corticosteroid therapy. *Eur J Clin Pharmacol* 1997;52:183–189.

46. Lubenow N, Kempf R, Eichner A, et al. Heparin-induced thrombocytopenia: temporal pattern of thrombocytopenia in relation to initial use or reexposure to heparin. *Chest* 2002;122:37–42.

47. Warkentin TE, Kelton JG. Delayed-onset heparin-induced thrombocytopenia and thrombosis. *Ann Intern Med* 2001;135:502–506.

48. Rice L, Attisha WK, Drexler A, et al. Delayed-onset heparin-induced thrombocytopenia. *Ann Intern Med* 2002;136:210–215.

49. Warkentin TE, Bernstein RA. Delayed-onset heparin-induced thrombocytopenia and cerebral thrombosis after a single administration of unfractionated heparin [letter]. *N Engl J Med* 2003;348:1067–1069.

50. Warkentin TE, Kelton JG. A 14-year study of heparin-induced thrombocytopenia. *Am J Med* 1996;101:502–507.

51. Warkentin TE. Heparin-induced thrombocytopenia and vascular surgery. *Acta Chir Belg* 2004;104:257–265.

52. Warkentin TE. Heparin-induced thrombocytopenia: IgG-mediated platelet activation, platelet microparticle generation, and altered procoagulant/anticoagulant balance in the pathogenesis of thrombosis and venous limb gangrene complicating heparin-induced thrombocytopenia. *Transfus Med Rev* 1996;10:249–258.

53. Smythe MA, Warkentin TE, Stephens JL, et al. Venous limb gangrene during overlapping therapy with warfarin and a direct thrombin inhibitor for immune heparin-induced thrombocytopenia. *Am J Hematol* 2002;71:50–52.

54. Srinivasan AF, Rice L, Bartholomew JR, et al. Warfarin-induced skin necrosis and venous limb gangrene in the setting of heparin-induced thrombocytopenia. *Arch Intern Med* 2004;164:66–70.

55. Warkentin TE, Sikov WM, Lillicrap DP. Multicentric warfarin-induced skin necrosis complicating heparin-induced thrombocytopenia. *Am J Hematol* 1999;62:44–48.

56. Warkentin TE. Heparin-induced skin lesions. *Br J Haematol* 1996;92: 494–497.

57. Fontana P, Bodmer A, Gruel Y, et al. Skin necrosis is a clinical manifestation of low-molecular-weight heparin-induced thrombocytopenia. *Thromb Haemost* 2004;91:196–197.

58. Warkentin TE. Heparin-induced thrombocytopenia, heparin-induced skin lesions, and arterial thrombosis [abstract]. *Thromb Haemost* 1997; 77(Suppl.):562.

59. Warkentin TE, Hirte HW, Anderson DR, et al. Transient global amnesia associated with acute heparin-induced thrombocytopenia. *Am J Med* 1994;97:489–491.

60. Popov D, Zarrabi MH, Foda H, et al. Pseudopulmonary embolism: acute respiratory distress in the syndrome of heparin-induced thrombocytopenia. *Am J Kidney Dis* 1997;29:449–452.

61. Warkentin TE. Platelet count monitoring and laboratory testing for heparin-induced thrombocytopenia: recommendations of the College of American Pathologists. *Arch Pathol Lab Med* 2002;126:1415–1423.

62. Warkentin TE, Greinacher A. Laboratory testing for heparin-induced thrombocytopenia. In: Warkentin TE, Greinacher A, eds. *Heparin-induced thrombocytopenia*, 3rd ed. New York: Marcel Dekker Inc, 2004: 271–311.

63. Warkentin TE. New approaches to the diagnosis of heparin-induced thrombocytopenia. *Chest* 2005;127(Suppl. 2):35S–45S.

64. Sheridan D, Carter C, Kelton JG. A diagnostic test for heparin-induced thrombocytopenia. *Blood* 1986;67:27–30.

65. Chong BH, Burgess J, Ismail F. The clinical usefulness of the platelet aggregation test for the diagnosis of heparin-induced thrombocytopenia. *Thromb Haemost* 1993;69:344–350.

66. Warkentin TE, Hayward CPM, Smith CA, et al. Determinants of donor platelet variability when testing for heparin-induced thrombocytopenia. *J Lab Clin Med* 1992;120:371–379.

67. Greinacher A, Michels I, Kiefel V, et al. A rapid and sensitive test for diagnosing heparin-associated thrombocytopenia. *Thromb Haemost* 1991;66: 734–736.

68. Lee DH, Warkentin TE, Denomme GA, et al. A diagnostic test for heparin-induced thrombocytopenia: detection of platelet microparticles using flow cytometry. *Br J Haematol* 1996;95:724–731.

69. Greinacher A, Amiral J, Dummel V, et al. Laboratory diagnosis of heparin-associated thrombocytopenia and comparison of platelet aggregation test, heparin-induced platelet activation test, and platelet factor 4/heparin enzyme-linked immunosorbent assay. *Transfusion* 1994;34: 381–385.

70. Warkentin TE, Sheppard JI, Horsewood P, et al. Impact of the patient population on the risk for heparin-induced thrombocytopenia. *Blood* 2000;96:1703–1708.

71. Amiral J, Marfaing-Koka A, Wolf M, et al. Presence of autoantibodies to interleukin-8 or neutrophil-activating peptide-2 in patients with heparin-associated thrombocytopenia. *Blood* 1996;88:410–416.

72. Regnault V, de Maistre E, Carteaux JP, et al. Platelet activation induced by human antibodies to interleukin-8. *Blood* 2003;101:1419–1421.

73. Visentin GP, Malik M, Cyganiak KA, et al. Patients treated with unfractionated heparin during open heart surgery are at high risk to form antibodies reactive with heparin:platelet factor 4 complexes. *J Lab Clin Med* 1996;128:376–383.

74. Meyer O, Salama A, Pittet N, et al. Rapid detection of heparin-induced platelet antibodies with particle gel immunoassay (ID-HPF4). *Lancet* 1999;354:1525–1526.

75. Eichler P, Raschke R, Lubenow N, et al. The new ID-heparin/PF4 antibody test for rapid detection of heparin-induced antibodies in comparison with functional and antigenic assays. *Br J Haematol* 2002;116:887–891.

76. Alberio L, Kimmerle S, Baumann A, et al. Rapid determination of anti-heparin/platelet factor 4 antibody titers in the diagnosis of heparin-induced thrombocytopenia. *Am J Med* 2003;114:528–536.

77. Warkentin TE, Greinacher A. Heparin-induced thrombocytopenia: recognition, treatment, and prevention. The Seventh ACCP Conference on Antithrombotic and Thrombolytic Therapy. *Chest* 2004;126(Suppl. 3): 311S–337S.

78. Lewis BE, Wallis DE, Berkowitz SD, et al. Argatroban anticoagulant therapy in patients with heparin-induced thrombocytopenia. *Circulation* 2001;103:1838–1843.

79. Farner B, Eichler P, Kroll H, et al. A comparison of danaparoid and lepirudin in heparin-induced thrombocytopenia. *Thromb Haemost* 2001;85: 950–957.

80. Warkentin TE. Heparin-induced thrombocytopenia: yet another treatment paradox? *Thromb Haemost* 2001;85:947–949.

81. Warkentin TE. Bivalent direct thrombin inhibitors: hirudin and bivalirudin. *Best Pract Res Clin Haematol* 2004;17:105–125.

82. Greinacher A, Lubenow N. Recombinant hirudin in clinical practice: focus on lepirudin. *Circulation* 2001;103:1479–1484.

83. Greinacher A. Lepirudin for the treatment of heparin-induced thrombocytopenia. In: Warkentin TE, Greinacher A, eds. *Heparin-induced thrombocytopenia*, 3rd ed. New York: Marcel Dekker Inc, 2004:397–436.

84. Greinacher A. Lepirudin: a bivalent direct thrombin inhibitor for anticoagulation therapy. *Expert Rev Cardiovasc Ther* 2004;2:339–357.

85. Eichler P, Friesen HJ, Lubenow N, et al. Antihirudin antibodies in patients with heparin-induced thrombocytopenia treated with lepirudin: incidence, effects on aPTT, and clinical relevance. *Blood* 2000;96:2373–2378.

86. Greinacher A, Eichler P, Lubenow N. Anaphylactic and anaphylactoid reactions associated with lepirudin in patients with heparin-induced thrombocytopenia. *Circulation* 2003;108:2062–2065.

87. Lewis BE, Hursting MJ. Argatroban therapy in heparin-induced thrombocytopenia. In: Reinacher A, ed. *Heparin-induced thrombocytopenia*, 3rd ed. New York: Marcel Dekker Inc, 2004:437–474.

88. Arpino PA, Hallisey RK. Effect of renal function on pharmacodynamics of argatroban. *Ann Pharmacother* 2004;38:25–29.

89. Warkentein TE, Greinacher A, Craven S, et al. Four direct thrombin inhibitors (DTIs) variably increase the prothrombin time: a consequence of differing therapeutic molar concentrations? [Abstract] *J Thromb Haemost* 2005 (*in press*).

90. Lewis BE, Matthai WH Jr, Cohen M et al., ARG-216/310/311 Study Investigators. Argatroban anticoagulation during percutaneous coronary intervention in patients with heparin-induced thrombocytopenia. *Catheter Cardiovasc Interv* 2002;57:177–184.

91. Maraganore JM, Bourdon P, Jablonski J, et al. Design and characterization of hirulogs: a novel class of bivalent peptide inhibitors of thrombin. *Biochemistry* 1990;29:7095–7101.

92. Bartholomew JR. Bivalirudin for the treatment of heparin-induced thrombocytopenia. In: Reinacher A, ed. *Heparin-induced thrombocytopenia*, 3rd ed. New York: Marcel Dekker Inc, 2004:475–507.

93. Francis JL, Drexler A, Gwyn G, et al. Bivalirudin, a direct thrombin inhibitor, is a safe and effective treatment for heparin-induced thrombocytopenia [abstract]. *Blood* 2003;102(Suppl. 1):164a.

94. Warkentin TE, Barkin RL. Newer strategies for the treatment of heparin-induced thrombocytopenia. *Pharmacotherapy* 1999;19:181–195.

95. Chong BH, Magnani HN. Danaparoid for the treatment of heparin-induced thrombocytopenia. In: reinacher A, ed. *Heparin-induced thrombocytopenia*, 3rd ed. New York: Marcel Dekker Inc, 2004:371–396.

96. Warkentin TE. Danaparoid (Orgaran®) for the treatment of heparin-induced thrombocytopenia (HIT) and thrombosis: effects on *in vivo* thrombin and cross-linked fibrin generation, and evaluation of the clinical significance of *in vitro* cross-reactivity (XR) of danaparoid for HIT-IgG (abstract). *Blood* 1996;88(Suppl. 1):626a.

97. Chong BH, Gallus AS, Cade JF, et al. Prospective randomised open-label comparison of danaparoid with dextran 70 in the treatment of heparin-induced thrombocytopaenia with thrombosis: a clinical outcome study. *Thromb Haemost* 2001;86:1170–1175.

98. Warkentin TE, Poncz M, Cines DB. Heparin-induced thrombocytopenia. In: Young NS, Gerson SL, High KA, eds. *Clinical hematology*. Philadelphia: Elsevier/Mosby, 2006 (*in press*).

99. Warkentin TE, Cook RJ, Marder VJ, et al. Comparison of heparin-induced thrombocytopenia antibody (HIT-Ab) generation and *in vitro* cross-reactivity after elective hip or knee replacement surgery in patients receiving antithrombotic prophylaxis with fondaparinux or enoxaparin. *Blood* 2003;102(Suppl. 1):164a.

100. Kuo KHM, Kovacs MJ. Successful treatment of heparin induced thrombocytopenia (HIT) with fondaparinux [abstract]. *Blood* 2003;102(Suppl. 1):319a.

101. Greinacher A, Eichler P, Lubenow N, et al. Heparin-induced thrombocytopenia with thromboembolic complications: meta-analysis of 2 prospective trials to assess the value of parenteral treatment with lepirudin and its therapeutic aPTT range. *Blood* 2000;96:846–851.

102. Lubenow N, Eichler P, Lietz T, et al. Lepirudin in patients with heparin-induced thrombocytopenia: results of the third prospective study (HAT-3) and a combined analysis of HAT-1, HAT-2, and HAT-3. *J Thromb Haemost* 2005 (in press).

103. Lubenow N, Eichler P, Greinacher A. Results of a large drug monitoring program confirms the safety and efficacy of Refludan (lepirudin) in patients with immune-mediated heparin-induced thrombocytopenia [abstract]. *Blood* 2000;100(Suppl. 1):502a.

104. Lewis BE, Wallis DE, Leya F et al., Argatroban-915 Investigators. Argatroban anticoagulation in patients with heparin-induced thrombocytopenia. *Arch Intern Med* 2003;163:1849–1856.

105. Lubenow N, Eichler P, Leitz T, et al. Lepirudin for prophylaxis of thrombosis in patients with acute isolated heparin-induced thrombocytopenia: an analysis of 3 prospective studies. *Blood* 2004;104:3072–3077.

106. Greinacher A, Michels I, Mueller-Eckhardt C. Heparin-associated thrombocytopenia: the antibody is not heparin specific. *Thromb Haemost* 1992;67:545–549.

# CHAPTER 115 ■ COUMARIN-INDUCED SKIN NECROSIS AND VENOUS LIMB GANGRENE

THEODORE E. WARKENTIN

Thrombotic events that result from coumarin administration are incongruous but well-documented complications of anticoagulant therapy. The key role of coumarin (vitamin K antagonist) in causing thrombosis and necrosis is by the depletion of one or both vitamin K–dependent natural anticoagulants, protein C and protein S. In this chapter, *coumarin-induced necrosis* denotes both (central) skin necrosis and (acral) venous limb gangrene syndromes. *Coumarin-induced skin necrosis* (CISN) was first recognized by Verhagen (1), who described 13 cases in 1954, noting features such as its female predominance, characteristic localization of lesions, and typical onset within a few days of initiating coumarin. CISN is characterized by infarction and necrosis of the skin and underlying subcutaneous tissues (2,3). A related syndrome, *coumarin-induced venous limb gangrene*, is linked to warfarin treatment of acute deep vein thrombosis (DVT) complicating certain hypercoagulability disorders, most notably immune heparin-induced thrombocytopenia (HIT) and adenocarcinoma (4–7).

## COUMARINS

The *coumarins* are a group of naturally occurring lactones that are produced by a number of plants and microbes. Ironically, the least complex member, *coumarin* (1,2-benzopyrone), has no anticoagulant action despite its synonymous designation for those chemically related molecules that possess anticoagulant activity (8). Warfarin (Coumadin), a 4-hydroxycoumarin derivative, is the most widely used oral anticoagulant in North America (2). Therefore, most instances of CISN in North America are warfarin-induced. However, the syndrome can be caused by other coumarin congeners (e.g., phenprocoumon, acenocoumarol, and nicoumalone), as well as by the rarely used phenindione group of oral anticoagulants (9,10). Phenprocoumon (Marcumar) is widely used in continental Europe. Because its half-life is longer than that of warfarin (6 vs. 1.5 days), relatively large loading doses are often given; however, whether these differences result in a lesser or greater frequency of CISN, compared with warfarin, is unknown. The coumarins interfere with vitamin K epoxide reductase (11), producing posttranslational modifications of four procoagulant and two anticoagulant vitamin K–dependent factors (12).

## PATHOGENESIS

Several observations suggest that the fundamental pathobiology of coumarin necrosis is a transient disturbance in procoagulant/anticoagulant balance that leads to microthrombosis in susceptible tissue sites. First, coumarin necrosis has a characteristic temporal profile, usually occurring within 1 week of initiating oral anticoagulant therapy (5–7,9,13–16). During this interval, functional levels of protein C decline much more quickly than the major procoagulant factor, prothrombin (17,18), because of differences in their half-lives (12) (see Table 115-1). Second, the pathology is that of noninflammatory, small-vessel thrombosis affecting the dermal and subcutaneous postcapillary venules and small veins (5,15). This is consistent with the role of the protein C anticoagulant pathway in preventing thrombosis of these small vessels (19). Third, a relatively high proportion of patients with CISN (although not venous limb gangrene) have a hereditary abnormality of the protein C anticoagulant pathway, which predisposes such patients to further, potentially dangerous reductions in protein C during the first few days of oral anticoagulant treatment. Fourth, the clinical and pathologic appearance of CISN resembles that of neonatal purpura fulminans caused by severe congenital protein C deficiency (20). Fifth, skin necrosis can be a feature of acquired deficiency of protein C or protein S due to infection, autoimmunity, or the antiphospholipid syndrome (21–23) or functional inhibition of protein C or protein S by antiphospholipid antibodies (24,25). Sixth, coumarin necrosis (particularly venous limb gangrene) is associated with increased thrombin generation (4–6,26).

## COUMARIN-INDUCED SKIN NECROSIS

CISN refers to *central* (nonacral) necrosis of skin and subcutaneous tissues (see Fig. 115-1) (4); it occurs more often in women (3:1 ratio), with mean age being 50 to 55 years, and most commonly involves sites with substantial underlying fatty tissues, such as the breast, anterior abdomen, buttocks, hips, thighs, and calves, less commonly the flank, back, penis, legs, arms, and face (3,9,13–16). Multiple (sometimes symmetric) lesions are observed in about one third of patients. CISN is rare, occurring in only two of approximately 20,000 patients (0.01%) who received warfarin (3).

The typical temporal onset between 3 and 6 days of oral anticoagulant therapy occurs in 90% of patients (9,13–16), although late onset after weeks or months has been reported (27,28). Localized pain, induration, and erythema progresses over hours to central purplish black skin discoloration, usually with blistering, and ultimately evolving to well-demarcated, full-thickness necrosis of the skin and subdermal tissues (see Fig. 115-2). With or without surgical debridement, there usually is a permanent region of depressed skin that reflects the loss of underlying tissues. The necrotic skin also presents the real possibility of secondary fatal sepsis (28,29).

**TABLE 115-1**

HALF-LIVES OF THE VITAMIN K–DEPENDENT PROCOAGULANT AND ANTICOAGULANT FACTORS

| Procoagulant factors (half-life, h) | Anticoagulant factors (half-life, h) |
|---|---|
| Factor II (prothrombin, 60 h) | Protein C (9 h) |
| Factor X (40 h) | Protein S (60 h) |
| Factor IX (24 h) | |
| Factor VII (4–6 h) | |

There are six vitamin K–dependent hemostatic factors: four with procoagulant activity and two with anticoagulant activity. Treatment with coumarin anticoagulants reduces functional levels of these factors. The paradoxic procoagulant effect of warfarin can be explained by the different half-lives (12) of these factors following onset of action of coumarin—the time to a therapeutically significant reduction of the major procoagulant factor, prothrombin (half-life, ≈60 h), is much longer than the time to a clinically important reduction in the major anticoagulant factor, protein C (half-life, ≈9 h). Thus, within the first several days of coumarin anticoagulation, and under certain clinical circumstances (see text), there can arise a transient, but clinically important, disturbance in procoagulant—anticoagulant balance.

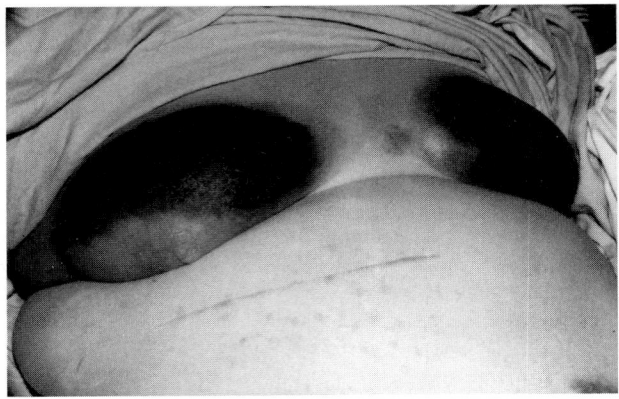

FIGURE 115-2. Coumarin-induced skin necrosis. Breast necrosis necessitating bilateral mastectomies occurred during the use of warfarin to treat pulmonary embolism complicating heparin-induced thrombocytopenia (HIT). Follow-up studies showed no congenital deficiency in protein C, protein S, or antithrombin. Factor V$_{Leiden}$ and the prothrombin G → A20210 variant were not present. (Reprinted with permission from Warkentin TE, Sikov WM, Lillicrap DP. Multicentric warfarin-induced skin necrosis complicating heparin-induced thrombocytopenia. *Am J Hematol* 1999;62:44–48.)

The earliest stages of CISN can resemble subcutaneous hemorrhage. Incipient skin necrosis is suggested by (a) recent initiation of coumarin, (b) typical location of lesions, (c) absence of trauma, and (d) an international normalized ratio (INR) that is within (in 33% to 60% of patients) or above the therapeutic range (13,14). CISN that occurs when the INR is within the therapeutic range suggests that the patient has a preexisting abnormality of the protein C natural anticoagulant pathway, as noted in four family members with hereditary protein S deficiency (30). In contrast, when warfarin-induced venous limb gangrene complicates disorders associated with disseminated intravascular coagulation (DIC), such as HIT or adenocarcinoma, there typically is a *supra*therapeutic INR. This reflects the special susceptibility of factor VII and protein C to severe depletion during coumarin therapy in DIC. In such patients, congenital abnormalities of the protein C natural anticoagulant pathway are usually not present (5,6,29).

Often, multiple risk factors can be identified in individual patients (see Table 115-2) (5–7,26,29–58). An example is the concurrence of postpartum DVT, antiphospholipid syndrome, "loading doses" of warfarin, and premature discontinuation of heparin in one patient (34).

Abnormalities of the protein C natural anticoagulant pathway are a relatively common finding in patients with CISN. Indeed, congenital deficiency of protein C was the first hemostatic abnormality identified in some patients with CISN (although reports do not always distinguish hereditary deficiency from the reversible reduction expected in a patient receiving coumarin) (50,51). Congenital deficiency of protein S (33,36,53) and of antithrombin (56) also has been observed, as has been the deficiency of factor V$_{Leiden}$ (33,37,46,54,55), a common mutation that renders factor V less susceptible to proteolytic degradation by activated protein C. Most patients with CISN have acute DVT (rather than a nonthrombotic indication such as atrial fibrillation) (39) as their indication for oral anticoagulants (3), suggesting that associated clinical factors (perhaps thrombin generation related to an acute thrombus) are relevant in CISN pathogenesis.

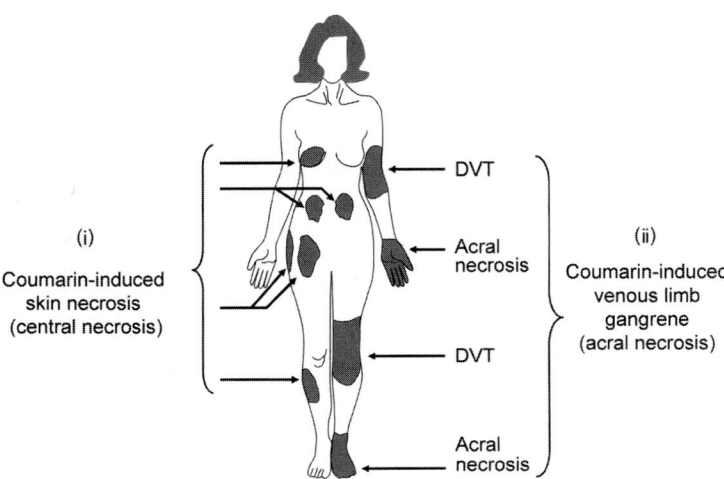

FIGURE 115-1. Two syndromes of coumarin-induced necrosis. (i) Coumarin-induced skin necrosis (CISN) and (ii) coumarin-induced venous limb gangrene. CISN most often affects the breast, abdomen, thigh, buttock, and calf, and often is symmetrical; it is usually associated with congenital or acquired abnormalities in the protein C natural anticoagulant pathway. In contrast, venous limb gangrene occurs in patients with disseminated intravascular coagulation (DIC) associated with immune heparin-induced thrombocytopenia (HIT) or adenocarcinoma. This syndrome is characterized by microvascular thrombosis in a limb affected by deep vein thrombosis (DVT) that leads to acral ischemic necrosis. (Reprinted, with modifications, with permission from Warkentin TE. Heparin-induced thrombocytopenia: IgG-mediated platelet activation, platelet microparticle generation, and altered procoagulant/anticoagulant balance in the pathogenesis of thrombosis and venous limb gangrene complicating heparin-induced thrombocytopenia. *Transfus Med Rev* 1996;10:249–258.)

**TABLE 115-2**

MULTIFACTORIAL NATURE OF COUMARIN NECROSIS

**LOCAL RISK FACTORS**
Sites of increased subcutaneous fat[a] (e.g., breast, abdomen, thigh, calf; obesity is common; lesions often are symmetric, e.g., bilateral thighs) (29,31–35)
Deep vein thrombosis[a,b] (29,31–34,36,37)
Peripheral vasospasm, e.g., Raynaud phenomenon (38,39)

**COUMARIN PHARMACOKINETICS (OFTEN RESULTING IN SUPRATHERAPEUTIC INR)**
"Loading doses" of warfarin[a] (29,31–35,37,40)
Drugs enhancing pharmacologic effect of warfarin (41,42)
Hepatic dysfunction (e.g., congestive heart failure) (42,43)
Vitamin K deficiency (44,45)
Premature discontinuation of heparin (or DTI) during coumarin overlap[c] (29,31,34,38,46,47)
Cytochrome P-450 mutations (CYP2C9*2, CYP2CP9*3) affecting coumarin pharmacokinetics (48,49)[d]

**DISORDERS ASSOCIATED WITH DIC[e]**
Heparin-induced thrombocytopenia[a] (5,26,33,36,38,47)
Adenocarcinoma[a] (6,7,31,38)

**CONGENITAL OR ACQUIRED HYPERCOAGULABILITY DISORDERS**
Abnormalities of the protein C natural anticoagulant pathway
    Congenital protein C deficiency[a] (37,50–52)
    Congenital or acquired protein S deficiency[a] (30,32,33,35,36,53)
    Factor V$_{Leiden}$ (heterozygous or homozygous)[a] (33,37,46,54,55)
    Antiphospholipid syndrome[a] (29,34)
Miscellaneous
    Postpartum state[a] (33–36)
    Antithrombin deficiency (56,57)
    Prothrombin gene mutation G20210A (58)
    Methyltetrahydrofolate reductase C677T polymorphism (hyperhomocysteinemia) (32)
The multifactorial nature of coumarin necrosis is illustrated by four or more risk factors in many patients (31–38).

INR, international normalized ratio; DTI, direct thrombin inhibitor; DIC, disseminated intravascular coagulations.
[a]Common association with coumarin necrosis that is likely of pathogenetic significance.
[b]Deep vein thrombosis (DVT) also predisposes to subtending acral limb necrosis, that is, venous limb gangrene.
[c]Early protein C depletion is more likely to be clinically significant if heparin is prematurely discontinued during heparin–coumarin overlap for treatment of thrombosis.
[d]Theoretical risk factor for coumarin necrosis that is not established.
[e]Disseminated intravascular coagulation (DIC) predisposes more strongly to venous limb gangrene than to Coumarin-induced skin necrosis (CISN).

# COUMARIN-INDUCED VENOUS LIMB GANGRENE

A form of coumarin necrosis known as *venous limb gangrene* affects acral tissues such as toes/feet/legs or fingers/hands/arms (see Fig. 115-1 and Fig. 115-3A, B, C) (4,5). Tissue necrosis occurs in the limb with acute DVT, sometimes with a discernible prodrome of phlegmasia cerulea dolens (5,29,59,60) (see Fig. 115-3D). Manifestations of acral tissue necrosis range from sloughing of skin of the toes or fingers that does not require amputation to extensive gangrene that requires below the knee or even above the knee amputation. In contrast, necrosis in CISN is limited to skin and subcutaneous tissues.

Two hypercoagulability disorders have been linked to coumarin-induced venous limb gangrene: immune HIT (5,26, 29) and DIC associated with adenocarcinoma (6,7,31,61,62). Occasionally, CISN and venous limb gangrene occur in the same patient (5,26,59,60).

Clinical and laboratory data support a pathogenic role for coumarin in the pathogenesis of venous limb gangrene complicating HIT. First, a case–control study (5) of patients with HIT observed a higher frequency of warfarin use coinciding with the onset of venous limb gangrene than in control patients with limb ischemia secondary to arterial thrombosis (eight of eight vs. three of 10; $P = 0.004$). Additional analysis showed that patients with HIT, DVT, and venous limb gangrene had a significantly greater median INR (5.8 vs. 3.1; $P < 0.001$) than control patients with HIT who had DVT and who were also treated with warfarin but did not develop limb gangrene.

Laboratory studies corroborated an important role for warfarin in the pathogenesis of venous limb gangrene (see Figs. 115-4A and B). Compared with controls, plasma from patients with venous limb gangrene had a higher ratio of thrombin–antithrombin complex (a marker of *in vivo* thrombin generation) to protein C activity during warfarin treatment (Fig. 115-4B). Analysis of individual cases showed that the onset of venous limb gangrene coincided with a fall in protein C activity to very low levels (Fig. 115-4A). No hereditable abnormalities in the protein C anticoagulant pathway were seen in any patient. Thrombosis of subcutaneous venules characteristic of this syndrome is consistent with the role of the protein C anticoagulant pathway to downregulate thrombin generated in the microvasculature (15,19). The normal INR values before initiation of warfarin therapy, as well as normal (or elevated) levels of factors V and VIII during warfarin

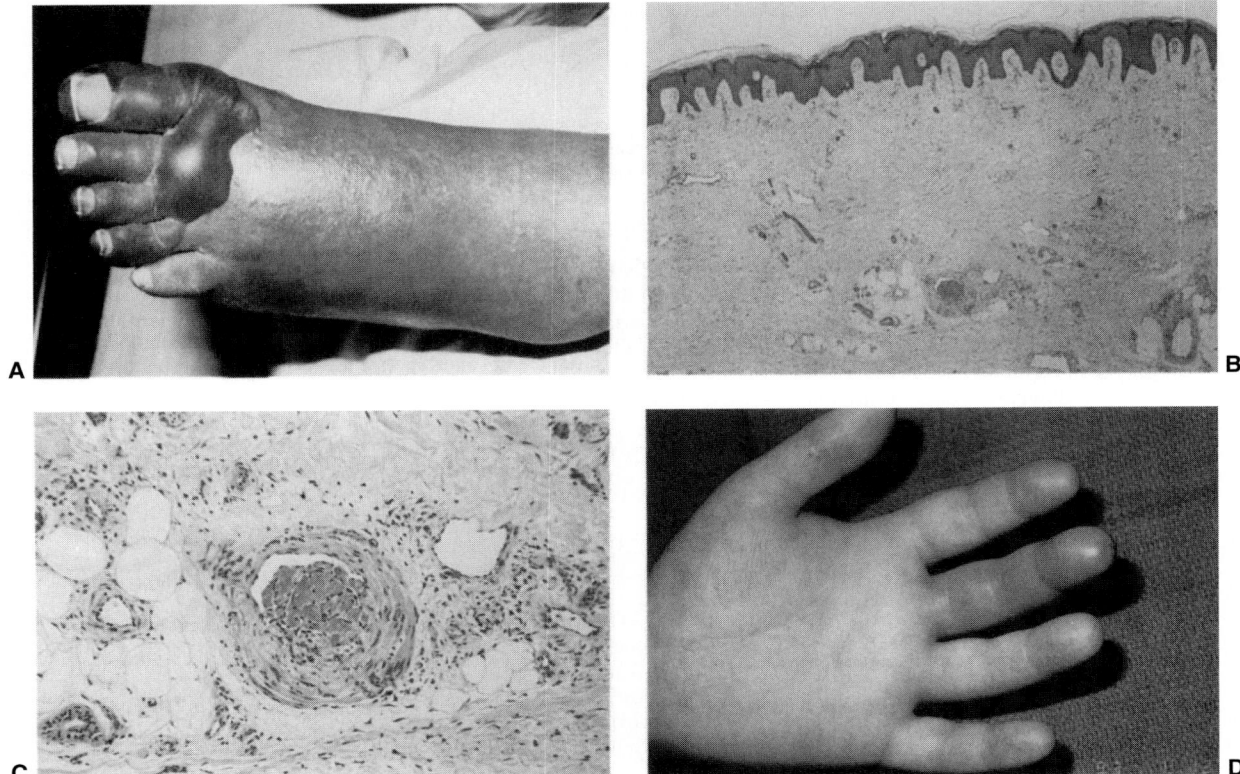

**FIGURE 115-3. A:** Warfarin-induced venous limb gangrene complicating heparin-induced thrombocytopenia (HIT). **B:** An occluding thrombus can be seen in a subcutaneous venule (original magnification, × 40). **C:** High-power view (original magnification, ×100) of the subcutaneous venule from part (**B**). **D:** Warfarin-associated phlegmasia cerulea dolens complicating HIT (see Color Fig. 115-3). [Photograph from patient 4, reported previously (5)]. (Figs. 115A-C from Warkentin TE, Elavathil LJ, Hayward CPM, et al. The pathogenesis of venous limb gangrene associated with heparin-induced thrombocytopenia. *Ann Intern Med* 1997;127:804–812, with permission.)

treatment, rule out DIC as the sole explanation for the elevated INR values (6).

Venous limb gangrene usually presents as a characteristic clinical triad (4–6): (a) an acute DVT involving the limb subsequently affected by necrosis, (b) a supratherapeutic INR, and (c) thrombocytopenia associated with a procoagulant disorder such as HIT or adenocarcinoma. Figure 115-5 summarizes the pathogenesis of warfarin-induced venous limb gangrene in relation to this clinical triad.

Typically, acral necrosis occurs in a limb with a concurrent symptomatic *acute DVT*. In the study of venous limb gangrene complicating HIT (5), this complication occurred in 10 limbs (among eight patients). Symptomatic lower limb DVT was present in all 10 limbs within the previous week; necrosis did not occur in upper or contralateral lower limbs unaffected by DVT. These observations suggest a role for large vein thrombosis in predisposing to ipsilateral involvement of small veins and venules, either by direct extension of thrombosis from large to progressively smaller veins or by venous stasis predisposing to microvascular thrombosis.

An *elevated INR* is the laboratory hallmark of this syndrome. Patients with venous limb gangrene typically have an INR that is at least 4.0 (4–7,29,31,61). The high INR is a surrogate marker for severe protein C depletion that reflects similar depletion in factor VII (6).

*Increased thrombin generation and platelet activation*, clinically manifesting as thrombocytopenia, are characteristic of coumarin-induced venous limb gangrene (5,6). Platelet activation by HIT antibodies produces a marked platelet procoagulant response, as shown by *in vitro* and *in vivo* generation of procoagulant, platelet-derived microparticles (63), leading to increased thrombin generation in patients with HIT, with the potential for impaired procoagulant–anticoagulant balance during coumarin treatment.

Table 115-3 lists reasons why physicians may not recognize the role of coumarin in contributing to venous limb gangrene (5). Clinicians should suspect oral anticoagulation as the explanation for progressive acral ischemia when an otherwise typical DVT worsens in association with a rise in the INR to above 3.5, especially if the patient has thrombocytopenia suggestive of HIT or DIC (4–6).

*Warfarin-induced digital necrosis* affecting multiple digits occurred in a patient with adenocarcinoma, HIT, and Raynaud phenomenon; the absence of DVT in three limbs affected by digital ischemia and necrosis suggested that vasospasm predisposed to this unusual presentation of multiple digital gangrene (38). Raynaud phenomenon was also a feature of warfarin-associated multiple digital necrosis in a patient with protein S deficiency (39).

## TREATMENT

Vitamin K may reverse incipient CISN or phlegmasia cerulea dolens if given in the earliest stages of the disease (5,29,64). Often, however, the diagnosis is not made until

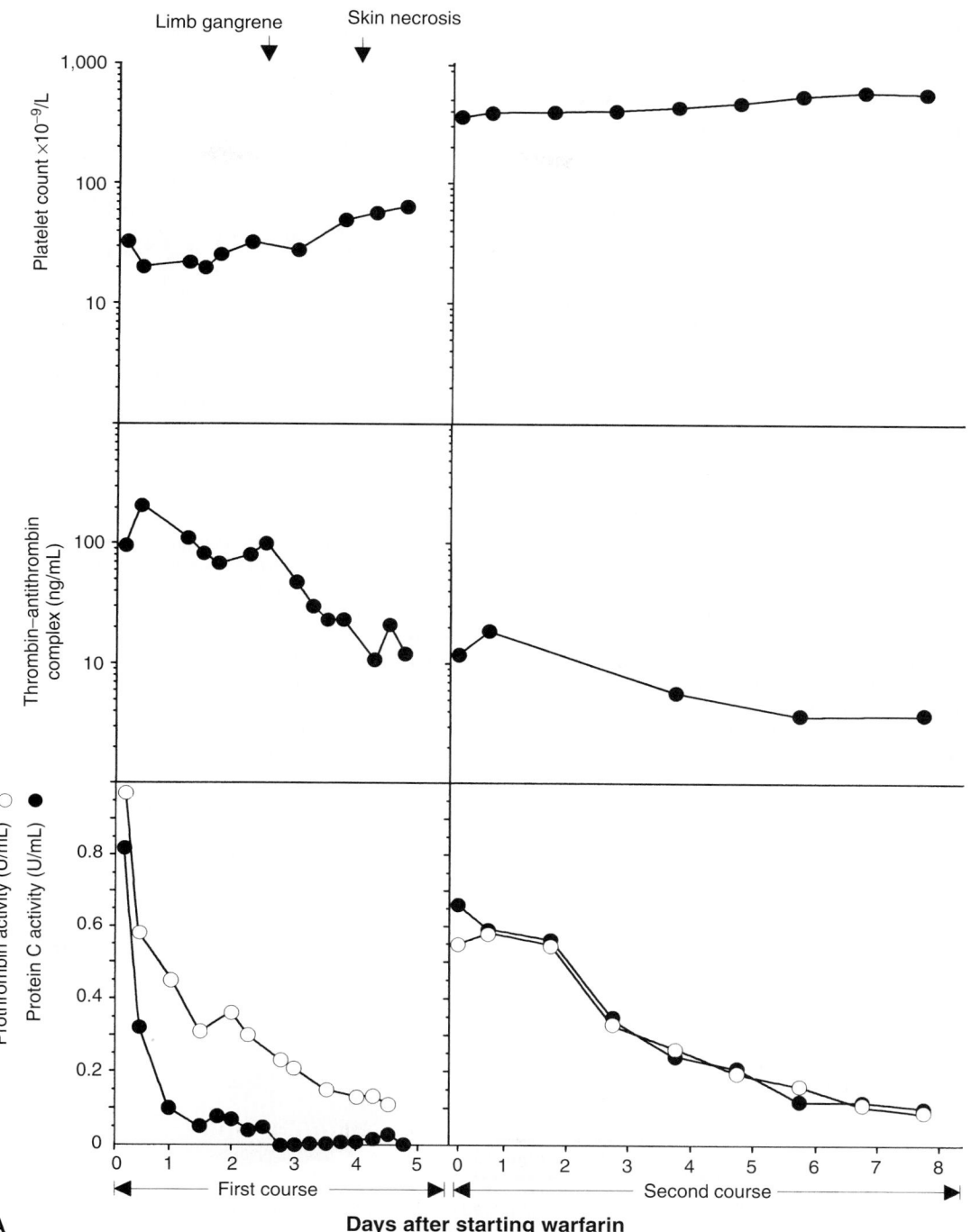

**A**    **Days after starting warfarin**

**FIGURE 115-4.** Coumarin-induced venous limb gangrene: a disturbance in procoagulant–anticoagulant balance. **A:** Hemostatic markers in relation to clinical course in patients with warfarin-induced venous limb gangrene. Venous limb gangrene and central skin necrosis occurred when warfarin was given during acute heparin-induced thrombocytopenia (HIT); the international normalized ratio (INR) rose to 7.2 at this time (first course of therapy, **left**). No adverse sequelae occurred when warfarin was given after thrombocytopenia resolved (second course of therapy, **right**). **B:** Thrombin–antithrombin complexes compared with protein C activity in patients with HIT. Each data point represents thrombin–antithrombin complexes and protein C activity per single treatment day per patient. In both panels, *open symbols* represent patients who developed venous limb gangrene (*n* = 3) or cerulea phlegmasia dolens (*n* = 1). The *diagonal line* indicates an arbitrary ratio of thrombin–antithrombin complex to protein C of 40. **Left:** Results obtained when HIT was first diagnosed and before warfarin therapy began for two patients (*open symbols*) who developed venous limb gangrene or severe venous ischemia and for eight patients (*closed circles*) who subsequently received warfarin for deep vein thrombosis (DVT) without developing venous limb gangrene. For comparison, results obtained when HIT was diagnosed in 15 patients (*closed squares*) without clinically suspected DVT who did not subsequently receive warfarin are shown. **Right:** Results in 16 patients who were receiving warfarin for HIT, including four patients (*open symbols*) who developed venous limb gangrene or phlegmasia cerulea dolens and 12 patients (*closed circles*) (nine of whom had DVT) who received warfarin without developing venous limb gangrene. More than one data points is shown for patients from whom plasma samples were available on more than 1 day of warfarin treatment. (Reprinted with permission from Warkentin TE, Elavathil LJ, Hayward CPM, et al. The pathogenesis of venous limb gangrene associated with heparin-induced thrombocytopenia. *Ann Intern Med* 1997;127:804–812.)

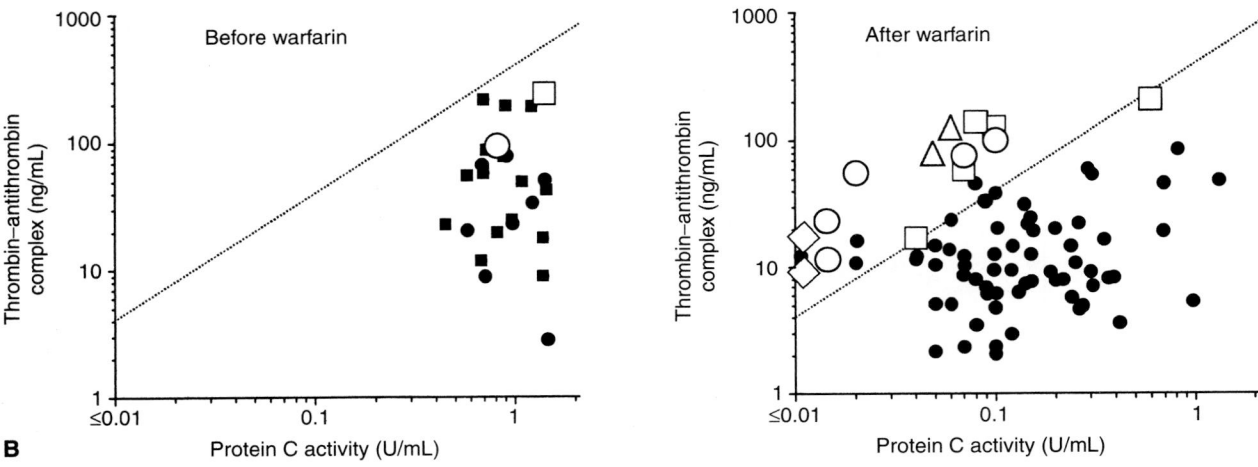

**FIGURE 115-4.** Continued.

extensive microthrombosis has occurred and necrosis is inevitable. It is not known whether vitamin K, plasma, protein C (65,66), or activated protein C concentrates, alter the natural history at this point. Amputation or skin grafting is required in about half of the patients with coumarin necrosis.

In the original report of CISN by Verhagen (1), the coumarin was usually continued despite the occurrence of tissue necrosis, and it was the author's view that tissue injury nevertheless did not progress beyond the level at which it was already clinically apparent. An alternative view is that intravenous vitamin K and

effective parenteral anticoagulation are important in avoiding progressive macrothrombosis and microthrombosis in a patient with coumarin-associated phlegmasia or venous limb gangrene complicating HIT or cancer. The reasoning is that unlike the transient disturbance of procoagulant–anticoagulant balance seen in some patients with CISN, ongoing consumption of the vitamin K–dependent factors can persist if the underlying hypercoagulability state is uncontrolled. Anticoagulation involves either heparin (or low-molecular-weight heparin) for cancer-associated DIC, or a nonheparin anticoagulant (e.g.,

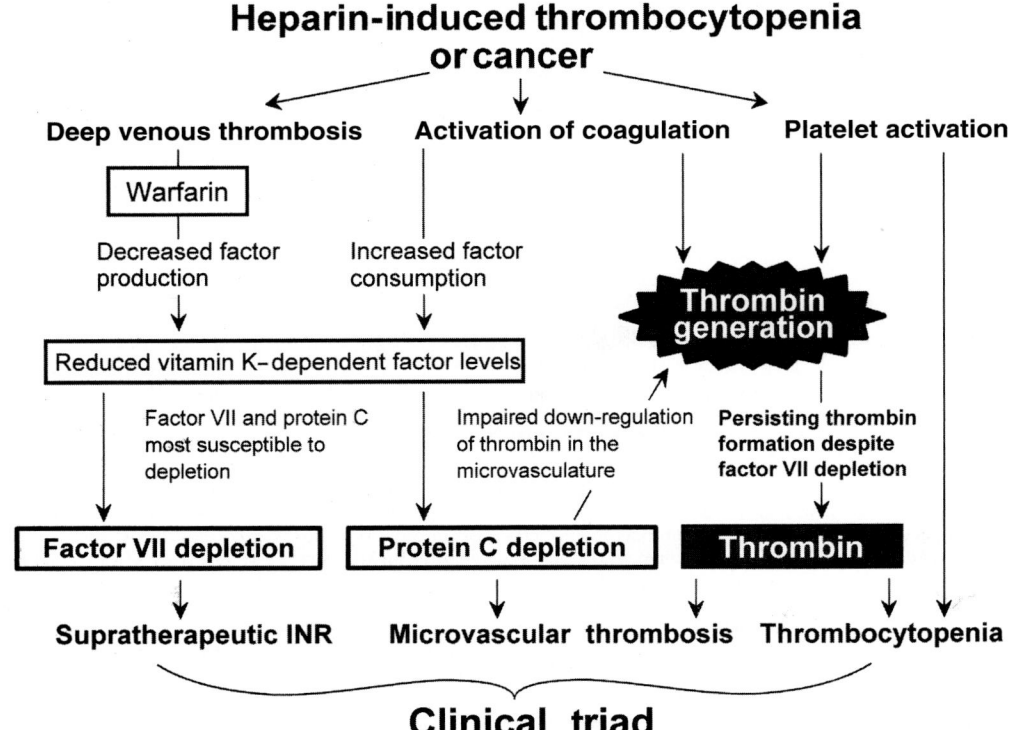

**FIGURE 115-5.** Proposed pathogenesis of coumarin-induced venous limb gangrene complicating either immune heparin-induced thrombocytopenia (HIT) or adenocarcinoma. INR, international normalized ratio. (From Warkentin TE. Venous limb gangrene during warfarin treatment of cancer-associated deep venous thrombosis. *Ann Intern Med* 2001;135:589–593, with permission.)

**TABLE 115-3**

**REASONS WHY VENOUS LIMB GANGRENE IS OFTEN NOT RECOGNIZED AS BEING CAUSED BY WARFARIN OR OTHER ORAL ANTICOAGULANTS**

1. Limb necrosis primarily blamed on associated illness alone (e.g., HIT, malignancy) rather than on warfarin
2. DVT usually precedes use of warfarin
3. Classic clinical features of CISN are usually lacking (e.g., central skin necrosis involving breast, abdomen, or thigh is usually not present)
4. Classic laboratory features of CISN are usually lacking (i.e., congenital abnormality of the protein C anticoagulant pathway usually is not found)

HIT, heparin-induced thrombocytopenia; DVT, deep vein thrombosis; CISN, coumarin-induced skin necrosis.
From WarkentinTE, Elavathil LJ, Hayward CPM, et al. The pathogenesis of venous limb gangrene associated with heparin-induced thrombocytopenia. *Ann Intern Med* 1997;127:804–812.

lepirudin, argatroban, danaparoid), if HIT is the diagnosis. A relevant issue is that ongoing vitamin K antagonism tends to prolong the activated partial thromboplastin time (aPTT), thereby complicating the monitoring of anticoagulation with heparin or a DTI (67), underscoring the importance of giving vitamin K.

## PREVENTION AND MANAGEMENT OF FURTHER ANTICOAGULATION

A cautious approach to further use of coumarin anticoagulants in acute HIT or DIC secondary to malignancy should be adopted. Warfarin should be started only in patients with acute HIT who are adequately anticoagulated with a nonheparin anticoagulant, and preferably only after the platelet count has recovered to more than $150 \times 10^9$ per L (67) (see Chapter 114). Low-molecular-weight heparin rather than warfarin should be considered for patients with cancer-associated DVT (62,68) who have laboratory evidence for DIC.

Routinely avoiding loading doses of oral anticoagulants may reduce the frequency of coumarin necrosis. A maximum of 5 mg for the first dose (even less in case of an elderly patient) is appropriate (69,70). Harrison et al. (17) performed a randomized clinical trial comparing 5 mg versus 10 mg warfarin as an initial "loading" dose for typical patients undergoing initial warfarin anticoagulation. The probability of achieving therapeutic anticoagulation (target INR, 2.0 to 3.0) at 5 days was similar in both patient groups (approximately 70%). However, the group that received the lower dose of warfarin had significantly higher levels of protein C at 36 and 60 hours after initiation of warfarin and were less likely to have early excess anticoagulation (as measured by the INR). Therefore, there is no clinical advantage to giving a relatively high initial dose of warfarin, but there is an advantage to using the lower dose (avoidance of protein C deficiency and an associated disturbance in procoagulant/anticoagulant balance) (17,71). The manufacturer of Coumadin advocates avoiding loading doses: "It is recommended that COUMADIN therapy be initiated with a dose of 2 to 5 mg per day with dosage adjustments based on the results of PT/INR determinations"

(72). An important reason to avoid loading doses of warfarin, although it is safe in most patients, is because it is unsafe in the *minority* of patients who have one or more risk factors for coumarin necrosis, the presence of which is generally unknown when warfarin is commenced (69).

For patients with a history of CISN or venous limb gangrene, it is acceptable to reintroduce oral anticoagulants with appropriate precautions (5,34,56). This is because coumarin necrosis is often related to dynamic and transient clinical and biochemical factors that may not exist later. It is prudent to start with low doses of warfarin (e.g., 1 to 2 mg per day for 3 to 4 days), gradually increasing the INR into the target range over 1 to 2 weeks. However, even higher initial doses (2 to 5 mg per day) are reported to be safe (73). Unless HIT is suspected, combined treatment with therapeutic-dose heparin is recommended (74) as thrombin inhibition theoretically reduces risk of coumarin necrosis. Plasma or protein C concentrates have been given to some patients with known congenital protein C deficiency during initiation of warfarin. The risk of recurrence of necrosis despite using any of these precautions is unknown, but likely is low.

## COUMARIN-ASSOCIATED "PURPLE TOE" AND CHOLESTEROL EMBOLISM SYNDROMES

Use of oral anticoagulants may contribute to the development of "purple" or "blue" toes in patients with severe atherosclerosis. This syndrome was first described by Feder and Auerbach (75), who reported six patients who developed blue-purple discoloration of the feet, especially the plantar surfaces and sides of the first two toes, that began 3 to 8 weeks after starting a coumarin. Other clinical features included pain and tenderness of the toes, blanching on moderate pressure, and persistence of these features despite stopping oral anticoagulation. Because these patients were male with peripheral vascular disease, it was suggested that "purple toe syndrome" could be explained by cholesterol microembolization (76,77), a concept that is gaining acceptance (78). However, some patients do not have other clinical features of cholesterol embolism syndrome.

Classically, cholesterol (or atheromatous) embolism syndrome is characterized by a variety of peripheral ischemic signs (livedo reticularis, "blue" toes, focal digital necrosis); renal failure may also occur (77,79,80). Pedal pulses are usually palpable, consistent with the histopathologic findings of biconvex clefts in small arteries and arterioles indicative of preceding microembolism of cholesterol crystals. Although advanced atherosclerosis is conspicuous, there is often a history of recent vascular injury (e.g., cardiac surgery, arteriography) (77) or of disruption of adherent thrombus (e.g., postthrombolytic therapy) (81).

Only about 20% to 50% of patients who are clinically diagnosed with cholesterol embolism syndrome are receiving anticoagulants (82,83). Theoretically, coumarins could cause or exacerbate this syndrome by contributing to a gradual loss over weeks of a protective fibrin layer overlying an ulcerated atherosclerotic plaque, facilitating cholesterol microembolization (84). Fibrin dissolution could also explain the occurrence of this syndrome following thrombolysis (81). However, any causal role for coumarin or other anticoagulants is speculative. Therefore, the physician must balance the risks of stopping warfarin with the uncertain potential for improvement. Although resolution of cholesterol embolism syndrome might seem improbable, there are well-documented reports of clinical improvement after stopping warfarin (80).

# MISCELLANEOUS CUTANEOUS EFFECTS OF ORAL ANTICOAGULANTS

In addition to ecchymotic purpura related to the anticoagulant effects of warfarin and other oral anticoagulants, a few patients may develop macular, papular, vesicular, or urticarial lesions, presumably of an allergic origin (85,86). Alopecia of varying severity in relation to oral anticoagulation has also been described. Use of a different oral anticoagulant agent may permit further anticoagulation with resolution of these adverse effects.

Calcific uremic arteriopathy (or arteriolopathy), also known as *calciphylaxis*, occurs in patients with severe chronic renal failure and is characterized by livedo reticularis and multicentric skin necrosis associated with microvascular thrombosis resembling that seen in coumarin necrosis (87,88). Mehta et al. (87) observed reduced protein C activity in patients with this disorder. Some patients develop this complication while receiving warfarin and may benefit from substituting oral anticoagulation by low-molecular-weight heparin (88).

## *References*

1. Verhagen H. Local haemorrhage and necrosis of the skin and underlying tissues, during anti-coagulant therapy with dicumarol or dicumacyl. *Acta Med Scand* 1954;148:453–462.
2. Hirsh J. Oral anticoagulant drugs. *N Engl J Med* 1991;324:1865–1875.
3. Comp PC. Coumarin-induced skin necrosis. Incidence, mechanisms, management and avoidance. *Drug Saf* 1993;8:128–135.
4. Warkentin TE. Heparin-induced thrombocytopenia: IgG-mediated platelet activation, platelet microparticle generation, and altered procoagulant/anticoagulant balance in the pathogenesis of thrombosis and venous limb gangrene complicating heparin-induced thrombocytopenia. *Transfus Med Rev* 1996;10:249–258.
5. Warkentin TE, Elavathil LJ, Hayward CPM, et al. The pathogenesis of venous limb gangrene associated with heparin-induced thrombocytopenia. *Ann Intern Med* 1997;127:804–812.
6. Warkentin TE. Venous limb gangrene during warfarin treatment of cancer-associated deep venous thrombosis. *Ann Intern Med* 2001;135:589–593.
7. Klein L, Galvez A, Klein O, et al. Warfarin-induced venous gangrene in the setting of lung adenocarcinoma. *Am J Hematol* 2004;76:176–179.
8. Marshall ME, Butler K, Metcalfe M, et al. Coumarin necrosis or Coumadin necrosis? [letter]. *Surgery* 1989;105:237–238.
9. Nalbandian RM, Mader IJ, Barrett JL, et al. Petechiae, ecchymoses, and necrosis of skin induced by coumarin congeners. *JAMA* 1965;192:603–608.
10. Ellbrück D, Wankmüller H, Rasche H, et al. Klinischer verlauf bei cumarinnekrose. *Dtsch Med Wochenschr* 1991;116:1307–1312.
11. Li T, Chang CY, Jin DY, et al. Identification of the gene for vitamin K epoxide reductase. *Nature* 2004;427:541–544.
12. Stirling Y. Warfarin-induced changes in procoagulant and anticoagulant proteins. *Blood Coagul Fibrinolysis* 1995;6:361–373.
13. Horn JR, Danziger LH, Davis RJ. Warfarin-induced skin necrosis: report of four cases. *Am J Hosp Pharm* 1981;38:1763–1768.
14. Cole MS, Minifee PK, Wolma FJ. Coumarin necrosis-a review of the literature. *Surgery* 1988;103:271–277.
15. Comp PC, Elrod JP, Karzenski S. Warfarin-induced skin necrosis. *Semin Thromb Hemost* 1990;16:293–298.
16. Eby CS. Warfarin-induced skin necrosis. *Hematol/Oncol Clin N Am* 1993;7:1291–1300.
17. Harrison L, Johnston M, Massicotte MP, et al. Comparison of 5-mg and 10-mg loading doses in initiation of warfarin therapy. *Ann Intern Med* 1997;126:133–136.
18. Vigano-D'Angelo S, Comp PC, Esmon CT, et al. Relationship between protein C antigen and anticoagulant activity during oral anticoagulation and in selected disease states. *J Clin Invest* 1986;77:416–425.
19. Esmon CT. Protein C anticoagulant pathway and its role in controlling microvascular thrombosis and inflammation. *Crit Care Med* 2001;29(Suppl. 7):S48–S51.
20. Marciniak E, Wilson HD, Marlar RA. Neonatal purpura fulminans: a genetic disorder related to the absence of protein C in blood. *Blood* 1985;65:15–20.
21. Smith OP, White B. Infectious purpura fulminans: diagnosis and treatment. *Br J Haematol* 1999;104:202–207.
22. Zenz W, Muntean W. Cutaneous necrosis associated with acquired severe protein S deficiency [letter]. *Thromb Haemost* 1994;71:396.
23. Combemale P, Amiral J, Estival JL, et al. Cutaneous necrosis revealing the coexistence of an antiphospholipid syndrome with acquired protein S deficiency, factor V Leiden and hyperhomocysteinemia. *Eur J Dermatol* 2002;12:278–282.
24. Cariou R, Tobelem G, Belluci S, et al. Effect of lupus anticoagulant on antithrombogenic properties of endothelial cells–inhibition of thrombomodulin-dependent protein C activation. *Thromb Haemost* 1988;60:54–58.
25. Malia RG, Kitchen S, Greaves M, et al. Inhibition of activated protein C and its cofactor protein S by antiphospholipid antibody. *Br J Haematol* 1990;76:101–107.
26. Warkentin TE, Sikov WM, Lillicrap DP. Multicentric warfarin-induced skin necrosis complicating heparin-induced thrombocytopenia. *Am J Hematol* 1999;62:44–48.
27. Essex DW, Wynn SS, Jin DK. Late-onset warfarin-induced skin necrosis: case report and review of the literature. *Am J Hematol* 1998;57:233–237.
28. Scarff CE, Baker C, Hill P, et al. Late-onset warfarin necrosis. *Australas J Dermatol* 2002;45:202–206.
29. Srinivasan AF, Rice L, Bartholomew JR, et al. Warfarin-induced skin necrosis and venous limb gangrene in the setting of heparin-induced thrombocytopenia. *Arch Intern Med* 2004;164:66–70.
30. Sallah S, Abdallah JM, Gagnon GA. Recurrent warfarin-induced skin necrosis in kindreds with protein S deficiency. *Haemostasis* 1998;28:25–30.
31. Everett RN, Jones FL Jr. Warfarin-induced skin necrosis. A cutaneous sign of malignancy? *Postgrad Med* 1986;79:97–103.
32. Byrne JS, Abdul Razak AR, Patchett S, et al. Warfarin skin necrosis associated with protein S deficiency and a mutation in the methylenetetrahydrofolate reductase gene. *Clin Exp Dermatol* 2004;29:35–36.
33. Ng T, Tillyer ML. Warfarin-induced skin necrosis associated with factor V Leiden and protein S deficiency. *Clin Lab Haematol* 2001;23:261–264.
34. Stewart AJ, Penman ID, Cook MK, et al. Warfarin-induced skin necrosis. *Postgrad Med J* 1999;75:233–235.
35. Cheng A, Scheinfeld NS, McDowell B, et al. Warfarin skin necrosis in a postpartum woman with protein S deficiency. *Obstet Gynecol* 1997;90:671–672.
36. Gailani D, Reese EP Jr. Anticoagulant-induced skin necrosis in a patient with hereditary deficiency of protein S. *Am J Hematol* 1999;60:231–236.
37. Zimbelman J, Lefkowitz J, Schaeffer C, et al. Unusual complications of warfarin therapy: skin necrosis and priapism. *J Pediatr* 2000;137:266–268.
38. Warkentin TE, Whitlock RP, Teoh KHT. Warfarin-associated multiple digital necrosis complicating heparin-induced thrombocytopenia and Raynaud's phenomenon after aortic valve replacement for adenocarcinoma-associated thrombotic endocarditis. *Am J Hematol* 2004;75:56–62.
39. Piccoli GB, Quaglia M, Quaglino P, et al. Acute digital gangrene in a long-term dialysis patient–a diagnostic challenge. *Med Sci Monit* 2002;8:CS83–CS89.
40. Wynn SS, Jin DK, Essex DW. Warfarin-induced skin necrosis occurring four days after discontinuation of warfarin. *Haemostasis* 1997;27:246–250.
41. Cameron A, van Berkel W, Sixma J. Skin necrosis after three years of treatment with acenocoumarin. *Ned Tijdschr Geneeskd* 1974;118:505–507.
42. Visser LE, Penning-van Beest FJA, Kasbergen AAH, et al. Overanticoagulation associated with combined use of antibacterial drugs and acenocoumarol or phenprocoumon anticoagulants. *Thromb Haemost* 2002;88:705–710.
43. Teepe R, Broekmans A, Vermeer B, et al. Recurrent coumarin-induced skin necrosis in a patient with an acquired functional protein C deficiency. *Arch Dermatol* 1986;122:1408–1412.
44. Hofmann V, Frick PG. Repeated occurrence of skin necrosis twice following coumarin intake and subsequently during decrease of vitamin K dependent coagulation factors associated with cholestasis. *Thromb Haemost* 1982;48:245–246.
45. Humphries JE, Gardner JH, Connelly JE. Warfarin skin necrosis: recurrence in the absence of anticoagulant therapy. *Am J Hematol* 1991;37:197–200.
46. Ad-El DD, Meirovitz A, Weinberg A, et al. Warfarin skin necrosis: local and systemic factors. *Br J Plast Surg* 2000;53:624–626.
47. Smythe MA, Warkentin TE, Stephens JL, et al. Venous limb gangrene during overlapping therapy with warfarin and a direct thrombin inhibitor for immune heparin-induced thrombocytopenia. *Am J Hematol* 2002;71:50–52.
48. Takahashi H, Echizen H. Pharmacogenetics of warfarin elimination and its clinical implications. *Clin Pharmacokinet* 2001;40:587–603.
49. Shikata E, Ieiri I, Ishiguro S, et al. Association of pharmacokinetic (CYP2C9) and pharmacodynamic (*factors* II, VII, IX, and X; *proteins* S and C; and *γ-glutamyl carboxylase*) gene variants with warfarin sensitivity. *Blood* 2004;103:2630–2635.
50. Broekmans AW, Bertina RM, Loeliger EA, et al. Protein C and the development of skin necrosis during anticoagulant therapy [letter]. *Thromb Haemost* 1983;49:251.
51. Rose VL, Kwaan HC, Williamson K, et al. Protein C antigen deficiency and warfarin necrosis. *Am J Clin Pathol* 1986;86:653–655.
52. Conlan MG, Bridges A, Williams E, et al. Familial type II protein C deficiency associated with warfarin-induced skin necrosis and bilateral adrenal hemorrhage. *Am J Hematol* 1988;29:226–229.
53. Anderson DR, Brill-Edwards P, Walker I. Warfarin-induced skin necrosis in 2 patients with protein S deficiency: successful reinstatement of warfarin therapy. *Haemostasis* 1992;22:124–128.
54. Freeman B, Schmieg RE Jr, McGrath S, et al. Factor V Leiden in a patient with warfarin-associated skin necrosis. *Surgery* 2000;127:595–596.

55. Makris M, Bardhan G, Preston FE. Warfarin induced skin necrosis associated with activated protein C resistance [letter]. *Thromb Haemost* 1995; 75:523–524.

56. Kiehl R, Hellstern P, Wenzel E. Hereditary antithrombin III (AT III) deficiency and atypical localization of a coumarin necrosis [letter]. *Thromb Res* 1987;45:191–193.

57. Colman RW, Rao AK, Rubin RN. Warfarin skin necrosis in a 33-year-old woman. *Am J Hematol* 1993;43:300–303.

58. Yang Y, Algazy KM. Warfarin-induced skin necrosis in a patient with a mutation of the prothrombin gene [letter]. *N Engl J Med* 1999;340:735.

59. Celoria GM, Steingart RH, Banson B, et al. Coumarin skin necrosis in a patient with heparin-induced thrombocytopenia–a case report. *Angiology* 1988;39:915–920.

60. Cohen DJ, Briggs R, Head HD, et al. Phlegmasia cerulea dolens and its association with hypercoagulable states: case reports. *Angiology* 1989;40:498–508.

61. Campbell R, Clanton TO, Heckman JD. Necrosis and gangrene as a complication of coumarin therapy. *J Bone Joint Surg* 1980;62A:1016–1017.

62. Warkentin TE. Pseudo-heparin-induced thrombocytopenia. In: Warkentin TE, Greinacher A, eds. *Heparin-induced Thrombocytopenia*, 3rd ed. New York: Marcel Dekker Inc, 2004:313–334.

63. Warkentin TE, Hayward CPM, Boshkov LK, et al. Sera from patients with heparin-induced thrombocytopenia generate platelet-derived microparticles with procoagulant activity: an explanation for the thrombotic complications of heparin-induced thrombocytopenia. *Blood* 1994;84:3691–3699.

64. Van Amstel WJ, Boekhout-Mussert MJ, Loeliger EA. Successful prevention of Coumarin-induced hemorrhagic skin necrosis by timely administration of vitamin K$_1$. *Blut* 1978;36:89–93.

65. Schramm W, Spannagl M, Bauer KA, et al. Treatment of coumarin-induced skin necrosis with a monoclonal antibody purified protein C concentrate. *Arch Dermatol* 1993;129:753–756.

66. Gatti L, Carnelli V, Rusconi R, et al. Heparin-induced thrombocytopenia and warfarin-induced skin necrosis in a child with severe protein C deficiency: successful treatment with dermatan sulfate and protein C concentrate. *J Thromb Haemost* 2003;1:387–388.

67. Warkentin TE, Greinacher A. Heparin-induced thrombocytopenia: recognition, treatment, and prevention. The Seventh ACCP Conference on Antithrombic and Thrombolytic Therapy. *Chest* 2004;126(Suppl. 3):311S–337S.

68. Lee AY, Levine MN, Baker RI, et al. Randomized comparison of low-molecular-weight heparin versus oral anticoagulant therapy for the prevention of recurrent venous thromboembolism in patients with cancer (CLOT) investigators. *N Engl J Med* 2003;349:146–153.

69. Warkentin TE. Randomized trial of warfarin nomograms [letter]. *Ann Intern Med* 2004;140:490–491.

70. Gage BF, Fihn SD, White RH. Management and dosing of warfarin therapy. *Am J Med* 2000;109:481–488.

71. Crowther MA, Ginsberg JB, Kearon C, et al. A randomized trial comparing 5-mg and 10-mg warfarin loading doses. *Arch Intern Med* 1999;159:46–48.

72. Coumadin® *Physicians' Desk Reference*, 56th ed. Montvale, NJ: Thompson PDR. 2002:1247.

73. Jillella AP, Lutcher CL. Reinstituting warfarin in patients who develop warfarin skin necrosis. *Am J Hematol* 1996;52:117–119.

74. Zauber NP, Stark MW. Successful warfarin anticoagulation despite protein C deficiency and a history of warfarin necrosis. *Ann Intern Med* 1986;104:659–660.

75. Feder W, Auerbach R. "Purple toes": an uncommon sequela of oral coumarin drug therapy. *Ann Intern Med* 1961;55:911–917.

76. Hyman BT, Landas SK, Ashman RF, et al. Warfarin-related purple toes syndrome and cholesterol microembolization. *Am J Med* 1987;82:1233–1237.

77. Colt HG, Begg RJ, Saporito JJ, et al. Cholesterol emboli after cardiac catheterization. Eight cases and a review of the literature. *Medicine* 1988;67:389–400.

78. Sallah S, Thomas DP, Roberts HR. Warfarin and heparin-induced skin necrosis and the purple toe syndrome: infrequent complications of anticoagulant treatment. *Thromb Haemost* 1997;78:785–790.

79. Moldveen-Geronimus M, Merriam JC Jr. Cholesterol embolization. From pathological curiosity to clinical entity. *Circulation* 1967;35:946–953.

80. Bruns FJ, Segel DP, Adler S. Control of cholesterol embolization by discontinuation of anticoagulant therapy. *Am J Med Sci* 1978;275:105–108.

81. Geraets DR, Hoehns JD, Burke TG, et al. Thrombolytic-associated cholesterol emboli syndrome: case report and literature review. *Pharmaotherapy* 1995;15:441–450.

82. Dahlberg PJ, Frecentese DF, Cogbill TH. Cholesterol embolism: experience with 22 histologically proven cases. *Surgery* 1989;105:737–746.

83. Fine MJ, Kapoor W, Falanga V. Cholesterol crystal embolization: a review of 221 cases in the English literature. *Angiology* 1987;38:769–784.

84. Bols A, Nevelsteen A, Verhaughe R. Atheromatous embolization precipitated by oral anticoagulants. *Int Angiol* 1994;13:271–273.

85. Kwong P, Roberts P, Prescott SM, et al. Dermatitis induced by warfarin. *JAMA* 1978;239:1884–1885.

86. Gallerani M, Manfredini R, Moratelli S. Non-hemorrhagic adverse reactions of oral anticoagulant therapy. *Int J Cardiol* 1995;49:1–7.

87. Mehta RL, Scott G, Sloand JA, et al. Skin necrosis associated with acquired protein C deficiency in patients with renal failure and calciphylaxis. *Am J Med* 1990;88:252–257.

88. Coates T, Kirkland GS, Dymock RB, et al. Cutaneous necrosis from calcific uremic arteriolopathy. *Am J Kidney Dis* 1998;32:384–391.

# CHAPTER 116 ■ ANTICOAGULANT THERAPY FOR MAJOR ARTERIAL AND VENOUS THROMBOEMBOLISM

HUYEN A. M. TRAN AND JEFFREY S. GINSBERG

Arterial and venous thromboembolism are common causes of morbidity and mortality in the world. The former includes emboli associated with atrial fibrillation (AF), prosthetic heart valves, other valvular heart disease and cardiomyopathies, as well as acute coronary syndromes (ACS), stroke, and peripheral vascular disease. The latter includes deep vein thrombosis (DVT) and pulmonary embolism (PE). Treatment of affected patients with anticoagulants has the potential to be beneficial, both in preventing thrombus growth and in reducing the risk of recurrent thromboembolism. However, all antithrombotic agents have the potential to cause bleeding, and individual agents have the potential to cause adverse effects that are drug or "drug-class" specific. In this chapter, the pharmacology and clinical application of anticoagulant drugs available for treatment of major arterial and venous thrombosis, including novel agents currently being developed, are reviewed.

## HEPARINS AND HEPARINOIDS

### Unfractionated Heparin

Although low-molecular-weight heparin (LMWH) therapy has replaced unfractionated heparin (UFH) for many indications, it is still relevant to highlight key studies of UFH that have elucidated concepts about the management of arterial and venous thrombosis. UFH is effective and is indicated for the prevention of venous thromboembolism (VTE); treatment of DVT, PE, and ACS; patients undergoing cardiac surgery using cardiac bypass, vascular surgery, or coronary angioplasty; and patients with coronary stents.

#### Pharmacology

Heparin is a heterogeneous group of molecules, which vary in molecular weight, anticoagulant activity, and pharmacokinetic properties. It is derived from porcine intestine and bovine lung (1). UFH has a mean molecular weight of 15,000 Da (range of 3,000 to 30,000 Da). Its anticoagulant activity varies because only approximately one third of heparin molecules contain the high-affinity pentasaccharide required for anticoagulant function (2). UFH binds to heparin-neutralizing proteins, and its clearance is influenced by the chain length of the molecules; the higher molecular weight species are cleared from the circulation more rapidly than the lower molecular weight species.

The anticoagulant effect of heparin is mediated through binding of pentasaccharide-containing molecules to antithrombin (AT), facilitating the inactivation of thrombin (factor IIa) and factors Xa, IXa, and XIIa. By inactivating thrombin, heparin not only prevents fibrin formation but also inhibits thrombin-catalyzed activation of factors V and VIII (3). At greater concentrations than those that are usually used clinically, UFH binds to heparin cofactor II, catalyzing its inactivation of thrombin. UFH also inhibits thrombin-related platelet function, contributing to its hemorrhagic potential.

Heparin clearance involves a combination of a rapid saturable and a much slower first-order mechanism. The mechanism of the saturable phase of heparin clearance is through binding to receptors on endothelial cells and macrophages, where it is depolymerized, while the slower nonsaturable mechanism is through the kidneys. When therapeutic doses are given, heparin is cleared predominantly through the rapid, saturable dose-dependent mechanism, and its anticoagulant effects are nonlinear with both the intensity and the duration of the effect rising disproportionately with increasing dose. With therapeutic intravenous doses of heparin, the half-life of UFH is approximately 60 minutes.

UFH should be administered parenterally, usually intravenously as a bolus dose followed by a continuous infusion. Provided sufficient starting doses are used ($\geq$30,000 U per day) and therapeutic activated partial thromboplastin time (aPTT) results are quickly achieved (within 48 hours), subcutaneous UFH administration is also effective (4). Although effective, intermittent intravenous heparin causes excessive bleeding (5). The efficacy of continuous intravenous heparin therapy depends on the starting dose; after an initial bolus dose of 5,000 U, at least 30,000 U per day should be infused because lower doses result in higher recurrence rates (6,7). The infusion should be adjusted to a therapeutic range using laboratory tests because heparin has a narrow therapeutic window and patients vary in their responsiveness to it; some of the variability results from different plasma concentrations of heparin-binding proteins, including histidine-rich glycoprotein, platelet factor 4, vitronectin, fibronectin, and von Willebrand factor (8). These proteins bind to and neutralize heparin. In addition, high levels of factor VIII can cause a "falsely" subtherapeutic aPTT response; the elevated factor VIII levels "pull down" the aPTT relative to the heparin level, resulting in falsely low aPTT results.

#### Monitoring

Heparin should be monitored by measurement of the aPTT or heparin concentration, the latter measured using protamine sulfate (PS) titration assays or anti–factor Xa chromogenic assays. Plasma heparin concentrations of 0.2 to 0.4 U per mL by PS titration are equivalent to concentrations of 0.35 to 0.70 U per mL by anti–factor Xa assays, both corresponding to the therapeutic range (9). An aPTT ratio of 1.5 to 2.5 times control is recommended as a target therapeutic range for heparin. The lower limit derives partly from results of a cohort study in which the recurrence rate was increased in UFH-treated patients with acute VTE whose aPTT results were below 1.5 times control (9,10). However, different aPTT reagents with ratios of 1.5 to 2.5 times control reflect different plasma heparin concentrations (11). Further, aPTT values 1.5 times control consistently correspond to subtherapeutic heparin concentrations (11). To address this problem, the aPTT values equivalent to plasma heparin concentrations of 0.2 to 0.4 U per ml by protamine titration (or 0.35 to 0.70 anti–factor Xa units) should be established for each reagent.

Patients receiving intravenous heparin who have subtherapeutic aPTT values in the first 24 hours could have increased (15-fold) recurrence rates (9). However, two overviews of clinical trials evaluating UFH regimens in patients with VTE in whom the starting infusion rates were over 30,000 U per day showed that the risk of recurrence was not significantly higher when the aPTT results were subtherapeutic in the first 24 to 48 hours than when they were not (12,13). Nevertheless,

achieving therapeutic aPTT results quickly is desirable because continual subtherapeutic results almost certainly increase recurrence risk.

When initiating intravenous heparin, one of three approaches that simplify heparin administration by standardizing starting doses and using nomograms for dose adjustment should be used (see Table 116-1) (7,14,15).

## Heparin Resistance

Most patients with heparin resistance (arbitrarily defined as requirement of over 40,000 U per day) have increased plasma concentrations of both factor VIII and heparin-binding proteins (16). Increased factor VIII concentrations, often elevated in sick patients, cause dissociation between aPTT and plasma heparin values, whereby the former are subtherapeutic and the latter therapeutic. Monitoring heparin-resistant patients with anti–factor Xa heparin assays (target range 0.35 to 0.70 U per mL) results in less dose escalation than monitoring with the aPTT (16) and is therefore recommended. LMWHs bind less to heparin-binding proteins, thereby obviating heparin resistance.

## TABLE 116-1

### THREE PUBLISHED HEPARIN DOSING SCHEMES

**A: Weight-based nomogram[a]; the initial dose was an 80 U/kg bolus followed by a starting infusion rate of 18 U/kg/h; aPTTs were performed every 6 hours and the heparin dose adjusted as follows:**

| | |
|---|---|
| aPTT <35 s (<1.2 × control) | 80 U/kg bolus, then increase infusion by 4U/kg/h |
| aPTT 35 to 45 s (1.2 to 1.5 × control) | 40U/kg bolus, then increase infusion by 2U/kg/h |
| aPTT 46 to 70 s (1.5 to 2.3 × control) | No change |
| aPTT 71 to 90 s (2.3 to 3 × control) | Decrease infusion rate by 2U/kg/h |
| aPTT >90 s (>3 × control) | Hold infusion 1 h, then decrease infusion rate by 3U/kg/h |

**B: Starting dose of 5,000 U bolus followed by 1,280 U/h (14)[b]**

| aPTT | Bolus (U) | Hold (min) | Rate change (mL/h)[c] | Repeat aPTT |
|---|---|---|---|---|
| <50[d] | 5,000 | 0 | +3 | In 6 h |
| 50–59 | 0 | 0 | +3 | In 6 h |
| 60–85 | 0 | 0 | 0 | Next morning |
| 86–95 | 0 | 0 | −2 | Next morning |
| 96–120 | 0 | 30 | −2 | In 6 h |
| >120 | 0 | 60 | −4 | In 6 h |

**C: Intravenous heparin dose-titration; nomogram for aPTT—starting dose = 5,000 U bolus followed by 40,000 U/24 h (low bleeding risk) or 30,000 U/24 h (high bleeding risk) (15)[e] IV infusion**

| aPTTs | Rate change (mL/h) | Dose change (U/24 h)[g] | Additional action |
|---|---|---|---|
| <45 | +6 | +5,760 | Repeat aPTT in 4 to 6 h |
| 46 to 54 | +3 | +2,880 | Repeat aPTT in 4 to 6 h |
| 55 to 85 | 0 | 0 | None[f] |
| 8 to 110 | −3 | −2,880 | Stop heparin for 1 h; repeat aPTT 4 to 6 h after restarting heparin treatment |
| >110 | −6 | −5760 | Stop heparin for 1 h; repeat aPTT 4 to 6 h after restarting heparin treatment |

aPTT, activated partial thromboplastin time; IV, intravenous.
[a]From Raschke RA, Reilly BM, Guidry JR, et al. The weight-based heparin dosing nomogram compared with a "standard care" nomogram. A randomized controlled trial. *Ann Intern Med* 1993;119(9):874–881, with permission.
[b]From Cruickshank MK, Levine MN, Hirsh J, et al. A standard heparin nomogram for the management of heparin therapy. *Arch Intern Med* 1991;151(2):333–337, with permission.
[c]mL/h = 40 U/h.
[d]If the aPTT was subtherapeutic despite a heparin dose of 1,440 U/h (36 mL/h) or greater at any time during the first 48 hours of therapy, the response to an aPTT of less than 50 seconds was a heparin bolus of 5,000 U and a rate increase of 5 mL/h.
[e]From Hull RD, Raskob GE, Rosenbloom D, et al. Optimal therapeutic level of heparin therapy in patients with venous thrombosis. *Arch Intern Med* 1992;152(8):1589–1595, with permission.
[f]During the first 24 hours, repeated aPTT in 4 to 6 hours. Thereafter, the aPTT will be determined once daily, unless therapeutic.
[g]Heparin sodium concentration, 20,000 U in 500 mL = 40 U/mL.

## Low-Molecular-Weight Heparin

LMWHs are effective and indicated for the prevention of TE, treatment of acute DVT and PE, and early treatment of non–ST segment elevation myocardial infarction. Long-term outpatient treatment with LMWH is used when anticoagulant therapy is indicated in pregnancy, in patients with VTE and cancer, and in patients who develop recurrent VTE while being treated with appropriate doses of oral anticoagulants.

### Pharmacology

LMWHs are derived from heparin by enzymatic (e.g., tinzaparin) or chemical (e.g., dalteparin and enoxaparin) depolymerization of UFH. They have a mean molecular weight of 4,500 to 5,000 Da (range of 1,000 to 10,000 Da), one third the size of UFH. The pharmacokinetic, anticoagulant, and biological differences between UFH and LMWH can be partly explained by lack of interaction of LMWH with acute-phase proteins in blood. Like UFH, LMWHs facilitate AT's anticoagulant effect (17). Compared to UFH, LMWH has reduced anti–factor IIa activity because the smaller fragments do not bind simultaneously with AT and thrombin to form ternary complexes. However, because bridging between AT and factor Xa is not crucial for anti–factor Xa activity, the smaller fragments inactivate factor Xa, as well as do larger molecules. LMWH is cleared principally by the renal route, and its biological half-life is prolonged in patients with renal failure (18,19).

LMWHs have several advantages over UFH, most importantly regarding their superior pharmacokinetic profile. Their half-lives are longer, and the antithrombotic dose-responses are more predictable, allowing administration in fixed doses without need for laboratory monitoring. In experimental animals, they cause less bleeding with equivalent antithrombotic effect than UFH (20,21), although this has not been borne out in human studies. They also cause less heparin-induced thrombocytopenia (HIT) and osteoporosis than UFH (22,23). LMWHs administered once or twice daily subcutaneously are at least as effective and safe as UFH for initial treatment of venous thrombosis (19,24). A metaanalysis of trials involving over 3,000 patients reported a risk reduction for recurrent VTE of about 15% in favor of LMWH and a risk reduction in major bleeding of about 40% (P = 0.05) also in favor of LMWH (25,26). Similar studies comparing the efficacy and safety of twice-daily dosing regimens of LMWH with UFH in patients with unstable angina show beneficial short-term results (27,28).

### Monitoring of Low-Molecular-Weight Heparin in Patients with Renal Failure, Obesity, and Pregnancy

Monitoring of LMWH therapy is usually unnecessary. However, in certain clinical situations, such as obesity, renal failure, and pregnancy, the optimum dose of LMWH can be difficult to determine. In pregnant subjects, for example, the half-life of LMWH might be different compared with nonpregnant subjects because of increased volume of distribution and increased renal blood flow, which may lead to increased clearance of LMWH. These physiologic changes are dynamic throughout pregnancy, and the pharmacokinetics might be trimester-specific. Pharmacokinetic studies and all randomized trials of LMWH have excluded pregnant patients, morbidly obese patients (>130 kg), and patients with renal failure (or failed to specify whether such patients were recruited). When LMWH is administered to these patients in therapeutic doses, it is prudent to monitor the anti–factor Xa levels periodically to guide dosing.

The chromogenic anti–factor Xa assay is the most widely available and frequently used assay for LMWH monitoring.

Although the anti–factor Xa level was inversely related to thrombus propagation in some studies (29,30), the minimal therapeutic level has not been accurately defined. Conversely, high anti–factor Xa levels at steady state in patients receiving therapeutic doses of LMWH have been associated with bleeding in some studies (31,32). The usual time to measure the anti–factor Xa levels (if indicated) is 4 hours after subcutaneous injection of a weight-adjusted dose of LMWH. For twice-daily regimens, the current recommended therapeutic range is 0.5 to 1.0 IU per mL (33,34). In patients treated with LMWH once daily, the target range at 4 hours is less clear, but 1.0 to 2.0 IU per mL is reasonable (34).

### Reversal of Anticoagulant Effect of Heparin

PS, a cationic protein derived from salmon sperm, can rapidly neutralize the anticoagulant effect of UFH. PS binds strongly to (anionic) heparin in a ratio of approximately 100 U UFH per milligram; 50 mg is needed to counteract the anticoagulant effect of 5,000 U of heparin given immediately as an intravenous bolus. When infused, only the heparin given during the preceding several hours should be included in the dose calculation because the half-life of heparin is approximately 60 minutes. About 30 mg of PS is needed in a patient receiving an infusion of 1,250 U per hour. A prolonged infusion or repeated injections of PS may be needed to neutralize a subcutaneous dose of heparin because plasma recovery of heparin following subcutaneous administration can be variable. A fall in aPTT can be used to confirm heparin neutralization. PS should be administered over 1 to 3 minutes to reduce the risk of severe adverse reactions, such as hypotension and bradycardia. Allergic reactions including anaphylaxis are associated with hypersensitivity to fish and previous exposure to PS-containing insulin. PS neutralizes the AT activity of LMWH but incompletely neutralizes the anti–factor Xa activity (35–37). The clinical impact of incomplete anti–factor Xa neutralization by protamine is unclear, and there have been no published studies demonstrating a beneficial effect of PS in bleeding patients who have been treated with LMWH.

### Heparin-Induced Thrombocytopenia

HIT is an adverse reaction to heparin, which results in a transient hypercoagulable state and can cause venous and arterial thrombosis (see Chapter 114). The clinicopathologic syndrome of HIT is characterized usually by an unexplained fall in platelet count of greater than 50% (even if the nadir is >150 × 10⁹ per L) with or without new thrombosis and by a positive test for HIT antibodies.

HIT occurs when heparin exposure causes formation of pathogenic antibodies (usually IgG class) that recognize multimolecular complexes of platelet factor 4 (PF4) and heparin on platelet surfaces and bind to platelet FcγIIa receptors, leading to in vivo platelet activation. Thrombin generation in patients with HIT results from procoagulant platelet-derived microparticles (38) and possibly from tissue factor exposed on endothelium and monocytes (39). The marked thrombin generation explains the prothrombotic state associated with venous and arterial thrombosis and the progression of DVT to gangrene in some patients with HIT who are treated with warfarin (40). The latter results from an imbalance between procoagulant and anticoagulant states during warfarin therapy; warfarin causes severe acquired protein C deficiency while failing to control thrombin generation (40).

The frequency of HIT varies widely, depending on the type of heparin (UFH more common than LMWH) and on the patient population (surgical patients more likely than medical and obstetrical patients) (41).

HIT antibodies are detected using either platelet "activation" (functional) assays or PF4-dependent "antigen" assays (42), including a rapid particle gel assay that utilizes PF4 coated onto spheres (43).

Isolated HIT has an unfavorable natural history; 25% to 50% of these patients develop thrombosis after stopping heparin (with or without warfarin replacement), and the risk of fatal thrombosis is 4% to 5% (44–46). Therefore, in patients who are strongly suspected of having HIT, even when there is no clinically apparent thrombosis, all heparin therapy should be stopped and (usually) an alternative anticoagulant started and continued until the platelet count recovers. Nonheparin alternatives include direct thrombin inhibitors (DTIs) such as argatroban, lepirudin, or bivalirudin, and a nonheparin glycosaminoglycan with mainly anti–factor Xa activity, danaparoid sodium (no longer available). Fondaparinux, a novel anticoagulant with anti–factor Xa activity, should be safe in patients with HIT, but experience is limited and optimal dosing has not been established (see Table 116-2). Because comparative studies are lacking and the relative efficacy of these agents is uncertain, drug selection should be based on availability and physician experience.

### Heparin-Induced Osteoporosis

Long-term (1 month or more) UFH therapy, used primarily during pregnancy, causes osteoporosis. Although the risk of fractures is low (2% to 3%), a partly reversible reduction in bone density that might increase susceptibility to future fractures occurs in approximately 30% of patients receiving long-term heparin therapy (47–49). There is evidence from experimental studies and a randomized controlled trial that the risk of osteoporosis is lower with LMWH than with UFH (23,50).

### Danaparoid

Danaparoid is derived from porcine and bovine mucosa. It is a heterogeneous mixture of heparan sulfate (84%), dermatan sulfate (12%), and chondroitin sulfate (4%), all of which are polysulfated glycosaminoglycans with structural similarities to heparin. The main anticoagulant effect of danaparoid is due to heparan sulfate, which facilitates antithrombin-mediated inactivation of thrombin and factor Xa in a manner similar to heparin. Approximately 10% of the anticoagulant effect of the drug is due to dermatan sulfate–mediated inhibition of thrombin by heparin cofactor II. This drug is no longer available.

Danaparoid is given either subcutaneously (sc) or by continuous IV infusion. The peak anticoagulant effect after intravenous administration occurs within minutes; after sc injection, the peak anticoagulant effect is delayed, and bioavailability is nearly 100% (51). The half-life of the anti–factor Xa effect of danaparoid is 24.5 hours, whereas its AT effect has a half-life of 4.3 hours (51). Renal excretion accounts for 40% to 50% of plasma clearance of anti–factor Xa activity of danaparoid, and hepatic disease does not affect its pharmacokinetics (52). Danaparoid significantly reduces the risk of both proximal DVT and total DVT when compared with UFH in patients with thrombotic stroke (53). For treatment of patients with acute thrombosis, danaparoid was significantly more effective than UFH (54). For treatment of isolated HIT with or without complicating thrombosis, an intravenous regimen has been used adjusted according to anti–factor Xa levels (55). Laboratory monitoring is usually not necessary when danaparoid is administered subcutaneously, but its anticoagulant activity can be monitored using anti–factor Xa activity, a therapeutic level similar to that required for LMWH (0.5 to 1.0 anti–factor Xa U per mL). Major or life-threatening bleeding in a patient who has received danaparoid is problematic, given its prolonged anti–factor Xa half-life. PS partially reverses the anti–factor IIa effect, but does not affect the anti–factor Xa anticoagulant activity (56).

### Coumarin Derivatives (Warfarin)

Coumarins are vitamin K antagonists that are used for long-term treatment of venous and arterial thrombosis; warfarin is the most widely used coumarin in North America and Asia, whereas acenocoumarol is used in some European countries. Warfarin doses are adjusted according to the prothrombin time (PT), expressed as the international normalized ratio (INR). In patients with VTE, warfarin should be started within 24 to 48 hours of initiation of heparin with a goal of achieving INR results between 2.0 and 3.0 because higher values are associated with more bleeding but no better efficacy. A higher target INR of 3.0 to 4.0 was previously thought to be necessary in patients with antiphospholipid antibody syndrome (APS) who developed thrombosis (57,58), but a recent study does not support this contention (59). Warfarin, with a target INR of 2.0 and 3.0, is considered adequate in preventing arterial complications, with the exception

| TABLE 116-2 | | | |
| --- | --- | --- | --- |

**NEW ANTICOAGULANT DRUGS**

| Anticoagulant drug | Class | Approved or likely appropriate indications | Contraindications |
| --- | --- | --- | --- |
| Fondaparinux/ Idraparinux | Synthetic factor Xa Inhibitor | Prophylaxis in high-risk patients; treatment of VTE | Unknown |
| Lepirudin | Hirudin derivative | HIT with thrombosis | Thrombocytopenia other than HIT |
| Bivalirudin | Hirudin derivative | Percutaneous coronary intervention | Unknown |
| Argatroban | Direct thrombin inhibitor | HIT with thrombosis | Thrombocytopenia other than HIT |
| Ximelagatran | Oral direct thrombin inhibitor | Atrial fibrillation; treatment of VTE | Unknown |

VTE, venous thromboembolism; HIT, heparin-induced thrombocytopenia.

of patients who have mechanical prosthetic valves; in general, a target range INR of 2.5 to 3.5 is considered appropriate in these patients.

## Mechanism of Action: Effect on Coagulation Factor Synthesis and Thrombosis

All coumarin compounds have the same mechanism of action, but different pharmacokinetics and pharmacodynamics. Coumarins produce their anticoagulant effect by inhibiting the hepatic synthesis of the four vitamin K–dependent coagulation proteins: prothrombin and factors VII, IX, and X. They induce their anticoagulant effect by interfering with the cyclic interconversion of vitamin K and its 2,3 epoxide (vitamin K 2,3 epoxide) (60). This process leads to intracellular depletion of the reduced form of vitamin K and limits γ-carboxylation of glutamic acid residues (61,62) and limits the carboxylation of vitamin K–dependent natural anticoagulant proteins C and S. The antithrombotic and anticoagulant effects of warfarin are dissociated during the initiation phase of treatment. After an oral dose, there is a delay in anticoagulant effect. This delay represents the time needed for decarboxylated vitamin K–dependent clotting factors to replace the normal clotting factors as the latter are cleared from the circulation. The early anticoagulant effect is caused by loss of fully carboxylated factor VII, which has a short half-life (approximately 6 hours) (61–64) and is associated with a rise in the INR. However, the reduction in factor VII does not produce an antithrombotic effect. Rather, the antithrombotic effect of warfarin requires similar reductions in the other vitamin K–dependent coagulation proteins, factors II, IX, and X. Because these coagulation factors have considerably longer half-lives than does factor VII, up to 60 hours is needed to achieve a therapeutic reduction in their levels. Support for the hypothesis that reduction in factor VII alone might not produce an antithrombotic effect comes from several studies. Using a stasis model in rabbits, Wessler and Gitel demonstrated that the antithrombotic effect of vitamin K antagonists was delayed for 6 days, whereas an anticoagulant effect was observed after 2 days (65). Similarly, Zivelin et al. demonstrated in animal studies that reductions in levels of factor II and to a lesser extent X, but not factor VII, produced an antithrombotic effect (66). Using fibrinopeptide A as an index of thrombin activity, Patel et al. demonstrated that clots formed from plasma with reduced prothrombin concentrations produced significantly less fibrinopeptide A than did clots formed in the presence of normal concentrations of prothrombin (67).

The delay in achieving an antithrombotic effect despite prolonged clotting times has clinical importance because during this period, patients can have a paradoxical prothrombotic state. This results from the decline of protein C at the same rate as factor VII (half-life also approximately 6 hours) and could contribute to the observation that treatment of acute venous thrombosis with oral anticoagulants alone (without concomitant heparin) results in a high rate of extension and early recurrence of thrombosis (6,68). Further, the rapid decrease in proteins C and S, while levels of prothrombin and factor X remain near normal, could contribute to warfarin-induced skin necrosis.

The concept that the antithrombotic effect of warfarin reflects its ability to lower prothrombin and factor X levels has clinical importance. First, it provides a rationale for overlapping heparin with warfarin treatment until the prothrombin level is lowered into the therapeutic range. Because prothrombin has a half-life of approximately 60 hours, an overlap of at least 4 days of heparin treatment is necessary to achieve this. Second, it supports the use of a maintenance dose of warfarin (approximately 5 mg) to initiate warfarin therapy because studies indicate that the rate of lowering prothrombin levels is similar whether warfarin treatment is initiated with a 5 mg or 10 mg dose (63,69). On the other hand, the level of the anticoagulant, protein C, is reduced more rapidly with the higher doses, producing a potential hypercoagulable state (63). Third, it supports the contention of Furie et al. that levels of native prothrombin antigen more closely reflect the antithrombotic activity of warfarin than does the PT (INR) (70).

### Pharmacodynamics and Pharmacokinetics

Warfarin is a racemic mixture of two optically active isomers, the R and S forms, in roughly equal proportions, although S-warfarin is five times more potent, and they are cleared by different pathways (71). Therefore, inhibition of the metabolic clearance of the S-isomer by drugs enhances the anticoagulant effect of warfarin more so than does inhibition of the R-isomer.

Warfarin is almost always given orally, although an injectable preparation is available. It has high bioavailability, is rapidly absorbed from the gastrointestinal tract, and reaches maximal blood concentrations in healthy volunteers 90 minutes after oral administration. In healthy volunteers, warfarin has a half-life of 47 hours, with a prolonged dose-dependent terminal phase of elimination associated with detectable levels of warfarin after 120 hours (72). Warfarin circulates bound to plasma proteins (mainly albumin) and rapidly accumulates in the liver, where it is metabolized into products that have little anticoagulant activity (73). Coumarins show variable intraindividual and interindividual anticoagulant response. Therefore, the coumarin dosage must be closely monitored to prevent overdosing or underdosing. The dose-response of warfarin is influenced by both pharmacokinetic and pharmacodynamic factors, variability in INR response, including inaccuracies in laboratory testing and reporting, poor patient compliance, and poor communication between patient and physician.

### Alterations of Pharmacokinetics and Pharmacodynamics

The pharmacokinetics and pharmacodynamics of warfarin are influenced by metabolic clearance of warfarin, by vitamin K intake and absorption, by rates of synthesis and clearance of vitamin K–dependent clotting factors, and by drugs or disorders that impair blood coagulation or platelet function. The events leading to altered pharmacokinetics or pharmacodynamics occur in the gastrointestinal tract, the liver, the circulation, and at the site of hemostatic plug formation.

Subjects receiving warfarin therapy are sensitive to fluctuating levels of vitamin K caused by variability in dietary intake and in gastrointestinal absorption of vitamin K (74,75). Dietary vitamin K is provided predominantly by phylloquinone in plant material (75). Phylloquinone acts through the warfarin-insensitive reductase reaction. Important fluctuations in vitamin K intake occur in both apparently healthy and sick patients (76). Increased dietary intake of vitamin K, sufficient to reduce the anticoagulant response of warfarin, occurs in patients on weight-reduction diets consuming green vegetables and in patients treated with intravenous supplements containing vitamin K. Reduced dietary vitamin K intake potentiates the anticoagulant effect of warfarin in sick patients treated with antibiotics and intravenous fluids without vitamin K supplementation, and in states associated with fat malabsorption. The liver can both potentiate and oppose the anticoagulant effect of coumarins because it plays a central role in modulating the anticoagulant effect of vitamin K antagonists. It is the site of the pharmacologic action of coumarins, metabolic clearance of coumarins and coagulation proteins, and synthesis of coagulation factors, including the vitamin K–dependent coagulation factors.

The anticoagulant response of warfarin can be affected by genetic factors. Mutation of allelic variants of CYP2C9 in the gene coding for cytochrome P-450, the hepatic enzyme responsible for oxidative metabolism of the S-isomer of warfarin (77,78), contributes to the variability in dose response to warfarin among healthy subjects (79). Hereditary resistance to warfarin has been described in rats (80) and humans (81), and is attributed to altered affinity of the receptor for warfarin. Patients with genetic warfarin resistance require doses fivefold to 20-fold higher than average to achieve an anticoagulant effect.

A mutation in the propeptide of factor IX can cause bleeding without excessive prolongation of the INR, which is not affected by the concentration of factor IX (82,83). Analysis revealed two different missense mutations involving the propeptide region that are expressed as a selective increase in the sensitivity of coumarin-mediated reduction of factor IX (83). When patients with this disorder are treated with warfarin, levels of factor IX fall precipitously to 1% to 3%, while the levels of other vitamin K–dependent factors decrease to approximately 30% to 40%. The mutation occurs in less than 1.5% of the population.

Many drugs have the potential to interact with coumarins and alter the INR. Although convincing evidence of causal association is lacking in most reports (84), it is prudent to increase the frequency of INR monitoring when prescribing new medications, changing the dose of a currently administered drug, or discontinuing a drug in patients treated with oral anticoagulants. The anticoagulant effect of warfarin is potentiated by drugs that inhibit metabolic clearance through stereoselective (affect oxidative metabolism of S-isomer or R-isomer of warfarin) or nonselective pathways (71,85). The metabolic clearance of the more potent S-warfarin isomer is inhibited by trimethoprim-sulfamethoxazole and sulfinpyrazone, both of which potentiate the anticoagulant effect of warfarin (84). In contrast, cimetidine and omeprazole inhibit clearance of the less potent R-isomer and have only a moderate potentiating effect on warfarin. Amiodarone inhibits the metabolic clearance of both the S- and R-isomers through a nonstereospecific pathway and has a potentiating effect on warfarin (84). In a case–control study, low to moderate doses of acetaminophen (9 or more 1,000 mg tablets per week) were associated with a tenfold risk of INR greater than 6.0 (86). Hepatic impairment can potentiate the response to warfarin through impaired synthesis of coagulation factors. Hypermetabolic states produced by fever, hyperthyroidism, or treatment with thyroxine potentiate the effects of warfarin, probably by increasing the catabolism of vitamin K–dependent coagulation factors (87). Rifampicin, barbiturates, and carbamazepine inhibit the anticoagulant effect of warfarin by increasing its metabolic clearance and inducing hepatic mixed oxidase activity (88). Although chronic alcohol use has the potential to increase the clearance of warfarin through a similar mechanism, relatively large amounts of wine do not influence the INR in patients treated with warfarin (89).

Drugs that inhibit platelet function can potentiate the hemorrhagic effect of coumarins. The most commonly used drugs include aspirin, ticlopidine, clopidogrel, other nonsteroidal antiinflammatory drugs, high doses of penicillins, and moxalactam. Of these, aspirin is the most important because of its widespread use and prolonged effect on hemostasis. Unlike the nonsteroidal antiinflammatory drugs, aspirin produces an irreversible inhibition of platelet function by blocking platelet cyclooxygenase. Aspirin can also produce gastric erosions that increase the risk of serious upper gastrointestinal bleeding. The risk of clinically important bleeding is increased when high doses of aspirin are used, particularly in combination with high-intensity warfarin therapy (INR range 3.0 to 4.5) (90,91).

## Monitoring Warfarin Therapy

The PT is sensitive to reductions in three of the four vitamin K–dependent coagulation factors (prothrombin, factor VII, and factor X). During the first few days of warfarin therapy, the prolongation of the PT reflects mainly a reduction of factor VII; with prolonged warfarin therapy, it also reflects a reduction of prothrombin and factor X. The PT assay is performed by adding calcium and thromboplastin to citrated plasma. Thromboplastin is a phospholipid–protein extract of tissue, usually lung, brain, or placenta, containing both the tissue factor and phospholipid necessary to promote the activation of factor X by factor VII. Thromboplastins vary in their responsiveness to the anticoagulant effects of warfarin depending on their source, phospholipid content, and preparation (92–96). A responsive thromboplastin produces a greater prolongation of the PT for a given reduction in vitamin K–dependent clotting factors than an unresponsive thromboplastin. The responsiveness of a thromboplastin can be measured by assessing its international sensitivity index (ISI); a highly sensitive thromboplastin such as a recombinant human preparation consisting of replicated synthetic tissue factor has an ISI of approximately 1.0 (97).

In the past, PT monitoring of warfarin treatment was imprecise because the PT was expressed in seconds or as a simple ratio of the patient's results divided by the normal control value. Differences in responsiveness of thromboplastins caused clinically important differences in oral anticoagulant dosing, recognition of which led to the adoption of the INR for monitoring oral anticoagulant therapy. The INR is calculated as follows:

$$INR = (\text{patient PT/mean normal PT})^{ISI}$$

where ISI (international sensitivity index) denotes thromboplastin activity used at the local laboratory (98).

The INR system is based on ISI values derived from the plasma of patients stabilized on warfarin therapy for at least 6 weeks and may be less reliable early in the course of warfarin therapy. However, the INR is much more reliable than the PT and is recommended during both initiation and maintenance of warfarin treatment (99,100). There is a relationship between the ISI value and interlaboratory variability, with higher ISI reagents causing a higher interlaboratory coefficient of variation (CV). Using a *manual* method of clot detection, the INR system is based on a mathematical relationship between the PT ratio obtained with test thromboplastin and the World Health Organization Standard. However, because most laboratories now use automated clot detectors, a new variable has been introduced that affects the accuracy of the INR system (101,102). The variance in the ISI determinations is reduced significantly by calibrating the instrument with lyophilized plasma calibrants prepared by depleting plasma of vitamin K–dependent clotting factors. On the basis of these observations, the College of American Pathologists has recommended that laboratories use reagent/instrument combinations for which the ISI has been established. The ISI value provided by the manufacturer for each new batch of thromboplastin reagent may also be incorrect (103,104).

Concerns have been raised about the validity of the prothrombin time–international normalized ratio (PT-INR) in monitoring oral anticoagulant treatment in patients with the APS and lupus anticoagulant (LA). This results from the variable responsiveness of thromboplastins to LA, in particular with some recombinant thromboplastins. Spurious prolongation of the INR without adequate reductions in the levels of coagulation factors II and X might lead to systematic underdosing of warfarin, with an associated increase in the risk of thrombosis. Although the optimum method of monitoring patients with LA is uncertain, Tripodi et al. found that LA interference of the PT-INR measured with the majority of commercial thromboplastins is not enough to cause concern if insensitive thromboplastins are properly calibrated to assign them an instrument-specific ISI (105).

## Warfarin Initiation

Years ago, large warfarin doses (up to 40 mg) were used to reduce the time to achieve a "therapeutic" anticoagulant response. O'Reilly et al. demonstrated that such doses of warfarin are unnecessary (106). In two separate randomized trials, Harrison et al. and Crowther et al. (63,69) showed that the practice of initiating warfarin starting with an average maintenance dose of 5 mg warfarin and adjusting the dose according to the INR usually results in a value of at least 2.0 in 4 to 5 days. A 5 mg starting dose of warfarin (rather than 10 mg) reduced the likelihood of early excessive anticoagulation, ameliorated a precipitous decline in protein C, and did not delay achievement of a therapeutic INR. Kovacs et al. (107) demonstrated that 10 mg of warfarin in the first 2 days of therapy for outpatients with acute VTE allows more rapid achievement of a therapeutic INR than does a 5 mg dosage, producing effective anticoagulation without an increase in supratherapeutic INR results (>5.0). Therefore, although a 5 mg warfarin starting dose is appropriate for most patients (108), it is reasonable to use 10 mg in select outpatients. Starting doses of less than 5 mg might be appropriate in the elderly (109), in patients with liver disease or nutritional deficiency, in those at high risk of bleeding (110,111), and in patients who are more sensitive to warfarin (112).

INR monitoring can be performed daily or every other day until the results are in the therapeutic range for at least 24 hours. With the advent of routine outpatient treatment of VTE with LMWHs, which do not require monitoring of their anticoagulant effect, there has been a push to develop warfarin dosing regimens that reduce the need for initial INR monitoring. Smaller doses of warfarin reduce the need for more frequent INR monitoring because fewer patients develop INR values greater than 3.0 in the early days of warfarin therapy. Kovacs et al. demonstrated that algorithm-guided warfarin initiation in outpatients that requires INR measurements only on days 3 and 5 is safe (107,108).

After initial dosing, warfarin can be monitored two or three times per week for 1 to 2 weeks, and then less frequently, depending on the stability of INR results, up to intervals as long as 4 to 6 weeks. If dose adjustment is needed, the cycle of more frequent monitoring is repeated until a stable dose-response is again achieved.

## Discontinuation of Warfarin Therapy

Similar to the initiation phase of warfarin, in the period immediately after warfarin is discontinued, the INR might not be an accurate reflection of the degree of coagulation impairment because the initial fall in the INR is likely due to the discrepant faster rise in coagulation factor VII (owing to its shorter half-life) relative to factors II and X. Whether this results in a clinically important "rebound transient hypercoagulable state" is unclear. White et al. (113) demonstrated that normal coagulation is not reliably achieved for at least 4 days after the last dose of warfarin, and there is substantial interindividual variation in the rate of fall of the INR.

## Improving Warfarin Control

Because the effectiveness and safety of warfarin are dependent on the INR result, every effort should be made to maintain the INR within the therapeutic range. This is facilitated by targeting an INR level in the middle of the INR range (i.e., 2.5 for a designated range of 2.0 to 3.0, and 3.0 for a designated range

of 2.5 to 3.5). There is a sharp increase in the risk of bleeding when the INR is above the upper limit of the therapeutic range (114–116), and the risk of thromboembolism increases when the INR falls below the lower limit (115,117). The importance of maintaining good anticoagulant control was shown by an "on-treatment" reanalysis of the primary prevention trials in AF (118). The results of this analysis showed that both bleeding and thromboembolic events were decreased by maintaining good anticoagulant control.

A variety of programs has been developed aimed at increasing "the time in the therapeutic range" (TTR). These programs include anticoagulant-monitoring clinics with dedicated personnel, the use of point-of-care monitors that allow patients to self-test and self-manage dose adjustments, and use of computerized programs to assist in dose adjustments (119–125). Home monitoring of warfarin therapy is accurate, feasible, and associated with a greater TTR and improved quality of life for the patient, but it requires special patient education and training to implement and should be overseen by a knowledgeable provider.

## Adverse Effects of Warfarin

Bleeding is the main complication of oral anticoagulant therapy. Randomized studies have demonstrated that the risk of bleeding increases steadily as the INR rises, doubling for each one-point increase in the INR (110,126,127). Hylek et al. (115) showed that five of 114 (4%) asymptomatic patients with an INR greater than 6.0 developed life-threatening bleeding within 2 weeks of their elevated INR value. Risk factors that have been associated with warfarin-induced bleeding include age greater than 65 years, previous stroke or gastrointestinal bleeding, AF, serious comorbidity (such as renal or hepatic failure), and concomitant antiplatelet therapy (5). When warfarin-treated patients bleed at a time when the INR is below 3.0, an underlying lesion is often found (127).

## Management of Supratherapeutic International Normalized Ratio Values in Asymptomatic Patients

In typical outpatient practices, patients have INRs outside the target range 50% of the time (128,129). Of all INR determinations, 18% are above the therapeutic range (126), accounting for 14% of total patient-time on anticoagulation therapy (130). This can be due to drug interaction with concomitant medications, dietary changes, presence of comorbid illnesses, or for no apparent reason. Frequent elevated INR results above the therapeutic target range of 2.0 to 3.0 is an independent predictor for major hemorrhage (131–133).

Patients receiving warfarin who present with an elevated INR should be screened for bleeding. Patients with active, major bleeding should receive plasma in combination with intravenous vitamin K to lower the INR into the normal range. Because of the risks and cost of plasma therapy, it should be used only in patients with an acute indication for the immediate reversal of the anticoagulant effect of warfarin, in combination with parenteral vitamin K. Plasma should not be used to correct a moderately prolonged INR in a nonbleeding patient, and its use in any nonbleeding patient should be discouraged given the effectiveness of intravenous and oral vitamin K for the rapid reversal of prolonged INR values. Activated recombinant factor VIIa (rFVIIa) has been reported to be safe and effective in correcting prolonged INRs, as well as in averting or reversing bleeding associated with warfarin therapy (134).

There is no generally accepted method to reduce an excessively prolonged INR in nonbleeding patients receiving warfarin therapy. This is because studies have used elevated INR results as a surrogate marker for the risk of bleeding, and to date, there are few published data to support the hypothesis that rapid return of an elevated INR to the desired range is associated with a reduction in bleeding. The most simple and widely used approach is to withhold warfarin and allow the INR to fall into the desired range, at which point warfarin is reinstituted, often at a reduced dose. Two large case series have examined the safety of this approach (135,136).

To hasten the decrease in INR toward the desired range, vitamin K can be administered intravenously, subcutaneously, or orally. Parenteral vitamin K can cause adverse effects, including warfarin resistance (136–138), anaphylactoid reactions (139–141), and skin reactions (142), and furthermore is inconvenient and requires a visit to a health care provider. Intravenous vitamin K, 0.5 to 1.0 mg, rapidly and reliably reduces excessively prolonged INR values to normal (138,143), but it is underutilized because of a concern about anaphylactoid reactions. Although frequently reported, and likely more common in patients who receive large intravenous doses administered rapidly, the true frequency of this complication is likely low. Slow intravenous administration (i.e., 1 to 2 mg over 20 to 30 minutes) of vitamin K is associated with a low risk of anaphylaxis.

Subcutaneous vitamin K is relatively ineffective in reducing the INR. Nee et al. conducted a randomized, clinical trial in which patients with INR values between 6.0 and 20.0 received either subcutaneous or intravenous vitamin K (144). Independent of the route of administration, patients with INR values between 6 and 10 received 0.5 mg of vitamin K, while those with values between 10 and 20 received 3 mg of vitamin K. Twenty-four hours after administration, 45% of patients in the subcutaneous vitamin K group had an INR less than 4.5, compared with 95% of patients in the intravenous vitamin K group. After 72 hours, overcorrection of the INR occurred more frequently in the subcutaneous vitamin K group (42%) than in the intravenous group (23%). Similar results were reported by Raj et al. (145). Taken together, these studies support the use of intravenous vitamin K for rapid reduction in the INR. To avoid the inconvenience and toxicity of parenteral vitamin K, recent interest has focused on the use of *oral* vitamin K for the treatment of warfarin-associated coagulopathy. Studies have demonstrated that low-dose (1 mg to 2.5 mg) oral vitamin K reduces the INR to acceptable limits within 24 hours in 33% to 74% of patients (67,146–149).

In conclusion, for patients receiving warfarin therapy with a target INR between 2.0 and 3.0, 1.0 mg of oral vitamin K is an appropriate choice when the INR result is 4.5 to 10.0. Higher doses of oral vitamin K (2.5 mg to 5 mg) or 0.5 to 1.0 mg of intravenous vitamin K should be considered in patients with INR values of more than 10.0.

### Management of Hemorrhage (with or without High International Normalized Ratio Values)

Management of oral anticoagulant–associated bleeding should be individualized, depending on the location and severity of bleeding, the INR at the time of bleeding, and the risk of recurrent thrombosis. For patients who have relatively minor bleeding from an external site, such as epistaxis or wound bleeding, local compression with or without a reduction or discontinuation of warfarin may suffice. Patients with major hemorrhage, such as that into a critical organ, require more aggressive therapy. Cessation of anticoagulant therapy and combined administration of intravenous vitamin K, alone or with fresh frozen plasma or prothrombin complex concentrate, will normalize the INR. Doses of vitamin K as small as 1 mg used in combination with plasma or prothrombin complexes are effective (138). For patients with life-threatening hemorrhage, the use of prothrombin complex concentrate is preferable to fresh frozen plasma because the concentrates allow for a more rapid and complete INR reversal (150,151). Recombinant activated factor VII also has

been reported to stop life-threatening oral anticoagulant–associated bleeding (134,152,153).

The long-term management of patients who have suffered a major bleeding episode while taking oral anticoagulant therapy and who require ongoing thromboprophylaxis is problematic. If bleeding occurs when the INR is above the therapeutic range, warfarin can often be restarted when bleeding stops and the cause of bleeding corrected. If bleeding occurs while the INR is in the therapeutic range, treatment is more difficult. For patients with AF or an episode of idiopathic proximal DVT or PE (and persisting increased bleeding risk), the anticoagulant target range can be reduced from 2.0 to 3.0, to 1.5 to 2.0 with the expectation that efficacy will be reduced but not abolished (130,154). For patients with AF, aspirin can be used instead of warfarin. For patients with mechanical heart valves (and persisting increased bleeding risk), it is reasonable to aim for a less intense INR range of 2.0 to 2.5 (instead of 2.5 to 3.5).

### Warfarin-Induced Skin Necrosis

This is an uncommon but important complication of warfarin, caused by extensive thrombosis of the venules and capillaries within the subcutaneous fat, usually observed on day 3 to 8 after starting warfarin therapy (155) (see Chapter 115). An association between warfarin-induced skin necrosis and protein C deficiency (156,157), and less commonly protein S deficiency (158), has been reported, but it also occurs in nondeficient individuals and patients with HIT complicated by thrombosis. A pathophysiologic role for protein C deficiency is supported by similarity of the lesions to those seen in neonatal purpura fulminans that complicates homozygous protein C deficiency. The management of patients with warfarin-induced skin necrosis who need long-term oral anticoagulant therapy is problematic. Warfarin must be used with extreme caution and long-term UFH (or LMWH) use is inconvenient and may be associated with osteoporosis. Warfarin can be restarted at low doses with concomitant therapeutic doses of UFH or LMWH and the dosage increased slowly over several weeks. Heparin can be stopped once INR has been in the therapeutic range for at least 24 hours. This approach is safe because it avoids an abrupt reduction in protein C levels before the reduction in prothrombin and factor IX and X levels (157,159).

### Warfarin-Associated "Blue Toe" Syndrome and Miscellaneous Cutaneous Effects of Warfarin

In patients with severe atherothrombosis, use of warfarin might contribute to the development of "blue" or "purple" toes. Although cholesterol microembolization is thought to be the cause, not all patients with this syndrome have clinical features of cholesterol embolism syndrome. The causal role of warfarin is speculative. Therefore, physicians must balance the risk of stopping warfarin with the uncertain potential for improvement.

Alopecia of varying severity has been described. Ecchymoses, as well as cutaneous rash, presumably allergic in origin, may develop (160). Use of a different oral anticoagulant might permit resolution of these adverse effects while maintaining anticoagulation.

## FACTOR Xa INHIBITORS

LMWH and coumarin derivatives are effective and safe for the prevention of recurrent thrombosis in patients with VTE. However, there remains room for improvement, particularly in the long-term treatment of VTE and the prevention of VTE in high-risk situations, such as orthopedic surgery. Fondaparinux, the first synthetic pentasaccharide, acts by specific inhibition of factor Xa (FXa) without activity against thrombin.

## Fondaparinux

### Pharmacology

Fondaparinux sodium is a sulfated pentasaccharide with specificity for factor Xa. Its structure is based on the minimal oligosaccharide sequence in heparin that interacts with AT. Unlike UFH and LMWH, which are heterogeneous and derived from animal sources, fondaparinux is synthesized and has uniform chemical composition (161). Binding to AT facilitates inhibition of factor Xa (700 U per mg) approximately 300-fold, but the short chain length renders it incapable of inactivating thrombin (162). Fondaparinux produces a predictable antithrombotic effect because it does not bind to platelet factor 4 or other plasma proteins (163).

Fondaparinux is completely absorbed following subcutaneous administration and results in a peak concentration in 2 to 3 hours. The plasma elimination half-life is 17 to 21 hours and is independent of dose. There is no significant metabolism of the molecule, and up to 84% of the injected dose is eliminated by the kidneys, which explains why once-daily dosing is sufficient and that laboratory monitoring is unnecessary (164–166). Fondaparinux does not induce release of tissue factor pathway inhibitor and does not affect platelet function or fibrinolysis. Fondaparinux has minimal effects on the PT and aPTT; plasma activity requires an anti–factor Xa assay with a fondaparinux calibration curve. Concomitant use of aspirin neither changes the pharmacokinetic properties of fondaparinux nor increases the bleeding time. There is no interaction with warfarin or piroxicam (nonsteroidal antiinflammatory drug) (167,168).

### Management of Bleeding

There is no specific antidote for fondaparinux; it is not neutralized by PS. In case of bleeding complication, plasma and prothrombin complex concentrates can be administered, although supporting data are lacking. Recombinant FVIIa (rFVIIa) normalizes the prolonged thrombin-generation time and prevents the decrease in plasma levels of prothrombin fragment 1 + 2 induced by fondaparinux in healthy volunteers (169), so it can be considered in the management of patients with serious bleeding.

### Indication for Use

The safety and efficacy of fondaparinux have been studied in large clinical phase II and III trials of prophylaxis (170–173) and treatment of VTE (174,175). It has been recently approved for clinical use to prevent VTE in patients undergoing orthopaedic procedures, after hip fracture, and as initial treatment of DVT and PE.

## Idraparinux (Long-Acting Pentasaccharide)

With the development of a long-acting pentasaccharide, such as idraparinux, once-weekly dosing strategies will be possible for the long-term treatment of venous and arterial thrombosis, assuming that current phase III trials show favorable efficacy and safety results.

### Pharmacology

Several chemical modifications to fondaparinux, such as replacement of N-sulphated groups from sulphated esters and the methylation of hydroxylated groups, increase affinity to AT and prolong half-life. Idraparinux, an O-methyl, O-sulphate pentasaccharide, has an expected half-life of 80 hours (176) and has been or is under current study in a phase II DVT trial

and phase III studies in DVT, PE, and AF. Given the long half-life of idraparinux, there are concerns regarding the management of patients who bleed while receiving this drug, particularly because there is no proven antidote.

# DIRECT THROMBIN INHIBITORS

## Argatroban

### Pharmacology

Argatroban is a potent and selective synthetic DTI derived from L-arginine (177) using rational drug design through substrate mimicry of thrombin. Argatroban exerts its anticoagulant effects by inhibiting free and clot-bound thrombin (178,179). Argatroban is 500 times more potent than r-hirudin in its ability to inhibit clot-bound versus free thrombin; but unlike r-hirudin, the interaction between argatroban and thrombin is reversible. The ability to effectively inhibit clot-bound thrombin may be beneficial in treating hypercoagulable states such as HIT and in reducing extension of existing thrombosis.

Argatroban has predictable pharmacodynamics and pharmacokinetics. It has a rapid onset of action and is rapidly eliminated via hepatic metabolism (180,181). Liver microsomal cytochrome P-450 3A4/5 is not important for metabolism of argatroban (182). The plasma clearance rate is approximately 5.1 mL/min/kg for infusion doses of up to 40 $\mu$g/kg/minute, and elimination half-life is 39 to 51 minutes (181). Patients with moderate hepatic impairment (Child-Hugh score >6), have an approximate fourfold decrease in drug clearance and threefold increase in drug elimination half-life compared with healthy volunteers; a fourfold reduction in argatroban dosage is required for individuals with moderate liver dysfunction. Age and renal function cause no clinically important effects on the pharmacodynamic and pharmacokinetic of argatroban, and no adjustment in argatroban dosage is necessary for these variables.

Argatroban is usually administered as an intravenous infusion. An anticoagulant effect is attained quickly, and steady-state levels and anticoagulant effect are usually achieved within 1 to 3 hours and maintained until the dosage is adjusted or the infusion stopped. With argatroban doses of up to 40 $\mu$g/kg/minute, plasma drug concentrations increase proportionately and correlate well with steady state anticoagulant effects. Upon stopping the infusion, plasma argatroban levels and the anticoagulant effect fall rapidly to pretreatment values (181).

### Monitoring

The anticoagulant effect of argatroban is routinely monitored using the aPTT. A higher level of argatroban anticoagulation than that used to treat patients with HIT is required during procedures such as percutaneous coronary interventions. The anticoagulant effect of argatroban during such procedures is monitored using the activated clotting time (ACT). In a dose-dependent fashion, argatroban increases the PT/INR, thrombin time (TT), and ecarin clotting time (ECT). Because argatroban is a DTI, concomitant use of argatroban and warfarin results in prolongation of the PT/INR beyond that produced by warfarin alone (183). This is problematic during the overlap period when argatroban would be replaced by warfarin anticoagulation. Sheth et al. (183) showed that the relationship between INR results on cotherapy (combined argatroban and warfarin) and those on warfarin therapy alone can be used to reliably estimate the INR effect of warfarin during the transition period. The INR results on cotherapy can be used most reliably to predict the INR prolongation attributable to warfarin alone when

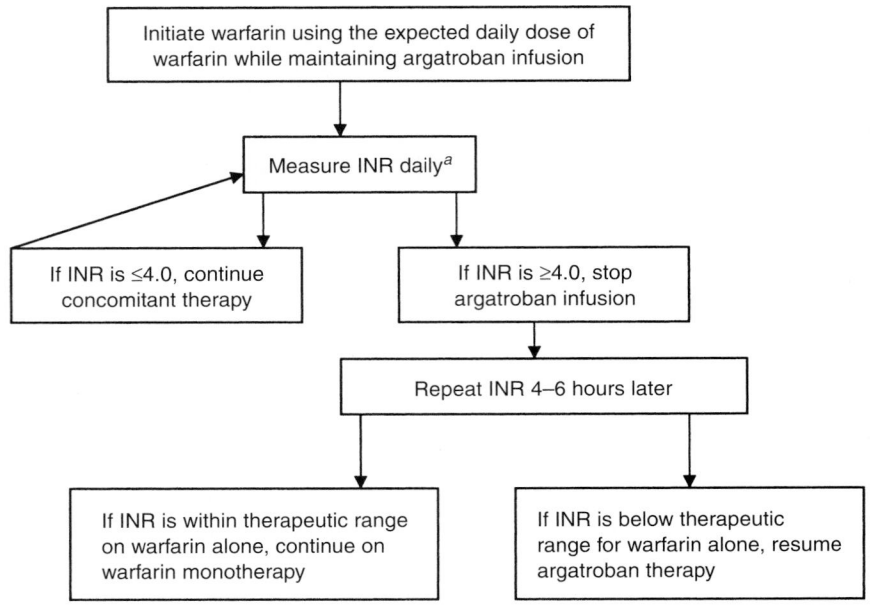

**FIGURE 116-1.** Conversion from argatroban to oral anticoagulant therapy.
[a]If the dose of argatroban is >2 μg/kg/minute, temporarily reduce to a dose of 2 μg/kg/minute 4 to 6 hours prior to measuring the international normalized ratio (INR).
(From Warkentin TE, Greinacher A, ed. *Heparin induced thrombocytopenia*, 2nd ed. New York: Marcel Dekker Inc, 2001, with permission.)

argatroban is infused at doses of up to 2 μg/kg/minute, using thromboplastins with ISIs of 0.88 to 2.13 (183). Guidelines for conversion from argatroban to warfarin therapy have been published by Warkentin et al. (184) (see Fig. 116-1).

### Management of Bleeding

There is no antidote to argatroban. Excessive anticoagulation, with or without bleeding, may be controlled by discontinuing argatroban or decreasing the infusion rate. Anticoagulant parameters should return to baseline within 2 to 4 hours after discontinuation of the drug. In patients with hepatic impairment, this reversal takes longer (6 hours to >20 hours). Argatroban should be ceased immediately and symptomatic supportive therapy given if life-threatening bleeding occurs.

### Indication for Use

Argatroban is approved for treatment of isolated HIT (with or without complicating thrombosis) in the United States and Canada. The starting dose of argatroban of 2 μg/kg/minute via continuous intravenous infusion should be adjusted (not to exceed 10 μg/kg/minute) to achieve a steady state aPTT of 1.5 to 3.0 times the baseline value (not to exceed 100 seconds). The dosage should be reduced in patients with hepatobiliary compromise.

## Hirudin

Hirudin is an antithrombotic produced by the salivary gland of the medicinal leech, *Hirudo medicinalis*. The most important recombinant hirudins, lepirudin (Refludan) and desirudin (Revasc), are derived from yeast cells using recombinant biotechnology. Although minor structural differences between natural hirudin and the recombinant forms result in a tenfold reduction in activity, there is no clinically relevant difference.

### Pharmacology

Hirudin is a potent and specific thrombin inhibitor. It acts independently of the cofactors AT and heparin cofactor II (185). Hirudin forms noncovalent, irreversible 1:1 complexes with thrombin, thereby inhibiting all biological activities of thrombin.

By doing so, hirudin inhibits the positive feedback loop of thrombin-induced activation of factor V and VIII (186). Hirudin also inhibits clot-bound thrombin and thrombin bound to fibrin split products (187,188).

Hirudins must be given parenterally. Effective antithrombotic drug levels can be reached by intravenous infusion or subcutaneous administration. After intravenous injection of bolus lepirudin doses of 0.01 to 0.5 mg per kg, the elimination half-life is 0.8 to 1.7 hour. After continuous infusions over 6 hours, the half-life is 1.1 to 2.0 hours. With subcutaneous administration, bioavailability is almost 100%, and the peak lepirudin concentration occurs 3 to 4 hours after subcutaneous injection. The pharmacokinetic profile of lepirudin does not change after repeated intravenous or subcutaneous doses, suggesting that there is no accumulation. Renal clearance accounts for approximately 90% of systemic clearance, and the elimination half-life of lepirudin is lengthened dramatically with deterioration of renal function.

### Monitoring

The best method for monitoring hirudin treatment has not been determined. Although therapy is typically monitored and dose adjusted based on aPTT results, this method shows considerable variability between patients and its correlation with plasma hirudin levels is not linear; at higher hirudin plasma levels and aPTT values greater than 70 seconds, the hirudin concentration versus aPTT curve flattens and correlation is poor (189,190). The ECT has been suggested as the method of choice for monitoring hirudin treatment in patients requiring high hirudin doses, such as during cardiopulmonary bypass surgery (191). However, prospective trials comparing ECT and aPTT monitoring of hirudin are lacking, and it remains unclear whether the ECT is more useful than the aPTT in predicting bleeding in high-risk patients.

### Adverse Effects

Antilepirudin antibodies may develop because r-hirudin is a nonhuman protein (192,193). In a small proportion of patients, development of antilepirudin antibodies results in an increase in anticoagulant effect, as indicated by a suprertherapeutic aPTT. In such instances, the hirudin doses have to be adjusted to maintain the aPTT within the target range. The enhanced anticoagulant effect might be a result of decreased renal elimination of hirudin–antihirudin antibody complex. Conversely, in some patients, the development of antihirudin antibodies is paralleled by a reduction in the aPTT (193). As a result, aPTT monitoring is recommended when using hirudin. To date, however, no major neutralizing effect or any correlation between antihirudin antibodies and adverse clinical outcomes has been observed (193).

### Indication for Use

Lepirudin is approved for the treatment of HIT complicated by thrombosis. An intravenous bolus of 0.4 mg per kg should be given followed by continuous infusion of 0.15 mg/kg/hour adjusted to target values relative to the patient's baseline aPTT or laboratory normal baseline. Because stable therapeutic levels are usually reached within 30 to 60 minutes, a bolus, which may cause overdosage and anaphylaxis, should only be given in cases of severe thromboembolic complication.

## Bivalirudin

### Pharmacology

Bivalirudin is a 20–amino acid synthetic polypeptide analog of hirudin in which the amino-terminal D-Phe-Pro-Arg-Pro sequence, which binds to the active site of thrombin, is connected via four Gly residues to a carboxy-terminal dodecapeptide that interacts with exosite 1 on thrombin. Like hirudin, bivalirudin forms a 1:1 stoichiometric complex with thrombin. Unlike hirudin, bivalirudin produces only transient inhibition of the active site of thrombin because once bound, thrombin cleaves the Pro-Arg bond within the amino-terminal of bivalirudin, thereby allowing recovery of thrombin activity. This property might result in bivalirudin being safer than hirudin. Bivalirudin has a plasma half-life of 25 minutes after intravenous injection (194) and only a fraction is excreted via the kidneys (195); the predominant pathway of elimination is enzymatic degradation by proteases, including thrombin.

### Indication for Use

Bivalirudin is approved as an alternative to heparin in patients with unstable angina undergoing percutaneous coronary angioplasty and stenting based on the results of a phase III study that compared bivalirudin (1.0 mg per kg bolus dose, followed by a 4-hour infusion at a rate of 2.5 mg/kg/hour, and 14 to 20 hour infusion at a rate of 0.2 mg/kg/hour) with heparin in 4,098 patients (196). Bivalirudin in patients undergoing percutaneous coronary interventions is associated with less bleeding and appears to obviate the need for adjunctive GP IIb/IIIa antagonists in most patients (197,198). The long-term clinical outcome (over 6 months and 1 year) of bivalirudin is comparable with that of heparin plus planned GP IIb/IIIa inhibition during contemporary protein C inhibitor (PCI) (199).

## Oral Direct Thrombin Inhibitors

Coumarin derivatives, such as warfarin, have long been the only available oral anticoagulant for patients who need long-term anticoagulation. However, their drawbacks include a narrow therapeutic index, need for careful routine monitoring, and consequent dose adjustments to avoid over dosing and underdosing, with associated risks of hemorrhage and thrombosis respectively. Consequently, there is a need for a new oral anticoagulant with more predictable pharmacokinetics and pharmacodynamics without the need for frequent coagulation monitoring.

## Ximelagatran

### Pharmacology

Ximelagatran is a prodrug and the first new extensively evaluated oral anticoagulant in more than 60 years. Structurally, the active form, melagatran, is a dipeptide with a molecular weight of about 430 Da. Melagatran binds competitively and reversibly to thrombin, providing specific inhibition of thrombin-mediated activation of coagulation factors and platelets. Melagatran produces thrombin inhibition by binding directly to the active site of thrombin; because of its small molecular mass, it penetrates thrombus to inhibit clot-bound thrombin.

Oral ximelagatran is rapidly absorbed and converted to its active form melagatran, which is the dominant form in plasma. Bioavailability is independent of dose administered. Melagatran is not metabolized or bound to plasma proteins, and its elimination occurs mainly by renal excretion (approximately 80%). Clearance of melagatran correlates with creatinine clearance (200,201); it has a half-life of 3 hours in young healthy subjects (202,203) and 4 to 5 hours in older patients due to age-related deterioration in renal function (204). The pharmacokinetic properties of ximelagatran are amenable to twice-daily administration.

Experimental data indicate that melagatran has a substantially wider difference between antithrombotic effect and bleeding than warfarin. In a comparison of the antithrombotic effects of warfarin and melagatran in a rat carotid artery thrombosis model (205,206), a twofold increase in warfarin dose resulted in a substantial increase in its antithrombotic effect, while a 10-fold increase in melagatran dose was required to achieve an equivalent increase in antithrombotic effect. Conversely, at doses of twice those required to produce an 80% antithrombotic effect, melagatran had little or no effect on bleeding time, while in the same dose range, a marked increase in bleeding time was observed with warfarin (205).

The pharmacokinetic and pharmacodynamic variability of ximelagatran is relatively low (201,203,207–209). Because ximelagatran is not metabolized by cytochrome P-450 system in the liver, many of the food and drug interactions found with warfarin are avoided (210). No dose adjustment is needed in young and elderly, obese patients, and those of different ethnic origins. The stable and predictable action of ximelagatran makes it possible to offer fixed-dose treatment with no need for coagulation monitoring.

### Adverse Effects

The interpretation of studies of long-term therapy with ximelagatran must take into consideration the problem of transaminase elevation. Asymptomatic, transient elevations of alanine aminotransferase (ALT) above three times the upper limit of normal were seen in 4.2% of patients treated with ximelagatran and in none of the patients treated with warfarin in SPORTIF II, the first long-term study with ximelagatran in which patients with AF were treated for 3 months (211). Also, in the long-term study of secondary prevention of VTE (THRIVE III), transient elevations of ALT above three times the upper limit of normal occurred with a cumulative risk of 6.4% in patients treated with ximelagatran versus 1.2% with placebo (212). Short-term studies in VTE prevention following orthopedic surgery show a lower incidence of ALT increase with ximelagatran (213). The clinical implications of these transaminase elevations are unclear because levels may decrease to normal with continued treatment. However, this side effect may require routine monitoring of liver function tests.

There is no proven antidote for rapid reversal of its anticoagulant effect. However, given its half-life of 3 to 5 hours, this is unlikely to be problematic unless ximelagatran is used in patients with poor renal function. Nevertheless, activated prothrombin complex concentrates dose-dependently reduce bleeding produced by high concentrations of melagatran. In animal models, activated coagulation factor VII was less effective, but this may be a reflection of the low tissue factor exposure in the models (214).

Ximelagatran and melagatran are not approved for clinical use, but have been evaluated in phase III clinical trials for the prophylaxis and treatment of VTE (212,215–217) and prevention of thromboembolism in patients with AF (218).

## References

1. Warda M, Gouda EM, Toida T, et al. Isolation and characterization of raw heparin from dromedary intestine: evaluation of a new source of pharmaceutical heparin. *Comp Biochem Physiol C Toxicol Pharmacol* 2003; 136(4):357–365.
2. Anderson LO, Barrowcliffe T, Holmer MK. Anticoagulant properties of heparin fractionated by affinity chromatography on matrix-bound antithrombin III and by gel filtration. *Thromb Res* 1976;9:575–583.
3. Ofosu FA, Sie P, Modi GJ, et al. The inhibition of thrombin-dependent positive-feedback reactions is critical to the expression of the anticoagulant effect of heparin. *Biochem J* 1987;243(2):579–588.
4. Hommes DW, Bura A, Mazzolai L, et al. Subcutaneous heparin compared with continuous intravenous heparin administration in the initial treatment of deep vein thrombosis. A meta-analysis. *Ann Intern Med* 1992; 116(4):279–284.
5. Levine MN, Raskob G, Landefeld S, et al. Hemorrhagic complications of anticoagulant treatment. *Chest* 1995;108(Suppl. 4):276S–290S.
6. Brandjes DP, Heijboer H, Buller HR, et al. Acenocoumarol and heparin compared with acenocoumarol alone in the initial treatment of proximal-vein thrombosis. *N Engl J Med* 1992;327(21):1485–1489.
7. Raschke RA, Reilly BM, Guidry JR, et al. The weight-based heparin dosing nomogram compared with a "standard care" nomogram. A randomized controlled trial. *Ann Intern Med* 1993;119(9):874–881.
8. Young E, Prins M, Levine MN, et al. Heparin binding to plasma proteins, an important mechanism for heparin resistance. *Thromb Haemost* 1992;67(6):639–643.
9. Hull RD, Raskob GE, Hirsh J, et al. Continuous intravenous heparin compared with intermittent subcutaneous heparin in the initial treatment of proximal-vein thrombosis. *N Engl J Med* 1986;315(18):1109–1114.
10. Basu D, Gallus A, Hirsh J, et al. A prospective study of the value of monitoring heparin treatment with the activated partial thromboplastin time. *N Engl J Med* 1972;287(7):324–327.
11. Brill-Edwards P, Ginsberg JS, Johnston M, et al. Establishing a therapeutic range for heparin therapy. *Ann Intern Med* 1993;119(2):104–109.
12. Anand S, Ginsberg JS, Kearon C, et al. The relation between the activated partial thromboplastin time response and recurrence in patients with venous thrombosis treated with continuous intravenous heparin. *Arch Intern Med* 1996;156(15): 1677–1681.
13. Anand SS, Bates S, Ginsberg JS, et al. Recurrent venous thrombosis and heparin therapy: an evaluation of the importance of early activated partial thromboplastin times. *Arch Intern Med* 1999;159(17):2029–2032.
14. Cruickshank MK, Levine MN, Hirsh J, et al. A standard heparin nomogram for the management of heparin therapy. *Arch Intern Med* 1991;151(2):333–337.
15. Hull RD, Raskob GE, Rosenbloom D, et al. Optimal therapeutic level of heparin therapy in patients with venous thrombosis. *Arch Intern Med* 1992;152(8):1589–1595.
16. Levine MN, Hirsh J, Gent M, et al. A randomized trial comparing activated thromboplastin time with heparin assay in patients with acute venous thromboembolism requiring large daily doses of heparin. *Arch Intern Med* 1994;154(1):49–56.
17. Casu B, Oreste P, Torri G, et al. Chemical and 13C Nuclear-Magnetic-Resonance Studies. The structure of heparin oligosaccharide fragments with high anti-(factor Xa) activity containing the minimal antithrombin III-binding sequence. *Biochem J* 1981;197(3):599–609.
18. Palm M, Mattsson C. Pharmacokinetics of heparin and low molecular weight heparin fragment (Fragmin) in rabbits with impaired renal or metabolic clearance. *Thromb Haemost* 1987;58(3):932–935.
19. Siragusa S, Cosmi B, Piovella F, et al. Low-molecular-weight heparins and unfractionated heparin in the treatment of patients with acute venous thromboembolism: results of a meta-analysis. *Am J Med* 1996;100(3):269–277.
20. Holmer E, Mattsson C, Nilsson S. Anticoagulant and antithrombotic effects of heparin and low molecular weight heparin fragments in rabbits. *Thromb Res* 1982;25(6):475–485.
21. Andriuoli G, Mastacchi R, Barbanti M, et al. Comparison of the antithrombotic and haemorrhagic effects of heparin and a new low molecular weight heparin in rats. *Haemostasis* 1985;15(5):324–330.
22. Warkentin TE, Levine MN, Hirsh J, et al. Heparin-induced thrombocytopenia in patients treated with low-molecular-weight heparin or unfractionated heparin. *N Engl J Med* 1995;332(20):1330–1335.
23. Monreal M, Lafoz E, Olive A, et al. Comparison of subcutaneous unfractionated heparin with a low molecular weight heparin (Fragmin) in patients with venous thromboembolism and contraindications to coumarin. *Thromb Haemost* 1994;71(1):7–11.
24. Lensing AW, Prins MH, Davidson BL, et al. Treatment of deep venous thrombosis with low-molecular-weight heparins. A meta-analysis. *Arch Intern Med* 1995;155(6):601–607.
25. Gould MK, Dembitzer AD, Doyle RL, et al. Low-molecular-weight heparins compared with unfractionated heparin for treatment of acute deep venous thrombosis. A meta-analysis of randomized, controlled trials. *Ann Intern Med* 1999;130(10):800–809.
26. Dolovich LR, Ginsberg JS, Douketis JD, et al. A meta-analysis comparing low-molecular-weight heparins with unfractionated heparin in the treatment of venous thromboembolism: examining some unanswered questions regarding location of treatment, product type, and dosing frequency. *Arch Intern Med* 2000;160(2):181–188.
27. Cohen M, Demers C, Gurfinkel EP, et al. Efficacy and Safety of Subcutaneous Enoxaparin in Non-Q-Wave Coronary Events Study Group. A comparison of low-molecular-weight heparin with unfractionated heparin for unstable coronary artery disease. *N Engl J Med* 1997;337(7):447–452.
28. Klein W, Buchwald A, Hillis SE, et al. Fragmin in Unstable Coronary Artery Disease Study (FRIC). Comparison of low-molecular-weight heparin with unfractionated heparin acutely and with placebo for 6 weeks in the management of unstable coronary artery disease. *Circulation* 1997; 96(1):61–68.
29. Levine MN, Planes A, Hirsh J, et al. The relationship between anti-factor Xa level and clinical outcome in patients receiving enoxaparine low molecular weight heparin to prevent deep vein thrombosis after hip replacement. *Thromb Haemost* 1989;62(3):940–944.
30. Alhenc-Gelas M, Jestin-Le Guernic C, Vitoux JF, et al. Fragmin-Study Group. Adjusted versus fixed doses of the low-molecular-weight heparin fragmin in the treatment of deep vein thrombosis. *Thromb Haemost* 1994; 71(6):698–702.
31. Albada J, Nieuwenhuis HK, Sixma JJ. Results of a Double-Blind Randomized Study. Treatment of acute venous thromboembolism with low molecular weight heparin (Fragmin). *Circulation* 1989;80(4):935–940.
32. Nieuwenhuis HK, Albada J, Banga JD, et al. Identification of risk factors for bleeding during treatment of acute venous thromboembolism with heparin or low molecular weight heparin. *Blood* 1991;78(9): 2337–2343.
33. Abbate R, Gori AM, Farsi A, et al. Monitoring of low-molecular-weight heparins in cardiovascular disease. *Am J Cardiol* 1998;82(5B):33L–36L.
34. Laposata M, Green D, Van Cott EM, et al. College of American Pathologists Conference XXXI on laboratory monitoring of anticoagulant therapy: the clinical use and laboratory monitoring of low-molecular-weight heparin, danaparoid, hirudin and related compounds, and argatroban. *Arch Pathol Lab Med* 1998; 122(9):799–807.
35. Gram J, Mercker S, Bruhn HD. Does protamine chloride neutralize low molecular weight heparin sufficiently? *Thromb Res* 1988;52(5):353–359.
36. Sugiyama T, Itoh M, Ohtawa M, et al. Study on neutralization of low molecular weight heparin (LHG) by protamine sulfate and its neutralization characteristics. *Thromb Res* 1992;68(2):119–129.
37. Wolzt M, Weltermann A, Nieszpaur-Los M, et al. Studies on the neutralizing effects of protamine on unfractionated and low molecular weight heparin (Fragmin) at the site of activation of the coagulation system in man. *Thromb Haemost* 1995;73(3): 439–443.
38. Warkentin TE, Sheppard JI. Generation of platelet-derived microparticles and procoagulant activity by heparin-induced thrombocytopenia IgG/serum and other IgG platelet agonists: a comparison with standard platelet agonists. *Platelets* 1999;10:319–326.
39. Pouplard C, Iochmann S, Renard B, et al. Induction of monocyte tissue factor expression by antibodies to heparin-platelet factor 4 complexes developed in heparin-induced thrombocytopenia. *Blood* 2001;97(10): 3300–3302.
40. Warkentin TE, Elavathil LJ, Hayward CP, et al. The pathogenesis of venous limb gangrene associated with heparin-induced thrombocytopenia. *Ann Intern Med* 1997;127(9):804–812.
41. Warkentin TE, Sheppard JA, Horsewood P, et al. Impact of the patient population on the risk for heparin-induced thrombocytopenia. *Blood* 2000;96(5):1703–1708.
42. Warkentin TE. Platelet count monitoring and laboratory testing for heparin-induced thrombocytopenia. *Arch Pathol Lab Med* 2002;126(11): 1415–1423.
43. Eichler P, Raschke R, Lubenow N, et al. The new ID-heparin/PF4 antibody test for rapid detection of heparin-induced antibodies in comparison with functional and antigenic assays. *Br J Haematol* 2002;116(4):887–891.
44. Warkentin TE. Heparin-induced thrombocytopenia: pathogenesis and management. *Br J Haematol* 2003;121(4):535–555.
45. Warkentin TE, Kelton JG. A 14-year study of heparin-induced thrombocytopenia. *Am J Med* 1996;101(5):502–507.
46. Wallis DE, Quintos R, Wehrmacher W, et al. Safety of warfarin anticoagulation in patients with heparin-induced thrombocytopenia. *Chest* 1999;116(5):1333–1338.

47. Ginsberg JS, Kowalchuk G, Hirsh J, et al. Heparin effect on bone density. *Thromb Haemost* 1990;64(2):286–289.

48. Dahlman TC. Osteoporotic fractures and the recurrence of thromboembolism during pregnancy and the puerperium in 184 women undergoing thromboprophylaxis with heparin. *Am J Obstet Gynecol* 1993;168(4):1265–1270.

49. Douketis JD, Ginsberg JS, Burrows RF, et al. A Prospective Matched Cohort Study. The effects of long-term heparin therapy during pregnancy on bone density. *Thromb Haemost* 1996;75(2):254–257.

50. Shaughnessy SG, Young E, Deschamps P, et al. The effects of low molecular weight and standard heparin on calcium loss from fetal rat calvaria. *Blood* 1995;86(4):1368–1373.

51. Danhof M, de Boer A, Magnani HN, et al. Pharmacokinetic considerations on Orgaran (Org 10172) therapy. *Haemostasis* 1992;22(2):73–84.

52. De Boer A, Stiekema JC, Danhof M, et al. The influence of Org 10172, a low molecular weight heparinoid, on antipyrine metabolism and the effect of enzyme induction on the response to Org 10172. *Br J Clin Pharmacol* 1991;32(1):23–29.

53. Turpie AG, Levine MN, Hirsh J, et al. Double-blind randomised trial of Org 10172 low-molecular-weight heparinoid in prevention of deep-vein thrombosis in thrombotic stroke. *Lancet* 1987;1(8532):523–526.

54. de Valk HW, Banga JD, Wester JW, et al. Comparing subcutaneous danaparoid with intravenous unfractionated heparin for the treatment of venous thromboembolism. A randomized controlled trial. *Ann Intern Med* 1995;123(1):1–9.

55. Farner B, Eichler P, Kroll H, et al. A comparison of danaparoid and lepirudin in heparin-induced thrombocytopenia. *Thromb Haemost* 2001;85(6):950–957.

56. Stiekema JC, Wijnand HP, ten Cate H, et al. Partial *in vivo* neutralisation of plasma anticoagulant effects of Lomoparan (Org 10172) by protamine chloride. *Thromb Res* 1991;63(1):157–167.

57. Khamashta MA, Cuadrado MJ, Mujic F, et al. The management of thrombosis in the antiphospholipid-antibody syndrome. *N Engl J Med* 1995;332(15):993–997.

58. Rosove MH, Brewer PM. Antiphospholipid thrombosis: clinical course after the first thrombotic event in 70 patients. *Ann Intern Med* 1992;117(4):303–308.

59. Crowther MA, Ginsberg JS, Julian J, et al. A comparison of two intensities of warfarin for the prevention of recurrent thrombosis in patients with the antiphospholipid antibody syndrome. *N Engl J Med* 2003;349(12):1133–1138.

60. Wallin R, Martin LF. Vitamin K-dependent carboxylation and vitamin K metabolism in liver. Effects of warfarin. *J Clin Invest* 1985;76(5):1879–1884.

61. Malhotra OP. Dicoumarol-induced prothrombins containing 6, 7, and 8 gamma-carboxyglutamic acid residues: isolation and characterization. *Biochem Cell Biol* 1989;67(8):411–421.

62. Malhotra OP. Dicoumarol-induced 9-gamma-carboxyglutamic acid prothrombin: isolation and comparison with the 6-, 7-, 8-, and 10-gamma-carboxyglutamic acid isomers. *Biochem Cell Biol* 1990;68(4):705–715.

63. Harrison L, Johnston M, Massicotte MP, et al. Comparison of 5-mg and 10-mg loading doses in initiation of warfarin therapy. *Ann Intern Med* 1997;126(2):133–136.

64. Marder VJ, Shulman NR. Clinical aspects of congenital factor VII deficiency. *Am J Med* 1964;37:182–194.

65. Wessler S, Gitel SN. Warfarin. From bedside to bench. *N Engl J Med* 1984;311(0):645–652.

66. Zivelin A, Rao LV, Rapaport SI. Mechanism of the anticoagulant effect of warfarin as evaluated in rabbits by selective depression of individual procoagulant vitamin K-dependent clotting factors. *J Clin Invest* 1993;92(5):2131–2140.

67. Patel RJ, Witt DM, Saseen JJ, et al. Randomized, placebo-controlled trial of oral phytonadione for excessive anticoagulation. *Pharmacotherapy* 2000;20(10):1159–1166.

68. Vigano S, Mannucci PM, Solinas S, et al. Decrease in protein C antigen and formation of an abnormal protein soon after starting oral anticoagulant therapy. *Br J Haematol* 1984;57(2):213–220.

69. Crowther MA, Ginsberg JB, Kearon C, et al. A randomized trial comparing 5-mg and 10-mg warfarin loading doses. *Arch Intern Med* 1999;159(1):46–48.

70. Furie B, Diuguid CF, Jacobs M, et al. Randomized prospective trial comparing the native prothrombin antigen with the prothrombin time for monitoring oral anticoagulant therapy. *Blood* 1990;75(2):344–349.

71. Breckenridge A, Orme M, Wesseling H, et al. Pharmacokinetics and pharmacodynamics of the enantiomers of warfarin in man. *Clin Pharmacol Ther* 1974;15(4):424–430.

72. King SY, Joslin MA, Raudibaugh K, et al. Dose-dependent pharmacokinetics of warfarin in healthy volunteers. *Pharm Res* 1995;12(12):1874–1877.

73. Sutcliffe FA, MacNicoll AD, Gibson GG. Aspects of anticoagulant action: a review of the pharmacology, metabolism and toxicology of warfarin and congeners. *Rev Drug Metab Drug Interact* 1987;5(4):225–272.

74. O'Reilly RA, Rytand DA. "Resistance" to warfarin due to unrecognized vitamin K supplementation. *N Engl J Med* 1980;303(3):160–161.

75. Suttie JW, Mummah-Schendel LL, Shah DV, et al. Vitamin K deficiency from dietary vitamin K restriction in humans. *Am J Clin Nutr* 1988;47(3):475–480.

76. Booth SL, Charnley JM, Sadowski JA, et al. Dietary vitamin K1 and stability of oral anticoagulation: proposal of a diet with constant vitamin K1 content. *Thromb Haemost* 1997;77(3):504–509.

77. Aithal GP, Day CP, Kesteven PJ, et al. Association of polymorphisms in the cytochrome P450 CYP2C9 with warfarin dose requirement and risk of bleeding complications. *Lancet* 1999;353(9154):717–719.

78. Mannucci PM. Genetic control of anticoagulation. *Lancet* 1999;353(9154):688–689.

79. Harris JE. Interaction of dietary factors with oral anticoagulants: review and applications. *J Am Diet Assoc* 1995;95(5):580–584.

80. O'Reilly RA, Pool JG, Aggeler PM. Hereditary resistance to coumarin anticoagulant drugs in man and rat. *Ann N Y Acad Sci* 1968;151(2):913–931.

81. Alving BM, Strickler MP, Knight RD, et al. Hereditary warfarin resistance. Investigation of a rare phenomenon. *Arch Intern Med* 1985;145(3):499–501.

82. Chu K, Wu SM, Stanley T, et al. A mutation in the propeptide of Factor IX leads to warfarin sensitivity by a novel mechanism. *J Clin Invest* 1996;98(7):1619–1625.

83. Oldenburg J, Quenzel EM, Harbrecht U, et al. Missense mutations at ALA-10 in the factor IX propeptide: an insignificant variant in normal life but a decisive cause of bleeding during oral anticoagulant therapy. *Br J Haematol* 1997;98(1):240–244.

84. Wells PS, Holbrook AM, Crowther NR, et al. Interactions of warfarin with drugs and food. *Ann Intern Med* 1994;121(9):676–683.

85. O'Reilly RA. Studies on the optical enantiomorphs of warfarin in man. *Clin Pharmacol Ther* 1974;16(2):348–354.

86. Hylek EM, Heiman H, Skates SJ, et al. Acetaminophen and other risk factors for excessive warfarin anticoagulation. *Jama* 1998;279(9):657–662.

87. Owens JC, Neely WB, Owen WR. Effect of sodium dextrothyroxine in patients receiving anticoagulants. *N Engl J Med* 1962;266:76–79.

88. O'Reilly RA. Stereoselective interaction of trimethoprim-sulfamethoxazole with the separated enantiomorphs of racemic warfarin in man. *N Engl J Med* 1980;302(1):33–35.

89. O'Reilly RA. Lack of effect of fortified wine ingested during fasting and anticoagulant therapy. *Arch Intern Med* 1981;141(4):458–459.

90. Dale J, Myhre E, Loew D. Bleeding during acetylsalicylic acid and anticoagulant therapy in patients with reduced platelet reactivity after aortic valve replacement. *Am Heart J* 1980;99(6):746–752.

91. Chesebro JH, Fuster V, Elveback LR, et al. Trial of combined warfarin plus dipyridamole or aspirin therapy in prosthetic heart valve replacement: danger of aspirin compared with dipyridamole. *Am J Cardiol* 1983;51(9):1537–1541.

92. Poller L, Taberner DA. Dosage and control of oral anticoagulants: an international collaborative survey. *Br J Haematol* 1982;51(3):479–485.

93. Poller L. Thromboplastin and oral anticoagulant control. *Br J Haematol* 1987;67(1):116–117.

94. Poller L. INR—calibration of the therapeutic range. *Adv Exp Med Biol* 1987;214:95–112.

95. Poller L. Laboratory control of oral anticoagulants. *Br Med J (Clin Res Ed)* 1987;294(6581):1184.

96. Latallo ZS, Thomson JM, Poller L. An evaluation of chromogenic substrates in the control of oral anticoagulant therapy. *Br J Haematol* 1981;47(2):307–318.

97. Tripodi A, Chantarangkul V, Braga M, et al. Results of a multicenter study assessing the status of standardization of a recombinant thromboplastin for the control of oral anticoagulant therapy. *Thromb Haemost* 1994;72(2):261–267.

98. Poller L. International Normalized Ratios (INR): the first 20 years. *J Thromb Haemost* 2004;2(6):849–860.

99. Johnston M, Harrison L, Moffat K, et al. Reliability of the international normalized ratio for monitoring the induction phase of warfarin: comparison with the prothrombin time ratio. *J Lab Clin Med* 1996;128(2):214–217.

100. Kovacs MJ, Wong A, MacKinnon K, et al. Assessment of the validity of the INR system for patients with liver impairment. *Thromb Haemost* 1994;71(6):727–730.

101. Poggio M, van den Besselaar AM, van der Velde EA, et al. The effect of some instruments for prothrombin time testing on the International Sensitivity Index (ISI) of two rabbit tissue thromboplastin reagents. *Thromb Haemost* 1989;62(3):868–874.

102. Ray MJ, Smith IR. The dependence of the International Sensitivity Index on the coagulometer used to perform the prothrombin time. *Thromb Haemost* 1990;63(3):424–429.

103. Ng VL, Levin J, Corash L, et al. Failure of the International Normalized Ratio to generate consistent results within a local medical community. *Am J Clin Pathol* 1993;99(6):689–694.

104. Kazama M, Suzuki S, Abe T, et al. Evaluation of international normalized ratios by a controlled field survey with 4 different thromboplastin reagents. *Thromb Haemost* 1990;64(4):535–541.

105. Tripodi A, Chantarangkul V, Clerici M, et al. Results of a Collaborative Study Involving Nine Commercial Thromboplastins. Laboratory control of oral anticoagulant treatment by the INR system in patients with the antiphospholipid syndrome and lupus anticoagulant. *Br J Haematol* 2001;115(3):672–678.

106. O'Reilly RA, Aggeler PM. Studies on coumarin anticoagulant drugs. Initiation of warfarin therapy without a loading dose. *Circulation* 1968;38(1):169–177.

107. Kovacs MJ, Rodger M, Anderson DR, et al. Comparison of 10-mg and 5-mg warfarin initiation nomograms together with low-molecular-weight heparin for outpatient treatment of acute venous thromboembolism. A randomized, double-blind, controlled trial. *Ann Intern Med* 2003;138(9):714–719.

108. Kovacs MJ, Cruickshank M, Wells PS, et al. Randomized assessment of a warfarin nomogram for initial oral anticoagulation after venous thromboembolic disease. *Haemostasis* 1998;28(2):62–69.

109. O'Connell MB, Kowal PR, Allivato CJ, et al. Evaluation of warfarin initiation regimens in elderly inpatients. *Pharmacotherapy* 2000;20(8):923–930.

110. Landefeld CS, Goldman L. Major bleeding in outpatients treated with warfarin: incidence and prediction by factors known at the start of outpatient therapy. *Am J Med* 1989;87(2):144–152.

111. Beyth RJ, Quinn LM, Landefeld CS. Prospective evaluation of an index for predicting the risk of major bleeding in outpatients treated with warfarin. *Am J Med* 1998;105(2):91–99.

112. Ageno W, Turpie AG. Exaggerated initial response to warfarin following heart valve replacement. *Am J Cardiol* 1999;84(8):905–908.

113. White RH, McKittrick T, Hutchinson R, et al. Temporary discontinuation of warfarin therapy: changes in the international normalized ratio. *Ann Intern Med* 1995;122(1):40–42.

114. Anticoagulants in the Secondary Prevention of Events in Coronary Thrombosis (ASPECT) Research Group. Effect of long-term oral anticoagulant treatment on mortality and cardiovascular morbidity after myocardial infarction. *Lancet* 1994;343(8896):499–503.

115. Hylek EM, Singer DE. Risk factors for intracranial hemorrhage in outpatients taking warfarin. *Ann Intern Med* 1994;120(11):897–902.

116. The Stroke Prevention in Reversible Ischemia Trial (SPIRIT) Study Group. A randomized trial of anticoagulants versus aspirin after cerebral ischemia of presumed arterial origin. *Ann Neurol* 1997;42(6):857–865.

117. Halperin B, Kron J, Wynn M, et al. Adjusted-dose warfarin versus low-intensity, fixed-dose aspirin plus aspirin for high-risk patients with atrial fibrillation: stroke prevention in atrial fibrillation III randomised clinical trial. *Lancet* 1996;348(9028):633–638.

118. Albers GW. Atrial fibrillation and stroke. Three new studies, three remaining questions. *Arch Intern Med* 1994;154(13):1443–1448.

119. Rose PE, Gilbert M. Computer control of anticoagulant dose. *BMJ* 1989;299(6714):1529.

120. Wyld PJ, West D, Wilson TH. Computer dosing in anticoagulant clinics—the way forward? *Clin Lab Haematol* 1988;10(2):235–236.

121. Ryan PJ, Gilbert M, Rose PE. Computer control of anticoagulant dose for therapeutic management. *BMJ* 1989;299(6709):1207–1209.

122. Poller L, Wright D, Rowlands M. Prospective comparative study of computer programs used for management of warfarin. *J Clin Pathol* 1993;46(4):299–303.

123. Poller L, Shiach CR, MacCallum PK, et al. Multicentre randomised study of computerised anticoagulant dosage. European concerted action on anticoagulation. *Lancet* 1998; 352(9139):1505–1509.

124. Cromheecke ME, Levi M, Colly LP, et al. Oral anticoagulation self-management and management by a specialist anticoagulation clinic: a randomised cross-over comparison. *Lancet* 2000;356(9224):97–102.

125. Ansell J, Hirsh J, Dalen J, et al. Managing oral anticoagulant therapy. *Chest* 2001;119 (Suppl. 1):22S–38S.

126. Oden A, Fahlen M. Oral anticoagulation and risk of death: a medical record linkage study. *BMJ* 2002;325(7372):1073–1075.

127. Landefeld CS, Rosenblatt MW, Goldman L. Bleeding in outpatients treated with warfarin: relation to the prothrombin time and important remediable lesions. *Am J Med* 1989;87(2):153–159.

128. Samsa GP, Matchar DB, Goldstein LB, et al. Quality of anticoagulation management among patients with atrial fibrillation: results of a review of medical records from 2 communities. *Arch Intern Med* 2000;160(7):967–973.

129. McMahan DA, Smith DM, Carey MA, et al. Risk of major hemorrhage for outpatients treated with warfarin. *J Gen Intern Med* 1998;13(5):311–316.

130. Kearon C, Ginsberg JS, Kovacs MJ, et al. Comparison of low-intensity warfarin therapy with conventional-intensity warfarin therapy for long-term prevention of recurrent venous thromboembolism. *N Engl J Med* 2003;349(7):631–639.

131. Hull R, Hirsh J, Jay R, et al. Different intensities of oral anticoagulant therapy in the treatment of proximal-vein thrombosis. *N Engl J Med* 1982;307(27):1676–1681.

132. Stein PD, Alpert JS, Bussey HI, et al. Antithrombotic therapy in patients with mechanical and biological prosthetic heart valves. *Chest* 2001; 119(Suppl. 1):220S–227S.

133. Levine M, Hirsh J, Gent M, et al. Double-blind randomised trial of a very-low-dose warfarin for prevention of thromboembolism in stage IV breast cancer. *Lancet* 1994;343(8902):886–889.

134. Deveras RA, Kessler CM. Reversal of warfarin-induced excessive anticoagulation with recombinant human factor VIIa concentrate. *Ann Intern Med* 2002;137(11):884–888.

135. Glover JJ, Morrill GB. Conservative treatment of overanticoagulated patients. *Chest* 1995;108(4):987–990.

136. Lousberg TR, Witt DM, Beall DG, et al. Evaluation of excessive anticoagulation in a group model health maintenance organization. *Arch Intern Med* 1998;158(5):528–534.

137. Whitling AM, Bussey HI, Lyons RM. Comparing different routes and doses of phytonadione for reversing excessive anticoagulation. *Arch Intern Med* 1998;158(19):2136–2140.

138. Shetty HG, Backhouse G, Bentley DP, et al. Effective reversal of warfarin-induced excessive anticoagulation with low dose vitamin K1. *Thromb Haemost* 1992;67(1):13–15.

139. de la Rubia J, Grau E, Montserrat I, et al. Anaphylactic shock and vitamin K1. *Ann Intern Med* 1989;110(11):943.

140. Havel M, Muller M, Graninger W, et al. Tolerability of a new vitamin K1 preparation for parenteral administration to adults: one case of anaphylactoid reaction. *Clin Ther* 1987;9(4):373–379.

141. Martinez-Abad M, Delgado F, Palop V, et al. Vitamin K1 and anaphylactic shock. *Dicp* 1991;25(7-8):871–872.

142. Wilkins K, DeKoven J, Assaad D. Cutaneous reactions associated with vitamin K1. *J Cutan Med Surg* 2000;4(3):164–168.

143. Andersen P, Godal HC. Predictable reduction in anticoagulant activity of warfarin by small amounts of vitamin K. *Acta Med Scand* 1975;198(4):269–270.

144. Nee R, Doppenschmidt D, Donovan DJ, et al. Intravenous versus subcutaneous vitamin K1 in reversing excessive oral anticoagulation. *Am J Cardiol* 1999;83(2):286–288, A6–7.

145. Raj G, Kumar R, McKinney WP. Time course of reversal of anticoagulant effect of warfarin by intravenous and subcutaneous phytonadione. *Arch Intern Med* 1999;159(22):2721–2724.

146. Crowther MA, Douketis JD, Schnurr T, et al. Oral vitamin K lowers the international normalized ratio more rapidly than subcutaneous vitamin K in the treatment of warfarin-associated coagulopathy. A randomized, controlled trial. *Ann Intern Med* 2002;137(4):251–254.

147. Crowther MA, Donovan D, Harrison L, et al. Low-dose oral vitamin K reliably reverses over-anticoagulation due to warfarin. *Thromb Haemost* 1998;79(6):1116–1118.

148. Crowther MA, Julian J, McCarty D, et al. Treatment of warfarin-associated coagulopathy with oral vitamin K: a randomised controlled trial. *Lancet* 2000;356(9241):1551–1553.

149. Duong TM, Plowman BK, Morreale AP, et al. Retrospective and prospective analyses of the treatment of overanticoagulated patients. *Pharmacotherapy* 1998;18(6):1264–1270.

150. Cartmill M, Dolan G, Byrne JL, et al. Prothrombin complex concentrate for oral anticoagulant reversal in neurosurgical emergencies. *Br J Neurosurg* 2000;14(5):458–461.

151. Makris M, Greaves M, Phillips WS, et al. Emergency oral anticoagulant reversal: the relative efficacy of infusions of fresh frozen plasma and clotting factor concentrate on correction of the coagulopathy. *Thromb Haemost* 1997;77(3):477–480.

152. Lin J, Hanigan WC, Tarantino M, et al. The use of recombinant activated factor VII to reverse warfarin-induced anticoagulation in patients with hemorrhages in the central nervous system: preliminary findings. *J Neurosurg* 2003;98(4):737–740.

153. Sorensen B, Johansen P, Nielsen GL, et al. Reversal of the International Normalized Ratio with recombinant activated factor VII in central nervous system bleeding during warfarin thromboprophylaxis: clinical and biochemical aspects. *Blood Coagul Fibrinolysis* 2003;14(5):469–477.

154. Hylek EM, Skates SJ, Sheehan MA, et al. An analysis of the lowest effective intensity of prophylactic anticoagulation for patients with non-rheumatic atrial fibrillation. *N Engl J Med* 1996;335(8):540–546.

155. Verhagen H. Local hemorrhage and necrosis of the skin and underlying tissues at starting therapy with dicumarol or dicymacyl. *Acta Med Scand* 1954;148:455–467.

156. Broekmans AW, Bertina RM, Loeliger EA, et al. Protein C and the development of skin necrosis during anticoagulant therapy. *Thromb Haemost* 1983;49(3):251.

157. Zauber NP, Stark MW. Successful warfarin anticoagulation despite protein C deficiency and a history of warfarin necrosis. *Ann Intern Med* 1986;104(5):659–660.

158. Grimaudo V, Gueissaz F, Hauert J, et al. Necrosis of skin induced by coumarin in a patient deficient in protein S. *BMJ* 1989;298(6668):233–234.

159. Samama M, Horellou MH, Soria J, et al. Successful progressive anticoagulation in a severe protein C deficiency and previous skin necrosis at the initiation of oral anticoagulant treatment. *Thromb Haemost* 1984;51(1):132–133.

160. Kwong P, Roberts P, Prescott SM, et al. Dermatitis induced by warfarin. *Jama* 1978;239(18):1884–1885.

161. Petitou M, van Boeckel CA. Chemical synthesis of heparin fragments and analogues. *Fortschr Chem Org Naturst* 1992;60:143–210.

162. Olson ST, Bjork I, Sheffer R, et al. Role of the antithrombin-binding pentasaccharide in heparin acceleration of antithrombin-proteinase reactions. Resolution of the antithrombin conformational change contribution to heparin rate enhancement. *J Biol Chem* 1992;267(18):12528–12538.

163. Amiral J, Lormeau JC, Marfaing-Koka A, et al. Absence of cross-reactivity of SR90107A/ORG31540 pentasaccharide with antibodies to heparin-PF4 complexes developed in heparin-induced thrombocytopenia. *Blood Coagul Fibrinolysis* 1997;8(2):114–117.

164. Donat F, Duret JP, Santoni A, et al. The pharmacokinetics of fondaparinux sodium in healthy volunteers. *Clin Pharmacokinet* 2002; 41(Suppl. 2):1–9.

165. Donat F, Duret JP, Santoni A. Pharmacokinetics of Org 31540/Sr90107A in young and elderly healthy subjects: a highly favourable pharmacokinetic profile. *Thromb Haemost* 2001;(Suppl. 1);1:3094 (CD-ROM).

166. Herbert JM, Petitou M, Lormeau JC. SR 90107A/Org 31540, a novel anti-factor Xa antithrombotic agent. *Cardiovasc Drug Rev* 1997;15:1–26.

167. Ollier C, Faaij RA, Santoni A, et al. Absence of interaction of fondaparinux sodium with aspirin and piroxicam in healthy male volunteers. *Clin Pharmacokinet* 2002;41(Suppl. 2):31–37.

168. Faaij RA, Burggraaf J, Schoemaker RC, et al. The synthetic pentasaccharide fondaparinux sodium does not interact with oral warfarin. *Clin Pharmacokinet* 2002;41(Suppl.2):27–29.

169. Bijsterveld NR, Moons AH, Boekholdt SM, et al. Ability of recombinant factor VIIa to reverse the anticoagulant effect of the pentasaccharide fondaparinux in healthy volunteers. *Circulation* 2002;106(20):2550–2554.

170. Lassen MR, Bauer KA, Eriksson BI, et al. Postoperative fondaparinux versus preoperative enoxaparin for prevention of venous thromboembolism in elective hip-replacement surgery: a randomised double-blind comparison. *Lancet* 2002; 359(9319):1715–1720.

171. Turpie AG, Bauer KA, Eriksson BI, et al. Postoperative fondaparinux versus postoperative enoxaparin for prevention of venous thromboembolism after elective hip-replacement surgery: a randomised double-blind trial. *Lancet* 2002;359(9319):1721–1726.

172. Eriksson BI, Bauer KA, Lassen MR, et al. Fondaparinux compared with enoxaparin for the prevention of venous thromboembolism after hip-fracture surgery. *N Engl J Med* 2001;345(18):1298–1304.

173. Bauer KA, Eriksson BI, Lassen MR, et al. Fondaparinux compared with enoxaparin for the prevention of venous thromboembolism after elective major knee surgery. *N Engl J Med* 2001;345(18):1305–1310.

174. Buller HR, Davidson BL, Decousus H, et al. Fondaparinux or enoxaparin for the initial treatment of symptomatic deep venous thrombosis: a randomized trial. *Ann Intern Med* 2004;140(11):867–873.

175. Buller HR, Davidson BL, Decousus H, et al. Subcutaneous fondaparinux versus intravenous unfractionated heparin in the initial treatment of pulmonary embolism. *N Engl J Med* 2003;349(18):1695–1702.

176. Herbert JM, Herault JP, Bernat A, et al. Biochemical and pharmacological properties of SANORG 34006, a potent and long-acting synthetic pentasaccharide. *Blood* 1998;91(11):4197–4205.

177. Okamoto S, Hijikata A, Kikumoto R, et al. Potent inhibition of thrombin by the newly synthesized arginine derivative No. 805. The importance of stereo-structure of its hydrophobic carboxamide portion. *Biochem Biophys Res Commun* 1981; 101(2):440–446.

178. Okamoto S, Hijikata-Okunomiya A. Synthetic selective inhibitors of thrombin. *Methods Enzymol* 1993;222:328–340.

179. Berry C, Girardot C, Lecoffre C. Effects of the synthetic thrombin inhibitor argatroban on fibrin- or clot-incorporated thrombin: comparison with heparin and recombinant hirudin. *Thromb Haemost* 1994;72:381–386.

180. Izawa O, Katsuki M, Komatsu T. (MD-805) in humans: concentrations of argatroban and its metabolites in plasma, urine and feces during and after drip intravenous infusion. *Jpn Pharmacol Ther* 1986;14:251–263.

181. Swan SK, Hursting MJ. The pharmacokinetics and pharmacodynamics of argatroban: effects of age, gender, and hepatic or renal dysfunction. *Pharmacotherapy* 2000;20(3):318–329.

182. Tran JQ, Di Cicco RA, Sheth SB, et al. Assessment of the potential pharmacokinetic and pharmacodynamic interactions between erythromycin and argatroban. *J Clin Pharmacol* 1999;39(5):513–519.

183. Sheth SB, DiCicco RA, Hursting MJ, et al. Interpreting the International Normalized Ratio (INR) in individuals receiving argatroban and warfarin. *Thromb Haemost* 2001;85(3):435–440.

184. Warkentin TE, Greinacher A, eds. *Heparin induced thrombocytopenia*, 2nd ed. New York: Marcel Dekker Inc, 2001.

185. Markwardt F. Hirudin: the promising antithrombotic. *Cardiovasc Drug Rev* 1992;10:211–232.

186. Pieters J, Lindhout T, Hemker HC. In situ-generated thrombin is the only enzyme that effectively activates factor VIII and factor V in thromboplastin-activated plasma. *Blood* 1989;74(3):1021–1024.

187. Weitz JI, Hudoba M, Massel D, et al. Clot-bound thrombin is protected from inhibition by heparin-antithrombin III but is susceptible to inactivation by antithrombin III-independent inhibitors. *J Clin Invest* 1990;86(2):385–391.

188. Weitz JI, Leslie B, Hudoba M. Thrombin binds to soluble fibrin degradation products where it is protected from inhibition by heparin-antithrombin but susceptible to inactivation by antithrombin-independent inhibitors. *Circulation* 1998;97(6):544–552.

189. Nurmohamed MT, Berckmans RJ, Morrien-Salomons WM, et al. Monitoring anticoagulant therapy by activated partial thromboplastin time: hirudin assessment. An evaluation of native blood and plasma assays. *Thromb Haemost* 1994;72(5):685–692.

190. Potzsch B, Madlener K, Seelig C, et al. Monitoring of r-hirudin anticoagulation during cardiopulmonary bypass—assessment of the whole blood ecarin clotting time. *Thromb Haemost* 1997;77(5):920–925.

191. Nowak G, Bucha E. Quantitative determination of hirudin in blood and body fluids. *Semin Thromb Hemost* 1996;22(2):197–202.

192. Song X, Huhle G, Wang L, et al. Generation of anti-hirudin antibodies in heparin-induced thrombocytopenic patients treated with r-hirudin. *Circulation* 1999; 100(14):1528–1532.

193. Eichler P, Friesen HJ, Lubenow N, et al. Antihirudin antibodies in patients with heparin-induced thrombocytopenia treated with lepirudin: incidence, effects on aPTT, and clinical relevance. *Blood* 2000;96(7):2373–2378.

194. Fox I, Dawson A, Loynds P, et al. Anticoagulant activity of Hirulog, a direct thrombin inhibitor, in humans. *Thromb Haemost* 1993;69(2):157–163.

195. Robson R. The use of bivalirudin in patients with renal impairment. *J Invasive Cardiol* 2000;12(Suppl. F):33F–336.

196. Bittl JA, Strony J, Brinker JA, et al. Hirulog Angioplasty Study Investigators. Treatment with bivalirudin (Hirulog) as compared with heparin during coronary angioplasty for unstable or postinfarction angina. *N Engl J Med* 1995;333(12):764–769.

197. Lincoff AM, Kleiman NS, Kottke-Marchant K, et al. Bivalirudin with planned or provisional abciximab versus low-dose heparin and abciximab during percutaneous coronary revascularization: results of the Comparison of Abciximab Complications with Hirulog for Ischemic Events Trial (CACHET). *Am Heart J* 2002;143(5):847–853.

198. Lincoff AM, Bittl JA, Harrington RA, et al. Bivalirudin and provisional glycoprotein IIb/IIIa blockade compared with heparin and planned glycoprotein IIb/IIIa blockade during percutaneous coronary intervention: REPLACE-2 randomized trial. *JAMA* 2003;289(7):853–863.

199. Lincoff AM, Kleiman NS, Kereiakes DJ, et al. Long-term efficacy of bivalirudin and provisional glycoprotein IIb/IIIa blockade vs. heparin and planned glycoprotein IIb/IIIa blockade during percutaneous coronary revascularization: REPLACE-2 randomized trial. *JAMA* 2004;292(6):696–703.

200. Eriksson H, Eriksson UG, Frison L, et al. Pharmacokinetics and pharmacodynamics of melagatran, a novel synthetic LMW thrombin inhibitor, in patients with acute DVT. *Thromb Haemost* 1999;81(3):358–363.

201. Johansson LC, Frison L, Logren U, et al. Influence of age on the pharmacokinetics and pharmacodynamics of ximelagatran, an oral direct thrombin inhibitor. *Clin Pharmacokinet* 2003;42(4):381–392.

202. Eriksson UG, Bredberg U, Gislen K, et al. Pharmacokinetics and pharmacodynamics of ximelagatran, a novel oral direct thrombin inhibitor, in young healthy male subjects. *Eur J Clin Pharmacol* 2003;59(1):35–43.

203. Eriksson UG, Bredberg U, Hoffmann KJ, et al. Absorption, distribution, metabolism, and excretion of ximelagatran, an oral direct thrombin inhibitor, in rats, dogs, and humans. *Drug Metab Dispos* 2003;31(3):294–305.

204. Eriksson UG, Mandema JW, Karlsson MO, et al. Pharmacokinetics of melagatran and the effect on *ex vivo* coagulation time in orthopaedic surgery patients receiving subcutaneous melagatran and oral ximelagatran: a population model analysis. *Clin Pharmacokinet* 2003;42(7):687–701.

205. Elg M, Gustafsson D, Carlsson S. Antithrombotic effects and bleeding time of thrombin inhibitors and warfarin in the rat. *Thromb Res* 1999; 94(3):187–197.

206. Elg M, Gustafsson D, Deinum J. The importance of enzyme inhibition kinetics for the effect of thrombin inhibitors in a rat model of arterial thrombosis. *Thromb Haemost* 1997;78(4):1286–1292.

207. Gustafsson D, Nystrom J, Carlsson S, et al. The direct thrombin inhibitor melagatran and its oral prodrug H 376/95: intestinal absorption properties, biochemical and pharmacodynamic effects. *Thromb Res* 2001; 101(3):171–181.

208. Johansson LC, Andersson M, Fager G, et al. No influence of ethnic origin on the pharmacokinetics and pharmacodynamics of melagatran following oral administration of ximelagatran, a novel oral direct thrombin inhibitor, to healthy male volunteers. *Clin Pharmacokinet* 2003;42(5):475–484.

209. Sarich TC, Teng R, Peters GR, et al. No influence of obesity on the pharmacokinetics and pharmacodynamics of melagatran, the active form of the oral direct thrombin inhibitor ximelagatran. *Clin Pharmacokinet* 2003; 42(5):485–492.

210. Bredberg E, Andersson TB, Frison L, et al. Ximelagatran, an oral direct thrombin inhibitor, has a low potential for cytochrome P450-mediated drug-drug interactions. *Clin Pharmacokinet* 2003;42(8):765–777.

211. Petersen P, Grind M, Adler J. SPORTIF II: A Dose-Guiding, Tolerability, and Safety Study. Ximelagatran versus warfarin for stroke prevention in patients with nonvalvular atrial fibrillation. *J Am Coll Cardiol* 2003; 41(9):1445–1451.

212. Schulman S, Wahlander K, Lundstrom T, et al. Secondary prevention of venous thromboembolism with the oral direct thrombin inhibitor ximelagatran. *N Engl J Med* 2003;349(18):1713–1721.

213. Eriksson BI, Bergqvist D, Kalebo P, et al. Ximelagatran and melagatran compared with dalteparin for prevention of venous thromboembolism after total hip or knee replacement: the METHRO II randomised trial. *Lancet* 2002;360(9344):1441–1447.

214. Elg M. Factor VIIa reversed the prolonged bleeding time induced by a direct thrombin inhibitor in anaesthetised rats pre-treated with lipopolysaccharide. *Blood* 2001;98(11):P176, (abstract).

215. Eriksson BI, Agnelli G, Cohen AT, et al. Direct thrombin inhibitor melagatran followed by oral ximelagatran in comparison with enoxaparin for prevention of venous thromboembolism after total hip or knee replacement. *Thromb Haemost* 2003;89(2):288–296.

216. Eriksson BI, Agnelli G, Cohen AT, et al. The direct thrombin inhibitor melagatran followed by oral ximelagatran compared with enoxaparin for

the prevention of venous thromboembolism after total hip or knee replacement: the EXPRESS study. *J Thromb Haemost* 2003;1(12): 2490–2496.

217. Colwell CW Jr., Berkowitz SD, Davidson BL, et al. A Randomized, Double-Blind Study. Comparison of ximelagatran, an oral direct thrombin inhibitor, with enoxaparin for the prevention of venous thromboembolism following total hip replacement. *J Thromb Haemost* 2003;1(10): 2119–2130.

218. Olsson SB. Stroke prevention with the oral direct thrombin inhibitor ximelagatran compared with warfarin in patients with non-valvular atrial fibrillation (SPORTIF III): randomised controlled trial. *Lancet* 2003; 362(9397):1691–1698.

# CHAPTER 117 ■ ANTICOAGULATION CLINICS

RENE QUIROZ AND SAMUEL Z. GOLDHABER

## HISTORY OF ANTICOAGULATION CLINICS

Warfarin's narrow therapeutic index, numerous medication and dietary interactions, and genetic and physiologic variations in metabolism have spurred the development of specialized health care services to maximize effectiveness and safety of oral anticoagulation. The first thrombosis center specifically dedicated to managing oral anticoagulant therapy was based at the University of Utrecht, utilizing a model created by Professor S. C. Jordan in 1949. In the 1950s, internists and surgeons at the University of Michigan developed the first US anticoagulation clinic (1). In 1959, Sevitt and Gallagher proposed formal recognition of an anticoagulant unit in the United Kingdom (2).

The Dutch Federation of Thrombosis Centers, founded in 1971, currently encompasses 70 anticoagulation clinics, including two centers in Spain for vacationing patients (3), and serves more than 95% of the Dutch population. Approximately 270,000 patients and 3.5 million blood samples are monitored annually (3), and specialized software provides computerized dosage calculations and a database for research [Anticoagulants in the Secondary Prevention of Events in Coronary Thrombosis (ASPECT) (4) and Leiden Artificial Valves and Anticoagulation (LAVA) study (5)]. A quality control program for prothrombin time (PT) testing in collaboration with the RELAC (Reference Laboratory for Anticoagulant Control, Netherlands) laboratory has reduced the coefficient of variation among laboratories from 10% to 6% (3). Self-testing has become an important aspect of patient management. Since 2003, insurance reimburses for self-testing coagulation meters, testing strips, and patient education (6).

In Italy, the patient group AIPA (Associazione Italiana Pazienti Anticoagulati) was formed in 1987 and joined with FEDER (Federazione Italiana per l'Assistenza) in 1995. FEDER–AIPA comprises 235 anticoagulation clinics and manages more than 140,000 patients. The Italian Federation of Centers for the Surveillance of Anticoagulation Therapies was founded in 1989, consists of more than 200 centers, and has made important contributions to the field of venous thromboembolism (VTE) research (2,7–9). Similar patient organizations exist in Denmark (AK-Patientforeningen), Spain (FESAN), and the United Kingdom (Anticoagulation Europe Organization).

The Anticoagulation Forum (www.acforum.org), based in the United States, has a membership of approximately 3,000 individuals representing more than 1,100 anticoagulation clinics (1). A survey of 233 participating member clinics revealed that median patient enrollment is 250, with a median clinic age of 4 years, duration (10). The two principal indications for anticoagulation are heart valve replacement and atrial fibrillation.

Reduction in adverse clinical outcomes has led to lower hospitalization costs, thereby making anticoagulation clinics a cost-effective alternative to conventional care (11–13). The American College of Chest Physicians (ACCP) currently recommends (grade 1C) "physicians who manage oral anticoagulation therapy do so in a systematic and coordinated fashion, incorporating patient education, systematic international normalized ratios (INR) testing, tracking, follow-up, and good patient communication of results and dosing decisions" (14).

## A REPRESENTATIVE ANTICOAGULATION SERVICE

The multidisciplinary Anticoagulation Service at Brigham and Women's Hospital maximizes the effectiveness and safety of anticoagulant therapy by organized programs of education, coordination, monitoring, and communication between patients and health care workers (see Table 117-1). The service manages more than 1,700 patients, is supervised by a physician and staffed by five full-time equivalents, including physician assistants, pharmacists, a nurse, and an administrative assistant. The service has 24-hour coverage (including weekends and holidays) for cardiac surgery, cardiology, vascular surgery, thoracics, orthopedics, neurology, neurosurgery, internal medicine, and the primary care practices of the hospital. Indications for anticoagulation are atrial fibrillation (30%), VTE (24%), heart valve replacement or repair (15%), orthopedic surgery (15%), and miscellaneous (16%).

Inpatients are visited by staff daily to reinforce anticoagulation education, and an information sheet is placed in front of each patient's chart upon discharge.

Long-term anticoagulation management is optimized with electronic monitoring (Standing Stone), using software that includes patient demographics and documentation, anticoagulant doses, laboratory results, follow-up procedures, drug–drug and drug–food interactions, patient adherence, and adverse events. The software can track dates when patients are due for testing, whether appointments have been missed, bleeding and thrombotic complications, out-of-range INRs, and the number of new and discharged patients each month. This information facilitates monitoring outcomes, making timely adjustments in patient management, and providing a database for research endeavors.

Patient safety, satisfaction, education, and communication are the most important factors for a successful anticoagulation clinic, and the anticoagulation service helps to provide a seamless transition from the inpatient to the community setting.

**TABLE 117-1**

BRIGHAM AND WOMEN'S HOSPITAL
ANTICOAGULATION SERVICE MISSION STATEMENT

Maximize effectiveness and safety of anticoagulation by
providing:
1. Careful monitoring and dosing of injectable and oral anticoagulants among hospitalized patients and outpatients
2. Facilitating and coordinating anticoagulation care among
   inpatient providers, phlebotomists, laboratories, skilled
   nursing facilities, and private residences, and keeping the
   primary care provider informed of changes
3. Bridging anticoagulation management between the home
   and hospital settings
4. Educating patients, families, and professionals about the
   most recent developments in anticoagulation therapy
5. Continuous quality improvement to minimize thromboembolic and hemorrhagic complications, including tracking
   and critique of each complication that does occur
6. Organizing and participating in clinical research projects,
   including registries and clinical trials

# MEMBERS OF THE ANTICOAGULATION SERVICE

Most US anticoagulation clinics are affiliated with teaching or
community hospitals and managed by nurses and pharmacists,
with a supervising physician. In general, one full-time provider
is assigned to approximately 300 patients. The provider
requires specialized training (15–17), a reliable follow-up or
patient tracking system, INR monitoring, patient education,
and a communication system (14,18,19). The ACCP Consensus Conference on Antithrombotic Therapy has endorsed anticoagulation clinics (14,20) and concludes that failure to use
such services may increase the risk of legal liability (21).

A variety of different anticoagulation clinic structures exists
(22–26). Depending on the circumstance, clinics may be composed primarily of pharmacists (12,15,17,27–38), integrated
physician–physician assistant–pharmacist groups (38–43), or
telephone-based services (44–47). Choosing an appropriate anticoagulation clinic structure depends on local factors such as
patient population, community- or university-based hospital,
and liability, and adjustments should be made accordingly.

Although anticoagulation clinics are widespread (48), caution must be advised to preserve a stable doctor–patient relationship (49), especially in clinics that depend completely on a
telephone-based service (50), which is vulnerable to inadequate
patient education and poor compliance (51,52). In general, patients and physicians describe receiving helpful information
from anticoagulation clinics (46,53) and satisfaction with having anticoagulation clinics manage warfarin therapy (54). Physicians who enroll patients tend to be satisfied and recommend
the service to other colleagues (46,53,55), although there remains some skepticism toward the universal application (49)
of clinical practice guidelines (56–60).

Computerized systems have offered substantial advantages
to health care providers (61). These systems facilitate access to
patient records, alert practitioners for noncompliant patients
and INR values outside defined criteria, provide dosage guidelines, and represent a potential database for clinical research
(24,61–64). In a study by Ryan et al. hospital anticoagulant control was improved with a computerized decision support system,
from approximately 50% of INR results in range prior to its introduction, to 80% in range after its implementation (65).

# ANTICOAGULATION CLINIC MANAGEMENT VERSUS CONVENTIONAL CARE

Various studies have evaluated different models of patient anticoagulation (5,7,8,12,13,15–17,38,64,66–82). Some studies
indicate that anticoagulation clinics provide better anticoagulant care than do family physicians (11–13,15,38,64,77–84),
resulting in improved management and fewer thrombotic and
hemorrhagic complications (see Table 117-2). Under anticoagulation clinic care, major hemorrhage rates have ranged from
5.0% (68) to 8.1% (67) per patient-year of therapy, although
a uniform definition of major hemorrhage was not used.

Chiquette et al. compared outcomes in 142 patients (102
patient-years) receiving conventional care with 176 patients
(123 patient-years) receiving anticoagulation clinic management (13). Although there was no difference between both
groups in target therapeutic range (TTR) for patients receiving
lower-range anticoagulation therapy, patients under the Anticoagulation Service management receiving higher-range anticoagulation therapy had significantly more INRs within
therapeutic range. A 50% and 80% reduction in major or
fatal bleeding and thromboembolic events, respectively, was
observed in the anticoagulation clinic managed group. Hospitalizations and emergency department visits related to anticoagulation were reduced by 73% in the anticoagulation service
group, yielding an annual savings of more than $132,000 per
100 patients. Anticoagulation clinics are also more cost-effective
by reducing hospitalizations for complications of anticoagulant therapy (11–13,91), suggesting a savings of approximately
$1,500 per patient-year of therapy (13,14).

Although most studies report major benefits from anticoagulation clinic management, two randomized controlled trials
show no substantial benefit in TTR between anticoagulation
clinics and conventional care (64,83), perhaps due to patient
referral bias or a high patient turnover (14,83). Neither RCT
was powered to detect statistically significant differences between anticoagulation clinics and conventional care models
(64,83). Patients tended to be more satisfied when anticoagulation therapy was managed through anticoagulation clinics
than by conventional care (64), although manner of monitoring was a leading source of dissatisfaction (91). Byeth et al.
compared anticoagulation clinics to usual care and showed a
higher proportion of patients in TTR under anticoagulation
clinic care, although death and recurrent VTE occurred with
similar frequency in both groups (85). The intention-to-treat
analysis showed a borderline significant reduction ($P = 0.0498$)
in major bleeding in the anticoagulation clinic group, and after
6 months, major bleeding occurred with similar frequency in
both groups.

# PATIENT SELF-TESTING

Patient self-testing offers the potential for simplifying oral anticoagulation management both in the patient's home and in
the physician's office (92). Point-of-care (POC) monitors (see
Table 117-3) measure a thromboplastin-mediated clotting time
from a fingerstick sample of capillary whole blood or from
unanticoagulated venous whole blood (93). A microprocessor
converts the result to a plasma PT equivalent, expressed as a
PT or INR. Each manufacturer establishes the conversion formula by comparing the fingerstick sample to an established
laboratory method and reagent traceable to the international
reference thromboplastin (14).

Although several monitors have been developed over the
last 15 years, the original methodology was incorporated into

## TABLE 117-2

### HEMORRHAGIC AND VENOUS THROMBOEMBOLISM EVENTS IN SELECTED TRIALS

| Study | Trial | | Usual care | | Anticoagulation service | | |
|---|---|---|---|---|---|---|---|
| | | | Major bleed | VTE | TTR | Major bleed | VTE |
| Beyth et al. (85) | RCT | 32 | 12.0[a] | 13.0[a] | 56 | 5.6[a] | 8.6[a] |
| Matchar et al. (83) | RCT | NA | 1.6 | 4.2 | NA | 1.7 | 3.5 |
| Wilson et al. (64) | RCT | 59 | 3.7 | 7.3 | 63 | 7.1 | 3.6 |
| Kortke et al. (86) | RCT[b] | 60 | 2.6 | 2.1 | 78 | 1.7 | 1.2 |
| Sawicki et al. (87) | RCT[b] | 43 | 2.4 | 4.9 | 53 | 2.4 | 0 |
| Azar et al. (88) | RCT | — | — | — | NA | 1.5 | 3.7 |
| Gadisseur et al. (89) | RCT[b] | 66 | 4.5 | 0 | 64 | 1.3 | 0 |
| White et al. (81) | RCT[b] | 93 | 0 | 0 | 75 | 0 | 0 |
| Garabedian-Ruffialo et al. (15) | RC | 64 | 12.5 | 6.3 | 86 | 2.4 | 0 |
| Gottlieb et al. (90) | RC | 50 | 0.7 | 1.3 | 76 | 1.1 | 1.5 |
| Cortelazzo et al. (77) | RC | NA | 4.7 | 6.6 | 70 | 1.0 | 0.6 |
| Chiquette et al. (13) | IC | 30 | 1.6 | 3.3 | 32 | 3.9 | 11.8 |

Rates are expressed as percent per patient-year.
VTE, venous thromboembolism; TTR, time in therapeutic range; RCT, randomized clinical trial; NA, not available; RC, retrospective cohort; IC, inception cohort.
[a]6-month cumulative incidence.
[b]Anticoagulation service group is self-monitored.

## TABLE 117-3

### SELF-TESTING INSTRUMENTS IN THE UNITED STATES

| Instrument | Manufacturer | Clot detection methodology | Type of sample | US home use approval |
|---|---|---|---|---|
| ProTIME Monitor 1,000 | Biotrack | Clot initiation: thromboplastin | Capillary | No |
| Coumatrak | Dupont Pharma | Clot detection: cessation of blood flow through capillary channel | Venous | No |
| CoaguChek Plus, Pro, Pro/DM | Roche Diagnostics | Clot detection: cessation of blood flow through capillary channel | Venous | No |
| CoaguChek | Roche Diagnostics | Clot initiation: thromboplastin | Capillary | Yes |
| CoaguChek S | Roche Diagnostics | Clot detection: cessation of movement of iron particles | Venous | Yes |
| Thrombolytic Assessment System | PharmaNetis | Clot detection: cessation of movement of iron particles | Plasma | Yes |
| Rapidpoint Coag | Bayer Diagnostics | Clot detection: cessation of movement of iron particles | Plasma | Yes |
| ProTIME Monitor | International Technidyne Corporation | Clot initiation: thromboplastin | Capillary | Yes |
| Hemochron Jr | International Technidyne Corporation | Clot detection: cessation of blood flow through capillary channel | Venous | Yes |
| AvoSure Pro+ | Avocet | Clot initiation: thromboplastin | Capillary | Yes |
| AvoSure Pro, AvoSure PT | Avocet | Clot detection: thrombin generation detected by fluorescent thrombin probe | Venous | Yes |
| Harmony | Lifescan | Clot initiation: thromboplastin | Capillary | Yes |
| | | Clot detection: cessation of blood flow through capillary channel | Venous | Yes |
| INRatio | HemoSense | Clot initiation: thromboplastin | Capillary | Yes |
| | | Clot detection: change in electrical impedance in sample | Venous | Yes |

From Ansell J, Hirsh J, Poller L, et al. The pharmacology and management of the vitamin K antagonists: the Seventh ACCP Conference on Antithrombotic and Thrombolytic Therapy. *Chest* 2004;126(Suppl. 3):222S.

the Biotrack instrument (Coumatrak; Biotrack, Inc.), a finger-stick procedure that provides an accurate correlation coefficient between reference plasma PT and capillary whole blood PT (94–96).

Despite offering convenience to both the physician and the patient, there are limitations to the accuracy and precision of POC machines (97–100). Because anticoagulated plasmas are compared using different instrument/thromboplastin combinations, the ensuing lack of correlation in INR results may have led to different dosing decisions in comparative studies (101–107). Although variation between INR values obtained with POC devices and laboratory testing undoubtedly exists, a similar variation may be obtained between different laboratories measuring an INR value from a single sample (108).

## PATIENT SELF-MANAGEMENT

Self-testing and self-management allow patients greater independence from laboratory testing, offer the possibility of extended travel, reduce the need for frequent visits to anticoagulation clinics, and improve compliance (16,109–112). Patients or caregivers must be compliant, motivated, and have sufficient manual dexterity and visual abilities to manage POC testing. Patients must also have a basic comprehension of the disease process, therapy, side effects, benefits, and rationale for anticoagulation.

Cohort studies (82,96,113,114) show self-management to be a feasible option in select populations, and randomized trials show that self-managed patients are more likely to be within therapeutic ranges (89) and therefore have fewer thrombotic and hemorrhagic complications (86,87). A long-term study following patient self-monitoring and adjustment of anticoagulation found that patients achieve a degree of therapeutic effectiveness equivalent to that of anticoagulation clinic management while maintaining an adequate safety profile (82). Self-management of anticoagulation is also cost-effective (115).

A randomized controlled crossover study in 50 patients on long-term anticoagulant therapy found patient satisfaction to be higher in self-managed groups than in those receiving conventional care (109). Potential self-managed patients must be selected with caution, and validation of a self-management algorithm must be carefully supervised to assure a safe alternative to anticoagulation service management.

## OUTPATIENT TREATMENT OF VENOUS THROMBOEMBOLISM

Randomized clinical trials have compared low-molecular-weight-heparins (LMWH) to unfractionated heparin (UFH) for the treatment of acute deep vein thrombosis (DVT) in hospitalized patients (116–123), and the guidelines from the ACCP recommend outpatient treatment of DVT when feasible (124). Two randomized clinical trials proved outpatient management of symptomatic DVT with LMWH to be as effective and safe as inpatient UFH management (120,125). LMWH has a longer plasma half-life than UFH (126), a reduced incidence of thrombocytopenia and osteopenia, and allows a cost-effective outpatient alternative to inpatient treatment of DVT with intravenous UFH (117,127–130).

Heparin is usually started with concomitant oral anticoagulation and discontinued when the INR stabilizes at greater than 2.0. There is currently no preference for initial dosing of either 5 mg (131,132) or 10 mg of warfarin (133). Lower doses are recommended in patients with liver failure or congestive heart disease and in elderly individuals (14).

Successful outpatient management of DVT includes a clear patient understanding of the disease and the rationale behind

treatment (134). Potential adverse effects, proper administration of LMWH, and particular emphasis on patient compliance must be reviewed carefully, preferably in lay terms with diagrams to facilitate understanding (135–137). Caution is especially crucial during the first few days of therapy to assure compliance and to monitor for hemorrhage or extension of thrombus. If self-administration of LMWH is not feasible, patients either resume hospitalization, initiate home health nursing services, or arrange for administration of LMWH by a trained family member or friend. Graduated elastic stockings may be prescribed to minimize the symptoms of postphlebitic syndrome (138,139).

Dosing modifications are often applied to patients who are pregnant or obese, or to those with impaired renal function (124, 140–143). Peak anti-Xa levels obtained 3 to 4 hours following subcutaneous injection of LMWH may help to adjust the dose in these patients (144–147).

Twice-daily or once-daily (119,148) administration is acceptable (144). LMWH is also effective in the long-term management of patients with cancer and acute DVT (149) and is currently the recommended anticoagulant modality (144). For patients with nonmassive acute pulmonary embolism, LMWH is comparable to UFH (121,150–153).

## FREQUENCY OF MONITORING

Patients are divided into normal and high-risk groups depending on comorbidities, previous hemorrhagic or thrombotic complications, or prothrombotic conditions. After initiating warfarin anticoagulation, daily INR monitoring may be performed after the third dose until a therapeutic INR is obtained. Weekly or twice-weekly INR monitoring is obtained until the patient is stable and may be extended to once-monthly testing. If the patient takes a medication that interferes with warfarin metabolism, more frequent testing is recommended to ensure adequate anticoagulation.

Noncompliant patients pose a particular challenge. An electronic computerized alert service will detect when a patient has missed a scheduled INR test and enables closer patient monitoring. Diet, alcohol consumption, malabsorption, changes in vitamin K intake, and inadequate dosing adjustments may all modify INR levels and prompt more frequent monitoring (14).

## MANAGEMENT OF NONTHERAPEUTIC INTERNATIONAL NORMALIZED RATIO LEVELS

Management of nontherapeutic INR levels is done on a largely empirical basis, although formulas (65) and nomograms (82, 154,155) may facilitate dosing (see Fig. 117-1). Adjustment of warfarin levels by modifying doses in small increments is the most common practice for patients with slight deviations from intended ranges. When patients are excessively anticoagulated (INR >1 U of the intended range), the warfarin dose can be reduced by half or withheld for 1 to 2 days. With greater elevations in INR or with patients at a particular risk of hemorrhage, the weekly warfarin dose should be reduced and INR monitored until the patient is appropriately anticoagulated. In cases of impending or acute hemorrhage, vitamin K (156,157) and/or fresh frozen plasma (158), prothrombin concentrates (159), or recombinant factor VIIa (160) may be administered. Oral, intravenous infusion, or subcutaneous injection of vitamin K are all effective (161–166), although intravenous injections may cause anaphylaxis (167,168).

If the international normalized ratio (INR) >120% of target (mean of therapeutic range):

$$Dose = \left( \sqrt[3]{(target + 20\%)/(today's\ INR)} \right) \times previous\ dose$$

If the INR <80% of target (mean of therapeutic range):

$$Dose = \left( \sqrt[3]{(target - 20\%)/(today's\ INR)} \right) \times previous\ dose$$

**FIGURE 117-1.** Warfarin dosing formula [international normalized ratio (INR)–based].

Subtherapeutic INR levels are generally increased by a fraction of the weekly dose when patients are initiating therapy, and a "booster" is given when stable patients have a lower INR. The booster is generally a 1- or 2-day increased dose to reach and maintain therapeutic levels. Weekly dosing is generally not modified unless the patient continues to have subtherapeutic INRs. It is important to rule out erroneous results obtained from samples that have not been processed rapidly, and a repeat INR should be obtained when this is suspected.

# BRIDGING

The number of patients with atrial fibrillation, mechanical heart valves, and VTE increases as the population ages. For those requiring invasive procedures such as colonoscopy with potential polyp removal or surgery, health care providers have the challenge of preventing thromboembolism while minimizing the periprocedural risk of hemorrhage from anticoagulation. The process of transitioning a chronically anticoagulated patient on warfarin to intravenous or subcutaneous heparin is called *bridging*. Ideal bridging allows outpatient periprocedural treatment with minimal laboratory monitoring and effective anticoagulation without increasing the risk of hemorrhagic complications.

Previous bridging strategies hospitalized patients 3 to 4 days before and after surgery to administer intravenous UFH (169–171), although adjusted-dose subcutaneous UFH and LMWH are now more frequently utilized. LMWH has shown particular promise in bridging (172–175) because of its efficacy, safety, ease of outpatient administration, cost-effectiveness (176), and decreased need for laboratory monitoring (124). Current bridging strategies are described in Table 117-4.

Options for bridging in patients with mechanical heart valves include the use of intravenous UFH, adjusted-dose subcutaneous UFH, and LMWH. The aim is to prevent the 15% mortality rate associated with valve thrombosis (177), particularly with high-risk caged-ball prosthetic mitral valves or in patients with two prosthetic valves (178). If one interpolates the 9% to 22% risk of a thromboembolic event in patients with prosthetic heart valves without anticoagulant therapy (179, 180), an absolute risk of 0.17% to 0.42% is obtained (181).

Generally, oral anticoagulant therapy should be discontinued 4 to 5 days before a procedure and the INR allowed to drift to a subtherapeutic level before bridging is initiated (14,182). If adjusted-dose subcutaneous UFH is used, the partial thromboplastin time is targeted to a range of 50 to 90 seconds with laboratory determinations at the halfway point between dosing intervals. LMWH is effective (173,174,183–185) and offers the advantage of minimal laboratory monitoring.

Criteria for thromboembolic risk classification are well established for patients with chronic atrial fibrillation (186, 187). Bridging with LMWH is recommended (184,188) for those patients with nonvalvular atrial fibrillation who ordinarily take warfarin and who also have additional risk factors for stroke (182).

After VTE, elective surgery and invasive procedures should be delayed for at least 3 months, if possible, because the risk for recurrent VTE is highest during this interval (189,190). However, if surgery or an invasive procedure is required, bridging with LMWH or intravenous continuous infusion UFH is advisable (182).

Oral anticoagulation is discontinued 4 to 5 days before the procedure, and in high-risk patients, a therapeutic dose of LMWH is administered 24 hours after the last dose of warfarin. Irreversible inhibited platelet function (191) from antiplatelet drugs may be controlled by withholding the antiplatelet agent starting 7 days before the procedure. In most cases, LMWH should be discontinued at least 12 hours before the procedure (124). If epidural anesthesia is planned, LMWH should be discontinued at least 24 hours earlier, to reduce the risk of epidural hematoma. LMWH should be discontinued approximately 48 hours before neurosurgical procedures, with LMWH and warfarin initiated 12 to 24 hours after the procedure (182). An INR should be checked twice weekly after the procedure, and

## TABLE 117-4

CURRENT BRIDGING PROTOCOLS IN THE UNITED STATES

| Bridging strategy | Administered by | Preoperative days − 3 − 2 − 1 | Day of procedure | Postoperative days + 1 + 2 + 3 + 4 |
|---|---|---|---|---|
| Enoxaparin 1.0 mg/kg twice daily | Patient | Bridging therapy self-administered by the patient at home | No bridging | Bridging self-administered by the patient at home[a] |
| Enoxaparin 1.5 mg/kg once daily | Nurse | Bridging therapy administered by a nurse in the patient's home | No bridging | Bridging administered by a nurse in the patient's home[a] |
| Intravenous unfractionated heparin | In-hospital | Patient hospitalized for bridging therapy | No bridging | Patient remains in hospital for bridging, even if already recovered from surgery |

[a]Unless in-hospital recovering from surgery.

LMWH continued for a minimum of 5 days or until a therapeutic INR is achieved. Particular attention should be given to the surgical wound site, where more than 90% of major bleeding episodes occur (192–194). No further anticoagulation is required prior to initiating the procedure. Postprocedure, oral anticoagulation with warfarin is resumed when hemostasis has been achieved.

# THE FUTURE OF ANTICOAGULATION CLINICS

Establishment of effective anticoagulation services is limited by the availability of knowledgeable providers and funds to support clinical operation (19). Reimbursement is often minimal, and most clinics use telephone or electronic communication rather than face-to-face visits. The benefiting institution generally subsidizes most or all anticoagulation clinic costs. New medications such as fixed-dose direct thrombin inhibitors (195,196) may offer an alternative to vitamin-K antagonists and reduce the demand for anticoagulation clinics (1). Until these new medications demonstrate long-term safety and effectiveness, and are accepted by health care professionals, anticoagulation clinics will continue to play a vital role in managing patients receiving anticoagulation.

## *References*

1. Nutescu EA. The future of anticoagulation clinics. *J Thromb Thrombolysis* 2003;16(1-2):61–63.
2. Berrettini M. Anticoagulation clinics: the Italian experience. *Haematologica* 1997;82(6):713–717.
3. Breukink-Engbers WG. Monitoring therapy with anticoagulants in the Netherlands. *Semin Thromb Hemost* 1999;25(1):37–42.
4. Anticoagulants in the Secondary Prevention of Events in Coronary Thrombosis (ASPECT) Research Group. Effect of long-term oral anticoagulant treatment on mortality and cardiovascular morbidity after myocardial infarction. *Lancet* 1994;343(8896):499–503.
5. Cannegieter SC, Rosendaal FR, Wintzen AR, et al. Optimal oral anticoagulant therapy in patients with mechanical heart valves. *N Engl J Med* 1995;333(1):11–17.
6. Schaefer C. Patient advocacy in INR self-monitoring. *Anticoagulation Forum* 2003;7(3):1–3.
7. Palareti G, Leali N, Coccheri S, et al. Bleeding complications of oral anticoagulant treatment: an inception-cohort, prospective collaborative study (ISCOAT). Italian Study on Complications of Oral Anticoagulant Therapy. *Lancet* 1996;348(9025):423–428.
8. Palareti G, Manotti C, DA A, et al. Thrombotic events during oral anticoagulant treatment: results of the inception-cohort, prospective, collaborative ISCOAT study: ISCOAT study group (Italian Study on Complications of Oral Anticoagulant Therapy). *Thromb Haemost* 1997;78(6):1438–1443.
9. Berrettini M, Agnelli G. Management of oral anticoagulant therapy in Italy. *Semin Thromb Hemost* 1999;25(1):27–31.
10. Sam C, Speckman J, Moskowitz M, et al. The management of warfarin therapy by anticoagulation clinics: results of a forum survey. *Anticoagulation Forum* 2000;5(2):1–3.
11. Gray DR, Garabedian-Ruffalo SM, Chrétien SD. Cost-justification of a clinical pharmacist-managed anticoagulation clinic. *Drug Intell Clin Pharm* 1985; 19(7-8):575–580.
12. Wilt VM, Gums JG, Ahmed OI, et al. Outcome analysis of a pharmacist-managed anticoagulation service. *Pharmacotherapy* 1995;15(6):732–739.
13. Chiquette E, Amato MG, Bussey HI. Comparison of an anticoagulation clinic with usual medical care: anticoagulation control, patient outcomes, and health care costs. *Arch Intern Med* 1998;158(15):1641–1647.
14. Ansell J, Hirsh J, Poller L, et al. The pharmacology and management of the vitamin K antagonists: The Seventh ACCP Conference on Antithrombotic and Thrombolytic Therapy. *Chest* 2004;126(Suppl. 3):204S–233S.
15. Garabedian-Ruffalo SM, Gray DR, Sax MJ, et al. Retrospective evaluation of a pharmacist-managed warfarin anticoagulation clinic. *Am J Hosp Pharm* 1985;42(2):304–308.
16. van der Meer FJ, Rosendaal FR, Vandenbroucke JP, et al. Bleeding complications in oral anticoagulant therapy. An analysis of risk factors. *Arch Intern Med* 1993;153(13):1557–1562.
17. Conte RR, Kehoe WA, Nielson N, et al. Nine-year experience with a pharmacist-managed anticoagulation clinic. *Am J Hosp Pharm* 1986;43(10): 2460–2464.
18. Ansell JE, Buttaro ML, Thomas OV, et al. Consensus guidelines for coordinated outpatient oral anticoagulation therapy management. Anticoagulation Guidelines Task Force. *Ann Pharmacother* 1997;31(5): 604–615.
19. Macik BG. The future of anticoagulation clinics. *J Thromb Thrombolysis* 2003;16(1-2):55–59.
20. Hirsh J, Dalen J, Anderson DR, et al. Oral anticoagulants: mechanism of action, clinical effectiveness, and optimal therapeutic range. *Chest* 2001; 119(Suppl. 1):8S–21S.
21. McIntyre KM. Medicolegal implications of consensus statements. *Chest* 1995;108(Suppl. 4):502S–505S.
22. Norton JL, Gibson DL. Establishing an outpatient anticoagulation clinic in a community hospital. *Am J Health Syst Pharm* 1996;53(10):1151–1157.
23. Grasso-Correnti N, Goldszer RC, Goldhaber SZ. The critical pathways of an anticoagulation service. *Crit Pathways Cardiol* 2003;2(1):41–45.
24. Makris M. Alternative models of delivery of anticoagulant services. *Semin Thromb Hemost* 1999;25(1):33–36.
25. Kroner BA. Anticoagulation Clinic in the VA Pittsburgh Healthcare System. *Pharm Pract Manag Q* 1998;18(3):17–33.
26. Askey JM, Cherry CB. Thromboembolism associated with auricular fibrillation; continuous anticoagulant therapy. *J Am Med Assoc* 1950;144(2): 97–100.
27. Bond CA, Raehl CL. Pharmacist-provided anticoagulation management in United States hospitals: death rates, length of stay, Medicare charges, bleeding complications, and transfusions. *Pharmacotherapy* 2004;24(8): 953–963.
28. Anderson RJ. Cost analysis of a managed care decentralized outpatient pharmacy anticoagulation service. *J Manag Care Pharm* 2004;10(2):159–165.
29. Ernst ME, Brandt KB. Evaluation of 4 years of clinical pharmacist anticoagulation case management in a rural, private physician office. *J Am Pharm Assoc (Wash DC)* 2003;43(5):630–636.
30. Witt DM, Tillman DJ. Clinical pharmacy anticoagulation services in a group model health maintenance organization. *Pharm Pract Manag Q* 1998;18(3): 34–55.
31. Witt DM, Humphries TL. A retrospective evaluation of the management of excessive anticoagulation in an established clinical pharmacy anticoagulation service compared to traditional care. *J Thromb Thrombolysis* 2003;15(2):113–118.
32. Farnsworth FA, Kim KY, Jacobs MR, et al. Centralized, pharmacist-managed anticoagulation service for a university-based health system. *Am J Health Syst Pharm* 2001;58(1):77–78.
33. Dager WE, Branch JM, King JH, et al. Optimization of inpatient warfarin therapy: impact of daily consultation by a pharmacist-managed anticoagulation service. *Ann Pharmacother* 2000;34(5):567–572.
34. Mehlberg J, Wittkowsky AK, Possidente C. National survey of training and credentialing methods in pharmacist-managed anticoagulation clinics. *Am J Health Syst Pharm* 1998;55(10):1033–1036.
35. Dedden P, Chang B, Nagel D. Pharmacy-managed program for home treatment of deep vein thrombosis with enoxaparin. *Am J Health Syst Pharm* 1997;54(17):1968–1972.
36. Kershaw B, White RH, Mungall D, et al. Computer-assisted dosing of heparin. Management with a pharmacy-based anticoagulation service. *Arch Intern Med* 1994;154(9):1005–1011.
37. McCurdy M. Oral anticoagulation monitoring in a community pharmacy. *Am Pharm* 1993;NS33(10):61–70; quiz 70–72.
38. Chenella FC, Klotz TA, Gill MA, et al. Comparison of physician and pharmacist management of anticoagulant therapy of inpatients. *Am J Hosp Pharm* 1983;40(10):1642–1645.
39. Fitzmaurice DA, Murray ET, Gee KM, et al. Does the Birmingham model of oral anticoagulation management in primary care work outside trial conditions? *Br J Gen Pract* 2001;51(471):828–829.
40. Lafata JE, Martin SA, Kaatz S, et al. The cost-effectiveness of different management strategies for patients on chronic warfarin therapy. *J Gen Intern Med* 2000;15(1):31–37.
41. Wieland KA, Ewy GA, Wise M. Quality assessment and improvement in a university-based anticoagulation management service. *Pharm Pract Manag Q* 1998;18(3):56–78.
42. Mamdani MM, Racine E, McCreadie S, et al. Clinical and economic effectiveness of an inpatient anticoagulation service. *Pharmacotherapy* 1999; 19(9):1064–1074.
43. Davis FB, Estruch MT, Samson-Corvera EB, et al. Management of anticoagulation in outpatients: experience with an anticoagulation service in a municipal hospital setting. *Arch Intern Med* 1977;137(2):197–202.
44. Lieder TR. Telephone aids in anticoagulation management. *Am J Health Syst Pharm* 2000;57(23):2126, 2130.
45. Waterman AD, Milligan PE, Banet GA, et al. Establishing and running an effective telephone-based anticoagulation service. *J Vasc Nurs* 2001;19(4): 126–132; quiz 133–134.
46. Waterman AD, Banet G, Milligan PE, et al. Patient and physician satisfaction with a telephone-based anticoagulation service. *J Gen Intern Med* 2001;16(7):460–463.
47. Moherman LJ, Kolar MM. Complication rates for a telephone-based anticoagulation service. *Am J Health Syst Pharm* 1999;56(15):1540–1542.
48. Foss MT, Schoch PH, Sintek CD. Efficient operation of a high-volume anticoagulation clinic. *Am J Health Syst Pharm* 1999;56(5):443–449.

49. Harrold LR, Gurwitz JH, Tate JP, et al. Physician attitudes concerning anticoagulation services in the long-term care setting. *J Thromb Thrombolysis* 2002;14(1):59–64.

50. Bodenheimer T. Disease management—promises and pitfalls. *N Engl J Med* 1999;340(15):1202–1205.

51. Arnsten JH, Gelfand JM, Singer DE. Determinants of compliance with anticoagulation: a case-control study. *Am J Med* 1997;103(1):11–17.

52. Pubentz MJ, Calcagno DE Jr, Teeters JL. Improving warfarin anticoagulation therapy in a community health system. *Pharm Pract Manag Q* 1998;18(3):1–16.

53. Lewis SM, Kroner BA. Patient survey of a pharmacist-managed anticoagulation clinic. *Manag Care Interface* 1997;10(11):66–70.

54. Calcagno D, Pubentz M, Carey R. Improving patient satisfaction with warfarin manaagement. *Am J Manag Care* 1996;2:804–810.

55. Taylor F, Ramsay M, Voke J, et al. Anticoagulation in patients with atrial fibrillation. GPs not prepared for monitoring anticoagulation. *BMJ* 1993;307(6917):1493.

56. Beyth RJ, Antani MR, Covinsky KE, et al. Why isn't warfarin prescribed to patients with nonrheumatic atrial fibrillation? *J Gen Intern Med* 1996;11(12):721–728.

57. Chang HJ, Bell JR, Deroo DB, et al. Physician variation in anticoagulating patients with atrial fibrillation. Dartmouth primary care COOP project. *Arch Intern Med* 1990;150(1):83–86.

58. Kutner M, Nixon G, Silverstone F. Physicians' attitudes toward oral anticoagulants and antiplatelet agents for stroke prevention in elderly patients with atrial fibrillation. *Arch Intern Med* 1991;151(10):1950–1953.

59. York M, Agarwal A, Ezekowitz M. Physicians' attitudes and the use of oral anticoagulants: surveying the present and envisioning future. *J Thromb Thrombolysis* 2003;16(1-2):33–37.

60. McCrory DC, Matchar DB, Samsa G, et al. Physician attitudes about anticoagulation for nonvalvular atrial fibrillation in the elderly. *Arch Intern Med* 1995;155(3):277–281.

61. Kent L, Galloway MJ. Use of computers in anticoagulant clinics. *J Clin Pathol* 1992;45(6):549.

62. British Committee for Standards in Haematology, Haemostasis and Thrombosis Task Force. Guidelines on oral anticoagulation: third edition. *Br J Haematol* 1998;101(2):374–387.

63. Rose PE, Fitzmaurice D. New approaches to the delivery of anticoagulant services. *Blood Rev* 1998;12(2):84–90.

64. Wilson SJ, Wells PS, Kovacs MJ, et al. Comparing the quality of oral anticoagulant management by anticoagulation clinics and by family physicians: a randomized controlled trial. *CMAJ* 2003;169(4):293–298.

65. Ryan PJ, Gilbert M, Rose PE. Computer control of anticoagulant dose for therapeutic management. *BMJ* 1989;299(6709):1207–1209.

66. Landefeld CS, Goldman L. Major bleeding in outpatients treated with warfarin: incidence and prediction by factors known at the start of outpatient therapy. *Am J Med* 1989;87(2):144–152.

67. Gitter MJ, Jaeger TM, Petterson TM, et al. Bleeding and thromboembolism during anticoagulant therapy: a population-based study in Rochester, Minnesota. *Mayo Clin Proc* 1995;70(8):725–733.

68. Beyth RJ, Quinn LM, Landefeld CS. Prospective evaluation of an index for predicting the risk of major bleeding in outpatients treated with warfarin. *Am J Med* 1998;105(2):91–99.

69. Steffensen FH, Kristensen K, Ejlersen E, et al. Major haemorrhagic complications during oral anticoagulant therapy in a Danish population-based cohort. *J Intern Med* 1997;242(6):497–503.

70. Forfar JC. Prediction of hemorrhage during long-term oral coumarin anticoagulation by excessive prothrombin ratio. *Am Heart J* 1982;103(3):445–446.

71. Errichetti AM, Holden A, Ansell J. Management of oral anticoagulant therapy. Experience with an anticoagulation clinic. *Arch Intern Med* 1984;144(10):1966–1968.

72. Petty GW, Lennihan L, Mohr JP, et al. Complications of long-term anticoagulation. *Ann Neurol* 1988;23(6):570–574.

73. Charney R, Leddomado E, Rose DN, et al. Anticoagulation clinics and the monitoring of anticoagulant therapy. *Int J Cardiol* 1988;18(2):197–206.

74. Bussey HI, Rospond RM, Quandt CM, et al. The safety and effectiveness of long-term warfarin therapy in an anticoagulation clinic. *Pharmacotherapy* 1989;9(4):214–219.

75. Seabrook GR, Karp D, Schmitt DD, et al. An outpatient anticoagulation protocol managed by a vascular nurse-clinician. *Am J Surg* 1990;160(5):501–505.

76. Fihn SD, McDonell M, Martin D, et al. Risk factors for complications of chronic anticoagulation. A multicenter study. Warfarin Optimized Outpatient Follow-up Study Group. *Ann Intern Med* 1993;118(7):511–520.

77. Cortelazzo S, Finazzi G, Viero P, et al. Thrombotic and hemorrhagic complications in patients with mechanical heart valve prosthesis attending an anticoagulation clinic. *Thromb Haemost* 1993;69(4):316–320.

78. Pell JP, McIver B, Stuart P, et al. Comparison of anticoagulant control among patients attending general practice and a hospital anticoagulant clinic. *Br J Gen Pract* 1993;43(369):152–154.

79. Chamberlain MA, Sageser NA, Ruiz D. Comparison of anticoagulation clinic patient outcomes with outcomes from traditional care in a family medicine clinic. *J Am Board Fam Pract* 2001;14(1):16–21.

80. Holden J, Holden K. Comparative effectiveness of general practitioner versus pharmacist dosing of patients requiring anticoagulation in the community. *J Clin Pharm Ther* 2000;25(1):49–54.

81. White RH, McCurdy SA, von Marensdorff H, et al. Home prothrombin time monitoring after the initiation of warfarin therapy. A randomized, prospective study. *Ann Intern Med* 1989;111(9):730–737.

82. Ansell JE, Patel N, Ostrovsky D, et al. Long-term patient self-management of oral anticoagulation. *Arch Intern Med* 1995;155(20):2185–2189.

83. Matchar DB, Samsa GP, Cohen SJ, et al. Improving the quality of anticoagulation of patients with atrial fibrillation in managed care organizations: results of the managing anticoagulation services trial. *Am J Med* 2002;113(1):42–51.

84. Cohen IA, Hutchison TA, Kirking DM, et al. Evaluation of a pharmacist-managed anticoagulation clinic. *J Clin Hosp Pharm* 1985;10(2):167–175.

85. Beyth RJ, Quinn L, Landefeld CS. A multicomponent intervention to prevent major bleeding complications in older patients receiving warfarin. A randomized, controlled trial. *Ann Intern Med* 2000;133(9):687–695.

86. Kortke H, Korfer R. International normalized ratio self-management after mechanical heart valve replacement: is an early start advantageous? *Ann Thorac Surg* 2001;72(1):44–48.

87. Sawicki PT. A structured teaching and self-management program for patients receiving oral anticoagulation: a randomized controlled trial. Working Group for the Study of Patient Self-Management of Oral Anticoagulation. *JAMA* 1999;281(2):145–150.

88. Azar AJ, Cannegieter SC, Deckers JW, et al. Optimal intensity of oral anticoagulant therapy after myocardial infarction. *J Am Coll Cardiol* 1996;27(6):1349–1355.

89. Gadisseur AP, Breukink-Engbers WG, van der Meer FJ, et al. Comparison of the quality of oral anticoagulant therapy through patient self-management and management by specialized anticoagulation clinics in the Netherlands: a randomized clinical trial. *Arch Intern Med* 2003;163(21):2639–2646.

90. Gottlieb LK, Salem-Schatz S. Anticoagulation in atrial fibrillation. Does efficacy in clinical trials translate into effectiveness in practice? *Arch Intern Med* 1994;154(17):1945–1953.

91. Hamby L, Weeks WB, Malikowski C. Complications of warfarin therapy: causes, costs, and the role of the anticoagulation clinic. *Eff Clin Pract* 2000;3(4):179–184.

92. Hirsh J, Fuster V, Ansell J, et al. American Heart Association/American College of Cardiology Foundation guide to warfarin therapy. *Circulation* 2003;107(12):1692–1711.

93. Ansell JE, Leaning KE. Capillary whole blood prothrombin time monitoring: instrumentation and methodologies. In: Ansell J, Oertel LB, Wittkowsky AK, eds. *Managing oral anticoagulation therapy: clinical and operational guidelines*. New York: Aspen Publishers, 1997:6.

94. Lucas FV, Duncan A, Jay R, et al. A novel whole blood capillary technic for measuring the prothrombin time. *Am J Clin Pathol* 1987;88(4):442–446.

95. Yano Y, Kambayashi J, Murata K, et al. Bedside monitoring of warfarin therapy by a whole blood capillary coagulation monitor. *Thromb Res* 1992;66(5):583–590.

96. Anderson DR, Harrison L, Hirsh J. Evaluation of a portable prothrombin time monitor for home use by patients who require long-term oral anticoagulant therapy. *Arch Intern Med* 1993;153(12):1441–1447.

97. Jennings I, Luddington RJ, Baglin T. Evaluation of the ciba corning biotrack 512 coagulation monitor for the control of oral anticoagulation. *J Clin Pathol* 1991;44(11):950–953.

98. McCurdy SA, White RH. Accuracy and precision of a portable anticoagulation monitor in a clinical setting. *Arch Intern Med* 1992;152(3):589–592.

99. Tripodi A, Arbini AA, Chantarangkul V, et al. Are capillary whole blood coagulation monitors suitable for the control of oral anticoagulant treatment by the international normalized ratio? *Thromb Haemost* 1993;70(6):921–924.

100. Tripodi A, Chantarangkul V, Clerici M, et al. Determination of the international sensitivity index of a new near-patient testing device to monitor oral anticoagulant therapy—overview of the assessment of conformity to the calibration model. *Thromb Haemost* 1997;78(2):855–858.

101. Lind SE, Pearce LA, Feinberg WM, et al. Clinically significant differences in the international normalized ratio measured with reagents of different sensitivities. SPAF investigators. Stroke prevention in atrial fibrillation. *Blood Coagul Fibrinolysis* 1999;10(5):215–227.

102. Poggio M, van den Besselaar AM, van der Velde EA, et al. The effect of some instruments for prothrombin time testing on the International Sensitivity Index (ISI) of two rabbit tissue thromboplastin reagents. *Thromb Haemost* 1989;62(3):868–874.

103. D'Angelo A, Seveso MP, D'Angelo SV, et al. Comparison of two automated coagulometers and the manual tilt-tube method for the determination of prothrombin time. *Am J Clin Pathol* 1989;92(3):321–328.

104. Poller L, Thomson JM, Taberner DA. Effect of automation on prothrombin time test in NEQAS surveys. *J Clin Pathol* 1989;42(1):97–100.

105. Ray MJ, Smith IR. The dependence of the international sensitivity index on the coagulometer used to perform the prothrombin time. *Thromb Haemost* 1990;63(3):424–429.

106. Thomson JM, Taberner DA, Poller L. Automation and prothrombin time: a United Kingdom field study of two widely used coagulometers. *J Clin Pathol* 1990;43(8):679–684.

107. Finck KM, Doetkott C, Miller DR. Clinical impact of interlaboratory variation in international normalized ratio determinations. *Am J Health Syst Pharm* 2001;58(8):684–688.

108. Kaatz SS, White RH, Hill J, et al. Accuracy of laboratory and portable monitor international normalized ratio determinations. Comparison with a criterion standard. *Arch Intern Med* 1995;155(17):1861–1867.

109. Cromheecke ME, Levi M, Colly LP, et al. Oral anticoagulation self-management and management by a specialist anticoagulation clinic: a randomised cross-over comparison. *Lancet* 2000;356(9224):97–102.

110. Levine MN, Raskob G, Landefeld S, et al. Hemorrhagic complications of anticoagulant treatment. *Chest* 1998;114(Suppl. 5):511S–523S.

111. Landefeld CS, Beyth RJ. Anticoagulant-related bleeding: clinical epidemiology, prediction, and prevention. *Am J Med* 1993;95(3):315–328.

112. van der Meer FJ, Briet E, Vandenbroucke JP, et al. The role of compliance as a cause of instability in oral anticoagulant therapy. *Br J Haematol* 1997; 98(4):893–900.

113. Erdman S, Vidne B, Levy MJ. A self control method for long term anticoagulation therapy. *J Cardiovasc Surg (Torino)* 1974;15(4):454–457.

114. Ansell J, Holden A, Knapic N. Patient self-management of oral anticoagulation guided by capillary (fingerstick) whole blood prothrombin times. *Arch Intern Med* 1989;149(11):2509–2511.

115. Taborski U, Wittstamm FJ, Bernardo A. Cost-effectiveness of self-managed anticoagulant therapy in Germany. *Semin Thromb Hemost* 1999;25 (1): 103–107.

116. Wells PS, Kovacs MJ, Bormanis J, et al. Expanding eligibility for outpatient treatment of deep venous thrombosis and pulmonary embolism with low-molecular-weight heparin: a comparison of patient self-injection with homecare injection. *Arch Intern Med* 1998;158(16):1809–1812.

117. Tillman DJ, Charland SL, Witt DM. Effectiveness and economic impact associated with a program for outpatient management of acute deep vein thrombosis in a group model health maintenance organization. *Arch Intern Med* 2000;160(19):2926–2932.

118. Lensing AW, Prins MH, Davidson BL, et al. Treatment of deep venous thrombosis with low-molecular-weight heparins. A meta-analysis. *Arch Intern Med* 1995;155(6):601–607.

119. Merli G, Spiro TE, Olsson CG, et al. Subcutaneous enoxaparin once or twice daily compared with intravenous unfractionated heparin for treatment of venous thromboembolic disease. *Ann Intern Med* 2001;134(3): 191–202.

120. Levine M, Gent M, Hirsh J, et al. A comparison of low-molecular-weight heparin administered primarily at home with unfractionated heparin administered in the hospital for proximal deep-vein thrombosis. *N Engl J Med* 1996;334(11):677–681.

121. Simonneau G, Sors H, Charbonnier B, et al. A comparison of low-molecular-weight heparin with unfractionated heparin for acute pulmonary embolism. The THESEE Study Group. Tinzaparine ou Heparine Standard: Evaluations dans l'Embolie Pulmonaire. *N Engl J Med* 1997;337 (10): 663–669.

122. Hull RD, Raskob GE, Pineo GF, et al. Subcutaneous low-molecular-weight heparin compared with continuous intravenous heparin in the treatment of proximal-vein thrombosis. *N Engl J Med* 1992;326(15): 975–982.

123. Lindmarker P, Holmstrom M. Use of low molecular weight heparin (dalteparin), once daily, for the treatment of deep vein thrombosis. A feasibility and health economic study in an outpatient setting. Swedish Venous Thrombosis Dalteparin Trial Group. *J Intern Med* 1996;240(6):395–401.

124. Hirsh J, Raschke R. Heparin and low-molecular-weight heparin: the Seventh ACCP Conference on Antithrombotic and Thrombolytic Therapy. *Chest* 2004;126(Suppl. 3):188S–203S.

125. Koopman MM, Prandoni P, Piovella F, et al. Treatment of venous thrombosis with intravenous unfractionated heparin administered in the hospital as compared with subcutaneous low-molecular-weight heparin administered at home. The Tasman Study Group. *N Engl J Med* 1996; 334(11):682–687.

126. Weitz JI. Low-molecular-weight heparins. *N Engl J Med* 1997;337(10): 688–698.

127. O'Brien B, Levine M, Willan A, et al. Economic evaluation of outpatient treatment with low-molecular-weight heparin for proximal vein thrombosis. *Arch Intern Med* 1999;159(19):2298–2304.

128. McGarry LJ, Thompson D, Weinstein MC, et al. Cost effectiveness of thromboprophylaxis with a low-molecular-weight heparin versus unfractionated heparin in acutely ill medical inpatients. *Am J Manag Care* 2004; 10(9):632–642.

129. Spyropoulos AC, Hurley JS, Ciesla GN, et al. Management of acute proximal deep vein thrombosis: pharmacoeconomic evaluation of outpatient treatment with enoxaparin vs. inpatient treatment with unfractionated heparin. *Chest* 2002;122(1):108–114.

130. Hull RD, Raskob GE, Rosenbloom D, et al. Treatment of proximal vein thrombosis with subcutaneous low-molecular-weight heparin vs. intravenous heparin. An economic perspective. *Arch Intern Med* 1997;157(3): 289–294.

131. Harrison L, Johnston M, Massicotte MP, et al. Comparison of 5-mg and 10-mg loading doses in initiation of warfarin therapy. *Ann Intern Med* 1997;126(2):133–136.

132. Crowther MA, Ginsberg JB, Kearon C, et al. A randomized trial comparing 5-mg and 10-mg warfarin loading doses. *Arch Intern Med* 1999;159 (1):46–48.

133. Kovacs MJ, Rodger M, Anderson DR, et al. Comparison of 10-mg and 5-mg warfarin initiation nomograms together with low-molecular-weight heparin for outpatient treatment of acute venous thromboembolism. A randomized, double-blind, controlled trial. *Ann Intern Med* 2003;138(9):714–719.

134. ASHP Therapeutic Position Statement on the Use of Low-Molecular-Weight Heparins for Adult Outpatient Treatment of Acute Deep-Vein Thrombosis. *Am J Health Syst Pharm* 2004;61(18):1950–1955.

135. Goldhaber SZ, Fanikos J. Cardiology patient pages. Prevention of deep vein thrombosis and pulmonary embolism. *Circulation* 2004;110(16): e445–e447.

136. Goldhaber SZ, Morrison RB. Cardiology patient pages. Pulmonary embolism and deep vein thrombosis. *Circulation* 2002;106(12):1436–1438.

137. Goldhaber SZ, Grasso-Correnti N. Cardiology patient pages. Treatment of blood clots. *Circulation* 2002;106(20):e138–e140.

138. Brandjes DP, Buller HR, Heijboer H, et al. Randomised trial of effect of compression stockings in patients with symptomatic proximal-vein thrombosis. *Lancet* 1997;349(9054):759–762.

139. Ginsberg JS, Hirsh J, Julian J, et al. Prevention and treatment of postphlebitic syndrome: results of a 3-part study. *Arch Intern Med* 2001;161 (17):2105–2109.

140. Litin SC, Heit JA, Mees KA. Use of low-molecular-weight heparin in the treatment of venous thromboembolic disease: answers to frequently asked questions. The thrombophilia center investigators. *Mayo Clin Proc* 1998; 73(6):545–550; quiz 551.

141. Kessler CM. Low molecular weight heparins: practical considerations. *Semin Hematol* 1997;34(Suppl. 4):35–42.

142. Abbate R, Gori AM, Farsi A, et al. Monitoring of low-molecular-weight heparins in cardiovascular disease. *Am J Cardiol* 1998;82(5B):33L–36L.

143. Samama MM, Poller L. Contemporary laboratory monitoring of low molecular weight heparins. *Clin Lab Med* 1995;15(1):119–123.

144. Buller HR, Agnelli G, Hull RD, et al. Antithrombotic therapy for venous thromboembolic disease: the Seventh ACCP Conference on Antithrombotic and Thrombolytic Therapy. *Chest* 2004;126(Suppl.3): 401S–428S.

145. Laposata M, Green D, Van Cott EM, et al. College of American Pathologists Conference XXXI on Laboratory Monitoring of Anticoagulant Therapy: the Clinical Use and Laboratory Monitoring of Low-Molecular-Weight Heparin, Danaparoid, Hirudin and Related Compounds, and Argatroban. *Arch Pathol Lab Med* 1998;122(9):799–807.

146. Boneu B. Low molecular weight heparin therapy: is monitoring needed? *Thromb Haemost* 1994;72(3):330–334.

147. Bara L, Billaud E, Gramond G, et al. Comparative pharmacokinetics of a low molecular weight heparin (PK 10 169) and unfractionated heparin after intravenous and subcutaneous administration. *Thromb Res* 1985;39(5): 631–636.

148. Charbonnier BA, Fiessinger JN, Banga JD et al, FRAXODI Group. Comparison of a once daily with a twice daily subcutaneous low molecular weight heparin regimen in the treatment of deep vein thrombosis. *Thromb Haemost* 1998;79(5):897–901.

149. Lee AY, Levine MN, Baker RI, et al. Low-molecular-weight heparin versus a coumarin for the prevention of recurrent venous thromboembolism in patients with cancer. *N Engl J Med* 2003;349(2):146–153.

150. Hull RD, Raskob GE, Brant RF, et al. Low-molecular-weight heparin vs. heparin in the treatment of patients with pulmonary embolism. American-Canadian Thrombosis Study Group. *Arch Intern Med* 2000;160(2): 229–236.

151. de Valk HW, Banga JD, Wester JW, et al. Comparing subcutaneous danaparoid with intravenous unfractionated heparin for the treatment of venous thromboembolism. A randomized controlled trial. *Ann Intern Med* 1995;123(1):1–9.

152. Meyer G, Brenot F, Pacouret G, et al. Subcutaneous low-molecular-weight heparin fragmin versus intravenous unfractionated heparin in the treatment of acute non massive pulmonary embolism: an open randomized pilot study. *Thromb Haemost* 1995;74(6):1432–1435.

153. The Columbus Investigators. Low-molecular-weight heparin in the treatment of patients with venous thromboembolism. *N Engl J Med* 1997;337 (10):657–662.

154. Fredriks DA, Coleman RW. Nomogram for dosing warfarin at steady state. *Clin Pharm* 1991;10(12):923–927.

155. Anderson DR, Wilson SJ, Blundell J, et al. Comparison of a nomogram and physician-adjusted dosage of warfarin for prophylaxis against deep-vein thrombosis after arthroplasty. *J Bone Joint Surg Am* 2002;84-A(11): 1992–1997.

156. Crowther MA, Julian J, McCarty D, et al. Treatment of warfarin-associated coagulopathy with oral vitamin K: a randomised controlled trial. *Lancet* 2000;356(9241):1551–1553.

157. Shetty HG, Backhouse G, Bentley DP, et al. Effective reversal of warfarin-induced excessive anticoagulation with low dose vitamin K1. *Thromb Haemost* 1992;67(1):13–15.

158. Makris M, Greaves M, Phillips WS, et al. Emergency oral anticoagulant reversal: the relative efficacy of infusions of fresh frozen plasma and clotting factor concentrate on correction of the coagulopathy. *Thromb Haemost* 1997;77(3):477–480.

159. Nitu IC, Perry DJ, Lee CA. Clinical experience with the use of clotting factor concentrates in oral anticoagulation reversal. *Clin Lab Haematol* 1998; 20(6):363–367.

160. Deveras RA, Kessler CM. Reversal of warfarin-induced excessive anticoagulation with recombinant human factor VIIa concentrate. *Ann Intern Med* 2002;137(11):884–888.

161. Whitling AM, Bussey HI, Lyons RM. Comparing different routes and doses of phytonadione for reversing excessive anticoagulation. *Arch Intern Med* 1998;158(19):2136–2140.

162. Raj G, Kumar R, McKinney WP. Time course of reversal of anticoagulant effect of warfarin by intravenous and subcutaneous phytonadione. *Arch Intern Med* 1999;159(22):2721–2724.

163. Crowther MA, Douketis JD, Schnurr T, et al. Oral vitamin K lowers the international normalized ratio more rapidly than subcutaneous vitamin K in the treatment of warfarin-associated coagulopathy. A randomized, controlled trial. *Ann Intern Med* 2002;137(4):251–254.

164. Pengo V, Banzato A, Garelli E, et al. Reversal of excessive effect of regular anticoagulation: low oral dose of phytonadione (vitamin K1) compared with warfarin discontinuation. *Blood Coagul Fibrinolysis* 1993;4(5):739–741.

165. Schirger A, Spittel JA Jr, Ragen PA. Small doses of vitamin K1 for correction of reduced prothrombin activity. *Mayo Clin Proc* 1959;34:453–458.

166. Weibert RT, Le DT, Kayser SR, et al. Correction of excessive anticoagulation with low-dose oral vitamin K1. *Ann Intern Med* 1997;126(12):959–962.

167. Martin JC. Anaphylactoid reactions and vitamin K. *Med J Aust* 1991;155(11-12):851.

168. Fiore LD, Scola MA, Cantillon CE, et al. Anaphylactoid reactions to vitamin K. *J Thromb Thrombolysis* 2001;11(2):175–183.

169. Madura JA, Rookstool M, Wease G. The management of patients on chronic Coumadin therapy undergoing subsequent surgical procedures. *Am Surg* 1994;60(7):542–546. discussion 546-7.

170. Busuttil WJ, Fabri BM. The management of anticoagulation in patients with prosthetic heart valves undergoing non-cardiac operations. *Postgrad Med J* 1995;71(837):390–392.

171. Bryan AJ, Butchart EG. Prosthetic heart valves and anticoagulant management during non-cardiac surgery. *Br J Surg* 1995;82(5):577–578.

172. Manley HJ, Smith JA, Garris RE. Subcutaneous enoxaparin for outpatient anticoagulation therapy in a patient with an aortic valve replacement. *Pharmacotherapy* 1998;18(2):408–412.

173. Spandorfer JM, Lynch S, Weitz HH, et al. Use of enoxaparin for the chronically anticoagulated patient before and after procedures. *Am J Cardiol* 1999;84(4):478–480, A10.

174. Tinmouth AH, Morrow BH, Cruickshank MK, et al. Dalteparin as periprocedure anticoagulation for patients on warfarin and at high risk of thrombosis. *Ann Pharmacother* 2001;35(6):669–674.

175. Douketis JD, Johnson JA, Turpie AG. Low-molecular-weight heparin as bridging anticoagulation during interruption of warfarin: assessment of a standardized periprocedural anticoagulation regimen. *Arch Intern Med* 2004;164(12):1319–1326.

176. Goldstein JL, Larson LR, Yamashita BD, et al. Low molecular weight heparin versus unfractionated heparin in the colonoscopy peri-procedure period: a cost modeling study. *Am J Gastroenterol* 2001;96(8):2360–2366.

177. Husebye DG, Pluth JR, Piehler JM, et al. Reoperation on prosthetic heart valves. An analysis of risk factors in 552 patients. *J Thorac Cardiovasc Surg* 1983;86(4):543–552.

178. Vongpatanasin W, Hillis LD, Lange RA. Prosthetic heart valves. *N Engl J Med* 1996;335(6):407–416.

179. Baudet EM, Oca CC, Roques XF, et al. A 5 1/2 year experience with the St. Jude medical cardiac valve prosthesis. Early and late results of 737 valve replacements in 671 patients. *J Thorac Cardiovasc Surg* 1985;90(1):137–144.

180. Cannegieter SC, Rosendaal FR, Briet E. Thromboembolic and bleeding complications in patients with mechanical heart valve prostheses. *Circulation* 1994;89(2):635–641.

181. Douketis JD. Perioperative anticoagulation management in patients who are receiving oral anticoagulant therapy: a practical guide for clinicians. *Thromb Res* 2002;108(1):3–13.

182. Piazza G, Goldhaber SZ. Periprocedural management of the chronically anticoagulated patient: critical pathways for bridging therapy. *Crit Pathways Cardiol* 2003;2(2):96–103.

183. Montalescot G, Polle V, Collet JP, et al. Low molecular weight heparin after mechanical heart valve replacement. *Circulation* 2000;101(10):1083–1086.

184. Johnson J, Turpie AG. Temporary discontinuation of oral anticoagulation: role of low molecular weight heparin (Dalteparin) [abstract]. *Circulation* 2000;102(Suppl. 18):II-826.

185. Ferreira I, Dos L, Tornos P, et al. Experience with enoxaparin in patients with mechanical heart valves who must withhold acenocumarol. *Heart* 2003;89(5):527–530.

186. Atrial Fibrillation Investigators. Risk factors for stroke and efficacy of antithrombotic therapy in atrial fibrillation. Analysis of pooled data from five randomized controlled trials. *Arch Intern Med* 1994;154(13):1449–1457.

187. Hart RG, Pearce LA, McBride R, et al. Factors associated with ischemic stroke during aspirin therapy in atrial fibrillation: analysis of 2012 participants in the SPAF I-III clinical trials. The Stroke Prevention in Atrial Fibrillation (SPAF) investigators. *Stroke* 1999;30(6):1223–1229.

188. Omran H, Hammerstingl C, Schmidt H. A prospective and randomized comparison of low molecular weight heparin and unfractionated heparin in chronically anticoagulated patients prior to cardiac catheterization [abstract]. *J Am Coll Cardiol* 2002;39(Suppl. A):234A.

189. Douketis JD, Foster GA, Crowther MA, et al. Clinical risk factors and timing of recurrent venous thromboembolism during the initial 3 months of anticoagulant therapy. *Arch Intern Med* 2000;160(22):3431–3436.

190. Heit JA, Mohr DN, Silverstein MD, et al. Predictors of recurrence after deep vein thrombosis and pulmonary embolism: a population-based cohort study. *Arch Intern Med* 2000;160(6):761–768.

191. Patrono C, Coller B, FitzGerald GA, et al. Platelet-active drugs: the relationships among dose, effectiveness, and side effects: the Seventh ACCP Conference on Antithrombotic and Thrombolytic Therapy. *Chest* 2004;126(Suppl. 3):234S–264S.

192. Turpie AG, Bauer KA, Eriksson BI, et al. Fondaparinux vs. enoxaparin for the prevention of venous thromboembolism in major orthopedic surgery: a meta-analysis of 4 randomized double-blind studies. *Arch Intern Med* 2002;162(16):1833–1840.

193. Mismetti P, Laporte S, Darmon JY, et al. Meta-analysis of low molecular weight heparin in the prevention of venous thromboembolism in general surgery. *Br J Surg* 2001;88(7):913–930.

194. Koch A, Ziegler S, Breitschwerdt H, et al. Low molecular weight heparin and unfractionated heparin in thrombosis prophylaxis: meta-analysis based on original patient data. *Thromb Res* 2001;102(4):295–309.

195. Dager WE, Vondracek TG, McIntosh BA, et al. Ximelagatran: an oral direct thrombin inhibitor. *Ann Pharmacother* 2004;38(11):1881–1897.

196. Olsson SB. Stroke prevention with the oral direct thrombin inhibitor ximelagatran compared with warfarin in patients with non-valvular atrial fibrillation (SPORTIF III): randomised controlled trial. *Lancet* 2003;362(9397):1691–1698.

# CHAPTER 118 ■ DRUG INTERACTIONS WITH ORAL ANTICOAGULANTS

ANN K. WITTKOWSKY

Warfarin is highly susceptible to interactions with prescription drugs, nonprescription drugs, and herbal products. More interactions have been reported for warfarin than for any other commercial drug. Over 200 specific agents that may interfere with warfarin are listed in the product information (1). Through a variety of mechanisms, these agents may increase or decrease the international normalized ratio (INR) and potentially result in significant adverse events, including hemorrhagic complications, thromboembolic recurrence, and death. In a study of 225 hospitalized patients treated with oral anticoagulants, 5.63% developed over-anticoagulation (INR >5.0), and two thirds of those patients had recently been started on new medications that interfere with warfarin metabolism, particularly antibiotics, antifungal agents, and amiodarone (2). A 5.1% mortality rate from hemorrhage was observed in the patients who were over-anticoagulated. Warfarin drug interactions may also increase length of stay and increase laboratory monitoring, both of which lead to higher health care costs (3).

The frequency of drug interactions with warfarin is difficult to quantify. A retrospective, longitudinal cohort study that evaluated pharmacy claims data for 65 million members found 134,833 patients receiving long-term warfarin, of whom 81.6% were prescribed one or more potentially interacting drugs during a 1-year period (4). However, a retrospective evaluation of the frequency and causes of over- and under-anticoagulation in patients treated with warfarin and managed in an anticoagulation clinic found that interactions with prescription, nonprescription, or herbal agents accounted for only 3.3% of out-of-range INRs less than 2.0, and only 10.3% of out-of-range INRs greater than 4.0 (5). Anticoagulation clinic management typically involves extensive education regarding avoidance of interacting drugs and reporting of changes in medications, as well as timely intervention to avoid adverse events when potentially interacting agents are added or discontinued. Therefore, the frequency of significant interactions in patients who are not managed in an anticoagulation setting may be much higher.

## GENERAL PRINCIPLES

Interactions occur between an object or index drug (the drug that is altered) and a precipitant or interacting drug (the drug that causes the change) (6). Interactions that influence the absorption, distribution, metabolism, or excretion of the object drug are characterized as pharmacokinetic interactions (e.g., fluconazole inhibits warfarin metabolism). Pharmacodynamic interactions are those in which the precipitant drug alters the patient's response to the object drug without altering the pharmacokinetics of the object drug (e.g., broad-spectrum antibiotics impair vitamin K production by gut flora). When warfarin is the object drug, either type of interaction may lead to a measurable pharmacodynamic response, specifically an increase or decrease in the INR. However, some pharmacodynamic interactions do not alter the INR (e.g., antiplatelet agents increase bleeding risk in patients taking warfarin).

## Drug Interaction Reporting Methods

Drug interactions may be identified through formal drug interaction studies. In 1999, the Center for Drug Evaluation and Research (CDER), a component of the U.S. Food and Drug Administration, issued a guidance for conducting drug interaction studies during new drug development (7). This guidance recognized that the study design (randomized crossover, one-sequence crossover, or parallel design), drug dosing sequence (single dose/single dose, single dose/multiple dose, multiple dose/single dose, or multiple dose/multiple dose), and population studied (healthy volunteers or patients) should be selected on the basis of the likely acute or chronic use of the object or precipitant drug, the pharmacokinetic and pharmacodynamic characteristics of each drug, and safety considerations. The Pharmaceutical Research and Manufacturers of America Drug Metabolism and Clinical Pharmacology Technical Working Groups subsequently defined best practices for *in vitro* and *in vivo* pharmacokinetic drug interaction studies in a white paper published in 2003 (8).

In general, both the quality and the quantity of drug interaction studies for new drug applications have improved over the years (9). However, the clinical importance of drug interactions as assessed in drug interaction studies may not be applicable to individual patients. The time course of an interaction may take longer to manifest than was evaluated in an experimental setting. Patients may respond differently than healthy volunteers. The sequence of drug administration and the dosing of the object and/or precipitant drugs may influence response. Although an average response for the population studied is typically reported, the range of responses for individual subjects should also be evaluated. These potential weaknesses should be considered when evaluating drug interaction studies.

Drug interactions may also be described in case reports. Although case reports offer an opportunity to assess drug interactions as they occur in patients in clinical practice, this reporting method is limited by selective reporting and may overestimate the clinical importance of certain interactions in that only the most dramatic cases are reported. The quality of case reports varies significantly. High-quality case reports typically include confirmation of prior stability of the object drug before the interaction occurred, an objective measurement of patient response, exclusion of confounding factors that might have led to a similar response, evidence of remission when the interacting substance was discontinued, and formal causality assessment. For warfarin drug interactions, causality can be

**TABLE 118-1**

WARFARIN DRUG INTERACTION PROBABILITY SCALE

| Questions | Yes | No | N/A |
|---|---|---|---|
| 1. Are there previous reports of this interaction in humans? | +1 | 0 | 0 |
| 2. Is the observed interaction consistent with the known interactive properties of the interacting drug? | +1 | −1 | 0 |
| 3. Is the observed interaction consistent with the known interactive properties of warfarin? | +1 | −1 | 0 |
| 4. Is the event consistent with the known or reasonable time course of the interaction? | +1 | −1 | 0 |
| 5. Did the interaction remit when the interacting drug was stopped? | +1 | −2 | 0 |
| 6. Did the interaction reappear when the interacting drug was readministered in the presence of continued use of warfarin? | +2 | −1 | 0 |
| 7. Are there alternative reasonable causes for the event other than a drug interaction? | −1 | +1 | 0 |
| 8. Was there a change in the international normalized ratio associated with the drug interaction? | +1 | 0 | 0 |
| 9. Did the interaction result in a clinical outcome consistent with the effects of anticoagulation (thrombosis or hemorrhage)? | +1 | 0 | 0 |
| 10. Was the reaction greater when the dose of the interacting drug was increased, or less when the dose of the interacting drug was decreased? | +1 | −1 | 0 |

Scoring: Highly probable &gt;8
Probable        5–8
Possible        2–4
Doubtful        &lt;2

Modified from Naranjo CA, Busto U, Sellers EM, et al. A method for estimating the probability of adverse drug reactions. *Clin Pharmacol Ther* 1981;30:239–245.

measured by using a modification of the Naranjo adverse drug reaction probability scale (see Table 118-1) (10). Unfortunately, many case reports lack adequate controls, and quality criteria for the publication of case reports are lacking (11).

## Drug Interaction Classification Schemes

In many instances, negative drug interaction studies may suggest that an interaction will not occur, whereas positive case reports confirm that it does. Owing to the strengths and weaknesses of various reporting methods, a thorough understanding of potential interactions is gained by evaluating all available evidence. On the basis of available evidence from both drug interaction studies and case reports, drug interactions have been rated according to various classification systems. Drug interactions may be classified by a significance rating scale, which considers both the severity of an interaction and the documentation supporting it (6). They may also be rated according to how an interaction should be managed to avoid adverse events (12). Two drug interaction classification systems are described in Table 118-2.

## Variability in Patient Response

Considerable variability among patients occurs with respect to susceptibility to a particular interaction, the magnitude of the response, the time of onset, and the duration of the effect (13). Numerous underlying patient characteristics influence these variables, including age, underlying disease states, alcohol use, smoking, dietary vitamin K intake, activity, and environmental factors. In patients taking warfarin,

these characteristics may influence clotting factor synthesis and degradation, the pharmacokinetics and/or pharmacodynamics of the interacting drug, as well as the pharmacokinetics and/or pharmacodynamics of the R- and S-enantiomers of warfarin (14). Genetic expression of the hepatic microsomal enzymes responsible for the metabolism of warfarin is known to influence warfarin dosing requirements and may also influence the risk and/or severity of warfarin drug interactions (15).

## Risk Factors for Adverse Outcomes

Drug interactions may occur when an interacting drug is added to stable warfarin therapy, discontinued during stable warfarin therapy, or used intermittently during oral anticoagulation. The clinical significance of an interaction is dependent on the change in the hypoprothrombinemic effect of warfarin and the patient's physiologic response to that change. Drug interactions that cause elevations in the INR may or may not lead to hemorrhagic complications. Similarly, interactions that cause reductions in the INR may or may not lead to thromboembolism. The risk of an adverse clinical outcome is dependent on underlying risk factors for thrombosis or hemorrhage, just as these factors influence the risk associated with over- and under-anticoagulation caused by other variables. Nonetheless, the concurrent use of warfarin with potentially interacting drugs is not absolutely contraindicated. Prevention of clinically significant adverse events is dependent on careful management of patients, including anticipating the likely response, making appropriate warfarin dosing adjustments, and increasing the frequency of INR monitoring until a new steady state is achieved.

## TABLE 118-2

### DRUG INTERACTION CLASSIFICATION SYSTEMS

| Rating | Criteria |
|---|---|
| **DRUG INTERACTION FACTS** | |
| 0 | Not listed |
| 1 | Potentially severe or life-threatening interaction; occurrence suspected, established, or probable in well-controlled studies; contraindicated drugs may also have this number |
| 2 | Interaction may cause deterioration in a patient's clinical status; occurrence suspected, established, or probable in well-controlled studies |
| 3 | Interaction causes minor effects; occurrence suspected, established, or probable in well-controlled studies |
| 4 | Interactions may cause moderate to major effects; data are very limited |
| 5 | Interaction may cause minor to major effects; occurrence is unlikely or no good evidence of an altered clinical effect exists |
| **DRUG INTERACTIONS ANALYSIS AND MANAGEMENT** | |
| 0 | Not listed |
| 1 | Avoid combination |
| 2 | Usually avoid combination |
| 3 | Minimize risk |
| 4 | No action needed |
| 5 | No interaction |

From Tatro DS, ed. *Drug interaction facts.* St. Louis, MO: Wolters Kluwer, 2005; Hansten P, Horn J. *Drug interactions analysis and management.* St. Louis, MO: Wolters Kluwer, 2005.

# WARFARIN DRUG INTERACTIONS

Drugs and drug classes with the potential for clinically significant drug interactions with warfarin are listed in Table 118-3, organized by proposed mechanism of interaction and including significance and management classifications (6,12,16,17).

## Pharmacokinetic Interactions

### Inhibition of Warfarin Absorption

Warfarin is rapidly and extensively absorbed from the stomach and small intestine and does not appear to be particularly susceptible to inhibition of absorption by other agents (18). The bile acid–binding resins, cholestyramine and, to a lesser extent, colestipol have been reported to bind to warfarin in the gastrointestinal tract, inhibiting oral absorption (19,20). Similarly, sucralfate has also been reported to inhibit warfarin absorption, although controlled studies have not demonstrated an interaction (21). However, these interactions can be minimized by administering the anticoagulant more than 2 hours before, or more than 6 hours after the administration of the interacting agents. Interestingly, sevelamir, a phosphate-binding polymer that exhibits bile acid–binding properties, does not interact with warfarin (22).

### Displacement of Warfarin from Protein-Binding Sites

Warfarin is extensively bound to plasma proteins, primarily albumin (18). Displacement of warfarin from protein-binding sites may transiently increase plasma warfarin concentrations and elevate the anticoagulant response (23). However, as with all protein-binding displacement interactions, a corresponding increase in elimination diminishes the clinical significance of this transient change.

## Induction of Warfarin Metabolism

Warfarin is a racemic mixture of R- and S-enantiomers, which differ in their elimination half-lives, potency, and routes of metabolism (18) (see Table 118-4). S-warfarin, the more potent of the enantiomers, is primarily eliminated by oxidative metabolism involving cytochrome P-450 (CYP)2C9 and, to a lesser extent, CYP3A4. R-warfarin is approximately 40% reduced to alcohols and undergoes 60% oxidation, primarily by CYP1A2, with additional contributions by CYP3A4 and CYP2C19. Induction of hepatic microsomal enzymes promotes hepatic metabolism of certain object drug compounds by increasing the amount and activity of drug-metabolizing enzymes (24). The clearance of the object drug is increased, leading to a reduction in plasma concentrations and a reduction in its therapeutic effect.

A number of potent enzyme inducers have been reported to interact significantly with warfarin (Table 118-3). Although highly variable, these interactions generally tend to have a fairly slow onset of effect, requiring gradual increases in warfarin dosage to maintain therapeutic anticoagulation (25). After discontinuation of the inducing agent, the offset of these interactions is also slow, with gradual increases in warfarin dosage over several weeks required to prevent over-anticoagulation.

Interactions between warfarin and enzyme inducers have been reported to increase warfarin dosing requirements as much as twofold over several weeks. Conversely, bleeding complications and profound elevations in INR have been reported when inducers are discontinued without corresponding reductions in warfarin dose in response to INR monitoring.

Several other drugs, including the thiazolidinediones, troglitazone and pioglitazone (26), and the antiretrovirals, evavirenz and nevirapine (27), have been reported to induce hepatic microsomal enzymes. Although no specific interactions between these agents and warfarin have been reported, the possibility of interactions should be considered when they are used concurrently.

## TABLE 118-3

### CLINICALLY SIGNIFICANT WARFARIN DRUG INTERACTIONS

| Mechanism | Effect on INR | Drugs/Drug classes | Significance (6) | Management (12) |
|---|---|---|---|---|
| Increased synthesis of clotting factors | Decreased | ■ Vitamin K | 2 | 3 |
| Reduced catabolism of clotting factors | Decreased | ■ Methimazole | 1 | 3 |
| | | ■ Propylthiouracil | 1 | 3 |
| Induction of warfarin metabolism | Decreased | ■ Alcohol (chronic use) | 4 | 3 |
| | | ■ Aminoglutethamide | 2 | 3 |
| | | ■ Barbiturates | 1 | 2 |
| | | ■ Bosentan | 2 | 3 |
| | | ■ Carbamazepine | 2 | 3 |
| | | ■ Dicloxacillin | 2 | 4 |
| | | ■ Ethchlorvynol | 2 | 3 |
| | | ■ Fosphenytoin[a] | 2 | 3 |
| | | ■ Glutethimide | 2 | 2 |
| | | ■ Griseofulvin | 2 | 3 |
| | | ■ Nafcillin | 2 | 3 |
| | | ■ Phenytoin[a] | 2 | 3 |
| | | ■ Primidone | 1 | 2 |
| | | ■ Rifampin | 2 | 2 |
| Reduced absorption of warfarin | Decreased | ■ Cholestyramine | 2 | 3 |
| | | ■ Colestipol | 2 | 3 |
| | | ■ Sucralfate | 5 | 3 |
| Unexplained mechanisms | Decreased | ■ Ascorbic acid | 5 | 3 |
| | | ■ Azathioprine | 2 | 3 |
| | | ■ Corticosteroids | 4 | 4 |
| | | ■ Cyclosporin | 4 | 4 |
| | | ■ Mercaptopurine | 2 | 3 |
| Increased catabolism of clotting factors | Increased | ■ Thyroid hormones | 1 | 3 |
| Protein-binding displacement | Increased | ■ Chloral hydrate | 3 | 3 |
| Decreased synthesis of clotting factors | Increased | ■ Cefamandole | 2 | 2 |
| | | ■ Cefotetan | 2 | 2 |
| | | ■ Cefmetazole | 2 | 2 |
| | | ■ Cefoperazone | 2 | 2 |
| | | ■ Moxalactam | 2 | 2 |
| | | ■ Vitamin E | 1 | 3 |
| Impaired vitamin K production by gastrointestinal flora | Increased | ■ Broad-spectrum antibiotics | 2 | 3 |
| Inhibition of warfarin metabolism | Increased | ■ Acetaminophen | 2 | 3 |
| | | ■ Alcohol (acute use) | 4 | 3 |
| | | ■ Allopurinol | 4 | 3 |
| | | ■ Amiodarone | 1 | 3 |
| | | ■ *Azole antifungals* | 1 | 3 |
| | | ■ Capecitabine | 2 | 0 |
| | | ■ Celecoxib | 4 | 4 |
| | | ■ Chloramphenicol | 2 | 2 |
| | | ■ Cimetidine | 1 | 2 |
| | | ■ Disulfiram | 2 | 2 |
| | | ■ *Fluoroquinolone antibiotics* | 2 | 3 |
| | | ■ Fluorouracil | 2 | 3 |
| | | ■ Fosphenytoin | 2 | 3 |
| | | ■ Isoniazid | 4 | 3 |
| | | ■ *Macrolide antibiotics* | 1 | 3 |

(continued)

**TABLE 118-3**

CONTINUED

| Mechanism | Effect on INR | Drugs/Drug classes | Significance (6) | Management (12) |
|---|---|---|---|---|
| | | ■ Metronidazole | 1 | 2 |
| | | ■ Omeprazole | 4 | 4 |
| | | ■ Phenytoin | 2 | 3 |
| | | ■ Propafenone | 4 | 3 |
| | | ■ Quinidine | 1 | 3 |
| | | ■ Rofecoxib | 4 | 4 |
| | | ■ *SSRIs* | 4 | 3 |
| | | ■ *Statins* | 2 | 3 |
| | | ■ Sulfa antibiotics | 1 | 3 |
| | | ■ Zafirlukast | 0 | 3 |
| Additive anticoagulant response | Increased | ■ Direct thrombin inhibitors | 0 | 0 |
| | | ■ Heparin | 0 | 0 |
| | | ■ Low-molecular-weight heparins | 0 | 0 |
| | | ■ Thrombolytic agents | 0 | 0 |
| Unexplained mechanisms | Increased | ■ Androgens | 1 | 2 |
| | | ■ Clofibrate | 1 | 2 |
| | | ■ Cyclophosphamide | 2 | 3 |
| | | ■ Fenofibrate | 1 | 2 |
| | | ■ Gemcitabine | 2 | 3 |
| | | ■ Gemfibrozil | 1 | 2 |
| | | ■ Influenza virus vaccine | 4 | 4 |
| | | ■ Mesalamine | 4 | 3 |
| Increased bleeding risk | No effect | ■ Aspirin/acetylated salicylates | 1 | 4 |
| | | ■ Clopidogrel/ticlopidine | 0 | 4 |
| | | ■ Cyclooxygenase 2 inhibitors | 4 | 4 |
| | | ■ Glycoprotein IIb/IIIa antagonists | 0 | 0 |
| | | ■ NSAIDs | 2 | 2 |

INR, international normalized ratio; NSAIDs, nonsteroidal antiinflammatory drugs.
*Reported to both increase and decrease prothrombin time/INR.
Data extracted from Tatro DS, ed. *Drug interaction facts*. St. Louis, MO: Wolters Kluwer, 2005; Hansten P, Horn J. *Drug interactions analysis and management*. St. Louis, MO: Wolters Kluwer, 2005; Wells PS, Holbrook AM, Crowther NR, et al. Interactions of warfarin with drugs and food. *Ann Intern Med* 1994;121:676–683; Harder S, Thurmann P. Clinically important drug interactions with warfarin. An update. *Clin Pharmacokinet* 1996;30:416–444.

## Inhibition of Warfarin Metabolism

Most warfarin drug interactions are the result of inhibition of warfarin metabolism by precipitant drugs. Enzyme inhibition usually involves competition between the object drug and the precipitant drug for binding sites on the metabolizing enzyme (28). Successful binding of the precipitant drug to the isozyme prevents binding of the object drug, resulting in reduced metabolism and increased serum concentrations, which can lead to adverse events. Noncompetitive inhibition may also occur, in which the precipitant drug binds to the enzyme–object drug complex, thereby suspending effective metabolism.

The inhibiting drug may or may not be metabolized by the same enzyme that it inhibits. Whether two drugs interact is dependent on numerous factors, including the relative affinity of each drug for the binding sites on the metabolizing enzyme, the free drug concentration available for binding, and the availability

of other pathways for elimination. The magnitude of the effect and the clinical consequences are highly variable and dependent on numerous interindividual and drug-related factors (29). Drugs that selectively inhibit the metabolism of S-warfarin, for example, may have a more significant effect on overall warfarin metabolism due to the higher potency of S-warfarin and the greater impact of oxidative metabolism on its elimination. Despite significant variability, drug interactions caused by enzyme inhibition tend to reach maximal intensity relatively quickly and reverse rapidly when the interacting drug is discontinued.

Numerous inhibitors of the hepatic microsomal enzymes responsible for R- and S-warfarin metabolism can lead to clinically significant interactions (Table 118-3). The metabolic and inhibitory characteristics of individual agents within certain classes often result in differences in drug interaction potential. For the selective serotonin reuptake inhibitors (SSRIs) and HMG-CoA reductase inhibitors (statins), differences in the potential

TABLE 118-4

PHARMACOKINETIC CHARACTERISTICS OF
WARFARIN ENANTIOMERS

|  | S-warfarin | R-warfarin |
|---|---|---|
| Half-life | 29 h | 45 h |
| Potency | 2.7–3.8×R-warfarin | 1.0 (reference point) |
| Metabolism | 10% reduction to alcohols | 40% reduction to alcohols |
|  | 90% oxidation by CYP2C9 > CYP3A4 | 60% oxidation by CYP1A2 > CYP3A4 > CYP2C19 |

CYP, cytochrome P-450.
Data extracted from Wittkowsky AK. Warfarin and other coumarin derivatives: pharmacokinetics, pharmacodynamics, and drug interactions. *Semin Vasc Med* 2003;3:221–230.

for warfarin drug interactions among drugs within the class is dependent on their propensity to inhibit CYP enzymes, as well as their metabolic characteristics (see Table 118-5) (30,31).

All agents within the azole antifungal class have been reported to interact with warfarin (fluconazole, miconazole, ketoconazole, itraconazole, miconazole, terbinafine) (32). The macrolide antibiotics have been ranked according to their CYP3A4 inhibitor potency (troleandomycin > erythromycin > clarithromycin > azithromycin) (33). Yet, troleandomycin, with the highest potency, has not been reported to interact with warfarin, whereas several warfarin–azithromycin interaction cases have been reported (34). The CYP1A2 inhibitory potency of the older fluoroquinolones has been ranked (enoxacin > ciprofloxacin > norfloxacin > ofloxacin) (35), although ciprofloxacin and norfloxacin are also able to inhibit CYP3A4 (36). CYP enzymes contribute little to the metabolism

of the newer fluoroquinolones levofloxacin, moxifloxacin, and gatifloxacin (37), yet all have been reported to interact with warfarin (38–40).

## Pharmacodynamic Interactions

### Effects on Clotting Factor Synthesis and Degradation

Synthesis of the vitamin K–dependent clotting factors II, VII, IX, and X is increased by exogenous vitamin K intake in the form of food products, multivitamin preparations, and chewing tobacco (41). Conversely, broad-spectrum antibiotics may deplete normal gastrointestinal flora, which typically act as a secondary source of endogenous vitamin K.

Thyroid function significantly impacts oral anticoagulation, as can medications that alter thyroid status (42). Hyperthyroidism increases the catabolism of clotting factors, and the addition of thyroid replacement therapy, which causes a relative hyperthyroidism, has been noted to increase the sensitivity to warfarin. Conversely, the antithyroid medications methimazole and propylthiouracil cause a relative hypothyroid state, resulting in a reduction in clotting factor catabolism and temporary warfarin resistance until warfarin dosing is increased.

### Increased Bleeding Risk

Other antithrombotic agents, including heparins, direct thrombin inhibitors, and thrombolytic agents, can increase the risk of bleeding in patients taking warfarin due to additive anticoagulant activity. The impact of these agents on INR is drug-specific (43). Agents with antiplatelet activity, including aspirin and other nonacetylated salicylates, nonsteroidal antiinflammatory agents, cyclooxygenase-2 inhibitors, clopidogrel and ticlopidine, and glycoprotein IIb/IIIa antagonists, may also increase bleeding risk in patients taking warfarin without any evident change in INR (44).

For most pharmacokinetic and pharmacodynamic interactions, the impact of the interaction can be monitored by the

TABLE 118-5

WARFARIN DRUG INTERACTION POTENTIAL FOR AGENTS WITHIN
DRUG CLASSES

| Drug class | Agent | Metabolized by | Inhibitor of | Relative warfarin interaction risk |
|---|---|---|---|---|
| Selective serotonin reuptake inhibitors (SSRIs) | Citalopram | CYP2C19 | – | Lowest |
|  | Fluoxetine | – | CYP3A4, 2C19 | Moderate |
|  | Fluvoxamine | CYP1A2 | CYP1A2, 3A4, 2C9 | Highest |
|  | Paroxetine | – | CYP1A2 | Moderate |
|  | Sertraline | CYP3A4 | – | Low |
| HMG-CoA reductase inhibitors (statins) | Atorvastatin | CYP3A4 | – | Low |
|  | Cerivastatin | CYP2C8 > CYP3A4 | – | Low |
|  | Fluvastatin | CYP2C9 > CYP3A4 | CYP2C9 | Highest |
|  | Lovastatin | CYP3A4 | – | Low |
|  | Pravastatin | non-CYP | – | None |
|  | Rosuvastatin | CYP2C9 (<10%) | – | Lowest |
|  | Simvastatin | CYP3A4 | – | Low |

CYP, cytochrome P-450.
Data extracted from Wittkowsky AK. Drug interactions update: drugs, herbs and oral anticoagulation. *J Thromb Thrombolysis* 2001;12:67–71; Williams D, Feely J. Pharmacokinetic-pharmacodynamic drug interactions with HMG-CoA reductase inhibitors. *Clin Pharmacokinet* 2002;41:343–370.

### TABLE 118-6

INTERACTIONS BETWEEN WARFARIN AND DIETARY SUPPLEMENTS

| Mechanism | Effect | Supplements |
|---|---|---|
| Inhibition of warfarin metabolism | Increased INR | Chinese wolfberry |
| | | Cranberry juice |
| | | Grapefruit juice |
| Contain coumarin derivatives | Increased INR | Danshen |
| | | Dong quai |
| | | Fenugreek |
| Unknown | Increased INR | Curbicin |
| | | Devil's claw |
| | | Glucosamine-chondroitin |
| | | Melatonin |
| | | Papaya extract |
| | | Quilinggao |
| Inhibition of platelet aggregation | Increased bleeding | Garlic |
| | | Ginger |
| | | Ginkgo |
| Contain vitamin K derivatives | Decreased INR | Coenzyme q10 |
| | | Green tea |
| | | Some multivitamins |
| Induction of CYP3A4 | Decreased INR | St. John's wort |
| Unknown | Decreased INR | Ginseng |
| | | Melatonin |

INR, international normalized ratio; CYP, cytochrome P-450.
Data extracted from Heck AM, DeWitt BA, Lukes AL. Potential interactions between alternative therapies and warfarin. *AM J Health Syst Pharm* 2000;57:1221–1227; Greenblagg DJ, von Moltke LL. Interaction of warfarin with drugs, natural substances, and foods. *J Clin Pharmacol* 2005;45:127–132; Vaes LP, Chyka PA. Interactions of warfarin with garlic, ginger, ginkgo and ginseng: nature of the evidence. *Ann Pharmacother* 2000;34:1478–1482.

effect on INR, and warfarin doses can be adjusted to maintain the intensity of anticoagulation within the appropriate therapeutic range. However, because interactions with antiplatelet agents increase the risk of bleeding without any effect on oral anticoagulation, concurrent use of warfarin and these agents must be managed carefully and in some situations may be relatively contraindicated.

## Interactions with Dietary Supplements

The use of dietary supplements, including vitamins, minerals, amino acids, and herbal medicinals (botanicals), has risen dramatically in the last decade (45). Unlike legend drug products, dietary supplements are not tested before marketing for safety, efficacy, dosing requirements, or drug interactions. In addition, these products are not regulated with respect to labeling, tablet contents, or tablet content uniformity (30). For these reasons, little is known about the risk of using these products in patients taking warfarin or other oral anticoagulants. Numerous case reports and some clinical studies have documented significant interactions between oral anticoagulants and dietary supplements, as described in Table 118-6 (46–48).

# MANAGING WARFARIN DRUG INTERACTIONS

## Preventing Adverse Outcomes

The most assured method to avoid adverse outcomes associated with drug interactions is simply to avoid concurrent use of potentially interacting drugs. When noninteracting alternatives are available and appropriate, they should be preferentially selected. In many circumstances, however, noninteracting alternatives are not available. When potentially interacting agents must be used concurrently with warfarin, adverse outcomes can be avoided by increasing the frequency of monitoring and adjusting warfarin doses appropriately. The frequency of monitoring is guided by the pharmacokinetic and pharmacodynamic characteristics of warfarin and of the interacting drug, evaluation of the characteristics of the interaction in similar patients, consideration of the expected time course associated with the presumed mechanism of the interaction, and assessment of the underlying risks for thrombosis or hemorrhage in the individual patient. For example, interactions involving enzyme inhibition typically occur rapidly. In such cases, the first monitoring INR might be checked 2 to 3 days after the interacting agent is added to warfarin therapy. Enzyme induction interactions tend to occur more slowly. Checking the INR within the first week after addition of the interacting drug might be appropriate. However, there are no guidelines for drug interaction management. Each case must be handled individually because of the expected variability in susceptibility, magnitude of response, onset of effect, and duration of response.

## Educating Patients

The prevention of adverse events associated with drug interactions is also supported by detailed, ongoing education of patients treated with warfarin (14). These patients must be counseled about the possibility of significant adverse outcomes when interacting drugs are added, discontinued, or used on an intermittent basis. They should be encouraged to report their status as anticoagulation patients to all their health care providers, to report all medication changes to their anticoagulation management team, and to obtain professional assistance in selecting over-the-counter medications and dietary supplements.

Current medication use should be thoroughly investigated at each anticoagulation clinic visit, regardless of whether the INR is within or outside the therapeutic range (14). Open-ended questions should be used to assess name, dosage form, dose, frequency, indication, compliance, and prescriber for all current medications. In addition, it is useful to determine whether and why doses of certain agents may be missed or duplicated and how current medications are used if the symptoms for which they are prescribed, change. In some instances, it may be necessary to visually inspect all current medications. Patients may be asked to bring in all prescription and nonprescription medications, as well as all dietary supplements. Labeled instructions should be compared to actual use, and administration devices or other reminder techniques should also be evaluated. These methods can assist in uncovering suspected interactions.

# CONCLUSION

Despite the best efforts of patients and anticoagulation clinic personnel, interacting drugs continue to be prescribed for patients taking warfarin, and significant interactions may occur. Adverse events can be minimized by careful INR monitoring, assessment of patient response, and appropriate warfarin dosing adjustments.

## *References*

1. Bristol-Myers Squibb Company. Coumadin (warfarin) package insert. Princeton, NJ, 2002.
2. Siguret V, Esquirol C, Debray M, et al. Excess antivitamin K in elderly hospitalised patients aged over 70. A one-year prospective survey. *Presse Med* 2003;32:972–977.
3. Jankel CA, McMillan JA, Martin BC. Effect of drug interactions of patients receiving warfarin or theophylline. *Am J Hosp Pharm* 1994;51:661–666.
4. Wittkowsky AK, Boccuzzi SJ, Wogen J, et al. Frequency of concurrent use of warfarin with potentially interacting drugs. *Pharmacotherapy* 2004;24: 1668–1674.
5. Wittkowsky AK, Devine EB. Frequency and causes of overanticoagulation and underanticoagulation in patients treated with warfarin. *Pharmacotherapy* 2004;24:1311–1316.
6. Tatro DS, ed. *Drug interaction facts*. St. Louis, MO: Wolters Kluwer, 2005.
7. CDER. Guidance for industry: *in vivo* drug metabolism/drug interaction studies: study design, data analysis and recommendations for dosing and labeling. November 1999. Available at http://www.fda.gov/cder/guidance/2635fnl.htm. Accessed March 2005.
8. Bjornsson TD, Callaghan JT, Einolf HJ, et al. The conduct of *in vitro* and *in vivo* drug-drug interaction studies: a PhRMA perspective. *J Clin Pharmacol* 2003;43:443–469.
9. Marroum PJ, Uppoor RS, Parmelee T, et al. *In vivo* drug-drug interaction studies: a survey of all new molecular entities approved from 1987 to 1997. *Clin Pharmacol Ther* 2000;68:280–285.
10. Naranjo CA, Busto U, Sellers EM, et al. A method for estimating the probability of adverse drug reactions. *Clin Pharmacol Ther* 1981;30: 239–245.
11. Kienle GS, Hamre HJ, Portalupi E, et al. Improving the quality of therapeutic reports of single cases and case series in oncology: criteria and checklist. *Altern Ther Health Med* 2004;10:68–72.
12. Hansten P, Horn J. *Drug interactions analysis and management*. St. Louis, MO: Wolters Kluwer, 2005.
13. Hansten P, Horn J. Principals of oral anticoagulant drug interactions. *Drug interactions and updates quarterly*. Vancouver, WA; Applied Therapeutics, 1993.
14. Wittkowsky AK. Warfarin drug interactions: detection, prediction, prevention. *J Thromb Thrombolysis* 1996;2:295–299.
15. Daly AK, Aithal GP. Genetic regulation of warfarin metabolism and response. *Semin Vasc Med* 2003;3:231–237.
16. Wells PS, Holbrook AM, Crowther NR, et al. Interactions of warfarin with drugs and food. *Ann Intern Med* 1994;121:676–683.
17. Harder S, Thurmann P. Clinically important drug interactions with warfarin. An update. *Clin Pharmacokinet* 1996;30:416–444.
18. Wittkowsky AK. Warfarin and other coumarin derivatives: pharmacokinetics, pharmacodynamics, and drug interactions. *Semin Vasc Med* 2003; 3:221–230.
19. Jahnchen E. Enhanced elimination of warfarin during treatment with cholestyramine. *Br J Clin Pharmacol* 1978;5:437–440.
20. Harvengt C, Dasager JP. Effect of colestipol, a new bile acid sequestrant, on the absorption of phenprocoumon in man. *Eur J Clin Pharmacol* 1973; 6:19–21.
21. Parrish RH, Waller B, Gondalia BG. Sucralfate-warfarin interaction. *Ann Pharmacother* 1992;26:1015–1016.
22. Burke S, Amin N, Incerti C, et al. Sevelamer hydrochloride (Renagel), a nonabsorbed phosphate-binding polymer, does not interfere with digoxin or warfarin pharmacokinetics. *J Clin Pharmacol* 2001;41:193–198.
23. Griner PF, Raisz LG, Rickles FR, et al. Chloral hydrate and warfarin interaction: clinical significance. *Ann Intern Med* 1971;74(4):540–543.
24. Okey AB. Enzyme induction in the cytochrome p450 system. *Pharmacotherapy* 1990;45:241–298.
25. Cropp JS, Bussey HI. A review of enzyme induction of warfarin metabolism with recommendations for patient management. *Pharmacotherapy* 1997; 17:917–928.
26. Sahi J, Black CB, Hamilton GA, et al. Comparative effects of thiazolidinediones on *in vitro* P450 enzyme induction and inhibition. *Drug Metab Dispos* 2003;31:439–446.
27. Barry M, Mulcahy F, Merry C, et al. Pharmacokinetics and potential interactions amongst antiretroviral agents used to treat patients with HIV infection. *Clin Pharmacokinet* 1999;36:289–304.
28. Murray M. Mechanisms and significance of inhibitory drug interactions involving cytochrome p450 enzymes. *Int J Mol Med* 1999;3:227–238.
29. Lin JH, Lu AYH. Interindividual variability in inhibition and induction of cytochrome p450 enzymes. *Annu Rev Pharmacol Toxicol* 2001;41:535–567.
30. Wittkowsky AK. Drug interactions update: drugs, herbs and oral anticoagulation. *J Thromb Thrombolysis* 2001;12:67–71.
31. Williams D, Feely J. Pharmacokinetic-pharmacodynamic drug interactions with HMG-CoA reductase inhibitors. *Clin Pharmacokinet* 2002;41: 343–370.
32. Venkatakrishnan K, von Moltke LL, Greenblatt DJ. Effects of the antifungal agents on oxidative drug metabolism. Clinical relevance. *Clin Pharmacokinet* 2000;38:111–180.
33. Periti P, Mazzei T, Mini E, et al. Pharmacokinetic drug interactions of macrolides. *Clin Pharmacokinet* 1992;23:106–131.
34. Shrader SP, Fermo JD, Dzikowski AL. Azithromycin and warfarin interaction. *Pharmacotherapy* 2004;24:945–949.
35. Fuhr U, Anders EM, Mahr G, et al. The inhibitory potency of quinolone antibacterial agents against cytochrome p4501A2 activity *in vivo* and *in vitro*. *Antimicrob Agents Chemother* 1992;14:272–284.
36. McLellan RA, Drobitch RK, Monshouwer M, et al. Fluoroquinolone antibiotics inhibit cytochrome p450-mediated microsomal drug metabolism in rat and human. *Drug Metab Dispos* 1996;24:1134–1138.
37. Aminimanizani A, Beringer P, Jelliffe R. Comparative pharmacokinetics and pharmacodynamics of the newer fluoroquinolone antibacterials. *Clin Pharmacokinet* 2001;40:169–168.
38. Jones CB, Fugate SE. Levofloxacin and warfarin interaction. *Ann Pharmacother* 2002;36:1554–1557.
39. Eble DH, Chang SW. Moxifloxacin-warfarin interaction: a series of five case reports. *Ann Pharmacother* 2002;36:1554–1557.
40. Artymowicz RJ, Cino BJ, Rossi JG, et al. Possible interaction between gatifloxacin and warfarin. *Am J Health Syst Pharm* 2002;59:1205–1206.
41. Khan T, Wynne H, Wood P, et al. Dietary vitamin K influences intra-individual variability in anticoagulant response to warfarin. *Br J Haematol* 2004;124:348–354.
42. Demirkan K, Stephens MA, Newman KP, et al. Response to warfarin and other oral anticoagulants: effects of disease states. *South Med J* 2000;93: 448–454.
43. Gosselin RC, Dager WE, King JH, et al. Effect of direct thrombin inhibitors, bivalirudin, lepirudin, and argatroban, on prothrombin time and INR values. *Am J Clin Pathol* 2004;121:593–599.
44. Chan TY. Adverse interactions between warfarin and nonsteroidal anti-inflammatory drugs: mechanisms, clinical significance, and avoidance. *Ann Pharmacother* 1995;29:1274–1283.
45. Eisenberg DM, Davis RB, Ettner SL, et al. Trends in alternative medicine use in the United States 1990-1997: results of a follow-up national survey. *JAMA* 1998;280:1569–1575.
46. Heck AM, DeWitt BA, Lukes AL. Potential interactions between alternative therapies and warfarin. *Am J Health Syst Pharm* 2000;57:1221–1227.
47. Greenblagg DJ, von Moltke LL. Interaction of warfarin with drugs, natural substances, and foods. *J Clin Pharmacol* 2005;45:127–132.
48. Vaes LP, Chyka PA. Interactions of warfarin with garlic, ginger, ginkgo and ginseng: nature of the evidence. *Ann Pharmacother* 2000;34: 1478–1482.

# CHAPTER 119 ■ HEMORRHAGIC COMPLICATIONS OF ANTICOAGULATION

MARK LEVINE, CLIVE KEARON, AND REBECCA J. BEYTH

The major complication of anticoagulant therapy is bleeding. In this chapter, the incidence of hemorrhage in patients receiving anticoagulant therapy and the clinical and laboratory risk factors that predispose to bleeding are discussed. The focus is on major bleeding and fatal bleeding. Details of the method used to select relevant articles can be found in the seven previous symposia of the American College of Chest Physicians (ACCP) (1–7). Bleeding was generally classified as major if it was intracranial or retroperitoneal, if it led directly to death, or if it resulted in hospitalization or transfusion (1,2). However, there was variation among studies for the definition of bleeding. Although bleeding is the major side effect of anticoagulant therapy, it should not be considered in isolation of potential benefit, that is, reduction in thromboembolism. This chapter focuses on bleeding related to heparin and vitamin K antagonists. First, risk factors for bleeding related to these agents are considered, and then bleeding rates for specific clinical conditions are presented. Bleeding related to new emerging antithrombotic agents is also briefly discussed.

## DETERMINANTS OF BLEEDING

### Heparin

Heparin has the potential to induce bleeding by inhibiting blood coagulation, by impairing platelet function (8), and by increasing capillary permeability (9). Heparin can also produce thrombocytopenia, but this is rarely an important cause of bleeding.

#### Relation Between Risk of Bleeding and Heparin Dose-Response

Since the anticoagulant response to heparin [measured by a test of blood coagulation, for example, the activated partial thromboplastin time (aPTT)] is influenced by the heparin dose, it is not possible from reported studies to separate the effects of these two variables (dose and laboratory response) on hemorrhagic rates. To our knowledge, there have been no randomized trials in patients with established venous thromboembolism (VTE) directly comparing different doses of heparin. In a study evaluating prophylaxis in patients with recent-onset traumatic spinal cord injuries, the incidence of bleeding was significantly greater in patients randomized to receive heparin adjusted to maintain the aPTT at 1.5 times control than compared with heparin, 5,000 U twice daily (10). The mean dose of heparin for the adjusted-dose regimen was 13,200 U twice daily. Bleeding occurred in seven adjusted-dose patients compared with none in the fixed-dose group.

Subgroup analysis of randomized trials and prospective cohort studies provide suggestive evidence for an association between the incidence of bleeding and the anticoagulant response.

In the Urokinase Pulmonary Embolism Trial (11), bleeding occurred in 20% of patients assigned to heparin whose whole blood clotting time was greater than 60 minutes compared to 5% of those whose whole blood clotting time was less than 60 minutes (relative risk, 4.0). Norman and Provan reported five major bleeds in 10 patients whose aPTT was prolonged to more than twice the upper limit of their therapeutic range for at least 50% of their assays, but in only one of 40 patients whose aPTT remained therapeutic (relative risk, 20.0) (12). Wilson described 80 nonsurgical patients receiving heparin monitored by the whole blood clotting time (13). Fifty-six percent who received "excessive heparin" bled, whereas only 16% who did not receive "excessive heparin" bled (relative risk, 3.5). Anand examined the relation between the aPTT and bleeding in 5,058 patients with acute coronary syndrome who received intravenous heparin in the Organisation to Assess Strategies for Ischemic Syndromes (OASIS)-2 trial (14). For every 10 second increase in the aPTT, the major bleeding was increased by 7%, $P = 0.0004$.

Although none of the studies were designed to compare the effects on bleeding of either different doses of heparin or different levels of heparin response, there is a suggestion that bleeding is more likely to occur when an *in vitro* test of coagulation is prolonged excessively, but this evidence is by no means definitive. In addition, there is good evidence that serious bleeding during heparin treatment can occur when the anticoagulant response is in the therapeutic range. Finally, the results of Global Utilization of Streptokinase and TPA for occluded coronary arteries (GUSTO) IIa and the Thrombolysis in Myocardial Infarction (TIMI) 9A studies in patients with ischemic coronary syndromes indicated that a 20% increase in the intravenous heparin dose above the 1,000 U per hour that was used in the GUSTO I study increased the risk of intracranial bleeding when combined with thrombolytic therapy (15,16).

#### Relation Between Risk of Bleeding and Method of Administering Heparin

The evidence for a relation between the risk of bleeding and the method of administering heparin comes from randomized trials in which unfractionated heparin was either administered by continuous intravenous (IV) infusion with intermittent IV injection (13,17–21), continuous IV heparin with subcutaneous heparin (22–25), continuous IV heparin for approximately 10 days with a shorter course (4 to 5 days) (26,27), continuous IV heparin and oral anticoagulants compared with oral anticoagulants alone (28), continuous IV heparin given on a weight-adjusted basis with a standard clinical approach (5,000 U bolus, 1,000 U per hour) (29), and continuous IV heparin monitored using either the aPTT or a heparin assay.

In summary, there was an increased rate of major bleeding with intermittent IV heparin compared with continuous IV infusion; continuous IV heparin caused less bleeding than intermittent IV heparin; continuous IV heparin and subcutaneous heparin were associated with a similar amount of bleeding; and continuous IV heparin for approximately 10 days and 5 days caused a similar amount of bleeding.

## Relation Between the Risk of Bleeding and Patient Risk Factors

Comorbid conditions, particularly recent surgery or trauma, are very important risk factors for heparin-induced bleeding (20,30,31). This association was demonstrated in the study by Hull et al. in patients with proximal vein thrombosis (31). Patients without clinical risk factors for bleeding were treated with a starting dose of 40,000 U per 24 hour of heparin by continuous infusion, whereas those with well-recognized risk factors for bleeding (recent surgery, trauma) received a starting dose of 30,000 U per 24 hour. Bleeding occurred in one of 88 low-risk patients (1%) who received 40,000 U initially and 12 of 111 high-risk patients (11%) who received 30,000 U.

The concomitant use of acetylsalicyclic acid (ASA) was identified as a risk factor in early retrospective studies (32) and corroborated by Sethi et al. (33). In their study in patients undergoing aortocoronary bypass surgery, the preoperative use of ASA caused excessive operative bleeding in patients who receive very high doses of heparin as part of the routine for bypass procedures. Although the concomitant use of ASA is associated with heparin-induced bleeding, this combination is used frequently in the initial treatment of acute coronary artery syndromes without serious bleeding. The risk of heparin-associated bleeding increases with concomitant thrombolytic therapy (4) or glycoprotein (GP) IIb/IIIa antagonists (34,35). In a retrospective analysis of 5,216 patients undergoing percutaneous coronary intervention using unfractionated heparin, bleeding complications incrementally increased at all activated clotting times greater than 200 seconds (36).

Renal failure and patient gender have also been implicated as risk factors for heparin-induced bleeding (37,38). The reported association with female gender has not been consistent among studies and remains in question.

Other studies have reported that older patients had a higher risk of heparin-induced bleeding (37,39). In an analysis of a randomized trial, age above 70 years was associated with a clinically important increased risk of major bleeding (40).

## Vitamin K Antagonists

The major determinants of oral vitamin K antagonist–induced bleeding are the intensity of the anticoagulant effect, patient characteristics, the concomitant use of drugs that interfere with hemostasis, and the length of therapy.

### Intensity of Anticoagulant Effect

There is a strong relation between the intensity of anticoagulant therapy and the risk of bleeding that has been reported in patients with deep vein thrombosis (DVT) (41), tissue heart valves (42), mechanical heart valves (43–47), ischemic stroke (48), and atrial fibrillation (49–51). In randomized clinical trials for these indications (41–44), the frequency of major bleeding in patients randomly assigned to warfarin therapy at a targeted international normalized ratio (INR) of approximately 2.0 to 3.0 has been less than half the frequency in patients randomly assigned to warfarin therapy at a targeted INR greater than 3.0. The intensity of anticoagulant effect is probably the most important risk factor for intracranial hemorrhage, independent of the indication for therapy, with the risk increasing dramatically with an INR greater than 4.0 to 5.0 (48,52,53). In a case–control study, the risk of intracerebral hemorrhage doubled for each increase of approximately 1 in the INR (53).

In five randomized trials in patients with atrial fibrillation, the annual incidence of major bleeding averaged 1.3% in patients randomly assigned to warfarin therapy (targeted INR generally 2.0 to 3.0) compared with 1.0% in patients randomly assigned to treatment with placebo (54). In patients with atrial fibrillation, an INR of 2.5 (range 2.0 to 3.0) minimizes the risk of either hemorrhage or thromboembolism (55,56). Similarly, among patients with antiphospholipid antibody syndrome and prior thrombosis there was a trend for lower major bleeding in patients treated with warfarin at a targeted INR of 2.0 to 3.0 compared to those treated with warfarin at a targeted INR of 3.1 to 4.0 (2.2% vs. 3.6%, respectively) (57).

Warfarin regimens (targeted INR <2.0) have been investigated and found to be safe in the primary prevention of thrombosis in patients with malignancy. In two randomized trials in patients with malignancy, warfarin therapy, 1 mg warfarin daily (58) and 1 mg for 6 weeks followed by adjustment to an INR of 1.3 to 1.9 (59), did not increase the frequency of hemorrhage while still preventing thrombosis.

Increased variation in the anticoagulant effect, manifested by variation in the INR, is associated with an increased frequency of hemorrhage independent of the mean INR (49,60,61). This effect is probably attributable to increased frequency and degree of marked elevations in the INR. Approaches to improve anticoagulant control (minimize INR fluctuations) could improve the safety and effectiveness of vitamin K antagonists. Anticoagulation management services (AMS) or clinics and point-of-care INR testing are two such approaches. Two recent randomized trials (62,63) did not show a difference in quality of anticoagulant control or bleeding between AMS and routine medical care. Results from four observational studies (64–67) showed AMS was beneficial and associated with less bleeding than usual care.

Point-of-care testing with either patient self-testing or patient self-management is another model for potentially improving outcomes and also for convenience. Patient self-testing provided better quality of anticoagulation control compared to routine medical care in one trial (time in therapeutic range 56% vs. 32%, P <0.001 and bleeding 5.6% vs. 12% respectively, P = 0.05 after 6 months of follow up) (68), but no convincing difference compared with AMS in two other studies (69,70). Similarly, studies of patient self-management report better quality of anticoagulant control compared to routine medical care (71–73) versus AMS (74–76). Therefore, no definite recommendations about the optimal approach for maintaining anticoagulation control can be made.

### Patient Characteristics

The risk of major bleeding during warfarin therapy can be related to specific comorbid conditions or patient characteristics. An increasing body of evidence supports age as an independent risk factor for major bleeding (30,77–94). For example, Pengo et al. (93) evaluated the relation of age and other risk factors to the incidence of major bleeding. Major bleeding occurred more frequently in patients older than 75 years of age (5.1% per year) than in younger patients (1% per year). Multivariate analysis indicated that age greater than 75 years was the only variable independently related to primary bleeding (i.e., bleeding unrelated to organic lesion). Also, risk for intracranial hemorrhage may be increased among older patients, especially those older than 75 years when the INR is above therapeutic levels (53,54,77,95). The mechanism of how aging causes anticoagulant-related bleeding is not known.

A history of prior bleeding has been reported as a risk factor for subsequent bleeding (96–98), but this observation has not been consistent (49,77,99). A history of nonbleeding peptic ulcer disease, however, has not been associated with subsequent gastrointestinal bleeding (60,87,99).

Other comorbid diseases have been associated with bleeding during warfarin therapy; these include treated hypertension (80,81,83,85,100), cerebrovascular disease (77), ischemic stroke (55,78), serious heart disease (77,82), and renal insufficiency (60,77,96,97,101). The presence of malignancy was a significant predictor of major bleeding in several studies (87,89,90,97,99, 102). In two of these studies, overanticoagulation was not the explanation for an increased risk of bleeding (87,102), whereas in one study the severity of the cancer was identified as a risk factor (102). Another study (101) did not confirm that malignancy predisposed to bleeding, whereas others (81,103) excluded patients with malignancies.

Although many other patient characteristics have been associated with bleeding during warfarin therapy, the data supporting these findings are not compelling. For example, some studies noted an increased frequency of bleeding among women treated with warfarin (60,81,82,84,86), but others have not (30,81,83, 104,105). Although most experienced clinicians believe that either alcoholism or liver disease increases the risk of bleeding during long-term warfarin therapy, two studies did not find such an association (80,81), whereas a large population-based study did (97).

Occult pathologic lesions may also precipitate warfarin-related bleeding. In one study, 73% of adequately evaluated patients with a prothrombin time ratio less than 1.5 at the time of bleeding had an underlying pathologic lesion compared to 16% of patients with a prothrombin time ratio greater than or equal to 1.5 ($P < 0.05$) (79). However, pathologic lesions were found to be associated with gastrointestinal or genitourinary bleeding in 30% of patients with prothrombin time ratio greater than or equal to 2.5.

### Concomitant Drugs

Concomitant use of ASA has been associated with a higher frequency of bleeding even in patients treated with warfarin therapy with a mean INR of 1.5 (106–109). In a large randomized trial comparing the combination of low-dose warfarin therapy and ASA 80 mg per day to ASA 160 mg per day in patients with a history of myocardial infarction, the frequency of spontaneous major hemorrhage during the first year of therapy was increased to 1.4% in patients treated with warfarin 3 mg (INR <2.0) and ASA 80 mg daily, compared with 0.7% in patients treated with ASA 160 mg daily ($P = 0.01$) (107). In a large trial of primary prevention in persons at high risk for ischemic heart disease, the rate of hemorrhagic stroke was 0.09% per year in those treated with low-dose warfarin (target INR 1.5) plus ASA 75 mg daily, 0.01% per year with low-dose warfarin alone and 0.02% per year with ASA alone, and none in the placebo group (108). Similarly, in a trial which compared warfarin (INR 1.5 to 2.5) plus 81 mg of ASA to 162 mg ASA alone in patients postmyocardial infarction, major bleeding was more common in the warfarin and ASA group than in the ASA-only group (1.28 vs. 0.72 events per 100 person-years of follow-up, respectively; $P < 0.001$) (109). A number of drugs can interact with warfarin and thereby lead to excessive prolongation of the INR. This can increase the potential for bleeding. A discussion of warfarin interactions is beyond the scope of this chapter.

### Risk of Bleeding and the Length of Time Relative to When Anticoagulant Therapy Started

Four studies reported higher frequencies of bleeding early in the course of therapy (60,80,81,87). In one of these studies, for example, the frequency of major bleeding decreased from 3.0% during the first month of outpatient warfarin therapy to 0.8% per month during the rest of the first year of therapy, and to 0.3% per month thereafter (80). Other descriptive studies have supported this observation (110–113), although some have not (100,114).

### Estimating Bleeding Risk

Models have been developed for estimating the risk for major bleeding during vitamin K–antagonist anticoagulant therapy. These models are based on the identification of independent risk factors for warfarin-related bleeding, such as a history of stroke, history of gastrointestinal bleeding, aged 65 years or older, and higher levels of anticoagulation (60,84,86,87,89, 96,115). Such prediction rules can be useful in clinical practice because although physicians' estimates of risk for anticoagulant-related bleeding are reasonably accurate during hospitalization, they are inaccurate during long-term outpatient therapy (96,115).

Two prediction models have been developed and validated in outpatients treated with warfarin. Beyth et al. identified four independent risk factors for bleeding: aged 65 years or greater, history of gastrointestinal bleeding, history of stroke, and one or more of four specific comorbid conditions (96). This model was validated in another cohort of patients treated in another city; the cumulative incidence of major bleeding at 48 months was 53% in high-risk patients (three or four risk factors), 12% in middle-risk patients (one or two risk factors), and 3% in low-risk patients (no risk factors). Kuijer et al. developed another prediction model based on age, gender, and the presence of malignancy (89). In patients classified at high-, middle-, and low-risk, the frequency of major bleeding was 7%, 4%, and 1%, respectively, after 3 months of therapy. These prediction models should not be the sole criteria for deciding whether to initiate therapy but should be used in conjunction with other assessments, such as the patient's functional and cognitive status, likelihood of compliance to therapy, risk of thrombosis, and personal preference (116). Clinicians can use these prediction models to help weigh the risks and benefits of coumarin therapy, potentially adjusting the intensity, type, or length of therapy or the frequency of INR monitoring. These assessments can be reviewed at the initiation of therapy and periodically assessed throughout the course of coumarin treatment.

## RISK OF HEMORRHAGE AND CLINICAL DISORDERS

### Ischemic Cerebrovascular Disease–Acute Stroke: Heparin Versus Control

Approximately 20, mostly small studies have compared early anticoagulant therapy with control in patients with acute ischemic stroke. The finding of studies that were published by 1999 (about 23,000 patients) has been combined in a Cochrane Systematic Review by Gubitz et al. (117). The trials in this overview evaluated unfractionated heparin, low-molecular-weight heparin (LMWH), heparinoid, oral anticoagulants, and direct thrombin inhibitors given in differing doses (e.g., prophylactic doses for VTE; therapeutic doses for stroke) and by different routes (e.g., subcutaneously or intravenously). In relation to bleeding, the review found that acute anticoagulation (a) increased symptomatic intracranial bleeding approximately 2.5-fold (an excess of nine per 1,000 patients); and (b) increased major extracranial bleeding approximately threefold (an excess of nine per 1,000 patients). Because the International Stroke Trial (IST), with more than 19,000 patients, accounted for more than 75% of patients in the analysis, it will be considered further (118).

**TABLE 119-1**

INTERNATIONAL STROKE TRIAL (118) RISK OF INTRACRANIAL AND MAJOR EXTRACRANIAL BLEEDING (14 DAYS) FOR SC HEPARIN IN ACUTE ISCHEMIC STROKE

| Treatment | No. of patients | Bleeding | | | |
|---|---|---|---|---|---|
| | | Total | Intracranial | Extracranial | Fatal |
| Heparin 12,500 U b.i.d. +ASA 300 mg o.d. | 2,430 | 75 (3.1%) | 42 (1.7%) | 33 (1.4%) | 10 (0.4%) |
| Heparin 5,000 U b.i.d. +ASA 300 mg o.d. | 2,431 | 39 (1.6%) | 19 (0.8%) | 20 (0.8%) | 9 (0.4%) |
| Heparin 12,500 U b.i.d. | 2,426 | 76 (3.2%) | 43 (1.8%) | 33 (1.4%) | 12 (0.5%) |
| Heparin 5,000 U b.i.d. | 2,429 | 26 (1.1%) | 16 (0.7%) | 10 (0.4%) | 9 (0.4%) |
| ASA 300 mg o.d. | 4,858 | 49 (1.0%) | 26 (0.5%) | 23 (0.5%) | 13 (0.3%) |
| Control | 4,859 | 29 (0.6%) | 15 (0.3%) | 14 (0.3%) | 5 (0.1%) |

ASA, acetylsalicylic acid.
From Group ISTC. The International Stroke Trial (IST): a randomized trial of aspirin, subcutaneous heparin, both or neither among 19,435 patients with acute ischaemic stroke. *Lancet* 1997;349:1569–1581, with permission.

In the IST, patients with acute ischemic stroke were treated with ASA (300 mg daily), subcutaneous heparin (5,000 or 12,500 U b.i.d.), both, or neither (see Table 119-1) (118). Heparin was associated with a dose-dependent increase of both intracranial and extracranial bleeding (all major bleeds: control, 0.6%; heparin 5,000 b.i.d., 1.1%; heparin 12,500 b.i.d., 3.2%) which, at the higher dose, more than offset antithrombotic benefit. Patients who had the highest risk of recurrent ischemic stroke also had the highest risk of intracerebral bleeding. For example, in patients with acute ischemic stroke and atrial fibrillation, although the frequency of hemorrhagic stroke after 14 days was 2.1% (32/1,557) with heparin therapy (either dose) compared with 0.4% (7/1,612) without heparin therapy, there was no difference in the combined endpoint of recurrent ischemic or hemorrhagic stroke.

More recently, the Therapy of Patients with Acute Stroke (TOPAS) study compared four doses of an LMWH (Certoparin) in 400 patients with ischemic stroke and found a trend to more major bleeding with the highest dose compared to the three lower doses combined (9.0% vs. 2.0%) (119).

## Ischemic Cerebrovascular Disease–Acute Stroke: Heparin Versus Antiplatelet Agents

Four trials have compared anticoagulants with antiplatelet agents in patients with acute ischemic stroke (118, 120–122). Unfractionated heparin (118,122) and LMWH (120,121) in low doses (118,122) or high doses (118,120,121) were compared with ASA (118,120,121) or ASA and dipyridamole (122). Three trials included cardioembolic and noncardioembolic strokes (118,121,122), whereas one was confined to cardioembolic strokes (120). The findings of these four studies, with data from more than 16,000 patients (88% from IST) (118), have been combined in a Cochrane Systematic Review by Berge and Sandercock (123). The review found that, compared to antiplatelet therapy, acute anticoagulation increased symptomatic intracranial hemorrhage 2.3-fold (an excess of 10 per 1,000 patients) and increased major extracranial hemorrhage 1.9-fold (an excess of five per 1,000 patients treated). The increase in major bleeding with anticoagulants was mostly confined to high-dose regimens (123).

## Ischemic Cerebrovascular Disease: Vitamin K Antagonists

Randomized trials have compared vitamin K antagonists with a placebo or nontreatment group (124–129), a very low-dose vitamin K antagonist group (130,131), or an antiplatelet group (48,132–136), after an acute episode of ischemic cerebrovascular disease of presumed arterial origin (for details of earlier studies see Fourth ACCP Consensus Conference on Antithrombotic Therapy) (4). In all but four of these studies (130–133,135), the intensity of vitamin K antagonist was high (middle of PT target corresponded to an INR of >4). Vitamin K antagonists were associated with increased bleeding in all of these studies, with a frequency of major bleeding (often intracerebral) varying from 2% to 13% during a mean duration of follow-up of 6 to 30 months. In addition to use of high intensities of anticoagulation, unsuspected initial intracerebral hemorrhage (pre–computerized tomography era), suboptimal control of hypertension, and initiation of anticoagulation in the setting of acute stroke may have contributed to high rates of bleeding in early studies. However, there is recent evidence (see subsequent text) that ischemic stroke not due to cardioembolism is associated with a much higher risk of anticoagulant-induced intracranial bleeding than strokes that are due to embolism (e.g., with atrial fibrillation) (132,137).

Algra et al. combined the findings of five studies (approximately 4,000 patients) that compared vitamin K antagonists with antiplatelet therapy after transient ischemic attack or minor stroke of presumed arterial origin in a Cochrane Systematic Review (updated 2002) (136). The authors estimated a risk of major bleeding with vitamin K antagonists compared with antiplatelet therapy of 1.3 [95% confidence intervals (CI), 0.8 to 2.0] for INR 1.4 to 2.8, of 1.2 (95% CI, 0.6 to 2.4) for INR 2.1 to 3.6, and of 9.0 (95% CI, 3.9 to 21.0) for INR 3.0 to 4.5. Because two studies (SPIRIT and WARSS) accounted for 86% of the patients in this review and were recently published, they will be considered further (48,133).

In the Stroke Prevention in Reversible Ischemia Trial (SPIRIT), 1,316 patients with a transient ischemia attack or minor ischemic stroke were randomized to 30 mg ASA daily or warfarin therapy at a targeted INR of 3.0 to 4.5 (48).

There was a statistically significant increase in major bleeding associated with warfarin; 53 (8.1%) major bleeding complications (27 intracranial, 17 fatal) versus six (0.9%) with ASA (three intracranial, one fatal) during a mean follow-up of 14 months. Bleeding increased by a factor of 1.4 for each 0.5-U increase of the INR. Previous stroke has not been identified as a risk factor for intracerebral bleeding in vitamin K antagonist–treated patients with atrial fibrillation (INR, 1.4 to 4.5) (54,77,78,138). An analysis of data from individual patients who were allocated to vitamin K antagonist in the European Atrial Fibrillation Trial (EAFT) (78) (stroke with atrial fibrillation; INR 2.5 to 4.0) and in SPIRIT (48) (stroke without atrial fibrillation; INR 3.0 to 4.5) found that, independent of other risk factors and achieved intensity of anticoagulation, risk of intracranial bleeding was at least 10 times higher if stroke was not due to atrial fibrillation (hazard ratio of 19 for intracranial, and only 1.9 for major extracranial bleeding) (137).

In the Warfarin-Aspirin Recurrent Stroke Study (WARSS), 2,206 patients were randomized to 325 mg aspirin daily or warfarin targeted to an INR of 1.4 to 2.8 (mean achieved INR was 2.1) within 30 days of an ischemic stroke (not including cardioembolism) (133). There was a nonsignificant trend for an increase in major bleeding with warfarin (44 vs. 30 events; seven vs. four associated with death) and a statistically significant increase in minor bleeding (21% vs. 13%) during 2 years of follow-up (number of intracranial bleeds were not reported) (133). The relative safety of oral anticoagulant therapy in WARSS compared with SPIRIT is consistent with intensity of anticoagulation having a major influence on risk of bleeding in patients with ischemic stroke.

## Prosthetic Heart Valves: Vitamin K Antagonists

Bleeding rates in patients receiving different regimens with long-term vitamin K antagonist therapy for prosthetic heart valves have been reported from 14 randomized clinical trials (43–46,139–148). The targeted intensity of oral anticoagulant therapy was not defined with the INR (139–143) in the first five trials.

In all nine randomized trials of long-term vitamin K–antagonist therapy in patients with mechanical heart valves since 1990, the targeted intensity of anticoagulation was reported using the INR (43–46,144–148). The rates of major bleeding reported in these trials (see Table 119-2) are, however, based on somewhat different definitions, and the time within the target INR range varied from 35% to 86%. In the study by Altman et al. 1991, major bleeding was not defined (44), and in the study by Pruefer et al., numerical data are not provided by treatment group (148). (Hence, these trials are not included in Table 119-2.) In three trials, different intensities of vitamin K antagonists were compared (43,45,145). Saour et al. (43) randomized patients to either warfarin therapy at a targeted INR of 2.65 or very high-intensity warfarin therapy (targeted INR 9.0). The rate of major bleeding in the former treatment arm was 3.3% compared with 7.2% in the latter arm during 3.5 years of follow-up ($P = 0.27$). In the trial conducted by Acar et al., 380 patients were randomized to treatment with acenocoumarol at a targeted INR of 2.0 to 3.0 or the same medication at a targeted INR of 3.0 to 4.5 (145). The rate of major bleeding in the lower-intensity group was 9.0% compared with 12.0% in the higher-intensity

## TABLE 119-2

### PROSTHETIC HEART VALVES

| Study | Treatment | No. of patients (patient-years) | Bleeding events | | |
|---|---|---|---|---|---|
| | | | Major (% per year) | Fatal (% per year) | Intracranial (% per year) |
| Saour (43) | Warfarin (INR 2.65) | 122 (421) | 1.0 | 0 | 0 |
| | Warfarin (INR 9.0) | 125 (436) | 2.1 | 0.5 | 0.5 |
| Turpie (144) | Warfarin (INR 3.0–4.5) + placebo | 184 (≈462)[a] | 4.1 | 0.7 | 0.7 |
| | Warfarin (INR 3.0–4.5) +ASA 100 mg | 186 (≈462)[a] | 5.2 | 0.6 | 1.5 |
| Altman (146) | Acenocoumarol (INR 2.0–3.0) +ASA 100 mg | 207 (416) | 3.6 | 0.5 | 0.2 |
| | Acenocoumarol (INR 2.0–3.0) +ASA 650 mg | 202 (366) | 5.2 | 0.3 | 0.3 |
| Acar (145) | Acenocoumarol (INR 2.0–3.0) | 188 (414) | 4.1 | 0.2 | 0.5 |
| | Acenocoumarol (INR 3.0–4.5) | 192 (422) | 5.5 | 0.2 | 0.7 |
| Pengo (45) | Warfarin (INR 2.5–3.5) | 104 (333) | 1.2[b] | 0 | 0.3 |
| | Warfarin (INR 3.5–4.5) | 101 (289) | 3.8 | 0.3 | 0.3 |
| Meschengieser (46) | Acenocoumarol (INR 2.5–3.5) +ASA 100 mg | 258 (529) | 1.1 | 0 | 0 |
| | Acenocoumarol (INR 3.5–4.5) | 245 (471) | 2.3 | 0.2 | 0.6 |
| Laffort (147) | Vitamin K antagonist (INR 2.5–3.5) | 120 (120) | 8.3[c] | 3 | 0 |
| | Vitamin K antagonist (INR 2.5–3.5) + ASA 200 mg | 109 (109) | 19.2 | 3 | 0 |

INR, international normalized ratio; ASA, acetylsalicylic acid.
[a]Estimated from mean follow-up.
[b]$P < 0.05$.
[c]$P = 0.02$.

group over 2.2 years ($P = 0.29$). In a trial conducted by Pengo et al. (45), 205 patients were randomized to treatment with either warfarin or acenocoumarol at a targeted INR of 2.5 to 3.5 or the same medications at a targeted INR of 3.5 to 4.5 and followed for a mean of 3 years. The rate of major bleeding was 3.8% in the former group compared with 11% in the latter group ($P = 0.019$). Therefore, the results of these trials suggest that by lowering the intensity of anticoagulation, the rate of major hemorrhage can be reduced.

The addition of ASA to vitamin K antagonists has been studied in four trials. In a double-blind trial, Turpie et al. (144) compared warfarin (INR, 3.0 to 4.5) with warfarin plus 100 mg ASA. The rate of major bleeding was 10.3% in the warfarin-alone group compared with 12.9% in the warfarin plus ASA group after 2.5 years of follow-up ($P = 0.043$). Altman et al. (146) compared two different doses of ASA (100 mg daily vs. 650 mg daily) in patients receiving acenocoumarol at an INR of 2.0 to 3.0 followed for an average of 24.1 and 21.7 months, respectively. The rate of major bleeding in the lower-dose ASA group was 7.2% compared with 9.4% in the higher-dose group ($P = 0.4$). Meschengieser et al. compared acenocoumarol alone (INR 3.5 to 4.5) with a combination of acenocoumarol at a lower intensity (INR, 2.5 to 3.5) plus 100 mg ASA (46). The rate of major bleeding was 4.5% in the monotherapy group compared with 2.3% in the combination therapy group after a median follow-up of 23 months ($P = 0.27$). The trial of Laffort et al. is unique in its homogeneity, because only patients with St. Jude Medical valve prosthesis in the mitral position were included (147). Treatment with vitamin K antagonists alone (INR 2.5 to 3.5) was compared with a combination of vitamin K antagonist and ASA (200 mg daily) for 1 year, starting immediately after surgery. This may explain the high rate of major bleeding, which was 8.3% with monotherapy and 19.2% with the combination ($P = 0.02$).

Three metaanalyses on studies including only patients with prosthetic heart valves on long-term vitamin K antagonist therapy have been performed (149–151). Two of the analyses aimed at evaluating risks and benefits of a combination of vitamin K antagonist and antiplatelet agent with anticoagulant alone and included five (149) and 10 studies (150), respectively. In the metaanalysis by Cappelleri et al. the combined regimen increased the risk of any hemorrhage by 65% and of major hemorrhage by 49%, but only the former difference was statistically significant (149). In the metaanalysis by Massel et al. the risk of major hemorrhage was increased by the addition of antiplatelet regimens ($P = 0.033$), but there was sufficient evidence that 100 mg of ASA compared to higher doses provided a safer combination (150). A metaanalysis by Pouleur et al. based on six trials evaluating the efficacy and safety of adding dipyridamole to anticoagulant therapy, showed that the risk of hemorrhage was identical in the two groups (151). The studies included in these analyses differed regarding the targeted intensity of anticoagulation (in many of the studies based on a best guess of the reagents used to perform the prothrombin time), the antiplatelet agent (ASA or dipyridamole), and the dose of ASA (100, 500, or 1,000 mg), which increases the heterogeneity of the findings.

The annual bleeding rates (percentage per year) regarding major, fatal, or intracranial hemorrhage are shown in Table 119-2. Cannegieter et al. (152) reported the results of a retrospective study in 1,608 patients who received vitamin K–antagonist therapy for mechanical heart valves. The rate of intracranial and spinal bleeding was 0.57% per year, and the rate of major extracranial bleeding was 2.1% per year. Cannegieter et al. also published the results of a metaanalysis of 46 studies (randomized trials and case series) in which patients received vitamin K antagonists for mechanical valves. The incidence of major bleeding was 1.4% per year (153).

## Atrial Fibrillation: Vitamin K Antagonists

The efficacy of warfarin in preventing stroke in patients with nonvalvular atrial fibrillation has been consistently demonstrated in a number of randomized clinical trials and in metaanalyses of randomized trials (49–51,63,78,138,154–169). Overall, the rates of warfarin-related bleeding in these studies has been low (see Table 119-3). In two metaanalyses of 12 trials of warfarin for stroke prevention, warfarin increased the odds of major bleeding; the odds ratio (OR) was 1.90 (162) and the relative risk 2.4 (164), respectively; the absolute risk increase was 0.3% per year (162). Although intracranial bleeding was more frequent in patients treated with warfarin in these trials (0.3% per year vs. 0.1% per year in patients not treated with warfarin or ASA), the absolute difference was small and overwhelmed by the substantial reduction in the frequency of stroke.

More recently, two metaanalyses have evaluated the relative risks and benefits of oral anticoagulant therapy versus antiplatelet therapy in patients with atrial fibrillation (166,167). Oral anticoagulant therapy was associated with increased major bleeding [OR, 1.45 (167) and hazard ratio, 1.71 (166)]; the increased risk of oral anticoagulant therapy was offset by reduced nonfatal stroke (OR, 0.68) (167), all strokes (hazard ratio, 0.55) (166), and all cardiovascular events (hazard ratio, 0.71) (166). The analysis by Taylor et al. (167) did not include the Stroke Prevention in Atrial Fibrillation (SPAF) I and III studies (49,155) or the EAFT study (55). The analysis by van Walraven et al. used the pooled individual patient data from all published trials comparing oral anticoagulants with ASA for atrial fibrillation (166). Oral anticoagulant therapy was associated with increased major bleeding (hazard ratio, 1.71, absolute increase 0.9 events per 100 patient-years, $P = 0.02$); the corresponding hazard ratios and absolute increases in rates per 100 patient-years for all hemorrhagic stroke were 1.84 and 0.2, ($P = 0.19$) and for fatal bleeding were 2.15 and 0.2 ($P = 0.32$). This analysis concluded that treating 1,000 patients with atrial fibrillation for 1 year with oral anticoagulants rather than ASA would prevent 23 ischemic strokes while causing 9 additional major bleeds (166).

Because 50% or more of patients with atrial fibrillation are older than age 75, the risk-benefit of oral anticoagulant therapy in this clinical subgroup is of particular interest. One study (SPAF II) raised concern that the risk for warfarin-related bleeding, especially intracranial hemorrhage, may be increased substantially in patients aged 75 years and older (Table 119-3) (169). The rate of major bleeding while receiving warfarin was 2.3% per year compared with 1.1% per year for patients receiving ASA 325 mg daily. However, the rate of major warfarin-related bleeding was 4.2% per year in patients aged 75 years and older, compared with 1.7% per year in younger patients; the corresponding rates for intracranial bleeding were 1.8% per year and 0.6% per year, respectively. The reason these rates are substantially higher than those observed in the other clinical trials of warfarin in patients with atrial fibrillation is likely related to the intensity of anticoagulant therapy: Virtually all intracranial hemorrhages in SPAF II, as in the other clinical trials, were associated with an INR greater than 3.0 (169). In contrast, in the SPAF III trial (targeted INR, 2.0 to 3.0), the mean age was 71 years and the rate of intracranial hemorrhage was 0.5% per year (49).

There have been two trials evaluating a fixed low dose of warfarin (1.25 mg per day) in atrial fibrillation (50,138,159). These trials were stopped early because of the SPAF III trial results, which demonstrated that low-intensity warfarin (i.e., INR <1.5) was insufficient for stroke prevention (49). The rates of major bleeding were low in these studies (Table 119-3).

## TABLE 119-3

### ATRIAL FIBRILLATION

| Study | Treatment | No. of patients | Bleeding Major (%) | Bleeding Fatal (%) |
|-------|-----------|-----------------|---------------------|---------------------|
| Petersen (156) | Warfarin (INR 2.8–4.2) | 335 | [a] | 1 (0.3) |
| | ASA (75 mg) | 336 | [a] | 0 |
| | Placebo | 336 | [a] | 0 |
| SPiAF (155) | Warfarin (INR 2.0–3.5) | 201 | 1.7%/yr | [a] |
| | ASA (325 mg) | 192 | 0.9%/yr | [a] |
| | Placebo | 195 | 1.2%/yr | [a] |
| Boston (154) | Warfarin (INR 1.5–2.7) | 212 | 8 (3.8) | 1 (0.5) |
| | No Rx | 208 | 8 (3.8) | 1 (0.5) |
| CAFA (158) | Warfarin (INR 2.0–3.0) | 187 | 5 (2.7) | 2 (1.1) |
| | Placebo | 191 | 1 (0.5) | 0 |
| SPAF II (169) | Warfarin ≤75 yr (INR 2.0–4.5) | 358 | 1.7%/yr | [a] |
| | ASA ≤75 yr | 357 | 0.9%/yr | [a] |
| | Warfarin >75 yr (INR 2.0–4.5) | 197 | 4.2%/yr[c] | [a] |
| | ASA >75 yr | 188 | 1.6%/yr | [a] |
| European (78) | Warfarin (INR 2.5–4.0) | 225 | 13 (5.8) | 3 (1.3) |
| | Placebo | 230 | 3 (1.3) | 1 (0.4) |
| | ASA (300 mg) | 404 | 6 (1.5) | 2 (0.5) |
| Veterans Affairs (157) | Warfarin (INR 1.4–2.8) | 260 | 6 (2.3) | 0 |
| | Placebo | 265 | 4 (1.5) | 1 (0.4) |
| SPAF III (49) | Warfarin (INR 1.2–1.5) + ASA (325 mg) | 521 | 13 (2.4%/yr) | 3 (0.6%/yr) |
| | Warfarin (INR 2.0–3.0) | 523 | 12 (2.1%/yr) | 2 (0.4%/yr) |
| Morocutti (160) | Warfarin (INR 2.0–3.5) | 454 | 6.0%/yr | 1.0%/yr |
| | Indobufen | 462 | 1.0%/yr | 0 |
| Gullov (50,138) | Warfarin (INR 2.0–3.0) | 170 | 1.1%/yr | 0.3%/yr |
| | Warfarin (1.25 mg) | 167 | 0.8%/yr | 0 |
| | Warfarin+ASA (1.25 mg + 300 mg) | 171 | 0.3%/yr | 0 |
| | ASA (300 mg) | 169 | 1.4%/yr | 0.3%/yr |
| Pengo (159) | Warfarin (INR 2.0–3.0) | 153 | 2.6%/yr | [a] |
| | Warfarin (1.25 mg) | 150 | 1.0%/yr | [a] |
| Hellemons (161) | Phenprocoumon/Acenocoumarol (INR 2.5–3.5) | 131 | 0.5%/yr | [a] |
| | Phenprocoumon/Acenocoumarol (INR 1.1–1.6) | 122 | 1.4%/yr | [a] |
| | ASA (150 mg) | 141 | 1.4%/yr | [a] |
| Yamaguchi (51) | Warfarin (INR 1.5–2.1) | 60 | 0%/yr | – |
| | Warfarin (INR 2.2–3.5) | 55 | 6 (6.6%/yr) | – |
| Matcher (63) | Warfarin (INR 2.0–3.0) | 572 | 6 | 0 |
| | Warfarin (INR 2.0–3.0) | 593 | 7 | 1 |

SPAF, Stroke Prevention in Atrial Fibrillation; CAFA, Canadian Atrial Fibrillation Anticoagulation; INR, international normalized ratio; ASA, acetylsalicylic acid.
[a]Not reported in publications.
[b]P <0.04.

The relative risk-benefit of warfarin therapy at a targeted INR of 1.5 to 2.1 compared with warfarin therapy at a targeted INR of 2.2 to 3.5 has been evaluated in a randomized trial in patients with atrial fibrillation (51). Major bleeding occurred in 6 of 55 patients in the conventional-intensity group (rate 6.6% per year), compared with none of the 60 patients (0% per year) in the low-intensity group (P = 0.01). The six patients with major bleeding were all elderly (mean 74 years) and older than the other 109 patients without major bleeding (mean 66 years) (P <0.01). The INR before bleeding was less than 3.0 in four patients and was 3.1 and 3.6 in the remaining two patients. The annual rate of ischemic stroke was low in both the conventional-intensity group (1.1% per year) and in the low-intensity group (1.7% per year); however, the 95% CI for these rates overlap widely, and the study is too small to make definitive conclusions about the relative effectiveness of these two different intensities of anticoagulation.

A systematic review compared the rates of stroke, intracranial bleeding, and major bleeding from studies of patients treated in actual clinical practice with the pooled data from randomized clinical trials (168). Patients in clinical practice were older and had more comorbid conditions than the patients in clinical trials. Nevertheless, the rates of ischemic stroke were similar between clinical practice and the clinical trials (1.8 and 1.4 per 100 patient-years, respectively), as were the corresponding rates of intracranial bleeding (0.1 and 0.3 per 100 patient-years, respectively) and major bleeding (1.1 and 1.3 per 100 patient-years respectively) (168). There was a higher rate of minor bleeding in clinical practice (12.0 per 100 patient-years) than in clinical trials (7.9 per 100 patient-years ) ($P = 0.002$).

## Atrial Fibrillation: Oral Thrombin Inhibitors

The direct thrombin inhibitor ximelagatran has been compared to warfarin in patients with nonvalvular atrial fibrillation. In the SPORTIF II trial, 257 patients were randomized to receive one of three twice-daily doses of ximelagatran (20, 40, or 60 mg) or warfarin (INR 2.0 to 3.0) for 3 months. There were no major bleeds in the ximelagatran group and one in the warfarin group (170). In the SPORTIF III trial, 3,407 patients with nonvalvular atrial fibrillation received ximelagatran 36 mg twice daily or warfarin (INR 2.0 to 3.0) (171). The rates of major bleeding were 1.3% and 1.8%, respectively. This difference was not statistically significant.

## Ischemic Heart Disease: Heparin

There have been two trials in which patients with ischemic coronary artery disease were randomized to treatment with heparin or no heparin (172,173), one trial in which heparin was compared with ASA (172), and one trial in which high-dose heparin therapy was compared with a lower dose of heparin (174). The results of these trials have shown that heparin administered alone in patients with coronary artery disease (without concurrent thrombolytic therapy) is not associated with an increased risk of major bleeding (4).

LMWH has been compared with a no-treatment control or IV unfractionated heparin in several trials in patients with unstable coronary artery disease (175–178). The bleeding outcomes from these clinical trials are shown in Table 119-4. For IV unfractionated heparin, the rates of major bleeding range from 0% to 6.3% during the initial 8 days of treatment and from 0.3% to 3.2% during the long-term treatment phase between approximately 1 week and 3 months. For several of the trials, explicit data for the incidence of fatal bleeding were not reported. The data in Table 119-4 support the inference that LMWH does not result in an increased risk of major bleeding compared with IV unfractionated heparin. The absolute rates of major bleeding were higher in more recent trials (179–181) than were observed in the initial large trials of LMWH (176, 177). This is probably due to inclusion in the more recent studies of patients who undergo cardiac catheterization or coronary bypass surgery; much of the major bleeding in these trials was associated with invasive vascular procedures or coronary bypass surgery (179–181). In contrast, the earlier studies (176,177) excluded patients for whom catheterization, angioplasty, or coronary bypass surgery was planned. A recent meta-analysis of randomized trials comparing unfractionated heparin or LMWH with placebo or untreated control, or comparing unfractionated heparin with LMWH, for the short-term and long-term management of patients with acute coronary syndrome without ST elevation identified 12 trials, involving a total of 17,157 patients (182). Long-term LMWH (>7 days) was associated with a significantly increased risk of major bleeding [OR, 2.26; 95% CI, 1.63 to 3.14]; $P$ <0.0001], which is equivalent to 12 major bleeds per 1,000 patients treated. In a multicenter, double-blind, placebo-controlled trial to examine the efficacy and safety of twice-daily

## TABLE 119-4

LOW-MOLECULAR-WEIGHT HEPARIN VERSUS UNFRACTIONATED HEPARIN FOR ACUTE ISCHEMIC CORONARY SYNDROMES

| Study | Regimens | Treatment duration | No. of patients | Major bleeding | Fatal bleeding |
|-------|----------|--------------------|-----------------|----------------|----------------|
| Gurfinkel et al. (175) | ASA alone | 5–7 d | 73 | 0 | 0 |
| | IV heparin aPTT ratio 2.0 | 5–7 d | 70 | 2 (2.9) | 0 |
| | Nadroparin 214 U/kg sc b.i.d. | 5–7 d | 68 | 0 | 0 |
| FRISC (176) | Placebo sc b.i.d. | 0–6 d | 760 | 4 (0.5) | 1 (0.1%) |
| | Dalteparin 120 U/kg sc b.i.d. | 0–6 d | 746 | 6 (0.8) | 0 |
| | Placebo sc o.d. | 6–45 d | 614 | 2 (0.3) | 0 |
| | Dalteparin 7,500 U sc o.d. | 6–45 d | 619 | 2 (0.3) | 0 |
| FRIC (177) | IV heparin aPTT ratio 1.5 | 0–6 d | 731 | 7 (1.0) | NR |
| | Dalteparin 120 U/kg sc b.i.d. | 0–6 d | 751 | 8 (1.1) | NR |
| | Placebo sc o.d. | 6–45 d | 565 | 2 (0.4) | NR |
| | Dalteparin 7,500 U sc o.d. | 6–45 d | 567 | 3 (0.5) | NR |
| TIMI IIA (179) | Enoxaparin 1.25 mg/kg sc q12h | 14 d | 321 | 21 (6.5) | NR |
| | Enoxaparin 1.0 mg/kg sc q12h | 14 d | 309 | 6 (1.9) | NR |
| ESSENCE (178) | IV heparin aPTT ratio 55 to 85 s | 2–8 d | 1,564 | 107 (6.8) | NR |
| | Enoxaparin 1.0 mg/kg sc q12h | 2–8 d | 1,607 | 102 (6.3) | NR |
| FRISC II (180) | Placebo sc b.i.d. | 3 mo | 1,056 | 16 (1.5) | NR |
| | Dalteparin 120 U/kg sc b.i.d. | 3 mo | 1,049 | 34 (3.2) | NR |
| TIMI IIB (181) | IV heparin aPTT ratio 1.5 to 2.5 | hospital (8 d) | 1,957 | 19 (1.0) | 4 (0.2%) |
| | Enoxaparin 1.0 mg/kg sc q12h | hospital (8 d) | 1,953 | 29 (1.5) | 4 (0.2%) |
| | Placebo sc q12h | 43 d | 1,185 | 18 (1.5) | NR |
| | Enoxaparin 40 mg or 60 mg sc o.d. | 43 d | 1,179 | 34 (2.9) | NR |

FRISC, Fragmin during Instability in Coronary Artery Disease; FRIC, Fragmin in Unstable Coronary Artery Disease; TIMI, Thrombolysis in Myocardial Infarction; ESSENCE, Efficacy and Safety of Subcutaneous Enoxaparin on Q wave Coronary Events; ASA, acetylsalicylic acid; aPTT, activated partial thromboplastin time; NR, not reported.

injections of weight-adjusted enoxaparin or placebo for 14 days after stenting in patients at high risk for stent thrombosis (183), the groups had comparable rates of major bleeding (3.3% for enoxaparin, 1.6% for placebo, $P = 0.08$), but minor bleeding was increased with enoxaparin (25% vs. 5.1%, $P \leq 0.001$).

## Ischemic Heart Disease–Myocardial Infarction: Vitamin K Antagonists

There are 13 published randomized trials of long-term oral anticoagulant therapy in patients with acute myocardial infarction (see Table 119-5) (104,107,109,184–195). These 13 trials compared the following regimens: Anticoagulant therapy was compared with placebo or control ($n = 7$) (104,184–186,189–193); anticoagulant therapy with ASA ($n = 1$) (187); anticoagulant therapy with ASA or placebo ($n = 1$) (188); fixed low doses of warfarin (1 or 3 mg) combined with ASA were compared with

ASA alone ($n = 1$) (107); anticoagulant therapy alone, or combined with ASA, was compared with ASA alone ($n = 1$) (194); and anticoagulant therapy with ASA was compared with ASA ($n = 1$) (109). The frequency of major bleeding ranged from 0% to 10%, and fatal bleeding ranged from 0% to 2.9%.

Smith et al. (184) reported the results of a randomized trial that renewed interest in the long-term use of oral anticoagulants after myocardial infarction. The targeted INR was 2.8 to 4.8. Five patients in the warfarin group (0.8%) had intracranial hemorrhages, and three of these were fatal. Eight (1.3%) warfarin-treated patients experienced major extracranial bleeds. There were no major bleeds in the placebo group.

In a trial conducted by the Anticoagulants in the Secondary Prevention of Events in Coronary Thrombosis 1 (ASPECT 1) investigators, patients who had sustained a myocardial infarction were randomized to either oral anticoagulant therapy at a targeted INR of 2.8 to 4.8 or placebo (193). The mean follow up was 37 months. Seventy-three patients (4.3%) in the

## TABLE 119-5

### ISCHEMIC HEART DISEASE–MYOCARDIAL INFARCTION

| Study | Treatment | No. of patients | Bleeding Major (%) | Fatal (%) |
|---|---|---|---|---|
| Sixty-plus (185,186) | Acenocoumarin (INR 2.2–5.0) | 439 | 18 (4.1) | 6 (1.4) |
| EPSIM group (187) | Placebo | 439 | 1 (0.2) | 1 (0.2) |
| Breddin et al. (188) | Oral anticoagulants[a] | 652 | 21 (3.2) | 8 (1.2) |
| Meuwissen et al. (104) | ASA (500 mg t.i.d.) | 651 | 5 (0.8) | 4 (0.6) |
| Loeliger et al. (189) | Phenprocoumon (INR 2.0–5.0) | 320 | NR | 0 |
| Bjerkelund et al. (190,191) | ASA (500 mg t.i.d.) | 317 | NR | 0 |
| Harvald et al. (192) | Placebo | 309 | NR | 0 |
| Smith et al. (184) | Phenprocoumon (INR 1.9–5.0) | 68 | 0 | 0 |
| | Placebo | 70 | 0 | 0 |
| | Phenprocoumon (INR 2.0–5.0) | 128 | 1 (0.8) | 0 |
| | Placebo | 122 | 1 (0.8) | 1 (0.8) |
| | Dicumarol (INR 1.3–2.1) | 138 | 20 (14.5) | 4 (2.9) |
| | No Rx | 139 | 5 (3.6) | 1 (0.7) |
| | Dicumarol (INR 1.5–2.1) | 145 | 28 (19.3) | 1 (0.7) |
| | Placebo | 170 | 0 | 0 |
| | Warfarin (INR 2.8–4.8) | 607 | 13 (2.1) | 3 (0.5) |
| | Placebo | 607 | 0 | 0 |
| ASPECT (193) | Nicoumalone/phenprocoumon (INR 2.8–4.8) | 1,700 | 73 (4.3)[b] | 11 (0.6)[b] |
| | Placebo | 1,704 | 19 (1.1) | 0 |
| CARS (107) | Warfarin 3 mg (INR 1.2)[c] + ASA 80 mg | 3,382 | 75 (2.2) | NR |
| | Warfarin 3 mg (INR 1.0)[c] + ASA 80 mg | 2,082 | 42 (1.7) | NR |
| | ASA 160 mg | 3,393 | 57 (1.5) | NR |
| ASPECT-2 (194) | ASA | 336 | 3 (1) | NR |
| | Phenprocoumon/acenocoumarol | 325 | 3 (1) | NR |
| | ASA+Phenprocoumon/ acenocoumarol | 332 | 7 (2) | NR |
| CHAMP (109) | Warfarin (INR 1.5–2.5) + ASA 81 mg | 2,522 | 0.72/100 pt-yr | NR |
| | ASA 162 mg | 2,537 | 1.28/100 pt-yr | NR |
| WARIS II (195) | Warfarin (INR 2.8–4.2) | | | |
| | ASA 160 mg | 1,216 | 0.68/pt-yr | 5 (0.4) |
| | | 1,206 | 0.17/pt-yr | 0 |
| | Warfarin (INR 2.0–2.5) + ASA 75 mg | 1,208 | 0.57/pt-yr | 6 (0.5) |

ASPECT, Anticoagulants in the Secondary Prevention of Events in Coronary Thrombosis; CARS, Coumadin Aspirin Reinfarction Study; CHAMP, Combination Hemotherapy and Mortality Prevention; WARIS, Warfarin Aspirin Reinfarction Study; ASA, acetylsalicylic acid; INR, international normalized ratio.
[a]A number of different oral anticoagulants.
[b]$P < 0.01$.
[c]Median INR at 6 months of treatment. Warfarin was given as a fixed dose (1 or 3 mg).

anticoagulant group experienced major bleeding compared with 19 placebo-treated patients (1.1%). Three extracranial bleeds in the anticoagulant group were fatal; all were gastrointestinal in origin. Cerebral hemorrhage was more common in patients who had been treated with anticoagulants [17 cases (1%)], eight of which were fatal, compared with two, none of which were fatal in placebo-treated patients. The rate of major bleeding in the anticoagulant-treated group was 1.5% per year compared with 0.2% per year in the placebo-treated group. This difference was statistically significant.

The Coumadin Aspirin Reinfarction Study (CARS) (107) compared long-term treatment using fixed low doses of warfarin (1 or 3 mg) combined with ASA, 80 mg, to treatment with ASA alone (160 mg) using a randomized double-blind study design. The median follow up was 14 months. The median INR values 4 weeks and 6 months after beginning treatment were 1.27 and 1.19, respectively, for patients given 3 mg warfarin with 80 mg ASA. Major hemorrhage, including those related to invasive procedures, occurred in 75 patients (2.0% per year) given 3 mg warfarin with 80 mg ASA, 42 patients (1.7% per year) given 1 mg warfarin with 80 mg ASA, and 57 patients (1.5% per year) given ASA alone. For spontaneous major hemorrhage (not procedure related), annual rates were 1.4% in the 3 mg warfarin plus 80 mg ASA group, 1.0% in the 1 mg warfarin plus 80 mg ASA group, and 0.74% in the 160 mg ASA alone group.

The Combination Hemotherapy and Mortality Prevention (CHAMP) study (109) compared the efficacy of warfarin (target INR 1.5 to 2.5) with 81 mg of ASA to 162 mg of ASA alone in patients with postmyocardial infarction who were followed for a median of 2.7 years. Major bleeding occurred more frequently in the combination therapy group than in the ASA alone group (1.28 vs. 0.72 events per 100 patient-years; $P < 0.001$).

ASPECT 2 trial (194) compared 80 mg ASA, high-intensity (INR 3.0 to 4.0) vitamin K antagonist or combination 80 mg ASA, and moderated intensity (INR 2.0 to 2.5) vitamin K antagonist in patients who had survived acute coronary events; the median follow up was 12 months. Major bleeding rates were 1%, 1%, and 2% per patient-year in the ASA, coumadin, and combination groups, respectively. The frequency of minor bleeding was 5%, 8%, and 15% per patient-years in the ASA, coumadin, and combination groups, respectively.

The Warfarin Aspirin Reinfarction Study (WARIS II) trial (195) compared the efficacy and safety of warfarin (target INR 2.8 to 4.2), ASA (160 mg), and the two combined (75 mg ASA with warfarin with target INR 2.0 to 2.5) in a long-term, randomized, unblinded multicenter study involving 3,606 patients after acute myocardial infarction (1,202 in each treatment group). The mean duration of follow-up was 4 years. Major nonfatal bleeding occurred in 0.62% of patients per treatment-year in both warfarin groups and in 0.17% of patients receiving ASA ($P < 0.001$). Anand conducted a meta-analysis of trials evaluating vitamin K antagonists in patients with coronary artery disease (196). Trials were stratified based on the intensity of the vitamin K antagonist and on the use of aspirin. In 16 trials (10,056 patients) of high-intensity therapy (INR 2.8 to 4.8), the reduction in mortality and thromboembolic complications was offset by a sixfold (95% CI, 4.4- to 8.2-fold) increase in major bleeding. For moderate intensity therapy (INR 2 to 3) versus control (four trials, 1,365 patients), the relative risk for major bleeding was 7.7 (95% CI, 3.3 to 18). For moderate- to high-intensity therapy (INR ≥2) versus ASA (seven trials, 3,457 patients), there was a relative risk of 2.4 (95% CI, 1.6 to 3.6) for increase in major bleeding. For low-intensity therapy (INR <2.0) and ASA versus ASA alone (three trials, 8,435 patients), the relative risk for major bleeding was 1.3 (95% CI, 1.0 to 1.8)

with no statistically significant reductions in mortality or cardiovascular events.

## Ischemic Heart Disease–Myocardial Infarction: Oral Thrombin Inhibitors

Oral direct thrombin inhibition with ximelagatran at doses of 24 mg, 36 mg, 48 mg, or 60 mg twice daily plus 160 mg aspirin daily was compared to 160 mg daily aspirin alone in a recent multicenter blinded trial (197) for secondary prevention of myocardial infarction. There were 1,883 patients followed for a 6-month treatment period. The rates of major bleeding did not differ between treatment groups (1% for ASA alone vs. 2% for combined ximelagatran doses), but patients in the combined ximelagatran groups were three times more likely to stop therapy due to bleeding (hazard ratio, 3.35; 95% CI, 1.87 to 6.01). In addition, any bleeding (major and minor) was more frequent in the combined ximelagatran group (22%) compared with the ASA alone group (13%) (hazard ratio, 1.76; 95% CI, 1.38 to 2.25).

## Venous Thromboembolism Initial Therapy: Heparin

Trials that have evaluated acute treatment of VTE with different heparin regimens have generally compared fixed-dose LMWH with adjusted-dose unfractionated heparin given IV (198–210) or subcutaneously (202,211) (see Table 119-6). The results of these studies have been combined in a number of recent metaanalyses (212–214). In relation to major bleeding, the findings of these studies and metaanalyses can be summarized as follows. Overall, LMWH has generally been associated with less bleeding than unfractionated heparin (e.g., OR, 0.60; 95% CI, 0.39 to 0.93) (214). It is not clear if between-study differences in the relative frequency of bleeding with LMWH and unfractionated heparin reflect differences in LMWH regimens, differences in unfractionated heparin regimens, or occurred by chance.

Once-daily and twice-daily administrations of the same LMWH has been directly compared in six studies (the same total daily dose of LMWH has not always been compared within studies) (215,216,219–222). A metaanalysis of five of these studies (216,219–222) that had unconfounded comparisons found no increase in major bleeding with once-daily treatment (OR, 1.2; 95% CI, 0.4 to 3.2) (223).

Outpatient administration and inpatient administration of LMWH (three preparations were used) were compared in a single study of 201 patients: Two major bleeds occurred in each group (224).

Tinzaparin and dalteparin, each given once daily, have been compared for outpatient treatment of VTE in a study of 497 patients; there was no difference in major bleeding (five with tinzaparin, three with dalteparin) (225).

In another study of 80 patients that compared 10,000 U unfractionated heparin with 5,000 IU dalteparin, each administered subcutaneously twice daily for 3 months after acute VTE, there was no difference in the frequency of total bleeding and no episodes of major bleeding in either group (226).

## Venous Thromboembolism Initial Therapy: Pentasaccharide

The synthetic pentasaccharide, fondaparinux, has been evaluated for acute treatment of pulmonary embolism and DVT

**TABLE 119-6**

LOW-MOLECULAR-WEIGHT HEPARIN VERSUS UNFRACTIONATED HEPARIN
FOR THE TREATMENT OF VENOUS THROMBOEMBOLISM

| Study | Regimens | No. of patients | Major bleeding | Fatal bleeding |
|---|---|---|---|---|
| Duroux et al. (198) | Nadroparin sc b.i.d. (weight-adjusted) | 85 | 2 (2.4%) | 0 |
|  | IV heparin aPTT ratio 1.5–2.0 | 81 | 4 (4.9%) | 0 |
| Prandoni et al. (200) | Nadroparin sc b.i.d. (weight-adjusted) versus | 85 | 1 (1%) | 0 |
|  | IV heparin aPTT ratio 1.5–2.0 | 85 | 3 (4%) | 0 |
| Hull et al.[a] (201) | Tinzaparin 175 Xa U/kg sc o.d. versus | 213 | 1 (0.5%) | 0 |
|  | IV heparin aPTT ratio 1.5–2.5 | 219 | 11 (5.0%) | 2 (0.9%) |
| Lopaciuk et al. (211) | Nadroparin 92 Xa U/kg sc b.i.d. versus | 74 | 0 | 0 |
|  | sc heparin aPTT ratio 1.5–2.5 | 72 | 1 (1%) | 0 |
| Simonneau et al. (202) | Enoxaparin 1 mg/kg sc b.i.d versus | 67 | 0 | 0 |
|  | IV heparin aPTT ratio 1.5–2.5 | 67 | 0 | 0 |
| Lindmarker et al. (203) | Dalteparin 200 Xa U/kg sc o.d versus | 101 | 0 | 0 |
|  | IV heparin aPTT ratio 1.5–3.0 | 103 | 0 | 0 |
| Fiessinger et al. (204) | Dalteparin 200 Xa U/kg sc o.d. versus | 127 | 0 | 0 |
|  | IV heparin aPTT ratio 1.5–3.0 | 133 | 2 (2%) | 0 |
| Levine et al.[b] (205) | Enoxaparin 1 mg/kg sc b.i.d. versus | 247 | 5 (2%) | 2 (0.8%) |
|  | IV heparin aPTT 60–85 s | 253 | 3 (1%) | 0 |
| Koopman et al.[b] (206) | Nadroparin sc b.i.d. (weight-adjusted) versus | 202 | 1 (0.5%) | 0 |
|  | IV heparin aPTT ratio 1.5–2.0 | 198 | 4 (2%) | 2 (1%) |
| COLUMBUS Study[b] (207) | Reviparin 3,500 to 6,300 Xa U sc b.i.d. (weight-adjusted) versus | 510 | 16 (3%) | 0 |
|  | IV heparin aPTT ratio 1.5–2.5 | 511 | 12 (2%) | 2 (0.4%) |
| Simonneau et al.[c] (208) | Tinzaparin 175 Xa U/kg sc o.d. versus | 304 | 0 | 0 |
|  | IV heparin aPTT ratio 2.0–3.0 | 308 | 1 (0.3%) | 1 (0.3%) |
| Decousus et al. (209) | Enoxaparin 1 mg/kg sc b.i.d. | 195 | 7 (3.6%) | 1 (0.5%) |
|  | IV heparin aPTT ratio 1.5–2.0 | 205 | 8 (3.9%) | 1 (0.5%) |
| Kirchmaier et al. (210) | Certoparin 8,000 IU sc b.i.d. | 128 | 1 (0.8%) | 0 |
|  | IV certoparin | 128 | 9 | 1 (0.8%) |
|  | IV heparin aPTT ratio 2.0–3.0 | 131 | 4 | 0 |
| Harenberg et al. (199) | Certoparin 8,000 IU sc b.i.d. | 265 | 4 (1.5%) | 0 |
|  | IV heparin aPTT ratio 2.0–3.0 | 273 | 12 (4.5%) | 2 (0.7 %) |
| Breddin et al. (215) | Reviparin 7,000–12,600 IU sc o.d. | 388 | 1 (0.3%) | 0 |
|  | Reviparin 7,000–12,600 IU sc q.d. × 21 d | 374 | 1 (0.3%) | 0 |
|  | IV heparin aPTT ratio 1.5–2.5 | 375 | 2 (0.5%) | 0 |
| Merli et al. (216) | Enoxaparin 1 mg/kg sc b.i.d. | 312 | 4 | 0 |
|  | Enoxaparin 1.5 mg/kg sc q.d. | 298 | 5 | 1 |
|  | IV heparin aPTT ratio 1.5–2.5 | 290 | 6 | 0 |
| Riess et al. (217) | Certoparin 8,000 I.S. sc b.i.d. × 12 d | 627 | 6 (1.0%) | 0 |
|  | IV heparin aPTT ratio 1.5–2.5 | 593 | 5 (0.8%) | 0 |
| Kakkar (218) | Bemiparin 115 IU/kg sc o.d. | 126 | 0 | 0 |
|  | IU heparin aPTT ratio 1.5–2.5 | 126 | 1 (0.8%) | 0 |

IV, intravenous; aPTT, activated partial thromboplastin time; sc, subcutaneous.
[a]Double-blind.
[b]Included home treatment with low-molecular-weight heparin.
[c]Pulmonary embolism.

(Matisse studies) (227,228). In the Matisse-PE trial, 2,213 patients were treated with a single subcutaneous dose of fondaparinux (7.5 mg if 50 to 100 kg) or IV unfractionated heparin (aPTT ratio 1.5 to 2.5) for at least 5 days using an open-label design (227). Major bleeding occurred in 1.3% of fondaparinux patients and 1.1% of unfractionated heparin patients during the initial treatment period (227).

In the Matisse-DVT trial, 2,205 patients were treated with a single subcutaneous dose of fondaparinux (7.5 mg if 50 to 100 kg) or twice-daily subcutaneous LMWH (enoxaparin 1 mg/kg) for at least 5 days using a double-blind design (228). Major bleeding occurred in 1.1% of fondaparinux and 1.2% of patients with LMWH during the initial treatment period (228).

## Venous Thromboembolism Extended Therapy: Vitamin K Antagonists

There have been 16 randomized trials in patients with VTE in which vitamin K antagonists were compared with various subcutaneous heparin regimens, usually over a 3-month period (see Table 119-7) (217,218,229–243). In one study, two intensities of vitamin K–antagonist therapy were compared following initial heparin therapy (Table 119-7) (41). Higher intensities of anticoagulation (i.e., INR 2.6 to 4.4) were evaluated in earlier studies (229–231) than in more recent trials (i.e., INR 2.0 to 3.0) (41,217,218,232–242). The higher-intensity regimens were consistently associated with more total bleeding than the

**TABLE 119-7**

VENOUS THROMBOEMBOLISM

| Study | Treatment | No. of patients | Bleeding (approximately 3 mo) (%) | |
|---|---|---|---|---|
| | | | Major[a] | Fatal[a] |
| Bynum and Wilson (229) | Warfarin (INR 2.6–4.4) | 24 | 4 (16.7) | 0 |
| | Heparin (5,000 U sc b.i.d.) | 24 | 0 | 0 |
| Hull et al. (230) | Warfarin (INR 2.6–4.4) | 33 | 4 (12.1) | 0 |
| | Heparin (5,000 U sc b.i.d.) | 35 | 0 | 0 |
| Hull et al. (231) | Warfarin (INR 2.6–4.4) | 53 | 3 (5.7) | 0 |
| | Heparin (≈10,000 U sc b.i.d.) | 53 | 0 | 0 |
| Hull et al. (41) | Warfarin (INR 2.6–4.5) | 49 | 2 (4.1) | 0 |
| | Warfarin (INR ≈2.2) | 47 | 2 (4.3) | 0 |
| Pini et al. (232) | Warfarin (INR 2.7) | 94 | 12 (12.8) | 0 |
| | Enoxaparin (4,000 IU sc o.d.) | 93 | 3 (3.2) | 0 |
| Das et al. (233) | Warfarin (INR 2.0–3.0) | 55 | 0 | 0 |
| | Dalteparin (5,000 IU sc o.d.) | 50 | 0 | 0 |
| Hamman et al. (235) | Phenprocoumon (INR 2.0–3.0) | 100 | 2 (2) | not available |
| | Dalteparin (5,000 IU sc o.d.) | 100 | 0 | |
| Lopaciuk et al. (234) | Acenocoumarol (INR 2.0–3.0) | 95 | 2 (2.1) | 0 |
| | Nadroparin (85 IU/kg sc o.d.) | 98 | 1 (1.0) | 0 |
| Gonzalez-Fajardo et al. (236) | Warfarin (INR 2.0–3.0) | 80 | 2 (2.5) | 0 |
| | Enoxaparin (4,000 IU sc o.d.) | 85 | 1 (1.2) | 0 |
| Veiga et al. (237) | Acenocoumarol (INR 2.0–3.0) | 50 | 2 (4.0) | 1 |
| | Enoxaparin (4,000 IU sc o.d.) | 50 | 1 (2.0) | 0 |
| Lopez-Beret et al. (238) | Acenocoumarol (INR 2.0–3.0) | 77 | 4.7 (5.2) | 0 |
| | Nadroparin (approx. 102 IU/kg sc b.i.d.) | 81 | 0 | 0 |
| Meyer et al. (239) | Warfarin (INR 2.0–3.0) | 75[b] | 12 (16) | 6 |
| | Enoxaparin (150 IU/kg sc o.d.) | 71[b] | 5 (7.0) | 0 |
| Hull et al. (240) | Warfarin (INR 2.0–3.0) | 239 | 2 (0.8) | not reported |
| | Tinzaparin (175 IU/kg sc o.d.) | 233 | 1 (0.4) | |
| Hull et al. (241) | Warfarin (INR 2.0–3.0) | 368 | 17 (4.6) | not reported |
| | Tinzaparin (175 IU/kg sc o.d.) | 369 | 12 (3.3) | |
| Lee et al. (242) | Warfarin (INR 2.0–3.0) | 335[b] | 12 (3.6)[c] | 0 |
| | Dalteparin (200 IU/kg sc o.d. first month) 150 IU/kg sc o.d. second–sixth month | 338[b] | 19 (5.6)[c] | 1 () |
| Kakkar (218) | Vitamin K antagonist (INR 2.0–3.0) | 246 | 1 (0.4) | 0 |
| | Bemiparin (3,500 IU o.d.) | 111 | 1 (0.9) | 1 () |

INR, international normalized ratio; sc, subcutaneous; approx., approximately.
[a]Data are presented as No. (%).
[b]All patients had cancer.
[c]Six-month follow-up.

comparison arms, with a similar trend for major bleeding (Table 119-7). In the study that compared two intensities of oral anticoagulation, the frequency of total bleeding was also substantially lower with the less intense regimen (4% vs. 22%), without being associated with a loss of antithrombotic efficacy (41).

The 12 most recent of these studies compared oral anticoagulant therapy at a targeted INR of 2.0 to 3.0 anticoagulation with widely differing regimens of three LMWH preparations (Table 119-7) (232–242,218). The daily LMWH dose was as low as 4,000 IU (232,236) to as high as 200 IU per kg (238, 242), approximately a 3.5-fold difference. Two metaanalyses of studies that compared LMWH with vitamin K antagonist, each given for 3 months after initial heparin therapy, have been performed (243,244). In the analysis by Lorio et al., which includes seven studies (232–234,236–238,240) and a total of 1,379 patients, there was a trend toward less bleeding with long-term LMWH therapy (OR, 0.45; 95% CI, 0.2 to 1.1)

(244). Importantly, the relative frequency of major bleeding with LMWH therapy was dose-dependent, varying from an OR of approximately 0.2 at a dose of approximately 4,000 IU per day to an OR of approximately 0.7 at a dose of approximately 12,000 IU per day ($P = 0.03$).

Linkins et al. performed a metaanalysis of 33 prospective studies to determine how often major episodes of bleeding that occurred during vitamin K antagonist therapy for VTE were fatal (target INR 2.0 to 3.0) (245). Most of the 10,757 patients included in the analysis were initially treated with unfractionated or LMWH and received vitamin K antagonists for 3 months (245). Of 275 major bleeds, 37 were fatal for an overall case-fatality of 13%. Case-fatality with intracranial bleeds was 46% and for major extracranial bleeds was 10%. Extracranial bleeds, which accounted for 81% of major bleeding episodes, caused approximately two thirds of the deaths from bleeding. Although the risk of bleeding was higher during the first 3 months of anticoagulant therapy than subsequently, case-fatality with major bleeding was similar during the acute and long-term phases of treatment (245).

The results of randomized trials in which patients with VTE were treated with less intense oral anticoagulation (not part of primary comparison) following initial treatment with either unfractionated or LMWH generally have found an overall frequency of major bleeding of approximately 3% or less during 3 months of therapy (212), with higher rates among patients with cancer (239,242).

Four randomized trials have compared 4 weeks (246,247) or 6 weeks (248,249) with 3 months (246,247) or 6 months (248,249), and three have compared 3 months (249–251) with 6 months (249,251) or 12 months (250,251) of oral anticoagulation (INR approximately 2.0 to 3.0) for the treatment of VTE. Following the initial phase of treatment during which all patients were treated with anticoagulants, major bleeding occurred infrequently without convincing evidence of more bleeding with the longer durations of therapy (246–250). Two randomized trials have evaluated long-term oral anticoagulation for the prevention of recurrent VTE following an acute episode (252,253). Schulman et al. (252) randomized 227 patients to regimens of either 6 months or 4 years of anticoagulation (INR 2.0 to 2.85) after a second episode of VTE. Major bleeding occurred more frequently in patients who were treated with long-term anticoagulation (2.4% vs. 0.7% per year). Kearon et al. (253) randomized 162 patients with a first episode of idiopathic VTE to remain on a regimen of warfarin (INR 2.0 to 3.0), or to receive placebo, for a further 2 years after an initial 3 months of anticoagulation. Major bleeding occurred more frequently in patients who continued to receive anticoagulants (3.8% vs. 0% per year).

A reasonable interpretation of the findings of these studies is that, for patients without a high risk of bleeding (i.e., such as those entered in clinical trials), differences in duration of anticoagulation do not translate into clinically important differences in frequencies of major bleeding until duration of therapy differs by a year or longer.

The Extended Low-intensity Anticoagulation (ELATE) trial, which compared warfarin therapy with INR 1.5 to 1.9 and INR 2.0 to 3.0 for long-term prevention of recurrent unprovoked VTE in 738 patients who had completed at least 3 months of initial treatment with INR 2.0 to 3.0, found no difference in the frequency of major bleeding between the two groups during an average of 2.4 years of follow-up [INR 1.5 to 1.9 vs. INR 2.0 to 3.0: 1.1% vs. 0.9% per year; hazard ratio, 1.2 (95% CI, 0.4 to 3.0)] (94). The Prevention of Recurrent Venous Thromboembolism (PREVENT) trial, which compared warfarin therapy with INR 1.5 to 2.0 and placebo in 508 patients who had completed at least 3 months of warfarin treatment with INR 2.0 to 3.0, found no statistically significant difference in the rate of major bleeding between the two groups during an average of 2.1 years of follow up [INR 1.5 to 2.0 vs. placebo: 0.9% vs. 0.4% per year; hazard ratio, 2.5 (95% CI, 0.5 to 13.0)] (254).

## Venous Thromboembolism: Oral Thrombin Inhibitors

Ximelagatran has been evaluated for both acute and long-term treatment of VTE [Thrombin Inhibitors in Venous Thromboembolism (THRIVE) studies] (255,256). In the acute treatment study, 2,491 patients with acute DVT were treated for 6 months with ximelagatran, 36 mg twice daily, or LMWH followed by vitamin K antagonist therapy (INR 2.0 to 3.0), using a blinded design. An "on treatment" analysis suggested less major bleeding with ximelagatran (1.3% vs. 2.2%; 95% CI for difference −20% to +0.2%); "intention to treat" analyses have not been reported for bleeding (256).

In a long-term treatment study, 18 months of ximelagatran, 24 mg twice daily, was compared with placebo in 1,224 patients with DVT or pulmonary embolism who had completed 6 months of initial treatment with vitamin K antagonists (255). There was no apparent increase of major bleeding with ximelagatran [0.7 % per year; hazard ratio, 1.2 (95% CI, 0.4 to 3.8)].

## SUMMARY

Bleeding is the major complication of anticoagulant therapy. The criteria for defining the severity of bleeding varied considerably between studies, accounting in part for the variation in the rates of bleeding reported. There is some evidence to suggest that bleeding risk with unfractionated heparin increases with the heparin dosage and age (>70 years).

The major determinants of vitamin K antagonist-induced bleeding are the intensity of the anticoagulant effect, underlying patient characteristics, and the length of therapy. There is good evidence that vitamin K antagonist therapy at a targeted INR of 2.5 (range, 2.0 to 3.0) is associated with a lower risk of bleeding than therapy targeted at an INR of greater than 3.0. There is no convincing evidence indicating that long-term secondary prevention of VTE with vitamin K antagonists targeted to INR values of 1.5 to 1.9 compared to INRs of 2.0 to 3.0 reduces the frequency of bleeding.

The risk of bleeding associated with IV unfractionated heparin in patients with acute VTE is less than 3% in recent trials. LMWH is associated with less major bleeding compared with unfractionated heparin in acute VTE. Unfractionated heparin and LMWH are not associated with an increase in major bleeding in ischemic coronary syndromes, but extended administration of LMWH in these patients is associated with increased bleeding. Acute treatment of ischemic stroke with therapeutic-dose LMWH or unfractionated heparin is associated with an increased risk of major bleeding and intracranial bleeding.

Recently, information on bleeding associated with the newer generation of antithrombotic agents has begun to emerge. Long-term primary prevention of atrial fibrillation and secondary prevention of myocardial infarction and VTE with ximelagatran are associated with a low risk of bleeding. Acute treatment of VTE with fondaparinux is associated with a frequency of bleeding similar to that of treatment with LMWH or unfractionated heparin.

In terms of treatment decision making for anticoagulant therapy, bleeding risk cannot be considered alone; that is, the potential decrease in thromboembolism must be balanced against the potential increased bleeding risk.

### References

1. Levine MN, Raskob G, Hirsh J. Hemorrhagic complications of long-term anticoagulant therapy. *Chest* 1986;89:16–25.
2. Levine MN, Raskob G, Hirsh J. Hemorrhagic complications of long-term anticoagulant therapy. *Chest* 1989;95:26–36.
3. Levine MN, Hirsh J, Landefeld CS, et al. Hemorrhagic complications of anticoagulant treatment. *Chest* 1992;102:352–363.
4. Levine MN, Raskob G, Landefeld CS, et al. Hemorrhagic complications of anticoagulant treatment. *Chest* 1995;108:276–290.
5. Levine MN, Raskob G, Landefeld CS, et al. Hemorrhagic complications of anticoagulant treatment. *Chest* 1998;114:511–523.
6. Levine MN, Raskob G, Landefeld CS, et al. Hemorrhagic complications of anticoagulant treatment. *Chest* 2001;119:108–121.
7. Levine MN, Raskob G, Beyth RJ, et al. Hemorrhagic complications of anticoagulant treatment: the Seventh ACCP Conference on Antithrombotic and Thrombolytic Therapy. *Chest* 2004;126:287S–310S.
8. Fernandez F, Nguyen P, van Ryn J, et al. Hemorrhagic doses of heparin and other glycosaminoglycans induce a platelet defect. *Thromb Res* 1986:43:491–495.

9. Blajchman MA, Young E, Ofosu FA. Effects of unfractionated heparin, dermatan sulfate and low molecular weight heparin on vessel wall permeability in rabbits. *Ann N Y Acad Sci* 1989;556:245–253.

10. Green D, Lee MY, Ito VY, et al. Fixed vs adjusted-dose heparin in the prophylaxis of thromboembolism in spinal cord injury. *JAMA* 1988;260: 1255–1258.

11. Urokinase Pulmonary Embolism Trial. Morbidity and Mortality. *Circulation* 1973;158:66–71.

12. Norman CS, Provan JL. Control and complications of intermittent heparin therapy. *Surg Gynecol Obstet* 1977;145:338–342.

13. Wilson JE, Bynum LJ, Parkey RW. Heparin therapy in venous thromboembolism. *Am J Med* 1981;70:808–816.

14. Anand SS, Yusuf S, Pogue J, et al. Relationship of activated partial thromboplastin time to coronary events and bleeding in patients with acute coronary syndromes who receive heparin. *Circulation* 2003;107:2884–2888.

15. Investigators GI. Randomized trial of intravenous heparin versus recombinant hirudin for acute coronary syndromes. *Circulation* 1994;90: 1631–1637.

16. Investigators TA. Hirudin in acute myocardial infarction. *Circulation* 1994; 90:1624–1630.

17. Salzman EW, Deykin D, Shapiro RM, et al. Management of heparin therapy. *N Engl J Med* 1975;292:1046–1050.

18. Glazier RL, Corwell EB. Randomized prospective trial of continuous vs intermittent heparin therapy. *JAMA* 1976;236:1365–1367.

19. Mant MJ, O'Brien BD, Thong KL, et al. Haemorrhagic complications of heparin therapy. *Lancet* 1977;1:1133.

20. Wilson JR, Lampman J. Heparin therapy: a randomized prospective study. *Am Heart J* 1979;97:155–158.

21. Fagher B, Lundh B. Heparin treatment of deep vein thrombosis. *Acta Med Scand* 1981;210:357–361.

22. Bentley PG, Kakkar VV, Scully MF, et al. An objective study of alternative methods of heparin administration. *Thromb Res* 1980;18:177–187.

23. Andersson G, Fagrell B, Holmgren K, et al. Subcutaneous administration of heparin: a randomized comparison with intravenous administration of heparin to patients with deep vein thrombosis. *Thromb Res* 1982;27: 631–639.

24. Doyle DJ, Turpie AGG, Hirsh J, et al. Adjusted subcutaneous heparin or continuous intravenous heparin in patients with acute deep vein thrombosis: a randomized trial. *Ann Intern Med* 1987;107:441–445.

25. Pini M, Pattacini C, Quintavalla R, et al. Subcutaneous vs intermittent heparin in the treatment of deep vein thrombosis: a randomized clinical trial. *Thromb Haemost* 1990;64:222–226.

26. Hull R, Raskob G, Hirsh J, et al. Continuous intravenous heparin compared with intermittent subcutaneous heparin in the initial treatment of proximal-vein thrombosis. *N Engl J Med* 1986;18:1109–1114.

27. Gallus AS, Jackaman J, Tillett J, et al. Safety and efficacy of warfarin started early after submassive venous thrombosis or pulmonary embolism. *Lancet* 1986;2:1293–1296.

28. Brandjes DPM, Heijboer H, Buller HR, et al. Acenocoumarol and heparin compared with acenocoumarol alone in the initial treatment of proximal-vein thrombosis. *N Engl J Med* 1992;327:1485–1489.

29. Raschke RA, Reilly BM, Gguidry J, et al. The weight-based heparin nomogram compared with a 'standard care' nomogram: a randomized controlled trial. *Ann Intern Med* 1993;119:874–881.

30. Coon WW, Willis PW. Hemorrhagic complications of anticoagulant therapy. *Arch Intern Med* 1974;133:386–392.

31. Hull RD, Raskob G, Rosenbloom D, et al. Heparin for 5 days as compared with 10 days in the initial treatment or proximal venous thrombosis. *N Engl J Med* 1990;322:1260–1264.

32. Yett HS, Skillman JJ, Salzman EW. The hazards of heparin plus aspirin. *N Engl J Med* 1978;298:1092.

33. Sethi GK, Copeland JG, Goldman S, et al. Implications of preoperative administration of aspirin in patients undergoing coronary artery bypass grafting. *J Am Coll Cardiol* 1990;15:15–20.

34. Investigators E. Use of a monoclonal antibody directed against the platelet glycoprotein IIb/IIIa receptor in high-risk coronary angioplasty. *N Engl J Med* 1994;330:956–961.

35. Investigators E. Platelet glycoprotein IIb/IIIa receptor blockage and low dose heparin during percutaneous coronary revascularization. *N Engl J Med* 1997;336:1689–1696.

36. Chew D, Bhatt D, Lincoff A, et al. Defining the optimal activated clotting time during percutaneous coronary intervention: aggregate results from 6 randomized controlled trials. *Circulation* 2001;103:961–966.

37. Jick H, Slone D, Borda IT, et al. Efficacy and toxicity of heparin in relation to age and sex. *N Engl J Med* 1968;279:284–286.

38. Levine MN, Hirsh J, Kelton JG. Heparin-induced bleeding. In: Lane DA, Lindahl U, eds. *Heparin: chemical and biological properties clinical applications*. London: Edward Arnold, 1989:517–532.

39. Basu D, Gallus AS, Hirsh J, et al. A prospective study of the value of monitoring heparin treatment with the activated partial thromboplastin time. *N Engl J Med* 1972;287:324–327.

40. Campbell NR, Hull R, Brant R, et al. Aging and heparin-related bleeding. *Arch Intern Med* 1996;156:857–860.

41. Hull R, Hirsh J, Jay R, et al. Different intensities of oral anticoagulant therapy in the treatment of proximal-vein thrombosis. *N Engl J Med* 1982; 307:1671–1681.

42. Turpie AGG, Gunstensen J, Hirsh J, et al. Randomized comparison of two intensities of oral anticoagulant therapy after tissue heart valve replacement. *Lancet* 1988;1:1242–1245.

43. Saour JN, Sieck JO, Mamo LAR, et al. Trial of different intensities of anticoagulation in patients with prosthetic heart valves. *N Engl J Med* 1990;322:428–432.

44. Altman R, Rouvier J, Gurfinkel E, et al. Comparison of two levels of anticoagulant therapy in patients with substitute heart valves. *J Thorac Cardiovasc Surg* 1991;101:427–431.

45. Pengo V, Barbero F, Banzato A, et al. A comparison of a moderate with moderate-high intensity oral anticoagulant treatment in patients with mechanical heart valve prostheses. *Thromb Haemost* 1997;77:839–844.

46. Meschengieser SS, Fondevila CG, Frontroth J, et al. Low-intensity oral anticoagulation plus low-dose aspirin versus high-intensity oral anticoagulation alone: a randomized trial in patients with mechanical prosthetic heart valves. *J Thorac Cardiovasc Surg* 1997;113:910–916.

47. Horstkotte D, Schulte HD, Bircks W, et al. Lower intensity anticoagulation therapy results in lower complication rates with the St. Jude medical prosthesis. *J Thorac Cardiovasc Surg* 1994;107:1136–1145.

48. Algra A, Franke CL, Koehler PJJ, et al. A randomized trial of anticoagulants versus aspirin after cerebral ischemia of presumed arterial origin. *Ann Neurol* 1997;42:857–865.

49. *Lancet*. Adjusted-dose warfarin versus low-intensity, fixed-dose warfarin plus aspirin for high-risk patients with atrial fibrillation: Stroke Prevention in Atrial Fibrillation III randomised clinical trial. see comments 1996; 348:633–638.

50. Gullov AL, Koefoed BG, Petersen P. Bleeding during warfarin and aspirin therapy in patients with atrial fibrillation: the AFASAK 2 study. *Arch Intern Med* 1999;159:1322–1328.

51. Yamaguchi T, Japanese Nonvalvular Atrial Fibrillation-Embolism Secondary Prevention Cooperative Study Group. Optimal intensity of warfarin therapy for secondary prevention of stroke in patients with nonvalvular atrial fibrillation: a multicenter, prospective, randomized trial. *Stroke* 2000; 31:817–821.

52. Cannegieter SC, Rosendaal FR, Wintzen AR, et al. Optimal oral anticoagulant therapy in patients with mechanical heart valves. *N Engl J Med* 1995; 333:11–17.

53. Hylek EM, Singer DE. Risk factors for intracranial hemorrhage in outpatients taking warfarin. *Ann Intern Med* 1994;120:897–902.

54. Atrial Fibrillation Investigators. Risk factors for stroke and efficacy of antithrombotic therapy in atrial fibrillation: analysis of pooled data from five randomized controlled trials. *Arch Intern Med* 1994;154:1449–1457.

55. European Atrial Fibrillation Trial (EAFT) Study Group. Secondary prevention in non-rheumatic atrial fibrillation after transient ischemic attack or minor stroke. *Lancet* 1993;342:1255–1262.

56. Hylek EM, Skates SJ, Sheehan MA, et al. An analysis of the lowest effective intensity of prophylactic anticoagulation for patients with nonrheumatic atrial fibrillation. *N Engl J Med* 1996;335:540–546.

57. Crowther MA, Ginsberg JS, Julian J, et al. A comparison of two intensities of warfarin for the prevention of recurrent thrombosis in patients with antiphospholipid antibody syndrome. *N Engl J Med* 2003;349:1138.

58. Bern MM, Lokich JJ, Wallach SR, et al. Very low doses of warfarin can prevent thrombosis in central vein catheters: a randomized prospective trial. *Ann Intern Med* 1990;112:423–428.

59. Levine M, Hirsh J, Gent M. Double-blind randomized trial of very low dose warfarin for prevention of thromboembolism in stage IV breast cancer. *Lancet* 1994;343:886–889.

60. Fihn SD, McDonnel M, Martin D, et al. Risk factors for complications of chronic anticoagulation: a multi-centre study. *Ann Intern Med* 1993;118: 511–520.

61. Casais P, Luceros AS, Meschengieser S, et al. Bleeding risk factors in chronic oral anticoagulation with acenocoumarol. *Am J Hematol* 2000; 63:192–196.

62. Anderson DR, Wilson JE, Wells PS, et al. Anticoagulant clinic vs family physician based warfarin monitoring: a randomized controlled trial. *Blood* 2000;96:846a.

63. Matcher D, Samsa G, Cohen S, et al. Improving the quality of anticoagulation of patients with atrial fibrillation in managed care organizations: results of managing anticoagulation services trial. *Am J Med* 2002;113:42–51.

64. Chiquette E, Amato MG, Bussey HI. Comparison of an anticoagulation clinic with usual medical care. Anticoagulation control, patient outcomes, health care costs. *Arch Intern Med* 1998;158:1641–1647.

65. Cortelazzo S, Finazzi P, Viero P, et al. Thrombotic and hemorrhagic complications in patients with mechanical heart valve prosthesis attending an anticoagulation clinic. *Thromb Haemost* 1993;69:316–320.

66. Garabedian-Rufalo SM, Gray DR, Sax MJ, et al. Retrospective evaluation of a pharmacist-managed warfarin anticoagulation clinic. *Am J Hosp Pharm* 1985;42:304–308.

67. Wilt VM, Gums JG, Ahmed OI, et al. Outcome analysis of a pharmacist-managed anticoagulation service. *Pharmacotherapy* 1995;15:732–739.

68. Beyth RJ, Quinn LM, Landefeld CS. A multicomponent intervention to prevent major bleeding complications in older patients receiving warfarin: a randomized clinical trial. *Ann Intern Med* 2000;133:687–695.

69. Elston-Lafata J, Martin SA, Kaatz S, et al. The cost effectiveness of different management strategies for patients on chronic warfarin therapy. *J Gen Intern Med* 2000;15:31–37.

70. White RH, McCurdy SA, von Marensdorff H, et al. Home prothrombin time monitoring after the initiation of warfarin therapy. A randomized, prospective study. *Ann Intern Med* 1989;111:730–737.

71. Hasenkam JM, Kimose HH II, Knudson L, et al. Self-management of oral anticoagulant therapy after heart valve replacement. *Eur J Cardiothorac Surg* 1997;11:935–942.

72. Sawicki PT, Working Group for the Study of Patient Self-Management of Oral Anticoagulation. A structured teaching and self-management program for patients receiving oral anticoagulation: a randomized controlled trial. *JAMA* 1999;281:145–150.

73. Korke H, Korfer R. International normalized ratio self-management after mechanical heart valve replacement: is an early start advantageous? *Ann Thorac Surg* 2001;72:44–48.

74. Ansell J, Patel N, Ostrovsky D, et al. Long-term patient self-management of oral anticoagulation. *Arch Intern Med* 1995;155:2185–2189.

75. Watzke HH, Forberg E, Svolba G, et al. A prospective controlled trial comparing weekly self-testing and self-dosing with the standard management of patients on stable oral anticoagulation. *Thromb Haemost* 2000; 83:661–665.

76. Cromheecke ME, Levi M, Coly LP, et al. Oral anticoagulation self-management and management by a specialist anticoagulation clinic: a randomized cross-over comparison. *Lancet* 2000;356:97–102.

77. Stroke Prevention in Atrial Fibrillation Investigators. Bleeding during antithrombotic therapy in patients with atrial fibrillation. *Arch Intern Med* 1996;156:409–416.

78. European Atrial Fibrillation Trial (EAFT) Study Group. Optimal oral anticoagulant therapy in patients with nonrheumatic atrial fibrillation and recent cerebral ischemia. *N Engl J Med* 1995;333:5–10.

79. Landefeld CS, Rosenblatt MW, Goldman L. Bleeding in outpatients treated with warfarin: relation to the prothrombin time and important remediable lesions. *Am J Med* 1989;87:153–159.

80. Landefeld CS, Goldman L. Major bleeding in outpatients treated with warfarin: incidence and prediction by factors known at the start of outpatient therapy. *Am J Med* 1989;87:144–152.

81. Petitti D, Strom B, Melmon K. Duration of warfarin anticoagulation therapy and the probabilities of recurrent thromboembolism and hemorrhage. *Am J Med* 1986;81:255–259.

82. Peyman MA. The significance of hemorrhage during treatment of patients with coumarin anticoagulants. *Acta Med Scand* 1958;162: 1–62.

83. Launbjerg J, Egeblad H, Heaf J, et al. Bleeding complications to oral anticoagulant therapy: multivariate analysis of 1,010 treatment years in 551 outpatients. *J Intern Med* 1991;229:351–355.

84. Roos J, van Joost HE. The cause of bleeding during anticoagulant treatment. *Acta Med Scand* 1965;178:129–131.

85. Pollard JW, Hamilton MJ, Christensen NA, et al. Problems associated with long-term anticoagulant therapy. *Circulation* 1962;25:386–392.

86. van der Meer FJ, Rosendaal FR, Van Den Broucke JP, et al. Bleeding complications in oral anticoagulant therapy: an analysis of risk factors. *Arch Intern Med* 1993;153:1557–1562.

87. Palareti G, Leali N, Coccheri S, et al. Bleeding complications of oral anticoagulant treatment: an inception-cohort, prospective collaborative study (ISCOAT). *Lancet* 1996;348:423–428.

88. Steffensen FH, Kristensen K, Ejlersen E, et al. Major haemorrhagic complications during oral anticoagulant therapy in a Danish population-based cohort. *J Intern Med* 1997;242:497–503.

89. Kuijer PM, Hutten BA, Prins MH, et al. Prediction of the risk of bleeding during anticoagulant treatment for venous thromboembolism. *Arch Intern Med* 1999;159:457–460.

90. Hutten BA, Lensing AW, Kraaijenhagen RA, et al. Safety of treatment with oral anticoagulants in the elderly. A systematic review. *Drugs Aging* 1999;14:303–312.

91. Chenhsu RT, Chiang SC, Chou MH, et al. Long-term treatment with warfarin in Chinese population. *Ann Pharmacother* 2000;34:1395–1401.

92. Yasaka MK, Minematsu K, Yamaguchi T. Optimal intensity of international normalized ratio in warfarin therapy for secondary prevention of stroke in patients with non-valvular atrial fibrillation. *Intern Med* 2001; 40:1183–1188.

93. Pengo V, Legnani C, Noventa F, et al. on behalf of the ISCOAT Study Group. Oral anticoagulant therapy in patients with nonrheumatic atrial fibrillation and risk of bleeding. A Multicenter Inception Cohort Study. *Thromb Haemost* 2001;85:418–422.

94. Kearon C, Ginsberg JS, Kovacs MJ, et al. Comparison of low-intensity warfarin therapy with conventional-intensity warfarin therapy for long-term prevention of recurrent venous thromboembolism. *N Engl J Med* 2003;349:631–639.

95. Albers GW. Atrial fibrillation and stroke: three new studies three remaining questions. *Arch Intern Med* 1994;154:1443–1448.

96. Beyth RJ, Quinn LM, Landefeld CS. Prospective evaluation of an index for predicting risk of major bleeding in outpatients treated with warfarin. *Am J Med* 1998;105:91–99.

97. White RH, Beyth RJ, Zhou H, et al. Major bleeding after hospitalization for deep vein thrombosis. *Am J Med* 1999;107:414–424.

98. White R, McKittrick T, Takakuwa J, et al. Management and prognosis of life-threatening bleeding during warfarin therapy. *Arch Intern Med* 1996; 156:1197–1201.

99. Gitter MJ, Jaeger TM, Petterson TM, et al. Bleeding and thromboembolism during anticoagulant therapy: a population-based study in Rochester, Minnesota. *Mayo Clin Proc* 1995;70:725–733.

100. Lundstrom T, Ryden L. Hemorrhagic and thromboembolic complications in patients with atrial fibrillation on anticoagulant prophylaxis. *J Intern Med* 1989;225:137–142.

101. McMahan DA, Smith DM, Carey MA, et al. Risk of major hemorrhage for outpatients treated with warfarin. *J Gen Intern Med* 1998;13:311–316.

102. Prandoni P, Lensing AWA, Piccioli A, et al. Recurrent venous thromboembolism and bleeding complications during anticoagulant treatment in patients with cancer and venous thrombosis. *Blood* 2002;100:3484–3488.

103. Schulman S. Quality of oral anticoagulant control and treatment in Sweden. *J Int Med* 1994;236:143–152.

104. Meuwissen O, Vervoom AC, Cohen O, et al. Double blind trial of long term anticoagulant treatment after myocardial infarction. *Acta Med Scand* 1969;186:361–368.

105. Davis FB, Estruch MT, Samson-Corvera EB, et al. Management of anticoagulation in outpatients: experience with an anticoagulation service in a municipal hospital setting. *Arch Intern Med* 1977;137:197–202.

106. Blackshear JL, Baker VS, Holland A, et al. Fecal hemoglobin excretion in elderly patients with atrial fibrillation: combined aspirin and low-dose warfarin vs conventional warfarin therapy. *Arch Intern Med* 1996;156: 658–660.

107. Coumadin Aspirin Reinfarction Study (CARS) Investigators. Randomised double-blind trial of fixed low-dose warfarin with aspirin after myocardial infarction. *Lancet* 1997;350:389–396.

108. The Medical Research Council's General Practice Research Framework. Thrombosis prevention trial: randomised trial of low-intensity oral anticoagulation with warfarin and low-dose aspirin in the primary prevention of ischaemic heart disease in men at increased risk. *Lancet* 1998;351:233–241.

109. Fiore LD, Ezekowitz MD, Brophy MT, et al. Department of veterans affairs cooperative studies program clinical trial comparing combined warfarin and aspirin with aspirin alone in survivors of acute myocardial infarction: primary results of the CHAMP study. *Circulation* 2002;105: 557–563.

110. McInnes GT, Helenglass G. The performance of clinics for outpatient control of anticoagulation. *J R Coll Physicians Lond* 1987;21:42–45.

111. Fuller JA, Melb MB. Experiences with long-term anticoagulant treatment. *Lancet* 1959;2:489–491.

112. Mosley DH, Schatz IJ, Breneman GM, et al. Long-term anticoagulant therapy. *JAMA* 1963;186:914–916.

113. Torn M, Algra A, Rosendaal FR. Oral anticoagulation for cerebral ischemia of arterial origin: high initial bleeding risk. *Neurology* 2001;57: 1933–1939.

114. Forfar JC. A 7-year analysis of hemorrhage in patients in long-term anticoagulant treatment. *Br Heart J* 1979;42:128–132.

115. Landefeld CS, McGuire E, Rosenblatt MW. A bleeding risk index for estimating the probability of major bleeding in hospitalized patients starting anticoagulant therapy. *Am J Med* 1990;89:569–578.

116. Gage BF, Cardinalli AB, Owens DK. Cost-effectiveness of preference-based antithrombotic therapy for patients with nonvalvular atrial fibrillation. *Stroke* 1998;29:1083–1091.

117. Gubitz G, Counsell C, Sandercock PAG, et al. Anticoagulants for acute ischaemic stroke (Cochrane Review). *The Cochrane Library*, Oxford: Update Software, 2002.

118. Group ISTC. The International Stroke Trial (IST): a randomized trial of aspirin, subcutaneous heparin, both or neither among 19,435 patients with acute ischaemic stroke. *Lancet* 1997;349:1569–1581.

119. Diener HC, Ringelstein EB, Von Kummer R, et al. Therapy of Patients with Acute Stroke (TOPAS) Investigators. Treatment of acute ischemic stroke with the low-molecular-weight heparin certoparin: results of the TOPAS trial. *Stroke* 2001;32:22–29.

120. Berge E, Abdelnoor M, Nakstad PH, et al. HAEST Study Group. Heparin in Acute Embolic Stroke Trial. Low molecular-weight heparin versus aspirin in patients with acute ischaemic stroke and atrial fibrillation: a double-blind randomised study. *Lancet* 2000;355:1205–1210.

121. Bath PM, Lindenstrom E, Boysen G, et al. Tinzaparin in acute ischaemic stroke (TAIST): a randomised aspirin-controlled trial. *Lancet* 2001;358: 702–710.

122. Prince J Thromboses veineuses des membres inferieurs et embolies pulmonaries au cours des accidents vasculaires cerebraux. *A Propos D'un Essai Comparatif De Traitment Preventif (These pour le doctorat d'etat en medicine)*. Toulouse: Universite Paul Sabatier, 1981.

123. Berge E, Sandercock P. Anticoagulants versus antiplatelet therapy agents for acute ischaemic stroke (Cochrane Review), 2002. Available at http://www.update-software.com/. Accessed May 24, 2004.

124. Enger E, Boyesen S. Long-term anticoagulant therapy in patients with cerebral infarction. *Acta Med Scand* 1965;178:7–55.

125. McDowell F, McDevitt E, Wright IS. Anticoagulant therapy: five years experience with the patient with an established cerebrovascular accident. *Arch Neurol* 1963;8:209–214.

126. Baker RN, Broward JA, Fang HC, et al. An evaluation of anticoagulant therapy in the treatment of cerebrovascular disease: report of the Veterans Administration Cooperative study of atherosclerosis. *Neurology* 1961;11: 132–138.

127. Baker RN, Broward JA, Fang HC, et al. Anticoagulant therapy in cerebral infarction: report on cooperative study. *Neurology* 1962;12:823–835.

128. Fisher CM. Anticoagulant therapy in cerebral thrombosis and cerebral embolism. *Neurology* 1961;11:119–131.

129. Ginsberg JS, Bates SM, Oczkowski W, et al. Low-dose warfarin in rehabilitating stroke survivors. *Thromb Res* 2003;107:287–290.

130. Hill AB, Marshall J, Shaw DA. A controlled clinical trial of long-term anticoagulant therapy in cerebrovascular disease. *Q J Med* 1960;29:597–609.

131. Hill AB, Marshall J, Shaw DA. Cerebrovascular disease: trial of long-term anticoagulant therapy. *BMJ* 1962;53:1003–1006.

132. Olsson JE, Brechter C, Backlund H, et al. Anticoagulant vs antiplatelet therapy as prophylactic against cerebral infarction in transient ischemic attacks. *Stroke* 1980;11:4–9.

133. Mohr JP, Thompson JL, Lazar RM, et al. A comparison of warfarin and aspirin for prevention of recurrent ischemic stroke. *N Engl J Med* 2001;345:1444–1451.

134. Garde A, Samuelsson K, Fahlgen H, et al. Treatment after transient ischemic attacks: a comparison between anticoagulant drug and inhibition of platelet aggregation. *Stroke* 1983;14:677–681.

135. Stewart B, Shuaib A, Veloso F. Stroke Prevention with Warfarin or Aspirin Trial (SWAT). *Stroke* 1998;29:304 (Abstract page 9).

136. Algra A, De Schryver ELLM, van Gijn J, et al. Oral anticoagulants versus antiplatelet therapy for preventing further vascular events after transient ischaemic attack or minor stroke of presumed arterial origin (Cochrane Review). *The Cochrane Library*, Vol. 3. Oxford: Update Software, 2003.

137. Gorter JW, Stroke Prevention in Reversible Ischemia Trial (SPIRIT). European Atrial Fibrillation Trial (EAFT) study groups. Major bleeding during anticoagulation after cerebral ischemia: patterns and risk factors. *Neurology* 2001;1999:1319–1327.

138. Gullov AL, Koefoed BG, Petersen P, et al. Fixed minidose warfarin and aspirin alone and in combination vs adjusted-dose warfarin for stroke prevention in atrial fibrillation: second Copenhagen Atrial Fibrillation, Aspirin and Anticoagulation Study. *Arch Intern Med* 1998;158:1513–1521.

139. Sullivan JM, Harken DE, Gorlin R. Pharmacologic control of thromboembolic complications of cardiac-valve replacement. *N Engl J Med* 1971; 284:1391–1394.

140. Altman R, Boullon F, Rouvier J, et al. Aspirin and prophylaxis of thromboembolic complications in patients with substitute heart valves. *J Thorac Cardiovasc Surg* 1976;72:127–129.

141. Dale J, Myhre E, Storstein O, et al. Prevention of arterial thromboembolism with acetylsalicylic acid: a controlled study in patients with aortic ball valves. *Am Heart J* 1977;94:101–111.

142. Dale J, Myhre E, Loew D. Bleeding during acetylsalicylic acid and anticoagulant therapy in patients with reduced platelet reactivity after aortic valve replacement. *Am Heart J* 1980;99:746–751.

143. Chesebro JH, Fuster V, Elveback LR, et al. Trial of combined warfarin plus dipyridamole or aspirin therapy in prosthetic heart valve replacement: danger of aspirin compared with dipyridamole. *Am J Cardiol* 1983; 51: 1537–1541.

144. Turpie AG, Gent M, Laupacis A, et al. A comparison of aspirin with placebo in patients treated with warfarin after heart-valve replacement. comment. *N Engl J Med* 1993;329:524–529.

145. Acar J, Iung B, Boissel JP, et al. AREVA: multicenter randomized comparison of low-dose versus standard-dose anticoagulation in patients with mechanical prosthetic heart valves. *Circulation* 1996;94:2107–2112.

146. Altman R, Rouvier J, Gurfinkel E, et al. Comparison of high-dose with low-dose aspirin in patients with mechanical heart valve replacement treated with oral anticoagulant. *Circulation* 1996;94:2113–2116.

147. Laffort P, Roudaist R, Rogues X, et al. Early and long-term (one-year) effects of the association of aspirin and oral anticoagulant on thrombi and morbidity after replacement of the mitral valve with the St. Jude medical prosthesis. *J Am Coll Cardiol* 2000;35:739–746.

148. Pruefer D, Dahm M, Dohmen G, et al. Intensity of oral anticoagulation after implantation of St. Jude medical mitral or multiple valve replacement: lessons learned from GELIA (GELIA 5). *Eur Heart J* 2001;3:Q39–Q43.

149. Cappelleri JC, Fiore LD, Brophy MT, et al. Efficacy and safety of combined anticoagulant and antiplatelet therapy versus anticoagulant monotherapy after mechanical heart-valve replacement: a metaanalysis. *Am Heart J* 1995; 130:547–552.

150. Massel D, Little SH. Risks and benefits of adding anti-platelet therapy to warfarin among patients with prosthetic heart valves: a meta-analysis. *J Am Coll Cardiol* 2001;37:569–578.

151. Pouleur H, Buyse M. Effects of dipyridamole in combination with anticoagulant therapy on survival and thromboembolic events in patients with prosthetic heart valves: a meta-analysis of the randomized trials. *J Thorac Cardiovasc Surg* 1995;110:463–472.

152. Cannegieter SC, Rosendaal FR, Wintzen AR, et al. Optimal oral anticoagulant therapy in patients with mechanical heart valves. comment. *N Engl J Med* 1995;333:11–17.

153. Cannegieter SC, Rosendaal FR, Briet E. Platelets/thromboembolism: thromboembolic and bleeding complications in patients with mechanical heart valve prostheses. *Circulation* 1994;89:635–641.

154. Boston Area Anticoagulation Trial for Atrial Fibrillation Investigators. The effect of low dose warfarin on the risk of stroke in patients with non-rheumatic atrial fibrillation. *N Engl J Med* 1990;323:1505–1511.

155. Special Report. Preliminary report of the stroke prevention in atrial fibrillation study. *N Engl J Med* 1990;322:863–868.

156. Petersen P, Boysan G, Godtfredsen J, et al. Placebo-controlled randomized trial of warfarin and aspirin for prevention of thromboembolic complications in chronic atrial fibrillation: the Copenhagen AFASAK study. *Lancet* 1989;1:175–179.

157. Ezekowitz MD, Bridgers SL, James KE, et al. Warfarin in the prevention of stroke associated with non-rheumatic atrial fibrillation. *N Engl J Med* 1992;327:1406–1412.

158. Connolly SJ, Laupacis A, Gent M, et al. Canadian atrial fibrillation anticoagulation trial. *J Am Coll Cardiol* 1991;18:349–355.

159. Pengo V, Zasso A, Barbero F, et al. Effectiveness of fixed minidose warfarin in the prevention of thromboembolism and vascular death in nonrheumatic atrial fibrillation. *Am J Cardiol* 1998;82:433–437.

160. Morocutti C, Amabile G, Fattapposta F, et al. SIFA (Studio Italiano Fibrillazione Atriale) Investigators. Indobufen versus warfarin in the secondary prevention of major vascular events in nonrheumatic atrial fibrillation. *Stroke* 1997;28:1015–1021.

161. Hellemons BS, Langenberg M, Lodder J, et al. Primary prevention of arterial thromboembolism in non-rheumatic atrial fibrillation in primary care: randomised controlled trial comparing two intensities of coumarin with aspirin. *BMJ* 1999;319:958–964.

162. Segal JB, McNamara RL, Miller MR, et al. Prevention of thromboembolism in atrial fibrillation. A meta-analysis of trials of anticoagulants and antiplatelet drugs. *J Gen Intern Med* 2000;15:56–67.

163. Hart RG, Benavente O, McBride R, et al. Antithrombotic therapy to prevent stroke in patients with atrial fibrillation: a meta-analysis. *Ann Intern Med* 1999;131:492–501.

164. Ezekowitz MD, Levine JA. Preventing stroke in patients with atrial fibrillation. *JAMA* 1999;281:1830–1835.

165. Lechat P, Lardoux H, Mallet A, et al. Anticoagulant (fluindione)-aspirin combination in patients with high risk atrial fibrillation. *Cerebrovasc Dis* 2001;12:245–252.

166. van Walraven C, Hart RG, Singer DE, et al. Oral anticoagulants versus aspirin in nonvalvular atrial fibrillation. An individual patient meta-analysis. *JAMA* 2002;288:2441–2448.

167. Taylor F, Cohen H, Ebrahim S. Systematic review of long-term anticoagulation or antiplatelet treatment in patients with non-rheumatic atrial fibrillation. *BMJ* 2001;322:321–326.

168. Evans A, Kalra L. Are the results of randomized controlled trials on anticoagulation in patients with atrial fibrillation generalizable to clinical practice. *Arch Intern Med* 2001;161:1443–1447.

169. Investigators SPiAF. Warfarin versus aspirin for prevention of thromboembolism in atrial fibrillation: stroke prevention in atrial fibrillation II study. *Lancet* 1994;343:687–691.

170. SPORTIF II Investigators. Ximelagatran versus warfarin for stroke prevention in patients with non-valvular atrial fibrillation. *J Am Coll Cardiol* 2003;41:1445–1451.

171. SPORTIF III Investigators. A long-term randomized trial comparing ximelagatran with warfarin for prevention of stroke and systemic embolism in patients with non-valvular atrial fibrillation. *Lancet* 2003;362:1691–1698.

172. Theroux P, Ouimet H, McCans J, et al. Aspirin, heparin or both to treat acute unstable angina? *N Engl J Med* 1988;319:1105–1111.

173. Seneri GGN, Roveli F, Gensini GF, et al. Effectiveness of low-dose heparin in prevention of myocardial reinfarction. *Lancet* 1987;1:937–942.

174. Turpie AGG, Robinson JG, Doyle DJ, et al. Comparison of high dose with low-dose subcutaneous heparin to prevent left ventricular mural thrombosis in patients with acute transmural anterior myocardial infarction. *N Engl J Med* 1989;320:352–394.

175. Gurfinkel E, Manos EJ, Mejail RI, et al. Low molecular weight heparin versus regular heparin or aspirin in the treatment of unstable angina and silent ischemia. *J Am Coll Cardiol* 1995;26:313–318.

176. Fragmin during instability in coronary artery diseae (FRISC) study group. Low molecular weight heparin during instability in coronary artery disease. *Lancet* 1996;347:561–568.

177. Klein W, Buchwald A, Hillis SE, et al. Comparison of low molecular weight heparin with unfractionated heparin acutely and with placebo for 6 weeks in the management of unstable coronary artery disease: fragmin in unstable coronary artery disease study. *Circulation* 1997;96:61–68.

178. Cohen M, Demers C, Gurfinkel E, et al. A comparison of low molecular weight heparin with unfractionated heparin for unstable angina: results of TIMI IIA. *J Am Coll Cardiol* 1997;29:1471–1482.

179. Investigators TTIMITIT. Dose-ranging trial of enoxaparin for unstable angina: results of TIMI IIA. *J Am Coll Cardiol* 1997;29:1471–1482.

180. Fragmin and Fast Revascularization during Instability in Coronary Artery Disease (FRISC II) Investigators. Long term low molecular mass heparin in unstable coronary artery disease: FRISC II prospective randomized multicentre study. *Lancet* 1999;354:701–707.

181. Antman EM, McCabe CH, Gurfinkel E, et al. Enoxaparin prevents death and cardiac ischemic events in unstable angina/non Q wave myocardial infarction: results of the Thrombolysis in Myocardial Infarction (TIMI) IIB trial. *Circulation* 1999;100:1593–1601.

182. Eikelboom JW, Anand SS, Malmberg K, et al. Unfractionated heparin and low-molecular-weight heparin in acute coronary syndrome without ST elevation: a meta-analysis. *Lancet* 2000;355:1936–1942.

183. Batchelor WB, Mahaffey KW, Berger PB, et al. A randomized, placebo-controlled trial of enoxaparin after high-risk coronary stenting: the ATLAST trial. *J Am Coll Cardiol* 2001;38:1608–1613.

184. Smith P, Arnesen H, Holme I. The effect of warfarin on mortality and re-infarction after myocardial infarction. *N Engl J Med* 1990;323:147–152.

185. Sixty-Plus Reinfarction Study Research Group. A double-blind trial to assess long-term anticoagulant therapy in elderly patients after myocardial infarction. *Lancet* 1980;2:989–994.

186. Sixty-Plus Reinfarction Study Research Group. Risks of long-term oral anticoagulant therapy in elderly patients after myocardial infarction. *Lancet* 1982;1:62–68.

187. Group ER. A controlled comparison of aspirin and oral anticoagulants in prevention of death after myocardial infarction. *N Engl J Med* 1982;307:701–708.

188. Breddin K, Loew D, Lechner K, et al. Secondary prevention of myocardial infarction: a comparison of acetylsalicylic acid, placebo and phenprocoumon. *Haemostasis* 1980;9:325–344.

189. Loeliger EA, Hensen A, Kroes F, et al. A double blind trial of long term anticoagulant treatment after myocardial infarction. *Acta Med Scand* 1967;182:549–566.

190. Bjerkelund CJ. The effect of long term treatment with dicumarol in myocardial infarction. *Acta Med Scand* 1957;158:1–212.

191. Bjerkelund CJ. Therapeutic level in long term anticoagulant therapy after myocardial infarction: its relation to recurrent infarction and sudden death. *Am J Cardiol* 1963;1:158–163.

192. Harvald B, Hilden T, Lund E. Long term anticoagulant therapy after myocardial infarction. *Lancet* 1962;2:626–630.

193. ASPECT Research Group. Effect of long-term oral anticoagulant treatment on mortality and cardiovascular morbidity after myocardial infarction. *Lancet* 1994;343:499–503.

194. Van Es RF, Jonker JJC, Verheugt FWA, et al. Aspirin and coumadin after acute coronary syndromes (the ASPECT-2 study): a randomised controlled trial. *Lancet* 2002;360:109–113.

195. Hurlen M, Smith P, Arnesen H, The WARIS-II (Warfarin-Aspirin Reinfarction Study) design. Effects of warfarin, aspirin and the two combined, on mortality and thromboembolic morbidity after myocardial infarction. *Scand Cardiovasc J* 2000;34:168–171.

196. Anand SS, Yusuf S. Oral anticoagulant therapy in patients with coronary artery disease: a meta-analysis. *JAMA* 1999;282:2058–2067.

197. Wallentin L, Wilcox RG, Weaver WD, et al. Oral ximelagatran for secondary prophylaxis after myocardial infarction: the ESTEEM randomized controlled trial. *Lancet* 2003;362:789–797.

198. Duroux P, A collaborative European multicentre study. A randomised trial of subcutaneous low molecular weight heparin (CY 216) compared with intravenous unfractionated heparin in the treatment of deep vein thrombosis. *Thromb Haemost* 1991;65:251–256.

199. Harenberg J, Schmidt JA, Koppenhagen K, et al. EASTERN Investigators. Fixed-dose, body weight-independent subcutaneous LMW heparin versus adjusted dose unfractionated intravenous heparin in the initial treatment of proximal venous thrombosis. *Thromb Haemost* 2000;83:652–656.

200. Prandoni P, Lensing AW, Buller HR, et al. Comparison of subcutaneous low molecular weight heparin with intravenous standard in proximal deep vein thrombosis. *Lancet* 1992;339:441–445.

201. Hull RD, Raskob G, Pineo GF, et al. Subcutaneous low molecular weight heparin compared with continuous intravenous heparin in the treatment of proximal vein thrombosis. *N Engl J Med* 1992;326:975–982.

202. Simonneau G, Charbonnier B, Decousus H, et al. Subcutaneous low molecular weight heparin compared with continuous intravenous unfractionated heparin in the treatment of proximal deep vein thrombosis. *Arch Intern Med* 1993;153:1541–1546.

203. Lindmarker P, Holmstrom M, Granqvist S, et al. Comparison of once-daily subcutaneous fragmin with continuous intravenous unfractionated heparin in the treatment of deep venous thrombosis. *Thromb Haemost* 1994;72:186–190.

204. Fiessinger JN, Lopez-Fernandez M, Gatterer E, et al. Once daily subcutaneous dalteparin, a low molecular weight heparin, for the initial treatment of acute deep vein thrombosis. *Thromb Haemost* 1996;76:195–199.

205. Levine M, Gent M, Hirsh J, et al. A comparison of low-molecular-weight heparin administered primarily at home with unfractionated heparin administered in the hospital for proximal deep-vein thrombosis. *N Engl J Med* 1996;334:677–681.

206. Koopman MMW, Prandoni P, Piovella F, et al. Treatment of venous thrombosis with intravenous unfractionated heparin administered in the hospital as compared with subcutaneous low-molecular-weight heparin administered at home. *N Engl J Med* 1996;334:683–687.

207. Investigators TC. Low molecular weight heparin is an effective and safe treatment for deep-vein thrombosis and pulmonary embolism. *N Engl J Med* 1997;337:657–662.

208. Simonneau G, Sors H, Charbonnier B, et al. A comparison of low-molecular-weight heparin with unfractionated heparin for acute pulmonary embolism. *N Engl J Med* 1997;337:663–669.

209. Decousus H, Leizorovicz A, Parent F, et al. A clinical trial of vena caval filters in the prevention of pulmonary embolism in patients with proximal deep-vein thrombosis. *N Engl J Med* 1998;338:409–415.

210. Kirchmaier CM, Wolf H, Schafer H, et al. Efficacy of a low molecular weight heparin administered intravenously or subcutaneously in comparison with intravenous unfractionated heparin in the treatment of deep venous thrombosis. *Int Angiol* 1998;17:135–145.

211. Lopaciuk S, Meissner AJ, Filipecki S, et al. Subcutaneous low molecular weight heparin versus subcutaneous unfractionated heparin in the treatment of deep vein thrombosis: a polish multicenter trial. *Thromb Haemost* 1992;68:14–18.

212. Dolovich LR, Ginsberg JS, Douketis JD, et al. A meta-analysis comparing low molecular weight heparins with unfractionated heparin in the treatment of venous thromboembolism. *Arch Intern Med* 2000;60:181–188.

213. Gould MK, Dembitzer A, Doyle R, et al. Low molecular weight heparins compared with unfractionated heparin for treatment of acute deep venous thrombosis. A meta-analysis of randomized controlled trials. *Ann Intern Med* 1999;130:800–809.

214. Van den Belt AGM, Prins MH, Lensing AWA, et al. Fixed dose subcutaneous low molecular weight heparin versus adjusted dose unfractionated heparin for venous thromboembolism (Cochrane Review). *The Cochrane Library*, Oxford: Update Software, 2002.

215. Breddin HK, Hach-Wunderle V, Nakov R, et al. Effects of a low-molecular-weight heparin on thrombus regression and recurrent thromboembolism in patients with deep-vein thrombosis. *N Engl J Med* 2001;344: 626–631.

216. Merli G, Spiro TE, Olsson CG, et al. Subcutaneous enoxaparin once or twice daily compared with intravenous unfractionated heparin for treatment of venous thromboembolic disease. *Ann Intern Med* 2001;134: 191–202.

217. Riess H, Koppenhagen K, Tolle A, et al. Fixed-dose, body weight-independent subcutaneous low molecular weight heparin certoparin compared with adjusted-dose intravenous unfractionated heparin in patients with proximal deep venous thrombosis. *Thromb Haemost* 2003;90: 252–259.

218. Kakkar VV, Gebska M, Kadziola Z, et al. Low-molecular-weight heparin in the acute and long-term treatment of deep vein thrombosis. *Thromb Haemost* 2003;89:674–680.

219. Siegbahn A, Hassan S, Boberg J, et al. Subcutaneous treatment of deep venous thrombosis with low molecular weight heparin. A dose finding study with LMWH-Novo. *Thromb Res* 1989;55:767–778.

220. Holmstrom M, Berglund L, Granqvist S, et al. Fragmin once or twice daily subcutaneously in the treatment of deep venous thrombosis of the leg. *Thromb Res* 1992;67:49–55.

221. Partsch H, Kechavarz B, Mostbeck A, et al. Frequency of pulmonary embolism in patients who have iliofemoral deep vein thrombosis and are treated with once- or twice- daily low-molecular-weight heparin. *J Vasc Surg* 1996;24:774–782.

222. Charbonnier BA, Flessinger JN, Banga JD, et al. Comparison of a once daily with a twice daily subcutaneous low molecular weight heparin regimen in the treatment of deep vein thrombosis. *Thromb Haemost* 1998;79:897–901.

223. Couturaud F, Julian JA, Kearon C, et al. Low molecular weight heparin administered once versus twice daily in patients with venous thromboembolism: a meta-analysis. *Thromb Haemost* 2001;86:980–984.

224. Boccalon H, Elias A, Chale JJ, et al. Clinical outcome and cost of hospital vs home treatment of proximal deep vein thrombosis with a low-molecular-weight heparin: the Vascular Midi-Pyrenees study. *Arch Intern Med* 2000;160:1769–1773.

225. Kovacs MJ, Wells PS, Rodger M, et al. A randomized trial comparing low molecular weight heparins for the outpatient treatment of DVT or PE. *Blood* 2001;98:1116a.

226. Monreal M, Lafoz E, Olive A, et al. Comparison of subcutaneous unfractionated heparin with a low molecular weight heparin (fragmin) in patients with venous thromboembolism and contraindications to coumarin. *Thromb Haemost* 1994;71:7–11.

227. The Matisse Investigators. Subcutaneous fondaparinux versus intravenous unfractionated heparin in the initial treatment of pulmonary embolism. *N Eng J Med* 2003;349:1695–1702.

228. The Matisse Investigators. Fondaparinux or enoxaparin for the initial treatment of symptomatic deep venous thrombosis. A randomized trial. *Ann Intern Med* 2004;140:867–873.

229. Bynum LJ, Wilson JE. Low dose heparin therapy in the long term management of venous thromboembolism. *Am J Med* 1979;67:553–556.

230. Hull R, Delmore T, Genton E. Warfarin sodium versus low dose heparin in the long term treatment of venous thromboembolism. *N Engl J Med* 1979;301:855–858.

231. Hull R, Delmore T, Carter C, et al. Adjusted subcutaneous heparin versus warfarin sodium in the long term treatment of venous thrombosis. *N Engl J Med* 1982;306:189–194.

232. Pini M, Aiello S, Manotti C, et al. Low molecular weight heparin versus warfarin for the prevention of recurrence after deep vein thrombosis. *Thromb Haemost* 1994;72:191–197.

233. Das SK, Cohen AT, Edmondson RA, et al. Low-molecular-weight heparin versus warfarin for prevention of recurrence venous thromboembolism: a randomized trial. *World J Surg* 1996;20:521–527.

234. Lopaciuk S, Bielska-Falda H, Noszcyk W, et al. Low molecular weight heparin versus acenocoumarol in the secondary prophylaxis of deep vein thrombosis. *Thromb Haemost* 1999;81:26–31.

235. Hamman H. Rezidivprophylaxe nach plebothrombose – orale antikoagulation oder nidermolelulares heparin subkutan. *Vasomed* 1998;10:133–136.

236. Gonzalez-Fajardo JA, Arreba E, Castrodexa J, et al. Venographic comparison of subcutaneous low-molecular weight heparin with oral anticoagulant therapy in the long-term treatment of deep venous thrombosis. *J Vasc Surg* 1999;30:283–292.

237. Veiga F, Escriba A, Maluenda MP, et al. Low molecular weight heparin (enoxaparin) versus oral anticoagulant therapy (acenocoumarol) in the long-term treatment of deep venous thrombosis in the elderly: a randomized trial. *Thromb Haemost* 2000;84:559–564.

238. Lopez-Beret P, Orgaz A, Fontcuberta J, et al. Low molecular weight heparin versus oral anticoagulants in the long-term treatment of deep venous thrombosis. *J Vasc Surg* 2001;33:77–90.

239. Meyer G, Marjanovic Z, Valcke J, et al. Comparison of low-molecular-weight heparin and warfarin for the secondary prevention of venous thromboembolism in patients with cancer: a randomized controlled study. *Arch Intern Med* 2002;162:1729–1735.

240. Hull R, Pineo GF, Mah A, et al. Long-term low molecular weight heparin treatment versus oral anticoagulant therapy for proximal deep vein thrombosis. *Blood* 2000;96:449a.

241. Hull R, Pineo GF, Mah A, et al. A randomized trial evaluating long-term low-molecular weight heparin therapy for three months versus intravenous heparin followed by warfarin. *Blood* 2003;100:556a.

242. Lee AYY, Levine MN, Baker RI, et al. Low-molecular-weight heparin versus a coumarin for the prevention of recurrent venous thromboembolism in patients with cancer. *N Engl J Med* 2003;349:146–153.

243. Van der Heijden JF, Hutten BA, Buller HR, et al. Vitamin K antagonists or low molecular weight heparin for the long term treatment of symptomatic venous thromboembolism (Cochrane Review). *The Cochrane Library*. Oxford: Update Software, 2002.

244. Lorio A, Guercini F, Pini M. Low-molecular-weight heparin for the long-term treatment of symptomatic venous thromboembolism: meta-analysis of the randomized comparisons with oral anticoagulants. *J Thromb Haemost* 2003;1:1906–1913.

245. Linkins L, Choi PT, Douketis JD. Clinical impact of bleeding in patients taking oral anticoagulant therapy for thromboembolism: a meta-analysis. *Ann Intern Med* 2003;139:893–900.

246. Research Committee of the British Thoracic Society. Optimum duration of anticoagulation for deep-vein thrombosis and pulmonary embolism. *Lancet* 1992;340:873–876.

247. Levine MN, Hirsh J, Gent M, et al. Optimal duration of oral anticoagulant therapy: a randomized trial comparing four weeks with three months of warfarin in patients with proximal deep vein thrombosis. *Thromb Haemost* 1995;74:606–611.

248. Schulman S, Rhedin A-S, Lindmarker P, et al. A comparison of six weeks with six months of oral anticoagulant therapy after a first episode of venous thromboembolism. *N Engl J Med* 1995;332:1661–1665.

249. Pinede L, Ninet J, Duhaut P, et al. Comparison of 3 and 6 months of oral anticoagulant therapy after a first episode of proximal deep vein thrombosis or pulmonary embolism and comparison of 6 and 12 weeks of therapy after isolated calf deep vein thrombosis. *Circulation* 2001;103: 2453–2460.

250. Agnelli G, Prandoni P, Santamaria MG, et al. Three months versus one year of oral anticoagulant therapy for idiopathic deep vein thrombosis. *N Engl J Med* 2001;345:165-169.

251. Agnelli G, Prandoni P, Becattini C, et al. Extended oral anticoagulant therapy after a first episode of pulmonary embolism. *Ann Intern Med* 2003; 139:19–25.

252. Schulman S, Granqvist S, Holmstrom M, et al. The duration of oral anticoagulant therapy after a second episode of venous thromboembolism. *N Engl J Med* 1997;336:393–398.

253. Kearon C, Gent M, Hirsh J, et al. A comparison of three months of anticoagulation with extended anticoagulation for a first episode of idiopathic venous thromboembolism. *N Engl J Med* 1999;340:901–907.

254. Ridker PM, Goldhaber SZ, Danielson E, et al. Long-term, low-intensity warfarin therapy for the prevention of recurrent venous thromboembolism. *N Engl J Med* 2003;348:1425–1434.

255. Schulman S, Wahlander K, Lundstrom T, et al. THRIVE III Investigators. Secondary prevention of venous thromboembolism with the oral direct thrombin inhibitor ximelagatran. *N Engl J Med* 2003;349:1713–1721.

256. Fiessinger JN, Huisman MV, Davidson BL, et al. Ximelagatran vs. low-molecular-weight heparin and warfarin for the treatment of deep vein thrombosis. A randomized trial. *JAMA* 2005;293:681–689.

# CHAPTER 120 ■ ANTIPLATELET THERAPY

GERALD J. ROTH

"I take aspirin for my heart," is a common statement from patients, reflecting the widespread acceptance of aspirin as a useful agent to prevent heart attacks and related manifestations of atherothrombotic disease (1). This chapter reviews current therapy that targets platelets, with aspirin and clopidogrel as the mainstays of *oral* treatment, and abciximab and eptifibatide as the major *intravenous* therapies that block platelet function (2,3). These two main categories of antiplatelet therapy (oral vs. intravenous) differ markedly in several respects, including their mechanisms of action (covalent modification vs. competitive binding), time courses (chronic vs. acute), and propensities to induce thrombocytopenia (rare with oral vs. more frequent with intravenous).

## ORAL AGENTS

### Aspirin

This common drug (inexpensive, generally nontoxic, readily available) has been studied intensively as an antithrombotic agent and is now accepted as a fundamental part of the management of arterial thrombosis (2,3). This discussion focuses on the fact that a daily "baby tablet" of oral aspirin (81 mg) usually provides the most available, most effective, and least toxic regimen (4).

#### Background

Aspirin has been used for a century as an analgesic and antipyretic (5), but its use as an antithrombotic began with the observation that the drug caused bleeding in some patients, particularly gastrointestinal (GI) bleeding (6). Reasoning that a drug that causes bleeding might also prevent thrombosis in patients with atherosclerotic disease, Craven, in the 1950s, studied the incidence of arterial thrombosis in patients taking aspirin and concluded that the drug prevented myocardial infarction (MI) (7). A wealth of subsequent studies has explored the manner in which aspirin alters prostaglandin (PG) synthesis, inhibits platelet function, and prevents thrombi in patients. A set of central facts has emerged: First, aspirin blocks a single enzyme [cyclooxygenase-1, (COX-1)] of PG synthesis in platelets; second, the inhibitory event is permanent, irreversible, and essentially complete (saturable) with uniquely small doses of the oral drug (minimum of approximately 30 mg daily); and third, this single event, covalent blockade of platelet COX-1, underpins all the evidence that aspirin prevents adverse effects due to atherothrombosis, directing the amount, interval, and indications for use in patients (2–4), as follows.

#### The Mechanism of Action

As shown in Figure 120-1, different cells, such as platelets and endothelial cells, synthesize different PG products (8). For example, thromboxane A₂ (TxA₂) is made by platelets, whereas prostacyclin₂ (PGI₂) is produced by endothelium. However, all PG synthesis proceeds through a similar "common" initial pathway catalyzed by a cyclooxygenase (COX) and associated peroxidase that produces the unstable compound, PGH₂, from arachidonate. PGH₂ is the essential intermediate that is subsequently used by "cell-specific" pathways to give individual end products in different cells with distinct, and at times, opposing, effects (TxA₂, PGI₂, PGE₂, etc.).

A series of early publications defined the nature of PGs; much of the work was done by Samuelsson et al. (9–11), accompanied by the original, groundbreaking observation of Vane on the ability of aspirin to block PG synthesis (12). With the identification of PGH2 synthase/COX as the enzyme inhibited by aspirin (13), subsequent studies defined the ability of aspirin to acetylate and covalently modify a single serine residue present in the lining of the "substrate channel" of COX-1, as shown in Figure 120-2 (14–17). Therefore, the critical target for aspirin as an antithrombotic agent is a specific amino acid residue, serine 529, in human platelet COX-1 (16). Transfer of an acetyl group from aspirin to this single site completely blocks access of the substrate, arachidonic acid, to the heme group/active site of the enzyme (Fig. 120-2) (17). As a result, an aspirin-modified, covalently acetylated molecule of COX-1 is permanently and irreversibly inactivated, because the acetyl group cannot be readily removed from the site under *in vivo*, physiologic conditions (14,15). From this starting point of a single modified amino acid, one can trace subsequent work to determine the dose of oral aspirin required to influence platelet COX-1, to explore the role of COX-2 (18,19), to define the functional inhibition that results from such a modification in platelets (20) both *in vitro* and *in vivo*, and finally, to demonstrate the antithrombotic effect of the drug in clinical trials (2–4). The clinical use of aspirin, therefore, stands as an example of an exceptionally well-understood action of a drug: starting from a single amino acid and leading, in turn, to a single enzyme, a clear effect on cellular function in platelets, and, finally, to a measurable clinical effect on the manifestations of systemic vascular disease (4).

#### The Unique Quality of the Aspirin–Platelet Relation

Both basic and clinical researchers have been struck by the remarkable ability of low levels of aspirin to inhibit platelet function *in vitro* (14) and to prevent adverse vascular events *in vivo* (2–4). Perhaps the most dramatic example of the "low-dose" phenomenon was the Dutch transient ischemic attack (TIA) trial, which showed a clear-cut ability of 30 mg of oral aspirin per day to prevent stroke (21). The dose of 30 mg was selected based on *ex vivo* work showing that miniscule amounts, 5 mg orally per day, caused significant decreases in serum TxB₂ levels and that 30 mg daily gave nearly maximal inhibition after several days of continual ingestion (22). These low doses are consistent with the umolar concentrations of aspirin that block the enzyme either in purified form in solution (15) or within normal platelets and endothelial cells (23). However, 30 mg of

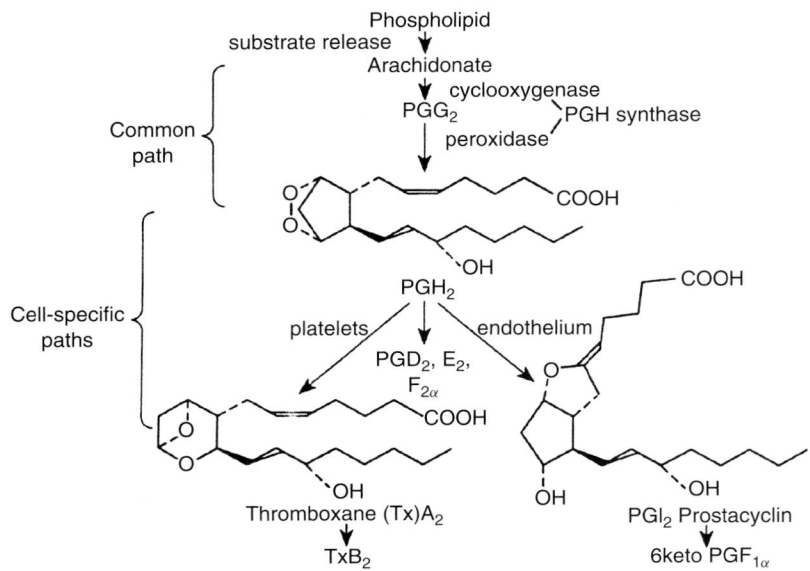

**FIGURE 120-1.** Prostaglandin synthesis. The four steps of prostaglandin (PG) synthesis. First, the unsaturated fatty acid substrate, arachidonate (20:4), is released from phospholipid stores such as phosphatidyl choline in response to an agonist that activates a phospholipase $A_2$. Second, substrate oxygenation, rearrangement, and peroxidation are accomplished through the common pathway that initiates PG synthesis in all cells capable of PG production. The enzyme, termed both $PGH_2$ synthase and COX, possesses two distinct catalytic properties: oxygenation (forming $PGG_2$) and peroxidation ($PGG_2$ to $PGH_2$), and two forms of the enzyme are now characterized (COX-1, constitutive; COX-2, inducible). Third, a variety of different cells, all with enzyme complements suitable for PG formation, metabolize the common intermediate, $PGH_2$, into a variety of end products with remarkably diverse functional activities. For example, platelets form thromboxane $A_2$ ($TxA_2$) with a short half-life and platelet aggregatory and vasoconstrictive effects, whereas endothelium forms prostacyclin ($PGI_2$), also with a short half-life, but with inhibitory effects on platelet aggregation and vasodilatory properties. These cell-specific pathways form both unstable ($TxA_2$, $PGI_2$) and stable (PGs E,F,D) PGs. Fourth, the active compounds are altered and inactivated, leading to metabolic breakdown compounds such as $TxB_2$ and 6 keto $PGF_{1\alpha}$. (From Roth GJ, Calverley DC. Aspirin, platelets and thrombosis. Theory and practice. *Blood* 1994;83:885–898, with permission).

oral aspirin is far below the dose (two adult tablets, 648 mg total) used for headache and fever (24). Therefore, certain unique properties must distinguish the platelet from other aspirin targets such as those related to headache and fever (4); and indeed, these unique qualities are well described: first, the platelet's lack of a nucleus due to its origin as a cytoplasmic fragment from marrow megakaryocytes (25), which precludes almost all new protein synthesis, and second, the fact that the platelet circulates in the blood and is thereby exposed in portal blood to newly ingested aspirin (26,27) (see Fig. 120-3).

**The "Anucleate" Quality of Platelets.** Because a platelet cannot replace its aspirin-acetylated, permanently inhibited COX-1 by new protein synthesis, an aspirin-treated platelet is "stuck with" its blocked enzyme for the rest of its circulating lifespan of 10 days (28), a situation that differs markedly from that of cerebral cells related to headache or of endothelial cells synthesizing $PGI_2$. These latter cells are nucleated, capable of new protein synthesis, and able to replace quickly any aspirin-inhibited COX-1 by making new, unacetylated, active enzyme (24). This anucleate aspect of platelets is responsible for the cumulative nature of oral aspirin inhibition of platelet COX-1; low daily doses exert a consistently increasing effect over several days because the previous day's dose blocked a fraction of platelets, and these platelets persist through their normal lifespan (22). The anucleate quality of platelets, coupled with the permanence of the enzyme modification, results in the long-lived effect of aspirin and explains why surgeons wait several days for the bleeding risk from aspirin ingestion to "wear off" in previously treated patients before surgery (29).

**Exposure of Platelets to Aspirin in the Portal Circulation.** Oral aspirin is absorbed over approximately 1 hour, with peak plasma levels occurring at approximately 30 minutes postingestion (26). The entire mass of circulating platelets appears to enter the portal circulation with about the same time course (3). As shown in Figure 120-3, the "balanced" nature of circulating platelets and absorbed aspirin both entering the portal circulation at about the same rate and with similar duration maximizes the effect of the oral drug on platelets in comparison to cells outside the portal system. Also, the absorbed aspirin is transported to the liver through portal blood, and a significant fraction of the drug is metabolized in the hepatic parenchyma and inactivated by hydrolysis (the "first phase/first pass" effect of hepatic metabolism on oral drugs) (30). This "presystemic" acetylation effect enhances aspirin's antiplatelet effect in comparison to its influence on cells downstream from the liver, such as vascular endothelium (27).

### The "Modest" Antiplatelet Effect of Aspirin: Aspirin Resistance

Patients taking aspirin do not have a severe bleeding diathesis, and aspirin is known to exert only modest effects on platelet function and bleeding times (31). The PG-$TxA_2$ pathway augments platelet aggregation to "weak" agonists such as collagen and epinephrine (32), but inhibition of platelet $TxA_2$ synthesis by aspirin will not alter responsiveness to "strong" responses, such as the primary wave of aggregation induced by adenosine 5′-diphosphate (ADP) and the response to even relatively low concentrations of thrombin (33). A number of platelet

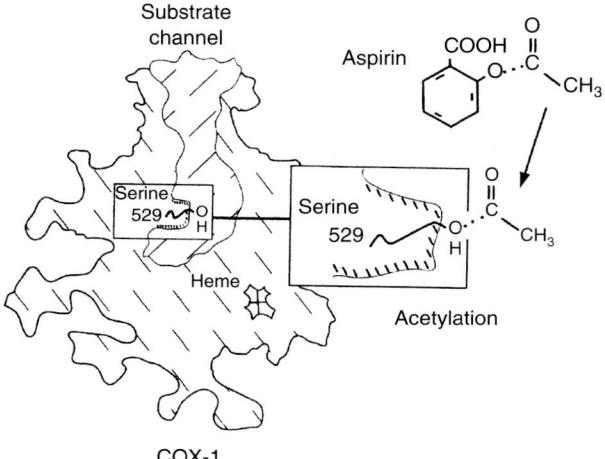

COX-1

FIGURE 120-2.   The molecular mechanism for aspirin-mediated inhibition of platelet prostaglandin synthesis: site-specific acetylation.

Aspirin (acetylsalicylic acid, ASA) transfers an acetyl group to a single serine residue that forms part of the substrate channel of both COX-1 and COX-2 (16,17). The drug has a substantially greater binding affinity for COX-1 as compared to COX-2, and, as a result, is a more effective inhibitor of COX-1 than COX-2. This diagram provides an outline of the COX-1 crystal structure (17) and its internal substrate channel through which the arachidonate substrate gains access to the active site heme group and undergoes oxygenation. Aspirin, as the intact acetylsalicylate molecule, shown at the upper right, possesses a reactive acetyl group ($-COCH_3$) that comes into close proximity to serine 529 when intact aspirin first binds in a reversible, competitive manner within the COX-1 substrate channel. Through nucleophilic attack, the oxygen atom of serine ($-O \cdots H$) forms a covalent bond ($-O \cdots C-$) with the first carbon atom of the acetyl moiety as indicated, and the resultant bound, bulky acetyl group, irreversibly linked to serine 529, blocks the substrate channel and, in turn, abolishes enzymatic activity.

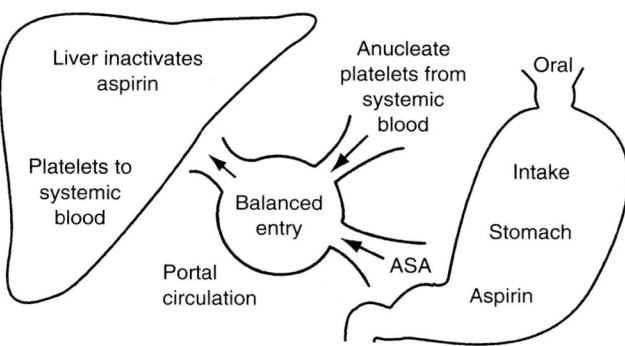

FIGURE 120-3.   Exposure of platelets in portal blood to orally ingested aspirin (acetylsalicylic acid, ASA). Two points are illustrated in this diagram. First, the time course of circulating platelets (termed *anucleate* because, as a cytoplasmic fragment, they lack a nucleus and are incapable of new protein synthesis) entering the portal circulation appears to be about the same (balanced) as that of absorption of newly ingested aspirin into the portal blood from the stomach and upper gastrointestinal tract. Each time course is approximately 30 minutes to 1 hour. Second, exposure of platelets to aspirin in the portal circulation takes place prior to aspirin inactivation in the liver parenchyma (the "first phase/first pass" effect of hepatic metabolism of drugs). Both aspects maximize the ability of oral aspirin to affect platelets to a greater extent than noncirculating cells that lie downstream from the liver, such as vascular endothelial cells.

signaling and amplification pathways are known, such as the influence of protein kinase C, calcium fluxes, granule release, and ADP secretion (4,25). The multifaceted nature of platelet responsiveness to agonists suggests that a number of alternative processes and intermediates can substitute for the $TxA_2$ system and provide nearly normal platelet function in the face of aspirin treatment. This suggestion is confirmed by studies that show many normal individuals will have relatively normal platelet aggregation profiles and bleeding times despite aspirin treatment (34,35). The wide variation in individual response to aspirin can be termed "treatment failure" or "aspirin resistance" (36,37), but the lack of response to aspirin is not due to failure to acetylate platelet COX-1 as assessed by arachidonate-induced platelet aggregation and urinary $TxA_2$ $B_2$ levels (38,39). Certainly, nonsteroidal antiinflammatory drugs (NSAIDs), such as ibuprofen, can compete with aspirin for platelet COX-1 and block aspirin's effect. However, this interference can be avoided by taking the NSAID 30 minutes *after* the daily aspirin tablet (40). The phenomenon of "resistance" to aspirin is generally detected by nonspecific means, such as the bleeding time, or as the occurrence of a thrombotic event in an aspirin-treated patient (41), and the challenge arises immediately to explore this issue further, identify patients with a reduced response to aspirin (by any one of a number of means), and investigate whether or not such individuals should receive an alternate antiplatelet agent, such as clopidogrel (42). From the earliest clinical studies, it was known that aspirin prevents only a few secondary vascular events (25% to 30%) and deaths (15%) and that the drug is only a moderately effective (but quite tolerable) antithrombotic (4). These considerations

suggest that aspirin resistance can be termed "normal variation" or "treatment failure" in at least some clinical situations.

Regardless of the previous arguments, aspirin resistance is a current topic of considerable interest. Intriguing data have been published suggesting that a patient's responsiveness to aspirin can wane with chronic therapy, perhaps due to the induction of platelet COX-2–dependent synthesis of $TxA_2$, which would be relatively resistant to inhibition by aspirin (43). If COX-2 were involved, then higher aspirin doses would be needed to block this source of platelet $TxA_2$ (44). Also, the optimal method for detecting individual variations in aspirin responsiveness is not entirely clear, although devices such as the PFA-100 are useful in this regard (45). The PFA-100 instrument measures the "closure time" by platelets following agonist stimulation, and the epinephrine-dependent system is fairly consistent in its sensitivity to aspirin and may prove to be a practical and relevant measure of aspirin responsiveness. However, the relation between this *in vitro* testing and the use of aspirin *in vivo* requires more study (45).

### Use in Patients: The "Flat Dose–Response" Curve and Its Implication

The data in Figure 120-4 show the results of the five larger, randomized clinical trials that directly compared lower to higher doses of aspirin as an antithrombotic in coronary or cerebral vascular disease (21,46–49). The dose–response relation in Figure 120-4 is "flat," demonstrating that low doses are at least equal to higher doses in preventing vascular events; and this fact, that low doses are effective, is the most telling *in vivo* evidence that aspirin acts solely through its effect on platelet COX-1, because no other known aspirin effect occurs at such low concentrations, including measures of shear-dependent platelet activation, fibrinolysis, and thrombin generation *in vitro* (50–52). Depending on the trials under consideration, one can find evidence that lower doses are *more* effective (2,44). The trend is in favor of lower rather than higher dose aspirin for use in patients (44), probably because higher doses tend to reduce prostacyclin synthesis from vascular cells (53–55), consistent with animal studies showing that a reduction in prostacyclin increases the likelihood

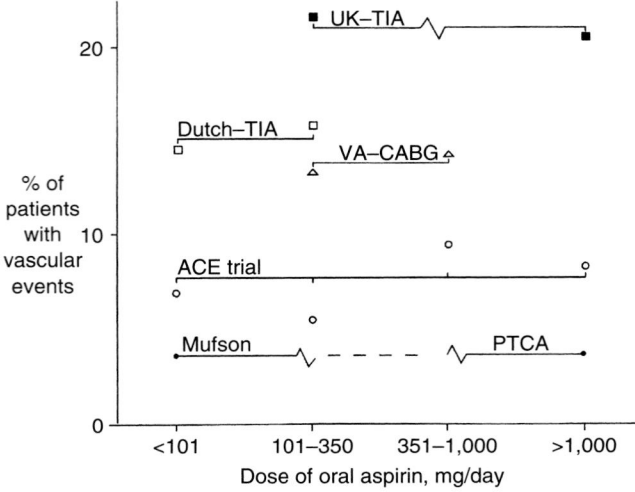

**FIGURE 120-4.** Low doses of oral aspirin are at least as effective as higher doses in preventing atherothrombotic events. The most direct evidence that low-dose aspirin is at least as effective as (and probably more effective than) higher doses comes from the five randomized, relatively large patient trials, the results of which are summarized here (21,46–49), graphing the daily oral dose of aspirin on the horizontal axis (<101,101 to 350, 351 to 1,000, >1,000 mg) and the percentage of enrolled patients in each dose group in whom a vascular event (e.g., myocardial infarction, transient ischemic attack, cerebrovascular accident) occurred on the vertical axis. The incidence of vascular events is slightly lower with lower doses of aspirin. The data are taken from the following studies: the Mufson Percutaneous Transluminal Coronary Angioplasty (PTCA) study (46): 253 patients received 80 mg/242 patients, 1,500 mg, for 6 months (o); the Aspirin in Carotid Endarterectomy (ACE) trial (47): 698 patients received 81 mg/697 patients, 325 mg/703 patients, 650 mg/706 patients, 1,300 mg, for 3 months (o); Veterans Affairs–Coronary Artery Bypass Grafting (VA-CABG) (48); 134 patients received 325 mg/128 patients, 975 mg, for 12 months (Δ); Dutch-TIA (21): 1,555 patients received 30 mg/1,576 patients, 283 mg, for 31 months (□); UK (United Kingdom)–TIA (49): 806 patients received 300 mg/815 patients, 1,200 mg, for 50 months (■). The flat lines show that no dose–response relation exists in these data, suggesting the low doses are at least as effective as higher doses, and in all probability, the lower doses are more effective and certainly cause less bleeding.

of thrombus formation (56). Lower doses are also less toxic in terms of causing GI bleeding (6).

The previously mentioned "trend" favoring lower dose aspirin also impacts on the aspirin resistance issue: Some authors have implied that aspirin resistance might be overcome by increasing the aspirin dosage to 500 mg daily or more (37). These higher doses may be counterproductive and even detrimental in causing GI bleeding and reducing vascular $PGI_2$ production without any additional beneficial effect on platelet $TxA_2$ synthesis, although the possibility of COX-2–dependent $TxA_2$ formation in platelets (43,44) would argue for such higher doses. Therefore, more data are needed to document the effectiveness of higher dose aspirin.

## Summary

**Setting the Stage for a Review of the Clinical Trials of Aspirin in Patients with Vascular Disease.** Aspirin's antiplatelet effect *saturates* (reaches a maximum) at low doses, and all of the drug's antithrombotic potency derives from the single *saturable* modification of platelet COX-1. The distinctions between different doses of aspirin for differing indications is summarized in Table 120-1, comparing three distinct uses for aspirin: first, antithrombotic, second, analgesic/antipyretic, and third, antirheumatic indications (4). The emphasis of Table 120-1 is on the unique features of the platelet as an aspirin target for prevention of thrombosis, along with a list of the remarkable differences that exist in the three uses for the drug.

**Clinical Trials in Patients with Vascular Disease.**

*Secondary prevention data in chronic coronary and cerebral disease.* Many trials involving aspirin have been performed in settings of chronic coronary or cerebral vascular disease. On the basis of multiple, high-quality studies of significant duration, a broad consensus has been reached in these instances that aspirin prevents approximately 20% to 30% of vascular events and 10% to 15% of deaths (2). Table 120-2 includes recent meta-analysis data (57).

*Prevention of recurrent myocardial infarction.* Six randomized double-blind trials in 11,000 total patients over an average of 2 years, testing aspirin alone as the active agent, demonstrated a 31% decline in all cardiac events and a 17% decline in mortality (58–63). When additional similar trials are considered (Table 120-2), combining aspirin with additional agents and/or using a variety of endpoints and durations, aspirin appears to be

---

**TABLE 120-1**

### CLINICAL USE OF ASPIRIN, PAST AND PRESENT: THREE MARKEDLY DIFFERENT INDICATIONS

| | Antithrombotic | Analgesic, Antipyretic | Antirheumatic |
|---|---|---|---|
| Dose, 10 × differences | Approximately 60 mg, 30–100 mg | Approximately 600 mg, two 324-mg tabs | Approximately 6,000 mg, g doses |
| Distinct aspects | Platelet-specific | Time-worn agent for headache and fever | Mechanism of action unclear |
| Toxicity | Mild bruising ± GI upset | GI upset, bleeding, Reye syndrome | GI upset, bleeding, tinnitus |
| Other agents supersede | Probably not, now tested in combinations | Yes NSAIDs, COX-2 inhibitors | Yes Many others, for example, methotrexate |
| Summary | THE FUTURE OF ASPIRIN MAY BE: Almost exclusive use as an inexpensive, specific, and potent antithrombotic agent, often employed at low dosages | | |

GI, gastrointestinal; NSAIDs, nonsteroidal antiinflammatory drugs; COX, cyclooxygenase.

## TABLE 120-2

ABILITY OF ANTIPLATELET REGIMENS (PREDOMINANTLY ASPIRIN) TO PREVENT VASCULAR EVENTS IN HIGH-RISK PATIENTS, SUBDIVIDED BY DISEASE CATEGORY

| Disease category | No. of trials | No. (%) of vascular events | | Observed/Expected | % Odds reduction |
|---|---|---|---|---|---|
| | | Antiplatelet | Control | | |
| Previous MI | 12 | 1,345/9,984 (13.5%) | 1,708/10,022 (17.0%) | −159.8 | 25 |
| Acute MI | 15 | 1,007/9,658 (10.4) | 1,370/9644 (14.2) | −181.5 | 30 |
| Previous CVA/TIAs | 21 | 2,045/11,493 (17.8) | 2464/11,527 (21.4) | −152.1 | 22 |
| Acute CVA | 7 | 1,670/20,418 (8.2) | 1,858/20,403 (9.1) | −94.6 | 11 |
| Stable angina | 7 | 144/1,448 (9.9) | 206/1,472 (14.1) | −30.7 | 33 |
| Unstable angina | 12 | 199/2,497 (8.0) | 336/2,534 (13.3) | −64.8 | 46 |
| Coronary angioplasty | 9 | 43/1,592 (2.7) | 89/1,620 (5.5) | −18.7 | 53 |
| Intermittent claudication | 26 | 201/3,123 (6.4) | 249/3,140(7.9) (6.4) | −22.3 | 23 |

MI, myocardial infarction; CVA, cerebrovascular accident; TIA, transient ischemic attack.
From Antithrombotic Trialists Collaboration. Collaborative meta-analysis of randomized trials of antiplatelet therapy for prevention of death, myocardial infarction, and stroke in high-risk patients. *Br Med J* 2002;324:71–86, with permission.

slightly less effective, and most authors summarize the aspirin benefit as a 25% to 30% reduction in vascular events and a 15% drop in mortality (57,64). The minimal dose used in these trials has been 75 mg per day, which is somewhat more effective than higher doses, consistent with the earlier discussion and, indeed, with all the available data (43,57,64).

*Use in patients with stroke.* Aspirin and related antiplatelet therapy is somewhat less effective in preventing recurrent stroke than in preventing MI, although the reason for the difference remains unclear. Several trials show a clear-cut benefit from aspirin (65,66), but the discussion has been clouded by the contention that much higher doses of aspirin are required in cerebral than in coronary disease (67,68). This question has been addressed in the ACE trial in which a significantly improved result was demonstrated with low-dose aspirin in carotid artery disease (47) (Table 120-2).

*Trials in acute settings such as unstable angina and acute stroke.* Although fewer studies and enrolled patients are available in these often brief trials, results indicate that aspirin is remarkably effective in altering an evolving thrombus (Table 120-2).

For example, several trials in crescendo or unstable angina involving 3,100 patients with an average follow-up of 4 months show a 50% to 70% decline in the risk of MI and cardiac death (4,69). Aspirin is a "standard of care" now in acute coronary syndromes, although higher initial doses, such as 324 mg oral aspirin, are required to rapidly alter platelet COX-1 in these acute situations, and heparin is often added to the initial regimen (2,70,71). Two recent trials in acute ischemic stroke, involving approximately 40,000 patients treated within 48 hours of the event and continued for approximately 1 month, showed approximately a 10% reduction in vascular events. A small increase in cerebral hemorrhage was associated with aspirin use (72,73).

*Primary prevention studies.* Several "primary" prevention studies have been conducted in individuals with risk factors for atherothrombosis, but without prior infarction/angina/TIA (74–80) (see Table 120-3), and the consensus has been reached that the incidence of adverse vascular events is often low in this group and that many patients will be treated without demonstrable benefit (74–82). The rate of adverse events in

## TABLE 120-3

USE OF ASPIRIN FOR PRIMARY PREVENTION OF VASCULAR EVENTS

| Trial | Subjects (no.) | Dose mg | Years | Placebo events %/yr | RR aspirin |
|---|---|---|---|---|---|
| US Phys. (74) | Healthy men (22,071) | 325 qod | 5.0 | 0.7 | 0.82 |
| PPP (80) | High risk (4,495) | 100 qd | 3.6 | 0.8 | 0.71 |
| HOT (78) | Hypertensive (18,790) | 75 qd | 3.8 | 1.1 | 0.85 |
| UK Doc. (76) | Healthy men (5,139) | 500 qd | 5.8 | 1.4 | 1.03 |
| TPT (79) | High-risk men (5,085) | 75 qd | 6.3 | 1.6 | 0.83 |

PPP, Collaborative Group of the Primary Prevention Project; HOT, Hypertension Optimal Treatment; RR aspirin, risk reduction by aspirin; TPT, Thrombosis Prevention Trial.
From Patrono C, Coller B, FitzGerald GA, et al. Platelet-active drugs: the relationships among dose, effectiveness and side effects. *Chest* 2004;126(Suppl. 3):234S–264S, with permission.

the control, untreated placebo groups ranges between 0.7% and 1.6% per year, and, therefore, prevention of such rare events by aspirin requires many "patient-years." Approximately one to three vascular events *per year* are prevented *per 1,000* treated individuals (see Fig. 120-5). This low degree of prevention can be compared to the results of the Swedish Angina Pectoris Aspirin Test (SAPAT) trial in stable angina in which 12 events per 1,000 were prevented in this *secondary* cohort with a control rate of 3.7% (83) (Fig. 120-5). The use of aspirin as a *primary* preventative requires some discretion (44,81). For example, recent work demonstrates a gender difference in aspirin's effect with a reduction in stroke, but not in MI or cardiovascular death in women, and the *converse* in men (74,75). In addition, the distinction between patients with and without demonstrable symptomatic manifestations of vascular disease may be difficult, and antiplatelet therapy is only one aspect of management, which includes attention to blood pressure, cholesterol, blood glucose, smoking, and weight. High-risk patients without actual angina or TIA are often treated with aspirin, but bleeding caused by aspirin is always a concern, and the risk–benefit ratio may be hard to judge. For example, several severe hemorrhagic strokes occurred in the US Physicians' trial in the aspirin-treated group, and although the strokes may have occurred by chance alone, their occurrence gives one pause in treating asymptomatic individuals (74).

**Other Indications for Aspirin Use Related to Thrombosis.** Aspirin has been studied as an antithrombotic in atrial fibrillation, deep venous thrombosis, and placental insufficiency in formal trials that have revealed quite modest or no beneficial effects.

Patients with atrial fibrillation are usually best managed with adjusted-dose warfarin to prevent thrombosis, particularly embolic stroke (84); but certain individuals with "lone" atrial fibrillation and those who cannot take warfarin become candidates for aspirin (85). One can expect aspirin to prevent approximately 25% of thrombi in this disorder, whereas careful warfarin management will prevent 50% to 67% of such episodes (86). An ongoing trial of clopidogrel added to aspirin in atrial fibrillation will, when complete, provide additional insight into the efficacy of antiplatelet therapy in this setting.

Aspirin is a relatively ineffective drug for deep vein thrombosis (DVT), and the somewhat sparse data suggest that it will be used only infrequently for this indication (87,88). The most impressive result with aspirin in this regard was a 36% reduction in DVT or pulmonary embolism (PE) in 13,000 patients with hip fracture (89). Overall, aspirin is much less effective than anticoagulants in DVT/PE (87).

Although the role of thrombosis in placental insufficiency and preeclampsia is somewhat unclear, aspirin has been studied in detail in this regard and found to be moderately effective (90,91). A broad overview of the data shows that aspirin reduces preeclampsia by 15% and fetal/near-term infant deaths by 14% (91).

### Toxicity Due to Aspirin

This discussion acknowledges that a bleeding risk is inescapable in all aspirin-treated patients simply because of the antiplatelet effect of the drug, and the risk is substantially increased if the individual has an underlying hemostatic defect such as hemophilia (92). Nonhematologic disease, with hypertension as an example, may not increase the extracranial bleeding risk to any appreciable extent, as shown in the Hypertension Optimal Treatment (HOT) trial (78). In regard to intracranial bleeding, at least two large trials suggest that aspirin can cause rare but significant intracranial bleeds, perhaps in individuals with some modest but undetected hemostatic disorder (4,74,93).

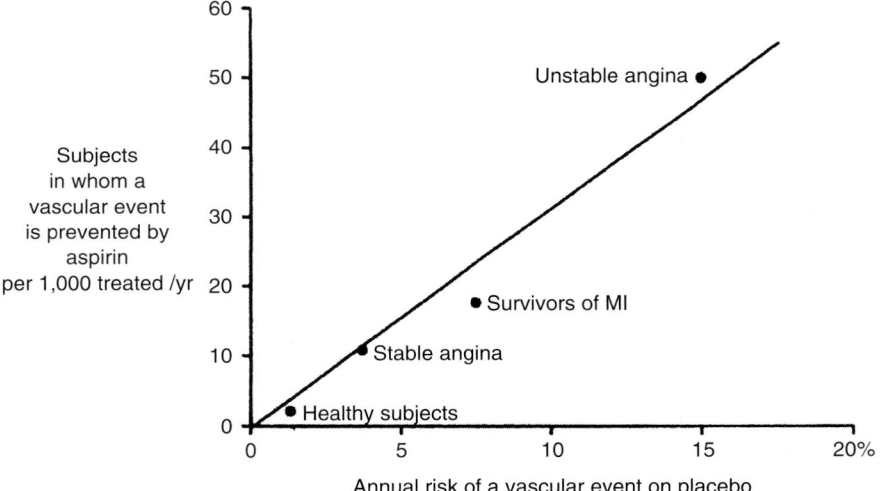

**FIGURE 120-5.** The potential benefit from aspirin is directly proportional to the risk posed by the vascular disease that is present. The graph plots the number of individuals per 1,000 aspirin-treated patients per year who avoid a vascular event (vertical axis) versus the percentage (%) of patients annually in a particular clinical grouping [i.e., normal individuals, stable angina, survivors of myocardial infarction (MI) unstable angina (UA)] in whom such an episode occurs (vertical axis). Individuals who have risk factors for atherothrombotic disease (e.g., smoking, hypertension, diabetes, elevated lipids) but in whom an actual vascular event (MI, cerebrovascular accident) has not occurred or exhibited a clear-cut vascular symptom (angina, transient ischemic attack) have annual risk levels of approximately 1% or 2%. As a result, one might treat 1,000 such "healthy" patients with aspirin for a year in order to prevent one or two vascular events, whereas the incidence of significant bleeding in these 1,000 persons might be one or two per thousand. The conclusion is that treating generally healthy patients with aspirin has a questionable benefit–risk ratio. On the other hand, in the case of unstable angina, with a 15% annual risk level, one could expect to prevent 50 vascular episodes while causing perhaps one or two major gastrointestinal bleeds, an obviously excellent benefit–risk ratio. [From Patrono C, Coller B, Dalen JE, et al. Platelet-active drugs. The relationships among dose, effectiveness, and side effects. Chest 2001;119(Suppl. 1):39S–63S, with permission.]

The major toxicity of aspirin is upper gastrointestinal bleeding, probably related to both a reduction in local PG synthesis and the irritant effect of the compound itself on the GI mucosa (94). A number of studies demonstrate that the likelihood of GI bleeding is dose-dependent with considerable increases in risk as the daily oral dose of aspirin is raised from 75 to 1,500 (95,96). This is in direct contrast to the lack of dose dependency of the therapeutic effect. The GI bleeding risk is a major reason to use low-dose aspirin, in the range of 30 to 100 mg per day, in order to avoid such bleeding (6,94). However, even the lowest doses of aspirin, approximately 75 mg per day, are well known to cause GI bleeding (6,65,94), and the practitioner must be aware that any dose of aspirin, even low doses, can induce major and perhaps even fatal GI bleeding because the fatality rate for the complication remains on the order of 5% to 10% (97). The problem of upper GI bleeding is a main point in restricting prophylactic aspirin therapy to individuals who have a clear-cut increased risk of atherothrombotic complications such as angina, TIA, or history of MI, and avoiding the drug in persons with only risk factors, which are often well managed by other measures and are associated with a low incidence of yearly events. This point is emphasized in Fig. 120-5, which demonstrates the obvious: that aspirin works only in those patients who can benefit from it, namely, those within a group whose vascular disease is associated with significant risk for clinically relevant adverse events, perhaps 1.5% to 2% per year or higher. Enteric-coated and slow-release forms of aspirin do not alter the GI bleeding risk (98), although omeprazole and treatment of a *Helicobacter pylori* infection will reduce the incidence (99,100). The adverse effects of aspirin on renal function and blood pressure appear to be minimal and are not of great concern with low antithrombotic dosages (101).

## Reversible Aspirinlike Drugs Such as Nonsteroidal Antiinflammatory Drugs and Coxibs

The NSAIDs, excluding aspirin, are competitive, as opposed to irreversible inhibitors of COX-1 and COX-2, and have not found a place in antithrombotic therapy. Most of these agents will bind within the substrate channel of platelet COX-1, block function transiently, and interfere with aspirin, but their inhibitory effect on the platelet enzyme is insufficient to warrant many clinical trials in atherothrombosis (102,103). Nonetheless, some study has been done, particularly on indobufen, demonstrating its modest ability to influence vascular events, an ability that probably falls short of aspirin (104,105). Triflusal, fluriprofen, and sulfinpyrazone have also been evaluated in randomized clinical trials, and all three have modest activity (57,106–108).

The coxibs, as relatively selective inhibitors of the inducible COX, COX-2, would be expected to lie outside the purview of aspirin and platelet COX-1 issues. However, these agents suppress prostacyclin production and could influence atherothrombosis (109). A large randomized trial of a selective agent, rofecoxib, in patients with rheumatoid arthritis showed an *increased* incidence of MI in individuals taking the coxib (110). In view of the broad acceptance of coxibs in clinical practice, the problem that these drugs may cause thromboembolism is of concern and poses a significant question. The findings of the VIGOR (Vioxx GI Outcomes Research) trial (110) were initially attributed to chance or to the ability of the comparative agent, naproxen, to prevent vascular events. The issue has now been revisited with an additional published trial (111) and editorial comment (112,113), and the data indicate that rofecoxib increases the risk of myocardial infarction and thrombotic stroke. The effect of the related coxibs (celecoxib, valdecoxib, and lumiracoxib) on vascular events will now be scrutinized more fully.

## Thienopyridines: Ticlopidine and Clopidogrel

Compared to aspirin, both ticlopidine and clopidogrel are somewhat superior agents in patients with cerebral and peripheral vascular disorders as contrasted to coronary disease (114). This suggests that platelet activation may use somewhat different pathways in different circulations. Although still hypothetical, one might conclude that ADP release and activation are more critical outside the coronary vessels because the thienopyridines (as ADP inhibitors) are more effective in vascular beds outside the heart (115). Conversely, the effect of $TxA_2$ may be more important within the heart because aspirin (which blocks $TxA_2$) is more active in this locale. Both ticlopidine and clopidogrel require prior metabolic activation in order to affect platelet activity through covalent modification, both cause thrombotic thrombocytopenic purpura (TTP) in rare patients, and both are more expensive than aspirin (114–116). Individual discussions follow.

Ticlopidine is metabolized by the liver to a 2-keto, thiol-contained active compound, which modifies the platelet $P2Y_{12}$ (ADP) receptor through a disulfide link (117,118). The recommended dose of 250 mg twice daily is rapidly absorbed but requires several days to exert an antiplatelet effect, which is cumulative, and reaches a steady state after approximately 1 week, resulting in approximately 60% blockade of platelet $P2Y_{12}$ receptor activity. A number of studies document the activity of ticlopidine in stroke and TIA (119), coronary disease and bypass grafting (120), and peripheral arterial disease (121). However, ticlopidine is also associated with significant neutropenia in approximately 2% of treated patients and, because of this toxicity and suspected effects on cholesterol and marrow function (122), most practitioners now use clopidogrel in preference to ticlopidine.

Clopidogrel shares many properties with ticlopidine, but it does not appear to cause neutropenia or marrow suppression and has a lower incidence of associated TTP (which, if it occurs, usually appears within 2 weeks of starting the drug) (114,116). It is metabolized to an active carboxylic derivative that covalently modifies the platelet $P2Y_{12}$ receptor (118,123), and the effect persists for the remaining lifespan of the altered platelet. The standard dose of 75 mg per day produces a cumulative antiplatelet effect after several days, and currently, a higher loading dose of 300 mg is employed to suppress platelet function more rapidly, within hours. The major clinical trial of clopidogrel involved three patient groups with recent stroke, MI, or symptoms of peripheral vascular disease; compared to aspirin, clopidogrel was clearly superior only in those patients with peripheral vascular disease while showing slightly more activity in stroke patients and less in coronary disease (115). However, clopidogrel is now approved for use in all three forms of vascular disease and is widely accepted as a slightly more potent agent than aspirin, often used as an additive to aspirin. In view of expense, many practitioners start appropriate patients on aspirin alone, then add clopidogrel if symptoms appear or persist. A number of current trials test the combination of agents (124,125). For example, recent studies of clopidogrel and aspirin in unstable angina and post percutaneous coronary intervention (PCI) have shown superior results in these settings, and the two drugs are widely used in combination at this time (126,127). Another study in patients with carotid endarterectomy shows the benefit of aspirin plus clopidogrel, initiated before surgery (128), and a variety of ongoing related studies of clopidogrel combined with aspirin will add to this information.

## Additional Oral Agents: Dipyridamole, Platelet Glycoprotein IIb/IIIa Inhibitors

Dipyridamole has been used extensively in patients for decades, but the database supporting its use has been questioned despite knowledge of the drug's effect on cyclic adenosine monophosphate and adenosine levels (129,130). To a large extent, dipyridamole had been dismissed as a somewhat inactive agent until the development of a modified release form and publication of this form's effectiveness in patients with stroke (131). Termed the European Stroke Prevention Study-2 (EPS-2) trial, which compared dipyridamole, aspirin, and the combination in 6,600 patients, dipyridamole prevented 18% of recurrent stroke when used alone and 37% when used in combination with aspirin. The quality, size, and duration of EPS-2 all suggest that dipyridamole has clear-cut activity and a role in the management of patients with cerebrovascular disease (132). The main differences between EPS-2 and earlier trials are the improved availability of the modified release form of the drug and its higher daily dose (400 mg instead of 225 mg) in EPS-2. A combination of modified release dipyridamole and low-dose aspirin (Aggrenox-Boehringer) is now FDA-approved.

In view of the dramatic success of intravenous glycoprotein (GP) IIb/IIIa inhibitors postcoronary angioplasty and stenting (133), which is discussed in a later section, considerable efforts were made to develop and test oral agents directed against the same target (134). However, despite the emergence of several highly active compounds that successfully block receptor function *in vitro*, the *in vivo* clinical trials have been disappointing (135,136). Some of the studies indicate a higher mortality in treated patients, perhaps because a drug that binds and inhibits GP IIb/IIIa may also activate the receptor and, in turn, the platelet. Such activation can lead to thrombocytopenia and thrombotic complications (137). The trials have been large and well designed with adequate size and duration (138–140), but they have almost invariably led to the conclusion that this form of antiplatelet therapy failed with the currently available agents, dosages, and dose schedules.

A variety of additional compounds inhibit platelet function and may have a role as antiplatelet agents. For example, thromboxane receptor antagonist-S 18886 is orally active and alters platelet activation (141). Two related agents, sulotroban and ifetroban, have shown relatively little activity in clinical trials (142). In addition, a competitive, reversible inhibitor (AR-C69931MX) of the platelet ADP receptor ($P2Y_{12}$) has been developed and studied in patients (143). Prostacyclin itself and its stable analog, iloprost, have useful properties but cause major side effects, such as hypotension (144). The search for additional agents and targets is ongoing.

# INTRAVENOUS AGENTS

## Inhibitors of Glycoprotein IIb/IIIa: Abciximab, Eptifibatide, Tirofiban

Platelet aggregation depends on the activation and ligand-binding properties of the major platelet surface integrin, termed GP IIb/IIIa, which interacts with fibrinogen and von Willebrand factor (VWF). As a dominant surface membrane protein, present in approximately 80,000 copies per platelet, GP IIb/IIIa is a logical target for antiplatelet therapy; and elimination of its activity would be expected to have a dramatic inhibitory effect on platelet function, although bleeding would be an immediate concern (145). Therefore, in contrast to the drugs discussed previously, such as aspirin, which block only

one of many intraplatelet activation pathways, the anti–GP IIb/IIIa inhibitors can cause almost complete platelet paralysis when given in sufficient dosages.

With the publication of the Second International Study of Infarct Survival (ISIS-2) trial in 1988 (70), the powerful effect of an antiplatelet agent, namely aspirin, was demonstrated in acute coronary disease; and with the development of a potent GP IIb/IIIa monoclonal antibody, 7E3, the idea of essentially complete blockade of the integrin in patients undergoing PCI (percutaneous coronary intervention) was tested in patients (133,145). The first large trial, termed 7E3 in Preventing Ischemic Complications study (EPIC) and published in 1994, showed that such therapy was both practical and effective, but was associated with episodes of major bleeding (146). A decade later, major progress has been made in understanding this type of therapy more fully, and extensive studies have explored additional agents, settings, and ancillary management in both PCI and acute coronary disease.

### The Agents in Current Use

**Abciximab.** Marketed under the trade name ReoPro (Lilly, Indianapolis), this is a "humanized" mouse–human chimeric monoclonal directed against GP IIb/IIIa, which is FDA-approved for use in PCI settings and in acute coronary syndromes when immediate PCI is planned. The original mouse monoclonal, c7E3, proved to have remarkable potency, both *in vitro* and *in vivo*, in suppressing GP IIb/IIIa function, inhibiting platelet aggregation completely at 80% receptor occupancy, and prolonging the bleeding time at 90% (133,147). The antibody is usually administered as a 0.25 mg per kg bolus followed by a 10 $\mu$g per minute constant 12-hour infusion, and the concentration of the free antibody falls rapidly when therapy is begun as it binds to platelets. The bolus/constant infusion approach will maintain nearly complete platelet inhibition for the entire infusion period, declining to approximately 50% of the peak effect after 24 hours and essentially disappearing after 48 hours (148). In addition to GP IIb/IIIa receptor effect, abciximab also inhibits platelet surface thrombin generation, an effect that may contribute to the antithrombotic potential of the drug (149).

Abciximab causes thrombocytopenia in approximately 1% or 2 % of treated patients, and the platelet count must be followed-up closely during and following a course of treatment (150). In addition, abciximab therapy carries a considerable risk of both intra and extracranial bleeding, although lowering of the heparin dosages and improved vascular sheath management have led to a drop in bleeding complications (146,151).

**Eptifibatide.** Eptifibatide (Integrilin, Key Pharmaceuticals) is a disulfide-containing, seven–amino acid, cyclic peptide based on the KGD (Lys-Gly-Asp) peptide sequence of the snake venom disintegrin, *barbourin*, which inhibits the vitronectin receptor $\alpha_V\beta_3$ slightly, but exerts most of its effect on platelet GP IIb/IIIa (152). The appropriate dosage for eptifibatide was not clarified initially (153,154), and later studies used a somewhat higher "double bolus" protocol to enhance effectiveness (155). Patients now receive an initial bolus of 180 $\mu$g per kg and an infusion of 2 $\mu$g/kg/min thereafter, with a second 180 $\mu$g per kg bolus 10 minutes after the first, which together provide substantial inhibition of ADP-induced platelet aggregation for approximately 12 hours (155,156). Like abciximab, eptifibatide inhibits platelet-surface thrombin generation, an effect that may contribute to its antithrombotic activity (149). Unlike abciximab, eptifibatide is generally not associated with thrombocytopenia (154,156,157).

**Tirofiban.** This is a tyrosine-based compound with almost total selectivity for platelet GP IIb/IIIa as opposed to other integrin targets (158). Marketed as Aggrastat (Merck,

West Point, Pennsylvania), tirofiban blocks *in vitro* ADP-induced aggregation with an IC50 of 9nM (159) and, following a bolus of 10 $\mu$g per kg and an 0.15 $\mu$g/kg/min infusion in patients, rapidly and nearly completely inhibits *ex vivo* ADP aggregation (160). Its effects on platelet function and bleeding time dissipate relatively rapidly upon cessation of the drug, and its plasma half-life is only 1.6 hours (160,161).

## The Randomized Trials in Percutaneous Coronary Intervention

A series of relatively large trials has tested the efficacy of anti–GP IIb/IIIa therapy in approximately 15,000 patients undergoing percutaneous coronary interventions (PCI) such as balloon angioplasty with or without stent placement and atherectomy, and all demonstrate the usefulness of these drugs, which is, at times, extraordinary. The major endpoint is generally death or MI at 30 days postprocedure, and abciximab has shown remarkable effectiveness in lowering risks by approximately 20% to 55%. In the case of abciximab, a series of related and sequential questions were asked and then answered in three trials. First, does the agent have activity (EPIC, 136)? Second, can the risk of bleeding be minimized [Evaluation in PTCA to Improve Long-term Outcome with Abciximab Glycoprotein IIb/IIIa Blockage (EPILOG) 141]? Third, is the drug useful in the setting of stent placement in a target artery [Evaluation of Platelet IIb/IIIa Inhibitor for Stenting (EPISTENT), 152]? The answer was yes in each instance.

The first major trial, EPIC (146), involved 2,099 patients and demonstrated a 35% reduction in 30-day death, MI, or recurrent ischemia with treatment (12.8% control vs. 8.3% inhibitor). However, considerable bleeding accompanied the treatment (162), and the next trial explored approaches that might mitigate bleeding, namely, a decrease in concomitant heparin and more timely removal of the femoral artery sheath. This second trial, EPILOG (151), excluded patients with ongoing ischemia and was discontinued (at 2,792 patients) before full enrollment (4,800 patients) was reached because of the clear-cut benefit of lower dose heparin and abciximab, resulting in a risk reduction of approximately 55%. This second trial demonstrated that abciximab was useful even in patients without evolving ischemia and that bleeding risk could be minimized with appropriate changes in management. The third trial, EPISTENT (163), enrolled 2,399 patients and was designed to study the evolving use of stent placement to prevent restenosis following PCI. A risk reduction of approximately 50% was observed at 1 month, and abciximab was shown to reduce restenosis even in the absence of stent placement, consistent with the concept that platelet deposition is part of the restenotic process (164). The 6-month follow-up data in all three trials consistently documented a longer term benefit of the antibody. These early trials established abciximab and/or related GP IIb/IIIa inhibitors, as discussed subsequently, as critically important agents in minimizing adverse events following PCI.

Three additional trials, two involving eptifibatide (156,165) and one with tirofiban (166), have shown that these agents also have a role in PCI management, particularly in view of their lower cost compared to abciximab. A third agent, lamifiban, has been shown to have activity, but its development has been discontinued (167). The first trial of eptifibatide, Integrilin to Minimise Platelet Aggregation and Combat Thrombosis in Acute Myocardial Infarction (IMPACT) II with 4,010 patients, gave somewhat disappointing results, probably because of inadequate doses of the drug. Risk reduction in IMPACT II was less than 20% at 1 month and undetectable at 6 months, clearly inferior to the results with abciximab. However, the later study, European and Australian Stroke Prevention in Reversible Ischaemic Trial (ESPRIT) (156) with 2,604 patients, double bolus infusions of eptifibatide, and more effective suppression of platelet function, showed 37% risk reduction at 48 hours and 35% at 1 month, similar to the benefit conferred by abciximab.

The tirofiban trial, Randomised Efficacy Study of Tirotiban for Outcomes and Restenosis (RESTORE) (166) with 2,139 patients, demonstrated a 20% to 25% risk reduction with this agent that occasionally induces thrombocytopenia (157). More recently, a direct comparison of tirofiban with abciximab, Therapeutic Arthritis Research and Gastrointestinal Event Trial (TARGET) (168), was completed, and the data favored abciximab as the more active drug in the study reported. However, one cannot make absolute distinctions at this point, on the bases of the current evidence, in selecting one of these three drugs—abciximab, eptifibatide, tirofiban—as clearly superior. Each trial related to this type of decision was different, with different patient groups, analyses, and exclusions; and at present, each of these approved agents may find a role in the management of specific patients in specific settings that include PCI. A metaanalysis of these trials has been published (169).

## Trials in Acute Coronary Syndromes Managed Medically and Related Issues

In contrast to the data reviewed previously in patients with acute coronary syndromes managed by PCI, the intravenous GP IIb/IIIa inhibitors have not yet found a definite place in the medical management of acute coronary disease, despite considerable study. Both positive and negative results have been obtained with the same agents. For example, the c7E3 Fab Antiplatelet Therapy in Unstable Refractory Angina (CAPTURE) trial with abciximab, with the data analyzed before the PCI step, demonstrated a benefit from the monoclonal (170), whereas the later Global Utilization of Streptokinase and TPA for Occluded arteries (GUSTO-IV) study indicated slightly better risk reduction with placebo (171). Similar conflicting results were obtained with tirofibin and the Platelet Receptor Inhibition in Ischemic Syndrome Management (PRISM)/PRISM-Plus studies in which earlier inspection of the data at 48 hours or 7 days gave opposite findings (172,173). Finally, the large Platelet Glycoprotein IIb/IIIa in Unstable Angina Receptor Suppression Using Integrilin Therapy (PURSUIT) trial with eptifibatide indicated a modest benefit from the drug (174). At this point, one must await the results of ongoing work in acute MI managed without PCI. This is an active area of investigation in which additional regimens are explored, such as the usefulness of clopidogrel (175) or low-molecular-weight heparin (176) and various combinations of fibrinolytic agents with GP IIb/IIIa inhibitors (177–179).

Finally, in even less well-characterized situations, the GP IIb/IIIa inhibitors are being assessed in stroke, peripheral vascular disease, and carotid artery disease (180–182). No conclusions or recommendations are appropriate at this stage for these patients in these settings.

## Summary of Intravenous Glycoprotein IIb/IIIa Antagonists

The intravenous GP IIb/IIIa drugs have opened a new era in antiplatelet therapy, that of essentially complete blockade of platelet activity in life-threatening settings. The data all support the use of these agents in patients undergoing coronary interventions, whereas their use in MI and related conditions remains less clear. The bleeding associated with these agents remains a critically important issue along with their cost.

# *References*

1. Shahar E, Folsom AR, Romm FJ, et al. Patterns of aspirin use in middle-aged adults: the Atherosclerosis Risk in Communities (ARIC) Study. *Am Heart J* 1996;131:915–922.

2. Antiplatelet Trialists' Collaboration. Collaborative overview of randomized trials of antiplatelet therapy- I: prevention of death, myocardial infarction, and stoke by prolonged antiplatelet therapy in various categories of patients. *Br Med J* 1994;308:81–106.

3. Patrono C, Coller B, Dalen JE, et al. Platelet-active drugs. The relationships among dose, effectiveness, and side effects. *Chest* 2001; 119(Suppl. 1): 39S–63S.

4. Roth GJ, Calverley DC. Aspirin, platelets and thrombosis. Theory and practice. *Blood* 1994;83:885–898.

5. Mann CC, Plummer ML. *The aspirin wars: money, medicine and 100 years of rampant competition.* New York: Knopf, 1991.

6. Roderick PJ, Wilkes HC, Meade TW. The gastrointestinal toxicity of aspirin: An overview of randomized controlled trials. *Br J Clin Pharmacol* 1993; 35:219–226.

7. Craven LL. Prevention of coronary and cerebral thrombosis. *Miss Valley Med J* 1956;78:213–215.

8. Oliw E, Granstrom E, Anggard E. The prostaglandins and essential fatty acids. In: Pace-Asciak C, Granstrom E, eds. *Prostaglandins and related substances,* Chap. 1. Amsterdam: Elsevier, 1983:1–44.

9. Samuelsson B, Granstrom E, Green K, et al. Prostaglandins. *Annu Rev Biochem* 1975;44:669–701.

10. Hamberg M, Svensson J, Samuelsson B. Thromboxanes: a new group of biologically active compounds derived from prostaglandin endoperoxides. *Proc Natl Acad Sci U S A* 1975;72:2994–2998.

11. Moncada S, Gryglewski R, Bunting S, et al. An enzyme isolated from arteries transforms prostaglandin endoperoxides to an unstable substance that inhibits platelet aggregation. *Nature* 1976;263:663–667.

12. Vane JR. Inhibition of prostaglandin synthesis as a mechanism of action for aspirin-like drugs. *Nat New Biol* 1971;231:232–235.

13. Smith WL, Lands WEM. Stimulation and blockade of prostaglandin biosynthesis. *J Biol Chem* 1971;246:6700–6708.

14. Roth GJ, Majerus PW. The mechanism of the effect of aspirin on human platelets. I Acetylation of a particulate fraction protein. *J Clin Invest* 1975; 56:624–632.

15. Roth GJ, Stanford N, Majerus PW. Acetylation of prostaglandin synthase by aspirin. *Proc Natl Acad Sci U S A* 1975;72:3073–3077.

16. Roth GJ, Machuga ET, Ozols J. Isolation and covalent structure of the aspirin-modified, active-site region of prostaglandin synthetase. *Biochemistry* 1983;22:4672–4676.

17. Picot D, Loll PJ, Garavito M. The X-ray crystal structure of the membrane protein prostaglandin H2 synthase-1. *Nature* 1994;367:243–249.

18. Kujubu DA, Fletcher BS, Varnum BC, et al. TIS10, a phorbol ester tumor promoter-inducible mRNA from Swiss 3T3 cells, encodes a novel prostaglandin synthase / cyclo-oxygenase homologue. *J Biol Chem* 1992; 266:12866–12872.

19. FitzGerald GA, Patrono C. The coxibs, selective inhibitors of cyclo-oxygenase-2. *N Engl J Med* 2001;345:433–442.

20. Weiss HJ. The discovery of the antiplatelet effect of aspirin: a personal reminiscence. *J Thromb Haemost* 2003;1:1869–1875.

21. The Dutch TIA Trial Study Group. A comparison of two doses of aspirin (30 mg versus 283 mg a day) in patients after a transient ischemic attack or minor stroke. *N Engl J Med* 1991;325:1261–1266.

22. Patrignani P, Filabozzi P, Patrono C. Selective, cumulative inhibition of platelet thromboxane production by low-dose aspirin in healthy subjects. *J Clin Invest* 1982;69:1366–1372.

23. Jaffe EA, Weksler BB. Recovery of endothelial cell prostacyclin production after inhibition by low doses of aspirin. *J Clin Invest* 1979;63:532–539.

24. Roberts LJ II, Morrow JD. Analgesic-antipyretic and anti-inflammatory agents and drugs employed in the treatment of gout. In: Hardman JG, Limbird LE, Gilman AG, eds. *Goodman & Gilman's the pharmacological basis of therapeutics,* Chap. 27, 10th ed. New York: McGraw-Hill, 2001: 687–731.

25. Kaushansky K, Roth GJ. Megakaryocytes and platelets. In: Greer SP, Foerster J, Lukens JN, et al. eds. *Wintrobe's clinical hematology,* Chap. 19, 11th ed. Philadelphia, PA: Lippincott Williams & Wilkins, 2004:605–650.

26. Levy G. Clinical pharmacokinetics of salicylates: a reassessment. *Br J Pharmacol* 1980;10(Suppl. 1):285S–294S.

27. Pedersen AK, FitzGerald GA. Dose-related kinetics of aspirin. Presystemic acetylation of platelet cyclo-oxygenase. *N Engl J Med* 1984;311:1206–1212.

28. Harker LA, Finch CA. Thrombokinetics in man. *J Clin Invest* 1969;48: 963–974.

29. Jiminez AH, Stubbs GH, Tofler K, et al. Rapidity and duration of platelet suppression by enteric-coated aspirin in healthy young men. *Am J Cardiol* 1992;69:258–262.

30. Watkins PB. Mechanisms of drug-induced liver injury. In: Schiff ER, Sorrell MF, Maddrey WC, eds. *Schiff's diseases of the liver,* Chap. 39. Philadelphia, PA: Lippincott Williams & Wilkins, 2003:1129–1145.

31. Weiss HJ, Aledort LM, Kochwa S. The effect of salicylates on the hemostatic properties of platelets in man. *J Clin Invest* 1968;47:2169–2180.

32. Hamberg M, Svensson J, Wakabayshi T, et al. Isolation and structure of two prostaglandin endoperoxides that cause platelet aggregation. *Proc Natl Acad Sci U S A* 1974;71:345–349.

33. Evans G, Packham MA, Nishizawa ED, et al. The effect of acetylsalicylic acid on platelet function. *J Exp Med* 1968;128:877–894.

34. Metha J, Metha P, Burger C, et al. Platelet aggregation studies in coronary artery disease. *Atherosclerosis* 1978;31:169–175.

35. Buchanan MR, Brister SJ. Individual variation in the effects of ASA on platelet function: implications for the use of ASA clinically. *Can J Cardiol* 1995;11:221–227.

36. Helgason CM, Tortorice KL, Winkler SR, et al. Aspirin response and failure in cerebral infarction. *Stroke* 1993;24:345–350.

37. Helgason CM, Bolin LD, Hoff JA, et al. Development of aspirin resistance in persons with previous ischemic stroke. *Stroke* 1994;25:2331–2336.

38. Hillarp A, Lethagen S, Mattiasson I. Aspirin resistance is not a common biochemical phenotype explained by unblocked cyclo-oxygenase-1 activity. *J Thromb Haemost* 2003;1:196–197.

39. Eikelboom JW, Hirsh J, Weitz JI, et al. Aspirin-resistant thromboxane biosynthesis and the risk of myocardial infarction, stroke, or cardiovascular death in patients at high risk for cardiovascular events. *Circulation* 2002; 105:1650–1655.

40. Catella-Lawson F, Reilly MP, Kapoor SC, et al. Cyclooxygenase inhibitors and the antiplatelet effects of aspirin. *N Engl J Med* 2001;345:1809–1815.

41. McKee SA, Sane DC, Deliargyris EN. Aspirin resistance in cardiovascular disease: a review of prevalence, mechanisms, and clinical significance. *Thromb Haemost* 2002;88:711–715.

42. Patrono C. Aspirin resistance: definition, mechanisms and clinical readouts. *J Thromb Haemost* 2003;1:1710–1713.

43. Pulcinelli FM, Pignaelli P, Celestini A, et al. Inhibition of platelet aggregation by aspirin progressively decreases in long-term treated patients. *J Am Coll Cardiol* 2004;43:979–984.

44. Patrono C, Coller B, FitzGerald GA, et al. Platelet-active drugs: the relationships among dose, effectiveness and side effects. *Chest* 2004;126(Suppl. 3): 234S–264S.

45. Francis JL. Platelet function analyzer (PFA)-100. In: Michelson AD, ed. *Platelets.* San Diego, CA: Academic Press, 2002:325–335.

46. Mufson L, Black A, Roubin G, et al. A randomized trial of aspirin in PTCA. Effect of high vs. low dose aspirin on major complications and restenosis. *J Am Coll Cardiol* 1988;11:236–244.

47. Taylor DW, Barnett HJM, Haynes RB, et al. Low dose and high dose acetylsalicylic acid for patients undergoing carotid endarterectomy. *Lancet* 1999; 353:2179–2184.

48. Goldman S, Copeland J, Moritz T, et al. Saphenous vein graft patency 1 year after coronary artery bypass surgery and effects of antiplatelet therapy: results of a Veterans Administration cooperative study. *Circulation* 1989; 80: 1190–1197.

49. UK-TIA Study Group. The United Kingdom transient ischaemic attack (UK-TIA) aspirin trial: final results. *J Neurol Neurosurg Psychiatry* 1991; 54:1044–1054.

50. Ratnatunga CP, Edmondson SF, Rees GM, et al. High-dose aspirin inhibits shear-induced platelet reaction involving thrombin generation. *Circulation* 1992;85:1077–1082.

51. Bjornsson TD, Schneider DE, Berger H. Aspirin acetylates fibrinogen and enhances fibrinolysis: fibrinolytic effect is independent of changes in plasminogen activator levels. *J Pharmacol Exp Ther* 1988;250:154–160.

52. Szczeklik A, Krzanowski M, Gora P, et al. Antiplatelet drugs and generation of thrombin in clotting blood. *Blood* 1992;80:12006–12011.

53. FitzGerald GA, Oates JA, Hawiger J, et al. Endogenous biosynthesis of prostacyclin and thromboxane and platelet function during chronic administration of aspirin in man. *J Clin Invest* 1983;71:678–688.

54. Weksler BB, Pett SB, Alonso D, et al. Differential inhibition by aspirin of vascular and platelet prostaglandin synthesis in atherosclerotic patients. *N Engl J Med* 1983;308:800–805.

55. Clarke RJ, Mayo G, Price P, et al. Suppression of thromboxane A2 but not systemic prostacyclin by controlled-release aspirin. *N Engl J Med* 1991; 325:1137–1141.

56. Murata T, Ushikubi F, Matsuoka T, et al. Altered pain perception and inflammatory response in mice lacking prostacyclin receptor. *Nature* 1997; 388:678–682.

57. Antithrombotic Trialists Collaboration. Collaborative meta-analysis of randomized trials of antiplatelet therapy for prevention of death, myocardial infarction, and stroke in high-risk patients. *Br Med J* 2002;324:71–86.

58. Elwood RC, Cochrane AL, Burr ML, et al. A randomized controlled trial of acetylsalicylic acid in the secondary prevention of mortality from myocardial infarction. *Br Med J* 1974;1:436–447.

59. Coronary Drug Project (CDP) Research Group. Aspirin in coronary heart disease. *J Chronic Dis* 1976;29:625–633.

60. Bredin K, Loew D, Lechner K, et al. Secondary prevention of myocardial infarction: a comparison of acetylsalicylic acid, placebo and phenprocoumon. *Haemostasis* 1980;9:325–334.

61. Elwood PC, Sweetnam PM. Aspirin and secondary mortality after myocardial infarction. *Lancet* 1979;2:1313–1319.

62. Aspirin Myocardial Infarction Study (AMIS) Research Group. A randomized, controlled trial of aspirin in persons recovered from myocardial infarction. *J Am Med Assoc* 1980;243:661–669.

63. The Persantine-Aspirin Reinfarctrion Study Group. Persantine and aspirin in coronary heart disease. *Circulation* 1980;62:449–455.

64. Patrono C. Aspirin as an antiplatelet drug. *N Engl J Med* 1994;330:1287–1294.

65. The SALT Collaborative Group. Swedish aspirin low-dose trial (SALT) of 75 mg aspirin as secondary prophylaxis after cerebrovascular ischaemic events. *Lancet* 1991;338:1345–1354.

66. Fields WE, Lemak NA, Frankowshi RF, et al. Controlled trial of aspirin in cerebral ischemia. *Stroke* 1977;8:301–309.

67. Dyken ML, Barnett HJM, Easton JD, et al. Low-dose aspirin and stroke. "It ain't necessarily so." *Stroke* 1992;23:1395–1399.

68. Patrono C, Roth GJ. Aspirin in ischemic cerebrovascular disease. How strong is the case for a different dosing regimen? *Stroke* 1996;27:756–760.

69. The RISC Group. Risk of myocardial infarction and death during treatment with low dose aspirin and intravenous heparin in men with unstable coronary artery disease. *Lancet* 1990;336:827–830.

70. ISIS-2 (Second International Study of Infarct Survival) Collaborative Group. Randomized trial of intravenous streptokinase, oral aspirin, both, or neither among 17,187 cases of suspected acute myocardial infarction. *Lancet* 1988;2:349–360.

71. Oler A, Whooley MA, Oler J, et al. Adding heparin to aspirin reduces the incidence of myocardial infarction and death in patients with unstable angina: a meta-analysis. *J Am Med Assoc* 1996;272:811–815.

72. International Stroke Trial Collaborative Group. The International Stroke Trial (IST): a randomized trial of aspirin, subcutaneous heparin, both, or neither among 19,435 patients with acute ischemic stroke. *Lancet* 1997;349:1569–1581.

73. CAST (Chinese Acute Stroke Trial) Collaborative Group. CAST: randomized placebo-controlled trial of early aspirin use in 20,000 patients with acute ischemic stroke. *Lancet* 1997;349:1641–1649.

74. Steering Committee of the Physicians' Health Study Research Group. Final report on the aspirin component of the ongoing Physicians' Health Study. *N Engl J Med* 1989;321:129–135.

75. Ridker PM, Cook NR, Lee I, et al. A randomized trial of low-dose aspirin in the primary prevention of cardiovascular disease in women. *N Engl J Med* 2005;352:1293–1304.

76. Peto R, Gray R, Collins R, et al. Randomized trial of prophylactic daily aspirin in British male doctors. *Br Med J* 1988;296:313–316.

77. Hennekens CH, Buring JE, Sandercock P, et al. Aspirin and other antiplatelet agents in the secondary and primary prevention of cardiovascular disease. *Circulation* 1989;80:749–756.

78. Hansson L, Zanchetti A, Carruthers SG, et al. Effects of intensive blood-pressure lowering and low-dose aspirin in patients with hypertension: principal results of the Hypertension Optimal Treatment (HOT) randomized trial. *Lancet* 1998;352:1755–1762.

79. The Medical Research Council's General Practice Research Framework. Thrombosis prevention trial: randomized trial of low-intensity oral anticoagulation with warfarin and low-dose aspirin in the primary prevention of ischemic heart disease in men at increased risk. *Lancet* 1998;351:233–241.

80. Collaborative Group of the Primary Prevention Project (PPP). Low-dose aspirin and vitamin E in people at cardiovascular risk: a randomized trial in general practice. *Lancet* 2001;357:89–95.

81. US Preventive Services Task Force. Aspirin for the primary prevention of cardio-vascular events: recommendation and rationale. *Ann Intern Med* 2002;136:157–160.

82. Lauer MS. Aspirin for primary prevention of coronary events. *N Engl J Med* 2002;346:1468–1474.

83. Juul-Moller S, Edvardsson N, Jahnmatz B, et al. Double-blind trial of aspirin in primary prevention of myocardial infarction in patients with stable chronic angina pectoris. *Lancet* 1992;340:1421–1425.

84. Stroke Prevention in Atrial Fibrillation Investigators. Adjusted-dose warfarin versus low-intensity, fixed dose warfarin plus aspirin for high-risk patients with atrial fibrillation: Stroke prevention in atrial fibrillation III randomized clinical trial. *Lancet* 1996;348:633–638.

85. Stroke Prevention in Atrial Fibrillation Investigators. Patients with nonvalvular atrial fibrillation at low risk of stroke during treatment with aspirin: Stroke prevention in atrial fibrillation III study. *J Am Med Assoc* 1998;279:1273–1277.

86. Stroke Prevention in Atrial Fibrillation Study. Final results. *Circulation* 1991;84:727–739.

87. Antiplatelet Trialists' Collaboration. Collaborative overview of randomized trials of antiplatelet therapy: III Reduction in venous thrombosis and pulmonary embolism by antiplatelet prophylaxis among surgical and medial patients. *Br Med J* 1994;308:235–243.

88. Sors H, Meyer G. Place of aspirin in prophylaxis of venous thromboembolism. *Lancet* 2000;355:1288–1289.

89. Pulmonary Embolism Prevention (PEP) Trial Collaborative Group. Prevention of pulmonary embolism and deep vein thrombosis with low dose aspirin. Pulmonary Embolism Prevention (PEP) trial. *Lancet* 2000;355:1295–1302.

90. Caritis S, Sibai B, Hauth J, et al. Low-dose aspirin to prevent pre-eclampsia in women at high risk. *N Engl J Med* 1998;338:701–705.

91. Duley L, Henderson-Smart D, Knight M, et al. Antiplatelet drugs for prevention of pre-eclampsia and its consequences: systematic review. *Br Med J* 2001;322:329–333.

92. Arun B, Kessler CM. Clinical manifestations and therapy of the hemophilias. In: Colman RW, Hirsh J, Marder VJ et al., eds. *Hemostasis and thrombosis. Basic principles and clinical practice.* 4th ed. Philadelphia, PA: Lippincott Williams & Wilkins, 2001:815–824.

93. Iso H, Hennekens CH, Stampfer MJ, et al. Prospective study of aspirin use and risk of stroke in women. *Stroke* 1999;30:1764–1771.

94. Graham DY. The relationship between nonsteroidal anti-inflammatory drug use and peptic ulcer disease. *Gastroenterol Clin North Am* 1990;19:171–199.

95. Weil J, Colin-Jones D, Langman M, et al. Prophylactic aspirin and risk of peptic ulcer bleeding. l. *Br Med J* 1995;310:827–830.

96. Garcia Rodriguez LA, Hernandez-Diaz S, de Abajo FJ. Association between aspirin and upper gastrointestinal complications: systematic review of epidemio-logic studies. *Br J Clin Pharmacol* 2001;52:563–571.

97. Wolfe MM, Lichtenstein DR, Singh G. Gastrointestinal toxicity of nonsteroidal anti-inflammatory drugs. *N Engl J Med* 1999;340:1888–1899.

98. De Abajo FJ, Garcia Rodriguez LA. Risk of upper gastrointestinal bleeding and perforation associated with low-dose aspirin as plain and enteric-coated pre-parations. *BMC Clin Pharmacol* 2001;1:1.

99. Hawkey CJ, Karrasch JA, Szczepanski L, et al. Omeprazole compared with misoprostol for ulcers associated with nonsteroidal anti-inflammatory drugs. *N Engl J Med* 1998;338:727–734.

100. Chan FKL, Chung SCS, Suen BY, et al. Preventing recurrent upper gastro-intestinal bleeding in patients with *Helicobacter pylori* infection who are taking low-dose aspirin or naproxen. *N Engl J Med* 2001;344:967–973.

101. Mene P, Pugliese F, Patrono C. The effects of nonsteroidal anti-inflammatory drugs on human hypertensive vascular disease. *Semin Nephrol* 1995;15:244–252.

102. Reilly IAG, FitzGerald GA. Inhibition of thromboxane formation *in vivo* and *ex vivo*: implications for therapy with platelet inhibitory drugs. *Blood* 1987;69:180–186.

103. Garcia-Rodriguez LA, Varas C, Patrono C. Differential effects of aspirin and non-aspirin nonsteroidal anti-inflammatory drugs in primary prevention of myocardial infarction in postmenopausal women. *Epidemiology* 2000;11:382–387.

104. Fornaro G, Rossi P, Mantica P, et al. Indobufen in the prevention of thrombo-embolic complications in patients with heart disease. *Circulation* 1993;87:162–164.

105. Morocutti C, Amabile G, Fattapposta F, et al. Indobufen versus warfarin in the secondary prevention of major vascular events in nonrheumatic atrial fibrillation. *Stroke* 1997;28:1015–1021.

106. Cruz-Fernandez JM, Lopez-Bescos L, Garcia-Dorado D, et al. Randomized comparative trial of triflusal and aspirin following acute myocardial infarction. *Eur Heart J* 2000;21:457–465.

107. Brochier ML. Evaluation of flurbiprofen for prevention of reinfarction and reocclusion after successful thrombolysis or angioplasty in acute myocardial infarction. The Flurbiprofen French Trial. *Eur Heart J* 1993;14:951–957.

108. Report from the Anturane Reinfarction Italian Study. Sulfinpyrazone in post myocardial infarction. *Lancet* 1982;1:237–283.

109. FitzGerald GA. COX-2 and beyond: approaches to prostaglandin inhibition in human disease. *Nat Rev Drug Discov* 2003;2:879–890.

110. Bombardier C, Laine L, Reicin A, et al. Comparison of upper gastrointestinal toxicity of rofecoxib and naproxen in patients with rheumatoid arthritis. *N Engl J Med* 2000;343:1520–1528.

111. Farkouh ME, Kirshner H, Harrington RA, et al. Comparison of lumiracoxib with naproxen and ibuprofen in the Therapeutic Arthritis Research and Gastrointestinal Event Trial (TARGET), cardiovascular outcomes: randomized controlled trial. *Lancet* 2004;364:675–684.

112. Topol EJ. Failing the public health – Rofecoxib, Merck, and the FDA. *N Engl J Med* 2004;351:1707–1708.

113. FitzGerald GA. Coxibs and cardiovascular disease. *N Engl J Med* 2004;351:1709–1711.

114. Quinn MJ, FitzGerald GA. Ticlopidine and clopidogrel. *Circulation* 1999;100:1667–1672.

115. CAPRIE Steering Committee. A randomized, blinded, trial of clopidogrel versus aspirin in patients at risk of ischemic events. (CAPRIE). *Lancet* 1996;348:1329–1339.

116. Bennet CL, Davidson CJ, Raisch DW, et al. Thrombotic thrombocytopenic purpura associated with ticlopidine in the setting of coronary artery stents and stroke prevention. *Arch Intern Med* 1999;159:2524–2528.

117. Schror K. The basic pharmacology of ticlopidine and clopidogrel. *Platelets* 1993;4:252–264.

118. Hollopeter G, Jantzen HM, Vincent D, et al. Identification of the platelet ADP receptor targeted by antithrombotic drugs. *Nature* 2001;409:202–207.

119. Hass WK, Easton JD, Adams HP, et al. A randomized trial comparing ticlopidine hydrochloride with aspirin for the prevention of stroke in high-risk patients. *N Engl J Med* 1989;321:501–507.

120. Balsano F, Rizzon P, Violi F, et al. Antiplatelet treatment with ticlopidine in unstable angina: a controlled multi-center trial. *Circulation* 1990;82:17–26.

121. Arcan JC, Blanchard J, Boissel JP, et al. Multicenter double blind study of ticlopidine in the treatment of intermittent claudication and the prevention of its complicatioins. *Angiology* 1988;38:802–811.

122. Yeh SP, Hsueh EJ, Wu H, et al. Ticlopidine associated aplastic anemia: a case report and review of the literature. *Ann Hematol* 1998;76:87–90.

123. Herbert JM, Frehel D, Vallee E, et al. Clopidogrel, a novel antiplatelet and antithrombotic drug. *Cardiovasc Drug Rev.* 1993;11:180–198.

124. Hankey GJ. Ongoing and planned trials of antiplatelet therapy in the acute and long-term management of patients with ischaemic brain syndromes: setting a new standard of care. *Cerebrovasc Dis* 2004;17(Suppl .3):11–16.

125. Lange RA, Hillis LD. Antiplatelet therapy for ischemic heart disease. *N Engl J Med* 2004;350:232–238.

126. The Clopidogrel in Unstable Angina to Prevent Recurrent Events Trial Investigators. Effects of clopidgrel in addition to aspirin in patients with acute coronary syndromes without ST-segment elevation. *N Engl J Med* 2001; 345:494–502.

127. Steinhubl SR, Berger PB, Tift Mann J III, et al. Early and sustained dual oral antiplatelet therapy following percutaneous coronary intervention. A randomized controlled trial. *J Am Med Assoc* 2002;288:2411–2420.

128. Payne DA, Jones CI, Hayes PD, et al. Beneficial effects of clopidogrel combined with aspirin in reducing cerebral emboli in patients undergoing carotid endarterectomy. *Circulation* 2004;113:1476–1481.

129. Eisert WG. Dipyridamole. In: Michelson A, ed. Platelets. London: Academic Press; 2002:803-815.

130. Fitzgerald GA. Dipyridamole. *N Engl J Med* 1987;316:1247–1257.

131. Diener HC, Cunha L, Forbes C, et al. European Stroke Prevention Study 2. Dipyridamole and acetylsalicylic acid in the secondary prevention of stroke. *J Neurol Sci* 1996;143:1–13.

132. Albers GW. Choice of endpoints in antiplatelet trials. *Neurology* 2000;54: 1022–1028.

133. Coller BS. GP IIb/IIIa antagonists: pathophysiologic and therapeutic insights from studies of c7E3 Fab. *Thromb Haemost* 1997;78:730–735.

134. Simpfendorfer C, Kottke-Marchant K, Lowrie M, et al. First chronic platelet glycoprotein IIb/IIIa integrin blockade: a randomized, placebo-controlled study of xemilofiban in unstable angina with percutaneous coronary interventions. *Circulation* 1997;96:76–81.

135. Chew DP, Bhatt DL, Sapp S, et al. Increased mortality with oral platelet glycoprotein IIb/IIIa antagonists: A meta-analysis of phase III multicenter randomized trials. *Circulation* 2001;103:201–206.

136. Leebeck FWG, Boersma E, Cannon CP, et al. Oral glycoprotein IIb-IIIa receptor inhibitors in patients with cardiovascular disease: why were the results so unfavorable? *Eur Heart J* 2002;23:444–457.

137. Cox D, Smith R, Quinn M, et al. Evidence of platelet activation during treatment with a GP IIb/IIIa antagonist in patients presenting with acute coronary syndromes. *J Am Coll Cardiol* 2000;36:1514–1519.

138. O'Neill WW, Serruys P, Knudtson M, et al. Long-term treatment with a platelet glycoprotein-receptor antagonist after percutaneous coronary revascularization. *N Engl J Med* 2000;342:1316–1324.

139. Cannon CP, McCabe CH, Wilcox RG, et al. Oral glycoprotein IIb/IIIa inhibition with orbofiban in patients with unstable coronary syndromes (OPUS-TIMI 16) trial. *Circulation* 2000;102:149–156.

140. Second SYMPHONY Investigators. Randomized trial of aspirin, sibrafiban, or both for secondary prevention after acute coronary syndromes. *Circulation* 2001;103:1727–1733.

141. Osende JI, Shimbo D, Fuster V, et al. Antithrombotic effects of S 18886, a novel orally active thromboxane A2 receptor antagonist. *J Thromb Haemost* 2004;2:492–498.

142. Joseph JE, Machin SJ. New anti-platelet drugs. *Blood Rev* 1997;11:178–188.

143. Storey RK, Oldroyd K, Wilcox R. Open multicentre study of the P2T receptor antagonist AR-C69931MX assessing safety, tolerability and activity in patients with acute coronary syndromes. *Thromb Haemost* 2001;85: 401–407.

144. Grant SM, Goa K. Iloprost. A review of its pharmacodynamic and pharmacokinetic properties, and therapeutic potential in peripheral vascular disease, myocardial ischaemia and extra-corporeal circulation procedures. *Drugs* 1992;43:889–903.

145. Coller BS. Platelet GP IIb/IIIa antagonists; the first anti-integrin receptor therapeutics. *J Clin Invest* 1997;99:1467–1471.

146. The EPIC Investigators. Use of a monoclonal antibody directed against the platelet glycoprotein IIb/IIIa receptor in high-risk coronary angioplasty. *N Engl J Med* 1994;330:956–961.

147. Coller BS, Peerschke EL, Scudder LE, et al. A murine monoclonal antibody that completely blocks the binding of fibrinogen to platelets produces a thromb-asthenic-like state in normal platelets and binds to glycoproteins IIb and/or IIIa. *J Clin Invest* 1983;72:325–338.

148. Mascelli MA, Lance ET, Damaraju L, et al. Pharmacodynamic profile of a short-term abciximab treatment demonstrates prolonged platelet inhibition with gradual recovery from GP IIb/IIIa receptor blockade. *Circulation* 1998;97:1680–1688.

149. Reverter JC, Beguin S, Kessels H, et al. Inhibition of platelet-mediated, tissue factor-induced thrombin generation by the mouse/human chimeric 7E3 anti-body: potential implications for the effect c7E3 Fab treatment on acute thrombosis and 'clinical restenosis'. *J Clin Invest* 1996;98: 863–874.

150. Abrams CS, Cines DB. Thrombocytopenia after treatment with platelet glycoprotein IIb/IIIa inhibitors. *Curr Hematol Rep* 2004;3:143–147.

151. The EPILOG Investigators. Platelet glycoprotein IIb/IIIa receptor blockade and low-dose heparin during percutaneous coronary revascularization. *N Engl J Med* 1997;336:1689–1696.

152. Scarborough RM, Naughton MA, Teng W, et al. Design of potent and specific integrin antagonists: Peptide antagonists with high specificity for glycoprotein IIb-IIIa. *J Biol Chem* 1993;268:1066–1073.

153. Phillips DR, Teng W, Arfsten A, et al. Effect of Ca2+ on GpIIb/IIIa interactions with integrilin enhanced GP IIb/IIIa binding and inhibition of platelet aggregation by reductions in the concentration of ionized calcium in plasma anti-coagulated with citrate. *Circulation* 1997;96:1488–1494.

154. Tcheng JE, Harrington RA, Kottke-Marchant K, et al. Multicenter, randomized, double-blind, placebo-controlled trial of the platelet integrin glycoprotein IIb/IIIa blocker integrelin in elective coronary intervention. *Circulation* 1995;91:2151–2157.

155. O'Shea JC, Madan M, Cantor WJ, et al. Design and methodology of the ESPRIT trial. Evaluating a novel dosing regimen of eptifibatide in percutaneous coronary intervention. *Am Heart J* 2000;140:834–839.

156. The ESPRIT Investigators. Novel dosing regimen of eptifibatide in planned coronary stent implantation (ESPRIT): a randomized, placebo-controlled trial. *Lancet* 2000;356:2037–2044.

157. Madan M, Berkowitz SD. Understanding thrombocytopenia and antigenicity with glycoprotein IIb-IIIa inhibitors. *Am Heart J* 1999;138:317–326.

158. Hartman GD, Egbertson MS, Halczenko W, et al. Non-peptide fibrinogen receptor antagonists: and design of exosite inhibitors. *J Med Chem* 1992; 35:4640–4642.

159. Egbertson MS, Chang CT, Duggan ME, et al. Non-peptide fibrinogen receptor antagonists: II. Optimization of a tyrosine template as a mimic for Arg-Gly-Asp. *J Med Chem* 1994;37:2537–2551.

160. Barrett JS, Murphy G, Peerlinck K, et al. Pharmacokinetics and pharmacodynamics of MK-383, a selective non-peptide platelet glycoprotein – IIb/IIIa receptor antagonist, in healthy men. *Clin Pharmacol Ther* 1994;56:377–388.

161. Peerlinck K, DeLepeleire I, Goldberg M, et al. MK-383 (L-700,462). A selective nonpeptide platelet glycoprotein IIb/IIIa antagonist, is active in man. *Circulation* 1993;88:1512–1517.

162. Harker LA. Platelets and vascular thrombosis. *N Engl J Med* 1994;330: 1006–1007.

163. The EPISTENT Investigators. Randomized placebo-controlled and balloon-angioplasty-controlled trial to assess safety of coronary stenting with use of platelet glycoprotein IIb-IIIa blockade. *Lancet* 1998;352: 87–92.

164. Ross R. The pathogenesis of atherosclerosis: a perspective for the 1990s. *Nature* 1993;362:801–809.

165. The IMPACT II Investigators. Randomized placebo-controlled trial of effect of eptifibatide on complications of percutaneous coronary intervention: IMPACT-II. *Lancet* 1997;349:1422–1428.

166. The RESTORE Investigators. Effects of platelet glycoprotein IIb/IIIa blockade with tirofiban on adverse cardiac events in patients with unstable angina or acute myocardial infarction undergoing coronary angioplasty. *Circulation* 1997;96:1445–1453.

167. The PARAGON Investigators. International, randomized, controlled trial of lamifiban (a platelet glycoprotein IIb/IIIa inhibitor), heparin, or both in unstable angina. *Circulation* 1998;97:2386–2395.

168. Topol EJ, Moliterno DJ, Herrmann ER, et al. Comparison of two platelet glycoprotein IIb/IIIa inhibitors, tirofian and abciximab, for the prevention of ischemic events with percutaneous coronary revascularization. *N Engl J Med* 2001;344:1888–1894.

169. Boersma E, Harrington RA, Moliterno DJ, et al. Platelet glycoprotein IIb/IIIa inhibitors in acute coronary syndromes: a meta analysis of all major randomized clinical trials. *Lancet* 2002;359:189–198.

170. The CAPTURE Investigators. Randomized placebo-controlled trial of abciximab before and during intervention in refractory unstable angina: the CAPTURE study. *Lancet* 1997;349:1429–1435.

171. The GUSTO IV-ACS Investigators. Effect of glycoprotein IIb/IIIa receptor blocker abciximab on outcome in patients with acute coronary syndromes without early coronary revascularization: the GUSTO IV-ACS randomized trial. *Lancet* 2001;357:1915–1924.

172. The PRISM Study Investigators. A comparison of aspirin plus tirofiban with aspirin plus heparin for unstable angina. *N Engl J Med* 1998;338: 1498–1505.

173. The PRISM-PLUS Study Investigators. Inhibition of the platelet glycoprotein IIb/IIIa receptor with tirofiban in unstable angina and non-Q-wave myocardial infarction. Platelet receptor inhibition in ischemic syndrome management in patients limited by unstable signs and symptoms. *N Engl J Med* 1998;338:1488–1497.

174. The PURSUIT Investigators. Inhibition of the platelet glycoprotein IIb/IIIa with eptifibatide in patients with acute coronary syndromes without persistent ST-segment elevation. *N Engl J Med* 1998;339:436–443.

175. Kastrati A, Mehilli J, Schuhlen H, et al. A clinical trial of abciximab in elective percutaneous coronary intervention after pretreatment with clopidogrel. *N Engl J Med* 2004;350:232–238.

176. Ferguson JJ, Antman EM, Bates ER, et al. Combining enoxaparin and glycoprotein IIb/IIIa antagonists for the treatment of acute coronary syndromes: final results of the National Investigators Collaborating on Enoxaparin –3 (NICE-3) study. *Am Heart J* 2003;146:628–634.

177. Antman EM, Giugliano RP, Gibson CM, et al. Abciximab facilitates the rate and extent of thrombolysis – results of the thrombolysis in myocardial infarction (TIMI) 14 trial. *Circulation* 1999;99:2720–2732.

178. The GUSTO V Investigators. Reperfusion therapy for acute myocardial infarction with fibrinolytic therapy or combination reduced fibrinolytic

therapy and platelet glycoprotein IIb/IIIa inhibition: the GUSTO V randomized trial. *Lancet* 2001;357:1905–1914.

179. Giugliano RP, Roe MT, Harrington RA, et al. Combination reperfusion therapy with eptifibatide and reduced dose tenecteplase for ST-elevation myocardial infarction: results of the integrilin and tenecteplase in acute myocardial infarction (INTEGRITI) Phase II Angiographic Trial. *J Am Coll Cardiol* 2003;41:1251–1260.

180. Ischemic Stroke Investigators. Abciximab in acute ischemic stroke: a randomized, double-blind, placebo-controlled, dose-escalation study. The Abciximab in Ischemic Stroke Investigators. *Stroke* 2000;31:601–609.

181. Burkart DJ, Borsa JJ, Anthony JP, et al. Thrombolysis of acute peripheral arterial and venous disease: a pilot study. *J Vasc Interv Radiol* 2003;14:729–733.

182. Wholey MH, Eles G, Toursakissian B, et al. Evaluation of glycoprotein IIb/IIIa inhibitors in carotid angioplasty and stenting. *J Endovasc Ther* 2003;10:33–41.

# CHAPTER 121 ■ FOUNDATIONS OF THROMBOLYTIC THERAPY

VICTOR J. MARDER

Thrombolytic therapy represents a conjoint approach to vascular reperfusion, based primarily on the use of fibrinolytic agents delivered systemically or directly into the offending thrombus and complemented by anticoagulation, antiplatelet, and even mechanical strategies. Theoretically, any major thrombosed vessel that is the cause of a clinically significant disease is amenable to this therapeutic approach, and the decision to utilize thrombolytic therapy requires an informed choice between the potential for clinical benefit and the risk for serious complication. In actuality, thrombolytic therapy represents an acute phase of a prolonged antithrombotic management plan, and the decision about the benefit:risk ratio relates to this usually brief but more aggressive approach to vascular occlusion (1–14). This review describes the properties of thrombolytic agents (see Chapter 18), the physiopathology of thrombolysis and bleeding complications, and the effects of treatment on blood coagulation and fibrinolytic parameters (see Chapter 69).

## FIBRINOLYTIC AGENTS

### Mode of Action

All of the currently used thrombolytic agents are plasminogen activators (PA), which induce plasmin action on fibrin contained within a thrombus, and an associated greater or lesser degree of plasma fibrinogenolysis (lytic state). Degradation of fibrin produces the beneficial effect of reducing thrombus size (thrombolysis), but at the same time, the activators may lyse hemostatic plugs (4) or induce matrix degradation at sites of vascular injury or abnormality (see Table 121-1). Rethrombosis of the vessel may follow initial reperfusion, generally as a result of a persistent local vascular lesion and a predisposing state of plasma hypercoagulability. The relation of these biologic actions of thrombolysis, loss of vascular integrity, rethrombosis, and the plasma lytic state control the effectiveness and safety of thrombolytic treatment. Figure 121-1 illustrates the molecular interactions by which such treatment is locally augmented at sites of thrombi (3,4,15,16). Plasminogen and PA bind to or react in contiguity with fibrin in the thrombus. Fibrin facilitates the conversion of plasminogen to plasmin, because plasminogen activator inhibitor-1 (PAI-1) and $\alpha_2$-plasmin inhibitor are not efficient for inhibiting thrombus-bound plasminogen activator and plasmin. Plasmin in turn degrades fibrin to fibrin degradation products (FDPs). Under physiologic conditions, systemic fibrinogenolysis does not occur, because tissue-type plasminogen activator (tPA) and plasmin are efficiently inhibited by PAI-1 and $\alpha_2$-plasmin inhibitor in the blood, respectively. However, upon administration of therapeutic dosages of PA, susceptible plasma substrates such as fibrinogen are degraded to some degree; at the same time, PA converts thrombus-bound plasminogen to plasmin, resulting in accelerated thrombolysis.

## Available Plasminogen Activators and New Thrombolytic Approaches

Six PAs have been previously approved by the US Food and Drug Administration (FDA) for use in major thrombotic diseases: streptokinase (SK) (17), urokinase (UK) (18,19), alteplase (tPA) (20,21), anistreplase [anisoylated plasminogen streptokinase (APSAC)] (22), reteplase (23), and tenecteplase (TNK-tPA) (24), although UK is no longer available in the United States, and anistreplase is rarely utilized. New PA variants have been synthesized by recombinant DNA technology in attempts to attain improved properties such as greater activity, prolonged half-life, or a lessened lytic state (see Chapter 122). For example, reteplase, which consists of the second kringle and the protease domain of alteplase, has a prolonged half-life (from 5 minutes to 15 minutes) that allows for administration in a double bolus regimen (25), and tenecteplase (24), altered at three specific tPA amino acid sites, is effective as a single bolus injection (26). Recombinant forms of UK (27), saruplase (pro-UK, scu-PA) (28), staphylokinase (29), and BAT-PA (30) (from the salivary gland of *Desmodus rotundus*), and fascinating chimerics of tPA and pro-UK (31), and bifunctional agents composed of antifibrin or antiplatelet antibodies complexed to PA (32) show encouraging results at various stages of testing.

The major distinctions between PAs relate to their origin (antigenicity), half-life, potential for inducing a lytic state, and hemorrhagic potential (see Table 121-2). Those PAs that are derived from a human protein (UK, alteplase, reteplase, saruplase, tenecteplase, lanoteplase) are minimally or nonantigenic, whereas those from a bacterial species, whether purified from the *Streptococcus* as SK, complexed with human plasminogen as anistreplase, or prepared by recombinant technology from *Staphylococci* as staphylokinase (33), can induce antibody formation and present a potential for allergic response that could preclude prolonged or follow-up administration. Modified recombinant forms of staphylokinase with lessened antigenicity and retained thrombolytic potency have been developed and tested in patients (34), and similar species of SK are also feasible (35).

The half-life of each PA determines whether it can be administered as a bolus injection, short infusion, or continuous infusion. The most suitable agents for bolus injections are anistreplase (half-life, approximately 40 minutes) (36), reteplase (37), tenecteplase (38), and lanoteplase (39), and the least suitable is alteplase (half-life, 5 minutes) (40), which best utilizes a continuous infusion for therapy. Clinical results suggest that some of the newer agents will have less of a plasma lytic state, for example, tenecteplase (41), but to date, all PAs are associated with a significant bleeding risk. The rate of bleeding is roughly equivalent for all agents, except for the higher rate of intracranial hemorrhage (ICH) with tPA (42) or tPA mutant derivatives (37,43), relative to results using SK.

**TABLE 121-1**

PRINCIPAL BIOLOGIC EFFECTS OF THROMBOLYSIS THERAPY

| Clinical result | Process | Cellular and biochemical events |
|---|---|---|
| Benefit | Thrombolysis | Degradation of fibrin and disruption of platelets in the thrombus |
| Side effect | Systemic lytic state | Plasma fibrinogenolysis and derangement of platelet function |
| Complications | Bleeding | Degradation of fibrin in hemostatic plugs and of matrix in abnormal vessels, plus blood hypocoagulability |
| | Rethrombosis | Persistent local vascular lesions plus permissive status of blood coagulation |

The anticipation of greater safety with a new PA, based on biochemical studies must be considered cautiously, because no agent has yet been shown to be free of hemorrhagic risk.

Recently, a recombinant plasminogen that is activated by thrombin, rather than by a PA, has been developed as an agent that would work only at sites of fresh thrombus formation (44). Theoretically, such a mode of action would spare stabilized, quiescent hemostatic plugs, and therefore avoid hemorrhagic complications, but this approach still needs to be tested critically in patients.

An old approach has recently been reactivated as a safe method of inducing therapeutic thrombolysis, namely, by use of the direct thrombolytic enzyme plasmin (45). The potential for safety is based upon regional administration of agent by catheter. After successful thrombolysis, the agent would be quickly neutralized by plasma inhibitors, thereby preventing its circulation to sites of vascular injury, and avoiding bleeding that could result from hemostatic plug degradation (46,47). Animal studies are supportive of this hypothesis, showing that more than sixfold the therapeutic dose of plasmin does not induce bleeding, whereas tPA causes bleeding at the therapeutic dose, but also even at dosages as low as 25% of the optimal therapeutic amount (48). A recombinant derivative of plasmin ("miniplasmin") has been synthesized and tested in animal

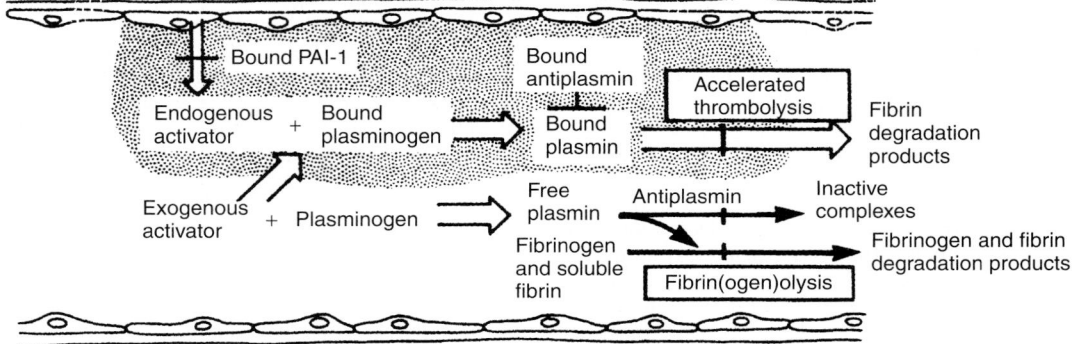

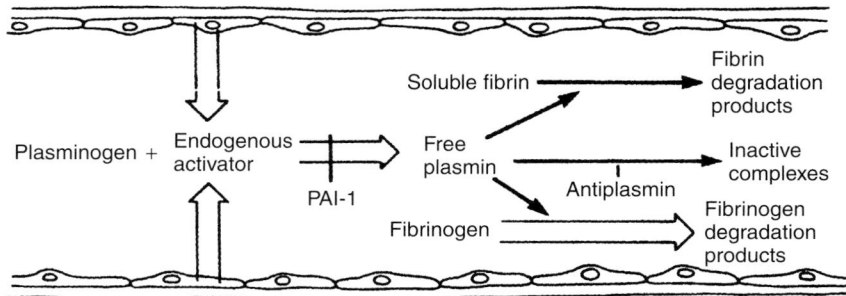

**FIGURE 121-1.** Molecular interactions of physiologic and therapeutic thrombolysis. In the **top panel**, therapeutic administration of plasminogen activator accelerates thrombolysis. Free plasmin in the blood exceeds the capacity of antiplasmin to neutralize the protease activity, resulting in fibrinogen degradation and the so-called plasma proteolytic state. In the **bottom panel**, tissue-type plasminogen activator (tPA) is released from endothelial cells in response to a variety of stimuli, mimicking therapeutic administration of plasminogen activator. Free plasmin degrades fibrinogen and soluble fibrin, producing both fibrinogen and fibrin degradation products. PAI-1, plasminogen activator inhibitor 1.

## TABLE 121-2

**COMPARISON OF PLASMINOGEN ACTIVATORS**

| Agent | Source | Antigenic | Half-life (min) | Regimen | Lytic state | Bleeding |
|-------|--------|-----------|-----------------|---------|-------------|----------|
| Streptokinase | *Streptococcus* | Yes | 20 | Infusion | 4+ | 4+ |
| Urokinase | Cell culture | No | 15 | Infusion | 4+ | 4+ |
| Alteplase | Recombinant | No | 5 | Infusion | 2+ | 4+ |
| Anistreplase | *Streptococcus* + plasma product | No | 70 | Bolus | 4+ | 4+ |
| Reteplase | Recombinant | No | 15 | Double bolus | 3+ | 4+ |
| Saruplase (scuPA) | Recombinant | No | 5 | Infusion | 1−3+ | 4+ |
| Staphylokinase | Recombinant | Yes | 6 | Infusion | 1+ | 4+ |
| Tenecteplase | Recombinant | No | 15 | Bolus | 1+ | 4+ |
| BAT-PA | Recombinant | Minimal | 17 | Infusion | 1+ | Probable |
| Lanoteplase | Recombinant | No | 30 | Bolus | 2+ | 4+ |

scuPA, single-chain urokinase-type plasminogen activator.

models of ischemic stroke (49). The safety profile in animals suggests that clinical usage of plasmin will be possible with a much reduced risk of bleeding.

## Adjunctive Antithrombotic Agents

Inadequate response to PA therapy occurs if a thrombosed vessel does not manifest full reperfusion or if reocclusion quickly follows initial success. Generally, tPA and recombinant derivatives have potent thrombolytic activity and achieve early vascular patency with relatively mild effect on blood coagulation, but are vulnerable to early reocclusion. Agents such as SK elicit a greater effect on plasma coagulation factors and reperfuse vessels more gradually but tend to maintain vascular patency. Acknowledging that early and persistent patency is a principal objective of treatment, considerable effort has been directed to adjunctive management with antithrombins and antiplatelet agents.

The first definitive demonstration of antiplatelet efficacy in the treatment of an acute thrombotic event was with the use of a simple aspirin regimen of 160 mg per day for 30 days, to decrease mortality after acute myocardial infarction (AMI) (Second International Study of Infarct Survival, ISIS-2) (50). In patients treated within 6 hours, aspirin reduced the 35-day mortality by 23%, equal to the reduction achieved by SK alone, and both agents together had an additive effect amounting to a 39% relative risk reduction compared to patients who received neither thrombolytic nor aspirin. The Global Use of Strategies to Open Occluded Coronary Arteries (GUSTO) study (51) documented that early intravenous heparin is no more effective than delayed subcutaneous heparin in patient survival at 30 days after AMI. Coronary artery patency studies show that intravenous heparin in addition to SK or APSAC (plus adequate aspirin), does not increase the incidence of vascular patency (52,53) but does increase bleeding complications (53). Although the use of delayed subcutaneous heparin in addition to aspirin is relatively safe, Collins et al. (10) conclude that "there is little evidence of any additional clinical advantage with subcutaneous or with intravenous heparin" added to PA therapy. When the dosage of aspirin is 160 mg per day or more, heparin produces either no increase in patency (54,55) or a marginal improvement (56). With 80 mg per day or less of aspirin, heparin exerts a marked effect on vascular patency (57,58) (see Fig. 121-2). Although there is general agreement that heparin does not contribute significantly to a regimen of SK plus aspirin (10,59), physicians in the United States still use intravenous heparin in concert with tPA and aspirin (59,60).

The recommendation of the 7th Conference of the American College of Chest Physicians (ACCP) is to use weight-adjusted heparin with tPA (14); these guidelines suggest routine unfractionated heparin (UFH) for use with SK, but caution should be exercised if such patients are also treated with aspirin (10). The Assessment of the Safety and Efficacy of a New Thrombolytic Regimen (ASSENT)-3 PLUS trial (61), which assessed low-molecular-weight heparin (LMWH) versus UFH in combination with tenecteplase, showed advantage in the composite efficacy endpoint (mortality, reinfarction, ischemia), but a higher rate of ICH for LMWH. These data were sufficient to allow recommendation by the ACCP for 7 days of enoxaparin in patients who are younger than 75 years and with preserved renal function (14).

Among the potential adjunctive agents, two groups have received the most attention, these being the hirudin family of agents or small molecule inhibitors of thrombin (62–65), and inhibitors of the glycoprotein (GP) IIb/IIIa platelet fibrinogen receptor (66–69). Pilot studies in patients with AMI showed

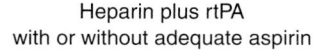

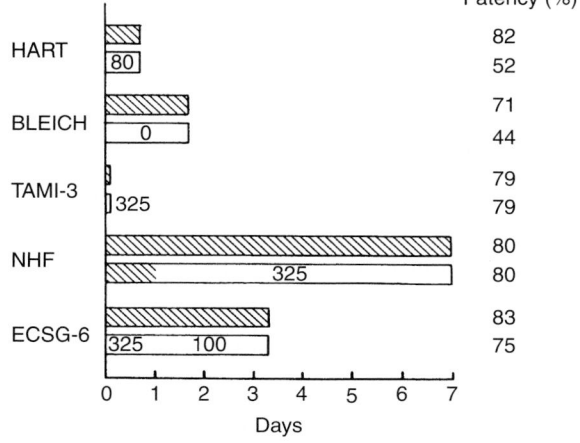

**FIGURE 121-2.** Coronary artery patency studies comparing heparin (*shaded areas*) with no heparin. The dose of aspirin given to patients who did not receive heparin is noted in the *clear bars*. The patency rates (%) noted with each treatment are indicated at the right. The length of the *horizontal bar* indicates the timing for angiographic demonstration of vascular patency, relative to the time of onset of plasminogen activator infusion. rtPA, recombinant tissue-type plasminogen activator.

encouraging increases in 90-minute patency rates with hirudin rather than heparin (70–72), but the relatively high dosages of anticoagulant resulted in unacceptable rates of ICH (73–75). With a scaled-back dosage regimen of anticoagulant in patients receiving tPA or SK along with aspirin, a large patient trial of 3,002 patients (TIMI-9B) showed no significant difference in clinical outcome using heparin or hirudin (76). On the basis of promising results of Hirulog in patients with unstable angina (77), and a small patency study showing greater reperfusion with Hirulog than with heparin used with SK for AMI (78), a patency study of 412 patients showed significantly greater TIMI-3 patency at 90 minutes (48% vs. 35%) and less bleeding using Hirulog (bivalirudin) rather than heparin after SK therapy (79). More emphatically, retrospective analysis of the GUSTO-IIb trial (80) showed that hirudin has a dramatic mortality benefit over heparin in AMI in the patients treated with SK but not in the patients treated with tPA. Prior analysis of the GUSTO-IIb data (81) and the TIMI-9B trial (82), both of which assessed the combined SK and tPA treatment groups, failed to show an advantage for hirudin over heparin. It is possible that the relatively high 90-minute patency rate attained with tPA plus heparin and aspirin approaches a maximal response, whereas the slower reperfusion that occurs with SK plus heparin and aspirin can be ameliorated by the more effective anticoagulant action of hirudin. A definitive study of 17,000 patients with AMI [Hirulog Early Reperfusion/Occlusion (HERO) 2] assessed whether such increased coronary artery patency is translated to a lower mortality using Hirulog rather than heparin (plus aspirin) before SK therapy (83). However, no difference in mortality was shown, despite the advantage of bivalirudin for inducing a higher 90-minute patency than heparin; a slight (insignificant) increase in ICH occurred with bivalirudin use. Other antithrombin strategies, such as LMWH (dalteparin) with SK (84), efegatran with SK (85), and argatroban with tPA (86) have been tested for effect on coronary artery patency, but without convincing data.

Effective GP IIb/IIIa inhibition can be achieved by the monoclonal antibody 7E3 [Abciximab (Centocor Inc., Malvern, PA)] and by small molecule inhibitors, which effectively block fibrinogen binding to platelets and prevent the cascade of biochemical events leading to aggregation. These agents are effective in preventing adverse outcome after unstable angina and angioplasty (87,88), and appropriate dosing of concomitant anticoagulant therapy prevents the excessive bleeding associated with these procedures (89). Considering that small molecule inhibitors of the fibrinogen receptor can accelerate reperfusion of coronary arteries in patients with AMI (90), it is not unreasonable to anticipate that platelet inhibitors will ultimately find a role as adjunctive therapy to PAs. The rationale for this approach would be that passivation of arterial wall by a long-acting or bound GP IIb/IIIa inhibitor could prevent vascular reocclusion, especially that which follows tPA therapy (91). A phase II trial that compared reteplase with low-dose reteplase plus abciximab showed enhanced Thrombolysis in Myocardial Infarction (TIMI) 3 flow using the combination regimen, but with increased major bleeding (92). Abciximab plus low-dose tPA versus tPA alone also demonstrated better flow results, without increased bleeding, in the combination regimen (93). In the ASSENT-3 mortality trial, tenecteplase plus LMWH or UFH showed the same mortality and ICH rates, as did reduced dose tenecteplase administered with lower dose UFH and abciximab (94). The GUSTO-V trial showed no difference in mortality between low-dose reteplase plus abciximab versus standard reteplase, but there was a higher rate of ICH in elderly patients (older than 75 years of age) in the combination therapy group (95). The ACCP guidelines recommend against various reduced dosage regimens of tenecteplase or reteplase with abciximab, in comparison with standard dosages of these thrombolytic agents (14).

## Other Adjunctive Approaches to Thrombolysis

### Plasminogen Supplementation

Because fibrinolysis depends on conversion of plasminogen to plasmin, the rate is determined at least in part by the plasminogen concentration incorporated into a clot (96). A decrease in plasma plasminogen is less striking with fibrinogen-sparing agents such as alteplase, saruplase, reteplase, and BAT-PA (97), and enrichment of plasminogen enhances the thrombolytic rate in vitro (98) and in animal models (99). Despite the theoretical advantage of supplemental plasminogen administration, clear-cut clinical benefit has not been obtained (100–102).

### Ultrasound

Ultrasound has been applied to thrombolysis, alone by remote or direct application, and with or without targeted delivery of microbubbles (103). Direct application by thin wire (104) is effective but less amenable for many thrombi, and appropriate conditions of frequency and energy can mechanically disrupt and disintegrate clots (105). Percutaneous, transvascular ultrasonic disruption of a femoral artery thrombus has been reported in animals (106,107) and patients (108). The mechanism whereby ultrasound may produce its accentuation of PA-mediated lysis is not known, but such therapy could potentially be achieved locally at the same time that systemic hemorrhagic complications may be avoided. Experiments suggest that transcutaneous ultrasound may induce thrombolysis when combined with systemic infusion of microbubbles, even in the absence of PA administration (106); another potential mechanism of action may involve accelerated transport of plasminogen into the thrombus (109). The role of ultrasound as adjunct to tPA administration has been assessed in patients with acute ischemic stroke, with short-term patency advantage, albeit with uncertain long-term clinical benefit (110).

### Catheter-Directed (Regional) Infusion

A recurrent issue concerns the administration of PA directly through a catheter onto or into a thrombus. The rationale for such regional therapy is compelling for arterial occlusions, because the thrombus is usually localized to a single vessel downstream from the catheter tip, and the catheter also provides a means for angiographic documentation of progress. Regional treatment of arterial thrombi does achieve better thrombolysis than systemic therapy, but activity of the PA is not restricted to the region in question. During the period of infusion, the lytic state may be comparable to that following systemic administration, and bleeding or ICH may complicate therapy (111). Local therapy for venous thromboembolic disease has a less compelling rationale, but this approach does achieve an impressive degree of vascular reperfusion (112–114), although bleeding complications, including ICH, are not avoided (115). For the treatment of thrombotic stroke, most studies have utilized systemic treatment to save time, but results of a trial using a local approach have been reported (116).

The main decision about regional treatment is the clinical exigency of the patient. For example, although regional infusion into the coronary artery may dissolve clots more effectively, systemic administration is more efficient for first-line treatment of the at-risk population with myocardial infarction. Still, with maximization of effort such as has been applied to early angioplasty for AMI (117), mechanical revascularization therapy may render the question of local coronary artery delivery of thrombolytic agent obsolete (118). Regional treatment of slower-progressing illnesses such as peripheral arterial occlusion (PAO) or deep vein thrombosis (DVT) has the luxury of time required for this approach, and it is most applicable for dissolving thrombi in occluded catheters.

### Plasmin

The potential of the direct fibrinolytic agent, plasmin, as described earlier, offers special opportunity for regionally administered therapy (13). Studies in animal models support the operational hypothesis of hemostatic safety of plasmin at thrombolytic dosages, in distinction from tPA, which causes hemorrhage from stable vascular injury sites at even subtherapeutic dosages (48). Thrombolysis under conditions of limited plasminogen content (restricted blood flow) indicate superior results with plasmin than are obtained with tPA (46) because the latter and not the former requires a replenished supply of this plasminogen for continued thrombolytic action (47).

---

# EFFECTS OF THROMBOLYTIC TREATMENT ON THE BLOOD

## Lytic State

The lytic state is a general description of the effects of plasmin activity on the circulation (119) (see Table 121-3; Fig. 121-3), beginning with a shortening of the euglobulin lysis time that measures free activator in the circulation. Laboratory parameters reflect the biochemical events that culminate in the degradation of plasma fibrinogen and a striking hypocoagulable state. The simplest and most physiologic definition of the lytic state is a clear-cut demonstration of a decrease in plasma fibrinogen that cannot be the result of laboratory artifact (3), for example, caused by the presence of heparin in the sample.

Free plasmin also decreases platelet aggregation induced by adenosine diphosphate (120), cleaves the platelet glycoprotein receptor for von Willebrand factor, and reduces ristocetin-induced platelet aggregation (121). Platelet hyperactivity and hyperaggregability may result from initial exposure of activator to platelets (122), and exposure of fresh thrombus surface or underlying vascular lesions may actually induce increased local coagulation. Therefore, a patient may experience sequential hypercoagulability and hypocoagulability or even the simultaneous occurrence of these opposite influences, depending upon the phase of lytic state that exists.

---

## Predictive Value of Laboratory Changes

Laboratory markers of hematologic events that occur after PA administration have potential relevance for predicting vascular

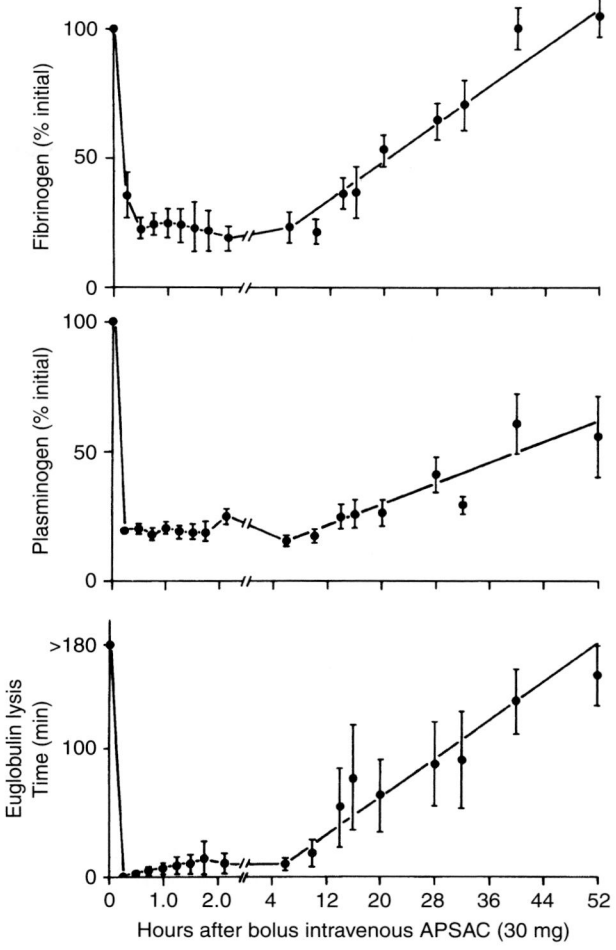

**FIGURE 121-3.** Plasma euglobulin lysis time and plasminogen and fibrinogen concentrations (mean ± standard error) measured before and after treatment of 15 patients with 30 mg anisoylated plasminogen streptokinase (APSAC) (anistreplase). (From Marder VJ, Rothbard RL, Fitzpatrick PG, et al. Rapid lysis of coronary artery thrombi with anisoylated plasminogen: streptokinase activator complex. Treatment by bolus intravenous injection. *Ann Intern Med* 1986;104:304, with permission.)

events (see Table 121-4). According to the concept that the actions of PAs in the blood and on the thrombus are separate events, successful dissolution of the pathologic thrombus through fibrin degradation would not necessarily correlate

---

**TABLE 121-3**

### DEVELOPMENT OF THE PLASMA PROTEOLYTIC (LYTIC) STATE

| Biochemical state | Laboratory parameter |
|---|---|
| Circulating plasminogen activator | Short euglobulin lysis time, variable platelet hyperreactivity |
| Plasminogen converted to plasmin | Decreased plasminogen |
| Antiplasmin complexes with plasmin and inhibits plasmin | Plasmin–antiplasmin complexes, decreased antiplasmin |
| | Free plasmin |
| Direct action | Increased plasma fibrin lysis and chromogenic activity |
| Degradation of fibrinogen | Decreased clottable protein, increased degradation products |
| Action on platelets | Glycoprotein cleavage, decreased aggregation |
| Hypocoagulable state | Prolonged coagulation tests (thrombin time) and bleeding time |

## TABLE 121-4

**RELATION OF VASCULAR AND HEMATOLOGIC PARAMETERS OF THROMBOLYSIS AND THE POTENTIAL FOR LABORATORY MARKERS OF RELATED EVENTS**

| Vascular | Hematologic | Potential marker |
|---|---|---|
| Reperfusion | Thrombolysis | Hypofibrinogenemia, elevated D-dimer, fibrin degradation products |
| Bleeding | Hemostatic plug or matrix disruption | Long bleeding time, hypofibrinogenemia |
| No reperfusion or occlusion | Hypercoagulable vessel thrombogenicity | Increased fibrinopeptide, prothrombin 1 + 2, thrombin–antithrombin complexes, soluble fibrin, persistent high fibrinogen |
| Late bleeding (with new injury) | Hypocoagulable state | Long bleeding time, persistent lytic state |
| Lasting patency | Hypocoagulable state, vascular passivation | Hypofibrinogenemia, long bleeding time, abnormal platelet function |

with the extent of fibrinogenolysis (lytic state). Likewise, bleeding that would result from hemostatic plug disruption or vascular matrix degradation could occur independently of changes in blood hemostatic measurements (3,4). An ongoing question is whether the degree of hypocoagulable state contributes to hemorrhagic events. Proponents of this thesis would state that a PA with fibrinogen-sparing properties causes less bleeding, because the induced hypocoagulability is minimized. Similar questions have been asked about the effect of blood changes on vascular reperfusion and reocclusion. The potential markers of bleeding could include any change in the lytic state cascade, including a decrease in plasminogen, hypofibrinogenemia, increased fibrinogen degradation products, prolonged bleeding time, and deranged platelet aggregation. Markers of vascular reperfusion as a surrogate of clinical recovery could potentially utilize lytic state markers, including changes in platelet function, or direct reflections of thrombolytic degradation of fibrin, such as increased D-dimer levels (see Fig. 121-4) (123).

## Bleeding Events

Although patients who receive thrombolytic agents are at risk of bleeding, such complications are at best only weakly correlated with laboratory parameters of the lytic state. For example, UK or SK treatment of pulmonary embolism (PE) or DVT regularly induces the lytic state, but the changes in fibrinogen concentration, plasminogen, or euglobulin lysis time are not

significantly different in patients with or without a hemorrhagic complication (124,125). The direct comparison of tPA and SK in the TIMI trial–phase I showed significantly lower fibrinogen values with SK than with tPA, but the incidence of major and minor bleeding complications was the same with both treatments (126). Furthermore, patients with ischemic (thrombotic) or hemorrhagic cerebrovascular accident (CVA) who were treated with tPA had the same nadir concentration of fibrinogen (127). The only predictive blood value for hemorrhagic complication during tPA treatment is the plasma tPA concentration (3.4 μg per mL in bleeders vs. 2.2 μg per mL; $P = 0.002$) (128). The higher value noted in those who bled suggests that tPA has a direct effect on susceptible hemostatic plugs or vascular sites, more with higher concentrations, independent of changes in fibrinogen concentration. This effect helps to explain the higher rate of ICH with high therapeutic dosages of tPA (129) and supports the concept that bleeding occurs independent of PA effect on blood coagulation, probably the result of action at sites of vascular injury or malformation (4). A retrospective analysis of more than 40,000 patients in the GUSTO-I study found independent predictors of hemorrhage to be of older age, lighter body weight, female sex, and of African origin, rather than the degree of laboratory derangement (130).

The template bleeding time is prolonged during thrombolytic therapy, either as a direct result of the PA or as a result of concomitant aspirin therapy, but there is no distinction in patients with or without hemorrhagic complication (131). Thrombocytopenia of less than $100 \times 10^9$ per L has been noted in 2.4% to 3.9% of patients undergoing coronary artery angioplasty and receiving abciximab, with approximately one fourth of these patients having severe decreases of less than $50 \times 10^9$ per L (132). Thrombocytopenia was associated with more unfavorable outcomes, including bleeding episodes, and with lower baseline counts, increasing age, and decreased weight.

The occurrence of ICH with PA treatment is relatively infrequent but of great clinical importance, in that more than 50% of patients have lethal outcomes or significant neurologic deficits. Although major hemorrhagic complications other than ICH are induced with approximately equal frequency by all of the PAs, the more potent agents such as tPA have a consistently higher risk of inducing ICH. The reason is not clear; it is not likely to reflect the presence of a fresh hemostatic plug that is dissolved, but may be related to a vascular abnormality associated with amyloid deposition (133). As with other bleeding complications, the degree of lytic state does not explain the event, as the fibrinogen is the same in patients with ICH or with a thrombotic (ischemic) CVA (127). Subcutaneous heparin added to aspirin during PA infusion increases the risk slightly (0.6% vs. 0.4%) (8), but the use of tPA is a most important

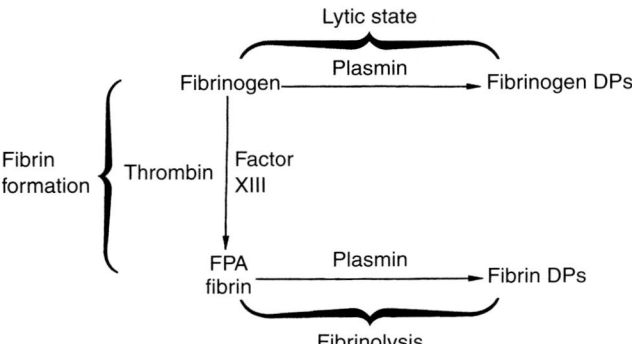

**FIGURE 121-4.** Biochemical actions of thrombin, plasmin, and factor XIII, or combinations of these enzymes on fibrinogen and fibrin substrates, as a foundation for laboratory monitoring of clinical events. DP, degradation products; FPA, fibrinopeptide A.

## TABLE 121-5

RATE OF INTRACRANIAL HEMORRHAGE IN FOUR STUDIES OF ACCELERATED REGIMEN ALTEPLASE (tPA)

| | GUSTO-I (1990–1993) | | GUSTO-III (1995–1997) | | COBALT | | ASSENT-2 | |
| | SK (17,804) | tPA (9,039) | Reteplase (10,138) | tPA (4,921) | Bolus tPA (3,585) | tPA (3,585) | Bolus tenecteplase (8,461) | tPA (8,488) |
|---|---|---|---|---|---|---|---|---|
| Age <75 yr | 0.4 | 0.5 | 0.7 | 0.8 | 0.7 | 0.6 | 0.8 | — |
| Age >75 yr | 1.2 | 2.5 | 2.5 | 1.7 | 3.6 | 2.6 | 1.7 | 2.6 |
| Overall | 0.5 | 0.7 | 0.9 | 0.9 | 1.1 | 0.8 | 0.93 | 0.94 |

GUSTO, Global Use of Strategies to Open Occluded Coronary Arteries; COBALT, Continuous Infusion Versus Double-Bolus Administration of Alteplase; ASSENT, Assessment of the Safety and Efficacy of a New Thrombolytic Regimen; SK, streptokinase; tPA, tissue-type plasminogen activator.

predictor (42), along with age greater than 65, weight less than 70 kg, hypertension on admission, and a prior history of transient ischemic attack or CVA (129). A retrospective comparison of SK (41,000 patients), anistreplase (21,000 patients), and tPA (41,000 patients) showed the incidence of ICH to be 0.2%, 0.6%, and 0.6%, respectively (13). Recent observations of accelerated regimen tPA versus SK, reteplase, or double bolus tPA show an overall risk of approximately 0.8% for accelerated tPA, with the risk in elderly patients (older than 75 years of age) being significantly higher (2.1%) (see Table 121-5) (51,134,135).

### Vascular Patency and Reocclusion

Laboratory results also do not predict vascular reperfusion or degree of patency. In the Urokinase Pulmonary Embolism Trial (UPET) study in which a large systemic dose of UK was administered, there was no correlation of laboratory results with decrease of embolus size (124), and DVT trials also showed a lack of correlation of venographic change after PA therapy with degrees of alteration in fibrinogen, thrombin time, plasminogen, and FDP (125). Even intracoronary administration of SK for treatment of AMI showed no difference in nadir plasma fibrinogen in patients who did or did not reperfuse (136), and similar measurements in patients with AMI receiving tPA also failed to show a correlation with posttreatment coronary artery patency (128). Although there is no universal agreement, the data does suggest that changes in blood coagulation or fibrinolytic assays following PA administration do not directly reflect the degree of thrombus dissolution.

A reasonable hypothesis for noninvasive measurement of successful thrombolysis would be to measure plasma levels of cross-linked FDPs, but the data so far are not conclusive, with some showing high predictability for successful vascular reperfusion (137) whereas others fail to document such a correlation (138). Prediction of coronary artery reocclusion in an individual patient is problematic, but trials using tPA provide instructive information (128). Among 55 patients with reocclusion, the decrease in fibrinogen was less (120 vs. 180 mg per dL) than in patients whose vessels stayed patent. The data suggest that a more profound lytic state protects against reocclusion and may partially explain the lower tendency for reocclusion with SK, UK, and anistreplase than with tPA (51,139,140).

### Laboratory Monitoring

Unlike treatment regimens with antithrombin agents such as heparin, the PA dosage regimens are standardized, on either a total dosage or weight-adjusted basis, and only the duration of infusion leaves room for variation. Therefore, the major role for monitoring thrombolytic therapy using a PA would be to document that a given dosage of agent has achieved a lytic state. Time constraints in patients with AMI allow little chance to react to a laboratory result during the acute phase of the illness. Once a lytic state has been attained, there is no need to regulate the dose of PA, because alterations based on laboratory markers would neither improve the chance of thrombolysis nor decrease the risk of hemorrhagic complication. On the other hand, in patients who are anticipated to receive more than bolus injections or short infusions, the absence of a lytic state might reasonably be the cause for discontinuation of therapy and initiation of standard anticoagulation. The exception to this rule is for therapy using direct thrombolytic agents such as plasmin, for which there is a direct relation of dose with plasma fibrinogen, and an apparent threshold of plasma fibrinogen above which hemostatic safety is anticipated (48).

# MANAGEMENT OF BLEEDING COMPLICATIONS

## Prevention of Bleeding

The absolute contraindications to PA therapy are those that may result in ICH or massive, life-threatening hemorrhage (see Table 121-6). The risks of minor bleeding or even of the

## TABLE 121-6

ABSOLUTE CONTRAINDICATIONS TO FIBRINOLYTIC THERAPY

| Risk | Condition |
|---|---|
| Intracranial bleeding | Hemorrhagic cerebrovascular accident, intracranial neoplasm, recent cranial surgery or trauma (within 10 d), uncontrolled severe hypertension |
| Massive hemorrhage | Major surgery of thorax or abdomen (within 10 d), prolonged cardiopulmonary resuscitation, current severe bleeding site (e.g., gastrointestinal tract) |

need for blood transfusion are not absolute contraindications. Decisions about PA use must weigh the expected severity of the complication with the potential benefit associated with accelerated thrombolysis. Therefore, some patients with obvious life-threatening thrombotic disease, for example, massive PE with profound shock or a large anterior wall AMI, may warrant potentially life-saving thrombolytic therapy even in the face of "absolute" contraindications. On the other hand, patients with a relatively less threatening thrombotic disease such as DVT would reasonably not receive PA therapy if there is a relevant history that significantly increases the risk of ICH, for example, transient ischemic attack, prior thrombotic stroke, or current hypertension. The risk of major bleeding after recent surgery of the head, thorax, or abdomen is obvious, but the risk of serious bleeding following brief and relatively nontraumatic cardiopulmonary resuscitation is probably less than feared. Some clinical situations are associated with an increased risk of symptomatic but not serious bleeding, for example, patients with superficial wounds, arteriotomy or venotomy, active menses, and minor surgical or biopsy procedures.

The elderly patients have a higher risk of bleeding, especially those with ICH, but they also have a higher risk of death from AMI than do younger patients. Therefore, the survival benefit in patients older than 70 years is relatively more than in patients younger than 60 years (80 vs. 25 lives saved per 1,000 treated) (50,141).

## Management of Acute Bleeding and Posttreatment Surgery

In patients who have life-threatening bleeding or sudden emergencies that require surgical intervention, normal hemostasis can quickly be reestablished by discontinuing PA infusion, replenishing plasma fibrinogen with either whole plasma or cryoprecipitate, and providing fresh platelets to correct a prolonged bleeding time (see Table 121-7). If the PA is not yet cleared from the circulation, fibrinolytic activity can be neutralized by infusion of fibrinolytic inhibitors such as ε-aminocaproic acid or aprotinin.

There are cases of coronary artery bypass graft surgery after SK usage indicating that the operation can be performed immediately (142,143), but that such therapy may result in bleeding complications and the need for blood transfusion (144). Such results are relevant for invasive procedures after tPA treatment as well, even if performed after a delay of 12 and sometimes 24 hours (145). In the TIMI-IIA study (128), angioplasty performed immediately after stopping tPA resulted in a considerably greater need for blood transfusion than if

performed 18 to 48 hours later. The reason for bleeding, coincident with interventional procedures after tPA, which is cleared quickly from the circulation, is that the nadir fibrinogen remains low for 24 hours (128). Plasma fibrinogen concentrations are ultimately achieved by hepatic synthesis of fresh fibrinogen, a process that requires 24 to 36 hours to accomplish, irrespective of the PA that was administered.

In anticipation of invasive surgery immediately after PA treatment, it is reasonable to replenish fibrinogen with cryoprecipitate because essentially no normal fibrinogen is present during SK (146) or tPA infusion (147), and to restore platelet function with fresh platelet transfusion for up to 24 hours after PA administration. In addition, antifibrinolytic therapy should be administered prophylactically if activator is still circulating, an expected situation for variable times after the infusion is stopped (148). Most bleeding complications can be anticipated by careful clinical evaluation. Recent and unhealed vascular trauma sites are susceptible to bleeding for approximately 10 days. Depending upon their location, the bleeding complication can be unimportant (ecchymoses, hematuria), bothersome and requiring transfusion (duodenal ulcer, accessible surgical site), or life-threatening (thoracic or cranial surgery, recent or even remote stroke).

Once a patient is to be treated with a PA, unnecessary trauma to the patient should be avoided. One should administer medication by mouth or intravenously, but not intramuscularly. Phlebotomy sites should be compressed for 5 or 10 minutes, unnecessary arteriotomy should be postponed or avoided, and rough manual manipulation of the patient should be minimized. Treatment of some thrombotic conditions requires concomitant antiplatelet or antithrombotic treatment, especially certain arterial occlusions, but for DVT and PE such therapies usually increase the risk of bleeding without adding to the clinical result. The use of intravenous or subcutaneous heparin in addition to aspirin and a PA increases the risk of bleeding.

Bleeding that occurs during PA infusion should be managed appropriately with blood replacement and, if necessary and possible, by discontinuing the PA treatment. If bleeding is to be controlled immediately, the PA must be neutralized by an afibrinolytic inhibitor, and cryoprecipitate and platelets should be transfused. If surgical intervention is required within the first 24 hours after PA administration, the hemostatic mechanisms of the patient should be maximized to avoid operative bleeding. Depending on the half-life of the activator, fibrinolytic inhibitor may or may not be required, but fresh fibrinogen replacement and platelet transfusion will often be required to ensure hemostasis, because plasma fibrinogen concentration does not recover spontaneously until 24 to 36 hours after discontinuing PA treatment. This pertains to

### TABLE 121-7

MANAGEMENT OF HYPOCOAGULABLE STATE INDUCED BY PLASMINOGEN ACTIVATORS

|  | During treatment | Immediately after treatment | 6–36 h after treatment |
|---|---|---|---|
| Plasma fibrinogen | Low | Nadir | Progressive recovery |
| Need for cryoprecipitate | Yes | Yes | Yes |
| Bleeding time | Long | Variable | Normal[a] |
| Need for platelets | Yes | Yes | No |
| Circulating activator | Present | Variable | Absent |
| Need for antifibrinolytics | Yes | Yes | Yes |

[a]Unless aspirin is also administered, in which case the potential for bleeding may persist.

## TABLE 121-8

### CURRENT OR PRIOR FOOD AND DRUG ADMINISTRATION APPROVALS OF PLASMINOGEN ACTIVATORS

| Agent | Clinical indication | FDA-approved regimen | Common usage |
|---|---|---|---|
| Urokinase (Abbokinase) | PE | 12-h IV infusion | Agent not currently available |
| | Acute MI | Intracoronary only | Agent not currently available |
| | PAO, DVT | Not approved | Widespread usage by regional route, but agent currently not available |
| | Thrombosed central line or shunt | 5,000 U in 1 mL | — |
| Streptokinase (Streptase) | Acute MI | IV or IC | Used primarily by IV route |
| | PE | IV over 12 h | Effective given for shorter courses, even 2 h |
| | DVT | IV for up to 36 h | Shorter infusions safer, e.g., over 18 h |
| | PAO | IV | IV route not as effective as regionally |
| | Thrombosed arteriovenous cannulae | Local installation | |
| Reteplase (Retavase) | Acute MI | Two bolus injections 30 min apart | Approved, 1999 |
| | PAO | Not approved | Usage "off-label" regionally |
| Alteplase (Activase) | Acute MI | 3 h or 90 min | Accelerated dosage used most often |
| | Acute ischemic stroke | 90 mg over 1 h | Limited usage, as must be applied within 3 h of onset |
| | PE | 100 mg/2 h | Urokinase over 2 h, equal efficacy |
| Anistreplase (Eminase) | Acute MI | 30 U over 2–5 min | Infrequently used |
| Tenecteplase (TNKase) | Acute MI | Single-bolus, weight-adjusted | Approved, 2000 |

FDA, U.S. Food and Drug Administration; PE, pulmonary embolism; IV, intravenous; MI, myocardial infarction; PAO, peripheral arterial occlusion; DVT, deep vein thrombosis; IC, intracutaneous.
Based on *Physicians' Desk Reference*. Montvale, NJ: Medical Economics Co., 2000.

## TABLE 121-9

### NATURAL HISTORY AND ANTICIPATED CLINICAL BENEFIT OF THROMBOLYTIC TREATMENT OF ACUTE THROMBOSIS

| Thrombotic disorder | Natural history (with antithrombotics) | Potential benefit of thrombolytics | Clinical decisions |
|---|---|---|---|
| DVT | Slow resolution, subclinical PE frequent, postphlebitic syndrome in 25%–50% with proximal thrombi | Treatment within 7 d, complete lysis in half the cases; decreased incidence of postphlebitic syndrome | Treat large proximal thrombi, especially with coexistent PE; catheter delivery (urokinase, alteplase, reteplase) in wide usage, but still under study |
| PE | Slow (1 wk) reduction of pulmonary hypertension; overall mortality 7%, up to 30% with massive PE and hypotension | Earlier treatment (within 48 h) induces rapid thrombolysis and accelerates reversal of pulmonary hypertension; possible increased survival in patients with clinical shock | Thrombolytics for massive PA with shock, coexistent cardiopulmonary disease, or submassive PE if no contraindications |
| PAO | Major surgical intervention in 95%, cardiopulmonary complications in 50%, loss of limb in 20%, 1-yr mortality up to 40% | Striking thrombolysis in 70%, surgery avoided in 35%, no change in limb salvage but potential for decrease in 1-yr mortality | Catheter delivery of PA superior to systemic infusion; thrombolytic preferred over surgery, for initial therapy for the ischemic but salvageable limb |
| MI | Overall mortality 11.5% versus 8.0% for inferior MI, 17.0% for anterior MI | Overall mortality reduced by by 20%–50% most striking in patients with anterior MI treated within 4 h after symptom onset | Indicated for most patients within 6 h of symptoms; angioplasty offers advantages and is increasingly utilized |
| CVA | Irreversible deficits and risk of death depending on location; hemorrhagic transformation relatively infrequent (3%) | Good results only if treatment initiated within 3 h, reversal of neurologic deficit at a cost of increased parenchymal hematoma | Clear-cut functional benefit without increased mortality risk if treatment before 3 h, but with increased risk of hemorrhagic transformation |

DVT, deep vein thrombosis; PE, pulmonary embolism; PA, plasminogen activator; PAO, peripheral arterial (or graft) occlusion; MI, myocardial infarction; CVA, cerebrovascular accident.

both the long- and short-acting agents, and also those that induce a potent or a mild fibrinolytic state.

## Other Side Effects and Complications

Termination of treatment may be necessitated by allergic or pyrogenic side effects, which could also be managed with corticosteroids, antihistamines or adrenergic agents for anaphylaxis, and antipyretics for fever. Allergic reactions are three to five times more frequent using bacterial-derived products than tPA– type derivatives, but patients who receive tPA rarely manifest allergic reactions such as bronchospasm or angioneurotic edema (149,150). A second side effect is hypotension, especially in patients with AMI, occurring in approximately 12% of patients exposed to SK or anistreplase and 7% of those exposed to tPA, in comparison with only 1.5% of patients not exposed to a PA (151).

Embolic phenomena of clinical importance are distinctly unusual in patients with venous thromboembolic disease who received PA treatment. In the UPET trial (124), recurrent PE occurred in 15% of patients who received either UK or heparin. A venous thrombus breaking off to become a fatal pulmonary embolus is distinctly unusual and may have alternative explanations other than lysis of a vulnerable, free-floating thrombus. On the other hand, distal systemic embolization from a cardiac source during PA treatment, although unusual, is clinically apparent, and up to 20% of patients with PAO are affected by sudden new ischemia of the distal extremity (152). In this circumstance, the best treatment mode is continued local instillation of PA, which usually succeeds in dissolving the new embolus. Rarely, systemic treatment with PA results in cholesterol crystal embolization, usually in the setting of extensive preexisting atherosclerotic disease (153).

## CLINICAL APPLICATIONS

Table 121-8 summarizes the FDA-approved agents in the major categories of vascular thrombotic disease, namely myocardial infarction, PAO, DVT, PE, acute ischemic stroke (CVA), and catheter occlusion. These approvals are based on pivotal clinical trials, but actual practice may reflect an evolution of dosage schedules or mode of administration. Table 121-9 summarizes the clinical benefit anticipated with the use of PA in patients with major vessel occlusions.

## References

1. Fletcher AP, Alkjaersig N, Sherry S. Fibrinolytic mechanisms and the development of thrombolytic therapy. *Am J Med* 1962;33:738.
2. Verstraete M. Biochemical and clinical aspects of thrombolysis. *Semin Hematol* 1978;15:35.
3. Marder VJ. The use of thrombolytic agents: choice of patient, drug administration, laboratory monitoring. *Ann Intern Med* 1979;90:802.
4. Marder VJ, Sherry S. Thrombolytic therapy: current status. *N Engl J Med* 1988;18:1512,1585.
5. Sherry S. The origin of thrombolytic therapy. *J Am Coll Cardiol* 1989;14:1085.
6. White HD, Van de Werf FJJ. Thrombolysis for acute myocardial infarction. *Circulation* 1998;97:1632.
7. Goldhaber SZ. Contemporary pulmonary embolism thrombolysis. *Chest* 1995;107:45S.
8. Fibrinolytic Therapy Trialists Collaborative Group. Indications for fibrinolytic therapy in suspected acute myocardial infarction: collaborative overview of early mortality and major morbidity results from all randomised trials of more than 1000 patients. *Lancet* 1994;343:311.
9. Simoons ML, Arnold AE. Tailored thrombolytic therapy. A perspective. *Circulation* 1993;88:2556.
10. Collins R, Peto R, Baigent C, et al. Aspirin, heparin, and fibrinolytic therapy in suspected acute myocardial infarction. *N Engl J Med* 1997;336:847.
11. Baker WF. Thrombolytic therapy: clinical applications. *Hematol Oncol Clin North Am* 2003;17:283–311.
12. Wardlaw JM, Warlow CP, Counsell C. Systematic review of evidence of thrombolytic therapy for acute ischemic stroke. *Lancet* 1997;350:607.
13. Marder VJ, Stewart D. Towards safer thrombolytic therapy. *Semin Hematol* 2002;39:206–216.
14. Menon V, Harrington RA, Hochman JS, et al. Thrombolysis and adjunctive therapy in acute myocardial infarction. The Seventh ACCP Conference on Antithrombotic and Thrombolytic Therapy. *Chest* 2004;126:549S–575S.
15. Francis CW, Marder VJ. Physiologic regulation and pathologic disorders of fibrinolysis. In: Colman RW, Hirsh J, Marder VJ et al., eds. *Hemostasis and thrombosis: basic principles and clinical practice*, 4th ed. Philadelphia, PA: Lippincott Williams & Wilkins, 2001:975.
16. Wiman B, Collen D. Molecular mechanisms of physiologic fibrinolysis. *Nature* 1978;272:549.
17. Tillett WS, Garner RL. Fibrinolytic activity of hemolytic streptococci. *J Exp Med* 1933;58:485.
18. White WF, Barlow GH, Mozen MM. The isolation and characterization of plasminogen activators (urokinase) from human urine. *Biochemistry* 1966;5:2160.
19. Bernik MB, Kwaan HC. Plasminogen activator activity in cultures from human tissue: an immunological and histochemical study. *J Clin Invest* 1969;48:1740.
20. Rijken DC, Collen D. Purification and characterization of the plasminogen activator secreted by human melanoma cells in cultures. *J Biol Chem* 1981;256:7035.
21. Pennica D, Holmes WE, Kohn WJ, et al. Cloning and expression of human tissue-type plasminogen activator cDNA in E. coli. *Nature* 1983;301:214.
22. Smith RAG, Dupe RJ, English PD, et al. Fibrinolysis with acyl enzymes: a new approach to thrombolytic therapy. *Nature* 1981;290:505.
23. Kohnert U, Rudolph R, Verheijen JH, et al. Biochemical properties of the kringle 2 and protease domains are maintained in the refolded t-PA deletion variant BM 06.022. *Protein Eng* 1992;5:93.
24. Keyt BA, Paoni NF, Refino CJ, et al. A faster-acting and more potent form of tissue plasminogen activator. *Proc Natl Acad Sci U S A* 1994;91: 3670.
25. Martin U, Sponer G, Konig R, et al. Double bolus administration of the novel recombinant plasminogen activator BM 06.022 improves coronary blood flow after reperfusion in a canine model of coronary thrombosis. *Blood Coagul Fibrinolysis* 1992;3:139.
26. Cannon CP, Gibson CM, McCabe CH, et al. Thrombolysis in Myocardial Infarction (TIMI) 10B Investigators. TNK-tissue plasminogen activator compared with front-loaded alteplase in acute myocardial infarction: results of the TIMI 10B trial. *Circulation* 1998;98:2805.
27. Ratzkin B, Lee SG, Schrenk WJ, et al. Expression in *Escherichia coli* of biologically active enzyme by a DNA sequence coding for the human plasminogen activator urokinase. *Proc Natl Acad Sci U S A* 1981;78:3313.
28. Husain S, Gurewich V, Lipinski B. Purification and partial characterization of a single-chain high-molecular-weight form of urokinase from human urine. *Arch Biochem Biophys* 1983;220:31.
29. Sako T, Sawaki S, Sakurai T, et al. Cloning and expression of the streptokinase gene of *Staphylococcus aureus* in *Escherichia coli*. *Mol Gen Genet* 1983;190:271.
30. Gardell SL, Duong LT, Diehl RE, et al. Isolation, characterization and cDNA cloning of a vampire bat salivary plasminogen activator. *J Biol Chem* 1989;264:17947.
31. Collen D, Lu HR, Lijnen HR, et al. Thrombolytic and pharmacokinetic properties of chimeric tissue-type and urokinase-type plasminogen activators. *Circulation* 1991;84:1216.
32. Runge MS, Quertermous T, Haber E. Plasminogen activators: the old and the new. *Circulation* 1989;79:217.
33. Behnke D, Gerlach D. Cloning and expression in *Escherichia coli*, *Bacillus subtilis*, and *Streptococcus sanguis* of a gene for staphylokinase: a bacterial plasminogen activator. *Mol Gen Genet* 1987;210:528.
34. Collen D, Moreau H, Stockx L, et al. Recombinant staphylokinase variants with altered immunoreactivity. II. Thrombolytic properties and antibody induction. *Circulation* 1996;94:207.
35. The TERIMA group investigators. Multicenter, randomized, comparative study of recombinant vs. natural streptokinases in acute myocardial infarct (TERIMA). Thrombolysis with Recombinant Streptokinase in Acute Myocardial Infarct. *Thromb Haemost* 1999;82:1605.
36. Staniforth DH, Smith RAG, Hibbs M. Streptokinase and anisoylated streptokinase plasminogen complex—their action on haemostasis in human volunteers. *Eur J Clin Pharmacol* 1983;24:751.
37. Bode C, Smalling RW, Berg G, et al. The RAPID II Investigators. Randomized comparison of coronary thrombolysis achieved with double-bolus reteplase (recombinant plasminogen activator) and front-loaded, accelerated alteplase (recombinant tissue plasminogen activator) in patients with acute myocardial infarction. *Circulation* 1996;94:891.
38. Modi NB, Eppler S, Breed J, et al. Pharmacokinetics of a slower clearing tissue plasminogen activator variant, TNK-t-PA, in patients with acute myocardial infarction. *Thromb Haemost* 1998;79:134.
39. Nordt TK, Moser M, Kohler B, et al. Pharmacokinetics and pharmacodynamics of lanoteplase (n-PA). *Thromb Haemost* 1999;82(Suppl. 1):121.
40. Korninger C, Matsuo O, Suy R, et al. Thrombolysis with human extrinsic (tissue-type) plasminogen activator in dogs with femoral vein thrombosis. *J Clin Invest* 1982;69:573.

41. Cannon CP, McCabe CH, Gibson CM, et al. TNK-tissue plasminogen activator in acute myocardial infarction. Results of the Thrombolysis in Myocardial Infarction (TIMI) 10A dose-ranging trial. *Circulation* 1997; 95:351.

42. Simoons ML, Maggioni AP, Knatterud G, et al. Individual risk assessment for intracranial haemorrhage during thrombolytic therapy. *Lancet* 1993; 342:1523.

43. InTIME-II Investigators. Intravenous NPA for the treatment of infarcting myocardium early: InTIME-II, a double-blind comparison of single-bolus lanoteplase vs. accelerated alteplase for the treatment of patients with acute myocardial infarction. Eur Heart J 2000;21:2005.

44. Comer MB, Cackett KS, Gladwell S, et al. Thrombolytic activity of BB-10153, a thrombin-activatable plasminogen. *J Thromb Haemost* 2005;3: 146–153.

45. Novokhatny V, Taylor K, Zimmerman TP. Thrombolytic potency of acid-stabilized plasmin: superiority over tissue-type plasminogen activator in an *in vitro* model of catheter-assisted thrombolysis. *J Thromb Haemost* 2003;1:1034–1041.

46. Marder VJ, Landskroner K, Novokhatny V, et al. Plasmin induces local thrombolysis without causing hemorrhage: a comparison with tissue plasminogen activator in the rabbit. *Thromb Haemost* 2001;86:739–745.

47. Novokhatny VV, Jesmok GJ, Landskroner KA, et al. Locally delivered plasmin: why should it be superior to plasminogen activators for direct thrombolysis? *Trends Pharmacol Sci* 2004;25:72–75.

48. Stewart D, Kong M, Novokhatny V, et al. Distinct dose-dependent effects of plasmin and TPA on coagulation and hemorrhage. *Blood* 2003;101: 3002–3007.

49. Nagai N, De Mol M, Van Hoef B, et al. Depletion of circulating á2-antiplasmin by intravenous plasmin or immunoneutralization reduces focal cerebral ischemic injury in the absence of arterial recanalization. *Blood* 2001;97:3086–3092.

50. ISIS-2 (Second International Study of Infarct Survival) Collaborative Group. Randomized trial of intravenous streptokinase, oral aspirin, both, or neither among 17,187 cases of suspected acute myocardial infarction. *Lancet* 1988;2:349.

51. The GUSTO Investigators. An international randomized trial comparing four thrombolytic strategies for acute myocardial infarction. *N Engl J Med* 1993;329:673.

52. Col JJ, Dol-De Beys CM, Renkin JP, et al. Pharmacokinetics, thrombolytic efficacy and hemorrhagic risk of different streptokinase regimens in heparin-treated acute myocardial infarction. *Am J Cardiol* 1989;63:1185.

53. O'Connor CM, Meese R, Carney R, et al. A randomized trial of intravenous heparin in conjunction with anistreplase (anisoylated plasminogen streptokinase activator complex) in acute myocardial infarction: the Duke University Clinical Cardiology Study (DUCCS) I. *J Am Coll Cardiol* 1994;23:11.

54. TAMI 7 Group. A randomizes controlled trial of intravenous tissue plasminogen activator and early intravenous heparin in acute myocardial infarction. *Circulation* 1992;79:281.

55. National Heart Foundation of Australia Coronary Thrombolysis Group. A randomized comparison of intravenous heparin with oral aspirin and dipyridamole 24 hours after recombinant tissue-type plasminogen activator for acute myocardial infarction. *Circulation* 1991;83:1534.

56. European Cooperative Study Group. Effect of early intravenous heparin on coronary patency, infarct size and bleeding complications after alteplase thrombolysis. Results of a randomized double- blind European Cooperative Group trial. *Br Heart J* 1992;67:122.

57. Hsia J, Hamilton WP, Kleinman N, et al. A comparison between heparin and low-dose aspirin as adjunctive therapy with tissue plasminogen activator for acute myocardial infarction. *N Engl J Med* 1990;323:1433.

58. Bleich SD, Nichols TC, Schumacher RR, et al. Effect of heparin on coronary arterial patency after thrombolysis with tissue plasminogen activator in acute myocardial infarction. *Am J Cardiol* 1990;66:1412.

59. Metz BK, Topol EJ. Heparin as an adjuvant to thrombolytic therapy in acute myocardial infarction. *Biomed Pharmacother* 1996;50:243.

60. Mahaffey KW, Granger CB, Collins R, et al. Overview of randomized trials of intravenous heparin in patients with acute myocardial infarction treated with thrombolytic therapy. *Am J Cardiol* 1996;77:551.

61. Wallentin L, Goldstein P, Armstrong PW, et al. Efficacy and safety of tenecteplase in combination with the low-molecular-weight heparin enoxaparin or unfractionated heparin in the prehospital setting. The Assessment of the Safety and Efficacy of a New Thrombolytic Regimen (ASSENT)-3 PLUS Randomized Trial in Acute Myocardial Infarction. *Circulation* 2003; 108:135–142.

62. Markwardt F. Development of hirudin as an antithrombotic agent. *Semin Thromb Hemost* 1989;15:269.

63. Maraganore JM, Bourdon P, Jablonski J, et al. Design and characterization of Hirulogs: a novel class of bivalent peptide inhibitors of thrombin. *Biochemistry* 1990;29:7095.

64. Lefkovits J, Topol EJ. Direct thrombin inhibitors in cardiovascular medicine. *Circulation* 1994;90:1522.

65. Jang I-K, Gold HK, Ziskind AA, et al. Prevention of platelet-rich thrombosis by selective thrombin inhibition. *Circulation* 1990;81:219.

66. Coller BS. Platelets and thrombolytic therapy. *N Engl J Med* 1990;322:33.

67. Coller BS, Folt JD, Scudder LE, et al. Antithrombotic effect of a monoclonal antibody to the platelet glycoprotein IIb/IIIa receptor in an experimental animal model. *Blood* 1986;68:783.

68. Topol EJ, Byzova TV, Plow EF. Platelet GPIIb-IIIa blockers. *Lancet* 1999; 353:227.

69. Vogt A. Antiplatelet drugs plus thrombolysis in myocardial infarction. Where are we now? *BioDrugs* 1999;11:377.

70. Cannon CP, McCabe CH, Henry TD, et al. A pilot trial of recombinant desulfatohirudin compared with heparin in conjunction with tissue-type plasminogen activator and aspirin for acute myocardial infarction: results of the Thrombolysis in Myocardial Infarction (TIMI) 5 trial. *J Am Coll Cardiol* 1994;23:993.

71. Lee LV. Initial experience with hirudin and streptokinase in acute myocardial infarction: results of the Thrombolysis in Myocardial Infarction (TIMI) 6 trial. *Am J Cardiol* 1995;75:7.

72. Zymer U, von Essen R, Tebbe U, et al. Recombinant hirudin and front-loaded alteplase in acute myocardial infarction: final results of a pilot study. HIT-1 (Hirudin for the improvement of thrombolysis). *Eur Heart J* 1995;16(Suppl. D):22.

73. The Global Use of Strategies to Open Occluded Coronary Arteries (GUSTO) IIa Investigators. Randomized trial of intravenous heparin versus recombinant hirudin for acute coronary syndromes. *Circulation* 1994; 90:1631.

74. Neuhaus KL, von Essen R, Tebbe U, et al. Safety observations from the pilot phase of the randomized r-Hirudin for Improvement of Thrombolysis (HIT-III) Study. A study of the Arbeitsgemeinschaft Leitender Kardiologischer Krankenhausarzte (ALKK). *Circulation* 1994;90:1638.

75. Antman EM. Hirudin in acute myocardial infarction. Study report from the Thrombolysis and Thrombin Inhibition in Myocardial Infarction (TIMI) 9A trial. *Circulation* 1994;90:1624.

76. Antman EM. Hirudin in acute myocardial infarction. Thrombolysis and Thrombin Inhibition in Myocardial Infarction (TIMI) 9B Trial. *Circulation* 1996;94:911.

77. Fuchs J, Cannon CP. Hirulog in treatment of unstable angina. Results of the Thrombin Inhibition in Myocardial Ischemia (TIMI) 7 Trial. *Circulation* 1995;92:727.

78. Theroux P, Perez-Villa F, Waters D, et al. Randomized double-blind comparison of two doses of Hirulog with heparin as adjunctive therapy to streptokinase to promote early patency of the infarct-related artery in acute myocardial infarction. *Circulation* 1995;98:2132.

79. White HD, Aylward PE, Frey MJ, et al. Randomized, double-blind comparison of Hirulog versus heparin in patients receiving streptokinase and aspirin for acute myocardial infarction (HERO). Hirulog Early Reperfusion/Occlusion (HERO) Trial Investigators. *Circulation* 1997; 96:2155.

80. Metz BK, White HD, Granger CB, et al. Randomized comparison of direct thrombin inhibition versus heparin in conjunction with fibrinolytic therapy for acute myocardial infarction: results from the GUSTO-IIb Trial. Global Use of Strategies to Open Occluded Coronary Arteries in Acute Coronary Syndromes (GUSTO-IIb) Investigators. *J Am Coll Cardiol* 1998;31:1493.

81. The Global Use of Strategies to Open Occluded Coronary Arteries (GUSTO IIb) Investigators. A comparison of recombinant hirudin with heparin for the treatment of acute coronary syndromes. *N Engl J Med* 1996;335:775.

82. Antman EM. Hirudin in acute myocardial infarction. Thrombolysis and Thrombin Inhibition in Myocardial Infarction (TIMI) 9B trial. *Circulation* 1996;94:911.

83. White HD. Thrombin-specific anticoagulation with bivalirudin versus heparin in patients receiving fibrinolytic therapy for acute myocardial infarction: the HERO-2 randomized trial. *Lancet* 2001;358:1855–1863.

84. Frostfeldt G, Ahlberg G, Gustafsson G, et al. Low molecular weight heparin (dalteparin) as adjuvant treatment of thrombolysis in acute myocardial infarction—a pilot study: biochemical markers in acute coronary syndromes (BIOMACS II). *J Am Coll Cardiol* 1999;33:627.

85. Fung AY, Lorch G, Cambier PA, et al. Efegatran sulfate as an adjunct to streptokinase versus heparin as an adjunct to tissue plasminogen activator in patients with acute myocardial infarction. ESCALAT Investigators. *Am Heart J* 1999;138:696.

86. Jang IK, Brown DF, Giugliano RP, et al. A multicenter, randomized study of argatroban versus heparin as adjunct to tissue plasminogen activator (TPA) in acute myocardial infarction: myocardial infarction with novastan and TPA (MINT) study. *J Am Coll Cardiol* 1999;33:1879.

87. Topol EJ, Ferguson JJ, Weisman HF, et al. Long-term protection from myocardial ischemic events in a randomized trial of brief integrin beta3 blockade with percutaneous coronary intervention. EPIC Investigator Group. Evaluation of Platelet IIb/IIIa Inhibition for Prevention of Ischemic Complication. *JAMA* 1997;278:479.

88. The RESTORE Investigators. Randomized Efficacy Study of Tirofiban for Outcomes and Restenosis: effects of platelet glycoprotein IIb/IIIa blockade with tirofiban on adverse cardiac events in patients with unstable angina or acute myocardial infarction undergoing coronary angioplasty. *Circulation* 1997;96:1445.

89. The EPILOG Investigators. Platelet glycoprotein IIb/IIIa receptor blockade and low-dose heparin during percutaneous coronary revascularization. *N Engl J Med* 1997;336:1689.

90. Ohman EM, Kleiman NS, Gacioch G, et al. IMPACT-AMI Investigators. Combined accelerated tissue-plasminogen activator and platelet glycoprotein IIb/IIIa integrin receptor blockade with Integrelin in acute myocardial

infarction. Results of a randomized, placebo-controlled, dose- ranging trial. *Circulation* 1997;95:846.

91. Topol EJ. Toward a new frontier in myocardial reperfusion therapy. Emerging platelet preeminence. *Circulation* 1998;97:211.

92. Strategies for Patency Enhancement in the Emergency Department (SPEED) Group. Trial of abciximab with and without low-dose reteplase for acute myocardial infarction. *Circulation* 2000;101:2788–2794.

93. Antman EM, Giugliano RP, Gibson CM et al, The TIMI 14 Investigators. Abciximab facilitates the rate and extent of thrombolysis: results of the thrombolysis in myocardial infarction (TIMI) 14 Trial. *Circulation* 1999;99:2720–2732.

94. The Assessment of the Safety and Efficacy of a New Thrombolytic Regimen (ASSENT)-3 Investigators. efficacy and safety of tenecteplase in combination with enoxaparin, abciximab, or unfractionated heparin: the ASSENT-3 randomized trial in acute myocardial infarction. *Lancet* 2001;358:605–613.

95. Topol EJ. Reperfusion therapy for acute myocardial infarction with fibrinolytic therapy or combination reduced fibrinolytic therapy and platelet glycoprotein IIb/IIIa inhibition: The GUSTO V randomized trial. *Lancet* 2001;357:1905–1914.

96. Alkjaersig N, Fletcher AP, Sherry S. The mechanism of clot dissolution by plasmin. *J Clin Invest* 1959;38:1086.

97. Lijnen HR, Collen D. Fibrinolytic agents: mechanisms of activity and pharmacology. *Thromb Haemost* 1995;74:387–390.

98. Onundarson PT, Francis CW, Marder VJ. Depletion of plasminogen *in vitro* or during thrombolytic therapy limits fibrinolytic potential. *J Lab Clin Med* 1992;120:120.

99. Badylak SF, Voytik SL, Henkin J, et al. Enhancement of the thrombolytic efficacy of prourokinase by lys-plasminogen in a dog model of arterial thrombosis. *Thromb Res* 1991;62:115.

100. Kakkar VV, Sagar S, Lewis M. Treatment of deep vein thrombosis with intermittent streptokinase and plasminogen infusion. *Lancet* 1975;2:674.

101. Giraud CL, Joffre F, Tasrini J, et al. Indications et resultats de l'association urokinase-lys plasminogene dans la pathologie ischemique aigue des membres inferieurs. *J Mal Vascul (Paris)* 1985;10:321.

102. deProst D, Guerot C, Laffay N, et al. Intra-coronary thrombolysis with streptokinase or lys-plasminogen/ urokinase in acute myocardial infarction: effects on recanalization and blood fibrinolysis. *Thromb Haemost* 1983;50:792.

103. Tsutsui JM, Grayburn PA, Xie F, et al. Drug and gene delivery and enhancement of thrombolysis using ultrasound and microbubbles. *Cardiol Clin* 2004;223:1291–1314.

104. Ariani M, Fishbein MC, Chae JS, et al. Dissolution of peripheral arterial thrombi by ultrasound. *Circulation* 1988;84:1680.

105. Everbach EC, Francis CW. Cavitational mechanisms in ultrasound-accelerated thrombolysis at 1 MHz. *Ultrasound Med Biol* 2000;26:1153–1160.

106. Birnbaum Y, Luo H, Nagai T, et al. Noninvasive *in vivo* clot dissolution without a thrombolytic drug. Recanalization of thrombosed ileofemoral arteries by transcutaneous ultrasound combined with intravenous infusion of microbubbles. *Circulation* 1998;97:130.

107. Suchkova VN, Baggs RB, Francis CW. Effect of 40 kHz ultrasound on acute thrombotic ischemia in a rabbit femoral artery thrombosis model: enhancement of thrombolysis and improvement in capillary muscle perfusion. *Circulation* 2000;101:2296–2301.

108. Rosenschein U, Rozenszajn LA, Kraus L, et al. Ultrasonic angioplasty in totally occluded peripheral arteries. Initial clinical, histological and angiographic results. *Circulation* 1991;83:1976.

109. Sakharov DV, Barrertt-Bergshoeff M, Hekkenberg RT, et al. Fibrin-specificity of a plasminogen activator affects the efficiency of fibrinolysis and responsiveness to ultrasound: comparison of nine plasminogen activators *in vitro*. *Thromb Haemost* 1999;81:605–612.

110. Alexandrov AV, Molina CA, Grotta JC, et al. Ultrasound-enhanced systemic thrombolysis for acute ischemic stroke. *N Engl J Med* 2004;351:2170–2178.

111. Ouriel K, Veith FJ, Sasahara AA. A comparison of recombinant urokinase with vascular surgery as initial treatment for acute arterial occlusion of the legs. *N Engl J Med* 1998;338:1105–1111.

112. Schweizer J, Kirch W, Koch R, et al. Short-and long-term results after thrombolytic treatment of deep venous thrombosis. *J Am Coll Cardiol* 2000;36:1336–1343.

113. Mewissen MW, Seabrook GR, Meissner MH, et al. Catheter-directed thrombolysis for lower extremity deep venous thrombosis: report of a national multicenter registry. *Radiology* 1999;211:39–49.

114. Comerota AJ, Throm RC, Mathias SD, et al. Catherter-directed thrombolysis for iliofemoral deep venous thrombosis improves health-related quality of life. *J Vasc Surg* 2000;32:130–137.

115. Ouriel K, Gray B, Clair DG, et al. Complications associated with the use of urokinase and recombinant tissue plasminogen activator for catheter-directed peripheral arterial and venous thrombolysis. *J Vasc Interv Radiol* 2000;11:295–298.

116. Furlan A, Higashida R, Wechsler L, et al. Intra-arterial prourokinase for acute ischemic stroke. The PROACT II Study: a randomized controlled trial. *JAMA* 1999;282:2003.

117. Anderson HR, Nielsen TT, Rasmussen K, et al. A comparison of coronary angioplasty with fibrinolytic therapy in acute myocardial infarction. *N Engl J Med* 2003;349:733–742.

118. Jacobs AK. Primary angioplasty for acute myocardial infarction—is it worth the wait? *N Engl J Med* 2003;349:798–800.

119. Sherry S, Fletcher AP, Alkjaersig N. Fibrinolysis and fibrinolytic activity in man. *Physiol Rev* 1959;39:343.

120. Loscalzo J, Vaughan DE. Tissue plasminogen activator promotes platelet disaggregation in plasma. *J Clin Invest* 1987;79:1749.

121. Adelman B, Michelson AD, Loscalzo J, et al. Plasmin effect on platelet glycoprotein IB-von Willebrand factor interactions. *Blood* 1985;65:32.

122. Rudd MA, George D, Amarante P, et al. Temporal effect of thrombolytic agents on platelet function *in vivo* and their modulation by prostaglandins. *Circ Res* 1990;67:1175.

123. Marder VJ. Relevance of changes in blood fibrinolytic and coagulation parameters during thrombolytic therapy. *Am J Med* 1987;83:15.

124. The Urokinase Pulmonary Embolism Trial. A national cooperative study. *Circulation* 1973;47(Suppl. II):1.

125. Marder VJ, Soulen RL, Atichartakarn V, et al. Quantitative venographic assessment of deep vein thrombosis in the evaluation of streptokinase and heparin therapy. *J Lab Clin Med* 1977;89:1018.

126. Rao AK, Pratt C, Berke A, et al. Thrombolysis in MI (TIMI) Trial—Phase I: hemorrhagic manifestations and changes in plasma fibrinogen and the fibrinolytic system in patients treated with recombinant tissue plasminogen activator and streptokinase. *J Am Coll Cardiol* 1988;11:1.

127. Gore JM, Sloan M, Price TR, et al. Intracerebral hemorrhage, cerebral infarction, and subdural hematoma after acute myocardial infarction and thrombolytic therapy in the thrombolysis in myocardial infarction study. *Circulation* 1991;83:448.

128. Stump DC, Califf RM, Topol EJ, et al. Pharmacodynamics of thrombolysis with recombinant tissue-type plasminogen activator. Correlation with characteristics of and clinical outcomes in patients with acute myocardial infarction. *Circulation* 1989;80:1222.

129. Carlson SE, Aldrich MS, Greenberg HS, et al. Intracerebral hemorrhage complicating intravenous tissue plasminogen activator treatment. *Arch Neurol* 1988;45:1070.

130. Berkowitz SD, Granger CB, Pieper KS, et al. Incidence and predictors of bleeding after contemporary thrombolytic therapy for myocardial infarction. The Global Utilization of Streptokinase and Tissue Plasminogen activator for Occluded coronary arteries (GUSTO) I Investigators. *Circulation* 1997;95:2508.

131. Bernardi MM, Califf RM, Kleiman N et al, The TAMI Study Group. Lack of usefulness of prolonged bleeding times in predicting hemorrhagic events in patients receiving the 7E3 glycoprotein IIb/IIIa platelet antibody. *Am J Cardiol* 1993;72:1121.

132. Berkowitz SD, Sane DC, Sigmon KN et al, Evaluation of c7E3 for the Prevention of Ischemic Complications (EPIC) Study Group. Occurrence and clinical significance of thrombocytopenia in a population undergoing high-risk percutaneous coronary revascularization. *J Am Coll Cardiol* 1998;32:311.

133. Sloan MA, Price TR, Petito CK, et al. Clinical features and pathogenesis of intracerebral hemorrhage after rt-PA and heparin therapy for acute myocardial infarct: the Thrombolysis in Myocardial Infarction (TIMI) II Pilot and Randomized Clinical Trial combined experience. *Neurology* 1995;45:649.

134. The Continuous Infusion Versus Double-Bolus Administration of Alteplase (COBALT) Investigators. A comparison of continuous infusion of alteplase with double-bolus administration for acute myocardial infarction. *N Engl J Med* 1997;337:1124.

135. The Global Use of Strategies to Open Occluded Coronary Arteries (GUSTO III) Investigators. A comparison of reteplase with alteplase for acute myocardial infarction. *N Engl J Med* 1997;337:1118.

136. White CW, Schwartz JL, Ferguson DW, et al. Systemic markers of fibrinolysis after unsuccessful intracoronary streptokinase thrombolysis for acute myocardial infarction: does nonreperfusion indicate failure to achieve a systemic lytic state? *Am J Cardiol* 1984;54:712.

137. Lawler CM, Bovill EG, Stump DC, et al. Fibrin fragment D-dimer and fibrinogen B beta peptides in plasma as markers of clot lysis during thrombolytic therapy in acute myocardial infarction. *Blood* 1990;76:1341.

138. Brenner B, Francis CW, Fitzpatrick PG, et al. Relation of plasma D- dimer concentrations to coronary artery reperfusion before and after thrombolytic treatment in patients with acute myocardial infarction. *Am J Cardiol* 1989;63:1179.

139. Chesebro JH, Knatterud G, Roberts R, et al. Thrombolysis in Myocardial Infarction (TIMI) Trial, phase 1: a comparison between intravenous tissue plasminogen activator and intravenous streptokinase. Clinical findings through hospital discharge. *Circulation* 1987;76:142.

140. Neuhaus KL, Tebbe U, Gottwik M, et al. Intravenous recombinant tissue plasminogen activator (rt-PA) and urokinase in acute myocardial infarction: results of the German Activator Urokinase Study (GAUS). *J Am Coll Cardiol* 1988;12:581.

141. Gruppo Italiano per lo Studio Della Streptochinase Nell'infarto Miocardico. Effectiveness of intravenous thrombolytic treatment in acute myocardial infarction. *Lancet* 1986;1:397.

142. Skinner JR, Phillips SJ, Zeff RJ, et al. Immediate coronary bypass following failed streptokinase infusion in evolving myocardial infarction. *J Thorac Cardiovasc Surg* 1984;87:567.

143. Anderson JL, Battistessa SA, Clayton PD, et al. Coronary bypass surgery early after thrombolytic therapy for acute myocardial infarction. *Ann Thorac Surg* 1986;41:176.

144. Lee KF, Mandell J, Rankin JS, et al. Immediate versus delayed coronary grafting after streptokinase treatment. Post-operative blood loss and clinical results. *J Thorac Cardiovasc Surg* 1988;95:216.

145. TIMI Research Group. Immediate vs. delayed catheterization and angioplasty following thrombolytic therapy for acute MI: TIMI IIA results. *JAMA* 1988;260:2849.

146. Mentzer RL, Budzynski AZ, Sherry S. High-dose, brief-duration intravenous infusion of streptokinase in acute myocardial infarction: description of effects in the circulation. *Am J Cardiol* 1986;57:1220.

147. Owen J, Friedman KD, Grossman BA, et al. Quantitation of fragment X formation during thrombolytic therapy with streptokinase and tissue plasminogen activator. *J Clin Invest* 1987;79:1642.

148. Nunn B, Esmail R, Fears R, et al. Pharmacokinetic properties of anisoylated plasminogen streptokinase activator complex and other thrombolytic agents in animals and in humans. *Drugs* 1987;33(Suppl. 3):88.

149. Goldhaber SZ, Heit J, Sharma GVRK, et al. Randomised controlled trial of recombinant tissue plasminogen activator versus urokinase in the treatment of acute pulmonary embolism. *Lancet* 1988;2:293.

150. Francis CW, Brenner B, Leddy JP, et al. Angioedema during therapy with recombinant tissue plasminogen activator. *Br J Haematol* 1991;77:562.

151. Third International Study of Infarct Survival Collaborative Group. ISIS-3: a randomized comparison of streptokinase vs. aspirin alone among 41,299 cases of suspected acute myocardial infarction. *Lancet* 1992;1:753.

152. Sicard GA, Schier JJ, Totty WG, et al. Thrombolytic therapy for acute arterial occlusion. *J Vasc Surg* 1985;2:65.

153. Queen M, Biem HJ, Moe GW, et al. Development of cholesterol embolization syndrome after intravenous streptokinase for acute myocardial infarction. *Am J Cardiol* 1990;65:1042.

# CHAPTER 122 ■ NEW THROMBOLYTIC AGENTS

H. ROGER LIJNEN AND DÉSIRÉ COLLEN

## ABSTRACT

Thrombolytic agents are plasminogen activators that induce fibrinolysis. The clinical benefits of thrombolytic therapy in patients with acute myocardial infarction (AMI) are well documented, and a close correlation between early coronary artery recanalization and clinical outcome is established. However, all currently used thrombolytic agents have considerable shortcomings, including the need for large therapeutic doses, limited fibrin-specificity, and significant associated bleeding tendency and reocclusion. Newly developed thrombolytic agents, mutants, and variants of the serine proteinases tissue-type plasminogen activator (tPA) or urokinase-type plasminogen activator (uPA), have reduced plasma clearance and lower reactivity with proteinase inhibitors, and maintained or enhanced plasminogen activator potency and/or fibrin-specificity. The nonenzyme bacterial plasminogen activator staphylokinase has also shown promise for fibrin-specific thrombolysis, although neutralizing antibodies are elicited in most patients. Furthermore, the use of adjunctive agents to thrombolytic therapy enhances benefit, whereas intravascular mechanical interventions increase long-term benefit. The therapeutic value of these new agents and approaches is presently being evaluated in large-scale randomized efficacy and safety studies in patients with thromboembolic disease.

## INTRODUCTION

Thrombolysis consists of the pharmacologic dissolution of a blood clot by intravenous infusion of plasminogen activators that activate the fibrinolytic system. The fibrinolytic system includes a proenzyme, plasminogen, which is converted by plasminogen activators to the active enzyme, plasmin, which in turn digests fibrin to soluble degradation products. Inhibition of the fibrinolytic system occurs by plasminogen activator inhibitors (mainly plasminogen activator inhibitor-1, PAI-1) and by plasmin inhibitors (mainly $\alpha_2$-antiplasmin). Presently available thrombolytic agents include streptokinase, recombinant tissue-type plasminogen activator (rtPA or alteplase), rtPA derivatives such as reteplase, lanoteplase, monteplase, and tenecteplase, anisoylated plasminogen-streptokinase activator complex (APSAC or anistreplase), two-chain urokinase-type plasminogen activator (tcuPA or urokinase), recombinant single-chain uPA (scuPA or pro-urokinase, saruplase), and recombinant staphylokinase and derivatives. Fibrin-selective agents (e.g., rtPA and derivatives, staphylokinase and derivatives and to a lesser extent scuPA) which digest the clot in the absence of systemic plasminogen activation are distinguished from non fibrin-selective agents (streptokinase, tcuPA, and APSAC) which activate systemic and fibrin-bound plasminogen relatively indiscriminately (see Fig. 122-1) (1,2). Some of these newer derivatives are under clinical investigation, mainly in patients with AMI, and also in patients with deep vein thrombosis, peripheral arterial occlusion, ischemic stroke, and pulmonary embolism. In patients with AMI, the addition of a variety of adjunctive agents to thrombolytic therapy enhances benefit with acceptable risk, and addition of intravascular angioplasty and stenting increases the potential long-term benefit (3–5). This chapter reviews the main properties of some of these newer agents with therapeutic potential for the treatment of patients with AMI.

## PHYSICOCHEMICAL PROPERTIES

### Tissue-Type Plasminogen Activator and Variants

Wild-type recombinant tPA (alteplase) was first obtained as a single-chain serine proteinase of 70 kDa, consisting of 527 amino acids with Ser as the $NH_2$-terminal amino acid; native tPA actually contains an $NH_2$-terminal extension of three amino acids, but in general, the initial numbering system has been maintained (see Fig. 122-2). Limited plasmic hydrolysis of the Arg275-Ile276 peptide bond converts tPA to a two-chain molecule (A chain comprising the $NH_2$-terminal and B chain comprising the COOH-terminal part) held together by one interchain disulfide bond. The tPA molecule contains four domains: (a) an $NH_2$-terminal region of 47-residues (residues 4 to 50) which is homologous with the finger domains of fibronectin; (b) residues 50 to 87 which are homologous with epidermal growth factor; (c) two kringle regions comprising residues 87 to 176 and 176 to 262 which are homologous with the five kringles of plasminogen; and (d) a serine proteinase domain (B chain, residues 276 to 527) with the active site residues His322, Asp371, and Ser478. There are three potential N-glycosylation sites, at Asn117, Asn184, and Asn448 (6). In contrast to the single-chain precursor form of most serine proteinases, single-chain tPA is enzymatically active. The normal plasma concentration of endogenous tPA is approximately 5 to 10 ng per mL, but varies strongly under different physiologic and pathologic conditions (2). Alteplase is obtained by expression in Chinese hamster ovary cells.

Structure–function analysis has revealed specific functions for the tPA domains. Therefore, high-affinity binding of tPA to fibrin is mediated by the finger and kringle 2 domains; stimulation of its activity by fibrin also involves the finger, (possibly also kringle 1) and kringle 2 domains; in vivo clearance is regulated by the finger and growth factor domains and by the carbohydrate side chains; rapid inhibition by PAI-1 requires a

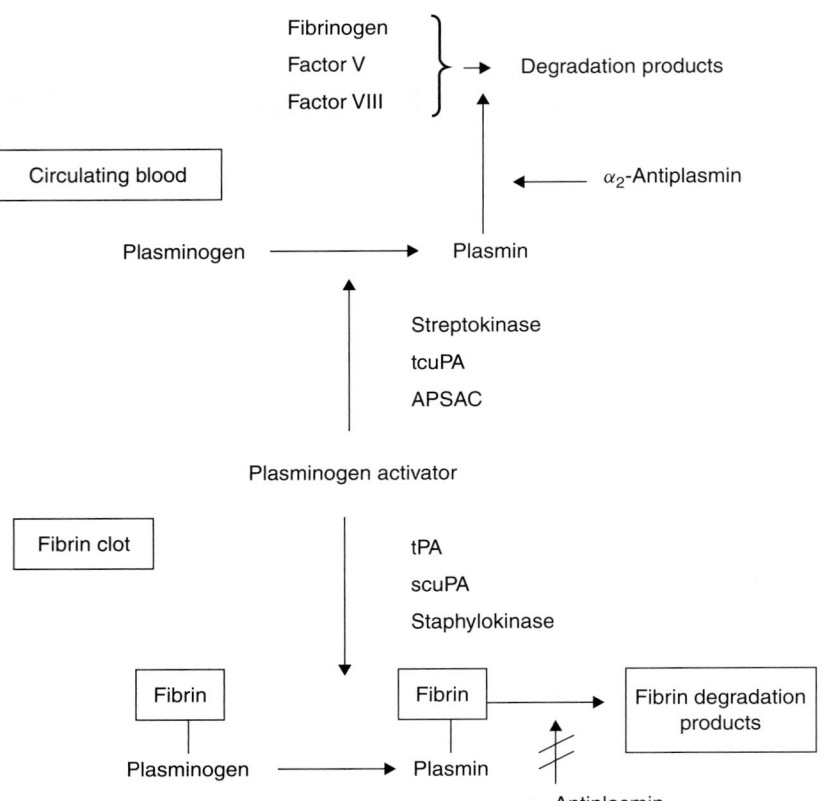

**FIGURE 122-1.** Schematic representation of the fibrinolytic system and of molecular interactions determining the fibrin-selectivity of plasminogen activators. The proenzyme plasminogen is activated to the active enzyme plasmin by plasminogen activators. Plasmin degrades fibrin into soluble fibrin degradation products. Inhibition of the fibrinolytic system may occur by plasminogen activator inhibitors (mainly PAI-1) or by plasmin inhibitors (mainly $\alpha_2$-antiplasmin). Nonfibrin-selective plasminogen activators [streptokinase, two-chain urokinase-type plasminogen activator (tcuPA), anisoylated plasminogen streptokinase activator complex (APSAC)] activate both plasminogen in the circulating blood and fibrin-associated plasminogen. Generated plasmin is rapidly inactivated by $\alpha_2$-antiplasmin and will, after saturation of the inhibitor, degrade other plasma proteins. Fibrin-selective plasminogen activators [tissue-type plasminogen activator (tPA), single-chain urokinase-type plasminogen activator (scuPA) and staphylokinase] preferentially active fibrin-associated plasminogen. Generated plasmin remains associated with fibrin and is protected from rapid inhibition by $\alpha_2$-antiplasmin.

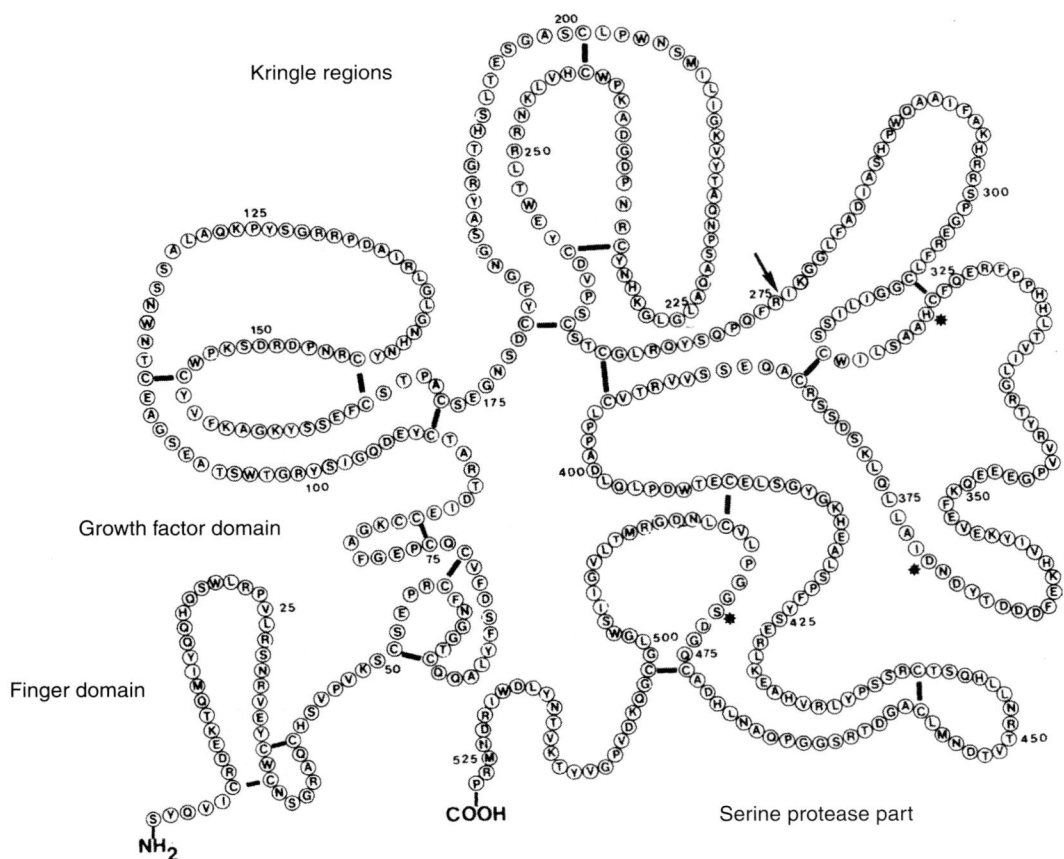

**FIGURE 122-2.** Schematic representation of the primary structure of recombinant tissue-type plasminogen activator (rtPA). The amino acids are represented by their single letter symbols and *black bars* indicate disulphide bonds. The active site residues are indicated with an *asterisk*. The *arrow* indicates the plasmin cleavage site for conversion of single-chain to two-chain rtPA.

second-site interaction with the positively charged amino acid sequence at position 296–304; and the enzymatic activity resides in the serine proteinase domain (2). By deletion or substitution of such functional domains, by site-specific point mutations, and/or by altering the carbohydrate composition, mutants of rtPA have been produced with higher fibrin-specificity, more zymogenicity, slower clearance from the circulation, and resistance to plasma proteinase inhibitors.

Reteplase (Rapilysin or Ecokinase) is a single-chain nonglycosylated deletion variant consisting only of the kringle 2 and the proteinase domain of human tPA; it contains amino acids 1–3 and 176–527 (deletion of Val4-Glu175); the Arg275-Ile276 plasmin cleavage site is maintained (7). In tenecteplase (TNK-rtPA), replacement of Asn117 with Gln (N117Q) deletes the glycosylation site in kringle 1, whereas substitution of Thr[103] by Asn (T103N) reintroduces a glycosylation site in kringle 1, but at a different locus; these modifications substantially decrease the plasma clearance rate. In addition, the amino acids Lys296-His297-Arg298-Arg299 are each replaced with Ala, which confers resistance to inhibition by PAI-1 (8). Lanoteplase is a deletion mutant of rtPA (without the finger and growth factor domains) in which glycosylation at Asn117 is lacking (9). Monteplase has a single amino acid substitution in the growth factor domain (Cys84 to Ser) (10); pamiteplase has deletion of the kringle 1 domain and substitution of Arg275 to Glu (rendering it resistant to conversion to a two-chain molecule by plasmin) (11).

In addition, different molecular forms of the Desmodus salivary plasminogen activator (DSPA) have been characterized. Two high $M_r$ forms, DSPA$\alpha_1$ (43 kDa) and DSPA$\alpha_2$ (39 kDa) show approximately 85% homology with human tPA, but contain neither a kringle 2 domain nor a plasmin-sensitive cleavage site. DSPA$\beta$ lacks the finger domain and DSPA$\gamma$ lacks the finger and growth factor domains (12).

## Urokinase-Type Plasminogen Activator Moieties

uPA is secreted as a 54-kDa single-chain molecule (scuPA, pro-urokinase) that can be converted to a two-chain form (tcuPA). uPA is a serine proteinase of 411 amino acids, with active site triad His204, Asp255, and Ser356 located in the serine proteinase (COOH-terminal) domain (see Fig. 122-3). The molecule contains an NH$_2$-terminal growth factor domain and one kringle structure homologous to the kringles of plasminogen and tPA (13); it contains only one N-glycosylation site (at Asn302), and is fucosylated at Thr18. Conversion of scuPA to tcuPA occurs after proteolytic cleavage at position Lys158–Ile159 by plasmin, but also by kallikrein, trypsin, cathepsin B, human T cell associated serine proteainse-1 and thermolysin. A fully active tcuPA derivative is obtained after additional proteolysis by plasmin at position Lys135–Lys136. A low $M_r$ form of scuPA generated by cleavage of the Glu143–Leu144 peptide bond has also been recognized. Recombinant scuPA (saruplase) is expressed in *Escherichia coli* and obtained as a 45-kDa nonglycosylated molecule.

Amediplase, a recombinant chimeric plasminogen activator consisting of the kringle 2 domain of the tPA, A chain and the COOH-terminal region of scuPA, is being evaluated for bolus administration to patients with AMI (14).

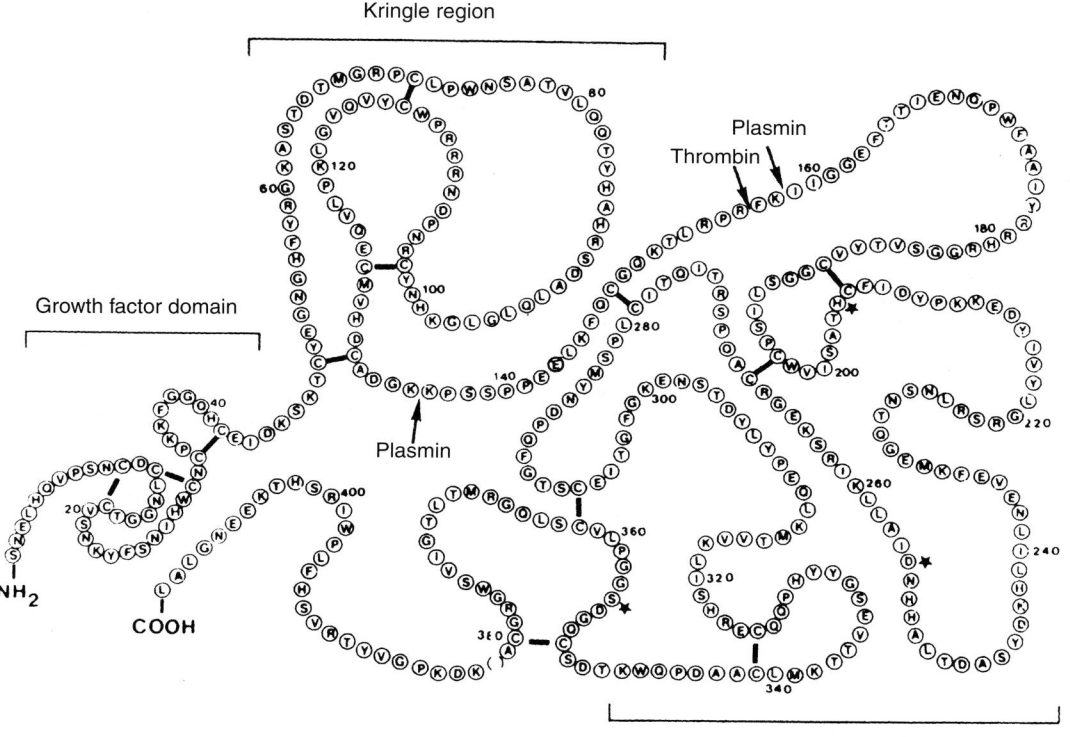

**FIGURE 122-3.** Schematic representation of the primary structure of single-chain urokinase-type plasminogen activator (scuPA). The amino acids are represented by their single letter symbols and *black bars* indicate disulphide bonds. The active site residues are indicated with an *asterisk*. The *arrows* indicate the plasmin cleavage sites for conversion of 54-kDa scuPA to 54-kDa tcuPA and of 54-kDa two-chain urokinase-type plasminogen activator (tcuPA) to 33-kDa tcuPA, and for conversion to inactive 54-kDa tcuPA by thrombin.

## Staphylokinase and Derivatives

Staphylokinase (Sak) is a 135–amino acid protein (comprising 45 charged amino acids, no cysteine residues nor glycosylation), secreted by *Staphylococcus aureus* strains after lysogenic conversion or transformation with bacteriophages. The primary structure of Sak shows no homology with that of other plasminogen activators. Staphylokinase folds into a compact ellipsoid structure in which the core of the protein is composed exclusively of hydrophobic amino acids. It is folded into a mixed five-stranded, slightly twisted β-sheet which wraps around a central α-helix and has two additional short two-stranded β-sheets opposing the central sheet (15). Recombinant Sak is obtained by expression in *Escherichia coli* (16–18).

Being a heterologous protein, Sak is immunogenic in humans. Wild-type Sak contains three immunodominant epitopes. A comprehensive site-directed mutagenesis program resulted in the identification of variants with reduced antigenicity, but maintained fibrinolytic potency and fibrin-specificity, such as SakSTAR (K35A, E65Q, K74R, D82A, S84A, T90A, E99D, T101S, E108A, K109A, K130T, K135R) (code SY 155) and SakSTAR (K35A, E65Q, K74R, E80A, D82A, T90A, E99D, T101S, E108A, K109A, K130T, K135R) (code SY 161). (19). Furthermore, SY 161 with Ser in position 3 mutated into Cys, was derived with maleimide-substituted polyethylene glycol (P) with molecular weights of 5,000 Da (P5), 10,000 Da (P10) or 20,000 Da (P20), and characterized *in vitro* and *in vivo* (20).

# MECHANISM OF ACTION

## Tissue-Type Plasminogen Activator and Variants

tPA is a poor enzyme in the absence of fibrin, but the presence of fibrin strikingly enhances the activation rate of plasminogen (21). Activation of plasminogen to plasmin occurs after proteolytic cleavage of the Arg561–Val562 peptide bond. During fibrinolysis, fibrinogen and fibrin are continuously modified by cleavage with thrombin or plasmin, yielding a diversity of reaction products (22). Optimal stimulation of tPA is only obtained after early plasmin cleavage in the COOH-terminal Aα chain and the NH2-terminal Bβ chain of fibrin, yielding fragment X-polymer. Kinetic data support a mechanism in which fibrin provides a surface to which tPA and plasminogen adsorb in a sequential and ordered way, yielding a cyclic ternary complex (21). Formation of this complex results in an enhanced affinity of tPA for plasminogen, yielding up to three orders of magnitude higher catalytic efficiencies for plasminogen activation. This is mediated at least in part by COOH-terminal lysine residues generated by plasmin cleavage of fibrin. Plasmin formed at the fibrin surface has both its lysine binding sites and active site occupied and is therefore only slowly inactivated by α2-antiplasmin (half-life of approximately 10 to 100 seconds); in contrast, free plasmin, when formed, is rapidly inhibited by α2-antiplasmin (half-life of approximately 0.1 second) (23). These molecular interactions mediate the fibrin-specificity of tPA (Fig. 122-1).

Reteplase has a similar plasminogenolytic activity as wild-type rtPA in the absence of a stimulator, but its activity in the presence of a stimulator is fourfold lower, and its binding to fibrin is fivefold lower. Reteplase and rtPA are inhibited by PAI-1 to a similar degree (7). Tenecteplase (TNK-rtPA) has a similar ability as wild-type rtPA to bind to fibrin, and lyses fibrin clots in a plasma milieu with enhanced fibrin-specificity and delayed inhibition by PAI-1 (8). DSPAα1 and DSPAα2 exhibit a specific activity *in vitro* that is equal to or higher than that of rtPA, a relative PAI-1 resistance, and a greatly enhanced fibrin-specificity with a strict requirement for polymeric fibrin as a cofactor (12).

## Urokinase-Type Plasminogen Activator Moieties

In contrast to tcuPA, scuPA displays very low activity toward low-molecular-weight chromogenic substrates, but it appears to have some intrinsic plasminogen activating potential, which represents 0.5% or less of the catalytic efficiency of tcuPA (24,25). In plasma, in the absence of fibrin, scuPA is stable and does not activate plasminogen; however, in the presence of a fibrin clot, scuPA, but not tcuPA, induces fibrin-specific clot lysis (24). This was explained by the findings that scuPA is an inefficient activator of plasminogen bound to internal lysine residues on intact fibrin, but has a higher activity toward plasminogen bound to newly generated COOH-terminal lysine residues on partially degraded fibrin (26,27).

Amediplase, containing the tPA kringle 2, displays a lower fibrin binding than rtPA, but has a higher clot-penetrating potency, similar to that of tcuPA (28).

## Staphylokinase and Derivatives

Sak forms a 1:1 stoichiometric complex with plasmin. It is not an enzyme, and generation of an active site in its equimolar complex with plasminogen requires conversion of plasminogen to plasmin. In plasma, in the absence of fibrin, there are no significant amounts of plasmin. Sak complexes are generated because traces of plasmin are inhibited by α2-antiplasmin. In the presence of fibrin, generation of the active complex is facilitated because traces of fibrin-bound plasmin are protected from α2-antiplasmin, and inhibition of the complex by α2-antiplasmin at the clot surface is delayed more than 100-fold. Furthermore, Sak does not bind to a considerable extent to plasminogen in circulating plasma, but binds with high affinity to plasmin and to plasminogen which is bound to partially degraded fibrin (29–31). During the activation process, the 10 NH2-terminal amino acids of Sak are cleaved off. With SY 161-P5, this results in the removal of the polyethylene glycol moiety.

# THROMBOLYTIC PROPERTIES

## Tissue-Type Plasminogen Activator and Variants

Because of its fibrin-specific mechanism of plasminogen activation, tPA has been developed for thrombolytic therapy. Following several pilot studies with natural tPA produced by Bowes melanoma cells, rtPA was administered to patients with AMI (1). It was shown to be effective and to be cleared from the circulation with an initial half-life of 4 to 8 minutes (32). Numerous clinical trials have since compared the thrombolytic properties of rtPA (alteplase, Activase, Actilyse) with those of other agents, culminating in the Global Use of Strategies to Open Occluded Coronary Arteries (GUSTO) trial and its angiographic substudy (33,34) which conclusively established the potential and limitations of rtPA for thrombolytic therapy in patients with AMI.

In the GUSTO trial, a dose of 15 mg intravenous bolus of alteplase followed by 0.75 mg per kg over 30 minutes (not to exceed 50 mg) and then 0.50 mg per kg over 60 minutes (not to exceed 35 mg) was utilized. In the Continuous Infusion Versus Double-Bolus Administration of Alteplase (COBALT) trial, double bolus administration of rtPA (50 mg given 30 minutes apart) was evaluated in patients with myocardial infarction (MI) (35). Whichever regimen is used, it is important to coadminister intravenous heparin during and after alteplase treatment.

The rapid *in vivo* clearance of rtPA, necessitating the use of large therapeutic doses, and the occurrence of bleeding complications and reocclusion, has triggered the search for improved rtPA moieties. Mutants of rtPA with higher fibrin-specificity, more zymogenicity, slower clearance from the circulation and resistance to plasma proteinase inhibitors have been constructed (reviewed in 36,37), and are presently under investigation in pilot studies, mainly in patients with AMI. The main advantage of these newer agents appears to be their prolonged half-life, allowing bolus administration [reviewed in (38–40)].

Therefore, reteplase has an initial half-life of 14 to 18 minutes. In the GUSTO-III trial, approximately 15,000 patients with AMI were randomly assigned to receive reteplase [two boluses of 10 million units (MU) given 30 minutes apart] or 100 mg alteplase over 90 minutes. No clinical benefit of reteplase over alteplase was demonstrated, in terms of 30-day mortality or frequency of hemorrhagic stroke, leading to the conclusion that both agents are equivalent (41). Feasibility and timing of prehospital administration of reteplase in patients with AMI is under investigation (42,43).

Tenecteplase has an initial half-life of $17 \pm 7$ minutes in patients with AMI (44,45). In the TIMI-10B trial, a phase II efficacy trial, a single bolus of 40 mg tenecteplase yielded similar TIMI-3 flow rates at 90 minutes as accelerated rtPA, with faster and more complete reperfusion (46). In the Assessment of the Safety and Efficacy of a New Thrombolytic Regimen (ASSENT)-2 study (approximately 17,000 patients with AMI of less than 6 hours) 0.53 mg per kg bolus tenecteplase yielded similar 30-day mortality and rate of intracranial bleeding as front-loaded alteplase (47). This weight-adjusted dose was determined after evaluation of efficacy and safety in dose-ranging studies (48,49). One year after randomization, mortality rates were still similar in patients treated with tenecteplase or alteplase (50). Furthermore, it was shown that single bolus administration of tenecteplase did not increase the risk of intracranial hemorrhage, but was associated with less noncerebral bleeding, especially among high-risk patients (51). A prospective electrocardiograph substudy revealed that the extent of ST resolution at 24 to 36 hours after treatment was influenced by time to treatment and inversely related to 1-year mortality rates (52). In another substudy of ASSENT-2, the antiplatelet properties (inhibition of aggregation and function) of tenecteplase were more pronounced than those of rtPA; this may be relevant to studies on combination therapy with thrombolytic and antiplatelet agents in patients with AMI (53). The thrombolytic properties of tenecteplase in patients with AMI have been reviewed in detail (54).

With lanoteplase, given as a single bolus in the "Intravenous n-PA for Treating Infarcting Myocardium Early (InTIME-2)" trial (approximately 15,000 patients), the 30-day mortality was similar to that obtained with front-loaded alteplase, but the rate of intracerebral hemorrhage was considerably increased in the lanoteplase group (55). Following single bolus administration of lanoteplase, a plasma half-life of approximately 35 minutes was observed, and at a dose of 120 kU per kg the plasminogen activator activity persisted for 6 hours as compared with less than 4 hours after 100 mg alteplase (56).

Monteplase has a half-life of 23 minutes following bolus injection of 0.22 mg per kg (57,58). In the Fibrinolysis And Subsequent Transluminal (FAST) trial, the efficacy and safety of thrombolysis with monteplase and subsequent transluminal therapy for the early achievement of TIMI-3 flow was evaluated in patients with AMI. The intervention resulted in significant reduction of the time to reach TIMI-3 flow as compared to thrombolysis with monteplase alone, without complications or effects on 30-day mortality. TIMI-3 flow was achieved at an earlier stage with a single bolus of monteplase as compared with an accelerated infusion of rtPA (59). Patency rates obtained with monteplase in patients with AMI, were found to be independent of the PAI-1 levels (60).

Pamiteplase has a half-life of 30 to 47 minutes following single bolus injection of 0.5 to 4 mg in human volunteers (61); it was investigated in a dose-finding study in patients with AMI (62), but no large-scale trial on safety or mortality was reported.

In several animal models of thrombolysis, $DSPA\alpha_1$ (desmoteplase) has a 2.5 times higher potency and four- to eightfold slower clearance than rtPA ( 36,37). Pilot studies have been performed in patients with AMI, but at present desmoteplase is mainly investigated in patients with stroke or pulmonary embolism. Desmoteplase In Acute ischemic Stroke (DIAS) and Dose Escalation Study of Desmoteplase in Acute ischemic Stroke (DEDAS) are placebo-controlled double blind and randomized phase II studies in ischemic stroke; Desmoteplase in Pulmonary Thromboembolism (DEPTH) is an open randomized phase II study in patients with massive pulmonary embolism. Results from these studies are not published at present.

## Urokinase-Type Plasminogen Activator Moieties

The main mechanism of removal of uPA from the blood is by hepatic clearance. scuPA is taken up in the liver by a recognition site on parenchymal cells and is subsequently degraded in the lysosomes (63). Following intravenous infusion of natural or recombinant scuPA in patients with AMI, a biphasic disappearance was observed with initial half-lives in plasma (postinfusion) of 4 minutes or 8 minutes, respectively (64,65).

With a preparation containing 160,000 IU per mg of saruplase, the dose used successfully in patients with AMI (PRIMI, Pro-urokinase in Myocardial Infarction Study) was 20 mg given as a bolus and 60 mg over the next 60 minutes, immediately followed by an intravenous heparin infusion (20 IU/kg/hour) for 72 hours (66). Early patency rate at 60 minutes [Thrombolysis in Myocardial Infarction (TIMI) grade 2 and 3 flow] was significantly higher with saruplase (71.8%) than with streptokinase 48%. A 5-year follow up of the PRIMI trial indicated similar long-term outcome in terms of mortality and cardiovascular events in patients treated with saruplase or streptokinase, and somewhat lower reinfarction rates but higher stroke rates in the streptokinase group (67). In the Study in Europe with Saruplase and Alteplase in Myocardial Infarction (SESAM), 60-minute patency rates were 79.9% with saruplase versus 75.3% with alteplase, and 90-minute patency rates were 79.9% versus 81.4%, respectively (68). In the Liquaemin in Myocardial Infarction during Thrombolysis with Saruplase (LIMITS) study in patients with AMI, the same dose regimen of saruplase was used, but with a prethrombolytic heparin bolus of 5,000 IU and an intravenous heparin infusion for 5 days starting 30 minutes after completion of thrombolysis (69). The reocclusion rates within 24 to 40 hours were between 0.9% and 2.4% in the saruplase studies. In the Pro-urokinase and tPA Enhancement of Thrombolysis (PATIENT) trial, sequential combination of low-dose rtPA (5 to 10 mg bolus and reduced dose prourokinase (90 minutes infusion at 40 mg per hour), produced high TIMI-2 or -3 patency rate (77%), was well tolerated and was associated with low 24-hour reocclusion rate (70). A recombinant glycosylated form of pro-urokinase (A-74187) has also been evaluated in patients with AMI using 60 or 80 mg monotherapy or 60 mg primed with a preceding bolus of 250,000 IU of recombinant tcuPA, always combined with aspirin and intravenous heparin (71).

Recombinant prourokinase has also been evaluated for intraarterial administration to patients with middle cerebral artery occlusion treated within 6 hours of stroke onset. The clinical efficiency and safety has been demonstrated in the Prolyse in Acute Cerebral Thromboembolism (PROACT) I and II trials (72,73).

## Staphylokinase and Derivatives

Intravenous staphylokinase (10 or 20 mg), combined with heparin and aspirin, was shown to be a potent, rapidly acting, and highly fibrin-selective thrombolytic agent in patients with AMI (29–31). The Collaborative Angiographic Patency Trial Of Recombinant Staphylokinase (CAPTORS) studied the optimal dose (15 to 45 mg) required to achieve TIMI-3 flow at 90 minutes with an acceptable safety profile (74). Surprisingly, TIMI-3 patency rates were independent of the dose given.

A multicenter randomized trial compared the effects of double bolus staphylokinase administration versus accelerated and weight-adjusted rtPA on early coronary artery patency in patients with AMI (75). Patients randomized to double bolus staphylokinase were given 15 mg over 5 minutes, with a second bolus of 15 mg 30 minutes later. Sixty eight percent of the patients receiving double bolus staphylokinase had TIMI-3 flow after 90 minutes, versus 57% after rtPA administration. At 24 hours, TIMI perfusion grade 3 rates were 100% in the staphylokinase group, and 79% in the tPA-treated group ($P = 0.005$). This difference at 24 hours is possibly related to the low procoagulant and proaggregatory side effects of staphylokinase (76). The rates of hemorrhagic, mechanical, and electrical complications did not considerably differ between treatment groups. Double bolus administration of staphylokinase also preserved plasma fibrinogen, plasminogen, and $\alpha_2$-antiplasmin levels to a higher degree than rtPA.

However, most patients developed high titers of neutralizing specific IgG after infusion of staphylokinase, which would predict therapeutic refractoriness upon repeated administration. Efforts have been undertaken to reduce the immunogenicity of staphylokinase by site-directed mutagenesis and to reduce the plasma clearance by derivation with polyethylene glycol. Staphylokinase-related antigen following bolus injection of SY161-P5, SY161-P10 or SY161-P20 in patients disappeared from plasma with an initial half-life of 13, 30, and 120 minutes and was cleared at a rate of 75, 43, and 8 mL per minute, respectively, as compared to an initial half-life of 3 minutes and a clearance of 360 mL per minute for wild-type staphylokinase (20). Intravenous bolus injection of 5 mg of SY161-P5, in 18 patients with AMI, restored TIMI-3 flow at 60 minutes in 14 patients. In a multicenter dose-range finding angiographic trial (CAPTORS II), doses of 0.01 to 0.05 mg per kg SY161-P5 yielded similar 60 minute TIMI-2 or -3 patency rates as rtPA (77). Further studies with (pegylated) staphylokinase variants will be required to define the optimal efficacy and safety profile in patients with AMI.

# ADJUNCTIVE THERAPY TO THROMBOLYSIS WITH PLASMINOGEN ACTIVATORS

In the absence of adjunctive therapy, a substantial number of patients with AMI successfully treated with thrombolytic agents, will develop reocclusion (1). Platelet activation and aggregation contribute to rethrombosis. Therefore, antiplatelet agents, such as aspirin, ticlopidine, and clopidogrel, alone or in combination are used after coronary angioplasty or successful thrombolysis. Platelet aggregation is mediated by activation of the platelet membrane GP IIb/IIIa receptor and subsequent cross-linking with fibrinogen. Pharmacologic blockade of GP IIb/IIIa will interfere with the final common pathway for arterial thrombus formation, irrespective of the mode of platelet activation. The first platelet GP IIb/IIIa receptor antagonist was the chimeric 7E3 (ReoPro) monoclonal antibody (78). Several antiplatelet agents (e.g., abciximab or 7E3, eptifibatide, tirofiban, ticlopidine, clopidogrel), with mechanisms differing from that of aspirin, show efficacy in reducing the incidence of thrombotic occlusion after restoration of arterial blood flow (79). In patients with AMI, combination reperfusion therapy with half-dose reteplase and abciximab did not considerably reduce 30-day or 1-year mortality (GUSTO V) compared with full-dose reteplase (80,81). The combination therapy led to a consistent reduction in secondary complications of MI including reinfarction, which was, however, partly counterbalanced by increased nonintracranial bleeding complications (80). In patients who underwent prior coronary artery bypass grafting, combination therapy also led to a consistent reduction in recurrent ischemia and a trend toward reduced urgent revascularization (82). Recently, the Integrelin and Tenecteplase in Acute Myocardial Infarction (INTEGRITI) phase II angiographic trial revealed that double bolus eptifibatide plus half-dose tenecteplase tended to improve angiographic flow and ST segment resolution compared with tenecteplase monotherapy, but this strategy was associated with more transfusions and noncerebral bleeding (83). Bioavailability and short pharmacologic half-life represent main problems for the clinical use of low $M_r$ GP IIb/IIIa receptor antagonists (84).

The pivotal role of thrombin in the initiation and propagation of intracoronary thrombus formation has stimulated the development of therapies that block thrombin generation or activity (85). Direct thrombin inhibitors are theoretically likely to be more effective than indirect thrombin inhibitors, such as unfractionated heparin or low-molecular-weight heparin (LMWH), because the heparins block only circulating thrombin, whereas direct thrombin inhibitors block both circulating and clot-bound thrombin. Several initial phase III trials did not demonstrate a convincing benefit of direct thrombin inhibitors over unfractionated heparin. However, the Direct Thrombin Inhibitor Trialists' Collaboration metaanalysis confirmed the superiority of direct thrombin inhibitors, particularly hirudin and bivalirudin, over unfractionated heparin for the prevention of death or MI during treatment in patients with acute coronary syndromes, primarily due to a reduction in MI (odds ratio 0.80; 95% confidence interval 0.70 to 0.91) with little impact on death. The absolute risk reduction in the composite of death or MI at the end of treatment (0.8%) was similar at 30 days (0.7%), indicating no loss of benefit after cessation of therapy. Supportive evidence for the superiority of direct thrombin inhibitors over heparin derives from the Hirulog and Early Reperfusion or Occlusion (HERO)-2 randomized trial with ST segment elevation acute coronary syndromes, which demonstrated a similar benefit of bivalirudin over heparin for the prevention of death or MI at 30 days (absolute risk resolution 1.0%), again primarily due to a reduction in MI during treatment (odds ratio, 0.70; 95% confidence interval, 0.56 to 0.87), with little impact on death (86).

Indirect antithrombin therapy with unfractionated heparin depends on its anti-IIa (thrombin) and anti-Xa activity. The current guidelines for treating patients with ST segment elevation MI undergoing thrombolysis with alteplase recommend a dose of adjunctive unfractionated heparin, 60 IU per kg bolus, administered on initiation of alteplase. This should be followed by an initial maintenance dose of approximately 12 IU/kg/hour adjusted to maintain an activated partial thromboplastin time of 1.5 to two times control (50 to 70 seconds) for 48 hours, or longer if there is a pronounced risk of thromboembolism.

Unfractionated heparin has several pharmacologic and practical disadvantages, such as the need for laboratory monitoring due to lack of predictability of anticoagulant response. The use of unfractionated heparin has also been associated with side effects (e.g., thrombocytopenia), so that alternative antithrombotics such as LMWH and the pentasaccharides have been evaluated. The advantages of LMWH over unfractionated heparin include greater ease of administration, more favorable anti-Xa to anti-IIa activity ratios, and more predictable pharmacokinetics, which eliminates the need for laboratory monitoring and subsequent dose-adjustment in many patients.

Efficacy and safety of tenecteplase in combination with LMWH (enoxaparin), unfractionated heparin or abciximab in patients with AMI was evaluated in the ASSENT-3 study (87). The tenecteplase plus enoxaparin or abciximab regimens reduced the frequency of ischemic complications as compared to unfractionated heparin. Also in a prehospital setting the combination of tenecteplase with enoxaparin reduced early ischemic events, but the optimal dose of enoxaparin especially in older patients still needs to be determined (88). The ENTIRE-TIMI 23 trial confirmed that the combination of tenecteplase with enoxaparin presented advantages over unfractionated heparin with respect to ischemic events through 30 days while achieving similar early TIMI-3 flow rates and similar risk of major hemorrhage (89). The evolution of thrombolytic therapy and adjunctive antithrombotic regimens in acute ST segment elevation MI (90) and the specific roles of LMWH (91) have recently been reviewed.

A quantitative review of 23 randomized trials comparing primary percutaneous transluminal coronary angioplasty (PTCA) versus intravenous thrombolytic therapy for AMI concluded that primary PTCA is more effective for the treatment of ST-segment elevation AMI (4). The TIMI-14 trial concluded that a combination regimen including abciximab and early adjunctive percutaneous coronary intervention (PCI) is associated with improved ST segment resolution after thrombolysis with alteplase or reteplase (5). Current perspectives in integrating pharmacologic and mechanical reperfusion strategies for treatment of acute ST segment elevation MI have been extensively reviewed (92).

## PLASMIN AND DERIVATIVES

Plasmin cleaves fibrinogen and fibrin directly, preferentially after Lys and Arg residues. The main plasmin inhibitor is $\alpha_2$-antiplasmin, a 70-kDa single-chain glycoprotein containing approximately 13% carbohydrate and 464 amino acids. $\alpha_2$-antiplasmin is a serpin with reactive site peptide bond Arg376–Met377. Its concentration in normal human plasma is approximately 7 mg per 100 mL (approximately 1 $\mu$M). $\alpha_2$-antiplasmin forms an inactive 1:1 stoichiometric complex with plasmin. The inhibition of plasmin (P) by $\alpha_2$-antiplasmin (A) can be represented by two consecutive reactions: a fast, second-order reaction producing a reversible inactive complex (PA), which is followed by a slower first-order transition resulting in an irreversible complex (PA'). This model can be represented by: $P + A \rightleftarrows PA \rightarrow PA'$. The second-order rate constant of the inhibition of plasmin by $\alpha_2$-antiplasmin is very high (2 to $4 \times 10^7$/M/second),but this high inhibition rate is dependent both on the presence of a free lysine binding site and active site in the plasmin molecule and on the availability of a plasminogen-binding site and reactive site peptide bond in the inhibitor (93). The half-life of plasmin molecules on the fibrin surface, which have both their lysine binding sites and active site occupied, is estimated to be 2 to 3 orders of magnitude longer than that of free

plasmin (94). Also plasmin moieties lacking the lysine binding sites in kringles 1 to 4 show significantly reduced inhibition rates by $\alpha_2$-antiplasmin.

Because of the rapid inhibition of plasmin by $\alpha_2$-antiplasmin and the limited substrate specificity of excess circulating plasmin, systemic administration of plasmin for thrombolytic therapy is generally not considered to be a valid option. In the 1950s and 1960s intravenous plasmin for thrombolytic therapy had been investigated in pilot studies in humans. Although plasmin was generally well tolerated, these studies were discontinued, probably because of a lack of understanding of the kinetics of the inhibition of plasmin in plasma ($\alpha_2$-antiplasmin was not yet discovered), the unavailability of local catheter delivery, and the lack of adequate methods for the production of stable plasmin devoid of plasminogen activators (95,96). However, recently reexamination of local administration of plasmin for arterial and venous thrombolysis was suggested. This was triggered by the report by Marder et al. showing that plasmin-induced local thrombolysis without causing hemorrhage in the rabbit (95). Hypothetical advances of plasmin over plasminogen activators would be: (a) no activation is needed; (b) local delivery allows it to attach to and lyse thrombi; and (c) after thrombolysis circulating plasmin is rapidly neutralized by $\alpha_2$-antiplasmin (95,96). These considerations would suggest that local plasmin administration would not cause rebleeding from performed hemostatic plugs and be efficient and safe for the dissolution of long, and retracted blood clots (95,97).

Development of adequate methods to produce highly purified and stable natural human plasmin (98) or recombinant human microplasmin (99) preparations have made it possible to reinvestigate the potential of plasmin or derivatives thereof as a fibrinolytic agent. Studies in animal models indicate that plasmin or derivatives may be useful for treatment of deep vein thrombosis and arterial occlusion (95,100), and ischemic stroke (99,101,102). Nagai et al. reported a reduction in infarct size in mice with a permanent ligation of the middle cerebral artery, with a bolus of human plasmin, which was associated with the neutralization of plasma $\alpha_2$-antiplasmin (101). The studies of Stewart et al. (103) suggest that plasmin has a sixfold margin of safety (absence of bleeding complication) over the thrombolytic dosage, in contrast with tPA, which causes bleeding even at half of the usual thrombolytic dosage.

## References

1. Collen D. Thrombolytic therapy. *Thromb Haemost* 1997;78:742–746.
2. Lijnen HR, Collen D. Tissue-type plasminogen activator. In: Barrett AJ, Rawlings ND, Woessner JF, eds. *Handbook of proteolytic enzymes*. London: Academic Press, 1998:184–190.
3. Baker WF Jr. Thrombolytic therapy. *Clin Appl Thromb Hemost* 2002;8:291–314.
4. Keeley EC, Boura JA, Grines CL. Primary angioplasty versus intravenous thrombolytic therapy for acute myocardial infarction: a quantitative review of 23 randomised trials. *Lancet* 2003;361:13–20.
5. de Lemos JA, Gibson CM, Antman EM, et al. Abciximab and early adjunctive percutaneous coronary intervention are associated with improved ST-segment resolution after thrombolysis. Observations from the TIMI 14 trial. *Am Heart J* 2001;141:592–598.
6. Pennica D, Holmes WE, Kohr WJ, et al. Cloning and expression of human tissue-type plasminogen activator cDNA in E. coli. *Nature* 1983;301:214–221.
7. Kohnert U, Rudolph R, Verheijen JH, et al. Biochemical properties of the kringle 2 and protease domains are maintained in the refolded t-PA deletion variant BM 06.022. *Protein Eng* 1992;5:93–100.
8. Paoni NF, Keyt BA, Refino CJ, et al. A slow clearing, fibrin-specific, PAI-1 resistant variant of t-PA (T103N,KHRR296-299AAAA). Thromb Haemost 1993;70:307–312.s
9. Den Heijer P, Vermeer F, Ambrosioni E, et al. Evaluation of a weight-adjusted single-bolus plasminogen activator in patients with myocardial infarction: a double-blind, randomized angiographic trial of lanoteplase versus alteplase. *Circulation* 1998;98:2117–2125.
10. Suzuki S, Saito M, Suzuki N, et al. Thrombolytic properties of a novel modified human tissue-type plasminogen activator (E6010): a bolus injection

of E6010 has equivalent potency of lysing young and aged canine coronary thrombi. *J Cardiovasc Pharmacol* 1991;17:738–746.

11. Katoh M, Suzuki Y, Miyamoto T, et al. Biochemical and pharmacokinetic properties of YM866, a novel fibrinolytic agent (Abstract 1794). *Thromb Haemost* 1991;65:1193.

12. Krätzschmar J, Haendler B, Langer G. The plasminogen activator family from the salivary gland of the vampire bat Desmodus rotundus: cloning and expression. *Gene* 1991;105:229–237.

13. Holmes WE, Pennica D, Blaber M, et al. Cloning and expression of the gene for pro-urokinase in Escherichia coli. *Biotechnology* 1985;3:923–929.

14. Amediplase: CGP 42935, K2tu-PA, MEN 9036. *BioDrugs* 2002;16:378–379.

15. Rabijns A, De Bondt HL, De Ranter C. Three-dimensional structure of staphylokinase, a plasminogen activator with therapeutic potential. *Nat Struct Biol* 1997;4:357–360.

16. Sako T, Tsuchida N. Nucleoticle sequence of the staphylokinase gene from Staphylococcus aureus. *Nucleic Acids Res* 1983;11:7679–7693.

17. Behnke D, Gerlach D. Cloning and expression in Escherichia coil, Bacillus subtilis and Streptococcus sanguis of a gene for staphylokinase: a bacterial plasminogen activator. *Mol Gen Genet* 1987;210:528–534.

18. Collen D, Zhao ZA, Holvoet P, et al. Primary structure and gene structure of staphylokinase. *Fibrinolysis* 1992;6:226–231.

19. Laroche Y, Heymans S, Capaert S, et al. Recombinant staphylokinase variants with reduced antigenicity due to elimination of B-lymphocyte epitopes. *Blood* 2000;96:1425–1432.

20. Collen D, Sinnaeve P, Demarsin E, et al. Polyethylene glycol-derivatized cysteine-substitution variants of recombinant staphylokinase for single-bolus treatment of acute myocardial infarction. *Circulation* 2000;102:1766–1772.

21. Hoylaerts M, Rijken DC, Lijnen HR, et al. Kinetics of the activation of plasminogen by human tissue plasminogen activator. Role of fibrin. *J Biol Chem* 1982;257:2912–2919.

22. Thorsen S. The mechanism of plasminogen activation and the variability of the fibrin effector during tissue-type plasminogen activator-mediated fibrinolysis. *Ann N Y Acad Sci* 1992;667:52–63.

23. Collen D. On the regulation and control of fibrinolysis. *Thromb Haemost* 1980;43:77–89.

24. Gurewich V, Pannell R, Louie S, et al. Effective and fibrin-specific clot lysis by a zymogen precursor form of urokinase (pro-urokinase). A study *in vitro* and in two animal species. *J Clin Invest* 1984;73:1731–1739.

25. Lijnen HR, Van Hoef B, Nelles L, et al. Plasminogen activation with single-chain urokinase-type plasminogen activator (scu-PA). Studies with active site mutagenized plasminogen (Ser740 → Ala) and plasmin-resistant scu-PA (Lys158 → Glu). *J Biol Chem* 1990;265:5232–5236.

26. Liu JN, Gurewich V. Fragment E-2 from fibrin substantially enhances pro-urokinase-induced Glu-plasminogen activation. A kinetic study using the plasmin-resistant mutant pro-urokinase Ala-158-rpro-UK. *Biochemistry* 1992;31:6311–6317.

27. Fleury V, Lijnen HR, Anglès-Cano E. Mechanism of the enhanced intrinsic activity of single-chain urokinase-type plasminogen activator during ongoing fibrinolysis. *J Biol Chem* 1993;268:18554–18559.

28. Rijken DC, Barrett-Bergshoeff MM, Jie AF, et al. Clot penetration and fibrin binding of amediplase, a chimeric plasminogen activator (K2 tu-PA). *Thromb Haemost* 2004;91:52–60.

29. Lijnen HR, Collen D. Staphylokinase, a fibrin-specific bacterial plasminogen activator. *Fibrinolysis* 1996;10:119–126.

30. Collen D. Staphylokinase: a potent, uniquely fibrin-selective thrombolytic agent. *Nat Med* 1998;4:279–284.

31. Collen D. The plasminogen (fibrinolytic) system. *Thromb Haemost* 1999;82:259–270.

32. Garabedian HD, Gold HK, Leinbach RC, et al. Comparative properties of two clinical preparations of recombinant human tissue-type plasminogen activator in patients with acute myocardial infarction. *J Am Coll Cardiol* 1987;9:599–607.

33. The GUSTO Investigators. An international randomized trial comparing four thrombolytic strategies for acute myocardial infarction. *N Engl J Med* 1993;329:673–682.

34. GUSTO Angiographic Investigators. The effects of tissue plasminogen activator, streptokinase or both on coronary-artery patency, ventricular function, and survival after acute myocardial infarction. *N Engl J Med* 1993;329:1615–1622.

35. The COBALT Investigators. A comparison of continuous infusion of alteplase with double-bolus administration for acute myocardial infarction. *N Engl J Med* 1997;337:1124–1130.

36. Lijnen HR, Collen D. Strategies for the improvement of thrombolytic agents. *Thromb Haemost* 1991;66:88–110.

37. Lijnen HR, Collen D. New thrombolytic strategies and agents. *Haematologica* 2000;85(Suppl. 2):106–109.

38. Verstraete M. Search for more effective and safe thrombolytic agents. *Biomed Prog* 2001;13:68–74.

39. Llevadot J, Giugliano RP, Antman EM. Bolus fibrinolytic therapy in acute myocardial infarction. *JAMA* 2001;286:442–449.

40. Armstrong PW, Granger C, Van de Werf F. Bolus fibrinolysis; risk, benefit and opportunities. *Circulation* 2001;103:1171–1173.

41. The GUSTO-III investigators. A comparison of reteplase with alteplase for acute myocardial infarction. *N Engl J Med* 1997;337:1118–1123.

42. Rosenberg DG, Levin E, Lausell A, et al. Feasibility and timing of prehospital administration of reteplase in patients with acute myocardial infarction. *J Thromb Thrombolysis* 2002;13:147–153.

43. Morrow DA, Antman EM, Sayah A, et al. Evaluation of the time saved by prehospital initiation of reteplase for ST-elevation myocardial infarction: results of the Early Retavase-Thrombolysis in Myocardial Infarction (ER-TIMI) 19 trial. *J Am Coll Cardiol* 2002;40:71–77.

44. Cannon CP, McCabe CH, Gibson CM, et al. TNK-tissue plasminogen activator in acute myocardial infarction: results of the Thrombolysis in Myocardial Infarction (TIMI) 10A dose-ranging trial. *Circulation* 1997;95:351–356.

45. Tanswell P, Modi N, Combs D, et al. Pharmacokinetics and pharmacodynamics of tenecteplase in fibrinolytic therapy of acute myocardial infarction. *Clin Pharmacokinet* 2002;41:1229–1245.

46. Cannon CP, Gibson MC, McCabe CH, et al. TNK-tissue plasminogen activator compared with front-loaded tissue plasminogen activator in acute myocardial infarction: results of the TIMI-10B trial. *Circulation* 1998;98:2805–2814.

47. Assessment of the Safety and Efficacy of a New Thrombolytic Regimen (ASSENT-2) Investigators. Single-bolus tenecteplase compared with front-loaded alteplase in acute myocardial infarction: the ASSENT-2 double-blind randomised trial. *Lancet* 1999;354:716–722.

48. Wang-Clow F, Fox NL, Cannon CP, et al. Determination of a weight-adjusted dose of TNK-tissue plasminogen activator. *Am Heart J* 2001;141:33–40.

49. Angeja BG, Alexander JH, Chin R, et al. Safety of the weight-adjusted dosing regimen of tenecteplase in the ASSENT-Trial. *Am J Cardiol* 2001;88:1240–1245.

50. Sinnaeve P, Alexander J, Belmans A, et al. One-year follow-up of the ASSENT-2 trial: a double-blind, randomized comparison of single-bolus tenecteplase and front-loaded alteplase in 16,949 patients with ST-elevation acute myocardial infarction. *Am Heart J* 2003;146:27–32.

51. Van de Werf F, Barron HV, Armstrong PW, et al. Incidence and predictors of bleeding events after fibrinolytic therapy with fibrin-specific agents: a comparison of TNK-tPA and rt-PA. *Eur Heart J* 2001;22:2253–2261.

52. Fu Y, Goodman S, Chang WC, et al. Time to treatment influences the impact of ST-segment resolution on one-year prognosis: insights from the assessment of the safety and efficacy of a new thrombolytic (ASSENT-2) trial. *Circulation* 2001;104:2653–2659.

53. Serebruany VL, Malinin AI, Callahan KP, et al. Effect of tenecteplase versus alteplase on platelets during the first 3 hours of treatment for acute myocardial infarction: the Assessment of the Safety and Efficacy of a New Thrombolytic Agent (ASSENT-2) platelet substudy. *Am Heart J* 2003; 145:636–642.

54. Guerra DR, Karha J, Gibson CM. Safety and efficacy of tenecteplase in acute myocardial infarction. *Expert Opin Pharmacother* 2003;4:791–798.

55. The InTime-II Investigators. Intravenous nPA for the treatment of infarcting myocardium early: InTime-II, a double blind comparison of single bolus lanoteplase vs. accelerated alteplase for the treatment of patients with acute myocardial infarction. *Eur Heart J* 2000;21:2005–2013.

56. Kostis JB, Dockens RC, Thadani U, et al. Comparison of pharmacokinetics of lanoteplase and alteplase during acute myocardial infarction. *Clin Pharmacokinet* 2002;41:445–452.

57. Kawai C, Hosada S, Kimata S. Coronary thrombolysis in acute myocardial infarction of E6010 (novel modified t-PA): a multicenter, double-blind dose-finding study. *Jpn Pharmacol Ther* 1994;22:3925–3950.

58. Kawai C, Yui Y, Hosada S, et al. A prospective, randomized, double-blind multicenter trial of a single bolus injection of the novel modified t-PA E6010 in the treatment of acute myocardial infarction: comparison with native t-PA. *J Am Coll Cardiol* 1997;29:1447–1453.

59. Nagao K, Hayashi K, Kanmatsuse K, et al. An early and complete reperfusion strategy for acute myocardial infarction using fibrinolysis and subsequent transluminal therapy – The FAST trial. *Circ J* 2002;66:576–582.

60. Inoue T, Yaguchi I, Takayanagi K, et al. A new thrombolytic agent, monteplase, is independent of the plasminogen activator inhibitor in patients with acute myocardial infarction: initial results of the Combining Monteplase with Angioplasty (COMA) trial. *Am Heart J* 2002;144:E5.

61. Hashimoto K, Oikawa K, Miyamoto I. Phase I study of a novel modified t-PA. *Jpn J Med Pharm Sci* 1996;36:623–646.

62. Yui Y, Haze K, Kawai C. Randomized, double-blind multicenter trial of YM866 (modified t-PA) by intravenous bolus injection in patients with acute myocardial infarction in comparison with tisokinase (native t-PA). *Jpn J New Remedies Clin.* 1996;45:2175–2221.

63. Kuiper J, Rijken DC, de Munk GAW, et al. *In vivo* and *in vitro* interaction of high and low molecular weight single-chain urokinase-type plasminogen activator with rat liver cells. *J Biol Chem* 1992;267:1589–1595.

64. Van de Werf F, Nobuhara M, Collen D. Coronary thrombolysis with human single chain urokinase-type plasminogen activator (scu-PA) in patients with acute myocardial infarction. *Ann Intern Med* 1986;104:345–348.

65. Van de Werf F, Vanhaecke J, De Geest H, et al. Coronary thrombolysis with recombinant single-chain urokinase-type plasminogen activator (rscu-PA) in patients with acute myocardial infarction. *Circulation* 1986; 74:1066–1070.

66. PRIMI Trial Study Group. Randomised double-blind trial of recombinant pro-urokinase against streptokinase in acute myocardial infarction. *Lancet* 1989;1:863–868.

67. Spiecker M, Windeler J, Vermeer F, et al. Thrombolysis with saruplase versus streptokinase in acute myocardial infarction: five-years results of the PRIMI trial. *Am Heart J* 1999;138:518–524.

68. Bar FW, Meyer J, Vermeer F, et al. Comparison of saruplase and alteplase in acute myocardial infarction. SESAM Study Group. The study in europe with saruplase and alteplase in myocardial infarction. *Am J Cardiol* 1997; 79:727–732.

69. Tebbe U, Windeler J, Boesl I, et al. On behalf of the LIMITS Study Group. Thrombolysis with recombinant unglycosylated single-chain urokinase-type plasminogen activator (Saruplase) in acute myocardial infarction: influence on early patency rate (LIMITS Study). *J Am Coll Cardiol* 1995;26: 365–373.

70. Zarich SW, Kowalchuk GJ, Weaver WD, et al. Sequential combination thrombolytic therapy for acute myocardial infarction: results of the Pro-Urokinase and t-PA Enhancement of Thrombolysis (PATENT) trial. *J Am Coll Cardiol* 1995;26:374–379.

71. Weaver WD, Hartmann JR, Anderson JL, et al. Prourokinase Study Group. New recombinant glycosylated prourokinase for treatment of patients with acute myocardial infarction. *J Am Coll Cardiol* 1994;24:1242–1248.

72. del Zoppo GJ, Higashida RT, Furlan AJ, et al. PROACT: a phase II randomized trial of recombinant pro-urokinase by direct arterial delivery in acute middle cerebral artery stroke. PROACT Investigators. Prolyse in acute cerebral thromboembolism. *Stroke* 1998;29:4–11.

73. Furlan AJ, Abou-Chebi A. The role of recombinant pro-urokinase (r-pro-UK) and inra-arterial thrombolysis in acute ischaemic stroke: the PROACT trials. Prolyse in acute cerebral thromboembolism. *Curr Med Res Opin* 2002;18(Suppl. 2):s44–s47.

74. Armstrong P, Burton J, Palisaitis D, et al. Collaborative angiographic patency trial of recombinant staphylokinase (CAPTORS). *Am Heart J* 2000; 139:820–823.

75. Vanderschueren S, Collen D, Van de Werf F. A pilot study on bolus administration of recombinant staphylokinase for coronary artery thrombolysis. *Thromb Haemost* 1996;76:541–544.

76. Okada K, Lijnen HR, Moreau H, et al. Procoagulant properties of intravenous staphylokinase versus tissue-type plasminogen activator. *Thromb Haemost* 1996;76:857–859.

77. Armstrong PW, Burton J, Pakola S, et al. CAPTORS II Investigators. Collaborative angiographic patency trial of recombinant staphylokinase (CAPTORS II). *Am Heart J* 2003;146:484–488.

78. Coller BS. A new murine monoclonal antibody reports an activation dependent change in the conformation and/or microenvironment of the platelet GPIIb/IIIa complex. *J Clin Invest* 1985;75:101–108.

79. Spinler SA, Hilleman DE, Cheng JW, et al. New recommendations from the 1999 American College of Cardiology/American Heart Association acute myocardial infarction guidelines. *Ann Pharmacother* 2001;35:589–617.

80. Topol EJ for the GUSTO V Investigators. Reperfusion therapy for acute myocardial infarction with fibrinolytic therapy or combination reduced fibrinolytic therapy and platelet glycoprotein IIb/IIIa inhibition: the GUSTO V randomised trial. *Lancet* 2001;357:1905–1914.

81. Lincoff AM, Califf RM, Van de Werf F, et al. Mortality at 1 year with combination platelet glycoprotein IIb/IIIa inhibition and reduced-dose fibrinolytic therapy vs. conventional fibrinolytic therapy for acute myocardial infarction: GUSTO V randomized trial. *JAMA* 2002;288:2130–2135.

82. Mukherjee D, Gurm H, Tang WH, et al. Outcome of acute myocardial infarction in patients with prior coronary artery bypass grafting treated with combination reduced fibrinolytic therapy and abciximab. *Am J Cardiol* 2002;90:1198–1203.

83. Giugliano RP, Roe MT, Harrington RA, et al. Combination reperfusion therapy with eptifibatide and reduced-dose tenecteplase for ST-elevation myocardial infarction: results of the integrilin and tenecteplase in acute myocardial infarction (INTEGRITI) Phase II Angiographic Trial. *J Am Coll Cardiol* 2003;41:1251–1260.

84. Hong TT, Driscoll EM, White AJ, et al. Glycoprotein IIb/IIIa receptor antagonist 2(S)-2-[(2-Naphtylsulfonyl)amino]-3-[[2-([4-(4-piperidinyl)-2-[2-(4-piperidinyl)ethyl]butanoyl]amino)acetyl]amino]propanoic acid dihydrochloride (CRL 42796), in combination with aspirin and/or enoxaparin, prevents coronary artery rethrombosis after successful thrombolytic therapy by recombinant tissue plasminogen activator. *J Pharmacol Exp Ther* 2003;306:616–623.

85. Hirsh J, Weitz JI. New antithrombotic agents. *Lancet* 1999;353:1431–1436.

86. Eikelboom J, White H, Yusuf S. The evolving role of direct thrombin inhibitors in acute coronary syndromes. *J Am Coll Cardiol* 2003;41:70S–78S.

87. The Assessment of the Safety and Efficacy of a New Thrombolytic Regimen-ASSENT-3 Investigators. Efficacy and safety of tenecteplase in combination with enoxaparin, abciximab, or unfractionated heparin: the ASSENT-3 randomized trial in acute myocardial infarction. *Lancet* 2001; 358: 605–613.

88. Wallentin L, Goldstein P, Armstrong PW, et al. Efficacy and safety of tenecteplase in combination with the low-molecular-weight heparin enoxaparin or unfractionated heparin in the prehospital setting: the Assessment of the Safety and Efficacy of a New Thrombolytic Regimen (ASSENT)-3 PLUS randomized trial in acute myocardial infarction. *Circulation* 2003; 108:135–142.

89. Antman EM, Louwerenburg HW, Baars HF, et al. Enoxaparin as adjunctive antithrombin therapy for ST-elevation myocardial infarction: results of the ENTIRE-Thrombolysis in Myocardial Infarction (TIMI) 23 trial. *Circulation* 2002;105:1642–1649.

90. Cohen M, Arjomand H, Pollack CV Jr. The evolution of thrombolytic therapy and adjunctive antithrombotic regimens in acute ST-segment elevation myocardial infarction. *Am J Emerg Med* 2004;22:14–23.

91. Brieger D. Optimizing adjunctive antithrombotic therapy in the treatment of acute myocardial infarction: a role for low-molecular-weight heparin. *Clin Cardiol* 2004;27:3–8.

92. Walters RE II, Mahaffey KW, Granger CB, et al. Current perspectives on reperfusion therapy for acute ST-segment elevation myocardial infarction: integrating pharmacologic and mechanical reperfusion strategies. *Am Heart J* 2003;146:958–968.

93. Wiman B, Collen D. On the mechanism of the reaction between human $\alpha$2-antiplasmin and plasmin. *J Biol Chem* 1979;254: 9291–9297.

94. Wiman B, Collen D. On the kinetics of the reaction between human antiplasmin and plasmin. *Eur J Biochem* 1978;84:573–578.

95. Marder VJ, Landskroner K, Novokhatny V, et al. Plasmin induces local thrombolysis without causing hemorrhage: a comparison with tissue plasminogen activator in the rabbit. *Thromb Haemost* 2001;86:739–745.

96. Collen D. Revival of plasmin as a therapeutic agent. *Thromb Haemost* 2001; 86:731–732.

97. Novokhatny VV, Jesmok GJ, Landskroner KA, et al. Locally delivered plasmin: why should it be superior to plasminogen activators for direct thrombolysis? *Trends Pharmacol Sci* 2004;25:72–75.

98. Novokhatny V, Taylor K, Zimmerman TP. Thrombolytic potency of acid-stabilized plasmin: superiority over tissue-type plasminogen activator in an *in vitro* model of catheter-assisted thrombolysis. *J Thromb Haemost* 2003; 1:1034–1041.

99. Nagai N, Demarsin E, Van Hoef B, et al. Recombinant human microplasmin: production and potential therapeutic properties. *J Thromb Haemost* 2003;1:307–313.

100. Jesmok G, Landskroner K, Taylor K. The effect of restricted blood flow on the thrombolytic activity of locally delivered plasmin: comparison with TPA in rabbit models of venous and arterial thrombosis. In: Vossoughi J, Fareed J, Mousa SA et al., eds. *Thrombosis research and treatment: bench to bedside*, Chap. 23. Washington, DC: Medical and Engineering Publishers, 2004:415–428.

101. Nagai N, De Mol M, Van Hoef B, et al. Depletion of circulating $\alpha_2$-antiplasmin by intravenous plasmin or immunoneutralization reduces focal cerebral ischemic injury in the absence of arterial recanalization. *Hemost Thromb Vasc Biol* 2001;97:3086–3092.

102. Nagai N, De Mol M, Lijnen HR, et al. Role of plasminogen system components in focal cerebral ischemic infarction. A gene targeting and gene transfer study in mice. *Circulation* 1999;99:2440–2444.

103. Stewart D, Kong M, Novokhatny V, et al. Relevance of plasma coguation for safety during plasmin administration: comparison with TPA in a model of fibrinolytic hemorrhage. *Blood* 2003;101:3002–3007.

# CHAPTER 123 ■ NEW ANTITHROMBOTIC DRUGS

SHANNON M. BATES AND JEFFREY I. WEITZ

Antithrombotic drugs that are currently available include antiplatelet agents that inhibit platelet activation and aggregation, anticoagulants that attenuate fibrin formation, and fibrinolytic agents that catalyze the generation of plasmin, which then degrades the fibrin component of thrombi. Because arterial thrombi consist of platelet aggregates held together by small amounts of fibrin (1), strategies to inhibit arterial thrombogenesis focus mainly on drugs that block platelet function but often include anticoagulants to prevent fibrin deposition. Anticoagulants also are used for prevention of cardioembolic events in patients with atrial fibrillation or mechanical heart valves. In contrast, because venous thrombi are composed mainly of fibrin (1), anticoagulants are the drugs of choice for their prevention and treatment. Fibrinolytic drugs are used for treatment of patients with acute myocardial infarction or acute ischemic stroke to rapidly restore antegrade flow in the occluded artery. For these indications, fibrinolytic drugs are usually given systemically. Patients with massive pulmonary embolism (PE) also benefit from systemic administration of fibrinolytic agents. In contrast, when used to effect lysis of proximal thrombi in the deep veins of the legs, fibrinolytic drugs are infused directly into the thrombus using a catheter-directed approach, although clear clinical benefit of such treatment is yet to be demonstrated.

Currently available antithrombotic agents have limitations. Although aspirin produces a 25% reduction in the risk of cardiovascular death, myocardial infarction, and stroke in patients with atherosclerotic disease (2), it remains a suboptimal antiplatelet agent because despite its use, thrombotic events occur in a substantial cohort of patients. The thienopyridine derivatives, ticlopidine and clopidogrel, and newer orally active platelet adenosine diphosphate (ADP) receptor antagonists, are only modestly more effective than aspirin (2–4). The recognition that the limited efficacy of aspirin and ADP receptor antagonists likely reflects the existence of alternative pathways for platelet activation provided the rationale for the development of inhibitors of glycoprotein (GP) IIb/IIIa, the receptor responsible for platelet aggregation, irrespective of the agonist. GP IIb/IIIa receptor antagonists have proven to be a powerful class of antiplatelet drugs, and parenteral forms of these agents are widely used in patients undergoing percutaneous coronary interventions and in those with unstable angina (5,6). However, their oral counterparts have not been shown to be safe or effective. Consequently, there remains a need for orally active antiplatelet drugs that are more potent inhibitors of platelet aggregation than aspirin or the thienopyridines.

When considering the anticoagulants in current use, low-molecular-weight heparin (LMWH) is gradually replacing unfractionated heparin for the treatment of most patients with venous thromboembolism (VTE) and acute coronary syndromes because LMWH has similar efficacy but is more convenient and cost-effective than heparin in these patients (7–13).

Despite the advances with LMWH, however, more potent parenteral anticoagulants are still required. Likewise, there is also a need for safer oral anticoagulants that do not require routine coagulation monitoring. Coumarin derivatives have a narrow therapeutic window (14), and their metabolism is influenced by dietary factors and concomitant medications. Consequently, time-consuming and expensive monitoring is required to ensure that a therapeutic anticoagulant effect is achieved. Moreover, even with close monitoring, warfarin dosing can be problematic.

Focusing on new antithrombotic agents, this chapter (a) reviews arterial and venous thrombogenesis, highlighting the targets for new antiplatelet and anticoagulant strategies, (b) describes new antiplatelet and anticoagulant drugs in more advanced stages of development, focusing on their mechanism of action and the results of clinical trials evaluating their utility, and (c) provides clinical perspective on the unmet needs in antithrombotic therapy for prevention and treatment of venous and arterial thrombosis.

## THROMBOGENESIS

Arterial thrombosis usually is initiated by spontaneous or mechanical rupture of atherosclerotic plaque, a process that exposes thrombogenic material in the lipid-rich core of the plaque to the blood (15). Typically, thrombi that form at the sites of plaque disruption extend both into the plaque and into the vessel lumen. If the intraluminal thrombus is nonocclusive, and if blood flow remains rapid, the thrombus may embolize downstream or it may organize and become incorporated into the vessel wall. With more extensive intraluminal thrombosis, however, blood flow diminishes and shear increases. Higher shear can promote further platelet and fibrin deposition that may result in the formation of an occlusive thrombus that obstructs blood flow to organs, such as the heart or brain, or to the extremities. Alternatively, vascular obstruction may reflect explosive thrombosis at sites of severe plaque disruption.

Venous thrombi, which occur when procoagulant stimuli overwhelm natural protective mechanisms, typically develop under low-flow conditions and usually originate in the muscular veins of the calf or in the valve cusp pockets of the deep calf veins (16). Because the venous valve cusps are avascular, they depend on the circulating blood for their oxygen and nutrient supply. With venous stasis, there is local hypoxemia, which can induce tissue factor expression in the valve cusps. Coagulation in the veins also can be initiated by vascular trauma, such as that associated with major hip or knee surgery (17) or with indwelling central venous catheters. Congenital and acquired thrombophilic disorders promote coagulation. Patients with congenital deficiencies of antithrombin, protein C, or protein S are prone to thrombosis because naturally occurring anticoagulant pathways are compromised. Patients with the factor $V_{Leiden}$ mutation have increased thrombin generation because the abnormal factor V protein, once activated, is resistant to degradation by activated protein C (APC). Increased thrombin generation also may underlie the propensity to thrombosis in patients with the prothrombin gene mutation, a defect that results in increased levels of prothrombin, or in those with elevations of other clotting factors, including factors VIII, IX, and X.

## Role of the Platelet in Thrombogenesis

Blood constituents normally do not interact with intact endothelium. When endothelial cells are activated by inflammatory cytokines or products of coagulation, such as thrombin, they express adhesion molecules on their surface. These adhesion molecules tether leukocytes and platelets. Adherent monocytes synthesize tissue factor that can trigger coagulation, whereas tethered neutrophils can compound vascular injury by generating free radicals and releasing hydrolytic enzyme. Platelets that deposit on the endothelium become activated, a process that causes flip-flop of membrane phospholipids to expose negatively charged phospholipids onto which coagulation factors bind.

More severe denuding injury to the vessel wall also triggers platelet adhesion and activation. Platelet adhesion at these sites is mediated by the interaction of constitutively expressed receptors on the platelet surface with exposed subendothelial matrix proteins (18). Collagen and von Willebrand factor (VWF) are the most important subendothelial proteins to which platelets adhere (19,20), but other matrix components, such as fibronectin, laminin, vitronectin, and thrombospondin, also may mediate platelet adhesion. Although a number of platelet GPs interact with collagen, GP Ia/IIa ($\alpha_2\beta_1$) and GP VI appear to be the physiologic collagen receptors because platelets isolated from patients lacking these GPs exhibit defective collagen-induced adhesion and aggregation (21–24). Under high shear conditions, platelet adhesion to subendothelium is mediated primarily by VWF (25,26). VWF, an elongated multimeric GP, binds to the GP Ib/V/IX receptor complex on nonactivated platelets and to GP IIb/IIIa on activated platelets. Although VWF is found in the plasma, circulating VWF does not interact with GP Ib/IX and conformational changes that occur after VWF binds to extracellular matrix are needed to promote the interaction of VWF with GP Ib/V/IX (27). Shear stress may also promote this interaction; under high shear conditions, immobilized VWF binds to GP Ib/V/IX and binds the platelet to the subendothelium. This bond is transient, however, unless there is concomitant binding of VWF to GP IIb/IIIa (28).

Occupancy of platelet receptors generates contractile cytoskeleton assembly and fusion of the storage granules with the surface such that their contents exit the cell. Once platelets are activated, they recruit additional platelets to sites of vascular injury by three coordinated mechanisms. First, the membrane surface of activated platelets is transformed, causing an increase in the content of anionic phospholipid that enables the membrane surface to support the assembly of intrinsic "tenase" (the factor X–activating complex) and prothrombinase (the prothrombin-activating complex), thereby markedly amplifying thrombin generation (18). Thrombin plays a key role in thrombosis both by inducing fibrin deposition and by serving as the most potent physiologic platelet agonist. Thrombin activates platelets by interacting with a class of transmembrane protease-activated receptors (PAR), found on vascular cells and cells within the central nervous system, as well as on platelets. After binding to an acidic region in the amino-terminal extracellular domain of the receptor, thrombin cleaves a peptide bond, thereby generating a new amino-terminus (29). This newly formed amino-terminus acts as a tethered ligand that, by

folding back on itself, binds to the receptor and triggers G protein–coupled signal transduction pathways that induce platelet activation. Second, ADP and serotonin secreted from storage granules of activated platelets stimulate nearby platelets. Third, activated platelets synthesize and release thromboxane A$_2$, another platelet agonist.

Platelet activation by thrombin, ADP, thromboxane A$_2$, or other agonists, induces conformational changes in the GP IIb/IIIa ($\alpha_{2b}\beta_3$) platelet receptor such that it becomes a functional receptor for fibrinogen as well as for other adhesive molecules, such as VWF, fibronectin, and thrombospondin (19,20, 30). Although fibrinogen is the preferred ligand for this receptor because its concentration in plasma is higher than that of other adhesive proteins, in vessels with high shear, VWF may also play a role in platelet-to-platelet cohesion (31,32). All of the adhesive molecules that interact with GP IIb/IIIa contain the Arg-Gly-Asp (RGD) sequence that serves as the minimal recognition sequence for the receptor (19,20,30–32). In addition to the RGD sequence on each of its A$\alpha$ chains, fibrinogen contains a specific dodecapeptide on the carboxyl terminals of the $\lambda$ chains that also interacts with GP IIb/IIIa (33). Binding of bivalent fibrinogen molecules to GP IIb/IIIa on adjacent platelets links them together, thereby forming platelet aggregates.

## Role of Coagulation in Thrombogenesis

Initiation of coagulation in arteries or veins is triggered by tissue factor, a cellular receptor for activated factor VII (factor VIIa), which is exposed with vessel wall injury (34). Although a small fraction of circulating factor VII is activated, factor VIIa has little or no enzymatic activity until it is bound to tissue factor. Most nonvascular cells express tissue factor in a constitutive fashion, whereas *de novo* tissue factor synthesis can be induced in monocytes (35,36). Lipid-laden macrophages in the core of atherosclerotic plaques are particularly rich in tissue factor (15), thereby explaining the propensity for arterial thrombus formation at sites of plaque disruption.

Once bound to tissue factor, factor VIIa activates factor IX and factor X, leading to the generation of factor IXa and factor Xa, respectively. Factor Xa converts small amounts of prothrombin to thrombin (37). This low concentration of thrombin is sufficient to activate platelets (38), factors V and VIII (key cofactors for coagulation) (34), and platelet-bound factor XI, thereby leading to further factor Xa generation (39). All of these steps are essential for propagation of coagulation.

Propagation is effected when factor IXa binds to factor VIIIa on the surface of activated platelets to form intrinsic tenase, a complex that efficiently activates factor X. Factor Xa then binds to factor Va on the activated platelet surface to form prothrombinase, thereby increasing the rate of factor Xa–mediated conversion of prothrombin to thrombin over 300,000-fold. The resultant burst of thrombin results in rapid conversion of fibrinogen to fibrin monomer at sites of vascular damage (18,37). These fibrin monomers polymerize to form the fibrin mesh that is stabilized and cross-linked by factor XIIIa, a thrombin-activated transglutaminase.

# NEW ANTITHROMBOTIC AGENTS

Although most new antithrombotic strategies have focused on development of more potent inhibitors of platelets and coagulation, strategies to enhance natural anticoagulant pathways or to increase endogenous fibrinolysis are also under investigation (see Fig. 123-1).

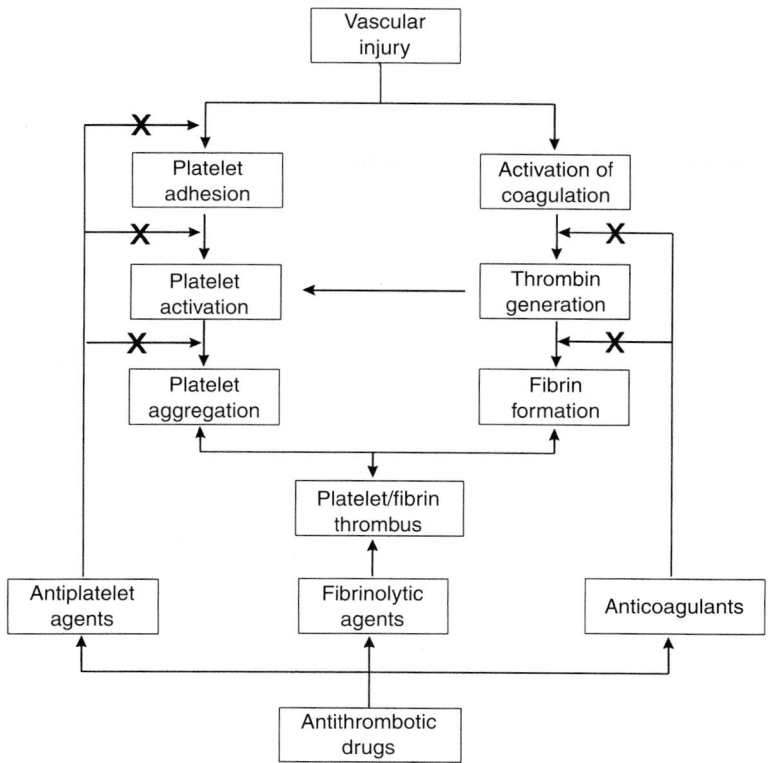

**FIGURE 123-1.** Targets of new antithrombotic drugs. Thrombosis occurs at sites of vascular injury by coordinated processes that result in platelet activation and activation of the coagulation system. Formation of the platelet plug represents the first step in hemostasis. Subsequent thrombin generation amplifies the platelet response because thrombin is a potent platelet agonist. Thrombin also converts fibrinogen to fibrin, and the fibrin strands stabilize the platelet aggregates, thereby forming a platelet/fibrin thrombus. Given the importance of platelets and fibrin in thrombogenesis, new antithrombotic agents target these components. New antiplatelet strategies focus on blocking platelet adhesion, activation, or aggregation. Novel anticoagulants, which target various coagulation enzymes, are geared at inhibiting thrombin generation or thrombin activity. Finally, fibrinolytic agents digest the fibrin component of the thrombus, thereby causing thrombus dissolution.

# PLATELET INHIBITORS

In the past, efforts to develop platelet inhibitors focused on agents that block the biochemical reactions involved in platelet activation. However, by targeting a single pathway in the platelet activation process, these drugs only partially inhibit platelet aggregation at sites of vascular injury. Therefore, the thrombotic events that occur despite aspirin therapy likely reflect platelet activation through thromboxane $A_2$–independent pathways that are not blocked by this drug. Similarly, the inability of ticlopidine and clopidogrel to completely block ADP-mediated platelet aggregation (40,41) may explain why these agents are only marginally more effective than aspirin (2–4). To overcome this problem, recent attention has focused on blocking the interaction of GP IIb/IIIa with its ligands based on the premise that the cross-linking of adjacent platelets that occurs after fibrinogen binds to this receptor represents the final common pathway for platelet aggregation (5,6). Although parenteral GP IIb/IIIa antagonists represent a major advance, their oral counterparts have not proven to be effective. Consequently, new strategies to inhibit platelets have focused on blocking platelet adhesion to the damaged endothelial surface or preventing platelet recruitment at sites of vascular injury (see Fig. 123-2).

## Inhibitors of Platelet Adhesion

Blocking the interaction of platelets with subendothelial adhesive proteins exposed at sites of vascular injury may represent a novel antithrombotic approach. Anti–GP VI monoclonal antibody-derived Fab fragments impair platelet adhesion and prevent thrombi formation under arterial growth (42). A number of strategies designed to block the interaction of VWF with GP Ib/IX have also been investigated. First, monoclonal antibodies against GP Ib or the GP Ib/IX complex can block VWF

receptors on unactivated platelets (43,44). In baboon arterial thrombosis models, the monoclonal antibody 6B4-Fab was able to disrupt platelet adhesion and prevent thrombus formation (45,46). However, there are significant challenges associated with the development of GP Ib inhibitors, including problems associated with antibody-induced thrombocytopenia (46) and potential pathogenic effects on megakaryocytes (47,48), as well as poor cross-species reactivity of anti–GP Ib antibodies. Second, peptide fragments containing the GP Ib/IX–binding domain of VWF can be used to compete with intact VWF for receptor occupancy (49). These substances block ristocetin-induced platelet agglutination *ex vivo* without causing thrombocytopenia but are less effective than GP IIb/IIIa antagonists in laboratory animal models of thrombosis. Third, GP Ib–binding proteins, such as those isolated from the venom of *Bothrops jararaca* (50,51) or *Crotalus atrox* (52,53), compete with VWF for GP Ib binding. The recombinant protein saratin, which is derived from the saliva of the medicinal leech, is able to prevent binding of VWF to collagen (54). This agent also decreased platelet adhesion, intimal hyperplasia, luminal stenosis, and thrombosis after carotid endarterectomy in rats (55). A fourth approach has been the use of agents directed against VWF. Neutralizing antibodies to VWF (56–58) and aurintricarboxylic acid, a heterogeneous mixture of polycarboxylic and polyaromatic polymers that bind VWF and prevent its interaction with GP Ib, have antithrombotic activity in animal models (59). However, they are less potent than GP IIb/IIIa receptor antagonists. None of these agents has been tested in humans.

## Inhibitors of Platelet Recruitment

Strategies to block this process have targeted thromboxane $A_2$ synthesis, the thromboxane $A_2$ receptor, the ADP receptor, ADP, or thrombin receptors on platelets (Fig. 123-2).

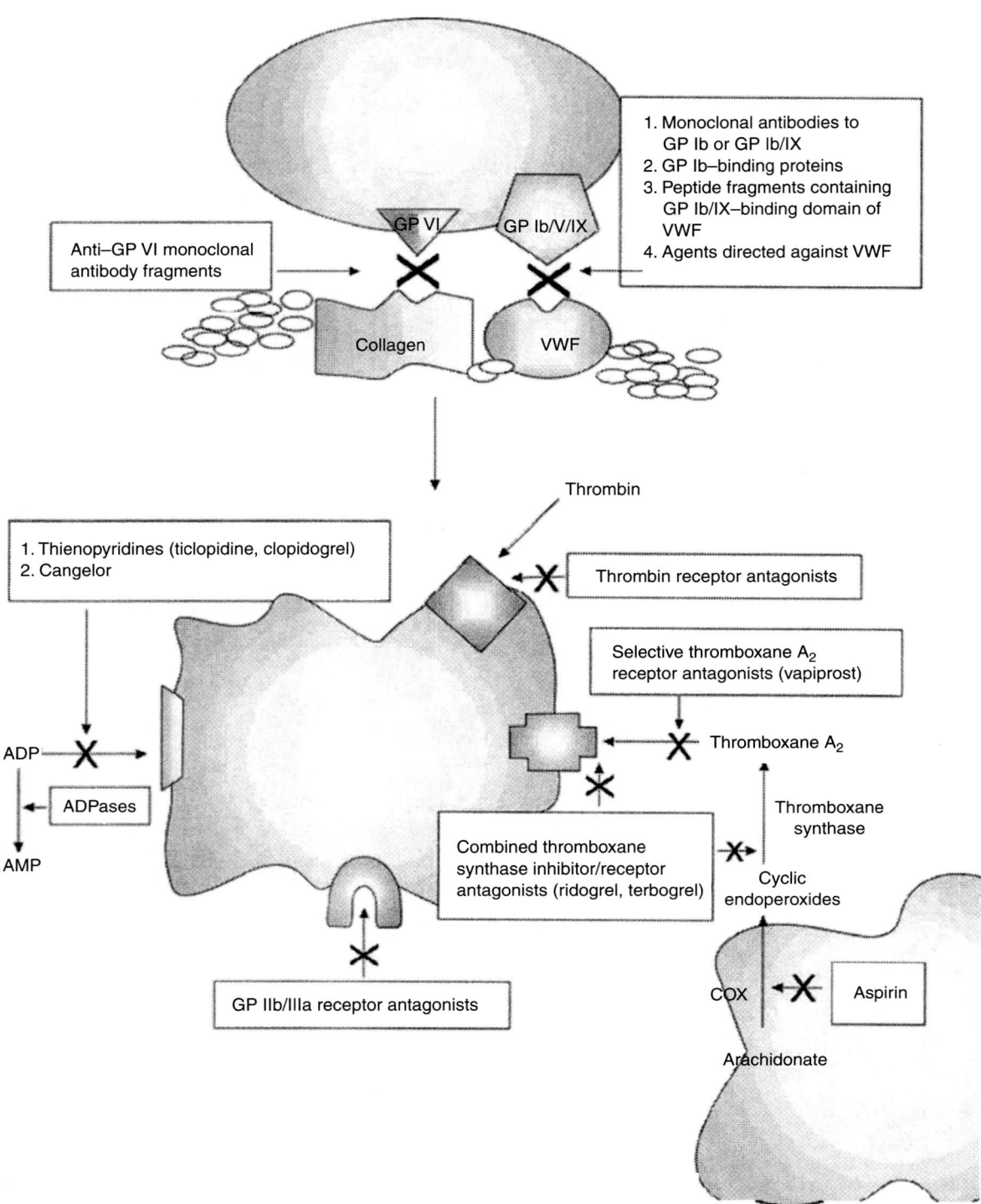

**FIGURE 123-2.** Sites of action of antiplatelet drugs. Platelets adhere to subendothelial collagen and von Willebrand factor (VWF) through glycoprotein (GP) VI and GP Ib/V/IX, respectively (**top panel**). These interactions can be blocked by monoclonal antibodies directed against the GP receptors on platelets. The interaction of VWF with GP Ib/V/IX also can be inhibited by GP Ib–binding proteins, VWF fragments, or agents directed against VWF that block its interaction with platelets. Adherent platelets become activated and release thromboxane $A_2$ and adenosine diphosphate (ADP), substances that activate adjacent platelets. By irreversibly inhibiting cyclooxygenase-1 (COX), aspirin blocks thromboxane $A_2$ synthesis. Combined thromboxane synthase inhibitors and thromboxane $A_2$ receptor antagonists have dual effects by blocking thromboxane $A_2$ synthesis and by inhibiting the thromboxane $A_2$ receptor. The latter action is important because the cyclic endoperoxide intermediates that accumulate after thromboxane synthase blockade also can activate the thromboxane $A_2$ receptor. Thienopyridines (ticlopidine and clopidogrel) and cangrelor prevent platelet recruitment by inhibiting $P2Y_{12}$, one of the key ADP receptors on platelets, whereas ADPases convert ADP, a platelet agonist, into adenosine monophosphate (AMP), which does not activate platelets. Thrombin, the most potent platelet agonist, binds to thrombin receptors on the platelet surface. Thrombin receptor antagonists block this interaction. Regardless of the agonist, the final common pathway of platelet aggregation is by GP IIb/IIIa. Once functionally activated, GP IIb/IIIa ligates fibrinogen and, under high shear, VWF. Bound fibrinogen and VWF link adjacent platelets to form platelet aggregates. This pathway is blocked by GP IIb/IIIa receptor antagonists.

## Thromboxane Synthetase Inhibitors and Thromboxane A₂ Receptor Antagonists

By inhibiting cyclooxygenase in platelets and endothelial cells, aspirin prevents the synthesis of both thromboxane $A_2$ and prostacyclin, an endothelial-derived platelet inhibitor (60). Because inhibition of prostacyclin synthesis has the potential to promote thrombogenesis, agents more selective for thromboxane $A_2$, such as thromboxane synthetase inhibitors and thromboxane $A_2$ receptor antagonists, have been developed.

In studies in laboratory animals, inhibitors of thromboxane synthetase, which block thromboxane $A_2$ generation without affecting prostacyclin synthesis, have not demonstrated superiority over aspirin. The limited efficacy of these agents may reflect the fact that the thromboxane $A_2$ precursors, prostaglandins $G_2$ and $H_2$, accumulate and can be released to serve as agonists for platelet thromboxane $A_2$ receptors (61).

Results with selective thromboxane $A_2$ receptor antagonists have also been disappointing. Although laboratory and animal data suggested that one such agent, vapiprost, might be a useful antithrombotic agent (62–64), this drug failed to prevent restenosis or improve clinical outcome in patients undergoing coronary angioplasty (65). Likewise, compared with aspirin, vapiprost did not reduce the frequency of chest pain in patients with prolonged chest discomfort and ST segment depression (66). S18886, a new orally active thromboxane $A_2$ receptor antagonist, exhibits antithrombotic effects superior to those of aspirin in perfusion chamber experiments done in pigs (67). However, under high and low shear conditions, the efficacy of S18886 was no better than that of clopidogrel, and the agent is yet to be tested in humans.

These findings raised the possibility that combined inhibition of thromboxane synthesis and the thromboxane receptor might be necessary to block thromboxane $A_2$–mediated platelet aggregation. Ridogrel, an agent with both of these properties, was shown to be effective in canine models of coronary thrombosis and to shorten the time to reperfusion when given in conjunction with tissue-type plasminogen activator (tPA) (68,69). However, when ridogrel was compared with aspirin in patients with acute myocardial infarction receiving streptokinase, ridogrel administration did not improve patency of the infarct-related artery, the primary study endpoint (70). On post hoc analysis, the frequency of recurrent ischemic events (myocardial infarction or ischemic stroke) was 13% in the ridogrel group, compared with 19% in those receiving aspirin ($P < 0.025$). The frequency of bleeding events was similar in the two patient groups. Terbogrel, an orally active combined thromboxane $A_2$ synthetase inhibitor and thromboxane receptor antagonist (71), also showed promise in early phase studies (71–74). However, its clinical development was halted because of severe leg pain associated with its use (74).

## Adenosine Diphosphate–Receptor Antagonists

The established ADP-receptor antagonists, ticlopidine and clopidogrel, inhibit platelet function by irreversibly blocking the $P2Y_{12}$ (or $P2Y_{AC}$) subtype of platelet ADP receptor (40,41, 75,76), which is responsible for amplification of platelet aggregation and secretion of thrombotic mediators. There are two other subtypes of platelet ADP receptors. The $P2X_1$ receptor mediates ADP-induced calcium influx (77), which leads to changes in platelet shape and platelet aggregation (77). The $P2Y_1$ receptor induces platelet shape change and transient aggregation by coupling to GP and mobilization of intracellular calcium (78).

Cangrelor (AR-C9931MX) is a selective $P2Y_{12}$ antagonist that is administered intravenously and has a rapid onset and offset of action (79). These properties are particularly attractive for patients undergoing percutaneous coronary interventions because reversible $P2Y_{12}$ antagonists provide immediate

ADP-receptor blockade, but their effects can be readily reversed should the patient require urgent surgery. In canine models, cangrelor prevents the development of occlusive arterial thrombus formation (80) and enhances coronary artery recanalization and myocardial tissue perfusion following thrombolytic therapy (81). In two small phase II studies, cangrelor was well tolerated when given as an adjunct to aspirin and heparin in patients with acute coronary syndromes (82,83). Studies are underway to evaluate this agent in patients undergoing percutaneous coronary interventions.

### CD39 (ectoADPase)

CD39, a component of the endothelial surface, hydrolyzes ADP released from activated platelets into adenosine monophosphate (AMP) (84), thereby exerting an antithrombotic effect by removing a major stimulus of platelet aggregation. Given that ADP and adenosine triphosphate (ATP) also have a role in leukocyte activation, CD39 has antiinflammatory properties (85). Recombinant soluble human CD39 inhibits *ex vivo* platelet aggregation in response to ADP (86). In a mouse model, it reduced cerebral infarct volumes after transient middle cerebral artery occlusion, without increasing intracerebral hemorrhage (86). This agent has not yet been tested in humans.

### Thrombin Receptor Antagonists

Thrombin's interaction with this receptor is mediated by its anion-binding exosite (exosite 1). This is the same site that mediates thrombin's interaction with other substrates. Thrombin receptor cleavage is effected by the enzyme's active site (87). Because all of the direct thrombin inhibitors (see subsequent text) bind to exosite 1 and/or the active site, these agents block thrombin-mediated platelet activation in addition to all other catalytic activities of thrombin (88).

At least four distinct receptors in the PAR class have been identified. The first, PAR-1, is the principal platelet receptor responsible for mediating thrombin's actions. PAR-2 is activated by trypsin, tryptase, and factor Xa, but not by thrombin, whereas PAR-3 is a thrombin-activated receptor found only on mouse platelets. PAR-4 is a second type of thrombin receptor identified on human platelets (89). Platelets from mice deficient in PAR-4 do not aggregate in response to thrombin but aggregate normally with collagen, ADP, or epinephrine (90). PAR-4–deficient mice exhibit a prolonged bleeding time and reduced thrombosis at sites of arterial injury. These findings highlight the importance of thrombin in hemostasis and thrombosis.

Strategies for selective inhibition of the thrombin receptor include prevention of receptor activation by the new amino-terminus that is generated on receptor cleavage or inhibition of specific downstream signal transduction pathways triggered by thrombin receptor activation. The potential for this therapeutic approach was highlighted when it was shown that an antibody against the thrombin-binding site on PAR-1 inhibits arterial thrombosis in monkeys (91). Although specific PAR-1 antagonist peptides have been developed (92–96), none has sufficient potency for clinical use (85). Thrombostatin, a five–amino acid degradation product of bradykinin, also inhibits thrombin-induced platelet activation (96) and attenuates platelet deposition after vascular injury by binding to PAR-1, thrombin, or both.

Although PAR-1 antagonists block platelet activation triggered by low concentrations of thrombin, platelets still can be activated with high thrombin concentrations by PAR-4 (97). A synthetic nonpeptide compound, YD-3 (1-benzyl-3-[ethoxycarbonylphenyl]-indazole) selectively blocks PAR-4 and disrupts platelet aggregation (98). Combined PAR-1 and PAR-4 inhibition results in additive antithrombotic effects (99), and new antiplatelet strategies are focusing on agents that block both PAR-1 and PAR-4.

## Inhibitors of Platelet Aggregation

Because the final common pathway of platelet aggregation in response to all agonists involves conformational activation of GP IIb/IIIa, considerable attention has been focused on development of GP IIb/IIIa antagonists (5,6). The parenteral agents abciximab, eptifibatide, and tirofiban have been shown to be effective in patients undergoing percutaneous coronary revascularization and in some patients with acute coronary syndromes, with maximum benefit seen in those with high-risk features (e.g., elevated troponin levels or diabetes mellitus) and those managed with percutaneous coronary intervention (100). In contrast, results with the oral GP IIb/IIIa inhibitors (xemilofiban, orbofiban, and sibrafiban) have been disappointing. Phase III trials found that these agents caused an excess of major bleeding without any significant benefit (even in high-risk patients), and a metaanalysis of four trials found an increase in all-cause mortality associated with their use (101). Potential mechanisms advanced to explain these findings include suboptimal inhibition of platelet aggregation, partial platelet agonist activity at trough concentrations, lack of responsiveness in patients with certain genetic polymorphisms, and promotion of cardiac myocyte apoptosis (102). With these clinical findings, further development of this class of drugs has been curtailed.

## NEW ANTICOAGULANTS

Anticoagulant strategies to inhibit thrombogenesis have focused on inhibiting thrombin, preventing thrombin generation, or blocking initiation of coagulation. Direct thrombin inhibitors block thrombin activity, whereas agents that target clotting enzymes higher in the coagulation pathways prevent thrombin generation. Coagulation factors that have been targeted for inactivation include factor Xa, factor IXa, and the factor VIIa/tissue factor complex (see Fig. 123-3). Another approach to attenuating thrombogenesis is to enhance endogenous anticoagulant pathways rather than to block specific clotting factors.

## Inhibitors of Initiation of Coagulation

Because the factor VIIa/tissue factor complex initiates coagulation, strategies targeting this pathway have received much attention. Inhibition of the factor VIIa/tissue factor complex is effected by tissue factor pathway inhibitor (TFPI) (103). A bivalent, Kunitz-type inhibitor, TFPI acts in a two-step manner (see Fig. 123-4). First, TFPI binds and inactivates factor Xa to form a TFPI/factor Xa complex. TFPI within this complex then inactivates tissue factor–bound factor VIIa as the second step. Because formation of the TFPI/factor Xa complex is a prerequisite for efficient inactivation of factor VIIa, the system ensures that some factor Xa generation occurs before factor VIIa–mediated initiation of coagulation system is halted. Propagation of coagulation occurs because TFPI concentrations are low. In addition, factor XI, which is efficiently activated by thrombin when bound to the activated platelet surface (104), generates factor IXa. A key component of the intrinsic tenase complex, factor IXa triggers the formation of sufficient amounts of factor Xa to propagate coagulation.

Most circulating TFPI is bound to lipoproteins. TFPI also is found in platelet α-granules and on the endothelial cell surface (103). TFPI bound to endothelium is released when therapeutic doses of heparin or LMWH are given, suggesting that TFPI binds to endogenous glycosaminoglycans on the endothelial wall surface (103). It is uncertain, however, whether released TFPI contributes to the antithrombotic properties of these agents.

Drugs targeting the factor VIIa/tissue factor complex that have reached advanced clinical testing include recombinant TFPI, recombinant nematode anticoagulant peptide (NAPc2), and active-site–blocked factor VIIa (factor VIIai).

### Tifacogin

A recombinant form of TFPI, tifacogin, has been evaluated in patients with sepsis. In a phase II trial (105) of 210 septic patients randomized to receive one of the two doses of tifacogin by continuous infusion (25 or 50 g/kg/hour) or placebo for 4 days, tifacogin produced a 20% relative reduction in all-cause

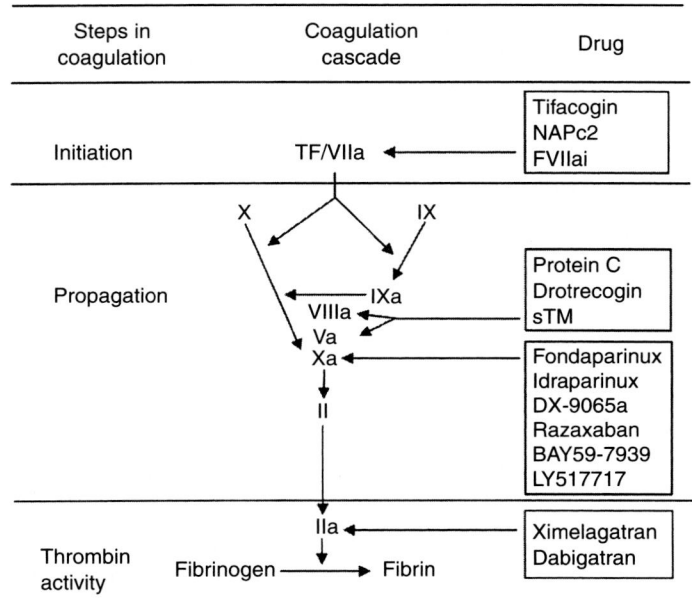

| Steps in coagulation | Coagulation cascade | Drug |
|---|---|---|
| Initiation | TF/VIIa | Tifacogin NAPc2 FVIIai |
| Propagation | X    IX<br>IXa<br>VIIIa<br>Va<br>Xa<br>II | Protein C Drotrecogin sTM<br><br>Fondaparinux Idraparinux DX-9065a Razaxaban BAY59-7939 LY517717 |
| Thrombin activity | IIa<br>Fibrinogen → Fibrin | Ximelagatran Dabigatran |

FIGURE 123-3. Sites of action of new anticoagulants. Coagulation is initiated by the tissue factor/factor VIIa (TF/VIIa) complex, which activates factors IX and X (IX and X, respectively). The process is propagated by activated factors IX and X (IXa and Xa, respectively) which, together with their cofactors, activated factors VIIIa and Va (VIIIa and Va, respectively), assemble on the surface of activated platelets to form intrinsic tenase and prothrombinase, respectively. Intrinsic tenase activates factor X, whereas prothrombinase converts prothrombin (II) to thrombin (IIa). In the final step, IIa converts fibrinogen to fibrin. Tifacogin, nematode anticoagulant protein (NAPc2), and active-site–blocked factor VIIa (FVIIai) inhibit the TF/VIIa complex. The cofactors FVIIIa and Va are inactivated by recombinant activated protein C (drotrecogin). The generation of activated protein C can be promoted by administering protein C or soluble thrombomodulin (sTM). Fondaparinux and indraparinux are indirect inhibitors of Xa that act by catalyzing antithrombin. In contrast, DX-9065a, razaxaban, BAY59-7939, and LY517717 are direct Xa inhibitors that interact with the active site of Xa. Ximelagatran and dabigatran are direct thrombin inhibitors. These agents interact with the active site of IIa and block its catalytic activity.

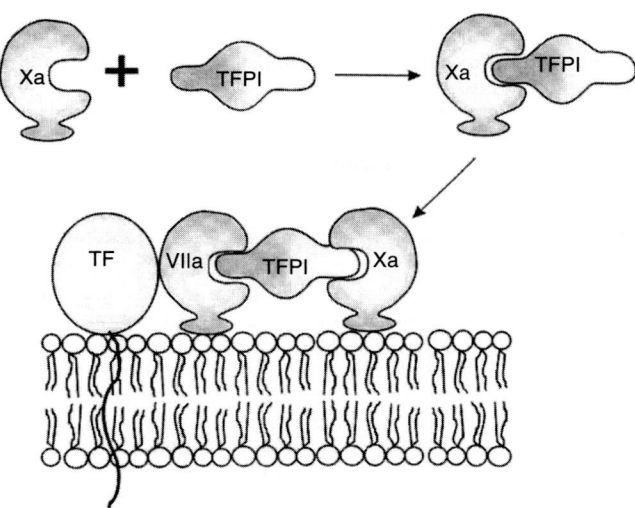

**FIGURE 123-4.** Mechanism of action of tissue factor pathway inhibitor (*TFPI*). A divalent inhibitor, TFPI first binds and inactivates activated factor X (*Xa*). The TFPI/Xa complex then inhibits factor VIIa (*VIIa*) bound to tissue factor (*TF*). By forming the quaternary Xa/TFPI/VIIa/TF complex, TFPI inhibits the activation of coagulation by the TF/VIIa complex.

mortality at 28 days compared with placebo. Major bleeding occurred in 9% of patients treated with tifacogin and 6% of those given placebo, a difference that was not significant. Building on these results, a phase III trial compared tifacogin with placebo in 1,754 patients with severe sepsis (106). The primary endpoint, all-cause mortality at 28 days, was similar in both groups (34.2% and 33.9% with tifacogin and placebo, respectively), and the rate of bleeding was significantly higher with tifacogin than with placebo (6.5% and 4.8%, respectively). The utility of tifacogin is currently being evaluated in patients with severe community acquired pneumonia.

### Nematode Anticoagulant Protein

Recombinant NAPc2, an 85–amino acid polypeptide originally isolated from the canine hookworm, *Ancylostoma caninum* (107), can be expressed in yeast. NAPc2 binds to a noncatalytic site on factor X or factor Xa (108), and the resulting NAPc2/factor Xa complex then inhibits factor VIIa within the factor VIIa/tissue factor complex (see Fig. 123-5). Because it binds to factor X with high affinity, as well as to factor Xa, NAPc2 has a half-life of approximately 50 hours after subcutaneous injection.

Initial clinical trials with NAPc2 focused on venous thromboprophylaxis. In a phase II dose-finding study (109) of 293 patients undergoing elective knee arthroplasty, patients were given subcutaneous NAPc2 1 to 12 hours after surgery, and every second day thereafter to a maximum of four doses. A NAPc2 dose of 3.0 g per kg administered 1 hour after surgery appeared most effective. With this dose, the overall rate of venographically detected deep vein thrombosis (DVT) in the operated leg was 12%, whereas the rate of proximal DVT was 1%. Major bleeding occurred in 2% of these patients. When compared with historical controls (17), the efficacy and safety of NAPc2 are similar to those with LMWH. However, prospective randomized trials are needed to confirm these findings.

Current phase II studies with NAPc2 are focusing on arterial thrombosis, and this agent is being evaluated in patients with unstable angina or non–ST elevation myocardial infarction and in those undergoing percutaneous coronary interventions.

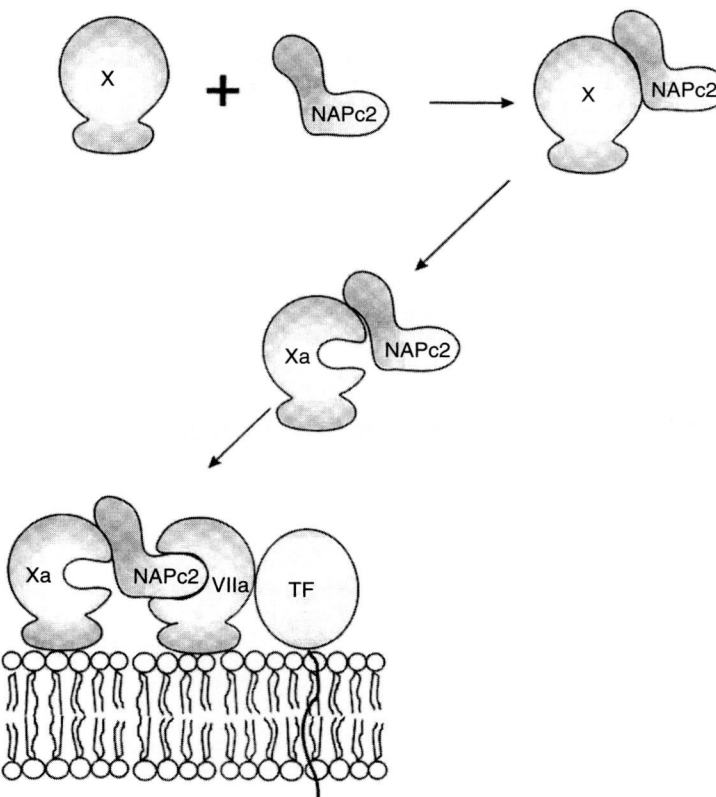

**FIGURE 123-5.** Mechanism of action of nematode anticoagulant protein (*NAPc2*). NAPc2 binds to a noncatalytic site of factor X (*X*) to form the X/NAPc2 complex. Once factor X is activated, the Xa/NAPc2 complex inactivates tissue factor (*TF*)-bound factor VIIa (*VIIa*). Because it binds X as well as Xa, NAPc2 has a long plasma half-life.

## Factor VIIai

Active-site–blocked factor VIIa (factor VIIai) attenuates initiation of coagulation by the factor VIIa/tissue factor complex by competing with factor VIIa for tissue factor binding. On the basis of promising results in animal models of thrombosis (110,111), factor VIIai, in doses ranging from 50 to 400 g per kg with or without adjunctive heparin, was compared with heparin alone in 491 patients undergoing elective percutaneous coronary interventions (112). Factor VIIai, with or without adjunctive heparin, was no more effective than heparin alone in reducing the primary endpoint, a composite of death, myocardial infarction, need for urgent revascularization, abrupt vessel closure, or bailout use of GP IIb/IIIa antagonists or heparin at day 7 or at hospital discharge. Rates of major bleeding were similar with factor VIIai and heparin. Because of these disappointing results, factor VIIai has not been developed further for treatment of arterial thrombosis.

## Inhibitors of Propagation of Coagulation

Drugs that block factor IXa, factor Xa, or their respective cofactors, factor VIIIa and factor Va, inhibit the propagation of coagulation. Strategies to block factor IXa include active-site–blocked factor IXa, which competes with factor IXa for incorporation into the intrinsic tenase complex that assembles on the surface of activated platelet and with monoclonal antibodies against factor IX/IXa. Factor IXa inhibitors have yet to reach phase II clinical testing.

New factor Xa inhibitors include agents that block factor Xa indirectly or directly. New indirect inhibitors act by catalyzing factor Xa inhibition by antithrombin but have features that distinguish them from LMWH (see Table 123-1). In contrast, direct factor Xa inhibitors bind directly to the active site of factor Xa, thereby blocking its interaction with its substrates. Unlike the heparin/antithrombin complex, direct factor Xa inhibitors not only inhibit free factor Xa, but also inactivate factor Xa bound to platelets within the prothrombinase complex (113,114). This property may endow these agents with an advantage over indirect factor Xa inhibitors. Fondaparinux and idraparinux are two new parenteral indirect factor Xa inhibitors. A parenteral (DX-9065a) and several orally active direct factor Xa inhibitors (razaxaban, BAY59-7939, and LY517717) are currently undergoing phase II clinical testing.

Inhibition of factors Va and VIIIa is effected by APC. From a therapeutic standpoint, this can be achieved by directly administering recombinant APC or its precursor, protein C. Recombinant soluble thrombomodulin (sTM), another means of generated APC, also is under evaluation.

## Indirect Factor Xa Inhibitors

**Fondaparinux.** A synthetic analog of the antithrombin-binding pentasaccharide sequence found in heparin and LMWH, fondaparinux binds antithrombin and enhances its reactivity with factor Xa (115). Because it is too short to bridge antithrombin to thrombin, fondaparinux has no activity against thrombin.

In plasma, fondaparinux binds to antithrombin without detectable binding to other plasma proteins. It has excellent bioavailability after subcutaneous injection and a plasma half-life of approximately 17 hours that permits once-daily subcutaneous administration. The drug is excreted unchanged in the urine. Consequently, dose adjustments are necessary in patients with renal insufficiency, and fondaparinux should not be used in those with renal failure.

Fondaparinux does not bind to platelets or platelet factor 4 (PF4). Because it does not induce the formation of heparin/PF4 complexes that serve as the antigenic target for the antibodies that cause heparin-induced thrombocytopenia, this condition is unlikely to occur with fondaparinux.

Fondaparinux also fails to interact with protamine sulfate (116), the antidote for heparin. With a half-life of approximately 17 hours, this could be problematic in a patient with life-threatening bleeding. If uncontrolled bleeding occurs with fondaparinux, a procoagulant, such as recombinant factor VIIa, might be effective (117). However, recombinant factor VIIa is not available in all hospitals, and the drug is expensive and can cause thrombotic complications. Although heparinase degrades fondaparinux into inactive disaccharides (118), heparinase is not available for clinical use.

Fondaparinux has been evaluated for prevention and treatment of VTE (see Table 123-2) and for treatment of arterial thrombosis.

*Venous thromboprophylaxis.* On the basis of four large phase III trials comparing fondaparinux with enoxaparin for thromboprophylaxis in patients undergoing surgery for hip fracture or elective hip or knee arthroplasty, fondaparinux has been licensed for these indications (119–122). In these trials, more than 7,300 patients were randomly assigned to receive fondaparinux (2.5 mg once daily) or fixed-dose enoxaparin. Overall, fondaparinux was found to reduce the risk of VTE by approximately 55%, compared with enoxaparin. Major bleeding occurred more frequently in the fondaparinux-treated group ($P = 0.008$), but the incidence of bleeding leading to death, reoperation, or occurring in a critical organ was not significantly different between the two groups (126). It is possible that the increase in major bleeding with fondaparinux relative to enoxaparin reflects the fact that fondaparinux was started 6 hours after surgery, whereas enoxaparin was initiated 12 to 24 hours after surgery, with or without a dose 12 hours before

---

**TABLE 123-1**

COMPARISON OF PROPERTIES OF FONDAPARINUX, IDRAPARINUX, AND LOW-MOLECULAR-WEIGHT HEPARIN

| Property | Fondaparinux | Idraparinux | LMWH |
|---|---|---|---|
| Factor Xa inhibition | Yes | Yes | Yes |
| Thrombin inhibition | No | No | Yes |
| Half-life (h) | 17 | 80 | 4 |
| Clearance | Renal | Renal | Renal |
| Reversal with protamine sulfate | No | No | Partial |

LMWH, low-molecular-weight heparin.

**TABLE 123-2**

PHASE III STUDIES EVALUATING FONDAPARINUX FOR THROMBOPROPHYLAXIS
AND TREATMENT OF VENOUS THROMBOEMBOLISM

| Study | Population | N | Fondaparinux dosing | Control dosing | Results |
|---|---|---|---|---|---|
| **THROMBOPROPHYLAXIS** | | | | | |
| PENTHIFRA (119) | Prophylaxis hip fracture | 1,250 | Fondaparinux 2.5 mg sc daily starting 6 ± 2 h after surgery | Enoxaparin 40 mg sc daily starting 12 ± 2 h before surgery | *Venographic DVT and Documented Symptomatic DVT or PE by Day 11:* Fondaparinux: 8.3%; Enoxaparin 19.1% ($P$ <0.001) *Major Bleeding:* Fondaparinux: 2.2%; Enoxaparin: 2.3% |
| EPHESUS (120) | Prophylaxis elective hip replacement | 1,827 | Fondaparinux 2.5 mg sc daily starting 6 ± 2 h after surgery | Enoxaparin 40 mg sc daily starting 12 h before surgery | *Venographic DVT and Documented Symptomatic DVT or PE by Day 11:* Fondaparinux: 4.1%; Enoxaparin 9.2% ($P$ <0.001) *Major Bleeding:* Fondaparinux: 4.1%; Enoxaparin: 2.8% |
| PENTATHLON 2000 (121) | Prophylaxis elective hip replacement | 1,584 | Fondaparinux 2.5 mg sc daily starting 6 ± 2 h after surgery | Enoxaparin 30 mg sc b.i.d. starting 12–24 h after surgery | *Venographic DVT and Documented Symptomatic DVT or PE by Day 11:* Fondaparinux: 6.1%; Enoxaparin: 8.3% *Major Bleeding:* Fondaparinux: 1.7%; Enoxaparin: 1.0% |
| PENTAMAKS (122) | Prophylaxis elective total knee replacement | 724 | Fondaparinux 2.5 mg sc daily starting 6 ± 2 h after surgery | Enoxaparin 30 mg sc b.i.d. starting 12–24 h after surgery | *Venographic DVT and Documented Symptomatic DVT or PE by Day 11:* Fondaparinux: 12.5%; Enoxaparin: 27.8% ($P$ <0.001) *Major Bleeding:* Fondaparinux: 2.1%; Enoxaparin: 0.2% ($P$ <0.006) |
| PENTHIFRA-Plus (123) | Extended prophylaxis hip fracture | 428 | Fondaparinux 2.5 mg sc daily for 19 to 23 d following 6 to 8 d of postoperative fondaparinux | Placebo for 19 to 23 d following 6 to 8 d of postoperative fondaparinux | *Venographic DVT and Documented Symptomatic DVT or PE:* Fondaparinux: 1.4%; Placebo: 35.09% ($P$ <0.001) *Major Bleeding:* Fondaparinux: 2.4%; Placebo: 0.6% |
| **TREATMENT OF VTE** | | | | | |
| MATISSE DVT (124) | Acute symptomatic DVT | 2,205 | Fondaparinux 5 mg (if <50 kg), 7.5 mg (if 50–100 kg), or 10 mg (if >100 kg) sc daily followed by warfarin (INR 2.0–3.0) | Enoxaparin (1 mg/kg sc b.i.d.) followed by warfarin (INR 2.0–3.0) | *Symptomatic Recurrent VTE at 3 mo:* Fondaparinux/warfarin: 3.9% Enoxaparin/warfarin: 4.1% *Major Bleeding:* Fondaparinux/warfarin: 1.1% Enoxaparin/warfarin: 1.2% |
| MATISSE PE (125) | Acute symptomatic PE | 2,213 | Fondaparinux 5 mg (if <50 kg), 7.5 mg (if >50–100 kg), or 10 mg (if >100 kg) sc daily followed by warfarin (INR 2.0–3.0) | Intravenous unfractionated heparin (activated partial thromboplastin time 1.5–2.5 × control) followed by warfarin (INR 2.0–3.0) | *Symptomatic Recurrent VTE at 3 mo:* Fondaparinux/warfarin: 2.8% Heparin/warfarin: 5.0% *Major Bleeding:* Fondaparinux/warfarin: 1.3% Heparin/warfarin: 1.1% |

PENTHIFRA, Pentasaccharide in Hip-Fracture surgery; sc, subcutaneously; EPHESUS, Eplerenone Post-AMI Heart Failure Efficacy and Survival Study; PENTATHLON, Pentasaccharide in the Prophylaxis and Treatment of Venous Thromboembolism; PENTAMAKS, Pentasaccharide in Major Knee Surgery; b.i.d., twice daily; DVT, deep-vein thrombosis; PE, pulmonary embolism; VTE, venous thromboembolism; INR, international normalized ratio.

surgery. It also is unclear whether the asymmetry in the timing of initiation of prophylaxis accounts for the superior efficacy of fondaparinux relative to enoxaparin.

Extended thromboprophylaxis with fondaparinux was studied in a phase III (Pentasaccharide in Hip-Fracture surgery) PENTHIFRA-Plus trial of 656 patients undergoing surgery for hip fracture (123). All patients received 2.5 mg of fondaparinux subcutaneously once daily for 7 days and were then randomized to receive continuing fondaparinux or to receive placebo for an additional 3 weeks, at which time routine venography was performed. Fondaparinux treatment decreased the rate of venographically diagnosed DVT from 35% to 1.4% ($P <0.001$). More importantly, the rate of symptomatic venous thromboembolic events also was reduced from 2.7% to 0.3% with extended fondaparinux treatment ($P = 0.021$).

Fondaparinux has also been evaluated for thromboprophylaxis in general medical and general surgical patients. In the double-blind ARTEMIS (Arixtra for Thromboembolism Prevention in Medical Indications Study) in which 849 medical patients 65 years or older who were randomly assigned to receive subcutaneous fondaparinux (2.5 mg once daily) or placebo for 6 to 14 days (127), the primary endpoint (a composite of venographically diagnosed DVT, symptomatic DVT, and nonfatal and fatal PE at day 15) occurred in 5.6% of patients randomized to fondaparinux and 10.5% of those given placebo ($P = 0.03$). There were no fatal pulmonary emboli in the fondaparinux arm and five in patients randomized to placebo. Major bleeding while on therapy was infrequent and occurred in 0.2% of patients in both groups. In a double-blind phase III trial of 2,297 patients undergoing abdominal surgery, participants were randomly assigned to receive subcutaneous fondaparinux (2.5 mg once daily, starting 6 hours after surgery) or dalteparin (2,500 U preoperatively and 5,000 U postoperatively) for 5 to 9 days (128). The primary endpoint, a composite of venographically documented DVT, symptomatic DVT, and nonfatal and fatal PE at postoperative day 30, occurred in 4.6% of those randomized to fondaparinux and in 6.1% of those given dalteparin ($P = 0.14$). Symptomatic VTE occurred in 0.4% of those given fondaparinux and in 0.3% of those treated with dalteparin, whereas major bleeding occurred in 3.4% of patients treated with fondaparinux and 2.4% of patients receiving dalteparin; differences that are not statistically significant. In the subgroup of patients with cancer, fondaparinux reduced the composite endpoint from 7.7% to 4.6% ($P = 0.02$).

*Treatment of venous thromboembolism.* Fondaparinux also has been evaluated for initial treatment of established VTE in two randomized phase III clinical trials. On the basis of these studies, the drug has been licensed for the initial treatment of VTE.

The double-blind MATISSE DVT trial enrolled 2,205 patients with DVT who were randomized to receive either fondaparinux (5, 7.5, or 10 mg subcutaneously once daily in those weighing <50 kg, 50 to 100 kg, or more than 100 kg, respectively) or enoxaparin (1 mg per kg subcutaneously twice daily) for 5 days followed by a minimum of a 3-month course of treatment with an oral vitamin K antagonist (124). At 3 months, rates of recurrent symptomatic VTE with fondaparinux or enoxaparin were 3.9% and 4.1%, respectively; whereas major bleeding rates were 1.1% and 1.2%, respectively. None of these differences are statistically significant.

The MATISSE Pulmonary Embolism trial was an open-label study of 2,213 patients with PE who were randomized to receive either fondaparinux (5, 7.5, or 10 mg subcutaneously once daily in patients weighing <50 kg, 50 to 100 kg, or >100 kg, respectively) or unfractionated heparin (by continuous infusion) for 5 days, followed by a minimum of a 3-month course of therapy with an oral vitamin K antagonist (125). At 3 months, rates of

recurrent symptomatic VTE with fondaparinux or unfractionated heparin were 3.8% and 5.0%, respectively; whereas major bleeding rates were 1.3% and 1.1%, respectively. On the basis of these two trials, fondaparinux appears to be as effective and safe as LMWH or unfractionated heparin for initial treatment of VTE.

*Treatment of acute coronary syndromes.* Fondaparinux has been evaluated for treatment of acute coronary syndromes in two phase II studies. In the (pentasaccharide as an adjunct to fibrinolysis in ST elevation acute myocardial infarction) PENTALYSE trial, an open-label dose-finding study, coadministration of varying doses of fondaparinux with alteplase in ST segment elevation myocardial infarction produced similar angiographic patency rates at 90 minutes, as did unfractionated heparin and alteplase (129). Bleeding rates were also similar in those receiving fondaparinux and in those randomized to heparin.

Fondaparinux also compared favorably with enoxaparin in a large phase II trial of patients with acute coronary syndrome without ST segment elevation. The (Pentasaccharide in Unstable Angina) PENTUA trial randomized 1,134 patients with unstable angina to subcutaneous fondaparinux (in once-daily doses ranging from 2.5 to 12 mg) or enoxaparin (1 mg per kg twice daily) (130). Overall, the primary outcome, a composite of death, myocardial infarction, or recurrent angina at day 9, occurred in 37% of those given any dose of fondaparinux and in 40.2% of patients treated with enoxaparin. There was no evidence of a dose-response with fondaparinux. In fact, the lowest dose appeared to produce the best results. Bleeding was similar in all treatment groups. On the basis of these phase II results, phase III trials with fondaparinux are underway in patients with ST elevation and non–ST elevation myocardial infarction.

**Idraparinux.** This more negatively charged derivative of fondaparinux binds antithrombin with such high affinity that its plasma half-life of 80 hours approximates that of antithrombin (131). Because of its long half-life, idraparinux can be given subcutaneously on a once-weekly basis. As with fondaparinux, there is no antidote for idraparinux. A neutralizing agent may be particularly important for this agent because of its long half-life. Idraparinux is not degraded by heparinase. Although procoagulants, such as factor VIIa, reverse the anticoagulant effects of idraparinux in healthy volunteers (132), their utility in patients treated with idraparinux with a major bleed is yet to be determined. Table 123-1 contains a comparison of the properties of fondaparinux, idraparinux, and LMWH.

In a phase II trial, idraparinux was compared with warfarin in 659 patients with proximal DVT (133). After 5 to 7 days of initial treatment with enoxaparin, patients were randomized to receive once-weekly subcutaneous idraparinux (2.5, 7.5, or 10 mg) or warfarin for 12 weeks. The primary endpoint, changes in compression ultrasound and perfusion lung scan findings, was similar in all idraparinux groups and did not differ from that in the warfarin group. However, there was a clear dose-response for major bleeding in patients given idraparinux, with an unacceptably high frequency in those given the 10-mg dose. In two patients, who received 5 mg of idraparinux once weekly, a fatal bleed occurred. Patients given the lowest dose of idraparinux had less bleeding than those randomized to warfarin ($P = 0.029$). On the basis of these results, a once-weekly 2.5-mg dose of idraparinux is being evaluated in a phase III clinical trial.

## Direct Factor Xa Inhibitors

**DX-9065a.** This nonpeptidic arginine derivative binds reversibly to the active site of factor Xa and has been shown to be effective in thrombosis models in laboratory animals (134). DX-9065a exhibits oral bioavailability in animals but must be given in high doses to produce an antithrombotic effect (134).

In a small phase II trial performed to assess safety, four different doses of DX-9065a were given as a continuous intravenous infusion to 73 patients with stable coronary artery disease. There were no major bleeds with DX-9065a (135). In the Xa Neutralization for Atherosclerotic Disease Understanding-Percutaneous Coronary Intervention (XANADU-PCI) pilot study (136), which randomized 175 patients undergoing percutaneous coronary interventions to different doses of DX-9065a or to heparin, DX-9065a appeared to be a promising alternative to heparin. This possibility requires confirmation in phase III clinical trials.

**Razaxaban.** An orally active agent, razaxaban is given twice daily. In a phase II dose-finding study, razaxaban was compared with enoxaparin in 656 patients undergoing elective knee arthroplasty (137). Patients were randomized to oral razaxaban (in doses ranging from 25 mg to 100 mg twice daily starting 8 hours after surgery) or to subcutaneous enoxaparin (30 mg twice daily starting 12 to 24 hours after surgery) for 10 days. The primary endpoint, a composite of venographically detected DVT and symptomatic VTE, occurred in 8.6% of patients randomized to the lowest dose of razaxaban and in 15.9% of those given enoxaparin. Major bleeding occurred in 0.7% of patients given this dose of razaxaban and in none of those treated with enoxaparin. The three higher-dose razaxaban arms of the study were stopped prematurely because of increased rates of major bleeding. Further phase II studies are underway to identify the optimal dose of this agent.

*BAY59-7939 and LY-517717.* These orally active, small-molecule direct factor Xa inhibitors are currently undergoing phase II testing for thromboprophylaxis in patients undergoing elective knee arthroplasty.

### Modulators of the Protein C Pathway

APC is a naturally occurring anticoagulant that is generated when the thrombin–thrombomodulin complex activates protein C. By proteolytically degrading and inactivating factors Va and VIIIa, APC (along with its cofactor protein S) blocks thrombin-induced autocatalysis (138). Strategies aimed at enhancing the protein C anticoagulant pathway include administration of recombinant activated protein C, protein C concentrates, or sTM (see Fig. 123-6).

**Activated Protein C.** In a phase III clinical trial, recombinant APC, drotrecogin alfa (activated), was compared with placebo in 1,690 patients with severe sepsis (139). When given as an infusion of 24 g/kg/hour over 96 hours, APC produced a 19% reduction in 28-day mortality (from 30.8% to 24.7%; $P = 0.005$). The rate of major bleeding was higher with APC than with placebo (3.5% and 2%, respectively; $P = 0.06$). On the basis of these results and economic analyses supporting the benefits of recombinant APC (140), this agent has been licensed in North America for treatment of patients with severe sepsis.

**Protein C.** Although promising results with protein C concentrates have been reported in patients with meningococcemia (141,142), additional studies are needed. For theoretical reasons, APC may be a better choice than protein C in patients with severe sepsis because inflammatory cytokines downregulate thrombomodulin (TM) and endothelial protein C receptor (the receptor that binds protein C and presents it to the thrombin/thrombomodulin complex) expression on the endothelial surface. This phenomenon may explain the results of immunohistochemical analyses of skin biopsies from patients with meningococcemia, which revealed reduced TM and endothelial protein C receptor staining (143).

**Soluble Thrombomodulin.** A recombinant analog of the extracellular domain of thrombomodulin, sTM binds thrombin and induces a conformational change in the active site of the enzyme that abolishes its procoagulant activity and converts it into a potent activator of protein C (144). This agent has a half-life of 2 to 3 days after subcutaneous injection. In an open-label, dose-escalation study, sTM attenuated coagulation abnormalities in patients with disseminated intravascular coagulation (145). In a phase II dose-ranging study of 312 patients undergoing elective hip arthroplasty (146), study participants were given subcutaneous TM (at a dose of 0.3 or 0.45 mg per kg) 2 to 4 hours after surgery; those given the lower dose of TM received a second injection 5 days later. The primary endpoint, a composite of venographically detected DVT and symptomatic VTE, occurred in 4.3% of the 94 patients given the lower dose of sTM and in none of the 99 patients receiving the higher dose. Major bleeding occurred in 1.6% and 5.7% of patients receiving the low or high dose of sTM, respectively. Phase III clinical trials are necessary to compare sTM with other forms of thromboprophylaxis, such as LMWH or fondaparinux.

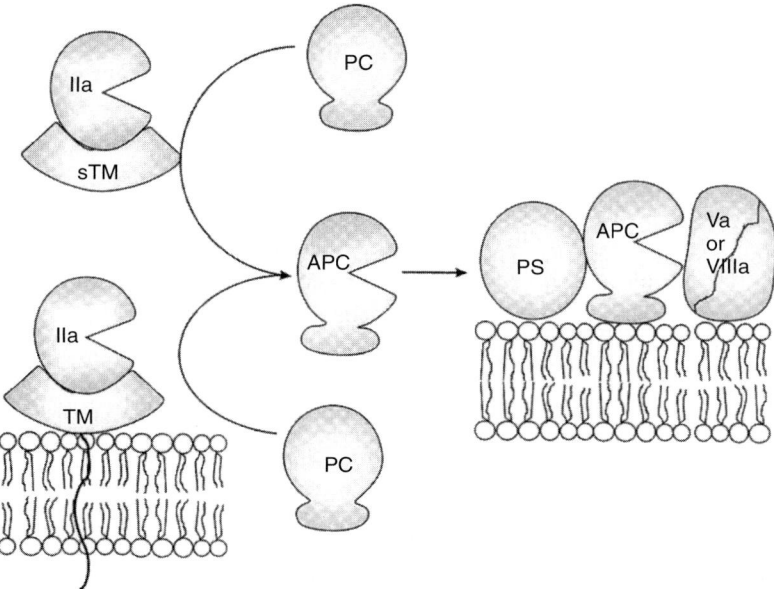

**FIGURE 123-6.** The protein C pathway. Protein C (*PC*) is converted to activated protein C (*APC*) by thrombin (*IIa*) bound either to thrombomodulin (*TM*) or to the soluble, extracellular portion of TM (*sTM*). APC acts as an anticoagulant by degrading and inactivating factors Va and VIIIa (*Va and VIIIa*), key cofactors in coagulation. Protein S (*PS*) serves as a cofactor in this inactivation reaction.

## Inhibitors of Thrombin Activity

Because of its central role in coagulation and hemostasis, thrombin is an ideal target for new anticoagulants. This enzyme can be inhibited indirectly or directly. Indirect thrombin inhibitors, such as unfractionated heparin, LMWH, and dermatan sulfate act by catalyzing the naturally occurring thrombin inhibitors, antithrombin and/or heparin cofactor II (7,147,148). In contrast, direct inhibitors bind directly to thrombin and block its interaction with substrates. All of the new agents that block fibrin formation are direct thrombin inhibitors.

Direct thrombin inhibitors have properties that give them potential mechanistic advantages over indirect thrombin inhibitors, such as heparin (149,150). Direct thrombin inhibitors produce a more predictable anticoagulant response because they do not bind to plasma proteins. Unlike heparin (151), direct thrombin inhibitors do not bind to PF4, and as a result, the anticoagulant activity of direct thrombin inhibitors is unaffected by the large quantities of PF4 released in the vicinity of platelet-rich thrombi. Whereas thrombin bound to fibrin or fibrin degradation products is relatively protected from inactivation by heparin (152–154), direct thrombin inhibitors inactivate fibrin-bound thrombin as well as fluid-phase thrombin (149,150,153,154). Unlike the heparin/antithrombin complex (155), direct thrombin inhibitors are able to readily access and inactivate thrombin bound to platelets, thereby blocking thrombin-mediated platelet aggregation. Three parenteral direct thrombin inhibitors (hirudin, argatroban, and bivalirudin) have been licensed in North America for limited indications. Ximelagatran, the first oral direct thrombin inhibitor, has undergone phase III clinical evaluation for prevention and treatment of VTE and for prevention of cardioembolic events in patients with atrial fibrillation. This agent is of particular interest because it has potential advantages over vitamin K antagonists (see Table 123-3).

**Hirudin.** Recombinant hirudin (156,157) has been studied for use in patients with acute coronary syndromes (158,159) as an adjunct to thrombolysis in patients with ST segment elevation myocardial infarction (160–166), for prevention of restenosis after percutaneous coronary angioplasty (167), for prophylaxis of VTE following hip arthroplasty (168,169), in the treatment of VTE (170), and as an alternative anticoagulant in patients with heparin-induced thrombocytopenia (171–173). Hirudin is at least as effective as heparin in unstable angina and non–ST elevation

and ST elevation myocardial infarction, and is more effective than LMWH and unfractionated heparin for the prevention of venous thrombosis in patients undergoing elective hip arthroplasty. Because of its narrow therapeutic window and associated bleeding risk, however, it is unlikely that hirudin will ever be approved for treatment of acute coronary syndromes. Although hirudin appears promising for prevention and treatment of venous thrombosis, clinical development of the drug for these indications has not been pursued. Hirudin has been used successfully to treat patients with arterial and venous thromboembolic complications of heparin-induced thrombocytopenia and as an alternative to heparin during cardiopulmonary bypass in a small number of patients with heparin-induced thrombocytopenia (174,175). On the basis of these data, hirudin has been approved by the US Food and Drug Administration for the treatment of patients with heparin-induced thrombocytopenia.

**Bivalirudin.** A synthetic 20–amino acid analog of hirudin, bivalirudin has been evaluated in patients undergoing percutaneous coronary interventions (176–179) and as an adjunct to streptokinase in patients with acute myocardial infarction (180). With its predictable anticoagulant response and short half-life (181–185), bivalirudin is a convenient drug to use in patients undergoing percutaneous coronary interventions. In this setting, bivalirudin appears to be at least as effective as heparin and produces less bleeding. For patients undergoing percutaneous coronary interventions without an adjunctive GP IIb/IIIa antagonist, bivalirudin may be a better choice than heparin. In patients with acute ST elevation myocardial infarction, bivalirudin can be used in place of heparin as an adjunct to streptokinase. In this setting, bivalirudin may reduce the risk of reinfarction, compared with heparin. However, bivalirudin therapy requires monitoring when used in conjunction with thrombolytic therapy, and dose adjustment appears necessary to reduce the risk of bleeding. At present, bivalirudin is licensed as an alternative to heparin in patients undergoing percutaneous coronary interventions.

**Argatroban.** A small-molecule, active-site–directed inhibitor of thrombin, argatroban has been investigated as a treatment of patients with heparin-induced thrombocytopenia and is currently licensed for this indication (186,187). Although phase II trials have evaluated argatroban for treatment of unstable angina (188), as an adjunct to thrombolysis (189), and as an alternative to heparin in patients undergoing coronary angioplasty (190), the studies are small and none have shown definitive advantages of argatroban over heparin.

**Ximelagatran.** The first orally available direct thrombin inhibitor, ximelagatran is a prodrug of the active-site–directed thrombin inhibitor, melagatran. Ximelagatran is absorbed from the small intestine, with bioavailability of approximately 20% (191). Ximelagatran levels peak in the blood 30 minutes after oral administration. Once in the blood, ximelagatran undergoes rapid biotransformation to melagatran by two intermediate metabolites, H338/57 and H415/04. Melagatran levels peak in the blood within 2 hours. Because melagatran has a plasma half-life of 3 to 4 hours in healthy volunteers and 4 to 5 hours in patients, ximelagatran is administered orally twice daily. To date, no foods or drugs have been documented to influence its absorption. Ximelagatran does not inhibit cytochrome P-450 enzymes (192) and therefore has a low potential for drug–drug interactions. Because ximelagatran produces such a predictable anticoagulant response, coagulation monitoring is unnecessary. Melagatran, the active agent, is eliminated through the kidneys. Consequently, dose adjustments may be needed in the elderly and in patients with renal insufficiency (191,193,194).

Ximelagatran is being evaluated for thromboprophylaxis in high-risk orthopedic patients, treatment of VTE, prevention of cardioembolic events in patients with nonvalvular atrial fibrillation, and prevention of recurrent ischemia in patients with recent myocardial infarction (see Table 123-4).

---

### TABLE 123-3

**POTENTIAL ADVANTAGES OF XIMELAGATRAN OVER WARFARIN AND THEIR CONSEQUENCES**

| Advantage | Consequence |
|---|---|
| Rapid onset of action | No need for overlap with a parenteral anticoagulant when initiating treatment of VTE |
| Predictable anticoagulant response | No need for routine coagulation monitoring |
| No drug, food, or alcohol interactions | Can be given in fixed doses |
| Wide therapeutic window | No need for routine coagulation monitoring |
| Short half-life | Overcomes lack of an antidote |

VTE, venous thromboembolism.

**TABLE 123-4**

PHASE III STUDIES EVALUATING XIMELAGATRAN FOR THROMBOPROPHYLAXIS AND VENOUS THROMBOEMBOLISM OR FOR PREVENTION OF CARDIOEMBOLIC EVENTS IN PATIENTS WITH ATRIAL FIBRILLATION

| Study | Population dosing | N | Ximelagatran | Control dosing | Results |
|---|---|---|---|---|---|
| **THROMBOPROPHYLAXIS** | | | | | |
| METHRO III (195) | Prophylaxis total hip or knee arthroplasty | 2,788 | Melagatran 3 mg sc postoperatively, then ximelagatran 24 mg b.i.d. | Enoxaparin 40 sc daily starting 12 h before surgery | *Proximal DVT by venogram and PE:* Ximelagatran: 5.6%; Enoxaparin 6.2% *Major Bleeding:* Ximelagatran: 1.4%; Enoxaparin: 1.7% |
| EXPRESS (196) | Prophylaxis total hip or knee replacement | 2,764 | Melagatran 2 mg sc preoperatively, then 3 mg sc given the evening after surgery followed by ximelagatran 24 mg b.i.d. | Enoxaparin 40 mg sc daily starting 12 h before surgery | *Venographic Proximal DVT and PE:* Ximelagatran: 2.3%; Enoxaparin 6.3% ($P$ <0.001) *Major Bleeding:* Ximelagatran: 3.3%; Enoxaparin: 1.2% ($P$ <0.001) |
| Platinum-hip (197) | Prophylaxis total hip replacement | 1,838 | Ximelagatran 24 mg b.i.d. starting after surgery | Enoxaparin 30 mg sc b.i.d. starting after surgery | *Venographic Proximal DVT and PE:* Ximelagatran: 3.6%; Enoxaparin: 1.2% ($P$ <0.05) *Major Bleeding:* Ximelagatran: 0.8%; Enoxaparin: 0.9% |
| Platinum-knee (198) | Prophylaxis total knee replacement | 680 | Ximelagatran 24 mg b.i.d. starting after surgery | Warfarin (INR 1.8–3.0) | *Venographic Proximal DVT and PE:* Ximelagatran: 3.3%; Warfarin: 5.0% *Major Bleeding:* Ximelagatran: 1.7%; Warfarin: 0.9% |
| EXULT A (199) | Prophylaxis total knee replacement | 2,301 | Ximelagatran 24 mg or 36 mg b.i.d. starting after surgery | Warfarin (INR 1.8–3.0) | *Total VTE or Death:* Ximelagatran (36 mg): 20.3% (vs. warfarin, $P$ = 0.003) Ximelagatran (24 mg): 24.9% Warfarin: 27.6% *Major Bleeding:* Ximelagatran (either dose): 0.8% Warfarin: 0.7% |
| EXULT B (200) | Prophylaxis total knee replacement | 2,303 | Ximelagatran 36 mg b.i.d. starting after surgery | Warfarin (INR 1.8–3.0) | *Total VTE or Death:* Ximelagatran: 22.5%; Warfarin: 31.9% ($P$ <0.001) *Major Bleeding:* Ximelagatran: 1.0%; Warfarin: 0.4% |
| **VTE FOR PREVENTION OF CARDIOEMBOLIC EVENTS IN PATIENTS WITH ATRIAL FIBRILLATIONS** | | | | | |
| THRIVE Treatment (201) | Acute VTE | 2,489 | Ximelagatran 36 mg b.i.d. × 6 mo | Enoxaparin (1 mg/kg sc b.i.d.) followed by warfarin (INR 2.0–3.0) | *Symptomatic Recurrent VTE:* Ximelagatran: 2.1% Enoxaparin/warfarin: 2.0% *Major Bleeding:* Ximelagatran: 1.3% Enoxaparin/warfarin: 2.2% |
| THRIVE III (202) | VTE, following 6 mo of conventional therapy | 1,233 | Ximelagatran 24 mg b.i.d. × 18 mo | Placebo | *Symptomatic Recurrent VTE:* Ximelagatran: 2.8%; Placebo 12.6% ($P$ <0.001) *Major Bleeding:* Ximelagatran: 1.1%; Placebo: 1.3% |
| SPORTIF III (203) | Atrial fibrillation | 3,407 | Ximelagatran 36 mg b.i.d. | Warfarin (INR 2.0–3.0) | *All Stroke and Systemic Embolism:* Ximelagatran: 1.6%; Warfarin: 2.3% *Major Bleeding:* Ximelagatran: 1.3%; Warfarin: 1.8% |
| SPORTIF V (204) | Atrial fibrillation | 3,922 | Ximelagatran 36 mg b.i.d. | Warfarin (INR 2.0–3.0) | *All Stroke and Systemic Embolism:* Ximelagatran: 1.6%; Warfarin: 1.2% *Major Bleeding:* Ximelagatran: 2.4%; Warfarin: 3.1% |

METHRO, melagatran for thrombin inhibition in orthopaedic surgery; sc, subcutaneously; b.i.d., twice daily; DVT, deep-vein thrombosis; EXPRESS, expanded prophylaxis evaluation surgery; PE, pulmonary embolism; EXULT, exanta used to lessen thrombosis A and B; VTE, venous thromboembolism; THRIVE, Thrombin Inhibitors in Venous Thromboembolism; SPORTIF, Stroke Prevention in Oral direct Thrombin Inhibitor ximelagatran in atrial Fibrillation; INR, international normalized ratio.

*Venous thromboprophylaxis.* For thromboprophylaxis, ximelagatran in combination with subcutaneous melagatran, or as monotherapy, has been compared with LMWH and warfarin. In the METHRO II (melagatran for thrombin inhibition in orthopaedic surgery) study (205), subcutaneous melagatran (given preoperatively and twice daily for 1 to 3 days postoperatively) followed by oral ximelagatran (in various doses) was compared with subcutaneous dalteparin (5000 U once daily starting the evening before surgery) in patients undergoing elective hip or knee arthroplasty. A highly significant dose-response for both effectiveness and safety was seen with the ximelagatran/melagatran combination.

Because a trend for excess bleeding at the operative site was seen in the METHRO II study, an attempt was made to omit the preoperative melagatran dose in the subsequent phase III trial. Consequently, the METHRO III trial (195) randomized 2,788 patients undergoing hip or knee arthroplasty to receive either subcutaneous melagatran (3 mg) postoperatively followed by oral ximelagatran (24 mg twice daily) or subcutaneous enoxaparin (40 mg once daily) starting 12 hours before surgery. Although the rates of venographically detected proximal DVT and symptomatic PE were similar in patients given melagatran/ximelagatran or enoxaparin (5.7% and 6.2%, respectively), rates of total VTE were slightly higher in the melagatran/ximelagatran group (31% and 27.3%, respectively). Rates of bleeding did not differ between the two groups. On the basis of these unfavorable results, a subsequent phase III trial again started melagatran treatment preoperatively.

The EXPRESS (expanded prophylaxis evaluation surgery) study (196) randomized 2,764 patients undergoing hip or knee arthroplasty to melagatran/ximelagatran or enoxaparin. Subcutaneous melagatran (2 mg) was given immediately before surgery with a subsequent 3-mg subcutaneous dose given on the evening after surgery. This was followed by oral ximelagatran (24 mg twice daily). In the enoxaparin group, subcutaneous enoxaparin (40 mg) was given once daily, starting the evening before surgery. The primary endpoint, a composite of venographically detected proximal DVT and symptomatic PE, occurred in 2.3% and 6.3% of patients treated with melagatran/ximelagatran and enoxaparin, respectively (P <0.001). Symptomatic venous thrombosis was rare, occurring in eight patients in the melagatran/ximelagatran group and 12 given enoxaparin. Although bleeding was more common with ximelagatran/melagatran than with enoxaparin (3.3% and 1.2%, respectively), there was no difference in the rates of fatal bleeding, critical organ bleeding, or bleeding requiring reoperation. Therefore, melagatran started immediately before surgery followed by postoperative ximelagatran reduces the incidence of proximal DVT and PE by 63% compared with enoxaparin.

In North America, thromboprophylaxis is started postoperatively in patients affected orthopedically because many patients have spinal anesthesia. To evaluate the utility of ximelagatran in this setting, the Platinum–Hip trial (197) randomized 1,838 patients undergoing total hip arthroplasty to receive oral ximelagatran (24 mg twice daily) or enoxaparin (30 mg twice daily) for 7 to 12 days. Both drugs were started the morning after surgery. The overall rates of venographically detected DVT in the operated leg and symptomatic PE by day 12 were 7.9% and 4.6% in patients given ximelagatran and enoxaparin, respectively (P <0.05); whereas the rates of proximal DVT and PE were 3.6% and 1.2%, respectively (P <0.05). Rates of major bleeding were similar in the two treatment groups (0.8% and 0.9%, respectively). Therefore, when started postoperatively, a 24-mg twice-daily dose of ximelagatran appears less effective than enoxaparin in patients undergoing total hip arthroplasty.

The same dose of ximelagatran also has been compared with warfarin for thromboprophylaxis in patients undergoing elective knee arthroplasty. The Platinum–Knee trial (198) randomized 680 such patients to receive postoperative ximelagatran (24 mg twice daily) or warfarin [in doses sufficient to produce an international normalized ratio (INR) of 1.8 to 3.0]. Rates of total DVT with ximelagatran and warfarin were 19.2% and 25.7%, respectively (P = 0.07), whereas rates of proximal DVT or symptomatic PE were 3.3% and 5.0%, respectively (P >0.2). There was no significant difference in the rate of major bleeding in the ximelagatran and warfarin groups (1.7% and 0.9%, respectively).

To determine whether the 24-mg twice-daily dose of ximelagatran is optimal for postoperative thromboprophylaxis, the first phase of the EXULT (exanta used to lessen thrombosis A and B) trial (199) randomized 2,301 patients undergoing elective knee arthroplasty to one of the two doses of unmonitored ximelagatran (24 or 36 mg twice daily) or warfarin (in doses sufficient to produce an INR of 1.8 to 3.0). Ximelagatran was started in the morning after surgery, whereas the first dose of warfarin was given in the evening of the day of surgery. The primary endpoint, a composite of total VTE and all-cause mortality, was significantly lower with the 36-mg dose of ximelagatran than with warfarin (20.3% and 27.6%, respectively; P = 0.003). Likewise, the point estimate for proximal venous thrombosis and all-cause mortality also was lower (2.7% and 4.1%, respectively), although this difference did not reach statistical significance. Major bleeding occurred in 4.8% and 5.3% of patients given low- or high-dose ximelagatran, respectively, and in 4.5% of those treated with warfarin, differences that were not statistically significant. On the basis of these data, the second phase of the EXULT trial randomized an additional 2,300 patients to ximelagatran (36 mg twice daily) or warfarin (200). The frequency of the primary efficacy endpoint (total VTE and death) was lower in those patients randomized to ximelagatran than in those given warfarin (22.5% and 31.9%, respectively; P <0.001). Major bleeding occurred in 1.0% and 0.4% of patients treated with ximelagatran and warfarin, respectively, a difference that was not statistically significant.

Therefore, data available to date suggest that (a) the combination of subcutaneous melagatran started before surgery followed by oral ximelagatran postoperatively is more effective than enoxaparin for thromboprophylaxis after hip or knee arthroplasty, but may cause more bleeding, and (b) postoperative ximelagatran, at a dose of 36 mg twice daily, is more effective than warfarin for thromboprophylaxis after knee arthroplasty. Unlike warfarin, however, ximelagatran does not require coagulation monitoring. Consequently, ximelagatran may be particularly useful for extended out-of-hospital prophylaxis in high-risk patients, a concept that will require testing in future studies.

*Treatment of venous thrombosis.* In THRIVE (Thrombin Inhibitors in Venous Thromboembolism) I, a phase II dose-ranging study (206), 350 patients with venous thrombosis were randomized to monotherapy with ximelagatran (in doses ranging from 24 to 60 mg twice daily) or subcutaneous dalteparin followed by warfarin for 2 weeks. On the basis of follow-up venograms, the rate of thrombus regression plus changes in clinical symptoms were similar in both groups. There was a trend for more thrombus progression with ximelagatran than with dalteparin (8% and 3%, respectively), but this difference was not statistically significant. Rates of bleeding were similar in both treatment groups.

Building on this information, a phase III trial comparing oral ximelagatran monotherapy (36 mg twice daily) for 6 months with enoxaparin (1 mg per kg subcutaneously twice daily) followed by warfarin (in doses sufficient to produce an INR of 2 to 3) for 6 months (THRIVE Treatment trial) was performed (201). A total of 2,498 patients with VTE were entered in the trial; 1,249 were randomized to ximelagatran and 1,249 to enoxaparin followed by warfarin. The primary endpoint, objectively documented recurrent VTE, occurred in 2.1% and 2.0% of those randomized to ximelagatran or enoxaparin/warfarin, respectively. Major bleeding occurred in 1.3% and 2.2% of those randomized to ximelagatran or enoxaparin/warfarin, respectively, differences that were not statistically significant. Elevations in serum alanine transaminase of greater than three times the upper limit of normal occurred in 9.6% of patients receiving ximelagatran versus 2.0% of those receiving enoxaparin/warfarin. All-cause mortality rates were 2.3% and 3.4% in the ximelagatran and enoxaparin/warfarin groups, respectively.

This study suggests that oral ximelagatran is as effective and safe as conventional anticoagulation with LMWH followed by warfarin for initial treatment of patients with VTE. Unlike LMWH, ximelagatran can be given orally, and in contrast to warfarin, ximelagatran does not require anticoagulation monitoring. Consequently, ximelagatran is more convenient to administer than conventional treatment. However, more information about the long-term sequelae of the liver transaminase increase is required.

Ximelagatran also has been evaluated for prevention of recurrent thrombosis in patients with VTE. The THRIVE III trial (202) randomized 1,233 patients who had completed a 6-month course of anticoagulant therapy for treatment of VTE to ximelagatran (24 mg twice daily) or placebo for an additional 18 months. Recurrent VTE, the primary endpoint, occurred in 2.8% of patients given ximelagatran and in 12.6% of those randomized to placebo (hazard ratio, 0.16; $P$ <0.001). Major bleeding occurred in 1.1% of patients treated with ximelagatran and in 1.3% of those given placebo (hazard ratio, 1.16; $P$ = NS), and there were no fatal or intracranial bleeds.

*Atrial fibrillation.* Ximelagatran has been compared with warfarin in patients with nonvalvular atrial fibrillation. In the SPORTIF (Stroke Prevention in Oral direct Thrombin Inhibitor ximelagatran in atrial Fibrillation) II trial (203), 257 patients were randomized to receive one of three doses of ximelagatran (20, 40, or 60 mg twice daily) or warfarin (in doses sufficient to produce an INR of 2.0 to 3.0). Ximelagatran was given without coagulation monitoring. At 12 weeks, fewer patients in the ximelagatran group had transient ischemic attacks (0.5% and 3%, respectively), and one patient in the ximelagatran group had an ischemic stroke, compared with none in those given warfarin. There were no major bleeds in any of the ximelagatran groups, but one major, non-intracranial bleed was observed in a patient receiving warfarin. The ongoing SPORTIF IV trial (207) is an open-label continuation of this trial comparing a fixed dose of unmonitored ximelagatran (36 mg twice daily) with warfarin.

The promising results of the SPORTIF II trial prompted two phase III trials comparing ximelagatran with warfarin. The SPORTIF III trial, which used an open-label design, was conducted in Europe, whereas the double-blind SPORTIF V trial was performed in North America. Both trials enrolled patients with atrial fibrillation and at least one additional risk factor for stroke. SPORTIF III (208) randomized 3,407 such patients to receive ximelagatran (36 mg twice daily) or warfarin (in doses sufficient to produce an INR of 2.0 to 3.0) for 12 to 26 months. The primary event rate (all strokes, both ischemic and hemorrhagic, and systemic embolic events) was similar in those given ximelagatran and warfarin (1.6% per year and 2.3% per year, respectively; $P$ = 0.10). Rates of major bleeding also were similar with ximelagatran and warfarin (1.3% and 1.8% per year, respectively), whereas the rate of major plus minor bleeding was significantly lower with ximelagatran than with warfarin (25.5% and 29.5% per year, respectively; $P$ = 0.003). All-cause mortality was 3.2% per year in both treatment groups.

The SPORTIF V trial enrolled 3,922 patients (204). The primary event rate with ximelagatran was 1.6% per year, a rate identical to that observed with ximelagatran in the SPORTIF III trial, whereas the rate with warfarin was 1.2% per year ($P$ = 0.13). Rates of major bleeding were similar in patients randomized to ximelagatran or warfarin (2.4% and 3.1% per year, respectively; $P$ = 0.16), and intracranial hemorrhage occurred in 0.06% of participants in both treatment groups. The rate of combined major plus minor bleeding was lower with ximelagatran than with warfarin (37% and 47% per year, respectively; $P$ <0.001 ).

Differences in the primary efficacy endpoint in patients randomized to warfarin in the SPORTIF V and SPORTIF III studies likely reflect chance. Entry criteria were the same in both studies, and bias from lack of blinding in the SPORTIF III study is unlikely because of the "hard" endpoints used in these trials. INR control was very good, and similar, in both trials.

When the results of the SPORTIF III and SPORTIF V are combined, the absolute difference in the rate of stroke and systemic embolic events is 0.3% lower in those given ximelagatran, a difference that is not significant. There was a 0.6% absolute difference in the rates of major bleeding favoring ximelagatran ($P$ = 0.54). Therefore, these studies indicate that unmonitored ximelagatran is as effective and safe as dose-adjusted warfarin. It is important to note that warfarin control was excellent in the two SPORTIF trials. Using an expanded therapeutic INR range of 1.8 to 3.2, 81% and 83% of INR values were within range in SPORTIF III and V, respectively. In contrast, reports suggest that less than 50% of INR values are therapeutic when warfarin is managed in the community setting. Therefore, the SPORTIF trials compare ximelagatran with optimally controlled warfarin.

*Myocardial infarction.* In the phase II Efficacy and Safety of Oral Direct Thrombin Inhibitor Ximelagatran in Patients with Recent Myocardial Damage (ESTEEM) trial (209), ximelagatran was compared with placebo in 1,883 patients with ST elevation or non–ST elevation myocardial infarction within the past 14 days. Study participants were randomized to receive oral ximelagatran (in doses of 24, 36, 48, or 60 mg twice daily) or placebo for 6 months. All patients were given aspirin (160 mg daily) and optimal medical management that included statins and angiotensin-converting enzyme (ACE) inhibitors. Compared with placebo, all four ximelagatran doses significantly reduced the frequency of the primary endpoint, a composite of all-cause mortality, recurrent myocardial infarction, and severe recurrent ischemia, by approximately 4% with no evidence of a dose-response. When placebo was compared with the four combined ximelagatran dose groups, ximelagatran produced a statistically significant 24% reduction in the composite endpoint from 16.3% to 12.7% [hazard ratio, 0.76; 95% confidence intervals (CI) of 0.59 to 0.98; $P$ = 0.036]. Mortality was low and similar between the groups. Post hoc analysis, using the composite endpoint of all-cause mortality, myocardial infarction, and stroke, demonstrated a reduction from 11.1% to 7.4% with ximelagatran compared with placebo (hazard ratio, 0.66; 95% CI of 0.48 to 0.90). Major bleeding occurred in 1% of patients treated with placebo and in 2% of those given ximelagatran, a difference that was not statistically different. Building on this information, a phase III trial using the 24-mg twice-daily dose of ximelagatran is under consideration.

Although ximelagatran has many advantages over the currently available anticoagulants, it also has potential limitations. As with other direct thrombin inhibitors, there is no antidote for ximelagatran. Fortunately, the short half-life of ximelagatran makes it unlikely that this will be a substantial problem. The most important side effect of ximelagatran is elevation in the levels of liver enzymes, specifically alanine aminotransferase. This complication appears to be dose-related. Elevations in levels of alanine aminotransferase of greater than three times the upper limit of normal occur in approximately 6.7% (range 5%

to 10%) of patients treated with long-term ximelagatran. Typically, increases in alanine aminotransferases levels occur after 6 weeks to 4 months of treatment. The increase in alanine aminotransferase level is usually asymptomatic and reversible, even if the medication is continued. Concomitant elevation in serum bilirubin level is rare. For comparison purposes, elevation in levels of transaminases occurs in approximately 4% to 8% of patients treated with heparin or LMWH (210) and in 1% of those given warfarin. Although the increase in levels of transaminases with ximelagatran appears to be benign, more information is needed. In the 7,000 patients treated with long-term ximelagatran, there were three deaths due to liver failure. One, and possibly two, of these deaths were related to the drug. Consequently, more information is needed about the long-term hepatic effects of this agent. If ximelagatran is approved for long-term use, liver function tests will need to be monitored when initiating therapy.

### Dabigatran Etexilate

Dabigatran etexilate, another oral direct thrombin inhibitor, is in a less advanced state of clinical development than ximelagatran. Its oral bioavailability is lower than that of ximelagatran (5% vs. 20%). Once absorbed, dabigatran etexilate is converted to its active metabolite, dabigatran (BIBR 953), which has a half-life of approximately 12 hours and is eliminated through the kidneys (211). Dabigatran and dabigatran etexilate have been demonstrated to be effective in animal models of venous thrombosis (212,213). Although early clinical studies are promising (214,215), further work is needed to establish the safety and efficacy of this agent.

# MODULATION OF ENDOGENOUS FIBRINOLYTIC ACTIVITY

Although traditional antithrombotic strategies have been aimed at inhibiting platelet function or blocking coagulation, a better understanding of physiologic fibrinolysis has identified potential methods to enhance endogenous fibrinolytic activity. These include inhibitors of type 1 plasminogen activator (PAI-1), activated thrombin-activatable fibrinolysis inhibitor (TAFIa), and activated factor XIII (factor XIIIa). These drugs are all in early stages of development.

Fibrinolysis, a system that removes intravascular fibrin and restores blood flow, is initiated by plasminogen activators that convert plasminogen to plasmin, which then degrades fibrin into soluble fibrin degradation products. Two immunologically distinct plasminogen activators are found in blood; tPA and urokinase-type plasminogen activator (uPA). Both plasminogen activators are synthesized and released from endothelial cells (216).

Intravascular plasminogen activation is initiated by tPA. Plasminogen activation is targeted to fibrin because plasminogen and tPA bind to fibrin and the enzymatic activity of tPA is enhanced by fibrin (216). Endothelial cells also support plasminogen activation by expressing annexin II, a coreceptor for tPA and plasminogen that promotes plasmin generation on their surface (217).

The fibrinolytic system is regulated at two levels. Plasminogen activator inhibitors, the most important of which is endothelial cell-derived PAI-1, regulate tPA and uPA, whereas $\alpha_2$-antiplasmin inhibits plasmin (216). Although $\alpha_2$-antiplasmin rapidly complexes and inactivates free plasmin, fibrin-bound plasmin is relatively protected from inactivation so that fibrinolysis can occur despite physiologic levels of this inhibitor (216).

TAFI, a procarboxypeptidase B-like enzyme, is activated by the thrombin/thrombomodulin complex and attenuates fibrinolysis by cleaving carboxyl-terminal lysine residues from fibrin (218,219). Removal of these lysine residues decreases plasminogen and plasmin binding to fibrin, thereby retarding the lytic process.

## Plasminogen Activator Inhibitor Type-1

Inhibition of PAI-1, the major physiologic inhibitor of tPA and uPA, results in increased endogenous fibrinolytic activity. PAI-1 activity can be reduced by decreasing PAI-1 gene expression or by reducing PAI-1 activity either by converting active PAI-1 into a nonreactive form or by directly blocking PAI-1 activity (220). Although extensive research has been carried out with respect to PAI-1 inhibition, none of the identified PAI-1 inhibitors has yet been evaluated in humans.

Lipid-lowering drugs, such as niacin and fibrates (221, 222), decrease PAI-1 synthesis in vitro. These agents are not specific for PAI-1, however, and also affect the synthesis of other proteins. It has been reported that a butadiene derivative, T-686, is able to attenuate the augmentation of PAI-1 activity that is associated with vascular injury (223). Likewise, systemic administration of antisense oligonucleotides directed against the signal peptide of PAI-1 in rats has been shown to reduce PAI-1 activity in blood and platelets (224) and to delay the time to occlusion after arterial injury (225).

Various monoclonal antibodies directed against human PAI-1 block its inhibitory activity either by (a) preventing PAI-1 from complexing its target proteinases, (b) inducing substrate behavior in PAI-1, or (c) accelerating conversion of PAI-1 to its latent form (220). Peptides, analogs of portions of the reactive center loop of PAI-1, have been shown to attenuate PAI-1 activity either by preventing insertion of the reactive center loop into the body of the inhibitor (226) or by converting PAI-1 into its latent conformation (227). However, the effectiveness of these agents has yet to be tested in vivo. More promising are small-molecule PAI-1 inhibitors, which inhibit PAI-1 by inducing its transition to its nonreactive conformation (220). Some of these agents have been reported to exhibit antithrombotic activity in vivo. For example, XR334, XR1853, and XR5082 enhanced endogenous fibrinolysis in an electrolytic injury model in the rat carotid artery (228). Likewise, XR115 has been shown to increase tPA activity and to slow arterial thrombus growth in rats (229) and rabbits by reducing plasma PAI-1 activity (230,231).

## Activated Thrombin-Activatable Fibrinolysis Inhibitor

Inhibitors of TAFIa enhance fibrinolytic activity, a concept supported by studies in dogs and rabbits demonstrating that a potato-derived TAFIa inhibitor increases plasminogen activator-induced thrombolysis (232,233). These observations have prompted development of small-molecule TAFIa inhibitors. A potential limitation of some such agents is paradoxical enhancement of TAFIa activity at low doses (234,235). Presumably, this reflects allosteric modulation at the active site of the enzyme. If this phenomenon is common to all TAFIa inhibitors, optimal dosing of these agents may be problematic.

## Factor XIIIa Inhibitors

A thrombin-activated transglutaminase, factor XIIIa cross-links the $\alpha$ and $\lambda$ chains of fibrinogen to form $\alpha$-polymers and $\lambda$-dimers, respectively. Crosslinking stabilizes the fibrin network and renders it more refractory to degradation by plasmin (236). Inhibition of factor XIIIa therefore has the potential to increase the susceptibility of the thrombus to lysis (236).

Tridegin, a peptide isolated from the giant Amazon leech, *Haementeria ghilianti*, is a specific inhibitor of factor XIIIa and enhances fibrinolysis *in vitro* when added before clotting of fibrinogen (237,238). Destabilase, a leech enzyme that hydrolyzes crosslinks, also provides a promising approach to reversing the consequences of factor XIIIa–mediated fibrin crosslinking (239,240). Neither of these agents has been tested in humans.

# CONCLUSIONS AND FUTURE DIRECTIONS

Although several promising new antithrombotic agents are under development, few have been approved. None of the new antiplatelet agents has yet been licensed, and only cangelor is nearing phase III evaluation. In contrast, there are more advances in the development of new anticoagulants. Fondaparinux is licensed for thromboprophylaxis in patients undergoing major orthopedic surgery and for the initial treatment of VTE. Ongoing studies will determine the utility of fondaparinux in patients with acute coronary syndromes.

Ximelagatran is superior to warfarin for prevention of VTE after knee replacement surgery. Therefore, ximelagatran has the potential to simplify prophylaxis because it can be given in fixed doses without coagulation monitoring. Ximelagatran may be particularly useful for extended prophylaxis in these patients, a concept that has yet to be tested. The THRIVE treatment study suggests that ximelagatran is as effective and safe as LMWH followed by warfarin for VTE treatment. If these results are confirmed in other studies, ximelagatran has the potential to streamline anticoagulant therapy by obviating the need for initial treatment with a parenteral anticoagulant and the coagulation monitoring that is required with warfarin administration. On the basis of the results of the SPORTIF III and V trials, ximelagatran also is a promising alternative to warfarin for stroke prevention in patients with atrial fibrillation. With no need for coagulation monitoring, ximelagatran is more convenient than warfarin, a feature that may increase anticoagulant use in high-risk patients. Although promising, more information is needed about the long-term sequelae of the liver transaminase increase that can occur in patients treated with ximelagatran for a month or more.

In addition to ximelagatran, other oral direct thrombin inhibitors and factor Xa inhibitors are under development. Some of the newer agents have the potential for once-daily administration. Yet to be determined is the long-term effect of these drugs on tests of liver function. However, given the large number of agents under study, it is likely that there will soon be an effective and safe alternative to the vitamin K antagonists.

# ACKNOWLEDGMENTS

Dr. Weitz is the recipient of a Career Investigator Award from the Heart and Stroke Foundation of Canada and holds the Heart and Stroke Foundation of Ontario/J. Fraser Mustard Chair in Cardiovascular Research and the Canada Research Chair in Thrombosis at McMaster University. Dr. Bates is a recipient of a New Investigator Award from the Canadian Institutes of Health Research University-Industry (bioMérieux) Program.

## *References*

1. Freidman DG. The structure of thrombi. In: Colman RW, Hirsh J, Marder V et al., eds. *Hemostasis and thrombosis: basic principles and clinical practice*, 2nd ed., Chap. 72. Philadelphia, PA: JB Lippincott Co, 1987.

2. Antithrombotic Trialists' Collaboration. Collaborative meta-analysis of randomised trials of antiplatelet therapy for prevention of death, myocardial infarction and stroke in high risk patients. *BMJ* 2002;324:71–86.

3. Haas WK, Easton JD, Adams HP Jr, et al. A randomized trial comparing ticlopidine hydrochloride with aspirin for the prevention of stroke in high-risk patients. *N Engl J Med* 1989;321:501–507.

4. CAPRIE Steering Committee. A randomised blinded trial of clopidogrel versus aspirin in patients at risk of ischemic events (CAPRIE). *Lancet* 1996;348:1329–1339.

5. Coller BS. Platelet GP IIb/IIIa antagonists: the first anti-integrin receptor therapeutics. *J Clin Invest* 1997;99:1467–1471.

6. Topol EJ, Byzova TV, Plow EF. Platelet GP IIb/IIIa blockers. *Lancet* 1999;353:223–227.

7. Weitz JI. Low-molecular-weight heparins. *N Engl J Med* 1997;337:688–698.

8. Gould MK, Dembitzer AD, Doyle RL, et al. Low-molecular-weight heparins compared with unfractionated heparin for treatment of acute deep venous thrombosis. A meta-analysis of randomized controlled trials. *Ann Intern Med* 1999;130:800–809.

9. Gould MK, Dembitzer AD, Sanders GD, et al. Low-molecular-weight heparins compared with unfractionated heparin for treatment of acute deep venous thrombosis. A cost-effectiveness analysis. *Ann Intern Med* 1999;130:789–799.

10. Cohen M, Demers C, Gurfinkel EP, et al. Efficacy and Safety of Subcutaneous Enoxaparin in Non-Q-Wave Coronary Events Study. A comparison of low-molecular-weight heparin with unfractionated heparin for unstable coronary artery disease. *N Engl J Med* 1997;337:447–452.

11. Eikelboom MW, Anand SS, Malmberg K, et al. Unfractionated heparin and low-molecular-weight heparin in acute coronary syndrome without ST-elevation: a meta-analysis. *Lancet* 2000;355:1936–1942.

12. Klein W, Buchwald A, Hillis SE, et al. Fragmin in Unstable Coronary Artery Disease Study. Comparison of low-molecular-weight heparin with unfractionated heparin acutely and with placebo for 6 weeks in the management of unstable coronary artery disease. *Circulation* 1997;96:61–68.

13. Mark DB, Cowper PA, Berkowitz SD, et al. Economic assessment of low-molecular-weight heparin (enoxaparin) versus unfractionated heparin in acute coronary patients: results from the ESSENCE randomized trial. Efficacy and Safety of Subcutaneous Enoxaparin in Non-Q-wave Coronary Events (unstable angina or non-Q-wave myocardial infarction). *Circulation* 1998;97:1702–1707.

14. Hirsh J. Oral anticoagulant drugs. *N Engl J Med* 1991;324:1865–1875.

15. Fuster V, Badimon L, Badimon JJ, et al. The pathogenesis of coronary artery disease and the acute coronary syndromes. *N Engl J Med* 1992;326:242–250.

16. Nicolaides AN, Kakkar VV, Field ES, et al. The origin of deep vein thrombosis: a venographic study. *Br J Radiol* 1971;44:653–663.

17. Geerts WH, Pineio GF, Heit JA, et al. Prevention of venous thromboembolism. *Chest* 2004;126:338S–400S.

18. Furie B, Furie BC. Molecular and cellular biology of blood coagulation. *N Engl J Med* 1992;326:800–806.

19. Plow EF, McEver RP, Coller BS, et al. Related binding mechanisms for fibrinogen, fibronectin, von Willebrand factor, and thrombospondin on thrombin-stimulated human platelets. *Blood* 1985;66:724–727.

20. Hynes RO. Integrins: versatility, modulation, and signaling in cell adhesion. *Cell* 1992;69:11–25.

21. Moroi M, Jung SM, Okuma M, et al. A patient with platelets deficient in glycoprotein VI that lack both collagen-induced aggregation and adhesion. *J Clin Invest* 1989;4:1440–1445.

22. Arai M, Yamamoto N, Moroi M, et al. Platelets with 10% of the normal amount of glycoprotein VI have an impaired response to collagen that results in a mild bleeding tendency. *Br J Haematol* 1995;89:124–130.

23. Nieuwenhuis HK, Akkerman JW, Houdijk WP, et al. Human blood platelets showing no response to collagen fail to express surface glycoprotein Ia. *Nature* 1985;318:47–42.

24. Kehrel B, Wierwille S, Clemetson KJ, et al. Glycoprotein VI is a major collagen receptor for platelet activation: it recognizes the platelet-activating quaternary structure of collagen, whereas CD36, glycoprotein IIb/IIIa and von Willebrand factor do not. *Blood* 1998;91:491–499.

25. Turitto VT, Weiss HJ, Zimmerman TS, et al. Factor VIII/von Willebrand factor in subendothelium mediates platelet adhesion. *Blood* 1985; 65:823–831.

26. Ruggeri ZM, DeMarco L, Gatti L, et al. Platelets have more than one binding site for von Willebrand factor. *J Clin Invest* 1983;72:1–12.

27. Lopez JA, Andrews RK, Afshar-Kharghan V, et al. Bernard-Soulier syndrome. *Blood* 1998;91:4397–4418.

28. Ruggeri ZM. Mechanisms initiating platelet thrombus formation. *Thromb Haemost* 1997;78:611–616.

29. Vu T-KH, Hung DT, Wheaton VI, et al. Molecular cloning of a functional thrombin receptor reveals a novel proteolytic mechanisms of receptor activation. *Cell* 1991;64:1057–1068.

30. Phillips DR, Charo EF, Scarborough RM. GP IIb/IIIa: the responsive integrin. *Cell* 1991;65:359–362.

31. Peterson DM, Stathopoulos NA, Giogio TD, et al. Shear-induced platelet aggregation requires von Willebrand factor and platelet membrane glycoproteins Ib and IIb-IIIa. *Blood* 1987;69:625–628.

32. Ikeda Y, Handa M, Kawano K, et al. The role of von Willebrand factor and fibrinogen in platelet aggregation under varying shear stress. *J Clin Invest* 1991;87:1234–1240.

33. Kloczewiak M, Timmons S, Lukas TL, et al. Platelet receptor recognition site on human fibrinogen: synthesis and structure function relationship of peptides corresponding to the carboxy-terminal segment of the gamma chain. *Biochem* 1984;23:1767–1774.

34. Kumar R, Beguin S, Hemker C. The influence of fibrinogen and fibrin on thrombin generation-evidence for feedback activation of the clotting system by clot-bound thrombin. *Thromb Haemost* 1994;72:713–721.

35. van den Eijnden MM, Steenhauer SI, Reitsma PH, et al. Tissue factor expression during monocyte-macrophage differentiation. *Thromb Haemost* 1997;77:1129–1136.

36. Neumann FJ, Ott I, Marx N, et al. Effect of human recombinant interleukin-6 and interleukin-8 on monocyte procoagulant activity. *Arterioscler Thromb Vasc Biol* 1997;17:3399–3405.

37. Mann KG, Butenas S, Brummel K. The dynamics of thrombin formation. *Arterioscler Thromb Vasc Biol* 2003;23:17–25.

38. Kumar R, Beguin S, Hemker C. The effect of fibrin clots and clot-bound thrombin on the development of platelet procoagulant activity. *Thromb Haemost* 1995;74:962–968.

39. Gailani D, Broze GJ Jr. Factor XI activation by thrombin and factor XIa. *Semin Thromb Hemos* 1993;19:396–404.

40. Geiger J, Honig-Liedl P, Schanzenbacher P, et al. Ligand specificity and ticlopidine effects distinguish three platelet receptors. *Eur J Pharmacol* 1998;351:235–246.

41. Geiger J, Brich J, Honig-Liedl P, et al. Specific impairment of human platelet P2$Y_{AC}$ ADP receptor-mediated signaling by the antiplatelet drug clopidogrel. *Arterioscl Thromb Vasc Biol* 1999;19:2007–2011.

42. Lecut C, Feeney LA, Kinsbury G, et al. Human platelet glycoprotein Ib function is antagonized by monoclonal antibody-derived Fab fragments. *J Thromb Haemost* 2003;112:2653–2662.

43. Miller JL, Thlam-Cisse M, Drouel LO. Reduction in thrombus formation by PG-1F(ab)2, an anti-guinea pig platelet glycoprotein Ib monoclonal antibody. *Arterioscler Thromb* 1991;11:1231–1236.

44. Yeh CH, Chang MC, Peng HC, et al. Pharmacological characterization and antithrombotic effect of agkistin, a platelet glycoprotein Ib antagonists. *Br J Pharmacol* 2001;132:843–850.

45. Wu D, Meiring M, Kotze HF, et al. Inhibition of platelet glycoprotein Ib, glycoprotein IIb/IIIa, or both by monoclonal antibodies prevent arterial thrombosis in baboons. *Arterioscler Thromb Vasc Biol* 2002;22: 323–328.

46. Cauwenberghs N, Meiring M, Vauterin S, et al. Antithrombotic effect of platelet glycoprotein Ib-blocking monoclonal antibody Fab fragments in nonhuman primates. *Arterioscler Thromb Vasc Biol* 2000;20: 1347–1353.

47. Takahasi R, Sekine N, Nakatake T. Influence of monoclonal antiplatelet glycoprotein antibodies on *in vitro* human megakaryocyte colony formation and proplatelet formation. *Blood* 1999;93:1951–1958.

48. Alimardani G, Guichard J, Fichelson S, et al. Pathogenic effects of antiglycoprotein Ib antibodies on megakaryocytes and platelets. *Thromb Haemost* 2002;88:1039–1046.

49. Handa M, Titani K, Holland LZ, et al. The von willebrand factor-binding domain of platelet membrane glycoprotein Ib. *J Biol Chem* 1986;261: 12579–12585.

50. Fujimura Y, Ikeda Y, Miuira S, et al. Isolation and characterization of jararaca GP Ib-BP, a snake venom antagonist specific to platelet glycoprotein Ib. *Thromb Haemost* 1995;74:743–750.

51. Nypalm Y, Puranen JS, Nyholm TK, et al. Jararhagin-derived RKKH peptides induce structural changes in alpha1Idomain of human integrin alpha1beta1. *J Biol Chem* 2004;279:7962–7970.

52. Chang MC, Lin HK, Peng HC, et al. Antithrombotic effect of crotalin, a platelet membrane glycoprotein Ib antagonist from venom to Crotalus atrox. *Blood* 1998;91:1582–1589.

53. Wu WB, Peng HC, Huang TF. Crotalin, a VWF and GP Ib cleaving metalloproteinase from venom of Crotalus atrox. *Thromb Haemost* 2001;86: 1501–1511.

54. Barnes CS, Krafft B, Frech M, et al. Production and characterization of saratin, an inhibitor of von Willebrand factor-dependent platelet adhesion to collagen. *Semin Thromb Hemost* 2001;27:337–348.

55. Cruz CP, Eidt J, Drouilhet J, et al. Saratin, an inhibitor of von Willebrand factor-dependent platelet adhesion, decreases platelet aggregation and intimal hyperplasia in a rat carotid endarterectomy model. *J Vasc Surg* 2001;34:724–729.

56. Bellinger DA, Hichols TC, Read MS, et al. Prevention of occlusive coronary artery thrombosis by murine monoclonal antibody to procine von Willebrand factor. *Proc Natl Acad Sci U S A* 1987;85:8100–8104.

57. Krupski WC, Bass A, Cadroy Y, et al. Antihemostatic and antithrombotic effects of monoclonal antibodies against von Willebrand factor (VWF) in nonhuman primates. *Surgery* 1992;112:433–440.

58. Wu D, Vanhoorelbeke K, Cauwenberghs N, et al. Inhibition of the von Willebrand (VWF)-collagen interaction by antihuman VWF monoclonal antibody results in abolition of *in vivo* arterial platelet thrombus formation in baboons. *Blood* 2002;99:3623–3628.

59. Strony J, Song A, Rusterholtz L, et al. Aurintricarboxylic acid prevents acute rethrombosis in a canine model of arterial thrombosis. *Arterioscler Thromb Vasc Biol* 1995;15:359–366.

60. Patrono C. Aspirin as an antiplatelet drug. *N Engl J Med* 1994;330: 1287–1294.

61. Hornby EJ, Skidmore IF. Evidence that prostaglandin endoperoxides can induce platelet aggregation in the absence of thromboxane A$_2$ production. *Biochem Pharmacol* 1982;31:1153–1160.

62. Takiguchi Y, Wada K, Nakashima M. Comparison of the inhibitory effects of the TxA2 receptor antagonist, vapiprost, and other antiplatelet drugs on arterial thrombosis in rats: possible role of TXA2. *Thromb Haemost* 1992;67:460–463.

63. Umemura K, Kawai H, Ishihara H, et al. Inhibitory effect of clopidogrel, vapiprost and argatroban on the middle cerebral artery thrombosis in the rat. *Jpn J Pharmacol* 1995;67:253–258.

64. Horie S, Yamada M, Satoh M, et al. The potent inhibition of vapiprost, a novel thromboxane A2 receptor antagonist, on the secondary aggregation and ATP release of human platelets. *Biol Pharm Bull* 1997;20:625–631.

65. Serruys PW, Rutsch W, Heyndrickx GR et al. Coronary Artery Restenosis Prevention on Repeated Thromboxane-Antagonism Study (CARPORT). Prevention of restenosis after percutaneous transluminal coronary angioplasty with thromboxane A$_2$-receptor blockade. A randomized, double-blind placebo-controlled trial. *Circulation* 1991;84:1568–1580.

66. Norris RM, White HE, Hart HH, et al. Comparison of aspirin with a thromboxane antagonist for patients with prolonged chest pain and ST segment depression. *N Z Med J* 1996;109:278–280.

67. Osende JI, Shimbo D, Fuster V, et al. Antithrombotic effects of S18886, a novel orally active thromboxane A2 receptor antagonist. *J Thromb Haemost* 2004;2:492–498.

68. Yasuda T, Gold HK, Raoitia H, et al. Antithrombotic effects of ridogrel, a combined thromboxane A2 synthase inhibitor and prostaglandin endoperoxide-receptor antagonist in platelet-mediated coronary artery occlusion preparation in the dog. *Coron Artery Dis* 1991;2:1103–1110.

69. Golino P, Rosolowsky M, Yao S-K, et al. Endogenous prostaglandin endoperoxides and prostacyclin modulate the thrombolytic activity of tissue plasminogen activator: effects of simultaneous inhibition of thromboxane A2 synthase and blockade of thromboxane A2/prostaglandin H2 receptors in a canine model of coronary thrombosis. *J Clin Invest* 1990;86: 1095–1102.

70. The RAPT Investigators. Randomized trial of ridogrel, a combined thromboxane A2 synthase inhibitor and thromboxane A2/prostaglandin endoperoxide receptor antagonist, versus aspirin as adjunct to thrombolysis in patients with acute myocardial infarction: the Ridogrel versus Aspirin Patency Trial (RAPT). *Circulation* 1994;89:588–595.

71. Michaux C, Norberg B, Dogne JM, et al. Terbogrel, a dual-acting agent for thromboxane receptor antagonism and thromboxane synthase inhibition. *Acta Crystallogr C* 2000;56:1265–1266.

72. Muck S, Webber A, Schror K. Effects of terbogrel on platelet function and prostaglandin endoperoxide transfer. *Eur J Pharmacol* 1998;344:45–48.

73. Soyka R, Guth BD, Weisenberger HM, et al. Guanidine derivatives as combined thromboxane A2 receptor antagonists and synthase inhibitors. *J Med Chem* 1999;42:1235–1249.

74. Langleben D, Christman BW, Barst RJ, et al. Effects of the thromboxane synthetase inhibitor and receptor antagonist terbogrel in patients with primary pulmonary hypertension. *Am Heart J* 2002;143:E4.

75. Ito M, Smith AR, Lee ML. Ticlopidine: a new platelet aggregation inhibitor. *Clin Pharm* 1992;11:603–617.

76. Herbert JM, Frehel D, Vallee B, et al. Clopidogrel, a novel antiplatelet and antithrombotic agent. *Cardiovasc Drug Rev* 1993;11:180–198.

77. Oury C, Toth-Zsamboki E, Vermylen J, et al. P2X(1)-mediated activation of extracellular signal-regulated kinase 2 contributes to platelet secretion and aggregation by collagen. *Blood* 2002;100:2499–2505.

78. Ohlmann P, Eckly A, Freund M, et al. ADP induces partial platelet aggregation without shape change and potentiates collagen-induced aggregation in the absence of G alpha-q. *Blood* 2000;96:2134–2139.

79. Ingall AH, Dixon J, Bailey A, et al. Antagonists of the platelet P2T receptor: a novel approach to antithrombotic therapy. *J Med Chem* 1999;42: 213–220.

80. Huang J, Driscoll EM, Gonzales ML, et al. Prevention of arterial thrombosis by intravenously administered platelet P2T receptor antagonist AR-C66931MX in a canine model. *J Pharmacol Exp Ther* 2000;295: 492–499.

81. Wang K, Zhou X, Zhou Z, et al. Blockade of the platelet P2Y12 receptor by AR-C69931MX sustains coronary artery recanalization and improves the myocardial tissue perfusion in a canine thrombosis model. *Arterioscler Thromb Vasc Biol* 2003;23:357–362.

82. Storey RF, Oldroyd KG, Wilcox RG. Open multicentre study of the P2T receptor antagonist AR-C69931MX assessing safety, tolerability, and activity in patients with acute coronary syndromes. *Thromb Haemost* 2001; 85:401–407.

83. Jacobsson F, Swahn E, Wallentin L, et al. Safety profile and tolerability of intravenous AR— C69931MX, a new antiplatelet drug, in unstable angina pectoris and non-Q-wave myocardial infarction. *Clin Ther* 2002;24: 752–765.

84. Brass S. Cardiovascular biology. Small cells, big issues. *Nature* 2001; 409: 145–147.

85. Bhatt DL, Topol EJ. Scientific and therapeutic advances in antiplatelet therapy. *Nature Rev* 2003;2:15–28.

86. Pinsky DJ, Borekman MJ, Peschon JJ, et al. Elucidation of the thromboregulatory role of CD39/ectoapyrase in the ischemic brain. *J Clin Invest* 2002;109:1031–1040.

87. Vu T-KH, Wheaton VI, Hung DT, et al. Domains specifying thrombin-receptor interaction. *Nature* 1991;353:674–677.

88. Seiler SM, Goldenberg HJ, Michel IM, et al. Multiple pathways of thrombin-induced platelet activation differentiated by desensitization and a thrombin exosite inhibitor. *Biochem Biophys Res Commun* 1991;181:636–643.

89. Kahn ML, Nakanishi-Matsui M, Shapiro MJ, et al. Protease-activated receptors 1 and 4 mediate activation of human platelets by thrombin. *J Clin Invest* 1999;103:879–887.

90. Sambrano GR, Weiss EJ, Zheng YW, et al. Role of thrombin signaling in platelets in haemostasis and thrombosis. *Nature* 2001;413:74–78.

91. Cook JJ, Sitko GR, Bednar B, et al. An antibody against the exosite of the cloned thrombin receptor inhibits experimental arterial thrombosis in the African green monkey. *Circulation* 1995;91:2961–2971.

92. Vassallo RR Jr, Kieber-Emmons T, Cichowski K, et al. Structure-function relationships in the activation of platelet thrombin receptors by receptor-derived peptides. *J Biol Chem* 1992;267:6081–6085.

93. Hung DT, Vu TK, Wheaton VI, et al. "Mirror image" antagonists of thrombin-induced platelet activation based on thrombin receptor structure. *J Clin Invest* 1992;89:444–450.

94. Seiler SM. Thrombin-receptor antagonists. *Semin Thromb Hemost* 1996;22:223–232.

95. Derian CK, Addo MF, Darrow AL, et al. A potent peptide-mimetic antagonist for the tethered-ligand receptor protease-activated receptor-1. *Thromb Haemost* 1999;82(Suppl.):483, (Abstract 1525).

96. Hasan Aak, Amenta S, Schmaier AH. Bradykinin and its metabolites, Arg-Pro-Pro-Gly-Phe, are selective inhibitors of alpha-thrombin-induced platelet activation. *Circulation* 1996;94:517–528.

97. Coughlin SR. Protease-activated receptors and platelet function. *Thromb Haemost* 1999;82:353–356.

98. Wu CC, Hwant TL, Liao CH, et al. Selective inhibition of protease-activated receptor 4-dependent platelet activation by YD-3. *Thromb Haemost* 2002;87:1026–1033.

99. Kahn ML, Nakanishi-Matsui M, Shapiro MJ, et al. Protease-activated receptors 1 and 4 mediate activation of human platelets by thrombin. *J Clin Invest* 1999;103:879–879.

100. Bhatt DL, Topol EJ. Current role of platelet glycoprotein IIb/IIIa inhibitors in acute coronary syndromes. *JAMA* 2000;284:1549–1558.

101. Chew DP, Bhatt DL, Sapp S, et al. Increased mortality with oral platelet glycoprotein IIb/IIIa antagonists: a meta-analysis of phase III multicenter randomized trials. *Circulation* 2001;103:201–206.

102. Chew DP, Bhatt DL, Topol EJ. Oral glycoprotein IIb/IIIa inhibitors: why don't they work? *Am J Cardiovasc Drugs* 2001;1:421–428.

103. Broze GJ Jr. Tissue factor pathway inhibitor. *Thromb Haemost* 1995;74:90–93.

104. Walsh PN. Roles of platelets and factor XI in the initiation of blood coagulation by thrombin. *Thromb Haemost* 2001;86:75–82.

105. Abraham E, Reinhart K, Svoboda P, et al. Assessment of the safety of recombinant tissue factor pathway inhibitor in patients with severe sepsis: a multicenter, randomized, placebo-controlled, single-blind, dose escalation study. *Crit Care Med* 2001;29:2081–2089.

106. Abraham E, Reinhart K, Opal S, et al. OPTIMIST Trial Study Group. Efficacy and safety of tifacogin (recombinant tissue factor pathway inhibitor) in severe sepsis: a randomized controlled trial. *JAMA* 2003;290:238–247.

107. Cappello M, Vlasuk GP, Bergum PW, et al. *Ancylostoma caninum* anticoagulant peptide: a hookworm-derived inhibitor of human coagulation factor Xa. *Proc Natl Acad Sci U S A* 1995;92:6152–6156.

108. Bergum PW, Gansemans Y, Stanssens P, et al. Anticoagulant repertoire of the hookworm *Ancylostoma caninum*. *Proc Natl Sci U S A* 1996;93:2149–2154.

109. Lee A, Agnelli G, Buller H, et al. Dose-response study of recombinant factor VIIa/tissue factor inhibitor recombinant nematode anticoagulant protein c2 in prevention of postoperative venous thromboembolism in patients undergoing total knee replacement. *Circulation* 2001;104:74–78.

110. Taylor FB Jr. Role of tissue factor and factor VIIa in the coagulant and inflammatory response to LD100 *Escherichia coli* in the baboon. *Haemostasis* 1996;26:83–91.

111. Jang Y, Guzman LA, Lincoff AM, et al. Influence of blockade at specific levels of the coagulation cascade on restenosis in a rabbit atherosclerotic femoral artery injury model. *Circulation* 1995;92:3041–3050.

112. Lincoff AM. First clinical investigation of a tissue-factor inhibitor administered during percutaneous coronary revascularization: a randomized, double-blinded, dose-escalation trial- assessing safety and efficacy of FFR-FVIIa in percutaneous transluminal coronary angioplasty (ASIS) trial. *J Am Coll Cardiol* 2000;36:312, (Abstract).

113. Rezaie AR. Prothrombin protects factor Xa in the prothrombinase complex from inhibition by the heparin-antithrombin complex. *Blood* 2001;97(8):2308–2313.

114. Brufatto N, Nesheim ME. The use of prothrombin (S525C) labeled with fluorescein to directly study the inhibition of prothrombinase by antithrombin during prothrombin activation. *J Biol Chem* 2001;276:17663–17671.

115. Boneu B, Necciari J, Cariou R, et al. Pharmacokinetics and tolerance of the natural pentasaccharide (SR90107/ORG31540) with high affinity to antithrombin III in man. *Thromb Haemost* 1995;74:1468–1473.

116. Walenga JM, Jeske WP, Samama MM, et al. Fondaparinux: a synthetic heparin pentasaccharide as a new antithrombotic agent. *Expert Opin Investig Drugs* 2002;11:397–404.

117. Bijsterveld NR, Moons AH, Boekholdt SM, et al. Ability of recombinant factor VIIa to reverse the anticoagulant effect of the pentasaccharide fondaparinux in healthy volunteers. *Circulation* 2002;106:2550–2554.

118. Daud AN, Ahsan A, Iqbal O, et al. Synthetic heparin pentasaccharide depolymerization by heparinase. I: molecular and biological implications. *Clin Appl Thromb Hemost* 2001;7:58–64.

119. Eriksson BI, Bauer KA, Lassen MR, et al. Steering Committee of the Pentasaccharide in Hip Fracture Study. Fondaparinux compared with enoxaparin for the prevention of venous thromboembolism after hip-fracture surgery. *N Engl J Med* 2001;345:1298–1304.

120. Lassen MR, Bauer KA, Eriksson BI, et al. European Pentasaccharide Elective Surgery Study (EPHESUS) Steering Committee. Postoperative fondaparinux versus preoperative enoxaparin for prevention of venous thromboembolism in elective hip-replacement surgery: a randomised double-blind comparison. *Lancet* 2002;359:1715–1720.

121. Turpie AG, Bauer KA, Eriksson BI, et al. PENTATHLON 2000 Study Steering Committee. Postoperative fondaparinux versus postoperative enoxaparin for prevention of venous thromboembolism after elective hip-replacement surgery: a randomised double-blind trial. *Lancet* 2002;359:1721–1726.

122. Bauer KA, Eriksson BI, Lassen MR, et al. Steering Committee of the Pentasaccharide in Knee Replacement Study. Fondaparinux compared with enoxaparin for the prevention of venous thromboembolism after elective major knee surgery. *N Engl J Med* 2001;345:1305–1310.

123. Eriksson BI, Lassen MR, PENTasaccharide in Hip-FRAture Surgery Plus Investigators. Duration of prophylaxis against venous thromboembolism with fondaparinux after hip fracture surgery: a multicenter, randomized, placebo-controlled, double-blind study. *Arch Intern Med* 2003;163:1337–1342.

124. Buller HR, Davidson BL, Decousus H, et al. Matisse Investigators. Fondaparinux or enoxaparin for the initial treatment of symptomatic deep venous thrombosis: a randomized trial. *Ann Intern Med* 2004;140(11):867–873.

125. The MATISSE Investigators. Subcutaneous fondaparinux versus intravenous unfractionated heparin in the initial treatment of pulmonary embolism. *N Engl J Med* 2003;349:1695–1702.

126. Turpie AGG, Bauer KA, Eriksson BI, et al. Steering Committees of the Pentasaccharide Orthopedic Prophylaxis Studies. Fondaparinux vs. enoxaparin for the prevention of venous thromboembolism in major orthopedic surgery: a meta-analysis of 4 randomized double-blind studies. *Arch Intern Med* 2002;162:1833–1840.

127. Cohen AT, Gallus AS, Lassen MR, et al. Fondaparinux vs. placebo for the prevention of venous thromboembolism in acutely ill medical patients (ARTEMIS). *J Thromb Haemost* 2003;(Suppl. 1), (Abstract P2046).

128. Agnelli, G, Bergqvist D, Cohen A, et al. A randomized double-blind study to compare the efficacy and safety of fondaparinux with dalteparin in the prevention of venous thromboembolism after high-risk abdominal surgery: the Pegasus Study. *J Thromb Haemost* 2003;(Suppl. 1), (Abstract OC006).

129. Coussement PK, Bassand JP, Convens C, et al. PENTALYSE Study. A synthetic factor-Xa inhibitor (ORG31540/SR9017A) as an adjunct to fibrinolysis in acute myocardial infarction. The PENTALYSE Study. *Eur Heart J* 2001;22:1716–1724.

130. Simoons ML, Bobbink IW, Boland J, et al. A dose-finding study of fondaparinux in patients with non-ST segment elevation acute coronary syndromes, the Pentasaccharide in Unstable Angina (PENTUA) Study. *J Am Coll Cardio* 2004;43:2183–2190.

131. Herbert JM, Herault JP, Bernat A, et al. Biochemical and pharmacological properties of SANORG 34006, a potent and long-acting synthetic pentasaccharide. *Blood* 1998;91:4197–4205.

132. Bijsterveld NR, Vink R, van Aken BE, et al. Recombinant factor VIIa reverses the anticoagulant effect of the long-acting pentasaccharide idraparinux in health volunteers. *Br J Haematol* 2004;124:653–658.

133. PERSIST Investigators. A novel long-acting synthetic factor Xa inhibitor (idraparinux sodium) to replace warfarin for secondary prevention in deep vein thrombosis: a phase II evaluation. *Blood* 2002;100:301, (Abstract).

134. Herbert JM, Bernat A, Dol F, et al. DX-9065a, a novel synthetic selective and orally active inhibitor of factor Xa: *in vitro* and *in vivo* studies. *J Pharmacol Exp Ther* 1996;276:1030–1038.

135. Dyke CK, Becker RC, Kleiman NS, et al. First experience with direct factor Xa inhibition in patients with stable coronary disease: a pharmacokinetic and pharmacodynamic evaluation. *Circulation* 2002;105:2385–2391.

136. Alexander JH, Dyke CK, Yang H, et al. The XaNADU-PCI PILOT Investigators. *J Thromb Haemost* 2004;2:234–241.

137. Lassen MR, Davidson BL, Gallus A, et al. A phase II randomized, double-blind, five-arm, parallel-group, dose-response study of a new oral directly-acting factor Xa inhibitor, Razaxaban, for the prevention of deep vein thrombosis in knee replacement surgery. *Blood* 2003;102:15a, (Abstract 41).

138. Esmon CT, Ding W, Yasuhiro K, et al. The protein C pathway: new insights. *Thromb Haemost* 1997;78:70–74.

139. Bernard GR, Vincent JL, Laterre PF, et al. Recombinant Human Protein C Worldwide Evaluation in Severe Sepsis (PROWESS) Study Group. Efficacy and safety of recombinant human activated protein C for severe sepsis. *N Engl J Med* 2001;344:699–709.

140. Manns BJ, Lee H, Doig CJ, et al. An economic evaluation of activated protein C treatment for severe sepsis. *N Engl J Med* 2002;347:993–1000.

141. Ettingshausen CE, Veldmann A, Beeg T, et al. Replacement therapy with protein C concentrate in infants and adolescents with meningococcal sepsis and purpura fulminans. *Semin Thromb Hemost* 1999;25:537–531.

142. White B, Livingstone W, Murphy C, et al. An open-label study of the role of adjuvant hemostatic support with protein C replacement therapy in purpura fulminans-associated meningococcemia. *Blood* 2000;96:3719–3724.

143. Faust SN, Levin M, Harrison OB, et al. Dysfunction of endothelial protein C activation in severe meningococcal sepsis. *N Engl J Med* 2001;345: 408–416.

144. Sadler JI. Thrombomodulin structure and function. *Thromb Haemost* 1997;78:392–395.

145. Maruyama I. Recombinant thrombomodulin and activated protein C in the treatment of disseminated intravascular coagulation. *Thromb Haemost* 1999;82:718–721.

146. Kearon C, Comp P, Douketis J, et al. Dose-response study of recombinant human soluble thrombomodulin (ART-123) in the prevention of venous thromboembolism after total hip replacement. *J Thromb Haemost* 2005; 3:962–968.

147. Hirsh J. Heparin. *N Engl J Med* 1991;324:1565–1574.

148. Tollefsen DM. Insight into the mechanism of action of heparin cofactor II. *Thromb Haemost* 1995;74:1209–1214.

149. Weitz JI, Buller HR. Direct thrombin inhibitors in acute coronary syndromes: present and future. *Circulation* 2002;105:1004–1011.

150. Weitz JI, Crowther M. Direct thrombin inhibitors. *Thromb Res* 2002; 106:V275–V284.

151. Lane DA, Pejler J, Flynn AM, et al. Neutralization of heparin-related saccharides by histidine-rich glycoprotein and platelet factor 4. *J Biol Chem* 1986;261:39280–39286.

152. Hogg PI, Jackson CM. Fibrin monomer protects thrombin from inactivation by heparin-antithrombin III: implications for heparin efficacy. *Proc Natl Acad Sci U S A* 1989;86:3619–3623.

153. Weitz J, Leslie B, Hudoba M. Thrombin binds to soluble fibrin degradation products where it is protected from inhibition by heparin-antithrombin but susceptible to inactivation by anti-thrombin-independent inhibitors. *Circulation* 1998;97:544–552.

154. Weitz JI, Hudoba M, Massel D, et al. Clot-bound thrombin is protected from inhibition by heparin-antithrombin III but is susceptible to inactivation by antithrombin III-dependent inhibitors. *J Clin Invest* 1990;86: 385–391.

155. De Cristofaro R, De Candia E, Rutella S, et al. The Asp$^{272}$-Glu$^{282}$ region of platelet glycoprotein Ibα interacts with heparin-binding site α-thrombin and protects the enzyme from heparin-catalyzed inhibition by antithrombin III. *J Biol Chem* 2000;275:3887–3895.

156. Wallis RB. Hirudins: from leeches to man. *Semin Thromb Hemost* 1996; 22:185–196.

157. Toschi V, Lettino M, Gallo R, et al. Biochemistry and biology of hirudin. *Coron Artery Dis* 1996;7:420–428.

158. Organization to Assess Strategies for Ischemic Syndromes (OASIS) Investigators. Comparison of the effects of two doses of recombinant hirudin compared with heparin in patients with acute myocardial ischemia without ST elevation: a pilot study. *Circulation* 1997;96:769–777.

159. *Lancet*. Effects of recombinant hirudin (lepirudin) compared with heparin on death, myocardial infarction, refractory angina, and revascularization procedures in patients with acute myocardial ischaemia without ST elevation: a randomised trial Organization to Assess Strategies for Ischemic Syndromes (OASIS-2) Investigators 1999;353:429–438.

160. Antman EM, TIMI 9A Investigators. Hirudin in acute myocardial infarction. Safety report from the Thrombolysis and Thrombin Inhibition in Myocardial Infarction (TIMI) 9A Trial. *Circulation* 1994;90:1624–1630.

161. Neuhaus KL, von Essen R, Tebbe U, et al. Safety observations from the pilot phase of the randomized r-Hirudin for Improvement of Thrombolysis (HIT-III) study. A study of the Arbeitsgemeinschaft Leitender Kardiologischer Krankenhausarzte (ALKK). *Circulation* 1994;90: 1638–1642.

162. The GUSTO IIa Investigators. Randomized trial of intravenous heparin versus recombinant hirudin for acute coronary syndromes. The Global Use of Strategies to Open Occluded Coronary Arteries (GUSTO) IIa Investigators. *Circulation* 1994;90:1631–1637.

163. The GUSTO Investigators. An international randomized trial comparing four thrombolytic strategies for acute myocardial infarction. The GUSTO Investigators. *N Engl J Med* 1993;329:673–682.

164. The GUSTO IIb Investigators. A comparison of recombinant hirudin with heparin for the treatment of acute coronary syndromes. The Global Use of Strategies to Open Occluded Coronary Arteries (GUSTO) IIb Investigators. *N Engl J Med* 1996;335:775–782.

165. Metz BK, White HD, Granger CB, et al. Global Use of Strategies to Open Occluded Coronary Arteries in Acute Coronary Syndromes (GUSTO-IIb) Investigators. Randomized comparison of direct thrombin inhibition versus heparin in conjunction with fibrinolytic therapy for acute myocardial infarction: results from the GUSTO-IIb Trial. *J Am Coll Cardiol* 1998;31: 1493–1498.

166. Antman EM, TIMI 9B Investigators. Hirudin in acute myocardial infarction. Thrombolysis and Thrombin Inhibition in Myocardial Infarction (TIMI) 9B trial. *Circulation* 1996;94:911–921.

167. Serruys PW, Herrman JP, Simon R, et al. Helvetica Investigators. A comparison of hirudin with heparin in the prevention of restenosis after coronary angioplasty. *N Engl J Med* 1995;333:757–763.

168. Eriksson BI, Ekman S, Lindbratt S, et al. Prevention of thromboembolism with use of recombinant hirudin. Results of a double-blind, multicenter trial comparing the efficacy of desirudin (Revasc) with that of unfractionated heparin in patients having a total hip replacement. *J Bone Joint Surg Am* 1997;79:326–333.

169. Eriksson BI, Wille-Jorgensen P, Kalebo P, et al. A comparison of recombinant hirudin with a low-molecular-weight heparin to prevent thromboembolic complications after total hip replacement. *N Engl J Med* 1997; 337:1329–1335.

170. Schiele F, Lindgaerde F, Eriksson H, et al. International Multicentre Hirudin Study Group. Subcutaneous recombinant hirudin (HBW 023) versus intravenous sodium heparin in treatment of established acute deep vein thrombosis of the legs: a multicentre prospective dose-ranging randomized trial. *Thromb Haemos* 1997;77:834–838.

171. Greinacher A, Janssens U, Berg G, et al. Heparin-Associated Thrombocytopenia Study (HAT) Investigators. Lepirudin (recombinant hirudin) for parenteral anticoagulation in patients with heparin-induced thrombocytopenia. *Circulation* 1999;100:587–593.

172. Greinacher A, Volpel H, Janssens U, et al. HIT Investigators Group. Recombinant hirudin (lepirudin) provides safe and effective anticoagulation in patients with heparin-induced thrombocytopenia. A prospective study. *Circulation* 1999;99:73–80.

173. Farner B, Eichler P, Kroll H, et al. A comparison of danaparoid and lepirudin in heparin-induced thrombocytopenia. *Thromb Haemost* 2001;85: 950–957.

174. Reiss FC, Lower C, Seelig C. Recombinant hirudin as a new anticoagulant during cardiac operations instead of heparin: successful for aortic valves replacement in man. *J Thorac Cardiovasc Surg* 1995;11:265–267.

175. Potzsch B, Iversen S, Reiss FC. Recombinant hirudin as an anticoagulant in open-heart surgery: a case report. *Ann Hematol* 1994;68:A53.

176. Bittl JA, Strony J, Brinker JA, et al. Hirulog Angioplasty Study Investigators. Treatment with bivalirudin (Hirulog) as compared with heparin during coronary angioplasty for unstable or post infarction angina. *N Engl J Med* 1995;333:764–769.

177. Bittl JA, Chaitman BR, Feit F, et al. Bivalirudin versus heparin during coronary angioplasty for unstable or post-infarction angina: the final report of the Bivalirudin Angioplasty Study. *Am Heart J* 2001;142: 952–959.

178. Lincoff AM, Kleiman NS, Kottke-Marchant K, et al. Bivalirudin with planned or provisional abciximab versus low-dose heparin and abciximab during percutaneous coronary revascularization: results of the Comparison of Abciximab Complications with Hirulog for Ischemic Events Trial (CACHET). *Am Heart J* 2002;143:847–853.

179. Lincoff AM, Bittl JA, Harrington RA, et al. Bivalirudin and provisional GP IIb/IIIa blockade compared with heparin and planned GP IIb/IIIa blockade during percutaneous coronary intervention: REPLACE-2 randomized trial. *JAMA* 2003;289:853–863.

180. White H, The Hirulog and Early Reperfusion or Occlusion (HERO)-2 Trial Investigators. Thrombin-specific anticoagulation with bivalirudin versus heparin in patients receiving fibrinolytic therapy for acute myocardial infarction: the HERO-2 randomised trial. *Lancet* 2001;348(9296):1855–1863.

181. Maraganore JM, Bourdon P, Jablonski J, et al. Design and characterization of hirulogs: a novel class of bivalent peptide inhibitors of thrombin. *J Clin Invest* 1990;29:7095–7101.

182. Skrzypczak-Jankun E, Carperos VE, Ravichandran KL, et al. Structure of the hirugen and hirulog 1 complexes of alpha-thrombin. *J Mol Biol* 1991;221:1379–1393.

183. Witting JI, Bourdon P, Maraganore JM, et al. Hirulog-1 and -B2 thrombin specificity. *Biochem J* 1992;287:663–664.

184. Fox I, Dawson A, Loynds P, et al. Anticoagulant activity of Hirulog, a direct thrombin inhibitor, in humans. *Thromb Haemost* 1993;69:157–163.

185. Robson R. The use of bivalirudin in patients with renal impairment. *J Invasive Cardiol* 2000;12:33F–36F.

186. Lewis BE, Wallis DE, Berkowitz SD, et al. ARG 911 Study Investigators. Argatroban anticoagulant therapy in patients with heparin-induced thrombocytopenia. *Circulation* 2001;103:1838–1843.

187. Lewis BE, Wallis DE, Leya F, et al. The Argatroban-915 Investigators. Argatroban anticoagulation in patients with heparin-induced thrombocytopenia. *Arch Intern Med* 2003;163:1849–1856.

188. Gold HK, Torres FW, Garabedian HD, et al. Evidence for a rebound coagulation phenomenon after cessation of a 4-hour infusion of a specific thrombin inhibitor in patients with unstable angina pectoris. *J Am Coll Cardiol* 1993;21:1039–1047.

189. Vermeer F, Vahanian A, Fels PW, et al. ARGAMI Study Group. Argatroban and alteplase in patients with acute myocardial infarction: the ARGAMI Study. *J Thromb Thrombolysis* 2000;10:233–240.

190. Herrman JP, Suryapranata H, den Heijer P, et al. Argatroban during percutaneous transluminal coronary angioplasty: results of a dose-verification study. *J Thromb Thrombolysis* 1996;3:367–375.

191. Gustafsson D, Nystrom JE, Carlsson S, et al. The direct thrombin inhibitor melagatran and its oral prodrug H 376/95: intestinal absorption properties, biochemical and pharmacodynamic effects. *Thromb Res* 2001; 101:171–181.

192. Bredberg E, Andersson TB, Frison L, et al. Ximelagatran, an oral direct thrombin inhibitor, has a low potential for cytochrome P450-mediated drug-drug interactions. *Clin Pharmacokinet* 2003;42:765–777.

193. Eriksson UG, Johansson S, Attman PO, et al. Influence of severe renal impairment on the pharmacokinetics and pharmacodynamics of oral ximelgatran and subcutaneous melagatran. *Clin Pharmacokinet* 2003;42:743–753.

194. Johansson LC, Frison L, Logren U, et al. Influence of age on the pharmacokinetics and pharmacodynamics of ximelgatran, an oral direct thrombin inhibitor. *Clin Pharmacokinet* 2003;42:381–392.

195. Eriksson BI, Agnelli G, Cohen AT, et al. METHRO III Study Group. Direct thrombin inhibitor melagatran followed by oral ximelagatran in comparison with enoxaparin for prevention of venous thromboembolism after total hip or knee joint replacement. *Thromb Haemost* 2003;89:288–296.

196. Eriksson BI, Agnelli G, Cohen AT, et al. EXPRESS Study Group. The oral direct thrombin inhibitor ximelagatran, and its subcutaneous form melagatran, compared with enoxaparin for prophylaxis of venous thromboembolism in total hip or total knee replacement: the EXPRESS Study. *Blood* 2001;100:299, (Abstract).

197. Colwell CW, Berkowitz SD, Davidson BL, et al. Randomized, double-blind, comparison of ximelagatran, an oral direct thrombin inhibitor, and enoxaparin to prevent venous thromboembolism after total hip arthroplasty. *Blood* 2001;98:706a, (Abstract 2952).

198. Heit JA, Colwell CW, Francis CW, et al. AstraZeneca Arthroplasty Study Group. Comparison of the oral direct thrombin inhibitor ximelagatran with enoxaparin as prophylaxis against venous thromboembolism after total knee replacement. *Arch Intern Med* 2001;161:2215–2221.

199. Francis CW, Berkowitz SD, Comp PC, et al. EXULT A Study Group. Comparison of ximelagatran with warfarin for prevention of venous thromboembolism after total knee replacement. *N Engl J Med* 2003;349: 1703–1712.

200. Colwell CW, Berkowz SC, Comp PC, et al. EXULT B Investigators. Randomized double-blind comparison of ximelagatran, an oral direct thrombin inhibitor, and warfarin to prevent venous thromboembolism (VTE) after total knee replacement. *Blood* 2003;102:14, (Abstract 39).

201. Francis CW, Ginsberg JS, Berkowitz SD, et al. THRIVE Treatment Study Investigators. Efficacy and safety of the oral direct thrombin inhibitor ximelagatran compared with current standard therapy for acute symptomatic deep vein thrombosis, with or without pulmonary embolism: the THRIVE Treatment Study. *Blood* 2003;102:6a, (Abstract 7).

202. Schulman S, Wahlander K, Lundstrom T, et al. Thrive III Investigators. Secondary prevention of venous thromboembolism with the oral direct thrombin inhibitor ximelagatran. *N Engl J Med* 2003;349:1713–1721.

203. Petersen P, Grind M, Adler J, SPORTIF II Investigators. Ximelagatran versus warfarin for stroke prevention in patients with nonvalvular atrial fibrillation. SPORTIF II: a dose-guiding tolerability, and safety study. *J Am Coll Cardiol* 2003;41:1445–1451.

204. Halperin JL. *Efficacy and safety study of oral direct thrombin inhibitor ximelagatran compared with dose-adjusted warfarin in the prevention of stroke and systemic embolic events in patients with atrial fibrillation: SPORTIF V.* Orlando, FL: American Heart Association Scientific Sessions, November, 2003.

205. Eriksson BI, Bergqvist D, Kalebo P, et al. Melagatran for Thrombin Inhibition in Orthopedic Surgery Study Group. Ximelagatran and melagatran compared with dalteparin for prevention of venous thromboembolism after total hip or knee replacement: the METHRO II randomised trial. *Lancet* 2002;360:1441–1447.

206. Eriksson H, Wahlander K, Gustafsson D, et al. THRIVE Investigators. A randomized, controlled, dose-guiding study of the oral direct thrombin inhibitor ximelagatran compared with standard therapy for the treatment of acute deep vein thrombosis: THRIVE I. *J Thromb Haemost* 2003;1:41–47.

207. Petersen P. A long-term follow-up of ximelagatran as an oral anticoagulant for the prevention of stroke and systemic embolism in patients with atrial fibrillation. *Blood* 2001;98:706a, (Abstract 2953).

208. Executive Steering Committee on behalf of the SPORTIF III Investigators. Stroke prevention with the oral direct thrombin inhibitor, ximelagatran compared with warfarin in patients with non-valvular atrial fibrillation (SPORTIF III): randomised controlled trial. *Lancet* 2003;362: 1691–1698.

209. Wallentin L, Wilcox RG, Weaver WD, et al. ESTEEM Investigators. Oral ximelagatran for secondary prophylaxis after myocardial infarction: the ESTEEM randomised controlled trial. *Lancet* 2003;362:789–792.

210. Guevara A, Labarca J, Gonzalez-Martin G. Heparin-induced transaminase elevations: a prospective study. *Int J Clin Pharmacol Ther Toxicol* 1993;31:137–141.

211. Gustafsson D. Oral direct thrombin inhibitors in clinical development. *J Int Med* 2003;254:322–334.

212. Wienen W, Nar H, Ries UJ, et al. Antithrombotic effects of the direct thrombin inhibitor BIBR953ZW and its orally active prodrug BIBR1048MS in a model of venous thrombosis in rabbits. *Thromb Haemost* 2001, (Abstract OC583).

213. Wienen W, Nar H, Ries UJ, et al. Effects of the direct thrombin inhibitor BIBR953ZW and its orally active prodrug BIBR1048MS on experimentally-induced clot formation and template bleeding time in rats. *Thromb Haemost* 2001;12, (Abstract P761).

214. Strangier J, Nehmiz G, Liesenfeld KN, et al. Pharmacokinetics of BIBR 953ZW, the active form of the oral direct thrombin inhibitor dagibatran etexilate, in patients undergoing hip replacment. *J Thromb Haemost* 2003;1(Suppl. 1), (Abstract P1916).

215. Stangier J, Liesenfeld KH, Troconiz CH, et al. The effect of BIBR 953ZW, the active form of the oral direct thrombin inhibitor BIBR 1048, on the prolongation of the aPTT and ECT in orthopedic patients: a population pharmacodynamic study. *J Thromb Haemost* 2003;1(Suppl. 1), (Abstract P1917).

216. Collen D. The plasminogen (fibrinolytic) system. *Thromb Haemost* 1999; 82:259–270.

217. Kim J, Hajjar KA. Annexin II: a plasminogen-plasminogen activator co-receptor. *Front Biosci* 2002;7:d341–d348.

218. Bajzar L, Morser J, Nesheim M. TAFI, or plasma procarboxypeptidase B, couples the coagulation and fibrinolytic cascades through the thrombin-thrombomodulin complex. *J Biol Chem* 1996;271:16603–16608.

219. Sakharov DV, Plow EF, Rijken DC. On the mechanism of the antifibrinolytic activity of plasma carboxypeptidase B. *J Biol Chem* 1997;272:14477–14482.

220. Gils A, Declerck PJ. The structural basis for the pathophysiological relevance of PAI-1 in cardiovascular diseases and the development of potential PAI-1 inhibitors. *J Thromb Haemost* 2004;91:425–437.

221. Fujii S, Sawa H, Sobel BE. Inhibition of endothelial cell expression of plasminogen activator inhibitor type-1 by gemfibrozil. *Thromb Haemost* 1993;70:642–647.

222. Brown SL, Sobel BE, Fujii S. Attenuation of the synthesis of plasminogen activator inhibitor type 1 by niacin: a potential link between lipid lowering and fibrinolysis. *Circulation* 1995;92:767–772.

223. Vinogradsky B, Bell SP, Woodcock-Mitchell J, et al. A new butadiene derivative, T-686, inhibits plasminogen activator inhibitor type-1 production *in vitro* by cultured human vascular endothelial cells and development of atherosclerotic lesions *in vivo* in rabbits. *Thromb Res* 1997;85:305–314.

224. Pawlowska Z, Chabielska E, Kobylanska A, et al. Regulation of PAI-1 concentration in platelets by systemic administration of antisense oligonucleotides to rats. *Thromb Haemost* 2001;85:1086–1089.

225. Pawlowska Z, Pluskota E, Chabielska E, et al. Phosphorothioate oligodeoxyribonucleotides antisense to PAI-1 mRNA increase fibrinolysis and modify experimental thrombosis in rats. *Thromb Haemost* 1998;79: 348–353.

226. Kvassman J, Lawrence D, Shore J. The acid stabilization of plasminogen activator inhibitor-1 depends on protonation of a single group that affects loop insertion into ∃-sheet A. *J Biol Chem* 1995;270:27942–27947.

227. Eitzman DT, Fay WP, Lawrence DA, et al. Peptide-mediated inactivation of recombinant and platelet plasminogen activator inhibitor-1 *in vitro*. *J Clin Invest* 1995;95:2416–2420.

228. Charlton PA, Faint RW, Collins M, et al. Evaluation of a low molecular weight modulator of human plasminogen activator inhibitor-1 activity. *Thromb Haemost* 1996;75:808–815.

229. Charlton P, Faint R, Barnes C, et al. XR5118, a novel modulator of plasminogen activator inhibitor (PAI-1) increases endogenous t-PA activity in the rat. *Fibrinol Proteol* 1997;11:51–56.

230. Friederich P, Levi M, Biemond B, et al. Low-molecular-weight inhibitor of PAI-1 (XR5118) promotes endogenous fibrinolysis and reduces postthrombolysis thrombus growth in rabbits. *Circulation* 1997;96:916–921.

231. Einholm AP, Pedersen KE, Wind T, et al. Biochemical mechanism of action of a diketopiperazine inactivator of plasminogen activator inhibitor-1. *Biochem J* 2003;373:723–732.

232. Redlitz A, Nicolini FA, Malycky JL, et al. Inducible carboxypeptidase activity: a role in clot lysis *in vivo*. *Circulation* 1996;93:1328–1330.

233. Klement P, Liao P, Bajzar L. A novel approach to arterial thrombolysis. *Blood* 1999;94:2735–2743.

234. Schneider M, Nesheim M. Reversible inhibitors of TAFIa can both promote and inhibit fibrinolysis. *J Thromb Haemost* 2003;1:147–144.

235. Walker J, Hughes B, James I, et al. Stabilization versus inhibition of TAFIa by competitive inhibitors *in vitro*. *J Biol Chem* 2003;278:8913–8921.

236. Mosesson MW. The roles of fibrinogen and fibrin in hemostasis and thrombosis. *Semin Hematol* 1992;29:177–178.

237. Muszbek L, Adany R, Mikkola H. Novel aspects of blood coagulation factor XIII. I. Structure, distribution, activation, and function. *Crit Rev Clin Lab Sci* 1996;33:357–421.

238. Seale L, Finney S, Sawyer RT, et al. Tridegin, a novel peptidic inhibitor of factor XIIIa from the leech, *Haementeria ghilianii*, enhances fibrinolysis *in vitro*. *Thromb Haemost* 1997;77:959–963.

239. Finney S, Seale L, Sawyer RT, et al. Tridegin, a new peptidic inhibitor of factor XIIIa, from the blood-sucking leech *Haementeria ghilianii*. *Biochem J* 1997;324:797–805.

240. Baskova IP, Nikonov GI. Destabilase, the novel epsilon-(gamma-Glu)-Lys isopeptidase with thrombolytic activity. *Blood Coagul Fibrinolysis* 1991; 2:167–172.